WILLIAMS TEXTBOOK OF
ENDOCRINOLOGY

ELSEVIER

WILLIAMS TEXTBOOK OF ENDOCRINOLOGY

Shlomo Melmed, MBChB, MACP
Professor of Medicine
Senior Vice President and Dean of the Medical Faculty
Cedars-Sinai Medical Center
Los Angeles, California

Kenneth S. Polonsky, MD
Richard T. Crane Distinguished Service Professor
Dean of the Division of the Biological Sciences and the Pritzker School of Medicine
Executive Vice President for Medical Affairs
The University of Chicago
Chicago, Illinois

P. Reed Larsen, MD, FRCP
Professor of Medicine
Harvard Medical School
Senior Physician
Division of Endocrinology, Diabetes, and Metabolism
Brigham and Women's Hospital
Boston, Massachusetts

Henry M. Kronenberg, MD
Professor of Medicine
Harvard Medical School
Chief, Endocrine Unit
Massachusetts General Hospital
Boston, Massachusetts

ELSEVIER

ELSEVIER

1600 John F. Kennedy Blvd.
Ste 1800
Philadelphia, PA 19103-2899

WILLIAMS TEXTBOOK OF ENDOCRINOLOGY,
13TH EDITION

ISBN: 978-0-323-29738-7

Previous editions copyrighted 2011, 2008, 2003, 1998, 1992, 1985, 1981, 1974, 1968, 1962, 1955, 1950 by Saunders, an affiliate of Elsevier Inc.
Copyright renewed 1990 by A.B. Williams, R.I. Williams
Copyright renewed 1983 by William H. Daughaday
Copyright renewed 1978 by Robert H. Williams

Library of Congress Cataloging-in-Publication Data

Williams textbook of endocrinology / [edited by] Shlomo Melmed, Kenneth S. Polonsky, P. Reed Larsen, Henry M. Kronenberg.—Thirteenth edition.
    p. ; cm.
  Textbook of endocrinology
  Includes bibliographical references and index.
  ISBN 978-0-323-29738-7 (pbk.)
  I. Melmed, Shlomo, editor. II. Polonsky, Kenneth S., editor. III. Larsen, P. Reed, editor. IV. Kronenberg, Henry, editor. V. Title: Textbook of endocrinology.
  [DNLM: 1. Endocrine Glands. 2. Endocrine System Diseases. WK 100]
  RC648
  616.4–dc23
                                                              2015036469

Associate Content Strategist: Katy Meert
Content Development Specialist: Margaret Nelson
Publishing Services Manager: Patricia Tannian
Senior Project Manager: Sharon Corell
Manager, Art and Design: Julia Dummitt

Printed in Canada.

Last digit is the print number: 9 8 7 6 5 4 3 2 1

Contributors

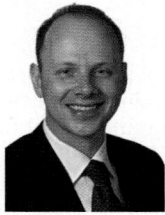

John C. Achermann, MB, MD, PhD
Wellcome Trust Senior
Fellow in Clinical Science
UCL Institute of Child Health
Honorary Consultant in Pediatric
Endocrinology
Great Ormond Street Hospital
NHS Foundation Trust
London, Great Britain

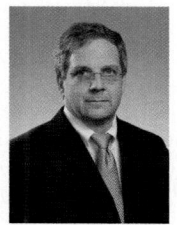

Lloyd P. Aiello, MD, PhD
Professor
Ophthalmology
Harvard Medical School
Director
Beetham Eye Institute
Joslin Diabetes Center
Boston, Massachusetts

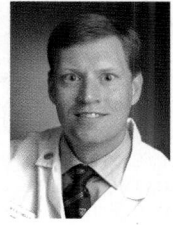

Erik K. Alexander, MD
Physician and Associate Professor
of Medicine
Brigham and Women's Hospital and
Harvard Medical School
Boston, Massachusetts

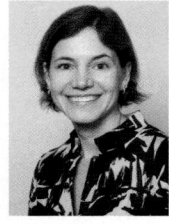

Rebecca H. Allen, MD, MPH
Assistant Professor
Obstetrics and Gynecology
The Warren Alpert Medical School of
Brown University
Providence, Rhode Island

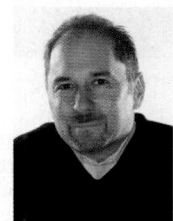

David Altshuler, MD, PhD
Deputy Director and Chief
Academic Officer
Broad Institute of Harvard and MIT
Professor of Biology (Adjunct)
Massachusetts Institute of
Technology
Cambridge, Massachusetts
Professor of Genetics and
of Medicine
Massachusetts General Hospital
Harvard Medical School
Boston, Massachusetts

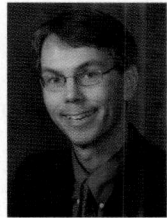

Mark S. Anderson, MD, PhD
Professor
Director
UCSF Medical Scientist Training
Program
Robert B. Friend and Michelle M.
Friend Endowed Chair in Diabetes
Research
University of California
San Francisco Diabetes Center
San Francisco, California

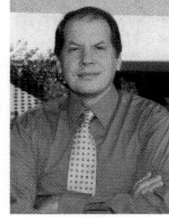

Mark A. Atkinson, PhD
American Diabetes Association
Eminent Scholar for
Diabetes Research
Pathology and Pediatrrics
Jeffrey Keene Family Professor
Director
UF Diabetes Institute
The University of Florida
Gainesville, Florida

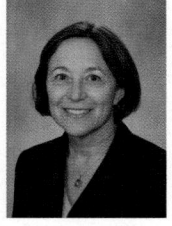

Rebecca S. Bahn, MD
Professor of Medicine
Endocrinology, Metabolism,
and Nutrition
Mayo Clinic
Rochester, Minnesota

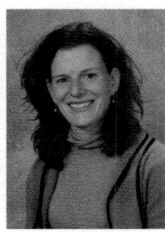

Jennifer M. Barker, MD
Associate Professor
Pediatrics
University of Colorado
Aurora, Colorado

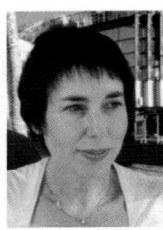

Rosemary Basson, MD, FRCP(UK)
Clinical Professor
Psychiatry
Obstetrics and Gynecology
University of British Columbia
Vancouver, British Columbia,
Canada

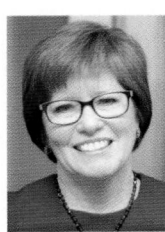

Sarah L. Berga, MD
Professor and Chair of OB/GYN
Vice President of Women's Health
Associate Dean of Women's
Health Research
Obstetrics and Gynecology
Wake Forest School of Medicine and
Wake Forest Baptist Medical Center
Winston-Salem, North Carolina

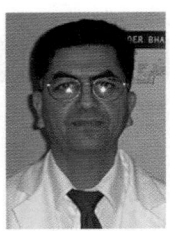

Shalender Bhasin, MD
Research Program in Men's Health:
Aging and Metabolism
Brigham and Women's Hospital
Harvard Medical School
Boston, Massachusetts

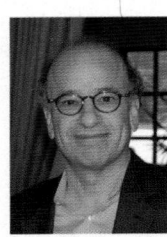

Morris J. Birnbaum, MD, PhD
Senior Vice President and Chief
Scientific Officer
CVMED
Pfizer, Inc.
Cambridge, Massachusetts

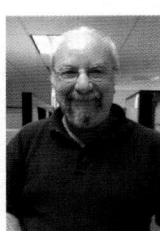

Dennis M. Black, PhD
Professor
Epidemiology and Biostatistics
University of California,
San Francisco
San Francisco, California

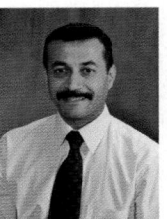

Anirban Bose, MD
Associate Professor of Medicine
Nephrology
University of Rochester Medical
Center
Rochester, New York

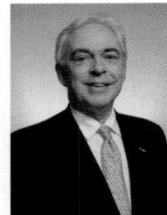

Andrew J. M. Boulton, MD, FACP,
FRCP
Professor
Centre for Endocrinology
and Diabetes
University of Manchester
Manchester, Great Britain
Visiting Professor
Endocrinology, Metabolism,
and Diabetes
University of Miami
Miami, Florida

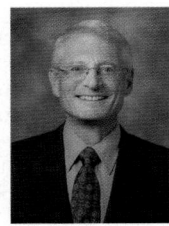

Glenn D. Braunstein, MD
The James R. Klinenberg, MD,
Professor of Medicine
Vice President for
Clinical Innovation
Cedars-Sinai Medical Center
Los Angeles, California

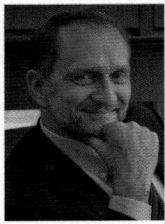

William J. Bremner, MD, PhD
Professor and Chair
Robert G. Petersdorf Endowed Chair
Medicine
University of Washington School
of Medicine
Chair
Medicine
University of Washington
Medical Center
Seattle, Washington

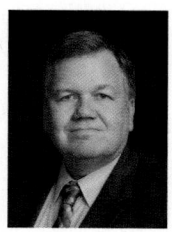

Gregory A. Brent, MD
Professor
Medicine and Physiology
David Geffen School of Medicine
at UCLA
Chair
Medicine
VA Greater Los Angeles
Healthcare System
Los Angeles, California

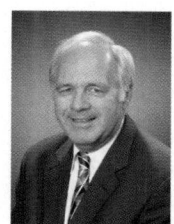

F. Richard Bringhurst, MD
Physician
Medicine
Massachusetts General Hospital
Boston, Massachusetts

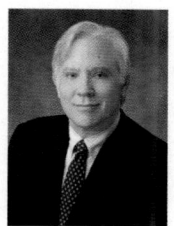

Michael Brownlee, MD
Anita and Jack Saltz Chair in
Diabetes Research
Associate Director for
Biomedical Sciences
Einstein Diabetes Research Center
Professor of Medicine and Pathology
Albert Einstein College of Medicine
Bronx, New York

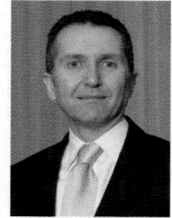

Serdar E. Bulun, MD
John J. Sciarra Professor of
Obstetrics and Gynecology
Chair
Obstetrics and Gynecology
Northwestern University
Feinberg School of Medicine
Chicago, Illinois

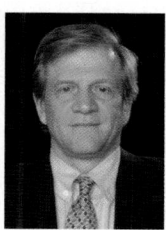

Charles F. Burant, MD, PhD
Professor
Internal Medicine
University of Michigan
Ann Arbor, Michigan

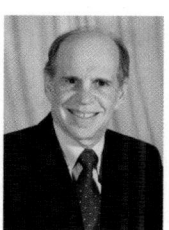

David A. Bushinsky, MD
Professor
Medicine, Pharmacology, and
Physiology
University of Rochester
Rochester, New York

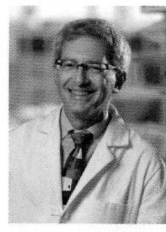

Roger D. Cone, PhD
Joe C. Davis Chair in
Biomedical Science
Professor and Chairman
Molecular Physiology and Biophysics
Director
Vanderbilt Institute for Obesity and
Metabolism
Vanderbilt University Medical Center
Nashville, Tennessee

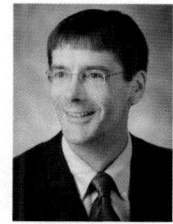

David W. Cooke, MD
Associate Professor
Pediatrics
The Johns Hopkins University
School of Medicine
Baltimore, Maryland

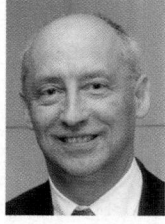

Mark E. Cooper, MB BS, PhD,
FRACP
Deputy Director and Chief Scientific
Officer
Baker IDI Heart and
Diabetes Institute
Melbourne, Victoria, Australia

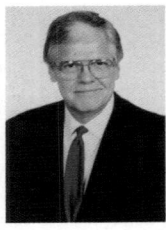

Philip E. Cryer, MD
Irene E. and Michael M. Karl
Professor of Endocrinology and
Metabolism in Medicine
Division of Endocrinology,
Metabolism, and Lipid Research
Washington University School
of Medicine
St. Louis, Missouri

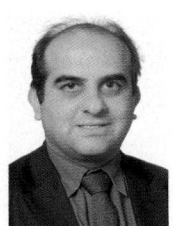

Mehul T. Dattani, MBBS, DCH,
FRCPCH, FRCP, MD
Professor
Developmental Endocrinology
Research Group
UCL Institute of Child Health
London, Great Britain

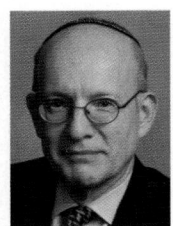

Terry F. Davies, MD, FRCP
Baumritter Professor of Medicine
Endocrinology, Diabetes,
and Bone Diseases
Icahn School of Medicine
at Mount Sinai
New York, New York
Director
Section of Endocrinology
and Metabolism
James J. Peters VA Medical Center
Bronx, New York

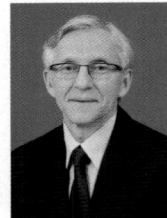

Francisco J. A. de Paula, MD, PhD
Associate Professor
Internal Medicine
Ribeirão Preto Medical School
University of São Paulo
Ribeirao Preto, São Paulo, Brazil

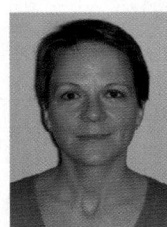

Marie B. Demay, MD
Professor of Medicine
Endocrine Unit
Harvard Medical School
Physician
Massachusetts General Hospital
Boston, Massachusetts

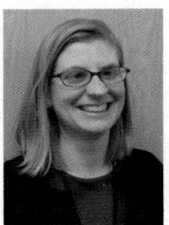

Sara A. DiVall, MD
Assistant Professor
Pediatrics
The Johns Hopkins University
Baltimore, Maryland

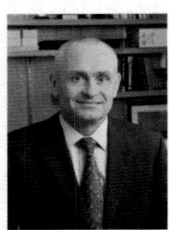

Joel K. Elmquist, DVM, PhD
Professor and Director
Division of Hypothalamic Research
Internal Medicine and Pharmacology
University of Texas Southwestern
Medical Center at Dallas
Dallas, Texas

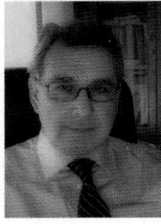

Sebastiano Filetti, MD
Professor of Internal Medicine
Internal Medicine
Sapienza Universita' di Roma
Chief
Internal Medicine
Policlinico Umberto I
Rome, Italy

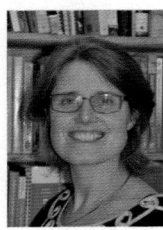

Evelien F. Gevers, MD, PhD
Barts Health NHS Trust
Royal London Hospital
Queen Mary University
William Harvey Research Institute
London, Great Britain

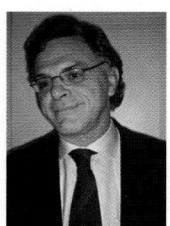

Ezio Ghigo, MD
Professor
Division of Endocrinology,
Diabetology, and Metabolism
Department of Medical Sciences
University of Turin
Turin, Italy

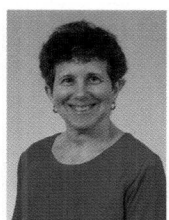

Anne C. Goldberg, MD
Associate Professor of Medicine
Division of Endocrinology,
Metabolism, and Lipid Research
Internal Medicine
Washington University School
of Medicine
St. Louis, Missouri

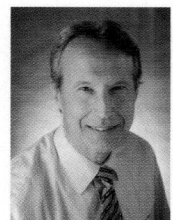

Ira J. Goldberg, MD
Director
Division of Endocrinology, Diabetes,
and Metabolism
New York University Langone
Medical Center
New York, New York

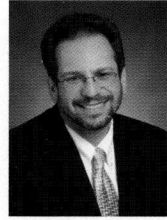

Peter A. Gottlieb, MD
Departments of Pediatrics and
Medicine
Barbara Davis Center
University of Colorado School of
Medicine
Aurora, Colorado

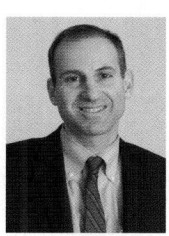

Steven K. Grinspoon, MD
Professor of Medicine
Harvard Medical School
Director
Program In Nutritional Metabolism
Massachusetts General Hospital
Co-Director
Nutrition Obesity Research Center at
Harvard University
Boston, Massachusetts

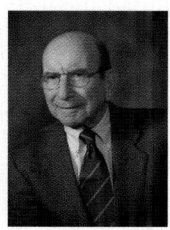

Melvin M. Grumbach, MD, DM
Hon causa (Geneva), D Hon causa
(Rene Descartes, Paris 5), D Hon
causa (Athens)
Edward B. Shaw Distinguished
Professor of Pediatrics and
Emeritus Chairman
Pediatrics
University of California
San Francisco
Attending Physician
Pediatrics
University of San Francisco Medical
Center
University of California
San Francisco Children's Hospital
San Francisco, California

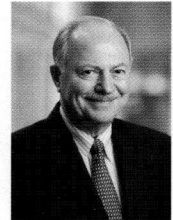

Ian D. Hay, MD, PhD
Professor of Medicine
Internal Medicine
The Dr. R.F. Emslander Professor of
Endocrine Research
Endocrinology
Consultant in Endocrinology
Internal Medicine
Mayo Clinic College of Medicine
Rochester, Minnesota

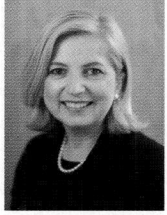

Frances J. Hayes, MB, BCh, BAO
Clinical Director
Reproductive Endocrine Associates
Co-Director
Turner Syndrome Clinic
Massachusetts General Hospital
Boston, Massachusetts

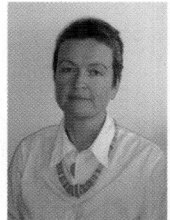

Martha Hickey, BA(Hons), MSc,
MBChB, FRCOG, FRANZCOG, MD
Professsor of Obstetrics and
Gynaecology
University of Melbourne
Head of Menopause Unit
Gynaecology
The Royal Women's Hospital
Melbourne, Victoria, Australia

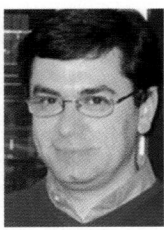

Joel N. Hirschhorn, MD, PhD
Concordia Professor
Department of Pediatrics
Professor
Department of Genetics
Boston Children's Hospital/Harvard
Medical School
Boston, Massachusetts
Senior Associate Member
Broad Institute
Cambridge, Massachusetts

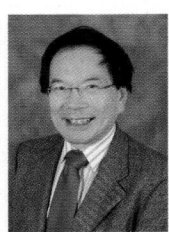

Ken K. Y. Ho, FRACP, FRCP (UK),
MD
Professor of Medicine
University of Queensland
Chair
Centres for Health Research
Princess Alexandra Hospital
Brisbane, Queensland, Australia

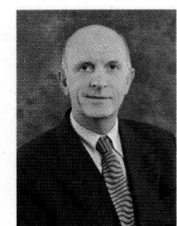

Ieuan A. Hughes, MA, MD, FRCP,
FRCP(C), FRCPCH F Med Sci
Emeritus Professor of Paediatrics
University of Cambridge
Honorary Consultant Paediatrician
Cambridge University Hospitals NHS
Foundation Trust
Cambridge, Great Britain

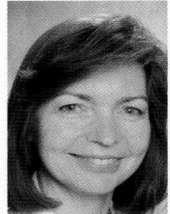

Ursula Kaiser, MD
Chief
Division of Endocrinology
Medicine
Brigham and Women's Hospital
Professor of Medicine
Harvard Medical School
Boston, Massachusetts

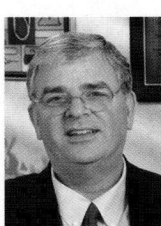

Andrew M. Kaunitz, MD
Professor and Associate Chairman
Obstetrics and Gynecology
University of Florida
College of Medicine, Jacksonville
Jacksonville, Florida

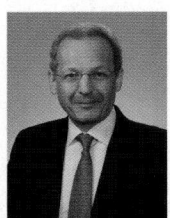

Samuel Klein, MD, MS
William H. Danforth Professor of
Medicine and Nutritional Science
Internal Medicine
Director
Center for Human Nutrition
Director
Center for Applied Research Sciences
Chief
Division of Geriatrics and
Nutritional Science
Internal Medicine
Washington University School
of Medicine
St. Louis, Missouri

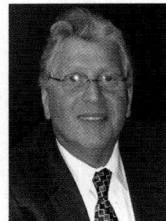

David Kleinberg, MD
Chief of Endocrinology
Veterans Administration Medical
Center
Department of Medicine
New York University
New York, New York

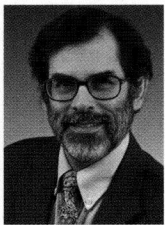

Henry M. Kronenberg, MD
Professor of Medicine
Harvard Medical School
Chief
Endocrine Unit
Massachusetts General Hospital
Boston, Massachusetts

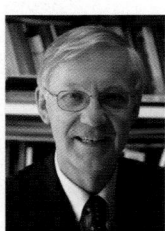

Steven W. J. Lamberts, MD, PhD
Professor
Internal Medicine
Erasmus Medical Center
Rotterdam, The Netherlands

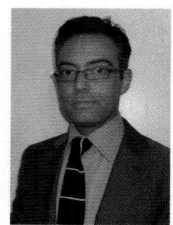

Fabio Lanfranco, MD, PhD
Division of Endocrinology,
Diabetology, and Metabolism
Department of Medical Sciences
University of Turin
Turin, Italy

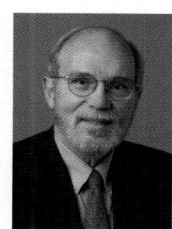

P. Reed Larsen, MD, FRCP
Professor of Medicine
Harvard Medical School
Senior Physician
Division of Endocrinology, Diabetes,
and Metabolism
Brigham and Women's Hospital
Boston, Massachusetts

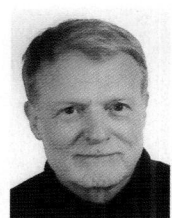

Peter Laurberg, MD
Professor of Endocrinology and
Internal Medicine
Endocrinology Clinical Medicine
Aalborg University Hospital
Aalborg, Denmark

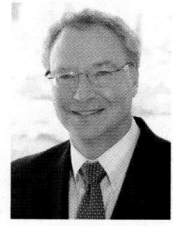

Mitchell A. Lazar, MD, PhD
Sylvan Eisman Professor of Medicine
Institute for Diabetes, Obesity,
and Metabolism
Perelman School of Medicine at the
University of Pennsylvania
Philadelphia, Pennsylvania

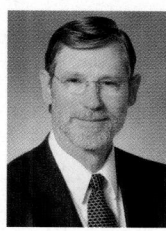

Lynn Loriaux, MD, PhD
Professor
Internal Medicine
Oregon Health and Science
University
Portland, Oregon

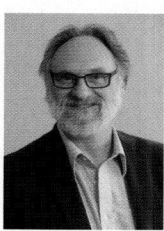

Malcolm J. Low, MD, PhD
Professor
Molecular and Integrative Physiology
Department of Internal Medicine
Division of Metabolism,
Endocrinology, and Diabetes
University of Michigan
Medical School
Ann Arbor, Michigan

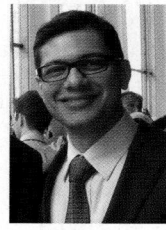

Amit R. Majithia, MD
Assistant Professor in Medicine
Endocrine Division
Massachusetts General Hospital
Instructor
Harvard Medical School
Boston, Massachusetts

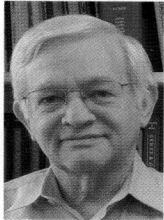

Stephen J. Marx, MD
Chief
Genetics and Endocrinology
National Institute of Diabetes,
Digestive, and Kidney Diseases
Bethesda, Maryland

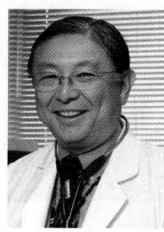

Alvin M. Matsumoto, MD
Professor
Medicine
University of Washington School
of Medicine
Associate Director
Geriatric Research
Education and Clinical Center
VA Puget Sound Health Care System
Seattle, Washington

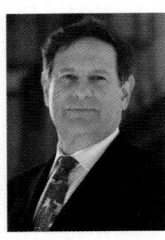

Shlomo Melmed, MBChB, MACP
Professor of Medicine
Senior Vice President and Dean of
the Medical Faculty
Cedars-Sinai Medical Center
Los Angeles, California

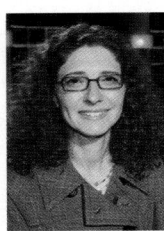

Rebeca D. Monk, MD
Associate Professor of Medicine
Nephrology
Program Director
Nephrology Fellowship
University of Rochester
Rochester, New York

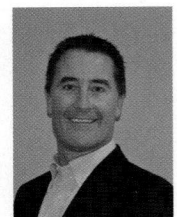

Robert D. Murray, MD
Consultant Endocrinologist and
Honorary Clinical Associate Professor
Department of Endocrinology
Leeds Teaching Hospitals NHS Trust
Leeds, Great Britain

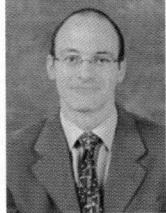

John D. C. Newell-Price, MA, PhD
FRCP
Reader in Endocrinology
Human Metabolism
University of Sheffield
Sheffield, Great Britain

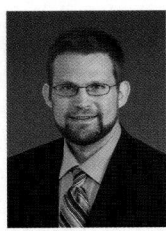

Joshua F. Nitsche, MD, PhD
Obstetrics and Gynecology
Maternal Fetal Medicine
Wake Forest School of Medicine and
Wake Forest Baptist Medical Center
Winston-Salem, North Carolina

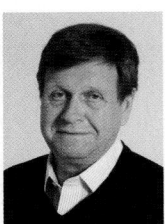

Kjell Öberg, MD, PhD
Professor
Endocrine Oncology
University Hospital
Uppsala, Sweden
Adjunct Professor
Surgery
Vanderbilt University
Nashville, Tennessee

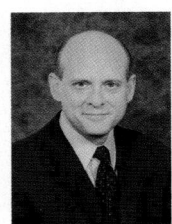

Jorge Plutzky, MD
Director
The Vascular Disease Prevention
Program
Co-Director
Preventive Cardiology
Brigham and Women's Hospital
Harvard Medical School
Boston, Massachusetts

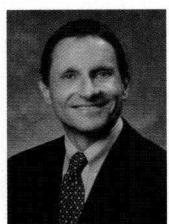

Kenneth S. Polonsky, MD
Richard T. Crane Distinguished
Service Professor
Dean of the Division of the
Biological Sciences and the Pritzker
School of Medicine
Executive Vice President for
Medical Affairs
The University of Chicago
Chicago, Illinois

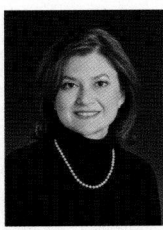

Sally Radovick, MD
The Johns Hopkins University
School of Medicine
The Johns Hopkins Hospital
Baltimore, Maryland

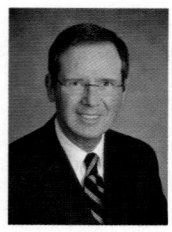

Alan G. Robinson, MD
Associate Vice Chancellor
Senior Associate Dean
Distinguished Professor of Medicine
David Geffen School of Medicine
at UCLA
University of California, Los Angeles
Los Angeles, California

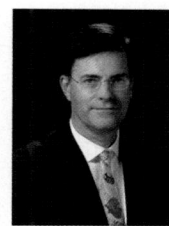

Johannes A. Romijn, MD, PhD
Professor of Medicine
Academic Medical Center
University of Amsterdam
Amsterdam, The Netherlands

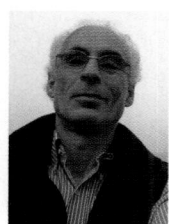

Clifford J. Rosen, MD
Center for Clinical and Translational
Research
Maine Medical Center Research
Institute
Scarborough, Maine

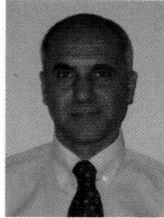

Domenico Salvatore, MD, PhD
Clinical Medicine and Surgery
University of Naples "Federico II"
Naples, Italy

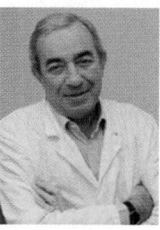

Martin-Jean Schlumberger, MD
Professor of Oncology
Université Paris Sud
Chair
Nuclear Medicine and Endocrine
Oncology
Institut Gustave Roussy
Villejuif, France

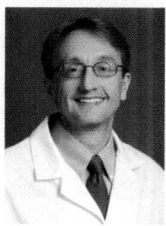

Clay F. Semenkovich, MD
Herbert S. Gasser Professor
Chief
Division of Endocrinology,
Metabolism, and Lipid Research
Washington University
St. Louis, Missouri

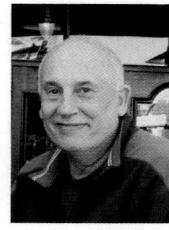

Patrick M. Sluss, PhD
Associate Director
Clinical Pathology Core
Pathology Service
Massachusetts General Hospital
Associate Professor
Pathology
Harvard Medical School
Boston, Massachusetts

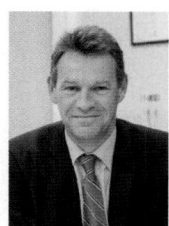

Paul M. Stewart, MD, FRCP,
F Med Sci
Dean and Professor of Medicine
University of Leeds
Leeds, Great Britain

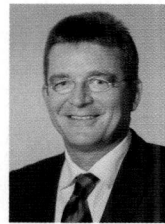

Christian J. Strasburger, MD
Department of Medicine
Division of Clinical Endocrinology
Charité Campus Mitte
Berlin, Germany

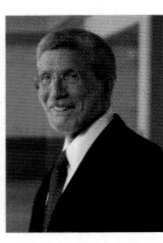

Dennis M. Styne, MD
Yocha Dehe Chair of Pediatric
Endocrinology
Professor
Pediatrics
University of California
Sacramento, California

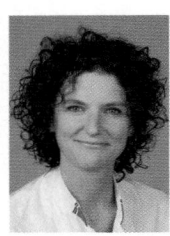

Annewieke W. van den Beld,
MD, PhD
Internal Medicine
Groene Hart Hospital
Gouda, The Netherlands

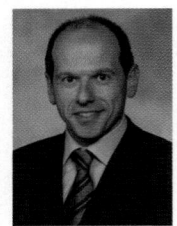

Adrian Vella, MD
Professor of Medicine
Endocrinology and Metabolism
Mayo Clinic
Rochester, Minnesota

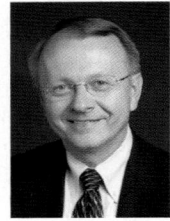

Joseph G. Verbalis, MD
Professor
Medicine
Georgetown University
Chief
Endocrinology and Metabolism
Georgetown University Hospital
Washington, DC

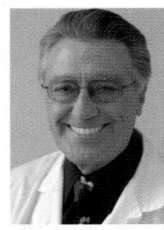

Aaron I. Vinik, MD, PhD
Professor of Medicine, Pathology,
and Neurobiology
Director of Research and
Neuroendocrine Unit
Strelitz Diabetes Center
Internal Medicine
Eastern Virginia Medical School
Norfolk, Virginia

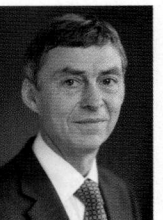

Anthony P. Weetman, MD, DSc
Professor of Medicine
Human Metabolism
University of Sheffield
Sheffield, Great Britain

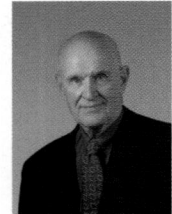

Samuel A. Wells, Jr., MD
Senior Investigator
Cancer Genetics Branch
National Cancer Institute
Bethesda, Maryland

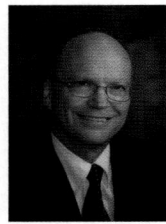

William F. Young, Jr., MD, MSc
Professor of Medicine
Tyson Family Endocrinology
Clinical Professor
Division of Endocrinology, Diabetes,
Metabolism, and Nutrition
Mayo Clinic
Rochester, Minnesota

Preface

The Editors are delighted to welcome you to the 65th anniversary thirteenth edition of *Williams Textbook of Endocrinology*. In this new edition we have strived to maintain Robert Williams' original 1950 mandate to publish "a condensed and authoritative discussion of the management of clinical endocrinopathies based upon the application of fundamental information obtained from chemical and physiological investigation." With the passing of the decades, our scholarly goal has been further enriched by the addition of genetic, molecular, cellular, and population sciences, which underpin our understanding of both the pathogenesis and management of endocrine disorders. This textbook is geared toward providing a cogent navigation through the wealth of scholarly information that emanates from the remarkable and continuously advancing medical discoveries of our times. Our challenge remains to be both concise and didactic, while still covering all relevant biomedical endocrine science in an accessible and comprehensive fashion.

With these goals in mind, we have once again assembled a team of outstanding authorities in the field who each contribute their unique expertise in the synthesis of current knowledge for each area. For this edition, we have added new chapters on the genetics of endocrinology and on population health, and several new authors also now provide fresh perspectives on their rapidly evolving fields. These new contributions reflect the changing emphasis of endocrine practice today. Each section has undergone significant revision and updating to bring the most current information to our readers.

We are deeply appreciative of the valued co-workers in our respective offices, including Lynn Moulton, Grace Labrado, and Sharon Sain, for their dedicated efforts. We also thank our colleagues at Elsevier—Helene Caprari, Margaret Nelson, Jennifer Ehlers, and Sharon Corell—for shepherding the entire production process so professionally. The final product of this exemplary text is due to their skilled navigation of the medical publishing world. We are confident that our combined efforts have succeeded in achieving the high standards set by previous editions that have made *Williams* the classic "go to" book for all those interested in endocrinology.

Note from the Editors

In July 2014, the prestigious medical journal *The Lancet* published an Open Letter online regarding the Gaza conflict that caused significant consternation among respected members of the academic community. The letter, authored by Paola Manducca et al., made a number of what many endocrinologists viewed as unsubstantiated and defamatory claims about that conflict. Their concerns also included use of the pages of *The Lancet* to advance a nonscientific agenda and the publication of opinions used on hate group websites.

The response to the Open Letter was passionate, with many academics across the world expressing outrage that *The Lancet* would publish what they viewed as a one-sided, overtly political letter. *The Lancet* defended publication of the letter, asserting that it was not political but dealt with issues directly relating to global health. *The Lancet* published a large number of response letters on both sides of the issue. (See http://www.thelancet.com/gaza-letter-2014 -responses.)

How does this matter relate to the thirteenth edition of *Williams Textbook of Endocrinology*? Elsevier is the publisher of both *The Lancet* and *Williams*. The events described above were playing out in the summer and fall of 2014 at a time when preparations for the thirteenth edition were at an advanced stage, with commitments from editors and authors to complete this comprehensive endocrine text in a timely manner. Because of these commitments and our view of the significant value of the textbook to the field, we resisted advice from colleagues who called upon us to withdraw from participating in the thirteenth edition of *Williams*, since this would have jeopardized publication of the book. We concluded that the commitments we had made, particularly to authors who had already submitted completed manuscripts, should take precedence and that we should not jeopardize the timely publication of the book.

We should point out that two of the authors who had agreed to coauthor chapters elected to remove their names from the list of coauthors of those chapters because of these events. Thus Chapters 31 and 32 do not list John Buse as a coauthor and Chapter 38 does not list Daniel Drucker as a coauthor, even though they made substantial contributions to the respective chapters.

As editors, we were disappointed that Elsevier did not put in place what we view as appropriate controls to ensure that a biomedical publication adds scientific knowledge rather than promotes what we view as the nonscientific agendas of editors and authors.

We, the editors of the *Williams Textbook of Endocrinology*, as well as Elsevier, are committed to producing the highest quality scholarly work strongly embedded in the principles of unfettered integrity of medical publication.

Henry M. Kronenberg
P. Reed Larsen
Shlomo Melmed
Kenneth S. Polonsky

Contents

SECTION IX: Polyendocrine and Neoplastic Disorders

Section I

Hormones and Hormone Action

CHAPTER 1

Principles of Endocrinology

HENRY M. KRONENBERG • SHLOMO MELMED • P. REED LARSEN • KENNETH S. POLONSKY

KEY POINTS

- Endocrinology is a scientific and medical discipline with a unique focus on hormones and features a multidisciplinary approach to understanding hormones and their diseases.
- Endocrine and paracrine systems differ in important respects that illustrate the evolutionary pressures on these distinct cell signaling strategies.
- Hormone-secreting cells are designed to efficiently synthesize hormones and secrete them in a regulated way.
- Hormones in the bloodstream often are associated with binding proteins to allow their solubility, keep them from degradation and renal excretion, and regulate their stability in the extracellular space.
- Hormones either act on receptors on the plasma membranes of target cells or move into cells to bind to intracellullar receptors; in either case, the target cell is not a passive recipient of signals but rather has key roles in regulating the responses to hormones.
- Control of hormone secretion involves multiple inputs from distant targets, nervous system inputs, and local paracrine and autocrine factors, all leading to complex patterns of circadian secretion, pulsatile secretion, secretion driven by homeostatic stimuli, or stimuli that lead to secular changes over the lifespan.
- Endocrine diseases fall into broad categories of hormone over- or underproduction, altered tissue response to hormones, or tumors arising from endocrine tissue.
- Hormones and synthetic molecules designed to interact with hormone receptors are administered to diagnose and treat diseases.

About a hundred years ago, Starling coined the term *hormone* to describe secretin, a substance secreted by the small intestine into the bloodstream to stimulate pancreatic secretion. In his Croonian Lectures, Starling considered the endocrine and nervous systems as two distinct mechanisms for coordination and control of organ function. Thus, endocrinology found its first home in the discipline of mammalian physiology.

Work over the next several decades by biochemists, physiologists, and clinical investigators led to the characterization of many hormones secreted into the bloodstream from discrete glands or other organs. These investigators showed that diseases such as hypothyroidism and diabetes could be treated successfully for the first time by replacing specific hormones. These initial triumphs formed the foundation of the clinical specialty of endocrinology.

Advances in cell biology, molecular biology, and genetics over the ensuing years began to explain the mechanisms of endocrine diseases and of hormone secretion and action. Even though these advances have embedded endocrinology in the framework of molecular cell biology, they have not changed the essential subject of endocrinology—the signaling that coordinates and controls the functions of multiple organs and processes. Herein we survey the general themes and principles that underpin the diverse approaches used by clinicians, physiologists, biochemists, cell biologists, and geneticists to understand the endocrine system.

THE EVOLUTIONARY PERSPECTIVE

Hormones can be defined as chemical signals secreted into the bloodstream that act on distant tissues, usually in a regulatory fashion. Hormonal signaling represents a special case of the more general process of signaling between cells. Even unicellular organisms, such as baker's yeast, *Saccharomyces cerevisiae*, secrete short peptide mating factors that act on receptors of other yeast cells to trigger mating between the two cells. These receptors resemble the ubiquitous family of seven membrane-spanning mammalian receptors that respond to ligands as diverse as photons and glycoprotein hormones. Because these yeast receptors trigger activation of heterotrimeric G proteins just as mammalian receptors do, this conserved signaling pathway must have been present in the common ancestor of yeast and humans.

Signals from one cell to adjacent cells, so-called paracrine signals, often use the same molecular pathways used by hormonal signals. For example, the sevenless receptor controls the differentiation of retinal cells in the *Drosophila* eye by responding to a membrane-anchored signal from an adjacent cell. Sevenless is a membrane-spanning receptor with an intracellular tyrosine kinase domain that signals in a way that closely resembles the signaling by hormone receptors such as the insulin receptor tyrosine kinase. Because paracrine factors and hormones can share

Regulation of signaling: endocrine

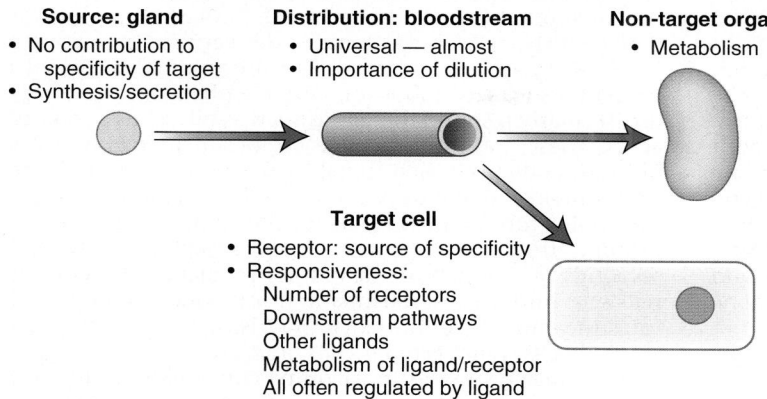

Source: gland
- No contribution to specificity of target
- Synthesis/secretion

Distribution: bloodstream
- Universal — almost
- Importance of dilution

Non-target organ
- Metabolism

Target cell
- Receptor: source of specificity
- Responsiveness:
    Number of receptors
    Downstream pathways
    Other ligands
    Metabolism of ligand/receptor
    All often regulated by ligand

Regulation of signaling: paracrine

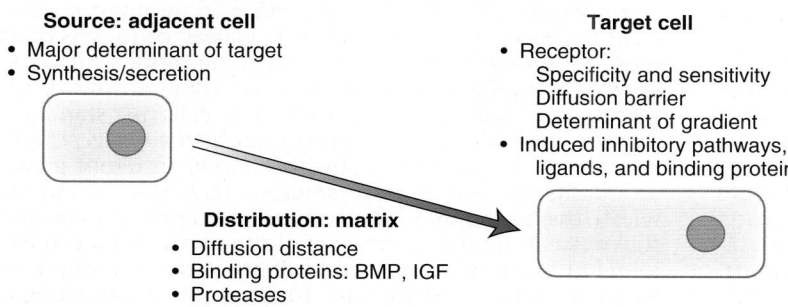

Source: adjacent cell
- Major determinant of target
- Synthesis/secretion

Target cell
- Receptor:
    Specificity and sensitivity
    Diffusion barrier
    Determinant of gradient
- Induced inhibitory pathways, ligands, and binding proteins

Distribution: matrix
- Diffusion distance
- Binding proteins: BMP, IGF
- Proteases
- Matrix components

Figure 1-1 Comparison of determinants of endocrine and paracrine signaling. BMP, bone morphogenetic protein; IGF, insulin-like growth factor.

signaling machinery, it is not surprising that hormones can, in some settings, act as paracrine factors. Testosterone, for example, is secreted into the bloodstream but also acts locally in the testes to control spermatogenesis. Insulin-like growth factor 1 (IGF-1) is a polypeptide hormone secreted into the bloodstream from the liver and other tissues but is also a paracrine factor made locally in most tissues to control cell proliferation. Furthermore, one receptor can mediate actions of a hormone, such as parathyroid hormone (PTH), and of a paracrine factor, such as parathyroid hormone–related protein. In some cases, the paracrine actions of "hormones" have functions quite unrelated to the hormonal functions. For example, macrophages synthesize the active form of vitamin D, 1,25-dihydroxyvitamin D_3 (1,25[OH]$_2$D$_3$), which can then bind to vitamin D receptors in the same cells and stimulate production of antimicrobial peptides.[1] The vitamin D 1α-hydroxylase responsible for activating 25-hydroxyvitamin D is synthesized in multiple tissues in which it has functions unrelated to the calcium homeostatic actions of the 1,25(OH)$_2$D$_3$ hormone. One can speculate that the hormonal actions of vitamin D might have evolved well after the paracrine vitamin D system provided the raw materials for the hormonal system.

Target cells respond similarly to signals that reach them from the bloodstream (hormones) or from the cell next door (paracrine factors); the cellular response machinery does not distinguish the sites of origin of signals. The shared final common pathways used by hormonal and paracrine signals should not, however, obscure important differences between hormonal and paracrine signaling

systems (Fig. 1-1). Paracrine signals do not travel very far; consequently, the specific site of origin of a paracrine factor determines where it will act and provides specificity to that action. When the paracrine factor bone morphogenetic protein 4 (BMP4) is secreted by cells in the developing kidney, BMP4 regulates the differentiation of renal cells; when the same factor is secreted by cells in bone, it regulates bone formation. Thus, the site of origin of BMP4 determines its physiologic role. In contrast, because hormones are secreted into the bloodstream, their sites of origin are often divorced from their functions. Like BMP4, thyroid hormone, for example, acts in many tissues, but the site of origin of thyroid hormone in a gland in the neck has nothing to do with the sites of action of the hormone.

Because the specificity of paracrine factor action is so dependent on its precise site of origin, elaborate mechanisms have evolved to regulate and constrain the diffusion of paracrine factors. Paracrine factors of the hedgehog family, for example, are covalently bound to cholesterol to constrain the diffusion of these molecules in the extracellular milieu. Most paracrine factors interact with binding proteins that block their action and control their diffusion. Chordin, noggin, and many other distinct proteins all bind to various members of the BMP family to regulate their action, for example. Proteases such as tolloid then destroy the binding proteins at specific sites to liberate BMPs so that they can act on appropriate target cells.

Hormones have rather different constraints. Because they diffuse throughout the body, they must be synthesized in enormous amounts relative to the amounts of paracrine factors needed at specific locations. This synthesis usually occurs in specialized cells designed for that specific purpose. Hormones must then be able to travel in the bloodstream and diffuse in effective concentrations into tissues. Therefore, for example, lipophilic hormones bind to soluble proteins that allow them to travel in the aqueous media of blood at relatively high concentrations. The ability of hormones to diffuse through the extracellular space means that the local concentration of hormone at target sites will rapidly decrease when glandular secretion of the hormone stops. Because hormones diffuse throughout extracellular fluid quickly, hormonal metabolism can occur in specialized organs such as the liver and kidney in a manner that determines the effective hormone concentration in other tissues.

Thus, paracrine factors and hormones use several distinct strategies to control their biosynthesis, sites of action, transport, and metabolism. These differing strategies probably explain partly why a hormone such as IGF-1, unlike its close relative, insulin, has multiple binding proteins that control its action in tissues. IGF-1 exhibits a double life as both a hormone and a paracrine factor. Presumably, the local actions of IGF-1 mandate an elaborate binding protein apparatus to enable appropriate hormone signaling.

All the major hormonal signaling programs—G protein–coupled receptors, tyrosine kinase receptors, serine/threonine kinase receptors, ion channels, cytokine receptors, nuclear receptors—are also used by paracrine factors. In contrast, several paracrine signaling programs are used only by paracrine factors and probably not by hormones. For example, Notch receptors respond to membrane-based ligands to control cell fate, but no blood-borne ligands use Notch-type signaling (at least, none is currently known). Perhaps the intracellular strategy used by Notch, which involves cleavage of the receptor and subsequent nuclear actions of the receptor's cytoplasmic portion, is too inflexible to serve the purposes of hormones.

The analyses of the complete genomes of multiple bacterial species, the yeast *S. cerevisiae,* the fruit fly *Drosophila melanogaster,* the worm *Caenorhabditis elegans,* the plant *Arabidopsis thaliana,* humans, and many other species have allowed a comprehensive view of the signaling machinery used by various forms of life. As noted already, *S. cerevisiae* uses G protein–linked receptors; this organism, however, lacks tyrosine kinase receptors and nuclear receptors that resemble the estrogen/thyroid receptor family. In contrast, the worm and fly share with humans the use of each of these signaling pathways, although with substantial variation in numbers of genes committed to each pathway. For example, the *Drosophila* genome encodes 20 nuclear receptors, the *C. elegans* genome encodes 270, and the human genome encodes 48. These patterns suggest that ancient multicellular animals must have already established the signaling systems that are the foundation of the endocrine system as we know it in mammals.

Even before the sequencing of the human genome, sequence analyses had made clear that many receptor genes are found in mammalian genomes for which no clear ligand or function was known. The analyses of these "orphan" receptors have succeeded in broadening the current understanding of hormonal signaling. For example, the liver X receptor (LXR) was one such orphan receptor found when searching for unknown nuclear receptors. Subsequent experiments showed that oxygenated derivatives of cholesterol are the ligands for LXR, which regulates genes involved in cholesterol and fatty acid metabolism.[2] The examples of LXR and many others raise the question of what constitutes a hormone. The classic view of

hormones is that they are synthesized in discrete glands and have no function other than activating receptors on cell membranes or in the nucleus. Cholesterol, which is converted in cells to oxygenated derivatives that activate the LXR receptor, in contrast, uses a hormonal strategy to regulate its own metabolism. Other orphan nuclear receptors similarly respond to ligands such as bile acids and fatty acids. These "hormones" have important metabolic roles quite separate from their signaling properties, although the hormone-like signaling serves to allow regulation of the metabolic function. The calcium-sensing receptor is an example from the G protein–linked receptor family that responds to a nonclassic ligand, ionic calcium. Calcium is released into the bloodstream from bone, kidney, and intestine and acts on the calcium-sensing receptor on parathyroid cells, renal tubular cells, and other cells to coordinate cellular responses to calcium. Thus, many important metabolic factors have taken on hormonal properties as part of a regulatory strategy.

ENDOCRINE GLANDS

Hormone formation may occur either in localized collections of specific cells, the endocrine glands, or in cells that have additional roles. Many protein hormones, such as growth hormone (GH), PTH, prolactin (PRL), insulin, and glucagon, are produced in dedicated cells by standard protein synthetic mechanisms common to all cells. These secretory cells usually contain specialized secretory granules designed to store large amounts of hormone and to release the hormones in response to specific signals. Formation of small hormone molecules initiates with commonly found precursors, usually in specific glands such as the adrenals, gonads, or thyroid. In the case of the steroid hormones, the precursor is cholesterol, which is modified by various hydroxylations, methylations, and demethylations, all using cytochrome P450-based reactions to form the glucocorticoids, androgens, estrogens, and their biologically active derivatives.

However, not all hormones are formed in dedicated and specialized endocrine glands. For example, the protein hormone leptin, which regulates appetite and energy expenditure, is formed in adipocytes, thus providing a specific signal reflecting the nutritional state of the organism to the central nervous system. The cholesterol derivative, 7-dehydrocholesterol, the precursor of vitamin D, is produced in skin keratinocytes by a photochemical reaction. The enteroendocrine system comprises a unique hormonal system in which peptide hormones that regulate metabolic and other responses to oral nutrients are produced and secreted by specialized endocrine cells scattered throughout the intestinal epithelium.

Thyroid hormone synthesis occurs via a unique pathway. The thyroid cell synthesizes a 660,000-kDa homodimer, thyroglobulin, which is then iodinated at specific iodotyrosines. Certain of these "couple" to form the iodothyronine molecule within thyroglobulin, which is then stored in the lumen of the thyroid follicle. In order for this to occur, the thyroid cell must concentrate the trace quantities of iodide from the blood and oxidize it via a specific peroxidase. Release of thyroxine (T_4) from the thyroglobulin requires its phagocytosis and cathepsin-catalyzed digestion by the same cells.

Hormones are synthesized in response to biochemical signals generated by various modulating systems. Many of these systems are specific to the effects of the hormone product; for example, PTH synthesis is regulated by the concentration of ionized calcium. Insulin synthesis is regulated by the concentration of glucose. For others, such as gonadal, adrenal, and thyroid hormones, control of hormone synthesis is achieved by the hormonostatic function of the hypothalamic-pituitary axis. Cells in the hypothalamus and pituitary monitor the circulating hormone concentration and secrete trophic hormones, which activate specific pathways for hormone synthesis and release. Typical examples are luteinizing hormone, follicle-stimulating hormone, thyroid-stimulating hormone, and adrenocorticotropic hormone (LH, FSH, TSH, and ACTH, respectively).

These trophic hormones increase rates of hormone synthesis and secretion, and they may induce target cell division, thus causing enlargement of the various target glands. For example, in hypothyroid individuals living in iodine-deficient areas of the world, TSH secretion causes a marked hyperplasia of thyroid cells. In such regions, the thyroid gland may be 20 to 50 times its normal size. Adrenal hyperplasia occurs in patients with genetic deficiencies in cortisol formation. Hypertrophy and hyperplasia of parathyroid cells, in this case initiated by an intrinsic response to the stress of hypocalcemia, occur in patients with renal insufficiency or calcium malabsorption.

Hormones may be fully active when released into the bloodstream (e.g., GH or insulin), or they may require activation in specific cells to produce their biologic effects. These activation steps are often highly regulated. For example, the T_4 released from the thyroid cell is a prohormone that must undergo a specific deiodination to form the active 3,5,3'-triiodothyronine (T_3). This deiodination reaction can occur in target tissues, such as in the central nervous system; in the thyrotrophs, where T_3 provides feedback regulation of TSH production; or in hepatic and renal cells, from which it is released into the circulation for uptake by all tissues. A similar postsecretory activation step catalyzed by a 5α-reductase causes tissue-specific activation of testosterone to dihydrotestosterone in target tissues, including the male urogenital tract and genital skin as well as in liver. Vitamin D undergoes hydroxylation at the 25 position in the liver and in the 1 position in the kidney. Both hydroxylations must occur to produce the active hormone, 1,25-hydroxyvitamin D. The activity of the 1α-hydroxylase, but not the 25-hydroxylase, is stimulated by PTH and reduced plasma phosphate but is inhibited by calcium, 1,25-hydroxyvitamin D, and fibroblast growth factor 23 (FGF23).

Hormones are synthesized as required on a daily, hourly, or minute-to-minute basis with minimal storage, but there are significant exceptions. One is the thyroid gland, which contains enough stored hormone to last for about 2 months. This storage permits a constant supply of this hormone despite significant variations in the availability of iodine. However, if iodine deficiency is prolonged, the normal reservoirs of T_4 can be depleted.

The various feedback signaling systems exemplified earlier enable the hormonal *homeostasis* characteristic of virtually all endocrine systems. Regulation may include the central nervous system or local signal recognition mechanisms in the glandular cells, such as the calcium-sensing receptor of the parathyroid cell. Superimposed, centrally programmed increases and decreases in hormone secretion or activation through neuroendocrine pathways also occur. Examples include the circadian variation in the secretion of ACTH directing the synthesis and release of cortisol. The monthly menstrual cycle exemplifies a system with much longer periodicity that requires a complex synergism between central and peripheral axes of the endocrine glands. Disruption of hormonal homeostasis due to glandular or central regulatory system dysfunction has both clinical and laboratory consequences. Recognition and correction of these are the essence of clinical endocrinology.

TRANSPORT OF HORMONES IN BLOOD

Protein hormones and some small molecules, such as the catecholamines, are water-soluble and are readily transported via the circulatory system. Others are nearly insoluble in water (e.g., the steroid and thyroid hormones) and their distribution presents special problems. Such molecules are bound to 50- to 60-kDa carrier plasma glycoproteins such as thyroxine-binding globulin (TBG), sex hormone–binding globulin (SHBG), and corticosteroid-binding globulin (CBG) as well as to albumin. These ligand-protein complexes serve as reservoirs of these hormones, ensure ubiquitous distribution of their water-insoluble ligands, and protect the small molecules from rapid inactivation or excretion in the urine or bile. The protein-bound hormones exist in rapid equilibrium with the often-minute quantities of hormone in the aqueous plasma. It is this "free" fraction of the circulating hormone that is taken up by the target cell. It has been shown, for example, that if tracer thyroid hormone is injected into the portal vein in a protein-free solution, it is bound to hepatocytes at the periphery of the hepatic sinusoid. When the same experiment is repeated with a protein-containing solution, there is a uniform distribution of the tracer hormone throughout the hepatic lobule.[3] Despite the very high affinity of some of the binding proteins for their ligands, one specific protein may not be essential for hormone distribution. For example, in humans with a congenital deficiency of TBG, other proteins, transthyretin (TTR) and albumin, subsume its role. Because the affinity of these secondary thyroid hormone transport proteins is several orders of magnitude lower than that of TBG, it is possible for the hypothalamic-pituitary feedback system to maintain free thyroid hormone in the normal range at a much lower total hormone concentration. The fact that the free hormone concentration is normal in subjects with TBG deficiency indicates that it is this free moiety that is defended by the hypothalamic-pituitary axis and is the active hormone.[4]

The availability of gene targeting techniques has allowed specific tests of the physiologic role of several hormone-binding proteins. For example, mice with targeted inactivation of the vitamin D–binding protein (DBP) have been generated.[5] Although the absence of DBP markedly reduces the circulating concentration of vitamin D, the mice are otherwise normal. However, they do show enhanced susceptibility to a vitamin D–deficient diet because of the reduced reservoir of this sterol. In addition, the absence of DBP markedly reduces the half-life of 25-hydroxyvitamin D by accelerating its hepatic uptake, making the mice less susceptible to vitamin D intoxication.

In rodents, TTR carries retinol-binding protein and is also the principal thyroid hormone–binding protein. This protein is synthesized in the liver and in the choroid plexus. It is the major thyroid hormone–binding protein in the cerebrospinal fluid of both rodents and humans and was thought to perhaps serve an important role in thyroid hormone transport into the central nervous system. This hypothesis has been disproved by the fact that mice without TTR have normal concentrations of T_4 in the brain as well as free T_4 in the plasma.[6,7] To be sure, the serum concentrations of vitamin A and total T_4 are decreased, but the knockout mice have no signs of vitamin A deficiency or hypothyroidism. Such studies suggest that these proteins primarily serve distributive and reservoir functions.

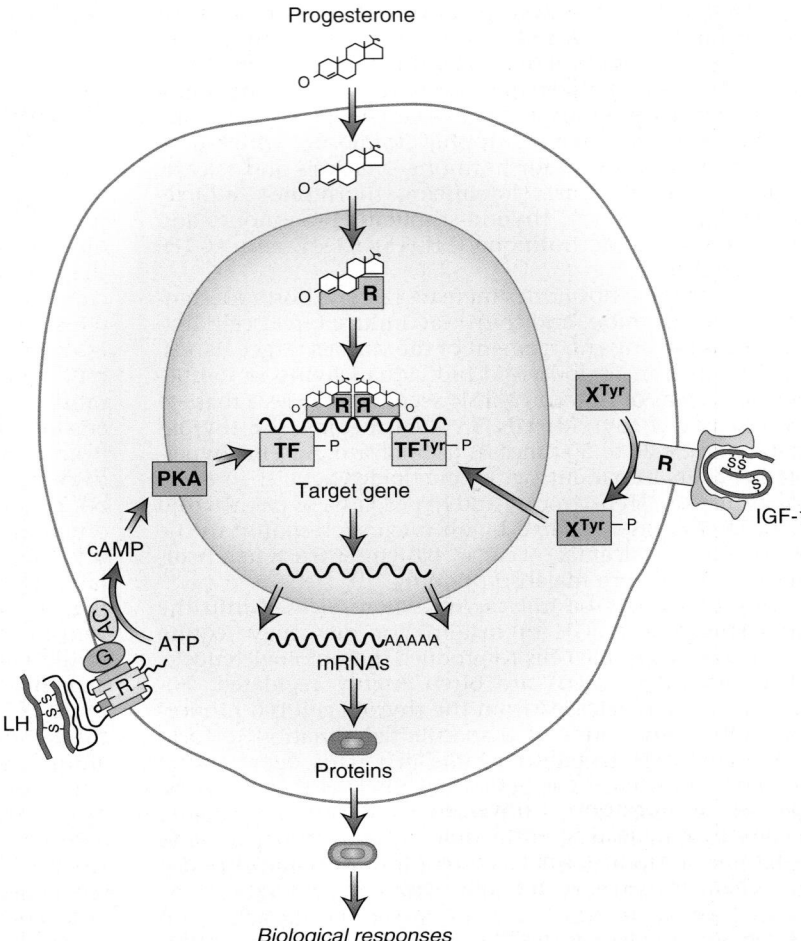

Figure 1-2 Hormonal signaling by cell-surface and intracellular receptors. The receptors for the water-soluble polypeptide hormones, luteinizing hormone (LH), and insulin-like growth factor 1 (IGF-1) are integral membrane proteins located at the cell surface. They bind the hormone-utilizing extracellular sequences and transduce a signal by the generation of second messengers: cyclic adenosine monophosphate (cAMP) for the LH receptor and tyrosine-phosphorylated substrates for the IGF-1 receptor. Although effects on gene expression are indicated, direct effects on cellular proteins (e.g., ion channels) are also observed. In contrast, the receptor for the lipophilic steroid hormone progesterone resides in the cell nucleus. It binds the hormone and becomes activated and capable of directly modulating target gene transcription. AC, adenylate cyclase; ATP, adenosine triphosphate; G, heterotrimeric G protein; mRNAs, messenger RNAs; PKA, protein kinase A; R, receptor molecule; TF, transcription factor; Tyr, tyrosine found in protein X; X, unknown protein substrate. (From Mayo K. Receptors: molecular mediators of hormone action. In: Conn PM, Melmed S, eds. *Endocrinology: Basic and Clinical Principles*. Totowa, NJ: Humana Press; 1997:11.)

Protein hormones and some small ligands (e.g., catecholamines) produce their effects by interacting with cell-surface receptors. Others, such as the steroid and thyroid hormones, must enter the cell to bind to cytosolic or nuclear receptors. In the past, it has been thought that much of the transmembrane transport of hormones was passive. Evidence now shows that there are specific transporters involved in cellular uptake of thyroid hormone.[7] This activity may be found to be the case for other small ligands as well, revealing yet another mechanism for ensuring the distribution of a hormone to its site of action. Studies in mice missing megalin, a large, cell-surface protein in the low-density lipoprotein (LDL) receptor family, suggest that estrogen and testosterone, bound to SHBG, use megalin to enter certain tissues while still bound to SHBG.[8] In this case, therefore, the hormone bound to SHBG, rather than "free" hormone, is the active moiety that enters cells. It is unclear how generally this apparent exception to the "free hormone" hypothesis occurs.

TARGET CELLS AS ACTIVE PARTICIPANTS

Hormones determine cellular target actions by binding with high specificity to receptor proteins. Whether or not a peripheral cell is hormonally responsive depends to a large extent on the presence and function of specific and selective hormone receptors. Receptor expression thus determines which cells will respond, as well as the nature of the intracellular effector pathways activated by the hormone signal. Receptor proteins may be localized to the cell membrane, cytoplasm, or nucleus. Broadly, polypeptide hormone receptors are cell membrane–associated, but steroid hormones selectively bind soluble intracellular proteins (Fig. 1-2).

Membrane-associated receptor proteins usually consist of extracellular sequences that recognize and bind ligand, transmembrane-anchoring hydrophobic sequences, and intracellular sequences, which initiate intracellular signaling. Intracellular signaling is mediated by covalent modification and activation of intracellular signaling molecules (e.g., signal transducers and activators of transcription [STAT] proteins) or by generation of small molecule second messengers (e.g., cyclic adenosine monophosphate) through activation of heterotrimeric G proteins. Subunits of these G proteins (α-, β-, and γ-subunits) activate or suppress effector enzymes and ion channels that generate the second messengers. Some of these receptors may in fact exhibit constitutive activity and have been shown to signal in the absence of added ligand.

Several growth factors and hormone receptors (e.g., for insulin) behave as intrinsic tyrosine kinases or activate intracellular protein tyrosine kinases. Ligand activation may cause receptor dimerization (e.g., GH) or heterodimerization (e.g., interleukin 6), followed by activation of intracellular phosphorylation cascades. These activated proteins ultimately determine specific nuclear gene expression.

Both the number of receptors expressed per cell, as well as their responses, are also regulated, thus providing a further level of control for hormone action. Several mechanisms account for altered receptor function. Receptor endocytosis causes internalization of cell-surface receptors; the hormone-receptor complex is subsequently dissociated, resulting in abrogation of the hormone signal. Receptor trafficking may then result in recycling back to the cell surface (e.g., as for insulin), or the internalized receptor may undergo lysosomal degradation. Both these mechanisms triggered by activation of receptors effectively lead to impaired hormone signaling by downregulation of these receptors. The hormone signaling pathway may also be downregulated by receptor desensitization (e.g., as for epinephrine); ligand-mediated receptor phosphorylation leads to a reversible deactivation of the receptor. Desensitization mechanisms can be activated by a receptor's ligand (homologous desensitization) or by another signal (heterologous desensitization), thereby attenuating receptor signaling in the continued presence of ligand. Receptor function may also be limited by action of specific phosphatases (e.g., Src homology phosphatase [SHP]) or by intracellular negative regulation of the signaling cascade (e.g., suppressor of cytokine signaling [SOCS] proteins inhibiting Janus kinase/signal transducers and activators of transcription [JAK-STAT] signaling). Certain ligand-receptor complexes may also translocate to the nucleus.

Mutational changes in receptor structure can also determine hormone action. Constitutive receptor activation may be induced by activating mutations (e.g., TSH receptor) leading to endocrine organ hyperfunction, even in the absence of hormone. Conversely, inactivating receptor mutations may lead to endocrine hypofunction (e.g., testosterone or vasopressin receptors). These syndromes are well characterized and are well described in this volume (Table 1-1).

The functional diversity of receptor signaling also results in overlapping or redundant intracellular pathways. For example, both GH and cytokines activate JAK-STAT signaling, whereas the distal effects of these stimuli clearly differ. Thus, despite common signaling pathways, hormones elicit highly specific cellular effects. Tissue- or cell-type genetic programs or receptor-receptor interactions at the cell surface (e.g., dopamine D2 with somatotropin release–inhibiting factor [SRIF] receptor hetero-oligomerization) may also confer specific cellular response to a hormone and provide an additive cellular effect.[9]

CONTROL OF HORMONE SECRETION

Anatomically distinct endocrine glands are composed of highly differentiated cells that synthesize, store, and secrete hormones. Circulating hormone concentrations are a function of glandular secretory patterns and hormone clearance rates. Hormone secretion is tightly regulated to attain circulating levels that are most conducive to elicit the appropriate target tissue response. For example, longitudinal bone growth is initiated and maintained by exquisitely regulated levels of circulating GH, yet mild GH hypersecretion results in gigantism, and GH deficiency causes growth retardation. Ambient circulating hormone concentrations are not uniform, and secretion patterns determine appropriate physiologic function. Thus, insulin secretion occurs in short pulses elicited by nutrient and other signals; gonadotropin secretion is episodic, determined by a hypothalamic pulse generator; and PRL secretion appears to be relatively continuous, with secretory peaks elicited during suckling.

TABLE 1-1			
Diseases Caused by Mutations in G Protein–Coupled Receptors			
Condition*	**Receptor**	**Inheritance**	**Δ Function†**
Retinitis pigmentosa	Rhodopsin	AD/AR	Loss
Nephrogenic diabetes insipidus	Vasopressin V2	X-linked	Loss
Isolated glucocorticoid deficiency	ACTH	AR	Loss
Color blindness	Red/green opsins	X-linked	Loss
Familial precocious puberty	LH	AD (male)	Gain
Familial hypercalcemia	Ca²⁺ sensing	AD	Loss
Neonatal severe parathyroidism	Ca²⁺ sensing	AR	Loss
Dominant form hypocalcemia	Ca²⁺ sensing	AD	Gain
Congenital hyperthyroidism	TSH	AD	Gain
Resistance to thyroid hormone	TSH	AR (comp het)	Loss
Hyperfunctioning thyroid adenoma	TSH	Somatic	Gain
Metaphyseal chondrodysplasia	PTH-PTHrP	Somatic	Gain
Hirschsprung disease	Endothelin-B	Multigenic	Loss
Coat color alteration (*E* locus, mice)	MSH	AD/AR	Loss and gain
Dwarfism (*little* locus, mice)	GHRH	AR	Loss

*All are human conditions with the exception of the final two entries, which refer to the mouse.
†Loss of function refers to inactivating mutations of the receptor, and gain of function to activating mutations.
ACTH, adrenocorticotropic hormone; AD, autosomal dominant inheritance; AR, autosomal recessive inheritance; FSH, follicle-stimulating hormone; GHRH, growth hormone–releasing hormone; LH, luteinizing hormone; MSH, melanocyte-stimulating hormone; PTH-PTHrP, parathyroid hormone and parathyroid hormone–related peptide; TSH, thyroid-stimulating hormone.
From Mayo K. Receptors: molecular mediators of hormone action. In: Conn PM, Melmed S, eds. *Endocrinology: Basic and Clinical Principles.* Totowa, NJ: Humana Press; 1997:27.

Hormone secretion also adheres to rhythmic patterns. Circadian rhythms serve as adaptive responses to environmental signals and are controlled by a circadian timing mechanism.[10] Light is the major environmental cue adjusting the endogenous clock. The retinohypothalamic tract entrains circadian pulse generators situated within hypothalamic suprachiasmatic nuclei. These signals subserve timing mechanisms for the sleep-wake cycle and determine patterns of hormone secretion and action. Disturbed circadian timing results in hormonal dysfunction and may also be reflective of entrainment or pulse generator lesions. For example, adult GH deficiency due to a damaged hypothalamus or pituitary is associated with elevations in integrated 24-hour leptin concentrations, decreased leptin pulsatility, and yet preserved circadian rhythm of leptin. GH replacement restores leptin pulsatility, followed by loss of body fat mass.[11] Sleep is also an important cue regulating hormone pulsatility. About 70% of overall GH secretion occurs during slow-wave sleep, and increasing age is associated with declining slow-wave sleep and concomitant decline in GH and elevation of cortisol secretion.[12] Most pituitary hormones are secreted in a circadian (day-night) rhythm, best exemplified by ACTH peaks before 9 AM, whereas ovarian steroids follow a 28-day menstrual rhythm. Disrupted episodic rhythms are often a hallmark

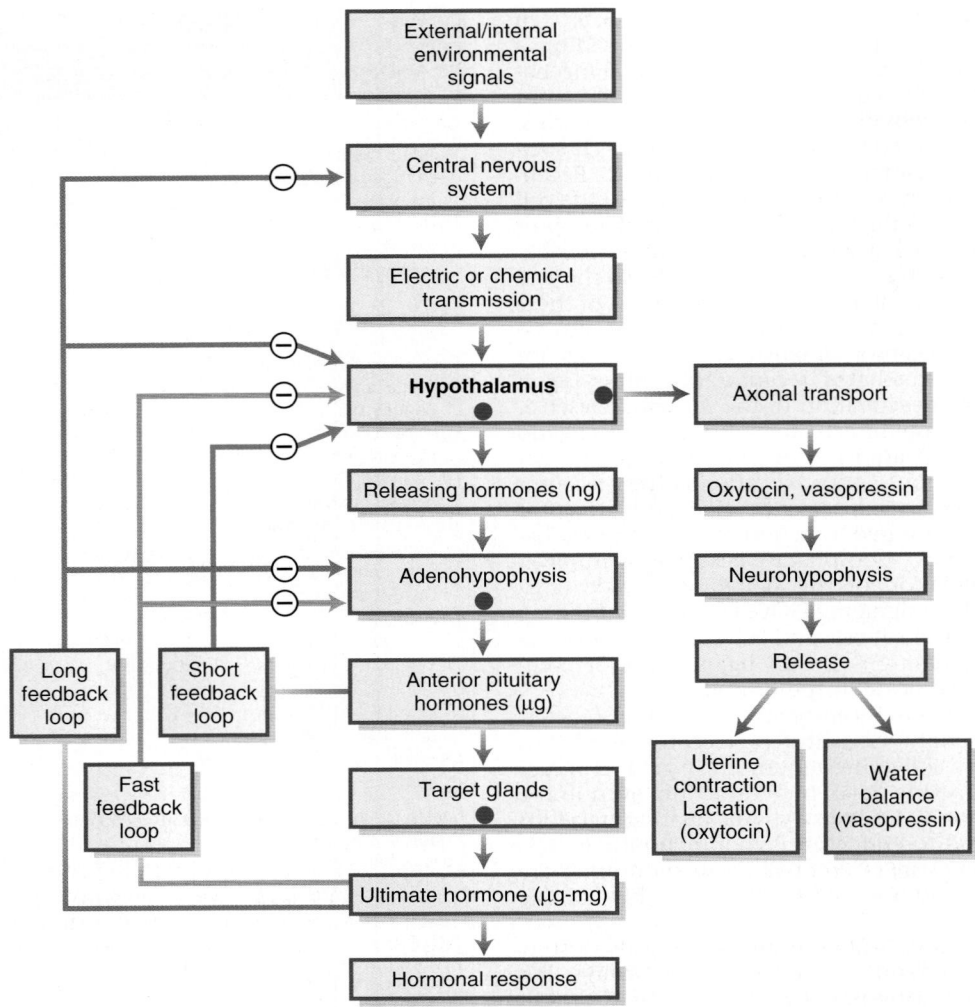

Figure 1-3 Peripheral feedback mechanism and a million-fold amplifying cascade of hormonal signals. Environmental signals are transmitted to the central nervous system, which innervates the hypothalamus, which responds by secreting nanogram amounts of a specific hormone. Releasing hormones are transported down a closed portal system, pass the blood-brain barrier at either end through fenestrations, and bind to specific anterior pituitary cell membrane receptors to elicit secretion of micrograms of specific anterior pituitary hormones. These hormones enter the venous circulation through fenestrated local capillaries, bind to specific target gland receptors, trigger release of micrograms to milligrams of daily hormone amounts, and elicit responses by binding to receptors in distal target tissues. Peripheral hormone receptors enable widespread cell signaling by a single initiating environmental signal, thus facilitating intimate homeostatic association with the external environment. *Arrows* with a large dot at their origin indicate a secretory process. (From Normal AW, Litwack G. *Hormones*, 2nd ed. New York: Academic Press; 1997:14.)

of endocrine dysfunction. Thus, loss of circadian ACTH secretion with high midnight cortisol levels is a feature of Cushing disease.

Hormone secretion is induced by multiple specific biochemical and neural signals. Integration of these stimuli results in the net temporal and quantitative secretion of the hormone (Fig. 1-3). Thus, signals elicited by hypothalamic hormones (growth hormone–releasing hormone [GHRH], SRIF), peripheral hormones (IGF-1, sex steroids, thyroid hormone), nutrients, adrenergic pathways, stress, and other neuropeptides all converge on the somatotroph cell, resulting in the ultimate pattern and quantity of GH secretion. Networks of reciprocal interactions allow for dynamic adaptation and shifts in environmental signals. These regulatory systems embrace the hypothalamic pituitary and target endocrine glands, as well as the adipocytes and lymphocytes. Peripheral inflammation and stress elicit cytokine signals that interface with the neuroendocrine system, resulting in hypothalamic-pituitary axis activation. The parathyroid and pancreatic secreting cells are less tightly controlled by the hypothalamus, but their func-

tions are tightly regulated by the effects they elicit. Thus, PTH secretion is induced when serum calcium levels fall, and the signal for sustained PTH secretion is abrogated by rising calcium levels.

Several tiers of control subserve the ultimate net glandular secretion. First, central nervous system signals including stress, afferent stimuli, and neuropeptides signal the synthesis and secretion of hypothalamic hormones and neuropeptides (Fig. 1-4). Four hypothalamic-releasing hormones (GHRH, corticotropin-releasing hormone [CRH], thyrotropin-releasing hormone [TRH], and gonadotropin-releasing hormone [GnRH]) traverse the hypothalamic portal vessels and impinge upon their respective transmembrane trophic hormone-secreting cell receptors. These distinct cells express GH, ACTH, TSH, and gonadotropins. In contrast, hypothalamic somatostatin and dopamine suppress GH, PRL, and TSH secretion. Trophic hormones also maintain the structural-functional integrity of endocrine organs, including the thyroid and adrenal glands and the gonads. Target hormones, in turn, serve as powerful negative feedback regulators of their respective

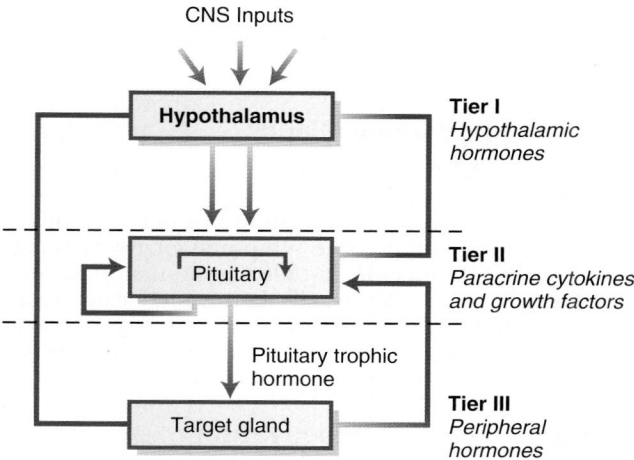

CNS Inputs

Hypothalamus — **Tier I** *Hypothalamic hormones*

Pituitary — **Tier II** *Paracrine cytokines and growth factors*

Pituitary trophic hormone

Target gland — **Tier III** *Peripheral hormones*

Figure 1-4 Model for regulation of anterior pituitary hormone secretion by three tiers of control. Hypothalamic hormones impinge directly on their respective target cells. Intrapituitary cytokines and growth factors regulate trophic cell function by paracrine (and autocrine) control. Peripheral hormones exert negative feedback inhibition of respective pituitary trophic hormone synthesis and secretion. CNS, central nervous system. (From Ray D, Melmed S. Pituitary cytokine and growth factor expression and action. *Endocrin Rev.* 1997;18:206-228.)

trophic hormone; they often also suppress secretion of hypothalamic-releasing hormones. In certain circumstances (e.g., during puberty), peripheral sex steroids may positively induce the hypothalamic-pituitary-target gland axis. Thus, LH induces ovarian estrogen secretion, which feeds back positively to induce further LH release. Pituitary hormones themselves, in a short feedback loop, may also regulate their own respective hypothalamic-controlling hormone. Hypothalamic-releasing hormones are secreted in nanogram amounts and have short half-lives of a few minutes. Anterior pituitary hormones are produced in microgram amounts and have longer half-lives, but peripheral hormones can be produced in up to milligram amounts daily, with much longer half-lives.

A further level of secretion control occurs within the gland itself. Thus, intraglandular paracrine or autocrine growth peptides serve to autoregulate pituitary hormone secretion, as exemplified by epidermal growth factor (EGF) control of PRL or IGF-1 control of GH secretion. Molecules within the endocrine cell may also subserve an intracellular feedback loop. Thus, corticotrope SOCS-3 induction by gp130-linked cytokines serves to abrogate the ligand-induced JAK-STAT cascade and block pro-opiomelanocortin (POMC) transcription and ACTH secretion. This rapid on-off regulation of ACTH secretion provides a plastic endocrine response to changes in environmental signaling and serves to maintain homeostatic integrity.[13]

In addition to the central nervous system–neuroendocrine interface mediated by hypothalamic chemical signal transduction, the central nervous system directly controls several hormonal secretory processes. Posterior pituitary hormone secretion occurs as direct efferent neural extensions. Postganglionic sympathetic nerves also regulate rapid changes in renin, insulin, and glucagon secretion, and preganglionic sympathetic nerves signal to adrenal medullary cells eliciting adrenaline release.

HORMONE MEASUREMENT

Endocrine function can be assessed by measuring levels of basal circulating hormone, evoked or suppressed hormone,

or hormone-binding proteins. Alternatively, peripheral hormone receptor function can be assessed. When a feedback loop exists between the hypothalamic-pituitary axis and a target gland, the circulating level of the pituitary trophic hormone, such as TSH or ACTH, is typically an exquisitely sensitive index of deficient or excessive function of the thyroid or the adrenal cortex, respectively. Meaningful strategies for timing hormonal measurements vary from system to system. In some cases, circulating hormone concentrations can be measured in randomly collected serum samples. This measurement, when standardized for fasting, environmental stress, age, and gender, is reflective of true hormone concentrations only when levels do not fluctuate appreciably. For example, thyroid hormone, PRL, and IGF-1 levels can be accurately assessed in fasting morning serum samples. On the other hand, when hormone secretion is clearly episodic, timed samples may be required over a defined time course to reflect hormone bioavailability. Thus, early morning and late evening cortisol measurements are most appropriate. Twenty-four–hour sampling for GH measurements, with samples collected every 2, 10, or 20 minutes, is expensive and cumbersome, yet may yield valuable diagnostic information. Random sampling may also reflect secretion peaks or nadirs, thus confounding adequate interpretation of results.

In general, confirmation of failed glandular function is made by attempting to evoke hormone secretion by recognized stimuli. Thus, testing of pituitary hormone reserve may be accomplished by injecting appropriate hypothalamic releasing hormones. Injection of trophic hormones, including TSH and ACTH, evokes specific target gland hormone secretion. Pharmacologic stimuli (e.g., metoclopramide for induction of PRL secretion) may also be useful tests of hormone reserve. In contrast, hormone hypersecretion can be diagnosed by suppressing glandular function. Thus, failure to appropriately suppress GH levels after a standardized glucose load implies inappropriate GH hypersecretion. The failure to suppress insulin secretion in response to hypoglycemia indicates inappropriate hypersecretion of insulin and should prompt a search for the cause, such as an insulin-secreting tumor.

Radioimmunoassays use highly specific antibodies that uniquely recognize the hormone, or a hormone fragment, to quantify hormone levels. Enzyme-linked immunosorbent assays (ELISAs) employ enzymes instead of radioactive hormone markers, and enzyme activity is reflective of hormone concentration. This sensitive technique has allowed ultrasensitive measurements of physiologic hormone concentrations. Hormone-specific receptors may be employed in place of the antibody in a radioreceptor assay.

ENDOCRINE DISEASES

Endocrine diseases fall into four broad categories: (1) hormone overproduction, (2) hormone underproduction, (3) altered tissue responses to hormones, and (4) tumors of endocrine glands. An additional fifth category is so far exemplified by one kind of hypothyroidism in which overexpression of a hormone-inactivating enzyme in a tumor leads to thyroid hormone deficiency.

Hormone Overproduction

Occasionally, hormones are secreted in increased amounts because of genetic abnormalities that cause abnormal regulation of hormone synthesis or release. For example, in glucocorticoid-remediable hyperaldosteronism, an abnormal chromosomal crossing over event puts the aldosterone synthetase gene under the control of the ACTH-regulated 11β-hydroxylase gene. More often, diseases of hormone overproduction are associated with an increase in the total number of hormone-producing cells. For example, the hyperthyroidism of Graves disease, in which antibodies mimic TSH and activate the TSH receptors on thyroid cells, is associated with dramatic increase in thyroid cell proliferation, as well as with increased synthesis and release of thyroid hormone from each thyroid cell. In this example, the increase in thyroid cell number represents a polyclonal expansion of thyroid cells, in which large numbers of thyroid cells proliferate in response to an abnormal stimulus. However, most endocrine tumors are not polyclonal expansions, but instead represent monoclonal expansions of one mutated cell. Pituitary and parathyroid tumors, for example, are usually monoclonal expansions in which somatic mutations in multiple tumor suppressor genes and proto-oncogenes occur. These mutations lead to an increase in proliferation or survival of the mutant cells. Sometimes, this proliferation is associated with abnormal secretion of hormone from each tumor cell as well. For example, mutant $G_s\alpha$ proteins in somatotrophs can lead to both increased cellular proliferation and increased secretion of GH from each tumor cell.

Hormone Underproduction

Underproduction of hormone can result from a wide variety of processes, ranging from surgical removal of parathyroid glands during neck surgery, to tuberculous destruction of adrenal glands, or to iron deposition in β cells of islets in hemochromatosis. A frequent cause of destruction of hormone-producing cells is autoimmunity. Autoimmune destruction of β cells in type 1 diabetes mellitus or of thyroid cells in Hashimoto thyroiditis are two of the most common disorders treated by endocrinologists. More uncommonly, a host of genetic abnormalities can also lead to decreased hormone production. These disorders can result from abnormal development of hormone-producing cells (e.g., hypogonadotropic hypogonadism caused by *KAL* gene mutations), from abnormal synthesis of hormones (e.g., deletion of the GH gene), or from abnormal regulation of hormone secretion (e.g., the hypoparathyroidism associated with activating mutations of the parathyroid cell's calcium-sensing receptor).

Altered Tissue Responses

Resistance to hormones can be caused by a variety of genetic disorders. Examples include mutations in the GH receptor in Laron dwarfism and mutations in the $G_s\alpha$ gene in the hypoparathyroidism of pseudohypoparathyroidism type 1A. The insulin resistance in muscle and liver central to the cause of type 2 diabetes mellitus is complex in origin, resulting from inherited variations in many genes, as well as from theoretically reversible physiologic stresses. Type 2 diabetes is also an example of a disease in which end-organ insensitivity is worsened by signals from other organs, in this case by signals originating in fat cells. In other cases, the target organ of hormone action is more directly abnormal, as in the PTH resistance of renal failure.

Increased end-organ function can be caused by mutations in signal reception and propagation. For example, activating mutations in TSH, LH, and PTH receptors can cause increased activity of thyroid cells, Leydig cells, and osteoblasts, even in the absence of ligand. Similarly, activating mutations in the $G_s\alpha$ protein can cause precocious puberty, hyperthyroidism, and acromegaly in McCune-Albright syndrome.

Tumors of Endocrine Glands

Tumors of endocrine glands, as noted previously, often result in hormone overproduction. Some tumors of endocrine glands produce little if any hormone but cause disease by causing local compressive symptoms or by metastatic spread. Examples include so-called nonfunctioning pituitary tumors, which are usually benign but can cause a variety of symptoms due to compression on adjacent structures, and thyroid cancer, which can spread throughout the body without causing hyperthyroidism.

Excessive Hormone Inactivation or Destruction

Although most enzymes important for endocrine systems activate a prohormone or precursor protein, there are also those whose function is to inactivate the hormone in a physiologically regulated fashion. An example is the type 3 iodothyronine deiodinase (D3), which inactivates T_3 and T_4 by removing an inner ring iodine atom from the iodothyronine, blocking its nuclear receptor binding. Large infantile hepatic hemangiomas express high D3 levels, causing "consumptive hypothyroidism," so named because thyroid hormone is inactivated at a more rapid rate than it can be produced.[14,15] Furthermore, D3 may also be induced in other tumors by tyrosine kinase inhibitors. In theory, accelerated destruction of other hormones could occur from similar processes, but no examples have been reported to date.

DIAGNOSTIC AND THERAPEUTIC USES OF HORMONES

In general, hormones are employed pharmacologically for both their replacement or suppressive effects. Hormones may also be used for diagnostic stimulatory effects (e.g., hypothalamic hormones) to evoke target organ responses, or to diagnose endocrine hyperfunction by suppressing hormone hypersecretion (e.g., T_3). Ablation of endocrine gland function due to genetic or acquired causes can be restored by hormone replacement therapy. In general, steroid and thyroid hormones are replaced orally, whereas peptide hormones (e.g., insulin, GH) require injection. Gastrointestinal absorption and first-pass kinetics determine oral hormone dosage and availability. Physiologic replacement can achieve both appropriate hormone levels (e.g., thyroid) as well as approximate hormone secretory patterns (e.g., GnRH delivered intermittently via a pump). Hormones can also be used to treat diseases associated with glandular hyperfunction. Long-acting depot preparations of somatostatin analogues suppress GH hypersecretion in acromegaly or 5-hydroxyindoleacetic acid (5-HIAA) hypersecretion in carcinoid syndrome. Estrogen receptor antagonists (e.g., tamoxifen) are useful for some patients with breast cancer, and GnRH analogues may downregulate the gonadotropin axis and benefit patients with prostate cancer.

Novel formulations of receptor-specific hormone ligands are now being clinically developed (e.g., estrogen agonists/antagonists, somatostatin receptor subtype ligands), resulting in more selective therapeutic targeting. Modes of hormone injection (e.g., for PTH) may also determine therapeutic specificity and efficacy. Improved hormone delivery systems, including computerized minipumps, intranasal sprays (e.g., for desmopressin [DDAVP]), pulmonary inhalers, depot intramuscular injections, and oral peptide formulations, will also enhance patient compliance and improve ease of administration. Insulin delivered by inhalation has already been approved for use, and inhaled GH and oral octreotide are under investigation. Cell-based therapies using the reprogramming of human cells to perform differentiated functions, either through differentiation of induced pluripotent stem cells or directed differentiation of one somatic cell type into another, are under active investigation.[16] Novel technologies offer promise of marked prolongation in the half-life of peptide hormones, thereby requiring infrequent administration. For example, a once weekly preparation of exenatide, a glucagon-like peptide-1 (GLP-1) analogue currently used in the treatment of type 2 diabetes, is currently undergoing clinical trials.

Tremendous progress has been made in the therapeutic use of hormones. Although the delivery of insulin still requires frequent administration by injection and close monitoring by the patient, the purity of the insulin preparations has been vastly improved, thereby almost entirely eliminating the occurrence of uncomfortable local reactions at the injection site. Preparations with differing pharmacokinetics allow the normal physiology of insulin secretion to be more closely mimicked. Continuous administration via subcutaneous pump infusion greatly enhances therapeutic effectiveness in carefully selected patients. Closed-loop systems, in which the dose of insulin could be regularly adjusted depending on blood glucose concentrations, are being actively studied. The implementation of such systems in the future would substantially reduce the burden of this disease. Hormones are biologically powerful molecules that exert therapeutic benefit and effectively replace pathologic deficits. They should not be prescribed without clear-cut indications and should not be administered without careful evaluation by an appropriately qualified medical practitioner.

WHAT WE DON'T KNOW (YET)

An introduction to the principles underlying endocrinology should end by emphasizing the rapidly changing dynamics of discovery in this field and attempting to foresee what remains to be discovered. New hormones are continually being discovered, from the recent focus on major regulators of metabolism and phosphate homeostasis (FGF19, -21, and -23) to the continued quest to identify ligands for "orphan" nuclear and G protein–coupled receptors.[17] Presumably, other equally important hormones remain to be discovered. The observation that nuclear receptors, like most transcription factors, bind to thousands of specific sites within the cell's nucleus stresses how little we understand about hormone action. Many of our diagnostic tests are severely limited by both technology as well as our ability to foresee novel diagnostic targets. For example, the "disappearance" of isolated GH deficiency when many children with that diagnosis achieve adulthood means either that we have little understanding of the etiology/pathogenesis of that deficiency or that our diagnostic tools today have many false-positive results. Although endocrinologists pride themselves with having logical treatments for many diseases, these treatments seldom address their underlying causes. We have no satisfactory tools for preventing autoimmune endocrine deficiencies or for preventing the benign tumors that underlie many diseases characterized by hormone excess. Treatments for diseases such as type 1 diabetes, although highly effective, are still very obtrusive in the lives of patients with this disease.

Although the primary rationale for this new edition is to communicate the major advances that have been made in our field over the past 5 years, large gaps in our knowledge about endocrinology remain. While this realization is sobering, we hope that it will be viewed by our readers as an exciting challenge for the future. That is the spirit underlying this text.

REFERENCES

1. Liu PT, Stenger S, Li H, et al. Toll-like receptor triggering of a vitamin D-mediated human antimicrobial response. *Science*. 2006;311:1770-1773.
2. Chawla A, Repa JJ, Evans RM, et al. Nuclear receptors and lipid physiology: opening the X-files. *Science*. 2001;294:1866-1870.
3. Mendel CM, Weisiger RA, Jones AL, Cavalieri RR. Thyroid hormone-binding proteins in plasma facilitate uniform distribution of thyroxine within tissues: a perfused rat liver study. *Endocrinology*. 1987;120(5):1742-1749.
4. Mendel CM. The free hormone hypothesis: physiologically based mathematical model. *Endocr Rev*. 1989;10(3):232-274.
5. Safadi FF, Thornton P, Magiera H, et al. Osteopathy and resistance to vitamin D toxicity in mice null for vitamin D binding protein. *J Clin Invest*. 1999;103:239-251.
6. Palha JA, Fernandes R, de Escobar GM, et al. Transthyretin regulates thyroid hormone levels in the choroid plexus, but not in the brain parenchyma: study in a transthyretin-null mouse model. *Endocrinology*. 2000;141:3267-3272.
7. Mayerl S, Müller J, Bauer R, et al. Transporters MCT8 and OATP1C1 maintain murine brain thyroid hormone homeostasis. *J Clin Invest*. 2014;124:1987-1999.
8. Hammes A, Andreassen TK, Spoelgen R, et al. Role of endocytosis in cellular uptake of sex steroids. *Cell*. 2005;122:751-762.
9. Rocheville M, Lange DC, Kumar U, et al. Receptors for dopamine and somatostatin: formation of hetero-oligomers with enhanced functional activity. *Science*. 2000;288:154-157.
10. Moore RY. Circadian rhythms: basic neurobiology and clinical applications. *Annu Rev Med*. 1997;48:253-266.
11. Aftab MA, Guzder R, Wallace AM, et al. Circadian and ultradian rhythm and leptin pulsatility in adult GH deficiency: effects of GH replacement. *J Clin Endocrinol Metab*. 2001;86:3499-3506.
12. Cauter EV, Leproult R, Plat L. Age-related changes in slow wave sleep and REM sleep and relationship with growth hormone and cortisol levels in healthy men. *JAMA*. 2000;284:861-868.
13. Melmed S. The immuno-neuroendocrine interface. *J Clin Invest*. 2001;108:1563-1566.
14. Huang SA, Tu HM, Harney JW, et al. Severe hypothyroidism caused by type 3 iodothyronine deiodinase (D3) in infantile hemangiomas. *N Engl J Med*. 2000;343:185-189.
15. Bianco AC, Salvatore D, Gereben B, et al. Biochemistry, cellular and molecular biology, and physiological roles of the iodothyronine selenodeiodinases. *Endocr Rev*. 2002;23:38-89.
16. Pagliuca FW, Melton DA. How to make a functional β-cell. *Development*. 2013;140:2472-2483.
17. Evans RM, Mangelsdorf DJ. Nuclear receptors. RXR, and the Big Bang. *Cell*. 2014;157:255-266.

CHAPTER 2

Clinical Endocrinology: A Personal View

LYNN LORIAUX

KEY POINTS

- Endocrinology is a consultative practice. It is the antipode of the general medical continuity approach to practice.
- All consultative requests should be met within 1 week or so, but only for patients who can benefit from the encounter.
- The fundamental elements of medical professionalism promote an environment of trust for patients.
- One of the most important variables in patient satisfaction is the number of people interspersed between patient and physician. Satisfaction is inversely related to this number.
- In addition to an examination focused on the findings of the endocrine disease, the essential physical examination expected of a competent internist is required.
- Endocrine diagnoses require two things: a clinical presentation compatible with the disease and a laboratory demonstration of the causative biochemical abnormality.

What follows is my approach to the endocrine patient, developed over 45 years of practice. My fundamental biases are these: the endocrinologist must continue to be an excellent general internist, the endocrinologist must be an expert in all of the content areas expected of the subspecialty, and the endocrinologist must constantly strive to teach and inspire all associated professionals, including nurses, nutritionists, pharmacists, students, house staff, and fellows. I am aware that there are many ways of practicing endocrinology and that many will find fault with my approach. In any case, I hope all readers find something of value here that can make their practice better.

THE PRACTICE

Endocrinology is a consultative practice. It is the antipode of the general medical continuity practice. A busy, fully occupied generalist should have a patient panel of 1200 to 1500 patients. The endocrinologist's list should have 100 to 200 patients. The generalist sees the entire panel every year or so in perpetuity. The endocrinologist sees his or her patients once, twice, maybe three times, and the patients are returned to the referring physician, preferably the primary care physician. Most of the endocrinologist's patients in any clinic session should be new patients. If the endocrinology patient panel is 1500, as an example, the new patient will become a rarity in that practice, and the value of that practitioner to the profession approaches nil. You may say, "Primary care physicians cannot do what is required for these patients." I reply, "Teach them." They are willing and able learners. Consider this: there are about 5000 board-certified endocrinologists in the United States. There will be 100 million type 2 diabetics in the United States by 2025. If all these patients were cared for by an endocrinologist, which is what we and they generally want, each of us will have a panel of 20,000 diabetics. Primary care will be the best we can do, and even that will be a big stretch.

Patients for whom 95% of their medical problems derive from their endocrine disease should be on the endocrinologist continuity panel. Brittle diabetes, medullary carcinoma of the thyroid, extreme insulin resistance, metastatic adrenal carcinoma, metastatic insulinoma, and metastatic thyroid cancer are good examples.

THE RULES OF ENGAGEMENT

There is a current sentiment among the practice management people that all consultative requests should be met within 1 week or so. This is true, but only for the patients who can benefit from the encounter. If the consultation poses a problem such as "This diabetic patient needs your help in managing plasma glucose in emotionally stressful situations, particularly piano recitals," you can help. If the consultation poses a problem such as "This poor lady cannot sleep and I suspect something hormonal," the patient is unlikely to benefit from the consultation. If the consultation is done, there is always the danger of false hope, or worse, a protracted search using an array of endocrine tests that, in the end, will be inconclusive after many thousands of dollars are spent. You do not have to see every patient, but you must discuss the situation and come to some consensus with the referring physician. After all, Maimonides, one of medicine's heroes, and perhaps our best exemplar of objective compassion, refused to see Richard "The Lion Heart" at Acre when Richard suffered debilitating dyspepsia, probably scorbutic, after beheading 2700 Muslim men of military age. You don't have to see every consultation.

On the other hand, if the consultation poses an answerable question, should all such be seen? Suppose the question concerned a 5-year-old boy with ambiguous genitalia, unilateral cryptorchidism, and episodic hematuria. If he were your son, would you want you for his physician? If your answer is yes, see the patient. If the answer is no, explain the problem to the referring physician and help him find the doctor you would want for your son. If this cannot be done, then it is usually better to see the patient than not, like the Good Samaritan. However, you must be aware that you are working at the edge of, or even outside, your competence. This admission must be part of the discussion with the referring physician and patient.

THE COVENANT

If you accept the patient for consultation, what should happen next is spelled out in the Oath of Hippocrates. It is what is meant by professionalism. Hippocrates wrote in "The Law, part 1" of the Hippocratic Corpus:

> Medicine is the most distinguished of all the arts, but through the ignorance of those who practice it, and those who casually judge such practitioners, it is now, of all the arts, by far the least esteemed.

At the beginning of Hippocrates' work, almost all physicians were temple priests. At the end of his time, the beginning of the Hippocratic revolution, the ratio of priests to physicians was probably closer to 1:1. In any case, there was basically no way for patients to tell the two types of physicians apart: the Divine Intervention practitioners did not divulge their lack of formal medical training. Hippocrates proposed to remedy this problem with the oath.

The Original Oath

> I swear by Apollo, the healer, Asklepios, and Panacea, and I take to witness all the gods, and all the goddesses to keep, according to my ability and my judgment, the following Oath and agreement:
>
> To consider dear to me, as my parents, him who taught me this art; to live in common with him, and, if necessary, to share my goods with him; to look upon his children as my own brothers, to teach them this art; and that by my teaching, I will impart a knowledge of this art to my own sons, and to my teacher's sons, and to disciples bound by an indenture and oath according to the medical laws, and no others.
>
> I will prescribe regimens for the good of my patients according to my ability and my judgment and never do harm to anyone.
>
> I will give no deadly medicine to anyone if asked, nor suggest any such counsel; and similarly I will not give women a pessary to cause an abortion.
>
> But I will preserve the purity of my life and my arts.
>
> I will not cut for stone, even for patients in whom all disease is manifest; I will leave this operation to be performed by practitioners, specialists in this art.
>
> In every house where I come I will enter only for the good of my patients, keeping myself far from all intentional ill-doing and all seduction especially from the pleasures of love with women or men, be they free or slaves.
>
> All that may come to my knowledge in the exercise of my profession or in daily commerce with men, which ought not to be spread abroad, I will keep secret and will never reveal.

> If I keep this oath faithfully, may I enjoy my life and practice my art, respected by all humanity and in all times; but if I swerve from it or violate it, may the reverse be my lot.

Here are the fundamental elements of medical professionalism. They are the guide to the patient-physician encounter:

You are expected to teach.

The oath must be taken before teaching can begin (the white coat ceremony).

You will always work in the best interest of your patient, even when doing so is not in your best interest.

You will not prescribe poisons in any case.

You will not prescribe, for anybody, things that have the potential to do more harm than good (e.g., bladder stone surgery).

You will be trustworthy in every way, including avoiding any sexual liaison with the patient or the patient's family.

You will hold all information, shared in a clinical setting, in the strictest confidence.

You will pay attention to the criticisms of your peers.

Put into action, these principles promote an environment of trust in which patients can divulge their secrets, take off their clothes in your presence, and allow you to examine them in a highly vulnerable state without fear. This covenant between two people exists in no other venue in Western civilization. It is unique.

Two thousand four hundred years after Hippocrates wrote his oath, Robert Louis Stevenson could say this about the profession in his dedication to Underwoods:[1]

> There are men and classes of men that stand above the common herd: the soldier, sailor, and shepherd not infrequently; the artist rarely; rarer still, the clergyman; the physician almost as a rule. He is the flower (such as it is) of our civilization; and when that age of man is done, and only to be marveled at in history, he will be thought to have shared as little as any in the defects of the period, and most notably exhibited the virtues of the race. Generosity he has, such as is possible to those who practice an art, never to those who drive a trade; discretion, tested by a hundred secrets, tact, tried in a thousand embarrassments; and what are more important, Herculean cheerfulness and courage. So that he brings air and cheer into the sick room, and often enough, though not so often as he wishes, brings healing.

Most physicians profess the oath a few times in their lives. Almost none has any idea about what he or she is professing and what it means to the profession. It should be on every doctor's office wall and in the clinics and hospitals. It defines the rules of engagement. Violate them at your peril.

THE ENCOUNTER

One of the most important variables in determining patient satisfaction is the number of people interspersed between patient and physician. Satisfaction is inversely related to this number. Optimally, the doctor will meet the patient in the waiting room, escort him or her to the examining room, wash hands, and start with the chief complaint while taking the vital signs.

In this era of the electronic medical record (EMR), the challenge is to talk with the patient and not the computer screen. I find that the best approach is to save the record keeping until the encounter is closed.

This is a good time to introduce a third person into the encounter. This is easy to accomplish in the academic world when there are omnipresent students, house staff, and fellows. It is not so easy in the private practice setting. The third person is a powerful force in promoting consensus about the facts of the history and physical examination, treatment, and assessment. This presence is also a powerful deterrent to misconduct of any kind.

Endocrine histories tend to focus on the question in the referral. In analyzing the incoming data, the physician should keep in mind the following principles:

First, it should be remembered that Ockham's razor begins to fail at 60 years of age. It is no longer safe to assume that all of the findings can be attributed to a single disease process. At 70 or 80 years of age, it is a safe assumption that there are two or three diseases present, which greatly complicates achieving an accurate diagnosis and makes it impossible to satisfy the principle of Ockham's razor.

Second, it is safe to assume that the medication list in the EMR is wrong. I have never found it to be right. It is also safe to assume that the patient either does not know exactly what medicines he or she is taking or will not reveal the entire list. The only antidote for this is to have the significant other, if there is one, bring in all of the medications in a paper bag. Somebody needs to do the reconciliation. Nurses are excellent at this. It can take a while. This reconciliation should occur before you see the patient, or you will have to do it, and your attention should be elsewhere.

Third, physicians give medications in part because patients expect it. It is also true that physicians rarely take a medication away. One of the most important things that can happen in a consultation is to pare the medication list down to its manageable essentials. How many medications can a patient safely be taking? A useful rule of thumb is that the number should not exceed the square root of the patient's age. There are exceptions: transplantation and cystic fibrosis come to mind. For the rest, the square root of age should be your target.

I see many patients who come in taking 20 to 30 medications. The possible drug-drug interactions for 30 drugs is greater than Avogadro's number. It simply cannot be managed by patient or physician. The place to start is with agonist-antagonist pairs. Florinef and spironolactone is a common pair. Nobody will argue with this deletion.

Physical Examination

In addition to an examination focused on the findings of the endocrine disease, the essential physical examination expected of a competent internist is required. A careful examination of the heart, lungs, abdomen, and neurologic systems is expected by the patient and the referring physician. As William Osler famously said, "It is the responsibility of the consultant to do the rectal examination." The endocrinologist's examination of the heart should be better than that of the average cardiologist, the examination of the chest better than that of the average pulmonologist, and the examination of the abdominal organs at least comparable to that of the average gastroenterologist. The general opinion of most referring physicians is that endocrinologists are also complete internists. I agree with that expectation. I often find that I am the only doctor who has carefully listened to the heart, percussed the lungs, and examined the external genitalia. I am often the first doctor to diagnose Parkinson disease in a referred patient and virtually always the first to diagnose clinical depression or early dementia. Mastering the physical examination will dramatically enhance your ability to define and manage the endocrine diseases you diagnose.

The general examination should include the vital signs and the essential examination noted previously. This should be followed by a careful search for the physical findings associated with the disorder in question. Using Cushing syndrome as a model, mood should be assessed, determining proximal muscle strength is critical, and skin thickness, striae, skin color, and any evidence of insulin resistance such as acanthosis nigricans should be noted.

Visual fields by confrontation should be second nature to the endocrinologist.

THE DIAGNOSIS

Endocrine diagnoses require two things: a clinical presentation compatible with the disease and a laboratory demonstration of the causative biochemical abnormality. The corollary is this: if the clinical picture is not compatible, no laboratory studies should be done. This is by far the most common mistake made in the practice of endocrinology.

Fundamental Lemma

If the results of a test will not change what you do, it should not be done. This is the second most common mistake made in the practice of endocrinology.

Unnecessary Tests

Unnecessary testing is the third most common mistake in the practice of endocrinology. Too many tests are ordered. Keep the number down to the essential tests, those that dictate the course of the evaluation. The critic may say that this approach excludes the possibility of an early diagnosis of any endocrine disease. I counter that if the disease is so mild that it cannot be recognized clinically, it does not need to be diagnosed. An excellent example of this is the patient referred for suspicion of Cushing syndrome with an elevated urine cortisol level measured in a person who does not have convincing clinical signs of Cushing syndrome. The urine cortisol should never have been measured (more about this later). Endocrine diseases progress with time. The diagnosis can and should wait until it can be made with confidence; no screening tests are ever indicated. The screening test for Cushing syndrome is the physical examination.

If the patient has a clinical picture compatible with the disease, the evaluation should progress to the most appropriate and powerful laboratory test available. Using my example of Cushing syndrome, the only reliable test that can be ordered is the 24-hour urinary free cortisol excretion. Measurement of the cortisol production rate using tritiated or deuterated cortisol infused to a constant plasma concentration is even better and the only test possible in patients with renal failure. This test is almost never available to the clinician. Because cortisol has a diurnal secretory pattern, even when caused by an adrenal adenoma, only a test that can integrate plasma free cortisol over a 24-hour period is useful. The results of this test dictate what comes next. No other test will do that; hence, no other tests should be ordered. Plasma cortisol, salivary cortisol, dehydroepiandrosterone (DHEA), adrenocorticotropic hormone (ACTH) stimulation test, and any of the urinary tests such as Porter-Sibler chromogens and 17-keto steroids should not be measured. Instead, do the indicated test more than once!

The interpretation of the clinical picture coupled with the urinary free cortisol is shown in Figure 2-1. No signs

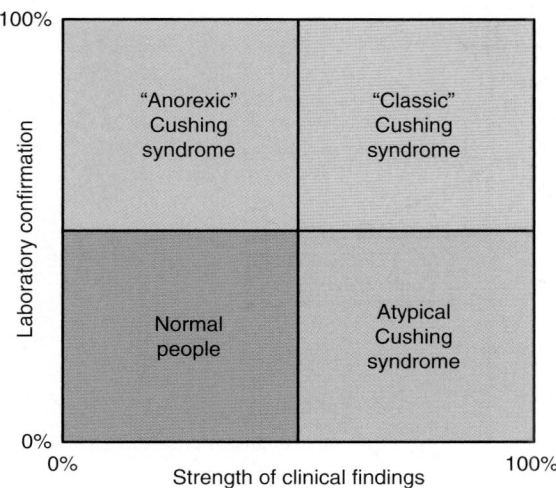

Figure 2-1 Diagnosis of Cushing syndrome. This chart illustrates the interplay between the clinical presentation and the laboratory test for the disease. Deciding when to make the call is an example of the art of medicine (inductive logic).

of the disease and a normal urinary free cortisol should end the search. High urinary free cortisol and classic clinical features define Cushing syndrome as first described.[2] Classic clinical features of the disease and no elevation of levels of urinary free cortisol are always caused by the exogenous administration of glucocorticoid. On occasion, a high urinary free cortisol will be found in a person with no signs of Cushing syndrome. This is usually discovered in the course of an evaluation for hypertension. The elevated levels of urinary free cortisol unaccompanied by classic clinical signs of Cushing syndrome occur in two settings. First is the ectopic secretion of ACTH from an occult malignancy. The development of the classic signs of Cushing syndrome are almost always associated with weight gain. If weight gain is prevented, as by the anorexia associated with an occult malignancy, the classic signs of Cushing syndrome cannot appear, but the mineralocorticoid action of cortisol will be fully expressed. The second scenario is the syndrome of generalized glucocorticoid resistance. A useful guideline in interpreting urinary free cortisol levels is that the normal hypothalamic pituitary adrenal axis, under maximum stress, cannot exceed about 250 µg/day. It is safe to say that levels above 300 µg/day are enough to make the diagnosis of Cushing syndrome in the absence of a convincing clinical picture, which can often be found in the syndrome of ectopic ACTH secretion.

If the diagnosis of Cushing syndrome is secure, tests of differential diagnosis can be deployed (Fig. 2-2): plasma ACTH, inferior petrosal sinus sampling for ACTH, computed tomography (CT), and magnetic resonance imaging (MRI) of the hypothalamus/pituitary or of the adrenal glands. These are the only tests used in the differential diagnoses of Cushing syndrome. If any of these tests is applied to a person who does not have glucocorticoid excess, the diagnosis of Cushing disease will be made. The treatments that follow are futile and, in the worst case, will result in an otherwise normal person who has no pituitary or adrenal glands. You will be surprised how often this iatrogenic nightmare happens. Every medical center has an example or two. It is the result of too many tests and a deficient understanding of the pathophysiology of the disease.

The arch offender in this catastrophe is the dexamethasone suppression test. The dexamethasone suppression test was developed by Grant Liddle and his group at Vanderbilt in 1960. He showed in 54 normal volunteers that 0.5 mg dexamethasone, every 6 hours by mouth, would suppress the excretion of urinary 17-hydroxycorticoids in urine to less than 3 mg in the second day of administration. The normal basal excretion of 17-hydroxycorticoids ranged between 3 and 12 mg/day. Applying the test to a group of 27 patients who had Cushing syndrome showed that none of them suppressed urinary 17-hydroxycorticoids to less than 3 mg/day. On the basis of these data, they concluded that suppression of urinary 17-hydroxycorticoid to less than 3 mg/day excludes Cushing syndrome caused by a pituitary microadenoma or an adrenal tumor, the only causes of Cushing syndrome known at the time. It was true then, and it is usually true now.

The corollary to this conclusion, that the failure to suppress 17-hydroxyglucocorticoids to less than 3 mg/day with dexamethasone, however, is diagnostic of Cushing syndrome, however, is not true. It was not true then, and it is not true now. Unfortunately, that is how the test currently is being used.

We now know that there are many situations in which dexamethasone at 2 mg/day will not suppress cortisol secretion. Such situations include obesity, physical and mental stress, depression, and psychosis.

The futility of this approach to the diagnoses of Cushing syndrome follows. The prevalence of obesity is 30%: 20 million people in the United States. Nine percent of these people, at any given time, have clinical depression: 10 million people. Of these, conservatively 50% will fail to suppress plasma cortisol following dexamethasone: 5 million people. The prevalence of noniatrogenic Cushing syndrome is 5 to 10 cases per 1 million people; let us say, 5000 people. Assume that all of these people fail to suppress plasma cortisol after an oral dose of dexamethasone. The positive predictive value (PPV) of the test will be:

$$PPV = \frac{\text{True positive tests}}{\text{False-positive tests} + \text{True-positive tests}}$$
$$= \frac{5000}{5,000,000 + 5000}$$
$$= 0.001$$

The performance of the test for detecting cortisol secretion by an incidental adrenal adenoma is not much better. The prevalence of the incidental adrenal adenoma is about 5%, 15 million people. Thirty percent are obese (5 million people), and 10% are depressed (500,000 people). Assume that all people with Cushing syndrome began as an incidental adenoma, and it requires 3 years to be large enough to detect. Assume they all fail to suppress plasma cortisol following dexamethasone. The prevalence will be 15,000. The PPV will be 0.03, or 3%. Not good enough.

The dexamethasone test has only a single remaining venue: dexamethasone suppressible hypertension. Because a positive test defines the disorder, the PPV = 1.0. Otherwise, it is the wrong test for the wrong reason. It needs to go the way of the protein-bound iodine, 17-ketosteroids, and the rabbit test for pregnancy.

The critic will say that this claim needs to be tested by a randomized trial. Not all things need a randomized trial (the parachute is a good example).

A Digression into Test Technology

Endocrinologists love ordering and interpreting tests. In order for the tests to be helpful, however, several performance characteristics must be known. First is the

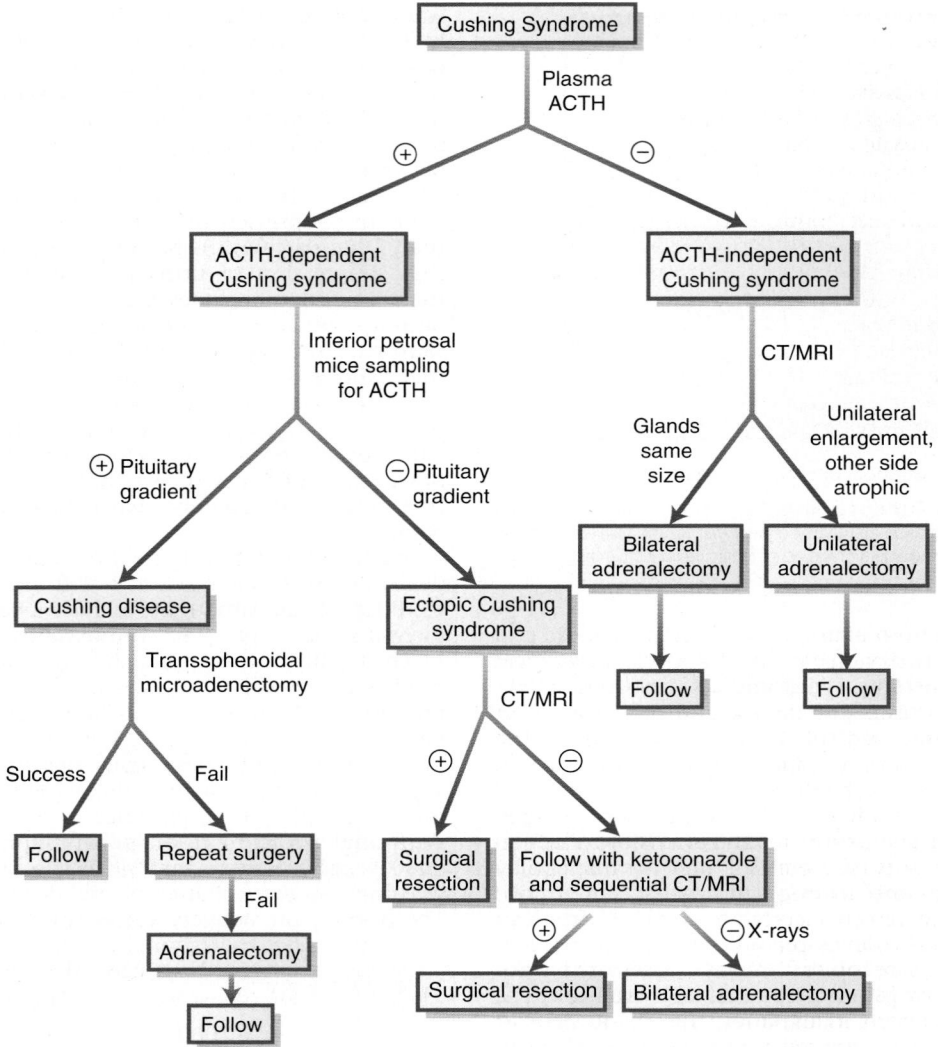

Figure 2-2 Differential diagnosis of Cushing syndrome. This algorithm illustrates the sequential application of the tests of differential diagnosis. There are only four tests: plasma ACTH, petrosal sinus sampling for ACTH, CT, and MRI. This is a good example of the application of the experimental method in medicine (deductive logic). ACTH, adrenocorticotropic hormone; CT, computed tomography; MRI, magnetic resonance imaging.

extinction point, or *blank* of the assay. It is the lowest measurable value that can be differentiated from zero. Plasma cortisol is a good example. The average plasma cortisol level in adults is 9 µg/dL ± 2 µg/dL. The blank for most clinically available tests is 5 µg/dL. In other words, half of the range between 0 and 10 is invisible. Plasma cortisol can never be used to diagnose adrenal insufficiency, yet it is commonly employed in this way.

Second is the coefficient of variation (the standard deviation in percent) of the test. This number should be as low as possible in the range of the test we are most interested in. A good example is a plasma glucose level of 50 mg/dL. If the coefficient of variation is 5%, then numbers falling between 40 mg/dL and 60 mg/dL are not different from each other with 95% confidence. The cutoff point for hypoglycemia is right in the middle of this range. We need a test with more precision for the 50-mg/dL target. Endocrinologists use a value of 18 µg/dL as a cutoff for an abnormal response to the Cortrosyn stimulation test. If the precision for this level of plasma cortisol is 5%, the 95% confidence interval around 18 µg/dL is 15.4 to 21.6 µg/dL. Where do we make the call? Virtually all hormone assays

are competitive binding assays. The most precise portion of the binding curve is when 50% of the ligand is bound. This "sweet spot" can be moved up or down by increasing or decreasing the antibody concentration. Using cortisol as an example, the test should be tuned to 18 µg/dL. Usually the assay is tuned for the middle of the normal range, 9 µg/dL in our example, a number the clinician almost never needs to know.

Sometimes the laboratory can tell you these parameters, but usually not. Sometimes the laboratory will respond to your need for a given value to be as precise as possible, but not often. Nonetheless, the endocrinologist should be able to know when two values are different from each other.

THE THERAPY

Replacement Therapy

1. The guidelines are these: always replace a hormone deficiency with the hormone that is missing. This is

possible with cortisol, thyroxine, growth hormone, and the gonadotropins. All of the other hormones have been modified, usually to enable oral administration. Why is this important? Cortisol, as an example, has a tightly regulated metabolic clearance rate with a half-life of 80 minutes. This leads to an oral dose of 12 to 15 mg/m^2 per day in all people. The half-life of dexamethasone varies between 60 and 360 minutes, making it virtually impossible to find the appropriate replacement dose. Most patients end up being overtreated. This goes for prednisone as well. Neither has measurable mineralocorticoid effects. Half of our daily mineralocorticoid effect comes from cortisol, another reason to use the natural hormone.

2. Use a once-a-day regimen, in the morning, if possible. Almost all hormones can be given this way. The plasma half-life of the hormone is short, but its biologic response is long. It optimizes compliance. Any other regimen leads to reduced compliance.
3. When the optimum replacement dose and frequency are established, stick with it. Patients on the ideal replacement regimen will still have good days and bad days, just like anyone. They will attribute their bad days to improper replacement and often try to change the plan. Never agree to chase the malaise with dose and schedule changes. If you do, the patient will attribute any unpleasantness to the change, which is, of course, a non sequitur. Once they make a change, they will never again be on the right dose.

Surgery

Surgery is the mainstay for the treatment of most disorders of hormone excess. It is not so clear that the same applies to disorders of hormone deficiency. Disorders of hormone deficiency can be treated effectively with hormone replacement. Therefore, the apology for surgery must depend on something else. This becomes a major issue in the treatment of nonsecretory pituitary tumors, as an example. The cost/benefit analysis for surgical interventions in this case depends on the natural history of the *chromophobe adenoma*.

The older data, before CT and MRI, and several current studies suggest that nonsecreting pituitary macroadenomas, once discovered, do not always progress. In fact, in three studies, over a 3- to 4-year follow-up, only half progressed.[4-7] This knowledge should be weighed against the known complications of transsphenoidal resection, such as new hormone deficiencies, diabetes insipidus, leak of cerebrospinal fluid, arterial vasospasm, worsened visual fields, and the known mortality risk of anesthesia. Far too many of these tumors are operated on. It is much safer to wait until progression can be documented with increase in tumor size or worsening of the visual fields.

Finally, endocrine surgery, taken as a whole, is a delicate and sophisticated activity. Everybody is familiar with the horrendous complications associated with the botched operation. The gifted endocrine surgeons are scattered across the country, but all can be reached. Ask yourself, "Which surgeon would you send *your* mother to?" He or she is the surgeon you must get to see your patient. "How will you train new surgeons?" ask the critics! "Not our problem," I reply. The surgeons are responsible for their own quality control, and we have all professed to do the best that we can for our patients. They depend on it. This is one of the most important ways.

PARTING THOUGHTS

1. Beware of guidelines. Everybody is familiar with the *confederacy of dunces*. A confederacy of dunces causes the wrong things to happen. A *confederacy of experts*, however, usually prevents the right thing from happening. Think for yourself.
2. Remember, medicine is not a business. Businesses strive to make their products as alike to each other as possible. Physicians strive to understand how their products are different, and they are all different. Business principles do not apply. The business folk will not understand this. Medicine is an art, the art of applied science. It is a high-stakes game.
3. To paraphrase an old American proverb, "Never be the first, nor the last, to incorporate a new idea into your practice."

Criticism

A through Z. The author is aware that there has been a goodly sprinkling of metaphysics among this recording of some experimental facts; he is very well aware that the deductions will not stand the test of time; he does hope, however, that thoughts will be stimulated by this presentation—if not by truths, why then by errors; apologia are there none.[6]

REFERENCES

1. Stevenson RL. *Underwoods*, 1887. First paragraph—Dedication.
2. Cushing H. *The Pituitary Body and its Disorders: Clinical States Produced by Disorders of the Hypophysis Cerebri*. Philadelphia: JB Lippincott; 1912.
3. Liddle GW. Tests of pituitary-adrenal supressibility in the diagnosis of Cushing's Syndrome. *J Clin Endo Metab*. 1960;20:1539-1560.
4. Weisberg L. Asymptomatic enlargement of the sella tarcica. *Arch Neurol*. 1975;32:483-485.
5. Dekkers O, Hammer S, de Keizer R, et al. The natural course of nonfunctioning pituitary macroadenomas. *Eur J Endocrinol*. 2007;156(2):217-224.
6. Karavitaki N, Collison K, Halliday J. What is the natural history of nonoperable, non-functioning pituitary adenomas. *Clin Endocrinol (Oxf)*. 2007;67(6):938-943.
7. Albright F. Cushing's syndrome. *Harvey Lecture Series*. 1942-1943;38:123.

CHAPTER 3

Principles of Hormone Action

MITCHELL A. LAZAR • MORRIS J. BIRNBAUM

KEY POINTS

- Hormones signal to target cells via receptors on the cell surface or in the cell nucleus.
- Polypeptide hormones act at the cell surface and trigger a cascade of events in the cytoplasm as well as in the nucleus that alter the function of their target cells.
- In addition to polypeptide hormones, many nonpolypeptide hormones such as catecholamines signal via cell surface receptors.
- There are multiple classes of cell surface receptors, including G protein–coupled receptors, protein tyrosine kinases, and Janus kinase (JAK) family members.
- Some receptors have intrinsic catalytic activity, whereas others depend on interaction with other signaling proteins.
- Steroid and thyroid hormones signal via nuclear receptors.
- The family of nuclear receptors includes molecules that transduce signals from other ligands, including vitamins, metabolites, and drugs, to regulate nearly every biologic process including reproduction, growth, and metabolism.
- These receptors work directly in the cell nucleus to regulate gene transcription, acting at the genome and recruiting coregulator proteins called corepressors and coactivators.
- Hormone action results from a conformational change in the receptor that occurs upon binding and favors the recruitment of coactivators to the specific genes that are regulated.

INTRODUCTION TO HORMONE SIGNALING

The fundamental purpose of hormones in human biology is to allow communication from one organ to another, ultimately transferring information from the outside of the cell to its interior to modulate cellular function. This information flow deals crucially with issues of sensitivity to low levels of signal and the specificity of the information sensed and the corresponding cellular responses to that information. In order for an extracellular substance to influence cellular activity, what is initially detected as a static concentration must be transformed into a change in cellular activity, a process generally known as *signal transduction*. The strategies used by hormones to affect cellular function are analogous and in many cases identical to those employed by other extracellular agents such as neurotransmitters, drugs, and even metabolites. However, classic endocrinology defines itself as the process by which signaling molecules use the bloodstream to travel from the organ of origin to the target tissue. By its nature this process invariably results in dilution of the secreted molecule in the intravascular space, and thus with rare exception the target cell must be capable of detecting and responding to very low concentrations of hormone.

In spite of the vanishingly small concentrations of hormones present in the circulation, classic endocrine organs are usually uniquely equipped to secrete substantial amounts of hormone. Much of the history of endocrinology is defined by purification of hormones from these specialized secretory tissues. In the earliest days, the discovery of a hormone usually followed a stereotypical course of events: (1) a syndrome, often resembling some human disease, was associated with removal of an endocrine gland; (2) the abnormal phenotype would be corrected by the reimplantation of the absent organ; (3) the same cure would be accomplished by administration of an extract from the organ of interest; (4) the active principal would be purified from the organ. The discovery of insulin represents the prototype for this series of observations, but the same process led to the identification of hormones such as thyroid hormone and cortisol. Remarkably, the first use of the term *hormone* had to await the discovery of secretin.[1]

Hormones can be divided into two groups on the basis of where they function in a target cell. The first group includes hormones that do not enter cells; instead, they carry out their actions by means of signals initiated by interactions with receptors at the cell surface. All polypeptide hormones (e.g., growth hormone), monoamines (e.g., serotonin), and prostaglandins (e.g., prostaglandin E_2), use cell surface receptors. The second group includes hormones that can enter cells. These hormones bind to intracellular receptors that function in the nucleus of the target cell to regulate gene expression. Classic hormones that use intracellular receptors include thyroid and steroid hormones.

LIGANDS THAT ACT THROUGH CELL SURFACE RECEPTORS

The impermeability of the plasma membrane to peptides and small, water-soluble, charged molecules engenders the need to locate the receptors that recognize such hormones on the outer surface of the cell. The limiting membrane of a typical eukaryotic cell is a 5- to 8-nm structure composed of proteins embedded in a sea of phospholipid and cholesterol, forming the so-called fluid-mosaic membrane. The phospholipid polar head groups face outward from the membrane, interacting with the hydrophilic milieu that comprises the extracellular fluid and the cytoplasm. Buried between this two-charged surface are the hydrophobic lipid tails made up of acyl groups, the long chains of hydrocarbons derived from fatty acids. The strongly nonpolar environment prevents the diffusion of water-soluble molecules, including many hormones, across the membrane, and thus surface proteins are needed to detect the presence of extracellular ligands that cannot diffuse and are not transported into the cell. Information from this hormone-binding process must then be transmitted across the plasma membrane so that intracellular signaling can commence.

Classic Peptide Hormones

Most notable among the hormones that bind to cell surface receptors are the peptide hormones, which vary in size from a handful to hundreds of amino acids; examples of peptide hormones include the glycoproteins and the growth hormone family of proteins secreted by the pituitary, the pancreatic hormones glucagon and insulin, and numerous peptides secreted from nonglandular organs, such as leptin from adipocytes and atrial natriuretic peptide from the heart (Table 3-1). Insulin-like growth factor 1 (IGF-1) enters the bloodstream from the liver and circulates to its target tissues, but it is also produced by target tissues, closer to its site of action, to exert its effects on neighboring cells. The peptidergic neurotransmitters exert their actions via cell surface receptors not only on postsynaptic membranes but also on non-neuronal tissues when these same peptides function as classic endocrine hormones.

The rate of secretion of hormone is closely tailored to its lifetime in the circulation and to its time course of action. In general, peptide hormones are released from endocrine glands quickly, as they are stored in a specialized compartment of the cell, the secretory vesicle or granule. In the course of synthesis of peptide hormones, they are diverted from the normal, constitutive secretory pathway to secretory vesicles in a regulated secretory pathway (Fig. 3-1). Endocrine glands containing such secretory vesicles, like the endocrine pancreas, the anterior pituitary, and parathyroid glands, display the characteristic feature on thin section transmission electron microscopy of a cytoplasm filled with 200-nm electron-dense granules that represent the packaged hormone awaiting secretion. Just as secretion of hormones stored within secretory vesicles can be evoked quickly, often within milliseconds, release can usually be terminated abruptly with great efficiency. Peptide hormones released in such a way also have very short lives within the circulation, allowing their levels to be adjusted promptly in response to changes in secretion. Last, the rapidity of changes in secretion and blood concentrations has to be mirrored by equally swift initiation of signaling, which translates into the need for high *on rates* for hormone binding to receptors. Because the need to detect low levels of hormone requires a high equilibrium binding constant, the *off rate* is often slow and there must

TABLE 3-1

Hormones That Work on the Cell Surface

Peptides and Proteins

Adrenocorticotropic hormone (ACTH)
Anterior pituitary thyrotropin or thyroid-stimulating hormone (TSH)
Antidiuretic hormone (ADH)
Atrial natriuretic peptide (ANP)
Calcitonin
Cholecystokinin
Corticotropin-releasing hormone (CRH)
Follicle-stimulating hormone (FSH)
Gastrin
Glucagon
Gonadotropin-releasing hormone (GnRH)
Growth hormone (GH)
Growth hormone–releasing hormone (GHRH)
Insulin
Insulin-like growth factor 1 (IGF-1)
Luteinizing hormone (LH)
Oxytocin
Parathyroid hormone (PTH)
Prolactin (PRL)
Secretin
Somatostatin (SS)
Thyrotropin-releasing hormone (TRH)

Molecules Derived From Amino Acids

Dopamine (inhibits prolactin)
Epinephrine (also called adrenaline)
Norepinephrine (also called noradrenaline)
Serotonin

Eicosanoids

Prostaglandins: PGA_1, PGA_2, PGE_2

exist mechanisms other than simple diffusion off the receptor for turning off the hormonal signal.

A notable exception to the rule that peptide hormones turn over quickly and have short durations of action is provided by IGF-1. This hormone was originally identified by two parallel lines of investigation: its ability to mimic the actions of insulin at high concentration and its profound positive regulation of growth. IGF-1 is also unusual in that it behaves like a classic hormone, secreted by the liver to act on distant sites, but is also produced in other tissues such as osteocytes, chondrocytes, and muscle to act in a autocrine (i.e., acting on the cell of origin) or paracrine (i.e., acting on adjacent cells) manner. IGF-1 is not stored in liver but is transcribed, translated, and synthesized as needed for release under the positive influence of growth hormone, itself secreted from the pituitary gland. Unlike most peptide hormones, IGF-1 circulates in the bloodstream bound to one of a small family of binding proteins; this has two important consequences. First, the concentration of total IGF-1 in blood is much greater than that of the unbound, biologically active hormone. Second, the lifetime of IGF-1 is greatly extended, such that circulating levels of the hormone change slowly over the course of hours or days. As predicted by these properties, IGF-1 primarily influences phenotypes that are modified over extended periods, such as growth and differentiation, and in marked contrast to its cousin insulin, most of the cellular targets of IGF-1 are transcriptional.

Nonclassic Peptide Hormones

Numerous other signaling molecules share with hormones the ability to convey environmental information to target cells and evoke specific biologic responses. Not all of these

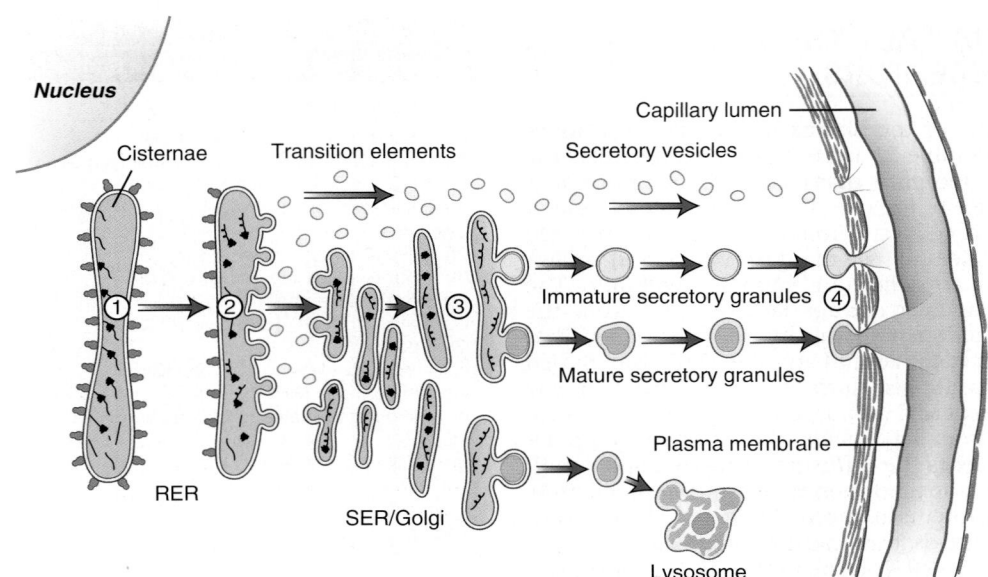

Figure 3-1 Subcellular organelles involved in transport and secretion of polypeptide hormones or other secreted proteins within a protein-secreting cell. (1) Synthesis of proteins on polyribosomes attached to rough endoplasmic reticulum (RER) and vectorial discharge of proteins through the membrane into the cisterna. (2) Formation of shuttling vesicles (transition elements) from endoplasmic reticulum followed by their transport to and incorporation by the Golgi complex. (3) Formation of secretory granules in the Golgi complex. (4) Transport of secretory granules to the plasma membrane, fusion with the plasma membrane, and exocytosis resulting in the release of granule contents into the extracellular space. Notice that secretion may occur by transport of secretory vesicles and immature granules or by transport of mature granules. Some granules are taken up and hydrolyzed by lysosomes (crinophagy). Golgi, Golgi complex; SER, smooth endoplasmic reticulum. (From Habener JF. Hormone biosynthesis and secretion. In: Felig P, Baxter JD, Broadus AE, et al, eds. *Endocrinology and Metabolism.* New York, NY: McGraw-Hill; 1981:29-59.)

molecules are produced in glandular tissues. Although some signaling molecules, such as classic endocrine hormones, arrive at target tissues through the bloodstream, others have paracrine functions or autocrine functions. Notable among these are the cytokines produce by cells of the immune system and the highly related peptides secreted by fat cells, which have been termed *adipokines*. Discovery of these hormones has led to the recognition that many tissues that are not classic secretory glands produce peptides or lipids that act locally or travel through the bloodstream to act at distance. Examples of these substances include atrial natriuretic peptide, which is unusual in being stored within secretory granules in atrial cardiomyocytes; the adipocyte hormones leptin, adiponectin, and resistin; and myostatin, which is secreted by muscle.[2-4]

Nonpeptide Hormones That Act at Cell Surface Receptors

In addition to peptide hormones, the major group of small, hydrophilic hormones is also related to monoamine neurotransmitters. They include the adrenergic agents such as norepinephrine as well as other amino acid–derived water-soluble molecules such as melatonin, serotonin, and histamine. These hormones can also be stored in dense secretory vesicles, but are more typically packaged into small, approximately 50-nm electron-lucent vesicles that are quite similar morphologically to those in neural and neuroendocrine cells, the major difference being that in the presynaptic cleft the vesicles are arrayed in a tightly packed array at the membrane. There exists a third class of secretory vesicles, the synaptic-like vesicles (SSVs), which can be found in more classic endocrine cell types like the insulin-secreting beta cells of the pancreas and are possibly involved in the secretion of γ-aminobutyric acid (GABA).[5]

Interestingly, there is at least one class of lipid that breaks the off-cited rule that lipophilic molecules have intracellular receptors. Eicosanoids are a class of extracel-

TABLE 3-2	
Receptors for Metabolites	
Metabolite	**Receptor**
Lactate	GPR81
Ketone bodies	GPR109A
3-Hydroxyoctanoate	GPR109B
Succinate	GPR91
α-Ketoglutarate	GPR80/99
Long-chain fatty acids	GPR40, GPR120
Medium-chain fatty acids	GPR84
Short-chain fatty acids	GPR41, GPR43

lular signaling molecules that includes the leukotrienes and prostanoids and are derived from 20-carbon fatty acids. Many of the biologically active eicosanoids bind to cell surface receptors, which initiate their typically paracrine and autocrine functions.[6]

One of the more interesting recent additions to the assortment of hormone-like molecules has been the circulating metabolites, such as lactate, ketone bodies, and succinate[7] (Table 3-2). An even more distant modification of the original definition of *hormone* is the idea that metabolites produced by microbes in the gut, like short-chain fatty acids, could signal by binding to cell surface receptors.[8] The recent expansion of messenger types and novel modes of interorgan communication have dramatically changed the traditional view of endocrinology such that all cell types can potentially send messages as well as receive them.

BINDING PROPERTIES OF CELL SURFACE RECEPTORS

When a hormone or extracellular signaling molecule arrives at a target cell, at least two critical components are required to induce the appropriate biologic response. First, there has to be recognition of the hormone as different from all other components of the extracellular milieu. This issue concerns *specificity*, that is, the ability to distinguish the hormone from other structurally related molecules, and *selectivity*, the property of recognizing the quantity of hormone among the multitude of potentially interfering substances. Second, the initial recognition step must be converted into a single action or a defined set of cellular events. The initial step of hormone recognition is mediated by cellular receptors. The origin of the modern understanding of receptor biology dates to pharmacologic experiments in the latter 19th and early 20th centuries.[9] Paul Ehrlich coined the maxim that still guides all endocrinology: "*corpora non agunt nisi fixate*," which can be translated as "a substance cannot act unless it is bound (fixed)." Ultimately, studies of the binding properties of hormones and neurotransmitters crystallized into a fundamental rule governing the action of extracellular agents: a biologic effect is directly proportional to the ligand occupancy of the receptor. A subtle but important modification to occupancy theory is the notion of *spare receptors*, which describes the situation in which a maximal biologic response is transduced by occupancy of a minor fraction of available receptors. One consequence of the existence of spare receptors is that a decrease in the number of cellular receptors results in a change in the ED_{50} (effective dose for 50% of the group) for a hormone but does not necessarily alter the maximal biologic response, as described in some detail for insulin.[10,11]

As noted previously, the fundamental characteristic of a cell surface receptor is the ability to bind extracellular hormone with high selectivity and high affinity. In practical terms, any receptor that functions in physiologic systems must display two cardinal, experimentally verifiable properties: specificity and saturability. These characteristics are established experimentally by assessing the binding of ligands to receptors, studies made possible by the development of radioactive ligands capable of binding specifically and with high affinity to receptors.[12] Authentic physiologic receptors for a given hormone will display a greater affinity for the cognate hormone than other potentially competing circulating molecules. In addition, the half maximal binding for a hormone to its real receptor will always be in the range of the circulating free concentration of that hormone.

CELL SURFACE HORMONE RECEPTORS

Cell surface receptors can be grouped conveniently into four classes: ion channel receptors, G protein–linked receptors, receptors with intrinsic enzymatic activity, and receptors that associate with enzymes.

Ligand-Gated Ion Channels

The simplest form of a cell surface signaling system is one in which both the hormone-binding and signal-generating functions are provided by a single protein or complex of proteins. Ligand-gated ion channels represent such a species. They are made up of two key components: a ligand-binding domain accessible from the surface of the cell and a transmembrane domain containing the permeation channel. Binding of ligand to the exofacial surface of the receptor generates a conformational change that results in opening of a pore, allowing ions to travel across the plasma membrane (Fig. 3-2).

The prototype and founding member of the family of ligand-gated ion channels is the nicotinic acetylcholine receptor, which is present on some neurons and on the postsynaptic membrane of the neuromuscular junction.[13] When a nerve impulse arrives at the presynaptic terminal, depolarization leads to an increase in cytosolic calcium and secretion of acetylcholine. This binds to its receptor on the muscle, increasing the permeability to cations, which leads to depolarization and muscle contraction. It was the observation that curare, which binds the acetylcholine receptor, blocks muscle contraction induced by nerve stimulation but not electrical stimulus applied directly to the muscle that led to first use of the phrase *receptive substance* to describe the recipient of the nerve stimulus.[14] Much of the understanding of the acetylcholine receptor derives from studies using the electric organ of the fish, *Electrophorus electricus*, which has an extraordinary number of nicotinic synapses.[15] The acetylcholine receptor is made of four different peptides that constitute five subunits, defining a family of receptors that also includes the

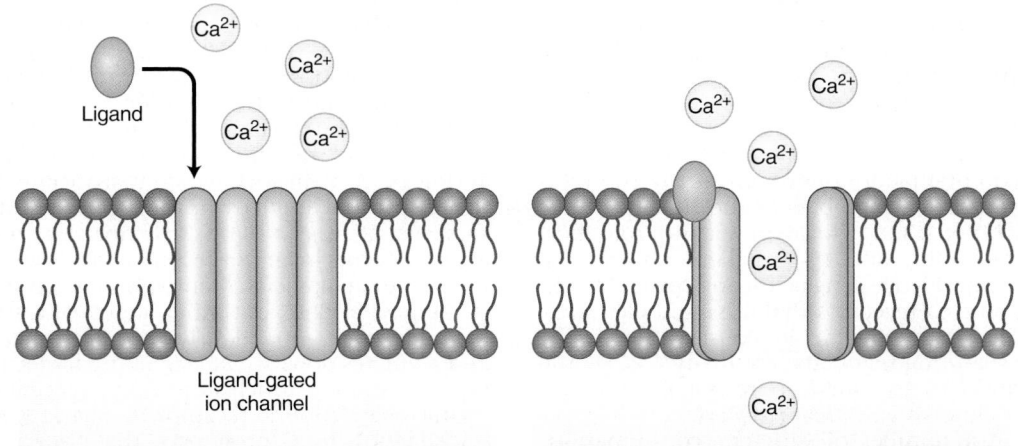

Figure 3-2 Ligand-gated ion channels are transmembrane proteins that comprise at least two domains, a ligand-binding domain and a membrane-spanning domain capable of functioning as a pore. When ligand binds, it induces a conformational change in the receptor such that the pore opens to the passage of ions, in this case calcium ions, down their electrochemical gradient.

5-hydroxytryptamine type 3 (5-HT$_3$R), glycine, and inhibitory GABA type A receptors. Another shared characteristic of pentameric receptors is a conserved 15–amino acid dicysteine loop in the extracellular ligand-binding domain (LBD), giving this family its alternative name, the *cys-loop receptors*.[16] Binding of acetylcholine to its receptor elicits a conformational change that opens the pore, which allows sodium and potassium ions to pass in and out of the cell, respectively.

In general, most ligand-gated ion channels serve as neurotransmitter receptors rather than receptors for classic hormones, probably in response to the need for microsecond signal transduction at the synapse. A notable exception involves the receptors for hypothalamic releasing factors, which are discharged from hypothalamic neurons into the portal circulation to regulate secretion of hormones from the anterior pituitary. For example, it is likely that serotonin regulates release of prolactin by binding to 5-HT$_3$R in lactotrophs in the anterior pituitary.[17] Similarly, glycine and GABA receptors are present in the pituitary gland, but their physiologic functions appear complex and remain imperfectly understood. Another class of ligand-gated ion channel, involving the purinergic cation receptors, is also expressed in the pituitary and most likely functions in an autocrine/paracrine fashion in response to extracellular adenosine triphosphate (ATP).

G Protein–Linked Receptors

The largest family of cell surface receptors is defined by their use of heterotrimeric G proteins for signaling, leading to their designation, *G protein–coupled receptors* (GPCRs). The conserved topology of these receptors is that they include seven 25–amino acid α-helical segments passing through the plasma membrane seven times with the amino (N)-terminus and carboxy (C)-terminus outside the cell and in the cytoplasm, respectively, leading to the name of *seven transmembrane* (7TM) proteins.[18] Whole genome sequencing defined the size of the GPCR family as over 800, with the vast majority being olfactory receptors. The diversity of ligands capable of being bound to 7TM receptors is remarkable, ranging from a single photon to large proteins and including ions, odorants, amines, peptides, lipids, nucleotides, and metabolic intermediates. The smaller hormones, including catecholamines, bind to their receptors within the transmembrane-spanning region, oriented parallel to the cell surface, whereas larger hormones bind to the extracellular N-terminus, which itself can range in size from 10 to 600 amino acids,[3] in addition to interacting with the transmembrane-spanning region (Fig. 3-3). The GPCR family can be divided into five subfamilies based on primary sequence and phylogeny, named glutamate, rhodopsin, adhesion, frizzled/taste2, and secretin families.[19] Many hormones, including some hypothalamic releasing factors, the glycoprotein hormones secreted by the pituitary, and the amines, are members of the rhodopsin-like family. On the other hand, glucagon, parathyroid hormone (PTH), calcitonin, and hypothalamic hormones, such as growth hormone–releasing factor and corticotropin-releasing factor, bind to receptors that are more like secretin receptors. The greatest region of conservation is the transmembrane-spanning segments. For many GPCRs, the endogenous ligand and its function are not known, and they are therefore known as *orphan receptors*.

GPCRs assume a number of different conformations based on interactions with other molecules, the immediate chemical environment, and their state of oligomerization. Dynamic changes in receptor configurations promoted by hormone binding are responsible for increased association with and activation of target G proteins. Like many GPCRs, the β$_2$-adrenergic receptor exhibits significant activity in the basal, unbound state, likely a reflection of its existence in multiple, interconverting conformations. In all likelihood, binding of epinephrine stimulates a tilting of several transmembrane-spanning helices, changing the conformation of G$_s$ on the cytoplasmic face of the receptor.

Signaling by Heterotrimeric G Proteins

An important advance in the understanding of GPCRs occurred when Bourne and associates took advantage of the lethality of cyclic adenosine monophosphate (cAMP) toward lymphoma cells to select mutant lines resistant to the actions of the β-adrenergic agent isoproterenol.[20] Because the mutant cell lines lost responsiveness to a number of agonists, it was clear that the genetic lesion did not reside in the β-adrenergic receptor but rather in a downstream component. When the signaling module that restored hormone responsiveness to the deficient membranes was purified, it turned out to be a heterotrimeric G protein complex, now known as G$_s$.[21] G$_s$ binds a single guanosine triphosphate (GTP) to its α-subunit, which dissociates from the β/γ-subunits upon binding of guanine nucleotide. Moreover, the GTP-bound α-subunit of G$_s$α is necessary and sufficient for activation of its downstream target, adenylyl cyclase. Sixteen distinct genes encode about 20 different G protein α-subunits, which can be divided into four groups based on both structure and function: G$_s$, G$_i$, G$_{q/11}$, and G$_{12}$.[18] The G$_s$ family has only two members, G$_s$ and the G protein for the olfactory receptor, G$_{olf}$; both couple to activation of adenylyl cyclase. The G$_i$ group includes three G$_i$ proteins, all of which inhibit adenylyl cyclase; two G$_0$ proteins, abundant brain proteins whose multiple targets still are not completely defined; two G$_t$ proteins that couple photoreceptors to cAMP phosphodiesterase (PDE); and G$_z$, which inhibits potassium channels. The G$_{q/11}$ subfamily consists of six members, all of which activate the enzyme phospholipase C beta (PLCβ), generating the second messengers diacylglycerol (DAG) and inositol triphosphate (IP$_3$). G$_{12}$ and G$_{13}$, which inhibit and activate the guanine exchange factor, RhoGEF, respectively, form the final group. The combinational possibilities are also complex, with 5 β-subunit isoforms and over 12 γ-subunit isoforms.

The key operational feature of G protein signaling is that the system behaves like a timed switch. Engagement of hormone with its cognate receptor promotes its association with a heterotrimeric G protein already complexed to its effector protein (Fig. 3-4). This stimulates dissociation of guanosine diphosphate (GDP) from the α-subunit, allowing GTP to bind to the unoccupied site, solely as a result of its greater intracellular concentration compared to GDP. The occupied receptor then detaches and searches for another G protein with which to associate. GTP loading of the G protein induces its dissociation into α- and β/γ-subunits, at least in vitro; it is not clear that dissociation actually occurs in an intact cell. In most cases, the α-subunit modulates an associated amplifier, which in the case of G$_s$ is adenylyl cyclase, but other targets of α-subunits include those referred to previously. The β/γ-dimer interacts with and regulates downstream signaling molecules, most notably potassium channels following engagement of the muscarinic acetylcholine receptor by ligand. Critical to signal transduction by G proteins is that they remain active as long as GTP is bound. It is the rate conversion of nucleotide to GDP that determines the timing for reassembly of subunits and inactivation of signaling. Thus, the G protein can exist in two distinct states: bound to GTP and active or

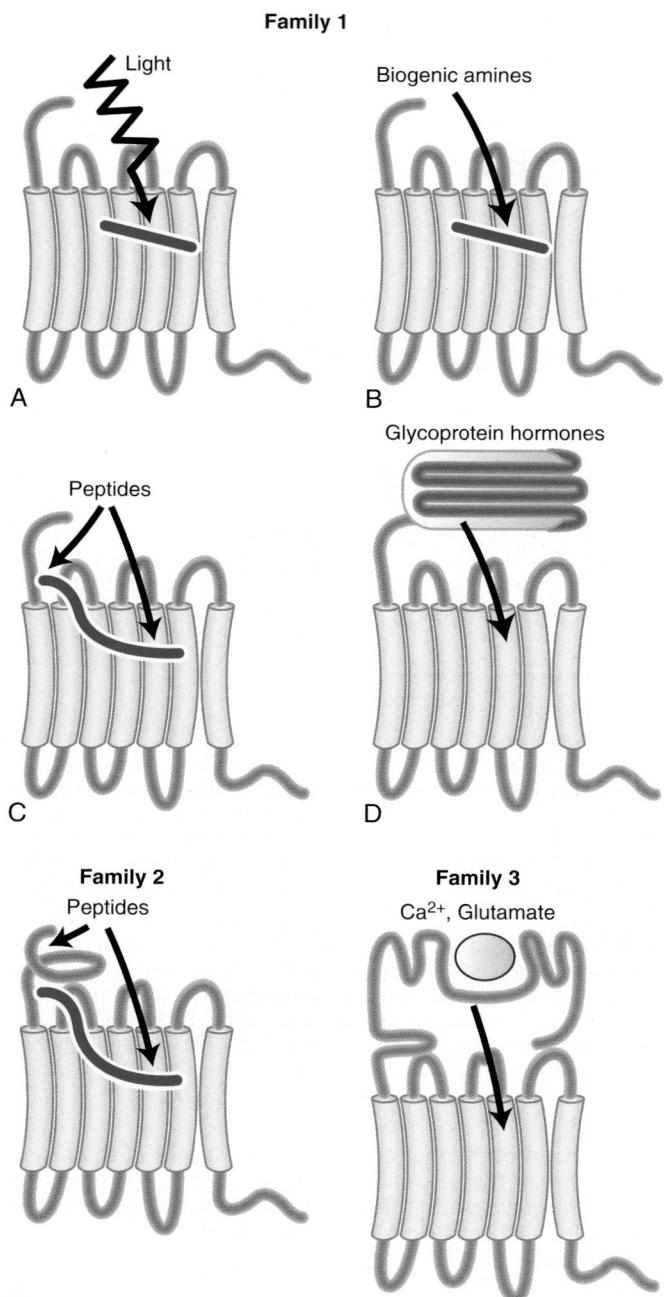

Family 1

Light

Biogenic amines

A

B

Glycoprotein hormones

Peptides

C

D

Family 2
Peptides

Family 3
Ca²⁺, Glutamate

E

F

Figure 3-3 The G protein–coupled receptor (GPCR) superfamily: diversity in ligand binding and structure. Each panel depicts members of the GPCR superfamily. The seven-membrane-spanning α-helices are shown as cylinders, with the extracellular amino (N)-terminus and three extracellular loops above them and the intracellular carboxy (C)-terminus and three intracellular loops below. The superfamily can be divided into three subfamilies on the basis of amino acid sequence conservation within the transmembrane helices. Family 1 includes the opsins (**A**), in which light *(arrow)* causes isomerization of retinal covalently bound within the pocket created by the transmembrane helices *(bar)*; monoamine receptors (**B**), in which agonists *(arrow)* bind noncovalently within the pocket created by the transmembrane helices *(bar)*; receptors for peptides such as vasopressin (**C**), in which agonist binding *(arrow)* may involve parts of the extracellular N-terminus and loops and the transmembrane helices *(bar)*; and glycoprotein hormone receptors (**D**), in which agonists *(oval)* bind to the large extracellular N-terminus, activating the receptor through undefined interactions with the extracellular loops or transmembrane helices *(arrow)*. **E,** Family 2 includes receptors for peptide hormones such as parathyroid hormone and secretin. Agonists *(arrow)* may bind to residues in the extracellular N-terminus and loops and to transmembrane helices *(bar)*. **F,** Family 3 includes the extracellular Ca²⁺-sensing receptor and metabotropic glutamate receptors. Agonists *(circle)* bind in a cleft of the Venus flytrap–like domain in the large extracellular N-terminus, activating the receptor through undefined interactions with the extracellular loops or transmembrane helices *(arrow)*. (From Spiegel AM, Carter-Su C, Taylor SI, et al. Mechanism of action of hormones that act at the cell surface. In: Melmed S, Polonsky KS, Larsen PR, et al, eds. *Williams Textbook of Endocrinology*, 12th ed. Philadelphia, PA: Elsevier; 2011:62-82.)

GDP and inactive, and the time spent in each condition defines the strength of signaling. G protein α-subunits have low levels of intrinsic GTPase activity, but this can be enhanced by association with the regulators of G protein signaling (RGS) proteins, which also can compete for binding to effector proteins.[22] Thus, RGS proteins serve to shorten the duration of signaling by G proteins, providing another important site of regulation. Many members of the large family of RGS proteins contain within their primary sequences canonical domains indicative of other functions and undergo complex post-translational modification. Modulation of the levels of RGS proteins affords a mechanism for signaling pathways to communicate with each other. For example, both thyroid-stimulating hormone (TSH, thyrotropin) and PTH signal though a G_s-cAMP path-

way to increase expression of RGS2, which feeds back to inhibit G_s and also to antagonize other pathways that depend on G_q.

Another GPCR regulatory system involves a family of proteins called arrestins (see Fig. 3-4). Ligand binding to a GPCR signals the dissociation of the G protein complex as described earlier but also promotes a conformational change that often leads to phosphorylation of the receptor by a G protein receptor kinase (GRK).[23] GRKs are represented by a family of seven related kinases, of which GRK1 and 7 are involved in phosphorylation of photoreceptors. Phosphorylation of the GPCR at serine and threonine residues is insufficient to inactivate the GPCR, but rather allows the binding of an arrestin, which displaces the G protein, terminating the signal. Binding to the receptor

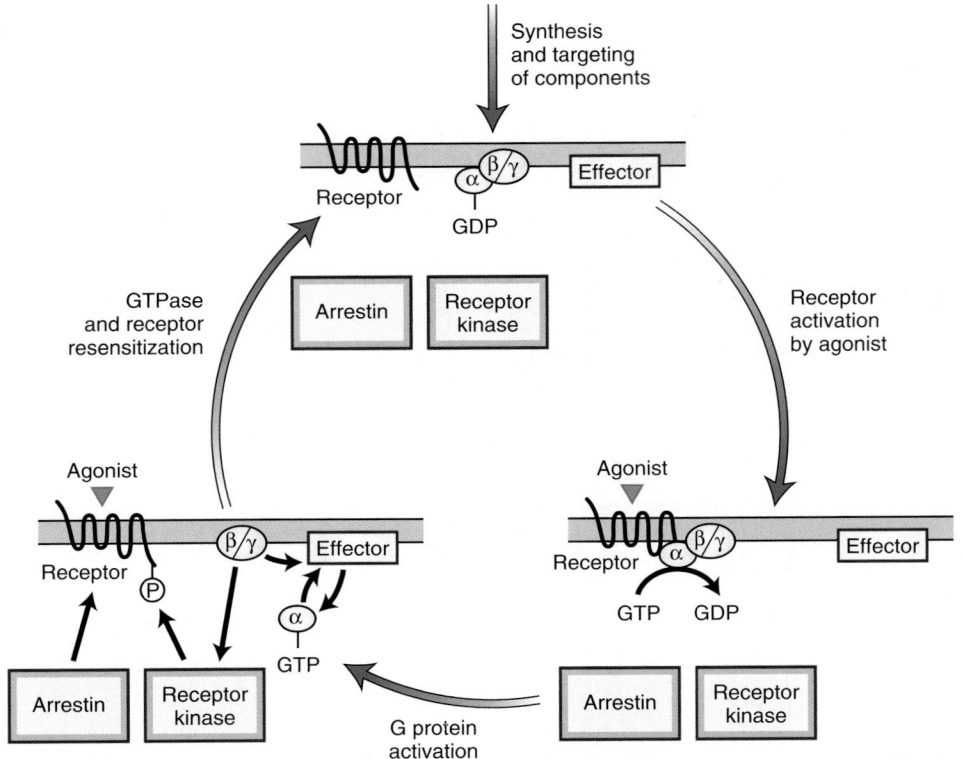

Figure 3-4 The G protein guanosine triphosphatase (GTPase) and G protein–coupled receptor (GPCR) desensitization-resensitization cycle. In each panel, the *shaded area* denotes the plasma membrane, with the extracellular region above and the intracellular region below. In the basal state, the G protein is a heterotrimer with guanosine diphosphate (GDP) tightly bound to the α-subunit. The agonist-activated GPCR catalyzes release of GDP, which permits guanosine triphosphate (GTP) to bind. The GTP-bound α-subunit dissociates from the βγ-dimer. *Arrows* from the α-subunit to the effector and from the βγ-dimer to the effector indicate regulation of effector activity by the respective subunits. The *arrow* from effector to the α-subunit indicates regulation of its GTPase activity by effector interaction. Under physiologic conditions, effector regulation by G protein subunits is transient and is terminated by the GTPase activity of the α-subunit. The latter converts bound GTP to GDP, thereby returning the α-subunit to its inactivated state with high affinity for the βγ dimer, which reassociates to form the heterotrimer in the basal state. In the basal state, the receptor kinase and arrestin are shown as cytosolic proteins. Dissociation of the GTP-bound α-subunit from the βγ-dimer permits the dimer to facilitate binding of receptor kinase to the plasma membrane (*arrow* from βγ-dimer to receptor kinase). Plasma membrane binding permits the receptor kinase to phosphorylate the agonist-bound GPCR (P, depicted here as occurring on the carboxy-terminal tail of the GPCR, although sites on intracellular loops are also possible). GPCR phosphorylation facilitates arrestin binding to the GPCR, resulting in desensitization. Endocytic trafficking of arrestin-bound GPCR and recycling to the plasma membrane during resensitization are not shown. (From Spiegel AM, Carter-Su C, Taylor SI, et al. Mechanism of action of hormones that act at the cell surface. In: Melmed S, Polonsky KS, Larsen PR, et al, eds. *Williams Textbook of Endocrinology*, 12th ed. Philadelphia, PA: Elsevier; 2011:62-82.)

also alters the conformation of the arrestin such that it interacts with components of the endocytosis system such as clathrin.[24] The GPCR is escorted to the sorting endosome where it either recycles back to the cell surface or is targeted to the lysosome for degradation. This system provides an efficient mechanism for homologous desensitization, in which there is receptor-specific downregulation of signaling pathways. This mechanism stands in contrast to negative regulation by second messenger–dependent protein kinases, which phosphorylate and inhibit all susceptible GPCRs whether or not occupied by ligand. In addition to its role in the modulation of G protein signaling, β-arrestin has a well-defined function as a signaling intermediate. Initially identified in this regard as a scaffold for the proto-oncogene c-SRC, β-arrestin is now recognized to bind multiple members of the SRC family as well as other proteins.[25,26] Similarly, mitogen-activated protein kinase (MAPK) was the first downstream kinase shown to be regulated by β-arrestin, but currently known targets include phosphoinositide 3-kinase (PI3K), Akt, PDE4, and c-Jun N-terminal kinase-3.

One of the most interesting aspects of GPCR signaling is their ability to undergo functional selectivity (also known as biased signaling), defined as the ability of ligands to stimulate distinct signaling pathways, presumably due to stabilization of distinct conformational states of the receptor.[27] Most of the research activity around biased signaling has taken place in the pharmaceutical industry, where the principle has been used in attempts to develop more specific therapeutics. For example, attempts have been made to develop opioid agonists that activate G protein signaling but are devoid of arrestin-dependent desensitization and tolerance.[28,29] A similar strategy is being attempted to dissociate opioid analgesia from constipation and respiratory depression, as the latter are also signaled through the arrestin pathway.[28,29] Biased signaling is not limited to synthetic drug products, as it has also been implicated in the action of the hormone ghrelin and by fragments of PTH.

Receptor Tyrosine Protein Kinases as Cell Surface Receptors

The receptors that make up the receptor tyrosine protein kinase (RTK) family use a number of strategies to accomplish the same goal: to convert the binding of ligand to the exofacial portion of the receptor to a change in the activity of a tyrosine protein kinase domain residing in the interior of the cell. All of these receptors are type I transmembrane proteins with an N-terminus and the hormone-binding domain on the outside, a 25–amino acid hydrophobic

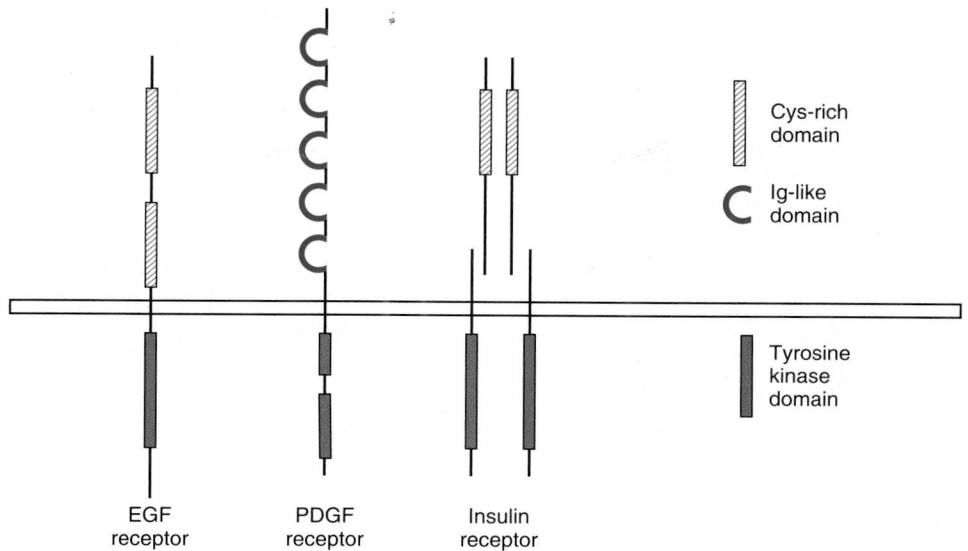

Figure 3-5 Receptor tyrosine kinases. Three of the 16 families of receptor tyrosine kinases are represented. All receptor tyrosine kinases possess an extracellular domain containing the ligand-binding site, a single transmembrane domain, and an intracellular portion containing the tyrosine kinase domain. Several structural motifs (i.e., cysteine-rich domain, immunoglobulin-like domain, tyrosine kinase domain) in these receptor tyrosine kinases are indicated on the right side of the figure. Cys, cysteine; EGF, epidermal growth factor; Ig, immunoglobulin; PDGF, platelet-derived growth factor. (From Spiegel AM, Carter-Su C, Taylor SI, et al. Mechanism of action of hormones that act at the cell surface. In: Melmed S, Polonsky KS, Larsen PR, et al, eds. *Williams Textbook of Endocrinology*, 12th ed. Philadelphia, PA: Elsevier; 2011:62-82.)

segment that spans the membrane (the transmembrane domain), and the carboxy portion of the protein containing a kinase domain extending into the cytoplasm[30] (Fig. 3-5). The intracellular catalytic domain transfers phosphate from ATP to tyrosine residues in proteins, including the receptor itself. The 58 RTKs expressed in humans can be divided into about 20 subfamilies based on structural features. One of these groups is defined by the insulin receptor, which unlike other RTKs, exists as a disulfide-linked tetramer in the basal state. All other receptors, including those for fibroblast growth factor, platelet-derived growth factors (PDGFs), and epidermal growth factor (EGF), exist as monomers, though there is evidence that some might associate noncovalently into larger structures in the basal state.

For insulin, or any other peptide hormone, to carry out its actions, four events must transpire: (1) the hormone must be recognized by the receptor; (2) the hormone must alter the state of the receptor; (3) the extracellular signal must be transmitted across the plasma membrane to the cytoplasm; and (4) the receptor must engage intracellular signaling pathways. Biochemical experiments involving affinity cross-linking and biosynthetic labeling identified the structure of the insulin receptor and that of the highly related IGF-1 receptor as a heterotetramer, composed of two 125-kDa α-subunits and two 90-kDa β-subunits linked by disulfide bonds.[31,32] The receptor is synthesized as a single peptide with a cleavable signal sequence directing insertion cotranslationally into the membrane and is glycosylated and cleaved into the alpha and beta chains in the Golgi complex.[33] Even though they exist as two separate peptides in the mature protein, each pair of alpha and beta chains behaves much like a receptor monomer found in other growth factor receptors. Affinity labeling by insulin shows cross-linking to both the α- and β-subunits, indicating that both are partly found on the exofacial surface of the cell. Insulin binding has been long recognized to exhibit *negative cooperativity*, in which, as a population of receptors binds more ligand, the affinity for additional hormone decreases.[34] In structural terms this is explained by the presence of four binding sites on each holoreceptor—two of low affinity and two of high affinity. Insulin initially binds to a low-affinity site before binding to a high-affinity site on the contralateral α/β-dimer, thus effectively cross-linking the two halves of the receptor such that the stoichiometry of this high-affinity complex is one insulin molecule per insulin receptor. This stable structure prevents binding of hormone to the second high-affinity site, thus reducing the affinity of the receptor for any subsequently bound insulin molecules. Solution by x-ray crystallography of the structure of the ectodomain of the insulin receptor in the unoccupied and bound states has confirmed this general model and added molecular detail, assigning the initial binding site to a leucine-rich (L1) domain and the second to the C-terminus of the alpha chain.[35,36] This structural organization for binding is largely conserved in the association of IGF-1 with its receptor.[37] Other classes of RTKs use alternative strategies for receptor binding. For example, even though the EGF and insulin receptor share structural motifs such as two leucine-rich domains separated by a cysteine-rich domain, EGF binds to the outer surface of the receptors, whereas the two monomers interact directly with each other so that there is a stoichiometry of one molecule of ligand per receptor monomer.[38]

In general, most ligands for RTKs activate their cognate receptors by inducing dimerization.[30] In its simplest form, this is accomplished by a bivalent ligand binding two receptor monomers and bringing them into close apposition (Fig. 3-6). Examples of ligands that act this way include PDGF, vascular endothelial growth factor, and nerve growth factor. However, even among these ligands there is some diversity in binding mechanisms; in some cases the receptor monomers also make contact with each other, stabilizing the interaction. The EGF family uses a markedly different strategy for inducing dimerization of its receptor, in that all of the contacts are provided by the receptor and the ligand provides no bridging function. Binding of EGF to two sites on a single receptor induces a conformational change that leads to exposure of a previously buried

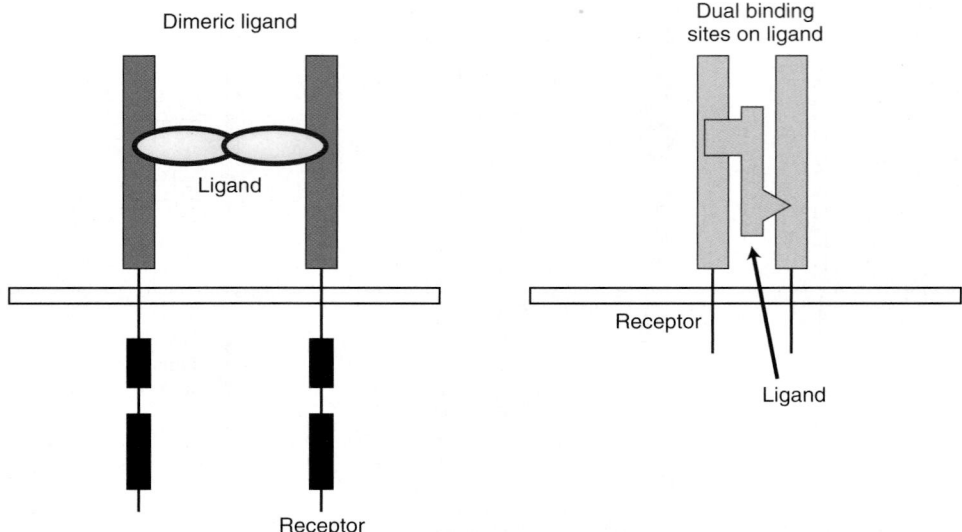

Figure 3-6 Molecular mechanisms of ligand-induced dimerization of receptors. In the example of platelet-derived growth factor *(left)*, the ligand is dimeric and contains two receptor-binding sites. In the case of growth hormone *(right)*, a single ligand molecule contains two binding sites so that it can bind simultaneously to two receptor molecules. (From Spiegel AM, Carter-Su C, Taylor SI, et al. Mechanism of action of hormones that act at the cell surface. In: Melmed S, Polonsky KS, Larsen PR, et al, eds. *Williams Textbook of Endocrinology*, 12th ed. Philadelphia, PA: Elsevier; 2011:62-82.)

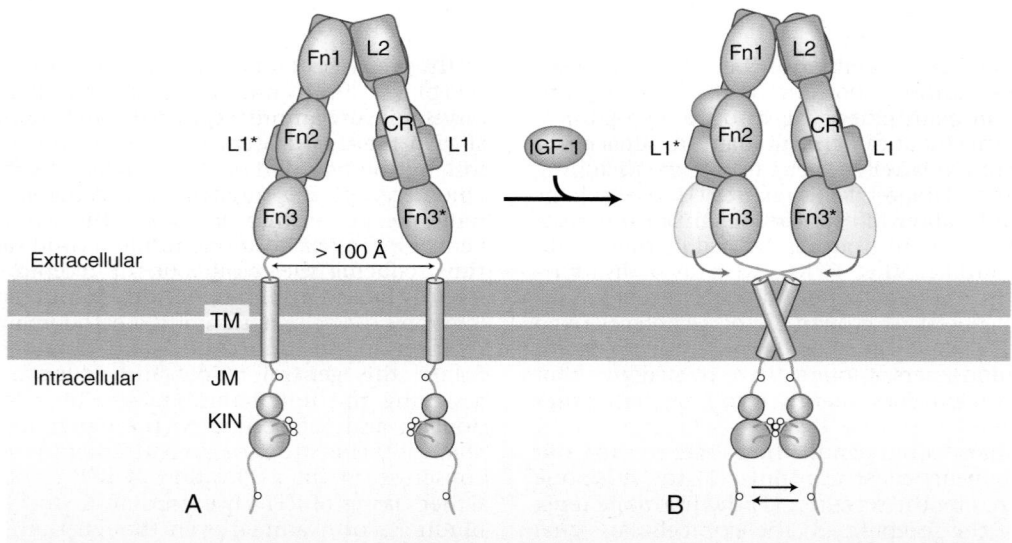

Figure 3-7 How insulin-like growth factor 1 (IGF-1) activates its receptor. Each IGF-1 receptor is made of two half-receptors, which are linked by disulfide bonds (not shown). The six domains in the extracellular region of the first half-receptor (orange) are L1, CR, L2, Fn1, Fn2, and Fn3; the domains in the second half-receptor (green) are the same and labeled with an asterisk. The L1, CR, L2, and Fn1 are in the α-chain, and the Fn3 and the transmembrane and intracellular domains make up the β-chain of each half-receptor; the Fn2 domain is made up of contributions from both chains. The intracellular region comprises the juxtamembrane region (JM) and the tyrosine kinase domain (KIN). Sites of transphosphorylation are shown as circles. **A,** When IGF-1 is not bound to the receptor, an interaction between L1* of the second half-receptor and Fn2 and Fn3 of the first half-receptor (and vice versa) is thought to maintain a large separation between the transmembrane (TM) helices *(double arrow)*. **B,** When IGF-1 binds to L1* (or to L1), it disrupts the L1*-Fn2 (or L1-Fn2*) interaction. This allows Fn2 and Fn3 of each half-receptor to pivot *(curved arrows)* toward each other (the previous positions of Fn2 and Fn3 are shown semitransparently). This in turn facilitates the dimerization of the TM helices in the membrane, which juxtaposes the kinase domains for efficient transphosphorylation *(black arrows)*. Binding of a single IGF-1 molecule (shown as binding to the left side) is sufficient to activate the receptor, but exactly how this asymmetry affects the conformational changes in the receptor is unclear. It is believed that the same mechanism also applies to activation of the insulin receptor. (Redrawn from Hubbard SR, Miller WT. Closing in on a mechanism for activation. *eLife*. 2014;3:e04909.)

dimerization motif; when two of these domains interact, they allow formation of a stable, EGF receptor dimer.

Because the insulin receptor exists as a functional dimer composed of two α/β pairs in the basal state, it is clear that dimerization is not sufficient to activate RTKs; indeed, there must also be some fundamental change in the interaction between the two halves of the receptor. In the inactive state, the extracellular portions of the insulin and

IGF-1 receptors exist in an inverted V conformation formed by the α-subunits and part of the β-subunits.[36] The base is continuous with and anchored by the transmembrane domains of the β-subunits. Insulin binding to its low-affinity site removes a brake on a molecular hinge, allowing the V to close and bring the transmembrane domains closer to each other[39,40] (Fig. 3-7). This conformational change is transmitted to the cytoplasmic domains, where it has the effect of bringing the two kinase domains into closer proximity. In the basal state, each kinase domain is inactive due to an intramolecular peptide, the so-called activation loop, which is buried in the catalytic cleft and sterically hinders entry of substrates.[41] When the two cytoplasmic portions of the receptor domains are brought sufficiently close together, the kinase domain of one β-subunit phosphorylates the other on a cluster of tyrosine residues in the activation loop, forcing it out of the catalytic cleft, thus converting the kinase domain into an active kinase.[42] This is possible because of kinetic nature of the receptor's inactive state, in which the catalytic site is always alternating between open and closed conformations, though in the basal state the activation loop is inaccessible for most of the time. However, when the contralateral kinase domain is brought sufficiently close, it can phosphorylate the activation loop during the brief period it is in the extended position, converting this to the more stable conformation. In this way, phosphorylation of one half of the receptor increases its activity, allowing it to phosphorylate the other half and, ultimately, exogenous substrates.[43] Proximity-driven phosphorylation and activation of one monomer by the other are common features of RTK activation, but again the precise strategies utilized to achieve this vary. Thus, although the active conformations of all tyrosine protein kinases are similar, with a bilobed structure analogous to that of a serine/threonine kinase, the configurations of the inactive states differ enormously. An exception to the rule of activation by transphosphorylation is provided by the EGF receptor, in which activation depends on allosteric regulation of one kinase domain by the other monomer, once again brought about by a conformational change bringing the two domains into adjacency. The critical interaction is between the C lobe of the activator kinase and the N lobe of the receiver kinase, which disrupts an autoinhibitory interaction present in the inactive monomer.[44]

Signaling by Receptor Tyrosine Protein Kinases

Because the insulin receptor is an enzyme with catalytic activity residing on the cytoplasmic surface of the plasma membrane, it stands to reason that it would transmit its signal by phosphorylating protein substrates within the cell. Yet, though autophosphorylation sites within and outside the cytoplasmic kinase domain of the β-subunit have been long recognized, it has proved difficult to identify robust, physiologically significant phosphorylation of tyrosine residues in other proteins. This seeming paradox is explained by the underlying mechanism of activation of signaling pathways by RTKs, which do not in general signal via a phosphorylation cascade akin to that utilized by a number of serine/threonine kinases, as described later. Instead, signaling is initiated by the assembly of a stable multimeric signaling complex, usually as a result of initial autophosphorylation or the phosphorylation of a scaffolding protein by the receptor. The most important phosphorylation-dependent binding motif is the Src homology 2 (SH2) domain, named after the founder of the family, the SH2 domain in the proto-oncogene c-Src.[45] Under basal conditions, c-Src is maintained in an inactive configuration via two intramolecular interactions: the SH2 domain binds a phosphorylated tyrosine residue in the C-terminus of the protein and an SH3 domain associates with a cluster of proline residues located between the SH2 and kinase domains.[46] c-Src can be activated by dephosphorylation of C-terminal tyrosine and displacement of the SH3 by another, competing protein. These same intramolecular SH2 and SH3 protein-protein interactions utilized by c-Src and other related nonmembrane tyrosine kinases to remain inactive are coopted by RTKs to assemble a signal transduction complex. The SH2 domain is the most versatile interaction cassette, as its association with a receptor is dependent on phosphorylation of a tyrosine residue in a specific context.[45] A phosphorylated tyrosine residue in concert with the amino acids 1 and 3 positions C-terminal to the phosphotyrosine serves as the binding interface for SH2 domains and therefore provides much of the specificity of the interaction. For example, after a PDGF receptor binds its ligand, autophosphorylation of tyrosines in a context defined by the sequence tyrosine-methionine-any amino acid-methionine (YMXM) generates a binding site for the SH2 domains of PI3K.[47] PI3K comprises a catalytic subunit and regulatory subunit containing two SH2 domains in tandem. Recruitment of PI3K to a phosphorylated receptor brings it into proximity to its major physiologic substrate, the lipid phosphatidylinositol 4,5-bisphosphate (PI4,5P$_2$), which resides on the inner surface of the plasma membrane. PI3K phosphorylates PI4,5P$_2$ on the 3'-position of its inositol ring, generating phosphatidylinositol 3,4,5-trisphosphate (PIP$_3$), a potent signaling molecule by virtue of its ability to recruit to the membrane protein kinases and other signaling molecules. The important principle that governs RTK signaling is that initiation of intracellular events is driven primarily by the spatial relationship of proteins and lipids rather than changes in the specific activity of assembled components. Although in some cases the hormone-bound receptor will modulate the activity of target protein by phosphorylation, nonetheless the more important event is the establishment of adjacency between two or more critical signaling molecules, such as PI3K and its substrate, PI4,5P$_2$. An additional example of this signaling mechanism is provided by activation of another proto-oncogene, c-ras. In this case, signaling is initiated by recruitment of the adapter protein, growth factor receptor—bound protein 2 (GRB2) via its SH2 domain. GRB2 is a 217–amino acid protein, the only other feature of note being two SH3 domains that remain constitutively bound to a polyproline sequence in the son of sevenless (SOS) protein, which is thus, in turn, carried to the plasma membrane.[48,49] Association of SOS with the plasma membrane is necessary and sufficient for activation of RAS.[50] SOS, a guanine nucleotide exchange (GEF) protein for ras, removes GDP from the inactive small G protein to allow binding of GTP and activation. As noted earlier, the critical event that determines the state of GTP-binding to ras and accordingly its activity is the positioning of its GEF protein, SOS, in proximity.[51,52]

Insulin and IGF-1 receptors signal via a variant of that described previously for the PDGF receptor (Fig. 3-8). Rather than assembling a signaling complex on the cytoplasmic domain of the receptor, they do so on members of a family of scaffolds, insulin receptor substrate (IRS) proteins.[53] There are at least four members of this family, but IRS1 and IRS2 are most important to physiologic signaling by insulin and IGF-1. Like other members of the group, IRS1 and 2 lack intrinsic enzymatic activity but serve solely as docking proteins to bring signaling molecules together into a multimeric complex. IRS1 and 2 are heavily tyrosine phosphorylated by the insulin receptor, generating binding sites for the SH2 domains of PI3K, Grb2, and the SH2 domain-containing protein phosphotyrosine phosphatase, SHP-2. A pleckstrin homology (PH) and phosphotyrosine binding (PTB) domain located at the N-terminus of IRS1/2 are instrumental in bringing the protein to its receptor.[54] Upon ligand engagement of the insulin or IGF-1 receptor, IRS1/2 is rapidly phosphorylated on tyrosine residues and

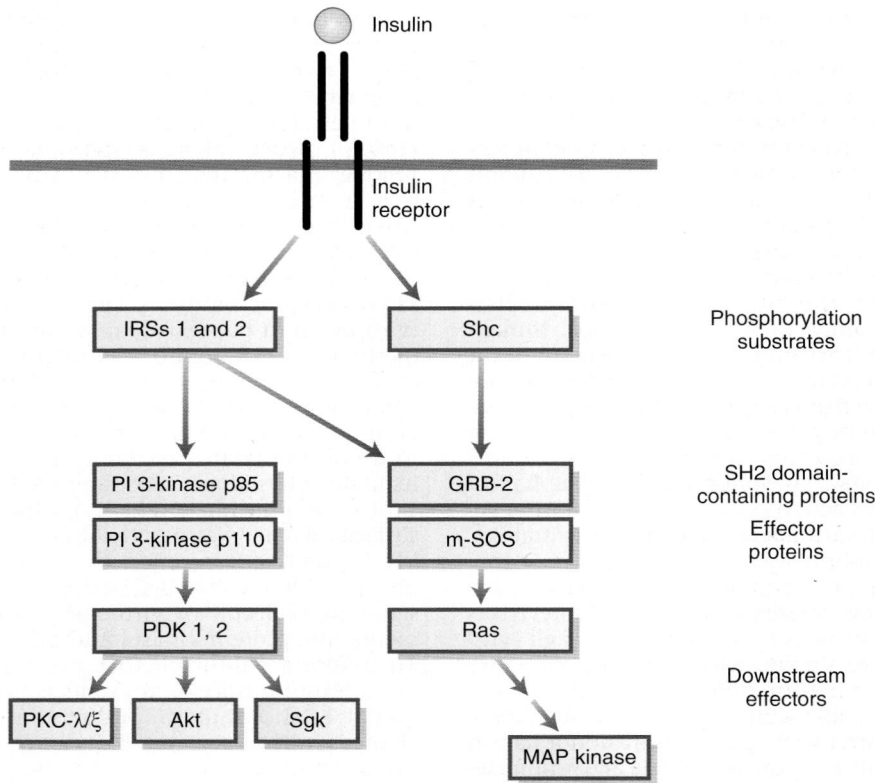

Figure 3-8 Simplified model of signaling pathways downstream from the insulin receptor. Insulin binds to the insulin receptor, activating the receptor tyrosine kinase to phosphorylate tyrosine residues on insulin receptor substrates (IRSs) including IRS1 and IRS2. The phosphotyrosine residues in the IRS molecules bind to SRC homology 2 (SH2) domains in molecules such as growth factor receptor–binding protein 2 (GRB-2) and the p85 regulatory subunit of phosphoinositide (PI) 3-kinase (PI3K). These SH2 domain–containing proteins initiate two distinct branches of the signaling pathway. Activation of PI3K leads to activation of phosphoinositide-dependent kinases (PDKs) 1 and 2, which activate multiple protein kinases, including Akt/protein kinase B, atypical protein kinase C (PKC) isoforms, and serum- and glucocorticoid-induced protein kinases (Sgk). GRB-2 interacts with m-SOS, a guanine nucleotide exchange factor that activates Ras. Activation of Ras triggers a cascade of protein kinases, leading to activation of mitogen-activated protein (MAP) kinase. Shc, SRC homology domain–containing protein. (From Spiegel AM, Carter-Su C, Taylor SI, et al. Mechanism of action of hormones that act at the cell surface. In: Melmed S, Polonsky KS, Larsen PR, et al, eds. *Williams Textbook of Endocrinology*, 12th ed. Philadelphia, PA: Elsevier; 2011:62-82.)

more slowly on serine/threonine residues, the latter by a number of cytoplasmic kinases including protein kinase C (PKC), c-Jun N-terminal kinase (Jnk), and pp70 S6 protein kinase. Serine/threonine phosphorylation of IRS provides a strong negative feedback signal as it blocks further tyrosine phosphorylation and in some cases induces degradation of the protein. There has been considerable interest in the idea that phosphorylation of IRS1/2 by some of these kinases describes the mechanism leading to defects in response to insulin that frequently accompany obesity, as increased serine/threonine phosphorylation of IRS is often associated with insulin-resistant states. However, this model has thus far not been supported by genetic experiments in mice, and it remains possible that such phosphorylation is a result of the hyperinsulinemia of insulin resistance rather than its cause.

There is some evidence that insulin receptor is capable of signaling through scaffolds other than the IRS proteins, though the physiologic significance of these pathways remains unclear. The insulin receptor recruits SRC homology 2 domain-containing protein (SHC) to a phosphotyrosine motif via SHC's PTB domain and phosphorylates SHC to generate a docking site for the SH2 domain of GRB2; this leads to activation of ras as described above.[55] GRB2-associated binder-1 (GAB-1) is an IRS protein in all but name and its phosphorylation by the insulin receptor results in recruitment of PI3K and generation of PIP_3.[56] GRB10, and most likely its close relative GRB14, is an SH2-containing protein that binds to the insulin receptor with high affinity.[57] However, unlike the IRS proteins, GRB10 binds to the three phosphorylated tyrosine residues in the activation loop and blocks the activity of the insulin receptor, inhibiting the insulin-dependent production of PIP_3.[58] GRB10 is stabilized via phosphorylation by mammalian (mechanistic) target of rapamycin complex 1 (mTORC1), itself activated downstream of insulin, providing another form of negative feedback.[59,60] Disruption of GRB10 in mice yields embryonic overgrowth, consistent with its being a negative regulator of IGF-1 signaling.[61] SH2B2, formerly known as APS, also binds directly to phosphorylated insulin receptor and acts a negative regulator.[58]

Receptor Serine/Threonine Protein Kinases

One of the more interesting variants on signaling by intracellular protein kinases is provided by a class of integral membrane receptors possessing intrinsic serine/threonine protein kinase activity. Ligands for these receptors are members of the transforming growth factor-β (TGF-β) family of first messengers. These 42 agonists encoded in the human genome can be classified into distinct groups typified by TGF-β itself, bone morphogenetic protein/growth and differentiation factor (GDF), activin, inhibin, nodal, myostatin, and antimüllerian hormone. Each is composed of a dimer of two peptides joined by hydrophobic interactions and often disulfide bonds. Inhibin was isolated as an activity produced by gonadal tissue that blocks the secretion of follicle-stimulating hormone (FSH) from the pituitary.[62] Like other members of the TGF-β family, it is composed of two chains, an α-subunit and one of two related β-subunits. The hormone activin is formed by the assembly of homodimers of the β-subunit; as its name suggests, activin promotes the release of FSH.[63] Activin was also originally identified as a product of the gonads but is now known to be secreted by many tissues and to function in an autocrine or paracrine manner as well. The first indication that the TGF-β family of ligands exerted its actions via membrane protein kinases arose from the cloning of a complementary DNA encoding the activin receptor and recognition of a canonical kinase domain.[64] Like all receptors for ligands in the TGF-β superfamily, the activin receptor (ActR) is composed of two transmembrane glycoproteins related in primary structure, the major difference being an insertion in the ActR-I cytoplasmic domain preceding the kinase domain of a conserved 30–amino acid sequence rich in glycine and serine (the GS domain), which binds the immunophilin, FKBP12. Activin interacts initially with ActR-II and brings the two receptors into proximity so that ActR-II can phosphorylate the GS domain of its partner. This alleviates steric hindrance of the ActR-I kinase catalytic site and releases FKBP12, the two changes working in concert to activate ActR-II and allow phosphorylation of target substrates.[65] Inhibin exerts its inhibitory action by recruiting the transmembrane glycoprotein betaglycan (also called the type III receptor) to form a stable complex with ActR-II, thus sequestering it and preventing activation of ActR-I.[66]

The major intracellular signaling mechanism utilized by all members of the TGF-β family involves SMAD proteins, which function as the major substrate for type I receptors, being phosphorylated at two serine residues at their C-terminal tail (Fig. 3-9). There are now recognized eight human genes coding for SMAD proteins. Five of the human SMAD proteins, termed the R-SMADS, contain the Ser-X-Ser phosphorylation site and thus serve as substrates for the type I receptors. The activin receptor phosphorylates SMAD3 (and possibly SMAD2), which then forms a trimer with the common mediator SMAD4 for transport to the nucleus.[67] It is likely that other SMAD isoforms contribute to activin regulation of gene expression in a tissue-specific manner in vivo. Upon import into the nucleus, SMAD proteins are modified at their so-called linker domains by a complex set of phosphorylations that serve both to enhance binding to transcriptional regulatory proteins and to target them for ubiquitin-dependent proteasomal degradation. SMAD proteins bind directly to DNA through a conserved N-terminal domain and interact with other transcription factors, in concert exerting control over a transcriptional network defined by the cell type and activating ligand.

One particularly interesting member of the TGF-β family is the hormone myostatin, formerly known as GDF-8. Myostatin is secreted by skeletal muscle and negatively regulates muscle growth through binding to ActR-IIB and the type I receptors ALK4 and ALK5, which phosphorylate SMAD2 and SMAD3.[68] A deficiency of myostatin is responsible for the "double-muscled" phenotype of Belgian Blue and Piedmontese cattle, and deletion of its gene in mice leads to massive muscle hypertrophy and hyperplasia.[69]

Signaling by Receptors That Associate With Enzymes

Another mode of signal transduction across the plasma membrane is provided by receptors with no intrinsic catalytic activity but with an association with a cytoplasmic,

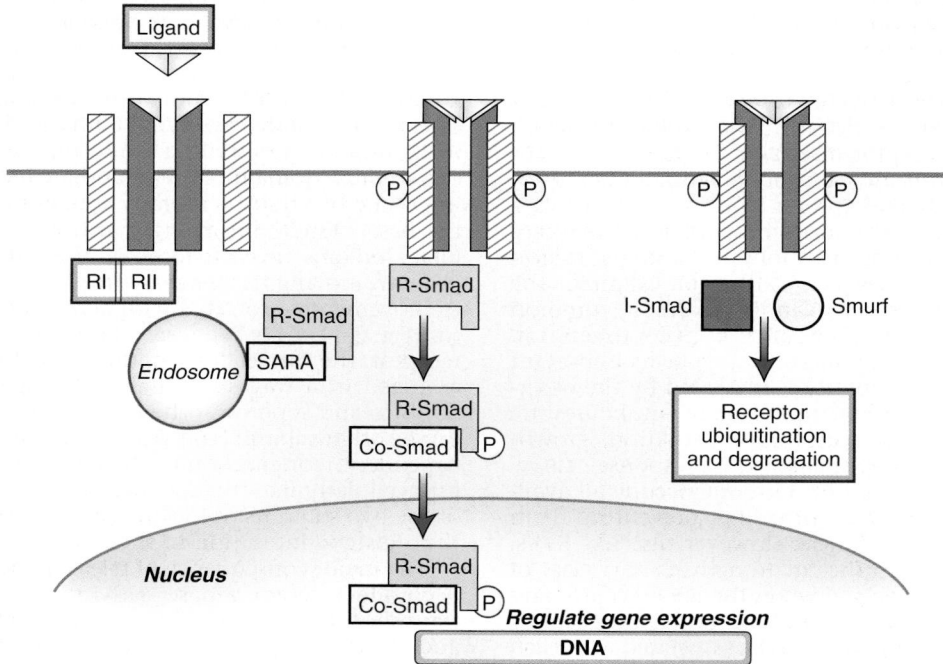

Figure 3-9 Mechanism of action for receptor serine kinases. Binding of dimeric ligand to the type II receptor (RII) subunit triggers assembly of the receptor into the heterotetrameric [(RI)₂(RII)₂] state. RII transphosphorylates the type I receptor (RI), thereby activating phosphorylation of the receptor-regulated SMAD (R-Smad) protein that is bound to the SMAD anchor for receptor activation (SARA) in endosomes. The phosphorylated R-Smad associates with a co-mediator SMAD (Co-Smad). Eventually, the R-Smad is translocated into the nucleus, where it binds to DNA, enabling it to regulate gene transcription. The inhibitory SMAD (I-Smad) also can bind to the activated receptor, promoting ubiquitination and degradation of the receptor. P, phosphorylation; Smurf, SMAD ubiquitination regulatory factor. (From Spiegel AM, Carter-Su C, Taylor SI, et al. Mechanism of action of hormones that act at the cell surface. In: Melmed S, Polonsky KS, Larsen PR, et al, eds. *Williams Textbook of Endocrinology*, 12th ed. Philadelphia, PA: Elsevier; 2011:62-82.)

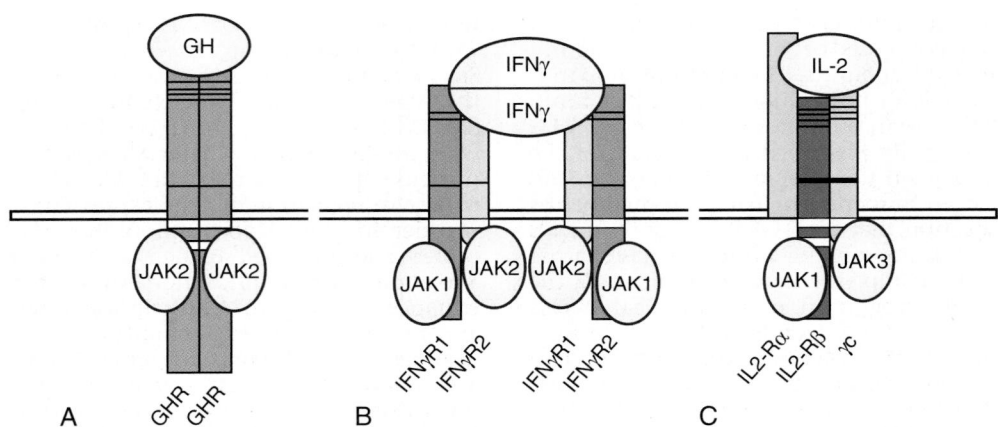

Figure 3-10 Cytokine receptors are composed of multiple subunits and bind to one or more members of the Janus kinase (JAK) family of tyrosine kinases. **A,** Growth hormone (GH), like prolactin and leptin, binds to growth hormone receptor (GHR) homodimers and activates JAK2. **B,** Interferon-γ (IFNγ) homodimers bind to their ligand-binding γR1 subunits. The γR2 subunits are then recruited, leading to activation of JAK1, which binds to the γR1 subunit, and JAK2, which binds to the γR2 subunit. Both subunits and both JAKs are necessary for responses to IFNγ. **C,** Interleukin 2 (IL-2) binds to receptors composed of three subunits: a γc subunit shared with receptors for IL-4, -7, -9, -15, and -21; an IL2-Rβ subunit shared with the IL-15 receptor; and a noncytokine receptor subunit, IL2-Rα. IL-2 activates JAK3, bound to the γc subunit, and JAK1, bound to IL2-Rβ. Extracellular regions of homology are indicated by the black lines and colored patterns. Intracellular regions of homology are indicated by the small white boxes. Identical subunits are indicated by identical colors. (From Spiegel AM, Carter-Su C, Taylor SI, et al. Mechanism of action of hormones that act at the cell surface. In: Melmed S, Polonsky KS, Larsen PR, et al, eds. *Williams Textbook of Endocrinology*, 12th ed. Philadelphia, PA: Elsevier; 2011:62-82.)

non–membrane-spanning tyrosine kinase. The best example of this is the family of class I cytokine receptors, which are type 1 transmembrane proteins with the N-terminus on the outside of the cell and a cytoplasmic C-terminus (Fig. 3-10). As for RTKs, dimerization appears important to activation of the receptor. In many cases, including the growth hormone receptor, a single ligand molecule containing two distinct recognition sequences interacts with different motifs on the outer portion of the receptor. The initial binding is to a high-affinity site 1 followed by a second lower affinity association with site 2 located on a second, associated monomer. Thus, binding has the effect of cross-linking the receptor. In addition, the two monomers that compose the activated receptor make significant contacts with each other, again in the exofacial domain close to where the receptor inserts in the membrane. For growth hormone, prolactin, thrombopoietin, and erythropoietin (EPO), the active receptor is a homodimer with two identical subunits. However, for some cytokines, the receptors consist of a ligand-specific monomer and a common transmembrane chain (see Fig. 3-10). For example, the interleukin 2 (IL-2) receptor family shares a common IL-2Rγc, and the IL-6 receptors all use glycoprotein 130 (GP130). As with RTKs, oligomerization appears important to activation of these receptors, as indicated by the observation that bivalent but not monovalent antibodies are capable of activating the receptors. In addition, growth hormone displays a bell-shaped dose-response curve, because high concentrations of hormone occupy all available receptors on the high-affinity sites, preventing them from forming productive dimers. However, also like RTKs, dimerization alone is insufficient to activate this class of receptors. This was recognized when the EPO receptor and subsequently the growth hormone and prolactin receptors were examined in situ and found to be associated with each other even in the basal state.[70]

Proximal to the membrane on the inside of the cell, the class I cytokine receptors have a conserved sequence often referred to as Box 1 that is critical to binding a protein tyrosine kinase of the JAK family. There are four members of this family: JAK1, JAK2, JAK3, and TYK2 (tyrosine kinase 2), with JAK3 largely restricted to cells of the hematopoietic

lineage.[71] For those receptors that function as homodimers, JAK2 is the predominant isoform involved in signaling. The JAK proteins associate with receptors in the absence of SH2 domains, but they do have a conserved domain structure unique to this family. The N-terminal contains a FERM domain (named for its presence in Band 4.1 protein, ezrin, radixin, and moesin) and most often is found in proteins that associate with the cytoskeleton, but in JAK this domain is responsible for binding to a cytoplasmic, juxtamembrane portion of the transmembrane receptor.[72] The carboxy half of JAK consists of two homologous regions in tandem, a kinase followed by a pseudokinase domain. The latter has many of the conserved sequences that define a protein kinase, but it also has mutations of amino acids that are essential for catalytic activity. Binding of growth hormone to its receptor results in a conformational change in the extracellular domain of the receptor, which leads to a crossing of the two transmembrane domains that are parallel in the basal state.[73] Surprisingly, this results in the intracellular domains in each receptor monomer that bind JAK proteins moving farther away from each other, in contrast to movements associated with activation of insulin receptor (Fig. 3-11). It is believed that in the non–ligand-bound receptor, the intracellular portions the two monomers are arranged in a way such that each pseudokinase domain binds to and suppresses the catalytic activity of the kinase on the other subunit, and vice versa. The growth hormone-dependent reorientation of the receptor induces a motion intracellularly like the opening of scissors, causing sliding of the two subunits of JAK in opposite directions, relieving the allosteric inhibition of the kinases.[74]

The major consequence of releasing the block to growth hormone receptor kinase activity is the JAK2-catalyzed transphosphorylation of the contralateral receptor subunit and its associated JAK2.[71] This serves to bind the SH2 domains of a number of signaling molecules, including PI3K, SHC, and PLC, thus recruiting them to the receptor and plasma membrane.[75] However, more important than these to growth hormone's physiologic actions are members of the signal transducers and activators of the transcription (STAT) family (Fig. 3-12). The growth hormone receptor binds a number of STAT isoforms, but STAT5 is

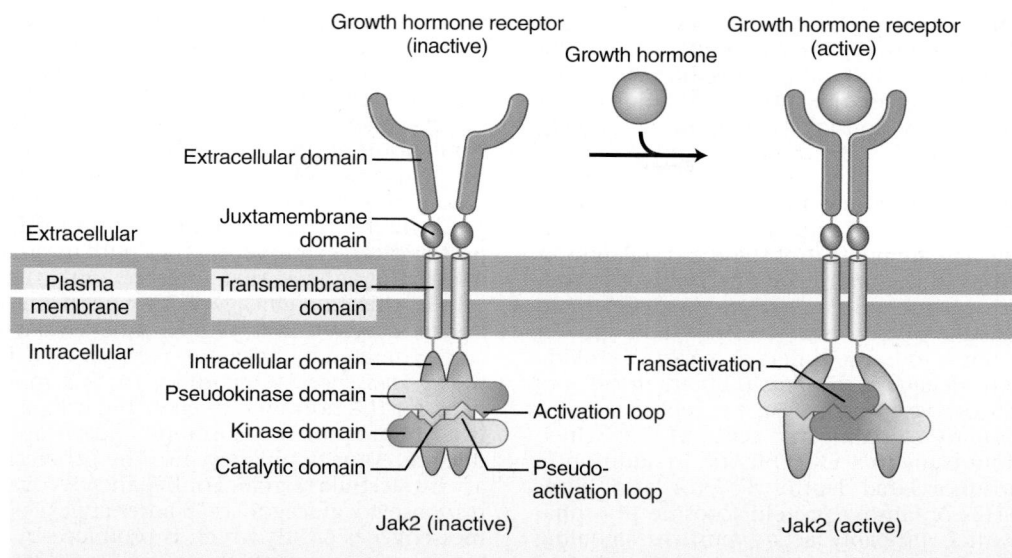

Figure 3-11 Scissor model for activation of the human growth hormone (hGH) receptor. In the basal state, the hGH receptor exists as an inactive dimer in which the two subunits are held together through weak interactions in the transmembrane membrane domain (TMD) and poised in the inactive state through electrostatic repulsion in the extracellular juxtamembrane domain (JMD) and pseudokinase inhibition in the associated Jak2 dimer *(left)*. Binding of hGH to the receptor *(right)* clamps the JMD such that it avoids the electrostatic repulsion and mechanically alters the TMD such that the intracellular domain is splayed outward. Splaying pulls on the Jak2 molecules to align their kinase domains. This triggers a wave of phosphorylation events including the STAT proteins critical to receptor signaling. (Redrawn from Wells JA, Kossiakoff AA. New tricks for an old dimer. *Science.* 2014;344:703.)

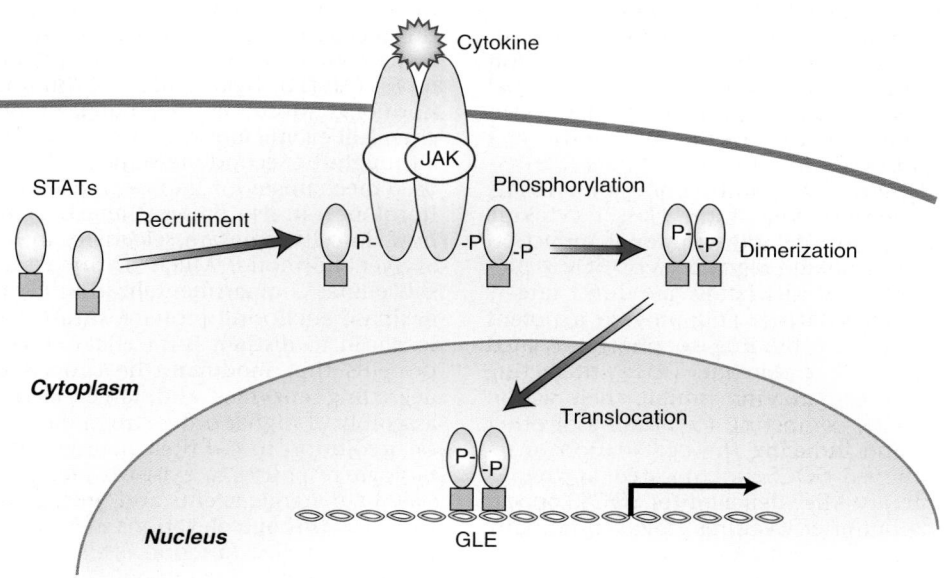

Figure 3-12 Cytokines activate signal transducers and activators of transcription (STATs). STAT proteins are latent cytoplasmic transcription factors. STATs bind through SRC homology 2 (SH2) domains to one or more phosphorylated tyrosines (P) in activated receptor–Janus kinase (JAK) complexes. Once bound, STATs themselves are tyrosyl phosphorylated, presumably by the receptor-associated JAKs. STATs then dissociate from the receptor-JAK complex, homodimerize or heterodimerize with other STAT proteins, move to the nucleus, and bind to gamma-activated sequence-like elements (GLEs) in the promoters of cytokine-responsive genes. P, phosphorylation. (Adapted from J. Herrington, used with permission.)

most critical to its physiologic actions. There are seven STAT isoforms with shared domain structure. The N-terminus is composed of four helical coils that function in binding to other proteins, followed by a DNA-binding domain (DBD).[76] The carboxy half of the proteins consists of a linker region, a SH2 domain, and a transcriptional transactivation domain. Among the tyrosine residues in

the growth hormone receptor that get phosphorylated in response to ligand binding, several serve as docking sites for STAT5. Once recruited to the receptor, STAT5 is itself phosphorylated, resulting in dimerization with each STAT5 molecule binding to its partner's SH2 domain. At the same time, STAT5 dissociates from the receptor and translocates into the nucleus, where it can regulate gene transcription.

In addition to this basic pathway, there are numerous other layers of regulation. Serine/threonine protein kinases such as MAPK and PKC also phosphorylate STAT proteins, and in some cases this phosphorylation is required for maximal transcriptional activation; employing a different mechanism, SH2B1 binds to and enhances JAK2 activity.[75,77]

Another important hormone that uses the JAK/STAT signaling pathway is leptin. Leptin is secreted by adipocytes to act on the arcuate nucleus of the hypothalamus as well as other regions in the brain to suppress appetite and, in rodents, increase metabolic rate. Humans deficient in leptin display massive obesity early in life.[78] Like growth hormone, leptin binds to homodimers of a class I cytokine receptor called the *long-form receptor* (LRb in mice) and activates JAK2.[79] However, in contrast, the leptin receptor recruits as its primary signaling molecule STAT3, which binds to phosphotyrosine in a YXXQ motif, in addition to STAT5. The phosphorylated leptin receptor also binds GRB2 and the SH2-containing protein tyrosine phosphatase 2 (SHP2), which probably acts a positive signaling module.[80] On the other hand, the tyrosine phosphatase PTP-1B dephosphorylates the receptor and inhibits leptin action, and thus its deletion in mouse brain leads to obesity and insulin resistance.[81] JAK2 also phosphorylates IRS1, thereby engaging the PI3K pathway. The roles of the different signaling pathways activated downstream of leptin and JAK2 has been investigated using mice in which specific tyrosine residues in the receptor have been mutated. Replacement of tyrosine 1138 by serine completely blocks recruitment of STAT3, generating mice similar in their degree of obesity to those with leptin receptor knockout, showing that STAT3 signaling is critical to the regulation of appetite and energy metabolism.[82] However, normal reproduction is largely preserved, indicating that leptin modulates at least some neuroendocrine functions via a pathway independent of STAT3.

In addition to dephosphorylation of phosphotyrosine as described earlier, termination of the class I cytokine signal is also promoted by the transcriptional induction of the suppressors of cytokine signaling, or SOCS proteins. The eight members of this family are direct targets of the STAT transcription factors and provide a potent negative feedback signal by binding to phosphorylated tyrosines via the SOCS SH2 domain. Once interacting with the receptors, SOCS proteins inhibit their action by reducing JAK activity, competing for binding of other signaling molecules and inducing the degradation of receptor via the conserved SOCS box located at the C-terminus of the protein.[83] Mice deficient for SOCS2 appear normal when young but after weaning grow substantially larger that their wild-type littermates, consistent with enhanced growth hormone signaling due to loss of negative feedback.[84]

COUPLING OF CELL SURFACE RECEPTORS TO INTRACELLULAR SIGNALING

Second Messengers

In order for the many hormones that bind exclusively to the outer surface of cells to carry out their actions, there must be some means of translating the extracellular signal into an intracellular response. The first example of a transduction system that was understood in some detail derived from investigating one of the key features of the fight-or-flight response, the mobilization of stored carbohydrate in the liver. The physiologic response to stress requires a supply of readily consumable energy, best provided in the form of blood glucose, which is stored as the polysaccharide glycogen at the highest levels in the liver. β-Adrenergic stimulation of hepatocytes by epinephrine leads rapidly to the hydrolysis of glycogen and the release of free sugar; glucagon also stimulates the breakdown of hepatic glycogen. The mechanism used to transmit this response is the prototypical example of a second messenger system, in which the agonist that interacts with the outside of the cell, in this case glucagon or epinephrine, is considered a *first messenger*, and a soluble, intracellular signaling molecule generated by hormone-receptor association is called a *second messenger*.[85] According to this model, there is no need for the hormone to enter the cell; all that is required is a receptor for the hormone and an apparatus to transduce receptor occupancy into the generation of a secondary intracellular signal. For hepatic glycogen breakdown in response to glucagon or β-adrenergic agents, the second messenger is cAMP, which is produced by a plasma membrane enzyme, adenylyl cyclase, from ATP (Fig. 3-13). Adenylyl cyclase is a direct target of G_s, which becomes GTP-loaded and active in response to receptor occupancy. cAMP is degraded to AMP and phosphate by a specific PDE, and the balance between these two activities determines the levels of the cyclic nucleotide.

The scope and diversity of hormones and other extracellular signals that activate adenylyl cyclase and increase the level of intracellular cAMP are remarkably extensive. Included in the long list of hormones that signal through this mechanism are β-adrenergic agents, glycoprotein hormones such as TSH, glucagon, adrenocorticotropic hormone (ACTH), hypothalamic hormones, and antidiuretic hormone. Moreover, the range of physiologic and biochemical events modulated by cAMP is equally vast. Thus, although the second messenger cAMP defines a commonly used mechanism for transducing signals from extracellular hormones, it also presents another problem in signaling: how do cells maintain selectivity in how they respond to a given hormone? Much of this is accomplished by the subcellular compartmentalization of signaling complexes. A-kinase anchoring proteins (AKAPs), which are scaffolds localized to distinct intracellular sites, bind a number of proteins that modulate the actions of cAMP, including degrading enzymes and target kinases.[86] The regulated assembly of higher order structures confers a spatiotemporal resolution to cAMP signaling that can allow multiple biologic responses to exist within the same cell. For example, β-adrenergic agents and prostaglandin E_1 both act on the heart through elevations in cAMP, but each regulates a different cardiac function. This is accomplished through stimulation of distinct populations of cAMP target kinases, such that β-adrenergic agents are more potent than prostaglandins in their effects on the particulate fractions of the heart cell.[87] It is likely that AKAPs confer this specificity to the cardiomyocyte.

Although hormones generally use adenylyl cyclase as the means for modulating cAMP level within the cell, the PDEs also provide an additional site of regulation.[88] The cyclic nucleotide PDEs are a large and complex family of enzymes, whose diversity in both tissue and subcellular localization has made them favorite targets for the development of therapeutics. Caffeine and theophylline were two of the first drugs recognized to be inhibitors of PDE, but more recently selective inhibitors of PDE5, an enzyme that degrades cyclic guanosine monophosphate (cGMP), have been widely used for the treatment of erectile dysfunction. In addition, PDE inhibitors are either currently

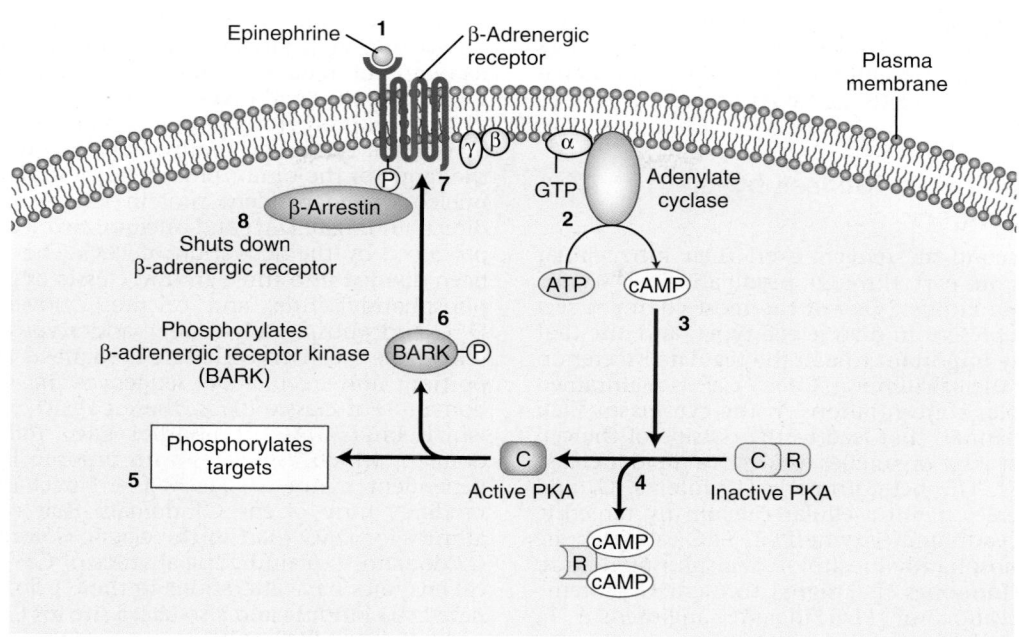

Figure 3-13 Adenylate cyclase, protein kinase A (PKA), and β-adrenergic receptor kinase (BARK) activation by epinephrine. Step 1: Upon binding of epinephrine to the β-adrenergic receptor, G_s is activated. Step 2: $G_s\alpha$ binds to and stimulates adenylate cyclase. Step 3: Adenylate cyclase catalyzes the conversion of ATP to cAMP. Step 4: cAMP binds to the regulatory subunit (R) of PKA, releasing free catalytic subunit (C), which is active. Step 5: C phosphorylates a number of intracellular substrates in a manner determined by its location in the cell. Step 6: C phosphorylates serine and threonine residues on BARK. Step 7: BARK, itself a serine/threonine kinase, phosphorylates serine and threonine residues on the β-adrenergic receptor. Step 8: β-Arrestin binds to the phosphorylated receptor, which blocks further activation of G_s. β-Arrestin also initiates signaling cascades, which are not shown.

being used or are in development for the treatment of a wide variety of diseases, including asthma, neurologic diseases, and pulmonary hypertension.

Many additional second messengers have been identified since the discovery of cAMP. These include cGMP, calcium, inositol polyphosphates, DAG, and nitric oxide.

Downstream Signaling by Cyclic Adenosine Monophosphate

The study of glycogen metabolism in liver and muscle provided the initial conceptual framework for understanding signal transduction by protein phosphorylation, which stands as one of the most used regulatory mechanisms in human biology. The state of a phosphoprotein is regulated dynamically, being a product of phosphorylation and dephosphorylation by protein kinases and phosphatases, respectively. In most cases, the turnover of the phosphate is rapid, allowing regulation by either the kinase or phosphatase, or in many instances both coordinately. Numerous endocrine signals exert control over intracellular metabolism, growth, and other function via modulation of protein kinase activity. Originally, protein kinases were found to phosphorylate proteins on serine and threonine residues, but, as described earlier, tyrosine phosphorylation has emerged as another mode of signaling.

A common mode of signaling initiated by second messengers is via activation of intracellular protein kinases arranged in linear cascades. Examples of such pathways include those involving MAPK and the regulation of glycogen breakdown by protein kinase A. The advantage of such series of kinases has been postulated to be signal amplification. cAMP binds to the heterotetrameric protein kinase A (PKA) via two regulatory subunits, which upon associating with cyclic nucleotide dissociate from two catalytic subunits. A domain in the regulatory subunit resem-

bles a PKA phosphorylation sequence but with the critical serine replaced by an alanine, which lacks the hydroxyl group required for transfer of the gamma phosphate from ATP. When assembled into a heterotetramer of two regulatory subunits and two catalytic subunits, this pseudosubstrate on the regulatory subunit interacts with the catalytic site of the catalytic subunit, preventing it from phosphorylating target proteins.[89] Displacement or dissociation of intramolecular pseudosubstrate or substrate sites represents a recurrent mechanism used for the activation of protein kinases, including PKC and myosin light chain kinase. PKA phosphorylates and activates glycogen phosphorylase kinase, which in turn phosphorylates and activates glycogen phosphorylase. In muscle, phosphorylase kinase is also stimulated by calcium, which is released from the sarcoplasmic reticulum during electrical stimulation and contraction.

In addition to glycogen metabolism, PKA mediates the effects of a number of hormones in various tissues, including the positive inotropic and chronotropic effects of epinephrine on the heart, the trophic effects of the anterior pituitary hormones TSH and ACTH, and the effects of antidiuretic hormone on the permeability of the renal collecting duct to water. PKA also translocates into the nucleus to regulate gene transcription.[90] The best studied nuclear target of PKA is the cAMP-response element–binding protein (CREB), though it is still not clear how many of the physiologic actions of cAMP require this transcription factor to be phosphorylated. PKA also phosphorylates a number of coregulatory proteins, which also contribute to transcriptional outputs.

Importantly, there also exist actions of cAMP that are independent of PKA. One of these is the direct regulation of ion channels but more recently discovered is the cAMP target exchange protein activated by cAMP, or EPAC, which functions as a guanine nucleotide exchange factor for the small GTP-binding protein Rap1.[91] Regulation of insulin secretion from pancreatic beta cells by glucagon-like peptide-1 (GLP-1) and stabilization of the endothelial barrier by β-adrenergic agents are two processes thought to be mediated by EPAC.

Regulation of Protein Kinases by Second Messengers

A number of second messengers exert their intracellular actions at least in part through modulation of serine/ threonine protein kinases. One of the most common second messengers present in diverse cell types, and one that has a particularly important role in the regulated secretion of hormones, is the calcium ion, Ca^{2+}.[92] Ca^{2+} is maintained at low micromolar concentrations in the cytoplasm such that opening channels that lead to the outside of the cell or intracellular storage organelles results in a rapid increase in cytosolic Ca^{2+}. The heterotrimeric G proteins, G_q and G_{11}, cause increases in intracellular calcium by targeting the membrane-associated enzyme PLC. PLC catalyzes the hydrolysis of phosphatidylinositol 4′,5′-bisphosphate into DAG and IP_3. Hormones that signal through G protein–dependent activation of PLC include angiotensin II, α-adrenergic catecholamines, growth hormone–releasing hormone, and vasopressin. IP_3 binds to a receptor located on the cytoplasmic face of the endoplasmic reticulum, leading to the release of stored Ca^{2+}. Ca^{2+} also interacts with the IP_3 receptor, further stimulating calcium discharge from the endoplasmic reticulum and providing a strong positive feedback loop. Another source of cytoplasmic Ca^{2+} is entry through receptor-operated channels, such as those activated by noradrenaline, endothelin, or histamine via heterotrimeric G proteins.

Ca^{2+} transmits its signal via a number of effectors including protein kinases, in most cases through the intermediary binding protein, calmodulin, or its relative, troponin C. Calmodulin is a small, acidic protein that contains four copies of a canonical calcium-binding motif.[93] Calmodulin associates with and regulates in a Ca^{2+}-dependent manner glycogen phosphorylase kinase, but also myosin light chain kinase and members of the family of calcium/ calmodulin-dependent kinases. In addition to protein kinases, other calcium/calmodulin-dependent enzymes include the serine/threonine protein phosphatase, calcineurin, some adenylate cyclase and PDE isoforms, and nitric oxide

synthase. Calcium interacts directly and independently of calmodulin with targets such as the protease calpain, the regulator of neurotransmitter and hormone exocytosis, synaptotagmin, and cytoskeletal proteins.

An important group of protein kinases directly activated by calcium is the PKC family. PKC, originally identified at the target of the tumor promoter, phorbol ester, is a cyclic nucleotide-independent protein kinase regulated by the direct binding of DAG and calcium, two second messengers produced by the activation of PLC. The PKC family has been divided into three groups: classic (regulated by DAG, phosphatidylserine, and calcium), novel (regulated by DAG and phosphatidylserine), and atypical. All PKC proteins have a conserved kinase domain in their C-terminal portion and regulatory sequences in the N-terminal domain. For classic PKCs, these consist of a C1 domain, which binds DAG or phorbol ester, followed by a C2 domain, which associates with anionic lipids in a Ca^{2+}-dependent manner[94] (Fig. 3-14). Novel isoforms have a modified form of the C1 domain that confers a higher affinity for DAG than in the classic isoforms but lack the C2 domain, explaining the absence of Ca^{2+} binding. Atypical enzymes have alterations in the C1 domain that eliminate DAG binding and also lack a site for Ca^{2+} binding. The regulation of PKC isoforms is complex, involving such covalent modifications as phosphorylation and proteolysis, as well as interaction with lipids and hydrophilic molecules other than those traditionally associated with activation of classic PKC.[95]

Regulation of Protein Kinases by PI3K

A family of related proteins catalyzes generation of phosphoinositides phosphorylated on the 3′ position of the inositol ring.[96] All class I PI3K proteins comprise a catalytic protein associated with a regulatory subunit that uses $PI4,5P_2$ as a preferred substrate; these isoforms are most important to signaling by RTK, GPCRs, and tyrosine kinase oncogenes. Class II PI3K phosphorylates PI and PI4P in vivo and lacks stable regulatory subunits but probably associates with other proteins as modulating factors. They have been implicated as mediating a diverse set of actions, but the downstream targets are largely unknown. Class III PI3K, which has one catalytic member also known as vacuolar protein sorting 34 (Vps34), binds tightly to the regulatory protein Vps15, uses exclusively PI as a substrate, and

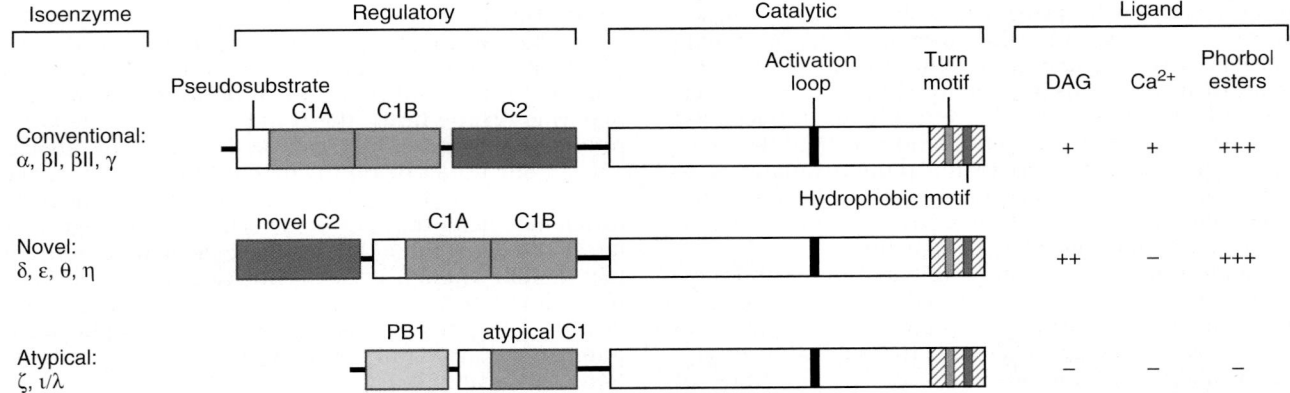

Figure 3-14 Domain structure and ligands of protein kinase C (PKC). The PKC family can be divided into three classes: the conventional, or classic, PKCs (cPKCs); the novel PKCs (nPKCs); and the atypical PKCs (aPKCs). The C1 domains bind diacylglycerol (DAG) or phorbol ester; the C2 domain binds calcium. A novel C2 domain in nPKCs does not bind calcium but mediates protein-protein interactions. Similarly, a PB1 domain in aPKCs is involved in protein-protein interactions. The aPKCs possess only one C1 domain and thus do not bind diacylglycerol. The conserved pseudosubstrate motif is represented by the white boxes in the regulatory domain. The activation loop and the turn and hydrophobic motifs are sites of regulatory phosphorylation.

is involved primarily in membrane protein trafficking such as relates to endocytosis and phagocytosis, but has been strongly implicated in the regulation of autophagy. Class IA PI3Ks are defined by their association with regulatory subunits containing SH2 domains, which target them to activated RTKs. The heterotrimeric G protein subunit pair $G_{\beta\gamma}$, when free, activates those class I PI3Ks containing regulatory subunits not bearing SH2 domains.

Class IA PI3K is most important to the actions of hormones, particularly insulin and IGF-1.[97] Activation of either receptor leads to phosphorylation of IRS1 or IRS2 at sites specialized for docking with SH2 domains in the p85 regulatory subunit associated with the p110α catalytic subunit of PI3K. The bound PI3K catalyzes the production of PIP_3 and possibly $PI3,4P_2$, which serve to recruit additional proteins including protein kinases to the membrane by binding their PH domains, named after the homologous sequences in pleckstrin, the major PKC substrate in platelets.[98] The PH domain is a conserved protein-lipid interaction module similar in structure to the PTB domain but designed to bind primarily to phosphoinositides. The serine/threonine protein kinase Akt, also named *protein kinase B* because of its structural similarities to PKA and PKC, contains an N-terminal PH domain that preferentially binds to PIP_3 and $PI3,4P_2$.[99] When insulin acts upon a target cell, the PH domain of Akt associates with the PIP3 generated on the cytoplasmic face of the plasma membrane, serving two purposes: to recruit Akt to the membrane and to remove the PH domain from its steric hindrance of Akt's phosphorylation sites and catalytic domain. Also at the plasma membrane via its own PH domain is the enzyme 3-phosphoinositide-dependent protein kinase (PDK1), which phosphorylates Akt on a threonine in its activation loop (Fig. 3-15). mTORC2 also phosphorylates Akt but on a serine in its C-terminus, and the two phosphorylation events confer full activity to Akt. mTORC2 appears to be regulated by insulin, but the mechanism is unknown.

Akt is essential to many of the metabolic actions of insulin and growth affects of IGF-1.[100,101] There are three Akt isoforms encoded by separate genes. Akt1 is the most widely expressed isoform and seems to be critical to the regulation of growth, whereas Akt2 is enriched in insulin target tissues and thus is more important to the control of metabolism. Akt3 is expressed primarily in the brain, where it controls growth.[102] Some downstream targets of Akt are known, though many remain to be elucidated. Indirect activation of mTORC1 by Akt and suppression of forkhead box (FOX)O-driven transcription are two of the critical targets for promoting organ growth, the Akt/mTORC1 pathway being particularly engaged in the regulation of cell size.[103] Members of the Rab GTPase-activating protein family, TBCD4 (also known as AS160) in fat cells and TBC1D1 in both muscle and fat, are phosphorylated and inhibited by Akt, contributing to the activation of glucose transport.[104]

Regulation of Protein Kinases by RAS

Routes to activation of RAS by GRB-SOS, in addition to RTKs, include GPCRs acting through β-arrestin.[105] GTP-bound RAS recruits to the plasma membrane several effectors including the serine/threonine kinase RAF, which is activated by dimerization and a series of phosphorylation/dephosphorylation events.[106] RAF then phosphorylates MAPK/ERK kinase (MEK1), a tyrosine and serine/threonine-dual specificity protein kinase, initiating a protein kinase cascade centered on extracellular signal-regulated kinases 1 and 2 (ERK1/2). This represents one of four MAPK cascades, the others involving c-Jun N-terminal kinase (Jnk), the 38-kDa stress-activated kinases (p38), and ERK5. Specificity for MAPKs is conferred by scaffold proteins that bind most or all members of a given pathway, ensuring that each member phosphorylates only its appropriate target kinase.[107] Gonadotropin-releasing hormone, PTH, growth hormone, angiotensin, and gastrin are just a few of the many hormones believed to signal through regulation of MAPKs.

DISEASE CAUSED BY DEFECTIVE CELL SURFACE RECEPTORS

Numerous diseases develop as a result of dysfunctional binding to or signaling by hormone receptors. These *hormone resistance syndromes* invariably have the hallmark of mimicking the phenotype of the hormone-deficient state but presenting with high levels of biologically active

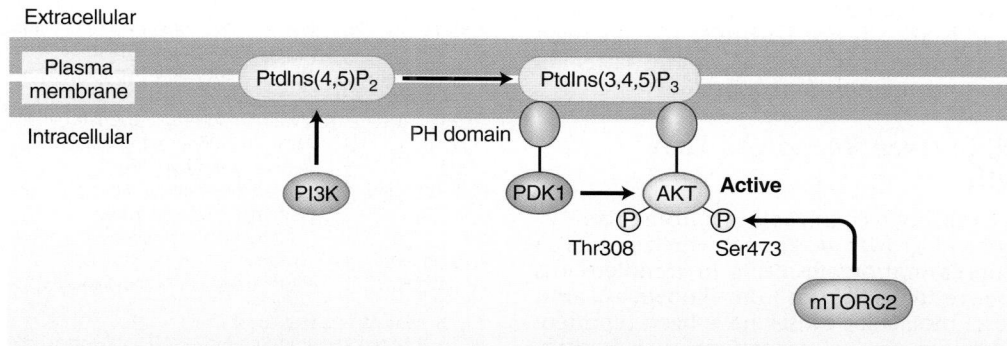

Figure 3-15 Mechanism of AKT activation. When phosphatidylinositol-3,4,5-trisphosphate (PtdIns(3,4,5)P_3) levels are low in the plasma membrane, AKT is in an inactive conformation in the cytoplasm and cannot be phosphorylated by the upstream activating 3-phosphoinositide-dependent protein kinase 1 (PDK1) (not shown). PtdIns(3,4,5)P_3 levels increase in the plasma membrane following the insulin-dependent recruitment to IRS1 and 2 of phosphoinositide 3-kinase (PI3K), which phosphorylates phosphatidylinositol-4,5-bisphosphate (PtdIns(4,5)P_2). AKT binds PIP$_3$ through its pleckstrin homology (PH) domain and induces a conformational change within the AKT kinase domain, allowing PDK1 to phosphorylate the critical residue in the activation loop required for AKT kinase activity, threonine 308 (Thr308). Mammalian target of rapamycin complex 2 (mTORC2) also phosphorylates AKT at the carboxy-terminal serine 473 (Ser473) site to fully activate its kinase activity. PDK1 has a PH domain that can bind PtdIns(3,4,5)P_3 but this interaction is not essential for PDK1 catalytic activity. (Redrawn from Finlay D, Cantrell DA. Metabolism, migration and memory in cytotoxic T cells. *Nat Rev Immunol.* 2011;11:109.)

hormone in the circulation and being unaffected by hormone administration.

Insulin-Resistance Syndromes

The best studied inherited disease of hormone resistance is that caused by mutations in the insulin receptor. In addition to hyperinsulinism and the expected abnormalities in metabolism, patients with severe insulin resistance invariably also display acanthosis nigricans (hyperpigmentation primarily in the skin folds) and often hyperandrogenism.[108] Beyond that, there is a range of syndromes that correlate with the degree of insulin signaling impairment. The strongest loss-of-function mutations result in leprechaunism, in which there are severe developmental defects presenting at birth. The mechanisms by which insulin receptor gene mutations occur are far-reaching, covering all aspects of the signal transduction system. They include a decrease in the number of receptors, in most but not all cases accompanied by a decrease in the mRNA, and mutations adversely affecting hormone binding or the function of the kinase domain.[108] In contrast to insulin resistance caused by mutations in the receptor gene, sometimes referred to as type A insulin resistance, type B resistance differs in presenting at middle age, often with signs of autoimmunity such as vitiligo, alopecia, and arthritis.[109] This syndrome is defined by the presence of antibodies directed against the insulin receptor; the levels of antibody correlate with the severity of the disease.

In many ways, the use of insulin resistance to describe the common syndrome associated with obesity or polycystic ovary syndrome (PCOS) is a misnomer. The term *resistance* was originally coined to describe the situation of hyperglycemia in the face of elevated concentrations of insulin in the blood.[110,111] However, the recognition that insulin has numerous physiologic actions in addition to those on carbohydrate metabolism has led to ambiguity in nomenclature. On the one hand, the term *insulin resistance* is often applied to abnormalities in insulin signaling to all outputs from the receptor; this typically occurs with mutations of the insulin receptor. However, in the insulin resistance of obesity or PCOS, some actions of insulin are preserved. This is demonstrated nicely by a comparison of the phenotype of individuals with type 2 diabetes mellitus to those with genetically encoded partial defects in insulin receptor function.[112] Both groups share hyperglycemia, but only those with type A insulin resistance display defects in the regulation of hepatic lipid metabolism by insulin. Thus, the metabolic phenotype associated with type A inherited insulin resistance is not faithfully phenocopied by the insulin resistance of obesity, as in the latter all actions of the hormone are not impeded.

Defects in Cell Surface Receptors That Control Growth

One of the most clinically recognizable syndromes is resistance to the actions of growth hormone, which results in shortness of stature. Mutations resulting in complete loss of growth hormone result in the syndrome known as Laron dwarfism.[113] Diverse molecular causes have been reported, including large deletions as well as missense, frameshift, and splicing mutations. Similar syndromes of decreased growth can also result from deficiency in IGF-1 or defects in IGF-1 signaling. Recently, a syndrome has been described in which mutations in the *PIK3R1* gene, which encodes the p85alpha regulatory subunit of class I PI3K, lead to the SHORT syndrome, which includes dysmorphic facial features and defects in growth (short stature, hyperextensibil-

ity, ocular depression, Rieger anomaly, and teething delay).[114] As might be expected by the similarities in insulin and IGF-1 signaling, individuals with SHORT syndrome also display lipodystrophy and insulin resistance.[115]

Diseases Caused by Mutations in GPCRs and G Proteins

A number of endocrine diseases can be attributed to mutations in the GPCR-G protein signaling system.[116,117] For GPCRs, many mutations are associated with some degree of loss of function and are inherited in a recessive manner (Table 3-3). Some examples include hypothyroidism from mutations in the thyrotropin-releasing hormone or TSH receptor, glucocorticoid deficiency from mutations in the melanocortin 2 receptor, extreme obesity from dysfunction of melanocortin 4 receptor, and infertility due to mutations in the receptor for luteinizing hormone or FSH. Gain-of-function mutations include those in the TSH receptor causing hyperthyroidism, in the α_2-adrenergic receptor leading to diabetes mellitus, and in the calcium-sensing receptor resulting in hypoparathyroidism. Somatic activating mutations have been reported in the luteinizing hormone and TSH receptors.[116] Only two heterotrimeric G proteins are known to have mutations that cause human disease, and in both cases they affect the α-subunit. Mutation of the transducin gene is associated with night blindness. Dominant, activating mutations of $G\alpha_s$ cause pituitary adenomas, most often secreting growth hormone, and more rarely tumors of the thyroid, parathyroid, and adrenal glands.[117] Patients who inherit a loss of a functional allele in $G\alpha_s$ develop Albright hereditary osteodystrophy (AHO); those who inherit the mutant allele from their mothers also have pseudohypoparathyroidism type 1a in addition to AHO. This is due to imprinting of the $G\alpha_s$ gene, such that it is expressed preferentially from the maternal allele in a number of hormone target tissues but biallelically in most cell types.

TABLE 3-3

Diseases Caused by G Protein–Coupled Receptor Loss-of-Function Mutations

Receptor	Disease	Inheritance
V$_2$ vasopressin	Nephrogenic diabetes insipidus	X-linked
ACTH	Familial ACTH resistance	AR
GHRH	Familial GH deficiency	AR
GnRH	Hypogonadotropic hypogonadism	AR
GPR54	Hypogonadotropic hypogonadism	AR
Prokineticin receptor 2	Hypogonadotropic hypogonadism	AD*
FSH	Hypergonadotropic ovarian dysgenesis	AR
LH	Male pseudohermaphroditism	AR
TSH	Familial hypothyroidism	AR
Ca^{2+} sensing	Familial hypocalciuric hypercalcemia	AD
	Neonatal severe primary hyperparathyroidism	AR
Melanocortin 4	Obesity	AR
PTH/PTHrP	Blomstrand chondrodysplasia	AR

*With incomplete penetrance.
ACTH, adrenocorticotropic hormone; AD, autosomal dominant; AR, autosomal recessive; FSH, follicle-stimulating hormone; GH, growth hormone; GHRH, growth hormone–releasing hormone; GnRH, gonadotropin-releasing hormone; GPR54, orphan G protein–coupled receptor 54; LH, luteinizing hormone; PTH, parathyroid hormone; PTHrP, parathyroid hormone–related protein; TSH, thyroid-stimulating hormone.
From Spiegel AM, Carter-Su C, Taylor SI, et al. Mechanism of action of hormones that act at the cell surface. In: Melmed S, Polonsky KS, Larsen PR, et al, eds. *Williams Textbook of Endocrinology*, 12th ed. Philadelphia, PA: Elsevier; 2011:62-82.

LIGANDS THAT ACT THROUGH NUCLEAR RECEPTORS

Many signaling molecules share with thyroid and steroid hormones the ability to function in the nucleus to convey intercellular and environmental signals. Not all of these molecules are produced in glandular tissues. Although some signaling molecules, such as classic endocrine hormones, arrive at target tissues through the bloodstream, others have paracrine functions (i.e., acting on adjacent cells) or autocrine functions (i.e., acting on the cell of origin).

In addition to the classic steroid and thyroid hormones, lipophilic signaling molecules that use nuclear receptors include derivatives of vitamins A and D, endogenous metabolites such as oxysterols and bile acids, and non-natural chemicals encountered in the environment (i.e., xenobiotics). These molecules are referred to as *nuclear receptor ligands*. The nuclear receptors for all of these signaling molecules are structurally related and are collectively referred to as the *nuclear receptor superfamily*. The study of these receptors is a rapidly evolving field, and more detailed information can be obtained by visiting the Nuclear Receptor Signaling Atlas website.[118,119]

General Features of Nuclear Receptor Ligands

Unlike polypeptide hormones that function through cell surface receptors, no ligands for nuclear receptors are directly encoded in the genome. All nuclear receptor ligands are small (molecular mass <1000 Da) and lipophilic, enabling them to enter cells by passive diffusion, although in some cases a membrane transport protein is involved. For example, several active and specific thyroid hormone transporters have been identified, including monocarboxylate transporter 8 (MCT8), MCT10, and organic anion transporting polypeptide 1C1 (OATP1C1).[120]

In addition, all naturally occurring nuclear receptor ligands are derived from dietary, environmental, or metabolic precursors. In this sense, the function of these ligands and their receptors is to translate cues from the external and internal environments into changes in gene expression. Their critical role in maintaining homeostasis in multicellular organisms is highlighted by the fact that nuclear receptors are found in all vertebrates and insects but not in single-cell organisms such as yeast.[121]

Because nuclear receptor ligands are lipophilic, most are readily absorbed from the gastrointestinal tract. This makes nuclear receptors excellent targets for pharmaceutical interventions. In addition to natural ligands, many drugs in clinical use target nuclear receptors, ranging from those used to treat specific hormone deficiencies to those used to treat common multigenic conditions such as inflammation, cancer, and type 2 diabetes.

Subclasses of Nuclear Receptor Ligands

One classification of nuclear receptor ligands is outlined in Table 3-4 and is described in the following paragraphs.

Classic Hormones

The classic hormones that use nuclear receptors for signaling are thyroid hormone and steroid hormones. Steroid hormones include cortisol, aldosterone, estradiol, progesterone, and testosterone. In some cases (e.g., thyroid hormone receptor α and β genes [*THRA* and *THRB*],

TABLE 3-4	
Nuclear Receptor Ligands and Their Receptors	
Ligand	**Receptor**
Classic Hormones	
Thyroid hormone	Thyroid hormone receptor (TR), subtypes α, β
Estrogen	Estrogen receptor (ER), subtypes α, β
Testosterone	Androgen receptor (AR)
Progesterone	Progesterone receptor (PR)
Aldosterone	Mineralocorticoid receptor (MR)
Cortisol	Glucocorticoid receptor (GR)
Vitamins	
1,25-(OH)$_2$-Vitamin D$_3$	Vitamin D receptor (VDR)
All-*trans*-retinoic acid	Retinoic acid receptor, subtypes α, β, γ
9-*cis*-Retinoic acid	Retinoid X receptor (RXR), subtypes α, β, γ
Metabolic Intermediates and Products	
Fatty acids	Peroxisome proliferator-activated receptor (PPAR), subtypes α, δ, γ
Oxysterols	Liver X receptor (LXR), subtypes α, β
Bile acids	Bile acid receptor (BAR, also called FXR)
Heme	Rev-Erb subtypes α, β
Phospholipids	Liver receptor homologue-1 (LRH-1)
	Steroidogenic factor-1 (SF-1)
Xenobiotics	Pregnane X receptor (PXR)
	Constitutive androstane receptor (CAR)

estrogen receptor α and β genes [*ESR1* and *ESR2*]), more than one gene exists, encoding multiple receptors. Each gene may in turn encode additional receptors for the same hormone by alternative promoter usage or by alternative splicing (e.g., *THRB1* and *THRB2*).

Some receptors can mediate the signals of multiple hormones. For example, the mineralocorticoid receptor, also known as the aldosterone receptor, has equal affinity for cortisol and probably functions as a glucocorticoid receptor in some tissues, such as the brain.[122] Likewise, the androgen receptor binds and responds to both testosterone and dihydrotestosterone (DHT).[123]

Vitamins

Vitamins are essential constituents of a healthful diet. Two fat-soluble vitamins, A and D, are precursors of important signaling molecules that function as ligands for nuclear receptors.

Precursors of vitamin D are synthesized and stored in skin and activated by ultraviolet light; vitamin D can also be derived from dietary sources. Vitamin D is then converted in the liver to 25(OH)D (25-hydroxyvitamin D, calcidiol) and in the kidney to 1,25(OH)$_2$ D$_3$ (1,25-dihydroxyvitamin D$_3$, calcitriol), the most potent natural ligand of the vitamin D receptor (VDR).[124] The 1-hydroxylation of calcidiol is tightly regulated, and calcitriol acts as a circulating hormone.

Vitamin A is stored in the liver and is activated by metabolism to all-*trans*-retinoic acid, which is a high-affinity ligand for retinoic acid receptors (RARs).[125] Retinoic acid is likely to function as a signaling molecule in paracrine as well as endocrine pathways. Retinoic acid is also converted to its 9-*cis*-isomer, which is a ligand for another nuclear receptor, the retinoid X receptor (RXR).[126] These retinoids and their receptors are essential for normal development of multiple organs and tissues, and they have pharmaceutical utility for conditions ranging from skin diseases to leukemia.[127]

Metabolic Intermediates and Products

Certain nuclear receptors respond to naturally occurring endogenous metabolic products. The peroxisome proliferator-activated receptors (PPARs) constitute the best defined subfamily of metabolite-sensing nuclear receptors.[128] All three PPAR subtypes are activated by polyunsaturated fatty acids, and although specific lipid species may act as selective PPAR ligands, the PPARs may also function as integrators of the concentration of a number of fatty acids.[129]

The natural ligand for PPARα may be a fatty acid derived from lipolysis.[130,131] The fibrate class of lipid-lowering pharmaceuticals are potent ligands for PPARα, and the very name of this receptor is derived from its ability to induce the proliferation of peroxisomes in the liver.[132] Indeed, stimulation of fatty acid oxidation is an important physiologic role of PPARα.

The other PPARs (δ and γ) are structurally related but are not activated by peroxisome proliferators. PPARδ, also known as PPARβ, is ubiquitous, and its ligands—other than fatty acids—are not well characterized. Activation of PPARδ appears to increase oxidative metabolism in fat and skeletal muscle.[133] PPARγ is expressed primarily in adipocytes and is necessary for differentiation along the adipocyte lineage.[134] PPARγ is also expressed in other cell types, including colonocytes, macrophages, and vascular endothelial cells, where it may play physiologic and pathologic roles. The natural ligand for PPARγ is not known, but PPARγ is a major tissue target of thiazolidinedione (TZD) antidiabetic drugs that improve insulin sensitivity.[135,136] These pharmaceutical agents bind to PPARγ with nanomolar affinities, and non-TZD PPARγ ligands are also insulin sensitizers, further implicating PPARγ in this physiologic role.

Another metabolite-responsive nuclear receptor, the liver X receptor (LXR), is activated by oxysterol intermediates in cholesterol biosynthesis. Mice lacking LXRα have a dramatically impaired ability to metabolize cholesterol.[137] A receptor known as farnesyl X receptor (FXR) binds and is activated by bile acids, and it likely plays a role in regulation of bile synthesis and circulation in normal conditions and in disease states.[137]

Xenobiotics

Other nuclear receptors appear to function as integrators of exogenous environmental signals, including natural endobiotics (e.g., medicinal agents and toxins found in plants) and xenobiotics (i.e., compounds that are not naturally occurring). In these cases, the role of the activated nuclear receptor is to induce cytochrome P450 enzymes that facilitate detoxification of potentially dangerous compounds in the liver. Receptors in this class include sterol and xenobiotic receptor (SXR), also known as *pregnane X receptor* (PXR), and constitutive androstane receptor (CAR).[138]

Unlike other nuclear receptors that have high affinity for very specific ligands, xenobiotic receptors have low affinity for a large number of ligands, reflecting their function in defense against a varied and challenging environment. Although these xenobiotic compounds are not hormones in the classic sense, the function of these nuclear receptors is consistent with the general theme of helping the organism to cope with environmental challenges.

Orphan Receptors

The nuclear receptor superfamily is one of the largest families of transcription factors. The hormones and vitamins just described account for the functions of only a fraction of the total number of nuclear receptors. The remaining receptors have been designated as *orphan receptors* because their putative ligands are not known.[139]

From analyses of mice and humans with mutations in various orphan receptors, it is clear that many of them are required for life or for development of specific organs, ranging from brain nuclei to endocrine glands. Some orphan receptors appear to be active in the absence of any ligand (i.e., constitutively active) and may not respond to a natural ligand. Nevertheless, all of the receptors known to respond to metabolites and environmental compounds were originally discovered as orphans. Therefore, future research will likely find that additional orphan receptors function as receptors for physiologic, pharmacologic, or environmental ligands. For example, the nuclear receptor NR1D1 (also known as Rev-Erbα), which is a regulator of circadian rhythms,[24] has been shown to be a receptor for heme,[140,141] although the physiologic significance of this remains to be determined.

Variant Receptors

The C-terminus of the nuclear receptors is responsible for hormone binding. In a few nuclear receptors, including THRA and the glucocorticoid receptor, alternative splicing produces variant receptors with unique C-termini that do not bind ligand.[142,143] These variant receptors are normally expressed, but their biologic relevance is uncertain. They may modulate the action of the classic receptor to which they are related by inhibiting its function.

Other normally occurring variant nuclear receptors lack a classic DBD (discussed later). These types include NROB1 (also known as DAX1), which is mutated in human disease,[144] and PTPN6 (also known as SHP1).[145] Their ligands have not been identified, and it is likely that NROB1 and PTPN6 bind to and repress the actions of other receptors.

Rare, naturally occurring mutations of hormone receptors can cause hormone resistance in affected patients. Inheritance of the hormone resistance phenotype is dominant if the mutant receptor inhibits the action of the normal receptor, as occurs with resistance to thyroid hormone or PPARγ ligands.[146] Inheritance is recessive if the mutation results in a complete loss of receptor function, as with the syndrome of hereditary calcitriol-resistant rickets, which is caused by mutations in the VDR.[147] Inheritance can also be X-linked, as with the mutated androgen receptor in androgen insensitivity syndromes.[148]

Regulation of Ligand Levels

Ligand levels can be regulated in several ways (Table 3-5). A dietary precursor may not be available in required amounts (e.g., in hypothyroidism due to iodine deficiency). Pituitary hormones (e.g., TSH) regulate the synthesis and secretion of classic thyroid and steroid hormones. If the glands that synthesize these hormones fail, hormone deficiency can occur.

TABLE 3-5

Mechanisms Regulating Ligand Levels

Precursor availability
Synthesis
Secretion
Activation (prohormone → active hormone)
Deactivation (active hormone → inactive hormone)
Elimination (hepatic, renal clearance)

Many of the nuclear receptor ligands are enzymatically converted from inactive prohormones to biologically active hormones; examples include the 5′ deiodination of thyroxine (T_4) to triiodothyronine (T_3) (see Chapter 11). In other cases, one hormone is a precursor for another, as illustrated by the aromatization of testosterone to estradiol. Biotransformation may occur in a specific tissue that is not the main target of the hormone, as with renal 1-hydroxylation of vitamin D (see Chapter 28), or it may occur primarily in target tissues (e.g., 5α-reduction of testosterone to DHT; see Chapter 19). Deficiency or pharmacologic inhibition of such enzymes can reduce hormone levels.

Hormones can be inactivated by standard hepatic or renal clearance mechanisms or by more specific enzymatic processes. In the latter case, reduction in enzyme activity due to gene mutations or pharmacologic agents can result in symptoms of hormone excess, such as renal deactivation of cortisol by 11β-hydroxysteroid dehydrogenase (11β-HSD). Because cortisol can activate the mineralocorticoid receptor, insufficient 11β-HSD activity due to licorice ingestion, gene mutation, or extremely high cortisol levels causes syndromes of apparent mineralocorticoid excess.[149]

NUCLEAR RECEPTOR SIGNALING MECHANISMS

Nuclear receptors are multifunctional proteins that transduce the signals of their cognate ligands. General features of nuclear receptor signaling are illustrated in Figure 3-16.

For hormone action, the ligand and the nuclear receptor must both get into the nucleus. The nuclear receptor also must bind its ligand with high affinity. Because a major function of the receptor is to selectively regulate target gene transcription, it must recognize and bind to promoter elements in appropriate target genes. One discriminatory mechanism is dimerization of a receptor with a second copy of itself or with another nuclear receptor. The DNA-bound receptor must work in the context of chromatin to signal the basal transcription machinery to increase or decrease transcription of the target gene. In the regulation of signaling by nuclear receptors, some basic mechanisms

are used by many or all members of the nuclear receptor superfamily, whereas other mechanisms impart the specificity that is crucial to the vastly different biologic effects of the many hormones and ligands that use these related receptors.

Domain Structure of Nuclear Receptors

Nuclear receptors are proteins with molecular masses between 50,000 and 100,000 Da. They share a common series of domains, referred to as domains A through F (Fig. 3-17). This linear depiction is useful for describing and

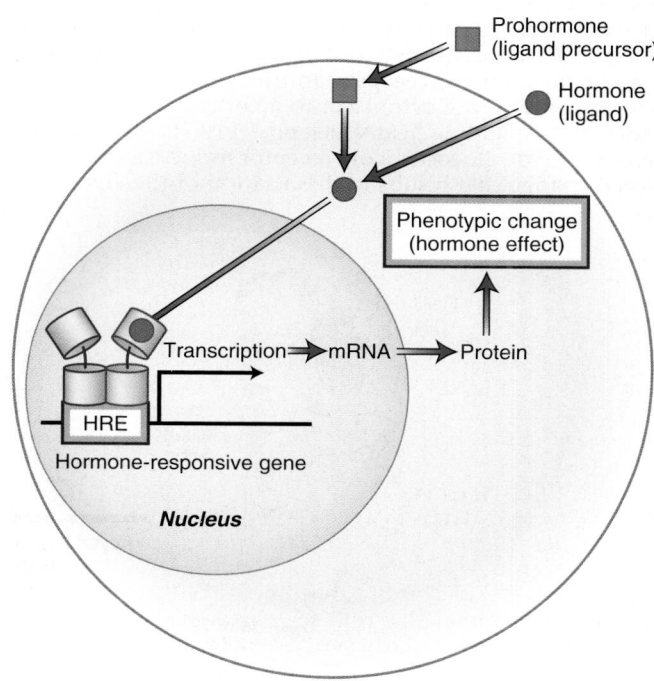

Figure 3-16 Mechanism of signal transduction by hormones and other ligands that act through nuclear receptors. HRE, hormone response element; mRNA, messenger ribonucleic acid.

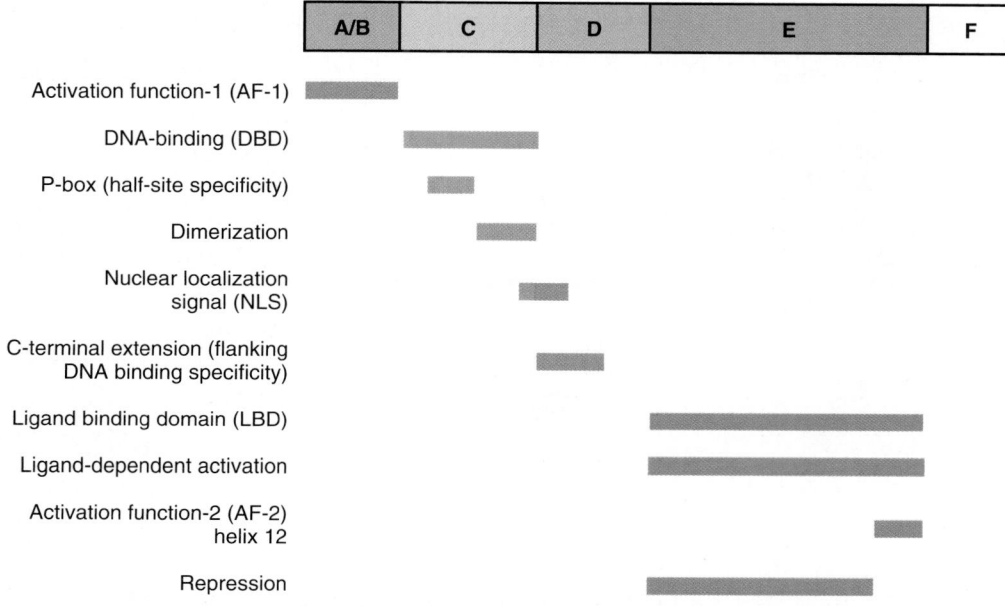

Figure 3-17 Domain structures of nuclear receptors.

comparing receptors, but it does not capture the roles of protein folding and tertiary structure in mediating various receptor functions. The structures of individual domains have now been solved for many receptors, as has the full-length structure of a more limited number of nuclear receptors.

Nuclear Localization

The nuclear receptors, like all cellular proteins, are synthesized on ribosomes that reside outside the nucleus. Import of the nuclear receptors into the nucleus requires the nuclear localization signal (NLS), which is located near the border of the C and D domains (see Fig. 3-17). As a result of their NLSs, most of the nuclear receptors reside in the nucleus, with or without their ligands. A major exception is the glucocorticoid receptor; in the absence of hormone, it is tethered in the cytoplasm to a complex of chaperone molecules, including heat shock proteins (HSPs). Hormone binding to the glucocorticoid receptor induces a conformational change that results in dissociation of the chaperone complex, allowing the hormone-activated glucocorticoid receptor to translocate to the nucleus by means of its NLS.

Hormone Binding

High-affinity binding of a lipophilic ligand is a shared characteristic of many nuclear receptors. This defining function of the receptor is mediated by the C-terminal ligand-binding domain (LBD), domains D and E in Figure 3-17. This region of the receptor has many other functions, including induction of dimerization and transcriptional regulation (see later discussions).

The structure of the LBD has been solved for a number of receptors. All share a similar overall structure consisting of 12 α-helical segments in a highly folded tertiary structure (Fig. 3-18A). The ligand binds within a hydrophobic pocket composed of amino acids in helices 3, 4, and 5 (H3, H4, and H5, respectively). The major structural change induced by ligand binding is an internal folding of the most C-terminal helix (H12), which forms a cap on the ligand-binding pocket (see Fig. 3-18B). Although the overall

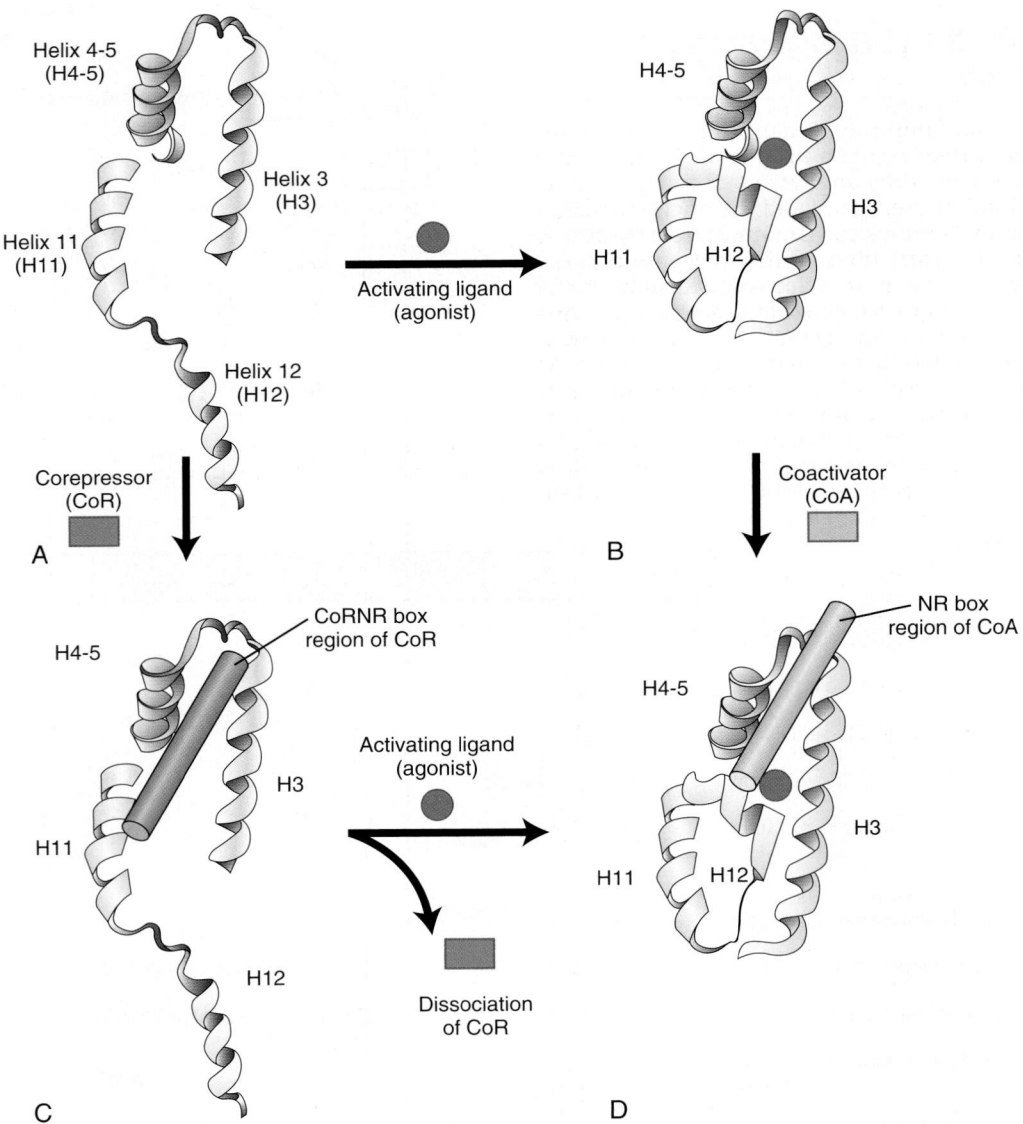

Figure 3-18 Structural basis of nuclear receptor ligand binding and cofactor recruitment. **A** and **B,** Apo-receptor (no ligand bound). **B** and **D,** Ligand-bound receptor. **C** and **D,** Structures showing the positional binding of a corepressor (CoR) in C or coactivator (CoA) in D. NR, nuclear receptor.

mechanism of ligand binding is similar for all receptors, the molecular details are essential for determining ligand specificity.[150,151] Ligand binding is the most critical determinant of receptor specificity.

Target Gene Recognition by Receptors

Another crucial specificity factor for nuclear receptors is their ability to recognize and bind to the subset of genes that is to be regulated by their cognate ligand. Target genes contain specific DNA sequences that are called *hormone response elements* (HREs). Binding to the HRE is mediated by the central C domain of the nuclear receptors (see Fig. 3-17). This region is typically composed of 66 to 68 amino acids, including two subdomains that are called *zinc fingers* because the structure of each subdomain is maintained by four cysteine residues coordinated with a zinc atom.

The first of these zinc-ordered modules contains basic amino acids that contact DNA; as with the LBD, the overall structure of the DBD is similar for all members of the nuclear receptor superfamily. The specificity of DNA binding is determined by multiple factors (Table 3-6). All steroid hormone receptors, except for the estrogen receptor, bind to the double-stranded DNA sequence AGAACA (Fig. 3-19).

By convention, the double-stranded sequence is described by the sequence of one of its complementary strands, with the bases ordered from the 5′ to the 3′ end. Other nuclear receptors recognize the sequence AGGTCA. The primary determinant of this specificity is a group of amino acid residues in the *P box* of the DBD (see Fig. 3-19). These hexamer DNA sequences are referred to as *half-sites*. The only difference between these hexameric half-sites is the central two base pairs (underlined in Fig. 3-19). For some nuclear receptors, the C-terminal extension of the DBD contributes specificity for extended half-sites containing additional, highly specific DNA sequences 5′ to the hexamer. Another source of specificity for target genes is the spacing and orientation of these half-sites, which in most cases are bound by receptor dimers.

Receptor Dimerization

The nuclear receptor DBD has affinity for the hexameric half-site or for extended half-sites; however, many HREs are composed of repeats of the half-site sequence, and most nuclear receptors bind these HREs as dimers.[152] Steroid receptors, including estrogen receptors, function primarily as homodimers, which preferentially bind to two half-sites

oriented toward each other (i.e., inverted repeats [IRs]) with three base pairs in between (IR3) (see Fig. 3-19A). The major dimerization domain in steroid receptors is within the C domain, although the LBD contributes. Ligand binding facilitates dimerization and DNA binding of steroid hormone receptors. Most other receptors, including THR, RAR, PPAR, LXR, and VDR, bind to DNA as heterodimers with RXR (see Fig. 3-19B).

Heterodimerization with RXR is mediated by two distinct interactions, one involving LBDs and the other involving DBDs. The receptor LBD mediates the strongest interaction, which occurs even in the absence of DNA. These receptor heterodimers bind to two half-sites arranged as direct repeats (DRs) with variable numbers of base pairs in between.

The spacing of the half-sites is a major determinant of target gene specificity, and it results from the second receptor-receptor interaction, which involves the DBDs and is highly sensitive to the spacing of the half-sites. For example, VDR/RXR heterodimers bind preferentially to DRs separated by three bases (DR3 sites), TR/RXR binds DR4, and RAR/RXR binds DR5 with highest affinity.[153]

Studies of isolated DBD binding to DNA have shown that these spacing requirements are related to the fact that

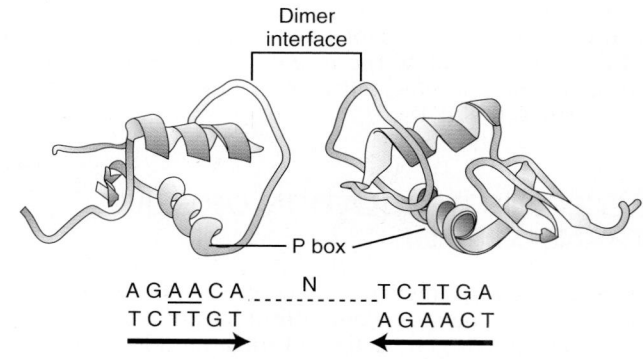

A   Steroid hormone receptor homodimer

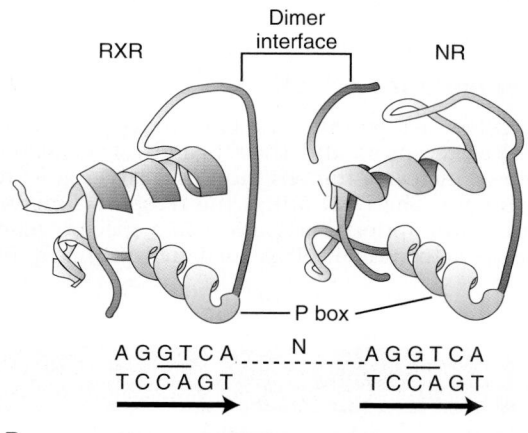

B   Nuclear receptor (NR)-RXR heterodimer

Figure 3-19 Structural basis for nuclear receptor (NR) DNA-binding specificity is shown in the ribbon diagrams of receptor DNA-binding domains (DBDs). **A,** Steroid hormone receptor binding as a homodimer to the inverted repeat *(arrows)* of the AGAACA half-site. The central base pairs are *underlined.* **B,** RXR-NR heterodimer binding to the direct repeat of AGGTCA. The position of the P box, the region of the DBD that makes direct contact with DNA, is shown. N, number of base pairs between the two half-sites; RXR, retinoid X receptor.

TABLE 3-6		
Determinants of Target Gene Specificity of Nuclear Receptors		
Specificity	**Region of Receptor**	
1. Binding to DNA	DBD (C domain)	
2. Binding to specific hexamer	P box in C domain (AGGTCA vs. AGAACA)	
3. Binding to sequences 5′ to hexamer	Carboxy-terminal extension of DBD	
4. Binding to hexamer repeats	Dimerization domain (C domain for steroid receptors; D, E, and F for others)	
5. Recognition of hexamer spacing	RXR heterodimerization domain (nonsteroid receptors, D/E domains)	
6. Cell-specific factors	Receptor-independent (cell-specific factors that open chromatin to permit receptor binding based on receptor-intrinsic properties above)	

DBD, DNA-binding domain; RXR, retinoid X receptor.

the RXR binds to the upstream half-site (i.e., farthest from the start of transcription). As a result of the periodicity of the DNA helix, each base pair separating the half-sites leads to a rotation of about 36 degrees of one half-site relative to the other. Subtle differences in the structure of the receptor DBDs make the interactions more or less favorable at different degrees of rotation.[154] Solution of the crystal structures of full-length nuclear receptor heterodimers bound to DNA has demonstrated remarkable diversity in that the PPARγ-RXR heterodimer forms a nonsymmetric complex, allowing the LBD of PPARγ to cooperate with both DBDs to enhance response element binding,[155] whereas the LXR-RXR heterodimer symmetrically binds to target sequence.[156] Additional structures will be required to better understand the spectrum of RXR heterodimer binding to DNA.

The discovery of nuclear receptor binding sites has been largely empiric, based on the finding of binding sites in small numbers of known target genes. Unbiased analysis of thousands of nuclear receptor binding locations in living cells using chromatin immunoprecipitation followed by next generation sequencing has confirmed the canonical binding sequences for many nuclear receptors, including those of the estrogen receptor,[157] the androgen receptor,[158,159] the glucocorticoid receptor,[160] and PPARγ/RXR heterodimers.[161,162] The complete set of cellular binding sites is referred to as the cistrome.[163] Although the sequence of the genome is the same in nearly all cells of the body, the cistromes are context-dependent owing to cooperation with factors that allow the receptors to bind by opening chromatin in a specific cell type or developmental stage, as illustrated by PPARγ.

RECEPTOR REGULATION OF GENE TRANSCRIPTION

Nuclear receptors mediate a variety of effects on gene transcription. The most common modes of regulation are ligand-dependent gene activation, ligand-independent repression of transcription, and ligand-dependent negative regulation of transcription (Table 3-7). Much of this regulation is mediated by interactions of nuclear receptors with proteins called *coregulators,* which include coactivators and corepressors.[164]

Ligand-Dependent Activation

Ligand-dependent activation is the best understood function of nuclear receptors and their ligands. The ligand-bound receptor increases transcription of a target gene to which it is bound. The DBD brings the receptor domains that mediate transcriptional activation to a specific gene. Transcriptional activation itself is mediated primarily by

the LBD, which can function as an independent unit even when it is transferred to a DNA-binding protein that is not related to nuclear receptors. The activation function (AF) of the LBD is referred to as *AF-2* (see Fig. 3-13).

Gene transcription is mediated by a large complex of factors that ultimately regulate the activity of ribonucleic acid (RNA) polymerase, the enzyme that uses the chromosomal DNA template to direct the synthesis of messenger RNA. Most mammalian genes are transcribed by RNA polymerase II using a large set of cofactor proteins that include basal transcription factors and associated factors collectively referred to as *general transcription factors* (GTFs). Details about GTFs are of fundamental importance and are available elsewhere.

The ligand-bound nuclear receptor communicates stimulatory signals to GTFs on the gene to which it is bound. Ligands specifically recruit a subset of the coregulators to the nuclear receptor LBD. Positively acting coregulators, called *coactivators,* specifically recognize the ligand-bound conformation of the LBD and bind to the nuclear receptor on DNA only when an activating (agonist) hormone or ligand is bound. A number of coactivator proteins that bind to liganded nuclear receptors have been described (Table 3-8).[165]

The most important determinant of coactivator binding is the position of H12, which changes dramatically when activating ligands bind receptors (see Fig. 3-18B). Along with H3, H4, and H5, H12 forms a hydrophobic cleft that is bound by short polypeptide regions of the coactivator molecules.[166-168] These polypeptides, called *NR boxes* (see Fig. 3-18D), have characteristic sequences of LxxLL, in which L is leucine and xx can be any two amino acids.[169]

Coactivators increase the rate of gene transcription. This is accomplished by enzymatic functions, including histone acetyltransferase (HAT) activity.[170] HAT activity is critically important for activation because chromosomal DNA is tightly wrapped in nucleosomal units composed of core histone proteins. Acetylation as well as other enzymatic modifications of histones opens up this chromatin structure.

The best understood class of coactivator proteins is the p160 family, whose name is based on their protein size (approximately 160 kDa). The family contains at least three such molecules, and each has many names (see Table 3-8).[171] These factors possess HAT activity and recruit other coactivators, such as CREB-binding protein (CBP) and p300, which are also HATs. A third HAT, p300/CBP-associated factor (PCAF, also designated TAF5L or TAF6L), is also recruited by liganded receptors. These HATs, along with a complex of SMARC molecules (SWI/

TABLE 3-7

Regulation of Gene Transcription by Nuclear Receptors

Mode of Regulation	Examples
1. Ligand-dependent gene activation	DNA binding and recruitment of coactivators
2. Ligand-independent gene repression	DNA binding and recruitment of corepressors
3. Ligand-dependent negative regulation of gene expression	DNA binding and recruitment of corepressors, or coactivator redistribution

TABLE 3-8

Nuclear Receptor Coregulators

Coactivators

Chromatin remodeling
SWI/SNF complex
Histone acetyltransferase
p160 family (SRCs)
p300/CBP
PCAF (p300/CBP-associated factor)
Mediator

Corepressors

NCoR (nuclear receptor corepressor)
SMRT (silencing mediator for retinoid and thyroid hormone receptors)

CBP, CREB-binding protein (CREB = cAMP-response element–binding protein).

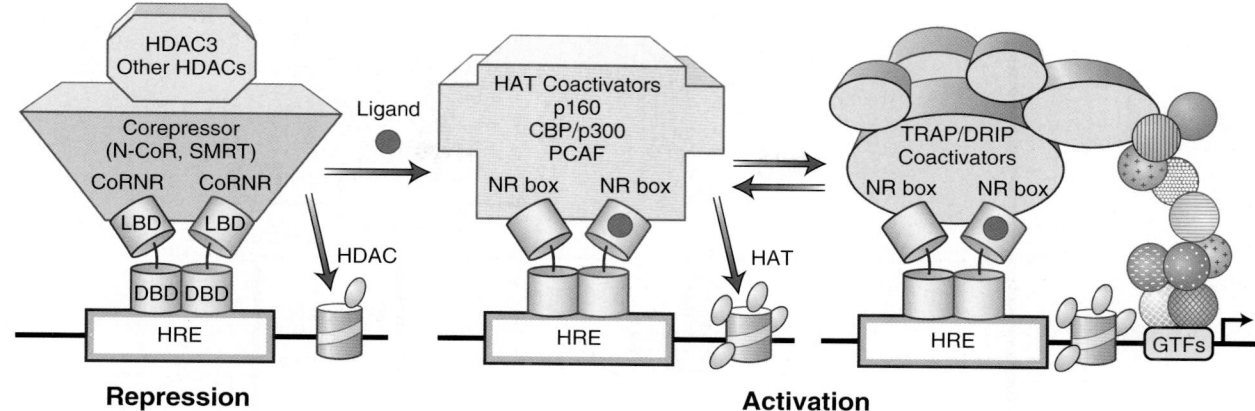

Figure 3-20 Coactivators and corepressors in transcriptional regulation by nuclear receptors. CBP, CREB-binding protein; CoRNR, coreceptor nuclear receptor box; DBD, DNA-binding domain; DRIP, vitamin D receptor–interacting protein; GTFs, general transcription factors; HAT, histone acetyltransferase; HDAC, histone deacetylase; HRE, hormone response element; LBD, ligand-binding domain; N-CoR, nuclear receptor corepressor; NR, nuclear receptor; PCAF, CBP/p300-associated factor; SMRT, silencing mediator of retinoid and thyroid receptors; TRAP, thyroid hormone receptor–associated protein.

SNF-related, matrix-associated, actin-dependent regulators of chromatin) that direct ATP-dependent DNA unwinding, create a chromatin structure that favors transcription (Fig. 3-20).[172]

Recruitment of multiple HATs may reflect different specificities for core histones and, potentially for some nonhistone proteins. Some HATs also interact directly with GTFs and further enhance their activities. The mediator complex, which has also been called the thyroid hormone receptor–associated protein (TRAP) complex, and the vitamin D receptor–interacting protein (DRIP) complex link nuclear receptors to GTFs.[173] The HATs and TRAP factors are recruited to the liganded, target gene–bound receptor in an ordered manner that also involves cycling on and off receptor gene targets with a time scale of minutes.[174] Nuclear receptor interactions with the genome are even more complex, with on-off rates that have been measured to be on the order of milliseconds.[175] These dynamics may allow multiple coactivators using similar NR boxes to contribute to gene regulation without binding to a single receptor simultaneously.

Repression of Gene Expression by Unliganded Receptor

Although DNA binding is ligand dependent for steroid hormone receptors, other nuclear receptors are bound to DNA even in the absence of their cognate ligand. Rather than passively waiting for hormone, the unliganded, DNA-bound receptor actively represses transcription of the target gene. By reducing the expression of the target gene, this repressive function of the receptor amplifies the magnitude of the subsequent activation by hormone or ligand. For instance, if the level of gene transcription in the repressed state is 10% of the basal level in the absence of a receptor, hormone activation to 10-fold above that basal level represents a 100-fold difference of transcription rate between hormone-deficient (repressed) genes and hormone-activated genes (Fig. 3-21).[176]

In many ways, the molecular mechanism of repression is the mirror image of ligand-dependent activation. The unliganded nuclear receptor recruits negatively acting coregulators, called *corepressors*, to the target gene. The two major corepressors are large (approximately 270 kDa) proteins: nuclear receptor corepressor (NCoR) and silencing mediator for retinoid and thyroid receptors (SMRT, also known as NCoR2).[177] NCoR and SMRT specifically recog-

nize the unliganded conformation of nuclear receptors and use an amphipathic helical sequence similar to the NR box of coactivators to bind to a hydrophobic pocket in the receptor.

For corepressors, the peptide responsible for receptor binding is called the *CoRNR box* (see Fig. 3-18C), and it contains the sequence (I or L)xx(I or V)I, in which I is isoleucine, L is leucine, V is valine, and xx represents any two amino acids.[178] The receptor uses helices 3 to 5 to form the hydrophobic pocket, as in coactivator binding, but H12 does not promote and even hinders corepressor binding. This negative function of H12 highlights the role of the ligand-dependent change in the position of H12 as the switch that determines repression and activation by nuclear receptors (see Fig. 3-20).[179]

The transcriptional functions of NCoR and SMRT are the opposite of those of the coactivators. The corepressors themselves do not possess enzyme activity but do recruit histone deacetylases (HDACs) to the target gene, thereby reversing the effects of histone acetylation described earlier and leading to a compact, repressed state of chromatin. Although the mammalian genome contains multiple HDACs, several of which may play a role in nuclear receptor function, the main one involved in repression is HDAC3, whose enzyme activity depends on interaction with NCoR or SMRT.[180] The ability of NCoR to bind and activate HDAC3 is required for normal metabolic and circadian physiology.[181] The corepressors interact directly with GTFs to inhibit their transcriptional activities, and they also exist in large, multiprotein complexes whose range of functions is not fully understood.

Ligand-Dependent Negative Regulation of Gene Expression: Transrepression

The ligand-dependent switch between repressed and activated receptor conformations explains how hormones activate gene expression. However, many important gene targets of hormones are turned off in the presence of the ligand. This is referred to as *ligand-dependent negative regulation of transcription*, or *transrepression*, to distinguish it from the repression of basal transcription by unliganded receptors.

The mechanism of negative regulation is less well understood than ligand-dependent activation, and there may be several mechanisms. One mechanism involves nuclear receptor binding to DNA-binding sites that reverse the

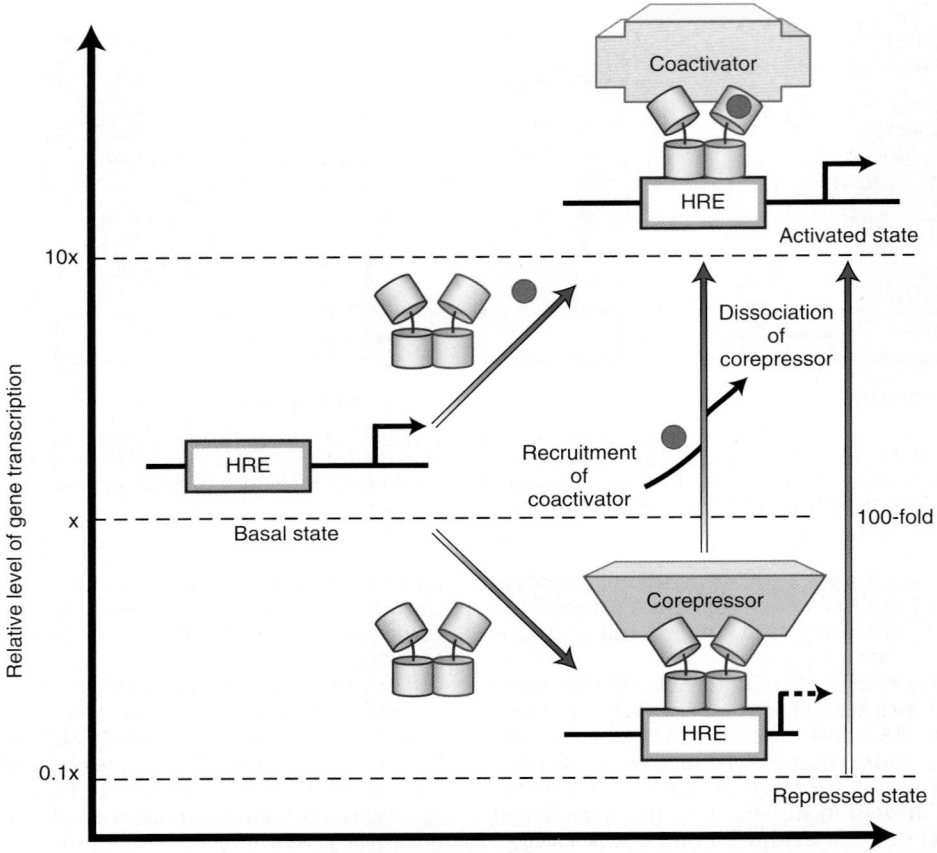

Figure 3-21 Repression and activation functions augment the dynamic range of transcriptional regulation by nuclear receptors. The magnitudes of activation and repression were arbitrarily set at 10-fold for this theoretical example. In cells, these magnitudes vary as a function of coactivator and corepressor concentration and in a target gene–specific manner. HRE, hormone response element.

paradigm of ligand-dependent activation (i.e., negative response elements). For example, when the unliganded thyroid receptor binds to the negative response element of the genes for the β-subunit of TSH or TSH-releasing hormone, transcription is activated,[182] although more recent studies suggest that the role and recruitment of coregulators in this process are complex.[183] In other cases, negative regulation may result from ligand binding to nuclear receptors that bind to other transcription factors without binding DNA. This interaction leads to redistribution of coactivators from the other transcription factors that positively regulate the gene. Recent evidence strongly supports this model, whereby inhibition of the activity of the positively acting factors results in the observed negative regulation.[184,185]

Roles of Other Nuclear Receptor Domains

The N-terminal A/B domain of the nuclear receptors is the most variable region among all members of the superfamily in terms of length and amino acid sequence. Subtypes of the same receptor often have completely different A/B domains. The function of this domain is the least defined of any. It is not required for unliganded repression or for ligand-dependent activation. In many receptors, the A/B domain contains positive transcriptional activity, often referred to as activation function 1 (AF-1) (see Fig. 3-17). Its activity is ligand independent but probably interacts with coactivators and may influence the magnitude of activation by agonists or partial agonists. This AF is

tissue-specific and tends to be more important for steroid hormone receptors, whose A/B domains are notably longer than those of other members of the superfamily.[186] The F domain of the nuclear receptors is hypervariable in length and sequence, and its function is not known.

Cross-Talk With Other Signaling Pathways

Hormones and cytokines that signal through cell surface receptors also regulate gene transcription, often by activating protein kinases that phosphorylate transcription factors such as cAMP-response element–binding protein (CREB). Such signals can also lead to phosphorylation of nuclear receptors. Multiple signal-dependent kinases can phosphorylate nuclear receptors, leading to conformational changes that regulate function.[187] Phosphorylation can lead to changes in DNA binding, ligand binding, or coactivator binding, depending upon the specific kinase, receptor, and domain of the receptor that is phosphorylated. The properties of coactivators and corepressors are also regulated by phosphorylation.[188]

Receptor Antagonists

Certain ligands function as receptor antagonists by competing with agonists for the ligand-binding site. In the case of steroid hormone receptors, the position of H12 in the antagonist-bound receptor is not identical to that in the unliganded receptor or in the agonist-bound receptor. H12, which has a sequence that resembles the NR box, binds to

TABLE 3-9
Factors Modulating Receptor Activity in Different Tissues

Concentration of receptor
Cell specificity
Variation within a given cell type
Post-translational modification of receptor (e.g., phosphorylation)
Regulation of intracellular ligand levels (see Table 3-5)
Tissue-specific factors that open chromatin
Function of ligand
    Agonist
    Partial agonist
    Antagonist
Concentration and types of coregulators
    Coactivators
    Corepressors

the coactivator-binding pocket of the receptor, and thereby prevents coactivator binding.[189] This antagonist-bound conformation of the receptor also favors corepressor binding to steroid hormone receptors.

Tissue Selectivity of Ligands Interacting With Nuclear Receptors

Many endogenous hormones that act through nuclear receptors do so in a tissue-specific manner. The most obvious mechanism is differential expression of the receptors, both in space (e.g., cell type specificity)[190] and in time (e.g., circadian variation).[191] Ligand levels may be regulated intracellularly (see earlier discussion and Table 3-5), and post-translational modification (e.g., phosphorylation) influences cell-specific receptor function. Although nuclear receptors bind at thousands of sites on genomic DNA, the specific binding sites are regulated in a cell type–specific manner. For example, the estrogen receptor binds to overlapping but clearly different sets of genomic sites in the uterus and in the breast, probably because of the differential actions of so-called pioneer transcription factors, including FOX proteins.[192]

Some ligands function as antagonists in certain tissues but as full or partial agonists in others. These selective receptor modulators include compounds such as tamoxifen, a selective estrogen receptor modulator (SERM). SERMs are estrogen receptor antagonists with respect to the functions of AF-2, including coregulator binding, and they require the AF-1 for their agonist activity.[193] This agonism, like AF-1 activity, tends to be tissue specific and therefore has great therapeutic utility.[194] Table 3-9 summarizes factors contributing to the tissue specificity of receptor activity.

REFERENCES

1. Henderson J. Ernest Starling and "Hormones": an historical commentary. *J Endocrinol.* 2005;184(1):5-10.
2. Brenner BM, Ballermann BJ, Gunning ME, Zeidel ML. Diverse biological actions of atrial natriuretic peptide. *Physiol Rev.* 1990;70(3):665-699.
3. Lee SJ. Regulation of muscle mass by myostatin. *Annu Rev Cell Dev Biol.* 2004;20(1):61-86.
4. Jackson MB, Ahima RS. Neuroendocrine and metabolic effects of adipocyte-derived hormones. *Clin Sci.* 2006;110(2):143-152.
5. Thomas-Reetz A, Hell JW, During MJ, et al. A gamma-aminobutyric acid transporter driven by a proton pump is present in synaptic-like microvesicles of pancreatic beta cells. *Proc Natl Acad Sci U S A.* 1993;90(11):5317-5321.
6. Hata AN, Breyer RM. Pharmacology and signaling of prostaglandin receptors: multiple roles in inflammation and immune modulation. *Pharmacol Ther.* 2004;103(2):147-166.
7. Blad CC, Tang C, Offermanns S. G protein-coupled receptors for energy metabolites as new therapeutic targets. *Nat Rev Drug Discov.* 2012;11(8):603-619.
8. Macia L, Tan J, Vieira AT, et al. Metabolite-sensing receptors GPR43 and GPR109A facilitate dietary fibre-induced gut homeostasis through regulation of the inflammasome. *Nat Commun.* 2015;6:6734.
9. Prüll CR. Part of a scientific master plan? Paul Ehrlich and the origins of his receptor concept. *Med Hist.* 2003;47(3):332-356.
10. Kono T, Barham FW. The relationship between the insulin-binding capacity of fat cells and the cellular response to insulin. Studies with intact and trypsin-treated fat cells. *J Biol Chem.* 1971;246(20):6210-6216.
11. Kahn CR. Insulin resistance, insulin insensitivity, and insulin unresponsiveness: a necessary distinction. *Metab Clin Exp.* 1978;27(12 Suppl 2):1893-1902.
12. Lefkowitz RJ. Historical review: a brief history and personal retrospective of seven-transmembrane receptors. *Trends Pharmacol Sci.* 2004;25(8):413-422.
13. Changeux JP. The nicotinic acetylcholine receptor: the founding father of the pentameric ligand-gated ion channel superfamily. *J Biol Chem.* 2012;287(48):40207-40215.
14. Bennett MR. The concept of transmitter receptors: 100 years on. *Neuropharmacology.* 2000;39(4):523-546.
15. Changeux JP, Kasai M, Lee CY. Use of a snake venom toxin to characterize the cholinergic receptor protein. *Proc Natl Acad Sci U S A.* 1970;67(3):1241-1247.
16. daCosta CJB, Baenziger JE. Gating of pentameric ligand-gated ion channels: structural insights and ambiguities. *Structure.* 2013;21(8):1271-1283.
17. Stojilkovic SS, Tabak J, Bertram R. Ion channels and signaling in the pituitary gland. *Endocr Rev.* 2013;31(6):845-915.
18. Katritch V, Cherezov V, Stevens RC. Structure-function of the G protein-coupled receptor superfamily. *Annu Rev Pharmacol Toxicol.* 2013;53:531-556.
19. Fredriksson R, Lagerström MC, Lundin LG, Schiöth HB. The G-protein-coupled receptors in the human genome form five main families. Phylogenetic analysis, paralogon groups, and fingerprints. *Mol Pharmacol.* 2003;63(6):1256-1272.
20. Bourne HR, Coffino P, Tomkins GM. Selection of a variant lymphoma cell deficient in adenylate cyclase. *Science.* 1975;187(4178):750-752.
21. Gilman AG. G proteins and regulation of adenylyl cyclase. *Biosci Rep.* 1995;15(2):65-97.
22. Ross EM, Wilkie TM. GTPase-activating proteins for heterotrimeric G proteins: regulators of G protein signaling (RGS) and RGS-like proteins. *Annu Rev Biochem.* 2000;69:795-827.
23. Homan KT, Tesmer JJ. Structural insights into G protein-coupled receptor kinase function. *Curr Opin Cell Biol.* 2014;27:25-31.
24. Kang DS, Tian X, Benovic JL. Role of β-arrestins and arrestin domain-containing proteins in G protein-coupled receptor trafficking. Role of β-arrestins and arrestin domain-containing proteins in G protein-coupled receptor trafficking. *Curr Opin Cell Biol.* 2014;27:63-71.
25. DeWire SM, Ahn S, Lefkowitz RJ, Shenoy SK. Beta-arrestins and cell signaling. *Annu Rev Physiol.* 2007;69:483-510.
26. Luttrell LM, Ferguson SS, Daaka Y, et al. Beta-arrestin-dependent formation of beta2 adrenergic receptor-Src protein kinase complexes. *Science.* 1999;283(5402):655-661.
27. Luttrell LM. Minireview: more than just a hammer: ligand "bias" and pharmaceutical discovery. *Mol Endocrinol.* 2014;28(3):281-294.
28. Charfi I, Audet N, Bagheri Tudashki H, Pineyro G. Identifying ligand-specific signalling within biased responses: focus on δ opioid receptor ligands. *Br J Pharmacol.* 2015;172(2):435-448.
29. Bohn LM, Lefkowitz RJ, Gainetdinov RR, et al. Enhanced morphine analgesia in mice lacking beta-arrestin 2. *Science.* 1999;286(5449):2495-2498.
30. Lemmon MA, Schlessinger J. Cell signaling by receptor tyrosine kinases. *Cell.* 2010;141(7):1117-1134.
31. Czech MP. Structural and functional homologies in the receptors for insulin and the insulin-like growth factors. *Cell.* 1982;31(1):8-10.
32. Jacobs S, Cuatrecasas P. Insulin receptors. *Annu Rev Pharmacol Toxicol.* 1983;23:461-479.
33. Hedo JA, Kahn CR, Hayashi M, et al. Biosynthesis and glycosylation of the insulin receptor. Evidence for a single polypeptide precursor of the two major subunits. *J Biol Chem.* 1983;258(16):10020-10026.
34. De Meyts P. Insulin and its receptor: structure, function and evolution. *Bioessays.* 2004;26(12):1351-1362.
35. Menting JG, Whittaker J, Margetts MB, et al. How insulin engages its primary binding site on the insulin receptor. *Nature.* 2013;493(7431):241-245.
36. McKern NM, Lawrence MC, Streltsov VA, et al. Structure of the insulin receptor ectodomain reveals a folded-over conformation. *Nature.* 2006;443(7108):218-221.
37. Menting JG, Lawrence CF, Kong GK, et al. Structural congruency of ligand binding to the insulin and insulin/type 1 insulin-like growth factor hybrid receptors. *Structure.* 2015;23(7):1271-1282.
38. Ward CW, Lawrence MC, Streltsov VA, et al. The insulin and EGF receptor structures: new insights into ligand-induced receptor activation. *Trends Biochem Sci.* 2007;32(3):129-137.
39. Kavran JM, McCabe JM, Byrne PO, et al. How IGF-1 activates its receptor. *eLife.* 2014;3:e03772.

40. Hubbard SR, Miller WT. Closing in on a mechanism for activation. *eLife.* 2014;3.

41. Hubbard SR, Wei L, Ellis L, Hendrickson WA. Crystal structure of the tyrosine kinase domain of the human insulin receptor. *Nature.* 1994;372(6508):746-754.

42. Favelyukis S, Till JH, Hubbard SR, Miller WT. Structure and autoregulation of the insulin-like growth factor 1 receptor kinase. *Nat Struct Biol.* 2001;8(12):1058-1063.

43. Murakami MS, Rosen OM. The role of insulin receptor autophosphorylation in signal transduction. *J Biol Chem.* 1991;266(33):22653-22660.

44. Zhang X, Gureasko J, Shen K, et al. An allosteric mechanism for activation of the kinase domain of epidermal growth factor receptor. *Cell.* 2006;125(6):1137-1149.

45. Pawson T. Specificity in signal transduction: from phosphotyrosine-SH2 domain interactions to complex cellular systems. *Cell.* 2004;116(2):191-203.

46. Martin GS. The hunting of the Src. *Nat Rev Mol Cell Biol.* 2001;2(6):467-475.

47. Cantley LC. The phosphoinositide 3-kinase pathway. *Science.* 2002;296(5573):1655-1657.

48. Egan SE, Giddings BW, Brooks MW, et al. Association of Sos Ras exchange protein with Grb2 is implicated in tyrosine kinase signal transduction and transformation. *Nature.* 1993;363(6424):45-51.

49. Rozakis-Adcock M, Fernley R, Wade J, et al. The SH2 and SH3 domains of mammalian Grb2 couple the EGF receptor to the Ras activator mSos1. *Nature.* 1993;363(6424):83-85.

50. Aronheim A, Engelberg D, Li N, et al. Membrane targeting of the nucleotide exchange factor Sos is sufficient for activating the Ras signaling pathway. *Cell.* 1994;78(6):949-961.

51. Chardin P, Camonis JH, Gale NW, et al. Human Sos1: a guanine nucleotide exchange factor for Ras that binds to GRB2. *Science.* 1993;260(5112):1338-1343.

52. Skolnik EY, Batzer A, Li N, et al. The function of GRB2 in linking the insulin receptor to Ras signaling pathways. *Science.* 1993;260(5116):1953-1955.

53. White MF. IRS proteins and the common path to diabetes. *Am J Physiol Endocrinol Metab.* 2002;283(3):E413-E422.

54. Myers MG, White MF. Insulin signal transduction and the IRS proteins. *Annu Rev Pharmacol Toxicol.* 1996;36:615-658.

55. Sasaoka T, Rose DW, Jhun BH, et al. Evidence for a functional role of Shc proteins in mitogenic signaling induced by insulin, insulin-like growth factor-1, and epidermal growth factor. *J Biol Chem.* 1994;269(18):13689-13694.

56. Lehr S, Kotzka J, Herkner A, et al. Identification of major tyrosine phosphorylation sites in the human insulin receptor substrate Gab-1 by insulin receptor kinase in vitro. *Biochemistry.* 2000;39(35):10898-10907.

57. Liu F, Roth RA. Grb-IR: a SH2-domain-containing protein that binds to the insulin receptor and inhibits its function. *Proc Natl Acad Sci U S A.* 1995;92(22):10287-10291.

58. Hubbard SR. The insulin receptor: both a prototypical and atypical receptor tyrosine kinase. *Cold Spring Harb Perspect Biol.* 2013;5(3):a008946.

59. Yu Y, Yoon SO, Poulogiannis G, et al. Phosphoproteomic analysis identifies Grb10 as an mTORC1 substrate that negatively regulates insulin signaling. *Science.* 2011;332(6035):1322-1326.

60. Hsu PP, Kang SA, Rameseder J, et al. The mTOR-regulated phosphoproteome reveals a mechanism of mTORC1-mediated inhibition of growth factor signaling. *Science.* 2011;332(6035):1317-1322.

61. Charalambous M, Smith FM, Bennett WR, et al. Disruption of the imprinted Grb10 gene leads to disproportionate overgrowth by an IGF2-independent mechanism. *Proc Natl Acad Sci U S A.* 2003;100(14):8292-8297.

62. Gregory SJ, Kaiser UB. Regulation of gonadotropins by inhibin and activin. *Semin Reprod Med.* 2004;22(3):253-267.

63. Ling N, Ying SY, Ueno N, et al. Pituitary FSH is released by a heterodimer of the beta-subunits from the two forms of inhibin. *Nature.* 1986;321(6072):779-782.

64. Mathews LS, Vale WW. Expression cloning of an activin receptor, a predicted transmembrane serine kinase. *Cell.* 1991;65(6):973-982.

65. Huse M, Muir TW, Xu L, et al. The TGF beta receptor activation process: an inhibitor-to substrate-binding switch. *Mol Cell.* 2001;8(3):671-682.

66. Lewis KA, Gray PC, Blount AL, et al. Betaglycan binds inhibin and can mediate functional antagonism of activin signalling. *Nature.* 2000;404(6776):411-414.

67. Fortin J, Ongaro L, Li Y, et al. Activin signaling in gonadotropes: what does the FOX say to the SMAD? *Mol Endocrinol.* 2015;29(7):963-977.

68. Rebbapragada A, Benchabane H, Wrana JL, et al. Myostatin signals through a transforming growth factor beta-like signaling pathway to block adipogenesis. *Mol Cell Biol.* 2003;23(20):7230-7242.

69. Bellinge RHS, Liberles DA, Iaschi SPA, et al. Myostatin and its implications on animal breeding: a review. *Anim Genet.* 2005;36(1):1-6.

70. Constantinescu SN, Keren T, Socolovsky M, et al. Ligand-independent oligomerization of cell-surface erythropoietin receptor is mediated by the transmembrane domain. *Proc Natl Acad Sci U S A.* 2001;98(8):4379-4384.

71. Waters MJ, Brooks AJ. JAK2 activation by growth hormone and other cytokines. *Biochem J.* 2015;466(1):1-11.

72. Babon JJ, Lucet IS, Murphy JM, et al. The molecular regulation of Janus kinase (JAK) activation. *Biochem J.* 2014;462(1):1-13.

73. Brooks AJ, Dai W, O'Mara ML, et al. Mechanism of activation of protein kinase JAK2 by the growth hormone receptor. *Science.* 2014;344(6185):1249783.

74. Wells JA, Kossiakoff AA. Cell biology. New tricks for an old dimer. *Science.* 2014;344(6185):703-704.

75. Herrington J, Smit LS, Schwartz J, Carter-Su C. The role of STAT proteins in growth hormone signaling. *Oncogene.* 2000;19(21):2585-2597.

76. Bromberg J, Darnell JE. The role of STATs in transcriptional control and their impact on cellular function. *Oncogene.* 2000;19(21):2468-2473.

77. Maures TJ, Kurzer JH, Carter-Su C. SH2B1 (SH2-B) and JAK2: a multifunctional adaptor protein and kinase made for each other. *Trends Endocrinol Metab.* 2007;18(1):38-45.

78. Farooqi IS, O'Rahilly S. Monogenic obesity in humans. *Annu Rev Med.* 2005;56:443-458.

79. Myers MG, Cowley MA, Münzberg H. Mechanisms of leptin action and leptin resistance. *Annu Rev Physiol.* 2008;70(1):537-556.

80. Zhang EE, Chapeau E, Hagihara K, Feng GS. Neuronal Shp2 tyrosine phosphatase controls energy balance and metabolism. *Proc Natl Acad Sci U S A.* 2004;101(45):16064-16069.

81. Bence KK, Delibegovic M, Xue B, et al. Neuronal PTP1B regulates body weight, adiposity and leptin action. *Nat Med.* 2006;12(8):917-924.

82. Bates SH, Stearns WH, Dundon TA, et al. STAT3 signalling is required for leptin regulation of energy balance but not reproduction. *Nature.* 2003;421(6925):856-859.

83. O'Sullivan LA, Liongue C, Lewis RS, et al. Cytokine receptor signaling through the Jak-Stat-Socs pathway in disease. *Mol Immunol.* 2007;44(10):2497-2506.

84. Metcalf D, Greenhalgh CJ, Viney E, et al. Gigantism in mice lacking suppressor of cytokine signalling-2. *Nature.* 2000;405(6790):1069-1073.

85. Sutherland EW. Studies on the mechanism of hormone action. *Science.* 1972;177(4047):401-408.

86. Smith FD, Langeberg LK, Scott JD. The where's and when's of kinase anchoring. *Trends Biochem Sci.* 2006;31(6):316-323.

87. Buxton IL, Brunton LL. Compartments of cyclic AMP and protein kinase in mammalian cardiomyocytes. *J Biol Chem.* 1983;258(17):10233-10239.

88. Azevedo MF, Faucz FR, Bimpaki E, et al. Clinical and molecular genetics of the phosphodiesterases (PDEs). *Endocr Rev.* 2014;35(2):195-233.

89. Kemp BE, Pearson RB, House C, et al. Regulation of protein kinases by pseudosubstrate prototopes. *Cell Signal.* 1989;1(4):303-311.

90. Mellon PL, Clegg CH, Correll LA, McKnight GS. Regulation of transcription by cyclic AMP-dependent protein kinase. *Proc Natl Acad Sci U S A.* 1989;86(13):4887-4891.

91. Gloerich M, Bos JL. Epac: defining a new mechanism for cAMP action. *Annu Rev Pharmacol Toxicol.* 2010;50:355-375.

92. Clapham DE. Calcium signaling. *Cell.* 2007;131(6):1047-1058.

93. Hook SS, Means AR. Ca(2+)/CaM-dependent kinases: from activation to function. Ca(2+)/CaM-dependent kinases: from activation to function. *Annu Rev Pharmacol Toxicol.* 2001;41:471-505.

94. Ohno S, Nishizuka Y. Protein kinase C isotypes and their specific functions: prologue. *J Biochem.* 2002;132(4):509-511.

95. Steinberg SF. Structural basis of protein kinase C isoform function. *Physiol Rev.* 2008;88(4):1341-1378.

96. Vanhaesebroeck B, Guillermet-Guibert J, Graupera M, Bilanges B. The emerging mechanisms of isoform-specific PI3K signalling. *Nat Rev Mol Cell Biol.* 2010;11(5):329-341.

97. Whiteman EL, Cho H, Birnbaum MJ. Role of Akt/protein kinase B in metabolism. *Trends Endocrinol Metab.* 2002;13(10):444-451.

98. Lemmon MA. Pleckstrin homology (PH) domains and phosphoinositides. *Biochem Soc Symp.* 2007;74:81-93.

99. Brazil DP, Hemmings BA. Ten years of protein kinase B signalling: a hard Akt to follow. *Trends Biochem Sci.* 2001;26(11):657-664.

100. Cho H, Thorvaldsen JL, Chu Q, et al. Akt1/PKBalpha is required for normal growth but dispensable for maintenance of glucose homeostasis in mice. *J Biol Chem.* 2001;276(42):38349-38352.

101. Cho H, Mu J, Kim JK, et al. Insulin resistance and a diabetes mellitus-like syndrome in mice lacking the protein kinase Akt2 (PKB beta). *Science.* 2001;292(5522):1728-1731.

102. Easton RM, Cho H, Roovers K, et al. Role for Akt3/protein kinase Bgamma in attainment of normal brain size. *Mol Cell Biol.* 2005;25(5):1869-1878.

103. Manning BD, Cantley LC. AKT/PKB signaling: navigating downstream. *Cell.* 2007;129(7):1261-1274.

104. Sakamoto K, Holman GD. Emerging role for AS160/TBC1D4 and TBC1D1 in the regulation of GLUT4 traffic. *Am J Physiol Endocrinol Metab.* 2008;295(1):E29-E37.

105. Mitin N, Rossman KL, Der CJ. Signaling interplay in Ras superfamily function. *Curr Biol.* 2005;15(14):R563-R574.

106. McCubrey JA, Steelman LS, Chappell WH, et al. Roles of the Raf/MEK/ERK pathway in cell growth, malignant transformation and drug resistance. *Biochim Biophys Acta.* 2007;1773(8):1263-1284.

107. Raman M, Chen W, Cobb MH. Differential regulation and properties of MAPKs. *Oncogene.* 2007;26(22):3100-3112.

108. Taylor SI, Kadowaki T, Kadowaki H, et al. Mutations in insulin-receptor gene in insulin-resistant patients. *Diabetes Care.* 1990;13(3):257-279.

109. Moller DE, Flier JS. Insulin resistance—mechanisms, syndromes, and implications. *N Engl J Med.* 1991;325(13):938-948.

110. Himsworth HP. Diabetes mellitus: its differentiation into insulin-sensitive and insulin-insensitive types. *Lancet.* 1936;227(5864):127-130. Available at: <http://eutils.ncbi.nlm.nih.gov/entrez/eutils/elink.fcgi?dbfrom=pubmed&id=22092505&retmode=ref&cmd=prlinks>.

111. Root HF. Insulin resistance and bronze diabetes. *N Engl J Med.* 1929;201(5):201-206.

112. Semple RK, Sleigh A, Murgatroyd PR, et al. Postreceptor insulin resistance contributes to human dyslipidemia and hepatic steatosis. *J Clin Invest.* 2009;119(2):315-322.

113. Hull KL, Harvey S. Growth hormone resistance: clinical states and animal models. *J Endocrinol.* 1999;163(2):165-172.

114. Dyment DA, Smith AC, Alcantara D, et al. Mutations in PIK3R1 cause SHORT syndrome. *Am J Hum Genet.* 2013;93(1):158-166.

115. Thauvin-Robinet C, Auclair M, Duplomb L, et al. PIK3R1 mutations cause syndromic insulin resistance with lipoatrophy. *Am J Hum Genet.* 2013;93(1):141-149.

116. Vassart G, Costagliola S. G protein-coupled receptors: mutations and endocrine diseases. *Nat Rev Endocrinol.* 2011;7(6):362-372.

117. Spiegel AM, Weinstein LS. Inherited diseases involving G proteins and G protein-coupled receptors. *Annu Rev Med.* 2004;55:27-39.

118. McKenna NJ, Cooney AJ, DeMayo FJ, et al. Minireview: evolution of NURSA, the Nuclear Receptor Signaling Atlas. *Mol Endocrinol.* 2009;23(6):740-746.

119. NURSA, the Nuclear Receptor Signaling Atlas website. Available at: <http://www.nursa.org>.

120. Visser WE, Friesema ECH, Visser TJ. Minireview: thyroid hormone transporters: the knowns and the unknowns. *Mol Endocrinol.* 2011;25(1):1-14.

121. Escriva H, Delaunay F, Laudet V. Ligand binding and nuclear receptor evolution. *Bioessays.* 2000;22(8):717-727.

122. Odermatt A, Atanasov AG. Mineralocorticoid receptors: emerging complexity and functional diversity. *Steroids.* 2009;74(2):163-171.

123. Haendler B, Cleve A. Recent developments in antiandrogens and selective androgen receptor modulators. *Mol Cell Endocrinol.* 2012;352(1–2):79-91.

124. Messa P, Alfieri C, Rastaldi MP. Recent insights into vitamin D and its receptor. *J Nephrol.* 2011;24:S30-S37.

125. Germain P, Chambon P, Eichele G, et al. International Union of Pharmacology. LXIII. Retinoid X receptors. *Pharmacol Rev.* 2006;58(4):760-772.

126. Evans RM, Mangelsdorf DJ. Nuclear receptors, RXR, and the big bang. *Cell.* 2014;157(1):255-266.

127. dos Santos GA, Kats L, Pandolfi PP. Synergy against PML-RARa: targeting transcription, proteolysis, differentiation, and self-renewal in acute promyelocytic leukemia. *J Exp Med.* 2013;210(13):2793-2802.

128. Michalik L, Auwerx J, Berger JP, et al. International Union of Pharmacology. LXI. Peroxisome proliferator-activated receptors. *Pharmacol Rev.* 2006;58(4):726-741.

129. Schupp M, Lazar MA. Endogenous ligands for nuclear receptors: digging deeper. *J Biol Chem.* 2010;285(52):40409-40415.

130. Haemmerle G, Moustafa T, Woelkart G, et al. ATGL-mediated fat catabolism regulates cardiac mitochondrial function via PPAR-alpha and PGC-1. *Nat Med.* 2011;17(9):1076-1085.

131. Ziouzenkova O, Perrey S, Asatryan L, et al. Lipolysis of triglyceride-rich lipoproteins generates PPAR ligands: evidence for an anti inflammatory role for lipoprotein lipase. *Proc Natl Acad Sci U S A.* 2003;100(5):2730-2735.

132. Issemann I, Green S. Activation of a member of the steroid-hormone receptor superfamily by peroxisome proliferators. *Nature.* 1990;347(6294):645-650.

133. Wagner KD, Wagner N. Peroxisome proliferator-activated receptor beta/delta (PPAR beta/delta) acts as regulator of metabolism linked to multiple cellular functions. *Pharmacol Ther.* 2010;125(3):423-435.

134. Lehrke M, Lazar MA. The many faces of PPAR gamma. *Cell.* 2005;123(6):993-999.

135. Lehmann JM, Moore LB, Smitholiver TA, et al. An antidiabetic thiazolidinedione is a high-affinity ligand for peroxisome proliferator-activated receptor gamma (PPAR-gamma). *J Biol Chem.* 1995;270(22):12953-12956.

136. Ahmadian M, Suh JM, Hah N, et al. PPAR gamma signaling and metabolism: the good, the bad and the future. *Nat Med.* 2013;19(5):557-566.

137. Calkin AC, Tontonoz P. Transcriptional integration of metabolism by the nuclear sterol-activated receptors LXR and FXR. *Nat Rev Mol Cell Biol.* 2012;13(4):213-224.

138. Wang YM, Ong SS, Chai SC, Chen TS. Role of CAR and PXR in xenobiotic sensing and metabolism. *Expert Opin Drug Metab Toxicol.* 2012;8(7):803-817.

139. Mullican SE, DiSpirito JR, Lazar MA. The orphan nuclear receptors at their 25-year reunion. *J Mol Endocrinol.* 2013;51(3):T115-T140.

140. Raghuram S, Stayrook KR, Huang PX, et al. Identification of heme as the ligand for the orphan nuclear receptors REV-ERB alpha and REV-ERB beta. *Nat Struct Mol Biol.* 2007;14(12):1207-1213.

141. Yin L, Wu N, Curtin JC, et al. Rev-erb alpha, a heme sensor that coordinates metabolic and circadian pathways. *Science.* 2007;318(5857):1786-1789.

142. Revollo JR, Cidlowski JA. Mechanisms generating diversity in glucocorticoid receptor signaling. *Ann N Y Acad Sci.* 2009;1179:167-178.

143. Brent GA. Mechanisms of thyroid hormone action. *J Clin Invest.* 2012;122(9):3035-3043.

144. Jadhav U, Harris RM, Jameson JL. Hypogonadotropic hypogonadism in subjects with DAX1 mutations. *Mol Cell Endocrinol.* 2011;346(1–2):65-73.

145. Seol W, Choi HS, Moore DD. An orphan nuclear hormone receptor that lacks a DNA binding domain and heterodimerizes with other receptors. *Science.* 1996;272(5266):1336-1339.

146. Gurnell M, Chatterjee VKK. Nuclear receptors and human disease: thyroid receptor beta peroxisome-proliferator-activated receptor gamma and orphan receptors. *Essays Biochem Nucl Receptor Superfamily.* 2004;40:169-189.

147. Malloy PJ, Tasic V, Taha D, et al. Vitamin D receptor mutations in patients with hereditary 1,25-dihydroxyvitamin D-resistant rickets. *Mol Genet Metab.* 2014;111(1):33-40.

148. Hughes IA, Werner R, Bunch T, Hiort O. Androgen insensitivity syndrome. *Semin Reprod Med.* 2012;30(5):432-442.

149. Chapman K, Holmes M, Seckl J. 11 β-hydroxysteroid dehydrogenases: intracellular gate-keepers of tissue glucocorticoid action. *Physiol Rev.* 2013;93(3):1139-1206.

150. Huang PX, Chandra V, Rastinejad F. Structural overview of the nuclear receptor superfamily: insights into physiology and therapeutics. *Annu Rev Physiol.* 2010;72:247-272.

151. Brelivet Y, Rochel N, Moras D. Structural analysis of nuclear receptors: from isolated domains to integral proteins. *Mol Cell Endocrinol.* 2012;348(2):466-473.

152. Germain P, Bourguet W. Dimerization of nuclear receptors. *Methods Cell Biol.* 2013;117:21-41.

153. Umesono K, Murakami KK, Thompson CC, Evans RM. Direct repeats as selective response elements for the thyroid-hormone, retinoic acid, and vitamin-D3 receptors. *Cell.* 1991;65(7):1255-1266.

154. Rastinejad F, Perlmann T, Evans RM, Sigler PB. Structural determinants of nuclear receptor assembly on DNA direct repeats. *Nature.* 1995;375(6528):203-211.

155. Chandra V, Huang PX, Hamuro Y, et al. Structure of the intact PPAR-gamma-RXR-alpha nuclear receptor complex on DNA. *Nature.* 2008;456(7220):350-356.

156. Lou XH, Toresson G, Benod C, et al. Structure of the retinoid X receptor α-liver X receptor β (RXR α-LXR β) heterodimer on DNA. *Nat Struct Mol Biol.* 2014;21(3):277-281.

157. Carroll JS, Meyer CA, Song J, et al. Genome-wide analysis of estrogen receptor binding sites. *Nat Genet.* 2006;38(11):1289-1297.

158. Bolton EC, So AY, Chaivorapol C, et al. Cell- and gene-specific regulation of primary target genes by the androgen receptor. *Genes Dev.* 2007;21(16):2005-2017.

159. Wang QB, Li W, Liu XS, et al. A hierarchical network of transcription factors governs androgen receptor-dependent prostate cancer growth. *Mol Cell.* 2007;27(3):380-392.

160. Wang JC, Derynck MK, Nonaka DF, et al. Chromatin immunoprecipitation (ChIP) scanning identifies primary glucocorticoid receptor target genes. *Proc Natl Acad Sci U S A.* 2004;101(44):15603-15608.

161. Lefterova MI, Zhang Y, Steger DJ, et al. PPAR gamma and C/EBP factors orchestrate adipocyte biology via adjacent binding on a genome-wide scale. *Genes Dev.* 2008;22(21):2941-2952.

162. Nielsen R, Pedersen TA, Hagenbeek D, et al. Genome-wide profiling of PPAR gamma: RXR and RNA polymerase II occupancy reveals temporal activation of distinct metabolic pathways and changes in RXR dimer composition during adipogenesis. *Genes Dev.* 2008;22(21):2953-2967.

163. Krum SA, Miranda-Carboni GA, Lupien M, et al. Unique ER alpha cistromes control cell type-specific gene regulation. *Mol Endocrinol.* 2008;22(11):2393-2406.

164. Lonard DM, O'Malley BW. Nuclear receptor coregulators: modulators of pathology and therapeutic targets. *Nat Rev Endocrinol.* 2012;8(10):598-604.

165. Bulynko YA, O'Malley BW. Nuclear receptor coactivators: structural and functional biochemistry. *Biochemistry.* 2011;50(3):313-328.

166. Feng WJ, Ribeiro RCJ, Wagner RL, et al. Hormone-dependent coactivator binding to a hydrophobic cleft on nuclear receptors. *Science.* 1998;280(5370):1747-1749.

167. Nolte RT, Wisely GB, Westin S, et al. Ligand binding and co-activator assembly of the peroxisome proliferator-activated receptor-gamma. *Nature.* 1998;395(6698):137-143.

168. Shiau AK, Barstad D, Loria PM, et al. The structural basis of estrogen receptor/coactivator recognition and the antagonism of this interaction by tamoxifen. *Cell.* 1998;95(7):927-937.

169. Heery DM, Kalkhoven E, Hoare S, Parker MG. A signature motif in transcriptional co-activators mediates binding to nuclear receptor. *Nature.* 1997;387(6634):733-736.

170. Berger SL. The complex language of chromatin regulation during transcription. *Nature.* 2007;447(7143):407-412.

171. Johnson AB, O'Malley BW. Steroid receptor coactivators 1, 2, and 3: critical regulators of nuclear receptor activity and steroid receptor modulator (SRM)-based cancer therapy. *Mol Cell Endocrinol.* 2012; 348(2):430-439.

172. Biddie SC, John S. Minireview: conversing with chromatin: the language of nuclear receptors. *Mol Endocrinol.* 2014;28(1):3-15.

173. Chen W, Roeder RG. Mediator-dependent nuclear receptor function. *Semin Cell Dev Biol.* 2011;22(7):749-758.

174. Shang YF, Hu X, DiRenzo J, et al. Cofactor dynamics and sufficiency in estrogen receptor-regulated transcription. *Cell.* 2000;103(6): 843-852.

175. Voss TC, Hager GL. Dynamic regulation of transcriptional states by chromatin and transcription factors. *Nat Rev Genet.* 2014;15(2): 69-81.

176. Hu X, Lazar MA. Transcriptional repression by nuclear hormone receptors. *Trends Endocrinol Metab.* 2000;11(1):6-10.

177. Privalsky ML. The role of corepressors in transcriptional regulation by nuclear hormone receptors. *Annu Rev Physiol.* 2004;66:315-360.

178. Hu X, Lazar MA. The CoRNR motif controls the recruitment of corepressors by nuclear hormone receptors. *Nature.* 1999;402(6757):93-96.

179. Glass CK, Rosenfeld MG. The coregulator exchange in transcriptional functions of nuclear receptors. *Genes Dev.* 2000;14(2):121-141.

180. Adams M, Montague CT, Prins JB, et al. Activators of peroxisome proliferator-activated receptor gamma have depot-specific effects on human preadipocyte differentiation. *J Clin Invest.* 1997;100(12): 3149-3153.

181. Alenghat T, Meyers K, Mullican SE, et al. Nuclear receptor corepressor and histone deacetylase 3 govern circadian metabolic physiology. *Nature.* 2008;456(7224):997-1000.

182. Tagami T, Madison LD, Nagaya T, Jameson JL. Nuclear receptor corepressors activate rather than suppress basal transcription of genes that are negatively regulated by thyroid hormone. *Mol Cell Biol.* 1997; 17(5):2642-2648.

183. Vella KR, Ramadoss P, Costa-e-Sousa RH, et al. Thyroid hormone signaling in vivo requires a balance between coactivators and corepressors. *Mol Cell Biol.* 2014;34(9):1564-1575.

184. Step SE, Lim HW, Marinis JM, et al. Anti-diabetic rosiglitazone remodels the adipocyte transcriptome by redistributing transcription to PPAR gamma-driven enhancers. *Genes Dev.* 2014;28(9):1018-1028.

185. Shlyueva D, Stelzer C, Gerlach D, et al. Hormone-responsive enhancer-activity maps reveal predictive motifs, indirect repression, and targeting of closed chromatin. *Mol Cell.* 2014;54(1):180-192.

186. Kumar R, Thompson EB. Transactivation functions of the N-terminal domains of nuclear hormone receptors: protein folding and coactivator interactions. *Mol Endocrinol.* 2003;17(1):1-10.

187. Trevino LS, Weigel NL. Phosphorylation: a fundamental regulator of steroid receptor action. *Trends Endocrinol Metab.* 2013;24(10): 515-524.

188. Han SJ, Lonard DM, O'Malley BW. Multi-modulation of nuclear receptor coactivators through posttranslational modifications. *Trends Endocrinol Metab.* 2009;20(1):8-15.

189. Gronemeyer H, Gustafsson JA, Laudet V. Principles for modulation of the nuclear receptor superfamily. *Nat Rev Drug Discov.* 2004;3(11): 950-964.

190. Bookout AL, Jeong Y, Downes M, et al. Anatomical profiling of nuclear receptor expression reveals a hierarchical transcriptional network. *Cell.* 2006;126(4):789-799.

191. Yang XY, Downes M, Yu RT, et al. Nuclear receptor expression links the circadian clock to metabolism. *Cell.* 2006;126(4):801-810.

192. Lupien M, Eeckhoute J, Meyer CA, et al. FoxA1 translates epigenetic signatures into enhancer-driven lineage-specific transcription. *Cell.* 2008;132(6):958-970.

193. Komm BS, Mirkin S. An overview of current and emerging SERMs. *J Steroid Biochem Mol Biol.* 2014;143:207-222.

194. Shang YF, Brown M. Molecular determinants for the tissue specificity of SERMs. *Science.* 2002;295(5564):2465-2468.

CHAPTER 4

Genetics of Endocrinology

AMIT R. MAJITHIA • DAVID ALTSHULER • JOEL N. HIRSCHHORN

KEY POINTS

- The genetic basis of each heritable endocrine disease/trait is quantified by its genetic architecture: (1) the number of genetic variants/genes, (2) their frequency in the population, and (3) their respective contributions to disease risk/phenotypic variation.
- Mendelian endocrine disorders are caused by few variants in few genes, found rarely in the population, and each has a large individual effect on disease risk.
- Common endocrine diseases/traits such as stature, type 2 diabetes, and serum lipids are polygenic—the result of combined, simultaneous effects of many variants in many genes, found frequently in the general population, and with each variant contributing a small individual effect.
- Genetic information enables endocrinologists to personalize therapy for patients.
- Comprehensive genetic testing (i.e., genome sequencing) can be standardized and automated, but drawing valid and clinically useful conclusions requires integration with patient history, physical examination, and other laboratory examinations.
- Genetic information is most likely to be of direct clinical use in patients with suspected mendelian syndromes.

THE ROLE OF GENETICS IN ENDOCRINOLOGY

The sequencing of the human genome has ushered in an era of genomic medicine. The catalog of protein-coding genes in humans is essentially complete, and the number of associations between genes and specific diseases is growing rapidly. Moreover, it is now feasible to identify nearly every genetic variant in an individual's protein-coding genes (whole-exome sequencing) or in his or her entire genome (whole-genome sequencing). The ability to interpret this variation is less advanced but is improving, as databases of variants and their clinical associations increase in both size and accuracy.

With the expanding reach of *precision medicine*—individualized diagnosis and therapy informed by genetics—we anticipate that increasing numbers of patients will have clinical indications for exome or genome sequencing, and others will come to clinical encounters with their sequences already in hand. Clinicians will be asked to interpret these genetic data to shed light on an individual's risk of developing disease, on diagnosis and prognosis for those already affected, on implications to family members, and on individualization of therapy. As such, it is critical that clinicians be able to draw valid and clinically useful connections between DNA sequence variation and human traits and diseases. Perhaps even more important, it is critical that clinicians understand the limits of such information.

In this chapter we present a guide to help clinicians appreciate and critically interpret the relationship between DNA sequence (genotype) and an individual's clinical presentation (phenotype). We first discuss principles of genetics to provide the framework for understanding and interpreting DNA variation in patients. We then focus on endocrine disorders, providing an overview of the genetics of endocrine diseases, with illustrative examples from both mendelian disorders (caused by mutations in single genes) and polygenic disorders (in which variation in many genes influences disease risk). Finally, we examine scenarios for clinical uses of genetic information in endocrinology and provide recommendations.

Most diseases, including endocrine disorders, are heritable, meaning that genetic variation contributes to disease risk in a population. These diseases range across the spectrum of rare, single-gene disorders, such as multiple endocrine neoplasia (Chapter 39), Carney complex (Chapter 15), and congenital adrenal hyperplasia (CAH) (Chapter 23), to polygenic diseases, such as type 2 diabetes (Chapter 31), Graves disease (Chapter 12), and osteoporosis (Chapter 28). The detailed discussions of the genetics of these and other disorders can be found throughout this textbook; this chapter will provide illustrative examples that illuminate key concepts and will refer the reader to those appropriate chapters for additional detail.

PRINCIPLES OF GENETICS

A Brief Historical Perspective

In Western conception, the relationship between inheritance and physical characteristics (disease and nonpathologic) has been recognized since the time of Aristotle (323 BC). But it was not until 1865 that the Austrian abbot

Gregor Mendel, after decades of careful experimentation in pea plants, posited and provided evidence for the modern genetic concept of *genes* (as coined by the botanist Wilhelm Johannsen in 1909).[1] Mendel deduced certain rules governing the passage of genotype (the collective versions of multiple genes in an individual) from parent to offspring, enabling the prediction of the resulting physical characteristics (phenotype) of the offspring. It was recognized in the early 20th century that certain human phenotypes, including diseases, were inherited according to the same rules that Mendel had described; these diseases are called *mendelian*.

Over the course of the next century, numerous breakthroughs established that genes were composed of DNA, physically connected on chromosomes, and encoded proteins. The first description of the molecular basis of a mendelian disease was made for sickle cell anemia, which involved a mutation in a single gene. In the 1970s, the ability to sequence DNA revealed natural and heritable sequence variation (genetic polymorphisms) in any given gene among different individuals. It was appreciated that the molecular basis of variation in the genotypes of individuals resulted from DNA sequence polymorphisms, which in turn effected alterations in phenotype. By tracing the transmission of these polymorphisms in families, it became possible to identify genes causing mendelian human disorders (those caused by altered function in a single gene and that consequently show distinctive patterns of inheritance in families).[2]

However, most human diseases and phenotypes are not mendelian. Biometricians had appreciated in the early 1900s that most continuous and commonly varying traits (such as height and blood pressure) did not follow mendelian patterns of inheritance. In 1918, R.A. Fisher[3] provided a general framework explaining continually varying traits as the consequence of polygenic inheritance; that is, polygenic phenotypes are a result of combined, small, and additive effects of variation in many genes simultaneously. In this framework, monogenic/mendelian traits were a special case. Despite this recognition, only a few genetic variants were convincingly connected with polygenic diseases/traits over the next 80 years. It would take a series of technologic advances, including the sequencing of the human genome (Human Genome Project 1990-2003) and the systematic cataloging of DNA sequence polymorphisms across diverse human populations (International HapMap Project 2002-

2005 Phase I), to systematically identify the genetic causes for common polygenic diseases.[4]

Heritability: An Estimate of the Importance of Genetic Factors to Disease Causation

Relatives resemble each other in many ways. Resemblance with respect to traits such as height or to diseases such as multiple endocrine neoplasia type 1 (MEN1) could be explained by shared genotypes passed down through generations, shared environments, and nonlinear interactions between genes and environment. Heritability quantifies, as a proportion, how much of this familial resemblance is due to genetic factors. A trait that has no genetic influence would have a heritability of 0%; a trait that is completely determined by inherited factors would have a heritability of 100%. Most clinically important traits have heritabilities ranging from 20% to 80% (Table 4-1). Appreciating the heritability of a trait is important when interpreting the contribution of genetic risk factors in disease: genetic factors are less influential for traits with low heritability and are likely to have more predictive or explanatory power for traits with high heritability.

In the past, the gold standard for heritability estimation was the comparison of monozygotic and dizygotic twin concordance rates for diseases/traits. Such studies relied on the rationale that an excess of disease correlation between genetically identical individuals (monozygotic twin pairs) as compared to those who share only 50% of their genes (dizygotic twin pairs) pointed to the role of genetic factors. However, the validity of comparing twin concordance rates across different families relied on the assumption that the effect of environment was the same for the twin pairs, regardless of whether they were monozygotic or dizygotic twins. More recent methods for heritability estimation can overcome some of these limitations by leveraging subtle fluctuations in genetic similarities between sibling pairs.[5]

Regardless of the methodology employed, it is critical to appreciate that heritability is not a fixed property of a disease/trait. The heritability estimate from any study must be interpreted in the context of the population in which it is being measured, including the historical period, and variability in environmental factors such as socioeconomic status and nutrition. These factors likely explain the wide range of heritability estimates for type 2 diabetes, ranging from 40% in Finland[6] to 80% in Japan.[7] An illustrative

---

TABLE 4-1

Heritable Endocrine Traits and Diseases

Common Form	Heritability	Reference*	Selected Mendelian Forms
Type 1 diabetes	80%	117	*KCNJ11, ABCC8* (permanent neonatal diabetes)
Type 2 diabetes	40-80%	29, 34, 118	*AGPAT2* (congenital generalized lipodystrophy), *LMNA* (familial partial lipodystrophy 1) *HNF4A, GCK, HNF1A* (MODY1-3)
Obesity	40-70%	119, 120	*MC4R, POMC*
Hypertension	30-70%	121	*MEN1, RET* (MEN2A/B), *VHL, SCNN1A* (Liddle syndrome)
Height	80%	30, 61	*GH1, FGFR3* (achondroplasia), *SHOX1* (Ullrich-Turner syndrome), *FBN1* (Marfan syndrome)
Pubertal timing	50-80%	122	*KAL1, KISS1R, FGFR1* (hypogonadotropic hypogonadism)
Graves disease	80%	123	*TSHR* (familial nonautonomous hyperthyroidism)
Hypothyroidism	67%	124	*TSHR, SLC5A5, TG, TPO,* and *TSHB* (congenital hypothyroidism)
Osteoporosis	50-85%	125, 126	*COL1A1, COL1A2, IFITM5* (osteogenesis imperfecta)
Serum calcium	40%	127, 128	*CASR* (familial hypocalciuric hypercalcemia), *HRPT2* (hyperparathyroid jaw-tumor syndrome)
Lipids	40-60%	81, 82	*LDL:* LDLR (familial hypercholesterolemia) *HDL:* CETP *Triglycerides:* APOE (familial dysbetalipoproteinemia)
Kidney stones	56%[129]	130	*CLCN5* (X-linked recessive nephrolithiasis), *NKCC2* (Bartter syndrome)

*Numbers in this column indicate references listed at the end of the chapter.

example of the importance of history can be drawn by examining type 1 diabetes rates across the Scandinavian region of Karelia. In 1940 this region was divided between Finland and the former Soviet Union with little contact between the two sections over the next 60 years. Finnish Karelians have a sixfold increased rate of type 1 diabetes compared to Russian Karelians.[8] As a result, heritability for type 1 diabetes will be different when estimated in the combined Karelian populations than when estimated in Finnish or Russian Karelians alone. The difference in diabetes rate is likely due to environmental factors, because both Karelian populations recently originated from a common ancestry and therefore likely have similar genetic risk factors for type 1 diabetes.[9]

Human DNA Sequence Variation: Molecular Forms and Biologic Effects

Each human has two versions of his or her genome (one from each parent); each version consists of a sequence of approximately 3 billion DNA bases. When comparing two versions of a human genome, either within the same person or between two different people, about 1/1000 of these bases vary (that is, 99.9% of them are the same) (Table 4-2). There are many possible ways in which DNA sequences can vary; several specific types of DNA sequence variants are frequently observed (Fig. 4-1).

The most frequent form of variation, the single nucleotide polymorphism (SNP), refers to the situation in which a single base in the sequence of one individual is different from the base seen at the same position in the sequence of another individual. SNPs can exert a wide range of biologic effects, depending on where the variant occurs and whether it alters the function of the DNA sequence. Some SNPs occur within the portions of genes that are transcribed into RNA and then translated into proteins (protein-coding regions). Synonymous SNPs occur in the protein-coding portion of DNA but both versions (alleles) of the SNP encode the same amino acid, and so this sort of variation

usually does not affect function. SNPs can be missense changes (alteration of a single amino acid in a protein-coding gene) as is the case of the C282Y mutation in the *HFE* gene responsible for autosomal recessive hereditary hemochromatosis (Chapter 19). Some missense SNPs greatly alter function, whereas others appear to have no consequences. SNPs can also alter splice sites, disrupting the structure of the mRNA that is transcribed from the DNA during gene expression. For example, the most common cause of autosomal dominant isolated growth hormone (GH) deficiency is single-base mutations that inactivate a splice donor site of intron 3 in the *GH1* gene, causing skipping of exon 3 in *GH1* (Chapter 24). SNPs can also introduce stop codons, leading to premature termination of translation and a truncated protein product. These nonsense variants typically dramatically impair or eliminate the function of the protein.

Changing the protein sequence is not the only way that SNPs (and other types of genetic variations) can alter gene function. Most of the human genome does not code for proteins (see Table 4-2) and most genetic variation occurs in this noncoding portion of the genome. For example, noncoding variants can alter the level, timing, or location of gene expression, without changing the sequence of the encoded protein. Noncoding variants often result in more subtle biologic effects, and the mechanisms are still being uncovered. For example, some SNPs subtly influence type 1 diabetes risk and lie in enhancers (noncoding DNA segments that activate gene transcription at a distance) that appear to affect gene expression only in lymphoid cells.[10]

Insertions and deletions (collectively called indels) refer respectively to the addition or removal of one or more bases in the DNA sequence. Indels in protein-coding sequences are called *frameshift mutations*, as long as the number of bases inserted or deleted is not a multiple of three. Because the genetic code is composed of triplets (every three bases encode one amino acid), a frameshift mutation alters how every subsequent base in the sequence is translated into a protein, resulting in profound molecular and clinical consequences. For example, classic salt-wasting CAH is often caused by frameshift deletions in the *CYP21A2* gene that ablate its function (Chapter 23). Repeat polymorphisms (often referred to as copy number variants, or CNVs, if the repeats are large) are a special case of indels in which DNA sequences are repeated in tandem and the number of copies of the repeated sequence varies. For example, the *AR* gene (encoding the androgen receptor) contains a repeat polymorphism in which a CAG codon, encoding glutamine, is repeated 11 to 31 times (Chapter 23). Structural variation can include both insertions and deletions as well as rearrangement of large chunks of DNA sequence (translocations and other complex forms of genomic variation). Structural variation causes familial hyperaldosteronism type 1; the adrenocorticotropic hormone (ACTH, corticotropin)-responsive promoter of the *CYP11B1* gene is incorrectly located adjacent to the aldosterone synthase gene (*CYP11B2*), causing aldosterone to be produced by ACTH stimulation (Chapter 16).

Factors Influencing the Biologic Impact of Genetic Variants in a Particular Gene

As discussed previously, the impact of a genetic variant on gene function will depend on the type of variant and its location with respect to the gene. For example, frameshift deletions in the *CYP21A2* gene completely eliminate 21-hydroxylase activity, whereas missense variants in *CYP21A2* often retain partial 21-hydroxylase activity (Chapter 23). However, even a single, specific variant may

TABLE 4-2

Characteristics of Human Genome Sequence Variation

Characteristic	Frequency
Length of the human genome sequence (base pairs)	3 billion
Number of human genes (estimated)	20,000
Fraction of base pairs that differ between the genome sequence of a human and a chimpanzee	1.3% (1 in 80)
Fraction of base pairs that vary between the genome sequence of any two humans	0.1% (1 in 1000)
Fraction of coding region base pairs that vary in a manner that substantially alters the sequence of the encoded protein	0.02% (1 in 5000)
Number of sequence variants present in each individual as heterozygous sites	3 million
Number of amino acid–altering variants present in each individual as heterozygous sites	12,000
Number of sequence variants in any given human population with frequency of >1%	10 million
Number of amino acid polymorphisms present in the human genome with a population frequency of >1%	75,000
Fraction of all human heterozygosity attributable to variants with a frequency of >1%	98%

Adapted from Altshuler D. The inherited basis of common diseases. In Goldman L, Schafer AI, eds. *Goldman's Cecil Medicine*, 24th ed. Philadelphia, PA: WB Saunders; 2012.

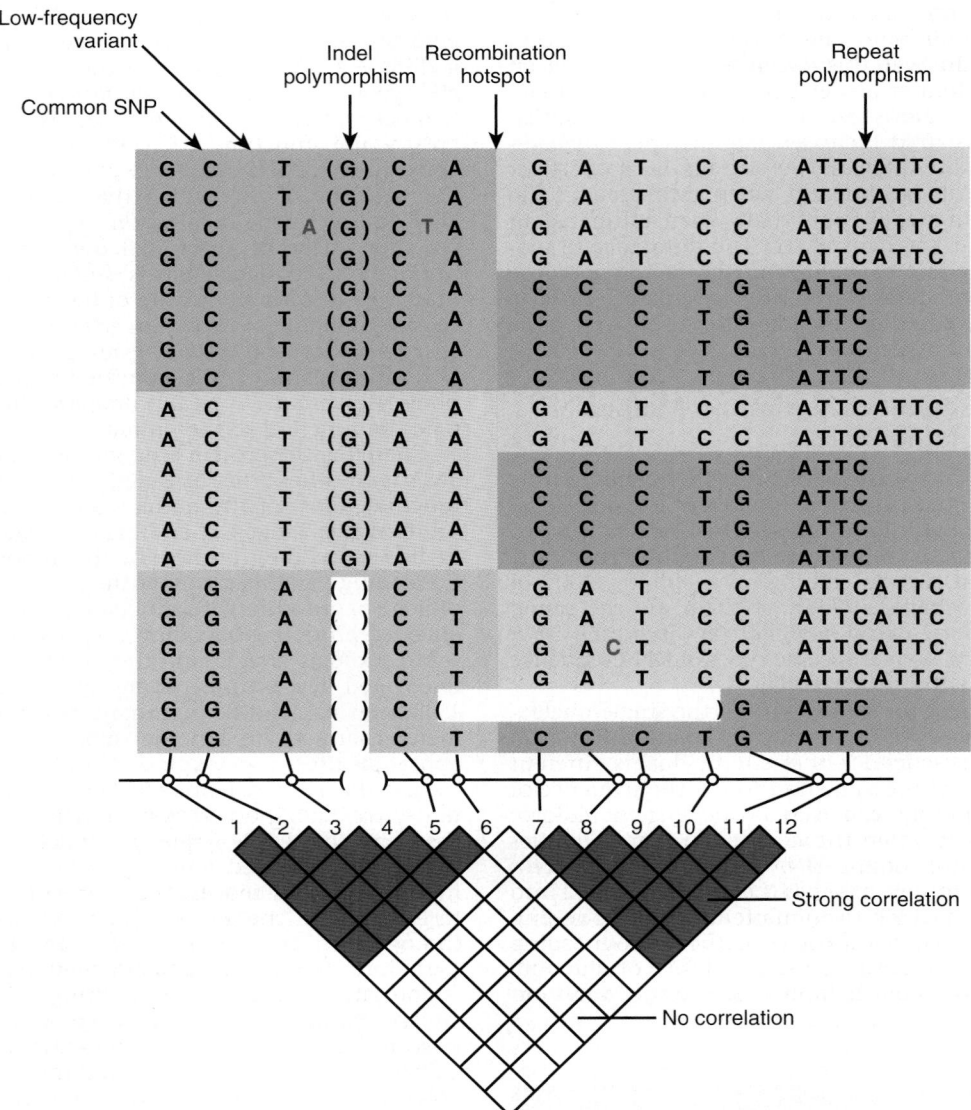

Figure 4-1 DNA sequence variation in the human genome. Common and rare genetic variation in 10 individuals, carrying 20 distinct copies of the human genome. The amount of variation shown here is typical for a 5-kb stretch of genome and is centered on a strong recombination hotspot. The 12 common variations include 10 single nucleotide polymorphisms (SNPs), an insertion-deletion polymorphism (indel), and a tetranucleotide repeat polymorphism. The six common polymorphisms on the left side are strongly correlated. Although these six polymorphisms could theoretically occur in 26 possible patterns, only three patterns are observed (indicated by pink, orange, and green). These patterns are called *haplotypes*. Similarly, the six common polymorphisms on the right side are strongly correlated and reside on only two haplotypes (indicated by blue and purple). The haplotypes occur because there has not been much genetic recombination between the sites. By contrast, there is little correlation between the two groups of polymorphisms because a hotspot of genetic recombination lies between them. In addition to the common polymorphisms, lower frequency polymorphisms occur in the human genome. Five rare SNPs are shown, with the variant nucleotide marked in red and the reference nucleotide not shown. In addition, on the second to last chromosome, a larger deletion variant is observed that removes several kilobases of DNA. Such larger deletion or duplication events (i.e., copy number variants [CNVs]) may be common and segregate as other DNA variants. (Redrawn from Altshuler D, Daly MJ, Lander ES. Genetic mapping in human disease. *Science.* 2008;322(5903):881-888.)

have different effects in different individuals. The effect of any given genetic variant (genotype) on phenotype can be modified by variants in other genes (gene-gene interactions) or by environmental factors (gene-environment interactions) or by random chance. It is usually not possible to measure or quantify these factors in any one person, but their combined effect can be quantified on a population level as *penetrance*, the proportion of individuals carrying a genetic variant who exhibit the phenotype. The penetrance of a genetic variant is highly context-dependent with respect to phenotypic definition. For example, the hemochromatosis-associated C282Y allele in the *HFE* gene exhibits high penetrance for the biochemical phenotype of high ferritin (>60% of homozygous carriers

manifest increased ferritin levels) but only 2% penetrance for the clinical phenotype of liver cirrhosis. Temporal context is also an important consideration, as disease incidence often increases with age. Carriers of mutations causing MEN1 have nearly 100% penetrance for parathyroid adenomas by age 40 but only 20% penetrance at age 20.

A common observation in members of a family carrying the same disease-causing genetic variant is that not all members of the family are equally affected. This range of phenotypic expression resulting from a particular genotype is referred to as variable *expressivity* and, as with penetrance, arises from the range of impacts of specific variants as well as modifying influences of genetic background (gene-gene interactions), environment (gene-environment interactions), and random chance. For example, the same mutation in the androgen receptor (*AR*, encoding an S703G substitution) resulted in a spectrum of clinical androgen insensitivity such that some individuals were raised as 46,XY females and others as males; other mutations in *AR* have different ranges of phenotypic effects (Chapter 23).

Mosaicism, whereby cells within a single individual have different genotypes, is another mechanism that leads to variable expressivity. Most mutations known to influence disease are *germline* mutations—inherited from the sperm or egg and present in every cell—but some diseases can be caused by somatic mutations that occur after fertilization and are present in only some cells, leading to mosaicism. In these cases, which tissues or organs carry the mutation will influence the clinical outcome. The most familiar class of disease caused in large part by somatic mutations is neoplasia, including endocrine tumor syndromes such as Conn syndrome and Cushing disease. Another classic example from endocrinology is the McCune-Albright syndrome, in which the same activating mutation in *GNAS1* exhibits variable expressivity because of postzygotic mosaicism. The phenotype of patients with McCune-Albright syndrome depends on which tissues and what fraction of cells carry the *GNAS1* mutation. A minority of affected individuals (24%) display the classic triad of café au lait spots, polyostotic fibrous dysplasia, and gonadotropin-releasing hormone (GnRH)-independent precocious puberty; the majority express two or fewer features of the classic triad (Chapter 25). The mechanism of variable expressivity likely maps to the zygotic stage in which the mutation arose: a mutation earlier in embryogenesis is present in more tissue lineages. Because mutations in a mosaic individual are not present in every cell, they can be hard to detect in DNA isolated from a blood sample if the cell in which the mutation occurred does not give rise to blood leukocytes. The *GNAS1* mutation responsible for the McCune-Albright syndrome is detected in only 8% to 46% of blood samples from affected individuals but is found in 90% of affected tissue sampled irrespective of clinical presentation (Chapter 25). Conversely, blood cells can contain somatic variation that is absent in other tissues or the germline.[11]

It is important to remember that the base pair composition of a DNA sequence is not the only molecular determinant of phenotypic expression (Table 4-3). DNA is subject to other forms of modification besides sequence variation (termed *epigenetic variation*), such as cytosine methylation or packaging into nucleosomes with various biochemically modified histones, each of which can alter gene expression and function. Thus, the same molecular form of DNA sequence variation can vary in its cellular and phenotypic effect through epigenetic modifications. Indeed, epigenetic modification is a normal part of development and is the reason why different cells have different properties even though they share the identical DNA sequence. A striking example of the effect of epigenetics is imprinting, the expression of a genetic variant in a parent-of-origin specific manner. For paternally imprinted genes, the copy that is inherited from the father is silenced, and only the mother's copy is expressed in the offspring. Imprinting can affect the impact of disease-causing mutations. Inactivating mutations in *SDHD* cause familial paraganglioma type 1 (Chapter 16). *SDHD* is maternally imprinted, so the mutation does not cause disease when inherited from the mother but is highly penetrant when inherited from the father. Imprinting can also be tissue-specific. A paternally inherited inactivating mutation in *GNAS1* causes Albright hereditary osteodystrophy (AHO, pseudopseudohypopara-

TABLE 4-3

Origins of DNA Sequence Variation in Human Populations: Common Versus Rare Variants

The type of genetic variant (missense, frameshift, noncoding, etc.) provides clues to its possible consequences; in addition, the population frequency of a variant, whether it is common or rare, can also provide information about its likely impact on phenotype. The relative balance between common and rare genetic variation is strongly influenced by evolution and human demographic history. Modern humans likely originated from a small population residing in Africa that had been evolving over millions of years. Within the past 50,000 years, members of this ancestral population migrated "out of Africa," settled the globe, and only recently, over the past 5000 to 10,000 years, multiplied exponentially.[12] As a consequence of this demographic history, most of the 3 million genetic variants an individual inherits from his or her parents are common (typically >1% frequency in the population), can be traced back to the ancient African population, and are shared in many unrelated individuals in the population. Individuals also inherit thousands of genetic variants unique to themselves and their relatives. These rare genetic variants arose more recently from spontaneous mutation in the past 10 millennia, after the migration of many humans out of Africa, and are typically observed infrequently (<0.1% of all chromosomes) in the population.

thyroidism, Chapter 28). The same mutation, when maternally inherited, manifests not only with AHO but also with hypocalcemia secondary to parathyroid hormone resistance (pseudohypoparathyroidism type 1b), because only the maternal copy of *GNAS1* is expressed in renal proximal tubules.

Evolution influences the frequency of variants that affect human phenotypes (such as endocrine diseases) through the process of natural selection. Variants that greatly increase the risk of a disease that is deleterious from a reproductive standpoint are less likely to be passed on to offspring and will be rare in the population (unless they have a compensatory benefit, such as malaria resistance in carriers of sickle cell disease). If a disease is at least mildly evolutionarily deleterious, then most common variants associated with that disease will only modestly increase disease risk. This is because those common variants, if they had strongly increased disease risk, would have then been subject to strong negative evolutionary selection and never would have risen in frequency to become common in the first place. By contrast, it is more plausible for rare/recent variants to exert strong effects on phenotype and greatly increase disease risk.

Finally, the number of genes that contribute to disease in a single individual (mendelian or polygenic disease) will be related to the strength of effect of any one variant on disease risk. By definition, variants that cause mendelian disorders have strong effects, whereas variants contributing to risk of polygenic diseases will typically have more modest effects. Thus, most variants with strong effects on disease will be rare, especially for those diseases that are clearly deleterious from an evolutionary standpoint (lethal before reproductive age). By contrast, common polygenic diseases and traits will have a much more substantial contribution from common genetic variants, although these considerations do not rule out an important role for rarer variants in polygenic phenotypes. As we will see later in this chapter, these patterns of genetic variation have important implications for identifying genetic variants that underlie disease and also for interpreting the impact of genetic variation on disease.

Summary

To summarize this introductory section, we have briefly described a number of basic principles of genetics. Heritability describes the proportion of a disease/trait that can be explained by genetic factors; the heritability of most endocrine diseases ranges between 20% and 80% (see Table 4-1). Genetic variants can take many forms ranging from single-base changes (SNPs) to translocations of entire chromosomes (see Fig. 4-1). The biologic effect of these variants depends on the type of variant, where in the DNA they are located (e.g., within coding sequence, splice sites, enhancers), how severely the variant affects function, and for somatic mutations, the cells and tissues that carry the mutation. Biologic impact can also be modified by the presence of genetic variants in other genes (gene-gene interactions), the individual organism's environment (gene-environment interactions), and random chance. The demographic history of modern human populations explains the presence of common and rare genetic variants in the human genome (see Table 4-2). Common variants are mostly ancient, and typically have relatively modest clinical effects, whereas rare variants tend to have arisen more recently and can exert larger clinical effects (Table 4-4).

GENETICS OF ENDOCRINE DISEASES

As described earlier, heritable diseases and traits, including endocrine phenotypes, span a range of genetic architectures ranging from single-gene mendelian disorders to common, polygenic diseases and traits. Mendelian and polygenic disorders represent two ends of a spectrum (see Fig. 4-2) of genetic architectures. While we distinguish between these two extremes of genetic architecture, it is important to appreciate that many disorders lie between these two extremes: rare variants of moderate effect can affect the common form of the disease, and genetic and nongenetic modifiers can strongly influence the outcome of mendelian disorders. Furthermore, many polygenic endocrine disorders also have rare mendelian forms (see Table 4-1).

The genes for a wide range of mendelian endocrine diseases have been mapped, revealing great mechanistic insight. Although mendelian diseases have offered valuable insights into pathophysiology, not all insights gained from mendelian forms of disease translate directly to the common forms of disease. For example, mendelian obesity caused by recessive inactivating mutations in the leptin receptor could be well treated by exogenous leptin, but this clinical insight did not apply to most obese individuals who actually demonstrate elevated leptin levels and do not respond to exogenous therapy with leptin (Chapter 36). Obesity as a common trait is highly heritable (heritability 40-80%),[19] and genome-wide association studies (GWAS) analysis has begun to identify risk variants for the common form. Although some of the risk variants overlap with those causing mendelian syndromes (as is also true for other diseases), GWAS have pointed to additional genetic contributions outside the mendelian genes. And, of course, the variants that have strong effects on quite rare genetic syndromes do not explain much, if any, of the risk of the common forms of disease. Thus, genetics of both mendelian forms and common polygenic forms will have important, often complementary impacts on our understanding of disease and on patient care.

The sections that follow discuss representative examples of mendelian and polygenic endocrine disorders that illustrate important concepts in gene discovery, understanding

TABLE 4-4
Performing and Interpreting Genetic Studies

For any heritable disease, the success of genetic mapping efforts, the strategy employed, and the clinical utility of any resulting genotype-phenotype map depend on its genetic architecture: (1) the number of genetic variants/genes, (2) their frequency in the population, and (3) their respective contributions to risk (i.e., penetrance). On one end of the spectrum lie mendelian diseases, such as multiple endocrine neoplasia type 1 (MEN1), characterized by (1) few variants often in a single gene, (2) extremely rare frequency in the population (<1:1000), and (3) high penetrance (>50-fold risk). On the other end of the spectrum lie the so-called common diseases, such as type 2 diabetes, characterized by (1) many variants in many genes (polygenic), (2) high frequency in the population (>1:20), and (3) low penetrance (<1.5-fold risk) (Fig. 4-2).

Owing to their simple genetic architectures, mendelian endocrine disorders were ideally suited for genetic mapping using the techniques of familial linkage mapping developed in the 1980s.[2] Because they are rare and have strong effects on phenotype, mendelian variants were typically identified in families. As a result, the genotype-phenotype correlations for these variants could not be generalized to the population at large. For example, penetrance of mendelian variants could be accurately estimated only if these variants were ascertained in the general population, rather than in selected families with a specific genetic background. Large-scale sequencing studies in the general population, which can identify all variants, rare and common, are now enabling such estimates. Such studies have found that, when ascertained in the general population, the so-called mendelian variants are less penetrant that was estimated from family-based studies.[13]

By contrast, the variants for common, polygenic disorders have been identified through genetic association studies in the general population. Genetic association studies do not require the identification of rare families segregating disease because they simply compared the frequency of a given genetic variant in disease cases and controls. Thus, they can be applied to identify genetic factors underlying diseases occurring in a population of unrelated individuals (i.e., common diseases). Unlike clinical risk factors/ biomarkers association studies, correlation in genetic association studies implies causation because genotype always precedes phenotype. Through the 1980s, genetic association studies were performed using single nucleotide polymorphisms (SNPs) at candidate genes selected by educated guessing. Such studies yielded a number of common disease associations but were poorly reproducible and confounded by false-positive results arising from population stratification. The development of modern sequencing and genotyping technologies along with the cataloging of over 10 million common variants (the International HapMap project[14]) enabled genome-wide association studies (GWAS), a systematic approach to simultaneously test all genes for associations that could account for population-based confounding.[4] GWAS have yielded a large number of reproducible genetic associations for diverse common/polygenic diseases/traits,[15] yielding insight into disease biology and genetic architecture.

When interpreting a result from any genetic study, it is important to bear in mind that the actual variant (usually a SNP) tested in the study marks a haplotype (a combination of genetic variants inherited together) that can span millions of bases. The causal variant, in the sense that it is molecularly responsible for alteration in gene function leading to cellular and disease phenotype, may lie anywhere on this haplotype. As with the chromosomal linkage studies of the past; identifying the causal variants/genes on a haplotype necessitates a combination of further association analysis (fine-mapping[16,17]) and functional experimentation in model systems.[18]

of the impact of genetic variation on disease, and implications for clinical care and insights into new biology. We discuss several classes of mendelian diseases and highlight three polygenic endocrine diseases/traits: (1) type 2 diabetes, (2) stature, and (3) serum lipids. In each section, we discuss what is known about the underlying genetic

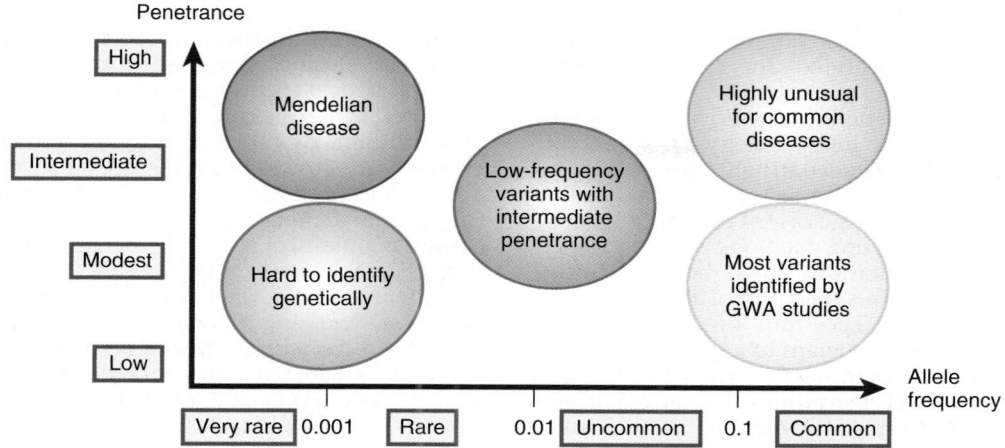

Figure 4-2 Genetic architecture of common and mendelian diseases. At one end of the spectrum are mendelian diseases cause by few variants in few genes each with a large individual effect on disease risk. On the other end of the spectrum are common diseases and traits that are caused by the combined effects of many variants, observed frequently in the population, each with a modest individual effect. (Redrawn from McCarthy MI, Abecasis GR, Cardon LR, et al. Genome-wide association studies for complex traits: consensus, uncertainty and challenges. *Nat Rev Genet.* 2008;9(5):356-369.)

contributors, the impact of genetics on our understanding of disease biology, and the translation into clinical care in the short and long term.

Mendelian Endocrine Diseases

Genetic Architecture

Mendelian diseases represent one extreme of a spectrum of possible genetic architectures (see Fig. 4-2). The alleles causing mendelian diseases are found in a *small number of genes*, are typically *rare* (<1 : 1000), are *highly penetrant*, and follow simple patterns of dominant and recessive inheritance. They are considered monogenic in that a mutation in a single gene causes disease in an individual or family. But as different families segregating the same mendelian disease are identified and the causal genetic variants mapped, *genetic heterogeneity* is often observed: different alleles in different genes can cause the same disease. Some mendelian disorders (e.g., MEN2) demonstrate recurrent mutations in the same gene, but of different molecular forms and locations, a phenomenon termed *allelic heterogeneity*. For other disorders (e.g., familial paraganglioma) multiple genes across different chromosomes are implicated, each causing the same/similar disease in different individuals. This phenomenon, variants in different genes causing the same disease, is termed *locus heterogeneity*. It is important to bear in mind that locus heterogeneity is intrinsically tied to the precision of disease definition. For example, CAH can be caused by defects in multiple genes encoding steroid biosynthetic enzymes (*CYP21A2, CYP11B1, CYP17A1, HSD3B2, POR, StAR*; Chapter 15). However, if the CAH phenotype is refined to include biochemical measurements (mineralocorticoid, sex hormone, and electrolyte levels), individual subtypes emerge, each of which possesses a simpler genetic architecture (i.e., decreased locus heterogeneity).

When contrasted with common polygenic diseases, mendelian disorders exhibit relatively less locus heterogeneity. In other words, an appreciable fraction of mendelian disease cases can be largely explained by mutations in one or a few genes. For example, recurrent mutations in a single gene (the eponymous *MEN1*) account for 70% of families segregating the MEN1 clinical syndrome. Even in this classic mendelian case, however, the genetic architecture remains incompletely defined, as 30% of cases have no

mutation in *MEN1*. Thus, much of the genetic architecture of mendelian diseases remains uncharted territory for genetic mapping. Modern sequencing technologies have facilitated a renaissance in mendelian disease gene mapping and will help improve our understanding of the genetic basis of mendelian disorders. For example, by exome sequencing two individuals in a kindred with familial combined hypolipidemia (Chapter 37), investigators identified two nonsense mutations in *ANGPTL3* that segregated with low serum lipoproteins when genotyped in other family members.[20] These mutations and the *ANGPTL3* gene were contained in the region identified by traditional linkage mapping[20] and could be quickly identified because the sequence of all exons in that region had been determined.

Disease Biology

Every endocrine organ ranging from the pituitary to adrenal is affected by well-described and less-described mendelian disorders. Mechanistic insight into disease biology has been gained from discovering the identities of the genes that lead to disease. When mutations in a number of different genes can all cause a disease (locus heterogeneity), additional mechanistic insight into molecular pathophysiology becomes possible. This makes intuitive sense in the context of a molecular understanding of genes as encoding proteins that act in concert to accomplish cellular functions. For example, Noonan syndrome (characterized endocrinologically by variable short stature, delayed puberty, and cryptorchidism in the setting of dysmorphic features and variable cardiac defects; Chapter 23) is typically caused by activating the RAS-MAPK (mitogen-activated protein kinase) signaling pathway. Dominant gain-of-function mutations in multiple pathway members (*PTPN11, SOS1, KRAS, RAF1, BRAF, NRAS*) have all been shown to cause Noonan syndrome. For other disorders, a more complex picture emerges in which multiple molecular pathways are implicated. For example, Kallmann syndrome (Chapter 25), which arises from failure of migration of GnRH neurons during fetal development, demonstrates X-linked (*KAL1*), autosomal dominant (*FGFR1*), and autosomal recessive (*PROK2*) inheritance. The gene product of *KAL1*, a secreted protein called *anosmin,* is thought to interact with the fibroblast growth factor (FGF) receptor, whereas the gene product of *PROK2*, the secreted protein prokineticin 2, interacts with a different receptor. Both signaling pathways are required for GnRH neuronal migration.

At the level of a single gene/locus, genotype-phenotype correlations mapping allelic heterogeneity to phenotypic heterogeneity can provide detailed insight into how alterations in gene function affect disease severity. CAH caused by *CYP21A2* deficiency is a classic case. A number of genetic variants including frameshifting deletions, splice site alterations, and missense mutations have been identified (Chapter 23) in *CYP21A2*. This spectrum of alleles has been mapped to a biochemical spectrum of 21-hydroxylase enzyme activity, which in turn maps to a spectrum of clinical features along the axes of mineralocorticoid sufficiency, androgen excess, and ACTH elevation (Chapter 23). In this disorder, it is possible to make predictions about clinical phenotype (categorized as salt-wasting, simple virilizing, and nonclassic) based on genotype. Notably, the positive predictive value (PPV, the strength of the genotype-phenotype correlation) is strongest for variants that severely affect *CYP21A2* gene function and are predicted to cause severe disease (salt-wasting, PPV ~100%). Predictive power is weaker for genetic variants that are expected to have more moderate effects on gene function and therefore result in milder disease (nonclassic, PPV ~60%). Some of this complexity is due to the potentially compensatory 21-hydroxylase enzyme activity of *CYP2C19* and *CYP3A4*, a form of gene-gene interaction.

Genotype-phenotype correlations must be established empirically and are not possible in many cases. Even when mutations of varying molecular severity are identified, they may not predictably affect phenotype. For example, many individuals with genetic variants in the *SRDA2* gene (encoding 5α-reductase) of differing molecular severity and location have been identified (Chapter 23), but no correlation between the genotype and the clinical degree of virilization is apparent.

The genetic causes of many mendelian disorders remain unknown, but advances in sequencing technology have accelerated the pace of discovery. The identification of gain-of-function mutations in the *KCNJ5* and *CACNA1D* genes as causes of hyperaldosteronism illustrates the potential of combining modern genome scale-sequencing with classical genetic study design.[21,22] By sequencing exomes in a series of aldosterone-producing adenomas from individuals with primary hyperaldosteronism (Conn syndrome) investigators identified missense mutations in the *KCNJ5* gene in about one third of tumors from unrelated individuals. They also identified a separate *KCNJ5* missense mutation in a mendelian family with hypertension, primary hyperaldosteronism, and massive adrenal hyperplasia. Follow-up biochemical and electrophysiologic studies showed that this series of somatic and inherited missense mutations eliminated ion selectivity in the *KCNJ5* gene product, a potassium channel. This caused membrane depolarization of adrenal cortical cells in the zona glomerulosa, stimulating aldosterone release and cell proliferation.

Whereas modern genome sequencing technologies facilitate the identification of causal mutations, translation of mutations into a disease mechanism requires relevant experimental model systems and close correlation with human phenotype. Pseudohypoparathyroidism 1a (PHP1a, Chapter 28) with gonadotropin-independent sexual precocity provides a classic example of the iterative relationship between mutations, human phenotypes, and laboratory experiments. Some individuals with PHP1a harbor the Ala366Ser missense mutation in a stimulatory G protein (G_s). This mutation destabilizes the protein, causing loss of function in most body tissues and thus hormone resistance. But these mutation carriers also exhibited paradoxical testotoxicosis consistent with gain of function in G_s. The paradox of the same mutation causing both loss and gain of function was resolved with a series of experiments showing that the Ala366Ser mutation caused a temperature-sensitive effect physiologically relevant to the normal temperature for Leydig cells. In most body tissues maintained at 37° C, the mutant G_s protein was destabilized, whereas in Leydig cells (maintained at a 3-5° C lower temperature), the mutant G_s demonstrated increased activity. Elucidating this mechanism required an appreciation of the discordant phenotype (testotoxicosis) and biochemical characterization in the relevant physiologic system (Leydig cells at a lower temperature).

Clinical Translation

Target discovery, risk prediction, and the tailoring of pharmacotherapy based on genotype are potential clinical applications of genotype-phenotype correlation. The existence of loss-of-function and gain-of-function variants in an allelic series and their concordance with opposing phenotypes can provide a rationale for therapeutically modulating gene function.[23] For example, inactivating mutations in the KISS1R receptor cause hypogonadotropic hypogonadism, whereas an Arg386Pro missense variant in *KISS1R* is associated with central precocious puberty. Kisspeptin, the agonist ligand of the KISS1R receptor, has shown promise as a fertility treatment.[24]

Genotype-phenotype correlation can be used to predict risk of disease in asymptomatic carriers. Prior to the identification and cloning of the *RET* proto-oncogene, MEN2 kindreds were monitored for evidence of medullary thyroid cancer (MTC) by calcitonin stimulation tests. Once mutations in *RET* were established as causing MEN2A/B and familial MTC, it became apparent that specific mutations could be mapped to the different syndromes. The *RET* gene product encodes a cell surface receptor tyrosine kinase. Mutations in the extracellular domain predispose to MEN2A (characterized by MTC, pheochromocytomas, and hyperparathyroidism), whereas mutations in the intracellular tyrosine kinase domain predispose to MEN2B (characterized by MTC, pheochromocytomas, and mucosal neuromas) (Chapter 39). The clinical aggressiveness of MTC, the sine qua non of all three syndromes, is greatest in MEN2B, then less in MEN2A, with familial MTC demonstrating the least propensity to grow and metastasize. A well-defined genotype-phenotype correlation between specific *RET* mutations and clinical aggressiveness of MTC now dictates the timing of lifesaving prophylactic thyroidectomy in carriers of *RET* mutations.[25] The key to establishing clinically robust risk prediction based on genotype-phenotype correlations is a well-differentiated allelic series derived from multiple individuals/families. The consensus genotype-phenotype correlation for prophylactic thyroidectomy in *RET* mutation carriers was derived from analysis of over 200 individuals from over 100 families (Chapter 39).

A genetic diagnosis in a number of mendelian disorders can also directly inform pharmacotherapies. A classic example includes obesity caused by leptin deficiency (Chapter 36), which can be treated by exogenous leptin injections. Other examples include *HNF1A* MODY (maturity-onset diabetes of the young) and neonatal diabetes (discussed in detail later) caused by genes whose properties predict excellent response to sulfonylureas. In the case of congenital hyperinsulinism, autosomal recessive mutations in *ABCC8* or *KCNJ11* correlate with diffuse disease on spectroscopic imaging and lack of responsiveness to medical therapy (diazoxide); such individuals require near-total pancreatectomy for control of hypoglycemia.[26]

Type 2 Diabetes
Genetic Architecture

Type 2 diabetes (T2D) is a multifactorial, polygenic disorder for which manifestation depends on multiple interacting genetic and environmental risk factors. Heritability estimates show strong evidence of familial clustering, ranging from 40%[6] to 80%.[7] Approximately 5% of diabetes cases that may be classified as type 2 (nonautoimmune) arise from a single-gene disorder, follow mendelian patterns of inheritance, and cluster into clinically defined syndromes. These mendelian diabetes syndromes include neonatal diabetes (Chapter 31), MODY (Chapter 31), and congenital lipodystrophies (Chapter 31).[27] To date, familial linkage studies have successfully implicated approximately 30 genes as monogenic causes of diabetes.[28]

The genetic factors underlying the majority of T2D cases (95% of cases) fit a polygenic model; genetic variants in multiple genes independently contribute to disease risk, each with a modest effect. The partial elucidation of these genetic risk factors required the advent of genetic association studies/GWAS and the assembly of cohorts of thousands of cases and control subjects.[29] As of 2014 about 70 loci have been identified from aggregated analysis on about 150,000 case controls. Taken together, these loci account for about 6% of heritability for T2D.[29] Of these loci, an SNP at *TCF7L2* (with the risk-increasing allele present at a frequency of ~30%) has the largest overall effect on risk, conferring a 1.4-fold increase in risk per allele.[29]

By contrast, type 1 diabetes shows a somewhat different genetic architecture, with common loci of large effect (a variant at the *HLA* locus found in 61% of the population confers a fivefold increase in risk,[30] and a common variant at the insulin gene confers a threefold increase in risk). This finding was consistent with prior studies from the 1980s estimating that 50% of the heritability of type 1 diabetes was explained by common haplotypes at the *HLA* locus.[31,32]

Notably, the genes implicated in monogenic causes of diabetes also contribute to polygenic forms, but through distinct genetic variants. Genes associated with mendelian diabetes syndromes, such as *KCNJ11* (neonatal diabetes, Chapter 31), *HNF1A* (MODY2, Chapter 31), and *PPARG* (familial partial lipodystrophy 3),[33] were found to harbor common variants that conferred risk for common T2D.[27,34] Conversely, genes first found associated with diabetes through GWAS have subsequently been identified as having rare, highly penetrant alleles. For example, noncoding common variants pointed to the *MTNR1B* gene (encoding the melatonin receptor) as a T2D-associated locus (1.15-fold risk).[35] Subsequently, large-scale resequencing studies identified multiple, rare coding variants of the same gene (present in <1:1000 individuals) that conferred a greater than fivefold increased risk of T2D.[36]

Mapping studies performed across various populations reveal both similarities and differences in the genetic risk factors contributing to diabetes among different ancestral groups. T2D GWAS performed in multiple populations/ancestries (European, South Asian, East Asian, Latino, African American)[37] reveal that many common variants are shared across populations with equivalent effects on disease risk, regardless of ancestry. This pattern is consistent with the origin of most common variants in an ancestral African population (see Table 4-3), but remarkable ancestry-specific effects have also been identified. A T2D GWAS performed in individuals of Latino and Mexican ancestry identified a common SNP at a locus containing the genes *SLC16A11/13* that confers a 1.25-fold increased risk of diabetes.[38] The same locus was identified by another T2D GWAS performed in Japanese individuals.[39] Because the associated SNPs were rare in Europeans, the locus had not been detected in GWAS in European-ancestry populations. Similarly, a common variant in *TBC1D4* in individuals from Greenland (present in 17% of Greenland's population) strongly increases risk of T2D (10-fold increased risk).[40] This variant, which causes a premature truncation and associates with elevated muscle insulin resistance, is extremely rare in continental Europe and likely became common in Greenland because it was present in founding ancestors of Greenland's current population.

In summary, genetic mapping studies over the past 3 decades have revealed a genetic architecture for T2D with widespread locus and allelic heterogeneity. With regard to effect size and allele frequency, T2D genetic architecture so far consists of some very rare variants of large effect, some common variants with small to moderate effects (1.2 to 1.5-fold increased risk), and a larger number of common variants with even more modest effects on disease risk, with rare and common genetic variants spread out across multiple loci in the genome. This genetic architecture has proved to be typical for other common diseases[30] (see Fig. 4-2) and reflects both the underlying genetic architecture of the disease and the ability of large GWAS to more readily detect common variants of modest effect.

Disease Biology

The past three decades of genetic discoveries in T2D have nucleated a molecular understanding of disease mechanisms, highlighted differences between glycemia and T2D, and implicated previously unknown physiology in disease pathogenesis.

Supporting the current physiologic conception of T2D as a disorder of decreased insulin production as well as decreased insulin sensitivity, genetic mapping has pointed to a molecular basis for both axes. Prediabetic individuals harboring T2D-associated variants in beta-cell genes (*SLC30A8, HNF1A*) and cell survival genes (*CDKAL1*) manifest with decreased insulin secretion (homeostatic model assessment [HOMA]-B; Chapter 31).[34] On the other hand, prediabetic individuals harboring T2D-associated variants in adipocyte genes *(PPARG, KLF14)* tend toward increases in insulin resistance (HOMA-IR; Chapter 31).[34] About 30% of T2D-associated SNPs point to insulin secretion/beta-cell function, and 15% point to insulin resistance.[28] Interestingly, the SNPs associating with insulin secretion in prediabetic individuals predict incident T2D but the SNPs associating with insulin resistance do not.[41] These findings from genetic epidemiology are consistent with beta-cell failure being a final common pathway for manifestation of hyperglycemia and diagnosis of T2D. Importantly, over half of associated SNPs and the genes they point to cannot be connected with either insulin secretion or sensitivity. Their pathogenic mechanisms remain to be elucidated by physiologic and functional investigation.

Even without a full understanding of their molecular/cellular mechanism of causation, the large number of T2D-associated loci (~70 as of 2014) have been deployed to refine disease classification. By examining quantitative glycemic traits (insulin production, sensitivity, processing, and fasting glucose) in nondiabetic individuals genotyped for 37 T2D-associated common genetic variants, investigators were able cluster genes with glycemic traits to define unique diabetes subtypes.[42] For example, individuals harboring variants in *MNTR1B* and *GCK* manifested a combination of fasting hyperglycemia and decreased insulin secretion, whereas those harboring variants in *SLC30A8*, *CDKN2A/B*, *TCF7L2*, and other genes manifested primarily with decreased insulin secretion. Notably, many genes did not cluster with predefined glycemic traits, again suggesting that the current physiologic description of T2D remains incomplete.

Genetic mapping has also corroborated the epidemiologically identified intersection between T2D and obesity. A SNP in the second intron of the *FTO* gene was identified in parallel in GWAS for T2D[43] as well as obesity.[44-46] The association signal for T2D entirely disappeared with correction for body mass index (BMI), indicating that this SNP increased T2D risk by increasing BMI. Interestingly, this locus illustrates some of the difficulties in proceeding from GWAS signal to function. Although this SNP was initially thought to exert its effect on BMI by affecting *FTO* gene function, detailed mechanistic studies have revealed that it may function by altering expression levels of *IRX3*, a gene over a million bases away.[47] Although initial studies in mice showed that increasing *Fto* gene dosage increased food intake leading to increased fat mass,[48] no connection has been found between the disease-associated SNPs and *Fto* expression level or function.[49]

Whereas T2D is diagnosed on the basis of hyperglycemia, genetic mapping has revealed that the genes that determine fasting glucose are partly distinct from those that are associated with T2D. Comparison of GWAS performed for blood glucose levels in nondiabetics versus in T2D case-control studies reveals that glycemia and T2D have distinct genetic associations.[50] Some genes harbor variants that increase blood glucose levels and T2D risk, but others alter blood glucose levels but do not confer T2D risk. Thus, the two phenotypes have both common and distinct biology. Additionally, it is important to bear in mind that the genetic basis for surrogate measures of glycemia do not always point to genes specifically altering glycemic physiology. A particularly salient example is the association of hexokinase 1 (*HK1*) with hemoglobin A_{1c} levels but not with fasting or dynamic glycemia.[51] It is thought that the genetic variant in *HK1* alters hemoglobin A_{1c} levels as a result of alteration of red blood cell life span and anemia.[51]

Clinical Translation

The principle of genetics pointing to important therapeutic targets in T2D is well validated. Both rare and common genetic variants link *PPARG*, the drug target of thiazolidines to syndromic and common T2D.[33] Similarly, rare variants in the sulfonylurea receptor (encoded by *ABCC8*) cause neonatal diabetes.[52] Although these oral hypoglycemics were identified in a pregenetic era, they point to an optimistic future of genetically guided drug discovery, one that will require detailed mechanistic understanding of the genes mapped by studies to date. A particularly attractive target nominated by genetics is *SLC30A8*, a gene that encodes a zinc transporter expressed almost exclusively in the endocrine pancreas. The common R325W missense variant in the protein encoded by the *SLC30A8* gene (present in ~1:3 individuals in most continental populations) was found to associate with protection from T2D (1.18-fold decreased risk).[53] Rare, protein-truncating variants in *SLC30A8* (present in ~2:1000 individuals) have also been associated with protection from T2D with a larger effect size (2.6-fold decreased risk).[54] The finding of human heterozygous knockouts for *SLC30A8* who are protected

from T2D and have no other deleterious phenotype offers a tantalizing therapeutic hypothesis that a chemical or antibody inhibitor of *SLC30A8* could treat diabetes and minimize side effects.

In the arena of risk prediction, genetics has not yet made a major impact on T2D because existing clinical risk factors already predict disease well. Common genetic variants, by virtue of their relatively high frequency, can explain a large part of heritability for a trait/disease but have small effects on the individual. For example, the common P12A variant in PPARG is associated with 1.25-fold risk of T2D.[55] Based on the high population frequency of the risk variant (85% P), if one were to theoretically substitute every P to A in the population, 20% of diabetes would be eliminated. Despite this incredible population-attributable risk, any given individual carrying the P variant only has a 25% increased risk of diabetes when compared to someone carrying the A variant. Given the high population frequency of common variants, many disease susceptibility variants are found in the same individual, each of which confers modest increases in risk. The progressive accessibility of genome sequencing makes it feasible to ascertain all known risk-conferring variants in an individual at once and combine these for potentially more clinically meaningful risk prediction. Investigators have attempted to combine common variants into a genetic risk score with modest success. For T2D, a risk score combining 18 common variants (including *PPARG* P12A) demonstrated 2.6-fold elevated risk in the high-risk versus low-risk group.[56] By contrast, simply reporting a family history of diabetes increases risk by threefold to sevenfold.[57]

Tailoring pharmacotherapy based on genotype has been successful in monogenic diabetes; the genome-sequencing era promises to bring this benefit to a wider group of individuals. The classic example of genotype guiding pharmacotherapy is that of individuals with MODY2 caused by autosomal dominant mutations in the *GCK* gene. Such individuals meet diagnostic criteria for diabetes but are able to regulate glycemia at a higher set-point, thus avoiding all secondary complications (Chapter 31). Thus, a genetic diagnosis of *GCK*-related diabetes can allow such individuals to avoid pharmacotherapy. Individuals with permanent neonatal diabetes cause by *ABCC8* or *KCNJ11* mutations can be safely treated with high-dose sulfonylureas in place of insulin.[58,59] It is likely that individuals with functional mutations in *ABCC8* or *KCNJ11* will be found who do not present with the classic neonatal syndrome and are classified as common T2D but who may still respond preferentially to sulfonylureas. Proving this will require identifying such individuals and performing prospective clinical trials. Prospective genotype-based intervention trials have been performed in individuals with MODY3 caused by *HNF1A* mutations and have shown the superiority of sulfonylureas over metformin.[60] Interestingly, exome sequencing of Latin American T2D case-control groups revealed the *HNF1A* E508K variant, previously annotated as MODY3, as conferring a fivefold risk of T2D in approximately 1:1000 individuals. These data demonstrate that the E508K is not fully penetrant; nevertheless, the individuals who carry it may still benefit preferentially from sulfonylurea treatment, as do their counterparts with clinically defined MODY3.

Short Stature
Genetic Architecture

Adult height is a polygenic quantitative trait with a heritability of 80%.[5] Many mendelian syndromes manifest

(Chapter 24) large phenotypic variations in stature, and more than 150 genes are associated with monogenic short stature or overgrowth. The effect sizes for these rare, highly penetrant alleles are typically large, up to 300 mm (3 standard deviations [SD]). The genetic factors underlying most of human height variation are polygenic. GWAS aggregating more than 250,000 European samples have identified over 400 independent loci associated with height[61] through common variant association. Common variants account for about 60% of heritability.[61,62] The effect sizes for these common alleles are in the range of 1 to 15 mm (0.01 to 0.15 SD). Taken together, these genetic mapping studies show that the genetics of height consists of the additive effects of common alleles with modest individual effects except in very short individuals (> 2 SD below the mean).[63] In extremely short individuals, it is likely that rare alleles of large effect play a larger role.[63]

Many genes harboring rare alleles causing monogenic alteration in stature also harbor common alleles that contribute to polygenic stature variations. Up to 30% of the genes in height-associated loci identified by GWAS also contain rare, monogenic alleles.[61] A classic example is *GH1* (isolated GH deficiency 1a, Chapter 24). This substantial overlap suggests that the genes in associated loci that have yet to demonstrate rare, large-effect alleles may be prime candidates for resequencing studies to discover new monogenic causes of alterations in stature.

Short stature, but not tall stature, has been associated with deletions in the genome. By systematically comparing CNVs across the genomes of over 4000 individuals with developmental delay and congenital abnormalities with 7000 population-based control subjects, investigators observed that individuals with short stature harbored an excess number of low-frequency (found in <5% of the population) deletions.[64] Individuals in the cohort clinically diagnosed with short stature demonstrated an average loss of 900,000 bp from their genomes.[64]

In summary, the genetic architecture of height is consistent with classical theory and animal models[65] for a polygenic, quantitative trait: thousands of genetic variants in hundreds of genes contribute to the genetic variability in height. Most of the genetic variation in height (97%) occurs from the additive effects of common variants, each contributing a modest effect. Rare variants of large effect often causing mendelian syndromes cluster at the short extreme of height variation.

Disease Biology

Genetic mapping of genes influencing both normal variation and the extremes of stature have revealed diverse molecular pathways operating in multiple tissue types that work through both endocrine and cell-autonomous mechanisms.

Genetic mapping in individuals with low GH levels and short stature have delineated multiple components of the GH/IGF-1 (insulin-like growth factor 1) axis as a key endocrine pathway in human height regulation (Chapter 24). These components include hormones, their receptors, binding proteins, and intracellular signaling proteins, such as GH1, GHR, GHRHR, STAT5B, IGFALS, IGF-1, and IGF-1R. Genetics has also pointed to the importance of the pituitary gland as a key endocrine organ regulating height, as mutations in genes that that encode transcriptional regulators of pituitary development such as *HESX1*, *PITX1*, *PITX2*, *PROP1*, *POU1F1*, and *LHX3* also lead to short stature when mutated in humans.[66] At the paracrine and cell-autonomous levels, genetic mapping has highlighted the importance of cellular proliferation, extracellular matrix deposition, and

cartilage/bone development. These cellular processes were first implicated by monogenic short stature syndromes caused by mutations in genes such as *FGFR3* (achondroplasia), *SHOX* (Langer mesomelic dysplasia), and *FBN1* (Marfan syndrome).

GWAS for height as a polygenic trait, combined with systematic clustering of genes in associated loci, have refined and expanded insights gained from mendelian genetics. Common variants associated with multiple members of the GH/IGF-1 axis demonstrate the importance of this pathway in height regulation within the normal range.[67] The association of TGF-β itself and of its binding proteins, LTBP1–3, complements the finding of *FBN1* mutations in Marfan syndrome in highlighting TGF-β signaling.[68] Similarly, the FGF signaling pathway is also highlighted, as common variants near *FGF4* are associated with height, complementing the finding of monogenic mutations in *FGFR3* causing achondroplasia. Clustering of GWAS-associated genes has also implicated hedgehog signaling (*GLI2*, *LAMA5*), Wnt signaling (*CTNNB1*, *FBXW11*, *WNT4*, *WNT5A*), and mammalian target of rapamycin (mTOR) signaling (*SMAD3*, *MTOR*) cascades in genetic control of height.[61] Many associated loci do not cluster with the pathways above or other known tissue/cellular processes such as bone/cartilage formation, implicating previously unknown biology in height regulation. A notable example is the microRNA cluster *MIR17HG*, which was also identified as a syndromic cause of short stature.[69] By cross-referencing GWAS-associated genes with gene-expression microarrays from thousands of human tissue samples, investigators have found height-associated genes are most highly expressed in cartilage and the growth plate and to a lesser extent in bone and endocrine organs.[61]

Clinical Translation

Gene mapping and functional characterization in monogenic stature disorders have motivated therapeutic advances for diseases of overgrowth and short stature. A classic example is that of Marfan syndrome, in which excess TGF-β signaling resulting from the effects of disruptive mutations in *FBN1* has led to the development of TGF-β antagonist therapies.[70] Human trials of the angiotensin receptor blocker losartan, which exhibit TGF-β antagonist properties in in vivo preclinical models, were begun in cohorts of Marfan syndrome patients.[71] Results three years after treatment showed a decrease in aortic root diameter but not more so than conventional therapy with beta blockers.[72] The identification of the activating G380N mutation in *FGFR3* that causes 95% of achondroplasia has motivated the development of inhibitors of the tyrosine kinase activity of *FGFR3* through small molecules[73] as well as through analogues of C-type natriuretic peptide.[74]

Diagnosis of short stature is an important application of genetic testing, particularly in pediatric populations. For example, the genotype-phenotype correlation of *SHOX* deficiency shows a clinical spectrum ranging from homozygous loss-of-function mutations causing the severe syndrome Langer mesomelic dysplasia to heterozygous defects found in patients with milder syndromic disease (Léri-Weill dyschondrosteosis, Ullrich-Turner syndrome) or idiopathic short stature.[75] Genetic diagnosis qualifies these patients for GH therapy. Genetic diagnosis also enables directed screening for comorbid conditions. For example, males with the likely underdiagnosed 3-M syndrome (caused by mutations in *CUL7*, *OBSL1*, or *CCDC8*), clinically defined by severe postnatal growth retardation, characteristic facies, and radiographic findings of skeletal abnormalities, are at high risk of primary hypogonadism and need to be monitored.[75] Similarly, individuals with short stature secondary to Noonan syndrome are also often underdiagnosed and are at higher risk for cardiac disease.[76]

Tailoring pharmacotherapy based on genotype is a useful adjunct to biochemical testing in stature disorders. Physiologic stimulation and serum biochemistry are the gold standards for assessing GH sensitivity and resistance guiding its pharmacologic use. But genetic information plays an important role in solidifying diagnoses suggested by biochemical testing and suggesting alternative pharmacologic therapy. For example, children with defects in the GH receptor or post-GH receptor signaling (STAT5B) will be candidates for treatment with biosynthetic IGF-1.[77] Children with defects in IGFALS, a serum protein that stabilizes IGFs, respond poorly to both medications.[78] GH therapy is used to treat short stature arising from certain genetic defects outside the GH/IGF-1 axis but is not indicated in many others. Given the variable expressivity in many syndromic stature disorders, clinically distinguishing among syndromes presenting with short stature can be challenging and imprecise. Genetic diagnosis can resolve ambiguity, particularly in children before all the features of a syndrome are present. For example, GH is contraindicated in chromosomal breakage disorders. Bloom syndrome (caused by loss-of-function mutations in *BLM*, which encodes a DNA helicase) is one such disorder presenting with short stature. In the absence of genetic diagnosis with only clinical and biochemical testing, there are case examples of children being treated for years with GH until their clinical presentation evolved and Bloom syndrome was diagnosed.[79]

Lipids and Coronary Artery Disease
Genetic Architecture

Serum lipid levels are a complex polygenic trait significantly influenced by environmental factors such as diet. Heritability estimates suggest a large role for genetic factors: approximately 40% to 60% for high-density lipoprotein cholesterol (HDL-C), about 40% to 50% for low-density lipoprotein cholesterol (LDL-C), and about 35% to 48% for triglycerides (TG).[80] Monogenic disorders causing extremes of dyslipidemia have been associated with around 20 genes. Mendelian dyslipidemia syndromes can present with single or combined lipoprotein abnormalities (Chapter 37). On the hyperlipidemic side these abnormalities include syndromes of elevated LDL (familial hypercholesterolemia, sitosterolemia), elevated TG (LPL deficiency, APOCII deficiency), elevated HDL (CETP deficiency), and combined LDL/TG elevation (familial combined hyperlipidemia, dysbetalipoproteinemia). Monogenic disorders manifesting with extremely low lipid levels have also been identified and include low LDL (familial hypobetalipoproteinemia, *PCSK9* mutations), low HDL (familial hypoalphalipoproteinemia, lecithin cholesterol acyltransferase [LCAT] deficiency, Tangier disease), and combined low cholesterol/TG (abetalipoproteinemia, chylomicron retention syndrome).

The genetic factors underlying most serum lipid variations are polygenic. GWAS aggregating approximately 200,000 multiethnic samples have identified more than 150 independent loci associated with serum lipids through common variant association accounting for about 15% of heritability.[81] The effect sizes of common variants on lipid levels range from less than 1 mg/dL to about 15 mg/dL (SNP rs964184 at *APOA1* and TG).[82]

Among the loci identified, many alter one of the lipoproteins identified, a few (*CETP, TRIB1, FADS1-2-3, APOA1*) alter all lipoprotein levels, and a subset alters various combinations of lipoproteins.[81] These overlaps are consistent with observations in mendelian disorders and corroborate the shared metabolism and lipoprotein constituents of LDL, HDL, and TG.

Many of the genes identified as monogenic causes of dyslipidemia also alter lipid levels in the general population through both common and rare variants. *LDLR*, encoding the LDL receptor, provides a case in point of how the allelic spectrum of genetic variation ranges from rare, mendelian alleles to common, small-effect alleles with effect sizes inversely proportional to variant frequency. Disruptive mutations (those that frameshift or prematurely terminate the protein) in *LDLR* like the ones found in familial hypercholesterolemia are found in 2:1000 to 7:1000 individuals and increase LDL levels by 150 to 200 mg/dL.[83] Missense variants that decrease function of LDLR in cell models are found in about 1:100 individuals and increase LDL levels by about 100 mg/dL.[84] A common, intronic SNP in *LDLR* found in 1:10 individuals decreases LDL levels by 7 mg/dL.[82]

In summary, the genetic architecture of serum lipids consists of a full spectrum of rare and common alleles in hundreds of genes throughout the genome acting in a polygenic fashion. Different variants at the same locus, based on varying impact on gene function, can alter lipid levels in a broad range. Variant frequency in the population is inversely correlated with the magnitude of effect on serum lipid levels. Many loci have an impact on multiple lipoprotein levels simultaneously.

Disease Biology

Genetic mapping for lipid traits has a rich history of synergizing with biochemical and physiologic investigation to reveal the molecular mechanisms of lipoprotein metabolism and its relationship to cardiovascular disease in humans.

Mendelian hyperlipidemia syndromes were the first to yield pathophysiologic insight, starting with Brown and Goldstein's classic studies showing that LDL failed to suppress HMG-CoA (3-hydroxy-3-methyl-glutaryl coenzyme A) reductase activity in fibroblasts from subjects with familial hypercholesterolemia.[85] Subsequent studies of families with severe hypercholesterolemia (*LDLR, APOB, ABCG5, ABCG8, ARH, PCSK9*) yielded insights into basic mechanisms of cholesterol absorption and biliary excretion as well as contributing to basic biologic understanding of receptor-mediated endocytosis, recycling, and feedback regulation.[86,87] The association between high LDL cholesterol and increased rates of myocardial infarction (MI) was also noticed in these families and complemented by observations of low rates of coronary disease in families segregating unusually low LDL levels (familial hypobetalipoproteinemia: *APOB, PCSK9, ANGPTL3*).[87] Epidemiologic association and the success of statin therapy in preventing coronary heart disease (CHD) extended the relationship of LDL and CHD to the general population,[88] as have common LDL-associated SNPs identified by GWAS.[82]

The large number of associated loci for LDL, HDL, and TG combined with clinical outcome data on population-sized cohorts of genotyped individuals has enabled causality testing for epidemiologic associations with important public health consequences. Elevated HDL cholesterol levels have been associated with protection from MI, but the causality of this association is controversial. Should public health efforts be made to raise HDL levels in the population? Should drugs that increase HDL levels continue to be developed after early clinical failures?[89] By leveraging common variants associated with HDL levels, the causality of HDL in heart disease can be tested using an approach called *mendelian randomization*.[90] As described earlier, genetic associations imply causality because genotype precedes phenotype, mitigating epidemiologic issues of confounding, bias, and reverse causation. Mendelian randomization can be conceived of as a clinical trial performed by nature in which the subjects are randomized at conception to genetic variants associated with a risk factor (e.g., SNPs increasing levels of HDL cholesterol). The subjects randomized to genotype are then assessed for the outcome (e.g., MI) and relative risk for the outcome compared in the treated and untreated arms. By utilizing a mendelian randomization approach with SNPs quantitatively associated with lipid levels, investigators found that genetic variants increasing HDL cholesterol were not protective for MI, whereas genetic variants decreasing LDL cholesterol were protective of MI.[91] These findings are consistent with drug trials showing that LDL-lowering agents protect from MI, whereas multiple agents aimed at increasing HDL do not.[92]

For TG, on the other hand, multiple lines of genetic evidence have supported a causal connection with CHD. First, rare, loss-of-function mutations in *APOC3* are associated with low levels of TG and are also protective for ischemic cardiovascular disease in European[93] and American cohorts.[94] Second, a mendelian randomization study showed that SNPs that raised serum TG levels also increased rates of CHD.[95] Finally, because of the interrelatedness of TG, LDL, and HDL, investigators have systematically examined all lipid-associated loci in cohorts phenotyped for CHD to dissect the contribution of TG to CHD risk apart from LDL and HDL.[81] By constructing a statistical framework to account for the pleiotropic effects of SNPs on all three lipoprotein levels, they demonstrated that (1) SNPs that alter LDL and TG in the same direction of effect are associated with CHD risk, (2) SNPs that exclusively alter TG levels are also associated with CHD, and (3) the strength of a SNP's effect on TG levels independently correlated with the magnitude of effect on CHD risk.[81]

Clinical Translation

In the area of therapeutics, mapping of genes that affect lipid levels has exemplified a promising approach to drug target identification: genes that protect from disease when inactivated by nature might be useful pharmacologic targets. Statins, which inhibit HMG-CoA reductase (encoded by *HMGCR*), are among the most therapeutically successful drugs in lowering LDL levels and decreasing risk for CHD in both primary and secondary prevention settings. GWAS did identify *HMGCR* as a locus altering LDL levels (with an effect size of about 3 mg/dL),[82] but how would this particular locus be prioritized as a therapeutic candidate among over 100 other associated loci? In some cases, experiments of nature (i.e., an allelic series) can be used to infer a dose-response curve of gene function that indicates how enhancement or suppression of the encoded protein's activity raises or lowers disease risk. In the well-known case of *PCSK9*, for instance, loss-of-function mutations decrease LDL and cardiovascular disease risk, whereas gain-of-function mutations increase LDL and cardiovascular disease risk.[96] Early clinical trials suggest that inhibiting the protein encoded by *PCSK9* is a promising strategy for lowering LDL and preventing cardiovascular disease.[97] Identifying genes that, when inactivated by nature, protect from disease offers several advantages for therapeutic targeting: (1) the target is already validated in humans, (2) designing inhibitors of gene/protein function is more tractable than

increasing gene/protein function, and (3) nature has performed a lifelong clinical trial of inhibiting gene function, and the side effects of doing so are known. In the case of *PCSK9*, individuals with loss-of-function mutations demonstrated no phenotypic abnormalities other than low LDL levels and decreased risk of heart attack. In a similar example, naturally occurring mutations that disrupt *NPC1L1* function, the inhibitory target of ezetimibe, were found to be associated with reduced plasma LDL cholesterol levels and a reduced risk of CHD.[98]

Genetic risk predictors of CHD based on lipid-associated loci alone add little to the excellent risk prediction already provided by clinical risk factors, but when combined with CHD-associated loci they can provide clinically meaningful CHD risk prediction. An early study utilized nine SNPs at loci known to alter lipid metabolism (*LDLR*, *APOB*, *HMGCR*, *PCSK9*, *CTEP*, *LPL*, *ABCA1*, *APOE*, and *LIPC*) to construct a genotype risk score and predict time to first cardiovascular event in a Swedish cohort.[99] Even when the baseline lipid levels were corrected for the genotype, the risk score was statistically associated with cardiovascular disease, indicating that the genotype-based score contained information not captured by serum lipid assessment.[99] However, when this nine-SNP risk score was added to a score derived from standard clinical risk factors, it did not improve risk prediction further. A subsequent study added SNPs associated directly with CHD from GWAS unrelated to lipid levels to create a 13-SNP genotype risk score.[100] This 13-SNP risk score also did not improve risk prediction over clinical risk factors alone.[100] By contrast, a 27-SNP risk score consisting of both lipid and CHD-associated loci provided a threefold reduction in the number needed to treat with statins to prevent a CHD event as compared to clinical risk factors alone.[101] This study was performed in high-risk primary prevention cohorts.[101]

Given the broad indications for statins in primary and secondary CHD prevention,[102] genetics can help to predict and elucidate side effects. GWAS has identified a few reproducible loci (*APOE*, *LPA*, *SLCO1B1*, and *SORT1/CELSR2/PSRC1*) for the trait of LDL response following statin therapy.[103] *SLCO1B1* encodes the organic anion transporter, OATP1B1, which has been shown to regulate the hepatic uptake of statins.[104] When exposed to a single dose of simvastatin, individuals carrying a missense variant in *SLCO1B1* (V174A), which causes loss-of-function, have up to a 2.5-fold increase in plasma levels of statin.[104] A GWAS for statin-induced myopathy performed in a secondary prevention cohort receiving high-dose simvastatin identified the same genetic signal (via a noncoding SNP within the same haplotype) at *SLCO1B1*, which conferred a 4.5-fold risk of myopathy for one allele and a 16.9-fold risk of myopathy in homozygous individuals.[105] The investigators estimated that 60% of the myopathy cases in their cohort were due to this variant at *SLCO1B1*.[105] They performed GWAS on only 200 case controls for myopathy, and it is likely that additional pharmacogenetically relevant loci like *SLCO1B1* will be identified in future studies with larger sample sizes. A number of observational and intervention studies have also associated statin therapy with increased T2D risk. An important question is whether this risk is mediated by an off-target effect of statins or an on-target effect via HMG-CoA reductase. An off-target effect suggests that new, more specific statins could be developed without this side effect, whereas an on-target effect implies that the development of more potent and specific statins would increase the risk of T2D. Genetics has begun to shed light on this question. Taking a mendelian randomization approach, investigators have found that SNPs at HMGCR that decrease LDL levels also increase BMI, insulin resistance, and risk for T2D, suggesting an on-target mechanism for statin-mediated T2D risk.

CONSIDERATIONS FOR CLINICAL USE OF GENETIC INFORMATION AND SEQUENCING IN ENDOCRINOLOGY

As detailed previously, the clinical applications of genetic information include diagnosis, prognosis, risk prediction, and personalized therapy (e.g., pharmacogenetics). In the past, the cost of DNA sequencing placed limitations on the use of genetic testing. Revolutionary advances in sequencing technologies (collectively referred to as next-generation sequencing [NGS]) have made it feasible to sequence every gene in the genomes of all individuals at low cost. With the barriers of cost and feasibility diminishing every year, we believe that the use of genetic information will become commonplace in clinical practice. To maximize benefits to patients while minimizing the burden of false-positive and false-negative results, clinicians will have to select the right patients, deploy the appropriate genetic testing technology, and interpret the results. Specific clinical algorithms for patient/genetic test selection are being proposed for various endocrine diseases (e.g., short stature),[75] but they will take time to validate. With this in mind, we present a series of broad patient scenarios ranging from those with no clinically apparent disease to affected individuals with clinically identifiable genetic syndromes, summarizing benefits and caveats of genetic testing in each scenario. We subsequently review issues related to targeted and genome-wide testing and provide some guidance for patient and test selection. Finally, we provide an overview of disease-relevant classification of genetic findings, examine the interpretation of genetic information as presented in a clinical laboratory report, and make suggestions for clinical decision making (Fig. 4-3).

Genome Screening in the General Population

Population-based screening for mendelian mutations known to cause disease would seem to be an advantageous application of genome sequencing. As mentioned earlier, certain mutations in the *RET* gene predispose to aggressive MTC with such high penetrance that the American Thyroid Association recommends prophylactic thyroidectomy in infants under 1 year of age.[25] As genome sequencing becomes commonplace, it seems reasonable that genomes from the general population (e.g., as part of newborn screening) might be examined for *RET* mutations causing this rare but potentially fatal disease. Cases of cancer might be prevented and lives saved. However, one must consider that the clinical data on *RET* gene mutations have been obtained from kindreds affected by MEN2A/B and familial MTC (Chapter 39). Are genotype-phenotype correlations between *RET* mutations and MTC, or between other gene mutations and risk of other diseases, applicable to someone from the general population with no family history of disease?

An investigation of mendelian diabetes mutations ascertained in the general population suggests that genotype-phenotype correlations identified in mendelian disease families may not generally hold for the population at large. As a case in point, genome sequencing of a population-based U.S. cohort phenotyped longitudinally for diabetes identified 25 individuals with mutations previously known to cause autosomal dominant diabetes (MODY). Despite harboring mutations from a curated catalog of disease genes (Human Gene Mutation Database Professional[106]) only one of these individuals met clinical criteria for MODY, and overall this group of MODY mutation carriers developed diabetes at a rate no different from that in the general population. As population-based sequencing becomes prevalent, it will become necessary to reexamine estimates of penetrance and genotype-phenotype correlations in the context of differing genetic backgrounds (e.g.,

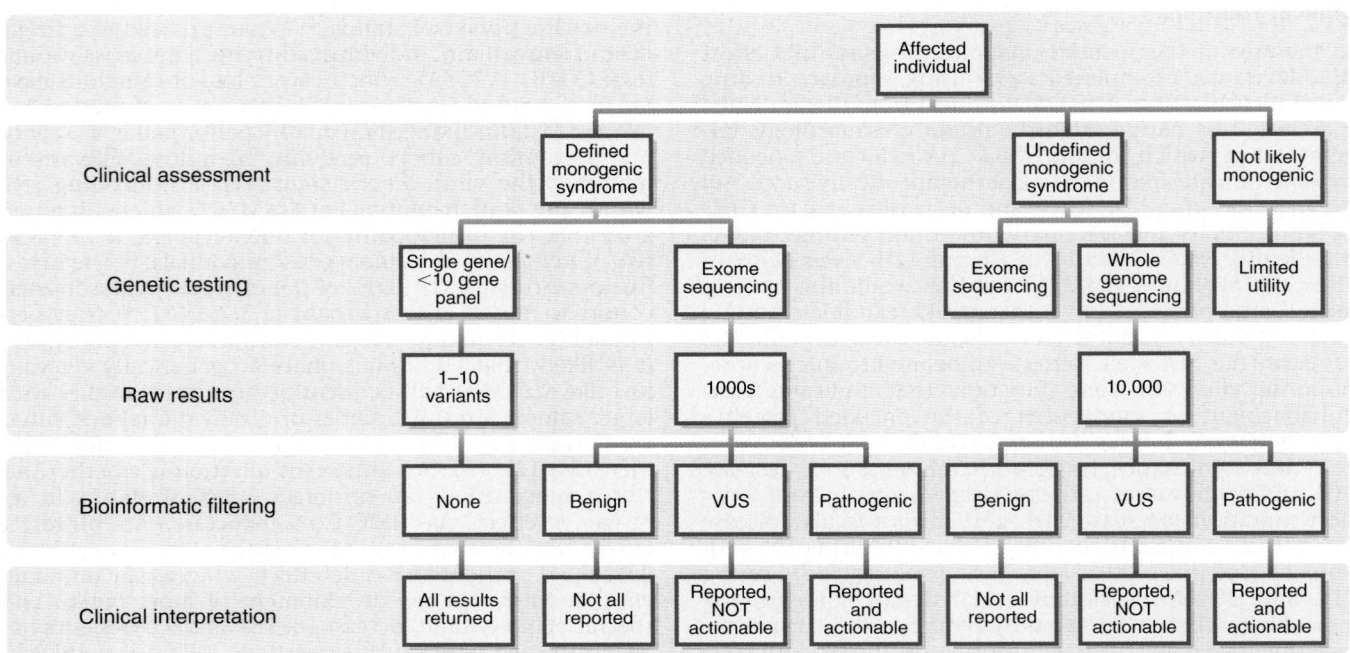

Figure 4-3 Suggested use of targeted and genome-wide genetic testing in individuals suspected of a harboring a monogenic/mendelian disease. VUS, variant of uncertain significance (see text).

ancestry) and environment. The current evidence and state of knowledge do not support genome sequencing for population-based screening.

Genetic Information and Sequencing in Individual Patients

Asymptomatic Individuals

Endocrinologists may be referred individuals with no apparent symptoms in whom risk of disease may be increased: (1) those with a family history of known genetic disease who have not yet been tested and (2) those without family history who were tested and found with an apparently pathogenic mutation (i.e., a genetic incidentaloma). As with any medical test, the implication of genetic testing with regard to the likelihood of developing disease in the individual depends on a combination of inherent test characteristics (quantified by sensitivity/specificity) and the pretest likelihood of disease. For individuals with a family history of genetic disease the pretest probability of disease can be as high as 1 in 2 for a highly penetrant autosomal dominant disorder or 1 in 4 for a sibling of an individual with a recessive disorder. Thus, for individuals with a family history of mendelian endocrine disease, genetic testing is often warranted (depending on the risks and benefits for the individual patient at hand, including psychosocial factors); this fits well with current clinical practice for asymptomatic individuals from families with mendelian disorders.

On the other hand, for individuals with no family history presenting with a mendelian-like genetic incidentaloma, the pretest likelihood of disease is that of the population (1 : 10,000 to 1 : 100,000). Even with a mutation conferring 50-fold increased risk, the individual is far more likely to remain free of disease. So what reassurance can be offered to such individuals who carry mendelian mutations? Population-based sequencing surveys reveal that, on average, the genome of an apparently healthy individual contains approximately 100 mendelian-like disruptive mutations (i.e., frameshifting indels and SNPs resulting in premature stop codons) up to 20 of which are homozygously inactivated.[107] Thus, even the protein-coding portion of the human genome (comprising only 1-2% of the total genome) contains unexpected redundancy that protects from disease. Depending on the severity of clinical consequences, and the estimate of penetrance in the general population, watchful waiting can be a prudent course of action.

Symptomatic Individuals

Individuals with symptomatic disease can present with clinically defined or unknown syndromes. In both cases, a genetic diagnosis can be of psychological benefit, inform family planning, and sometimes can direct therapeutic screening/intervention. The genotype-phenotype correlation of endocrine tumor syndromes (MEN1, MEN2; see previous discussion) are a classic example of the benefits of genetic diagnosis for directed screening and prophylactic interventions in both affected individuals and close relatives. For example, the genotype-phenotype correlation of *RET* oncogene mutations dictates the urgency of prophylactic thyroidectomy (ranging from <1 year old to >5 years old) in children.[25] Thus, even with a clinical diagnosis, genetic testing can have great prognostic value. Another example is the 3-M syndrome (clinically defined by short stature, facial dysmorphism, and skeletal abnormalities) caused by mutations in the *CUL7* gene (among others). Males with this syndrome are at high risk for hypogonad-

ism and should be screened more vigilantly as a result of the genetic diagnosis to prevent future infertility. Sometimes, a genetic diagnosis can allow a patient to avoid lifelong treatment and testing. Individuals with diabetes from *GCK* mutations (MODY2) manifest hyperglycemia but are still able to regulate their blood sugar levels such that they neither require hypoglycemic therapy nor are at elevated risk for secondary complications of diabetes. More generally, and especially for heterogeneous endocrine diseases such as diabetes, genetic classification has the potential to guide pharmacotherapy. An existing example of genetically guided pharmacotherapy can be found in individuals with diabetes caused by *HNF1A* mutations. In clinical trials, these *HNF1A* mutation carriers were much more sensitive to sulfonylureas than noncarriers and maintained more durable glycemic control without additional agents.[60]

As in the above-described cases, genetic testing of affected patients is most likely to be informative when a high penetrance genetic variant is identified (i.e., for rare mendelian-type diseases). We offer the following criteria and mnemonic (SSSS), which should raise clinical suspicion for a mendelian disorder: (1) severe—more severe than usual for the disease, (2) segregating—multiple affected family members or family history of consanguinity, (3) syndromic—features such as dysmorphism, developmental abnormalities, unusual biochemical phenotypes, etc.), and (4) too soon—early age of onset. The diagnostic yield of genetic testing is highly variable both due to technologic reasons and underlying genetic (locus) heterogeneity. Even for well-described mendelian syndromes such as MEN1, 30% of kindreds have no identifiable mutations identified by *MEN1* gene sequencing. For affected individuals with unknown syndromes, or for whom targeted sequencing has failed to make a diagnosis, systematic gene sequencing using NGS methods would be required, and diagnostic yields are typically lower. A National Institutes of Health (NIH) study of exome sequencing for rare disorders found a diagnosis in 20% of cases.[108]

Selection of Genetic Tests: Targeted Versus Genome-wide Approaches

If cost were no object, one might consider deploying whole genome sequencing to maximize sensitivity and find the "smoking gun" mutation in every case. Using genome sequencing in this way is tantamount to performing thousands of genetic tests at once and clinically analogous to ordering every possible hormone level for every endocrine patient. Intuitively, this approach is not pursued because every test carries with it the possibility of false-positive results. The more tests one orders, the more likely at least one result will be false. The same logic applies to genetic tests and genome sequencing. Even if genetic variants are identified with 100% analytical sensitivity and specificity, their clinical sensitivity and specificity for disease risk are much less, due to incomplete penetrance, variable expressivity, and our incomplete knowledge of genotype-phenotype correlations. Thus, targeted testing (either measuring variation in a requested set of genes or masking/only reporting back variation in the requested set of genes) can decrease false-positive results. In addition, clinical laboratories that focus on testing specific sets of genes may be particularly well versed in interpretation of variation in these genes, potentially improving sensitivity and specificity. Of course, when targeted testing is negative, then more comprehensive testing may be required to make a diagnosis.

However, even beyond the issue of false-positive findings, targeted testing may offer superior analytic performance. Detection of variants can be highly variable in current versions of genome-wide sequencing, in which millions of genetic variants are identified simultaneously.[109] There is often a tradeoff between the number of variants identified and the sensitivity/specificity for detecting and calling any individual variant. This analytic sensitivity/specificity relates to coverage, which is the depth of sequencing performed, or the number of independent times a particular nucleotide has been sequenced in a single test. Depth can vary greatly across the genome. For example, a clinical trial of whole-genome sequencing reported clinical grade genome sequencing at "30× coverage on average and at least 8× coverage for more than 95% of bases."[110] This means that of the 3 billion bases in the human genome, each base was sequenced independently 30 times on average, and more than 95% of bases were observed at least 8 times. However, 5% of the human genome was still poorly observed or missing. Thus, if clinical suspicion motivated examination of certain genes or genomic regions, a targeted approach might well have higher analytic sensitivity and specificity. The above-described clinical grade genome is sufficient for detecting variants at a frequency found with germline heterozygosity (on average 50% of the molecules sequenced would contain the variant base), but for disorders requiring detection below germline heterozygosity, such as somatic mutation testing in tumors, higher coverage would be required.

The molecular type of genetic variation (single-base changes or more complex variation such as insertions/deletions/duplications) strongly affects the analytic sensitivity and specificity. The most commonly used gene-panel and genome-wide tests rely on NGS technology, which is currently well suited for detecting single or multiple base variations, but poorly optimized for the detection of structural variants (chromosomal rearrangements), triplet repeat expansions, and CNVs. For example, all false-positive genetic variants identified in a pilot clinical-grade genome sequencing study were indels or were near repetitive DNA stretches.[110] As NGS technology and genome reconstruction algorithms improve, so will the ability to accurately detect these more complex genetic variants, reducing both false-negative and false-positive results. Currently, alternative modes of testing, such as chromosomal microarrays (array CGH), are used to identify large (>50 kb) structural and CNVs.[111]

Interpretation of Identified Genetic Variants

Once genetic variants are identified (from sequencing or otherwise), they must be interpreted for their impact on health and disease. This interpretation requires the integration of population data (to know whether a variant is seen at higher frequency than expected for a pathogenic variant), computational predictions, experimental evidence, and familial comparisons. Curated databases are being established to begin to accurately catalogue this information and assist in interpretation. The ClinVar archive aggregates information about genomic variation and its relationship to human health.[112]

Identified variants can be classified into three broad clinical categories: benign variants, pathogenic variants, and variants of uncertain significance (VUS), but intermediate categories have also been proposed.[113] In single-gene or disease-targeted testing, the number of identified variants is small enough to allow for the individual assessment of all variants in each patient, once common benign variations are curated. However, exome sequencing identifies tens of thousands of variants, and genome sequencing identifies several million in each individual.[114] Thus, automated filtering is necessary to point out a few pathogenic

variants in a haystack of benign ones. Based on the assumption that the testing was done for a highly penetrant, mendelian variant, most genetic variants can be filtered as benign based on having been observed at a frequency greater than 1% (or even lower thresholds for rare disorders) in suitable reference populations. Computational analysis can support a benign classification by showing a variant is *silent* (e.g., encodes the same amino acid as the reference base). Experimental data can provide evidence that a missense variant does not alter protein function in disease-relevant bioassays. In addition, family-based data can be extremely powerful for interpretation; for example, the vast majority of variants for dominant diseases can be classified as benign if they are also observed in healthy relatives. Typically, the filtering of benign variants results in a 100-fold to 1000-fold reduction in the number of variants, requiring further analysis to 30 to 300 variants.[12,110]

Among these, a similar hierarchy of evidence can support a *pathogenic* designation, or the evidence can remain inconclusive, resulting in a VUS designation. Computational analysis showing predicted gene disruption (premature stop or frameshift variants) in a gene known to cause disease when inactivated provides strong evidence of pathogenicity. Experiments in disease-relevant bioassays can demonstrate deleteriousness of a variant, and family-based data can increase the conclusiveness of findings by showing that a proposed pathogenic variant segregates with disease or that it is absent from both parents in de novo cases of disease. Presence of the variant in databases such as the Human Gene Mutation Database (HGMD) can also provide supportive evidence, but the quality of evidence can vary widely among variants. Before final reporting, variants classified as pathogenic are typically validated by resequencing using traditional methods (i.e., Sanger sequencing),[113] although this practice may shift depending on the state of sequencing technology. In a recent pilot case-control study of 20 cardiomyopathy patients and controls subjected to genome sequencing, 2 to 4 variants per individual (in both cases and controls) were classified as pathogenic,[110] illustrating the challenges in interpreting genetic variation in isolation.

Using a Genetics Laboratory Report to Make Clinical Decisions

In the clinic, genetic testing is used to identify or confirm the cause of disease and to help the physicians make individualized treatment decisions (Table 4-5). Given the complexity of genetic testing, especially at the genomic (exome or genome) scale, physicians and clinical laboratories will have to work collaboratively to achieve useful results. For example, when a laboratory finds a rare or novel variant in the course of genomic sequencing, the director cannot assume it is relevant to a patient just because it is rare, or novel. The context of the patient's history, physical examinations, and previous laboratory examinations are key to distinguishing among causal variants for the patient's disorder, incidental findings, and benign variants.

How should identified variants be used in clinical decision making? Variant analysis contains uncertainties that are implicitly defined in the three-part classification described earlier: benign, pathogenic, and VUS. American College of Medical Genetics (ACMG) guidelines[113] recommend that variants classified as pathogenic can be used in clinical decision making. However, genetic evidence should not be the only evidence of disease and should be used in conjunction with complementary clinical information when possible, especially as some pathogenic variants may be misclassified. Examples of corroborative clinical data

TABLE 4-5

Examining a Clinical Genetics Laboratory Report

A clinician considers several issues when examining a clinical genetics laboratory report:

Technical Summary of Genetic Testing

For targeted tests, the list of genes tested and coverage for each gene can be found at the Genetic Testing laboratory (http://www.ncbi.nlm.nih.gov/sites/GeneTests). For genomic tests, average coverage (e.g., >30×) and minimum coverage (e.g., >8× for 95% of bases) should be considered in evaluating test quality. Genes with poor coverage or no coverage should be listed. For both targeted and genomic testing, the specific limitations of detection for different molecular classes of genetic variants given the technology utilized (e.g., copy number variants are not well captured by next-generation sequencing) should be described.

Clinical Interpretation

With regard to the clinical indication for testing, was the test positive (an explanatory variant identified for the patient's condition), negative (no explanatory variants identified), or inconclusive (only variants of uncertain significance [VUS] identified)? Does the potential explanatory variant fit with the clinical scenario, or at least explain some of the patient's phenotypes? With regard to incidental findings, is there a carrier risk to future progeny or future risk of monogenic disease to the patient? A compendium of monogenic diseases and their patterns of inheritance can be found at the Online Mendelian Inheritance in Man (OMIM) website (www.omim.org/).

Variant Reporting and Classification

When applicable, the gene name, transcript, molecular form of variant (SNP, indel, etc.), base changes, amino acid change, zygosity, population frequency, and classification (benign, pathogenic, VUS) should be provided. Naming conventions are determined by the HUGO Gene Nomenclature Committee (http://www.genenames.org). Variant frequencies in the population can be found at the 1000 Genomes Project (http://www.1000genomes.org) and for exomes at the Exome Aggregation Consortium (http://exac.broadinstitute.org/). The justification for variant classifications should be provided, taking into account family-based data if available and information from clinical databases. Previously reported relationships among variants and phenotypes can be found at ClinVar (http://www.ncbi.nlm.nih.gov/clinvar).[112] The analytic accuracy of each reported variant in terms of coverage and validation (e.g., Sanger resequencing) should be reported.

include enzyme assays, physical findings, and imaging studies. VUS should generally not be used in clinical decision making. Efforts to resolve the classification of the variant as pathogenic or benign should be undertaken, and interpretation in the context of the patient's clinical scenario is critical. Variants classified as benign can usually be assumed not to cause the patient's disorder.

Detection of pathogenic variants incidental to the diagnostic motivation for sequencing, but of potential clinical relevance, will be an inevitable consequence of genomic testing. This scenario is analogous to the inevitable detection of adrenal masses in computed tomography scans or thyroid nodules on physical examination. A clinician ordering genomic testing should be aware of laboratory policies and current ethical guidelines regarding such incidental or secondary findings. Current recommendations are to offer the patient the option not to receive such incidental findings, and laboratories may vary in their reporting of such incidental findings. From both the clinician and patient perspective, incidental findings can also be specifically requested or declined. The laboratory should provide clear information about what constitutes a report-able incidental finding and how they may be requested or declined. Guidelines have been set forth in the ACMG recommendations for reporting of incidental findings in clinical exome and genome sequencing.[115]

Future Perspectives and Summary

In the future, we anticipate that a genome sequence will become a standard accompaniment to the medical chart; thus, the question Should we sequence? will transmute to What part of the sequence should we look at? A rational clinical approach will require the discipline to not look at all of it, or at least to rigorously interpret sequence data in the clinical context. As detailed previously, every human genome is littered with thousands of VUS and multiple variants classified as pathogenic; clinical suspicion is essential to help direct where to look and how to interpret genetic variation. This approach recapitulates current clinical algorithms for genetic testing. For example, familial paraganglioma shows locus heterogeneity as a mendelian disorder with cases attributable to mutations in multiple genes encoding proteins for the succinate dehydrogenase complex. The current genetic testing algorithm is hierarchical, starting with sequencing of the *SDHD* gene where the majority of causal mutations are found (Chapter 16). If no mutations in *SDHD* are found, other complex members are tested (e.g., *SDHC*). In a genome-sequencing era, a clinical algorithm might hierarchically look up mutations in the succinate dehydrogenase complex members from a sequenced individual with familial paraganglioma syndrome. No additional sequencing costs would be incurred as each gene is subsequently tested, but honing in on the appropriate and interpretable areas of the genome will reduce the clinical burden of false-positive results.

In summary, genetic information is most likely to be of clinical use in individuals with suspected mendelian syndromes (see 4S criteria enumerated earlier). For individuals with a clinically defined syndrome, for which targeted panels exist and are well validated, a targeted approach (single-gene or gene panel testing) is currently recommended as an initial approach. For example, genome-wide sequencing is likely not needed when MEN2B is suspected on clinical grounds; sequencing *RET* will usually make a diagnosis. If results from targeted genetic testing are uninformative, and the suspicion of a genetic disorder is high, exome or genome sequencing will make additional diagnoses in some patients (see Fig. 4-3). We recommend primary genome-wide approaches that assess both structural variation and sequence variation for individuals with clinically unclassifiable genetic syndromes or when targeted panels are not available or well validated. Depending on technologic progress, this may simply be an unmasking of data that had not been reported back in a targeted test or may require new sequencing. The exome comprises 1% to 2% of the genome yet contains nearly 85% of known disease-causing mutations.[116] Thus, given current technologies, exome sequencing supplemented with or following array CGH is a reasonable initial genome-wide approach. Many other best practices will improve the outcome of genetic diagnosis through sequencing. Ideally, DNA from both parents should be obtained, if possible, and DNA from additional relatives may also aid in interpretation. If unaffected and affected tissues are identified, paired affected tissue-blood samples should be obtained when possible. Identified variants can be classified as benign, pathogenic, or VUS based on cross referencing with databases of diseased and undiseased individuals as well as family members, computational analysis, and experimental evidence. Indeed, in order to maximize interpretability of any genomic approach, it will be vital to interpret variation in the context of massive numbers of genome sequences obtained in healthy individuals and in patients with disease. Finally, accurate classification will require physicians and clinical laboratories to work collaboratively, and the resulting genetic information should always be used in conjunction with complementary data (chemistries, imaging, etc.) for clinical decision making.

REFERENCES

1. Sturtevant AH. *A History of Genetics*. New York, NY: Harper & Row; 1965:165.
2. Botstein D, White RL, Skolnick M, Davis RW. Construction of a genetic linkage map in man using restriction fragment length polymorphisms. *Am J Hum Genet*. 1980;32(3):314-331.
3. Fisher RA. The causes of human variability. *Eugen Rev*. 1919;10(4):213-220.
4. Altshuler D, Daly MJ, Lander ES. Genetic mapping in human disease. *Science*. 2008;322(5903):881-888.
5. Visscher PM, Medland SE, Ferreira MAR, et al. Assumption-free estimation of heritability from genome-wide identity-by-descent sharing between full siblings. *PLoS Genet*. 2006;2(3):e41.
6. Kaprio J, Tuomilehto J, Koskenvuo M, et al. Concordance for type 1 (insulin-dependent) and type 2 (non-insulin-dependent) diabetes mellitus in a population-based cohort of twins in Finland. *Diabetologia*. 1992;35(11):1060-1067.
7. Diabetes mellitus in twins: a cooperative study in Japan. Committee on Diabetic Twins, Japan Diabetes Society. *Diabetes Res Clin Pract*. 1988;5(4):271-280.
8. Kondrashova A, Viskari H, Kulmala P, et al. Signs of beta-cell autoimmunity in nondiabetic schoolchildren: a comparison between Russian Karelia with a low incidence of type 1 diabetes and Finland with a high incidence rate. *Diabetes Care*. 2007;30(1):95-100.
9. Kondrashova A, Reunanen A, Romanov A, et al. A six-fold gradient in the incidence of type 1 diabetes at the eastern border of Finland. *Ann Med*. 2005;37(1):67-72.
10. Onengut-Gumuscu S, Chen WM, Burren O, et al. Fine mapping of type 1 diabetes susceptibility loci and evidence for colocalization of causal variants with lymphoid gene enhancers. *Nat Genet*. 2015;47(4):381-386.
11. Jaiswal S, Fontanillas P, Flannick J, et al. Age-related clonal hematopoiesis associated with adverse outcomes. *N Engl J Med*. 2014;371:2488-2498.
12. Tennessen JA, Bigham AW, O'Connor TD, et al. Evolution and functional impact of rare coding variation from deep sequencing of human exomes. *Science*. 2012;337(6090):64-69.
13. Flannick J, Beer NL, Bick AG, et al. Assessing the phenotypic effects in the general population of rare variants in genes for a dominant mendelian form of diabetes. *Nat Genet*. 2013;45(11):1380-1385.
14. International HapMap Consortium. The International HapMap Project. *Nature*. 2003;426(6968):789-796.
15. National Human Genome Research Institute. A Catalog of Published Genome-Wide Association Studies. Available at: <http://www.genome.gov/gwastudies/>.
16. Farh KK, Marson A, Zhu J, et al. Genetic and epigenetic fine mapping of causal autoimmune disease variants. *Nature*. 2015;518(7539):337-343.
17. Nejentsev S, Howson JM, Walker NM, et al. Localization of type 1 diabetes susceptibility to the MHC class I genes HLA-B and HLA-A. *Nature*. 2007;450(7171):887-892.
18. Musunuru K, Strong A, Frank-Kamenetsky M, et al. From noncoding variant to phenotype via SORT1 at the 1p13 cholesterol locus. *Nature*. 2010;466(7307):714-719.
19. O'Rahilly S, Farooqi IS. Human obesity: a heritable neurobehavioral disorder that is highly sensitive to environmental conditions. *Diabetes*. 2008;57(11):2905-2910.
20. Musunuru K, Pirruccello JP, Do R, et al. Exome sequencing, ANGPTL3 mutations, and familial combined hypolipidemia. *N Engl J Med*. 2010;363(23):2220-2227.
21. Choi M, Scholl UI, Yue P, et al. K+ channel mutations in adrenal aldosterone-producing adenomas and hereditary hypertension. *Science*. 2011;331(6018):768-772.
22. Scholl UI, Goh G, Stolting G, et al. Somatic and germline CACNA1D calcium channel mutations in aldosterone-producing adenomas and primary aldosteronism. *Nat Genet*. 2013;45(9):1050-1054.
23. Plenge RM, Scolnick EM, Altshuler D. Validating therapeutic targets through human genetics. *Nat Rev Drug Discov*. 2013;12(8):581-594.
24. Hameed S, Jayasena CN, Dhillo WS. Kisspeptin and fertility. *J Endocrinol*. 2011;208(2):97-105.
25. Kloos RT, Eng C, Evans DB, et al. Medullary thyroid cancer: management guidelines of the American Thyroid Association. *Thyroid*. 2009;19(6):565-612.
26. Kapoor RR, James C, Hussain K. Advances in the diagnosis and management of hyperinsulinemic hypoglycemia. *Nat Clin Pract Endocrinol Metab*. 2009;5(2):101-112.
27. O'Rahilly S. Human genetics illuminates the paths to metabolic disease. *Nature*. 2009;462(7271):307-314.
28. Bonnefond A, Froguel P. Rare and common genetic events in type 2 diabetes: what should biologists know? *Cell Metab*. 2015;21(3):357-368.
29. Morris AP, Voight BF, Teslovich TM, et al. Large-scale association analysis provides insights into the genetic architecture and pathophysiology of type 2 diabetes. *Nat Genet*. 2012;44(9):981-990.
30. Wellcome Trust Case Control Consortium. Genome-wide association study of 14,000 cases of seven common diseases and 3,000 shared controls. *Nature*. 2007;447(7145):661-678.
31. Todd JA, Bell JI, McDevitt HO. HLA-DQ beta gene contributes to susceptibility and resistance to insulin-dependent diabetes mellitus. *Nature*. 1987;329(6140):599-604.
32. Rotter JI, Landaw EM. Measuring the genetic contribution of a single locus to a multilocus disease. *Clin Genet*. 1984;26(6):529-542.
33. Jeninga EH, Gurnell M, Kalkhoven E. Functional implications of genetic variation in human PPARgamma. *Trends Endocrinol Metab*. 2009;20(8):380-387.
34. Voight BF, Scott LJ, Steinthorsdottir V, et al. Twelve type 2 diabetes susceptibility loci identified through large-scale association analysis. *Nat Genet*. 2010;42(7):579-589.
35. Bouatia-Naji N, Bonnefond A, Cavalcanti-Proenca C, et al. A variant near MTNR1B is associated with increased fasting plasma glucose levels and type 2 diabetes risk. *Nat Genet*. 2009;41(1):89-94.
36. Bonnefond A, Clement N, Fawcett K, et al. Rare MTNR1B variants impairing melatonin receptor 1B function contribute to type 2 diabetes. *Nat Genet*. 2012;44(3):297-301.
37. DIAbetes Genetics Replication And Meta-analysis (DIAGRAM) Consortium, Asian Genetic Epidemiology Network Type 2 Diabetes (AGEN-T2D) Consortium, South Asian Type 2 Diabetes (SAT2D) Consortium, et al. Genome-wide trans-ancestry meta-analysis provides insight into the genetic architecture of type 2 diabetes susceptibility. *Nat Genet*. 2014;46(3):234-244.
38. SIGMA Type 2 Diabetes Consortium, Williams AL, Jacobs SB, et al. Sequence variants in SLC16A11 are a common risk factor for type 2 diabetes in Mexico. *Nature*. 2014;506(7486):97-101.
39. Hara K, Fujita H, Johnson TA, et al. Genome-wide association study identifies three novel loci for type 2 diabetes. *Hum Mol Genet*. 2014;23(1):239-246.
40. Moltke I, Grarup N, Jorgensen ME, et al. A common Greenlandic TBC1D4 variant confers muscle insulin resistance and type 2 diabetes. *Nature*. 2014;512(7513):190-193.
41. Vassy JL, Hivert MF, Porneala B, et al. Polygenic type 2 diabetes prediction at the limit of common variant detection. *Diabetes*. 2014;63(6):2172-2182.
42. Dimas AS, Lagou V, Barker A, et al. Impact of type 2 diabetes susceptibility variants on quantitative glycemic traits reveals mechanistic heterogeneity. *Diabetes*. 2014;63(6):2158-2171.
43. Zeggini E, Weedon MN, Lindgren CM, et al. Replication of genome-wide association signals in UK samples reveals risk loci for type 2 diabetes. *Science*. 2007;316(5829):1336-1341.
44. Dina C, Meyre D, Gallina S, et al. Variation in FTO contributes to childhood obesity and severe adult obesity. *Nat Genet*. 2007;39(6):724-726.
45. Frayling TM, Timpson NJ, Weedon MN, et al. A common variant in the FTO gene is associated with body mass index and predisposes to childhood and adult obesity. *Science*. 2007;316(5826):889-894.
46. Scuteri A, Sanna S, Chen WM, et al. Genome-wide association scan shows genetic variants in the FTO gene are associated with obesity-related traits. *PLoS Genet*. 2007;3(7):e115.
47. Smemo S, Tena JJ, Kim KH, et al. Obesity-associated variants within FTO form long-range functional connections with IRX3. *Nature*. 2014;507(7492):371-375.
48. Church C, Moir L, McMurray F, et al. Overexpression of Fto leads to increased food intake and results in obesity. *Nat Genet*. 2010;42(12):1086-1092.
49. Wahlen K, Sjolin E, Hoffstedt J. The common rs9939609 gene variant of the fat mass- and obesity-associated gene FTO is related to fat cell lipolysis. *J Lipid Res*. 2008;49(3):607-611.
50. Dupuis J, Langenberg C, Prokopenko I, et al. New genetic loci implicated in fasting glucose homeostasis and their impact on type 2 diabetes risk. *Nat Genet*. 2010;42(2):105-116.
51. Bonnefond A, Vaxillaire M, Labrune Y, et al. Genetic variant in HK1 is associated with a proanemic state and A1C but not other glycemic control-related traits. *Diabetes*. 2009;58(11):2687-2697.
52. Vaxillaire M, Dechaume A, Busiah K, et al. New ABCC8 mutations in relapsing neonatal diabetes and clinical features. *Diabetes*. 2007;56(6):1737-1741.
53. Sladek R, Rocheleau G, Rung J, et al. A genome-wide association study identifies novel risk loci for type 2 diabetes. *Nature*. 2007;445(7130):881-885.

54. Flannick J, Thorleifsson G, Beer NL, et al. Loss-of-function mutations in SLC30A8 protect against type 2 diabetes. *Nat Genet.* 2014;46(4):357-363.

55. Altshuler D, Hirschhorn JN, Klannemark M, et al. The common PPAR-gamma Pro12Ala polymorphism is associated with decreased risk of type 2 diabetes. *Nat Genet.* 2000;26(1):76-80.

56. Meigs JB, Shrader P, Sullivan LM, et al. Genotype score in addition to common risk factors for prediction of type 2 diabetes. *N Engl J Med.* 2008;359(21):2208-2219.

57. Hariri S, Yoon PW, Qureshi N, et al. Family history of type 2 diabetes: a population-based screening tool for prevention? *Genet Med.* 2006; 8(2):102-108.

58. Sagen JV, Raeder H, Hathout E, et al. Permanent neonatal diabetes due to mutations in KCNJ11 encoding Kir6.2: patient characteristics and initial response to sulfonylurea therapy. *Diabetes.* 2004;53(10): 2713-2718.

59. Rafiq M, Flanagan SE, Patch AM, et al. Effective treatment with oral sulfonylureas in patients with diabetes due to sulfonylurea receptor 1 (SUR1) mutations. *Diabetes Care.* 2008;31(2):204-209.

60. Pearson ER, Starkey BJ, Powell RJ, et al. Genetic cause of hyperglycaemia and response to treatment in diabetes. *Lancet.* 2003;362(9392): 1275-1281.

61. Wood AR, Esko T, Yang J, et al. Defining the role of common variation in the genomic and biological architecture of adult human height. *Nat Genet.* 2014;46(11):1173-1186.

62. Yang J, Benyamin B, McEvoy BP, et al. Common SNPs explain a large proportion of the heritability for human height. *Nat Genet.* 2010; 42(7):565-569.

63. Chan Y, Holmen OL, Dauber A, et al. Common variants show predicted polygenic effects on height in the tails of the distribution, except in extremely short individuals. *PLoS Genet.* 2011;7(12): e1002439.

64. Dauber A, Yu Y, Turchin MC, et al. Genome-wide association of copy-number variation reveals an association between short stature and the presence of low-frequency genomic deletions. *Am J Hum Genet.* 2011; 89(6):751-759.

65. Valdar W, Solberg LC, Gauguier D, et al. Genome-wide genetic association of complex traits in heterogeneous stock mice. *Nat Genet.* 2006; 38(8):879-887.

66. Mullis PE. Genetic control of growth. *Eur J Endocrinol.* 2005;152(1): 11-31.

67. Weedon MN, Lango H, Lindgren CM, et al. Genome-wide association analysis identifies 20 loci that influence adult height. *Nat Genet.* 2008;40(5):575-583.

68. Lango Allen H, Estrada K, Lettre G, et al. Hundreds of variants clustered in genomic loci and biological pathways affect human height. *Nature.* 2010;467(7317):832-838.

69. de Pontual L, Yao E, Callier P, et al. Germline deletion of the miR-17 approximately 92 cluster causes skeletal and growth defects in humans. *Nat Genet.* 2011;43(10):1026-1030.

70. Neptune ER, Frischmeyer PA, Arking DE, et al. Dysregulation of TGF-beta activation contributes to pathogenesis in Marfan syndrome. *Nat Genet.* 2003;33(3):407-411.

71. Habashi JP, Judge DP, Holm TM, et al. Losartan, an AT1 antagonist, prevents aortic aneurysm in a mouse model of Marfan syndrome. *Science.* 2006;312(5770):117-121.

72. Lacro RV, Dietz HC, Sleeper LA, et al. Atenolol versus losartan in children and young adults with Marfan's syndrome. *N Engl J Med.* 2014;371(22):2061-2071.

73. Jonquoy A, Mugniery E, Benoist-Lasselin C, et al. A novel tyrosine kinase inhibitor restores chondrocyte differentiation and promotes bone growth in a gain-of-function Fgfr3 mouse model. *Hum Mol Genet.* 2012;21(4):841-851.

74. Yasoda A, Kitamura H, Fujii T, et al. Systemic administration of C-type natriuretic peptide as a novel therapeutic strategy for skeletal dysplasias. *Endocrinology.* 2009;150(7):3138-3144.

75. Dauber A, Rosenfeld RG, Hirschhorn JN. Genetic evaluation of short stature. *J Clin Endocrinol Metab.* 2014;99(9):3080-3092.

76. Wang SR, Carmichael H, Andrew SF, et al. Large-scale pooled next-generation sequencing of 1077 genes to identify genetic causes of short stature. *J Clin Endocrinol Metab.* 2013;98(8):E1428-E1437.

77. David A, Hwa V, Metherell LA, et al. Evidence for a continuum of genetic, phenotypic, and biochemical abnormalities in children with growth hormone insensitivity. *Endocr Rev.* 2011;32(4):472-497.

78. Domene HM, Hwa V, Argente J, et al. Human acid-labile subunit deficiency: clinical, endocrine and metabolic consequences. *Horm Res.* 2009;72(3):129-141.

79. Renes JS, Willemsen RH, Wagner A, et al. Bloom syndrome in short children born small for gestational age: a challenging diagnosis. *J Clin Endocrinol Metab.* 2013;98(10):3932-3938.

80. Weiss LA, Pan L, Abney M, Ober C. The sex-specific genetic architecture of quantitative traits in humans. *Nat Genet.* 2006;38(2): 218-222.

81. Global Lipids Genetics Consortium, Willer CJ, Schmidt EM, et al. Discovery and refinement of loci associated with lipid levels. *Nat Genet.* 2013;45(11):1274-1283.

82. Teslovich TM, Musunuru K, Smith AV, et al. Biological, clinical and population relevance of 95 loci for blood lipids. *Nature.* 2010;466(7307): 707-713.

83. Do R, Stitziel NO, Won HH, et al. Exome sequencing identifies rare LDLR and APOA5 alleles conferring risk for myocardial infarction. *Nature.* 2015;518(7537):102-106.

84. Thormaehlen AS, Schuberth C, Won HH, et al. Systematic cell-based phenotyping of missense alleles empowers rare variant association studies: a case for LDLR and myocardial infarction. *PLoS Genet.* 2015;11(2):e1004855.

85. Brown MS, Goldstein JL. Familial hypercholesterolemia: defective binding of lipoproteins to cultured fibroblasts associated with impaired regulation of 3-hydroxy-3-methylglutaryl coenzyme A reductase activity. *Proc Natl Acad Sci U S A.* 1974;71(3):788-792.

86. Brown MS, Goldstein JL. A receptor-mediated pathway for cholesterol homeostasis. *Science.* 1986;232(4746):34-47.

87. Kathiresan S, Srivastava D. Genetics of human cardiovascular disease. *Cell.* 2012;148(6):1242-1257.

88. Holmes MV, Harrison S, Talmud PJ, et al. Utility of genetic determinants of lipids and cardiovascular events in assessing risk. *Nat Rev Cardiol.* 2011;8(4):207-221.

89. Barter PJ, Caulfield M, Eriksson M, et al. Effects of torcetrapib in patients at high risk for coronary events. *N Engl J Med.* 2007;357(21): 2109-2122.

90. Smith GD, Ebrahim S. Mendelian randomization: prospects, potentials, and limitations. *Int J Epidemiol.* 2004;33(1):30-42.

91. Voight BF, Peloso GM, Orho-Melander M, et al. Plasma HDL cholesterol and risk of myocardial infarction: a mendelian randomisation study. *Lancet.* 2012;380(9841):572-580.

92. Keene D, Price C, Shun-Shin MJ, Francis DP. Effect on cardiovascular risk of high density lipoprotein targeted drug treatments niacin, fibrates, and CETP inhibitors: meta-analysis of randomised controlled trials including 117,411 patients. *BMJ.* 2014;349:g4379.

93. Jorgensen AB, Frikke-Schmidt R, Nordestgaard BG, Tybjaerg-Hansen A. Loss-of-function mutations in APOC3 and risk of ischemic vascular disease. *N Engl J Med.* 2014;371(1):32-41.

94. TG and HDL Working Group of the Exome Sequencing Project, National Heart, Lung, and Blood Institute, Crosby J, Peloso GM, et al. Loss-of-function mutations in APOC3, triglycerides, and coronary disease. *N Engl J Med.* 2014;371(1):22-31.

95. Holmes MV, Asselbergs FW, Palmer TM, et al. Mendelian randomization of blood lipids for coronary heart disease. *Eur Heart J.* 2015;36(9): 539-550.

96. Cohen JC, Boerwinkle E, Mosley TH Jr, Hobbs HH. Sequence variations in PCSK9, low LDL, and protection against coronary heart disease. *N Engl J Med.* 2006;354(12):1264-1272.

97. Blom DJ, Hala T, Bolognese M, et al. A 52-week placebo-controlled trial of evolocumab in hyperlipidemia. *N Engl J Med.* 2014;370(19):1809-1819.

98. Myocardial Infarction Genetics Consortium Investigators, Stitziel NO, Won HH, et al. Inactivating mutations in NPC1L1 and protection from coronary heart disease. *N Engl J Med.* 2014;371(22):2072-2082.

99. Kathiresan S, Melander O, Anevski D, et al. Polymorphisms associated with cholesterol and risk of cardiovascular events. *N Engl J Med.* 2008;358(12):1240-1249.

100. Ripatti S, Tikkanen E, Orho-Melander M, et al. A multilocus genetic risk score for coronary heart disease: case-control and prospective cohort analyses. *Lancet.* 2010;376(9750):1393-1400.

101. Mega JL, Stitziel NO, Smith JG, et al. Genetic risk, coronary heart disease events, and the clinical benefit of statin therapy: an analysis of primary and secondary prevention trials. *Lancet.* 2015;385(9984): 2264-2271.

102. Taylor F, Huffman MD, Macedo AF, et al. Statins for the primary prevention of cardiovascular disease. *Cochrane Database Syst Rev.* 2013; (1):CD004816.

103. Postmus I, Trompet S, Deshmukh HA, et al. Pharmacogenetic meta-analysis of genome-wide association studies of LDL cholesterol response to statins. *Nat Commun.* 2014;5:5068.

104. Wilke RA, Ramsey LB, Johnson SG, et al. The clinical pharmacogenomics implementation consortium: CPIC guideline for SLCO1B1 and simvastatin-induced myopathy. *Clin Pharmacol Ther.* 2012;92(1): 112-117.

105. Link E, Parish S, Armitage J, et al. SLCO1B1 variants and statin-induced myopathy—a genomewide study. *N Engl J Med.* 2008;359(8): 789-799.

106. Stenson PD, Mort M, Ball EV, et al. The Human Gene Mutation Database: 2008 update. *Genome Med.* 2009;1(1):13.

107. MacArthur DG, Balasubramanian S, Frankish A, et al. A systematic survey of loss-of-function variants in human protein-coding genes. *Science.* 2012;335(6070):823-828.

108. Gahl WA, Markello TC, Toro C, et al. The National Institutes of Health Undiagnosed Diseases Program: insights into rare diseases. *Genet Med.* 2012;14(1):51-59.

109. Rehm HL, Bale SJ, Bayrak-Toydemir P, et al. ACMG clinical laboratory standards for next-generation sequencing. *Genet Med.* 2013;15(9): 733-747.

110. McLaughlin HM, Ceyhan-Birsoy O, Christensen KD, et al. A systematic approach to the reporting of medically relevant findings from whole genome sequencing. *BMC Med Genet.* 2014;15:134.

111. Kearney HM, Thorland EC, Brown KK, et al. American College of Medical Genetics standards and guidelines for interpretation and reporting of postnatal constitutional copy number variants. *Genet Med.* 2011;13(7):680-685.

112. National Center for Biotechnology Information. ClinVar website. Available at: <http://www.ncbi.nlm.nih.gov/clinvar>.

113. Richards S, Aziz N, Bale S, et al. Standards and guidelines for the interpretation of sequence variants: a joint consensus recommendation of the American College of Medical Genetics and Genomics and the Association for Molecular Pathology. *Genet Med.* 2015;17(5): 405-424.

114. Rehm HL. Disease-targeted sequencing: a cornerstone in the clinic. *Nat Rev Genet.* 2013;14(4):295-300.

115. Green RC, Berg JS, Grody WW, et al. ACMG recommendations for reporting of incidental findings in clinical exome and genome sequencing. *Genet Med.* 2013;15(7):565-574.

116. Majewski J, Schwartzentruber J, Lalonde E, et al. What can exome sequencing do for you? *J Med Genet.* 2011;48(9):580-589.

117. Barrett JC, Clayton DG, Concannon P, et al. Genome-wide association study and meta-analysis find that over 40 loci affect risk of type 1 diabetes. *Nat Genet.* 2009;41(6):703-707.

118. Diabetes Genetics Initiative of Broad Institute of Harvard and MIT, Lund University, and Novartis Institutes of BioMedical Research, Saxena R, Voight BF, Lyssenko V, et al. Genome-wide association analysis identifies loci for type 2 diabetes and triglyceride levels. *Science.* 2007;316(5829):1331-1336.

119. Fall T, Ingelsson E. Genome-wide association studies of obesity and metabolic syndrome. *Mol Cell Endocrinol.* 2014;382(1):740-757.

120. Loos RJ, Lindgren CM, Li S, et al. Common variants near MC4R are associated with fat mass, weight and risk of obesity. *Nat Genet.* 2008; 40(6):768-775.

121. International Consortium for Blood Pressure Genome-Wide Association Studies, Ehret GB, Munroe PB, Rice KM, et al. Genetic variants in novel pathways influence blood pressure and cardiovascular disease risk. *Nature.* 2011;478(7367):103-109.

122. Dauber A, Hirschhorn JN. Genome-wide association studies in pediatric endocrinology. *Horm Res Paediatr.* 2011;75(5):322-328.

123. Chu X, Pan CM, Zhao SX, et al. A genome-wide association study identifies two new risk loci for Graves' disease. *Nat Genet.* 2011;43(9): 897-901.

124. Eriksson N, Tung JY, Kiefer AK, et al. Novel associations for hypothyroidism include known autoimmune risk loci. *PLoS ONE.* 2012;7(4): e34442.

125. Estrada K, Styrkarsdottir U, Evangelou E, et al. Genome-wide meta-analysis identifies 56 bone mineral density loci and reveals 14 loci associated with risk of fracture. *Nat Genet.* 2012;44(5):491-501.

126. Richards JB, Zheng HF, Spector TD. Genetics of osteoporosis from genome-wide association studies: advances and challenges. *Nat Rev Genet.* 2012;13(8):576-588.

127. Kapur K, Johnson T, Beckmann ND, et al. Genome-wide meta-analysis for serum calcium identifies significantly associated SNPs near the calcium-sensing receptor (CASR) gene. *PLoS Genet.* 2010;6(7):e1001035.

128. O'Seaghdha CM, Yang Q, Glazer NL, et al. Common variants in the calcium-sensing receptor gene are associated with total serum calcium levels. *Hum Mol Genet.* 2010;19(21):4296-4303.

129. Goldfarb DS, Fischer ME, Keich Y, Goldberg J. A twin study of genetic and dietary influences on nephrolithiasis: a report from the Vietnam Era Twin (VET) Registry. *Kidney Int.* 2005;67(3):1053-1061.

130. Urabe Y, Tanikawa C, Takahashi A, et al. A genome-wide association study of nephrolithiasis in the Japanese population identifies novel susceptible loci at 5q35.3, 7p14.3, and 13q14.1. *PLoS Genet.* 2012;8(3): e1002541.

CHAPTER 5

Health Care Reform, Population Health, and the Endocrinologist

GLENN D. BRAUNSTEIN

Man is a pliant animal, a being who gets accustomed to anything.

—Fyodor Dostoyevsky

KEY POINTS

- In 2010 U.S. health care legislation was passed to help improve quality, access, and delivery of health care to a large segment of the population while decreasing the rate of rise in health care costs.
- To reduce costs and variation in the delivery of health care, legislation now provides transparency about health insurance products and supports innovative approaches such as bundling payments to health care systems to care for a defined population of patients.
- Under a bundled payment system, such as with an Accountable Care Organization, coordination of care across the continuum of care is essential in order to increase efficiency and reduce waste. The old volume paradigm is being replaced with the value paradigm, which represents outcomes plus patient experience divided by cost.
- The clinical endocrinologist will be required to direct a multidisciplinary endocrine disease management team, oversee an endocrine disease registry, develop and implement evidence-based guidelines, provide direct and indirect clinical care, teach, and perform clinical research.
- There are many barriers to change that will need to be overcome. They include manpower issues; the aging patient population with an increased prevalence of chronic diseases; the dramatic rise in obesity and diabetes; the emergence of social networks, big data, an overabundance of information, and new technology; and cultural issues.

The American health care system consists of a medley of poorly coordinated microsystems that, for the most part, deliver fragmented, costly, and, at times, inadequate care to the public. Its evolution over the past century has been more the result of political, situational, competitive market forces and lobbying processes than of a rational design to deliver high-quality, cost-effective care to the entire population. It is not possible start over and implement a totally redesigned rational health care system, and therefore, we institute incremental changes and the occasional large disruptive ones such as the Patient Protection and Affordable Care Act (ACA).[1] The combination of legal mandates, cost, outcomes, technology advances, and consumerism together is bringing about unprecedented changes in the way we deliver medical care to the population. The roles of the primary care physician and subspecialist, including endocrinologists, are being redefined at a rapid rate with less emphasis on dealing with each patient in a vacuum, and more on improving and maintain health for all individuals within a population.[2] Some of the consequences will be discussed later in this chapter.

THE CHANGE IMPERATIVE THAT LED TO THE AFFORDABLE CARE ACT

Cost, outcomes, access, and delivery process were key forces that led to the passage of the ACA. Despite a variety of major and minor reforms, health care costs in the United States were rising at an unsustainable rate, accounting for approximately 17% of our gross domestic product—almost one third higher those of the next highest cost member (Netherlands) of the Organisation for Economic Co-operation and Development (OECD) countries, and close to twice the OECD average.[3] Since 2000, the vast majority of health care cost increase has been due to price increases for hospital charges, professional services, drugs and devices, and administrative costs.[4]

There are many reasons why our system is so expensive. One of the major factors is cultural. Until recently, neither physicians, health care systems, nor patients had a major incentive to curtail costs. With the exception of the inpatient Medicare DRG (diagnosis-related group) system on hospitals and fixed payments under the health maintenance organization (HMO) systems on physicians and hospitals, the systems rewarded volume. The more tests ordered and procedures that were performed, the more physicians and hospitals were paid, and this approach has contributed in part to the large amount of variation in Medicare expenditures and procedures performed in different regions of the country as elaborated upon by the Dartmouth Atlas of

Health Care project.[5] Patients also grew accustomed to having everything done without much consideration of cost, unless they had high deductible insurance plans or large co-payments. Additionally, unlike other markets, there has been little price transparency to allow consumers to perform a cost-benefit analysis or to comparison shop, which would be expected to drive down prices.[6]

Another major driver of costs has been the development of new technology. During my own career, I have witnessed the development of immunoassays; computed tomography (CT), magnetic resonance imaging, and positron emission tomography scans; decoding of the human genome; production of protein hormones through recombinant DNA technology; clinically useful molecular diagnostic tests (e.g., *RET* proto-oncogene mutations); laparoscopic, minimally invasive, and robotic surgery; targeted therapies based on genetic defects in tumors; and of course, the information revolution that the Internet has spawned. Once new technologies or therapies are introduced, they are rapidly deployed, whether warranted or not, and for the most part many are expensive and drive up the cost of health care. Rapid dissemination of information about new developments to physicians through publications, meetings, the Internet, and drug or device manufacture detailing along with direct-to-consumer marketing of disease information, tests, procedures, and therapies drive patients to want the latest state-of-the-art treatments and for physicians to provide them. Sometimes the data strongly support the adoption of a new product (e.g., imatinib for chronic myeloid leukemia) and sometimes the cost-benefit equation does not (e.g., robotic thyroidectomy).[7]

Fear of malpractice litigation also plays a role in the overuse of resources ("defensive medicine") and has been estimated to account for 5% to 10% of unnecessary tests and services.[8,9] As recently emphasized by the Choosing Wisely campaign, data have repeatedly shown that patients with headache without neurologic findings or other "red flags" do not benefit from a CT scan of the head.[10,11] Yet, this frequently is done to make sure that a small infarct or a brain tumor in not missed, even though the probability is very low. In fact, head CT scan overuse is very common in patients frequently admitted to medical services, with the vast majority of patients lacking clinically significant findings.[12] A recent meta-analysis determined that 30% of medical laboratory tests that are ordered are unnecessary or inappropriate, especially at the time of the initial evaluation of the patient.[13] Defensive medicine is also frequently practiced in end-of-life situations when the physician accedes to the patient's and family members' insistence that "everything be done" including another round of chemotherapy be administered, intubation and artificial ventilation, gastrostomy tube placement, dialysis, and cardiopulmonary resuscitation, even though the patient's condition and available data indicate that these measures are medically ineffective and will only increase pain and suffering (i.e., harm) at the end of life.[14-16]

ELEMENTS OF THE AFFORDABLE CARE ACT

Although the ACA falls short of providing true universal health care, it does increase the access to over 30 million of the 50-plus million previously uninsured citizens, as well as more of the "underinsured" population. In order to increase the number of patients covered and prevent exclusion of patients with preexisting conditions, it established a federal government-run exchange, supported the development of state-run health insurance exchanges, and set up systems to reduce cost through establishment of Accountable Care Organizations (ACOs) and other bundled care and payment programs that share risk and savings to a greater or lesser extent with providers. Thus, under a full risk, total cost-of-care contract, the provider including the physicians, pharmacies, hospitals, skilled nursing facilities, home health care, and all other elements of the health delivery system receive a single payment to cover cradle-to-grave health care for a population of patients, for a specific group of patients such as those with congestive heart failure, or for an episode of care (e.g., coronary artery bypass surgery). Such bundled payments are strong inducers for health care providers to coordinate the care, remove waste by eliminating unnecessary testing and excessive subspecialty consultation, use generic drugs rather than more expensive trade name medications, and to set up programs to keep patients from going to the emergency room for non-life-threatening conditions or being hospitalized.

This increased emphasis on population health, with the use of a global budget to care for a population of patients, means that there will be greater efforts to prevent disease. In order to discourage ACOs and health systems from withholding tests, procedures, and medications to reduce cost, the Centers for Medicare and Medicaid Services has incorporated quality metrics such as reduction in 30-day hospital readmission rates, the timing of prophylactic antibiotic use before surgery, and venous thrombosis prevention with payment penalties for poor performance as part of its Value-Based Purchasing Program.[17] The Physician Quality Reporting system also measures physician performance based on a variety of quality metrics. Examples include the proportion of diabetic patients with glycohemoglobin values less than 9%, low-density lipoprotein cholesterol less than 100 mg/dL, blood pressure lower than 140/90 mm Hg, tobacco education, and aspirin or clopidogrel use in patients with ischemic vascular disease. Patient satisfaction with health care, including satisfaction with the providers, the systems, and the environment of care, also is assessed and together with quality and outcome measures form the elements of hospital pay-for-performance as components of the Value-Based Purchasing Program. Systems that do not meet the quality and satisfaction metrics receive less payment than those that do, whether they are providing care through an ACO or the Medicare fee-for-service system.[18] A similar program at the physician level, the Physician Value-Based Payment Modifier, rewards physicians who provide high-quality, low-cost medical care. This program began in 2013 with a sample of physicians and is scheduled to begin affecting all physicians and their Medicare payments by 2017.[19]

The insurance industry has followed suit through the development of their own ACOs for their insured population with different risk models. Another development has been the emergence of narrow networks in which the insurance company chooses physicians and hospitals that they deem cost-effective. Patients who sign up for these networks pay a lower premium and cost deductible but must use prescribed medical providers or cover all costs out of pocket. Because consumers are receiving more information about what health plans offer, at what price, and standardized information about deductibles, co-payments, and out-of-pocket maximums to allow comparison shopping and because the cost of health insurance in the United States is high, this lower cost option with little flexibility is very attractive to many patients and employers. Indeed, many employers have moved from defined benefit insurance plans to defined contribution plans, giving their employees a set amount of funds for health insurance and allowing the employee to make the decision as to which plan to join.

The migration from volume to value is the tectonic shift that the ACA and the existing economics of health care delivery in the United States have brought about. Value is defined as outcomes plus patient experience divided by cost. So, in order to increase value, either outcomes or satisfaction must increase or costs must be reduced, and indeed, most of the care systems are working on both sides of the equation.[20]

HOW ACCOUNTABLE CARE ORGANIZATIONS AND OTHER SYSTEMS CAN INCREASE VALUE

Both quality and costs are enhanced through a holistic patient-centered systems approach that emphasizes coordination of patient care across the entire continuum of care through the use of a dynamic team approach, partnering with community resources, communication tools, evidence-based best practice treatment algorithms, systems-based approaches to quality and safety, and the provision of real-time actionable data (Table 5-1).[21-24] Today, much medicine is practiced by practitioners acting in silos. For instance, a man with polyuria, polydipsia, and weight loss may see a primary care physician who diagnoses diabetes mellitus. The patient is sent to the laboratory for evaluation of blood glucose, electrolytes, lipids, renal function, and glycohemoglobin. The patient may be referred to a dietitian for weight loss and dietary instruction and, depending on the level of the glucose abnormality, may be started on a

glucose-lowering drug. The patient is seen again in a few weeks and medication adjustments are made. Eventually other medications may be added. If the physician follows the American Diabetes Association guidelines, appointments will be made with an ophthalmologist and a podiatrist. If difficulties arise in achieving glucose control, the patient may be sent to an endocrinologist for assessment. The patient who develops an intercurrent infection such as a cellulitis requiring hospitalization may not be managed by the primary care physician. Increasingly, hospital care is provided by full-time hospitalists, and there may be minimal communication between the hospitalist and the primary care physician. The hospitalist may repeat the exact same tests that the primary care physician performed that day before sending the patient into the hospital. In order to achieve glucose control during the stress of the infection, insulin may have been substituted for the oral antidiabetic agent and the patient told to resume the oral agent at the time of discharge. In addition, upon hospital admission, preexisting ambulatory medications are changed to conform to the hospital's formulary, and at the time of discharge, there may be inadequate medication reconciliation. As a result the patient may be taking one statin prescribed in the hospital along with the statin that was prescribed before the hospitalization. The patient may have been told to follow up with the primary care physician, without being given an appointment, and there may not have been real-time communication with the primary care physician by the hospital staff at the time of the patient's discharge. This sequence is a setup for patient confusion, worsening diabetes control, and clinical deterioration requiring hospital readmission. This type of care is neither efficient nor effective and is costly for both the patient and the health care system.

Under a truly integrated system, medicine is not practiced in silos (see Table 5-1). Rather, it is a team endeavor with systems in place to optimally care for the most common medical conditions such as diabetes, asthma/chronic obstructive pulmonary disease, congestive heart failure, orthopedic issues, and pain management using the principles of a patient-centered medical home.[22] Our newly diagnosed diabetic patient will be managed by a team composed of the primary care physician and his or her team, augmented by a diabetes management team overseen by an endocrinologist. The members will include a nurse practitioner or advanced practice nurse, a dietitian, a pharmacist, and a patient navigator, whose primary function is to keep track of the patient, making sure that all appointments are made and kept (arranging transportation if necessary), tests obtained, and results are reviewed and acted upon in a timely fashion. The diabetes education and management follow established evidence-based, best practice protocols.[25] Medication titration is carried out under the direction of the clinical pharmacist, checklists are utilized by the navigator to make sure that appropriate tests and procedures are performed, and reminders for glycohemoglobin tests, microalbumin tests, eye and foot examinations, vaccinations, and general health maintenance are generated electronically through the electronic health record. The patient is entered into a diabetes registry to allow assessment of the status of care provided to all patients with diabetes in the health care system, as well as providing feedback about their performance to the individual primary care physician and the diabetic team. All members of the team communicate with each other through the electronic medical record and communicate directly with the patient through the patient's portal.[26] Patients are taught to monitor their glucose levels with home glucose monitoring and the data are electronically

---

TABLE 5-1
Elements of a Coordinated Health Care System

Patient-centered medical home
- Primary care team
- Disease- or organ-specific chronic care team

Shared decision making between patient and health care providers

Coordination of care across the continuum of care
- Health care navigator
- Checklists
- Algorithms for evidence-based diagnostic and treatment decisions
- Electronic medical record
  - Clinical decision support (provide actionable information at the time of order entry)
- Reminders for general health maintenance (e.g., vaccinations, mammograms)
- Reminders for disease-specific assessment (e.g., glycohemoglobin, eye examination)
- e-Consults (telemedicine)
- Handoffs between providers and venues of care requiring a confirmed "handshake" (e.g., primary care physician to hospitalist; hospitalist to primary care physician; hospitalist to skilled nursing faculty; primary care physician to home health care program)
- Multiple venues linked together (e.g., hospital, urgent care center, infusion center, Hospital-at-Home)
- Patient portals
- Coordination with community resources

Biometric monitoring

Mobile health applications with alerts to patient and health care providers

Commitment devices (e.g., gym membership to increase exercise)

Feedback about performance provided to all providers and their teams transmitted to the care team through mobile health technology, with alerts generated if control falls out of certain parameters or if the patient does not perform the necessary testing.[27] If deteriorating control is detected, the health care navigator will communicate directly with the patient to determine the reasons for the backsliding and an appointment will be made to see the primary care physician or nurse practitioner, dietitian, pharmacist, endocrinologist, or social worker, depending on the likely problem. Medication nonadherence may be addressed through the use of an electronic medication packaging device.[28] If an acute medical issue arises, the patient is seen the same day either at home, in the primary care physician's office, or at one of the health care system's urgent care centers close to the patient's home, avoiding a costly trip to the emergency room or hospital for an ambulatory-sensitive condition (e.g., management of diabetes going out of control before it is greatly out of control). In our cellulitis example, early diagnosis and treatment with antibiotics and daily observation and, if necessary, intravenous antibiotic administration can be carried out in an outpatient infusion center or at home with daily home health nursing visits. For a more severe infection, a Hospital at Home program pioneered by the Johns Hopkins University Schools of Medicine and Public Health may be initiated. Infusion and other necessary equipment and medications are delivered and set up at the patient's home, with full-time nursing care (provided for 24 hours/day 7 days a week) and daily physician visits until the patient is discharged.[29]

The patient receives general preventive services through the system, which includes vaccinations, weight management, exercise programs, advance care planning, depression screening, and other evidence-based screening procedures such as colonoscopies, whose frequency is determined in part by patient-specific factors including family history, risk profile, past results, and if known, predisposition based upon genetic testing (e.g., *RET* proto-oncogene for medullary carcinoma of the thyroid). Should the patient require inpatient hospitalization, coordination of care between the primary care physician and the hospitalist is essential and is managed either directly or through the patient navigator using a formal template in the electronic medical record as well as direct voice communication. The navigator will stay abreast of the patient's progress no matter where he or she resides in the system. Medication reconciliation is managed by the hospital-based clinical pharmacist using the medications that are used by the same formulary throughout the system. Unless there is compelling scientific evidence favoring the use of a specific trade name drug, all patients receive generic medications.

As part of the population health paradigm, the health care system will try to prevent their members from becoming overtly diabetic by educating families about good nutrition, exercise, and proven weight control methods. If necessary, "commitment devices," such as providing a gym membership, scheduling workouts with an exercise partner, having the patient put money in a deposit contract that is forfeited if a specific goal such as a 5-lb weight loss is not met, or reducing insurance premiums if a goal is achieved, may provide an added incentive to change behavior.[30] A proactive approach to risk reduction will be instituted for blood-related family members of the patient with diabetes in order to help mitigate the increased risk of diabetes due to genetic factors.

Role of the Endocrinologist

The endocrinologist plays several key roles in this coordinated, patient-centered paradigm (Table 5-2). First, he or

---

TABLE 5-2

Role of Clinical Endocrinologist in Population Health

Direct the endocrine disease management team
Oversee the Endocrine Disease Registry
Develop evidence-based guidelines for endocrine diseases
Consult on patients with endocrine disorders who have diagnostic or therapeutic issues that require special expertise
Co-manage difficult patients
Establish endocrine e-consult protocols and systems
Oversee the quality control and clinical effectiveness of clinical endocrine programs
Teach medical students, house staff, and fellows the principles and practice of endocrinology as well as procedural components
Teach primary care physicians and their team members how to manage patients with endocrine disease and when to refer to an endocrinologist
Bring latest knowledge about endocrine diseases to the accountable care organization
Perform clinical research

---

she should be responsible for the formation, staffing, and oversight of the diabetic and obesity disease management programs. With a third of our population being obese and about 9.3% having diabetes and another 27% with prediabetes, all health care systems involved in population management require a "diabesity" management program.[31] The endocrinologist must oversee the implementation of evidence-based management algorithms, keep them updated, and monitor the effectiveness of the program through trending and summative data analysis of glycohemoglobin, fasting blood sugar levels, lipid levels, blood pressure control, micro- and macrovascular complication rates; percentage of patients who receive eye, foot, and renal assessment; and patient satisfaction. The endocrinologist needs to be one of the major managers of the registries for endocrine diseases. In addition, the endocrinologist must be available to consult in individual, difficult-to-manage patients because not all patients can be successfully treated through even the best treatment algorithm. Minor management issues may be able to be effectively handled through informal curbside consults with the primary care physician or an e-consult mechanism in which the pertinent history, physical examination, laboratory studies, and clinical questions are summarized by the primary care physician, advance care or nurse practitioner, or patient navigator, sent electronically (through HIPAA [Health Insurance Portability and Accountability Act]-compliant secure encryption) to the endocrinologist who responds (ideally) within a day with suggestions or a request to see the patient.[32,33] Telemedicine can also be used directly with the patient, as has been done for patients with diabetes.[34] Of course, under any system, old or new, endocrinologists will be asked to formally consult and often co-manage patients with the vast array of endocrine problems. Ideally, under an integrated system, endocrinologists will only practice endocrinology and not serve as primary care physicians. This conforms to the concept that all health care providers including doctors should practice up to the top of their license and training. Under an ACO, the primary care physician and his or her team in the Medical Home should be the primary manager of each patient. This allows the endocrinologist (or any other specialist) to take part in the management of more patients in an efficient manner. Patients with special problems, such as the difficult-to-manage diabetic, or a patient with thyroid cancer should be co-managed with the primary care physician, with the majority of the nonendocrine-related issues being managed by the patient's primary team. This "multiplier effect" of having endocrinologists practice only endocrinology functionally should help relieve the shortage of endocrinologists available to manage patients.[35]

The endocrinologist will be essential as an educator both for the cognitive aspects of the discipline and for teaching procedures such as thyroid ultrasonography and aspiration biopsy, skeletal dual-energy x-ray absorptiometry interpretation, and management of insulin pumps and continuous glucose monitoring.[36] In addition to the traditional role in teaching medical students, house staff, and fellows, the endocrinologist in a coordinated health care system will need to educate the primary care teams about the current standards of disease management of the common endocrine conditions, the diagnostic and therapeutic algorithms, when to call for active involvement of the endocrinologist, and what types of information should be collected before the endocrinologist is called.

Another role for the practicing endocrinologist is to carry out clinical research. New diagnostic tests such as noninvasive glucose monitors or molecular markers performed on fine needle aspirations of thyroid nodules need to be tested in real world environments. Similarly, new endocrine medications need testing in large numbers of patients for efficacy and safety. An endocrinologist with an endocrine disease registry composed of hundreds or thousands of patients and a clinical research team are in an ideal position to carry out such research. Similarly, an endocrinologist in such a rich "clinical lab" environment is in an ideal position to perform health delivery research, such as comparing the effectiveness, efficiency, and overall costs of an e-consultation system versus traditional face-to-face consultations. Finally, endocrinologists should be tasked with keeping up with all current developments in applied endocrine research including new diagnostic and therapeutic modalities and cost-effective approaches to patient care in order to educate the entire ACO and implement changes that will enhance patient care, satisfaction, and cost-effectiveness.

CHALLENGES

Our health care delivery system faces a myriad of challenges (Table 5-3). First and foremost is the delivery of effective, efficient, and appropriate health care to more patients without a proportional increase in health care dollars. In order to care for more patients, more personnel

TABLE 5-3
Health Care Challenges

Providing more (more patients, more personnel, more prevention) for less

Increased prevalence of chronic diseases as population ages

Obesity and diabetes epidemic

Manpower issues

New technology (e.g., "omics" revolution leading to more personalized care)

Accurate analysis of "big data" utilizing social networking and multiple data sources

Academic medical center survival

   Teaching

   Research

   Faculty salaries

Internet and social network dissemination of information

Lack of universal health care—still have 20 to 30 million people without health care coverage

Misaligned economic incentives

Cultural barriers to change

need to be hired. Additionally, the aging of the population will result in more patients with the chronic diseases of aging—diabetes, heart disease, chronic obstructive pulmonary disease, cancer, dementia, and arthritis—which will need to be managed. At present there are not enough doctors to take care of this influx of patients and the longer duration of care for patients with chronic diseases that is required because of increased longevity. The United States has fewer physicians per 1000 population (2.5) than the OECD average (3.2),[3] and it has been estimated that there will be a shortage of 63,000 physicians by 2015 and twice that number by 2025.[35,37] Thus, it is inevitable that more coordinated systems of team-based care will evolve. Endocrinologists will certainly experience this problem with the influx of patients with diabetes mellitus and obesity, and they will be on the forefront of developing and implementing diabetes disease management programs that utilize nurses, dietitians, and pharmacists following algorithms, biometric monitoring, checklists, and electronic reminders. In 2011, there were 4841 clinical adult endocrinologists in the United States and about 27 million patients with diagnosed diabetes.[31,35] The average male adult endocrinologist works 42 hours each week and provides 3434 patient visits per year, and female endocrinologists provide an average of 2484 visits per year.[35] This works out to almost 5600 patients with diabetes per clinical endocrinologist. There are not enough hours in the day for the community of endocrinologists to see every diabetic patient even once per year, let alone see patients with other endocrine problems. In fact, only 15% of all diabetic care is provided by endocrinologists.[35] Thus, change as previously enunciated is inevitable if endocrinologists are going to be responsible and accountable for optimal care of such patients in a health system.

With insufficient funds to provide unlimited care for individuals and to use resources to enhance the overall health of the population, endocrinologists will be required to enhance their efficiency and appropriateness when providing direct medical care. In 2002, the American Board of Internal Medicine and the American College of Physicians, along with their foundations, redefined medical professionalism. They stated: "While meeting the needs of individual patients, physicians are required to provide health care that is based on the wise and cost-effective management of limited clinical resources. The provision of unnecessary services not only exposes patients to avoidable harm and expense but also diminishes the resources available for others."[2,38] The balance between caring for an individual patient and our responsibilities to preserving precious financial resources for the good of society as a whole is a difficult challenge, especially because our emphasis has generally been on the individual doctor-patient interaction.

The current models for reimbursement create roadblocks for change. In many of the fee-for-service plans, the patients must be seen directly by a physician, rather than another health care worker. Treatments at home or admission to chronic care facilities require physicians and patients to jump through bureaucratic hoops for approval, and this is time consuming and wasteful of resources. There is generally no reimbursement for phone, text, or e-mail correspondence between the patient, caregiver, and physician, and payment models for e-consults or virtual visits through videoconferencing between the patient and provider are in their infancy. In addition, major reform to allow interstate medical licensing is needed to help physicians extend their expertise to areas in the United States without specialty care.[39] Thus, there is a financial disincentive to use modern, efficient, and less time-consuming methodologies than a face-to-face visit to help deliver care. Of course, in a bundled care or global payment system, this barrier is eliminated.

The evolution of existing technology and introduction of new technologies also create a challenge. What is new is not always better, and it is incumbent upon us to evaluate all such new technology or therapies against the existing technology or therapy to see if the utilization of the new development substantially improves patient care and at what cost. In this regard, the United Kingdom's National Institute for Clinical Excellence (NICE) program provides an informative prototype. This independent, government-funded organization evaluates new technology and new medications for the British National Health System, initially for clinical effectiveness and then cost effectiveness using a metric of incremental cost over no treatment or treatment with an existing drug or technology per quality-adjusted life-year (QALY). In general, if the new technology or medication costs £20,000 (~$32,690) or less per QALY, it is approved. If it costs more than £30,000 (~$49,000), it generally is not approved (with exceptions such as care for orphan diseases and special risk-sharing relationships with pharmaceutical companies); between £20,000 and £30,000 there is a case-by-case assessment and decision.[40] The U.S. Congress specifically prohibited using cost effectiveness as a criterion for provision of care in the ACA.

One of the more interesting challenges is in the area of the "omics" revolution in biotechnology—genomics, transcriptomics, proteomics, and metabolomics—and the proliferation of diagnostic biomarkers. Soon we will have the ability to run an individual patient's genome relatively inexpensively and to use that information to predict which patients are at risk for certain diseases (e.g., *RET* proto-oncogene and medullary thyroid carcinoma), which drugs they may metabolize too rapidly, and which tumors with specific genetic mutations are likely to respond to a specific drug, along with other information, resulting in much more accurate "personalized medicine" (or "precision medicine"), which is the tailoring of medical treatment to the individual characteristics of each patient.[41-43]

As an example, the 2009 *Medullary Thyroid Cancer Management Guidelines* from the American Thyroid Association highlights the utility of using specific mutations of the *RET* proto-oncogene to help guide clinical decisions. Infants with *RET* mutations in codons 883 or 918 have a very high risk of developing medullary thyroid carcinoma and metastasis and, therefore, should undergo thyroidectomy as soon as possible within the first year of life, but those with a mutation in codons 768, 790, 791, 804, or 891 have a less aggressive clinical course, and thyroidectomy can be delayed until age 5 or later as long as the patient is carefully monitored.[44] In screening populations of patients with a strong family history of colon cancer, those who are found to have a genetic profile that places them at high risk can be advised to undergo a colonoscopy at an earlier age and more frequently than is currently recommended for the population at large. Those at lower risk for a disease may not need to be screened at all. Individuals who metabolize certain classes of drugs more rapidly than the average should be treated with a different class.[45] Indeed, there are currently over 150 Food and Drug Administration (FDA)-approved drugs that contain pharmacogenomics information in their labels.[46] This personalized approach based on data may ultimately reduce health care costs by getting rid of the "one size fits all" approach that currently often is used. However, in the near term, it is likely that there will be increased costs associated with the molecular testing as well as the translation into clinical care. There are issues with specificity and sensitivity of some of the newer diagnostics that have been marketed.[47] New pharmacotherapeutics will emerge to treat the various molecular defects that are identified. Enhanced decision support tools will be essential to provide guidance to clinicians on how to use this information to care for their patients. Another positive development to emerge from high-throughput genomic and information technologies is drug repurposing or repositioning based on mining of genomic information that suggests a novel use. The former refers to a new use of a drug during its development or after it has been approved and released for another purpose, and the latter refers to a compound that had been discarded but based on new genomic data could be developed for a novel use.[48]

The information revolution empowered by the Internet also raises multiple challenges. We have all experienced patients coming in with very recent information that they gleaned from the Internet of which we were not aware. In the YouTube and social network era, as soon as information is generated, it is available. Unfortunately, not all of the information is valid, so separating truth from fiction or hype can at times be difficult and certainly time consuming. Although social networks can be a source of misinformation that spreads rapidly, they are also important for learning about diseases and therapies. Social media sites allow individuals to share information about themselves that can be analyzed using computerized methods for text analysis that incorporates natural language processing technology. For instance, analyzing the contents of millions of public Twitter messages, investigators have been able to identify individual-level diurnal and seasonal mood rhythms in cultures around the world.[49] *Patients Like Me* allows patients to discuss their illness including their treatment experiences, use of alternative or unproven remedies, and the emotional aspects of their disease. Not only does monitoring these sites and patient-derived blogs provide information about what patients with a condition are actually doing, they also provide a glimpse about communication gaps between health professionals and patients.[50] Social media sites also have been used successfully for patient recruitment for research studies.[51] Analysis of Internet search volumes on certain topics can yield important epidemiologic information. For instance, in 2009, Google described the prototype for a flu tracking system that evolved into *Google Flu Trends*.[52] They developed an algorithm that monitored health-seeking behavior by examining online web search queries that are correlated with the percentage of physician visits in which a patient presents with flu-like symptoms from millions of users throughout the world to detect flu within a day, earlier than traditional surveillance systems which have a 1- to 2-week reporting lag. However, as was later documented, the Google system was overestimating the actual number of influenza cases, which has been attributed to "big data hubris" when large masses of data are considered a substitute rather than an adjunct to traditional data collection and analysis, as well as "algorithm dynamics" when there are ongoing changes made in the algorithms and changes in user behavior from media reports about the flu.[53] A number of public and private entities are integrating multiple databases, such as billing, laboratory, and pharmacy data, along with demographics and information from electronic medical records and genetic databases, to mine and analyze this "big data" to identify high-risk populations of patients, determine drug interactions and side effects, see which subpopulations of patients are likely to be "responders" or "nonresponders" to a drug, detect diagnostic test over- and underutilization, and answer many other questions.[54] An example is the FDA's Mini-Sentinel Distributed Database, which has data on 178 million members with 358 million person-years of observation time including 4.1 billion unique encounters, and data on 4 billion dispensations of medication, which the FDA mines for drug safety after drugs have been approved and are on the market.[46]

Another type of information that is becoming more widely available is price transparency. Information on prices is available from Healthcare Blue Book and insurance companies and on hospital and physician payments from Centers for Medicare and Medicaid Services.[6] Consumerism has led large retail supermarket and pharmacy companies to open low-cost clinics that provide medical care for common issues like upper respiratory infections, otitis media, and vaccinations.[55] Consumers also have access to quality metrics publicly reported for hospitals and physician groups and, in some areas of the country, on specific physicians.[55] Patients who look up information about their potential out-of-pocket costs for laboratory and imaging tests and clinician office visits before receiving the services pay lower prices for the services than those who do not seek out the information, confirming that consumers do alter their behavior based on price transparency.[56] Additionally, the Physician Payment Sunshine Act and the Open Payments Program allow patients the ability to look up data on pharmaceutical and device manufacture company payments to physicians, as do some websites such as *ProPublica*.[57]

There is a great deal of consolidation of hospitals to form locally integrated health systems.[58] These systems offer an advantage for quality improvement. For instance, studies have shown that the more thyroid and parathyroid surgeries that a head and neck surgeon does, the more laparoscopic adrenalectomies performed by endocrine surgeons, or the more pituitary surgeries a neurosurgeon performs, the better the outcome and the lower the complication rate.[59-63] Individual, independent hospitals may not be able to provide enough patient volume for any one surgeon to meet the evidence-based criteria for volume needed to have excellent outcomes. However, a consolidated health system may be able to provide a surgical team operating at only one of the system's institutions with that volume. This consolidation also allows the system to invest in a single infrastructure and equipment for highly specialized services without duplicating the service at each institution. The economies of scale that consolidation and integration within a system offer also should make it easier to engage in true population health. It will allow patients to see providers and be hospitalized close to their home in a system with uniform protocols, electronic health records, and data collection. It should also help outreach to community services such as homeless shelters, mental health agencies, schools, faith-based programs, and city planning for recreational facilities. The downside of this consolidation is that it may result in higher prices and less innovation because of less competition.[58]

Academic medical centers also care for a disproportionate proportion of the indigent population and have relied on cross-subsidy from payers to cover the true cost of patient care for this population. Although the ACA has increased the number of patients covered by insurance, there are still a substantial number of uninsured patients whose care will be delivered in large part under the aegis of academic medical centers. At a time when the National Institutes of Health budget is not rising as fast as inflation and is actually decreasing in terms of real dollars in comparison to prior years, funding of conferences by industry is being severely curtailed, and physician payments for direct patient care are being reduced, the funding of the academic enterprise will inevitably suffer. In addition, academic medical centers are often siloed by departments and

are resistant to integration.[64] Not only will this result in the loss of faculty from the institutions, but also it may serve as a major disincentive for new teachers and investigators to enter academic medicine. This may have the unfortunate effect of leading to a loss of America's preeminence in regard to new discoveries and innovation, as well as a decline in the quality of medical education. Recently, the Institute of Medicine has recommended that we should maintain the Medicare Graduate Medical Education support while we transition to modernize the payment method based on performance and needs (e.g., a more ambulatory team-based approach rather than one based on the percentage of time working in a hospital).[65]

Finally, in my opinion, the biggest challenge to change in medicine generally, and endocrinology specifically, is cultural. Patients, especially in the United States, are used to the status quo and are reluctant to change, although in order to keep payments affordable, many are being forced to join narrow insurance networks or programs on the state or federal government exchanges. Even with these changes, many patients harbor unrealistic expectations and demand procedures and treatments (especially at the end of life) that are unwarranted or ineffective. Changing patients' expectations is a major challenge. Similarly, changing the mindset of physicians is also a challenge. To a certain extent this is generational. Those who have been in practice for a long time are often unwilling to change. Some have entered concierge practices and some have planned to retire earlier than they had originally expected. Many argue against the change because they fear that they will be forced to practice "cookbook" medicine, will lose their autonomy, will lose the intimacy of the doctor-patient relationship, and will lose the ability to practice the way they wish, especially if they must join a large health care system to financially survive. The transparency and feedback that they will receive about their performance are also threatening. Nevertheless, I believe that endocrinologists' sense of professionalism and ethical responsibility will keep them doing what is in the best interest of their patients and, thus, will overcome the challenges and provide efficient, effective, appropriate, and less wasteful medical care.

REFERENCES

1. Hoffman A, Emanuel E. Reengineering US health care. *JAMA*. 2013; 309(7):661-662.
2. Sox H. Resolving the tension between population health and individual health care. *JAMA*. 2013;310:1933-1934.
3. Organisation for Economic Co-Operation and Development. OECD statistics, 2014. Available at: <http://stats.oecd.org>. Accessed October 6, 2014.
4. Moses HI, Matheson D, Dorsey E, et al. The anatomy of health care in the United States. *JAMA*. 2013;310(18):1947-1963.
5. The Dartmouth Institute. The Dartmouth atlas of health care, 2014. Available at: <www.dartmouthatlas.org>. Accessed October 6, 2014.
6. Reinhardt U. The disruptive innovation of price transparency in health care. *JAMA*. 2013;310(18):1927-1928.
7. Inabnet WI. Robotic thyroidectomy: must we drive a luxury sedan to arrive at our destination safely? *Thyroid*. 2012;22(10):988-990.
8. Baicker K, Fisher E, Chandra A. Malpractice liability costs and the practice of medicine in the Medicare program. *Health Aff*. 2007;26: 841-852.
9. Carrier E, Reschovsky J, Katz D, Mello M. High physician concern about malpractice risk predicts more aggressive diagnostic testing in office-based practice. *Health Aff*. 2013;32:1383-1391.
10. ABIM Foundation. Imaging tests for headaches, 2012. Available at: <www.choosingwisely-org/doctor-patient-lists/imaging-tests-for-headaches>. Accessed October 6, 2014.
11. Morden N, Colla C, Sequist T, Rosenthal MB. Choosing wisely—the politics and economics of labeling low-value services. *N Engl J Med*. 2014;370(7):589-592.
12. Owlia M, Yu L, Deible C, et al. Head CT scan overuse in frequently admitted medical patients. *Am J Med*. 2014;127:406-410.

13. Zhi M, Ding E, Theisen-Toupal J, et al. The landscape of inappropriate laboratory testing: a 15-year meta-analysis. *PLoS ONE.* 2013;8(11):1-8.
14. Kasman D. When is medical treatment futile? A guide for students, residents, and physicians. *J Gen Intern Med.* 2004;19:1053-1056.
15. Wright A, Zhang B, Ray A, et al. Associations between end-of-life discussions, patient mental health, medical care near death, and caregiver bereavement adjustment. *JAMA.* 2008;300(14):1665-1673.
16. Ebell MH, Jang W, Shen Y, Geocadin R. Development and validation of the Good Outcome Following Attempted Resuscitation (GO-FAR) score to predict neurologically intact survival after in-hospital cardiopulmonary resuscitation. *JAMA Intern Med.* 2013;173(20):1872-1878.
17. VanLare J, Conway P. Value-based purchasing—national programs to move from volume to value. *N Engl J Med.* 2012;367(4):292-295.
18. Centers for Medicare and Medicaid Services. Physician quality reporting system, 2014. Available at: <http://www.cms.gov/Medicare/Quality-Initiatives-Patient-Assessment-Instruments/PQRS/MeasuresCodes.html>. Accessed October 6, 2014.
19. Chien A, Rosenthal M. Medicare's Physician Value-Based Payment Modifier—will the tectonic shift create waves? *N Engl J Med.* 2013;369(22):2076-2078.
20. Spiro T, Lee E, Emanuel E. Price and utilization: why we must target both to curb health care costs. *Ann Intern Med.* 2012;157:586-590.
21. Jackson G, Powers B, Chatterjee R, et al. The patient-centered medical home. A systematic review. *Ann Intern Med.* 2013;158(3):169-178.
22. Doherty R, Crowley R. Principles supporting dynamic clinical care teams: an American College of Physicians position paper. *Ann Intern Med.* 2013;159:620-626.
23. Plumb J, Weinstein L, Brawer R, Scott K. Community-based partnerships for improving chronic disease management. *Prim Care Clin Office Pract.* 2012;39:433-447.
24. Pronovost P. Enhancing physicians' use of clinical guidelines. *N Engl J Med.* 2013;310(23):2501-2502.
25. American Diabetes Association. Standards of medical care in diabetes—2014. *Diabetes Care.* 2014;37(Suppl 1):S14-S80.
26. Goldzweig C, Orshansky G, Paige N, et al. Electronic patient portals: evidence on health outcomes, satisfaction, efficiency, and attitudes. *Ann Intern Med.* 2013;159:677-687.
27. Steinhubl S, Muse E, Topol E. Can mobile health technologies transform health care? *JAMA.* 2013;310(22):2395-2396.
28. Checchi K, Huybrechts K, Avorn J, Kesselheim A. Electronic medication packaging devices and medication adherence. A systematic review. *JAMA.* 2014;312(12):1237-1247.
29. Leff B, Burton L, Mader S, et al. Hospital at home: feasibility and outcomes of a program to provide hospital-level care at home for acutely ill older patients. *Ann Intern Med.* 2005;143:798-808.
30. Rogers T, Milkman K, Volpp K. Commitment devices. Using initiatives to change behavior. *JAMA.* 2014;311(20):2065-2066.
31. American Diabetes Association. Statistics about diabetes, 2014. Available at: <http://www.diabetes.org/diabetes-basics/statistics/>. Accessed September 29, 2014.
32. Cook D, Sorensen K, Wilkinson J. Value and process of curbside consultations in clinical practice: a grounded theory study. *Mayo Clin Proc.* 2014;89(5):602-614.
33. Chen A, Murphy E, Yee HJ. eReferral—a new model for integrated care. *N Engl J Med.* 2013;26:2450-2453.
34. Franc S, Daoudi A, Mounier S, et al. Telemedicine: what more is needed for its integration in everyday life? *Diabetes Metab.* 2011;37:S71-S77.
35. Vigersky R, Fish L, Hogan P, et al. The clinical endocrinology workforce: current status and future projections of supply and demand. *J Clin Endocrinol Metab.* 2014;99:3112-3121.
36. Ladenson P, Balasubramanyam A, Danoff A, Bhasin S. Defining, assessing, and certifying procedural competency in endocrinology, diabetes, and metabolism. *J Clin Endocrinol Metab.* 2014;99(8):2651-2653.
37. Kane G, Grever M, Kennedy J, et al. The anticipated physician shortage: meeting the nation's need for physician services. *Amer J Med.* 2009;122(12):1156-1162.
38. ABIM Foundation A-AF, European Federation of Internal Medicine. Medical professionalism in the new millennium: a physician charter. *Ann Intern Med.* 2002;136(3):243-246.
39. Steinbrook R. Interstate medical licensure. Major reform of licensing to encourage medical practice in multiple states. *JAMA.* 2014;312(7):695-696.
40. Steinbrook R. Saying no isn't NICE—the travails of Britain's National Institute for Health and Clinical Excellence. *N Engl J Med.* 2008;359(19):1977-1981.
41. President's Council of Advisors on Science and Technology. Priorities for personalized medicine, 2008. Available at: <http://www.whitehouse.gov/files/documents/ostp/PCAST/pcast_report_v2.pdf>. Accessed September 2014.
42. Mirnezami R, Nicholson J, Darzi A. Preparing for precision medicine. *N Engl J Med.* 2012;366(6):489-491.
43. Mega JL, Sabatine MS, Antman EM. Population and personalized medicine in the modern era. *JAMA.* 2014;312(19):1969-1970.
44. Kloos R, Eng C, Evans D, et al. Medullary thyroid cancer: management guidelines of the American Thyroid Association. *Thyroid.* 2009;19(6):565-612.
45. Wilke R, Dolan M. Genetics and variable drug response. *JAMA.* 2011;306(3):306-307.
46. Food and Drug Adminstration. Table of pharmacogenomic biomarkers in drug labeling, 2014. Available at: <http://www.fda.gov/Drugs/ScienceResearch/ResearchAreas/Pharmacogenetics/ucm083378.htm>. Accessed October 6, 2014.
47. Hamburg M, Collins F. The path to personalized medicine. *N Engl J Med.* 2010;363(4):301-304.
48. Power A, Berger A, Ginsburg G. Genomics-endabled drug repositioning and repurposing. Insights from an IOM roundtable activity. *JAMA.* 2014;311(20):2063-2064.
49. Golder S, Macy M. Diurnal and seasonal mood vary with work, sleep, and day length across diverse cultures. *Science.* 2011;333:1878-1881.
50. Gruzd A, Black F, Le T, Amos K. Investigating biomedical research literature in the blogosphere: a case study of diabetes and glycated hemoglobin (HbA1c). *J Med Libr Assoc.* 2012;100(1):34-42.
51. Balfe M, Doyle F, Conroy R. Using Facebook to recruit young adults for qualitative research projects: how difficult is it? *Comput Inform Nurs.* 2012;511-515.
52. Ginsberg J, Mohebbi M, Patel R, et al. Detecting influenza epidemics using search engine query data. *Nature.* 2009;457:1012-1015.
53. Lazer D, Kennedy R, King G, Vespignani A. The parable of Google flu: traps in big data analysis, 2013. Available at: <http://blogs.iq.harvard.edu/netgov/The%20Parable%20of%20Google%20Flu%20(WP-Final).pdf>. Accessed September 2014.
54. Schneeweiss S. Learning from big health care data. *N Engl J Med.* 2014;370(23):2161-2163.
55. Huckman R, Kelley M. Public reporting, consumerism, and patient empowerment. *N Engl J Med.* 2013;369:1875-1877.
56. Whaley C, Schneider Chafen J, Pinkard S, et al. Association between availability of health service prices and payments for these services. *JAMA.* 2014;312(16):1670-1676.
57. Kirschner N, Sulmasy L, Kesselheim A. Health policy basics: the Physician Payment Sunshine Act and the Open Payments Program. *Ann Intern Med.* 2014;161(7):519-521.
58. Cutler D, Morton F. Hospitals, market share, and consolidation. *JAMA.* 2013;310(18):1964-1970.
59. Sosa J, Bowman H, Tielsch J, et al. The importance of surgeon experience for clinical and economic outcomes from thyroidectomy. *Ann Surg.* 1998;228(3):320-330.
60. Wang T, Roman S, Sosa J. Predictors of outcomes following pediatric thyroid and parathyroid surgery. *Curr Opin Oncol.* 2008;21:23-28.
61. Villar J, Moreno P, Ortega J, et al. Results of adrenal surgery. Data of a Spanish National Survey. *Langenbecks Arch Surg.* 2010;395:837-843.
62. Ciric I, Ragin A, Baumgartner C, Pierce D. Complications of transsphenoidal surgery: results of a national survey, review of the literature, and personal experience. *Neurosurgery.* 1997;40:225-236.
63. Stavrakis A, Ituarte P, Ko C, Yeh M. Surgeon volume as a predictor of outcomes in inpatient and outpatient endocrine surgery. *Surgery.* 2007;142:887-899.
64. Washington A, Coye M, Feinberg D. Academic health centers and the evolution of the health care system. *JAMA.* 2013;18:1929-1930.
65. Eden JB, Berwick D, Wilensky G, Committee on the Governance and Financing of Graduate Medical Education, Board on Health Care Services, Institute of Medicine. Graduate medical education that meets the nation's health needs, 2014. Available at: <www.iom.edu/GME>. Accessed October 6, 2014.

CHAPTER 6

Laboratory Techniques for Recognition of Endocrine Disorders

PATRICK M. SLUSS • FRANCES J. HAYES

KEY POINTS

- The practice of endocrinology relies heavily on accurate laboratory measurements. Small changes in hormone levels, biomarkers, or molecular markers are often more specific and earlier indicators of disease than the appearance of physical symptoms.
- Analytic methods for assessing endocrine problems are continually expanding. Traditional measurement of endocrine factors, protein, and steroid hormones and related factors has been supplemented by a wide array of disease biomarkers, particularly with respect to endocrine cancers.
- Newer systems are often manufactured outside the laboratory. Although the configurations are generally more "user friendly," they also become more of a "black box," concealing most of the details of the system. Numeric values, especially when reported to several decimal places, can falsely suggest levels of accuracy and reproducibility beyond the technical limits of the technology employed.
- Understanding the basic principles of method validation and quality control is essential if endocrinologists are to be able to assess the reliability and robustness of numeric values reported and to work effectively with the laboratory to reconcile test values that do not match clinical presentations.
- Laboratory testing as practiced today contributes significantly, both directly and indirectly, to the cost of care, which over the past decade or so has increased faster than improvements in clinical outcomes. Clinicians and pathologists are increasingly required to understand the inner workings of laboratory medicine and work as a team in determining optimal management strategies to contain the costs of care without compromising quality.

Endocrinology is a practice of medicine that is highly dependent on accurate laboratory measurements. Small changes in hormone levels, biomarkers, or molecular markers often may be more specific and more sensitive for early disease detection (or risk) than the classic physical signs and symptoms. Most endocrinologists no longer have facilities to develop and validate laboratory assays. They must rely on centralized hospital or commercial reference laboratories. Understanding the nuances of laboratory testing can greatly aid the clinician in working with the laboratory, particularly when faced with disparate clinical observations and laboratory results.

Laboratory testing as practiced today contributes significantly, both directly and indirectly, to the cost of care, which over the past decade or so has increased faster than improvements in clinical outcomes.[1] Current treatment guidelines, especially in endocrine practice, rely heavily on early laboratory testing. Thus, clinicians and pathologists are increasingly required to understand the inner workings of laboratory medicine and work as a team in determining optimal management strategies to contain the costs of care without compromising quality.

This chapter provides an overview of the analytic techniques typically used for diagnosing and monitoring the progress of endocrine disorders. Historically the quantitative measurement of endocrine factors, protein, and steroid hormones and related factors, such as steroid binding proteins, in blood and urine has been the primary goal. More recently, a wide array of disease biomarkers, particularly with respect to endocrine cancers, have become valuable targets for measurement in the clinical laboratory. Analytic validation is then discussed. The parameters of analytic validation are not method specific, and principles are presented to help endocrinologists better assess the performance of the analytic systems that they are using. Techniques used by clinical laboratories to control and assure quality testing results and services follow to provide guidance in appreciating the reliability and robustness of numeric values reported and in working with the laboratory to reconcile test values that do not match clinical presentations. Finally, especially for the academic practitioner, the classes of assays are discussed to provide some clarity on the regulatory requirements laboratories are required to meet in providing test results for patient care, federally supported human studies, and federally regulated clinical trials.

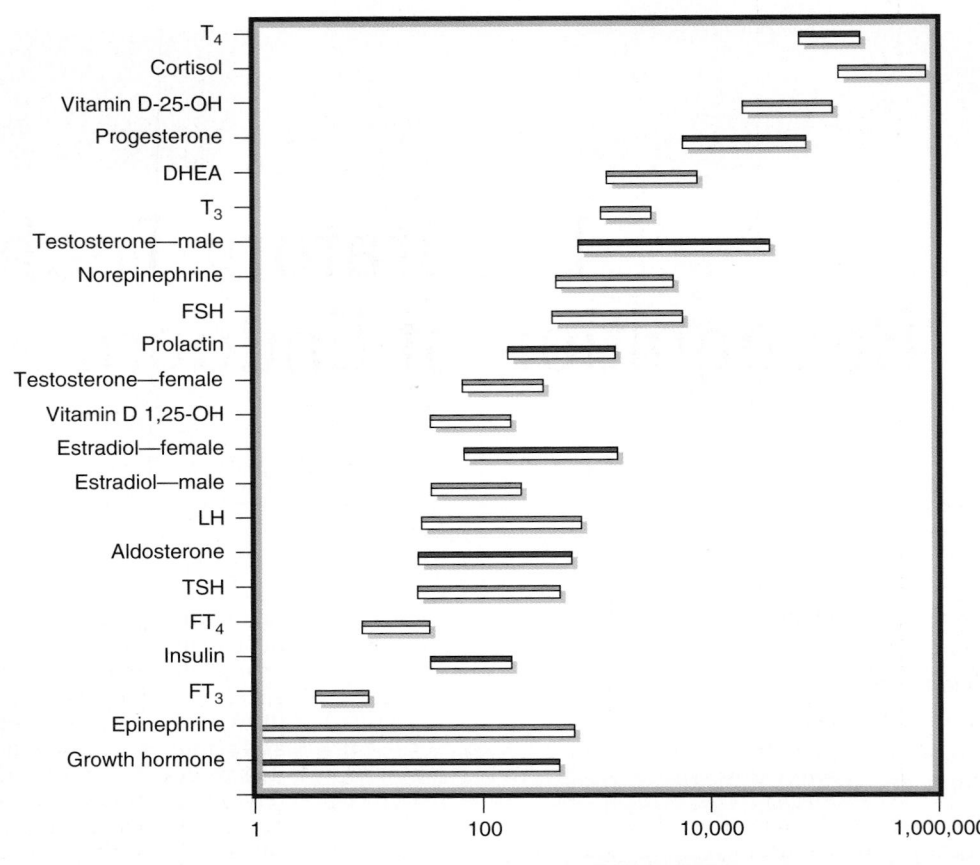

Figure 6-1 Six-logarithm range of normal plasma concentrations in endocrine tests. DHEA, dehydroepiandrosterone; FSH, follicle-stimulating hormone; FT_4, free thyroxine; FT_3, free triiodothyronine; LH, luteinizing hormone; T_3, triiodothyronine; T_4, thyroxine; TSH, thyrotropin.

LABORATORY METHODS

Historically, laboratory methods unique to the clinical practice of endocrinology were directed at the measurement of peripheral levels of hormones or hormone metabolites in urine. This measurement is analytically challenging because concentrations of most hormones are much lower than those of general chemistry analytes. Specialized techniques are necessary to measure these low concentrations that can be reported in molar units, mass units, or standardized units, such as the World Health Organization (WHO) International Unit (IU). Figure 6-1 illustrates the concentrations of representative hormones in plasma from healthy individuals. Expressed in molar units to allow direct comparisons, peripheral hormone levels range from 10^{-6} to 10^{-12} mol/L (i.e., micromolar to picomolar concentrations). Thus, clinically useful analytic methods must have exquisite sensitivity. Furthermore, as also illustrated in Figure 6-1, the range of concentrations is very broad (often several orders of magnitude), necessitating methods with a very wide dynamic range of measurement. Antibody-based methods are ideally suited to achieve sensitivity and wide dynamic ranges and were the first methods successfully used both to define endocrine systems and to be applied clinically in patient care. Because of their suitability for cost effectiveness, high throughput, and potential for automation, antibody methods replaced earlier chromatographic/mass spectrometric methods that were used in the discovery and characterization of hormones, particularly steroid hormones. Initially, competitive binding assays using polyclonal antibodies were utilized;

then with the development of monoclonal antibody technology in the 1980s immunometric, or double antibody, methods were utilized. Both of these analytic designs are automated and are in widespread use today: competitive binding assays are used for measuring small molecules and immunometric assay is used for measuring antigens containing multiple antibody-binding epitopes (i.e., protein hormones and biomarkers).

As will be discussed in detail later, antibody-based assays are subject to interference and lack of specificity that can result in inaccurate measurements. Even when a given assay has been well validated and reference intervals are known (see discussion under "Analytic Validation"), this limitation is manifest as producing measurements that are method specific, vitiating the ability of clinicians to compare measurements reported using different assays (e.g., assays from different laboratories) for the same hormone or biomarker. Although preanalytic methods such as extraction and chromatography have been tried to improve the accuracy of immunoassays used in research settings, these methods are very seldom utilized in clinical laboratories today because of their high cost, complexity, and lack of commercial availability; all are by definition laboratory developed tests (see "Classes of Assays").

Since the early 2000s, technological advances in mass spectrometry–based assay systems have led to the rapid and ongoing replacement of antibody-based methods for the clinical measurement of hormones and biomarkers relevant to the endocrine practice. Currently these more complex and expensive methods are utilized primarily by commercial reference and large academic hospital laboratories, but as the technology becomes more cost effective

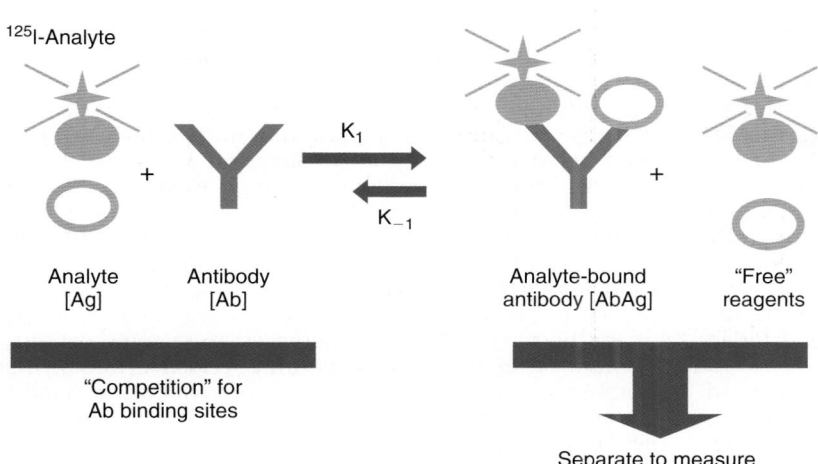

Antibody affinity $= K_1/K_{-1} = $ [AbAg]/[Ab][Ag]

^{125}I-Analyte

K_1
K_{-1}

Analyte [Ag]   Antibody [Ab]

Analyte-bound antibody [AbAg]   "Free" reagents

"Competition" for Ab binding sites

Separate to measure analyte-bound antibody

Figure 6-2 Components of a radioimmunoassay; a prototype competitive binding methodology.

and user friendly its use will clearly increase. Thus, it is important for clinicians to appreciate the principles of these assays as well as those of the older, albeit still widely used, antibody-based methods.

The final technologies considered in this section are molecular-based assays. These methods are not specifically designed for endocrine practice but are generic for identifying and in some cases quantifying genetic variance. Subsequent to the sequencing of the human genome and the continuing evolution of molecular methods and knowledge, these methods are rapidly penetrating endocrine practice. Although these methods are still in the early stages of clinical use and generally require specialized informatics and interpretative support, laboratories are increasingly providing molecular-based testing with respect to determining endocrine cancers, inherited disease, and individualized therapeutics.

Antibody-Based Methods

Classic Competitive Binding Immunoassays

The term *competitive binding assay* refers to a measurement method in which an analyte (e.g., a hormone or biomarker) in a specimen competes with labeled reagent analyte for a limited number of binding sites on a binding protein. The earliest clinical assays used for the measurement of circulating concentrations of endocrine hormones utilized radioisotope-labeled analyte and antibodies in the classic radioimmunoassay format illustrated in Figure 6-2. The three basic components of a competitive immunoassay are antibody, labeled analyte, and unlabeled analyte.[2,3] The basic principle of this methodology is to allow an equilibrium or steady-state condition (e.g., competition) to be established between a labeled analyte and the unlabeled analyte in calibrators or specimens binding to the antibody. The reaction obeys the law of mass action and is driven by the affinity of the antibody as shown in Figure 6-2. If the concentrations of antibody and labeled analyte are held constant, the amount of labeled analyte bound is inversely proportional to the concentration of the competing unlabeled analyte, as illustrated in Figure 6-3. By comparing the percentage of bound antigen (% [Bound/Total]) generated by an unknown specimen to the dose-response curve generated by known concentrations of analyte (see Fig. 6-3B), the amount of analyte in a specimen can be quantified.

Competitive binding

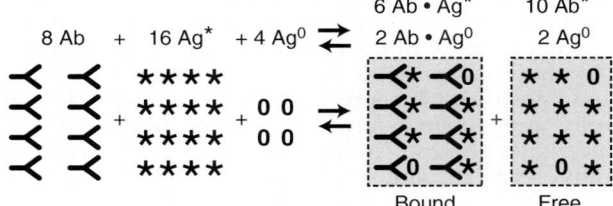

6 Ab • Ag*   10 Ab*
8 Ab + 16 Ag* + 4 Ag⁰ ⇌ 2 Ab • Ag⁰   2 Ag⁰

Bound   Free

Calibration of standards

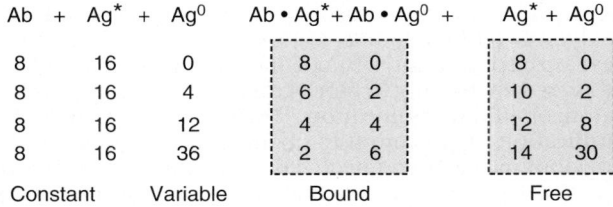

Ab	+ Ag*	+ Ag⁰	Ab • Ag* + Ab • Ag⁰ +		Ag* + Ag⁰	
8	16	0	8	0	8	0
8	16	4	6	2	10	2
8	16	12	4	4	12	8
8	16	36	2	6	14	30
Constant	Variable		Bound		Free	

A

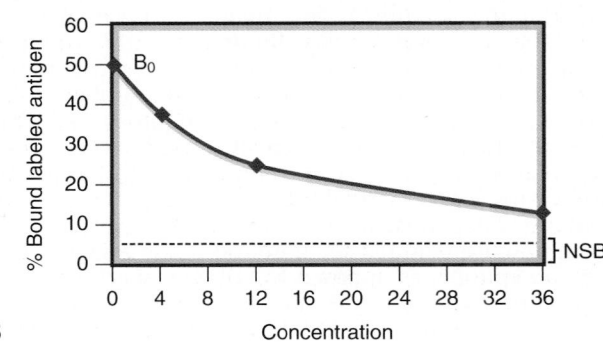

B

Figure 6-3 Quantitation using competitive binding assays. **A,** Principles of competitive binding assays. Ab, antibody; Ag*, labeled antigen; Ag⁰, native antigen. See text for details. **B,** Typical dose-response curve. The point on the curve labeled B₀ represents the percentage binding of the radiolabeled antigen when zero native antigen is present. The nonspecific binding (NSB) level is the minimal binding level of radiolabeled antigen at high concentrations of native antigen.

Competitive antibody-based assays are referred to generically as immunoassays. The analytic sensitivity of a competitive immunoassay is approximately inversely related to the affinity of the antiserum, such that an antiserum with an affinity constant of 10^9 L/M can be used to measure analytes in the nanomolar concentration range. This methodology has evolved significantly since the development of the prototypical radioimmunoassay in the late 1950s. Currently, although radioimmunoassays still have a role in the research laboratory, the immunoassays most widely utilized in clinical endocrine testing are fully automated, nonisotopic instrument systems whose manufacture and reagents are regulated by the Food and Drug Administration (FDA). Each of the component parts of the competitive immunoassay is discussed in detail later in this chapter.

Antibody. Antibodies are ideal as the binding component in a competitive binding assay that is highly specific and can measure very low concentrations of analyte in complex mixtures such as serum or plasma. Antibodies are inherently specific and both their specificity and affinity can be manipulated in developing immunoassays. Immunoassays developed prior to the mid-1980s relied upon polyclonal antiserum produced in animals. Limited quantities of high-affinity antisera that react primarily with the specific target antigen are obtained and can be used either as diluted antiserum or, most often, as purified immunoglobulins.

A polyclonal antiserum represents a composite of many immunologic clones, with each clone having a different affinity and different antigenic epitope specificity. Most clones have affinities in the 10^7 to 10^9 L/M range. The affinity of the antiserum or purified immunoglobulins for the analyte (i.e., the immunogen) is the sum of the affinities of all the various clones. Antisera used in immunoassays typically have affinity constants above the 10^{12} L/M range and can easily measure picomolar concentrations of analyte in biologic fluids. Various techniques are used to develop a specific antiserum. For example, the antigen may be altered chemically to block cross-reacting epitopes either before or after immunization. Historically, immunoaffinity purification of antiserum to obtain epitope-specific immunoglobulins has been effectively used, and this technology can also be applied to preanalytic assay steps to enhance the specificity of immunoassays as well as chromatographic or mass spectrometric assays by selecting or eliminating cross-reacting factors.[4-6] The major disadvantage of a polyclonal antiserum is the limited quantity produced. Commercial manufacturers require large quantities of immunoassay reagents to support a large number of laboratories, and these reagents require rigorous validation. Thus, the majority of commercial immunoassay systems available today are based on monoclonal antibodies that can be produced in virtually limitless quantities.

Monoclonal antisera are used in most current immunoassays and are required for immunometric assays because they are epitope, as opposed to antigen, specific and can be produced virtually without limit. These antibodies are obtained by immunizing animals using techniques similar to those used for polyclonal antisera. Instead of harvesting the antisera from the blood, lymphocytes from the spleen are fused with myeloma cells to make cells (hybridomas) that will grow in culture continuously and produce mono-specific antibodies.[7-10] These fused cells are separated into clones by means of serial plating techniques similar to those used in subculturing bacteria. The supernatant of these monoclonal cell lines (or ascites fluid if the cells are transplanted into carrier mice) contains monoclonal antisera. The selection processes used to separate the initial clones can be targeted to identify specific clones, producing

antibodies with high affinities and low cross-reactivity to related compounds.[11]

In addition to the ability to produce limitless quantities of antibody, the epitope specificity of monoclonal antibodies allows assays to be designed for large analytes (containing multiple nonoverlapping epitopes), which do not depend on competition; these immunometric assays are often referred to as *two-site* or *sandwich* assays (see later). However, the high specificity of monoclonal-based assays can cause problems for some endocrine assays. Many hormones circulate in the blood as heterogeneous mixtures of multiple biologically active forms. Some of these forms are caused by genetic differences in patients, and others are related to metabolic precursors and degradation products of the hormone. Genetic differences cause some patients to produce variant forms of a hormone such as luteinizing hormone (LH). These genetic differences can cause marked variations in measurements made using assays with specific monoclonals, compared with more uniform measurements made using assays with polyclonal antisera that cross-react with the multiple forms.[12] Well-characterized monoclonal antisera can be mixed together to make an *engineered polyclonal antiserum* with improved sensitivity and specificity.[13] Cross-reactivity with precursor forms of the analyte and with metabolic degradation products can cause major differences in assays. For example, cross-reactivity with six molecular forms of human chorionic gonadotropin (hCG) causes differences in hCG assays, and cross-reactivity with metabolic fragments causes differences in parathyroid hormone (PTH) assays.[14,15] Cortisol is another analyte for which major cross-reactivity with other steroids, such as corticosterone, 11-deoxycortisol, cortisone, and numerous synthetic steroids, causes significant immunoassay interferences.[16] Matrix effects with albumin also can cause major differences in cortisol immunoassays (see "Mass Spectrometry" for a more robust method for measuring steroids).[17]

Labeled Antigen. In radioimmunoassays, radioactive iodine (^{125}I or ^{131}I) was originally used to label the antigen. Subsequently, a large variety of methods have been developed to label the analytes.[18-23] Today most commercial kits and all automated immunoassays use nonisotopic signaling systems to measure hormone concentrations. These assays use colorimetric, fluorometric, or chemiluminescent signals rather than radioactivity to quantify the relative amount of antigen bound to the antibody used in the assay. The advantages of these nonisotopic labeling technologies include biosafety, longer reagent shelf life, ease of automation, and reduced cost. On the other hand, they can be more subject to matrix interferences than radioactive detection systems. Radioactivity is not affected by changes in protein concentration, hemolysis, color, or drugs (except for other radioactive compounds), whereas many of the current signal systems can yield spurious results when such interferences are present. Later in this chapter, potential troubleshooting steps are outlined to help clinicians evaluate the integrity of test measurements when spurious results are suspected.

Labeled antigen assays have the disadvantage that assay specificity and accuracy depend on the purity of the labeled antigen. Especially with respect to labeling small molecules, such as steroid hormones, purification of the labeled antigen can be challenging and certainly contributes to lot-to-lot variance in assay performance. Additionally, sensitivity in this assay design is influenced by the specific activity of the labeled product (i.e., the amount of label incorporated into the antigen on a molar basis). An alternative design for competition assays is to attach the antigen to a solid phase and label the antibody. A competitive binding assay is then achieved by allowing unlabeled antigen to compete with solid-phase antigen for labeled antibody binding. Currently this design is found in research-only tests available in the United States. Although it addresses issues associated with antigen labeling, this format is subject to similar issues associated with modification of antibody binding characteristics as the antigen is chemically attached to a solid-phase or due to restricting its conformation once the antigen is attached.

Unlabeled Antigen. The labeled and unlabeled antigens compete for this limited number of binding sites on the antiserum. The competition is not always equal because the labeled antigen (*tracer*) and the native antigen may react differently with the antibody. This disparity in reactivity may be caused by alteration of the antigen due to labeling, as discussed earlier, or by differences in the endogenous antigen compared with the form of the antigen used in the reagents. The latter is a problem often encountered with protein hormones or biomarkers that often exhibit a wide range of isoforms and degradation products in peripheral circulation. Because the assay can be calibrated with certified reference materials having known concentrations, differences in reactivity of labeled compared to unlabeled antigen do not prevent obtaining useful clinical measurements as long as the reactions are reproducible and appropriate reference intervals are established. Such differences do, however, result in method-specific measurements, and in this case assay results cannot be extrapolated among assays using different reagents.

Separation of Reactants/Automation. As illustrated in Figures 6-2 and 6-3, immunoassays depend on detecting only the labeled antigen bound by the antibody. Thus, the entire antibody component of the assay must be recovered and separated for any unbound reactants (i.e., labeled or unlabeled antigens not bound to antibody). Over the years since the introduction of radioimmunoassays a vast technology has been developed to accomplish this separation. Approaches vary from methods to precipitate immunoglobulins and recover them by centrifugation or filtration to very innovative ways to create solid-phase antibodies (i.e., antibodies attached to solid surfaces that can be washed to remove unreacted reagents after the binding process is completed).

Separation of immune complexes by precipitation and centrifugation is labor intensive and, like the use of radioactivity itself, not amenable to full automation. This approach is still widely used in research applications but seldom utilized in clinical testing. In contrast, solid-phase approaches are widely employed and can be batch or fully automated. Three frequently used solid-phase materials are microtiter plates, polystyrene or latex beads, and paramagnetic particles. Most recently the use of immunoassay systems at the point of care and miniaturization of assay systems are driving the development of novel methods of creating solid-phase antibody systems.[21,23-25] Separation of solid-phase immune complexes from the unbound moieties is accomplished by plate washers, bead washers, magnetic wash stations, or microfluidics. Centrifugation is not required, enabling full automation of the assay.

Antibodies can be attached to solid-phase materials directly or indirectly. Antibodies can be passively attached directly to plastic surfaces by hydrophobic interactions, and this method is often used in the manufacture of enzyme-linked immunosorbent assays (ELISA). Clinical assays, requiring more defined procedures and long reagent shelf lives, typically involve chemical procedures in which amino acid groups or carbohydrate groups on the Fc portion of immunoglobulins are covalently coupled to the solid phase. This can be achieved directly by coupling the antibody used in the assay to the solid phase or indirectly by covalently coupling a universal capture to the solid phase. Examples of universal capture systems are solid-phase particles with covalently attached streptavidin to capture biotinylated assay antibodies or solid-phase particles covalently coated with goat antimouse IgG as attachment moiety for mouse monoclonal-based assays. Another novel way of accomplishing this separation is to attach high-affinity linkers to antiserum, which then can be coupled to a complementary linker on the solid phase.

Quantitation. Figure 6-3 illustrates the principles of quantitative measurement using competitive immunoassay techniques. In the schematic diagram, 8 units of antibody react with 16 units of labeled antigen and 4 units of native antigen. At equilibrium (assuming equal reactivity), 6 units of label and 2 units of native antigen are bound to the limited supply of antibody. The antigen bound to the antibody is separated from the liquid antigen by any of several methods, and the amount of labeled antigen in the bound portion is quantified (see Fig. 6-3A). The assay is calibrated by measuring standards with known concentrations and cross-plotting the signal (i.e., counts of the gamma rays emitted from the radioactive label) versus the concentration of the standard to generate a dose-response curve. As the concentration increases, the signal decreases exponentially (Fig. 6-3B).

Statistical data-processing techniques are needed to translate the assay signals into concentrations. These dose-response curves typically are not linear, and numerous curve-fitting algorithms have been developed. Before the introduction of microprocessors, tedious, error-prone manual calculations were required to mathematically transform the data into linear models. Today, curve fitting usually is accomplished electronically with the use of programs that automatically test the robustness of fit of multiparameter curves after statistically eliminating discordant data points.[26,27] However, users of these systems must understand their limitations and should pay attention to any warnings presented by the programs during processing of the data. Commercial immunoanalyzers, used by the majority of clinical laboratories currently, are closed systems. The manufacturer validates not only the method (see "Analytic Validation") but also the curve-fitting software, which cannot be altered by the user. Thus, clinical laboratories and clinicians see only the final values for the signal generated and calculated analyte concentration for a given specimen.

In clinical practice today competitive assays are used primarily for this measurement of small molecules, such as steroid hormones or bioactive peptides, which present only one antigenic epitope. For molecules in which multiple epitopes are present, allowing more than one antibody to bind each molecule, two-site or immunometric assays are used. Immunometric assays, discussed in detail in the following section, are advantageous because they do not require the time-consuming establishment of a binding steady-state condition and thus can be performed much faster. Speed of test performance is an important factor in the clinical laboratory supporting acute care. Speed is also directly related to high testing throughput, which is an important cost factor to optimize in modern clinical laboratories.

Immunoassays, indeed any antibody-based method, measure concentrations rather than biologic activity. The reactive site for most antibodies is relatively small, about 5 to 10 amino acids for linear peptides. Some antibody reactions are specific for the tertiary structure that corresponds to unique molecular configurations. In either case, linear or conformational antigenic epitopes, the structural elements of the hormone involved in receptor activation and biologic signaling, are not necessarily identical to antigenic epitopes. The clinician must keep this in mind when interpreting the results of antibody-based assays. When measurements are ordered to identify abnormal secretion of hormones the possible disparity between antigenic and biologic epitopes is not as relevant as when measurements are ordered to assess the endocrine stimulus received by the target glands.

Epitope-Specific Immunometric Assays

As briefly mentioned earlier, for larger analytes that contain more than one nonoverlapping antigenic epitope, the development of methods to produce monoclonal antibodies facilitates a unique assay design in which two antibodies are used. This format is illustrated in Figure 6-4. The analyte in this example has four nonoverlapping epitopes: A, B, C, and D. A solid-phase monoclonal antibody (referred to as the capture antibody) that is specific to one site (in this example, A) can be used to bind the antigen in calibrators or specimens. Using a second, labeled monoclonal antibody (referred to as the detection antibody) that is specific to one of the other epitopes (in the example, D), the captured antigen can be quantified after washing away the unreacted reagents. Because there are four distinct antibody-binding sites on the analyte, 12 different assays can be configured using four monoclonal antibodies to each of these epitopes. It is important to realize that each of these 12 formats is a distinct assay with unique performance characteristics, each requiring validation. The detection systems employed include all the options discussed earlier for labeling protein antigens in immunoassay formats. Figure 6-5 illustrates one of the most common signaling systems used today in either fully automated clinical immunoanalyzers or as specialized plate assays for research and discovery testing. The detection antibody is covalently labeled with ruthenium (tris bipyridine), which can be excited by an electric circuit that draws an electron from the molecule, leading ultimately to a high-energy state that will emit light when it decays; this is an electrochemiluminescent signaling system.[28] The assay buffer contains an excess of the electron donor tripropylamine (TPA). The Ru^{2+} (tris bipyridine ruthenium metal cation) complex is used as the chemical luminescent label, and the TPA is used as the emitter. Ru^{2+} undergoes an electrochemical oxidation reaction on the electrode surface and transitions to an excited state to become Ru^{3+}. When the excited state returns to the ground state, light is emitted. The magnetic particles that are captured on the electrode are immunocomplexes that consist of sample and Ru metal complex (Ru^{2+}) and emit light at a specified voltage. The amount of light emitted is proportional to the weight of the immunocomplex and thus the weight of the sample. It can therefore be used for quantitative measurement. This design is typical of modern detection systems in that the signal generated is controlled in the analyzer (in this case light production initiated by activating the electrode), and a regenerating system (in this case TPA in the assay buffer) is employed to enhance the signal generated, hence achieving high sensitivity detection.

In contrast to competitive immunoassays, these assays use a large excess of antibody-binding sites compared with the concentration of antigen. The capture antibody immunoextracts the antigen from the sample, and the signal antibody binds to the capture antibody-antigen complex to form a tertiary complex. These assays are referred to as immunometric because the binding reaction is very fast (first-order kinetics due to excess antibody) and it is not necessary to establish a binding steady state (a requirement for competition assays) in the assay before quantifying the amount of label associated with the immune complex. Immunometric assay can be performed very quickly (5-15 minutes compared to 30 minutes to days for competition assays) and typically have very broad measuring ranges (several log orders).

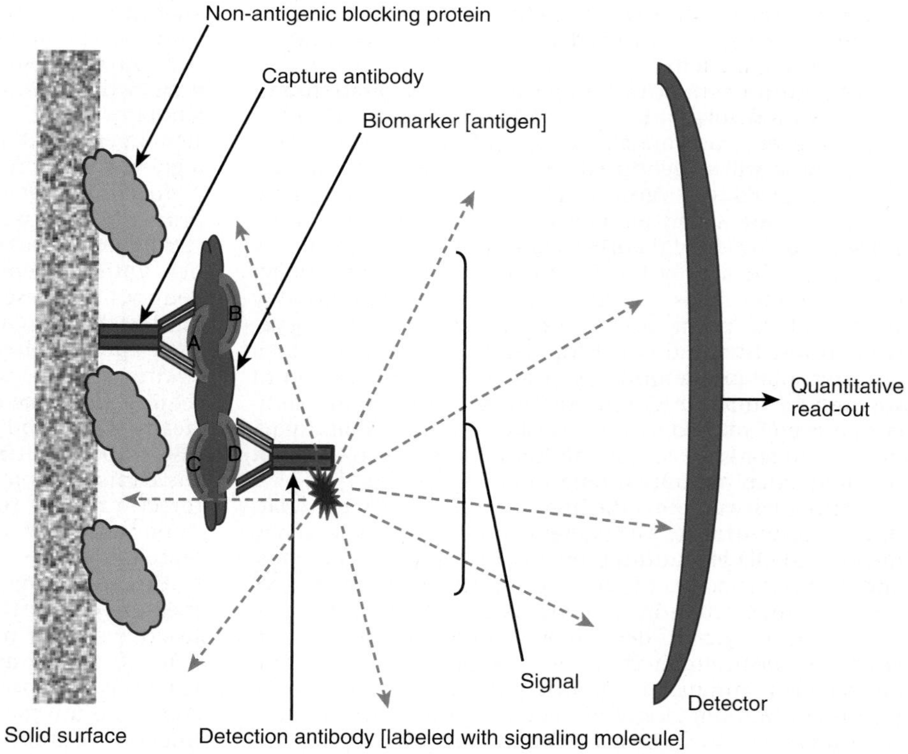

Figure 6-4 Components and design of an immunometric assay. See discussion in text. (From Sluss PM. Methodologies for measurement of cardiac markers. *Clin Lab Med.* 2014;34:167-185. Reproduced with permission from Elsevier Inc.)

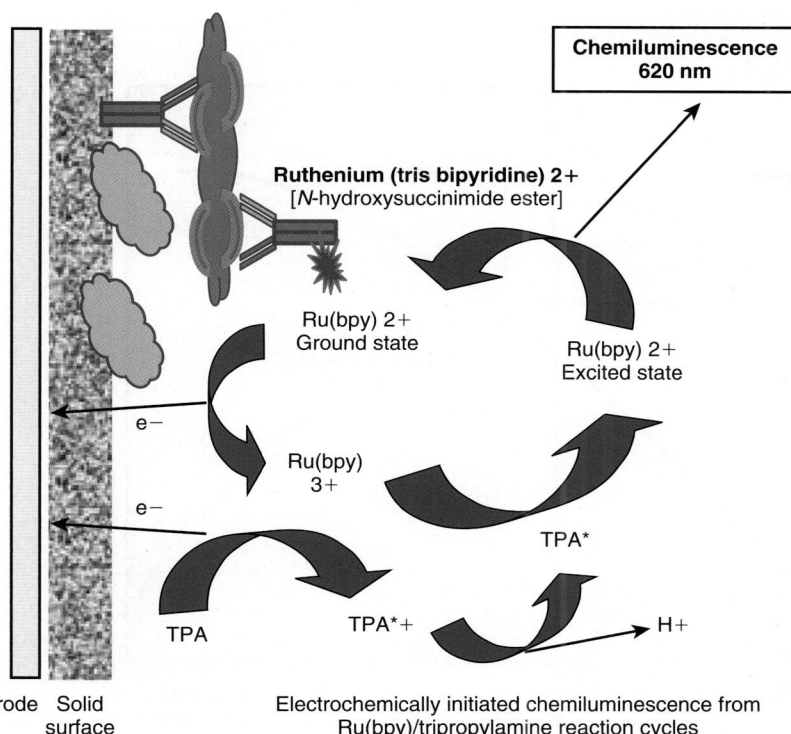

Chemiluminescence 620 nm

Ruthenium (tris bipyridine) 2+
[*N*-hydroxysuccinimide ester]

Ru(bpy) 2+
Ground state

Ru(bpy) 2+
Excited state

e−

Ru(bpy)
3+

e−

TPA*

TPA   TPA*+   → H+

Electrode   Solid
            surface

Electrochemically initiated chemiluminescence from
Ru(bpy)/tripropylamine reaction cycles

Figure 6-5 Electrochemiluminescence detection system as employed in an immunometric assay. See text for details. byp, bipyridine; TPA, tripropylamine. (From Sluss PM. Methodologies for measurement of cardiac markers. *Clin Lab Med.* 2014;34:167-185. Reproduced with permission from Elsevier Inc.)

In contrast to competition assays the dose-response curve generated in an immunometric assay is directly proportional to the analyte concentration (Fig. 6-6). The signal increases progressively with the concentration. For lower concentrations, the signal generated represents the amount of labeled antibody bound to the solid-phase immune complex after binding and washing steps are completed. The amount of labeled antibody bound increases proportionally to the amount of analyte present in the immune complex, which is directly proportional to the amount of analyte in the specimen or calibrator. Quantitative measurements are achieved in the same manner as those used in competition assays. The signal generated by the specimen (the "unknown" in Fig. 6-6) is compared to the calibration curve generated by known concentrations of the analyte (plotted on the x-axis in Fig. 6-6).

As with any assay, there is a minimum detection limit (referred to as the limit of detection, or LOD) at which the signal generated by the analyte is not statistically different from that generated in the absence of analyte (referred to as nonspecific signal). Note that for an immunometric assay the LOD is associated with a small signal, but in a competition assay the LOD is associated with a large signal (compare the dose-response curve in Fig. 6-6 to that illustrated in Fig. 6-3B). All antibody-based assays also have an upper limit of measurement associated with the maximum signal that can be generated by the assay. The working or dynamic range of the assay encompasses only analyte concentrations between the LOD and the maximum response. Analyte concentrations above the maximum response or below the LOD level do not generate signal changes (e.g., there is no dose-response relationship). Thus, the measurement variance across the dynamic range of an antibody-based assay is heteroscedastic. The insert in Figure 6-6 shows the measurement variance expressed as the percent coefficient of variance (CV) of repeated measurements of the same specimen. The CV is calculated as the standard deviation (SD) of the repeated measures divided by the

mean value of the measurements. The highest percent CV (e.g., CV × 100) will occur at the extremes of the measurement where the analyte dose response is lost. This point is critical when interpreting assay results or monitoring quality control performance. Variance determined in the middle of the dynamic range of an assay will always underestimate the variance at the extremes.

Although the laboratory can control variance associated with high analyte concentrations by determining at what level of analyte to dilute and retest the specimen, variance associated with relatively low concentrations cannot be altered for a given assay without changing the kinetics of the system (i.e., the concentrations of reagents and/or incubation conditions). Changing the kinetics of a commercial clinical assay is not possible because the systems are "locked" to comply with FDA manufacturing regulations.

The combined specificity of two antibodies can produce exquisitely sensitive and specific immunoassays. In the past, a common problem with early competitive immunoassays was cross-reactivity among the structurally similar gonadotropins: LH, follicle-stimulating hormone (FSH), thyrotropin (thyroid-stimulating hormone, or TSH), and hCG. The α-subunits of each of these hormones are almost identical, and the β-subunits have considerable structural homology. The polyclonal antisera used for measuring one of these hormones in many of the earlier immunoassays had significant cross-reactivity for the other gonadotropins. The cross-reactivity of a pair of antibodies is less than the cross-reactivity of each of the individual antibodies because any cross-reacting substance must contain both of the binding epitopes in order to simultaneously bind to both antibodies. For example, consider two antibodies for LH, each having 1% cross-reactivity with hCG. The cross-reactivity of the pair is less than the product of the two cross-reactivities or, in this case, less than 0.01%. Most current immunoassays for LH have a cross-reactivity of less than 0.01%. This low cross-reactivity is important, because

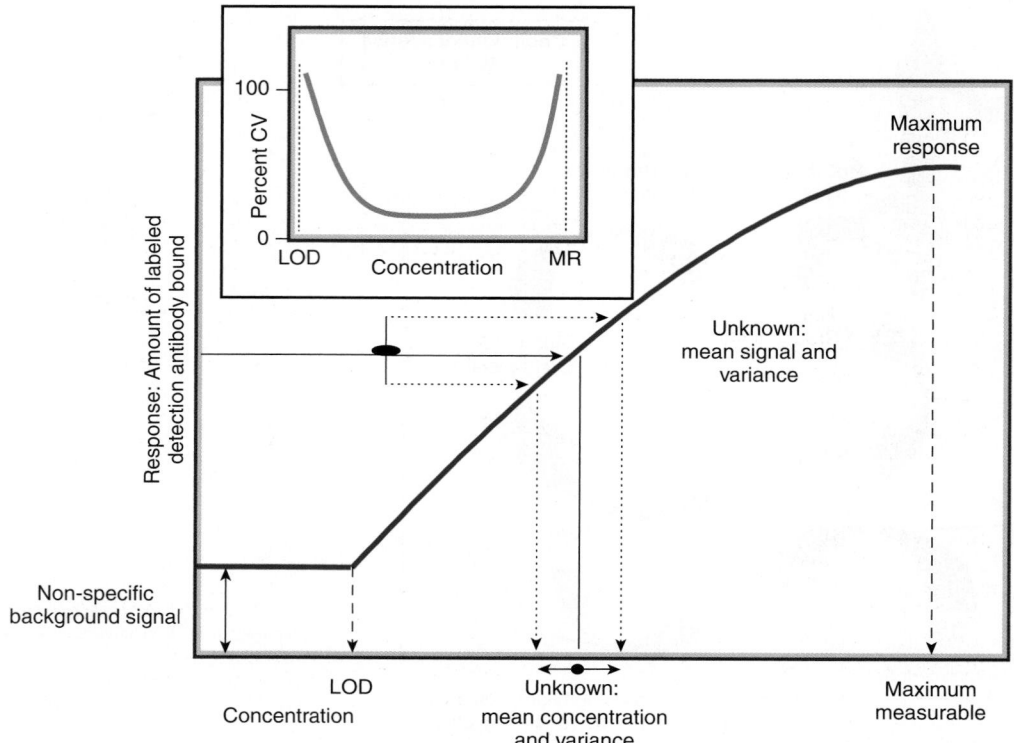

Figure 6-6 Characteristics of the signal generated by an immunometric assay. Signal generated by the amount of detection antibody bound to the capture-analyte complex is directly proportional to the concentration of analyte in an immunometric assay. The concentration can be extrapolated from response (signal measured) by measuring known concentrations of "calibrators." As shown in the inset, the variance associated with measurement is heteroscedastic and increases significantly as the upper or lower limits of the assay are approached. CV, coefficient of variance; LOD, limit of detection; MR, maximum response. (From Sluss PM. Methodologies for measurement of cardiac markers. *Clin Lab Med.* 2014;34:167-815. Reproduced with permission from Elsevier Inc.)

pregnant patients or patients with choriocarcinoma can have very high hCG concentrations that could interfere with measurements of the other gonadotropin hormones. Most hormones circulate in the blood in multiple forms. Some hormones (e.g., prolactin, growth hormone) circulate with macro forms, which can cause difficulty in their analysis if specimens are not pretreated.[29,30] For hormones composed of subunits (e.g., the gonadotropins), both the intact and the free subunits circulate in blood. Immunometric assays can be made specific for intact molecules by pairing an antibody specific for the α-β bridge site of the subunits with a second antibody specific for the β-subunit. Assays using these antibody pairs retain the two-antibody low cross-reactivity needed for measuring gonadotropins and do not react with the free subunit forms of the hormones.

The heterogeneous forms of circulating hormones and differences in specificity characteristics of immunoassays for these forms make calibration and harmonization difficult. Two immunoassays calibrated with the same reference preparation can give widely varying measurements on patient specimens. Consider the example of hCG in Table 6-1. The three assays are calibrated with a pure preparation of intact hCG, such as the WHO Third International Reference Preparation. The three assays differ in their cross-reactivity with free β-hCG (0%, 100%, and 200%, respectively). These assays give identical measurements for a specimen containing only intact hCG but progressively disparate values as the percentage of free β-hCG in the specimen increases. In reality, the standardization issue is much more complex, because multiple forms of hormones (i.e., intact hormone, free subunits, nicked forms, glyco-

TABLE 6-1			
Effect of Immunoassay Specificity on Calibration of Human Chorionic Gonadotropin (hCG) Assays			
hCG Sample	**Assay 1**	**Assay 2**	**Assay 3**
Specificity for intact hCG standard (%)	100	100	100
Cross-reactivity with free β-hCG (%)	0	100	200
Measured values (IU/L)			
Specimen with 0% free β-hCG	10.0	10.0	10.0
Specimen with 10% free β-hCG	9.0	10.0	11.0
Specimen with 50% free β-hCG	5.0	10.0	15.0

slyated forms, degradation products) circulate in patients, and each assay has different cross-reactivity characteristics with respect to these forms.[31-34]

Because of their speed, specificity, and sensitivity, immunometric assay designs have also been applied successfully to point-of-care testing devices. A typical design is shown in Figure 6-7. In this example, a laminar flow system is shown with two solid-phase monoclonal antibodies affixed to the flow device. One antibody is specific for the analyte and the other, located on a different section of the analytic strip, is directed at the capture antibody itself. This strip contains a reservoir of detection antibody covalently coupled to gold microparticles. A drop of specimen (blood, serum, plasma, urine, etc.) is placed on one end of the strip and carried across the analytic strip by laminar flow, passing first through the detection antibody reservoir and then over the capture antibodies in sequence. The final state, as illustrated in Figure 6-7, results in a band of gold particles over

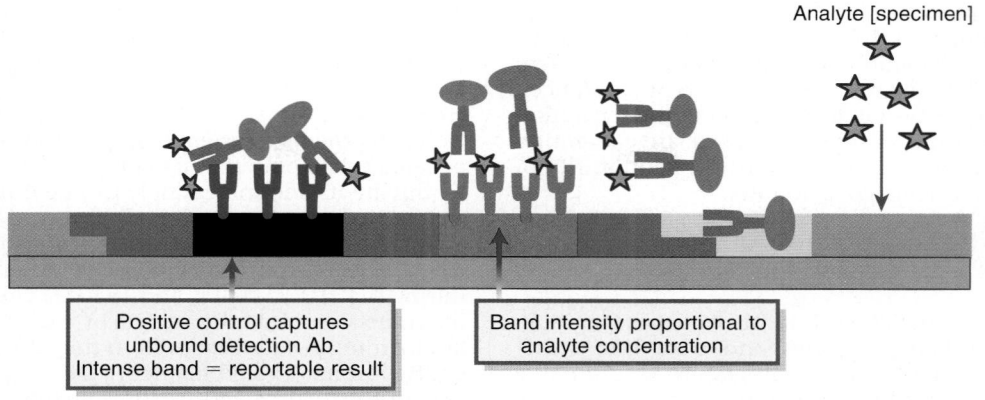

Figure 6-7 Laminar flow immunometric assay design. See discussion in text. Ab, antibody. (From Sluss PM. Methodologies for measurement of cardiac markers. *Clin Lab Med*. 2014;34:167-185. Reproduced with permission from Elsevier Inc.)

the capture antibody region that is proportional to the amount of analyte in the specimen and a positive control band of gold particles over the antidetection antibody region. Such tests are generally qualitative but with the use of a standardized meter for measuring the gold bands and calibrator can be quantitative. Increasingly these systems are being miniaturized and optimized for quantitative measures at the point of care and other nonlaboratory settings (e.g., field testing and low-resource settings). Although still primarily research tools, similar technologies are utilized in developing multiarray assays (e.g., "lab on a chip" assays) that will likely become part of the clinical laboratory's repertoire of tools in the future.[19,24,25,35,36]

Molecular Structure–Based Methods

Extraction Methods

Extraction of hormones from serum and urine specimens before measurement is a technique that can enhance both the sensitivity and the specificity of immunoassays and mass spectrometry–based assays. Generally extraction procedures applied to the measurement of steroids are based on the polarity or water solubility of the molecules. Extraction methods for proteins/peptides can be based on molecular size as well as polarity. It is essential in any extraction method that recovery (the amount of analyte extracted) is consistent across all specimens. If the extraction recovery is less than 100% but consistent, the method will produce biased yet usable, albeit method-specific, results. If the recovery is different among specimens and cannot be corrected by monitoring, the assay is not valid.

Numerous extraction systems have been developed, including organic-aqueous partitioning to remove water-soluble interferences seen with steroids, solid-phase extraction with absorption and selective elution from resins such as silica gels, and immunoaffinity chromatography. Early immunoassays for steroids relied heavily on extraction prior to assay and provided a basis for assessing interference in subsequent direct assays.[37,38] However, extraction before immunoassay is seldom used in clinical assays today. Extraction techniques are difficult to automate, require skills and equipment not available in many clinical laboratories, and generally require correction based on measuring recovery. Monitoring recovery in automated immunoassays is very difficult and creates issues with regulatory compliance (i.e., modification of manufacturer methods). In contrast, extraction methods are a key element in preanalytic processing for mass spectrometry–based assays (see later) in which it is possible to measure

recovery using an internal standard added to every specimen being tested. Extraction can also be applied to the measurement of proteins/peptides. Most current mass spectrometry assays for steroids involve deproteinization of the specimen (extraction of the steroids) prior to further extraction/purification preanalytically. Similarly, mass spectrometry–based assay of proteins/peptides generally utilizes a batch extraction based on molecular size or polarity. A good deal of progress has been made in developing preanalytic extraction methods prior to assay.[39-50]

Chromatographic Systems

The second major method of measuring hormone concentrations involves chromatographic separation of the various biochemical forms and quantitation of specific characteristics of the molecules. High-performance liquid chromatography (HPLC) systems use multiple forms of detection, including light absorption, fluorescence, and electrochemical properties.[51-53] Chromatography also is frequently combined with mass spectrometry (see later). There are two major advantages of these techniques: They can be used to simultaneously measure multiple forms of an analyte, and they are not dependent on unique immunologic reagents. Therefore, harmonization of measurements made with different assays is more feasible. The major disadvantages of these methods are their complexity and their limited availability.

Many chemical separation techniques are based on chromatography, but the two most commonly used for liquid chromatography are normal-phase HPLC and reverse-phase HPLC. In both systems, a bonded solid-phase column is made that interacts with the analytes as they flow past in a liquid solvent. In normal-phase HPLC, the functional groups of the stationary phase are polar (e.g., amino or nitrile ions) relative to the nonpolar stationary phase (e.g., hexane); in reverse-phase HPLC, a nonpolar stationary phase (e.g., C18 octadecylsilane molecules bonded to silica) is used. Polymeric packings made of mixed copolymers have been made with C4, C8, and C18 functional groups directly incorporated so that they are more stable over a wide pH range. The mobile and stationary phases are selected to optimize adherence of the analytes to the stationary phase. The adhered molecules can be eluted differentially from the solid phase, after washing to separate specific forms of the analyte from interfering substances. If the composition of the mobile phase remains constant throughout the run, the process is called an isocratic elution. If the mobile-phase composition is abruptly changed, a step elution occurs. If the composition is gradually changed throughout the run, a gradient elution occurs.

The efficiency of separation in a chromatography system is a function of the flow rates of the different substances. The resolution of the system is a measure of the separation of the two solute bands in terms of their relative retention volumes (V_f) and their bandwidths (ω). Resolution (R_s) of solutes A and B is calculated as follows:

$$R_s = \frac{2[V_f(B) - V_f(A)]}{\omega(A) + \omega(B)}$$

Values of R_s lower than 0.8 result in inadequate separation, and values greater than 1.25 correspond to baseline separation. The resolution of a chromatography column is a function of flow rates and thermodynamic factors.

HPLC remains the method of choice for clinical measurements of catecholamines in biologic fluids.[54,55] Simultaneous measurement of the three catecholamines (epinephrine, norepinephrine, and dopamine) can be obtained. Prior extraction by absorption on activated alumina and acid elution helps to improve specificity. Dihydroxybenzylamine, a molecule similar to endogenous catecholamines, can be used as an internal standard.

Mass Spectrometry

Mass spectrometry depends on the movement of charged particles through a magnetic field in order to separate and quantify them on the basis of their mass, or more rigorously their mass-to-charge ratio (m/z).[56] A mass spectrometer is an instrument designed to ionize analytes, accelerate them into a device (mass analyzer) that separates them based on their m/z, and quantifies their relative abundance. Figure 6-8 illustrates the components and principles of a generic mass spectrometer. The heart of the system is the mass analyzer, which utilizes adjustable magnetic fields to accelerate or deflect volatile (e.g., in gaseous form) ions, typically in a vacuum so that the ion's flight path is determined only by the magnetic field. A source is used to ionize and if necessary volatilize and fragment analytes in order to introduce them into the mass analyzer. Analytes are introduced into the source via an inlet that can be as simple as an injection port or as sophisticated as a laser-driven matrix desorption system or photo-ionization chamber. Charged particles passing through the mass analyzer are counted by a simple Faraday plate detector, which generates an electric current proportional in intensity to the frequency (abundance) of ions striking the detector. As will become apparent as the components are discussed in more detail later, mass spectrometers used in endocrine

clinical testing are quite complex, with analytes being delivered to the inlet via a chromatography system, subtle selection of ions with m/z characteristics unique to the analyte, and measurement based on system calibration and recovery of internal standards. All of these aspects are controlled by the data system (computer software), which also generates data outputs that comply with clinical reporting requirements and increasingly can be integrated into fully electronic laboratory and medical record systems.

Analytic mass spectrometry developed in tandem with the discovery and characterization of endocrine steroids during the 1930s, 1940s, and 1950s.[57] The source for these instruments ionized the analyte by electron impact (i.e., by bombarding gas molecules from the sample with electrons emitted from a heated filament), creating a full fragmentation of the analyte and multiple charged particles of each of the composite atoms. By determining the relative abundance and mass of each ionized particle the molecular structure of the steroid could be constructed. However, the methodology requires that the steroids, indeed any analyte, be purified and volatilized prior to fragmentation and ionization in the source. Most steroid hormones are easily heat damaged and must be derivatized with molecules that can be volatilized and ionized before mass analysis. This methodology was used in strictly research applications in which it was invaluable in delineating the physiology of reproductive steroids. The development of gas chromatography, in conjunction with electron impact mass analyzers (GC/MS), led to the clinical use of mass spectrometry, which was applied first to endocrine steroids and subsequently to other small biologically important molecules. GC/MS, using quadrupole analyzers in scanning mode (see later), remains a key technology in the research laboratory today and arguably is the method of choice for the study of steroid hormone metabolites.[58] GC/MS was replaced for clinical endocrine steroid testing by the cheaper, higher throughput antibody-based assays, which remain the primary method in all but very large academic hospital or reference laboratories. However, dramatic advances in mass spectrometry design have led to the availability of instruments that are rapidly replacing many antibody-based assays, especially competition immunoassays, in clinical laboratories.

The technological advances leading up to modern mass spectrometers involve primarily the source and the mass analyzer components. The most dramatic advance in sources, with respect to clinical applications of mass spectrometry in endocrine testing, was the development of electrospray ionization (ESI).[59,60] This technology underlies the direct connection of liquid chromatography systems to mass spectrometry and is currently the method of choice

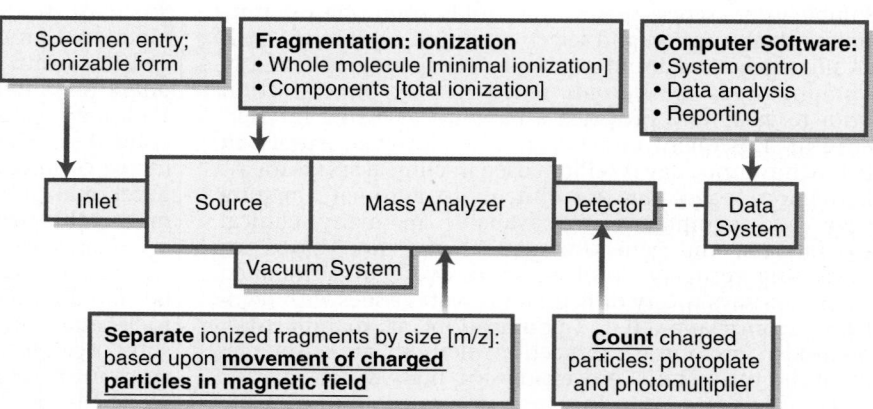

Figure 6-8 Components and principles of a generic mass spectrometer. See discussion in text. *m/z*, mass-to-charge ratio.

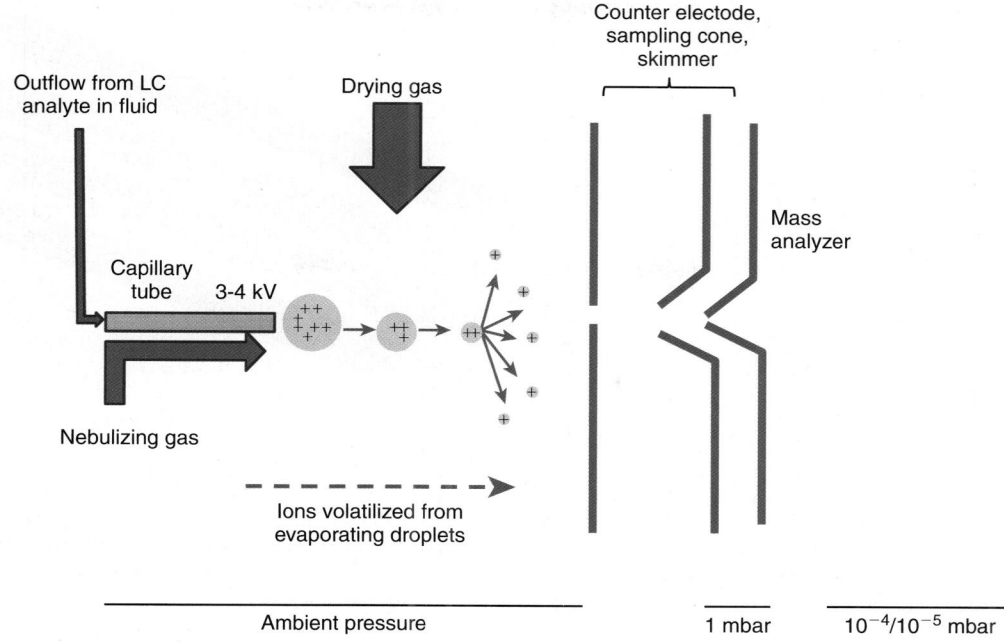

Figure 6-9 Principle of electrospray ionization for introducing analytes isolated by liquid chromatography (LC) directly into the mass spectrometer.

for measuring analytes relevant to endocrinology, such as steroid hormones, in biologic fluids. The principle of ESI is illustrated in Figure 6-9. The specimen to be measured in the effluent from a chromatography system is pushed at low speed through a capillary column into the source region of the spectrometer to create an aerosol when high voltage (positive or negative) is applied to the tube in the presence of a nebulizing gas. As the droplets in the aerosol dry, often with the aid of a drying gas, the molecules in the specimen become charged and volatilized. In gaseous form these molecules then enter the mass analyzer.

ESI has directly resulted in the development of systems that are rapidly replacing the antibody-based competition assays in the clinical laboratory. The most obvious advantage is that liquid chromatography systems can be coupled directly to the mass spectrometer. This system allows the extensive knowledge of steroid and peptide purification by liquid chromatography to be directly applied in mass spectrometry systems that for the first time can be automated and support high throughput testing. Because the analysis time (seconds) in a mass analyzer is much shorter than the time required for chromatographic separations (minutes) several independent liquid chromatography systems can be supported by one mass spectrometer. Thus, the technical advantages of the mass spectrometer (measurements based directly on the molecular composition of the analyte rather than indirect competition of the analyte for antibody binding) can be realized in the practical setting of clinical testing services.

The ionization achieved by ESI is also an important technological advance. Although the exact mechanisms are still unclear, ESI is characterized by ionization at low temperatures and pressures and results in relatively little fragmentation of the analyte so that a molecular ion is always generated. This procedure has allowed the development of exquisitely specific methods. Most significant with respect to current clinical testing is *tandem mass spectrometry*, especially triple quadrupole mass analyzers linked together.

The design of a quadrupole mass analyzer is illustrated in Figure 6-10. The analyzer is composed of four round

electrodes. Voltage of the same polarity is applied to directly opposite electrodes, and opposite voltage polarity is applied to adjacent ones. An oscillating electric field is generated within the quadrupole when an alternating current (voltage V, frequency ω, and time t) is applied with a superimposed direct current (voltage U). Thus, charged particles (ions) moving through the quadrupole follow oscillating paths and only ions with a specific m/z can pass through to the downstream detector. Ions with greater or lesser m/z collide with the electrodes and are not detected. By controlling the applied voltages the analyzer can be operated to select ions of specific m/z for detection (or transit). Because ions are moving rapidly and voltage can be controlled rapidly, the analysis time is very short. The analyzer thus can be operated in three distinct modes to (1) filter ion for the quantitation of only one m/z, (2) scan to sequentially quantify all ions by m/z, or (3) trap ions within the quadrupole.

Combining three quadrupole analyzers results in a very powerful system (Fig. 6-11), often referred to as the Triple Quad mass spectrometer and often just as LC/MS-MS or LC/tandem MS in the clinical literature. The molecular ions generated by ESI can be filtered by the first mass analyzer (quadrupole) to capture, in a second mass analyzer, a molecular ion whose m/z is consistent with that of the target analyte. The captured molecular ion is fragmented and ionized in the second analyzer, which becomes the source for the third analyzer that either analyzes all the fragments or selects one that is unique to the parent ion. By operating the first and second quadrupoles in various modes different analytic goals can be achieved. The primary approaches used for endocrine testing are multiple reaction monitoring and product ion scanning.

Multiple reaction monitoring mode allows both analytic analyzers (quadrupoles 1 and 3) to be fixed, selecting for a specific m/z. This adjustment increases specificity and sensitivity. This mode is used to monitor specific analytes and to confirm unambiguously the presence of a compound in a matrix. For example, two unique ions (first/second analyzer) for testosterone are 289.221/97.140 and 289.222/109.130. Because steroid hormones have well-known and

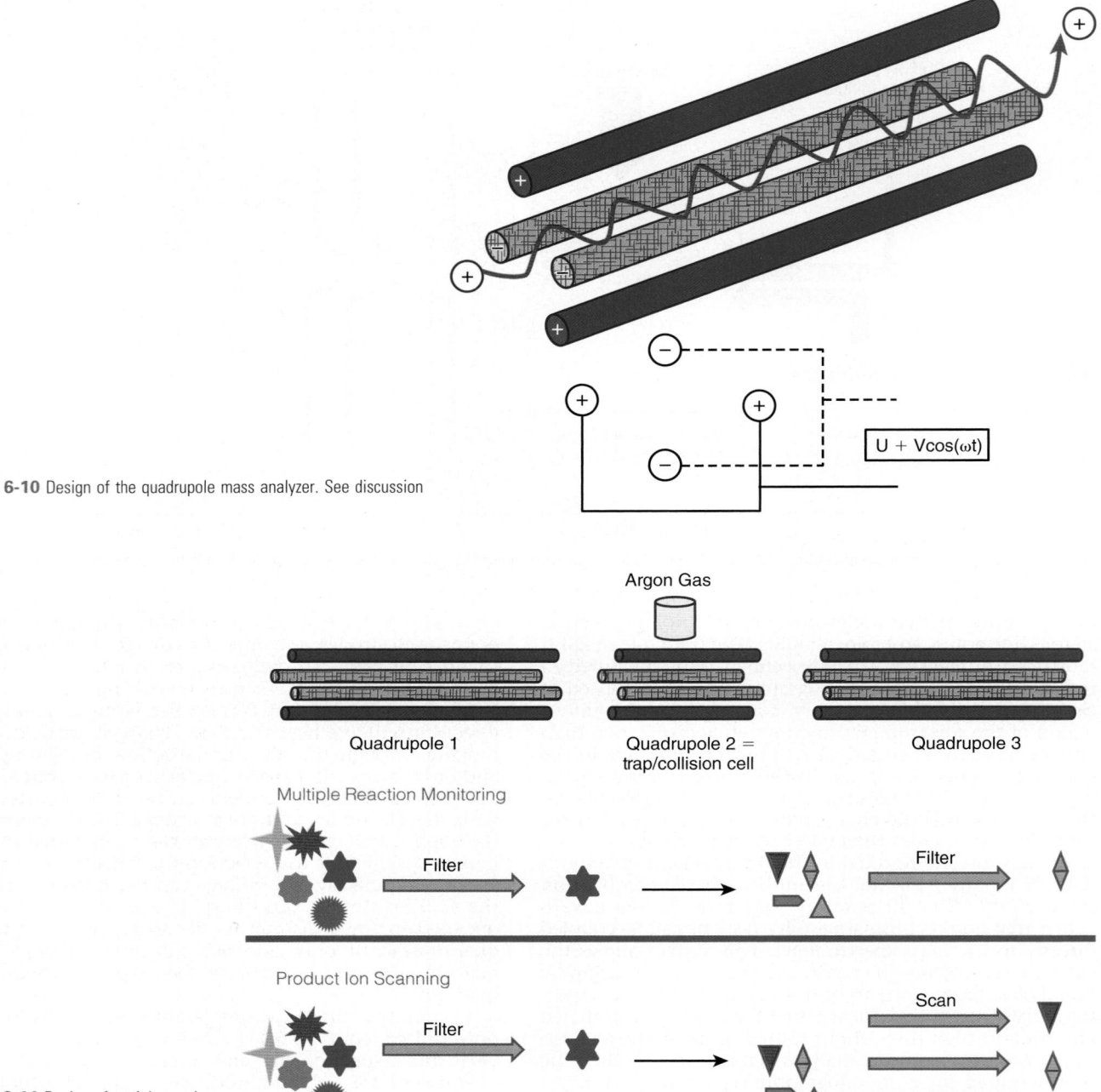

Figure 6-10 Design of the quadrupole mass analyzer. See discussion in text.

Figure 6-11 Design of a triple quadrupole mass analyzer and modes of operation useful in endocrine testing. See text discussion.

unique elution times from LC systems, this mode is also widely employed for steroid profiling, as illustrated in Figure 6-12.

Product ion scanning allows a parent or precursor ion to be selected in quadrupole 1, and the scan in quadrupole 3 measures all the product ions resulting from fragmentation of that ion. This is a particularly useful method of operation for providing structural information concerning small organic molecules or for generating peptide sequence information.

Mass analyzer design continues to evolve rapidly. Another system that deserves consideration with respect to endocrine clinical testing is time-of-flight mass spectrom-

eters (TOFMSs). As illustrated in Figure 6-13, TOFMSs are simple, albeit more highly engineered, instruments designed to determine m/z based on the time required to traverse a vacuum tube. The source is designed to align and accelerate ions after ionization so that they all enter the vacuum tube at the same time. The time required to traverse the vacuum tube is proportional to m/z (more precisely, the square root of the m/z; smaller or more highly charged ions will move faster to the detector. Most modern TOFMSs have electronic reflectors to effectively increase path length and thus resolution. The advantageous qualities of this type of analyzer include a very wide range of measurement, and it is compatible with pulse ionization

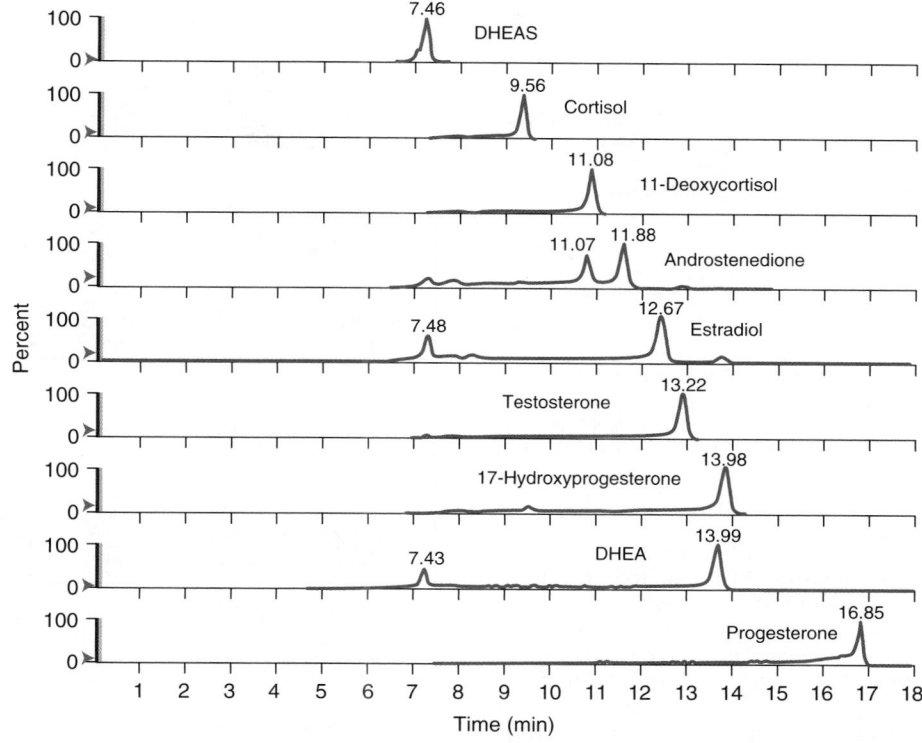

Figure 6-12 Liquid chromatography–tandem mass spectroscopy profiles of nine steroids. DHEA, dehydroepiandrosterone; DHEAS, dehydroepiandrosterone 3-sulfate.

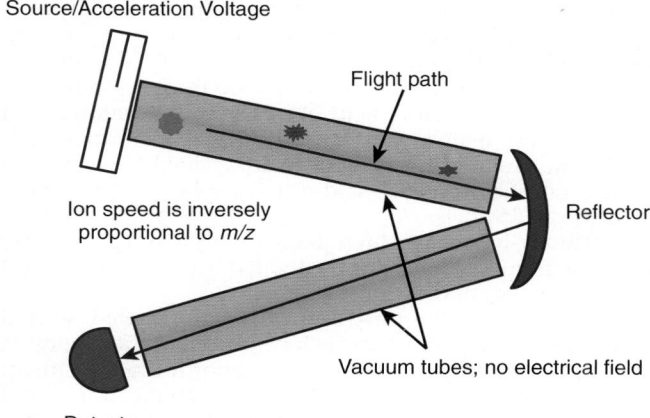

Source/Acceleration Voltage

Flight path

Ion speed is inversely proportional to m/z

Reflector

Vacuum tubes; no electrical field

Detector

Figure 6-13 Design of a time-of-flight mass spectrometer. m/z, mass-to-charge ratio.

TABLE 6-2

Circulating High-Affinity Protein Carriers of Steroid Hormones

Protein Carrier	Primary Ligand(s)	Note
Corticosteroid-binding globulin (CBG)	Glucocorticoids, mineralocorticoids	Also binds cell membranes
Sex hormone–binding globulin	Dihydrotestosterone, testosterone, estradiol	Also binds cell membranes
Thyroxine-binding globulin (TBG)	Thyroxine (T_4), triiodothyronine (T_3)	
Vitamin A–binding protein(s)	Vitamin A (retinol)	
Vitamin D–binding protein	25(OH) vitamin D_2, 25(OH) vitamin D_3, 1,25(OH) vitamin D_2, 1,25 vitamin D_3	Also binds cell membranes

sources such as matrix-assisted laser desorption/ionization (MALDI) methods. MALDI-TOFMS is widely used in proteomics and recently has become a powerful clinical tool in infectious disease testing. It is likely to find increasing applications in endocrine clinical laboratories for large protein measurements. For example, current antibody-based methods for proteins such as TSH, prolactin, and thyroglobulin are often inaccurate in the presence of endogenous antibody. Mass spectrometry, particularly the MALDI-TOFMS, given its ability to measure large proteins, is an attractive approach to addressing this issue.

Free Hormone Methods

The design of assays, either antibody or mass spectrometry based, to measure steroid hormones and sterols (such as

vitamin D) present special issues that warrant discussion. These analytes, which for the sake of simplicity will be discussed as steroid hormones, are extremely hydrophobic. In aqueous environments, particularly blood and blood-derived specimens in which measurement is intended, steroid hormones are associated with hydrophobic regions of proteins or bound tightly to high-affinity, specific transport proteins. The former includes albumin, prealbumin, transthyretin, and apolipoproteins, among others, and the latter include specific transport proteins listed in Table 6-2. Less than 5% to 10% of most steroid hormones circulate as free (unbound) analyte, and assay design requires that the protein-bound analyte be released or does not interfere in the assay in order to have an accurate measure of the total hormone present. Although not universally applicable, in many cases the physiologic effects of steroid hormones depend on the free hormone concentration rather than the total hormone concentration. Of course, under normal conditions the free and total hormone concentrations are directly related. This concept, known as the free

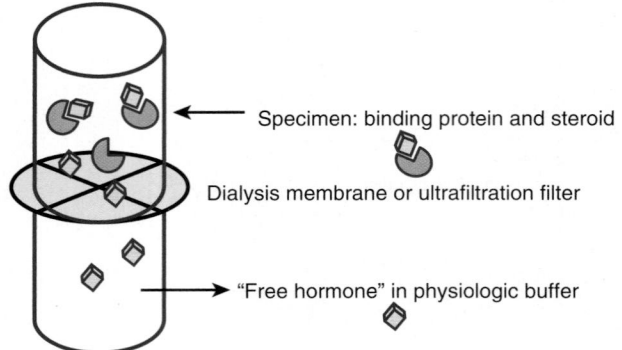

Figure 6-14 Free hormone assay design: Physical separation of free hormone. Dialysis membranes or ultrafiltration allow the separation of free hormone from protein-bound hormone prior to measurement of free hormone directly or by determining the percent distribution of labeled hormone added to the specimen before processing.

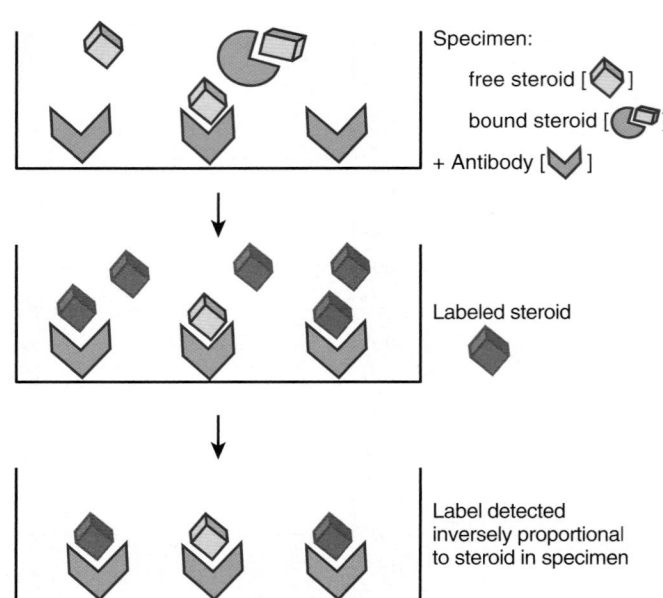

Figure 6-15 Free hormone assay design: Solid-phase, indirect immunoassay. Excess solid-phase antibody binds the free steroid hormone during step one of this method. After washing, incubation with labeled steroid hormone (step two) allows unbound antibody sites to be titrated. After a second wash, the amount of labeled steroid bound to the solid-phase antibody is inversely proportional to the amount of free hormone in the specimen. In figure symbol key, red indicates labeled antibody.

hormone hypothesis, is the basis for the design of methods specifically intended to measure just the free hormone levels.[61-66] The free hormone hypothesis itself is controversial and a critical discussion of it is beyond the scope of this chapter; however, the reader is directed to specific applications in the clinical chapters of this text. Here it is hoped that a technology-based discussion will give the reader an appreciation of the various methods that have been and are currently used to measure free hormones.

There are two basic types of assay designs for measuring free hormones: (1) assays based on the physical separation of bound and free hormone prior to measurement and (2) antibody-based binding assays designed to measure only the free hormone.

Figure 6-14 illustrates the design of assays based on physically separating bound from free steroid hormones. Classically a dialysis membrane was used to separate two fluid-filled chambers (e.g., tubes). The pore size of the dialysis membrane is specific to the analyte/binding proteins but in principle allows free movement of free steroid hormone while retaining the higher molecular weight binding proteins and conjugated binding protein-steroid hormone complexes. Thus, by placing the specimen in one chamber (top in Fig. 6-14) and matrix-appropriate buffer in the other and allowing the diffusion of free hormone to equilibrate, the free hormone can be measured directly by this *equilibrium dialysis* approach. Subsequent variations on the method include using an ultrafiltration membrane to allow faster (e.g., no need to wait for an equilibrium to be established) separation of bound from free steroid hormone (as illustrated in Fig. 6-14) or to chemically separate the high-molecular-weight bound hormone from the free hormone (e.g., precipitation of SHBG-bound steroid using ammonium sulfate). The biggest challenge associated with this approach, regardless of how separating bound from free steroid hormone was achieved, is the measurement of the very low concentrations of free steroid hormone after separation (e.g., in the dialysate or lower chamber in Fig. 6-14). Thus, a variation on the equilibrium dialysis design is to add labeled steroid hormone to the specimen prior to dialysis. High specific activity labels, such as radioisotopes, allow the detection of trace amounts of free hormone after dialysis. It is then possible to use the percentage of free hormone based on the distribution of labeled hormone to calculate the mass of free hormone from a direct measurement of total hormone by traditional methods.

One might easily get the misimpression, especially now that LC/MS-MS systems with sufficiently high sensitivity have been combined with it, that equilibrium dialysis is the method of choice or a gold standard method for measuring free hormones.[57,67,68] However, it must be emphasized that currently there is no established reference method for the measurement of free steroid hormones and that the vast majority of separation methods, including equilibrium dialysis, have not been applied in a fashion that is necessarily valid or directly applicable to in vivo conditions.[62,66,69-72]

Antibody-based binding assays designed to measure only the free hormone can be divided into two classes: (1) two-step assays and (2) one-step assays.

The two-step immunoassay relies on labeled steroid and is illustrated in Figure 6-15. Solid-phase antibody is used to capture the free hormone present in the specimen. The amount, if any, of bound hormone capture will depend on the relative affinity of the steroid for the antibody versus the binding protein. If the antibody affinity is much higher, the bound steroid will be stripped from the binding protein. If the antibody affinity is relatively low compared to the binding protein, only free hormone will be bound. In either case after washing the solid-phase antibody, unoccupied antibody-binding sites are titrated using labeled steroid, which after a second wash step can be quantified. The signal generated by the captured labeled steroid is inversely proportional to the amount of free hormone in the specimens. It is important to note that *free* in this assay format is defined by the relative affinity of the antibody used and the endogenous steroid binding proteins.

One-step immunoassays are designed using either labeled steroid or labeled antibody. The basic formats are illustrated in Figure 6-16. These assays are fast and easy to perform given their relatively simple format, which is also quite amenable to automation. The use of a labeled steroid analogue is summarized in Figure 6-16A. The labeled analogue is not recognized by the binding protein but is able

Labeled Analogue Assay   Labeled Antibody Assay

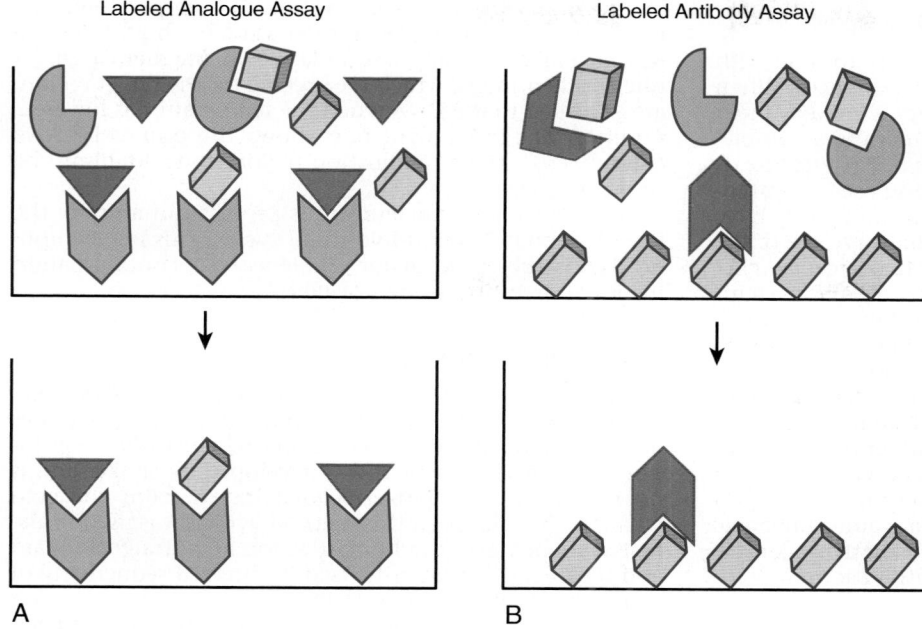

A   B

Figure 6-16 Free hormone assay design: One-step immunoassays. **A,** A labeled analogue steroid hormone that binds to antibody but not to binding proteins is used in a classical competitive binding format to measure only the free hormone in the specimen. **B,** Labeled antibody is used in a single-step competitive assay in which free steroid hormone in the specimen competes with solid-phase steroid hormone for antibody binding. The amount of labeled antibody bound to the solid phase after washing is inversely proportional to the amount of free steroid hormone in the specimen. (See Figs. 6-14 and 6-15 for symbol key.)

to compete with free hormone for antibody-binding sites on the solid phase. This type of assay depends on the validity of the assumption that the signal generated, which is inversely proportional to the concentration of free steroid in the specimen, is solely due to the competition with free hormone. This has been shown not to be true for free testosterone assays and is likely valid only over a limited range for binding protein concentrations for free thyroxine assays.[66,71,73-77] An alternative approach is shown in Figure 6-16B in which a labeled antibody is employed in an assay based upon its binding to solid-phase antigen (e.g., the analyte of interest). In this design the signal generated reflects the amount of labeled antibody bound to the solid phase which, after reaching a steady state, is inversely proportional to the concentration of free steroid hormone in the specimen. The advantage of this newer approach is that a relatively higher signal is measured (e.g., improved sensitivity and precision), and it is not necessary to alter the structure of the steroid (other than that which may be associated with attachment to the solid phase).

It is important to recognized that for free steroid assay designs, the kinetics of competition and binding are very complex given the variety of proteins interacting with steroid hormones over a wide range of affinities. Specimens with low concentrations of binding proteins, including low-affinity but high-capacity binders such as albumin, are particularly challenging. As is true for any assay, all of these free hormone measurement methods require careful validation and method-specific reference intervals to be clinically useful.[62,63,69,70,72,78,79]

Nucleic Acid–Based Methods

Nucleic acid–based assays are designed to identify variations in an individual's DNA or RNA sequence that reflect molecular variance (e.g., mutations, rearrangements) that alters gene expression, regulatory pathways, and bioactive molecules in a fashion relevant to human disease (i.e., early diagnosis or increased disease susceptibility). Genetic variance results in a range of alterations from whole chromosome effects visible by karyotyping/cytogenetics to point

mutations leading ultimately to changes in protein expression or functionality. As small molecules, such as steroid hormones, depend on protein enzymes, genetic alterations may affect all aspects of endocrine function and hence are important analytic targets. A plethora of analytic methods exist for the analysis of nucleic acids.

Discussion of the full range of methods is beyond the scope of this review, but these methods can be grouped into three major categories: (1) chromosome visualization methods, with or without application of sequence-selective enzymatic fragmentation, (2) assays based on binding of labeled nucleic acid probes, which obey Watson and Crick base-pairing rules and thus are sequence specific, and (3) direct sequencing of DNA or RNA. Methods in categories 2 and 3 are generally combined with methods for the amplification or selective enrichment of target sequences, but methods in category 1 generally depend on microscopy (whole chromosome analysis), fragmentation, gel electrophoresis, and blotting techniques (e.g., Southern blotting for DNA or Northern blotting for RNA). Thus, the key elements to appreciate are hybridization, restriction enzyme fragmentation, electrophoretic separation, amplification, and nucleic acid sequencing. Methods composed of various combinations of these principles are available for scanning DNA sequences for new variants, scoring DNA sequences for known variants, and expression analysis of DNA or RNA target sequences. Direct sequencing effectively scores known variants as well as identifies new variants.

Currently, molecular methods being utilized by clinical laboratories are primarily for well-known inherited diseases, cancer diagnostics and management, and increasingly in infectious disease applications. Based on developments in research laboratories, particularly with respect to next generation sequencing, these methods are likely to impact clinical endocrine testing in the very near future.[80-82] The majority of nucleic acid–based assays are laboratory-developed methods applied in research settings or highly specialized clinical reference laboratories. However, this picture is rapidly changing as devices suitable for use in hospital clinical laboratories are increasingly becoming available.

Hybridization Assays (Mutation Assays, Genotyping)

Nucleic acid molecules have a unique ability to bind with high affinity to complementary base-pair sequences. When a fragment of a known sequence (probe) is mixed under specific conditions with a specimen containing a complementary sequence, hybridization occurs. This feature is analogous to the antibody-antigen binding used in immunoassays. Many of the formats used for immunoassay have been adapted to nucleic acid assays, including some of the same signal systems (e.g., radioactivity, fluorescence, chemiluminescence) and the same solid-phase capture systems (e.g., magnetic beads, biotin-streptavidin binding). In situ hybridization, which involves the binding of probes to intact tissue and cells, provides information about morphologic localization analogous to that provided by immunohistochemistry. Combining hybridization methods with enzymatic procedures to amplify, extend, and ligate DNA targets or probes greatly enhances the analytic sensitivity and specificity of hybridization-based methods. Hybridization methods, like other binding assays, are quite amenable to automation and incorporation into relatively simple devices suitable for clinical laboratory utilization.

Restriction Fragmentation

DNA restriction enzymes break DNA strands at specific sites based on the nucleic acid sequence. Thus, digestion with a given restriction enzyme or combination of restriction enzymes will produce fragments of different lengths that are directly related to the DNA sequence. Mutations that alter the sequence of the enzyme cleavage site(s) will result in altered fragment size patterns, referred to as restriction fragment length polymorphisms (RFLPs), which can be visualized after fragment separation by gel electrophoresis or other separation methods. For known mutations the affected DNA sequence can be amplified (see later) prior to RFLP analysis (or by single-nucleotide extension if the mutation does not alter a restriction enzyme cleavage site). A large number of online tools are available to support researchers designing methods involving the use of restriction enzymes.[83,84] These tools can be useful in designing validation studies of commercially available assays for molecular variance.

Electrophoretic Separation

E.M. Southern invented an electrophoretic separation technique known as Southern blotting.[66] Restriction enzymes are used to digest a sample of DNA into fragments, and the product is subjected to electrophoresis. The separated bands of DNA are then transferred to a solid support and hybridized. Northern blotting is a similar technique in which RNA is used as the starting material. Western blotting refers to electrophoresis and transfer of proteins. Currently a wide range of methods for electrophoretic separation and blotting of DNA, RNA, and proteins are available and incorporated into clinically relevant methods. All are relatively complex laboratory-developed methods.

Amplification

Nucleic acid assays have an advantage in that low concentrations can be amplified in vitro before quantitation. The best-known amplification procedure is the polymerase chain reaction (PCR). The three steps in the process (denaturation, annealing, and elongation) occur rapidly at different temperatures. Each cycle of amplification can occur in less than 90 seconds by cycling the temperature. The target double-stranded DNA is denatured at high temperature to make two single-stranded DNA fragments. Oligonucleotide primers, which are specific for the target region, are annealed to the DNA when the temperature is lowered. Addition of DNA polymerase allows the primer DNA to extend across the amplification region, thus doubling the number of DNA copies.

At 85% to 90% efficiency, this process can amplify the DNA by about 250,000-fold in 20 cycles. This huge amplification is subject to major problems with contamination if special precautions are not taken.

Sequencing Methods

Traditionally sequencing was performed using DNA polymerase to selectively incorporate dideoxynucleotides (causing chain termination) during in vitro DNA replication. This method, which was developed by Sanger and is now referred to as Sanger sequencing, remains the gold standard.[85,86] Although this method, which was used in the first sequencing of the human genome, is straightforward and reliable, it is primarily used in directed sequencing of relatively small lengths of DNA.

Next-generation sequencing is a very different approach to sequencing and refers to a wide array of applications including whole genome sequencing, exon sequencing, DNA-protein interaction assays, and RNA sequencing.[80,87-89] These approaches hold tremendous clinical diagnostic potential because they are faster and cheaper than Sanger sequencing, are amenable to automation, and are rapidly being commercialized. Methods encompassed in next-generation sequencing are evolving very rapidly but currently include massively parallel signature sequencing, polony sequencing, pyrosequencing, dye sequencing (Illumina), and sequencing by ligation (Applied Biosystems).

ANALYTIC VALIDATION

In this section the basic elements of method validation are outlined and are applicable to any quantitative assay method discussed in the methods sections earlier. It is only the degree to which the parameters are determined and the frequency with which they are verified that vary from method to method or as a function of assay class. Clearly, to be clinically valuable an analytic method must be valid; that is, the results or measurements generated are accurate and reproducible within the context of use (i.e., specified concentration limits, specimen types, clinical settings). This is often expressed as demonstrating that the method is "fit for use." In more straightforward terms, any given method is valid only within specifications of use. In practical terms, methods are *validated*, or more accurately, their validity is verified, by clinical laboratories to the extent required by appropriate regulatory guidelines (see section on "Classes of Assays").

The validation process begins with the design and development of the method, regardless of the technical processes involved. Clinical laboratories approach validation differently depending on the technologies and reagents used. Commercial systems (instruments and reagents) are validated by the manufacturer, who is also responsible for quality control of subsequent reagent lots and instrument change. Clinical laboratories conduct limited studies to verify the validation. When using instruments and reagents made or modified by the clinical laboratory, full validation is necessary. In both settings the clinical laboratory relies on professional guidelines specific to the technology.

Failure to fully appreciate these subtleties can lead to very erroneous perspectives of the results reported by a given laboratory or obtained by a given method. For example, the majority of assays used to diagnose endocrine diseases are accurate only over specific ranges of analytes, only with reference to specific and generally nonstandardized calibration materials, and only when applied to specific specimen types. In many cases results that are essential to patient care are method-specific and cannot be extrapolated between methods and laboratories.

The basic elements of method validation are listed in Table 6-3 along with the typical studies conducted to characterize each parameter. The parameters that define an assay's analytic performance are dependent on the technology and reagents employed and are often referred to as intrinsic characteristics. These characteristics include sensitivity, specificity, precision, and accuracy. Validation must also include specification of the assay's utility and provide data to support the clinical interpretation of results generated by the assay; these are listed in Table 6-3 as utility and interpretation parameters. As illustrated in Figure 6-17, intrinsic parameters are interrelated. For example, as illustrated in Figure 6-18, accuracy and precision are related parameters and must be optimized and validated in conjunction with each other. In the context of method development, assay validation is typically an iterative as shown in Figure 6-19. It is after an assay optimized analytically for specificity, sensitivity, precision, and accuracy is applied to clinical testing that these parameters can be fully evaluated and interpretive specifications established.

Intrinsic Performance Parameters
Analytic Specificity

Analytic specificity can be simply defined as the ability of the assay to measure only the intended analyte. In other words, the value obtained from a measurement reflects only the concentration of the target analyte. Clearly, then, specificity is closely related to accuracy; an assay cannot be accurate if it is not specific. On the other hand, an assay may be specific but not accurate if, for example, the assay measures only the target analyte but produces a value that over- or underestimates its concentration due to calibration or recovery or other technical issues. From a more practical perspective specificity is often defined based on the signal generated in the assay (i.e., the signal produced in a specific assay is generated only by the target analyte). Few assays, regardless of the technology employed, are truly specific in this sense; typically the signal measured can be generated by components of the specimen or assay systems in addition to the target analyte. Thus, practical validation of specificity encompasses not only specificity per se but also interferences, such as matrix effects or ion suppression, that can alter the derived concentration, resulting in an inaccurate measurement. It is important to emphasize that interference can be specimen-specific and is a challenge to assay validation as well as quality control and quality assurance.

Cross-Reactivity. Assay cross-reactivity can be generically defined as signal generation by similar analytes. Typically it is a definable and predictable assay characteristic (e.g., any specimen containing cross-reacting analytes will not be accurately measured).

TABLE 6-3	
Parameters and Studies for Method Validation	
Parameter of Performance	**Validation Study**
Specificity	Cross-reactivity
	Interference
Sensitivity	Analytic sensitivity
	Limits
Precision	Intra-assay variance
	Inter-assay variance
Accuracy	Recovery
	Bias
	Linearity
	Carryover
Utility (robustness)	Specimen stability
	Reagent stability
	Assay stability
Interpretation	Reportable range
	Reference intervals
	Diagnostic power

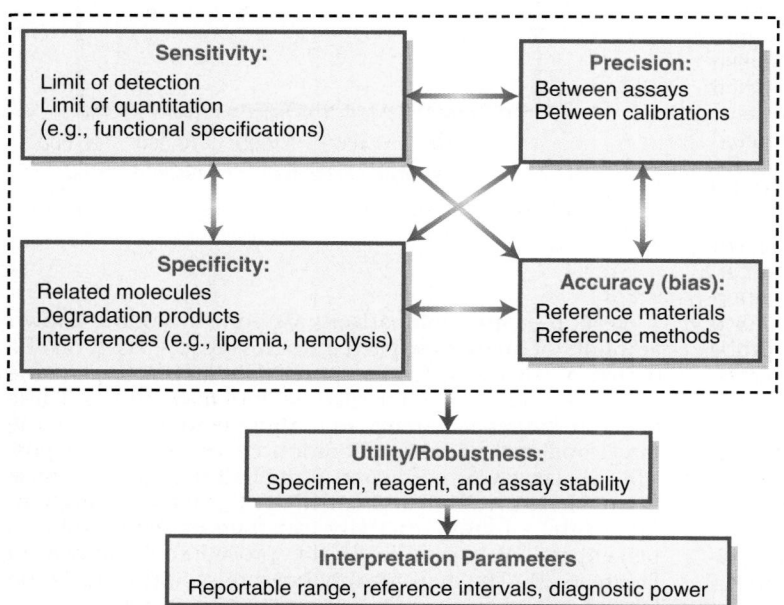

Figure 6-17 Relationships and sequencing of method validation parameters.

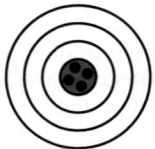

Accurate and Precise Assay

Accuracy =
correct (target) value
is measured

Precision =
measurement is reproducible

Possible results of validation testing of new assay

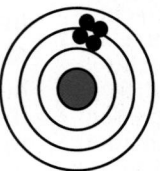
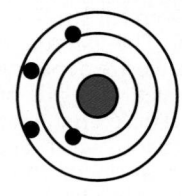
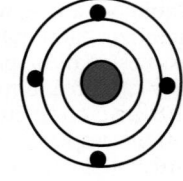

Precise but Inaccurate

**Systematic error (bias):
useful with reference
intervals, but results are
assay-specific**

**Inaccurate and
Imprecise**

**Accurate but
Imprecise**

**Random error:
not a useful assay**

Figure 6-18 Assay accuracy and precision are closely related parameters that must be optimized and validated together.

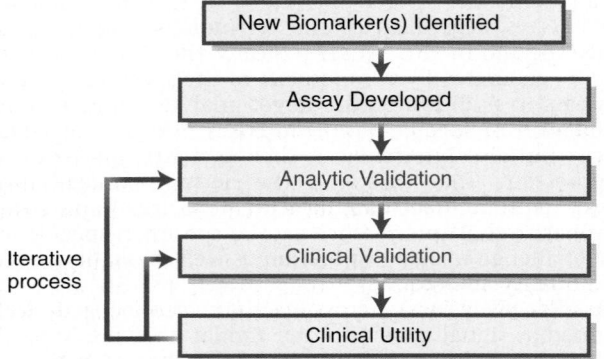

New Biomarker(s) Identified

↓

Assay Developed

↓

Analytic Validation

↓

Clinical Validation

↓

Clinical Utility

Iterative process

Figure 6-19 Iterative nature of the assay development and validation process.

Cross-reactivity in antibody-based assays is due primarily to the specificity of the antibody-binding sites employed in the assay. For example, steroids with similar structure may bind to the antibody and compete with the labeled analyte to produce the same signal (decrease in labeled analyte binding) as the target analyte. Similarly, proteins containing a binding epitope similar to the ones targeted in an immunometric assay can generate signal (i.e., increased binding of the detection antibody). Cross-reactivity is not a term typically used with respect to structural or nucleic acid–based assays, but the concept is applicable. For example, if the fragment ion used for quantification can be generated by more than one analyte, the signal generated is not specific. Similarly if the sequence target for a nucleic acid–binding assay is large, the detection probe may bind to more than one analyte. In all cases the cross-reactivity is not necessarily complete in that the cross-reacting analyte may generate the same, more, or less signal than the target analyte. Thus, the degree to which cross-reactivity vitiates assay measurements will be dependent on the concentration of cross-reacting analyte and the degree to which it cross-reacts.

Assays are validated with respect to cross-reactivity primarily by two approaches: (1) response curve comparison and (2) spiked specimen measurement.

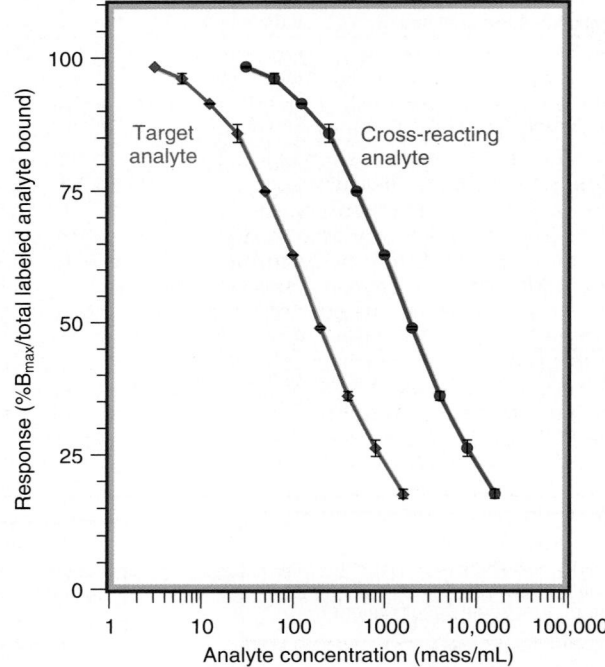

Figure 6-20 Method for determining analyte cross-reactivity. See discussion of cross-reactivity in text.

Response curve comparisons are done by adding known amounts of analytes expected to cross-react (based on the design of the assay) to the appropriate matrix to generate a dose-response curve for each analyte to be tested. These response curves are compared to those used to quantify the target analyte (e.g., the calibration curve). Whenever possible the curves are compared at the half-maximal response point where precision and sensitivity (see later) are highest. The degree of cross-reactivity can then be expressed as a percentage. An example of the procedure is shown in Figure 6-20. The half-maximal response (50% B_{max}/total labeled antibody bound) is generated by a concentration

TABLE 6-4

Example of Spiked Specimen Cross-Reactivity Data From a Commercial Immunoassay

Compound	Concentration (µg/dL)	Cross-Reactivity (%)
Aldosterone	1000	0
Beclomethasone	1000	0
Budesonide	1000	0
Canrenone	1000	0.1
Corticosterone	1000	0.9
Cortisol 21-glucuronide	1000	0.2
Cortisone	1000	2.7
β-Cortol	1000	0
β-Cortolone	1000	0
11-Deoxycorticosterone	100	0
11-Deoxycortisol	100	1.9
Dexamethasone	1000	0
DHEA	1000	0
DHEAS	1000	0
β-Estradiol	1000	0
Estriol	1000	0
Estrone	1000	0
Fludrocortisone	100	36.6
Fluticasone propionate	1000	0

DHEA, dehydroepiandrosterone; DHEAS, dehydroepiandrosterone 3-sulfate.

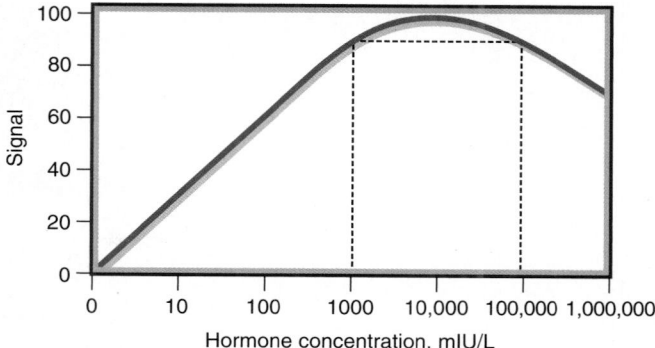

Figure 6-21 Immunometric high-dose hook effect. The response signal reaches a maximum and then decreases when the antigen concentration exceeds the limit of the assay.

of 200 mass/mL of the target analyte. In contrast, 2000 mass/mL of the cross-reacting analyte is required to generate a half-maximal response. Thus, the cross-reactivity of this cross-reacting analyte is 10% (i.e., percent cross-reactivity = [200/2000] × 100). It is important to appreciate that this approach is valid only if the response curves are parallel.

Spiked specimen measurement is often used to determine analyte cross-reactivity. This approach involves adding the cross-reacting analyte to a specimen that has been measured and then performing re-assay to determine if the added analyte cross-reacted. This approach is often seen in the package inserts of commercial assays. An example is shown in Table 6-4 for a commercial assay for the measurement of cortisol in human serum or plasma. The concentration achieved by spiking human serum is indicated for each potential cross-reactant listed. The unspiked human serum contained 12 µg/dL of endogenous cortisol as measured in the assay. Thus, a cross-reactivity of 36.6% for fludrocortisone means that a cortisol value of 16.4 µg/dL was measured after the addition of 100 µg/dL of fludrocortisone to the specimen. Spiked specimen cross-reactivity data must be interpreted carefully as it assumes that the percent of cross-reactivity will be the same at all levels of cross-reactant and that the concentrations of cross-reactant tested are clinically relevant.

Interference. As alluded to previously, interference is can be due to the influence of a specimen component on the signal generated by the target analyte or to the generation of signal by the interfering substance. In the latter case, what distinguishes interference from cross-reactivity is the lack of parallelism in the signal generation by interfering substances. The interfering substance or the mechanism of interference is something known; frequently encountered examples are given in the following paragraphs. In other cases neither the mechanism nor interfering substance is known; in this case interference is referred to as a *matrix effect*. Matrix effects are typically identified only during the validation of accuracy (see later). They can be specimen-specific in which case they are identified only during the investigation of results that are inconsistent with the clinical setting or other analytic results. It is critical that the clinical laboratory keep in mind that any analytic method

can be subject to specimen-specific interferences unknown to the laboratory or indicated by routine quality control monitoring. Thus, despite a numeric value, often to several decimal places, reported from a validated method, an analytic result from any single specimen must be interpreted in the overall clinical context.

Well-known interference with assays that depend on light or fluorescence signaling can be due to hemolyzed, lipemic, and icteric specimens. Interference can also be a function of physically influencing the system. For example, a severe degree of lipemia as can result in inaccurate measurement of water-soluble analytes. Interference can also be analyte-specific. Proteins sensitive to proteolysis are inaccurately measured in hemolyzed specimens (by the proteases released during hemolysis rather than color interference with light detection, which also occurs in hemolyzed specimens).

Two interferences well known to affect immunometric assays (but an issue to some extent for all antibody-based assays) are *hook effects* and *heterophile antibody interferences*.

The mechanism of the hook effect is illustrated in Figure 6-21. As the antigen concentration approaches the effective binding capacity of the capture antibody system, the signal no longer increases. At this point laboratory specifications for maximum reportable signal are exceeded and the specimen is diluted to obtain an accurate measurement. However, analyte concentrations vastly exceeding the binding capacity of the capture antibody result in also blocking the detection antibody, resulting in a decrease in signal back into the reportable range. Extending the principle to the extreme, it is theoretically possible to have so much analyte present that all the binding sites on both the capture and detection antibodies are occupied; in this case no detection antibody can be bound to the solid phase and the signal is baseline, which would be interpreted as no analyte present! Hook effects occur and are extremely important to recognize in the context of measuring hormones in patients with tumors that secret large quantities of the hormone. Hook effects have been extensively reported for prolactin, hCG, thyroglobulin, calcitonin, and α-fetoprotein.[29,30,90-98]

Heterophile antibody interference is, if not a misnomer, certainly a process that encompasses more than just the ability of endogenous antibodies to animal immunoglobulins to interfere in immunometric assays. The mechanism is simple and is illustrated in Figure 6-22. Any analyte-independent process that alters the amount of detection antibody bound to the solid will result in inaccurate assay values. As shown in Figure 6-22, endogenous antibodies

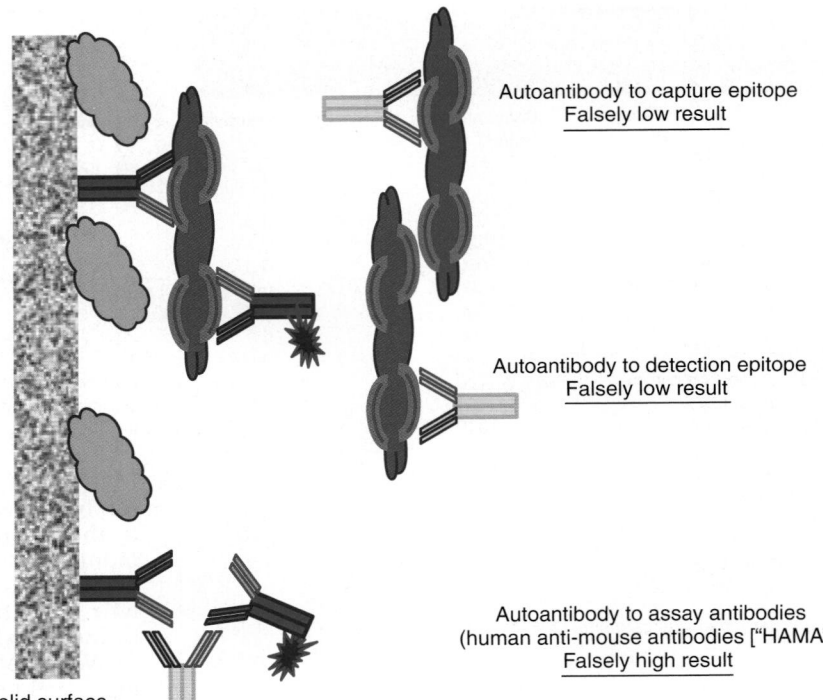

Autoantibody to capture epitope
Falsely low result

Autoantibody to detection epitope
Falsely low result

Autoantibody to assay antibodies
(human anti-mouse antibodies ["HAMA"])
Falsely high result

Solid surface

Figure 6-22 Heterophile antibody interference. See text for details. (From Sluss PM. Methodologies for measurement of cardiac markers. *Clin Lab Med.* 2014;34:167-185. Reproduced with permission from Elsevier Inc.)

(called heterophile antibodies) to animal immunoglobulins can, because antibodies are bivalent, link the detection antibody to the solid-phase capture antibody in the absence of analyte, resulting in a falsely high value reported. Animal immunoglobulins are foreign proteins, and thus the majority of humans are expected to have low titers of animal immunoglobulin antibodies. Immunometric assays are designed with blockers to eliminate heterophile antibody interference. However, some individuals have high titers of heterophile antibodies, which overcome the assay blockers and do result in accurate measurements. In some cases, such as patients treated with drugs containing animal immunoglobulins (e.g., monoclonal-based therapeutics), it is clear why the patient has high titers; in others it is difficult to identify a priori individuals whose specimens might be subject to this artifact.[99-109] Heterophiles are not the only form of endogenous antibody that can interfere with immunometric assays by this mechanism (e.g., antibody-based analyte-independent interference). Figure 6-22 shows that endogenous antibodies to epitopes on the target analyte can also result in inaccurate measurements, in this case falsely low results, because the endogenous antibodies block the quantitative detection of analyte. Although the protein hormones and biomarkers relevant to endocrine practice do not elicit the formation of endogenous antibodies in healthy individuals, patients with various autoimmune conditions or other disease processes may have endogenous antibodies that interfere with specific immunometric assays. A classic example of nonheterophile endogenous antibody interference is the interference in thyroglobulin assays by thyroglobulin antibodies in cancer patients.[110-112]

Endogenous antibodies and binding proteins can also interfere with the interpretation of values obtained from antibody-based assays. For example, endogenous antibodies bound to prolactin create what is referred to as *macroprolactin*. Macroprolactin is not biologically active but is measured in many immunometric assays. This results in

prolactin levels being reported that are discordant with clinical manifestations of hyperprolactinemia.[94,113] Another example is the ability of competition assays to measure small molecules, such as thyroid or sex hormones, that are inactive when bound to high-affinity carrier proteins, such as thyroxine-binding globulin or sex hormone–binding globulin. In this case, values reported by immunoassay can grossly overestimate the biologic signal represented by the hormone measurement.

Analytic Sensitivity

Strictly, analytic sensitivity is the slope of the response curve. It is determined simply as the change in signal as a function of the change in analyte concentration and represents the smallest change in analyte concentration that can be measured. An example calibration curve is shown in Figure 6-23. The slope of this calibration curve determined by least squares linear regression analysis was 1.01 pg/mL with a goodness of fit of $r^2 = 0.993$ and an intercept of 1.05. Thus the smallest difference that can be measured overall is 1.01 pg/mL with an LOD (intercept) of 1.08 pg/mL. This approach is useful only when the calibration curve is linear (or linearized by log transformation of the analyte concentrations) and the zero calibrator is accurately determined (i.e., there is no matrix effect on the blank measurement). Dose-response curves for clinical assays, regardless of technology employed, are seldom linear, and detector impression can be high. Thus, limits of detection and direct estimates of variance at clinically meaningful analyte concentrations are typically more meaningful in describing assay performance.

The analytic LOD, often less rigorously referred to as sensitivity, is a statistical definition of the lowest concentration that can be measured (i.e., distinguished for zero analyte in the assay system). This concentration is mathematically determined as the upper 95% limit of replicate measurements of the zero standard, calculated from the

This is a scientific figure showing a calibration curve.

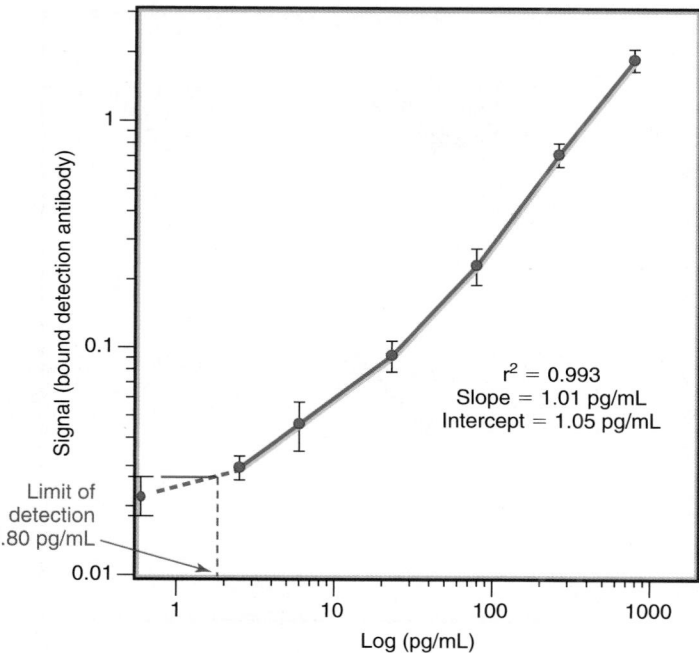

Figure 6-23 Determination of analytic sensitivity and limit of detection. See text for details.

average signal plus 2.0 SD. The LOD for the curve in Figure 6-23 is 1.80 pg/mL. This minimal detection limit is valid only for the average of multiple replicate measurements. When individual determinations are performed on a specimen having a true concentration exactly at the minimal detection limit, the probability that the measurement is above the noise level of the assay is only about 50%.

A second parameter for the lowest level of reliable measurement for an assay is the functional detection limit, or the limit of quantitation. For this value to be measured, multiple pools with low concentrations are made and analyzed in the replicate. A cross-plot of the coefficient of variation of the measurements versus concentration allows one to generate a precise profile. The concentration corresponding to a coefficient of variation of 20% is the functional detection limit. This term typically applies to across-assay variation, but it also can be calculated for within-assay variation if one uses the tests to evaluate results measured within one run (e.g., provocative and suppression tests).

Precision

Precision is a measure of the replication of repeated measurements of the same specimen; it is a function of the time between repeats and the concentration of the analyte. Both short-term precision (within a run or within a day) and long-term precision (across calibrations and across batches of reagents) should be documented at clinically appropriate concentration levels.[114] In general, normal-range, abnormally low range, and abnormally high range targets are chosen for precision studies; however, targets focused on critical medical decision limits may be more appropriate for some analytes.

Twenty measurements are generally considered minimal at each level for both short-term and long-term precision validations. Precision usually is expressed as the coefficient of variation, calculated as 100 times the SD divided by the average of the replicate measurements.[115] There is no universal agreement on the performance criteria for analytic precision, although numerous recommen-

dations have been put forth. Two major approaches to defining these criteria have been (1) comparison with biologic variation and (2) expert opinion of clinicians based on their perceived impact of laboratory variation on clinical decisions.

The total variation clinically observed in test measurements is a combination of the analytic and biologic variations. For instance, if the analytic SD is less than one fourth of the biologic SD, the analytic component increases the SD of the total error by less than 3%. If the analytic precision is less than one half of the biologic SD, the total error increases by only 12%. These observations have led to recommendations for maintaining precision of less than one fourth or one half of the biologic variation.

The expert opinion precision recommendations are based on estimates of the magnitude of change of a test value that would cause clinicians to alter their clinical decisions.

Accuracy

Two methods of assessing the recovery of assays are (1) measuring the proportional changes caused by mixing high-concentration and low-concentration specimens and (2) measuring the increase in test values after the reference analyte is added. Some analytes circulate in the blood in multiple forms, and some of these forms may be bound to carrier proteins. The recovery rate of pure substances added to a specimen may be low if the assay does not measure some of the bound forms. Mixtures of patient specimens may not be measured correctly if one of the specimens contains cross-reacting substances such as autoantibodies. A thorough understanding of the chemical forms of the analyte and their cross-reactivities in the assay is important during assessment of recovery data.

Measuring the proportional changes caused by mixing high-concentration and low-concentration specimens is referred to as a linearity validation. An example is shown in Figure 6-24. A specimen containing a relatively high analyte concentration is diluted with a specimen containing "no" analyte. Practically, "no" analyte means analyte

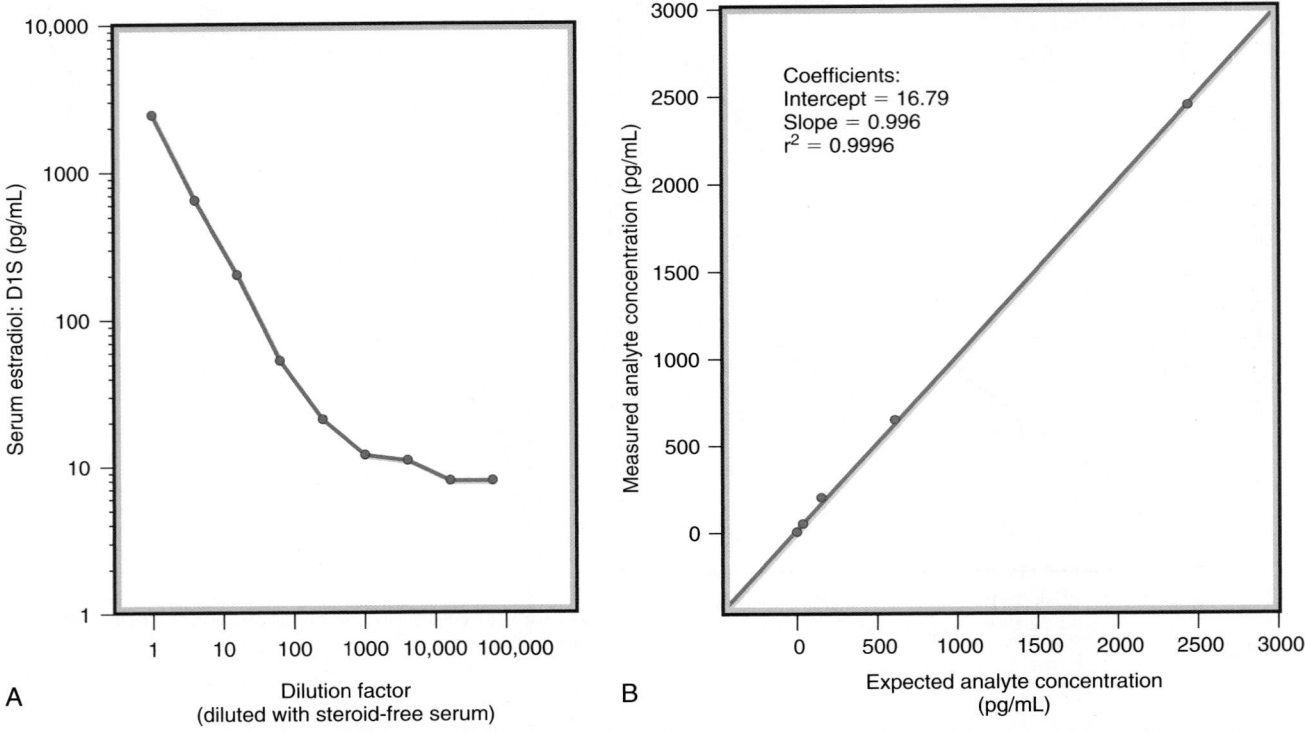

Figure 6-24 Determination of assay accuracy. **A,** Linear dilution recovery. **B,** Spike analyte recovery.

levels less than the detection limit of the assay as specimens with no analyte are typically not available. Figure 6-24A shows the measurement of diluted specimens as a function of dilution. The point at which concentration no longer changes with increasing dilution is called the limit of blank (in this example, 10 pg/mL). The limit of blank can be significantly higher than the LOD or the limit of quantitation in some assays. Dilution linearity data (as in Fig. 6-24A) can be replotted (as in Fig. 6-24B) to evaluate the accuracy of an assay in terms of the analytic recovery of added analyte. Usually data are fitted by a linear regression. Assuming that the x- and y-axes have identical scaling, the slope*100 is the percent analytic recovery. Analytic recoveries less than or more than 100 reflect the bias of measurement for a given assay.

Measuring the increase in test values after a reference analyte is added is referred to as a spiked recovery validation. The analytic approach is identical to that illustrated in Figure 6-24B except that the expected analytic concentration is based on the addition of analyte to specimens rather than calculated based on the dilution of specimens. The most appropriate analytes for use in analytic recovery studies are certified reference materials, such as those from the WHO or the National Institute of Standards and Technology (NIST), although such well-characterized materials are not available for all analytes. Ideally a rigorous method validation would also include comparison to a reference method (i.e., a method that has been carefully validated previously). These are generally performed by highly specialized laboratories, and reference methods do not yet exist for many analytes of interest in endocrine testing or for novel biomarkers.[116-124]

At a minimum, the evaluation of accuracy by any of the methods described previously should be conducted using specimens from healthy subjects and specimens from patients with the diseases being investigated.[125] Whenever possible, the assay should be traceable to established reference standards or methods. Between 100 and 200 different specimens distributed over the assay range are recommended for method comparisons.[126-130] Although acceptable performance criteria for method comparisons are not well established, some important characteristics to examine are as follows:

- Any grossly discordant test values
- The degree of scatter about the regression curve
- The size of the regression offset on the vertical axis
- The number of points crossing between the low, normal, and high reference intervals for the two methods

The European Union has enacted an In Vitro Diagnostics Directive that requires manufacturers marketing in the European Union to establish that their products are "traceable to reference standards and reference procedures of a higher order" when such references exist.[132] Hopefully, medically relevant performance characteristics that define the allowable ranges for differences between a specific assay's test values and the traceable standards will be linked with this traceability requirement. This combination of traceability and allowable error requirements could serve to harmonize many test methods worldwide, because most diagnostic companies market internationally. Standardization and harmonization of hormone assays have become priorities for quality health care.[119,124,131,132]

Carryover

Many diagnostic systems use automated sample-handling devices. If a specimen to be tested is preceded by a specimen with a very high concentration, a trace amount remaining from the first specimen may significantly increase the reported concentration in the second specimen. The choice of the concentration that should be tested for carryover depends on the pathophysiology of the disease, but high values may need to be tested because some endocrine disorders can produce high values. Validations also typically include assessing possible carryover from the sampling probe and for plate-based assays assessing detector carryover from nearby wells.

Utilization Parameters

Once an assay has been analytically validated, it is necessary to validate its utilization. The key aspects of utilization involve defining limits associated with specimen and reagent stability and ensuring that the assay is stable over time.

Specimen Stability

Validating specimen stability typically involves testing a series of aliquots taken to determine if the analyte measurement changes over time. This evaluation typically includes specimens representing the full range of specimen types to be tested (see later) and encompasses processing times and temperatures expected with respect to specimen collection and transport to the laboratory as well as stability during laboratory processing and on instrument time and during the assay itself. This is a critical aspect of method validation that can be very costly and labor intensive.

Reagent Stability

The stability of reagents used in the assay must also be defined. This includes both on-board stability and shelf-life stability for commercial, automated systems that are widely used in modern clinical laboratories. Although reagent expiration dates are determined and provided by commercial manufacturers, they must be verified under the actual working conditions of the laboratory and take into account workflow processes such as reconstituting lyophilized calibrators or refreezing calibrator/control aliquots. For laboratory-developed methods such as LC/MS-MS, the laboratory must also determine expiration dates for all reagent components and stock materials.

Robustness (Assay Stability)

Robustness is typically defined as the stability of measurement over time, which includes variance associated with reagent lot changes, equipment changes, and technologist performance.[133] Robustness validation provides the specifications for the reliability of the method during extended normal usage. These specifications become the basis for setting limits on variance, and it is critical that laboratories inform clinicians of changes that exceed these practice-relevant limits. For example, changes in antisera can cause significant changes in immunoassay performance, which in turn require revising reference interval and clinical decision points.

Interpretation Parameters

Reportable Range

The reportable range of an assay usually spans from the limit of quantitation to the concentration of the highest calibrator. Signal measured above the highest standard requires specimen dilution and retesting. This is typically done automatically in instrument systems but must be done manually in plate assay systems. In either case, an important aspect of method validation is to assess accuracy when a specimen must be diluted. Dilution is often associated with alternation of matrix effects and other interferences in an assay. Thus, an assay that is accurate over the calibration range may not be accurate over the full reportable range when dilutions are utilized to obtain quantitative measurements. The validity of the analytic range is documented by the linearity and recovery studies. Most clinical laboratories confirm the reportable range of each assay at least twice a year.

Reference Intervals

Reference intervals, also commonly referred to as normal ranges, describe the analyte values expected from a given assay when healthy individuals are tested.[134-136] This is in contrast to clinical decision points, or cutoff values, determined for identifying patients with specific disease conditions (see "Diagnostic Power" following). The development and validation of reference intervals for endocrine tests can be very complex tasks as they require defining the healthy population by clinical evaluation[137,138] and testing large numbers of healthy individuals,[134,136] which often involves obtaining informed consent and related costly activities. Manufacturers of commercially available assays are required to provide reference intervals, but these do not necessarily represent the subpopulation served by the laboratory.

The normal reference interval for most laboratory tests is based on estimates of the central 95 percentile limits of measurements in healthy subjects. A minimum of 120 subjects is needed to reliably define the 2.5 and 97.5 percentiles. Formal statistical consultation is usually required to determine the appropriate number of subjects to test and to develop statistical models for defining multivariate reference ranges.[139-141]

The reference intervals for many endocrine tests depend on gender, age, developmental status, and other test values. Figure 6-25 illustrates this complexity. Shown are the ranges of values (shaded areas) expected on a daily basis for hormone measurements in healthy young women across the menstrual cycle.

Diagnostic Power

Determining the clinical usefulness of the assay is typically the last step in validation. For commercially available assays the manufacturer is required to do this. The degree to which the assay is validated in this regard depends on specific FDA regulatory requirements (see "Classes of Assays" section later). Clinical laboratories using these assays are required to verify clinical utility claims depending on the specific requirements of the relevant accrediting organization, but generally the approach is to verify the clinical sensitivity and specificity of the assay using specimens from patients known to have or not have a specific clinical condition that the assay is designed to address. In contrast, for laboratory-developed methods, which include mass spectrometry and many molecular-based assays, the clinical laboratory is required to determine clinical decision points (cutoff values). In either case, good laboratory practice includes verification of clinical utility periodically as part of the laboratory's quality control (QC) and quality assurance (QA) programs. The details of clinical utility validation are beyond the scope of this chapter, but a high-level understanding of the processes is important because clinical sensitivity and specificity and cutoff parameters can help clinicians determine the relative weight to give assay results in the context of the entire clinical picture. Many excellent discussions have been published to provide in-depth details for interested readers.[142-146]

Clinical sensitivity and specificity are not to be confused with analytic sensitivity and specificity, which are assay

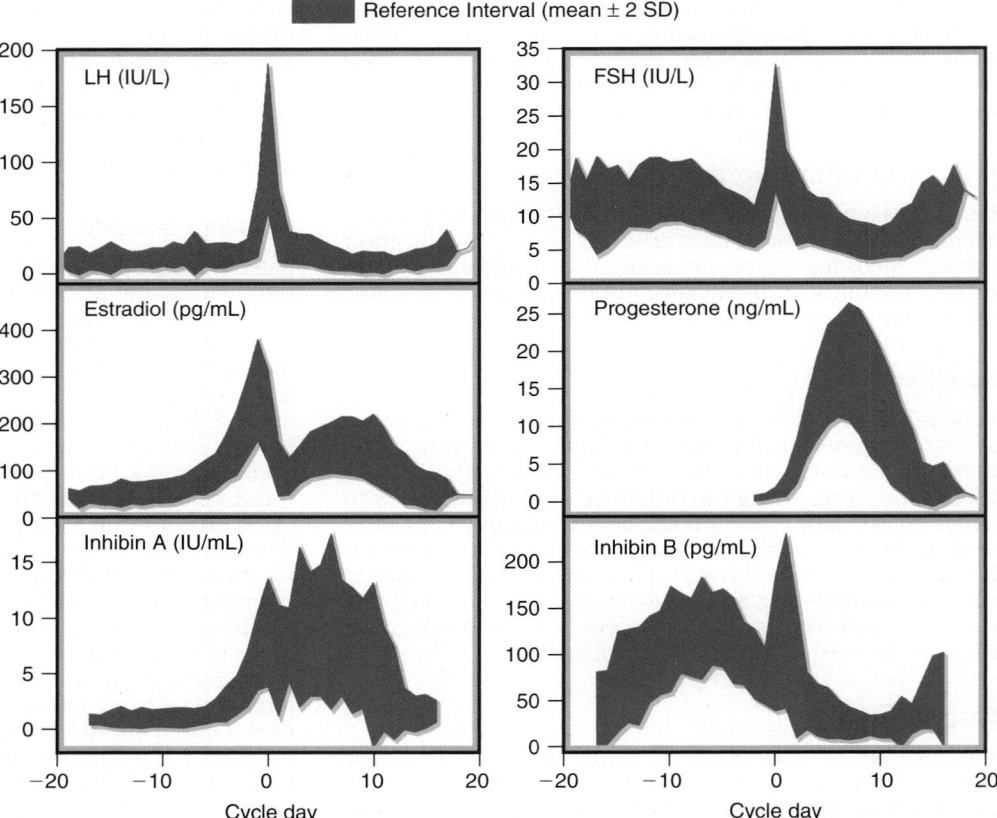

Figure 6-25 High-resolution reference intervals required for the interpretation of reproductive hormone measurements across the menstrual cycle. FSH, follicle-stimulating hormone; LH, luteinizing hormone; SD, standard deviation.

characteristics. In contrast, clinical sensitivity and specificity quantify the ability of the assay, or any clinical diagnostic procedure, to correctly identify disease states, and these parameters are expressed as percentages. Clinical sensitivity is the percentage of patients with positive test results who actually have the target condition (i.e., they have the disease the assay is intended to identify); it is the true rate of accurate diagnosis. Subtraction of the clinical sensitivity from 100 provides the rate of false-positive results for an assay (i.e., the percentage of patients with positive test results who do not have the disease).

Clinical specificity deals with patients with negative assay results. It is the percentage who actually do not have the disease (i.e., who are correctly identified as negative by the assay). Subtracting the clinical specificity from 100 gives the false-negative rate of the assay.

Clearly, to determine clinical sensitivity and specificity the laboratory must have two key things: (1) specimens from patients known to have or not have the disease and (2) either reference intervals or clinical cutoff points to provide a positive or negative interpretation to quantitative test results. Obtaining specimens from patients with known conditions for the purpose of assay validation/verification is challenging as the process requires accurate clinical information, Health Insurance Portability and Accountability Act (HIPAA) compliance, and specimens collected and handled in a fashion consistent with normal workflow. All these steps can be expensive and challenging and are best accomplished with the close collaboration of physicians who utilize the laboratory services.

Clinicians must appreciate that laboratory-derived clinical sensitivities and specificities are subject to many potential biases. First, in many cases laboratories rely on already

established assays to provide the disease status information; in other words, they are comparing to predicate device results rather than clinical information. Even when using clinically characterized individuals to provide the disease-positive specimens, bias can be incorporated if the healthy group is not age- or gender-matched. Finally, using either clinical cutoffs or reference intervals to define a positive versus negative assay result is subject to statistical biases, such as normal versus non-normal distribution of measurement.

Operational Parameters (Preanalytic Considerations)
Specimen Types

Many types of specimens are routinely used for the measurement of analytes in bodily fluids. The most common are whole blood, serum, plasma, urine, and saliva. Less frequently, fluids or cells derived from fine-needle aspirates are sent to the clinical laboratory for analysis. It is critical to understand that each type of specimen must be subjected to rigorous validation to ensure accurate measurements. Simply because an assay is valid for a given specimen type does not mean that it is valid for any specimen type. Even if an assay is capable of reproducible and specific measurement of an analyte in different specimen types, there may be clinically significant bias depending on the specimen type tested. Reference intervals and clinical cutoff values must be verified for each specimen type utilized.

Whole Blood. Whole blood specimens have both the limitation and the advantage of time dependency. The ability to detect rapid changes to a provocative stimulus is a strong advantage, whereas the unsuspected changes resulting from pulsatile secretions may be a major limitation. Whole blood is advantageous when the analyte is very labile as the specimen can be collected and tested quickly. The ability to test whole blood without processing at the point of care can be cost effective and enhance patient management as well as effectively address problems of specimen stability with respect to very labile analytes. Blood drops collected on filter paper from punctures of a finger or heel are a convenient system for collecting, transporting, and measuring hormones.[147,148]

If standardized collection conditions and extraction techniques are used, these measurements correlate well with serum measurements. Integration of immunochemistry with computer chip technology has also led to immunochips that can measure multiple analytes using a single drop of blood.[149]

The use of whole blood is severely limited by several factors: (1) whole blood must be prevented from clotting during analysis, necessitating the use of anticoagulants, which often interfere in assays, and (2) whole blood is a very complex mixture of components that can directly interfere with analytic methods. Solutions to these problems include (1) dilution of the whole blood specimen in the assay, which in turn requires that the analyte being measured is in relatively high concentration or that the assay is extremely sensitive, and (2) preanalytic processing to remove the cellular fraction or reduce the complexity of the specimen. Traditionally specimen types most often used for endocrine testing are serum or plasma for these reasons.

Serum. Serum is obtained from whole blood specimens simply by allowing the blood to clot. Allowing whole blood to clot in glass tubes allows the serum to be completely and easily separated from the clot by centrifugation. The resultant serum specimen is free of cells, and many of the proteins involved in the clotting process are also removed. This has been the method of choice for large protein analytes such as immunoglobulins or for very stable analytes such as steroid hormones. In some laboratories testing has involved replacing the glass phlebotomy tube with safer plastic ones that will not break during handling, especially in the newer fully automated laboratories. Unfortunately whole blood does not clot cleanly or quickly in plastic tubes and clot activators or enhancers are added to the tubes. These factors can interfere with many analytic methods and must be carefully validated.

Plasma. Plasma is obtained by chemically preventing the clotting process and then centrifuging to remove the cellular components of whole blood. There are a number of approaches to preventing clotting; most commonly, ethylenediaminetetra-acetic acid (EDTA), citrate, or heparin is added to prevent clotting. These chemicals, especially EDTA, have the additional advantage of inhibiting proteolysis and are thus also advantageous when testing labile analytes such as adrenocorticotropic hormone (ACTH) or PTH. Other additives are also added to stable plasma for specific tests; for example, sodium fluoride is added to EDTA tubes to inhibit glycolysis when glucose measurements are desired. Of course, all of these additives have the potential to interfere with specific assay methods.

Separation of the cellular elements in anticoagulated whole blood can be enhanced by the use of gel separators. This type of tube is often preferred in automated aliquoting systems. Unfortunately, the gel used can interfere directly or indirectly (e.g., by trapping analytes) in some analytic methods.

Phlebotomy tubes with additives also create special considerations when collecting blood in multiple tube types.

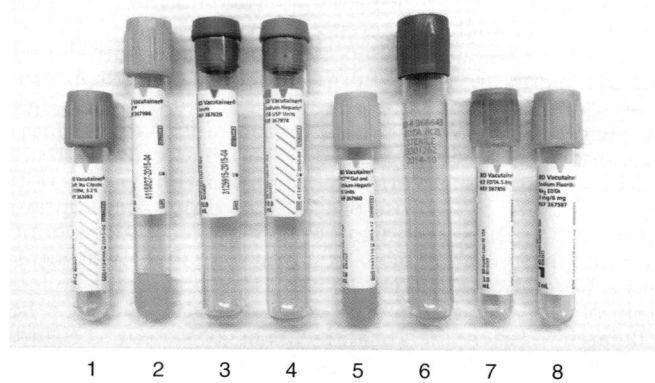

Figure 6-26 The order in which blood tubes containing no or various additives must be filled to avoid contamination and possible interference with accurate laboratory measurements. Tube types: 1, citrate; 2, clot tube (serum) with separator gel; 3, clot tube without separator gel; 4, heparin; 5, heparin with separator gel; 6 and 7, EDTA; 8, sodium floride/EDTA. (Courtesy of Michael Purugganan.)

Tubes must be drawn in a specific order to avoid contamination with additives that are known to interfere in standard laboratory tests. Failure to collect additive tubes in the proper order is not identifiable once the tubes are received in the laboratory and can lead to serious inaccuracies in test results. The correct order for drawing the most commonly used phlebotomy tubes is shown in Figure 6-26.[150] The stopper color is standardized to indicate what additives each tube contains. For example, the tube with a red stopper (3) contains only clot activators, and the yellow stopper tube (2) contains both clot activators and a separation gel. The lavender-topped tube (6) contains EDTA and must be drawn after a clot tube for serum (2 or 3) or tubes containing heparin (4 and 5).

Urine. Urine often contains not only the original hormone but also key metabolites that may or may not have biologic activity. The 24-hour urine specimen is used for many endocrine tests. Such urine specimens represent a time average that integrates over the multiple pulsatile spikes of hormone secretion occurring throughout the day. The 24-hour urine specimen also has the advantage of better analytic sensitivity for some hormones and metabolites.[55,151-158]

Drawbacks include the inconvenience of collecting the 24-hour specimen and delays in collection. Another limitation of urine specimens is uncertainty regarding the completeness of the collection. Measurement of urinary creatinine concentrations helps in monitoring collection completeness, especially when this value is compared with the patient's muscle mass. Many urinary hormones are conjugated to carrier proteins before excretion. Therefore, both hepatic function and, to a lesser degree, renal function may alter urinary hormone values.

Saliva. Saliva is an attractive alternative specimen for measuring non–protein-bound hormones and small molecules.[159-162] Small analytes in blood pass into oral fluid by crossing capillary walls and basement membranes and by passing through lipophilic membranes of epithelial cells.[163] This transport involves passive diffusion, ultrafiltration, active transport, or some combination of these processes. The concentration in saliva depends on the concentration of the non–protein-bound analyte in blood, the salivary pH, the acid dissociation constant (pKa) of the analyte, and the size of the analyte. Analytes entering saliva by passive diffusion usually are less than 500 Da in size, non–protein-bound, and nonionized. As with any specimen type, it is essential to fully validate the use of saliva in each analytic method and to establish the data needed for interpretation of test results, such as reference intervals.

Saliva measurements reportedly correlate with blood measurements for some hormones such as cortisol, progesterone, estradiol, and testosterone, but they do not correlate well for others (e.g., thyroid and pituitary hormones).[164-172] Multiple preanalytic variables can affect the salivary measurement. Stimulation of oral fluid production by chewing or by the use of candy or drops that contain stimulants such as citric acid can increase oral fluid volume and stabilize pH but may alter some analyte concentrations. Several commercial devices are available for collection of oral fluid; however, these devices need to be validated for each analyte and each assay system to ensure they adequately recover each of the analytes.

Saliva is also an effective specimen type for obtaining genomic DNA and other nucleic acid assay applications. Its use in this regard is now well established and rapidly advancing.[173-175]

Fluids and Tissue From Fine-Needle Aspiration. Fine-needle aspiration (FNA) involves the insertion of a hollow needle into tissue, typically a suspicious lump or inflamed tissue, to withdraw fluid or cells for diagnostic evaluation. The procedure is usually performed manually by the surgeon or a cytopathologist when a palpable lump is present or the tissue target can be seen (e.g., during a surgical procedure). Deep sampling can be achieved using x-ray or ultrasound guidance. Analysis of the cellular components of a FNA is done in the cytopathology laboratory and involves the examination of cells by histologic and immunohistologic procedures.

FNA fluids thus represent a unique specimen type for analysis of biomarkers by traditional immunoassays or by LC/MS-MS methods. However, FNA fluids present special considerations with respect to handling, stability, validation, and interpretation. Aspirated fluids are typically obtained in volumes too small to directly assay and often will clot due to contamination with whole blood. Analyte stability as well as assay parameter validation must be determined using aspirated fluid and diluents required to provide the necessary volume and anticoagulation prior to testing. Interpretation is often difficult because reference intervals applicable to individual patients are seldom available and often analytes, such as thyroglobulin in neck mass aspirates, are high enough to cause artifacts in assays (such as hook effects in antibody-based assays).

Aspirated cells can provide sufficient DNA and RNA for genetic analysis. Currently this is an area of intensive investigation that has only just begun to be applied by clinical laboratories. Typical methods being applied include expression arrays, real-time PCR, and DNA methylation assays as well as the widespread and traditional application of immunohistochemical assays for specific biomarkers.[177] For example, expression arrays can provide clinically valuable information for the 15% to 30% of thyroid nodules subjected to FNA and characterized as indeterminate by cytologic tests.[178]

Other current clinical applications of FNA in conjunction with diagnostic assays include chorionic villus sampling[179,180] and measurement of biomarkers in aspirates from pancreatic tumors.[181-183]

QUALITY CONTROL

Laboratory quality control procedures are intended to ensure that the tests are being performed within defined limits established during the validation of the assay.[184-188] The goal of these procedures is to identify circumstances when results obtained may not be accurate. They rely heavily on the testing of materials with known analyte concentrations. Quality control failures are meant to detect instrument problems (hardware or instrument failures), reagent or calibration failures, and human mistakes (improper handling of reagents or specimens, training problems, or shift change communication failures).

Statistically, there are two major forms of analytic errors: random and systematic. Random error relates to reproducibility; systematic error relates to the offset or bias of the test values from the target or reference value. Performance criteria can be defined for each of these parameters, and quality control systems can be programmed to monitor compliance with these criteria. Control systems must have low false-positive rates as well as high statistical power to detect assay deviations. The multirule algorithms developed by Westgard and colleagues use combinations of control rules—such as two consecutive controls outside warning limits, one control outside action limits, or moving average trend analyzers outside limits—to achieve good statistical error detection characteristics.[185-188] Traditionally, quality control programs have focused primarily on precision; however, analytic bias also can cause major clinical problems. If fixed decision levels are used to trigger clinical actions (e.g., therapy, additional investigations), changes in the analytic set-point of an assay can cause major changes in the number of follow-up cases. More modern quality control systems use moving averages of patient test values to help monitor changes in analytic bias. Increasing numbers of web-based systems are available for laboratories to share quality performance data, allowing better statistical evaluations (larger numbers of values to identify shifts and drifts in quality control measurements).

QUALITY ASSURANCE

Quality assurance procedures go beyond monitoring test values for control materials. Testing of quality control materials only identifies errors that occur during testing per se (i.e., the analytic phase of the overall process from ordering a test until the results are reported back to the physician). A look at when errors typically occur provides important insight into the issues. As illustrated in Figure 6-27, errors that occur during the analytic process represent less than a third of all errors associated with laboratory testing.

Quality assurance procedures are part of the regulatory requirements of a clinical laboratory. All laboratories have procedures to monitor things like specimen transport times and report accuracy, which are processes that can be established solely within the laboratory. A key element of quality assurance, and one that should be emphasized for clinicians who are critical to its success, is the identification and investigation of test values that are discordant. Some of these discordant test values may be analytically correct, but others may be erroneous. Clinicians must help identify and investigate these suspicious test values by requesting laboratories to perform a few simple validation procedures.

Repeated testing of the same specimen is a valuable first step. If the specimen has been stored under stable conditions, the absolute value of the difference between the initial and the repeated measurements should be less than 3 analytic SDs 95% of the time. Normally, the 95% confidence range is associated with the mean ± 2 SDs; with repeated laboratory tests, however, errors are associated with the first as well as the second measurement. The confidence interval for the uncertainty of the difference between two measurements can be calculated using the statistical rules for propagation of errors.

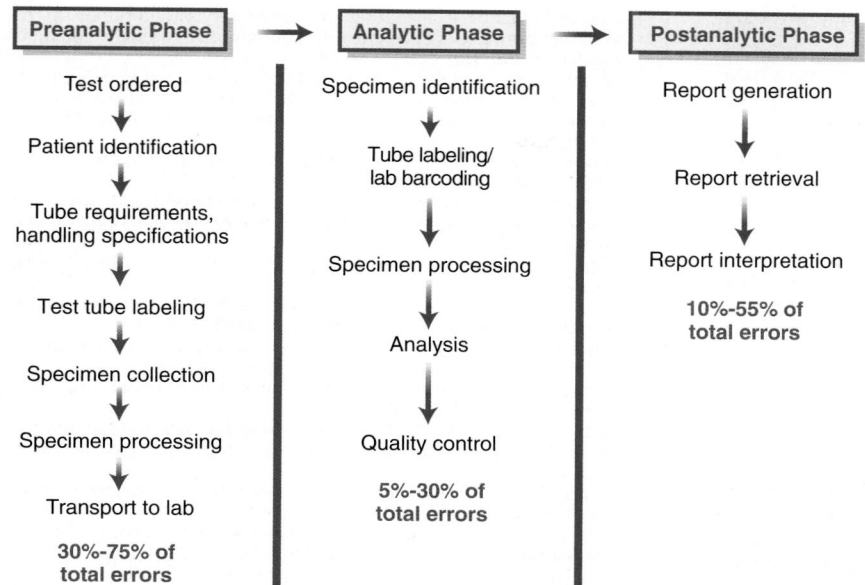

Figure 6-27 Distribution of errors during the entire process of clinical laboratory testing.

To better understand this propagation of error, consider:

$$D = X_1 - X_2$$

where X_1 is the first measurement, X_2 is the repeated measurement, and D is the difference.

$$\text{Variance (D)} = \text{Variance }(X_1) + \text{Variance }(X_2)$$
$$\text{Variance (D)} = 2\,\text{Variance (X)}$$
$$\text{SD (D)} = \sqrt{2\,\text{Variance (X)}}$$
$$\text{SD (D)} = \sqrt{2}\,\text{SD(X)}$$

The variance of D is the sum of the variance of X_1 and the variance of X_2. The SD of D is the square root of the variance of D, or the square root of twice the variance of X_1. The SD of D equates to the square root of 2 multiplied by SD(X). Therefore, 95% of the absolute values for D should be within square root of 2 times 2 SD(X), or approximately 3 SD(X). If a repeat measurement exceeds this 3 SD(X) limit, the initial (or reagent) measurement is probably in error.

Linearity and recovery are valuable techniques for evaluating test validity in individual specimens. If the initial test value is elevated, serial dilution of the specimen in the assay diluent and reassay should be considered. If the initial value is low, one may consider adding known quantities of the analyte to part of the specimen. Analyzing these spiked or diluted specimens with the original specimen allows one to evaluate both reproducibility and recovery. It may be helpful to analyze the linearity or recovery of the assay standards at the same time, to provide internal controls of the dilution or spiking procedures and the appropriateness of the diluent and spiking material. If the replication, dilution, or recovery experiment appears successful, further analytic troubleshooting will vary according to the method used. For example, immunoassays may be affected by interference caused by heterophile antibodies or hook effects as described earlier. Addition of nonimmune mouse serum or heterophile antibody-blocking solutions may neutralize these effects. Chromatographic assays are usually more robust than immunoassays but often lack the specificity. Specimens with suspected interference on one type of assay can be reanalyzed by means of an alternative methodology. Interferences with cross-reacting drugs and metabolic products can be minimized with selective extraction or identified by adding drug to nondiscordant specimens.

CLASSES OF ASSAYS

In the United States the regulations governing clinical laboratories fall into several categories based on the manufacture of assay components, the intended use of the assay, and how the assay service is billed. In order to be reimbursed by Medicare and other health insurance organizations laboratories must comply with federal legislation known as the Clinical Laboratory Improvement Amendments (CLIA). This legislation requires that laboratories be certified by specified organizations (e.g., the College of American Pathologists or the Joint Commission for the Accreditation of Hospital Organizations) and is administered by the Centers for Medicare & Medicaid Services (CMS) within the United States Department of Health and Human Services (DHHS). CMS also administers the HIPAA of 1996 and other quality standards that laboratories must comply with under federal law. CMS/CLIA certification requires quality inspections every 2 years to ensure that laboratories are meeting the standards outlined in the federal CLIA guidelines and the performance standards specified by the laboratory's inspecting agency. Inspecting agency standards are based on the CLIA guidelines.

In contrast, the manufacture and sale of assay reagents and instruments are regulated by guidelines called current Good Manufacturing Practices (cGMPs), which cover very specific topics and are periodically amended.[189-194] Compliance with cGMPs is enforced by the FDA under federal law.[195] Besides the manufacture and sale of instruments and reagents, laboratory-developed methods used in patient care are encompassed within the jurisdiction of the FDA. The FDA does not certify compliance and conducts its own quality inspections. Failure to comply with cGMPs is a violation of federal law (as opposed to reimbursement requirements under CLIA) and can result in laboratory closure as well as potential fines and legal actions. Sale of assay instruments and reagents requires premarket approval by the FDA or FDA clearance under Section 510(k), depending on the clinical use of the product and its potential impact on patient care.

Common elements to clinical laboratory standards and CLIA and cGMP guidelines include laboratory evaluation and documentation of validation verification for commercially available reagents and instruments, which have been 510(k) approved or preapproved by the FDA and whose continued manufacture is overseen by the FDA. Requirements for laboratory-developed methods, which include any modifications of FDA-approved/cleared commercial procedures, are more extensive, and validation per se is expected.

CONCLUSION

The analytic methods of assessing endocrine problems in patients are continually expanding. The newer systems are often based on analytic techniques similar to those outlined in this chapter, but the configurations are generally more user friendly. These advances make the systems more convenient, but they also become more of a "black box" that conceals most of the details of the system. The methods, their descriptions, and approach to their validation, as outlined in this chapter, are intended to provide the clinician with insights into the inner workings of these systems and to encourage a more detailed level of interaction with the clinical laboratory in its ever more challenging endeavors to provide cost-effective, yet high-quality support for patient care.

ACKNOWLEDGMENT

The authors gratefully acknowledge the work of George G. Klee, MD, PhD, who authored this chapter in the previous edition. The authors also thank Dr. Neal Lindeman and Dr. Kent Lewandrowski for reading the draft manuscript and for their helpful suggestions.

REFERENCES

1. Meyer GS, Demehin AA, Liu X, Neuhauser D. Two hundred years of hospital costs and mortality—MGH and four eras of value in medicine. *N Engl J Med.* 2012;366:2147-2149.
2. Thorell JI, Larson SM. *Radioimmunoassay and Related Techniques: Methodology and Clinical Applications.* St. Louis, MO: Mosby; 1978.
3. Price CP, Newman DJ, eds. *Principles and Practice of Immunoassay.* New York, NY: Stockton Press; 1996.
4. Moser AC, Hage DS. Immunoaffinity chromatography: an introduction to applications and recent developments. *Bioanalysis.* 2010;2:769-790.
5. Fitzgerald J, Leonard P, Darcy E, O'Kennedy R. Immunoaffinity chromatography. *Methods Mol Biol.* 2011;681:35-59.
6. Pfaunmiller EL, Paulemond ML, Dupper CM, Hage DS. Affinity monolith chromatography: a review of principles and recent analytical applications. *Anal Bioanal Chem.* 2013;405:2133-2145.
7. Nakamura RM. Monoclonal antibodies: methods and clinical laboratory applications. *Clin Physiol Biochem.* 1983;1:160-172.
8. Epstein N, Epstein M. The hybridoma technology: I. Production of monoclonal antibodies. *Adv Biotechnol Processes.* 1986;6:179-218.
9. Vetterlein D. Monoclonal antibodies: production, purification, and technology. *Adv Clin Chem.* 1989;27:303-354.
10. Burns R. Making hybridomas. *Methods Mol Biol.* 2005;295:41-54.
11. Underwood PA, Bean PA. The influence of methods of production, purification and storage of monoclonal antibodies upon their observed specificities. *J Immunol Methods.* 1985;80:189-197.
12. Pettersson KS, Soderholm JR. Individual differences in lutropin immunoreactivity revealed by monoclonal antibodies. *Clin Chem.* 1991;37:333-340.
13. Ehrlich PH, Moyle WR. Cooperative immunoassays: ultrasensitive assays with mixed monoclonal antibodies. *Science.* 1983;221:279-281.
14. Gao P, D'Amour P. Evolution of the parathyroid hormone (PTH) assay—importance of circulating PTH immunoheterogeneity and of its regulation. *Clin Lab.* 2005;51:21-29.
15. Bristow A, Berger P, Bidart JM, et al. Establishment, value assignment, and characterization of new WHO reference reagents for six molecular forms of human chorionic gonadotropin. *Clin Chem.* 2005;51:177-182.
16. Roberts RF, Roberts WL. Performance characteristics of five automated serum cortisol immunoassays. *Clin Biochem.* 2004;37:489-493.
17. Barnes SC, Swaminathan R. Effect of albumin concentration on serum cortisol measured by the Bayer Advia Centaur assay. *Ann Clin Biochem.* 2007;44:79-82.
18. Hempen C, Karst U. Labeling strategies for bioassays. *Anal Bioanal Chem.* 2006;384:572-583.
19. Chan CP, Cheung YC, Renneberg R, Seydack M. New trends in immunoassays. *Adv Biochem Eng Biotechnol.* 2008;109:123-154.
20. Fan A, Cao Z, Li H, et al. Chemiluminescence platforms in immunoassay and DNA analyses. *Anal Sci.* 2009;25:587-597.
21. Zhong W. Nanomaterials in fluorescence-based biosensing. *Anal Bioanal Chem.* 2009;394:47-59.
22. Roda A. Guardigli M. Analytical chemiluminescence and bioluminescence: latest achievements and new horizons. *Anal Bioanal Chem.* 2012;402:69-76.
23. Muzyka K. Current trends in the development of the electrochemiluminescent immunosensors. *Biosens Bioelectron.* 2014;54:393-407.
24. Tang D, Cui Y, Chen G. Nanoparticle-based immunoassays in the biomedical field. *Analyst.* 2013;138:981-990.
25. Han KN, Li CA, Seong GH. Microfluidic chips for immunoassays. *Annu Rev Anal Chem (Palo Alto Calif).* 2013;6:119-141.
26. Gosling JP. A decade of development in immunoassay methodology. *Clin Chem.* 1990;36:1408-1427.
27. Fomenko I, Durst M, Balaban D. Robust regression for high throughput drug screening. *Comput Methods Programs Biomed.* 2006;82:31-37.
28. Sluss PM. Methodologies for measurement of cardiac markers. *Clin Lab Med.* 2014;34:167-185.
29. Petakov MS, Damjanovic SS, Nikolic-Durovic MM, et al. Pituitary adenomas secreting large amounts of prolactin may give false low values in immunoradiometric assays. The hook effect. *J Endocrinol Invest.* 1998;21:184-188.
30. Schofl C, Schofl-Siegert B, Karstens JH, et al. Falsely low serum prolactin in two cases of invasive macroprolactinoma. *Pituitary.* 2002;5:261-265.
31. Cole LA. Human chorionic gonadotropin and associated molecules. *Expert Rev Mol Diagn.* 2009;9:51-73.
32. Cole LA. Hyperglycosylated hCG, a review. *Placenta.* 2010;31:653-664.
33. Cole LA. hCG, five independent molecules. *Clin Chim Acta.* 2012;413:48-65.
34. Harvey RA, Mitchell HD, Stenman UH, et al. Differences in total human chorionic gonadotropin immunoassay analytical specificity and ability to measure human chorionic gonadotropin in gestational trophoblastic disease and germ cell tumors. *J Reprod Med.* 2010;55:285-295.
35. Marquette CA, Corgier BP, Blum LJ. Recent advances in multiplex immunoassays. *Bioanalysis.* 2012;4:927-936.
36. Woolley CF, Hayes MA. Recent developments in emerging microimmunoassays. *Bioanalysis.* 2013;5:245-264.
37. Leung YS, Dees K, Cyr R, et al. Falsely increased serum estradiol results reported in direct estradiol assays. *Clin Chem.* 1997;43:1250-1251.
38. Fitzgerald RL, Herold DA. Serum total testosterone: immunoassay compared with negative chemical ionization gas chromatography-mass spectrometry. *Clin Chem.* 1996;42:749-755.
39. Krishna MV, Gorrepati M, Vusa R. Electromembrane extraction—a novel extraction technique for pharmaceutical, chemical, clinical and environmental analysis. *J Chromatogr Sci.* 2013;51:619-631.
40. Keevil BG. Novel liquid chromatography tandem mass spectrometry (LC-MS/MS) methods for measuring steroids. *Best Pract Res Clin Endocrinol Metab.* 2013;27:663-674.
41. Furey A, Moriarty M, Bane V, et al. Ion suppression; a critical review on causes, evaluation, prevention and applications. *Talanta.* 2013;115:104-122.
42. Rogeberg M, Malerod H, Roberg-Larsen H, et al. On-line solid phase extraction-liquid chromatography, with emphasis on modern bioanalysis and miniaturized systems. *J Pharm Biomed Anal.* 2014;87:120-129.
43. Michel T, Destandau E, Elfakir C. New advances in countercurrent chromatography and centrifugal partition chromatography: focus on coupling strategy. *Anal Bioanal Chem.* 2014;406:957-969.
44. Pan J, Zhang C, Zhang Z, Li G. Review of online coupling of sample preparation techniques with liquid chromatography. *Anal Chim Acta.* 2014;815:1-15.
45. Leong MI, Fuh MR, Huang SD. Beyond dispersive liquid-liquid microextraction. *J Chromatogr A.* 2014;1335:2-14.
46. Soares RR, Novo P, Azevedo AM, et al. On-chip sample preparation and analyte quantification using a microfluidic aqueous two-phase extraction coupled with an immunoassay. *Lab Chip.* 2014;14:4284-4294.

47. Barker SA. Matrix solid phase dispersion (MSPD). *J Biochem Biophys Methods.* 2007;70:151-162.

48. Luque-Garcia JL, Neubert TA. Sample preparation for serum/plasma profiling and biomarker identification by mass spectrometry. *J Chromatogr A.* 2007;1153:259-276.

49. Hennion MC, Pichon V. Immuno-based sample preparation for trace analysis. *J Chromatogr A.* 2003;1000:29-52.

50. Delaunay-Bertoncini N, Hennion MC. Immunoaffinity solid-phase extraction for pharmaceutical and biomedical trace-analysis-coupling with HPLC and CE-perspectives. *J Pharm Biomed Anal.* 2004;34: 717-736.

51. Anderson DJ. High-performance liquid chromatography in clinical analysis. *Anal Chem.* 1999;71:314R-327R.

52. Volin P. High-performance liquid chromatographic analysis of corticosteroids. *J Chromatogr B Biomed Appl.* 1995;671:319-340.

53. Kuronen P, Volin P, Laitalainen T. Reversed-phase high-performance liquid chromatographic screening method for serum steroids using retention index and diode-array detection. *J Chromatogr B Biomed Sci Appl.* 1998;718:211-224.

54. Bicker J, Fortuna A, Alves G, Falcao A. Liquid chromatographic methods for the quantification of catecholamines and their metabolites in several biological samples—a review. *Anal Chim Acta.* 2013; 768:12-34.

55. Grouzmann E, Lamine F. Determination of catecholamines in plasma and urine. *Best Pract Res Clin Endocrinol Metab.* 2013;27:713-723.

56. Clinical Laboratory Standards Institute, National Committee for Clinical Laboratory Standards. *Mass Spectrometry in the Clinical Laboratory: General Principles and Guidance; Approved Guideline, C50-A.* Wayne, PA: CLSI/NCCLS; 2007.

57. Shackleton C. Clinical steroid mass spectrometry: a 45-year history culminating in HPLC-MS/MS becoming an essential tool for patient diagnosis. *J Steroid Biochem Mol Biol.* 2010;121:481-490.

58. Krone N, Hughes BA, Lavery GG, et al. Gas chromatography/mass spectrometry (GC/MS) remains a pre-eminent discovery tool in clinical steroid investigations even in the era of fast liquid chromatography tandem mass spectrometry (LC/MS/MS). *J Steroid Biochem Mol Biol.* 2010;121:496-504.

59. Whitehouse CM, Dreyer RN, Yamashita M, Fenn JB. Electrospray interface for liquid chromatographs and mass spectrometers. *Anal Chem.* 1985;57:675-679.

60. Fenn JB, Mann M, Meng CK, et al. Electrospray ionization for mass spectrometry of large biomolecules. *Science.* 1989;246:64-71.

61. Thienpont LM. A major step forward in the routine measurement of serum free thyroid hormones. *Clin Chem.* 2008;54:625-626.

62. Midgley JE. Direct and indirect free thyroxine assay methods: theory and practice. *Clin Chem.* 2001;47:1353-1363.

63. Stockigt JR. Free thyroid hormone measurement. A critical appraisal. *Endocrinol Metab Clin North Am.* 2001;30:265-289.

64. Ekins RP, Edwards PR. Plasma protein-mediated transport of steroid and thyroid hormones. A critique. *Ann N Y Acad Sci.* 1988;538: 193-203.

65. Raff H, Sluss PM. Pre-analytical issues for testosterone and estradiol assays. *Steroids.* 2008;73:1297-1304.

66. Faix JD. Principles and pitfalls of free hormone measurements. *Best Pract Res Clin Endocrinol Metab.* 2013;27:631-645.

67. Van UK, Stockl D, Ross HA, Thienpont LM. Use of frozen sera for FT4 standardization: investigation by equilibrium dialysis combined with isotope dilution-mass spectrometry and immunoassay. *Clin Chem.* 2006;52:1817-1821.

68. Yue B, Rockwood AL, Sandrock T, et al. Free thyroid hormones in serum by direct equilibrium dialysis and online solid-phase extraction—liquid chromatography/tandem mass spectrometry. *Clin Chem.* 2008; 54:642-651.

69. Midgley JE. "All that glisters is not gold": ultrafiltration and free thyroxine measurement with apologies to W Shakespeare. *Clin Biochem.* 2011;44:151-153.

70. Nelson JC, Yoo EW, Wilcox RB. Accuracy issues in free thyroxine testing methods. *Semin Perinatol.* 2008;32:403-406.

71. Hoshikawa S, Mori K, Kaise N, et al. Artifactually elevated serum-free thyroxine levels measured by equilibrium dialysis in a pregnant woman with familial dysalbuminemic hyperthyroxinemia. *Thyroid.* 2004;14:155-160.

72. Kochansky CJ, McMasters DR, Lu P, et al. Impact of pH on plasma protein binding in equilibrium dialysis. *Mol Pharm.* 2008;5:438-448.

73. D'Herbomez M, Forzy G, Gasser F, et al. Clinical evaluation of nine free thyroxine assays: persistent problems in particular populations. *Clin Chem Lab Med.* 2003;41:942-947.

74. Fritz KS, Wilcox RB, Nelson JC. A direct free thyroxine (T4) immunoassay with the characteristics of a total T4 immunoassay. *Clin Chem.* 2007;53:911-915.

75. Fritz KS, McKean AJ, Nelson JC, Wilcox RB. Analog-based free testosterone test results linked to total testosterone concentrations, not free testosterone concentrations. *Clin Chem.* 2008;54:512-516.

76. Hackbarth JS, Hoyne JB, Grebe SK, Singh RJ. Accuracy of calculated free testosterone differs between equations and depends on gender and SHBG concentration. *Steroids.* 2011;76:48-55.

77. Vanbillemont G, Bogaert V, De BD, et al. Polymorphisms of the SHBG gene contribute to the interindividual variation of sex steroid hormone blood levels in young, middle-aged and elderly men. *Clin Endocrinol (Oxf).* 2009;70:303-310.

78. Nelson JC, Wang R, Asher DT, Wilcox RB. The nature of analogue-based free thyroxine estimates. *Thyroid.* 2004;14:1030-1036.

79. Shea JL, Wongt PY, Chen Y. Free testosterone: clinical utility and important analytical aspects of measurement. *Adv Clin Chem.* 2014;63: 59-84.

80. Emes RD, Farrell WE. Make way for the "next generation": application and prospects for genome-wide, epigenome-specific technologies in endocrine research. *J Mol Endocrinol.* 2012;49:R19-R27.

81. Ono M, Harley VR. Disorders of sex development: new genes, new concepts. *Nat Rev Endocrinol.* 2013;9:79-91.

82. Monticone S, Else T, Mulatero P, et al. Understanding primary aldosteronism: impact of next generation sequencing and expression profiling. *Mol Cell Endocrinol.* 2015;399:311-320.

83. Bioinformatics. Sequence extractor. Available at <http://www .bioinformatics.org/seqext/>.

84. BioTools. Restriction digestion of DNA. Available at <http://biotools .umassmed.edu/tacg4/>.

85. Sanger F, Coulson AR. A rapid method for determining sequences in DNA by primed synthesis with DNA polymerase. *J Mol Biol.* 1975; 94:441-448.

86. Sanger F, Nicklen S, Coulson AR. DNA sequencing with chain-terminating inhibitors. *Proc Natl Acad Sci U S A.* 1977;74:5463-5467.

87. Daber R, Sukhadia S, Morrissette JJ. Understanding the limitations of next generation sequencing informatics, an approach to clinical pipeline validation using artificial data sets. *Cancer Genet.* 2013;206: 441-448.

88. Nguyen L, Burnett L. Automation of molecular-based analyses: a primer on massively parallel sequencing. *Clin Biochem Rev.* 2014;35: 169-176.

89. Buermans HP, den Dunnen JT. Next generation sequencing technology: advances and applications. *Biochim Biophys Acta.* 2014;1842: 1932-1941.

90. Al Sifri SN, Raef H. The hook effect in prolactin immunoassays. *Saudi Med J.* 2004;25:656-659.

91. Falzarano R, Viggiani V, Michienzi S, et al. CLEIA CA125 evidences: good analytical performance avoiding "hook effect." *Tumour Biol.* 2013;34:387-393.

92. Fangous MS, Kerspern H, Moineau MP, et al. The hook effect in calcitonin immunoradiometric assay: a case report. *Ann Endocrinol (Paris).* 2012;73:552-555.

93. Fleseriu M, Lee M, Pineyro MM, et al. Giant invasive pituitary prolactinoma with falsely low serum prolactin: the significance of "hook effect." *J Neurooncol.* 2006;79:41-43.

94. Pereira O, Bevan JS. Preoperative assessment for pituitary surgery. *Pituitary.* 2008;11:347-351.

95. Spencer CA, Bergoglio LM, Kazarosyan M, et al. Clinical impact of thyroglobulin (Tg) and Tg autoantibody method differences on the management of patients with differentiated thyroid carcinomas. *J Clin Endocrinol Metab.* 2005;90:5566-5575.

96. Vilar L, Fleseriu M, Bronstein MD. Challenges and pitfalls in the diagnosis of hyperprolactinemia. *Arq Bras Endocrinol Metabol.* 2014;58:9-22.

97. Wilgen U, Pretorius CJ, Gous RS, et al. Hook effect in Abbott i-STAT beta-human chorionic gonadotropin (beta-hCG) point of care assay. *Clin Biochem.* 2014;47:1320-1322.

98. Yener S, Comlekci A, Arda N, et al. Misdiagnosis due to the hook effect in prolactin measurement. *Med Princ Pract.* 2008;17:429-431.

99. Preissner CM, Dodge LA, O'Kane DJ, et al. Prevalence of heterophilic antibody interference in eight automated tumor marker immunoassays. *Clin Chem.* 2005;51:208-210.

100. Ellis MJ, Livesey JH. Techniques for identifying heterophile antibody interference are assay specific: study of seven analytes on two automated immunoassay analyzers. *Clin Chem.* 2005;51:639-641.

101. Papapetrou PD, Polymeris A, Karga H, Vaiopoulos G. Heterophilic antibodies causing falsely high serum calcitonin values. *J Endocrinol Invest.* 2006;29:919-923.

102. Ross HA, Menheere PP, Thomas CM, et al. Interference from heterophilic antibodies in seven current TSH assays. *Ann Clin Biochem.* 2008; 45:616.

103. Liang Y, Yang Z, Ye W, et al. Falsely elevated carbohydrate antigen 19-9 level due to heterophilic antibody interference but not rheumatoid factor: a case report. *Clin Chem Lab Med.* 2009;47:116-117.

104. Cavalier E, Carlisi A, Chapelle JP, et al. Human anti-mouse antibodies interferences in Elecsys PTH assay after OKT3 treatment. *Transplantation.* 2009;87:451-452.

105. Altinier S, Varagnolo M, Zaninotto M, et al. Heterophilic antibody interference in a non-endogenous molecule assay: an apparent elevation in the tacrolimus concentration. *Clin Chim Acta.* 2009;402: 193-195.

106. Fritz BE, Hauke RJ, Stickle DF. New onset of heterophilic antibody interference in prostate-specific antigen measurement occurring during the period of post-prostatectomy prostate-specific antigen monitoring. *Ann Clin Biochem.* 2009;46:253-256.

107. Halsall DJ, English E, Chatterjee VK. Interference from heterophilic antibodies in TSH assays. *Ann Clin Biochem*. 2009;46:345-346.

108. Bolstad N, Warren DJ, Bjerner J, et al. Heterophilic antibody interference in commercial immunoassays; a screening study using paired native and pre-blocked sera. *Clin Chem Lab Med*. 2011;49:2001-2006.

109. Bolstad N, Warren DJ, Nustad K. Heterophilic antibody interference in immunometric assays. *Best Pract Res Clin Endocrinol Metab*. 2013;27: 647-661.

110. Spencer C, Petrovic I, Fatemi S. Current thyroglobulin autoantibody (TgAb) assays often fail to detect interfering TgAb that can result in the reporting of falsely low/undetectable serum Tg IMA values for patients with differentiated thyroid cancer. *J Clin Endocrinol Metab*. 2011;96:1283-1291.

111. Spencer C, Fatemi S. Thyroglobulin antibody (TgAb) methods—strengths, pitfalls and clinical utility for monitoring TgAb-positive patients with differentiated thyroid cancer. *Best Pract Res Clin Endocrinol Metab*. 2013;27:701-712.

112. Donegan D, McIver B, Algeciras-Schimnich A. Clinical consequences of a change in anti-thyroglobulin antibody assays during the follow-up of patients with differentiated thyroid cancer. *Endocr Pract*. 2014; 20(10):1032-1036.

113. Chahal J, Schlechte J. Hyperprolactinemia. *Pituitary*. 2008;11:141-146.

114. Petersen PH, Sandberg S, Fraser CG. Do new concepts for deriving permissible limits for analytical imprecision and bias have any advantages over existing consensus? *Clin Chem Lab Med*. 2011;49:637-640.

115. Clinical Laboratory Standards Institute, National Committee for Clinical Laboratory Standards. *Evaluation of Precision Performance of Quantitative Measurement Methods: Approved Guideline, EP05-A2*. Wayne, PA: CLSI/NCCLS; 2004.

116. Milton MJ, Wielgosz RI. Use of the international system of units (SI) in isotope ratio mass spectrometry. *Rapid Commun Mass Spectrom*. 2002;16:2201-2204.

117. Thienpont LM, Van UK, De Leenheer AP. Reference measurement systems in clinical chemistry. *Clin Chim Acta*. 2002;323:73-87.

118. Ward NS. The accuracy of clinical information systems. *J Crit Care*. 2004;19:221-225.

119. Miller WG, Tate JR, Barth JH, Jones GR. Harmonization: the sample, the measurement, and the report. *Ann Lab Med*. 2014;34:187-197.

120. Rose MP. Follicle stimulating hormone international standards and reference preparations for the calibration of immunoassays and bioassays. *Clin Chim Acta*. 1998;273:103-117.

121. Sturgeon CM, Ellis AR. Standardization of FSH, LH and hCG—current position and future prospects. *Mol Cell Endocrinol*. 2007;260-262: 301-309.

122. Bidlingmaier M. Problems with GH assays and strategies toward standardization. *Eur J Endocrinol*. 2008;159(Suppl 1):S41-S44.

123. Hilleman MR. International biological standardization in historic and contemporary perspective. *Dev Biol Stand*. 1999;100:19-30.

124. Vesper HW, Thienpont LM. Traceability in laboratory medicine. *Clin Chem*. 2009;55:1067-1075.

125. Clinical Laboratory Standards Institute, National Committee for Clinical Laboratory Standards. *Method Comparison and Bias Estimation Using Patient Samples: Approved Guideline, EP09-A2*. Wayne, PA: CLSI/NCCLS; 2002.

126. Clinical Laboratory Standards Institute, National Committee for Clinical Laboratory Standards. *Evaluation of the Linearity of Quantitative Measurement Procedures—A Statistical Approach: Approved Guideline, EP06-A*. Wayne, PA: CLSI/NCCLS; 2003.

127. Clinical Laboratory Standards Institute, National Committee for Clinical Laboratory Standards. *Evaluation of Matrix Effects: Proposed Guideline, EP14-P*. Wayne, PA: CLSI/NCCLS; 1998.

128. Kroll MH, Elin RJ. Interference with clinical laboratory analyses. *Clin Chem*. 1994;40(11 Pt 1):1996-2005.

129. Twomey PJ, Kroll MH. How to use linear regression and correlation in quantitative method comparison studies. *Int J Clin Pract*. 2008;62: 529-538.

130. Kroll MH, Emancipator K. A theoretical evaluation of linearity. *Clin Chem*. 1993;39:405-413.

131. Holden MJ, Madej RM, Minor P, Kalman LV. Molecular diagnostics: harmonization through reference materials, documentary standards and proficiency testing. *Expert Rev Mol Diagn*. 2011;11:741-755.

132. Dudal S, Baltrukonis D, Crisino R, et al. Assay formats: recommendation for best practices and harmonization from the global bioanalysis consortium harmonization team. *AAPS J*. 2014;16:194-205.

133. Cowan KJ. On assay robustness: the importance of early determination and science-driven decision-making. *Bioanalysis*. 2013;5:1317-1319.

134. Clinical Laboratory Standards Institute, National Committee for Clinical Laboratory Standards. *How to Define and Determine Reference Intervals in the Clinical Laboratory: Approved Guideline, C28-A2*. Wayne, PA: CLSI/NCCLS; 2000.

135. Sikaris K. Application of the Stockholm hierarchy to defining the quality of reference intervals and clinical decision limits. *Clin Biochem Rev*. 2012;33:141-148.

136. O'Brien PC, Dyck PJ. Procedures for setting normal values. *Neurology*. 1995;45:17-23.

137. Sikaris KA. Physiology and its importance for reference intervals. *Clin Biochem Rev*. 2014;35:3-14.

138. Solberg HE. Using a hospitalized population to establish reference intervals: pros and cons. *Clin Chem*. 1994;40(12):2205-2206.

139. Wellek S, Lackner KJ, Jennen-Steinmetz C, et al. Determination of reference limits: statistical concepts and tools for sample size calculation. *Clin Chem Lab Med*. 2014;52(12):1685-1694.

140. Solberg HE. The IFCC recommendation on estimation of reference intervals. The RefVal program. *Clin Chem Lab Med*. 2004;42:710-714.

141. Solberg HE, Lahti A. Detection of outliers in reference distributions: performance of Horn's algorithm. *Clin Chem*. 2005;51:2326-2332.

142. Batterton KA, Schubert CM. Confidence intervals around Bayes cost in multi-state diagnostic settings to estimate optimal performance. *Stat Med*. 2014;33:3280-3299.

143. Yin J, Tian L. Optimal linear combinations of multiple diagnostic biomarkers based on Youden index. *Stat Med*. 2014;33:1426-1440.

144. Moore HE, Andlauer O, Simon N, Mignot E. Exploring medical diagnostic performance using interactive, multi-parameter sourced receiver operating characteristic scatter plots. *Comput Biol Med*. 2014;47: 120-129.

145. Irwin RJ, Irwin TC. A principled approach to setting optimal diagnostic thresholds: where ROC and indifference curves meet. *Eur J Intern Med*. 2011;22:230-234.

146. Zurakowski D, Johnson VM, Lee EY. Biostatistics in clinical decision making for cardiothoracic radiologists. *J Thorac Imaging*. 2013;28: 368-375.

147. Howe CJ, Handelsman DJ. Use of filter paper for sample collection and transport in steroid pharmacology. *Clin Chem*. 1997;43:1408-1415.

148. Worthman CM, Stallings JF. Hormone measures in finger-prick blood spot samples: new field methods for reproductive endocrinology. *Am J Phys Anthropol*. 1997;104:1-21.

149. Guihen E. Recent advances in miniaturization—the role of microchip electrophoresis in clinical analysis. *Electrophoresis*. 2014;35:138-146.

150. Rosner W, Hankinson SE, Sluss PM, et al. Challenges to the measurement of estradiol: an Endocrine Society position statement. *J Clin Endocrinol Metab*. 2013;98:1376-1387.

151. Kuijper EA, Houwink EJ, van Weissenbruch MM, et al. Urinary gonadotropin measurements in neonates: a valuable non-invasive method. *Ann Clin Biochem*. 2006;43:320-322.

152. Kesner JS, Knecht EA, Krieg EF Jr, et al. Detecting pre-ovulatory luteinizing hormone surges in urine. *Hum Reprod*. 1998;13:15-21.

153. Demir A, Voutilainen R, Juul A, et al. Increase in first morning voided urinary luteinizing hormone levels precedes the physical onset of puberty. *J Clin Endocrinol Metab*. 1996;81:2963-2967.

154. Demir A, Alfthan H, Stenman UH, Voutilainen R. A clinically useful method for detecting gonadotropins in children: assessment of luteinizing hormone and follicle-stimulating hormone from urine as an alternative to serum by ultrasensitive time-resolved immunofluorometric assays. *Pediatr Res*. 1994;36:221-226.

155. Bona G, Petri A, Rapa A, et al. The impact of gender, puberty and body mass on reference values for urinary growth hormone (GH) excretion in normally growing non-obese and obese children. *Clin Endocrinol (Oxf)*. 1999;50:775-781.

156. Pirazzoli P, Mandini M, Zucchini S, et al. Urinary growth hormone estimation in diagnosing severe growth hormone deficiency. *Arch Dis Child*. 1996;75:228-231.

157. Hourd P, Edwards R. Current methods for the measurement of growth hormone in urine. *Clin Endocrinol (Oxf)*. 1994;40:155-170.

158. van Berkel A, Lenders JW, Timmers HJ. Diagnosis of endocrine disease: biochemical diagnosis of phaeochromocytoma and paraganglioma. *Eur J Endocrinol*. 2014;170:R109-R119.

159. Wood P. Salivary steroid assays—research or routine? *Ann Clin Biochem*. 2009;46:183-196.

160. Marti-Alamo S, Mancheno-Franch A, Marzal-Gamarra C, Carlos-Fabuel L. Saliva as a diagnostic fluid. Literature review. *J Clin Exp Dent*. 2012;4:e237-e243.

161. Raff H. Update on late-night salivary cortisol for the diagnosis of Cushing's syndrome: methodological considerations. *Endocrine*. 2013;44: 346-349.

162. Turpeinen U, Hamalainen E. Determination of cortisol in serum, saliva and urine. *Best Pract Res Clin Endocrinol Metab*. 2013;27:795-801.

163. Choo RE, Huestis MA. Oral fluid as a diagnostic tool. *Clin Chem Lab Med*. 2004;42:1273-1287.

164. Hankinson SE, Tworoger SS. Assessment of the hormonal milieu. *IARC Sci Publ*. 2011;163:199-214.

165. Papacosta E, Nassis GP. Saliva as a tool for monitoring steroid, peptide and immune markers in sport and exercise science. *J Sci Med Sport*. 2011;14:424-434.

166. Zolotukhin S. Metabolic hormones in saliva: origins and functions. *Oral Dis*. 2013;19:219-229.

167. Akuailou EN, Vijayagopal P, Imrhan V, Prasad C. Measurement and validation of the nature of salivary adiponectin. *Acta Diabetol*. 2013;50:727-730.

168. Stenman UH. Pitfalls in hormone determinations. *Best Pract Res Clin Endocrinol Metab*. 2013;27:743-744.

169. Voegtline KM, Granger DA. Dispatches from the interface of salivary bioscience and neonatal research. *Front Endocrinol (Lausanne)*. 2014; 5:25.
170. Vining RF, McGinley RA. The measurement of hormones in saliva: possibilities and pitfalls. *J Steroid Biochem*. 1987;27:81-94.
171. O'Rorke A, Kane MM, Gosling JP, et al. Development and validation of a monoclonal antibody enzyme immunoassay for measuring progesterone in saliva. *Clin Chem*. 1994;40:454-458.
172. Granger DA, Schwartz EB, Booth A, et al. Assessing dehydroepiandrosterone in saliva: a simple radioimmunoassay for use in studies of children, adolescents and adults. *Psychoneuroendocrinology*. 1999;24: 567-579.
173. Starke EM, Smoot JC, Wu JH, et al. Saliva-based diagnostics using 16S rRNA microarrays and microfluidics. *Ann N Y Acad Sci*. 2007;1098: 345-361.
174. Zimmermann BG, Park NJ, Wong DT. Genomic targets in saliva. *Ann N Y Acad Sci*. 2007;1098:184-191.
175. Pandeshwar P, Das R. Role of oral fluids in DNA investigations. *J Forensic Leg Med*. 2014;22:45-50.
176. Cuevas-Cordoba B, Santiago-Garcia J. Saliva: a fluid of study for OMICS. *OMICS*. 2014;18:87-97.
177. de Graaff AA, Delvoux B, Van de Vijver KK, et al. Paired-box gene 2 is down-regulated in endometriosis and correlates with low epidermal growth factor receptor expression. *Hum Reprod*. 2012;27:1676-1684.
178. Alexander EK, Kennedy GC, Baloch ZW, et al. Preoperative diagnosis of benign thyroid nodules with indeterminate cytology. *N Engl J Med*. 2012;367:705-715.
179. Ahmed S. Transabdominal chorionic villus sampling (CVS) for prenatal diagnosis of genetic disorders. *J Coll Physicians Surg Pak*. 2006;16: 204-207.
180. Spallina J, Anselem O, Haddad B, et al. [Transabdominal chorionic villus sampling using biopsy forceps or needle: pregnancy outcomes by technique used]. *J Gynecol Obstet Biol Reprod (Paris)*. 2013;43(9): 713-720.
181. Pinto MM, Emanuel JR, Chaturvedi V, Costa J. Ki-ras mutations and the carcinoembryonic antigen level in fine needle aspirates of the pancreas. *Acta Cytol*. 1997;41:427-434.
182. Ryu JK, Woo SM, Hwang JH, et al. Cyst fluid analysis for the differential diagnosis of pancreatic cysts. *Diagn Cytopathol*. 2004;31:100-105.
183. Belsley NA, Pitman MB, Lauwers GY, et al. Serous cystadenoma of the pancreas: limitations and pitfalls of endoscopic ultrasound-guided fine-needle aspiration biopsy. *Cancer*. 2008;114:102-110.
184. Aziz N, Zhao Q, Bry L, et al. College of American Pathologists' Laboratory Standards for Next-Generation Sequencing Clinical Tests. *Arch Pathol Lab Med*. 2014;[Epub ahead of print].
185. Westgard JO, Westgard SA. The quality of laboratory testing today: an assessment of sigma metrics for analytic quality using performance data from proficiency testing surveys and the CLIA criteria for acceptable performance. *Am J Clin Pathol*. 2006;125:343-354.
186. Westgard JO. Use and interpretation of common statistical tests in method comparison studies. *Clin Chem*. 2008;54:612.
187. Westgard JO. Statistical quality control procedures. *Clin Lab Med*. 2013;33:111-124.
188. Westgard JO. Perspectives on quality control, risk management, and analytical quality management. *Clin Lab Med*. 2013;33:1-14.
189. Medical devices; current good manufacturing practice (CGMP) final rule; quality system regulation—FDA. Final rule. *Fed Regist*. 1996;61: 52602-52662.
190. Medical devices; procedures for premarket notification, premarket approval, classification, performance standards establishment, banning devices, and availability of regulatory hearings—FDA. Final rule. *Fed Regist*. 1992;57:58400-58406.
191. Medical devices; 30-day notices and 135-day PMA (premarket approval application) supplement review—FDA. Direct final rule. *Fed Regist*. 1998;63(80 Pt 1):20530-20533.
192. Medical devices; reports of corrections and removals—FDA. Direct final rule. *Fed Regist*. 1998;63:42229-42233.
193. Medical devices; pediatric uses of devices; requirement for submission of information on pediatric subpopulations that suffer from a disease or condition that a device is intended to treat, diagnose, or cure; direct final rule. Direct final rule. *Fed Regist*. 2010;75:16347-16351.
194. Medical devices; exception from general requirements for informed consent. Final rule. *Fed Regist*. 2011;76:36989-36993.
195. Food, Drug, and Cosmetic Act, title 21, U.S. Code section 351, Adulterated drugs and devices.

Section II

Hypothalamus and Pituitary

Neuroendocrinology

MALCOLM J. LOW

KEY POINTS

- An underlying principle of neuroendocrinology is that peptide and monoamine signaling molecules are secreted from specialized neurons directly into the peripheral circulation.
- The secretion of anterior pituitary hormones and expression of the genes encoding these hormones is primarily regulated by releasing and inhibitory factors that are produced in hypophyseotropic hypothalamic neurons and secreted into the portal vessel system located in the median eminence.
- Homeostasis of each hypothalamic-pituitary axis is maintained by the complex integration of positive and negative feedback loops involving the pituitary hormones themselves, downstream signals including steroid hormones, and synaptic input from other brain areas onto the hypopyseotropic neurons.
- Hypothalamic neuropeptides are expressed in neurons throughout the brain to modulate the activity of neural circuits and coordinate a range of behavioral outputs that complement the hormonal actions of the hypothalamic-pituitary axes.
- A variety of mechanisms including gene mutations, epigenetic alterations, tumors, inflammatory states, infections, vascular abnormalities, trauma, and psychogenic states can produce neuroendocrine disease involving the hypothalamus.
- Hypothalamic disease can present with a variety of nonendocrine manifestations in addition to alterations in hypothalamic-pituitary function.

HISTORICAL PERSPECTIVE

The field of neuroendocrinology has expanded from its original focus on the control of pituitary hormone secretion by the hypothalamus to encompass multiple reciprocal interactions between the central nervous system (CNS) and endocrine systems in the control of homeostasis and physiologic responses to environmental stimuli. Although many of these concepts are relatively recent, the intimate interaction of the hypothalamus and the pituitary gland was recognized more than a century ago. For example, at the end of the 19th century clinicians including Alfred Fröhlich described an obesity and infertility condition referred to as *adiposogenital dystrophy* in patients with sellar tumors.[1] This condition subsequently became known as *Fröhlich syndrome* and was most often associated with the accumulation of excessive subcutaneous fat, hypogonadotrophic hypogonadism, and growth retardation.

Whether this syndrome was due to injury to the pituitary gland itself or to the overlying hypothalamus was extremely controversial. Several leaders in the field of endocrinology, including Cushing and his colleagues, argued that the syndrome was due to disruption of the pituitary gland.[2] However, experimental evidence began to accumulate that the hypothalamus was somehow involved in the control of the pituitary gland. For example, Aschner demonstrated in dogs that the precise removal of the pituitary gland without damage to the overlying hypothalamus did not result in obesity.[3] Later, seminal studies by Hetherington and Ranson demonstrated that stereotaxic destruction of the medial basal hypothalamus with electrolytic lesions, which spared the pituitary gland, resulted in morbid obesity and neuroendocrine derangements similar to those of the patients described by Fröhlich.[4] This and subsequent studies clearly established that an intact hypothalamus is required for normal endocrine function. However, the mechanisms by which the hypothalamus was involved in endocrine regulation remained unsettled for years to come. We now know that the phenotypes of Fröhlich syndrome and the ventromedial hypothalamic lesion syndrome are probably due to dysfunction or destruction of key hypothalamic neurons that regulate pituitary hormone secretion and energy homeostasis.

The field of neuroendocrinology took a major step forward when several groups, especially Ernst and Berta Scharrer, recognized that neurons in the hypothalamus were the source of the axons that constitute the neural lobe (see "Neurosecretion"). The hypothalamic control of the anterior pituitary gland remained unclear, however. For example, Popa and Fielding identified the pituitary portal vessels linking the median eminence of the hypothalamus and the anterior pituitary gland.[5] Although they appreciated the fact that this vasculature provided a link between hypothalamus and pituitary gland, they hypothesized at the time that blood flowed from the pituitary up to the brain. Anatomic studies by Wislocki and King supported the concept that blood flow was from the hypothalamus to the pituitary.[6] Later studies, including the seminal work of Geoffrey Harris, established the flow of blood from the hypothalamus at the median eminence to the anterior pituitary gland.[7] This supported the concept that the hypothalamus controlled anterior pituitary gland function indirectly and led to the now accepted hypophyseal-portal chemotransmitter hypothesis.

Subsequently, several important studies, especially those from Schally and colleagues and the Guillemin group, established that the anterior pituitary is tightly controlled by the hypothalamus.[8,9] Both groups identified several putative peptide hormone releasing factors (see later sections). These fundamental studies resulted in the awarding of the Nobel Prize in Medicine in 1977 to Andrew Schally and Roger Guillemin. We now know that these releasing factors are the fundamental link between the CNS and the control of endocrine function. Furthermore, these neuropeptides are highly conserved across species and are essential for reproduction, growth, and metabolism. The anatomy, physiology, and genetics of these factors constitute a major portion of this chapter.

Over the past 4 decades, work in the field of neuroendocrinology has continued to advance across several fronts. Cloning and characterization of the specific G protein–coupled receptors (GPCRs) used by the hypothalamic releasing factors have helped define signaling mechanisms utilized by the releasing factors. Characterization of the distribution of these receptors has universally demonstrated receptor expression in the brain and in peripheral tissues other than the pituitary, arguing for multiple physiologic roles for the neuropeptide releasing factors. Finally, there have been tremendous advances in our understanding of both regulatory neuronal and humoral inputs to the hypophyseotropic neurons.

The adipostatic hormone leptin, discovered in 1994,[10] is an example of a humoral factor that has profound effects on multiple neuroendocrine circuits.[11] Reduction in circulating leptin is responsible for suppression of the thyroid and reproductive axes during the starvation response. The subsequent discovery of ghrelin,[12] a stomach peptide that regulates appetite and also acts on multiple neuroendocrine axes, demonstrates that much remains to be learned regarding the regulation of the hypothalamic releasing hormones. Traditionally, it has been extremely difficult to study releasing factor gene expression or the specific regulation of the releasing factor neurons because of their small numbers and, in some cases, diffuse distribution. Transgenic experiments have produced mice in which expression of fluorescent marker proteins has been specifically targeted to gonadotropin-releasing hormone (GnRH) neurons[13] and arcuate pro-opiomelanocortin (POMC) neurons,[14] among many others. This technology will allow detailed study of the electrophysiologic properties of hypothalamic neurons in the more native context of slice preparations or organotypic cultures.

Although much of the field of neuroendocrinology has focused on hypothalamic releasing factors and their control of reproduction, growth, development, fluid balance, and the stress response through their control of pituitary hormone production, the term *neuroendocrinology* has come to mean the study of interaction of the endocrine and nervous systems in the regulation of homeostasis. The field of neuroendocrinology has been further expanded, however, because diverse areas of basic research have often been fundamental to understanding the neuroendocrine system and thus have been championed by its investigators. These areas include studies of neuropeptide structure, function, and mechanism of action; neural secretion; hypothalamic neuroanatomy; GPCR structure, function, and signaling; transport of substances into the brain; and the action of hormones on the brain. Moreover, homeostatic systems often involve integrated endocrine, autonomic, and behavioral responses. In many of these systems

(e.g., energy homeostasis, immune function), the classic neuroendocrine axes are important but not autonomous pathways, and these subjects are also often studied in the context of neuroendocrinology.

In this chapter, the concepts of neural secretion, the neuroanatomy of the hypothalamic-pituitary unit, and the CNS structures most relevant to the control of the neurohypophysis and adenohypophysis are presented. Then, each classic hypothalamic-pituitary axis is described, including a consideration of the immune system and its integration with neuroendocrine function. Finally, the pathophysiology of disorders of neural regulation of endocrine function are reviewed. The neuroendocrinology of energy homeostasis is fully considered in Chapter 35.

NEURAL CONTROL OF ENDOCRINE SECRETION

A fundamental principle of neuroendocrinology encompasses the regulated secretion of hormones, neurotransmitters, or neuromodulators by specialized cells.[15] Endocrine cells and neurons are prototypical secretory cells. Both have electrically excitable plasma membranes and specific ion conductances that regulate exocytosis of their signaling molecules from storage vesicles. Secretory cells are broadly classified by their topographic mechanisms of secretion. For example, *endocrine* cells secrete their contents directly into the bloodstream, allowing these substances to act globally as hormones. Cells classified as *paracrine* secrete their contents into the extracellular space and predominantly affect the function of closely neighboring cells. *Autocrine* secretory cells affect their own function by the local actions of their secretions. In contrast, secretory cells within *exocrine* glands secrete proteinaceous substances, including enzymes, and lipids into the lumen of ductal systems.

Neurosecretion

Neurons are excitable cells that send their axons throughout the nervous system to release their neurotransmitters and neuromodulators predominantly at specialized chemical synapses. Neurohumoral or neurosecretory cells constitute a unique subset of neurons whose axon terminals are not associated with classic synapses. Two examples of neurosecretory cells are neurohypophyseal and hypophyseotropic cells. The prototypical neurohypophyseal cells are the magnicellular neurons of the paraventricular and supraoptic nuclei in the hypothalamus (PVH, SON). Hypophyseotropic cells are neurons that secrete their products into the pituitary portal vessels at the median eminence (Fig. 7-1).

In the most basic sense, neurosecretory cells are neurons that secrete substances directly into the bloodstream to act as hormones. The theory of neurosecretion evolved from the seminal work of Scharrer and Scharrer,[15] who used morphologic techniques to identify stained secretory granules in the SON and PVH neurons. They found that cutting the pituitary stalk led to an accumulation of these granules in the hypothalamus, which led them to hypothesize that hypothalamic neurons were the source of substances secreted by the neural lobe (posterior pituitary). Although this concept initially raised great skepticism among contemporary researchers, it is now known that the axon terminals in the neural lobe arise from the SON and PVH magnicellular neurons that contain oxytocin and the antidiuretic hormone arginine vasopressin (AVP).

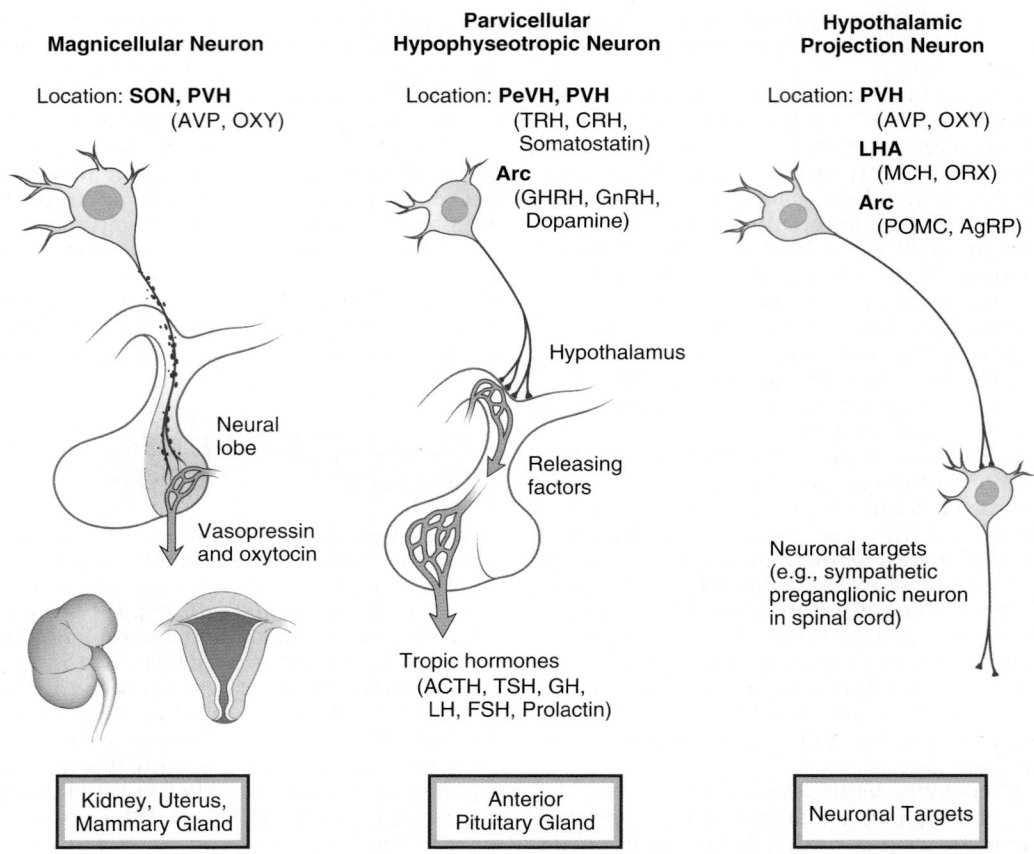

Figure 7-1 Three types of hypothalamic neurosecretory cells. *Left*, A magnicellular neuron that secretes arginine vasopressin (AVP) or oxytocin (OXY). The cell body, which is located in the supraoptic nucleus (SON) or paraventricular hypothalamic nucleus (PVH), projects its neuronal process into the neural lobe, and neurohormone is released from nerve endings. *Center*, Parvicellular peptidergic neurons are located in the medial basal hypothalamus in nuclear groups including the periventricular hypothalamic nucleus (PeVH), the PVH, and infundibular or arcuate nucleus of the hypothalamus (Arc). The neuropeptides in this case are released into the specialized blood supply to the pituitary to regulate its secretion. *Right*, A third category of hypothalamic peptidergic neurons terminates at chemical synapses on other neurons. These projection neurons are found in sites including the PVH, Arc, and lateral hypothalamic area (LHA) that innervate multiple central nervous system nuclei, including autonomic preganglionic neurons in the brainstem and spinal cord. Such substances act as neurotransmitters or neuromodulators. ACTH, corticotropin; AgRP, agouti-related peptide; CRH, corticotropin-releasing hormone; FSH, follicle-stimulating hormone; GH, growth hormone; GHRH, growth hormone–releasing hormone; GnRH, gonadotropin-releasing hormone; LH, luteinizing hormone; MCH, melanin-concentrating hormone; ORX, orexin/hypocretin; POMC, pro-opiomelanocortin; TRH, thyrotropin-releasing hormone; TSH, thyrotropin.

The modern definition of *neurosecretion* has evolved to include the release of any neuronal secretory product from a neuron. Indeed, a fundamental tenet of neuroscience is that all neurons in the CNS, including neurons that secrete AVP and oxytocin in the neural lobe, receive multiple synaptic inputs largely onto their dendrites and cell bodies. In addition, neurons have the basic ability to detect and integrate input from multiple neurons through specific receptors. They in turn fire action potentials that result in the release of neurotransmitters and neuromodulators into synapses formed with postsynaptic neurons. The vast majority of communications between neurons is accomplished by classic fast-acting neurotransmitters (e.g., glutamate, γ-aminobutyric acid [GABA], acetylcholine) and neuromodulators (e.g., dopamine, neuropeptides) acting at chemical synapses.[16,17] Neurosecretion represents a fundamental concept in understanding the mechanisms used by the nervous system to control behavior and maintain homeostasis.

In the era of optigenetics, multidimensional "omics," and personalized medicine, the importance of these early observations is often not fully appreciated. However, accounts of these early studies are illuminating and it is not an overstatement that the confirmation of the neurosecretion hypothesis represented one of the major advances in the field of neuroscience and neuroendocrinology. Indeed, this and other early experiments, including the pioneering work of Geoffrey Harris,[7] led to the fundamental concept that the hypothalamus releases hormones directly into the bloodstream (neurohypophyseal cells). These observations provided the principles on which the modern discipline of neuroendocrinology is built.

Contribution of the Autonomic Nervous System to Endocrine Control

Another major precept of neuroendocrinology is that the nervous system controls or modifies the function of both endocrine and exocrine glands. The exquisite control of the anterior pituitary gland is accomplished by the action of releasing factor hormones (see "Hypophyseotropic Hormones and Neuroendocrine Axes"). Other endocrine and exocrine organs (e.g., pancreas and adrenal, pineal, and salivary glands) are also regulated through direct innervation from the cholinergic and noradrenergic inputs from the autonomic nervous system. An appreciation of the functional anatomy and pharmacology of the parasympathetic and sympathetic nervous systems is fundamental in understanding the neural control of endocrine function.[18]

The efferent arms of the autonomic nervous system comprise the sympathetic and parasympathetic systems. They have similar wiring diagrams characterized by a preganglionic neuron that innervates a postganglionic neuron that in turn targets an end organ.[19] Preganglionic and postganglionic parasympathetic neurons are cholinergic. In contrast, preganglionic sympathetic neurons are cholinergic, and postganglionic neurons are noradrenergic (except for those innervating sweat glands, which are cholinergic). Another basic concept is that autonomic neurons coexpress several neuropeptides. This coexpression is a common feature of neurons in the central and peripheral nervous systems.[16] For example, postganglionic noradrenergic neurons coexpress somatostatin and neuropeptide Y (NPY). Postganglionic cholinergic neurons coexpress neuropeptides including vasoactive intestinal polypeptide (VIP) and calcitonin gene–related peptide (CGRP).

Most sympathetic preganglionic neurons lie in the intermediolateral cell column in the thoracolumbar regions of the spinal cord.[19] Most postganglionic neurons are located in sympathetic ganglia lying near the vertebral column (e.g., sympathetic chain and superior cervical ganglia). Postganglionic fibers innervate target organs. As a rule, sympathetic preganglionic fibers are relatively short and the postganglionic fibers are long. In contrast, the parasympathetic preganglionic neurons lie in the midbrain (perioculomotor area, long misidentified as the Edinger-Westphal nucleus[20]), the medulla oblongata (e.g., dorsal motor nucleus of the vagus and nucleus ambiguus), and the sacral spinal cord. Postganglionic neurons that innervate the eye and salivary glands arise from the ciliary, pterygopalatine, submandibular, and otic ganglia. Postganglionic parasympathetic neurons in the thorax and abdomen typically lie within the target organs including the gut wall and pancreas.[19] Consequently, the parasympathetic preganglionic fibers are relatively long and the postganglionic fibers are short.

The dual autonomic innervation of the pancreas illustrates the importance of coordinated neural control of endocrine organs. The endocrine pancreas receives sympathetic (noradrenergic) and parasympathetic (cholinergic) innervation.[19,21] The latter activity is provided by the vagus nerve (dorsal motor nucleus of the vagus) and is an excellent example of neural modulation because the cholinergic tone of the beta cells affects their secretion of insulin. For example, vagal input is thought to modulate insulin secretion before (cephalic phase), during, and after ingestion of food.[22] In addition, noradrenergic stimulation of the endocrine pancreas can alter the secretion of glucagon and inhibits insulin release.[21] Of course, a major regulator of insulin secretion is the extracellular concentration of glucose,[23] and glucose can induce insulin secretion in the absence of neural input. However, the exquisite control by the nervous system is illustrated by the fact that populations of neurons in the brainstem and hypothalamus, like the beta cell, have the ability to sense glucose levels in the bloodstream.[24] This information is integrated by the hypothalamus and ultimately results in alterations in the activity of the autonomic nervous system innervating the pancreas. Thus, neural control of the endocrine pancreas contributes significantly to the physiologic control of insulin secretion and likely contributes to the pathophysiology of disorders such as diabetes mellitus. Certainly, an increased understanding of this complex interplay between the CNS and endocrine function is necessary to diagnose and clinically manage endocrine disorders.

HYPOTHALAMIC-PITUITARY UNIT

The hypothalamus is one of the most evolutionarily conserved and essential regions of the mammalian brain. Indeed, the hypothalamus is the ultimate brain structure that allows mammals to maintain homeostasis, and its destruction is not compatible with life. Hypothalamic control of homeostasis stems from the ability of this collection of neurons to orchestrate coordinated endocrine, autonomic, and behavioral responses. A key principle is that the hypothalamus receives sensory inputs from the external environment (e.g., light, nociception, temperature, odorants) and information regarding the internal environment (e.g., blood pressure, blood osmolality, blood glucose levels). Of particular relevance to neuroendocrine control, hormones (e.g., glucocorticoids, gondal steroids, thyroid hormone, leptin) exert both negative and positive feedback directly on the hypothalamus.

The hypothalamus integrates diverse sensory and hormonal inputs and provides coordinated responses through motor outputs to key regulatory sites. These sites include the anterior pituitary gland, posterior pituitary gland, cerebral cortex, premotor and motor neurons in the brainstem and spinal cord, and parasympathetic and sympathetic preganglionic neurons. The patterned hypothalamic outputs to these effector sites ultimately result in coordinated endocrine, behavioral, and autonomic responses that maintain homeostasis. The hypothalamic control of the pituitary gland is an elegant system that underlies the ability of mammals to coordinate endocrine functions that are necessary for survival.

Development and Differentiation of Hypothalamic Nuclei

Tremendous advances in knowledge of the molecular and genetic basis for embryonic development of the hypothalamic-pituitary unit have occurred in the past 3 decades as a result of the genome sequencing projects and use of transgenic model systems. Pituitary development is discussed in detail in Chapter 8, and only a few key points most relevant to the physiology and pathophysiology of the neuroendocrine hypothalamus are presented here.

There has been considerable debate concerning the extent to which developmental studies in the rodent hypothalamic-pituitary system are applicable to the human. However, accumulating data suggest that the similarities outweigh the differences. Ontogenic analyses of the organization of the human hypothalamus utilizing a battery of neurochemical markers have reinforced its homologies to the better studied rat brain.[25] The cytoarchitectonic boundaries of hypothalamic nuclei are much more easily discerned in fetal human brain than in the adult brain, and for the most part correspond to homologous structures in the rodent hypothalamus. This finding has important implications for the validity of interspecies comparative analyses. Two examples further illustrate this point. First, the ventromedial nucleus of the hypothalamic core (ventromedial hypothalamus, or VMH), which plays a role in energy balance and female sexual behavior, differentiates from neuroblasts in both humans and rodents at a time-point intermediate to the earlier differentiation of lateral hypothalamic nuclei and later differentiation of the midline nuclei, including the suprachiasmatic nucleus (SCN), the arcuate nucleus, and the PVH.[25,26] Expression of the transcription factor SF1 (steroidogenic factor 1) has been shown to be restricted both temporally and spatially to cells in the VMH, and knockout of the *Sf1* gene in mice alters VMH development by influencing the migration of cells and hence their ultimate location.[26] A second example of interspecies homologies in hypothalamic development is the migration of GnRH-secreting neurons from their origins in rostral neuroepithelium to the anterior hypothalamus.[27] As discussed later, spontaneous and inherited mutations in genes that affect the migration of these neurons are an important cause of Kallmann syndrome or hypogonadotropic hypogonadism associated with anosmia.

In addition to SF1 and the genes associated with Kallmann syndrome, there is a growing list of genes primarily encoding transcription factors that have been implicated in human neuroendocrine disorders and characterized experimentally in rodent models (see Chapter 4).[28,29] This list includes the homeobox transcription factor OTP and the heterodimeric complex formed by the basic helix-loop-helix (bHLH) transcription factors SIM1 and ARNT2. These factors are required for the proper development of the PVH and SON and for expression of many key hypophyseotropic neuropeptide genes. The physiologic importance of SIM1 is illustrated by the development of an obesity phenotype in both mice and humans with a haploinsufficiency of SIM1 expression.[28] A major breakthrough in the understanding of factors controlling the development and terminal differentiation of human hypothalamic neurons is the ability to generate these neurons in vitro from induced pluripotential stem cells.[30,31]

Two key concepts involved in CNS development, which also apply to the hypothalamus, are the balance between neurogenesis and cell death in the establishment of nuclei and the role of circulating hormones in providing organizational signals that regulate cell number and synaptic remodeling. The most thoroughly characterized examples are the effects of sex steroid hormones on the developing brain that result in key sexual dimorphisms of functional importance in later reproductive behaviors.[32] This principle has been extended recently to include organizational effects of other classes of hormones. For example, leptin plays an important role in the development of medial-basal hypothalamic circuits important for energy homeostasis.[33]

Anatomy of the Hypothalamic-Pituitary Unit

The pituitary gland is regulated by three interacting elements: hypothalamic inputs (releasing factors or hypophyseotropic hormones), feedback effects of circulating hormones, and paracrine and autocrine secretions of the pituitary itself. In humans, the pituitary gland (hypophysis) can be divided into two major parts, the adenohypophysis and the neurohypophysis, which are easily distinguishable from each other by T1-weighted magnetic resonance imaging (MRI) (Fig. 7-2).[34] The adenohypophysis can be subdivided into three distinct lobes, the pars distalis (anterior lobe), pars intermedia (intermediate lobe), and pars tuberalis. Whereas a well-developed intermediate lobe is found in most mammals, only rudimentary vestiges of the intermediate lobe are detectable in adult humans, with the bulk of intermediate lobe cells being dispersed in the anterior lobe.

The neurohypophysis is composed of the pars nervosa (also known as the neural or posterior lobe), the infundibular stalk, and the median eminence. The infundibular stalk is surrounded by the pars tuberalis, and together they constitute the *hypophyseal stalk*. The pituitary gland lies in the sella turcica (Turkish saddle) of the sphenoid bone and underlies the base of the hypothalamus. This anatomic location explains the hypothalamic damage described by Fröhlich.[1] In humans, the base of the hypothalamus forms

a mound called the *tuber cinereum*, the central region of which gives rise to the median eminence (see Fig. 7-2).

The anterior and intermediate lobes of the pituitary derive from a dorsal invagination of the pharyngeal epithelium, called *Rathke's pouch*, in response to inductive signals from the overlying neuroepithelium of the ventral diencephalon. During development, precursor cells within the pouch undergo steps of organ determination, cell fate commitment to a pituitary phenotype, proliferation, and migration. The intermediate lobe is in direct contact with the neural lobe and is the least prominent of the three lobes. With age, the human intermediate lobe decreases in size to leave a small, residual collection of POMC cells. In nonprimate species, these cells are responsible for secreting the POMC-derived product α-melanocyte-stimulating hormone (α-MSH).[35]

The major component of the neural lobe is a collection of axon terminals arising from magnicellular secretory neurons located in the PVH and SON of the hypothalamus (Fig. 7-3; see Fig. 7-1).[36] These axon terminals are in close association with a capillary plexus, and they secrete substances including AVP and oxytocin into the hypophyseal veins and into the general circulation (Table 7-1). The blood supply to the neurohypophysis arises from the inferior hypophyseal artery (a branch of the internal carotid artery). Glial-like cells called pituicytes are scattered among the nerve terminals. As the source of AVP to the general circulation, the PVH and SON and their axon terminals in the neural lobe are the effector arms for the central regulation of blood osmolality, fluid balance, and blood pressure (see Chapter 10).

The secretion of oxytocin by magnicellular neurons is critical at parturition, resulting in uterine myometrial contraction. In addition, the secretion of oxytocin is regulated by the classic milk let-down reflex. Mechanosensory information from the nipple reaches the magnicellular neurons, directly or indirectly, from the dorsal horn of the spinal cord, resulting in a synchronized burst of action potentials in the whole population of oxytocin neurons followed by the release of oxytocin into the general circulation.[37] Oxytocin acts on receptors on myoepithelial cells in the mammary gland acini, leading to release of milk into the ductal system and ultimately the release of milk from the mammary gland.

The Median Eminence and Hypophyseotropic Neuronal System

The median eminence is the functional link between the hypothalamus and the anterior pituitary gland. It lies in the center of the tuber cinereum and is composed of an extensive array of blood vessels and nerve endings (Fig. 7-4; see Fig. 7-2).[38] Its extremely rich blood supply arises from the superior hypophyseal artery (a branch of the internal carotid artery), which sends off many small branches that form capillary loops. The small capillary loops extend into the internal and external zones of the median eminence, form anastomoses, and drain into sinusoids that become the pituitary portal veins that enter the vascular pool of the pituitary gland. The flow of blood in these short loops is thought to be predominantly (if not exclusively) in a hypothalamic-to-pituitary direction. This well-developed plexus results in a tremendous increase in the vascular surface area. In addition, the vessels are fenestrated, allowing diffusion of the peptide-releasing factors to their site of action in the anterior pituitary gland. Because this vascular complex in the base of the hypothalamus and its "arteriolized" venous drainage to the pituitary compose a circulatory system analogous to the portal vein system

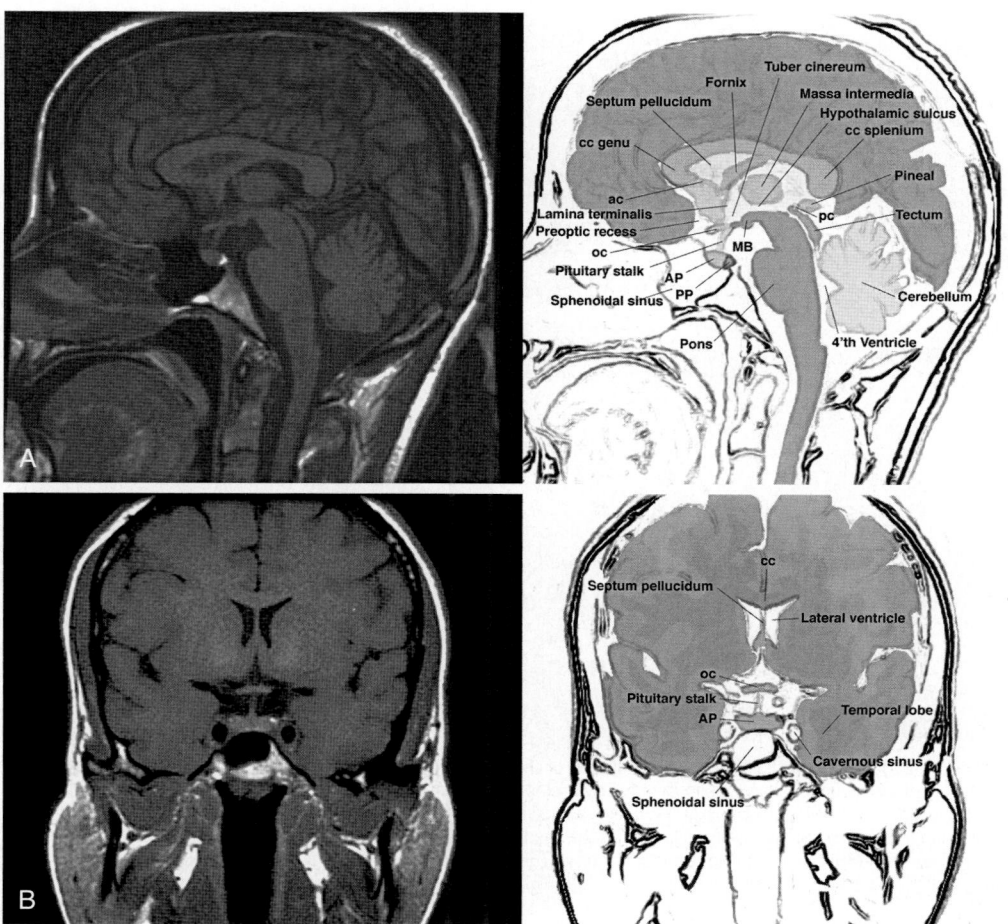

Figure 7-2 Normal anatomy of the human hypothalamic-pituitary unit in sagittal (**A**) and coronal planes (**B**). Structures that are visible in the T1-weighted magnetic resonance images *(left panels)* are identified in the corresponding diagrams *(right panels)*. The hypothalamus is bounded anteriorly by the optic chiasm, laterally by the sulci formed with the temporal lobes and posteriorly by the mammillary bodies (in which the mammillary nuclei are located). Dorsally, the hypothalamus is delineated from the thalamus by the hypothalamic sulcus. The smooth, rounded base of the hypothalamus is the tuber cinereum; the pituitary stalk descends from its central region, which is termed the *median eminence*. The median eminence stands out from the rest of the tuber cinereum because of its dense vascularity, which is formed by the primary plexus of the hypophyseal-portal system. The long portal veins run along the ventral surface of the pituitary stalk. Note the location of the pituitary stalk, the hyperintense signal *(white)* from the posterior pituitary (PP) (panel **A**, left), and the anatomic relationships of the pituitary gland to the optic chiasm (oc) and the sphenoidal and cavernous sinuses. ac, anterior commissure; AP, anterior pituitary; cc, corpus callosum; MB, mammillary body; pc, posterior commissure. (Magnetic resonance images courtesy of Dr. D. M. Cook.)

of the liver, it has been termed the *hypophyseal-portal circulation.*

Three distinct compartments of the median eminence are recognized: the innermost ependymal layer, the internal zone, and the external zone (see Fig. 7-4).[38] Ependymal cells form the floor of the third ventricle and are unique in that they have microvilli rather than cilia. Tight junctions at the ventricular pole of the ependymal cells prevent the diffusion of high-molecular-weight substances between the cerebrospinal fluid (CSF) and the extracellular space within the median eminence. The ependymal layer also contains specialized cells, called *tanycytes*,[39] that send processes into the other layers of the median eminence. Tight junctions between tanycytes at the lateral edges of the median eminence likely prevent the diffusion of releasing factors back into the medial basal hypothalamus.

The internal zone of the median eminence is composed of axons of the SON and PVH magnicellular neurons passing en route to the posterior pituitary (see Fig. 7-4C) and axons of the hypophyseotropic neurons destined for the external layer of the median eminence (see Fig. 7-4A and B). In addition, supporting cells populate this layer.

Finally, the external zone of the median eminence represents the exchange point of the hypothalamic releasing factors and the pituitary portal vessels.[38] Two general types of tuberohypophyseal dopaminergic (THDA) neurons project to the external zone: (1) peptide-secreting (peptidergic) neurons, including thyrotropin-releasing hormone (TRH), corticotropin-releasing hormone (CRH), and GnRH (see Fig. 7-1); and (2) neurons containing monoamines (e.g., dopamine, serotonin). Although the secretion of these substances into the portal circulation is an important control mechanism, some peptides and neurotransmitters in nerve endings are not released into the hypophyseal-portal circulation but instead function to regulate the secretion of other nerve terminals. The anatomic relationships of nerve endings, basement membranes, interstitial spaces, fenestrated (windowed) capillary endothelia, and glia in the median eminence are similar to those in the neural lobe. As in the case of neurohormone secretion from the neurohypophysis, depolarization of hypothalamic cells leads to the release of neuropeptides and monoamines at the median eminence.

Non-neuronal supporting cells in the hypothalamus also play a dynamic role in hypophyseotropic regulation. For example, nerve terminals in the neurohypophysis are enveloped by pituicytes; when the gland is inactive they surround the nerve endings, whereas they retract to expose

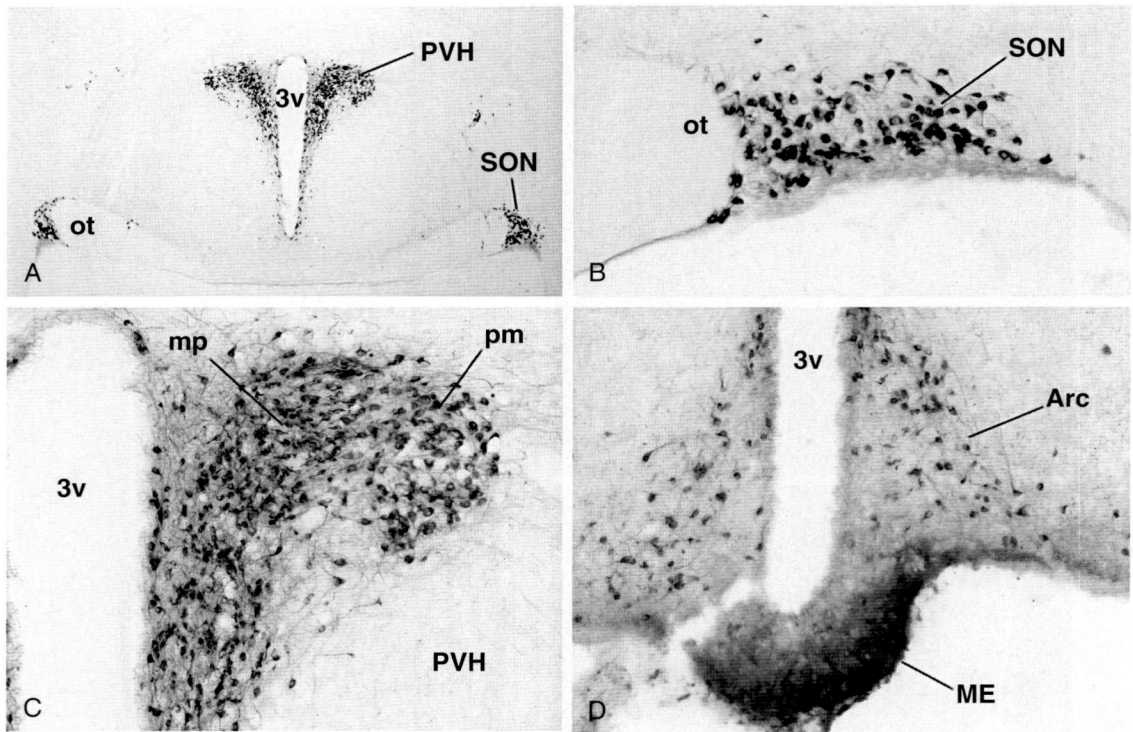

Figure 7-3 The tuberoinfundibular system is revealed by retrograde transport of cholera toxin subunit B (CtB). The location of hypothalamic cell bodies of neurons projecting to the median eminence (ME) and the posterior pituitary can be identified by microinjecting a small volume of the retrograde tracer CtB into the median eminence of the rat. **A,** Retrogradely labeled cells can be seen in the paraventricular (PVH) and supraoptic nuclei of the hypothalamus (SON). **B,** Magnicellular neurons are observed in the SON. **C,** Labeled neurons are found in the posterior magnicellular group (pm) as well as the medial parvicellular subdivision (mp). The labeled cells in the PVH include those that contain corticotropin-releasing hormone (CRH) and thyrotropin-releasing hormone (TRH). **D,** Retrogradely labeled cells are also found in the arcuate nucleus of the hypothalamus (Arc). These include neurons that release growth hormone–releasing hormone (GHRH) and dopamine. ot, optic tract; 3v, third ventricle. (Photomicrographs courtesy of Dr. R. M. Lechan.)

the terminals when vasopressin secretion is enhanced as in states of dehydration. Within the median eminence, GnRH nerve endings are enveloped by the tanycytes, which also cover or uncover neurons with changes in functional status.[40,41] Thus, supporting elements, with their own sets of receptors, can change the neuroregulatory milieu within the hypothalamus, median eminence, and pituitary.

The site of production, the genetics, and the regulation of synthesis and release of individual peptide-releasing factors are discussed in detail in later sections. Briefly, there are several cell groups in the medial hypothalamus that contain releasing factors that are secreted into the pituitary portal circulation (Table 7-2). These cell groups include the infundibular nucleus (called the *arcuate nucleus* in rodents) (see Fig. 7-3D), the PVH (see Fig. 7-3A and C), the periventricular nucleus, and a group of cells in the medial preoptic area near the organum vasculosum of the lamina terminalis (OVLT) (Fig. 7-5). As discussed earlier, magnicellular neurons in the SON and PVH send axons that predominantly traverse the median eminence to terminate in the neural lobe of the pituitary. In addition, a smaller number of magnicellular axons project directly to the external zone of the median eminence, but their functional significance is unknown.

The third structure often grouped as a component of the median eminence is a subdivision of the adenohypophysis called the *pars tuberalis*. It is a thin sheet of glandular tissue that lies around the infundibulum and pituitary stalk. In some animals, the epithelial component may make up as much as 10% of the total glandular tissue of the anterior pituitary. The pars tuberalis contains cells making pituitary

tropic hormones including luteinizing hormone (LH) and thyrotropin (thyroid-stimulating hormone, or TSH). A definitive physiologic function of the pars tuberalis is not established, but melatonin receptors are expressed in the pars tuberalis.

CIRCUMVENTRICULAR ORGANS

A guiding principle of neurophysiology and neuropharmacology is that the brain, including the hypothalamus, resides in an environment that is protected from humoral signals.[40,42] The exclusion of macromolecules is due to the structural vascular specializations that make up the blood-brain barrier.[43] These specializations include tight and adherens junctions of brain vascular endothelial cells that preclude the free passage of polarized macromolecules including peptides and hormones. In addition, astrocytic foot processes and perivascular microglial cells contribute to the integrity of the blood-brain barrier. However, to exert homeostatic control, the brain must assess key sensory information from the bloodstream including hormone levels, metabolites, and potential toxins. For example, to monitor key signals the brain has "windows on the circulation," or circumventricular organs (CVOs), that serve as a conduit of peripheral cues into key neuronal cell groups that maintain homeostasis.[42]

As the name implies, CVOs are specialized structures that lie on the midline of the brain along the third and fourth ventricles. These structures include the OVLT, subfornical organ (SFO), median eminence, neurohypophysis

TABLE 7-1

Neurotransmitters and Neuromodulators in the Paraventricular Nucleus and the Arcuate Nucleus of the Hypothalamus

Paraventricular Nucleus	Arcuate Nucleus
Magnicellular Division	Acetylcholine
	γ-Aminobutyric acid (GABA)
Angiotensin II	Agouti-related peptide (AgRP)
Cholecystokinin (CCK)	Cocaine- and amphetamine-
Dynorphins	regulated transcript (CART)
Glutamate	Dopamine
Nitric oxide (NO)	Dynorphin
Oxytocin	Endocannabinoids
Vasopressin (AVP)	Enkephalins
	Galanin
Parvicellular Divisions	Galanin-like peptide (GALP)
	Glutamate
γ-Aminobutyric acid (GABA)	Gonadotropin-releasing
Angiotensin II	hormone (GnRH)
Atrial natriuretic factor (ANF)	Growth hormone–releasing
Bombesin-like peptides	hormone (GHRH)
Cholecystokinin (CCK)	Kisspeptins
Corticotropin-releasing hormone	Melanocortins (ACTH, α-MSH,
(CRH)	β-MSH, γ-MSH)
Dopamine	Neurokinin B (NKB)
Endocannabinoids	Neuromedin U
Enkephalins	Neuropeptide Y (NPY)
Galanin	Neurotensin
Glutamate	Nociceptin/orphanin FQ (OFQ)
Interleukin 1 (IL-1)	Opioids (β-endorphin) peptides
Neuropeptide Y (NPY)	Pancreatic polypeptide
Neurotensin	Prolactin (PRL)
Nitric oxide (NO)	Pro-opiomelanocortin (POMC)
RFamide-related peptides (RFRP)	Pyro-glutamyl-RFamide
Somatostatin (SST)	peptide (QRFP)
Thyrotropin-releasing hormone	Somatostatin (SST)
(TRH)	Substance P
Vasopressin (AVP)	
Vasoactive intestinal peptide (VIP)	

TABLE 7-2

Structural Formulas of Principal Human Hypothalamic Peptides Directly Related to Pituitary Hormone Secretion*

Vasopressin

Cys-Tyr-Phe-Gln-Asn-*Cys*-Pro-Arg-Gly-NH$_2$ (MW = 1084.38)

Oxytocin

Cys-Tyr-Ile-Gln-Asn-*Cys*-Pro-Leu-Gly-NH$_2$ (MW = 1007.35)

Thyrotropin-Releasing Hormone

pGlu-His-Pro-NH$_2$ (MW = 362.42)

Gonadotropin-Releasing Hormone

pGlu-His-Trp-Ser-Tyr-Gly-Leu-Arg-Pro-Gly-NH$_2$ (MW = 1182.39)

Corticotropin-Releasing Hormone

Ser-Glu-Glu-Pro-Pro-Ile-Ser-Leu-Asp-Leu-Thr-Phe-His-Leu-Leu-Arg-Glu-Val-Leu-Glu-Met-Ala-Arg-Ala-Glu-Gln-Leu-Ala-Gln-Gln-Ala-His-Ser-Asn-Arg-Lys-Leu-Met-Glu-Ile-Ile-NH$_2$ (MW = 4758.14)

Growth Hormone–Releasing Hormone

Tyr-Ala-Asp-Ala-Ile-Phe-Thr-Asn-Ser-Tyr-Arg-Lys-Val-Leu-Gly-Gln-Leu-Ser-Ala-Arg-Lys-Leu-Leu-Gln-Asp-Ile-Met-Ser-Arg-Gln-Gln-Gly-Glu-Ser-Asn-Gln-Glu-Arg-Gly-Ala-Arg-Ala-Arg-Leu-NH$_2$ (MW = 5040.4)

Somatostatin

Ala-Gly-*Cys*-Lys-Asn-Phe-Phe-Trp-Lys-Thr-Phe-Thr-Ser-*Cys* (MW = 1638.12)

Vasoactive Intestinal Peptide

His-Ser-Asp-Ala-Val-Phe-Thr-Asp-Asn-Tyr-Thr-Arg-Leu-Arg-Lys-Gln-Met-Ala-Val-Lys-Lys-Tyr-Leu-Asn-Ser-Ile-Leu-Asn-NH$_2$ (MW = 3326.26)

*Disulfide bonds between pairs of cystines that produce cyclization of the peptides are indicated by their italicized cognate *Cys* residues.
MW, molecular weight; pGlu, pyro-glutamyl.

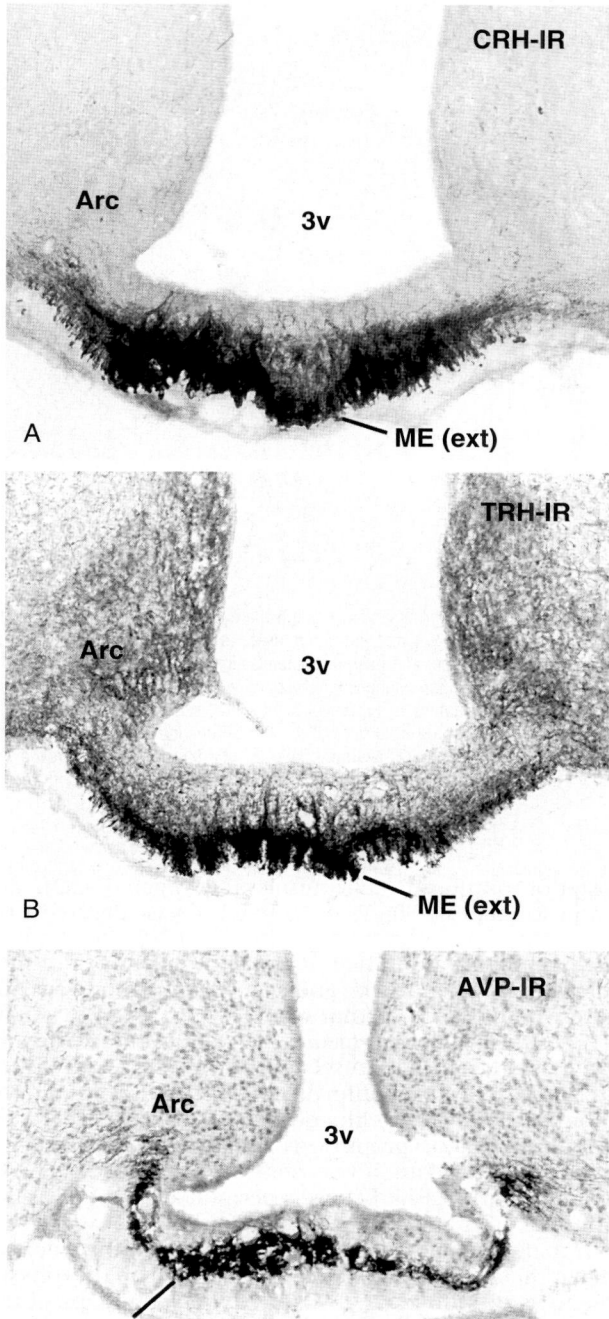

Figure 7-4 The median eminence is the functional connection between the hypothalamus and the pituitary gland. **A** and **B**, Distribution of corticotropin-releasing hormone and thyrotropin-releasing hormone immunoreactivity (CRH-IR and TRH-IR) in the external layer of the median eminence (ME ext) of the rat. CRH and TRH cell bodies reside in the medial division of the paraventricular hypothalamic nucleus. **C**, Arginine vasopressin immunoreactivity (AVP-IR) in nerve endings in the internal layer of the median eminence (ME int). Arc, arcuate nucleus; 3v, third ventricle. (Photomicrographs courtesy of Dr. R. M. Lechan.)

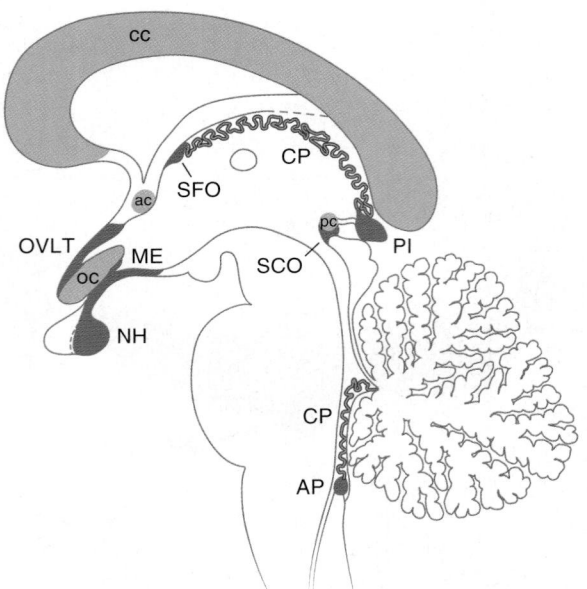

Figure 7-5 Median sagittal section through the human brain to show the circumventricular organs *(dark brown)*. Light brown areas are the optic chiasm (oc), corpus callosum (cc), anterior (ac) and posterior commissures (pc). AP, area postrema; CP, choroid plexus; ME, median eminence; NH, neurohypophysis; OVLT, organum vasculosum of the lamina terminalis; PI, pineal gland; SCO, subcommissural organ; SFO, subfornical organ. (Adapted from Weindl A. Neuroendocrine aspects of circumventricular organs. In: Ganong WF, Martini L, eds. *Frontiers in Neuroendocrinology*, vol 3. New York, NY: Oxford University Press; 1973:3-32.)

(posterior pituitary), subcommissural organ (SCO), and area postrema (see Fig. 7-5). Unlike the vasculature in the rest of the brain, the blood vessels in CVOs have fenestrated capillaries that allow relatively free passage of molecules such as proteins and peptide hormones. Thus, neurons and glial cells that reside within the CVOs have access to these macromolecules. In addition to the distinct nature of the vessels themselves, the CVOs have an unusually rich blood supply, allowing them to act as integrators at the interface of the blood-brain barrier. Several of the CVOs have major projections to hypothalamic nuclear groups that regulate homeostasis. Therefore, the CVOs serve as a critical link between peripheral metabolic cues, hormones, and potential toxins and cell groups within the brain that regulate coordinated endocrine, autonomic, and behavioral responses. Detailed discussion of the physiologic roles of individual CVOs is beyond the scope of this chapter, but several in-depth reviews have assessed the function of each.[42,44-46]

Median Eminence

The anatomic location of the median eminence places it in a position to serve as an afferent sensory organ as well as a functional link between the hypothalamus and the pituitary gland. Specifically, the median eminence is located adjacent to several neuroendocrine and autonomic regulatory nuclei at the tuberal level of the hypothalamus (see Fig. 7-3). These nuclear groups include the infundibular or arcuate, ventromedial, dorsomedial, and paraventricular nuclei.

A role of hypothalamic nuclei surrounding the median eminence as afferent sensory centers is supported by several observations. For example, toxins such as monosodium glutamate and gold thioglucose damage neurons in cell groups overlying the median eminence, resulting in obesity and hyperphagia. Experimental evidence suggests that the median eminence is a portal of entry for hormones such as leptin. Indeed, administration of radiolabeled leptin led to its accumulation around the median eminence. Moreover, leptin receptor messenger ribonucleic acid (mRNA) and leptin-induced gene expression are densely localized in the arcuate, ventromedial, dorsomedial, and ventral premammillary hypothalamic nuclei.[47] Leptin is an established mediator of body weight and neuroendocrine function that acts on several cell groups in the hypothalamus including POMC neurons that reside in the arcuate nucleus.[14,47,48] Thus, it is likely that the median eminence is involved in conveying information from humoral factors such as leptin to key hypothalamic regulatory neurons in the medial basal hypothalamus.[40]

Organum Vasculosum of the Lamina Terminalis and the Subfornical Organ

The OVLT and the SFO are located at the anterior wall of the third ventricle, the lamina terminalis. The OVLT and SFO lie, respectively, at the ventral and dorsal boundaries of the third ventricle (see Fig. 7-5). Because it lies at the rostral and ventral tip of the third ventricle, the OVLT is surrounded by cell groups of the preoptic region of the hypothalamus. Like other CVOs, the OVLT is composed of neurons, glial cells, and tanycytes. Axon terminals containing several neuropeptides and neurotransmitters including somatostatin, angiotensin, dopamine, norepinephrine, serotonin, acetylcholine, oxytocin, AVP, and TRH innervate the OVLT. In the rodent, neurons that contain GnRH surround the OVLT, and recent evidence suggests that they possess unique projections with combined properties of dendrites and axons, termed *dendrons*, that bridge the distance between the OVLT and median eminence.[49] In addition, the OVLT in the rat brain contains estrogen receptors, and the application of estrogen or electric stimulation at this site is capable of stimulating ovulation through GnRH-containing neurons that project to the median eminence.

The region of the hypothalamus that immediately surrounds the OVLT regulates a diverse array of autonomic processes. However, because the OVLT is potentially involved in the maintenance of so many processes, definitive studies ascribing specific functions to the OVLT are inherently difficult. For example, lesions of the OVLT and surrounding preoptic area led to altered febrile responses after immunologic stimulation and disruptions in fluid and electrolyte balance, blood pressure, reproduction, and thermoregulation. Large lesions of the OVLT attenuated lipopolysaccharide-induced fever.[50] Consistent with this finding, it has been demonstrated that receptors for prostaglandin E_2 are located within and immediately surrounding the OVLT.[51] Because prostaglandin E_2 is thought to be an obligate endogenous pyrogen, the OVLT may be a critical regulator of febrile responses.

The OVLT is also likely to be involved in sensing serum osmolality because lesions of the OVLT attenuate AVP and oxytocin secretion in response to osmotic stimuli. In addition, hypertonic saline administration to rats induced c-Fos (a marker of neuronal activation) in OVLT neurons.[52] The efferent projections of the OVLT are not well defined because of the fundamental difficulty of injecting this small structure with specific neuroanatomic tracers without contaminating surrounding preoptic nuclei. This limitation will likely be overcome in the near future using the latest set of genetic tracing tools that use Cre recombinase technology to target specific neuronal cell types.[53]

The SFO is located in the roof of the third ventricle below the fornix. This CVO critically regulates fluid homeostasis and contributes to blood pressure regulation.[42] Consistent with these functions, the SFO has receptors for angiotensin II and atrial natriuretic peptide.[54,55] In addition to expressing these key receptors, the SFO is thought to regulate fluid homeostasis because of its specific and massive projections to key hypothalamic regulatory sites. Notable among these are the inputs to oxytocin and AVP magnicellular neurons in the SON and PVH. Parvicellular neurons in the PVH concerned with neuroendocrine and autonomic control also receive innervation from the SFO. In addition, the SFO densely innervates the paramedian preoptic region of the hypothalamus (also known as the anteroventral third ventricular region) and other hypothalamic sites including the perifornical area of the lateral hypothalamus. A major cell group within the anteroventral third ventricular region is the median preoptic nucleus, which receives dense innervation from the SFO.[56] Several neuroanatomic studies have demonstrated that the median preoptic nucleus is a major source of afferents to the magnicellular neuroendocrine neurons in the PVH and SON.

In addition to the preceding neuroanatomic findings, physiologic evidence suggests that the SFO is critical in maintaining fluid balance. For example, Simpson and Routtenberg demonstrated that substances such as angiotensin II elicited drinking behavior when microinjected at low doses directly into the SFO.[57] Later studies demonstrated that SFO neurons have electrophysiologic responses to angiotensin II.[54] In addition, stimulation of the SFO elicited AVP secretion. Like the OVLT, the SFO expressed c-Fos after stimulation by hypertonic saline administration.[52] Importantly, the use of Cre recombinase technology combined with optogenetics has enabled researchers to demonstrate that the SFO contains genetically separable populations of neurons whose activation can either stimulate or inhibit thirst and drinking behavior.[58]

Area Postrema

The area postrema lies at the caudal end of the fourth ventricle adjacent to the nucleus of the tractus solitarius (NTS) (see Fig. 7-5). In rodents, it is a midline structure lying above the NTS.[42,59] However, in humans the area postrema is a bilateral structure. Because the area postrema overlies the NTS, it also receives direct visceral afferent input from the glossopharyngeal nerve and the vagus nerves. In addition, the area postrema receives direct input from several hypothalamic nuclei. The efferent projections of the area postrema include projections to the NTS, ventral lateral medulla, and parabrachial nucleus. Consistent with its role as a sensory organ, the area postrema is enriched with receptors for several neuropeptides including glucagon-like peptide-I and amylin.[60] It also contains chemosensory neurons that include osmoreceptors. The area postrema is thought to be critical in the detection of potential toxins and induction of vomiting in response to foreign substances. In fact, the area postrema is often referred to as the chemoreceptor trigger zone.[60]

The best described physiologic role of the area postrema is the coordinated control of blood pressure.[42] The area postrema contains binding sites for angiotensin II, AVP, and atrial natriuretic peptide. Lesions of the area postrema in rats blunt the rise in blood pressure induced by angiotensin II.[61] Finally, administration of angiotensin II induces the expression of c-Fos in neurons of the area postrema. The area postrema has also been hypothesized to play a role in responding to inflammatory cytokines during the acute febrile response, CNS glucose sensing, and the satiating effects of amylin.[60]

Subcommissural Organ

The SCO is located near the junction of the third ventricle and cerebral aqueduct below the posterior commissure and the pineal gland (see Fig. 7-5). It is composed of specialized ependymal cells that secrete a highly glycosylated protein of unknown function. The secretion of this protein leads to aggregation and formation of the so-called Reissner fibers.[62] The glycoproteins are extruded through the aqueduct, the fourth ventricle, and the spinal cord lumen to terminate in the caudal spinal canal. In humans, intracellular secretory granules are identifiable in the SCO but Reissner fibers are absent. The SCO secretion in humans is therefore presumed to be more soluble and to be absorbed directly from the CSF. Compared with other CVOs, the physiologic role of the SCO is largely unknown. Hypothesized roles for the SCO include clearance of substances including monoamines from the CSF.[62]

PINEAL GLAND

Descartes called the pineal gland the "seat of the soul." A more contemporary, although less colorful, viewpoint is that the pineal integrates information encoded by light into coordinated secretions that underlie biologic rhythmicity.[63] The pineal is both an endocrine gland and a CVO; it is derived from cells located in the roof of the third ventricle and lies above the posterior commissure near the level of the habenular complex and the sylvian aqueduct. The gland is composed of two cell types, pinealocytes and interstitial (glial-like) cells. Histologic studies suggest that the pineal gland cells are secretory in nature, and indeed the pineal is the principal source of melatonin in mammals.

The pineal gland is an epithalamic structure and consists of primordial photoreceptive cells. The gland retains its light sensitivity in lower vertebrates such as fish and amphibians but lacks direct photosensitivity in mammals and has evolved as a strictly secretory organ in higher vertebrates. However, neuroanatomic studies have established that light-encoded information is relayed to the pineal by a polysynaptic pathway.[64] This series of synapses ultimately results in innervation of the gland by noradrenergic sympathetic nerve terminals that are critical regulators of melatonin production and release. Specifically, retinal ganglion cells directly innervate the SCN of the hypothalamus through the retinohypothalamic tract. The SCN in turn provides input to the dorsal parvicellular PVH, a key cell group in neuroendocrine and autonomic control. This pathway consists of direct and indirect intrahypothalamic projections. The PVH in turn provides direct innervation to sympathetic preganglionic neurons in the intermediolateral cell column of the thoracic regions of the spinal cord. Sympathetic preganglionic neurons innervate postganglionic neurons in the superior cervical ganglion, ultimately supply the noradrenergic innervation to the pineal (see "Hypothalamic-Pituitary Unit"). This circuitous pathway represents the anatomic substrate for light to regulate the secretion of melatonin. In the absence of light input, the pineal gland rhythms persist but are not entrained to the external light-dark cycle.

The Pineal Is the Source of Melatonin

The predominant hormone secreted by the pineal gland is melatonin. However, the pineal contains other biogenic

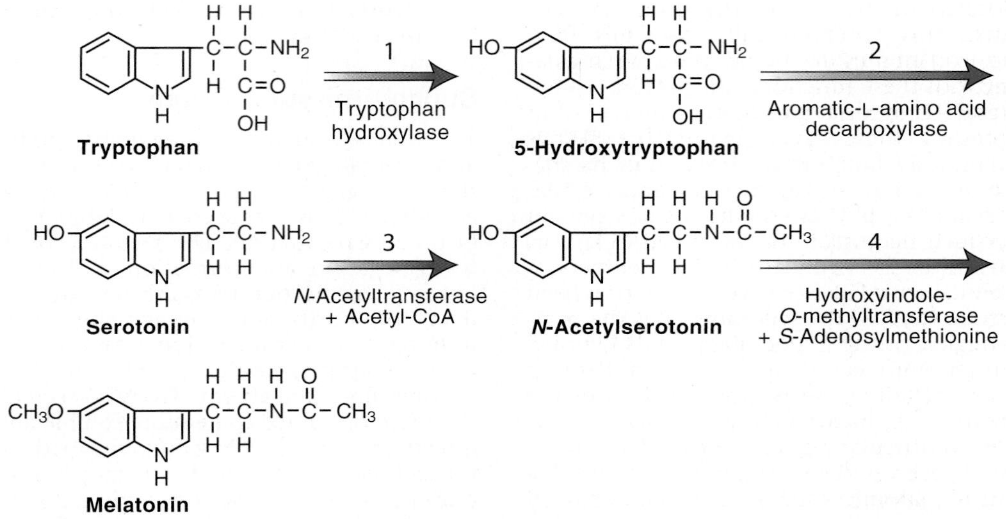

Figure 7-6 Biosynthesis of melatonin from tryptophan in the pineal gland. Step 1 is catalyzed by tryptophan hydroxylase, step 2 by aromatic-L-amino acid decarboxylase, step 3 by arylalkylamine *N*-acetyltransferase, and step 4 by hydroxyindole-*O*-methyltransferase. (From Wurtman RJ, Axelrod J, Kelly DE. Biochemistry of the pineal gland. In: Wurtman RJ, Axelrod J, Kelly DE, eds. *The Pineal.* New York, NY: Academic Press; 1968:47-75.)

amines, peptides, and GABA. Pineal-derived melatonin is synthesized from tryptophan, through serotonin, with the rate-limiting step catalyzed by the enzyme arylalkylamine *N*-acetyltransferase (AANAT) (Fig. 7-6).[65] Hydroxyindole-O-methyltransferase (HIOMT) catalyzes the final step of melatonin synthesis. Melatonin plays a key role in regulating a myriad of circadian rhythms, and a fundamental principle of circadian biology is that the synthesis of melatonin is exquisitely controlled.[66] AANAT mRNA levels, AANAT activity, and melatonin synthesis and release are regulated in a circadian fashion and are entrained by the light-dark cycle, with darkness thought to be the most important signal.[63,65] Melatonin and AANAT levels are highest during the dark and decrease sharply with the onset of light. Melatonin is not stored to any significant degree; it is released into blood or CSF directly after its biosynthesis in proportion to AANAT activity.

Lack of light ultimately results in the release of norepinephrine from postganglionic sympathetic nerve terminals that act on β-adrenergic receptors in pinealocytes, resulting in an increase in adenylyl cyclase activity and synthesis of cyclic adenosine monophosphate (cAMP) from adenosine triphosphate. Increased levels of intracellular cAMP activate downstream signal transduction cascades, including the catalytic subunits of protein kinase A and phosphorylation of cAMP response element (CRE) binding protein. CREs have been identified in the promoter of AANAT.[67] Therefore, light (or lack of it) acting through the sympathetic nervous system induces an increase in cAMP, representing a fundamental regulator of AANAT transcription and melatonin synthesis that ultimately results in a dramatic change of melatonin levels across the day.[64]

Physiologic Roles of Melatonin

One of the best characterized roles of melatonin is the regulation of the reproductive axis, including gonadotropin secretion[68] and the timing and onset of puberty (see "Gonadotropin-Releasing Hormone and Control of the Reproductive Axis"). The potent regulation of the reproductive axis by melatonin is established in rodents and domestic animals such as the sheep. It was observed experimentally with the demonstration that removal of the

pineal leads to precocious puberty. In addition, male rats exposed to constant darkness or blinded by enucleation display testicular atrophy and decreased levels of testosterone. These profound effects of gonadal involution are normalized by removal of the pineal gland.[64] The physiologic significance of melatonin is probably most important in species referred to as seasonal breeders. Indeed, the role of melatonin in regulating reproductive capacity in species such as the sheep and the horse is now established. This type of reproductive strategy probably evolved to synchronize the length of day with the gestational period of the species to ensure that the offspring are born at favorable times of the year and maximize the viability of the young. Interestingly, although there is a strong and consistent correlation between altered melatonin secretion, day length, and seasonal breeding in diverse species, the valence of the signal can be either positive or negative dependent on the ecologic niche for each species.

Despite the potent effects of day length on reproduction in these species, the exact mechanisms of melatonin regulation of GnRH release are unsettled. However, melatonin inhibits LH release from the rat pars tuberalis.[68] The role of the pineal in human reproduction is even less understood.[64]

Interspecies comparative studies of melatonin's physiologic function must be tempered by knowledge of key differences between rodent and human melatonin regulation. Significantly more light, as much as 4 log units, is required in humans to produce an equivalent nocturnal suppression of melatonin[69] and the control of AANAT is largely post-transcriptional in humans rather than transcriptional.[65]

Melatonin Receptors

Melatonin mediates some of its effects by acting on a family of GPCRs, which have been characterized by pharmacologic, neuroanatomic, and molecular approaches.[63,65,66] The first member of the family, MT1 (Mel$_{1a}$), is a high-affinity receptor that was isolated originally from *Xenopus* melanophores. The second, MT2 (Mel$_{1b}$), has approximately 60% homology with MT1. A third receptor in mammals, MT3, is not a GPCR but instead a high-affinity binding site on the cytosolic enzyme quinone reductase 2 that is involved in cellular detoxification and might explain some of melatonin's effects as an antioxidant.[63,65] Melatonin also acts directly as a free radical scavenger to detoxify reactive oxygen and nitrogen species.[64]

The mechanisms for melatonin's effects on regulating and entraining circadian rhythms are becoming increasingly understood. For example, melatonin inhibits the activity of neurons in the SCN of the hypothalamus, the master circadian pacemaker in the mammalian brain.[66,70,71] Melatonin can entrain several mammalian circadian rhythms, probably by the inhibition of neurons in the SCN. Neuroanatomic evidence suggests that many of the effects of melatonin on circadian rhythms involve actions on MT1 receptors in that the distribution of MT1 mRNA overlaps with radiolabeled melatonin binding sites in the relevant brain regions. These sites include the SCN, the retina, and the pars tuberalis of the adenohypophysis. The MT2 receptor is also expressed in retina and brain, particularly the SCN, but evidently at much lower levels.[65,66,70]

Genetic studies in mice have also helped to illuminate the relative roles of each melatonin receptor in mediating the effects of this hormone. Targeted deletion (knockout) of the MT1 but not the MT2 receptor abolished the ability of melatonin to inhibit the activity of SCN neurons.[71,72] Several studies have suggested that the inhibition of SCN neurons by melatonin is of great physiologic significance. Melatonin may underlie the mechanism by which light induces phase shifts. However, it should be noted that lack of the MT1 gene does not block the ability of melatonin to induce phase shifts. These unexpected and somewhat confusing results have resulted in the hypothesis that MT2 is involved in melatonin-induced phase shifts, as this receptor may be expressed in the SCN in human brain.[65]

Melatonin Therapy in Humans

Melatonin is purported to exert multiple beneficial functions that include slowing or reversing the progression of aging, protecting against ischemic damage after vascular reperfusion, and enhancing immune function.[63-65] However, the most studied and established role of melatonin in humans is that of phase shifting and resetting circadian rhythms. In this context, melatonin has been used to treat jet lag and may be effective in treating circadian-based sleep disorders.[73] In addition, melatonin administration has been shown to regulate sleep in humans. Specifically, melatonin has a hypnotic effect at relatively low doses. Melatonin therapy has also been suggested as a way to treat seasonal affective disorders. However, two recent meta-analyses of the published reports on melatonin for the treatment of either primary or secondary sleep disorders concluded that there is limited evidence for significant clinical efficacy, but melatonin is safe with short-term use ($\leq$3 months).[74,75]

HYPOPHYSEOTROPIC HORMONES AND NEUROENDOCRINE AXES

With the demonstration by the first half of the 1900s that pituitary secretion is controlled by hypothalamic hormones released into the portal circulation, the race was on to identify the hypothalamic releasing factors. The search for hypothalamic neurohormones with anterior pituitary regulating properties focused on extracts of stalk median eminence, neural lobe, and hypothalamus from sheep and pigs. To give some idea of the herculean nature of this effort, approximately 250,000 hypothalamic fragments were required to purify and characterize the first such factor, TRH.[9] Such hypophyseotropic substances were initially called *releasing factors* but are now more commonly called *releasing hormones*.

All of the principal hypothalamic-pituitary regulating hormones are peptides with the notable exception of dopamine, which is a biogenic amine and the major prolactin-inhibiting factor (PIF; see later discussion and Table 7-2). All are available for clinical investigations or diagnostic tests, and therapeutic analogues for dopamine, GnRH, and somatostatin are widely prescribed.

In addition to regulating hormone release, some hypophyseotropic factors control pituitary cell differentiation and proliferation and hormone synthesis. Some act on more than one pituitary hormone. For example, TRH is a potent releaser of prolactin (PRL) and of TSH and under some circumstances releases corticotropin (ACTH, adrenocorticotropic hormone) and growth hormone (GH). GnRH releases both LH and follicle-stimulating hormone (FSH). Somatostatin inhibits the secretion of GH, TSH, and a wide variety of nonpituitary hormones. The principal inhibitor of PRL secretion, dopamine, also inhibits secretion of TSH, gonadotropin, and under certain conditions, GH. Dual control is exerted by the interaction of inhibitory and stimulatory hypothalamic hormones. For example, somatostatin interacts with growth hormone–releasing hormone (GHRH) and TRH to control secretion of GH and TSH, respectively, and dopamine interacts with prolactin-releasing factors (PRFs) to regulate PRL secretion. Some hypothalamic hormones act synergistically; for example, CRH and AVP cooperatively regulate the release of pituitary ACTH.

Secretion of the releasing hormones in turn is regulated by neurotransmitters and neuropeptides released by a complex array of neurons synapsing with hypophyseotropic neurons. Control of secretion is also exerted through feedback control by hormones such as glucocorticoids, gonadal steroids, thyroid hormone, anterior pituitary hormones (short-loop feedback control), and hypophyseotropic factors themselves (ultrashort-loop feedback control).

The distribution of the hypophyseotropic hormones is not limited to the hypothalamus. Most are produced in nonhypophyseotropic hypothalamic neurons, in extrahypothalamic regions of the brain, and in peripheral organs where they mediate functions unrelated to pituitary regulation (e.g., effects on behavior or homeostasis). Most of the peptides, hormones, and neurotransmitters involved in the regulation of hypothalamic-pituitary control transduce their signals through members of the extensive GPCR family.

Feedback Concepts in Neuroendocrinology

In order to understand the regulation of each hypothalamic-pituitary-target organ axis, it is important to understand some basic concepts of homeostatic systems. A simplified account of feedback control in relation to neuroendocrine regulation is presented here. Hormonal systems form part of a feedback loop in which the controlled variable (generally the blood hormone level or some biochemical surrogate of the hormone) determines the rate of secretion of the hormone. In negative feedback systems the controlled variable inhibits hormone output, and in positive feedback control systems it increases hormone secretion. Both negative and positive endocrine feedback control systems can be part of a closed loop, in which regulation is entirely restricted to the interacting regulatory glands, or an open loop, in which the nervous system influences the feedback loop. All pituitary feedback systems have nervous system inputs that either alter the set-point of the feedback control system or introduce open-loop elements that can influence or override the closed-loop control elements.

In engineering formulations of feedback, three controlled variables can be identified: a sensing element that detects the concentration of the controlled variable, a reference input that defines the proper control levels, and an error signal that determines the output of the system. The reference input is the set-point of the system.

Hormonal feedback control systems resemble engineering systems in that the concentration of the hormone in the blood (or some function of the hormone) regulates the output of the controlling gland. However, hormonal feedback differs from engineering systems in that the sensor element and the reference input element are not readily distinguishable. The set-point of the controlled variable is determined by a complex cascade beginning with the kinetics of binding to a receptor and the activities of successive intermediate messengers. Sophisticated models incorporating control elements, compartmental analysis, and hormone production and clearance rates exist for many systems. In fact, this sort of modeling applied to developmental programming, intracellular signaling cascades, and neural circuits in addition to endocrine feedback systems is commonly referred to as *systems biology*.[76]

Endocrine Rhythms

Virtually all functions of living animals (regardless of their position on the evolutionary scale) are subject to periodic or cyclic changes, many of which are influenced primarily by the nervous system (Table 7-3).[77,78] Most periodic changes are free-running; that is, they are intrinsic to the organism, independent of the environment, and driven by a biologic clock.

Most free-running rhythms are coordinated (entrained) by external signals (cues), such as light-dark changes, meal patterns, cycles of the lunar periods, or the ratio of day length to night length. External signals of this type (*zeitgeber*, or time giver) do not bring about the rhythm but provide the synchronizing time cue. Many endogenous rhythms have a period of approximately 24 hours (circadian [around a day] or diurnal rhythms). Circadian changes follow an intrinsic program that is about 24 hours long, whereas diurnal rhythms can be either circadian or dependent on shifts in light and dark. Rhythms that occur more frequently than once a day are ultradian. Infradian rhythms have a period longer than 1 day, as in the approximately 27-day human menstrual cycle and the yearly breeding patterns of some animals.

Most endocrine rhythms are circadian (Fig. 7-7). The secretion of GH and PRL in humans is maximal shortly after the onset of sleep, and that of cortisol is maximal between 2 AM and 4 AM. TSH secretion is lowest in the morning between 9 AM and 12 noon and maximal between 8 PM and midnight. Gonadotropin secretion in adolescents is increased at night. Superimposed on the circadian cycle are ultradian bursts of hormone secretion. LH secretion during adolescence is characterized by rapid, high-amplitude pulsations at night, whereas in sexually mature individuals secretory episodes are lower in amplitude and occur throughout the 24 hours. GH, ACTH, and PRL are also secreted in brief, fairly regular pulses. The short-term fluctuations in hormonal secretion have important functional significance. In the case of LH, the normal endogenous rhythm of pituitary secretion reflects the pulsatile release of GnRH. The period of approximately 90 minutes between LH peaks corresponds to the optimal timing of GnRH pulses to induce maximal pituitary stimulation. Episodic secretion of GH also enhances its biopotency, but for many rhythms, the function is not clear. Most homeostatic activities are also rhythmic, including body temperature, water balance, blood volume, sleep, and activity.[79,80]

Assessment of endocrine function must take into account the variability of hormone levels in the blood. Thus, appropriately obtained samples at different times of day or night may provide useful dynamic indicators of hypothalamic-pituitary function. For example, the loss of diurnal rhythm of GH and ACTH secretion may be an early sign of hypothalamic dysfunction. Furthermore, the optimal timing for the administration of glucocorticoids to suppress ACTH secretion (as in therapy for congenital adrenal hyperplasia) must take into account the varying suppressibility of the axis at different times of day.

The best understood neural structures responsible for circadian rhythms are the SCNs, paired structures in the anterior hypothalamus above the optic chiasm.[77,80] In addition to the retinohypothalamic projection from the retina described earlier, the SCN receives neuronal input from many nuclei. Individual cells of the SCN have an intrinsic capacity to oscillate in a circadian pattern due to the existence of a cell-autonomous transcription-translation feedback loop involving the transcription factors CLOCK and BMAL1 that interact with the promoters of the *period* (*PER*) and *cryptochrome* (*CRY*) genes.[81] The SCN is organized to permit many reciprocal neuron-neuron interactions mediated by GABA at direct synaptic contacts. It is especially rich in neuropeptides, including AVP, VIP, gastrin-releasing peptide (GRP), and calretinin. The SCN also responds to the pineal hormone melatonin through melatonin receptors.[63,65] Studies have indicated that intrinsic pacemaker function is not unique to neurons of the SCN; circadian oscillators are also found in many peripheral tissues.[80]

Metabolic changes in the SCN, such as increased uptake of 2-deoxyglucose and an increased level of VIP, accompany circadian rhythms. This nucleus projects to the pineal gland indirectly via the PVH and the autonomic nervous

TABLE 7-3

Terms Used to Describe Cyclic Endocrine Phenomena

Term	Definition
Period	Length of the cycle
Circadian	About a day (24 hr)
Diurnal	Exactly a day
Ultradian	Less than a day (i.e., minutes or hours)
Infradian	Longer than a day (i.e., month or year)
Mean	Arithmetic mean of all values within a cycle
Range	Difference between the highest and lowest values
Nadir	Minimal level (inferred from mathematical curve-fitting calculations)
Acrophase	Time of maximal levels (inferred from curve fitting)
Zeitgeber	Time giver (German); the external cue, usually the light-dark cycle that synchronizes endogenous rhythms
Entrainment	The process by which an endogenous rhythm is regulated by a zeitgeber
Phase shift	Induced change in an endogenous rhythm
Intrinsic clock	Neural structures that possess intrinsic capacity for spontaneous rhythms; for circadian rhythms, these are located in the suprachiasmatic nucleus

Modified from Van Cauter E, Turek FW. Endocrine and other biological rhythms. In DeGroot LJ, ed. *Endocrinology*, 3rd ed. Philadelphia, PA: Saunders; 1995:2497-2548.

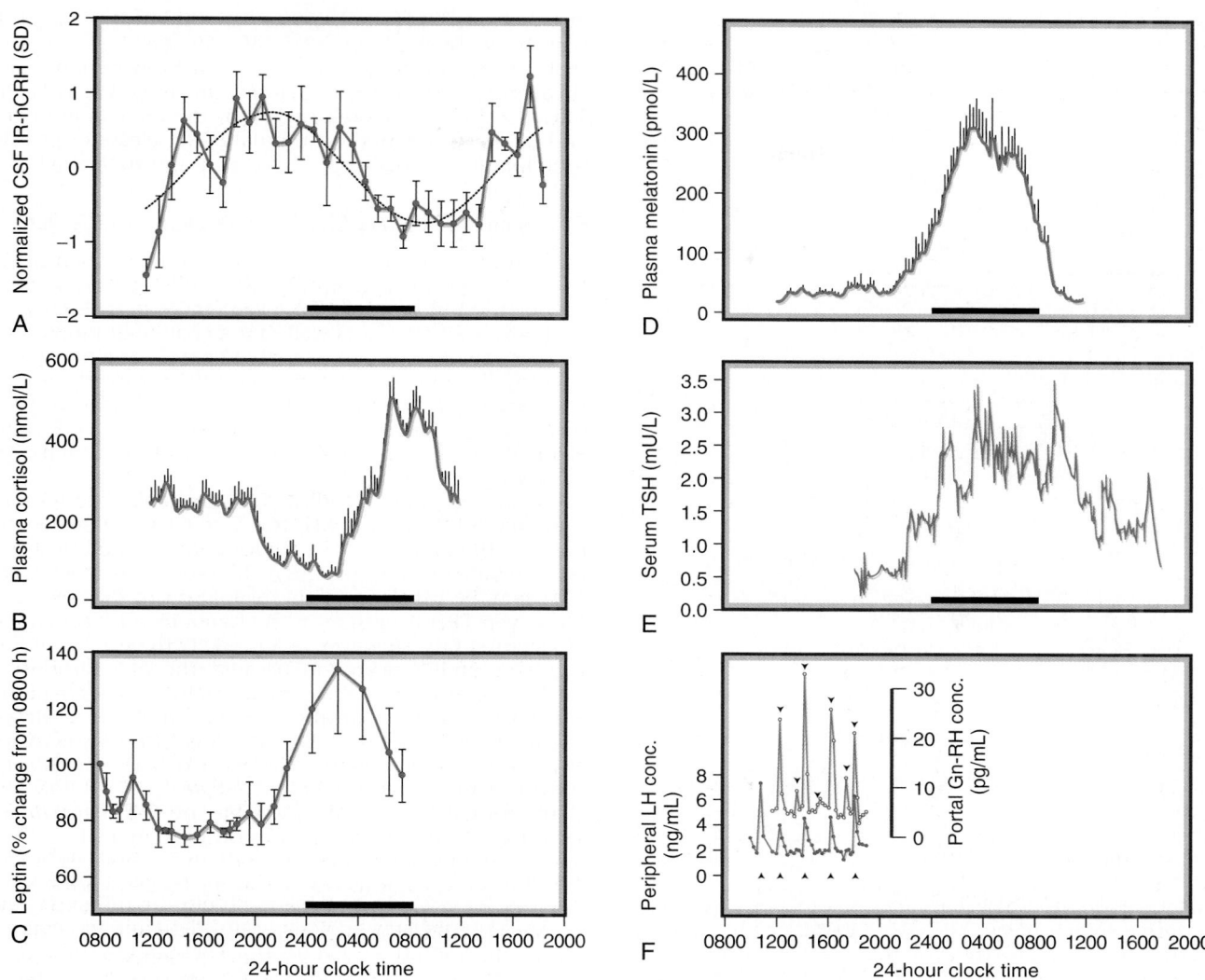

Figure 7-7 Diurnal rhythms of corticotropin-releasing hormone (CRH) (**A**), cortisol (**B**), leptin (**C**), melatonin (**D**), and thyrotropin (TSH) in humans (**E**), and the relationship between gonadotropin-releasing hormone (GnRH) and luteinizing hormone (LH) secretion in sheep (**F**). CSF, cerebrospinal fluid; IR, immunoreactive. (From Kling MA, DeBellis MD, O'Rourke DK, et al. Diurnal variation of cerebrospinal fluid immunoreactive corticotropin-releasing hormone levels in healthy volunteers. *J Clin Endocrinol Metab.* 1994;79:233-239, Fig. 3; van Coevorden A, Mockel J, Laurent E, et al. Neuroendocrine rhythms and sleep in aging men. *Am J Physiol.* 1991;260:E651-E661, Fig. 1A and C; Sinha MK, Ohannesian JP, Heiman ML, et al. Nocturnal rise of leptin in lean, obese,and non-insulin-dependent diabetes mellitus subjects. *J Clin Invest.* 1996;97:1344-1347, Fig. 2; Brabant G, Prank K, Ranft U, et al. Physiological regulation of circadian and pulsatile thyrotropin secretion in normal man and woman. *J Clin Endocrinol Metab.* 1990;70:403-409, Fig. 2B; and Clarke IJ, Cummins JT. The temporal relationship between gonadotropin-releasing hormone (GnRH) and luteinizing hormone (LH) secretion in ovariectomized ewes. *Endocrinology.* 1982;111:1737-1739, Fig. 2A.)

system (see earlier discussion) and regulates its activity.[77] However, the bulk of SCN outflow occurs in a trunk coursing dorsolaterally through the ventral subparaventricular zone and terminating in the dorsal medial hypothalamic nucleus. Polysynaptic pathways involving these latter structures are responsible for the actions of the SCN to produce the circadian rhythms in thermoregulation, glucocorticoid secretion, sleep, arousal, and feeding.[77,81]

Circadian rhythms during fetal life are regulated by maternal circadian rhythms.[82] Circadian changes can be detected 2 to 3 days before birth, and SCN from fetuses of this age display spontaneous rhythmicity in vitro. Maternal regulation of fetal circadian rhythms may be mediated by circulating melatonin or by cyclic changes in the food intake of the mother. The timing of the circadian pacemaker can be shifted in humans by the administration of triazolam, a short-acting benzodiazepine, or melatonin (described earlier) or by altered patterns of intense illumination.[69]

Thyrotropin-Releasing Hormone
Chemistry and Evolution

TRH, the short peptide hypophyseotropic hormone, is the tripeptide pyroGlu-His-Pro-NH$_2$. Six copies of the TRH peptide sequence are encoded within the human TRH preprohormone gene (Fig. 7-8).[83] The rat pro-TRH precursor contains five TRH peptide repeats flanked by dibasic residues (Lys-Arg or Arg-Arg), along with seven or more non-TRH peptides.[84] Two prohormone convertases, PC1 and PC2, cleave on the carboxy-terminal (COOH-terminal) side of these dibasic residues as the prohormone molecule transits the regulated secretory pathway. Carboxypeptidase E then removes the dibasic residues, leaving the sequence Gln-His-Pro-Gly. This peptide is then amidated at the COOH-terminus by peptidylglycine α-amidating monooxygenase (PAM), with Gly acting as the amide donor. The amino-terminal (NH$_2$-terminal) pyro-Glu residue results from cyclization of the Gln.

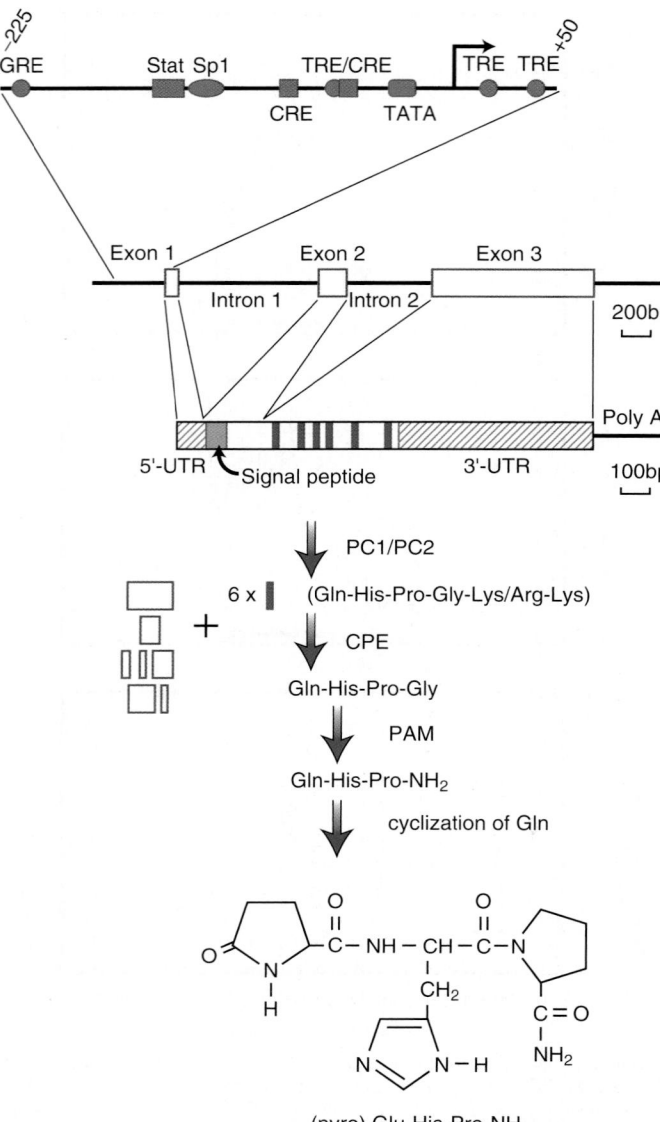

Figure 7-8 Structure of the human thyrotropin-releasing hormone (TRH) gene, messenger RNA, and prohormone, showing six repeats of the TRH peptide sequence encoded within exon 3. CPE, carboxypeptidase E; CRE, cyclic AMP response element; GRE, glucocorticoid response element; PAM, peptidylglycine α-amidating monooxygenase; PC1/PC2, prohormone convertases 1 and 2; Sp1, specificity protein 1 binding sequence; Stat, signal transducer and activator of transcription binding sequence; TATA, Goldstein-Hogness box involved in binding RNA polymerase; TRE, thyroid hormone response element; UTR, untranslated. (Adapted from data in Yamada M, Radovick S, Wondisford FE, et al. Cloning and structure of human genomic DNA and hypothalamic cDNA encoding human preprothyrotropin-releasing hormone. *Mol Endocrinol.* 1990;4:551-556.)

TRH is a phylogenetically ancient peptide; it has been isolated from primitive vertebrates such as the lamprey and even invertebrates such as the snail. TRH is widely expressed in both the CNS and periphery in amphibians, reptiles, and fishes but does not stimulate TSH release in these poikilothermic vertebrates. Therefore, TRH has multiple peripheral and central activities and was co-opted as a hypophyseotropic factor midway during the evolution of vertebrates, perhaps specifically as a factor needed for coordinated regulation of temperature homeostasis.

Although the TRH tripeptide is the only established hormone encoded within its large prohormone, rat pro-TRH yields seven additional peptides that have unique tissue

distributions.[85] Several biologic activities of these peptides have been observed: pro-TRH(160-169) may be a hypophyseotropic factor because it is released from hypothalamic slices and potentiates the TSH-releasing effects of TRH. Pro-TRH(178-199) is also released from the median eminence and has been reported to stimulate PRL release or possibly function as a corticotropin release-inhibiting factor.[86]

Effects on the Pituitary Gland and Mechanism of Action

After intravenous injection of TRH in humans, serum TSH levels rise within a few minutes,[87] followed by a rise in serum triiodothyronine (T_3) levels; there is an increase in thyroxine (T_4) release as well, but a change in blood levels of T_4 is usually not demonstrable because the pool of circulating T_4 (most of which is bound to carrier proteins) is so large. TRH action on the pituitary is blocked by previous treatment with thyroid hormone, which is a crucial element in the negative feedback control of pituitary TSH secretion.

TRH is also a potent PRF.[87] The time course of response of blood PRL levels to TRH, the dose-response characteristics, and the suppression by thyroid hormone pretreatment (all of which parallel changes in TSH secretion) suggest that TRH may be involved in the regulation of PRL secretion. Moreover, TRH is present in the hypophyseal-portal blood of lactating rats. However, it is unlikely to be a physiologic regulator of PRL secretion because the PRL response to nursing in humans is unaccompanied by changes in plasma TSH levels and mice lacking TRH have normal lactotrophs and basal PRL secretion.[88] Nevertheless, TRH may occasionally cause hyperprolactinemia (with or without galactorrhea) in patients with hypothyroidism.

In normal individuals, TRH has no influence on the secretion of pituitary hormones other than TSH and PRL, but it enhances the release of GH in acromegaly and of ACTH in some patients with Cushing disease. Furthermore, prolonged stimulation of the normal pituitary with GHRH can sensitize it to the GH-releasing effects of TRH. TRH also causes the release of GH in some patients with uremia, hepatic disease, anorexia nervosa, and psychotic depression and in children with hypothyroidism.[87] TRH inhibits sleep-induced GH release through its actions in the CNS (see later discussion).

Stimulatory effects of TRH are initiated by binding of the peptide to its GPCR on the plasma membrane of the thyrotroph.[89] Thyroid hormone and somatostatin antagonize the effects of TRH but do interfere with its binding. TRH action is mediated mainly through $G_{q/11}$ and hydrolysis of phosphatidylinositol, with phosphorylation of key protein kinases and an increase in intracellular free calcium (Ca^{2+}) as the crucial steps in postreceptor activation (see Chapter 3).[90] TRH effects can be mimicked by exposure to a Ca^{2+} ionophore and are partially abolished by a Ca^{2+}-free medium. TRH stimulates the formation of mRNAs coding for TSH and PRL in addition to regulating their secretion and stimulates the mitogenesis of thyrotrophs.

TRH is degraded to acid TRH and to the dipeptide histidylprolineamide, which cyclizes nonenzymatically to histidylproline diketopiperazine (cyclic His-Pro). Acid TRH has some behavioral effects in rats that are similar to those of TRH but has no other proven actions. Cyclic His-Pro is reported to act as a PRF and to have other neural effects, including reversal of ethanol-induced sleep (TRH is also effective in this system), elevation of brain cyclic guanosine monophosphate (cGMP) levels, an increase in stereotypical behavior, modification of body temperature, and inhibition of eating behavior. Some of the effects of TRH may be mediated through cyclic His-Pro, but the fact that cyclic His-Pro is abundant in some areas and is not proportional to the amount of TRH suggests that the peptide may not be derived solely from TRH. This latter assertion appears to be confirmed by the detection of substantial amounts of the dipeptide in brains of TRH knockout mice.[88]

Extrapituitary Function

TRH is present in virtually all parts of the brain: cerebral cortex, circumventricular structures, neurohypophysis, pineal gland, and spinal cord.[91] TRH is also found in pancreatic islet cells and in the gastrointestinal tract. Although it exists in low concentration, the total amount in extrahypothalamic tissues exceeds the amount in the hypothalamus.

The extensive extrahypothalamic distribution of TRH, its localization in nerve endings, and the presence of TRH receptors in brain tissue suggest that TRH serves as a neurotransmitter or neuromodulator outside the hypothalamus.[92,93] TRH is a general stimulant and induces hyperthermia on intracerebroventricular injection, suggesting a role in central thermoregulation.[91] Studies in TRH knockout mice may further clarify the nonhypophyseotropic actions of TRH.[88]

Clinical Applications

The use of TRH for the diagnosis of hyperthyroidism or to discriminate between hypothalamic and pituitary causes of TSH deficiency is uncommon since the development of ultrasensitive assays for TSH (see Chapter 11). TRH testing is also not of value in the differential diagnosis of causes of hyperprolactinemia but is useful for the demonstration of residual abnormal somatotropin-secreting cells in acromegalic patients who release GH in response to TRH before treatment.

Studies of the effect of TRH on depression have shown inconsistent results, possibly because of poor blood-brain barrier penetration and short half-life.[91,93] Although a role for TRH in depression is not established, many depressed patients have a blunted TSH response to TRH, and changes in TRH responsiveness correlate with the clinical course. The mechanism by which blunting occurs is unknown.

TRH has been evaluated for the treatment of diverse neurobiologic disorders (for review see Gary and colleagues[91]) including spinal muscle atrophy and amyotrophic lateral sclerosis; transient improvement in strength was reported in both disorders, but the combined experience at many centers using a variety of treatment protocols including long-term intrathecal administration failed to confirm efficacy. TRH administration also reduces the severity of experimentally induced spinal and ischemic shock; preliminary studies in humans suggest that TRH treatment may improve recovery after spinal cord injury and head trauma. TRH has been used to treat children with neurologic disorders including West syndrome, Lennox-Gastaut syndrome, early infantile epileptic encephalopathy, and intractable epilepsy.[94] TRH has been proposed to be an analeptic agent. Sleeping or drug-sedated animals were awakened by the administration of TRH, TRH reportedly reversed sedative effects of ethanol in humans, and TRH is said to have awakened a patient with a profound sleep disorder caused by a hypothalamic and midbrain eosinophilic granuloma.[91]

Regulation of Thyrotropin Release

The secretion of TSH is regulated by two interacting elements: negative feedback by thyroid hormone and open-loop neural control by hypothalamic hypophyseotropic factors (Fig. 7-9). TSH secretion is also modified by other hormones, including estrogens, glucocorticoids, and possibly GH, and is inhibited by cytokines in the pituitary and hypothalamus.[87,95] Aspects of the pituitary-thyroid axis are considered further in Chapter 11.

Feedback Control: Pituitary-Thyroid Axis

In the context of a feedback system, the level of thyroid hormone in blood or of its unbound fraction is the controlled variable and the set-point is the normal resting level of plasma thyroid hormone. The levels of thyroid hormone inversely regulate TSH secretion so that deviations from the set-point lead to appropriate changes in the rate of TSH secretion (Fig. 7-10). Factors that determine the rate of TSH secretion required to maintain a given level of thyroid hormone include the rate at which TSH and thyroid hormone disappear from the blood (turnover rate) and the rate at which T_4 is converted to its more active form, T_3.

Thyroid hormones act on both the pituitary and the hypothalamus.[95] Feedback control of the pituitary by thyroid hormone is remarkably precise. Administration of small doses of T_3 and T_4 inhibited the TSH response to TRH, and barely detectable decreases in plasma thyroid hormone levels were sufficient to sensitize the pituitary to TRH. TRH stimulates TSH secretion within a few minutes through its action on a GPCR, whereas thyroid hormone actions, mediated by intranuclear receptors, require several hours to take effect.

The secretion of hypothalamic TRH is also regulated by thyroid hormone feedback. Systemic injections of T_3 or implantations of tiny T_3 pellets in the PVH of hypothyroid rats[96] (Fig. 7-11A and B) reduced the concentration of TRH mRNA and TRH prohormone in TRH-secreting cells. The downregulation of TRH transcription by DNA binding of ligand-bound thyroid hormone receptors to TREs (see Fig. 7-8) is associated with paradoxical effects of the recruited coactivator steroid receptor coactivator 1 and nuclear corepressor 1.[95]

T_4 in the blood gains access to TRH-secreting neurons in the hypothalamus by way of the CSF. The hormone is taken up by epithelial cells of the choroid plexus of the lateral ventricle of the brain, bound within the cell to locally produced transthyretin (T_4-binding prealbumin), and then secreted across the blood-brain barrier.[97] Within the brain, T_4 is converted to T_3 by type II deiodinase, and T_3 interacts with subtypes of the thyroid hormone receptor ($TR\alpha_1$, $TR\beta_1$, and $TR\beta_2$) in the PVH and other brain cells. In this way, the set-point of the pituitary-thyroid axis is determined by thyroid hormone levels within the brain.[98] T_3 in the circulation is not transported into brain in this manner but presumably gains access to the paraventricular TRH neurons across the blood-brain barrier. The brain T_4 transport and deiodinase system account for the fact that higher blood levels of T_3 are required to suppress pituitary-thyroid function after administration of T_3 than after administration of T_4.[99,100]

Transthyretin is present in the brain of early reptiles and in addition is synthesized by the liver in warm-blooded animals.[97] During embryogenesis in mammals, transthyretin is first detected when the blood-brain barrier appears, ensuring thyroid hormone access to the developing nervous system.

Neural Control

The hypothalamus determines the set-point of feedback control around which the usual feedback regulatory

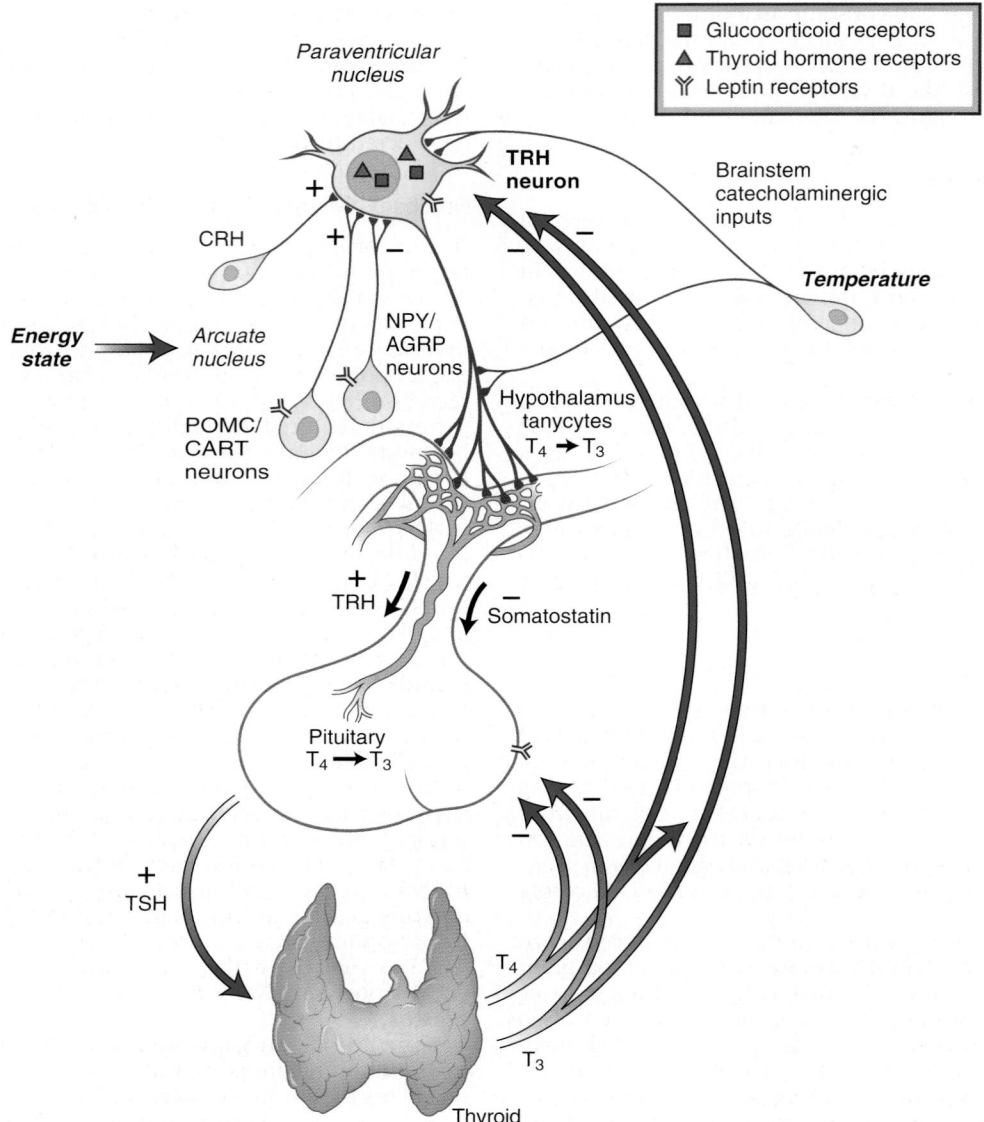

	Glucocorticoid receptors
▲	Thyroid hormone receptors
Υ	Leptin receptors

Paraventricular nucleus

TRH neuron

CRH

Brainstem catecholaminergic inputs

Temperature

Energy state → *Arcuate nucleus*

NPY/ AGRP neurons

POMC/ CART neurons

Hypothalamus tanycytes
$T_4 \rightarrow T_3$

+ TRH

− Somatostatin

Pituitary
$T_4 \rightarrow T_3$

+ TSH

T_4

T_3

Thyroid

Figure 7-9 Regulation of the hypothalamic-pituitary-thyroid axis. AGRP, agouti-related peptide; CART, cocaine- and amphetamine-regulated transcript; CRH, corticotropin-releasing hormone; NPY, neuropeptide Y; POMC, pro-opiomelanocortin; T_3, triiodothyronine; T_4, thyroxine; TRH, thyrotropin-releasing hormone; TSH, thyrotropin.

responses are elicited.[100] Lesions of the thyrotropic area lower basal thyroid hormone levels and make the pituitary more sensitive to inhibition by thyroid hormone, and high doses of TRH raise the levels of TSH and thyroid hormone. Synthesis of TRH in the paraventricular nuclei is regulated by feedback actions of thyroid hormone.[95,100] The hypothalamus can override normal feedback control through an open-loop mechanism involving neuronal inputs to the hypophyseotropic TRH neurons (see Fig. 7-9). For example, cold exposure causes a sharp increase in TSH release in animals and in human newborns. Circadian changes in TSH secretion are another example of brain-directed changes in the set-point of feedback control, but if thyroid hormone levels are sufficiently elevated, as in hyperthyroidism, TRH cannot overcome the inhibition.

Hypothalamic regulation of TSH secretion is also influenced by the inhibitory factor somatostatin. Antisomatostatin antibodies increase basal TSH levels and potentiate the response to stimuli that normally induce

TSH release in the rat, such as cold exposure and TRH administration.[101] Thyroid hormone in turn inhibits the release of somatostatin, implying coordinated, reciprocal regulation of TRH and somatostatin by thyroid hormone. GH stimulates hypothalamic somatostatin synthesis and can inhibit TSH secretion. However, the physiologic role of somatostatin in the regulation of TSH secretion in humans is uncertain.

Circadian Rhythm

Plasma TSH in humans is characterized by a circadian periodicity, with a maximum between 9 PM and 5 AM and a minimum between 4 PM and 7 PM (see Fig. 7-7E).[102] Smaller ultradian TSH peaks occur every 90 to 180 minutes, probably because of bursts of TRH release from the hypothalamus, and are physiologically important in controlling the synthesis and glycosylation of TSH. Glycosylation is a determinant of TSH potency.[103]

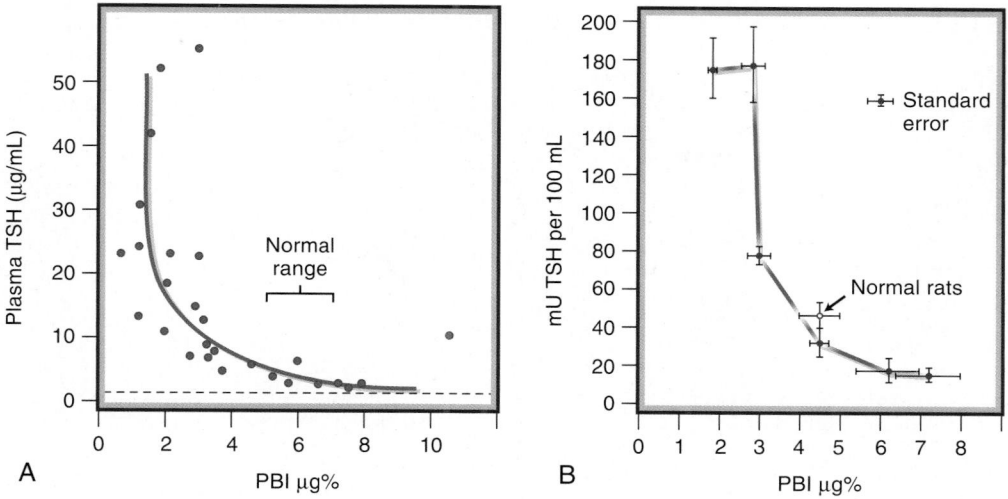

Figure 7-10 Relationship between plasma thyrotropin (TSH) levels and thyroid hormone as determined by plasma protein-bound iodine (PBI) measurements in humans and rats. These curves illustrate, in the human (**A**) and the rat (**B**), that plasma TSH levels are a curvilinear function of plasma thyroid hormone level. Human studies were carried out by giving myxedematous patients successive increments of thyroxine (T_4) at approximately 10-day intervals. Each point represents simultaneous measurements of plasma PBI and plasma TSH at various times in the six patients studied. The rat studies were performed by treating thyroidectomized animals with various doses of T_4 for 2 weeks before assay of plasma TSH and plasma PBI. These curves illustrate that the secretion of TSH is regulated over the entire range of thyroid hormone levels. At the normal set-point for T_4, the small changes above and below the control level are followed by appropriate increases or decreases in plasma TSH. (**A,** From Reichlin S, Utiger RD. Regulation of the pituitary thyroid axis in man: relationship of TSH concentration to concentration of free and total thyroxine in plasma. *J Clin Endocrinol Metab.* 1967;27:251-255, copyright by The Endocrine Society. **B,** From Reichlin S, Martin JB, Boshans RL, et al. Measurement of TSH in plasma and pituitary of the rat by a radioimmunoassay utilizing bovine TSH: effect of thyroidectomy or thyroxine administration on plasma TSH levels. *Endocrinology.* 1970;87:1022-1031, copyright by The Endocrine Society.)

Temperature

External cold exposure activates and high ambient temperature inhibits the pituitary-thyroid axis in animals, and analogous changes occur in humans under certain conditions.[104] Exposure of infants to cold at the time of delivery causes an increase in blood TSH levels, possibly because of alterations in the turnover and degradation of the thyroid hormones. Blood thyroid hormone levels are higher in the winter than in the summer among people living in cold climates but not in other climates. However, it is difficult to show that changes in environmental or body temperature in adults influence TSH secretion. For example, exposure to cold ambient temperature or central hypothalamic cooling does not modify TSH levels in young men. Behavioral changes, activation of the sympathetic nervous system, and shivering appear to be more important than the thyroid response for temperature regulation in adults.

The autonomic nervous system and the thyroid axis work together to maintain temperature homeostasis in mammals, and TRH plays a role in both pathways.[104] Hypothalamic TRH release is rapidly increased (30 to 45 minutes) in rats exposed to cold. Rapid inhibition of somatostatin release in the median eminence has also been documented, and both changes appear to play important roles in the rise in plasma TSH induced by cold exposure. TRH mRNA is elevated within an hour of cold exposure (see Fig. 7-11C and D). The regulation of hypophyseotropic TRH release and expression by cold is largely mediated by catecholamines. Noradrenergic and adrenergic fibers, originating in the brainstem, are found in close proximity to TRH nerve endings in the median eminence, and a rapid rise in TRH release occurs after norepinephrine treatment of hypothalamic fragments containing mainly median eminence. Brainstem adrenergic and noradrenergic fibers also make synaptic contacts with TRH neurons in the PVH (see Fig. 7-9),[105] so catecholamines are likely to be involved in the regulation of TRH gene expression by cold. TRH neurons

in the PVH are densely innervated by NPY terminals,[100] and a portion of the NPY terminals arising from the C1, C2, C3, and A1 cell groups of the brainstem and projecting to the PVH are known to be catecholaminergic. Somatostatin, dopamine, and serotonin also play a variety of roles in the regulation of TRH.

Stress

Stress is another determinant of TSH secretion.[106] In humans physical stress inhibits TSH release, as indicated by the finding that low levels of T_3 and T_4 in patients with the nonthyroidal illness syndrome do not cause compensatory increases in TSH secretion as would occur in normal individuals.[107]

A number of observations demonstrate interactions between the thyroid and adrenal axes.[106] Physiologically, the bulk of evidence suggests that glucocorticoids in humans and rodents act to blunt the thyroid axis through actions in the CNS.[108] Some actions may be direct because the TRH gene (see Fig. 7-8) contains a glucocorticoid response element consensus half-site,[84] and hypophyseotropic TRH neurons appear to contain glucocorticoid receptors.[109] The diurnal rhythm of cortisol is opposite that of TSH (see Fig. 7-7) and acute administration of glucocorticoids can block the nocturnal rise in TSH, but disruption of cortisol synthesis with metyrapone only modestly affects the TSH circadian rhythm.

Nevertheless, several lines of evidence identify conditions in which elevated glucocorticoids are associated with stimulation of the thyroid axis. Human depression is often associated with hypercortisolism and hyperthyroxinemia, and TRH mRNA levels are elevated by glucocorticoids in a number of cell lines as well as in cultured fetal hypothalamic TRH neurons from the rat. Thus, although glucocorticoids probably stimulate TRH production in TRH neurons, their overall inhibitory effect on the thyroid axis results from indirect glucocorticoid negative feedback on

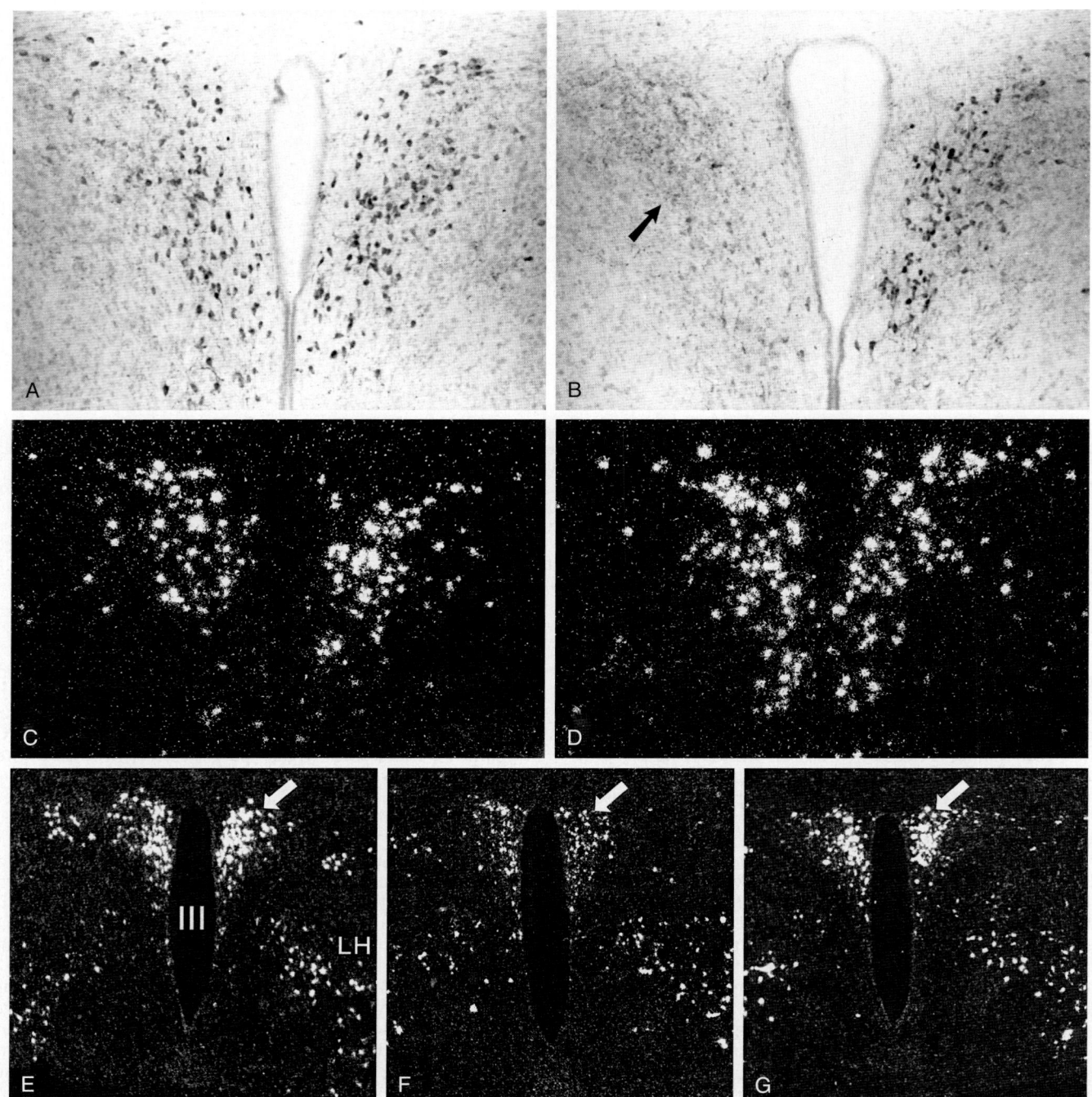

Figure 7-11 A and **B,** Direct effects of triiodothyronine (T$_3$) on thyrotropin-releasing hormone (TRH) synthesis in the rat hypothalamic paraventricular nucleus (parvicellular division) were shown in this experiment by immunohistochemical detection of pre-pro-TRH(25-50) after implantation of a pellet of either T$_3$ (**B**) or inactive diiodothyronine (T$_2$) as a control (**A**). The T$_2$ pellet had no effect on the concentration of pre-pro-TRH (**A**). In contrast, the TRH prohormone (**B**) concentrations were markedly reduced (*black arrow* indicates the unilateral pellet implantation). These studies indicate that thyroid hormone regulates the hypothalamic component of the pituitary-thyroid axis as well as the pituitary thyrotrope itself. **C** and **D,** Effects of 1 hour at 4° C on TRH messenger ribonucleic acid (mRNA). **E** to **G,** Effects on TRH mRNA levels of starvation (**F**) and leptin replacement during starvation (**G**). *White arrows* show the location of the paraventricular nucleus. III, 3rd ventricle; LH, lateral hypothalamus. (Photomicrographs in panels **A, B, E, F,** and **G,** courtesy of Dr. R. M. Lechan. From Dyess EM, Segerson TP, Liposits Z, et al. Triiodothyronine exerts direct cell-specific regulation of thyrotropin-releasing hormone gene expression in the hypothalamic paraventricular nucleus. *Endocrinology.* 1988;123:2291-2297, copyright by The Endocrine Society; photomicrographs in panels **C** and **D,** courtesy of Dr. P. Joseph-Bravo.)

structures such as the hippocampus. Disruption of hippocampal suppression of the hypothalamic-pituitary-adrenal (HPA) axis is proposed to be involved in the hypercortisolemia commonly seen in affective illness, and disruption of hippocampal inputs to the hypothalamus has been shown to produce a rise in hypophyseotropic TRH in the rat.[110]

Starvation

The thyroid axis is depressed during starvation, presumably to help conserve energy by depressing metabolism (Fig. 7-11E to G). In humans, reduced T$_3$, T$_4$, and TSH are seen during starvation or fasting.[100] There are also changes in the thyroid axis in anorexia nervosa, such as low blood levels of T_3 and low normal levels of T_4. Inappropriately low levels of TSH are found, suggesting defective activation of TRH production by low thyroid hormone levels. During starvation in rodents, reduced TRH release into hypophyseal portal blood and reduced pro-TRH mRNA levels are seen, despite lowered thyroid hormone levels.[111] Reduced basal TSH levels are also usually present.

The hypothyroidism seen in fasting or in the leptin-deficient *ob/ob* mouse can be reversed by administration of leptin,[112] and evidence suggests that the mechanism involves leptin's ability to upregulate TRH gene expression in the PVH (see Fig. 7-11E to G).[113] Leptin appears to act both directly through leptin receptors on hypophyseotropic TRH neurons and indirectly through its actions on other hypothalamic cell groups, such as arcuate nucleus POMC and NPY/agouti-related peptide (AgRP) neurons.[114,115] TRH neurons in the PVH receive dense NPY/AgRP and POMC projections from the arcuate and express NPY and melanocortin-4 receptors (MC4R),[116] and α-MSH administration partially prevents the fasting-induced drop in thyroid hormone levels.[114,115] Indeed, the TRH promoter contains a signal transducer and activator of transcription (STAT) response element and a CRE that have been demonstrated to mediate induction of TRH gene expression by leptin and α-MSH, respectively, in a heterologous cell system (see Fig. 7-8).[116] The regulation of TRH by metabolic state is likely to be under redundant control, however, because leptin-deficient children, unlike rodents, are euthyroid,[117] whereas both humans and rodents with MC4R deficiency are euthyroid.[118]

Infection and Inflammation

The molecular basis of infection- or inflammation-induced TSH suppression is partially established. TSH secretion is inhibited by sterile abscesses; by the injection of interleukin 1β (IL-1β), an endogenous pyrogen and secretory peptide of activated lymphocytes[119]; or by tumor necrosis factor α (TNF-α). IL-1β stimulates the secretion of somatostatin.[120] TNF-α inhibits TSH secretion directly and induces functional changes in the rat characteristic of the sick euthyroid state.[121] It is likely that the TSH inhibition in animal models of the sick euthyroid syndrome is due to cytokine-induced changes in hypothalamic and pituitary function.[122] IL-6, IL-1, and TNF-α contribute to the suppression of TSH in the nonthyroidal illness syndrome.[123] Other evidence suggests that bacterial lipopolysaccharide can directly stimulate tanycytes via their expression of toll-like receptor 4. The stimulated tanycytes express higher levels of type 2 deiodinase that in turn increases the levels of T_3 relative to T_4, causing feedback inhibition on TRH neurons.[100]

Corticotropin-Releasing Hormone
Chemistry and Evolution

The HPA axis is the humoral component of an integrated neural and endocrine system that functions to respond to internal and external challenges to homeostasis (stressors). The system comprises the neuronal pathways linked to release of catecholamines from the adrenal medulla (fight-or-flight response) and the hypothalamic-pituitary control of ACTH release. Pituitary ACTH secretion is stimulated primarily by CRH and to a lesser extent by AVP (see Chapter 8). The hypophyseotropic CRH neurons are located in the parvicellular division of the PVH and project to the median eminence (see Figs. 7-3 and 7-4).

In a broader context, the CRH system in the CNS is also vitally important in the behavioral response to stress. This complex system includes both nonhypophyseotropic CRH neurons, three additional CRH-like peptides (urocortin, urocortin 2 or stresscopin-related peptide, and urocortin 3 or stresscopin), at least two cognate GPCRs (CRH-R1 and CRH-R2), and a high-affinity CRH-binding protein, each with distinct and complex distributions in the CNS.

The Schally and Guillemin laboratories demonstrated in 1955 that extracts from the hypothalamus stimulated ACTH release from the pituitary. The primary active principle, CRH, was purified and characterized from sheep in 1981. Human CRH is an amidated 41–amino acid peptide that is cleaved from the COOH-terminus of a 196–amino acid pre-prohormone precursor by PC1 and PC2 (Fig. 7-12).[124] CRH is highly conserved phylogenetically; the human peptide is identical in sequence to the mouse and rat peptides but differs at seven residues from the ovine sequence. Mammalian CRH, the three urocortin peptides, fish urotensin, anuran sauvagine, and the insect diuretic peptides are members of an ancient family of peptides that evolved from an ancestral precursor early in the evolution of metazoans, approximately 500 million years ago.[125] Comparison of peptide sequences in vertebrates suggests a grouping of the peptides into two subfamilies, CRH-urotensin-urocortin-sauvagine and urocortin 2-urocortin 3 (Fig. 7-13).[126] Urocortin and sauvagine appear to represent tetrapod orthologues of fish urotensin. Sauvagine, isolated originally from *Phyllomedusa sauvagei*, is an osmoregulatory peptide produced in the skin of certain frogs; urotensin is an osmoregulatory peptide produced in the caudal neurosecretory system of the fish. Whereas isolation of CRH required 250,000 ovine hypothalami, the virtual cloning of urocortin II and III was accomplished by computer search of the human genome database.[126]

The CRH peptides signal by binding to CRH-R1[127] and CRH-R2[128] receptors that couple to the stimulatory G protein (G_s) and adenylyl cyclase. Two splice variants of the latter receptor that differ in the extracellular NH_2-terminal domain, CRH-R2α and CRH-R2β, have been found in both rodents and humans,[129] and a third NH_2-terminal splice variant, CRH-R2γ, has been reported in the human.[130]

CRH, urotensin, and sauvagine are potent agonists of CRH-R1; urocortin is a potent agonist of both receptors; and urocortins 2 and 3 are specific agonists of CRH-R2. CRH activation of the HPA axis is mediated exclusively through CRH-R1 expressed in the corticotroph. CRH neurons projecting to the median eminence are found mostly in the PVH (Fig. 7-14A). Some CRH fibers in the PVH also project to the brainstem, and nonhypophyseotropic CRH neurons are abundant elsewhere, primarily in limbic structures involved in processing sensory information and in regulating the autonomic nervous system. Sites include the prefrontal, insular, and cingulate cortices; amygdala; substantia nigra; periaqueductal gray; locus coeruleus; NTS; and parabrachial nucleus. In the periphery, CRH is found in human placenta, where it is upregulated 6- to 40-fold during the third trimester; in lymphocytes; in autonomic nerves; and in the gastrointestinal tract. Urocortin is expressed at highest levels in the nonpreganglionic Edinger-Westphal nucleus, the lateral superior olive, and the SON of the rodent brain, with additional sites including the substantia nigra, ventral tegmental area, and dorsal raphe (Fig. 7-14B). In the human, urocortin is widely distributed, with highest levels in the frontal cortex, temporal cortex, and hypothalamus,[131] and has also been reported in the nonpreganglionic Edinger-Westphal nucleus.[20] In the periphery, urocortin is seen in placenta, mucosal inflammatory cells of the gastrointestinal tract, lymphocytes, and cardiomyocytes. Urocortin 2 is expressed in hypothalamic neuroendocrine and stress-related cell

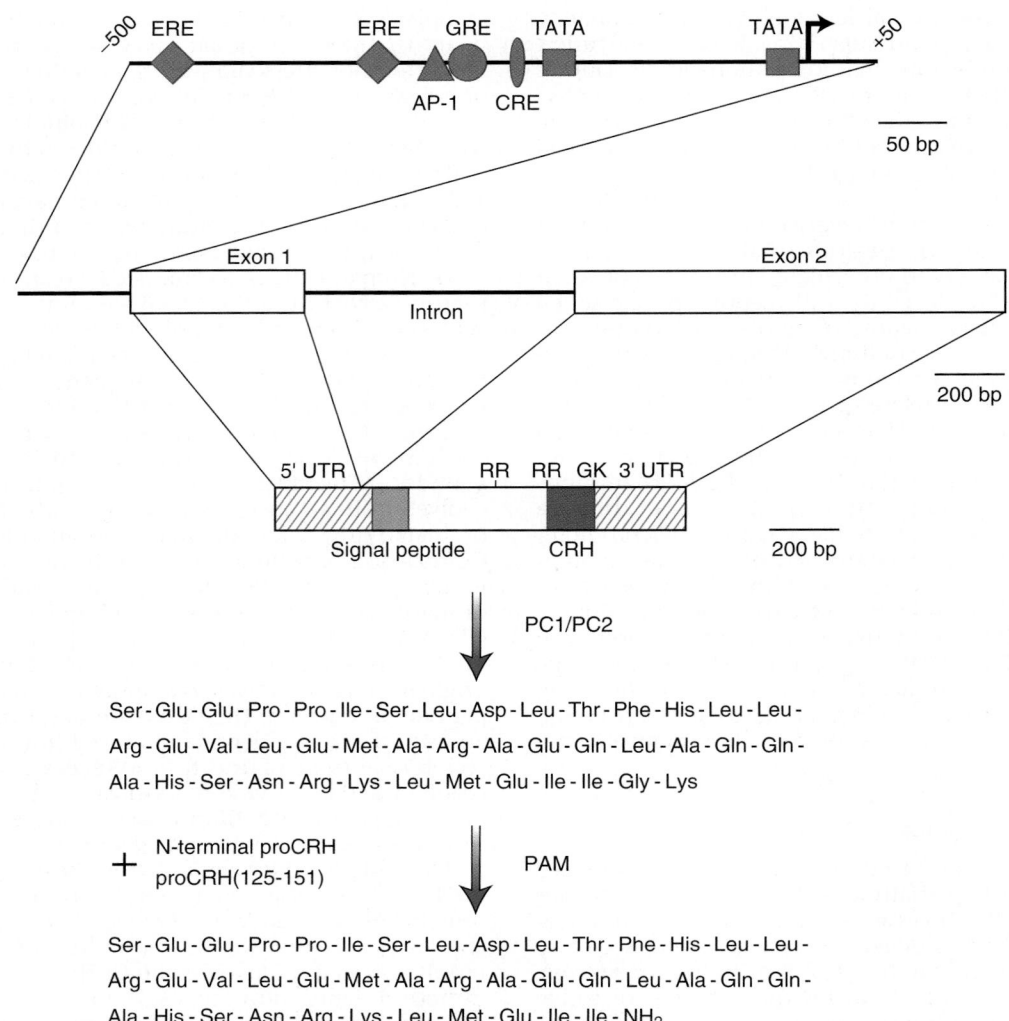

Figure 7-12 Structure of the human corticotropin-releasing hormone (CRH) gene, complementary DNA, and peptide. The sequence encoding CRH occurs at the carboxy-terminus of the prohormone. Dibasic amino acid cleavage sites (RR) and the penultimate Gly and terminal Lys (GK) are shown. AP-1, activator protein-1 binding sequence; CRE, cyclic adenosine monophosphate response element; ERE, estrogen response element; GRE, glucocorticoid response element; PAM, peptidylglycine α-amidating monooxygenase; PC1/PC2, prohormone convertases 1 and 2; TATA, Goldstein-Hogness box involved in binding RNA polymerase; UTR, untranslated. (Redrawn from data of Shibahara S, Morimoto Y, Furutani Y, et al. Isolation and sequence analysis of the human corticotropin-releasing factor precursor gene. *EMBO J.* 1983;2:775-779.)

```
Human  CRH                SEE**PPISLDLTF**HLLREV**LEMAR**AEQLAQ**QA**HS**NRK**L**ME**II
Human  urocortin              DN**P**S**LSIDLTF**HLLRTL**LE**L**AR**TQSQ**RERA**EQ**NRI**IFD**SV
Human  urocortin II(SRP) HPGSRIV**LSLDV**PIG**LL**QIL**LE**Q**AR**ARAA**REQA**TTN**ARI**LARV**GHC
Human  urocortin III(SCP)    TKFT**LSLDV**PTNIMNLLFNI**AK**AKNL**RAQA**AAN**AHL**MAQ**I**GRRK
Frog   sauvagine            QG**PPISIDLS**LELLRKM**IE**IEKQEKE**KQQA**ANN**RLLL**DTI
Carp   urotensin-I        NDD**PPISIDLTF**HLLRNM**IEMAR**NENQ**REQA**GL**NRK**YLD**EV
```

Figure 7-13 Sequence comparison of members of the corticotropin-releasing hormone (CRH) peptide family. Identical or highly conserved amino acids are indicated in boldface letters. SCP, stresscopin; SRP, stresscopin-related peptide.

groups in the mouse, including the locus coeruleus, whereas urocortin 3 is expressed in the hypothalamus and amygdala, and particularly in pancreatic islet beta cells.[132,133]

In addition to its expression in pituitary corticotrophs, CRH-R1 is found in the neocortex and cerebellar cortex, subcortical limbic structures, and amygdala, with little to no expression in the hypothalamus (Fig. 7-14C). CRH-R1 is also found in a variety of peripheral sites in humans, including ovary, endometrium, and skin. CRH-R2α is found mainly in the brain in rodents, with high levels of expression seen in the ventromedial hypothalamic nucleus and lateral septum (see Fig. 7-14C)[134]; CRH-R2β is found centrally in cerebral arterioles and peripherally in the gastrointestinal tract, heart, and muscle.[128,135] In humans, CRH-R2α is expressed in brain and periphery, whereas the β and γ subtypes are primarily central.[129,130] Little CRH-R2 message is seen in pituitary. Although CRH-R1 appears to be exclusively involved in regulation of pituitary ACTH

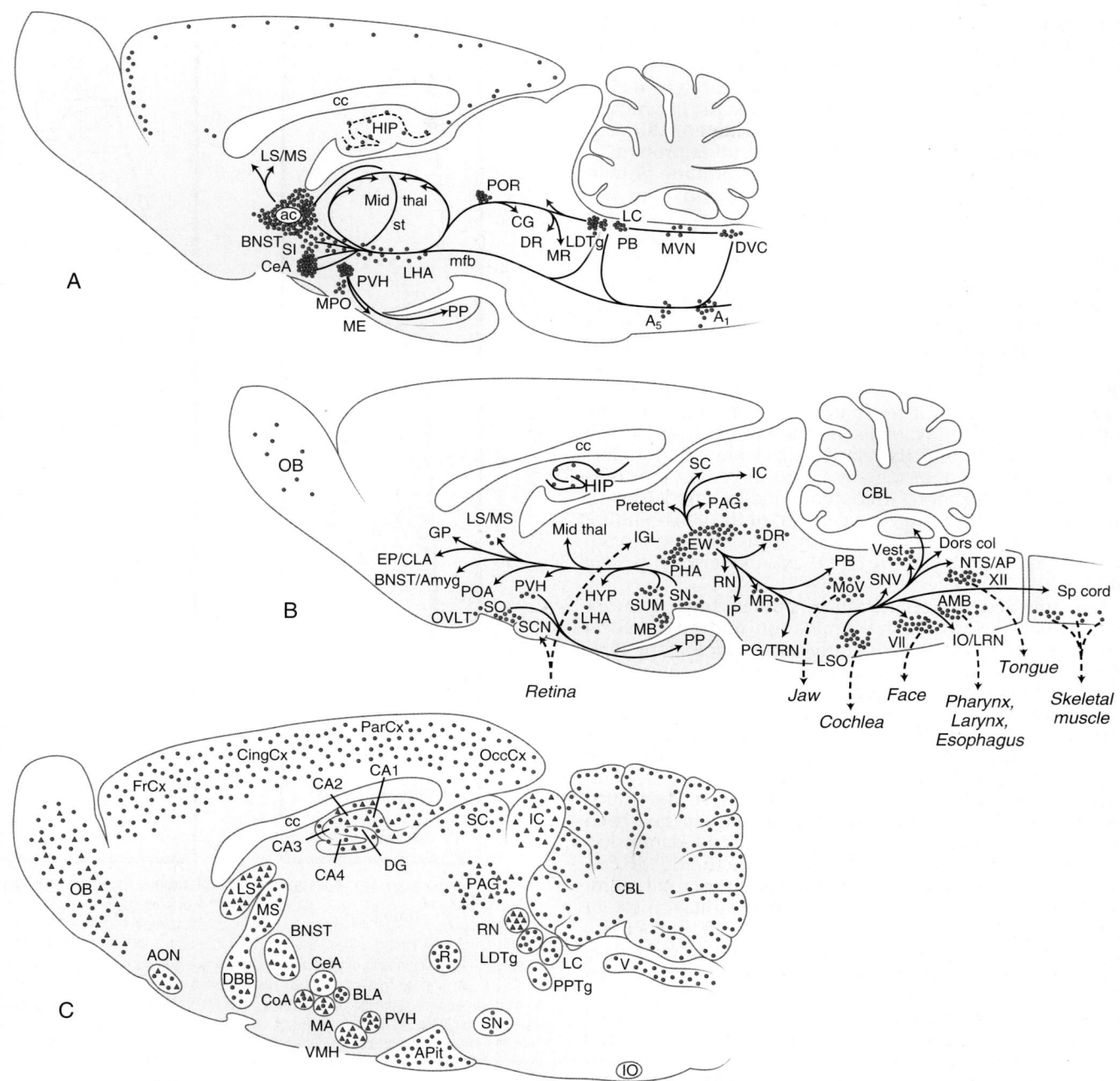

Figure 7-14 Distribution of messenger RNA sequences for corticotropin-releasing hormone (CRH) (**A**), urocortin (**B**), and the CRH receptor 1 (CRH-R1) (**C,** *circles*) and CRH-R2 (**C,** *triangles*) in the rat brain. A_1, noradrenergic cell group 1; A_5, noradrenergic cell group 5; ac, anterior commissure; AMB, nucleus ambiguus; APit, anterior pituitary; AP, area postrema; BLA, basolateral amygdala; BNST, bed nucleus of the stria terminalis; CBL, cerebellum; cc, corpus callosum; CeA, central nucleus amygdala; CG, central gray; DG, dentate gyrus; DR, dorsal raphe; DVC, dorsal vagal complex; EW, Edinger-Westphal nucleus, noncholinergic; HIP, hippocampus; IC, inferior colliculus; LC, locus coeruleus; LDTg, laterodorsal tegmental nucleus; LHA, lateral hypothalamic area; LS, lateral septum; MA, medial amygdala; ME, median eminence; mfb, medial forebrain bundle; Mid Thal, midline thalamic nuclei; MS, medial septum; MPO, medial preoptic area; MR, medial raphe; MVN, medial vestibular nucleus; OB, olfactory bulb; PAG, periaqueductal gray; PB, parabrachial nucleus; POR, perioculomotor nucleus; PP, posterior pituitary; PPTg, peripeduncular tegmental nucleus; PVH, paraventricular nucleus hypothalamus; R, raphe; RN, red nucleus; SC, superior colliculus; SI, substantia innominata; st, stria terminalis; V/Vest, vestibular nuclei; VMH, ventral medial nucleus hypothalamus. (From Swanson LW, Sawchenko PE, Rivier J, et al. Organization of ovine corticotropin-releasing factor immunoreactive cells and fibers in the rat brain: an immunohistochemical study. *Neuroendocrinology.* 1983;36:165-186; Bittencourt JC, Vaughan J, Arias C, et al. Urocortin expression in rat brain: evidence against a pervasive relationship of urocortin-containing projections with targets bearing type 2 CRF receptors. *J Comp Neurol.* 1999;415:285-312, Fig. 17; Steckler T, Holsboer F. Corticotropin-releasing hormone receptor subtypes and emotion. *Biol Psychol.* 1999;46:1480-1508, Fig. 1.)

synthesis and release, both receptors are expressed in the rodent adrenal cortex. Data suggest that this intra-adrenal CRH-ACTH system may be involved in fine-tuning of adrenocortical corticosterone release.

The CRH system is also regulated in both brain and periphery by a 37-kDa high-affinity CRH-binding protein.[136]

This factor was initially postulated from the observation that CRH levels rise dramatically during the second and third trimesters of pregnancy without activating the pituitary-adrenal axis. Among hypophyseotropic factors, CRH is the only one for which a specific binding protein (in addition to the receptor) exists in tissue or blood. The placenta is the principal source of pregnancy-related CRH-binding protein. Human and rat CRH-binding proteins are homologous (85% amino acid identity), but in the rat the protein is expressed only in brain and pituitary gland. The binding protein is species specific; bovine CRH, which is almost identical in sequence to rat and human CRH, has a lower binding affinity to the human binding protein.

The functional significance of the CRH-binding protein is not fully understood. CRH-binding protein does not bind to the CRH receptor but does inhibit CRH action. For this reason CRH-binding protein probably acts to modulate CRH actions at the cellular level. Corticotroph cells in the anterior pituitary have membrane CRH receptors and intracellular CRH-binding protein; conceivably, the binding protein acts to sequester or terminate the action of membrane-bound CRH. CRH-binding protein is present in many regions of the CNS, including cells that synthesize CRH and cells that receive innervation from CRH-containing neurons. The anatomic distribution of the protein, the variability of its location in relation to the presence of CRH, and its relative sparseness in the CRH THDA neuronal system suggest a control system that is as yet poorly understood. Transgenic mouse models with both overexpression and gene deletion of the CRH-binding protein have been produced with little effect on basal or stress activation of the HPA axis reviewed by Bale and Vale.[137]

Structure-activity relationship studies have demonstrated that COOH-terminal amidation and an α-helical secondary structure are both important for biologic activity of CRH. The first CRH antagonist described was termed α-helical CRH(9-41).[138] A second, more potent antagonist, termed *astressin*, has the structure cyclo(30-33)(D-Phe[12], Nle[12], Glu[12], Lys[12])hCRH(12-41).[139] Both peptides are somewhat nonspecific, antagonizing both CRH-R1 and CRH-R2. Because of the anxiogenic activity of CRH and urocortin, a number of pharmaceutical companies have developed small molecule CRH antagonists; several of these have been the subject of clinical trials for anxiety and depression (see later discussion). Thus far, this structurally diverse group of small molecule compounds, such as antalarmin, CP-154,526, and NBI27914, are potent antagonists of CRH-R1, with little activity at CRH-R2. The efficacy of these compounds across the entire behavioral, neuroendocrine, and autonomic repertoire of response to stress has been demonstrated in a number of laboratory animal studies. For example, oral administration of antalarmin in a social stress model in the primate (introduction of strange males) reduced behavioral measures of anxiety such as lack of exploratory behavior, decreased plasma ACTH and cortisol, and reduced plasma epinephrine and norepinephrine.[140] Other preclinical studies in rhesus monkeys have compared the pharmacologic profiles of astressin B and antalarmin.[141] A peptide antagonist with 100-fold selectivity for the CRH 2β receptor, (D-Phe[11], His[12])sauvagine(11-40) or antisauvagine-30, has also been described.[142]

Effects on the Pituitary and Mechanism of Action

Administration of CRH to humans causes prompt release of ACTH into the blood, followed by secretion of cortisol (Fig. 7-15) and other adrenal steroids including aldosterone. Most studies have used ovine CRH, which is more potent and longer acting than human CRH, but human and porcine CRHs appear to have equal diagnostic value. The effect of CRH is specific to ACTH release and is inhibited by glucocorticoids.

As mentioned before, CRH acts on the pituitary corticotroph primarily by binding to CRH-R1 and activating

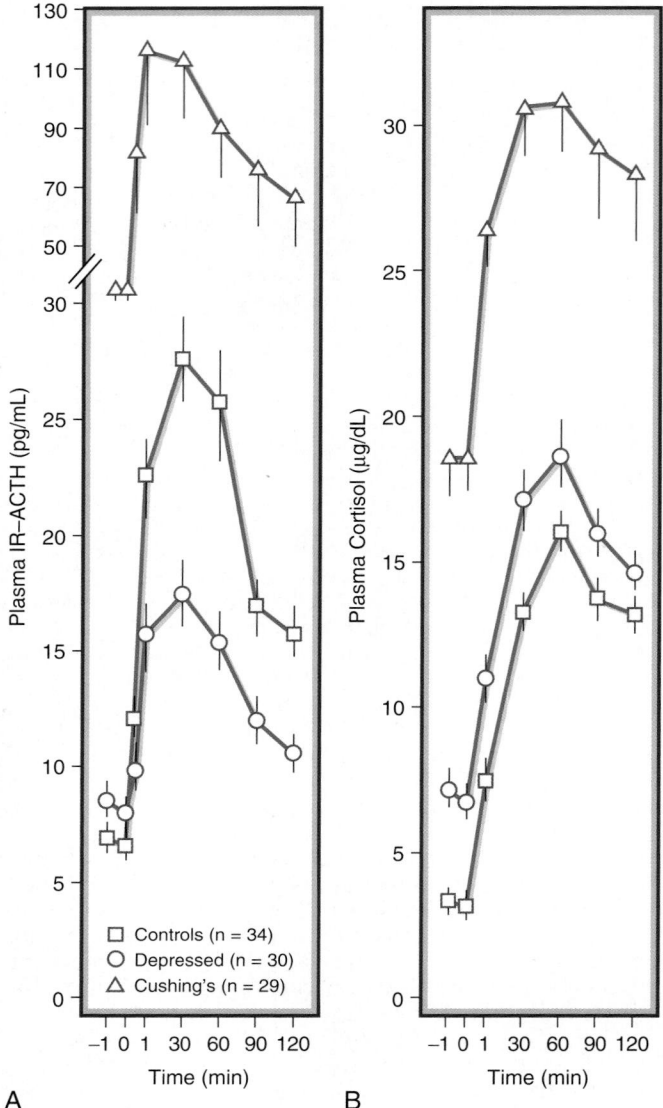

Figure 7-15 Comparison of plasma immunoreactive adrenocorticotropic hormone (IR-ACTH) (**A**) and plasma cortisol (**B**) responses to ovine corticotropin-releasing hormone in control subjects, patients with depression, and patients with Cushing disease. (From Gold PW, Loriaux DL, Roy A, et al. Responses to corticotropin-releasing hormone in the hypercortisolism of depression and Cushing's disease: pathophysiologic and diagnostic implications. *N Engl J Med*. 1986;314:1329-1335.)

adenylyl cyclase. The concentration of cAMP in the tissue is increased in parallel with the biologic effects and is reduced by glucocorticoids. The rate of transcription of the mRNA that encodes the ACTH prohormone POMC is also enhanced by CRH.

Extrapituitary Functions

CRH and the urocortin peptides have a wide range of biologic activities in addition to the hypophyseotropic role of CRH in regulating ACTH synthesis and release. Centrally, these peptides have behavioral activities in anxiety, mood, arousal, locomotion, reward, and feeding[143,144] and increase sympathetic activation. Many of the nonhypophyseotropic behavioral and autonomic functions of these peptides can be viewed as complementary to activation of the HPA axis in the maintenance of homeostasis under exposure to stress. In the periphery, activities have been reported in immunity, cardiac function, gastrointestinal function, and reproduction.[145]

Hyperactivity of the HPA axis is a common neuroendocrine finding in affective disorders (see Fig. 7-15).[143,146] Normalization of HPA regulation is highly predictive of successful treatment. Defective dexamethasone suppression of CRH release, implying defective corticosteroid receptor signaling, is seen not only in depressed patients but also in healthy subjects with a family history of depression.[147] Depressed patients also show elevated levels of CRH in the CSF.[148] Extensive behavioral testing in a variety of mutant mouse models with genetically altered expression of either the CRH ligands or receptors generally supports the hypothesis that activation of central CRH pathways is a critical neurobiologic substrate of anxiety and depressive states.[137,144]

Central administration of CRH or urocortin activates neuronal cell groups involved in cardiovascular control and increases blood pressure, heart rate, and cardiac output.[149] However, urocortin is expressed in cardiac myocytes, and intravenous administration of CRH or urocortin decreases blood pressure and increases heart rate in most species, including humans.[149] This hypotensive effect is probably mediated peripherally because ganglionic blockade did not disrupt the hypotensive effects of intravenous urocortin. Furthermore, high levels of CRH-R2β have been seen in the cardiac atria and ventricles,[128,135] and knockout of the *Crhr2* gene in the mouse eliminated the hypotensive effects of intravenous urocortin administration.[150]

Cytokines have an important role in extinguishing inflammatory responses through activation of CRH and AVP neurons in the PVH and subsequent elevation of anti-inflammatory glucocorticoids. Interestingly, CRH is generally proinflammatory in the periphery, where it is found in sympathetic efferents, in sensory afferent nerves, in leukocytes, and in macrophages in some species.[145,151] CRH also functions as a paracrine factor in the endometrium, where it may play a role in decidualization and implantation and act as a uterine vasodilator.[145]

The relative contributions of each of the CRH-urocortin peptides and receptors to the different biologic functions reported has been the topic of considerable analysis, given the receptor-specific antagonists already described as well as the CRH, CRH-R1, and CRH-R2 knockout mice available for study (reviewed by Bale and Vale[137] and Keck and colleagues[144]). Examination of three potent stressors—restraint, ether, and fasting—demonstrated that other ACTH secretagogues, such as AVP, oxytocin, and catecholamines, could not replace CRH in its role in mounting the stress response. In contrast, augmentation of glucocorticoid secretion by a stressor after prolonged stress was not defective in CRH knockout mice, implicating CRH-independent mechanisms.

Although CRH is a potent anxiogenic peptide, CRH knockout mice exhibit normal anxiety behaviors in, for example, conditioned fear paradigms (reviewed by Bale and Vale[137]). The nonpeptide CRH-R1–specific antagonist CP-154,526 was anxiolytic in a shock-induced freezing paradigm in both wild-type and CRH knockout mice, suggesting that the anxiogenic activity is a CRH-like peptide acting at the CRH-R1 receptor.

CRH and urocortin peptides also have potent anorexigenic activity, implicating the CRH system in stress-induced inhibition of feeding. However, studies utilizing CRH, CRH-R1, and CRH-R2 knockout mice have not fully unraveled the complex interactions of these peptides and receptor signaling pathways in the acute effects of stress on feeding behavior.

Additional gene knockout studies have suggested that urocortin 2 plays a physiologic role in female mice to dampen basal daily rhythms of the HPA axis and reduce behavioral coping mechanisms in response to chronic stress.[132] Urocortin 3 may have a primary action to augment insulin secretion in response to the metabolic stress of excessive calorie intake.[133]

Clinical Applications

No approved therapeutic application of CRH or CRH-like peptides exists, although the peptide has been demonstrated to have a number of activities in human and primate studies. For example, intravenous administration of CRH was found to stimulate energy expenditure but is an unlikely pharmaceutical target for inducing weight loss. The development of small-molecule, orally available, CRH-R1 antagonists has, however, produced considerable interest in their potential for treatment of anxiety and depression.[148,152] In particular, the compound R121919 was studied in phase I and IIa clinical trials before its discontinuance. These studies of 20 patients demonstrated significant reductions in scores of anxiety and depression, using ratings determined by either patient or clinician, and also demonstrated the compound's safety and favorable side-effect profile including a lack of effect on endocrine function or body weight gain.[153] Similarly, preclinical studies in relevant animal models have implicated the CRH/urocortin system in the neurobiology of addiction and as a therapeutic target.[154]

Feedback Control

The administration of glucocorticoids inhibits ACTH secretion, and conversely, removal of the adrenals (or administration of drugs that impair secretion of glucocorticoids) leads to increased ACTH release. The set-point of pituitary feedback is determined by the hypothalamus acting through hypothalamic releasing hormones CRH and AVP (see Chapter 8).[155-158] Glucocorticoids act on both the pituitary corticotrophs and the hypothalamic neurons that secrete CRH and AVP. These regulatory actions are analogous to the control of the pituitary-thyroid axis. However, whereas TSH becomes completely unresponsive to TRH when thyroid hormone levels are sufficiently high, severe neurogenic stress and large amounts of CRH can break through the feedback inhibition due to glucocorticoids. A still higher level of feedback control is exerted by glucocorticoid-responsive neurons in the hippocampus that project to the hypothalamus; these neurons affect the activity of CRH hypophyseotropic neurons and determine the set-point of pituitary responsiveness to glucocorticoids.[158] A comprehensive review of glucocorticoid effects on CRH and AVP and regulation of the HPA axis has emphasized the complexity of this control beyond that of a simple closed-loop feedback.[159]

Glucocorticoids are lipid soluble and freely enter the brain through the blood-brain barrier.[157] In brain and pituitary they can bind to two receptors: Type I (encoded by *NR3C1*) is called the *mineralocorticoid receptor* because it binds aldosterone and glucocorticoids with high affinity. Type II (*NR3C2*), the glucocorticoid receptor, has low affinity for mineralocorticoids.[156-158] Classic glucocorticoid action involves binding of the steroid-receptor complex to regulator sequences in the genome. Type I receptors are saturated by basal levels of glucocorticoids, whereas type II receptors are not saturated under basal conditions but approach saturation during peak phases of the circadian rhythm and during stress. These differences and differences in regional distribution within the brain suggest that type I receptors determine basal activity of the hypothalamic-pituitary axis and that type II receptors mediate stress responses.[160]

In the pituitary, glucocorticoids inhibit secretion of ACTH and the synthesis of POMC mRNA; in the hypothalamus they inhibit secretion of CRH and AVP and the synthesis of their respective mRNAs is inhibited, although with distinct temporal patterns.[157-159] Neuron membrane excitability and ion transport properties are suppressed by changes in glucocorticoid-directed synthesis of intracellular protein. Glucocorticoids can exert additional rapid signaling events in neurons including an endocannabinoid-mediated suppression of synaptic excitation.[161] These rapid events involve membrane-associated complexes and are independent of changes in gene transcription or acute protein translation, but the exact mechanisms and nature of the receptor(s) remain controversial.[162]

Glucocorticoids can block stress-induced ACTH release. The latency of the inhibitory effect is so short (<30 minutes) that it is likely that gene regulation is not the sole basis of the response.[162] However, long-term suppression (>1 hour) clearly acts through genomic mechanisms.

Glucocorticoid receptors are also found outside the hypothalamus in the septum and amygdala,[157,158] and these structures are involved in the psychobehavioral changes in hypercortisolism and hypocortisolism. It is worth noting that in all these areas, apart from CRH neurons of the PVH, glucocorticoids have either a stimulatory or a neutral effect on CRH gene expression.[159] Hippocampal neurons are reduced in number by prolonged elevation of glucocorticoids during chronic stress.[158]

Neural Control

Significant physiologic or psychological stressors evoke an adaptive response that commonly includes activation of both the HPA axis and the sympathoadrenal axis. The end products of these pathways then help to mobilize resources to cope with the physiologic demands in emergency situations, acutely through the fight-or-flight response, and over the long term through systemic effects of glucocorticoids on functions such as gluconeogenesis and energy mobilization. The HPA axis also has unique stress-specific homeostatic roles, the best example being the role of glucocorticoids in downregulating immune responses after infection and other events that stimulate cytokine production by the immune system.

The PVH is the primary hypothalamic nucleus responsible for providing the integrated whole-animal response to stress.[159,163,164] This nucleus contains within it three major types of effector neurons that are spatially distinct from one another: magnicellular oxytocin and AVP neurons that project to the posterior pituitary and participate in the regulation of blood pressure, fluid homeostasis, lactation, and parturition; neurons projecting to the brainstem and spinal cord that regulate a variety of autonomic responses including sympathoadrenal activation; and parvicellular CRH neurons that project to the median eminence and regulate ACTH synthesis and release. Many CRH neurons coexpress AVP, which acts synergistically with CRH by activating the V1b receptor subtype on corticotrophs. AVP is regulated quite differently in parvicellular versus magnicellular neurons but is also regulated somewhat differently from CRH by stressors in parvicellular cells that express both peptides.[159] Different stressors result in different patterns of activation of the three major visceromotor cell groups within the PVH, as measured by the general neuronal activation marker c-Fos (Fig. 7-16). For example, salt

loading downregulates CRH mRNA in parvicellular CRH cells, upregulates CRH in a small number of magnicellular CRH cells, but consistently activates magnicellular cells. Hemorrhage activates every division of the PVH, whereas cytokine administration primarily activates parvicellular CRH cells with some minor activation of magnicellular and autonomic divisions.

The synthesis and release of AVP, which regulates renal water absorption and vascular smooth muscle, are controlled mainly by the volume and tonicity of the blood. This information is relayed to the magnicellular AVP cell through the NTS and A1 noradrenergic cell group of the ventrolateral medulla and projections from a triad of CVOs lining the third ventricle, the SFO, the medial preoptic nucleus (MePO), and OVLT. Oxytocin is primarily involved in reproductive functions, such as parturition, lactation, and milk ejection, although it is cosecreted with AVP in response to osmotic and volume challenges, and oxytocin cells receive direct projections from the NTS as well as from the SFO, MePO, and OVLT. In contrast to the neurosecretory neurons functionally defined by the three peptides, CRH, oxytocin, and AVP, PVH neurons projecting to brainstem and spinal cord include neurons expressing each of these peptides.

In the rodent, a wide variety of stressors have been determined to activate parvicellular CRH neurons, including cytokine injection, salt loading, hemorrhage, adrenalectomy, restraint, foot shock, hypoglycemia, fasting, and ether exposure. In contrast to the relative simplicity of inputs to magnicellular cells (Fig. 7-17A), parvicellular CRH neurons receive a diverse and complex assortment of inputs (Fig. 7-18; see Fig. 7-17B). These inputs are divided into three major categories: brainstem, limbic forebrain, and hypothalamus. Because the PVH is not known to receive any direct projections from the cerebral cortex or thalamus, stressors involving emotional or cognitive processing must involve indirect relay to the PVH.

Visceral sensory input to the PVH involves primarily two pathways. The NTS, the primary recipient of sensory information from the thoracic and abdominal viscera, sends dense catecholaminergic projections to the PVH, both directly and through relays in the ventrolateral medulla. These brainstem projections account for about half of the NPY fibers present in the PVH. A second major input responsible for transducing signals from blood-borne substances derives from three CVOs adjacent to the third ventricle, the SFO, OVLT, and MePO. These pathways account for activation of CRH neurons by what are referred to as *systemic* or *physiologic stressors*.[164]

By contrast, what are termed *neurogenic, emotional*, or *psychological* stressors involve, in addition, nociceptive or somatosensory pathways as well as cognitive and affective brain centers. Using elevation of c-Fos as an indicator of neuronal activation, detailed studies have compared PVH-projecting neurons activated by IL-1 treatment (systemic stressor) versus foot shock (neurogenic stressor).[164] Only catecholaminergic solitary tract nucleus and ventrolateral medulla neurons were activated by moderate doses of IL-1. In contrast, foot shock activated neurons of the NTS and ventrolateral medulla but also cell groups in the limbic forebrain and hypothalamus. Notably, pharmacologic or mechanical disruption of the ascending catecholaminergic fibers blocked IL-1–mediated activation but not foot shock–mediated activation of the HPA axis. Data suggest that pathways activated by other neurogenic and systemic stressors may overlap significantly with those activated by foot shock and IL-1 treatment, respectively.[163,164]

Except for the catecholaminergic neurons of the NTS and ventrolateral medulla, parts of the bed nucleus of the

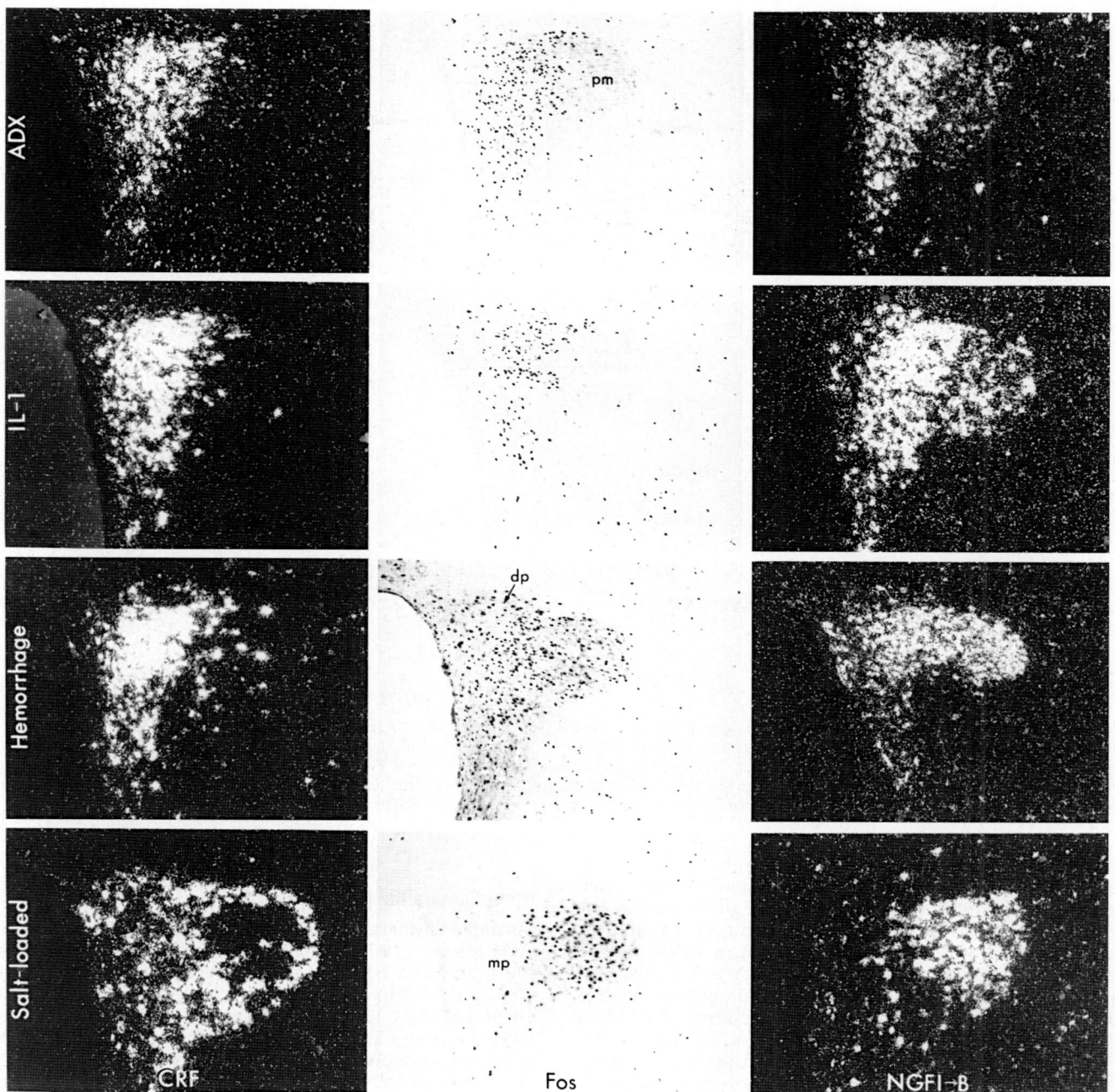

Figure 7-16 Regulation of neurons of the paraventricular nucleus (PVH) by diverse stressors. ADX, adrenalectomy; CRF, corticotropin-releasing factor in situ hybridization *(dark-field)*; dp, dorsal parvicellular; Fos, c-Fos immunoreactivity *(bright-field)*; IL-1, interleukin 1; mp, medial parvicellular; NGF1-β, nerve growth factor 1-β in situ hybridization *(dark-field)*; pm, posterior magnicellular. (From Sawchenko PE, Brown ER, Chan RK, et al. The paraventricular nucleus of the hypothalamus and the functional neuroanatomy of visceromotor responses to stress. *Prog Brain Res.* 1996;107:201-222.)

stria terminalis (BST), and the dorsomedial nucleus of the hypothalamus, many inputs to the PVH, such as those deriving from the prefrontal cortex and lateral septum, are thought to act indirectly through local hypothalamic glutamatergic[165] and GABAergic neurons[166] with direct synapses to the CRH neurons. The BST is the only limbic region with prominent direct projections to the PVH. With substantial projections from the amygdala, hippocampus, and septal nuclei, it may thus serve as a key integrative center for transmission of limbic information to the PVH.[163]

Inflammation and Cytokines

Stimulation of the immune system by foreign pathogens leads to a stereotyped set of responses orchestrated by the CNS. This constellation of stereotyped responses results from the complex interaction of the immune system and the CNS. They are mediated in large part by the hypothalamus and include coordinated autonomic, endocrine, and behavioral components with adapative consequences to restore homeostasis. It is now clear that cytokines produced by peripheral circulating cells of the immune system and

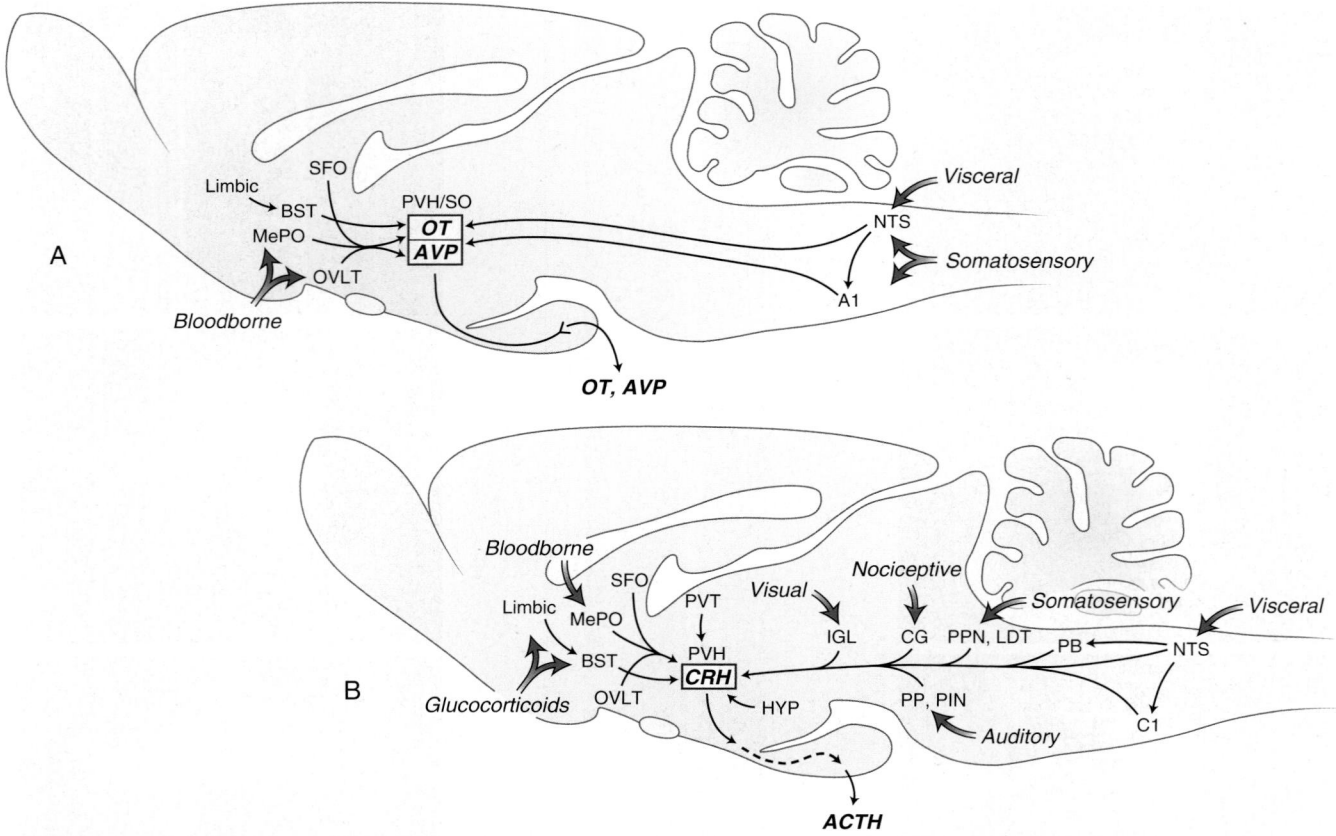

Figure 7-17 A, Neuronal inputs to magnicellular and, **B,** parvicellular neurons of the paraventricular nucleus (PVH). AVP, arginine vasopressin; BST, bed nucleus of the stria terminalis; CG, central gray; CRH, corticotropin-releasing hormone; HYP, hypothalamus; IGL, intergeniculate leaflet; LDT, laterodorsal tegmental nucleus; MePO, medial preoptic nucleus; NTS, nucleus of the tractus solitarius; OT, oxytocin; OVLT, organum vasculosum of the lamina terminalis; PB, parabrachial nucleus; PIN, posterior intralaminar nucleus; PP, peripeduncular nucleus; PPN, pedunculopontine nucleus; SFO, subfornical organ; SO, supraoptic nucleus. (From Sawchenko PE, Brown ER, Chan RK, et al. The paraventricular nucleus of the hypothalamus and the functional neuroanatomy of visceromotor responses to stress. *Prog Brain Res.* 1996;107:201-222.)

central glial cells mediate the CNS responses. Early evidence supporting this hypothesis was provided by the seminal observations that cytokines such as IL-1β can activate the HPA axis.[167-169] The resultant glucocorticoid secretion acts as a classical negative feedback to the immune system to dampen its response. In general, glucocorticoids inhibit most limbs of the immune response, including lymphocyte proliferation, production of immunoglobulins, cytokines, and cytotoxicity. These inhibitory reactions form the basis of the anti-inflammatory actions of glucocorticoids.

Glucocorticoid feedback on immune responses is regulatory and beneficial because loss of this function makes animals with adrenal insufficiency vulnerable to inflammation. However, this feedback response can have pathophysiologic consequences, as chronic activation of the HPA axis can certainly be detrimental.[170] Indeed, it is well established that chronic stress can lead to immunosuppression. The fact that products of inflammation such as IL-1β can activate the HPA axis suggests the operation of a negative feedback control loop to regulate the intensity of inflammation. The role of the hypothalamus in regulating pituitary-adrenal function is an excellent example of neuroimmunomodulation. Proposed models to explain how immune system signals might act upon the CNS to modulate homeostatic circuits by the integration of vagal input, peripheral cytokine interactions with receptors in the CVOs and cerebral blood vessels, and local production of cytokines within the CNS are explored in Chapter 35.

Other Factors Influencing Secretion of Corticotropin

Circadian Rhythms. Levels of ACTH and cortisol peak in the early morning, fall during the day to reach a nadir at about midnight, and begin to rise between 1 AM and 4 AM (see Fig. 7-7). Within the circadian cycle approximately 15 to 18 pulses of ACTH can be discerned, their height varying with the time of day.[171] The set-point of feedback control by glucocorticoids also varies in a circadian pattern. Pituitary-adrenal rhythms are entrained to the light-dark cycle and can be changed over several days by exposure to an altered light schedule. It has long been assumed that the rhythm of ACTH secretion is driven by CRH rhythms, and CRH knockout mice were found to exhibit no circadian rhythm in corticosterone production. Remarkably, however, a diurnal rhythm in corticosterone was restored by a constant infusion of CRH to CRH knockout mice,[172] suggesting that CRH is necessary to permit pituitary or adrenal responsiveness to another diurnal rhythm generator.

Growth Hormone–Releasing Hormone
Chemistry and Evolution

Evidence for neural control of GH secretion originated from studies of its regulation in animals with lesions of the hypothalamus and from the demonstration that hypothalamic extracts stimulate the release of GH from the pituitary. When it was shown that GH is released episodically,

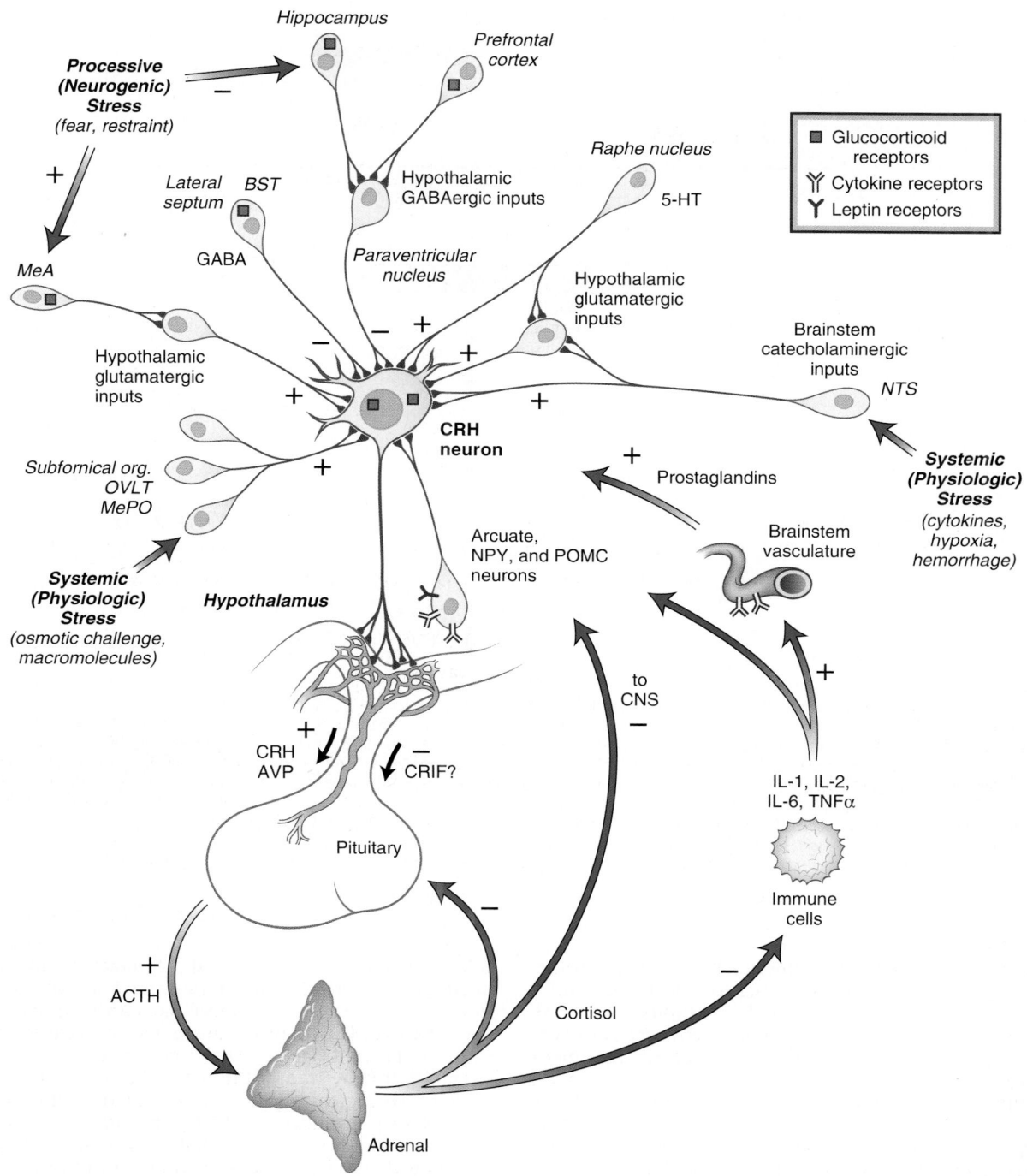

Figure 7-18 Regulation of the hypothalamic-pituitary-adrenal axis. ACTH, adrenocorticotropic hormone; AVP, arginine vasopressin; BST, bed nucleus of the stria terminalis; CNS, central nervous system; CRH, corticotropin-releasing hormone; CRIF, corticotropin release–inhibiting factor; GABA, γ-aminobutyric acid; 5-HT, 5-hydroxytryptamine; IL-1, interleukin 1; MeA, medial amygdala; MePO, medial preoptic nucleus; NPY, neuropeptide Y; NTS, nucleus of the tractus solitarius; OVLT, organum vasculosum of the lamina terminalis; POMC, pro-opiomelanocortin; TNF-α, tumor necrosis factor-α.

follows a circadian rhythm, responds rapidly to stress, and is blocked by pituitary stalk section, the concept of neural control of GH secretion became a certainty. However, it was only with the discovery of the paraneoplastic syndrome of ectopic GHRH secretion by pancreatic adenomas in humans that sufficient starting material became available for peptide sequencing and subsequent cloning of a complementary deoxyribonucleic acid (cDNA).[173-175]

Two principal molecular forms of GHRH occur in human hypothalamus: GHRH(1-44)-NH$_2$ and GHRH(1-40)-OH

(Fig. 7-19).[176] As with other neuropeptides, the various forms of GHRH arise from post-translational modification of a larger prohormone.[173] The NH$_2$-terminal tyrosine of GHRH (or histidine in rodent GHRHs) is essential for bioactivity, but a COOH-terminal NH$_2$ group is not. A circulating type IV dipeptidylpeptidase potently inactivates GHRH to its principal and more stable metabolite, GHRH(3-44)-NH$_2$,[177] which accounts for most of the immunoreactive peptide detected in plasma. As in the case of GnRH, there are species differences among GHRHs; the peptides

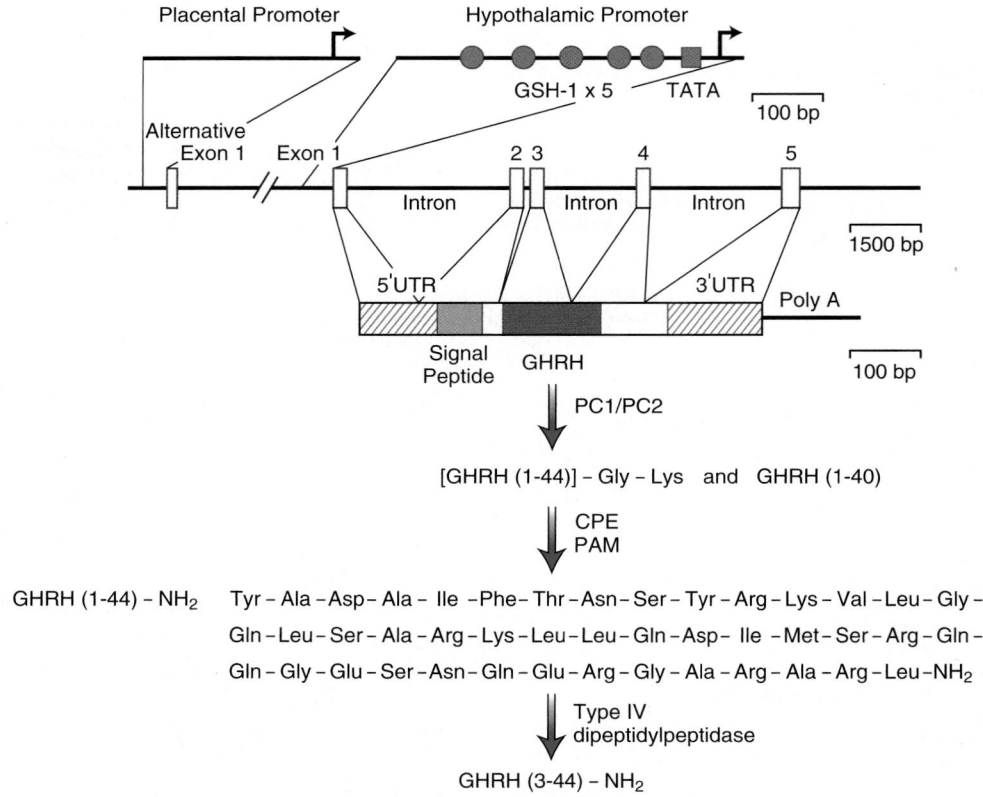

Figure 7-19 Diagram illustrating the genomic organization, messenger RNA structure, and post-translational processing of the human growth hormone–releasing hormone (GHRH) prohormone. Five GSH-1 homeodomain transcription factor-binding sites in the proximal promoter have been characterized in the rat gene. All of the amino acid residues required for bioactive GHRH peptides are encoded by exon 3. An amino-terminal exopeptidase that cleaves the Tyr-Ala dipeptide is primarily responsible for the inactivation of GHRH peptides in extracellular compartments. CPE, carboxypeptidase E; PAM, peptidylglycine α-amidating monooxygenase; PC1/PC2, prohormone convertases 1 and 2; TATA, Goldstein-Hogness box involved in binding RNA polymerase; UTR, untranslated region. (Compiled from data of Mayo KE, Cerelli GM, Lebo RV, et al. Gene encoding human growth hormone-releasing factor precursor: structure, sequence, and chromosomal assignment. *Proc Natl Acad Sci U S A.* 1985;82:63-67; Frohman LA, Downs TR, Chomczynski P, et al. Growth hormone-releasing hormone: structure, gene expression and molecular heterogeneity. *Acta Paediatr Scand Suppl.* 1990;367:81-86; González-Crespo S, Boronat A. Expression of the rat growth hormone-releasing hormone gene in placenta is directed by an alternative promoter. *Proc Natl Acad Sci U S A.* 1991;88:8749-8753; and Mutsuga N, Iwasaki Y, Morishita M, et al. Homeobox protein Gsh-1-dependent regulation of the rat GHRH gene promoter. *Mol Endocrinol.* 2001;15:2149-2156.)

from seven species range in sequence homology with the human peptide from 93% in the pig to 67% in the rat.[176] The COOH-terminal end of GHRH exhibits the most sequence diversity among species, consistent with the exon arrangement of the gene and dispensability of these residues for GHRH receptor binding.

Despite its importance for the elucidation of GHRH structure, ectopic secretion of the peptide is a rare cause of acromegaly.[178] Fewer than 1% of acromegalic patients have elevated plasma levels of GHRH (see Chapters 8 and 9). Approximately 20% of pancreatic adenomas and 5% of carcinoid tumors contain immunoreactive GHRH, but most are clinically silent.[179]

In addition to expression in the hypothalamus, the *GHRH* gene is expressed eutopically in human ovary, uterus, and placenta,[180] although its function in these tissues is not known. Studies in rat placenta indicate that an alternative transcriptional start site 10 kilobases upstream from the hypothalamic promoter is utilized together with an alternatively spliced exon 1a.[181]

Growth Hormone–Releasing Hormone Receptor

The GHRH receptor is a member of a subfamily of GPCRs that includes receptors for VIP, pituitary adenylyl cyclase–activating peptide, secretin, glucagon, glucagon-like pep-

tide 1, calcitonin, parathyroid hormone or parathyroid hormone–related peptide, and gastric inhibitory polypeptide.[182] GHRH elevates intracellular cAMP by its receptor coupling to a G_s, which activates adenylyl cyclase, increases intracellular free Ca^{2+}, releases preformed GH, and stimulates GH mRNA transcription and new GH synthesis.[183] GHRH also increases pituitary phosphatidylinositol turnover. Nonsense mutations in the human GHRH receptor gene are the cause of rare familial forms of GH deficiency[184] and indicate that no other gene product can fully compensate for the specific receptor in pituitary.

Effects on the Pituitary and Mechanism of Action

Intravenous administration of GHRH to individuals with normal pituitaries causes a prompt, dose-related increase in serum GH that peaks after 15 to 45 minutes, followed by a return to basal levels by 90 to 120 minutes (Fig. 7-20).[185] A maximally stimulating dose of GHRH is approximately 1 μg/kg, but the response differs considerably among individuals and within the same individual tested on different occasions, presumably because of endogenous cosecretagogue and somatostatin tone that exists at the time of GHRH injection. Repeated bolus administration or sustained infusions of GHRH over several hours cause a modest decrease in the subsequent GH secretory response

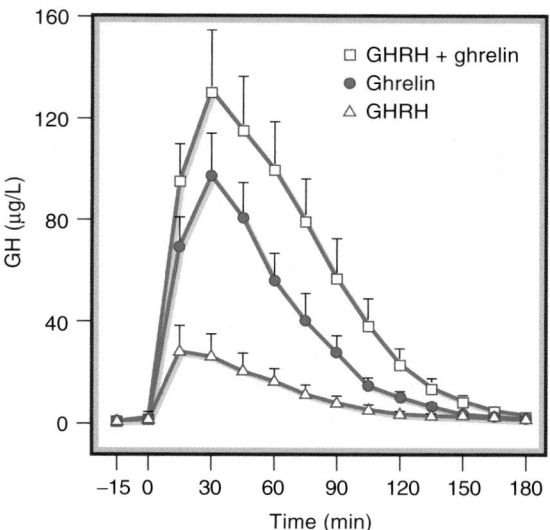

Figure 7-20 Response of normal men to growth hormone–releasing hormone (GHRH)(1-29) (1 µg/kg), ghrelin (1 µg/kg), or the combination of GHRH(1-29) and ghrelin administered by intravenous injection. Note the prompt release of GH, followed by a rather prolonged fall in hormone level in response to both secretagogues. Ghrelin alone was more efficacious than GHRH(1-29), and there was an additive effect from the two peptides administered simultaneously. (From Arvat E, Macario M, Di Vito L, et al. Endocrine activities of ghrelin, a natural growth hormone secretagogue (GHS), in humans: comparison and interactions with hexarelin, a nonnatural peptidyl GHS, and GH-releasing hormone. *J Clin Endocrinol Metab.* 2001;86:1169-1174.)

to acute GHRH administration. However, unlike the marked desensitization of the GnRH receptor and decline in circulating gonadotropins that occur in response to continuous GnRH exposure, pulsatile GH secretion and insulin-like growth factor 1 (IGF-1) production are maintained by constant GHRH in the human.[185] This response suggests the involvement of additional factors that mediate the intrinsic diurnal rhythm of GH, and these factors are addressed in the following sections.

The pituitary effects of a single injection of GHRH are almost completely specific for GH secretion, and there is minimal evidence for any interaction between GHRH and the other classical hypophyseotropic releasing hormones.[185] GHRH has no effect on gut peptide hormone secretion. The GH secretory response to GHRH is enhanced by estrogen administration, glucocorticoids, and starvation. Major factors known to blunt the response to GHRH in humans are somatostatin, obesity, and advancing age.

In addition to its role as a GH secretagogue, GHRH is a physiologically relevant growth factor for somatotrophs. Transgenic mice expressing a GHRH cDNA coupled to a suitable promoter developed diffuse somatotroph hyperplasia and eventually pituitary macroadenomas.[186] The intracellular signal transduction pathways mediating the mitogenic action of GHRH are not known with certainty but probably involve an elevation of adenylyl cyclase activity. Several lines of evidence support this conclusion, including the association of activating mutations of the $G_s\alpha$ polypeptide in many human somatotroph adenomas.[187]

Extrapituitary Functions

GHRH has few known extrapituitary functions. The most important may be its activity as a sleep regulator. The administration of nocturnal GHRH boluses to normal men

significantly increases the density of slow-wave sleep, as also shown in other species.[188] Furthermore, there is a striking correlation between the age-related declines in slow-wave sleep and daily integrated GH secretion in healthy men.[189] These and other data suggest that central GHRH secretion is under circadian entrainment and nocturnal elevations in GHRH pulse amplitude or frequency directly mediate sleep stage and sleep-induced increases in GH secretion.

GHRH has been reported to stimulate food intake in rats and sheep, but the effect is dependent on route of administration, time of administration, and macronutrient composition of the diet.[182] The neuropeptide's physiologic relevance to feeding in humans is unknown. Evidence suggests that nonpituitary GHRH modulates cell proliferation and promotes healing of skin wounds.[190]

Growth Hormone–Releasing Peptides

In studies of the opioid control of GH secretion, several peptide analogues of met-enkephalin were found to be potent GH secretagogues. These include the GH-releasing peptide GHRP-6 (Fig. 7-21), hexarelin (His-D2MeTrp-Ala-Trp-DPhe-Lys-NH$_2$), and other more potent analogues including cyclic peptides and modified pentapeptides.[182,191] Subsequently, a series of nonpeptidyl GHRP mimetics were synthesized with greater oral bioavailability, including the spiropiperidine MK-0677 and the shorter acting benzylpiperidine L-163,540 (see Fig. 7-21). Common to all these compounds, and the basis of their differentiation from GHRH analogues in pharmacologic activity screens, is their activation of phospholipase C and inositol 1,4,5-trisphosphate. This property was exploited in a cloning strategy that led to the identification of a novel GPCR GHS-R that is highly selective for the GH secretagogue class of ligands.[192] The GHS-R is unrelated to the GHRH receptor and is highly expressed in the anterior pituitary gland and multiple brain areas, including the medial basal hypothalamus, the hippocampus, and the mesencephalic nuclei that are centers of dopamine and serotonin production.

Peptidyl and nonpeptidyl GHSs are active when administered by intranasal and oral routes, are more potent on a weight basis than GHRH itself, are more effective in vivo than in vitro, synergize with coadministered GHRH and are almost ineffective in the absence of GHRH, and do not suppress somatostatin secretion.[182,185] Prolonged infusions of GHRP amplify pulsatile GH secretion in normal men. GHRP administration, like that of GHRH, facilitates slow-wave sleep. Patients with hypothalamic disease leading to GHRH deficiency have low or no response to hexarelin; similarly, pediatric patients with complete absence of the pituitary stalk have no GH secretory response to hexarelin.[193]

The potent biologic effects of GHRPs and the identification of the GHS-R suggested the existence of a natural ligand for the receptor that is involved in the physiologic regulation of GH secretion. The acylated peptide ghrelin, produced and secreted into the circulation from the stomach, is this ligand (Fig. 7-22).[12] The effects of ghrelin on GH secretion in humans are identical to or more potent than those of the non-natural GHRPs (see Fig. 7-20).[194] In addition, ghrelin acutely increases circulating PRL, ACTH, cortisol, and aldosterone levels.[194] There is debate concerning the extent and localization of ghrelin expression in the brain that must be resolved before the implications of gastric-derived ghrelin in the regulation of pituitary hormone secretion are fully understood. Furthermore, post-translational processing of pro-ghrelin gives rise to a second neuropeptide, obestatin, which may also have

GHRP-6: His–DTrp–Ala–Trp–DPhe–Lys–NH_2

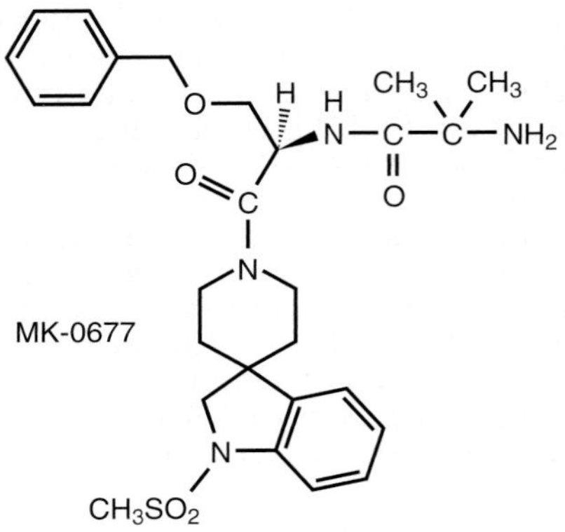

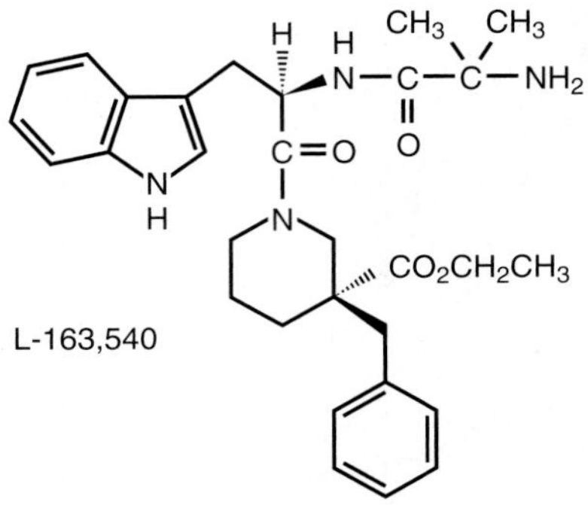

$O = C - (CH_2)_6 - CH_3$
|
O
|
Ghrelin: Gly - Ser - Ser - Phe - Leu - Ser - Pro - Glu - His - Gln - Arg - Val - Gln - Gln - Arg - Lys - Glu - Ser - Lys - Lys - Pro - Pro - Ala - Lys - Leu - Gln - Pro - Arg

Figure 7-21 Structure of a synthetic peptidyl growth hormone (GH) secretagogue (GH-releasing peptide 6, or GHRP-6) and nonpeptidyl growth hormone secretagogues (MK-0677 and L-163,540) and a natural ligand (ghrelin) that all bind and activate the growth hormone secretagogue (GHS) receptor. Ghrelin is an acylated 28–amino acid peptide. The *O-n*-octanoylation at Ser3 is essential for biologic activity and is a unique post-translational modification mediated enzymatically by ghrelin-*O*-acyltransferase (GOAT). (Adapted from Smith RG, Feighner S, Prendergast K, et al. A new orphan receptor involved in pulsatile growth hormone release. *Trends Endocrinol Metab.* 1999;10:128-135; Kojima M, Hosoda H, Date Y, et al. Ghrelin is a growth hormone-releasing acylated peptide from stomach. *Nature.* 1999;402:656-660.)

functional roles in activity of the GH/IGF-1 axis and metabolism.[195] A proposed role for pro-ghrelin peptides in appetite and the regulation of food intake is discussed in Chapter 35.

Clinical Applications

GHRH stimulates growth in children with intact pituitaries, but the optimal dosage, route, and frequency of administration, as well as possible usefulness by the nasal route, have not been determined. The availability of recombinant hGH (which requires less frequent injections than GHRH) and the development of the more potent GHSs with improved oral bioavailability have reduced enthusiasm for the clinical use of GHRH or its analogues. GHRH is not useful for the differential diagnosis of hypothalamic and pituitary causes of GH deficiency in children. Controversy remains concerning the ideal challenge test for the diagnosis of GH reserve in adults. GH release in response to the combination of GHRH and a GHRP is not influenced by age, sex, or body mass index, and the test has a wider margin of safety than an insulin tolerance test.[196] Others consider the combination of GHRH and arginine to be robust, but neither of these tests is relevant in the United States owing to the unavailability of GHRH.[197]

The potential clinical applications of GHSs including MK-0677 are still being explored.[182,191] An area of intense interest is the normal decline in GH secretion with age. GH administration in healthy older individuals has been associated with increased lean body mass, increased muscle strength, and decreased fat mass, although there is a high incidence of adverse side effects. The physiologic GH profile induced by MK-0677 may be better tolerated than GH injections. However, unlike treatment with GHRH, chronic administration of GHSs leads to significant desensitization of the GHS-R and attenuation of the GH response. The release of pituitary hormones other than GH may also limit the applicability of GHS therapy. Finally, apart from actions on GH secretion, both GHRH and GHSs are being investigated for the treatment of sleep disorders commonly associated with aging.

Neuroendocrine Regulation of Growth Hormone Secretion

GH secretion is regulated by hypothalamic GHRH and somatostatin interacting with circulating hormones and additional modulatory peptides at the level of both the pituitary and the hypothalamus (see Fig. 7-22).[182,185,195,198-200] Additional background on somatostatin and its functions other than control of GH secretion are presented in a later section (see "Somatostatin").

Feedback Control

Negative feedback control of GH release is mediated by GH itself and by IGF-1, which is synthesized in the liver and other tissues under the control of GH. Direct GH effects on the hypothalamus are produced by short-loop feedback, whereas those involving IGF-1 and other circulating factors influenced by GH, including free fatty acids and glucose, are long-loop systems analogous to the pituitary-thyroid and pituitary-adrenal axes. Control of GH secretion therefore includes two closed-loop systems (GH and IGF-1) and one open-loop regulatory system (neural).

Although most of the evidence for a direct role of GH in its own negative feedback has been derived from animals, an elegant study in normal men demonstrated that GH pretreatment blocks the subsequent GH secretory response to GHRH by a mechanism that is dependent on somatostatin.[201] The mechanism responsible for GH feedback through

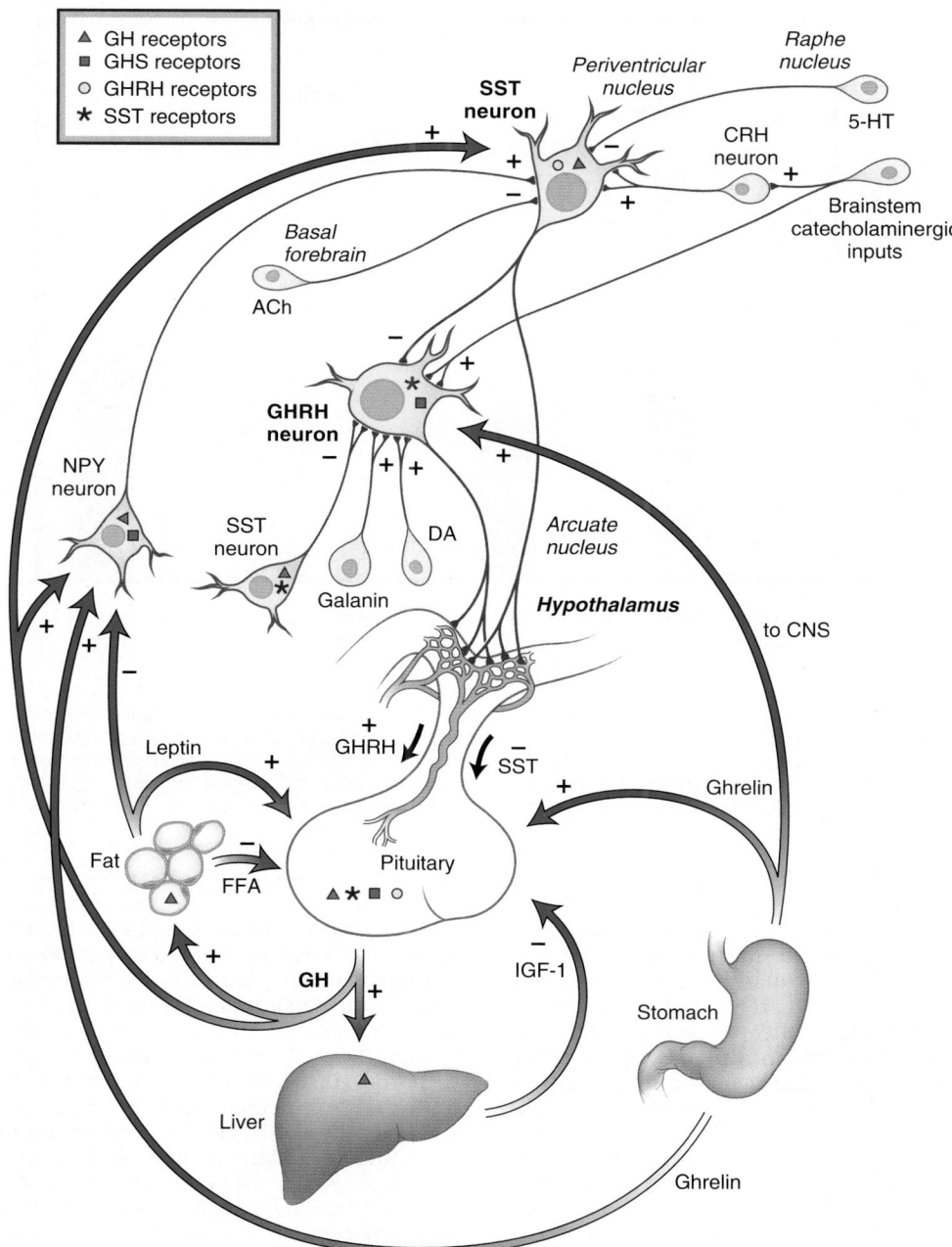

Figure 7-22 Regulation of the hypothalamic-pituitary-growth hormone (GH) axis. GH secretion by the pituitary is stimulated by GH-releasing hormone (GHRH) and is inhibited by somatostatin (SST). Negative feedback control of GH secretion is exerted at the pituitary level by insulin-like growth factor 1 (IGF-1) and by free fatty acids (FFA). GH itself exerts a short-loop negative feedback through activation of SST neurons in the hypothalamic periventricular nucleus. These SST neurons directly synapse on arcuate GHRH neurons and project axon collaterals to the median eminence. Neuropeptide Y (NPY) neurons in the arcuate nucleus also indirectly modulate GH secretion by integrating peripheral GH, leptin, and ghrelin signals and projecting to periventricular SST neurons. Ghrelin is secreted from the stomach and is a natural ligand for the GH secretagogue (GHS) receptor that stimulates GH secretion at both the hypothalamic and pituitary levels. On the basis of indirect pharmacologic data, it appears that release of GHRH is stimulated by galanin, γ-aminobutyric acid (GABA), α_2-adrenergic and dopaminergic inputs and inhibited by SST. Secretion of SST is inhibited by muscarinic acetylcholine (ACh) and 5-HT-1D receptor ligands, and increased by β_2-adrenergic stimuli and corticotropin-releasing hormone (CRH). CNS, central nervous system; DA, dopamine; 5-HT, serotonin (5-hydroxytryptamine).

the hypothalamus has been largely elucidated in rodent models. GH receptors are selectively expressed on somatostatin neurons in the hypothalamic periventricular nucleus and on NPY neurons in the arcuate nucleus. C-Fos gene expression is acutely elevated in both populations of GH receptor–positive neurons by GH administration, indicating an activation of hypothalamic circuitry that includes these neurons. Similarly, GHRH neurons in the arcuate nucleus are acutely activated by MK-0677 because of their

selective expression of the GHS-R. Zheng and colleagues[202] showed in the latter group of neurons that c-Fos induction after MK-0677 administration was blocked by pretreatment of mice with GH (Fig. 7-23). The effect must be indirect because there are no GH receptors on GHRH neurons. However, type 2 somatostatin receptors are expressed on GHRH neurons, and the somatostatin analogue octreotide also significantly blocked c-Fos activation in the arcuate nucleus by MK-0677. The inhibitory effects of either GH

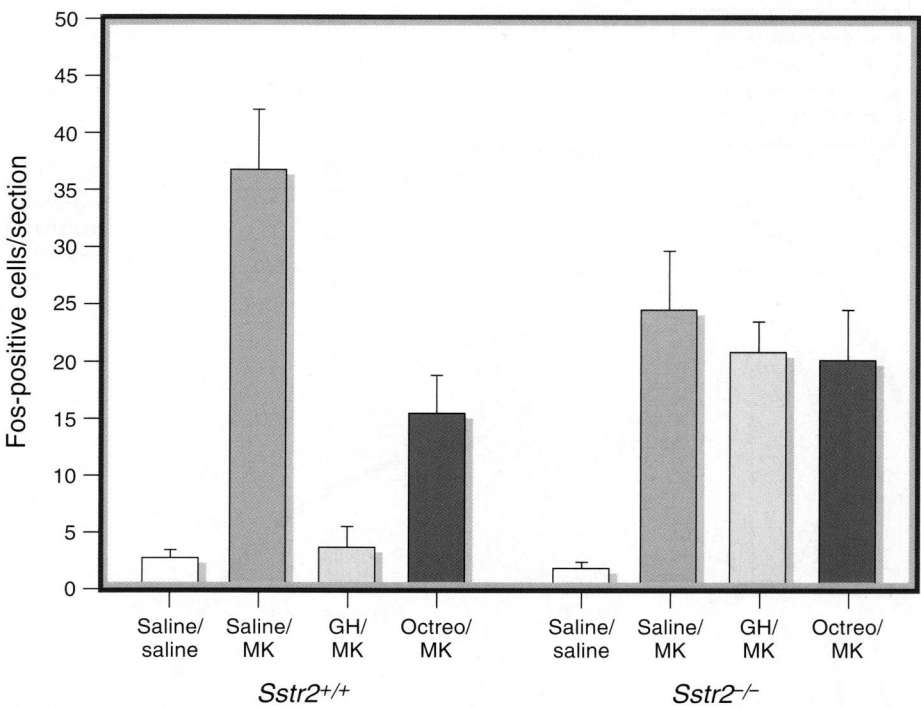

Figure 7-23 Somatostatin and the somatostatin receptor 2 subtype are involved in the short-loop inhibitory feedback of growth hormone (GH) on arcuate neurons. Activation of neurons in the arcuate nucleus was determined by the quantification of immunoreactive Fos-positive cells after administration of the growth hormone secretagogue MK-0677 (MK). Preliminary treatment of wild-type mice *(Sstr2+/+)* with either GH or the somatostatin analogue octreotide (Octreo) significantly attenuated the neuronal activation by MK-0677. In contrast, GH and octreotide had no effect on MK-0677 neuronal activation in somatostatin receptor 2-deficient mice *(Sstr2−/−)*. (Adapted from Zheng H, Bailey A, Jian M-H, et al. Somatostatin receptor subtype 2 knockout mice are refractory to growth hormone-negative feedback on arcuate neurons. *Mol Endocrinol.* 1997;11: 1709-1717.)

or octreotide pretreatment were abolished in knockout mice lacking the specific somatostatin receptor (see Fig. 7-23). Together with data from many other experiments, these results strongly support a model of GH negative feedback regulation that involves the primary activation of periventricular somatostatin neurons by GH. These tuberoinfundibular dopaminergic (TIDA) neurons then inhibit GH secretion directly by release of somatostatin in the median eminence, but they also indirectly inhibit GH secretion by way of collateral axonal projections to the arcuate nucleus that synapse on and inhibit GHRH neurons (see Fig. 7-22). It is probable from evidence in rodents that NPY and galanin also play a part in the short-loop feedback of GH secretion, but a definitive mechanism in humans is not yet established.

IGF-1 has a major inhibitory action on GH secretion at the level of the pituitary gland.[182] IGF-1 receptors are expressed on human somatotroph adenoma cells and inhibit both spontaneous and GHRH-stimulated GH release. In addition, gene expression of both GH and the pituitary-specific transcription factor PIT1 is inhibited by IGF-1. Conflicting data among species suggest that circulating IGF-1 may also regulate GH secretion by actions within the brain. The feedback effects of IGF-1 account for the fact that serum GH levels are elevated in conditions in which circulating levels of IGF-1 are low, such as anorexia nervosa, protein-calorie starvation,[203] and Laron dwarfism (the result of a defect in the GH receptor).

Neural Control

The predominant hypothalamic influence on GH release is stimulatory, and transection of the pituitary stalk or lesions of the basal hypothalamus cause reduction of basal and induced GH release.[182] When the somatostatinergic component is inactivated (e.g., by antisomatostatin antibody injection in rats), basal GH levels and GH responses to the usual provocative stimuli are enhanced.

GHRH-containing nerve fibers that terminate adjacent to portal vessels in the external zone of the median eminence arise principally from within, above, and lateral to the infundibular nucleus in human hypothalamus, corresponding to rodent arcuate and ventromedial nuclei.[204] Perikarya of the TIDA somatostatin neurons are located almost completely in the medial periventricular nucleus and parvicellular component of the anterior PVH.

Multiple extrahypothalamic brain regions provide efferent connections to the hypothalamus and regulate GHRH and somatostatin neuronal activity (Fig. 7-24; see Fig. 7-22). Somatosensory and affective information is integrated and filtered through the amygdaloid complex. The basolateral amygdala provides an excitatory input to the hypothalamus, and the central extended amygdala, which includes the central and medial nuclei of the amygdala together with the BST, provides a GABAergic inhibitory input. Many intrinsic neurons of the hypothalamus also release GABA, often with a peptide cotransmitter. Excitatory cholinergic fibers arise to a small extent from forebrain projection nuclei but mostly from hypothalamic cholinergic interneurons, which densely innervate the external zone of the median eminence. Similarly, the origin of dopaminergic and histaminergic neurons is local with their cell bodies located in the hypothalamic arcuate and tuberomammillary bodies, respectively. Two important ascending pathways to the medial basal hypothalamus regulate GH secretion and originate from serotoninergic

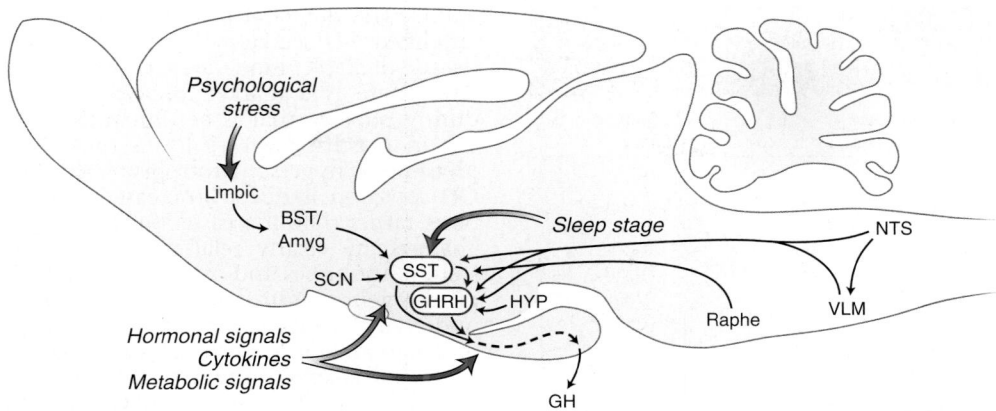

Figure 7-24 Neural pathways involved in growth hormone (GH) regulation. This diagram illustrates the varied pathways by which impulses from the limbic system and brainstem ultimately impinge on the hypothalamic periventricular and arcuate nuclei to regulate GH release by opposing effects of somatostatin (SST) and growth hormone–releasing hormone (GHRH). Psychological stress modulates hypothalamic function indirectly through the bed nucleus of the stria terminalis (BST) and amygdalar complex (Amyg). Circadian rhythms are entrained in part by projections from the suprachiasmatic nucleus (SCN). Cortex and subcortical nuclei are involved in complex reciprocal interactions between sleep stage and GHRH release, but the detailed mechanisms are not known. Dopaminergic and histaminergic afferents originate from neurons located in the arcuate and mammillary nuclei, respectively, of the hypothalamus (HYP). Ascending catecholaminergic projections arise in both the nucleus of the tractus solitarius (NTS) and ventral lateral medulla (VLM). Serotoninergic (5-HT) afferents are from the raphe nuclei. In addition to these neural pathways, a variety of peripheral hormonal and metabolic signals and cytokines influence GH secretion by actions within the medial basal hypothalamus and pituitary gland.

neurons in the raphe nuclei and adrenergic neurons in the NTS and ventral lateral nucleus of the medulla.

Both GHRH and somatostatin neurons express presynaptic and postsynaptic receptors for multiple neurotransmitters and peptides (Table 7-4). The α_2-adrenoreceptor agonist clonidine reliably stimulates GH release, and for this reason a clonidine test was a standard diagnostic tool in pediatric endocrinology. The stimulatory effect is blocked by the specific α_2-antagonist yohimbine and appears to involve a dual mechanism of action, inhibition of somatostatin neurons and activation of GHRH neurons. In addition, partial attenuation of the effects of clonidine by mixed serotonin 5-HT1 and 5-HT2 antagonists suggests that some of the relevant α_2-receptors are located presynaptically on serotoninergic nerve terminals and increase serotonin release. Both norepinephrine and epinephrine play physiologic roles in the adrenergic stimulation of GH secretion. The α_1-agonists have no effect on GH secretion in humans, but β_2-agonists such as the bronchodilator salbutamol inhibit GH secretion by stimulating the release of somatostatin from nerve terminals in the median eminence. These effects are blocked by propranolol, a nonspecific β-receptor antagonist. Dopamine generally has a net effect to stimulate GH secretion, but the mechanism is not clear because of multiple dopamine receptor subtypes and the apparent activation of both GHRH and somatostatin neurons.

Serotonin's effect on GH release in humans was difficult to decipher because of the large number of receptor subtypes. However, clinical studies with the receptor-selective agonist sumatriptan clearly implicated the 5-HT1D receptor subtype in the stimulation of basal GH levels.[205] The drug also potentiates the effect of a maximal dose of GHRH, suggesting the recurring theme of GH disinhibition by inhibition of hypothalamic somatostatin neurons in its mechanism of action. Histaminergic pathways acting through H1 receptors play only a minor, conditional stimulatory role in GH secretion in humans.

Acetylcholine appears to be an important physiologic regulator of GH secretion.[206] Blockade of muscarinic acetylcholine receptors reduces or abolishes GH secretory responses to GHRH, glucagon and arginine, morphine, and exercise. In contrast, drugs that potentiate cholinergic

transmission increase basal GH levels and enhance the GH response to GHRH in normal individuals or in subjects with obesity or Cushing disease. In vitro acetylcholine inhibits somatostatin release from hypothalamic fragments, and acetylcholine can act directly on the pituitary to inhibit GH release. There may even be a paracrine cholinergic control system within the pituitary. However, the sum of evidence suggests that the primary mechanism of action of M1 agonists is inhibition of somatostatin neuronal activity or the release of peptide from somatostatinergic terminals. Short-term cholinergic blockade with the M1 muscarinic receptor antagonist pirenzepine reduced the GH excess of patients with poorly controlled diabetes mellitus.[207] However, in the long term, cholinergic blockade did not prevent complications associated with the hypersomatotropic state.

Many neuropeptides in addition to GHRH and somatostatin are involved in the modulation of GH secretion in humans (see Table 7-4).[182,185] Among these, the evidence is most compelling for a stimulatory role of galanin acting in the human hypothalamus by a GHRH-dependent mechanism.[208] Many GHRH neurons are immunopositive for galanin as well as neurotensin and tyrosine hydroxylase. Galanin's actions may be explained, in part, by presynaptic facilitation of catecholamine release from nerve terminals and subsequent direct adrenergic stimulation of GHRH release.[209] Opioid peptides also stimulate GH release, probably by disinhibition of GHRH neurons, but under normal circumstances endogenous opioid tone in the hypothalamus is presumed to be low because opioid antagonists have little acute effect on GH secretion.

A larger number of neuropeptides are known or suspected to inhibit GH secretion in humans, at least under certain circumstances.[185] The list includes NPY, CRH, calcitonin, oxytocin, neurotensin, VIP, and TRH. Inhibitory actions of NPY are well established in the rat. The effect on GH secretion is secondary to stimulation of somatostatin neurons and is of particular interest because of the presumed role in GH autofeedback (discussed earlier) and the integration of GH secretion with regulation of energy intake and expenditure[200] (see "External and Metabolic Signals"). Finally, TRH has the well-established paradoxical effect of increasing GH secretion in patients with

TABLE 7-4

Factors That Change Growth Hormone (GH) Secretion in Humans

Physiologic Factors	Hormones and Neurotransmitters	Pathologic Factors
Stimulatory Factors		
Episodic, spontaneous release	Insulin hypoglycemia 2-Deoxyglucose Amino acid infusions	Acromegaly TRH GnRH
Exercise	Arginine, lysine	Glucose
Stress	Neuropeptides	Arginine
Physical	GHRH	Interleukins 1,
Psychological	Ghrelin	2, 6
Slow-wave sleep	Galanin	Protein depletion
Postprandial glucose decline	Opioids (μ-receptors) Melatonin	Starvation Anorexia
Fasting	Classic neurotransmitters	nervosa
	α$_2$-Adrenergic agonists	Renal failure
	β-Adrenergic antagonists	Liver cirrhosis
	M1 cholinergic agonists	Type 1 diabetes
	5-HT1D receptor agonists	mellitus
	H1 histamine agonists	
	GABA (basal levels)	
	Dopamine (? D$_2$ receptor)	
	Estrogen	
	Testosterone	
	Glucocorticoids (acute)	
Inhibitory Factors*		
Postprandial hyperglycemia	Glucose infusion Neuropeptides	Acromegaly L-Dopa
Elevated free fatty acids	Somatostatin Calcitonin	D$_2$ receptor DA agonists
Elevated GH levels	Neuropeptide Y (NPY[†])	Phentolamine
Elevated IGF-1 (pituitary)	CRH[†] Classic neurotransmitters	Galanin Obesity
REM sleep	α$_{1/2}$-Adrenergic	Hypothyroidism
Senescence, aging	antagonists	Hyperthyroidism
	β$_2$-Adrenergic agonists	
	H1 histamine antagonists	
	Serotonin antagonist	
	Nicotinic cholinergic agonists	
	Glucocorticoids (chronic)	

*In many instances, the inhibition can be demonstrated only as a suppression of GH release induced by a pharmacologic stimulus.
[†]The inhibitory actions of NPY and CRH on GH secretion are firmly established in the rodent and are secondary to increased somatostatin tone. Contradictory evidence exists in the human for both peptides, and further studies are required.
CRH, corticotropin-releasing hormone; DA, dopamine; GABA, γ-aminobutyric acid; GHRH, growth hormone–releasing hormone; GnRH, gonadotropin-releasing hormone; IGF-1, insulin-like growth factor type 1; REM, rapid eye movement; TRH, thyrotropin-releasing hormone.

acromegaly, type 1 diabetes mellitus, hypothyroidism, or hepatic and renal failure.

Other Factors Influencing Secretion of Growth Hormone

Human Growth Hormone Rhythms. The deciphering of rhythmic GH secretion has relied on a combination of technical innovations in sampling and GH assay, and sophisticated mathematical modeling including deconvolution analysis and the calculation of approximate entropy as a measure of orderliness or regularity in minute-to-minute secretory patterns.[185] At least three distinct categories of GH rhythms, which differ markedly in their time scales, can be considered here.

The daily GH secretion rate varies over two orders of magnitude from a maximum of nearly 2.0 mg/day in late puberty to a minimum of 20 μg/day in older or obese adults. The neonatal period is characterized by markedly amplified GH secretory bursts followed by a prepubertal decade of stable, moderate GH secretion of 200 to 600 μg/day. There is a marked increase in daily GH secretion during puberty that is accompanied by a commensurate rise in plasma IGF-1 to levels that constitute a state of physiologic hypersomatotropism. This pubertal increase in GH secretion is due to increased GH mass per secretory burst rather than increased pulse frequency. Although the changes are clearly related to the increases in gonadal steroid hormones and can be mimicked by administration of estrogen or testosterone to hypogonadal children, the underlying neuroendocrine mechanisms are not fully understood. One hypothesis is that decreased sensitivity of the hypothalamic-pituitary axis to negative feedback of GH and IGF-1 leads to increased GHRH release and action. Young adults have a return of daily GH secretion to prepubertal levels despite continued gonadal steroid elevation. The so-called somatopause is defined by an exponential decline in GH secretory rate with a half-life of 7 years starting in the third decade of life.

GH secretion in young adults exhibits a true circadian rhythm over a 24-hour period, characterized by a greater nocturnal secretory mass that is independent of sleep onset.[210] However, as discussed earlier, GH release is further facilitated when slow-wave sleep coincides with the normal circadian peak. Under basal conditions GH levels are low most of the time, with an ultradian rhythm of about 10 secretory pulses per 24 hours in men (20 in women) as calculated by deconvolution analysis.[211] Both sexes have an increased pulse frequency during the nighttime hours, but the fraction of total daily GH secretion associated with the nocturnal pulses is much greater in men. Overall, women have more continuous GH secretion and more frequent GH pulses that are of more uniform size than men.[199,211] A complementary study using approximate entropy analysis concluded that the nonpulsatile regularity of GH secretion is also significantly different in men and women.[212] These sexually dimorphic patterns in the human are actually quite similar to those in the rat, although the sex differences are not as extreme in humans.[185,212]

The neuroendocrine basis for sex differences in the ultradian rhythm of GH secretion is not fully understood. Gonadal sex steroids play both an organizational role during development of the hypothalamus and an activational role in the adult, regulating expression of the genes for many of the peptides and receptors central to GH regulation.[182,185] In the human, unlike the rat, the hypothalamic actions of testosterone appear to result predominantly from its aromatization to 17β-estradiol and interaction with estrogen receptors. Hypothalamic somatostatin appears to play a more prominent role in men than in women in the regulation of pulsatile GH secretion, and this difference is postulated to be a key factor in producing the sexual dimorphism.[211,213]

External and Metabolic Signals. The various peripheral signals that modulate GH secretion in humans are summarized in Table 7-4 (also see Figs. 7-22 and 7-24). Of particular importance are factors related to energy intake and metabolism because they provide a common signal between the peripheral tissues and hypothalamic centers regulating nonendocrine homeostatic pathways in addition to the classic hypophyseotropic neurons. It is also in this complex arena that species-specific regulatory responses are particularly prominent, making extrapolations between rodent experimental models and human GH regulation less reliable.[182,185]

Important triggers of GH release include the normal decrease in blood glucose level after intake of a carbohydrate-rich meal, absolute hypoglycemia, exercise, physical and emotional stress, and high intake of protein (mediated by amino acids). Some of the pathologic causes of elevated GH represent extremes of these physiologic signals and include protein-calorie starvation, anorexia nervosa, liver failure, and type 1 diabetes mellitus. A critical concept is that many of these GH triggers work through the same final common mechanism of somatostatin withdrawal and consequent disinhibition of GH secretion. In contrast, postprandial hyperglycemia, glucose infusion, elevated plasma free fatty acids, type 2 diabetes mellitus (with obesity and insulin resistance), and obesity are all associated with inhibition of GH secretion. The specific role of leptin in modulating GH release is complicated by its multiple sites of action and coexistent secretory environment. Similarly, other members of the cytokine family including IL-1, IL-2, IL-6, and endotoxin have been inconsistently shown to stimulate GH in humans.

The actions of steroid hormones on GH secretion are complex because of their multiple loci of action within the proximal hypothalamic-pituitary components in addition to secondary effects on other neural and endocrine systems.[214] Glucocorticoids in particular produce opposite responses that are dependent on the chronicity of administration. Moreover, glucocorticoid effects follow an inverted U-shaped dose-response curve. Both low and high glucocorticoid levels reduce GH secretion, the former because of decreased GH gene expression and somatotroph responsiveness to GHRH and the latter because of increased hypothalamic somatostatin tone and decreased GHRH. Similarly, physiologic levels of thyroid hormones are necessary to maintain GH secretion and promote GH gene expression. Excessive thyroid hormone is also inhibitory to the GH axis, and the mechanism is speculated to be a combination of increased hypothalamic somatostatin tone, GHRH deficiency, and suppressed pituitary GH production.

Somatostatin
Chemistry and Evolution

A factor that potently inhibited GH release from pituitary in vitro was unexpectedly identified during early efforts to isolate GHRH from hypothalamic extracts. Somatostatin, the peptide responsible for this inhibition of GH secretion and the inhibition of insulin secretion by a pancreatic islet extract, was eventually isolated from hypothalamus and sequenced by Brazeau and colleagues in 1973.[215] The term *somatostatin* was originally applied to a cyclic peptide containing 14 amino acids, also called *somatostatin-14* (SST-14) (Fig. 7-25). Subsequently, a second form, NH$_2$-terminal extended somatostatin-28 (SST-28), was identified as a secretory product. Both forms of somatostatin are derived by independent cleavage of a common prohormone by prohormone convertases.[216] In addition, the isolation of SST-28(1-12) in some tissues suggests that SST-14 can be secondarily processed from SST-28. SST-14 is the predominant form in the brain (including the hypothalamus), whereas SST-28 is the major form in the gastrointestinal tract, especially the duodenum and jejunum.

The name *somatostatin* is descriptively inadequate because the molecule also inhibits TSH secretion from the pituitary and has nonpituitary roles including activity as a neurotransmitter or neuromodulator in the central and peripheral nervous systems and as a regulatory peptide in gut and pancreas. As a pituitary regulator, somatostatin is a true neurohormone—that is, a neuronal secretory product that enters the blood (hypophyseal-portal circula-

tion) to affect cell function at remote sites. In the gut, somatostatin is present in the myenteric plexus, where it acts as a neurotransmitter, and in epithelial cells, where it influences the function of adjacent cells as a paracrine secretion. Somatostatin can influence its own secretion from delta cells (an autocrine function) in addition to acting as a paracrine factor in pancreatic islets. Gut exocrine secretion can be modulated by intraluminal action, so it is also a lumone. Because of its wide distribution, broad spectrum of regulatory effects, and evolutionary history, this peptide can be regarded as an archetypical pansystem modulator.

The genes that encode somatostatin in humans[217] (see Fig. 7-25) and a number of other species exhibit striking sequence homology, even in primitive fish such as the anglerfish. Furthermore, the amino acid sequence of SST-14 is identical in all vertebrates. Formerly, it was accepted that all tetrapods have a single gene encoding both SST-14 and SST-28, whereas teleost fish have two nonallelic pre-prosomatostatin genes (*PPSI* and *PPSII*), each of which encodes only one form of the mature somatostatin peptides. This situation implied that a common ancestral gene underwent a duplication event after the split of teleosts from the descendants of tetrapods.

However, both lampreys and amphibians, which predate and postdate the teleost evolutionary divergence, respectively, have now been shown to have at least two PPS genes.[218] A more distantly related gene has been identified in mammals that encodes cortistatin, a somatostatin-like peptide that is highly expressed in cortex and hippocampus.[219] Cortistatin-14 differs from SST-14 by three amino acid residues but has high affinity for all known subtypes of somatostatin receptors (see later discussion). The human gene sequence predicts a tripeptide-extended cortistatin-17 and a further NH$_2$-terminal extended cortistatin-29.[220] A revised evolutionary concept of the somatostatin gene family is that a primordial gene underwent duplication at or before the advent of chordates, and the two resulting genes underwent mutation at different rates to produce the distinct pre-prosomatostatin and pre-procortistatin genes in mammals.[218] A second gene duplication probably occurred in teleosts to generate *PPSI* and *PPSII* from the ancestral somatostatin gene.

Apart from its expression in neurons of the periventricular and arcuate hypothalamic nuclei and involvement in GH secretion (discussed earlier), somatostatin is highly expressed in the cortex, lateral septum, extended amygdala, reticular nucleus of the thalamus, hippocampus, and many brainstem nuclei. Cortistatin is present in the brain at a small fraction of the levels of somatostatin and in a more limited distribution primarily confined to the cortex and hippocampus. The molecular mechanisms underlying the developmental and hormonal regulation of somatostatin gene transcription have been most extensively studied in pancreatic islet cells.[221,222] Less is known concerning the regulation of somatostatin gene expression in neurons except that activation is strongly controlled by binding of the phosphorylated transcription factor CRE-binding protein to its cognate CRE contained in the promoter sequence.[223,224] Enhancer elements in the somatostatin gene promoter that bind complexes of homeodomain-containing transcription factors (PAX6, PBX, PREP1) and upregulate gene expression in pancreatic islets may actually represent gene silencer elements in neurons (see Fig. 7-25, promoter elements TSE$_{II}$ and UE-A). Conversely, another related *cis* element in the somatostatin gene (see Fig. 7-25, promoter element TSE$_I$) apparently binds a homeodomain transcription factor PDX1 (also called STF1/IDX1/IPF1) that is common to developing brain, pancreas, and

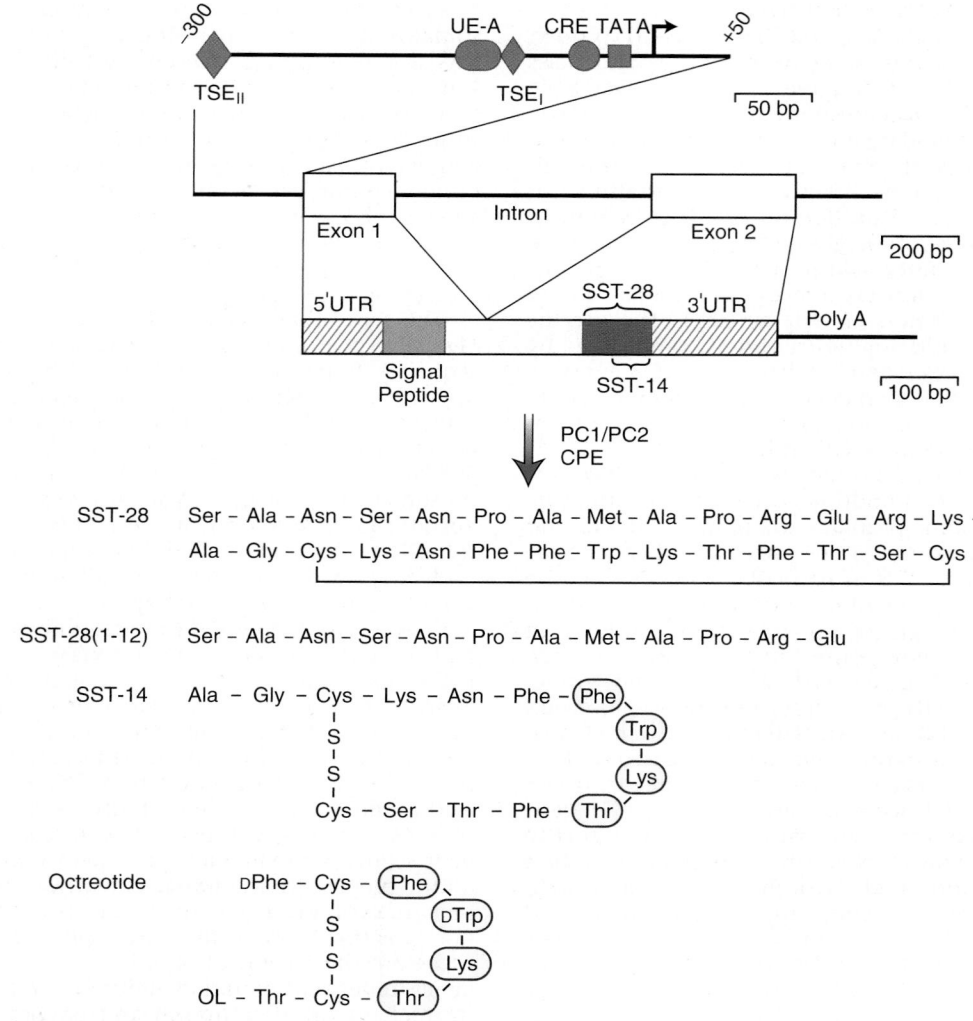

Figure 7-25 Diagram illustrating the genomic organization, messenger ribonucleic acid (mRNA) structure, and post-translational processing of the human somatostatin (SST) prohormone. Transcriptional regulation of the somatostatin gene, including the identification of tissue-specific elements (TSE), upstream elements (UE), and the cyclic adenosine monophosphate (cAMP) response element (CRE) that are binding sites for specific factors, has been studied extensively in pancreatic islet cell lines. It is not known whether all or some of these factors are also involved in the neural-specific expression of somatostatin. SST-28 and SST-14 are cyclic peptides containing a single covalent disulfide bond between a pair of cystine (Cys) residues. A β-turn containing the tetrapeptide Phe-Trp-Lys-Thr is stabilized by hydrogen bonds to produce the core receptor binding epitope. This minimal structure has been the model for conformationally restrained analogues of somatostatin including octreotide. CPE, carboxypeptidase E; PC1/PC2, prohormone convertases 1 and 2; TATA, Goldstein-Hogness box involved in binding RNA polymerase; UTR, untranslated region. (Compiled from data by Shen LP, Rutter WJ. Sequence of the human somatostatin 1 gene. *Science.* 1984;224:168-171; Goudet G, Delhalle S, Biemar F, et al. Functional and cooperative interactions between the homeodomain PDX1, Pbx, and Prep1 factors on the somatostatin promoter. *J Biol Chem.* 1999;274:4067-4073; and Milner-White EJ. Predicting the biologically active conformations of short polypeptides. *Trends Pharmacol Sci.* 1989;10:70-74.)

foregut and regulates gene expression in both the CNS and gut.[225]

The function of somatostatin in GH and TSH regulation is considered earlier in this chapter. Its actions in the extrahypothalamic brain and diagnostic and therapeutic roles are considered in the remainder of this section and in Chapter 8. An additional function of somatostatin in pancreatic islet cell regulation is described in Chapter 31, and the manifestations of somatostatin excess as in somatostatinoma are described in Chapter 38.

Somatostatin Receptors

Five somatostatin receptor subtypes (SSTR1 to SSTR5) have been identified by gene cloning techniques, and one of these (SSTR2) is expressed in two alternatively spliced forms.[226] These subtypes are encoded by separate genes

located on different chromosomes; they are expressed in unique or partially overlapping distributions in multiple target organs and differ in their coupling to second messenger signaling molecules and therefore in their range and mechanism of intracellular actions.[226] The subtypes also differ in their binding affinity to specific somatostatin analogues. Certain of these differences have important implications for the use of somatostatin analogues in therapy and in diagnostic imaging.

All SSTR subtypes are coupled to pertussis toxin–sensitive G proteins and bind SST-14 and SST-28 with high affinity in the low nanomolar range, although SST-28 has a uniquely high affinity for SSTR5. SSTR1 and SSTR2 are the two most abundant subtypes in the brain; they probably function as presynaptic autoreceptors in the hypothalamus and limbic forebrain, respectively, in addition to their postsynaptic actions. SSTR4 is most prominent in the hippocampus. All the subtypes are expressed in pituitary, but SSTR2 and SSTR5 are the most abundant subtypes on somatotrophs. They are also the most physiologically important in pancreatic islets, with SSTR5 responsible for inhibition of insulin secretion from beta cells and SSTR2 responsible for inhibition of glucagon from alpha cells in mice.[227]

Binding of somatostatin to its receptor leads to activation of one or more plasma membrane–bound inhibitory G proteins ($G_{i/o}$), which in turn inhibit adenylyl cyclase activity and lower intracellular cAMP. Other G protein–mediated actions common to all SSTRs are activation of a vanadate-sensitive phosphotyrosine phosphatase and modulation of mitogen-activated protein kinase (MAPK). Different subsets of SSTRs are also coupled to inwardly rectifying K^+ channels, voltage-dependent Ca^{2+} channels, an Na^+/H^+ exchanger, α-amino-3-hydroxy-5-methyl-4-isoxazole proprionic acid (AMPA)-kainate glutamate receptors, phospholipase C, and phospholipase A_2.[226] The lowering of intracellular cAMP and Ca^{2+} is the most important mechanism for inhibition of hormone secretion, and actions on phosphotyrosine phosphatase and MAPK are postulated to play a role in somatostatin's antiproliferative effect on tumor cells.

Effects on Target Tissues and Mechanism of Action

In the pituitary, somatostatin inhibits secretion of GH, TSH, and under certain conditions, PRL and ACTH. It exerts inhibitory effects on virtually all endocrine and exocrine secretions of the pancreas, gut, and gallbladder (Table 7-5). Somatostatin inhibits secretion by the salivary glands and, under some conditions, the secretion of parathyroid hormone and calcitonin. Somatostatin blocks hormone release in many endocrine-secreting tumors, including insulinomas, glucagonomas, VIPomas, carcinoid tumors, and some gastrinomas.

The physiologic actions of somatostatin in extrahypothalamic brain remain the subject of investigation.[228] In the striatum, somatostatin increases the release of dopamine from nerve terminals by a glutamate-dependent mechanism. It is widely expressed in GABAergic interneurons of limbic cortex and hippocampus, where it modulates the excitability of pyramidal neurons. Temporal

lobe epilepsy is associated with a marked reduction in somatostatin-expressing neurons in the hippocampus consistent with a putative inhibitory action on seizures.[229] A wealth of correlative data has linked reduced forebrain and CSF concentrations of somatostatin with Alzheimer disease, major depression, and other neuropsychiatric disorders, raising speculation about the role of somatostatin in modulating neural circuits underlying cognitive and affective behaviors.[230] A study using both genetic and pharmacologic methods to induce somatostatin deficiency in mice bolsters the hypothesis that the neuropeptide plays a physiologic role in the acquisition of contextual fear memory, possibly by altering long-term potentiaion in hippocampal circuits.[231]

Clinical Applications of Somatostatin Analogues

An extensive pharmaceutical discovery program has produced somatostatin analogues with receptor subtype selectivity and improved pharmacokinetics and oral bioavailability compared with the native peptide. Initial efforts focused on the rational design of constrained cyclic peptides that incorporated D-amino acid residues and included the Trp^8-Lys^9 dipeptide of somatostatin, which was shown by structure-function studies to be necessary for high-affinity binding to somatostatin receptors (see Fig. 7-25). Many such analogues have been studied in clinical trials including octreotide, lanreotide, vapreotide, seglitide, and pasireotide.[226] These compounds are agonists with similarly high-affinity binding to SSTR2 and SSTR5, moderate binding to SSTR3, and no (or low) binding to SSTR1 (except for pasireotide) and SSTR4. A combinatorial chemistry approach has now led to a new generation of nonpeptidyl somatostatin agonists that bind selectively and with subnanomolar affinity to each of the five SSTR subtypes.[232] In contrast to the marked success in development of potent and selective somatostatin agonists, there is a relative paucity of useful antagonists.[232]

The actions of octreotide (SMS 201-995 or Sandostatin) illustrate the general therapeutic potential of somatostatin analogues.[233] Octreotide controls excess secretion of GH in acromegaly in most patients and shrinks tumor size in about one third. It is also indicated for the treatment of recurrent TSH-secreting adenomas after surgery. It is used to treat other functioning metastatic neuroendocrine tumors, including carcinoid, VIPoma, glucagonoma, and insulinoma, but is seldom of use for the treatment of gastrinoma.[234] Octreotide is also useful in the management of many forms of diarrhea (acting on salt and water excretion mechanisms in the gut) and in reducing external secretions in pancreatic fistulas (thus permitting healing). A decrease in blood flow to the gastrointestinal tract is the basis for its use in bleeding esophageal varices, but it is not effective in the treatment of bleeding from a peptic ulcer.

The only major undesirable side effect of octreotide is reduction of bile production and of gallbladder contractility, leading to sludging of bile and an increased incidence of gallstones. Other common adverse effects including nausea, abdominal cramps, diarrhea secondary to malabsorption of fat, and flatulence usually subside spontaneously within 2 weeks of continued treatment. Impaired glucose tolerance is not associated with long-term octreotide therapy, despite an inhibitory effect on insulin secretion, because of compensating reductions in carbohydrate absorption and GH and glucagon secretion that are caused by the drug.

Somatostatin analogues labeled with a radioactive tracer have been used as external imaging agents for a wide range of disorders.[233,234] An indium-111 (^{111}In)-labeled analogue

TABLE 7-5

Biologic Actions of Somatostatin Outside the Central Nervous System

Hormone Secretion Inhibited (by Tissue)	Other Gastrointestinal Actions Inhibited
Pituitary gland	Gastric acid secretion
GH, thyrotropin, ACTH, prolactin	Gastric and jejunal fluid secretion
Gastrointestinal tract	Gastric emptying
Gastrin	Pancreatic bicarbonate secretion
Secretin	Pancreatic enzyme secretion
Motilin	Secretory diarrhea (stimulates
Glucagon-like peptide 1	intestinal absorption of water
Glucose-dependent	and electrolytes)
insulinotropic polypeptide	Gastrointestinal blood flow
Vasoactive intestinal peptide	AVP-stimulated water transport
Pancreas	Bile flow
Insulin	**Extragastrointestinal Actions Inhibited**
Glucagon	
Somatostatin	Inhibits the function of activated immune cells
Genitourinary tract	
Renin	Inhibition of tumor growth

ACTH, adrenocorticotropic hormone; AVP, arginine vasopressin; GH, growth hormone.

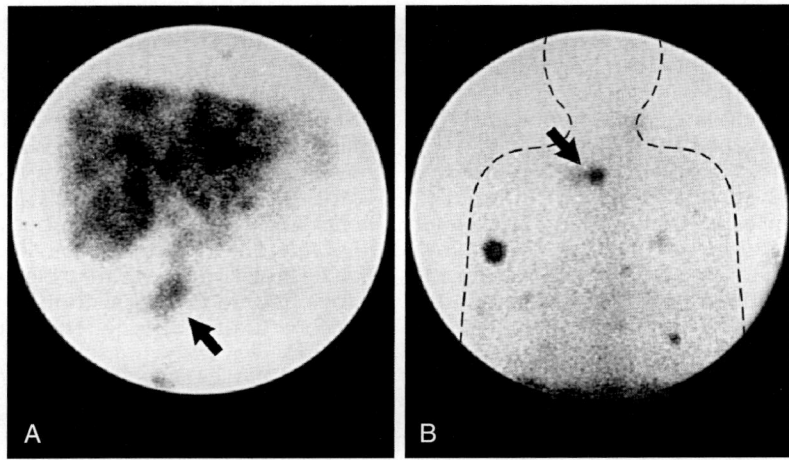

Figure 7-26 The use of ^{111}In-labeled diethylenetriaminepenta-acetic acid (DTPA)-octreotide (radioactive somatostatin analogue) and external imaging techniques to localize a carcinoid tumor expressing somatostatin receptors. Scans were obtained 24 hours after administration of labeled tracer. **A,** Anterior view of the abdomen showing nodular metastases in an enlarged liver and the primary carcinoid tumor *(arrow)* in the wall of the jejunum of a patient with severe flushing and diarrhea. **B,** Posterior view of the chest and neck showing a metastasis in a lymph node on the left side of the neck *(arrow)* and multiple metastases in the ribs and pleura. (Modified from Lamberts SWJ, Krenning EP, Reubi J-C. The role of somatostatin and its analogs in the diagnosis and treatment of tumors. *Endocrine Rev.* 1991;12:450-482. Copyright 1991, The Endocrine Society.)

of octreotide (OctreoScan) has been approved for clinical use in the United States and several other countries (Fig. 7-26). The majority of neuroendocrine tumors and many pituitary tumors that express somatostatin receptors are visualized by external imaging techniques after administration of this agent; a variety of nonendocrine tumors and inflammatory lesions are also visualized, all of which have in common the expression of somatostatin receptors. Such tumors include non–small cell cancer of the lung (100%), meningioma (100%), breast cancer (74%), and astrocytomas (67%). Because activated T cells of the immune system display somatostatin receptors, inflammatory lesions that take up the tracer include sarcoidosis, Wegener granulomatosis, tuberculosis, and many cases of Hodgkin disease and non-Hodgkin lymphoma. Although the tracer lacks specificity in differential diagnosis, its ability to identify the presence of abnormality and the extent of the lesion provides important information for management, including tumor staging. The use of a small hand-held radiation detector in the operating room makes it possible to ensure the completeness of removal of medullary thyroid carcinoma metastases.[235] New developments in the synthesis of tracers chelated to octreotide for positron emission tomography have allowed the sensitive detection of meningiomas only 7 mm in diameter and located beneath osseous structures at the base of the skull.[236]

The ability of somatostatin to inhibit the growth of normal and some neoplastic cell lines and to reduce the growth of experimentally induced tumors in animal models has stimulated interest in somatostatin analogues for the treatment of cancer. Somatostatin's tumoristatic effects may be a combination of direct actions on tumor cells related to inhibition of growth factor receptor expression, inhibition of MAPK, and stimulation of phosphotyrosine phosphatase. SSTR1, SSTR2, SSTR4, and SSTR5 can all promote cell cycle arrest associated with induction of the tumor suppressor retinoblastoma (Rb) and p21 (CDKN1A), and SSTR3 can trigger apoptosis accompanied by induction of the tumor suppressor p53 and the proapoptotic protein Bax.[226] In addition, somatostatin has indirect effects on tumor growth by its inhibition of circulating, paracrine, and autocrine tumor growth–promoting factors and it can modulate the activity of immune cells and influence

tumor blood supply. Despite this promise, the therapeutic utility of octreotide as an antineoplastic agent remains controversial.

Two new treatment approaches in preclinical trials may yet effectively utilize somatostatin receptors in the arrest of cancer cells.[233,234] The first is receptor-targeted radionuclide therapy using octreotide chelated to a variety of γ- or β-emitting radioisotopes. Theoretical calculations and empirical data suggest that radiolabeled somatostatin analogues can deliver a tumoricidal radiotherapeutic dose to some tumors after receptor-mediated endocytosis. A variation on this theme is the chelation of a cytotoxic chemotherapeutic agent, such as doxorubicin, to a somatostatin analogue. A second approach involves somatic cell gene therapy to transfect SSTR-negative pancreatic cancer cells with an SSTR gene.[237] Therapeutic results can be obtained with the creation of autocrine or paracrine inhibitory growth effects or the addition of targeted radionuclide treatments.

Prolactin-Regulating Factors
Dopamine

It is well known that PRL secretion, unlike the secretion of other pituitary hormones, is primarily under tonic inhibitory control by the hypothalamus (Fig. 7-27).[238] Destruction of the stalk median eminence or transplantation of the pituitary gland to ectopic sites causes a marked constitutive increase in PRL secretion, in contrast to a decrease in the release of GH, TSH, ACTH, and the gonadotropins. Many lines of evidence indicate that dopamine is the principal physiologic PIF released from the hypothalamus.[239] Dopamine is present in hypophyseal-portal vessel blood in sufficient concentration to inhibit PRL release; dopamine inhibits PRL secretion from lactotrophs both in vivo and in vitro; and dopamine D_2 receptors are expressed on the plasma membrane of lactotrophs. Mutant mice with a targeted disruption of the D_2 receptor gene uniformly developed lactotroph hyperplasia, hyperprolactinemia, and eventually lactotroph adenomas, further emphasizing the importance of dopamine in the physiologic regulation of lactotroph proliferation in addition to hormone secretion.[240]

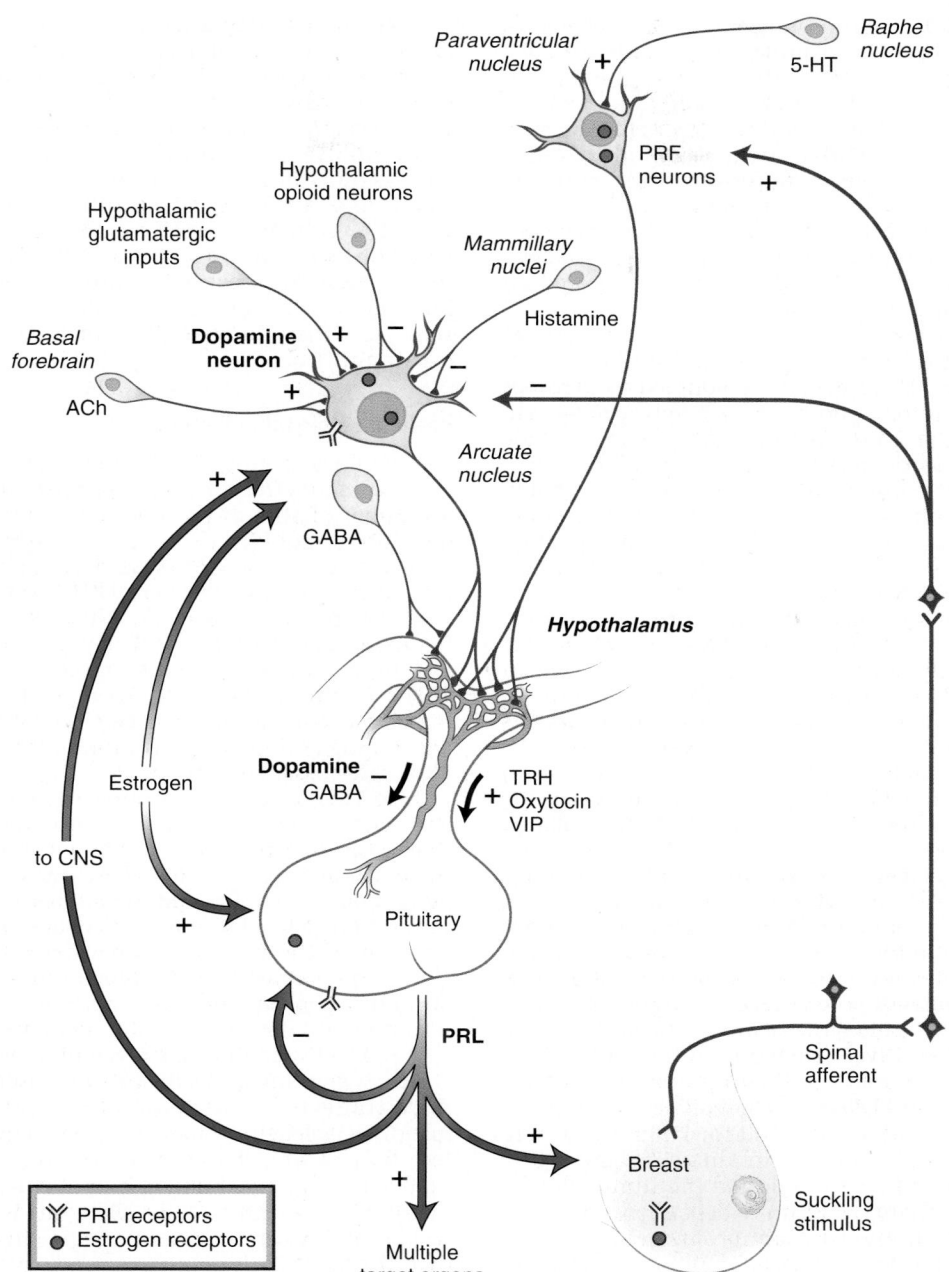

Figure 7-27 Regulation of the hypothalamic-pituitary-prolactin (PRL) axis. The predominant effect of the hypothalamus is inhibitory, mediated principally by the tuberohypophyseal dopaminergic neuron system and dopamine D_2 receptors on lactotrophs. The dopamine neurons are stimulated by acetylcholine (ACh) and glutamate and inhibited by histamine and opioid peptides. One or more prolactin-releasing factors (PRFs) probably mediate acute release of PRL (e.g., in suckling, during stress). There are several candidate PRFs, including thyrotropin-releasing hormone (TRH), vasoactive intestinal polypeptide (VIP), and oxytocin. PRF neurons are activated by serotonin (5-HT). Estrogen sensitizes the pituitary to release PRL, which feeds back on the pituitary to regulate its own secretion (ultrashort-loop feedback) and also influences gonadotropin secretion by suppressing the release of gonadotropin-releasing hormone (GnRH). Short-loop feedback is also mediated indirectly by prolactin receptor regulation of hypothalamic dopamine synthesis, secretion, and turnover. CNS, central nervous system; GABA, γ-aminobutyric acid.

The intrinsic dopamine neurons of the medial basal hypothalamus constitute a dopaminergic population with regulatory properties that are distinct from those in other areas of the brain. Notably, they lack D_2 autoreceptors but express PRL receptors, which are essential for positive feedback control (discussed in detail later). In the rat, these neurons are subdivided by location into the A12 group within the arcuate nucleus and the A14 group in the anterior periventricular nucleus. The caudal A12 dopamine neurons are further classified as TIDA because of their axonal projections to the external zone of the median eminence. THDA neuronal somata are located more rostrally in the arcuate nucleus and project to both the neural lobe and intermediate lobe through axon collaterals that are found in the internal zone of the median eminence. Finally, the A14 periventricular hypophyseal dopaminergic (PHDA) neurons send their axons only to the intermediate lobe of the pituitary gland.

Although the TIDA neurons are generally considered to be the major source of dopamine to the anterior lobe through the long portal vessels originating in the median eminence, dopamine can also reach the anterior lobe from the neural and intermediate lobes by the interconnecting short portal veins.[241] In addition to direct actions of dopamine on lactotrophs, central dopamine can indirectly affect PRL secretion by altering the activity of inhibitory interneurons that in turn synapse on the TIDA neurons. These effects are complicated by opposing intracellular signaling pathways linked to D_1 and D_2 receptors located on different populations of interneurons.[242]

The binding of dopamine or selective agonists such as bromocriptine to the D_2 receptor has multiple effects on lactotroph function. D_2 receptors are coupled to pertussis toxin–sensitive G proteins and inhibit adenylyl cyclase and decrease intracellular cAMP levels. Other effects include activation of an inwardly rectifying K^+ channel, increase of voltage-activated K^+ currents, decrease of voltage-activated Ca^{2+} currents, and inhibition of inositol phosphate production. Together, this spectrum of intracellular signaling events decreases free Ca^{2+} concentrations and inhibits exocytosis of PRL secretory granules.[243]

There is continuing debate concerning the mechanism by which D_2 receptor activation inhibits transcription of the PRL gene. Likely pathways involve the inhibition of MAPK or protein kinase C, with a resultant reduction in the phosphorylation of Ets family transcription factors. Ets factors are important for the stimulatory responses of TRH, insulin, and epidermal growth factor on PRL expression and they interact cooperatively with the pituitary-specific POU protein Pit1, which is essential for cAMP-mediated PRL gene expression.[244]

The second messenger pathways used by the D_2 receptor to inhibit lactotroph cell division are also unsettled.[245] A study using primary pituitary cultures from rats demonstrated that forskolin treatment, which activates protein kinase A and elevates intracellular cAMP, or insulin treatment, which activates a potent receptor tyrosine kinase, were both effective mitogenic stimuli for lactotrophs. Bromocriptine competitively antagonized the proliferative response caused by elevated cAMP. Furthermore, inhibition of MAPK signaling by PD98059 markedly suppressed the mitogenic action of both insulin and forskolin, suggesting an interaction of MAPK and protein kinase A signaling.[246]

Another line of study has implicated the stimulation of phospholipase D activity by a Rho A–dependent, pertussis toxin–insensitive pathway in the antiproliferative effects of D_2 receptor activation in both GH4C1 pituitary cells and NCI-H69 small cell lung cancer cells.[247] Activation of the extracellular signal-regulated kinase 1/2 pathway and inhibition of the AKT/protein kinase B pathway have also been implicated in the action of the D_2 receptor to reduce lactotroph mitogenesis.[248] Therefore, it is clear that dopamine actions on lactotrophs involve multiple different intracellular signaling pathways linked to activation of the D_2 receptor, but different combinations of these pathways are relevant for the inhibitory effects on PRL secretion, PRL gene transcription, and lactotroph proliferation.

The other major action of dopamine in the pituitary is the inhibition of hormone secretion from the POMC-expressing cells of the intermediate lobe[249]—although, as noted earlier, the adult human differs from most other mammals in the rudimentary nature of this lobe. THDA and PHDA axon terminals provide a dense plexus of synaptic-like contacts on melanotrophs. Dopamine release from these terminals is inversely correlated with serum MSH levels and also regulates POMC gene expression and melanotroph proliferation.

Other hypothalamic factors probably play a role secondary to that of dopamine as additional PIFs.[238] The primary reason to conjecture the existence of these PIFs is the frequent inconsistency between portal dopamine levels and circulating PRL in different rat models. GABA is the strongest candidate and most likely acts through $GABA_A$ inotropic receptors in the anterior pituitary. Melanotrophs, like lactotrophs, are inhibited by both dopamine and GABA but with the principal involvement of G protein–coupled, metabotropic $GABA_B$ receptors.[250] Because basal dopamine tone is high, the measurable inhibitory effects of GABA on PRL release are generally small under normal circumstances. Other putative PIFs include somatostatin and calcitonin.

Prolactin-Releasing Factors

Although tonic suppression of PRL release by dopamine is the dominant effect of the hypothalamus on PRL secretion, a number of stimuli promote PRL release, not merely by disinhibition of PIF effects but by causing release of one or more neurohormonal PRFs (see Fig. 7-27). The most important of the putative PRFs are TRH, oxytocin, and VIP, but vasopressin, angiotensin II, NPY, galanin, substance P, bombesin-like peptides, and neurotensin can also trigger PRL release under different physiologic circumstances.[238] TRH has already been discussed. In humans there is an imperfect correlation between pulsatile PRL and TSH release, suggesting that TRH cannot be the sole physiologic PRF under basal conditions.[251]

Like TRH, oxytocin, vasopressin, and VIP fulfill all the basic criteria for a PRF. They are produced in PVH neurons that project to the median eminence. Concentrations of the hormones in portal blood are much higher than in the peripheral circulation and are sufficient to stimulate PRL secretion in vitro. Moreover, there are functional receptors for each of the neurohormones in the anterior pituitary gland, and either pharmacologic antagonism or passive immunization against each hormone can decrease PRL secretion, at least under certain circumstances.[252]

AVP is released during stress and hypovolemic shock, as is PRL, suggesting a specific role for vasopressin as a PRF in these contexts. Similarly, another candidate PRF, peptide histidine isoleucine, may be specifically involved in the secretion of PRL in response to stress. Peptide histidine isoleucine and the human homologue peptide histidine methionine are structurally related to VIP and are synthesized from the same prohormone precursor in their respective species.[253] Both peptides are coexpressed with CRH in parvicellular PVH neurons, and presumably they are released by the same stimuli that cause release of CRH into the hypophyseal-portal vessels.[254]

Finally, reports of new PRFs continue to be published. Much excitement was generated by the isolation of a mammalian RFamide peptide from bovine hypothalamus named *prolactin-releasing peptide* (PrRP).[255] PrRP binds with high affinity to its GPCR GPR10, expressed in human pituitary; it selectively stimulates PRL release from rat pituitary cells with a potency lower than that of TRH, but synergistically stimulates PRL secretion in combination with TRH. However, PrRP is expressed predominantly in a subpopulation of noradrenergic neurons in the medulla and a small population of non-neurosecretory neurons of the VMH, raising the serious question of whether PrRP reaches the anterior pituitary and actually causes PRL secretion. Subsequent studies found no direct evidence for release of PrRP in the arcuate nucleus or median eminence, further suggesting that the peptide is not a hypophyseotropic neurohormone. PrRP probably does function as a neuromodulator within the CNS at sites expressing its receptor and may be involved in the neural circuitry mediating stress responses and satiety.[256,257]

Intrapituitary Regulation of Prolactin Secretion

Probably more than that of any other pituitary hormone, the secretion of PRL is regulated by autocrine-paracrine factors within the anterior lobe and by neurointermediate lobe factors that gain access to venous sinusoids of the anterior lobe by way of the short portal vessels. The wealth of local regulatory mechanisms within the anterior lobe has been reviewed extensively[238,258] and is also discussed in Chapter 8. Galanin, VIP, endothelin-like peptides, angiotensin II, epidermal growth factor, basic fibroblast growth factor, GnRH, and the cytokine IL-6 are among the most potent local stimulators of PRL secretion. Locally produced inhibitors include PRL itself, acetylcholine, transforming growth factor β, and calcitonin. Although none of these stimulatory or inhibitory factors plays a dominant role in the regulation of lactotroph function and much of the research in this area has not been directly confirmed in human pituitary, it seems apparent that the local milieu of autocrine and paracrine factors plays an essential modulatory role in determining the responsiveness of lactotrophs to hypothalamic factors in different physiologic states. Recent advancements in two-photon imaging of the pituitary and three-dimensional analyses of pituitary cell networks reinforce the importance of these local connections.[259]

Neuroendocrine Regulation of Prolactin Secretion

Secretion of PRL, like that of other anterior pituitary hormones, is regulated by hormonal feedback and neural influences from the hypothalamus.[238,239,260] Feedback is exerted by PRL itself at the level of the hypothalamus. PRL secretion is regulated by many physiologic states including the estrous and menstrual cycles, pregnancy, and lactation. Furthermore, PRL is stimulated by several exteroceptive stimuli including light, ultrasonic vocalization of pups (in rodents), olfactory cues, and various modalities of stress. Expression and secretion of PRL are also influenced strongly by estrogens at the level of both the lactotrophs and TIDA neurons[261] (see Fig. 7-27) and by paracrine regulators within the pituitary such as galanin and VIP.

Feedback Control

Negative feedback control of PRL secretion is mediated by a unique short-loop mechanism within the hypothalamus. PRL activates PRL receptors, which are expressed on all three subpopulations of A12 and A14 dopamine neurons, leading to increased tyrosine hydroxylase expression and increased dopamine synthesis and release.[261,262] Ames dwarf mice that secrete virtually no PRL, GH, or TSH have decreased numbers of arcuate dopamine neurons, and this hypoplasia can be reversed by neonatal administration of PRL, suggesting a trophic action on the neurons.[263] However, another mouse model of isolated PRL deficiency generated by gene targeting appears to have normal numbers of hypofunctioning dopamine neurons secondary to the loss of PRL feedback.[264]

Neural Control

Lactotrophs have spontaneously high secretory activity, and therefore the predominant effect of the hypothalamus on PRL secretion is tonic suppression, which is mediated by regulatory hormones synthesized by THDA neurons. Secretory bursts of PRL are caused by the acute withdrawal of dopamine inhibition, stimulation by PRFs, or combinations of both events. At any given moment, locally produced autocrine and paracrine regulators further modulate the responsiveness of individual lactotrophs to neurohormonal PIFs and PRFs.

Multiple neurotransmitter systems impinge on the hypothalamic dopamine and PRF neurons to regulate their neurosecretion[238] (see Fig. 7-27). Nicotinic cholinergic and glutamatergic afferents activate TIDA neurons, whereas histamine, acting predominantly through H_2 receptors, inhibits these neurons. An inhibitory peptidergic input to TIDA neurons of major physiologic significance is that associated with the endogenous opioid peptides enkephalin and dynorphin and their cognate μ- and κ-receptor subtypes.[265] Opioid inhibition of dopamine release has been associated with increased PRL secretion under virtually all physiologic conditions, including the basal state, different phases of the estrous cycle, lactation, and stress. Ascending serotoninergic inputs from the dorsal raphe nucleus are the major activator of PRF neurons in the PVH. There is still debate concerning the identity of the specific 5-HT receptors involved in this activation.

The PRL regulatory system and its monoaminergic control have been scrutinized in detail because of the frequent occurrence of syndromes of PRL hypersecretion (see Chapter 8). Both the pituitary and the hypothalamus have dopamine receptors, and the response to dopamine receptor stimulation and blockade does not distinguish between central and peripheral actions of the drug. Many commonly used neuroleptic drugs influence PRL secretion. Reserpine (a catecholamine depleter) and phenothiazines such as chlorpromazine and haloperidol enhance PRL release by disinhibition of dopamine action on the pituitary, and the PRL response is an excellent predictor of the antipsychotic effects of phenothiazines because of its correlation with D_2 receptor binding and activation.[266] The major antipsychotic neuroleptic agents act on brain dopamine receptors in the mesolimbic system and in the pituitary-regulating TIDA system. Consequently, treatment of such patients with dopamine agonists such as bromocriptine can reverse the psychiatric benefits of such drugs. A report of three patients with psychosis and concomitant prolactinomas recommended the combination of clozapine and quinagolide as the treatment of choice to manage both diseases simultaneously.[267]

Factors Influencing Secretion

Circadian Rhythm. PRL is detectable in plasma at all times during the day but is secreted in discrete pulses superimposed on basal secretion and exhibits a diurnal rhythm with peak values in the early morning hours.[268] In humans, this is a true circadian rhythm, because it is maintained in a constant environment independently of the sleep rhythm.[269] The combined body of data examining TIDA neuronal activity, dopamine concentrations in the median eminence, and manipulations of the SCN suggests that endogenous diurnal alterations in dopamine tone that are entrained by light constitute the major neuroendocrine mechanism underlying the circadian rhythm of PRL secretion.

External Stimuli. The suckling stimulus is the most important physiologic regulator of PRL secretion. PRL levels rise within 1 to 3 minutes of nipple stimulation, and they remain elevated for 10 to 20 minutes.[270] This reflex is distinct from the milk let-down, which involves oxytocin release from the neurohypophysis and contraction of mammary alveolar myoepithelial cells. These reflexes provide a mechanism by which the infant regulates both the production and the delivery of milk. The nocturnal rise in PRL secretion in nursing and non-nursing women may have evolved as a mechanism of milk maintenance during prolonged nonsuckling periods at night.

Pathways involved in the suckling reflex arise in nerves innervating the nipple, enter the spinal cord by way of spinal afferent neurons, ascend the spinal cord through spinothalamic tracts to the midbrain, and enter the hypothalamus by way of the median forebrain bundle (see Fig. 7-27). Neurons regulating the oxytocin-dependent milk let-down response accompany those involved in PRL regulation throughout most of this pathway and then separate at the level of the PVH nuclei. The suckling reflex brings about an inhibition of PIF activity and a release of PRFs, although an undisputed suckling-induced PRF has not been identified.

Although their significance for PRL regulation in humans is not certain, environmental stimuli from seasonal changes in light duration and auditory and olfactory cues are clearly of great importance to many mammalian species.[238] Seasonal breeders, such as the sheep, exhibit a reduction in PRL secretion in response to shortened days. The specific ultrasound vocalization of rodent pups is among the most potent stimuli for PRL secretion in lactating and virgin female rats. Olfactory stimuli from pheromones also have potent actions in rodents. A prime example is the Bruce effect or spontaneous abortion induced by exposure of a pregnant female rat to an unfamiliar male. It is mediated by a well-studied neural circuitry involving the vomeronasal nerves, the corticomedial amygdala, and the medial preoptic area of the hypothalamus, which results in activation of TIDA neurons and a reduction in circulating PRL that is essential for maintenance of luteal function in the first half of pregnancy.

Stress in many forms dramatically affects PRL secretion, although the teleologic significance is uncertain. It may be related to actions of PRL on cells of the immune system or some other aspect of homeostasis. Different stressors are associated with either a reduction or an increase in PRL secretion, depending on the local regulatory environment at the time of the stress. However, whereas well-documented changes in PRL are associated with relatively severe forms of stress in laboratory animal models, the relevance to human physiology is not well established.

Gonadotropin-Releasing Hormone and Control of the Reproductive Axis

Chemistry and Evolution

GnRH is the 10–amino acid hypothalamic neuropeptide that controls the function of the reproductive axis. It is synthesized as part of a larger precursor molecule that is enzymatically cleaved to remove a signal peptide from the NH$_2$-terminus and GnRH-associated peptide (GAP) from the COOH-terminus (Fig. 7-28).[271] All forms of the decapeptide have a pyroGlu at the NH$_2$-terminus and Gly-amide at the COOH-terminus, indicating the functional importance of the terminal residues throughout evolution.

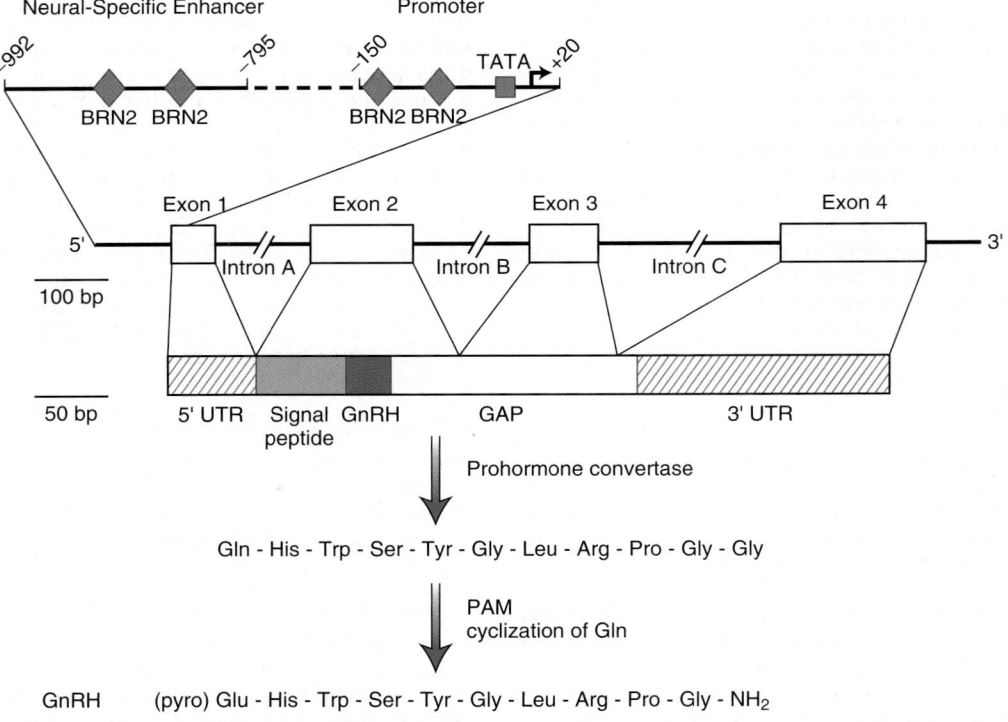

Figure 7-28 Schematic diagram of the human gene for gonadotropin-releasing hormone-1 *(GNRH1)*, the hypothalamic complementary deoxyribonucleic acid (cDNA), and post-translational processing of the GnRH prohormone. A cluster of binding sites for the homeodomain transcription factor BRN2 is present in both the proximal promoter and a distal enhancer region and is important for neuron-specific expression of the gene. Phylogenetically conserved homologous regions have been identified in the rat *Gnrh1* gene, but in that species the Oct1 transcription factor has been implicated in neuron-specific expression. The cDNA for GnRH-I isolated from human placenta has a longer 5′ untranslated region (UTR) because of differential splicing of the heterogeneous nuclear RNA (hnRNA) and inclusion of intron A sequences. GAP, GnRH-associated peptide; PAM, peptidylglycine α-amidating monooxygenase; TATA, Goldstein-Hogness box involved in binding RNA polymerase. (Compiled from data of Cheng CK, Leung PCK. Molecular biology of gonadotropin-releasing hormone (GnRH)-I, GnRH-II, and their receptors in humans. *Endocr Rev.* 2005;26:283-306; Wolfe A, Kim HH, Tobet S, et al. Identification of a discrete promoter region of the human GnRH gene that is sufficient for directing neuron-specific expression: a role for POU homeodomain transcription factors. *Mol Endocrinol.* 2002;16:435-449.)

Two genes encoding GnRH have been identified within mammals.[272,273] The first, *GNRH1*, encodes a 92–amino acid precursor protein. This form of GnRH is found in hypothalamic neurons and serves as a releasing factor to regulate pituitary gonadotroph function.[274] The second GnRH gene, *GNRH2*, encodes a decapeptide that differs from the first by three amino acids.[275] This form of GnRH is found in the midbrain region and serves as a neurotransmitter rather than as a pituitary releasing factor. Both GnRH-I and GnRH-II are found in phylogenetically diverse species, from fish to mammals, suggesting that these multiple forms of GnRH diverged from one another early in vertebrate evolution.[274] A third form of GnRH, GnRH-III, has been identified in neurons of the telencephalon in teleost fish. GnRH is also found in cells outside the brain. The roles of GnRH peptides produced outside the brain are not well understood but are an area of current investigation.

All GnRH genes have the same basic structure, with the pre-prohormone mRNA encoded in four exons. Exon 1 contains the 5′ untranslated region of the gene; exon 2 contains the signal peptide, GnRH, and the NH$_2$-terminus of GAP; exon 3 contains the central portion of GAP; and exon 4 contains the COOH-terminus of GAP and the 3′ untranslated region (see Fig. 7-28).[274] Among species, the nucleotide sequences encoding the GnRH decapeptide are highly homologous. This chapter focuses on the hypothalamic GnRH that is derived from *GNRH1* mRNA and plays an important role in the regulation of the hypothalamic-pituitary-gonadal axis.

Two transcriptional start sites have been identified in the rat *Gnrh1* gene, at the +1 and −579, with the +1 promoter being active in hypothalamic neurons and the other promoter active in placenta. The first 173 base pairs of the promoter are highly conserved among species. In the rat, this promoter region has been shown to contain two Oct1 binding sites; three regions that bind the POU domain family of transcription factors (Scip, Oct6, and Tst1); and three regions that can bind the progesterone receptor.[276] In addition, a variety of hormones and second messengers have been shown to regulate GnRH gene expression, and the majority of the *cis*-acting elements thus far characterized for hormonal control of GnRH transcription are located in the proximal promoter region.[277,278] The 5′ flanking region of the rodent and human *GNRH1* genes also contains a distal 300–base pair enhancer region that is 1.8 or 0.9 kb, respectively, upstream of the transcription start site.[278,279] Studies have implicated the homeodomain transcription factors OCT1, MSX, and DLX in the specification of neuron expression and developmental activation.[279,280]

Anatomic Distribution

GnRH neurons are small, diffusely located cells that are not concentrated in a discrete nucleus. They are generally bipolar and fusiform in shape, with slender axons projecting predominantly to the median eminence and infundibular stalk. The location of hypothalamic GnRH neurons is species-dependent. In the rat, hypothalamic GnRH neurons are concentrated in rostral areas including the medial preoptic area, the diagonal band of Broca, the septal areas, and the anterior hypothalamus. In humans and nonhuman primates, the majority of hypothalamic GnRH neurons are located more dorsally in the medial basal hypothalamus, the infundibulum, and periventricular region. Throughout the hypothalamus, neurohypophyseal GnRH neurons are interspersed with non-neuroendocrine GnRH neurons that extend their axons to other areas of the brain including other hypothalamic regions and various regions of the cortex. GnRH secreted from non-neuroendocrine neurons has been implicated in the control of sexual behavior in rodents but not in higher primates.[281]

Embryonic Development

GnRH neuroendocrine neurons are an unusual neuronal population in that they originate outside the CNS, from the epithelial tissue of the nasal placode.[282] During embryonic development, GnRH neurons migrate across the surface of the brain and into the hypothalamus, with the final hypothalamic location differing somewhat among species. Migration is dependent on a scaffolding of neurons and glial cells along which the GnRH neurons move, with neural cell adhesion molecules playing a critical role in guiding the migration process.

Failure of GnRH neurons to migrate properly leads to a clinical condition, Kallmann syndrome, in which GnRH neuroendocrine neurons do not reach their final destination and therefore do not stimulate pituitary gonadotropin secretion.[282,283] Patients with Kallmann syndrome do not enter puberty spontaneously. The X-linked form of Kallmann syndrome results from a deficiency of the *KAL1* gene, which encodes the extracellular glycoprotein termed *anosmin-1*. Loss of function mutations in the fibroblast growth factor receptor type 1 gene *(FGFR1)* produce an autosomal dominant form of Kallmann syndrome. This form, together with other known mutations in FGF8, prokinectin receptor 2 (PROKR2), and prokinectin-2 (PROK2), still accounts for only 30% of cases, and other lesions are yet to be characterized.[284] Administration of exogenous GnRH effectively treats this form of hypothalamic hypogonadism. Patients with Kallmann syndrome often have other congenital midline defects, including anosmia, which results from hypoplasia of the olfactory bulb and tracts.

Action at the Pituitary

Receptors. GnRH binds to a membrane receptor on pituitary gonadotrophs and stimulates both LH and FSH synthesis and secretion. The GnRH receptor is a seven-transmembrane-domain GPCR, but it lacks a typical intracellular COOH-terminal cytoplasmic domain.[278] Under physiologic conditions, GnRH receptor number varies and is usually directly correlated with the gonadotropin secretory capacity of pituitary gonadotrophs. For example, across the rat estrous cycle, a rise in GnRH receptors is seen just before the surge of gonadotropins that occurs on the afternoon of proestrus. GnRH receptor message levels are regulated by a variety of hormones and second messengers, including steroid hormones (estradiol can both suppress and stimulate; progesterone suppresses), gonadotropins (which suppress), and calcium and protein kinase C (which stimulate).[276,278]

$G_{q/11}$ is the primary guanosine triphosphate–binding protein mediating GnRH responses; however, there is evidence that GnRH receptors can couple to other G proteins including G_s and G_i.[278] With activation, the GnRH receptor couples to a phosphoinositide-specific phospholipase C, which leads to increases in calcium transport into gonadotrophs and calcium release from internal stores through a diacylglycerol-protein kinase C pathway. Increased calcium entry is a critical step in GnRH-stimulated release of gonadotropin secretion. However, GnRH also stimulates the MAPK cascade.

When there is a decline in GnRH stimulation to the pituitary, as occurs in a variety of physiologic conditions including states of lactation, undernutrition, or seasonal periods of reproductive quiescence, the number of GnRH receptors on pituitary gonadotrophs declines dramatically. Subsequent exposure of the pituitary to pulses of GnRH restores receptor number by a Ca^{2+}-dependent mechanism that requires protein synthesis.[285] The effect of GnRH to induce its own receptor is termed *upregulation* or *self-priming*. Only certain physiologic frequencies of pulsatile GnRH can augment GnRH receptor production, and these frequencies appear to differ among species.[286] Upregulation of GnRH receptors after a period of low GnRH stimulation to the pituitary can take hours to days of exposure to pulsatile GnRH, depending on the duration and extent of the prior decrease in GnRH. The self-priming effect of GnRH to upregulate its own receptors also plays a crucial role in the production of the gonadotropin surge that occurs at midcycle in females of spontaneously ovulating species and triggers ovulation. Just before the gonadotropin surge, two factors—the increased frequency of pulsatile GnRH release and a sensitization of the pituitary gonadotrophs by rising levels of estradiol—make the pituitary exquisitely sensitive to GnRH and allow an output of LH that is an order of magnitude greater than the release seen during the rest of the female reproductive cycle. This surge of LH triggers the ovulatory process at the ovary.

In contrast to upregulation of GnRH receptors by pulsatile regimens of GnRH, continuous exposure to GnRH leads to downregulation of GnRH receptors and an accompanying decrease in LH and FSH synthesis and secretion, termed *desensitization*.[287] Downregulation does not require calcium mobilization or gonadotropin secretion. It involves a rapid uncoupling of receptor from G proteins and sequestration of the receptors from the plasma membrane, followed by internalization and proteolytic degradation of the receptors.

The concept of downregulation has a number of clinical applications. For example, the most common current therapy for precocious puberty of hypothalamic origin (i.e., precocious GnRH secretion) is to treat it with a long-acting GnRH *superagonist* that downregulates pituitary GnRH receptors and effectively turns off the reproductive axis.[286,288] Children with precocious puberty can be maintained with long-acting GnRH agonists for years to suppress the premature activation of the reproductive axis, and at the normal age of puberty agonist treatment can be withdrawn, allowing reactivation of pituitary gonadotrophs and a downstream increase in gonadal steroid hormone production (also see Chapter 25). Long-acting GnRH agonists are also used in the treatment of forms of breast cancer that are estrogen-dependent and of other gonadal steroid-dependent cancers.[286] Long-acting antagonists of GnRH have been developed that can also be used for these therapies.[289] Antagonists have the advantage of not having a flare effect; that is, an acute stimulation of gonadotropin secretion that is seen during the initial treatment of individuals with superagonists.

Pulsatile Gonadotropin-Releasing Hormone Stimulation. Because a single pulse of GnRH stimulates the release of both LH and FSH and chronic exposure of the pituitary to pulsatile GnRH supports the synthesis of both LH and FSH, it is generally believed that there is only one releasing factor regulating the synthesis and secretion of LH and FSH. However, in a number of physiologic conditions there are divergent patterns of LH and FSH secretion, and thus a second FSH-releasing peptide has been proposed, but such a peptide has not been isolated to date. Other mechanisms, discussed in more detail later, are likely to account for the differential regulation of LH and FSH release.

The ensemble of GnRH neurons in the hypothalamus that send axons to the portal blood system in the median eminence fire in a coordinated, repetitive, episodic manner, producing distinct pulses of GnRH in the portal bloodstream. The pulsatile nature of GnRH stimulation to the pituitary leads to the release of distinct pulses of LH into the peripheral circulation. In experimental animals, in which it is possible to collect blood samples simultaneously from the portal and peripheral blood, GnRH and LH pulses have been found to correspond in about a 1 : 1 ratio at most physiologic rates of secretion.[290] Because the portal bloodstream is generally inaccessible in humans, the collection of frequent peripheral venous blood samples is used to define the pulsatile nature of LH secretion (i.e., frequency and amplitude of LH pulses), and pulsatile LH is used as an indirect measure of the activity of the GnRH secretory system. Indirect assessment of GnRH secretion by monitoring the rate of pulsatile LH secretion is also used in many animal studies examining the factors that govern the regulation of the pulsatile activity of the reproductive neuroendocrine axis. Unlike LH secretion, FSH secretion is not always pulsatile, and even when it is pulsatile, there is only partial concordance between LH and FSH pulses.

It is possible to place multiple-unit recording electrodes in the medial basal hypothalamus of monkeys and other species and detect spikes of electrical activity that are concordant with the pulsatile secretion of LH secretion.[291] However, it is unknown whether these bursts of electrical activity reflect the activity of GnRH neurons themselves or the activity of neurons that impinge on GnRH neurons and govern their firing. With the development of mice in which the gene for green fluorescent protein has been put under the regulation of the GnRH promoter, it has been possible to identify GnRH neurons in hypothalamic tissue slices using fluorescence microscopy, record from them intracellularly,[13] and simultaneously measure GnRH release from the median eminence by fast-scan cyclic voltammetry.[292] These studies have shown that many, but not all, GnRH neurons show a bursting pattern of electrical activity. A central, unsolved question in the field of reproductive neuroendocrinology is what causes GnRH neurons to pulse in a coordinated manner. Embryonic GnRH neurons from rhesus monkeys have shown intrinsic oscillatory changes in intracellular calcium concentration and synchronized calcium peaks among tens of neurons associated with GnRH release. A mathematical network model has been developed to further characterize this synchronization process.[293] The term *GnRH pulse generator* is often used to acknowledge the fact that GnRH secretion occurs in pulses and to refer to the central mechanisms responsible for pulsatile GnRH release.

A critical factor governing LH and FSH secretion is the rate of pulsatile GnRH stimulation of the gonadotrophs. Experimental studies in which the hypothalamus was lesioned and GnRH was replaced by pulsatile administration of exogenous GnRH showed that different frequencies of GnRH can lead to different ratios of LH to FSH secretion from the pituitary. Figure 7-29 shows that in a monkey with a hypothalamic lesion, replacement of one pulse of GnRH per hour led to a relatively low ratio of FSH to LH secretion. Subsequent institution of a slower pulse frequency (one pulse of GnRH every 3 hours) led to a decrease in LH secretion but an increase in FSH secretion so that the ratio of FSH to LH secretion was greatly elevated. It is likely that this effect of pulse frequency on the ratio of FSH to LH secretion accounts, at least in part, for the clinical finding that at times when the GnRH pulse generator is just turning on, such as at the onset of puberty and during recovery from chronic undernutrition, the ratio of FSH to LH is higher than when it is measured in adults experiencing regular reproductive function. As discussed later, steroid

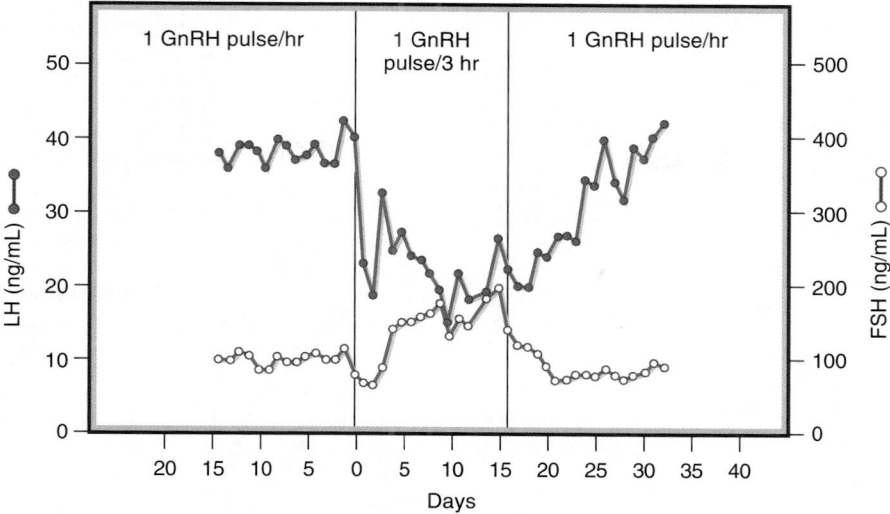

Figure 7-29 The influence of gonadotropin-releasing hormone (GnRH) pulse frequency on luteinizing hormone (LH) and follicle-stimulating hormone (FSH) secretion in a female rhesus monkey with an arcuate nucleus lesion ablating endogenous GnRH support of the pituitary. Decreasing the GnRH pulse frequency from 1 pulse every hour to 1 pulse every 3 hours led to a decrease in plasma LH concentrations but an increase in plasma FSH concentrations. (Redrawn from Wildt L, Haulser A, Marshall G, et al. Frequency and amplitude of gonadotropin-releasing hormone stimulation and gonadotropin secretion in the rhesus monkey. *Endocrinology.* 1981;109:376-385.)

hormones act at both the hypothalamus and pituitary to influence strongly the rate of pulsatile GnRH release and amount of LH and FSH secreted from the pituitary.

GnRH pulse frequency not only influences the rate of pulsatile gonadotropin release and the ratio of FSH to LH secretion but also plays an important role in modulating the structural makeup of the gonadotropins. LH and FSH are structurally similar glycoprotein hormones. Each of these hormones is made up of an α- and a β-subunit. LH, FSH, and TSH share a common α-subunit, and each has a unique β-subunit that conveys receptor specificity to the intact hormone. Before secretion of gonadotropins, terminal sugars are attached to each gonadotropin molecule.[103] The sugars include sialic acid, galactose, *N*-acetylglucosamine, and mannose, but the most important is sialic acid. The extent of glycosylation of LH and FSH is important for the physiologic function of these hormones.[103] Forms of gonadotropin with more sialic acid have a longer half-life because they are protected from degradation by the liver. Forms of gonadotropin with less sialic acid have more potent effects at their biologic receptors. Both the rate of GnRH stimulation and ovarian hormone feedback at the level of the pituitary regulate the degree of LH and FSH glycosylation. For example, slow frequencies of GnRH, seen during follicular development, are associated with greater degrees of FSH glycosylation, which would provide sustained FSH support to growing follicles. In contrast, faster frequencies of GnRH, seen just before the midcycle gonadotropin surge, are associated with lesser degrees of FSH glycosylation, providing a more potent but shorter lasting form of FSH at the time of ovulation.[294]

Regulatory Systems

Many neurotransmitter systems from the brainstem, limbic system, and other areas of the hypothalamus convey information to GnRH neurons (Fig. 7-30). These afferent systems include neurons that contain norepinephrine, dopamine, serotonin, GABA, glutamate, kisspeptin, endogenous opiate peptides, NPY, galanin, and a number of other peptide neurotransmitters. Glutamate and norepinephrine play

important roles in providing stimulatory drive to the reproductive axis, whereas GABA and endogenous opioid peptides provide a substantial portion of the inhibitory drive to GnRH neurons. Influences of specific neurotransmitter systems are discussed where appropriate in later sections on the physiologic regulation of GnRH neurons.

GnRH neurons are surrounded by glial processes, and only a small percentage of their surface area is available to receive dendritic contacts from afferent neurons. Changes in the steroid hormone milieu influence the degree of glial sheathing and may play important roles in regulating afferent input to GnRH neurons by this mechanism.[40] Some glial cells also secrete substances including transforming growth factor-α and prostaglandin E_2 that can modulate the activity of GnRH neurons.

Feedback Regulation

Steroid hormone receptors are abundant in the hypothalamus and in many neural systems that impinge on GnRH neurons, including noradrenergic, serotoninergic, kisspeptin, β-endorphin–containing, and NPY neurons. Early studies identifying regions of the brain that bound labeled estrogens showed that in rodents the preoptic area and VMH had the highest concentrations of estrogen receptors in the brain. Further localization studies, identifying estrogen receptors by immunocytochemistry or in situ hybridization, confirmed the strong presence of estrogen receptors in the hypothalamus and in brain areas with abundant connections to the hypothalamus, including the amygdala, septal nuclei, BST, medial part of the NTS, and lateral portion of the parabrachial nucleus.[295] In 1986, a new member of the steroid hormone receptor superfamily with high sequence homology to the classical estrogen receptor (now referred to as *estrogen receptor-α*) was isolated from rat prostate and named *estrogen receptor-β*. This novel estrogen receptor was shown to bind estradiol and to activate transcription by binding to estrogen response elements.[296]

In situ hybridization studies examining the localization of estrogen receptor-β mRNA have shown that these receptors are present throughout the rostral-caudal extent of the brain, with a high level of expression in the preoptic area,

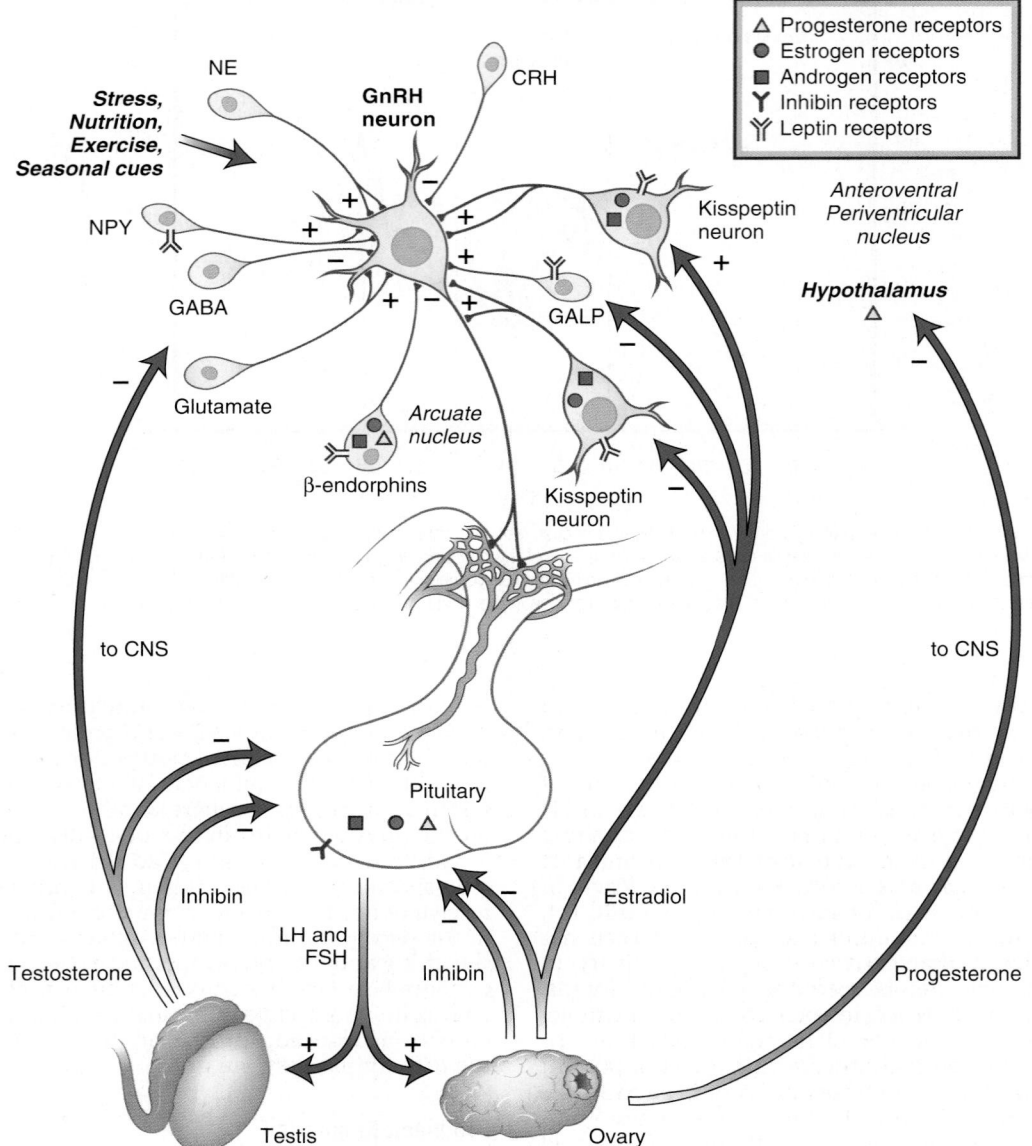

Figure 7-30 Regulation of the hypothalamic-pituitary-gonadal axis. Schematic diagram of the hypothalamic-pituitary-gonadal axis showing neural systems that regulate gonadotropin-releasing hormone (GnRH) secretion and feedback of gonadal steroid hormones at the level of the hypothalamus and pituitary. CNS, central nervous system; CRH, corticotropin-releasing hormone; FSH, follicle-stimulating hormone; GABA, γ-aminobutyric acid; GALP, galanin-like peptide; LH, luteinizing hormone; NE, norepinephrine; NPY, neuropeptide Y.

BST, PVH and SON, amygdala, and laminae II to VI of the cerebral cortex.[297] Specific receptors for progesterone are induced by estrogen in hypothalamic regions of the brain, including the preoptic area, the ventromedial and ventrolateral nuclei, and the infundibular-arcuate nucleus, although there is also evidence for constitutive expression of progesterone receptors in some regions.[298] Androgen receptor mapping studies have shown considerable overlap in the distribution of androgen and estrogen receptors throughout the brain. The highest density of androgen receptors was found in hypothalamic nuclei known to participate in the control of reproduction and sexual behaviors, including the arcuate nucleus, PVH, MePO, ventromedial nucleus, and brain regions with strong connections to the hypothalamus including the amygdala, nuclei of the septal region, BST, NTS, and lateral division of the parabrachial nucleus.[295] The anterior pituitary also contains receptors for all of the gonadal steroid hormones.

Steroid hormones can dramatically alter the pattern of pulsatile release of GnRH and of the gonadotropins through actions at both the hypothalamus and the pituitary. At the hypothalamus, estradiol, progesterone, and testosterone can all act to slow the frequency of GnRH release into the portal bloodstream as part of a closed negative feedback loop.[299] Because GnRH neurons have generally been shown to lack steroid hormone receptors, it is likely that the effects of steroid hormones on the firing rate of GnRH neurons are mediated by steroid hormone actions on other neural systems that provide afferent input to GnRH neurons. For example, progesterone-mediated negative feedback on GnRH secretion in primates appears to be regulated by β-endorphin–containing neurons in the hypothalamus, acting primarily through μ-opioid receptors. If a μ-receptor antagonist, such as naloxone, is administered along with progesterone, the negative feedback action of progesterone on GnRH secretion can be blocked.

Negative feedback of steroid hormones can also occur directly at the level of the pituitary. For example, estradiol has been shown to be capable of binding to the pituitary, decreasing LH and FSH synthesis and release, and decreasing the sensitivity of pituitary gonadotrophs to the actions of GnRH so that less LH and FSH are released when a pulse of GnRH stimulates the pituitary. Evidence for such a direct pituitary action of estradiol came from studies with rhesus monkeys that had been rendered deficient in endogenous GnRH by a lesion in the arcuate nucleus and showed a decline in endogenous gonadotropin secretion. When these monkeys received a pulsatile regimen of GnRH treatments, subsequent estradiol infusions dramatically suppressed the responsiveness of the pituitary to GnRH and suppressed the gonadotropin secretion that was being driven by the pulsatile administration of GnRH.[300] Similarly, in a compound mutant mouse model on a GnRH-deficient *(Hpg)* genetic background, expression of a human FSH-β transgene was inhibited by testosterone directly at the pituitary level.[301] In primate species including humans, there is considerable feedback of estradiol at the pituitary, but most of the progesterone and testosterone negative feedback occurs at the level of the hypothalamus.[299]

Most of the time, the hypothalamic-pituitary axis is under the negative feedback influence of gonadal steroid hormones. If the gonads are removed surgically or their normal secretion of steroid hormones is suppressed pharmacologically, there is a dramatic increase (10-fold to 20-fold) in circulating levels of LH and FSH secretion.[299] This type of *castration response* occurs normally at menopause in women, when ovarian follicular development and, therefore, ovarian production of large quantities of estradiol and progesterone decrease and eventually cease.

In addition to negative feedback, estradiol can have a positive feedback action at the level of the hypothalamus and pituitary to lead to a massive release of LH and FSH from the pituitary. This release of gonadotropins occurs once each menstrual cycle and is referred to as the *LH-FSH surge*. The positive feedback action of estradiol occurs as a response to the rising tide of estradiol that is produced during the process of dominant follicle development in the late follicular phase of the menstrual cycle. In women, elevated estradiol levels are generally maintained at about 300 to 500 pg/mL for about 36 hours before the stimulation of the gonadotropin surge.

Experiments have shown that both a critical concentration and duration of elevated estradiol are necessary to achieve positive feedback and a resulting gonadotropin surge. If supraphysiologic doses of estradiol are administered, the surge can occur as early as 18 hours after their administration. Because the ovary is responsible for the production of estradiol and the time course and magnitude of estradiol release control the rate of positive feedback, the ovary has been referred to as the *zeitgeber* of the menstrual cycle. The dependence of the positive feedback system on the magnitude of estradiol production helps explain the fact that the portion of the menstrual cycle that varies most in length is the follicular phase. Production of higher levels of estradiol by a dominant follicle in one cycle leads to a more rapid positive feedback action, with earlier ovulation and therefore a shorter follicular phase, compared with a cycle in which the dominant follicle produced lower levels of estradiol.

As with negative feedback in response to estradiol, the positive feedback actions of estradiol occur both at the hypothalamus, to increase GnRH secretion, and at the pituitary, to greatly enhance pituitary responsiveness to GnRH. Estradiol increases pituitary sensitivity to GnRH by increasing the synthesis of new GnRH receptors and by enhancing the responsiveness to GnRH at a postreceptor site of action. At the level of the hypothalamus in rodent species, estradiol appears to act at a *surge center* to induce the ovulatory surge of GnRH. Lesions in areas adjacent to the medial preoptic area, near the anterior commissure and septal complex, block the ability of estradiol to induce a surge in these species without blocking the negative feedback effects of estradiol.[302] In primate species, there does not appear to be a separate surge center mediating the positive feedback actions of estradiol.

Cellular mechanisms that mediate the switch from negative to positive feedback of estrogen are not fully understood, but there is support for the concept that estrogen induction of various transcription factors and receptors (notably progesterone receptors) may play an important role in mediating this switch.[303] The molecular mechanisms by which estradiol influences GnRH gene expression are also not well understood, but it is likely that these influences similarly occur through actions of neural systems afferent to GnRH neurons. The isolation of a novel mammalian RFamide-like peptide named *kisspeptin* as the natural ligand for the former orphan GPCR GPR54 has shed considerable light on this area.[256] Loss-of-function mutations in GPR54 (now termed *KISSR*) cause hypogonadotropic hypogonadism (HH), kisspeptin is expressed in subpopulations of arcuate and anteroventricular periventricular (AVPV) neurons that project to GnRH neurons, kisspeptin expression is regulated by estradiol and testosterone and is upregulated at the time of puberty, and intracerebroventricular administration of kisspeptin causes the secretion of GnRH and gonadotropins.[304,305] Furthermore, kisspeptin expression in the AVPV, but not the arcuate nucleus, is sexually diergic, with a much greater number of kisspeptin neurons in the female. This particular subpopulation of kisspeptin neurons is activated in an estrogen-dependent manner immediately preceding the GnRH surge, as detected by Fos expression, and is postulated to play a key role in the positive feedback effects of estradiol on GnRH release.[306] PRL inhibition of kisspeptin neurons is apparently responsible for the HH and anovulatory infertility associated with hyperprolactinemia.[307] Because of the coexpression of kisspeptin with neurokinin B and dynorphin, these neurons are commonly referred to as *KNDy* neurons.[308] Neurokinin B increases GnRH pulse frequency and dynorphin decreases GnRH pulse frequency in ovariectomized ewes.[308]

Regulation of the Ovarian Cycle

Cyclic activity in the ovary is controlled by an interplay between steroid hormones produced by the ovary and the hypothalamic-pituitary neuroendocrine components of the reproductive axis. The duration of each phase of the ovarian cycle is species dependent, but the general mechanisms controlling the cycle are similar in all species that have spontaneous ovarian cycles. In the human menstrual cycle, day 1 is designated as the first day of menstrual bleeding. At this time, small and medium-sized follicles are present in the ovaries, and only small amounts of estradiol are produced by the follicular cells. As a result, there is a low level of negative feedback to the hypothalamic-pituitary axis, LH pulse frequency is relatively fast (one pulse about every 60 minutes), and FSH concentrations are slightly elevated compared with much of the rest of the cycle (Fig. 7-31). FSH acts at the level of the ovarian follicles to stimulate development

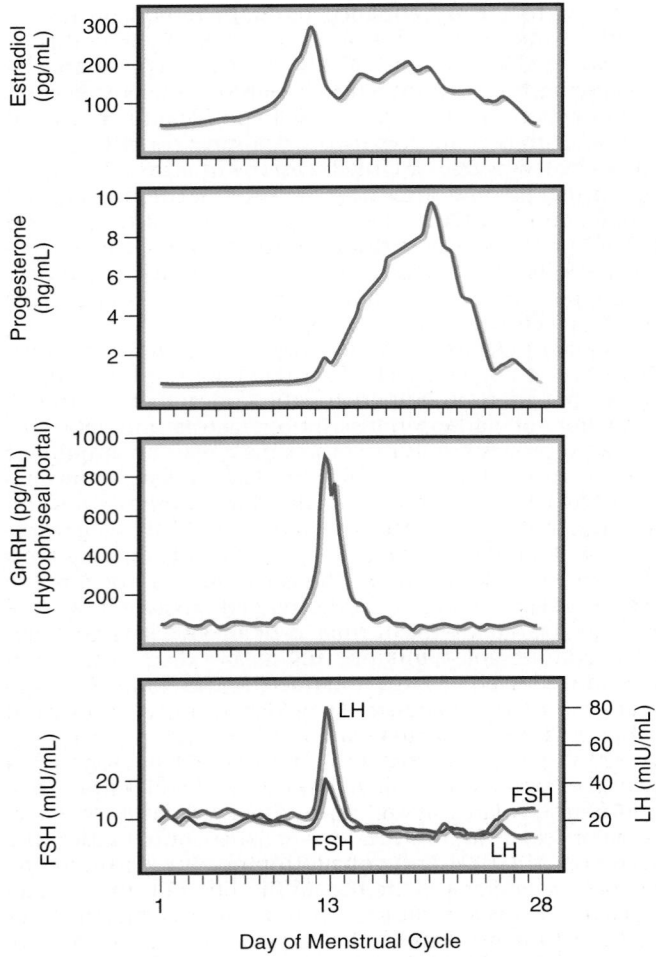

Figure 7-31 Diagrammatic representation of changes in plasma levels of estradiol, progesterone, luteinizing hormone (LH), and follicle-stimulating hormone (FSH) in portal levels of gonadotropin-releasing hormone (GnRH) over the human menstrual cycle.

diminishes. This reduces the negative feedback signals to the hypothalamus and pituitary and allows an increase in FSH and LH secretion. The fall in progesterone is also a withdrawal of steroid hormone support to the endometrial lining of the uterus; as a result the endometrium is shed as menses, and a new cycle begins.

In other species, the interplay between the neuroendocrine and ovarian hormones is similar but the timing of events is different and other factors, such as circadian and seasonal regulatory factors, play a role in regulating the cycle. The rat has a 4- or 5-day ovarian cycle with no menses (the endometrial lining is absorbed rather than shed). The rat also shows strong circadian rhythmicity in the timing of the LH-FSH surge, with the surge always occurring in the afternoon of the day of proestrus. The sheep is an example of a species that has a strongly seasonal pattern of ovarian cyclicity. During the breeding season, ewes have 15-day cycles, with a very short follicular phase and an extended luteal phase; during the nonbreeding season, signals relaying information about day length through the visual system, pineal, and SCN cause a dramatic suppression of GnRH neuronal activity, and cyclic ovarian function is prevented by a decrease in trophic hormonal support from the pituitary (see "Physiologic Roles of Melatonin").

Early Development and Puberty

Neuroendocrine stimulation of the reproductive axis is initiated during fetal development, and in primates in midgestation, circulating levels of LH and FSH reach values similar to those in castrated adults.[309] Later in gestational development, gonadotropin levels decline, restrained by rising levels of circulating gonadal steroids. The steroids that have this effect are probably placental in origin because after parturition there is a rise in circulating gonadotropin levels that is apparent for variable periods of the first year of life, depending on the species. The decline in reproductive hormone secretion in the postnatal period appears to be due to a decrease in GnRH stimulation of the reproductive axis because it occurs even in the castrated state and because gonadotropin and gonadal steroid secretion can be supported by the administration of pulses of GnRH.[310]

Pubertal reawakening of the reproductive axis occurs in late childhood and is marked initially by nighttime elevations in gonadotropin and gonadal steroid hormone levels.[310,311] The mechanisms controlling the pubertal reawakening of the GnRH pulse generator have been an area of intense investigation for more than 2 decades.[310,312] Although the mechanisms are not fully understood, significant progress has been made in identifying central changes in the hypothalamus that appear to play a role in this process. At puberty, there is both a decrease in transsynaptic inhibition to the GnRH neuronal system and an increase in stimulatory input to GnRH neurons.[310] One of the major inhibitory inputs to the GnRH system is provided by GABAergic neurons. Studies in rhesus monkeys have shown that hypothalamic levels of GABA decrease during early puberty and that blocking GABAergic input before puberty, by intrahypothalamic administration of antisense oligodeoxynucleotides against the enzymes responsible for GABA synthesis, results in premature activation of the GnRH neuronal system.

It has been suggested, on the basis of findings that a subset of glutamate receptors (i.e., kainate receptors) increase in the hypothalamus at puberty, that the pubertal decrease in GABA tone may be caused by an increase in glutamatergic transmission. Further evidence for a role for glutamate comes from studies showing that administration

and causes an increase in follicular estradiol production, which in turn provides increased negative feedback to the hypothalamic-pituitary unit.

A result of the increased negative feedback is a slowing of pulsatile LH secretion over the course of the follicular phase to a rate of about one pulse every 90 minutes. However, as the growing follicle (or follicles, depending on the species) secretes more estradiol, the positive feedback action of estradiol is triggered that leads to an increase in GnRH release and the LH-FSH surge. The surge of gonadotropins acts at the fully developed follicle to stimulate the dissolution of the follicular wall, leading to ovulation of the matured ovum into the nearby fallopian tube, where fertilization takes place if sperm are present. Ovulation results in a reorganization of the cells of the follicular wall, which undergo hypertrophy and hyperplasia and start to secrete large amounts of progesterone and some estradiol. Progesterone and estradiol have a negative feedback effect at the level of the hypothalamus and pituitary, so the LH pulse frequency becomes very slow during the luteal phase of the menstrual cycle. The corpus luteum has a fixed life span, and without additional stimulation in the form of human chorionic gonadotropin (hCG) from a developing embryo, the corpus luteum regresses spontaneously after about 14 days and progesterone and estradiol secretion

of N-methyl-DL-aspartic acid (NMDA) to prepubertal rhesus monkeys can drive the reawakening of the reproductive axis.[313] Increased stimulatory drive to the GnRH neuronal system also appears to come from increases in norepinephrine and NPY at the time of puberty.[310] Furthermore, as discussed earlier, there is evidence that growth factors act through release of prostaglandin from glial cells at puberty to play a role in stimulating GnRH neurons.[314]

Despite an increased understanding of the neural changes occurring at puberty, the question of what signals trigger the pubertal awakening of the reproductive axis is unanswered at this time.[312,315] However, the kisspeptin neuron system described earlier in the section on feedback regulation has become a prime integrative candidate for this function.[306] Also relevant to pubertal onset was galanin-like peptide (GALP), which is expressed specifically in the arcuate nucleus and binds with high affinity to galanin receptors. GALP is a potent central stimulator of gonadotropin release and sexual behavior in the rat and can reverse the decreased reproductive function associated with diabetes mellitus and hypoinsulinemia.[316] Both kisspeptin and GALP neurons are targets of leptin and are hypothesized to be involved in the well-known modulation of puberty and reproductive function by food availability and nutritional status (see the following section). Epigenetic mechanisms have been proposed to coordinate the changes in the expression of multiple genes that accompany the initiation of puberty.[312]

Reproductive Function and Stress

Many forms of physical stresses, such as energy restriction, exercise, temperature stress, infection, pain, and injury, as well as psychological stresses, such as being subordinate in a dominance hierarchy, can suppress the activity of the reproductive axis.[317] If the stress exposure is brief, there may be acute suppression of circulating gonadotropins and gonadal steroid hormones; in females disruption of normal menstrual cyclicity may be disrupted, but fertility is unlikely to be impaired.[317] In contrast, prolonged periods of significant stress exposure can lead to complete impairment of reproductive function, also characterized by low circulating levels of gonadotropins and gonadal steroids. Stress appears to decrease the activity of the reproductive axis by decreasing GnRH drive to the pituitary because in all cases in which it has been examined, administration of exogenous GnRH can reverse the effects of the stress-induced decline in reproductive hormone secretion.

In the case of foot shock stress in rats[318] or immune stress (i.e., injection of IL-1α) in primates,[319] the suppression of gonadotropin secretion that occurs was shown to be reversible by administration of a CRH antagonist, implying that endogenous CRH secretion mediates the effects of these stresses on GnRH neurons. In other studies, naloxone, a μ-opioid receptor antagonist, was shown to be capable of reversing restraint stress–induced suppression of gonadotropin secretion in monkeys; however, naloxone is ineffective in reversing the suppression of gonadotropin secretion that occurs during insulin-induced hypoglycemia.[320,321] In the case of metabolic stresses, multiple regulators appear to mediate changes in the neural drive to the reproductive axis.

Various metabolic fuels including glucose and fatty acids can regulate the function of the reproductive axis, and blocking cellular utilization of these fuels can lead to suppression of gonadotropin secretion and decreased gonadal activity. Leptin, a hormone produced by fat cells, can also modulate the activity of the reproductive axis. Mutant ob/ob mice that are deficient in leptin are infertile, and fertility can be restored to by administration of leptin.[322] Moreover, leptin administration has been shown to reverse the suppressive effects of undernutrition on the reproductive axis in some situations.[323] Leptin receptors are found in several populations that are known to have a strong influence on the reproductive axis, particularly NPY and kisspeptin neurons.[306]

In summary, it appears that a number of neural circuits can mediate effects of stress on the GnRH neuronal system and that the neural systems involved are at least somewhat specific to the type of stress that is experienced.

NEUROENDOCRINE DISEASE

Disease of the hypothalamus can cause pituitary dysfunction, neuropsychiatric and behavioral disorders, and disturbances of autonomic and metabolic regulation. In the diagnosis and treatment of suspected hypothalamic or pituitary disease, four issues must be considered: the extent of the lesion, the physiologic impact, the specific cause, and the psychosocial setting. The cause of hypothalamic neuroendocrine disorders categorized by age and syndrome is summarized in Tables 7-6 and 7-7.

Manifestations of pituitary insufficiency secondary to hypothalamic or pituitary stalk damage are not identical to those of primary pituitary insufficiency. Hypothalamic injury causes decreased secretion of most pituitary hormones but can cause hypersecretion of hormones normally under inhibitory control by the hypothalamus, as in hypersecretion of PRL after damage to the pituitary stalk and precocious puberty caused by loss of the normal restraint over gonadotropin maturation. Impairment of inhibitory control of the neurohypophysis can lead to the syndrome of inappropriate vasopressin (antidiuretic hormone) secretion (SIADH) (see Chapter 10). More subtle abnormalities in secretion can result from impairment of the control system. For example, loss of the normal circadian rhythm of ACTH secretion may occur before loss of pituitary-adrenal secretory reserve, and responses to physiologic stimuli may be paradoxical. Because hypophyseotropic hormone levels cannot be measured directly and pituitary hormone secretion is regulated by complex, multilayered controls, assay of pituitary hormones in blood does not necessarily give a meaningful picture of events at hypothalamic and higher levels. Rarely, tumors secrete excessive amounts of releasing peptides and cause hypersecretion of hormones from the pituitary.

Disorders of the hypothalamic-pituitary unit can result from lesions at several levels. Defects can arise from destruction of the pituitary (as by tumor, infarct, inflammation, or autoimmune disease) or from a hereditary deficiency of a particular hormone as in rare cases of isolated FSH, GH, or POMC deficiency. Selective loss of thyroid hormone receptors in the pituitary can give rise to increased TSH secretion and thyrotoxicosis. Furthermore, disorders can arise through disruption of the contact zone between the stalk and median eminence, the stalk itself, or the nerve terminals of the THDA system; such disruption occurs after surgical stalk section, with tumors involving the stalk, and in some inflammatory diseases. At a higher level, tonic inhibitory and excitatory inputs can be lost as manifested by absence of circadian rhythms or the development of precocious puberty. Physical stress, cytokine products of inflammatory cells, toxins, and reflex inputs from peripheral homeostatic monitors also impinge on the TIDA system. At the highest level of control, emotional stress and psychological disorders can activate the pituitary-adrenal stress response and suppress gonadotropin secretion (e.g.,

TABLE 7-6
Etiology of Hypothalamic Disease by Age

Premature Infants and Neonates

Intraventricular hemorrhage
Meningitis: bacterial
Tumors: glioma, hemangioma
Trauma
Hydrocephalus, kernicterus

Age 1 Month to 2 Years

Tumors: optic glioma, histiocytosis X, hemangioma
Hydrocephalus
Meningitis
Congenital disorders: Laurence-Moon-Biedl syndrome, Prader-Willi
    syndrome

Age 2 to 10 Years

Tumors: craniopharyngioma, glioma, dysgerminoma, hamartoma,
    leukemia, histiocytosis X, ganglioneuroma, ependymoma,
    medulloblastoma
Meningitis: bacterial, tuberculous
Encephalitis: viral (exanthematous demyelinating)
Congenital diabetes insipidus
Radiation therapy
Diabetic ketoacidosis
Moyamoya disease, circle of Willis

Age 10 to 25 Years

Tumors: craniopharyngioma, glioma, hamartoma, dysgerminoma,
    histiocytosis X, leukemia, dermoid, lipoma, neuroblastoma
Trauma
Vascular: aneurysm, subarachnoid hemorrhage, arteriovenous
    malformation
Inflammatory disease: meningitis, encephalitis, sarcoidosis, tuberculosis
Structural brain defects: chronic hydrocephalus, increased intracranial
    pressure

Age 25 to 50 Years

Nutritional: Wernicke disease
Tumors: glioma, lymphoma, meningioma, craniopharyngioma, pituitary
    tumors, plasmacytoma, angioma, colloid cysts, sarcoma,
    ependymoma, histiocytosis X
Inflammatory diseases: sarcoidosis, tuberculosis, viral encephalitis
Vascular: aneurysm, subarachnoid hemorrhage, arteriovenous
    malformation
Damage from pituitary radiation therapy

Age 50 Years and Older

Nutritional: Wernicke disease
Tumors: pituitary tumors, sarcoma, glioblastoma, ependymoma,
    meningioma, colloid cysts, lymphoma
Vascular disease: infarct, subarachnoid hemorrhage, pituitary apoplexy
Inflammatory disease: encephalitis, sarcoidosis, meningitis
Damage from radiation therapy for ear-nose-throat carcinoma, pituitary
    tumors

Adapted from Plum F, Van Uitert R. Nonendocrine diseases and disorders of
    the hypothalamus. In: Reichlin S, Baldessarini RJ, Martin JB, eds. *The
    Hypothalamus*, vol 56. New York, NY: Raven Press; 1978:415-473.

TABLE 7-7
Etiology of Endocrine Syndromes of Hypothalamic Origin

Hypophyseotropic Hormone Deficiency

Surgical pituitary stalk section
Inflammatory disease: basilar meningitis and granuloma, sarcoidosis,
    tuberculosis, sphenoid osteomyelitis, eosinophilic granuloma
Craniopharyngioma
Hypothalamic tumor: infundibuloma, teratoma (ectopic pinealoma),
    astrocytoma
Maternal deprivation syndrome, psychosocial dwarfism
Isolated GHRH deficiency
Hypothalamic hypothyroidism
Panhypophyseotropic failure

Disorders of Regulation of GnRH Secretion

Female
Precocious puberty: GnRH-secreting hamartoma, hCG-secreting
    germinoma
Delayed puberty
Neurogenic amenorrhea
Pseudocyesis
Anorexia nervosa
Functional amenorrhea and oligomenorrhea
Drug-induced amenorrhea

Male
Precocious puberty
Fröhlich syndrome
Kallmann syndrome (olfactory-genital dysplasia)

Disorders of Regulation of Prolactin-Regulating Factors

Tumor
Sarcoidosis
Drug-induced
Reflex
Herpes zoster of chest wall
Post-thoracotomy
Nipple manipulation
Spinal cord tumor
Psychogenic
Hypothyroidism
Carbon dioxide narcosis

Disorders of Regulation of CRH

Paroxysmal corticotropin discharge (Wolff syndrome)
Loss of circadian variation
Depression
CRH-secreting gangliocytoma

CRH, corticotropin-releasing hormone; hCG, human chorionic gonadotropin;
    GHRH, growth hormone–releasing hormone; GnRH, gonadotropin-releasing
    hormone.

psychogenic amenorrhea) or inhibit GH secretion (e.g.,
psychosocial dwarfism) (see Chapter 24). Intrinsic disease
of the anterior pituitary is reviewed in Chapters 8 and 9,
and disturbances in posterior pituitary function are discussed in Chapter 10. This chapter primarily considers
diseases of the hypothalamic-pituitary unit.

Pituitary Isolation Syndrome

Destructive lesions of the pituitary stalk, as occur with head
injury, surgical transection, tumor, or granuloma, produce
a characteristic pattern of pituitary dysfunction.[324,325]
Central diabetes insipidus (DI) develops in a large percent-

age of patients, depending on the level at which the stalk
has been sectioned. If the cut is close to the hypothalamus,
DI is almost always produced, but if the section is low on
the stalk, the incidence is lower. The extent to which nerve
terminals in the upper stalk are preserved determines the
clinical course. The classic triphasic syndrome of initial
polyuria followed by normal water control and then by
AVP deficiency over a period of 1 week to 10 days occurs
in fewer than half of the patients. The sequence is attributed to an initial loss of neurogenic control of the neural
lobe, followed by autolysis of the neural lobe with release
of AVP into the circulation, and finally by complete loss of
AVP. However, full expression of polyuria requires adequate
cortisol levels; if cortisol is deficient, AVP deficiency may
be present with only minimal polyuria. DI can also develop
after stalk injury without an overt transitional phase.
When DI occurs after head injury or operative trauma,
varying degrees of recovery can be seen even after months

or years. Sprouting of nerve terminals in the stump of the pituitary stalk may give rise to sufficient functioning tissue to maintain water balance. In contrast to the effects of stalk section, nondestructive injury to the neurohypophysis or stalk, as during surgical resection of sellar tumors, can sometimes give rise to transient or delayed SIADH.[326]

Although head injury, granulomas, and tumors are the most common causes of acquired DI, other cases develop in the absence of a clear-cut cause.[327] Autoimmune disease of the hypothalamus may be the cause in some instance, as was suggested by the finding of autoantibodies to neurohypophyseal cells in a third of cases of idiopathic DI in one series.[328] However, autoantibodies were also frequently found in association with histiocytosis X. Later reports suggested the importance of continued vigilance in cases of idiopathic DI. A definite cause is frequently uncovered in time, including a high proportion of occult germinomas, whose detection by MRI may be preceded by elevated levels of hCG in CSF.[329] Congenital DI can be part of a hereditary disease. DI in the Brattleboro rat is due to an autosomal recessive genetic defect that impairs production of AVP but not of oxytocin. In contrast, inherited forms of DI in humans have been attributed to mutations in the vasopressin V_2 receptor gene or less frequently in the aquaporin or the AVP genes.[330-332]

Menstrual cycles cease after stalk section, although gonadotropins may still be detectable, unlike the situation after hypophysectomy. Plasma glucocorticoid levels and urinary excretion of cortisol and 17-hydroxycorticoids decline after hypophysectomy and stalk section, but the change is slower after stalk section. A transient increase in cortisol secretion after stalk section is believed to be due to release of ACTH from preformed stores. The ACTH response to the lowering of blood cortisol is markedly reduced, but ACTH release after stress may be normal, possibly because of CRH-independent mechanisms. Reduction in thyroid function after stalk section is similar to that seen with hypophysectomy. The fall in GH secretion is said to be the most sensitive indication of damage to the stalk, but the insidious nature of this endocrinologic change in adults who have suffered traumatic brain injuries may cause it to be overlooked and therefore contribute to delayed rehabilitation.[333]

Humans with stalk sections or with tumors of the stalk region have widely varying levels of hyperprolactinemia and may have galactorrhea.[334] PRL responses to hypoglycemia and to TRH are blunted, in part because of loss of neural connections with the hypothalamus. PRL responses to dopamine agonists and antagonists in patients with pituitary isolation syndrome are similar to those in patients with prolactinomas. Interestingly, PRL secretion continues to show a diurnal variation in patients with either hypothalamic-pituitary disconnection or microprolactinoma.[268] Both forms of hyperprolactinemia are characterized by a similarly increased frequency of PRL pulses and a marked rise in nonpulsatile or basal PRL secretion, although the disruption is greater in the tumoral hyperprolactinemia.

An incomplete pituitary isolation syndrome may occur with the empty sella syndrome, intrasellar cysts, or pituitary adenomas.[335,336] Anterior pituitary failure after stalk section is in part due to loss of specific neural and vascular links to the hypothalamus and in part due to pituitary infarction.

Hypophyseotropic Hormone Deficiency

Selective pituitary failure can be due to a deficiency of specific pituitary cell types or a deficiency of one or more hypothalamic hormones. Isolated GnRH deficiency is the most common hypophyseotropic hormone deficiency. In Kallmann syndrome (gonadotropin deficiency commonly associated with hyposmia),[283] hereditary agenesis of the olfactory lobe may be demonstrable by MRI.[337] Abnormal development of the GnRH system is a result of defective migration of the GnRH-containing neurons from the olfactory nasal epithelium in early embryologic life (see earlier discussion). Other malformations of the cranial midline structures, such as absence of the septum pellucidum in septo-optic dysplasia (De Morsier syndrome), can cause HH or, less commonly, precocious puberty. A surprisingly large percentage of children with septo-optic dysplasia who otherwise have multiple hypothalamic-pituitary abnormalities actually retain normal gonadotropin function and enter puberty spontaneously.[338] The genetic basis of HH, including Kallmann syndrome, has now been established in approximately 15% of patients.[284,339] Mutations in *KAL1*, the Kallmann syndrome gene, and in *NROB1* (formerly *AHC* or *DAX1*), the gene that causes adrenal hypoplasia congenital with HH, produce X-linked recessive disease. Autosomal recessive HH has been associated with mutations in the genes encoding the GnRH receptor, KISS1 receptor, leptin, leptin receptor, FSH, LH, PROP1 (combined pituitary deficiency), and HESX (septo-optic dysplasia) genes, and deficient FGFR1 function causes an autosomal dominant form of HH. Mutations in *PROK2* and *PROKR2*, which encode prokinectin-2 and its receptor, have been associated with heterozygous, homozygous, compound heterozygous, and oligogenic patterns of genetic penetrance.

The GnRH response test is of little value in the differential diagnosis of HH. Most patients with GnRH deficiency show little or no response to an initial test dose but normal responses after repeated injection. This slow response has been attributed to downregulation of GnRH receptors in response to prolonged GnRH deficiency. In patients with intrinsic pituitary disease, the response to GnRH may be absent or normal. Consequently, it is not possible to distinguish between hypothalamic and pituitary disease with a single injection of GnRH. Prolonged infusions or repeated administration of GnRH agonists after hormone replacement therapy priming may aid in the diagnosis or provide therapeutic options for women with Kallmann syndrome who wish to become pregnant.[340,341]

Deficiency of TRH secretion gives rise to hypothalamic hypothyroidism, also called *tertiary hypothyroidism*, which can occur in hypothalamic disease or more rarely as an isolated defect.[342] Molecular genetic analyses have revealed infrequent autosomal recessive mutations in the TRH and TRH receptor genes in the cause of central hypothyroidism.[343] Hypothalamic and pituitary causes of TSH deficiency are most readily distinguished by imaging methods. Although it is theoretically reasonable to use the TRH stimulation test for the differentiation of hypothalamic disease from pituitary disease, the test is of limited value. The typical pituitary response to TRH administration in patients with TRH deficiency is an enhanced and somewhat delayed peak, whereas the response with pituitary failure is subnormal or absent. The hypothalamic type of response has been attributed to an associated GH deficiency that sensitizes the pituitary to TRH (possibly through suppression of somatostatin secretion), but GH also affects T_4 metabolism and may alter pituitary responses as well.[344] In practice, the responses to TRH in hypothalamic and pituitary disease overlap so much that they cannot be used reliably for a differential diagnosis. Persistent failure to demonstrate responses to TRH is good evidence for the presence of intrinsic pituitary disease, but the presence of a response does not mean that the pituitary is normal. Deficient TRH secretion leads to altered TSH biosynthesis by the pituitary, including impaired glycosylation. Poorly glycosylated TSH has low biologic activity, and dissociation of bioactive and immunoreactive TSH can lead to the paradox of normal or elevated levels of TSH in hypothalamic hypothyroidism.[342,345]

GHRH deficiency appears to be the principal cause of hGH deficiency in children with idiopathic dwarfism.[346] This condition is frequently associated with abnormal electroencephalograms, a history of birth trauma, and breech delivery, although a cause-and-effect relationship has not been established. MRI scans show that most children with isolated, idiopathic hGH deficiency have a normal-sized or only slightly reduced anterior pituitary; less common findings are ectopic posterior pituitary, anterior pituitary hypoplasia, or empty sella.[347] In contrast, children with idiopathic combined pituitary hormone deficiency are significantly more likely to have evidence of moderate to severe anterior pituitary hypoplasia, ectopic posterior pituitary, complete agenesis of the pituitary stalk (both nervous and vascular components), and a variety of associated midline cerebral malformations.[347] Human GH is the most vulnerable of the anterior pituitary hormones when the pituitary stalk is damaged. It can be difficult to differentiate between primary pituitary disease and GHRH deficiency by standard tests of GH reserve. However, a substantial GH secretory response to a single administration of hexarelin occurs only in the presence of at least a partially intact vascular stalk (Fig. 7-32).[193]

In many children with dwarfism, the anatomic abnormalities of the intrasellar contents and pituitary stalk together with the frequent occurrence of other midline defects, such as those in septo-optic dysplasia, are consistent with the alternative hypothesis of a developmental defect occurring in embryogenesis.[347] There has been a remarkable advance in our understanding of the molecular ontogeny of the hypothalamic-pituitary unit, much of it based on mutant mouse models.[348] Parallel genetic analyses have been conducted in children with isolated GH deficiency or combined pituitary hormone deficiencies. These studies have identified autosomal recessive mutations in both structural and regulatory genes including the genes encoding the GHRH receptor, PIT1, PROP1, HESX1, LHX3, and LHX4 that are responsible for a sizable proportion of congenital hypothalamic-pituitary disorders once considered idiopathic.[184,346,347,349]

Adrenal insufficiency is another manifestation of hypothalamic disease and rarely is caused by CRH deficiency.[350] Isolated ACTH deficiency is uncommon, but there is suggestive evidence in at least one family of genetic linkage to the *CRH* gene locus.[351] More recent investigations have revealed mutations in *TBX19*, the gene encoding TPIT, a T-box transcription factor expressed only in pituitary corticotrophs and melanotrophs, which is associated with the majority of cases of isolated ACTH deficiency in neonates.[352] The CRH stimulation test does not reliably distinguish hypothalamic from pituitary failure as a cause of ACTH deficiency.[353]

Apart from intrinsic diseases of the hypothalamus such as tumors and granulomas, two environmental causes of central hypophyseotropic deficiencies are of increasing clinical importance: trauma to the brain,[325,333] particularly from motor vehicle accidents, and the sequelae of chemotherapy and radiation therapy for intracranial lesions in children and adults.[345,354,355] Improved short-term survival from head injuries associated with coma and CNS malignancies has greatly increased the prevalence of long-term neuroendocrine consequences.

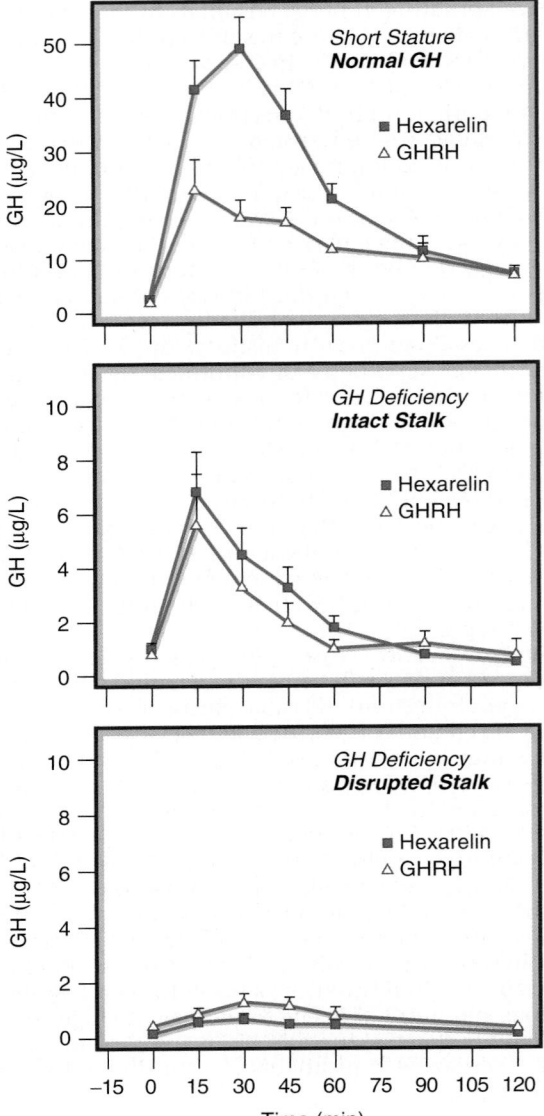

Figure 7-32 Effect of hypothalamic-pituitary disconnection on the growth hormone (GH) secretory responses to GH-releasing hormone (GHRH) (1 µg/kg) and the GH-secretagogue (GHS) receptor agonist hexarelin (2 µg/kg) administered intravenously to children with GH deficiency. *Top,* Mean responses in a group of 24 prepubertal children with short stature secondary to familial short stature or constitutional growth delay are shown. *Middle,* Children with GH deficiency and an intact vascular pituitary stalk as visualized by dynamic magnetic resonance imaging exhibited a clear, but blunted, GH response to both secretagogues. *Bottom,* In contrast, children with pituitary stalk agenesis (both vascular and neural components) had no response or a markedly attenuated response to both peptides. (From Maghnie M, Spica-Russotto V, Cappa M, et al. The growth hormone response to hexarelin in patients with different hypothalamic-pituitary abnormalities. *J Clin Endocrinol Metab.* 1998;83:3886-3889.)

Craniopharyngioma

Craniopharyngioma is the most common pediatric tumor occurring in the sellar and parasellar area (see Table 7-6). Because of their location these benign neoplasms frequently cause significant neuroendocrine dysfunction. The more common adamantinomatous tumors in children usually contain both a cystic component filled with a turbid, cholesterol-rich fluid and a solid component characterized by organized epithelial cells.[356] Roughly 25% of craniopharyngiomas are diagnosed in patients over the age of 25, and this subset of tumors is more typically papillary in nature, solid, and less likely to be calcified or cystic.[356] Both forms of craniopharyngiomas probably result from metaplastic changes in vestigial epithelial cell rests that originate in Rathke's pouch and the craniopahryngeal duct during fetal development.

Common presenting symptoms are those due to a mass intracranial lesion and increased intracranial pressure. Visual field defects, papilledema, and optic atrophy can occur from compression of the optic chiasm or nerves. Between 80% and 90% of affected children have signs and symptoms of endocrine dysfunction, although these are not usually the chief complaint. The most frequent hormone deficiencies are GH and gonadotropins. The latter is almost universal in adolescents and adults and likely also present, but undetected, in prepubertal children with craniopharyngiomas. TSH and ACTH deficiency are also common. Even if not present at initial diagnosis, endocrine dysfunction often occurs subsequent to treatment and necessitates long-term follow-up and retesting.[357]

MRI is the imaging modality of choice in cases of suspected craniopharyngioma.[358] A recommended examination includes T1-weighted thin sagittal and coronal sections through the sella and suprasellar regions, obtained before and after contrast administration. T2-weighted and fluid attenuation inversion recovery (FLAIR) images are useful to further delineate cysts and are hyperintense. Computed tomography scans can be useful to determine the presence of calcification.

Hypophyseotropic Hormone Hypersecretion

Pituitary hypersecretion is occasionally caused by tumors of the hypothalamus. GnRH-secreting hamartomas can cause precocious puberty.[359] CRH-secreting gangliocytomas can cause Cushing syndrome,[360] and GHRH-secreting gangliocytomas of the hypothalamus can cause acromegaly.[361] Although they do not arise from the hypothalamus, paraneoplastic syndromes can also cause pituitary hypersecretion, as with CRH-secreting tumors and GHRH-secreting tumors of the bronchi and pancreas. Bronchial carcinoids and pancreatic islet cell tumors are the usual causes of this phenomenon.

Neuroendocrine Disorders of Gonadotropin Regulation

Precocious Puberty

The term *precocious puberty* is used when physiologically normal pituitary-gonadal function appears at an early age (see also Chapter 25).[362] By convention, it is defined as the onset of androgen secretion, and spermatogenesis must occur before the age of 9 or 10 years in boys and the onset of estrogen secretion and cyclic ovarian activity before age 7 or 8 in girls.[363,364] Central precocious puberty is due to disturbed CNS function, which may or may not have an identifiable structural basis. Pseudoprecocious puberty refers to premature sexual development resulting from excessive secretion of androgens, estrogens, or hCG; it is caused by tumors (both gonadal and extragonadal), administration of exogenous gonadal steroids, or genetically determined activation of gonadotropin receptors (see Chapter 25). Central precocious puberty with neurogenic causes and pineal gland disease are discussed in this chapter.

Idiopathic Sexual Precocity. Familial occurrence of idiopathic sexual precocity is uncommon, but there is a hereditary form of idiopathic sexual precocity that is largely confined to boys. Abnormal electroencephalograms and

behavioral disturbances, suggesting the presence of brain damage, have been reported occasionally in girls with idiopathic precocious puberty. The pathogenesis may be related to the rate of hypothalamic development or other as yet undetermined nutritional, environmental, or psychosocial factors. Many cases previously thought to be idiopathic are caused by small hypothalamic hamartomas (see later discussion). It has been argued that localized activation of discrete cellular subsets connected to GnRH neurons may be sufficient to initiate puberty.[365]

Neurogenic Precocious Puberty. Approximately two thirds of hypothalamic lesions that influence the timing of human puberty are located in the posterior hypothalamus, but in the subset of patients who come to autopsy, damage is extensive. Specific lesions known to cause precocity include craniopharyngioma (although delayed puberty is far more common with these lesions), astrocytoma, pineal tumors, subarachnoid cysts, encephalitis, miliary tuberculosis, tuberous sclerosis or neurofibromatosis type 1, the Sturge-Weber syndrome, porencephaly, craniostenosis, microcephaly, hydrocephalus, empty sella syndrome, and Tay-Sachs disease.[366,367]

Hamartoma of the hypothalamus is an exception to the generalization that tumors of the brain cause precocious puberty by impairment of gonadotropin secretion (although hamartomas on occasion cause hypothalamic damage). A hamartoma is a tumor-like collection of normal-appearing nerve tissue lodged in an abnormal location. The parahypothalamic type consists of an encapsulated nodule of nerve tissue attached to the floor of the third ventricle or suspended from the floor by a peduncle; it is typically less than 1 cm in diameter. The intrahypothalamic or sessile type is enveloped by the posterior hypothalamus and can distort the third ventricle. These hamartomas tend to be larger than the pedunculated variety, grow in the interpeduncular cistern, and are frequently accompanied by seizures, mental retardation, and developmental delays. They result in precocious puberty with about half the incidence observed with the parahypothalamic lesions.[368,369] Before the development of high-resolution scanning techniques, this tumor was considered rare, but small ones can now be visualized. Miniature hamartomas of the tuber cinereum are common at autopsy. Precocious puberty occurs when the hamartoma makes connections with the median eminence and thus serves as an accessory hypothalamus. Peptidergic nerve terminals containing GnRH have been found in the tumors.[359] Early pubertal development is presumably due to unrestrained GnRH secretion, although the hamartomas almost certainly have an intrinsic pulse generator of GnRH secretion because pulsatility is required for stimulation of gonadotropin secretion (see earlier discussion).

Manifestations of premature puberty in patients with hamartomas are similar to those associated with other central causes of precocity. Hamartomas occur in both sexes and may be present as early as age 3 months. In the past most cases were thought to be fatal by age 20 years, but many hamartomas cause no brain damage and need not be excised.[368] The interpeduncular fossa of the brain is difficult to approach, and surgical experience is somewhat limited. Early in the course of illness, epilepsy manifested as "brief, repetitive, stereotyped attacks of laughter"[370] may provide a clue to the disease. Late in the course, hypothalamic damage can cause severe neurologic defects and intractable seizures.

Hypothyroidism. Hypothyroidism can cause precocious puberty in girls that is reversible with thyroid therapy. Hyperprolactinemia and galactorrhea may be present. One possibility is that elevated TSH levels (in children with thyroid failure) cross-react with the FSH receptor.[371]

Alternatively, low levels of thyroid hormone might simultaneously activate release of LH, FSH, and TSH. A third possibility is that hypothyroidism causes hypothalamic encephalopathy that impairs the normal tonic suppression of gonadotropin release by the hypothalamus. The high PRL levels that sometimes accompany this disorder may be due to a deficiency in PIF secretion, increased secretion of TRH, or increased sensitivity of the lactotrophs to TRH secretion.

Tumors of the Pineal Gland. Pineal gland tumors account for only a small percentage of intracranial neoplasms. They occur as a central midline mass with an enhancing lesion on MRI frequently accompanied by hydrocephalus. Pinealomas cause a variety of neurologic abnormalities. Parinaud syndrome, which consists of paralysis of upward gaze, pupillary areflexia (to light), paralysis of convergence, and a wide-based gait, occurs with about half of patients with pinealomas. Gait disturbances can also occur because of brainstem or cerebellar compression. Additional neurologic signs occurring with moderate frequency include spasticity, ataxia, nystagmus, syncope, vertigo, cranial nerve palsies other than VI and VIII, intention tremor, scotoma, and tinnitus.

Several discrete cytopathologic entities account for mass lesions in the pineal region (Table 7-8).[372] The most common non-neoplastic conditions are degenerative

pineal cysts, arachnoid cysts, and cavernous hemangioma. Pinealocytes give rise to primitive neuroectodermal tumors, the so-called *small blue-cell tumors* that are immunopositive for the neuronal marker synaptophysin and negative for the lymphocyte marker CD45. True pinealomas can be relatively well differentiated pineocytomas, intermediate mixed forms, or the less differentiated pineoblastomas,[372,373] which are essentially identical to medulloblastomas, neuroblastomas, and oat cell carcinomas of the lung.

The most common tumors of the pineal gland are actually germinomas (a form of teratoma), so designated because of their presumed origin in germ cells. Germinomas may also occur in the anterior hypothalamus or the floor of the third ventricle, where they are often associated with the clinical triad of DI, pituitary insufficiency, and visual abnormalities.[367] Identical tumors can be found in the testis and anterior mediastinum. Intracranial germinomas have a tendency to spread locally, infiltrate the hypothalamus, and metastasize to the spinal cord and CSF. Extracranial metastases (to skin, lung, or liver) are rare. Teratomas derived from two or more germ cell layers also occur in the pineal region. Chorionic tissue in teratomas and germinomas may secrete hCG in sufficient amounts to cause gonadal maturation, and some of these tumors have histologic and functional characteristics of choriocarcinomas. Diagnosis is confirmed by the combination of a mass lesion, cytologic analysis of CSF, and radioimmunoassay detection of hCG in the CSF.

Precocious puberty is a relatively unusual manifestation of pineal gland disease. When it occurs, neuroanatomic studies suggest that the cause is secondary to pressure or destructive effects of the pineal tumor on the function of the adjacent hypothalamus or to the secretion of hCG. Most patients have other evidence of hypothalamic involvement such as DI, polyphagia, somnolence, obesity, or behavioral disturbance. Choriocarcinoma of the pineal gland is associated with high plasma levels of hCG. The hCG can stimulate testosterone secretion from the testis but not estrogen secretion by the ovary; it therefore causes premature puberty almost exclusively in boys. The prevalence of elevated hCG levels in children with premature puberty related to tumors in the pineal region is unknown, but the fact that this phenomenon occurs further challenges the theory that nonparenchymal tumors cause precocious puberty by damaging the normal pineal gland. Rarely, pinealomas cause delayed puberty, raising speculation about a role of melatonin in inhibiting gonadotropin secretion in these cases.

Management of tumors in the pineal region is not straightforward.[372,374] Operative mortality rates can be high, but the rationale for an aggressive approach to the pineal region is based on the need to make a histologic diagnosis, the variety of lesions found in this region, the possibility of cure of an encapsulated lesion, and the effectiveness of chemotherapeutic agents for germinomas and choriocarcinoma. Stereotaxic biopsy of the pineal region provided diagnosis in 33 of 34 cases in one series, suggesting that this is a useful alternative to open surgical exploration for diagnostic purposes.[375] Long-term palliation or cure of many pineal region tumors is possible by combinations of surgery, radiation, gamma knife radiosurgery, or chemotherapy, depending on the nature of the lesion.[376]

Approach to the Patient with Precocious Puberty. Several groups have reviewed the diagnostic approach to suspected central precocious puberty (see Chapter 25).[377,378] Although guidelines differ, the index of suspicion is clearly inversely proportional to the age of the patient. A GnRH stimulation test to assess gonadotropin release and thereby differentiate between primed and inactive gonadotrophs

---

TABLE 7-8

Classification of Tumors of the Pineal Region

Germ Cell Tumors

Germinoma
    Posterior third ventricle and pineal lesions
    Anterior third ventricle, suprasellar, or intrasellar lesions
    Combined lesions in anterior and posterior third ventricle,
        apparently noncontiguous, with or without foci of cystic or solid
        teratoma
Teratoma
    Evidencing growth along two or three germ lines in varying
        degrees of differentiation
    Dermoid and epidermoid cysts with or without solid foci of
        teratoma
    Histologically malignant forms with or without differentiated foci of
        benign, solid, or cystic teratoma-teratocarcinoma,
        chorioepithelioma, embryonal carcinoma (endodermal–sinus
        tumor or yolk-sac carcinoma); combinations of these with or
        without foci of germinoma, chemodectoma

Pineal Parenchymal Tumors

Pinealocytes
    Pineocytoma
    Pineoblastoma
    Ganglioglioma and chemodectoma
    Mixed forms exhibiting transitions among these types
Glia
    Astrocytoma
    Ependymoma
    Mixed forms and other less frequent gliomas (e.g., glioblastoma,
        oligodendroglioma)

Tumors of Supporting or Adjacent Structures

Meningioma
Hemangiopericytoma

Nonneoplastic Conditions of Neurosurgical Importance

Degenerative cysts of pineal gland lined by fibrillary astrocytes
Arachnoid cysts
Cavernous hemangioma

From DeGirolami U. Pathology of tumors of the pineal region. In: Schmidek HH, ed. *Pineal Tumors.* New York, NY: Masson; 1977:1-19.

is probably the single most important endocrinologic measure. If LH and FSH levels are not stimulated and there is no evidence of gonadal germ cell maturation, the cause of precocious puberty lies outside the hypothalamic-pituitary axis, and the diagnostic process should focus on the adrenal glands and gonads (see Chapters 15 and 17). MRI studies are central to the workup for exclusion or characterization of organic lesions in the areas of the sella, optic chiasm, suprasellar hypothalamus, and interpeduncular cistern.[379]

Management of Sexual Precocity. Structural lesions of the hypothalamus are treated by surgery, radiation, chemotherapy, or combinations of these as indicated by the pathologic diagnosis and extent of disease. Endocrinologic manifestations of precocious puberty are best treated by GnRH agonists with the therapeutic goals of delaying sexual maturation to a more appropriate age and achieving optimal linear growth and bone mass, possibly with the combined use of GH treatment.[380,381] Other approaches include the use of cyproterone acetate, testolactone, or spironolactone to antagonize or inhibit gonadal steroid biosynthesis.[382,383] Precocious puberty is stressful to both the child and the parents, and it is essential that psychological support be provided.

Psychogenic Amenorrhea

Menstrual cycles can cease in young nonpregnant women with no demonstrable abnormalities of the brain, pituitary, or ovary in several situations,[384,385] including pseudocyesis (false pregnancy), anorexia nervosa, excessive exercise, psychogenic disorders, and hyperprolactinemic states (see Chapter 17). Psychogenic amenorrhea, the most common cause of secondary amenorrhea except for pregnancy, can occur with major psychopathology or minor psychic stress and is often temporary.

Exercise-induced amenorrhea may be a variant of psychogenic amenorrhea or may result from loss of body fat.[384,386] The syndrome is associated with intense and prolonged physical exertion such as running, swimming, or ballet dancing. Affected women are always below ideal body weight and have low stores of fat. If the activity is begun before puberty, normal sexual maturation can be delayed for many years. Fat mass may be a regulator of gonadotropin secretion with adipocyte-derived leptin as the principal mediator between peripheral energy stores and hypothalamic regulatory centers.[387] Studies in nonhuman primates showed a direct role of caloric intake in the pathogenesis of amenorrhea associated with long-distance running.[388] Exercise and psychogenic amenorrhea can have adverse effects because of the associated estrogen deficiency and accompanying osteopenia.[389]

Neurogenic Hypogonadism in Males

A discussion of neurogenic hypogonadism in males should begin with an account of Fröhlich syndrome (adiposogenital dystrophy), originally characterized as delayed puberty, hypogonadism, and obesity associated with a tumor that impinges on the hypothalamus.[1] It was subsequently recognized that either hypothalamic or pituitary dysfunction can induce hypogonadism and that the presence of obesity indicates that the appetite-regulating regions of the hypothalamus have been damaged. Several organic lesions of the hypothalamus can cause this syndrome, including tumors, encephalitis, microcephaly, Friedreich ataxia, and demyelinating diseases. Other important causes of HH are Kallmann syndrome and a subset of the Prader-Willi syndrome.[390]

However, most males with delayed sexual development do not have serious neurologic conditions. Furthermore, most obese boys with delayed sexual development have no structural damage to the hypothalamus but have constitutional delayed puberty, which is commonly associated with obesity. It is not known whether there is a functional disorder of the hypothalamus in this condition. It is thought that psychosexual development of brain maturation depends on the presence of androgens within a critical developmental window corresponding to puberty and therefore hypogonadism in boys (regardless of cause) should be treated by the middle teen years (15 years of age at the latest).

In adult men, hypogonadism (including reduced spermatogenesis) can be induced by emotional stress or severe exercise,[391] but this abnormality is seldom diagnosed because the symptoms are more subtle than menstrual cycle changes in similarly stressed women. Prolonged physical stress and sleep and energy deficiency can also decrease testosterone and gonadotropin levels.[392] Chronic intrathecal administration of opiates for the control of intractable pain syndromes is strongly associated with HH, and to a lesser extent with hypocorticism and GH deficiency, in both men and women.[393] Finally, critical illness with multiple causes is well known to be associated with hypogonadism and ineffectual altered pulsation of GnRH.[394]

Neurogenic Disorders of Prolactin Regulation

Neurogenic causes of hyperprolactinemia include irritative lesions of the chest wall (e.g., herpes zoster, thoracotomy), excessive tactile stimulation of the nipple, and lesions within the spinal cord (e.g., ependymoma).[395] Prolonged mechanical stimulation of the nipples by suckling or the use of a breast pump can initiate lactation in some women who are not pregnant, and neurologic lesions that interrupt the hypothalamic-pituitary connection can cause hyperprolactinemia, as discussed earlier. Hyperprolactinemia also occurs after certain forms of epileptic seizures. In one series, six of eight patients with temporal lobe seizures had a marked increase in PRL, whereas only one of eight patients with frontal lobe seizures developed hyperprolactinemia.[396] Agents that block D_2-like dopamine receptors (e.g., phenothiazines, later generation atypical antipsychotics) or prevent dopamine release (e.g., reserpine, methyldopa) must be excluded in all cases.

Because the nervous system exerts such profound effects on PRL secretion, patients with hyperprolactinemia (including those with adenomas) may have a deficit of PIF or an excess of PRF activity. In studies of PRL secretion in patients apparently cured of hyperprolactinemia by removal of a pituitary microadenoma, regulatory abnormalities persisted in some but not all patients. Persistence of regulatory abnormalities may be due to incomplete removal of tumor, abnormal function of the remaining part of the gland, or underlying hypothalamic abnormalities.[397]

Neurogenic Disorders of Growth Hormone Secretion

Hypothalamic Growth Failure

Loss of the normal nocturnal increase in GH secretion and loss of GH secretory responses to provocative stimuli occur early in the course of hypothalamic disease and may be the most sensitive endocrine indicator of hypothalamic dysfunction. As described earlier, anatomic malformations of midline cerebral structures are associated with abnormal GH secretion, presumably related to failure of the development of normal GH regulatory mechanisms. Such disorders include optic nerve dysplasia and midline prosencephalic malformations (absence of the septum pellucidum, abnormal third ventricle, and abnormal lamina terminalis). Certain complex genetic disorders including Prader-Willi syndrome also commonly involve reduced GH secretory capacity.[398] Idiopathic hypopituitarism with GH deficiency was considered earlier.

Maternal Deprivation Syndrome and Psychosocial Dwarfism

Infant neglect or abuse can impair growth and cause failure to thrive (the maternal deprivation syndrome). Malnutrition interacts with psychological factors to cause growth failure in children with the maternal deprivation syndrome, and each case should be carefully evaluated from this point of view. Older children with growth failure in a setting of abuse or severe emotional disturbance (termed *psychosocial dwarfism*) may also have abnormal circadian rhythms and deficient hGH release after insulin-induced hypoglycemia or arginine infusion (see Chapter 24).[399] Deficient release of ACTH and gonadotropins may also be present. A variant termed *hyperphagic short stature* has been identified.[400] These disorders can be reversed by placing the child in a supportive milieu; growth and neuroendocrine hGH responses rapidly return to normal.[401] The pathogenesis of altered GH secretion in children in response to deprivation is unknown. Furthermore, in the adult human, physical or emotional stress usually causes an increase in hGH secretion (see earlier discussion).

Neuroregulatory Growth Hormone Deficiency

The availability of biosynthetic hGH for treatment of short stature has brought into focus a group of patients who grow at low rates (<3rd percentile) and have low levels of serum IGF-1 but a normal hGH secretory reserve. Studies of 24-hour hGH secretion profiles indicate that many of these children do not have normal spontaneous hGH secretion (i.e., abnormal ultradian and circadian rhythms or decreased number or amplitude of secretory bursts, or both). These children with idiopathic short stature may have a functional regulatory disturbance of the hypothalamus and appear to grow normally when given exogenous hGH.[402]

There is considerable uncertainty about the criteria for the diagnosis of neuroregulatory hGH deficiency. Many normally growing children have profiles of hGH secretion that are indistinguishable from those in children with the postulated syndrome.[403] Patterns of hGH secretion do not predict which child will benefit from therapy, and there is a poor correlation between hGH secretion and growth. Furthermore, the results of repeated tests in children show considerable variability. It has been suggested that specific genetic defects may underlie the pathogenesis of a subset of children with this heterogeneous syndrome of growth failure.[404] The prevalence of an hGH neuroregulatory deficiency syndrome is thus unclear, and the decision to treat short children with hGH should be made cautiously.[405,406]

Neurogenic Hypersecretion of Growth Hormone

Diencephalic Syndrome. Children and infants with tumors in and around the third ventricle frequently become cachectic, which is often associated with elevated hGH levels and paradoxical GH secretory responses to glucose and insulin.[407] GH hypersecretion may be due to a hypothalamic abnormality or to malnutrition. Deficits of pituitary-adrenal regulation are less common. A striking feature is an alert appearance and seeming euphoria despite the profound emaciation. A variety of associated neurologic abnormalities may be present, including nystagmus, irritability, hydrocephalus, optic atrophy, tremor, and excessive sweating. CSF abnormalities include increased protein and the presence of abnormal cells. Most cases are due to chiasmatic-hypothalamic gliomas, with the majority classified as astrocytomas.[407] Treatment options include surgical resection, radiation therapy, and chemotherapy.[408]

Growth Hormone Hypersecretion Associated With Metabolic Disturbances. Apparently inappropriate hGH hypersecretion occurs with uncontrolled diabetes mellitus, hepatic failure, uremia, anorexia nervosa, and protein-calorie malnutrition. Nutritional factors are probably important in this response, because in normal persons obesity inhibits and fasting stimulates episodic GH hypersecretion.[409] In diabetes mellitus, cholinergic blockers reverse the abnormality,[207] possibly by inhibiting hypothalamic somatostatin secretion (see earlier discussion). Loss of inhibition of GH secretion by IGF-1 may also play a role, because most disorders in which this syndrome occurs are associated with low IGF-1 levels.

Neurogenic Disorders of Corticotropin Regulation

Hypothalamic CRH hypersecretion is the likely cause of sustained pituitary-adrenal hyperfunction in at least two situations: Cushing syndrome caused by the rare CRH-secreting gangliocytomas of the hypothalamus[410] and severe depression. Severe depression is associated with pituitary-adrenal abnormalities, including inappropriately elevated ACTH levels, abnormal cortisol circadian rhythms, and resistance to dexamethasone suppression.[143,147,148,411] The dexamethasone suppression test has, in fact, been used as an aid to the diagnosis of depressive illness. Another possible example of disordered neurogenic control of CRH associated with stress is the dysmetabolic syndrome.[412,413] This syndrome is characterized by mild hypercortisolism, blunted dexamethasone suppression of the HPA axis, visceral obesity, and hypertension and may be strongly associated with greater risks for cardiovascular disease and stroke.

A unique syndrome of ACTH hypersecretion termed *periodic hypothalamic discharge* (Wolff syndrome) has been described in one young man. The patient had a recurring cyclic disorder characterized by high fever, paroxysms of glucocorticoid hypersecretion, and electroencephalographic abnormalities.[414]

Nonendocrine Manifestations of Hypothalamic Disease

The hypothalamus is involved in the regulation of diverse functions and behaviors (Table 7-9). Psychological abnormalities in hypothalamic disease include antisocial behavior; attacks of rage, laughing, and crying; disturbed sleep patterns; excessive sexuality; and hallucinations. Both somnolence (with posterior lesions) and pathologic wakefulness (with anterior lesions) occur, as do bulimia and profound anorexia. The abnormal eating patterns are analogous to the syndromes of hyperphagia produced in rats by destruction of the VMH or of connections to the PVH. Lateral hypothalamic damage causes profound anorexia. A more complete discussion of imbalance in energy homeostasis (both obesity and cachexia) associated

TABLE 7-9
Neurologic Manifestations of Nonendocrine Hypothalamic Disease

Disorders of Temperature Regulation

Hyperthermia
Hypothermia
Poikilothermia

Disorders of Food Intake

Hyperphagia (bulimia)
Anorexia nervosa, aphagia
Cachexia

Disorders of Water Intake

Compulsive water drinking
Adipsia
Essential hypernatremia

Disorders of Sleep and Consciousness

Narcolepsy/cataplexy
Somnolence
Sleep rhythm reversal
Akinetic mutism
Coma
Delirium

Periodic Disease of Hypothalamic Origin

Diencephalic epilepsy
Kleine-Levin syndrome
Periodic discharge syndrome of Wolff

Disorders of Psychic Function

Rage behavior
Hallucinations
Hypersexuality

Disorders of the Autonomic Nervous System

Pulmonary edema
Cardiac arrhythmias
Sphincter disturbance

Congenital Hypothalamic Disease

Prader-Willi syndrome
Laurence-Moon-Biedl syndrome

Miscellaneous

Diencephalic syndrome of infancy
Cerebral gigantism

with hypothalamic dysfunction and neuropeptides is presented in Chapter 35.

Patients with hypothalamic damage may experience hyperthermia, hypothermia, unexplained fluctuations in body temperature, and poikilothermy. Disturbances of sweating, acrocyanosis, loss of sphincter control, and diencephalic epilepsy are occasional manifestations. Hypothalamic damage also causes loss of recent memory, believed to be due to damage of the mammillothalamic pathways. Severe memory loss, obesity, and personality changes (e.g., apathy, loss of ability to concentrate, aggressive antisocial behavior, severe food craving, inability to work or attend school) may occur with suprasellar extension of pituitary tumors, hypothalamic radiation, or damage incurred from surgical removal of parasellar tumors. Hypothalamic tumors grow slowly and may reach a large size while producing minimal disturbance of behavior or visceral homeostasis, whereas surgery of limited extent can produce striking functional abnormalities. Presumably, this is because slowly growing lesions permit compensatory responses to develop. These potential consequences should

be weighed carefully with the neurosurgeon, patient, and patient's family in planning the therapeutic approach. Adverse effects of treatment have led to more conservative surgical guidelines for the treatment of craniopharyngioma. A recent review from the University of Pittsburgh summarizes their individualized treatment program that includes microsurgical tumor resection, intracavitary ^{32}P radiotherapy, and gamma knife stereotactic radiosurgery to produce maximal benefit with minimal morbidity.[415]

Narcolepsy

A convergence of functional genomics from two animal species, the dog and mouse, has dramatically refocused attention on neuropeptide circuits of the hypothalamus in the control of sleep and wakefulness. Positional cloning was used to identify mutations in the hypocretin-orexin receptor 2 as a cause of canine narcolepsy.[416] Subsequently, knockout of the gene encoding the orexin-hypocretin peptide precursor produced an equivalent narcoleptic syndrome in mice,[417] further establishing this neuropeptide system as a major component of sleep-modulating neural circuits. The additional role of orexin-hypocretin in coordinating arousal states and feeding behavior is discussed in Chapter 35. These new discoveries add to the list of other hypothalamic neuropeptides including GHRH, somatostatin, cortistatin, CRH, galanin, ghrelin, and NPY that have established functions in modulation of the sleep cycle.

Histaminergic neurons of the tuberomammillary nucleus express both forms of the orexin receptor and make reciprocal synaptic connections with orexin neurons in the lateral hypothalamus. Furthermore, orexin is an excitatory transmitter for the histamine neurons, suggesting that the two populations cooperate in the regulation of rapid eye movement sleep.[418] A recent study suggested that the two populations of neurons also play complementary, but distinct, roles in the maintenance of wakefulness.[419] Targeted ablation of orexin neurons in the lateral hypothalamus of rats by means of a hypocretin receptor 2–saporin conjugate produced narcoleptic-like sleep behavior,[420] closely paralleling the clinical findings and profound reduction in numbers of orexin-hypocretin neurons in the lateral hypothalamus of humans with narcolepsy.[421]

In summary, most cases of spontaneous narcolepsy with cataplexy result from a degenerative hypothalamic disorder, most likely autoimmune in pathogenesis, that produces a selective destruction of neuropeptidergic neurons. The absence of immunoreactive orexin-hypocretin in CSF is a sensitive diagnostic test for the disease. Future development of bioavailable, orexin-hypocretin receptor-selective compounds may provide a specific treatment alternative or adjunct to the stimulant and antidepressant drugs currently used for management of symptoms. More generally, these recent discoveries suggest the possibility that other cryptic hypothalamic disorders could be caused by selective disturbances in other neuropeptidergic circuits.

ACKNOWLEDGMENTS

The author is highly indebted to Dr. Seymour Reichlin, not only for material he shared from the ninth edition of this text but also for the inspiration and mentorship he has provided to the current generation of neuroendocrinologists. Thanks are also due to Drs. Roger Cone, Joel Elmiquist, and Judy Cameron for their respective contributions to the tenth edition of this text.

REFERENCES

1. Fröhlich A. Ein Fall von Tumor der Hypophysis cerebri ohne Akromegalie. *Wein Klin Rundsch.* 1901;15:883.
2. Crowe S, Cushing H, Homans J. Experimental hypophysectomy. *Bull Johns Hopkins Hosp.* 1910;21:128-169.
3. Aschner B. Uber die Funktion der Hypophyse. *Pflugers Arch Physiol.* 1912;146:1.
4. Hetherington AW, Ranson SW. Hypothalamic lesions and adiposity in the rat. *Anat Rec.* 1940;78:149-172.
5. Popa G, Fielding U. A portal circulation from the pituitary to the hypothalamic region. *J Anat.* 1930;65:88.
6. Wislocki GB, King LS. Permeability of the hypophysis and hypothalamus to vital dyes, with study of hypophyseal blood supply. *Am J Anat.* 1936;58:421-472.
7. Harris G. Neural control of the pituitary. *Physiol Rev.* 1948;28:139-179.
8. Schally AV, Redding TW, Bowers CY, et al. Isolation and properties of porcine thyrotropin-releasing hormone. *J Biol Chem.* 1969;244:4077-4088.
9. Burgus R, Dunn TF, Desiderio D, et al. Characterization of ovine hypothalamic hypophysiotropic TSH-releasing factor. *Nature.* 1970;226:321-325.
10. Zhang Y, Proenca A, Maffei M, et al. Positional cloning of the mouse obese gene and its human homologue. *Nature.* 1994;372:425-434.
11. Park HK, Ahima RS. Physiology of leptin: energy homeostasis, neuroendocrine function and metabolism. *Metabolism.* 2015;64:24-34.
12. Kojima M, Hosoda H, Date Y, et al. Ghrelin is a growth-hormone-releasing acylated peptide from stomach. *Nature.* 1999;402:656-660.
13. Spergel DJ, Kruth U, Hanley DF, et al. GABA- and glutamate-activated channels in green fluorescent protein-tagged gonadotropin-releasing hormone neurons in transgenic mice. *J Neurosci.* 1999;19:2037-2050.
14. Cowley MA, Smart JL, Rubinstein M, et al. Leptin activates anorexigenic POMC neurons through a neural network in the arcuate nucleus. *Nature.* 2001;411:480-484.
15. Scharrer B. Neurosecretion: beginnings and new directions in neuropeptide research. *Annu Rev Neurosci.* 1987;10:1-17.
16. Hokfelt T, Johansson O, Ljungdahl A, et al. Peptidergic neurons. *Nature.* 1980;284:515-521.
17. Marder E. Neuromodulation of neuronal circuits: back to the future. *Neuron.* 2012;76:1-11.
18. Ondicova K, Mravec B. Multilevel interactions between the sympathetic and parasympathetic nervous systems: a minireview. *Endocr Regul.* 2010;44:69-75.
19. Loewy AD. Anatomy of the autonomic nervous system: an overview. In: Loewy AD, Spyer KM, eds. *Central Regulation of Autonomic Function.* New York, NY: Oxford University Press; 1990:3-16.
20. Ryabinin AE, Tsivkovskaia NO, Ryabinin SA. Urocortin 1-containing neurons in the human Edinger-Westphal nucleus. *Neuroscience.* 2005;134:1317-1323.
21. Ahren B. Autonomic regulation of islet hormone secretion: implications for health and disease. *Diabetologia.* 2000;43:393-410.
22. Berthoud HR, Fox EA, Powley TL. Localization of vagal preganglionics that stimulate insulin and glucagon secretion. *Am J Physiol.* 1990;258:R160-R168.
23. Saltiel AR. New perspectives into the molecular pathogenesis and treatment of type 2 diabetes. *Cell.* 2001;104:517-529.
24. Levin BE, Dunn-Meynell AA, Routh VH. Brain glucose sensing and body energy homeostasis: role in obesity and diabetes. *Am J Physiol.* 1999;276:R1223-R1231.
25. Koutcherov Y, Mai JK, Paxinos G. Hypothalamus of the human fetus. *J Chem Neuroanat.* 2003;26:253-270.
26. McClellan KM, Parker KL, Tobet S. Development of the ventromedial nucleus of the hypothalamus. *Front Neuroendocrinol.* 2006;27:193-209.
27. Whitlock KE. Origin and development of GnRH neurons. *Trends Endocrinol Metab.* 2005;16:145-151.
28. Caqueret A, Yang C, Duplan S, et al. Looking for trouble: a search for developmental defects of the hypothalamus. *Horm Res.* 2005;64:222-230.
29. Pearson CA, Placzek M. Development of the medial hypothalamus: forming a functional hypothalamic-neurohypophyseal interface. *Curr Top Dev Biol.* 2013;106:49-88.
30. Wang L, Meece K, Williams DJ, et al. Differentiation of hypothalamic-like neurons from human pluripotent stem cells. *J Clin Invest.* 2015;125:796-808.
31. Merkle FT, Maroof A, Wataya T, et al. Generation of neuropeptidergic hypothalamic neurons from human pluripotent stem cells. *Development.* 2015;142:633-643.
32. Forger NG. Cell death and sexual differentiation of the nervous system. *Neuroscience.* 2006;138:929-938.
33. Simerly RB. Wired on hormones: endocrine regulation of hypothalamic development. *Curr Opin Neurobiol.* 2005;15:81-85.
34. Fujisawa I. Magnetic resonance imaging of the hypothalamic-neurohypophyseal system. *J Neuroendocrinol.* 2004;16:297-302.
35. Evans VR, Manning AB, Bernard LH, et al. Alpha-melanocyte-stimulating hormone and N-acetyl-beta-endorphin immunoreactivities are localized in the human pituitary but are not restricted to the zona intermedia. *Endocrinology.* 1994;134:97-106.
36. Leng G, Pineda Reyes R, Sabatier N, et al. The posterior pituitary: from Geoffrey Harris to our present understanding. *J Endocrinol.* [Epub 2015 Apr 21].
37. Crowley WR. Neuroendocrine regulation of lactation and milk production. *Compr Physiol.* 2015;5:255-291.
38. Knigge KM, Scott DE. Structure and function of the median eminence. *Am J Anat.* 1970;129:223-243.
39. Bolborea M, Dale N. Hypothalamic tanycytes: potential roles in the control of feeding and energy balance. *Trends Neurosci.* 2013;36:91-100.
40. Rodriguez EM, Blazquez JL, Pastor FE, et al. Hypothalamic tanycytes: a key component of brain-endocrine interaction. *Int Rev Cytol.* 2005;247:89-164.
41. Parkash J, Messina A, Langlet F, et al. Semaphorin7A regulates neuroglial plasticity in the adult hypothalamic median eminence. *Nat Commun.* 2015;6:6385.
42. Ganong WF. Circumventricular organs: definition and role in the regulation of endocrine and autonomic function. *Clin Exp Pharmacol Physiol.* 2000;27:422-427.
43. Abbott NJ, Ronnback L, Hansson E. Astrocyte-endothelial interactions at the blood-brain barrier. *Nat Rev Neurosci.* 2006;7:41-53.
44. Coble JP, Grobe JL, Johnson AK, et al. Mechanisms of brain renin angiotensin system-induced drinking and blood pressure: importance of the subfornical organ. *Am J Physiol Regul Integr Comp Physiol.* 2015;308:R238-R249.
45. Mimee A, Smith PM, Ferguson AV. Circumventricular organs: targets for integration of circulating fluid and energy balance signals? *Physiol Behav.* 2013;121:96-102.
46. Rodriguez EM, Rodriguez S, Hein S. The subcommissural organ. *Microsc Res Tech.* 1998;41:98-123.
47. Schwartz MW, Seeley RJ, Campfield LA, et al. Identification of targets of leptin action in rat hypothalamus. *J Clin Invest.* 1996;98:1101-1106.
48. Elias CF, Aschkenasi C, Lee C, et al. Leptin differentially regulates NPY and POMC neurons projecting to the lateral hypothalamic area. *Neuron.* 1999;23:775-786.
49. Herde MK, Iremonger KJ, Constantin S, et al. GnRH neurons elaborate a long-range projection with shared axonal and dendritic functions. *J Neurosci.* 2013;33:12689-12697.
50. Blatteis CM. Role of the OVLT in the febrile response to circulating pyrogens. *Prog Brain Res.* 1992;91:409-412.
51. Oka T. Prostaglandin E2 as a mediator of fever: the role of prostaglandin E (EP) receptors. *Front Biosci.* 2004;9:3046-3057.
52. Oldfield BJ, Bicknell RJ, McAllen RM, et al. Intravenous hypertonic saline induces Fos immunoreactivity in neurons throughout the lamina terminalis. *Brain Res.* 1991;561:151-156.
53. Wouterlood FG, Bloem B, Mansvelder HD, et al. A fourth generation of neuroanatomical tracing techniques: exploiting the offspring of genetic engineering. *J Neurosci Methods.* 2014;235:331-348.
54. Ferguson AV, Bains JS. Actions of angiotensin in the subfornical organ and area postrema: implications for long term control of autonomic output. *Clin Exp Pharmacol Physiol.* 1997;24:96-101.
55. Standaert DG, Saper CB. Origin of the atriopeptin-like immunoreactive innervation of the paraventricular nucleus of the hypothalamus. *J Neurosci.* 1988;8:1940-1950.
56. Saper CB, Levisohn D. Afferent connections of the median preoptic nucleus in the rat: anatomical evidence for a cardiovascular integrative mechanism in the anteroventral third ventricular (AV3V) region. *Brain Res.* 1983;288:21-31.
57. Simpson JB, Routtenberg A. Subfornical organ: a dipsogenic site of action of angiotensin II. *Science.* 1978;201:379-381.
58. Oka Y, Ye M, Zuker CS. Thirst driving and suppressing signals encoded by distinct neural populations in the brain. *Nature.* 2015;520:349-352.
59. Miller AD, Leslie RA. The area postrema and vomiting. *Front Neuroendocrinol.* 1994;15:301-320.
60. Riediger T. The receptive function of hypothalamic and brainstem centres to hormonal and nutrient signals affecting energy balance. *Proc Nutr Soc.* 2012;71:463-477.
61. Osborn JW, Collister JP, Carlson SH. Angiotensin and osmoreceptor inputs to the area postrema: role in long-term control of fluid homeostasis and arterial pressure. *Clin Exp Pharmacol Physiol.* 2000;27:443-449.
62. Rodriguez S, Caprile T. Functional aspects of the subcommissural organ-Reissner's fiber complex with emphasis in the clearance of brain monoamines. *Microsc Res Tech.* 2001;52:564-572.
63. Dubocovich ML, Markowska M. Functional MT1 and MT2 melatonin receptors in mammals. *Endocrine.* 2005;27:101-110.
64. Reiter RJ, Tan DX, Galano A. Melatonin: exceeding expectations. *Physiology (Bethesda).* 2014;29:325-333.
65. Boutin JA, Audinot V, Ferry G, et al. Molecular tools to study melatonin pathways and actions. *Trends Pharmacol Sci.* 2005;26:412-419.
66. Reppert SM. Melatonin receptors: molecular biology of a new family of G protein-coupled receptors. *J Biol Rhythms.* 1997;12:528-531.

67. Foulkes NS, Borjigin J, Snyder SH, et al. Rhythmic transcription: the molecular basis of circadian melatonin synthesis. *Trends Neurosci.* 1997;20:487-492.
68. Nakazawa K, Marubayashi U, McCann SM. Mediation of the short-loop negative feedback of luteinizing hormone (LH) on LH-releasing hormone release by melatonin-induced inhibition of LH release from the pars tuberalis. *Proc Natl Acad Sci U S A.* 1991;88:7576-7579.
69. Rea MS, Figueiro MG, Bullough JD, et al. A model of phototransduction by the human circadian system. *Brain Res Brain Res Rev.* 2005; 50:213-228.
70. Shibata S, Cassone VM, Moore RY. Effects of melatonin on neuronal activity in the rat suprachiasmatic nucleus in vitro. *Neurosci Lett.* 1989;97:140-144.
71. Liu C, Weaver DR, Jin X, et al. Molecular dissection of two distinct actions of melatonin on the suprachiasmatic circadian clock. *Neuron.* 1997;19:91-102.
72. Jin X, von Gall C, Pieschl RL, et al. Targeted disruption of the mouse Mel(1b) melatonin receptor. *Mol Cell Biol.* 2003;23:1054-1060.
73. Arendt J. Melatonin, circadian rhythms, and sleep. *N Engl J Med.* 2000;343:1114-1116.
74. Buscemi N, Vandermeer B, Hooton N, et al. The efficacy and safety of exogenous melatonin for primary sleep disorders. A meta-analysis. *J Gen Intern Med.* 2005;20:1151-1158.
75. Buscemi N, Vandermeer B, Hooton N, et al. Efficacy and safety of exogenous melatonin for secondary sleep disorders and sleep disorders accompanying sleep restriction: meta-analysis. *Br Med J.* 2006;332: 385-393.
76. Castiglione F, Pappalardo F, Bianca C, et al. Modeling biology spanning different scales: an open challenge. *Biomed Res Int.* 2014;2014:902545.
77. Saper CB, Lu J, Chou TC, et al. The hypothalamic integrator for circadian rhythms. *Trends Neurosci.* 2005;28:152-157.
78. Reppert SM, Weaver DR. Coordination of circadian timing in mammals. *Nature.* 2002;418:935-941.
79. Perreau-Lenz S, Pevet P, Buijs RM, et al. The biological clock: the bodyguard of temporal homeostasis. *Chronobiol Int.* 2004;21:1-25.
80. Gachon F, Nagoshi E, Brown SA, et al. The mammalian circadian timing system: from gene expression to physiology. *Chromosoma.* 2004;113:103-112.
81. Tonsfeldt KJ, Chappell PE. Clocks on top: the role of the circadian clock in the hypothalamic and pituitary regulation of endocrine physiology. *Mol Cell Endocrinol.* 2012;349:3-12.
82. Reppert SM. Pre-natal development of a hypothalamic biological clock. *Prog Brain Res.* 1992;93:119-131, discussion 132.
83. Yamada M, Radovick S, Wondisford FE, et al. Cloning and structure of human genomic DNA and hypothalamic cDNA encoding human prepro thyrotropin-releasing hormone. *Mol Endocrinol.* 1990;4: 551-556.
84. Lee SL, Stewart K, Goodman RH. Structure of the gene encoding rat thyrotropin releasing hormone. *J Biol Chem.* 1988;263:16604-16609.
85. Perello M, Nillni EA. The biosynthesis and processing of neuropeptides: lessons from prothyrotropin releasing hormone (proTRH). *Front Biosci.* 2007;12:3554-3565.
86. Engler D, Redei E, Kola I. The corticotropin-release inhibitory factor hypothesis: a review of the evidence for the existence of inhibitory as well as stimulatory hypophysiotropic regulation of adrenocorticotropin secretion and biosynthesis. *Endocr Rev.* 1999;20:460-500.
87. Jackson IM. Thyrotropin-releasing hormone. *N Engl J Med.* 1982;306: 145-155.
88. Yamada M, Satoh T, Mori M. Mice lacking the thyrotropin-releasing hormone gene: what do they tell us? *Thyroid.* 2003;13:1111-1121.
89. Straub RE, Frech GC, Joho RH, et al. Expression cloning of a cDNA encoding the mouse pituitary thyrotropin-releasing hormone receptor. *Proc Natl Acad Sci U S A.* 1990;87:9514-9518.
90. Sun Y, Lu X, Gershengorn MC. Thyrotropin-releasing hormone receptors—similarities and differences. *J Mol Endocrinol.* 2003;30: 87-97.
91. Gary KA, Sevarino KA, Yarbrough GG, et al. The thyrotropin-releasing hormone (TRH) hypothesis of homeostatic regulation: implications for TRH-based therapeutics. *J Pharmacol Exp Ther.* 2003;305:410-416.
92. Yarbrough GG, Kamath J, Winokur A, et al. Thyrotropin-releasing hormone (TRH) in the neuroaxis: therapeutic effects reflect physiological functions and molecular actions. *Med Hypotheses.* 2007;69: 1249-1256.
93. Khomane KS, Meena CL, Jain R, et al. Novel thyrotropin-releasing hormone analogs: a patent review. *Expert Opin Ther Pat.* 2011;21: 1673-1691.
94. Takeuchi Y, Takano T, Abe J, et al. Thyrotropin-releasing hormone: role in the treatment of West syndrome and related epileptic encephalopathies. *Brain Dev.* 2001;23:662-667.
95. Costa-e-Sousa RH, Hollenberg AN. Minireview: The neural regulation of the hypothalamic-pituitary-thyroid axis. *Endocrinology.* 2012;153: 4128-4135.
96. Dyess EM, Segerson TP, Liposits Z, et al. Triiodothyronine exerts direct cell-specific regulation of thyrotropin-releasing hormone gene expression in the hypothalamic paraventricular nucleus. *Endocrinology.* 1988; 123:2291-2297.

97. Schreiber G, Southwell BR, Richardson SJ. Hormone delivery systems to the brain-transthyretin. *Exp Clin Endocrinol Diabetes.* 1995;103: 75-80.
98. Lechan RM, Kakucska I. Feedback regulation of thyrotropin-releasing hormone gene expression by thyroid hormone in the hypothalamic paraventricular nucleus. *Ciba Found Symp.* 1992;168:144-158, discussion 158-164.
99. Lechan RM, Fekete C. Role of thyroid hormone deiodination in the hypothalamus. *Thyroid.* 2005;15:883-897.
100. Fekete C, Lechan RM. Central regulation of hypothalamic-pituitary-thyroid axis under physiological and pathophysiological conditions. *Endocr Rev.* 2014;35:159-194.
101. Arimura A, Schally AV. Increase in basal and thyrotropin-releasing hormone (TRH)-stimulated secretion of thyrotropin (TSH) by passive immunization with antiserum to somatostatin in rats. *Endocrinology.* 1976;98:1069-1072.
102. Brabant G, Prank K, Ranft U, et al. Physiological regulation of circadian and pulsatile thyrotropin secretion in normal man and woman. *J Clin Endocrinol Metab.* 1990;70:403-409.
103. Fares F. The role of O-linked and N-linked oligosaccharides on the structure-function of glycoprotein hormones: development of agonists and antagonists. *Biochim Biophys Acta.* 2006;1760:560-567.
104. Arancibia S, Rage F, Astier H, et al. Neuroendocrine and autonomous mechanisms underlying thermoregulation in cold environment. *Neuroendocrinology.* 1996;64:257-267.
105. Shioda S, Nakai Y, Sato A, et al. Electron-microscopic cytochemistry of the catecholaminergic innervation of TRH neurons in the rat hypothalamus. *Cell Tissue Res.* 1986;245:247-252.
106. Joseph-Bravo P, Jaimes-Hoy L, Charli JL. Regulation of TRH neurons and energy homeostasis-related signals under stress. *J Endocrinol.* 2015; 224:R139-R159.
107. Mebis L, van den Berghe G. The hypothalamus-pituitary-thyroid axis in critical illness. *Neth J Med.* 2009;67(10):332-340.
108. Kakucska I, Qi Y, Lechan RM. Changes in adrenal status affect hypothalamic thyrotropin-releasing hormone gene expression in parallel with corticotropin-releasing hormone. *Endocrinology.* 1995;136: 2795-2802.
109. Cintra A, Fuxe K, Wikstrom AC, et al. Evidence for thyrotropin-releasing hormone and glucocorticoid receptor-immunoreactive neurons in various preoptic and hypothalamic nuclei of the male rat. *Brain Res.* 1990;506:139-144.
110. Shi ZX, Levy A, Lightman SL. Hippocampal input to the hypothalamus inhibits thyrotrophin and thyrotrophin-releasing hormone gene expression. *Neuroendocrinology.* 1993;57:576-580.
111. Blake NG, Eckland DJ, Foster OJ, et al. Inhibition of hypothalamic thyrotropin-releasing hormone messenger ribonucleic acid during food deprivation. *Endocrinology.* 1991;129:2714-2718.
112. Ahima RS, Prabakaran D, Mantzoros C, et al. Role of leptin in the neuroendocrine response to fasting. *Nature.* 1996;382:250-252.
113. Legradi G, Emerson CH, Ahima RS, et al. Leptin prevents fasting-induced suppression of prothyrotropin-releasing hormone messenger ribonucleic acid in neurons of the hypothalamic paraventricular nucleus. *Endocrinology.* 1997;138:2569-2576.
114. Lechan RM, Fekete C. Feedback regulation of thyrotropin-releasing hormone (TRH): mechanisms for the non-thyroidal illness syndrome. *J Endocrinol Invest.* 2004;27:105-119.
115. Lechan RM, Fekete C. Role of melanocortin signaling in the regulation of the hypothalamic-pituitary-thyroid (HPT) axis. *Peptides.* 2006;27: 310-325.
116. Harris M, Aschkenasi C, Elias CF, et al. Transcriptional regulation of the thyrotropin-releasing hormone gene by leptin and melanocortin signaling. *J Clin Invest.* 2001;107:111-120.
117. Montague CT, Farooqi IS, Whitehead JP, et al. Congenital leptin deficiency is associated with severe early-onset obesity in humans. *Nature.* 1997;387:903-908.
118. Farooqi IS, Yeo GS, Keogh JM, et al. Dominant and recessive inheritance of morbid obesity associated with melanocortin 4 receptor deficiency. *J Clin Invest.* 2000;106:271-279.
119. Dubuis JM, Dayer JM, Siegrist-Kaiser CA, et al. Human recombinant interleukin-1 beta decreases plasma thyroid hormone and thyroid stimulating hormone levels in rats. *Endocrinology.* 1988;123:2175-2181.
120. Scarborough DE, Lee SL, Dinarello CA, et al. Interleukin-1 beta stimulates somatostatin biosynthesis in primary cultures of fetal rat brain. *Endocrinology.* 1989;124:549-551.
121. Pang XP, Hershman JM, Mirell CJ, et al. Impairment of hypothalamic-pituitary-thyroid function in rats treated with human recombinant tumor necrosis factor-alpha (cachectin). *Endocrinology.* 1989;125: 76-84.
122. Koenig JI, Snow K, Clark BD, et al. Intrinsic pituitary interleukin-1 beta is induced by bacterial lipopolysaccharide. *Endocrinology.* 1990;126: 3053-3058.
123. Spath-Schwalbe E, Schrezenmeier H, Bornstein S, et al. Endocrine effects of recombinant interleukin 6 in man. *Neuroendocrinology.* 1996;63:237-243.

124. Shibahara S, Morimoto Y, Furutani Y, et al. Isolation and sequence analysis of the human corticotropin-releasing factor precursor gene. *EMBO J.* 1983;2:775-779.

125. Lovejoy DA, Balment RJ. Evolution and physiology of the corticotropin-releasing factor (CRF) family of neuropeptides in vertebrates. *Gen Comp Endocrinol.* 1999;115:1-22.

126. Hsu SY, Hsueh AJ. Human stresscopin and stresscopin-related peptide are selective ligands for the type 2 corticotropin-releasing hormone receptor. *Nat Med.* 2001;7:605-611.

127. Chen R, Lewis KA, Perrin MH, et al. Expression cloning of a human corticotropin-releasing-factor receptor. *Proc Natl Acad Sci U S A.* 1993; 90:8967-8971.

128. Stenzel P, Kesterson R, Yeung W, et al. Identification of a novel murine receptor for corticotropin-releasing hormone expressed in the heart. *Mol Endocrinol.* 1995;9:637-645.

129. Valdenaire O, Giller T, Breu V, et al. A new functional isoform of the human CRF2 receptor for corticotropin-releasing factor. *Biochim Biophys Acta.* 1997;1352:129-132.

130. Kostich WA, Chen A, Sperle K, et al. Molecular identification and analysis of a novel human corticotropin-releasing factor (CRF) receptor: the CRF2gamma receptor. *Mol Endocrinol.* 1998;12:1077-1085.

131. Takahashi K, Totsune K, Sone M, et al. Regional distribution of urocortin-like immunoreactivity and expression of urocortin mRNA in the human brain. *Peptides.* 1998;19:643-647.

132. Chen A, Zorrilla E, Smith S, et al. Urocortin 2-deficient mice exhibit gender-specific alterations in circadian hypothalamus-pituitary-adrenal axis and depressive-like behavior. *J Neurosci.* 2006;26:5500-5510.

133. Li C, Chen P, Vaughan J, et al. Urocortin 3 regulates glucose-stimulated insulin secretion and energy homeostasis. *Proc Natl Acad Sci U S A.* 2007;104:4206-4211.

134. Chalmers DT, Lovenberg TW, De Souza EB. Localization of novel corticotropin-releasing factor receptor (CRF2) mRNA expression to specific subcortical nuclei in rat brain: comparison with CRF1 receptor mRNA expression. *J Neurosci.* 1995;15:6340-6350.

135. Lovenberg TW, Chalmers DT, Liu C, et al. CRF2 alpha and CRF2 beta receptor mRNAs are differentially distributed between the rat central nervous system and peripheral tissues. *Endocrinology.* 1995;136: 4139-4142.

136. Westphal NJ, Seasholtz AF. CRH-BP: the regulation and function of a phylogenetically conserved binding protein. *Front Biosci.* 2006;11: 1878-1891.

137. Bale TL, Vale WW. CRF and CRF receptors: role in stress responsivity and other behaviors. *Annu Rev Pharmacol Toxicol.* 2004;44:525-557.

138. Rivier J, Rivier C, Vale W. Synthetic competitive antagonists of corticotropin-releasing factor: effect on ACTH secretion in the rat. *Science.* 1984;224:889-891.

139. Maecker H, Desai A, Dash R, et al. Astressin, a novel and potent CRF antagonist, is neuroprotective in the hippocampus when administered after a seizure. *Brain Res.* 1997;744:166-170.

140. Habib KE, Weld KP, Rice KC, et al. Oral administration of a corticotropin-releasing hormone receptor antagonist significantly attenuates behavioral, neuroendocrine, and autonomic responses to stress in primates. *Proc Natl Acad Sci U S A.* 2000;97:6079-6084.

141. Broadbear JH, Winger G, Rivier JE, et al. Corticotropin-releasing hormone antagonists, astressin B and antalarmin: differing profiles of activity in rhesus monkeys. *Neuropsychopharmacology.* 2004;29: 1112-1121.

142. Ruhmann A, Bonk I, Lin CR, et al. Structural requirements for peptidic antagonists of the corticotropin-releasing factor receptor (CRFR): development of CRFR2beta-selective antisauvagine-30. *Proc Natl Acad Sci U S A.* 1998;95:15264-15269.

143. Claes SJ. Corticotropin-releasing hormone (CRH) in psychiatry: from stress to psychopathology. *Ann Med.* 2004;36:50-61.

144. Keck ME, Holsboer F, Muller MB. Mouse mutants for the study of corticotropin-releasing hormone receptor function: development of novel treatment strategies for mood disorders. *Ann N Y Acad Sci.* 2004;1018:445-457.

145. Gravanis A, Margioris AN. The corticotropin-releasing factor (CRF) family of neuropeptides in inflammation: potential therapeutic applications. *Curr Med Chem.* 2005;12:1503-1512.

146. Gold PW. The organization of the stress system and its dysregulation in depressive illness. *Mol Psychiatry.* 2015;20:32-47.

147. Modell S, Lauer CJ, Schreiber W, et al. Hormonal response pattern in the combined DEX-CRH test is stable over time in subjects at high familial risk for affective disorders. *Neuropsychopharmacology.* 1998;18: 253-262.

148. Nemeroff CB, Vale WW. The neurobiology of depression: inroads to treatment and new drug discovery. *J Clin Psychiatry.* 2005;66(Suppl 7): 5-13.

149. Parkes DG, Weisinger RS, May CN. Cardiovascular actions of CRH and urocortin: an update. *Peptides.* 2001;22:821-827.

150. Coste SC, Kesterson RA, Heldwein KA, et al. Abnormal adaptations to stress and impaired cardiovascular function in mice lacking corticotropin-releasing hormone receptor-2. *Nat Genet.* 2000;24: 403-409.

151. Jessop DS, Harbuz MS, Lightman SL. CRH in chronic inflammatory stress. *Peptides.* 2001;22:803-807.

152. Seymour PA, Schmidt AW, Schulz DW. The pharmacology of CP-154,526, a non-peptide antagonist of the CRH1 receptor: a review. *CNS Drug Rev.* 2003;9:57-96.

153. Holsboer F, Ising M. Central CRH system in depression and anxiety: evidence from clinical studies with CRH1 receptor antagonists. *Eur J Pharmacol.* 2008;583:350-357.

154. Zorrilla EP, Logrip ML, Koob GF. Corticotropin releasing factor: a key role in the neurobiology of addiction. *Front Neuroendocrinol.* 2014;35: 234-244.

155. Keller-Wood ME, Dallman MF. Corticosteroid inhibition of ACTH secretion. *Endocr Rev.* 1984;5:1-24.

156. Arriza JL, Simerly RB, Swanson LW, et al. The neuronal mineralocorticoid receptor as a mediator of glucocorticoid response. *Neuron.* 1988;1: 887-900.

157. de Kloet ER, Oitzl MS, Joels M. Functional implications of brain corticosteroid receptor diversity. *Cell Mol Neurobiol.* 1993;13:433-455.

158. Sapolsky RM, Krey LC, McEwen BS. The neuroendocrinology of stress and aging: the glucocorticoid cascade hypothesis. *Endocr Rev.* 1986;7: 284-301.

159. Watts AG. Glucocorticoid regulation of peptide genes in neuroendocrine CRH neurons: a complexity beyond negative feedback. *Front Neuroendocrinol.* 2005;26:109-130.

160. Berardelli R, Karamouzis I, D'Angelo V, et al. Role of mineralocorticoid receptors on the hypothalamus-pituitary-adrenal axis in humans. *Endocrine.* 2013;43:51-58.

161. Malcher-Lopes R, Di S, Marcheselli VS, et al. Opposing crosstalk between leptin and glucocorticoids rapidly modulates synaptic excitation via endocannabinoid release. *J Neurosci.* 2006;26:6643-6650.

162. Dallman MF. Fast glucocorticoid actions on brain: back to the future. *Front Neuroendocrinol.* 2005;26:103-108.

163. Herman JP, Figueiredo H, Mueller NK, et al. Central mechanisms of stress integration: hierarchical circuitry controlling hypothalamo-pituitary-adrenocortical responsiveness. *Front Neuroendocrinol.* 2003;24: 151-180.

164. Sawchenko PE, Li HY, Ericsson A. Circuits and mechanisms governing hypothalamic responses to stress: a tale of two paradigms. *Prog Brain Res.* 2000;122:61-78.

165. Ziegler DR, Cullinan WE, Herman JP. Organization and regulation of paraventricular nucleus glutamate signaling systems: N-methyl-D-aspartate receptors. *J Comp Neurol.* 2005;484:43-56.

166. Roland BL, Sawchenko PE. Local origins of some GABAergic projections to the paraventricular and supraoptic nuclei of the hypothalamus in the rat. *J Comp Neurol.* 1993;332:123-143.

167. Sapolsky R, Rivier C, Yamamoto G, et al. Interleukin-1 stimulates the secretion of hypothalamic corticotropin-releasing factor. *Science.* 1987; 238:522-524.

168. Berkenbosch F, van Oers J, del Rey A, et al. Corticotropin-releasing factor-producing neurons in the rat activated by interleukin-1. *Science.* 1987;238:524-526.

169. Besedovsky H, del Rey A, Sorkin E, et al. Immunoregulatory feedback between interleukin-1 and glucocorticoid hormones. *Science.* 1986;233: 652-654.

170. Bellavance MA, Rivest S. The neuroendocrine control of the innate immune system in health and brain diseases. *Immunol Rev.* 2012; 248:36-55.

171. Gudmundsson A, Carnes M. Pulsatile adrenocorticotropic hormone: an overview. *Biol Psychiatry.* 1997;41:342-365.

172. Muglia LJ, Jacobson L, Weninger SC, et al. Impaired diurnal adrenal rhythmicity restored by constant infusion of corticotropin-releasing hormone in corticotropin-releasing hormone-deficient mice. *J Clin Invest.* 1997;99:2923-2929.

173. Mayo K, Vale W, Rivier J, et al. Expression-cloning and sequence of a cDNA encoding human growth hormone-releasing factor. *Nature.* 1983;306:86-88.

174. Rivier J, Speiss J, Thorner M, et al. Characterisation of a growth hormone-releasing factor from a human pancreatic islet tumour. *Nature.* 1982;300:276-278.

175. Guillemin R, Barazeau P, Bohlen P, et al. Growth hormone-releasing factor from a human pancreatic tumor that caused acromegaly. *Science.* 1981;218:585-587.

176. Frohman LA, Downs TR, Chomczynski P, et al. Growth hormone-releasing hormone: structure, gene expression and molecular heterogeneity. *Acta Paediatr Scand Suppl.* 1990;367:81-86.

177. Frohman LA, Downs TR, Heimer EP, et al. Dipeptidylpeptidase IV and trypsin-like enzymatic degradation of human growth hormone-releasing hormone in plasma. *J Clin Invest.* 1989;83:1533-1540.

178. Ghazi AA, Amirbaigloo A, Dezfooli AA, et al. Ectopic acromegaly due to growth hormone releasing hormone. *Endocrine.* 2013;43: 293-302.

179. Dayal Y, Lin H, Tallberg K, et al. Immunocytochemical demonstration of growth hormone-releasing factor in gastrointestinal and pancreatic endocrine tumors. *Am J Clin Pathol.* 1986;85:13-20.

180. Khorram O, Garthwaite M, Grosen E, et al. Human uterine and ovarian expression of growth hormone-releasing hormone messenger RNA in

benign and malignant gynecologic conditions. *Fertil Steril.* 2001;75:174-179.

181. Gonzalez-Crespo S, Boronat A. Expression of the rat growth hormone-releasing hormone gene in placenta is directed by an alternative promoter. *Proc Natl Acad Sci U S A.* 1991;88:8749-8753.
182. Muller EE, Locatelli V, Cocchi D. Neuroendocrine control of growth hormone secretion. *Physiol Rev.* 1999;79:511-607.
183. Mayo KE, Godfrey PA, Suhr ST, et al. Growth hormone-releasing hormone: synthesis and signaling. *Recent Prog Horm Res.* 1995;50:35-73.
184. Wajnrajch MP, Gertner JM, Harbison MD, et al. Nonsense mutation in the human growth hormone-releasing hormone receptor causes growth failure analogous to the *little (lit)* mouse. *Nat Genet.* 1996;12:88-90.
185. Giustina A, Veldhuis JD. Pathophysiology of the neuroregulation of growth hormone secretion in experimental animals and the human. *Endocr Rev.* 1998;19:717-797.
186. Mayo KE, Hammer RE, Swanson LW, et al. Dramatic pituitary hyperplasia in transgenic mice expressing a human growth hormone-releasing factor gene. *Mol Endocrinol.* 1988;2:606-612.
187. Vallar L, Spada A, Giannattasio G. Altered Gs and adenylate cyclase activity in human GH-secreting pituitary adenomas. *Nature.* 1987;330:566-568.
188. Obal F Jr, Krueger JM. GHRH and sleep. *Sleep Med Rev.* 2004;8:367-377.
189. Van Cauter E, Leproult R, Plat L. Age-related changes in slow wave sleep and REM sleep and relationship with growth hormone and cortisol levels in healthy men. *JAMA.* 2000;284:861-868.
190. Kiaris H, Chatzistamou I, Papavassiliou AG, et al. Growth hormone-releasing hormone: not only a neurohormone. *Trends Endocrinol Metab.* 2011;22:311-317.
191. Smith RG, Feighner S, Prendergast K, et al. A new orphan receptor involved in pulsatile growth hormone release. *Trends Endocrinol Metab.* 1999;10:128-135.
192. Howard AD, Feighner SD, Cully DF, et al. A receptor in pituitary and hypothalamus that functions in growth hormone release. *Science.* 1996;273:974-977.
193. Maghnie M, Spica-Russotto V, Cappa M, et al. The growth hormone response to hexarelin in patients with different hypothalamic-pituitary abnormalities. *J Clin Endocrinol Metab.* 1998;83:3886-3889.
194. Arvat E, Maccario M, Di Vito L, et al. Endocrine activities of ghrelin, a natural growth hormone secretagogue (GHS), in humans: comparison and interactions with hexarelin, a nonnatural peptidyl GHS, and GH-releasing hormone. *J Clin Endocrinol Metab.* 2001;86:1169-1174.
195. Zizzari P, Hassouna R, Grouselle D, et al. Physiological roles of preproghrelin-derived peptides in GH secretion and feeding. *Peptides.* 2011;32:2274-2282.
196. Baldelli R, Otero XL, Camina JP, et al. Growth hormone secretagogues as diagnostic tools in disease states. *Endocrine.* 2001;14:95-99.
197. Andersen M. The robustness of diagnostic tests for GH deficiency in adults. *Growth Horm IGF Res.* 2015;25(3):108-114.
198. Veldhuis JD, Anderson SM, Shah N, et al. Neurophysiological regulation and target-tissue impact of the pulsatile mode of growth hormone secretion in the human. *Growth Horm IGF Res.* 2001;11(Suppl A):S25-S37.
199. Goldenberg N, Barkan A. Factors regulating growth hormone secretion in humans. *Endocrinol Metab Clin North Am.* 2007;36:37-55.
200. Steyn FJ. Nutrient sensing overrides somatostatin and GHRH to control pulsatile GH release. *J Neuroendocrinol.* 2015;27(7):577-587.
201. Ross RJ, Tsagarakis S, Grossman A, et al. GH feedback occurs through modulation of hypothalamic somatostatin under cholinergic control: studies with pyridostigmine and GHRH. *Clin Endocrinol (Oxf).* 1987;27:727-733.
202. Zheng H, Bailey A, Jiang MH, et al. Somatostatin receptor subtype 2 knockout mice are refractory to growth hormone-negative feedback on arcuate neurons. *Mol Endocrinol.* 1997;11:1709-1717.
203. Soliman AT, El Zalabany MM, Salama M, et al. Serum leptin concentrations during severe protein-energy malnutrition: correlation with growth parameters and endocrine function. *Metabolism.* 2000;49:819-825.
204. Bloch B, Gaillard RC, Brazeau P, et al. Topographical and ontogenetic study of the neurons producing growth hormone-releasing factor in human hypothalamus. *Regul Pept.* 1984;8:21-31.
205. Mota A, Bento A, Penalva A, et al. Role of the serotonin receptor subtype 5-HT1D on basal and stimulated growth hormone secretion. *J Clin Endocrinol Metab.* 1995;80:1973-1977.
206. Muller EE. Cholinergic function and neural control of GH secretion. A critical re-appraisal. *Eur J Endocrinol.* 1997;137:338-342.
207. Atiea J, Creagh F, Page M, et al. Early morning hyperglycemia in insulin-dependent diabetes: acute and sustained effects of cholinergic blockage. *J Clin Endocrinol Metab.* 1989;69:390-395.
208. Giustina A, Licini M, Schettino M, et al. Physiological role of galanin in the regulation of anterior pituitary function in humans. *Am J Physiol.* 1994;266:E57-E61.
209. Cella SG, Locatelli V, De Gennaro V, et al. Epinephrine mediates the growth hormone-releasing effect of galanin in infant rats. *Endocrinology.* 1988;122:855-859.
210. Van Cauter E, Kerkhofs M, Caufriez A, et al. A quantitative estimation of growth hormone secretion in normal man: reproducibility and relation to sleep and time of day. *J Clin Endocrinol Metab.* 1992;74:1441-1450.
211. Jaffe CA, Ocampo-Lim B, Guo W, et al. Regulatory mechanisms of growth hormone secretion are sexually dimorphic. *J Clin Invest.* 1998;102:153-164.
212. Pincus SM, Gevers EF, Robinson IC, et al. Females secrete growth hormone with more process irregularity than males in both humans and rats. *Am J Physiol.* 1996;270:E107-E115.
213. Low MJ, Otero-Corchon V, Parlow AF, et al. Somatostatin is required for masculinization of growth hormone-regulated hepatic gene expression but not of somatic growth. *J Clin Invest.* 2001;107:1571-1580.
214. Mazziotti G, Giustina A. Glucocorticoids and the regulation of growth hormone secretion. *Nat Rev Endocrinol.* 2013;9:265-276.
215. Brazeau P, Vale W, Burgus R, et al. Hypothalamic polypeptide that inhibits the secretion of immunoreactive pituitary growth hormone. *Science.* 1973;179:77-79.
216. Galanopoulou AS, Kent G, Rabbani SN, et al. Heterologous processing of prosomatostatin in constitutive and regulated secretory pathways. Putative role of the endoproteases furin, PC1, and PC2. *J Biol Chem.* 1993;268:6041-6049.
217. Shen LP, Rutter WJ. Sequence of the human somatostatin I gene. *Science.* 1984;224:168-171.
218. Conlon JM, Tostivint H, Vaudry H. Somatostatin- and urotensin II-related peptides: molecular diversity and evolutionary perspectives. *Regul Pept.* 1997;69:95-103.
219. de Lecea L, Criado JR, Prospero-Garcia O, et al. A cortical neuropeptide with neuronal depressant and sleep-modulating properties. *Nature.* 1996;381:242-245.
220. Fukusumi S, Kitada C, Takekawa S, et al. Identification and characterization of a novel human cortistatin-like peptide. *Biochem Biophys Res Commun.* 1997;232:157-163.
221. Andersen FG, Jensen J, Heller RS, et al. Pax6 and Pdx1 form a functional complex on the rat somatostatin gene upstream enhancer. *FEBS Lett.* 1999;445:315-320.
222. Goudet G, Delhalle S, Biemar F, et al. Functional and cooperative interactions between the homeodomain PDX1, Pbx, and Prep1 factors on the somatostatin promoter. *J Biol Chem.* 1999;274:4067-4073.
223. Capone G, Choi C, Vertifuille J. Regulation of the preprosomatostatin gene by cyclic-AMP in cerebrocortical neurons. *Brain Res Mol Brain Res.* 1998;60:247-258.
224. Montminy M, Brindle P, Arias J, et al. Regulation of somatostatin gene transcription by cyclic adenosine monophosphate. *Metabolism.* 1996;45:4-7.
225. Schwartz PT, Perez-Villamil B, Rivera A, et al. Pancreatic homeodomain transcription factor IDX1/IPF1 expressed in developing brain regulates somatostatin gene transcription in embryonic neural cells. *J Biol Chem.* 2000;275:19106-19114.
226. Rai U, Thrimawithana TR, Valery C, et al. Therapeutic uses of somatostatin and its analogues: current view and potential applications. *Pharmacol Ther.* 2015;152:98-110.
227. Strowski MZ, Parmar RM, Blake AD, et al. Somatostatin inhibits insulin and glucagon secretion via two receptors subtypes: an in vitro study of pancreatic islets from somatostatin receptor 2 knockout mice. *Endocrinology.* 2000;141:111-117.
228. Blake AD, Badway AC, Strowski MZ. Delineating somatostatin's neuronal actions. *Curr Drug Targets CNS Neurol Disord.* 2004;3:153-160.
229. Mathern GW, Babb TL, Pretorius JK, et al. Reactive synaptogenesis and neuron densities for neuropeptide Y, somatostatin, and glutamate decarboxylase immunoreactivity in the epileptogenic human fascia dentata. *J Neurosci.* 1995;15:3990-4004.
230. Dulcis D, Jamshidi P, Leutgeb S, et al. Neurotransmitter switching in the adult brain regulates behavior. *Science.* 2013;340:449-453.
231. Kluge C, Stoppel C, Szinyei C, et al. Role of the somatostatin system in contextual fear memory and hippocampal synaptic plasticity. *Learn Mem.* 2008;15(4):252-260.
232. Hannon JP, Nunn C, Stolz B, et al. Drug design at peptide receptors: somatostatin receptor ligands. *J Mol Neurosci.* 2002;18:15-27.
233. Slooter GD, Mearadji A, Breeman WA, et al. Somatostatin receptor imaging, therapy and new strategies in patients with neuroendocrine tumours. *Br J Surg.* 2001;88:31-40.
234. Baldelli R, Barnabei A, Rizza L, et al. Somatostatin analogs therapy in gastroenteropancreatic neuroendocrine tumors: current aspects and new perspectives. *Front Endocrinol (Lausanne).* 2014;5:7.
235. Schirmer WJ, O'Dorisio TM, Schirmer TP, et al. Intraoperative localization of neuroendocrine tumors with 125I-TYR(3)-octreotide and a hand-held gamma-detecting probe. *Surgery.* 1993;114:745-751, discussion 751-742.
236. Henze M, Schuhmacher J, Hipp P, et al. PET imaging of somatostatin receptors using [^{68}Ga]DOTATOC. *J Nucl Med.* 2001;42:1053-1056.
237. Rochaix P, Delesque N, Esteve JP, et al. Gene therapy for pancreatic carcinoma: local and distant antitumor effects after somatostatin receptor sst2 gene transfer. *Hum Gene Ther.* 1999;10:995-1008.
238. Freeman ME, Kanyicska B, Lerant A, et al. Prolactin: structure, function, and regulation of secretion. *Physiol Rev.* 2000;80:1523-1631.

239. Ben-Jonathan N, Hnasko R. Dopamine as a prolactin (PRL) inhibitor. *Endocr Rev.* 2001;22:724-763.

240. Asa SL, Kelly MA, Grandy DK, et al. Pituitary lactotroph adenomas develop after prolonged lactotroph hyperplasia in dopamine D2 receptor-deficient mice. *Endocrinology.* 1999;140:5348-5355.

241. Lerant A, Herman ME, Freeman ME. Dopaminergic neurons of periventricular and arcuate nuclei of pseudopregnant rats: semicircadian rhythm in Fos-related antigens immunoreactivities and in dopamine concentration. *Endocrinology.* 1996;137:3621-3628.

242. Durham RA, Johnson JD, Eaton MJ, et al. Opposing roles for dopamine D1 and D2 receptors in the regulation of hypothalamic tuberoinfundibular dopamine neurons. *Eur J Pharmacol.* 1998;355:141-147.

243. Vallar L, Meldolesi J. Mechanisms of signal transduction at the dopamine D2 receptor. *Trends Pharmacol Sci.* 1989;10:74-77.

244. Day RN, Liu J, Sundmark V, et al. Selective inhibition of prolactin gene transcription by the ETS-2 repressor factor. *J Biol Chem.* 1998;273:31909-31915.

245. Booth AK, Gutierrez-Hartmann A. Signaling pathways regulating pituitary lactotrope homeostasis and tumorigenesis. *Adv Exp Med Biol.* 2015;846:37-59.

246. Suzuki S, Yamamoto I, Arita J. Mitogen-activated protein kinase-dependent stimulation of proliferation of rat lactotrophs in culture by 3′,5′-cyclic adenosine monophosphate. *Endocrinology.* 1999;140:2850-2858.

247. Senogles SE. D2 dopamine receptor-mediated antiproliferation in a small cell lung cancer cell line, NCI-H69. *Anticancer Drugs.* 2007;18:801-807.

248. Radl D, De Mei C, Chen E, et al. Each individual isoform of the dopamine D2 receptor protects from lactotroph hyperplasia. *Mol Endocrinol.* 2013;27:953-965.

249. Low MJ. Neural control of the intermediate lobe of the pituitary gland (pars intermedia) and proopiomelanocortin. In: Fink G, Pfaff D, Levine J, eds. *Handbook of Neuroendocrinology.* Amsterdam: Academic Press; 2012:157-174.

250. Chronwall BM, Davis TD, Severidt MW, et al. Constitutive expression of functional GABA(B) receptors in mIL-tsA58 cells requires both GABA(B(1)) and GABA(B(2)) genes. *J Neurochem.* 2001;77:1237-1247.

251. Samuels MH, Veldhuis J, Ridgway EC. Copulsatile release of thyrotropin and prolactin in normal and hypothyroid subjects. *Thyroid.* 1995;5:369-372.

252. Samson WK, Taylor MM, Baker JR. Prolactin-releasing peptides. *Regul Pept.* 2003;114:1-5.

253. Itoh N, Obata K, Yanaihara N, et al. Human preprovasoactive intestinal polypeptide contains a novel PHI-27- like peptide, PHM-27. *Nature.* 1983;304:547-549.

254. Hokfelt T, Fahrenkrug J, Tatemoto K, et al. The PHI (PHI-27)/corticotropin-releasing factor/enkephalin immunoreactive hypothalamic neuron: possible morphological basis for integrated control of prolactin, corticotropin, and growth hormone secretion. *Proc Natl Acad Sci U S A.* 1983;80:895-898.

255. Tachibana T, Sakamoto T. Functions of two distinct "prolactin-releasing peptides" evolved from a common ancestral gene. *Front Endocrinol (Lausanne).* 2014;5:170.

256. Fukusumi S, Fujii R, Hinuma S. Recent advances in mammalian RFamide peptides: the discovery and functional analyses of PrRP, RFRPs and QRFP. *Peptides.* 2006;27:1073-1086.

257. Takayanagi Y, Matsumoto H, Nakata M, et al. Endogenous prolactin-releasing peptide regulates food intake in rodents. *J Clin Invest.* 2008;118:4014-4024.

258. Schwartz J, Van de Pavert S, Clarke I, et al. Paracrine interactions within the pituitary gland. *Ann N Y Acad Sci.* 1998;839:239-243.

259. Le Tissier PR, Hodson DJ, Lafont C, et al. Anterior pituitary cell networks. *Front Neuroendocrinol.* 2012;33:252-266.

260. Voogt JL, Lee Y, Yang S, et al. Regulation of prolactin secretion during pregnancy and lactation. *Prog Brain Res.* 2001;133:173-185.

261. DeMaria JE, Livingstone JD, Freeman ME. Ovarian steroids influence the activity of neuroendocrine dopaminergic neurons. *Brain Res.* 2000;879:139-147.

262. Arbogast LA, Voogt JL. Prolactin (PRL) receptors are colocalized in dopaminergic neurons in fetal hypothalamic cell cultures: effect of PRL on tyrosine hydroxylase activity. *Endocrinology.* 1997;138:3016-3023.

263. Phelps CJ, Hurley DL. Pituitary hormones as neurotrophic signals: update on hypothalamic differentiation in genetic models of altered feedback. *Proc Soc Exp Biol Med.* 1999;222:39-58.

264. Phelps CJ, Horseman ND. Prolactin gene disruption does not compromise differentiation of tuberoinfundibular dopaminergic neurons. *Neuroendocrinology.* 2000;72:2-10.

265. Callahan P, Klosterman S, Prunty D, et al. Immunoneutralization of endogenous opioid peptides prevents the suckling-induced prolactin increase and the inhibition of tuberoinfundibular dopaminergic neurons. *Neuroendocrinology.* 2000;71:268-276.

266. Creese I, Burt DR, Snyder SH. Dopamine receptor binding predicts clinical and pharmacological potencies of antischizophrenic drugs. *Science.* 1976;192:481-483.

267. Melkersson K, Hulting AL. Prolactin-secreting pituitary adenoma in neuroleptic treated patients with psychotic disorder. *Eur Arch Psychiatry Clin Neurosci.* 2000;250:6-10.

268. Veldman RG, Frolich M, Pincus SM, et al. Basal, pulsatile, entropic, and 24-hour rhythmic features of secondary hyperprolactinemia due to functional pituitary stalk disconnection mimic tumoral (primary) hyperprolactinemia. *J Clin Endocrinol Metab.* 2001;86:1562-1567.

269. Waldstreicher J, Duffy JF, Brown EN, et al. Gender differences in the temporal organization of proclactin (PRL) secretion: evidence for a sleep-independent circadian rhythm of circulating PRL levels—a clinical research center study. *J Clin Endocrinol Metab.* 1996;81:1483-1487.

270. Diaz S, Seron-Ferre M, Cardenas H, et al. Circadian variation of basal plasma prolactin, prolactin response to suckling, and length of amenorrhea in nursing women. *J Clin Endocrinol Metab.* 1989;68:946-955.

271. Seeburg PH, Adelman JP. Characterization of cDNA for precursor of human luteinizing hormone releasing hormone. *Nature.* 1984;311:666-668.

272. Urbanski HF, White RB, Fernald RD, et al. Regional expression of mRNA encoding a second form of gonadotropin-releasing hormone in the macaque brain. *Endocrinology.* 1999;140:1945-1948.

273. Sherwood NM, Lovejoy DA, Coe IR. Origin of mammalian gonadotropin-releasing hormones. *Endocr Rev.* 1993;14:241-254.

274. Fernald RD, White RB. Gonadotropin-releasing hormone genes: phylogeny, structure, and functions. *Front Neuroendocrinol.* 1999;20:224-240.

275. Pawson AJ, Morgan K, Maudsley SR, et al. Type II gonadotrophin-releasing hormone (GnRH-II) in reproductive biology. *Reproduction.* 2003;126:271-278.

276. Lee VH, Lee LT, Chow BK. Gonadotropin-releasing hormone: regulation of the GnRH gene. *FEBS J.* 2008;275:5458-5478.

277. Hapgood JP, Sadie H, van Biljon W, et al. Regulation of expression of mammalian gonadotrophin-releasing hormone receptor genes. *J Neuroendocrinol.* 2005;17:619-638.

278. Cheng CK, Leung PC. Molecular biology of gonadotropin-releasing hormone (GnRH)-I, GnRH-II, and their receptors in humans. *Endocr Rev.* 2005;26:283-306.

279. Givens ML, Kurotani R, Rave-Harel N, et al. Phylogenetic footprinting reveals evolutionarily conserved regions of the gonadotropin-releasing hormone gene that enhance cell-specific expression. *Mol Endocrinol.* 2004;18:2950-2966.

280. Givens ML, Rave-Harel N, Goonewardena VD, et al. Developmental regulation of gonadotropin-releasing hormone gene expression by the MSX and DLX homeodomain protein families. *J Biol Chem.* 2005;280:19156-19165.

281. Phoenix CH, Chambers KC. Sexual performance of old and young male rhesus macaques following treatment with GnRH. *Physiol Behav.* 1990;47:513-517.

282. Wierman ME, Kiseljak-Vassiliades K, Tobet S. Gonadotropin-releasing hormone (GnRH) neuron migration: initiation, maintenance and cessation as critical steps to ensure normal reproductive function. *Front Neuroendocrinol.* 2011;32:43-52.

283. MacColl G, Quinton R, Bouloux PM. GnRH neuronal development: insights into hypogonadotrophic hypogonadism. *Trends Endocrinol Metab.* 2002;13:112-118.

284. Hardelin JP, Dode C. The complex genetics of Kallmann syndrome: KAL1, FGFR1, FGF8, PROKR2, PROK2, et al. *Sex Dev.* 2008;2:181-193.

285. Clayton RN. Mechanism of GnRH action in gonadotrophs. *Hum Reprod.* 1988;3:479-483.

286. Conn PM, Crowley WF Jr. Gonadotropin-releasing hormone and its analogs. *Annu Rev Med.* 1994;45:391-405.

287. Rispoli LA, Nett TM. Pituitary gonadotropin-releasing hormone (GnRH) receptor: structure, distribution and regulation of expression. *Anim Reprod Sci.* 2005;88:57-74.

288. Lahlou N, Carel JC, Chaussain JL, et al. Pharmacokinetics and pharmacodynamics of GnRH agonists: clinical implications in pediatrics. *J Pediatr Endocrinol Metab.* 2000;13(Suppl 1):723-737.

289. Reissmann T, Schally AV, Bouchard P, et al. The LHRH antagonist cetrorelix: a review. *Hum Reprod Update.* 2000;6:322-331.

290. Clarke IJ, Cummins JT. The temporal relationship between gonadotropin releasing hormone (GnRH) and luteinizing hormone (LH) secretion in ovariectomized ewes. *Endocrinology.* 1982;111:1737-1739.

291. Mori Y, Nishihara M, Tanaka T, et al. Chronic recording of electrophysiological manifestation of the hypothalamic gonadotropin-releasing hormone pulse generator activity in the goat. *Neuroendocrinology.* 1991;53:392-395.

292. Glanowska KM, Venton BJ, Moenter SM. Fast scan cyclic voltammetry as a novel method for detection of real-time gonadotropin-releasing hormone release in mouse brain slices. *J Neurosci.* 2012;32:14664-14669.

293. Krupa M, Vidal A, Clement F. A network model of the periodic synchronization process in the dynamics of calcium concentration in GnRH neurons. *J Math Neurosci.* 2013;3(1):4.

294. Chappel SC, Ulloa-Aguirre A, Coutifaris C. Biosynthesis and secretion of follicle-stimulating hormone. *Endocr Rev.* 1983;4:179-211.

295. Simerly RB, Chang C, Muramatsu M, et al. Distribution of androgen and estrogen receptor mRNA-containing cells in the rat brain: an in situ hybridization study. *J Comp Neurol.* 1990;294:76-95.

296. Kuiper GG, Shughrue PJ, Merchenthaler I, et al. The estrogen receptor beta subtype: a novel mediator of estrogen action in neuroendocrine systems. *Front Neuroendocrinol.* 1998;19:253-286.

297. Shughrue PJ, Lane MV, Merchenthaler I. Comparative distribution of estrogen receptor-alpha and -beta mRNA in the rat central nervous system. *J Comp Neurol.* 1997;388:507-525.

298. Bethea CL, Brown NA, Kohama SG. Steroid regulation of estrogen and progestin receptor messenger ribonucleic acid in monkey hypothalamus and pituitary. *Endocrinology.* 1996;137:4372-4383.

299. Plant TM. Gonadal regulation of hypothalamic gonadotropin-releasing hormone release in primates. *Endocr Rev.* 1986;7:75-88.

300. Nakai Y, Plant TM, Hess DL, et al. On the sites of the negative and positive feedback actions of estradiol in the control of gonadotropin secretion in the rhesus monkey. *Endocrinology.* 1978;102:1008-1014.

301. Kumar TR, Low MJ. Hormonal regulation of human follicle-stimulating hormone-beta subunit gene expression: GnRH stimulation and GnRH-independent androgen inhibition. *Neuroendocrinology.* 1995;61: 628-637.

302. Bishop W, Kalra PS, Fawcett CP, et al. The effects of hypothalamic lesions on the release of gonadotropins and prolactin in response to estrogen and progesterone treatment in female rats. *Endocrinology.* 1972;91:1404-1410.

303. Levine JE, Chappell PE, Schneider JS, et al. Progesterone receptors as neuroendocrine integrators. *Front Neuroendocrinol.* 2001;22:69-106.

304. Seminara SB. Metastin and its G protein-coupled receptor, GPR54: critical pathway modulating GnRH secretion. *Front Neuroendocrinol.* 2005;26:131-138.

305. Dungan HM, Clifton DK, Steiner RA. Minireview: kisspeptin neurons as central processors in the regulation of gonadotropin-releasing hormone secretion. *Endocrinology.* 2006;147:1154-1158.

306. Popa SM, Clifton DK, Steiner RA. The role of kisspeptins and GPR54 in the neuroendocrine regulation of reproduction. *Annu Rev Physiol.* 2008;70:213-238.

307. Bernard V, Young J, Chanson P, et al. New insights in prolactin: pathological implications. *Nat Rev Endocrinol.* 2015;11:265-275.

308. Goodman RL, Hileman SM, Nestor CC, et al. Kisspeptin, neurokinin B, and dynorphin act in the arcuate nucleus to control activity of the GnRH pulse generator in ewes. *Endocrinology.* 2013;154:4259-4269.

309. Kaplan SL, Grumbach MM, Aubert ML. The ontogenesis of pituitary hormones and hypothalamic factors in the human fetus: maturation of central nervous system regulation of anterior pituitary function. *Recent Prog Horm Res.* 1976;32:161-243.

310. Plant TM. Neurobiological bases underlying the control of the onset of puberty in the rhesus monkey: a representative higher primate. *Front Neuroendocrinol.* 2001;22:107-139.

311. Boyar RM, Rosenfeld RS, Kapen S, et al. Human puberty. Simultaneous augmented secretion of luteinizing hormone and testosterone during sleep. *J Clin Invest.* 1974;54:609-618.

312. Lomniczi A, Wright H, Castellano JM, et al. A system biology approach to identify regulatory pathways underlying the neuroendocrine control of female puberty in rats and nonhuman primates. *Horm Behav.* 2013;64:175-186.

313. Gay VL, Plant TM. Sustained intermittent release of gonadotropin-releasing hormone in the prepubertal male rhesus monkey induced by N-methyl-DL-aspartic acid. *Neuroendocrinology.* 1988;48:147-152.

314. Ojeda SR, Ma YJ, Lee BJ, et al. Glia-to-neuron signaling and the neuroendocrine control of female puberty. *Recent Prog Horm Res.* 2000;55: 197-223, discussion 223-194.

315. Ebling FJ. The neuroendocrine timing of puberty. *Reproduction.* 2005; 129:675-683.

316. Stoyanovitch AG, Johnson MA, Clifton DK, et al. Galanin-like peptide rescues reproductive function in the diabetic rat. *Diabetes.* 2005;54: 2471-2476.

317. Cameron JL. Stress and behaviorally induced reproductive dysfunction in primates. *Semin Reprod Endocrinol.* 1997;15:37-45.

318. Rivier C, Rivier J, Vale W. Stress-induced inhibition of reproductive functions: role of endogenous corticotropin-releasing factor. *Science.* 1986;231:607-609.

319. Feng YJ, Shalts E, Xia LN, et al. An inhibitory effect of interleukin-1a on basal gonadotropin release in the ovariectomized rhesus monkey: reversal by a corticotropin-releasing factor antagonist. *Endocrinology.* 1991;128:2077-2082.

320. Chen MD, O'Byrne KT, Chiappini SE, et al. Hypoglycemic "stress" and gonadotropin-releasing hormone pulse generator activity in the rhesus monkey: role of the ovary. *Neuroendocrinology.* 1992;56:666-673.

321. Norman RL, Smith CJ. Restraint inhibits luteinizing hormone and testosterone secretion in intact male rhesus macaques: effects of concurrent naloxone administration. *Neuroendocrinology.* 1992;55: 405-415.

322. Chehab FF. 20 years of leptin: leptin and reproduction: past milestones, present undertakings, and future endeavors. *J Endocrinol.* 2014;223(1):T37-T48.

323. Schneider JE, Zhou D, Blum RM. Leptin and metabolic control of reproduction. *Horm Behav.* 2000;37:306-326.

324. Honegger J, Buchfelder M, Fahlbusch R. Surgical treatment of craniopharyngiomas: endocrinological results. *J Neurosurg.* 1999;90: 251-257.

325. Benvenga S, Campenni A, Ruggeri RM, et al. Clinical review 113: hypopituitarism secondary to head trauma. *J Clin Endocrinol Metab.* 2000;85:1353-1361.

326. Hussain NS, Piper M, Ludlam WG, et al. Delayed postoperative hyponatremia after transsphenoidal surgery: prevalence and associated factors. *J Neurosurg.* 2013;119:1453-1460.

327. Maghnie M, Cosi G, Genovese E, et al. Central diabetes insipidus in children and young adults. *N Engl J Med.* 2000;343:998-1007.

328. Scherbaum WA, Wass JA, Besser GM, et al. Autoimmune cranial diabetes insipidus: its association with other endocrine diseases and with histiocytosis X. *Clin Endocrinol (Oxf).* 1986;25:411-420.

329. Al-Agha AE, Thomsett MJ, Ratcliffe JF, et al. Acquired central diabetes insipidus in children: a 12-year Brisbane experience. *J Paediatr Child Health.* 2001;37:172-175.

330. Nagasaki H, Ito M, Yuasa H, et al. Two novel mutations in the coding region for neurophysin-II associated with familial central diabetes insipidus. *J Clin Endocrinol Metab.* 1995;80:1352-1356.

331. Morello JP, Bichet DG. Nephrogenic diabetes insipidus. *Annu Rev Physiol.* 2001;63:607-630.

332. Nielsen S, Frokiaer J, Marples D, et al. Aquaporins in the kidney: from molecules to medicine. *Physiol Rev.* 2002;82:205-244.

333. Lieberman SA, Oberoi AL, Gilkison CR, et al. Prevalence of neuroendocrine dysfunction in patients recovering from traumatic brain injury. *J Clin Endocrinol Metab.* 2001;86:2752-2756.

334. Smith MV, Laws ER Jr. Magnetic resonance imaging measurements of pituitary stalk compression and deviation in patients with nonprolactin-secreting intrasellar and parasellar tumors: lack of correlation with serum prolactin levels. *Neurosurgery.* 1994;34:834-839, discussion 839.

335. Voelker JL, Campbell RL, Muller J. Clinical, radiographic, and pathological features of symptomatic Rathke's cleft cysts. *J Neurosurg.* 1991;74:535-544.

336. Zucchini S, Ambrosetto P, Carla G, et al. Primary empty sella: differences and similarities between children and adults. *Acta Paediatr.* 1995;84:1382-1385.

337. Klingmuller D, Dewes W, Krahe T, et al. Magnetic resonance imaging of the brain in patients with anosmia and hypothalamic hypogonadism (Kallmann's syndrome). *J Clin Endocrinol Metab.* 1987;65: 581-584.

338. Nanduri VR, Stanhope R. Why is the retention of gonadotrophin secretion common in children with panhypopituitarism due to septo-optic dysplasia? *Eur J Endocrinol.* 1999;140:48-50.

339. Bhagavath B, Podolsky RH, Ozata M, et al. Clinical and molecular characterization of a large sample of patients with hypogonadotropic hypogonadism. *Fertil Steril.* 2006;85:706-713.

340. Chryssikopoulos A, Gregoriou O, Vitoratos N, et al. The predictive value of double Gn-RH provocation test in unprimed Gn-RH-primed and steroid-primed female patients with Kallmann's syndrome. *Int J Fertil Womens Med.* 1998;43:291-299.

341. Hayes FJ, Seminara SB, Crowley WF Jr. Hypogonadotropic hypogonadism. *Endocrinol Metab Clin North Am.* 1998;27:739-763, vii.

342. Samuels MH, Ridgway EC. Central hypothyroidism. *Endocrinol Metab Clin North Am.* 1992;21:903-919.

343. Winter WE, Signorino MR. Review: molecular thyroidology. *Ann Clin Lab Sci.* 2001;31:221-244.

344. Jorgensen JO, Pedersen SA, Laurberg P, et al. Effects of growth hormone therapy on thyroid function of growth hormone-deficient adults with and without concomitant thyroxine-substituted central hypothyroidism. *J Clin Endocrinol Metab.* 1989;69:1127-1132.

345. Rose SR. Cranial irradiation and central hypothyroidism. *Trends Endocrinol Metab.* 2001;12:97-104.

346. Argente J, Abusrewil SA, Bona G, et al. Isolated growth hormone deficiency in children and adolescents. *J Pediatr Endocrinol Metab.* 2001; 14(Suppl 2):1003-1008.

347. Maghnie M, Ghirardello S, Genovese E. Magnetic resonance imaging of the hypothalamus-pituitary unit in children suspected of hypopituitarism: who, how and when to investigate. *J Endocrinol Invest.* 2004;27:496-509.

348. Zhu X, Gleiberman AS, Rosenfeld MG. Molecular physiology of pituitary development: signaling and transcriptional networks. *Physiol Rev.* 2007;87:933-963.

349. Baumann G, Maheshwari H. The Dwarfs of Sindh: severe growth hormone (GH) deficiency caused by a mutation in the GH-releasing hormone receptor gene. *Acta Paediatr Suppl.* 1997;423:33-38.

350. Nishihara E, Kimura H, Ishimaru T, et al. A case of adrenal insufficiency due to acquired hypothalamic CRH deficiency. *Endocr J.* 1997; 44:121-126.

351. Kyllo JH, Collins MM, Vetter KL, et al. Linkage of congenital isolated adrenocorticotropic hormone deficiency to the corticotropin releasing hormone locus using simple sequence repeat polymorphisms. *Am J Med Genet.* 1996;62:262-267.

352. Vallette-Kasic S, Brue T, Pulichino AM, et al. Congenital isolated adrenocorticotropin deficiency: an underestimated cause of neonatal death, explained by TPIT gene mutations. *J Clin Endocrinol Metab.* 2005;90:1323-1331.

353. Fukata J, Shimizu N, Imura H, et al. Human corticotropin-releasing hormone test in patients with hypothalamo-pituitary-adrenocortical disorders. *Endocr J.* 1993;40:597-606.

354. Gleeson HK, Shalet SM. Endocrine complications of neoplastic diseases in children and adolescents. *Curr Opin Pediatr.* 2001;13:346-351.

355. Arlt W, Hove U, Muller B, et al. Frequent and frequently overlooked: treatment-induced endocrine dysfunction in adult long-term survivors of primary brain tumors. *Neurology.* 1997;49:498-506.

356. Prabhu VC, Brown HG. The pathogenesis of craniopharyngiomas. *Childs Nerv Syst.* 2005;21:622-627.

357. Halac I, Zimmerman D. Endocrine manifestations of craniopharyngioma. *Childs Nerv Syst.* 2005;21:640-648.

358. Curran JG, O'Connor E. Imaging of craniopharyngioma. *Childs Nerv Syst.* 2005;21:635-639.

359. Hochman HI, Judge DM, Reichlin S. Precocious puberty and hypothalamic hamartoma. *Pediatrics.* 1981;67:236-244.

360. Asa SL, Kovacs K, Tindall GT, et al. Cushing's disease associated with an intrasellar gangliocytoma producing corticotrophin-releasing factor. *Ann Intern Med.* 1984;101:789-793.

361. Asa SL, Scheithauer BW, Bilbao JM, et al. A case for hypothalamic acromegaly: a clinicopathological study of six patients with hypothalamic gangliocytomas producing growth hormone-releasing factor. *J Clin Endocrinol Metab.* 1984;58:796-803.

362. Lee PA. Central precocious puberty. An overview of diagnosis, treatment, and outcome. *Endocrinol Metab Clin North Am.* 1999;28:901-918, xi.

363. De Sanctis V, Corrias A, Rizzo V, et al. Etiology of central precocious puberty in males: the results of the Italian Study Group for Physiopathology of Puberty. *J Pediatr Endocrinol Metab.* 2000;13(Suppl 1): 687-693.

364. Cisternino M, Arrigo T, Pasquino AM, et al. Etiology and age incidence of precocious puberty in girls: a multicentric study. *J Pediatr Endocrinol Metab.* 2000;13(Suppl 1):695-701.

365. Ojeda SR, Heger S. New thoughts on female precocious puberty. *J Pediatr Endocrinol Metab.* 2001;14:245-256.

366. Virdis R, Sigorini M, Laiolo A, et al. Neurofibromatosis type 1 and precocious puberty. *J Pediatr Endocrinol Metab.* 2000;13(Suppl 1):841-844.

367. Rivarola MA, Belgorosky A, Mendilaharzu H, et al. Precocious puberty in children with tumours of the suprasellar and pineal areas: organic central precocious puberty. *Acta Paediatr.* 2001;90:751-756.

368. Arita K, Ikawa F, Kurisu K, et al. The relationship between magnetic resonance imaging findings and clinical manifestations of hypothalamic hamartoma. *J Neurosurg.* 1999;91:212-220.

369. Debeneix C, Bourgeois M, Trivin C, et al. Hypothalamic hamartoma: comparison of clinical presentation and magnetic resonance images. *Horm Res.* 2001;56:12-18.

370. Berkovic SF, Andermann F, Melanson D, et al. Hypothalamic hamartomas and ictal laughter: evolution of a characteristic epileptic syndrome and diagnostic value of magnetic resonance imaging. *Ann Neurol.* 1988;23:429-439.

371. Anasti JN, Flack MR, Froehlich J, et al. A potential novel mechanism for precocious puberty in juvenile hypothyroidism. *J Clin Endocrinol Metab.* 1995;80:276-279.

372. Fauchon F, Jouvet A, Paquis P, et al. Parenchymal pineal tumors: a clinicopathological study of 76 cases. *Int J Radiat Oncol Biol Phys.* 2000;46:959-968.

373. Jouvet A, Saint-Pierre G, Fauchon F, et al. Pineal parenchymal tumors: a correlation of histological features with prognosis in 66 cases. *Brain Pathol.* 2000;10:49-60.

374. Baumgartner JE, Edwards MS. Pineal tumors. *Neurosurg Clin North Am.* 1992;3:853-862.

375. Popovic EA, Kelly PJ. Stereotactic procedures for lesions of the pineal region. *Mayo Clin Proc.* 1993;68:965-970.

376. Dahlborg SA, Petrillo A, Crossen JR, et al. The potential for complete and durable response in nonglial primary brain tumors in children and young adults with enhanced chemotherapy delivery. *Cancer J Sci Am.* 1998;4:110-124.

377. Chalumeau M, Chemaitilly W, Trivin C, et al. Central precocious puberty in girls: an evidence-based diagnosis tree to predict central nervous system abnormalities. *Pediatrics.* 2002;109:61-67.

378. Iughetti L, Predieri B, Ferrari M, et al. Diagnosis of central precocious puberty: endocrine assessment. *J Pediatr Endocrinol Metab.* 2000; 13(Suppl 1):709-715.

379. Argyropoulou MI, Kiortsis DN. MRI of the hypothalamic-pituitary axis in children. *Pediatr Radiol.* 2005;35:1045-1055.

380. Klein KO, Barnes KM, Jones JV, et al. Increased final height in precocious puberty after long-term treatment with LHRH agonists: the National Institutes of Health experience. *J Clin Endocrinol Metab.* 2001;86:4711-4716.

381. Tato L, Savage MO, Antoniazzi F, et al. Optimal therapy of pubertal disorders in precocious/early puberty. *J Pediatr Endocrinol Metab.* 2001; 14(Suppl 2):985-995.

382. Laron Z, Kauli R. Experience with cyproterone acetate in the treatment of precocious puberty. *J Pediatr Endocrinol Metab.* 2000;13(Suppl 1): 805-810.

383. Feuillan P, Merke D, Leschek EW, et al. Use of aromatase inhibitors in precocious puberty. *Endocr Relat Cancer.* 1999;6:303-306.

384. Warren MP, Fried JL. Hypothalamic amenorrhea. The effects of environmental stresses on the reproductive system: a central effect of the central nervous system. *Endocrinol Metab Clin North Am.* 2001;30: 611-629.

385. Yen SS. Female hypogonadotropic hypogonadism. Hypothalamic amenorrhea syndrome. *Endocrinol Metab Clin North Am.* 1993;22: 29-58.

386. Cannavo S, Curto L, Trimarchi F. Exercise-related female reproductive dysfunction. *J Endocrinol Invest.* 2001;24:823-832.

387. Moschos S, Chan JL, Mantzoros CS. Leptin and reproduction: a review. *Fertil Steril.* 2002;77:433-444.

388. Williams NI, Helmreich DL, Parfitt DB, et al. Evidence for a causal role of low energy availability in the induction of menstrual cycle disturbances during strenuous exercise training. *J Clin Endocrinol Metab.* 2001;86:5184-5193.

389. Hobart JA, Smucker DR. The female athlete triad. *Am Fam Physician.* 2000;61(11):3357-3364, 3367.

390. Goldstone AP. Prader-Willi syndrome: advances in genetics, pathophysiology and treatment. *Trends Endocrinol Metab.* 2004;15:12-20.

391. Hackney AC. Endurance exercise training and reproductive endocrine dysfunction in men: alterations in the hypothalamic-pituitary-testicular axis. *Curr Pharm Des.* 2001;7(4):261-273.

392. Opstad K. Circadian rhythm of hormones is extinguished during prolonged physical stress, sleep and energy deficiency in young men. *Eur J Endocrinol.* 1994;131:56-66.

393. Abs R, Verhelst J, Maeyaert J, et al. Endocrine consequences of long-term intrathecal administration of opioids. *J Clin Endocrinol Metab.* 2000;85:2215-2222.

394. Vanhorebeek I, Van den Berghe G. The neuroendocrine response to critical illness is a dynamic process. *Crit Care Clin.* 2006;22:1-15, v.

395. Biller BM, Luciano A, Crosignani PG, et al. Guidelines for the diagnosis and treatment of hyperprolactinemia. *J Reprod Med.* 1999;44: 1075-1084.

396. Meierkord H, Shorvon S, Lightman S, et al. Comparison of the effects of frontal and temporal lobe partial seizures on prolactin levels. *Arch Neurol.* 1992;49:225-230.

397. Molitch ME. Diagnosis and treatment of prolactinomas. *Adv Intern Med.* 1999;44:117-153.

398. Burman P, Ritzen EM, Lindgren AC. Endocrine dysfunction in Prader-Willi syndrome: a review with special reference to GH. *Endocr Rev.* 2001;22:787-799.

399. Gohlke BC, Khadilkar VV, Skuse D, et al. Recognition of children with psychosocial short stature: a spectrum of presentation. *J Pediatr Endocrinol Metab.* 1998;11:509-517.

400. Gilmour J, Skuse D. A case-comparison study of the characteristics of children with a short stature syndrome induced by stress (hyperphagic short stature) and a consecutive series of unaffected "stressed" children. *J Child Psychol Psychiatry.* 1999;40:969-978.

401. Albanese A, Hamill G, Jones J, et al. Reversibility of physiological growth hormone secretion in children with psychosocial dwarfism. *Clin Endocrinol (Oxf).* 1994;40:687-692.

402. Bercu BB, Diamond FB Jr. Growth hormone neurosecretory dysfunction. *Clin Endocrinol Metab.* 1986;15:537-590.

403. Lin TH, Kirkland RT, Sherman BM, et al. Growth hormone testing in short children and their response to growth hormone therapy. *J Pediatr.* 1989;115:57-63.

404. Attie KM. Genetic studies in idiopathic short stature. *Curr Opin Pediatr.* 2000;12:400-404.

405. Voss LD. Short normal stature and psychosocial disadvantage: a critical review of the evidence. *J Pediatr Endocrinol Metab.* 2001;14:701-711.

406. Mehta A, Hindmarsh PC. The use of somatropin (recombinant growth hormone) in children of short stature. *Paediatr Drugs.* 2002;4:37-47.

407. Poussaint TY, Barnes PD, Nichols K, et al. Diencephalic syndrome: clinical features and imaging findings. *Am J Neuroradiol.* 1997;18: 1499-1505.

408. Gropman AL, Packer RJ, Nicholson HS, et al. Treatment of diencephalic syndrome with chemotherapy: growth, tumor response, and long term control. *Cancer.* 1998;83:166-172.

409. Ho KY, Veldhuis JD, Johnson ML, et al. Fasting enhances growth hormone secretion and amplifies the complex rhythms of growth hormone secretion in man. *J Clin Invest.* 1988;81:968-975.

410. Saeger W, Puchner MJ, Ludecke DK. Combined sellar gangliocytoma and pituitary adenoma in acromegaly or Cushing's disease. A report of 3 cases. *Virchows Arch.* 1994;425:93-99.

411. Posener JA, DeBattista C, Williams GH, et al. 24-Hour monitoring of cortisol and corticotropin secretion in psychotic and nonpsychotic major depression. *Arch Gen Psychiatry.* 2000;57:755-760.

412. Chrousos GP. The role of stress and the hypothalamic-pituitary-adrenal axis in the pathogenesis of the metabolic syndrome: neuroendocrine and target tissue-related causes. *Int J Obes Relat Metab Disord.* 2000;24(Suppl 2):S50-S55.

413. Bjorntorp P, Rosmond R. The metabolic syndrome: a neuroendocrine disorder? *Br J Nutr*. 2000;83(Suppl 1):S49-S57.
414. Wolff S, Adler R, Buskirk E, et al. A syndrome of periodic hypothalamic discharge. *Am J Med*. 1964;36:956-967.
415. Albright AL, Hadjipanayis CG, Lunsford LD, et al. Individualized treatment of pediatric craniopharyngiomas. *Childs Nerv Syst*. 2005;21:649-654.
416. Lin L, Faraco J, Li R, et al. The sleep disorder canine narcolepsy is caused by a mutation in the hypocretin (orexin) receptor 2 gene. *Cell*. 1999;98:365-376.
417. Chemelli RM, Willie JT, Sinton CM, et al. Narcolepsy in orexin knock-out mice: molecular genetics of sleep regulation. *Cell*. 1999;98:437-451.
418. Eriksson KS, Sergeeva O, Brown RE, et al. Orexin/hypocretin excites the histaminergic neurons of the tuberomammillary nucleus. *J Neurosci*. 2001;21:9273-9279.
419. Anaclet C, Parmentier R, Ouk K, et al. Orexin/hypocretin and histamine: distinct roles in the control of wakefulness demonstrated using knock-out mouse models. *J Neurosci*. 2009;29:14423-14438.
420. Gerashchenko D, Kohls MD, Greco M, et al. Hypocretin-2-saporin lesions of the lateral hypothalamus produce narcoleptic-like sleep behavior in the rat. *J Neurosci*. 2001;21:7273-7283.
421. Thannickal TC, Moore RY, Nienhuis R, et al. Reduced number of hypocretin neurons in human narcolepsy. *Neuron*. 2000;27(3):469-474.

CHAPTER 8

Pituitary Physiology and Diagnostic Evaluation

URSULA KAISER • KEN K. Y. HO

KEY POINTS

- The pituitary gland orchestrates endocrine system integrity through central hypothalamic and peripheral hormonal signals.
- Pituitary gland cells are organized into structural and functional networks formed during embryonic development but modified throughout life.
- Differentiated lactotrophs, somatotrophs, gonadotrophs, corticotrophs, and thyrotrophs are each regulated by system-specific factors.
- The growth hormone axis controls growth in childhood while regulating energy and substrate metabolism throughout life.
- Prolactin, responsible primarily for milk production during pregnancy and lactation, is uniquely under tonic inhibitory hypothalamic control by dopamine.
- The hypothalamic-pituitary-adrenal axis is the pivotal system subserving stress and survival, elaborated through effects on energy supply, fuel metabolism, immunity, and cardiovascular function.
- The hypothalamic-pituitary-gonadal axis plays a pivotal role in puberty, reproductive function, and fertility, controlling both gametogenesis and sex steroid hormone production.
- The hypothalamic-pituitary-thyroid axis plays a critical role in development, growth, and cellular metabolism, mediated by thyroid hormones.
- Pituitary gland failure can arise from developmental, heritable, and acquired disorders and is diagnosed by baseline and provocative pituitary and target gland hormone testing.

ANATOMY, DEVELOPMENT, AND OVERVIEW OF CONTROL OF HORMONE SECRETION

The pituitary gland, situated within the sella turcica, derives its name from the Greek *ptuo* and Latin *pituita*,

meaning *phlegm*, reflecting its nasopharyngeal origin. Galen hypothesized that nasal phlegm originated from the brain and drained via the pituitary gland. It is now clear that together with the hypothalamus, the pituitary orchestrates the structural integrity and function of endocrine glands including the thyroid, adrenal, and gonads, in addition to target tissues including liver, cartilage, and breast. The pituitary stalk serves as an anatomic and functional connection to the hypothalamus. Preservation of the hypothalamo-pituitary unit is critical for integration of systemic and central nervous system inputs for anterior pituitary control of sexual function and fertility, linear and organ growth, lactation, stress responses, energy, appetite, and temperature regulation, and secondarily for carbohydrate and mineral metabolism.

Integration of vital body functions by the brain was first proposed by Descartes in the 17th century. In 1733, Morgagni recorded the absence of adrenal glands in an anencephalic neonate, providing early evidence for a developmental and functional connection between the brain and the adrenal glands. In 1849, Claude Bernard set the stage for the subsequent advances in neuroendocrinology by demonstrating that central lesions to the area of the fourth ventricle resulted in polyuria.[1] Subsequent studies led to the identification and chemical isolation of pituitary hormones, and astute clinical observations led to the realization that pituitary tumors were associated with functional hypersecretory syndromes, including acromegaly and Cushing disease.[2-4] In 1948, Geoffrey Harris, the father of modern neuroendocrinology, reviewed the control of anterior pituitary gland hormones and proposed their hypothalamic regulation, predicting the subsequent discovery of specific hypothalamic regulating hormones.[5]

Anatomy

The pituitary gland comprises the predominant anterior lobe, the posterior lobe, and a vestigial intermediate lobe (Fig. 8-1). The gland is situated within the bony sella turcica and is overlain by the dural diaphragma sella through which the stalk connects to the median eminence of the hypothalamus. The adult pituitary weighs approximately 600 mg (range 400-900 mg) and measures approximately 13 mm in the longest transverse diameter, 6 to 9 mm in vertical height and about 9 mm anteroposteriorly. Structural variation may occur in multiparous women, and gland volume also changes during the menstrual cycle. During pregnancy these measurements may be increased in either dimension, with pituitary weight increasing up to

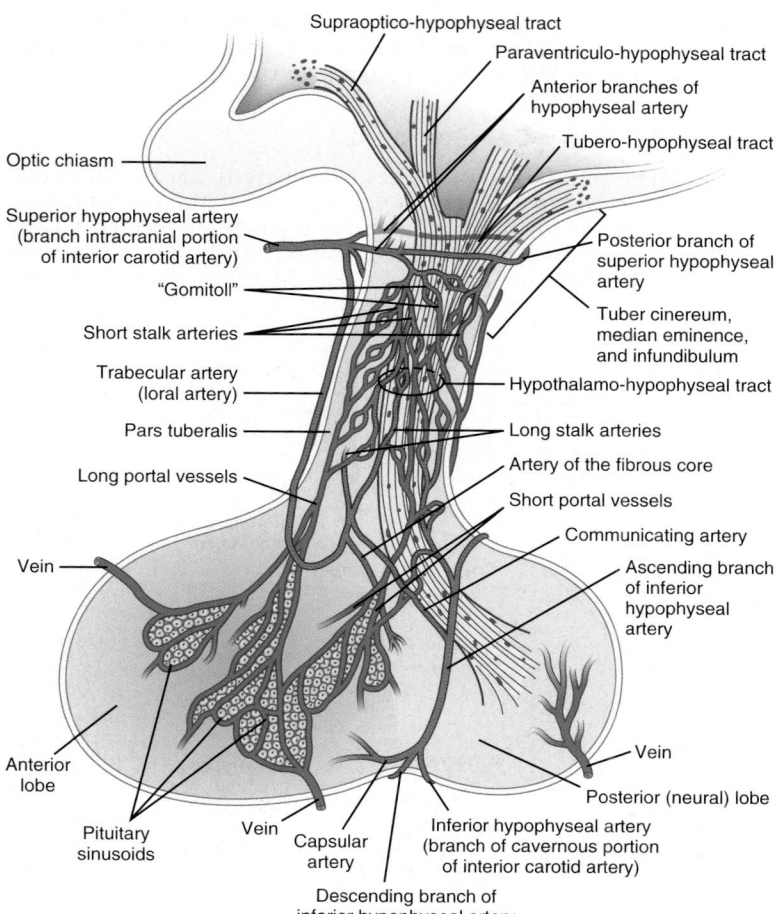

Supraoptico-hypophyseal tract
Paraventriculo-hypophyseal tract
Anterior branches of hypophyseal artery
Tubero-hypophyseal tract
Optic chiasm
Superior hypophyseal artery (branch intracranial portion of interior carotid artery)
"Gomitoll"
Short stalk arteries
Trabecular artery (loral artery)
Pars tuberalis
Long portal vessels
Vein
Anterior lobe
Pituitary sinusoids
Vein
Capsular artery
Inferior hypophyseal artery (branch of cavernous portion of interior carotid artery)
Descending branch of inferior hypophyseal artery
Posterior branch of superior hypophyseal artery
Tuber cinereum, median eminence, and infundibulum
Hypothalamo-hypophyseal tract
Long stalk arteries
Artery of the fibrous core
Short portal vessels
Communicating artery
Ascending branch of inferior hypophyseal artery
Vein
Posterior (neural) lobe

Figure 8-1 Schematic representation of the blood supply of the hypothalamus and pituitary. (From Scheithauer BW. The hypothalamus and neurohypophysis. In: Kovacs K, Asa SL, eds. *Functional Endocrine Pathology.* Oxford, UK: Blackwell Scientific; 1991.)

1 g. Pituitary hypertrophy without evidence for the presence of an adenoma was described in seven eugonadal women with pituitary height greater than 9 mm and a convex upper gland boundary observed on magnetic resonance imaging (MRI).[6]

The sella turcica, located at the base of the skull, forms the thin bony roof of the sphenoid sinus. The lateral walls comprise either bony or dural tissue about the cavernous sinuses, which are traversed by the third, fourth, and six cranial nerves and internal carotid arteries. Thus, the cavernous sinus contents are vulnerable to intrasellar expansion. The dural roofing protects the gland from compression by fluctuant cerebrospinal fluid (CSF) pressure. The optic chiasm, located anterior to the pituitary stalk, is directly above the diaphragma sella. The optic tracts and central structures are therefore vulnerable to pressure effects by an expanding pituitary mass, which typically follows the path of least tissue resistance. The posterior pituitary gland, in contrast to the anterior pituitary, is directly innervated by the supraopticohypophyseal and tuberohypophyseal nerve tracts of the posterior stalk. Hypothalamic neuronal lesions, stalk disruption, or systemically derived metastases to the hypothalamus are therefore often associated with attenuated vasopressin (diabetes insipidus) or oxytocin secretion.

The hypothalamus contains, among other neuronal populations, nerve cell bodies that synthesize hypophysiotropic releasing and inhibiting hormones, as well as the neurohypophyseal hormones of the posterior pituitary (arginine vasopressin [AVP] and oxytocin). Five distinct hormone-secreting cell types are present in the mature anterior pituitary gland:

1. Corticotroph cells express pro-opiomelanocortin (POMC) peptides including adrenocorticotropic hormone (ACTH).
2. Somatotroph cells express growth hormone (GH).
3. Thyrotroph cells express the common glycoprotein α-subunit and the specific thyroid-stimulating hormone (TSH, thyrotropin) β-subunit.
4. Gonadotroph cells express the α- and β-subunits for both follicle-stimulating hormone (FSH) and luteinizing hormone (LH).
5. Lactotroph cells express prolactin (PRL).

Each cell type is under highly specific signal controls that regulate their respective differentiated gene expression.

Pituitary Blood Supply

The pituitary gland enjoys an abundant blood supply derived from several sources (see Fig. 8-1). The superior hypophyseal arteries branch from the internal carotid arteries to supply the hypothalamus, where they form a capillary network in the median eminence, external to the blood-brain barrier. Both long and short hypophyseal portal vessels originate from infundibular plexuses and the stalk, respectively. These vessels form the hypothalamic-portal circulation, the predominant blood supply to the anterior pituitary gland. They deliver hypothalamic releasing and inhibiting hormones to the trophic hormone-producing cells of the adenohypophysis, without significant systemic dilution, allowing the pituitary cells to be sensitively regulated by timed hypothalamic hormone secretion. Vascular transport of hypothalamic hormones is also locally regulated by a contractile internal capillary plexus (gomitoli), derived from stalk branches of the superior hypophysial arteries.[7] Retrograde blood flow toward the median eminence also occurs, facilitating bidirectional functional hypothalamic-pituitary interactions.[8] Systemic arterial blood supply is maintained by inferior hypophyseal arterial branches, which predominantly supply the posterior pituitary. Disruption of stalk integrity may lead to compromised pituitary portal blood flow, depriving the anterior pituitary cells of hypothalamic hormone access.

Pituitary Development

The pituitary gland arises from within the rostral neural plate. Rathke's pouch, a primitive ectodermal invagination anterior to the roof of the oral cavity, is formed by the fourth or fifth week of gestation[9] and gives rise to the anterior pituitary gland[10,11] (Fig. 8-2). The pouch is directly

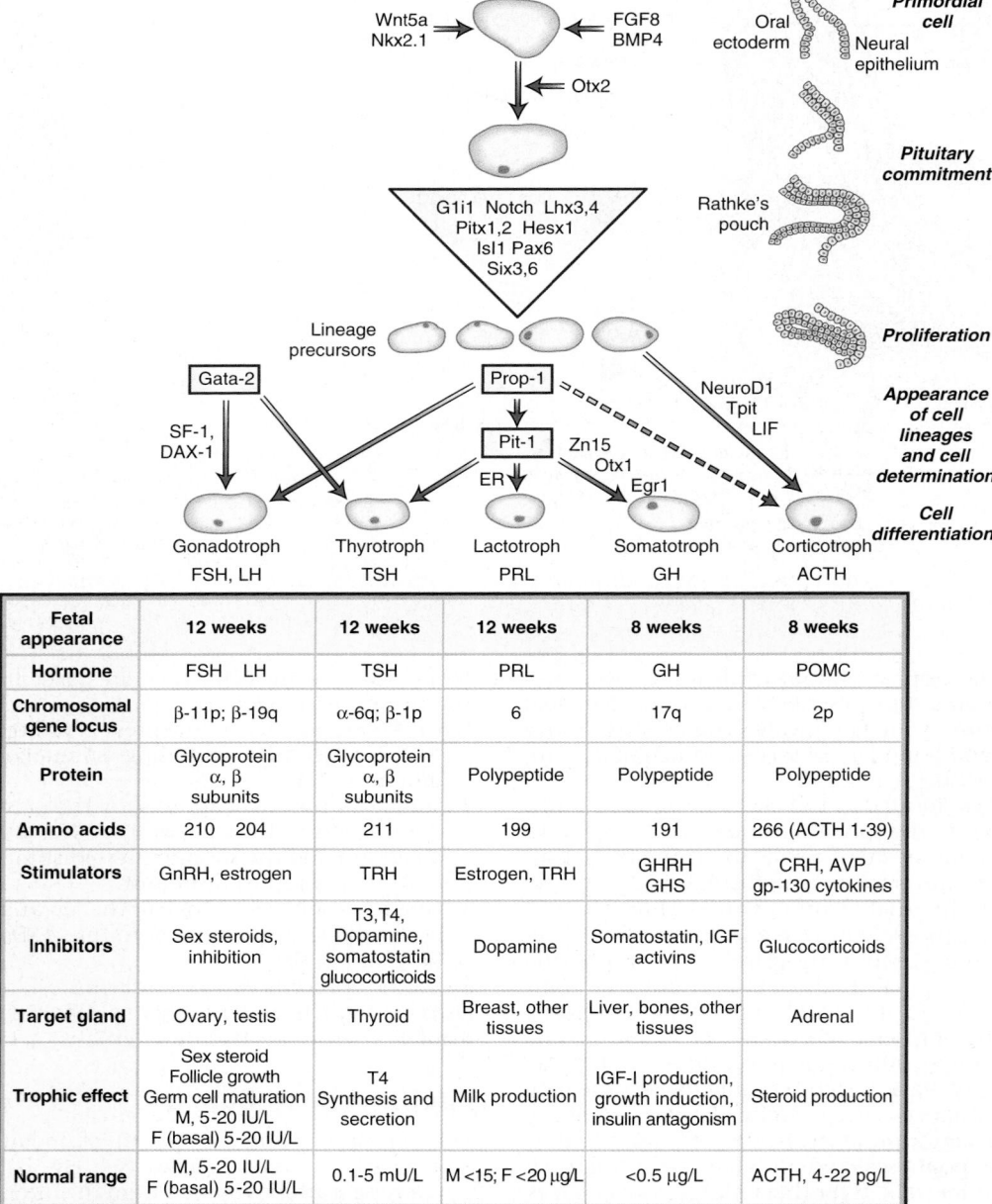

Fetal appearance	12 weeks	12 weeks	12 weeks	8 weeks	8 weeks
Hormone	FSH LH	TSH	PRL	GH	POMC
Chromosomal gene locus	β-11p; β-19q	α-6q; β-1p	6	17q	2p
Protein	Glycoprotein α, β subunits	Glycoprotein α, β subunits	Polypeptide	Polypeptide	Polypeptide
Amino acids	210 204	211	199	191	266 (ACTH 1-39)
Stimulators	GnRH, estrogen	TRH	Estrogen, TRH	GHRH GHS	CRH, AVP gp-130 cytokines
Inhibitors	Sex steroids, inhibition	T3,T4, Dopamine, somatostatin glucocorticoids	Dopamine	Somatostatin, IGF activins	Glucocorticoids
Target gland	Ovary, testis	Thyroid	Breast, other tissues	Liver, bones, other tissues	Adrenal
Trophic effect	Sex steroid Follicle growth Germ cell maturation M, 5-20 IU/L F (basal) 5-20 IU/L	T4 Synthesis and secretion	Milk production	IGF-I production, growth induction, insulin antagonism	Steroid production
Normal range	M, 5-20 IU/L F (basal) 5-20 IU/L	0.1-5 mU/L	M <15; F <20 μg/L	<0.5 μg/L	ACTH, 4-22 pg/L

Figure 8-2 Model for development of the human anterior pituitary gland and cell lineage determination by a cascade of transcription factors. Trophic cells are depicted with transcription factors known to determine cell-specific human or murine gene expression. ACTH, adrenocorticotropic hormone; AVP, arginine vasopressin; CRH, corticotropin-releasing hormone; ER, estrogen receptor; F, female; FSH, follicle-stimulating hormone; GH, growth hormone; GHRH, growth hormone–releasing hormone; GHS, growth hormone secretagogue; GnRH, gonadotropin-releasing hormone; IGF, insulin-like growth factor; LH, luteinizing hormone; M, male; POMC, pro-opiomelanocortin; PRL, prolactin; T_3, triiodothyronine; T_4, thyroxine; TRH, thyrotropin-releasing hormone; TSH, thyrotropin. (Adapted from Shimon I, Melmed S. Anterior pituitary hormones. In: Conn P, Melmed S, eds. *Scientific Basis of Endocrinology.* Totowa, NJ: Humana Press; 1996; and Amselem S. Perspectives on the molecular basis of developmental defects in the human pituitary region. In: Rappaport R, Amselem S, eds. *Hypothalamic-Pituitary Development.* Basel, Switzerland: Karger; 2001; and Dasen JS, O'Connell SM, Flynn SE, et al. Reciprocal interactions of Pit1 and GATA2 mediate signaling gradient-induced determination of pituitary cell types. *Cell.* 1999;97:587-598.)

connected to the stalk and hypothalamic infundibulum, and ultimately becomes distinct from the oral cavity and nasopharynx. Rathke's pouch proliferates toward the third ventricle, where it fuses with the diverticulum, and subsequently obliterates its lumen, which may persist as Rathke's cleft. The anterior lobe is formed from Rathke's pouch, and the diverticulum gives rise to the adjacent posterior lobe. Remnants of pituitary tissue may persist in the nasopharyngeal midline and rarely give rise to functional ectopic hormone-secreting tumors in the nasopharynx. The neurohypophysis arises from neural ectoderm associated with third ventricle development.[12]

Functional development of the anterior pituitary cell types involves complex spatiotemporal regulation of cell lineage–specific transcription factors expressed in pluripotential pituitary stem cells, as well as dynamic gradients of locally acting soluble factors.[13-16] Critical neuroectodermal signals for organizing the dorsal gradient of pituitary morphogenesis include infundibular bone morphogenetic protein 4 (BMP4) required for the initial pouch invagination,[11] fibroblast growth factor 8 (FGF8), FGF10, Wnt5, and Wnt4.[17] Subsequent ventral developmental patterning and transcription factor expression are determined by spatial and graded expression of factors including BMP2 and sonic hedgehog (SHH) protein, which appear critical for directing early patterns of cell proliferation.[18]

The human fetal Rathke's pouch is evident at 3 weeks, and the pituitary grows rapidly in utero. By 7 weeks, the anterior pituitary vasculature begins to develop, and by 20 weeks, the entire hypophyseal portal system is established. The anterior pituitary undergoes major cellular differentiation during the first 12 weeks, by which time all the major secretory cell compartments are structurally and functionally intact, except for lactotrophs. Totipotential pituitary stem cells give rise to acidophilic (mammosomatotroph, somatotroph, and lactotroph) and basophilic (corticotroph, thyrotroph, and gonadotroph) differentiated pituitary cell types, which appear at clearly demarcated developmental stages. At 6 weeks, corticotroph cells are morphologically identifiable, and immunoreactive ACTH is detectable by 7 weeks. At 8 weeks, somatotroph cells are evident with abundant immunoreactive cytoplasmic GH expression. Glycoprotein hormone–secreting cells express a common α-subunit, and at 12 weeks, differentiated thyrotrophs and gonadotrophs express immunoreactive β-subunits for TSH, LH, and FSH, respectively.[19] Fully differentiated PRL-expressing lactotrophs are only evident late in gestation (after 24 weeks). Prior to that time, immunoreactive PRL is only detectable in mixed mammosomatotrophs, also expressing GH, reflecting the common genetic origin of these two hormones.[20]

Pituitary Transcription Factors

Determination of anterior pituitary cell type lineages results from a temporally regulated cascade of homeodomain transcription factors.[13] Although most pituitary developmental information has been acquired from murine models,[21] histologic and pathogenetic observations in human subjects largely corroborate these developmental mechanisms (see Fig. 8-2; Tables 8-1 and 8-2). Early cell differentiation requires intracellular Hesx1 and Pitx expression. Rathke's pouch expresses several transcription factors of the LIM homeodomain family, including Lhx3, Lhx4, and Isl1,[21] which are early determinants of functional pituitary development and are required for progenitor cell survival and proliferation. In contrast, activated *Notch2* delays murine gonadotroph differentiation,[22] underscoring the role of Notch signaling pathways in the developmental

TABLE 8-1
Etiology of Inherited Pituitary Deficiency

Mutation	Hormone Deficit
Receptor	
GHRH receptor	GH
CRH receptor	ACTH
GnRH receptor	FSH, LH
TRH receptor	TSH
Structural	
Pituitary aplasia	Any
Pituitary hypoplasia	Any
CNS masses; encephalocele	Any
Transcription Factor Defect	
HESX1	GH, PRL, TSH, LH, FSH, ACTH
SOX2/3	GH, PRL, TSH, LH, FSH, ACTH
LHX3/4	GH, PRL, TSH, LH, FSH
PITX2	GH
PROP1	GH, PRL, TSH, LH, FSH, ACTH
POU1F1	PRL, GH, TSH
IGSF1	PRL, GH, TSH
TBX19	ACTH
NR5A1	LH, FSH
NR0B1	LH, FSH
Hormone Mutation	
GH1	GH
Bioinactive GH	GH
FSHβ	FSH
LHβ	LH
TSHβ	TSH
POMC	ACTH
POMC processing defect	ACTH
PC1	ACTH, FSH, LH

ACTH, adrenocorticotropic hormone; CNS, central nervous system; CRH, corticotropin-releasing hormone; FSH, follicle-stimulating hormone; GH, growth hormone; GHRH, growth hormone–releasing hormone; GnRH, gonadotropin-releasing hormone; GPR, orphan G protein–coupled receptor; LH, luteinizing hormone; POMC, pro-opiomelanocortin; PRL, prolactin; TSH, thyroid-stimulating hormone; TRH, thyrotropin-releasing hormone.

cascade. Diversity of pituitary cell type determination is mediated by binary Wnt/β-catenin signaling, leading to suppression of Hesx1 and induction of Prophet of Pit 1 (PROP1).[23] These specific anterior pituitary transcription factors participate in a highly orchestrated cascade, ultimately leading to the commitment of the five differentiated cell types (see Fig. 8-2). The major proximal determinant of pituitary cell lineage is PROP1, which determines subsequent development of POU1F1(Pit1)-dependent and gonadotroph cell lineages, whereas corticotroph cell commitment is directed by Tpit protein.[24,25]

The bicoid homeodomain proteins, Pitx1 and Pitx2, behave as universal pituitary regulators and activate transcription of all of the major anterior pituitary hormones.[26,27] Pitx1 is expressed in the oral ectoderm, and subsequently in all pituitary cell types, particularly those arising ventrally.[28] Rieger syndrome, characterized by defective eye, tooth, umbilical cord, and pituitary development, is caused by mutations in Pitx2.[29] Lhx3 determines GH, PRL, and TSH cell differentiation, and PROP1, a member of the paired-like family of homeodomain transcription factors, is expressed early in the development of Rathke's pouch and behaves as a prerequisite for Pit1. Pit1 is a POU homeodomain transcription factor, which determines development and appropriate temporal and spatial expression of GH, PRL, and TSH, binding to specific DNA motifs to activate and regulate somatotroph, lactotroph, and thyrotroph

TABLE 8-2

Hereditary Pituitary Deficiency Caused by Transcription Factor Mutations

Gene	Chromosome	Pituitary Deficiency	MRI	Associated Malformations	Inheritance Mode
POU1F1	3p11	GH, PRL, ± TSH	Normal or hypoplastic anterior pituitary		Recessive, Dominant
PROP1	5q35	GH, PRL, TSH, LH, FSH, ± ACTH	Normal, hypoplastic, hyperplastic or cystic anterior pituitary		Recessive
HESX1	3p21	GH, PRL, TSH, LH, FSH, ACTH Posterior defects	Hypoplastic or hyperplastic anterior pituitary; normal or ectopic posterior pituitary	Septo-optic dysplasia	Recessive
PITX2	4q25	GH, PRL, TSH, FSH, LH		Rieger Syndrome	Dominant
LHX3	9q34	GH, PRL, TSH, LH, FSH	Hypoplastic or hyperplastic anterior pituitary	Stubby neck with rigid cervical spine	Recessive
LHX4	1q25	GH, TSH, ACTH	Hypoplastic anterior pituitary Ectopic posterior pituitary		Dominant
TBX19	1q23	ACTH	Normal		Recessive
OTX2		GH, PRL, TSH, LH, FSH, ACTH	Hypoplastic anterior pituitary Ectopic posterior pituitary	Eye malformations	Dominant/Negative
SIX6	14q22		Hypoplastic pituitary Absent chiasm	Brachio-otorenal and oculoauriculo-vertebral syndromes	Haplo-insufficiency
SOX2	3q26	GH, FSH, LH	Anterior pituitary hypoplasia Mid-brain defects	Anopthalmia Esophageal atresia	
SOX3	Xq27	GH, TSH, ACTH, FSH, LH	Anterior pituitary hypoplasia Ectopic posterior pituitary		X-lined recessive
IGSF1	Xq25	GH, PRL, TSH		Testicular enlargement	X-linked recessive
NR5A1	9q33	FSH, LH		Adrenal insufficiency, gonadal defects, XY sex reversal	Dominant, recessive
NR0B1	Xp21.3	FSH, LH		Adrenal hypoplasia congenital, gonadal defects, XY sex reversal	X-linked dominant

Genes involved in pituitary development, or in maintaining integrity of the hypothalamic-pituitary axis. Functional defects include missense or frameshifts leading to truncated or deleted protein, DNA binding abnormality.

development and mature secretory function. Signal-dependent coactivating factors cooperate with Pit1 to determine specific hormone expression. Thus, in POU1F1-containing cells, high estrogen receptor levels induce a commitment to express PRL, and thyrotroph embryonic factor (TEF) favors TSH expression. Selective pituitary cell type specificity is also perpetuated by binding of Pit1 to its own DNA regulatory elements, as well as those contained within the GH, PRL, and TSH genes. Steroidogenic factor 1 (SF1) and DAX1 determine gonadotroph development.[30,31] TSH and gonadotropin-expressing cells share a common α-subunit (αGSU) expression under developmental control of Gata2.[32] Foxl2, a forkhead transcription factor, regulates differentiation of cell types expressing αGSU, including gonadotrophs and thyrotrophs, and transcription of αGSU and FSHβ.[17,33-36] Corticotroph cell commitment, occurring earliest during fetal development, is independent of PROP1-determined lineages, and Tpit protein is a prerequisite for POMC expression.[37] Hereditary mutations arising within these transcription factors may result in isolated or combined pituitary hormone failure syndromes (see later).[38]

Pituitary Stem Cells

The adult pituitary gland exhibits plastic and regenerative trophic properties, which allow maintenance of homeostatic functions.[39] This characteristic is exemplified by pituitary lactotroph expansion during pregnancy, and pituitary trophic hormone cell hyperplasia occurring after target organ ablation. Mechanisms underlying adult pituitary cell renewal and expansion are as yet unclear and may include intrinsic pituitary transdifferentiation, differentiation of previously uncommitted "null" cells, or expansion of already differentiated cells.

Several lines of evidence support the existence of cells with stem or progenitor characteristics in the adult pituitary gland.[40-44] Pituitary progenitor cells exhibit several characteristics of a stem cell phenotype including an undifferentiated gene profile, clonality, the ability to form colonies, and expression of known stem cell markers including Sca1 and CD133. Other markers, including Notch, Wnt, and SHH, are essential transcription factors for cell type determination and expansion of pituitary cell lineages. Evidence has emerged that SOX2, SOX9, and OCT4 are markers of pituitary progenitors with properties for multipotent pituitary cell differentiation,[45] and a population of nestin-expressing murine pituitary cells fulfill criteria consistent with organ-specific multipotent stem cells.[44] These cells form differentiated pituitary-expressing progeny and contribute to an adult pituitary stem cell population distinct from embryonic precursor cells. Expression of potential stem cell markers such as nestin in the marginal zone around Rathke's cleft has suggested that the stem cell population may exist in this marginal zone.[46] Cell-lineage tracing analysis has demonstrated that SOX2- and SOX9-expressing progenitors can self-renew and give rise to pituitary endocrine cells in vivo, supporting the model of these as tissue stem cells. Moreover, these cells can become mobilized and differentiate toward a specific cell fate in response to physiologic stress.[47,48] Advances have also been made toward recapitulation of pituitary differentiation in vitro—three-dimensional (3D) cultures of embryonic stem cells have been stimulated to differentiate into Rathke's pouch–like 3D structures, and various endocrine cells including functional corticotrophs and somatotrophs were subsequently produced, opening new avenues for the application of pluripotent stem cells to treat hypopituitarism.[49] Interestingly, adamantinomatous craniopharyngiomas share expression of stem cell markers with pituitary progenitor/stem cells, suggesting a common origin.[50]

Pituitary Control

The endocrine and nonendocrine cells of the pituitary gland are organized into structural and functional networks formed during embryonic development but modified throughout life. Structural mapping of the various endocrine cell types has highlighted the existence of distinct network motifs and spatial relationships with the vasculature that can explain the marked secretory capacity not evident from those observed from dispersed cells in culture.[51] The functional characterization of the network activity of GH, PRL, and gonadotropin have provided firm evidence for cell organization in gene regulation, in magnitude, and in temporal facets of hormone secretion. As such, the existence of these endocrine cell networks confers the pituitary as more than a gland that simply responds to external regulation, but rather, it acts as an oscillator that can imprint memory and adapt to coordinated networks' responses to hypothalamic inputs.[51]

Three levels of control subserve the regulation of anterior pituitary hormone secretion (Fig. 8-3). Hypothalamic control is mediated by adenohypophysiotropic hormones secreted into the hypothalamic portal system to impinge directly upon anterior pituitary cell surface receptors. G protein–coupled cell surface membrane binding sites are highly selective and specific for each of the hypothalamic hormones and elicit positive or negative signals mediating pituitary hormone gene transcription and secretion. Peripheral hormones also participate in mediating pituitary cell function, predominantly by negative feedback regulation of trophic hormones by their respective target hormones. Intrapituitary paracrine and autocrine soluble growth factors and cytokines act to locally regulate neighboring cell development and function. The net result of these three tiers of complex intracellular signals is the controlled pulsatile secretion of the six pituitary trophic hormones—ACTH, GH, PRL, TSH, FSH, and LH (Fig. 8-4). Temporal and quantitative control of pituitary hormone secretion is critical for physiologic integration of peripheral hormonal systems, as exemplified by the menstrual cycle, which relies on complex and precisely regulated hormonal pulse control.

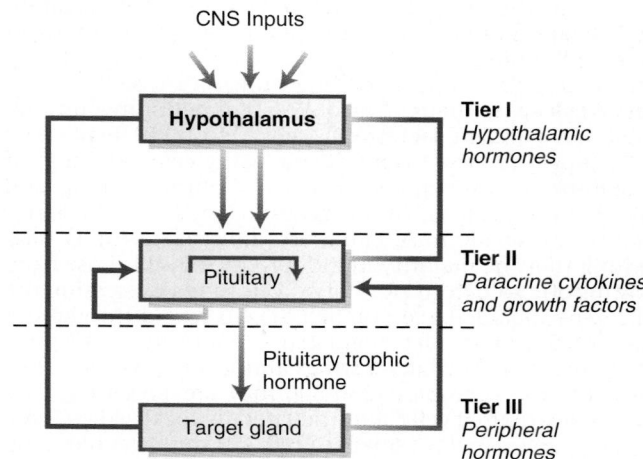

Figure 8-3 Model for regulation of anterior pituitary hormone secretion by three tiers of control. Hypothalamic hormones traverse the portal system and impinge directly upon their respective target cells. Intrapituitary cytokines and growth factors regulate tropic cell function by paracrine (and autocrine) control. Peripheral hormones exert negative feedback inhibition of respective pituitary trophic hormone synthesis and secretion. (From Ray D, Melmed S. Pituitary cytokine and growth factor expression and action. *Endocr Rev.* 1997;18:206-228.)

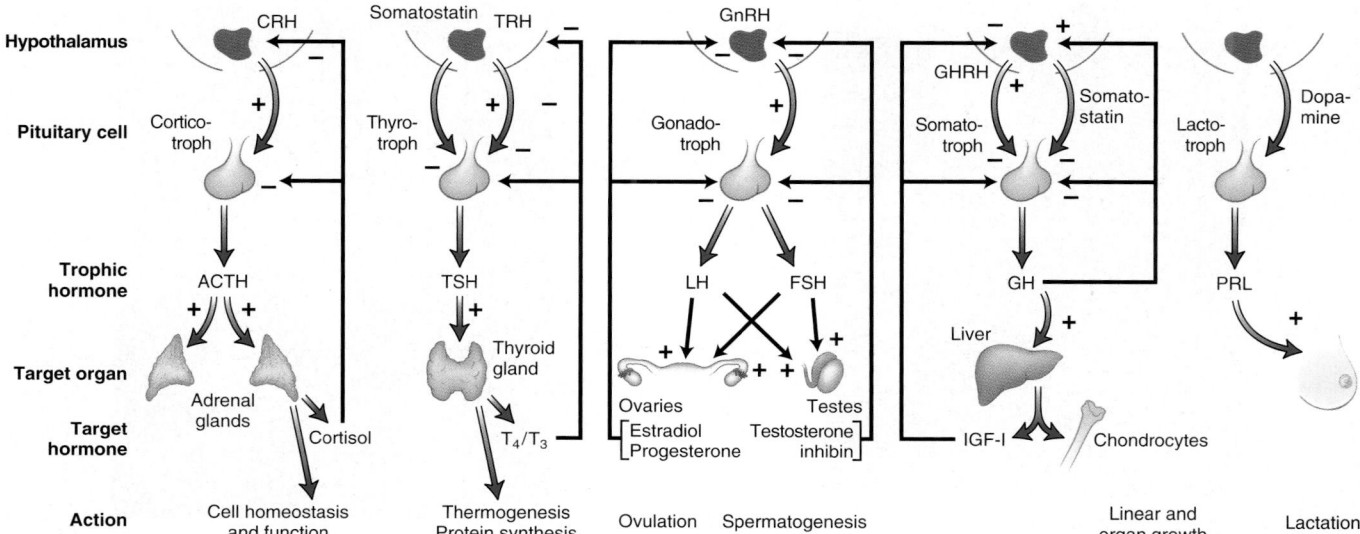

Figure 8-4 Control of hypothalamic-pituitary target organ axes. ACTH, adrenocorticotropic hormone; CRH, corticotropin-releasing hormone; FSH, follicle-stimulating hormone; GH, growth hormone; GHRH, growth hormone–releasing hormone; GnRH, gonadotropin-releasing hormone; IGF, insulin-like growth factor; LH, luteinizing hormone; PRL, prolactin; T_3, triiodothyronine; T_4, thyroxine; TRH, thyrotropin-releasing hormone; TSH, thyroid-stimulating hormone. (Adapted from Melmed S. Mechanisms for pituitary tumorigenesis: the plastic pituitary. *J Clin Invest.* 2003;112:1603-1618.)

PHYSIOLOGY AND DISORDERS OF PITUITARY HORMONE AXES

Prolactin

Physiology

The identification of PRL in humans was elusive until 1970 because human GH is highly lactogenic and active in bioassays used to isolate and measure PRL.[52] Furthermore, GH is present in human pituitary glands in much higher concentrations (5 to 10 mg) than PRL (approximately 100 μg).[53] To distinguish human PRL from GH, lactogenic activity was neutralized with GH antiserum; sera from postpartum women and patients with galactorrhea had high lactogenic activity in the presence of GH antibodies.[54,55] Purification and isolation of PRL by Friesen and development of a specific radioimmunoassay underscored the utility of PRL measurements in understanding human disease.[56,57]

Lactotroph Cells. About 15% to 25% of functioning anterior pituitary cells are lactotroph cells. Most PRL-expressing cells appear to arise from GH-producing cells. Ablation of somatotrophs by expression of GH-diphtheria toxin and GH-thymidine kinase fusion genes inserted into the germline of transgenic mice eliminates most lactotrophs, suggesting that the majority of PRL-producing cells arise from postmitotic somatotrophs.[58] Two cell forms expressing the PRL gene include large polyhedral cells found throughout the gland and smaller angulated or elongated cells clustered mainly in the lateral wings and median wedge. Large PRL secretory granules (250-800 nm) are present in the evenly distributed cells, and the laterally localized cells are sparsely populated by smaller (200-350 nm) granules (Fig. 8-5). Occasional mammosomatotroph cells cosecrete both PRL and GH, often stored within the same granule (Fig. 8-6). In animal models, lactotroph cell function is heterogeneous. Thus, dopamine or thyrotropin-releasing hormone (TRH) responsiveness, and shifting proportions of PRL versus GH secreting cells, may depend on cell localization within the pituitary, as well as the surrounding hormonal milieu, especially that of estrogen.[59] Although their absolute number does not change with age, lactotroph hyperplasia does occur during pregnancy and lactation[60] and resolves within several months of delivery (Fig. 8-7).

Prolactin Structure. The human PRL gene, located on chromosome 6,[61] arose from a single common ancestral gene,

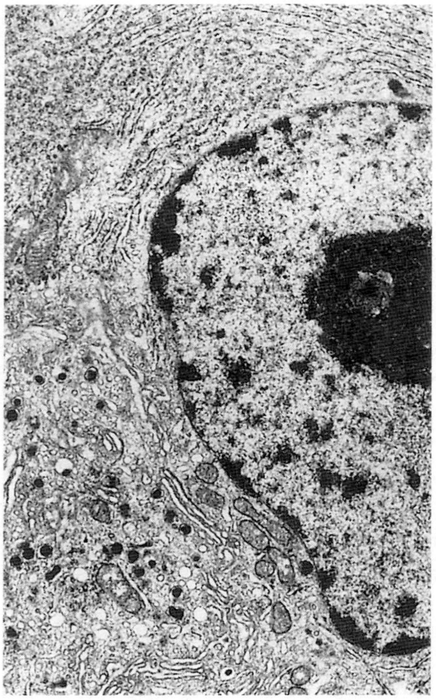

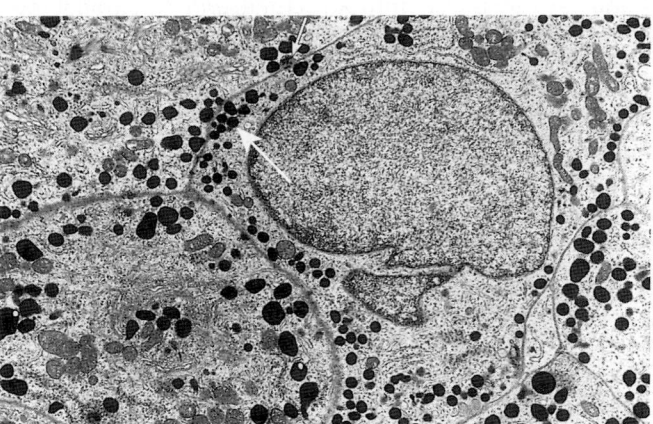

Figure 8-6 Normal mammosomatotroph. Occasional cells resembling densely granulated somatotrophs exhibit atypical features consistent with prolactin secretion: the secretory granules are highly pleomorphic and there is misplaced exocytosis, i.e., extrusion of secretory material along the lateral cell border *(arrow)*. (From Asa SL. Tumors of the pituitary gland. In: Rosai J, ed. *Atlas of Tumor Pathology*, Series III, Fascicle 22. Washington, DC: Armed Forces Institute of Pathology; 1997:17.)

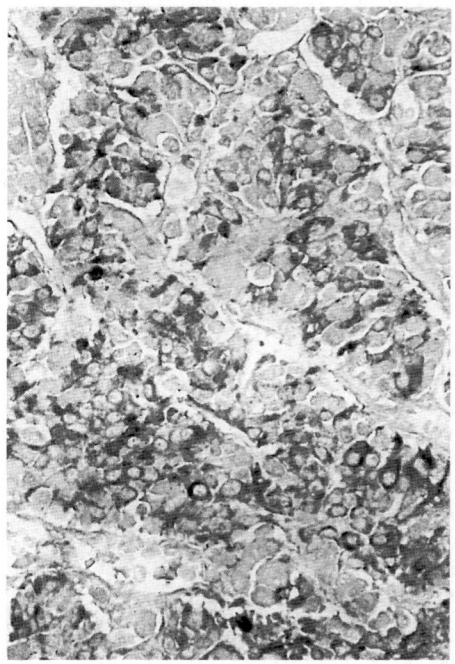

Figure 8-7 Prolactin cell hyperplasia. In the third trimester of pregnancy, prolactin cell hyperplasia occurs; cells containing immunoreactive prolactin make up almost 50% of the cell population of the gland. (From Asa SL. Tumors of the pituitary gland. In: Rosai J, ed. *Atlas of Tumor Pathology*, Series III, Fascicle 22. Washington, DC: Armed Forces Institute of Pathology; 1997:15.)

Figure 8-5 Electron micrograph of a normal lactotroph shows a well-developed rough endoplasmic reticulum that forms concentric whorls. A prominent Golgi complex is seen in a juxtanuclear location and harbors forming pleomorphic secretory granules. The cytoplasm is otherwise sparsely granulated. (From Asa SL. Tumors of the pituitary gland. In: Rosai J, ed. *Atlas of Tumor Pathology*, Series III, Fascicle 22. Washington, DC: Armed Forces Institute of Pathology; 1997:16.)

which gave rise to the relatively homologous PRL, GH, and placental lactogen-related proteins.[62] Several factors influence PRL gene expression, including estrogen, dopamine, TRH, and thyroid hormones.[63] PRL is a 199–amino acid polypeptide containing three intramolecular disulfide bonds. It circulates in blood in various sizes—monomeric PRL ("little prolactin"; 23 kDa), dimeric PRL ("big prolactin"; 48-56 kDa), and polymeric forms (also known as "big, big prolactin"; >100 kDa).[64-66] The monomeric form is the most bioactive PRL. In response to TRH; the proportion of the monomeric form increases. A glycosolated form of PRL identified in pituitary extracts is less biologically active than little PRL.[67] Monomeric PRL is cleaved into 8- and 16-kDa forms,[68] and the 16-kDa variant is antiangiogenic.[69,70] Indeed, this 16-kDa PRL cleavage product has been implicated in peripartum cardiomyopathy.[71] The mechanism underlying this association was recently shown to occur via actions of the 16-kDa PRL on capillary endothelial cells, stimulating the production of miR-146a, which in turn acts through a paracrine mechanism on cardiomyocytes to inhibit metabolism by blocking the activity of ERBB4, a tyrosine kinase receptor, and impairing cardiomyocyte function. Cardiac dysfunction could be improved by treatment with the dopamine agonist bromocriptine, which resulted in a fall in miR-146a levels in parallel with an improvement in cardiac function.[72-74]

Regulation. PRL secretion is under the inhibitory control of dopamine, which is largely produced by the tuberoinfundibular (TIDA) cells and the hypothalamic tuberohypophyseal dopaminergic system.[75,76] Dopamine reaches the lactotrophs via the hypothalamic pituitary portal system and inhibits PRL secretion by binding to the type 2 dopamine (D_2) receptors on pituitary lactotrophs.[77] PRL, in turn, participates in negative feedback to control its release by increasing tyrosine hydroxylase activity and thereby dopamine synthesis in the TIDA neurons.[76] In PRL-deficient animals, dopamine is decreased in the median eminence.[78] Mice lacking the D_2 receptor develop hyperprolactinemia and lactotroph proliferation.[77] Many other factors modulate PRL secretion, although their physiologic or clinical relevance remains in large part unresolved. Factors other than dopamine inhibit PRL secretion, including endothelin-1 and TGF-β1, which act as paracrine PRL inhibitors,[79,80] and calcitonin, which may be derived from the hypothalamus.[81] Several substances act as PRL-releasing factors. Basic FGF and epidermal growth factor induce PRL synthesis and secretion. Vasoactive intestinal polypeptide (VIP) stimulates PRL synthesis via cyclic adenosine monophosphate (cAMP).[82] A hypothalamic prolactin-releasing peptide (PrRP) produced in the hypothalamus acts through a specific receptor[83] in normal pituitary glands and in a subset of PRL-secreting tumors.[84] TRH stimulates PRL secretion.[85] Estrogen stimulates PRL gene transcription and secretion,[86] explaining why women have higher PRL levels, particularly during the periovulatory menstrual phase.[87] The physiologic roles of γ-aminobutyric acid (GABA), neurotensin, substance P, bombesin, and cholecystokinin (CCK) in regulating human PRL secretion are unresolved.[76]

Serotonin may be additive with VIP in releasing PRL, and infusion of 5-hydroxytryptophan, a serotonin precursor, elicits PRL release. Nocturnal PRL secretion is attenuated by cyproheptadine. Thus, serotonin may mediate nocturnal PRL secretion and also participate with VIP in the suckling reflex. Opiates acutely induce PRL release, although naloxone does not consistently suppress PRL levels. GH-releasing hormone (GHRH), when administered at high doses, moderately induces PRL secretion, and patients harboring ectopic GHRH-producing tumors have mild to moderate hyperprolactinemia. Although posterior pituitary hormones have been shown to regulate rat PRL secretion,[88] the role of vasopressin or oxytocin or other neurohypophyseal molecules in regulating human PRL remains unresolved. Histamine may act on the hypothalamus to regulate PRL, and histamine H_2 blockers induce PRL secretion.

Prolactin Secretion. The calculated production rate of PRL ranges from 200 to 536 µg/day/m², and the metabolic clearance rate ranges from 40 to 71 mL/minute/m².[89] PRL is cleared rapidly, with a calculated disappearance half-life ranging from 26 to 47 minutes. PRL secretion occurs episodically in 4 to 14 secretory pulses over 24 hours, each lasting 67 to 76 minutes,[90,91] with the highest levels achieved during sleep and the lowest occurring between 10 AM and noon.[92] The nocturnal elevation is sleep entrained, and a temporal relationship exists between rapid eye movement (REM) and non-REM sleep cycles.[93] PRL levels decline with age in both men and women. In older men, less PRL is produced with each secretory burst than in younger men.[94] Likewise, postmenopausal women have lower mean serum PRL levels and PRL pulse frequency than do premenopausal women, suggesting a stimulatory effect of estrogen on both these parameters.[87]

Prolactin Action. The PRL receptor gene is a member of the cytokine receptor superfamily,[95] localized to chromosome 5p13, with an extracellular domain, a hydrophobic transmembrane domain, and an intracytoplasmic region homologous to the GH receptor[96] (Fig. 8-8). PRL receptor dimerization occurs in both ligand-dependent and ligand-independent manners, with a single PRL molecule binding to both components of the receptor dimer, with phosphorylation of intracellular Janus kinase/signal transducers and activators of transcription (JAK-STAT) molecules subsequent to PRL binding. Two ligand-receptor binding sites are critical for formation of the trimeric ligand-receptor complex and subsequent signaling.[97-99] PRL receptor induces protein tyrosine phosphorylation and activation of JAK2 and STAT1-5.[100,101] STAT5 phosphorylation mediates transcriptional activation of the β-casein gene.[102]

PRL receptors are expressed in breast tissue and in many other tissues including pituitary, liver, adrenal cortex, kidneys, prostate, ovary, testes, intestine, epidermis, pancreatic islets, lung, myocardium, brain, and lymphocytes. Regulation of milk production occurs via a cascade of intracellular events. Homozygous mice in which the PRL receptor has been inactivated are infertile.[97] A gain-of-function mutation conferring constitutive activity of the PRL receptor is present in a subset of patients with multiple breast fibroadenomas.[103] PRL receptor antagonists have been developed for targeting the receptor in PRL-sensitive disturbances, including resistant prolactinomas, breast tumors, and prostate tumors.[99,104]

Prolactin Function. PRL is essential for human species survival, because it is responsible for milk production during pregnancy and lactation. Additional biologic functions ascribed to PRL include reproductive and metabolic effects, mammary development, freshwater survival, melanin synthesis, molting, and parental behavior.[105] Although PRL and its receptor are clearly crucial in lower animals,[106] the impact of PRL on maternal behavior in humans has not been fully delineated.

Mammary Gland Development and Lactation

Puberty. PRL is not essential for pubertal mammary development, which appears to require GH, the action of which is mediated by insulin-like growth factor 1 (IGF-1).[107-109] At birth, the rodent mammary gland consists of a fat pad with small areas of ductal anlagen, which differentiate into pubertal mammary glandular elements under the influence

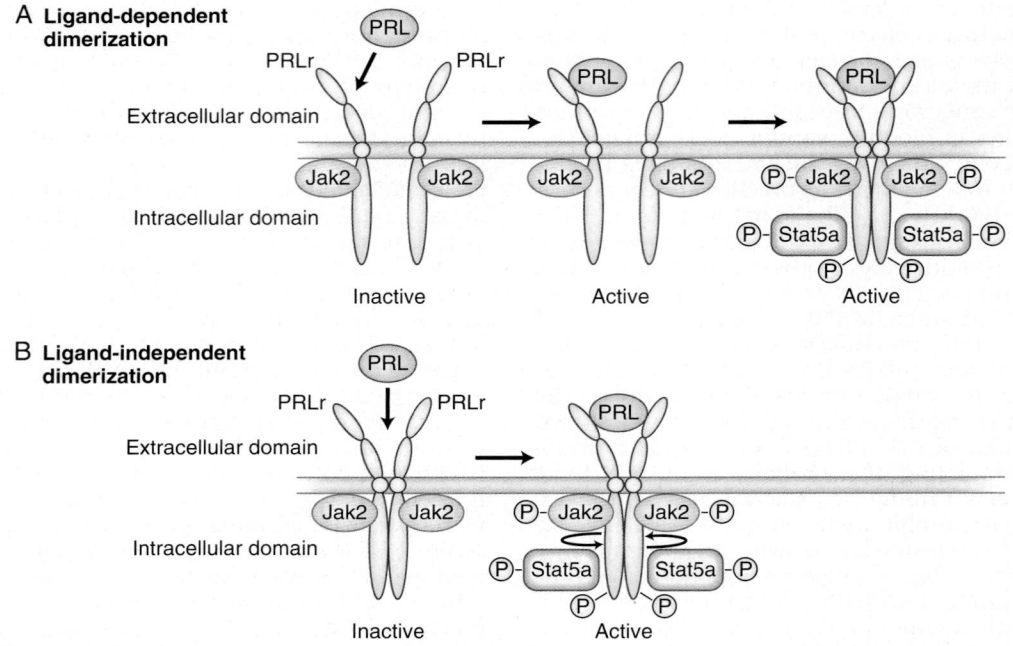

Figure 8-8 Ligand-dependent and -independent dimerization of the prolactin (PRL) receptor (PRLr). **A,** Ligand-dependent dimerization model. PRLr is in monomeric form at the cell membrane. One molecule of PRL first binds to one PRLr monomer via binding site 1, and this 1:1 complex then recruits the second PRLr via binding site 2. Dimerization of the two PRLrs leads to activating changes in the intracellular domain, leading to PRL signal transduction, such as phosphorylation (P) of Janus kinase 2 (Jak2), phosphorylation of the PRLr, and the recruitment and phosphorylation of the signal transducer and activator of transcription (Stat5). **B,** Ligand-independent model. PRLr exists in dimeric form at the cell membrane in the absence of ligand. The receptors are held in an inactive form until binding of PRL to this preformed complex induces activating changes in the intracellular domain, leading to phosphorylation of Jak2, phosphorylation of the PRLr, and recruitment and phosphorylation of Stat5a. (From Clevenger C, Gadd SL, Zheng J. New mechanisms for PRLr action in breast cancer. *Trends Endocrinol Metab.* 2009;20:223-229.)

of estrogen, GH, and IGF-1. At puberty, a surge of estrogen begins the developmental process. Terminal end buds form and lead the process of mammary development by branching and extending into the substance of the mammary fat pad, leaving in its wake a network of ducts that virtually fill the mouse mammary fat pad.[110,111] GH acts on the mammary stoma compartment to produce IGF-1, which, in turn, stimulates formation of terminal end buds and ducts in synergy with estrogen.[109,112] Parathyroid hormone–related protein is essential for fetal mammary development,[113] and epidermal growth is essential for pubertal mammary development.[114] Progesterone, possibly in association with GH and PRL, causes formation of lobular "decorations" along ducts, which are precursors to true glands.[115] Pubertal mammary development begins in girls between the ages of 8 and 13 (see developmental scale of Tanner, Chapter 23). Once fully developed, the pubertal mammary gland remains quiescent until pregnancy, although cyclic changes occur during the menstrual cycle.

In pregnancy, alveolar elements proliferate and begin to produce milk proteins and colostrum. At 3 to 4 weeks of gestation, terminal ductal sprouting occurs, followed by lobular-alveolar formation, and true alveoli form at the end of the first trimester. Glandular elements proliferate further and secretory products appear in the alveolar lumina. During the third trimester, fat droplets are seen within alveolar cells, and the glands fill with colostrum.[116] A combination of estrogen, PRL, progesterone, and possibly IGF-1 and placental hormones are largely responsible for this phase of mammary development.[117] In mice with targeted disruption of the PRL gene, formation of alveolar structures is impaired.[77] Likewise, women with isolated PRL deficiency are unable to lactate.[118] Similarly, in mice lacking the progesterone receptor, lobular-alveolar formation does not occur.[119] Interestingly, only a minority of women have

expressible milk during pregnancy, most likely due to inhibitory effects of estradiol[120] and progesterone[121] on PRL-induced milk production.

Lactation. Active lactation is due in part to attenuation of estrogen and progesterone levels and elevation of PRL levels after delivery. Suckling also increases milk production after parturition and is essential for continued lactation because of its distal effect on pituitary hormone production and because it empties the mammary gland of milk.[122] Milk accumulation inhibits milk synthesis, explaining why a certain level of nursing activity is necessary for successful breastfeeding. In the absence of suckling, PRL concentrations, which rise throughout gestation, return to normal by 7 days post partum.[123] Although PRL is essential for milk production, the milk yield does not correlate closely with serum PRL levels.[124] Suckling also stimulates posterior pituitary oxytocin release and, unlike PRL, oxytocin responses to suckling do not decline for up to 6 months if nursing continues. Mothers who breastfed exclusively had mean stimulated oxytocin levels significantly higher during late versus early lactation.[125] Oxytocin induces myoepithelial cell contraction, thereby causing milk ejection.[126] Oxytocin also has important effects on alveolar proliferation.[127] Mice deficient in oxytocin are unable to nurse their young, and oxytocin replacement permits these dams to nurse.

Reproductive Function. Lactation results in amenorrhea and secondary infertility, and this natural form of contraception depends upon the frequency and duration of breastfeeding. The Kung hunter-gatherer women suckle their infants approximately four times an hour and at will during the night, and women bear a mean of 4.7 children during their reproductive years.[128] In contrast, the Hutterites of North America bear a mean of 10.6 children during their lifetimes, presumably because they nurse according to a rigid schedule, use supplemental feedings, and wean at 1 year. Amenorrhea and infertility result from PRL-mediated inhibitory effects on hypothalamic gonadotropin-releasing hormone (GnRH) neurons and on the pituitary to reduce secretion of the gonadotropins, LH, and FSH, resulting in a reduction in both amplitude and frequency of LH pulses (Fig. 8-9).[129] In a hyperprolactinemic mouse model, hypothalamic kisspeptin immunoreactivity was reduced, and administration of kisspeptin restored estrous cyclicity, ovulation, and circulating LH and FSH levels. In addition, kisspeptin neurons have been shown to express PRL receptors.[130] Taken together, these data suggest that kisspeptin may be the missing link between hyperprolactinemia and the associated hypogonadotropic hypogonadism, anovulation, and infertility.[131,132] During lactation, additional metabolic factors induced by negative energy balance may also contribute to disruption of pulsatile GnRH and LH secretion.

Immune Function. Early evidence indicated that PRL regulates immune function. However, some evidence indicates that PRL may not be important for immune function,[133] as innate immunity was not altered in transgenic mice devoid of either the PRL receptor (PRLR[-/-]) or PRL (PRL[-/-]).[77,134] On the other hand, PRL has been shown to have protective effects against inflammation-induced chondrocyte apoptosis, with potential to reduce joint damage and inflammation in rheumatoid arthritis.[135]

Prolactin Assays. Modern PRL immunoassays are highly specific in distinguishing PRL from GH. The serum concentration of PRL can be given in mass concentration (µg/L or ng/mL), molar concentration (nmol/L or pmol/L), or international units (typically mIU/L). The current IU is calibrated against the Third International Standard for Prolactin, IS 84/500.[136] As these samples are usually assayed at

a single dilution, extremely high PRL concentrations may saturate their ability to detect very high PRL levels, resulting in a falsely low value being reported.[137] This "hook effect" may result in PRL-secreting macroadenomas diagnosed as clinically nonfunctioning adenomas, with "normal" PRL levels reported in about 5% of patients. In patients harboring macroadenomas with clear-cut clinical features of hyperprolactinemia, serum samples should be subjected to at least 1:100 dilution prior to assay.

Hyperprolactinemia

Causes. The causes of hyperprolactinemia may be physiologic, pathologic, or drug-induced[138,139] (Table 8-3).

Physiologic Causes

Pregnancy. During pregnancy, the normal pituitary gland may double or more in size,[60] the result of a marked increase in the number of PRL-producing cells and a relative decrease in other hormone-secreting cells. Serum PRL concentrations rise to 10 times normal during pregnancy,[123] and amniotic fluid PRL concentrations are 100 times those of maternal or fetal blood.[123]

Suckling. Suckling increases serum PRL levels approximately 8.5-fold in actively nursing mothers.[140,141] As nursing continues, PRL concentrations fall, but each suckling episode continues to cause a subsequent episodic rise in serum PRL. Mean serum concentrations were 162 µg/L at 2 to 4 weeks post partum, 130 µg/L at 5 to 14 weeks, and 77 µg/L at 15 to 24 weeks.[125] It is unclear why active milk production continues despite progressively lower PRL levels following parturition.

Idiopathic Hyperprolactinemia. An elevated circulating PRL level in patients in whom no cause is identified is considered idiopathic, and these patients are relatively resistant to dopamine agonist therapy. Mean serum PRL levels in patients with idiopathic hyperprolactinemia are usually less than 100 µg/L.[142]

Macroprolactinemia. PRL is a 23-kDa single-chain polypeptide but may also circulate in high-molecular-weight forms (50 kDa and 150 kDa). High-molecular-weight PRL variants may in some situations represent 85% or more of total PRL, but under usual circumstances the 23-kDa variety predominates. Macroprolactinemia reflects these larger circulating PRL molecules (particularly the 150-kDa variety), which exhibit markedly reduced bioactivity. Few of the expected clinical abnormalities usually associated with hyperprolactinemia (sexual dysfunction, hypogonadism, galactorrhea, osteoporosis) occur in patients with macroprolactinemia.[143] Screening for macroprolactinemia can be accomplished by polyethylene glycol precipitation of serum samples. In a 2005 survey, macroprolactinemia was detected in 22% of 2089 hyperprolactinemia samples.[144]

Pathologic Causes. Pathologic hyperprolactinemia may be caused by a prolactinoma, pituitary or sellar tumors that inhibit dopamine because of pressure on the pituitary stalk, or interruption of the vascular connections between the pituitary and hypothalamus. In a large series of histologically confirmed cases, serum PRL level greater than 2000 mUL (~100 µg/L) was almost never encountered from stalk dysfunction.[145] However, prolactinomas can present with any level of PRL elevation.

Breast stimulation has only a minimal effect on serum PRL levels. In 18 normal women serum PRL levels rose from a mean of 10 µg/L to 15 µg/L during breast pump stimulation.[140] *Chest wall lesions,* for example, in association with herpes zoster (shingles), can also be associated with mild hyperprolactinemia as a result of activation of neurogenic pathways that inhibit dopamine. Up to 20% of patients with *hypothyroidism* have elevated PRL levels.[146] Treatment of hypothyroidism with thyroid hormone normalizes

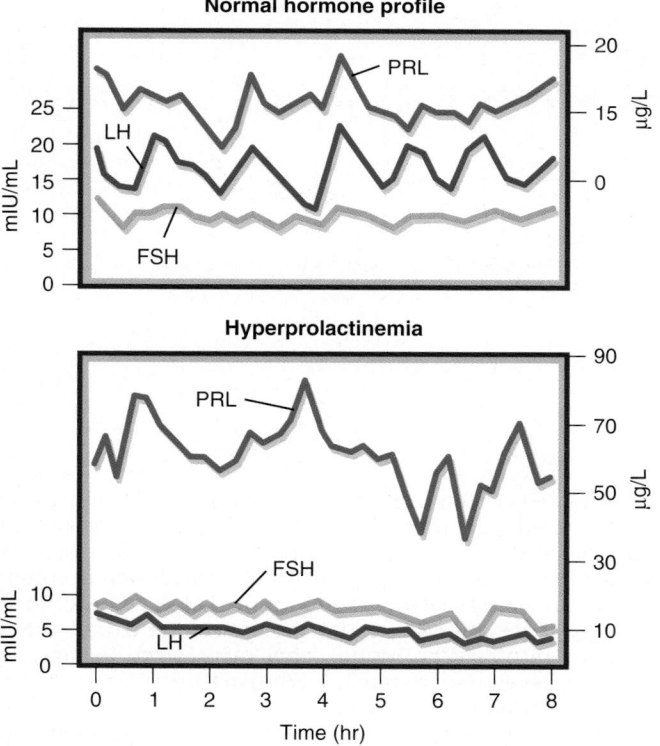

Figure 8-9 Effect of hyperprolactinemia on suppressing follicle-stimulating hormone (FSH) and luteinizing hormone (LH) secretory patterns leading to hypogonadotrophism in a female patient. PRL, prolactin. (Adapted from Tolis G. Prolactin: physiology and pathology. *Hosp Pract.* 1980;15:85-95.)

TABLE 8-3
Etiology of Hyperprolactinemia

Physiologic	*Dopamine Synthesis Inhibitors* α-Methyldopa
Pregnancy Sucking Stress Sleep Coitus Exercise	*Catecholamine Depleters* Reserpine *Cholinergic Agonists* Physostigmine
Pathologic	*Antihypertensives* Labetolol Reserpine Verapamil
Hypothalamic-Pituitary Stalk Damage Tumors Craniopharyngioma Suprasellar pituitary mass extension Meningioma Dysgerminoma Hypothalamic metastases Granulomas Infiltrations Rathke's cyst Irradiation Trauma: pituitary stalk section, sellar surgery, head trauma	*H₂ Antihistamines* Cimetidine Ranitidine *Estrogens* Oral contraceptives Oral contraceptive withdrawal *Anticonvulsants* Phenytoin
Pituitary Prolactinoma Acromegaly Macroadenoma (compressive) Idiopathic Plurihormonal adenoma Lymphocytic hypophysitis Parasellar mass Macroprolactinemia	*Neuroleptics* Chlorpromazine Risperidone Promazine Promethazine Trifluoperazine Fluphenazine Butaperazine Perphenazine Thiethylperazine Thioridazine Haloperidol Pimozide Thiothixene Molindone
Systemic Disorders Chronic renal failure Polycystic ovary syndrome Cirrhosis Pseudocyesis Epileptic seizures Cranial irradiation Chest: neurogenic, chest wall trauma, surgery, herpes zoster	
Genetic Inactivating prolactin receptor mutation	*Opiates and Opiate Antagonists* Heroin Methadone Apomorphine Morphine
Pharmacologic	
Neuropeptides Thyrotropin-releasing hormone	*Antidepressants* Tricyclic antidepressants: chlorimipramine, amitriptyline Selective serotonin reuptake inhibitors: fluoxetine
Drug-Induced Hypersecretion *Dopamine Receptor Blockers* Phenothiazines: chlorpromazine, perphenazine Butyrophenones: haloperidol Thioxanthenes Metoclopramide	

serum PRL if the hyperprolactinemia is due to thyroid hormone deprivation.

PRL is moderately elevated (mean 28 μg/L) in patients with *chronic renal failure* and those on dialysis.[147] The increase is largely a result of an increase in PRL cleavage products, due in part to decreased glomerular filtration rate. Sexual dysfunction is common in men on dialysis, and reducing PRL with dopamine agonists improves sexual function[148] but does not normalize menses in women.[149] Side effects of dopamine agonists in patients with renal failure may be exacerbated because of fluid shifts and multiple medication interactions. PRL levels rise in response to *stress*, correlate with the degree of stress, and generally return to normal as stress abates. Mean peak serum PRL

level in 19 women undergoing general anesthesia was 39 μg/L immediately prior to surgery, 173 μg/L at surgery, and still elevated 24 hours after surgery at 47 μg/L.[150] Severe *head trauma* can also result in hyperprolactinemia, often accompanied by diabetes insipidus or SIADH (syndrome of inappropriate antidiuretic hormone secretion) and other anterior pituitary hormone deficiencies. Fifty percent of patients develop moderate hyperprolactinemia after *cranial and hypothalamic irradiation*.[151]

Hyperprolactinemia was reported in association with an *inactivating prolactin receptor mutation* in three sisters with oligomenorrhea.[152] The mutation disrupted ligand binding and downstream signaling, demonstrated in vitro. The presence of hyperprolactinemia in these affected women suggested central negative feedback by prolactin on its secretion in humans, as previously demonstrated in animal studies.[77,78] Affected women were all heterozygous for the mutation; the presence of hyperprolactinemia suggests that the mutant receptor may interfere with signaling by the normal receptor, encoded by the wild-type allele, to result in PRL insensitivity. As the occurrence of oligomenorrhea and the ability to lactate is contrary to what might be predicted from a state of prolactin insensitivity, the function of PRL and its receptor in humans requires further study.[73]

Drug-Induced Hyperprolactinemia. A variety of *medications* cause minimal or moderate prolactin elevations. Neuroleptic drugs elevate PRL because of their dopamine receptor antagonist properties, as do atypical antipsychotics that act by antagonizing both serotonin and dopamine receptors. Clozapine and olanzapine weakly induce PRL, and risperidone is a potent PRL stimulator.[153]

Unless patients exhibit hypogonadism, related osteoporosis, or troublesome galactorrhea, treatment of drug-induced hyperprolactinemia may not be necessary.[154] It should not always be assumed that hyperprolactinemia in patients on drugs known to elevate PRL is, in fact, due to those medications. Prolactinoma, other sellar lesions,[155] hypothyroidism, and renal failure should be considered as possible causes of hyperprolactinemia requiring active management. In patients taking neuroleptic medications, if the clinical situation permits, temporary drug withdrawal might be considered to determine if PRL levels normalize. If PRL levels do not normalize or medication withdrawal is not possible, a pituitary MRI should be performed. When neuroleptics elevate PRL levels, switching to olanzapine may be attempted because the medication has minimal effects on PRL levels. In determining whether to discontinue a drug or whether to use alternative medication, the benefits should be weighed against the risks of drug replacement or cessation.[156] Although combined use of dopamine antagonists and dopamine agonists is not usually advised because of an increased risk of side effects, such as postural hypotension or exacerbation of the underlying psychosis, some advocate the use of both formulations simultaneously.[157]

Clinical Features. Galactorrhea and reproductive dysfunction are the hallmarks of pathologic hyperprolactinemia. Women present with galactorrhea associated with a range of menstrual disturbances including infertility, oligomenorrhea, and amenorrhea, and men present with symptoms of hypogonadism and of tumor mass effects, with galactorrhea occurring infrequently.

Galactorrhea and amenorrhea were reported in the 19th century by Chiari and Frommel.[158] The Chiari-Frommel syndrome comprises postpartum galactorrhea, amenorrhea, and "utero-ovarian atrophy" in patients not nursing. This disorder is usually self-limiting, and fertility eventually returns after normalization of PRL levels, sometimes without an intervening menstrual period. Patients with postpartum amenorrhea, hyperprolactinemia, and galactorrhea have sometimes subsequently been found to harbor prolactinomas. In the 1950s, Argonz and del Castillo[159] and Forbes and colleagues[160] associated galactorrhea and amenorrhea with pituitary tumors. In a report of 18 such patients, galactorrhea and amenorrhea were reported for up to 11 years after parturition with a mean PRL level of 45 µg/L.[146]

Galactorrhea. Inappropriate nipple secretion of milk-like substances[161] may persist after childbirth or discontinuation of nursing for as long as 6 months. Thereafter, continued milk production is considered abnormal, and other causes for galactorrhea should be investigated. Galactorrhea can occur in either women or men and may be unilateral or bilateral, can be profuse or sparse, and can vary in color and thickness. If blood is present in the galactorrhea fluid, it could be the harbinger of an underlying pathologic process, such as a ductal papilloma or carcinoma, and mammography or sonography is indicated. Twenty-nine of 48 patients with pituitary tumors and galactorrhea had PRL concentrations less than 200 µg/L, likely on the basis of stalk compression, suggesting that they harbored pituitary tumors other than prolactinomas.[146] It is likely that most patients with so-called idiopathic galactorrhea with amenorrhea harbor microprolactinomas. Fifty percent of patients with acromegaly also have galactorrhea, even in the absence of hyperprolactinemia, because human GH is a potent lactogen and can cause galactorrhea when elevated.[162] Normoprolactinemic galactorrhea with regular menses represents the most frequent single cause of galactorrhea. In two thirds of these patients, galactorrhea persists after parturition, despite the resumption of menses, and likely does not represent a pathologic entity. Normal PRL levels may still permit milk production, because treatment of such patients with dopamine agonists alleviates galactorrhea. Galactorrhea may also develop transiently after surgical procedures to the chest wall, including mammoplasty, arising from neural reflexes due to intercostal nerve stimulation.[163] The optimal management of galactorrhea should be determined by identifying and treating the underlying cause. Regardless of the cause, galactorrhea associated with hyperprolactinemia responds to correction of hyperprolactinemia.

Prolactin Deficiency. Congenital PRL deficiency can occur in association with mutations in transcription factors involved in lactotroph lineage development, including POU1F1, PROP1, LHX3, LHX4, and HESX1 (see Tables 8-1 and 8-2). In these cases, deficiencies in other anterior pituitary hormones occur in conjunction with PRL deficiency, with the spectrum of pituitary hormone deficiencies depending on the gene affected.[45] PRL deficiency has also been reported in conjunction with central hypothyroidism in a subset of patients with the immunoglobulin superfamily member 1 (IGSF1) deficiency syndrome.[164]

The only known clinical manifestation of PRL deficiency is the inability to lactate after delivery. Isolated PRL deficiency is rare but has been reported in association with autoantibodies directed specifically against PRL-secreting pituitary cells.[165] Most patients with acquired PRL deficiency have evidence of other pituitary hormone deficiencies in association with pituitary injury.[166] Infarction of the pituitary gland after postpartum hemorrhage, known as Sheehan syndrome, has long been recognized as a cause of hypopituitarism.[167] In developed countries, postpartum hemorrhage now less often results in Sheehan syndrome than previously, largely due to improvements in obstetric care. No commercially available PRL preparation is available for these women, although studies with recombinant human PRL administration have been shown to increase milk volume in women with PRL deficiency or lactation insufficiency.[168]

Growth Hormone

Physiology

Somatotroph Cells. Mammosomatotroph cells expressing both PRL and GH arise from the acidophilic stem cell and immunostain mainly for PRL. Somatotrophs are located predominantly in the lateral wings of the anterior pituitary gland and comprise 35% to 45% of pituitary cells (Fig. 8-10). These ovoid cells contain prominent secretory granules up to 700 µm in diameter. Juxtanuclear Golgi structures are particularly prominent with secretory granules in

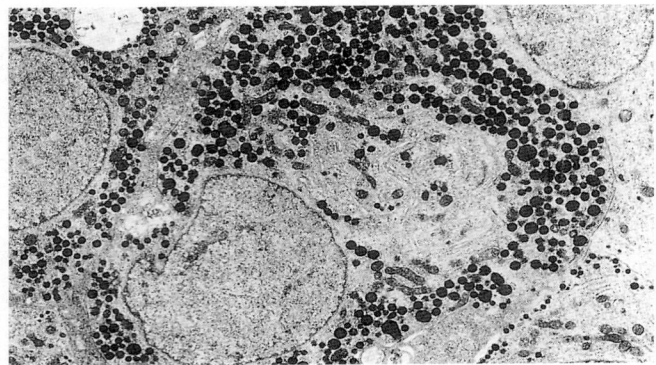

Figure 8-10 Normal somatotroph. A somatotroph in the nontumorous pituitary is large, round to ovoid, and contains numerous electron-dense secretory granules that range from 250 to 700 μm in diameter. Short profiles of rough endoplasmic reticulum are scattered throughout the cytoplasm. The juxtanuclear Golgi complex is prominent and harbors forming secretory granules. (From Asa SL. Tumors of the pituitary gland. In: Rosai J, ed. *Atlas of Tumor Pathology*, Series III, Fascicle 22. Washington, DC: Armed Forces Institute of Pathology; 1997:14.)

formation. The gland contains a total of 5 to 15 mg of GH.[169]

Biosynthesis. The human growth hormone (hGH) genome locus spans approximately 66 kb and contains a cluster of five highly conserved genes located on the long arm of human chromosome 17q22-24.[170] It encodes the following forms of hGH and human chorionic somatomammotropin (hCS): hGH-N, hCS-L, hCS-A, hGH-V, and hCS-B,[171] all of which consist of five exons separated by four introns.

The hGH-N gene is selectively transcribed in pituitary somatotrophs and codes for a 22-kDa (191–amino acid) protein.[172] Approximately 10% of pituitary GH is a 20-kDa variant lacking amino acid residues 32 through 46 formed from alternate slicing. The hCS-A and hCS-B genes are expressed in placental trophoblasts.[173] hGH-V, expressed in placental syncytiotrophoblasts, encodes a 22-kDa protein that emerges from midgestation as hGH-V2. When hGH-V levels are elevated, hGH-N declines progressively, suggesting feedback regulation of the maternal hypothalamic-pituitary axis. Postpartum circulating hGH-V levels drop rapidly and are undetectable 1 hour after delivery.[174] hCS-L is found in placental villi but has been considered a pseudogene.

The hGH promoter region contains *cis* elements that mediate both pituitary-specific and hormone-specific signaling. The POUIFI transcription factor confers tissue-specific GH expression and a second, ubiquitous factor binds to a distal Pit-1 site containing a consensus sequence for the Sp1 transcription factor. Pit-1 and Sp1 both contribute to GH promoter activation, as mutation of the Sp1 binding site attenuates promoter activity.[175] DNase hypersensitive sites of a locus control region (LCR) located 14.5 kb upstream of the hGH-N promoter confers and restricts the expression of GH only to somatotrophs and mammosomatotrophs among the Pit-1 positive cell population during development.[176] This distant locus also plays a major role in sustaining the level of hGH gene expression in somatotrophs. GH synthesis and release are under control of a variety of hormonal agents, including GHRH, somatostatin, ghrelin, IGF-1, thyroid hormone, and glucocorticoids. GHRH stimulates GH synthesis and release mediated by cAMP. cAMP-response element binding (CREB) protein (CBP) is phosphorylated by protein kinase A and is a cofactor for Pit-1–dependent human GH activation. IGF-1 attenuates basal and stimulated GH gene expression.

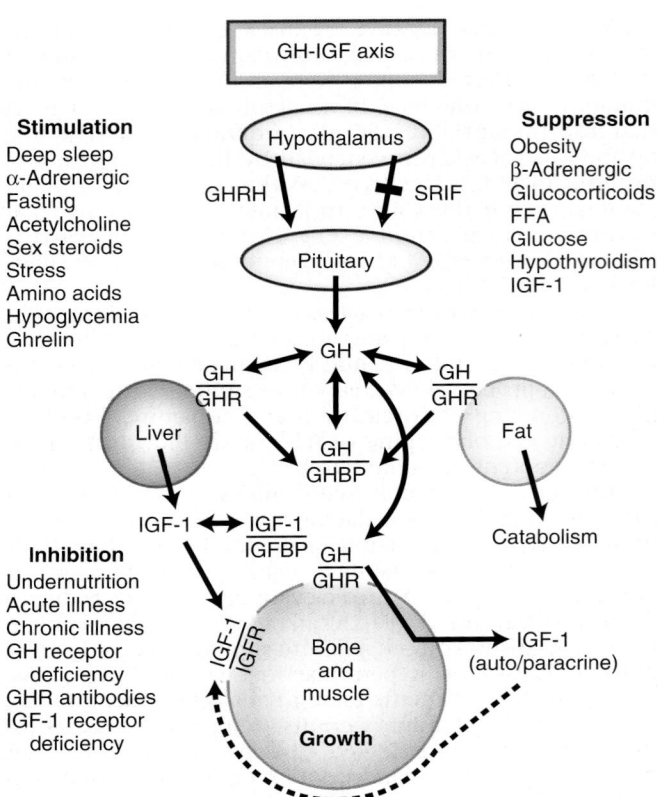

Figure 8-11 The growth hormone/insulin-like growth factor (GH-IGF) axis. Simplified diagram of GH axis involving hypophysiotropic hormones controlling pituitary GH release, circulating GH-binding protein (GHBP) and its GH receptor (GHR) source, IGF-1 and its largely GH-dependent binding proteins (IGFBP), and cellular responsiveness to GH and IGF-1 interacting with their specific receptors. GHRH, growth hormone–releasing hormone; IGFR, IGF-1 receptor; FFA, free fatty acids; SRIF, somatotropin release–inhibiting factor (somatostatin). (From Rosenbloom A. Growth hormone insensitivity: physiologic and genetic basis, phenotype and treatment. *J Pediatr.* 1999; 135:280-289.)

The GH molecule, a single-chain polypeptide hormone consisting of 191 amino acids, is synthesized, stored, and secreted by somatotroph cells. The crystal structure of hGH reveals four α-helixes.[177] Circulating GH molecules comprise several heterogeneous forms: 22- and 20-kDa monomers, an acetylated 22-kDa form, and two desamino GH molecules. The 22-kDa peptide is the major physiologic GH component, accounting for 75% of pituitary GH secretion. Amino acids 32 through 46 are deleted by alternative splicing of the GH gene to yield 20-kDa GH, accounting for approximately 10% of pituitary GH. The 20-kDa GH has a slower metabolic clearance.[178]

Regulation. Neuropeptides, neurotransmitters, and opiates impinge on the hypothalamus and modulate release of GHRH and somatostatin (somatotropin release–inhibiting factor, or SRIF). Integrated effects of these complex neurogenic influences determine the final secretory pattern of GH (Fig. 8-11). Apomorphine, a central dopamine receptor agonist, stimulates GH secretion,[179] as does levodopa (L-dopa). Oral L-dopa administration evokes a brisk serum GH response within an hour in healthy young subjects. Norepinephrine increases GH secretion via α-adrenergic pathways and inhibits GH release via β-adrenergic pathways. Insulin-induced hypoglycemia, clonidine, arginine administration, exercise, and L-dopa facilitate GH secretion by α-adrenergic effects.[180] β-Adrenergic blockade increases GHRH-induced GH release, possibly due to a direct pituitary action or by decreasing hypothalamic somatostatin release. Endorphins and enkephalins stimulate GH and may account for GH release during severe physical stress and extreme exercise[180] (see Fig. 8-11). Galanin, a 29–amino acid neuropeptide, induces GH release and enhances responses to GHRH. Cholinergic and serotoninergic neurons and several neuropeptides stimulate GH, including neurotensin, VIP, motilin, cholecystokinin, and glucagon.

GHRH and SRIF Interaction. The somatotroph cell expresses specific receptors for GHRH,[181] GH secretagogues, and SRIF receptor subtypes 2 and 5, which mediate GH secretion.[182,183] GHRH selectively induces GH gene transcription and hormone release.[184] GHRH administered to normal adults elicits a prompt rise in serum GH levels, with higher levels occurring in female subjects.[185] SRIF suppresses both basal and GHRH-stimulated GH pulse amplitude and frequency but does not affect GH biosynthesis.

Hypothalamic SRIF and GHRH are secreted in independent waves and interact together with additional GH secretagogues to generate pulsatile GH release. The rat hypothalamus releases GHRH and SRIF 180 degrees out of phase every 3 to 4 hours, resulting in pulsatile GH levels. SRIF antibody administration elevates GH levels, with intact intervening GH pulses,[186] implying that hypothalamic SRIF secretion generates GH troughs. Similarly, GHRH antibodies eliminate spontaneous GH surges. In humans, GH pulsatility persists when GHRH is tonically elevated, as in ectopic tumor GHRH production or during GHRH infusion,[187] suggesting that hypothalamic SRIF is largely responsible for GH pulsatility. However, GHRH antagonists inhibit GH pulses, indicating an important role in the generation of pulsatile secretion in humans.[188] The periodic, pulsatile GH release is the result of coordinated SRIF and GHRH secretion and action.

Chronic GHRH stimulation, either by continuous infusion or repeated bolus administration, eventually desensitizes GH release in vitro and in vivo, possibly due to depletion of a GHRH-sensitive pool of GH. GHRH pretreatment also decreases somatotroph GHRH binding sites.[189] GH stimulates hypothalamic SRIF, GHRH and SRIF autoregulate their own respective secretion, and GHRH stimulates SRIF release.[190] GH secretion is further regulated by its target growth factor, IGF-1, which participates in a hypothalamic-pituitary peripheral regulatory feedback system.[191,192] IGF-1 stimulates hypothalamic SRIF release and inhibits pituitary GH gene transcription and secretion.

Growth Hormone Secretagogues and Ghrelin. The isolation of ghrelin has implicated an additional control system for regulating GH secretion (see Chapter 7). Ghrelin is a 28–amino acid peptide which binds the growth hormone secretagogue (GHS) receptor[193] to induce hypothalamic GHRH and pituitary GH.[194] A unique n-octanoylated serine 3 residue confers GH-releasing activity to the molecule. Ghrelin is synthesized in peripheral tissues, especially gastric mucosal neuroendocrine cells, as well as centrally in the hypothalamus. Ghrelin administration dose-dependently evokes GH release and also induces food intake (Fig. 8-12). Hypothalamic ghrelin likely controls GH secretion interacting with GHRH and SRIF,[195] and peripheral sources exhibit additional complex nutritional effects (see Chapter 7). Plasma ghrelin levels are suppressed after gastric bypass surgery,[196] and mice with disrupted ghrelin or GHS receptor are resistant to diet-induced obesity.[197] Control of GH secretion thus requires hypothalamic GHRH/SRIF as well as ghrelin.[195]

Synthetic hexapeptides (artificial GH secretagogues) recognize the GHS (ghrelin) receptor and induce potent and reproducible GH release (Fig. 8-12). GHSs stimulate GH secretion acting through receptors and intracellular signal-

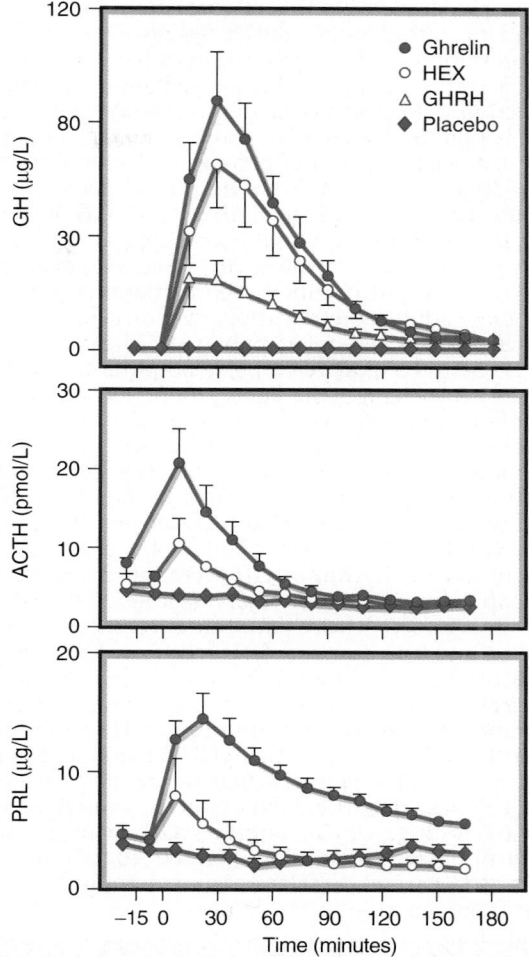

Figure 8-12 Effect of GH secretagogues on secretion of GH, adrenocorticotropic hormone (ACTH), and prolactin (PRL) in healthy subjects. Mean (± standard error of the mean [SEM]) curve responses after administration of ghrelin (1.0 µg/kg), hexarelin (HEX, 1.0 µg/kg), growth hormone–releasing hormone (GHRH) (1.0 µg/kg), or placebo. (Adapted from Arvat E, Maccario M, Di Vito L, et al. Endocrine activities of ghrelin, a natural growth hormone secretagogue [GHS], in humans: comparison and interactions with hexarelin, a nonnatural peptidyl GHS, and GH-releasing hormone. *J Clin Endocrinol Metab.* 2001;86(3):1169-1174.)

ing pathways distinct from GHRH on somatotroph subpopulations. However, GHRH also acts as an allosteric co-agonist for the ghrelin receptor.[198] Ghrelin agonists require the presence of GHRH to evoke GH release, as evidenced in patients with intact pituitary but disordered hypothalamic function, when GHS does not induce GH.[199] GHS agonists also potentiate GH release in response to a maximal stimulating dose of exogenous GHRH, and after a saturating dose of GHRH, subsequent GHRH administration is ineffective, although GHS agonists remain effective.[188]

GHSs are now used as pharmacologic tools in the diagnosis of adult growth hormone deficiency (GHD). An advantage of GHSs relates to their lack of side effects, unlike the insulin tolerance test (ITT). Modest increases in PRL and ACTH/cortisol occur with some GHSs (Fig. 8-12); however, more selective GH secretagogues have been developed.[200]

Secretion. GH secretion is episodic and exhibits a diurnal rhythm with approximately two thirds of the total daily GH secretion produced at night triggered by the onset of slow-wave sleep. Major GH secretory pulses accounting for up to 70% of daily GH secretion occur with the first episode of slow-wave sleep.[201] Normal GH secretion is characterized by secretary episodes separated by troughs of minimal basal secretion during which GH is undetectable. For more than 50% of a 24-hour period GH levels remain below the level of detection of conventional immunoassays. GH concentration is high in the fetal circulation, peaking at approximately 150 µg/L during midgestation. Neonatal levels are lower (~30 µg/L), possibly reflecting the negative feedback control by rising levels of circulating IGF-1. GH output falls to a stable level during childhood, rising at the onset of puberty to peak at a twofold to threefold level at late puberty. GH output declines exponentially in both sexes at the young adulthood transition, declining to one quarter of the values achieved in late puberty.[180] The decline in GH status occurs by a change in pulse amplitude rather than frequency. On average, the daily production of GH in the in the prepubertal state is 200 to 600 µg/day, rising to 1000 to 1800 µg/day at the peak of puberty.[180] In adulthood production rates range from approximately 200 to 600 µg/day with rates higher in women than in men.[180,202] Adiposity accounts for a significant component of declining GH output with increasing age[203] (Table 8-4).

The ultradian rhythm of GH secretion is generated by coordinated interaction of many factors. "Jet lag" transiently increases GH peak amplitude, resulting in a transient increase of 24-hour GH secretion. Exercise and physical stress, including trauma with hypovolemic shock and sepsis, increase GH levels.[180] Emotional deprivation and endogenous depression suppresses GH secretion.

Nutrition plays a major role in GH regulation. Malnutrition increases GH secretion, whereas obesity decreases GH secretion. These nutritional effects occur acutely, as exemplified by fasting, which amplifies GH secretion within 12 hours[204] (Fig. 8-13), and glucose ingestion, which suppresses GH secretion. Central glucoreceptors appear to sense glucose fluctuations, rather than absolute levels. Intravenous (IV) administration of single amino acids, such as arginine and leucine, stimulate GH secretion. Free fatty acids blunt the effects of arginine infusion, sleep, L-dopa, exercise, and GHRH on GH release.[205] Leptin plays a key role in regulation of food intake and energy expenditure[206] and may act as a metabolic signal in stimulating GH secretion[207] by interactions with somatostatin, GHRH, and the neuropeptide Y (NPY) system.

Interaction With Other Hormone Axes. There are complex and sometimes opposing interactions between GH and other pituitary hormone axes. Acute glucocorticoid administration stimulates GH secretion, but chronic steroid treatment inhibits GH. Three hours after acute glucocorticoid administration, GH levels rise and remain elevated for 2 hours.[208] Glucocorticoids administered to normal subjects dose-dependently inhibit GHRH-simulated GH secretion.[208]

Thyroid hormones are required for the function of the GH system. GH response to stimulation is impaired in hypothyroidism and normalized when thyroid status is restored.

Gonadal steroids regulate GH secretion and GH action in men and women. Testosterone administration to hypogonadal men stimulates GH secretion, an effect that is mediated centrally and dependent on prior aromatization to estrogen.[209] In women, estrogen stimulates GH secretion, evident only with oral but not parenteral administration because the oral route reduces first-pass hepatic inhibition of IGF-1 production[210] such that the stimulatory effect on GH secretion is indirect and is facilitated by reduction in IGF-1 feedback inhibition.

However, in women, endogenous GH secretion is driven centrally by aromatization of androgens. This is unmasked by central estrogen receptor blockade with tamoxifen, which blunts GH secretion in women. Thus in women, estrogens act centrally in a paracrine manner in stimulating but act peripherally in an endocrine manner in enhancing GH secretion through reduced IGF-1 feedback inhibition.[211]

Growth Hormone–Binding Proteins. Two high- and low-affinity circulating GH–binding proteins (GHBPs) include a 20-kDa low-affinity GHBP and a 60-kDa high-affinity GHBP, which corresponds to the extracellular domain of the GH receptor (GHR) and binds half of the circulating 22-kDa GH form.[212,213] The high-affinity GHBP in humans is generated by proteolytic cleavage through the action of tumor necrosis factor-α–converting enzyme, a metalloprotease.[214] The 20-kDa GH binds preferentially to the low-affinity binding protein, which is unrelated to the GHR. It has been proposed that the circulating level of GHBP reflects global GHR expression in the body.

The GHBPs dampen the acute oscillations in serum GH levels associated with pulsatile pituitary GH secretion, and plasma GH half-life is prolonged by decreased renal GH clearance of bound GH. The high-affinity binding protein also competes with GH for binding to surface GHRs and as such alters GH pharmacokinetics and distribution.

GHBP concentrations are unaffected by GH status such as in GHD or acromegaly.[215] Some patients with Laron dwarfism have absent or reduced levels of GHBP, reflecting mutations that result in absent translation of the GHR or the extracellular domain.[216] Serum concentrations of GHBP are low in some children with idiopathic short stature[217] and in African pygmies, suggesting abnormalities in the gene for the GHR.[218] GHBP levels are increased in obesity, during pregnancy, and in subjects undergoing refeeding,[218] and they are increased by oral estrogen administration.[210] Levels are reduced in malnutrition, cirrhosis, and hypothyroidism and by glucocorticoids and androgens.[219]

TABLE 8-4

Adult Growth Hormone Secretion[*]

Interval	Young Adult	Fasting	Obesity	Middle Age
24-h secretion (µg/24 h)	540 ± 44	2171 ± 333	77 ± 20	196 ± 65
Secretory bursts (number in 24 h)	12 ± 1	32 ± 2	3 ± 0.5	10 ± 1
GH burst (µg)	45 ± 4	64 ± 9	24 ± 5	10 ± 6

*Deconvolution analysis of growth hormone (GH) secretion in adult males.
From Thorner MO, Vance ML, Horvath E, Kovacs K. The anterior pituitary. In: Wilson JD, Foster D, eds. *Williams Textbook of Endocrinology*, 8th ed. Philadelphia: WB Saunders; 1992:221-310.

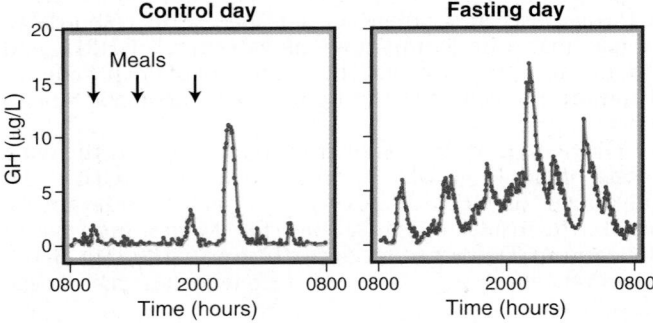

Figure 8-13 Effect of fasting on growth hormone (GH) secretion patterns in a healthy male subject. (From Hartman ML, Veldhuis JD, Johnson ML, et al. Augmented growth hormone [GH] secretory burst frequency and amplitude mediate enhanced GH secretion during a two-day fast in normal men. *J Clin Endocrinol Metab.* 1992; 74:757-765.)

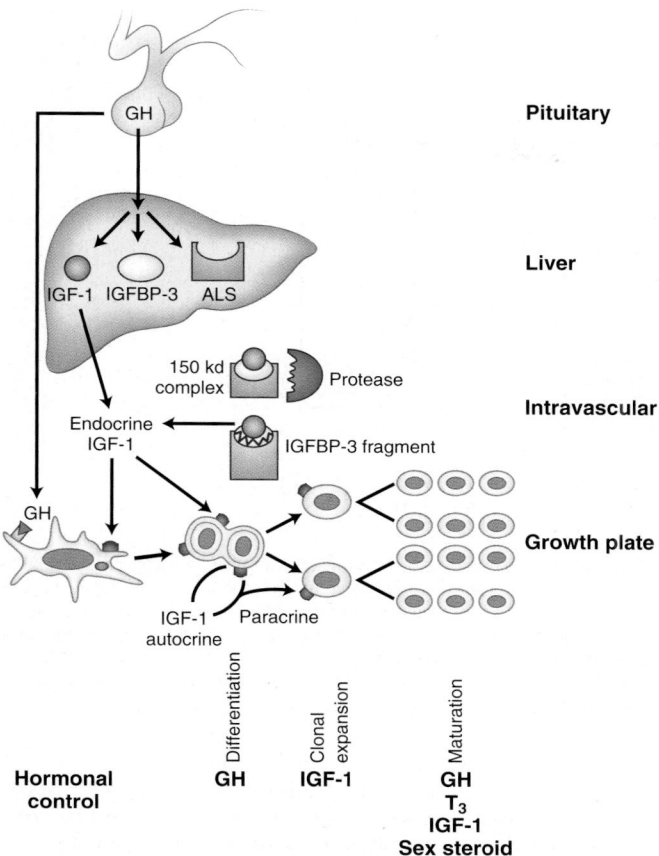

Figure 8-14 Integrated model of the GH-IGFBP-IGF axis in the growth process. Three mechanisms are proposed: (1) Growth hormone (GH) stimulates insulin-like growth factor 1 (IGF-1) production; circulating IGF-1 (endocrine IGF-1) acts at the growth plate. (2) GH regulates hepatic production of IGF-binding protein 3 (IGFBP-3) and acid-labile subunit (ALS): IGF-1 binds to IGFBP-3 and thereafter with ALS, forming the 150-kDa ternary complex; proteases cleave into fragments that release IGFBP-3 into fragments that release IGF-1 in the intravascular space and at the growth plate. (3) GH induces differentiation of local IGF-1 production, and IGF-1 acts via an autocrine and paracrine mechanism to stimulate cell division. T_3, triiodothyronine. (From Spagnol A, Rosenfeld RG. The mechanism by which GH brings about growth. The relative contributions of GH and insulin-like growth factors. *Endocrinol Metab Clin North Am.* 1996;25(3):615-631; and Clemmons DR, Van Wyk JJ, Ridgway EC, et al. Evaluation of acromegaly by radioimmunoassay of somatomedin-C. 1979;301: 1138-1142.)

Action. GH acts to mediate growth and metabolic functions (Fig. 8-14).

Signaling. GH elicits intracellular signaling though a peripheral receptor, initiating a phosphorylation cascade involving the JAK-STAT pathway.[220] The liver contains abundant GHRs, and several peripheral tissues also express modest amounts of receptor, including muscle and fat[221] (Fig. 8-15). The GHR is a 620–amino acid 70-kDa protein of the class I cytokine/hematopoietin receptor superfamily consisting of an extracellular ligand-binding domain, a single membrane-spanning domain, and a cytoplasmic signaling component.[222] The GHR superfamily is homologous with receptors for PRL, interleukin 2 (IL-2) through IL-7, erythropoeitin, interferon, and colony-stimulating factor. GH complexes with two predimerized GHR components, resulting in the apposition of complementary JAK2 domains that triggers signaling[223,224] (see Fig. 8-15). JAK2 (tyrosine kinase) activation leads to phosphorylation of intracellular signaling molecules, including the signal transducing activators of transcription proteins (STATs 1,

3, and 5), critical signaling components for GH action.[225] Phosphorylated STAT proteins are directly translocated to the cell nucleus, where they elicit GH-specific target gene expression by binding to nuclear DNA. STAT1 and STAT5 may also interact directly with the GHR molecule.[225] GH also induces c-fos induction, insulin receptor substrate 1 phosphorylation, and insulin synthesis. Additional intracellular signaling pathways induced by GH include mitogen-activated protein kinase (MAPK), protein kinase C, SH2-β, SHP-2, SIRPA, SHC, FAK, CrKll, C-SRC, paxillin, and tensin. How these seemingly overlapping pathways converge to integrate the net cellular effects of GH are at present unclear. Intracellular GH signaling is abrogated by suppressor of cytokine signaling (SOCS) proteins, which disrupt the JAK-STAT pathway and thus disrupt GH action.[226] In transgenic mice with deletion of SOCS-2, gigantism develops, presumably due to unrestrained GH action. As SOCS proteins are also induced by proinflammatory cytokines, critically ill patients, or those with renal failure may develop GH resistance due to cytokine-induced SOCS.[227] Unraveling STAT/SOCS regulation in syndromes associated with disordered GH signaling will likely yield mechanistic insights for dysregulated GH action.

The pattern of GH secretion also determines tissue responses to GH in addition to the absolute amount secreted. Gender-specific patterns of GH secretion profiles determine sex-specific expression of cytochrome P450 enzymes. In turn, circulating steroids regulate neuroendocrine release of GH. SRIF, by suppressing interpulse GH levels, serves to masculinize the ultradian GH rhythm. In mice harboring a disrupted SRIF gene, plasma GH secretory patterns are elevated and liver enzyme induction loses its gender-specific dimorphism, but these animals retain sexually dimorphic growth patterns.[228] Linear growth patterns and liver enzyme induction are phenotypically gender-specific, driven by higher GH pulse frequency rates involving STAT5B mediation. STAT5B is sensitive to repeated pulses of injected GH,[229] unlike other GH-induced responses, which are desensitized by repeated GH administration. Disruption of STAT5B in transgenic mice impairs male pattern body growth[230] associated with female pattern IGF-1 and testosterone levels. Appropriate GH pulsatility drives body growth mediated by STAT5B[231,232] but not metabolic GH effects. In humans, GH secretion is also sexually dimorphic and regulates the P450 liver enzymes.[232] A flatter pattern appears to evoke a higher IGF-1 response and a lesser degree of lipolysis.[234]

IGF-1 mediates growth-promoting activities of GH[191] in an endocrine or paracrine manner.[235] In mice, paracrine IGF-1 produced in extrahepatic tissues is critical for growth, which persists even when hepatic IGF-1 is deleted.[236] GHR mutations are associated with partial or complete GH insensitivity and growth failure. These syndromes are associated with normal or high circulating GH levels, decreased circulating GHBP levels, and low levels of circulating IGF-1. Multiple homozygous or heterozygous exonic and intronic GHR mutations have been described. These occur mostly in the extracellular ligand-binding receptor domain (see Chapter 24).

Metabolic Action. GH functions as a major metabolic hormone in the adult by optimizing body composition and physical function as well as regulating energy and substrate metabolism. Metabolic actions of GH also closely interact with those of insulin in the control of fat, glucose, and protein metabolism during fasted and fed states.

GH promotes fat metabolism by enhancing lipolysis and fatty acid oxidation. This function is particularly important during the fasted state when GH secretion is enhanced, resulting in the partitioning of fuel utilization toward fat

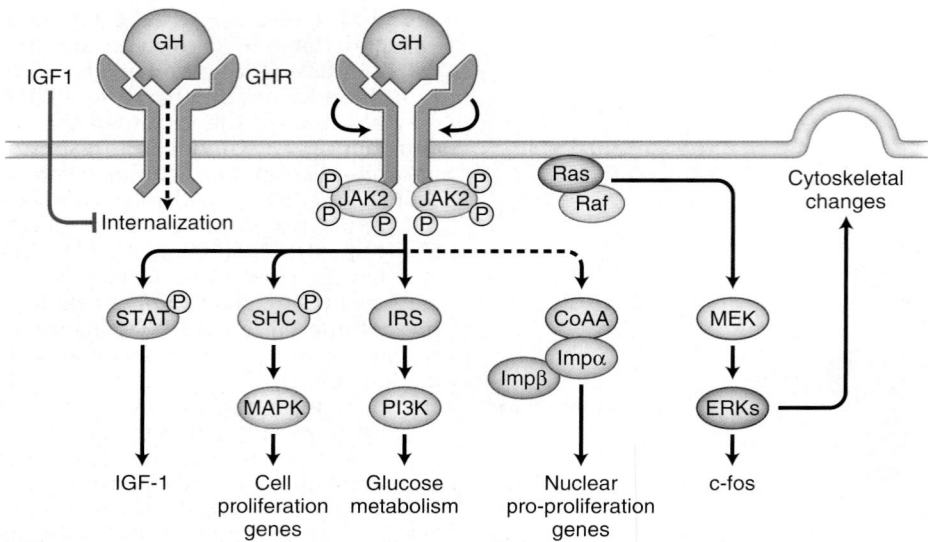

Figure 8-15 Growth hormone (GH) action. GH binds to the growth hormone receptor (GHR) dimer, which undergoes internal rotation, resulting in Janus kinase 2 (JAK2) phosphorylation (P) and subsequent signal transduction. GH signaling is mediated by JAK2 phosphorylation of depicted signaling including Src/ERK pathways. Ligand binding to a preformed GHR dimer results in internal rotation and subsequent phosphorylation cascades. GH targets include insulin-like growth factor 1 (IGF1), c-fos, cell proliferation genes, glucose metabolism, and cystoskeletal proteins. GHR internalization and translocation *(dotted lines)* induce nuclear pro-proliferation genes via importin α/β(Impα/Impβ) coactivator (CoAA) signaling. IGF-1 may also block GHR internalization, acting in a feedback loop. ERK, extracellular signal-related kinase; IRS, insulin receptor substrate; MAPK, mitogen-activated protein kinase; MEK, dual specifying mitogen-activated kinase 2. (From Lupu F, Terwilliger JD, Lee K, et al. Roles of growth hormone and insulin-like growth factor 1 in mouse postnatal growth. *Dev Biol.* 2001;229:141; and Melmed S. Acromegaly pathogenesis and treatment. *J Clin Invest.* 2009;119:3189-3202.)

with the sparing of protein. Stimulation of lipolysis occurs indirectly through potentiating the activity of hormone-sensitive lipase by β-adrenergic stimulation. GH also regulates lipoprotein metabolism by enhancing low-density lipoprotein (LDL) clearance by activating expression of hepatic LDL receptors.[237,238] The atherogenic profile of lipoproteins is increased in GHD and reduced by GH therapy.[239]

GH exerts profound effects on glucose metabolism either directly or by antagonizing insulin action. GH enhances glucose uptake and utilization in cells, referred to as its *insulin-like* effects.[240] At the whole-body level, GH suppresses glucose oxidation and utilization while enhancing hepatic glucose production subserving the nonoxidative[240] use of glucose. The target tissues or the biochemical fate of this glucose surplus are unclear. As GH is an important counterregulatory hormone, it is conceivable that this function protects against hypoglycemia.

Protein anabolism is a signature property of GH that reduces urea synthesis and urea excretion. Some of the effects of GH are not IGF-1 mediated. However, GH also acutely stimulates amino acid uptake and incorporation into protein in vitro.[241] Arteriovenous measurements in the forearm report an acute increase in protein synthesis over a few hours of GH infusion, suggesting a direct effect.[242] Whole-body studies in humans using isotopes have consistently shown that GH reduces protein oxidation and stimulates protein synthesis.[144] The protein-sparing effect of GH is coupled to the availability and increased parallel utilization of free fatty acids, whereas pharmacologic reduction of free fatty acids during fasting augments the rate of protein breakdown.[240]

Growth Hormone Deficiency

GH is the most abundant hormone in the adult pituitary gland, and it plays an important role in maintaining the metabolic process and the integrity and function of many tissues and systems after the cessation of growth. Life

expectancy is reduced in hypopituitary patients with GHD[243-245] largely as a consequence of cardiovascular and cerebrovascular events, especially in female subjects.[246]

Pathophysiology. Adult GHD may be acquired or congenital. Of the acquired causes, 50% arise from pituitary tumors, one fifth from extrapituitary tumors, 5% from inflammatory or infiltrative lesions, with up to 15% of cases being idiopathic[247] (Table 8-5). Surgical or radiation treatment of pituitary and parasellar tumors is the most common cause of GHD, accounting for nearly two thirds of cases. The frequency of causes differs between patients with childhood-onset and adult-onset GHD.[247,248] Idiopathic causes, representing the most commonly encountered group in childhood-onset GHD, likely represent a heterogeneous collection of congenital developmental abnormalities, including mutations of *PROP1* or *POU1F1* genes, causing GHD with other pituitary hormone deficiencies[249] (see Table 8-1). Isolated GHD may be complete or partial, and up to 67% of children initially diagnosed with idiopathic GHD had normal GH responses when subsequently retested as adults for GHD following cessation of GH treatment.[250] Children with GHD should be retested before GH treatment is continued into adulthood unless they have clearly documented panhypopituitarism or a defined genetic or developmental abnormality that causes complete and irreversible GHD. Mutations in the GH[251] and GHRH receptor genes,[252] and GH insensitivity as a result of primary GHR dysfunction,[253] result in a selective lack of GH action.

Presentation. GHD in adults is a recognized entity (Table 8-6). Symptoms of GHD are nonspecific and include fatigue, lack of energy, social isolation, low mood, poor concentration, and reduced physical capacity.[254] The signs are also nonspecific and include general and central adiposity and reduced lean tissue and bone mineral density (BMD), along with unfavorable biochemical changes such as hyperlipidemia[255,256] and glucose intolerance.[254] Some patients have established evidence of macrovascular disease such as increased carotid intimal thickness.[257,258] GHD may

TABLE 8-5

Causes of Acquired Pituitary Insufficiency

Traumatic	Functional
Surgical resection	Nutritional
Radiation damage	Caloric restriction
Traumatic brain injury	Malnutrition
Infiltrative/Inflammatory	Excessive exercise
	Critical illness
Primary hypophysitis	Acute illness
Lymphocytic	Chronic renal failure
Granulomatous	Chronic liver failure
Xanthomatous	Hormonal
Secondary hypophysitis	Hyperprolactinemia
Sarcoidosis	Hypothyroidism
Histiocytosis X	Drugs
Infections	Anabolic steroids
Wegener granulomatosis	Glucocorticoid excess
Takayasu disease	GnRH agonists
Hemochromatosis	Estrogen
Infections	Dopamine
	Somatostatin analogue
Tuberculosis	Thyroid hormone excess
Pneumocytis jirovecii infection	**Causes of Acquired Growth Hormone Deficiency in 1034 Hypopituitary Adult Patients**
Fungal (histoplasmosis, aspergillosis)	
Parasites (toxoplasmosis)	
Viral (cytomegalovirus)	Pituitary tumor (53.9%)
Vascular	Craniopharyngioma (12.3%)
	Idiopathic (10.2%)
Pregnancy-related	CNS tumor (4.4%)
Aneurysm	Empty sella syndrome (4.2%)
Apoplexy	Sheehan syndrome (3.1%)
Diabetes	Head trauma (2.4%)
Hypotension	Hypophysitis (1.6%)
Arteritis	Surgery* (1.5%)
Sickle cell disease	Granulomatous diseases (1.3%)
Neoplastic	Irradiation* (1.1%)
	CNS malformation (1.0%)
Pituitary adenoma	Perinatal trauma or infection (0.5%)
Parasellar mass	Other (2.5%)
Rathke's cyst	
Dermoid cyst	
Meningioma	
Germinoma	
Ependymoma	
Glioma	
Craniopharyngioma	
Hypothalamic harmatoma, gangliocytoma	
Pituitary metastatic deposits	
Hematologic malignancy	
Leukemia	
Lymphoma	

*Other than for pituitary treatment.
From Abs R, Bengtsson BA, Hernberg-Stahl E, et al. GH replacement in 1034 growth hormone deficient hypopituitary adults: demographic and clinical characteristics, dosing and safety. *Clin Endocrinol (Oxf)*. 1999;50:703-713.

also be associated with heart abnormalities including reduced left ventricular mass.[259-261] Cardiovascular risk abnormalities are often less pronounced in adults with childhood-onset GHD than in those acquiring the deficiency during adulthood who have more pronounced disordered quality of life, lipids, and body composition.[262,263]

Although the features of GHD are recognizable, they are not particularly distinct and mimic body compositional and biochemical changes of the aging process. Thus, clinical suspicion must be confirmed by accurate biochemical diagnosis to ensure that GH-deficient patients are accurately identified and treated.

Subjects with isolated GHD or inactivating mutation of the GHR manifest some features that contrast with those of GHD as a component of multiple pituitary hormone deficits. Patients with selective absence of GH action display reduced insulin resistance, lower prevalence of diabetes, absence of premature atherosclerosis, and normal life expectancy[264-266] (Fig. 8-16). These findings suggest that the observed increased mortality rate in hypopituitary adults with GHD arises in part from suboptimal replacement regimens and coexisting comorbid conditions.

Evaluation. GHD is diagnosed biochemically within an appropriate clinical context. Biochemical testing for GHD occurs with a high probability in patients with a history of organic hypothalamic-pituitary dysfunction, cranial irradiation, known childhood-onset GHD, and traumatic brain injury (TBI).[267]

Provocative Testing. The diagnosis of adult GHD is established by provocative testing of GH secretion (Table 8-7). Patients should be adequately replaced for other pituitary hormonal deficits before testing. Several provocative tests include ITT, arginine, glucagon, clonidine, growth hormone–releasing peptide (GHRP), and GHRH, alone or

TABLE 8-6

Adult Somatotropin Deficiency

Clinical Consequence	Effect of GH Replacement
Body Composition	
General and central adiposity	Decrease
Reduced lean mass	Increase
Reduced bone mass	Increase
Function	
Reduced exercise capacity	Improve
Muscle weakness	Increase
Impaired cardiac function	Improve
Hypohydrosis	Increase
Quality of Life	
Low mood	Improve
Fatigue	Improve
Low motivation	Improve
Reduced satisfaction	Improve
Cardiovascular Risk Profile	
Abnormal lipid profile	Improve
Insulin resistance	No change
Increased inflammatory markers	Decrease
Intimal media thickening	Decrease
Laboratory	
Blunted peak GH to stimulation (see Table 8-7)	Increase
Low IGF-1 (in 50-60%)	Increase
Hyperinsulinemia	Improve
High LDL and low HDL cholesterol	Improve

GH, growth hormone; HDL, high-density lipoprotein; IGF-1, insulin-like growth factor 1; LDL, low-density lipoprotein.

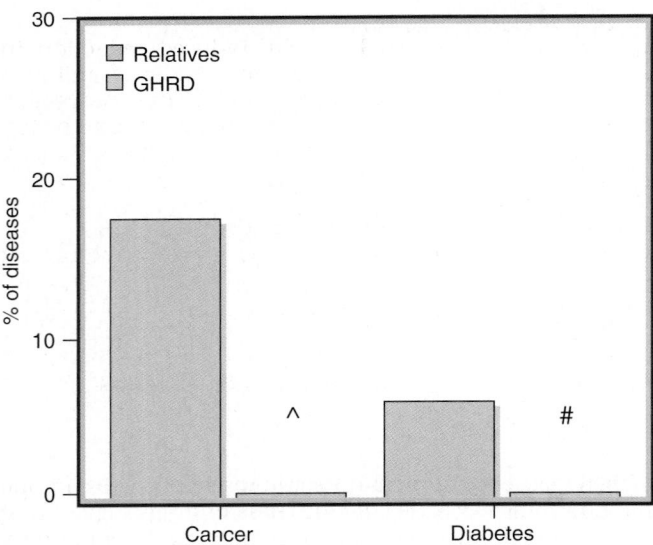

Figure 8-16 Percentage of cancer and type 2 diabetes in patients with growth hormone receptor deficiency (GHRD) and in unaffected relatives in a large Ecuadorian cohort. Data are shown as a percentage of all diagnosed/reported diseases. ^ = 1 case of cancer and # = no case of diabetes was recorded. (From Guevara-Aguirre J, Balasubramanian P, Guevara-Aguirre M, et al. Growth hormone receptor deficiency is associated with a major reduction in pro-aging signaling, cancer, and diabetes in humans. *Sci Transl Med.* 2011;3(70):70ra13.)

TABLE 8-7

Validated Diagnostic Tests for the Diagnosis of Growth Hormone Deficiency in Adults

Test	Subject Numbers Normal/GHD	GH Threshold (µg/L)	Reference
Insulin-induced* Hypoglycemia	35/23	<5	Hoffman et al[272]
Arginine-GHRH*	74/49	<9	Aimaretti et al[270]
GHRP 6-GHRH*	125/125	<15	Popovic et al[271]
GHRP 2-GHRH*	30/36	<17	Mahajan et al[274]
GHRP 2	77/58	<15	Chihara et al[276]
Glucagon*	46/73	<3	Gomez et al[275]
Low IGF-1 and ≥3 PHDs*	785	N/A	Hartman et al[285]

*Recommended by the Growth Hormone Research Society and the Endocrine Society

GH, growth hormone; GHD, growth hormone deficiency; GHRH, growth hormone–releasing hormone; GHRP, growth hormone–releasing peptide; IGF-1, insulin-like growth factor 1; N/A, not applicable; PHD, pituitary hormone deficiency.

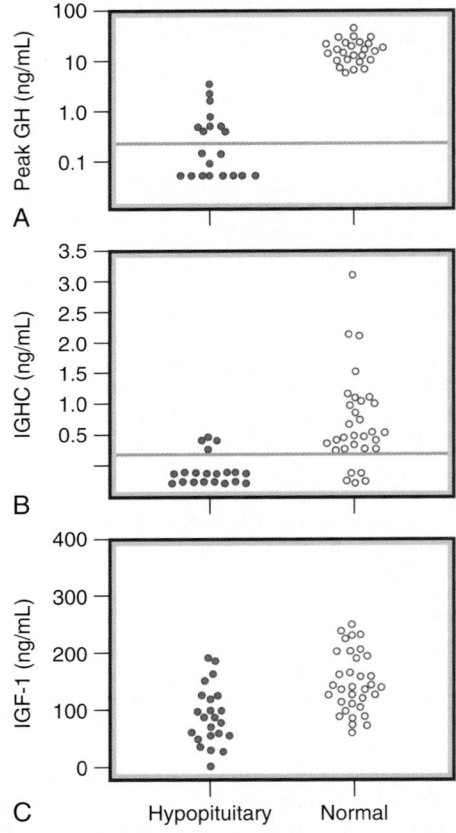

Figure 8-17 Comparison of peak growth hormone (GH) concentration obtained during an insulin-tolerance test (**A**), integrated GH concentration (IGHC) obtained from blood samples withdrawn every 20 minutes over 24 hours (**B**), and insulin-like growth factor 1 (IGF-1) concentrations (**C**) in patients with organic hypopituitarism and sex-matched normal subjects. Horizontal lines represent the limit of reading. (Modified from Hoffman DM, O'Sullivan AJ, Baxter RC, Ho KKY. Diagnosis of growth hormone deficiency in adults. *Lancet.* 1994;343:1064-1068.)

in combination with arginine or pyridostigmine. GHRPs are synthetic analogues of ghrelin. As provocative tests vary in the ability to evoke GH release, a single value cannot be applied as a diagnostic threshold across different tests.[268] ITT is a more potent stimulator of GH release than arginine, clonidine, or L-dopa, whereas combinations such

as arginine plus GHRH, or GHRP plus GHRH are more potent than ITT alone.[269-271]

The ITT is the gold standard test for GHD. Normal subjects respond to insulin-induced hypoglycemia with peak GH concentrations of more than 5 µg/L[272] (Fig. 8-17). Severe GHD is defined by a peak GH response to hypoglycemia of less than 3 μg/L.[273] These cutoff values have been defined using GH assays employing polyclonal competitive radioimmunoassays.[273] The test is contraindicated in patients with electrocardiographic evidence, or history of, ischemic heart disease and in patients with seizure disorders.

Alternative tests that have been validated for the diagnosis of GHD are GHRH plus arginine,[270] GHRH plus GHRP,[271,274] glucagon,[275] and GHRP2.[276] The diagnostic thresholds for these tests are shown in Table 8-7. The recent unavailability of GHRH has brought glucagon greater attention as a simple diagnostic test for GHD when the ITT is not desirable.[277] The ITT evaluates the integrity of the hypothalamic-pituitary axis and has the added advantage of also stimulating ACTH secretion. Diagnostic tests employing GHRH or GHRP, both of which directly stimulate GH release from the pituitary gland, may not identify GHD caused by hypothalamic disease.[278] This is exemplified by studies in patients treated with cranial irradiation, when the ITT shows the greatest sensitivity and specificity within the first 5 years after irradiation.[279] If peak GH levels are normal during a GHRH plus arginine test in patients who have received irradiation, then an ITT should also be performed. In irradiated patients as well as those with inflammatory and infiltrative parasellar lesions, GHD may develop many years after the initial insult. Therefore, this group of patients should be followed in the long term with repeat testing as clinically indicated. Obesity confounds the diagnostic testing of GHD as it blunts the peak GH response.[280] Body mass index–adjusted reference ranges are available for the combined arginine-GHRH test.[281]

Growth Hormone–Responsive Markers. These markers include IGF-1, IGF binding protein 3 (IGFBP3), and the acid-labile subunit of the IGFBP complex. IGF-1 is useful for diagnosis only when age-adjusted normal ranges are used. Although IGF-1 levels are reduced in adult GHD, a normal concentration does not exclude the diagnosis[272] (see Fig. 8-17). A subnormal IGF-1 level in an adult patient with coexisting pituitary hormone deficits is strongly suggestive of GHD, particularly in the absence of conditions known to reduce IGF-1 levels, such as malnutrition, liver disease, poorly controlled diabetes mellitus, and hypothyroidism. The separation of IGF-1 values between GH-deficient and normal subjects is greatest in the young. As IGF-1 levels decline with aging in normal subjects, IGF-1 measurements become less reliable as a biochemical marker of GHD in patients older than 50 years when the values merge with those of normal age-matched subjects.[282] Measurement of IGFBP3 or the acid-labile subunit does not offer diagnostic advantage over IGF-1.[267,283]

In patients with organic hypothalamic-pituitary disease, the prevalence of GHD is strongly linked to the number of pituitary hormone deficits, ranging from approximately 25% to 40% in those with no other deficit to virtually 95% to 100% when more than three pituitary hormone deficiencies are present.[284] Patients with three or more pituitary hormone deficiencies and an IGF-1 level below the reference range have a greater than 97% chance of being GH deficient (see Table 8-7)[285] and therefore do not require GH stimulation testing.[267,283]

Spontaneous GH Secretion. As pituitary GH secretion occurs episodically, accurate quantification of integrated GH secretion requires continuous measurement of secretion over 24 hours. This procedure requires insertion of a continuous withdrawal pump or patent indwelling catheter for frequent sampling. Continuous 24-hour GH measurement in the diagnosis of GHD is not superior to provocative testing[272] (see Fig. 8-17) and is cumbersome and expensive.

Growth Hormone Assays. Plasma GH is measured by radioimmunoassay (RIA; polyclonal or monoclonal) or by immunoradiometric assay (IRMA; dual monoclonal), but considerable differences exist in the results of GH measurements between assays by a factor of as much as 3.[286] These differences are due mainly to heterogeneity in assay components and characteristics. An important contributor is the use of different calibrator materials.[287] Not all assays are calibrated to a recombinant international GH reference preparation (98/574). Heterogeneous analytes pose an additional problem. Circulating GH, for example, consists of various forms, including monomers, dimers, and other post-translational modified products, the detection of which varies among assays. The different types of antibodies vary in their specificity for the different molecular forms of GH. The reporting of assay results also varies. GH assay results are expressed in mass units but also in international units, which have been arbitrarily defined and do not have a clear relationship to mass.[287] Many factors interfere with GH measurements, including GHBP, which binds approximately 50% of circulating GH. The inhomogeneity of GH immunoassay results poses a challenge in the definition of accepted standards for diagnosis of GHD. Clinicians should be aware of the nature of the GH assay employed and how values compare to those previously obtained by polyclonal RIA.

Growth Hormone Replacement Therapy. The effects of GH replacement were first reported in 1989. GH replacement induces profound effects on protein, fat, and energy metabolism, which result in increased lean body mass and decreased fat mass without a significant change in body weight within months[288] (Fig. 8-18). The greatest reduction of body fat occurs in abdominal and visceral adipose tissue[289] (Fig. 8-19). Significant increases in extracellular water also occur as a consequence of the dose-dependent antinatriuretic properties of GH.[290] GH-induced reduction in abdominal and visceral fat is accompanied by a significant shift of lipoprotein metabolism to a less atherogenic profile. Most studies report an improvement in the cholesterol and in HDL-cholesterol ratio with little or no change in triglycerides.[239] Long-term experience of more than 10 years indicates that treatment provides sustained benefits in body composition and metabolic risk markers[291] (Fig. 8-20). GH treatment reduces intimal media thickness of the carotid arteries.[257] Proinflammatory factors such as C-reactive protein and IL-6, strongly implicated in the pathogenesis of vascular disease, fall significantly with GH treatment.[255]

GH replacement increases bone density[292] which is accompanied by activation of both bone formation and bone resorption.[293] Markers of bone turnover increase over the first 12 months but return to baseline after 3 to 4 years.[294] BMD continues to increase for up to 10 years in the lumbar spine, whereas a decline that occurs in the femoral neck may start sooner[295] (Fig. 8-21).

GH replacement improves exercise capacity and performance in parallel with an increase in maximal oxygen uptake[296,297] and in cardiac output and diastolic function.[298,299] Several, but not all, studies report improved muscle strength. Most studies assessing GH effects beyond 12 months have reported a significant improvement in muscle strength and muscle mass,[300,301] whereas trials of less than 6 months' duration have not shown this effect.[302,303] The collective evidence indicates that GH increases muscle strength by increasing muscle mass.[304]

Most trials with GH replacement report improved quality of life.[305] Discrepant results may relate to varying study tools, with some being generic health questionnaires on perceived health status and subjective well-being and others being developed specifically for patients with GHD.

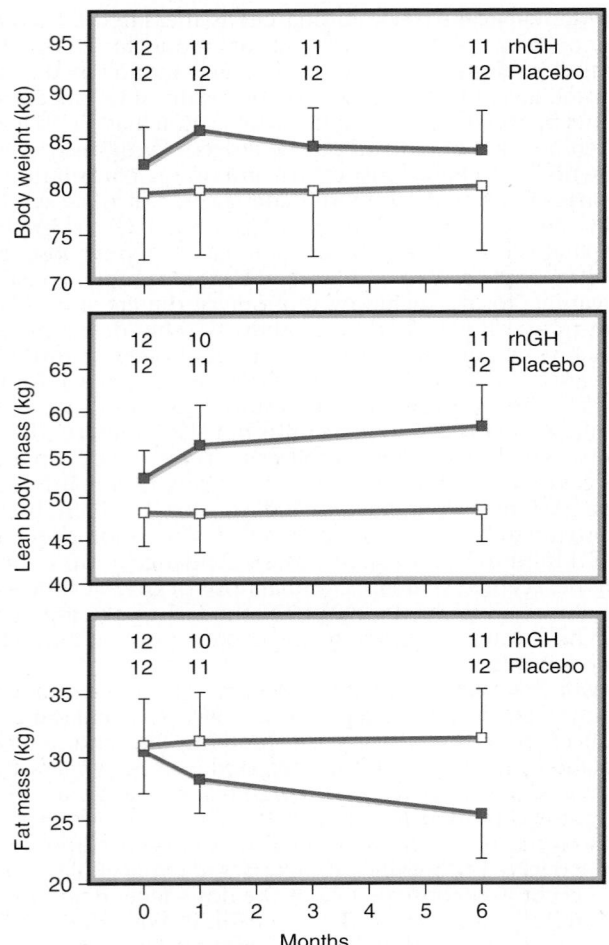

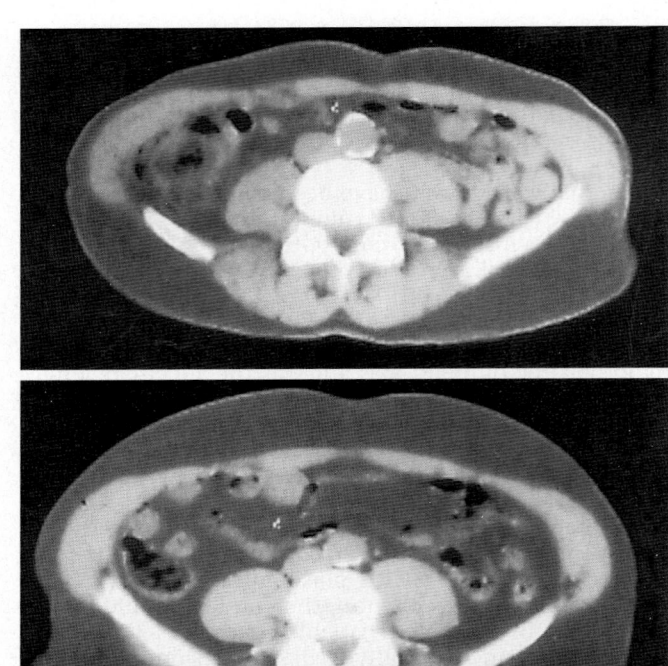

Figure 8-19 Computed tomography scan through the abdomen before *(top)* and after treatment with human growth hormone (hGH) *(bottom)* in a GH-deficient patient. (Courtesy of B.A. Bengtsson.)

Figure 8-18 Effects of growth hormone (GH) replacement on lean body mass and fat mass in adults with GH deficiency. Effect of GH replacement on lean body mass and fat mass in 24 adults with GH deficiency. rhGH, recombinant human growth hormone. (From Salomon F, Cuneo RC, Hesp R, et al. The effects of treatment with recombinant human growth hormone on body composition and metabolism in adults with growth hormone deficiency. *N Engl J Med.* 1989;321:1797-1803.)

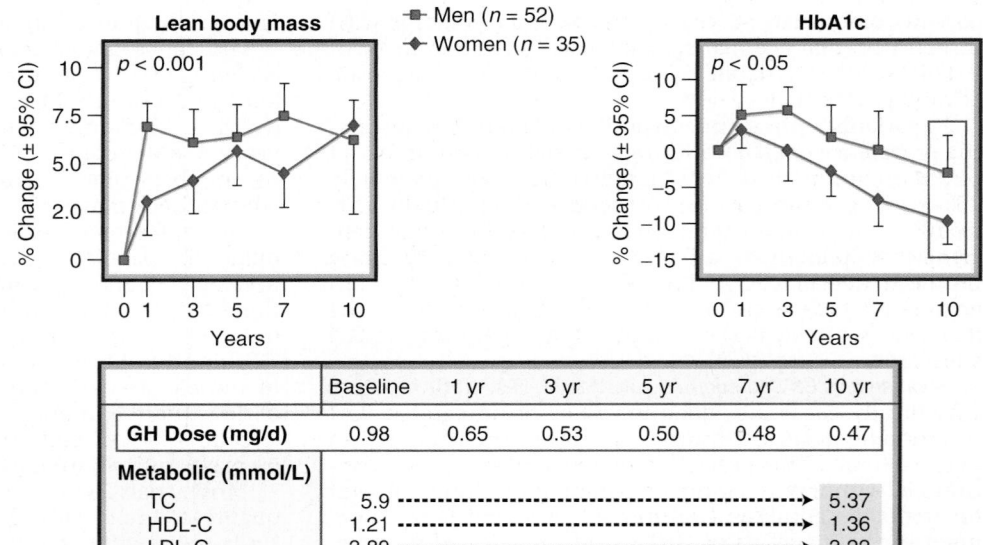

Figure 8-20 Ten-year growth hormone (GH) therapy in 87 GH-deficient adults.[291] CI, confidence interval; HbA1c, hemoglobin A_{1c}; HDL-C, high-density lipoprotein-cholesterol; LDL-C, low-density lipoprotein-cholesterol; TC, total cholesterol. (Modified from Melmed S. Update in pituitary disease. *J Clin Endocrinol Metab.* 2008;93:331-338.)

	Baseline	1 yr	3 yr	5 yr	7 yr	10 yr
GH Dose (mg/d)	0.98	0.65	0.53	0.50	0.48	0.47
Metabolic (mmol/L)						
TC	5.9				→	5.37
HDL-C	1.21				→	1.36
LDL-C	3.89				→	3.22
Glucose	4.00				→	4.96

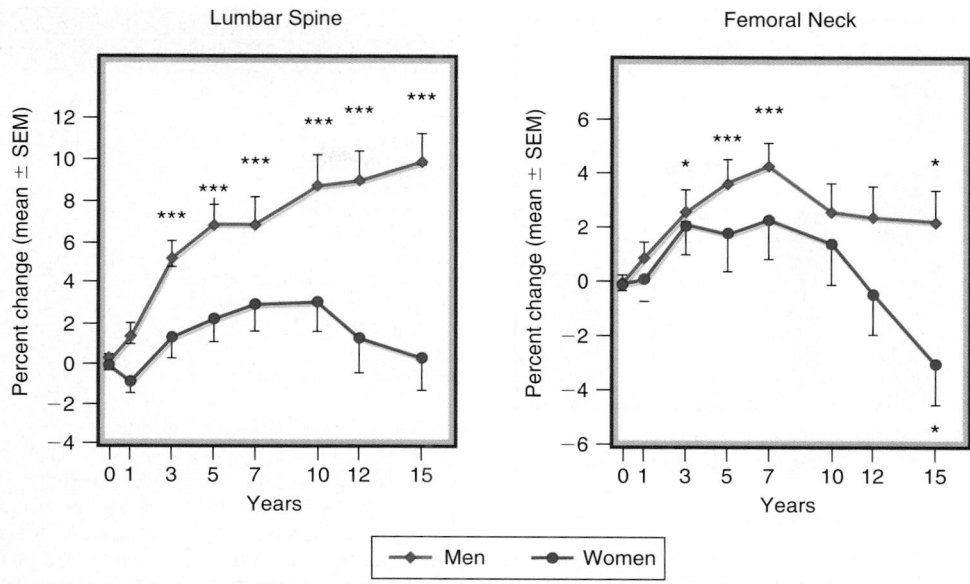

Figure 8-21 Fifteen years of growth hormone (GH) replacement on bone mineral densities at the lumbar (L2-L4) spine *(left)* and femur neck *(right)* in adult men and women with GH deficiency. The results are shown as percent change from baseline. The vertical bars indicate the SEM (standard error of the mean) values shown. *$p < 0.05$; ***$p < 0.001$ versus baseline. $p < 0.01$ for men versus women. (From Elbornsson M, Gotherstrom G, Bosaeus I, et al. Fifteen years of GH replacement increases bone mineral density in hypopituitary patients with adult-onset GH deficiency. *Eur J Endocrinol.* 2012;166(5):787-795.)

Domains of energy and emotional reaction tend to show the greatest improvements in generic health questionnaires. Disease-specific tools have reported unequivocal improvement in measures of life satisfaction after GH treatment.[306] A large survey of 304 patients showed improved quality of life, and significant reduction in the numbers of sick leave days and doctor visits during 12 months of GH therapy.[307] A latency period of up to 3 months is required before patients recognize benefits of hGH replacement, which are also most obvious in those with the most profound symptoms and signs of GHD.[308]

Growth Hormone Administration. GH secretion is greater in the young and greater in women than in men. It is recommended that the starting dose of GH in young men and women be 0.2 and 0.3 mg/day, respectively, and in older individuals 0.1 mg/day,[283,267] which is then titrated according to serum IGF-1 concentrations and at a rate that minimizes side effects[309] (Fig. 8-22). If side effects occur, the dose should be reduced, and if no side effects are reported, the therapeutic goal is to maintain IGF-1 levels in the normal age- and gender-matched range, while avoiding levels in the upper quintile or above. Dose determination based on body weight is not recommended because there is a lack of evidence that a larger replacement is required for heavier adults and that GH secretion is reduced in the obese.[267,283] GH is administered by nightly subcutaneous injection to mimic the greater secretion of GH at night. Side effects of GH in children are considerably fewer than those observed in adults.

Women with GHD require higher doses of hGH when also receiving oral rather than transdermal estrogen[310,311] because of the first-pass hepatic effect. Fifty percent more GH was required during oral estrogen treatment to maintain an IGF-1 level equivalent to that achieved during transdermal administration; the waste is even greater when contraceptive instead of replacement doses are prescribed[312] (Fig. 8-23). In contrast, androgens enhance metabolic effects of GH.[144] The divergent effects of estrogens and androgens on GH action are a likely explanation for the observation that women are less responsive than men to GH.[291]

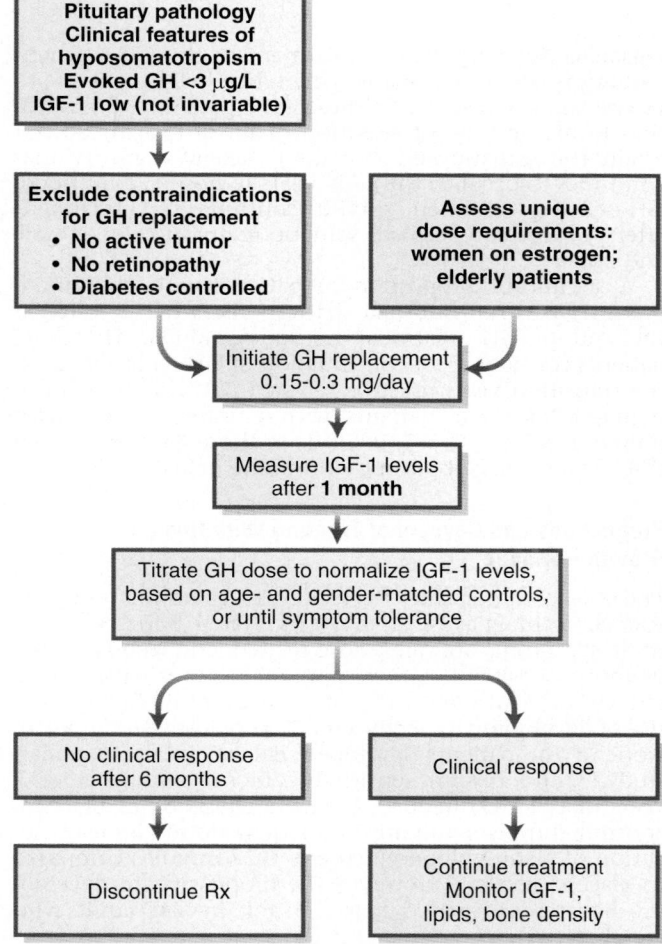

Figure 8-22 Management of somatotropin deficiency in adults. Patients older than 60 years require lower maintenance doses. Women receiving transdermal estrogen require lower doses than those receiving oral estrogen preparations. GH, growth hormone; IGF-1, insulin-like growth factor 1; Rx, treatment.

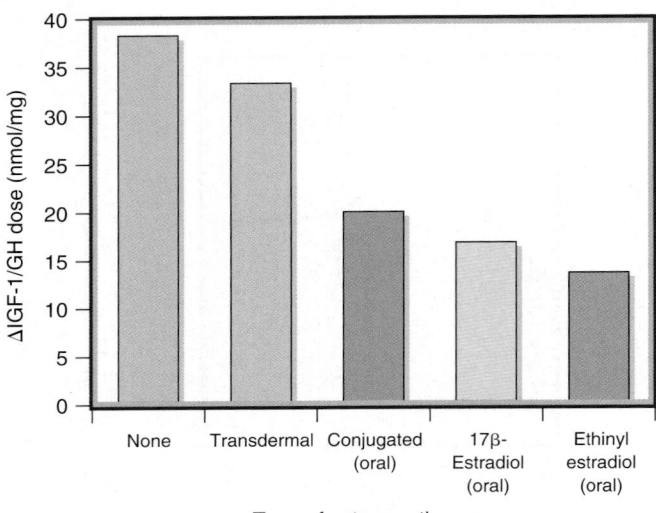

Figure 8-23 The effect of route and type of estrogen therapy on the sensitivity of growth hormone (GH) therapy in women with hypopituitarism. The GH sensitivity index was calculated as change in insulin-like growth factor 1 (IGF-1) level (nmol/L) by dose of GH (mg). Created using data from several studies.[310,313,314] (From Birzniece V, Ho KK. Growth and development: patching up a better pill for GH-deficient women. *Nat Rev Endocrinol.* 2012;8(4):197-198.)

Transition Age Patients. GH treatment of the GH-deficient child normally is terminated when final height and epiphysis closure are reached.[315] These GHD patients who transition from the time of cessation of linear growth do not attain the somatic and structural skeletal maturity that continues to occur in the early years of normal adulthood. GH-deficient children should continue GH treatment after puberty to complete somatic maturation of muscle and bone.[315]

A significant proportion of patients with childhood-onset GHD exhibit normal GH response when retested at the end of GH treatment as young adults. Therefore, patients considered for continuation of GH replacement in the transition years must be retested. GH retesting is not required for those patients with a transcription factor mutation (e.g., POU1F1, PROP-1) or those with more than three demonstrated pituitary hormone deficits.[267,283]

Precautions and Caveats of Treating With Human Growth Hormone

The most common side effects of hGH replacement include edema, arthralgias, and myalgias (Table 8-8). However, these symptoms are mild, dose related, and resolve in the majority of patients either spontaneously or with dosage reduction.[309] Although GH antagonizes insulin action, the risk of developing hyperglycemia is very low (see Fig. 8-20). None of 166 patients developed diabetes in an Australian study,[316] and insulin sensitivity did not change after 7 years of GH treatment.[317] A meta-analysis of 13 placebo-controlled trials involving 511 patients found a mean elevation of fasting blood glucose of 0.22 mmol/L compared to placebo levels.[239] However, the propensity for developing diabetes is increased up to eightfold in GHD adults who are obese.[318]

Patients with active malignancies should not be treated with GH. The possibility that hGH might initiate new cancers or stimulate growth of preexisting benign tumors is an important theoretical issue. The incidence of cancer

TABLE 8-8
Side Effects of Adult Growth Hormone Treatment
Edema
Arthralgias
Myalgias
Muscle stiffness
Paresthesias
Carpal tunnel syndrome
Atrial fibrillation
Headache
Benign intracranial hypertension
Increase in melanocytic nevi
Hyperglycemia
Sleep apnea
Iatrogenic acromegaly

is markedly reduced among subjects with inactivating mutations of the GHR[266] (see Fig. 8-16). A number of epidemiologic studies have reported association between higher, albeit normal, IGF-1 levels and later risk of developing prostate cancer,[319] breast cancer in premenopausal women,[320] and colon and lung cancer.[321] In contrast, patients with acromegaly do not have an increased incidence of either breast or prostate cancer or cancer in general. The overall risk for cancer in acromegaly is lower than expected. However, these patients have a significantly increased mortality risk from colon cancer.[322-324] Pediatric experience shows no convincing evidence for a causal link between GH treatment and tumor recurrence or the development of neoplasia including leukemia.[325,326] When comparing the relative risk of brain tumor recurrence in 180 children treated with hGH versus 891 who did not receive hGH, the risk of recurrence after a mean of 6.4 years was lower in the treated group than in those not receiving hGH.[327] GH treatment does, however, increase the risk of radiation-induced second tumor formation, especially meningiomas.[328] Nevertheless, long-term surveillance with adequate control groups and avoidance of high IGF-1 levels in adults being treated for adult GHD are required to assure that adult GH replacement does not increase the incidence of new cancers or growth of existing benign tumors.

Investigational Uses of Growth Hormone

Catabolic States. The anabolic actions of GH have prompted use of GH in catabolic states including surgery, trauma, burns, parenteral nutrition, and organ failure. These potential indications for GH are not approved in the United States. The negative nitrogen balance in critically ill patients is partly attributable to GH resistance as well as to decreased IGF-1 production and action.[329] GH administered to postsurgical patients, normal subjects receiving hypocaloric diets, or elderly malnourished patients with IV alimentation results in reversion to positive nitrogen balance.[330]

Beneficial effects of GH have been reported in patients with extensive burns, in those receiving chronic high-dose glucocorticoid treatment, in those with chronic obstructive pulmonary disease, and in patients with cardiac failure. There is some evidence that GH treatment in people with large burns results in more rapid healing of the burn wound and donor sites, and in reduced length of hospital stay, without increased risk of mortality or scarring, but there is an increased risk of hyperglycemia.[331] A study in which critically ill patients received very high doses of GH (up to 7 mg/day) was prematurely terminated due to increased unexplained fatality.[332] It has been suggested that GH may have had an adverse effect on acute-phase protein synthesis in these patients.[333] Caution is advised for nonapproved uses of GH in adults.[334]

Osteoporosis. There is strong evidence that GH administered to otherwise healthy subjects with idiopathic osteoporosis improves bone mineral mass.[335] A double-blind placebo-controlled treatment study for 18 months observed improvements in bone mineral content at the lumbar spine, in the femoral neck, and of the whole skeleton by up to 14%, which was sustained at 4 years.[336] Unclear long-term side effects, cost, and lack of comparative studies with other therapies for osteoporosis limit the potential use of GH in treating osteoporosis.

Human Immunodeficiency Virus Infection. GH is Food and Drug Administration (FDA)-approved for administration to adult patients with human immunodeficiency virus (HIV)-associated cachexia, and results in positive nitrogen balance, increased lean body mass, decreased body fat, and improved work output.[337] One large study using supraphysiologic GH doses of 4 mg/day has reported impairment in glucose tolerance.[338] A study using a physiologic dosing approach to maintain IGF-1 in the high-normal range has reported beneficial body compositional changes of lesser magnitude, reduced triglycerides, and lowered diastolic blood pressure but impaired glucose tolerance.[339] Treatment with a GH releasing factor analogue for 26 weeks improved visceral fat and lipid profiles.[340] However, long-term beneficial effects of GH on survival and quality of life in those with HIV infection have not yet been reported.

Sports. The public policy issues of GH abuse in competitive sports has received much attention. GH has been widely abused by athletes to enhance performance.[341] A systematic review concluded that claims that GH enhances physical performance are not supported by the scientific literature evaluating effects on aerobic capacity, strength, and power[342] and that more research is needed to conclusively determine the effects of GH on athletic performance. A double-blind placebo-controlled study has reported that GH enhances anaerobic sprint capacity, but not aerobic capacity, strength, or power in recreational athletes.[343]

Aging. There has been considerable interest in the use of GH as an antiaging hormone to prevent body composition changes and physical decline of the aging process, which superficially recapitulates the features of adults with organic GHD for which beneficial effects of GH replacement have been demonstrated. A systematic review of literature published on randomized, controlled trials in the healthy elderly indicates that GH supplementation is associated with small changes in body composition, no functional benefit, and increased rates of adverse events. On the basis of the evidence, GH cannot be recommended as an antiaging therapy.[344] GH is increasingly marketed and distributed for antiaging therapy under "off-label" use. Such off-label marketing of GH as antiaging therapy is not approved by the FDA in the United States.[334]

Adrenocorticotropic Hormone

Physiology

The hypothalamic-pituitary-adrenal (HPA) axis is the major system subserving stress and survival. Key components of the stress response are aimed at providing adequate amounts of glucocorticoids, which exert vital pleotrophic effects on energy supply, fuel metabolism, immunity, and cardiovascular function.

Corticotroph Cells. Corticotroph cells comprise about 20% of functional anterior pituitary cells and are the earliest detectable human fetal pituitary cell type, appearing by the eighth week of gestation. Corticotrophs are clustered mainly in the central median pituitary wedge. They are

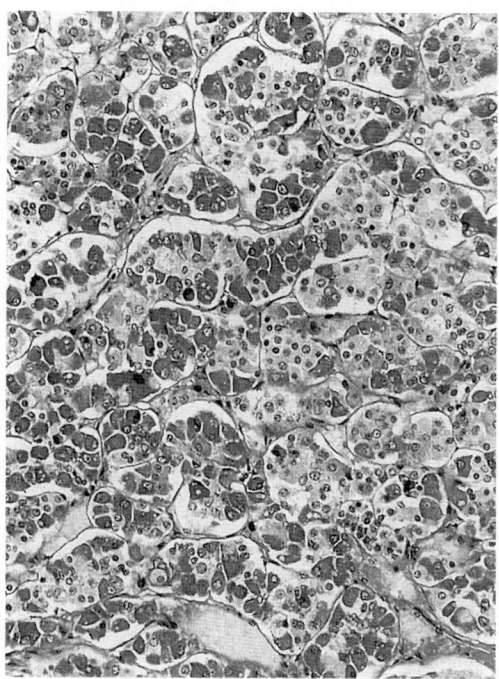

Figure 8-24 Corticotroph cell. The periodic acid–Schiff stain documents the presence of corticotrophs in the normal pituitary, reflecting glycosylation of the ACTH peptide. Some cells have clear cytoplasmic vacuoles corresponding to the enigmatic body. ACTH, adrenocorticotropic hormone. (From Asa SL. Tumors of the pituitary gland. In: Rosai J, ed. *Atlas of Tumor Pathology*, Series III, Fascicle 22. Washington, DC: Armed Forces Institute of Pathology; 1997:21.)

large irregular cells, and their ultrastructural features include prominent neurosecretory granules (150-400 nm), endoplasmic reticulum, and Golgi bodies[345] (Fig. 8-24). These cells produce the POMC gene products, including ACTH(1-39), β-lipotropin (LPH), and endorphins. Because of the rich carbohydrate moiety of these molecules, the cells are strongly positive for periodic acid–Schiff (PAS). In the presence of excess glucocorticoid, characteristic hyaline deposits develop (Fig. 8-25). In normal human pituitary, POMC is expressed only in corticotroph cells. Most mammals possess an intermediate lobe comprising POMC-expressing melanotroph cells; however, this lobe is not developed in adult humans. Tpit, now referred to as Tbx19, has been identified[37] as a critical transcriptional factor for corticotroph cell differentiation during pituitary development and for transcription of the POMC gene.[37]

Structure. POMC is the precursor for ACTH, which acts on the adrenal glands to induce synthesis and secretion of adrenal steroids. The primary translation product of POMC is a 266–amino acid pre-prohormone molecule encoding corticotrophic, opioid, and melanotropic peptides. The peptide contains a leader sequence, and multiple dibasic proteolytic cleavage sites for glycosylation, acetylation, and amidation. Products of this processing include ACTH(1-39) and β-LPH, which in turn give rise to α-LPH and β-endorphin, also containing metenkephalin. ACTH itself may also be cleaved to α-melanocyte-stimulating hormone (MSH)(1-13) and corticotropin-like intermediate lobe peptide (CLIP)(18-39).

The 8-kb human POMC gene, located on chromosome 2p23,[37,346] consists of 3 exons interspersed with 2 intervening introns (Fig. 8-26). The first exon encodes a leader sequence, the second encodes the signal initiation sequence and the amino-terminal (N-terminal) portion of the POMC

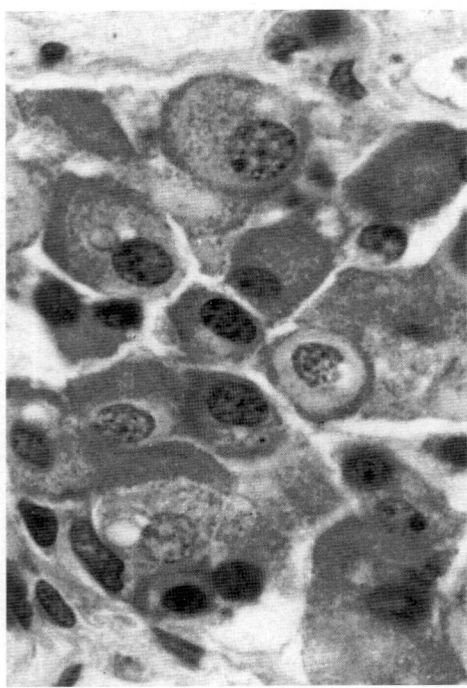

Figure 8-25 Crooke's hyalinization. Pituitary corticotrophs subjected to glucocorticoid excess develop cytoplasmic hyalinization that displaces ACTH-positive secretory material to the cell periphery. The clear vacuoles correspond to complex lysosomes known as enigmatic bodies. ACTH, adrenocorticotropic hormone. (From Asa SL. Tumors of the pituitary gland. In: Rosai J, ed. *Atlas of Tumor Pathology*, Series III, Fascicle 22. Washington, DC: Armed Forces Institute of Pathology; 1997:23.)

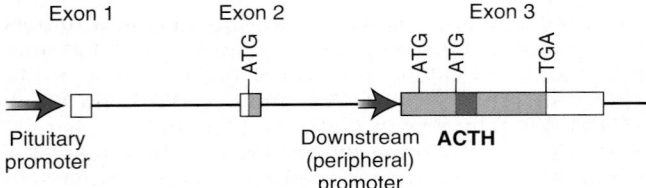

Figure 8-26 Structure of POMC gene. Exon 1 encodes the RNA leader sequence, and exon 2 encodes the initiator methionine (ATG), the signal peptide, and several N-terminal residues of the precursor peptide, the remainder of which is encoded by exon 3. Corticotroph expression is determined by the upstream pituitary promoter *(longer arrowhead)*, whereas peripheral expression of the short POMC mRNA is determined by the downstream promoter *(shorter arrowhead)*. Translation of these shorter transcripts initiates from the initiator methionines (ATG) indicated in exon 3. The precursor peptide coding region is lightly shaded, and the ACTH coding region is darkly shaded. (From Adrian JL, Clark AJL, Swords FM. Molecular pathology of corticotroph function. In: Rappaport R, Amselem S, eds. *Hypothalamic-Pituitary Development*. Basel, Switzerland: Karger; 2001.)

peptide, and the third exon encodes most of the mature peptide sequences including ACTH and β-LPH.[347] The POMC gene is expressed in pituitary and nonpituitary tissues including brain, skin, placenta, gonads, gastrointestinal tissues, liver, kidney, adrenal medulla, lung, and lymphocytes.

In corticotroph cells, a pituitary-selective promoter region for POMC generates a POMC messenger RNA (mRNA) transcript of approximately 1200 nucleotides. The 800 nucleotides of the coding region are translated into a pre-POMC molecule that includes a 26–amino acid signal peptide, which is rapidly cleaved. The parent POMC protein of 241 amino acids enters the secretory pathway for subsequent processing.

In extrapituitary tissues, POMC gene expression is regulated differently from that in the pituitary. An upstream promoter generates a longer transcript of approximately 1350 nucleotides. A downstream promoter generates short truncated transcripts of approximately 800 nucleotides arising from the 5′ end of exon 3. In the brain, however, neurons in the arcuate nucleus express POMC mRNA that is identical to that of the pituitary.[348] In these neurons, POMC serves as a precursor to brain β-endorphin, α-MSH, and other peptides, which have important brain functions, including a major role in energy homeostasis.

Transcriptional Regulation

Multiple signals act in synergy to activate POMC gene expression, including corticotropin-releasing hormone (CRH), cytokines, AVP, catecholamines, and VIP. Elements of the promoter regions mediate POMC regulation by glucocorticoids, cAMP, activator protein-1 (AP1), and STAT signaling molecules.[349]

The CRH type 1 receptor is predominantly expressed on the corticotroph[350] and receptor activation increases cAMP, protein kinase A, and CREB induction of CRH-binding protein (CRHBP) to the promoter, leading to POMC transcription.[351] CRH also activates an AP1 site within the first exon by an MAPK-mediated pathway. In addition to mediating ACTH secretion, this receptor also appears critical for fear and anxiety responses, possibly by a related ligand, urocortin.[352] The type 2 CRH receptor predominantly regulates cardiovascular function.[353] Leukemia inhibitory factor (LIF), a proinflammatory cytokine also expressed in the pituitary and hypothalamus, signals via the JAK-STAT pathway and acts in synergy with CRH potentiating POMC expression.[354] This represents a mechanism of immunoneuroendocrine interfacing that facilitates stimulation of ACTH secretion by inflammation-derived STAT-inducing cytokines.

Glucocorticoid receptor activation leads to transcriptional suppression via two cooperative binding sites. The intracellular glucocorticoid receptor binds directly to 5′-regulatory elements to suppress POMC transcription.[348] CRH action is also potentiated by vasopressin and β-adrenergic catecholamines, by either enhancing POMC mRNA levels, increasing ACTH secretion, or both. The net effects of these intracellular signals are to regulate POMC gene transcription, peptide synthesis, and ACTH secretion for mediating appropriate neuroendocrine responses.[349]

POMC Processing. Several post-translational POMC modification steps are required for ultimate polypeptide hormone secretion (Fig. 8-27). First, the N-terminal signal sequence is removed, followed by glycosylation via an O-linkage to Thr45 and N-linkage to Asn65.[355] Serine-phosphorylation then occurs within the Golgi apparatus. After being transported to secretory vesicles the constituent peptides are cleaved at dibasic amino acid residues, and ACTH-related peptides are stored in dense secretory granules for ultimate regulated release. Some POMC products also undergo carboxy-terminal (C-terminal) amidation mediated by peptidylglycine-amidating monooxygenase (PAM), peptidylhydroxyglycine-amidating lyase (PAL),[356] and N-terminal acetylation.

POMC proteolytic processing occurs at Lys-Arg or Arg-Arg residues by enzymes called prohormone convertases (PCs), which are a superfamily of subtilisin/kexin proteinases. They play a critical role in determining function of the peptides at the tissue level through site-specific cleavages. PC1 is most abundant in the pituitary and hypothalamus, whereas PC2 is present in the CNS, skin, and pancreatic islets, but is absent in the pituitary. In

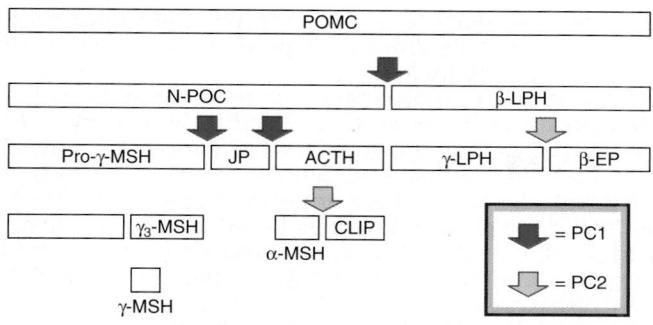

Figure 8-27 Processing and cleavage of pro-opiomelanocortin (POMC). The mature POMC precursor peptide is sequentially cleaved by prohormone convertase 1 (PC1) in the anterior pituitary corticotroph. In the neurointermediate lobe and other cell types, cleavage by PC2 allows release of β-MSH or β-endorphin or both. Carboxypeptidase H (not shown) removes residual basic amino acids at cleavage sites. ACTH, adrenocorticotropic hormone; CLIP, corticotropin-like intermediate lobe peptide; EP, endorphin; JP, joining peptide; LPH, lipotropin; MSH, melanocyte-stimulating hormone; N-POC, N-terminal pro-POMC fragment. (From Clark AJL, Swords FM. Molecular pathology of corticotroph function. In: Rappaport R, Amselem S, eds. *Hypothalamic-Pituitary Development*. Basel, Switzerland: Karger; 2001.)

corticotrophs, PC1 expression results in cleavage limited to four sites, with ACTH being a major end product (see Fig. 8-27). In the hypothalamus and CNS, both PC1 and PC2 allow coordinated proteolysis, resulting in the generation of smaller fragments such as α-, β-, and γ-MSH and CLIP. Heterozygous mutations of the PC1 gene have been associated with childhood obesity, adrenal insufficiency, hyperproinsulinemia, and postprandial hypoglycemia[357] with elevated levels of plasma ACTH precursors.

Biologic Actions of POMC-Derived Peptides

POMC products in blood are derived from corticotrophs and are secreted in equimolar amounts; however, circulating concentrations differ in accordance with respective half-lives of each molecule.

Adrenal Action. Full-length ACTH is the only POMC-derived peptide with adrenocorticotroph function, and it is the ligand of the melanocortin receptor type 2 receptor (MC2R). MC2R activation results in production of adrenal glucocorticoids, androgenic steroids, and to a lesser extent, mineralocorticoids. There is evidence that the N-terminal peptide POMC(1-28) exerts an independent mitogenic and growth-sustaining effect on the adrenal gland.[358]

Skin Pigmentation. Melanocyte stimulation occurs through the activation of MC1R. ACTH, β-LPH, and γ-LPH produced from the corticotroph share a common heptapeptide sequence (Met-Glu-His-Phe-Arg-Trp-Gly) required to activate MC1R. These peptides are responsible for inducing skin pigmentation in Addison disease because the other melanostimulating peptides, α-MSH and β-MSH, are not produced in the pituitary. There is also evidence for a paracrine system regulating skin pigmentation. Local production of ACTH and α-MSH occurs in melanocytes and keratinocytes and is stimulated by cytokines and ultraviolet irradiation in parallel with PC1 and PC2 expression.[359]

Appetite Regulation. POMC-derived peptides and in particular α-MSH play a critical role in the central regulation of appetite. The melanocortin system mediates feedback suppression of appetite by leptin through activation of MC3R and MC4R by α-MSH in the hypothalamus. Genetic and pharmacologic abrogation of the melanocortin system causes profound obesity. POMC-deficient mice and humans are hyperphagic, but intraventricular infusion of α-MSH or synthetic agonists induces weight loss.[360,361]

Immune Modulation. α-MSH influences the inflammatory process by modulating the function of antigen-presenting cells and T cells. It suppresses fever induced by IL-6 and inhibits macrophage function and leukocyte migration.[362]

Analgesia. β-Endorphin is produced by corticotrophs and circulating concentrations may be high in Addison disease. The peptide exerts a potent analgesic effect through opiate receptors. However, these effects are unlikely to be of physiologic significance because the peptide does not cross the blood-brain barrier.

Placenta-Derived POMC Peptides. Full-length pituitary-like POMC mRNA is expressed in human placenta along with ACTH, LPH, endorphin, and α-MSH. Intact POMC is not detectable in the nonpregnant state, but becomes measurable in early gestation, rising 3- to 10-fold in the second trimester, plateauing thereafter, and returning to prepregnancy levels within 3 days after delivery.[363] The physiologic function of this placental molecule is unknown, and blood levels do not correlate with those of ACTH or cortisol, both of which also increase during pregnancy.

Ectopic ACTH Synthesis

POMC is also expressed in the gonads, lung, skin, gastrointestinal and adrenal medullary neuroendocrine cells, and white blood cells. Nevertheless, the overwhelming source of circulating ACTH is derived from the anterior pituitary or from neuroendocrine tumor ectopic production. Nonpituitary tumors demonstrate a spectrum of altered POMC gene expression and processing. The ectopic ACTH syndrome occurs in tumors capable of generating high amounts of the pituitary-like 1072-nucleotide mRNA. Appropriate processing may not occur because of the lack of PC enzyme or may result in preferential generation of smaller fragments such as CLIP and β-MSH.[363] Small cell lung cancers preferentially release intact POMC, but carcinoid tumors tend to process the precursor, releasing ACTH and smaller peptides.[363] Defective POMC processing indicates an impaired state of neuroendocrine differentiation in poorly differentiated tumors.

Extrapituitary neuroendocrine tumors associated with ectopic ACTH secretion do not process the prohormone efficiently because of a general defect in PC expression. As ACTH is synthesized in nontumorous neuroendocrine cells, ectopic tumor hormone production may in fact reflect inappropriate ACTH processing. These patients also exhibit a higher ratio of circulating ACTH precursors, as well as smaller peptides, including CLIP.

ACTH Regulation

The complex control of ACTH reflects the integrated neuroendocrine control of stress homeostasis. Similar to other anterior pituitary hormones, ACTH regulation is subserved by at least three tiers of control. First, the brain and hypothalamus release regulatory molecules (including CRH, vasopressin, and dopamine) that traverse the portal system and directly regulate corticotroph function. Second, intrapituitary cytokines and growth factors act locally to regulate ACTH, either in concert with hypothalamic factors or independently. These paracrine controls often overlap and induce sensitive intracellular molecules that limit the ACTH response, preventing chronic ACTH hypersecretion. Third, glucocorticoids maintain regulatory feedback control of corticotroph secretion by rapidly inhibiting hypothalamic CRH and pituitary ACTH secretion. After chronic glucocorticoid exposure (>24 hours), HPA suppression may persist for days or longer. In a short feedback loop, pituitary ACTH inhibits hypothalamic CRH, and in an ultrashort loop, it may also suppress the corticotroph itself.

Normal pituitary corticotrophs express somatostatin receptors. Of the five subtypes, subtypes 2 and 5 are predominantly expressed. Somatostatin inhibits ACTH secretion, but the sensitivity is strongly regulated by glucocorticoids, which nullify the inhibition via downregulating somatostatin receptor expression.[364] Dopamine receptors (DRs) are involved in the regulation of the HPA axis. Among five DR subtypes rodent studies show D2R is the predominant subtype in melanotroph cells of the intermediate lobe, where they play a role in PC expression, which determines the processing of POMC.[365] DRs have not been characterized in normal human corticotrophs, although they are expressed in tumorous corticotrophs.[366]

Stress Response. The HPA stress response occurs in the context of a wide variety of peripheral and central adaptors to stress, including vasovagal and catecholamine activation, and cytokine secretion and action. A tightly controlled immuno-neuroendocrine interface regulates the ACTH response to peripheral stressors, which include pain, infection, inflammation, hemorrhage, hypovolemia, trauma, psychological stress, and hypoglycemia. These signals vary in their ability to generate ACTH secretion and to sensitize the glucocorticoid response to ACTH. In addition to CRH, peripheral and centrally released pro-inflammatory cytokines potently induce POMC transcription and ACTH secretion.[349] Sensitive intracellular signals within the corticotroph also serve to override the ACTH response to stress, thus preventing persistent and chronic hypercortisolemia.

Cytokines such as IL-6 and LIF activate the HPA axis and enhance glucocorticoid production, protecting the organism against lethality by constraining the inflammatory response.[354] Thus, mice with inactivated CRH or LIF genes mount an inadequate neuroendocrine response to stress, inflammation, or endotoxins. During stress, glucocorticoid inhibition of ACTH is also prevented by nuclear factor κB activation, which interferes with pituitary glucocorticoid receptor function, thus further exaggerating enhanced ACTH secretion.[367]

Exercise is a physiologic stimulus of ACTH release. Exercising to 90% of maximum oxygen capacity causes a significant elevation of ACTH, similar to levels observed during surgery or hypoglycemia.[368] Levels may remain elevated for up to 6 minutes after the cessation of exercise. Although lower intensity exercise does not evoke ACTH,[369] well-trained athletes exhibit hypercortisolism, possibly due to decreased adrenal ACTH sensitivity.

ACTH Secretion. The hormone is secreted with both circadian periodicity and ultradian pulsatility under the control of the suprachiasmatic nucleus. This centrally controlled pattern is influenced by peripheral corticosteroids. The circadian pattern of ACTH secretion typically begins at about 4 AM, peaking before 7 AM, with both ACTH and adrenal steroid levels reaching their nadir between 11 PM and 3 AM. Within this overall 24-hour diurnal cycle, periodic ACTH secretory bursts occur at a frequency of 40 pulses per 24 hours; amplitude rather than frequency modulation contributes to diurnal changes in ACTH profile.[370,371] ACTH circadian rhythm is entrained by visual cues and the light-dark cycle and is centrally controlled by CRH and other factors.[372] The mode of CRH signal determines ACTH response, with a continuous signal desensitizing the ACTH response and a pulsatile CRH signal restoring cortisol secretion without depleting the pituitary ACTH pool.[373] Daily ACTH but not cortisol secretion is higher in males, who also exhibit higher pulse frequency and peak amplitudes.[374] Endogenous and exogenous stress, including hypoglycemia, act centrally to increase ACTH pulse amplitude, but corticosteroids directly suppress basal or stimulated ACTH pulse amplitude.[375]

Action. ACTH is a polypeptide of 39 amino acids with a molecular weight of 4.5 kDa. The highly conserved 12 N-terminal amino acid residues are critical for adrenal gland steroid synthesis. The primary action of ACTH is to maintain adrenal gland size, structure, and function; ACTH induces adrenal steroidogenesis by MC2R on the adrenal cortex. ACTH signals via adenyl cyclase to regulate P450 enzyme transcription of cortisol, aldosterone (10%), 17-hydroxyprogesterone, and to a lesser extent, adrenal androgens.[376] ACTH stimulates mitochondrial cholesterol transport and regulates the rate-limiting side-chain cleavage of cholesterol to pregnenolone.[377] Secretory cortisol pulses follow ACTH pulses within 5 to 10 minutes, with a linear dose dependency that is especially evident after physiologic CRH stimulation.[378] Adrenal cortisol response to ACTH is sensitive to the background ambient ACTH milieu. In states of chronic ACTH deficiency, adrenal reserve is compromised, although during ongoing ACTH hypersecretion, the gland is primed such that a given ACTH bolus elicits a higher cortisol response. Both basal and stimulated (e.g., by CRH) ACTH secretion is blunted by glucocorticoids. Conversely, low or absent circulating glucocorticoids (e.g., after adrenalectomy) result in exaggerated ACTH secretion[379,380] and in corticotroph cell hyperplasia.[381]

Disorders of ACTH Secretion

ACTH Deficiency

Causes. Congenital ACTH deficiency may occur as an isolated pituitary defect or as a component of a wider spectrum of multiple pituitary hormone deficiencies. A mutation of *TBX19*, encoding Tpit, a transcription factor involved in corticotroph differentiation, has been identified as a cause of isolated ACTH deficiency (see Tables 8-1 and 8-2).[37] Mutations of transcription factors involved in early stages of pituitary cell differentiation or midline brain development may also give rise to ACTH deficiency as a component of multiple hormone deficiencies. These genes with mutations include *LHX4* and *HESX1* (see Table 8-2). Secondary causes include pituitary tumors, sellar mass lesions, trauma, irradiation, and lymphocytic hypophysitis, which may be associated with other autoimmune manifestations (see Table 8-5).

Clinical Features. The manifestations of ACTH deficiency are clinically indistinguishable from glucocorticoid deficiency of any cause. Glucorticorticoids exert pleotrophic effects on metabolism, appetite, cardiovascular function, fluid homeostasis, and inflammation. The clinical features are dependent on severity, the time of onset, and clinical context. In the newborn, ACTH deficiency may present as hypoglycemia and failure to thrive. In the adult, there is slowly progressive weight and appetite loss, anorexia, and generalized fatigue mimicking a wasting syndrome. As adrenal mineralocorticoid secretion is largely unimpaired, salt wasting, volume contraction, and hyperkalemia, commonly encountered features in Addison disease, are not manifest. Furthermore, hyperpigmentation, usually associated with exuberant ACTH-related peptide secretion in the face of adrenal damage, does not occur.

Evaluation. Diagnostic evaluation of adrenal insufficiency requires concurrent measurement of glucocorticoid and ACTH levels. Morning serum cortisol levels lower than 3 µg/dL suggest ACTH deficiency, but basal morning cortisol levels higher than 18 µg/dL usually indicate normal ACTH reserve. Patients with ACTH deficiency have low to normal serum cortisol levels and low to normal plasma ACTH levels. Blunted responses to provocative tests such as insulin-induced hypoglycemia or metyrapone are required to document a partial deficiency. As cortisol is highly bound to cortisol-binding globulin (CBG), the level of CBG may confound interpretation of cortisol values. Cirrhosis and hyperthyroidism lower CBG concentrations whereas estrogens elevate them.

ACTH Excess

Causes. Excessive ACTH production can arise from a corticotroph adenoma or from an extrapituitary ectopic tumor source. Small cell lung carcinomas, bronchial carcinoids, and neuroendocrine tumors are common causes of ectopic ACTH production.

Clinical Features. ACTH-induced adrenal hyperfunction causes a syndrome of hypercortisolism and of androgen excess in women. Manifestations arise from appetite stimulation (weight gain), altered fat distribution (moon facies, buffalo hump, central obesity), catabolism (skin thinning, muscle wasting), mood disturbance (depression, anxiety), sodium retention (hypertension), and androgen excess (menstrual irregularity, hirsutism, acne, and oily skin). The evaluation and management of patients with Cushing disease is fully described in Chapter 15.

Measurement of ACTH

Measurements of plasma ACTH are extremely useful in the diagnosis of both Cushing syndrome and adrenal insufficiency. ACTH assays have evolved considerably since the first radioimmunoassay. Current commercially available two-site immunometric assays display high specificity and analytic sensitivity of less than 0.5 ng/L.[382] However, significant variability in precision and performance exists between commercial assays.[383] ACTH and other POMC-derived peptides such as α-MSH, β-LPH, or β-endorphin can also be measured with precision with current assays. Awareness of the assay peptide specificity may be especially critical when evaluating ectopic POMC products secreted by lung tumors. Ideally, nonstressed resting subjects should have venous blood withdrawn between 6 and 9 AM. As ACTH is relatively unstable at room temperature, and has a propensity to adhere to glass, plasma samples should immediately be separated in iced siliconized glass tubes containing ethylenediaminetetra-acetic acid (EDTA), and stored below –20° C for transport. Morning (8 AM) plasma ACTH levels range from 8 to 25 ng/L. Episodic secretion and short plasma half-life result in wide and rapid fluctuation of plasma measurements. Cortisol values at 4 PM are about half those of morning levels, and at 11 PM levels are usually less than 5 μg/dL. Plasma ACTH levels fluctuate broadly within the same individual and are highly sensitive to stress, time of collection, and gender. Pregnant females have higher ambient ACTH levels, possibly because of placental CRH secretion.[384]

Dynamic Testing for ACTH Reserve

Hypothalamic Testing. Insulin hypoglycemia is a potent endogenous stressor that evokes ACTH secretion as well as GH release. Insulin (0.1-0.15 U/kg) is injected intravenously after an overnight fast to achieve symptomatic hypoglycemia and a blood glucose level of less than 40 mg/dL. This test must be performed under supervision. Normal HPA response to this stressor evokes cortisol levels higher than 20 μg/dL. As hypoglycemia acts centrally, a normal response implies integrity of all three tiers of HPA axis control. Some patients may require up to 0.3 U/kg insulin or more to achieve adequate hypoglycemia.[385] Venous samples are collected at –15, 0, 15, 30, 45, 60, 90, and 120 minutes for measurement of glucose, ACTH, and cortisol

levels. After the test, oral glucose should be administered. Both intraindividual variations in blood glucose levels attained by a given dose of insulin, as well as fluctuations in central sensitivity to glucose and activation of catecholamines, may lead to difficulties in reproducibility. The test is contraindicated in subjects with a history of seizures or active coronary or cerebral ischemia and during pregnancy. Importantly, if pronounced adrenal insufficiency is likely, insulin injection may provoke an adrenal crisis as a result of inadequate adrenal reserve, and hydrocortisone (100 mg) should be available for urgent IV use, if required.

Metyrapone blocks cortisol synthesis by inhibiting adrenal 11β-hydroxylase. Thus, the drug releases the HPA axis from negative feedback by cortisol, normally resulting in an ACTH surge and elevated levels of 11-deoxycortisol. A single oral dose (2-3 g) is given at midnight and serum levels of ACTH, 11-deoxycortisol, and cortisol are measured at 8 AM the following day. The test is only valid in the face of documented suppressed cortisol levels to less than 10 μg/dL. In normal subjects, peak ACTH values higher than 200 ng/L are achieved. Side effects include nausea, gastrointestinal upset, and insomnia.[386] False-positive results may be obtained with phenytoin, which prevents adequate enzymatic blockade. This test should be performed under observation in a hospital because acute adrenal insufficiency may ensue.

Pituitary Stimulation. Pituitary ACTH secretion may be evoked by injecting either CRH or AVP. Ovine or human CRH (100 μg or 1 μg/kg) is administered intravenously, and cortisol and ACTH are measured at –5, –1, 0, 15, 30, 60, 90, and 120 minutes. Normally, maximal ACTH responses (twofold to fourfold above baseline) are evoked at 30 minutes,[387] and cortisol levels peak (over 20 μg/dL) at 60 minutes or increase more than 10 μg/dL above baseline. Although CRH readily induces ACTH secretion and may demonstrate corticotroph ACTH deficiency or ACTH excess, the wide variation of responses observed has limited the utility of this test. A useful application of the CRH test is in making the diagnosis of Cushing disease, with or without dexamethasone pretreatment, and in the context of petrosal venous sampling for diagnosing the presence of an ACTH-secreting pituitary adenoma. CRH injection allows a sensitive and specific central to peripheral ACTH gradient to be established, which effectively distinguishes peripheral from pituitary sources of excess ACTH secretion.[388] A pseudo-Cushing state is defined as the presence of some clinical features of Cushing syndrome with biochemical evidence of hypercortisolism that has arisen from some other cause. The most commonly associated conditions are alcoholism, depression, and obesity itself. Some investigators have advocated combining the CRH test with the dexamethasone suppression test. The combined dexamethasone-CRH test administers dexamethasone 0.5 mg every 6 hours for 48 hours starting at noon and ending at 6 AM, followed by CRH administered intravenously at 8 AM.[389] An initial report showed high diagnostic accuracy. Subsequent reports have shown that this test does not reliably discriminate between Cushing disease and pseudo-Cushing disorders[390] (see Chapter 15).

Adrenal Stimulation. The acute response of the adrenal gland to a bolus ACTH injection reflects ambient ACTH concentrations to which the gland has been exposed. Thus, the cortisol response to an acute ACTH injection will be blunted if the subject has experienced chronic pituitary ACTH hyposecretion, with resultant adrenal atrophy and diminished cortisol reserve. Conversely, persistently elevated ACTH levels lead to adrenal hypertrophy and augmented cortisol responses.[391] The utility of this test in diagnosing diminished pituitary ACTH reserve has been challenged as the commonly employed dose of 250 µg ACTH(1-24) (Cortrosyn) or Synacthen is pharmacologic and may evoke a "normal" cortisol response in hypopituitary subjects. An unacceptably high false-negative rate (about 65%) has been determined in a large series,[392] although peak cortisol levels at 30 minutes correlate well with peak responses to ITT.[393]

A normal cortisol response is greater than 20 µg/dL, or a doubling of baseline values. Basal cortisol levels correlate inversely with the incremental response to ACTH.[394] Low-dose stimulation with 1 µg Synacthen evokes maximal serum cortisol levels at 30 minutes, and these correlate well with values observed after insulin or high-dose ACTH administration.[393] A cutoff value of more than 500 nmol/L provides almost 100% sensitivity and a specificity of 80% to 100%.[395] Failure to respond to low-dose ACTH should be corroborated by a standard dose of insulin or ACTH stimulation.

Test: 250 µg ACTH(1-24) (Cortrosyn) is injected intramuscularly or intravenously, and cortisol levels are measured before, 30 minutes after, and 60 minutes after injection. Cortisol values greater than 20 µg/dL reflect a normal adrenal reserve response.

Adrenal Steroid Replacement

Hydrocortisone is widely used for glucocorticoid replacement. The normal secretory rate of cortisol is 15 to 20 mg/day, which is the recommended total daily dose. As plasma circulating half-life of cortisol is less than 2 hours, three times daily dosing of a total daily requirement of 10 to 20 mg (5-10 mg in the morning, 2.5-5 mg at noon, and 2.5-5 mg in the evening) is recommended.[396] Other synthetic glucocorticoids, including prednisolone (2.5-5 mg/day) and dexamethasone (0.25-0.5 mg/day) are suitable alternatives. Having longer half-lives, they can be administered once daily but are difficult to monitor biochemically. There is no consensus for monitoring treatment. Central diabetes insipidus may be unmasked after initial glucocorticoid replacement. Mineralocorticoid replacement is not required for treating secondary hypoadrenalism. Adrenal androgen replacement with dehydroepiandrosterone (DHEA) at doses of 25 mg/day may improve the sense of well-being, relieve fatigue, and improve sexual function in patients with primary and secondary adrenal insufficiency.[397,398]

However, conventional regimens do not recapitulate the physiologic pattern of cortisol release and may explain the high prevalence of poor quality of life and osteoporosis in these patients.[399] Two modified release formulations aimed at mimicking diurnal profiles have been introduced for clinical trials.[400,401] One of these, a dual-release hydrocortisone tablet (DuoCort), containing an immediate-release coating and an extended-release core, was approved by the European Medicines Agency for once-daily therapy of adrenal insufficiency in 2012. In a 12-week randomized crossover study of 64 patients with adrenal insufficiency, DuoCort exhibited improved weight, glucose, and blood pressure control compared to conventional thrice-daily hydrocortisone dosing at the same total daily dose.[400] Thus, modified-release preparations mimicking cortisol diurnal profiles represent a potential advance in the management of glucocorticoid insufficiency.

Gonadotropins

Physiology

Gonadotroph Cells. Gonadotroph cells secrete FSH and LH. The hypothalamic-pituitary-gonadal (HPG) axis plays a critical role in reproductive development, puberty, and fertility. Reproduction is a tightly regulated function, influenced by genetic, nutritional, environmental, and socioeconomic factors. For example, owing to the elevated energy requirements of reproduction, metabolic factors exert a pivotal role in the control of the HPG axis. LH and FSH act on the ovaries and testes to direct gametogenesis and sex steroid hormone synthesis. Befitting their important roles, the synthesis and secretion of LH and FSH are under complex regulation by hypothalamic input (e.g., gonadotropin-releasing hormone, or GnRH), by positive and negative feedback from gonadal sex steroid and peptide hormones, and by paracrine modulation from local factors produced within the pituitary gland itself (e.g., activins, inhibins, follistatin).[33]

Gonadotroph cells comprise about 10% to 15% of the functional anterior pituitary cells. Gonadotrophs are a heterogeneous cell population, with large round cell bodies with prominent rough endoplasmic reticulum and Golgi apparatus. Two classes of electrodense secretory granules are evident; large (350 to 450 nm) and smaller (150 to 250 nm) granules are packaged in vesicles (Figs. 8-28 and 8-29). Immunocytochemical studies have demonstrated the presence of both bihormonal and monohormonal groups of gonadotrophs. Cells with LH secretory granules often accumulate peripherally, and their Golgi structures may be less prominent. Gonadotrophs are characterized also by GnRH receptor expression and by SF1 and DAX1 nuclear receptors, which contribute to gonadotroph-specific gene expression.

Gonadotropin Structure. FSH and LH function to regulate gonadal steroid hormone biosynthesis and initiate and maintain germ cell development in concert with peripheral hormones and paracrine soluble factors. The four heterodimeric glycoprotein hormones—LH, FSH, TSH, and hCG—share structural homology, having evolved from a common ancestral gene. Although both the homologous LH and FSH molecules are cosecreted by gonadotrophs, their regulatory mechanisms are not uniformly concordant. The αGSU, LHβ, and FSHβ subunits are encoded by different genes, located on chromosomes 6, 11, and 19, respectively (Fig. 8-30; see also Fig. 8-2). The heterodimeric structure of the common—and unique—subunit of LH and FSH is essential for biologic activity. Disulfide linkages within

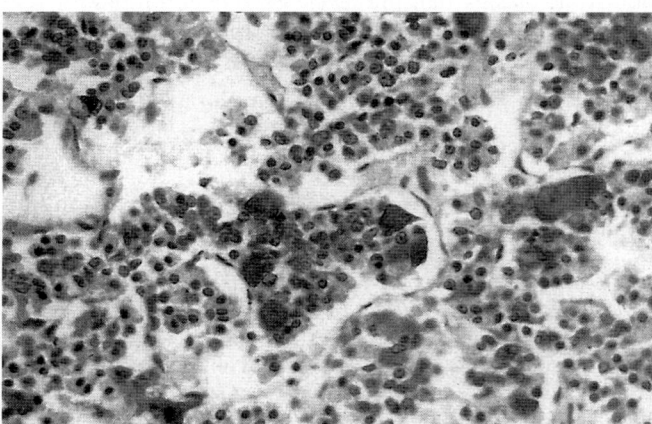

Figure 8-28 Normal gonadotroph cells contain immunoreactive β-follicle-stimulating hormone scattered throughout acini of the nontumorous pituitary. These round cells have evenly dispersed cytoplasmic immunoreactivity for α and β gonadotropic subunits. (From Asa SL. Tumors of the pituitary gland. In: Rosai J, ed. *Atlas of Tumor Pathology*, Series III, Fascicle 22. Washington, DC: Armed Forces Institute of Pathology; 1997:26.)

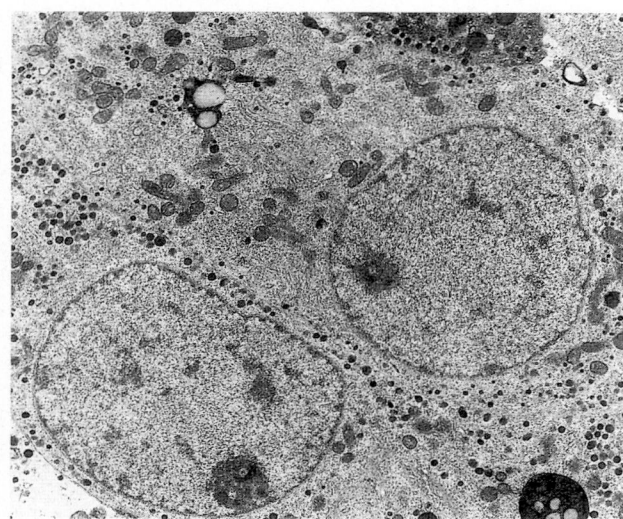

Figure 8-29 Electron micrograph of gonadotroph cell showing large round to elongated cells with ovoid nuclei with occasional nucleoli. Short profiles of rough endoplasmic reticulum are scattered throughout the cytoplasm and are dilated and frequently contain electron-lucent material. The Golgi complex is usually well developed and in a juxtanuclear location. Secretory granules are highly variable in size, shape, and electron density, and lysosomes are prominent. (From Asa SL. Tumors of the pituitary gland. In: Rosai J, ed. *Atlas of Tumor Pathology*, Series III, Fascicle 22. Washington, DC: Armed Forces Institute of Pathology; 1997:26.)

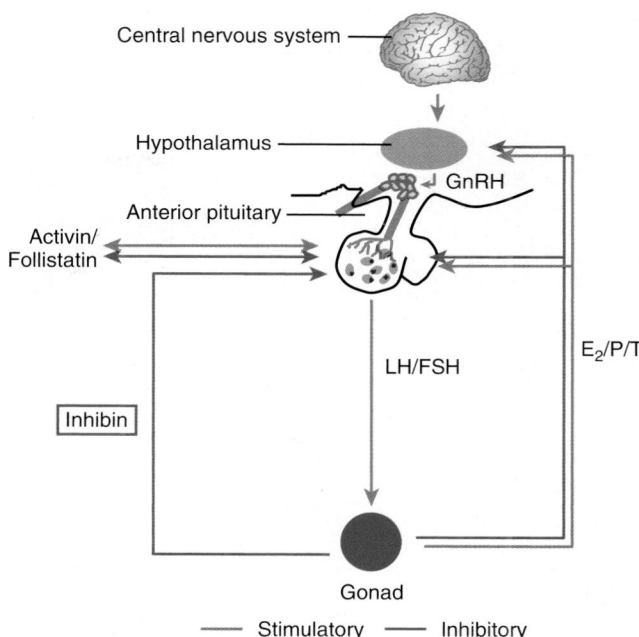

Figure 8-31 The hypothalamic-pituitary-gonadal axis. See text for discussion. E_2/P/T, estrogen/progesterone/testosterone; GnRH, gonadotropin-releasing hormone; FSH, follicle-stimulating hormone; LH, luteinizing hormone. (From Kaiser UB. Gonadotrophin hormones. In: Melmed S, ed. *The Pituitary*, 3rd ed. San Diego, CA: Elsevier; 2011:205-260.)

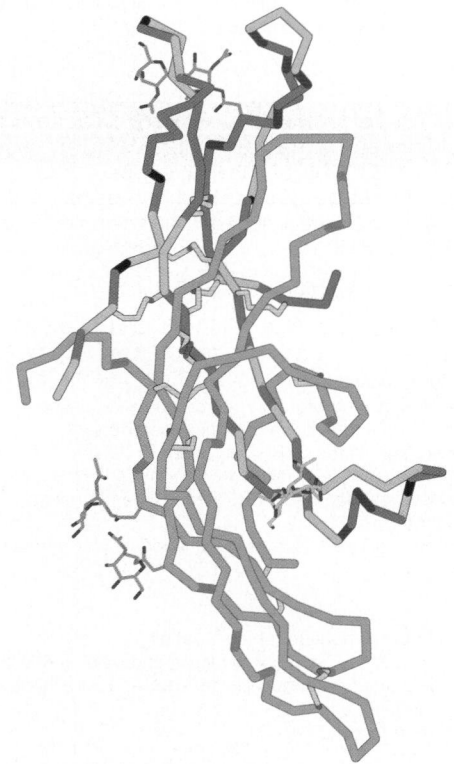

Figure 8-30 The subunit structure and glycosylation sites of the four glycoprotein hormone heterodimers (α-subunit, blue; β-subunit, green). (From the University of Glasgow protein crystallography website. Available at http://www.chem.gla.ac.uk/protein/glyco/GPH.html.)

each subunit result in a tertiary structure that enables and maintains noncovalent heterodimerization, which also determines the ultrastructure of the mature folded molecule to facilitate specific ligand-receptor interaction.[402] Glycosylation of the subunits occurs by the transfer of oligosac-

charide complexes to asparaginylasparagine residues.[403] Post-translational processing of carbohydrate side chains is critical for hormone signaling and may be species specific, distinct for LH and FSH, and may even vary physiologically to influence biologic activity and metabolic clearance rates.[403,404] The human LH/CG β gene cluster comprises seven genes, arising from gene duplication, of which one gene encodes LHβ, one encodes CGβ, and the remainder are pseudogenes. Unlike LH, hCG is present only in primate and equine species and is expressed primarily in the placenta. The LHβ and CGβ genes have different promoters and transcriptional start sites, accounting for their different tissue distribution patterns of expression.[405] LHβ includes a 24–amino acid signal peptide followed by a 121–amino acid mature protein. In contrast, the mature hCGβ protein is 145 amino acids in length and does not include a leader peptide, but contains a 24–amino acid C-terminal extension important for the longer biologic half-life of hCG.[406,407] The FSHβ gene, on chromosome 11, is organized similarly to the other glycoprotein hormone β genes, encoding a mature peptide of 111 amino acids, with two glycosylation sites, and like LHβ, it is expressed only in gonadotrophs.

Regulation

LH and FSH secretion patterns reflect the integration of sensitive complex hypothalamic signals (mediated primarily via GnRH), paracrine intrapituitary factors (primarily activin and follistatin), and peripheral feedback (both gonadal sex steroids and gonadal peptide hormones) (Fig. 8-31).

Gonadotropin-Releasing Hormone. Hypothalamic control of gonadotropin secretion occurs primarily through actions of GnRH. Hypothalamic GnRH neurons represent the pivotal integrators of peripheral signals in regulation of the pituitary-gonadal axis. Insights into the mechanisms that regulate GnRH secretion have been provided by the identification and study of genetic abnormalities in patients

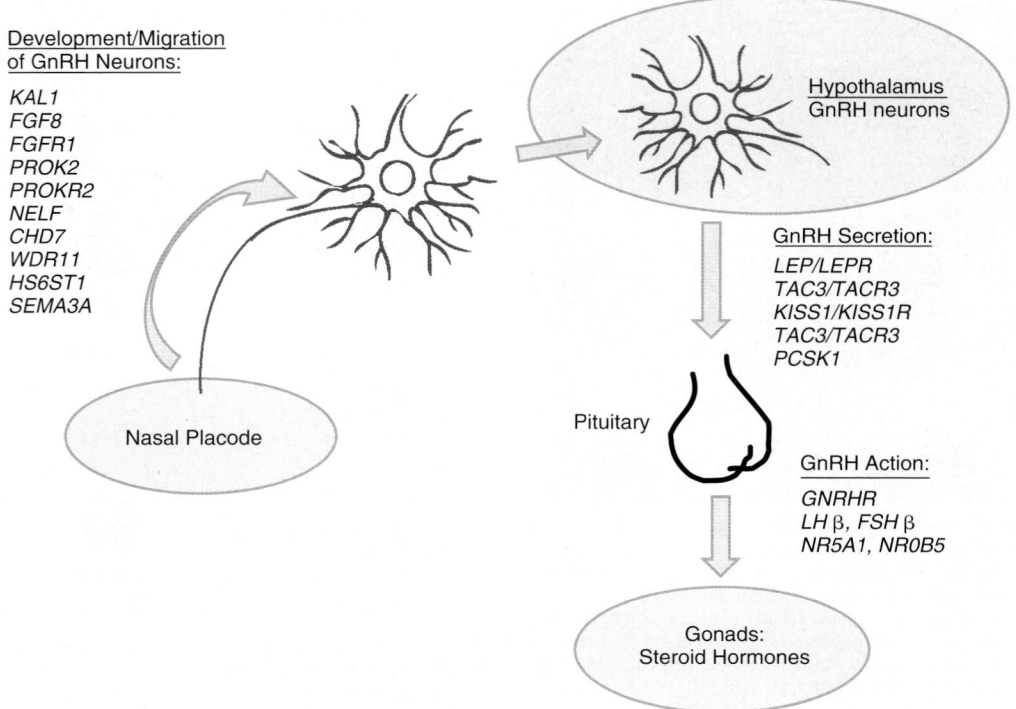

Figure 8-32 Genetic and molecular basis of gonadotropin-releasing hormone (GnRH) neuronal development and migration, GnRH secretion, and GnRH action. (From Bianco SD, Kaiser UB. The genetic and molecular basis of idiopathic hypogonadotrophic hypogonadism. *Nat Rev Endocrinol.* 2009;5:569-576.)

TABLE 8-9

Genetics of Hypogonadotropic Hypogonadism

Phenotype/Mechanism	Gene*	Inheritance	Function
Kallmann syndrome/neuronal development and migration	KAL1[448]	X-linked	Anosmin required for cell surface signaling, adhesion and migration
	FGFR1[408]	AD	Role in axonal development and guidance
	FGF8[409]	AD	Endogenous ligand of FGFR1
	PROK2[410] PROKR2[410]	AD, AR	Development of olfactory bulb and migration of GnRH neurons
	NELF[411]	?	Encoding nasal embryonic LHRH factor
	SEMA3A[457]	AD	Axonal pathfinding
	HS6ST1[412]	AD	Modifications of extracellular sugars
	CHD7[413]	AD	Chromodomain helicase DNA binding protein 7, chromatin remodeling
	WDR11[414]	AD	WD repeat domain protein interacts with transcription factor EMX1
Normosmic hypogonadotropic hypogonadism/GnRH synthesis, secretion, or action	KISS1[415]	AR	Hypothalamic neuropeptide, stimulates GnRH secretion
	KISS1R[419,420]	AR	Receptor for kisspeptin
	TAC3[423]	AR	Encodes neurokinin B, a neuropeptide that stimulates kisspeptin release
	TACR3[423]	AR	Encodes neurokinin B receptor
	LEP[416]	AR	Encodes leptin, derived from adipose tissue to signal adequacy of nutritional status
	LEPR[416]	AR	Encodes leptin receptor
	PCSK1[357]	AR	Processes GnRH
	GNRH1[417,529]	AR	Encodes GnRH
	GNRHR[419]	AR	Receptor for GnRH, stimulation of gonadotropin secretion
	NR5A1	AD	Transcription factor for hypothalamic, pituitary, gonadal, and adrenal development
	NR0B5	X-linked	Transcriptional repressor; hypothalamic, pituitary, gonadal, and adrenal development
	LHB	AR	Encodes luteinizing hormone β-subunit
	FSHB	AR	Encodes follicle-stimulating hormone β-subunit

*Superscript numbers refer to references at the end of this chapter.
AD, autosomal dominant; AR, autosomal recessive; FGF, fibroblast growth factor; GNRH, gonadotropin-releasing hormone; GPR, orphan G protein–coupled receptor; IHH, isolated hypogonadotropic hypogonadism; KAL, Kallmann syndrome; KISS, KiSS metastasis suppressor; LHRH, luteinizing hormone–releasing hormone; NELF, nasal embryonic LHRH factor; PROK, prokineticin.

with pubertal disorders or infertility as well as by the use of animal models. Molecular defects that manifest as GnRH deficiency, or hypogonadotropic hypogonadism (HH), can be classified as defects in GnRH neuronal development, defects in control of GnRH secretion, and defects in GnRH action (Fig. 8-32 and Table 8-9). Conversely, a genetic defect in *MKRN3* was found to cause premature reactivation of GnRH secretion and central precocious puberty. This gene encodes a putative ubiquitin ligase and appears to act as a repressor or inhibitor of GnRH secretion during childhood.[418] Many neurotransmitters directly or indirectly modulate GnRH secretion, including norepinephrine, dopamine, serotonin, GABA, glutamate, opiates, NPY, and galanin, among others. Glutamate and norepinephrine provide stimulatory drive, whereas GABA and opioid peptides are inhibitory. Kisspeptins, encoded by the *KISS1* gene, and their cognate receptor, KISS1R, were identified as key GnRH secretagogues.[419,420] Administration of kisspeptin to normal men increases FSH, LH, and testosterone concentrations, and in normal women the peptide stimulates gonadotropin release most potently during the preovulatory surge.[421] Neurokinin B (NKB), a member of the substance P–related tachykinin family, is coexpressed with kisspeptin in the hypothalamus and appears to act through control of kisspeptin secretion to modulate GnRH release.[422,423] Substance P, another tachykinin family member, has also been shown to modulate GnRH secretion. Leptin, a product of peripheral adipose tissue, is a positive regulator of the HPG axis. This adipokine enables a pivotal link between body fat and reproduction, signaling energy availability centrally.[424] Nutritional, metabolic, stress, and circadian inputs all appear to act through these peptides to modulate GnRH, gonadotropin secretion, and the activity of the HPG axis.[418]

The hallmark of hypothalamic GnRH secretion is the pulsatile rather than continuous release into the hypophyseal portal circulation, resulting in episodic stimulation of the gonadotroph.[425] In patients with GnRH deficiency, restoration of gonadotropin secretion can be achieved after exogenous pulsatile GnRH treatment, whereas continuous GnRH exposure suppresses gonadotropin secretion.[426] GnRH signaling initiates with recognition by its cognate receptor, GnRHR, which belongs to the rhodopsin G protein–coupled receptor family. GnRHR activation increases calcium mobilization and stimulates influx of extracellular calcium to induce pituitary LH and FSH secretion.[427] The pattern of GnRH signaling is important in determining the quantity and quality of gonadotropins secreted[428,429] (Fig. 8-33). The amplitude, frequency, and contour of GnRH pulses can all vary, and each of these characteristics can influence gonadotroph responses, providing a mechanism for the differential synthesis and secretion of the two gonadotropins, LH and FSH. These alterations in GnRH pulse pattern are one mechanism by which two functionally distinct gonadotropins can be differentially regulated by a single hypothalamic-releasing hormone.

Inhibins and Activins. The hypothesis that a peptide of gonadal origin selectively regulates FSH secretion dates back to at least 1932.[430] It took over 50 years to isolate and characterize the structure of inhibin and its related peptides.[431] Inhibin-related peptides, members of the transforming growth factor-β family, are dimeric proteins covalently linked by a disulfide bridge and consisting of a common α-subunit and one of two highly homologous β-subunits, β_A or β_B (Fig. 8-34). In addition, the β-subunits can form dimers, called activins, to stimulate FSH synthesis and secretion.[432] A structurally unrelated, monomeric polypeptide, follistatin, was also identified, based on its ability to inhibit FSH.[432,433] These three peptides (inhibins, activins, and follistatin) are considered to be relatively selective for FSH in terms of their effects on gonadotropins and serve as an additional mechanism for the differential control of FSH and LH. Although inhibins act primarily as classic circulating endocrine hormones, originating in the gonads and acting on the pituitary to regulate FSH, activins play an important role as regulators of growth and differentiation in diverse tissues and are produced and act locally in the pituitary as autocrine/paracrine factors. In the human male, inhibin B is produced in the testes in response to FSH stimulation and circulates systemically to provide feedback inhibition of FSH. In women, inhibin A is secreted by dominant ovarian follicles and corpora lutea, contributing to the high circulating levels during the late follicular and luteal phases. Inhibin B is reciprocally elevated during the late luteal and early follicular phases of the menstrual cycle.

Activin receptors are heteromeric complexes comprising type I (ActRI) and type II (ActRII) serine-threonine kinase receptors. Activin binds to the type II receptors, thereby increasing association with the type I receptor and stimulating its phosphorylation, which in turn results in the activation by phosphorylation of intracellular signaling Smad proteins, resulting in translocation of the Smad complex to the nucleus, where it binds to gene regulatory elements and interacts with other transcription factors (such as FoxL2) to regulate gene transcription, thereby influencing cell fate and function.[33] Follistatin and inhibin act as extracellular modulators of activin through distinct mechanisms.[434] Follistatin, an activin-binding protein, inhibits activin action by interfering with activin binding to its receptor. Inhibins compete for binding to type II activin receptors, preventing recruitment of type I receptors and thereby blocking activin signaling. Additional

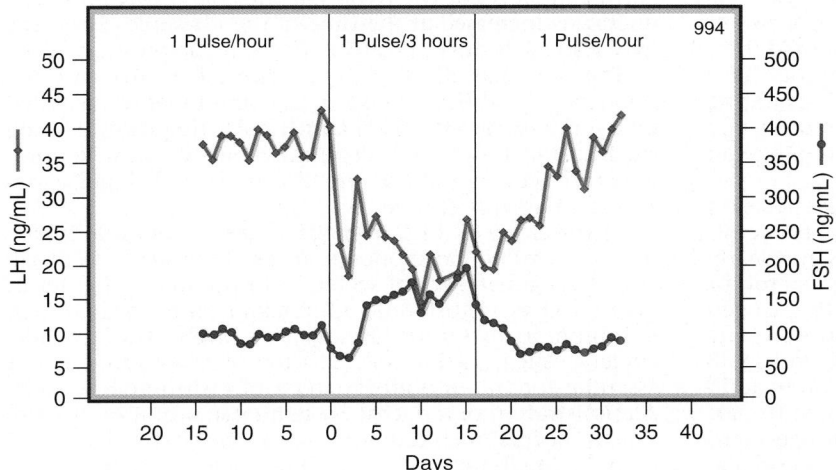

Figure 8-33 Knobil's experiments: the frequency of pulsatile gonadotropin-releasing hormone (GnRH) administration has differential effects on gonadotropin secretion—more rapid GnRH pulse frequencies favor luteinizing hormone (LH) secretion, whereas slower pulse frequencies favor follicle-stimulating hormone (FSH). (From Wildt L, Hausler A, Marshall G, et al. Frequency and amplitude of gonadotropin-releasing hormone stimulation and gonadotropin secretion in the rhesus monkey. *Endocrinology.* 1981;109:376-385.)

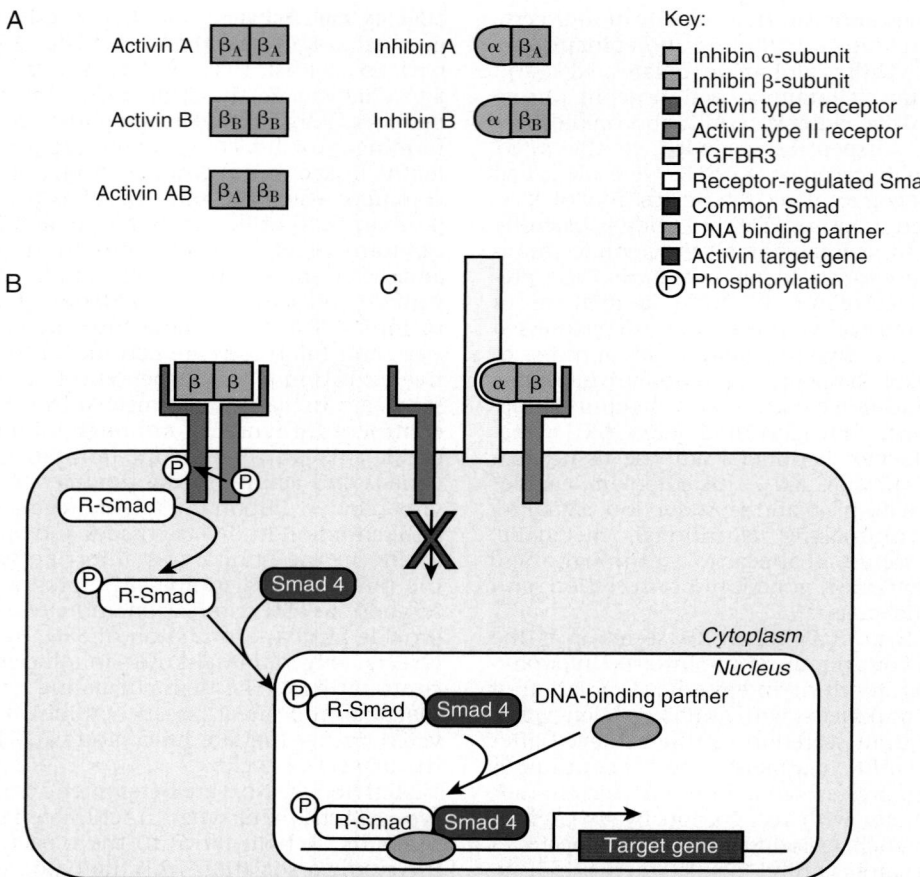

Figure 8-34 Activins and inhibins and their mechanism of action. **A,** Inhibins and activins are dimeric proteins made up of two subunits. Inhibins are made up of an α-subunit linked to one of two β-subunits, whereas activins are made up by dimerization of two β-subunits. **B,** Activin signaling pathway. Activins bind to specific sets of serine–threonine kinase type I and type II receptors on the cell surface. Upon ligand binding, the type II receptor phosphorylates and thereby activates the type I receptor, which in turn phosphorylates downstream signaling molecules, the receptor-regulated S-Smads (R-Smads). Once phosphorylated, the R-Smads associate with the common co-Smad (Smad 4) and translocate to the nucleus where, in combination with cell type–specific binding partners, they bind to the promoter sequences of target genes to regulate gene transcription and cellular function. **C,** Inhibins bind to activin type II receptors and block the recruitment of type I receptors, thereby blocking R-Smad activation and activin signaling. The presence of TGFBR3, a TGF-β superfamily accessory receptor also known as betaglycan, enhances the binding of inhibins to type II receptors, thereby enhancing the antagonistic actions of inhibins. (From Stenvers KL, Findlay JK. Inhibins: from reproductive hormones to tumor suppressors. *Trends Endocrinol Metab.* 2010;21:174-180.)

extracellular and intracellular proteins and mechanisms also serve to modulate the local activin signal.

Sex Steroids. Gonadal steroid hormones include estrogens, progesterones, and androgens. Effects on gonadotropins occur both directly at the level of the gonadotroph and indirectly via effects at the hypothalamus that modulate GnRH secretion. Estrogen, androgen, and progesterone receptors have been identified in gonadotrophs, consistent with direct actions of these peripheral sex steroid hormones. Within the hypothalamus, these receptors have been identified in multiple neuronal cell types, suggesting that alterations in GnRH release largely occur indirectly through modulation of neuronal systems that impinge on GnRH neurons.

In women, estrogens can exert dual feedback effects on gonadotropin secretion, depending on the reproductive state. The negative feedback effects of estrogens are clearly demonstrated by the elevated LH and FSH levels that follow ovariectomy or menopause but that reverse with estrogen replacement. Negative feedback effects of estrogens are observed at the level of α-subunit and at LHβ and FSHβ mRNA levels through effects on gene transcription in addition to effects on LH and FSH secretion, mediated in part directly at the level of the pituitary gland. Estrogen also has negative feedback effects at the levels of the hypothala-

mus, mediated in large part through effects on kisspeptin neurons.[435] On the other hand, during the late follicular phase of the menstrual cycle, the feedback effects of estrogens shift from negative to positive, triggering the midcycle ovulatory surge of LH and FSH secretion. Positive feedback effects of estrogen are mediated at least in large part at the level of the hypothalamus, as GnRH pulse frequency is increased at the time of the LH surge. Estrogens may also elicit direct positive effects at the pituitary level.

The principal effect of progesterone is to decrease the frequency of gonadotropin pulses, presumably mediated by hypothalamic effects on GnRH pulse frequency. During the luteal phase of the human menstrual cycle, when progesterone concentrations are the highest, LH pulse frequency markedly slowed.

Testosterone and its aromatized derivative estradiol are the two steroid hormones that exert negative feedback effects on gonadotropin secretion in the male. The net in vivo effect of testosterone administration to normal men is inhibition of serum LH and FSH levels. The available evidence suggests that 5α-reduction of testosterone is not essential for the inhibitory effects of testosterone on LH. Administration of a potent 5α-reductase inhibitor, finasteride, to normal men did not result in elevated LH and FSH levels.[436] Much like the effects of estrogen, these inhibitory effects are felt to occur largely at the hypothalamic level, by kisspeptin neurons, mediated by both androgen and estrogen receptors (AR and ERα). Mechanisms for testosterone feedback are complex, as testosterone also exerts a stimulatory effect on FSHβ mRNA levels.[437]

Secretion

In light of the episodic, pulsatile nature of LH and FSH secretion, there was a need to develop discrete pulse-detection algorithms. Santen and Bardin developed an algorithm that defined a peak as a 20% increase in the hormone concentration in a single sample over the preceding sample, which was subsequently modified to define the pulse based on a chosen multiple of the assay coefficient of variation. Because of its simplicity of use and apparent freedom from assumptions, this program is still widely used, although a number of refinements and alternative algorithms have also been developed. Application of deconvolution to pulse analysis made it possible to determine the instantaneous real-time secretory rates. The characteristic secretory episodes characterized for LH and FSH indicate daily production rates of 1000 IU and 200 IU, respectively, and a disappearance half-life of 90 and 500 minutes for each respective β-subunit.[438,439] The longer circulating half-life of FSH makes the pulsatile secretory pattern of this gonadotropin less clear than that of LH, although differences in secretory pathways for FSH and LH may also contribute.[440]

Action

The primary targets of FSH and LH are the gonads, and thus, targets and effects differ in the male and female (Fig. 8-35). The actions of FSH and LH in the male and female are presented briefly here but are discussed in greater detail in Chapters 17 and 18.

Female. FSH acts on FSH receptors in granulosa cells to facilitate follicular growth and estradiol biosynthesis (see Fig. 8-35).[441] The initiation of follicular growth can occur independently of gonadotropin stimulation, after which further maturation requires FSH. At these more advanced stages of development, follicles convert theca cell–derived androstenedione to estradiol (E2) by the induction of aromatase activity in response to FSH.[442] FSH also controls granulosa cell production of inhibin during the follicular phase and induces LH receptor expression in granulosa cells of large preovulatory follicles. At the same time that FSH promotes the development of the dominant follicle, it also initiates the recruitment of the next generation of follicles that will enlarge during subsequent cycles.

LH, acting on LH receptors in ovarian theca cells, is a major regulator of ovarian steroid synthesis. LH stimulates estrogen production by promoting synthesis of androgen precursors in theca cells, which then diffuse into neighboring granulosa cells, where they are aromatized into estrogens under the control of FSH.[407] LH increases cholesterol availability for ovarian steroidogenesis by inducing the steroidogenic acute regulatory (StAR) protein,[443] which mediates cholesterol transfer from the outer to the inner membrane, where it becomes available for steroidogenesis. LH also enhances cytochrome P450-linked enzyme activity to synthesize pregnenolone and induces synthesis of 3β-hydroxysteroid dehydrogenase, 17α-hydroxylase, and 17,20-lyase. The midcycle LH surge stimulates resumption of oocyte meiosis and maturation in the preovulatory follicle, initiates the rupture of the ovulatory follicle and ovulation, and induces conversion of the follicle wall into the corpus luteum (luteinization).[441,442] LH stimulates the expression of progesterone receptors in the granulosa cells of the dominant follicle, which promotes luteinization. In addition, LH helps to sustain luteinization by stimulating progesterone synthesis.

Male. LH acts on LH receptors in Leydig cells to induce intratesticular testosterone synthesis, mediated by enhanced cAMP production. FSH in the male is involved in spermatogenesis (see Fig. 8-35), although the precise role in the spermatogenic process remains unclear.[444] FSH binds to FSH receptors on Sertoli cells and stimulates the production of inhibins, androgen-binding protein, androgen receptor, and other proteins. FSH mediates the maturation of spermatids into mature spermatozoa in concert with testosterone.[445]

Gonadotropin Assays

Because of the high homology of the glycoprotein hormones, development of highly specific assays, especially those distinguishing free α-subunit from intact hormones, has been challenging. Heterogeneity of circulating LH and FSH molecules, insufficient assay sensitivity to distinguish normal from low levels, and lack of rigorously pure reference preparations have hampered assay development. Two-site–directed immunofluorometric and immunochemiluminescent LH and FSH assays have much improved sensitivity, are able to detect LH with a sensitivity of 0.1 mIU/mL, and have resolved prior challenges with cross-reactivity.[446] Differences in carbohydrate moieties result in isoelectric charge heterogeneity for LH, accounting for some observed disparities in biologic and immunoreactive LH ratios observed after GnRH agonist treatment, acute critical illness, or aging.

α-Subunit Assays. Both GnRH and TRH increase circulating levels of free α-subunit derived from either gonadotrophs or thyrotrophs, especially in patients with hypothyroidism, after castration, and during menopause. GnRH agonist treatment, TSH-secreting tumors, or nonfunctioning pituitary adenomas may result in discordant circulating ratios of free α-subunit from intact LH dimers.

GnRH Stimulation Test. A single bolus of GnRH (25-100 µg) dose-dependently evokes serum LH and FSH levels within 20 and 30 minutes. LH rises more abundantly than FSH,

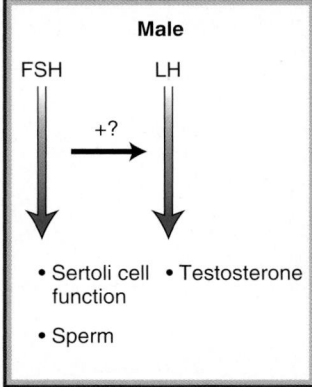
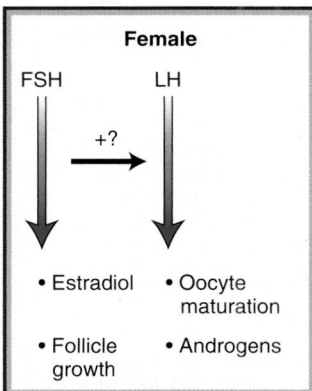

Figure 8-35 Actions of follicle-stimulating hormone (FSH) and luteinizing hormone (LH) in the male and female. The plus signs and horizontal arrows indicate potentially unrecognized new functions of FSH since the discovery of FSHβ gene mutations. (Modified from Layman LC. Genetics of human hypogonadotropic hypogonadism. *Am J Med Genet (Semin Med Genet)*. 1999;89:240-248; Richards JS, Pangas SA. The ovary: basic biology and clinical implications. *J Clin Invest*. 2010;120:963-972; and Bhasin S, Fisher CE, Sverdloff RS. Follicle-stimulating hormone and luteinizing hormone. In: Melmed S, ed. *The Pituitary*, 2nd ed. Malden, MA: Blackwell Science; 2002:216-278.)

and peak values range from 8 to 34 mIU/mL. In contrast, patients with HH and no demonstrable hypothalamic-pituitary lesion have blunted LH responses and reversal of the LH:FSH ratio. The test, however, cannot adequately distinguish hypothalamic from pituitary lesions, and similar patterns are observed in patients with anorexia nervosa. Repetitive GnRH pulses may in fact normalize responses, as would be expected from an intact hypothalamic-pituitary unit. GnRH responses may vary during the stages of puberty, reflecting altered pituitary sensitivity. This test is most frequently used in the assessment of pubertal status, for the diagnosis of HH, or for evaluation of central precocious puberty.[447]

Clomiphene Stimulation Test. Clomiphene (100 mg), administered daily for up to 4 weeks, usually doubles LH levels, but FSH increases by about 50% over baseline. Because an abnormal or absent response does not distinguish hypothalamic from pituitary lesions, the utility of this test is limited.

Gonadotropin Deficiency

Causes. Gonadotropin deficiency may be congenital or acquired and may arise from hypothalamic or pituitary disorders. Congenital causes include gene mutations governing the processes of development and migration of GnRH neurons, the control of GnRH secretion, the development of the gonadotroph, or the regulation of LH and FSH secretion. Acquired HH may arise from functional or organic disorders. Functional causes are frequently encountered and include stress, malnutrition, chronic illness, depression, excessive exercise, and low body weight. Several centrally acting drugs including opiates, glucocorticoids, sex steroids, GnRH agonists and antagonists, tranquilizers, antidepressants, and antipsychotic medications suppress gonadotropin secretion, either directly or indirectly via induction of hyperprolactinemia. Organic causes include malignant disease, developmental disorders, tumors, infiltrative disease, trauma, and hypothalamic or pituitary damage from surgery or radiotherapy. Congenital and acquired causes of central hypogonadism are considered more fully in Chapters 23 to 25.

Hypogonadotropic Hypogonadism. The genetic basis of HH was recognized over 60 years ago with the description by Kallmann of hypogonadism and anosmia in two families. It was not until 1991 that anosmin, a glycoprotein encoded by the *KAL1* gene, was identified as a cause of X-linked Kallmann syndrome.[448] The realization that *KAL1* gene defects only accounted for a small proportion of patients with classic Kallmann syndrome has led to genotype-phenotype studies that have provided important insights into the molecular genetics underlying HH. Gene mutations affecting the olfactory bulb and GnRH neuronal migration tend to give rise to the Kallmann phenotype. Multiple genetic defects have been associated with Kallmann syndrome, which in many cases can be distinguished clinically based on well-established nonreproductive phenotypes. On the other hand, defects in genes involved in regulating GnRH secretion or GnRH action are usually associated with normosmia, and in some cases the clinical phenotype is solely that of isolated HH (for details, see Table 8-9 and Fig. 8-32).

Kallmann Syndrome. Kallmann syndrome consists of defective GnRH neuronal development, with olfactory nerve agenesis or hypoplasia and variable anosmia. Associated developmental disorders include optic atrophy, color blindness, sensorineural deafness, cleft palate, renal agenesis, cryptorchidism, and movement disorders.[449] This X-linked recessive disorder has been ascribed to a defective *KAL1* gene located on chromosome Xp22.3.[450] The encoded anosmin protein mediates hypothalamic migration of GnRH cells from the primitive olfactory placode, and its absence leads to defective GnRH synthesis and anosmia.[451,452] Both autosomal recessive and dominant forms of the disorder have since been described, with multiple additional genetic causes identified (see Table 8-9 and Fig. 8-32).

These patients are exposed to low or absent sex steroids from birth. Consequently, females are tall and present with primary amenorrhea and absent secondary sexual development and males have delayed puberty and micropenis.[453] Absent GnRH secretory pulses result in characteristically low LH and FSH levels in the face of very low concentrations of estradiol or testosterone. Because the nonprimed normal pituitary may not respond initially to GnRH stimulation, this test is of little value in distinguishing a hypothalamic from a pituitary defect. In some patients, repetitive GnRH priming may elicit pituitary LH and FSH responses, indicating a hypothalamic defect in GnRH secretion.

Prader-Willi Syndrome. These patients have marked hyperphagia and obesity with retarded mental development, muscle hypotonia, and diabetes mellitus.[454] The condition results from the absence of expression of genes on the paternally inherited chromosome 15q11.2-q13, which can arise from deletions, maternal uniparental disomy, or rare imprinting center defects. Patients usually have hypogonadism, which can be primary or hypothalamic in origin, and premature adrenarche and central precocious puberty have also been reported in a subset of patients.[455] Interestingly, the gene implicated in central precocious puberty, *MKRN3*, lies within the Prader-Willi syndrome critical region on chromosome 15.[418] Other endocrine abnormalities commonly associated with Prader-Willi syndrome include type 2 diabetes, GHD, central hypothyroidism, and central adrenal insufficiency.[456]

Clinical Features. Gonadotropin deficiency causes hypogonadism with decreased sex steroid production of varying degree, depending upon the severity of the insult (Table 8-10). This disorder may occur at any stage of life. In its

---

TABLE 8-10
Clinical Features of Hypogonadotropism

Prepubertal Onset

High-pitched voice
Absent terminal facial hair
Decreased or absent body hair
Eunuchoidal body proportions
Female escutcheon
Testicular volume < 6 cm³
Testicular length < 2.5 cm
Cryptorchidism may be present
Penile length < 5 cm
Hypopigmented scrotum with absent rugae
Small prostate
Decreased libido
Decreased muscle and bone mass

Postpubertal Onset

Decreased libido
Decreased spontaneous erections
Slow beard growth
Decreased body hair
Testicular atrophy if long-standing
Decreased muscle and bone mass

Normal
Voice pitch
Skeletal proportions
Penis length
Scrotal rugae
Prostate size

congenital form, primary amenorrhea and total absence of development of secondary sexual characteristics may occur. Onset later in life may present with a varying spectrum of reproductive dysfunction, ranging from luteal phase abnormalities with subfertility to oligomenorrhea or amenorrhea in women. Women exhibit secondary amenorrhea, infertility, decreased vaginal secretion, dyspareunia, hot flashes, decreased bone density, and breast tissue atrophy.

Males with congenital HH have small testes (<4 mL) and absence of secondary sexual characteristics. Tall stature with eunuchoid habitus may be present as a result of delayed or absent epiphyseal closure. Cryptorchidism and microphallus may be present, reflecting the absence of activity of the HPG axis during fetal development.[457] Men with gonadotropin deficiency later in life present with loss of libido, potency, and fertility. They may have impotence, testicular atrophy, decreased libido, low energy, infertility, loss of secondary sexual characteristics, decreased muscle strength and mass, decreased bone mass, decreased facial and body hair, and fine facial wrinkling.[458]

In both men and women, serum gonadotropin levels are inappropriately low in the face of decreased sex steroid levels. In women with amenorrhea or oligomenorrhea, serum LH, FSH, and estradiol levels should be measured. Endogenous estrogen sufficiency can also be assessed by the response to a progesterone challenge (100 mg intramuscularly or 10 mg medroxyprogesterone acetate orally daily for 5-10 days). Men should have serum LH, FSH, and testosterone levels measured in a morning sample.

Hypothalamic and pituitary disorders are the most common endocrine cause of male subfertility. Because normal secretion of both FSH and LH is required for quantitatively and qualitatively normal spermatogenesis, any disease that affects hypothalamic secretion of GnRH or pituitary secretion of FSH or LH will impair spermatogenesis.[459] As FSH is required for normal spermatogenesis, isolated FSH deficiency is associated with oligospermia or azoospermia. Men with inactivating FSHβ mutations are azoospermic, but some have normal puberty associated with normal to low-normal testosterone levels and high LH levels, whereas another presented with a low testosterone concentration and absent puberty.[460-462] Inactivating FSHβ mutations have also been characterized in women and resulted in a phenotype of delayed puberty, absent or incomplete breast development, primary amenorrhea, and infertility, with low levels of estradiol and progesterone, undetectable FSH, and high LH.[460,461]

Mutations that abolish the activity of LH, resulting in isolated LH deficiency, have also been reported.[463,464] Isolated LH deficiency in males may manifest with delayed or absent puberty, with eunuchoidal body proportions as a result of low testosterone levels. Low LH levels in these patients lead to low intratesticular testosterone concentrations with resultant decreased spermatogenesis. A female with isolated LH deficiency due to an LH mutation had normal pubertal development and menarche but secondary amenorrhea and infertility.

Management. The goals of therapy are to replace or restore sex steroid hormones and to induce and maintain normal reproductive function. If fertility is not an immediate objective, sex steroid hormone replacement is usually sufficient. For induction of gametogenesis in those desiring fertility, therapy with gonadotropins or GnRH is usually required.

Evaluation. In evaluating hypogonadal patients in the absence of an obvious pituitary or gonadal disorder, the primary diagnostic challenge is to distinguish constitutional pubertal delay from other causes of hypogonadotropism.[331,465] When puberty is delayed after 14 years of age,

a primary developmental disorder, HH, should be considered in the absence of acquired causes. Cryptorchidism or micropenis are suggestive of congenital HH, whereas low patient height relative to the parent's height suggests constitutional delay of puberty (CDP) rather than congenital HH, in which height tends to be normal or even increased, and possibly with eunuchoidal proportions. No single test clearly distinguishes constitutional delayed puberty and true HH, and expectant follow-up is often helpful as many patients enter puberty spontaneously. To enable androgenization, testosterone replacement should be provided intermittently until age 18, with periodic interruptions to unmask physiologic pubertal advance.

Sex Steroid Replacement Therapy. Estrogen or testosterone replacement is required for inducing and maintaining primary and secondary sexual characteristics, to minimize cardiovascular risk factors, and to maintain normal body composition and integrity of BMD and muscle mass. For patients not seeking fertility, sex steroid therapy is warranted to correct central hypogonadism. However, monitoring of LH and FSH responses does not accurately reflect adequate steroid hormonal replacement, as basal gonadotropin levels are already low or undetectable.

Estrogens are available as a tablet, patch, gel, or implant. Initiation of puberty can begin with any type or route of exogenous estrogen, oral or transdermal. One traditional regimen that has been used is conjugated equine estrogens, beginning with 0.3 mg/day and increasing gradually and progressively to the lowest dose that produces normal menses, or up to 1.25 mg/day. Initial therapy should consist of estrogen alone to maximize breast growth and to induce uterine and endometrial proliferation. Initiation of puberty with transdermal 17β-estradiol, 0.08 to 0.12 µg/kg body weight, is an alternative regimen. A progestin eventually needs to be added to prevent endometrial hyperplasia but should be avoided before completion of breast development, because it is likely to reduce ultimate breast size. In premenopausal women, oral estrogens or transdermal estradiol delivering 50 to 100 mg daily can be used, with concomitant cyclic progesterone therapy (e.g., medroxyprogesterone acetate 5-10 mg) for women with an intact uterus to prevent unopposed endometrial proliferation. Although early sex steroid replacement lessens the risk of developing osteoporosis, effects of estrogen replacement on cardiovascular function are unresolved. In patients with hypopituitarism, estrogen replacement should be maintained until the age of 50, whereafter continuation should be determined on an individual basis by assessing risks and benefits, especially in terms of bone mineral integrity, cardiovascular function, and cancer risk. Estrogen treatment may be associated with thromboembolic disease, breast tenderness, and possibly enhanced risk for breast cancer.

For men, androgen replacement is available as intramuscular gel, patch, or oral preparations. Intramuscular injection of testosterone enanthate or testosterone cypionate is usually administered at 200- to 300-mg doses every 2 or 3 weeks.[458] Administration of lower doses on a more frequent basis (e.g., 100 mg weekly) may stabilize fluctuations of hormone levels. Elderly males require lower doses, as do boys with delayed puberty. Testosterone undecanoate provides long-term replacement for 3 to 4 months after each injection with improved pharmacokinetic profiles, but rare cases of pulmonary oil microembolism and anaphylaxis have been reported, and it must be administered in an office or hospital setting by a trained health care provider and the patient monitored for 30 minutes afterward for adverse reactions. Transdermal testosterone patch and gel systems deliver 4 to 6 mg and sustain testosterone profiles.

Patch sites may develop skin irritation, blisters, and vesicles in approximately 25% of patients.[466] There is no apparent cost-benefit advantage of patch delivery over intramuscular injection. Oral androgen replacement therapy is generally not recommended because of nonuniform absorption and hepatotoxicity. Testosterone may cause acne, gynecomastia, prostatic hypertrophy, and polycythemia. Although there is no compelling evidence that testosterone replacement causes prostate cancer, benign prostatic hypertrophy can be exacerbated, especially in elderly patients. Testosterone replacement should not be administered to men with diagnosed prostate cancer. Target serum hormone levels, which benefit lean mass, muscle strength, and sexual function without inducing undesirable adverse consequences, vary, and in the future, individual targets may guide the treatment of hypogonadism in men.[467]

Fertility. In patients with HH, fertility may be achieved with gonadotropin or GnRH therapy. In males, even relatively low sperm counts may be adequate for impregnation when fertility is induced by gonadotropins or GnRH. As testosterone therapy may suppress spermatogenesis, the steroid should be discontinued prior to initiating treatment. Partial rather than complete hypogonadism predicts a more favorable response to treatment, whereas persistence of cryptorchidism beyond the age of 1 year reduces the likelihood of successful fertility induction. hCG is administered subcutaneously or intramuscularly (1000-2000 IU two to three times weekly) to induce spermatogenesis, with the dose titrated according to testosterone levels.[468] If necessary, after 6 months, human menopausal gonadotropin (hMG) or purified FSH (75 IU three times weekly) should be added to improve sperm quantity, and doses may be doubled after a further 6 months. An increase in testicular volume correlates well with induction of spermatogenesis. If testosterone levels are increased, subsequent conversion to estradiol may result, leading to gynecomastia, oily skin, and acne. Therefore, both testosterone and estradiol levels should be monitored.

Pulsatile GnRH therapy is an alternative treatment for patients with normal pituitary function (i.e., those with idiopathic HH or Kallmann syndrome). GnRH is infused subcutaneously by continuous mini-pump (5 mg every 2 hours), with the dose titrated to maintain normal gonadotropin and testosterone levels. This approach may be marginally more effective than treatment with gonadotropins and may cause less gynecomastia. These approaches require strong patient commitment, as adequate spermatogenesis may not be attained for 2 years or longer despite normalized testosterone levels. Aliquots of successfully generated sperm samples should be frozen for future impregnation.

Clomiphene citrate is a weak estrogen receptor antagonist that stimulates gonadotropin secretion in normal women and men. Clomiphene has been used to increase spermatogenesis in men with partial hypogonadotropism with oligospermia or azoospermia and normal to mildly low serum testosterone concentrations, particularly in men with functional hypogonadism, with variable results.

In women with HH, fertility may be effectively achieved by pulsatile GnRH administration or by gonadotropin therapy (fully discussed in Chapter 17). Although ovulation is often induced and pregnancy achieved by gonadotropin treatment, a high rate of multiple follicle development remains a concern.[469] If residual pituitary gonadotroph reserve is sufficiently robust, GnRH therapy is more likely to result in ovulation of a single rather than multiple follicles, thereby reducing the chances of multiple gestation.[470] Therapy with kisspeptin or kisspeptin analogues is an area of current investigation, and holds promise

for further reducing the chances of multiple gestation or the risks of ovarian hyperstimulation[471] (see Chapter 17).

Thyroid-Stimulating Hormone
Physiology

The hypothalamic-pituitary-thyroid system plays a critical role in development, growth, and cellular metabolism with thyroid hormone availability and action controlled by complex mechanisms at the tissue level.

Thyrotroph Cells. Thyrotroph cells comprise approximately 5% of the functional anterior pituitary cells and are situated predominantly in the anteromedial areas of the gland. They are smaller than the other cell types and are irregularly shaped with flattened nuclei and relatively small secretory granules ranging from 120 to 150 μm (Figs. 8-36 and 8-37).

Structure. TSH is a glycoprotein hormone comprising a 28-kDa heterodimer of two noncovalently linked α- and β-subunits.[472] The tertiary TSH structure comprises three hairpin loops separated by central disulfide bonds, with the longer loop straddling one side.[473,474] The α-subunit is common to TSH, LH, FSH, and hCG, whereas the β-subunit is unique and confers specificity of action.[475] The α-subunit is the earliest hormone gene expressed embryonically, but activation of the β-subunit gene occurs later under the influence of GATA2 and Pit1.[476] The 13.5-kb α-subunit gene is located on chromosome 6 and comprises four exons and three introns.[477] Although the α-subunit gene is expressed in thyrotroph, gonadotroph, and placental cells, its regulation is uniquely cell-specific. The downstream promoter region (−200 and below) is required for placental expression, intermediate sequences are required for gonadotroph expression, and upstream promoter elements are required for thyrotroph-specific expression.[478] α-Subunit transcription is inhibited by triiodothyronine (T$_3$) at regions close

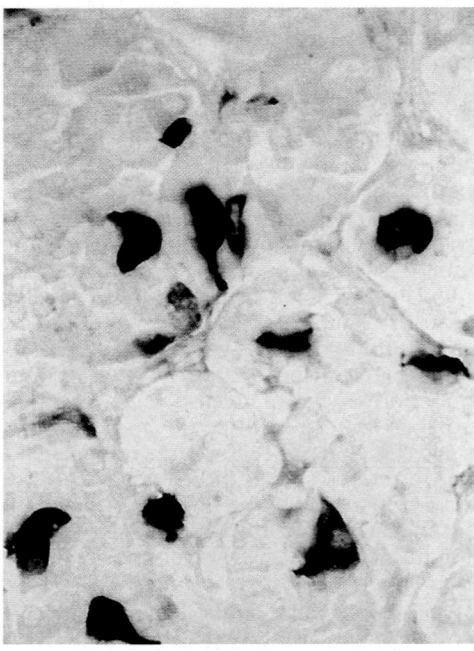

Figure 8-36 Normal thyrotrophs have angular cell bodies with elongated processes. (From Asa SL. Tumors of the pituitary gland. In: Rosai J, ed. *Atlas of Tumor Pathology,* Series III, Fascicle 22. Washington, DC: Armed Forces Institute of Pathology; 1997:19.)

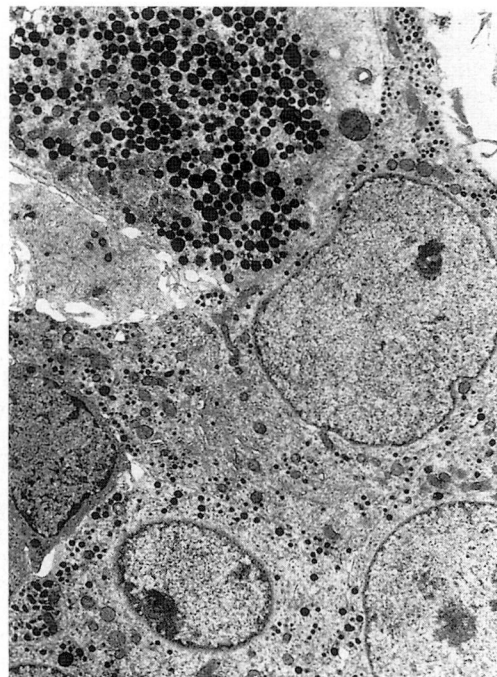

Figure 8-37 Electron micrograph of normal thyrotrophs shows angular cell bodies with elongated processes. (From Asa SL. Tumors of the pituitary gland. In: Rosai J, ed. *Atlas of Tumor Pathology*, Series III, Fascicle 22. Washington, DC: Armed Forces Institute of Pathology; 1997:19.)

to the transcriptional initiation site, in concert with other nuclear corepressors.[479] The 4.9-kb TSH β-subunit gene located on chromosome 1 comprises three exons and two introns.[480] Pit-1 binds directly to the gene promoter to confer tissue-specific expression.[481] TSH-β gene transcription is suppressed by the thyroid hormone receptor (TR) acting directly on exon 1.[482] This potent suppression is evident within 30 minutes of T_3 exposure and is a critical determinant of TSH synthesis and ultimate secretion. Both α- and β-TSH subunit gene transcription are induced by TRH and suppressed by dopamine.[483] Intrapituitary TSH is stored in secretory granules and the mature hormone is released primarily in response to hypothalamic TRH.

Production of the mature heterodimeric TSH molecule requires complex cotranslational glycosylation and folding of nascent α- and β-subunits.[475] After subunit translation and signal peptide cleavage, glycosylation occurs at asparagine 23 on the β-subunit and at two asparagine residues, 52 and 78, on the α-subunit.[484] Appropriate glycosylation is required for accurate molecular folding and subsequent combination of α- and β-subunits within the rough endoplasmic reticulum and Golgi apparatus. Both TRH and T_3 regulate TSH glycosylation, albeit in opposite directions. TRH exposure or T_3 deprivation enhances oligosaccharide addition to the TSH molecule.[485]

Secretion

Daily TSH production is approximately 100 to 400 mU[486] with a calculated circulating half-life of approximately 50 minutes. Secretion rates are enhanced up to 15-fold in hypothyroidism and are suppressed in hyperthyroidism. The degree of TSH glycosylation determines both metabolic clearance rate as well as bioactivity, and in hypothyroidism, the molecule appears highly sialylated, enhancing bioactivity.[484] Immunoreactive fetal pituitary TSH is detect-

able by 12 weeks. Immediately after full-term birth, there is a brisk rise in TSH, which remains elevated for up to 5 days before stabilizing at adult levels.[487] TSH secretion is pulsatile; however, the low pulse amplitudes and long TSH half-life result in modest circulating variances that are amplified in hypothyroidism and abrogated in critical illness.[488] Secretory pulses every 2 to 3 hours are interspersed with periods of tonic, nonpulsatile TSH secretion.[489] Circadian TSH secretion peaks between 11 PM and 5 AM, mainly due to increased pulse amplitude that is not sleep-entrained.[490] The 24-hour TSH secretion is stable and robust and not influenced by sex, body mass index, and age.[491] Thyroid hormones suppress tonic TSH secretion and pulse amplitude.

Regulation

The TRH neuron plays a central role in determining the set-point of the hypothalamic-pituitary thyroid axis by regulating pituitary TSH release.[492] Three main neuronal groups mediate the effects of other physiologic stimuli on hypothalamic TRH neurons, which are located in the paraventricular nucleus. The first is adrenergic input from the medulla that mediates the stimulatory effects of cold exposure on the TRH neuron. Catecholamines increase the set-point for inhibition of TRH gene expression by T_3, permitting high circulating levels of thyroid hormone to contribute to increased thermogenesis.[493] Second, TRH neurons receive projections from the arcuate nucleus that contain two leptin-responsive groups regulating energy homeostasis: the POMC system that promotes weight loss and the NPY/agouti-related protein (AGRP) system that promotes weight gain.[493] Fasting results in reduction of TRH expression, which is mediated by suppression of the POMC system and stimulation of the NPY/AGRP system. Third, the hypothalamic dorsomedial nucleus projects to the paraventricular nucleus and represents alternative pathways by which leptin acts to regulate TRH neurons.[493]

Feedback regulation by thyroid hormones on TRH and TSH are elaborated through a complex system of paracrine control. The effects of thyroid hormones are mediated by thyroid hormone receptors (TRs), which are members of a superfamily of nuclear hormone receptors. TRs exist as two major isoforms, TRα and TRβ. TRα is the key TR isoform responsible for T_3-mediated negative-feedback regulation by hypophysiotropic TRH neurons.[473] The local availability of T_3, is determined by deiodinase 2 and deiodinase 3, respectively, which provides and deactivates T_3.[492]

Deiodinase 2 is expressed in surrounding glial cells of the hypothalamus[494] and in tanycytes (lining the third ventricles), which generate T_3 from circulating thyroxine (T_4). Tanycytes appear to be the main contributor to the negative feedback regulation of the hypothalamic-pituitary-thyroid axis.[492] The expression by the TRH neuron of deiodinase 3, which inactivates T_3, points to the existence of an important local level of TRH regulation. T_3 suppresses hypothalamic TRH synthesis and decreases pituitary TRH receptor number.

In the anterior pituitary gland, deiodinase 2 is found in folliculo-stellate cells, whereas TRs and deiodinase 3 are expressed in thyrotrophs.[494] These findings indicate an important role for folliculo-stellate cells in processing and activating T_4. Production and action of local T_3 occurs in separate cell types of the hypothalamus and anterior pituitary gland resulting in setting the level of TSH output.

Transporters of thyroid hormone play a key role in regulating the TRH neuron. The two most important transporter families that are involved in thyroid hormone transport in the brain are the organic anion transporting polypeptide (OATP) and the monocarboxylate transporter (MCT).[492] Among these, OATP14 is highly expressed in the paraventricular nucleus and OATP8 in brain neurons.[495] In humans, mutations in the MCT8 gene, located on the X chromosome, result in males with neurologic abnormalities with elevated T_3 levels and decreased T_4 levels in the presence of a normal TSH secretion.[496]

Other Factors. SRIF inhibits TSH pulse amplitude and blocks the nocturnal TSH surge[497] directly at the pituitary level, and may also suppress TRH release and possibly TRH receptor abundance.[498] Although SRIF analogues are used to treat TSH-secreting pituitary adenomas (see later), long-term SRIF treatment for acromegaly does not lead to hypothyroidism in adult subjects. However, T_4 levels may be lowered within the normal range.[499] Dopamine infusions suppress TSH pulse amplitude by 70% and abrogate the nocturnal TSH surge.[500] Prolonged use of dopamine agonists, however, does not result in hypothyroidism. Glucocorticoids suppress TSH secretion. Nonsteroidal anti-inflammatory agents, especially meclofenamate and fenclofenac, decrease serum TSH levels, albeit still within the normal range. The mechanism may involve displacement of thyroid hormone ligands from their binding proteins or a direct inhibition of pituitary TSH.[501]

TSH Action. TSH induces thyroid hormone synthesis and release and maintains trophic thyroid cell integrity.[502] The TSH G protein–coupled receptor is located on the thyrocyte plasma membrane and is encoded by a gene on chromosome 11q31. Its regulation is comprehensively described in Chapter 11.

Disorders of TSH Secretion

TSH Deficiency

Causes. Congenital isolated TSH deficiency may arise from mutational defects of the TSH and TRH receptor genes. Genetic disorders of pituitary gland development involved in cell differentiation give rise to TSH deficiency as a component of multiple pituitary hormone deficiencies. These genes with mutations include *LHX3*, *PROP1*, and *POU1F1* (see Table 8-2). Pituitary damage may result in functional TSH deficiency, often without a clearly demonstrable reduction in serum TSH levels.

Clinical Features. The consequences of TSH deficiency are those of thyroid hormone deficiency, which causes childhood mental and growth retardation, and in adults is associated with a broad spectrum of clinical features including hypothermia, fluid retention, voice and skin changes, and ultimately, if untreated, frank myxedema and death.

TSH Assays. Most thyrotroph disorders can be diagnosed by measuring basal TSH and thyroid hormone levels. Modern sensitive and specific TSH assays distinguish circulating TSH levels in euthyroid subjects from both hyperthyroid and hypothyroid patients with little or no cross-reactivity with other glycoprotein hormones.[503,504] The most sensitive commercially available third-generation assays have a functional sensitivity of 0.01 to 0.02 mU/L, whereas newer fourth-generation assays portend greatly enhanced sensitivity (0.001-0.002 mU/L). Levels of free α-subunit (normal range 0.1-1.6 µg/L) are elevated in patients harboring TSH-secreting or nonfunctional pituitary adenomas, choriocarcinoma, and several malignancies.

TSH measurement is not helpful in diagnosing central hypothyroidism, which is identified by concurrent measurement of thyroid hormone levels. Only about one third of patients with secondary hypothyroidism have subnormal basal TSH levels.[505] TSH deficiency is thus associated with low T_4 levels concomitant with low, normal, or even minimally elevated TSH levels. Importantly, this biochemical profile may also be encountered in critically

ill patients with low TSH and T_4 levels without evidence of pituitary disease.

However, TSH measurements evoked by TRH may be required to fully assess the integrity of the hypothalamic-pituitary-thyroid axis.[506] In a stimulation test, TRH (200-500 µg) is administered intravenously, and TSH levels are measured at –15, 0, 15, 30, 60, and 120 minutes. In euthyroid subjects, peak TSH levels (up to 22-fold higher than basal) are observed after 30 minutes.[504] Because feedback suppression by elevated thyroid hormone levels on TSH overrides stimulation by the hypothalamus, hyperthyroid subjects have undetectable basal TSH levels that do not respond to TRH. In subjects with secondary thyroid failure due to pituitary disease, TSH levels do not change in response to TRH. Within hours of T_3 administration, basal TSH levels fall, and TRH-evoked TSH levels are attenuated. Thyroid hormones suppress tonic TSH secretion and pulse amplitude but do not appear to regulate TSH pulse frequency.

Treatment. L-Thyroxine is used for replacement therapy, and dosing variables are similar to those required for treating primary hypothyroidism. Hypothyroid features are effectively ameliorated by T_4 (0.075-0.25 mg/day). The molecule is converted peripherally into the active T_3 and has a 7-day half-life with stable blood levels. The dose of T_4 in hypopituitary patients is titrated to achieve midnormal serum free T_4 levels because serum TSH levels are low or undetectable in patients with impaired pituitary function. Measurement of TSH levels is not useful in determining thyroid hormone replacement because the damaged thyrotroph is unlikely to adequately reflect appropriate feedback suppression. As many women with pituitary failure also likely receive estrogen replacement, free instead of total T_4 level is measured to avoid the confounding effects of increased TBG levels. T_4 overdosing may lead to bone demineralization and cardiac arrhythmias. Thyroid hormone replacement accelerates cortisol metabolism and requirements and may therefore exacerbate primary hypoadrenalism or precipitate adrenal crisis in patients with perturbed adrenal function. Therefore, in pituitary patients suspected of having ACTH deficiency, thyroid hormone replacement should not be initiated until adrenal status has been evaluated and treated.

DEVELOPMENTAL AND GENETIC CAUSES OF PITUITARY FAILURE

Developmental Disorders

Congenital pituitary gland absence (aplasia), partial hypoplasia, or ectopic tissue rudiments are rarely encountered. Pituitary development follows midline cell migration from Rathke's pouch and impaired midline anomalies, including failed forebrain cleavage and anterior commissure and corpus collosum defects, lead to structural pituitary anomalies. Craniofacial developmental anomalies, including anencephaly, result in cleft lip and palate, basal encephalocele, hypertelorism, and optic nerve hypoplasia with varying degrees of pituitary dysplasia and aplasia. If these infants survive, lifelong appropriate pituitary hormone replacement is required. With sensitive MRI techniques for pituitary visualization, several anatomic features characteristic of hypopituitarism are now apparent. Evidence for acquired pituitary damage or destruction is often clearly visible on MRI, and patients presenting with hypopituitarism of undetermined cause may exhibit decreased gland volume, partial or complete empty sella, disturbed sella turcica architecture, absent or transected pituitary stalk, and an absent or ectopic posterior pituitary bright intensity signal.[507] Lesions of the pituitary stalk can arise from congenital maldevelopment causing stalk interruption (see later) or from acquired diseases involving the infundibulum. Among 92 patients with pituitary stalk lesions, 32% were found incidentally. About 15% were due to congenital (ectopic posterior pituitary, Rathke's cyst), 33% to inflammatory (sarcoidosis, histiocytosis, hypophysitis), and over 50% to neoplastic (craniopharyngioma, pituitary adenoma, metastatic disease) causes.[508] An absent infundibulum noted on MRI is associated with pituitary hormone deficits, and approximately 40% of patients with GHD of unclear cause show imaging evidence of mild stalk defects, reflecting a midline developmental anomaly.

Congenital basal encephalocele may result in the pituitary herniating through the sphenoid sinus roof, resulting in pituitary failure and diabetes insipidus.

Heritable Disorders

Mutations at each level of pituitary function, including hormones, receptors, and transcription factors that determine anterior pituitary development, may lead to pituitary deficiency syndromes[509] (see Table 8-1). Furthermore, mutations in specific pituitary genes, including those for GH, POMC, TSH, LH, and FSH, all lead to single hormone deficiencies. Patients heretofore diagnosed with idiopathic isolated or polyhormonal pituitary failure may in fact harbor a mutation, and as the transcriptional control of pituitary development is clarified, increasing numbers of mutant genes have become apparent (see Table 8-2).

HESX1, SOX2, SOX3, and OTX2

HESX1 (also known as RPX), one of the earliest transcriptional markers of the primitive pituitary, with expression restricted to Rathke's pouch, is a paired-like homeodomain transcription factor that acts as a transcriptional repressor.[510] Coincidentally with appearance of specific pituitary cell types, HESX1 expression declines and is extinguished in the mature anterior pituitary,[511] leading to PROP1 activation. The heterogeneous syndrome of septo-optic dysplasia (hypoplastic optic nerves, absent corpus callosum and septum pellucidum, and hypopituitarism) is associated with mutations in HESX1.[512] Hypopituitarism ranges from panhypopituitarism to isolated GHD. Although the mutant molecule exhibits reduced DNA binding, panhypopituitarism may also occur secondary to profound anatomic defects in midline development. Mutations in HESX1 have also been associated with pituitary stalk interruption syndrome (PSIS), a congenital defect of the pituitary gland characterized by a very thin, interrupted pituitary stalk, an ectopic or absent posterior pituitary gland, and hypoplasia or aplasia of the anterior pituitary gland, visible on MRI.[513] Mutated SOX2, a member of the SRY-related high mobility group box (Sox) genes, is also associated with septo-optic dysplasia, anophthalamia or microphthalmia, and anterior pituitary hypoplasia, frequently associated with HH and GHD, and other forebrain defects.[514] SOX3 mutations are associated with X-linked hypopituitarism and mental retardation. Affected males have GHD and may also have deficient gonadotropins, TSH, or ACTH. Both SOX3 duplications and loss of function mutations show similar phenotypes, suggesting that SOX3 dosage is critical for normal pituitary development.[515,516]

Mutations in OTX2 have also been implicated in anophthalmia/microphthalmia syndromes in humans. These mutations are associated with severe ocular and neurologic phenotypes, including developmental delay and seizures. Panhypopituitarism occurs, perhaps as a result of failure to activate transcription of HESX1 and POU1F1.[516]

LHX3 and LHX4

LHX3 is expressed early during anterior pituitary development, with strong uniform expression within Rathke's pouch. Expression persists into adulthood. Missense and deletion mutations of LHX3, a LIM-type homeodomain transcription factor essential for pituitary development, are associated with failure of pituitary gland morphogenesis with reduced numbers of all cell types and multiple anterior pituitary hormone deficits, affecting all axes except for largely intact ACTH reserve.[434] Most missense mutations identified in patients have diminished capacity to activate transcription of the promoters of several potential LHX3 target genes, including those encoding αGSU, PRL, FSHβ, TSHβ, and POU1F1.[517] These patients also exhibit defective neck rotation ability due to a rigid cervical spine and variable sensorineural hearing loss.[518]

LHX4 is closely related to LHX3 and is also expressed throughout the invaginating Rathke's pouch, but unlike LHX3, its expression is transient and not maintained in the adult pituitary. Patients with LHX4 mutations exhibit GHD and associated short stature, with variable additional endocrine deficits, particularly TSH and ACTH deficiency, and extrapituitary abnormalities. LHX4 mutations associated with anterior pituitary hypoplasia, an ectopic posterior pituitary, and with PSIS are unable to activate both PROP1 and POU1F1, and these result in pituitary failure.[516,519]

PITX1 and PITX2

PITX1 and PITX2, members of the class of bicoid homeodomain proteins, show a high degree of homology and are expressed in an overlapping pattern during pituitary development. PITX1 is expressed in all five anterior pituitary lineages in both the fetal and adult pituitary gland and is able to activate the expression of all six of the major anterior pituitary hormones, including LH and FSH, frequently acting in synergy with other pituitary transcription factors. Mutations in PITX2 cause Rieger syndrome, characterized by defects in the eyes and teeth and a protuberant umbilicus as well as pituitary hormone deficiencies.[26,27,520]

PROP1

Mutations in PROP1 (OMIM 601538) are the most common genetic cause of combined pituitary hormone deficiency (CPHD) (Fig. 8-38).[521] The role of this gene was first uncovered from studies of the Ames dwarf mouse, which harbors a missense PROP1 mutation and exhibits a hypoplastic pituitary gland with combined GH, PRL, and TSH deficiency. This mutation abrogates POU1F1 activation and results in failed development of POU1F1-dependent cell lineages.[522] Similarly, human PROP1 mutations are associated with deficiencies in POU1F1-dependent lineages (GH, PRL, and TSH). Impaired FSH and LH secretion, associated with delayed or absent puberty, HH, and infertility in females and in some males, is also frequently present.[523] ACTH deficiency can also occur, frequently with a later onset, suggesting a role in maintenance of corticotroph function and emphasizing the necessity for complete and continued clinical assessment of patients with PROP1 mutations.[249] Inheritance modes of PROP1 mutations

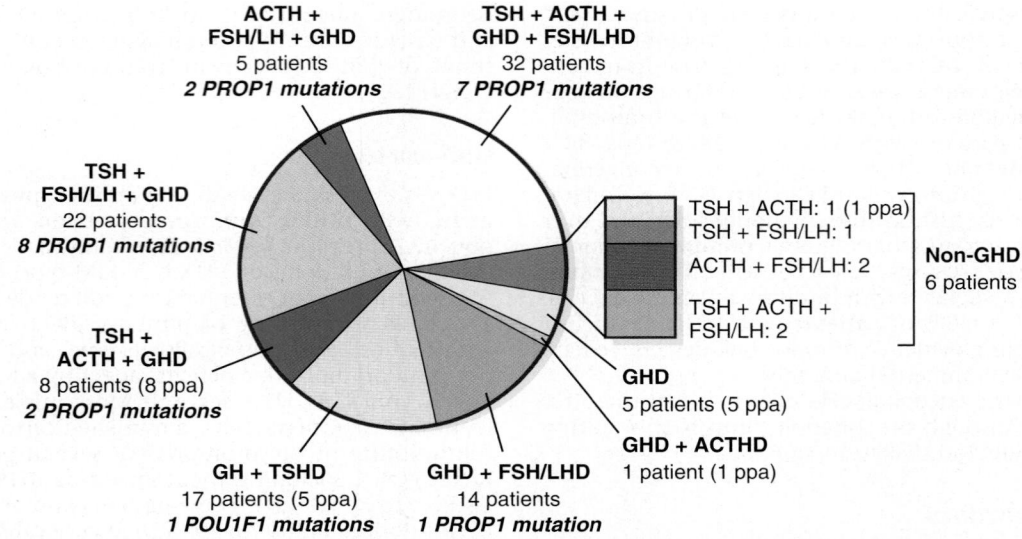

Figure 8-38 Pituitary hormone deficiencies repartition in 110 unrelated patients affected by congenital pituitary deficiency without stalk pituitary interruption or septo-optic dysplasia. Patients were studied for *PROP1*, *POUF1*, or *LHX3* according to hormonal deficit phenotype. Twenty mutations of *PROP1* and one mutation of *POU1F1* were found. Gonadotroph function was unavailable for prepubertal age (ppa) patients. ACTH, adrenocorticotropic hormone; ACTHD, ACTH deficiency; FSH, follicle-stimulating hormone; GH, growth hormone; GHD, growth hormone deficiency; LH, luteinizing hormone; LHD, luteinizing hormone deficiency; TSH, thyroid-stimulating hormone; TSHD, thyroid-stimulating hormone deficiency. (From Reynaud R, Gueydan M, Saveanu A, et al. Genetic screening of combined pituitary hormone deficiency: experience in 195 patients. *J Clin Endocrinol Metab.* 2006;91:3326-3329.)

usually reflect autosomal recessive patterns. Thus, patients are usually homozygous for either deletion or missense frameshift mutations leading to truncated PROP1 protein products devoid of functional activity. The most commonly encountered mutation is a 2–base pair deletion at position 296 (301-302delAG), resulting in early translational termination and a nonfunctional protein product.[462]

The clinical spectra of CPHD associated with PROP1 mutations are variable and temporal. The phenotype varies with both the type of mutation as well as the age of the patient.[516] The onset of clinically evident pituitary failure is usually first manifest with slowing of linear growth (GHD, ~80%), then thyroid failure (TSH deficiency, ~20%), followed by hypogonadism, and later subclinical or overt adrenal insufficiency.[524] The pituitary gland size is usually small or normal. Combined hypothalamic hormone stimulation (GnRH, TRH, CRH, and GHRH) or insulin-evoked hypoglycemia reveals blunted responses consistent with varying degrees of pituitary hormone deficiencies. Serum IGF-1 and IGFBP3 levels are usually low, but peripheral thyroid hormone levels are low or at the lower limits of normal ranges. In the face of low or absent TSH responses, these findings are consistent with secondary hypothyroidism. Most older patients also exhibit blunted cortisol responses to CRH and ACTH or insulin stimulation.[523]

POU1F1

The POU1F1 gene (OMIM 173110) encodes a POU homeobox protein, PIT1, which activates transcription of the GH, PRL, TSHβ, and GHRH receptor genes.[525] PIT1 also partners with coactivators including thyroid hormone, estrogen, and retinoic acid receptors, as well as other transcription factors including CREB, P-LIM, PITX1, HESX1, and ZN-15. PIT1 autoregulates its own expression. Because of the absolute requirement of PIT1 for somatotroph, lactotroph, and thyrotroph development and specific gene expression, inactivating mutations of the gene result in a spectrum of pituitary hormone deficiencies.[526] The Snell and Jackson dwarf mouse strains both harbor POU1F1 gene muta-

tions.[527] Both autosomal recessive (loss of function) and autosomal dominant (dominant negative action) POU1F1 mutations have been identified.

Some POU1F1 mutations exhibit characteristic clinical phenotypes, depending on the spectrum of loss of DNA binding, transcriptional activation, or interaction with partner proteins affected.[307,528] Both CBP/p300 protein recruitment as well as PIT1 dimerization are required for appropriate PIT1 activation of target hormone genes.[529] LHX4 appears to activate POU1F1 and mutations of LHX4 also lead to growth retardation.[519] Interestingly, adult-onset combined GH, PRL, and TSH deficiencies have also been reported in association with circulating autoantibodies directed against the PIT1 protein.[530]

IGSF1

Loss-of-function mutations have been identified in *IGSF1* in association with X-linked congenital central hypothyroidism, often in association with variable PRL deficiency and GHD and with testicular enlargement.[164] IGSF1 is a membrane glycoprotein highly expressed in the anterior pituitary gland, and the patients with mutations appear to have impaired pituitary TRH signaling.

TBX19

TBX19 (also referred to as TPIT) mutations result in early-onset isolated ACTH deficiency and hypocortisolism[37] (see Table 8-2). Associated phenotypes, including those for POMC deficiency, may include obesity, red hair pigmentation, and other associated pituitary deficiencies. Patients are homozygous or compound heterozygous for TBX19/TPIT mutations, indicating an autosomal recessive mode of inheritance. Mutations in this gene appear to be the principal molecular cause of congenital neonatal isolated ACTH deficiency.[531] Interestingly, among 22 patients with isolated ACTH deficiency, diagnosed between ages 5 and 15 years, and no identified mutation of TBX19/TPIT, three had common variable immunodeficiency (CVID), characterized by defective immunoglobulin production and recurrent infections, diagnosed at age 2 to 8 years. This has led to the proposal of a new syndrome linking these two rare disorders: deficient anterior pituitary function and variable immune deficiency, or DAVID.[532]

NR5A1 and NR0B1

NR5A1 encodes SF1, a member of the nuclear receptor family expressed throughout the reproductive axis (hypothalamus, pituitary, and gonads) and in the adrenal gland. It is a key transcriptional regulator of many genes involved in sexual differentiation, steroidogenesis, and reproduction, including the pituitary genes encoding αGSU, LHβ, FSHβ, and GnRHR. Patients with mutations in SF1 have been described with varying degrees of XY sex reversal, testicular dysgenesis, ovarian insufficiency, adrenal failure, and impaired pubertal maturation with HH.[56,533,534]

NR0B1 encodes DAX1 (*d*osage-sensitive sex-reversal *a*drenal hypoplasia critical region on the *X* chromosome protein 1), a nuclear receptor transcription factor related to SF1, with a similar distribution pattern of expression. Mutations in NR0B1 are associated with X-linked HH and adrenal hypoplasia congenita,[30] with the majority of mutations causing truncations or frameshifts rendering the protein nonfunctional. HH is often mild, revealing itself as failure to undergo puberty or as incomplete puberty. The hypogonadism appears to be a due to variable and combined hypothalamic and pituitary function. DAX1 is a transcriptional repressor and has been shown to inhibit SF1-mediated transcription of an array of target genes, including LHβ. How the loss of function in these two opposing genes, SF1 and DAX1, results in similar phenotypes is still not well understood. The HH is likely due to a developmental defect of the hypothalamus and pituitary, suggesting a role for DAX1 in proper development of these organs.[535]

Pituitary Stalk Interruption Syndrome

PSIS is a congenital defect of the pituitary gland characterized by a thin or interrupted pituitary stalk, anterior pituitary hypoplasia, and an ectopic posterior pituitary. Patients may present with an isolated pituitary hormone deficiency or with combined hypothalamic-pituitary hormone deficiencies. Accompanying midline defects and eye abnormalities suggest involvement of developmental processes. Mutations or single nucleotide variants in HESX1, LHX4, OTX2, SOX3, and PROKR2 have been associated with PSIS. A homozygous missense mutation was identified in a family with PSIS in GPR161, an orphan G protein–coupled receptor expressed in the hypothalamus and pituitary and implicated in the SHH signaling pathway.[536] Mutations have been identified in less than 5% of patients with PSIS, suggesting that there is much more to be learned about the pathogenesis of this disorder.

Acquired Disorders

In the absence of demonstrable hypothalamic-pituitary anatomic damage, and after excluding genetic and syndromic causes of pituitary insufficiencies, acquired, often transient, causes of pituitary failure should be considered (see Table 8-5). Causes of pituitary insufficiency including pituitary tumors, parasellar masses, hypophysitis, aneurysms, and pituitary apoplexy were discussed earlier. Hypothalamic damage reflected by the presence of a large parasellar mass leading to decreased GnRH production results in muscle wasting, obesity, and central hypogonad-

ism with low levels of FSH and LH (Fig. 8-39). Marked caloric restriction, anorexia,[537,538] weight loss of other causes, and strenuous exercise may attenuate GnRH secretion and action. HH may occur in both men and women (see Chapters 17 and 19). Exogenous anabolic steroid and glucocorticoid therapy suppresses the reproductive and adrenal axes, respectively. Patients with severe critical illnesses or chronic debilitating disease (including cirrhosis) may have impaired GH/IGF-1, adrenal, and gonadal axes. Hyperprolactinemia causes sexual dysfunction by inhibiting GnRH pulsatility via a short feedback loop. Hypothyroidism, hypoadrenalism, or hypogonadism cause hyperplasia of specific trophic cells due to lack of negative feedback and sometimes actual pituitary tumor formation.[539] Acquired immunodeficiency syndrome (AIDS) is associated with suppressed pituitary function that is independent of other associated infections.[540] Drugs such as estrogens, which suppress FSH and LH, and GnRH analogues used for treating prostate cancer inhibit gonadotropin action. In addition to pituitary apoplexy, other vascular accidents such as aneurysms, strokes, cavernous sinus thrombosis, and arteritis can cause pituitary hormone insufficiency. Isolated hormone pituitary hormone deficiencies may also occur as a manifestation of vascular abnormalities including arteritis or subarachnoid hemorrhage (Table 8-11).

Head Trauma

The pituitary may be partially or totally damaged by birth trauma, cranial hemorrhage, fetal asphyxia, or breech delivery. Head trauma may lead to direct pituitary damage by a sella turcica fracture, pituitary stalk section, trauma-induced vasospasm, or ischemic infarction following blunt trauma.[546] The most common traumatic cause of compromised pituitary function in the adult is iatrogenic neurosurgical trauma. Pituitary manipulation or damage during surgery leads to transient or permanent diabetes insipidus and varying degrees of anterior pituitary dysfunction. Hypopituitarism following head trauma usually manifests within a year after the insult. Seventy-five percent of patients with posttraumatic pituitary failure are young men under age 40 years involved in a motor vehicle accident. Virtually all patients with subsequent pituitary failure have a history of loss of consciousness following trauma, and half of all such patients have documented skull fracture.[546] One third of these patients have demonstrable signs of hypothalamic or posterior pituitary hemorrhage or anterior lobe infarction on MRI. Diabetes insipidus is the most common endocrine disorder, encountered in about 30% of these patients.[547] As pituitary function can recover after trauma, the prevalence and extent of dysfunction vary and depend on the time of evaluation. A meta-analysis of over 700 adult patients in 2007 reported that up to 35% of subjects acquired some impairment to pituitary function evaluated at least 5 months after major TBI.[548] GHD was found in 11%, gonadotropin deficiency in 13%, ACTH deficiency in 11%, TSH deficiency in 6%, and multiple deficits in 9%. There are sparse data of the pituitary consequences of TBI in children. A large prospective French study of 87 children, mean age of 6.7 years, has reported a prevalence of 7% for GHD, 2% for thyroid, and 1% adrenal insufficiency evaluated 5 months after TBI.[549]

Klose and associates have questioned the accuracy of the frequency of adult GHD from previous studies because of methodologic issues arising from the use of different diagnostic tests, assays, and criteria based on published guidelines.[550] Using normative data drawn from over 100 healthy control subjects, the authors observed that the prevalence of GHD among 439 patients with TBI was

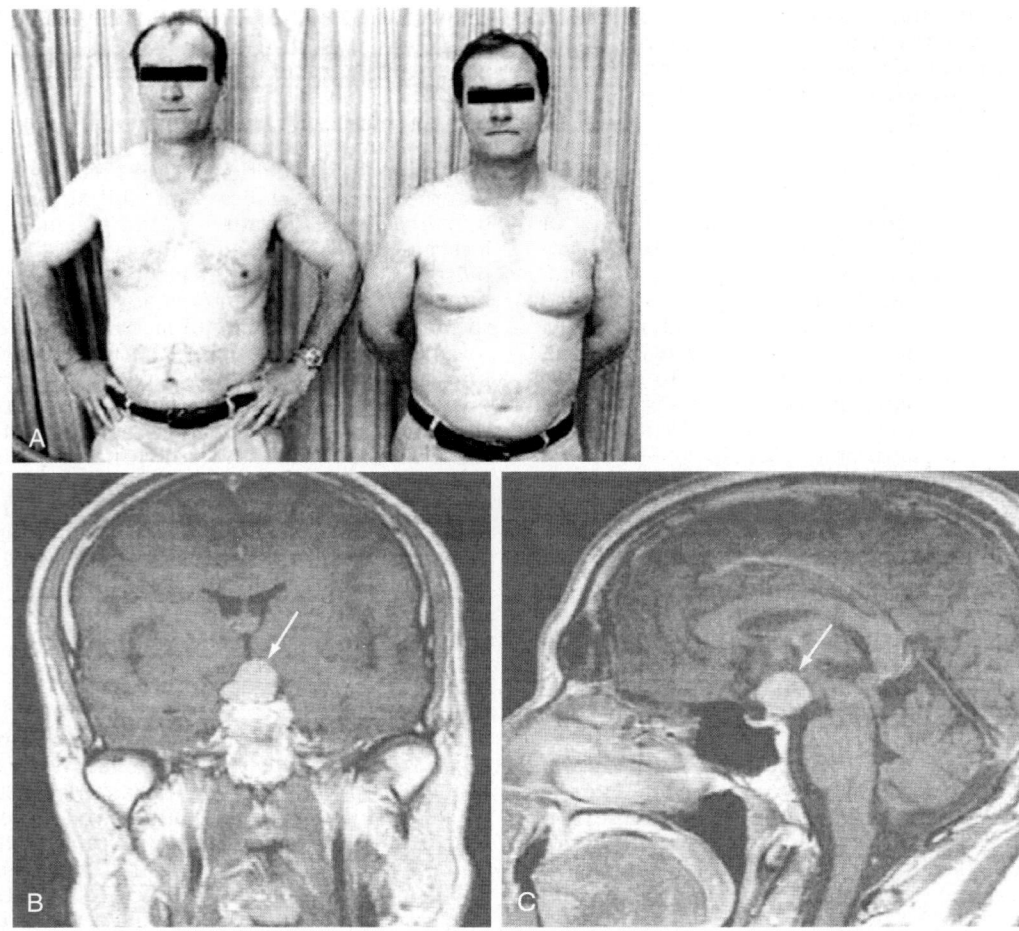

Figure 8-39 Features of hypopituitarism and hypogonadism, including central adiposity, proximal muscle wasting, loss of body hair, and gynecomastia. Note the contrast between the hypogonadal patient (panel **A,** right side) and his unaffected identical twin (left side). Laboratory tests confirmed secondary hypogonadism, with testosterone level of 0.4 ng/mL (normal range, 2.9 to 8.0 ng/mL), follicle-stimulating hormone level of 2.8 IU/L (normal range, 1.5 to 12.4 IU/L), and luteinizing hormone level of 1.5 IU/L (normal range, 1.7 to 8.6 IU/L). Magnetic resonance imaging showed a lobulated, contrast-enhancing suprasellar mass (coronal view in panel **B** *[arrow]* and sagittal view in panel **C** *[arrow]*). Pathologic analysis confirmed the diagnosis of pituicytoma. (From Newnham HH, Rivera-Woll LM. Images in clinical medicine: hypogonadism due to pituicytoma in an identical twin. *N Engl J Med.* 2008;359:2824.)

TABLE 8-11
Hypopituitarism After Subarachnoid Hemorrhage

Reference	Number of Patients	Any Degree of Hypopituitarism (*n*)	Multiple Deficiencies (*n*)	GH (*n*)	LH/FSH (*n*)	ACTH (*n*)	TSH (*n*)	Remarks
Kelly et al, 2000[541]	2	2	0	2	0	0	0	
Brandt et al, 2004[542]	10	5	0	1	4	0	0	
Aimaretti et al, 2004[543]	40	15	4	10	5	1	3	No stimulation test for ACTH
Kreitschmann-Andermahr et al, 2004[544]	40	22	3	8	0	16	1	
Dimopoulou et al, 2004[545]	30	14	4	11	4	3	2	No stimulation test for GH (11 patients low IGF-1)
Total number (%)	122 (100)	58 (48)	11 (9)	32 (26)	13 (11)	20 (16)	6 (5)	

ACTH, adrenocorticotropic hormone; GH, growth hormone; IGF-1, insulin-like growth factor 1; LH, luteinizing hormone; FSH, follicle-stimulating hormone; TSH, thyroid-stimulating hormone.
Modified from Schneider H, Aimaretti G, Kreitschmann-Andermahr I, et al. Hypopituitarism. *Lancet.* 2007;369:1461-1470.

highly dependent on choice of local or guideline-derived cutoffs, on diagnostic tests, and on the use of either single or confirmatory testing. They reported a prevalence of GHD of 4% with the ITT and 12% with the combined pyridostigmine-GHRH test and of isolated GHD in just 1% confirmed from these two tests.[547,551-553]

Radiation

Pituitary irradiation, usually indicated for pituitary adenoma therapy, will directly cause atrophy of the gland, in addition to the damaging impact of irradiation on hypothalamic synthesis of hypophysiotropic hormones.[554]

Pituitary function in children and adolescents is particularly sensitive to head and neck therapeutic irradiation.[555] Radiation dose exposure, time interval after completion of radiotherapy, and distance of the pituitary or hypothalamus from the central energy field correlate with the development of pituitary hormone deficits (Figs. 8-40 and 8-41). After a median dose of 5000 rads directed at the skull base, nasopharynx, or cranium, up to 75% of patients will develop pituitary insufficiency within 10 years.[556] Later manifestations of pituitary failure usually reflect hypotha-

lamic damage, rather than atrophy of irradiated pituitary cells. Although the degree of hormone loss after radiation is variable, the pattern of loss usually occurs sequentially: GH > FSH and LH followed by ACTH and TSH.[557] Thus, evidence for secondary thyroid or adrenal failure usually implies that the GH and gonadotropin axes are also compromised. Stereotactic radiosurgery directed to the pituitary gland also results in 23% of patients exhibiting pituitary deficits within 48 to 96 months.[558] Previously irradiated patients should therefore undergo lifelong periodic anterior pituitary hormone testing. Ideally, rigorous long-term screening should unmask incipient pituitary failure prior to onset of morbidity.[559]

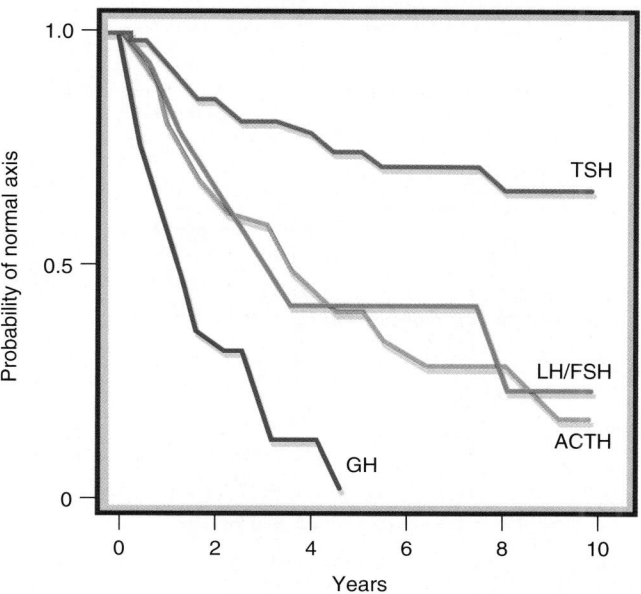

Figure 8-40 Life-table analysis indicating probabilities of initially normal hypothalamic-pituitary-target gland axes remaining normal after radiotherapy (3750 to 4250 cGy). Growth hormone (GH) secretion is the most sensitive of the anterior pituitary hormones to the effects of external radiotherapy, and thyroid-stimulating hormone (TSH) secretion is the most resistant. In two thirds of patients, gonadotropin deficiency develops before adrenocorticotropic hormone (ACTH) deficiency. The reverse occurs in the remaining third. FSH, follicle-stimulating hormone, LH, luteinizing hormone. (From Littley MD, Shalet SM, Beardwell CG, et al. Hypopituitarism following external radiotherapy for pituitary tumors in adults. *Q J Med.* 1989;70: 145-160.)

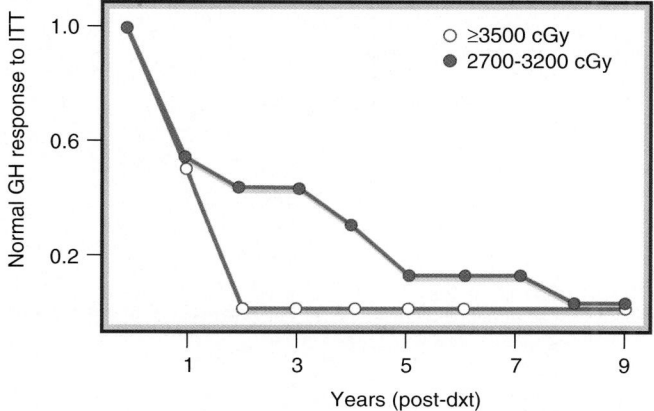

Figure 8-41 The incidence of growth hormone (GH) deficiency in children receiving 27 to 32 Gy or 35 Gy of cranial irradiation for a brain tumor in relation to time from irradiation (dxt). This illustrates that the speed at which individual pituitary hormone deficits develop is dose-dependent; the higher the radiation dose, the earlier GH deficiency occurs. ITT, insulin tolerance test. (Courtesy of the Department of Medical Illustrations, Wilkington Hospital, Manchester, England. From Shalet S. Pituitary failure. In: DeGroot LJ, Jameson JL, eds. *Endocrinology.* Philadelphia, PA: WB Saunders; 2001.)

Empty Sella Syndrome

Damage to the sellar diaphragm may lead to arachnoid herniation into the sellar space. An empty sella may develop as a consequence of a primary congenital weakness of the diaphragm in those patients in whom no secondary cause is evident. Up to 50% of patients with primary empty sella have associated benign intracranial hypertension.[560] A secondary empty sella may develop subsequent to infarction of a pituitary adenoma, or surgical or radiation-induced damage to the sellar diaphragm. These patients usually exhibit demonstrable pituitary tissue compressed against the sellar floor, with lateral stalk deviation visible on MRI. Although an empty sella is usually an incidental finding, if more than 90% of pituitary tissue is compressed or atrophied, pituitary failure usually occurs. About 10% of patients may develop small GH- or PRL-secreting adenomas within the narrow rim of compressed pituitary tissue.

Clinical Features of Hypopituitarism

Patients with pituitary failure, regardless of cause, have excessive mortality rates, primarily due to vascular disease.[245] Age at diagnosis, female gender, and history of craniopharyngioma were the most striking determinants of increased fatality. The spectrum of clinical features of pituitary insufficiency depends on several factors. In acquired pituitary insufficiency the clinical spectrum depends upon the degree of hormone deficiency, the number of hormones impaired, and the rapidity of onset. In congenital forms, the earlier the age of onset, the greater the severity of thyroid, gonadal, adrenal, growth, or water disturbances. Heritable genetic disorders invariably exhibit the most severe phenotypic changes, although later changes may also occur in these disorders, as seen with PROP1 mutations. The resilience of the individual pituitary cell lineages to compressive, inflammatory, vascular, radiation, and invasive insults also differs. The lactotroph cell is often hyperfunctional as a result of decreased tonic inhibitory signals. PRL deficiency is thus exceedingly rare, except for complete pituitary destruction or genetic syndromes. The order of diminished trophic hormone reserve function by pituitary compression usually is as follows: GH > FSH > LH > TSH > ACTH. The corticotroph cell appears particularly resistant to hypothalamic or pituitary destruction and is usually the last cell to lose function. The qualitative phenotypic manifestations of pituitary failure are determined by which specific trophic hormones are lost (see earlier for description of individual hormone deficiencies).

Screening for Pituitary Failure

As the onset of hypopituitarism may be extremely slow, subclinical pituitary failure is often not apparent to the patient or physician. Screening for pituitary dysfunction

TABLE 8-12

Assessment of Anterior Pituitary Function

Test	Dose	Normal Response	Side Effects
ACTH			
Insulin tolerance	0.1-0.15 U/kg IV	Peak cortisol response > 18 µg/dL, or increase by 7 µg/dL	Sweating, palpitation, tremor
Metyrapone	Oral administration of 30 mg/kg at 11 PM	Peak 11-DOC ≥ 7 µg/dL Peak cortisol ≤ 7 µg/dL Peak ACTH > 75 pg/mL	Nausea, insomnia, adrenal crisis
CRH stimulation	100 µg IV	Peak ACTH ≥ two- to fourfold Peak cortisol ≥ 20 µg/dL or ↑ ≥ 7 µg/dL	Flushing
ACTH stimulation	250 µg IV or IM or 1 µg IV	Peak cortisol ≥ 20 µg/dL	Rare
TSH			
Serum T_4 (free T_4) Total T_3 TSH—third generation TRH stimulation	200-500 µg IV	Peak TSH ≥ 2.5-fold or ↑ ≥ 5-6 mU/L (females), ↑ ≥ 2-3 mU/L (males)	Flushing, nausea, urge to micturate
PRL			
Serum PRL TRH stimulation	200-500 µg IV	PRL ≥ 2.5-fold	Flushing, nausea, urge to micturate
LH/FSH			
Serum LH and FSH Serum testosterone GnRH stimulation	100 µg IV	Elevated in menopause and in men with primary testicular failure 300-900 ng/mL LH ≥ two- to threefold, or by 10 IU/L FSH 1.5-2-fold, or by 2 IU/L	Rare
GH			
Insulin tolerance L-Arginine	0.1-0.15 U/kg 0.5 g/kg (max 30 g) IV over 30-120 min	GH peak > 5 µg/L	Sweating, palpitation, tremor Nausea
L-Arginine plus GHRH	1-5 µg/kg	GH peak > 5 µg/L	Flushing

ACTH, adrenocorticotropic hormone; CRH, corticotropin-releasing hormone; 11-DOC, 11-deoxycorticosterone; FSH, follicle-stimulating hormone; GH, growth hormone; GHRH, growth hormone–releasing hormone; GnRH, gonadotropin-releasing hormone; IM, intramuscular; IV, intravenous; LH, luteinizing hormone; PRL, prolactin; T_3, triiodothyronine; T_4, thyroxine; TSH, thyroid-stimulating hormone; TRH, thyrotropin-releasing hormone.

TABLE 8-13

Replacement Therapy for Adult Hypopituitarism*

Deficient Hormone	Treatment
ACTH	Hydrocortisone, 10-20 mg daily in divided doses Cortisone acetate, 15-25 mg/day in divided doses
TSH	L-Thyroxine, 0.05-0.2 mg daily according to T_4 levels
FSH/LH	*Males:* Testosterone enanthate, 200 mg IM every 2-3 weeks Testosterone skin patch, 2.5-5.0 mg/day—can increase dose up to 7.5 mg/day Testosterone gel, 3-6 g daily For fertility: hCG three times weekly, or hCG + FSH or menopausal gonadotropin or GnRH *Females:* Conjugated estrogen, 0.65 mg daily Micronized estradiol, 1 mg daily Estradiol valerate, 2 mg Piperazine estrone sulfate, 1.25 mg Ethinyl estradiol, 0.02-0.05 mg Estradiol skin patch, 4-8 mg, twice weekly Estradiol + testosterone All of the estrogens are administered with progesterone or progestin sequentially or in combination if uterus present For fertility: menopausal gonadotropin and hCG or GnRH
GH	*Adults:* Somatotropin, 0.2-1.0 mg SC daily *Children:* Somatotropin, 0.02-0.05 mg/kg/day
Vasopressin	Intranasal desmopressin, via rhinal tube, 5-20 µg twice daily Oral DDAVP, 300-600 µg daily, usually in divided doses

*Doses shown should be individualized and reassessed during stress, surgery, or pregnancy. Male and female fertility management is fully discussed in Chapter 20.

ACTH, adrenocorticotropic hormone; DDAVP, desmopressin acetate; FSH, follicle-stimulating hormone; GH, growth hormone; GnRH, gonadotropin-releasing hormone; hCG, human chorionic gonadotropin; IM, intramuscularly; SC, subcutaneously; T_4, thyroxine.

should be undertaken in patients with hypothalamic or pituitary mass lesions, developmental craniofacial abnormalities, inflammatory disorders, brain granulomatous disease, prior head or neck irradiation, head trauma, prior skull base surgery, those with newly discovered empty sella, and those who have previously experienced pregnancy-associated hemorrhage or blood pressure changes.[561]

As hypopituitarism may develop insidiously and is often not readily clinically apparent, screening of appropriate patients is important to prevent long-term morbidity. Therefore, all patients harboring hypothalamic or pituitary masses should be screened for hypopituitarism (Table 8-12). PRL should be measured because many patients with hypopituitarism may also present with secondary hyperprolactinemia. Up to two thirds of patients harboring pituitary macroadenomas, craniopharyngiomas, and other parasellar lesions have compromised pituitary reserve function. Less commonly, patients with intrasellar aneurysms, pituitary metastases, parasellar meningiomas, optic gliomas, and hypothalamic astrocytomas may also have pituitary failure. Although about a third of patients with hypopituitarism undergoing pituitary surgery recover function after decompression, about 25% of patients experience further loss of pituitary function after surgery and therefore should be screened annually. Treatment of pituitary failure is described in Table 8-13.

REFERENCES

1. Bernard C. Physiologie; chiens rendus diabetiques. *C R Soc Biol.* 1849; 1:60.
2. Marie P. On two cases of acromegaly: marked hypertrophy of the upper and lower limbs and the head. *Rev Med.* 1886;6:297-333.
3. Cushing H. Partial hypophysectomy for acromegaly: with remarks on the function of the hypophysis. *Ann Surg.* 1909;50:1002-1017.
4. Cushing H. Surgical experiences with pituitary disorders. *JAMA.* 1914;63:1515-1525.
5. Harris GW. Neural control of pituitary gland. *Physiol Rev.* 1948;28: 139-179.
6. Chanson P, Daujat F, Young J, et al. Normal pituitary hypertrophy as a frequent cause of pituitary incidentaloma: a follow-up study. *J Clin Endocrinol Metab.* 2001;86:3009-3015.
7. Stanfield JP. The blood supply of the human pituitary gland. *J Anat.* 1960;94:257-273.
8. Bergland RM, Page RB. Pituitary-brain vascular relations: a new paradigm. *Science.* 1979;204:18-24.
9. Rathke H. Ueber die Entsehung der glandula. *Arch Anat Physio Wissened.* 1838;482-485.
10. Etchevers HC, Vincent C, Le Douarin NM, Couly GF. The cephalic neural crest provides pericytes and smooth muscle cells to all blood vessels of the face and forebrain. *Development.* 2001;128:1059-1068.
11. Takuma N, Sheng HZ, Furuta Y, et al. Formation of Rathke's pouch requires dual induction from the diencephalon. *Development.* 1998; 125:4835-4840.
12. Gleiberman AS, Fedtsova NG, Rosenfeld MG. Tissue interactions in the induction of anterior pituitary: role of the ventral diencephalon, mesenchyme, and notochord. *Dev Biol.* 1999;213:340-353.
13. Scully KM, Rosenfeld MG. Pituitary development: regulatory codes in mammalian organogenesis. *Science.* 2002;295:2231-2235.
14. Zhu X, Wang J, Ju BG, Rosenfeld MG. Signaling and epigenetic regulation of pituitary development. *Curr Opin Cell Biol.* 2007;19:605-611.
15. Pulichino AM, Lamolet B, Vallette-Kasic S, et al. Tpit-/-NeuroD1-/- mice reveal novel aspects of corticotroph development. *Endocr Res.* 2004;30:551-552.
16. Ward RD, Stone BM, Raetzman LT, Camper SA. Cell proliferation and vascularization in mouse models of pituitary hormone deficiency. *Mol Endocrinol.* 2006;20:1378-1390.
17. Davis SW, Ellsworth BS, Peréz Millan MI, et al. Pituitary gland development and disease: from stem cell to hormone production. *Curr Top Dev Biol.* 2013;106:1-47.
18. Treier M, Gleiberman AS, O'Connell SM, et al. Multistep signaling requirements for pituitary organogenesis in vivo. *Genes Dev.* 1998;12: 1691-1704.
19. Asa SL, Kovacs K, Laszlo FA, et al. Human fetal adenohypophysis. Histologic and immunocytochemical analysis. *Neuroendocrinology.* 1986;43:308-316.
20. Dubois PM, Hemming FJ. Fetal development and regulation of pituitary cell types. *J Electron Microsc Tech.* 1991;19:2-20.
21. Zhu X, Lin CR, Prefontaine GG, et al. Genetic control of pituitary development and hypopituitarism. *Curr Opin Genet Dev.* 2005;15: 332-340.
22. Raetzman LT, Wheeler BS, Ross SA, et al. Persistent expression of Notch2 delays gonadotrope differentiation. *Mol Endocrinol.* 2006;20: 2898-2908.
23. Olson LE, Tollkuhn J, Scafoglio C, et al. Homeodomain-mediated beta-catenin-dependent switching events dictate cell-lineage determination. *Cell.* 2006;125:593-605.
24. Carriere C, Gleiberman A, Lin CR, Rosenfeld MG. From panhypopituitarism to combined pituitary deficiencies: do we need the anterior pituitary? *Rev Endocr Metab Disord.* 2004;5:5-13.
25. Pulichino A-M, Vallette-Kasic S, Drouin J. Transcriptional regulation of pituitary gland development: binary choices for cell differentiation. *Curr Opin Endocrinol Metab.* 2004;11:13-17.
26. Suh H, Gage PJ, Drouin J, Camper SA. Pitx2 is required at multiple stages of pituitary organogenesis: pituitary primordium formation and cell specification. *Development.* 2002;129:329-337.
27. Tremblay JJ, Lanctot C, Drouin J. The pan-pituitary activator of transcription, Ptx1 (pituitary homeobox 1), acts in synergy with SF-1 and Pit1 and is an upstream regulator of the Lim-homeodomain gene Lim3/Lhx3. *Mol Endocrinol.* 1998;12:428-441.
28. Lanctot C, Gauthier Y, Drouin J. Pituitary homeobox 1 (Ptx1) is differentially expressed during pituitary development. *Endocrinology.* 1999;140:1416-1422.
29. Lu MF, Pressman C, Dyer R, et al. Function of Rieger syndrome gene in left-right asymmetry and craniofacial development. *Nature.* 1999; 401:276-278.
30. Muscatelli F, Strom TM, Walker AP, et al. Mutations in the DAX-1 gene give rise to both X-linked adrenal hypoplasia congenita and hypogonadotropic hypogonadism. *Nature.* 1994;372:672-676.
31. Tabarin A, Achermann JC, Recan D, et al. A novel mutation in DAX1 causes delayed-onset adrenal insufficiency and incomplete hypogonadotropic hypogonadism. *J Clin Invest.* 2000;105:321-328.
32. Charles MA, Saunders TL, Wood WM, et al. Pituitary-specific Gata2 knockout: effects on gonadotrope and thyrotrope function. *Mol Endocrinol.* 2006;20:1366-1377.
33. Coss D, Mellon PL, Thackray VG. A FoxL in the Smad house: activin regulation of FSH. *Trends Endocrinol Metab.* 2010;21:562-568.
34. Ellsworth BS, Egashira N, Haller JL, et al. FOXL2 in the pituitary: molecular, genetic, and developmental analysis. *Mol Endocrinol.* 2006; 20:2796-2805.
35. Justice NJ, Blount AL, Pelosi E, et al. Impaired FSHbeta expression in the pituitaries of Foxl2 mutant animals. *Mol Endocrinol.* 2011;25: 1404-1415.
36. Lamba P, Fortin J, Tran S, et al. A novel role for the forkhead transcription factor FOXL2 in activin A-regulated follicle-stimulating hormone beta subunit transcription. *Mol Endocrinol.* 2009;23:1001-1013.
37. Lamolet B, Pulichino AM, Lamonerie T, et al. A pituitary cell-restricted T box factor, Tpit, activates POMC transcription in cooperation with Pitx homeoproteins. *Cell.* 2001;104:849-859.
38. Reynaud R, Gueydan M, Saveanu A, et al. Genetic screening of combined pituitary hormone deficiency: experience in 195 patients. *J Clin Endocrinol Metab.* 2006;91:3329-3336.
39. Melmed S. Mechanisms for pituitary tumorigenesis: the plastic pituitary. *J Clin Invest.* 2003;112:1603-1618.
40. Castinetti F, Davis SW, Brue T, Camper SA. Pituitary stem cell update and potential implications for treating hypopituitarism. *Endocr Rev.* 2011;32:453-471.
41. Lepore DA, Roeszler K, Wagner J, et al. Identification and enrichment of colony-forming cells from the adult murine pituitary. *Exp Cell Res.* 2005;308:166-176.
42. Fauquier T, Rizzoti K, Dattani M, et al. SOX2-expressing progenitor cells generate all of the major cell types in the adult mouse pituitary gland. *Proc Natl Acad Sci U S A.* 2008;105:2907-2912.
43. Chen J, Crabbe A, Van Duppen V, Vankelecom H. The notch signaling system is present in the postnatal pituitary: marked expression and regulatory activity in the newly discovered side population. *Mol Endocrinol.* 2006;20:3293-3307.
44. Gleiberman AS, Michurina T, Encinas JM, et al. Genetic approaches identify adult pituitary stem cells. *Proc Natl Acad Sci U S A.* 2008;105: 6332-6337.
45. Alatzoglou KS, Kelberman D, Dattani MT. The role of SOX proteins in normal pituitary development. *J Endocrinol.* 2009;200:245-258.
46. Garcia-Lavandeira M, Quereda V, Flores I, et al. A GRFa2/Prop1/stem (GPS) cell niche in the pituitary. *PLoS ONE.* 2009;4:e4815.
47. Rizzoti K, Akiyama H, Lovell-Badge R. Mobilized adult pituitary stem cells contribute to endocrine regeneration in response to physiological demand. *Cell Stem Cell.* 2013;13:419-432.
48. Andoniadou CL, Matsushima D, Mousavy Gharavy SN, et al. Sox2(+) stem/progenitor cells in the adult mouse pituitary support organ homeostasis and have tumor-inducing potential. *Cell Stem Cell.* 2013;13:433-445.
49. Suga H, Kadoshima T, Minaguchi M, et al. Self-formation of functional adenohypophysis in three-dimensional culture. *Nature.* 2011;480: 57-62.

50. Garcia-Lavandeira M, Saez C, Diaz-Rodriguez E, et al. Craniopharyngiomas express embryonic stem cell markers (SOX2, OCT4, KLF4, and SOX9) as pituitary stem cells but do not coexpress RET/GFRA3 receptors. *J Clin Endocrinol Metab.* 2012;97:E80-E87.

51. Le Tissier PR, Hodson DJ, Lafont C, et al. Anterior pituitary cell networks. *Front Neuroendocrinol.* 2012;33:252-266.

52. Wilhelmi AE. Fractionation of human pituitary glands. *Can J Biochem.* 1961;39:1659-1668.

53. Suganuma N, Seo H, Yamamoto N, et al. Ontogenesis of pituitary prolactin in the human fetus. *J Clin Endocrinol Metab.* 1986;63:156-161.

54. Kleinberg DL, Frantz AG. A sensitive in vitro assay for prolactin. Program of the 51st Meeting of the Endocrine Society. 1969 Abstract 32.

55. Frantz AG, Kleinberg DL. Prolactin: evidence that it is separate from growth hormone in human blood. *Science.* 1970;170:745-747.

56. Hwang P, Guyda H, Friesen H. A radioimmunoassay for human prolactin. *Proc Natl Acad Sci U S A.* 1971;68:1902-1906.

57. Friesen HG. The discovery of human prolactin: a very personal account. *Clin Invest Med.* 1995;18:66-72.

58. Burrows HL, Birkmeier TS, Seasholtz AF, Camper SA. Targeted ablation of cells in the pituitary primordia of transgenic mice. *Mol Endocrinol.* 1996;10:1467-1477.

59. Boockfor FR, Hoeffler JP, Frawley LS. Estradiol induces a shift in cultured cells that release prolactin or growth hormone. *Am J Physiol.* 1986;250:E103-E105.

60. Scheithauer BW, Sano T, Kovacs KT, et al. The pituitary gland in pregnancy: a clinicopathologic and immunohistochemical study of 69 cases. *Mayo Clin Proc.* 1990;65:461-474.

61. Owerbach D, Rutter WJ, Cooke NE, et al. The prolactin gene is located on chromosome 6 in humans. *Science.* 1981;212:815-816.

62. Cooke NE, Coit D, Weiner RI, et al. Structure of cloned DNA complementary to rat prolactin messenger RNA. *J Biol Chem.* 1980;255:6502-6510.

63. Lamberts SW, Macleod RM. Regulation of prolactin secretion at the level of the lactotroph. *Physiol Rev.* 1990;70:279-318.

64. Farkouh NH, Packer MG, Frantz AG. Large molecular size prolactin with reduced receptor activity in human serum: high proportion in basal state and reduction after thyrotropin-releasing hormone. *J Clin Endocrinol Metab.* 1979;48:1026-1032.

65. Sinha YN. Structural variants of prolactin: occurrence and physiological significance. *Endocr Rev.* 1995;16:354-369.

66. Suh HK, Frantz AG. Size heterogeneity of human prolactin in plasma and pituitary extracts. *J Clin Endocrinol Metab.* 1974;39:928-935.

67. Lewis UJ, Singh RN, Sinha YN, VanderLaan WP. Glycosylated human prolactin. *Endocrinology.* 1985;116:359-363.

68. Mittra I. A novel "cleaved prolactin" in the rat pituitary: Part I. Biosynthesis, characterization and regulatory control. *Biochem Biophys Res Commun.* 1980;95(4):1750-1759.

69. Lee H, Struman I, Clapp C, et al. Inhibition of urokinase activity by the antiangiogenic factor 16K prolactin: activation of plasminogen activator inhibitor 1 expression. *Endocrinology.* 1998;139:3696.

70. Ferrara N, Clapp C, Weiner R. The 16K fragment of prolactin specifically inhibits basal or fibroblast growth factor stimulated growth of capillary endothelial cells. *Endocrinology.* 1991;129:896-900.

71. Hilfiker-Kleiner D, Kaminski K, Podewski E, et al. A cathepsin D-cleaved 16 kDa form of prolactin mediates postpartum cardiomyopathy. *Cell.* 2007;128:589-600.

72. Halkein J, Tabruyn SP, Ricke-Hoch M, et al. MicroRNA-146a is a therapeutic target and biomarker for peripartum cardiomyopathy. *J Clin Invest.* 2013;123:2143-2154.

73. Ho KK. The year in pituitary 2014. *J Clin Endocrinol Metab.* 2014;99(12):4449-4454.

74. Yang Y, Rodriguez JE, Kitsis RN. A microRNA links prolactin to peripartum cardiomyopathy. *J Clin Invest.* 2013;123:1925-1927.

75. Liu JW, Ben Jonathan N. Prolactin-releasing activity of neurohypophysial hormones: structure-function relationship. *Endocrinology.* 1994;134:114-118.

76. Horseman ND. Prolactin. In: DeGroot LJ, Jameson JL, eds. *Endocrinology.* 4th ed. Philadelphia, PA: WB Saunders; 2001:209-220.

77. Horseman ND, Zhao W, Montecino-Rodriguez E, et al. Defective mammopoiesis, but normal hematopoiesis, in mice with targeted disruption of the prolactin gene. *EMBO J.* 1997;16:6926-6935.

78. Steger RW, Chandrashekar V, Zhao W, et al. Neuroendocrine and reproductive functions in male mice with targeted disruption of the prolactin gene. *Endocrinology.* 1998;139:3691-3695.

79. Kanyicska B, Lerant A, Freeman ME. Endothelin is an autocrine regulator of prolactin secretion. *Endocrinology.* 1998;139:5164-5173.

80. Sarkar DK, Kim KH, Minami S. Transforming growth factor-beta 1 messenger RNA and protein expression in the pituitary gland: its action on prolactin secretion and lactotropic growth. *Mol Endocrinol.* 1992;6:1825-1833.

81. Shah GV, Pedchenko V, Stanley S, et al. Calcitonin is a physiological inhibitor of prolactin secretion in ovariectomized female rats. *Endocrinology.* 1996;137:1814-1822.

82. Ben Jonathan N. Regulation of prolactin secretion. In: Imura H, ed. *The Pituitary Gland.* 2nd ed. New York, NY: Raven Press; 1994:261-283.

83. Hinuma S, Habata Y, Fujii R, et al. A prolactin-releasing peptide in the brain [see comments] [published erratum appears in *Nature.* 1998;394(6690):302]. *Nature.* 1998;393:272-276.

84. Rubinek T, Hadani M, Barkai G, et al. Prolactin (PRL)-releasing peptide stimulates PRL secretion from human fetal pituitary cultures and growth hormone release from cultured pituitary adenomas. *J Clin Endocrinol Metab.* 2001;86:2826-2830.

85. Reichlin S. TRH: historical aspects. *Ann N Y Acad Sci.* 1989;553:1-6.

86. Cooke NE. Prolactin: normal synthesis, regulation, and actions. In: DeGroot LJ, Besser GM, Cahill GFJ, eds. *Endocrinology.* Philadelphia, PA: WB Saunders; 1989:384-407.

87. Katznelson L, Riskind PN, Saxe VC, Klibanski A. Prolactin pulsatile characteristics in postmenopausal women. *J Clin Endocrinol Metab.* 1998;83:761-764.

88. Peters LL, Hoefer MT, Ben-Jonathan N. The posterior pituitary: regulation of anterior pituitary prolactin secretion. *Science.* 1981;213:659-661.

89. Cooper DS, Ridgway EC, Kliman B, et al. Metabolic clearance and production rates of prolactin in man. *J Clin Invest.* 1979;64:1669-1680.

90. Veldhuis JD, Johnson ML. Operating characteristics of the hypothalamo-pituitary-gonadal axis in men: circadian, ultradian, and pulsatile release of prolactin and its temporal coupling with luteinizing hormone. *J Clin Endocrinol Metab.* 1988;67:116-123.

91. Greenspan SL, Klibanski A, Rowe JW, Elahi D. Age alters pulsatile prolactin release: influence of dopaminergic inhibition. *Am J Physiol.* 1990;258:E799-E804.

92. Sassin JF, Frantz AG, Weitzman ED, Kapen S. Human prolactin: 24-hour pattern with increased release during sleep. *Science.* 1972;177:1205-1207.

93. Parker DC, Rossman LG, Vanderlaan EF. Relation of sleep-entrained human prolactin release to REM-nonREM cycles. *J Clin Endocrinol Metab.* 1974;38:646-651.

94. Iranmanesh A, Mulligan T, Veldhuis JD. Mechanisms subserving the physiological nocturnal relative hypoprolactinemia of healthy older men: dual decline in prolactin secretory burst mass and basal release with preservation of pulse duration, frequency, and interpulse interval—a General Clinical Research Center study. *J Clin Endocrinol Metab.* 1999;84:1083-1090.

95. Bazan JF. Structural design and molecular evolution of a cytokine receptor superfamily. *Proc Natl Acad Sci U S A.* 1990;87:6934-6938.

96. Hu ZZ, Zhuang L, Meng J, et al. The human prolactin receptor gene structure and alternative promoter utilization: the generic promoter hPIII and a novel human promoter hP(N). *J Clin Endocrinol Metab.* 1999;84:1153-1156.

97. Bole-Feysot C, Goffin V, Edery M, et al. Prolactin (PRL) and its receptor: actions, signal transduction pathways and phenotypes observed in PRL receptor knockout mice. *Endocr Rev.* 1998;19:225-268.

98. de Vos AM, Ultsch M, Kossiakoff AA. Human growth hormone and extracellular domain of its receptor: crystal structure of the complex. *Science.* 1992;255:306-312.

99. Clevenger CV, Gadd SL, Zheng J. New mechanisms for PRLr action in breast cancer. *Trends Endocrinol Metab.* 2009;20:223-229.

100. Gao J, Hughes JP, Auperin B, et al. Interactions among JANUS kinases and the prolactin (PRL) receptor in the regulation of a PRL response element. *Mol Endocrinol.* 1996;10:847-856.

101. Hynes NE, Cella N, Wartmann M. Prolactin mediated intracellular signaling in mammary epithelial cells. *J Mammary Gland Biol Neopl.* 1997;19-27.

102. Goffin V, Kelly PA. The prolactin/growth hormone receptor family: structure/function relationships. *J Mammary Gland Biol Neopl.* 1997;2:7-17.

103. Bogorad RL, Courtillot C, Mestayer C, et al. Identification of a gain-of-function mutation of the prolactin receptor in women with benign breast tumors. *Proc Natl Acad Sci U S A.* 2008;105:14533-14538.

104. Jomain JB, Tallet E, Broutin I, et al. Structural and thermodynamic bases for the design of pure prolactin receptor antagonists, x-ray structure of Del1-9-G129R-hPRL. *J Biol Chem.* 2007;282:33118-33131.

105. Riddle O. Prolactin in vertebrate function and organization. *J Nat Cancer Inst.* 1963;31:1039-1110.

106. Lucas BK, Ormandy CJ, Binart N, et al. Null mutation of the prolactin receptor gene produces a defect in maternal behavior. *Endocrinology.* 1998;139:4102-4107.

107. Kleinberg DL, Ruan W, Catanese V, et al. Non-lactogenic effects of growth hormone on growth and insulin-like growth factor-I messenger ribonucleic acid of rat mammary gland [published erratum appears in *Endocrinology.* 1990;127(4):1977]. *Endocrinology.* 1990;126:3274-3276.

108. Feldman M, Ruan WF, Cunningham BC, et al. Evidence that the growth hormone receptor mediates differentiation and development of the mammary gland. *Endocrinology.* 1993;133:1602-1608.

109. Ruan W, Catanese V, Wieczorek R, et al. Estradiol enhances the stimulatory effect of insulin-like growth factor-I (IGF-I) on mammary development and growth hormone-induced IGF-I messenger ribonucleic acid. *Endocrinology.* 1995;136:1296-1302.

110. Cunha GR. Role of mesenchymal-epithelial interactions in normal and abnormal development of the mammary gland and prostate. *Cancer.* 1994;74:1030-1044.

111. Ruan W, Monaco ME, Kleinberg DL. Progesterone stimulates mammary gland ductal morphogenesis by synergizing with and enhancing insulin-like growth factor-I action. *Endocrinology.* 2005;146:1170-1178.

112. Walden PD, Ruan W, Feldman M, Kleinberg DL. Evidence that growth hormone acts on stromal tissue to stimulate pubertal mammary gland development. Program 79th Annual Meeting of the Endocrine Society. 1997 Abstract P1-120.

113. Wysolmerski JJ, Stewart AF. The physiology of parathyroid hormone-related protein: an emerging role as a developmental factor. *Annu Rev Physiol.* 1998;60:431-460.

114. Wiesen JF, Young P, Werb Z, Cunha GR. Signaling through the stromal epidermal growth factor receptor is necessary for mammary ductal development. *Development.* 1999;126:335-344.

115. Anderson TJ, Battersby S, King RJB, et al. Oral contraceptive use influences resting breast proliferation. *Hum Pathol.* 1989;20:1139-1144.

116. Vorherr H. Hormonal and biochemical changes of pituitary and breast during pregnancy. *Semin Perinat.* 1979;3:193-198.

117. Richert MM, Wood TL. The insulin-like growth factors (IGF) and the IGF type I receptor during postnatal growth of the murine mammary gland: sites of messenger ribonucleic acid expression and potential functions. *Endocrinology.* 1999;140:454-461.

118. Falk RJ. Isolated prolactin deficiency: a case report. *Fertil Steril.* 1992; 58:1060-1062.

119. Humphreys RC, Lydon J, O'Malley BW, Rosen JM. Mammary gland development is mediated by both stromal and epithelial progesterone receptors. *Mol Endocrinol.* 1997;11:801-811.

120. Kleinberg DL, Boyd AEII, Wardlaw S, et al. Pergolide for the treatment of pituitary tumors secreting prolactin or growth hormone. *N Engl J Med.* 1983;309:704-709.

121. Graham JD, Clarke CL. Physiological action of progesterone in target tissues. *Endocr Rev.* 1997;18:502-519.

122. Vorherr H. Galactopoiesis, galactosecretion, and onset of lactation. In: Vorherr H, ed. *The Breast.* New York, NY: Academic Press; 1974: 71-127.

123. Tyson JE, Hwang P, Guyda H. Studies of prolactin secretion in human pregnancy. *Am J Obstet Gynecol.* 1972;113:14-20.

124. Howie PW, McNeilly AS, McArdle T, et al. The relationship between suckling-induced prolactin response and lactogenesis. *J Clin Endocrinol Metab.* 1980;50:670-673.

125. Johnston JM, Amico JA. A prospective longitudinal study of the release of oxytocin and prolactin in response to infant suckling in long term lactation. *J Clin Endocrinol Metab.* 1986;62:653-657.

126. Leite V, Cowden EA, Friesen HG. Endocrinology of lactation and nursing: disorders of lactation. In: DeGroot LJ, ed. *Endocrinology.* 3rd ed. Philadelphia, PA: WB Saunders; 1995:2224-2233.

127. Wagner KU, Young WS, Liu X, et al. Oxytocin and milk removal are required for post partum mammary-gland development. *Genes Funct.* 1997;1:233-244.

128. Short RV. Breast feeding. *Sci Am.* 1984;250:35-41.

129. Matsuzaki T, Azuma K, Irahara M, et al. Mechanism of anovulation in hyperprolactinemic amenorrhea determined by pulsatile gonadotropin-releasing hormone injection combined with human chorionic gonadotropin. *Fertil Steril.* 1994;62:1143-1149.

130. Kokay IC, Petersen SL, Grattan DR. Identification of prolactin-sensitive GABA and kisspeptin neurons in regions of the rat hypothalamus involved in the control of fertility. *Endocrinology.* 2011;152:526-535.

131. Kaiser UB. Hyperprolactinemia and infertility: new insights. *J Clin Invest.* 2012;122:3467-3468.

132. Sonigo C, Bouilly J, Carré N, et al. Hyperprolactinemia-induced ovarian acyclicity is reversed by kisspeptin administration. *J Clin Invest.* 2012;122:3791-3795.

133. Richards SM, Murphy WJ. Use of human prolactin as a therapeutic protein to potentiate immunohematopoietic function. *J Neuroimmunol.* 2000;109:56-62.

134. Ormandy CJ, Camus A, Barra J, et al. Null mutation of the prolactin receptor gene produces multiple reproductive defects in the mouse. *Genes Dev.* 1997;11:167-178.

135. Adán N, Guzmán-Morales J, Ledesma-Colunga MG, et al. Prolactin promotes cartilage survival and attenuates inflammation in inflammatory arthritis. *J Clin Invest.* 2013;123:3902-3913.

136. Schulster D, Gaines Das RE, Jeffcoate SL. International Standards for human prolactin: calibration by international collaborative study. *J Endocrinol.* 1989;121:157-166.

137. Barkan AL, Chandler WF. Giant pituitary prolactinoma with falsely low serum prolactin: the pitfall of the "high-dose hook effect": case report. *Neurosurgery.* 1998;42:913-915.

138. Chahal J, Schlechte J. Hyperprolactinemia. *Pituitary.* 2008;11:141-146.

139. Molitch ME. Pathologic hyperprolactinemia. *Endocrinol Metab Clin North Am.* 1992;21:877-901.

140. Noel GL, Suh HK, Frantz AG. Prolactin release during nursing and breast stimulation in postpartum and nonpostpartum subjects. *J Clin Endocrinol Metab.* 1974;38:413-423.

141. Diaz S, Seron-Ferre M, Cardenas H, et al. Circadian variation of basal plasma prolactin, prolactin response to suckling, and length of amenorrhea in nursing women. *J Clin Endocrinol Metab.* 1989;68:946-955.

142. Berinder K, Stackenas I, Akre O, et al. Hyperprolactinaemia in 271 women: up to three decades of clinical follow-up. *Clin Endocrinol (Oxf).* 2005;63:450-455.

143. McKenna TJ. Should macroprolactin be measured in all hyperprolactinaemic sera? *Clin Endocrinol (Oxf).* 2009;71:466-469.

144. Gibney J, Smith TP, McKenna TJ. The impact on clinical practice of routine screening for macroprolactin. *J Clin Endocrinol Metab.* 2005;90: 3927-3932.

145. Karavitaki N, Thanabalasingham G, Shore HC, et al. Do the limits of serum prolactin in disconnection hyperprolactinaemia need re-definition? A study of 226 patients with histologically verified nonfunctioning pituitary macroadenoma. *Clin Endocrinol (Oxf).* 2006;65: 524-529.

146. Kleinberg DL, Noel GL, Frantz AG. Galactorrhea: a study of 235 cases, including 48 with pituitary tumors. *N Engl J Med.* 1977;296:589-600.

147. Travaglini P, Moriondo P, Togni E, et al. Effect of oral zinc administration on prolactin and thymulin circulating levels in patients with chronic renal failure. *J Clin Endocrinol Metab.* 1989;68:186-190.

148. Ramirez G, Butcher DE, Newton JL, et al. Bromocriptine and the hypothalamic hypophyseal function in patients with chronic renal failure on chronic hemodialysis. *Am J Kidney Dis.* 1985;6:111-118.

149. Lim VS, Henriquez C, Sievertsen G, Frohman LA. Ovarian function in chronic renal failure: evidence suggesting hypothalamic anovulation. *Ann Intern Med.* 1980;93:21-27.

150. Noel GL, Suh HK, Stone JG, Frantz AG. Human prolactin and growth hormone release during surgery and other conditions of stress. *J Clin Endocrinol Metab.* 1972;35:840-851.

151. Agha A, Sherlock M, Brennan S, et al. Hypothalamic-pituitary dysfunction after irradiation of nonpituitary brain tumors in adults. *J Clin Endocrinol Metab.* 2005;90:6355-6360.

152. Newey PJ, Gorvin CM, Cleland SJ, et al. Mutant prolactin receptor and familial hyperprolactinemia. *N Engl J Med.* 2013;369:2012-2020.

153. Szarfman A, Tonning JM, Levine JG, Doraiswamy PM. Atypical antipsychotics and pituitary tumors: a pharmacovigilance study. *Pharmacotherapy.* 2006;26:748-758.

154. Misra M, Papakostas GI, Klibanski A. Effects of psychiatric disorders and psychotropic medications on prolactin and bone metabolism. *J Clin Psychiatry.* 2004;65:1607-1618, quiz 1590, 1760-1761.

155. Bonert V, Melmed S. Acromegaly with moderate hyperprolactinemia caused by an intrasellar macroadenoma. *Nat Clin Pract Endocrinol Metab.* 2006;2:408-412, quiz following 412.

156. Johnsen E, Kroken RA, Abaza M, et al. Antipsychotic-induced hyperprolactinemia: a cross-sectional survey. *J Clin Psychopharmacol.* 2008; 28:686-690.

157. Tollin SR. Use of the dopamine agonists bromocriptine and cabergoline in the management of risperidone-induced hyperprolactinemia in patients with psychotic disorders. *J Endocrinol Invest.* 2000;23: 765-770.

158. Sharp EA. Historical review of a syndrome embracing utero-ovarian atrophy with persistent lactation (Frommel's disease). *Am J Obstet Gynecol.* 1935;30:411-414.

159. Argonz J, del Castillo EB. A syndrome characterized by estrogenic insufficiency, galactorrhea and decreased urinary gonadotropin. *J Clin Endocrinol Metab.* 1953;13:79-87.

160. Forbes AP, Henneman PH, Griswold GC, Albright F. Syndrome characterized by galactorrhea, amenorrhea and low urinary FSH: comparison with acromegaly and normal lactation. *J Clin Endocrinol Metab.* 1954; 14:265-271.

161. Kleinberg DL. Endocrinology of mammary development, lactation and galactorrhea. In: DeGroot LJ, Jameson JL, eds. *Endocrinology.* 4th ed. Philadelphia, PA: WB Saunders; 2000:2464-2475.

162. Kleinberg DL, Lieberman A, Todd J, et al. Pergolide mesylate: a potent day-long inhibitor of prolactin in rhesus monkeys and patients with Parkinson's disease. *J Clin Endocrinol Metab.* 1980;51:152-154.

163. MacFarlane IA, Rosin MD. Galactorrhoea following surgical procedures to the chest wall: the role of prolactin. *Postgrad Med J.* 1980;56: 23-25.

164. Joustra SD, Schoenmakers N, Persani L, et al. The IGSF1 deficiency syndrome: characteristics of male and female patients. *J Clin Endocrinol Metab.* 2013;98:4942-4952.

165. Iwama S, Welt CK, Romero CJ, et al. Isolated prolactin deficiency associated with serum autoantibodies against prolactin-secreting cells. *J Clin Endocrinol Metab.* 2013;98:3920-3925.

166. Mukherjee A, Murray RD, Columb B, et al. Acquired prolactin deficiency indicates severe hypopituitarism in patients with disease of the hypothalamic-pituitary axis. *Clin Endocrinol.* 2003;59:743-748.

167. Keleştimur F. Sheehan's syndrome. *Pituitary.* 2003;6:181-188.

168. Powe CE, Allen M, Puopolo KM, et al. Recombinant human prolactin for the treatment of lactation insufficiency. *Clin Endocrinol.* 2010;73: 645-653.

169. Frohman LA, Burek L, Stachura MA. Characterization of growth hormone of different molecular weights in rat, dog and human pituitaries. *Endocrinology.* 1972;91:262-269.

170. Ho Y, Liebhaber SA, Cooke NE. Activation of the human GH gene cluster: roles for targeted chromatin modification. *Trends Endocrinol Metab*. 2004;15:40-45.

171. Miller WL, Eberhardt NL. Structure and evolution of the growth hormone gene family. *Endocr Rev*. 1983;4:97-130.

172. Ho Y, Elefant F, Liebhaber SA, Cooke NE. Locus control region transcription plays an active role in long-range gene activation. *Mol Cell*. 2006;23:365-375.

173. Kimura AP, Sizova D, Handwerger S, et al. Epigenetic activation of the human growth hormone gene cluster during placental cytotrophoblast differentiation. *Mol Cell Biol*. 2007;27:6555-6568.

174. Frankenne F, Closset J, Gomez F, et al. The physiology of growth hormones (GHs) in pregnant women and partial characterization of the placental GH variant. *J Clin Endocrinol Metab*. 1988;66:1171-1180.

175. Parks JS, Brown MR, Hurley DL, et al. Heritable disorders of pituitary development. *J Clin Endocrinol Metab*. 1999;84:4362-4370.

176. Ho Y, Liebhaber SA, Cooke NE. The role of the hGH locus control region in somatotrope restriction of hGH-N gene expression. *Mol Endocrinol*. 2011;25:877-884.

177. Cunningham BC, Ultsch M, De Vos AM, et al. Dimerization of the extracellular domain of the human growth hormone receptor by a single hormone molecule. *Science*. 1991;254:821-825.

178. Baumann G, MacCart JG, Amburn K. The molecular nature of circulating growth hormone in normal and acromegalic man: evidence for a principal and minor monomeric form. *J Clin Endocrinol Metab*. 1983;56:946-952.

179. Lal S, Martin JB, De la Vega CE, Friesen HG. Comparison of the effect of apomorphine and L-DOPA on serum growth hormone levels in normal men. *Clin Endocrinol (Oxf)*. 1975;4:277-285.

180. Giustina A, Veldhuis JD. Pathophysiology of the neuroregulation of growth hormone secretion in experimental animals and the human. *Endocr Rev*. 1998;19:717-797.

181. Mayo KE, Miller T, DeAlmeida V, et al. Regulation of the pituitary somatotroph cell by GHRH and its receptor. *Recent Prog Horm Res*. 2000;55:237-266.

182. Shimon I, Taylor JE, Dong JZ, et al. Somatostatin receptor subtype specificity in human fetal pituitary cultures. Differential role of SSTR2 and SSTR5 for growth hormone, thyroid-stimulating hormone, and prolactin regulation. *J Clin Invest*. 1997;99:789-798.

183. Shimon I, Yan X, Taylor JE, et al. Somatostatin receptor (SSTR) subtype-selective analogues differentially suppress in vitro growth hormone and prolactin in human pituitary adenomas. Novel potential therapy for functional pituitary tumors. *J Clin Invest*. 1997;100:2386-2392.

184. Barinaga M, Yamonoto G, Rivier C, et al. Transcriptional regulation of growth hormone gene expression by growth hormone-releasing factor. *Nature*. 1983;306:84-85.

185. Gelato MC, Pescovitz O, Cassorla F, et al. Effects of a growth hormone releasing factor in man. *J Clin Endocrinol Metab*. 1983;57:674-676.

186. Tannenbaum GS, Ling N. The interrelationship of growth hormone (GH)-releasing factor and somatostatin in generation of the ultradian rhythm of GH secretion. *Endocrinology*. 1984;115:1952-1957.

187. Vance ML, Cragun JR, Reimnitz C, et al. CV205-502 treatment of hyperprolactinemia. *J Clin Endocrinol Metab*. 1989;68:336-339.

188. Jaffe CA, Friberg RD, Barkan AL. Suppression of growth hormone (GH) secretion by a selective GH-releasing hormone (GHRH) antagonist. Direct evidence for involvement of endogenous GHRH in the generation of GH pulses. *J Clin Invest*. 1993;92:695-701.

189. Bilezikjian LM, Seifert H, Vale W. Desensitization to growth hormone-releasing factor (GRF) is associated with down-regulation of GRF-binding sites. *Endocrinology*. 1986;118:2045-2052.

190. Kineman RD, Teixeira LT, Amargo GV, et al. The effect of GHRH on somatotrope hyperplasia and tumor formation in the presence and absence of GH signaling. *Endocrinology*. 2001;142:3764-3773.

191. LeRoith D, Buler A. What is the role of circulating IGF-I? *Trends Endocrinol Metab*. 2001;12:48-52.

192. Yamashita S, Melmed S. Insulin regulation of rat growth hormone gene transcription. *J Clin Invest*. 1986;78:1008-1014.

193. Howard AD, Feighner SD, Cully DF, et al. A receptor in pituitary and hypothalamus that functions in growth hormone release. *Science*. 1996;273:974-977.

194. Kojima M, Hosoda H, Date Y, et al. Ghrelin is a growth-hormone-releasing acylated peptide from stomach. *Nature*. 1999;402:656-660.

195. Tannenbaum GS, Epelbaum J, Bowers CY. Interrelationship between the novel peptide ghrelin and somatostatin/growth hormone-releasing hormone in regulation of pulsatile growth hormone secretion. *Endocrinology*. 2003;144:967-974.

196. Cummings DE, Weigle DS, Frayo RS, et al. Plasma ghrelin levels after diet-induced weight loss or gastric bypass surgery. *N Engl J Med*. 2002;346:1623-1630.

197. Grove KL, Cowley MA. Is ghrelin a signal for the development of metabolic systems? *J Clin Invest*. 2005;115:3393-3397.

198. Casanueva FF, Camina JP, Carreira MC, et al. Growth hormone-releasing hormone as an agonist of the ghrelin receptor GHS-R1a. *Proc Natl Acad Sci U S A*. 2008;105:20452-20457.

199. Popovic V, Damjanovic S, Micic D, et al. Blocked growth hormone-releasing peptide (GHRP-6)-induced GH secretion and absence of the synergic action of GHRP-6 plus GH-releasing hormone in patients with hypothalamopituitary disconnection: evidence that GHRP-6 main action is exerted at the hypothalamic level. *J Clin Endocrinol Metab*. 1995;80:942-947.

200. Smith RG, Jiang H, Sun Y. Developments in ghrelin biology and potential clinical relevance. *Trends Endocrinol Metab*. 2005;16:436-442.

201. Van Cauter E, Plat L, Copinschi G. Interrelations between sleep and the somatotropic axis. *Sleep*. 1998;21:553-566.

202. Taylor AL, Finster JL, Mintz DH. Metabolic clearance and production rates of human growth hormone. *J Clin Invest*. 1969;48:2349-2358.

203. Vahl N, Jorgensen JO, Jurik AG, Christiansen JS. Abdominal adiposity and physical fitness are major determinants of the age associated decline in stimulated GH secretion in healthy adults. *J Clin Endocrinol Metab*. 1996;81:2209-2215.

204. Ho KY, Veldhuis JD, Johnson ML, et al. Fasting enhances growth hormone secretion and amplifies the complex rhythms of growth hormone secretion in man. *J Clin Invest*. 1988;81:968-975.

205. Casanueva FF, Dieguez C. Neuroendocrine regulation and actions of leptin. *Front Neuroendocrinol*. 1999;20:317-363.

206. Carro E, Senaris R, Considine RV, et al. Regulation of in vivo growth hormone secretion by leptin. *Endocrinology*. 1997;138:2203-2206.

207. Watanobe H, Habu S. Leptin regulates growth hormone-releasing factor, somatostatin, and alpha-melanocyte-stimulating hormone but not neuropeptide Y release in rat hypothalamus in vivo: relation with growth hormone secretion. *J Neurosci*. 2002;22:6265-6271.

208. Casanueva FF, Burguera B, Muruais C, Dieguez C. Acute administration of corticoids: a new and peculiar stimulus of growth hormone secretion in man. *J Clin Endocrinol Metab*. 1990;70:234-237.

209. Weissberger AJ, Ho KKY. Activation of the somatotropic axis by testosterone in adult males: evidence for the role of aromatization. *J Clin Endocrinol Metab*. 1993;76:1407-1412.

210. Leung KC, Johannsson G, Leong GM, Ho KK. Estrogen regulation of growth hormone action. *Endocr Rev*. 2004;25:693-721.

211. Birzniece V, Sata A, Sutanto S, Ho KK. Paracrine regulation of growth hormone secretion by estrogen in women. *J Clin Endocrinol Metab*. 2010;95:3771-3776.

212. Herington AC, Ymer S, Stevenson J. Identification and characterization of specific binding proteins for growth hormone in normal human sera. *J Clin Invest*. 1986;77:1817-1823.

213. Leung DW, Spencer SA, Cachianes G, et al. Growth hormone receptor and serum binding protein: purification, cloning and expression. *Nature*. 1987;330:537-543.

214. Schantl JA, Roza M, Van Kerkhof P, Strous GJ. The growth hormone receptor interacts with its sheddase, the tumour necrosis factor-alpha-converting enzyme (TACE). *Biochem J*. 2004;377:379-384.

215. Ho KY, Valiontis E, Waters MJ, Rajkovic IA. Regulation of growth hormone binding protein in man: comparison of gel chromatography and immunoprecipitation methods. *J Clin Endocrinol Metab*. 1993;76:302-308.

216. Daughaday W, Trivedi B. Absence of serum growth hormone binding protein in patients with growth hormone receptor deficiency (Laron dwarfism). *Proc Natl Acad Sci U S A*. 1987;84:4636-4640.

217. Goddard AD, Covello R, Luoh SM, et al. Mutations in the growth hormone receptor in children with idiopathic short stature. The Growth Hormone Insensitivity Study Group. *N Engl J Med*. 1995;333:1093-1098.

218. Baumann G, Shaw MA, Merimee TJ. Low levels of high-affinity growth hormone binding protein in African pigmies. *N Engl J Med*. 1989;320:1705-1709.

219. Ip TP, Hoffman DM, Leung KC, Ho KKY. Do androgens regulate growth hormone binding protein in man? *J Clin Endocrinol Metab*. 1995;80:1278-1282.

220. Carter-Su C, Schwartz J, Smit LS. Molecular mechanism of growth hormone action. *Annu Rev Physiol*. 1996;58:187-207.

221. Brown RJ, Adams JJ, Pelekanos RA, et al. Model for growth hormone receptor activation based on subunit rotation within a receptor dimer. *Nat Struct Mol Biol*. 2005;12:814-821.

222. Leung KC, Waters MJ, Markus I, et al. Insulin and insulin-like growth factor-I acutely inhibit surface translocation of growth hormone receptors in osteoblasts: a novel mechanism of growth hormone receptor regulation. *Proc Natl Acad Sci U S A*. 1997;94:11381-11386.

223. Brooks AJ, Wooh JW, Tunny KA, Waters MJ. Growth hormone receptor; mechanism of action. *Int J Biochem Cell Biol*. 2008;40:1984-1989.

224. Brooks AJ, Dai W, O'Mara ML, et al. Mechanism of activation of protein kinase JAK2 by the growth hormone receptor. *Science*. 2014;344:1249783.

225. Xu BC, Wang X, Darus CJ, Kopchick JJ. Growth hormone promotes the association of transcription factor STAT5 with the growth hormone receptor. *J Biol Chem*. 1996;271:19768-19773.

226. Starr R, Hilton DJ. SOCS: suppressors of cytokine signalling. *Int J Biochem Cell Biol*. 1998;30:1081-1085.

227. Greenhalgh CJ, Rico-Bautista E, Lorentzon M, et al. SOCS2 negatively regulates growth hormone action in vitro and in vivo. *J Clin Invest*. 2005;115:397-406.

228. Low MJ, Otero-Corchon V, Parlow AF, et al. Somatostatin is required for masculinization of growth hormone-regulated hepatic gene expression but not of somatic growth. *J Clin Invest.* 2001;107:1571-1580.

229. Ram PA, Park SH, Choi HK, Waxman DJ. Growth hormone activation of Stat 1, Stat 3, and Stat 5 in rat liver. Differential kinetics of hormone desensitization and growth hormone stimulation of both tyrosine phosphorylation and serine/threonine phosphorylation. *J Biol Chem.* 1996;271:5929-5940.

230. Teglund S, McKay C, Schuetz E, et al. Stat5a and Stat5b proteins have essential and nonessential, or redundant, roles in cytokine responses. *Cell.* 1998;93:841-850.

231. Davey HW, Park SH, Grattan DR, et al. STAT5b-deficient mice are growth hormone pulse-resistant. Role of STAT5b in sex-specific liver p450 expression. *J Biol Chem.* 1999;274:35331-35336.

232. Park SH, Liu X, Hennighausen L, et al. Distinctive roles of STAT5a and STAT5b in sexual dimorphism of hepatic P450 gene expression. Impact of STAT5a gene disruption. *J Biol Chem.* 1999;274:7421-7430.

233. Erturk E, Jaffe CA, Barkan AL. Evaluation of the integrity of the hypothalamic-pituitary-adrenal axis by insulin hypoglycemia test. *J Clin Endocrinol Metab.* 1998;83:2350-2354.

234. Surya S, Horowitz JF, Goldenberg N, et al. The pattern of growth hormone delivery to peripheral tissues determines insulin-like growth factor-1 and lipolytic responses in obese subjects. *J Clin Endocrinol Metab.* 2009;94(8):2828-2834.

235. LeRoith D, Bondy C, Yakar S, et al. The somatomedin hypothesis: 2001. *Endocr Rev.* 2001;22:53-74.

236. Yakar S, Liu JL, Stannard B, et al. Normal growth and development in the absence of hepatic insulin-like growth factor I. *Proc Natl Acad Sci U S A.* 1999;96:7324-7329.

237. Rudling M, Norstedt G, Olivecrona H, et al. Importance of growth hormone for the induction of hepatic low density lipoprotein receptors. *Proc Natl Acad Sci U S A.* 1992;89:6983-6987.

238. Rudling M, Olivecrona H, Eggertsen G, Angelin B. Regulation of rat hepatic low density lipoprotein receptors. In vivo stimulation by growth hormone is not mediated by insulin-like growth factor I. *J Clin Invest.* 1996;97:292-299.

239. Maison P, Griffin S, Nicoue-Beglah M, et al. Impact of growth hormone (GH) treatment on cardiovascular risk factors in GH-deficient adults: a metaanalysis of blinded, randomized, placebo-controlled trials. *J Clin Endocrinol Metab.* 2004;89:2192-2199.

240. Moller N, Jorgensen JO. Effects of growth hormone on glucose, lipid, and protein metabolism in human subjects. *Endocr Rev.* 2009;30:152-177.

241. Cameron CM, Kostyo JL, Adamafio NA, et al. The acute effects of growth hormone on amino acid transport and protein synthesis are due to its insulin-like action. *Endocrinology.* 1988;122:471-474.

242. Fryburg DA, Barrett EJ. Growth hormone acutely stimulates skeletal muscle but not whole-body protein synthesis in humans. *Metabolism.* 1993;42:1223-1227.

243. Rosen T, Bengtsson BA. Premature mortality due to cardiovascular disease in hypopituitarism. *Lancet.* 1990;336:285-288.

244. Bates AS, Van't Hoff W, Jones PJ, Clayton RN. The effect of hypopituitarism on life expectancy. *J Clin Endocrinol Metab.* 1996;81:1169-1172.

245. Tomlinson JW, Holden N, Hills RK, et al. Association between premature mortality and hypopituitarism. West Midlands Prospective Hypopituitary Study Group. *Lancet.* 2001;357:425-431.

246. Bulow B, Hagmar L, Eskilsson J, Erfurth EM. Hypopituitary females have a high incidence of cardiovascular morbidity and increased prevalence of cardiovascular risk factors. *J Clin Endo Metab.* 2000;85:574-584.

247. Ho KKY. Growth hormone deficiency in adults. In: DeGroot LJ, Jameson JL, eds. *De Groot's Textbook of Endocrinology.* 5th ed. Philadelphia, PA: WB Saunders; 2004:550-558.

248. Webb SM, Strasburger CJ, Mo D, et al; HypoCCS International Advisory Board. Changing patterns of the adult growth hormone deficiency diagnosis documented in a decade-long global surveillance database. *J Clin Endocrinol Metab.* 2009;94:392-399.

249. Wu W, Cogan JD, Pfaffle RW, et al. Mutations in PROP1 cause familial combined pituitary hormone deficiency. *Nature Gen.* 1998;18:147-149.

250. Tauber M, Moulin P, Pienkowski C, et al. Growth hormone retesting and auxological data in 131 GH-deficient patients after completion of treatment. *J Clin Endocrinol Metab.* 1997;82:352-356.

251. Cogan JD, Phillips JA, Schenkman SS, et al. Familial growth hormone deficiency: a model of dominant and recessive mutations affecting a monomeric protein. *J Clin Endocrinol Metab.* 1994;79:1261-1265.

252. Baumann G. Mutations in the growth hormone releasing hormone receptor: a new form of dwarfism in humans. *Growth Horm IGF Res.* 1999;9(Suppl B):24-29, discussion 29-30.

253. Rosenfeld RG, Rosenbloom AL, Guevara-Aguirre J. Growth hormone (GH) insensitivity due to primary GH receptor deficiency. *Endocr Rev.* 1994;15:369-390.

254. Carroll PV, Christ ER, Bengtsson BA, et al. Growth hormone deficiency in adulthood and the effects of growth hormone replacement: a review. *J Clin Endocrinol Metab.* 1998;83:382-395.

255. Sesmilo G, Biller BM, Llevadot J, et al. Effects of growth hormone administration on inflammatory and other cardiovascular risk markers in men with growth hormone deficiency. A randomized, controlled clinical trial. *Ann Intern Med.* 2000;133:111-122.

256. Attanasio AF, Lamberts SWJ, Matranga AMC, et al. Adult growth hormone (GH)-deficient patients demonstrate heterogeneity between childhood onset and adult onset before and during human GH treatment. *J Clin Endocrinol Metab.* 1997;82:82-88.

257. Pfeifer M, Verhovec R, Zizek B, et al. Growth hormone (GH) treatment reverses early atherosclerotic changes in GH-deficient adults [see comments]. *J Clin Endocrinol Metab.* 1999;84:453-457.

258. Borson-Chazot F, Serusclat A, Kalfallah Y, et al. Decrease in carotid intima-media thickness after one year growth hormone (GH) treatment in adults with GH deficiency. *J Clin Endocrinol Metab.* 1999;84:1329-1333.

259. Merola B, Cittadini A, Colao A, et al. Cardiac structural and functional abnormalities in adult patients with growth hormone deficiency. *J Clin Endocrinol Metab.* 1993;77:1658-1661.

260. Amato G, Carella C, Fazio S, et al. Body composition, bone metabolism, and heart structure and function in growth hormone (GH)-deficient adults before and after GH replacement therapy at low doses. *J Clin Endocrinol Metab.* 1993;77:1671-1676.

261. Klibanski A. Growth hormone and cardiovascular risk markers. *Growth Horm IGF Res.* 2003;13(Suppl A):S109-S115.

262. Aimaretti G, Colao A, Corneli G, et al. The study of spontaneous GH secretion after 36-h fasting distinguishes between GH-deficient and normal adults. *Clin Endocrinol (Oxf).* 1999;51:771-777.

263. Murray RD, Skillicorn CJ, Howell SJ, et al. Dose titration and patient selection increases the efficacy of GH replacement in severely GH deficient adults. *Clin Endocrinol (Oxf).* 1999;50:749-757.

264. Aguiar-Oliveira MH, Oliveira FT, Pereira RM, et al. Longevity in untreated congenital growth hormone deficiency due to a homozygous mutation in the GHRH receptor gene. *J Clin Endocrinol Metab.* 2010;95:714-721.

265. Menezes Oliveira JL, Marques-Santos C, Barreto-Filho JA, et al. Lack of evidence of premature atherosclerosis in untreated severe isolated growth hormone (GH) deficiency due to a GH-releasing hormone receptor mutation. *J Clin Endocrinol Metab.* 2006;91:2093-2099.

266. Guevara-Aguirre J, Balasubramanian P, Guevara-Aguirre M, et al. Growth hormone receptor deficiency is associated with a major reduction in pro-aging signaling, cancer, and diabetes in humans. *Sci Transl Med.* 2011;3:70ra13.

267. Molitch ME, Clemmons DR, Malozowski S, et al. Evaluation and treatment of adult growth hormone deficiency: an Endocrine Society clinical practice guideline. *J Clin Endocrinol Metab.* 2011;96:1587-1609.

268. Biller BM, Samuels MH, Zagar A, et al. Sensitivity and specificity of six tests for the diagnosis of adult GH deficiency. *J Clin Endocrinol Metab.* 2002;87(5):2067-2079.

269. Rahim A, Toogood AA, Shalet SM. The assessment of growth hormone status in normal young adult males using a variety of provocative agents. *Clin Endocrinol.* 1996;45:557-562.

270. Aimaretti G, Cornelli G, Razzore P, et al. Comparison between insulin-induced hypoglycemia and the growth hormone (GH) releasing hormone + arginine as provocative tests for the diagnosis of GH deficiency. *J Clin Endocrinol Metab.* 1998;83:1615-1618.

271. Popovic V, Leal A, Micic D, et al. GH-releasing hormone and GH-releasing peptide-6 for diagnostic testing in GH-deficient adults. *Lancet.* 2000;356:1137-1142.

272. Hoffman DM, O'Sullivan AJ, Baxter RC, Ho KKY. Diagnosis of growth hormone deficiency in adults. *Lancet.* 1994;343:1064-1068.

273. Growth Hormone Research Society Workshop on Adult Growth Hormone Deficiency. Consensus guidelines for the diagnosis and treatment of adults with growth hormone deficiency: summary statement. *J Clin Endocrinol Metab.* 1998;83:379-381.

274. Mahajan T, Lightman SL. A simple test for growth hormone deficiency in adults. *J Clin Endocrinol Metab.* 2000;85:1473-1476.

275. Gomez JM, Espadero RM, Escobar-Jimenez F, et al. Growth hormone release after glucagon as a reliable test of growth hormone assessment in adults. *Clin Endocrinol (Oxf).* 2002;56:329-334.

276. Chihara K, Shimatsu A, Hizuka N, et al. A simple diagnostic test using GH-releasing peptide-2 in adult GH deficiency. *Eur J Endocrinol.* 2007;157:19-27.

277. Yuen KC, Biller BM, Molitch ME, Cook DM. Clinical review: is lack of recombinant growth hormone (GH)-releasing hormone in the United States a setback or time to consider glucagon testing for adult GH deficiency? *J Clin Endocrinol Metab.* 2009;94:2702-2707.

278. Leal-Cerro A, Garcia E, Astorga R, et al. Growth hormone (GH) responses to the combined administration of GH-releasing peptide 6 in adults with GH deficiency. *Eur J Endocrinol.* 1995;132:712-715.

279. Darzy KH, Aimaretti G, Wieringa G, et al. The usefulness of the combined growth hormone (GH)-releasing hormone and arginine stimulation test in the diagnosis of radiation-induced GH deficiency is dependent on the post-irradiation time interval. *J Clin Endocrinol Metab.* 2003;88:95-102.

280. Bonert VS, Elashoff JD, Barnett P, Melmed S. Body mass index determines evoked growth hormone (GH) responsiveness in normal healthy

male subjects: diagnostic caveat for adult GH deficiency. *J Clin Endocrinol Metab.* 2004;89:3397-3401.

281. Corneli G, Di Somma C, Baldelli R, et al. The cut-off limits of the GH response to GH-releasing hormone-arginine test related to body mass index. *Eur J Endocrinol.* 2005;153:257-264.

282. Ghigo E, Aimaretti G, Gianotti L, et al. New approach to the diagnosis of growth hormone deficiency in adults. *Eur J Endocrinol.* 1996;134: 352-356.

283. Ho KK. Consensus guidelines for the diagnosis and treatment of adults with GH deficiency II: a statement of the GH Research Society in association with the European Society for Pediatric Endocrinology, Lawson Wilkins Society, European Society of Endocrinology, Japan Endocrine Society, and Endocrine Society of Australia. *Eur J Endocrinol.* 2007;157:695-700.

284. Toogood AA, Beardwell C, Shalet SM. The severity of growth hormone deficiency in adults with pituitary disease is related to the degree of hypopituitarism. *Clin Endocrinol.* 1994;41:511-516.

285. Hartman ML, Crowe BJ, Biller BM, et al. Which patients do not require a GH stimulation test for the diagnosis of adult GH deficiency? *J Clin Endocrinol Metab.* 2002;87:477-485.

286. Granada ML, Sanmarti A, Lucas A, et al. Assay-dependent results of immunoassayable spontaneous 24-hour growth hormone secretion in short children. *Acta Paediatr Scand.* 1990;370:63-70.

287. Clemmons DR. Consensus statement on the standardization and evaluation of growth hormone and insulin-like growth factor assays. *Clin Chem.* 2011;57:555-559.

288. Salomon F, Cuneo RC, Hesp R, Sonksen PH. The effects of treatment with recombinant human growth hormone on body composition and metabolism in adults with growth hormone deficiency. *N Engl J Med.* 1989;321:1797-1803.

289. Bengtsson B-A, Eden S, Lonn L, et al. Treatment of adults with growth hormone (GH) deficiency with recombinant human GH. *J Clin Endocrinol Metab.* 1993;76:309-317.

290. Hoffman DM, Crampton L, Sernia C, Ho KKY. Short term growth hormone (GH) treatment of GH deficient adults increases body sodium and extracellular water but not blood pressure. *J Clin Endocrinol Metab.* 1996;81:1123-1128.

291. Gotherstrom G, Bengtsson BA, Bosaeus I, et al. A 10-year, prospective study of the metabolic effects of growth hormone replacement in adults. *J Clin Endocrinol Metab.* 2007;92:1442-1445.

292. Baum HB, Biller BM, Finkelstein JS, et al. Effects of physiologic growth hormone therapy on bone density and body composition in patients with adult-onset growth hormone deficiency. A randomized, placebo-controlled trial. *Ann Intern Med.* 1996;125:883-890.

293. Kotzmann H, Riedl M, Bernecker P, et al. Effect of long-term growth-hormone substitution therapy on bone mineral density and parameters of bone metabolism in adult patients with growth hormone deficiency. *Calcif Tissue Int.* 1998;62:40-46.

294. Valimaki MJ, Salmela PI, Salmi J, et al. Effects of 42 months of GH treatment on bone mineral density and bone turnover in GH-deficient adults. *Eur J Endocrinol.* 1999;140:545-554.

295. Elbornsson M, Gotherstrom G, Bosaeus I, et al. Fifteen years of GH replacement increases bone mineral density in hypopituitary patients with adult-onset GH deficiency. *Eur J Endocrinol.* 2012;166: 787-795.

296. Cuneo RC, Salomon F, Wiles CM, et al. Growth hormone treatment of growth hormone deficient adults. II. Effects on exercise performance. *J Appl Physiol.* 1991;70:695-700.

297. Nass R, Huber RM, Klauss V, et al. Effect of growth hormone (hGH) replacement therapy on physical work capacity and cardiac and pulmonary function in patients with hGH deficiency acquired in adulthood. *J Clin Endocrinol Metab.* 1995;80:552-557.

298. Boger RH, Skamira C, Bode-Boger SM, et al. Nitric oxide may mediate the hemodynamic effects of recombinant growth hormone in patients with acquired growth hormone deficiency. A double-blind, placebo-controlled study. *J Clin Invest.* 1996;98:2706-2713.

299. Colao A, Marzullo P, Di Somma C, Lombardi G. Growth hormone and the heart. *Clin Endocrinol (Oxf).* 2001;54:137-154.

300. Gotherstrom G, Elbornsson M, Stibrant-Sunnerhagen K, et al. Ten years of growth hormone (GH) replacement normalizes muscle strength in GH-deficient adults. *J Clin Endocrinol Metab.* 2009;94: 809-816.

301. Janssen YJ, Doornbos J, Roelfsema F. Changes in muscle volume, strength, and bioenergetics during recombinant human growth hormone (GH) therapy in adults with GH deficiency. *J Clin Endocrinol Metab.* 1999;84:279-284.

302. Jorgensen JO, Pedersen SA, Thuesen L, et al. Beneficial effects of growth hormone treatment in GH-deficient adults. *Lancet.* 1989;1: 1221-1225.

303. Woodhouse LJ, Asa SL, Thomas SG, Ezzat S. Measures of submaximal aerobic performance evaluate and predict functional response to growth hormone (GH) treatment in GH-deficient adults. *J Clin Endocrinol Metab.* 1999;84:4570-4577.

304. Chikani V, Ho KKY. Action of GH on skeletal muscle function: molecular and metabolic mechanisms. *J Mol Endocrinol.* 2013;52(1): R107-R123.

305. Hazem A, Elamin MB, Bancos I, et al. Body composition and quality of life in adults treated with GH therapy: a systematic review and meta-analysis. *Eur J Endocrinol.* 2012;166:13-20.

306. Rosilio M, Blum WF, Edwards DJ, et al. Long-term improvement of quality of life during growth hormone (GH) replacement therapy in adults with GH deficiency, as measured by questions on life satisfaction-hypopituitarism (QLS-H). *J Clin Endocrinol Metab.* 2004; 89:1684-1693.

307. Hernberg-Stahl E, Luger A, Abs R, et al. Healthcare consumption decreases in parallel with improvements in quality of life during GH replacement in hypopituitary adults with GH deficiency. *J Clin Endocrinol Metab.* 2001;86:5277-5281.

308. Drake WM, Howell SJ, Monson JP, Shalet SM. Optimizing GH therapy in adults and children. *Endocr Rev.* 2001;22:425-450.

309. de Boer H, Blok GJ, Popp-Snijders C, et al. Monitoring of growth hormone replacement therapy in adults, based on measurement of serum markers. *J Clin Endocrinol Metab.* 1996;81:1371-1377.

310. Wolthers T, Hoffman DM, Nugent AG, et al. Oral estrogen therapy impairs the metabolic effects of growth hormone (GH) in GH deficient women. *Am J Physiol.* 2001;281:E1191-E1196.

311. Cook DM, Ludlam WH, Cook MB. Route of estrogen administration helps to determine growth hormone (GH) replacement dose in GH-deficient adults. *J Clin Endocrinol Metab.* 1999;84:3956-3960.

312. Birzniece V, Ho KK. Growth and development: patching up a better pill for GH-deficient women. *Nat Rev Endocrinol.* 2012;8:197-198.

313. Mah PM, Webster J, Jonsson P, et al. Estrogen replacement in women of fertile years with hypopituitarism. *J Clin Endocrinol Metab.* 2005; 90:5964-5969.

314. Phelan N, Conway SH, Llahana S, Conway GS. Quantification of the adverse effect of ethinylestradiol containing oral contraceptive pills when used in conjunction with growth hormone replacement in routine practice. *Clin Endocrinol (Oxf).* 2012;76(5):729-733.

315. Clayton PE, Cuneo RC, Juul A, et al; European Society of Paediatric Endocrinology. Consensus statement on the management of the GH-treated adolescent in the transition to adult care. *Eur J Endocrinol.* 2005;152:165-170.

316. Cuneo RC, Judd S, Wallace JD, et al. The Australian multicentre trial of growth hormone treatment in GH-deficient adults. *J Clin Endocrinol Metab.* 1998;83:107-116.

317. Svensson J, Fowelin J, Landin K, et al. Effects of seven years of GH-replacement therapy on insulin sensitivity in GH-deficient adults. *J Clin Endocrinol Metab.* 2002;87:2121-2127.

318. Attanasio AF, Jung H, Mo D, et al. Prevalence and incidence of diabetes mellitus in adult patients on growth hormone replacement for growth hormone deficiency: a surveillance database analysis. *J Clin Endocrinol Metab.* 2011;96:2255-2261.

319. Chan JM, Stampfer MJ, Giovannucci E, et al. Plasma insulin-like growth factor-I and prostate cancer risk: a prospective study. *Science.* 1998;279:563-566.

320. Hankinson SE, Willett WC, Colditz GA, et al. Circulating concentrations of insulin-like growth factor-I and risk of breast cancer. *Lancet.* 1998;351:1393-1396.

321. Yu H, Rohan T. Role of the insulin-like growth factor family in cancer development and progression. *J Natl Cancer Inst.* 2000;92:1472-1489.

322. Orme S, McNally RJQ, Cartwright RA, Belchetz PE. Mortality and cancer incidence in acromegaly: a retrospective cohort study. *J Clin Endocrinol Metab.* 1998;83:2730-2734.

323. Melmed S. Acromegaly and cancer: not a problem? *J Clin Endocrinol Metab.* 2001;86:2929-2934.

324. Renehan AG, Bhaskar P, Painter JE, et al. The prevalence and characteristics of colorectal neoplasia in acromegaly. *J Clin Endocrinol Metab.* 2000;85:3417-3424.

325. Allen D. National Cooperative Growth Study safety symposium: safety of human growth hormone therapy. *J Pediatr.* 1996;128:S8-S13.

326. Sklar C. Paying the price for cure-treating cancer survivors with growth hormone. *J Clin Endocrinol Metab.* 2000;85:4441-4443.

327. Swerdlow AJ, Reddingius RE, Higgins CD, et al. Growth hormone treatment of children with brain tumors and risk of tumor recurrence. *J Clin Endocrinol Metab.* 2000;85:4444-4449.

328. Ergun-Longmire B, Mertens AC, Mitby P, et al. Growth hormone treatment and risk of second neoplasms in the childhood cancer survivor. *J Clin Endocrinol Metab.* 2006;91:3494-3498.

329. Jenkins RC, Ross RJ. Growth hormone therapy for protein catabolism. *Q J Med.* 1996;89:813-819.

330. Chu LW, Lam KS, Tam SC, et al. A randomized controlled trial of low-dose recombinant human growth hormone in the treatment of malnourished elderly medical patients. *J Clin Endocrinol Metab.* 2001;86: 1913-1920.

331. Breederveld RS, Tuinebreijer WE. Recombinant human growth hormone for treating burns and donor sites. *Cochrane Database Syst Rev.* 2012;(12):CD008990.

332. Takala J, Ruokonen E, Webster NR, et al. Increased mortality associated with growth hormone treatment in critically ill adults. *N Engl J Med.* 1999;341:785-792.

333. Hoiden-Guthenberg I, Flores-Morales A, Norstedt G, Fryklund L. *Anabolic actions of growth hormone in catabolic states: analysis of differential*

gene expression in rats treated with GH and LPS using cDNA microarrays. *83rd Annual of The Endocrine Society, 2001: Abstract P2-601.* Denver, CO: The Endocrine Society; 2001:423.

334. Perls TT, Reisman NR, Olshansky SJ. Provision or distribution of growth hormone for "antiaging": clinical and legal issues. *JAMA.* 2005;294:2086-2090.

335. Holloway L, Kohlmeier L, Kent K, Marcus R. Skeletal effects of cyclic recombinant human growth hormone and salmon calcitonin in osteopenic postmenopausal women. *J Clin Endocrinol Metab.* 1997; 82:1111-1117.

336. Landin-Wilhelmsen K, Nilsson A, Bosaeus I, Bengtsson B. Growth hormone increases bone mineral content in postmenopausal osteoporosis: a randomized placebo-controlled trial. *J Bone Miner Res.* 2003; 18:393-405.

337. Schambelan M, Mulligan K, Grunfeld C, et al. Recombinant human growth hormone in patients with HIV-associated wasting. A randomized, placebo-controlled trial. Serostim Study Group. *Ann Intern Med.* 1996;125:873-882.

338. Grunfeld C, Thompson M, Brown SJ, et al. Recombinant human growth hormone to treat HIV-associated adipose redistribution syndrome: 12 week induction and 24-week maintenance therapy. *J Acquir Immune Defic Syndr.* 2007;45:286-297.

339. Lo J, You SM, Canavan B, et al. Low-dose physiological growth hormone in patients with HIV and abdominal fat accumulation: a randomized controlled trial. *JAMA.* 2008;300:509-519.

340. Falutz J, Allas S, Blot K, et al. Metabolic effects of a growth hormone-releasing factor in patients with HIV. *N Engl J Med.* 2007;357: 2359-2370.

341. Nelson AE, Ho KK. Abuse of growth hormone by athletes. *Nat Clin Pract Endocrinol Metab.* 2007;3:198-199.

342. Liu H, Bravata DM, Olkin I, et al. Systematic review: the effects of growth hormone on athletic performance. *Ann Intern Med.* 2008; 148:747-758.

343. Meinhardt U, Nelson AE, Hansen JL, et al. The effects of growth hormone on body composition and physical performance in recreational athletes: a randomized trial. *Ann Intern Med.* 2010;152:568-577.

344. Liu H, Bravata DM, Olkin I, et al. Systematic review: the safety and efficacy of growth hormone in the healthy elderly. *Ann Intern Med.* 2007;146:104-115.

345. Scheithauer BW, Horvath E, Lloyd RV, Kovacs K. Pathology of pituitary adenomas and pituitary hyperplasia. In: Thapar K, Kovacs K, Scheithauer BW, Lloyd RV, eds. *Diagnosis and Management of Pituitary Tumors.* Totowa, NJ: Humana Press; 2001:91-154.

346. Zabel BU, Naylor SL, Sakaguchi AY, et al. High-resolution chromosomal localization of human genes for amylase, proopiomelanocortin, somatostatin, and a DNA fragment (D3S1) by in situ hybridization. *Proc Natl Acad Sci U S A.* 1983;80:6932-6936.

347. Cochet M, Chang AC, Cohen SN. Characterization of the structural gene and putative 5'-regulatory sequences for human proopiomelanocortin. *Nature.* 1982;297:335-339.

348. Gee CE, Chen CL, Roberts JL, et al. Identification of proopiomelanocortin neurones in rat hypothalamus by in situ cDNA-mRNA hybridization. *Nature.* 1983;306:374-376.

349. Jenks BG. Regulation of proopiomelanocortin gene expression: an overview of the signaling cascades, transcription factors, and responsive elements involved. *Ann N Y Acad Sci.* 2009;1163:17-30.

350. Arai M, Assil IQ, Abou-Samra AB. Characterization of three corticotropin-releasing factor receptors in catfish: a novel third receptor is predominantly expressed in pituitary and urophysis. *Endocrinology.* 2001;142:446-454.

351. Jin WD, Boutillier AL, Glucksman MJ, et al. Characterization of a corticotropin-releasing hormone-responsive element in the rat proopiomelanocortin gene promoter and molecular cloning of its binding protein. *Mol Endocrinol.* 1994;8:1377-1388.

352. Weninger SC, Dunn AJ, Muglia LJ, et al. Stress-induced behaviors require the corticotropin-releasing hormone (CRH) receptor, but not CRH. *Proc Natl Acad Sci U S A.* 1999;96:8283-8288.

353. Coste SC, Kesterson RA, Heldwein KA, et al. Abnormal adaptations to stress and impaired cardiovascular function in mice lacking corticotropin-releasing hormone receptor-2. *Nat Genet.* 2000;24: 403-409.

354. Bousquet C, Zatelli MC, Melmed S. Direct regulation of pituitary proopiomelanocortin by STAT3 provides a novel mechanism for immunoneuroendocrine interfacing. *J Clin Invest.* 2000;106:1417-1425.

355. Seidah NG, Chretien M. Complete amino acid sequence of a human pituitary glycopeptide: an important maturation product of proopiomelanocortin. *Proc Natl Acad Sci U S A.* 1981;78:4236-4240.

356. Fenger M, Johnsen AH. Alpha-amidated peptides derived from proopiomelanocortin in normal human pituitary. *Biochem J.* 1988;250: 781-788.

357. Jackson RS, Creemers JW, Ohagi S, et al. Obesity and impaired prohormone processing associated with mutations in the human prohormone convertase 1 gene. *Nat Genet.* 1997;16:303-306.

358. Bicknell AB, Lomthaisong K, Woods RJ, et al. Characterization of a serine protease that cleaves pro-gamma-melanotropin at the adrenal to stimulate growth. *Cell.* 2001;105:903-912.

359. Scholzen TE, Kalden DH, Brzoska T, et al. Expression of proopiomelanocortin peptides in human dermal microvascular endothelial cells: evidence for a regulation by ultraviolet light and interleukin-1. *J Invest Dermatol.* 2000;115:1021-1028.

360. Krude H, Biebermann H, Luck W, et al. Severe early-onset obesity, adrenal insufficiency and red hair pigmentation caused by POMC mutations in humans. *Nat Genet.* 1998;19:155-157.

361. Yaswen L, Diehl N, Brennan MB, Hochgeschwender U. Obesity in the mouse model of pro-opiomelanocortin deficiency responds to peripheral melanocortin. *Nat Med.* 1999;5:1066-1070.

362. Catania A, Delgado R, Airaghi L, et al. Alpha-MSH in systemic inflammation. Central and peripheral actions. *Ann N Y Acad Sci.* 1999;885: 183-187.

363. Raffin-Sanson ML, de Keyzer Y, Bertagna X. Proopiomelanocortin, a polypeptide precursor with multiple functions: from physiology to pathological conditions. *Eur J Endocrinol.* 2003;149:79-90.

364. Gatto F, Hofland LJ. The role of somatostatin and dopamine D2 receptors in endocrine tumors. *Endocr Relat Cancer.* 2011;18:R233-R251.

365. Saiardi A, Borrelli E. Absence of dopaminergic control on melanotrophs leads to Cushing's-like syndrome in mice. *Mol Endocrinol.* 1998;12:1133-1139.

366. Boschetti M, Gatto F, Arvigo M, et al. Role of dopamine receptors in normal and tumoral pituitary corticotropic cells and adrenal cells. *Neuroendocrinology.* 2010;92(Suppl 1):17-22.

367. Clark AR. Anti-inflammatory functions of glucocorticoid-induced genes. *Mol Cell Endocrinol.* 2007;275:79-97.

368. Kanaley JA, Weltman JY, Pieper KS, et al. Cortisol and growth hormone responses to exercise at different times of day. *J Clin Endocrinol Metab.* 2001;86:2881-2889.

369. Luger A, Deuster PA, Kyle SB, et al. Acute hypothalamic-pituitary-adrenal responses to the stress of treadmill exercise. Physiologic adaptations to physical training. *N Engl J Med.* 1987;316:1309-1315.

370. Veldhuis JD, Iranmanesh A, Johnson ML, Lizarralde G. Twenty-four-hour rhythms in plasma concentrations of adenohypophyseal hormones are generated by distinct amplitude and/or frequency modulation of underlying pituitary secretory bursts. *J Clin Endocrinol Metab.* 1990;71:1616-1623.

371. Veldhuis JD, Iranmanesh A, Johnson ML, Lizarralde G. Amplitude, but not frequency, modulation of adrenocorticotropin secretory bursts gives rise to the nyctohemeral rhythm of the corticotropic axis in man. *J Clin Endocrinol Metab.* 1990;71:452-463.

372. Gomez MT, Magiakou MA, Mastorakos G, Chrousos GP. The pituitary corticotroph is not the rate limiting step in the postoperative recovery of the hypothalamic-pituitary-adrenal axis in patients with Cushing syndrome. *J Clin Endocrinol Metab.* 1993;77:173-177.

373. Desir D, Van Cauter E, Beyloos M, et al. Prolonged pulsatile administration of ovine corticotropin-releasing hormone in normal man. *J Clin Endocrinol Metab.* 1986;63:1292-1299.

374. Horrocks PM, Jones AF, Ratcliffe WA, et al. Patterns of ACTH and cortisol pulsatility over twenty-four hours in normal males and females. *Clin Endocrinol (Oxf).* 1990;32:127-134.

375. Dorin RI, Ferries LM, Roberts B, et al. Assessment of stimulated and spontaneous adrenocorticotropin secretory dynamics identifies distinct components of cortisol feedback inhibition in healthy humans. *J Clin Endocrinol Metab.* 1996;81:3883-3891.

376. Keeney DS, Waterman MR. Regulation of steroid hydroxylase gene expression: importance to physiology and disease. *Pharmacol Ther.* 1993;58:301-317.

377. Ilvesmaki V, Voutilainen R. Interaction of phorbol ester and adrenocorticotropin in the regulation of steroidogenic P450 genes in human fetal and adult adrenal cell cultures. *Endocrinology.* 1991;128: 1450-1458.

378. Orth DN. Corticotropin-releasing hormone in humans. *Endocr Rev.* 1992;13:164-191.

379. Debold CR, Jackson RV, Kamilaris TC, et al. Effects of ovine corticotropin-releasing hormone on adrenocorticotropin secretion in the absence of glucocorticoid feedback inhibition in man. *J Clin Endocrinol Metab.* 1989;68:431-437.

380. Sonino N, Zielezny M, Fava GA, et al. Risk factors and long-term outcome in pituitary-dependent Cushing's disease. *J Clin Endocrinol Metab.* 1996;81:2647-2652.

381. Kubota T, Hayashi M, Kabuto M, et al. Corticotroph cell hyperplasia in a patient with Addison disease: case report. *Surg Neurol.* 1992; 37:441-447.

382. Talbot JA, Kane JW, White A. Analytical and clinical aspects of adrenocorticotrophin determination. *Ann Clin Biochem.* 2003;40: 453-471.

383. Pecori Giraldi F, Saccani A, Cavagnini F. Assessment of ACTH assay variability: a multicenter study. *Eur J Endocrinol.* 2011;164:505-512.

384. Allolio B, Gunther RW, Benker G, et al. A multihormonal response to corticotropin-releasing hormone in inferior petrosal sinus blood of patients with Cushing's disease. *J Clin Endocrinol Metab.* 1990;71: 1195-1201.

385. Lee P, Greenfield JR, Ho KK. Factors determining inadequate hypoglycaemia during insulin tolerance testing (ITT) after pituitary surgery. *Clin Endocrinol (Oxf).* 2009;71:82-85.

386. Hartzband PI, Van Herle AJ, Sorger L, Cope D. Assessment of hypothalamic-pituitary-adrenal (HPA) axis dysfunction: comparison of ACTH stimulation, insulin-hypoglycemia and metyrapone. *J Endocrinol Invest.* 1988;11:769-776.

387. Streeten DH, Anderson GH Jr, Dalakos TG, et al. Normal and abnormal function of the hypothalamic-pituitary-adrenocortical system in man. *Endocr Rev.* 1984;5:371-394.

388. Oldfield EH, Doppman JL, Nieman LK, et al. Petrosal sinus sampling with and without corticotropin-releasing hormone for the differential diagnosis of Cushing's syndrome. *N Engl J Med.* 1991;325:897-905.

389. Yanovski JA, Cutler GB Jr, Chrousos GP, Nieman LK. Corticotropin-releasing hormone stimulation following low-dose dexamethasone administration. A new test to distinguish Cushing's syndrome from pseudo-Cushing's states. *JAMA.* 1993;269:2232-2238.

390. Nieman LK, Biller BM, Findling JW, et al. The diagnosis of Cushing's syndrome: an Endocrine Society Clinical Practice Guideline. *J Clin Endocrinol Metab.* 2008;93:1526-1540.

391. L'Allemand D, Penhoat A, Lebrethon MC, et al. Insulin-like growth factors enhance steroidogenic enzyme and corticotropin receptor messenger ribonucleic acid levels and corticotropin steroidogenic responsiveness in cultured human adrenocortical cells. *J Clin Endocrinol Metab.* 1996;81:3892-3897.

392. Hurel SJ, Thompson CJ, Watson MJ, et al. The short Synacthen and insulin stress tests in the assessment of the hypothalamic-pituitary-adrenal axis. *Clin Endocrinol (Oxf).* 1996;44:141-146.

393. Rasmuson S, Olsson T, Hagg E. A low dose ACTH test to assess the function of the hypothalamic-pituitary-adrenal axis. *Clin Endocrinol (Oxf).* 1996;44:151-156.

394. Kukreja SC, Williams GA. Corticotrophin stimulation test: inverse correlation between basal serum cortisol and its response to corticotrophin. *Acta Endocrinol (Copenh).* 1981;97:522-524.

395. Shankar RR, Jakacki RI, Haider A, et al. Testing the hypothalamic-pituitary-adrenal axis in survivors of childhood brain and skull-based tumors. *J Clin Endocrinol Metab.* 1997;82:1995-1998.

396. Howlett TA. An assessment of optimal hydrocortisone replacement therapy. *Clin Endocrinol (Oxf).* 1997;46:263-268.

397. Arlt W, Callies F, van Vlijmen JC, et al. Dehydroepiandrosterone replacement in women with adrenal insufficiency. *N Engl J Med.* 1999;341:1013-1020.

398. Johannsson G, Burman P, Wiren L, et al. Low dose dehydroepiandrosterone affects behavior in hypopituitary androgen-deficient women: a placebo-controlled trial. *J Clin Endocrinol Metab.* 2002;87:2046-2052.

399. Hahner S, Loeffler M, Fassnacht M, et al. Impaired subjective health status in 256 patients with adrenal insufficiency on standard therapy based on cross-sectional analysis. *J Clin Endocrinol Metab.* 2007;92:3912-3922.

400. Johannsson G, Nilsson AG, Bergthorsdottir R, et al. Improved cortisol exposure-time profile and outcome in patients with adrenal insufficiency: a prospective randomized trial of a novel hydrocortisone dual-release formulation. *J Clin Endocrinol Metab.* 2012;97:473-481.

401. Whitaker MJ, Debono M, Huatan H, et al. An oral multiparticulate, modified-release, hydrocortisone replacement therapy that provides physiological cortisol exposure. *Clin Endocrinol (Oxf).* 2014;80:554-561.

402. Gharib SD, Wierman ME, Shupnik MA, Chin WW. Molecular biology of the pituitary gonadotropins. *Endocr Rev.* 1990;11:177-199.

403. Sairam MR, Bhargavi GN. A role for glycosylation of the alpha subunit in transduction of biological signal in glycoprotein hormones. *Science.* 1985;229:65-67.

404. Fares F. The role of O-linked and N-linked oligosaccharides on the structure-function of glycoprotein hormones: development of agonists and antagonists. *Biochim Biophys Acta.* 2006;1760:560-567.

405. Albanese C, Colin IM, Crowley WF, et al. The gonadotropin genes: evolution of distinct mechanisms for hormonal control. *Recent Prog Horm Res.* 1996;51:23-58.

406. Talmadge K, Vamvakopoulos NC, Fiddes JC. Evolution of the genes for the beta subunits of human chorionic gonadotropin and luteinizing hormone. *Nature.* 1984;307:37-40.

407. Themmen APN, Huhtaniemi IT. Mutations of gonadotropins and gonadotropin receptors: elucidating the physiology and pathophysiology of pituitary-gonadal function. *Endocr Rev.* 2000;21:551-583.

408. Dode C, Levilliers J, Dupont JM, et al. Loss-of-function mutations in FGFR1 cause autosomal dominant Kallmann syndrome. *Nat Genet.* 2003;33:463-465.

409. Falardeau J, Chung WC, Beenken A, et al. Decreased FGF8 signaling causes deficiency of gonadotropin-releasing hormone in humans and mice. *J Clin Invest.* 2008;118:2822-2831.

410. Dode C, Teixeira L, Levilliers J, et al. Kallmann syndrome: mutations in the genes encoding prokineticin-2 and prokineticin receptor-2. *PLoS Genet.* 2006;2:e175.

411. Miura K, Acierno JS Jr, Seminara SB. Characterization of the human nasal embryonic LHRH factor gene, NELF, and a mutation screening among 65 patients with idiopathic hypogonadotropic hypogonadism (IHH). *J Hum Genet.* 2004;49:265-268.

412. Tornberg J, Sykiotis GP, Keefe K, et al. Heparan sulfate 6-O-sulfotransferase 1, a gene involved in extracellular sugar modifications, is mutated in patients with idiopathic hypogonadotrophic hypogonadism. *Proc Natl Acad Sci U S A.* 2011;108:11524-11529.

413. Kim HG, Kurth I, Lan F, et al. Mutations in CHD7, encoding a chromatin-remodeling protein, cause idiopathic hypogonadotropic hypogonadism and Kallmann syndrome. *Am J Hum Genet.* 2008;83:511-519.

414. Kim HG, Ahn JW, Kurth I, et al. WDR11, a WD protein that interacts with transcription factor EMX1, is mutated in idiopathic hypogonadotropic hypogonadism and Kallmann syndrome. *Am J Hum Genet.* 2010;87:465-479.

415. Topaloglu AK, Tello JA, Kotan LD, et al. Inactivating KISS1 mutation and hypogonadotropic hypogonadism. *N Engl J Med.* 2012;366:629-635.

416. Farooqi IS, Wangensteen T, Collins S, et al. Clinical and molecular genetic spectrum of congenital deficiency of the leptin receptor. *N Engl J Med.* 2007;356:237-247.

417. Bouligand J, Ghervan C, Tello JA, et al. Isolated familial hypogonadotropic hypogonadism and a GNRH1 mutation. *N Engl J Med.* 2009;360:2742-2748.

418. Abreu AP, Dauber A, Macedo DB, et al. Central precocious puberty caused by mutations in the imprinted gene MKRN3. *N Engl J Med.* 2013;368:2467-2475.

419. de Roux N, Genin E, Carel JC, et al. Hypogonadotropic hypogonadism due to loss of function of the KiSS1-derived peptide receptor GPR54. *Proc Natl Acad Sci U S A.* 2003;100:10972-10976.

420. Seminara SB, Messager S, Chatzidaki EE, et al. The GPR54 gene as a regulator of puberty. *N Engl J Med.* 2003;349:1614-1627.

421. Dhillo WS, Chaudhri OB, Thompson EL, et al. Kisspeptin-54 stimulates gonadotropin release most potently during the preovulatory phase of the menstrual cycle in women. *J Clin Endocrinol Metab.* 2007;92:3958-3966.

422. Navarro VM, Gottsch ML, Chavkin C, et al. Regulation of gonadotropin-releasing hormone secretion by kisspeptin/dynorphin/neurokinin B neurons in the arcuate nucleus of the mouse. *J Neurosci.* 2009;29:11859-11866.

423. Topaloglu AK, Reimann F, Guclu M, et al. TAC3 and TACR3 mutations in familial hypogonadotropic hypogonadism reveal a key role for Neurokinin B in the central control of reproduction. *Nat Genet.* 2009;41:354-358.

424. Moschos S, Chan JL, Mantzoros CS. Leptin and reproduction: a review. *Fertil Steril.* 2002;77:433-444.

425. Belchetz PE, Plant TM, Nakai Y, et al. Hypophysial responses to continuous and intermittent delivery of hypothalamic gonadotropin-releasing hormone. *Science.* 1978;202:631-633.

426. Crowley WF Jr, Whitcomb RW, Jameson JL, et al. Neuroendocrine control of human reproduction in the male. *Recent Prog Horm Res.* 1991;47:27-62.

427. Naor Z. Signaling by G-protein-coupled receptor (GPCR): studies on the GnRH receptor. *Front Neuroendocrinol.* 2009;30:10-29.

428. Knobil E. The neuroendocrine control of the menstrual cycle. *Recent Prog Horm Res.* 1980;36:53-88.

429. Ciccone NA, Kaiser UB. The biology of gonadotroph regulation. *Curr Opin Endocrinol Diabetes Obes.* 2009;16:321-327.

430. McCullagh DR. Dual endocrine activity of the testes. *Science.* 1932;76:19-23.

431. Mason AJ, Hayflick JS, Ling N, et al. Complementary DNA sequences of ovarian follicular fluid inhibin show precursor structure and homology with transforming growth factor-beta. *Nature.* 1985;318:659-663.

432. Ying SY. Inhibins, activins, and follistatins: gonadal proteins modulating the secretion of follicle-stimulating hormone. *Endocr Rev.* 1988;9:267-293.

433. Vale W, Rivier C, Hsueh A, et al. Chemical and biological characterization of the inhibin family of protein hormones. *Recent Prog Horm Res.* 1988;44:1-34.

434. Kristrom B, Zdunek AM, Rydh A, et al. A novel mutation in the LIM homeobox 3 gene is responsible for combined pituitary hormone deficiency, hearing impairment, and vertebral malformations. *J Clin Endocrinol Metab.* 2009;94:1154-1161.

435. Dungan HM, Clifton DK, Steiner RA. Kisspeptin neurons as central processors in the regulation of gonadotropin-releasing hormone secretion. *Endocrinology.* 2006;147:1154-1158.

436. Gormley GJ. Chemoprevention strategies for prostate cancer: the role of 5 alpha-reductase inhibitors. *J Cell Biochem Suppl.* 1992;16H:113-117.

437. Bhasin S, Fielder TJ, Swerdloff RS. Testosterone selectively increases serum follicle-stimulating hormonal (FSH) but not luteinizing hormone (LH) in gonadotropin-releasing hormone antagonist-treated male rats: evidence for differential regulation of LH and FSH secretion. *Biol Reprod.* 1987;37(1):55-59.

438. Santen RJ, Bardin CW. Episodic luteinizing hormone secretion in man. Pulse analysis, clinical interpretation, physiologic mechanisms. *J Clin Invest.* 1973;52:2617-2628.

439. Veldhuis JD, Keenan DM, Pincus SM. Motivations and methods for analyzing pulsatile hormone secretion. *Endocr Rev.* 2008;29:823-864.

440. McNeilly AS, Crawford JL, Taragnat C, et al. The differential secretion of FSH and LH: regulation through genes, feedback and packaging. *Reprod Suppl.* 2003;61:463-476.

441. Richards JS, Pangas SA. The ovary: basic biology and clinical implications. *J Clin Invest.* 2010;120:963-972.

442. Macklon NS, Stouffer RL, Giudice LC, Fauser BC. The science behind 25 years of ovarian stimulation for in vitro fertilization. *Endocr Rev.* 2006;27:170-207.

443. Stocco DM. Tracking the role of a star in the sky of the new millennium. *Mol Endocrinol.* 2001;15:1245-1254.

444. Plant TM, Marshall GR. The functional significance of FSH in spermatogenesis and the control of its secretion in male primates. *Endocr Rev.* 2001;22:764-786.

445. Ruwanpura SM, McLachlan RI, Meachem SJ. Hormonal regulation of male germ cell development. *J Endocrinol.* 2010;205:117-131.

446. Jaakkola T, Ding YQ, Kellokumpu-Lehtinen P, et al. The ratios of serum bioactive/immunoreactive luteinizing hormone and follicle-stimulating hormone in various clinical conditions with increased and decreased gonadotropin secretion: reevaluation by a highly sensitive immunometric assay. *J Clin Endocrinol Metab.* 1990;70:1496-1505.

447. Brito VN, Batista MC, Borges MF, et al. Diagnostic value of fluorometric assays in the evaluation of precocious puberty. *J Clin Endocrinol Metab.* 1999;84:3539-3544.

448. Franco B, Guioli S, Pragliola A, et al. A gene deleted in Kallmann's syndrome shares homology with neural cell adhesion and axonal path-finding molecules. *Nature.* 1991;353:529-536.

449. Kallmann F, Schonfeld WA, Barrera WS. Genetic aspects of primary eunuchoidism. *Am J Ment Defic.* 1944;48:203.

450. Rugarli EI, Ballabio A. Kallmann syndrome. From genetics to neurobiology. *JAMA.* 1993;270:2713-2716.

451. Hardelin JP, Levilliers J, Young J, et al. Xp22.3 deletions in isolated familial Kallmann's syndrome. *J Clin Endocrinol Metab.* 1993;76:827-831.

452. Prager D, Braunstein GD. X-chromosome-linked Kallmann's syndrome: pathology at the molecular level. *J Clin Endocrinol Metab.* 1993;76:824-826.

453. Lieblich JM, Rogol AD, White BJ, Rosen SW. Syndrome of anosmia with hypogonadotropic hypogonadism (Kallmann syndrome): clinical and laboratory studies in 23 cases. *Am J Med.* 1982;73:506-519.

454. Bray GA, Dahms WT, Swerdloff RS, et al. The Prader-Willi syndrome: a study of 40 patients and a review of the literature. *Medicine (Baltimore).* 1983;62:59-80.

455. Eldar-Geva T, Hirsch HJ, Benarroch F, et al. Hypogonadism in females with Prader-Willi syndrome from infancy to adulthood: variable combinations of a primary gonadal defect and hypothalamic dysfunction. *Eur J Endocrinol.* 2010;162:377-384.

456. Emerick JE, Vogt KS. Endocrine manifestations and management of Prader-Willi syndrome. *Int J Pediatr Endocrinol.* 2013;2013(1):14.

457. Hanchate NK, Giacobini P, Lhuillier P, et al. SEMA3A, a gene involved in axonal pathfinding, is mutated in patients with Kallmann syndrome. *PLoS Genet.* 2012;8:e1002896.

458. Basaria S. Male hypogonadism. *Lancet.* 2014;383:1250-1263.

459. Anawalt BD. Approach to male infertility and induction of spermatogenesis. *J Clin Endocrinol Metab.* 2013;98:3532-3542.

460. Layman LC, Lee EJ, Peak DB, et al. Delayed puberty and hypogonadism caused by mutations in the follicle-stimulating hormone beta-subunit gene. *N Engl J Med.* 1997;337:607-611.

461. Layman LC, Porto AL, Xie J, et al. FSH beta gene mutations in a female with partial breast development and a male sibling with normal puberty and azoospermia. *J Clin Endocrinol Metab.* 2002;87:3702-3707.

462. Cogan JD, Wu W, Phillips J 3rd, et al. The PROP1 2-base pair deletion is a common cause of combined pituitary hormone deficiency. *J Clin Endocrinol Metab.* 1998;83:3346-3349.

463. Valdes-Socin H, Salvi R, Daly AF, et al. Hypogonadism in a patient with a mutation in the luteinizing hormone beta-subunit gene. *N Engl J Med.* 2004;351:2619-2625.

464. Weiss J, Axelrod L, Whitcomb RW, et al. Hypogonadism caused by a single amino acid substitution in the beta subunit of luteinizing hormone. *N Engl J Med.* 1992;326:179-183.

465. Anawalt BD, Bremner WJ. Diagnosis and treatment of male gonadotropin insufficiency. In: Lamberts SW, ed. *The Diagnosis and Treatment of Pituitary Insufficiency.* Bristol, UK: BioScientifica; 1997:163-207.

466. Handelsman DJ, Conway AJ, Boylan LM. Pharmacokinetics and pharmacodynamics of testosterone pellets in man. *J Clin Endocrinol Metab.* 1990;71:216-222.

467. Finkelstein JS, Lee H, Burnett-Bowie SA, et al. Gonadal steroids and body composition, strength, and sexual function in men. *N Engl J Med.* 2013;369:1011-1022.

468. Bhasin S, Salehian B. Gonadotropin therapy of men with hypogonadotropic hypogonadism. *Curr Ther Endocrinol Metab.* 1997;6:349-352.

469. Balen AH, Braat DD, West C, et al. Cumulative conception and live birth rates after the treatment of anovulatory infertility: safety and efficacy of ovulation induction in 200 patients. *Hum Reprod.* 1994;9:1563-1570.

470. Martin KA, Hall JE, Adams JM, Crowley WF Jr. Comparison of exogenous gonadotropins and pulsatile gonadotropin-releasing hormone for induction of ovulation in hypogonadotropic amenorrhea. *J Clin Endocrinol Metab.* 1993;77:125-129.

471. Jayasena CN, Abbara A, Comninos AN, et al. Kisspeptin-54 triggers egg maturation in women undergoing in vitro fertilization. *J Clin Invest.* 2014;124:3667-3677.

472. Pierce JG, Parsons TF. Glycoprotein hormones: structure and function. *Annu Rev Biochem.* 1981;50:465-495.

473. Abel ED, Kaulbach HC, Campos-Barros A, et al. Novel insight from transgenic mice into thyroid hormone resistance and the regulation of thyrotropin. *J Clin Invest.* 1999;103:271-279.

474. Beck-Peccoz P, Persani L. Variable biological activity of thyroid-stimulating hormone. *Eur J Endocrinol.* 1994;131:331-340.

475. Grossmann M, Weintraub BD, Szkudlinski MW. Novel insights into the molecular mechanisms of human thyrotropin action: structural, physiological, and therapeutic implications for the glycoprotein hormone family. *Endocr Rev.* 1997;18:476-501.

476. Dasen JS, O'Connell SM, Flynn SE, et al. Reciprocal interactions of Pit1 and GATA2 mediate signaling gradient-induced determination of pituitary cell types. *Cell.* 1999;97:587-598.

477. Fiddes JC, Goodman HM. The gene encoding the common alpha subunit of the four human glycoprotein hormones. *J Mol Appl Genet.* 1981;1:3-18.

478. Sarapura VD, Strouth HL, Wood WM, et al. Activation of the glycoprotein hormone alpha-subunit gene promoter in thyrotropes. *Mol Cell Endocrinol.* 1998;146:77-86.

479. Tagami T, Madison LD, Nagaya T, Jameson JL. Nuclear receptor corepressors activate rather than suppress basal transcription of genes that are negatively regulated by thyroid hormone. *Mol Cell Biol.* 1997;17:2642-2648.

480. Wondisford FE, Radovick S, Moates JM, et al. Isolation and characterization of the human thyrotropin beta-subunit gene. Differences in gene structure and promoter function from murine species. *J Biol Chem.* 1988;263:12538-12542.

481. Steinfelder HJ, Hauser P, Nakayama Y, et al. Thyrotropin-releasing hormone regulation of human TSHB expression: role of a pituitary-specific transcription factor (Pit-1/GHF-1) and potential interaction with a thyroid hormone-inhibitory element. *Proc Natl Acad Sci U S A.* 1991;88:3130-3134.

482. Bodenner DL, Mroczynski MA, Weintraub BD, et al. A detailed functional and structural analysis of a major thyroid hormone inhibitory element in the human thyrotropin beta-subunit gene. *J Biol Chem.* 1991;266:21666-21673.

483. Ross DS, Downing MF, Chin WW, et al. Changes in tissue concentrations of thyrotropin, free thyrotropin beta, and alpha-subunits after thyroxine administration: comparison of mouse hypothyroid pituitary and thyrotropic tumors. *Endocrinology.* 1983;112:2050-2053.

484. Lania A, Persani L, Ballare E, et al. Constitutively active Gs alpha is associated with an increased phosphodiesterase activity in human growth hormone-secreting adenomas. *J Clin Endocrinol Metab.* 1998;83:1624-1628.

485. Papandreou MJ, Persani L, Asteria C, et al. Variable carbohydrate structures of circulating thyrotropin as studied by lectin affinity chromatography in different clinical conditions. *J Clin Endocrinol Metab.* 1993;77:393-398.

486. Ridgway EC, Weintraub BD, Maloof F. Metabolic clearance and production rates of human thyrotropin. *J Clin Invest.* 1974;53:895-903.

487. Vanhole C, Aerssens P, Naulaers G, et al. L-thyroxine treatment of preterm newborns: clinical and endocrine effects. *Pediatr Res.* 1997;42:87-92.

488. Van den Berghe G, de Zegher F, Veldhuis JD, et al. Thyrotrophin and prolactin release in prolonged critical illness: dynamics of spontaneous secretion and effects of growth hormone-secretagogues. *Clin Endocrinol (Oxf).* 1997;47:599-612.

489. Samuels MH, Henry P, Kleinschmidt-DeMasters BK, et al. Pulsatile glycoprotein hormone secretion in glycoprotein-producing pituitary tumors. *J Clin Endocrinol Metab.* 1991;73:1281-1288.

490. Goichot B, Weibel L, Chapotot F, et al. Effect of the shift of the sleep-wake cycle on three robust endocrine markers of the circadian clock. *Am J Physiol.* 1998;275:E243-E248.

491. Roelfsema R, Pijl H, Kok P, et al. Thyrotropin secretion in healthy subjects is robust and independent of age and gender, and only weakly dependent on body mass index. *J Clin Endocrinol Metab.* 2014;99:570-578.

492. Chiamolera MI, Wondisford FE. Minireview: Thyrotropin-releasing hormone and the thyroid hormone feedback mechanism. *Endocrinology.* 2009;150:1091-1096.

493. Lechan RM, Fekete C. The TRH neuron: a hypothalamic integrator of energy metabolism. *Prog Brain Res.* 2006;153:209-235.

494. Fliers E, Unmehope UA, Alkemade A. Functional neuroanatomy of thyroid hormone feedback in the human hypothalamus and pituitary gland. *Mol Cell Endocrinol.* 2006;251:1-8.

495. Trajkovic M, Visser TJ, Mittag J, et al. Abnormal thyroid hormone metabolism in mice lacking the monocarboxylate transporter 8. *J Clin Invest.* 2007;117:627-635.

496. Dumitrescu AM, Liao XH, Best TB, et al. A novel syndrome combining thyroid and neurological abnormalities is associated with mutations

in a monocarboxylate transporter gene. *Am J Hum Genet*. 2004;74: 168-175.

497. Samuels MH, Henry P, Ridgway EC. Effects of dopamine and somatostatin on pulsatile pituitary glycoprotein secretion. *J Clin Endocrinol Metab*. 1992;74:217-222.

498. Siler TM, Yen SC, Vale W, Guillemin R. Inhibition by somatostatin on the release of TSH induced in man by thyrotropin-releasing factor. *J Clin Endocrinol Metab*. 1974;38:742-745.

499. Newman CB, Melmed S, Snyder PJ, et al. Safety and efficacy of long-term octreotide therapy of acromegaly: results of a multicenter trial in 103 patients—a clinical research center study. *J Clin Endocrinol Metab*. 1995;80:2768-2775.

500. Cooper DS, Klibanski A, Ridgway EC. Dopaminergic modulation of TSH and its subunits: in vivo and in vitro studies. *Clin Endocrinol (Oxf)*. 1983;18:265-275.

501. Wang R, Nelson JC, Wilcox RB. Salsalate administration: a potential pharmacological model of the sick euthyroid syndrome. *J Clin Endocrinol Metab*. 1998;83:3095-3099.

502. Rapoport B, Chazenbalk GD, Jaume JC, McLachlan SM. The thyrotropin (TSH) receptor: interaction with TSH and autoantibodies. *Endocr Rev*. 1998;19:673-716.

503. Nicoloff JT, Spencer CA. Clinical review 12: the use and misuse of the sensitive thyrotropin assays. *J Clin Endocrinol Metab*. 1990;71: 553-558.

504. Spencer CA, Schwarzbein D, Guttler RB, et al. Thyrotropin (TSH)-releasing hormone stimulation test responses employing third and fourth generation TSH assays. *J Clin Endocrinol Metab*. 1993;76: 494-498.

505. Beck-Peccoz P, Persani L. TSH-producing adenomas. In: DeGroot LJ, Jameson JL, eds. *Endocrinology*. 5th ed. Philadelphia, PA: Elsevier Saunders; 2006:475-484.

506. Faglia G. The clinical impact of the thyrotropin-releasing hormone test. *Thyroid*. 1998;8:903-908.

507. Root AW. Neonatal screening for 21-hydroxylase deficient congenital adrenal hyperplasia: the role of CYP21 analysis. *J Clin Endocrinol Metab*. 1999;84:1503-1504.

508. Turcu AF, Erickson BJ, Lin E, et al. Pituitary stalk lesions: the Mayo Clinic experience. *J Clin Endocrinol Metab*. 2013;98:1812-1818.

509. Mehta A, Dattani MT. Developmental disorders of the hypothalamus and pituitary gland associated with congenital hypopituitarism. *Best Pract Res Clin Endocrinol Metab*. 2008;22:191-206.

510. Dattani MT, Martinez-Barbera JP, Thomas PQ, et al. Mutations in the homeobox gene HESX1/Hesx1 associated with septo-optic dysplasia in human and mouse. *Nat Genet*. 1998;19:125-133.

511. Thomas PQ, Dattani MT, Brickman JM, et al. Heterozygous HESX1 mutations associated with isolated congenital pituitary hypoplasia and septo-optic dysplasia. *Hum Mol Genet*. 2001;10:39-45.

512. Sobrier ML, Maghnie M, Vie-Luton MP, et al. Novel HESX1 mutations associated with a life-threatening neonatal phenotype, pituitary aplasia, but normally located posterior pituitary and no optic nerve abnormalities. *J Clin Endocrinol Metab*. 2006;91:4528-4536.

513. Reynaud R, Albarel F, Saveanu A, et al. Pituitary stalk interruption syndrome in 83 patients: novel HESX1 mutation and severe hormonal prognosis in malformative forms. *Eur J Endocrinol*. 2011;164:457-465.

514. Ragge NK, Lorenz B, Schneider A, et al. SOX2 anophthalmia syndrome. *Am J Med Genet*. 2005;135:1-7.

515. Woods KS, Cundall M, Turton J, et al. Over and under dosage of SOX3 is associated with infundibular hypoplasia and hypopituitarism. *Am J Hum Genet*. 2005;76:833-849.

516. Kelberman D, Rizzoti K, Lovell-Badge R, et al. Genetic regulation of pituitary gland development in human and mouse. *Endocr Rev*. 2009;30:790-829.

517. Savage JJ, Hunter CS, Clark-Sturm SL, et al. Mutations in the LHX3 gene cause dysregulation of pituitary and neural target genes that reflect patient phenotypes. *Gene*. 2007;400:44-51.

518. Netchine I, Sobrier ML, Krude H, et al. Mutations in LHX3 result in a new syndrome revealed by combined pituitary hormone deficiency. *Nat Genet*. 2000;25:182-186.

519. Machinis K, Amselem S. Functional relationship between LHX4 and POU1F1 in light of the LHX4 mutation identified in patients with pituitary defects. *J Clin Endocrinol Metab*. 2005;90:5456-5462.

520. Saadi I, Semina EV, Amendt BA, et al. Identification of a dominant negative homeodomain mutation in Rieger syndrome. *J Biol Chem*. 2001;276:23034-23041.

521. Cohen LE, Radovick S. Molecular basis of combined pituitary hormone deficiencies. *Endocr Rev*. 2002;23:431-442.

522. Sornson MW, Wu W, Dasen JS, et al. Pituitary lineage determination by the prophet of Pit-1 homeodomain factor defective in Ames dwarfism. *Nature*. 1996;384:327-333.

523. Reynaud R, Barlier A, Vallette-Kasic S, et al. An uncommon phenotype with familial central hypogonadism caused by a novel PROP1 gene mutant truncated in the transactivation domain. *J Clin Endocrinol Metab*. 2005;90:4880-4887.

524. Rosenbloom AL, Almonte AS, Brown MR, et al. Clinical and biochemical phenotype of familial anterior hypopituitarism from mutation of the PROP1 gene. *J Clin Endocrinol Metab*. 1999;84:50-57.

525. Voss JW, Rosenfeld MG. Anterior pituitary development: short tales from dwarf mice. *Cell*. 1992;70:527-530.

526. Andersen B, Rosenfeld MG. POU domain factors in the neuroendocrine system: lessons from developmental biology provide insights into human disease. *Endocr Rev*. 2001;22:2-35.

527. Li S, Crenshaw EB 3rd, Rawson EJ, et al. Dwarf locus mutants lacking three pituitary cell types result from mutations in the POU-domain gene pit-1. *Nature*. 1990;347:528-533.

528. Turton JP, Reynaud R, Mehta A, et al. Novel mutations within the POU1F1 gene associated with variable combined pituitary hormone deficiency. *J Clin Endocrinol Metab*. 2005;90:4762-4770.

529. Cohen RN, Brue T, Naik K, et al. The role of CBP/p300 interactions and Pit-1 dimerization in the pathophysiological mechanism of combined pituitary hormone deficiency. *J Clin Endocrinol Metab*. 2006;91: 239-247.

530. Yamamoto M, Iguchi G, Takeno R, et al. Adult combined GH, prolactin, and TSH deficiency associated with circulating PIT-1 antibody in humans. *J Clin Invest*. 2011;121:113-119.

531. Vallette-Kasic S, Brue T, Pulichino AM, et al. Congenital isolated adrenocorticotropin deficiency: an underestimated cause of neonatal death, explained by TPIT gene mutations. *J Clin Endocrinol Metab*. 2005;90:1323-1331.

532. Quentien MH, Delemer B, Papadimitriou DT, et al. Deficit in anterior pituitary function and variable immune deficiency (DAVID) in children presenting with adrenocorticotropin deficiency and severe infections. *J Clin Endocrinol Metab*. 2012;97:E121-E128.

533. Ingraham HA, Lala DS, Ikeda Y, et al. The nuclear receptor steroidogenic factor 1 acts at multiple levels of the reproductive axis. *Genes Dev*. 1994;8:2302-2312.

534. Schimmer BP, White PC. Minireview: steroidogenic factor 1: its roles in differentiation, development, and disease. *Mol Endocrinol*. 2010;24: 1322-1337.

535. Jadhav U, Harris RM, Jameson JL. Hypogonadotropic hypogonadism in subjects with DAX1 mutations. *Mol Cell Endocrinol*. 2011;346:65-73.

536. Karaca E, Buyukkaya R, Pehlivan D, et al. Whole exome sequencing identifies homozygous GPR161 mutation in a family with pituitary stalk interruption syndrome. *J Clin Endocrinol Metab*. 2015;100(1): E140-E147.

537. Stoving RK, Hangaard J, Hansen-Nord M, Hagen C. A review of endocrine changes in anorexia nervosa. *J Psychiatr Res*. 1999;33:139-152.

538. Stoving RK, Veldhuis JD, Flyvbjerg A, et al. Jointly amplified basal and pulsatile growth hormone (GH) secretion and increased process irregularity in women with anorexia nervosa: indirect evidence for disruption of feedback regulation within the GH-insulin-like growth factor I axis. *J Clin Endocrinol Metab*. 1999;84:2056-2063.

539. Kleinberg DL. Pituitary tumors and failure of endocrine target organs. *Arch Intern Med*. 1979;139:969-970.

540. Mulroney SE, McDonnell KJ, Pert CB, et al. HIV gp120 inhibits the somatotropic axis: a possible GH-releasing hormone receptor mechanism for the pathogenesis of AIDS wasting. *Proc Natl Acad Sci U S A*. 1998;95:1927-1932.

541. Kelly DF, Gonzalo IT, Cohan P, et al. Hypopituitarism following traumatic brain injury and aneurysmal subarachnoid hemorrhage: a preliminary report. *J Neurosurg*. 2000;93:743-752.

542. Brandt L, Saveland H, Valdemarsson S, et al. Fatigue after aneurysmal subarachnoid hemorrhage evaluated by pituitary function and 3D-CBF. *Acta Neurol Scand*. 2004;109:91-96.

543. Aimaretti G, Ambrosio MR, Di Somma C, et al. Traumatic brain injury and subarachnoid haemorrhage are conditions at high risk for hypopituitarism: screening study at 3 months after the brain injury. *Clin Endocrinol (Oxf)*. 2004;61:320-326.

544. Kreitschmann-Andermahr I, Hoff C, Saller B, et al. Prevalence of pituitary deficiency in patients after aneurysmal subarachnoid hemorrhage. *J Clin Endocrinol Metab*. 2004;89:4986-4992.

545. Dimopoulou I, Kouyialis AT, Tzanella M, et al. High incidence of neuroendocrine dysfunction in long-term survivors of aneurysmal subarachnoid hemorrhage. *Stroke*. 2004;35:2884-2889.

546. Benvenga S, Campenni A, Ruggeri RM, Trimarchi F. Clinical review 113: hypopituitarism secondary to head trauma. *J Clin Endocrinol Metab*. 2000;85:1353-1361.

547. Agha A, Thornton E, O'Kelly P, et al. Posterior pituitary dysfunction after traumatic brain injury. *J Clin Endocrinol Metab*. 2004;89: 5987-5992.

548. Schneider HJ, Aimaretti G, Kreitschmann-Andermahr I, et al. Hypopituitarism. *Lancet*. 2007;369:1461-1470.

549. Personnier C, Crosnier H, Meyer P, et al. Prevalence of pituitary dysfunction after severe traumatic brain injury in children and adolescents: a large prospective study. *J Clin Endocrinol Metab*. 2014;99: 2052-2060.

550. Klose M, Stochholm K, Janukonyte J, et al. Prevalence of posttraumatic growth hormone deficiency is highly dependent on the diagnostic set-up: results from The Danish National Study on Posttraumatic Hypopituitarism. *J Clin Endocrinol Metab*. 2014;99:101-110.

551. Schneider HJ, Schneider M, Saller B, et al. Prevalence of anterior pituitary insufficiency 3 and 12 months after traumatic brain injury. *Eur J Endocrinol*. 2006;154:259-265.

552. Agha A, Rogers B, Sherlock M, et al. Anterior pituitary dysfunction in survivors of traumatic brain injury. *J Clin Endocrinol Metab.* 2004;89: 4929-4936.

553. Aimaretti G, Ambrosio MR, Di Somma C, et al. Residual pituitary function after brain injury-induced hypopituitarism: a prospective 12-month study. *J Clin Endocrinol Metab.* 2005;90:6085-6092.

554. Brada M, Jankowska P. Radiotherapy for pituitary adenomas. *Endocrinol Metab Clin North Am.* 2008;37:263-275.

555. Constine LS, Woolf PD, Cann D, et al. Hypothalamic-pituitary dysfunction after radiation for brain tumors. *N Engl J Med.* 1993;328:87-94.

556. Clayton PE, Shalet SM. Dose dependency of time of onset of radiation-induced growth hormone deficiency. *J Pediatr.* 1991;118:226-228.

557. Rose SR, Lustig RH, Pitukcheewanont P, et al. Diagnosis of hidden central hypothyroidism in survivors of childhood cancer. *J Clin Endocrinol Metab.* 1999;84:4472-4479.

558. Castinetti F, Nagai M, Morange I, et al. Long-term results of stereotactic radiosurgery in secretory pituitary adenomas. *J Clin Endocrinol Metab.* 2009;94:3400-3407.

559. Toogood AA. Endocrine consequences of brain irradiation. *Growth Horm IGF Res.* 2004;14(Suppl A):S118-S124.

560. De Marinis L, Bonadonna S, Bianchi A, et al. Primary empty sella. *J Clin Endocrinol Metab.* 2005;90:5471-5477.

561. Prabhakar VK, Shalet SM. Aetiology, diagnosis, and management of hypopituitarism in adult life. *Postgrad Med J.* 2006;82:259-266.

CHAPTER 9

Pituitary Masses and Tumors

SHLOMO MELMED • DAVID KLEINBERG

KEY POINTS

- Sellar masses arise from intrapituitary or parasellar tissues, and most are classified as benign pituitary adenomas.
- Nonpituitary sellar masses are rare and are usually infiltrations, inflammatory processes, or metastatic deposits or may arise from adjacent structures including aneurysms, meningiomas, or chordomas.
- Nonsecreting pituitary adenomas are usually of gonadotroph or null cell origin and present with compressive features or are diagnosed as incidentalomas.
- Secreting pituitary adenomas exhibit unique syndromes due to excess production of prolactin (prolactinomas), growth hormone (acromegaly/gigantism), adrenocorticotropic hormone (Cushing disease), or rarely, thyrotropin or gonadotropins.
- Management of these masses includes surgery, radiation, and specific targeted medical therapies.

PITUITARY MASSES

Pituitary Mass Effects

An expanding pituitary mass may inexorably alter the sellar size and shape by bony erosion and remodeling (Fig. 9-1). Although the exact time course for this process is unknown, it appears to be slowly progressive over years or decades. The tumor may invade soft tissue, and the dorsal sellar roof presents the least resistance to expansion from within the confines of the bony sella. Nevertheless, both suprasellar and parasellar compression and invasion may occur with an enlarging mass, with resultant clinical manifestations (Table 9-1). As sellar masses impinge upon the optic chiasm they may interfere with vision. Because of the anatomy of the chiasm, pressure from below affects temporal visual fields, starting superiorly and ultimately extending to the entire temporal field. Continued growth and pressure on the optic apparatus can extend visual loss to the nasal field and may result in blindness. Long-standing optic chiasmal pressure results in optic disc pallor. Extension of pituitary lesions laterally may also impinge on or invade the dural wall of the cavernous sinus. Despite invasion, these lesions only rarely affect function of the third, fourth, and sixth cranial nerves, as well as the ophthalmic and maxillary branches of the fifth cranial nerve. Although tumors in the cavernous sinus often surround the internal carotid artery, clinical vascular sequelae are rarely encountered. Varying degrees of diplopia, ptosis, ophthalmoplegia, and decreased facial sensation may occur infrequently, depending on the extent of neural involvement by the cavernous sinus mass. In contrast to cavernous invasion by slow tumor progression, sudden insults to the cavernous sinus by hemorrhage or infarction of a pituitary tumor occur more frequently and may affect nerves coursing through the sinus. Downward extension into the sphenoid sinus indicates that the parasellar mass has eroded the bony sellar floor. Aggressive tumors may also invade the roof of the palate and cause nasopharyngeal obstruction, infection, and cerebrospinal fluid (CSF) leakage. Infrequently, temporal or frontal lobes may be invaded, causing uncinate seizures, personality disorders, and anosmia. In addition to the anatomic lesions caused by the expanding mass, direct hypothalamic involvement of the encroaching mass may lead to important metabolic sequelae discussed in Chapter 8.

Intrasellar tumors commonly present with headaches, even in the absence of demonstrable suprasellar extension. Small changes in intrasellar pressure caused by a microadenoma within the confined sella are sufficient to stretch the dural plate with resultant headache. Headache severity does not correlate with the size of the adenoma or the presence of suprasellar extension.[1] Relatively minor diaphragmatic distortions or dural impingement may be associated with persistent headache. Successful medical management of small functional pituitary tumors with dopamine agonists or somatostatin analogues is often accompanied by remarkable headache improvement. In a retrospective assessment of transsphenoidal surgery for microadenomas, headaches resolved or disappeared in 90% of patients with nonfunctioning tumors and in 56% with functioning tumors.[2] Regardless of cause or size, pituitary masses, including adenomas, may be associated with compression of surrounding healthy pituitary tissue and resultant hypopituitarism. In 49 patients undergoing transsphenoidal resection of pituitary adenomas, mean intrasellar pressure was elevated twofold to threefold in patients with associated pituitary failure. Furthermore, prevalence of headache and elevated prolactin (PRL) levels correlate positively with intrasellar pressure levels,[3] suggesting interrupted portal delivery of hypothalamic hormones. Thus,

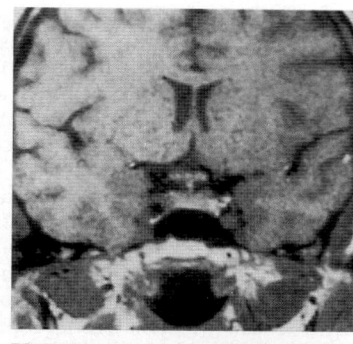

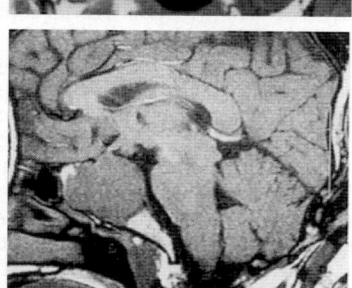

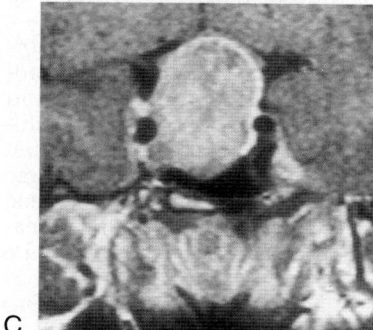

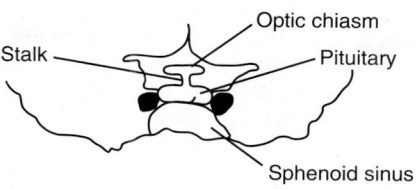

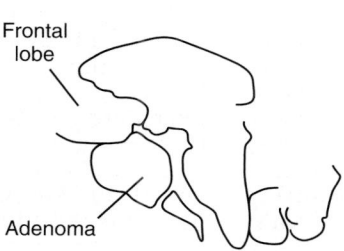

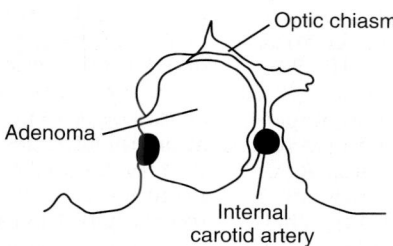

Figure 9-1 Magnetic resonance images of the pituitary. **A,** Coronal section of a normal pituitary gland. **B,** Sagittal view of a large pituitary adenoma lifting and distorting the optic chiasm and invading the sphenoid sinus and impinging the frontal lobe. **C,** Coronal view of a large macroadenoma elevating the optic chiasm and invading the right cavernous sinus.

TABLE 9-1
Local Effects of an Expanding Pituitary, Parasellar, or Hypothalamic Mass

Impacted Structure	Clinical Effect
Pituitary	Growth failure, adult hyposomatotropism, hypogonadism, hypothyroidism, hypoadrenalism
Optic tract	Loss of red perception, bitemporal hemianopia, superior or bitemporal field defect, scotoma, blindness
Hypothalamus	Temperature dysregulation, obesity, diabetes insipidus; thirst, sleep; appetite, behavioral, and autonomic nervous system dysfunctions
Cavernous sinus	Ptosis, diplopia, ophthalmoplegia, facial numbness
Temporal lobe	Uncinate seizures
Frontal lobe	Personality disorder, anosmia
Central	Headache, hydrocephalus, psychosis, dementia, laughing seizures
Neuro-ophthalmologic tract	*Field defects:*
	Bitemporal hemianopia (50%), amaurosis with hemianopia (12%), contralateral or monocular hemianopia (7%)
	Scotomas—junctional; monocular central, arcuate, altitudinal; hemianopic
	Homonymous hemianopia
	Acuity loss:
	Snellen
	Contrast sensitivity
	Color vision
	Visual evoked potential
	Pupillary abnormality:
	Impaired light reactivity
	Afferent defect
	Optic atrophy:
	Papilledema
	Cranial nerve palsy—oculomotor, trochlear, abducens, sensory trigeminal
	Nystagmus
	Visual hallucinations
	Postfixation blindness

Adapted from Snyder P, Melmed S. Clinically nonfunctioning sellar masses. In: DeGroot L, Jameson JL, eds. *Endocrinology*, 5th ed. Philadelphia: Elsevier; 2010:312-323; Arnold A. Neuroophthalmologic evaluation of pituitary disorders. In: Melmed S, ed. *The Pituitary*, 2nd ed. Boston, MA: Blackwell; 2002.

surgical decompression of a sellar mass may lead to recovery of compromised anterior pituitary function. In patients who do not recover pituitary function postoperatively, ischemic necrosis of residual pituitary tissue is likely to have occurred. Stalk compression may result in pituitary failure caused by encroachment of the portal vessels that normally provide pituitary access to the hypothalamic hormones. Stalk compression also usually leads to hyperprolactinemia and concomitant failure of other pituitary trophic hormones.

Evaluation of Pituitary Masses
Approach to the Patient Harboring a Pituitary Mass

Most pituitary masses are adenomas. Ninety-one percent of 1120 patients undergoing transsphenoidal surgery for sellar masses were diagnosed as harboring pituitary adenomas.[4] In a series of 2598 patients undergoing pituitary magnetic resonance imaging (MRI), pituitary adenomas accounted for 82% of visible lesions. Most commonly encountered nonadenomatous lesions include Rathke's cleft cyst, craniophargyioma, and meningioma,[5] with Rathke's cysts accounting for up to 40% of all such masses.[6] Thus, the differential diagnosis of a pituitary mass should be aimed at excluding the diagnosis of a pituitary adenoma before considering the presence of other rare sellar lesions. Pituitary adenomas arise from differentiated cells secreting trophic hormones including growth hormone (GH), PRL, adrenocorticotropin, thyroid-stimulating hormone (TSH, thyrotropin), or gonadotropins. These tumors may hypersecrete respective hormones or may be clinically nonsecreting (Fig. 9-2). The management and prognosis of anterior pituitary adenomas differ markedly from those for other nonpituitary masses, and an important diagnostic challenge is to effectively distinguish a pituitary adenoma from other parasellar masses. Several physiologic states are associated with pituitary enlargement. Lactotroph hyperplasia occurs during pregnancy, and thyrotroph, gonadotroph, or rarely corticotroph hyperplasias occur in the presence of long-standing primary thyroid, gonadal, or adrenal failure, respectively.[7] Pituitary enlargement may also occur as a result of ectopic GH-releasing hormone (GHRH) or corticotropin-releasing hormone (CRH) secretion, from carcinoid tumors or hypothalamic gangliocytomas, with resultant hyperplasia of somatotroph or corticotroph cells. Autopsy series show that up to 20% of subjects harbor an incidental clinically silent pituitary adenoma (incidentaloma). With the widespread use of sensitive imaging techniques for nonpituitary indications including head trauma, chronic sinusitis, or headaches, previously inapparent pituitary lesions are being identified with increasing frequency. Incidental pituitary cysts, hemorrhages, and infarctions are also discovered at autopsy. Pituitary abnormalities compatible with the diagnosis of microadenoma are detectable in about 10% of the normal adult population undergoing MRI studies.[8] Recognizing that approximately 90% of observed pituitary lesions represent pituitary adenomas, initial assessment should determine whether the mass is hormonally functional and whether local mass effects are apparent at the time of diagnosis or likely to develop in the future.

As the onset of clinical features associated with disordered hormone secretion is insidious and may be unnoticed for years or decades, endocrine function should always be tested at presentation (Table 9-2). Clinical evaluation for changes compatible with hyper- or hyposecretion of GH, gonadotropins, PRL, or adrenocorticotropic hormone (ACTH) may reveal unique long-term sequelae requiring distinct therapies. In the absence of clinical features of a humoral hypersecretory syndrome, cost-effective

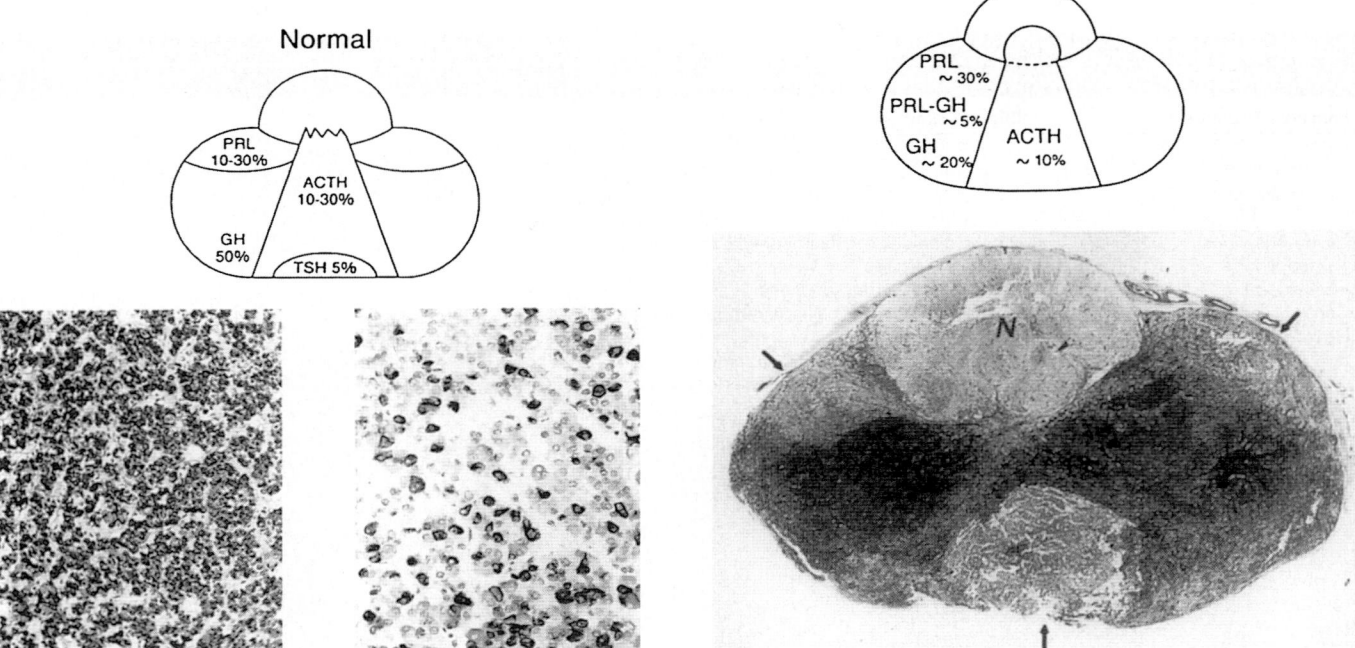

Figure 9-2 Distribution of normal adenohypophyseal cells is reflected in pituitary adenomas. Nonfunctioning tumors, on the other hand, are typically macroadenomas that efface pituitary landmarks. The localization and frequency of functioning microadenomas reflect the maximal concentration of their corresponding normal pituitary cells. Left panels show normal pituitary with GH cells in lateral wings *(lower left)* compared with diseased pituitary *(lower right)*. Right panels depict adenoma distribution with multiple incidental adenomas shown by arrows. ACTH, adrenocorticotropic hormone; GH, growth hormone; N, neurohypophysis; PRL, prolactin; TSH, thyroid-stimulating hormone (thyrotropin). (From Scheithauer BW, Horvath E, Lloyd RV, Kovacs K. Pathology of pituitary adenomas and pituitary hyperplasia. In: Thapar K, Kovacs K, Scheithauer BW, Lloyd RV, eds. *Diagnosis and Management of Pituitary Tumors.* Totowa, NJ: Humana Press; 2001.)

TABLE 9-2

Screening Tests for Functional Pituitary Adenomas

Disorder	Test	Comments
Acromegaly	IGF-1	Interpret IGF-1 relative to age- and gender-matched control subjects.
	OGTT with GH obtained at 0, 30, and 60 min	Normal subjects should suppress GH to <1 µg/L.
Prolactinoma	Serum PRL level	A level >500 µg/L is pathognomonic for macroprolactinoma.
		If >200 µg/L, prolactinoma is likely.*
Cushing disease	24-hr UFC	Ensure that urine collection is total and accurate by measuring urinary creatinine. Free salivary cortisol reflects circadian rhythm, and elevated levels may indicate Cushing disease.
	Nighttime salivary cortisol	
	Dexamethasone (1 mg) at 11 PM and fasting plasma cortisol measured at 8 AM	Normal subjects suppress to <1.8 µg/dL.
		Distinguishes adrenal adenoma from ectopic ACTH secretion or Cushing disease.
	ACTH assay	
TSH-secreting tumor	TSH measurement	If T_4 or T_3 is elevated and TSH is measurable or elevated, a TSH-secreting tumor may be present.
	Free T_4 by dialysis	
	Total T_3	

*Risperidol may result in prolactin levels >200 µg/L.

ACTH, adrenocorticotropic hormone; GH, growth hormone; IGF-1, insulin-like growth factor type 1; OGTT, oral glucose tolerance test; PRL, prolactin; T_3, triiodothyronine; T_4, thyroxine; TSH, thyroid-stimulating hormone; UFC, urinary free cortisol.

laboratory screening should be performed. Serum PRL levels greater than 200 µg/L strongly suggest the presence of a micro- or macroprolactinoma. Any elevation in serum PRL from minimal to high can occur when a microadenoma is present. A minimal to moderate elevation can also indicate secondary stalk interruption by a pituitary mass (usually a nonfunctioning macroadenoma). A PRL level greater than 500 ng/mL in a nonpregnant individual is considered pathognomonic of a prolactinoma, as significant PRL elevations can be caused by drugs such as risperidol.[9] Elevated age- and gender-matched insulin-like growth factor 1 (IGF-1) levels indicate the presence of GH-secreting adenoma, and a high 24-hour urinary free cortisol level or elevated nighttime salivary cortisol[10] is an effective screen for most patients with Cushing disease. Nevertheless, the incidence of functional hormone-secreting tumors in asymptomatic subjects with incidentally discovered pituitary masses is low. The presence of, or the potential for, local compressive effects must also be considered. Because the risk for microadenoma progression to a compressive macroadenoma is low, no direct intervention may be warranted. For parasellar masses of uncertain origin, histologic examination of surgically excised tissue may be the best approach to yield an accurate diagnosis. Clearly, the benefits versus risks of surgery should be considered in such cases, especially for lesions that are not growing or not causing a functional deficit. Although MRI or computed tomography (CT) imaging features may be helpful in diagnosing the cause of a nonpituitary sellar mass, the final diagnosis may remain elusive until pathologic confirmation is obtained.

Parasellar masses include neoplastic and non-neoplastic lesions and manifest clinically by local compression of surrounding vital structures or as a result of metabolic or hormonal derangements. Rarely, sellar masses or infiltrative processes may be the presenting feature of a previously undiagnosed systemic disorder such as lymphoma, tuberculosis, sarcoidosis,[11] or histiocytosis.[12] Fever with or without associated sterile or septic meningitis may rarely be caused by fluid leakage into the subarachnoid space from Rathke's cleft, dermoid and epidermoid cysts, craniopharyngioma, and apoplexy.[13,14] Pituitary masses may present with hemorrhage and infarction, especially during pregnancy (see earlier discussion), when there is a pituitary tumor or when elderly individuals with unsuspected pituitary tumors become hypotensive because of another illness. Rarely, these adenomas present with CSF leak, which may predispose to meningitis. Pituitary masses may also undergo silent infarction leading to development of a partial or totally empty pituitary sella, with normal pituitary reserve, implying that the surrounding rim of pituitary tissue is fully functional. Large sellar cysts may be mistaken for an empty sella. Rarely, functional pituitary adenomas may arise within the remnant pituitary tissue, and these tumors may not be visible by sensitive MRI (i.e., <2 mm in diameter), despite their endocrine hyperactivity. More than one kind of tumor may be found in the same patient, such as a pituitary tumor and a meningioma[15] or pituitary adenoma with a craniopharyngioma component.[16] Acute or chronic infection with abscess formation may rarely occur within the mass. Compromised pituitary hormone hyposecretion may be due to direct pressure effects of the expanding mass on hormone-secreting cells or parasellar pressure effects that attenuate synthesis or secretion of hypothalamic hormones, with resultant pituitary failure.

Imaging

Tumors of the pituitary gland are best diagnosed with MRI, because the technique has better resolution than other radiologic modalities for identifying soft tissue changes (see Fig. 9-1). When a pituitary tumor or other parasellar mass is suspected, an MRI specifically focused on the pituitary should be requested, as more widely spaced cuts during a routine brain MRI are often inadequate to visualize relatively small pituitary tumors.[17] This technique permits high-contrast detailed visualization of tumor mass effects on neighboring soft tissue structures, including the cavernous sinus or optic chiasm. A pituitary MRI includes images of the optic chiasm, hypothalamus, pituitary stalk, and cavernous and sphenoid sinuses.[18] High-resolution T1-weighted sections in the coronal and sagittal plane both before and after gadolinium pentetic acid contrast administration will distinguish most pituitary masses. Slice thickness should be less than 3 mm to obtain a pixel of 1 mm. Contiguous sections are therefore required to diagnose lesions of 1 to 3 mm. If necessary, especially for diagnosing high-signaling hemorrhage, T2-weighted images will provide additional diagnostic information. MRI thus clearly delineates the pituitary gland, stalk, optic tracts, and surrounding soft tissues. The gland may be concave, convex, or flat. The posterior pituitary lobe exhibits a discrete bright spot of high signal intensity on T1-weighted images, which declines with age and is absent in diabetes insipidus and most posterior pituitary lesions. This T1 shortening may reflect the presence of antidiuretic hormone (ADH) localized within neurosecretory vesicles.[19] The pituitary gland may transiently enlarge during adolescence, pregnancy, and post partum, with teenage girls exhibiting increasing gland convexity during the menstrual cycle. During pregnancy, the gland should normally not exceed 10 to 12 mm, and the stalk should not exceed 4 mm in diameter. Pregnant women may rarely develop visual field deficits due to an enlarging pituitary gland even in the absence of a pituitary tumor. A thickened stalk may indicate the presence of hypophysitis, granuloma, or chordoma. After gadolinium injection, microadenomas usually appear hypodense compared to the normal gland, especially when multiple thin section echo sequences are examined in the first few minutes after contrast agent injection. It has been suggested that this hypointensity may reflect compromised microadenoma vasculature.[20] Microadenomas may also cause gland asymmetry or stalk deviation. In contrast, macroadenomas, which are significantly more vascular than microadenomas, have a higher affinity for gadolinium. They often enlarge the sella turcica by remodeling the bony fossa, suggesting a gradual long-term process. These tumors can grow upward toward the optic apparatus and cause draping of the nerves over the tumor, often accompanied by visual field abnormalities. Tumors can also extend into the sphenoid sinus and not infrequently invade connective tissue separating the pituitary from the cavernous sinus. Radiologically, visible tumor tissue surrounding the carotid artery confirms cavernous sinus invasion. Infrequently, these patients infrequently develop palsies of the third, fourth, or sixth cranial nerves. MRI may readily distinguish pituitary adenomas from other masses, including hyperplasias, craniopharyngiomas, meningiomas, chordomas, cysts, and metastatic lesions. Visualization of a distinct pituitary gland adjacent to a parasellar mass (Fig. 9-3) suggests that the mass is not of pituitary origin. Secondary distinguishing features such as visualization of noninvolved pituitary tissue, mass consistency, calcification, hemorrhage, and suprasellar involvement usually allow an imaging diagnosis of these masses, which can often only be confirmed by direct cranial histologic diagnosis. Preoperative localization of carotid artery aneurysms can also be confirmed by MRI or MR angiography. Administration of gadolinium may be contraindicated in patients with impaired renal function because it may cause acute renal failure or be associated with nephrogenic systemic fibrosis.[21]

Pituitary CT allows visualization of bony structures, including the sellar floor and clinoid bones, and identifies bony invasion. CT also recognizes calcifications that characterize craniopharyngiomas, meningiomas, and rarely aneurysms that are not evident on MRI. Rarely, pituitary adenomas may calcify. Pituitary CT scan is indicated for discovery of hemorrhagic lesions, metastatic deposits, chordomas, and evidence of calcification.

Receptor Imaging. As prolactinomas express dopamine 2 (D_2) receptors, they can be imaged with a radiolabeled D_2 receptor antagonist by using ^{123}I-iodobenzamine single-photon emission scanning. Failure to visualize nonfunctioning tumors by this technique has led some to advocate its use to distinguish the two tumor types.[22] Radiolabeled indium-pentetreotide has been used for in vivo tumor imaging. Most pituitary adenomas express somatostatin receptor subtypes to a varying degree, thus limiting the specificity of the procedure. As the sensitivity of single-photon emission CT (SPECT) is about 1 cm, and also detects normal pituitary tissue receptor expression, its use is limited for pituitary tumor detection, but it may be helpful for imaging ectopic ACTH-secreting tumors.

Neuro-ophthalmologic Assessment of Pituitary Masses

The optic tracts are particularly vulnerable to compression by expanding pituitary masses. Accurate neuro-ophthalmologic evaluation is helpful for tumor diagnosis, determining pretreatment baseline visual status for posttreatment monitoring, or detection of mass recurrence.[23] The relationship of the optic chiasm and the intracranial components of the optic nerves with the pituitary gland and surrounding vessels are depicted in Figure 9-4. A 10-mm posteriorly angled gap separates the optic chiasm and diaphragma sellae (Fig. 9-5). Therefore, extensive suprasellar mass extension is required before visual function is compromised. Decussation of neural fibers originating from the nasal half of each retina occurs at the chiasm, and those originating from the temporal retinal halves are situated ipsilaterally.[24] Fibers from the superior and inferior retinal aspect are segregated in the corresponding chiasmal regions. Local vascular compromise and chiasmal stretching contribute to the pathogenesis of selective visual compromise. Reversibility of visual effects may correlate inversely with acuteness of the compressive insult.

Visual Symptoms. An abnormal visual examination may unmask the presence of a pituitary mass in an asymptomatic patient. Prior to the availability of sophisticated assay and imaging techniques, virtually all pituitary masses presented with visual loss. Currently, fewer than 10% of patients present with visual loss and most harbor clinically nonfunctioning pituitary adenomas often detected by incidental imaging. Unilateral or bilateral temporal or central visual loss is often asymmetric and may be quite insidious, remitting or recurring. Rarely, sudden visual loss occurs in a previously asymptomatic patient. Other symptoms include diplopia, impaired depth perception, and very rarely, visual hallucinations.[25]

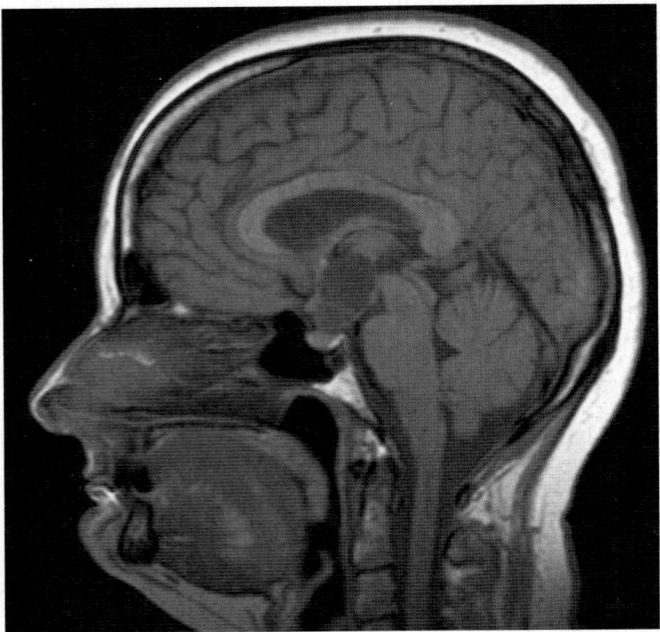

Figure 9-3 Sagittal magnetic resonance image of a craniopharyngioma, with cystic and solid components. The tumor is in the suprasellar area sitting above a normal pituitary gland. The presence of a separate pituitary gland indicates that the suprasellar tumor is not of pituitary origin. (Courtesy of N. Karavitaki.)

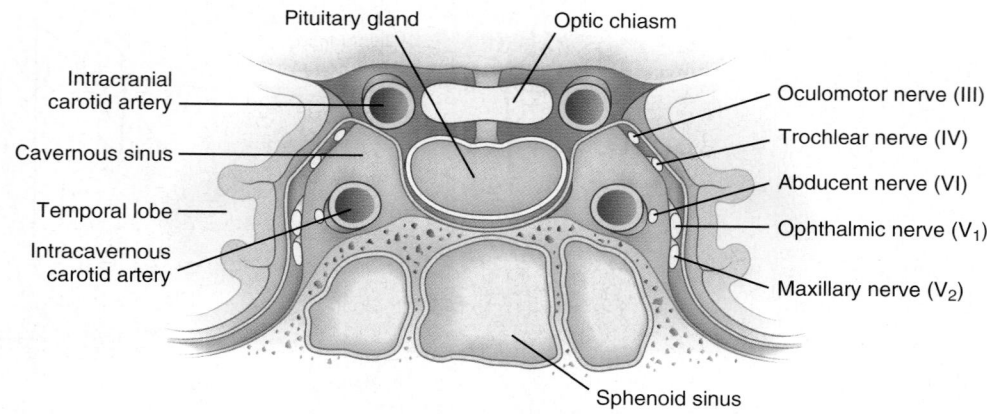

Figure 9-4 Coronal section of the sellar structures and cavernous sinus showing the relationship of the oculomotor (III) and trochlear (IV) cranial nerves to the pituitary gland. (From Silver SI, Sharpe JA. Neuro-ophthalmologic evaluation of pituitary tumors. In: Thapar K, Kovacs K, Scheihauer BW, Lloyd RV, eds. *Diagnosis and Management of Pituitary Tumors.* Totowa, NJ: Humana Press; 2001:173-200.)

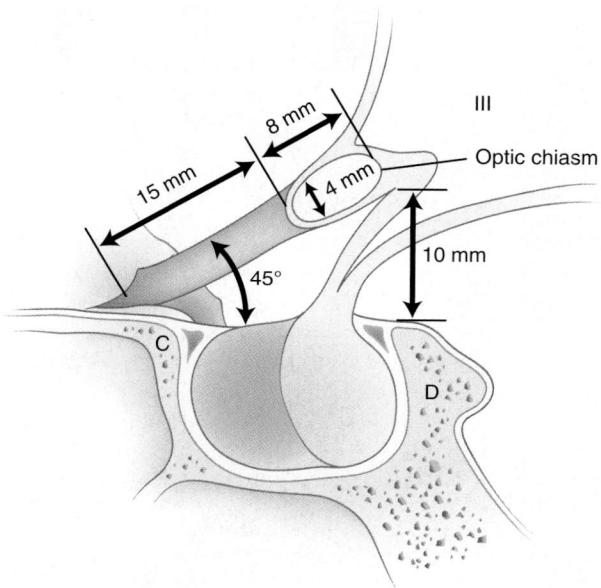

Figure 9-5 Relationship of the pituitary gland to the optic chiasm. The intracranial optic nerve/chiasmal complex lies up to 10 mm above the diaphragma sellae. C, anterior clinoid process; D, dorsum of the sella turcica. (From Miller NR. *Walsh and Hoyt's Clinical Neuro-Ophthalmology,* 4th ed, vol 1. Baltimore, MD: Williams & Wilkins; 1985:60-69.)

Clinical Signs

Impingement of the inferior crossing chiasmal fibers leads to bitemporal visual loss, especially in the superior field portions, accounting for most pituitary-related visual defects (Fig. 9-6). Rarely tumors can compress the optic chiasm from above and cause inferior temporal compromise. As damage to the optic chiasm becomes more extreme, field cuts can extend into the nasal field and also cause optic atrophy. Isolated impairment of nasal visual fields is mostly seen in patients with glaucoma. Pituitary-related defects preferentially marginate at the vertical field midline[23] in contrast to other causes of bitemporal defects, which tend to occur away from the midline. Despite prominent field defects, many of which can be directly correlated with defined tumor location by MRI, visual acuity in the remaining fields is invariably normal in most patients. Anterior tumor extension may damage central visual

acuity, and this is detected using the Snellen chart or by loss of color discrimination, especially in the red-green spectrum. Rarely, pupillary abnormalities, optic atrophy, papilledema, cranial nerve palsies, and nystagmus may be encountered. Visual fields are assessed by bedside confrontational testing, Goldmann perimetry, the Amsler grid, and automated quantitative perimetry. As red vision is lost prior to white, a small pin (<10-mm diameter) with the two colors can be employed. The patient should be asked to cover one eye so that the examiner can evaluate both temporal and nasal fields without compromise.

Management of Pituitary Masses

Although pituitary masses are usually benign, they may compress local structures or invade brain tissue (Fig. 9-7). The goals of therapy are to alleviate local compressive mass effects and to suppress hormone hypersecretion or relieve hormone hyposecretion, while maintaining intact pituitary trophic function. Three modes of available therapy include surgical, radiotherapeutic, and medical approaches. In general, the benefits of each type of therapy should be weighed against their respective risks, and comprehensive physician and patient awareness is required to individualize treatment approaches.

Surgical Management of Pituitary Tumors and Sellar Masses

Pituitary surgery is indicated for excision of mass lesions causing central pressure effects, including visual compromise, primary correction of hormonal hypersecretion, or functional tumor resection in patients resistant or not immediately responsive to medical treatment. Unusual sellar lesions may require diagnostic tissue evaluation, and rarely, primary or secondary parasellar malignancies require wide excision.

In 1904, Horsley reported the surgical resection of a pituitary tumor by a lateral middle fossa approach.[26] The first successful transsphenoidal approach for pituitary tumor resection was reported by Schloffer in 1907[27] and subsequently refined by Cushing, who between 1910 and 1925 operated on 231 patients harboring pituitary tumors with a remarkably low 5.6% mortality rate.[26] Cushing used a sublabial incision to enable an endonasal approach for removing the septum and improved visualization using Kanavel's headlight. Hardy later improved the technique by using the operating microscope and intraoperative

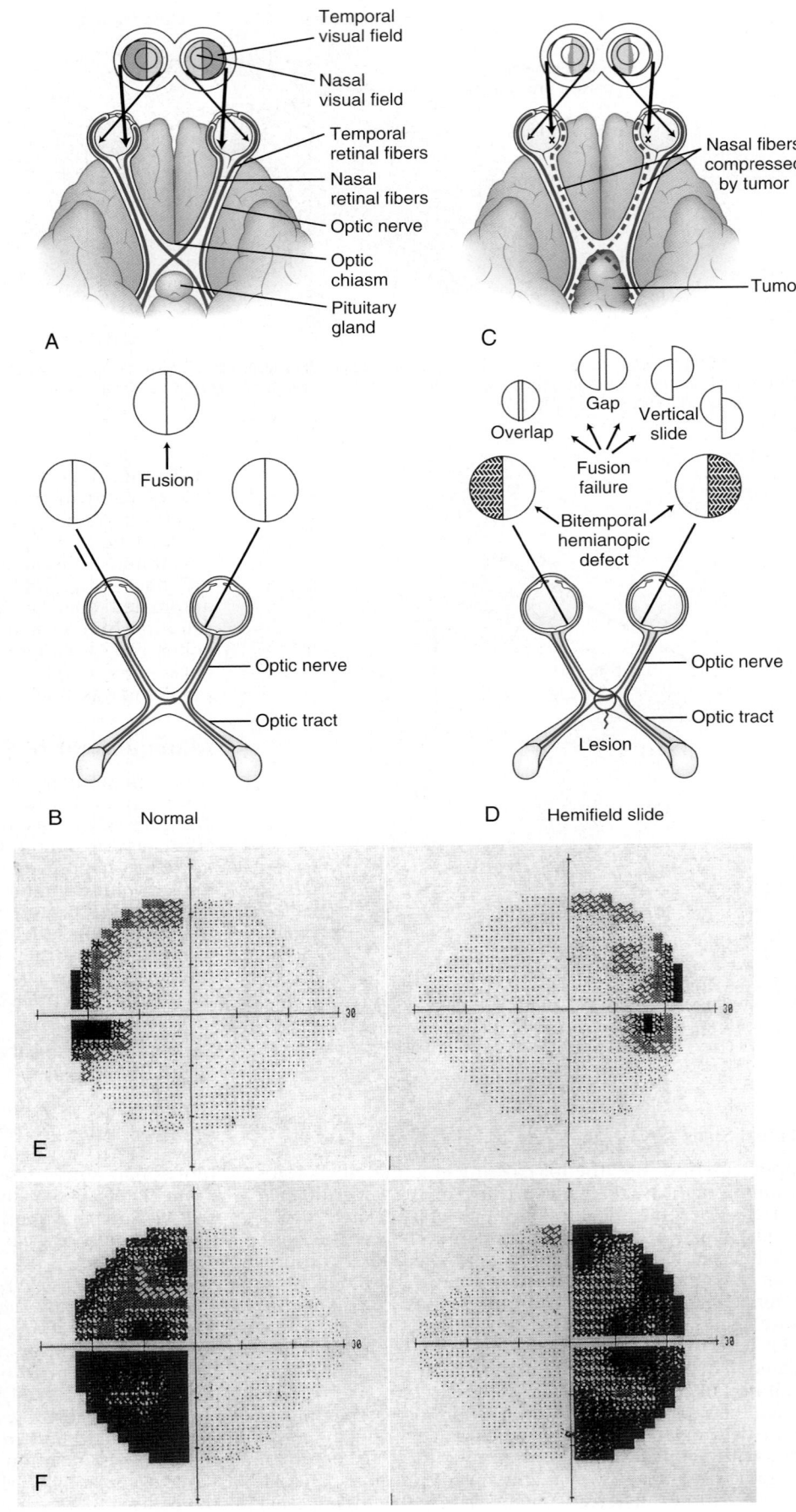

Figure 9-6 A to **D,** Local effects of an expanding pituitary tumor causing visual field defects. **A,** Normal vision; **C,** bitemporal hemianopia. **B** and **D,** Hemifield slide phenomena arising in the setting of bitemporal hemianopia and from fusion instability. The nasal and temporal fields lose their linkage, resulting in overlap of the preserved visual fields. **E** and **F,** Threshold field test showing superior bitemporal hernianopia in a patient with pituitary tumor compressing the optic chiasma (**E**) which later advanced to bitemporal hemianopia (**F**). (A and C from Newell-Price J. Endocrine assessment. In: Sheaves R, Jenkins PJ, Wass JAH, eds. *Clinical Endocrinology Oncology.* Boston, MA: Blackwell Science; 1977. B and D from Stiver SI, Sharpe JA. Neuro-ophthalmologic evaluation of pituitary tumors. In: Thapar K, Kovacs K, Scheithauer BW, Lloyd RV, eds. *Diagnosis and Management of Pituitary Tumors.* Totowa, NJ: Humana Press; 2001.)

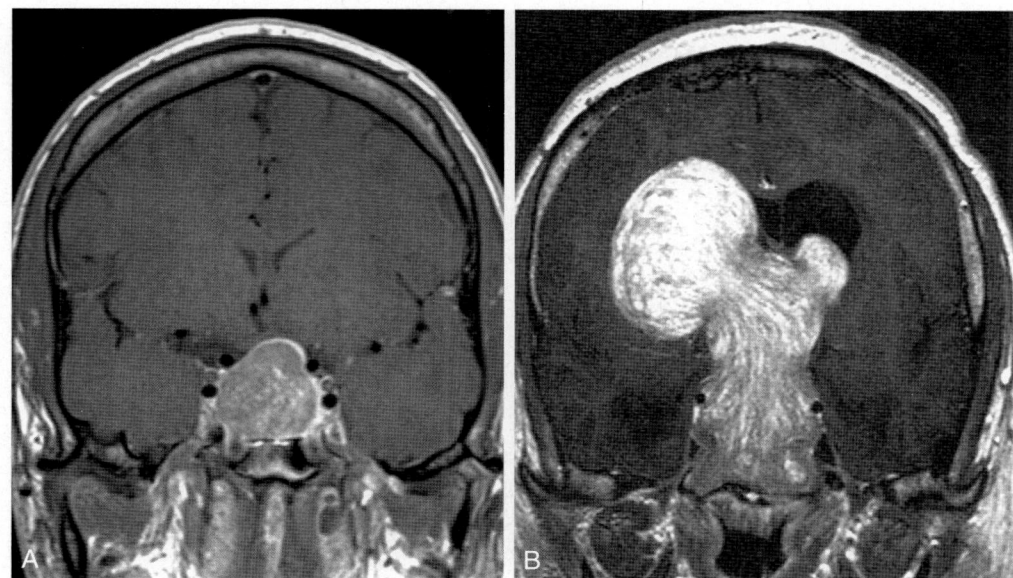

Figure 9-7 A, Pituitary macroadenoma invading laterally and elevating the optic chiasm dorsally. **B,** Large invasive macroadenoma invading brain tissue. (**B** from Li-Ng M, Sharma M. Invasive pituitary adenoma. *J Clin Endocrinol Metab.* 2008;93:3284-3285.)

fluoroscopy, resulting in markedly reduced morbidity and mortality rates compared to those usually encountered with craniotomy, and his approach became the mainstay surgical technique for resecting these tumors.

The transsphenoidal approach avoids invasion of the cranial cavity and precludes the need for brain tissue manipulation required during a subfrontal surgical approach (Fig. 9-8). A ventral sphenoid approach for resection of pituitary masses likewise does not violate the cranial fossa. Thus, transsphenoidal surgery is associated with minimal morbidity and mortality rates, most patients are ambulatory within 6 to 9 hours, and the hospital stay is generally about 3 days. Furthermore, the transsphenoidal approach allows for a clearly visible operative field with high magnification and internal illumination. Normal pituitary can be clearly distinguished from tumor tissue, facilitating microdissection and small tumor resection (Fig. 9-9). The use of the transsphenoidal approach has been greatly enhanced by several technologic advances, including head immobilization techniques, microinstrumentation development, and novel angled endoscopes. Enhanced MRI sensitivity and precision, as well as intraoperative use of MRI, allow for clear delineation of tumor location, size, and invasiveness, all critical determinants of surgical success.

The endoscopic surgical technique has enabled an approach to both intrapituitary and some extrasellar masses.[28] Most approaches are endonasal[29] but some traverse the cranial base, and suprasellar lesions are reached by transposing the pituitary to access the lesion. In experienced hands, the endoscopic technique results in similar complication rates and outcomes, as compared to the traditional transsphenoidal approach.[30]

Craniotomy is indicated for the rare invasive suprasellar masses extending into the frontal or middle cranial fossa, optic nerves, or extensive posterior clival invasion. Suprasellar extension contained by a small diaphragmatic aperture ("hour-glass configuration") may also require a transcranial approach. Very rarely, tumors that are too solid to be removed transsphenoidally may require a combination of transsphenoidal and intracranial surgery.

Goals of Surgery. The goal of pituitary surgery is for total resection limited to the lesion, without compromising

postoperative endogenous pituitary function.[31] Careful selective mass resection may be difficult for poorly encapsulated lesions, those embedded deeply within the gland body, and those extending into the wall or the body of the cavernous sinuses or suprasellar lesions. However, suprasellar tumors (e.g., craniopharygiomas) may also be successfully removed via a transnasal approach. Poor operative field visibility also limits precise resection. Excision of normal pituitary tissue and intraoperative gland manipulation should be avoided unless critical for effective tumor dissection. Occasionally, hemihypophysectomy or even nonselective total gland resection may be indicated for multifocal tumors if the surrounding normal gland is necrotic or if no mass lesion is discernible despite an accurate clinical and biochemical diagnosis (especially for ACTH-cell tumors). Successful surgery should decompress central visual defects and compromised trophic hormone secretion. For children and young adults the consideration of adequate normal tissue for subsequent growth patterns and reproductive function is an important determinant for intraoperative decision making. Nevertheless, especially for functional tumors, small residual remnants attached to the dura are difficult to access but remain hypersecretory with persistent clinical progression. Thus, the skilled neurosurgeon will carefully balance maximally effective tumor removal with the requirement to preserve nontumorous pituitary trophic function.

Recent advances have enabled improved surgical results, and long-term outcomes using new techniques have been rigorously compared to standard operations performed by skilled surgeons.[31,32] Image-guided approaches enable intraoperative surgical neuronavigation by three-dimensional imaging. Intraoperative ultrasound and MRI technologies allow for real-time assessment of the dimensions and extent of the pituitary mass and the progress of surgery. Intraoperative MRI is performed while the surgical field is still open, thus allowing the surgeon to directly assess the need for further dissection, and provides an excellent baseline for postoperative follow-up. If there is suspicion of a vascular lesion, carotid and intracranial angiography is indicated prior to surgery. In contrast, postoperative image stabilization may not be evident for months after surgery,

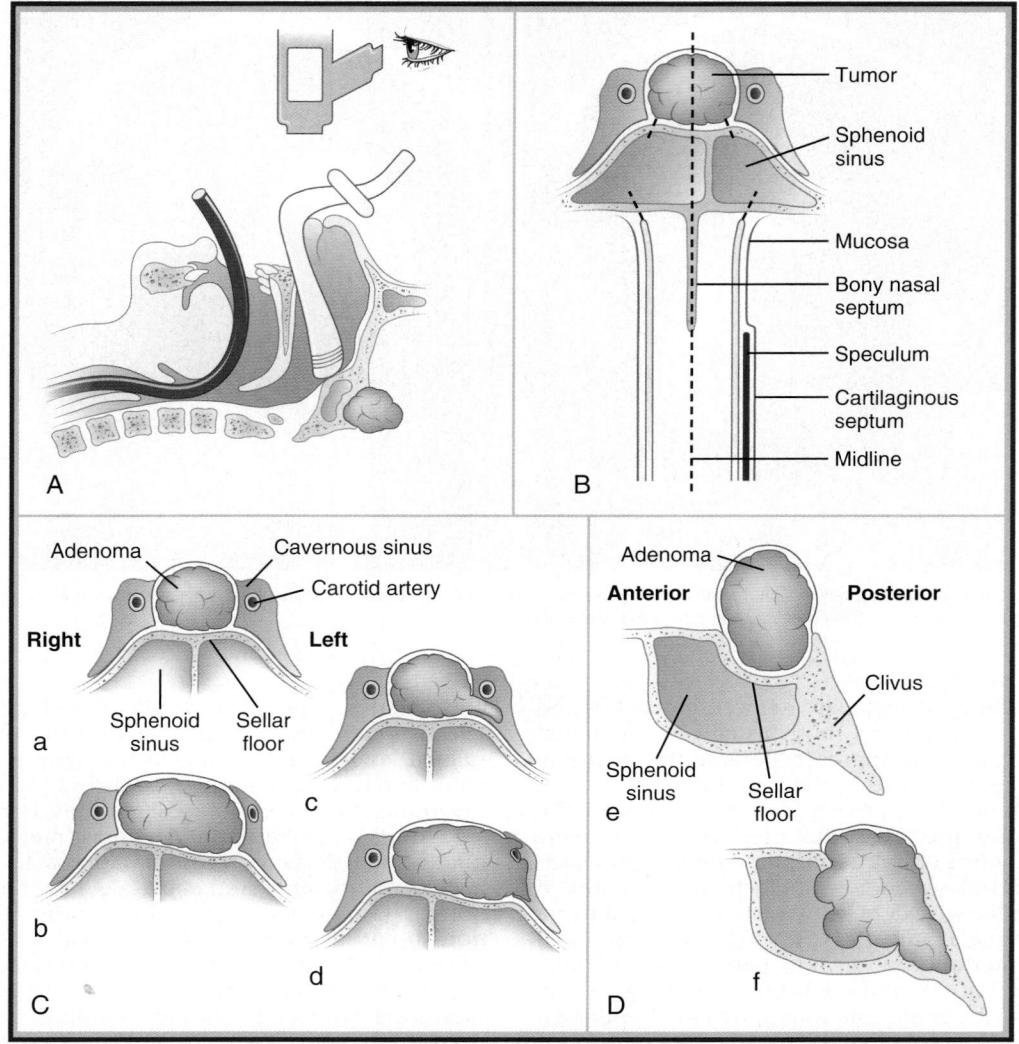

Figure 9-8 Transsphenoidal pituitary surgery. **A,** Route of the transsphenoidal approach (lateral view) and surgical corridor of the transsphenoidal approach and positioning of the retractor. **B,** The extent of removal of bone structures is indicated (shaded areas). **C,** Parasellar extensions of pituitary adenomas (coronal sections) are shown: *a,* intrasellar adenoma; *b,* displacement of the cavernous sinus; *c,* focal invasion of the cavernous sinus; *d,* diffuse invasion of the cavernous sinus by the adenoma. **D,** Extensions of a pituitary adenoma (sagittal sections): *e,* suprasellar extension; *f,* invasion of the sphenoid sinus and of the clivus. (Adapted from Honegger J, Buchfelder M, Fahlbusch R. Surgery for pituitary tumors. In: Sheaves R, Jenkins PJ, Wass JAH, eds. *Clinical Endocrinology Oncology.* Boston, MA: Blackwell Science; 1977.)

and MRI may be useful only after 1 year or longer, especially after resection of secretory tumors with measurable serum biomarkers.[33] Endonasal transsphenoidal endoscopy avoids use of a retractor or speculum, does not require nasal packing, and sometimes leads to a shorter operating time, allowing for reduced postoperative morbidity and a shorter hospital stay (Fig. 9-10). The advantages of the technique include a clear panoramic view of bony landmarks and the ability to access suprasellar and parasellar tumor extensions into the cavernous sinuses.[30] Disadvantages of this approach include the management of perioperative intrasellar bleeding and CSF leaks. Combining both techniques may allow the advantages of both approaches. **Indications for Transsphenoidal Surgery.** A pituitary mass that may or may not be compressing local vital structures should be evaluated for surgical resection (Table 9-3). Although surgical resection offers a rapid resolution of hormone hypersecretion and many of the resultant clinical features of functioning adenomas, indications for the procedure differ, depending on tumor type (see later). In general, patients who are intolerant or resistant to

medical therapy require surgery. Surgery is primarily indicated for patients with well-circumscribed GH-secreting adenomas, TSH-secreting adenomas, all ACTH-secreting tumors, and nonfunctioning macroadenomas that require surgery. Surgery may also be indicated when tissue histologic confirmation is required for diagnosing the nature of an enigmatic sellar mass. Progressive compressive features including visual field loss, compromised pituitary function, or other central nervous system functional change are indications for surgical debulking and sellar decompression. Hemorrhage into the encased bony sella turcica, usually occurring within a known or previously unknown adenoma, may require immediate surgical decompression. Urgent surgical decompression is required for acute pituitary hemorrhage, especially in patients who have developed sudden visual field compromise. Hypopituitarism due to increased portal vessel pressure may recover shortly after decompressive surgery.[34] When pituitary function after surgery was assessed in 234 patients, 52 patients developed new trophic hormone dysfunction, and 45 of 93 patients with preoperative evidence for hypopituitarism recovered

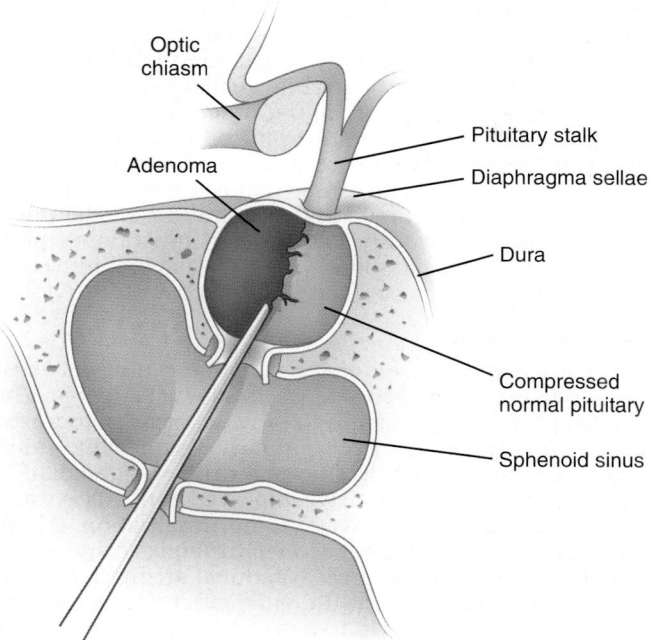

Figure 9-9 Transsphenoidal resection of pituitary adenoma.

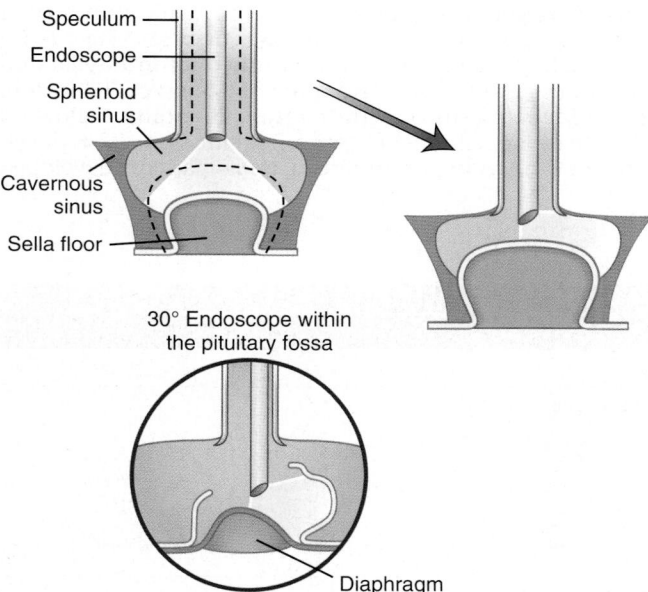

Figure 9-10 Endoscope-assisted microsurgery provides a panoramic view of the sphenoid sinus. Using a 30-degree endoscope, a view "around the corner" is possible. Parasellar structures can be visualized and residual tumor detected and resected. (From Fahlbush R, Buchfelder M, Kreutzer J, Nomikos P. Surgical management of acromegaly. In: Wass J, ed. *Handbook of Acromegaly*. Bristol, UK: BioScientifica; 2001.)

TABLE 9-3
Transsphenoidal Pituitary Surgery

Primary Indications

General
Visual tract or central nervous compression arising from within sella
Relief of compressive hypopituitarism by presenting, residual, or recurrent tumor tissue
Tumor recurrence after surgery or irradiation
Pituitary hemorrhage
Cerebrospinal fluid leak
Resistance to medical therapy
Intolerance of medical therapy
Personal choice
Desire for immediate pregnancy with macroadenoma
Requirement for diagnostic tissue histology

Specific
Acromegaly
Cushing disease
Clinically nonfunctioning macroadenoma
Prolactinoma
Nelson syndrome
TSH-secreting adenoma

Side Effects

Transient
Diabetes insipidus
Cerebrospinal fluid leak and rhinorrhea
Inappropriate ADH secretion
Arachnoiditis
Meningitis
Postoperative psychosis
Local hematoma
Arterial wall damage
Epistaxis
Local abscess
Pulmonary embolism
Narcolepsy

Permanent (up to 10%)
Diabetes insipidus
Total or partial hypopituitarism
Visual loss
Inappropriate ADH secretion
Vascular occlusion
CNS damage—oculomotor palsy, hemiparesis, encephalopathy
Nasal septum perforation

Surgery-Related Mortality (up to 1%)

Brain, hypothalamic injury
Vascular damage
Postoperative meningitis
Cerebrospinal fluid leak
Pneumocephalus
Acute cardiopulmonary disease
Anesthesia-related
Seizure

ADH, antidiuretic hormone; CNS, central nervous system; TSH, thyroid-stimulating hormone.

between one and three previously suppressed axes. Significant factors determining restoration of postoperative pituitary function were no visible tumor remnants as assessed by MRI and no tumor invasion as determined both by the neurosurgeon as well as by pathologic examination of surrounding tissue.[35] Therefore, as some patients with preoperative pituitary failure recover function, depending on the clinical circumstance, patients should be considered for retesting of pituitary reserve prior to initiating

postoperative substitution therapy, except for adrenal steroid replacement, which requires greater caution. Indications for second surgery in the same patient include tumor recurrence, persistent hormonal hypersecretion by tumor remnants, and repair of a CSF leak.

After surgery, patients should be kept at bedrest at an angle of 30 to 45 degrees, and urine and serum osmolality and serum electrolytes are measured every 6 hours. Indications for postoperative vasopressin replacement include polyuria, especially with elevated serum sodium and osmolality and inappropriately low urine osmolality. Postoperative polyuria alone is not an indication for vasopressin replacement, unless it is a reflection of compromised posterior pituitary function. Excess fluid given intraoperatively may also result in postoperative polyuria. Requirements for fluid replacement should take into consideration both fluid intake and urine output.

Side Effects. The success of surgery is largely determined by the skill and experience of the neurosurgeon. Higher volume pituitary centers and experienced surgeons report superior postoperative outcomes and shorter hospital stays.[36,37] Tumor size, degree of invasiveness, preoperative hormone levels, or previous pituitary surgery are all determinants of surgical outcome.[38] Overall, the most significant predictors of postoperative recurrence of hormone-secreting tumors is the postoperative basal hormone level.[39,40] CSF leakage, transient diabetes insipidus, and inappropriate ADH secretion are the most commonly encountered transient side effects, occurring in up to 20% of patients (see Table 9-3). Local damage may also result in arachnoiditis, vascular bleeding, hematoma formation, and epistaxis. Rarely, pulmonary embolism, narcolepsy, and local abscess have been reported. Iatrogenic hypopituitarism, diabetes insipidus, or syndrome of inappropriate antidiuretic hormone secretion (SIADH) is reported in up to 10% of patients. Rarely, the central nervous system may be permanently damaged with hemiparesis, cranial nerve palsies, or encephalopathy.

Three phases of postoperative diabetes insipidus have been described when the transient disorder is followed by an interphase on days 6 to 11 with no polydipsia or polyuria. During this second phase, hyponatremia with features of inappropriate ADH secretion have also been reported, even in patients with no signs and symptoms of diabetes insipidus after surgery.[41] The third phase is return of polyuria, polydipsia, and reduced ability to concentrate urine. Cognitive dysfunction, including anterograde memory deficits and executive function, has been reported

in several retrospective studies after transsphenoidal surgery.[42] Fatality has been reported in up to 1% of patients undergoing pituitary surgery and may be related to direct hypothalamic or cerebrovascular damage, meningitis, pneumocephalus formation, or anesthetic complications. Surgical failure may result from a non–pituitary-related event including anesthesia-related complication or bleeding disorder. Incomplete tumor removal may also be due to inaccurate preoperative MRI localization or identification. Rarely, a previously undiagnosed functioning pituitary tumor or ectopic source of ACTH may be unmasked after initially unsuccessful pituitary surgery.

Pituitary Radiation

Principles. High energy ionizing radiation can be delivered to deep tissues by megavoltage techniques (Table 9-4). The challenge of this approach is to provide maximal localized necrotizing radiation to the pituitary lesion while minimally exposing surrounding normal structures to radiation damage. Several advances have improved both efficacy and safety, including highly precise tumor localization, a high voltage (6 to 15 MeV) linear accelerator, and accurate simulation models with isocentric rotational arcing that allow repeat head positioning at the same exact points for each recurrent patient visit. Up to a maximum of 5000 rads are administered as 180-rad daily fractions for about 5 to 6 weeks. High-precision techniques such as stereotactic confocal radiotherapy, gamma knife using focused cobalt-60 emissions, and proton beam allow delivery of high energy directly targeting the pituitary lesion, while minimizing radiation exposure to surrounding tissues[43] (Fig. 9-11). Gamma knife radiosurgery is best suited for intrasellar and cavernous lesions distant from the optic nerves (Table 9-5). In a long-term study with a mean 96-month follow-up of 76 patients, about half were in remission, 23% developed new-onset hypopituitarism, and 3 patients developed

---

TABLE 9-4
Pituitary Irradiation

Indications
Pituitary adenoma—acromegaly, Cushing disease, nonfunctioning adenoma, prolactinoma
Craniopharyngioma
Nelson syndrome
Nonadenomatous invasive sellar mass
Tumor recurrence
Hormone hypersecretion recurrence

Side Effects
Hypopituitarism—deficient growth hormone, gonadotropin, TSH, and ACTH reserve
Eye—visual loss, optic neuritis
Brain—brain necrosis, temporal lobe deficits, cognitive dysfunction

Relative Risk of Second Brain Tumor					
Second Tumor	**Observed Incidence**	**Expected Incidence**	**SIR**	**95% CI**	**References**
Astrocytoma (2) Meningioma (1) Meningeal sarcoma (1)	5	0.53	9.43	3.05-21.98	Brada et al, 1992
Gliomas	4	0.25	16	4.4-41	Tsang et al, 1993
Astrocytoma (2) Meningioma (1)	3	1.13	2.7	0.55-7.76	Erfurth et al, 2001*
Meta-analysis	12	1.96	6.1	3.16-10.69	

*Excludes patients with acromegaly.
ACTH, adrenocorticotropic hormone; CI, confidence interval; SIR, standardized incidence ratio for person-years at risk; TSH, thyroid-stimulating hormone.
Adapted from Erfurth EM, Bulow B, Mikoczy Z, et al. Incidence of a second tumor in hypopituitary patients operated for pituitary tumors. *J Clin Endocrinol Metab.* 2001;86:659-662; Brada M, Ford D, Ashley S, et al. Risk of second brain tumour after conservative surgery and radiotherapy for pituitary adenoma. *BMJ.* 1992;304:1343-1346; Tsang RW, Laperriere NJ, Simpson WJ, et al. Glioma arising after radiation therapy for pituitary adenoma. A report of four patients and estimation of risk. *Cancer.* 1993;72:2227-2233.

oculomotor palsies.[44] Whether or not stereotactic radiosurgery exhibits superior long-term efficacy or safety over fractionated treatments remains unresolved.[45]

Indications. The use of radiation for treating pituitary tumors is highly individualized, and depends on the expertise of the treating center, conviction of the treating physician in weighing the potential benefits and risks of the procedure, and patient preference based upon informed choice (see Table 9-5).[46] In general, radiation techniques are indicated for persistent hormone hypersecretion or residual mass effects after surgery or when surgery of a compressive mass is contraindicated. As GH-secreting and PRL-secreting tumors are generally amenable to medical therapy, indications for their irradiation are rare. Most indications for radiation are adjuvant to either surgical or medical treatment. Radiation may be indicated after resection of a potentially recurring or inadequately resected pituitary mass, such as nonfunctioning pituitary adenoma, craniopharyngioma, or chordoma. In acromegaly, use of radiation as primary treatment is generally not recommended and is usually reserved as adjuvant to surgery or medical treatments,[47] but for aggressively growing prolactinomas that are resistant to medical therapy, the procedure may prevent further local invasion. Recurrent pituitary-dependent Cushing disease appears to be particularly suited for radiation, especially in younger patients.

Side Effects

Hypopituitarism. Pituitary failure occurs commonly in patients who have received pituitary irradiation (Table 9-6). Within 10 years after radiation, up to 80% of patients may have gonadotroph, somatotroph, thyrotroph, or corticotroph deficits.[44] The mechanism for hypopituitarism appears to involve damage to hypothalamic hormone–releasing cells as well as direct pituitary damage. These patients require lifelong endocrine follow-up for pituitary reserve testing and hormone replacement when appropriate.

Second Brain Tumors. Glioma has been reported after conventional pituitary radiation for adenomas and craniopharyngioma with a mean latency period of 11.5 years[48] (see Table 9-4). In patients irradiated for pituitary tumors, it appears that the standardized incidence ratio (SIR) for second brain tumors is approximately 6 (confidence interval 3.16-10.69), with a latency of 6 to 24 years in separate

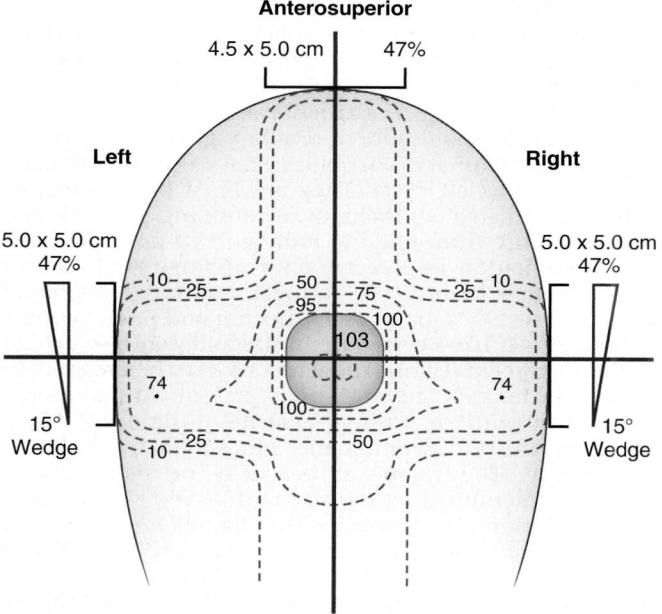

Figure 9-11 Pituitary radiotherapy. An 8-mV x-ray isodosimetric plan is used. The three fields restrict high-dose volume to the target. Numbered areas reflect radiation exposure. (Redrawn from Plowman PN. Pituitary radiotherapy: techniques and potential complications. In: Sheaves R, Jenkins PJ, Wass JAH, eds. *Clinical Endocrinology Oncology.* Boston, MA: Blackwell Science, 1997:185-188.)

TABLE 9-5

Effects of Gamma Knife Stereotactic Radiosurgery in Patients with Secreting Pituitary Adenomas

Study*	Number of Patients	Marginal Dose (Gy)	Mean Follow-up (months)	Remission Rate[†] (%)	Time to Remission (months)	Predictive Factors of Remission	Rate of Hypopituitarism (%)
Acromegaly							
Castinetti et al[44] (2009)[‡]	43	26	96	42	50	Initial hormone levels	21
Ronchi et al[393] (2009)	35	20	114	43	144	Initial hormone levels	8.5
Jagannathan et al (2008)	95	22	57	53	29.8	SSA	34
Losa et al[392] (2008)	83	21.5	69	60	NA	Initial hormone levels	8.5
Vik-Mo et al (2007)	53	26.5	66	17	NA	None	18
Pollack et al (2007)	46	20	63	50	36	Initial hormone levels, SSA	33
Jezkova et al (2006)	96	32	54	50	NA	Initial hormone levels	27
Cushing Disease							
Castinetti et al (2009)[‡]	18	28.5	96	46	24	Initial hormone levels	28
Jagannathan et al (2007)	90	23	42	53	13	Tumor volume	22
Kobayashi et al (2002)	20	40	60	35	NA	NA	NA
Hoybye et al (2001)	18	NA	204	83	NA	NA	66
Prolactinomas							
Castinetti et al (2009)[‡]	15	26	86	43	28	Initial hormone levels	13.3
Jezkova et al (2008)	35	34	75	37	96	None	14.3
Pouratian et al (2006)	23	18.6	58	26	24.5	Use of dopamine agonists at time of surgery, tumor volume	29

*Studies with >15 patients and follow-up >48 months, except for Jagannathan et al.
[†]Remission after withdrawal of somatostatin analogues.
[‡]Only patients with a follow-up >60 months were reported in this study.
NA, not available; SSA, withdrawal of somatostatin agonists at the time of gamma knife radiosurgery considered as a predictive factor of remission.
From Castinetti F, Regis J, Dufour H, Brue T. Role of stereotactic radiosurgery in the management of pituitary adenomas. *Nat Rev Endocrinol.* 2010;6:214-223.

cohorts.[49-51] As patients harboring pituitary tumors are more likely to undergo routine brain imaging during follow-up, it is not entirely clear whether observed meningiomas are coincidental findings. Because this complication, which occurs in fewer than 5% of patients, also appears to be dose related, fractionated doses not exceeding 5000 rads should be given. Use of confocal radiation techniques to irradiate a smaller tissue volume, including radiosurgery, fractionated stereotactic radiotherapy, and proton beam, may minimize this adverse effect, but prospectively controlled surveillance studies are required to rigorously evaluate this critical question.

Cerebrovascular Disease. Mortality rate from cerebrovascular disease appears higher in previously irradiated pituitary-deficient patients.[52,53] The direct causality of this relationship is as yet unclear, but direct effects on cerebral vasculature, including atherosclerotic occlusive lesions, have been reported.[54]

Visual Damage. The risk of visual damage (and very rarely blindness) is minimized by fractionating dosages to less than 200 rads per treatment session for conventional radiotherapy. The incidence of reported new visual damage in patients undergoing radiosurgery is approximately 4%.[55]

Brain Necrosis. Dose-related radiation-induced brain necrosis was documented by MRI in 14 of 45 patients, with temporal lobe atrophy and cystic and diffuse cerebral atrophy reported. Cognitive dysfunction, especially memory loss, has also been reported.[56]

Medical Management

Pituitary tumors often express receptors mediating hypothalamic control of hormone secretion, and appropriate therapeutic ligands for dopamine D_2 receptor and the somatotropin release–inhibiting factor (SRIF) receptor subtype 2 (SSTR2) are employed to effectively suppress PRL, GH, and TSH hypersecretion; to block tumor growth; and often to shrink tumor size. Medical ablation of target gland function, including thyroid and adrenal, may also be useful in mitigating the deleterious impact of pituitary tumor trophic hormone hypersecretion. Thus, peripheral antagonists block GH or cortisol action without targeting the respective pituitary tumor source. These medical approaches are considered later in this chapter.

PARASELLAR MASSES

Hypothalamic masses are described in Chapter 7, and causes of parasellar masses are depicted in Table 9-7.

Types of Parasellar Masses

Rathke's Cyst

The anterior and intermediate lobes of the pituitary gland arise embryologically from Rathke's pouch. Inadequate pouch obliteration results in cysts or cystic remnants at the interface between the anterior and posterior pituitary lobes found in about 20% of pituitary glands at autopsy[57] (Fig. 9-12). Pituitary adenomas may also occasionally contain small cleft cysts. They are lined by cuboidal or columnar ciliated epithelium surrounding mucoid cyst fluid and arise from midline rudiments of failed Rathke's cyst invagination and account for approximately 3% of pituitary mass lesions.[58] In contrast, pituitary epidermoid cysts are lined by squamous epithelium and rarely become malignant. Rathke's cysts vary in size and may also extend to the suprasellar region. These lesions have heterogeneous MRI characteristics and may rarely present with panhypopituitarism with or without diabetes insipidus.[59] Most, however, are not symptomatic and should be followed expectantly. The extent of headache or visual disturbance is determined by the size and location of the cyst. Cyst formation is associated with sellar enlargement. MRI reveals hyperdense or hypodense masses on either T1- or T2-weighted images, and CT scan shows homogeneous hypodense areas that may be distinguished from pituitary adenomas.[59] These patients should all be evaluated for hypopituitarism. After surgical resection or drainage, MRI should be performed during long-term follow-up for signs of cyst recurrence.[57,58]

Arachnoid, epidermoid, and dermoid cysts develop mainly in the cerebellopontine angle but may also arise in the suprasellar region. Dermoid cysts containing greasy sebaceous products or hair follicles are rarely encountered in the pituitary, and the cyst lining may be calcified.

TABLE 9-6
Complications After Stereotactic Radiosurgery

Complication	No. of Patients (%)
Patients w/ new cranial nerve (CN) dysfunction*	41 of 422 (9.3)
CN II	29 (6.6)
CN III	6 (1.36)
CN IV	1 (0.23)
CN V	4 (0.90)
CN VI	2 (0.45)
CN VII	1 (0.23)
Any new worsened hypopituitarism	92 of 435 (21.1)
Cortisol	29 of 293 (9.9)
Thyroid	40 of 246 (16.3)
Gonadotropin	24 of 288 (8.3)
Growth hormone	31 of 269 (8.4)
Diabetes insipidus	6 of 422 (1.4)
Further tumor growth	31 of 469 (6.6)
Further surgery or radiation therapy	34 of 444 (7.7)

*Forty-one patients had 43 deficits.

From Sheehan JP, Starke RM, Mathieu D, et al. Gamma Knife radiosurgery for the management of nonfunctioning pituitary adenomas: a multicenter study. *J Neurosurg.* 2013;119:446-456.

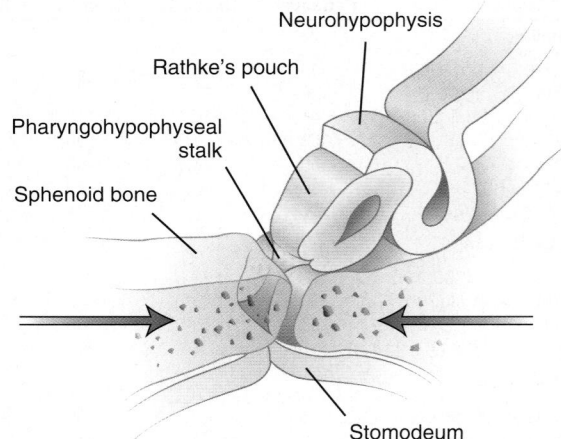

Figure 9-12 Pathogenesis of Rathke's cysts. Schematic of the embryologic progenitors of sellar and parasellar structures. Rathke's pouch arises from an outpocketing of stomodeum (ectoderm) and gives rise to the adenohypophysis. The pharyngohypophyseal stalk, which connects the stomodeum and Rathke's pouch, is divided by the sphenoid bone as it grows together (*arrows*), isolating Rathke's pouch and the neurohypophysis within the sella. (From Harrison MJ, Morgello S, Post KD. Epithelial cystic lesions of the sellular and parasellular region: a continuum of ectodermal derivates? *J Neurosurg.* 1994;80:1018-1025.)

TABLE 9-7

Results of Diagnostic Pituitary Magnetic Resonance Imaging of Parasellar Masses*

Diagnosis	Total	Diagnosis	Total
Anterior Pituitary Tumors		**Infectious**	
Prolactinoma	395	Pseudomonas aeruginosa	1
Nonfunctioning adenoma	364	Syphilis	1
GH adenoma	127	**Metastases**	
ACTH adenoma	84		
GH/prolactin mixed adenoma	4	Breast	3
Nelson syndrome	2	CNS lymphoma, to pituitary stalk	1
Pituitary carcinoma	2	Nasopharyngeal lymphoma	1
LH/FSH functioning adenoma	1	Liver epithelioid hemangioendothelioma	1
TSH adenoma	1	Lung, adenocarcinoma	1
GH/TSH mixed adenoma	1	Pineal germinoma/dysgerminoma	1
Cysts		Plasmacytoma	1
		Prostate, adenocarcinoma	1
Rathke cleft cyst	42	Sinusoidal squamous cell carcinoma	1
Craniopharyngioma	33	**Vascular**	
Arachnoid	2		
Epidermoid	1	Apoplexy with masses	16
Pineal cyst	1	Carotid aneurysm	4
Nonadenomatous Neoplasms		Hypothalamic cavernous angioma	1
		Hypothalamic interpeduncular hematoma	1
Meningioma	32	**Miscellaneous**	
Chordoma	3		
Pituitary lymphoma	2	Empty sella	21
Chondrosarcoma	1	Hyperplasia	14
Embryonal rhabdomyosarcoma	1	Ectopic pituitary gland	4
Germinoma	1	Fibrous dysplasia	3
Granular cell tumor	1	Lipoma	1
Hemangiopericytoma, malignant	1	**Hypothalamic**	
Leiomyosarcoma	1		
Mucoepidermoid carcinoma	1	Astrocytoma	2
Pituicytoma	1	Germinoma	1
Xanthogranuloma	1	Hamartoma	1
Inflammatory and Vasculitides		**Undiagnosed Masses**	159
Lymphocytic hypophysitis	3	**Normal Pituitary**	1242
Hypophysitis, unspecified type	2		
Lymphocytic infundibulitis	1		
Amyloidosis, primary	1		
Sarcoidosis	1		
Wegener granulomatosis	1		

*Diagnosis in 2598 patients undergoing pituitary magnetic resonance imaging.
ACTH, adrenocorticotropic hormone; CNS, central nervous system; FSH, follicle-stimulating hormone; GH, growth hormone; LH, luteinizing hormone; TSH, thyroid-stimulating hormone (thyrotropin).
Modified from Famini P, Maya MM, Melmed S. Pituitary magnetic resonance imaging for sellar and parasellar masses: ten-year experience in 2598 patients. *J Clin Endocrinol Metab.* 2011;96:1633-1641.

Acquired pituitary cysts may arise secondarily to intrapituitary hemorrhage, usually associated with an underlying adenoma, and these rarely cause pituitary failure. Cyst compression causes internal hydrocephalus, visual disturbances, GH or ACTH deficiency, hyperprolactinemia, and diabetes insipidus. Rarely squamous cell carcinoma may arise in the cyst.[60]

Granular Cell Tumors

Pituitary choristomas, or schwannomas, usually present only after the age of 20. Their abundant cytoplasmic granules do not contain pituitary hormones, but these lesions may present with diabetes insipidus. Pituitary adenomas are occasionally coincidentally associated with these tumors.[61]

Chordomas

These slow growing cartilaginous tumors arise from midline notochord remnants, are locally invasive, and may metastasize.[62] Most arise from the vertebrae and about one third involve the clivus region. Chordomas contain a mucin-rich matrix that allows diagnosis by fine-needle aspiration. They present with headaches, asymmetric visual disturbances, hormone deficiency, and occasional nasopharyngeal obstruction. The tumor mass is associated with osteolytic bony erosion and calcification, and MRI may allow the normal pituitary gland to be distinguished from the very heterogeneous and often flocculent tumor mass. At surgery, the tumors are rough, heterogeneous, and lobular. Markers for epithelial cells, including cytokeratin and vimentin, are present. Recurrences commonly occur after surgical excision, with mean patient survival time of about 5 years. Rarely, chordomas undergo sarcomatous transformation with an aggressive natural history and require extensive surgical dissection.[63] Because of their anatomic location, the endoscopic endonasal approach may be preferable for chordoma surgical resection.[64]

Craniopharyngiomas

This parasellar tumor constitutes about 3% of all intracranial tumors and up to 10% of childhood brain tumors.

The tumors are commonly diagnosed during childhood and adolescence.[65] However, they show a bimodal age distribution, occurring in children between 5 and 14 years old and adults from 50 to 74 years of age.[66] Tumors arise from embryonic squamous remnants of Rathke's pouch extending dorsally toward the diencephalon and may be large (>10 cm in diameter) and invade the third ventricle and associated brain structures. Over 60% arise from within the sella, and others arise from parasellar cell rests.[67,68] When intrasellar, they can often be distinguished from pituitary adenomas by separate visible rim of normal pituitary tissue seen on MRI (see Fig. 9-1A). The cystic mass is usually filled with cholesterol-rich viscous fluid, which may leak into the CSF, causing aseptic meningitis. They may also contain calcifications and immunoreactive human chorionic gonadotropin (hCG). Histologic appearance shows these tumors comprising two cell populations: cysts are lined with a squamous epithelium containing islands characterized by columnar cells, and a mixed inflammatory reaction may also occur with calcification. Adamantinomatous craniopharyngiomas have a greater propensity to relapse than the less aggressive papillary variant.[69] Although large craniopharyngiomas may obstruct CSF flow, they rarely undergo malignant transformation. Increased intracranial pressure results in headache, projectile vomiting, papilledema, and somnolence, especially in children. Only about one third of patients are over 40 years of age, and they commonly present with asymmetric visual disturbances, including papilledema, optic atrophy, and field deficits. If cavernous sinus invasion is present, other cranial nerves may also be involved. On CT imaging, most children and about half of all adults exhibit characteristic flocculent or convex calcifications. Rarely, however, pituitary adenomas, other parasellar tumors, and vascular lesions within the sella are also calcified. In contrast to pituitary adenomas, where it is rarely encountered, diabetes insipidus is often the earliest feature of craniopharyngioma. These patients may also develop partial or complete pituitary deficiency. GH deficiency with short stature, diabetes insipidus, and gonadal failure is common. Pituitary stalk compression or damage to hypothalamic dopaminergic neurons results in hyperprolactinemia. Thus, craniopharygioma may mimic a prolactinoma by intrapituitary imaging, presence of hyperprolactinemia, and favorable biochemical response to dopamine agonists.

Treatment of primary or recurrent craniopharyngiomas may involve radical surgery, radiotherapy, or a combination of these modalities.[66,68] A major side effect associated with such surgery is postoperative obesity, which can be mitigated by surgery that spares the hypothalamus.[70] The more complicated the surgical treatment, the more visual problems are encountered. Patients with diabetes insipidus have higher rates of anterior pituitary hormone deficits and subsequent obesity.[71] Treatment outcome appears to be related to hypothalamic involvement of the tumor, and hypothalamus-sparing surgery followed by local radiation therapy is recommended. Although survival rates are high (92%) recurrences and progressions are frequent.[65] Although transsphenoidal surgery has also been successfully employed for intrasellar craniopharyngiomas,[72] the expanded endoscopic transnasal approach has been successfully crafted to approach suprasellar tumors.[65] Stereotactic irradiation has also successfully been employed. Postoperative recurrence may occur in about 20% of patients undergoing radical surgical excision, but there are no compelling differences in outcome in those who undergo subtotal surgical excision followed by radiotherapy.

Life-complicating obesity that occurs after craniopharyngioma resection is associated with increased appetite (often insatiable), as well as altered food intake–regulating hormones leptin and ghrelin.[73] Preoperative treatment with glucagon-like peptide-1 (GLP-1) analogues led to weight loss in 5 of 8 patients.[74]

Meningiomas

Meningiomas arise from arachnoid and meningioendothelial cells, and those occurring in the sellar and parasellar region account for about one fifth of all meningiomas.[75] Sellar meningiomas are usually well circumscribed and do not attain the size of craniopharyngiomas. Suprasellar meningiomas may invade the pituitary ventrally, and intrasellar tumor origins are rare.[76] Coexisting functional pituitary adenomas have been described in patients with parasellar meningiomas. Secondary hyperprolactinemia occurs in up to half of these patients, who usually present with local mass effects including headache and progressive visual disturbances accompanied by optic atrophy. The differential distinction of a suprasellar meningioma with downward extension from an upwardly extending pituitary adenoma may be difficult. On MRI, meningiomas are isodense on both T1- and T2-weighted imaging, in contrast to other parasellar lesions, which are usually hyperdense on T2-weighted imaging. Dural calcification may be evident on CT scanning. Because of their rich vascularization, these tumors pose an intraoperative risk for hemorrhage and a resultant higher surgical mortality rate than is usually encountered for pituitary adenoma resection.

Gliomas

Optic gliomas and low-grade astrocytomas arise from within the optic chiasm or optic tract, they often infiltrate the optic nerve, and less than one third are intraorbital. Von Recklinghausen disease is the underlying cause in about one third of these patients, and occasionally these tumors may be associated with growth retardation and delayed or precocious puberty and mass effects including visual disturbances, diencephalic syndrome, diabetes insipidus, and hydrocephalus. Rarely, gliomas arise within the sella associated with hyperprolactinemia and should be considered in the uncommon differential diagnosis of a PRL-secreting pituitary adenoma.[77] Important distinguishing features include the young age of these patients (80% are <10 years old), relatively intact pituitary function, gross visual disturbances, and localization of the mass as visualized on MRI. Gliomas, unlike hamartomas, usually enhance after contrast injection.

Mucocele

Mucoceles are expanding accumulations of fluid within the sphenoid sinus and may compress parasellar structures. Headaches, visual disturbances (usually unilateral), and exophthalmos are characteristic features. On MRI, the homogeneous sphenoid mass may be quite prominent but may be distinguished from the pituitary gland dorsally.

Parasellar Aneurysms

A parasellar aneurysm may mimic a pituitary adenoma, and intraoperative rupture may be catastrophic, underlying the absolute need for preoperative diagnosis. Differentiating features of aneurysms from other pituitary masses may be subtle, including eye pain, very intense headaches, and relatively sudden onset of cranial nerve palsies (Fig. 9-13). Although imaging techniques usually distinguish blood and hemorrhage from solid tumor or tissue, a

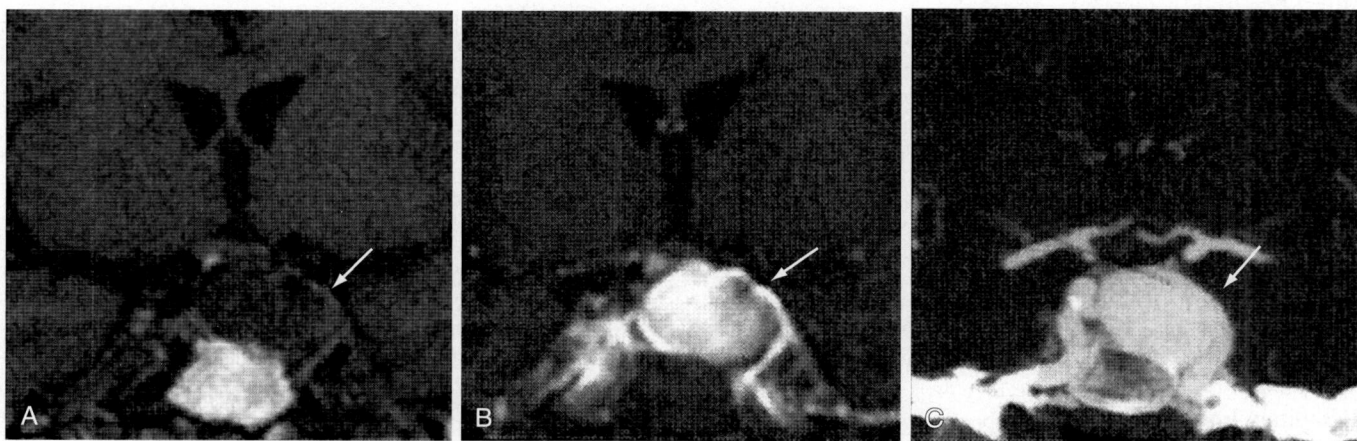

Figure 9-13 Left internal carotid artery giant cavernous aneurysm. **A,** Coronal T1-weighted magnetic resonance imaging (MRI) without intravenous contrast. A mildly hypointense mass is seen within the sella and left cavernous sinus. **B,** Coronal T1-weighted MRI after gadolinium contrast. The mass enhances heterogeneously. **C,** Computed tomography angiogram with maximum intensity projection reconstruction. The arrow in each image indicates the origin of a left internal carotid artery giant cavernous aneurysm. (From Lawson EA, Buchbinder BR, Daniels GH. Image in endocrinology: hypopituitarism associated with a giant aneurysm of the internal carotid artery. *J Clin Endocrinol Metab.* 2008;93:4616.)

highly vascular meningioma may be confused with an aneurysm.

Pituitary Infections

Acute pituitary abscesses, and perisellar arachnoiditis, are encountered with sinus infections, especially after transsphenoidal surgery. Pituitary abscess may develop from hematogenous or direct local spread of infectious agents or may arise within a preexisting pituitary adenoma and may be difficult to distinguish from an adenoma, as these patients may not have fever or signs of meningitis. They often present with diabetes insipidus and headache, and some have pituitary insufficiency.[78,79] On MRI, an isointense central cavity with surrounding ring enhancement is characteristic for an abscess.[4] In 33 consecutive patients with pituitary abscess, most presented with a mass associated with pituitary failure, and 5 had undergone previous surgery. Typical MRI features included a sellar cystic mass with an enhanced rim.[80] Gram-positive streptococci or staphylococci may originate from nasopharyngeal passages. Disseminated *Entamoeba histolytica*, *Pneumocystis jirovecii*, or *Klebsiella* may also seed to the pituitary.[81,82] Immunosuppressed patients may develop pituitary infections including cytomegalovirus, toxoplasmosis, aspergillosis, histoplasmosis, and coccidiosis. Syphilitic gumma may also lead to pituitary damage and insufficiency. Common viral infections, including influenza, measles, mumps, and herpes, are rarely associated with pituitary damage and insufficiency. Although tuberculosis is rarely confined to the pituitary gland, most of the fewer than 20 reported patients exhibited suprasellar extension of the pituitary mass, compromised pituitary function, and visual defects. Although systemic tuberculosis is usually present, isolated sellar tuberculomas have been described.[83]

Hematologic Malignancies

Primary central nervous system lymphomas are usually β-cell non-Hodgkin types, and fewer than 20 such patients with pituitary lymphoma have been described.[84-86] The pituitary mass may be an isolated presentation of the underlying disease. The disorder is usually diagnosed by histologic finding of tissue obtained by excision biopsy. Six

of nine patients had headache, and five had cranial nerve abnormalities with varying degrees of hypopituitarism. MRI reveals cavernous sinus invasion and isotense T1- and T2-weighted images, which enhance after gadolinium. Patients with solitary pituitary plasmacytomas have been reported who may or may not develop classical multiple myeloma. Acute lymphoblastic leukemia may be associated with periglandular pituitary infiltrates with minimal pituitary dysfunction.

Pituicytoma

Pituicytoma is a rare benign suprasellar glial cell tumor that presents with mass effects or hypopituitarism.[87] The tumor arises from cells in the neurohypophysis and stains for vimentin, S100 protein, and glial fibrillar acidic protein.[88]

Sarcoidosis

Hypothalamic granulomatous involvement is commonly encountered in patients with central nervous system sarcoidosis and may be the sole manifestation of the disease.[89] The hypothalamus, pituitary stalk, and posterior pituitary are diffusely invaded by noncaseating granulomas, consisting of giant cells, macrophages, and lymphocytes. These patients may present with varying degrees of anterior pituitary failure with or without diabetes insipidus.[90] Onset of diabetes insipidus with no obvious features of a pituitary disorder should alert the physician to exclude hypothalamic sarcoid deposits especially in the face of a thickened stalk on MRI.[91] In 24 patients with hypothalamic-pituitary sarcoid, all but 2 had anterior pituitary dysfunction (gonadotropin deficiency 21/24, TSH deficiency 15/24, and hyperprolactinemia in 12/24 cases), and 12 had diabetes insipidus. Imaging studies showed pituitary stalk thickness and involvement of the infundibulum and pituitary gland, which improved or disappeared in 50% of patients. After steroid treatment, 2 patients experienced reversal of hypopituitarism.[92]

Langerhans Cell Histiocytosis

The disorder may be associated with granulomatous damage to the hypothalamus and/or posterior pituitary, with characteristic diabetes insipidus occurring in about 25% of children with this disorder.[93] Sleep disorders, adipsia, morbid obesity axillary skin rash, history of recurrent pneumothorax, and classic bony lesions can occur.[94] Pituitary lesions comprise dendritic Langerhans cells, and pituitary MRI may reveal stalk thickening or a diminished posterior pituitary bright spot. Adults with the disorder should be carefully evaluated for anterior pituitary hormone deficits and appropriately replaced. Multisystem Langerhans cell histiocytosis causes long-term morbidity extending into adulthood.[95] Although surgery and radiation were, for many years, the mainstay treatments, a chemotherapeutic approach using cladripine has been successful in some patients.[96]

Hereditary Iron Storage Diseases

Hemochromatosis and hemosiderosis result in predominantly gonadotroph cell damage.

Idiopathic Retroperitoneal Fibrosis

Idiopathic retroperitoneal fibrosis may also be associated with a suprasellar mass and hypothalamic panhypopituitarism.[97]

Metastases to the Pituitary Region

Pituitary metastases are found in up to 3.5% of cancer patients,[98] especially in older patients with diffuse malignant disease. As the vascular supply to the posterior pituitary is derived directly from the systemic circulation via the internal carotid arteries, the posterior pituitary is the preferred site for bloodborne metastatic spread.[99] Over one third of carcinomas that metastasize to the pituitary are breast metastases (37.2% of 425 reported cases), followed by lung (24.2%), prostate (5.2%), renal (4.9%), and 28 other sites.[100] Diabetes insipidus is a common presenting sign and cranial nerve palsies and hypopituitarism may occur as well.[101] If extensive bony erosion is present and disease onset is rapid, the diagnosis is more readily apparent. However, pituitary imaging may not clearly distinguish metastatic deposits from a pituitary adenoma, and these lesions may masquerade as an adenoma, and the diagnosis only made by histologic study of the resected specimen.[102] When the diagnosis is clear cut in the presence of a primary cancer, relatively low-dose pituitary radiation may be sufficient to shrink the metastasis and improve morbidity.

Evaluation of Parasellar Lesions

Because the differential diagnosis of parasellar lesions covers a wide spectrum of neoplastic, vascular, inflammatory, and infectious processes, patient age and sex, relevant clinical history and symptoms, and other comorbid conditions can often help narrow down the differential diagnosis. MRI with gadolinium is essential in defining the exact location of the lesion, the gadolinium enhancement pattern, the presence of vascular voids or cystic regions, and associated vasogenic edema in surrounding brain tissue. Other imaging studies are often used in select cases: CT scan identifies calcification in craniopharyngiomas; CT angiogram, MR angiogram, or other angiography may be used when vascular lesions are suspected; and positron emission tomography may occasionally be used to identify metabolically active and rapidly growing lesions.

In a subset of lesions, serum molecular markers may be helpful in the diagnostic workup. For example,

nongerminomatous germ cell tumors, which often localize to the suprasellar space, can be diagnosed by elevation of characteristic tumor markers, including β-hCG or α-fetoprotein (AFP). Furthermore, if the lesion is suspected to cause pituitary or hypothalamic dysfunction, pituitary function testing is useful in characterizing potential endocrine dysfunction. As parasellar lesions often impinge on the optic apparatus, due to their anatomic proximity, neuro-ophthalmologic evaluation, including Humphrey visual fields test, is required. The decision to resect a parasellar lesion depends on factors related to the patient (age, neurologic status, medical comorbid conditions) and the lesion itself (size, anatomic location, vascular pattern, benign or malignant growth pattern, sensitivity to radiotherapy or chemotherapy, sensitivity to medical therapy).

If resection is pursued, a number of surgical approaches can be used, including craniotomies (pterional, supraorbital, subfrontal), as well as endoscopic transnasal approaches. Minimally invasive transnasal endoscopy is useful for resection of select parasellar lesions, with excellent surgical outcomes and potentially fewer complications than those observed after conventional craniotomy.[28]

Primary Hypophysitis

Pituitary mass lesions composed of inflammatory cells may arise as primary disorders of the anterior and posterior pituitary glands or the neurohypophysis.[103,104] At least five clinicopathologic forms have been described.

Lymphocytic Hypophysitis

This apparently autoimmune inflammatory disorder occurs during or shortly after parturition[105] but has also been reported after menopause,[104] and approximately 15% of reported cases occur in males.[106] Of the 57% of patients developing the disorder in association with pregnancy, most often the disorder occurs during the last month of pregnancy or during the first 2 months post partum.[104] It is characterized by a lymphocytic and plasma cell pituitary infiltrate, which may be isolated or associated with other recognized endocrinopathies. Circulating antipituitary antibodies have occasionally been reported, and the presence of isolated pituitary hormone deficiency may imply a selectively targeted autoimmune process to pituitary cell types. Although the natural history is often short-lived, the few comprehensive pathologic evaluations suggest that secondary adenohypophyseal cell atrophy, with a resultant empty sella, is a frequent outcome. Pathologic criteria for diagnosis include islands of anterior pituitary cells surrounded by diffuse lymphocytic (T and B cell) infiltrates. The defining feature is lymphocytic infiltration comprising T and B lymphocytes; plasma cells were found in 53%, eosinophils in 12%, and macrophage histiocytes and neurophils in 6% of cases,[104] and mast cells have also been identified.

Clinical Features. Over half the patients with lymphocytic hypophysitis present with headache, visual field impairment, and hyperprolactinemia,[104] and pituitary deficiency accounts for the remaining cases. Fifty-six percent of patients have secondary hypoadrenalism, followed in frequency by hypothyroidism, hypogonadism, and GH or PRL deficiency. Hypothyroidsim may occur later, even after 9 months. MRI reveals a pituitary mass, often indistinguishable from an adenoma. Both intrasellar and suprasellar pituitary enlargement occur, and the pituitary stalk may be thickened, especially when diabetes insipidus is present.[103] The inflammatory process often resolves with time, and initially abnormal pituitary function may be restored as well or may remain chronically compromised. Diabetes insipidus, which is encountered in up to 20% of patients, has been attributed to posterior pituitary or stalk infiltration of the inflammatory process.[107] In a study of 95 patients with autoimmune hypopituitarism and positive antipituitary antibodies, those with central diabetes insipidus had antihypothalamic antibodies, suggesting autoimmune involvement of the hypothalamus rather than expansion of the pituitary inflammatory process.[108] In one third of patients, other autoimmune conditions, including thyroiditis, hypoadrenalism, parathyroid failure, atrophic gastritis, systemic lupus erythematosus, or Sjögren syndrome, are also present.[109] The differential diagnosis includes prolactinoma and other sellar masses, and careful history and demonstrated loss of the posterior pituitary "bright spot" on MRI are useful for supporting the diagnosis.

Laboratory Findings. The erythrocyte sedimentation rate is often elevated; antibodies to a 49-kDa cytosolic protein were detected in 70% of patients with histologically confirmed lymphoytic hypophysitis and in 10% of control subjects.[110] PRL levels are usually elevated in both female and male patients. Hyperprolactinemia is expected during pregnancy and during the early postpartum period, and the mass effect may contribute to stalk compression and secondary hyperprolactinemia in the others. GH and ACTH responses to hypothalamic hormone challenges may be blunted. Rarely, the disorder may be associated with isolated ACTH or TSH deficiencies.

Treatment. If the diagnosis is convincingly supported, then in the absence of compressive visual field disturbances, surgical therapy should be withheld, pituitary hormone deficits appropriately replaced, and spontaneous resolution of the inflammatory mass expectantly followed. Treatment with adrenal steroids is mainstay, often resolving the sellar mass and improving endocrine dysfunction. Steroids are also indicated if adrenal reserve is compromised. Transsphenoidal or endoscopic surgical resection may be required to confirm a tissue diagnosis and may also relieve compression symptoms,[111] but the degree of surgical resection should be constrained by the need to conserve viable pituitary tissue, particularly in view of frequent spontaneous resolution.

Granulomatous Hypophysitis

Granulomatous hypophysitis is not usually associated with pregnancy, but in a systematic review comprising 82 patients, females predominated.[112] Rarely, the condition may coexist with lymphocytic hypophysitis in the same gland.[111] Pituitary histologic appearance shows features of chronic inflammation and granuloma with histiocytes and multinucleated giant cells. Patients present with headache and may have aseptic meningitis. Fever, nausea, or vomiting at presentation and histologic evidence of necrosis correlate with reduced time to presentation. Panhypopituitarism at presentation is predictive of the requirement for long-term replacement therapy.[112] MRI shows pituitary enlargement. Suprasellar extension occurs in about 60% of patients, often with extension to or compression of the optic chiasm (25.7%). The condition may reflect an underlying systemic disorder such as sarcoidosis[113] or Takayasu disease.[114]

Xanthomatous Hypohysitis

This rare primary pituitary inflammatory process occurs at equal frequency in both sexes and comprises lipid-laden macrophages. MRI often reveals a highly cystic lesion,

possibly reflecting an inflammatory response to a ruptured pituitary cyst.

Necrotizing Infundibulo-Hypophysitis

This rare form of hypophysitis has been reported in patients with an enlarged sellar mass. They present with diabetes insipidus and hypopituitarism, and severe headache may occur[115] (Fig. 9-14).

Ipilimumab-Induced Hypophysitis

This form of hypophysitis is caused by exposure to an antibody, ipilimumab, used to treat metastatic cancer. The drug blocks the cytotoxic T-lymphocyte antigen 4 (CTLA4), which is also expressed on pituitary tissue[116] (Table 9-8). In a single-center analysis of 211 tested patients with advanced melanoma, an 8% overall incidence of hypophysitis was reported. Presenting symptoms include headache, nausea, vomiting, extreme fatigue, diarrhea, arthralgias, and mental status changes.[117] The median time to onset following drug administration was 4 months, but a delay in up to 19 months after treatment was also observed. The most common endocrine deficit encountered was secondary adrenal insufficiency (84%). In contrast to other forms of hypophysitis, no patients receiving ipilimumab developed diabetes insipidus.[118] Many also had evidence of hypothyroidism/thyroiditis (6%). Eleven of 19 patients had biochemical evidence consistent with central hypothyroidism (low free T_4 [thyroxine] and normal or low TSH). Pituitary MRIs were clearly abnormal in most patients with diffuse enlargement. Treatment with high-dose steroids initially, followed by replacement doses in those with sustained secondary adrenal insufficiency, is effective. However, few patients exhibit return of normal endocrine function.[119] Azathioprine has been found effective in some patients.[120]

Hemorrhage and Infarction

Intrapituitary hemorrhage and infarction are usually caused by ischemic damage to the hypophyseal-portal system and may be catastrophic. These acute events cause significant damage to the pituitary gland, and small clinically silent microinfarcts are found in up to 5% of unselected autopsies. Pituitary cells are relatively resilient to vascular insult,

TABLE 9-8

Features of Ipilimumab-Induced Hypophysitis

Measurement	Result
Incidence	10%
Ipilimumab dose	3 or 10 mg/kg
M:F ratio	2:1
Time until hypophysitis diagnosis	7-16 weeks
Anterior hypopituitarism	All affected patients
Central hypothyroidism	60-100%
Adrenal insufficiency	50-84%
Thyroiditis	Up to 25%
Hyponatremia	Up to 50 %
Prolactin	Usually low
Testosterone	Usually low

Adapted from retrospective analyses of 365 patients treated for melanoma in Faje AT, Sullivan R, Lawrence D, et al. Ipilimumab-induced hypophysitis: a detailed longitudinal analysis in a large cohort of patients with metastatic melanoma. *J Clin Endocrinol Metab.* 2014;99(11):4078-4085; and Ryder M, Callahan M, Postow MA, et al. Endocrine-related adverse events following ipilimumab in patients with advanced melanoma: a comprehensive retrospective review from a single institution. *Endocr Relat Cancer.* 2014;21:371-381.

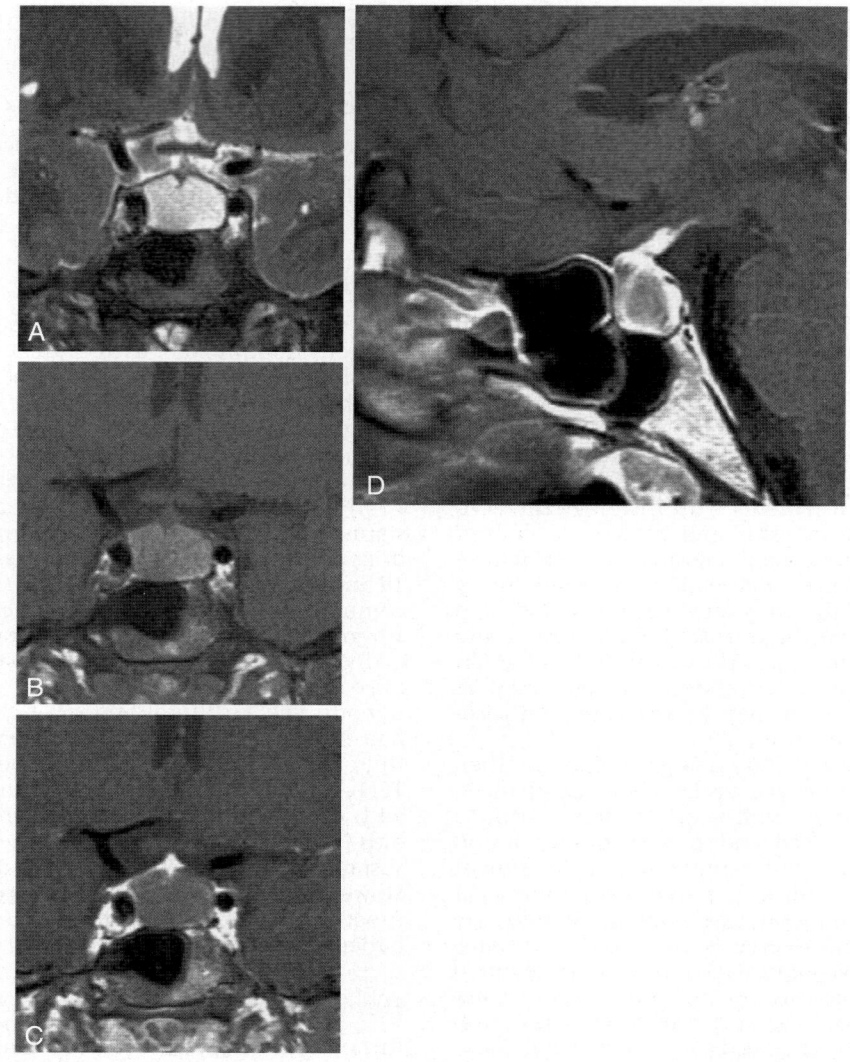

Figure 9-14 Infundibulo-hypophysitis depicted by preoperative magnetic resonance imaging. The 22 × 20 × 16-mm pituitary mass is iso- to hyperintense on T2-weighted image with suprasellar extension (**A**) and hypointense in T1-weighted, nonenhanced image (**B**). After intravenous contrast (**C**), only slight to moderate and inhomogeneous enhancement occurs, most pronounced at the periphery of the mass. The pituitary stalk and infundibulum are slightly thickened, showing avid enhancement (**D**). (From Gutenberg A, Caturegli P, Metz I, et al. Necrotizing infundibulo-hypophysitis: an entity too rare to be true? *Pituitary.* 2012;15:202-208.)

and pituitary insufficiency is only clinically apparent when approximately 75% of the gland is ischemically damaged. Ten percent residual functional pituitary cell mass appears sufficient to mask complete pituitary failure. Ischemic damage is limited to the anterior lobe, and posterior pituitary function usually remains intact, reflecting the predominant neural control of oxytocin and ADH secretion. Acute intrapituitary hemorrhage can cause significant life-threatening damage to the pituitary and its surrounding vital structures.[13]

Postpartum Pituitary Infarction

During pregnancy, the pituitary gland normally enlarges in response to estrogen stimulation. The hypervascular gland is thus particularly vulnerable to arterial pressure changes and prone to hemorrhage. Sheehan syndrome classically described after severe postpartum hemorrhage is now less commonly encountered with the advent of modern obstetric care,[121] but it occurs much more frequently in developing countries.[122,123] The presentation varies from development of hypovolemic shock resulting

in adenohypophyseal vessel vasospasm and pituitary necrosis to the gradual onset of partial to complete pituitary insufficiency over months to years. Initial presentations also include hyponatremia, asthenia, and weight loss. Most prominent among symptoms are inability to nurse and postpartum amenorrhea.[122] Pituitary autoimmunity has been implicated in gland failure after postpartum hemorrhage.[124]

Pituitary Apoplexy

Pituitary apoplexy may result from spontaneous hemorrhage into a pituitary adenoma (pituitary tumor apoplexy) or may occur after head trauma, with skull base fracture, or in association with hypertension and diabetes mellitus, sickle cell anemia, or acute hypovolemic shock[125] (Table 9-9). Precipitating factors include major surgery, pregnancy, gamma knife irradiation, anticoagulant therapy, coagulopathy secondary to liver failure,[126] and administration of thyrotropin-releasing hormone (TRH), gonadotropin-releasing hormone (GnRH) agonists, bromocriptine, and cabergoline.[127,128]

TABLE 9-9
Features of Pituitary Apoplexy

Feature	Bills et al (1993)	Randeva et al (1999)	Lubina et al (2005)
No. patients	37	35	40
No. males/females	25/12	21/14	27/13
Mean age (yr)	56.6	49.8	51.2
No. not operated	1	4	6
Symptoms			
Headache (%)	95	97	63
Visual defects (%)	64	71	61
Ophthalmoplegia (%)	78	69	40
Adenoma Type			
NFPA (%)	52	61	63
PRL cell (%)	17	6.6	31
Visual fields improvement (%)		76	81
Ocular palsy improvement (%)		91	71
Hormone Deficiency			
Central hypocortisol (%)	82	58	40
Central hypothyroid (%)	89	45	54
Hypogonadism (%)	64	43	79
Diabetes insipidus (%)	11	6	8

NFPA, nonfunctioning pituitary adenoma; PRL, prolactin.
Data from Bills DC, Meyer FB, Laws ER Jr, et al. A retrospective analysis of pituitary apoplexy. *Neurosurgery*. 1993;33:602-608; discussion 608-609; Randeva HS, Schoebel J, Byrne J, et al. Classical pituitary apoplexy: clinical features, management and outcome. *Clin Endocrinol (Oxf)*. 1999;51(2):181-188; Lubina A, Olchovsky D, Berezin M, et al. Management of pituitary apoplexy: clinical experience with 40 patients. *Acta Neurochir (Wien)*. 2005;147:151-157; discussion 157.

Clinical Features. Pituitary apoplexy is often an endocrine emergency.[14] The condition may evolve over 1 to 2 days, usually presenting with severe headache and ocular palsies or visual field defects. Cardiovascular collapse, change in consciousness, neck stiffness, and sometimes hypoglycemia may occur. Bilateral cerebral infarction may also occur.[129] Acute adrenal insufficiency is a frequent occurrence due to loss of ACTH. It may also be superimposed owing to disordered intravascular clotting disorders, heparin administration, or acute effects of central nervous system hemorrhage. Pituitary imaging without contrast (CT or MRI) usually reveals signs of intrapituitary or intra-adenoma hemorrhage, stalk deviation, compression of normal pituitary tissue, and in severe cases, signs of parasellar hemorrhage.[130] In a study on 13 consecutive patients with pituitary apoplexy, baseline serum cortisol was below 5 µg/dL in 7, between 5 and 15 µg/dL in 4, and above 15 µg/dL in 2 patients. Five patients also had low T_4 levels, and all 13 had evidence of gonadal dysfunction. Thus, these patients with underlying pituitary tumors likely had preexisting pituitary insufficiency.[131] Apoplexy, like Sheehan syndrome, is one of the few pituitary tumor presentations in which hyperprolactinemia is not a feature unless the infarction occurs within a prolactinoma. Patient characteristics, signs and symptoms, and outcomes in 112 patients in three series are shown in Table 9-9.[14]

Management. Patients with visual field compromise require emergency transsphenoidal surgery. Others may recover spontaneously but may develop long-term pituitary insufficiency. Patients who are fully alert and conscious with no visual symptoms may be observed. The decision to initiate therapy with high-dose glucocorticoids depends on the clinical status,[13] but the high incidence of adrenal dysfunction either before or after treatment indicates a need for replacement or stress doses of cortisone in most. Ophthalmoplegia, which is common, may resolve spontaneously over time.[13] Postoperative recovery of visual function correlates inversely with the time elapsed subsequent to the acute hemorrhage.[132] Cranial nerve palsies, however, often improve whether or not surgery is undertaken. Pituitary function does not commonly recover after resolution of the acute hemorrhage, and adrenal, thyroid, and gonadal steroid hormone replacement may be required. The subsequent atrophy of infarcted pituitary tissue often results in the development of a complete or partially empty sella evident on MRI.

Pituitary Adenomas
Pathogenesis
Pituitary tumors account for about 15% of all intracranial neoplasms and are commonly encountered at autopsy.[133] The Brain Tumor Registry of Japan reports that 15.8% of 28,424 cases were histologically confirmed pituitary adenomas.[134] The prevalence of pituitary tumors in Belgium is 1 in 1064 inhabitants,[135] and in Banbury, U.K., 63 pituitary tumors were noted in 89,334 inhabitants, a population prevalence of approximately 77 cases per 100,000. Of these, 57% were prolactinomas, 28% were nonfunctioning adenomas, 11% were GH-secreting adenomas, and 2% were Cushing adenomas. The median age of onset was 37 years, but nonfunctioning tumors were most commonly encountered in patients older than 60 years.[136] Employing large and comprehensive population-based cancer registries, the annual pituitary tumor incidence rate in the United States was reported to increase from 2.52 per 100,000 population in 2004 to 3.13 in 2009.[137] Whether or not this increase is due to an inherent actual tumor increase or to enhanced reporting, awareness, and diagnosis is yet unclear. These benign monoclonal adenomas may express and secrete hormones autonomously, leading to hyperprolactinemia, acromegaly, Cushing disease, and hyperthyroidism, or they may be functionally silent and initially diagnosed as a sellar mass. Although almost invariably benign, the neoplastic features of these adenomas represent a unique tumor biology, which is reflected in their important local and systemic manifestations. These neoplasms have a slow doubling time, and rarely resolve spontaneously. Nevertheless, they can be aggressive and locally invasive or compressive to vital central structures. Two classifications, Hardy and Knosp, are used to characterize adenoma mass characteristics (Fig. 9-15). Pituitary adenomas usually express a single gene product, but polyhormonal expression may reflect a primitive stem cell or mature bimorphous cellular origin.

Pituitary Trophic Activity
Benign Adenomas. Several transgenic animal models have been described in which pituitary growth factors or genes have been overexpressed or deleted to recapitulate both functional and nonfunctional pituitary adenomas (Table 9-10). For example, a transgenic zebrafish expressing corticotroph-targeted pituitary tumor-transforming gene *(PTTG)* recapitulates a Cushing phenotype with pituitary adenoma growth and hypercortisolism.[138] Benign human monoclonal pituitary adenomas arise from differentiated pituitary cells (see Fig. 9-2). Pituitary trophic signals may enhance or restrain expansion of a monoclonal tumor cell population by regulating the intrapituitary milieu.[139,140]

Normal and hyperplastic pituitary tissues are polyclonal, and pituitary adenomas arise as the result of monoclonal pituitary cell proliferation. Using X-chromosomal inactivation analysis, the monoclonal origin of GH-, PRL-,[141] and

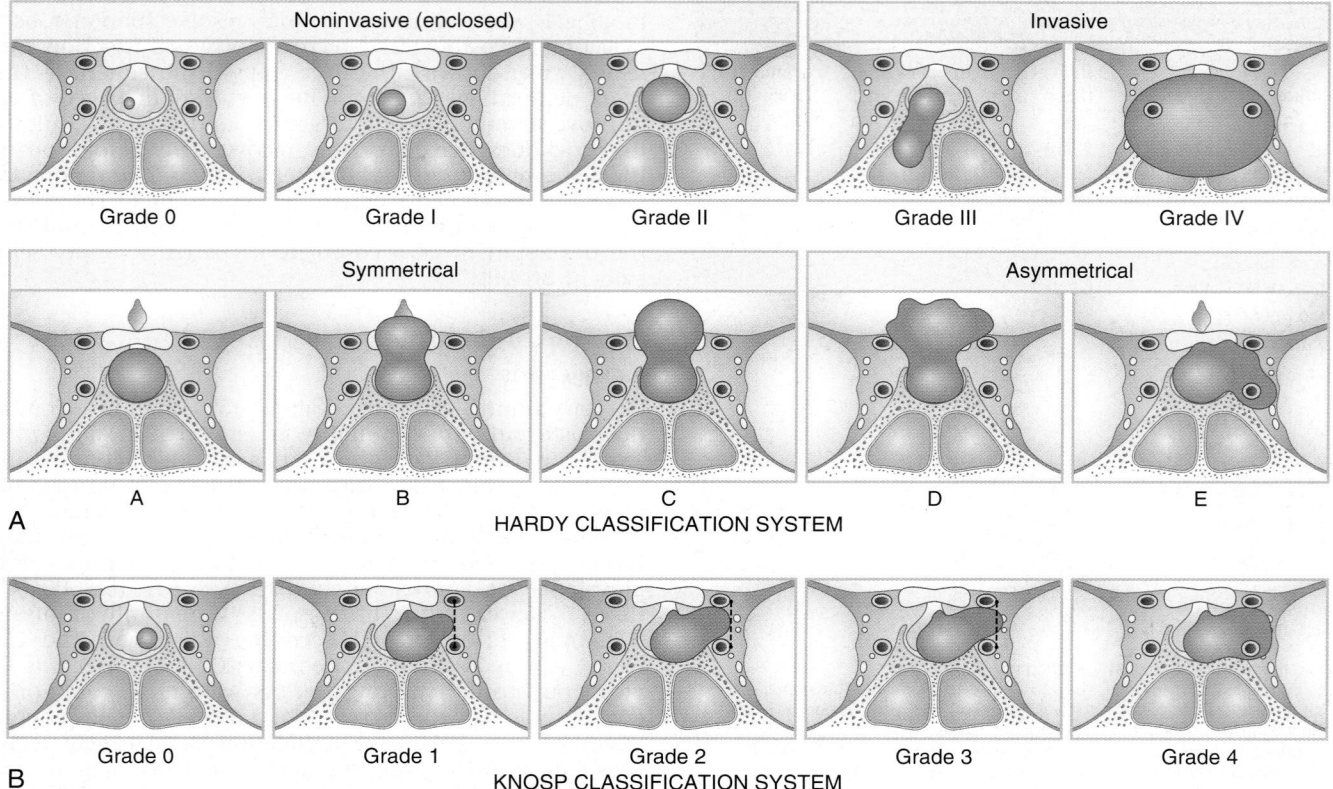

Figure 9-15 Classification systems characterizing pituitary adenomas. **A,** *Hardy classification system.* Sella turcica tumors can be noninvasive (grade 0, intact with normal contour; grade I, intact with bulging floor; or grade II, intact, enlarged fossa) or invasive (grade III, localized sellar destruction; or grade IV, diffuse destruction). Suprasellar tumors can be symmetrical (grade A, suprasellar cistern only; grade B, recess of the third ventricle; or grade C, whole anterior third ventricle) or asymmetrical (grade D, intracranial extradural; or grade E, extracranial extradural [cavernous sinus]). **B,** *Knosp classification system* used to quantify invasion of the cavernous sinus, in which only grades 3 and 4 define true invasion of the tumor into the cavernous sinus. Grade 0, no cavernous sinus involvement; grades 1 and 2, the tumor pushes into the medial wall of the cavernous sinus but does not go beyond a hypothetical line extending between the centers of the two segments of the internal carotid artery (grade 1) or it goes beyond such a line but without passing a line tangent to the lateral margins of the artery itself (grade 2); grade 3, the tumor extends laterally to the internal carotid artery within the cavernous sinus; grade 4, total encasement of the intracavernous carotid artery. (Modified from Di Ieva A, Rotondo F, Syro LV, et al. Aggressive pituitary adenomas: diagnosis and emerging treatments. *Nat Rev Endocrinol.* 2014;10:423-435, used with permission.)

ACTH-secreting adenomas[142,143] and nonfunctioning pituitary tumors was confirmed in female patients heterozygous for variant alleles of the X-linked genes hypoxanthine phosphoribosyl transferase *(HPRT)* and phosphoglycerate kinase *(PGK).* Thus, an intrinsic somatic pituitary cell genetic alteration likely gives rise to clonal expansion of a single cell, resulting in adenoma formation (Table 9-11).

The pituitary gland responds to central and peripheral signals that regulate both hormone production and cell proliferation ranging from microadenoma to aggressive adenoma (Fig. 9-16). For example, during pregnancy hypothalamic and peripheral hormones act to regulate pituitary trophic activity resulting in increased pituitary volume, and prolonged target gland failure (e.g., hypothyroidism) can cause pituitary hyperplasia by releasing the gland from negative feedback inhibition. There is, however, no compelling or direct evidence in humans that pituitary hyperplasia is a prerequisite for tumor development. Thus, lactotroph hyperplasia occurring with pregnancy and lactation does not lead to increased frequency of prolactinomas. Oral contraception use is also not associated with pituitary adenoma development, and somatotroph hyperplasia caused by ectopic GHRH production[144] is not commonly associated with true adenoma formation. Adenohypophyseal tissue surrounding pituitary tumors is usually not hyperplastic, supporting the notion that hypothalamic hormones, pituitary growth factors, and sex steroid hormones enable a permissive environment, which potentiates cell mutation and subsequent tumor growth.

Hormonal Factors. Hypothalamic factors may have a specific role in the pathogenesis of pituitary tumors, in addition to regulating pituitary hormone gene expression and secretion (see Table 9-11). Ectopic GHRH-secreting tumors (bronchial carcinoids, pancreatic islet cell tumors, or small cell lung carcinomas) result in GH hypersecretion and acromegaly with somatotroph hyperplasia.[144,145] In transgenic mice overexpressing a GHRH transgene, the pituitary size increases dramatically due to somatotroph hyperplasia, and older mice develop GH-secreting adenomas.[146] However, adenomatous hormonal secretion is usually independent of physiologic hypothalamic control, and the surgical resection of small well-defined adenomas usually results in definitive cure of hormonal hypersecretion. These observations imply that these tumors do not arise because of excessive polyclonal pituitary cell proliferation due to generalized hypothalamic stimulation. However, hypothalamic factors may promote and maintain growth of already transformed adenomatous pituitary cells (Fig. 9-17).

Genetic Factors. Activating mutations of the stimulatory G protein (G_s) are present in up to 40% of human GH-secreting

TABLE 9-10
Transgenic Mouse Models for Pituitary Tumors

Genes	Hyperplasia/Adenoma*
Gene Overexpression†	
CMV.HMGA1	GH, PRL
CMV.HMGA2	GH, PRL
Ubiquitin C.hCG	PRL
αGSU.bLH	Pit1 lineage
GH.galanin	GH, PRL
PRL.galanin	PRL‡
PRL.TGFα	PRL
αGSU.PTTG1	LH, GH, TSH
αGSU.Prop1	Nonfunctioning
PRL.pdt-FGFR4	PRL
Gene Inactivation	
p27/Kip1−/−	ACTH, αMSH
p18/INK4c−/−	ACTH, αMSH
Rb+/−	ACTH, αMSH
	αGSU, GH, βTSH
D2R-deficient	PRL
MEN1+/−	PRL
PRL−/−	Nonfunctioning

*Hormone immunoreactivity/secreting profile.
†Genes are listed in bold and are preceded by the promoter that determines transcriptional control.
‡Pituitary hyperplasia, with no tumor formation.
ACTH, adrenocorticotropic hormone; bLH, bovine active luteinizing hormone; CMV, cytomegalovirus; D2R, dopamine 2 receptor; GH, growth hormone; αGSU, glycoprotein α-subunit; hCG, human chorionic gonadotropin; HMGA, high mobility group A; pdt-FGFR4, pituitary tumor-derived fibroblast growth factor receptor 4; MEN1, multiple endocrine neoplasia type 1; MSH, melanocyte-stimulating hormone; p18/INK4c, cyclin-dependent kinase inhibitor 2C; p27/Kip1, cyclin-dependent kinase inhibitor 1B; PRL, prolactin; Prop1, prophet of Pit1 (paired-like homeodomain transcription factor); PTTG, pituitary tumor-transforming gene; Rb, retinoblastoma; TGF, transforming growth factor; TSH, thyroid-stimulating hormone.
Modified from Melmed S. Pathogenesis of pituitary tumors. *Nat Rev Endocrinol.* 2011;7:257-266.

TABLE 9-11
Factors Involved in Pituitary Tumor Pathogenesis

Hereditary

MEN1
Transcription factor defect (e.g., PROP1 excess)
Carney complex
AIP mutations

Hypothalamic

Excess GHRH or CRH production
Receptor activation
Dopamine deprivation

Pituitary

Signal transduction mutations or constitutive activation (e.g., GSP, CREB, McCune-Albright syndrome)
Disrupted paracrine growth factor or cytokine action (e.g., FGF2, FGF4, LIF, BMP, EGF)
Activated oncogene or cell cycle disruption (e.g., PTTG, RAS, P27, HMG)
Intrapituitary paracrine hypothalamic hormone action (e.g., GHRH, TRH)
Loss of tumor suppressor gene function with LOH (11q13, 13, GADD45γ)

Environmental

Estrogens
Irradiation

Peripheral

Target failure (ovary, thyroid, adrenal)
Ectopic hypothalamic hormone secretion

Evidence for an Intrinsic Pituitary Defect in the Pathogenesis of Pituitary Tumors

Pituitary adenomas are monoclonal.
There is no hyperplasia surrounding the adenomas.
Surgical resection of well-circumscribed small adenomas leads to control in ~75% of patients.
Unrestrained pituitary hormonal hypersecretion persists independently of feedback regulation by elevated target hormones.
Hormonal pulsatility pattern is often restored after adenoma resection.

AIP, aryl hydrocarbon receptor–interacting protein; BMP, bone morphogenetic protein; CREB, cyclic adenosine monophosphate response element–binding protein; CRH, corticotropin-releasing hormone; EGF, epidermal growth factor; FGF, fibroblast growth factor; GADD45γ, growth arrest and DNA damage–inducible gamma gene; GHRH, growth hormone–releasing hormone; GSP, stimulatory G protein α-subunit oncogene; HMG, high mobility group; LIF, leukemia inhibitory factor; LOH, loss of heterozygosity; MEN1, multiple endocrine neoplasia type 1; P27, cyclin-dependent kinase inhibitor 1B; PROP1, prophet of Pit1 (paired-like homeodomain transcription factor); PTTG, pituitary tumor-transforming gene; RAS, RAS family of oncogenes; TRH, thyrotropin-releasing hormone.
Modified from Melmed S. Acromegaly pathogenesis and treatment. *J Clin Invest.* 2009;119:3189-3202; and Melmed S. Pathogenesis of pituitary tumors. *Nat Rev Endocrinol.* 2011;7:257-266.

adenomas (Table 9-12). These somatic heterozygous activating point mutations of the G protein α-subunit (G$_s$α) gene involving either arginine 201 (replaced by cysteine or histidine) or glutamine 227 (replaced with arginine or leucine) constitutively activate the G$_s$α protein and convert it into an oncogene *(GSP)*. This G protein activation increases cyclic adenosine monophosphate (cAMP) levels; activates protein kinase A, which in turn phosphorylates the cAMP response element-binding protein (CREB); and leads to sustained constitutive GH hypersecretion and cell proliferation. *GSP*-bearing adenomas are smaller, have mildly lower GH levels and enhanced intratumoral cAMP, do not respond briskly to GHRH, and are sensitive to the inhibitory effect of somatostatin.[147] *GSP*-activating mutations do not occur in PRL-secreting and in TSH-producing adenomas and are very rarely present in nonfunctioning pituitary tumors or ACTH-secreting tumors (<10%). Similar early postzygotic somatic mutations in codon 201 of the G$_s$α were identified in tissues derived from patients with McCune-Albright syndrome.[148] Transgenic mice overexpressing an inactive pituitary CREB mutant exhibit a dwarf phenotype and somatotroph hypoplasia.[149] Thus, cAMP likely stimulates somatotroph proliferation mediated by CREB phosphorylation. This was borne out by the observation that 15 human GH-secreting pituitary adenomas were shown to express elevated levels of phosphorylated CREB.[150] However, only four of these tumors also contained the mutant *GSP* oncogene, and CREB phosphorylation was also demonstrated in adenomas overexpressing wild-type

G$_s$α protein, suggesting a trophic role of CREB, independent of G protein actions. Other signaling pathways overexpressed in pituitary tumors include those for AKT and mitogen-activated protein kinase (MAPK).[151]

Mice with heterozygous *Rb1* inactivation develop pituitary tumors with high penetrance, but mice with deregulated pituitary E2F activity develop tissue hyperplasia without progression to tumor formation, likely because sustained E2F activity ultimately triggers premature senescence in a pRB-, p16-, and p19-dependent fashion.[152] About 15% of spontaneous pituitary adenomas exhibit loss of heterozygosity (LOH) for chromosomes 11q13, 13, and 9, often correlating with tumor size and invasiveness. Although highly invasive pituitary tumors and pituitary metastases exhibit LOH of region 13q14 *(RB1* locus), no

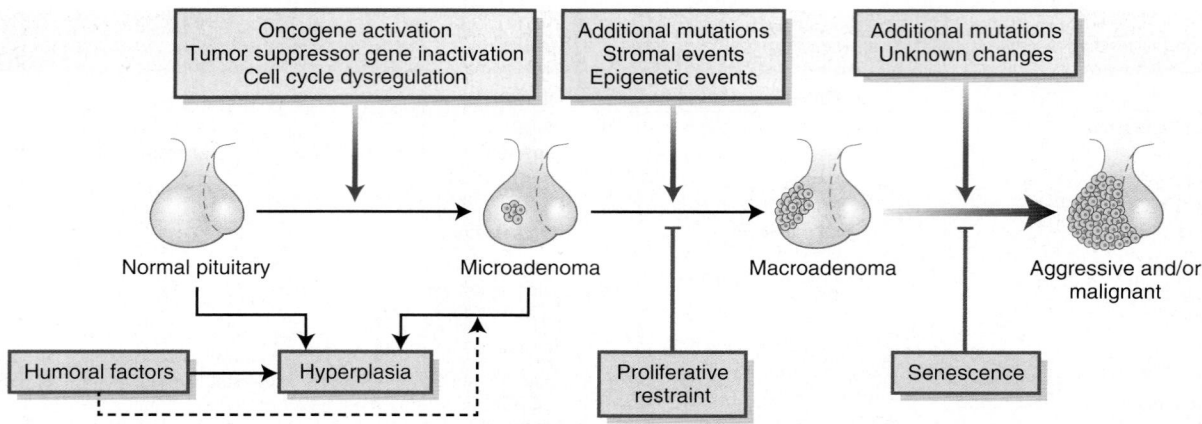

Figure 9-16 Cascade of pituitary tumorigenesis. Pituitary hyperplasia is usually reversible, as exemplified by the situation that occurs during pregnancy. (Modified from Melmed S. Pathogenesis of pituitary tumors. *Nat Rev Endocrinol.* 2011;7:257-266; and Di leva A, Rotondo F, Syro LV, et al. Aggressive pituitary adenomas: diagnosis and emerging treatments. *Nat Rev Endocrinol.* 2014;10:423-435, used with permission.)

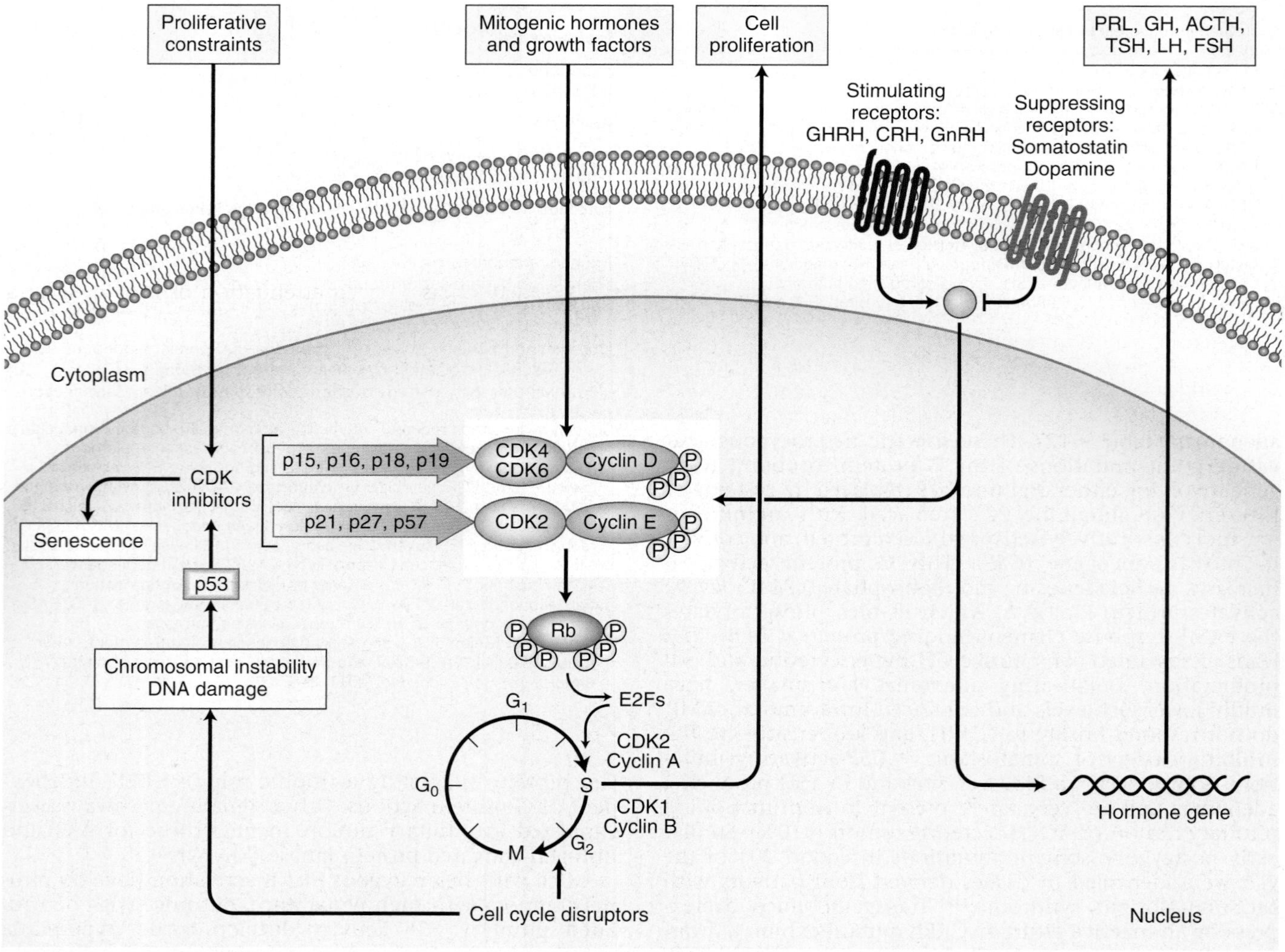

Figure 9-17 Pituitary tumorigenesis. Transcription of hormone genes in a differentiated cell and cell proliferation are mostly induced by pituitary mitogenic factors including hypothalamic hormones and transcription factors, as well as endocrine hormones. Pituitary proliferative constraints include somatotropin release-inhibiting factor and tumor suppressor genes. Cell cycle progression through G1 to S phase is mediated by CDK–cyclin complexes that phosphorylate Rb and cause it to release E2F, which drives cell proliferation. CDK inhibitors block kinase phosphorylation, thereby restraining the cell cycle. Chromosomal instability, DNA damage, and senescence may act to constrain malignant transformation of pituitary tumors. ACTH, adrenocorticotropic hormone; CDK, cyclin-dependent kinase; CRH, corticotropin-releasing hormone; FSH, follicle-stimulating hormone; GnRH, gonadotropin-releasing hormone; GH, growth hormone; GHRH, growth hormone–releasing hormone; LH, luteinizing hormone; PRL, prolactin; TSH, thyroid-stimulating hormone. (Modified from the American Society for Clinical Investigation © Melmed S. Acromegaly pathogenesis and treatment. *J Clin Invest.* 2009;119:3189-3202, used with permission.)

TABLE 9-12

Selected Genes Associated with Molecular Pathogenesis of Pituitary Adenomas

Gene	Function	Mode of Activation or Inactivation	Clinical Context
GNAS	Oncogene	Activating, imprinting	Nonfamilial, syndromic or sporadic
CREB	Transcription factor	Constitutive phosphorylation	Sporadic
AIP	Tumor suppressor	Inactivating	Familial, syndromic
MEN1	Tumor suppressor	Inactivating	Familial, syndromic
PRKAR1A	Tumor suppressor	Inactivating	Familial, syndromic
H-Ras	Oncogene	Activating	Invasive or malignant
CCNB2	Cyclin	Induced by HMGA	Sporadic
CCND1	Oncogene	Overexpression	Sporadic
CDKNIB	Cyclin-dependent kinase inhibitor	Inactivating	Sporadic, syndromic
HMGA2	Oncogene	Overexpression	Sporadic
FGFR4	Oncogene	Alternative transcription	Sporadic
PTTG	Securin	Overexpression	Sporadic
Rb	Tumor suppressor	Epigenetic silencing	Sporadic
CDKN2A	Cyclin-dependent kinase inhibitor	Epigenetic silencing	Sporadic
BRG1	Tumor suppressor	Glucocorticoid receptor function	Sporadic
GADD45G	Proliferation inhibitor	Epigenetic silencing	Sporadic
MEG3	Proliferation inhibitor	Epigenetic silencing	Sporadic

Modified from Melmed S. Acromegaly pathogenesis and treatment. *J Clin Invest.* 2009;119(11):3189-3202; used with permission of the American Society for Clinical Investigation.

distinct tumor suppressor gene has yet been identified for sporadic pituitary tumors.[153] Nevertheless approximately 25% of GH-secreting adenomas do exhibit loss of pRB expression, likely associated with promoter hypermethylation.[154] p53 gene mutations have not been detected in pituitary adenomas or in pituitary carcinomas and their metastases.[155]

PTTG, isolated from experimental pituitary tumors, is abundant in all pituitary tumor types, especially prolactinomas.[156,157] *PTTG*, a mammalian securin homolog, also induces fibroblast growth factor (FGF) production and angiogenesis and is upregulated by estrogen.[158] *PTTG* overexpression may lead to dysregulated chromatid separation and cell aneuploidy,[159,160] and pituitary targeted *PTTG* transgene expression in mice leads to hormone-secreting adenomas.[161] *PTTG* mutations have not been identified in pituitary tumors, but tumor *PTTG* abundance correlates with VEGF and VEGFR receptors, which both colocalize with *PTTG*.[162,163]

Cyclin D1, D2, and D3 are upregulated when quiescent cells enter the cell cycle and cyclin-dependent kinase (CDK) complexes lead to pRB phosphorylation, releasing E2F to promote cell cycle progresssion. Allelic imbalance at the *CCND1* locus encoding cyclin D1 is frequently observed in invasive, nonfunctioning pituitary adenomas.[164] The CDK4 and CDK6 inhibitor p16INK4a, encoded by the *CDKN2A* gene, maintains RB in the unphosphorylated state. In nonfunctioning pituitary tumors, the p16INK4a promoter is hypermethylated and consequently not expressed; less frequently the *CDKN2B* gene that encodes p15INK4b is also silenced. Mice deficient in p18INK4c develop features of gigantism with intermediate lobe pituitary hyperplasia and tumors.[165] When the CDK1 and CDK2 inhibitor p27Kip1 is knocked out, multiorgan hyperplasia occurs with development of intermediate lobe pro-opiomelanocortin (POMC) cell pituitary tumors.[166]

Basic FGF (FGF2) is abundantly expressed in the pituitary, and pituitary PTTG and bFGF expression is increased in a time- and dose-dependent manner in estrogen-treated rats.[158] A truncated FGF receptor isoform is expressed in prolactinomas and induces PRL secretion from normal and pituitary adenoma cells.[167] Human prolactinomas express FGF4, and transfected FGF4 enhances PRL secretion and tumor vascularity.[168]

Epidermal growth factor (EGF) exhibits potent mitogenic activity in pituitary cells, and both EGF and its receptor EGFR are overexpressed in pituitary tumors, particularly in nonfunctioning adenomas. Both ErbB2 and ErbB3 are expressed in aggressive, recurrent prolactinomas.[169] Gefitinib, the EGFR antagonist, decreases experimental prolactinoma cell proliferation and PRL secretion in vitro and in vivo, associated with abrogated EGFR/ERK signaling.[170] In a pilot study, two patients with dopamine-resistant aggressive prolactinomas showed attenuation of PRL levels and stabilization of tumor growth after treatment with lapatinib, a tyrosine kinase inhibitor.[171]

The growth arrest and DNA damage–inducible protein γ (GADD45-γ), a tumor growth suppressor, is silenced in most pituitary adenomas, likely by methylation of CpG islands in the gene promoter.[172] An isoform of *MEG3* containing an extra exon *(MEG3a)* is undetectable in both nonfunctioning and GH-secreting pituitary adenomas, conferring a tumor growth advantage, likely due to hypermethylation of the promoter region.[173]

Transgenic *HMGA1* and *HMGA2* overexpression results in murine GH-secreting adenomas and prolactinomas, and chromosome 12 trisomy, the locus for *HMGA2*, is frequently encountered in human PRL-secreting pituitary adenomas. *HMGA2* was overexpressed in 38 of 98 (39%) pituitary adenomas, being found in 15 of 22 FSH/LH-secreting adenomas (68%), 5 of 15 prolactinomas (31%), and 12 of 18 ACTH-secreting adenomas (18%). However, *HMGA2* was rarely detected in GH-secreting adenomas.[174] *HMGA2* levels correlate with tumor size, invasiveness, and proliferation markers. *HMGA2* tumorigenic effects may also be mediated by inducing cyclin B2 expression[175] and activation of the E2F pathway. *HMGA2* is suppressed by *Let-7* microRNA, and *HMGA2* and *Let-7* expression correlates inversely in human pituitary adenoma samples.[174]

Frequent epigenetic changes are encountered in all pituitary tumor types, and novel targeted therapies to reverse disrupted epigenomic events have been proposed.[176]

Pituitary Senescence

Cellular senescence, or cell growth arrest, is induced by age-linked telomere shortening, DNA damage, oxidative stress, and oncogene activation. Oncogene-induced premature cell cycle arrest is protective of the cellular response to oncogenic events, is largely irreversible, and is mediated through upregulation of cell cycle inhibitors including p16INK4A, p15INK4B, p21CIP1, and p53. p21Cip1 induction and senescence markers were elevated in all of the 38 GH-secreting adenomas tested.[177] In contrast, p21 was undetectable in pituitary carcinomas, nonsecreting pituitary oncocytomas, and in null cell adenomas. Senescence-associated β-galactosidase activity (SA-β-gal), a marker of senescence, is also strongly positive in GH-secreting adenomas (Fig. 9-18). As cellular senescence is protective for malignant transformation,[178] this process may underlie the invariably benign nature of pituitary adenomas.[152]

Familial Syndromes

These rare syndromes are summarized in Table 9-13 and include the following types.

Multiple Endocrine Neoplasia Type 1

Multiple endocrine neoplasia type 1 (MEN1) is an autosomal dominant hereditary disorder characterized by tumor formation or hyperfunction of parathyroid, pancreatic islets, anterior pituitary, and less commonly, carcinoid, thyroid, and adrenal tumors.[179,180] The MEN1 syndrome (fully described in Chapter 39), is associated with germ cell inactivation of the *MEN1* gene *(MENIN)* located on chromosome 11q13.[181] Unlike pituitary tumors in the MEN1 syndrome, *MEN1* gene mutations were not identified in non-MEN1 familial pituitary adenomas.[182] Mutations of other genes may also confer an MEN1 clinical syndrome. Approximately 20% of patients with a clinical diagnosis of MEN1 do not exhibit identifiable *MEN1* mutations, and rarely the gene for p27Kip1 *(CDKN1B)* is mutated in patients with clinical features of MEN1 but with no *MEN1* mutations.[183]

Familial Isolated Pituitary Adenomas

Less than 5% of prolactinomas and GH-secreting tumors are inherited on a familial basis.[184] In familial acromegaly, about 25% of afflicted individuals are diagnosed as teenagers or young adults, usually with gigantism. These patients have been linked to LOH at the 11q13.1-11q13.3 locus.[185] Germline mutations of the aryl hydrocarbon receptor–interacting protein (AIP) were found to predispose to familial pituitary tumors.[184,186] Eleven of 73 families with familial isolated pituitary adenomas were found to have 10 germline AIP gene mutations associated mainly with GH- and PRL-secreting tumors.[187,188] AIP mutations are rarely encountered in patients with sporadic tumors and have been reported mainly in the youngest patients with acromegaly or gigantism.[189,190] When patients under the age of 30 with sporadic macroadenomas were tested, 11.7% were found to harbor germline AIP mutations. In young

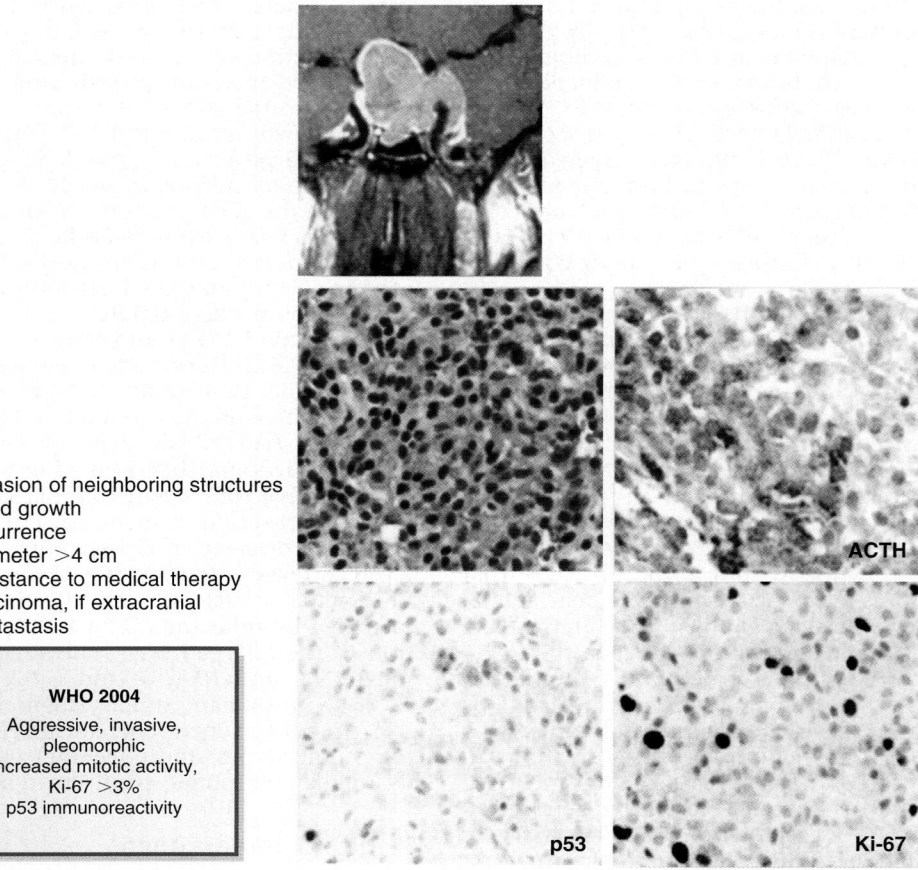

- invasion of neighboring structures
- rapid growth
- recurrence
- diameter >4 cm
- resistance to medical therapy
- carcinoma, if extracranial metastasis

WHO 2004

Aggressive, invasive, pleomorphic increased mitotic activity, Ki-67 >3% p53 immunoreactivity

Figure 9-18 Atypical pituitary adenomas. Criteria for diagnosis as proposed by World Health Organization (WHO). Histologic panels depict atypical adrenocorticotropic hormone (ACTH)-expressing adenoma. (From Zada G, Woodmansee WW, Ramkissoon S, et al. Atypical pituitary adenomas: incidence, clinical characteristics, and implications. *J Neurosurg.* 2011;114:336-344.)

TABLE 9-13

Genes Associated with Familial Pituitary Tumor Syndromes

Syndrome	Gene (Locus)	Most Frequent Mutation(s)	Pituitary Features	Other Key Features	Animal Model
MEN1	*MEN1* (11q13)	c.249-252delGTCT, an exon 2 predicted frameshift, in 4.5%	Pituitary adenoma in 30-40% (PRL 60%, NFA 15%, GH 10%, ACTH 5%, TSH rare)	Primary hyperparathyroidism, pancreatic tumors, foregut carcinoid tumors, adreno-cortical tumors (usually nonfunctional), rarely pheochromocytomas, skin lesions (facial angiomas, collegenomas, and lipomas)	*MEN1* null mouse embryonic lethal (engineered mutant) Heterozygote mutant: pituitary adenomas, parathyroid, pancreatic, adrenal, and thyroid tumors; Leydig cell tumors, ovary sex cord stromal tumors
MEN1-like (MEN4)	*CDKN1B* (12p13)	Only two reported cases	Pituitary adenoma[a]	Primary hyperparathyroidism and single cases reported of renal angiomyolipoma, neuroendocrine cervical carcinoma	*MENX* rat: pheochromocytomas, paragangliomas, parathyroid adenomas, thyroid C cell hyperplasia, endocrine pancreas hyperplasia, cataracts, pituitary hyperplasia and multifocal adenomas Mouse *Cdkn1b* knockout: intermediate-lobe pituitary tumors sole tumor phenotype P27^{CK-} mouse model[b]: pituitary tumors, adrenal, retinal, spleen, lung, and ovarian hyperplasia and/or tumors
Carney complex	*PRKAR1A* (17q23-24)	c.491-492delTG in exon 5	Pituitary hyperplasia in most patients Adenoma in ~10% (GH and PRL)	Atrial myxomas, lentigines, Schwann cell tumors, adrenal hyperplasia	*Prkar1a* decreased expression: no consistent pituitary phenotype; *Prkar1a* pituitary-specific knockout: GH axis abnormalities, pituitary tumors
Familial, isolated pituitary adenomas	*AIP*[c] (11q13.3)	Gln14X nonsense mutation[d]	Pituitary adenoma (majority GH, PRL, or mixed GH and PRL)	NR	Pituitary knockout model not yet described

[a]Only two reported cases to date: one GH-secreting adenoma and one ACTH-secreting adenoma.
[b]p27^{CK-} is a mouse model, in which p27^{Kip1} contains four amino acid substitutions.
[c]*AIP* mutations reported in 15% of individuals with familial isolated pituitary adenoma and 50% of those with isolated familial somatotropinomas.
[d]This is the most commonly identified mutation but is likely to be overrepresented secondary to a Finnish founder effect.
ACTH, adrenocorticotropic hormone; GH, growth hormone; MEN1, multiple endocrine neoplasia type 1; NFA, nonfunctioning adenoma; NR, not reported; PRL, prolactin.
From Elston MS, McDonald KL, Clifton-Bligh RJ, Robinson BG. Familial pituitary tumor syndromes. *Nat Rev Endocrinol.* 2009;5(8):453-461.

acromegaly patients, the frequency of AIP mutations ranged from 2.3% to 5.5% with no apparent differences in patients with or without mutations.[191]

Carney Complex

Carney complex is an autosomal dominant disorder comprising benign mesenchymal tumors including cardiac myxomas, schwannomas, thyroid adenomas, and pituitary adenomas associated with spotty skin pigmentation.[192] The disorder has been mapped to chromosome 17q24 and results from a mutated type 1α regulatory subunit (R1α) of the cAMP-dependent protein kinase A (PRKAR1A).[193] These patients may have elevated levels of GH, IGF-1, or PRL, and 10% exhibit clinical acromegaly with GH-secreting tumor formation associated with inactivating mutations of *PRKAR1A*, leading to constitutive protein kinase A catalytic subunit activation. In some patients, the wild-type *PRKAR1A* allele is retained in tumor tissue, and haploinsufficiency may be sufficient for tumorigenesis. A 17-miRNA signature for pituitary tumors was identified on the background of pituitary hyperplasia and *PRKARIA* mutations. In GH-secreting tumors miR-26b and miR-128 appear to regulate the PTEN-AKT pathway.[194] These defects provide attractive potential subcellular therapeutic targets.

In summary, multifactorial mechanisms subserve the multistep pathogenetic process of pituitary adenoma formation, including early initiating chromosomal mutations that result in mutated pituitary stem or progenitor cells. The transformed pituitary cell is subjected to signals facilitating clonal expansion, and permissive factors, including hypothalamic hormone receptor signals, intrapituitary growth factors, and disordered cell cycle regulation may determine the ultimate biologic fate of the tumor. Autonomous anterior pituitary hormone production and secretion and cell proliferation, which are the hallmarks of pituitary adenomas, result. However, proximal subcellular events initiating the formation of most sporadic pituitary adenomas have yet to be elucidated.

CLASSIFICATION OF PITUITARY TUMORS

Pituitary tumors arise from hormone-secreting adenohypophyseal cells, and their secretory products depend upon the cell of origin (Table 9-14). Pathologic classification enables accurate clinical correlates and identifies cell-type origin.[195-197] Previously clinically inapparent pituitary adenomas are found in about 11% of autopsies (Table 9-15). They localize to unique areas of the gland, reflecting relative cell-type abundance and intragland distribution (see Fig. 9-2). Although 46% of a subset of these immunostain for PRL,[198] expectant management may still be indicated.[199] In a study on 100 normal volunteers, 10 were found to

TABLE 9-14
Clinical and Pathologic Characteristics of Pituitary Adenomas

Adenoma Type	Incidence Pathologic (%)	Clinical (%)	Annual Incidence (New Cases/10⁶)	Prevalence (Total Cases/10⁶)	Messenger RNA Expression	Immunohistochemistry	Electron Microscopic Secretory Granules (nm)	Clinical Syndrome
Lactotroph		29	6-10	60-100				
Sparsely granulated	28				PRL	PRL	150-500	Hypogonadism, galactorrhea
Densely granulated	1				PRL	PRL	400-1200	
Somatotroph		15	4-6	40-60				
Sparsely granulated	5				GH	GH	100-250	Acromegaly or gigantism
Densely granulated	5				GH	GH	300-700	
Combined GH/PRL cell		8						
Mixed GH/PRL	5				GH/PRL	GH/PRL	100-600	
Mammosomatotroph	1				GH/PRL	GH/PRL	350-2000	Hypogonadism, acromegaly, galactorrhea
Acidophil stem cell	3				GH/PRL	GH/PRL	50-300	
Corticotroph			2-3	20-30				
Cushing disease	10	10			POMC	ACTH	250-700	Cushing disease
Silent corticotroph	3	6			POMC	ACTH	Variable	None
Nelson syndrome	2				POMC	ACTH	250-700	Local signs
Thyrotroph	1	0.9			TSH	TSH	50-250	Hyperthyroidism
Plurihormonal	10	4			GH/PRL	GH/PRL/glycoprotein	Mixed	Mixed
Nonfunctioning/null cell/gonadotroph		27	7-9	70-90				
Nononcocytic	14				FSH/LHα	Glycoprotein	<25% of cells 100-250	Silent or pituitary failure
Oncocytic	6				FSH/LHα	Glycoprotein	<25% of cells 100-250, many mitochondria	Silent or pituitary failure
Gonadotroph	7-15				FSH/LH	FSH/LH	50-200	Silent or pituitary failure

Hardy Classification of Pituitary Tumors

Extension—Extrasellar

Suprasellar (Symmetric)
A. Suprasellar cistern
B. Recesses of third ventricle
C. Whole anterior third ventricle

Parasellar (Asymmetric)
D. Intracranial intradural
   1. Anterior
   2. Midline
   3. Posterior
E. Extracranial extradural (lateral cavernous sinus)

Spread/Invasion

Radiologic	Anatomic	Surgical
Grade 0	Intact, normal contour	Micro enclosed
Grade I	Intact, focal bulging	Micro enclosed
Grade II	Intact, enlarged	Macro enclosed
Grade III	Destroyed, partially	Macro invasive
Grade IV	Destroyed, totally	Macro invasive
Grade V	Distant spread via CSF or blood	Macro carcinoma

ACTH, adrenocorticotropic hormone; CSF, cerebrospinal fluid; FSH, follicle-stimulating hormone; GH, growth hormone; LHα, luteinizing hormone α-subunit; PRL, prolactin; TSH, thyroid-stimulating hormone (thyrotropin).
Data from Clayton RN. Sporadic pituitary tumours: from epidemiology to use of databases. *Best Pract Res Clin Endocrinol Metab*. 1999;13:451 (study of a relatively stable 1 million catchment population surrounding Stoke-on-Trent, UK) and from Kovacs and Horvath (1987)[222]; Scheithauer (1994); Mindermann and Wilson (1994)[470]; Asa (1993).

have focal abnormalities on MRI consistent with microadenomas; they measured from 3 to 6 mm in diameter.[8] Such tumors have been termed *incidentalomas*. In a survey of 506 patients harboring incidentalomas, 20% were nonfunctioning, and of these, 20% increased in size during a mean follow-up of 50 months.[198] When larger, particularly nonfunctioning tumors are encountered inadvertently, pituitary function should be assessed, including measuring PRL, IGF-1, luteinizing hormone (LH), follicle-stimulating hormone (FSH), and sex steroids. A 24-hour urinary free

TABLE 9-15
Frequency of Pituitary Adenomas Found at Autopsy

Study	No. Pituitaries Examined	No. Adenomas Found	Frequency (%)
Susman	260	23	9
Costello	1,000	225	23
Sommers	400	26	7
McCormick	1,600	140	9
Kovacs	152	20	13
Landolt	100	13	13
Mosca	100	24	24
Burrow	120	32	27
Parent	500	42	8
Muhr	205	3	2
Schwezinger	5,100	485	9
Coulon	100	10	10
Chambers	100	14	14
Siqueira	450	39	9
El-Hamid	486	97	20
Scheithauer	251	41	16
Marin	210	35	16
Mosca	111	13	11
Sano	166	15	9
Teramoto	1,000	51	5
Buurman	3,048	334	11
Totals	15,459	1,742	11

Modified from Molitch ME. Pituitary incidentalomas. In: de Herder WW, ed. *Functional and Morphological Imaging of the Endocrine System*. Norwell, MA: Kluwer Academic; 2000:59-70; and Buurman H, Saeger W. Subclinical adenomas in postmortem pituitaries: classification and correlations to clinical data. *Eur J Endocrinol*. 2006;154:753-758.

TABLE 9-16
Aggressive Pituitary Adenoma Cell Types

Adenoma	Cell Characteristics
Crooke cell adenomas	Characterized by cells that undergo massive accumulation of perinuclear cytokeratin filaments in response to glucocorticoid excess as seen in Cushing disease
Gonadotroph adenomas	Generally do not cause hormonal disturbances; clinically silent until growing mass invades surrounding structures
Sparsely granulated somatotroph adenomas	Express GH and have low secretory granule density
Densely granulated lactotroph adenomas	High density of PRL secretory granules
Acidophil stem cell adenomas	Rapidly growing undifferentiated cell adenomas immunopositive for PRL and GH
Thyrotroph adenomas	Produce TSH; very rare cause of hyperthyroidism
Plurihormonal adenomas	Produce more than one pituitary hormone (atypical combinations, such as TSH, FSH, and GH, or PRL and TSH)
Silent adenomas	Immunohistochemical evidence of hormone production without biochemical or clinical features
Null cell adenomas	Immunostain negatively for all trophic hormones

FSH, follicle-stimulating hormone; GH, growth hormone; PRL, prolactin; TSH, thyroid-stimulating hormone (thyrotropin).
Modified from Di Ieva A, Rotondo F, Syro LV, et al. Aggressive pituitary adenoma—diagnosis and emerging treatments. *Nat Rev Endocrinol*. 2014;10:423-435.

cortisol or salivary cortisol measurement may exclude Cushing disease. In a study of 52 patients with macroadenomas that were incidentally discovered by CT or MRI, 22 were gonadotroph cell adenomas, 21 were null cell adenomas, and 9 were clinically nonfunctioning but immunostained for various pituitary hormones.[163] Radiologic and surgical classifications are based upon tumor localization, size, and degree of invasiveness (see Fig. 9-15). Microadenomas are intrasellar and generally smaller than 10 mm in widest diameter. Macroadenomas are 10 mm or larger and usually impinge upon adjacent sellar structures. Specific tumor types are considered below for each respective cell type. Immunocytochemistry detects pituitary cell gene products at both the light and electron microscopic levels, and allows classification of pituitary tumors based on their function. Unlike the corticotroph, somatotroph, lactotroph, and thyrotroph cell tumors, which hypersecrete their respective hormones, gonadotroph cell tumors, however, are usually clinically silent and do not efficiently secrete their gene products.[200] Double immunostaining identifies mixed tumors expressing combinations of hormones; they are often macroadenomas secreting GH concomitantly with PRL or TSH or ACTH. Generally, immunohistochemical identification of pituitary hormones correlates with tumor-specific messenger RNA (mRNA) markers measured either in whole tissue extracts by Northern analysis or at the single cell level by in situ hybridization techniques.[201] With the exception of the glycoprotein α-subunit, immunohistochemical positivity of greater than 5% of cells composing the tumor is usually reflective of peripheral circulating hormone levels. Quantification of immunostaining intensity is subjective, and a scale of intensity should also include a description of the extent of staining, such as whether occasional, scattered, or most tumor cells express the immunodetectable

protein. Electron microscopy is useful for assessing the ultrastructure of hormone secretory granules, their size, and distribution. Other subcellular features important for diagnosis include visualizing large mitochondria in nonfunctioning oncocytomas and the secretory nature of Golgi and endoplasmic reticulum, especially for prolactinomas. Peroxidase or colloid gold particles of different diameters are also sensitive electron microscopic markers for identifying and localizing intracellular hormone signals. Because even invasive pituitary tumors are slow growing, mitotic markers including proliferating cell nuclear antigen (PCNA) and Ki-67 are of limited use.[200]

Atypical Adenomas

True pituitary carcinoma with demonstrable extrapituitary metastases is exceedingly rare.[202,203] However, diagnostic criteria for aggressive atypical adenomas include an invasive tumor with an MIB-1 proliferative index greater than 3%, abundant p53 immunoreactivity, and increased mitotic activity[201] (see Fig. 9-18). In a series of 121 consecutive patients undergoing transsphenoidal pituitary tumor resection, 18 were classified as "atypical."[204] These tumors grow aggressively and often persist or recur after surgery. They may arise from any of the pituitary cell types, and about half actively secrete GH, PRL, or rarely ACTH. Several histologic types are particularly prone to aggressive growth (Table 9-16). For example, silent corticotroph adenomas are inherently more aggressive, and many are classified as atypical.[171] No controlled prospective studies have assessed the postoperative recurrence rates of these tumors, and the utility of MIB-1 or p53 as prognostic markers has also been questioned. There is also no compelling evidence that these tumors undergo true malignant transformation. Nevertheless, frequently recurring or persistent invasive adenomas with high Ki-67 indices should raise awareness to consider the rare diagnosis of malignancy by excluding the presence of metastasis.[205]

Malignant Pituitary Tumors

Very rarely, pituitary tumors may metastasize either outside the central nervous system or as a separate focus within the brain.[206] Because no cell markers clearly distinguish aggressive invasiveness from malignancy, demonstration of extracranial metastasis is a prerequisite for diagnosis of pituitary malignancy.[207] When they occur, these cancers most often secrete either ACTH or PRL. As *ras* mutations are rarely encountered in distant metastatic pituitary carcinomas, but not in their respective primary pituitary tumors or in noninvasive adenomas,[155,208] these mutations may be important in the very rare progression to malignancy.

Temozolomide, an alkylating agent that induces DNA damage to disrupt gene transcription, has been used to treat aggressive pituitary tumors in patients who have failed to respond to other therapies or who have evidence of pituitary carcinoma.[209] Although O^6-methylguanine-DNA methyltransferase (MGMT) may interfere with drug efficacy, assessing MGMT expression in pituitary tumor samples has been reported to have variable use.[210-214]

PROLACTIN-SECRETING ADENOMAS

Prolactinomas are the most frequently encountered secretory pituitary tumors, occurring with an annual incidence of approximately 30 per 100,000 population.[136] This incidence would be much higher if the estimate included microadenomas discovered in approximately 11% of pituitaries at autopsy, 46% of which immunostain positively for PRL.[198] The female/male ratio for microprolactinomas is 20:1, and for macroadenomas the gender ratio is roughly equivalent. Both PRL levels and tumor size generally remain stable, although in some patients, PRL levels fall over time and microadenomas may disappear after discontinuing dopamine agonist therapy, although 7% to 14% of microadenomas continue to grow.[215] Additionally, smaller prolactinomas may sometimes regress after pregnancy and lactation.[216]

Macroprolactinomas have a greater propensity to grow and tumor size correlates with serum PRL levels (Fig. 9-19), so a PRL level higher than 200 ng/mL is strongly indicative of a PRL-secreting pituitary tumor. Although prolactinomas account for more than 75% of all female pituitary adenomas,[136] men harbor larger tumors. In 45 men and 51 women with prolactinomas mean serum PRL was 2789 ± 572 ng/mL versus 292 ± 74 ng/mL, respectively. Prolactinomas are larger in men than in women (26 ± 2 mm vs. 10 ± 1 mm), are more invasive, and show histologic evidence of more rapid growth.[217] Giant prolactinomas have been characterized as being larger than 4 cm in diameter with a serum PRL of higher than 1000 ng/mL, and they occur more commonly in men.[218,219]

PRL levels higher than 200 ng/mL are not always indicative of a prolactinoma and may reflect use of a drug such as risperidol, but levels higher than 500 ng/mL are exclusively observed in patients with prolactinomas.[220] In contrast, a PRL concentration of less than 200 ng/mL in a patient harboring a macroadenoma indicates that the tumor is likely not producing PRL, but hyperprolactinemia may occur as a result of mass pressure on the pituitary

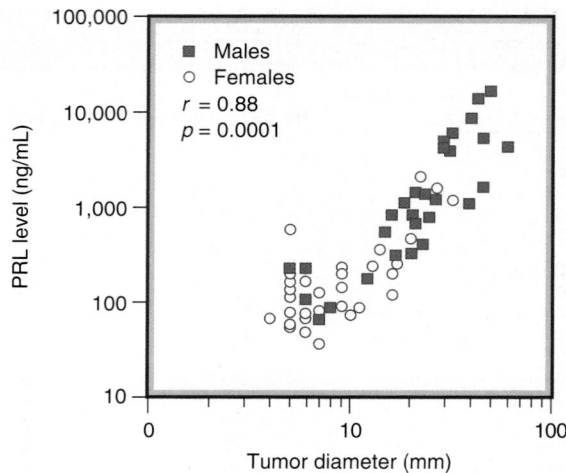

Figure 9-19 Prolactin (PRL)-secreting tumors are more often macroadenomas in men ($n = 31$) versus women ($n = 45$). Serum prolactin levels highly correlate with tumor size. (Adapted from Danila DC, Klibanski A. Prolactin secreting pituitary tumors in men. *Endocrinologist.* 2001;11:105-111.)

stalk or portal circulation, likely interrupting inhibitory control by dopamine.[221] Importantly, microprolactinomas can be associated with PRL levels ranging from minimal elevations to hundreds of nanograms per milliliter. However, when a patient with a small macroadenoma and a PRL level approximately 200 ng/mL is first encountered, it is prudent to first treat medically. If the tumor is indeed a prolactinoma, dopamine agonist treatment should lower PRL levels and shrink the tumor. If the tumor does not shrink, the mass is likely not secretory, and the hyperprolactinoma is caused by compressive stalk effect.

Pathology and Pathogenesis

Although more than 99% of prolactinomas are benign and often sharply demarcated without evidence of invasion, about half invade local structures[222] (Fig. 9-20). Invasive tumors may have higher mitotic activity and are more cellular and pleomorphic. Invasion into adjacent dura, bone, or venous structures may represent an intermediate form of prolactinoma between the sharply demarcated benign variety and the exceedingly rare malignant tumor. Invasive tumors that do not metastasize are considered benign. Immunostaining for PRL confirms the diagnosis of prolactinoma, which is usually distinct from the adjacent normal pituitary but is not truly encapsulated. These tumors have a "pseudocapsule" composed of compressed adenohypophyseal cells and a reticulin fiber network. About 20% of macroprolactinomas contain areas of hemorrhage not usually associated with features of apoplexy, and these areas may resolve.[223]

Prolactinomas are mostly slow growing, arise sporadically, usually occur singly, and are the most common pituitary tumors associated with MEN1, occurring in approximately 20% of a large kindred.[224] Familial prolactinomas have been described with no other features of MEN1,[225] and rarely prolactinomas also occur in patients with germline AIP mutations.[226]

Clinical Features

Prolactinomas usually come to attention because of symptoms or signs associated with hyperprolactinemia or with tumor size or invasiveness (Table 9-17).

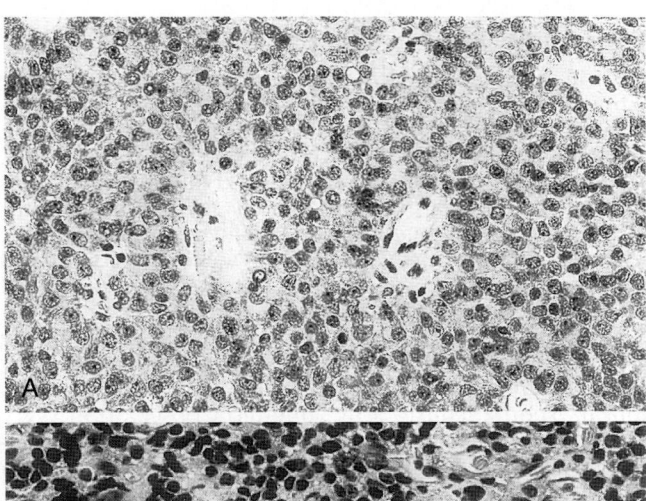
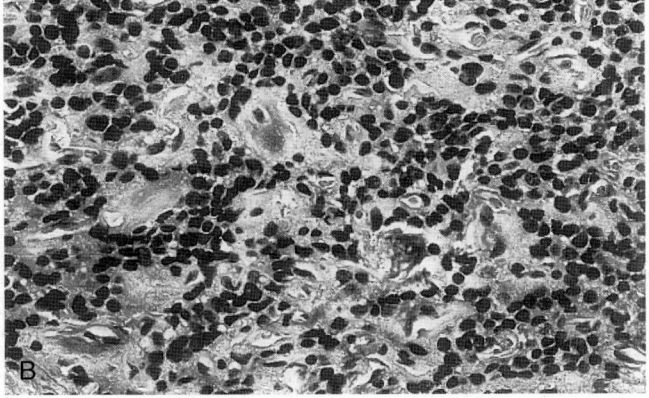

Figure 9-20 A, Densely granulated prolactin-secreting adenoma. **B,** Prolactin-producing pituitary adenoma removed by surgery from a patient treated with dopamine agonist in the preoperative period. The adenoma cells are small, possessing dark nuclei and a narrow rim of cytoplasm. Mild accumulation of interstitial connective tissue is apparent. (Hematoxylin-eosin stain; original magnification ×400.) (Photomicrograph kindly provided by Dr. Kalman Kovacs. University of Toronto, Toronto, Canada.)

TABLE 9-17	
Signs and Symptoms of Prolactinomas	
Signs and Symptoms Associated with Tumor Mass	**Signs and Symptoms Associated with Hyperprolactinemia**
Visual field abnormalities	Amenorrhea, oligomenorrhea, infertility
Blurred vision or decreased visual acuity	Decreased libido, impotence, premature ejaculation, erectile dysfunction, oligospermia
Symptoms of hypopituitarism	
Headaches	
Cranial nerve palsies	Galactorrhea
Pituitary apoplexy	Osteoporosis
Seizures (temporal lobe)	
Hydrocephalus (rare)	
Unilateral exophthalmos (rare)	

Hyperprolactinemia

Both large and small PRL-secreting tumors can present with signs and symptoms of hyperprolactinemia. Menstrual irregularities, sexual dysfunction, galactorrhea,[227] osteopenia,[228] and impaired quality of life[229] are attributable to elevated PRL levels and presence of a tumor. Elevated PRL causes sexual dysfunction via a short loop feedback effect on gonadotropin pulsatility, presumably inhibiting GnRH[230] and LH pulse frequency and amplitude. High PRL also directly inhibits ovarian and testicular function.

Women with prolactinomas may present with primary or secondary amenorrhea, oligomenorrhea, menorrhagia, delayed menarche, or regular menses with a short luteal phase that may cause infertility. Patients may also report changes in libido and vaginal dryness. Sexual dysfunction in men usually manifests as loss or decrease in libido, impotence, premature ejaculation or intracoital erection loss, oligospermia, or azospermia.[231]

Up to 50% of women and 35% of men with prolactinomas have galactorrhea; this difference may occur because male mammary tissue is less susceptible to lactogenic effects of hyperprolactinemia. Galactorrhea can be overlooked unless actively elicited. Bone density may decrease in both men and women as a result of hyperprolactinemia-induced sex steroid deficiency, and an increase in vertebral fractures detected radiologically has been reported in women.[232]

Tumor Mass Effects

Prolactinomas may present as a result of tumor size or invasiveness. Microadenomas range from entirely asymptomatic tumors found at autopsy as small as 2 to 3 mm in diameter to larger ones that are still less than 10 mm in diameter. These tumors can be invasive despite their small size. In contrast, macroadenomas range in size from non-invasive or diffuse tumors approximately 1 cm in diameter to huge tumors that may impinge upon parasellar structures. Signs and symptoms caused by large or invasive tumors are often related to compressive effects on visual structures. The most frequent ophthalmic complaint in a series of 1000 patients with tumors was "loss of vision."[233] Objective findings are superior bitemporal defects, bitemporal hemianopia, and decreased visual acuity. Headaches are common, but seizures (a result of extension into the temporal lobe) and hydrocephalus[234] are rarely encountered, as is unilateral exophthalmos. Many tumors invade the cavernous sinuses and yet cranial nerve palsies are rare. A sudden insult, such as pituitary apoplexy, is the more common cause of such palsies and may be a presenting symptom. Prolactinomas can also be found inadvertently on an MRI or CT scan performed for another purpose.

Evaluation

Patients with pituitary tumors should all have serum PRL levels measured. Conversely, patients with elevated serum PRL levels not fully explicable by an obvious cause (such as pregnancy or exposure to neuroleptic medications) should be evaluated for the presence of a pituitary tumor. Prolactinomas may also coexist with another cause of hyperprolactinemia, such as neuroleptic drug administration (see Chapter 8). Even minimal to moderate PRL elevations are important to investigate because they may indicate the presence of a large pituitary tumor that does not secrete PRL. PRL levels correlate with tumor size and are usually higher in male patients. Occasionally, a patient with a very high serum PRL level might have a "normal" result reported if serum dilutions are not assayed, a phenomenon called the "high-dose hook effect."[235] In contrast, serum PRL may be elevated by the presence high-molecular-weight PRL, which is a weaker lactogen than the monomeric PRL molecule. Although usually clinically inactive, macroprolactinemia can also occur in patients with pituitary tumors. Pituitary adenomas are diagnosed in approximately 20% of patients with macroprolactinemia, some of which are associated with galactorrhea, oligo- or amenorrhea, or erectile dysfunction and decreased libido. Thus, assessment of macroprolactinemia by polyethyleneglycol precipitation should be performed in patients with reported high levels of PRL and few or absent clinical features of hyperprolactinemia.[236]

A careful history will often unmask symptoms or signs of a space-related mass such as visual field abnormalities, impaired visual acuity, blurred or double vision, CSF rhinorrhea, headaches, diabetes insipidus, and hypopituitarism. Patients should also be questioned carefully about sexual history including onset of menarche, regularity of menses, fertility, libido, potency, and ability to maintain an erection. A history of galactorrhea should also be ascertained. The coexistence of galactorrhea and amenorrhea suggests a diagnosis of pituitary adenoma until otherwise proven.

PRL is also elevated in up to 50% of patients with acromegaly.[237] Patients in the early stages of acromegaly or with mild disease or those harboring acidophilic stem cell adenomas may have few obvious signs of GH excess. Because the human GH molecule has similar lactogenic properties similar to those of PRL,[238] signs and symptoms of a prolactinoma may be mimicked by a purely GH-secreting tumor, and serum IGF-1 should be measured. Elevated PRL levels are occasionally encountered in patients with TSH-secreting tumors. Other pituitary hormone functions should be ascertained to determine the presence of hypopituitarism. An MRI is required to establish a definitive diagnosis of prolactinoma.

Treatment

Optimal treatment outcomes for a prolactinoma include normalization of PRL levels (and associated signs and symptoms) and complete tumor removal or shrinkage with a reversal of tumor-mass effects (Table 9-18). Specifically, previously abnormal sexual function and fertility should be restored, galactorrhea stopped, impaired bone density improved, tumor eliminated or reduced in size without impairing pituitary or hypothalamic function, and vision normalized, if impaired.

TABLE 9-18

Dopamine Agonist Treatment of Prolactinomas*

	Bromocriptine[†] (2.5-7.5 mg/day)	Cabergoline[†] (0.5-1 mg twice weekly)
Microadenomas		
PRL normalized	70	80
Menses resumed	70	80
Macroadenomas		
PRL normalized	65	70
Menses resumed	85	80
Tumor Shrinkage		
None	20	20
Up to 50%	40	55
50% or more	40	25
Visual Field Improvement	90	70
Drug Intolerance	15	5

*Long-acting cabergoline has improved patient compliance and has fewer gastrointestinal side effects. For fertility, bromocriptine is preferred as it is short-acting and can be discontinued immediately on pregnancy confirmation.
†Values = % of patients.
Data from Webster J, Piscatelli G, Polli A, et al. A comparison of cabergoline and bromocriptine in the treatment of hyperprolactinemic amenorrhea. Cabergoline Comparative Study Group. *N Engl J Med.* 1994;331:904-909; and Verhelst J, Abs R, Maiter D, et al. Cabergoline in the treatment of hyperprolactinemia: a study in 455 patients. *J Clin Endocrinol Metab.* 1999;84:2518-2522.

Medical Treatment

Medical management of prolactinomas with dopamine agonist drugs has been widely recommended as the treatment of choice.

Bromocriptine. Bromocriptine, a semisynthetic ergot alkaloid dopamine agonist, lowers elevated PRL levels, restores abnormal menstrual function in 80% to 90% of patients, shrinks prolactinomas, restores impaired sexual function, and resolves galactorrhea.[239] Improvement in visual field abnormalities occurs in approximately 90% of affected patients.[240] Drug withdrawal can result in rapid tumor expansion.[241] Occasionally, tumors that shrink during bromocriptine therapy do not enlarge following drug withdrawal. In a subset of patients hyperprolactinemia disappears spontaneously after long-term observation. Very occasionally, bromocriptine lowers PRL levels despite continued tumor expansion, although when tumors grow during dopamine agonist therapy there is usually a simultaneous PRL elevation.

Despite high doses of bromocriptine, some patients are entirely or partially resistant to its effects and to those of cabergoline as well.[242] Not infrequently, it is difficult to completely normalize PRL levels in patients with initially very high levels, although these patients respond to treatment with impressive tumor shrinkage and sometimes improved sexual function. Although higher doses or a change in the form of dopamine agonist has been reported to further normalize PRL in some cases,[242] many such patients remain with elevated PRL levels regardless of treatment employed. Resistance to dopamine agonists may reflect reduced D_2 receptor binding sites or receptor gene polymorphisms.[243]

Bromocriptine shrinks prolactinomas by shrinking tumor cell size, including cytoplasmic, nuclear, and nucleolar areas.[244] Histologic sections appear very dense as a result of small cell size and clumping of nuclei (see Fig. 9-20). PRL mRNA and PRL synthesis are inhibited, exocytoses are reduced, PRL secretory granules decrease, and rough endoplasmic reticulum and Golgi apparatus involute. The net effect is reduced cell volume. Tumor necrosis may also occur.[245]

Perivascular fibrosis observed in prolactinomas derived from patients treated with bromocriptine has been attributed to difficulty in tumor removal. However, there is no effect of prior treatment with bromocriptine on surgical success rates,[246] and bromocriptine was a helpful adjunct to transsphenoidal microsurgery for macroprolactinomas.[247] Even the largest tumors or those with the highest PRL levels respond well to treatment with up to 2.5 mg bromocriptine three times daily. Higher doses are often not more effective. Once positive effects on tumor size and amenorrhea and galactorrhea are established, some patients can be satisfactorily maintained with lower doses but rarely without medication.

Cabergoline. Because cabergoline has a longer duration of action than bromocriptine and is usually administered once or twice weekly, it has surpassed bromocriptine as the first-line therapeutic choice for most patients, unless pregnancy is desired.[240] The long half-life of cabergoline is a result of its high affinity for lactotroph D_2 receptors on lactotrophs and a greater propensity of the drug to remain in pituitary tissue. In pharmacokinetic studies, cabergoline lowered PRL levels in a dose-related manner.[248] PRL levels were normalized in 83% of 459 women with hyperprolactinemia treated with cabergoline (0.5 to 1 mg twice weekly) and in 52% of women on bromocriptine (2.5 to 5 mg twice daily). Cabergoline was also more effective than bromocriptine in restoring ovulatory cycles and fertility (72% vs.

52%; $p < 0.001$), was better tolerated than bromocriptine, and caused fewer but similar side effects (Fig. 9-21). Tumor size decreased in 11 of 15 patients with macroadenomas, and menses resumed in 3 of 4 premenopausal women.[249] In 85 patients with macroprolactinomas treated with cabergoline (0.25 mg to 10.5 mg per week) PRL concentrations were normalized in 61% of patients and decreased by at least 75% in an additional 24 patients, and tumor size decreased in 66% of patients. Nine patients were resistant to cabergoline despite doses of up to 7 mg per week.[242] Despite the continued experience that a subset of hyperprolactinemic patients are resistant to dopamine agonists, cabergoline normalized PRL level in 15 of 19 patients with macroprolactinomas previously resistant to other dopamine agonists. Cabergoline also may result in dramatic improvement of prolactinoma-associated headache.

Prolactinomas completely or substantially resistant to medication are infrequently encountered. Most "resistant" patients have only partial resistance (i.e., tumors shrink and PRL levels are lowered but do not normalize). With the tumor growth controlled on treatment, persistently elevated PRL levels should be addressed by evaluating and treating specific disorders caused by hyperprolactinemia.

Administration. Attention to the mode of dopamine agonist administration may avoid or minimize potential adverse effects (Fig. 9-22). Usual starting doses are 1.25 mg bromocriptine (daily) or 0.25 mg cabergoline (weekly). Doses of medication are either increased gradually, as tolerated, or decreased depending on tolerability and should be initiated with a small dose with food before bedtime. Patients should initially avoid activities that cause peripheral vasodilatation (e.g., hot baths), thereby decreasing the risk of postural hypotension. If side effects are troublesome, the subsequent dose should be halved, and doses increased gradually thereafter to achieve effective levels. Switching from one medication to another may be beneficial. Application of intravaginal bromocriptine administration has been advocated to alleviate adverse gastrointestinal events.[250]

Adverse Effects of Dopamine Agonists. Side effects of dopamine agonists are common. Nausea occurs in up to 50% of patients; nasal stuffiness, depression, and digital vasospasm occur, the latter more frequently with higher doses, as seen in patients with Parkinson disease. Postural hypotension can cause loss of consciousness, occurs infrequently, and is usually avoided by careful dosing. Signs and symptoms of psychosis or exacerbation of preexisting psychosis can be encountered in up to 1.3% of patients receiving bromocriptine.[251] Psychosis also occurs with other dopamine agonists, including cabergoline (personal experience). A history of psychotic symptoms should raise concerns about using these medications. If psychosis occurs in a patient in whom dopamine agonists are clearly the treatment of choice, the judicious combination of this agent and antipsychotic medication can be effective. A neuroleptic that is not a potent PRL stimulator, such as olanzapine, is preferred. CSF rhinorrhea occurs during dopamine agonist treatment in up to 6.1% of patients with macroadenomas, some of which are more resistant to dopamine agonists.[252] Other rarely reported serious side effects include hepatic dysfunction and cardiac arrythmias. Retroperitoneal fibrosis, pleural effusions and thickening, and restrictive mitral regurgitation have been reported in patients taking high doses of bromocriptine.[253,254]

High doses of dopamine agonists with serotoninergic properties have been associated with a risk for heart valve regurgitation.[255] In patients with Parkinson disease high doses of ergot-derived dopamine agonists may lead to increase of moderate to severe regurgitation in at least one valve.[255] Clinically significant heart valve regurgitation (moderate to severe, grade 3 to 4) was observed in pergolide-(23.4%) or cabergoline-treated (28.6%) patients.[256] These observations in patients receiving high ergot doses raise concern for patients with pituitary tumors who mostly take far lower drug doses. Although increased mild tricuspid regurgitation in patients receiving cabergoline for hyperprolactinemia was reported,[257] several reports have not shown evidence that low doses of cabergoline place patients at risk for significant valve disease.[258-260] More recent reports, however, have raised the possibility that heart valve disease might be associated with standard endocrine doses of cabergoline used for patients with prolactinomas. In patients treated with dopamine agonists for at least a year an increased prevalence in valvular calcification with no change in valvular function was observed.[261] Increased subclinical cardiac valve fibrosis was also noted in patients receiving cabergoline.[262] In a study of 51 patients receiving cabergoline for at least 1 year, the prevalence of trace mitral and tricuspid regurgitation and mild tricuspid regurgitation was increased.[263] Until a randomized controlled trial more firmly establishes the safety of low-dose cabergoline, physicians might consider ordering periodic echocardiograms for patients receiving cabergoline.

Radiation Therapy

Linear accelerator radiotherapy is effective in controlling or reducing the size of prolactinomas. However, this therapy takes years to achieve maximal effect. The usual recommended radiation dose is 4500 to 4600 centigray (cGy), and normalization of PRL was achieved in 18 of 36 patients at a mean of 7.3 years after treatment.[264] Hypopituitarism occurs as a side effect of radiation. In 36 patients with prolactinomas, of whom 83% had normal GH responses to insulin-induced hypoglycemia before therapy, 34 were GH deficient at 9 to 12 years after radiotherapy.[264] Gamma knife stereotactic radiosurgery is often effective in treating prolactinomas resistant to or intolerant of dopamine agonists.[265]

Surgery

The success rate of pituitary surgery correlates inversely with tumor size and serum PRL concentrations.[246] In a compilation of results in 31 published surgical series, serum PRL was normalized in 71% of 1224 patients

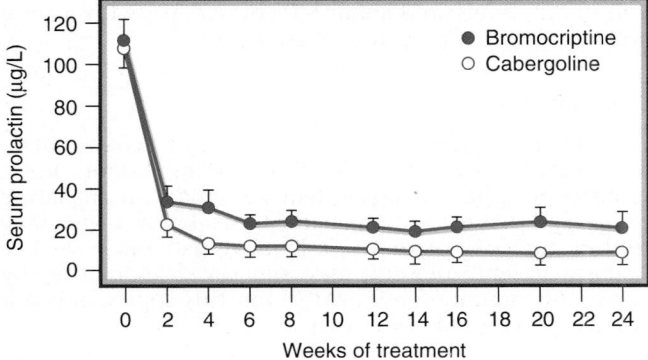

Figure 9-21 Comparison of bromocriptine and cabergoline in suppressing prolactin levels in women with hyperprolactinemia. (From Webster J, Piscitelli G, Polli A, et al. A comparison of cabergoline and bromocriptine in the treatment of hyperprolactinemic amenorrhea. *N Engl J Med.* 1996;331:904-909.)

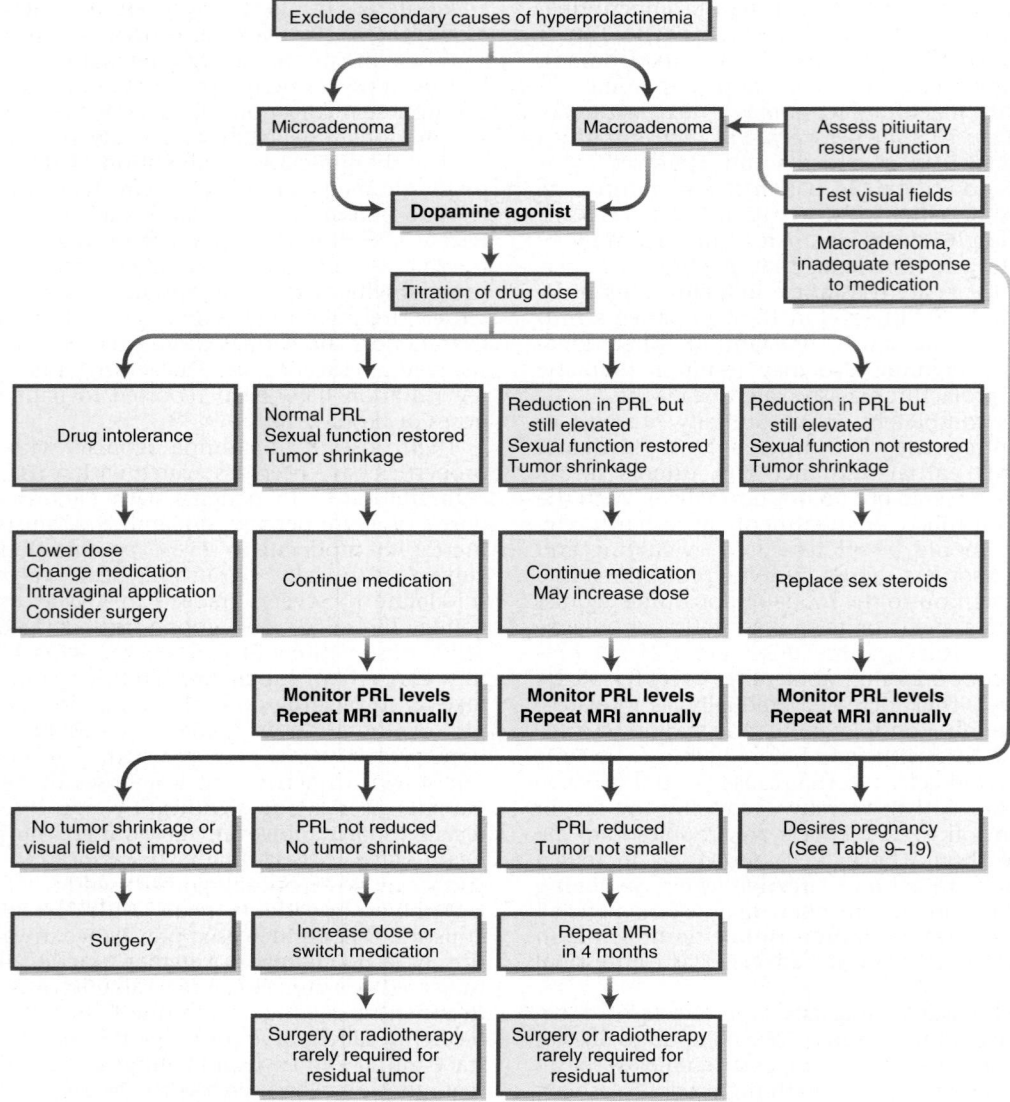

Figure 9-22 Prolactinoma management. After secondary causes of hyperprolactinemia have been excluded, subsequent management decisions are based on clinical imaging and biochemical criteria. MRI, magnetic resonance imaging; PRL, prolactin.

with microprolactinomas. Although surgical cure rates for microprolactinomas are high, the rate of hyperprolactinemia recurrence is also relatively high,[266] estimated at about 17% of patients initially considered cured.[267] In contrast, complete resection of macroprolactinomas, especially large invasive tumors, is difficult to achieve, and postoperative serum PRL level is normalized in only 32% of patients, with a 19% recurrence rate. The experience of the surgeon is of major importance, as the cure rate is not as favorable in the hands of neurosurgeons who perform only a limited number of procedures.

Although results of medical therapy are superior to those of surgery, there remains a role for surgery in these patients. Patients with prolactinomas who are resistant to dopamine agonist therapy are particularly well suited for surgery. If tumor removal is only partial, adjunctive radiation therapy should be considered. Prophylactic transsphenoidal surgery should also be considered in women whose prolactinomas are large enough to potentially threaten vision during pregnancy. A subset of patients cannot tolerate available dopamine agonists, and others prefer surgery

and refuse medication. Endoscopic endonasal transsphenoidal surgery has been used to resect prolactinomas. Most patients with microprolactinomas experience normalization of PRL levels, and about 50% of patients with macroprolactinoma are in remission after surgery.

Chemotherapy

There has been growing interest in employing chemotherapeutic agents for aggressive PRL-secreting tumors unresponsive to other therapies. Temozolomide, an alkylating compound that readily crosses the blood-brain barrier, may control tumor growth in individual patients.[268-270] The response to temozolomide may sometimes be predicted by low tumor staining for MGMT,[271] but this approach is not uniformly accepted (see earlier).

Pregnancy

The normal pituitary enlarges during pregnancy and prolactinomas may also increase in size during pregnancy. The

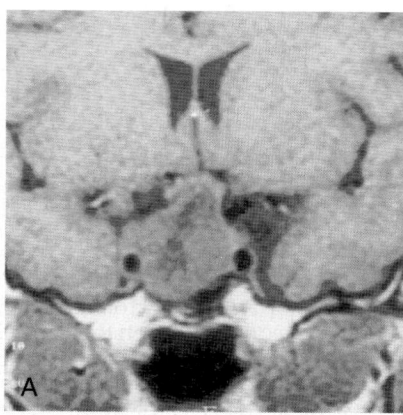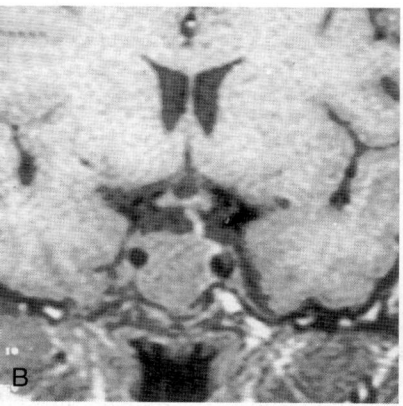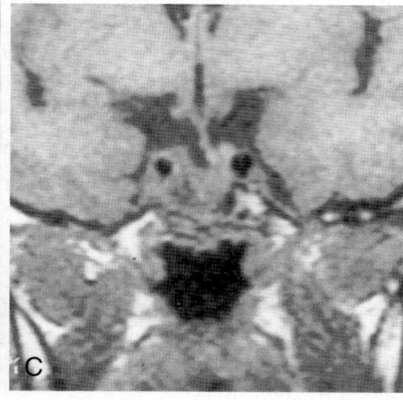

Figure 9-23 Shrinkage of macroadenoma by cabergoline in a woman harboring a macroadenoma at 22 weeks of gestation (**A**), when prolactin was 488 μg/L (**B**), and further reduction at 3 weeks postpartum (**C**). (Reproduced from Liu C, Tyrrell JB. Successful treatment of large macroprolactinoma with cabergoline during pregnancy. *Pituitary.* 2001;4:179-185.)

TABLE 9-19

Management of Patients with Prolactinomas Planning Pregnancies

Microadenoma	Macroadenoma
Discontinue dopamine agonist when pregnancy test is positive	Consider surgery before pregnancy
Periodic visual field examinations during pregnancy	Ensure bromocriptine sensitivity before pregnancy
Postpartum magnetic resonance imaging (MRI) after 6 weeks*	Monitor visual fields expectantly and frequently
	Administer bromocriptine if vision becomes compromised
	Or continue bromocriptine throughout pregnancy if tumor previously affected vision
	Consider high-dose steroids or surgery during pregnancy if vision is threatened or adenoma hemorrhage occurs
	Postpartum MRI after 6 weeks

*Pituitary MRI may be performed during pregnancy if deemed necessary.

incidence of pregnancy-associated tumor enlargement, as determined by development of abnormal visual fields, has been estimated to occur in 1.4% of women with microadenomas and 16% of women with macroadenomas.[272] In other reports, the risk for macroadenoma enlargement has been estimated to be as high as 36%. In a prospective analysis in which 57 patients with microprolactinomas were followed by formal visual field examinations during pregnancy, none developed visual disturbances. In contrast, 6 of 8 primiparous women with macroadenomas developed visual loss.[273] The results on patients with macroadenomas are likely skewed because these patients had been recommended for surgery prior to pregnancy.

Although dopamine agonists have been used during pregnancy to prevent tumor growth (Fig. 9-23),[274] it seems prudent to reduce fetal exposure to medication if possible. It is recommended that menstrual periods be allowed to occur naturally for a period of time (3-4 months) long enough to predict that a missed period might be a result of pregnancy (Table 9-19). Barrier contraception is recommended during this period. Within several days to a week of obtaining a positive hCG test, medication should be discontinued. Of 6239 pregnancies managed in this manner, bromocriptine therapy was not associated with increased abortions or terminations, prematurity, multiple

births, or infant malformations above that expected in the control population. There is no compelling evidence that other dopamine agonists are less safe, but pregnancy exposure to the other agonist forms are less comprehensively documented. Treatment options for patients harboring prolactinomas whose vision becomes impaired during pregnancy include administering bromocriptine during pregnancy, high-dose steroids, and surgical resection.[272] Of 53 pregnant women receiving bromocriptine mean offspring birth weight was normal, congenital abnormalities occurred in four babies, and physical and intellectual development of children was normal for up to 9 years. In an observational report on 380 pregnancies in women treated with cabergoline, early fetal exposure did not increase the risk of miscarriage or fetal malformation.[275] In 91 patients with hyperprolactinemia treated with cabergoline prior to pregnancy (*n* = 143), the medication was discontinued at 6 weeks of gestation, and no increase in miscarriages or fetal malformations was observed when monitored for up to 60 months.[276]

To avoid neurologic complications of tumor enlargement during pregnancy, it is recommended that women with prolactinomas be tested for sensitivity to dopamine agonists before proceeding with a pregnancy. If tumors are insensitive to dopamine agonist–related tumor shrinkage, prophylactic surgery could be appropriate. If the tumor is a macroadenoma approximating the optic chiasm, the likelihood of visual difficulties is greater and therefore undertaking surgery prior to pregnancy could be prudent.[277]

NONFUNCTIONING PITUITARY TUMORS

Nonfunctioning pituitary tumors comprise approximately 25% to 35% of pituitary tumors.[278] These tumors are clinically silent (i.e., do not actively secrete hormones), but they arise from pituitary cells capable of expressing hormones, including LH and FSH, ACTH, and TSH.

Gonadotroph Cell Tumors

Most nonfunctioning or hormonally silent tumors arise from gonadotroph cells, and they most frequently present as clinically nonfunctioning masses and are not associated with elevated serum gonadotropins. Yet, they usually express gonadotropin subunits detectable by immunohistochemistry. In a series of nonfunctioning adenomas, 42% of tumors immunostained for TSH β-subunit, 83% for LH β-subunit, 75% for FSH β-subunit, and 92% for α-subunit.[279] Although LH, FSH, and α-subunit are released from these nonfunctioning tumors when maintained in culture, production is usually not sufficient to elevate blood levels. These tumors are classified as null cell adenomas when they do not express glycoprotein subunits. A small subset of tumors do secrete sufficient hormone to elevate serum gonadotropin or α-subunit levels, which occasionally cause clinical syndromes.

Presentation

Clinically nonfunctioning tumors generally come to attention because of their large size or they are detected incidentally (incidentaloma) (Table 9-20). Of 506 incidentally discovered pituitary masses, 324 were clinically nonfunctioning tumors, and the remainder were cystic or parasellar masses.[280] A gradual visual deficit arising from optic chiasmal compression is common, and patients are often unaware of the disturbance. Recognition of visual field deficits is often delayed because formal visual fields are not routinely evaluated unless a defect is suspected clinically. In the absence of associated space-occupying or hormonal disorders these large tumors may go unrecognized for many years and be inadvertently detected on scans or radiographs performed for other purposes (incidentaloma). Sinusitis evaluation, pituitary apoplexy, or performance of a brain MRI for an unrelated indication (e.g., head trauma) may bring these tumors to clinical attention. Although not often the initial presenting complaint, these patients are commonly deficient in one or more pituitary hormones, as noted in two thirds of 56 patients with nonfunctioning macroadenomas.[35] Although the most commonly encountered endocrine symptoms are related to gonadotropin deficiency, quality of life may be decreased[281] or not altered, and daytime somnolence has also been reported.[282]

A very small subset of gonadotroph adenomas producing elevated serum FSH, LH, and α-subunit concentrations are considered functioning adenomas and may be associated with specific endocrine syndromes. Most of these are macroadenomas, and imaging may also reveal ovarian cysts or increased testicular volumes.[283] High serum FSH level, usually with a low LH level, is usually the only sign that a pituitary tumor secretes FSH. Female patients with such tumors may present with pelvic pain due to ovarian hyperstimulation.[284] High gonadotropin levels associated with menopause or testicular failure may complicate interpretation of gonadotropin levels, but both LH and FSH are high in primary gonadal failure (Table 9-21). LH-producing tumors are exceedingly rare and in males may cause elevations in serum testosterone with acne and skin oiliness. Very rarely, isosexual precocious puberty may be a presenting feature in children. Paradoxically, these patients may sometimes present with hypogonadism due to gonadal downregulation.

Evaluation

MRI, visual field examination, and pituitary hormones should be evaluated, the latter not only to detect hypopituitarism but also to exclude hormone overproduction that may not be clinically apparent. LH, FSH, α-subunit, PRL, T_4, triiodothyronine (T_3), TSH, cortisol, and IGF-1 levels should be measured. A serum cortisol at 8 AM, cortisol response to cosyntropism, or an insulin tolerance test can be helpful in excluding secondary adrenal insufficiency. Measurement of dehydroepiandrosterone sulfate (DHEAS) and DHEA may also be helpful in assessing adrenal function in these patients, for a low DHEAS may predate an actual lowering of cortisol levels. The extent of hormonal evaluation requires clinical judgment. When LH or FSH is elevated, the values must be interpreted in light of the patient's physiologic state. Elevated serum FSH in a woman with regular menstrual cycles would be interpreted differently from those detected in a menopausal patient; gonadotropin elevations in patients with primary gonadal failure are not generally limited to one hormone, and circulating α-subunit elevation is consistent with a pituitary tumor but not gonadal failure. TRH stimulation may differentiate elevated gonadotropin levels ascribed to end-organ failure or to independent tumor production. In patients harboring gonadotroph adenomas, increased FSH, LH, LH β-subunit, or α-subunit are evoked in response to TRH.[285] Calculating the molar ratio of LH or FSH to α-subunit may assist in the diagnosis.

Treatment

Clinical judgment should be used in determining appropriate therapy including surgery, surgery followed by radiotherapy, radiotherapy alone, or expectant observation (Fig. 9-24). No reliable tumor marker is predictive of mass growth or recurrence.

Surgery. If tumors threaten vision or are macroadenomas whose size threatens vital structures, transsphenoidal microscopic or endoscopic endonasal transsphenoidal surgery is recommended[286] (Table 9-22). Gross total mass removal was reported after surgery in 137 of 173 patients with

---

TABLE 9-20
Presentation of Gonadotroph Adenomas

Common	Uncommon
Clinically nonfunctioning macroadenoma	Intact gonadotrophin overproduction
Immunostain for gonadotrophin subunits (usually more than one)	Immunostain for subunits or intact hormone being hypersecreted
Usually discovered because of space-occupying effects or inadvertently	Usually discovered because of space-occupying effects or inadvertently
Pituitary deficiency	May cause clinical syndrome due to hormone overproduction
	Other pituitary hormones may be deficient

TABLE 9-21
Comparison of Characteristics of Gonadotroph Adenomas and Primary Hypogonadism in Men

Parameter	Gonadotroph Adenoma	Primary Hypogonadism
Puberty	Normal	Often incomplete
Fertility history	Normal	Decreased
Testicular size	Normal	Small
Serum testosterone level	Low to high	Low to normal
Testosterone response to hCG (when basal value is subnormal)	Brisk to well within normal range	Subnormal
Serum FSH level	High	High
Serum LH level	Usually normal or slightly high	High if testosterone is low
α-subunit level	High to very high	High
FSH response to TRH	Common	Absent
LHβ response to TRH	Very common	Absent

FSH, follicle-stimulating hormone; hCG, human chorionic gonadotropin; LH, luteinizing hormone; TRH, thyrotropin-releasing hormone.
Modified from Snyder PJ. Gonadotroph adenomas. In Melmed S, ed. *The Pituitary.* Philadelphia, PA: Elsevier; 1995:559-575.

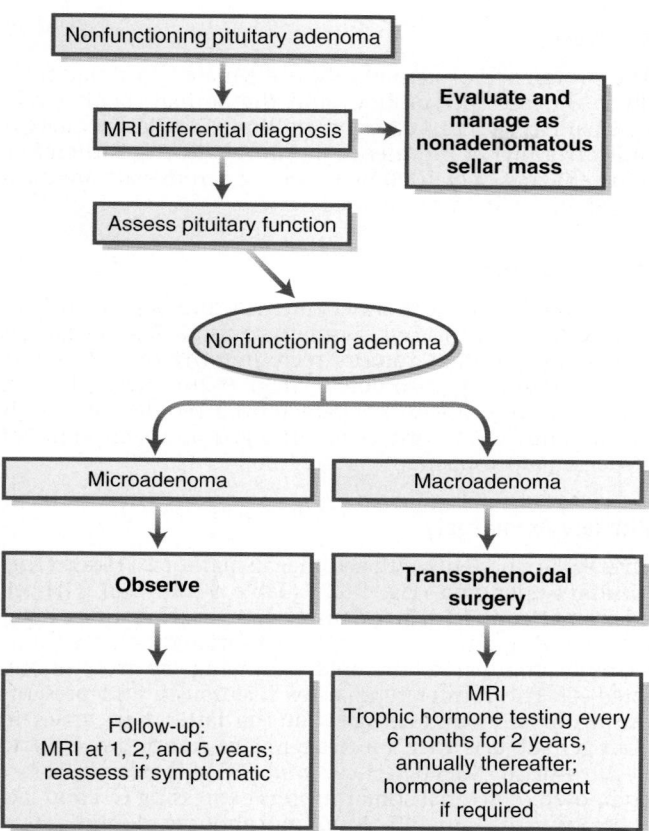

Figure 9-24 Management of nonfunctioning pituitary adenomas. Skilled magnetic resonance imaging (MRI) interpretation is crucial to diagnose nonadenomatous mass (e.g., meningioma, aneurysm, or other sellar lesion).

TABLE 9-22

Outcomes of Transsphenoidal Surgery for Nonfunctioning Pituitary Tumors

Outcomes	Risk (95% CI)	No. of Patients	I^2 (%)
Complete removal	0.20 (0.09-0.38)	1207	95
Surgical death	0.01 (0.01-0.02)	1232	0
CSF leakage/fistula	0.03 (0.02-0.06)	868	44
Meningitis	0.01 (0.01-0.03)	547	0
Transient diabetes insipidus	0.11 (0.04-0.27)	774	95
Persistent diabetes insipidus	0.05 (0.03-0.07)	622	14
New anterior pituitary deficits	0.09 (0.03-0.23)	850	87
Pituitary function improvement	0.30 (0.12-0.57)	714	89
New visual field defects	0.03 (0.02-0.04)	1032	0
Visual field defect improvement	0.78 (0.62-0.89)	795	93
Recurrence after surgery alone	0.18 (0.12-0.26)	734	79
ACTH improvement	0.37 (0.22-0.54)	145	64
ACTH worsening	0.39 (0.26-0.53)	49	0
TSH improvement	0.22 (0.07-0.51)	46	58
TSH worsening	0.17 (0.09-0.28)	160	31
LH/FSH improvement	0.23 (0.13-0.28)	190	71
LH/FSH worsening	0.10 (0.01-0.71)	143	89

Median follow-up was 4.29 years after surgery.
ACTH, adrenocorticotropic hormone; CSF, cerebrospinal fluid; FSH, follicle-stimulating hormone; LH, luteinizing hormone; TSH, thyroid-stimulating hormone (thyrotropin).
From Murad MH, Fernandez-Balsells MM, Barwise A, et al. Outcomes of surgical treatment for nonfunctioning pituitary adenomas: a systematic review and meta-analysis. Clin Endocrinol. 2010;73:777-791.

nonfunctioning pituitary adenomas,[286] and in another study gross total resection was achieved in 65.3% of 359 patients with improved vision or normalization of visual loss in 80.2% of affected patients.[287] In a comprehensive meta-analysis of surgical treatment for nonfunctioning adenomas[288] median follow-up was 4.29 years. Newer flap techniques have reduced the incidence of CSF leaks, and permanent diabetes insipidus occurs in up to 1.4% of patients.[30]

Postoperative Radiotherapy. An expectant follow-up of 65 patients after pituitary surgery for nonfunctioning adenomas showed that 32% of patients not receiving postoperative radiotherapy exhibited tumor regrowth during a mean follow-up period of 76 months.[289] Similar recurrence rates were observed in a retrospective follow-up of 212 patients.[290] In another study, tumor recurrence or regrowth occurred in 6% to 46% of patients not receiving radiotherapy after transsphenoidal surgery, and patients having received radiotherapy had a recurrence rate of 0% to 36%.[291] Nevertheless, despite the relatively high incidence of postoperative tumor regrowth, even after apparently complete resection, many neurosurgeons avoid routine postoperative radiation therapy. This approach requires advising careful follow-up, with periodic annual MRIs and visual evaluations, and encouraging patients to maintain medical follow-up.

Radiation can be offered if the tumor mass reexpands. In a retrospective study of 62 patients with nonfunctioning pituitary tumors treated with gamma knife radiosurgery, 60% experienced decreased tumor size, and 37% of tumors remained unchanged. However, the risk of developing new anterior pituitary hormone deficits at 5 years was 32%.[292]

In 140 consecutive patients undergoing gamma knife radiosurgery, the tumor mass was stabilized or decreased in 90% and median time to tumor progression was 14.5 years, with delayed hypopituitarism observed in 30% of patients.[293] In a large multicenter outcomes analysis of 512 patients undergoing gamma knife radiosurgery for nonfunctioning pituitary adenomas, median follow-up was 36 months. Progression-free tumor survival was associated with smaller tumor size and absence of suprasellar extension. New or aggravated pituitary failure was encountered in 21% of patients.[294] Because patients experience tumor regrowth even after radiation therapy, they too should undergo periodic posttreatment MRIs, albeit less frequently.[281]

Expectant Observation. For nonfunctioning microadenomas or small macroadenomas (incidentalomas), patients may be followed expectantly.[295] Some tumors do not grow over years or even decades. Nonfunctioning adenomas may grow insidiously postoperatively and are usually asymptomatic until such time that they are large enough to affect vision (Fig. 9-25). As 20% of tumor regrowth occurs more than 10 years after surgery, performing serial MRIs, perhaps indefinitely, is suggested.[296] Periodic, but less frequent, endocrine evaluation is also suggested because hypopituitarism occurs frequently and may be challenging to detect. A recent study has proposed testing for secondary adrenal insufficiency with low-dose cosyntropin (1 μg) together with measurement of cortisol, DHEA, and DHEAS, which enhance sensitivity of the test.[297]

Pregnancy

Microadenomas only very rarely lead to impaired vision during pregnancy, as opposed to macroadenomas, which do so with greater frequency.[298] Because macroadenomas do not usually shrink on medical therapy the risks of visual impairment arising during pregnancy must be weighed carefully and tumor resection may be indicated prior to pregnancy.

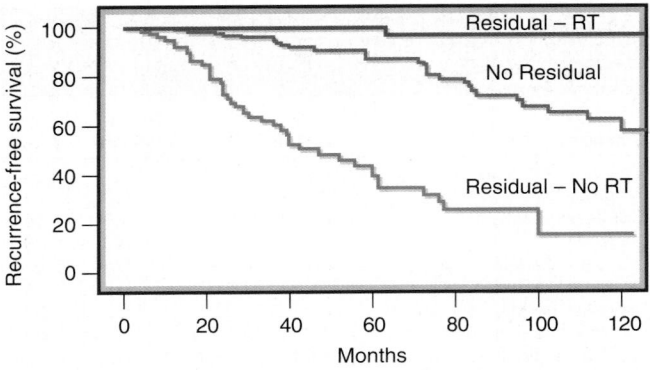

Figure 9-25 Recurrence-free survival by Kaplan-Meier plots in 436 patients with silent (clinically nonfunctioning) pituitary adenomas according to the presence or absence of residual adenoma after surgery and with or without radiation therapy (RT). (Adapted from Losa M, Mortini P, Barzaghi R, et al. Early results of surgery in patients with nonfunctioning pituitary adenoma and analysis of the risk of tumor recurrence. *J Neurosurg.* 2008;108(3):525-532. As adapted in Mayson SE, Snyder PJ. Silent (clinically nonfunctioning) pituitary adenomas. *J Neurooncol.* 2014;117:429-436.)

Medications

Medications are not usually effective in reducing tumor size and visual compromise. Although GnRH antagonists and somatostatin analogues modestly shrink tumors in a very few patients, they are not sufficiently effective to be recommended as therapy. Rarely, dopamine agonists have been reported to shrink some nonfunctioning tumors or to prevent regrowth.[299]

Silent ACTH-Producing Tumors

Tumors that immunostain for ACTH but are clinically silent are more aggressive than nonfunctioning tumors of pure gonadotroph cell origin. A subset of these hormonally silent yet aggressive tumors may actually express genetic markers of both corticotroph as well as gonadotroph lineages.[300] A review of 20 cases of silent ACTH-producing macroadenomas reported visual dysfunction as the most common presenting complaint (38%), and 13% presented with pituitary apoplexy.[301] Regular MRI follow-up is necessary for those tumors immunostaining positively for ACTH because recurrences occur more frequently in these tumors (see later).[302]

ACROMEGALY

In 1886 Pierre Marie published the first clinical description of disordered somatic growth and proportion and proposed the name "acromegaly." He also recognized cases previously described by others.[303] When relation of this syndrome to a pituitary tumor was later recognized, Benda showed in 1900 that these tumors comprise mainly adenohypophyseal eosinophilic cells, which he proposed to be hyperfunctioning.[304] Cushing, Davidoff, and Bailey documented the clinicopathologic features of acromegaly and demonstrated clinical remission of soft tissue signs after adenoma resection.[305] Evans and Long induced gigantism in rats injected with anterior pituitary extracts, confirming the association of a pituitary factor with somatic growth.[306] Establishment of the unequivocal pathophysiologic link between hyperfunctioning adenoma and acromegaly was the earliest example of a pituitary disorder to be clinically and pathologically recognized and appropriately managed by surgical excision of a hypersecreting source.

Incidence

The prevalence of acromegaly is estimated to range from 38 to 80 cases per million, and the annual incidence of new patients is 3 to 4 cases per million.[307-310] Recent surveys indicate a higher prevalence in Europe.[135,136] It is therefore apparent that over 1000 new cases of acromegaly are diagnosed annually in the United States.

Pathogenesis

GH and IGF-1 act both independently and dependently to induce features of hypersomatotropism. Acromegaly is caused by pituitary tumors secreting GH or very rarely by extrapituitary disorders[311] (Fig. 9-26). Regardless of the cause, the disease is characterized by elevated levels of GH and IGF-1 with resultant signs and symptoms of hypersomatotropism.

Pituitary Acromegaly

Over 95% of patients with acromegaly harbor a GH-secreting pituitary adenoma (Fig. 9-27) (Table 9-23). Pure GH-cell adenomas contain either densely or sparsely staining cytoplasmic GH granules, and these two variants are either slow (densely granulated) or rapidly growing (sparsely granulated).[312] The former type arises insidiously and presents during or after middle age, but the latter type arises in younger subjects with more aggressive tumor growth and florid disease. Mixed GH-cell and PRL-cell adenomas are composed of distinct somatotrophs expressing GH and lactotrophs expressing PRL. Monomorphous acidophilic stem cell adenomas arise from the common GH and PRL stem cell and often contain giant mitochondria and misplaced GH granule exocytosis. They grow rapidly, are invasive, and present with predominant features of hyperprolactinemia. Monomorphous mammosomatotroph cell adenomas express both GH and PRL from a single cell, but plurihormonal tumors may express GH with any combination of PRL, TSH, ACTH, and α-subunit. These patients present with clinical features of acromegaly as well as hyperprolactinemia, Cushing disease, or rarely hyperthyroxinemia. Somatotroph hyperplasia is difficult to distinguish from a GH-cell adenoma, and silver staining displays a well-preserved reticulin network without a surrounding pseudocapsule. The rigorous morphologic diagnosis of GH-cell hyperplasia is usually associated with stimulation by ectopic GHRH derived from an extrapituitary tumor causing acromegaly. *Silent somatotroph adenomas* immunostain positively for GH and are apparently clinically nonfunctional, although GH and PRL levels may in fact be modestly elevated in over half these patients.[313]

Pathogenesis of Somatotroph Cell Adenomas. Both pituitary as well as hypothalamic factors influence pituitary tumor pathogenesis. Even when exhibiting marked nuclear pleomorphism, mitotic activity, and invasiveness, these tumors are invariably benign.

Disordered GHRH Secretion or Action. Adenomas express receptors for GHRH, ghrelin,[314] and SRIF but activating mutations of either the GHRH or SRIF receptor have not been reported. GHRH directly stimulates GH gene expression and also induces somatotroph mitotic activity. Transgenic GHRH expression causes somatotroph hyperplasia and ultimately adenoma. Clinically, GHRH production by hypothalamic, abdominal, or chest neuroendocrine tumors causes somatotroph hyperplasia, and rarely adenoma, with resultant unrestrained GH secretion and acromegaly.[145] However, histologic examination of most pituitary GH-cell adenoma tissue specimens does not show hyperplastic

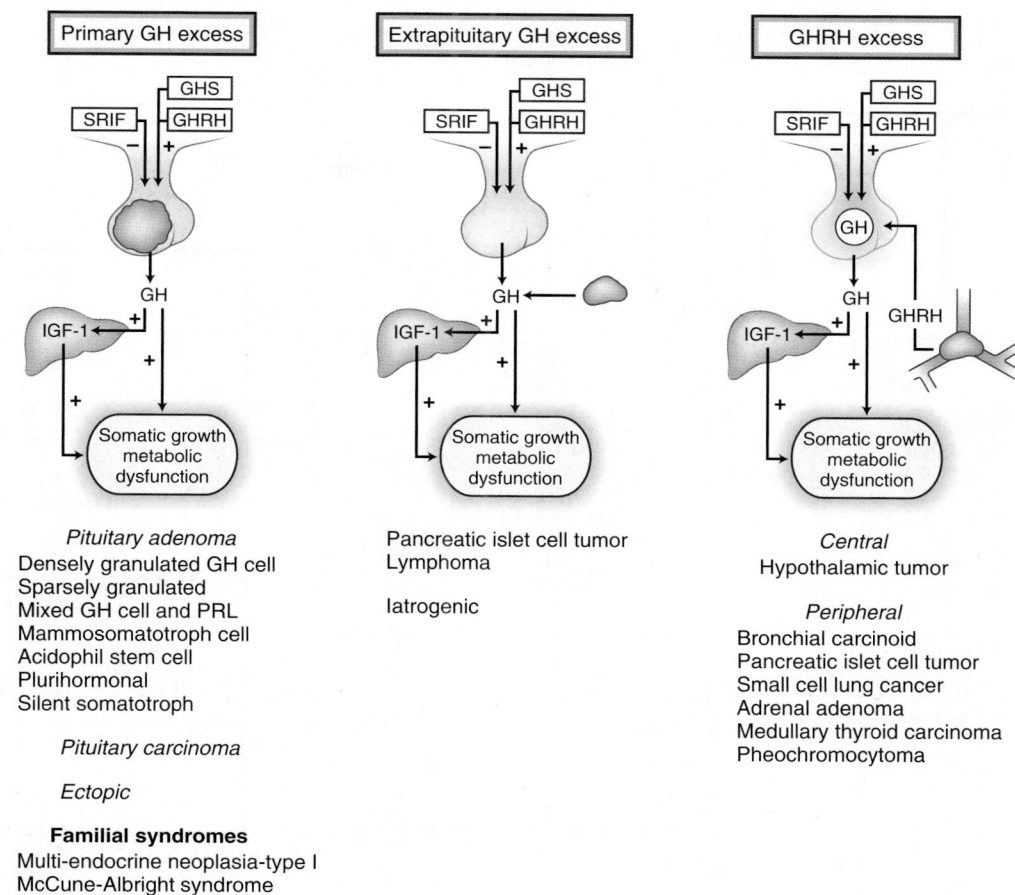

Figure 9-26 Pathogenesis of acromegaly. GH, growth hormone; GHRH, growth hormone–releasing hormone; GHS, growth hormone secretagogue; IGF-1, insulin-like growth factor type 1; PRL, prolactin; SRIF, somatotropin release–inhibiting factor. (From Melmed S. Medical progress: acromegaly. *N Engl J Med.* 2006;355:2558-2573.)

somatotroph tissue surrounding the adenoma, implying no generalized hypothalamic overstimulation. Failure to downregulate GH secretion during prolonged GHRH stimulation also points to a role for GHRH in maintaining persistent GH hypersecretion. Furthermore, a GHRH antagonist reduced human growth hormone production in 50 patients with acromegaly, suggesting a role for endogenous GHRH.[315] Expression of intra-adenomatous GHRH correlates with tumor size and activity, implying a paracrine role for GHRH in mediating adenoma growth.[316] GHRH modestly stimulates PRL secretion and up to 40% of patients with acromegaly also have hyperprolactinemia. Complete surgical resection of well-defined GH-secreting microadenomas usually results in a definitive cure of excess hormone secretion with very low postoperative tumor recurrence rates, strongly suggestive of intact hypothalamic function in these patients. Although basal GH levels are usually high in acromegaly, the episodic pulsatile pattern of GH release is intact, and the nocturnal GH surge usually preserved.[317]

Disordered Somatotroph Cell Function. A somatotroph mutation may be a prerequisite for the abnormal growth response to disordered GHRH secretion or action (see earlier). Monoclonal origin of somatotroph adenomas was determined by X-chromosome inactivation analysis of somatotroph tumor DNA.[141] An altered $G_s(\alpha)$ protein identified in a subset of GH-secreting pituitary adenomas leads to high levels of intracellular cAMP and GH hypersecretion.[147] Point mutations in two critical sites, Arg201, the site for adenosine diphosphate ribosylation, and Gly227, the guanosine triphosphate (GTP)-binding domain of $G_s(\alpha)$ proteins, prevent GTPase activity and result in constitutive adenyl cyclase activation. This dominant *GSP* mutant mimics GHRH effects, results in elevated cAMP levels, and is present in about 30% of GH-secreting tumors. Germline inactivating mutations of AIP have been found in a subset of familial somatotropinomas,[188,226] especially in younger patients with acromegaly or gigantism. However, no defined tumor suppressor gene has been identified for sporadic nonfamilial GH-secreting tumors.

Multiple Endocrine Neoplasia. GH-cell pituitary adenoma is a well-documented component of the autosomal dominant MEN1 syndrome, which also includes parathyroid and pancreatic tumors (see Chapter 41). MEN1, associated with germ cell inactivation of the *MENIN* tumor suppressor gene,[181] appears intact in sporadic GH-cell adenomas. Rarely, functional pancreatic tumors in patients with MEN1 also express GHRH.

The sequence of events leading to somatotroph clonal expansions appears multifactorial (see earlier). An activated oncogene may be required for initiating tumorigenesis, and promotion of tumor growth may require GHRH and other growth factor stimulation. The cellular mutation may not be sufficient to provide a growth advantage for a GH-secreting adenoma without additional disordered hypothalamic or paracrine growth factor signaling.

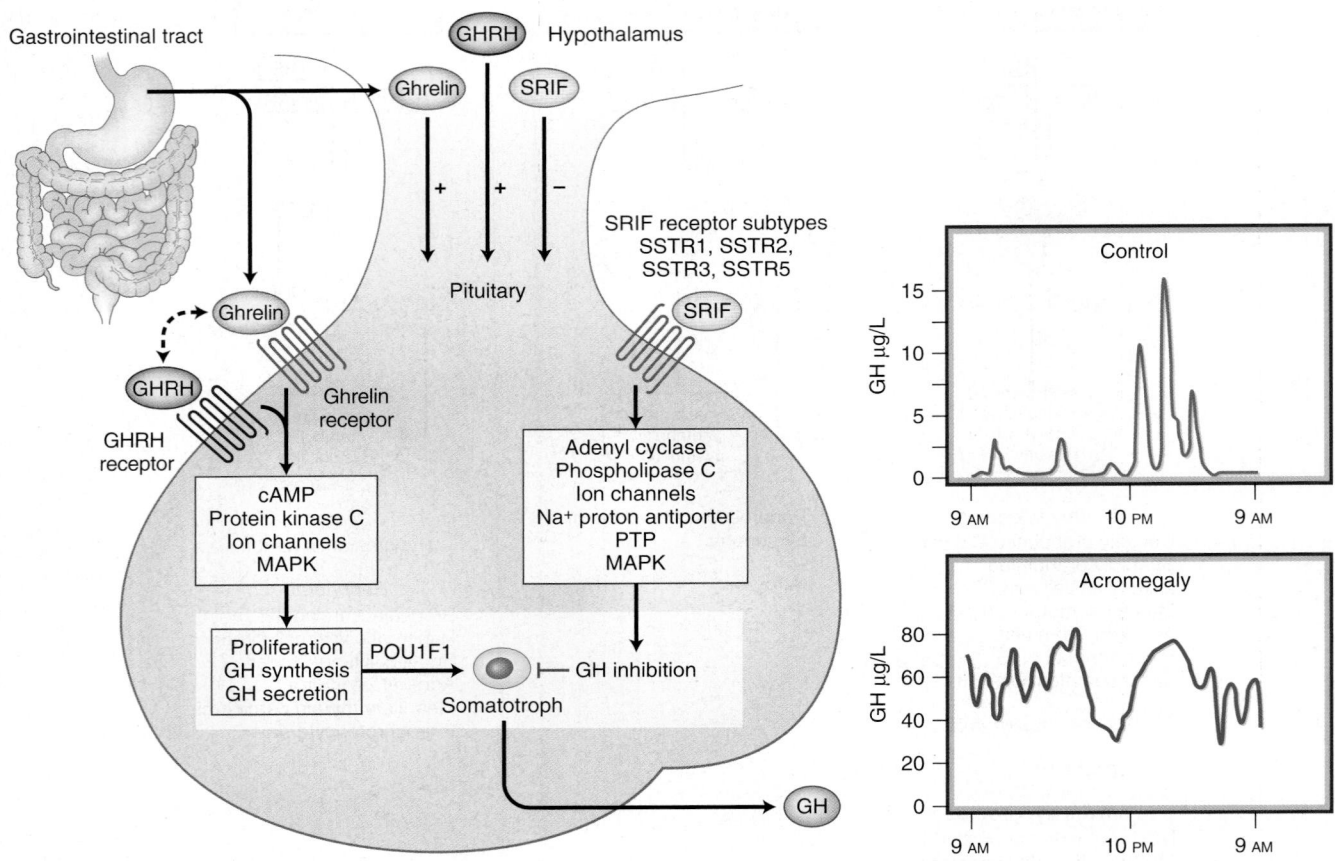

Figure 9-27 Normal and disrupted GHRH–GH–IGF-1 axis and molecular targets for therapy. Normal and disrupted GHRH–GH–IGF-1 axis in GH-secreting somatotroph adenomas, pituitary somatotroph cell development, and gene expression are determined by the POU1F1 transcription factor. Net GH secretion is determined by integration of hypothalamic, nutritional, hormonal, and intrapituitary signals. GH synthesis and secretion are induced by hypothalamic GHRH and gut-derived ghrelin. Hypothalamic SRIF suppresses GH secretion mainly by high-affinity binding to SSTR2 and SSTR5 receptor subtypes expressed on somatotrophs. SRIF ligands (SRLs) signal through SSTR2 and SSTR5 to control GH hypersecretion and shrink tumor mass. GH secretion patterns in a normal subject and in acromegaly are depicted in the insets showing secretory bursts (mainly at night) and daytime troughs. cAMP, cyclic adenosine monophosphate; GH, growth hormone; GHRH, growth hormone–releasing hormone; IGF-1, insulin-like growth factor type 1; MAPK, mitogen-activated protein kinase; PTP, protein tyrosine phosphatase; SRIF, somatotropin release–inhibiting factor; SSTR, SRIF receptor subtypes. (Modified from Melmed S. Acromegaly pathogenesis and treatment. *J Clin Invest.* 2009;119:3189-3202, used with permission.)

Extrapituitary Acromegaly

The source of excess GH secretion in acromegaly may not necessarily be of pituitary origin. Because management of ectopic acromegaly differs from that for pituitary-dependent GH hypersecretion, rigorous clinical and biochemical criteria should be fulfilled to confirm the diagnosis of ectopic acromegaly.[318] These criteria include demonstration of elevated circulating GHRH or GH levels in the absence of a primary pituitary lesion, a significant arteriovenous hormone gradient across the ectopic tumor source, biochemical and clinical cure of acromegaly after resection of the ectopic hormone-producing tumor, as well as normalization of the GHRH/GH/IGF-1 axis. Finally, GHRH or GH gene product expression should be shown. Patients with nonconclusive imaging or biochemical or clinical features of pituitary acromegaly may inadvertently be diagnosed as harboring a nonpituitary source of excess GH secretion, and then may be inappropriately treated.

GHRH Hypersecretion. Hypothalamic tumors, including hamartomas, choristomas, gliomas, and gangliocytomas, may produce GHRH with subsequent somatotroph hyperplasia, or even a pituitary GH-cell adenoma and resultant acromegaly[145] (see Fig. 9-26). Primary mammosomatotroph hyperplasia with no evidence for pituitary adenoma or an extrapituitary tumor source of GHRH has been described in gigantism.[319] The structure of hypothalamic GHRH was in fact elucidated from material extracted from pancreatic GHRH-secreting tumors in patients with acromegaly.[144] GHRH immunoreactivity is detectable in about 25% of carcinoid tumor samples, and bronchial carcinoids comprise most tumors associated with ectopic GHRH secretion.[320] Acromegaly in carcinoid patients, however, is uncommon. In a retrospective survey of 177 patients with acromegaly, only a single patient was identified with elevated plasma GHRH levels.[321] Rare pancreatic cell tumors, small cell lung cancers, adrenal adenoma, pheochromocytoma, and medullary thyroid, endometrial, and breast cancer express GHRH and may cause acromegaly.[322,323] Surgical resection of the tumor secreting ectopic GHRH should reverse the GH hypersecretion, and pituitary surgery is not required in these patients. Carcinoid syndrome with ectopic GHRH secretion can also be managed with somatostatin analogues, which lower GH and IGF-1 levels and suppress ectopic tumor elaboration of GHRH.[324]

Ectopic Pituitary Adenomas. GH-secreting adenomas may arise from ectopic pituitary remnants in the sphenoid sinus, petrous temporal bone, or nasopharyngeal cavity.[325] Very rarely, pituitary carcinoma may spread to the meninges, CSF, or cervical lymph nodes, resulting in functional GH-secreting metastases, which may be diagnosed by radiolabeled octreotide imaging (Octreoscan).[326]

TABLE 9-23

Causes of Acromegaly

Cause	Prevalence (%)	Hormonal Products	Clinical Features	Pathologic Characteristics
Excess GH Secretion				
Pituitary	98			
Densely granulated GH cell adenoma	30	GH	Slow growing, clinically insidious	Resemble normal somatotrophs, numerous large secretory granules
Sparsely granulated adenoma	30	GH	Rapidly growing, often invasive	Cellular pleomorphism, characteristic ultrastructure
Mixed GH cell and PRL cell adenoma	25	GH and PRL	Variable	Densely granulated somatotrophs, sparsely granulated lactotrophs
Mammosomatotroph cell adenoma	10	GH and PRL	Common in children; gigantism, mild hyperprolactinemia	Both GH and PRL in same cell, often same secretory granule
Acidophil stem cell adenoma		PRL and GH	Rapidly growing, invasive, hyperprolactinemia dominant	Distinctive ultrastructure, giant mitochondria
Plurihormonal adenoma		GH (PRL with αGSU, FSH/LH, TSH, or ACTH)	Often secondary hormonal products are clinically silent	Variable; either monomorphous or plurimorphous
GH cell carcinoma or metastases		GH	Usually aggressive	Documented metastasis
MEN1 (adenoma)		GH or PRL	Pancreatic, parathyroid, or pituitary tumors	Adenoma
McCune-Albright syndrome		GH, PRL	Classic triad	Hyperplasia
Ectopic sphenoid or parapharyngeal sinus pituitary adenoma		GH	Ectopic mass	Adenoma
Familial acromegaly		GH	Young patients	Large adenomas
Carney syndrome		GH	Classic syndrome	Adenoma
Extrapituitary Tumor				
Pancreatic islet-cell tumor	<1			Small pituitary
Excess GHRH Secretion				
Central—hypothalamic hamartoma, choristoma, ganglioneuroma	<1		Hypothalamic mass	Somatotroph hyperplasia
Peripheral—bronchial carcinoid, pancreatic islet cell tumor, small cell lung cancer, adrenal adenoma, medullary thyroid carcinoma, pheochromocytoma	1	GH, PRL	Systemic features	Somatotroph hyperplasia, rarely adenoma

ACTH, adrenocorticotropic hormone; FSH, follicle-stimulating hormone; GH, growth hormone; GHRH, growth hormone–releasing hormone; αGSU, glycoprotein α-subunit; LH, luteinizing hormone; MEN1, multiple endocrine neoplasia type 1; PRL, prolactin; TSH, thyroid-stimulating hormone.
Adapted from Melmed S. Acromegaly. *N Engl J Med.* 2006;355:2558-2573; and Melmed S, Braunstein GD, Horvath E, et al. Pathophysiology of acromegaly. *Endocr Rev.* 1983;4:271-290.

Peripheral Growth Hormone–Secreting Tumors. Lung adenocarcinoma, breast cancer, and ovarian tissues contain immunoreactive GH without clinical evidence of acromegaly. Rarely, GH-secreting intramesenteric pancreatic islet cell tumor[318] or a non-Hodgkin lymphoma[327] may cause acromegaly. These patients have a normal-sized or small pituitary gland on MRI, no GH response to TRH injection, and normal levels of circulating plasma GHRH.

Acromegaloidism. Rarely, patients who exhibit soft tissue and skin changes usually associated with acromegaly but normal baseline and dynamic GH and IGF-1 with no demonstrable pituitary or extrapituitary tumor have been termed *acromegaloid*. Pachydermoperiostosis should be considered in the differential diagnosis. Insulin resistance and defective IGF-1 binding have been demonstrated in cells derived from some patients with acanthosis nigricans, and treatment is symptomatic.

McCune-Albright Syndrome. This rare hypersecretory syndrome consists of polyostotic fibrous dysplasia, cutaneous pigmentation, sexual precocity, hyperthyroidism, hypercortisolism, hyperprolactinemia, and acromegaly due to somatotroph hyperplasia. In a comprehensive review of 112 patients published worldwide, acromegaly was reported in up to 30% of patients with the syndrome and was invariably associated with skull base fibrous dysplasia.[328]

About half of these patients have definitive imaging evidence for a pituitary adenoma. $G_s\alpha$ mutations have been detected in both endocrine and nonendocrine tissues.[148] GH hypersecretion is very rarely controlled by surgery, and these patients require somatostatin analogues, GH receptor antagonist, or pituitary irradiation.

Clinical Features

Manifestations of acromegaly are caused by either central pressure effects of the pituitary mass or peripheral actions of excess GH and IGF-1. Central features of the expanding pituitary mass are common to all pituitary masses and have already been described. In acromegaly, headache is often severe and debilitating. Local signs are especially important presenting features because a higher preponderance of macroadenomas (>65%) is encountered in acromegaly, as compared to mostly microadenomas for PRL-secreting tumors.[329]

Gigantism

Tall stature may be caused by a GH-secreting pituitary tumor or hyperplasia associated with several specific syndromes.[330] AIP mutations (see earlier) have been traced in the lineage of patients with gigantism.[331] About 20%

of patients have the McCune-Albright syndrome, with somatotroph hyperplasia or rarely pituitary adenomas. Somatotroph hyperplasia and acidophilic stem cell adenomas (with hyperprolactinemia) may rarely cause gigantism during infancy or early childhood, suggesting early hypersecretion of GHRH or disordered pituicyte cell differentiation.[319] Pituitary gigantism should be considered in children who are more than 3 standard deviations above normal mean height for age, or more than 2 standard deviations over their adjusted mean parental height. The biochemical diagnosis is similar to that for acromegaly (i.e., GH levels are in excess of 1 µg/L after a glucose load and serum IGF-1 concentrations are elevated). In children undergoing pubertal growth spurts, GH responses to glucose may be paradoxical and serum IGF-1 concentrations are often physiologically elevated. Thus, the diagnosis requires clear-cut MRI evidence for a pituitary lesion. The differential diagnosis includes familial tall stature,

redundancy of Y chromosomes, Marfan syndrome, and homocystinuria. Aggressive control of the tumor mass as well as hormone hypersecretion is important to mitigate long-term tissue damage from excess GH and IGF-1. Surgery is recommended as primary therapy, and postoperative somatostatin receptor ligands (SRLs) and the GH receptor antagonist have been used effectively.[332,333] Radiation therapy should be followed by life-long serial evaluation of pituitary function.

Clinical Features of Acromegaly

Effects of hypersomatotropism on acral and soft tissue growth and metabolic function occur insidiously over several years (Table 9-24)[334] (Figs. 9-28 and 9-29). As a result, acromegaly remains underrecognized; the slow onset and elusive symptomatology often result in delayed diagnosis, ranging from 6.6 to 10.2 years, with a mean

---

TABLE 9-24

Clinical Features of Acromegaly*

Local Tumor Effects	Endocrine-Metabolic Effects
Pituitary enlargement Visual field defects Cranial nerve palsy Headache	*Reproductive* Menstrual abnormalities Galactorrhea Decreased libido, impotence, low sex hormone–blinding globulin
Somatic Effects	
Acral Enlargement Thickening of soft tissues in hands and feet	*Multiple Endocrine Neoplasia Type 1 (MEN1)* Hyperparathyroidism Pancreatic islet cell tumors
Musculoskeletal Gigantism Prognathism Jaw malocclusion Arthralgias and arthritis Carpal tunnel syndrome Acroparesthesia Proximal myopathy Hypertrophy of frontal bones	*Carbohydrates* Impaired glucose tolerance Insulin resistance and hyperinsulinemia Diabetes mellitus
Skin Hyperhidrosis Oily Skin tags	*Lipids* Hypertriglyceridemia
Colon Polyps	*Minerals* Hypercalciuria, increased 1,25-hydroxyvitamin D$_3$ Urinary hydroxyproline
Cardiovascular Left ventricular hypertrophy Asymmetric septal hypertrophy Cardiomyopathy Hypertension Congestive heart failure	*Electrolytes* Low renin Increased aldosterone
Pulmonary Sleep disturbances Sleep apnea—central and obstructive Narcolepsy	*Thyroid* Low thyroxine-binding globulin Goiter
Visceromegaly Tongue Thyroid Salivary gland Liver Spleen Kidney Prostate	

*Most soft tissue and metabolic changes are reversible by tight hormonal control. Bony changes, hypertension, and central sleep apnea are generally not reversible.
Modified from Bonert V, Melmed S. Acromegaly. In: Bar S, ed. *Contemporary Endocrinology*. Totowa, NJ: Humana Press; 2002:201-228.

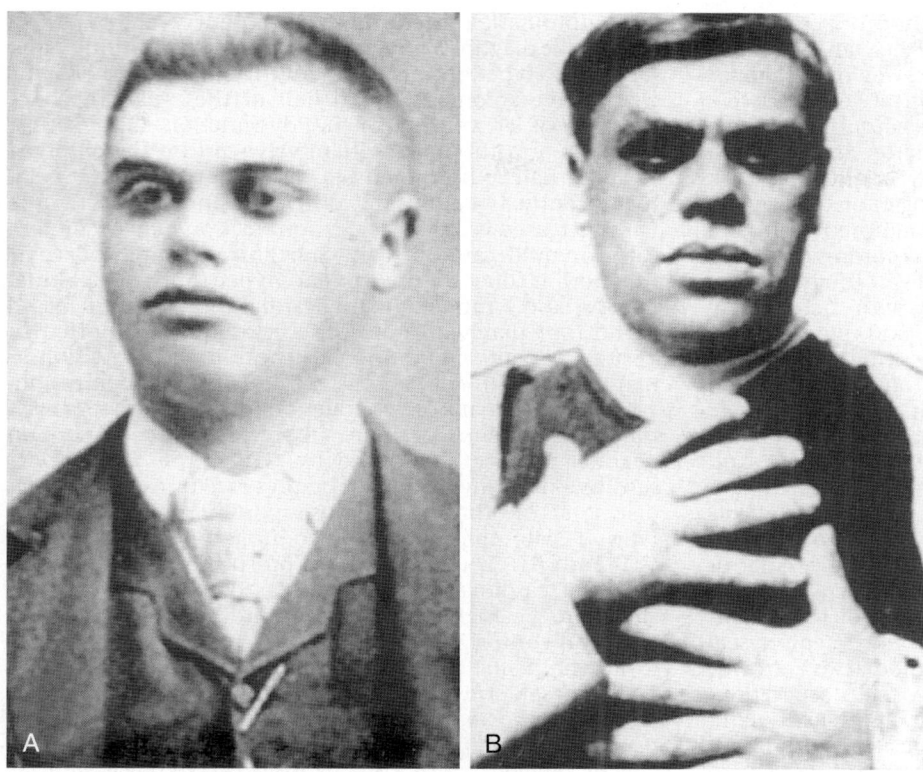

Figure 9-28 Harvey Cushing's first acromegaly patient. **A,** Some years before presentation and (**B**) at admission. (From Jane JA, Laws ER. History of acromegaly. In: Wass J, ed. *Handbook of Acromegaly.* Bristol, UK: BioScientifica; 2001:3-15.)

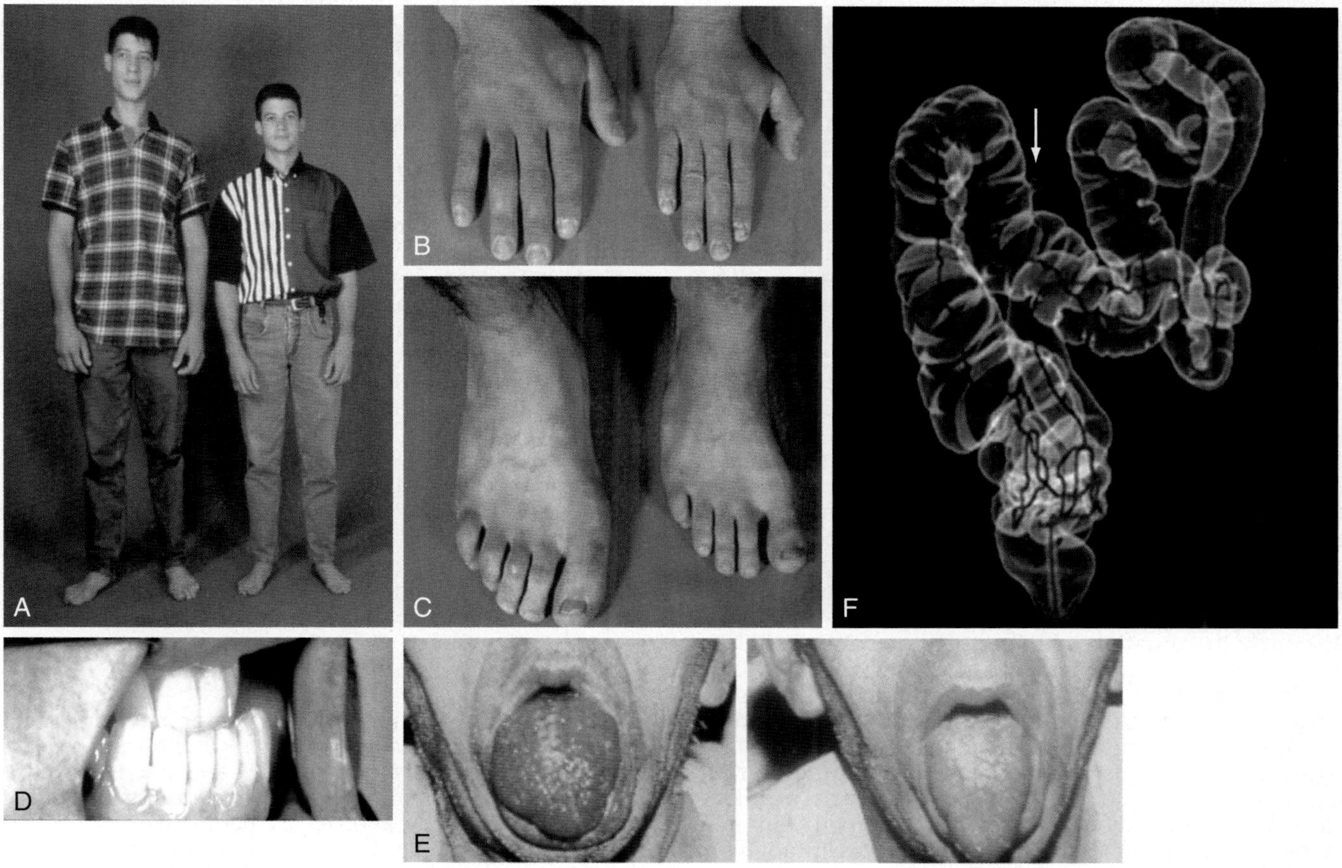

Figure 9-29 Clinical features of acromegaly. **A** to **C,** Features of acromegaly/gigantism in identical twins. A 22-year-old man with gigantism due to excess growth hormone is shown to the left of his identical twin. The increased height and prognathism (**A**) and enlarged hand (**B**) and foot (**C**) of the affected twin are apparent. Their clinical features began to diverge at the age of approximately 13 years. **D,** Increased incisor spacing and prognathism in patient with acromegaly. **E,** Macroglossia (*left*) and a normal tongue (*right*). **F,** Dolicomegacolon in acromegaly as visualized by computed tomography colonography. (A-C from Gagel R, McCutcheon IE. Images in clinical medicine: pituitary gigantism. *N Engl J Med.* 1999;324:524, used with permission. D and E from Turner HE. Clinical features, investigation and complications of acromegaly. In: Wass J, ed. *Handbook of Acromegaly.* Bristol, UK: BioScientifica; 2001, used with permission. F from Resmini E, Tagliafico A, Bacigalupo L, et al. Computed tomography colonography in acromegaly. *J Clin Endocrinol Metab.* 2009;94:218-222, used with permission.)

delay of almost 9 years.[335] In a comparison of acromegaly features observed between 1981 and 1994, and between 1995 and 2006, the delay in diagnosis was quite similar (5.9 vs. 5.2 years). Although biochemical features were also remarkably similar, sleep apnea and colon polyps were more frequently encountered in the latter time frames, likely reflecting enhanced awareness.[336] Patients may seek care for dental, orthopedic, rheumatologic, or cardiac disorders. Only 13% of 256 patients diagnosed during a 20-year period presented with primary symptoms of altered facial appearance or enlarged extremities.[337] In a review of several hundred patients presenting with acromegaly worldwide, 98% had acral enlargement, and hyperhidrosis was prominent in 70%.[334] When presenting early, facial and peripheral features are usually not obvious and serial review of old photographs often accentuates the progress of subtle physical changes. Characteristic features include large fleshy lips and nose, spadelike hands, frontal skull bossing, and cranial ridges. Enlarged tongue, bones, salivary glands, thyroid, heart, liver, and spleen are the effects of generalized visceromegaly. Clinically apparent hepatosplenomegaly, however, is rare. Increase in shoe, ring, or hat size is commonly reported. Progressive acral changes may lead to facial coarsening and skeletal disfigurement especially if excess GH secretion begins prior to epiphyseal closure.[338] These changes include mandibular overgrowth with prognathism, maxillary widening, teeth separation, jaw malocclusion overbite, large nose, and coarse oily skin. Sonorous voice deepening occurs in association with laryngeal hypertrophy and enlarged paranasal sinuses. Up to half of patients may experience joint symptoms severe enough to limit daily activities. Arthropathy occurs in about 70% of patients, most of whom exhibit joint swelling, hypermobility, and cartilaginous thickening.[339] These signs may often persist after complete remission.[340] Local periarticular fibrous tissue thickening may cause joint stiffening or deformities and nerve entrapment. Knees, hips, shoulders, lumbosacral joints, elbows, and ankles are affected as monoarticular or polyarticular arthritides, but joint effusions rarely develop. Spinal involvement includes osteophytosis, disk space widening, and increased anteroposterior vertebral length, which may result in dorsal kyphosis. Neural enlargement and wrist tissue swelling may lead to carpal tunnel syndrome in up to half of all patients. Both median and ulnar nerve cross-sectional areas increase and nerve conduction is abnormal.[341] Chondrocyte proliferation with increased joint space occurs early, and ulcerations and fissures of weight-bearing cartilage areas are often accompanied by new bone formation. Debilitating osteoarthritis may result in bone remodeling, osteophyte formation, subchondral cysts, narrowed joint spaces, and lax periarticular ligaments. Vertebral fractures occur with increasing frequency, and osteophytes commonly occur at the phalangeal tufts and over the anterior aspects of spinal vertebrae.[342-344] Ligaments may ossify and periarticular calcium pyrophosphate deposition occurs. Although the duration of hypersomatotropism correlates with clinical severity of the joint changes, it is unclear whether higher GH levels correlate with increased articular disease activity. Therapeutic responses usually depend on the degree of irreversible bony changes already in place. Hyperhidrosis and malodorous oily skin are common early signs, occurring in up to 70% of patients. Facial wrinkles, nasolabial folds, and heel pads thicken, and body hair may become coarsened,[345] attributed to glycosaminoglycan deposition and increased connective tissue collagen production. Skin tags are common and may be markers for the adenomatous colonic polyps. Raynaud's phenomenon is reported in up to one third of patients.

Symptomatic cardiac disease is present in about 20% of patients at diagnosis and is a major cause of morbidity and fatality.[346] Hypertension is present in about 50% of patients with active acromegaly, and half of these patients have evidence of left ventricular (LV) dysfunction. LV hypertrophy with or without regurgitant valve disease[347] is observed in about half of normotensive patients. Asymmetric septal hypertrophy is commonly observed, and cardiac failure with increased ventricular ejection fraction may occur with early or mild cardiomegaly. Subclinical LV diastolic dysfunction is due to myocardial hypertrophy, interstitial fibrosis, and lymphocytic myocardial infiltrates. Increased aortic root diameter and aortic ectasia were reported in 26% of patients.[348] Resting electrocardiograms are abnormal in about 50% of patients, with ST-segment depression, T-wave abnormalities, conduction defects, and arrhythmias. Plasma renin levels are suppressed, and renal sodium channel activity is induced by GH at the aldosterone-sensitive distal nephron.[349] The presence of cardiovascular disease at the time of diagnosis portends high mortality rates despite improved cardiac function after effective GH and IGF-1 control. In a prospective study of 30 patients, cardiovascular responses to SRL therapy were shown to be highly variable, despite attainment of biochemical control.[350]

Prognathism, thick lips, macroglossia, and hypertrophied nasal structures may obstruct airways. Irregular laryngeal mucosa, cartilage hypertrophy, tracheal calcification, and cricoarytenoid joint arthropathy lead to unilateral or bilateral vocal cord fixation or laryngeal stenosis with voice changes. Tracheal intubation may be particularly difficult in patients undergoing anesthesia, and tracheostomy may be required. Both central respiratory depression and airway obstruction lead to paroxysmal daytime sleep (narcolepsy), sleep apnea, and habitual excessive snoring. Obstructive sleep apnea, characterized by excessive daytime sleepiness with at least five episodes of apnea per hour of sleep, causes daytime somnolence, especially in men with acromegaly, who also may have a ventilation-perfusion defect with hypoxemia. Sleep apnea may also be central in origin and associated with higher GH and IGF-1 levels.[351]

Synovial edema leads to hyperplastic wrist ligaments and tendons that contribute to painful median nerve compression. Peripheral acroparesthesias and symmetric peripheral neuropathy should be distinguished from diabetic neuropathy, which may occur secondarily to acromegaly.[352] Proximal myopathy may also be accompanied by myalgias, cramps, and nonspecific electromyogram myopathic changes. Exophthalmos may be present but may be masked by frontal bossing. Hypertrophied tissue surrounding the canal of Schlemm may impede aqueous filtration, leading to open-angle glaucoma. Progressive facial and bodily disfigurement often leads to lowered self-esteem. Depression and mood swings may occur secondarily to physical deformity, with impaired quality of life.[353]

Growth Hormone and Tumor Formation

The early practice of hypophysectomy for managing metastatic carcinoma was based on evidence implicating GH as a factor in tumor development. GH and IGF-1 as well as insulin may exhibit direct or indirect mitogenic effects on mammalian cells and act as permissive cell growth stimulators.[354,355] Nevertheless, a compelling cause-and-effect relationship of acromegaly with cancer has not been established.[356,357] Overall, benign colon polyps have been reported in 45% of 678 patients in 12 prospective studies (Table 9-25). However, a controlled prospective study in

TABLE 9-25

Colon Polyps in Acromegaly*

No. Patients	No. Males/Females	Mean Age (yr)	Adenoma	Hyperplastic	Total	Carcinoma	Reference
17	10/7	49	5	3	8	2	Klein (1982)
12	11/11	56	2	1	3	2	Ituarte (1984)
29	NA	NA	4	0	4	2	Brunner (1990)
23	12/11	47	8	1	9	0	Ezzat (1991)
54	26/28	47	5	11	19	0	Ladas (1994)
50	25/25	25-70	11	12	23	1	Colao (1997)
49	30/19	54	11	5	16	0	Vasen (1994)
31	11/20	52	11	8	16	0	Terzolo (1994)
103	49/54	51	23	25	48	0	Delhougne (1995)[356]
129	68/60	57	33	42	75	6	Jenkins (1997)
115	63/69	54.8‡	27	18	45	3	Renehan (2000)[358]
66†	NA	32.7	25	18	43	1	Jenkins (2000)
Totals							
678			165 (24%)	144 (21%)	309 (45%)	17 (2.5%)	

*Incidence of colonic lesions in 678 patients prospectively evaluated in 12 studies. Of note, up to 45% of asymptomatic males age >50 years harbored colon adenomas.
†Repeat colonoscopy.
‡Median age.
NA, not available.
From Lieberman DA. Use of colonoscopy to screen asymptomatic adults for colorectal cancer. *N Engl J Med.* 2000;343:162-168; derived from Melmed S. Acromegaly and cancer: not a problem? *J Clin Endocrinol Metab.* 2001;86:2929-2934.

161 patients showed no increased colon polyp incidence in acromegaly.[358] More than three skin tags in patients aged over 50 may be peripheral markers for the presence of adenomatous colon polyps, unrelated to GH or IGF-1 serum levels. Hypertrophic mucosal folds and colonic hypertrophy are commonly present, and dolicomegacolon may be visualized by CT colonography.[359] Markedly increased incidence of gallbladder polyps[360] and benign prostate hypertrophy with no appreciable increase in prostate cancer rates[361] have been reported. Analysis of nine retrospective reports (1956-1998) encompassing 21,470 person-years at risk, yielded no significant overall increased cancer incidence.[362] Cancer incidence was in fact lower than expected in 1362 patients with acromegaly in the United Kingdom, and the enhanced colon cancer mortality rate observed in this study correlated with GH levels rather than increased incidence.[357] In contrast, subsequent studies have reported increased incidence of thyroid, bladder, and kidney cancers.[363,364] Thus, although disordered cell proliferation and increased risk for promotion of coexisting neoplasms could be anticipated from elevated GH and IGF-1 levels, a significantly enhanced cancer incidence has not been reported consistently in acromegaly. Colon cancer appears to be of particular concern, and screening colonoscopy should be performed at diagnosis in all patients. As patients are now living longer as a result of improved biochemical control, long-term prospective controlled studies are required to resolve this question in an aging population.

Endocrine Complications

About 30% of patients exhibit elevated serum PRL levels (up to 100 μg/L or more), with or without galactorrhea. Functional pituitary stalk compression by a pituitary mass prevents lactotroph access of hypothalamic dopamine, releasing the cell from tonic hypothalamic inhibition. GH-secreting adenoma subtypes may also concomitantly secrete PRL. As GH behaves as an agonist for breast PRL-binding sites, the tumor may cause galactorrhea in the face of normal PRL levels. Tumor mass compressing surrounding normal pituitary tissue may also cause hypopituitarism. Over half of all patients have amenorrhea or impo-

tence,[329,365] and secondary thyroid or adrenal failure is present in about 20% of patients. Gonadal dysfunction may result in bone loss and vertebral fractures.[343,344] The direct anti-insulin effect of GH causes carbohydrate intolerance and patients may also develop insulin-requiring diabetes mellitus. Carbohydrate intolerance and insulin requirements improve rapidly on lowering GH after surgery or somatostatin analogue therapy. Hypertriglyceridemia (type IV), hypercalciuria, and hypercalcemia also occur. Thyroid dysfunction in acromegaly may be associated with diffuse or nodular toxic or nontoxic goiter or Graves disease, especially as IGF-1 is a major determinant of thyroid cell growth.[366] Associated MEN1 features may be present in affected individuals, including hypercalcemia with hyperparathyroidism or pancreatic tumors.

Morbidity and Mortality

In a meta-analysis of 16 studies, overall mortality rate was reported to be increased in acromegaly with a standardized mortality ratio of 1.72. Higher mortality rates were observed prior to 1993, likely reflecting the positive impact of introduction of somatostatin analogues, improved surgical technique, and enhanced cardiac therapies.[367] Cardiovascular disease, respiratory disorders, and diabetes contribute to enhanced (threefold) mortality rate in acromegaly.[368,369] Cardiovascular disease is the leading cause of death followed by respiratory disease (18%) and cerebrovascular disease (14%). Diabetes mellitus, occurring in 20% of patients, is associated with 2.5 times the predicted mortality rate, and hypertension is present in about half of all patients[369] (Fig. 9-30). The most significant mortality rate determinants are GH levels greater than 2.5 μg/L, elevated IGF-1 levels, the presence of coexisting hypertension and cardiac disease, older age, a history of pituitary irradiation, and inadequately replaced ACTH-dependent adrenal insufficiency.[53] Importantly, overtreatment of adrenal insufficiency with doses of hydrocortisone that are more than 25 mg daily also is predictive of mortality rate.[53] In the large U.K. West Midlands acromegaly registry comprising 501 patients, a last available recorded GH level of 1 ng/mL or less versus 1 ng/mL or more was highly predictive of mortality rate. However, when summated over time in an

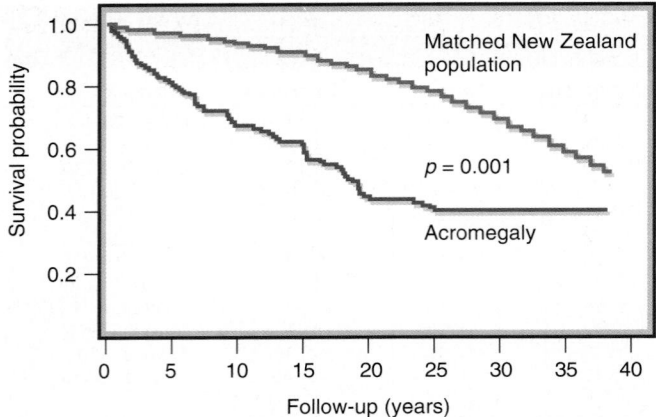

Figure 9-30 Documented determinants of mortality rate outcome in retrospective studies of acromegaly. (Data integrated from Holdaway IM, Rajasoorya RC, Wong J, et al. The natural history of treated functional pituitary adenomas. In: Webb S, ed. *Pituitary Tumors.* Bristol, UK: BioScientifica; 1998:31-42.)

unbiased fashion, the relative risk of fatality appeared to be associated with a GH cutoff level of 5 ng/mL.[370] Moreover, control of GH levels to less than 2.5 µg/L and normal IGF-1 levels after surgery or medical treatments is associated with significant reductions of both morbidity and mortality rates.[369]

Diagnosis

Measurement of Growth Hormone and IGF-1 Levels

The diagnosis of acromegaly requires measurement of a GH nadir during a 75-g glucose load of less than 0.4 ng/mL using ultrasensitive GH assays or GH less than 1.0 ng/mL using standard assays with an accompanying elevated IGF-1 level[371-373] (Fig. 9-31). In healthy subjects serum GH levels initially fall after oral glucose administration and subsequently increase as plasma glucose declines. However, in patients with acromegaly, oral glucose fails to suppress GH; GH levels may increase, remain unchanged, or fall modestly in approximately one third of patients. Basal morning (AM) and random GH levels are usually elevated in acromegaly. Because of the episodic nature of GH secretion, however, serum concentrations may normally fluctuate from "undetectable" up to 30 µg/L. Unlike the largely undetectable nadir GH levels in normal subjects, those with acromegaly sampled over 24 hours contain detectable levels of GH (>2 µg/L).[373] Evoked GH responses to GHRH administration are not of diagnostic use. A higher episodic GH pulse frequency occurs, which often persists after surgical adenoma resection. Random GH levels measured with sensitive assays in acromegaly may be as low as 0.37 µg/L with persistently elevated postoperative IGF-1 levels.[374] Serum IGF-1 levels are high[375,376] and correlate with clinical features (Fig. 9-32). Basal GH levels determine ambient circulating IGF-1 levels in a log-linear fashion.[377] Age- and gender-matched IGF-1 elevations may persist for several months after GH levels are biochemically controlled after surgery. Elevated IGF-1 levels are also encountered during pregnancy and late puberty. A high IGF-1 level is thus highly specific for acromegaly and correlates with clinical indices of disease activity. IGF-binding protein 3 (IGFBP3) levels are also elevated, but provide little added diagnostic value. GH-secreting adenomas exhibit discordant GH responses to TRH and GnRH administration in up to 50% of patients, but these adjunctive tests are rarely required to confirm the diagnosis.

Differential Diagnosis of Acromegaly

The overwhelming majority of patients with acromegaly harbor a GH-cell pituitary adenoma; rarely extrapituitary acromegaly should be considered. Nevertheless, distinguishing pituitary versus extrapituitary acromegaly is important for planning effective management. Regardless of the cause of unrestrained GH secretion, IGF-1 levels are invariably elevated and GH levels fail to suppress (<1 µg/L) after an oral glucose load. When clinical features of acromegaly are associated with normal GH and IGF-1 levels, "burned out" or "silent" acromegaly associated with an infarcted pituitary adenoma, often with a secondary empty sella, should be considered.[378] About 5% of consecutive patients with proven GH-cell adenomas have "normal" GH and elevated IGF-1 levels. It is likely that improved GH assay sensitivity will unmask abnormal GH secretion in these patients. Dynamic pituitary testing (to TRH, dopamine) does not distinguish patients with pituitary adenomas from those harboring extrapituitary tumors. Plasma GHRH levels are invariably elevated in patients with peripheral GHRH-secreting tumors but are normal or low in patients with pituitary adenomas.[321] GHRH plasma level measurement is precise and cost-effective for the diagnosis of excess ectopic GHRH production. Peripheral GHRH levels are not elevated in patients with hypothalamic GHRH-secreting tumors, presumably because eutopic hypothalamic GHRH secretion into the hypophyseal portal system does not appreciably enter the systemic circulation.

Encountering unique or unexpected clinical features, including respiratory wheezing or dyspnea, facial flushing, peptic ulcers, or renal stones, will sometimes indicate the diagnosis of a nonpituitary endocrine tumor. Hypoglycemia, hyperinsulinemia, hypergastrinemia, and rarely hypercortisolism, all not usually encountered in pituitary acromegaly, should justify an evaluation for an extrapituitary source of GH excess. MRI and CT scanning are employed to localize pituitary or extrapituitary tumor. Routine abdominal or chest imaging of all patients will yield a very low incidence of true positive cases of ectopic tumor, and such screening is not recommended as cost effective. A normal-sized or small pituitary gland, or clinical and biochemical features of other tumors known to be associated with extrapituitary acromegaly and elevated circulating GHRH levels, are indications for extrapituitary imaging. An enlarged pituitary is, however, often present in patients with peripheral GHRH-secreting tumors, and the radiologic diagnosis of a pituitary adenoma may be difficult to exclude. The McCune-Albright syndrome should be considered after definitive exclusion of pituitary and extrapituitary tumors.

Treatment

Aims

A comprehensive strategy for treating patients with acromegaly should aim to manage the pituitary mass, suppress GH and IGF-1 hypersecretion, and prevent long-term clinical sequelae of hypersomatotropism while maintaining normal anterior pituitary function[379,380]. As elevated GH levels per se are associated with a threefold increased morbidity rate and account for the single most important determinant of mortality rate[368,381], it is important to reverse the mortality rate to that of age-matched healthy subjects, by aiming for tight GH control.[382] Serum GH levels should be suppressed to at least 1 µg/L or less after an oral glucose load, and age- and gender-matched serum IGF-1 levels should be normalized. A controlled patient should also have a "normal" 24-hour integrated secretion

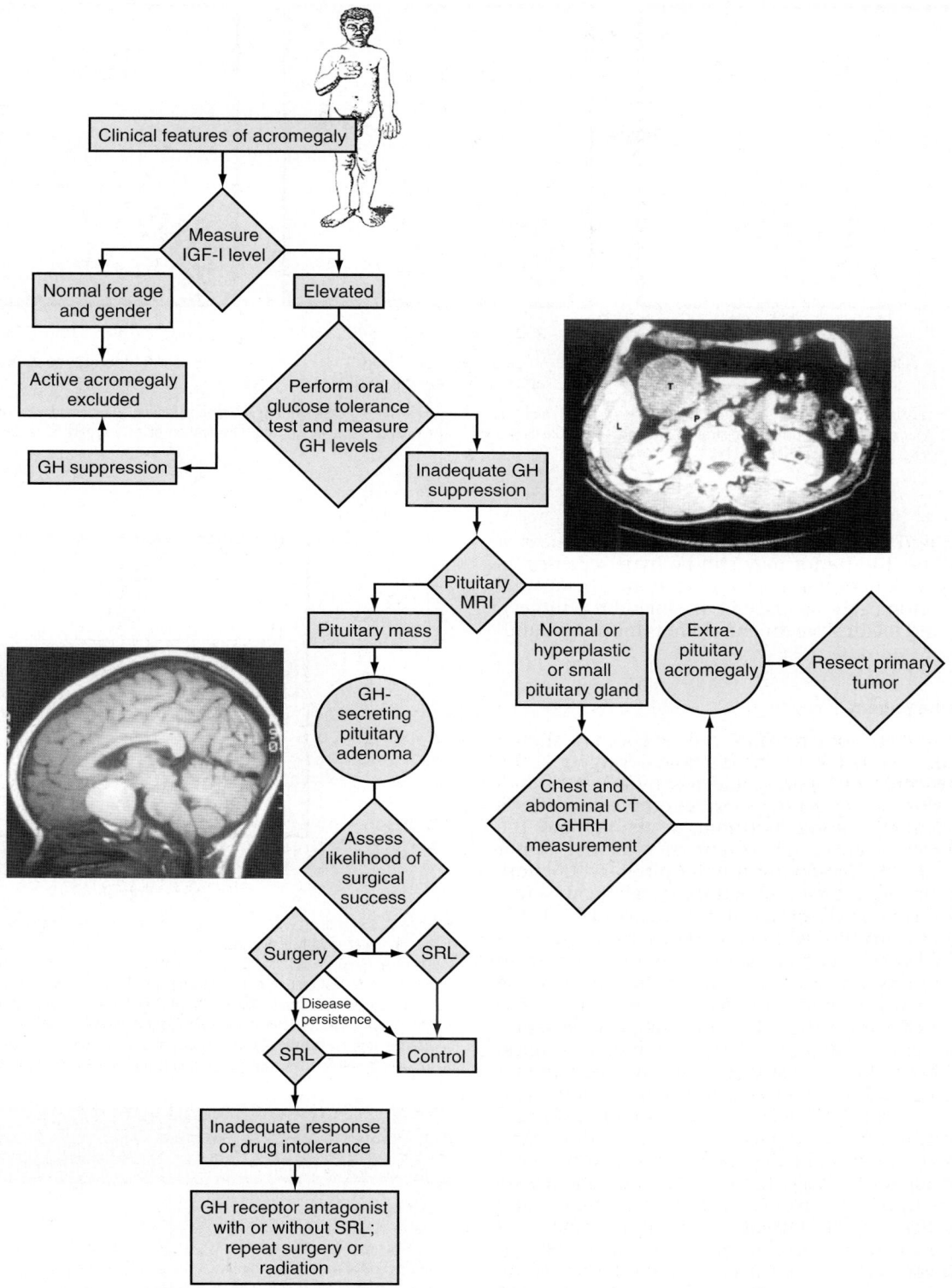

Figure 9-31 Diagnosis and treatment of acromegaly. Oral glucose tolerance test (OGTT) is performed with 75 g glucose and growth hormone (GH) measured during 2 hours. Disease control implies nadir GH level of less than 1 μg/L after OGTT, and age- and gender-matched normal insulin-like growth factor type 1 (IGF-1) level. CT, computed tomography; GHRH, growth hormone–releasing hormone; MRI, magnetic resonance imaging; SRL, somatostatin receptor ligand. Inset on left depicts pituitary adenoma. Inset on the right shows extrapituitary acromegaly: L, liver; P, pancreas; T, tumor-secreting GH. (From Melmed S. Acromegaly. *N Engl J Med.* 2006;355:2558-2573. Clinical features figure from Minkowski O. Ueber einen Fal von Akromegalie Berliner. *Klin Wochenschr.* 1887;21:371-374.)

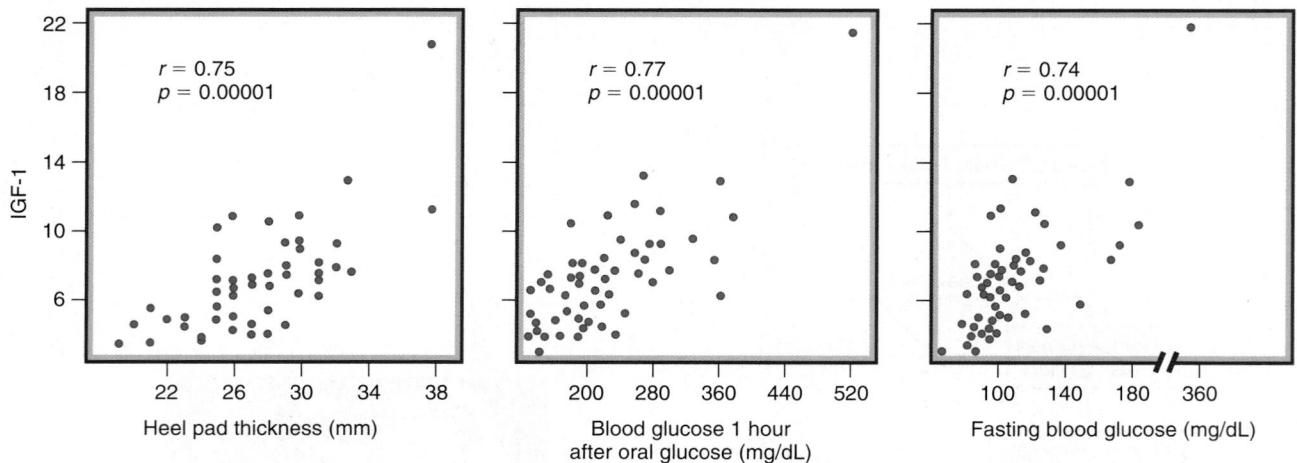

Figure 9-32 Correlation between insulin-like growth factor type 1 (IGF-1) and clinical indexes linear regression analysis between fasting somatomedin C (IGF-1) and growth hormone levels 1 hour after oral glucose administration. (Adapted from Clemmons DR, Van Wyk JJ, Ridgway EC, et al. Evaluation of acromegaly by radioimmunoassay of somatomedin-C. *N Engl J Med.* 1979;301:1138-1142.)

of GH (<2.5 μg/L). GH may not be measurable for most of the day and yet the tumor may still be hypersecreting as reflected by elevated IGF-1 levels. Current therapeutic modes for acromegaly management, including surgery, irradiation, and medical treatment, do not uniformly fulfill these goals.[383]

Surgical Management

Well-circumscribed somatotroph cell adenomas should preferably be resected by transsphenoidal surgery using either microscopic or laparoscopic techniques.[384-386] Successful resection alleviates preoperative compression effects and compromised trophic hormone secretion, and the skilled surgeon balances the extent of maximal tumor tissue removal while preserving anterior pituitary function. Within 2 hours of successful resection, metabolic dysfunction and soft tissue swelling start improving, and GH levels are sometimes controlled within an hour. Surgical outcome correlates well with adenoma size and preoperative serum GH levels and particularly with the experience of the surgeon.[36] Smaller tumors (less than 5 mm) and those totally confined within the sella, and preoperative serum GH levels lower than 40 μg/L, portend a favorable surgical outcome. About 90% of patients with microadenomas achieve postoperative GH levels lower than 2.5 μg/L, and less than 50% of all-sized macroadenomas had postoperative GH levels lower than 2 μg/L after glucose administration. Less than one third of all patients are controlled after resection of adenomas larger than 10 mm, and about 75% of patients with preoperative GH levels lower than 5 μg/L have normalized IGF-1. Overall, in multiple reports of endoscopic and microscopic surgical outcomes, 38% to 83% of patients achieve normalized IGF-1 levels. Fewer patients with macroadenomas are controlled. Of 2665 patients from a single center, 72% with microadenomas and 50% harboring macroadenomas had GH levels lower than 1.0 μg/L during glucose loading and normal serum IGF-1 levels.[387] When remission was rigorously defined as a normal IGF-1 and either a nadir glucose-suppressed GH level less than 0.4 ng/mL or a random GH level less than 1 ng/mL, all 14 of 14 patients with microadenomas and 28 of 46 with macroadenomas achieved remission[384] (Fig. 9-33). Smaller tumor size, lower Knosp score, and lower preoperative IGF-1 and GH levels are predictive of

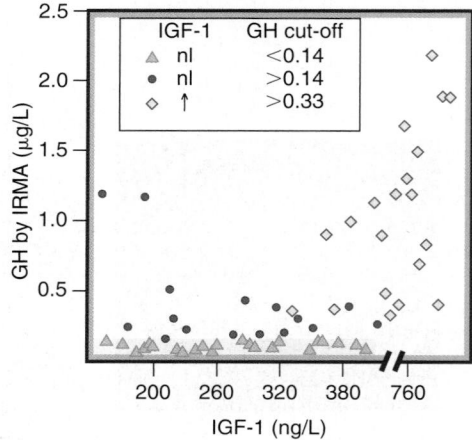

Figure 9-33 Nadir growth hormone (GH) as measured by IRMA (immunoradiometric assay) in subjects with active disease (◆), subjects in remission with normal GH suppression (group I; ▲), and subjects in remission with abnormal GH suppression (group II; ○) in relation to the normal range of GH suppression (mean ± 2 SD of the healthy subjects' responses, ■) versus the insulin-like growth factor type 1 (IGF-1) level. nl, normal. (Adapted from Freda PU, Post KD, Powell JS, Wardlaw SL. Evaluation of disease status with sensitive measures of growth hormone secretion in 60 postoperative patients with acromegaly. *J Clin Endocrinol Metab.* 1998;83:3808.)

TABLE 9-26

Significant Predictors of Postoperative Biochemical Remission by Multivariate Analysis in Acromegaly Patients

Older age
Smaller tumor size
Lower Knosp grade
Lower preoperative GH level
Lower preoperative IGF-1 level

GH, growth hormone; IGF-1, insulin-like growth factor 1.
Modified from Sun H, Brzana J, Yedinak CG, et al. Factors associated with biochemical remission after microscopic transsphenoidal surgery for acromegaly. *J Neurol Surg B Skull Base.* 2014;75(1):47-52.

postsurgical remission (Table 9-26). Postoperative GH levels measured within 24 hours of surgery are significant outcome determinants (Fig. 9-34).[40] Difficulties in endotracheal intubation due to macroglossia or severe kyphosis may rarely necessitate tracheostomy for anesthesia.

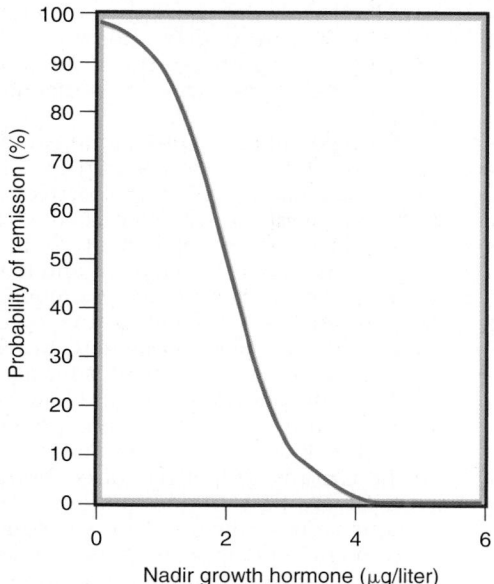

Nadir GII level (μg/L)	Remission (%)
0.1	98
0.3	97.1
0.5	95.7
0.7	93.7
0.9	90.8
1	88.9
1.2	84.2
1.4	78
1.6	70.2
1.8	61.1
2	51.1
2.1	46
2.3	36.2
2.5	27.4
2.7	20
2.9	14.3
3	12
4	1.7
5	0.2

Figure 9-34 Postoperative GH monitoring. The probability of surgical remission according to the nadir growth hormone (GH) level in a 1-week postoperative oral glucose tolerance test (OGTT). When the nadir GH level on the 1-week postoperative OGTT is around 1 μg/L, an 88.9% probability of surgical remission is expected. However, if it is greater than 4 μg/L, it is unlikely that the patients will achieve delayed surgical remission. (Derived from Kim, Oh MC, Lee EJ, Kim SH. Predicting long-term remission by measuring immediate postoperative growth hormone levels and oral glucose tolerance test in acromegaly. *Neurosurgery.* 2012;70:1106-1113.)

Side Effects. Although often transient, surgical complications may require lifelong pituitary hormone replacement. New hypopituitarism develops in up to approximately 20% of patients, reflecting operative damage to the surrounding normal pituitary tissue.[388] Permanent diabetes insipidus, CSF leaks, hemorrhage, and meningitis occur in up to 10% of patients (see Table 9-3). Although adrenal insufficiency is an important determinant of acromegaly mortality rate,[389] the incidence of postoperative adrenal failure is only 2/1000 person-years in acromegaly patients in remission.[390] The extent and prevalence of local complications depend upon tumor size and invasiveness. Experienced pituitary surgeons report more favorable postoperative complication rates.[36,37] Biochemical or anatomic recurrence (~7% over 10 years) or postoperative tumor persistence may indicate incomplete resection of adenomatous tissue, surgically inaccessible cavernous sinus tissue, or nesting of functional tumor tissue within the dura.

Radiation Therapy

Primary or adjuvant radiation of GH-secreting tumors may be achieved by conventional external deep x-ray therapy as well as heavy-particle (proton-beam) or gamma knife radiosurgery. Maximal tumor radiation should ideally be attained with minimal soft tissue damage. Precise MRI localization, accurate simulation, isocentral rotational techniques, and high-voltage (6-15 MeV) delivery have improved radiation efficacy. Radiation is a highly individualized choice, depending on the expertise and experience of the treating radiotherapist, and includes careful physician and patient consideration of the benefits of therapy weighed against potential risks. Up to 5000 rads are administered in split doses of 180-rad fractions divided over 6 weeks. Radiation arrests tumor growth and most pituitary adenomas ultimately shrink. GH levels fall gradually during the first year after treatment, and after 10 years, levels are lower than 10 μg/L in 70% of patients[391] (Fig. 9-35). Accordingly, during the initial years after irradiation, most patients are still exposed to unacceptably

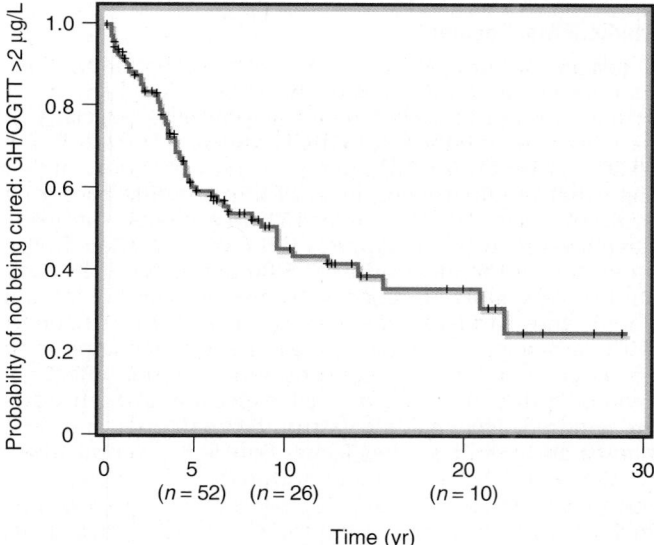

Figure 9-35 Long-term effects of radiation therapy on growth hormone (GH) secretion using a GH nadir after oral glucose load below 2 μg/L as the cure criterion and the probability of not being cured with time after radiotherapy. The numbers of patients not cured at 5, 10, and 20 years after pituitary irradiation are indicated in parentheses. Each step represents one cure; each cross (+) denotes a patient not cured at the latest follow-up. (From Barrande G, Pittino-Lungo M, Coste J, et al. Hormonal and metabolic effects of radiotherapy in acromegaly: long term results in 128 patients followed in a single center. *J Clin Endocrinol Metab.* 2000; 85:3779-3785.)

high levels of circulating GH and IGF-1. Stereotactic radiosurgery (gamma knife) treatment of GH-secreting adenomas effectively focuses on the adenoma, thereby sparing normal surrounding structures.[47,392-395] Of 136 patients followed for a median 61.5 months, 65% achieved normalized IGF-1 levels or nadir GH level less than 1 ng/mL after an oral glucose load.[47] Both higher radiation doses as well as lower initial IGF-1 levels portend a significantly more favorable outcome.

Side Effects. After 10 years, about half of all patients receiving radiotherapy have signs of pituitary trophic hormone disruption, and this prevalence increases annually thereafter, requiring gonadal steroids, thyroid hormone, or cortisone replacement. Side effects of conventional radiation including hair loss, cranial nerve palsies, tumor necrosis with hemorrhage, and rarely loss of vision or pituitary apoplexy have been documented in up to 2% of patients. Lethargy, impaired memory, and personality changes may also occur. The incidence and extent of local complications have been markedly diminished by use of highly reproducible simulators, precise rotational isocentric arc capability, and doses of less than 5000 rad. Proton-beam therapy is contraindicated in patients with suprasellar tumor extension due to unacceptable optic tract exposure to the radiation field. The rare development of second brain tumors in these patients has been reported at a cumulative risk frequency of 1.9% over 20 years.[51] In a 10-year follow-up study of 35 patients treated with gamma knife radiosurgery, half the patients developed pituitary hormone deficiencies (40% hypoadrenalism, 11% hypothyroidism, 13% hypogonadism, and 6% GH deficiency).[393] In another study, new pituitary hormone deficits were reported in 31% of patients within 61.5 months; however, visual deterioration and new cranial nerve palsies were rarely observed.[47] Because of side effects and slow onset of efficacy, radiation therapy should be employed as an adjuvant for patients not controlled by surgery or medical management or for those who do not consent to these therapies.

Medical Management

Dopamine Agonists. D_2 receptor agonists, including bromocriptine, and cabergoline, have been used as either primary or adjuvant therapy for acromegaly, especially in patients with mildly elevated GH and IGF-1 levels.[396] Up to 20 mg/day bromocriptine may lower GH, a dose higher than that required to suppress PRL in patients harboring prolactinomas. Approximately 15% of patients worldwide have been reported to suppress GH levels less than 5 µg/L when taking the medication (7.5-80 mg daily).[397] In open studies, cabergoline is reported to suppress GH to less than 2 µg/L and normalize IGF-1 in up to a third of patients with acromegaly.[396] Dopamine agonist efficacy appears to be independent of PRL concentrations.[398] Side effects of bromocriptine are more marked, especially as high doses are required. They include gastrointestinal upset, transient nausea and vomiting, headache, transient postural hypotension with dizziness, nasal stuffiness, and rarely, cold-induced peripheral vasospasm. Side effects of cabergoline include gastrointestinal symptoms, dizziness, headache, and mood disorders.

SRIF Receptor Ligands. Of the five SRIF receptor subtypes, SSTR2 and SSTR5 are preferentially expressed on somatotroph and thyrotroph cell surfaces and mediate suppression of GH and TSH secretion.[399,400] Several SRIF ligands (SRLs) have been safely employed as approved or investigational drugs for acromegaly (Fig. 9-36). Octreotide (D-Phe-Cys-Phe-D-Trp-Lys-Thr-Cys-Thr-OH), an octapeptide SRIF analogue, binds predominantly to SSTR2 and less avidly to SSTR5[401] and inhibits GH secretion with a potency 45 times greater than native SRIF, but its potency for inhibiting insulin release is only 1.3-fold that of SRIF. The in vivo half-life of the analogue is prolonged (up to 2 hours) because of its relative resistance to enzymatic degradation. Rebound GH hypersecretion seen following SRIF infusion does not occur following octreotide injection. These properties are highly advantageous for long-term use in acromegaly.[402] In vivo Octreoscan imaging visualizing SRIF receptors demonstrates that GH responsiveness directly correlates with the abundance of pituitary receptors, and patients resistant to octreotide do not have visible in vivo receptor binding sites.[403] Transfection of the *SSTR2* gene to somatotrophs enhances responsiveness to somatostatin analogues.[404]

A single subcutaneous administration (50 or 100 µg) suppresses GH secretion for up to 5 hours. In a double-blind, placebo-controlled trial octreotide (injections every 8 hours) significantly attenuated GH and IGF-1 levels overall in over 90% of patients.[405] In patients harboring microadenomas, integrated GH and IGF-1 levels are almost invariably normalized but the response in larger tumors is less pronounced. A combination of octreotide and bromocriptine or cabergoline may provide added efficacy. Increasing the frequency of administration more effectively suppresses GH levels, and continuous subcutaneous infusion (up to 600 µg/day) provides sustained GH control.[406] Elderly male patients are particularly sensitive to the GH-lowering effects of octreotide, and in the long term, desensitization does not occur.[407]

Long-acting somatostatin analogue formulations are convenient, enhance compliance, and allow sustained biochemical control. Serum levels of long-acting release (LAR) octreotide (20-30 mg/intramuscularly), a sustained release octreotide depot preparation,[408] peak at 28 days, with integrated GH levels effectively suppressed for up to 49 days. Monthly injections for 9 years reduced integrated serum GH levels to less than 2 µg/L in over 75% of patients.[409]

Lanreotide is a slow-release (SR) long-acting depot SRL, administered as a fixed 30-mg injectable dose every 7, 10, or 14 days. GH levels lower than 2.5 µg/L were achieved in 60% of 56 patients treated for 48 weeks and to less than 2.5 µg/L in about one third of 22 patients treated for up to 3 years, and IGF-1 levels were normalized in almost two thirds of patients.[410] A longer-acting preparation of lanreotide (lanreotide autogel) is administered by monthly deep subcutaneous injection. In a randomized, placebo-controlled, multicenter study with a 52-week open extension, serum GH levels decreased by more than 50% from baseline in 63% of patients receiving lanreotide autogel, compared with 0% of control subjects, and was effective throughout the trial.[411]

Pasireotide, a multireceptor-targeting SRL, exhibits highest affinity for SSTR5 more than SSTR2.[412] Both subcutaneous[413] and long-acting pasireotide formulations[414] exhibit superior efficacy over octreotide (Fig. 9-37). Reported side effects included those expected for SRLs as well as hyperglycemia noted in 57% of patients.

Oral octreotide formulated with a transient permeability enhancer attenuates basal and GHRH-elicited GH levels in healthy volunteers.[415] Oral octreotide is also effective in controlling and maintaining GH and IGF-1 levels in acromegaly; 65% of subjects were controlled after being switched from injectable long-acting SRLs and about 90% of subjects maintained responsiveness for up to 13 months. As oral octreotide safety is consistent with the known safety profile of octreotide, with no safety signals related to a different formulation and route of administration, the drug although not yet approved, may offer an alternative treatment option for acromegaly patients.[416]

Effects of SRLs on Pituitary Adenoma. Tumors rarely grow but patients receive depot preparations of SRIF analogues. Significant decrease in tumor size has been reported in 52% of patients on primary therapy.[417] A critical analysis of 14 studies reported that 37% of patients treated primarily by SRL experience significant tumor shrinkage.[418] Tumor shrinkage was reported in 75% and 78% of patients receiving octreotide LAR or somatuline depot, respectively, for up to 5 years.[419] In a comprehensive meta-analysis, 59% of

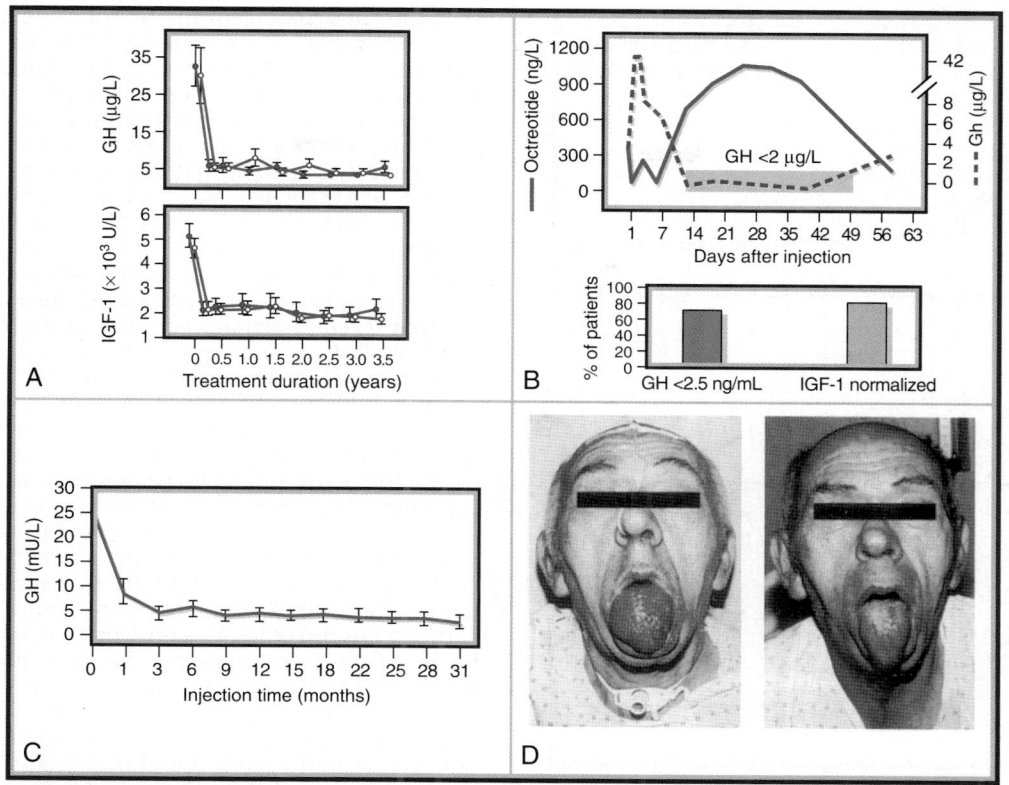

Figure 9-36 A, Growth hormone (GH) and insulin-like growth factor 1 (IGF-1) concentrations with long-term octreotide treatment. Comparison of primary octreotide treatment in 25 previously untreated patients and in 80 patients who had previously undergone surgical resection or irradiation. **B,** Pharmacodynamics of octreotide LAR (long-acting release) 12-hour mean serum octreotide and GH concentrations in a representative patient treated with a single 30-mg injection of Sandostatin LAR and followed for 60 days. After injection, drug levels peak at 28 days, and nadir GH levels are sustained for 4 weeks. **C,** Mean GH concentration with octreotide (long-acting release) long-term treatment. Serum GH levels in acromegaly following monthly LAR octreotide injections in 12 patients for 1 year and 8 patients for 31 months. **D,** Clinical impact of octreotide in reducing soft tissue swelling. Acromegaly in a patient suffering from obstructive sleep apnea before octreotide. Note the macroglossia, tracheotomy for airway obstruction, and intranasal feeding tube. After 6 months' treatment with octreotide, tongue size was reduced by half. Tracheotomy and nasal tube have been removed and sleep apnea has resolved. (A from Newman C, Melmed S, George A, et al. Octreotide as primary therapy for acromegaly. *J Clin Endocrinol Metab.* 1998;83:3034-3040. B adapted from Lancranjan I, Bruns C, Grass P, et al. Sandostatin LAR: a promising therapeutic tool in the management of acromegalic patients. *Metabolism.* 1996;45[8 Suppl 1]:67-71. C from Davies PH, Stewart SE, Lancranjan I, et al: Long-term therapy with long-acting octreotide [Sandostatin-LAR] for the management of acromegaly. *Clin Endocrinol.* 1998;48:311-316. D courtesy of Seymour Reichlin, University of Arizona, Treson.)

patients were reported to experience a 50% reduction of tumor mass, and this effect generally correlates with controlled GH and IGF-1 levels.[420] When patients undergoing pituitary surgery received preoperative octreotide for 3 to 6 months, moderately improved postoperative outcomes were observed, especially for larger tumors.[421-423]

Effects on Clinical Features. Over 70% of patients experience improved general well-being, and soft tissue swelling dissipates within several days of treatment. Headache, a common symptom in acromegaly, usually resolves within minutes of injection of octreotide,[424] likely reflecting a specific central analgesic effect. Asymptomatic patients experience decreased heart rate and diminished LV wall thickness. In patients with cardiac failure SRLs reversibly reduce systemic arterial resistance, oxygen consumption, and fluid volume and restore functional activity. In 30 patients, improved LV ejection fraction, with unchanged diastolic filling, was associated with octreotide-induced GH suppression to less than 2.5 µg/L. Control of IGF-1 and GH levels is associated with improved LV ejection function, but in those patients not controlled, cardiac performance worsened.[425] Joint function improves and crepitus is reduced, ultrasound shows evidence of bone or cartilage repair, and after several months, sleep apnea resolves.[361]

Determinants of SRL Responsiveness. In a critical analysis octreotide LAR and lanreotide autogel were shown to be

equivalent in the control of acromegaly symptoms and biochemical markers[426] (Fig. 9-38). In 166 patients with acromegaly, results of oral glucose tolerance tests were concordant for appropriate diagnosis and establishing efficacy of surgery and radiotherapy but were not helpful in evaluating effectiveness of medical SRL therapy. Measurement of serum IGF-1 levels was sufficient to assess the effectiveness of SRL therapy.[427] In results of prospective studies, IGF-1 levels are normalized in up to 35% of patients.[411,414,417,428-430] However, in earlier studies, use of SRL formulations were reported to control GH and IGF-1 in most patients. More favorable results reported in earlier studies may reflect clinical trial design, subject heterogeneity, and possibly selection of responsive patients. Increasing the monthly dose of Sandostatin LAR to as high as 40 to 60 mg may improve efficacy.[431,432] In a meta-analysis of 4464 patients treated with an SRL, average GH control rates and IGF-1 normalization rates were 56% and 55%, respectively (Fig. 9-39).[433]

Efficacy of octreotide action is determined by frequency of drug administration, total daily dose, tumor size, degree of tumor granularity, and pretreatment GH levels. The most important determinant of therapeutic responsiveness is the tumor expression of SSTR2.[434] Thus, less abundant SSTR2 expression as assessed by immunochemistry is associated with drug insensitivity or nonresponsiveness.[435]

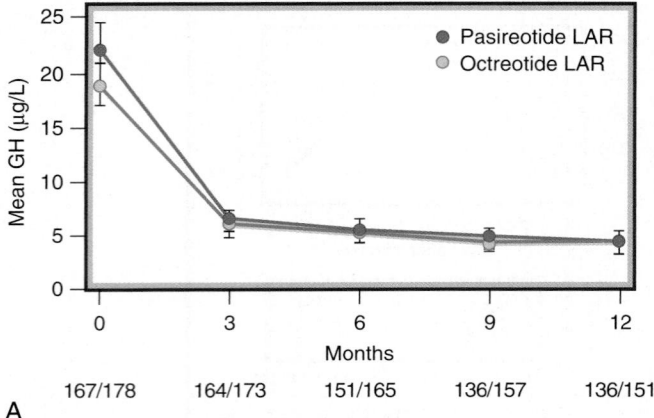

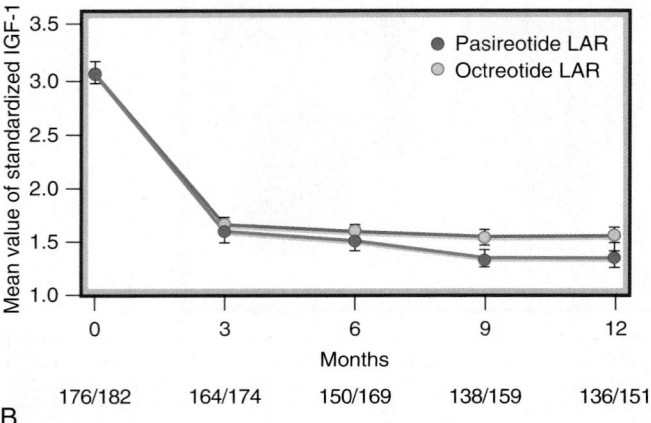

Figure 9-37 Comparison of pasireotide and octreotide efficacy. Mean + SE growth hormone (GH) levels (**A**) and standardized insulin-like growth factor type 1 (IGF-1) levels (**B**) over time by treatment group. The numbers at the bottom of each graph are the numbers of patients in the pasireotide long-acting release (LAR)/octreotide LAR treatment groups. Standardized IGF-1 is the IGF-1 value divided by the upper limit of normal range. (From Colao A, Bronstein M, Freda P, et al. Pasireotide versus octreotide in acromegaly: a head-to-head superiority study. *J Clin Endocrinol Metab.* 2014;99:791-799.)

Tumors containing more densely packed GH granules are more responsive than sparsely granulated adenomas.[436] Similarly, hypointense T2-weighted MRI tumor images portend SRL responsiveness, likely reflective of a denser tumor granularity.[437] Overall, older patients with lower GH and IGF-1 levels and smaller tumor masses tend to respond more favorably.

Side Effects. SRLs are generally safe and well tolerated. Gastrointestinal side effects predominate, occur early, and include transient loose stools, nausea, cramps, mild malabsorption, and flatulence, reported in about one third of patients. Hypoglycemia or hyperglycemia are not commonly encountered, and insulin requirements in diabetic patients with acromegaly are dramatically reduced within hours of receiving octreotide, concomitant with GH lowering. Overall, SRLs do not cause major effects on glucose homeostasis, and hyperglycemia may also be associated with uncontrolled underlying disease.[438] The drugs attenuate gallbladder contractility, and delayed emptying leads to reversible sludge formation evidenced by ultrasonography in up to 25% of patients.[439] Cholecystitis is very rarely reported in these patients. The incidence of gallbladder sludge or stones is geographically variable, with higher rates reported in China, Australia, and the United Kingdom.

In the United States, up to 30% of patients have demonstrable evidence of echogenic gallbladder deposits within the first 18 months of treatment. Thereafter, further sludge formation is not usually encountered.[408] Octreotide may interact with several drugs including cyclosporine, enhancing transplant rejection risk. SRL dose adjustments should be carefully titrated in patients requiring insulin or oral hypoglycemic agents, calcium channel blockers, and beta blockers. Asymptomatic sinus bradycardia has also been recognized.

Growth Hormone Receptor Antagonist. GH action through the surface membrane GH receptor is mediated by ligand-induced receptor signaling.[440] The postreceptor GH signal is not elicited if the receptor is bound (Fig. 9-40) by pegvisomant, a GH-receptor antagonist, which blocks subsequent IGF-1 generation.[441] The drug blocks peripheral GH action and does not target the pituitary tumor. IGF-1 measurement is the appropriate marker of patient responsiveness, and measuring GH is therefore not an efficacy marker. Earlier studies showed that daily injections (up to 40 mg daily) normalize IGF-1 levels in over 90% of patients, and dose-dependently improves fatigue, decreases soft tissue swelling as assessed by ring size, and diminishes perspiration.[442] In a subsequent drug surveillance report of 1288 patients, control of IGF-1 was reported in 63% of patients,[443] likely reflecting submaximal dose titration as compared to controlled dosing of a clinical trial. Accordingly, in a 91-month follow-up (median 18 months), IGF-1 levels were controlled in 95% of patients treated in two centers.[444] The drug is particularly useful in patients resistant to SRL therapy, because it effectively normalizes IGF-1 levels in these patients.[445,446] There is a concern that the loss of IGF-1 negative feedback control on tumor proliferation may theoretically lead to rebound mass expansion. However, rebound tumor enlargement rarely occurs and may reflect discontinuing somatostatin analogues, yet tumor growth while receiving pegvisomant should be monitored, especially if the residual tumor mass abuts the visual tracts.[447-450] The GH receptor antagonist likely enhances insulin sensitivity and is therefore particularly suited for patients with coexisting diabetes.[444,451]

Side Effects. Because elevated (threefold or higher) hepatic transaminases have been reported,[452] liver enzymes should be measured every 6 months. Local injection site inflammation and lipodystrophy have been reported.[453] Levels of GH rise as IGF-1 negative feedback on the pituitary is lost.

SRIF Receptor Ligand and GH Receptor Antagonist Combination. Combination treatment for acromegaly is most effective in patients in whom there has been tumor shrinkage on somatostatin analogue with reduction, albeit inadequate, in GH or IGF-1 levels (Fig. 9-41). In 11 such uncontrolled patients, dual blockade of the GH axis with pegvisomant and SRLs has been shown to exhibit greater efficacy than either drug alone.[454] Monthly doses of long-acting somatostatin analogue have been successfully combined with weekly doses of pegvisomant.[455] A study in 63 patients showed that 4 years of combination treatment was safe, but 23 patients developed elevated liver enzymes, especially if they were diabetic.[456]

Choice of Therapy

Tight control of GH secretion and normalization of IGF-1 levels should be achieved as adverse mortality rates correlate strongly with GH levels. Discordant GH and IGF-1 results after treatment should necessitate repeating the respective assay(s) in a reputable laboratory using rigorous assay standardizations and appropriate sensitivity cutoffs.[376] Furthermore, assessment of clinical activity may indicate

Comparing Octreotide LAR and Lanreotide ATG

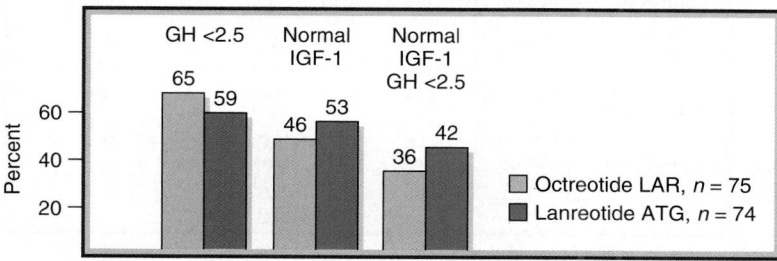

	SRIF Analog	n	GH <2.5 µg/L (n)	Normal IGF-1 (n)	Normal IGF-1 GH <2.5 µg/L	Mean dose (mg/4 wks)
Alexopoulou 2004	OCT	25	16	13	9	25
	LAN	25	12	13	8	108
Ashwell 2004	OCT	10	9	6	6	20
	LAN	10	9	8	8	93
Van Thiel 2004	OCT	7	4	3	3	24
	LAN	7	3	3	3	111
Andries 2007	OCT	10	10	5	5	—
	LAN	10	7	6	5	—
Ronchi 2007	OCT	23	10	8	4	24
	LAN	22	13	9	7	96

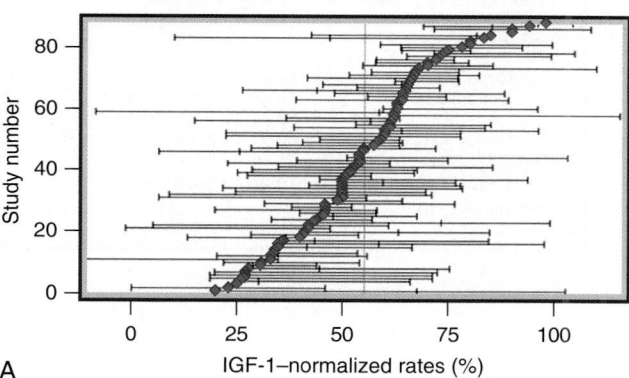

Figure 9-38 Comparing octreotide long-acting release (LAR) and lanreotide autogel (ATG). Summary of biochemical end points of studies comparing efficacy of octreotide LAR and lanreotide ATG. GH, growth hormone; IGF-1, insulin-like growth factor type 1; OCT, octreotide; OCT to LAN, initial treatment with octreotide LAR followed by lanreotide ATG; SRIF, somatotropin release–inhibiting factor. (Adapted from Murray R, Melmed S. A critical analysis of clinically available somatostatin analog formulations for therapy of acromegaly. *J Clin Endocrinol Metab.* 2008;93:2957-2968.)

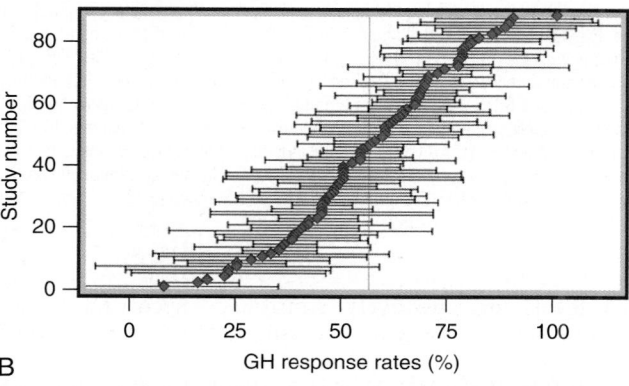

Figure 9-39 Meta-analysis of somatostatin receptor ligand (SRL) responsiveness in acromegaly. **A,** Insulin-like growth factor type 1 (IGF-1) response rates and 95% confidence intervals for 90 analyzed cohorts. **B,** Growth hormone (GH) response rates and 95% confidence intervals for the 90 analyzed cohorts. Median response rates for GH and IGF-1 noted by the vertical lines. Figures are sorted from least to greatest percent response rate. (From Carmichael J, Bonert VS, Nuno M, et al. Acromegaly clinical trial methodology impact on reported biochemical efficacy rates of somatostatin receptor ligand treatments: a meta-analysis. *J Clin Endocrinol Metab.* 2014; 99:1825-1833.)

mild disease with suppressed GH and residual elevated IGF-1 levels. Alternatively, normal or low IGF-1 levels may be encountered with systemic disease or malnutrition, and GH elevations reflecting persistent disease activity. Each treatment modality has respective advantages and disadvantages that should be assessed to individualize patient care (Fig. 9-42; Table 9-27).[457] Counterintuitively, features of GH deficiency may be encountered after effective therapy, and judicious GH replacement may be required to reverse adverse quality of life and lipid disorders.[458]

Selective surgical excision of a well-defined pituitary mass is recommended for most patients with microadenomas.[459] Remission rates are unacceptably low for patients with macroadenomas and locally invasive tumors. Attempted medical debulking of the sellar mass prior to surgery would be intuitively desirable, and limited controlled prospective studies appear to confirm the validity of this approach to improve surgical morbidity and possibly enhance subsequent postoperative outcomes, especially for patients with surgically inaccessible tumor tissue and cavernous sinus invasion.[423] Surgical debulking may also improve subsequent responsiveness to SRL therapy.[460] Postoperatively, patients with mild GH elevations can also be treated with cabergoline; although the efficacy of this drug is low, it is relatively inexpensive and free of major side effects. For uncontrolled patients a long-acting SRL should be administered.[380] Gallbladder ultrasonography should be performed in symptomatic patients, and those with symptomatic gallstones may require prophylactic anticholelilithogenic agents or laparoscopic cholecystectomy.

Primary therapy with SRLs may be offered to those patients in whom complete tumor removal is not likely or to those who refuse surgery or in whom the risks of surgery or anesthesia are unacceptable (Fig. 9-43). Invasive macroadenomas will invariably hypersecrete GH postoperatively and require SRL treatment. In patients whose pituitary lesion does not compress vital structures, primary

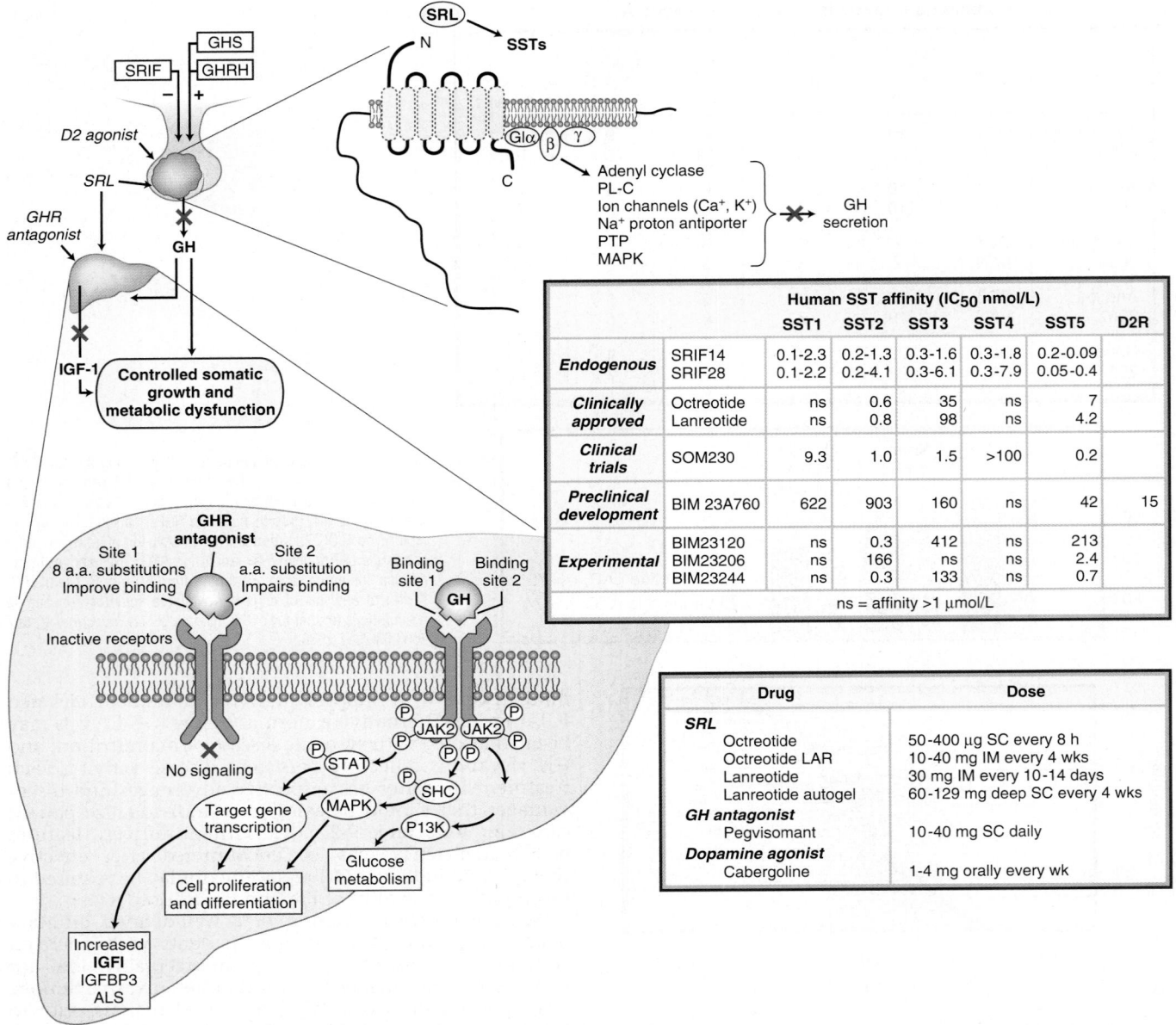

		Human SST affinity (IC$_{50}$ nmol/L)					
		SST1	**SST2**	**SST3**	**SST4**	**SST5**	**D2R**
Endogenous	SRIF14	0.1-2.3	0.2-1.3	0.3-1.6	0.3-1.8	0.2-0.09	
	SRIF28	0.1-2.2	0.2-4.1	0.3-6.1	0.3-7.9	0.05-0.4	
Clinically approved	Octreotide	ns	0.6	35	ns	7	
	Lanreotide	ns	0.8	98	ns	4.2	
Clinical trials	SOM230	9.3	1.0	1.5	>100	0.2	
Preclinical development	BIM 23A760	622	903	160	ns	42	15
Experimental	BIM23120	ns	0.3	412	ns	213	
	BIM23206	ns	166	ns	ns	2.4	
	BIM23244	ns	0.3	133	ns	0.7	

ns = affinity >1 µmol/L

Drug	**Dose**
SRL	
Octreotide	50-400 µg SC every 8 h
Octreotide LAR	10-40 mg IM every 4 wks
Lanreotide	30 mg IM every 10-14 days
Lanreotide autogel	60-129 mg deep SC every 4 wks
GH antagonist	
Pegvisomant	10-40 mg SC daily
Dopamine agonist	
Cabergoline	1-4 mg orally every wk

Figure 9-40 Action of growth hormone receptor (GHR) antagonist, somatostatin receptor ligands (SRLs), and dopamine (D$_2$) agonists. Normally a single molecule of GH binds two GH receptors through sites 1 and 2, and the GH signal transduction pathway is activated. Pegvisomant increases binding of GHR to site 1 and blocks binding at site 2 to prevent functional GHR dimerization, initiation of GH action, and induction of insulin-like growth factor type 1 (IGF-1) synthesis and secretion. The peripheral effects of excess GH are antagonized at the cellular level, independent of the presence of somatostatin (SST) or dopamine receptors on the pituitary tumor. SRLs inhibit GH secretion and IGF-1 synthesis and suppress pituitary tumor growth. GH-secreting adenomas express predominantly SST2 and SST5. Figure depicts affinities for SST receptor subtypes and for D$_2$ receptor. a.a., amino acid; ALS, acid-labile subunit; C, carboxyl terminal; GHRH, gonadotropin hormone–releasing hormone; GHS, gonadotropin hormone secretagogue; IC$_{50}$, 50% inhibitory concentration; IGFBP3, insulin-like growth factor–binding protein 3; JAK2, Janus kinase 2 tyrosine kinase; MAPK, mitogen-activated protein kinase; N, amino terminal; ns, not significant; P, elemental phosphorus; PI3K, phosphoinositide 3 kinase; PL-C, phospholipase C; PTP, protein tyrosine phosphatase; SHC, Src homology–containing protein; SRIF, somatotropin release–inhibiting factor (somatostatin); STAT, signal transducer and activator or transcription. (Adapted from Melmed S. Acromegaly. *N Engl J Med.* 2006;355:2558-2573; and Heaney AP, Melmed S. Molecular targets in pituitary tumours. *Nat Rev Cancer.* 2004;4:285-295.)

medical management may therefore be an appropriate therapeutic option.[419,429,461,462] Preoperative SRL treatment may also enhance subsequent surgical outcomes, especially for macroadenomas,[422] but long-term analyses have not shown significant differences for long-term outcomes.[423,463] Pegvisomant, either alone or in combination with an SRL, should be offered to resistant patients. Radiation should be administered to patients who are resistant to or cannot tolerate medications, who prefer not to receive long-term injections, or those who cannot afford medication. After irradiation, medications are required for several years until

GH levels are effectively controlled. Recurring tumors despite medical therapy or irradiation may rarely require reoperation.

Although tight GH control is critical, these patients also require counseling for anxiety engendered by disfigurements and interpretation of laboratory test results. Patients should be followed quarterly until biochemical control is achieved; thereafter, hormone evaluation is performed semiannually. In those patients who are biochemically in remission and in whom no residual tumor tissue is present, MRI should be repeated every 1 to 2 years. Follow-up

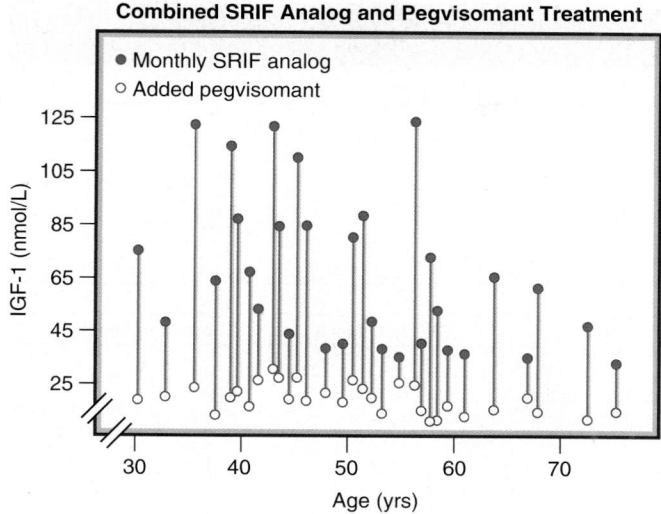

Combined SRIF Analog and Pegvisomant Treatment

● Monthly SRIF analog
○ Added pegvisomant

Figure 9-41 Combined somatotropin release–inhibiting factor (SRIF) analogue and pegvisomant treatment. Insulin-like growth factor type 1 (IGF-1) concentration in serum of 31 patients with acromegaly before (●) and after (○) 138 (35-149) weeks of combined therapy. Shaded area indicates age-dependent normal range for IGF-1. (From Neggers S, van Aken M, Janssen JA, et al. Long-term efficacy and safety of combined treatment of somatostatin analogs and pegvisomant in acromegaly. *J Clin Endocrinol Metab.* 2007;92:4598-4601.)

evaluation includes documenting and treating new skin tag and lipoma growth, nerve entrapments, and jaw overbites; rheumatologic, dental, and cardiac evaluations; and metabolic assessment. Visual field perimetry (for macroadenomas) and pituitary reserve testing should be repeated semiannually, and pituitary MRI is performed annually, especially in patients with residual tumor or in those requiring hormone replacement or medical treatment. Mammography and colonoscopy should be performed as clinically indicated for patients over age 50 or those harboring polyps. Maximal and sustained long-term GH and IGF-1 control should ameliorate the deleterious effects of these hormones by judicious use of available treatment modalities.

ACTH-SECRETING TUMORS (CUSHING DISEASE)

The evaluation and management of patients with ACTH-secreting pituitary tumor (Cushing disease) is fully described in Chapter 15. Briefly, the diagnosis of an ACTH-secreting pituitary tumor is suggested by features of hypercortisolism, elevated 24-hour urinary free cortisol levels, and elevated late night salivary cortisol values, together with

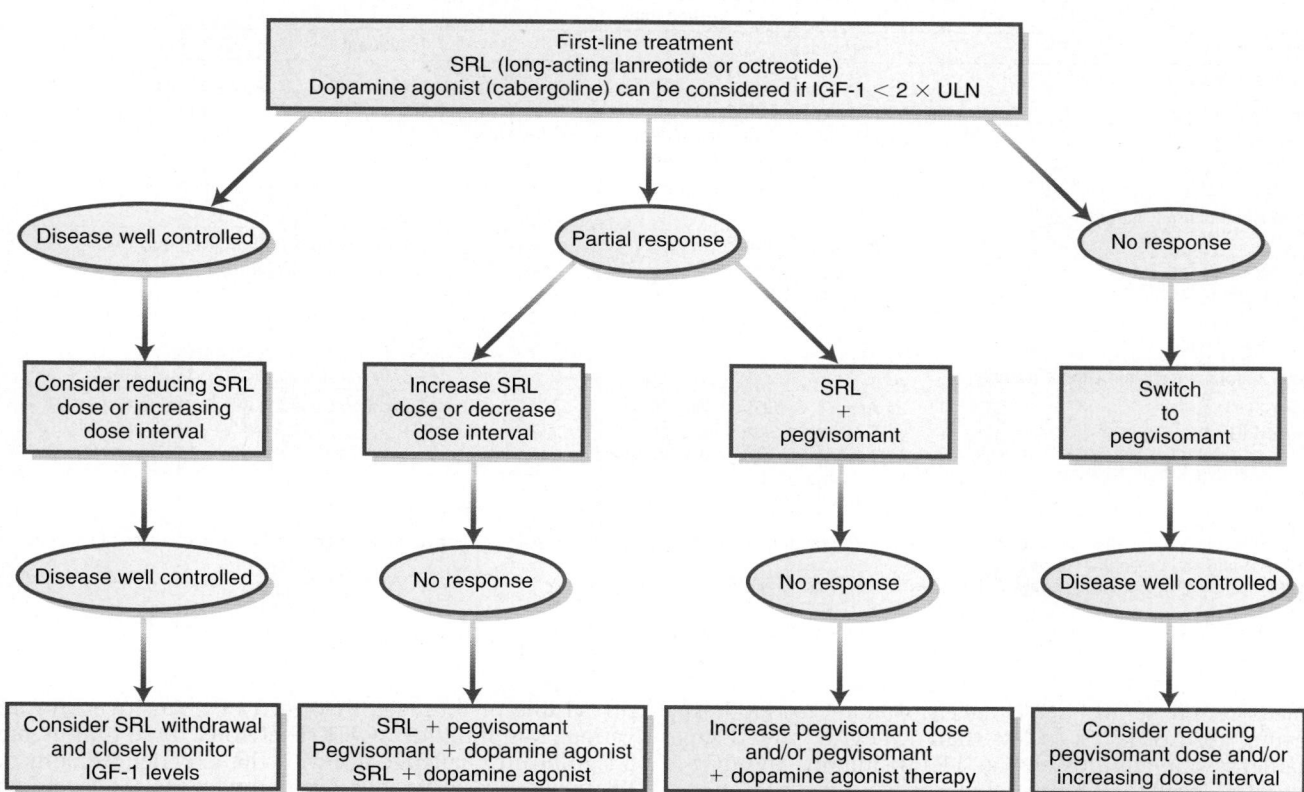

Figure 9-42 Consensus guidelines for medical management of patients with acromegaly. A proposed algorithm for the medical management of acromegaly after surgery or as primary treatment strategy when surgery is inappropriate. Radiation therapy as rescue therapy is not considered in this algorithm as its use is usually determined by a multidisciplinary management team. IGF-1, insulin-like growth factor 1; SRL, somatostatin receptor ligand; ULN, upper limit of normal. (Adapted from Giustina A, Chanson P, Kleinberg D, et al. Expert consensus document: a consensus on the medical treatment of acromegaly. *Nat Rev Endocrinol.* 2014;10:243-248.)

TABLE 9-27

Management of Acromegaly

Goals
Control GH and IGF-1 secretion
Control tumor growth
Relieve central compressive effects, if present
Preserve or restore pituitary trophic hormone function
Treat comorbidities (hypertension, cardiac failure, hyperglycemia, sleep apnea, arthritis)
Normalize mortality rates
Prevent biochemical recurrence

			Treatments		
Characteristic	**Surgery**	**Radiotherapy**	**SRL**	**GHR Antagonist**	**Dopamine Agonist**
Advantages					
Mode	Transsphenoidal resection	Noninvasive	Monthly injection	Daily injection	Oral
Biochemical control GH < 2.5 µg/L	Macroadenomas, <50% Microadenomas, >80%	~35% in 10 yr	~80%	Increases	<15%
IGF-1 normalized		<30%	~70%	>90%	<15%
Onset	Rapid	Slow (years)	Rapid	Rapid	Slow (weeks)
Patient compliance	One-time consent	Good	Must be sustained	Must be sustained	Good
Tumor mass	Debulked or resected	Ablated	Growth constrained or shrinks ~50%	Unknown	Unchanged
Disadvantages					
Cost	One-time	One-time	Ongoing	Ongoing	Ongoing
Hypopituitarism	~10%	>50%	None	Very low IGF-1 if overtreated	None
Other	Tumor persistence or recurrence, 6% Diabetes insipidus, 3% Local complications, 5%	Local nerve damage Second brain tumor Visual and CNS disorders, ~2% Cerebrovascular risk	Gallstones, 20% Nausea, diarrhea	Elevated liver enzymes (rare)	Nausea, ~30% Sinusitis High dose required

	Outcomes	
Feature	**Evaluation**	**Treatment**
Safe Biochemical Activity		
Nadir GH < 0.4 µg/L Age-matched normal IGF-1 Asymptomatic No comorbidities	Assess GH/IGF-1 axis Evaluate adrenal, thyroid, and gonadal axes Periodic but less frequent MRI	None or no change in current treatment
Unsafe Biochemical Activity		
Nadir GH > 0.4 µg/L Elevated IGF-1 Discordant GH and IGF-1 Asymptomatic No comorbidities	Assess GH/IGF-1 axis Evaluate pituitary function Periodic MRI	Weigh treatment benefit vs. risks Consider new treatment if being treated
Unsafe Biochemical and Clinical Activity		
Nadir GH > 1 µg/L Elevated IGF-1 Clinically active tumor growing	Assess GH/IGF-1 axis Evaluate pituitary function Assess cardiovascular, metabolic, and tumoral comorbidity Periodic MRI	Actively treat or change treatment

CNS, central nervous system; GH, growth hormone; GHR, growth hormone receptor; IGF-1, insulin-like growth factor type 1; MRI, magnetic resonance imaging; SRL, somatostatin receptor ligand.
Modified from Melmed S. Acromegaly. *N Engl J Med.* 2006;355:2558-2573.

nonsuppressed serum ACTH levels. Failure to suppress morning cortisol levels to less than 1.8 µg/dL after 1 mg dexamethasone administered at 11 PM supports the diagnosis.[464] In healthy subjects, glucocorticoid feedback suppresses CRH and ACTH, attenuating cortisol secretion. Surgical resection of an ACTH-secreting adenoma is the treatment of choice. As these tumors are usually small, sometimes less than 2 mm diameter, they may be either not visible or localized incorrectly by sensitive MRI and venous sampling for ACTH. Therefore, these tumors pose a significant challenge even for the experienced surgeon. Bilateral petrosal venous sampling for ACTH levels and cavernous sinus venography should ideally be performed prior to surgery. However, if sellar venous sinus drainage is predominantly unilateral, left-right ACTH gradients may not reliably lateralize the lesion. If an ACTH gradient is

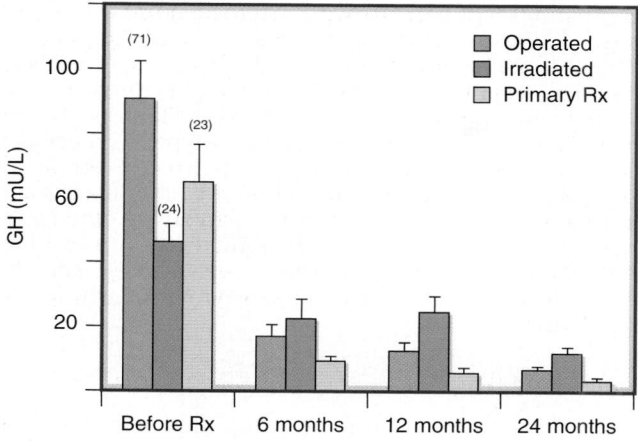

Figure 9-43 Primary medical therapy in acromegaly patients. Control with medical therapy compared to surgery or radiation. Plasma growth hormone (GH) levels (mean ± SEM) in the group of patients (*n* = 118) before and during long-term treatment with lanreotide. Rx, treatment; SEM, standard error of the mean. (Data from Baldelli R, Colao A, Razzore P, et al. Two-year follow-up of acromegalic patients treated with slow release lanreotide (30 mg). *J Clin Endocrinol Metab.* 2000;85(11):4099-4103.)

indeed detected with normal venous drainage patterns, hemihypophysectomy may in fact be curative in most patients with clearly defined biochemical features of ACTH-dependent Cushing disease. Meticulous surgical exploration of both anterior and posterior lobes is required for these tiny tumors, which are often off-white and speckled by petechiae, and may be inadvertently suctioned. Even carefully performed preoperative lateralization is not infallible, and the so-called "normal" side should also be carefully explored.

Assessment of Surgical Outcome

Transsphenoidal adenoma resection is the preferred treatment for these adenomas.[465] After selective adenomectomy of a clearly identifiable adenoma, remission was achieved in 75% of 295 patients. However, partial hypophysectomy performed in patients in whom an adenoma cannot be identified may result in biochemical remission in some patients.[466] On the third postoperative day, 1 mg dexamethasone can be given at 10 PM, and cortisol levels are measured the following morning, prior to initiating hydrocortisone therapy. If the immediate postoperative cortisol level is less than 3 μg/dL, a 95% 5-year remission rate can be expected. In 21 of 27 patients tested prior to glucocorticoid administration, postoperative cortisol levels less than 10 mg/dL or less than those obtained from preoperative midnight sampling were predictive of remission.[467]

Medical Treatment

Pasireotide, an SRL, has been approved for treating ACTH hypersecretion associated with Cushing disease.[468] About 20% of patients exhibit normalized urinary free cortisol levels, associated with improved clinical features. Up to 50% of patients may develop hyperglycemia, and blood sugars should be aggressively monitored. Mefipristone, a glucocorticoid receptor antagonist, is approved to ameliorate hyperglycemia associated with Cushing disease.[469] Side effects include adrenal failure, hypokalemia, and excessive vaginal bleeding.

Silent Corticotroph Adenoma

These basophilic tumors are generally nonfunctional and yet exhibit POMC product immunoreactivity. ACTH secretion is unaltered, with no associated clinical or biochemical features of hypercortisolism, although these tumors are morphologically indistinguishable from adenomas associated with Cushing disease. A mixed corticotroph-gonadotroph cell origin may underlie the primitive tumor cell type, with associated aggressive growth.[300] These tumors may represent up to 7% of all surgically removed adenomas and are usually hemorrhagic and invariably macroadenomas. Unlike Cushing disease, they have a 2 : 1 male preponderance, often present with mass effects, and about one third have preoperative evidence for pituitary insufficiency. About half exhibit cavernous sinus or bony invasion, hemorrhage, necrosis, and cyst formation. These tumors often recur and postoperative radiation and reoperation are required to eradicate tumor regrowth or residual mass.[301] Unless appropriate immunostaining is performed, many of these tumors remain undiagnosed and are inadvertently classified as recurrent nonfunctioning macroadenomas.

THYROTROPIN-SECRETING TUMORS

TSH-producing pituitary tumors are rare. During 1979 to 1992, Mindermann and Wilson analyzed tumor type by immunohistochemistry and found that the overall prevalence of TSH-secreting tumors was 19/2225 (0.85%). Between 1989 and 1991, the same group found a prevalence of 2.8% of pituitary adenomas.[470] It is not clear whether newer more sensitive TSH assays account for this or whether the tumor type frequency is increasing. TSH-secreting tumors can also cosecrete other hormones including GH, PRL, and rarely ACTH and can cause elevated serum IGF-1 or PRL levels.[471]

Pathology

These tumors are invasive, but for the most part benign, and distant metastases are extremely rare. The secretory pattern is determined by a panel of immunoreactive antibodies to TSH-β, α-subunit, GH, PRL, and ACTH. Twenty-four-hour sampling indicates that pulse frequency of TSH is increased and diurnal rhythm was preserved at a higher mean hormone level.[472] TSH-secreting tumors exhibit positive immunostaining for α-subunit and TSH-β in up to 75% of cells and for the pituitary-specific transcription factor, Pit-1. These tumors express SSTR2 mRNA and, in some cases, SSTR3 and SSTR5 mRNA.[473]

Presentation

Patients with TSH-secreting tumors present with symptoms due to tumor growth (including visual field abnormalities, cranial nerve palsies, or headache) or to hormone overproduction. Signs and symptoms of hyperthyroidism including palpitations, arrhythmias, weight loss, tremor and nervousness, or goiter are common. Very rarely, periodic paralysis and postoperative thyroid storm have been reported.[474,475] Serum TSH is often, but not invariably, elevated. In those cases, the combination of abnormally high thyroid hormone levels and a TSH value within the normal range points to a TSH-producing pituitary tumor. A relatively long period of hyperthyroidism, initially thought to be Graves disease and treated accordingly, often predates the realization that the hyperthyroidism is indeed a result of a TSH-secreting pituitary tumor. Alternatively, thyroid hormone insensitivity can also present with similar laboratory profiles.[476] TSH-secreting tumors are usually large, and in one series, 88% were macroadenomas, and 12% microadenomas. Over 60% were also locally invasive.[477] In another series, 70% were reported as macroadenomas.[478] From analysis of 10 reports on a total of 153 patients, it appears that TSH is frankly elevated in 58% of patients, with the remainder having normal albeit inappropriately elevated TSH levels. Patients previously treated with radioactive iodine for presumed Graves disease present with significantly higher TSH levels than patients not previously radioablated (mean: 56 mU/L vs. 9 mU/L, respectively). An ectopic TSH-producing tumor has also been reported.[479] Serum T_4 is high in the majority of patients, as is the glycoprotein hormone α-subunit. Approximately two thirds[480] of patients with TSH-producing pituitary tumors have goiters with elevated radioactive iodine uptake. Rarely, patients with TSHomas and differentiated thyroid cancer have been reported.[481] About 30% of TSHomas cosecrete GH or PRL.[471] Consequently, features of acromegaly or hyperprolactinemia may also be present.

Evaluation

Serum T_4, T_3, TSH (by high sensitivity assay), and α-subunit should be measured. The combination of high T_4, T_3, and α-subunit; high or inappropriately normal TSH; and a pituitary tumor strongly confirms the diagnosis of a TSH-producing pituitary adenoma. TRH stimulation can differentiate between TSH overproduction by a TSH-secreting tumor and thyroid hormone insensitivity. In TSH-secreting tumors, the TSH response elicited by TRH is blunted. In contrast, TSH usually rises in response to TRH in thyroid hormone insensitivity and in normal subjects. Concomitant measurement of α-subunit at each point during the TRH test is helpful because the molar ratio of α-subunit to TRH is high (>1) in almost 85% of patients with TSH-secreting tumors. A T_3 suppression test is helpful in that complete inhibition of TSH does not occur in patients with TSH-secreting tumors. This test can also differentiate subclinical hypothyroidism in patients previously treated with radioactive iodine for hyperthyroidism but found to have an incidental pituitary tumor. TSH elevation may also result from inadequate thyroid hormone replacement. A pituitary MRI should be performed, and IGF-1 and PRL levels determined to exclude acromegaly or hyperprolactinemia. Expression of other pituitary hormones in immunostained histologic sections does not necessarily imply elevated serum levels.

Importantly, the degree of hyperthyroidism should be assessed to determine whether control of these signs and symptoms should be undertaken prior to further evaluation or treatment of the pituitary tumor. Hyperthyroidism in this condition has been characterized as being severe in 14 of 25 patients, and having been present in most patients for years before the diagnosis was made.[477] Perioperative deaths in patients with TSH-secreting tumors have been reported, which might be attributed to poorly controlled hyperthyroidism.

Management
Surgery

The European Thyroid Association guidelines suggest surgery as first-line therapy. Cures are achieved for most patients with microadenomas, but remission is achieved in less than 60% of patients with macroadenomas.[482] After a mean follow-up of 64.4 months, 75% of 70 patients achieved biochemical control, and 58% normalized both pituitary imaging and thyroid function, but surgical cures occur in fewer than 40% of patients[478] (Table 9-28; Fig. 9-44). However, the rarity of this tumor type has precluded large controlled studies. Most patients have cavernous or sphenoid sinus invasion, and tumors are often fibrous and unusually hard. About one third of patients require radiotherapy to achieve biochemical normalization. Nine percent developed pituitary hormone deficiencies, and 3% had recurrence of tumor or hyperthyroidism within the first 2 years.[478]

Radiation Therapy

There are no large series reporting treatment of TSH-secreting tumors with radiotherapy alone. Radiation has mostly been employed as adjunctive therapy to surgery, especially when the latter was not curative.

Somatostatin Analogues

Octreotide, used as either primary or adjunctive treatment, normalizes T_4 and T_3 and reduces TSH levels by half.[483] Overall, tumors shrink in about a third of patients. In 18 patients with TSH-secreting adenomas, lanreotide (30 mg every 10 or 14 days) significantly decreased TSH levels from 2.72 to 1.89 mU/L, decreased T_4 levels, but did not shrink tumors. Octreotide LAR (up to 30 mg monthly) responsiveness appeared similar to that observed for the subcutaneous preparation in 7 patients.[484] In another report, octreotide suppressed TSH in 90% of patients with TSH-secreting tumors and reduced tumor size in 50% of these patients.[485] Somatostatin analogues are effective in more than 90% of patients with TSHomas,[482] but tachyphylaxis may occasionally occur.

Preoperative Management

Unless vision is threatened, patients should be evaluated to determine whether clinical signs of hyperthyroidism warrant immediate treatment. Propranolol, radioactive iodine thyroid ablation, thyroidectomy, antithyroid medications including tapazol, and somatostatin analogues are employed. Both radioactive iodine and antithyroid medications are targeted to the thyroid gland rather than the pituitary seat of the disorder. This approach also inhibits the negative feedback of T_3 on TSH and leads to increased tumor TSH production. Surgery and somatostatin analogues simultaneously treat hyperthyroidism and tumor TSH hypersecretion. Somatostatin analogues lower TSH, α-subunit, and T_4 and are recommended as first-line drugs in the initial control of hyperthyroidism due to TSH-secreting tumors because their onset of action is faster than other therapeutic approaches, and tumor shrinkage occurs in up to 40% of patients. When invasive tumor tissue persists, patients continue to have abnormal TSH responses to TRH and require somatostatin analogue therapy.

Silent TSH-Secreting Tumors

A subset of TSH-secreting tumors immunostain positively for but do not hypersecrete TSH or cause thyrotoxicosis. Of 29 tumors that immunostained positively for TSH, 9 were not associated with hyperthyroidism.[486]

TABLE 9-28

Features of TSH-Secreting Adenomas

Study	No. of Patients	Microadenoma	Macroadenoma	Extrasellar Extension	Visual Field Deficit	Histologic Stain	Radiation	Euthyroid on Somatostatin Analogue
Grisoli (1987)[487]	6	0/6	6/6	4/6	3/6	4/4 TSH	3/6	
Gesundheit (1989)[488]	9	2/9	7/9			2/4 TSH, PRL 5/7 TSH 3/7 α-subunit	3/8	NA
McCutcheon (1990)[489]	8	1/8	7/8	6/7	4/8	6/7 TSH	3/8	NA
Beckers (1991)[490]	7	1/7	6/7			2/7 PRL 2/7 pure TSH 1/7 TSH, PRL 1/7 TSH, PRL, GH		Octreotide 3/3
Chanson (1993, 1992)[491,492]	52	5	47	Most of the macroadenomas			9/52	Octreotide 38/52
Mindermann (1993)[470]	19	0/19	19/19	12/19	6/19	6/14 pure TSH 4/14 TSH, GH, PRL, ACTH 1/14 TSH, GH, PRL 1/14 TSH, PRL 1/14 TSH, GH	9/19 E	NA
Losa (1996)[493]	17	3/17	14/17	10/14	3/17	1/14 TSH, ACTH 14 TSH 2 GH 3 PRL 1 LH 13/14 α-subunit		NA
Brucker-Davis (1999)[477]	25	2/25	23/25	20/25	7/18	5/25 GH 4/25 PRL 3/25 FSH	11	Octreotide 5/6
Kuhn (2000)[494]	16	5/16	11/16	8/11		10/11 TSH 1 TSH, PRL	0/4	Lanreotide 13/16
Caron (2001)[484]	11	2	9	9/11		2/5 TSH + GH 1/5 TSH, GH, ACTH, FSH, PRL 1/2 GH + TSH 1/2 β-TSH 2/5 TSH + AI 1/5 TSH 2/5 GH		Octreotide 10/11
Ness-Abramov (2007)[495]	11	1	10	10/11	6/11		0/11	Lanreotide 10/11
Roelfsema (2009)[471]	6	1/6	5/6	NA	1/6		2/6	Octreotide 5/6
Elston (2010)[496]	6	1	4	3/4	3/6		3/6	Octreotide 3/3
Zhang (2012)[497]	15	0	15	NA		10/15 TSH 3/4 TSH + GH 1/15 1/1 TSH + PRL	0/15	14/15 normalization of TSH after 2 months of octreotide LAR
Totals (%)	208	24/193 (12%)	178/193 (92%)	82/108 (75%)	33/91 (36%)		43/160 (27%)	102/121 (84%)

ACTH, adrenocorticotropic hormone; FSH, follicle-stimulating hormone; GH, growth hormone; LAR, long-acting release; LH, luteinizing hormone; NA, not available; PRL, prolactin; TSH, thyroid-stimulating hormone (thyrotropin).

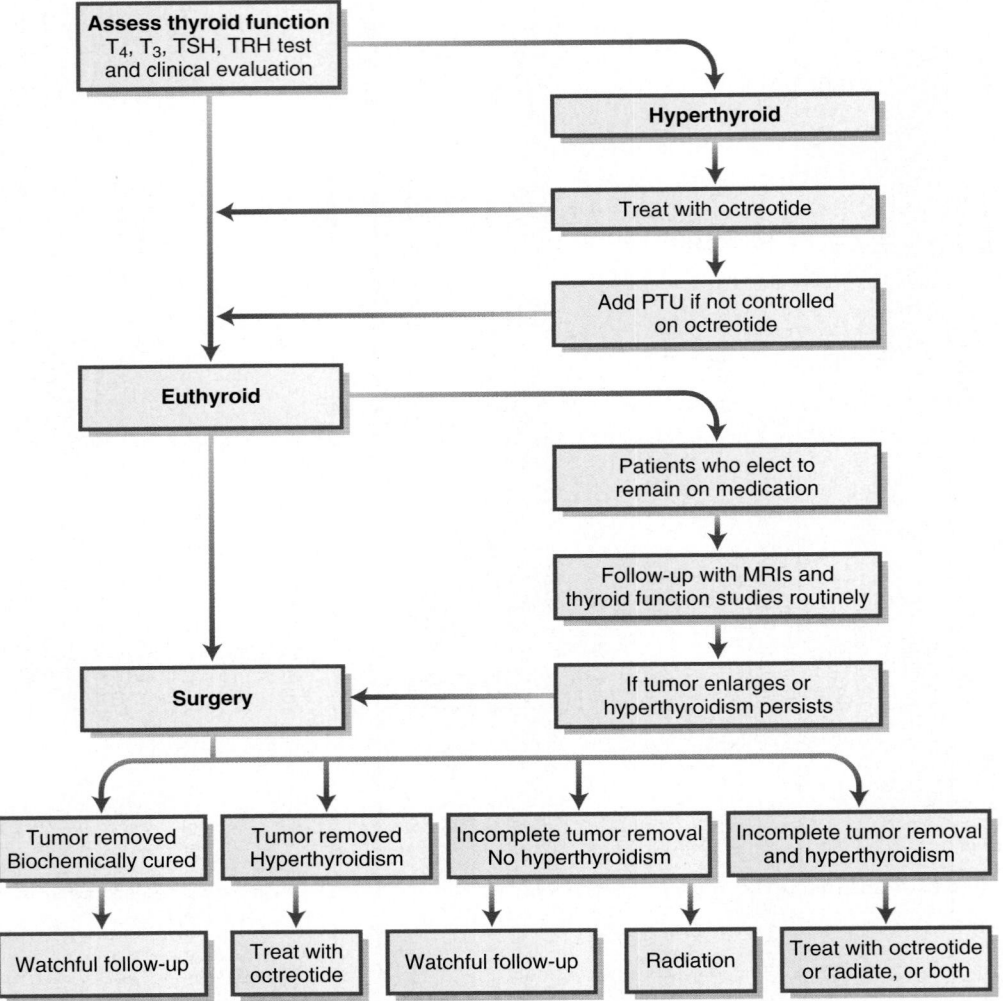

Figure 9-44 Management of thyrotropin (TSH)-secreting pituitary tumors. MRI, magnetic resonance imaging; PTU, propylthiouracil; T_3, triiodothyronine; T_4, thyroxine; TRH, thyrotropin-releasing hormone.

REFERENCES

1. Musolino NR, Marino R Jr, Bronstein MD. Headache in acromegaly: dramatic improvement with the somatostatin analogue SMS 201-995. *Clin J Pain.* 1990;6:243-245.
2. Fleseriu M, Yedinak C, Campbell C, Delashaw JB. Significant headache improvement after transsphenoidal surgery in patients with small sellar lesions. *J Neurosurg.* 2009;110:354-358.
3. Arafah BM, Prunty D, Ybarra J, et al. The dominant role of increased intrasellar pressure in the pathogenesis of hypopituitarism, hyperprolactinemia, and headaches in patients with pituitary adenomas. *J Clin Endocrinol Metab.* 2000;85:1789-1793.
4. Freda PU, Post KD. Differential diagnosis of sellar masses. *Endocrinol Metab Clin North Am.* 1999;28:81-117, vi.
5. Famini P, Maya MM, Melmed S. Pituitary magnetic resonance imaging for sellar and parasellar masses: ten-year experience in 2598 patients. *J Clin Endocrinol Metab.* 2011;96:1633-1641.
6. Valassi E, Biller BM, Klibanski A, Swearingen B. Clinical features of nonpituitary sellar lesions in a large surgical series. *Clin Endocrinol (Oxf).* 2010;73:798-807.
7. Kleinberg DL. Pituitary tumors and failure of endocrine target organs. *Arch Intern Med.* 1979;139:969-970.
8. Hall WA, Luciano MG, Doppman JL, et al. Pituitary magnetic resonance imaging in normal human volunteers: occult adenomas in the general population. *Ann Intern Med.* 1994;120:817-820.
9. Karavitaki N, Thanabalasingham G, Shore HC, et al. Do the limits of serum prolactin in disconnection hyperprolactinaemia need re-definition? A study of 226 patients with histologically verified nonfunctioning pituitary macroadenoma. *Clin Endocrinol (Oxf).* 2006; 65:524-529.
10. Yaneva M, Mosnier-Pudar H, Dugue MA, et al. Midnight salivary cortisol for the initial diagnosis of Cushing's syndrome of various causes. *J Clin Endocrinol Metab.* 2004;89:3345-3351.
11. Lam KS, Sham MM, Tam SC, et al. Hypopituitarism after tuberculous meningitis in childhood. *Ann Intern Med.* 1993;118:701-706.
12. Makras P, Alexandraki KI, Chrousos GP, et al. Endocrine manifestations in Langerhans cell histiocytosis. *Trends Endocrinol Metab.* 2007;18:252-257.
13. Maccagnan P, Macedo CL, Kayath MJ, et al. Conservative management of pituitary apoplexy: a prospective study. *J Clin Endocrinol Metab.* 1995;80:2190-2197.
14. Lubina A, Olchovsky D, Berezin M, et al. Management of pituitary apoplexy: clinical experience with 40 patients. *Acta Neurochir (Wien).* 2005;147:151-157, discussion 157.
15. Rehman HU, Atkin SL. Growth hormone-secreting pituitary macroadenoma and meningioma in a woman—a case report and review of the literature. *Endocrinologist.* 2001;11:335-337.
16. Gokden M, Mrak RE. Pituitary adenoma with craniopharyngioma component. *Hum Pathol.* 2009;40:1189-1193.
17. Witte RJ, Mark LP, Daniels DL, Haughton VM. Radiographic evaluation of the pituitary and anterior hypothalamus. In: DeGroot LJ, Jameson JL, eds. *Endocrinology.* 4th ed. Philadelphia, PA: WB Saunders; 2001: 257-268.
18. Wolpert SM, Molitch ME, Goldman JA, Wood JB. Size, shape, and appearance of the normal female pituitary gland. *AJR Am J Roentgenol.* 1984;143:377-381.
19. Kucharczyk W, Lenkinski RE, Kucharczyk J, Henkelman RM. The effect of phospholipid vesicles on the NMR relaxation of water: an explanation for the MR appearance of the neurohypophysis? *AJNR Am J Neuroradiol.* 1990;11:693-700.

20. Turner HE, Nagy Z, Gatter KC, et al. Angiogenesis in pituitary adenomas and the normal pituitary gland. *J Clin Endocrinol Metab*. 2000; 85:1159-1162.
21. Issa N, Poggio ED, Fatica RA, et al. Nephrogenic systemic fibrosis and its association with gadolinium exposure during MRI. *Cleve Clin J Med*. 2008;75:95-97, 103-104, 6 passim.
22. de Herder WW, Reijs AE, Kwekkeboom DJ, et al. In vivo imaging of pituitary tumours using a radiolabelled dopamine D2 receptor radioligand. *Clin Endocrinol (Oxf)*. 1996;45:755-767.
23. Arnold A. Neuroophthalmologic evaluation of pituitary disorders. In: Melmed S, ed. *The Pituitary*. 2nd ed. Boston, MA: Blackwell Sciences; 2001.
24. Hoyt WF. Correlative functional anatomy of the optic chiasm, 1969. *Clin Neurosurg*. 1970;17:189-208.
25. Poon A, McNeill P, Harper A, O'Day J. Patterns of visual loss associated with pituitary macroadenomas. *Aust N Z J Ophthalmol*. 1995;23: 107-115.
26. Cushing H. Surgical experiences with pituitary disorders. *JAMA*. 1914; 63:1515-1525.
27. Schloffer H. Erfolgreiche operation eines hypohysentumors auf nasalem wege. *Wien Klin Wochenschr*. 1907;20:621-624.
28. Graffeo CS, Dietrich AR, Grobelny B, et al. A panoramic view of the skull base: systematic review of open and endoscopic endonasal approaches to four tumors. *Pituitary*. 2014;17:349-356.
29. Gondim JA, Schops M, de Almeida JP, et al. Endoscopic endonasal transsphenoidal surgery: surgical results of 228 pituitary adenomas treated in a pituitary center. *Pituitary*. 2010;13:68-77. [Epub 2009 Aug 21].
30. Tabaee A, Anand VK, Barron Y, et al. Endoscopic pituitary surgery: a systematic review and meta-analysis. *J Neurosurg*. 2009;111:545-554.
31. Swearingen B. Update on pituitary surgery. *J Clin Endocrinol Metab*. 2012;97:1073-1081.
32. Laws ER. Surgery for acromegaly: evolution of the techniques and outcomes. *Rev Endocr Metab Disord*. 2009;9:67-70.
33. Zirkzee EJ, Corssmit EP, Biermasz NR, et al. Pituitary magnetic resonance imaging is not required in the postoperative follow-up of acromegalic patients with long-term biochemical cure after transsphenoidal surgery. *J Clin Endocrinol Metab*. 2004;89:4320-4324.
34. Arafah BM, Kailani SH, Nekl KE, et al. Immediate recovery of pituitary function after transsphenoidal resection of pituitary macroadenomas. *J Clin Endocrinol Metab*. 1994;79:348-354.
35. Webb SM, Rigla M, Wagner A, et al. Recovery of hypopituitarism after neurosurgical treatment of pituitary adenomas. *J Clin Endocrinol Metab*. 1999;84:3696-3700.
36. Barker FG 2nd, Klibanski A, Swearingen B. Transsphenoidal surgery for pituitary tumors in the United States, 1996-2000: mortality, morbidity, and the effects of hospital and surgeon volume. *J Clin Endocrinol Metab*. 2003;88:4709-4719.
37. Gittoes NJ, Sheppard MC, Johnson AP, Stewart PM. Outcome of surgery for acromegaly—the experience of a dedicated pituitary surgeon. *Q J Med*. 1999;92:741-745.
38. Berker M, Hazer DB, Yucel T, et al. Complications of endoscopic surgery of the pituitary adenomas: analysis of 570 patients and review of the literature. *Pituitary*. 2012;15:288-300.
39. Roelfsema F, Biermasz NR, Pereira AM. Clinical factors involved in the recurrence of pituitary adenomas after surgical remission: a structured review and meta-analysis. *Pituitary*. 2012;15:71-83.
40. Kim EH, Oh MC, Lee EJ, Kim SH. Predicting long-term remission by measuring immediate postoperative growth hormone levels and oral glucose tolerance test in acromegaly. *Neurosurgery*. 2012;70:1106-1113, discussion 1113.
41. Nemergut EC, Dumont AS, Barry UT, Laws ER. Perioperative management of patients undergoing transsphenoidal pituitary surgery. *Anesth Analg*. 2005;101:1170-1181.
42. Guinan EM, Lowy C, Stanhope N, et al. Cognitive effects of pituitary tumours and their treatments: two case studies and an investigation of 90 patients. *J Neurol Neurosurg Psychiatry*. 1998;65:870-876.
43. Castinetti F, Regis J, Dufour H, Brue T. Role of stereotactic radiosurgery in the management of pituitary adenomas. *Nat Rev Endocrinol*. 2010; 6:214-223.
44. Castinetti F, Nagai M, Morange I, et al. Long-term results of stereotactic radiosurgery in secretory pituitary adenomas. *J Clin Endocrinol Metab*. 2009;94:3400-3407.
45. Minniti G, Gilbert DC, Brada M. Modern techniques for pituitary radiotherapy. *Rev Endocr Metab Disord*. 2009;10:135-144.
46. Loeffler JS, Shih HA. Radiation therapy in the management of pituitary adenomas. *J Clin Endocrinol Metab*. 2011;96:1992-2003.
47. Lee CC, Vance ML, Xu Z, et al. Stereotactic radiosurgery for acromegaly. *J Clin Endocrinol Metab*. 2014;99:1273-1281.
48. Simmons NE, Laws ER Jr. Glioma occurrence after sellar irradiation: case report and review. *Neurosurgery*. 1998;42:172-178.
49. Erfurth EM, Bulow B, Mikoczy Z, Hagmar L. Incidence of a second tumor in hypopituitary patients operated for pituitary tumors. *J Clin Endocrinol Metab*. 2001;86:659-662.
50. Tsang RW, Laperriere NJ, Simpson WJ, et al. Glioma arising after radiation therapy for pituitary adenoma. A report of four patients and estimation of risk. *Cancer*. 1993;72:2227-2233.
51. Minniti G, Traish D, Ashley S, et al. Risk of second brain tumor after conservative surgery and radiotherapy for pituitary adenoma: update after an additional 10 years. *J Clin Endocrinol Metab*. 2005;90:800-804.
52. Erfurth EM, Bulow B, Svahn-Tapper G, et al. Risk factors for cerebrovascular deaths in patients operated and irradiated for pituitary tumors. *J Clin Endocrinol Metab*. 2002;87:4892-4899.
53. Sherlock M, Reulen RC, Alonso AA, et al. ACTH deficiency, higher doses of hydrocortisone replacement, and radiotherapy are independent predictors of mortality in patients with acromegaly. *J Clin Endocrinol Metab*. 2009;94:4216-4223.
54. O'Connor MM, Mayberg MR. Effects of radiation on cerebral vasculature: a review. *Neurosurgery*. 2000;46:138-149, discussion 50-51.
55. Cifarelli CP, Schlesinger DJ, Sheehan JP. Cranial nerve dysfunction following Gamma Knife surgery for pituitary adenomas: long-term incidence and risk factors. *J Neurosurg*. 2012;116:1304-1310.
56. Tooze A, Gittoes NJ, Jones CA, Toogood AA. Neurocognitive consequences of surgery and radiotherapy for tumours of the pituitary. *Clin Endocrinol (Oxf)*. 2009;70:503-511.
57. el-Mahdy W, Powell M. Transsphenoidal management of 28 symptomatic Rathke's cleft cysts, with special reference to visual and hormonal recovery. *Neurosurgery*. 1998;42:7-16, discussion 17.
58. Freda PU, Wardlaw SL, Post KD. Unusual causes of sellar/parasellar masses in a large transsphenoidal surgical series. *J Clin Endocrinol Metab*. 1996;81:3455-3459.
59. Mukherjee JJ, Islam N, Kaltsas G, et al. Clinical, radiological and pathological features of patients with Rathke's cleft cysts: tumors that may recur. *J Clin Endocrinol Metab*. 1997;82:2357-2362.
60. Lewis AJ, Cooper PW, Kassel EE, Schwartz ML. Squamous cell carcinoma arising in a suprasellar epidermoid cyst. Case report. *J Neurosurg*. 1983;59:538-541.
61. Schaller B, Kirsch E, Tolnay M, Mindermann T. Symptomatic granular cell tumor of the pituitary gland: case report and review of the literature. *Neurosurgery*. 1998;42:166-170, discussion 170-171.
62. Volpe R, Mazabraud A. A clinicopathologic review of 25 cases of chordoma (a pleomorphic and metastasizing neoplasm). *Am J Surg Pathol*. 1983;7:161-170.
63. Rosenberg AE, Nielsen GP, Keel SB, et al. Chondrosarcoma of the base of the skull: a clinicopathologic study of 200 cases with emphasis on its distinction from chordoma. *Am J Surg Pathol*. 1999;23:1370-1378.
64. Stippler M, Gardner PA, Snyderman CH, et al. Endoscopic endonasal approach for clival chordomas. *Neurosurgery*. 2009;64:268-277, discussion 277-278.
65. Muller HL. Craniopharyngioma. *Endocr Rev*. 2014;35:513-543.
66. Karavitaki N, Wass JA. Craniopharyngiomas. *Endocrinol Metab Clin North Am*. 2008;37:173-193, ix-x.
67. Karavitaki N, Brufani C, Warner JT, et al. Craniopharyngiomas in children and adults: systematic analysis of 121 cases with long-term follow-up. *Clin Endocrinol (Oxf)*. 2005;62:397-409.
68. Honegger J, Buchfelder M, Fahlbusch R. Surgical treatment of craniopharyngiomas: endocrinological results. *J Neurosurg*. 1999;90:251-257.
69. Holsken A, Stache C, Schlaffer SM, et al. Adamantinomatous craniopharyngiomas express tumor stem cell markers in cells with activated Wnt signaling: further evidence for the existence of a tumor stem cell niche? *Pituitary*. 2013;17:546-556.
70. Elowe-Gruau E, Beltrand J, Brauner R, et al. Childhood craniopharyngioma: hypothalamus-sparing surgery decreases the risk of obesity. *J Clin Endocrinol Metab*. 2013;98:2376-2382.
71. Yuen KC, Koltowska-Haggstrom M, Cook DM, et al. Primary treatment regimen and diabetes insipidus as predictors of health outcomes in adults with childhood-onset craniopharyngioma. *J Clin Endocrinol Metab*. 2014;99:1227-3125.
72. Honegger J, Tatagiba M. Craniopharyngioma surgery. *Pituitary*. 2008; 11:361-373.
73. Roemmler-Zehrer J, Geigenberger V, Stormann S, et al. Food intake regulating hormones in adult craniopharyngioma patients. *Eur J Endocrinol*. 2014;170:627-635.
74. Zoicas F, Droste M, Mayr B, et al. GLP-1 analogues as a new treatment option for hypothalamic obesity in adults: report of nine cases. *Eur J Endocrinol*. 2013;168:699-706.
75. Nozaki K, Nagata I, Yoshida K, Kikuchi H. Intrasellar meningioma: case report and review of the literature. *Surg Neurol*. 1997;47:447-452, discussion 452-454.
76. Beems T, Grotenhuis JA, Wesseling P. Meningioma of the pituitary stalk without dural attachment: case report and review of the literature. *Neurosurgery*. 1999;45:1474-1477.
77. Collet-Solberg PF, Sernyak H, Satin-Smith M, et al. Endocrine outcome in long-term survivors of low-grade hypothalamic/chiasmatic glioma. *Clin Endocrinol (Oxf)*. 1997;47:79-85.
78. Ciappetta P, Calace A, D'Urso PI, De Candia N. Endoscopic treatment of pituitary abscess: two case reports and literature review. *Neurosurg Rev*. 2008;31:237-246, discussion 246.
79. Dalan R, Leow MK. Pituitary abscess: our experience with a case and a review of the literature. *Pituitary*. 2008;11:299-306.
80. Liu F, Li G, Yao Y, et al. Diagnosis and management of pituitary abscess: experiences from 33 cases. *Clin Endocrinol (Oxf)*. 2011;74: 79-88.

81. Telzak EE, Cote RJ, Gold JW, et al. Extrapulmonary *Pneumocystis carinii* infections. *Rev Infect Dis.* 1990;12:380-386.
82. Danilowicz K, Sanz CF, Manavela M, et al. Pituitary abscess: a report of two cases. *Pituitary.* 2008;11:89-92.
83. Freda PU. Tuberculosis of the pituitary and sellar region. *Pituitary.* 2002;5:147-148.
84. Capra M, Wherrett D, Weitzman S, et al. Pituitary stalk thickening and primary central nervous system lymphoma. *J Neurooncol.* 2004;67:227-231.
85. Giustina A, Gola M, Doga M, Rosei EA. Clinical review 136: primary lymphoma of the pituitary: an emerging clinical entity. *J Clin Endocrinol Metab.* 2001;86:4567-4575.
86. Moshkin O, Muller P, Scheithauer BW, et al. Primary pituitary lymphoma: a histological, immunohistochemical, and ultrastructural study with literature review. *Endocr Pathol.* 2009;20:46-49.
87. Brat DJ, Scheithauer BW, Staugaitis SM, et al. Pituicytoma: a distinctive low-grade glioma of the neurohypophysis. *Am J Surg Pathol.* 2000;24:362-368.
88. Chen KT. Crush cytology of pituicytoma. *Diagn Cytopathol.* 2005;33:255-257.
89. Bell NH. Endocrine complications of sarcoidosis. *Endocrinol Metab Clin North Am.* 1991;20:645-654.
90. Newman LS, Rose CS, Maier LA. Sarcoidosis. *N Engl J Med.* 1997;336:1224-1234.
91. Pitale SU, Camacho PM, Gordon DL. Central nervous system involvement in sarcoidosis presenting as a recurrent pituitary mass. *Endocrinologist.* 2000;10:429-431.
92. Langrand C, Bihan H, Raverot G, et al. Hypothalamo-pituitary sarcoidosis: a multicenter study of 24 patients. *Q J Med.* 2012;105:981-995.
93. Braunstein GD, Kohler PO. Pituitary function in Hand-Schuller-Christian disease. Evidence for deficient growth-hormone release in patients with short stature. *N Engl J Med.* 1972;286:1225-1229.
94. Marchand I, Barkaoui MA, Garel C, et al. Central diabetes insipidus as the inaugural manifestation of Langerhans cell histiocytosis: natural history and medical evaluation of 26 children and adolescents. *J Clin Endocrinol Metab.* 2011;96:E1352-E1360.
95. Nanduri VR, Pritchard J, Levitt G, Glaser AW. Long term morbidity and health related quality of life after multi-system Langerhans cell histiocytosis. *Eur J Cancer.* 2006;42:2563-2569.
96. Dhall G, Finlay JL, Dunkel IJ, et al. Analysis of outcome for patients with mass lesions of the central nervous system due to Langerhans cell histiocytosis treated with 2-chlorodeoxyadenosine. *Pediatr Blood Cancer.* 2008;50:72-79.
97. Braun J, Schuldes H, Berkefeld J, et al. Panhypopituitarism associated with severe retroperitoneal fibrosis. *Clin Endocrinol (Oxf).* 2001;54:273-276.
98. Komninos J, Vlassopoulou V, Protopapa D, et al. Tumors metastatic to the pituitary gland: case report and literature review. *J Clin Endocrinol Metab.* 2004;89:574-580.
99. Post KD. Pituitary metastases: what is the role of surgery? *World Neurosurg.* 2013;79:251-252.
100. He W, Chen F, Dalm B, et al. Metastatic involvement of the pituitary gland: a systematic review with pooled individual patient data analysis. *Pituitary.* 2015;18(1):159-168.
101. Chamarthi B, Morris CA, Kaiser UB, et al. Clinical problem-solving. Stalking the diagnosis. *N Engl J Med.* 2010;362:834-839.
102. Sidiropoulos M, Syro LV, Rotondo F, et al. Melanoma of the sellar region mimicking pituitary adenoma. *Neuropathology.* 2013;33:175-178.
103. Rivera JA. Lymphocytic hypophysitis: disease spectrum and approach to diagnosis and therapy. *Pituitary.* 2006;9:35-45.
104. Caturegli P, Newschaffer C, Olivi A, et al. Autoimmune hypophysitis. *Endocr Rev.* 2005;26:599-614.
105. Leung GK, Lopes MB, Thorner MO, et al. Primary hypophysitis: a single-center experience in 16 cases. *J Neurosurg.* 2004;101:262-271.
106. Bellastella A, Bizzarro A, Coronella C, et al. Lymphocytic hypophysitis: a rare or underestimated disease? *Eur J Endocrinol.* 2003;149:363-376.
107. Lee YJ, Lin JC, Shen EY, et al. Loss of visibility of the neurohypophysis as a sign of central diabetes insipidus. *Eur J Radiol.* 1996;21:233-235.
108. De Bellis A, Sinisi AA, Pane E, et al. Involvement of hypothalamus autoimmunity in patients with autoimmune hypopituitarism: role of antibodies to hypothalamic cells. *J Clin Endocrinol Metab.* 2012;97:3684-3690.
109. Muir A, Maclaren NK. Autoimmune diseases of the adrenal glands, parathyroid glands, gonads, and hypothalamic-pituitary axis. *Endocrinol Metab Clin North Am.* 1991;20:619-644.
110. Crock PA. Cytosolic autoantigens in lymphocytic hypophysitis. *J Clin Endocrinol Metab.* 1998;83:609-618.
111. Honegger J, Fahlbusch R, Bornemann A, et al. Lymphocytic and granulomatous hypophysitis: experience with nine cases. *Neurosurgery.* 1997;40:713-722, discussion 722-723.
112. Hunn BH, Martin WG, Simpson S Jr, McLean CA. Idiopathic granulomatous hypophysitis: a systematic review of 82 cases in the literature. *Pituitary.* 2014;17:357-365.
113. Hayashi H, Yamada K, Kuroki T, et al. Lymphocytic hypophysitis and pulmonary sarcoidosis. Report of a case. *Am J Clin Pathol.* 1991;95:506-511.
114. Toth M, Szabo P, Racz K, et al. Granulomatous hypophysitis associated with Takayasu's disease. *Clin Endocrinol (Oxf).* 1996;45:499-503.
115. Gutenberg A, Caturegli P, Metz I, et al. Necrotizing infundibulo-hypophysitis: an entity too rare to be true? *Pituitary.* 2012;15:202-208.
116. Iwama S, De Remigis A, Callahan MK, et al. Pituitary expression of CTLA-4 mediates hypophysitis secondary to administration of CTLA-4 blocking antibody. *Sci Transl Med.* 2014;6:230ra45.
117. Ryder M, Callahan M, Postow MA, et al. Endocrine-related adverse events following ipilimumab in patients with advanced melanoma: a comprehensive retrospective review from a single institution. *Endocr Relat Cancer.* 2014;21:371-381.
118. Faje AT, Sullivan R, Lawrence D, et al. Ipilimumab-induced hypophysitis: a detailed longitudinal analysis in a large cohort of patients with metastatic melanoma. *J Clin Endocrinol Metab.* 2014;99(11):4078-4085.
119. Dillard T, Yedinak CG, Alumkal J, Fleseriu M. Anti-CTLA-4 antibody therapy associated autoimmune hypophysitis: serious immune related adverse events across a spectrum of cancer subtypes. *Pituitary.* 2010;13:29-38.
120. Caputo C, Bazargan A, McKelvie PA, et al. Hypophysitis due to IgG4-related disease responding to treatment with azathioprine: an alternative to corticosteroid therapy. *Pituitary.* 2014;17:251-256.
121. Kovacs K. Sheehan syndrome. *Lancet.* 2003;361:520-522.
122. Kelestimur F. Sheehan's syndrome. *Pituitary.* 2003;6:181-188.
123. Sanyal D, Raychaudhuri M. Varied presentations of Sheehan's syndrome at diagnosis: a review of 18 patients. *Indian J Endocrinol Metab.* 2012;16:S300-S301.
124. Goswami R, Kochupillai N, Crock PA, et al. Pituitary autoimmunity in patients with Sheehan's syndrome. *J Clin Endocrinol Metab.* 2002;87:4137-4141.
125. Arafah BM, Harrington JF, Madhoun ZT, Selman WR. Improvement of pituitary function after surgical decompression for pituitary tumor apoplexy. *J Clin Endocrinol Metab.* 1990;71:323-328.
126. Semple PL, Jane JA Jr, Laws ER Jr. Clinical relevance of precipitating factors in pituitary apoplexy. *Neurosurgery.* 2007;61:956-961, discussion 961-962.
127. Hands KE, Alvarez A, Bruder JM. Gonadotropin-releasing hormone agonist-induced pituitary apoplexy in treatment of prostate cancer: case report and review of literature. *Endocr Pract.* 2007;13:642-646.
128. Balarini Lima GA, Machado Ede O, Dos Santos Silva CM, et al. Pituitary apoplexy during treatment of cystic macroprolactinomas with cabergoline. *Pituitary.* 2008;11:287-292.
129. Banerjee C, Snelling B, Hanft S, Komotar RJ. Bilateral cerebral infarction in the setting of pituitary apoplexy: a case presentation and literature review. *Pituitary.* 2015;18(3):352-358.
130. Elsasser Imboden PN, De Tribolet N, Lobrinus A, et al. Apoplexy in pituitary macroadenoma: eight patients presenting in 12 months. *Medicine (Baltimore).* 2005;84:188-196.
131. Zayour DH, Selman WR, Arafah BM. Extreme elevation of intrasellar pressure in patients with pituitary tumor apoplexy: relation to pituitary function. *J Clin Endocrinol Metab.* 2004;89:5649-5654.
132. Ayuk J, McGregor EJ, Mitchell RD, Gittoes NJ. Acute management of pituitary apoplexy—surgery or conservative management? *Clin Endocrinol (Oxf).* 2004;61:747-752.
133. Melmed S. Mechanisms for pituitary tumorigenesis: the plastic pituitary. *J Clin Invest.* 2003;112:1603-1618.
134. Sano K. Incidence of primary tumors (1969-1983). In: *Brain Tumor Registry of Japan. Neurol Med Chir (Tokyo).* 1992;37(special issue):391-441.
135. Daly AF, Jaffrain-Rea ML, Ciccarelli A, et al. Clinical characterization of familial isolated pituitary adenomas. *J Clin Endocrinol Metab.* 2006;91:3316-3323.
136. Fernandez A, Karavitaki N, Wass JA. Prevalence of pituitary adenomas: a community-based, cross-sectional study in Banbury (Oxfordshire, UK). *Clin Endocrinol (Oxf).* 2010;72:377-382.
137. Gittleman H, Ostrom QT, Farah PD, et al. Descriptive epidemiology of pituitary tumors in the United States, 2004-2009. *J Neurosurg.* 2014;121(3):527-535.
138. Liu NA, Jiang H, Ben-Shlomo A, et al. Targeting zebrafish and murine pituitary corticotroph tumors with a cyclin-dependent kinase (CDK) inhibitor. *Proc Natl Acad Sci U S A.* 2011;108:8414-8419.
139. Quereda V, Malumbres M. Cell cycle control of pituitary development and disease. *J Mol Endocrinol.* 2009;42:75-86.
140. Melmed S. Pathogenesis of pituitary tumors. *Nat Rev Endocrinol.* 2011;7:257-266.
141. Herman V, Fagin J, Gonsky R, et al. Clonal origin of pituitary adenomas. *J Clin Endocrinol Metab.* 1990;71:1427-1433.
142. Schulte HM, Oldfield EH, Allolio B, et al. Clonal composition of pituitary adenomas in patients with Cushing's disease: determination by X-chromosome inactivation analysis. *J Clin Endocrinol Metab.* 1991;73:1302-1308.
143. Alexander JM, Biller BM, Bikkal H, et al. Clinically nonfunctioning pituitary tumors are monoclonal in origin. *J Clin Invest.* 1990;86:336-340.
144. Thorner MO, Perryman RL, Cronin MJ, et al. Somatotroph hyperplasia. Successful treatment of acromegaly by removal of a pancreatic islet

tumor secreting a growth hormone-releasing factor. *J Clin Invest.* 1982;70:965-977.

145. Sano T, Asa SL, Kovacs K. Growth hormone-releasing hormone-producing tumors: clinical, biochemical, and morphological manifestations. *Endocr Rev.* 1988;9:357-373.

146. Mayo KE, Hammer RE, Swanson LW, et al. Dramatic pituitary hyperplasia in transgenic mice expressing a human growth hormone-releasing factor gene. *Mol Endocrinol.* 1988;2:606-612.

147. Landis CA, Harsh G, Lyons J, et al. Clinical characteristics of acromegalic patients whose pituitary tumors contain mutant Gs protein. *J Clin Endocrinol Metab.* 1990;71:1416-1420.

148. Weinstein LS, Shenker A, Gejman PV, et al. Activating mutations of the stimulatory G protein in the McCune-Albright syndrome. *N Engl J Med.* 1991;325:1688-1695.

149. Struthers RS, Vale WW, Arias C, et al. Somatotroph hypoplasia and dwarfism in transgenic mice expressing a non-phosphorylatable CREB mutant. *Nature.* 1991;350:622-624.

150. Bertherat J, Chanson P, Montminy M. The cyclic adenosine 3′,5′-monophosphate-responsive factor CREB is constitutively activated in human somatotroph adenomas. *Mol Endocrinol.* 1995;9: 777-783.

151. Grossman AB. The molecular biology of pituitary tumors: a personal perspective. *Pituitary.* 2009;12:265-270.

152. Lazzerini Denchi E, Attwooll C, Pasini D, Helin K. Deregulated E2F activity induces hyperplasia and senescence-like features in the mouse pituitary gland. *Mol Cell Biol.* 2005;25:2660-2672.

153. Pei L, Melmed S, Scheithauer B, et al. Frequent loss of heterozygosity at the retinoblastoma susceptibility gene (RB) locus in aggressive pituitary tumors: evidence for a chromosome 13 tumor suppressor gene other than RB. *Cancer Res.* 1995;55:1613-1616.

154. Simpson DJ, Hibberts NA, McNicol AM, et al. Loss of pRb expression in pituitary adenomas is associated with methylation of the RB1 CpG island. *Cancer Res.* 2000;60:1211-1216.

155. Herman V, Drazin NZ, Gonsky R, Melmed S. Molecular screening of pituitary adenomas for gene mutations and rearrangements. *J Clin Endocrinol Metab.* 1993;77:50-55.

156. Pei L, Melmed S. Isolation and characterization of a pituitary tumor-transforming gene (PTTG). *Mol Endocrinol.* 1997;11:433-441.

157. Zhang X, Horwitz GA, Heaney AP, et al. Pituitary tumor transforming gene (PTTG) expression in pituitary adenomas. *J Clin Endocrinol Metab.* 1999;84:761-767.

158. Heaney AP, Horwitz GA, Wang Z, et al. Early involvement of estrogen-induced pituitary tumor transforming gene and fibroblast growth factor expression in prolactinoma pathogenesis. *Nat Med.* 1999;5: 1317-1321.

159. Zou H, McGarry TJ, Bernal T, Kirschner MW. Identification of a vertebrate sister-chromatid separation inhibitor involved in transformation and tumorigenesis. *Science.* 1999;285:418-422.

160. Yu R, Heaney AP, Lu W, et al. Pituitary tumor transforming gene causes aneuploidy and p53-dependent and p53-independent apoptosis. *J Biol Chem.* 2000;275:36502-36505.

161. Abbud RA, Takumi I, Barker EM, et al. Early multipotential pituitary focal hyperplasia in the alpha-subunit of glycoprotein hormone-driven pituitary tumor-transforming gene transgenic mice. *Mol Endocrinol.* 2005;19:1383-1391.

162. McCabe CJ, Boelaert K, Tannahill LA, et al. Vascular endothelial growth factor, its receptor KDR/Flk-1, and pituitary tumor transforming gene in pituitary tumors. *J Clin Endocrinol Metab.* 2002;87: 4238-4244.

163. Suzuki M, Minematsu T, Oyama K, et al. Expression of proliferation markers in human pituitary incidentalomas. *Endocr Pathol.* 2006;17: 263-275.

164. Hibberts NA, Simpson DJ, Bicknell JE, et al. Analysis of cyclin D1 (CCND1) allelic imbalance and overexpression in sporadic human pituitary tumors. *Clin Cancer Res.* 1999;5:2133-2139.

165. Franklin DS, Godfrey VL, Lee H, et al. CDK inhibitors p18(INK4c) and p27(Kip1) mediate two separate pathways to collaboratively suppress pituitary tumorigenesis. *Genes Dev.* 1998;12:2899-2911.

166. Kiyokawa H, Kineman RD, Manova-Todorova KO, et al. Enhanced growth of mice lacking the cyclin-dependent kinase inhibitor function of p27(Kip1). *Cell.* 1996;85:721-732.

167. Ezzat S, Zheng L, Zhu XF, et al. Targeted expression of a human pituitary tumor-derived isoform of FGF receptor-4 recapitulates pituitary tumorigenesis. *J Clin Invest.* 2002;109:69-78.

168. Shimon I, Huttner A, Said J, et al. Heparin-binding secretory transforming gene (hst) facilitates rat lactotrope cell tumorigenesis and induces prolactin gene transcription. *J Clin Invest.* 1996;97: 187-195.

169. Vlotides G, Cooper O, Chen YH, et al. Heregulin regulates prolactinoma gene expression. *Cancer Res.* 2009;69:4209-4216.

170. Vlotides G, Siegel E, Donangelo I, et al. Rat prolactinoma cell growth regulation by epidermal growth factor receptor ligands. *Cancer Res.* 2008;68:6377-6386.

171. Cooper O, Mamelak A, Bannykh S, et al. Prolactinoma ErbB receptor expression and targeted therapy for aggressive tumors. *Endocrine.* 2014;46:318-327.

172. Zhang X, Sun H, Danila DC, et al. Loss of expression of GADD45 gamma, a growth inhibitory gene, in human pituitary adenomas: implications for tumorigenesis. *J Clin Endocrinol Metab.* 2002;87: 1262-1267.

173. Gejman R, Batista DL, Zhong Y, et al. Selective loss of MEG3 expression and intergenic differentially methylated region hypermethylation in the MEG3/DLK1 locus in human clinically nonfunctioning pituitary adenomas. *J Clin Endocrinol Metab.* 2008;93:4119-4125.

174. Qian ZR, Asa SL, Siomi H, et al. Overexpression of HMGA2 relates to reduction of the let-7 and its relationship to clinicopathological features in pituitary adenomas. *Mod Pathol.* 2009;22:431-441.

175. De Martino I, Visone R, Wierinckx A, et al. HMGA proteins up-regulate CCNB2 gene in mouse and human pituitary adenomas. *Cancer Res.* 2009;69:1844-1850.

176. Farrell WE. Epigenetics of pituitary tumours: an update. *Curr Opin Endocrinol Diabetes Obes.* 2014;21:299-305.

177. Chesnokova V, Zonis S, Kovacs K, et al. p21(Cip1) restrains pituitary tumor growth. *Proc Natl Acad Sci U S A.* 2008;105:17498-17503.

178. Kuilman T, Michaloglou C, Vredeveld LC, et al. Oncogene-induced senescence relayed by an interleukin-dependent inflammatory network. *Cell.* 2008;133:1019-1031.

179. Brandi ML, Gagel RF, Angeli A, et al. Guidelines for diagnosis and therapy of MEN type 1 and type 2. *J Clin Endocrinol Metab.* 2001;86:5658-5671.

180. Trouillas J, Labat-Moleur F, Sturm N, et al. Pituitary tumors and hyperplasia in multiple endocrine neoplasia type 1 syndrome (MEN1): a case-control study in a series of 77 patients versus 2509 non-MEN1 patients. *Am J Surg Pathol.* 2008;32:534-543.

181. Chandrasekharappa SC, Guru SC, Manickam P, et al. Positional cloning of the gene for multiple endocrine neoplasia-type 1. *Science.* 1997;276:404-407.

182. Tanaka C, Yoshimoto K, Yamada S, et al. Absence of germ-line mutations of the multiple endocrine neoplasia type 1 (MEN1) gene in familial pituitary adenoma in contrast to MEN1 in Japanese. *J Clin Endocrinol Metab.* 1998;83:960-965.

183. Pellegata NS, Quintanilla-Martinez L, Siggelkow H, et al. Germ-line mutations in p27Kip1 cause a multiple endocrine neoplasia syndrome in rats and humans. *Proc Natl Acad Sci U S A.* 2006;103:15558-15563.

184. Beckers A, Aaltonen LA, Daly AF, Karhu A. Familial isolated pituitary adenomas (FIPA) and the pituitary adenoma predisposition due to mutations in the aryl hydrocarbon receptor interacting protein (AIP) gene. *Endocr Rev.* 2013;34:239-277.

185. Gadelha MR, Une KN, Rohde K, et al. Isolated familial somatotropinomas: establishment of linkage to chromosome 11q13.1-11q13.3 and evidence for a potential second locus at chromosome 2p16-12. *J Clin Endocrinol Metab.* 2000;85:707-714.

186. Vierimaa O, Georgitsi M, Lehtonen R, et al. Pituitary adenoma predisposition caused by germline mutations in the AIP gene. *Science.* 2006;312:1228-1230.

187. Daly AF, Vanbellinghen JF, Khoo SK, et al. Aryl hydrocarbon receptor-interacting protein gene mutations in familial isolated pituitary adenomas: analysis in 73 families. *J Clin Endocrinol Metab.* 2007;92: 1891-1896.

188. Leontiou CA, Gueorguiev M, van der Spuy J, et al. The role of the aryl hydrocarbon receptor-interacting protein gene in familial and sporadic pituitary adenomas. *J Clin Endocrinol Metab.* 2008;93: 2390-2401.

189. Vasilev V, Daly A, Naves L, et al. Clinical and genetic aspects of familial isolated pituitary adenomas. *Clinics (Sao Paulo).* 2012;67(Suppl 1): 37-41.

190. Korbonits M, Storr H, Kumar AV. Familial pituitary adenomas—who should be tested for AIP mutations? *Clin Endocrinol (Oxf).* 2012;77: 351-356.

191. Schofl C, Honegger J, Droste M, et al. Frequency of AIP gene mutations in young patients with acromegaly: a registry-based study. *J Clin Endocrinol Metab.* 2014;99(12):E2789-E2793.

192. Casey M, Vaughan CJ, He J, et al. Mutations in the protein kinase A R1alpha regulatory subunit cause familial cardiac myxomas and Carney complex. *J Clin Invest.* 2000;106:R31-R38.

193. Kirschner LS, Sandrini F, Monbo J, et al. Genetic heterogeneity and spectrum of mutations of the PRKAR1A gene in patients with the Carney complex. *Hum Mol Genet.* 2000;9:3037-3046.

194. Palumbo T, Faucz FR, Azevedo M, et al. Functional screen analysis reveals miR-26b and miR-128 as central regulators of pituitary somato-mammotrophic tumor growth through activation of the PTEN-AKT pathway. *Oncogene.* 2013;32:1651-1659.

195. Trouillas J, Roy P, Sturm N, et al. A new prognostic clinicopathological classification of pituitary adenomas: a multicentric case-control study of 410 patients with 8 years post-operative follow-up. *Acta Neuropathol.* 2013;126:123-135.

196. Mete O, Asa SL. Clinicopathological correlations in pituitary adenomas. *Brain Pathol.* 2012;22:443-453.

197. Sav A, Rotondo F, Syro LV, et al. Biomarkers of pituitary neoplasms. *Anticancer Res.* 2012;32:4639-4654.

198. Molitch ME. Nonfunctioning pituitary tumors and pituitary incidentalomas. *Endocrinol Metab Clin North Am.* 2008;37:151-171, xi.

199. Chanson P, Young J. Pituitary incidentalomas. *Endocrinologist.* 2003; 13:124-135.
200. Osamura RY, Kajiya H, Takei M, et al. Pathology of the human pituitary adenomas. *Histochem Cell Biol.* 2008;130:495-507.
201. Al-Shraim M, Asa SL. The 2004 World Health Organization classification of pituitary tumors: what is new? *Acta Neuropathol.* 2006;111:1-7.
202. Oh MC, Tihan T, Kunwar S, et al. Clinical management of pituitary carcinomas. *Neurosurg Clin North Am.* 2012;23:595-606.
203. Scheithauer BW, Kurtkaya-Yapicier O, Kovacs KT, et al. Pituitary carcinoma: a clinicopathological review. *Neurosurgery.* 2005;56:1066-1074, discussion 1074.
204. Zada G, Woodmansee WW, Ramkissoon S, et al. Atypical pituitary adenomas: incidence, clinical characteristics, and implications. *J Neurosurg.* 2011;114:336-344.
205. Dudziak K, Honegger J, Bornemann A, et al. Pituitary carcinoma with malignant growth from first presentation and fulminant clinical course—case report and review of the literature. *J Clin Endocrinol Metab.* 2011;96:2665-2669.
206. Kaltsas GA, Nomikos P, Kontogeorgos G, et al. Clinical review: diagnosis and management of pituitary carcinomas. *J Clin Endocrinol Metab.* 2005;90:3089-3099.
207. Heaney AP. Clinical review: pituitary carcinoma: difficult diagnosis and treatment. *J Clin Endocrinol Metab.* 2011;96:3649-3660.
208. Pei L, Melmed S, Scheithauer B, et al. H-ras mutations in human pituitary carcinoma metastases. *J Clin Endocrinol Metab.* 1994;78:842-846.
209. Raverot G, Castinetti F, Jouanneau E, et al. Pituitary carcinomas and aggressive pituitary tumours: merits and pitfalls of temozolomide treatment. *Clin Endocrinol (Oxf).* 2012;76:769-775.
210. Whitelaw BC, Dworakowska D, Thomas NW, et al. Temozolomide in the management of dopamine agonist-resistant prolactinomas. *Clin Endocrinol (Oxf).* 2012;76:877-886.
211. Bush ZM, Longtine JA, Cunningham T, et al. Temozolomide treatment for aggressive pituitary tumors: correlation of clinical outcome with O(6)-methylguanine methyltransferase (MGMT) promoter methylation and expression. *J Clin Endocrinol Metab.* 2010;95:E280-E290.
212. Hirohata T, Asano K, Ogawa Y, et al. DNA mismatch repair protein (MSH6) correlated with the responses of atypical pituitary adenomas and pituitary carcinomas to temozolomide: the national cooperative study by the Japan Society for Hypothalamic and Pituitary Tumors. *J Clin Endocrinol Metab.* 2013;98:1130-1136.
213. Raverot G, Sturm N, de Fraipont F, et al. Temozolomide treatment in aggressive pituitary tumors and pituitary carcinomas: a French multicenter experience. *J Clin Endocrinol Metab.* 2010;95:4592-4599.
214. Syro LV, Ortiz LD, Scheithauer BW, et al. Treatment of pituitary neoplasms with temozolomide: a review. *Cancer.* 2011;117:454-462.
215. Colao A, Di Sarno A, Cappabianca P, et al. Withdrawal of long-term cabergoline therapy for tumoral and nontumoral hyperprolactinemia. *N Engl J Med.* 2003;349:2023-2033.
216. Domingue ME, Devuyst F, Alexopoulou O, et al. Outcome of prolactinoma after pregnancy and lactation: a study on 73 patients. *Clin Endocrinol (Oxf).* 2014;80:642-648.
217. Delgrange E, Trouillas J, Maiter D, et al. Sex-related difference in the growth of prolactinomas: a clinical and proliferation marker study. *J Clin Endocrinol Metab.* 1997;82:2102-2107.
218. Moraes AB, Silva CM, Vieira Neto L, Gadelha MR. Giant prolactinomas: the therapeutic approach. *Clin Endocrinol (Oxf).* 2013;79:447-456.
219. Delgrange E, Raverot G, Bex M, et al. Giant prolactinomas in women. *Eur J Endocrinol.* 2014;170:31-38.
220. Vilar L, Freitas MC, Naves LA, et al. Diagnosis and management of hyperprolactinemia: results of a Brazilian multicenter study with 1234 patients. *J Endocrinol Invest.* 2008;31:436-444.
221. Arafah BM, Nekl KE, Gold RS, Selman WR. Dynamics of prolactin secretion in patients with hypopituitarism and pituitary macroadenomas. *J Clin Endocrinol Metab.* 1995;80:3507-3512.
222. Kovacs K, Horvath E. Pathology of pituitary tumors. *Endocrinol Metab Clin North Am.* 1987;16:529-551.
223. Sarwar KN, Huda MS, Van de Velde V, et al. The prevalence and natural history of pituitary hemorrhage in prolactinoma. *J Clin Endocrinol Metab.* 2013;98:2362-2367.
224. Burgess JR, Shepherd JJ, Parameswaran V, et al. Spectrum of pituitary disease in multiple endocrine neoplasia type 1 (MEN 1): clinical, biochemical, and radiological features of pituitary disease in a large MEN 1 kindred. *J Clin Endocrinol Metab.* 1996;81:2642-2646.
225. Berezin M, Karasik A. Familial prolactinoma. *Clin Endocrinol (Oxf).* 1995;42:483-486.
226. Cazabat L, Bouligand J, Salenave S, et al. Germline AIP mutations in apparently sporadic pituitary adenomas: prevalence in a prospective single-center cohort of 443 patients. *J Clin Endocrinol Metab.* 2012;97:E663-E670.
227. Kleinberg DL, Noel GL, Frantz AG. Galactorrhea: a study of 235 cases including 48 with pituitary tumors. *N Engl J Med.* 1977;296:589-600.
228. Klibanski A, Neer RM, Beitins IZ, et al. Decreased bone density in hyperprolactinemic women. *N Engl J Med.* 1980;303:1511-1514.
229. Andela CD, Niemeijer ND, Scharloo M, et al. Towards a better quality of life (QoL) for patients with pituitary diseases: results from a focus group study exploring QoL. *Pituitary.* 2015;18(1):86-100.
230. Milenkovic L, D'Angelo G, Kelly PA, Weiner RI. Inhibition of gonadotropin hormone-releasing hormone release by prolactin from GT1 neuronal cell lines through prolactin receptors. *Proc Natl Acad Sci U S A.* 1994;91:1244-1247.
231. Ciccarelli A, Guerra E, De Rosa M, et al. PRL secreting adenomas in male patients. *Pituitary.* 2005;8:39-42.
232. Mazziotti G, Mancini T, Mormando M, et al. High prevalence of radiological vertebral fractures in women with prolactin-secreting pituitary adenomas. *Pituitary.* 2011;14:299-306.
233. Hollenhorst RW, Younge BR. Ocular manifestations produced by adenomas of the pituitary gland: analysis of 1000 cases. In: Kohler PO, Ross GT, eds. *Diagnosis and Treatment of Pituitary Tumors.* New York: Elsevier; 1973:53-64.
234. Zikel OM, Atkinson JL, Hurley DL. Prolactinoma manifesting with symptomatic hydrocephalus. *Mayo Clin Proc.* 1999;74:475-477.
235. Barkan AL, Chandler WF. Giant pituitary prolactinoma with falsely low serum prolactin: the pitfall of the "high-dose hook effect": case report. *Neurosurgery.* 1998;42:913-915.
236. Hattori N, Ishihara T, Saiki Y. Macroprolactinaemia: prevalence and etiologies in a large group of hospital workers. *Clin Endocrinol (Oxf).* 2009;71:702-708.
237. Kleinberg DL, Todd J, Groves ML. Studies on human α-lactalbumin: radioimmunoassay measurements in normal human breast and breast cancer. *J Clin Endocrinol Metab.* 1977;45:1238-1250.
238. Kleinberg DL, Todd J. Evidence that human growth hormone is a potent lactogen in primates. *J Clin Endocrinol Metab.* 1980;51:1009-1015.
239. Thorner MO, Martin WH, Rogol AD, et al. Rapid regression of pituitary prolactinomas during bromocriptine treatment. *J Clin Endocrinol Metab.* 1980;51:438-445.
240. Colao A, Vitale G, Cappabianca P, et al. Outcome of cabergoline treatment in men with prolactinoma: effects of a 24-month treatment on prolactin levels, tumor mass, recovery of pituitary function, and semen analysis. *J Clin Endocrinol Metab.* 2004;89:1704-1711.
241. Thorner MO, Perryman RL, Rogol AD, et al. Rapid changes of prolactinoma volume after withdrawal and reinstitution of bromocriptine. *J Clin Endocrinol Metab.* 1981;53:480-483.
242. Colao A, Di Sarno A, Sarnacchiaro F, et al. Prolactinomas resistant to standard dopamine agonists respond to chronic cabergoline treatment. *J Clin Endocrinol Metab.* 1997;82:876-883.
243. Shimazu S, Shimatsu A, Yamada S, et al. Resistance to dopamine agonists in prolactinoma is correlated with reduction of dopamine D2 receptor long isoform mRNA levels. *Eur J Endocrinol.* 2012;166:383-390.
244. Bassetti M, Spada A, Pezzo G, Giannattasio G. Bromocriptine treatment reduces the cell size in human macroprolactinomas: a morphometric study. *J Clin Endocrinol Metab.* 1984;58:268-273.
245. Hallenga B, Saeger W, Ludecke DK. Necroses of prolactin-secreting pituitary adenomas under treatment with dopamine agonists: light microscopical and morphometric studies. *Exp Clin Endocrinol.* 1988;92:59-68.
246. Tyrrell JB, Lamborn KR, Hannegan LT, et al. Transsphenoidal microsurgical therapy of prolactinomas: initial outcomes and long-term results. *Neurosurgery.* 1999;44:254-261.
247. Fahlbusch R, Buchfelder M, Schrell U. Short-term preoperative treatment of macroprolactinomas by dopamine agonists. *J Neurosurg.* 1987;67:807-815.
248. Webster J, Piscitelli G, Polli A, et al. A comparison of cabergoline and bromocriptine in the treatment of hyperprolactinemic amenorrhea. Cabergoline Comparative Study Group. *N Engl J Med.* 1994;331:904-909.
249. Biller BM, Molitch ME, Vance ML, et al. Treatment of prolactin-secreting macroadenomas with the once-weekly dopamine agonist cabergoline. *J Clin Endocrinol Metab.* 1996;81:2338-2343.
250. Kletzky OA, Vermesh M. Effectiveness of vaginal bromocriptine in treating women with hyperprolactinemia. *Fertil Steril.* 1989;51:269-272.
251. Turner TH, Cookson JC, Wass JA, et al. Psychotic reactions during treatment of pituitary tumours with dopamine agonists. *Br Med J (Clin Res Ed).* 1984;289:1101-1103.
252. Suliman SG, Gurlek A, Byrne JV, et al. Nonsurgical cerebrospinal fluid rhinorrhea in invasive macroprolactinoma: incidence, radiological, and clinicopathological features. *J Clin Endocrinol Metab.* 2007;92:3829-3835.
253. Melmed S, Braunstein GD. Bromocriptine and pleuropulmonary disease. *Arch Intern Med.* 1989;149:258-259.
254. Pinero A, Marcos-Alberca P, Fortes J. Cabergoline-related severe restrictive mitral regurgitation. *N Engl J Med.* 2005;353:1976-1977.
255. Antonini A, Poewe W. Fibrotic heart-valve reactions to dopamine-agonist treatment in Parkinson's disease. *Lancet Neurol.* 2007;6:826-829.
256. Zanettini R, Antonini A, Gatto G, et al. Valvular heart disease and the use of dopamine agonists for Parkinson's disease. *N Engl J Med.* 2007;356:39-46.
257. Colao A, Galderisi M, DiSarno A, et al. Increased prevalence of tricuspid regurgitation in patients with prolactinomas chronically treated with cabergoline. *J Clin Endocrinol Metab.* 2008;93:3777-3784.

258. Devin JK, Lakhani VT, Byrd BF III, Blevins LS Jr. Prevalence of valvular heart disease in a cohort of patients taking cabergoline for management of hyperprolactinemia. *Endocr Pract.* 2008;14:672-677.

259. Lancellotti P, Livadariu E, Markov M, et al. Cabergoline and the risk of valvular lesions in endocrine disease. *Eur J Endocrinol.* 2008; 159:1-5.

260. Vallette S, Serri K, Rivera J, et al. Long-term cabergoline therapy is not associated with valvular heart disease in patients with prolactinomas. *Pituitary.* 2009;12:153-157.

261. Delgado V, Biermasz NR, van Thiel SW, et al. Changes in heart valve structure and function in patients treated with dopamine agonists for prolactinomas, a 2-year follow-up study. *Clin Endocrinol (Oxf).* 2012; 77:99-105.

262. Elenkova A, Shabani R, Kalinov K, Zacharieva S. Increased prevalence of subclinical cardiac valve fibrosis in patients with prolactinomas on long-term bromocriptine and cabergoline treatment. *Eur J Endocrinol.* 2012;167:17-25.

263. Boguszewski CL, dos Santos CM, Sakamoto KS, et al. A comparison of cabergoline and bromocriptine on the risk of valvular heart disease in patients with prolactinomas. *Pituitary.* 2012;15:44-49.

264. Tsagarakis S, Grossman A, Plowman PN, et al. Megavoltage pituitary irradiation in the management of prolactinomas: long-term follow-up. *Clin Endocrinol (Oxf).* 1991;34:399-406.

265. Liu X, Kano H, Kondziolka D, et al. Gamma knife stereotactic radiosurgery for drug resistant or intolerant invasive prolactinomas. *Pituitary.* 2013;16:68-75.

266. Serri O, Rasio E, Beauregard H, et al. Recurrence of hyperprolactinemia after selective transsphenoidal adenomectomy in women with prolactinoma. *N Engl J Med.* 1983;309:280-283.

267. Molitch ME. Management of prolactinomas. *Annu Rev Med.* 1989;40: 225-32:225-232.

268. Kovacs K, Horvath E, Syro LV, et al. Temozolomide therapy in a man with an aggressive prolactin-secreting pituitary neoplasm: morphological findings. *Hum Pathol.* 2007;38:185-189.

269. Fadul CE, Kominsky AL, Meyer LP, et al. Long-term response of pituitary carcinoma to temozolomide. Report of two cases. *J Neurosurg.* 2006;105:621-626.

270. Neff LM, Weil M, Cole A, et al. Temozolomide in the treatment of an invasive prolactinoma resistant to dopamine agonists. *Pituitary.* 2007; 10:81-86.

271. McCormack AI, McDonald KL, Gill AJ, et al. Low O6-methylguanine-DNA methyltransferase (MGMT) expression and response to temozolomide in aggressive pituitary tumours. *Clin Endocrinol (Oxf).* 2009; 71:226-233.

272. Molitch ME. Pregnancy and the hyperprolactinemic woman. *N Engl J Med.* 1985;312:1364-1370.

273. Kupersmith MJ, Rosenberg C, Kleinberg D. Visual loss in pregnant women with pituitary adenomas. *Ann Intern Med.* 1994;121:473-477.

274. Liu C, Tyrrell JB. Successful treatment of a large macroprolactinoma with cabergoline during pregnancy. *Pituitary.* 2001;4:179-185.

275. Colao A, Abs R, Barcena DG, et al. Pregnancy outcomes following cabergoline treatment: extended results from a 12-year observational study. *Clin Endocrinol (Oxf).* 2008;68:66-71.

276. Auriemma RS, Perone Y, Di Sarno A, et al. Results of a single-center observational 10-year survey study on recurrence of hyperprolactinemia after pregnancy and lactation. *J Clin Endocrinol Metab.* 2013; 98:372-379.

277. Laws ER Jr, Fode NC, Randall RV, et al. Pregnancy following transsphenoidal resection of prolactin-secreting pituitary tumors. *J Neurosurg.* 1983;58:685-688.

278. Horvath E, Kovacs K. Ultrastructural diagnosis of human pituitary adenomas. *Microsc Res Tech.* 1992;20:107-135.

279. Samuels MH, Henry P, Kleinschmidt-DeMasters BK, et al. Pulsatile glycoprotein hormone secretion in glycoprotein-producing pituitary tumors. *J Clin Endocrinol Metab.* 1991;73:1281-1288.

280. Sanno N, Oyama K, Tahara S, et al. A survey of pituitary incidentaloma in Japan. *Eur J Endocrinol.* 2003;149:123-127.

281. Dekkers OM, van der Klaauw AA, Pereira AM, et al. Quality of life is decreased after treatment for nonfunctioning pituitary macroadenoma. *J Clin Endocrinol Metab.* 2006;91:3364-3369.

282. van der Klaauw AA, Dekkers OM, Pereira AM, et al. Increased daytime somnolence despite normal sleep patterns in patients treated for nonfunctioning pituitary macroadenoma. *J Clin Endocrinol Metab.* 2007;92: 3898-3903.

283. Ntali G, Capatina C, Grossman A, Karavitaki N. Functioning gonadotroph adenomas. *J Clin Endocrinol Metab.* 2014;99(12): 4423-4433.

284. Cooper O, Geller JL, Melmed S. Ovarian hyperstimulation syndrome caused by an FSH-secreting pituitary adenoma. *Nat Clin Pract Endocrinol Metab.* 2008;4:234-238.

285. Daneshdoost L, Gennarelli TA, Bashey HM, et al. Recognition of gonadotroph adenomas in women. *N Engl J Med.* 1991;324: 589-594.

286. Mamelak AN, Carmichael J, Bonert VH, et al. Single-surgeon fully endoscopic endonasal transsphenoidal surgery: outcomes in three-hundred consecutive cases. *Pituitary.* 2013;16:393-401.

287. Paluzzi A, Fernandez-Miranda JC, Tonya Stefko S, et al. Endoscopic endonasal approach for pituitary adenomas: a series of 555 patients. *Pituitary.* 2014;17:307-319.

288. Murad MH, Fernandez-Balsells MM, Barwise A, et al. Outcomes of surgical treatment for nonfunctioning pituitary adenomas: a systematic review and meta-analysis. *Clin Endocrinol (Oxf).* 2010;73:777-791.

289. Turner HE, Stratton IM, Byrne JV, et al. Audit of selected patients with nonfunctioning pituitary adenomas treated without irradiation: a follow-up study. *Clin Endocrinol (Oxf).* 1999;51:281-284.

290. O'Sullivan EP, Woods C, Glynn N, et al. The natural history of surgically treated but radiotherapy-naive nonfunctioning pituitary adenomas. *Clin Endocrinol (Oxf).* 2009;71:709-714.

291. Dekkers OM, Pereira AM, Romijn JA. Treatment and follow-up of clinically nonfunctioning pituitary macroadenomas. *J Clin Endocrinol Metab.* 2008;93:3717-3726.

292. Pollock BE, Cochran J, Natt N, et al. Gamma knife radiosurgery for patients with nonfunctioning pituitary adenomas: results from a 15-year experience. *Int J Radiat Oncol Biol Phys.* 2008;70:1325-1329.

293. Starke RM, Williams BJ, Jane JA Jr, Sheehan JP. Gamma knife surgery for patients with nonfunctioning pituitary macroadenomas: predictors of tumor control, neurological deficits, and hypopituitarism. *J Neurosurg.* 2012;117:129-135.

294. Sheehan JP, Starke RM, Mathieu D, et al. Gamma knife radiosurgery for the management of nonfunctioning pituitary adenomas: a multicenter study. *J Neurosurg.* 2013;119:446-456.

295. Greenman Y, Stern N. How should a nonfunctioning pituitary macroadenoma be monitored after debulking surgery? *Clin Endocrinol (Oxf).* 2009;70:829-832.

296. Reddy R, Cudlip S, Byrne JV, et al. Can we ever stop imaging in surgically treated and radiotherapy-naive patients with non-functioning pituitary adenoma? *Eur J Endocrinol.* 2011;165:739-744.

297. Sayyed Kassem L, El Sibai K, Chaiban J, et al. Measurements of serum DHEA and DHEA sulphate levels improve the accuracy of the low-dose cosyntropin test in the diagnosis of central adrenal insufficiency. *J Clin Endocrinol Metab.* 2012;97:3655-3662.

298. Wass JA, Karavitaki N. Nonfunctioning pituitary adenomas: the Oxford experience. *Nat Rev Endocrinol.* 2009;5:519-522.

299. Greenman Y, Tordjman K, Osher E, et al. Postoperative treatment of clinically nonfunctioning pituitary adenomas with dopamine agonists decreases tumour remnant growth. *Clin Endocrinol (Oxf).* 2005;63: 39-44.

300. Cooper O, Ben-Shlomo A, Bonert V, et al. Silent corticogonadotroph adenomas: clinical and cellular characteristics and long-term outcomes. *Horm Cancer.* 2010;1:80-92.

301. Alahmadi H, Lee D, Wilson JR, et al. Clinical features of silent corticotroph adenomas. *Acta Neurochir (Wien).* 2012;154:1493-1498.

302. Erickson D, Scheithauer B, Atkinson J, et al. Silent subtype 3 pituitary adenoma: a clinicopathologic analysis of the Mayo Clinic experience. *Clin Endocrinol (Oxf).* 2009;71:92-99.

303. Marie P. On two cases of acromegaly: marked hypertrophy of the upper and lower limbs and the head. *Rev Med.* 1886;6:297-333.

304. Benda C. Beitrage zur normalen und pathologischen histologischen der menschhchen hypophysis cerebri. *Klin Wochenschr.* 1900;36:1205.

305. Cushing H. Partial hypophysectomy for acromegaly: with remarks on the function of the hypophysis. *Ann Surg.* 1909;50:1002-1017.

306. Evans HM, Long JA. The effect of the anterior lobe of the pituitary administered intra-peritoneally upon growth, maturity and oestrus cycle of the rat. *Anat Rev.* 1921;21:62.

307. Alexander L, Appleton D, Hall R, et al. Epidemiology of acromegaly in the Newcastle region. *Clin Endocrinol (Oxf).* 1980;12:71-79.

308. Bengtsson BA, Eden S, Ernest I, et al. Epidemiology and long-term survival in acromegaly. A study of 166 cases diagnosed between 1955 and 1984. *Acta Med Scand.* 1988;223:327-335.

309. Ritchie CM, Atkinson AB, Kennedy AL, et al. Ascertainment and natural history of treated acromegaly in Northern Ireland. *Ulster Med J.* 1990;59:55-62.

310. Fernandez A, Karavitaki N, Wass JA. Prevalence of pituitary adenomas: a community-based, cross-sectional study in Banbury (Oxfordshire, UK). *Clin Endocrinol (Oxf).* 2010;72(3):377-382.

311. Melmed S. Medical progress: acromegaly. *N Engl J Med.* 2006;355: 2558-2573.

312. Cuevas-Ramos D, Carmichael JD, Cooper O, et al. A structural and functional acromegaly classification. *J Clin Endocrinol Metab.* 2015; 100(1):122-131.

313. Kovacs K, Lloyd R, Horvath E, et al. Silent somatotroph adenomas of the human pituitary. A morphologic study of three cases including immunocytochemistry, electron microscopy, in vitro examination, and in situ hybridization. *Am J Pathol.* 1989;134:345-353.

314. Howard AD, Feighner SD, Cully DF, et al. A receptor in pituitary and hypothalamus that functions in growth hormone release. *Science.* 1996;273:974-977.

315. Dimaraki EV, Chandler WF, Brown MB, et al. The role of endogenous growth-releasing hormone in acromegaly. *J Clin Endocrinol Metab.* 2006;91:2185-2190.

316. Thapar K, Kovacs K, Stefaneanu L, et al. Overexpression of the growth-hormone-releasing hormone gene in acromegaly-associated pituitary

tumors. An event associated with neoplastic progression and aggressive behavior. *Am J Pathol.* 1997;151:769-784.

317. Ho KY, Veldhuis JD, Johnson ML, et al. Fasting enhances growth hormone secretion and amplifies the complex rhythms of growth hormone secretion in man. *J Clin Invest.* 1988;81:968-975.

318. Melmed S, Ezrin C, Kovacs K, et al. Acromegaly due to secretion of growth hormone by an ectopic pancreatic islet-cell tumor. *N Engl J Med.* 1985;312:9-17.

319. Moran A, Asa SL, Kovacs K, et al. Gigantism due to pituitary mammosomatotroph hyperplasia. *N Engl J Med.* 1990;323:322-327.

320. Verrua E, Ronchi CL, Ferrante E, et al. Acromegaly secondary to an incidentally discovered growth-hormone-releasing hormone secreting bronchial carcinoid tumour associated to a pituitary incidentaloma. *Pituitary.* 2010;13(3):289-292. [Epub 2008 Oct 23].

321. Thorner MO, Frohman LA, Leong DA, et al. Extrahypothalamic growth-hormone-releasing factor (GRF) secretion is a rare cause of acromegaly: plasma GRF levels in 177 acromegalic patients. *J Clin Endocrinol Metab.* 1984;59:846-849.

322. Frohman LA, Szabo M, Berelowitz M, Stachura ME. Partial purification and characterization of a peptide with growth hormone-releasing activity from extrapituitary tumors in patients with acromegaly. *J Clin Invest.* 1980;65:43-54.

323. Vieira NL, Taboada GF, Correa LL, et al. Acromegaly secondary to growth hormone-releasing hormone secreted by an incidentally discovered pheochromocytoma. *Endocr Pathol.* 2007;18:46-52.

324. Drange MR, Melmed S. Long-acting lanreotide induces clinical and biochemical remission of acromegaly caused by disseminated growth hormone-releasing hormone-secreting carcinoid. *J Clin Endocrinol Metab.* 1998;83:3104-3109.

325. Ramirez C, Hernandez-Ramirez LC, Espinosa-de-los-Monteros AL, et al. Ectopic acromegaly due to a GH-secreting pituitary adenoma in the sphenoid sinus: a case report and review of the literature. *BMC Res Notes.* 2013;6:411.

326. Greenman Y, Woolf P, Coniglio J, et al. Remission of acromegaly caused by pituitary carcinoma after surgical excision of growth hormone-secreting metastasis detected by 111-indium pentetreotide scan. *J Clin Endocrinol Metab.* 1996;81:1628-1633.

327. Beuschlein F, Strasburger CJ, Siegerstetter V, et al. Acromegaly caused by secretion of growth hormone by a non-Hodgkin's lymphoma. *N Engl J Med.* 2000;342:1871-1876.

328. Salenave S, Boyce AM, Collins MT, Chanson P. Acromegaly and McCune-Albright syndrome. *J Clin Endocrinol Metab.* 2014;99:1955-1969.

329. Drange MR, Fram NR, Herman-Bonert V, Melmed S. Pituitary tumor registry: a novel clinical resource. *J Clin Endocrinol Metab.* 2000;85:168-174.

330. de Herder WW. Acromegaly and gigantism in the medical literature. Case descriptions in the era before and the early years after the initial publication of Pierre Marie (1886). *Pituitary.* 2009;12:236-244.

331. Chahal HS, Stals K, Unterlander M, et al. AIP mutation in pituitary adenomas in the 18th century and today. *N Engl J Med.* 2011;364:43-50.

332. Maheshwari HG, Prezant TR, Herman-Bonert V, et al. Long-acting peptidomimergic control of gigantism caused by pituitary acidophilic stem cell adenoma. *J Clin Endocrinol Metab.* 2000;85:3409-3416.

333. Goldenberg N, Racine MS, Thomas P, et al. Treatment of pituitary gigantism with the growth hormone receptor antagonist pegvisomant. *J Clin Endocrinol Metab.* 2008;93:2953-2956.

334. Molitch ME. Clinical manifestations of acromegaly. *Endocrinol Metab Clin North Am.* 1992;21:597-614.

335. Jadresic A, Banks LM, Child DF, et al. The acromegaly syndrome. Relation between clinical features, growth hormone values and radiological characteristics of the pituitary tumours. *Q J Med.* 1982;51:189-204.

336. Reid TJ, Post KD, Bruce JN, et al. Features at diagnosis of 324 patients with acromegaly did not change from 1981 to 2006: acromegaly remains under-recognized and under-diagnosed. *Clin Endocrinol (Oxf).* 2010;72:203-208.

337. Nabarro JD. Acromegaly. *Clin Endocrinol (Oxf).* 1987;26:481-512.

338. Colao A, Marzullo P, Ferone D, et al. Prostatic hyperplasia: an unknown feature of acromegaly. *J Clin Endocrinol Metab.* 1998;83:775-779.

339. Lieberman SA, Bjorkengren AG, Hoffman AR. Rheumatologic and skeletal changes in acromegaly. *Endocrinol Metab Clin North Am.* 1992;21:615-631.

340. Biermasz NR, Pereira AM, Smit JW, et al. Morbidity after long-term remission for acromegaly: persisting joint-related complaints cause reduced quality of life. *J Clin Endocrinol Metab.* 2005;90:2731-2739.

341. Tagliafico A, Resmini E, Nizzo R, et al. Ultrasound measurement of median and ulnar nerve cross-sectional area in acromegaly. *J Clin Endocrinol Metab.* 2008;93:905-909.

342. Scarpa R, De Brasi D, Pivonello R, et al. Acromegalic axial arthropathy: a clinical case-control study. *J Clin Endocrinol Metab.* 2004;89:598-603.

343. Mazziotti G, Bianchi A, Porcelli T, et al. Vertebral fractures in patients with acromegaly: a 3-year prospective study. *J Clin Endocrinol Metab.* 2013;98:3402-3410.

344. Brzana J, Yedinak CG, Hameed N, Fleseriu M. FRAX score in acromegaly: does it tell the whole story? *Clin Endocrinol (Oxf).* 2014;80:614-616.

345. Ben-Shlomo A, Melmed S. Skin manifestations in acromegaly. *Clin Dermatol.* 2006;24:256-259.

346. Colao A, Cuocolo A, Marzullo P, et al. Impact of patient's age and disease duration on cardiac performance in acromegaly: a radionuclide angiography study. *J Clin Endocrinol Metab.* 1999;84:1518-1523.

347. Pereira AM, van Thiel SW, Lindner JR, et al. Increased prevalence of regurgitant valvular heart disease in acromegaly. *J Clin Endocrinol Metab.* 2004;89:71-75.

348. Casini AF, Neto LV, Fontes R, et al. Aortic root ectasia in patients with acromegaly: experience at a single center. *Clin Endocrinol (Oxf).* 2011;75:495-500.

349. Kamenicky P, Viengchareun S, Blanchard A, et al. Epithelial sodium channel is a key mediator of growth hormone-induced sodium retention in acromegaly. *Endocrinology.* 2008;149:3294-3305.

350. Annamalai AK, Webb A, Kandasamy N, et al. A comprehensive study of clinical, biochemical, radiological, vascular, cardiac, and sleep parameters in an unselected cohort of patients with acromegaly undergoing presurgical somatostatin receptor ligand therapy. *J Clin Endocrinol Metab.* 2013;98:1040-1050.

351. Grunstein RR, Ho KY, Berthon-Jones M, et al. Central sleep apnea is associated with increased ventilatory response to carbon dioxide and hypersecretion of growth hormone in patients with acromegaly. *Am J Respir Crit Care Med.* 1994;150:496-502.

352. Jenkins PJ, Sohaib SA, Akker S, et al. The pathology of median neuropathy in acromegaly. *Ann Intern Med.* 2000;133:197-201.

353. Santos A, Resmini E, Martinez MA, et al. Quality of life in patients with pituitary tumors. *Curr Opin Endocrinol Diabetes Obes.* 2009;16:299-303.

354. Le Roith D. The insulin-like growth factor system. *Exp Diabesity Res.* 2003;4:205-212.

355. Clayton PE, Banerjee I, Murray PG, Renehan AG. Growth hormone, the insulin-like growth factor axis, insulin and cancer risk. *Nat Rev Endocrinol.* 2011;7:11-24.

356. Delhougne B, Deneux C, Abs R, et al. The prevalence of colonic polyps in acromegaly: a colonoscopic and pathological study in 103 patients. *J Clin Endocrinol Metab.* 1995;80:3223-3226.

357. Orme SM, McNally RJ, Cartwright RA, Belchetz PE. Mortality and cancer incidence in acromegaly: a retrospective cohort study. United Kingdom Acromegaly Study Group. *J Clin Endocrinol Metab.* 1998;83:2730-2734.

358. Renehan AG, Bhaskar P, Painter JE, et al. The prevalence and characteristics of colorectal neoplasia in acromegaly. *J Clin Endocrinol Metab.* 2000;85:3417-3424.

359. Resmini E, Tagliafico A, Bacigalupo L, et al. Computed tomography colonography in acromegaly. *J Clin Endocrinol Metab.* 2009;94:218-222.

360. Annamalai AK, Gayton EL, Webb A, et al. Increased prevalence of gallbladder polyps in acromegaly. *J Clin Endocrinol Metab.* 2011;96:E1120-E1125.

361. Colao A, Ferone D, Marzullo P, Lombardi G. Systemic complications of acromegaly: epidemiology, pathogenesis, and management. *Endocr Rev.* 2004;25:102-152.

362. Melmed S. Clinical perspective: acromegaly and cancer: not a problem? *J Clin Endocrinol Metab.* 2001;86:2929-2934.

363. Kauppinen-Makelin R, Sane T, Valimaki MJ, et al. Increased cancer incidence in acromegaly: a nationwide survey. *Clin Endocrinol (Oxf).* 2010;72:278-279.

364. dos Santos MC, Nascimento GC, Nascimento AG, et al. Thyroid cancer in patients with acromegaly: a case-control study. *Pituitary.* 2013;16:109-114.

365. Katznelson L, Kleinberg D, Vance ML, et al. Hypogonadism in patients with acromegaly: data from the multi-centre acromegaly registry pilot study. *Clin Endocrinol (Oxf).* 2001;54:183-188.

366. Kasagi K, Shimatsu A, Miyamoto S, et al. Goiter associated with acromegaly: sonographic and scintigraphic findings of the thyroid gland. *Thyroid.* 1999;9:791-796.

367. Dekkers OM, Biermasz NR, Pereira AM, et al. Mortality in acromegaly: a metaanalysis. *J Clin Endocrinol Metab.* 2008;93:61-67.

368. Rajasoorya C, Holdaway IM, Wrightson P, et al. Determinants of clinical outcome and survival in acromegaly. *Clin Endocrinol (Oxf).* 1994;41:95-102.

369. Holdaway IM, Bolland MJ, Gamble GD. A meta-analysis of the effect of lowering serum levels of GH and IGF-I on mortality in acromegaly. *Eur J Endocrinol.* 2008;159:89-95.

370. Sherlock M, Reulen RC, Aragon-Alonso A, et al. A paradigm shift in the monitoring of patients with acromegaly: last available growth hormone may overestimate risk. *J Clin Endocrinol Metab.* 2014;99:478-485.

371. Freda PU, Reyes CM, Nuruzzaman AT, et al. Basal and glucose-suppressed GH levels less than 1 microg/L in newly diagnosed acromegaly. *Pituitary.* 2003;6:175-180.

372. Melmed S. Acromegaly pathogenesis and treatment. *J Clin Invest.* 2009;119:3189-3202.

373. Ribeiro-Oliveira A Jr, Barkan A. The changing face of acromegaly—advances in diagnosis and treatment. *Nat Rev Endocrinol.* 2012; 8:605-611.
374. Freda PU, Wardlaw SL, Post KD. Long-term endocrinological follow-up evaluation in 115 patients who underwent transsphenoidal surgery for acromegaly. *J Neurosurg.* 1998;89:353-358.
375. Clemmons DR, Van Wyk JJ, Ridgway EC, et al. Evaluation of acromegaly by radioimmunoassay of somatomedin-C. *N Engl J Med.* 1979;301:1138-1142.
376. Bidlingmaier M, Friedrich N, Emeny RT, et al. Reference intervals for insulin-like growth factor-1 (IGF-1) from birth to senescence: results from a multicenter study using a new automated chemiluminescence IGF-1 immunoassay conforming to recent international recommendations. *J Clin Endocrinol Metab.* 2014;99(5):1712-1721.
377. Faje AT, Barkan AL. Basal, but not pulsatile, growth hormone secretion determines the ambient circulating levels of insulin-like growth factor-I. *J Clin Endocrinol Metab.* 2010;95:2486-2491.
378. Dimaraki EV, Jaffe CA, DeMott-Friberg R, et al. Acromegaly with apparently normal GH secretion: implications for diagnosis and follow-up. *J Clin Endocrinol Metab.* 2002;87:3537-3542.
379. Giustina A, Barkan A, Casanueva FF, et al. Criteria for cure of acromegaly: a consensus statement. *J Clin Endocrinol Metab.* 2000;85: 526-529.
380. Giustina A, Chanson P, Kleinberg D, et al. Expert consensus document: a consensus on the medical treatment of acromegaly. *Nat Rev Endocrinol.* 2014;10:243-248.
381. Holdaway IM, Rajasoorya RC, Gamble GD. Factors influencing mortality in acromegaly. *J Clin Endocrinol Metab.* 2004;89:667-674.
382. Melmed S. Tight control of growth hormone: an attainable outcome for acromegaly treatment. *J Clin Endocrinol Metab.* 1998;83:3409-3410.
383. Giustina A, Chanson P, Bronstein MD, et al. A consensus on criteria for cure of acromegaly. *J Clin Endocrinol Metab.* 2010;95:3141-3148.
384. Jane JA Jr, Starke RM, Elzoghby MA, et al. Endoscopic transsphenoidal surgery for acromegaly: remission using modern criteria, complications, and predictors of outcome. *J Clin Endocrinol Metab.* 2011; 96:2732-2740.
385. Starke RM, Raper DM, Payne SC, et al. Endoscopic vs microsurgical transsphenoidal surgery for acromegaly: outcomes in a concurrent series of patients using modern criteria for remission. *J Clin Endocrinol Metab.* 2013;98:3190-3198.
386. Hazer DB, Isik S, Berker D, et al. Treatment of acromegaly by endoscopic transsphenoidal surgery: surgical experience in 214 cases and cure rates according to current consensus criteria. *J Neurosurg.* 2013; 119:1467-1477.
387. Shimon I, Cohen ZR, Ram Z, Hadani M. Transsphenoidal surgery for acromegaly: endocrinological follow-up of 98 patients. *Neurosurgery.* 2001;48:1239-1243, discussion 1244-1245.
388. Kreutzer J, Vance ML, Lopes MB, Laws ER Jr. Surgical management of GH-secreting pituitary adenomas: an outcome study using modern remission criteria. *J Clin Endocrinol Metab.* 2001;86:4072-4077.
389. Ayuk J, Clayton RN, Holder G, et al. Growth hormone and pituitary radiotherapy, but not serum insulin-like growth factor-I concentrations, predict excess mortality in patients with acromegaly. *J Clin Endocrinol Metab.* 2004;89:1613-1617.
390. Burgers AM, Kokshoorn NE, Pereira AM, et al. Low incidence of adrenal insufficiency after transsphenoidal surgery in patients with acromegaly: a long-term follow-up study. *J Clin Endocrinol Metab.* 2011;96:E1163-E1170.
391. Jenkins PJ, Bates P, Carson MN, et al. Conventional pituitary irradiation is effective in lowering serum growth hormone and insulin-like growth factor-I in patients with acromegaly. *J Clin Endocrinol Metab.* 2006;91:1239-1245.
392. Losa M, Gioia L, Picozzi P, et al. The role of stereotactic radiotherapy in patients with growth hormone-secreting pituitary adenoma. *J Clin Endocrinol Metab.* 2008;93:2546-2552.
393. Ronchi CL, Attanasio R, Verrua E, et al. Efficacy and tolerability of gamma knife radiosurgery in acromegaly: a 10-year follow-up study. *Clin Endocrinol (Oxf).* 2009;71:846-852.
394. Pollock BE, Jacob JT, Brown PD, Nippoldt TB. Radiosurgery of growth hormone-producing pituitary adenomas: factors associated with biochemical remission. *J Neurosurg.* 2007;106:833-838.
395. Castinetti F, Taieb D, Kuhn JM, et al. Outcome of gamma knife radiosurgery in 82 patients with acromegaly: correlation with initial hypersecretion. *J Clin Endocrinol Metab.* 2005;90:4483-4488.
396. Sandret L, Maison P, Chanson P. Place of cabergoline in acromegaly: a meta-analysis. *J Clin Endocrinol Metab.* 2011;96:1327-1335.
397. Jaffe CA, Barkan AL. Treatment of acromegaly with dopamine agonists. *Endocrinol Metab Clin North Am.* 1992;21:713-735.
398. Sherlock M, Fernandez-Rodriguez E, Alonso AA, et al. Medical therapy in patients with acromegaly: predictors of response and comparison of efficacy of dopamine agonists and somatostatin analogues. *J Clin Endocrinol Metab.* 2009;94:1255-1263.
399. Shimon I, Yan X, Taylor JE, et al. Somatostatin receptor (SSTR) subtype-selective analogues differentially suppress in vitro growth hormone and prolactin in human pituitary adenomas. Novel potential therapy for functional pituitary tumors. *J Clin Invest.* 1997;100:2386-2392.
400. Weckbecker G, Lewis I, Albert R, et al. Opportunities in somatostatin research: biological, chemical and therapeutic aspects. *Nat Rev Drug Discov.* 2003;2:999-1017.
401. Lamberts SW, van der Lely AJ, de Herder WW, Hofland LJ. Octreotide. *N Engl J Med.* 1996;334:246-254.
402. Lamberts SW, Oosterom R, Neufeld M, del Pozo E. The somatostatin analog SMS 201-995 induces long-acting inhibition of growth hormone secretion without rebound hypersecretion in acromegalic patients. *J Clin Endocrinol Metab.* 1985;60:1161-1165.
403. Ur E, Mather SJ, Bomanji J, et al. Pituitary imaging using a labelled somatostatin analogue in acromegaly. *Clin Endocrinol (Oxf).* 1992;36: 147-150.
404. Acunzo J, Thirion S, Roche C, et al. Somatostatin receptor sst2 decreases cell viability and hormonal hypersecretion and reverses octreotide resistance of human pituitary adenomas. *Cancer Res.* 2008; 68:10163-10170.
405. Ezzat S, Snyder PJ, Young WF, et al. Octreotide treatment of acromegaly. A randomized, multicenter study. *Ann Intern Med.* 1992;117: 711-718.
406. Wang C, Lam KS, Arceo E, Chan FL. Comparison of the effectiveness of 2-hourly versus 8-hourly subcutaneous injections of a somatostatin analog (SMS 201-995) in the treatment of acromegaly. *J Clin Endocrinol Metab.* 1989;69:670-677.
407. Newman CB, Melmed S, Snyder PJ, et al. Safety and efficacy of long-term octreotide therapy of acromegaly: results of a multicenter trial in 103 patients. A clinical research center study. *J Clin Endocrinol Metab.* 1995;80:2768-2775.
408. Gillis JC, Noble S, Goa KL. Octreotide long-acting release (LAR). A review of its pharmacological properties and therapeutic use in the management of acromegaly. *Drugs.* 1997;53:681-699.
409. Cozzi R, Montini M, Attanasio R, et al. Primary treatment of acromegaly with octreotide LAR: a long-term (up to nine years) prospective study of its efficacy in the control of disease activity and tumor shrinkage. *J Clin Endocrinol Metab.* 2006;91:1397-1403.
410. Caron P, Morange-Ramos I, Cogne M, Jaquet P. Three year follow-up of acromegalic patients treated with intramuscular slow-release lanreotide. *J Clin Endocrinol Metab.* 1997;82:18-22.
411. Melmed S, Cook D, Schopohl J, et al. Rapid and sustained reduction of serum growth hormone and insulin-like growth factor-1 in patients with acromegaly receiving lanreotide autogel therapy: a randomized, placebo-controlled, multicenter study with a 52 week open extension. *Pituitary.* 2010;13:18-28.
412. Bruns C, Lewis I, Briner U, et al. SOM230: a novel somatostatin peptidomimetic with broad somatotropin release inhibiting factor (SRIF) receptor binding and a unique antisecretory profile. *Eur J Endocrinol.* 2002;146:707-716.
413. Petersenn S, Schopohl J, Barkan A, et al. Pasireotide (SOM230) demonstrates efficacy and safety in patients with acromegaly: a randomized, multicenter, phase II trial. *J Clin Endocrinol Metab.* 2010;95: 2781-2789.
414. Colao A, Bronstein M, Freda P, et al. Pasireotide versus octreotide in acromegaly: a head-to-head superiority study. *J Clin Endocrinol Metab.* 2014;99(3):791-799.
415. Tuvia S, Atsmon J, Teichman SL, et al. Oral octreotide absorption in human subjects: comparable pharmacokinetics to parenteral octreotide and effective growth hormone suppression. *J Clin Endocrinol Metab.* 2012;97:2362-2369.
416. Melmed SB, Bidlingmaier M, Mercado MA, et al. Safety and efficacy of oral octreotide in acromegaly; results of a multicenter phase III trial. *J Clin Endocrinol Metab.* 2015;100(4):1699-1708.
417. Bevan JS. Clinical review: the antitumoral effects of somatostatin analog therapy in acromegaly. *J Clin Endocrinol Metab.* 2005;90:1856-1863.
418. Melmed S, Sternberg R, Cook D, et al. A critical analysis of pituitary tumor shrinkage during primary medical therapy in acromegaly. *J Clin Endocrinol Metab.* 2005;90:4405-4410.
419. Colao A, Auriemma RS, Galdiero M, et al. Effects of initial therapy for five years with somatostatin analogs for acromegaly on growth hormone and insulin-like growth factor-I levels, tumor shrinkage, and cardiovascular disease: a prospective study. *J Clin Endocrinol Metab.* 2009;94:3746-3756.
420. Giustina A, Mazziotti G, Torri V, et al. Meta-analysis on the effects of octreotide on tumor mass in acromegaly. *PLoS ONE.* 2012;7:e36411.
421. Colao A, Auriemma RS, Rebora A, et al. Significant tumour shrinkage after 12 months of lanreotide autogel 120-mg treatment given first-line in acromegaly. *Clin Endocrinol (Oxf).* 2009;71:237-245.
422. Carlsen SM, Lund-Johansen M, Schreiner T, et al. Preoperative octreotide treatment in newly diagnosed acromegalic patients with macroadenomas increases cure short-term postoperative rates: a prospective, randomized trial. *J Clin Endocrinol Metab.* 2008;93:2984-2990.
423. Pita-Gutierrez F, Pertega-Diaz S, Pita-Fernandez S, et al. Place of preoperative treatment of acromegaly with somatostatin analog on surgical outcome: a systematic review and meta-analysis. *PLoS ONE.* 2013;8: e61523.
424. Pascual J, Freijanes J, Berciano J, Pesquera C. Analgesic effect of octreotide in headache associated with acromegaly is not mediated by opioid mechanisms. Case report. *Pain.* 1991;47:341-344.

425. Colao A, Cuocolo A, Marzullo P, et al. Is the acromegalic cardiomyopathy reversible? Effect of 5-year normalization of growth hormone and insulin-like growth factor I levels on cardiac performance. *J Clin Endocrinol Metab.* 2001;86:1551-1557.
426. Murray RD, Melmed S. A critical analysis of clinically available somatostatin analog formulations for therapy of acromegaly. *J Clin Endocrinol Metab.* 2008;93:2957-2968.
427. Carmichael JD, Bonert VS, Mirocha JM, Melmed S. The utility of oral glucose tolerance testing for diagnosis and assessment of treatment outcomes in 166 patients with acromegaly. *J Clin Endocrinol Metab.* 2009;94:523-527.
428. Caron PJ, Bevan JS, Petersenn S, et al. Tumor shrinkage with lanreotide autogel 120 mg as primary therapy in acromegaly: results of a prospective multicenter clinical trial. *J Clin Endocrinol Metab.* 2014;99:1282-1290.
429. Mercado M, Borges F, Bouterfa H, et al. A prospective, multicentre study to investigate the efficacy, safety and tolerability of octreotide LAR (long-acting repeatable octreotide) in the primary therapy of patients with acromegaly. *Clin Endocrinol (Oxf).* 2007;66:859-868.
430. Drake WM, Stiles CE, Howlett TA, et al. A cross-sectional study of the prevalence of cardiac valvular abnormalities in hyperprolactinemic patients treated with ergot-derived dopamine agonists. *J Clin Endocrinol Metab.* 2014;99:90-96.
431. Giustina A, Bonadonna S, Bugari G, et al. High-dose intramuscular octreotide in patients with acromegaly inadequately controlled on conventional somatostatin analogue therapy: a randomised controlled trial. *Eur J Endocrinol.* 2009;161:331-338.
432. Fleseriu M. Clinical efficacy and safety results for dose escalation of somatostatin receptor ligands in patients with acromegaly: a literature review. *Pituitary.* 2011;14:184-193.
433. Carmichael JD, Bonert VS, Nuno M, et al. Acromegaly clinical trial methodology impact on reported biochemical efficacy rates of somatostatin receptor ligand treatments: a meta-analysis. *J Clin Endocrinol Metab.* 2014;99:1825-1833.
434. Fougner SL, Borota OC, Berg JP, et al. The clinical response to somatostatin analogues in acromegaly correlates to the somatostatin receptor subtype 2a protein expression of the adenoma. *Clin Endocrinol (Oxf).* 2008;68:458-465.
435. Brzana J, Yedinak CG, Gultekin SH, et al. Growth hormone granulation pattern and somatostatin receptor subtype 2A correlate with postoperative somatostatin receptor ligand response in acromegaly: a large single center experience. *Pituitary.* 2013;16:490-498.
436. Fougner SL, Casar-Borota O, Heck A, et al. Adenoma granulation pattern correlates with clinical variables and effect of somatostatin analogue treatment in a large series of patients with acromegaly. *Clin Endocrinol (Oxf).* 2012;76:96-102.
437. Puig-Domingo M, Resmini E, Gomez-Anson B, et al. Magnetic resonance imaging as a predictor of response to somatostatin analogs in acromegaly after surgical failure. *J Clin Endocrinol Metab.* 2010;95:4973-4978.
438. Mazziotti G, Floriani I, Bonadonna S, et al. Effects of somatostatin analogs on glucose homeostasis: a metaanalysis of acromegaly studies. *J Clin Endocrinol Metab.* 2009;94:1500-1508.
439. Melmed S, Dowling RH, Frohman L, et al. Consensus statement: benefits vs. risks of medical therapy for acromegaly. *Am J Med.* 1994;97:468.
440. Waters MJ, Brooks AJ, Chhabra Y. A new mechanism for growth hormone receptor activation of JAK2, and implications for related cytokine receptors. *JAKSTAT.* 2014;3:e29569.
441. Kopchick JJ, Parkinson C, Stevens EC, Trainer PJ. Growth hormone receptor antagonists: discovery, development, and use in patients with acromegaly. *Endocr Rev.* 2002;23:623-646.
442. Trainer PJ, Drake WM, Katznelson L, et al. Treatment of acromegaly with the growth hormone-receptor antagonist pegvisomant. *N Engl J Med.* 2000;342:1171-1177.
443. van der Lely AJ, Biller BM, Brue T, et al. Long-term safety of pegvisomant in patients with acromegaly: comprehensive review of 1288 subjects in ACROSTUDY. *J Clin Endocrinol Metab.* 2012;97:1589-1597.
444. Higham CE, Rowles S, Russell-Jones D, et al. Pegvisomant improves insulin sensitivity and reduces overnight free fatty acid concentrations in patients with acromegaly. *J Clin Endocrinol Metab.* 2009;94:2459-2463.
445. Herman-Bonert VS, Zib K, Scarlett JA, Melmed S. Growth hormone receptor antagonist therapy in acromegalic patients resistant to somatostatin analogs. *J Clin Endocrinol Metab.* 2000;85:2958-2961.
446. Trainer PJ, Ezzat S, D'Souza GA, et al. A randomized, controlled, multicentre trial comparing pegvisomant alone with combination therapy of pegvisomant and long-acting octreotide in patients with acromegaly. *Clin Endocrinol (Oxf).* 2009;71:549-557.
447. van der Lely AJ, Muller A, Janssen JA, et al. Control of tumor size and disease activity during cotreatment with octreotide and the growth hormone receptor antagonist pegvisomant in an acromegalic patient. *J Clin Endocrinol Metab.* 2001;86:478-481.
448. Frohman LA, Bonert V. Pituitary tumor enlargement in two patients with acromegaly during pegvisomant therapy. *Pituitary.* 2007;10:283-289.
449. Marazuela M, Paniagua AE, Gahete MD, et al. Somatotroph tumor progression during pegvisomant therapy: a clinical and molecular study. *J Clin Endocrinol Metab.* 2011;96:E251-E259.
450. Buhk JH, Jung S, Psychogios MN, et al. Tumor volume of growth hormone-secreting pituitary adenomas during treatment with pegvisomant: a prospective multicenter study. *J Clin Endocrinol Metab.* 2010;95:552-558.
451. Barkan AL, Burman P, Clemmons DR, et al. Glucose homeostasis and safety in patients with acromegaly converted from long-acting octreotide to pegvisomant. *J Clin Endocrinol Metab.* 2005;90:5684-5691.
452. Biering H, Saller B, Bauditz J, et al. Elevated transaminases during medical treatment of acromegaly: a review of the German pegvisomant surveillance experience and a report of a patient with histologically proven chronic mild active hepatitis. *Eur J Endocrinol.* 2006;154:213-220.
453. Bonert VS, Kennedy L, Petersenn S, et al. Lipodystrophy in patients with acromegaly receiving pegvisomant. *J Clin Endocrinol Metab.* 2008;93(9):3515-3518.
454. Jorgensen JO, Feldt-Rasmussen U, Frystyk J, et al. Cotreatment of acromegaly with a somatostatin analog and a growth hormone receptor antagonist. *J Clin Endocrinol Metab.* 2005;90:5627-5631.
455. Feenstra J, de Herder WW, ten Have SM, et al. Combined therapy with somatostatin analogues and weekly pegvisomant in active acromegaly. *Lancet.* 2005;365:1644-1646.
456. Neggers SJ, de Herder WW, Janssen JA, et al. Combined treatment for acromegaly with long-acting somatostatin analogs and pegvisomant: long-term safety for up to 4.5 years (median 2.2 years) of follow-up in 86 patients. *Eur J Endocrinol.* 2009;160:529-533.
457. Marko NF, LaSota E, Hamrahian AH, Weil RJ. Comparative effectiveness review of treatment options for pituitary microadenomas in acromegaly. *J Neurosurg.* 2012;117:522-538.
458. Tritos NA, Johannsson G, Korbonits M, et al. Effects of long-term growth hormone replacement in adults with growth hormone deficiency following cure of acromegaly: a KIMS analysis. *J Clin Endocrinol Metab.* 2014;99:2018-2029.
459. Katznelson L, Laws ER Jr, Melmed S, et al. Acromegaly: an Endocrine Society Clinical Practice Guideline. *J Clin Endocrinol Metab.* 2014;99(11):3933-3951.
460. Jallad RS, Musolino NR, Kodaira S, et al. Does partial surgical tumour removal influence the response to octreotide-LAR in acromegalic patients previously resistant to the somatostatin analogue? *Clin Endocrinol (Oxf).* 2007;67:310-315.
461. Newman CB, Melmed S, George A, et al. Octreotide as primary therapy for acromegaly. *J Clin Endocrinol Metab.* 1998;83:3034-3040.
462. Maiza JC, Vezzosi D, Matta M, et al. Long-term (up to 18 years) effects on GH/IGF-1 hypersecretion and tumour size of primary somatostatin analogue (SSTa) therapy in patients with GH-secreting pituitary adenoma responsive to SSTa. *Clin Endocrinol (Oxf).* 2007;67:282-289.
463. Fougner SL, Bollerslev J, Svartberg J, et al. Preoperative octreotide treatment of acromegaly: long-term results of a randomised controlled trial. *Eur J Endocrinol.* 2014;171:229-235.
464. Nieman LK, Biller BM, Findling JW, et al. The diagnosis of Cushing's syndrome: an Endocrine Society Clinical Practice Guideline. *J Clin Endocrinol Metab.* 2008;93:1526-1540.
465. Biller BM, Grossman AB, Stewart PM, et al. Treatment of adrenocorticotropin-dependent Cushing's syndrome: a consensus statement. *J Clin Endocrinol Metab.* 2008;93:2454-2462.
466. Fahlbusch R, Honegger J, Paulus W, et al. Surgical treatment of craniopharyngiomas: experience with 168 patients. *J Neurosurg.* 1999;90:237-250.
467. Simmons NE, Alden TD, Thorner MO, Laws ER Jr. Serum cortisol response to transsphenoidal surgery for Cushing disease. *J Neurosurg.* 2001;95:1-8.
468. Colao A, Petersenn S, Newell-Price J, et al. A 12-month phase 3 study of pasireotide in Cushing's disease. *N Engl J Med.* 2012;366:914-924.
469. Fleseriu M, Biller BM, Findling JW, et al. Mifepristone, a glucocorticoid receptor antagonist, produces clinical and metabolic benefits in patients with Cushing's syndrome. *J Clin Endocrinol Metab.* 2012;97:2039-2049.
470. Mindermann T, Wilson CB. Thyrotropin-producing pituitary adenomas. *J Neurosurg.* 1993;79:521-527.
471. Roelfsema F, Kok S, Kok P, et al. Pituitary-hormone secretion by thyrotropinomas. *Pituitary.* 2009;12:200-210.
472. Roelfsema F, Pereira AM, Keenan DM, et al. Thyrotropin secretion by thyrotropinomas is characterized by increased pulse frequency, delayed diurnal rhythm, enhanced basal secretion, spikiness, and disorderliness. *J Clin Endocrinol Metab.* 2008;93:4052-4057.
473. Yoshihara A, Isozaki O, Hizuka N, et al. Expression of type 5 somatostatin receptor in TSH-secreting pituitary adenomas: a possible marker for predicting long-term response to octreotide therapy. *Endocr J.* 2007;54:133-138.
474. Alings AM, Fliers E, de Herder WW, et al. A thyrotropin-secreting pituitary adenoma as a cause of thyrotoxic periodic paralysis. *J Endocrinol Invest.* 1998;21:703-706.

475. Pappa T, Papanastasiou L, Markou A, et al. Thyrotoxic periodic paralysis as the first manifestation of a thyrotropin-secreting pituitary adenoma. *Hormones (Athens)*. 2010;9:82-86.

476. Beck-Peccoz P, Brucker-Davis F, Persani L, et al. Thyrotropin-secreting pituitary tumors. *Endocr Rev*. 1996;17:610-638.

477. Brucker-Davis F, Oldfield EH, Skarulis MC, et al. Thyrotropin-secreting pituitary tumors: diagnostic criteria, thyroid hormone sensitivity, and treatment outcome in 25 patients followed at the National Institutes of Health. *J Clin Endocrinol Metab*. 1999;84:476-486.

478. Malchiodi E, Profka E, Ferrante E, et al. Thyrotropin-secreting pituitary adenomas: outcome of pituitary surgery and irradiation. *J Clin Endocrinol Metab*. 2014;99:2069-2076.

479. Cooper DS, Wenig BM. Hyperthyroidism caused by an ectopic TSH-secreting pituitary tumor. *Thyroid*. 1996;6:337-343.

480. Beck-Peccoz P, Persani L. TSH-producing adenomas. In: DeGroot LJ, Jameson JL, eds. *Endocrinology*. 4th ed. Philadelphia: WB Saunders; 2001:321-328.

481. Unluturk U, Sriphrapradang C, Erdogan MF, et al. Management of differentiated thyroid cancer in the presence of resistance to thyroid hormone and TSH-secreting adenomas: a report of four cases and review of the literature. *J Clin Endocrinol Metab*. 2013;98:2210-2217.

482. Beck-Peccoz P, Lania A, Beckers A, et al. 2013 European Thyroid Association guidelines for the diagnosis and treatment of thyrotropin-secreting pituitary tumors. *Eur Thyroid J*. 2013;2:76-82.

483. Beck-Peccoz P, Mariotti S, Guillausseau PJ, et al. Treatment of hyperthyroidism due to inappropriate secretion of thyrotropin with the somatostatin analog SMS 201-995. *J Clin Endocrinol Metab*. 1989;68:208-214.

484. Caron P, Arlot S, Bauters C, et al. Efficacy of the long-acting octreotide formulation (octreotide-LAR) in patients with thyrotropin-secreting pituitary adenomas. *J Clin Endocrinol Metab*. 2001;86:2849-2853.

485. Colao A, Cappabianca P, Caron P, et al. Octreotide LAR vs. surgery in newly diagnosed patients with acromegaly: a randomized, open-label, multicentre study. *Clin Endocrinol (Oxf)*. 2009;70:757-768.

486. Wang EL, Qian ZR, Yamada S, et al. Clinicopathological characterization of TSH-producing adenomas: special reference to TSH-immunoreactive but clinically non-functioning adenomas. *Endocr Pathol*. 2009;20:209-220.

487. Grisoli F, Leclercq T, Winteler JP, et al. Thyroid-stimulating hormone pituitary adenomas and hyperthyroidism. *Surg Neurol*. 1986;25(4):361-368.

488. Gesundheit N, Petrick P, Nissim M, et al. Thyrotropin-secreting pituitary adenomas: clinical and biochemical heterogeneity: case reports and follow-up of nine patients. *Ann Intern Med*. 1989;111(10):827-835.

489. McCutcheon I, Weintraub B, Oldfield E. Surgical treatment of thyrotropin-secreting pituitary adenomas. *J Neurosurg*. 1990;73(5):674-683.

490. Beckers A, Abs R, Mahler C, et al. Thyrotropin-secreting pituitary adenomas: report of seven cases. *J Clin Endocrinol Metab*. 1991;72(2):477-483.

491. Chanson P, Weintraub BD, Harris AG. Octreotide therapy for thyroid-stimulating hormone-secreting pituitary adenomas: a follow-up of 52 patients. *Ann Intern Med*. 1993;119(3):236-240.

492. Chason P, Warnet A. Treatment of thyroid-stimulating hormone-secreting adenomas with octreotide. *Metabolism*. 1992;41(9 Suppl 2):62-65.

493. Losa M, Giovanelli M, Persani L, et al. Criteria of cure and follow-up of central hyperthyroidism due to thyrotropin-secreting pituitary adenomas. *J Clin Endocrinol Metab*. 1996;81(8):3084-3090.

494. Kuhn JM, Arlot S, Lefebver H, et al. Evaluation of the treatment of thyrotropin-secreting pituitary adenomas with a slow release formulation of the somatostatin analog lanreotide. *J Clin Endcrinol Metab*. 2000;85(4):1487-1491.

495. Ness-Abramof R, Ishay A, Harel G, et al. TSH-secreting pituitary adenomas: follow-up of 11 cases and review of the literature. *Pituitary*. 2007;10(3):307-310.

496. Elson MS, Conaglen JV. Clinical and biochemical characteristics of patients and thryroid-stimulating hormone-secreting pituitary adenomas from one New Zealand centre. *Intern Med J*. 2010;40(3):214-219.

497. Zhang CF, Liang D, Zhong LY. Efficacy of the long-acting octreotide formulation in patients with thyroid-stimulating hormone-secreting pituitary adenomas after incomplete surgery and octreotide treatment failure. *Chin Med J (Engl)*. 2012;125(15):2758-2763.

CHAPTER 10

Posterior Pituitary

ALAN G. ROBINSON • JOSEPH G. VERBALIS

KEY POINTS

- The posterior pituitary is neural tissue and consists only of the distal axons of the hypothalamic magnocellular neurons that make up the neurohypophysis.
- The control of hormone synthesis is at the level of transcription. Stimuli for secretion of vasopressin or oxytocin also stimulate transcription and increase the messenger ribonucleic acid (mRNA) content in the magnocellular neurons.
- The physiologic regulation of vasopressin synthesis and secretion involves two systems: osmotic and pressure/volume.
- Diabetes insipidus is a disorder of a large volume of urine (diabetes) that is hypotonic, dilute, and tasteless (insipid).
- The syndrome of inappropriate antidiuretic hormone secretion (SIADH) is produced when plasma levels of arginine vasopressin (AVP) are elevated at times when the physiologic secretion of vasopressin from the posterior pituitary would normally be osmotically suppressed.

ANATOMY

Normal

The posterior pituitary is neural tissue and consists only of the distal axons of the hypothalamic magnocellular neurons that make up the neurohypophysis. The perikarya (cell bodies) of these axons are located in paired paraventricular nuclei (PVN) and supraoptic nuclei (SON) of the hypothalamus. During embryogenesis[1] neuroepithelial cells of the lining of the third ventricle mature into magnocellular neurons while migrating laterally to and above the optic chiasm to form the supraoptic nuclei and to the walls of the third ventricle to form the paraventricular nuclei. In the posterior pituitary the axon terminals of the magnocellular neurons contain neurosecretory granules, membrane-bound packets of hormones stored for subsequent release. The blood supply for the anterior pituitary is via the hypothalamic/pituitary portal system, but the posterior pituitary is supplied directly from the inferior hypophyseal arteries, which are branches of the posterior communicating and internal carotid arteries. The drainage is into the cavernous sinus and internal jugular vein.

The hormones of the posterior pituitary, oxytocin and vasopressin, are for the most part synthesized in individual hormone-specific magnocellular neurons, although a small number of neurons (approximately 3%) express both peptides.[2] The supraoptic nucleus is relatively simple, with 80% to 90% of the neurons producing vasopressin[3] and virtually all axons projecting to the posterior pituitary.[1] The organization of the paraventricular nuclei, however, is much more complex and varies among species. In the human there are five subnuclei[3] and parvocellular (smaller cells) divisions that synthesize other peptides, such as corticotropin-releasing hormone (CRH), thyrotropin-releasing hormone (TRH), somatostatin,[4] and opioids.[5] The parvocellular neurons project to the median eminence, brainstem, and spinal cord,[6] where they play a role in a variety of neuroendocrine autonomic functions. The suprachiasmatic nucleus, which is located in the midline at the base of and anterior to the third ventricle, also synthesizes vasopressin and controls circadium rhythms as well as seasonal rhythms.[3]

The major stimulatory neurotransmitter in the neurohypophysis is glutamate with noradrenergic stimulatory inputs acting by stimulation of glutamate.[7,8] Glutamate receptors account for 25% of synapses on magnocellular neurons.[7] The major inhibitory input is γ-aminobutyric acid (GABA), which accounts for 20% to 40% of the synaptic input to the magnocellular neurons.[9] Phasic firing of vasopressin neurons is the most efficient activity pattern for release of vasopressin from axon terminals. Phasic activity is controlled by glutamate stimulation and opioid inhibition. Dynorphin is synthesized in vasopressin neurons and co-released with vasopressin from dendrites at the somatic level, where it acts in an autocrine fashion to inhibit the activity of the vasopressin neurons, contributing to the phasic firing pattern.[10,11]

One of the most remarkable aspects of the magnocellular system is the plasticity of the system in response to prolonged stimulation. This plasticity is of greatest import in humans during parturition and lactation.[9]

Ectopic Posterior Pituitary

With the development of magnetic resonance imaging (MRI) scans of the brain it was discovered that T1-weighted images with MRI produced a bright signal in the posterior pituitary.[12] This allowed the identification of children in whom there was abnormal anatomy of the posterior pituitary when the *bright spot* was recognized in the base of the hypothalamus. These cases are referred to as *ectopic posterior*

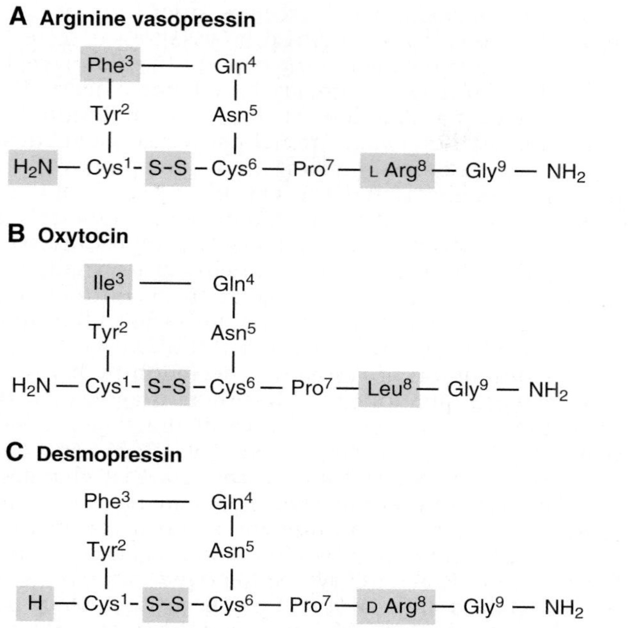

A Arginine vasopressin

```
         Phe³ ——— Gln⁴
          |          |
         Tyr²       Asn⁵
          |          |
H₂N — Cys¹- S-S – Cys⁶ — Pro⁷ — L Arg⁸ — Gly⁹ — NH₂
```

B Oxytocin

```
         Ile³ ——— Gln⁴
          |          |
         Tyr²       Asn⁵
          |          |
H₂N — Cys¹- S-S – Cys⁶ — Pro⁷ — Leu⁸ — Gly⁹ — NH₂
```

C Desmopressin

```
         Phe³ ——— Gln⁴
          |          |
         Tyr²       Asn⁵
          |          |
 H — Cys¹- S-S – Cys⁶ — Pro⁷ — D Arg⁸ — Gly⁹ — NH₂
```

Figure 10-1 Comparison of the chemical structures of arginine vasopressin (**A**), oxytocin (**B**), and desmopressin (**C**). The differences are illustrated by the shaded areas. Oxytocin differs from vasopressin in position 3 (Ile for Phe) and position 8 (Leu for Arg). Desmopressin differs from arginine vasopressin in that the terminal cystine is deaminated and the arginine in position 8 is a D- rather than an L-isomer. (From A.G. Robinson, University of California at Los Angeles, used with permission.)

pituitary or *pituitary stalk interruption*. Causes include traumatic delivery (these patients have a higher incidence of breech delivery and perinatal injuries) and genetic abnormalities of the transcription factors that regulate pituitary embryogenesis.[13] The latter is supported in cases in which abnormalities of the posterior pituitary or stalk are associated with extrapituitary malformations such as septo-optic dysplasia. Cases with malformations are more likely to have diabetes insipidus or other osmotic dysfunction than simple ectopic posterior pituitary.[14,15] Cases are recognized in children with growth retardation and anterior pituitary deficiency rather than posterior pituitary deficiency. The degree of anterior pituitary deficit depends on the persistence of a pituitary stalk and a retained portal vasculature from the hypothalamus to the anterior pituitary.[16-18] Deficiency of adrenocorticotropic hormone (ACTH) is common and should be investigated as the patients may not respond appropriately to stress.[13]

SYNTHESIS AND RELEASE OF NEUROHYPOPHYSEAL HORMONES

Vasopressin and oxytocin are nonapeptides consisting of a 6–amino acid ring with a cysteine-to-cysteine bridge and a 3–amino acid tail (Fig. 10-1). All mammals have arginine vasopressin (AVP) and oxytocin, as illustrated in Figure 10-1, with the exception of the pig, in which lysine is substituted for arginine in position 8, producing lysine vasopressin. Both genes are found on chromosome 20,[19] although they are situated in a tail-to-tail position and transcribed in opposite directions.[20] The hormones are synthesized as part of a precursor molecule consisting of the nonapeptide and a hormone-specific neurophysin and for vasopressin a glycopeptide.[21] The precursor is packaged in

neurosecretory granules and cleaved to the products during transport to the posterior pituitary.

When a stimulus for secretion of vasopressin or oxytocin acts on the appropriate magnocellular cell body, an action potential is generated and propagates down the long axon to the posterior pituitary. The action potential causes an influx of calcium, which induces neurosecretory granules to fuse with the cell membrane and extrude the entire contents of the neurosecretory granule into the perivascular space and subsequently into the capillary system of the posterior pituitary. At physiologic pH of plasma there is no binding of hormone (vasopressin or oxytocin) to their respective neurophysins, so each peptide circulates independently in the bloodstream.

The control of hormone synthesis is at the level of transcription. Stimuli for secretion of vasopressin or oxytocin also stimulate transcription and increase the mRNA content in the magnocellular neurons. This has been studied in most detail in rats where dehydration[22] accelerates transcription and increases the levels of vasopressin (and oxytocin) mRNA[23-25] and where hypoosmolality produces a decrease in the content of vasopressin mRNA.[26]

The transport of neurosecretory vesicles from the site of synthesis to the posterior pituitary along microtubule tracks[27] is also regulated. When synthesis is turned off, transport stops, and when synthesis is increased, transport is upregulated.[27] Thus, there is coordination of stimulated release of hormone, transport of hormone, and synthesis of new hormone. There is, however, asynchrony in the timing of these events. The asynchrony is demonstrated by changes in the content of vasopressin stored in the posterior pituitary. The absolute content varies considerably among species but is a remarkable store, generally equivalent to the amount of hormone required to sustain basal release for 30 to 50 days or maximum release for 5 to 10 days.[28] In animals, prolonged and intense stimulation of vasopressin release such as dehydration or salt loading produces a depletion of stored hormone in the posterior pituitary.[25,29,30] Then, when animals are returned to normal water intake, there is in 7 to 14 days a gradual recovery of pituitary content back to baseline. This phenomenon has been modeled by Fitzsimmons,[31] who provided experimental evidence that a long half-life of the vasopressin message, approximately 2 days, is (from a minimalist point of view) a plausible explanation of the events. When a strong or sustained stimulus releases vasopressin there is an immediate stimulus to transcription of new mRNA. However, several days are required for the peak level of mRNA to be reached, so although release of hormone is rapid, translation increases slowly. When the stimulus is removed, the elevated mRNA slowly declines while continuing to synthesize hormone that repletes the store in the posterior pituitary.

PHYSIOLOGY OF SECRETION OF VASOPRESSIN AND THIRST

The physiologic regulation of vasopressin synthesis and secretion involves two systems: osmotic and pressure/volume (Fig. 10-2). The functions of these two systems are so distinct that historically it was thought there were two hormones—an antidiuretic hormone and a vasopressor hormone. Hence, the two names are used interchangeably for (8-arginine) vasopressin. There are separate systems at the level of the receptors on the end organs of response. The V_{1a} receptors on blood vessels are distinct from V_2 receptors on renal collecting duct epithelia. These two

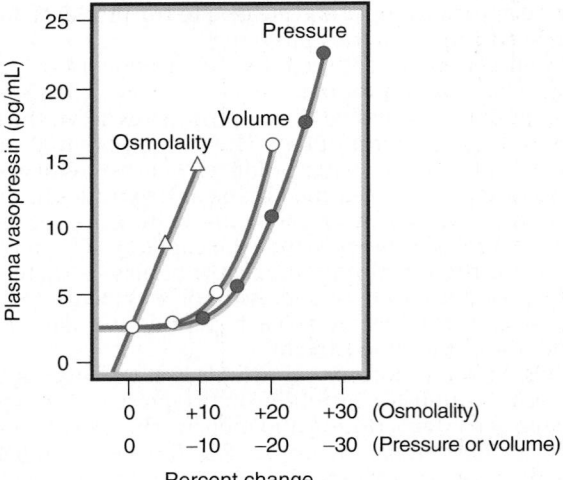

Figure 10-2 Comparison in humans of the release of vasopressin in response to increased osmolality *(open triangles)* or to decreased blood pressure *(filled circles)* or blood volume *(open circles)*. Plasma vasopressin is much more sensitive to change in osmolality, responding to as little as a 1% increase, whereas a change of 10% to 15% or greater in volume or pressure is required to stimulate release of vasopressin. (Redrawn from Robertson GL, Berl T. Water metabolism. In: Brenner B, Rector F Jr, eds. *The Kidney*, 3rd ed, vol 1. Philadelphia, PA: Elsevier; 1986:385. Figure by A.G. Robinson, University of California at Los Angeles, used with permission.)

vasopressin receptor subtypes are responsible for the main physiologic actions of vasopressin. A third receptor, V_{1b}, is responsible for the nontraditional biologic action of vasopressin to stimulate ACTH secretion from the anterior pituitary and has been found in numerous peripheral tissues and areas of the brain.[32] V_2 receptors also regulate the nontraditional action of vasopressin to stimulate factor VIII and von Willebrand factor production. Vasopressin is the main hormone involved in the regulation of water homeostasis and osmolality, and the renin-angiotensin-aldosterone system (RAAS) is mainly responsible for regulation of blood pressure and volume. Pathologic disorders of the neurohypophysis are primarily expressed as abnormalities of osmolality produced by abnormal excretion or retention of water. In the case of osmoregulation vasopressin secretion is relatively uncomplicated, with small increases in osmolality producing a parallel increase in vasopressin secretion and small decreases in osmolality causing a parallel decrease in vasopressin secretion. The regulation of volume and blood pressure is significantly more complicated (see review by Thrasher[33]), and experimental models of vasopressin and baroreceptor regulation in animals often involve inhibiting and measuring other concurrent sympathetic inputs to the system in order to ascertain direct effects of any stimulus on secretion of vasopressin (see Fig. 10-2). Other influences on secretion of vasopressin such as the inhibiting influence of glucocorticoids and the potent stimulus of nausea and vomiting are less important as physiologic regulators of vasopressin but may be important in pathologic situations.

Volume and Pressure Regulation

High-pressure arterial baroreceptors are located in the carotid sinus and aortic arch, and low-pressure volume receptors are located in the atria and pulmonary venous system.[33] The afferent signals from these receptors are carried from the chest to the brainstem through cranial nerves IX and X. Interruption of the vagal input by vagal cold block in dogs[34,35] and destruction in rabbits of the A1

area of the medulla, which receives input from nerves IX and X,[36-38] leads to an increase in vasopressin secretion. These and other data led to the concept that baroreceptors and volume receptors normally inhibit the magnocellular neurons and that decreases in this tonic inhibition result in release of vasopressin. Arterial and venous constriction induced by vasopressin action on V_{1a} receptors will contract the vessels around the existing plasma volume to effectively increase plasma volume and reestablish the inhibition of secretion of vasopressin. Vasopressin's action at the kidney to retain water will help replace volume, but in fact, the major hormonal regulation to control volume is the RAAS, which stimulates sodium reabsorption in the kidney (see Chapter 15, The Adrenal Cortex). The concept of tonic inhibition of vasopressin secretion by baroreceptors has been questioned,[33,39] but there is agreement that the volume/baroreceptor responses are much less sensitive than are the osmoreceptors (see Fig. 10-2). The lesser response has been attributed to the fact that changes in blood volume and central venous pressure have little effect to increase vasopressin in humans as long as arterial pressure can be maintained by alternative regulatory mechanisms such as RAAS and sympathetic reflexes.[33] When the hypovolemia is sufficient to cause a decrease in blood pressure there is a sudden and exponential increase in the level of vasopressin in plasma[33,40] (see Fig. 10-2). There is also agreement that changes in volume or pressure that are insufficient to cause direct increases in vasopressin can nonetheless modify the response of the vasopressin system to osmoregulatory inputs.[40,41] Increases in pressure and central volume will decrease the secretion of vasopressin,[42] but again, the response of the RAAS to cause sodium excretion is much more sensitive to increases of pressure and volume than is the response to decrease secretion of vasopressin.[33] Consequently, changes in blood pressure and volume involve both excitatory and inhibitory influences from the brainstem to magnocellular neurons, with the dominant depending on the physiologic circumstances.

Osmotic Regulation

The primary receptors for sensing changes in osmolality are located in the brain. Most of the brain is within the blood-brain barrier, which is generally impermeable to polar solutes. The osmostat is insensitive to urea and glucose, which readily cross cellular membranes but not the blood-brain barrier; this provides evidence that the osmoreceptors must be outside the blood-brain barrier. Experimental brain lesions in animals have strongly implicated cells in the organum vasculosum of the lamina terminalis (OVLT) and in areas of the anterior hypothalamus near the anterior wall of the third cerebral ventricle as the primary osmoreceptors. Because these and other circumventricular organs are perfused by fenestrated capillaries, they are outside the blood-brain barrier. Surgical destruction of the OVLT abolishes vasopressin secretion and thirst responses to hyperosmolality but not their responses to hypovolemia.[43] Patients with brain damage that destroys the region around the OVLT cannot maintain normal plasma osmolalities even under basal conditions.[44] In contrast, destruction of the magnocellular neurons of the supraoptic nuclei and paraventricular nuclei eliminates dehydration-induced secretion of vasopressin but does not alter thirst, clearly indicating that osmotically stimulated thirst must be generated at a site proximal to the magnocellular cells.

Extracellular fluid (ECF) osmolality (predominantly determined by sodium concentration) varies from 280 to 295 mOsm/kg H_2O in normal subjects, but in any individual it is maintained within a narrower range. The ability to maintain this narrow range is dependent on the sensitive response of plasma vasopressin to changes in plasma osmolality; the sensitive response of urine osmolality to changes in plasma vasopressin; and then the gain in the system by the response of urine volume to change in plasma vasopressin (Fig. 10-3). Basal plasma vasopressin is in the range of 0.5 to 2 pg/mL. As little as a 1% increase or decrease in plasma osmolality will cause a rapid increase or decrease of vasopressin released from the store of hormone in the posterior pituitary.[40] Rapid metabolism of vasopressin is also characteristic of the hormone, which circulates in plasma with a half-life of approximately 15 minutes, and this allows rapid changes in levels of vasopressin in plasma. Thus, small increases in plasma osmolality produce a concentrated urine, and small decreases produce a water diuresis. Figure 10-3 illustrates the linear relationship between plasma osmolality and plasma vasopressin that has been described in humans.[40] This linear relationship for osmolalities persists well above the normal excursion of osmolalities as demonstrated when the increase is induced by infusion of hypertonic saline or is observed during dehydration of patients with nephrogenic diabetes insipidus.[45] Similarly, Figure 10-3 illustrates that there is a sensitive and linear relationship between the level of vasopressin in plasma and the induced osmolality of the urine. Although plasma vasopressin may increase above the normal physiologic range, the urine osmolality plateaus at approximately 800 to 1200 mOsm/kg H_2O because the maximum concentration of fluid in the renal collecting duct is the osmolality of the inner medulla. Figure 10-3 also shows the relationship of plasma vasopressin to urine volume. This is a calculated relationship based on the urine volume necessary to excrete a fixed quantity of osmolytes (800 mOsm) at the urine osmolality produced by the change in plasma vasopressin. These graphs demonstrate the gain in the system when considering the changes in urine volume relative to plasma vasopressin. When vasopressin is absent, 18 to 20 L/day are excreted, but with an increase of vasopressin by as little as 0.5 to 1 pg/mL urine volume is reduced to less than 4 L/day. This illustrates the important point that at low plasma levels of vasopressin small changes of vasopressin are much larger determinants of polyuria than are greater changes at higher plasma levels.

In the kidney, water is conserved by the combined functions of the loop of Henle and the collecting duct. The loop of Henle generates a high osmolality in the renal medulla via the countercurrent multiplier system. Vasopressin acts in the collecting duct to increase water (and urea) permeability, thereby allowing osmotic equilibration between the urine and the hypertonic medullary interstitium. The net effect of this process is to extract water from the urine (which is removed from the medulla by interstitial blood vessels, the vasa recta), resulting in increased urine concentration and decreased urine volume (antidiuresis). Vasopressin produces antidiuresis by binding to V_2 receptors on the epithelial principal cells of the renal collecting tubule. Binding activates adenylate cyclase, increasing cyclic adenosine monophosphate (cAMP), which then stimulates protein kinase A. This leads to phosphorylation and activation of aquaporin 2 and movement of the water channels into the luminal membrane.[46] Aquaporin 2 is one of the widely expressed family of water channels that mediate rapid water transport across cell membranes.[47] In the kidney, water moves from the collecting duct into the hypertonic inner medulla and produces a concentrated urine.[48] In addition to moving constitutively synthesized aquaporin 2 from the cytoplasm to the luminal membrane,

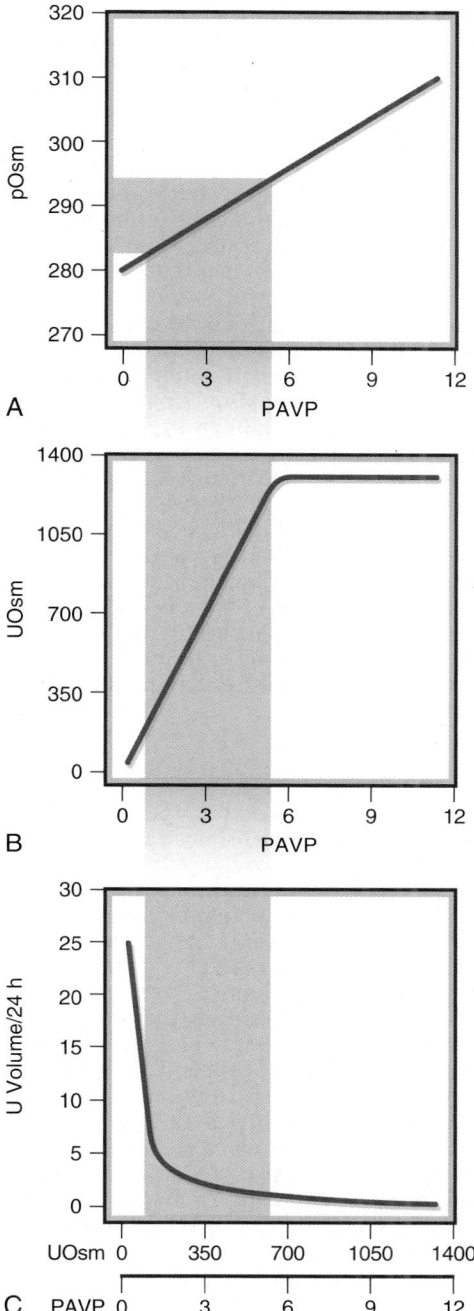

Figure 10-3 Effect of change in plasma osmolality (pOsm, in mOsm/kg of H_2O) on plasma arginine vasopressin (PAVP, in pg/mL) and consequent effects on urine osmolality (UOsm, in mOsm/kg of H_2O) and urine volume (L/day). The shaded area represents the normal range. **A,** Small changes in pOsm induce changes in PAVP, typically between less than 0.5 and 5 to 6 pg/mL. **B,** Changes in PVAP induce changes in UOsm through the full range, from maximally dilute to maximally concentrated urine. Although PAVP can rise to higher levels than 6 pg/mL, this does not translate into increased UOsm, which has a maximum determined by the osmolality of an inner medulla of the kidney. **C,** The relationship of urine volume to UOsm is logarithmic, assuming a constant osmolar load and the urine volume that would excrete that osmolar load at the UOsm indicated. As a result, urine volume changes relatively little with small changes in the other parameters until there is almost complete absence of PAVP, after which the urine volume increases dramatically. (Calculated from a formula presented in Robertson G, Shelton R, Athar S. The osmoregulation of vasopressin. *Kidney Int.* 1976;10:25-37. Figure by A.G. Robinson, University of California at Los Angeles, used with permission of Macmillan Publishers, Ltd.)

activation of the V_2 receptor also increases the synthesis of aquaporin 2 and the permeability of aquaporin 2 to water.[49] Aquaporins 3 and 4 are constitutively synthesized and are expressed at high levels in the basolateral plasma membranes of principal cells, where they are responsible for the high water permeability of the basolateral plasma membrane.[47,48] Dissociation of vasopressin from the V_2 receptor allows intracellular cAMP levels to decrease, and the water channels are then reinternalized, terminating the increased water permeability. The aquaporin-containing vesicles remain just below the apical membrane and can be quickly shuttled into and out of the membrane in response to changes in intracellular cAMP levels. This mechanism allows minute-to-minute regulation of renal water excretion in response to changes in ambient levels of vasopressin in plasma. There is also long-term regulation of collecting duct water permeability in response to prolonged high levels of circulating vasopressin. Chronically high levels of vasopressin induce increased synthesis of aquaporin 2 and aquaporin 3 water channels in the collecting duct principal cells and hence high levels of these proteins. This response requires at least 24 hours and is not rapidly reversible. Increased numbers of aquaporin 2 and 3 water channels, combined with the effect of vasopressin to insert aquaporin 2 into the apical plasma membrane, allow the collecting ducts to achieve extremely high water permeabilities and water conservation during prolonged dehydration.[47,48]

Thirst

Urine volume can be reduced to a minimum but not completely eliminated, and insensible water loss is a continuous process. To maintain water homeostasis water must also be consumed to replace the obligate urinary and insensible fluid losses. This is regulated by thirst. Similar to vasopressin, thirst can be stimulated by increases in osmolality of the ECF or by decreases in intravascular volume. Furthermore, there is evidence that the receptors are similar, that is, osmoreceptors in the anterior hypothalamus and low- and high-pressure baroreceptors in the chest mediate the thirst stimulus (with a likely contribution from circulating angiotensin II to stimulate thirst during more severe degrees of intravascular hypovolemia and hypotension).[50] Studies in humans using quantitative estimates of subjective symptoms of thirst have confirmed that increases in plasma osmolality of 2% to 3% are necessary to produce an unequivocal sensation described as "thirst."[44] Similar to vasopressin secretion, the threshold for producing thirst by hypovolemia is significantly higher.

Although osmotic changes clearly are effective stimulants of thirst, most humans consume the bulk of their ingested water as a result of the relatively unregulated components of fluid intake. Beverages are consumed with food for reasons of palatability or taken for desired secondary effects (e.g., caffeine), or for social or habitual reasons (e.g., sodas or alcoholic beverages), and as a result humans generally ingest volumes in excess of what can be considered to be an actual *need* for fluid. Consistent with this observation is the fact that under most conditions plasma osmolalities in humans remain within 1% to 2% of basal levels, levels generally thought to be below the threshold levels that stimulate thirst. This suggests that despite the obvious vital importance of thirst during pathologic situations of hyperosmolality and hypovolemia, under normal physiologic conditions water balance in humans is accomplished more by free water excretion regulated by vasopressin than by water intake regulated by thirst. This also explains why water intake must be consciously restricted

in cases of persistent unregulated secretion of vasopressin (see later discussion of SIADH).

Clinical Consequences of Osmotic and Volume Regulation

In most physiologic situations there are concurrence and synergy between the effect of increased osmolality and decreased volume to stimulate release of vasopressin. For example, with dehydration osmolality increases and volume decreases and each stimulates the release of vasopressin. Furthermore, there is good evidence that a decrease in volume shifts the plasma vasopressin/plasma osmolality response curve to the left, resulting in a greater release of vasopressin at any given osmolality.[33,51] Similarly, excess of fluid produces a decrease in osmolality and an increase in volume, and both will cause a decrease in vasopressin secretion.

The physiology of the relationships between plasma osmolality, plasma vasopressin, and especially urine volume determines some of the pathophysiology of decreased or increased secretion of vasopressin. Note in Figure 10-3 that a regular loss of vasopressin neurons that might decrease the secretory capacity of the neurohypophysis from that able to produce a blood level of 10 to 20 pg/mL of vasopressin down to a secretory capacity only sufficient to maintain a blood level of 5 pg/mL would not cause any significant change in the ability to attain a maximum urine osmolality. Below 5 pg/mL there is a linear decrease in the ability to maximally concentrate the urine. However, from the volume curve it can be seen that this results in only a modest increase in urine volume. Then, only when the last few vasopressinergic neurons are lost and the ability to maintain a maximum vasopressin drops from 1 to 0.5 pg/mL is there a large increase in urine volume. These responses therefore allow water conservation even with minimal ability to secrete vasopressin and may explain why patients with diabetes insipidus that has persisted for a relatively long period of time (e.g., after surgery or head injury) may eventually be able to discontinue treatment with vasopressin. The number of vasopressinergic neurons that need to recover to maintain an asymptomatic urine volume is small. The same pathophysiology is important in considering SIADH. For example, a patient who is unable to suppress vasopressin to less than 1 pg/mL can excrete 2 L/day at a standard osmolar load, but if fluid intake increases to greater than that which can be excreted with the fixed level of vasopressin, 1 pg/mL, then fluid will be retained and the sequence of events that causes hyponatremia in SIADH will be initiated.

An analysis of what is presently known about the regulation of thirst and secretion of vasopressin in humans demonstrates a simple but elegant system to maintain water balance. Under normal physiologic conditions, the sensitivity of the osmoregulatory system for secretion of vasopressin accounts for maintenance of plasma osmolality within narrow limits by adjusting renal water excretion in response to small changes in osmolality. Stimulated thirst does not represent a major regulatory mechanism under these conditions because unregulated fluid ingestion and water from metabolized food supply water in excess of true need. However, when unregulated water intake does not supply body needs even with maximal antidiuresis, plasma osmolality rises to levels that stimulate thirst, which produces water intake proportional to the elevation of osmolality. This arrangement has the advantage of freeing animals and humans from frequent episodes of thirst and water-seeking behavior when the water deficiency is sufficiently mild to be compensated for by renal water conservation, yet it does stimulate water ingestion when water deficiency reaches a potentially harmful level.

The Reset Osmostat During Pregnancy

Major shifts of fluid during normal pregnancy produce a decreased plasma osmolality of about 10 mmol/kg and an increase in plasma volume[52] and is the best example of a true resetting of the osmostat. The shift in osmotic threshold appears at about 5 to 8 weeks of gestation and persists throughout pregnancy, returning to normal by 2 weeks after delivery.[52] The physiology of the reset osmostat has been considered in relation to the expanded plasma volume. Total body water in pregnant women is increased by 7 to 8 L as a result of profound vasodilatation.[53] This volume is sensed as normal and vasopressin responds appropriately to decreases and increases of the expanded volume.[52,54] Both the changes in volume and the changes in osmolality have been reproduced by infusion of relaxin (a normal hormone of pregnancy that is a member of the insulin-like growth factor family) into virgin female and normal male rats[55,56] and reversed in pregnant rats by immunoneutralization of relaxin.[57] Increased nitric oxide by relaxin is reported to increase vasodilatation, and estrogens also increase nitric oxide synthesis.[58]

In women the placenta produces an enzyme, cysteine aminopeptidase, which is released into the plasma and is also known as oxytocinase.[52,59] This enzyme is equally potent in degrading oxytocin and vasopressin. The activity of oxytocinase (vasopressinase) increases markedly around 20 weeks of gestation and increases further to 40 weeks, returning slowly to normal over a few weeks after delivery.[60] The potential pathologic condition produced by oxytocinase is described later under "Diabetes Insipidus Due to Accelerated Metabolism of Vasopressin (Diabetes Insipidus of Pregnancy)."

Osmotic Regulation in Aging

Numerous studies have reported that elderly humans are at risk for both hypernatremia and hyponatremia.[61,62] In older subjects there is a decrease in glomerular filtration rate,[61] and the collecting duct in the aged kidney may be less responsive to vasopressin-stimulated increases in aquaporin 2 water channels, thus limiting the ability to excrete free water.[63] Elderly subjects are reported to have a lower nocturnal plasma level of AVP and a prolonged effect of administered desmopressin.[64] Many other abnormalities of fluid and electrolyte balance in the elderly are due to comorbid conditions and the numerous pharmacologic agents these patients are often taking.[65] Studies of responses to dehydration, osmolar stimulation, or volume stimulation in the elderly are complicated by the fact that by age 75 to 80 total body water declines to 50% of the level of normal young adults.[66] The elderly have a decreased thirst with dehydration and a lower fluid intake during recovery from dehydration.[67,68] At the other end of the spectrum, elderly patients have been found to excrete a water load less well than younger subjects, and at least part of this is due to decreased suppression of vasopressin.[69]

In summary, there are age-related changes in body volumes and renal function that predispose the elderly to abnormalities in water and electrolyte balance.[70] Diseases that are more common in the elderly aggravate this, and in addition, the therapies for these diseases affect water balance. Healthy elderly humans probably have at least a normal (or increased) ability to secrete vasopressin but a decreased appreciation for thirst and a decreased ability to achieve either a maximum concentration of urine to retain water or a maximum dilution of urine to excrete water. This demonstrates the necessity of paying attention to fluid balance problems in the elderly as undetected hypernatremia or hyponatremia can lead to increased morbidity and fatality.[71]

DIABETES INSIPIDUS

Diabetes insipidus is a disorder of a large volume of urine (diabetes) that is hypotonic, dilute, and tasteless (insipid). This is opposed to the hypertonic and sweet urine of diabetes mellitus (honey). Diabetes insipidus is caused by absence of the hormone vasopressin or inadequate response to vasopressin. Four syndromes of diabetes insipidus— primary polydipsia, hypothalamic/neurohypophyseal diabetes insipidus, diabetes insipidus of pregnancy, and nephrogenic diabetes insipidus—can be explained, respectively, by the pathophysiology of excess intake of water, decreased synthesis or secretion of vasopressin, accelerated metabolism of vasopressin, and lack of appropriate response to vasopressin by the kidney. The absence of vasopressin produces pathologic change related only to water, not blood pressure. Most patients have an intact thirst mechanism, so they do not become dehydrated but present with polyuria and polydipsia. Patients with diabetes insipidus who have inadequate thirst can rapidly become dehydrated and develop severe hypernatremia with devastating effects on the central nervous system (CNS). Hypertonic encephalopathy with obtundation, coma, and seizures may be produced by brain shrinkage. A decreased volume of the brain in the skull may lead to subarachnoid hemorrhage, intracerebral bleeding, or petechial hemorrhage.[72] Fortunately, problems associated with severe hypernatremia are usually not observed in patients with diabetes insipidus because of intact thirst. Hypernatremic encephalopathy is only a risk when a patient is unable to respond to thirst either because of age or level of consciousness.

To determine whether there is a large volume of urine one can measure a 24-hour urine volume, but because of the large volume it is easier in adults to keep a diary for 24 hours, recording the volume and time of each voided urine. Simultaneously, there is a determination of whether polyuria is due to an osmotic agent, such as glucose, or intrinsic renal disease. Usually routine laboratory studies and the clinical setting will distinguish these disorders from consideration of diabetes insipidus. There is universal agreement that the diagnosis of diabetes insipidus is made by some dehydration to stimulate the normal release of vasopressin but with a less than normal concentration of the urine. The gold standard is a dehydration test in a controlled environment followed by measure of vasopressin in plasma and response to administered vasopressin or the analogue desmopressin. The description that follows is for adults. Special attention is required in children and testing should be done only by a pediatrician; testing should not be done in infants.[46] In children care should be taken to prevent hyponatremia after administration of desmopressin.[46,73] If the adult patient has mild polyuria, the test may begin in the evening and the majority of dehydration carried out overnight. If the patient gives a history of large volumes of urine during the night, it is best to perform the test during the day when the patient can be observed.

The patient voids at the beginning of the test, and the starting weight is recorded. Serum sodium is obtained and nothing is allowed by mouth (certainly no fluid) during the test. Each voided urine is then recorded and urine osmolality measured. The patient is weighed after each liter of urine. When two consecutive measures of urine osmolality differ by no more than 10% and the patient has lost 2% of the body weight, plasma for Na+, osmolality, and vasopressin is drawn and the patient is given 2 µg of desmopressin intravenously or intramuscularly. Urine output and osmolality are recorded hourly for an additional 2 hours.[74,75] The dehydration is stopped and measurements taken if the patient loses greater than 3% of the body weight or at any time that the Na+ is elevated above the normal range. The duration of the test varies among patients. Patients with complete diabetes insipidus reach a maximum but low urine osmolality within a few hours, but patients with other disorders may take up to 18 hours. There is no difficulty determining the diagnosis in severe hypothalamic/neurohypophyseal diabetes insipidus or severe nephrogenic diabetes insipidus. In the former, urine osmolality will have minimal concentration in spite of dehydration and there is a marked increase in urine osmolality in response to administered desmopressin, at least a 50% increase but often increasing 200% to 400%. At the end of the test these patients will have undetectable vasopressin in plasma. In nephrogenic diabetes insipidus there will similarly be little concentration of the urine in spite of achieving dehydration, but urine osmolality will also show little or no increase to administered desmopressin. Patients with nephrogenic diabetes insipidus are unequivocally distinguished from hypothalamic/neurohypophyseal diabetes insipidus by high levels of vasopressin in plasma at the end of the dehydration, often greater than 5 pg/µL.

There may be difficulty in differentiating partial hypothalamic/neurohypophyseal diabetes insipidus from primary polydipsia. With dehydration both have some concentration of the urine, often above plasma osmolality, but the urine osmolality does not approach the level of 800 to 1200 mOsm/kg that is characteristic of normal subjects. In response to the administered desmopressin patients with partial hypothalamic/neurohypophyseal diabetes insipidus usually have a further concentration of the urine, of at least 10%, whereas patients with primary polydipsia have no further increase. The reliability of the response to desmopressin is debated. Some patients with primary polydipsia may achieve a plateau level in urine osmolality before reaching their maximum urine osmolality and hence respond to desmopressin. Alternatively, some patients with partial hypothalamic/neurohypophyseal diabetes insipidus may, with severe dehydration, secrete sufficient vasopressin to achieve the maximum attainable urine osmolality and will not have a further increase to administered desmopressin. Investigators who have a highly sensitive radioimmunoassay for vasopressin are able to distinguish between partial hypothalamic/neurohypophyseal diabetes insipidus and primary polydipsia by the measure of vasopressin at the end of the dehydration test[76,77] and further report that patients with one of these disorders may be inappropriately diagnosed as the alternate using the standard dehydration test. However, a longitudinal clinical study of patients with autoimmune hypothalamic/neurohypophyseal diabetes insipidus reported good correlation between results of the dehydration test and measured vasopressin to diagnose partial diabetes insipidus.[78] When the diagnosis is in doubt, patients should have adequate follow-up to ensure that a good therapeutic response to desmopressin is obtained and that the patients do not develop hyponatremia. This clinical follow-up and response are a continuation of the diagnosis with the trial of desmopressin as a test agent. If on follow-up desmopressin produces a decrease in polyuria, a decrease in thirst, and a normal sodium concentration, the patient almost certainly has partial hypothalamic/neurohypophyseal diabetes insipidus. However, if the poly-

dipsia does not improve and the patient develops hyponatremia, the patient has some abnormality of thirst and primary polydipsia.[76,79]

The clinical presentation is often helpful in the differential diagnosis. In a patient with onset of polyuria or polydipsia immediately after surgery in the hypothalamic/pituitary area or after head trauma (especially with skull fracture and loss of consciousness), the diagnosis of hypothalamic/neurohypophyseal diabetes insipidus is highly likely. Patients with hypothalamic/neurohypophyseal diabetes insipidus often have a sudden onset of symptoms and persistent thirst throughout the day and night associated with a desire for cold liquids.[80] Patients with diabetes insipidus usually have serum sodium in the high range of normal, and patients with primary polydipsia have serum sodium in the low range of normal. Blood urea nitrogen concentration is often low in both hypothalamic/neurohypophyseal diabetes insipidus and in primary polydipsia because of the high renal clearance, but there is a difference in serum uric acid concentrations. Serum uric acid is elevated in hypothalamic/neurohypophyseal diabetes insipidus both because of modest volume contraction and absence of the normal action of vasopressin on V_1 receptors in the kidney to increase urate clearance. A value greater than 5 µg/dL was reported to separate hypothalamic/neurohypophyseal diabetes insipidus from primary polydipsia. Presumably in patients with primary polydipsia, there is modest volume expansion and intermittent secretion of vasopressin to act on V_1 receptors to clear serum urate.[81] Urine volume greater than 18 L is highly suggestive of primary polydipsia because this exceeds the amount of urine delivered to the collecting duct. Most patients with hypothalamic/neurohypophyseal diabetes insipidus have modest dehydration, decreased glomerular filtration rate, and urine volumes in the range of 6 to 12 L/day.

Recently there have been publications about the measure of copeptin, the glycopeptide that with neurophysin and vasopressin is part of the prohormone for vasopressin. Copeptin is secreted equimolar to vasopressin and has the advantage of being stable in plasma and more readily measurable by radioimmunoassay than is vasopressin. Although the results of clinical testing are promising, the value of copeptin as a distinguishing measure in confusing cases of diabetes insipidus (or SIADH) is still uncertain.[82]

Imaging of the Neurohypophysis

On T1-weighted images the MRI produces a bright spot in the sella[12] caused by stored hormone in neurosecretory granules in the posterior pituitary.[29,83-86] The bright spot is present in approximately 80% of normal subjects[87,88] and is absent in most patients with diabetes insipidus. Some studies have reported a bright spot in patients with clinical evidence of diabetes insipidus.[89] For example, patients with familial hypothalamic/neurohypophyseal diabetes insipidus (see later) may have a bright spot early in the disease (especially when the diabetes insipidus is partial), but the bright spot disappears with increasing severity of the diabetes insipidus.[90] The role of stored oxytocin as a source of the pituitary bright spot has been ignored, and it is possible that a persistent bright spot in patients with diabetes insipidus is due to the pituitary content of oxytocin.

The posterior pituitary bright spot decreases with a prolonged stimulus to vasopressin secretion[91] and has been variably reported in other polyuric disorders. In primary polydipsia the bright spot usually is seen.[85,92] In nephrogenic diabetes insipidus the bright spot has been reported to be absent in some patients[85] but present in others.[85,93] Patients with nephrogenic diabetes insipidus have high levels of vasopressin in plasma and are chronically dehydrated, so the posterior pituitary might be depleted of vasopressin stores. Similarly, with the osmotic stress of untreated diabetes mellitus or the transient diabetes insipidus of pregnancy the posterior pituitary may be depleted and the bright spot lost, but then it returns with recovery.[91,94]

Imaging of the hypothalamus is also an important diagnostic tool for diseases of the neurohypophysis. As noted earlier, the hormones of the neurohypophysis are synthesized in the paired paraventricular nuclei located bilaterally in the walls of the third ventricle and supraoptic nuclei located at the extremes of the optic chiasm. Knowledge of this large area, coupled with the knowledge that 90% of the vasopressinergic neurons must be destroyed to produce symptomatic diabetes insipidus,[95,96] makes it apparent that for a mass lesion or a destructive lesion to produce diabetes insipidus it must either destroy a large area of the hypothalamus or be located where the tracks of these four nuclei converge at the base of the hypothalamus at the top of the pituitary stalk. Tumors confined within the sella do not cause diabetes insipidus.[96] The area of interest is the discrete area immediately above the sellar diaphragm. The hormones are synthesized in cell bodies and travel in axons to the posterior lobe. With section of the axons or pressure on the axons at the level of the posterior lobe there is a reaccumulation of neurosecretory material and the appearance of a posterior lobe above the site of injury.[91,97,98] The pituitary stalk can also be readily identified on MRI and has been an additional tool in the differential diagnosis of diseases of the neurohypophysis. Enlargement of the stalk is reported with the diseases listed in Table 10-1. When there is a diagnosis of central diabetes insipidus, thickening of the stalk is usually associated with absence of the posterior pituitary bright spot and a search for systemic diseases is indicated.[99] A thickened stalk with coexistent anterior pituitary deficiency is especially suggestive of etiologic systemic disease.[100,101] When the cause is still in doubt, MRI should be repeated every 3 to 6 months for the first 2 years, especially in children, in whom enlargement may indicate a germinoma.[100-103] When follow-up shows a decrease in size of the stalk, a likely diagnosis is infundibulolymphohypophysitis.[104]

Clinical Causes of Diabetes Insipidus

Diabetes Insipidus Due to Excess Intake (Primary Polydipsia)

Primary polydipsia and subsequent polyuria must be differentiated from diabetes insipidus and may also contribute to SIADH. Primary polydipsia may be induced by any organic structural lesion in the hypothalamus that causes hypothalamic/neurohypophyseal diabetes insipidus (described later) and may be especially associated with sarcoidosis of the hypothalamus.[105] It may also be produced by drugs that cause a dry mouth or by any peripheral disorder causing an elevation of renin or angiotensin.[106] When there is no identifiable pathologic cause, the disorder may be associated with psychiatric syndromes or be habitual throughout a lifetime. Series of polydipsic patients in psychiatric hospitals have shown an incidence as high as 42% of patients with some form of polydipsia and for greater than half of those there was no obvious explanation for the polydipsia.[107,108]

Treatment of Primary Polydipsia

When there is no structural lesion, these patients are usually refractory to treatment.[106] Propanolol has been used with some success presumably because of its ability to inhibit the renin/angiotensin system.[109]

Diabetes Insipidus Due to Decreased Synthesis or Secretion (Hypothalamic/ Neurohypophyseal Diabetes Insipidus)

Genetic Abnormalities of the Vasopressin Gene. Hypothalamic/neurohypophyseal diabetes insipidus is characterized by the onset of classic diabetes insipidus with polydipsia and polyuria in childhood or as a young adult, but during infancy they may be asymptomatic.[110,111] In contrast, in familial nephrogenic diabetes insipidus the defect is expressed as a polyuric disease at birth (see later description). A rare type of familial hypothalamic/neurohypophyseal diabetes insipidus may be present at birth in infants with homozygote mutation of the AVP hormone region of the preprohormone. This may produce excretion of an inactive vasopressin but no difficulty in folding of the preprohormone.[112] In the usual familial hypothalamic/neurohypophyseal diabetes insipidus, MRI findings are variable even within affected family members, but the most constant finding in children is the presence of a posterior pituitary bright spot, which progressively disappears with time.[113] The genetic defect is usually in the biologically inactive neurophysin or in the signal peptide of the preprohormone. Although genetically heterozygous with the defect expressed in only one allele, the clinical phenotype is autosomal dominant. Lack of normal cleavage of the signal peptide from the prohormone and abnormal folding of the vasopressin/neurophysin precursor are thought to produce fibrillar aggregations in the endoplasmic reticulum, which is cytotoxic to the neuron, explaining the dominant phenotype.[114,115] Autopsy studies have confirmed neuronal cell death.[116] Genetic testing of asymptomatic children in affected families will negate the need for repeated dehydration testing and allow early treatment.[117] Wolfram syndrome is a rare autosomal recessive disease with diabetes insipidus, diabetes mellitus, optic atrophy, and deafness (DIDMOAD). The genetic defect is for the protein wolframin that is found in the endoplasmic reticulum and is important for folding proteins.[118] Wolframin is localized to chromosome 4. It is involved in beta-cell proliferation and intracellular protein processing and calcium homeostasis, producing a wide spectrum of endocrine and CNS disorders. Diabetes insipidus is usually a late manifestation and is associated with decreased magnocellular neurons in the paraventricular and supraoptic nuclei.[113,119]

Malignancies. Some tumors such as craniopharyngioma and primary germ cell tumors in children characteristically occur in a suprasellar basal hypothalamic area and are

---

TABLE 10-1
Diseases Associated With Enlarged Infundibular Stalk

1. Germinoma
2. Craniopharyngioma
3. Metastases to the hypothalamus and long portal vessels (e.g., carcinoma of the breast or lung)
4. Granulomatosis diseases
   a. Langerhans cell histiocytosis
   b. Sarcoidosis
   c. Wegener granulomatosis
   d. Non–Langerhans cell histiocytosis (e.g., Erdheim-Chester disease)
5. Tuberculosis
6. Lymphocytic infundibulohypophysitis

regularly associated with diabetes insipidus.[120-122] It is not uncommon for diabetes insipidus to be the presenting complaint, although other evidence of hypopituitarism is often present. The MRI often shows a thickened stalk[123] and may show a hypothalamic mass. Tumor markers in plasma or cerebrospinal fluid (CSF) may confirm the tumor type in children, but absence of markers does not rule out any specific cause.[124]

Metastatic disease involving the pituitary is usually found in association with widespread metastatic disease and may be asymptomatic and only reported at autopsy. Metastases are twice as likely to involve the posterior pituitary as the anterior pituitary,[125,126] and this is thought to be due to a more direct arterial blood supply to the posterior pituitary.[127] Most primary tumors in the hypothalamic/pituitary area that cause diabetes insipidus are relatively slow growing, and any tumor in this area that shows rapid growth in a short period of time should be considered as a possible metastatic tumor.[128,129] Pituitary abscess is a rare cause of a pituitary mass and diabetes insipidus.[122,130]

Diabetes insipidus is reported with lymphomas in the hypothalamic/pituitary area.[131] There may be some increased incidence of lymphoma presenting with diabetes insipidus due to the increased incidence lymphoproliferative disease with human immunodeficiency virus (HIV) and hepatitis C infection.[132] Diabetes insipidus is also associated with leukemia. The mechanism is thought to be infiltration of the hypothalamus, thrombosis, or infection.[133,134] Diabetes insipidus is distinctly more common in nonlymphocytic leukemia.[135-137] MRI studies in leukemia may show infiltration or an infundibular mass[135] but often are normal even when leukemic cells are found in the CSF.[137]

Granulomatous Diseases. In most cases of diabetes insipidus caused by granulomatous disease there is clear evidence of characteristic disease elsewhere in the body.[99,138,139] The MRI will show involvement of the hypothalamus and absence of the posterior pituitary bright spot on T1-weighted images with widening of the stalk (see Table 10-1). Although there are occasional reports of resolution of the diabetes insipidus with appropriate therapy of the primary disease, in most cases, once it is established, diabetes insipidus is permanent.[140-142]

Infundibulohypophysitis. The forms of lymphocytic hypophysitis are classified by the tissues as adenohypophysitis, infundibuloneurohypophysitis, or panhypophysitis and may extend into the hypothalamus.[143] All of these forms are usually associated with a thickened stalk and loss of the pituitary bright spot on T1-weighted MRI. Adenohypophysitis often involves females around the time of a pregnancy, whereas infundibuloneurohypophysitis occurs in either sex. A recently recognized form of infundibuloneurohypophysitis occurs in middle-aged to elderly males and is associated with immunoglobulin G4 (IgG4)-related systemic disease. Various organs, especially the pancreas, are infiltrated with IgG4 plasma cells, and neurohypophysitis is only one manifestation of a multiorgan disease that may include other endocrine glands. This finding should be considered as a cause of diabetes insipidus based on age and sex at presentation and evidence of other systemic disease. The diagnosis can be established by elevated serum IgG4 level and characteristic histologic findings on biopsies. Response to steroids or other immunosuppressive drugs is characteristic.[144,145] When a definitive cause of diabetes insipidus is not found, most cases of diabetes insipidus will be labeled *idiopathic*, but an autoimmune process should always be considered.[146,147]

Surgery or Trauma of the Neurohypophyseal System. Although diabetes insipidus is well known to occur after hypothalamic or pituitary surgery, this diagnosis should be made with caution.[148,149] Vasopressin is normally secreted in the stress of surgical procedures and fluid may be retained, which is then excreted normally after surgery. Stress of surgery may also induce insulin resistance and exacerbate diabetes mellitus, producing an osmotic diuresis from glucose. The patterns of diabetes insipidus after surgery have been described in detail.[150,151] As many as 50% to 60% of patients will have some transient diabetes insipidus within 24 hours of pituitary surgery, and it will usually resolve (especially with transsphenoidal surgery in which the resection of a tumor is confined to the sella), with only a small number having permanent diabetes insipidus.[152] The introduction of endoscopic pituitary surgery has not increased the incidence of diabetes insipidus,[153] and there continues to be greater morbidity with surgery for craniopharyngioma.[154]

If there is complete stalk section patients may exhibit a pattern known as *triphasic diabetes insipidus* (Fig. 10-4). The first phase is diabetes insipidus with onset within the first 24 hours of surgery and is thought to be due to axon shock and inability of action potentials to be propagated from the cell body to the axon terminals in the posterior pituitary. The second phase is an antidiuretic phase, which was originally described as a *normal interphase* but is not normal and is thought to be due to unregulated release of vasopressin from the store of hormone in the degenerating axons of the posterior pituitary. Because the release of vasopressin in this phase is unregulated, excess administration of fluids will produce hyponatremia and SIADH. When the entire hormone content has been released diabetes insipidus returns, constituting the third phase. The course of diabetes insipidus may be permanent, or subsequently it may resolve to partial or clinically inapparent disease.

An important observation is that the second phase of the triphasic response (i.e., uncontrolled release of vasopressin due to axon trauma) may occur without preceding or subsequent diabetes insipidus.[155,156] This isolated phase has been reported clinically and has been produced experimentally in the rat by unilateral lesion of the supraopticohypophyseal tract.[156] The interpretation is that if the trauma has involved only some of the axons coursing to the posterior pituitary, then the remaining intact axons

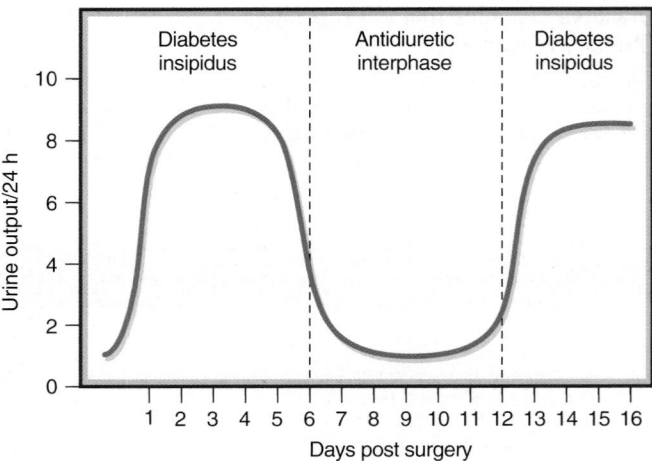

Figure 10-4 Typical triphasic response of urine volume after sectioning of the pituitary stalk induced by surgery or head trauma. The first phase of diabetes insipidus occurs immediately postoperatively and continues to day 6. The second phase of antidiuresis occurs from day 7 and continues to day 12. The third stage is the recurrence of diabetes insipidus on day 13. Durations vary; see text for detailed discussion. (From A.G. Robinson, University of California at Los Angeles, used with permission.)

will have sufficient vasopressin function to avoid the clinically apparent diabetes insipidus that is characteristic of the first and third phases of the triphasic response. However, the store of hormone in the posterior pituitary is sufficiently large that necrosis of even a fraction of these vasopressin neurons will cause enough uncontrolled release of vasopressin to produce hyponatremia if excess fluid is administered. The hyponatremia is often symptomatic, and patients present with headache, nausea, and emesis or seizure.[157] When all the vasopressin from the damaged neurons has been secreted the stimulus for water retention resolves and the retained water is excreted, producing recovery from the hyponatremia. Thus, the clinical picture is one of hyponatremia occurring around 7 to 10 days after pituitary surgery, persisting for a few days, and then returning to normal. This syndrome of transient hyponatremia has been referred to as *isolated second phase*[156] to emphasize the pathophysiologic cause. Isolated hyponatremia has been reported in 10% to 25% of patients after pituitary surgery.[150,158,159]

The same patterns of diabetes insipidus that occur after surgery can be seen in patients after closed-head trauma,[96] and the incidence may be increasing because of better care and increased survival of patients with severe head injury.[160] Patients with penetrating injury[160] and children[161] are especially at risk. Three quarters of these cases are due to motor vehicle accidents.[96,162] Computed tomography or MRI in a large group of patients with posttraumatic hypopituitarism including diabetes insipidus revealed hemorrhage in the hypothalamus or posterior pituitary in 55% of patients, and approximately 5% of patients had stalk resection or infarction of the posterior pituitary.[163]

There are several important clinical points to be made with regard to diabetes insipidus induced by head trauma. First, these patients are virtually always unconscious and will not have the normal ability to sense thirst. Second, it is a situation in which large volumes of fluid might be given because of blood loss or other volume deficits, and this fluid loss or stress might induce diabetes mellitus and an osmotic diuresis. Third, there may be a greater risk if the second phase is unrecognized because hyponatremia will produce cerebral edema, which may aggravate any edema due to trauma. Therefore, in administering desmopressin the effect of one dose should be allowed to wane before administering another dose to ensure that the patient has not entered the second phase.

There is a high incidence of anterior pituitary deficiency in association with diabetes insipidus induced by head trauma.[163] The possibility of cortisol deficiency should be considered immediately because this problem may be life threatening in these patients.[161] Cortisol deficiency should also be considered subsequently if diabetes insipidus appears to improve because of decreased polyuria. Cortisol deficiency alone decreases the ability to excrete water even in the absence of vasopressin.[96] Last, in a long-term follow-up of these patients partial diabetes insipidus may be found,[164,165] and there may be return of sufficient vasopressin function that under basal conditions the patient is no longer symptomatic from a large urine output.[96,164]

Absent Release of Vasopressin and Absent Thirst in Response to Osmotic Stimulation. Lack of thirst in response to increased osmolality indicates an abnormality of the osmostat. This may be seen in hypothalamic/neurohypophyseal diabetes insipidus when the initial lesion or surgical damage is so severe that the damage is not only to the neurohypophysis but also to the central anteriorly placed osmostat[166] or with isolated damage of the osmostat with intact baroreceptors described as essential hypernatremia. In the former there is no release of vasopressin in response to either osmotic or baroreceptor stimulation, but in the latter there is adequate synthesis of vasopressin and release with baroreceptor stimulation but no release with osmotic stimulation. Massive damage of the hypothalamus is necessary for the former and is most commonly seen in patients with craniopharyngioma or a pituitary tumor with extremely large supraseller extension, often with anterior pituitary deficiencies and other manifestations of hypothalamic syndrome (e.g., hyperphagia, sleep apnea, thermoregulation, seizures).[166,167] Abnormalities of thirst with primary hypothalamic lesions are most common with sarcoidosis, but the pattern of essential hypernatremia with absent osmostat and intact baroreceptor is most commonly reported after clipping of an anterior communicating artery aneurysm.[166,167] In these cases there is evidence that vasopressin is synthesized and stored in that maneuvers to stimulate baroreceptors increase secretion of vasopressin and concentration of the urine.[168,169] The pathophysiologic explanation of essential hypernatremia is that inadequate water intake and excess water excretion produce a degree of dehydration with hypernatremia; when the dehydration is sufficient to stimulate the baroreceptors, vasopressin is released, urine is concentrated, and the patient remains in a steady state of hypernatremia with modest dehydration. The increased concentration of sodium per se also causes sodium excretion to help maintain the new steady state.[170]

Diabetes Insipidus and Brain Death. Diabetes insipidus is reported in 50% to 90% of patients with brain death.[171,172] Although some aspects of hormonal treatment of organ donors are controversial, there is consensus that treatment of diabetes insipidus should be standard in donors with this disorder.[173]

Treatment of Hypothalamic/Neurohypophyseal Diabetes Insipidus

Mass Lesions of the Neurohypophysis: Malignancies, Granulomas, Infundibulitis. A major goal of therapy is to decrease the thirst and polyuria to a level that allows the patient to maintain a normal lifestyle. The timing and quantity of dosage should be individually prescribed and easy for the patient to accommodate. Safety of the prescribed agent and avoiding detrimental effects of overtreatment are primary considerations because of the relatively benign course of diabetes insipidus and the adverse consequences of hyponatremia. The therapeutic agents to treat diabetes insipidus are shown in Table 10-2. Water is considered a therapeutic agent because when taken in sufficient quantity there is no metabolic abnormality. Therapy is designed to reduce the

TABLE 10-2

Therapeutic Agents for Treatment of Diabetes Insipidus

1. Water
2. Water-retaining agents
   a. L-Arginine vasopressin
   b. Desmopressin, 1-(3-mercaptopropionic acid)-8-D-arginine vasopressin
   c. Chlorpropamide
   d. Carbamazepine*
   e. Clofibrate*
   f. Indomethacin
3. Natriuretic agents
   a. Thiazide diuretics
   b. Amiloride
   c. Indapamide

*Not recommended.

necessary water intake (and polyuria) to an acceptable level, but occasional lapses in pharmacologic therapy are not detrimental, may avoid overtreatment producing hyponatremia, and allow recognition of any spontaneous recovery.

The drug of choice is desmopressin,[76,174] a synthetic analogue of vasopressin in which the substitution of D-arginine markedly reduces pressor activity and removing the terminal amine increases the half-life (see Fig. 10-1). The two changes produce an agent nearly 2000 times more specific for antidiuresis than naturally occurring L-arginine vasopressin.[175] Desmopressin is available as tablets for oral administration, a lyophilisate for sublingual administration (oral melt), a solution for intranasal administration, and a solution for parenteral use.[176] Most patients prefer desmopressin tablets (0.1 and 0.2 mg), although many patients continue to be successfully treated with the intranasal spray. Desmopressin melt (60, 120, and 240 µg) is reported to be more acceptable in some children.[177] Because of the variability among patients it is desirable to determine the duration of action of individual doses in each patient.[178-180] The patient is first allowed to escape from the effects of any previous medication, and for each voided urine the time and volume are recorded and, if possible, osmolality is measured. A dose of desmopressin is given and the patient is allowed to drink fluid ad lib. A decrease in urine volume is noted in 1 to 2 hours, and the total duration of action will usually be 6 to 18 hours. When a dose is sufficient to elicit a stable therapeutic response, further increasing the dose (e.g., doubling the dose) produces only a moderate increase in duration of a few hours,[178,179] consistent with the half-life of desmopressin in plasma.[178] Usually a satisfactory schedule is achieved with a modest dose and the maximum dose rarely exceeds 0.2 mg orally or 20 µg intranasally (two sprays) given two or three times a day (usually three times a day for tablets and twice for intranasal spray).[179] Using the tablets allows considerable flexibility in dosage by using either whole or split tablets. For intranasally administered desmopressin there is less flexibility with the metered spray, which is fixed at 10 µg in 100 µL. For greater flexibility with intranasal administration the patient may be taught to use the rhinal catheter. Specific directions are described elsewhere.[174] Rarely is it necessary to resort to parenterally administered desmopressin (2 mL vials of 4 µg/mL) for ambulatory patients. If an intercurrent illness or allergy makes this desirable, a dose of 0.5 to 2.0 µg can be administered subcutaneously using an insulin (low dose if necessary) syringe and needle.[179] Parenterally administered desmopressin gives virtually identical therapeutic response when given as an intravenous bolus, intramuscularly, or subcutaneously,[179] and the parenteral administration is 5 to 20 times as potent as an intranasally administered dose.[174,179] Recent studies have reported an increased antidiuretic response to desmopressin in women and in the elderly.[181]

Therapeutic agents such as chlorpropamide or thiazide diuretics are especially useful when only a modest decrease in urine volume will make the patient asymptomatic. The major action of chlorpropamide is on the renal tubule to increase the hydroosmotic action of residual vasopressin,[182] but the agent can produce significant antidiuresis even in patients with severe hypothalamic/neurohypophyseal diabetes insipidus.[76] The usual dose is 250 to 500 mg/day with a response noted in 1 to 2 days and a maximum antidiuresis in 4 days.[76,174] This is an off-label use of the drug. This agent should not be used in pregnancy and is not recommended in children, especially with concurrent hypopituitarism, because of the possibility of severe hypoglycemia.

The therapeutic agents listed in Table 10-2 that induce water retention have other clinical indications and when used in patients with diabetes insipidus might augment the effect of administered desmopressin, exposing the patient to excess water retention and hyponatremia. This effect may be especially true of over-the-counter nonsteroidal anti-inflammatory drugs (NSAIDs), which inhibit the action of prostaglandin E_2. Prostaglandin E has a limiting action on vasopressin-induced water uptake by enhancing the retrieval of aquaporin 2 from the plasma membrane and returning it to the intracellular pool. NSAIDs inhibit prostaglandin E_2 and prolong the time the water channels remain in the membrane, thus increasing the duration of action of administered desmopressin.[183]

Hyponatremia is a rare complication of desmopressin therapy and only occurs if the patient is continually antidiuretic while maintaining a fluid intake sufficient to become volume expanded and natriuretic. Thirst may be protective; most patients on standard therapy are not continuously maximally antidiuretic or may occasionally delay a dose to excrete any excess retained water. Treatment of infants requires special attention and expertise. Infants consume a large part of their calories as liquid formula or breast milk and have corresponding high volume of dilute urine. Treatment with oral or intranasal desmopressin is reported to have broad swings of the serum sodium and the risk of symptomatic hyponatremia.[184] In Europe a lyophilisate of desmopressin is used orally[185] and in the United States pediatricians have used desmopressin subcutaneously or substituted a low solute formula with a thiazide diuretic.[184] In the earlier discussion of physiology it was noted that normal elderly persons have reduced ability both to concentrate their urine and to excrete a water load. Therefore, treatment of an elderly patient with diabetes insipidus requires special attention to avoid hyponatremia.[185] Because elderly persons may have an increased use of NSAIDs, patients with diabetes insipidus should be specifically informed of the risk of developing hyponatremia when taking an NSAID with desmopressin.[186]

Diabetes Insipidus After Hypothalamic or Pituitary Surgery or Injury. The surgeon often knows how severely the posterior pituitary or stalk was injured. Sometimes diuresis after surgery is the result of water retention during the procedure. Vasopressin is released during surgical procedures, and administered fluid may be retained. When the stress of surgery abates the vasopressin level falls and retained fluid is excreted. If an attempt is made to match the urine output with further fluid infusion, persistent polyuria might be mistaken for diabetes insipidus. If in doubt, fluid can be withheld until there is a modest increase in sodium. If the urine output decreases and the serum sodium remains normal, the polyuria was due to excretion of physiologically retained fluid. If the serum sodium begins to rise while urine osmolality is low and there is a positive response to administered desmopressin, the diagnosis of diabetes insipidus can be established.[148] Sometimes the duration of diabetes insipidus is quite transient and the surgeon may prefer to treat it only with fluid replacement parenterally or orally (if the patient is awake and able to respond to thirst). In treating diabetes insipidus desmopressin may be given parenterally 0.5 to 2 µg, subcutaneously, intramuscularly, or intravenously. The intravenous route may be preferable because there is no question about absorption. Urine output will be reduced in 1 to 2 hours and the duration of effect is 6 to 24 hours. If the patient is alert, thirst is a good guide to fluid replacement. Care should be taken that intravenous fluids (especially hypotonic) are not given excessively after administering desmopressin because this practice can lead to profound hyponatremia.[187] As the diabetes insipidus may be quite transient and some of these patients may develop the triphasic pattern described previously, it is desirable to allow polyuria to return before administering subsequent doses of desmopressin.[151]

Treatment of acute diabetes insipidus after blunt trauma to the head can be similar to postoperative care, except that the patient with head injury is more likely to be comatose and unable to respond to thirst and therefore is more likely to develop hypernatremia. Because a comatose patient must be given fluids parenterally some clinicians prefer to use a continuous infusion of low-dose vasopressin. The vasopressin can be added directly to the crystalloid solution that is being administered[188] or can be infused separately to maintain a constant antidiuresis while adjusting the fluid intake appropriate to any persistent polyuria and to cover insensible water loss. Doses of 0.25 to 2.7 mU/kg/hour have been described.[189-191] If this method is used, there is a potential to produce hyponatremia,[188,189] and serum sodium must be checked regularly. Of course, with continuous replacement one will not know whether there is return of normal function or whether a patient might be entering the second phase of the triphasic pattern described earlier.

Diabetes Insipidus With Inadequate Thirst. The high incidence of anterior pituitary deficiency in these patients should be considered in any treatment of diabetes insipidus.[192] With lack of thirst and continuing polyuria these patients will develop severe hypernatremia; if they are encouraged to drink and an antidiuretic agent is administered, they are at risk for hyponatremia. Therefore, these patients are subject to wide swings in osmolality, but most characteristically, they have persistent hypernatremia. The first therapeutic agent that might be tried is chlorpropamide off label because it is useful to treat diabetes insipidus and has been reported to increase the thirst response.[193,194] Again, this is off-label use of chlorpropamide. If chlorpropamide does not produce adequate control, treatment involves balancing desmopressin and fluid intake. The patients are not thirsty and it is difficult to balance water intake, so a better regimen is a rigid fixed dose of desmopressin to maintain chronic antidiuresis and a prescribed quantity of water that must be drunk every 6 to 8 hours.[167,195] Daily weight can be used to guide intake, and regular follow-up with measurement of serum sodium is essential to assure that these patients do not develop water intoxication with hyponatremia or recurrent dehydration with hypernatremia. This balance may be especially difficult to manage in infants. Desmopressin by injection and careful management of fluids with regular measurement of sodium have been used successfully.[196]

Organ Donors. As noted earlier, diabetes insipidus is a common accompaniment of brain death, and if these patients are candidates for organ donation, it has been suggested that maintaining fluid homeostasis is desirable for maintenance of the health of the organs. Continuous administration of low-dose vasopressin intravenously as described earlier for postsurgical diabetes insipidus may be easier than maintaining antidiuresis with intermittent doses of desmopressin.

Diabetes Insipidus Due to Accelerated Metabolism of Vasopressin (Diabetes Insipidus of Pregnancy)

An important clinical point is the expanded volume and decreased osmolality and serum sodium that occur in normal pregnancy, as described earlier in the discussion of physiology. Pregnant patients with polyuria may have serum sodium levels that would be in the normal range for a nonpregnant patient but would be indicative of diabetes insipidus in the pregnant patient and require evaluation. There are two types of transient diabetes insipidus in pregnancy, both caused by the enzyme cysteine aminopeptidase (oxytocinase).[197] In the first type the activity of cysteine aminopeptidase (which is also a vasopressinase) is extremely and abnormally elevated. This syndrome has been referred to as *vasopressin-resistant diabetes insipidus of pregnancy*.[198] It occurs with preeclampsia, acute fatty liver, and coagulopathies (e.g., HELLP [hemolysis, elevated liver enzymes and low platelets] syndrome). These patients have decreased metabolism of vasopressinase by the liver.[53,199-201] Usually in subsequent pregnancies these women have neither diabetes insipidus nor acute fatty liver. In the second type the accelerated metabolic clearance of vasopressin produces diabetes insipidus in a patient with borderline vasopressin function from a specific disease, such as mild nephrogenic diabetes insipidus or partial hypothalamic/neurohypophyseal diabetes insipidus.[59,202,203] Vasopressin is rapidly destroyed and the neurohypophysis is unable to keep up with the increased demand. Labor and parturition usually proceed normally, and patients have no trouble with lactation.[204] When diabetes insipidus is unrecognized in a pregnant woman, chronic and severe dehydration may pose a threat.[205] Patients with Sheehan syndrome have been reported to have asymptomatic partial diabetes insipidus,[206] but they rarely develop overt diabetes insipidus.[207]

Treatment of Diabetes Insipidus in Pregnancy

Desmopressin is the only therapy recommended for treatment of diabetes insipidus during pregnancy. Desmopressin has 2% to 25% the oxytocic activity of lysine vasopressin or AVP[175] and can be used with minimal stimulation of the oxytocin receptors in the uterus.[204,208] The physician must note the naturally occurring volume expansion and the reset osmostat that occur in pregnancy and give sufficient therapy to satisfy thirst and to maintain a serum sodium at the low level that is normal during pregnancy. Desmopressin is not destroyed by the cysteine aminopeptidase (oxytocinase) of pregnancy[204,209] and is reported to be safe for both the mother and the child.[210,211] During delivery these patients can maintain adequate oral intake and continue administration of desmopressin. Physicians should be cautious about overadministration of fluid parenterally during delivery because these patients will not be able to excrete the fluid and may develop water intoxication and hyponatremia. After delivery oxytocinase decreases in plasma and the patient may recover completely or be asymptomatic with regard to volume of fluid intake and urine excretion.

Diabetes Insipidus Due to Lack of Renal Response (Nephrogenic Diabetes Insipidus)

Genetic Abnormalities. Infants with nephrogenic diabetes insipidus present with vomiting, constipation, failure to thrive, fever, and polyuria. Symptoms usually occur during the first week of life,[212,213] and on testing the patients will be found to have hypernatremia and a low urine osmolality. The diagnosis is established by high levels of vasopressin in the plasma in the presence of hypotonic polyuria and then the absence of response to administered desmopressin. Special attention should be given if a dehydration test is used in children and the test should not be done in infants. Care should be taken to avoid hyponatremia when desmopressin is given at the end of the test as hypotonic fluid is the normal diet.[46] Considered here are disorders related directly to function of vasopressin, and no other inherited complex disorders of the kidney that cause loss of electrolytes as well as water.[214] Two causes of nephrogenic diabetes insipidus are mutations in the V_2 receptor and mutations of the aquaporin 2 water channels. The presentation is independent of the genotype.[212-214]

More than 90% of cases of nephrogenic diabetes insipidus are X-linked recessive disorders in males who have one of more than 200 individually different mutations of the V_2 receptor.[215] Three classes of mutations of the V_2 receptor have been described: type 1 disorders reach the cell surface but have impaired AVP binding; type 2 have defective transport and remain in the cell without reaching the cell surface; and type 3 are unstable and rapidly degraded.[215] Most of the reported cases are type 2.[216] In clinical series approximately 10% of the V_2 receptor defects causing congenital nephrogenic diabetes insipidus are thought to be de novo. Although most female carriers of the X-linked V_2 receptor defect have no clinical disease, some female carriers may have a decreased maximum urine osmolality in response to the plasma level of vasopressin that they achieve.[217] Rarely, heterozygous females have a defect as severe as males and this is thought to be due to inactivation of the normal X chromosome.[218,219]

When the proband is a female it is likely that the defect is a mutation of the aquaporin 2 water channel gene producing an autosomal recessive disease.[220] This should be especially considered when consanguinity is known in the family and the disease is expressed in males and females. The patients may be heterozygous for two different recessive mutations[221] or may be homozygous for the same abnormality from both parents.[222] Mutations of the aquaporin 2 protein may produce an autosomal dominant nephrogenic diabetes insipidus when the mutant aquaporin 2 protein associates with the wild-type normal protein to inhibit normal intracellular routing and function of the wild type.[223]

Acquired Nephrogenic Diabetes Insipidus. Producing a concentrated urine depends on maintaining hyperosmolality of the inner medulla of the kidney. Producing and maintaining hyperosmolality of the inner medulla requires that the kidney architecture be intact with an intact tubular structure of the loop of Henle, essential to the development of the countercurrent multiplier, and then a normal anatomy of the collecting duct to pass back through the inner medulla. The vascular structure must be anatomically intact so the hyperosmolality of the inner medulla is not washed away by normal blood flow. The broad definition of nephrogenic diabetes insipidus may include numerous chronic renal diseases that distort the architecture of the kidney. Vascular and anatomic causes of reduced concentration of urine are not considered here as diabetes insipidus because these are not disorders caused by abnormal function of vasopressin.[224] Acquired nephrogenic diabetes insipidus associated with hypokalemia, hypercalcemia, and release of bilateral urinary tract obstruction are all associated with downregulation of aquaporin 2 and decreased function of vasopressin.[220,223]

Administration of lithium to treat psychiatric disorders is the most common cause of drug-induced acquired nephrogenic diabetes insipidus and illustrates the mechanisms.[223] Lithium produces a decrease in urea transporters, reducing vasopressin-stimulated urea uptake and decreasing urea recycling, which reduces intermedullary osmolality.[220,225] Even more dramatic is the reduction in aquaporin 2 levels to decrease water transport in the collecting duct.[223] There is as much as a 95% decrease in aquaporin 2 content, and even the 5% of aquaporin 2 that persists is not normally transported to the renal principal cell membrane.[226] The defect of aquaporins with lithium is slow to correct

both in experimental animals and in humans and may be permanent.[223,227] Demeclocycline is another drug commonly recognized to cause nephrogenic diabetes insipidus and is used clinically to treat SIADH (discussed later). See the review by Bendz and Aurell[228] for a list of drugs that cause nephrogenic diabetes insipidus.

Treatment of Nephrogenic Diabetes Insipidus

Adequate water intake should always be maintained and may be lifesaving in congenital nephrogenic diabetes insipidus. By definition these forms of diabetes insipidus do not respond to vasopressin or desmopressin, although there may rarely be some partial defects with some response to high doses of desmopressin.[229,230] In congenital nephrogenic diabetes insipidus therapy is aimed at reducing symptomatic polyuria. This is done primarily by causing volume contraction with a low-sodium diet and a thiazide diuretic. The antidiuretic effect has been interpreted as due to contraction of ECF volume, decreased glomerular filtration rate, proximal sodium and water reabsorption, and decreased delivery of fluid to the collecting duct resulting in a decreased volume of urine.[231] Studies have also demonstrated that thiazide diuretics may increase aquaporin 2 independent of vasopressin.[232] All the thiazide diuretics appear to have similar effects. Potassium replacement or coadministration of a potassium-sparing antidiuretic may be desirable. There is an added effect obtained by coadministration of NSAIDs, but duodenal ulcer and gastrointestinal hemorrhage may be produced. Newer selective cyclooxygenase 2 inhibitors with less gastrointestinal effect have been reported to decrease water loss, but long-term safety has not been documented.[223]

Drug-induced nephrogenic diabetes insipidus should be treated by stopping the offending agent if possible. Persistence of nephrogenic diabetes insipidus can be treated by hydrochlorothiazide and amiloride. With the induced volume contraction, these patients should be closely followed for the development of renal or other toxicity of the drug that caused the diabetes insipidus.[233] For example, volume contraction produced by thiazide diuretics when used to treat lithium-induced nephrogenic diabetes insipidus may decrease lithium excretion and predispose to lithium toxicity.[228,234] The diuretic amiloride blocks Na^+ channels in the luminal membrane of the collecting duct cells and inhibits lithium reabsorption, a unique advantage in treating lithium-induced nephrogenic diabetes insipidus.[235] In animal studies of lithium-induced nephrogenic diabetes insipidus treatment with amiloride increased both the levels of aquaporin 2 and of urea transporters.[225]

Studies have reported the possibility of rescuing mutant receptors in nephrogenic diabetes insipidus. In autosomal dominant nephrogenic diabetes insipidus of type 2 the misfolded receptor protein is trapped in the quality control system of the endoplasmic reticulum. In some cases the defect may be transport rather than function, and were the receptor to reach the cell membrane, it would respond to vasopressin. V_2 receptor antagonists (vaptans) have been reported as pharmacologic chaperones that combine with the misfolded receptor, changing the confirmation to allow maturation and transport to the plasma membrane, where vasopressin (in excess of the vaptans) would cause the receptor to be activated.[236-238] Similar studies of rescue have recently been reported with the nonpeptide V_2 receptor agonists. These agonists combine with the mutant receptor trapped in the endoplasmic reticulum and allow the maturation of the mutant receptor. The rescued receptor is then inserted into the cell membrane and when stimulated by vasopressin or desmopressin generates sufficient cAMP to move aquaporin 2 from the cytoplasm to the cell membrane to enhance water transport.[237,238] Nonpeptide antagonists working as chaperones is a potential new treatment of nephrogenic diabetes insipidus, especially in patients with a partial disorder.[239]

Sequencing of genes in all families with nephrogenic diabetes insipidus is recommended because of the small size of the genes to be sequenced and because of the value of the information.[216] In X-linked disorders, carrier females can be distinguished from noncarrier females so it is known which sibling's children are at risk and require special observation at birth. Molecular testing of newborns will confirm the need for long-term treatment to avoid complications in the affected children and obviate the need for dehydration or other testing in unaffected children.[219,240]

Diabetes Insipidus in Association With Other Therapeutic Decisions

Routine Surgical Procedures

In all cases there should be preoperative consultation among the surgeon, the anesthesiologist, and the endocrinologist/nephrologist. For most routine surgical procedures the patient is not unconscious for a sufficiently long period to require anything more that administration of the usual dose of desmopressin and careful monitoring of fluids during the surgery to ensure against overhydration. If the patient has been taking desmopressin orally but is now NPO (taking nothing by mouth), a parenteral dose can be administered before the procedure. If the procedure is especially long, one might consider a low-dose vasopressin given continuously with fluid as described earlier for postoperative or trauma-induced hypothalamic/neurohypophyseal diabetes insipidus. Close monitoring of serum sodium is essential. In nephrogenic diabetes insipidus there might be a greater emphasis on fluid replacement to avoid dehydration and hypernatremia.[241]

Panhypopituitarism

Because hypothyroidism and adrenal insufficiency have a direct action on the kidney to inhibit the ability to excrete water, any patient who has anterior pituitary deficiency in association with diabetes insipidus is at risk to develop hyponatremia if treatment for diabetes insipidus is continued while treatment with thyroid hormone and (more dramatically) hydrocortisone is stopped. It is important that such patients maintain treatment of all anterior and posterior pituitary deficiencies continuously because the balance among these replacements is essential.

Promoting a Saline Diuresis

In certain clinical situations, such as chemotherapy or use of some contrast agents, diuresis is desirable to minimize renal toxicity. If desmopressin is continued and a large volume of normal saline is given, natriuresis and hyponatremia will be induced. Withholding desmopressin and replacing fluids with 5% dextrose in water (D5W) may lead to hyperglycemia, whereas replacing with normal saline may lead to hypernatremia. It has been reported that very low-dose vasopressin administered continuously intravenously (similar to that described earlier for comatose patients) can be used. In this case the dose of vasopressin is even lower (e.g., 0.08 to 0.1 mU/kg per hour) to allow a moderate and controlled diuresis.[242] As with any situation in which vasopressin is given continuously, serum sodium must be checked regularly and the amount of fluids infused monitored carefully.

Hypertonic Encephalopathy

Hypertonic encephalopathy is uncommon in diabetes insipidus and is only seen when there is inadequate fluid intake in an adipsic patient or in a patient who is unconscious and not receiving adequate fluid supplementation. Conditions other than diabetes insipidus are the more common causes of hypernatremic encephalopathy. It may be caused by loss of hypotonic fluids by the kidney or the gut or by insensible losses or may be secondary to administration of hypertonic sodium-containing fluids or hyperalimentation.[243] Sodium is mainly an extracellular electrolyte, and hypernatremia invariably leads to movement of water out of cells and cellular dehydration.

Studies indicate that in the brain so-called idiogenic osmoles are generated intracellularly, so the degree of cell shrinkage is less than would be expected based on the degree of hypernatremia. These idiogenic osmoles belong to three organic classes: polyols, trimethylamines, and amino acids and their derivatives.[244] Loss of water from the brain occurs in minutes, and electrolytes enter the brain in a few hours, but the increase in organic osmoles occurs over several days.[72] Similarly, when fluid is replaced, these intracellular organic osmoles decrease more slowly than the decrease in osmolality of ECF. This asynchrony increases the potential for cerebral edema and worsening of the neurologic condition with overzealous treatment of hypernatremia.[72] In most cases of diabetes insipidus seen immediately after surgery or diagnosed promptly after head injury the diagnosis will be made within a few hours and therapy may be instituted promptly. In cases in which the duration of the hypernatremia is not known, the degree of correction of hypernatremia should not exceed 0.5 mEq/L per hour to prevent cerebral edema and convulsions.[72,243]

THE SYNDROME OF INAPPROPRIATE ANTIDIURETIC HORMONE SECRETION

SIADH is produced when plasma levels of AVP are elevated at times when the physiologic secretion of vasopressin from the posterior pituitary would normally be osmotically suppressed. The clinical abnormality is a decrease in the osmotic pressure of body fluids, so the hallmark of SIADH is hypoosmolality. This finding led to the identification of the first well-described cases of this disorder in 1957[245] and the subsequent clinical investigations that resulted in delineation of the essential characteristics of the syndrome.[246] It is, therefore, necessary to review hypoosmolality and hyponatremia before discussing details that are specific to SIADH.

Hypoosmolality and Hyponatremia

Incidence

Hypoosmolality is the most common disorder of fluid and electrolyte balance encountered in hospitalized patients. The incidence and prevalence of hypoosmolar disorders depend on the nature of the patient population studied as well as on the laboratory methods and criteria used to diagnose hyponatremia. Most investigators have used the serum sodium concentration ([Na+]) to determine the clinical incidence of hypoosmolality. When hyponatremia is defined as a serum [Na+] of less than 135 mEq/L, prevalences as high as 15% to 38% have been observed in studies of both acutely and chronically hospitalized patients.[247,248] However, incidences decrease to the range of 1% to 4% when studies include only patients with serum [Na+] under

130 to 131 mEq/L, which represents a more appropriate level at which to define the occurrence of clinically significant cases of this disorder.[249] Even using these more stringent criteria, incidences from 7% to 53% have been reported in institutionalized geriatric patients.[250] Although hyponatremia and hypoosmolality are quite common, the majority of cases are relatively mild, and most are acquired during the course of hospitalization. Nonetheless, hyponatremia is important clinically because (1) severe hypoosmolality (serum [Na$^+$] levels <120 mEq/L) is associated with substantial morbidity and mortality rates[251]; (2) even relatively mild hypoosmolality can quickly progress to more dangerous levels during the course of therapeutic management of other disorders; (3) overly rapid correction of hyponatremia can itself cause severe neurologic morbidity and death[252]; and (4) it has been observed that mortality rates are much higher, from 3-fold to 60-fold higher, in patients with even asymptomatic degrees of hypoosmolality compared to normonatremic patients.[253,254]

Osmolality, Tonicity, and Serum Sodium Concentration

As discussed previously, the osmolality of body fluid normally is maintained within narrow limits for each individual by osmotically regulated vasopressin secretion and thirst. Plasma osmolality can be determined directly by measuring the freezing-point depression or the vapor pressure of plasma. Alternatively, it can be calculated indirectly from the concentrations of the three major solutes in plasma:

$$pOsm = 2[Na^+] + (glucose/18) + (BUN/2.8)$$

where plasma osmolality (pOsm) is measured in mOsm/kg H$_2$O, [Na$^+$] in mEq/L, plasma glucose concentration in mg/dL, and blood urea nitrogen (BUN) in mg/dL.

Direct measure and indirect calculation produce comparable results under most conditions. However, even though either of these methods will produce valid measures of *total* osmolality, this is not always equivalent to the *effective* osmolality, which is commonly referred to as the *tonicity* of the plasma. Only solutes such as Na$^+$ and Cl$^-$ that are impermeable to the cell membrane and remain relatively compartmentalized within the ECF space are effective solutes, because these solutes create osmotic gradients across cell membranes and regulate the osmotic movement of water between the intracellular fluid (ICF) compartment and the ECF compartment. Solutes that readily permeate cell membranes (e.g., urea, ethanol, methanol) are not effective solutes. Therefore, only the concentrations of effective solutes in plasma should be used to ascertain whether clinically significant hyperosmolality or hypoosmolality is present.

Sodium and its accompanying anions represent the major effective plasma solutes, so hyponatremia and hypoosmolality are usually synonymous. However, there are two situations in which hyponatremia will not reflect true hypoosmolality. The first is *pseudohyponatremia*, which is produced by marked elevations of either lipids or proteins in plasma. If serum [Na$^+$] is measured by flame photometry, the concentration of sodium per liter of plasma is artifactually decreased because of the larger relative proportion of plasma volume that is occupied by the excess lipids or proteins.[255] However, the increased protein or lipid will not appreciably change the total number of solute particles in solution, so the directly measured plasma osmolality will not be significantly affected. Measurement of serum [Na$^+$] by ion-specific electrodes, which is now commonly employed by most clinical laboratories, is less influenced by high concentrations of lipids or proteins than is

measurement of serum [Na$^+$] by flame photometry. However, this can still occur if the electrode measurement is done using a diluted sample of the serum.

The second situation in which hyponatremia does not reflect true plasma hypoosmolality occurs when high concentrations of effective solutes other than Na$^+$ are present in the plasma. The initial hyperosmolality produced by the additional solute causes an osmotic shift of water from the ICF to the ECF, which in turn produces a dilutional decrease in serum [Na$^+$]. Once equilibrium between both fluid compartments is achieved, the total effective osmolality remains relatively unchanged. This situation most commonly occurs with hyperglycemia and represents a frequent cause of hyponatremia in hospitalized patients, accounting for up to 10% to 20% of all cases.[253] Misdiagnosis of true hypoosmolality in such cases can be avoided by measuring plasma osmolality directly or, alternatively, by correcting the measured serum [Na$^+$] for the glucose elevation. Traditionally, this correction factor has been 1.6 mEq/L for each 100-mg/dL increase in serum glucose concentration above normal levels,[256] but some studies have shown a more complex relation between hyperglycemia and serum [Na$^+$] and reported that a more accurate correction factor is closer to 2.4 mEq/L.[257] When the plasma contains significant amounts of unmeasured solutes, such as osmotic diuretics, radiographic contrast agents, and some toxins (ethanol, methanol, and ethylene glycol), plasma osmolality cannot be calculated accurately, and in these situations osmolality must be ascertained by direct measurement.

Pathogenesis of Hypoosmolality

Water moves freely between the ICF and ECF, and consequently, osmolality will always be equivalent in both of these fluid compartments. Because the bulk of body solute comprises electrolytes, namely, the exchangeable Na$^+$ (Na^+_E) in the ECF and the exchangeable K$^+$ (K^+_E) in the ICF, along with their associated anions, total body osmolality (OSM$_T$) will largely be a function of these parameters:[258]

$$OSM_T = OSM_{ECF} = OSM_{ICF}$$

$$OSM_T = (ECF\ solute + ICF\ solute)/body\ water$$

$$OSM_T = (2[Na^+]_E + 2[K^+]_E + nonelectrolyte\ solute)/body\ water.$$

According to this definition, the presence of plasma hypoosmolality indicates a relative excess of water to solute in the ECF. This can be produced either by an excess of body water, resulting in a *dilution* of remaining body solute, or by a *depletion* of body solute, either Na$^+$ or K$^+$, relative to body water. This classification is an oversimplification, because most hypoosmolar states involve significant components of both solute depletion and water retention. Nonetheless, it is conceptually useful for understanding the mechanisms underlying the pathogenesis of hypoosmolality and as a framework for therapy of hypoosmolar disorders.

Solute Depletion. Depletion of body solute can result from any significant losses of ECF. Body fluid losses by themselves rarely cause hypoosmolality because excreted or secreted body fluids are usually isotonic or hypotonic relative to plasma and therefore tend to increase plasma osmolality. When hypoosmolality accompanies ECF losses, it is the result of replacement of body fluid losses by more hypotonic solutions either by drinking or by infusion, thereby diluting the remaining body solutes. If the solute losses are marked, these patients show signs of volume depletion (e.g., addisonian crisis). However, such patients often have a more deceptive clinical presentation because the volume deficits have been partially replaced. Moreover, they may not manifest signs or symptoms of cellular dehydration because osmotic gradients will draw water into the ICF, which is relatively hypertonic to the solute-depleted ECF. Therefore, clinical evidence of hypovolemia strongly supports solute depletion as the cause of plasma hypoosmolality, but absence of clinically evident hypovolemia never completely eliminates this as a possibility. Although ECF solute losses are responsible for most cases of depletion-induced hypoosmolality, ICF solute loss can also cause hypoosmolality as a result of osmotic water shifts from the ICF into the ECF. This mechanism contributes to some cases of diuretic-induced hypoosmolality in which depletion of total body K+ often occurs.[259]

Water Retention. Despite the importance of solute depletion in some patients, most cases of clinically significant hypoosmolality are caused by increases in total body water rather than by primary losses of extracellular solute. This can occur because of either impaired renal free water excretion or excessive free water intake. The former accounts for most hypoosmolar disorders because normal kidneys have sufficient diluting capacity to allow excretion of 18 to 24 L/day of free water. Intakes of this magnitude are occasionally seen in some psychiatric patients but not in most patients with SIADH in whom fluid intake averages 2 to 3 L/day.[260] Consequently, dilutional hypoosmolality usually is the result of an abnormality of renal free water excretion. The renal mechanisms responsible for impairments in free water excretion can be subgrouped according to whether the major impairment in free water excretion occurs in proximal or distal parts of the nephron, or both. Any disorder that leads to a decrease in glomerular filtration rate causes increased reabsorption of both Na+ and water in the proximal tubule. As a result, the ability to excrete free water is limited because of decreased delivery of tubular fluid to the distal nephron. Disorders that cause a decreased glomerular filtration rate in the absence of significant ECF fluid losses are, for the most part, edema-forming states associated with decreased effective arterial blood volume (EABV) and secondary hyperaldosteronism.[261] Even though these conditions are characterized by increased proximal reabsorption of both Na+ and fluid, water retention also results from increased distal reabsorption caused by nonosmotic baroreceptor-mediated stimulated increases in plasma vasopressin levels. Distal nephron impairments in free water excretion are characterized by an inability to dilute tubular fluid maximally. These disorders are usually associated with abnormalities in the secretion of vasopressin. Just as depletion-induced hypoosmolar disorders usually include an important component of secondary impairments of free water excretion, most dilution-induced hypoosmolar disorders also involve significant degrees of secondary solute depletion. This is described later with SIADH.

Some dilutional disorders do not fit well into either category, specifically the hyponatremia that sometimes occurs in patients who ingest large volumes of beer with little food intake for prolonged periods (beer potomania).[262] Even though the volume of fluid ingested may not seem sufficiently excessive to overwhelm renal diluting mechanisms, free water excretion is limited by very low urinary solute excretion, thereby causing water retention and dilutional hyponatremia.

Adaptation to Hyponatremia: ICF and ECF Volume Regulation

Many past studies have suggested that the combined effects of water retention plus urinary solute excretion cannot adequately explain the degree of plasma hypoosmolality observed in patients.[246,263] This observation led to the theory of *cellular inactivation of solute*, which suggested that as ECF osmolality falls, water moves into cells along osmotic gradients, thereby causing the cells to swell; at some point during this volume expansion, the cells theoretically osmotically inactivate some of their intracellular solutes as a defense mechanism to prevent continued cellular swelling with subsequent detrimental effects on cell function and survival. This effect would decrease the intracellular osmolality, allowing water to shift back out of the ICF into the ECF, thereby further worsening the dilution-induced hypoosmolality. Despite the appeal of this theory, its validity has never been demonstrated conclusively in either human or animal studies. An alternative theory is that cell volume is maintained under hypoosmolar conditions by extrusion of intracellular solutes such as potassium.[264] Whole brain volume regulation via electrolyte losses was first described by Yannet[265] and has long been recognized as the mechanism by which the brain is able to adapt to hyponatremia and limit brain edema to sublethal levels.[266] Following the recognition that low-molecular-weight organic compounds, called *organic osmolytes*, also constituted a significant osmotic component of a wide variety of cells, studies demonstrated the accumulation of these compounds in response to hyperosmolality in both kidney[267] and brain[268] tissue and conversely that the brain also loses organic osmolytes in addition to electrolytes during volume regulation to hypoosmolar conditions in experimental animals[269,270] and human patients.[271] These losses occur relatively quickly (within 24 to 48 hours in rats) and can account for as much as one third of the brain solute losses during hyponatremia.[272] Such coordinate losses of both electrolytes and organic osmolytes from brain cells allow effective regulation of brain volume during chronic hyponatremia.

Although recent studies of volume regulation during hyponatremia have focused on the brain, all cells regulate volume by cellular losses of both electrolyte and organic solutes to varying degrees. However, volume regulatory processes are not limited to cells. In most cases of hyponatremia induced by stimulated antidiuresis and water retention, natriuresis also regulates the volumes of the ECF and intravascular spaces. Both experimental and clinical observations are consistent with ECF volume regulation via secondary solute losses. First, the concentrations of most blood constituents other than Na+ and Cl- are not decreased in patients with SIADH,[273] suggesting that plasma volume is not nearly as expanded as would be predicted simply by the measured decreases in serum [Na+]. Second, an increased incidence of hypertension has never been observed in patients with SIADH, again evidence against significant expansion of the arterial blood volume. Third, results of animal studies in both dogs[274] and rats[275] have indicated that a significant component of chronic hyponatremia is attributable to secondary Na+ losses rather than water retention; the relative contributions from water retention versus sodium loss vary with the duration and severity of the hyponatremia: water retention was found to be the major cause of decreased serum [Na+] in the first 24 hours of induced hyponatremia in rats, but Na+ depletion then became the predominant etiologic factor after longer periods (7-14 days) of sustained hyponatremia, particularly at very low (<115 mEq/L) serum [Na+] levels.[275] Finally, multiple studies of body fluid compartment volumes in hyponatremic patients have not demonstrated either plasma or ECF expansion. For example, a report of body fluid space measurements using isotope dilution techniques in hyponatremic and normonatremic patients with

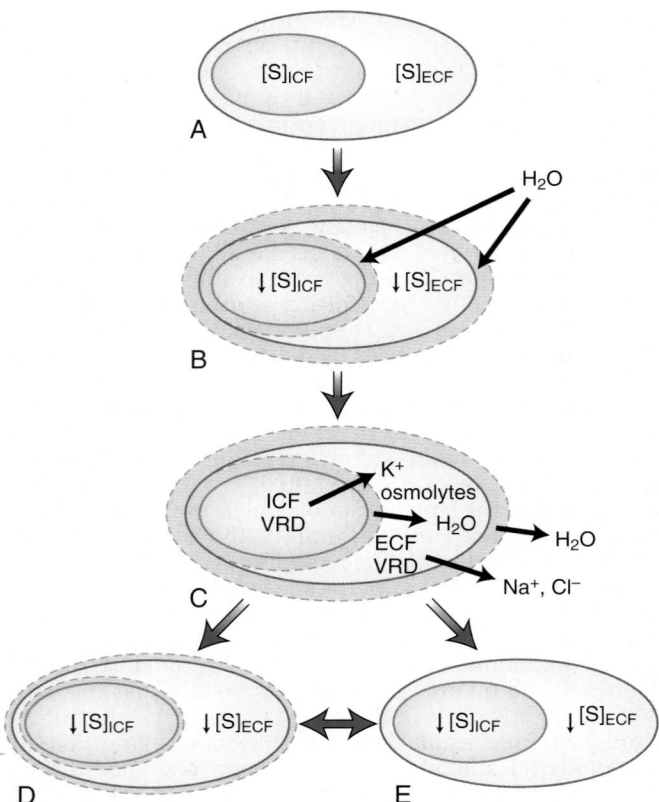

Figure 10-5 Schematic illustration of potential changes in whole-body fluid compartment volumes at various times during adaptation to hyponatremia. **A,** Under basal conditions, the concentrations of effective solutes in the extracellular fluid ($[S]_{ECF}$) and in the intracellular fluid ($[S]_{ICF}$) are in osmotic balance. **B,** During the first phase of water retention resulting from inappropriate antidiuresis, the excess water distributes across total body water, causing expansion of both ECF and ICF volumes *(dotted lines)*, with equivalent dilutional decreases in both $[S]_{ICF}$ and $[S]_{ECF}$. **C,** In response to the volume expansion, compensatory volume regulatory decreases (VRD) occur to reduce the effective solute content of the ECF (via pressure diuresis and natriuretic factors) and the ICF (via increased electrolyte and osmolyte extrusion mediated by stretch-activated channels and downregulation of synthesis of osmolytes and osmolyte uptake transporters). **D** and **E,** If both processes go to completion, such as under conditions of fluid restriction, a final steady state can be reached in which ICF and ECF volumes have returned to normal levels but $[S]_{ICF}$ and $[S]_{ECF}$ remain low. In most cases, this final steady state is not reached, and moderate degrees of ECF and ICF expansion persist, although they are significantly less than would be predicted from the decrease in body osmolality (**D**). Consequently, the degree to which hyponatremia is the result of dilution due to water retention versus solute depletion from volume regulatory processes can vary markedly, depending on which phase of adaptation the patient is in and the relative rates at which the different compensatory processes occur. For example, delayed ICF VRD can worsen hyponatremia because of shifts of intracellular water into the ECF as intracellular organic osmolytes are extruded and subsequently metabolized; this likely accounts for some component of the hyponatremia that was unexplained by the combination of water retention and sodium excretion in early clinical studies. (From Verbalis JG. Hyponatremia: epidemiology, pathophysiology, and therapy. *Curr Opin Nephrol Hypertens.* 1993;2:626-652.)

small cell lung carcinoma showed no differences between the two groups with regard to exchangeable sodium space, ECF volume by $^{35}SO_4$ distribution, or total body water.[276] Figure 10-5 schematically illustrates the volume regulatory processes that occur in response to water retention induced by inappropriate antidiuresis.

Differential Diagnosis of Hyponatremia and Hypoosmolality

Because of the multiplicity of disorders causing hypoosmolality and the fact that many involve more than one pathologic mechanism, a definitive diagnosis is not always possible at the time of initial presentation. Nonetheless, an approach based on clinical parameters of ECF volume status and urine sodium concentration generally allows a sufficient categorization for appropriate decisions regarding initial therapy and further evaluation.

Decreased Extracellular Fluid Volume. Clinically detectable hypovolemia always signifies total body solute depletion. A low urine [Na^+] indicates a nonrenal cause and an appropriate renal response. A high urine [Na^+] indicates that renal causes of solute depletion are more likely. Therapy with thiazide diuretics is the most common cause of renal solute losses,[259] particularly in the elderly,[277] but mineralocorticoid deficiency as a result of adrenal insufficiency or mineralocorticoid resistance must be considered as well as (less commonly) renal solute losses due to salt-wasting nephropathy (e.g., polycystic kidney disease, interstitial nephritis, or chemotherapy).

Increased Extracellular Fluid Volume. Clinically detectable hypervolemia always signifies total body Na^+ excess. In these patients hypoosmolality results from an even greater expansion of total body water caused by a marked reduction in the rate of water excretion (and sometimes an increased rate of water ingestion). The impairment in water excretion is secondary to a decreased EABV,[261] which increases the reabsorption of glomerular filtrate not only in the proximal nephron but also in the distal and collecting tubules by stimulated secretion of vasopressin. These patients generally have a low urine [Na^+] because of secondary hyperaldosteronism. However, under certain conditions urine [Na^+] may be elevated if there is concurrent diuretic therapy or a solute diuresis (e.g., glucosuria in diabetics) or after successful treatment of the underlying disease (e.g., improved cardiac output in patients with congestive heart failure).

Normal Extracellular Fluid Volume. Many different hypoosmolar disorders present with euvolemia, and measurement of urinary [Na^+] is an especially important first step in their assessment.[278] A high urine [Na^+] usually implies a distally mediated, dilution-induced hypoosmolality such as SIADH. However, glucocorticoid deficiency can mimic SIADH so closely that these two disorders are often indistinguishable in terms of water balance. Hyponatremia from diuretic use also can present without clinically evident hypovolemia, and the urine [Na^+] will usually be elevated.[259] A low urine [Na^+] suggests a depletion-induced hypoosmolality from ECF losses with subsequent volume replacement by water or other hypotonic fluids. The solute loss often is nonrenal, but an important exception is recent cessation of diuretic therapy, because urine [Na^+] can decrease to low values within 12 to 24 hours after discontinuation of the drug. A low urine [Na^+] also can also be seen during the recovery phase from SIADH.

Clinical Aspects of SIADH

SIADH is the most common cause of euvolemic hypoosmolality as well as the single most common cause of all types of hypoosmolality encountered in clinical practice, with prevalence rates from 20% to 40% among all hypoosmolar patients.[253,260] The clinical criteria necessary to diagnose SIADH remain basically those set forth by Bartter and Schwartz in 1967:[246]

1. Decreased effective osmolality of the ECF (plasma osmolality <275 mOsm/kg H_2O). Pseudohyponatremia or hyperglycemia alone must be excluded.
2. Inappropriate urinary concentration at some level of hypoosmolality. This does not mean that urine osmolality must be greater than plasma osmolality, only that it

is less than maximally dilute (i.e., urine osmolality >100 mOsm/kg H_2O). Also, urine osmolality need not be elevated inappropriately at all levels of plasma osmolality, because in the reset osmostat variant form of SIADH, vasopressin secretion can be suppressed with resultant maximal urinary dilution if plasma osmolality is decreased to sufficiently low levels.[279]

3. Clinical euvolemia, as defined by the absence of signs of hypovolemia (orthostasis, tachycardia, decreased skin turgor, dry mucous membranes) or hypervolemia (subcutaneous edema, ascites). Hypovolemia and hypervolemia strongly suggest different causes of hypoosmolality. Patients with SIADH can become hypovolemic or hypervolemic for other reasons, but in such cases it is impossible to diagnose the underlying inappropriate antidiuresis until the patient is rendered euvolemic and is found to have persistent hypoosmolality.

4. Elevated urinary sodium excretion with normal salt and water intake. This criterion is included because of its utility in differentiating between hypoosmolality caused by a decreased EABV, in which case renal Na^+ conservation occurs, and distal dilution-induced disorders, in which urine Na^+ excretion is normal or increased secondary to ECF volume expansion. Patients with SIADH can have low urine Na^+ excretion if they subsequently become hypovolemic or solute depleted, conditions that sometimes follow severe salt and water restriction. Consequently, a high urine Na^+ excretion is the rule in most patients with SIADH; thus, its presence does not guarantee this diagnosis, and its absence does not rule out the diagnosis.

5. Absence of other potential causes of euvolemic hypoosmolality, notably, hypothyroidism, hypocortisolism (Addison disease or pituitary ACTH insufficiency), and diuretic use.

Several other criteria support, but are not essential for, a diagnosis of SIADH. Volume expansion and vasopressin acting on V_1 receptors in the kidney increase the clearance of uric acid, so hypouricemia is found with SIADH. When patients are hyponatremic, values of uric acid are reported to be lower than 4 mg/dL (<0.24 mmol/L).[280] A water-loading test is of value when there is uncertainty regarding the cause of modest degrees of hypoosmolality in euvolemic patients, but it does not add useful information if the plasma osmolality is already lower than 275 mOsm/kg H_2O. Inability to excrete a standard water load normally (with normal excretion defined as a cumulative urine output of at least 90% of the administered water load within 4 hours and suppression of urine osmolality to <100 mOsm/kg H_2O) confirms the presence of an underlying defect in free water excretion. However, water excretion is abnormal in almost all disorders that cause hypoosmolality, whether dilutional or depletion-induced with secondary impairments in free water excretion. Two exceptions are primary polydipsia, in which hypoosmolality can rarely be secondary to excessive water intake alone, and the reset osmostat variant of SIADH, in which normal excretion of a water load can occur once plasma osmolality falls below the new set-point for vasopressin secretion.

Another supportive criterion is an inappropriately elevated plasma vasopressin level in relation to plasma osmolality. However, several factors limit the utility of vasopressin measurements to diagnose SIADH. First, although plasma vasopressin levels are elevated in most patients with this syndrome, the elevations generally remain within the normal physiologic range and are abnormal only in relation to plasma osmolality (Fig. 10-6). Second, 10% to 20% of patients with SIADH do not have measurably elevated plasma vasopressin levels and are at the limits of detection

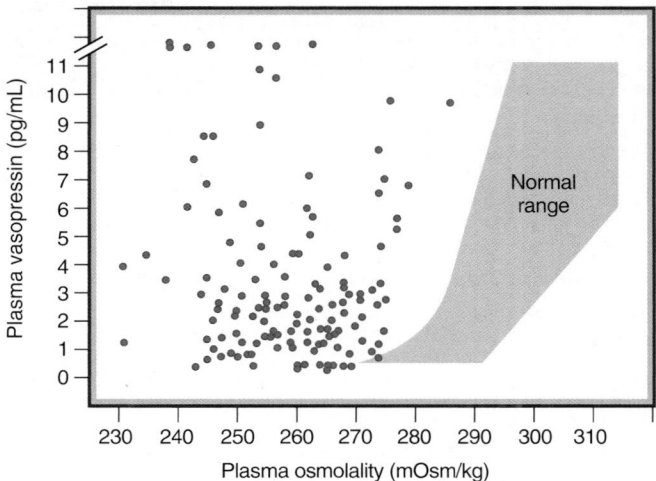

Figure 10-6 Plasma arginine vasopressin (AVP) levels in patients with the syndrome of inappropriate antidiuretic hormone secretion (SIADH) as a function of plasma osmolality. Each point depicts one patient at a single point in time. The shaded area represents AVP levels in normal subjects over physiologic ranges of plasma osmolality. The lowest measurable plasma AVP level that could be detected with this radioimmunoassay was 0.5 pg/mL. (From Robertson GL, Aycinena P, Zerbe RL. Neurogenic disorders of osmoregulation. *Am J Med.* 1982;2:339-353.)

by radioimmunoassay (see Fig. 10-6).[281] Third (and perhaps most important), most disorders causing solute and volume depletion or decreased EABV are associated with elevations of plasma vasopressin levels secondary to nonosmotic hemodynamic stimuli.

Etiology

Although the list of disorders associated with SIADH is long (Table 10-3), they can be divided into several major etiologic groups, including tumors, CNS disorders, drugs, and pulmonary disorders.

Tumors. The most common association of SIADH is with tumors. Many different types of tumors have been associated with SIADH, but bronchogenic carcinoma of the lung has been uniquely associated with SIADH since the first description of this disorder in 1957.[245] In virtually all cases, the bronchogenic carcinomas causing this syndrome have been of the small cell variety. The incidence of hyponatremia is reported to be as high as 11% among all patients with small cell carcinoma[282] and as high as 33% among those with more extensive disease.[283] The high incidence of small cell carcinoma of the lung makes it imperative that all adult patients presenting with an otherwise unexplained SIADH be investigated thoroughly and aggressively for a possible lung tumor. Head and neck cancers account for another group of malignancies associated with relatively higher incidences of SIADH,[284] and some of these tumors have clearly been shown to synthesize vasopressin.[285] A report from a large cancer hospital showed an incidence of hyponatremia for all malignancies of 3.7%, with approximately one third of these due to SIADH.[286]

Central Nervous System Disorders. A large number of different CNS disorders have been associated with SIADH, but there has been no common denominator linking them. This is not surprising when one considers the neuroanatomy described earlier. Magnocellular vasopressin neurons receive excitatory inputs from osmoreceptive cells located in the anterior hypothalamus, but also a major innervation from brainstem cardiovascular regulatory and emetic centers. Although various components of these pathways

TABLE 10-3

Common Causes of the Syndrome of Inappropriate Antidiuretic Hormone Secretion (SIADH)

Tumors

Pulmonary/mediastinal (bronchogenic carcinoma, mesothelioma, thymoma)
Nonchest (duodenal carcinoma, pancreatic carcinoma, ureteral/prostate carcinoma, uterine carcinoma, nasopharyngeal carcinoma, leukemia)

Central Nervous System Disorders

Mass lesions (tumors, brain abscesses, subdural hematoma)
Inflammatory diseases (encephalitis, meningitis, systemic lupus erythematosus, acute intermittent porphyria, multiple sclerosis)
Degenerative/demyelinative diseases (Guillain-Barré syndrome, spinal cord lesions)
Miscellaneous (subarachnoid hemorrhage, head trauma, acute psychosis, delirium tremens, pituitary stalk section, transsphenoidal adenomectomy, hydrocephalus)

Drug-Related

Stimulated release of AVP (nicotine, phenothiazines, tricyclics)
Direct renal effects or potentiation of AVP antidiuretic effects (dDAVP, oxytocin, prostaglandin synthesis inhibitors)
Mixed or uncertain actions (ACE inhibitors, carbamazepine and oxcarbazepine, chlorpropamide, clofibrate, clozapine, cyclophosphamide, 3,4-methylenedioxymethamphetamine [ecstasy], omeprazole; serotonin reuptake inhibitors, vincristine)

Pulmonary

Infections (tuberculosis, acute bacterial and viral pneumonia, aspergillosis, empyema)
Mechanical/ventilatory causes (acute respiratory failure, COPD, positive-pressure ventilation)

Other Causes

Acquired immunodeficiency syndrome (AIDS) and AIDS-related complex
Prolonged strenuous exercise (marathon, triathlon, ultramarathon, hot-weather hiking)
Senile atrophy
Idiopathic

ACE, angiotensin-converting enzyme; AVP, arginine vasopressin; COPD, chronic obstructive pulmonary disease; dDAVP, desmopressin.

have yet to be elucidated fully, many of them appear to have inhibitory as well as excitatory components. Consequently, any diffuse CNS disorder can potentially cause vasopressin hypersecretion either by nonspecifically exciting these pathways via irritative foci or, alternatively, by disrupting them and thereby decreasing the level of inhibition.

Drugs. Drug-induced hyponatremia is a common cause of hypoosmolality.[287] Table 10-3 lists some of the agents that have been associated with SIADH, but new drugs are added continually. Pharmacologic agents may stimulate secretion of vasopressin, activate renal V_2 receptors, or potentiate the antidiuretic effect of vasopressin. Not all of the drug effects are fully understood, and many appear to work through a combination of mechanisms. A particularly interesting, and clinically important, class of agents is the selective serotonin reuptake inhibitors (SSRIs). Hyponatremia following SSRI administration has been reported almost exclusively in the elderly, with rates as high as 22% to 28%, although in larger series the incidence was closer to 1 in 200.[288] A similar effect is likely also responsible for the recent reports of severe fatal hyponatremia caused by use of the recreational drug 3,4-methylenedioxymethamphetamine (MDMA, ecstasy), which possesses substantial serotoninergic activity.[289]

Pulmonary Disorders. A variety of pulmonary disorders have been associated with this syndrome, but other than tuberculosis, acute pneumonia, and advanced chronic obstructive lung disease, the occurrence of hypoosmolality has been noted only sporadically. Hypoxia stimulates secretion of vasopressin in animals,[290] but in humans hypercarbia is more associated with abnormal water retention. Elevated vasopressin may be limited to the initial days of hospitalization, when respiratory failure is most marked. Therefore, with SIADH in nontumor pulmonary disease the pulmonary disease is obvious with severe dyspnea or extensive radiographically evident infiltrates and the inappropriate antidiuresis will usually be limited to the period of respiratory failure. Mechanical ventilation can cause SIADH via inappropriate secretion of vasopressin via decreased venous return.

Other Causes. In acquired immunodeficiency syndrome (AIDS) or AIDS-related complex (ARC) and in patients with HIV infection, incidence of hyponatremia has been reported to be as high as 30% to 38% in adults and children.[291] Although there are many potential causes, including dehydration, adrenal insufficiency, and pneumonitis, from 12% to 68% of AIDS patients who develop hyponatremia appear to meet criteria for a diagnosis of SIADH.[291] Not unexpectedly, some of the medications used to treat these patients may cause the hyponatremia, either via direct renal tubular toxicity or induced SIADH.[292]

Elderly patients often develop SIADH without any apparent underlying cause, and the high incidence of hyponatremia in geriatric patients[250,293] suggests that the normal aging process may be accompanied by abnormalities of regulation of water balance and of secretion of vasopressin, as noted earlier. Such an effect could potentially account for the fact that drug-induced hyponatremia occurs much more frequently in elderly patients. In a series of 50 consecutive elderly patients meeting criteria for SIADH, 60% remained idiopathic despite rigorous evaluation, leading the authors to conclude that extensive diagnostic procedures were not warranted in such elderly patients if routine history, physical examination, and laboratory evaluation failed to suggest an underlying cause.[294]

Pathophysiology

Sources of Vasopressin Secretion. Elevated plasma levels of vasopressin can be broadly divided into those associated with paraneoplastic (ectopic) secretion of vasopressin or pituitary hypersecretion of vasopressin. There is substantial cumulative evidence that tumor tissue can, in fact, synthesize vasopressin,[295] but it is not certain that all tumors associated with SIADH do so, because only about half of small cell carcinomas have been found to contain vasopressin immunoreactivity, and many of the tumors listed in Table 10-3 have not been carefully studied.

Pituitary Vasopressin Secretion: Inappropriate Versus Appropriate. In the majority of cases of SIADH, the vasopressin secretion originates from the posterior pituitary. This is also true of more than 90% of all cases of hyponatremia, including patients with hypovolemic and hypervolemic hyponatremia.[253] This raises the question of what constitutes *inappropriate* secretion of vasopressin. Secretion of vasopressin in response to a hypovolemic stimulus is clearly physiologically appropriate, but when it leads to symptomatic hyponatremia it could be considered inappropriate for the ECF osmolality. Despite these semantic conundrums, the diagnosis of SIADH should be based on the original Schwartz-Bartter criteria[246] and specifically exclude other clinical conditions that cause known impairments in free water excretion even when these are mediated by a

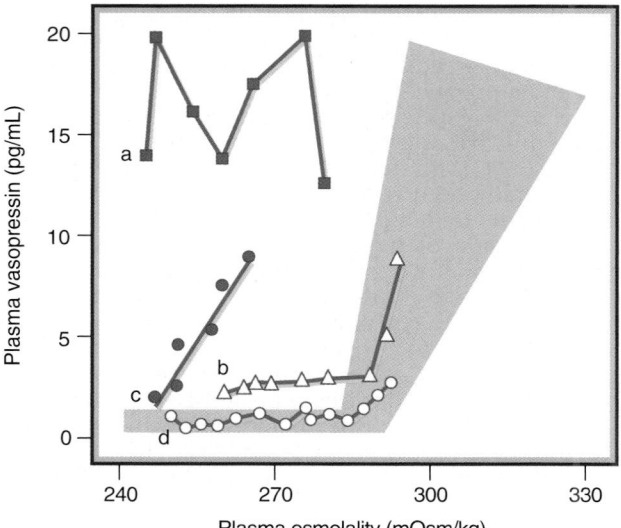

Figure 10-7 Schematic summary of four patterns of arginine vasopressin (AVP) secretion in patients with the syndrome of inappropriate antidiuretic hormone secretion (SIADH). Each line (*a* through *d*) represents the relation between plasma AVP and plasma osmolality in an individual patient in whom osmolality was increased by infusion of hypertonic NaCl. The shaded area represents plasma AVP levels in normal subjects over physiologic ranges of plasma osmolality. See text for details. (From Robertson GL. Thirst and vasopressin function in normal and disordered states of water balance. *J Lab Clin Med.* 1983;101:351-371.)

secondary nonosmotic physiologic stimulation of vasopressin secretion. Without maintaining these distinctions, arguable as some may be, the definition of SIADH becomes too broad to retain any practical clinical utility.

Patterns of Vasopressin Secretion. Studies of plasma vasopressin levels in patients with SIADH during graded increases in plasma osmolality produced by hypertonic saline administration have defined four patterns of secretion (Fig. 10-7): (1) random hypersecretion of vasopressin; (2) inappropriate nonsuppressible basal vasopressin release but normal secretion in response to osmolar changes above basal plasma osmolality; (3) a reset osmostat system, whereby vasopressin is secreted at an abnormally low threshold of plasma osmolality but otherwise displays a normal response to relative changes in osmolality; and (4) low or even undetectable plasma vasopressin levels despite classic clinical characteristics of SIADH.[281] The first pattern, unregulated vasopressin secretion, is often observed in patients exhibiting paraneoplastic vasopressin production. Resetting of the osmotic threshold for vasopressin secretion has been well described with volume depletion[296] and edema-forming states with EABV,[261] but most patients with a reset osmostat are clinically euvolemic[279] and may represent SIADH. The best physiologic example of a reset osmostat occurs in pregnancy, as discussed earlier. Perhaps the most perplexing aspect of the reset osmostat pattern is its occurrence in patients with tumors, which suggests that in some of these cases a tumor-related mechanism may affect pituitary vasopressin secretion.[281] The pattern of SIADH that occurs without measurable vasopressin secretion is not yet well understood, but the positive response of one such patient to a vasopressin V_2-receptor antagonist would suggest that this may represent increased renal sensitivity to low circulating levels of vasopressin.[297] Recent studies of pediatric patients with hyponatremia and unmeasurable plasma vasopressin levels led to the discovery of an activating mutation of the vasopressin V_2 receptor as the cause of

their inappropriate antidiuresis.[298] It is more appropriate to call these cases the *nephrogenic syndrome of inappropriate antidiuresis*, reserving SIADH only for those cases in which measured plasma vasopressin levels are really inappropriate. Although the incidence of nephrogenic syndrome of inappropriate antidiuresis in the general population is unknown, the description of Belgian kindred with this mutation suggests that it can present later in life as well as in childhood. It is surprising that no correlation has been found between any of these patterns of secretion of vasopressin and the various causes of SIADH.[281]

Contribution of Natriuresis to the Hyponatremia of SIADH. Since the original cases studied by Schwartz and Bartter, increased renal Na+ excretion has been one of the cardinal manifestations of SIADH, indeed one which later became embedded in the requirements for its diagnosis.[246] Demonstration that the natriuresis accompanying administration of antidiuretic hormone is not due to vasopressin itself but rather to the volume expansion produced as a result of water retention was unequivocally shown by Leaf and coworkers even before the description of the disorder.[299] Although a negative Na+ balance occurs during the development of hyponatremia in patients with SIADH, eventually urinary sodium excretion simply reflects daily sodium intake.[245] Thus, the term *renal sodium wasting* is used to describe continued excretion of sodium despite being hyponatremic, but in reality there is a new steady state in which patients are in neutral sodium balance. Studies of long-term antidiuretic-induced hyponatremia in both dogs and rats have indicated that a large proportion of the hyponatremia was attributable to secondary Na+ losses rather than to water retention,[274,275] but the natriuresis did not actually worsen the hyponatremia; rather, it allowed volume regulation of ECF.[300] Secondary natriuresis in patients with SIADH likely explains the failure to find expanded plasma or ECF volumes using tracer dilution techniques (see Fig. 10-5).[276]

Cerebral Salt Wasting. The degree to which hyponatremia might occur primarily as a result of primary natriuresis is controversial. Cerebral salt-wasting syndrome (CSWS) was proposed by Peters and colleagues in 1950[301] as an explanation for the natriuresis and hyponatremia that sometimes accompany intracranial disease, particularly subarachnoid hemorrhage, in which up to one third of patients often develop hyponatremia. After the description of SIADH in 1957, such patients were generally assumed to have hyponatremia secondary to vasopressin hypersecretion with a secondary natriuresis. However, over the past decade clinical and experimental data have been interpreted to indicate that some patients with subarachnoid hemorrhage and other intracranial diseases indeed have a primary natriuresis leading to volume contraction rather than SIADH,[302,303] and the elevated plasma vasopressin levels may be physiologically appropriate for the degree of volume contraction. With regard to the potential mechanisms of natriuresis, both plasma and CSF levels of atrial natriuretic peptide are elevated in many patients with subarachnoid hemorrhage and have been found to correlate variably with hyponatremia in patients with intracranial diseases.[304] However, clearly documented SIADH also is frequently associated with elevated plasma levels of atrial natriuretic peptide, so this finding does not prove causality. In other disorders of hyponatremia due to Na+ wasting (e.g., Addison disease) and diuretic-induced hyponatremia, infusion of saline restores normal ECF volume and plasma tonicity by shutting off the secondary vasopressin secretion. In subarachnoid hemorrhage, however, large volumes of isotonic saline sufficient to maintain plasma volume did not change the incidence of hyponatremia.[305]

Those authors who have distinguished CSWS from SIADH have emphasized that in CSWS the primary disorder, salt wasting, produces convincing evidence of decreased ECF volume.[306,307] There are only a few case reports of patients after traumatic brain injury or neurosurgery who while being observed in the hospital have acute onset of massive diuresis and natriuresis with clear evidence of volume contraction by weight loss, decreased central venous pressure, increased blood urea nitrogen, or increased hematocrit. Most of these cases have been in children[308,309] and have responded to replacement with normal or hypertonic saline, but concurrent treatment with fludrocortisone has also been advocated.[308,310] However, a recent study of 100 consecutive adult patients with acute nontraumatic aneurysmal subarachnoid hemorrhage found that the cause of the hyponatremia was attributable to SIADH in 71.4% and acute glucocorticoid deficiency in 8.2%, with the remaining cases caused by incorrect intravenous fluid administration or hypovolemia. Most significantly, no cases were found that met historically accepted criteria for a diagnosis of CSWS.[311] This suggests that CSWS is an exceedingly rare cause of hyponatremia with intracranial disorders.

Renal Escape From Antidiuresis. In addition to excreting osmoles to bring volumes back toward normal, there are intrarenal adaptations that allow excretion of more water. Chronic stimulation by vasopressin in SIADH produces dramatic increases of aquaporin 2 content and insertion into the collecting duct principal cell membranes, which increases the efficiency of water retention and aggravates the disease. However, the induced volume expansion and hypotonicity act on the tubular cells of the collecting duct to decrease the content and action of aquaporin 2 substantially, thus decreasing the amount of water resorbed in spite of high vasopressin levels. Experimental studies have suggested that this effect may be due to downregulation of vasopressin V_2 receptor expression in the kidney.[312] This renal "escape" therefore represents another (in addition to natriuresis) adaptation that allows patients with persistent SIADH to come into a new steady state of Na^+ and water balance despite low serum sodium concentrations.[313]

Clinical Manifestations of Hypoosmolar Disorders

Regardless of the cause of hypoosmolality, most clinical manifestations are similar. Non-neurologic symptoms are relatively uncommon, although a number of cases of rhabdomyolysis have been reported, presumably secondary to osmotically induced swelling of muscle fibers. Hypoosmolality is primarily associated with a broad spectrum of neurologic manifestations, ranging from mild nonspecific symptoms (e.g., headache, nausea) to more significant disorders (e.g., disorientation, confusion, obtundation, focal neurologic deficits, and seizures).[314] This neurologic symptom complex has been termed *hyponatremic encephalopathy*[315] and primarily reflects brain edema resulting from osmotic water shifts into the brain because of decreased effective plasma osmolality. Significant neurologic symptoms generally do not occur until serum $[Na^+]$ falls below 125 mmol/L and the severity of symptoms are roughly correlated with the degree of hypoosmolality.[314,316] However, individual variability is marked, and for any single patient, the level of serum $[Na^+]$ at which symptoms appear cannot be predicted.

The rate of fall of serum $[Na^+]$ is often more strongly correlated with morbidity and mortality than is the actual magnitude of the decrease.[314,316] The reason is that the volume-adaptation process takes a finite period of time to complete, and the more rapid the fall in serum $[Na^+]$, the more brain edema will be accumulated before the brain is able to volume-regulate. Thus, there is a much higher incidence of neurologic symptoms, as well as a higher mortality rate, in patients with acute hyponatremia than in those with chronic hyponatremia.[314] For example, the most dramatic cases of death due to hyponatremic encephalopathy have generally been reported in postoperative patients in whom hyponatremia develops rapidly as a result of intravenous infusion of hypotonic fluids.[314,317] In such cases nausea and vomiting are frequently overlooked as potential early signs of increased intracranial pressure. Critically ill patients with unexplained seizures also should be immediately evaluated for possible hyponatremia, because as many as one third of such patients have a serum $[Na^+]$ lower than 125 mEq/L as the cause of the seizure activity.[318] Underlying neurologic disease and non-neurologic metabolic disorders (e.g., hypoxia,[319] acidosis, hypercalcemia) can raise the level of plasma osmolality at which CNS symptoms occur.

In the most severe cases of hyponatremic encephalopathy, death results from respiratory failure after tentorial cerebral herniation and brainstem compression. One quarter of patients with severe postoperative hyponatremic encephalopathy manifested hypercapnic respiratory failure, the expected result of brainstem compression; but three quarters of these patients had pulmonary edema as the apparent cause of the hypoxia.[320] Studies of acute hyponatremia after marathon races have shown hypoxia and pulmonary edema in association with brain edema.[321] These results suggest the possibility that hypoxia from noncardiogenic pulmonary edema may represent an early sign of developing cerebral edema even before brainstem compression and tentorial herniation. Clinical studies have suggested that menstruating women[317] and young children[322] may be particularly susceptible to the development of neurologic morbidity and death during hyponatremia, especially in the acute postoperative setting.[315] However, other studies have failed to corroborate these findings.[323,324]

Once the brain has volume-regulated via solute losses, thereby reducing brain edema, neurologic symptoms are not as prominent and may even be virtually absent. This accounts for the fairly common finding of relatively asymptomatic patients even with severe levels of hyponatremia.[316,325] Despite this powerful adaptation process, chronic hyponatremia is frequently associated with neurocognitive symptoms, albeit milder and subtler in nature, such as headaches, nausea, mood disturbances, depression, difficulty concentrating, slowed reaction times, unstable gait, increased falls, confusion, and disorientation.[326,327] Even in patients adjudged to be asymptomatic by virtue of a normal neurologic examination, accumulating evidence suggests that there may be previously unrecognized adverse effects as a result of chronic hyponatremia, including gait instability and increased falls.[326] The clinical significance of the data on increased gait instability and falls in hyponatremic patients would be an increased fracture rate, which has now been documented in multiple international retrospective studies.[328-331] More recently published studies have shown that hyponatremia is also associated with increased bone loss in experimental animals and a significant increased odds ratio for osteoporosis of the femoral neck in humans over the age of 50 in the National Health and Nutrition Examination Survey (NHANES) III database.[332] Thus, the major clinical significance of chronic hyponatremia may lie in the increased morbidity and mortality rates associated with falls and fractures in the elderly population.

Therapy of SIADH and Other Hypoosmolar Disorders

General Principles

Correction of hyponatremia is associated with markedly improved neurologic outcomes in patients with severely symptomatic hyponatremia. In a retrospective review of patients who presented with severe neurologic symptoms and serum [Na+] lower than 125 mmol/L, prompt therapy with isotonic or hypertonic saline resulted in a correction in the range of 20 mEq/L over several days and neurologic recovery in almost all cases; in contrast, in patients who were treated with fluid restriction alone, there was very little correction over the study period (<5 mmol/L over 72 hours), and the neurologic outcomes were much worse, with most of these patients either dying or entering a persistent vegetative state.[333] Based on this and similar retrospective analyses, prompt therapy to rapidly increase the serum [Na+] represents the standard of care for treatment of patients presenting with severe symptoms of hyponatremia.

Brain herniation, the most dreaded complication of hyponatremia, is seen almost exclusively in patients with acute hyponatremia (usually <24 hours) or in patients with intracranial disease.[334] In postoperative patients and in patients with self-induced water intoxication associated with marathon running, psychosis, or use of MDMA, nonspecific symptoms such as headache, nausea, and vomiting or confusion can rapidly progress to seizures, respiratory arrest, and ultimately death or a permanent vegetative state as a complication of cerebral edema.[251] Hypoxia from noncardiogenic pulmonary edema or hypoventilation can exacerbate brain swelling caused by the low serum [Na+].[320,321] Although usually self-limited, hyponatremic seizures may be refractory to anticonvulsants.

As discussed earlier, chronic hyponatremia is much less symptomatic as a result of the process of brain volume regulation. Because of this adaptation process, chronic hyponatremia is arguably a condition that clinicians feel they may not need to be as concerned about, which has been reinforced by the common usage of the descriptor *asymptomatic hyponatremia* for many such patients. However, as discussed previously, it is clear that many such patients very often do have neurologic symptoms, even if milder and subtler in nature. Consequently, all patients with hyponatremia who manifest any neurologic symptoms that could possibly be related to the hyponatremia should be considered candidates for treatment of the hyponatremia, regardless of the chronicity of the hyponatremia or the level of serum [Na+]. An additional reason to treat even asymptomatic hyponatremia effectively is to prevent a lowering of the serum [Na+] to more symptomatic and dangerous levels during treatment of underlying conditions (e.g., increased fluid administration via parenteral nutrition, treatment of heart failure with diuretics).

Currently Available Therapies for Treatment of Hyponatremia

Conventional management strategies for hyponatremia range from saline infusion and fluid restriction to pharmacologic measures to adjust fluid balance. Although the number of available treatments for hyponatremia is large, some are not appropriate for correction of symptomatic hyponatremia because they work too slowly or inconsistently to be effective in hospitalized patients (e.g., demeclocycline, mineralocorticoids). Consideration of treatment options should always include an evaluation of the benefits as well as the potential toxicities of any therapy and must

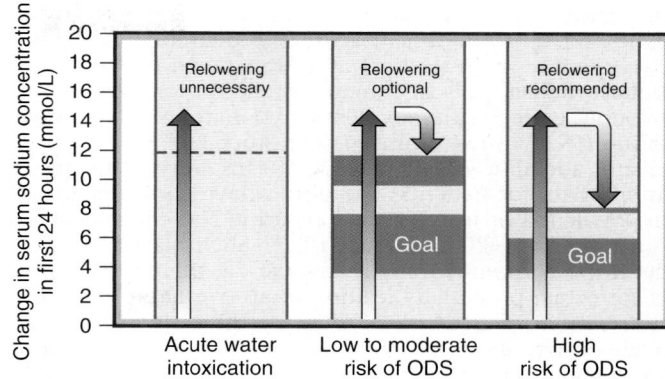

Figure 10-8 Recommended goals *(green)* and limits *(red)* for correction of hyponatremia based on risk of producing ODS and recommendations for relowering of serum sodium concentration ([Na+]) to goals for patients presenting with serum [Na+] lower than 120 mmol/L who exceed the recommended limits of correction in the first 24 hours. ODS, osmotic demyelination syndrome. (From Verbalis JG, Goldsmith SR, Greenberg A, et al. Diagnosis, evaluation, and treatment of hyponatremia: expert panel recommendations. *Am J Med.* 2013;126(10 Suppl 1):S1-42.)

be individualized for each patient.[327,335] For all therapies, careful attention should be paid to recommendations for goals and limits of correction of the serum [Na+] in order to reduce the risk of the osmotic demyelination syndrome (ODS)[327] (Fig. 10-8). It should also be remembered that sometimes simply stopping treatment with an agent that is associated with causing hyponatremia is sufficient to correct a low serum [Na+].

Hypertonic Saline. Acute hyponatremia presenting with severe neurologic symptoms is life threatening and should be treated promptly with hypertonic solutions, typically 3% NaCl ([Na+] = 513 mmol/L), as this represents the most reliable method to quickly raise the serum [Na+]. A continuous infusion of hypertonic NaCl is usually utilized in inpatient settings. Various formulas have been suggested for calculating the initial rate of infusion of hypertonic solutions,[334] but until now there has been no consensus regarding optimal infusion rates of 3% NaCl. One of the simplest methods to estimate an initial 3% NaCl infusion rate utilizes the following relationship:[327]

> Patient's weight (kg) × desired correction rate (mEq/L per hour)
> = infusion rate of 3% NaCl (mL/hour)

Depending on individual hospital policies, the administration of hypertonic solutions may require special considerations (e.g., placement in the intensive care unit, sign-off by a consultant), which each clinician needs to take into account in order to optimize patient care.

An alternative option for more emergent situations is administration of a 100-mL bolus of 3% NaCl, repeated twice if there is no clinical improvement in 30 minutes, which has been recommended by a consensus conference organized to develop guidelines for prevention and treatment of exercise-induced hyponatremia[336] and adopted as a general recommendation by an expert panel.[327] Injecting this amount of hypertonic saline intravenously raises the serum [Na+] by an average of 2 to 4 mmol/L, which is well below the recommended maximal daily rate of change of 10 to 12 mmol/L per 24 hours or 8 mmol/L per 24 hours for patients with increased risk factors for ODS (serum [Na+] ≤105 mmol/L), hypokalemia, advanced liver disease, malnutrition, or a history of alcoholism[327,337] (see Fig. 10-8). Because the adult brain can only accommodate an average increase of approximately 8% in brain volume before herniation occurs, quickly increasing the serum [Na$^+$] by as little as 2 to 4 mmol/L in acute hyponatremia can effectively reduce brain swelling and intracranial pressure.[338]

Isotonic Saline. The treatment of choice for depletional hyponatremia (i.e., hypovolemic hyponatremia) is isotonic saline ([Na$^+$] = 154 mmol/L) to restore ECF volume and ensure adequate organ perfusion. This initial therapy is appropriate for patients who either have clinical signs of hypovolemia or in whom a spot urine Na$^+$ concentration is lower than 20 to 30 mEq/L.[327] Such patients often develop a free water diuresis (*aquaresis*) as their ECF volume is corrected, potentially leading to an overly rapid correction with increased risk of ODS, so the serum [Na$^+$] and urine output should be followed carefully during the first 24 to 48 hours of therapy. However, isotonic saline is ineffective for dilutional hyponatremias such as SIADH,[245] and continued administration of isotonic saline to a euvolemic patient may worsen the hyponatremia[339] or cause fluid overload. Although saline may improve the serum [Na$^+$] in some patients with hypervolemic hyponatremia, the volume status will generally worsen with this therapy, so unless the hyponatremia is profound, both hypertonic and isotonic saline should be avoided.

Fluid Restriction. For patients with chronic hyponatremia, fluid restriction has been the most popular and most widely accepted treatment. When SIADH is present, fluids should generally be limited to 500 to 1000 mL/24 hours. Because fluid restriction increases the serum [Na$^+$] by underreplacing the excretion of fluid by the kidneys, some have advocated an initial restriction to 500 mL less than the 24-hour urine output.[340] When instituting fluid restriction, it is important for the nursing staff and the patient to understand that this includes all fluids that are consumed, not just water (Table 10-4). Generally the water content of ingested food is not included in the restriction because this is balanced by insensible water losses (perspiration, exhaled air, feces, etc.), but caution should be exercised with foods that have high fluid concentrations (such as fruits and soups). Restricting fluid intake can be effective when properly applied and managed in selected patients, but serum [Na$^+$] is generally increased only slowly (1-2 mmol/L per day) even with severe fluid restriction.[245] In addition, this therapy is often poorly tolerated because of an associated increase in thirst leading to poor compliance with long-term therapy.

Fluid restriction should not be used with hypovolemic patients and is particularly difficult to maintain in hospitalized patients with very elevated urine osmolalities secondary to high vasopressin levels; similarly, if the sum of

urine Na$^+$ and K$^+$ exceeds the serum [Na$^+$], most patients will not respond to a fluid restriction because an electrolyte-free water clearance will be difficult to achieve.[341,342] These and other known predictors of failure of fluid restriction are summarized in Table 10-4; the presence of any of these factors in hospitalized patients with symptomatic hyponatremia make this less than ideal as an initial therapy. In addition, fluid restriction is not practical for some patients, particularly patients in intensive care settings who often require administration of significant volumes of fluids as part of their therapies. Such patients are candidates for more effective pharmacologic or saline treatment strategies.

Arginine Vasopressin Receptor Antagonists. Conventional therapies for hyponatremia, although effective in specific circumstances, are suboptimal for many different reasons, including variable efficacy, slow responses, intolerable side effects, and serious toxicities. But perhaps the greatest deficiency of most conventional therapies is that most of these therapies do not directly target the underlying cause of most dilutional hyponatremias, namely, inappropriately elevated plasma vasopressin levels. A new class of pharmacologic agents, *vasopressin receptor antagonists*, also known as *vaptans*, that directly block vasopressin-mediated receptor activation have recently been approved for treatment of euvolemic (U.S. and EU approval) and hypervolemic (U.S. approval) hyponatremia.[343]

Conivaptan is a mixed antagonist of vasopressin V_{1a} and V_2 receptors. It is available only as an intravenous preparation and is given as a 20-mg loading dose over 30 minutes, followed by a continuous infusion of 20 or 40 mg/day.[344] Generally, the 20-mg continuous infusion is used for the first 24 hours to gauge the initial response. If the correction of serum [Na$^+$] is felt to be inadequate (e.g., <5 mmol/L), then the infusion rate can be increased to 40 mg/day. Therapy is limited to a maximum duration of 4 days because of drug-interaction effects with other agents metabolized by the CYP3A4 hepatic isoenzyme. For conivaptan and all other vaptans, it is critical that the serum [Na$^+$] is measured frequently during the active phase of correction of the hyponatremia—a minimum of every 6 to 8 hours for conivaptan but more frequently in patients with risk factors for ODS. If the correction exceeds 10 to 12 mmol/L in the first 24 hours, the infusion should be stopped and the patient monitored closely. Consideration should be given to administering sufficient water, either orally or as intravenous D5W, to avoid a correction of more than 10 to 12 mmol/L/day. The maximum correction limit should be reduced to 8 mmol/L over the first 24 hours in patients with risk factors for ODS (see Fig. 10-8). The most common side effects of conivaptan include headache, thirst, and hypokalemia.[345]

Tolvaptan is a selective antagonist of vasopressin V_2 receptors. In contrast to conivaptan, the availability of tolvaptan in tablet form allows both short- and long-term use.[346] Similar to conivaptan, tolvaptan treatment must be initiated in the hospital so that the rate of correction can be monitored carefully. In the United States, patients with a serum [Na$^+$] lower than 125 mmol/L are eligible for therapy with tolvaptan as primary therapy; if the serum [Na$^+$] is 125 mmol/L or higher, tolvaptan therapy is indicated only if the patient has symptoms that could be attributable to the hyponatremia and the patient is resistant to attempts at fluid restriction.[347] In the European Union, tolvaptan is approved only for the treatment of euvolemic hyponatremia, but any symptomatic euvolemic patient is eligible for tolvaptan therapy, regardless of the level of hyponatremia or response to previous fluid restriction. The starting dose of tolvaptan is 15 mg on the first day, and

---

TABLE 10-4

General Recommendations for Employment of Fluid Restriction and Predictors of the Increased Likelihood of Failure of Fluid Restriction

General Recommendations

- Restrict *all* intake that is consumed by drinking, not just water.
- Aim for a fluid restriction that is 500 mL/d *below* the 24-hour urine volume.
- Do *not* restrict sodium or protein intake unless indicated.

Predictors of the Likely Failure of Fluid Restriction

- High urine osmolality (≥500 mOsm/kg H_2O).
- Sum of the urine Na$^+$ and K$^+$ concentrations exceeds the serum Na$^+$ concentration.
- 24-hour urine volume <1500 mL/d.
- Increase in serum Na$^+$ concentration <2 mmol/L per day in 24 to 48 hours on a fluid restriction of ≥1 L/d.

the dose can be titrated to 30 mg and 60 mg at 24-hour intervals if the serum [Na$^+$] remains lower than 135 mmol/L or the increase in serum [Na$^+$] has been lower than 5 mmol/L in the previous 24 hours. As with conivaptan, it is essential that the serum [Na$^+$] is measured frequently during the active phase of correction of the hyponatremia, particularly in patients with risk factors for ODS. Goals and limits for safe correction of hyponatremia and methods to compensate for overly rapid corrections are the same as described previously for hypertonic saline and conivaptan (see Fig. 10-8). One additional factor that helps to avoid overly rapid correction with tolvaptan is the recommendation that fluid restriction not be used during the active phase of correction, thereby allowing the patient's thirst to compensate for an overly vigorous aquaresis. Side effects of tolvaptan include dry mouth, thirst, increased urinary frequency, dizziness, nausea, and orthostatic hypotension.[346,347]

Vaptans are not needed for treatment of hypovolemic hyponatremia, because simple volume expansion would be expected to abolish the nonosmotic stimulus to AVP secretion and lead to a prompt aquaresis. Furthermore, inducing increased renal fluid excretion via either a diuresis or an aquaresis can cause or worsen hypovolemia and hypotension in such patients. This possibility has resulted in the labeling of these drugs as contraindicated for hypovolemic hyponatremia.[348] Importantly, clinically significant hypotension was not observed in either the conivaptan or tolvaptan clinical trials in euvolemic and hypervolemic hyponatremic patients. Although vaptans are not contraindicated with decreased renal function, these agents generally will not be effective if the serum creatinine is higher than 3.0 mg/dL. Recent findings of hepatotoxicity in a small number of patients on high doses of tolvaptan in a clinical trial of polycystic kidney disease has led to Food and Drug Administration (FDA) warnings on the use of vaptans in patients with liver failure and a recommendation that they not be used longer than 30 days, though this decision should be based on a risk-benefit analysis individualized for specific patients.[327]

Urea. Urea has been described as an alternative oral treatment for SIADH and other hyponatremic disorders. The mode of action is to correct hypoosmolality not only by increasing solute-free water excretion but also by decreasing urinary sodium excretion. Doses of 15 to 60 g/day are generally effective; the dose can be titrated in increments of 15 g/day at weekly intervals as necessary to achieve normalization of the serum [Na$^+$]. It is advisable to dissolve the urea in orange juice or some other strongly flavored liquid to camouflage the bitter taste. Even if completely normal water balance is not achieved, it is often possible to allow the patient to maintain a less strict regimen of fluid restriction while receiving urea. The disadvantages associated with the use of urea include poor palatability, the development of azotemia at higher doses, and the unavailability of a convenient or FDA-approved form of the agent. Data suggest that blood urea concentrations may double during treatment,[349] but it is important to remember that this does not represent renal impairment.

Reports of retrospective, uncontrolled studies suggest that the use of urea has been effective in treating SIADH in patients with hyponatremia due to subarachnoid hemorrhage and in critical care patients,[350] and case reports have documented success in infants with chronic SIADH[351] and the nephrogenic syndrome of inappropriate antidiuresis.[352] More recent evidence from a short study in a small cohort of SIADH patients suggests that urea may have a comparable efficacy to vaptans in reversing hyponatremia due to chronic SIADH.[353]

Furosemide and NaCl. The use of furosemide (20 to 40 mg/day) coupled with a high sodium intake (200 mEq/day) represents an extension of the treatment of acute symptomatic hyponatremia[354] in selected cases.[355,356] However, the efficacy of this approach to correct symptomatic hyponatremia both promptly and within accepted goal limits (see Fig. 10-8) is unknown.

Hyponatremia Treatment Guidelines Based on Symptom Severity

Although various authors and groups have published recommendations on the treatment of hyponatremia,[327,334,348,356-359] no standardized treatment algorithms have yet been universally accepted. For all treatment recommendations, the initial evaluation includes an assessment of the ECF volume status of the patient, because treatment recommendations differ in hypovolemic, euvolemic, and hypervolemic hyponatremic patients.[327] Euvolemic patients, mainly patients with SIADH, represent a unique challenge because of the multiplicity of causes and presentations of patients with SIADH. Recent expert opinion recommendations are based primarily on the neurologic symptoms of hyponatremic patients rather than the serum [Na$^+$] or on the chronicity of the hyponatremia, which is often difficult to ascertain.[327] A careful neurologic history and assessment should always be done to identify potential causes for the patient's symptoms other than hyponatremia, although it will not always be possible to exclude an additive contribution from the hyponatremia to an underlying neurologic condition. In this algorithm, patients are divided into three groups based on their presenting symptoms.

Severe Symptoms. Coma, obtundation, seizures, respiratory distress or arrest, and unexplained vomiting usually imply a more acute onset or worsening of hyponatremia, requiring immediate active treatment. Therapies that will quickly raise serum [Na$^+$] are required to reduce cerebral edema and decrease the risk of potentially fatal brain herniation.

Moderate Symptoms. Altered mental status, disorientation, confusion, unexplained nausea, gait instability, and falls generally indicate some degree of brain volume regulation and absence of clinically significant cerebral edema. These symptoms can be either chronic or acute but allow more time to elaborate a deliberate approach to choice of treatment.

Mild or Absent Symptoms. Minimal symptoms such as difficulty concentrating, irritability, altered mood, depression, and unexplained headache, or a virtual absence of discernible symptoms, indicate that the patient may have chronic or slowly evolving hyponatremia. These symptoms necessitate a cautious approach, especially when patients have underlying comorbid conditions.

Patients with severe symptoms should be treated with hypertonic (3%) NaCl as first-line therapy, followed by fluid restriction with or without vaptan therapy. Because overly rapid correction of serum [Na$^+$] occurs in more than 10% of patients treated with hypertonic NaCl,[360] such patients are at risk for ODS unless carefully monitored. For this reason, some authors have proposed simultaneous treatment with desmopressin to reduce the rate of correction to only that produced by the hypertonic NaCl infusion itself.[361,362] Whether sufficient clinical data eventually prove that this approach is both effective and safe in larger numbers of patients remains to be determined. Only one case of ODS has been reported in a patient receiving a vaptan monotherapy, and two abstracts have reported ODS when vaptans were used directly following hypertonic saline administration within in the same 24-hour period.

Consequently, no active hyponatremia therapy should be administered until at least 24 hours following successful increases in serum [Na⁺] using hypertonic NaCl.

The choice of treatment for patients with moderate symptoms will depend on their ECF volume status. Hypovolemic patients should be treated with solute repletion, either via isotonic NaCl infusion or oral sodium replacement.[327] Euvolemic patients, typically with SIADH, will benefit from vaptan therapy, limited hypertonic saline administration, or in some cases urea, when available. This treatment can then be followed by fluid restriction or long-term vaptan therapy when the cause of the SIADH is expected to be chronic.[327] In hypervolemic patients with heart failure, vaptans are usually the best choice because fluid restriction is rarely successful in this group, saline administration can cause fluid retention with increased edema, and urea can lead to ammonia buildup in the gastrointestinal tract if hepatic function is impaired. Although moderate neurologic symptoms can indicate that a patient is in an early stage of acute hyponatremia, they more often indicate a chronically hyponatremic state with sufficient brain volume adaptation to prevent marked symptoms from cerebral edema. Because most patients with moderate hyponatremic symptoms have a more chronic form of hyponatremia, guidelines for goals and limits of correction should be followed closely (see Fig. 10-8), and close monitoring of these patients in a hospital setting is warranted until the symptoms improve or stabilize.

Patients with mild or absent symptoms should be managed initially with fluid restriction, although treatment with pharmacologic therapy, such as vaptans or urea, may be appropriate for a wide range of specific clinical conditions, foremost of which is a failure to improve the serum [Na⁺] despite reasonable attempts at fluid restriction, or the presence of clinical characteristics associated with poor responses to fluid restriction (see Table 10-4).

A special case is seen when spontaneous correction of hyponatremia occurs at an undesirably rapid rate as a result of the onset of a water diuresis, or aquaresis. This situation can occur following cessation of desmopressin therapy in a patient who has become hyponatremic, replacement of glucocorticoids in a patient with adrenal insufficiency, replacement of solutes in a patient with diuretic-induced hyponatremia, or spontaneous resolution of transient SIADH. Brain damage from ODS can clearly ensue in this setting if the preceding period of hyponatremia has been of sufficient duration (usually ≥48 hours) to allow brain volume regulation to occur. If the previously discussed correction parameters have been exceeded and the correction is proceeding more rapidly than planned (usually because of continued excretion of hypotonic urine), the risk of subsequent demyelination can be reduced by administration of hypotonic fluids, with or without desmopressin. Efficacy of this approach is suggested both from animal studies[363] as well as case reports in humans[358,364] even when patients are overtly symptomatic.[365] However, relowering the serum [Na⁺] after an initial overly rapid correction is only strongly recommended in patients who are at high risk of ODS, is considered optional in patients with low to moderate risk of ODS, and is unnecessary in patients with acute water intoxication (see Fig. 10-8).

Although this classification is based on presenting symptoms at the time of initial evaluation, it should be remembered that in some cases patients initially exhibit more moderate symptoms because they are in the early stages of hyponatremia. In addition, some patients with minimal symptoms are prone to develop more symptomatic hyponatremia during periods of increased fluid ingestion. In support of this, approximately 70% of 31 patients presenting to a university hospital with symptomatic hyponatremia and a mean serum [Na⁺] of 119 mmol/L had preexisting asymptomatic hyponatremia as the most common risk factor identified.[366] Consequently, therapy of hyponatremia should also be considered to prevent progression from lower to higher levels of symptomatic hyponatremia, particularly in patients with a past history of repeated presentations for symptomatic hyponatremia.

Monitoring the Serum [Na⁺] in Hyponatremic Patients

The frequency of serum [Na⁺] monitoring is dependent on both the severity of the hyponatremia and the therapy chosen. All patients undergoing active treatment with hypertonic saline for symptomatic hyponatremia should have frequent monitoring of serum [Na⁺], urine output, and ECF volume status (every 2-4 hours) to ensure that the serum [Na⁺] does not exceed the limits of safe correction during the active phase of correction,[327] because overly rapid correction of serum [Na⁺] will increase the risk of ODS.[252] Patients treated with vaptans for moderate or mild symptoms should have serum [Na⁺] monitored every 6 to 8 hours during the active phase of correction, which will generally be the first 24 to 48 hours of therapy. Active treatment with any therapy should be stopped when the patient's symptoms are no longer present, a safe serum [Na⁺] (usually >120 mmol/L) has been achieved, or the rate of correction has reached maximum limits of 10 to 12 mmol/L within 24 hours or 18 mmol/L within 48 hours[327,337] or 8 mmol/L over any 24-hour period in patients at high risk of ODS (see Fig. 10-8). In patients with a stable level of serum [Na⁺] treated with fluid restriction or therapies other than hypertonic saline, measurement of serum [Na⁺] daily is generally sufficient, because levels will not change that quickly in the absence of active therapy or large changes in fluid intake or administration.

Future of Hyponatremia Therapy

Despite the many advances made in understanding the manifestations and consequences of hyponatremia, and the availability of effective pharmacologic therapies for the treatment of hyponatremia, it is obvious that we do not yet have a uniformly accepted consensus on how and when this disorder should be treated. In particular, the indications for the use of vasopressin receptor antagonists by regulatory agencies differ substantially around the world, and various treatment guidelines published to date also differ substantially on appropriate hyponatremia management.[327,335,356] There are many reasons for this failure to achieve consensus, and until this is achieved via further clinical research studies, physicians must recognize the primary role that clinical judgment must continue to play in decision making about the management of hyponatremia in individual patients. Such judgments should take into account appropriate appraisals of evidence by authoritative experts in the field, the decisions of regulatory agencies that have based their approvals on a critical review of the efficacy and safety data for approved treatments for hyponatremia, and most important, the specialized needs of individual hyponatremic patients.[335]

In the meantime, clinical trials using vasopressin receptor antagonists will enable investigators to answer some long-standing questions about the role of vasopressin V₂ receptor activation in producing antidiuresis in various physiologic conditions (e.g., regulation of sweat production[367]), pathophysiologic states (e.g., hyponatremic patients without measurable vasopressin levels), and especially the potential reversibility of long-term adverse effects of hyponatremia that may account for the increased mortality rate and bone fracture rates of hyponatremic patients across multiple different comorbid conditions, as well as in subjects in the elderly community without known underlying diseases.

OXYTOCIN

Study of the normal physiologic regulation of oxytocin secretion and action is complicated by the fact that secretion and function of oxytocin vary markedly among different experimental mammals. The sites of synthesis in the ovary and in tissues of the uterus also vary among species. It is difficult to study pregnant women and human tissue, so physiologic regulation of oxytocin secretion and function is less well known in humans than in other species. The classic roles of oxytocin are smooth muscle activation promoting milk let-down with nursing and uterine myometrial contraction at parturition.

Lactation

A characteristic of all mammals is lactation, and all mammals secrete oxytocin to stimulate milk let-down associated with nursing.[368] The other hormone critical to lactation is prolactin. Each of these pituitary/hypothalamic hormones is importantly influenced and regulated by gonadal steroid hormones. The milk-producing unit of the breast is the alveolar system with multiple clusters of milk-producing cells surrounded by specialized myoepithelial cells. The alveoli are directly connected to ductules and then ducts converge and lead to the nipple. Milk is synthesized in the glandular cells of the alveoli.[369] Oxytocin receptors are localized on glandular cells and oxytocin in the systemic circulation acts on these receptors to cause myoepithelial contraction. Oxytocin also acts on myoepithelial cells along the duct to shorten and widen the ducts to enhance milk flow through the ducts to the nipple.[370]

When an infant begins sucking at the breast an afferent signal is transmitted from the mechanoreceptors or tactile receptors in the breast to the spinal cord and eventually ascends to the oxytocinergic magnocellular neurons in the supraoptic nucleus and the paraventricular nucleus.[370,371] Pulsatile release of oxytocin produces a pulsatile pumping action on the alveoli, which promotes maximum emptying of milk from the alveoli.[369] The importance of oxytocin in maintaining milk secretion is demonstrated by transgenic mice with a knockout gene that inhibits oxytocin synthesis. These animals deliver their young normally and have normal milk production, but there is no milk release in spite of normal suckling. The pups die of dehydration with no milk in the stomach.[372] Administration of oxytocin to these oxytocin-deficient mice rescues the ability to secrete milk and allows the pups to survive. Similarly, oxytocin may promote successful lactation in women who have difficulty with lactation and milk production.[373] If oxytocin is not secreted, only 20% to 30% of stored milk is released during nursing.[374]

As breastfeeding continues in humans the basal levels of oxytocin decrease, but pulses of oxytocin in response to suckling continue and may increase.[375] Humans with diabetes insipidus have been able to successfully breastfeed infants, and this finding has caused some to question the importance of oxytocin in humans.[376] However, oxytocin secretion may be preserved in the absence of vasopressin in patients with diabetes insipidus, even in those with traumatic section of the stalk.

Parturition

The isolation of oxytocin was followed quickly by the description of oxytocin to stimulate uterine contractions, and this was followed shortly by clinical use of oxytocin as a uterotonic agent.[377] Parturition in humans is much more complex than just the role of oxytocin.[378] In all species the uterus must grow during pregnancy and estrogen is a promoter of this growth. Levels of oxytocin in humans is not well defined in pregnancy, but it is not reported to increase until the expulsive stage at term.[378-380] The uterine myometrial cells have instrinsic contractile activity, but during pregnancy the uterus is maintained in a quiescent state by the actions of progesterone and relaxin (produced by the corpus luteum and decidual tissue).[381-383] The initiation of labor is accomplished by a relative increase in estrogen activation and decrease in progesterone activation. Changes in oxytocin receptors and oxytocin produced by the placenta may be more important than levels of oxytocin in the circulation. During early labor there is an upregulation in the uterus of oxytocin receptor mRNA, and oxytocin receptor numbers increase.[380,384] Oxytocin receptors are prominent in the fundus of the uterus, where they stimulate myometrial contraction, and in decidual cells, where they stimulate the production of prostaglandins. At parturition increased oxytocin activity in the fundus will push the fetus toward the cervix, which is thinned and relaxed by the effects of prostaglandins.[379,385] Prostaglandins play a key role in an inflammatory process that is important in the uterus at parturition. Cytokines induce enzymes that digest extracellular matrix to soften and ripen the cervix.[379] The role of progesterone in maintaining uterine quiescence is not only the action on oxytocin receptors but also by antagonizing the inflammatory response that is important for softening the lower uterus and cervix.[380]

Teleologically, it is appealing that the developing fetus when it reaches maturation would be a controlling factor in the initiation of labor. In sheep the action of the fetal hypothalamic/pituitary/adrenal axis is essential to initiating parturition, and in the human the role of CRH in human parturition has been extensively studied. CRH is synthesized by the placenta and increases exponentially throughout pregnancy with a peak during labor. CRH is secreted into the maternal plasma, where, as pregnancy advances, it stimulates ACTH and cortisol, although the feedback of cortisol on the pituitary and increased CRH binding proteins in plasma moderate the effect.[378] In the fetus stimulation of pituitary ACTH and cortisol promotes maturation of the fetal lungs. The fetal lung secretes surfactant proteins and lipids into amniotic fluid, which enhances the release of cytokines and progression of the inflammatory response.[386] In the human, parturition is a complicated cascade of agents and events that interact with each other and feed forward with cross-stimulation. It is not surprising that a physiologic event as important to the species as pregnancy and parturition would have many redundant systems to assure survival of the species. An obvious thing to note in all of these discussions is the lack of understanding of the role of cysteine aminopeptidase (oxytocinase) in the physiology of pregnancy in the human. If this enzyme developed as a protective mechanism, then one would assume that oxytocin secretion by the neurohypophysis was increased throughout pregnancy, but the very presence of this enzyme and the obvious inability to do studies of the hypothalamus in vivo make this possibility uncertain.

There are three situations in pregnancy in which a pharmacologic role of oxytocin is of interest. The first situation involves the most widely used role of oxytocin to induce and augment labor.[387] This situation has received increased interest in an effort to decrease the number of and morbidity of cesarean sections.[388] Oxytocin may be delivered alone or in combination with another pharmacologic agent such as propranolol or prostaglandins.[388,389] The second area of interest is preterm labor with an effort to prevent premature labor by decreasing contractile activity of the uterus and inhibiting the inflammatory response.[386] Peptide and nonpeptide oxytocin antagonists have been of especial interest to inhibit myometrial contractions, but widespread clinical use awaits the development of antagonists with better risk/benefit activity.[380] The third pharmacologic interest in oxytocin is as a uterotonic to decrease postpartum hemorrhage associated with uterine atony.[390] Postpartum hemorrhage is the major cause of maternal deaths worldwide and ranks second to embolism as a cause of maternal death in the United States.[391] Mechanical options in the active management of the third stage of labor include cord traction to reduce the risk of retained placenta and uterine massage, which has been augmented by pharmacologic agents, most commonly oxytocin and ergotamine.[390] Maternal deaths by postpartum hemorrhage are most significant in developing countries. Oxytocin is heat labile and requires a trained staff for appropriate administration,[392] prompting a search for other agents. The most promising results have been reported with prostaglandin analogues, especially misoprostol.[390,393,394]

Behavior

This chapter is about functions of vasopressin and oxytocin as traditional endocrine hormones secreted by the posterior pituitary. For further discussion related to these hormones in purported functions as neurotransmitters, especially with regard to influencing behavior, the reader is referred to Chapters 7 and 20.

REFERENCES

1. Makarenko IG, Ugrumov MV, Derer P, Calas A. Projections from the hypothalamus to the posterior lobe in rats during ontogenesis: 1,1'-dioctadecyl-3,3,3', 3'-tetramethylindocarbocyanine perchlorate tracing study. *J Comp Neurol.* 2000;422(3):327-337.
2. Gainer H. Cell-type specific expression of oxytocin and vasopressin genes: an experimental odyssey. *J Neuroendocrinol.* 2012;24(4):528-538.
3. Sofroniew MV. Morphology of vasopressin and oxytocin neurones and their central and vascular projections. *Prog Brain Res.* 1983;60:101-114.
4. Treier M, Rosenfeld MG. The hypothalamic-pituitary axis: co-development of two organs. *Curr Opin Cell Biol.* 1996;8(6):833-843.
5. Sawchenko PE, Swanson LW. The organization and biochemical specificity of afferent projections to the paraventricular and supraoptic nuclei. *Prog Brain Res.* 1983;60:19-29.
6. Swanson LW, Sawchenko PE. Paraventricular nucleus: a site for the integration of neuroendocrine and autonomic mechanisms. *Neuroendocrinology.* 1980;31(6):410-417.
7. Oliet SH. Functional consequences of morphological neuroglial changes in the magnocellular nuclei of the hypothalamus. *J Neuroendocrinol.* 2002;14(3):241-246.
8. Theodosis DT, Poulain DA. Maternity leads to morphological synaptic plasticity in the oxytocin system. *Prog Brain Res.* 2001;133:49-58.
9. Oliet SH, Piet R, Poulain DA, Theodosis DT. Glial modulation of synaptic transmission: insights from the supraoptic nucleus of the hypothalamus. *Glia.* 2004;47(3):258-267.
10. Israel JM, Poulain DA, Oliet SH. Glutamatergic inputs contribute to phasic activity in vasopressin neurons. *J Neurosci.* 2010;30(4):1221-1232.
11. Scott V, Bishop VR, Leng G, Brown CH. Dehydration-induced modulation of kappa-opioid inhibition of vasopressin neurone activity. *J Physiol.* 2009;587(Pt 23):5679-5689.
12. Mark L, Pech P, Daniels D, et al. The pituitary fossa: a correlative anatomic and MR study. *Radiology.* 1984;153(2):453-457.
13. Melo ME, Marui S, Carvalho LR, et al. Hormonal, pituitary magnetic resonance, LHX4 and HESX1 evaluation in patients with hypopituita-

14. Reynaud R, Albarel F, Saveanu A, et al. Pituitary stalk interruption syndrome in 83 patients: novel HESX1 mutation and severe hormonal prognosis in malformative forms. *Eur J Endocrinol.* 2011;164(4):457-465.
15. Secco A, Allegri AE, di Iorgi N, et al. Posterior pituitary (PP) evaluation in patients with anterior pituitary defect associated with ectopic PP and septo-optic dysplasia. *Eur J Endocrinol.* 2011;165(3):411-420.
16. Garel C, Leger J. Contribution of magnetic resonance imaging in non-tumoral hypopituitarism in children. *Horm Res.* 2007;67(4):194-202.
17. Maghnie M, Genovese E, Villa A, et al. Dynamic MRI in the congenital agenesis of the neural pituitary stalk syndrome: the role of the vascular pituitary stalk in predicting residual anterior pituitary function. *Clin Endocrinol (Oxf).* 1996;45(3):281-290.
18. Ultmann MC, Siegel SF, Hirsch WL, et al. Pituitary stalk and ectopic hyperintense T1 signal on magnetic resonance imaging. Implications for anterior pituitary dysfunction. *Am J Dis Child.* 1993;147(6):647-652.
19. Gainer H, Wray S. Cellular and molecular biology of oxytocin and vasopressin. In: Knobil E, Neill JD, eds. *The Physiology of Reproduction.* 2nd ed. New York, NY: Raven Press; 1994:1099-1129.
20. Chen LQ, Rose JP, Breslow E, et al. Crystal structure of a bovine neurophysin II dipeptide complex at 2.8 A determined from the single-wavelength anomalous scattering signal of an incorporated iodine atom. *Proc Natl Acad Sci U S A.* 1991;88(10):4240-4244.
21. Acher R. Evolution of neurohypophysial control of water homeostasis: integrative biology of molecular, cellular and organismal aspects. In: Saito T, Kurokawa K, Yoshida S, eds. *Neurohypophysis: Recent Progress of Vasopressin and Oxytocin Research.* Amsterdam: Elsevier; 1995:39-54.
22. Herman JP, Schafer MK, Watson SJ, Sherman TG. In situ hybridization analysis of arginine vasopressin gene transcription using intron-specific probes. *Mol Endocrinol.* 1991;5(10):1447-1456.
23. Majzoub J. Vasopressin biosynthesis. In: Schrier RW, ed. *Vasopressin.* New York, NY: Raven Press; 1985:465-474.
24. Sherman T, Akil H, Watson S. Vasopressin mRNA expression: a Northern and in situ hybridization analysis. In: Schrier RW, ed. *Vasopressin.* New York, NY: Raven Press; 1985:475-483.
25. Zingg HH, Lefebvre D, Almazan G. Regulation of vasopressin gene expression in rat hypothalamic neurons: response to osmotic stimulation. *J Biol Chem.* 1986;261(28):12956-12959.
26. Robinson AG, Roberts MM, Evron WA, et al. Hyponatremia in rats induces downregulation of vasopressin synthesis. *J Clin Invest.* 1990;86(4):1023-1029.
27. Roberts MM, Robinson AG, Hoffman GE, Fitzsimmons MD. Vasopressin transport regulation is coupled to the synthesis rate. *Neuroendocrinology.* 1991;53(4):416-422.
28. Lederis K, Jayasena K. Storage of neurohypophysial hormones and the mechanism for their release. In: Heller H, Pickering BT, eds. *Pharmacology of the Endocrine System and Related Drugs.* London: Pergamon; 1970:111-154.
29. Kurokawa H, Fujisawa I, Nakano Y, et al. Posterior lobe of the pituitary gland: correlation between signal intensity on T1-weighted MR images and vasopressin concentration. *Radiology.* 1998;207(1):79-83.
30. Sato N, Tanaka S, Tateno M, et al. Origin of posterior pituitary high intensity on T1-weighted magnetic resonance imaging. Immunohistochemical, electron microscopic, and magnetic resonance studies of posterior pituitary lobe of dehydrated rabbits. *Invest Radiol.* 1995;30(10):567-571.
31. Fitzsimmons MD, Roberts MM, Sherman TG, Robinson AG. Models of neurohypophyseal homeostasis. *Am J Physiol.* 1992;262(6 Pt 2):R1121-R1130.
32. Barberis C, Mouillac B, Durroux T. Structural bases of vasopressin/oxytocin receptor function. *J Endocrinol.* 1998;156(2):223-229.
33. Thrasher TN. Baroreceptor regulation of vasopressin and renin secretion: low-pressure versus high-pressure receptors. *Front Neuroendocrinol.* 1994;15(2):157-196.
34. Bishop VS, Thames MD, Schmid PG. Effects of bilateral vagal cold block on vasopressin in conscious dogs. *Am J Physiol.* 1984;246(4 Pt 2):R566-R569.
35. Thames MD, Schmid PG. Cardiopulmonary receptors with vagal afferents tonically inhibit ADH release in the dog. *Am J Physiol.* 1979;237(3):H299-H304.
36. Blessing WW, Sved AF, Reis DJ. Destruction of noradrenergic neurons in rabbit brainstem elevates plasma vasopressin, causing hypertension. *Science.* 1982;217(4560):661-663.
37. Blessing WW, Sved AF, Reis DJ. Arterial pressure and plasma vasopressin: regulation by neurons in the caudal ventrolateral medulla of the rabbit. *Clin Exp Hypertens A.* 1984;6(1–2):149-156.
38. Sved AF, Blessing WW, Reis DJ. Caudal ventrolateral medulla can alter vasopressin and arterial pressure. *Brain Res Bull.* 1985;14(3):227-232.
39. Schreihofer AM, Stricker EM, Sved AF. Chronic nucleus tractus solitarius lesions do not prevent hypovolemia-induced vasopressin secretion in rats. *Am J Physiol.* 1994;267(4 Pt 2):R965-R973.
40. Robertson GL. The regulation of vasopressin function in health and disease. *Recent Prog Horm Res.* 1976;33:333-385.

41. Callahan MF, Ludwig M, Tsai KP, et al. Baroreceptor input regulates osmotic control of central vasopressin secretion. *Neuroendocrinology.* 1997;65(4):238-245.

42. Pump B, Gabrielsen A, Christensen NJ, et al. Mechanisms of inhibition of vasopressin release during moderate antiorthostatic posture change in humans. *Am J Physiol.* 1999;277(1 Pt 2):R229-R235.

43. Johnson AK, Thunhorst RL. The neuroendocrinology of thirst and salt appetite: visceral sensory signals and mechanisms of central integration. *Front Neuroendocrinol.* 1997;18(3):292-353.

44. Baylis PH, Thompson CJ. Osmoregulation of vasopressin secretion and thirst in health and disease. *Clin Endocrinol (Oxf).* 1988;29(5):549-576.

45. Baylis PH. Investigation of suspected hypothalamic diabetes insipidus. *Clin Endocrinol (Oxf).* 1995;43(4):507-510.

46. Majzoub JA, Srivatsa A. Diabetes insipidus: clinical and basic aspects. *Pediatr Endocrinol Rev.* 2006;4(Suppl 1):60-65.

47. Nielsen S, Frokiaer J, Marples D, et al. Aquaporins in the kidney: from molecules to medicine. *Physiol Rev.* 2002;82(1):205-244.

48. Brown D. The ins and outs of aquaporin-2 trafficking. *Am J Physiol Renal Physiol.* 2003;284(5):F893-F901.

49. Eto K, Noda Y, Horikawa S, et al. Phosphorylation of aquaporin-2 regulates its water permeability. *J Biol Chem.* 2010;285(52):40777-40784.

50. Stocker SD, Sved AF, Stricker EM. Role of renin-angiotensin system in hypotension-evoked thirst: studies with hydralazine. *Am J Physiol Regul Integr Comp Physiol.* 2000;279(2):R576-R585.

51. Robertson G, Berl T. Water metabolism. In: Brenner BM, Rector FC Jr, eds. *The Kidney.* 3rd ed. Philadelphia, PA: WB Saunders; 1986:385-432.

52. Lindheimer MD, Davison JM. Osmoregulation, the secretion of arginine vasopressin and its metabolism during pregnancy. *Eur J Endocrinol.* 1995;132(2):133-143.

53. Lindheimer MD, Barron WM. Water metabolism and vasopressin secretion during pregnancy. *Baillieres Clin Obstet Gynaecol.* 1994;8(2):311-331.

54. Barron WM, Stamoutsos BA, Lindheimer MD. Role of volume in the regulation of vasopressin secretion during pregnancy in the rat. *J Clin Invest.* 1984;73(4):923-932.

55. Danielson LA, Kercher LJ, Conrad KP. Impact of gender and endothelin on renal vasodilation and hyperfiltration induced by relaxin in conscious rats. *Am J Physiol Regul Integr Comp Physiol.* 2000;279(4):R1298-R1304.

56. Danielson LA, Sherwood OD, Conrad KP. Relaxin is a potent renal vasodilator in conscious rats. *J Clin Invest.* 1999;103(4):525-533.

57. Novak J, Danielson LA, Kerchner LJ, et al. Relaxin is essential for renal vasodilation during pregnancy in conscious rats. *J Clin Invest.* 2001;107(11):1469-1475.

58. Schrier RW. Systemic arterial vasodilation, vasopressin, and vasopressinase in pregnancy. *J Am Soc Nephrol.* 2010;21(4):570-572.

59. Robinson AG, Fitzsimmons M. Diabetes insipidus. In: Mazzaferri EL, Bar RS, Kreisberg RA, eds. *Advances in Endocrinology and Metabolism.* St. Louis, MO: Mosby; 1994:261-296.

60. Davison JM, Sheills EA, Barron WM, et al. Changes in the metabolic clearance of vasopressin and in plasma vasopressinase throughout human pregnancy. *J Clin Invest.* 1989;83(4):1313-1318.

61. Davis PJ, Davis FB. Water excretion in the elderly. *Endocrinol Metab Clin North Am.* 1987;16(4):867-875.

62. Stout NR, Kenny RA, Baylis PH. A review of water balance in ageing in health and disease. *Gerontology.* 1999;45(2):61-66.

63. Tian Y, Serino R, Verbalis JG. Downregulation of renal vasopressin V2 receptor and aquaporin-2 expression parallels age-associated defects in urine concentration. *Am J Physiol Renal Physiol.* 2004;287(4):F797-F805.

64. Hvistendahl GM, Frokiaer J, Nielsen S, Djurhuus JC. Gender differences in nighttime plasma arginine vasopressin and delayed compensatory urine output in the elderly population after desmopressin. *J Urol.* 2007;178(6):2671-2676.

65. Schlanger LE, Bailey JL, Sands JM. Electrolytes in the aging. *Adv Chronic Kidney Dis.* 2010;17(4):308-319.

66. Fulop T Jr, Worum I, Csongor J, et al. Body composition in elderly people. II. Comparison of measured and predicted body composition in healthy elderly subjects. *Gerontology.* 1985;31(3):150-157.

67. Phillips PA, Johnston CI, Gray L. Disturbed fluid and electrolyte homoeostasis following dehydration in elderly people. *Age Ageing.* 1993;22(1):S26-S33.

68. Takamata A, Ito T, Yaegashi K, et al. Effect of an exercise-heat acclimation program on body fluid regulatory responses to dehydration in older men. *Am J Physiol.* 1999;277(4 Pt 2):R1041-R1050.

69. Crowe MJ, Forsling ML, Rolls BJ, et al. Altered water excretion in healthy elderly men. *Age Ageing.* 1987;16(5):285-293.

70. Sands JM. Urine concentrating and diluting ability during aging. *J Gerontol A Biol Sci Med Sci.* 2012;67(12):1352-1357.

71. Roberts MM, Robinson AG. Hyponatremia in the elderly: diagnosis and management. *Geriatr Nephrol Urol.* 1993;3(1):43-50.

72. Adrogue HJ, Madias NE. Hypernatremia. *N Engl J Med.* 2000;342(20):1493-1499.

73. Koskimies O, Pylkkanen J, Vilska J. Water intoxication in infants caused by the urine concentration test with vasopressin analogue (DDAVP). *Acta Paediatr Scand.* 1984;73(1):131-132.

74. Miller M, Dalakos T, Moses AM. Recognition of partial defects in antidiuretic hormone secretion. *Ann Intern Med.* 1970;73(5):721-729.

75. Baylis PH, Cheetham T. Diabetes insipidus. *Arch Dis Child.* 1998;79(1):84-89.

76. Robertson GL. Diabetes insipidus. *Endocrinol Metab Clin North Am.* 1995;24(3):549-572.

77. Zerbe RL, Robertson GL. A comparison of plasma vasopressin measurements with a standard indirect test in the differential diagnosis of polyuria. *N Engl J Med.* 1981;305(26):1539-1546.

78. De Bellis A, Colao A, Di Salle F, et al. A longitudinal study of vasopressin cell antibodies, posterior pituitary function, and magnetic resonance imaging evaluations in subclinical autoimmune central diabetes insipidus. *J Clin Endocrinol Metab.* 1999;84(9):3047-3051.

79. Baylis PH. Diabetes insipidus. *J R Coll Physicians Lond.* 1998;32(2):108-111.

80. Salata RA, Verbalis JG, Robinson AG. Cold water stimulation of oropharyngeal receptors in man inhibits release of vasopressin. *J Clin Endocrinol Metab.* 1987;65(3):561-567.

81. Decaux G, Prospert F, Namias B, Soupart A. Hyperuricemia as a clue for central diabetes insipidus (lack of V1 effect) in the differential diagnosis of polydipsia. *Am J Med.* 1997;103(5):376-382.

82. Morgenthaler NG, Struck J, Jochberger S, Dunser MW. Copeptin: clinical use of a new biomarker. *Trends Endocrinol Metab.* 2008;19(2):43-49.

83. Arslan A, Karaarslan E, Dincer A. High intensity signal of the posterior pituitary. A study with horizontal direction of frequency-encoding and fat suppression MR techniques. *Acta Radiol.* 1999;40(2):142-145.

84. Gudinchet F, Brunelle F, Barth MO, et al. MR imaging of the posterior hypophysis in children. *AJR Am J Roentgenol.* 1989;153(2):351-354.

85. Moses AM, Clayton B, Hochhauser L. Use of T1-weighted MR imaging to differentiate between primary polydipsia and central diabetes insipidus. *AJNR Am J Neuroradiol.* 1992;13(5):1273-1277.

86. Tien R, Kucharczyk J, Kucharczyk W. MR imaging of the brain in patients with diabetes insipidus. *AJNR Am J Neuroradiol.* 1991;12(3):533-542.

87. Brooks BS, el Gammal T, Allison JD, Hoffman WH. Frequency and variation of the posterior pituitary bright signal on MR images. *AJNR Am J Neuroradiol.* 1989;10(5):943-948.

88. Saeki N, Tokunaga H, Wagai N, et al. MRI of ectopic posterior pituitary bright spot with large adenomas: appearances and relationship to transient postoperative diabetes insipidus. *Neuroradiology.* 2003;45(10):713-716.

89. Maghnie M, Genovese E, Bernasconi S, et al. Persistent high MR signal of the posterior pituitary gland in central diabetes insipidus. *AJNR Am J Neuroradiol.* 1997;18(9):1749-1752.

90. Miyamoto S, Sasaki N, Tanabe Y. Magnetic resonance imaging in familial central diabetes insipidus. *Neuroradiology.* 1991;33(3):272-273.

91. Fujisawa I. Magnetic resonance imaging of the hypothalamic-neurohypophyseal system. *J Neuroendocrinol.* 2004;16(4):297-302.

92. Maghnie M, Villa A, Arico M, et al. Correlation between magnetic resonance imaging of posterior pituitary and neurohypophyseal function in children with diabetes insipidus. *J Clin Endocrinol Metab.* 1992;74(4):795-800.

93. Kubota T, Yamamoto T, Ozono K, Shimotsuji T. Hyperintensity of posterior pituitary on MR T1WI in a boy with central diabetes insipidus caused by missense mutation of neurophysin II gene. *Endocr J.* 2001;48(4):459-463.

94. Yamamoto T, Ishii T, Yoshioka K, et al. Transient central diabetes insipidus in pregnancy with a peculiar change in signal intensity on T1-weighted magnetic resonance images. *Intern Med.* 2003;42(6):513-516.

95. Heinbecker P, White HL. Hypothalamico-hypophysial system and its relation to water balance in the dog. *Am J Physiol.* 1941;133(3):582-593.

96. Verbalis J, Robinson A, Moses M. Postoperative and post-traumatic diabetes insipidus. In: Czernichow P, Robinson AG, eds. *Diabetes Insipidus in Man.* Basel, Switzerland: Karger; 1985:247-265.

97. Fujisawa I, Uokawa K, Horii N, et al. Bright pituitary stalk on MR T1-weighted image: damming up phenomenon of the neurosecretory granules. *Endocr J.* 2002;49(2):165-173.

98. Takahashi T, Miki Y, Takahashi JA, et al. Ectopic posterior pituitary high signal in preoperative and postoperative macroadenomas: dynamic MR imaging. *Eur J Radiol.* 2005;55(1):84-91.

99. Prosch H, Grois N, Prayer D, et al. Central diabetes insipidus as presenting symptom of Langerhans cell histiocytosis. *Pediatr Blood Cancer.* 2004;43(5):594-599.

100. Di Iorgi N, Allegri AE, Napoli F, et al. Central diabetes insipidus in children and young adults: etiological diagnosis and long-term outcome of idiopathic cases. *J Clin Endocrinol Metab.* 2014;99(4):1264-1272.

101. Di Iorgi N, Napoli F, Allegri AE, et al. Diabetes insipidus—diagnosis and management. *Horm Res Paediatr.* 2012;77(2):69-84.

102. Czernichow P, Garel C, Leger J. Thickened pituitary stalk on magnetic resonance imaging in children with central diabetes insipidus. *Horm Res.* 2000;53(Suppl 3):61-64.

103. Leger J, Velasquez A, Garel C, et al. Thickened pituitary stalk on magnetic resonance imaging in children with central diabetes insipidus. *J Clin Endocrinol Metab.* 1999;84(6):1954-1960.

104. Maghnie M. Diabetes insipidus. *Horm Res.* 2003;59(Suppl 1):42-54.

105. Bell NH. Endocrine complications of sarcoidosis. *Endocrinol Metab Clin North Am.* 1991;20(3):645-654.

106. Moses AM. Clinical and laboratory observations in the adult with diabetes insipidus and related syndromes. In: Czernichow P, Robinson AG, eds. *Diabetes Insipidus in Man.* Basel, Switzerland: Karger; 1985: 156-175.

107. de Leon J, Dadvand M, Canuso C, et al. Polydipsia and water intoxication in a long-term psychiatric hospital. *Biol Psychiatry.* 1996; 40(1):28-34.

108. Siegel AJ, Baldessarini RJ, Klepser MB, McDonald JC. Primary and drug-induced disorders of water homeostasis in psychiatric patients: principles of diagnosis and management. *Harv Rev Psychiatry.* 1998; 6(4):190-200.

109. Kishi Y, Kurosawa H, Endo S. Is propranolol effective in primary polydipsia? *Int J Psychiatry Med.* 1998;28(3):315-325.

110. Baylis PH, Robertson GL. Vasopressin function in familial cranial diabetes insipidus. *Postgrad Med J.* 1981;57(663):36-40.

111. Christensen JH, Rittig S. Familial neurohypophyseal diabetes insipidus: an update. *Semin Nephrol.* 2006;26(3):209-223.

112. Abu Libdeh A, Levy-Khademi F, Abdulhadi-Atwan M, et al. Autosomal recessive familial neurohypophyseal diabetes insipidus: onset in early infancy. *Eur J Endocrinol.* 2010;162(2):221-226.

113. Ghirardello S, Garre ML, Rossi A, Maghnie M. The diagnosis of children with central diabetes insipidus. *J Pediatr Endocrinol Metab.* 2007;20(3):359-375.

114. Birk J, Friberg MA, Prescianotto-Baschong C, et al. Dominant pro-vasopressin mutants that cause diabetes insipidus form disulfide-linked fibrillar aggregates in the endoplasmic reticulum. *J Cell Sci.* 2009;122(Pt 21):3994-4002.

115. Brachet C, Birk J, Christophe C, et al. Growth retardation in untreated autosomal dominant familial neurohypophyseal diabetes insipidus caused by one recurring and two novel mutations in the vasopressin-neurophysin II gene. *Eur J Endocrinol.* 2011;164(2):179-187.

116. Christensen JH, Siggaard C, Rittig S. Autosomal dominant familial neurohypophyseal diabetes insipidus. *APMIS Suppl.* 2003;(109): 92-95.

117. Chitturi S, Harris M, Thomsett MJ, et al. Utility of AVP gene testing in familial neurohypophyseal diabetes insipidus. *Clin Endocrinol (Oxf).* 2008;69(6):926-930.

118. Rohayem J, Ehlers C, Wiedemann B, et al. Diabetes and neurodegeneration in Wolfram syndrome: a multicenter study of phenotype and genotype. *Diabetes Care.* 2011;34(7):1503-1510.

119. Hilson JB, Merchant SN, Adams JC, Joseph JT. Wolfram syndrome: a clinicopathologic correlation. *Acta Neuropathol.* 2009;118(3):415-428.

120. Karavitaki N, Brufani C, Warner JT, et al. Craniopharyngiomas in children and adults: systematic analysis of 121 cases with long-term follow-up. *Clin Endocrinol (Oxf).* 2005;62(4):397-409.

121. Smith D, Finucane F, Phillips J, et al. Abnormal regulation of thirst and vasopressin secretion following surgery for craniopharyngioma. *Clin Endocrinol (Oxf).* 2004;61(2):273-279.

122. Vuillermet P, Cauliez B, Freger P, et al. Simultaneous suprasellar and pineal germ cell tumors in five late stage adolescents: endocrinological studies and prolonged follow-up. *J Pediatr Endocrinol Metab.* 2008; 21(12):1169-1178.

123. Alter CA, Bilaniuk LT. Utility of magnetic resonance imaging in the evaluation of the child with central diabetes insipidus. *J Pediatr Endocrinol Metab.* 2002;15(Suppl 2):681-687.

124. De Buyst J, Massa G, Christophe C, et al. Clinical, hormonal and imaging findings in 27 children with central diabetes insipidus. *Eur J Pediatr.* 2007;166(1):43-49.

125. Kovacs K. Metastatic cancer of the pituitary gland. *Oncology.* 1973; 27(6):533-542.

126. Max MB, Deck MD, Rottenberg DA. Pituitary metastasis: incidence in cancer patients and clinical differentiation from pituitary adenoma. *Neurology.* 1981;31(8):998-1002.

127. Basaria S, Westra WH, Brem H, Salvatori R. Metastatic renal cell carcinoma to the pituitary presenting with hyperprolactinemia. *J Endocrinol Invest.* 2004;27(5):471-474.

128. Fassett DR, Couldwell WT. Metastases to the pituitary gland. *Neurosurg Focus.* 2004;16(4):E8.

129. Komninos J, Vlassopoulou V, Protopapa D, et al. Tumors metastatic to the pituitary gland: case report and literature review. *J Clin Endocrinol Metab.* 2004;89(2):574-580.

130. Dutta P, Bhansali A, Singh P, Bhat MH. Suprasellar tubercular abscess presenting as panhypopituitarism: a common lesion in an uncommon site with a brief review of literature. *Pituitary.* 2006;9(1):73-77.

131. Pascual JM, Gonzalez-Llanos F, Roda JM. Primary hypothalamic-third ventricle lymphoma. Case report and review of the literature. *Neurocirugia (Astur).* 2002;13(4):305-310.

132. Agarwal S, Gockerman JP, Aldous MD, Swaim MW. Primary central nervous system lymphoma, presenting as diabetes insipidus, as a sequela of hepatitis C. *Am J Med.* 1999;107(3):303-304.

133. Castagnola C, Morra E, Bernasconi P, et al. Acute myeloid leukemia and diabetes insipidus: results in 5 patients. *Acta Haematol.* 1995;93(1):1-4.

134. Foresti V, Casati O, Villa A, et al. Central diabetes insipidus due to acute monocytic leukemia: case report and review of the literature. *J Endocrinol Invest.* 1992;15(2):127-130.

135. Dilek I, Uysal A, Demirer T, et al. Acute myeloblastic leukemia associated with hyperleukocytosis and diabetes insipidus. *Leuk Lymphoma.* 1998;30(5-6):657-660.

136. Nieboer P, Vellenga E, Adriaanse R, van de Loosdrecht AA. Central diabetes insipidus preceding acute myeloid leukemia with t(3;12) (q26;p12). *Neth J Med.* 2000;56(2):45-47.

137. Ra'anani P, Shpilberg O, Berezin M, Ben-Bassat I. Acute leukemia relapse presenting as central diabetes insipidus. *Cancer.* 1994;73(9): 2312-2316.

138. Demaerel P, Van Gool S. Paediatric neuroradiological aspects of Langerhans cell histiocytosis. *Neuroradiology.* 2008;50(1):85-92.

139. Donadieu J, Rolon MA, Thomas C, et al. Endocrine involvement in pediatric-onset Langerhans' cell histiocytosis: a population-based study. *J Pediatr.* 2004;144(3):344-350.

140. Abla O, Weitzman S, Minkov M, et al. Diabetes insipidus in Langerhans cell histiocytosis: when is treatment indicated? *Pediatr Blood Cancer.* 2009;52(5):555-556.

141. Amato MC, Elias LL, Elias J, et al. Endocrine disorders in pediatric-onset Langerhans cell histiocytosis. *Horm Metab Res.* 2006;38(11): 746-751.

142. Tabuena RP, Nagai S, Handa T, et al. Diabetes insipidus from neurosarcoidosis: long-term follow-up for more than eight years. *Intern Med.* 2004;43(10):960-966.

143. Bianchi A, Mormando M, Doglietto F, et al. Hypothalamitis: a diagnostic and therapeutic challenge. *Pituitary.* 2014;17(3):197-202.

144. Caputo C, Bazargan A, McKelvie PA, et al. Hypophysitis due to IgG4-related disease responding to treatment with azathioprine: an alternative to corticosteroid therapy. *Pituitary.* 2014;17(3):251-256.

145. Shimatsu A, Oki Y, Fujisawa I, Sano T. Pituitary and stalk lesions (infundibulo-hypophysitis) associated with immunoglobulin G4-related systemic disease: an emerging clinical entity. *Endocr J.* 2009; 56(9):1033-1041.

146. Abe T. Lymphocytic infundibulo-neurohypophysitis and infundibulo-panhypophysitis regarded as lymphocytic hypophysitis variant. *Brain Tumor Pathol.* 2008;25(2):59-66.

147. Maghnie M, Ghirardello S, De Bellis A, et al. Idiopathic central diabetes insipidus in children and young adults is commonly associated with vasopressin-cell antibodies and markers of autoimmunity. *Clin Endocrinol (Oxf).* 2006;65(4):470-478.

148. Bononi PL, Robinson AG. Central diabetes insipidus: management in the postoperative period. *Endocrinologist.* 1991;1(3):180-186.

149. Buonocore CM, Robinson AG. The diagnosis and management of diabetes insipidus during medical emergencies. *Endocrinol Metab Clin North Am.* 1993;22(2):411-423.

150. Kristof RA, Rother M, Neuloh G, Klingmuller D. Incidence, clinical manifestations, and course of water and electrolyte metabolism disturbances following transsphenoidal pituitary adenoma surgery: a prospective observational study. *J Neurosurg.* 2009;111(3):555-562.

151. Loh JA, Verbalis JG. Disorders of water and salt metabolism associated with pituitary disease. *Endocrinol Metab Clin North Am.* 2008;37(1):213-234, x.

152. Fatemi N, Dusick JR, Mattozo C, et al. Pituitary hormonal loss and recovery after transsphenoidal adenoma removal. *Neurosurgery.* 2008; 63(4):709-718, discussion 718-709.

153. Sigounas DG, Sharpless JL, Cheng DM, et al. Predictors and incidence of central diabetes insipidus after endoscopic pituitary surgery. *Neurosurgery.* 2008;62(1):71-78, discussion 78-79.

154. Gardner PA, Kassam AB, Snyderman CH, et al. Outcomes following endoscopic, expanded endonasal resection of suprasellar craniopharyngiomas: a case series. *J Neurosurg.* 2008;109(1):6-16.

155. Cusick JF, Hagen TC, Findling JW. Inappropriate secretion of antidiuretic hormone after transsphenoidal surgery for pituitary tumors. *N Engl J Med.* 1984;311(1):36-38.

156. Ultmann MC, Hoffman GE, Nelson PB, Robinson AG. Transient hyponatremia after damage to the neurohypophyseal tracts. *Neuroendocrinology.* 1992;56(6):803-811.

157. Olson BR, Rubino D, Gumowski J, Oldfield EH. Isolated hyponatremia after transsphenoidal pituitary surgery. *J Clin Endocrinol Metab.* 1995; 80(1):85-91.

158. Olson BR, Gumowski J, Rubino D, Oldfield EH. Pathophysiology of hyponatremia after transsphenoidal pituitary surgery. *J Neurosurg.* 1997;87(4):499-507.

159. Sata A, Hizuka N, Kawamata T, et al. Hyponatremia after transsphenoidal surgery for hypothalamo-pituitary tumors. *Neuroendocrinology.* 2006;83(2):117-122.

160. Hadjizacharia P, Beale EO, Inaba K, et al. Acute diabetes insipidus in severe head injury: a prospective study. *J Am Coll Surg.* 2008;207(4): 477-484.

161. Einaudi S, Bondone C. The effects of head trauma on hypothalamic-pituitary function in children and adolescents. *Curr Opin Pediatr.* 2007;19(4):465-470.

162. Boughey JC, Yost MJ, Bynoe RP. Diabetes insipidus in the head-injured patient. *Am Surg.* 2004;70(6):500-503.

163. Benvenga S, Campenni A, Ruggeri RM, Trimarchi F. Clinical review 113: hypopituitarism secondary to head trauma. *J Clin Endocrinol Metab.* 2000;85(4):1353-1361.

164. Agha A, Sherlock M, Phillips J, et al. The natural history of post-traumatic neurohypophysial dysfunction. *Eur J Endocrinol.* 2005;152(3):371-377.

165. Agha A, Thornton E, O'Kelly P, et al. Posterior pituitary dysfunction after traumatic brain injury. *J Clin Endocrinol Metab.* 2004;89(12):5987-5992.

166. Crowley RK, Sherlock M, Agha A, et al. Clinical insights into adipsic diabetes insipidus: a large case series. *Clin Endocrinol (Oxf).* 2007;66(4):475-482.

167. Mavrakis AN, Tritos NA. Diabetes insipidus with deficient thirst: report of a patient and review of the literature. *Am J Kidney Dis.* 2008;51(5):851-859.

168. DeRubertis FR, Michelis MF, Beck N, et al. "Essential" hypernatremia due to ineffective osmotic and intact volume regulation of vasopressin secretion. *J Clin Invest.* 1971;50(1):97-111.

169. Halter JB, Goldberg AP, Robertson GL, Porte D Jr. Selective osmoreceptor dysfunction in the syndrome of chronic hypernatremia. *J Clin Endocrinol Metab.* 1977;44(4):609-616.

170. Oh MS, Carroll HJ. Essential hypernatremia: is there such a thing? *Nephron.* 1994;67(2):144-145.

171. Dominguez-Roldan JM, Garcia-Alfaro C, Diaz-Parejo P, et al. Risk factors associated with diabetes insipidus in brain dead patients. *Transplant Proc.* 2002;34(1):13-14.

172. Saner FH, Kavuk I, Lang H, et al. Organ protective management of the brain-dead donor. *Eur J Med Res.* 2004;9(10):485-490.

173. Chamorro C, Falcon JA, Michelena JC. Controversial points in organ donor management. *Transplant Proc.* 2009;41(8):3473-3475.

174. Robinson AG, Verbalis JG. Diabetes insipidus. *Curr Ther Endocrinol Metab.* 1997;6:1-7.

175. Robinson AG. DDAVP in the treatment of central diabetes insipidus. *N Engl J Med.* 1976;294(10):507-511.

176. Oiso Y, Robertson GL, Norgaard JP, Juul KV. Clinical review: treatment of neurohypophyseal diabetes insipidus. *J Clin Endocrinol Metab.* 2013;98(10):3958-3967.

177. Juul KV, Van Herzeele C, De Bruyne P, et al. Desmopressin melt improves response and compliance compared with tablet in treatment of primary monosymptomatic nocturnal enuresis. *Eur J Pediatr.* 2013;172(9):1235-1242.

178. Lam KS, Wat MS, Choi KL, et al. Pharmacokinetics, pharmacodynamics, long-term efficacy and safety of oral 1-deamino-8-D-arginine vasopressin in adult patients with central diabetes insipidus. *Br J Clin Pharmacol.* 1996;42(3):379-385.

179. Richardson DW, Robinson AG. Desmopressin. *Ann Intern Med.* 1985;103(2):228-239.

180. Juul KV, Erichsen L, Robertson GL. Temporal delays and individual variation in antidiuretic response to desmopressin. *Am J Physiol Renal Physiol.* 2013;304(3):F268-F278.

181. Juul KV, Klein BM, Sandstrom R, et al. Gender difference in antidiuretic response to desmopressin. *Am J Physiol Renal Physiol.* 2011;300(5):F1116-F1122.

182. Pokracki FJ, Robinson AG, Seif SM. Chlorpropamide effect: measurement of neurophysin and vasopressin in humans and rats. *Metabolism.* 1981;30(1):72-78.

183. Zelenina M, Christensen BM, Palmer J, et al. Prostaglandin E(2) interaction with AVP: effects on AQP2 phosphorylation and distribution. *Am J Physiol Renal Physiol.* 2000;278(3):F388-F394.

184. Rivkees SA, Dunbar N, Wilson TA. The management of central diabetes insipidus in infancy: desmopressin, low renal solute load formula, thiazide diuretics. *J Pediatr Endocrinol Metab.* 2007;20(4):459-469.

185. Vande Walle J, Stockner M, Raes A, Norgaard JP. Desmopressin 30 years in clinical use: a safety review. *Curr Drug Saf.* 2007;2(3):232-238.

186. Verrua E, Mantovani G, Ferrante E, et al. Severe water intoxication secondary to the concomitant intake of non-steroidal anti-inflammatory drugs and desmopressin: a case report and review of the literature. *Hormones.* 2013;12(1):135-141.

187. Campigotto MJ, Koczmara C, Greenall J, Hyland S. Desmopressin (dDAVP) incident signals the need for enhanced monitoring protocols. *Dynamics.* 2008;19(3):34-36.

188. Ralston C, Butt W. Continuous vasopressin replacement in diabetes insipidus. *Arch Dis Child.* 1990;65(8):896-897.

189. Chanson P, Jedynak CP, Dabrowski G, et al. Ultralow doses of vasopressin in the management of diabetes insipidus. *Crit Care Med.* 1987;15(1):44-46.

190. Lee YJ, Yang D, Shyur SD, Chiu NC. Neurogenic diabetes insipidus in a child with fatal coxsackie virus B1 encephalitis. *J Pediatr Endocrinol Metab.* 1995;8(4):301-304.

191. Lugo N, Silver P, Nimkoff L, et al. Diagnosis and management algorithm of acute onset of central diabetes insipidus in critically ill children. *J Pediatr Endocrinol Metab.* 1997;10(6):633-639.

192. Arima H, Wakabayashi T, Nagatani T, et al. Adipsia increases risk of death in patients with central diabetes insipidus. *Endocr J.* 2014;61(2):143-148.

193. Bode HH, Harley BM, Crawford JD. Restoration of normal drinking behavior by chlorpropamide in patients with hypodipsia and diabetes insipidus. *Am J Med.* 1971;51(3):304-313.

194. Nandi M, Harrington AR. Successful treatment of hypernatremic thirst deficiency with chlorpropamide. *Clin Nephrol.* 1978;10(3):90-95.

195. Ball SG, Vaidja B, Baylis PH. Hypothalamic adipsic syndrome: diagnosis and management. *Clin Endocrinol (Oxf).* 1997;47(4):405-409.

196. Hameed S, Mendoza-Cruz AC, Neville KA, et al. Home blood sodium monitoring, sliding-scale fluid prescription and subcutaneous DDAVP for infantile diabetes insipidus with impaired thirst mechanism. *Int J Pediatr Endocrinol.* 2012;2012(1):18.

197. Oiso Y. Transient diabetes insipidus during pregnancy. *Intern Med.* 2003;42(6):459-460.

198. Barron WM, Cohen LH, Ulland LA, et al. Transient vasopressin-resistant diabetes insipidus of pregnancy. *N Engl J Med.* 1984;310(7):442-444.

199. Kennedy S, Hall PM, Seymour AE, Hague WM. Transient diabetes insipidus and acute fatty liver of pregnancy. *Br J Obstet Gynaecol.* 1994;101(5):387-391.

200. Krege J, Katz VL, Bowes WA Jr. Transient diabetes insipidus of pregnancy. *Obstet Gynecol Surv.* 1989;44(11):789-795.

201. Krysiak R. Kobielusz-Gembala I, Okopien B. Recurrent pregnancy-induced diabetes insipidus in a woman with hemochromatosis. *Endocr J.* 2010;57(12):1023-1028.

202. Hashimoto M, Ogura T, Otsuka F, et al. Manifestation of subclinical diabetes insipidus due to pituitary tumor during pregnancy. *Endocr J.* 1996;43(5):577-583.

203. Kalelioglu I, Kubat Uzum A, Yildirim A, et al. Transient gestational diabetes insipidus diagnosed in successive pregnancies: review of pathophysiology, diagnosis, treatment, and management of delivery. *Pituitary.* 2007;10(1):87-93.

204. Amico J. Diabetes insipidus and pregnancy. In: Czernichow P, Robinson AG, eds. *Diabetes Insipidus in Man.* Basel, Switzerland: Karger; 1985:266-277.

205. Sherer DM, Cutler J, Santoso P, et al. Severe hypernatremia after cesarean delivery secondary to transient diabetes insipidus of pregnancy. *Obstet Gynecol.* 2003;102(5 Pt 2):1166-1168.

206. Atmaca H, Tanriverdi F, Gokce C, et al. Posterior pituitary function in Sheehan's syndrome. *Eur J Endocrinol.* 2007;156(5):563-567.

207. Laway BA, Mir SA, Dar MI, Zargar AH. Sheehan's syndrome with central diabetes insipidus. *Arq Bras Endocrinol Metabol.* 2011;55(2):171-174.

208. Edwards CR, Kitau MJ, Chard T, Besser GM. Vasopressin analogue DDAVP in diabetes insipidus: clinical and laboratory studies. *Br Med J.* 1973;3(5876):375-378.

209. Davison JM, Sheills EA, Philips PR, et al. Metabolic clearance of vasopressin and an analogue resistant to vasopressinase in human pregnancy. *Am J Physiol.* 1993;264(2 Pt 2):F348-F353.

210. Kallen BA, Carlsson SS, Bengtsson BK. Diabetes insipidus and use of desmopressin (Minirin) during pregnancy. *Eur J Endocrinol.* 1995;132(2):144-146.

211. Ray JG. DDAVP use during pregnancy: an analysis of its safety for mother and child. *Obstet Gynecol Surv.* 1998;53(7):450-455.

212. Bichet DG. Nephrogenic diabetes insipidus. *Am J Med.* 1998;105(5):431-442.

213. van Lieburg AF, Knoers NV, Monnens LA. Clinical presentation and follow-up of 30 patients with congenital nephrogenic diabetes insipidus. *J Am Soc Nephrol.* 1999;10(9):1958-1964.

214. Bichet DG. Hereditary polyuric disorders: new concepts and differential diagnosis. *Semin Nephrol.* 2006;26(3):224-233.

215. Spanakis E, Milord E, Gragnoli C. AVPR2 variants and mutations in nephrogenic diabetes insipidus: review and missense mutation significance. *J Cell Physiol.* 2008;217(3):605-617.

216. Bichet DG. Physiopathology of hereditary polyuric states: a molecular view of renal function. *Swiss Med Wkly.* 2012;142:w13613.

217. Schoneberg T, Schulz A, Biebermann H, et al. V2 vasopressin receptor dysfunction in nephrogenic diabetes insipidus caused by different molecular mechanisms. *Hum Mutat.* 1998;12(3):196-205.

218. Satoh M, Ogikubo S, Yoshizawa-Ogasawara A. Correlation between clinical phenotypes and X-inactivation patterns in six female carriers with heterozygote vasopressin type 2 receptor gene mutations. *Endocr J.* 2008;55(2):277-284.

219. Wildin RS, Cogdell DE. Clinical utility of direct mutation testing for congenital nephrogenic diabetes insipidus in families. *Pediatrics.* 1999;103(3):632-639.

220. Sands JM, Bichet DG. Nephrogenic diabetes insipidus. *Ann Intern Med.* 2006;144(3):186-194.

221. Iolascon A, Aglio V, Tamma G, et al. Characterization of two novel missense mutations in the AQP2 gene causing nephrogenic diabetes insipidus. *Nephron Physiol.* 2007;105(3):33-41.

222. van Os CH, Deen PM. Aquaporin-2 water channel mutations causing nephrogenic diabetes insipidus. *Proc Assoc Am Physicians*. 1998; 110(5):395-400.

223. Robben JH, Knoers NV, Deen PM. Cell biological aspects of the vasopressin type-2 receptor and aquaporin 2 water channel in nephrogenic diabetes insipidus. *Am J Physiol Renal Physiol*. 2006;291(2): F257-F270.

224. Morello JP, Bichet DG. Nephrogenic diabetes insipidus. *Annu Rev Physiol*. 2001;63:607-630.

225. Bedford JJ, Leader JP, Jing R, et al. Amiloride restores renal medullary osmolytes in lithium-induced nephrogenic diabetes insipidus. *Am J Physiol Renal Physiol*. 2008;294(4):F812-F820.

226. Marples D, Frokiaer J, Knepper MA, Nielsen S. Disordered water channel expression and distribution in acquired nephrogenic diabetes insipidus. *Proc Assoc Am Physicians*. 1998;110(5):401-406.

227. Bendz H, Sjodin I, Aurell M. Renal function on and off lithium in patients treated with lithium for 15 years or more. A controlled, prospective lithium-withdrawal study. *Nephrol Dial Transplant*. 1996;11(3): 457-460.

228. Bendz H, Aurell M. Drug-induced diabetes insipidus: incidence, prevention and management. *Drug Saf*. 1999;21(6):449-456.

229. Faerch M, Christensen JH, Corydon TJ, et al. Partial nephrogenic diabetes insipidus caused by a novel mutation in the AVPR2 gene. *Clin Endocrinol (Oxf)*. 2008;68(3):395-403.

230. Postina R, Ufer E, Pfeiffer R, et al. Misfolded vasopressin V2 receptors caused by extracellular point mutations entail congenital nephrogenic diabetes insipidus. *Mol Cell Endocrinol*. 2000;164(1-2):31-39.

231. Magaldi AJ. New insights into the paradoxical effect of thiazides in diabetes insipidus therapy. *Nephrol Dial Transplant*. 2000;15(12): 1903-1905.

232. Loffing J. Paradoxical antidiuretic effect of thiazides in diabetes insipidus: another piece in the puzzle. *J Am Soc Nephrol*. 2004;15(11): 2948-2950.

233. Bendz H, Aurell M, Balldin J, et al. Kidney damage in long-term lithium patients: a cross-sectional study of patients with 15 years or more on lithium. *Nephrol Dial Transplant*. 1994;9(9):1250-1254.

234. Singer I, Oster JR, Fishman LM. The management of diabetes insipidus in adults. *Arch Intern Med*. 1997;157(12):1293-1301.

235. Nguyen MK, Nielsen S, Kurtz I. Molecular pathogenesis of nephrogenic diabetes insipidus. *Clin Exp Nephrol*. 2003;7(1):9-17.

236. Robben JH, Deen PM. Pharmacological chaperones in nephrogenic diabetes insipidus: possibilities for clinical application. *BioDrugs*. 2007; 21(3):157-166.

237. Jean-Alphonse F, Perkovska S, Frantz MC, et al. Biased agonist pharmacochaperones of the AVP V2 receptor may treat congenital nephrogenic diabetes insipidus. *J Am Soc Nephrol*. 2009;20(10):2190-2203.

238. Robben JH, Kortenoeven ML, Sze M, et al. Intracellular activation of vasopressin V2 receptor mutants in nephrogenic diabetes insipidus by nonpeptide agonists. *Proc Natl Acad Sci U S A*. 2009;106(29): 12195-12200.

239. Takahashi K, Makita N, Manaka K, et al. V2 vasopressin receptor (V2R) mutations in partial nephrogenic diabetes insipidus highlight protean agonism of V2R antagonists. *J Biol Chem*. 2012;287(3):2099-2106.

240. Bichet DG. Vasopressin receptor mutations in nephrogenic diabetes insipidus. *Semin Nephrol*. 2008;28(3):245-251.

241. Moug SJ, McKee RF, O'Reilly DS, et al. The perioperative challenge of nephrogenic diabetes insipidus: a multidisciplinary approach. *Surgeon*. 2005;3(2):89-94.

242. Bryant WP, O'Marcaigh AS, Ledger GA, Zimmerman D. Aqueous vasopressin infusion during chemotherapy in patients with diabetes insipidus. *Cancer*. 1994;74(9):2589-2592.

243. Bagshaw SM, Townsend DR, McDermid RC. Disorders of sodium and water balance in hospitalized patients. *Can J Anaesth*. 2009;56(2): 151-167.

244. Lien YH, Shapiro JI, Chan L. Effects of hypernatremia on organic brain osmoles. *J Clin Invest*. 1990;85(5):1427-1435.

245. Schwartz WB, Bennett W, Curelop S, Bartter FC. A syndrome of renal sodium loss and hyponatremia probably resulting from inappropriate secretion of antidiuretic hormone. *Am J Med*. 1957;23(4):529-542.

246. Bartter FC, Schwartz WB. The syndrome of inappropriate secretion of antidiuretic hormone. *Am J Med*. 1967;42(5):790-806.

247. Upadhyay A, Jaber BL, Madias NE. Incidence and prevalence of hyponatremia. *Am J Med*. 2006;119(7 Suppl 1):S30-S35.

248. Wald R, Jaber BL, Price LL, et al. Impact of hospital-associated hyponatremia on selected outcomes. *Arch Intern Med*. 2010;170(3): 294-302.

249. Hawkins RC. Age and gender as risk factors for hyponatremia and hypernatremia. *Clin Chim Acta*. 2003;337(1-2):169-172.

250. Miller M, Morley JE, Rubenstein LZ. Hyponatremia in a nursing home population. *J Am Geriatr Soc*. 1995;43(12):1410-1413.

251. Arieff AI. Hyponatremia, convulsions, respiratory arrest, and permanent brain damage after elective surgery in healthy women. *N Engl J Med*. 1986;314(24):1529-1535.

252. Sterns RH, Riggs JE, Schochet SS Jr. Osmotic demyelination syndrome following correction of hyponatremia. *N Engl J Med*. 1986;314(24): 1535-1542.

253. Anderson RJ, Chung HM, Kluge R, Schrier RW. Hyponatremia: a prospective analysis of its epidemiology and the pathogenetic role of vasopressin. *Ann Intern Med*. 1985;102(2):164-168.

254. Corona G, Giuliani C, Parenti G, et al. Moderate hyponatremia is associated with increased risk of mortality: evidence from a meta-analysis. *PLoS One*. 2013;8(12):e80451.

255. Weisberg LS. Pseudohyponatremia: a reappraisal. *Am J Med*. 1989; 86(3):315-318.

256. Katz MA. Hyperglycemia-induced hyponatremia—calculation of expected serum sodium depression. *N Engl J Med*. 1973;289(16): 843-844.

257. Hillier TA, Abbott RD, Barrett EJ. Hyponatremia: evaluating the correction factor for hyperglycemia. *Am J Med*. 1999;106(4):399-403.

258. Rose BD. New approach to disturbances in the plasma sodium concentration. *Am J Med*. 1986;81(6):1033-1040.

259. Spital A. Diuretic-induced hyponatremia. *Am J Nephrol*. 1999;19(4): 447-452.

260. Gross PA, Pehrisch H, Rascher W, et al. Pathogenesis of clinical hyponatremia: observations of vasopressin and fluid intake in 100 hyponatremic medical patients. *Eur J Clin Invest*. 1987;17(2):123-129.

261. Schrier RW. Body fluid volume regulation in health and disease: a unifying hypothesis. *Ann Intern Med*. 1990;113(2):155-159.

262. Demanet JC, Bonnyns M, Bleiberg H, Stevens-Rocmans C. Coma due to water intoxication in beer drinkers. *Lancet*. 1971;2(7734): 1115-1117.

263. Cooke CR, Turin MD, Walker WG. The syndrome of inappropriate antidiuretic hormone secretion (SIADH): pathophysiologic mechanisms in solute and volume regulation. *Medicine (Baltimore)*. 1979;58(3):240-251.

264. Grantham J, Linshaw M. The effect of hyponatremia on the regulation of intracellular volume and solute composition. *Circ Res*. 1984;54(5): 483-491.

265. Yannet H. Changes in the brain resulting from depletion of extracellular electrolytes. *Am J Physiol*. 1940;128(4):683-689.

266. Holliday MA, Kalayci MN, Harrah J. Factors that limit brain volume changes in response to acute and sustained hyper- and hyponatremia. *J Clin Invest*. 1968;47(8):1916-1928.

267. Garcia-Perez A, Burg MB. Renal medullary organic osmolytes. *Physiol Rev*. 1991;71(4):1081-1115.

268. Heilig CW, Stromski ME, Blumenfeld JD, et al. Characterization of the major brain osmolytes that accumulate in salt-loaded rats. *Am J Physiol*. 1989;257(6 Pt 2):F1108-F1116.

269. Lien YH, Shapiro JI, Chan L. Study of brain electrolytes and organic osmolytes during correction of chronic hyponatremia. Implications for the pathogenesis of central pontine myelinolysis. *J Clin Invest*. 1991;88(1):303-309.

270. Verbalis JG, Gullans SR. Hyponatremia causes large sustained reductions in brain content of multiple organic osmolytes in rats. *Brain Res*. 1991;567(2):274-282.

271. Videen JS, Michaelis T, Pinto P, Ross BD. Human cerebral osmolytes during chronic hyponatremia. A proton magnetic resonance spectroscopy study. *J Clin Invest*. 1995;95(2):788-793.

272. Gullans SR, Verbalis JG. Control of brain volume during hyperosmolar and hypoosmolar conditions. *Annu Rev Med*. 1993;44:289-301.

273. Graber M, Corish D. The electrolytes in hyponatremia. *Am J Kidney Dis*. 1991;18(5):527-545.

274. Smith MJ Jr, Cowley MJ Jr, Guyton AC, Manning RD Jr. Acute and chronic effects of vasopressin on blood pressure, electrolytes, and fluid volumes. *Am J Physiol*. 1979;237(3):F232-F240.

275. Verbalis JG. Pathogenesis of hyponatremia in an experimental model of the syndrome of inappropriate antidiuresis. *Am J Physiol*. 1994;267(6 Pt 2):R1617-R1625.

276. Southgate HJ, Burke BJ, Walters G. Body space measurements in the hyponatraemia of carcinoma of the bronchus: evidence for the chronic "sick cell" syndrome? *Ann Clin Biochem*. 1992;29(Pt 1):90-95.

277. Clark BA, Shannon RP, Rosa RM, Epstein FH. Increased susceptibility to thiazide-induced hyponatremia in the elderly. *J Am Soc Nephrol*. 1994;5(4):1106-1111.

278. Chung HM, Kluge R, Schrier RW, Anderson RJ. Clinical assessment of extracellular fluid volume in hyponatremia. *Am J Med*. 1987;83(5): 905-908.

279. Michelis MF, Fusco RD, Bragdon RW, Davis BB. Reset of osmoreceptors in association with normovolemic hyponatremia. *Am J Med Sci*. 1974; 267(5):267-273.

280. Beck LH. Hypouricemia in the syndrome of inappropriate secretion of antidiuretic hormone. *N Engl J Med*. 1979;301(10):528-530.

281. Zerbe R, Stropes L, Robertson G. Vasopressin function in the syndrome of inappropriate antidiuresis. *Annu Rev Med*. 1980;31:315-327.

282. List AF, Hainsworth JD, Davis BW, et al. The syndrome of inappropriate secretion of antidiuretic hormone (SIADH) in small-cell lung cancer. *J Clin Oncol*. 1986;4(8):1191-1198.

283. Maurer LH, O'Donnell JF, Kennedy S, et al. Human neurophysins in carcinoma of the lung: relation to histology, disease stage, response rate, survival, and syndrome of inappropriate antidiuretic hormone secretion. *Cancer Treat Rep*. 1983;67(11):971-976.

284. Ferlito A, Rinaldo A, Devaney KO. Syndrome of inappropriate antidiuretic hormone secretion associated with head neck cancers: review of the literature. *Ann Otol Rhinol Laryngol.* 1997;106(10 Pt 1): 878-883.

285. Kavanagh BD, Halperin EC, Rosenbaum LC, et al. Syndrome of inappropriate secretion of antidiuretic hormone in a patient with carcinoma of the nasopharynx. *Cancer.* 1992;69(6):1315-1319.

286. Berghmans T, Paesmans M, Body JJ. A prospective study on hyponatraemia in medical cancer patients: epidemiology, aetiology and differential diagnosis. *Support Care Cancer.* 2000;8(3):192-197.

287. Moses AM, Miller M. Drug-induced dilutional hyponatremia. *N Engl J Med.* 1974;291(23):1234-1239.

288. Wilkinson TJ, Begg EJ, Winter AC, Sainsbury R. Incidence and risk factors for hyponatraemia following treatment with fluoxetine or paroxetine in elderly people. *Br J Clin Pharmacol.* 1999;47(2):211-217.

289. Burgess C, O'Donohoe A, Gill M. Agony and ecstasy: a review of MDMA effects and toxicity. *Eur Psychiatry.* 2000;15(5):287-294.

290. Kelestimur H, Leach RM, Ward JP, Forsling ML. Vasopressin and oxytocin release during prolonged environmental hypoxia in the rat. *Thorax.* 1997;52(1):84-88.

291. Tang WW, Kaptein EM, Feinstein EI, Massry SG. Hyponatremia in hospitalized patients with the acquired immunodeficiency syndrome (AIDS) and the AIDS-related complex. *Am J Med.* 1993;94(2):169-174.

292. Yeung KT, Chan M, Chan CK. The safety of i.v. pentamidine administered in an ambulatory setting. *Chest.* 1996;110(1):136-140.

293. Miller M, Hecker MS, Friedlander DA, Carter JM. Apparent idiopathic hyponatremia in an ambulatory geriatric population. *J Am Geriatr Soc.* 1996;44(4):404-408.

294. Hirshberg B, Ben-Yehuda A. The syndrome of inappropriate antidiuretic hormone secretion in the elderly. *Am J Med.* 1997;103(4): 270-273.

295. Ishikawa S, Kuratomi Y, Saito T. A case of oat cell carcinoma of the lung associated with ectopic production of ADH, neurophysin and ACTH. *Endocrinol Jpn.* 1980;27(2):257-263.

296. Robertson GL, Athar S. The interaction of blood osmolality and blood volume in regulating plasma vasopressin in man. *J Clin Endocrinol Metab.* 1976;42(4):613-620.

297. Kamoi K. Syndrome of inappropriate antidiuresis without involving inappropriate secretion of vasopressin in an elderly woman: effect of intravenous administration of the nonpeptide vasopressin V2 receptor antagonist OPC-31260. *Nephron.* 1997;76(1):111-115.

298. Feldman BJ, Rosenthal SM, Vargas GA, et al. Nephrogenic syndrome of inappropriate antidiuresis. *N Engl J Med.* 2005;352(18):1884-1890.

299. Leaf A, Bartter FC, Santos RF, Wrong O. Evidence in man that urinary electrolyte loss induced by pitressin is a function of water retention. *J Clin Invest.* 1953;32(9):868-878.

300. Verbalis JG. Whole-body volume regulation and escape from antidiuresis. *Am J Med.* 2006;119(7 Suppl 1):S21-S29.

301. Peters JP, Welt LG, Sims EA, et al. A salt-wasting syndrome associated with cerebral disease. *Trans Assoc Am Physicians.* 1950;63:57-64.

302. Nelson PB, Seif S, Gutai J, Robinson AG. Hyponatremia and natriuresis following subarachnoid hemorrhage in a monkey model. *J Neurosurg.* 1984;60(2):233-237.

303. Wijdicks EF, Ropper AH, Hunnicutt EJ, et al. Atrial natriuretic factor and salt wasting after aneurysmal subarachnoid hemorrhage. *Stroke.* 1991;22(12):1519-1524.

304. Diringer MN, Lim JS, Kirsch JR, Hanley DF. Suprasellar and intraventricular blood predict elevated plasma atrial natriuretic factor in subarachnoid hemorrhage. *Stroke.* 1991;22(5):577-581.

305. Diringer MN, Wu KC, Verbalis JG, Hanley DF. Hypervolemic therapy prevents volume contraction but not hyponatremia following subarachnoid hemorrhage. *Ann Neurol.* 1992;31(5):543-550.

306. Cerda-Esteve M, Cuadrado-Godia E, Chillaron JJ, et al. Cerebral salt wasting syndrome: review. *Eur J Intern Med.* 2008;19(4):249-254.

307. Palmer BF. Hyponatremia in patients with central nervous system disease: SIADH versus CSW. *Trends Endocrinol Metab.* 2003;14(4): 182-187.

308. Kinik ST, Kandemir N, Baykan A, et al. Fludrocortisone treatment in a child with severe cerebral salt wasting. *Pediatr Neurosurg.* 2001; 35(4):216-219.

309. von Bismarck P, Ankermann T, Eggert P, et al. Diagnosis and management of cerebral salt wasting (CSW) in children: the role of atrial natriuretic peptide (ANP) and brain natriuretic peptide (BNP). *Childs Nerv Syst.* 2006;22(10):1275-1281.

310. Taplin CE, Cowell CT, Silink M, Ambler GR. Fludrocortisone therapy in cerebral salt wasting. *Pediatrics.* 2006;118(6):e1904-e1908.

311. Hannon MJ, Behan LA, O'Brien MM, et al. Hyponatremia following mild/moderate subarachnoid hemorrhage is due to SIAD and glucocorticoid deficiency and not cerebral salt wasting. *J Clin Endocrinol Metab.* 2014;99(1):291-298.

312. Tian Y, Sandberg K, Murase T, et al. Vasopressin V2 receptor binding is down-regulated during renal escape from vasopressin-induced antidiuresis. *Endocrinology.* 2000;141(1):307-314.

313. Verbalis JG, Murase T, Ecelbarger CA, et al. Studies of renal aquaporin-2 expression during renal escape from vasopressin-induced antidiuresis. *Adv Exp Med Biol.* 1998;449:395-406.

314. Arieff AI, Llach F, Massry SG. Neurological manifestations and morbidity of hyponatremia: correlation with brain water and electrolytes. *Medicine (Baltimore).* 1976;55(2):121-129.

315. Fraser CL, Arieff AI. Epidemiology, pathophysiology, and management of hyponatremic encephalopathy. *Am J Med.* 1997;102(1):67-77.

316. Daggett P, Deanfield J, Moss F. Neurological aspects of hyponatraemia. *Postgrad Med J.* 1982;58(686):737-740.

317. Ayus JC, Wheeler JM, Arieff AI. Postoperative hyponatremic encephalopathy in menstruant women. *Ann Intern Med.* 1992;117(11): 891-897.

318. Wijdicks EF, Sharbrough FW. New-onset seizures in critically ill patients. *Neurology.* 1993;43(5):1042-1044.

319. Vexler ZS, Ayus JC, Roberts TP, et al. Hypoxic and ischemic hypoxia exacerbate brain injury associated with metabolic encephalopathy in laboratory animals. *J Clin Invest.* 1994;93(1):256-264.

320. Ayus JC, Arieff AI. Pulmonary complications of hyponatremic encephalopathy. Noncardiogenic pulmonary edema and hypercapnic respiratory failure. *Chest.* 1995;107(2):517-521.

321. Ayus JC, Varon J, Arieff AI. Hyponatremia, cerebral edema, and noncardiogenic pulmonary edema in marathon runners. *Ann Intern Med.* 2000;132(9):711-714.

322. Arieff AI, Ayus JC, Fraser CL. Hyponatraemia and death or permanent brain damage in healthy children. *BMJ.* 1992;304(6836):1218-1222.

323. Wattad A, Chiang ML, Hill LL. Hyponatremia in hospitalized children. *Clin Pediatr (Phila).* 1992;31(3):153-157.

324. Wijdicks EF, Larson TS. Absence of postoperative hyponatremia syndrome in young, healthy females. *Ann Neurol.* 1994;35(5):626-628.

325. Sterns RH. Severe symptomatic hyponatremia: treatment and outcome. A study of 64 cases. *Ann Intern Med.* 1987;107(5):656-664.

326. Renneboog B, Musch W, Vandemergel X, et al. Mild chronic hyponatremia is associated with falls, unsteadiness, and attention deficits. *Am J Med.* 2006;119(1):71 e71-71 e78.

327. Verbalis JG, Goldsmith SR, Greenberg A, et al. Diagnosis, evaluation, and treatment of hyponatremia: expert panel recommendations. *Am J Med.* 2013;126(10 Suppl 1):S1-S42.

328. Gankam Kengne F, Andres C, Sattar L, et al. Mild hyponatremia and risk of fracture in the ambulatory elderly. *QJM.* 2008;101(7): 583-588.

329. Hoorn EJ, Rivadeneira F, van Meurs JB, et al. Mild hyponatremia as a risk factor for fractures: the Rotterdam Study. *J Bone Miner Res.* 2011;26(8):1822-1828.

330. Kinsella S, Moran S, Sullivan MO, et al. Hyponatremia independent of osteoporosis is associated with fracture occurrence. *Clin J Am Soc Nephrol.* 2010;5(2):275-280.

331. Sandhu HS, Gilles E, DeVita MV, et al. Hyponatremia associated with large-bone fracture in elderly patients. *Int Urol Nephrol.* 2009;41(3): 733-737.

332. Verbalis JG, Barsony J, Sugimura Y, et al. Hyponatremia-induced osteoporosis. *J Bone Miner Res.* 2010;25(3):554-563.

333. Ayus JC. Diuretic-induced hyponatremia. *Arch Intern Med.* 1986;146(7): 1295-1296.

334. Adrogue HJ, Madias NE. Hyponatremia. *N Engl J Med.* 2000;342(21): 1581-1589.

335. Verbalis JG, Grossman A, Hoybye C, Runkle I. Review and analysis of differing regulatory indications and expert panel guidelines for the treatment of hyponatremia. *Curr Med Res Opin.* 2014;30(7): 1201-1207.

336. Hew-Butler T, Ayus JC, Kipps C, et al. Statement of the Second International Exercise-Associated Hyponatremia Consensus Development Conference, New Zealand, 2007. *Clin J Sport Med.* 2008;18(2): 111-121.

337. Sterns RH, Cappuccio JD, Silver SM, Cohen EP. Neurologic sequelae after treatment of severe hyponatremia: a multicenter perspective. *J Am Soc Nephrol.* 1994;4(8):1522-1530.

338. Battison C, Andrews PJ, Graham C, Petty T. Randomized, controlled trial on the effect of a 20% mannitol solution and a 7.5% saline/6% dextran solution on increased intracranial pressure after brain injury. *Crit Care Med.* 2005;33(1):196-202, discussion 257-198.

339. Steele A, Gowrishankar M, Abrahamson S, et al. Postoperative hyponatremia despite near-isotonic saline infusion: a phenomenon of desalination. *Ann Intern Med.* 1997;126(1):20-25.

340. Robertson GL. Regulation of arginine vasopressin in the syndrome of inappropriate antidiuresis. *Am J Med.* 2006;119(7 Suppl 1):S36-S42.

341. Berl T. Impact of solute intake on urine flow and water excretion. *J Am Soc Nephrol.* 2008;19(6):1076-1078.

342. Furst H, Hallows KR, Post J, et al. The urine/plasma electrolyte ratio: a predictive guide to water restriction. *Am J Med Sci.* 2000;319(4): 240-244.

343. Greenberg A, Verbalis JG. Vasopressin receptor antagonists. *Kidney Int.* 2006;69(12):2124-2130.

344. Astellas Pharma US. Vaprisol (conivaptan hydrochloride injection). prescribing information. Deerfield, IL, 2006.

345. Zeltser D, Rosansky S, van Rensburg H, et al. Conivaptan Study G. Assessment of the efficacy and safety of intravenous conivaptan in euvolemic and hypervolemic hyponatremia. *Am J Nephrol.* 2007;27(5): 447-457.

346. Schrier RW, Gross P, Gheorghiade M, et al. Tolvaptan, a selective oral vasopressin V2-receptor antagonist, for hyponatremia. *N Engl J Med.* 2006;355(20):2099-2112.

347. Otsuka Pharmaceutical Company. Samsca (tolvaptan). Prescribing information. Tokyo, Japan, 2009.

348. Verbalis JG, Goldsmith SR, Greenberg A, et al. Hyponatremia treatment guidelines 2007: expert panel recommendations. *Am J Med.* 2007;120(11 Suppl 1):S1-S21.

349. Coussement J, Danguy C, Zouaoui-Boudjeltia K, et al. Treatment of the syndrome of inappropriate secretion of antidiuretic hormone with urea in critically ill patients. *Am J Nephrol.* 2012;35(3):265-270.

350. Decaux G, Andres C, Gankam Kengne F, Soupart A. Treatment of euvolemic hyponatremia in the intensive care unit by urea. *Crit Care.* 2010;14(5):R184.

351. Chehade H, Rosato L, Girardin E, Cachat F. Inappropriate antidiuretic hormone secretion: long-term successful urea treatment. *Acta Paediatr.* 2012;101(1):e39-e42.

352. Levtchenko EN, Monnens LA. Nephrogenic syndrome of inappropriate antidiuresis. *Nephrol Dial Transplant.* 2010;25(9):2839-2843.

353. Soupart A, Coffernils M, Couturier B, et al. Efficacy and tolerance of urea compared with vaptans for long-term treatment of patients with SIADH. *Clin J Am Soc Nephrol.* 2012;7(5):742-747.

354. Hantman D, Rossier B, Zohlman R, Schrier R. Rapid correction of hyponatremia in the syndrome of inappropriate secretion of antidiuretic hormone. An alternative treatment to hypertonic saline. *Ann Intern Med.* 1973;78(6):870-875.

355. Decaux G, Waterlot Y, Genette F, Mockel J. Treatment of the syndrome of inappropriate secretion of antidiuretic hormone with furosemide. *N Engl J Med.* 1981;304(6):329-330.

356. Spasovski G, Vanholder R, Allolio B, et al. Clinical practice guideline on diagnosis and treatment of hyponatraemia. *Nephrol Dial Transplant.* 2014;29(Suppl 2):i1-i39.

357. Ellison DH, Berl T. Clinical practice. The syndrome of inappropriate antidiuresis. *N Engl J Med.* 2007;356(20):2064-2072.

358. Sterns RH, Nigwekar SU, Hix JK. The treatment of hyponatremia. *Semin Nephrol.* 2009;29(3):282-299.

359. Verbalis JG. Hyponatremia and hypo-osmolar disorders. In: Greenberg A, Cheung AK, Coffman TM, et al., eds. *Primer on Kidney Diseases.* 5th ed. Philadelphia, PA: Saunders Elsevier; 2009:52-59.

360. Mohmand HK, Issa D, Ahmad Z, et al. Hypertonic saline for hyponatremia: risk of inadvertent overcorrection. *Clin J Am Soc Nephrol.* 2007;2(6):1110-1117.

361. Perianayagam A, Sterns RH, Silver SM, et al. DDAVP is effective in preventing and reversing inadvertent overcorrection of hyponatremia. *Clin J Am Soc Nephrol.* 2008;3(2):331-336.

362. Sterns RH, Hix JK, Silver S. Treating profound hyponatremia: a strategy for controlled correction. *Am J Kidney Dis.* 2010;56(4):774-779.

363. Soupart A, Penninckx R, Crenier L, et al. Prevention of brain demyelination in rats after excessive correction of chronic hyponatremia by serum sodium lowering. *Kidney Int.* 1994;45(1):193-200.

364. Goldszmidt MA, Iliescu EA. DDAVP to prevent rapid correction in hyponatremia. *Clin Nephrol.* 2000;53(3):226-229.

365. Oya S, Tsutsumi K, Ueki K, Kirino T. Reinduction of hyponatremia to treat central pontine myelinolysis. *Neurology.* 2001;57(10):1931-1932.

366. Bissram M, Scott FD, Liu L, Rosner MH. Risk factors for symptomatic hyponatraemia: the role of pre-existing asymptomatic hyponatraemia. *Intern Med J.* 2007;37(3):149-155.

367. Hew-Butler T, Hummel J, Rider BC, Verbalis JG. Characterization of the effects of the vasopressin V2 receptor on sweating, fluid balance, and performance during exercise. *Am J Physiol Regul Integr Comp Physiol.* 2014;307(4):R366-R375.

368. Insel TR, Gingrich BS, Young LJ. Oxytocin: who needs it? *Prog Brain Res.* 2001;133:59-66.

369. Glasier A, McNeilly AS. Physiology of lactation. *Baillieres Clin Endocrinol Metab.* 1990;4(2):379-395.

370. Uvnas-Moberg K, Eriksson M. Breastfeeding: physiological, endocrine and behavioural adaptations caused by oxytocin and local neurogenic activity in the nipple and mammary gland. *Acta Paediatr.* 1996;85(5):525-530.

371. Giraldi A, Enevoldsen AS, Wagner G. Oxytocin and the initiation of parturition: a review. *Dan Med Bull.* 1990;37(4):377-383.

372. Young WS 3rd, Shepard E, DeVries AC, et al. Targeted reduction of oxytocin expression provides insights into its physiological roles. *Adv Exp Med Biol.* 1998;449:231-240.

373. Renfrew MJ, Lang S, Woolridge M. Oxytocin for promoting successful lactation. *Cochrane Database Syst Rev.* 2000;(2):CD000156.

374. McNeilly AS, Tay CC, Glasier A. Physiological mechanisms underlying lactational amenorrhea. *Ann N Y Acad Sci.* 1994;709:145-155.

375. Johnston JM, Amico JA. A prospective longitudinal study of the release of oxytocin and prolactin in response to infant suckling in long term lactation. *J Clin Endocrinol Metab.* 1986;62(4):653-657.

376. De Coopman J. Breastfeeding after pituitary resection: support for a theory of autocrine control of milk supply? *J Hum Lact.* 1993;9(1):35-40.

377. Robinson A, Amico J. Remarks on the history of oxytocin. In: Robinson A, Amico J, eds. *Oxytocin: Clinical and Laboratory Studies/Proceedings of the Second International Conference on Oxytocin, Lac Beauport, Quebec, Canada.* Amsterdam: Excerpta Medica; 1985:xvii-xxiv.

378. Smith R. Parturition. *N Engl J Med.* 2007;356(3):271-283.

379. Terzidou V. Preterm labour: biochemical and endocrinological preparation for parturition. *Best Pract Res Clin Obstet Gynaecol.* 2007;21(5):729-756.

380. Vrachnis N, Malamas FM, Sifakis S, et al. The oxytocin-oxytocin receptor system and its antagonists as tocolytic agents. *Int J Endocrinol.* 2011;2011:350546.

381. Evans JJ. Oxytocin in the human: regulation of derivations and destinations. *Eur J Endocrinol.* 1997;137(6):559-571.

382. Hertelendy F, Zakar T. Prostaglandins and the myometrium and cervix. *Prostaglandins Leukot Essent Fatty Acids.* 2004;70(2):207-222.

383. Olson DM, Mijovic JE, Sadowsky DW. Control of human parturition. *Semin Perinatol.* 1995;19(1):52-63.

384. Terzidou V, Blanks AM, Kim SH, et al. Labor and inflammation increase the expression of oxytocin receptor in human amnion. *Biol Reprod.* 2011;84(3):546-552.

385. Lockwood CJ. The initiation of parturition at term. *Obstet Gynecol Clin North Am.* 2004;31(4):935-947, xii.

386. Mendelson CR. Minireview: fetal-maternal hormonal signaling in pregnancy and labor. *Mol Endocrinol.* 2009;23(7):947-954.

387. Smith JG, Merrill DC. Oxytocin for induction of labor. *Clin Obstet Gynecol.* 2006;49(3):594-608.

388. Moghadam AD, Jaafarpour M, Khani A. Comparison effect of oral propranolol and oxytocin versus oxytocin only on induction of labour in nulliparous women (a double blind randomized trial). *J Clin Diagn Res.* 2013;7(11):2567-2569.

389. Mozurkewich EL, Chilimigras JL, Berman DR, et al. Methods of induction of labour: a systematic review. *BMC Pregnancy Childbirth.* 2011;11:84.

390. Chelmow D. Postpartum haemorrhage: prevention. *BMJ Clin Evid.* 2011;2011:pii: 1410.

391. Grotegut CA, Paglia MJ, Johnson LN, et al. Oxytocin exposure during labor among women with postpartum hemorrhage secondary to uterine atony. *Am J Obstet Gynecol.* 2011;204(1):56.e1-6.

392. Afolabi EO, Kuti O, Orji EO, Ogunniyi SO. Oral misoprostol versus intramuscular oxytocin in the active management of the third stage of labour. *Singapore Med J.* 2010;51(3):207-211.

393. Firouzbakht M, Kiapour A, Omidvar S. Prevention of post-partum hemorrhage by rectal misoprostol: a randomized clinical trial. *J Nat Sci Biol Med.* 2013;4(1):134-137.

394. Prata N, Bell S, Weidert K. Prevention of postpartum hemorrhage in low-resource settings: current perspectives. *Int J Womens Health.* 2013;5:737-752.

Section III

Thyroid

CHAPTER 11

Thyroid Physiology and Diagnostic Evaluation of Patients With Thyroid Disorders

DOMENICO SALVATORE • TERRY F. DAVIES • MARTIN-JEAN SCHLUMBERGER • IAN D. HAY • P. REED LARSEN

KEY POINTS

- This chapter illustrates the principal events involved in the ontogeny and development of the thyroid gland in many life forms, ranging from invertebrates to humans.
- The thyroid gland anatomy and function and the pivotal role played by iodine in thyroid economy are described.
- The key molecular elements and mechanisms involved in thyroid hormone action and metabolism in peripheral tissues are reviewed.
- This chapter also dissects the mechanisms responsible for thyroid hormone homeostasis and function under physiologic and pathologic conditions.
- In addition, this chapter provides the physiologic rationale and expected results for the various tests that can be employed in the biochemical evaluation of patients with clinical thyroid dysfunction or disease.

Dysfunction and anatomic abnormalities of the thyroid are among the most common diseases of the endocrine glands. This chapter provides the physiologic and biochemical background and describes the various tests for evaluating patients with suspected thyroid disease based on the pathophysiology of these conditions.

PHYLOGENY, EMBRYOLOGY, AND ONTOGENY

Phylogeny

The phylogeny, embryogenesis, and certain aspects of thyroid function are closely interlinked with the gastrointestinal tract. The capacity of the thyroid to metabolize iodine and incorporate it into a variety of organic compounds occurs widely throughout the animal and plant kingdoms. However, the anatomy of the thyroid gland differs considerably among the vertebrate classes. Monoiodotyrosine (3'-monoiodo-L-tyrosine [MIT]) and diiodotyrosine (3,5-diiodo-L-tyrosine [DIT]) are present in a variety of invertebrate species, including mollusks, crustaceans, coelenterates, annelids, insects, and certain marine algae. In these lower forms, however, no recognizable thyroid tissue is present. Thyroid tissue is confined to, and is present in, all vertebrates. A close link to the thyroid of higher vertebrates is evident in the ammocoete, the larval form of the lamprey, where the ventral part of the pharynx is the origin of a structure present only during larval life, the endostyle. The epithelium of the endostyle is capable of carrying out iodinations, and these cells are fated to become follicular cells only after metamorphosis, when they will form classic thyroid follicles.[1]

The phylogenetic association of the thyroid gland and the gastrointestinal tract is evident in several functions. The salivary and gastric glands, like the thyroid, are capable of concentrating iodide in their secretions, although iodide transport in these sites is not responsive to stimulation by thyrotropin (TSH, thyroid-stimulating hormone). The salivary gland contains enzymes that are capable of iodinating tyrosine in the presence of hydrogen peroxide, although it forms insignificant quantities of iodoproteins under normal circumstances.

Structural Embryology

The morphogenesis of the thyroid gland, the anterior-most organ that buds from the gut tube, begins with a thickening of the endodermal epithelium in the foregut, which is referred to as the *thyroid anlage*. The human thyroid anlage is first recognizable at embryonic day 16 or 17. This median thickening deepens and forms first a small pit and then an outpouching of the endoderm adjacent to the developing myocardial cells. With continuing development, the median diverticulum is displaced caudally following the myocardial cells in their descent. The primitive stalk connecting the primordium with the pharyngeal floor elongates into the thyroglossal duct. During its caudal displacement, the primordium assumes a bilobate shape, coming into contact and fusing with the ventral aspect of the fourth pharyngeal pouch when it reaches its final position at about embryonic day 50. Normally the thyroglossal duct undergoes dissolution and fragmentation by about the second month after conception, leaving at its point of origin a small dimple at the junction of the middle and posterior thirds of the tongue, the *foramen caecum*. Cells of the lower portion of the duct differentiate into thyroid tissue, forming the pyramidal lobe of the gland. At this time, the lobes contact the ultimobranchial glands, leading to the incorporation of C cells into the thyroid. Concomitantly, histologic alterations occur throughout the gland. Complex interconnecting cordlike arrangements of cells interspersed with vascular connective tissue replace the solid epithelial mass and become tubule-like structures at about the third month of fetal life; shortly thereafter, follicular arrangements devoid of colloid appear, and by 13 to 14 weeks the follicles begin to fill with colloid. Investigations of thyroid gland development in mice using gene-targeting techniques are beginning to identify the critical factors that are required for normal thyroid gland development.[2,3] The role of these various proteins is currently being evaluated with respect to the potential for defects in the synthesis or formation of the thyroid gland (see Chapter 13).

Functional Ontogeny

The ontogeny of thyroid function and its regulation in the human fetus are fairly well defined.[4] Future follicular cells acquire the capacity to form thyroglobulin (Tg) as early as the 29th day of gestation, whereas the capacities to concentrate iodide and synthesize thyroxine (T_4) are delayed until about the 11th week. Radioactive iodine inadvertently given to the mother would be accumulated by the fetal thyroid soon thereafter. Early growth and development of the thyroid do not seem to be TSH-dependent, because the capacity of the pituitary to synthesize and secrete TSH is not apparent until the 14th week. Subsequently, rapid changes in pituitary and thyroid function take place. Probably as a consequence of hypothalamic maturation and increasing secretion of thyrotropin-releasing hormone (TRH), the serum TSH concentration increases between 18 and 26 weeks' gestation, after which levels remain higher than those in the mother.[4] The higher levels may reflect a higher set-point of the negative feedback control of TSH secretion during fetal life than at maturity. Thyroxine–binding globulin (TBG), the major thyroid hormone–binding protein in plasma, is detectable in the serum by the 10th gestational week and increases in concentration progressively to term. This increase in TBG concentration accounts in part for the progressive increase in the serum T_4 concentration during the second and third trimesters, but increased secretion of T_4 must also play a role because the concentration of free T_4 also rises.

Several aspects of thyroid development are of note from the clinical standpoint. Rarely, thyroid tissue may develop from remnants of the thyroglossal duct near the base of the tongue. Such lingual thyroid tissue may be the sole functioning thyroid present, and thus, its surgical removal will lead to hypothyroidism. More commonly, elements of the thyroglossal duct may persist and later give rise to thyroglossal duct cysts, or ectopic thyroid tissue may be present at any location in the mediastinum or, rarely, even in the heart.

ANATOMY AND HISTOLOGY

The thyroid is one of the largest of the endocrine organs, weighing approximately 15 to 20 g in North American adults. Moreover, the potential of the thyroid for growth is tremendous. The enlarged thyroid, commonly termed a *goiter,* can weigh many hundreds of grams. The normal thyroid is made up of two lobes joined by a thin band of tissue, the isthmus, which is approximately 0.5 cm thick, 2 cm wide, and 1 to 2 cm high. The individual lobes normally have a pointed superior pole and a poorly defined blunt inferior pole that merges medially with the isthmus. Each lobe is approximately 2.0 to 2.5 cm in thickness and width at its largest diameter and is approximately 4.0 cm in length. Occasionally, especially when the remainder of the gland is enlarged, a pyramidal lobe is discernible as a finger-like projection directed upward from the isthmus, generally just lateral to the midline, usually on the left. The right lobe is normally more vascular than the left, is often the larger of the two, and tends to enlarge more in disorders associated with a diffuse increase in gland size. Two pairs of vessels constitute the major arterial blood supply: the superior thyroid artery, arising from the external carotid artery, and the inferior thyroid artery, arising from the subclavian artery. Estimates of thyroid blood flow range from 4 to 6 mL/minute/g, well in excess of the blood flow to the kidney (3 mL/minute/g). In diffuse toxic goiter due to Graves disease, blood flow may exceed 1 L/minute and be associated with an audible bruit or even a palpable thrill.

The gland is composed of closely packed spherical units termed *follicles,* which are invested with a rich capillary network. The interior of the follicle is filled with the clear proteinaceous colloid that normally is the major constituent of the total thyroid mass. On cross section, thyroid tissue appears as closely packed ring-shaped structures consisting of a single layer of thyroid cells surrounding a lumen. The diameter of the follicles varies considerably, even within a single gland, but averages about 200 nm. The follicular cells vary in height with the degree of glandular stimulation, becoming columnar when active and cuboidal when inactive. The epithelium rests on a basement membrane that is rich with glycoproteins separating the follicular cells from the surrounding capillaries. From 20 to 40 follicles are demarcated by connective tissue septa to form a lobule supplied by a single artery. The function of a given lobule may differ from that of its neighbors.

On electron microscopy, the thyroid follicular epithelium has many features in common with other secretory cells and some peculiar to the thyroid. From the apex of the follicular cell, numerous microvilli extend into the colloid. It is at or near this surface of the cell that iodination, exocytosis, and the initial phase of hormone secretion, namely, colloid resorption, occur (Fig. 11-1). The nucleus has no distinctive features and the cytoplasm contains an extensive endoplasmic reticulum (ER) laden with microsomes. The ER is composed of a network of wide irregular tubules that contain the precursor of Tg. The carbohydrate component of Tg is added to this precursor in the Golgi apparatus, which is located apically. Lysosomes and mitochondria are scattered throughout the

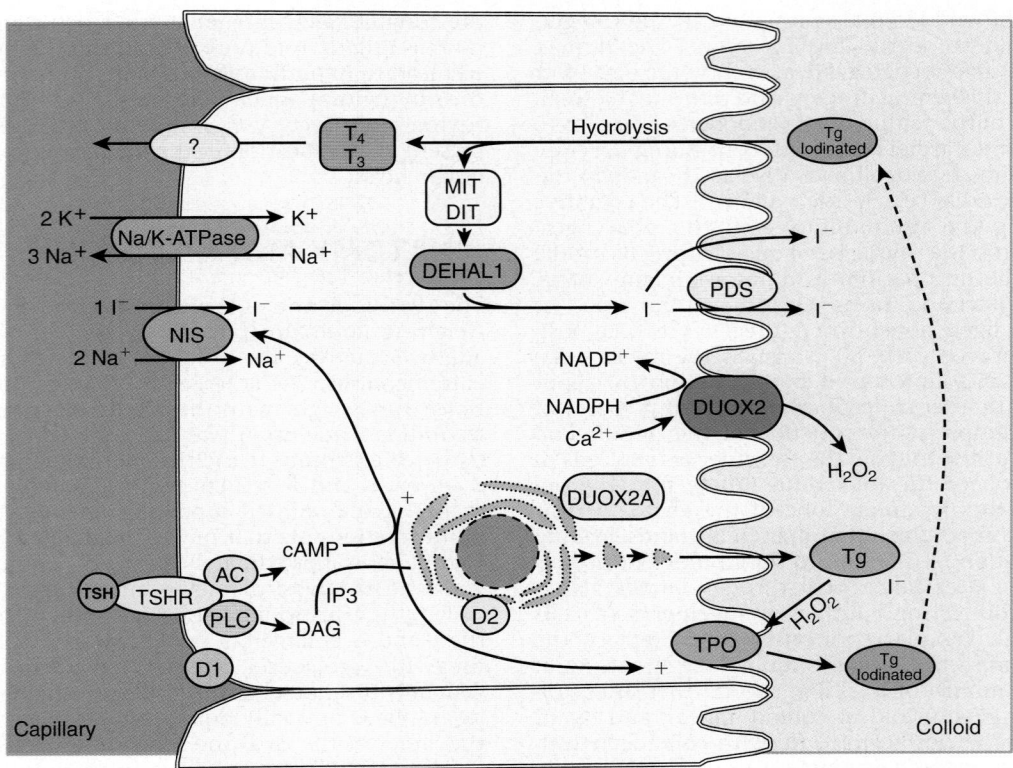

Figure 11-1 Schematic illustration of a follicular cell showing the key aspects of thyroid iodine transport and thyroid hormone synthesis. AC, adenyl cyclase; ATPase, adenosine triphosphatase; cAMP, cyclic adenosine monophosphate; D1, thyroidal deiodinase type 1; D2, thyroidal deiodinase type 2; DAG, diacylglycerol; DEHAL1, iodotyrosine dehalogenase 1 (IYD); DIT, diiodotyrosine; DUOX, dual oxidase; IP3, inositol triphosphate; MIT, monoiodotyrosine; NADP+, oxidized form of nicotinamide adenosine dinucleotide phosphate; NADPH, reduced nicotinamide adenosine dinucleotide phosphate; NIS, sodium-iodide symporter; PDS, pendrin (SLC26A4); PLC, phospholipase C; T_3, triiodothyronine; T_4, thyroxine; Tg, thyroglobulin; TPO, thyroid peroxidase; TSH, thyrotropin; TSHR, thyrotropin receptor.

cytoplasm. Stimulation by TSH results in enlargement of the Golgi apparatus, formation of pseudopodia at the apical surface, and the appearance in the apical portion of the cell of many droplets that contain colloid taken up from the follicular lumen (see Fig. 11-1).

The thyroid also contains parafollicular cells, or C cells, that bilaterally migrate from the neural crest and are the source of calcitonin. These cells originate during embryonic development from the last pair of pharyngeal pouches but ultimately come to rest either among the cells of the follicular epithelium or in the thyroid interstitium. They differ from the cells of the follicular epithelium in never bordering on the follicular lumen and in being rich in mitochondria. The C cells, detected also in human lingual thyroids,[5] undergo hyperplasia early in the syndrome of familial medullary carcinoma of the thyroid (multiple endocrine neoplasia type 2 [MEN2]) and give rise to this tumor in both its familial and its sporadic forms (see Chapter 39).

IODINE AND THE SYNTHESIS AND SECRETION OF THYROID HORMONES

The function of the thyroid is to generate the quantity of thyroid hormone necessary to meet the demands of the peripheral tissues. This action requires iodide uptake by the thyroidal sodium-iodide symporter (NIS), its transfer to the colloid, and its oxidation by thyroid peroxidase (TPO) to allow the synthesis of approximately 110 nmol/L (85 µg)

of T_4, which is 65% iodine by weight. This requires the synthesis of an approximately 330-kDa glycoprotein, Tg. Specific tyrosine residues of Tg homodimers are then iodinated at the apical border of the thyroid cell to form MIT and DIT (see Fig. 11-1). This requires formation of hydrogen peroxide (H_2O_2) by dual oxidase (DUOX1 and 2) and TPO, which catalyzes the oxidation of iodide and its transfer to tyrosine. TPO also catalyzes the coupling of two molecules of DIT or one of DIT and one of MIT, leading to formation of T_4 and triiodothyronine (T_3), respectively, which are then stored within the colloid, still as part of the Tg molecule. Pinocytosis of stored colloid leads to the formation of phagolysosomes, the colloid droplets in which Tg is digested by specific proteases to release T_4, T_3, DIT, and MIT as the droplet is translocated toward the basal portion of the cell. T_4 and T_3 are transported out of the phagolysosomes and across the basolateral cell membrane to exit the cell and enter circulation, whereas DIT and MIT are deiodinated by iodotyrosine dehalogenase (DEHAL1) to allow recycling of the iodide. The synthesis of thyroid hormones requires the expression of a number of thyroid cell–specific proteins. In addition to Tg and TPO, the TSH receptor (TSHR) is also required to transduce the effects of extracellular TSH for efficient hormone synthesis. A number of transcription factors, including thyroid transcription factors TTF-1 (NKX2-1) and TTF-2 (FOXE1), PAX8, and hepatocyte nuclear factor 3 (HNF-3 [FOXE2]), as well as TSH, are necessary to achieve functional differentiation of the thyroid follicular cells and the onset of hormonogenesis.[1,3] Transient overexpression of the transcription factors NKX2-1 and PAX8 is sufficient to direct mouse embryonic

TABLE 11-1

Recommended and Typical Values for Dietary Iodine Intake

Recommended Daily Intake	
Adults	150 µg
During pregnancy	200 µg
Children	90-120 µg
Typical Iodine Daily Intakes	
North America (1992)	75-300 µg
Chile (1981)	<50-150 µg
Belgium (1993)	50-60 µg
Germany (1993)	20-70 µg
Switzerland (1993)	130-160 µg

stem cell (mESC) differentiation into thyroid follicular cells that organize into three-dimensional follicular structures when treated with TSH and follicles showed significant iodide organification activity.[6] Although the biochemical details of these processes are beyond the scope of this discussion, those aspects with clinical relevance are reviewed in greater detail in the following section.

Dietary Iodine

Formation of normal quantities of thyroid hormone requires the availability of adequate quantities of exogenous iodine to allow thyroidal uptake of approximately 60 to 75 µg daily, taking into account the fecal losses of about 10 to 20 µg iodine of iodothyronines as glucuronides and about 100 to 150 µg as urinary iodine in iodine-sufficient populations.[7] Plasma iodide (I^-), the form of the element in biologic solutions, is completely filterable with about 60% to 70% of the filtered load reabsorbed passively. At least 100 µg of iodine per day is required to eliminate all signs of iodine deficiency (Table 11-1). In healthy adults, the absorption of iodide is greater than 90%. In North America, the daily dietary iodine intake is in the range of 150 to 300 µg daily, largely owing to the iodination of salt, whereas in Japan, where large quantities of foods rich in iodine are consumed, intakes may be as high as several milligrams per day. Notably, iodine intake in the United States is decreasing due to a reduction in salt consumption, with median urinary iodine of 160 µg/L but a low urinary iodine (<5 µg/dL) in 11% of the population.[8] The daily dietary intake of iodine varies widely throughout the world, depending on the iodine content of soil and water and on dietary practice (see Table 11-1). Even in a single area, iodine intake varies among different individuals and in the same individual from day to day. Iodine may also enter the body via medications, diagnostic agents, dietary supplements, and food additives. As discussed more extensively under "Regulation of Thyroid Function," iodine deficiency is common, especially in mountainous and formerly glaciated regions of the earth.[9] An estimated 1 billion individuals live in iodine-deficient areas of the world, and these people often develop TSH-induced compensatory enlargement of the thyroid *(endemic goiter)*. If iodine deficiency is severe during pregnancy, fetal thyroid hormone production falls with irreparable damage to the developing central nervous system (CNS). This damage is manifested by varying degrees of mental retardation and is termed *endemic cretinism*. Thus, iodine-deficiency disorders (IDDs), including endemic goiter and cretinism, are the most common thyroid-related human illnesses; indeed, they are the most common endocrine disorders worldwide.

Plasma iodide is partly replenished by that lost from the thyroid into the blood and by iodide liberated through deiodination of iodothyronines in peripheral tissues. Ultimately, however, the diet is its most important source. Iodine is ingested in both inorganic and organically bound forms. Iodide per se is rapidly and efficiently absorbed from the gastrointestinal tract (within 30 minutes), and little is lost in the stool. In the body, iodide is confined largely to the extracellular fluid. It is also found, however, in red blood cells and is concentrated in the intraluminal fluids of the gastrointestinal tract, notably the saliva and gastric juice, from which it is reabsorbed, thus reentering the extracellular fluid. Iodide is also concentrated in milk. Until oxidized and bound to tyrosyl residues in Tg, iodide entering the thyroid by active transport is in rapid equilibrium with the main iodide pool. The concentration of iodide in the extracellular fluid is normally 10 to 15 µg/L (~10^{-7} mol/L), and the content of the peripheral pool is approximately 250 µg. The thyroid contains the largest pool of body iodine, under normal circumstances approximately 8000 µg, most of which is in the form of DIT and MIT. Normally, this pool of iodine turns over slowly (about 1% per day).

Iodide Metabolism by the Thyroid Cell

Because the concentration of iodide in plasma is so low, a mechanism is required for the thyroid cell to concentrate the required amounts of this element. This process, iodide trapping, is accomplished by a membrane protein, the NIS, encoded by the gene *SLC5A*. Human NIS is a 643–amino acid glycoprotein with 13 membrane-spanning domains. The transport of iodide is an active process dependent on the presence of sodium gradient across the basal membrane of the thyroid cell such that downhill transport of two Na^+ ions results in the entry of one iodide atom against an electrochemical gradient (see Fig. 11-1). In addition to being expressed in the basolateral membrane of the thyroid cell, NIS has also been identified in other iodide-concentrating cells, including salivary and lactating mammary glands, choroid plexus, and gastric mucosa and in the cytotrophoblast and syncytiotrophoblast.[10,11] NIS is expressed also in the ovary and testis and in ovarian cancer and the majority of seminomas and embryonal testicular carcinomas.[12] In the lactating mammary gland, NIS plays an important role by concentrating iodide in the milk, thereby supplying newborns with iodide for thyroid hormone synthesis. The iodide transport system generates an iodide gradient of 20 to 40 over the cell membrane, and NIS will also transport pertechnetate (TcO_4^-), perchlorate (ClO_4^-), and thiocyanate (SCN^-), accounting for the utility of radioactive TcO_4^- as a thyroid scanning tool and the capacity of $KClO_4^-$ to block iodide uptake.[13,14] On the other hand, the affinity of NIS for iodide is much higher than it is for the other inorganic anions, such as bromide and chloride, accounting for the selectivity of the thyroid transport mechanism.[15]

Transcription of the NIS gene is increased by TSH, and TSH also prolongs NIS protein half-life and targets the protein to the cell membrane. That the iodide-concentrating mechanism is required for normal thyroid function has been known for decades in that its absence is associated with congenital hypothyroidism and goiter unless large quantities of inorganic iodide are provided.[16] A number of families have now been identified in which various mutations in the NIS gene are associated with congenital hypothyroidism and an iodide transport defect. Importantly, several studies have documented decreases in NIS expression in human thyroid adenomas and carcinomas that contribute to the loss of iodine uptake in neoplastic thyroid cells, which therefore present as "cold" nodules on radioisotopic imaging.[16] However, changes in the subcellular location of NIS may also explain this phenomenon. Pendrin is a highly hydrophobic membrane glycoprotein located at the apical membrane of thyrocytes where it could function as an apical iodide transporter in thyroid cells.[17] In addition to the thyroid, pendrin is also expressed in the kidney and in the inner ear.[18] In the kidney, pendrin plays an important role in acid-base metabolism as a chloride/bicarbonate exchanger.[19] In the inner ear, pendrin is important for generation of the endocochlear potential.[16]

Pendrin belongs to the SLC26A family and is encoded by the *SLC26A4* gene. Mutations in the *SLC26A4* gene lead to Pendred syndrome, an autosomal recessive disorder characterized by sensorineural deafness, goiter, and a partial defect in iodide organification.[20,21] Deafness or hearing impairment is the major phenotypic manifestation in Pendred syndrome. Goiter usually develops during childhood. There is, however, a substantial variation within and between families and different geographic regions. Curiously, targeted inactivation of *SLC26A4* does not result in thyroid dysfunction in mice.

This argues against a rate-limiting role for this protein for apical follicular transport at least in this animal. Localization of the chloride channel 5 (ClCn5) protein at the apical membrane of thyrocytes and a thyroidal phenotype of the *ClCn5*-deficient mice that is reminiscent of Pendred syndrome suggests that ClCn5 could be, possibly in conjunction with other chloride channels, involved in mediating apical iodide efflux or iodide/chloride exchange.[22]

In addition to the active transport of iodide from the extracellular fluid, intracellular iodide is also generated by the action of the DEHAL1 or iodotyrosine deiodinase (IYD) enzymes. IYD-catalyzed nicotinamide adenosine dinucleotide phosphate (NADPH)-dependent deiodination of MIT and DIT, with greater activity against MIT.[23] *Dhal1* transcription is stimulated by cyclic adenosine monophosphate (cAMP) and encodes a membrane protein concentrated at the apical cell surface, which catalyzes NADPH-dependent deiodination of MIT and DIT and recycles iodide. The iodide thereby released is immediately reconjugated to newly synthesized Tg after exiting the apical membrane of the cell. This process is interrupted by the thiourea class of antithyroid drugs that inhibit TPO, such as methimazole (MMI), carbimazole (CBZ), and propylthiouracil (PTU), thus causing intrathyroidal iodine deficiency in patients receiving these agents.[24] Mutations in homozygosity in the *IYD* gene have been identified in patients with hypothyroidism, goiter, and an elevated DIT level.[25] Functional studies revealed that the mutations abolished the capacity of IYD to deiodinate MIT and DIT.

Iodide Oxidation and Organification

Within the thyroid, iodide participates in a series of reactions that lead to the synthesis of the active thyroid hormones. The first of these involves oxidation of iodide and incorporation of the resulting intermediate into the hormonally inactive iodotyrosines MIT and DIT, a process termed *organification*. Iodide is normally oxidized rapidly, immediately appearing in organic combination with Tg. The iodinations that lead to formation of iodotyrosines occur within Tg, rather than on the free amino acids. Oxidation of thyroidal iodide is mediated by the heme-containing protein TPO and requires the H_2O_2 generated by the calcium-dependent DUOX1 and DUOX2 enzymes. The protein contains a membrane-spanning region near the carboxy-terminus, and it is oriented in the apical membrane of the thyroid cell with residues 1-844 in the follicular lumen in which iodination occurs (see Fig. 11-1). TPO

is the major thyroid microsomal antigen, and recombinant human TPO is now used for the detection of antithyroid microsomal antibodies commonly present in the serum of patients with Hashimoto thyroiditis. The evanescent product of the peroxidation of iodide (i.e., the active iodinating form) may be free hypoiodous acid (I_2) or iodinium (I^+).[26] The DUOX1 and 2 genes (also termed THOX1 and THOX2) encode glycoflavoproteins predominantly expressed at the apical thyrocyte membrane where they constitute the catalytic core of the H_2O_2 generator required for thyroid hormone synthesis (see Fig. 11-1).[27] They are Ca^{2+}, NADPH-dependent oxidases that catalyze the formation of the H_2O_2 required for TPO-catalyzed Tg iodination. DUOXA2, a resident ER protein, is required for the maturation, plasma membrane localization of DUOX2, and H_2O_2 generation.[28] Mice deficient in dual oxidase maturation factors are severely hypothyroid.[29] Iodide excess inhibits DUOX2 glycosylation, which may be an additional mechanism for the Wolff-Chaikoff effect. DUOX-generated H_2O_2 has been found to be an early event of the wound response in zebrafish larvae that is required for rapid requirement of leukocytes to the wound.[30]

The rate of organic iodinations is dependent on the degree of thyroid stimulation by TSH (see later). Congenital defects in the organic binding mechanism cause goitrous congenital hypothyroidism or, if less severe, goiter without hypothyroidism. In some families, the thyroidal TPO is absent.[31] Homozygous nonsense mutations in the *DUOX2* gene, as well as heterozygous mutations in the *DUOX2* gene that prematurely truncated the protein, have been found in patients with mild transient congenital hypothyroidism and a partial iodide organification defect.[32,33] Furthermore, a mutation in the *DUOXA2* gene has been found in a patient with congenital hypothyroidism and partial iodine organification defect (see Chapter 13).[34,35]

Iodothyronine Synthesis

The MIT and DIT are precursors of the hormonally active iodothyronines T_4 and T_3. Synthesis of T_4 from DIT requires the TPO-catalyzed fusion of two DIT molecules to yield a structure with two diiodinated rings linked by an ether bridge (the coupling reaction). Concomitantly, a residual dehydroalanine is formed at the site of the DIT residue contributing to the phenolic hydroxyl group.

Efficient synthesis of T_4 and T_3 in the thyroid requires Tg. The Tg messenger RNA (mRNA) is approximately 8.5 kb in length and encodes a 330-kDa (12S) subunit that is 10% carbohydrate by weight. There are 134 tyrosyl residues in the 660-kDa homodimer. Only 25 to 30 of these are iodinated, but only residues 5, 1290, and 2553 form T_4 and residue 2746, T_3.[36] The T_4-forming, readily iodinated, and iodothyronine-forming acceptor residues of Tg from different species are in a Glu/AspTyr or a Thr/SerTyrSer sequence, suggesting an important role of primary sequence in these reactions. There are three to four T_4 molecules in each molecule of human Tg under conditions of normal iodination (25 atoms per Tg molecule, approximately 0.5% iodine by weight), but only about one in five molecules of human Tg contains a T_3 residue. In Tg from patients with untreated Graves disease, the content of T_4 residues remains approximately the same, but the number of T_3 residues doubles to an average of 0.4 per molecule. This difference is independent of the iodination state of the Tg and is a consequence of thyroidal stimulation. Because the coupling reaction is catalyzed by TPO, virtually all agents that inhibit organic binding (e.g., the thiourea drugs) also inhibit coupling.

Storage and Release of Thyroid Hormone

The thyroid is unique among the endocrine glands by virtue of the large store of hormone it contains and the low rate at which the hormone turns over (1% per day). This aspect of thyroid hormone economy has homeostatic value in that the reservoir provides prolonged protection against depletion of circulating hormone in case synthesis ceases. In normal humans, the administration of antithyroid agents for as long as 2 weeks has little effect on serum T_4 concentrations. There are approximately 250 μg T_4 per gram of wet weight in normal human thyroid, or 5000 μg of T_4 in a 20-g gland.[24] This amount is sufficient to maintain a euthyroid state for at least 50 days. When released rapidly in an uncontrolled fashion during subacute or painless thyroiditis, this quantity of T_4 will cause significant transient thyrotoxicosis. Tg is present in the plasma of normal individuals at concentrations up to 80 ng/mL, probably leaving the thyroid through the lymphatics. However, peripheral hydrolysis of Tg does not contribute significantly to the thyroid hormones in the circulation, even during thyroiditis when large quantities of this protein are present.

The first step in thyroid hormone release is the endocytosis of colloid from the follicular lumen by two processes: macropinocytosis by pseudopods formed at the apical membrane and micropinocytosis by small coated vesicles that form at the apical surface (see Fig. 11-1). Both processes are stimulated by TSH, but the relative importance of the two pathways varies among species, with micropinocytosis thought to predominate in humans. Following endocytosis, endocytotic vesicles fuse with lysosomes, and proteolysis is catalyzed by cathepsin D and D-like thiol proteases, all of which are active at the acidic pH of the lysosome. The iodotyrosines released from Tg are rapidly deiodinated by the NADPH-dependent iodotyrosine deiodinase, and the released iodine is recycled. Thyroid hormones are released from Tg in the lysosome, but it is not clear how their transfer into the cytosol and subsequently the plasma is effected. Given the expression of the thyroid hormone transporter MCT8 in the thyroid gland (see later), it is possible that this transporter could be involved in the exit of T_4 and T_3 from the phagolysosome or thyroid cell. It has been shown that T_4 can be released from Tg within the thyroid cell with minimal disruption of its molecular weight. This presumably is a consequence of selective proteolysis, which is facilitated by the fact that the major hormonogenic peptides of the Tg molecule are located at the amino-terminus and the carboxy-terminus of the Tg monomer.

Presumably the T_4 becomes accessible to the thyroidal type 1 and 2 deiodinases (D1 and D2) because basal and TSH-stimulated conversion of T_4 to T_3 is readily demonstrated in the perfused dog thyroid. Because this conversion is inhibited by PTU, it is catalyzed by D1. The contribution of thyroidal T_4 deiodination to T_3 secretion in humans under physiologic conditions is not known. The fact that the ratio of T_4 to T_3 in human Tg is 15:1, although estimates of the molar ratio of T_4 to T_3 in thyroid secretion is approximately 10:1, suggests that this does occur. Stimulation of D1- and D2-catalyzed 5′-deiodination of T_4 in Graves thyroid may enhance that pathway and contribute to the marked increase of the ratio of T_3 to T_4 production in that condition.[37] An inhibition of the D1-catalyzed T_4 to T_3 conversion may contribute to the rapid effect of PTU to reduce circulating T_3 in the Graves patient (see Chapter 12).[37,38] That deiodinases in thyroid-derived cells can modulate the systemic conversion of T_4 to T_3 has been shown in several patients with metastatic thyroid carcinoma. The

high expression of D2 in one large mediastinal tumor mass was associated with a high normal T_3 and reduced T_4 with a normal TSH. Removal of the tumor reversed these abnormalities.[39]

T_4 release from the thyroid cells is inhibited by several agents, the most important of which is iodide. Inhibition of hormone release is responsible for the rapid improvement that iodide causes in hyperthyroid patients. The mechanism by which this effect is mediated is uncertain, but iodide inhibits the stimulation of thyroid adenylate cyclase by TSH and by the stimulatory immunoglobulins of Graves disease. Increasing iodination of Tg also increases its resistance to hydrolysis by acid proteases in the lysosomes. Lithium inhibits thyroid hormone release, although its mechanism of action is poorly understood and may differ from that of iodide.[40]

Role and Mechanism of Thyrotropin Effects

All steps in the formation and release of thyroid hormones are stimulated by TSH secreted by the pituitary thyrotrophs (see Chapter 8). Thyroid cells express the TSHR, a member of the glycoprotein G protein–coupled receptor family. This protein contains a large extracellular amino-terminal domain, seven membrane-spanning domains, and an intracellular domain that transduces the signal by promoting exchange of guanosine diphosphate (GDP) for guanosine triphosphate (GTP) on the α-subunit of G proteins.[1,3,41] In fact, the TSHR has been reported to couple to 11 different G protein α-subunits in vitro, and therefore, much remains to be learned about signaling through it. Although the TSHR mainly couples to G_s, when activated by high concentrations of TSH (100 times physiologic levels) it couples also to G_q/G_{11}, activating the inositol-phosphate diacylglycerol cascade. The induction of signal via the phospholipase C (PLC) and intracellular Ca^{2+} pathways regulates iodide efflux, H_2O_2 production, and Tg iodination, whereas the signal via the protein kinase A (PKA) pathways mediated by cAMP regulates iodine uptake and transcription of Tg, TPO, and the NIS mRNAs leading to thyroid hormone production (Table 11-2).[42,43] Although

TABLE 11-2
Thyroid Cell Functions Stimulated by Thyrotropin

Function Affected	General Mechanism
Iodide Metabolism	
Increase I⁻ in follicular lumen	PLC
Delayed increase in NIS expression	cAMP
Increase in thyroid blood flow	↑ Nitric oxide synthesis (↓ cellular iodide)
Increase in I⁻ efflux from thyroid cell	?
Thyroid Hormone Synthesis	
Hydrogen peroxide	PLC
Thyroglobulin and TPO synthesis	cAMP
NADPH via pentose-phosphate Pathway	?
Thyroid Hormone Secretion	
Pinocytosis of thyroglobulin	cAMP
Release of thyroglobulin into plasma via basolateral membrane	cAMP (?)
Mitogenesis	cAMP, PLC, and IGF-I⁻ and FGF-mediated kinase activation

cAMP, cyclic adenosine monophosphate; FGF, follicular growth factor; IGF, insulin-like growth factor; I⁻, plasma iodide; NADPH, nicotinamide adenosine dinucleotide phosphate; NIS, sodium-iodide symporter; PLC, phospholipase C; TPO, thyroid peroxidase.

the discovery that different mutations in various regions of the TSHR molecule resulted in intrinsic activation and the identification of important domains for intramolecular TSHR signal transduction (see Chapter 12), the precise mechanisms of receptor activation and the early events of TSHR signal transduction are not fully understood.[41] Studies using mutational analyses have suggested that the interactions between the ectodomain and the extracellular loops of the transmembrane domains in the TSHR may be critical for the maintenance of an inactive state with no constitutive activity. When these constraints are removed, an open conformation ensues. Therefore, it has been proposed that the TSHR exists in both a closed (inactive) and open (active) format. This model predicts that only the open format of the receptor would be able to bind ligand and become activated. Further support for this model came from the development of constitutive activation when the TSHR ectodomain was truncated, suggesting that its presence dampened a constitutively active α-subunit.

The TSHR, in addition to the TSH, also binds TSHR-stimulating antibody (TRAb), thyroid-blocking antibodies (TBAb), and neutral antibodies to the TSHR (see Chapter 12). The closely related luteinizing hormone (LH) and chorionic gonadotropin (CG) also bind to and activate TSHR signaling.[41] The latter accounts for the physiologic hyperthyroidism of early pregnancy. Besides the thyrocyte, the TSHR is also expressed in a variety of tissues such as osteoclasts, fibroblasts, and adipocytes, as well as retroorbital adipocytes and skin.[41,44] As discussed earlier, certain activating and inactivating mutations, either germline or somatic, have been identified in the membrane-spanning or intracellular portions of the TSHR molecule that cause generalized or nodular hyperfunction and congenital hypofunction.[41,45]

THYROID HORMONES IN PERIPHERAL TISSUES

Plasma Transport

The metabolic transformations of thyroid hormones in peripheral tissues determine their biologic potency and regulate their biologic effects. Consequently, an understanding of thyroid physiopathology requires knowledge of the pathways of thyroid hormone metabolism. A wide variety of iodothyronines and their metabolic derivatives exist in plasma. Of these, T_4 is highest in concentration and the only one that arises solely from direct secretion by the thyroid gland. In normal humans, T_3 is also released from the thyroid, but approximately 80% is derived from the peripheral tissues by the enzymatic removal of a single 5′ iodine atom (outer ring or 5′ monodeiodination) from T_4.[46] The remaining iodothyronines and their derivatives are generated in the peripheral tissues from T_4 and T_3. Principal among them are 3,3′,5′-triiodothyronine (reverse T_3, or rT_3) and 3,3′-diiodo-L-thyronine (3,3′-T_2) (Fig. 11-2).

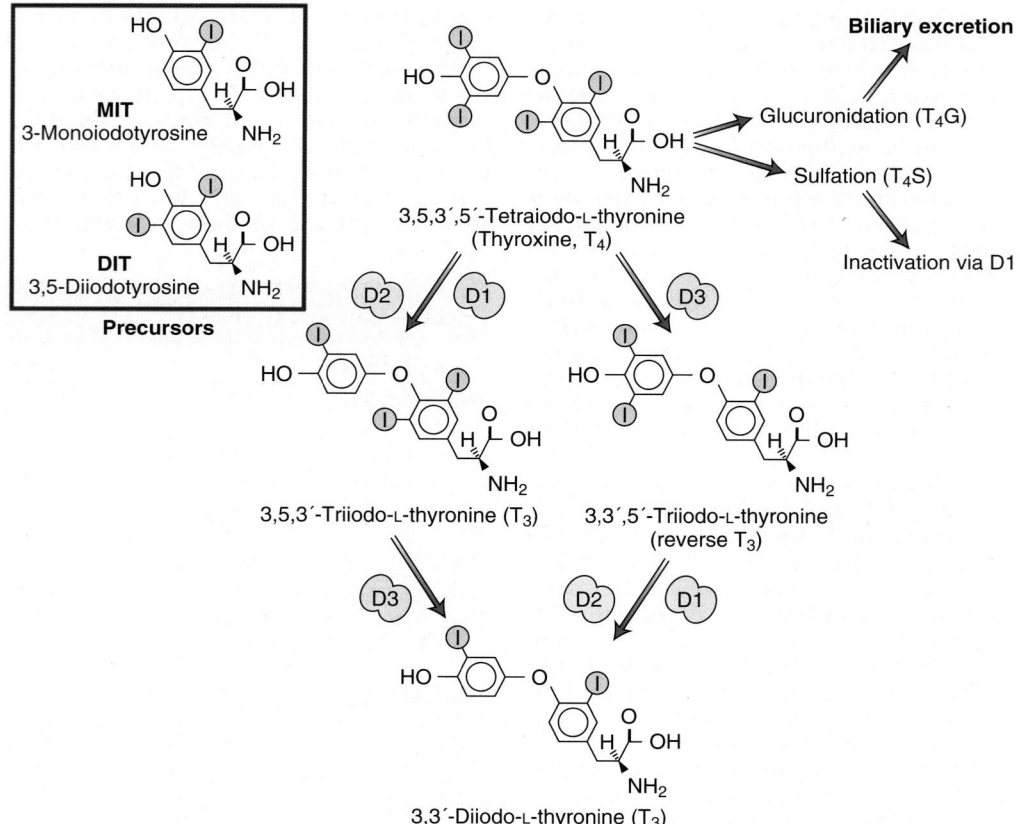

Figure 11-2 Major deiodinative and nondeiodinative pathways of thyroid hormone metabolism. The iodothyronine deiodinases are abbreviated D1, D2, and D3 for type 1, 2, and 3 deiodinases, respectively. *Arrows* refer to monodeiodination of the outer or inner ring of the iodothyronine nucleus, which are termed 5′ or 5 by convention. T_4 is activated by monodeiodination of the phenolic thyronine ring by D1 or D2 to form T_3. Deiodination of the tyrosyl ring by D1 or D3 inactivates T_4 and T_3. This inactivation pathway is markedly favored by sulfation of the phenolic hydroxyl to form T_4SO_4 (T_4S) or T_3SO_4 (T_3S). Glucuronidated T_4 and T_3 (T_4G and T_3G) are excreted into the bile but may be partially reabsorbed after deglucuronidation in the intestine.

TABLE 11-3

Comparison of the Major Human Thyroid Hormone–Binding Proteins

Parameter	Thyroxine-Binding Globulin	Transthyretin	Albumin
Molecular weight of holoprotein (kDa)	54,000	54,000 (4 subunits)	66,000
Plasma concentrations (μmol/L)	0.27	4.6	640
T_4 binding capacity as μg T_4/dL	21	350	50,000
Association constants of the major binding site (L/mol)			
T_4	1×10^{10}	7×10^7	7×10^5
T_3	5×10^8	1.4×10^7	1×10^5
Fraction of sites occupied by T_4 in euthyroid plasma	0.31	0.02	<0.001
Distribution volume (L)	7	5.7	7.8
Turnover rate (% day)	13	59	5
Distribution of iodothyronines (% protein)			
T_4	68	11	20
T_3	80	9	11

T_3, triiodothyronine; T_4, thyroxine.

Trace concentrations of other diiodothyronines, monoiodothyronines, and conjugates thereof with glucuronic or sulfuric acid are also present.[47,48] Deaminated derivatives of T_4 and T_3 that bear an acetic acid rather than an alanine side chain (tetrac and triac) are also present in low concentrations (see Fig. 11-2). 3-Iodothyronamine (T1AM) is an endogenous thyroid hormone derivative with unknown biosynthetic origins. Structural similarities have led to the hypothesis that T1AM is an extrathyroidal metabolite of T_4.[49]

The major iodothyronines are poorly soluble in water and thus bind reversibly to plasma proteins. The plasma proteins with which T_4 is mainly associated are TBG and transthyretin (TTR; formerly termed T_4-binding prealbumin [TBPA]) and albumin (Table 11-3). About 75% to 80% of T_3 is bound by TBG and the remainder by TTR and albumin.

Thyroxine-Binding Globulin

TBG is a glycoprotein with a molecular mass of about 54 kDa, about 20% of which is carbohydrate, encoded by a 3.8-kb transcript located on the X chromosome.[50] The protein sequence of TBG resembles that of the serpin family of serine antiproteases. Because there is one iodothyronine binding site per TBG molecule, the T_4 or T_3 binding capacity of TBG in normal human serum is equivalent to its concentration, which is approximately 270 nmol/L (1.5 μg/dL). The half-life of the protein in plasma is about 5 days. A congenital deficiency of TBG is common, occurring in 1/5000 newborns, and is associated with the complete absence of the protein in males. L-Asparaginase blocks the synthesis of TBG, which accounts for the low T_4 concentrations in patients receiving this agent.

The glycosylation of TBG influences its clearance from the plasma and its behavior during isoelectric focusing. In estrogen-treated patients, there is an increase in the prevalence of the more acidic bands of TBG. The more highly sialylated TBG is cleared more slowly from plasma than is the more positively charged TBG, because sialylation inhibits the hepatic uptake of glycoproteins. Sera from pregnant patients, women receiving oral contraceptives, and patients

with acute hepatitis have increased fractions of acidic TBG. Patients with inherited TBG excess have normal amounts of highly sialylated TBG, as do men and nonpregnant women. Because TBG is the principal T_4- and T_3-binding protein, changes in TBG or its binding are paralleled by changes in total plasma T_4 and T_3 even though T_4 and T_3 production is little changed.

Another post-translational modification affecting TBG occurs in septic patients or following cardiopulmonary bypass surgery.[51] TBG is subjected to cleavage by a serine protease released from polymorphonuclear leukocytes, resulting in the release of a 5-kDa carboxy-terminal loop with a consequent decrease in affinity for T_4. An analogous reaction has been described for cortisol-binding globulin, which releases cortisol at the site of inflammation.[52] It has been postulated that the released T_4 might play a critical role in the response to injury perhaps by providing a supply of iodine for antibacterial purposes.[51] The cleaved TBG of approximately 49 kDa circulates, and because it binds T_4 with lower avidity, it may explain the increased ratio of free to bound T_4 in acute illness, even when TBG saturation studies or immunoassays indicate TBG concentration is normal (see later section, "Thyroid Function During Fasting or Illness").

Transthyretin

TTR exists in part as a complex with retinol (vitamin A)-binding protein, hence its name. It consists of four identical polypeptide chains with a total molecular mass of approximately 55 kDa and is not glycosylated. Its concentration in plasma is approximately 4 mmol/L (250 μg/mL). Each mole of TTR binds 1 mole of T_4 with high affinity, and a second T_4 molecule is bound with lower affinity at high concentrations of T_4. Its half-life in plasma is normally about 2 days, but this decreases during illness. TTR is expressed in the choroid plexus and it is the major thyroid hormone-binding protein in the cerebrospinal fluid (CSF).[53] High levels of TTR have been detected in fetal serum, probably directly produced by placental cells.[54] Targeted TTR gene disruption in mice shows that there is no impairment of uptake of T_4 into the brain, leaving the role of TTR in CSF undefined in regard to thyroid physiology.[55,56]

Variant forms of TTR are associated with familial amyloidotic polyneuropathy.[57,58] In affected families, the TTR monomer has one of several different point mutations, and TTR accumulates in the amyloid tissue deposits. Neither thyroid dysfunction nor altered vitamin A metabolism has been reported, although there is altered affinity of some of the mutant proteins for T_4. Families with both high-affinity TTR and a few with increased TTR levels have been reported.

Competition for T_4 and T_3 Binding to TBG and TTR by Therapeutic Agents

The TBG binding site has an affinity for T_3 that is about 20-fold less than that for T_4 (see Table 11-3). Binding of T_4 and T_3 by TBG is inhibited by phenytoin,[59] salicylate,[60] salsalate, furosemide, fenclofenac, and mitotane. The affinity of these compounds for TBG is much weaker than is that of the iodothyronines, but their concentration in plasma is sufficiently high to compete with T_4 and T_3 binding and reduce total hormone levels, although free T_4 remains normal. Because all methods used for estimating the free fractions of T_4 and T_3 in human serum except ultrafiltration dilute the serum, euthyroid patients receiving these drugs may appear to have low total and free T_4 or T_3, whereas in vivo the free fraction is normal.

Albumin

The affinity of albumin for T_4 and T_3 binding is much lower than that of either TBG or TTR, but the high concentration of this protein results in the binding of 10% of the plasma thyroid hormones (see Table 11-3). Changes in albumin concentration per se have little influence on the total hormone levels, unless accompanied by alterations in TBG and TTR, all three of which are synthesized in the liver. Hepatic failure or nephrotic syndrome leads to decreases in the plasma concentration of all three, and the serum albumin concentration in patients with these illnesses may serve as a surrogate for estimating TBG concentrations.

The role of albumin in thyroid physiology becomes clinically important in patients with familial dysalbuminemic hyperthyroxinemia (FDH).[61,62] In this autosomal dominant disorder, the plasma contains high amounts of a usually minor albumin variant that binds T_4 (but not T_3) with increased avidity. This increases total T_4, but free T_4 and total and free T_3 remain normal in an otherwise euthyroid patient. However, such patients may have a confusing pattern of test results, especially when analogue methods or labeled T_3 are used to estimate the free T_4 or T_3 (see Chapter 6).

Other Plasma Thyroid Hormone–Binding Proteins

Between 3% and 6% of plasma T_4 and T_3 are bound to lipoproteins. The T_4-binding lipoprotein is a 27-kDa homodimer with an affinity for T_4 that is lower than that of TBG. This binding is of uncertain physiologic significance but could play a role in targeting T_4 delivery to specific tissues.

Free Thyroid Hormones

Because most of the circulating T_4 and T_3 is bound to TBG, its concentration and degree of saturation are the major determinants of the free fraction of T_4. Binding of the thyroid hormones to the plasma proteins alters their metabolism. The negligible urinary excretion of T_3 and T_4 is due to the limited filterability of the hormone-binding protein complexes at the glomerulus. In vitro, the interaction between the thyroid hormones and their binding proteins conforms to a reversible binding equilibrium that can be expressed by conventional equilibrium equations. For the formulations that follow, T_4 is used as the prototype, with the understanding that similar interactions apply in the case of T_3. The interaction between T_4 and TBG can be expressed as follows:

$$T_4 + TBG \xrightarrow{k_a} T_4 \cdot TBG$$

where TBG represents the *unoccupied* binding protein, k_a the equilibrium association constant for the interaction, and T_4 the concentration of *free* T_4; $T_4 \cdot TBG$ is T_4 bound to TBG (~68% of total T_4 is bound to TBG).

Rearranging, we can express this as:

$$\frac{T_4 \cdot TBG}{(T_4)(TBG)} = k_a$$

$$\frac{T_4}{T_4 \cdot TBG} = \frac{1}{(TBG)k_a}$$

Thus, the free fraction of T_4 ($T_4 / T_4 \cdot TBG$) is inversely proportional to the concentration of *unoccupied* TBG binding sites. Estimates of the free T_4 concentration in serum can be generated by direct or indirect assays. In normal serum, the free T_4 is approximately 0.02% of the total (about 20 pmol/L, 1.5 ng/dL). The approximately 20-fold lower affinity of TBG for T_3 results in a higher proportion of unbound T_3 (0.30%) (see Table 11-3).

It is the free hormone that is available to the tissues for intracellular transport and feedback regulation that induces its metabolic effects and that undergoes deiodination or degradation. The bound hormone acts merely as a reservoir. It follows that the concentration of the free hormone is the determinant of the metabolic state and it is this concentration that is defended by homeostatic mechanisms. If a change in TBG occurs, the free T_4 concentration and T_3 concentrations can be maintained at normal levels only if the bound hormone changes in the same direction. For example, when TBG concentrations are increased by administration of estrogen, the free T_4 reduction reduces T_4 clearance, allowing an increase in the plasma total T_4 concentration. This is an iterative process that eventually would normalize the free T_4 at a new equilibrium without a change in T_4 secretion rate. The transient decrease in free thyroid hormones also slightly reduces the negative feedback on the hypothalamic-pituitary-thyroid axis, which causes an increase in thyroid hormone production as an additional compensation.[63]

The preceding formulation is termed the *free thyroid hormone hypothesis*.[64,65] If it is free hormone that is available for cellular entry, what is the role, if any, of the hormone-binding proteins? Protein binding facilitates the distribution of the hydrophobic thyroid hormones throughout the vascular system. For example, if a protein-free solution containing tracer T_3 is perfused through rat liver via the portal vein, there is a steep concentration gradient with a decreasing quantity of T_3 in the solution as the distance from the center of the portal lobule increases. In fact, virtually all of the T_3 is taken up by the first cells to be contacted by the bolus. In contrast, if albumin is added to the perfusate, the distribution of tracer is uniform throughout the lobule. Both influx and efflux of thyroid hormone from tissues is rapid. Thus, intracellular free T_3 and T_4 are in equilibrium with the free hormone pool in plasma although transporter activity and metabolism will influence the magnitude of the ratio. In the steady state, the rate of T_3 and T_4 metabolism, not the dissociation rate from plasma proteins, is rate-limiting in the exit of hormones from the plasma.

T_4 and T_3 Transport Across Cell Membranes and Intracellular T_3 Binding

The progress in the field of transmembrane thyroid hormone transport has been truly astonishing. It has been assumed for a long time that transport of iodothyronines across the plasma membrane occurs by passive diffusion, but it has become increasingly clear that cellular uptake and efflux of thyroid hormone is mediated by transporter protein.[66] Several specific thyroid hormone transporters have been identified, including monocarboxylate transporter 8 (MCT8), MCT10, and organic anion transporting polypeptide 1C1 (OATP1C1). MCT8 and MCT10 are expressed in multiple tissues where they facilitate transport of T_3, T_4, rT_3, and T_2 across cell membranes; OATP1C1 is expressed predominantly in the brain and transports preferentially T_4, wherein it may mediate the entry of T_4 into the astrocytes. A defect in a single thyroid hormone transporter molecule, MCT8, has been shown to cause a severe developmental neurologic phenotype.[66,62] The Allan-Herndon-Dudley syndrome (AHDS) is an X-linked condition characterized by severe mental retardation, dysarthria, athetoid movements, muscle hypoplasia, and spastic paraplegia associated with an elevated serum T_3. All patients tested with this syndrome have mutations in the *MCT8* gene.[63,67] More than 200 individuals belonging to some 100 families of all races and diverse ethnic origins harboring more than 70 different mutations have been identified.[68] Although most mutations resulted in a complete functional inactivation of the MCT8 protein, significant residual activity was observed with a number of *MCT8* mutations, some of which associated with a milder clinical phenotype.[69] Surprisingly, MCT8-null mice, despite the presence of marked increased T_3 levels, lack any overt neurologic abnormalities, a rather unexpected finding in light of the severe human phenotype.[70,71] Coexistence of thyroid hormone excess and deprivation in different tissues is a distinct characteristic of this syndrome. Tissues expressing transporters other than MCT8, such as liver and kidney, respond to the high circulating T_3 levels resulting in a local hyperthyroid state, whereas tissues depending on MCT8 for thyroid hormone entry into cells, such as the brain, are hypothyroid.[68,72] Two therapeutic options, PTU combined with L-T_4[68] and a thyromimetic compound, diiodothyropropionic acid (DITPA), which is not dependent on MCT8 for cellular entry, have been used to treat several patients harboring *MCT8* gene mutations.[73]

Another transporter specific for T_4, OATP1C1 (a member of the organic anion transporting polypeptide family), is expressed in capillaries throughout the brain, suggesting it may be involved in the transport of T_4 across the blood-brain barrier.[66] Taken together, these results suggest that the supply of T_3 to neurons may occur according to the schema shown in Figure 11-3.[74] T_4 is transferred into the choroid plexus or into tanycytes via the action of OATP1C1, which is negatively regulated in brain capillaries by thyroid

hormone. In the tanycyte or astrocyte, T_4 is converted to T_3 by the type 2 iodothyronine deiodinase (D2) and exits the cell, possibly via the MCT8/MCT10 transporters, where it becomes available for neuronal uptake, also via MCT8.[75,76] Neurons express the type 3 deiodinase (D3), which prevents activation of T_4 and catalyzes degradation of T_3 (see "Iodothyronine Deiodination"). This would provide a logical explanation of the association of the mutations in MCT8 with the ADHD syndrome, although it still remains puzzling why the neurologic manifestations of this condition are so different from those seen in patients with untreated congenital hypothyroidism or severe iodine deficiency (see Chapter 13).

The transport field has become more complex as evidence accumulates of tissue-specific as well as generalized iodothyronine transporters belonging to a number of different transporter protein families. Each of these has many members with small variations in structure, which alter the specificity of the target substance. A thorough review of this topic is beyond the scope of this chapter, and the interested reader is referred to excellent reviews for further information.[66,77]

In most cells, about 90% of the intracellular T_3 is located in the cytosol. The known exception is in the pituitary, where approximately 50% of the intracellular T_3 is present in the nucleus. The mechanisms determining this distribution are still unknown, but it would not be surprising if there were active transport of thyroid hormones in and out of the nucleus and between other intracellular compartments. An intracellular T_3-binding protein (mu-crystallin) has been identified, which is expressed at high levels in

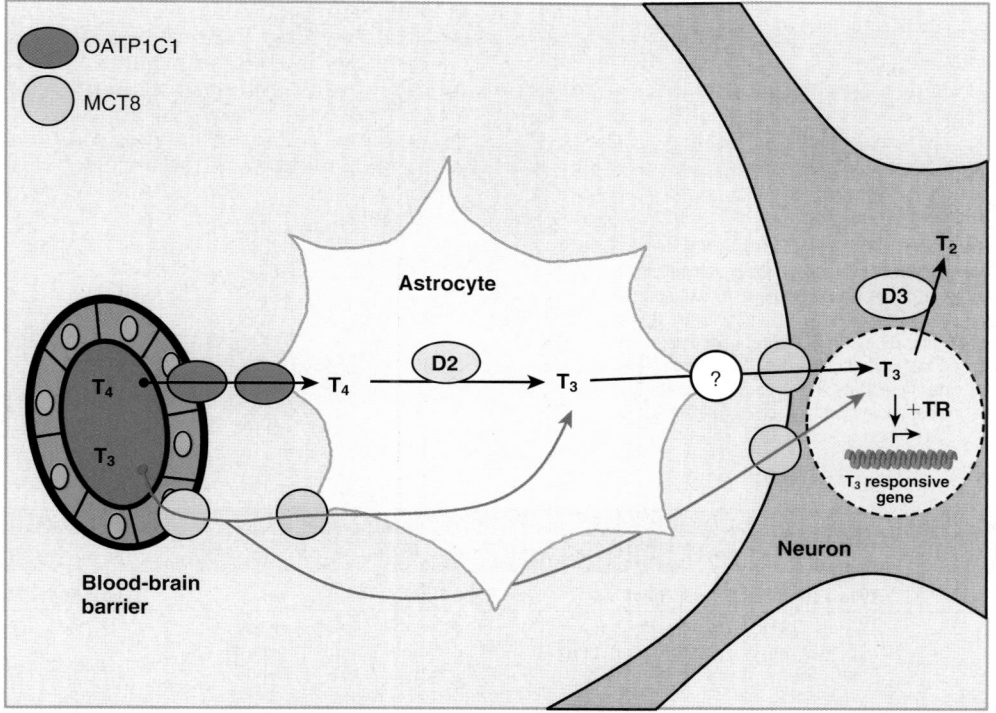

Figure 11-3 Potential pathways for entry of T_3 into the central nervous system. Thyroid hormones are transported through the blood-brain barrier (OATP) or the blood-CSF barrier (OATP and MCT8). In the astrocytes and tanycytes, T_4 is converted to T_3, which then enters the neurons, possibly through MCT8. In the neurons, both T_4 and T_3 are degraded by D3. T_3 from the tanycytes may reach the portal vessels in the median eminence. Other transporters may be present on the astrocyte or tanycyte membranes. In most cases the transport could be bidirectional, although only one direction is shown. The interaction of T_3 with the thyroid hormone receptor (TR) bound as a heterodimer with retinoid X receptor to the thyroid hormone–response element, often in the 5′ flanking region of a T_3-responsive gene, causes either an increase or a decrease in the transcription of that gene. This leads to parallel changes in the concentrations of critical proteins, thus producing the thyroid hormone response characteristic of a given cell. CSF, cerebrospinal fluid; D2 and D3, type 2 and type 3 iodothyronine deiodinases; MCT8, the monocarboxylate transporter 8; OATP, organic anion transporting polypeptide; T_2, diiodothyronine; T_3, triiodothyronine; T_4, thyroxine.

human brain and heart but is widely distributed. This or similar proteins may also play a role in the subcellular localization of the active hormone.

Iodothyronine Deiodination

The most important pathway for T_4 metabolism is its outer ring (5′) monodeiodination to the active thyroid hormone, T_3. This reaction is catalyzed by the type 1 and 2 deiodinases (D1 and D2) and is the source of more than 80% of the circulating T_3 in humans (see Fig. 11-2). Inner ring deiodination, an inactivating step, is catalyzed primarily by D3, which inactivates T_3 and prevents activation of T_4 by converting it to rT_3 (see Fig. 11-2).[46,78] The structures of the three human deiodinases are similar, all being homodimers and integral membrane proteins and all require a thiol cofactor for successful catalysis (Fig. 11-4). They contain the rare amino acid selenocysteine in the active catalytic center (Table 11-4). Selenocysteine has nucleophilic properties that make it ideal for catalysis of oxidoreductive reactions such as iodothyronine deiodination and the reduction of H_2O_2 by another family of selenoenzymes, the glutathione peroxidases.[79,80] The crystal structure of the catalytic domain of mouse deiodinase 3 (Dio3) revealed a close structural similarity to atypical 2-cysteine peroxiredoxin(s).[81] Selenium is thought to be the iodine acceptor during deiodination reactions. Mutagenesis of selenocysteine in D1 to cysteine, that is, replacing selenium with sulfur, reduces the enzyme velocity by approxi-

mately 200-fold. The presence of selenocysteine has implications beyond catalytic activity, considering that the cellular processes for synthesizing selenoproteins are complex and inefficient.[46] This is accomplished by a combination of a specific structural feature, the selenocysteine insertion sequence (SECIS) element, in the 3′ untranslated region of the mRNAs encoding these proteins together with a specific group of selenocysteine incorporating gene products. All these elements are required for the complex cellular function by which the normal STOP codon UGA is recognized as the specific codon for the insertion of the selenocysteine residue during protein translation.[82]

Enzymology and Regulation of the Selenodeiodinases

Although both D1 and D2 activate T_4, they have several important differences (see Table 11-4). D1 catalyzes both 5′ and 5 deiodination of T_4 to form T_3 and rT_3, respectively, although the Michaelis-Menten constant (K_m) for these reactions is approximately 3 orders of magnitude greater than that of D2 and D3 for this substrate. The preferred substrates of D1 are rT_3 (5′ deiodination) and T_3SO_4 (5 deiodination). D1 is inhibited by PTU, unlike D2 or D3. D1 also differs from D2 in being markedly increased by excess thyroid hormone through increased gene transcription, whereas D2 mRNA and protein are reduced by thyroid hormones. D2 has a half-life of only 20 to 30 minutes but that of D1 and D3 is more than 12 hours. This is due to the rapid ubiquitination of D2, a process that is accelerated

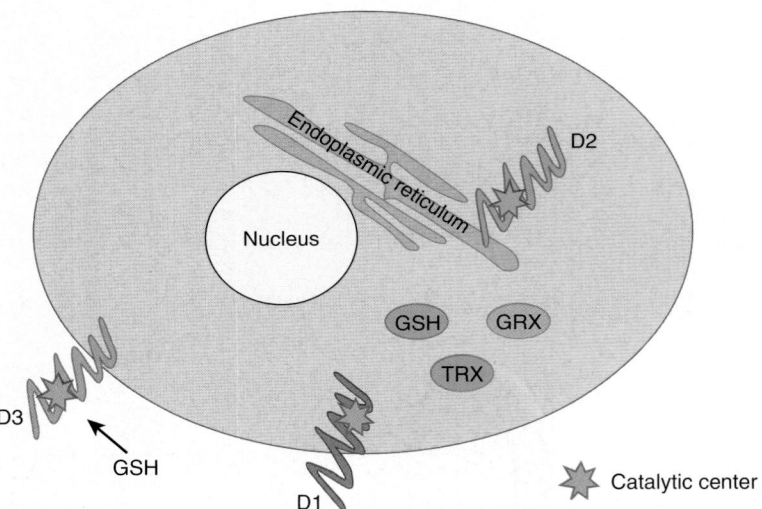

Figure 11-4 Predicted topologies of the three iodothyronine deiodinases. The deiodinases are integral membrane proteins that require a thiol cofactor for catalytic activity. The type 1 deiodinase (D1) is in the plasma membrane and type 2 (D2) is localized in the endoplasmic reticulum. The active centers of D1 and D2 are in the cytosol and depend on intracellular thiols such as reduced glutathione (GSH), thioredoxin (TRX), and glutaredoxin (GRX) for catalytic activity. The type 3 deiodinase (D3) is also anchored in the plasma membrane but has access to extracellular thiols.

TABLE 11-4
Human Iodothyronine Selenodeiodinases

Parameter	Type 1 (Outer and Inner Ring)	Type 2 (Outer Ring)	Type 3 (Inner Ring)
Physiologic role	rT_3 and T_3S degradation, the source of plasma T_3 in thyrotoxic patients	Provide intracellular T_3 in specific tissues, a source of plasma T_3	Inactivate T_3 and T_4
Tissue location	Liver, kidney, thyroid, pituitary (?) (not CNS)	CNS, pituitary, BAT, placenta thyroid, skeletal muscle, heart	Placenta, CNS, hemangiomas, fetal or adult liver, skeletal muscle
Subcellular location	Plasma membrane	Endoplasmic reticulum	Plasma membrane
Preferred substrates (position deiodinated)	rT_3 (5′), T_3S (5)	T_4, rT_3 (5′)	T_3, T_4 (5)
K_m	rT_3, 10^{-7}; T_4, 10^{-6}	10^{-9}	10^{-9}
Susceptibility to PTU	High	Absent	Absent
Response to increased T_4	↑	↓	↑

BAT, brown adipose tissue; CNS, central nervous system; K_m, Michaelis-Menten constant; PTU, 6-n-propylthiouracil; rT_3, reverse triiodothyronine; T_3, triiodothyronine; T_3S, T_3SO_4; T_4, thyroxine.

by interaction with its substrates T_4 or rT_3. D1 and D3 are not thought to be ubiquitinated.

The intracellular location of D2 close to the nucleus gives the T_3 formed by its catalytic action better access to the nucleus than that formed by D1.[83] The T_3 produced by D2 is especially effective in entering the nucleus and binding to thyroid hormone receptors (TRs), a property explained by its location in the ER (see Fig. 11-4). D1, on the other hand, is located in the plasma membrane, and the T_3 produced by this enzyme preferentially enters the plasma pool.[46] Studies with deiodinase inhibitors and cofactors differentially able to cross the cell membrane indicate that the D3 active center is outside the cell and that of D2 and D1 are intracellular (see Fig. 11-4).[84] This makes D2 especially important for regulating the hypothalamic-pituitary-thyroid axis, where its activity increases in response to a decrease in serum T_4 concentrations, such as occurs in iodine deficiency or early autoimmune thyroid disease, well before the serum T_3 falls. If the decrease in plasma T_4 is too great to be compensated for by the increase in D2 activity in the hypothalamus and thyrotrophs, an increase in TRH and TSH will occur to stimulate the thyroid. For this reason D2 has principally been thought of as an enzyme that provides intracellular T_3 but there is increasing evidence that D2 could also contribute to plasma T_3. On the other hand, in thyrotoxicosis, the threefold to fourfold increase in D1, particularly in the thyroid, and the reduced D2 make D1 the major extrathyroidal source of T_3. This explains why the D1-inhibitor PTU causes a much more rapid fall in circulating T_3 than does methimazole in the patient with Graves disease.[37,38]

A single-nucleotide polymorphism, A/G, in the *Dio2* gene, predicts a threonine (Thr) to alanine (Ala) substitution at codon 92 (D2 Thr92Ala). This is present in about 20% of the Caucasian population. This polymorphism has been found, in some studies, to be associated with insulin resistance in obese patients, bipolar mood disorder, psychological well-being, mental retardation, hypertension, and risk for osteoarthritis, although other studies failed to find such association. It is not yet clear whether this D2 polymorphism impairs its catalytic efficiency in vivo.[85]

In the opposite direction, D2 has been found overexpressed in a few follicular carcinomas. In these patients, a reduced T_4/T_3 ratio has been found and is likely due to the increased D2-mediated T_4 to T_3 conversion.[39]

D3 is the most important thyroid hormone–inactivating enzyme catalyzing deiodination of the inner ring of both T_3 and T_4.[86,87] D3 activity has been identified in only a limited number of postnatal tissues, including placenta and uterine endometrium, the CNS (in which it is primarily in neurons), and skin. Much higher D3 expression has been demonstrated in various fetal tissues such as liver, brain, placenta, uterus, and umbilical arteries and vein. In the adult, D3 has been identified in some malignant cell lines and in a number of human tumors, including astrocytomas, oligodendromas, gliosarcomas, glioblastomas, TSH-secreting pituitary adenomas, colon cancers,[88] and basal cell carcinomas.[89] Tumoral D3 activity can be robust, and the highest D3 activity reported in any human tissue to date has been in infantile hemangiomas. In infants with extensive hepatic hemangiomas, D3 may overwhelm the secretory capacity of the infant's thyroid, causing hypothyroidism, a syndrome termed *consumptive hypothyroidism*.[90] Although most patients with consumptive hypothyroidism have hemangiomas, it now has become evident that it can occur in other types of tumors, including gastrointestinal stromal tumors.[91] Patients with consumptive hypothyroidism may only represent the extreme of a clinical spectrum of hypothyroidism due to dysregulated thyroid hormone

metabolism in malignant tissues. *Dio3* gene expression is increased by thyroid hormone at a transcriptional level.[92]

Gene-targeting studies have begun to provide further insights into the physiologic roles of the deiodinases in mammals.[93] Inactivation of the *Dio2* gene results in a phenotypically normal mouse with an elevated serum T_4, normal serum T_3, and elevated serum TSH.[78,94] These animals have hypothalamic-pituitary resistance to T_4, impaired auditory function, impaired thermogenesis in response to cold stress, impaired muscle regeneration[95] and relatively subtle defects in neurologic function. These findings are all consistent with the expectations based on earlier studies indicating an important role for D2 in brown fat cell function, cochlear maturation, and neurologic development. The intracellular balance between D2 and D3 is dynamically regulated and plays a central role in controlling muscle homeostasis and regenerative potential.[96] Mice with targeted inactivation of *Dio1* are phenotypically normal but also have an elevated serum T_4 and a normal serum T_3 and but TSH is normal.[97] The most striking finding in the D1-deficient mouse is a marked shift in the T_4 clearance pathway from deiodinative to biliary/fecal clearance. Interestingly, mice lacking both of the activating deiodinases D1 and D2 are still capable (by increasing TSH and thyroidal T_3 secretion) of maintaining normal T_3 concentrations in serum and do not suffer from systemic hypothyroidism, indicating that thyroidal T_3 production can guarantee T_3 homeostasis at least in rodents.[78,94] Mice with targeted inactivation of the *Dio3* gene show profound abnormalities. They have impaired fertility and develop central hypothyroidism in adult life, presumably due to hypothalamic thyrotoxicosis during developmental programming.[98]

Quantitative and Qualitative Aspects of Thyroid Hormone Metabolism
Thyroid Hormone Turnover

In the normal adult, T_4 has a distribution volume of approximately 10 L (Table 11-5). Because the concentration of total T_4 in plasma is approximately 100 nmol/L (~8 µg/dL), the extrathyroidal T_4 pool is approximately 1 µmol (800 µg). In the adult, the fractional rate of turnover of T_4 in the periphery is about 10% per day (half-life, 6.7 days). Thus, about 1.1 L of the peripheral T_4 distribution space is cleared of hormone daily, a volume containing approximately 110 nmol (85 µg) of T_4.

The kinetics of T_3 metabolism differ from those of T_4, partly because of its 10- to 15-fold lower affinity for TBG.

TABLE 11-5

Comparison of Triiodothyronine (T_3) and Thyroxine (T_4) in Humans

Parameter	T_3	T_4
Production rate (nmol/day)	50	110
Fraction from thyroid	0.2	1.0
Relative metabolic potency	1.0	0.3
Serum concentration		
Total (nmol/L)	1.8	100
Free (pmol/L)	5	20
Fraction of total hormone in free form ($\times 10^{-2}$)	0.3	0.02
Distribution volume (L)	40	10
Fraction intracellular	0.64	0.15
Half-life (days)	0.75	6.7

To convert T_4 from nmol/L to µg/dL (total) or pmol/L to ng/dL (free), divide by 12.87. To convert T_3 from nmol/L to ng/dL (total) or pmol/L to pg/dL (free), multiply by 65.1.

The volume of distribution of T_3 in the normal adult is about 40 L, about four times that of T_4, and its fractional turnover rate is approximately 60% per day. At a mean normal serum T_3 concentration of 1.8 nmol/L (120 ng/dL), 50-fold lower than T_4, the daily production of T_3 is approximately 50 nmol (33 µg) or about 46% that of T_4 (see Table 11-5). The rapid metabolic clearance rate of the product of inner ring T_4 deiodination, rT_3, and the low concentration in plasma (0.25 nmol/L, 15 ng/dL) combine to yield daily production rates for rT_3 of about 45 nmol. Thus, about 80% of T_3 and all of rT_3 production in humans can be accounted for by peripheral deiodination of T_4, findings consonant with the high ratio of T_4 to T_3 (15 : 1) and rT_3 (100 : 1) in human Tg. Of the T_3 generated via T_4 5′ deiodination in euthyroid humans, only about 70% is inhibited by PTU consistent with a significant contribution of D2-dependent T_3 production.[99] Although much of the T_3 and rT_3 produced from T_4 in peripheral tissues exits those tissues and enters the blood, an uncertain fraction of both are degraded intracellularly before their exit. As discussed later, in some D2-containing tissues, such as the pituitary, a significant fraction of T_3 in the cell nucleus is derived from intracellular T_4 deiodination to T_3, rather than from the plasma. This is particularly true in the thyrotroph.[100]

Other pathways are also involved in T_4 and T_3 metabolism. In humans, T_4 undergoes glucuronidation of the phenolic hydroxyl by the uridine diphosphate glucuronyl transferases (UDPGTs), but only minimal amounts of T_3 undergo this process (see Fig. 11-2). This pathway is clinically significant because certain pharmacotherapeutic agents may enhance glucuronide conjugation through induction of UDPGT, leading to biliary excretion of T_4-glucuronide (T_4-G) into the intestine.[101] These agents include phenobarbital, phenytoin, rifampin, and, possibly, certain of the synaptosomal serotonin reuptake inhibitors, such as sertraline. Because T_4-glucuronide may not be easily reabsorbed from intestinal contents, the clinical significance of this pathway is that therapy with such agents will generally increase levothyroxine requirements. In patients with an intact thyroid, this will not be apparent because internal adjustments will increase the T_4 production rate to compensate for the accelerated biliary excretion. In patients with hypothyroidism, however, an increase in levothyroxine dosage will often be required.

Sources of Intracellular T_3

In view of the differential tissue distribution of the various deiodinases, their different K_m values, and differential regulation, it is not surprising that tissues may derive intracellular T_3 via different pathways (Fig. 11-5). In several rat tissues, including tissues expressing D1 such as kidney and liver, most of the nuclear T_3 is derived from plasma T_3. In D2-containing tissues, such as the rat cerebral cortex, pituitary, brown fat, and skeletal muscle, D2 functions as an additional intracellular source of T_3, such that the nuclear T_3 concentration will be higher given the combination of T_3 from the plasma and the T_3 that is locally converted from T_4. In these tissues, half or more of intracellular T_3 is generated locally from T_4 within the tissue. In the CNS, the D2-generated T_3 in neurons is likely to derive from paracrine sources in tanycytes and astrocytes (see Fig. 11-3). In the rat, the tissues that depend on D2 for nuclear T_3 are those in which a constant supply of thyroid hormone is critical for either normal development (cerebral cortex), thyroid gland regulation (pituitary), or survival during cold stress (brown adipose tissue). These tissues are also characterized by a high degree of saturation of the nuclear T_3 receptors in comparison to tissues such as liver and kidney

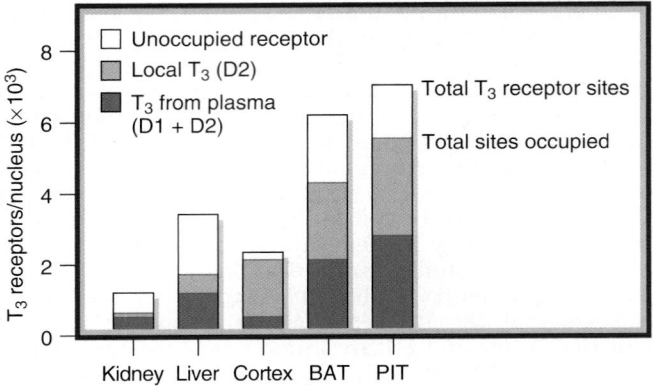

Figure 11-5 Schematic diagram of the origin of the specifically bound nuclear T_3 in various rat tissues. Data are derived from studies in which the sources of specifically bound nuclear T_3 in rat tissues were estimated using double-isotope labeling techniques. In tissues in which the receptor saturation is significantly greater than 50%, the additional T_3 is provided by D2-catalyzed conversion of thyroxine (T_4) to T_3. T_3 in rat plasma is derived from thyroid secretion (~40%) with the remainder from D1- and D2-catalyzed T_4 to T_3 conversion. BAT, brown adipose tissue; D1 and D2, type 1 and 2 iodothyronine deiodinases; PIT, pituitary; T_3, triiodothyronine.

in which nuclear T_3 receptor sites are only about 50% occupied at normal serum T_3 concentrations (see Fig. 11-5).

Intracellular D2-catalyzed T_3 production has important implications for thyroid hormone physiology. First, because the T_3 produced from T_4 occupies a significant fraction of the receptors in those tissues, changes in either serum T_4 or serum T_3 can change receptor occupancy. However, because a fall in T_4 will also increase D2 protein half-life by decreasing the rate of ubiquitination and its proteasomal degradation, a rise in D2 activity mitigates the impact of a reduction of serum T_4 in D2-expressing tissues, helping to maintain T_3 homeostasis.[46] The requirement for both T_3 and T_4 for normal saturation of pituitary and CNS T_3 receptors permits a response of the hypothalamic-pituitary axis to a reduction in plasma T_4, which is the earliest manifestation of iodine deficiency or primary hypothyroidism (see "Regulation of Thyroid Function"). Because the *Dio2* gene is positively regulated by cAMP, D2 activity and T_3 production increase rapidly in brown adipose tissue under stimulation by the sympathetic nervous system. This response is critical to adaptive thermogenesis during cold exposure in the human neonate and lifelong in the rodent.[102]

At the same time, tissues expressing D3 have lower T_3 concentrations than would be expected from the plasma contribution; thus, D3-expressing tissues have a gene expression profile similar to hypothyroid cells. This is explained by the inactivation of T_3 and T_4 that takes place immediately after these hormones enter the cell. The D3-mediated reduction in T_3 levels likely occurs in several physiologic (development, regeneration) or pathologic settings (cancer cells, inflammation, myocardial infarction) in which D3 is upregulated.[103]

Pharmacologic Agents Inhibiting Thyroid Hormone Deiodination

A number of commonly used pharmacologic agents have significant effects on thyroid hormone deiodination. PTU inhibition of D1 is mentioned earlier. The antiarrhythmic drug amiodarone shares sufficient structural similarity with T_4 that it can inhibit deiodination of T_4 and rT_3 by D1 and possibly by D2 (Fig. 11-6). This causes an increase in plasma T_4 to maintain serum T_3 in the normal range. Also, levels

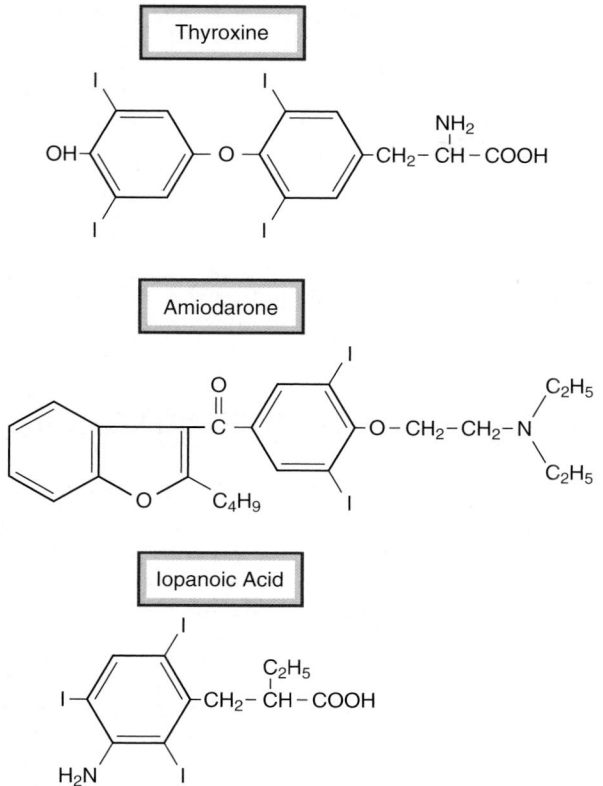

Figure 11-6 Comparison of the chemical structure of thyroxine (T$_4$) with that of two agents that block the deiodination of the iodothyronines. The inhibition of T$_4$-to-T$_3$ conversion, which occurs in patients receiving amiodarone, may be due to the drug itself or to a metabolic product. Iopanoic acid and related iodoanilines are competitive inhibitors of all three iodothyronine deiodinases. T$_3$, triiodothyronine.

of TSH increase within the first weeks of therapy but gradually return to normal as the thyroid axis reequilibrates.[104] The T$_4$ and rT$_3$ metabolic clearance rates are reduced by 20% to 25%, with a reduction in the fractional T$_4$ to T$_3$ conversion rate of about 50%. Amiodarone also inhibits the active transport of T$_4$ and T$_3$ into hepatocytes, and the drug or one of its degradation products may interfere with T$_3$ binding to TRs.[105]

The effects of amiodarone resemble those observed with the iodoaniline derivatives formerly used for gallbladder visualization (see Fig. 11-6). Iopanoic and iopodipic acid inhibit the deiodinases by competing with the iodothyronine substrates.[46] These agents are useful in the acute treatment of patients with severe hyperthyroidism, but they are no longer available for clinical use in the United States.

High dosages of glucocorticoids (10 times replacement) will acutely reduce the ratio of T$_3$ to T$_4$ in plasma, suggesting that conversion of T$_4$ to T$_3$ is blocked. The ratio of rT$_3$ to T$_4$ increases, raising the possibility that D3 action is also increased.[106] These effects resolve during long-term therapy such that thyroid function is little affected and thyroid hormone requirements are not increased by chronic glucocorticoid therapy.

Recombinant growth hormone increases circulating T$_3$/T$_4$ ratio. Growth hormone deficiency is associated with a decrease in the ratio of T$_3$ to T$_4$ in serum, possibly associated with a decrease in outer ring deiodination. As expected, dietary selenium deficiency also inhibits the synthesis of D1 in humans.[107]

Mechanism of Thyroid Hormone Action

Thyroid hormone acts by binding to a specific nuclear TR, which, in turn, binds to DNA usually as a heterodimer with retinoid X receptor (RXR) at specific sequences (thyroid hormone response elements, or TREs) dictated by the DNA binding-site preferences of the RXR-TR (or TR-TR) complex (Fig. 11-7). The general mechanism by which nuclear

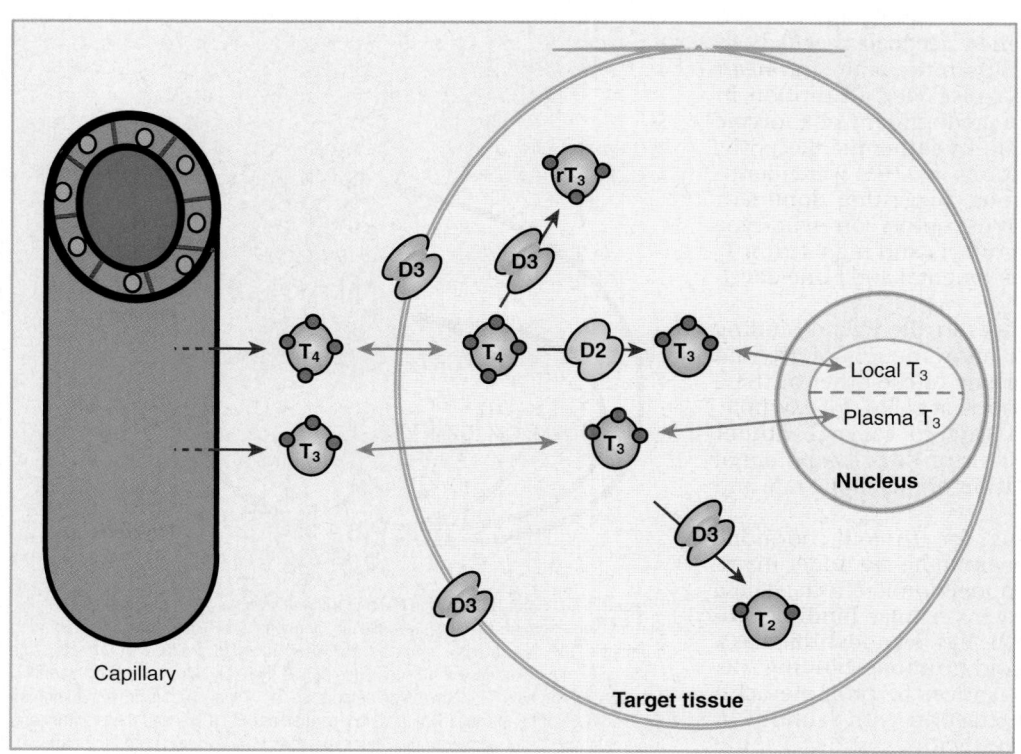

Figure 11-7 Schematic diagram of thyroid hormone activation and inactivation in a cell expressing the iodothyronine deiodinases D2 and D3. The triiodothyronine (T$_3$) that enters the cell can either be deiodinated to 3,3′-diiodothyronine (T$_2$) or enter the nucleus and bind to the thyroid hormone receptor. An additional source of T$_3$ is that generated by outer ring deiodination of thyroxine (T$_4$) within the cell. rT$_3$, reverse T$_3$.

receptor–activating ligands such as T_3 produce their effects is discussed in Chapter 3. T_3 has a 15-fold higher binding affinity for TRs than does T_4, explaining its function as the active thyroid hormone. In humans, there are two TR genes, α and β, found on different chromosomes (TRα, chromosome 17; TRβ, chromosome 3). Several alternatively spliced gene products from each of these genes form both active and inactive gene products. The active proteins are TRα_1 and TRs β_1, β_2, and β_3.[108] The protein structure of TRs includes three major functional domains, one binding DNA, one binding ligand, and a major transcriptional activation domain in the carboxy-terminus.

There are tissue-specific preferences in expression of the various TRs, suggesting that they subserve different functions in different tissues.[109] TRα_1 mRNA is expressed in the brain and brown adipose tissue and also in skeletal muscle, gastrointestinal tract, lungs, and heart. In general, TRβ, particularly TRβ_2, is thought to be important in the hypothalamus and pituitary, in which regulation of thyroid function occurs.[110] TRβ_1 is expressed in all tissues, although its mRNA is especially highly expressed in the kidney and liver. TRβ_2 is also expressed in the cochlea and the retina. TRβ_3 mRNA is expressed at very low levels but is more abundant in the liver, kidneys, and lungs in comparison with other tissues. In addition to differences in the amino-terminus between TRβ_1 and TRα_1, the two proteins are under the regulation of different promoters, which can function in tissue-specific patterns. TRβ_2 is downregulated by T_3, whereas TRα_1 mRNA expression is not affected.[111]

Experiments in which TRα and TRβ have been inactivated illuminate their different physiologic roles. Disruption of the TRβ gene (both TRβ_1 and TRβ_2) in mice causes deafness, a marked reduction in feedback sensitivity of the hypothalamic-pituitary-thyroid axis, and a decrease in hepatic D1. Thus, these mice have significant elevations in both TSH and thyroid hormones similar to those in families with resistance to thyroid hormone (RTH) in which TRβ mutations markedly reduce its binding affinity for T_3. This binding defect produces a TRβ_1 or TRβ_2 protein, which acts as a dominant negative inhibitor of the intact TRβ proteins encoded by the normal allele (see Chapters 3 and 13). Despite evidence of impaired feedback regulation, there is relatively little abnormality in the brain and heart of TRβ-deficient mice. The effect of a TRα_1 disruption in the mouse is quite different. The predominant phenotypic effects are modest bradycardia and hypothermia. Recently, the first four patients with mutations in *THRA* were identified. All patients are heterozygous, suggesting dominant negative effects of the mutant receptors on wild-type TRα. They presented with low serum T_4 and high serum T_3 levels, growth retardation, delayed mental and bone development, and constipation.[112,113]

It is likely that small differences in the ligand-binding domains of TRα and TRβ will allow design of thyroid hormone analogues selective for one or the other of these receptors. This may result in agents that could, for example, suppress TSH in patients with thyroid cancer, without inducing tachycardia, such as GC-1, or KB141, a potential treatment for obesity via stimulation of metabolic rate and oxygen consumption.[114]

Other potential mechanisms for thyroid hormone action by interaction with the membrane are under investigation and are referred to as nongenomic effects. These effects are most likely mediated by cellular binding proteins other than TRs. Integrin $\alpha_V\beta_3$ has been identified as a putative plasma membrane thyroid hormone–binding site. Previously, T_4, but not T_3, was shown to promote actin polymerization and integrin interaction with laminin in neural cells.[115] Continuing investigations show T_4 and

thyroid hormone analogues such as GC-1 can activate mitogen-activated protein kinase (MAPK) and have proangiogenic effects.[116] The MAPK signal results in serine phosphorylation of several nuclear proteins and occurs within minutes of exposure, analogous to the effects of 17β-estradiol. The physiologic relevance of these effects is not well characterized. Some of these proteins include plasma membrane associated T_3 transporters, calcium adenosine triphosphatase (ATPase), adenylate cyclase, and glucose transporters; an ER-associated protein, prolyl hydroxylase; and monomeric pyruvate kinase. The effect of T_4 per se to initiate the ubiquitination of D2 is perhaps the most important nongenomic effect of physiologic concentrations of free T_4.[46]

REGULATION OF THYROID FUNCTION

The Hypothalamic-Pituitary-Thyroid Axis

The thyroid participates with the hypothalamus and pituitary in a classical feedback control loop (Fig. 11-8). In addition, there is an inverse relationship between the iodine level in the thyroid and the fractional rate of hormone formation. Such autoregulatory mechanisms stabilize the rate of hormone synthesis despite fluctuations in the availability of iodine. Stability in hormone production is achieved in part because the large intraglandular store of hormone buffers the effect of acute increases or decreases in hormone synthesis. Autoregulatory mechanisms within the gland, in turn, tend to maintain a constant thyroid hormone pool. Finally, the hypothalamic-pituitary feedback mechanism senses variations in the availability of free thyroid hormones, however small, and acts to correct them. There is a close relationship between the hypothalamus, the anterior pituitary, the thyroid gland, and still higher centers in the brain, the function of the entire complex being modified in a typical negative-feedback manner by the availability of the thyroid hormones. In addition, other hormones and neuropeptides also influence this axis (see Chapters 7 and 8).

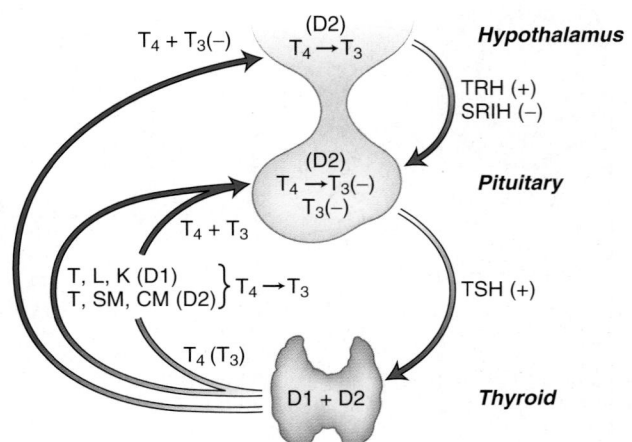

Figure 11-8 Roles of thyroxine (T_4) and triiodothyronine (T_3) in the feedback regulation of secretion of thyrotropin-releasing hormone (TRH) and thyroid-stimulating hormone (TSH). Secreted T_4 must be converted to T_3 to produce its effects. This conversion may take place in tissues such as the liver (L), kidney (K), and thyroid (T) catalyzed by the type 1 iodothyronine deiodinase, D1. Type 2 (D2) is present in human thyroid (T), skeletal muscle (SM), possibly cardiac muscle (CM), and the pituitary and hypothalamus. SRIH, somatotropin release-inhibiting factor (somatostatin hormone).

Thyrotropin-Releasing Hormone Synthesis and Secretion

TRH, a modified tripeptide (pyroglutamyl-histidyl-proline amide), is derived from a large prepro-TRH molecule of 29 kDa that contains five progenitor sequences. The TRH peptides are released from the prepro molecule by a peptidase that acts at flanking lysine/arginine residues. TRH is expressed in the hypothalamus, the brain, the C cells of the thyroid gland, the beta cells of the pancreas, the myocardium, the reproductive organs including prostate and testis, and the spinal cord. The parvocellular region of the paraventricular nuclei (PVN) of the hypothalamus is the source of the TRH that regulates TSH secretion. The 5' flanking region of the gene encoding TRH has sequences for mediating responses to glucocorticoids and cAMP. In addition, at least two elements in this region are responsible for the negative regulation of this gene by thyroid hormone.[117] TRH travels in the axons of the peptidergic neurons through the median eminence and is released close to the hypothalamic-pituitary portal plexus. The neuron bodies producing TRH are innervated by catecholamine, leptin, neuropeptide Y (NPY), agouti-related protein (AgRP) or melanocyte-stimulating hormone (MSH), and somatostatin-containing axons, all of which potentially influence the rate of synthesis of the prepro-TRH molecule (see Chapter 7). T_3 suppresses the levels of prepro-TRH mRNA in the hypothalamus,[118,119] but normal feedback regulation of prepro-TRH mRNA synthesis by thyroid hormone requires a combination of T_3 and T_4 in the circulation, the latter giving rise to T_3 via T_4 5' deiodination in the CNS in astrocytes and tanycytes (see Fig. 11-3). Another event in this feedback regulation may be the thyroid hormone–mediated induction of the TRH-inactivating pyroglutamyl peptidase II (PPII) in the hypothalamic tanycytes. This regulation is observed in vivo exclusively in the parvocellular division of the PVN, but in tissues outside the CNS expressing the TRH gene, negative regulation by thyroid hormone is absent. Thus, part of the negative feedback induced by T_4 may be generated at the median eminence/arcuate nucleus at a point where neuropeptides and T_3 enter the pituitary portal system.[120] Although D2 is also present in astrocytes in the median eminence and arcuate nucleus region, selective ablation of D2 from astrocytes in transgenic mice has no significant effect on feedback regulation of the hypophysiotropic TRH neurons, indicating that astrocytes have little or no role in the regulation of this response.[121] In addition to inhibiting the synthesis of prepro-TRH mRNA, thyroid hormone also blocks the capacity of TRH to stimulate TSH release from the thyrotroph.

TRH is rapidly inactivated within the CNS by a cell-surface peptidase called TRH-degrading ectoenzyme (TRH-DE), also termed protein peptidase II. TRH-DE is very specific: there is no other ectopeptidase known capable of degrading TRH, and TRH is the only known substrate of this unique enzyme.[122]

Thyrotropin Synthesis and Secretion

TSH is the major regulator of the morphologic and functional states of the thyroid. It is a glycoprotein secreted by the thyrotrophs in the anteromedial portion of the adenohypophysis (see Chapter 8). TSH is composed of an α-subunit of 14 kDa (92 amino acids) that is common to LH, follicle-stimulating hormone (FSH), human chorionic gonadotropin (hCG), and a specific β-subunit synthesized in thyrotrophs, which is a 112–amino acid protein. In normal thyrotrophs and in thyrotroph tumors, synthesis of α-subunit is in excess, indicating that the quantity of

β-subunit is rate-limiting for TSH secretion. Levels of α-subunit in serum range from 0.5 to 5 µg/L but are increased in postmenopausal women and patients with pituitary tumors. TRH increases and thyroid hormone suppresses the transcription of both subunits; these are the two most important influences on TSH synthesis.

The pretranslational regulation of TSH synthesis and secretion is a complex process. The physiologic glycosylation of TSH involves several post-translational steps including the excision of signal peptides from both subunits and cotranslational glycosylation with high mannose oligosaccharides.[123] The glycosylation of the subunits protects them from intracellular degradation and permits normal folding of the protein chains so that internal disulfide linkages are correctly formed. Glycosylation is required for full biologic activity.[124,125] TRH is required for this process as illustrated by the inappropriately low biologic activity of the TSH in the serum of patients with pituitary tumors or hypothalamic disorders is compared with immunologic activity due to TRH deficiency.

In normal serum, TSH is present at concentrations between 0.4 and 4.2 mU/L. The level is increased in primary hypothyroidism and reduced in thyrotoxicosis. The plasma TSH half-life is about 30 minutes, and production rates in humans are 40 to 150 mU/day. Circulating TSH displays both pulsatile and circadian variations. The former are characterized by fluctuations at 1- to 2-hour intervals. The magnitude of TSH pulsations is decreased during fasting, during illness, or after surgery. There is an acute reduction of TSH in fasted humans, associated with a fall in leptin levels. This is due to a decrease in the amplitude of the TSH pulses.[126] The circadian variation is characterized by a nocturnal surge that precedes the onset of sleep and appears to be independent of the cortisol rhythm and fluctuations in the serum and T_4 and T_3 concentrations.[127] When the onset of sleep is delayed, the nocturnal TSH surge is enhanced and prolonged, and the early onset of sleep results in a surge of lesser magnitude and shorter duration.

The degree of thyroid hypofunction after destruction of the hypothalamus is less severe than that which follows hypophysectomy, and residual thyroid function in the former circumstance can be altered by raising or lowering the concentration of thyroid hormones in the blood. Thus, both T_4 and T_3 mediate the feedback regulation of TSH secretion, and TRH determines its set-point (see Fig. 11-8). There is a linear inverse relationship between the serum free T_4 concentration and the log of the TSH (Fig. 11-9), making the serum TSH concentration an exquisitely sensitive indicator of the thyroid state of patients with an intact hypothalamic-pituitary axis. Gene-targeting studies show that TRH secretion is likely to be the dominant factor mediating the thyroid hormone feedback regulation of TSH secretion because the markedly elevated TSH secretion of mice with inactivation of TRβ cannot be sustained in mice lacking the TRH gene.[128] This is somewhat surprising given the less severe hypothyroidism associated with hypothalamic (as opposed to primary) hypothyroidism but may be explained by the absolute nature of the TRH deficiency achieved by the genetic manipulation as opposed to the clinical situation in humans with central hypothyroidism wherein the TRH deficiency is not likely to be complete.

Somatostatin (somatotropin release–inhibiting hormone [SRIH]), acting through inhibitory G protein (G_i), decreases TSH secretion in vitro and in vivo, but prolonged treatment with a somatostatin analogue does not cause hypothyroidism.[129,130] Similar acute effects occur during dopamine infusion and the administration of bromocriptine, a dopamine agonist. Both of these agents inhibit

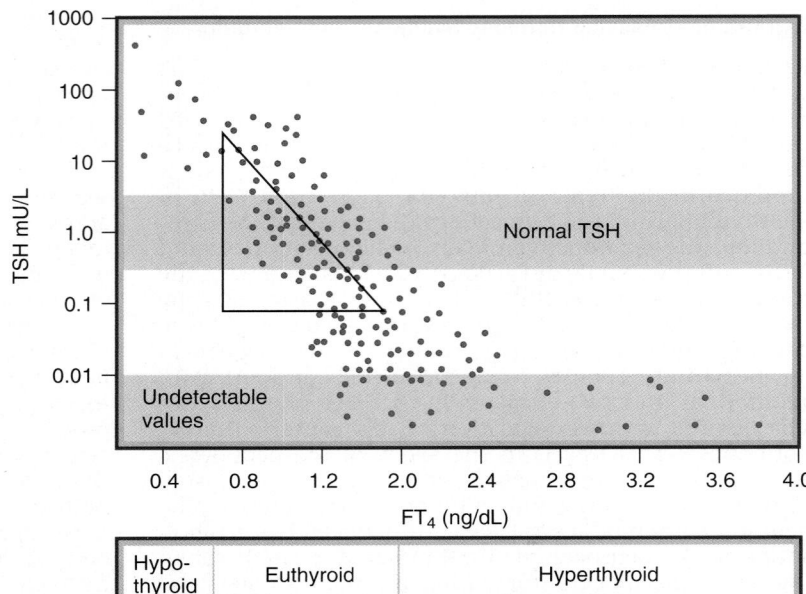

Figure 11-9 The log/linear relationship between thyroid-stimulating hormone (TSH) (on the vertical axis) and the free T_4 concentrations (FT_4). Typical free T_4 concentrations in hypothyroid, euthyroid, and hyperthyroid patients are shown.

TABLE 11-6

Endogenous and Exogenous Agents That May Stimulate or Inhibit Thyrotropin Secretion

Stimulatory Agents	Inhibitory Agents
Thyrotropin-releasing hormone (TRH)	Thyroid hormones and analogues
	Dopamine and dopamine agonists
Prostaglandins (?)	Gastrin
α-Adrenergic agonist (? via TRH)	Opioids (rat)
	Glucocorticoids (in vivo, high dose)
Opioids (humans)	Serotonin
Arginine vasopressin (AVP)	Cholecystokinin (CCK)
	Gastrin-releasing peptide (GRP)
Glucagon-like peptide 1 (GLP1)	Vasopressin (AVP)
	Neuropeptide Y (NPY)
Galanin	Interleukin 1β and 6
Leptin	Tumor necrosis factor α (TNF-α)
Glucocorticoids (in vitro)	Bexarotene (retinoid receptor agonist)
	Phenytoin
	Somatostatin and somatostatin analogues

adenylate cyclase. Conversely, blockade of the dopamine receptor by metoclopramide increases the basal serum TSH concentration in both euthyroid and hypothyroid patients. These findings indicate that dopamine is a regulator of TSH secretion, but chronic administration of dopamine agonists, for example, for the treatment of prolactinoma, do not cause central hypothyroidism, indicating that compensatory mechanisms negate these acute effects.[131]

A number of drugs or hormones may suppress or stimulate TSH secretion (Table 11-6). Glucocorticoids given in high doses transiently suppress TSH secretion, although prolonged therapy is not associated with central hypothyroidism.[129] Patients with Cushing disease have subnormal TSH production but with minimal effects on T_4 production.[129] Bexarotene, a RXR agonist used for treatment of T-cell lymphoma, suppresses TSH sufficiently to cause central hypothyroidism, presumably by reducing TSHβ gene transcription.[132,133]

Neurotransmitters are important direct and indirect modulators in TSH synthesis and secretion. A complex network of neurotransmitter neurons terminates on cell bodies of hypophysiotropic neurons, and several neurotransmitters (such as dopamine) are directly released into hypophyseal portal blood, exerting direct effects on anterior pituitary cells. Furthermore, many dopaminergic, serotoninergic, histaminergic, catecholaminergic, opioidergic, and GABAergic systems project from other hypothalamic/brain regions to the hypophysiotropic neurons involved in TSH regulation. These projections are important for a normal TSH circadian rhythm and response to stress and cold exposure, but basal TSH secretion is mainly regulated by intrinsic hypothalamic activity. An agonist of the TSHR, known as *thyrostimulin*, is a noncovalent heterodimer of two glycoprotein hormone-like proteins, α2 and β5. It is synthesized in the corticotrophs and placenta, has high affinity for TSHRs, and increases thyroid hormones in rats with a suppressed TSH.[134] Thyrostimulin was ineffective in activating either LH or FSH receptors. Thyrostimulin is expressed also in oocytes, in which it acts as a paracrine regulator to activate TSHR expressed in ovary.[135] Thyrostimulin, evolving before the appearance of gonadotropins, is considered the most ancestral glycoprotein hormone. Studies are currently under way to determine whether this protein is present in the circulation and how it is regulated.

Iodine Deficiency

The response of vertebrates to iodine deficiency is designed to conserve this limited resource and improve the efficiency of its utilization. These adjustments occur at the hypothalamic, pituitary, thyroid, and peripheral tissue levels. Removal of iodine from the diet causes a rapid decrease in serum T_4 concentrations and a simultaneous increase in serum TSH (Fig. 11-10).[136] Interestingly, no detectable decrease in T_3 occurs, suggesting that the signal to increase TSH must derive from a decrease in the T_3 generated intracellularly from T_4 in the pituitary, the hypothalamus, or both. TSH increases NIS, Tg, and TPO synthesis and iodine organification and Tg turnover (see Fig. 11-1). Because of the decrease in iodide supply and the ratio of DIT/MIT, the ratio of T_4 to T_3 in Tg decreases and the rate of thyroidal T_3 secretion may increase despite a fall in T_4 secretion. TSH also stimulates cell division, leading to

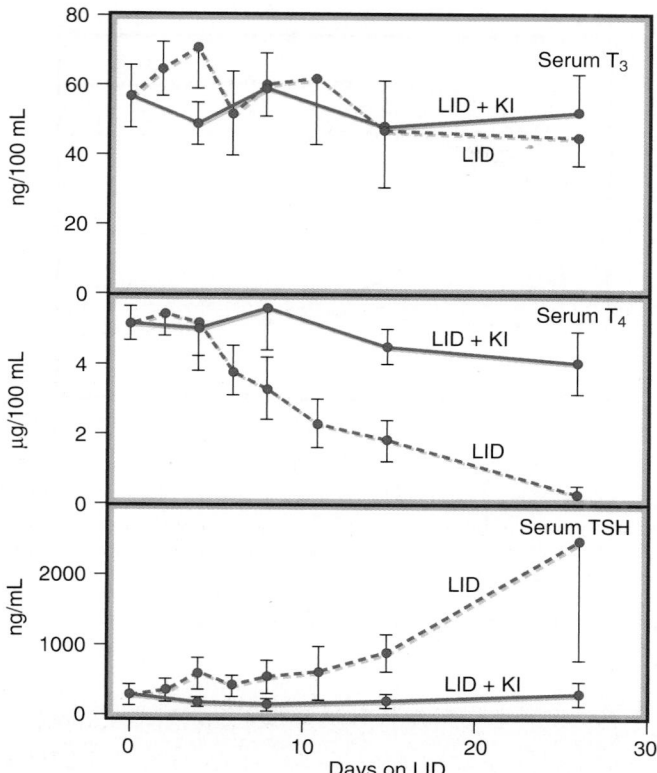

Figure 11-10 Effects of acute depletion of dietary iodine on serum triiodothyronine (T_3), thyroxine (T_4), and thyroid-stimulating hormone (TSH) in rats. Animals received a low iodine diet (LID) without or with supplementation of potassium iodide (KI) in drinking water. (From Riesco G, Taurog A, Larsen PR, et al. Acute and chronic responses to iodine deficiency in rats. *Endocrinology.* 1977;100:303-313.)

TABLE 11-7

Iodine Content of Various Iodinated Pharmaceuticals*

Agent	Iodine Content
Saturated solution of potassium iodide	38 mg/drop
Lugol's solution	6 mg/drop
Iodized salt (1 part KI/10,000 NaCl)	760 µg/10 g
Amiodarone	75-200 mg tablet
Iopanoate, ipodate	350 mg/tablet
Angiographic and CT dyes	400-4000 mg/dose
Povidone-iodine	10 mg/mL
Kelp tablets	150 µg/tablet
Prenatal vitamins	150 µg/tablet
Iodinated glycerol	25 mg/mL
Quantity of iodine required to suppress radioactive iodine to <2%	>30 mg/day

CT, Computed tomography; KI, potassium iodide; NaCl, sodium chloride.
*Typical iodide intake in the United States is 100 to 400 µg/day.

ciency of iodide trapping and organification is reduced in Hashimoto disease or in the patient with Graves disease receiving thiourea drugs.[24] The physiologic effects of this series of events are clear. T_3 has approximately 10 times the potency of the prohormone T_4 and contains only three iodine atoms. This results in a more efficient use of the iodine atom. Maintenance of normal circulating T_3 independent of serum T_4 concentrations should provide hormone for those tissues in which the nuclear T_3 is completely derived from the plasma such as liver and kidney (see Fig. 11-5).

Iodine Excess

The thyroid is also protected against an excess of iodide that might otherwise lead to hyperthyroidism. As with the response to iodine deficiency, there are multiple levels of defense against this eventuality. The usual source of excess iodine is pharmaceutical, with radiographic dyes, amiodarone, and povidone-iodine being the most common sources (Table 11-7).

Effects of Increased Iodine Intake on Thyroid Hormone Synthesis

The quantity of iodine organified in Tg, which includes T_4 and T_3, displays a biphasic response to increasing doses of iodide, at first increasing and then decreasing as a result of a relative blockade of organic binding. This decreasing yield of organic iodine from increasing doses of iodide, termed the *Wolff-Chaikoff effect*, results from a high concentration of inorganic iodide within the thyroid cell.[142] The susceptibility to the Wolff-Chaikoff effect can be increased either by stimulation of iodide trapping, as occurs in patients with Graves disease, or during persistent TSH stimulation by impairment of iodide organification in the human fetus, in patients with Hashimoto disease, or in thyroids previously irradiated by either ^{131}I or external beam therapy. In such situations, goiter and hypothyroidism (iodide myxedema) can develop if excess iodide is given for long periods. The mechanism for organification inhibition may involve inhibitory effects of high iodide concentrations on TPO and THOX2.

In normal subjects given iodide, the inhibition of iodothyronine formation is reduced over time. This escape or adaptation phenomenon occurs because iodide transport activity decreases probably through a decrease in NIS expression. Consequently, thyroidal iodide falls to levels insufficient to maintain the full Wolff-Chaikoff effect.[16,143]

goiter. In the rat model, the fall in plasma T_4 increases D2 from 5- to 20-fold in the CNS, hypothalamus, and pituitary, increasing the efficiency of T_4 conversion to T_3. With moderately severe iodine deficiency, D3 in the CNS is also reduced, prolonging the mean residence time of T_3 in that organ.[137] This permits serum T_3 to remain normal and the CNS T_3 to be only moderately reduced despite up to a 10-fold decrease in circulating T_4. Supporting an important role for D2 in humans is the positive association between mental retardation in an iodine-deficient region of China and two common single-nucleotide polymorphisms in the *Dio2* gene.[138]

Despite the TSH elevation and nearly undetectable serum T_4 in acutely iodine-deficient rodents, growth, O_2 consumption, and thermal homeostasis can be maintained.[139] However, if iodine deficiency is prolonged and severe, hypothyroidism will supervene. In humans, these compensatory alterations in thyroid function come into operation when total iodine intake falls below 75 µg/day (see Table 11-1). This situation can occur in some countries in Europe and South America as well as affect several hundred million individuals in China, India, Indonesia, and Africa.[140,141]

Changes in serum hormones seen in experimental animals have been well documented in humans in areas of iodine deficiency and in patients with NIS mutations.[14] However, they may not be seen in older members of the population when thyroid autonomy often develops. The physiologic response to iodine deficiency is similar to that which occurs during the development of primary hypothyroidism in humans. It is also reproduced when the effi-

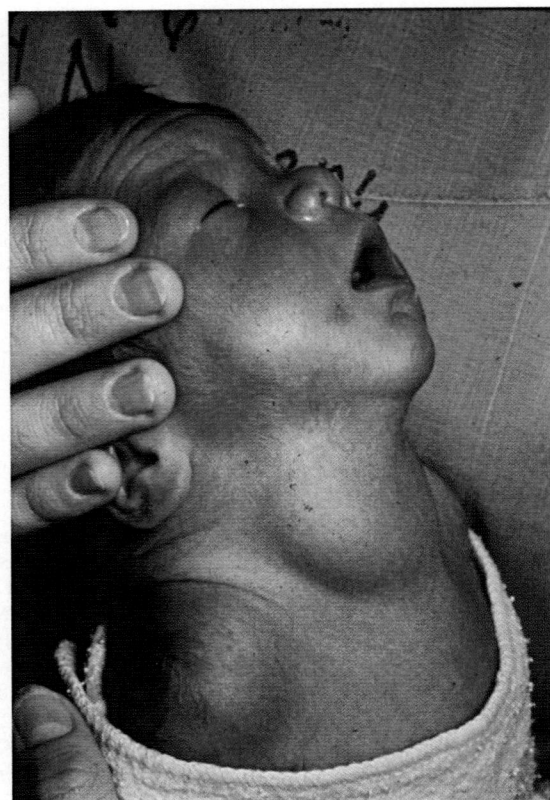

Figure 11-11 Newborn infant with iodide-induced goiter due to Lugol's solution treatment of the mother during the third trimester. This illustrates the danger of chronic excess iodide administration during pregnancy.

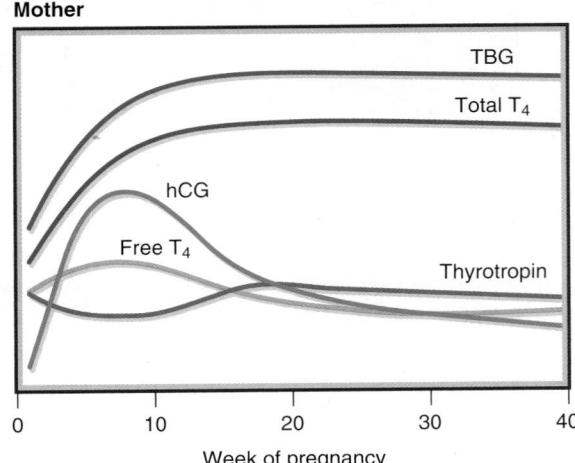

Figure 11-12 Changes in various critical components of the thyroid-pituitary axis during pregnancy. Note the early increase in free thyroxine (T_4), probably due to thyroidal stimulation by human chorionic gonadotropin (hCG), which causes a reciprocal modest suppression of serum thyroid-stimulating hormone (TSH) during the late first trimester. (From Burrow GN, Fisher DA, Larsen PR. Mechanisms of disease: maternal and fetal thyroid function. *N Engl J Med.* 1994;331:1072-1078.)

TABLE 11-8	
Effects of Pregnancy on Thyroid Physiology	
Physiologic Change	**Thyroid-Related Consequences**
↑ Serum thyroxine-binding globulin	↑ Total T_4 and T_3; ↑ T_4 production
↑ Plasma volume	↑ T_4 and T_3 pool size; ↑ T_4 production; ↑ cardiac output
D3 expression in placenta and (?) uterus	↑ T_4 production
First trimester ↑ in hCG	↑Free T_4; ↓ basal thyrotropin; ↑ T_4 production
↑ Renal I⁻ clearance	↑ Iodine requirements
↑ T_4 production; fetal T_4 synthesis during second and third trimesters	
↑ Oxygen consumption by fetoplacental unit, gravid uterus, and mother	↑ Basal metabolic rate; ↑ cardiac output

D3, type 3 iodothyronine deiodinase; I⁻, plasma iodide; hCG, human chorionic gonadotropin; T_3, triiodothyronine; T_4, thyroxine.

Importantly, it does *not* occur in the third trimester fetus, so chronic high iodine intake during pregnancy must be avoided because it will cause fetal hypothyroidism and compensatory potentially obstructive goiter in the newborn (Fig. 11-11).

Effects on Thyroid Hormone Release

An important practical effect of pharmacologic doses of iodide is the prompt inhibition of thyroid hormone release. This occurs to some extent normally but is especially apparent in patients with Graves disease or toxic nodules (see Chapter 12). The mechanism is unknown, but the effect is mediated at the thyroid cell level, rather than through an action on TSH. Iodine also diminishes the hypervascularity and hyperplasia that characterize the diffuse toxic goiter of Graves disease. This effect facilitates surgical therapy for the disorder.

Thyroid Function in Pregnancy and in the Fetus and Newborn

Pregnancy affects virtually all aspects of thyroid hormone economy (Table 11-8).[7,144,145] The total serum T_4 and T_3 concentrations rise to levels about 1.5-fold those of nonpregnant women owing to the increase in TBG concentration in the first trimester (Fig. 11-12). The markedly increased TBG extracellular pool must be filled steadily with increasing amounts of T_4 until a new equilibrium is reached. During normal pregnancy, the direct stimulatory effect of hCG on thyrocytes induces a small and transient increase in free T_4 levels near the end of the first trimester (peak circulating hCG), resulting in a partial TSH suppression. When tested in bioassays, normal hCG is only about 1/100 as potent as TSH. This weak thyrotropic activity explains why, in normal conditions, the effects of hCG remain largely unnoticed.[146] In addition to the increase in serum TBG, there is also an increased plasma volume as well as accelerated inactivation of T_3 and T_4 by D3 expression in the fetal-placental-uterine unit.[147] Based on the changes in requirements for levothyroxine during gestation in women with primary hypothyroidism, the estimated increase in T_4 production required during this period is 20% to 40%.

The requirement for increased T_4 secretion increases iodine requirements during pregnancy.[148] This need is compounded by the fact that the higher glomerular filtration rate during gestation enhances renal iodide clearance, leading to higher fractional urinary excretion of circulating iodide. In addition, maternal iodine intake must be increased to supply the requirements of the fetal thyroid during the second and third trimesters (see Table 11-8). If these increased requirements for iodide are not met, serum T_4 falls and TSH rises. This series of events is well documented in areas of endemic iodine deficiency or borderline iodine supply, such as Brussels, Belgium.[7] In that city, 70% of pregnant women carefully followed throughout pregnancy had a 20% or greater increase in thyroid volume during gestation due to increased TSH. After delivery, the changes in thyroid function gradually return to normal, and serum TBG values reach normal levels 6 to 8 weeks post partum.

During pregnancy, autoimmunity is suppressed, affecting patients with Graves and Hashimoto diseases (see Chapters 12 and 13). In general, TSHR antibody (TRAb)-mediated thyroid stimulation in the Graves disease patient is exacerbated during the first trimester and is attenuated during the second and third trimesters only to exacerbate in the first several months post partum. Thyroid autoantibody titers fall during gestation in patients with Hashimoto disease only to rise sharply post partum in association with a phase of acute T-cell–mediated thyroid cell destruction—postpartum thyroid disease (PPTD)—which occurs in about 30% of patients with Hashimoto disease and significant residual thyroid tissue.[149]

The basal metabolic rate (BMR) increases during the second trimester owing to the increase in the total mass of body tissue consequent to the pregnancy. The changes of pregnancy, together with the decreased peripheral vascular resistance, vasodilatation, and modest tachycardia, may suggest thyrotoxicosis (see Table 11-8). It is important to appreciate that such changes are physiologic in pregnancy, especially when managing the hyperthyroid pregnant patient.

Fetal Thyroid Function

The peripheral metabolism of T_4 in the human fetus differs markedly from that in the adult, both quantitatively and qualitatively. Overall, rates of production and degradation of T_4 in terms of units per body mass exceed those in the adult by 10-fold. In addition, D1 catalysis is reduced and D3 is enhanced, favoring the formation of the inactive rT_3 at the expense of T_3. D3 is highly expressed in fetal tissues including the liver, skin, tracheobronchial, urothelial, and gastrointestinal epithelia.[147] This condition results in a persistently subnormal serum T_3 concentration and an elevated serum rT_3. This change permits the highly regulatable conversion of T_4 to T_3 by D2 to be the major pathway for generating tissue T_3.[150]

Fetal thyroid function begins at about the end of the first trimester. Thereafter, there are steady increases in fetal TBG and total T_4 and T_3.[7,145] Throughout gestation, the serum TSH values are greater than are present in maternal circulation and higher than would be expected in adults with normal thyroid function. This indicates that there is increasing hypothalamic-pituitary resistance to T_4 during fetal development, which is speculated to be a consequence of increased TRH secretion.[151] Despite the low circulating T_3, the fetal free T_4 concentrations approximate those in the maternal circulation from gestational age of 28 weeks and onward.

Maternal-Fetal Interactions

The fetal pituitary-thyroid axis functions as a unit that is essentially independent from the mother.[4,151] Transplacental passage of TSH from mother to fetus is negligible, but the same is not true of maternal T_4. In infants with congenital hypothyroidism caused by either genetic TPO deficiency or athyreosis, serum concentrations of T_4 in cord

blood are usually one third to one half of normal.[31] Thus, at least when the maternal-fetal concentration gradient is high, significant transfer of maternal T_4 to the fetal circulation can occur. This transfer may be significant, given the capacity of the fetal brain to increase the efficiency of T_4-to-T_3 conversion. Furthermore, T_4 can be found in coelomic and amniotic fluids before the onset of thyroid function.[152] The major factor limiting T_4 and T_3 transfer from mother to fetus is the D3 expressed in the uterus, placenta, and fetal epithelium.

Thyroid Function in the Newborn

Mean total T_4 level in cord sera is 150 nmol/L (12 µg/dL). Serum TBG concentrations are elevated, but are not as high as in the maternal serum. At term, free T_4 concentrations are slightly lower than those in the mother. Cord serum T_3 concentrations are low (0.8 nmol/L, 50 ng/dL), and rT_3 and T_3SO_4 are elevated.[4,153,154] After delivery, the serum TSH level in the neonate increases rapidly to a peak at about 2 to 4 hours after birth, returning to its initial value within 48 hours.[153] Levels above 60 mU/L are typical. This neonatal TSH surge is thought to occur in response to the rapid reduction in environmental temperature after delivery. In response, the serum T_4, T_3, and Tg concentrations increase rapidly during the first few hours after delivery and are in the hyperthyroid range by 24 hours of life.[155] The TSH surge doubtless contributes to the increase in serum T_3 concentration, but enhancement of extrathyroidal conversion of T_4 to T_3 by D1 or D2 is thought to be a major factor as well.[46] The adrenergic stimulation of the *Dio2* gene and the reactivation of D2 by its deubiquitination in brown adipose tissue are likely to be major contributors to this increase.[156]

Premature infants have an immature hypothalamic-pituitary-thyroid axis with low T_4, T_3, and TSH.[153,157] Serum T_4, TBG, and free T_4 all tend to correlate with gestational age. Preterm infants also have an attenuated TSH surge after delivery. In addition, when prematurity is accompanied by complications, such as respiratory distress syndrome or nutritional problems, serum T_4, and especially T_3, may fall to low levels as a result of a combination of reduced TBG production, immaturity of the thyroid gland, suppression of the hypothalamic-pituitary axis due to illness, impairment of T_4-to-T_3 conversion, and increases in D3 activity.[158,159] These changes are, in many respects, similar to those in adults with severe illness. All of these issues need to be taken into account when evaluating the thyroid status of the preterm infant, particularly given the increased prevalence of congenital hypothyroidism in this age group.[157]

Thyroid hormone production rates are higher per unit of body weight in neonatal infants and children than in adults. The daily levothyroxine requirement is about 10 µg/kg in the newborn, decreasing progressively to about 1.6 µg/kg in the adult.[157]

Aging and the Thyroid

The thyroid gland undergoes several anatomic changes with age. There is a reduction in weight of the gland, in the size of follicles, and in the content of colloid, and there is increased fibrosis, often with marked lymphocytic infiltration. However, these changes do not correlate with thyroid function.[160] In the healthy elderly patient, there is a normal level of free T_4, but serum T_3 levels appear to be lower, although studies of selected healthy people indicated that T_3 levels are unaffected by aging.[161] TSH may increase or decrease with age in relation to the iodine

TABLE 11-9

Changes in Thyroid Hormone Levels During Illness

Severity of Illness	Free T$_3$	Free T$_4$	Reverse T$_3$	TSH	Probable Cause
Mild	↓	N	↑	N	↓ D2, D1
Moderate	↓↓	N, ↑↓	↑↑	N, ↓	↓↓ D2, D1, ? ↑ D3
Severe	↓↓↓	↓	↑	↓↓	↓↓ D2, D1, ↑ D3
Recovery	↓	↓	↑	↑	?

D1 through D3, iodothyronine deiodinases; N, no change; T$_3$, triiodothyronine; T$_4$, thyroxine; TSH, thyroid-stimulating hormone (thyrotropin).

intake.[162] Of note, population studies in humans and animal models show negative correlations between thyroid hormone levels and longevity, a finding that led to the hypothesis that constraints on thyroid hormone signaling at certain life stages, notably during maturity, are advantageous for optimal aging.[163]

Thyroid Function During Fasting or Illness

A number of changes take place in thyroid function during nutritional deprivation or illness. These changes consist of a central reduction in TSH secretion and a decrease in plasma T$_3$ levels and T$_4$ and T$_3$ binding in serum. This constellation of findings is termed the *low T$_3$ syndrome, the euthyroid sick syndrome,* or *nonthyroid illness.* The patterns of changes in circulating thyroid hormones and TSH during fasting and illness are quite similar. During fasting, there is a reduction of 50% or more in serum T$_3$ and an increase in serum rT$_3$ without initial changes in serum total or free T$_4$ (Table 11-9).[126,164] Although the role of specific deiodinases in causing these changes has not been documented at a tissue level in humans during fasting, several lines of evidence suggest that decreases in peripheral T$_4$-to-T$_3$ conversion by both D1 and D2 and a reduced clearance of rT$_3$ by D1 do play a role in this process. The finding of normal T$_3$ plasma levels in mice with the genetic absence of both D1 and D2 enzymes suggests that, under normal conditions, the thyroid gland by itself is able to compensate for impaired peripheral conversion to normalize serum T$_3$. This observation suggests that very powerful mechanisms are in place to maintain serum T$_3$ levels within the normal range, with the notable exceptions of when it is not meant to be in that range (i.e., during fasting or illness). In these circumstances, by a mechanism probably regulated by the hypothalamus, all compensatory mechanisms are reduced and serum T$_3$ may drop to almost undetectable levels.[83] Deiodination by D3 increases the generation of rT$_3$ from T$_4$ and converts T$_3$ to 3,3′-diiodothyronine (see Fig. 11-2), which exaggerates the changes resulting from the decrease in D1 and D2. The finding that D3-null mice can still develop the low T$_3$ syndrome suggests that D3 upregulation is not the only event occurring in this clinical state. It is not yet known if such an increase in D3 also occurs during caloric restriction. The attenuation of TSH secretion despite a fall in serum T$_3$ levels during fasting is discussed earlier (see "The Hypothalamic-Pituitary-Thyroid Axis").

During fasting, basal oxygen consumption and heart rate decline, and nitrogen balance, initially negative, returns toward normal.[165] In some studies, these changes in overall metabolism are partially reversed by replacement of exogenous T$_3$ while fasting continues. Thus, the decrease in T$_3$ during fasting (and presumably illness) can be viewed as a beneficial energy- and nitrogen-sparing adaptation. Chronic malnutrition such as occurs in anorexia nervosa is also associated with a reduction in serum T$_3$ and rarely

in free T$_4$.[166] TSH concentrations remain in the normal range, although again, they are inappropriately low in the context of the reductions in circulating T$_3$. In contrast, overfeeding, particularly with carbohydrate, increases T$_3$ production rates and the serum T$_3$ concentration, reduces serum rT$_3$, and increases basal thermogenesis.[167]

During illness, decreases in T$_3$ and pulsatile TSH release and increases in rT$_3$ also occur.[168] If illness progresses, the hypothalamic-pituitary-thyroid axis is even further suppressed, with a consequent reduction in the free T$_4$. Severe decreases in serum T$_4$ are associated with a high probability of death. This syndrome is associated with a decrease in TRH mRNA in the human PVN.[169] An increase in T$_3$ production by D2-catalyzed T$_4$-to-T$_3$ conversion in the tanycytes lining the third ventricle during illness may contribute to the blunted response of TSH to the reduced serum T$_3$, particularly during infections.[170] Cytokines, such as interleukin 6 (IL-6), also increase during illness and are coincident with the decrease in circulating T$_3$, although it is not clear whether this is the cause of the hypothalamic changes.[171] A 2011 in vitro study indicated that IL-6 causes an increase in intracellular and extracellular reactive oxygen species (ROS).[84] As mentioned earlier, the active centers of both D1 and D2 are intracellular, and that of D3 has access to extracellular thiols, which do not pass easily through the cell membrane (see Fig. 11-4). The increase in ROS reduces intracellular thiols such as GSH (glutathione) and presumably the GSH/NADPH-dependent thioredoxin and glutaredoxin. Thus, T$_4$-to-T$_3$ conversion by D1 and D2 is reduced while D3-mediated T$_3$ and T$_4$ inactivation continues. In addition to these cofactor changes, the increase in ROS and the activation of MAPK-dependent pathways due to IL-6 and ROS induce increases in the transcription of the deiodinases, especially D3.[84] In vitro, all these changes are reversed by addition of N-acetylcysteine (NAC) to the media, which rescues intracellular GSH synthesis. Interestingly, follow-up studies in patients with the low T$_3$ syndrome due to acute myocardial infarction show that the reduction in T$_3$ and the increase in rT$_3$ can be prevented by NAC infusions,[172] suggesting these in vitro results are relevant to sick patients. These endogenous changes may be further exaggerated by agents such as dopamine or glucocorticoids, which will also, at least transiently, suppress the TRH-TSH axis.[173] The changes in thyroid function are a continuum, with the abnormalities becoming progressively more severe in parallel with the patient's clinical condition (see Table 11-9). Postmortem studies show that hepatic D1 activity is reduced by about 50%, skeletal muscle D2 is absent, and D3 is present in liver and skeletal muscle.[174] No differences have been found in the T$_3$ transporter MCT8 in skeletal muscle or liver, and possible abnormalities in other thyroid hormone transporters have not been evaluated. Interestingly, the same global pattern of changes during acute medical illness has been described in patients with primary hypothyroidism receiving levothyroxine.[175] In such patients, serum T$_4$, T$_3$, and TSH concentrations all fell about 50% over the first 3 days, presumably due to a disruption of T$_4$ binding due to a decrease in TBG, TTR, and albumin, as well as to blockade of T$_4$-protein interactions due to circulating interfering substances. Contributing to this may be the translational modification of TBG due to a serpin-catalyzed release of a carboxy-terminal fragment of TBG in inflamed tissues discussed earlier (see "Thyroxine-Binding Globulin").

Therapies have been introduced in an attempt to ameliorate certain of the illness-related central abnormalities in the hypothalamic-pituitary axis (including decreases in growth hormone and gonadotropins). One of these, infusions of growth hormone–releasing peptide 2 (GHRP2) combined with TRH, has resulted in increases in TSH, T_3, and T_4, as well as insulin-like growth factor 1 (IGF-1), insulin, and the IGF binding proteins 1, 3, and 5.[176] Although the biochemical improvements were significant, the clinical state did not change, suggesting that the thyroid dysfunction is a marker of the severity of the illness rather than its cause.

Although serum TSH concentrations in severely ill patients are reduced, an increase in TSH above the normal range may appear during recovery, with the elevation in TSH concentration persisting until circulating free T_4 and T_3 levels return to normal.[177] This pattern can be confusing if the elevated TSH concentration is associated with the still-reduced concentrations of free T_4. Such patients meet all laboratory criteria for primary hypothyroidism with the exception of the clinical context. Follow-up generally reveals a normalization of TSH and T_4 within 1 to 2 months (see Table 11-9).

Despite the severity of the abnormalities, particularly in serum T_3, there is still disagreement as to whether or not therapeutic intervention should be initiated even in the most severely ill patients because most controlled studies have not shown beneficial effects of T_4 or T_3 supplementation in such individuals.[178] The one exception is a possible beneficial effect of T_3 therapy in patients after coronary artery bypass grafting, with one study showing a positive effect but a second study showing none.[179,180] In 2014 the cautious use of thyroid hormonal therapy in patients with low T_3 syndrome or a stunned myocardium was proposed.[181]

The Thyroid Axis and Neuropsychiatric Illness

Patients with neuropsychiatric disease can present with any of a number of abnormalities in thyroid function. Patients with bipolar disorders may show slight elevations in serum TSH and reductions in free T_4, whereas patients with severe depression have slight elevation in serum T_4 and reduced serum TSH. Other acutely psychotic patients may have either high or low serum TSH concentrations and tend to have elevations in free T_4.[182] The cause of these minor abnormalities is not clear, but such patients may have thyroid function test results resembling those in patients with primary thyroid disease from whom they must be differentiated.

Effects of Hormones on Thyroid Function
Glucocorticoids

The acute administration of pharmacologic doses of glucocorticoid eliminates pulsatile release of serum TSH concentrations in normal patients presumably by reducing TRH release. With continued administration, there is an escape from this suppression (Table 11-10). Pharmacologic doses of glucocorticoid decrease the serum T_3 concentration in normal and hyperthyroid patients as well as in hypothyroid patients maintained on levothyroxine. The latter finding and the accompanying increase in rT_3 production suggest that glucocorticoids may increase D3 activity.[106]

Primary adrenal insufficiency may be associated with reduced serum T_4 and elevated serum TSH concentrations, suggesting the coexistence of primary hypothyroidism. However, treatment of the adrenal insufficiency can lead to complete resolution of these abnormalities, suggesting that in some patients they are a consequence of glucocorticoid deficiency rather than primary thyroid disease.[183] Nevertheless, the prevalence of primary hypothyroidism is increased in patients with autoimmune hypoadrenalism, so the two causes must be differentiated (see Chapter 15).

TABLE 11-10
Effects of Hormones on Thyroid Function
Glucocorticoids
Excess
Decrease TSH, TBG, TTR (high-dose)
Decrease serum T_3/T_4 and increase rT_3/T_4 ratios
Increase rT_3 production (? ↑ D3)
Decrease T_4 and T_3 secretion in Graves disease
Deficiency
Increase TSH
Estrogen
Increase TBG sialylation and half-life in serum
Increase TSH in postmenopausal women
Increase T_4 requirement in hypothyroid patients
Androgen
Decrease TBG
Decrease T_4 turnover in women and reduce T_4 requirements in hypothyroid patients
Growth Hormone
Decrease D3 activity

D3, type 3 deiodinase; rT_3, reverse T_3; T_3, triiodothyronine; T_4, thyroxine; TBG, thyroxine-binding globulin; TSH, thyrotropin; TTR, transthyretin.

Likewise, patients successfully treated for Cushing disease can develop thyroid autoimmunity.

Gonadal Steroids

Estrogen increases TBG by mechanisms already mentioned.[184] Estrogen administration to postmenopausal women causes an increase of 15% to 20% in TSH.[185] Presumably this increases T_4 secretion, in that total T_4 increases and free T_4 is unchanged. Estrogen also increases the levothyroxine requirement in patients with primary hypothyroidism.[63] In contrast, administration of androgens to women decreases TBG and decreases T_4 turnover and levothyroxine requirements in patients with primary hypothyroidism.[186]

Growth Hormone

Growth hormone increases the serum free T_3 and decreases free T_4 in both levothyroxine-treated and normal individuals, suggesting either suppression of D3 activity or increased T_4-to-T_3 conversion.

PHYSICAL EVALUATION OF THE THYROID GLAND

Manifestations of thyroid disease are usually due to excessive or insufficient production of thyroid hormone, local symptoms in the neck (principally goiter but occasionally pain or compression of adjacent structures), or in the case of Graves disease, ophthalmopathy or dermopathy. A functional diagnosis of thyroid disease is based on a carefully taken history, a thorough search for the physical signs of hypothyroidism or thyrotoxicosis, and an appraisal of the results of laboratory tests. Although conditioned by the functional diagnosis, the anatomic diagnosis depends largely on the physical examination of the thyroid gland itself. The typical symptoms of an excess or a deficiency of thyroid hormone are discussed in Chapters 12 and 13.

Physical Examination

Examination of the neck is best accomplished with the patient seated in good light with the neck relaxed. The patient should be provided with a cup of water to facilitate swallowing. The physician should first inspect the neck, especially while the patient swallows, with the neck slightly extended. The presence of old surgical scars, distended veins, and redness or fixation of the overlying skin should be noted. The position of the trachea should be noted. If a mass is present, a determination should be made as to whether it moves with swallowing. A midline mass high in the neck, which rises further when the patient extends the tongue, is typical of a thyroglossal duct remnant or cyst. Movement on swallowing is a characteristic of the thyroid gland because it is ensheathed in the pretracheal fascia; this feature distinguishes a goiter from most other neck masses. However, if the thyroid is so large that it occupies all the available space in the neck, movement on swallowing may be lost. The physician should also inspect the posterior dorsum of the tongue, which is the origin of the thyroglossal duct and the location of lingual thyroid tissue.

Except when the thyroid enlargement is extreme, the thyroid examination can be readily performed with the physician facing the seated patient. The physician should use gentle pressure with his or her thumb to locate the thyroid isthmus just caudal to the cricoid cartilage. This provides a convenient starting point for the palpation of the lobes of the gland but an increase in the thickness of the isthmus or a firm texture will already suggest the presence of some generalized thyroid enlargement. To examine the right lobe, the right thumb is then moved laterally, without release of gentle pressure, to locate the lobe of the thyroid by pressing it against the trachea as the patient swallows sips of water. This strategy allows the palpating thumb to laterally displace the medial border of the sternocleidomastoid muscle, allowing direct access to the entire thyroid lobe. As the patient swallows with the thumb pressing the lobe against the trachea with sufficient tension to displace it slightly over the midline, it will slide up and down under the ball of the thumb. This permits an appreciation of the size and texture of the gland as well as the presence or absence of nodules. A similar strategy with the left thumb is employed for the left lobe. The thyroid may also be examined with the physician standing behind the seated patient, palpating with the fingertips of both hands.

The examiner should note the shape of the gland, its size in relation to normal, and its consistency, which is usually slightly greater than adipose tissue but less than muscle. The normal thyroid lobe has approximately the same size in frontal projection as the terminal phalanx of the patient's thumb. Whereas a diffuse goiter and the hyperplastic gland of the hyperthyroid patient with Graves disease may be softer than normal, the gland of Hashimoto disease is usually firm. Irregularities of the surface, variations in consistency, and tender areas should be noted. If nodules are palpated, their shape, size, position, translucency, and consistency in relation to the surrounding tissue should be determined. It is counterintuitive, but a firm nodule is more likely to be a cyst than a malignancy. A search should be made for the pyramidal lobe, which is a thin band of tissue extending upward from the isthmus to the thyroid cartilage to the right or left of the midline. A hypertrophied pyramidal lobe may be mistaken for a pretracheal lymph node that sometimes accompanies thyroid carcinoma or thyroiditis. It is usually palpable in patients with generalized thyroid disease, such as Hashimoto or Graves disease. During palpation, a vascular thrill may be felt that, in the absence of cardiac disease, is suggestive of hyperthyroidism. Finally, palpation should always include examination of the regional lymph nodes along the jugular vein, posterior to the sternocleidomastoids and in the supraclavicular region.

Auscultation of the neck may confirm the increased vascularity of an enlarged, hyperactive gland, suggesting Graves disease. A systolic or continuous bruit is sometimes heard over a hyperplastic gland. Care should be taken to distinguish a thyroid bruit from a murmur transmitted from the base of the heart or from a venous hum that can be obliterated by gentle compression of the external jugular vein or by turning the head. A venous hum is generally found in younger patients with high cardiac output, such as occurs in Graves disease or with severe anemia.

An arm-raising test is useful when a retrosternal goiter is suspected. The basis for this maneuver is that if the size of the thoracic inlet is already reduced by such a goiter, raising both arms until they touch the sides of the head further narrows the thoracic inlet and causes congestion and venous engorgement of the face and sometimes respiratory distress (*Pemberton sign*) or even (rarely) syncope.

In addition to examination of the thyroid gland and regional lymph nodes, evidence of compression or displacement of adjacent structures should be sought. Hoarseness may indicate compression of the recurrent laryngeal nerve, usually by a malignant thyroid neoplasm, and this should be confirmed by laryngoscopy. Displacement of the trachea may be evident, usually associated with a large nodule or nodules, and inspiratory stridor may indicate its compression.

It is likely that an ultrasound device will become a ubiquitous instrument in the endocrinologist's office or clinic in the coming years owing to its superior sensitivity for the detection of thyroid nodules. The use of ultrasound should enhance, not replace, the physical examination of the thyroid, the only endocrine gland accessible to physical examination.

LABORATORY ASSESSMENT OF THYROID STATUS

In considering the laboratory assessment of the patient with known or suspected thyroid disease, the physician should seek to arrive at both a functional and, when appropriate, an anatomic diagnosis. Laboratory determinations will confirm whether there is an excess, normal, or insufficient supply of thyroid hormone to verify the inferences from the clinical history and physical examination. Laboratory tests can be divided into five major categories: (1) those that assess the state of the hypothalamic-pituitary-thyroid axis; (2) estimates of the T_4 and T_3 concentrations in the serum; (3) tests that reflect the impact of thyroid hormone on tissues; (4) tests for the presence of autoimmune thyroid disease; and (5) tests that provide information about thyroidal iodine metabolism. The use of iodine and other isotopes for thyroid scanning is discussed in Chapter 14.

Tests of the Hypothalamic-Pituitary-Thyroid Axis

Thyroid-Stimulating Hormone

Although an inherently indirect reflection of thyroid hormone supply, tests that assess the state of the hypothalamic-pituitary-thyroid axis play a critical role in the diagnosis of thyroid disease. This is because the rate of

TSH secretion is exquisitely sensitive to the plasma concentrations of free thyroid hormones, thus providing a precise and specific barometer of the thyroid status of the patient (see Figs. 11-8 and 11-9). The rare exceptions to this rule are discussed later. Immunometric assay technology now makes it possible to define the normal range for serum TSH and hence to ascertain both when thyroid function is inadequate and when the hormone supply is excessive (see Chapter 6). This assay uses the TSH molecule to link a TSH antibody bound to an inert surface (e.g., particles, the side of a test tube) to a second antibody directed against a different TSH epitope that is labeled with a detectable marker (^{125}I, an enzyme, or a chemiluminescent reagent). Thus, the signal generated is proportional to the concentration of TSH in the serum. This technique is more specific, sensitive, and rapid than radioimmunoassay.

The normal range of the serum TSH concentration by immunometric assay varies slightly in different laboratories but is most commonly 0.4 to 4.2 mU/L. There has been discussion of adopting an even lower upper limit for the normal range, but the 4.2 value includes 96% of the disease- and risk-free population.[187,188] The lower limit of 0.4 is too high for pregnancy due to hCG-induced hyperthyroidism as discussed earlier.[146] It should be kept in mind that there is a diurnal variation of TSH secretion with peak values in the early morning and a nadir in the afternoon. A borderline abnormal value should always be repeated within a week or so to be certain that it is representative. A minimally suitable TSH assay should be able to quantitate concentrations of TSH of 0.1 mU/L with a coefficient of variation of less than 20%. Potential artifacts of these assays are discussed in Chapter 6.

The free α-subunit common to TSH, FSH, LH, and hCG is generally detectable in serum with a normal range of 1 to 5 μg/L, but the TSH β-subunit is not. When FSH and LH production are increased, as in postmenopausal women, or when TSH production is increased, as in primary hypothyroidism, the free α-subunit level is also increased. The α-subunit level may also be increased in patients with glycoprotein-producing tumors of the anterior pituitary (see Chapter 8). Its measurement may be useful in the rare patient with hyperthyroidism and a normal or elevated TSH to differentiate between neoplastic and non-neoplastic causes of TSH excess.[189,190]

TSH in Patients with Thyroid Dysfunction

Patients with hyperthyroidism (excess thyroid hormone secretion) or thyrotoxicosis (excess thyroid hormone from any cause) will virtually always have a subnormal TSH. The values fall into two general categories: those between the lower limit of normal and 0.1 mU/L, and those less than 0.1 mU/L. Individuals in the former category are often asymptomatic (*subclinical hyperthyroidism*), whereas those in the latter group usually have symptomatic thyrotoxicosis and a significant elevation in free T_4. Patients with hypothalamic or pituitary hypothyroidism often have normal or even slightly elevated serum TSH. The circulating TSH generally has reduced biologic activity due to abnormal glycosylation, reflecting the impaired access of TRH to the thyrotroph.[124,125] Patients with primary hypothyroidism have serum TSH concentrations that range from minimally elevated to 1000 mU/L. In general, the degree of TSH elevation correlates with the clinical severity of the hypothyroidism. Patients with serum TSH values in the range of 5 to 15 mU/L have few if any symptoms, and the serum free T_4 or free T_4 index (FT_4I) is typically low-normal whereas the serum free T_3 concentration is normal. Such individuals with modest TSH elevation are said to have *subclinical hypothyroidism* if the serum free T_4 is in the normal range. These findings indicate minor thyroidal failure with a compensatory increase in TSH secretion. A detailed discussion of the various conditions associated with abnormal serum TSH concentrations follows that describing the quantitation of serum thyroid hormones.

An elevation in both serum TSH and free T_4 is unusual and indicates either autonomous TSH production, as with a TSH-secreting pituitary tumor, *resistance to thyroid hormone* (RTH), or hyperthyroidism with an artifactual elevation in TSH. Differentiating between these diagnoses may require magnetic resonance imaging (MRI) of the hypothalamic-pituitary region or consultation with the clinical chemistry laboratory to rule out an assay artifact (see Chapter 6).

QUANTITATION OF SERUM THYROID HORMONE CONCENTRATIONS

Total T_4 and T_3

Quantitation of the circulating thyroid hormone concentrations is essential to confirm that the thyroid status abnormality suggested by an abnormal TSH result is accurate as well as documenting its severity. Sensitive and specific radioimmunoassays are available for measuring the total concentrations of T_4 and T_3 and some of their metabolic by-products (see Chapter 6). Because the thyroid status correlates with the free, rather than with the total, hormone concentration, the physician must also obtain some estimate of that (see following discussion). The degree of abnormality in the free T_4 generally correlates with the severity of the hormone excess or deficiency, whereas the serum TSH concentration is an indication of the impact of this abnormality in that specific patient. The normal range for total T_4 in healthy, euthyroid adults with a normal circulating TBG concentration is 64 to 142 nmol/L (5 to 11 μg/dL). Normal serum T_3 concentrations are 1.1 to 2.9 nmol/L (70 to 190 ng/dL). At birth (cord serum), T_3 concentrations are about 50% of those in normal adults, but within a few hours T_3 rises abruptly, peaking at about 24 hours at concentrations in the low thyrotoxic range for adults.

Radioimmunoassays for rT_3, T_3SO_4, triac, tetrac, and the diiodothyronines are of primary interest in the research setting because these iodothyronines are derived from the circulating T_4 or T_3, both of which can be easily quantitated.

Concentrations of Free T_4 and Free T_3

The most accurate and direct measurements of the concentrations of free T_4 and free T_3 in serum are performed by assay of these hormones in a dialysate or ultrafiltrate of serum. This assay is not practical for clinical purposes, so alternative strategies have been developed to estimate free thyroid hormone concentrations. In one method, serum is enriched with tracer amounts of the labeled hormone, and the concentration of the isotope in the dialysate or ultrafiltrate is expressed as a fraction of that in undiluted serum. The absolute concentration of free hormone is the product of the total hormone concentration and the fraction that is dialyzable or ultrafiltrable. About 0.02% of T_4 and 0.3% of T_3 is free or unbound (see Table 11-5). The normal range for free T_4 is 9 to 30 pmol/L (0.7 to 2.5 ng/dL), and for free T_3 the range is 3 to 8 pmol/L (0.2 to 0.5 ng/dL).

Because T_4 is the major secretory product of the thyroid and correlates most closely with the serum TSH, in most situations a free T$_4$ estimate is all that is required to ascertain the state of thyroid secretion or supply. An array of methods is used to quantitate free T$_4$ (or T$_3$) in whole serum using automated methods. Even though many such automated tests imply that they quantitate free T$_4$ directly, they do not, and results in sera with abnormal binding proteins are not generally absolute.[191] There are two general categories of methods: comparative free T$_4$ methods and so-called FT$_4$I methods. Three general approaches are used: (1) two-step labeled hormone methods, (2) one-step labeled analogue methods, and (3) labeled antibody approaches (see Chapter 6). In general, two-step labeled hormone back-titration methods are less subject to artifacts due to abnormal binding proteins, changes in albumin, TBG, or increases in free fatty acids than are one-step hormone analogue methods.[192,193] All general approaches are subject to artifacts from endogenous antibodies to T$_4$, abnormal binding proteins, or illness.[191,194] Thus, the clinician must be wary if the free T$_4$ result by *any* method does not agree with the clinical state and the TSH. In such cases, another method should be used to estimate the free T$_4$, the FT$_4$I should be measured, or the result should be ignored. For pregnant or severely ill patients, the automated methods typically give falsely low results, particularly if these are performed using one-step procedures. A reasonable alternative for pregnancy is to use the normal range for the serum T$_4$ concentration multiplied by 1.5 in lieu of an automated free T$_4$ assay.[144,195]

The Free T$_4$ Index

Particularly useful in estimating the free T$_4$ in severely ill patients is the determination of the thyroid hormone–binding ratio (THBR), multiplying this result by the total T$_4$ (or T$_3$) to obtain a free hormone index (FT$_4$I or FT$_3$I). In this test, a tracer quantity of labeled T$_4$ (or T$_3$) is added to serum, which is then exposed to a solid phase matrix coated with T$_4$ or T$_3$ antibody or to an inert matrix that binds the iodothyronine irreversibly. The proportion of labeled T$_4$ or T$_3$ bound by the solid phase is then quantitated. This value, like the free fraction of T$_4$ quantitated directly in a dialysate, varies inversely with the concentration of unoccupied TBG sites in the serum. When tracer T$_3$ is used, its binding to TBG is determined by the ratio of T$_4$, not T$_3$, to TBG in that T$_4$ is present in 50- to 60-fold higher concentrations than T$_3$, has a much higher affinity for TBG than does T$_3$, and therefore determines the ratio of unoccupied to occupied TBG.

The results of such assays are normalized by comparing them with those obtained simultaneously for standard control sera with normal TBG and serum T$_4$ concentrations. This step is generally performed by dividing the result for the unknown sample by that obtained for control sera in the same assay. The quotient is the THBR, which typically has a normal range of 0.85 to 1.10. Because the THBR is proportional to the free fraction of the endogenous thyroid hormones in the serum, it can be multiplied by the total T$_4$ (or T$_3$) concentration to estimate the free thyroid hormone concentration, termed the *free T$_4$* or *free T$_3$ index* (FT$_4$I or FT$_3$I). Because the midnormal THBR is 1.0, the FT$_4$I has a normal range in units that are identical to that of the total T$_4$ (or T$_3$)—for example, 64 to 142 nmol/L (SI units) and 5 to 11 µg/dL (gravimetric terms). A schematic demonstration of the relationships between total and free T$_4$, occupied and unoccupied TBG binding sites, and the THBR is shown in Figure 11-13 for euthyroid individuals with variations in TBG concentrations and in Figure 11-14 for subjects with a constant TBG and alterations in serum thyroid hormone production rates.

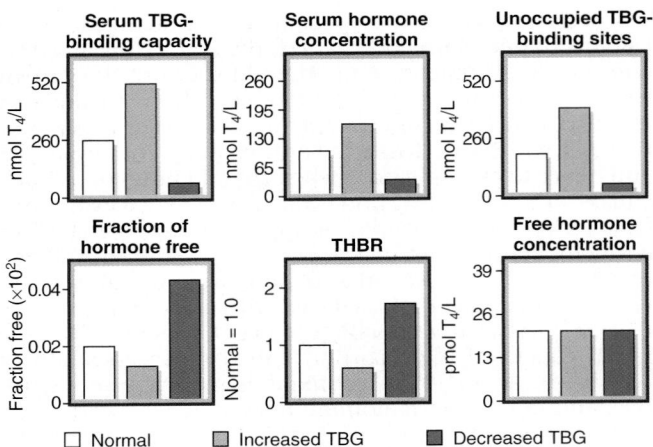

Figure 11-13 Pattern of changes in total serum thyroxine (T$_4$) concentrations and the thyroid hormone–binding ratio (THBR) in euthyroid patients with alterations in the circulating concentrations of thyroxine-binding globulin (TBG). To convert T$_4$ from nmol/L to µg/dL (total) or pmol/L (free), divide by 12.87.

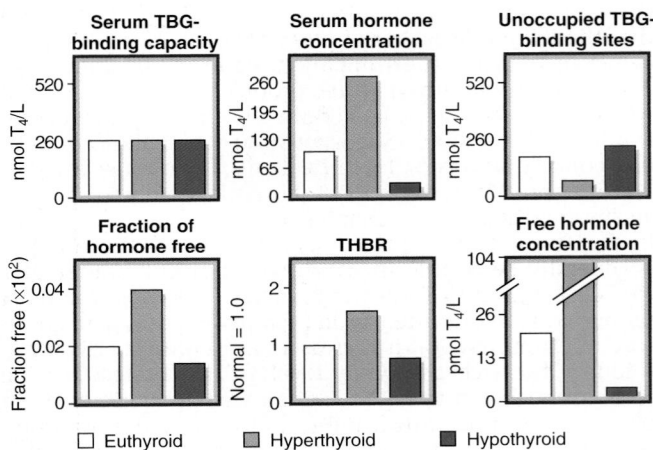

Figure 11-14 Pattern of changes in total serum thyroxine (T$_4$) concentration and thyroid hormone–binding ratio (THBR) in patients with hyperthyroidism or hypothyroidism with normal serum thyroxine-binding globulin (TBG) concentration.

Estrogen, pregnancy, and severe illness are more common causes of changes in total T$_4$ concentrations than are hyperthyroidism and hypothyroidism (Table 11-11). In the euthyroid person, only about one third of the available binding sites on TBG are occupied by T$_4$, and the free T$_4$ fraction is 2×10^{-4} of the total. During pregnancy, the TBG binding capacity, the serum T$_4$, and the number of unoccupied TBG binding sites approximately double, leading to an approximately 50% reduction of the free T$_4$ fraction. This change is reflected in a reduced THBR. If the reduced THBR (or free fraction) is multiplied by the increased total T$_4$, the FT$_4$I estimate is normal, an accurate reflection of the free T$_4$ concentration. In patients in whom the serum T$_4$ concentration is reduced owing to a low TBG, the concentration of unoccupied binding sites is reduced to an even greater extent. This reduction leads to an increase in the free T$_4$ (and T$_3$) fractions and the THBR, and both the free T$_4$ and the FT$_4$I remain in the normal range.

There is one caution when calculating the FT$_4$I using the product of the total T$_4$ and the THBR. The THBR is not linearly related to the free fraction of thyroid hormones at the extremes of its range. Therefore, it is important to consider both the calculated FT$_4$I and the pattern of the

TABLE 11-11

Circumstances Associated with Altered Binding of Thyroxine by Thyroxine-Binding Globulin

Increased Binding	Decreased Binding
Pregnancy	Androgens
Neonatal state	Large doses of glucocorticoids
Estrogens and hyperestrogenemic states	Active acromegaly
	Nephrotic syndrome
Tamoxifen	Major systemic illness
Oral contraceptives	Genetic factors
Acute intermittent porphyria	Asparaginase
Infectious and chronic active hepatitis	
Biliary cirrhosis	
Genetic factors	
Perphenazine	
Human immunodeficiency virus infection	

deviations of total hormone and THBR from normal to derive the maximum information. When concentrations of TBG are altered, the deviation of the total T_4 measurements from normal is in the opposite direction to that of the THBR (see central panels of Fig. 11-13). On the other hand, when the T_4 level is elevated due to increased T_4 secretion or overreplacement, the concentration of unoccupied TBG binding sites is reduced, and both the free fraction and the total T_4 are altered in the same direction (see Fig. 11-14). The changes in hypothyroidism are both in the opposite direction, although of lower magnitude. The reduced FT_4I of hypothyroidism is due predominantly to the decrease in T_4 rather than to a decrease in its free fraction.

Simultaneous abnormalities in both TBG and thyroid hormone production may also occur. One should suspect hyperthyroidism during pregnancy when the T_4 concentration is very high and the THBR is not *subnormal*. Likewise, a serum T_4 concentration in the lower portion of normal range for a nonpregnant individual accompanied by a significant reduction in the THBR indicates hypothyroidism. For pregnant patients, the best strategy may be to use the normal range for total T_4 for the assay being used multiplied by 1.5.

Several caveats should be kept in mind in the interpretation of these results. The use of labeled T_3 in some assays can produce difficulties in three situations: in cases of *familial dysalbuminemic hyperthyroxinemia* (FDH); in the presence of endogenous antibodies directed against T_3; and in sick patients, as already discussed. In FDH, the abnormal albumin binds T_4, but *not* T_3, with increased avidity. Therefore, these patients have an elevated total T_4 and reduced free fraction of T_4, *but not* T_3.[61]

An alternative approach to assessing the FT_4I is to measure TBG either by saturation analysis or radioimmunoassay. Normal concentrations of TBG by radioimmunoassay are about 270 nmol/L (1.0 to 1.5 mg/dL) and are only slightly higher in women than in men. However, it should be recalled (see TBG) that the elastase released from leukocytes during infection may reduce the binding affinity of TBG for T_4 (and T_3) but not change its immunoreactivity or its binding capacity.[196] In such patients, the gravimetric TBG concentration is not paralleled by its binding affinity for T_4 or T_3. With this proviso, the serum TBG concentration result can be employed in one of two ways. First, normalization of the T_4/TBG (or T_3/TBG) ratio yields values that correlate reasonably well with the FT_4I or FT_3I. Second, an FT_4I can be derived from the concentrations of TBG, total T_4, and the association constant for the interaction between the two. In most instances, values

calculated in this manner correlate with the FT_4I determined by other techniques, although the T_4/TBG ratio suggests a subnormal FT_4I in some euthyroid patients with an elevated TBG.[193]

Causes of Abnormal TSH or Thyroid Hormone Concentrations

Several causes of an abnormal TSH should be considered by the clinician (Table 11-12). The clinical status and free T_4 or FT_4I results allow evaluation of the cause for abnormal TSH levels. Assay of the FT_3I is rarely required but is included for completeness.

Causes of a Suppressed TSH

The most common cause of a reduction in serum TSH is an excess supply of thyroid hormone due to either increased endogenous thyroid hormone production or excessive exogenous thyroid hormone. Because the concentration of TSH is inversely proportional to the degree of thyroid hormone excess, patients with clinical symptoms almost invariably have serum TSH concentrations below 0.1 mU/L. Such patients nearly always have an increase in the serum free T_4. In rare patients with low iodine intake, with clinical thyrotoxicosis, the FT_4I is only high-normal despite a suppressed TSH. An FT_3I is required in those patients to establish a diagnosis of T_3 thyrotoxicosis. When thyroid hormone supply is only slightly in excess of the requirement for that patient, serum TSH is suppressed, but clinical manifestations are subtle or absent, and the FT_4I and FT_3I are in the high-normal range. Such minimal changes can occur with euthyroid Graves disease, autonomous thyroid hormone–producing adenomas, multinodular goiters, subacute or painless thyroiditis, and the ingestion of an amount of exogenous thyroid hormone slightly greater than that required for metabolic needs. This condition is termed *subclinical hyperthyroidism*.

The hypothalamic-pituitary axis may remain suppressed for up to 3 months after complete resolution of the thyrotoxic state.[197] The best test for assessing the physiologic state in such patients is the free T_4 or FT_4I. A common scenario for this pattern is during follow-up of patients receiving antithyroid drugs or ^{131}I for Graves disease. With time, the TSH feedback regulatory loop will normalize, and TSH secretion will return and become appropriate for the circulating free thyroid hormone concentration.

In severe illnesses, with or without dopamine infusion or excess glucocorticoid, TSH is suppressed, making assessment of thyroid functional status difficult (see earlier discussion). Because the FT_4I may also be reduced in such patients, astute clinical judgment is required to assign the thyroid status.

Because hCG can activate the TSHR, conditions in which hCG is elevated, such as in the first trimester of pregnancy, with twin pregnancies, during severe *hyperemesis gravidarum*, and in patients with hydatidiform mole or choriocarcinoma, the TSH concentration is often suppressed.[146] TSH returns to normal in the second and third trimesters in the euthyroid patient. A persistently suppressed TSH (<0.1 mU/L) in the pregnant patient after the first trimester suggests that the hyperthyroidism is due to autonomous thyroid function.

Changes in thyroid test results in patients with psychosis or depression, in the geriatric population, and with the use of long-term glucocorticoids were discussed earlier.

If the serum TSH is suppressed *and* the serum free T_4 is low, one should be suspicious that liothyronine (triiodothyronine) is being ingested. Desiccated thyroid also has a

TABLE 11-12

Thyroid Status and Free Thyroid Hormone Levels in Clinical States Associated With Abnormal Serum Thyrotropin (TSH) Concentrations*

	Expected TSH (mU/L)	Clinical Thyroid Status	Free T$_4$ Index	Free T$_3$ Index
Thyrotropin Reduced				
Hyperthyroidism of any cause	<0.1	↑	↑	↑
Euthyroid Graves disease	0.2-0.5	N, (↑)	N	N, (↑)
Autonomous nodule or multinodular goiter	0.2-0.5	N, (↑)	N	↑
Exogenous thyroid hormone excess	<0.1-0.5	N, ↑	N, ↑	↑
Thyroiditis (subacute or painless)	<0.1-0.5	N, ↑	N, ↑	↑, (N)
Recent thyrotoxicosis due to any cause	<0.1-0.5	↑, N, ↓	N, ↓	N, ↓
Illness with or without dopamine infusion	<0.1-5.0	N	↑, N, ↓	↓
First trimester of pregnancy	0.2-0.5	N, (↑)	N, (↑)	↑
Hyperemesis gravidarum	0.2-0.5	N, (↑)	↑, (N)	↑
Hydatidiform mole	0.1-0.4	↑	↑	↑
Acute psychosis or depression (rare)	0.4-10	N	N, (↑)	N, (↓ or↑)
Elderly (small fraction)	0.2-0.5	N	N	N
Glucocorticoids (acute, high dose)	0.1-0.5	N	N	↓
Congenital TSH deficiency				
a. Pit-I deficiency	0	↓	↓	↓
b. CAGYC mutant	0	↓	↓	↓
Thyrotropin Elevated				
Primary hypothyroidism	6-500	↓	↓	N, ↓
Recovery from severe illness	5-30	N, (?)	N, ↓	N, ↓
Iodine deficiency	6-150	N, ↓	↓	N
Thyroid hormone resistance	1-20	↑, N, ↓	↑	↑
Thyrotroph tumor	0.5-50	↑	↑	↑
Hypothalamic-pituitary disease	1-20	↓	↓	N, ↓
Psychiatric illnesses	0.4-10	N	N	N, ↓
Adrenal insufficiency	5-30	N	N	N, ↓
Artifact (endogenous antimouse γ-globulin antibodies)	10-500	N	N	N

*Arrows indicate the nature of the abnormality in the T$_4$ or T$_3$ index. Parentheses indicate that such a result is unusual but may occur.
N, no change; T$_3$, triiodothyronine; T$_4$, thyroxine.

high T$_3$/T$_4$ ratio and if given in excess may cause a similar abnormality.[198]

Causes of an Elevated TSH

Elevations in TSH nearly always imply a reduction in the supply of T$_4$ or T$_3$, which may be permanent or transient. Primary hypothyroidism is far and away the usual explanation. Other causes include acutely ill patients, such as those in renal insufficiency[199] or the asynchronous return of the hypothalamic-pituitary-thyroid axis to normal as critically ill patients recover.[200] Iodine deficiency is the most common cause of an elevation in TSH worldwide, but this does not occur in North America. The rare patient with RTH due to a mutation in the *THRB* gene (RTHβ) may be clinically hyperthyroid, euthyroid, or hypothyroid. The most common laboratory pattern is a serum TSH level that is normal in absolute terms but inappropriately high for the elevated free T$_4$. Individuals with a more marked pituitary than general RTH have symptoms suggesting hyperthyroidism, an elevated FT$_4$I, and a normal or even elevated serum TSH.[201,202] They must be differentiated from the patient with a thyrotroph tumor in whom the persistent secretion of TSH causes hyperthyroidism (see Chapters 9 and 12).[189] Patients with mutations in the *THRA* gene (RTHα) would be expected to have a normal TSH.

Patients with hypothalamic-pituitary dysfunction may have clinical and chemical hypothyroidism but low, normal, or even elevated serum TSH concentrations. The explanation for this paradox is that the biologic effectiveness of the circulating TSH is impaired as a result of abnormal glycosylation secondary to reduced TRH stimulation of the thyrotrophs. Nonetheless, the abnormal TSH is a suitable antigen in the immunometric assay. In adrenal insufficiency, TSH may be modestly elevated but returns to normal with glucocorticoid replacement.[183] This may reflect glucocorticoid-mediated amelioration of Hashimoto thyroiditis.

Despite the utility and general efficacy of the serum TSH measurement alone as a screening tool for identifying patients with thyroid dysfunction, a patient should not receive treatment solely on the basis of an abnormal TSH. The TSH assay is an *indirect reflection* of thyroid hormone supply and does not, by itself, permit a conclusive diagnosis of a specific disorder of thyroid hormone production. Accordingly, the TSH abnormality must be confirmed and the expected alteration in thyroid hormone concentrations documented before initiating treatment.

Tests That Assess the Metabolic Impact of Thyroid Hormones

Abnormalities in the supply of thyroid hormone to the peripheral tissues are associated with alterations in a number of metabolic processes that can be quantitated. Some of these may be useful in the rare patient in whom serum TSH is not an accurate barometer of thyroid status, such as those with RTHβ. These tests may be the sole means of evaluating the metabolic response of the peripheral tissues to thyroid hormones in such patients.

Basal Metabolic Rate

Thyroid hormones increase energy expenditure and heat production, as manifested by weight loss, increased caloric requirement, and heat intolerance. Because it is impractical to measure heat production directly, the BMR measures oxygen consumption under specified conditions of fasting, rest, and tranquil surroundings. Under these conditions, the energy equivalent of 1 L of oxygen is 4.83 kcal.

Under basal conditions, approximately 25% of oxygen consumption is due to energy expenditure in visceral organs, including the liver, kidneys, and heart; 10% occurs in the brain; 10% in respiratory activity; and the remainder in skeletal muscle. Because energy expenditure is related to functioning tissue mass, oxygen consumption is related to some index thereof, most often body surface area. Calculated in this way, basal oxygen consumption (resting energy expenditure) is higher in men than in women and declines rapidly from infancy to the third decade and more slowly thereafter. Values in patients, calculated as a percentage of established normal means for gender and age, normally range from −15% to +5%. In severely hypothyroid patients, values may be as low as −40%, and in thyrotoxic patients these values may reach +25% to +50%. Abnormal, usually elevated, values are seen during recovery in burn patients and in those with systemic disorders, such as febrile illnesses, pheochromocytoma, myeloproliferative disorders, anxiety, and disorders associated with involuntary muscular activity. Resting energy expenditure correlates very well with the free T_4 and TSH in hypothyroid patients given varying doses of exogenous levothyroxine.[203]

Biochemical Markers of Altered Thyroid Status

Occasionally a diagnosis of thyroid dysfunction is first suspected due to an abnormality in a laboratory result performed during an evaluation for an unrelated medical problem. Classic examples are a markedly elevated creatine kinase MM isoenzyme or low-density lipoprotein (LDL) cholesterol leading to the recognition of hypothyroidism.[204] Other similar markers are listed in Table 11-13. These tests are not useful in the diagnosis of thyroid disease, but some, such as sex hormone–binding globulin (SHBG), ferritin, or LDL cholesterol, have been used as end points in clinical studies of the responsivity of the liver to thyroid hormone in patients with thyroid hormone resistance.

TABLE 11-13
Biochemical Markers of Thyroid Status

Thyrotoxicosis

Increased
Osteocalcin
Urine pyridinium collagen cross-links
Alkaline phosphatase (bone or liver)
Atrial natriuretic hormone
Sex hormone–binding globulin
Ferritin
von Willebrand factor

Decreased
Low-density lipoprotein cholesterol
Lipoprotein(a)

Hypothyroidism

Increased
Creatine kinase (MM isoform)
Low-density lipoprotein cholesterol
Lipoprotein(a)
Plasma norepinephrine

Decreased
Vasopressin

Serum Thyroglobulin

The functional sensitivity of most Tg assays is 1 ng/mL or less.[205] The results can be artifactually altered by serum anti-Tg antibodies, and serum should be screened for Tg antibodies with a sensitive Tg-antibody immunoassay. In immunoradiometric assays, interferences lead to underestimations of Tg or false-negative values.

Tg is normally present in the serum, the concentration ranging up to 90 pmol/L (50 ng/mL); mean normal values vary with the assay used but are on the order of 30 pmol/L (20 ng/mL).[206] Concentrations are somewhat higher in women than in men and are elevated severalfold in pregnant women and in the newborn. Levels are elevated in three types of thyroid disorders: goiter and thyroid hyperfunction, inflammatory or physical injury to the thyroid, and differentiated follicular cell–derived thyroid tumors and especially in consumptive hypothyroidism.[90] Values are elevated in both endemic and sporadic nontoxic goiter, and the degree of elevation correlates with the thyroid size. Transient elevations occur in patients with subacute thyroiditis and as a result of trauma to the gland during thyroid surgery or after ^{131}I therapy. Subnormal or undetectable concentrations are found in patients with thyrotoxicosis factitia and aid in differentiating this disorder from other causes of thyrotoxicosis with a low thyroid radioiodine uptake (RAIU).

A major clinical value of measuring the level of serum Tg is in the management, but not in the diagnosis, of differentiated thyroid carcinoma.[205,207] Serum Tg concentrations are increased in patients with both benign and differentiated malignant follicular cell–derived tumors of the thyroid and do not serve to distinguish between the two. After total thyroid ablation for papillary or follicular thyroid carcinoma, Tg should not be detectable, and its subsequent appearance typically signifies the presence of persistent disease.[207] The serum Tg level is related to the mass of neoplastic tissue and may be undetectable in patients with small lymph node micrometastases (see Chapter 14). Secretion of Tg is TSH-dependent. Therefore, the serum Tg level may rise when suppressive therapy is withdrawn or after injections of rhTSH, which will increase the sensitivity of the marker for the detection of persistent or recurrent thyroid carcinoma, even when ^{131}I scans are negative (see Chapter 14). Supersensitive assays of Tg with a functional sensitivity less than 0.1 ng/mL improve the sensitivity during thyroid hormone treatment but at the expense of a decreased specificity.[208,209] This measurement is useful for the follow-up of patients treated with total thyroidectomy without radioactive iodine ablation.[210] Unfortunately, there is a major potential artifact in some patients due to the presence of autoantibodies binding to Tg. To overcome this, the potential use of a liquid chromatography-tandem mass spectrometry (LC-MS/MS) method for the measurement of serum Tg after tryptic digestion of serum samples has been explored. This assay will permit the accurate determination of Tg levels even in patients with Tg autoantibodies[211] even though its current sensitivity is lower than the normal assay.

In the hypothyroid newborn, serum Tg is undetectable in patients with thyroid agenesis and is usually elevated in those with ectopic thyroid tissue or goiter and in consumptive hypothyroidism due to infantile hemangioma.

Tests for Thyroid Autoantibodies

Graves disease and Hashimoto thyroiditis are well characterized and interrelated autoimmune thyroid disorders with a variety of clinical manifestations. The diagnostic

TABLE 11-14

Prevalence of Thyroid Autoantibodies

Group	TSHR-Ab (%)	hTg-Ab (%)	hTPO-Ab (%)
General population	0	5-20	8-27
Patients with Graves disease	80-95	50-70	50-80
Patients with autoimmune thyroiditis	10-20	80-90	90-100
Relatives of patients	0	40-50	40-50
Patients with IDDM	0	40	40
Pregnant women	0	14	14

IDDM, insulin-dependent diabetes mellitus; hTg-Ab, human thyroglobulin antibody; hTPO-Ab, human thyroid peroxidase antibody; TSHR-Ab, thyroid-stimulating hormone receptor antibody.

hallmark of the autoimmune thyroid disorders is the presence, in most patients, of circulating autoantibodies and reactive T cells against one or more thyroid antigens.[212] Three varieties of thyroid autoantibodies are in common use and widely available in clinical diagnostic laboratories (Table 11-14). In this section, autoantibodies to Tg and TPO are discussed. Antibodies directed against the TSHR, the cause of hyperthyroidism in patients with Graves disease, are covered in detail in Chapter 12.

Autoantibodies to Thyroid Peroxidase and Thyroglobulin

Current automated assay techniques for thyroid autoantibodies have good precision because they depend on direct measurement of the interaction between autoantibody and autoantigen (i.e., the interaction between thyroid antigen and the patient's serum). In general, the more sensitive an assay, the more precise and antigen-specific it is. However, many euthyroid individuals exhibit low levels of autoantibodies, and in this situation, the absolute concentration becomes important. The higher the concentration of autoantibody, the greater the clinical specificity (see Table 11-14).[213]

So that comparisons of thyroid antibody concentrations can be made from one office visit to the next, among different patients, and among laboratories, assays for thyroid autoantibodies have been standardized, with results expressed as standard units per milliliter. Of course, the actual standard serum preparation cannot be included in every assay. Instead, a serum pool is usually compared and normalized to the original standard. Autoantibodies differ considerably in their affinity and epitope recognition of antigen and so the slopes of different standard curves may vary. As a result, despite this attempt at standardization, assay results from different commercial assays may still vary considerably. Hence, when monitoring antibody titers (e.g., measuring Tg-Ab after the treatment of thyroid cancer), it is always best to use the same autoantibody assay consistently.

Do Thyroglobulin and Thyroid Peroxidase Antibodies Have a Pathogenic Role?

Tg-Ab and TPO autoantibodies (TPO-Ab) appear to be a secondary response to thyroid injury and are not thought to cause disease themselves, although they may contribute to its development and chronicity. Both types of antibodies are polyclonal, and although they are of the immunoglobulin G class, they are not restricted to one particular immunoglobulin G subclass. Polyclonality also mitigates against a primary role in disease pathogenesis.[214,215] For example, these thyroid antibodies cannot transfer disease from mother to fetus or between animals even though they can pass across the placenta. However, both antibodies may contribute to disease mechanisms. For example, TPO-Ab on the surface of B cells may be involved in antigen presentation, thus activating thyroid-specific T cells.[216] Such autoantibodies may have complement-fixing cytotoxic activity. And TPO-Ab, in particular, correlates well with thyroid damage and lymphocytic infiltration.

Thyroid Autoantibodies in Hashimoto Thyroiditis and Graves Disease

The disease most widely associated with Tg-Ab and TPO-Ab is autoimmune thyroiditis, or Hashimoto disease (terms that embrace both goitrous thyroiditis, as first described by Hashimoto, and atrophic thyroid failure, previously referred to as primary myxedema). Both Tg-Ab and TPO-Ab are found in almost 100% of such patients, but TPO-Ab has higher affinity and occurs in higher concentrations and so testing for TPO-Ab is the more helpful.

Tg-Ab and TPO-Ab are also detectable in 50% to 90% of patients with Graves disease, indicative of the associated thyroiditis that is evident histologically as a heterogeneous lymphocytic infiltration. Hence, Graves disease tends to develop on a background of autoimmune thyroiditis. Although the presence of such autoantibodies favors an autoimmune cause for the hyperthyroidism over other causes, the tests are neither sensitive nor specific in this setting and are interpretable only as part of the clinical scenario. Testing for TSHR antibodies remains the test of choice in hyperthyroid patients.

Thyroid Autoantibodies in Nonautoimmune Thyroid Disorders

Tg-Ab and TPO-Ab are more common in patients with sporadic goiter, multinodular goiter, or isolated thyroid nodules and cancer than in the general population. This finding usually represents an associated thyroiditis on histologic examination. Low levels of thyroid autoantibodies may occur transiently in patients with subacute (de Quervain) thyroiditis but correlate poorly with disease course and are probably a nonspecific response to thyroid injury. There is also a higher prevalence of thyroid autoantibodies in many other autoimmune diseases, particularly insulin-dependent diabetes mellitus.

Thyroid Autoantibodies in Pregnancy

Euthyroid women with thyroid autoantibodies have been shown to suffer from increased early pregnancy loss. The miscarriage rate in the presence of TPO-Ab is almost doubled in many studies,[217-219] and the cause is uncertain. This is likely a reflection of an immune diathesis rather than thyroid function, but the screening of pregnant women has been widely advocated.

The Normal Population

Although the prevalence of thyroid autoantibodies depends on the technique used for detection, Tg-Ab and TPO-Ab are common in the general population (see Table 11-14). At all ages, these antibodies are almost five times more common in women than in men. Selected groups at risk include younger women and relatives of patients with an autoimmune thyroid disorder, in whom the incidence is higher. The low levels of TPO-Ab and Tg-Ab found in many individuals are of uncertain significance in the presence of normal thyroid function; however, they remain a significant risk factor in families with autoimmune thyroid disorders.[220]

Radioiodine Uptake

The only direct test of thyroid function employs a radioactive isotope of iodine as a tag for the body's stable form of iodine, [127]I. Most often the test involves the measurement of the fractional uptake by the thyroid of a tracer (chemically inconsequential) dose of radioiodine. However, several factors make this test less frequently used than in the past. The first is the improvement in indirect methods for assessing thyroid status. The second is the decrease in normal values for thyroid RAIU consequent to the widespread increase in daily dietary iodine intake, reducing the utility of the test in the diagnosis of thyroid disorders.

[131]I (half-life 8.1 days) and [123]I (half-life 0.55 day) both emit gamma radiation, which permits their external detection and quantitation at sites of accumulation, such as the thyroid. These isotopes (abbreviated I* hereafter) are physiologically indistinguishable, not only from one another but also from the naturally occurring [127]I, which permits their use as valid tracers. The shorter half-life of ^{123}I is preferable because the radiation delivered to the thyroid per amount of administered ^{123}I is only about 1% of that delivered by [131]I.

Physiologic Basis

When tracer quantities of inorganic radioiodine are administered orally or intravenously, the isotope quickly mixes with the endogenous stable iodide in the extracellular fluid and begins to be removed by the two major sites of clearance, the thyroid and the kidneys. As this process continues, the plasma level of tracer iodide I* decreases exponentially. Low levels are reached by 24 hours, and inorganic I* is virtually undetectable in the plasma 72 hours after its administration. The thyroid content of I* increases rapidly during the early hours and then at a decreasing rate until a plateau is approached. The proportion of administered I* ultimately accumulated by the thyroid is a function of the clearance of iodide by the thyroid and kidneys. The relation is simply expressed by the following equation:

$$\text{RAIU at plateau} = \frac{C_T}{C_T + C_K}$$

where C_T represents the thyroid iodide clearance rate and C_K the renal iodide clearance rate. The normal thyroid iodide clearance rate is approximately 0.4 L/hour, and the renal iodide clearance rate is 2.0 L/hour, so the uptake of I* normally approximates 20% of the administered dose.

Measurements of RAIU are generally made at 24 hours, both as a matter of convenience and because the value at 24 hours is usually near the plateau but can be measured at 6 hours with appropriate determination of a normal range. The RAIU usually indicates the rate of thyroid hormone synthesis and, by inference, the rate of thyroid hormone release into the blood.

Radioactive Iodine Uptake

Little difference will be noted if the uptake is measured at any time during the day following that on which the isotope was administered, and for the calculation of therapeutic radioiodine doses in treating thyrotoxic Graves disease an early uptake at 3 to 6 hours may produce results comparable to those found at 20 to 28 hours.[221] With the

TABLE 11-15
Factors That Influence 24-Hour Thyroid Iodide Uptake
Factors That Increase Uptake
Increased Hormone Synthesis
Hyperthyroidism
Response to glandular hormone depletion
Recovery from thyroid suppression
Recovery from subacute thyroiditis
Antithyroid agents
Excessive hormone losses
Nephrotic syndrome
Chronic diarrheal states
Soybean ingestion
Normal Hormone Synthesis
Iodine deficiency
Dietary insufficiency
Excessive loss (dehalogenase defect, pregnancy)
Hormone biosynthetic defects
Factors That Decrease Uptake
Decreased Hormone Synthesis
Primary hypofunction
Primary hypothyroidism
Antithyroid agents
Hormone biosynthetic defects
Hashimoto disease
Subacute thyroiditis
Secondary hypofunction
Exogenous thyroid hormones
Not Reflecting Decreased Hormone Synthesis
Increased availability of iodine
Diet or drugs
Cardiac or renal insufficiency
Increased hormone release
Very severe hyperthyroidism (rare)

use of this modified early RAIU measurement, diagnosis and treatment of thyrotoxic Graves disease can be accomplished on the same day. In general, the range of normal values in North America is approximately 5% to 25%. Higher values are found in iodine-deficient regions or in patients with thyroid hyperfunction, but as with other procedures, patients with mild hyperthyroidism may display values at or just above the upper limit of the normal range (Table 11-15).

The Perchlorate Discharge Test

In normal individuals, more than 90% of thyroidal radioiodine is present as iodotyrosine and iodothyronine within minutes of its entry into the thyroid. It is then no longer in the intracellular iodide pool. In patients with Pendred syndrome or with other disorders that inhibit the iodination of tyrosine, such as Hashimoto thyroiditis, or those receiving thiourea drugs, this process is delayed, as shown by the exit (discharge) of more than 10% of the thyroidal radioiodine within 2 hours of administration of 500 mg of $KClO_4$.[10] Perchlorate inhibits NIS function by competing with iodide for NIS, eliminating the iodide gradient that is required for maintaining the radioiodide in the gland. This illustrates that both iodide transport by NIS at the basal pole of the thyrocyte and its efflux across the apical membrane by pendrin are required for thyroid hormone synthesis.

States Associated With Increased RAIU

Hyperthyroidism. Hyperthyroidism causes increased RAIU unless body iodide stores are increased. Such increases in uptake are always evident except in patients with severe thyrotoxicosis, in whom release of hormone can be so rapid that the thyroid content of I* has decreased to the normal range by the time the measurement is made. This condition is rare and is usually associated with obvious thyrotoxicosis.

Aberrant Hormone Synthesis. RAIU can be increased in the absence of hyperthyroidism in disorders in which iodine accumulation is normal but the secretion of hormone is impaired, such as in patients with abnormal Tg synthesis.[222] The magnitude of the increase in uptake and the time at which the plateau is achieved vary with the nature and severity of the disorder. Differentiation of the foregoing states from hyperthyroidism is generally not difficult, because in the former, clinical findings and laboratory evidence of hyperthyroidism are lacking, and indeed hypothyroidism may be present.

Iodine Deficiency. RAIU is increased in acute or chronic iodine deficiency, as demonstrated by measurement of urinary iodine excretion, with urinary iodine values lower than 100 µg/day, indicating deficiency. Chronic iodine deficiency is usually the result of an inadequate content of iodine in the food and water (endemic iodine deficiency). Patients with cardiac, renal, or hepatic disease may develop iodine deficiency if given diets severely restricted in salt, especially if diuretic agents are administered.

Response to Thyroid Hormone Depletion. Rebound increases in RAIU are seen after withdrawal of antithyroid therapy, after subsidence of transient or subacute thyroiditis, and after recovery from prolonged suppression of thyroid function by exogenous hormone. A striking increase in uptake occurs in patients with iodide-induced myxedema after cessation of iodide administration. The duration of the rebound depends on the time required to replenish thyroid hormone stores.

Excessive Hormone Losses. In nephrotic syndrome, excessive losses of hormone in the urine occurring in association with urinary loss of binding protein cause a compensatory increase in hormone synthesis and RAIU. A similar sequence may occur when losses of hormone via the gastrointestinal tract are abnormal, as in chronic diarrheal states or during ingestion of agents, such as soybean protein and cholestyramine, that bind T_4 in the gut.

States Associated With Decreased RAIU

A general increase in iodine intake has made values of the RAIU in hypothyroidism indistinguishable from those at the lower end of the normal range. Therefore, the major indication for measuring the RAIU is to establish whether thyrotoxicosis is due to hyperthyroidism (high RAIU) or thyroiditis (low RAIU).

Exogenous Thyroid Hormone: Thyrotoxicosis Factitia. Except in disorders in which homeostatic control is disrupted or overridden (e.g., Graves disease or autonomously functioning thyroid nodules), administration of exogenous thyroid hormone suppresses TSH secretion and reduces the RAIU, usually to values below 5%.

Low values of the RAIU in a patient who is clinically thyrotoxic may also indicate the presence of *thyrotoxicosis factitia*, the syndrome produced by the ingestion of excess thyroid hormone. The unmeasurably low level of Tg in serum differentiates thyrotoxicosis factitia from other causes of thyrotoxicosis with decreased RAIU.[223]

Disorders of Hormone Storage. The RAIU is usually low in the early phase of subacute thyroiditis and in chronic thyroiditis with transient hyperthyroidism. Here, inflammatory follicular disruption leads to loss of the normal storage function of the gland and leakage of hormone into the blood. In the early stage of subacute thyroiditis, leakage of hormone is usually sufficient to suppress TSH secretion and the RAIU. Transient hypothyroidism often occurs late in both diseases, when stores of preformed hormone are depleted; the RAIU may return to normal or increased values at that time.

Exposure to Excessive Iodine. Exposure to excessive iodine is a common cause of a subnormal RAIU. Such decreases are spurious in the clinical sense because they do not indicate decreased absolute iodine uptake or decreased hormone production but can be produced by the introduction of excessive iodine in any form: inorganic, organic, or elemental. Common offenders are organic iodinated dyes used as radiograph contrast media and amiodarone (see Table 11-7). The duration of suppression of the uptake varies among individuals and with the compound administered. In general, dyes used for pyelography or computed tomography scanning are cleared within a few months, whereas amiodarone may influence the uptake for up to 12 months because of its storage in fat. A single large dose of inorganic iodide can decrease uptake for several days, and chronic ingestion of iodide may depress the uptake for many weeks. Excessive quantities of iodine may also be present in vitamin and mineral preparations, vaginal or rectal suppositories, and iodinated antiseptics such as povidone (see Table 11-7).

The measurement of urinary iodine excretion is an invaluable means of establishing or excluding the existence of excessive body iodide stores; the 24-hour iodine excretion can be roughly extrapolated from the iodide-to-creatinine ratio in a random urine sample. Values in excess of 2 mg/day can account for a low RAIU value, whereas values less than 1 mg/day suggest that a low RAIU is due to one of the other disorders discussed in this section.

REFERENCES

1. De Felice M, Di Lauro R. Murine models for the study of thyroid gland development. *Endocr Dev.* 2007;10:1-14.
2. Kratzsch J, Pulzer F. Thyroid gland development and defects. *Best Pract Res Clin Endocrinol Metab.* 2008;22:57-75.
3. Park SM, Chatterjee VK. Genetics of congenital hypothyroidism. *J Med Genet.* 2005;42:379-389.
4. Burrow GN, Fisher DA, Larsen PR. Mechanisms of disease: maternal and fetal thyroid function. *N Engl J Med.* 1994;331:1072-1078.
5. Vandernoot I, Sartelet H, Abu-Khudir R, et al. Evidence for calcitonin-producing cells in human lingual thyroids. *J Clin Endocrinol Metab.* 2012;97:951-956.
6. Antonica F, Kasprzyk DF, Opitz R, et al. Generation of functional thyroid from embryonic stem cells. *Nature.* 2012;491:66-71.
7. Glinoer D. Clinical and biological consequences of iodine deficiency during pregnancy. *Endocr Dev.* 2007;10:62-85.
8. Caldwell KL, Miller GA, Wang RY, et al. Iodine status of the U.S. population, National Health and Nutrition Examination Survey 2003-2004. *Thyroid.* 2008;18:1207-1214.
9. Dohan O, De la Vieja A, Paroder V, et al. The sodium/iodide symporter (NIS): characterization, regulation, and medical significance. *Endocr Rev.* 2003;24:48-77.
10. Wolff J. Perchlorate and the thyroid gland. *Pharmacol Rev.* 1998; 50:89-105.
11. De La Vieja A, Dohan O, Levy O, et al. Molecular analysis of the sodium/iodide symporter: impact on thyroid and extrathyroid pathophysiology. *Physiol Rev.* 2000;80:1083-1105.
12. Riesco-Eizaguirre G, Leoni SG, Mendiola M, et al. NIS mediates iodide uptake in the female reproductive tract and is a poor prognostic factor in ovarian cancer. *J Clin Endocrinol Metab.* 2014;99:E1199-E1208.
13. Van Sande J, Massart C, Beauwens R, et al. Anion selectivity by the sodium iodide symporter. *Endocrinology.* 2003;144:247-252.
14. Wolff J. Congenital goiter with defective iodide transport. *Endocrinol Rev.* 1983;4:240.
15. Nicola JP, Carrasco N, Amzel LM. Physiological sodium concentrations enhance the iodide affinity of the Na+/I- symporter. *Nat Commun.* 2014;5:3948.
16. Bizhanova A, Kopp P. Minireview: the sodium-iodide symporter NIS and pendrin in iodide homeostasis of the thyroid. *Endocrinology.* 2009;150:1084-1090.

17. Everett LA, Green ED. A family of mammalian anion transporters and their involvement in human genetic diseases. *Hum Mol Genet.* 1999;8: 1883-1891.
18. Everett LA, Morsli H, Wu DK, et al. Expression pattern of the mouse ortholog of the Pendred's syndrome gene (Pds) suggests a key role for pendrin in the inner ear. *Proc Natl Acad Sci U S A.* 1999;96: 9727-9732.
19. Royaux IE, Wall SM, Karniski LP, et al. Pendrin, encoded by the Pendred syndrome gene, resides in the apical region of renal inter-calated cells and mediates bicarbonate secretion. *Proc Natl Acad Sci U S A.* 2001;98:4221-4226.
20. Morgans ME, Trotter WR. Association of congenital deafness with goitre; the nature of the thyroid defect. *Lancet.* 1958;1:607-609.
21. Kopp P, Pesce L, Solis SJ. Pendred syndrome and iodide transport in the thyroid. *Trends Endocrinol Metab.* 2008;19:260-268.
22. van den Hove MF, Croizet-Berger K, Jouret F, et al. The loss of the chloride channel, ClC-5, delays apical iodide efflux and induces a euthyroid goiter in the mouse thyroid gland. *Endocrinology.* 2006;147: 1287-1296.
23. Gnidehou S, Caillou B, Talbot M, et al. Iodotyrosine dehalogenase 1 (DEHAL1) is a transmembrane protein involved in the recycling of iodide close to the thyroglobulin iodination site. *FASEB J.* 2004;18: 1574-1576.
24. Larsen PR. Thyroidal triiodothyronine and thyroxine in Graves' disease: correlation with presurgical treatment, thyroid status, and iodine content. *J Clin Endocrinol Metab.* 1975;41:1098-1104.
25. Moreno JC, Klootwijk W, van Toor H, et al. Mutations in the iodoty-rosine deiodinase gene and hypothyroidism. *N Engl J Med.* 2008;358: 1811-1818.
26. Taurog A, Dorris ML, Doerge DR. Mechanism of simultaneous iodin-ation and coupling catalyzed by thyroid peroxidase. *Arch Biochem Biophys.* 1996;330:24-32.
27. Ris-Stalpers C. Physiology and pathophysiology of the DUOXes. *Anti-oxid Redox Signal.* 2006;8:1563-1572.
28. Grasberger H, Refetoff S. Identification of the maturation factor for dual oxidase. Evolution of an eukaryotic operon equivalent. *J Biol Chem.* 2006;281:18269-18272.
29. Grasberger H, De Deken X, Mayo OB, et al. Mice deficient in dual oxidase maturation factors are severely hypothyroid. *Mol Endocrinol.* 2012;26:481-492.
30. Niethammer P, Grabher C, Look AT, et al. A tissue-scale gradient of hydrogen peroxide mediates rapid wound detection in zebrafish. *Nature.* 2009;459:996-999.
31. Vulsma T, Gons MH, DeVijlder JMM. Maternal fetal transfer of thyrox-ine in congenital hypothyroidism due to a total organification defect of thyroid dysgenesis. *N Engl J Med.* 1989;321:13-16.
32. Moreno JC, Bikker H, Kempers MJ, et al. Inactivating mutations in the gene for thyroid oxidase 2 (THOX2) and congenital hypothyroidism. *N Engl J Med.* 2002;347:95-102.
33. Zamproni I, Grasberger H, Cortinovis F, et al. Biallelic inactivation of the dual oxidase maturation factor 2 (DUOXA2) gene as a novel cause of congenital hypothyroidism. *J Clin Endocrinol Metab.* 2008;93: 605-610.
34. Bakker B, Bikker H, Vulsma T, et al. Two decades of screening for congenital hypothyroidism in The Netherlands: TPO gene mutations in total iodide organification defects (an update). *J Clin Endocrinol Metab.* 2000;85:3708-3712.
35. Gerard AC, Daumerie C, Mestdagh C, et al. Correlation between the loss of thyroglobulin iodination and the expression of thyroid-specific proteins involved in iodine metabolism in thyroid carcinomas. *J Clin Endocrinol Metab.* 2003;88:4977-4983.
36. Dunn AD, Corsi CM, Myers HE, et al. Tyrosine 130 is an important outer ring donor for thyroxine formation in thyroglobulin. *J Biol Chem.* 1998;273:25223-25229.
37. Abuid J, Larsen PR. Triiodothyronine and thyroxine in hyperthyroid-ism. Comparison of the acute changes during therapy with antithyroid agents. *J Clin Invest.* 1974;54:201-208.
38. Bahn RS, Burch HS, Cooper DS, et al. The role of propylthiouracil in the management of Graves' disease in adults: report of a meeting jointly sponsored by the American Thyroid Association and the Food and Drug Administration. *Thyroid.* 2009;19:673-674.
39. Kim BW, Daniels GH, Harrison BJ, et al. Overexpression of type 2 iodothyronine deiodinase in follicular carcinoma as a cause of low circulating free thyroxine levels. *J Clin Endocrinol Metab.* 2003;88: 594-598.
40. Lazarus JH. The effects of lithium therapy on thyroid and thyrotropin-releasing hormone. *Thyroid.* 1998;8:909-913.
41. Davies TF, Ando T, Lin RY, et al. Thyrotropin receptor-associated dis-eases: from adenomata to Graves disease. *J Clin Invest.* 2005;115: 1972-1983.
42. Corvilain B, Van Sande J, Dumont JE, et al. Somatic and germline mutations of the TSH receptor and thyroid diseases. *Clin Endocrinol (Oxf).* 2001;55:143-158.
43. Saavedra AP, Tsygankova OM, Prendergast GV, et al. Role of cAMP, PKA and Rap1A in thyroid follicular cell survival. *Oncogene.* 2002;21: 778-788.
44. Cianfarani F, Baldini E, Cavalli A, et al. TSH receptor and thyroid-specific gene expression in human skin. *J Invest Dermatol.* 2010;130: 93-101.
45. Tonacchera M, Van Sande J, Parma J, et al. TSH receptor and disease. *Clin Endocrinol (Oxf).* 1996;44:621-633.
46. Bianco AC, Salvatore D, Gereben B, et al. Biochemistry, cellular and molecular biology and physiological roles of the iodothyronine sele-nodeiodinases. *Endocr Rev.* 2002;23:38-89.
47. Haugen BR. Drugs that suppress TSH or cause central hypothyroidism. *Best Pract Res Clin Endocrinol Metab.* 2009;23:793-800.
48. Findlay KA, Kaptein E, Visser TJ, et al. Characterization of the uridine diphosphate-glucuronosyltransferase-catalyzing thyroid hor-mone glucuronidation in man. *J Clin Endocrinol Metab.* 2000;85: 2879-2883.
49. Hackenmueller SA, Marchini M, Saba A, et al. Biosynthesis of 3-iodothyronamine (T1AM) is dependent on the sodium-iodide sym-porter and thyroperoxidase but does not involve extrathyroidal metab-olism of T4. *Endocrinology.* 2012;153:5659-5667.
50. Schussler GC. The thyroxine-binding proteins. *Thyroid.* 2000;10: 141-149.
51. Jirasakuldech B, Schussler GC, Yap MG, et al. A characteristic serpin cleavage product of thyroxine-binding globulin appears in sepsis sera. *J Clin Endocrinol Metab.* 2000;85:3996-3999.
52. Pemberton PA, Stein PE, Pepys MB, et al. Hormone binding globulins undergo serpin conformational change in inflammation. *Nature.* 1988; 336:257-258.
53. Dickson PW, Aldred AR, Marley PD, et al. Rat choroid plexus special-izes in the synthesis and secretion of transthyretin (prealbumin). *J Biol Chem.* 1985;261:3475.
54. Patel J, Landers KA, Li H, et al. Ontogenic changes in placental trans-thyretin. *Placenta.* 2011;32:817-822.
55. Palha JA, Episkopou V, Maeda S, et al. Thyroid hormone metabolism in a transthyretin-null mouse strain. *J Biol Chem.* 1994;269:32767.
56. Palha JA, Fernandes R, de Escobar GM, et al. Transthyretin regulates thyroid hormone levels in the choroid plexus, but not in the brain parenchyma: study in a transthyretin-null mouse model. *Endocrinol-ogy.* 2000;141:3267-3272.
57. Bartalena L. Recent achievements in studies on thyroid hormone-binding proteins. *Endocr Rev.* 1990;11:47-64.
58. Bartalena L. Thyroid hormone-binding proteins: update 1994. *Endocr Rev.* 1994;3:140-142.
59. Chin W, Schussler GC. Decreased serum free thyroxine concentration in patients treated with diphenylhydantoin. *J Clin Endocrinol.* 1968;28: 181-186.
60. Larsen PR. Salicylate-induced increases in free triiodothyronine in human serum. Evidence of inhibition of triiodothyronine binding to thyroxine-binding globulin and thyroxine-binding prealbumin. *J Clin Invest.* 1972;51:1125-1134.
61. Docter R, Bos G, Krenning EP, et al. Inherited thyroxine excess: a serum abnormality due to an increased affinity for modified albumin. *Clin Endocrinol.* 1981;15:363-371.
62. Mendel CM, Cavalieri RR. Thyroxine distribution and metabolism in familial dysalbuminemic hyperthyroxinemia. *J Clin Endocrinol Metab.* 1984;59:499-504.
63. Arafah BM. Increased need for thyroxine in women with hypothyroid-ism during estrogen therapy. *N Engl J Med.* 2001;344:1743-1749.
64. Robbins J, Rall JE. The interaction of thyroid hormones and protein in biological fluids. *Recent Prog Horm Res.* 1957;13:161.
65. Mendel CM. The free hormone hypothesis: a physiologically based mathematical model. *Endocr Rev.* 1989;10:232-274.
66. Heuer H, Visser TJ. Minireview: pathophysiological importance of thyroid hormone transporters. *Endocrinology.* 2009;150:1078-1083.
67. Mendel CM, Weisiger RA, Jones AL, et al. Thyroid hormone-binding proteins in plasma facilitate uniform distribution of thyroxine within tissues: a perfused rat liver study. *Endocrinology.* 1987;120:1742-1749.
68. Visser WE, Vrijmoeth P, Visser FE, et al. Identification, functional analysis, prevalence and treatment of monocarboxylate transporter 8 (MCT8) mutations in a cohort of adult patients with mental retarda-tion. *Clin Endocrinol (Oxf).* 2013;78:310-315.
69. Visser WE, Friesema EC, Jansen J, et al. Thyroid hormone transport in and out of cells. *Trends Endocrinol Metab.* 2008;19:50-56.
70. Dumitrescu AM, Liao XH, Weiss RE, et al. Tissue-specific thyroid hormone deprivation and excess in monocarboxylate transporter (MCT) 8-deficient mice. *Endocrinology.* 2006;147:4036-4043.
71. Trajkovic M, Visser TJ, Mittag J, et al. Abnormal thyroid hormone metabolism in mice lacking the monocarboxylate transporter 8. *J Clin Invest.* 2007;117:627-635.
72. Dumitrescu AM, Refetoff S. The syndromes of reduced sensitivity to thyroid hormone. *Biochim Biophys Acta.* 2013;1830:3987-4003.
73. Ferrara AM, Liao XH, Gil-Ibanez P, et al. Placenta passage of the thyroid hormone analog DITPA to male wild-type and MCT8-deficient mice. *Endocrinology.* 2014;155:4088-4093.
74. Bernal J. The significance of thyroid hormone transporters in the brain. *Endocrinology.* 2005;146:1698-1700.
75. Tu HM, Kim SW, Salvatore D, et al. Regional distribution of type 2 thyroxine deiodinase messenger ribonucleic acid in rat hypothalamus

and pituitary and its regulation by thyroid hormone. *Endocrinology.* 1997;138:3359-3368.

76. Guadano-Ferraz A, Escamez MJ, Rausell E, et al. Expression of type 2 iodothyronine deiodinase in hypothyroid rat brain indicates an important role of thyroid hormone in the development of specific primary sensory systems. *J Neurosci.* 1999;19:3430-3439.

77. Fu J, Refetoff S, Dumitrescu AM. Inherited defects of thyroid hormone-cell-membrane transport: review of recent findings. *Curr Opin Endocrinol Diabetes Obes.* 2013;20:434-440.

78. St Germain DL, Galton VA, Hernandez A. Minireview: defining the roles of the iodothyronine deiodinases: current concepts and challenges. *Endocrinology.* 2009;150:1097-1107.

79. Berry MJ, Banu L, Larsen PR. Type I iodothyronine deiodinase is a selenocysteine-containing enzyme. *Nature.* 1991;349:438-440.

80. Berry MJ, Larsen PR. The role of selenium in thyroid hormone action. *Endocr Rev.* 1992;13:207-219.

81. Schweizer U, Schlicker C, Braun D, et al. Crystal structure of mammalian selenocysteine-dependent iodothyronine deiodinase suggests a peroxiredoxin-like catalytic mechanism. *Proc Natl Acad Sci U S A.* 2014;111:10526-10531.

82. Berry MJ, Banu L, Chen YY, et al. Recognition of UGA as a selenocysteine codon in type I deiodinase requires sequences in the 3' untranslated region. *Nature.* 1991;353:273-276.

83. Gereben B, Zavacki AM, Ribich S, et al. Cellular and molecular basis of deiodinase-regulated thyroid hormone signaling. *Endocr Rev.* 2008;29:898-938.

84. Wajner SM, Goemann IM, Bueno AL, et al. IL-6 promotes nonthyroidal illness syndrome by blocking thyroxine activation while promoting thyroid hormone inactivation in human cells. *J Clin Invest.* 2011;121:1834-1845.

85. Verloop H, Dekkers OM, Peeters RP, et al. Genetics in endocrinology: genetic variation in deiodinases: a systematic review of potential clinical effects in humans. *Eur J Endocrinol.* 2014;171:R123-R135.

86. Huang SA. Physiology and pathophysiology of type 3 deiodinase in humans. *Thyroid.* 2005;15:875-881.

87. Salvatore D, Low SC, Berry M, et al. Type 3 iodothyronine deiodinase: cloning, in vitro expression, and functional analysis of the placental selenoenzyme. *J Clin Invest.* 1995;96:2421-2430.

88. Dentice M, Luongo C, Ambrosio R, et al. Beta-catenin regulates deiodinase levels and thyroid hormone signaling in colon cancer cells. *Gastroenterology.* 2012;143:1037-1047.

89. Dentice M, Ambrosio R, Salvatore D. Role of type 3 deiodinase in cancer. *Expert Opin Ther Targets.* 2009;13:1363-1373.

90. Huang SA, Tu HM, Harney JW, et al. Severe hypothyroidism caused by type 3 iodothyronine deiodinase in infantile hemangiomas. *N Engl J Med.* 2000;343:185-189.

91. Maynard MA, Marino-Enriquez A, Fletcher JA, et al. Thyroid hormone inactivation in gastrointestinal stromal tumors. *N Engl J Med.* 2014;370:1327-1334.

92. Hernandez A. Structure and function of the type 3 deiodinase gene. *Thyroid.* 2005;15:865-874.

93. St Germain DL, Hernandez A, Schneider MJ, et al. Insights into the role of deiodinases from studies of genetically modified animals. *Thyroid.* 2005;15:905-916.

94. Galton VA, Schneider MJ, Clark AS, et al. Life without thyroxine to 3,5,3'-triiodothyronine conversion: studies in mice devoid of the 5'-deiodinases. *Endocrinology.* 2009;150:2957-2963.

95. Dentice M, Marsili A, Ambrosio R, et al. The FoxO3/type 2 deiodinase pathway is required for normal mouse myogenesis and muscle regeneration. *J Clin Invest.* 2010;120:4021-4030.

96. Salvatore D, Simonides WS, Dentice M, et al. Thyroid hormones and skeletal muscle—new insights and potential implications. *Nat Rev Endocrinol.* 2014;10:206-214.

97. Schneider MJ, Fiering SN, Thai B, et al. Targeted disruption of the type 1 selenodeiodinase gene (dio1) results in marked changes in thyroid hormone economy in mice. *Endocrinology.* 2006;147:580-589.

98. Hernandez A, Martinez ME, Fiering S, et al. Type 3 deiodinase is critical for the maturation and function of the thyroid axis. *J Clin Invest.* 2006;116:476-484.

99. Saberi M, Sterling FH, Utiger RD. Reduction in extrathyroidal triiodothyronine production by propylthiouracil in man. *J Clin Invest.* 1975;55:218-223.

100. Christoffolete MA, Ribeiro R, Singru P, et al. Atypical expression of type 2 iodothyronine deiodinase in thyrotrophs explains the thyroxine-mediated pituitary TSH feedback mechanism. *Endocrinology.* 2006;147:1735-1743.

101. Wu SY, Green WL, Huang WS, et al. Alternate pathways of thyroid hormone metabolism. *Thyroid.* 2005;15:943-958.

102. Ribeiro MO, Carvalho SD, Schultz JJ, et al. Thyroid hormone-sympathetic interaction and adaptive thermogenesis are thyroid hormone receptor isoform-specific. *J Clin Invest.* 2001;108:97-105.

103. Huang SA, Bianco AC. Reawakened interest in type III iodothyronine deiodinase in critical illness and injury. *Nat Clin Pract Endocrinol Metab.* 2008;4:148-155.

104. Martino E, Bartalena L, Bogazzi F, et al. The effects of amiodarone on the thyroid. *Endocr Rev.* 2001;22:240-254.

105. Bogazzi F, Tomisti L, Bartalena L, et al. Amiodarone and the thyroid: a 2012 update. *J Endocrinol Invest.* 2012;35:340-348.

106. LoPresti JS, Eigen A, Kaptein E, et al. Alterations in 3,3'5'-triiodothyronine metabolism in response to propylthiouracil, dexamethasone, and thyroxine administration in man. *J Clin Invest.* 1989;84:1650-1656.

107. Schomburg L, Kohrle J. On the importance of selenium and iodine metabolism for thyroid hormone biosynthesis and human health. *Mol Nutr Food Res.* 2008;52:1235-1246.

108. Lazar MA. Thyroid hormone action: a binding contract. *J Clin Invest.* 2003;112:497-499.

109. Amma LL, Campos-Barros A, Wang Z, et al. Distinct tissue-specific roles for thyroid hormone receptors beta and alpha1 in regulation of type 1 deiodinase expression. *Mol Endocrinol.* 2001;15:467-475.

110. Abel ED, Kaulbach HC, Campos-Barros A, et al. Novel insight from transgenic mice into thyroid hormone resistance and the regulation of thyrotropin. *J Clin Invest.* 1999;103:271-279.

111. Forrest D, Golarai G, Connor J, et al. Genetic analysis of thyroid hormone receptors in development and disease. *Recent Prog Horm Res.* 1996;51:1-22.

112. Bochukova E, Schoenmakers N, Agostini M, et al. A mutation in the thyroid hormone receptor alpha gene. *N Engl J Med.* 2012;366:243-249.

113. van Mullem A, van Heerebeek R, Chrysis D, et al. Clinical phenotype and mutant TRalpha1. *N Engl J Med.* 2012;366:1451-1453.

114. Togashi M, Borngraeber S, Sandler B, et al. Conformational adaptation of nuclear receptor ligand binding domains to agonists: potential for novel approaches to ligand design. *J Steroid Biochem Mol Biol.* 2005;93:127-137.

115. Bassett JH, Harvey CB, Williams GR. Mechanisms of thyroid hormone receptor-specific nuclear and extra nuclear actions. *Mol Cell Endocrinol.* 2003;213:1-11.

116. Mousa SA, O'Connor LJ, Bergh JJ, et al. The proangiogenic action of thyroid hormone analogue GC-1 is initiated at an integrin. *J Cardiovasc Pharmacol.* 2005;46:356-360.

117. Hollenberg AN, Monden T, Flynn TR, et al. The human thyrotropin-releasing hormone gene is regulated by thyroid hormone through two distinct classes of negative thyroid hormone response elements. *Mol Endocrinol.* 1995;9:540-550.

118. Segerson TP, Kauer J, Wolfe H, et al. Thyroid hormone regulates TRH biosynthesis in the paraventricular nucleus of the rat hypothalamus. *Science.* 1987;238:78-80.

119. Dyess EM, Segerson TP, Liposits Z, et al. Triiodothyronine exerts direct cell-specific regulation of thyrotropin-releasing hormone gene expression in the hypothalamic paraventricular nucleus. *Endocrinology.* 1988;123:2291-2297.

120. Lechan RM, Fekete C. Role of thyroid hormone deiodination in the hypothalamus. *Thyroid.* 2005;15:883-897.

121. Fonseca TL, Correa-Medina M, Campos MP, et al. Coordination of hypothalamic and pituitary T3 production regulates TSH expression. *J Clin Invest.* 2013;123:1492-1500.

122. Heuer H, Schafer MK, Bauer K. The thyrotropin-releasing hormone-degrading ectoenzyme: the third element of the thyrotropin-releasing hormone-signaling system. *Thyroid.* 1998;8:915-920.

123. Magner JA. Thyroid-stimulating hormone: biosynthesis, cell biology and bioactivity. *Endocr Rev.* 1990;11:354.

124. Gesundheit N, Petrick PA, Nissim M, et al. Thyrotropin-secreting pituitary adenomas: clinical and biochemical heterogeneity. *Ann Intern Med.* 1989;11:827-835.

125. Beck-Peccoz P, Amir S, Menezes-Ferreira MM, et al. Decreased receptor binding of biologically inactive thyrotropin in central hypothyroidism: effect of treatment with thyrotropin-releasing hormone. *N Engl J Med.* 1985;312:1085-1090.

126. Chan JL, Heist K, DePaoli AM, et al. The role of falling leptin levels in the neuroendocrine and metabolic adaptation to short-term starvation in healthy men. *J Clin Invest.* 2003;111:1409-1421.

127. Brabant G, Frank K, Ranft U. Physiological regulation of circadian and pulsatile thyrotropin secretion in normal man and woman. *J Clin Endocrinol Metab.* 1990;70:403.

128. Nikrodhanond AA, Ortiga-Carvalho TM, Shibusawa N, et al. Dominant role of thyrotropin-releasing hormone in the hypothalamic-pituitary-thyroid axis. *J Biol Chem.* 2006;281:5000-5007.

129. Chiamolera MI, Wondisford FE. Minireview: thyrotropin-releasing hormone and the thyroid hormone feedback mechanism. *Endocrinology.* 2009;150:1091-1096.

130. Beck-Peccoz P, Brucker-Davis F, Persani L, et al. Thyrotropin-secreting pituitary tumors. *Endocr Rev.* 1996;17:610-638.

131. Biller BM, Molitch ME, Vance ML, et al. Treatment of prolactin-secreting macroadenomas with the once-weekly dopamine agonist cabergoline. *J Clin Endocrinol Metab.* 1996;81:2338-2343.

132. Sherman SI, Gopal J, Haugen BR, et al. Central hypothyroidism associated with retinoid X receptor-selective ligands. *N Engl J Med.* 1999;340:1075-1079.

133. Sharma V, Hays WR, Wood WM, et al. Effects of rexinoids on thyrotrope function and the hypothalamic-pituitary-thyroid axis. *Endocrinology.* 2006;147:1438-1451.

134. Nakabayashi K, Matsumi H, Bhalla A, et al. Thyrostimulin, a heterodimer of two new human glycoprotein hormone subunits, activates the thyroid-stimulating hormone receptor. *J Clin Invest.* 2002;109: 1445-1452.

135. Sun SC, Hsu PJ, Wu FJ, et al. Thyrostimulin, but not thyroid-stimulating hormone, acts as a paracrine regulator to activate thyroid-stimulating hormone receptor in the mammalian ovary. *J Biol Chem.* 2010;285: 3758-3765.

136. Riesco G, Taurog A, Larsen R, et al. Acute and chronic responses to iodine deficiency in rats. *Endocrinology.* 1977;100:303-313.

137. Peeters R, Fekete C, Goncalves C, et al. Regional physiological adaptation of the central nervous system deiodinases to iodine deficiency. *Am J Physiol Endocrinol Metab.* 2001;281:E54-E61.

138. Guo TW, Zhang FC, Yang MS, et al. Positive association of the DIO2 (deiodinase type 2) gene with mental retardation in the iodine-deficient areas of China. *J Med Genet.* 2004;41:585-590.

139. Pazos-Moura CC, Moura EG, Dorris ML, et al. Effect of iodine deficiency and cold exposure on thyroxine 5′-deiodinase activity in various rat tissues. *Am J Physiol.* 1991;260:E175-E182.

140. Zimmermann MB. Iodine deficiency. *Endocr Rev.* 2009;30:376-408.

141. Delange F. The disorders induced by iodine deficiency. *Thyroid.* 1994;4:107-128.

142. Wolff J, Chaikoff IL. Plasma inorganic iodide as a homeostatic regulator of thyroid function. *J Biol Chem.* 1948;174:555.

143. Eng PH, Cardona GR, Fang SL, et al. Escape from the acute Wolff-Chaikoff effect is associated with a decrease in thyroid sodium/iodide symporter messenger ribonucleic acid and protein. *Endocrinology.* 1999;140:3404-3410.

144. LeBeau SO, Mandel SJ. Thyroid disorders during pregnancy. *Endocrinol Metab Clin North Am.* 2006;35:117-136.

145. Glinoer D. The regulation of thyroid function during normal pregnancy: importance of the iodine nutrition status. *Best Pract Res Clin Endocrinol Metab.* 2004;18:133-152.

146. Dashe JS, Casey BM, Wells CE, et al. Thyroid-stimulating hormone in singleton and twin pregnancy: importance of gestational age-specific reference ranges. *Obstet Gynecol.* 2005;106:753-757.

147. Huang SA, Dorfman DM, Genest DR, et al. Type 3 iodothyronine deiodinase is highly expressed in the human uteroplacental unit and in fetal epithelium. *J Clin Endocrinol Metab.* 2003;88:1384-1388.

148. Alexander EK, Marqusee E, Lawrence J, et al. Timing and magnitude of increases in levothyroxine requirements during pregnancy in women with hypothyroidism. *N Engl J Med.* 2004;351:241-249.

149. Weetman AP. Autoimmune thyroid disease. *Autoimmunity.* 2004;37: 337-340.

150. Dentice M, Bandyopadhyay A, Gereben B, et al. The hedgehog-inducible ubiquitin ligase subunit WSB-1 modulates thyroid hormone activation and PTHrP secretion in the developing growth plate. *Nat Cell Biol.* 2005;7:698-705.

151. Fisher DA, Schoen EJ, La Franchi S, et al. The hypothalamic-pituitary-thyroid negative feedback control axis in children with treated congenital hypothyroidism. *J Clin Endocrinol Metab.* 2000;85:2722-2727.

152. Contempre B, Jauniaux E, Calvo R, et al. Detection of thyroid hormones in human embryonic cavities during the first trimester of pregnancy. *J Clin Endocrinol Metab.* 1993;77:1719-1722.

153. Stagnaro-Green A. Maternal thyroid disease and preterm delivery. *J Clin Endocrinol Metab.* 2009;94:21-25.

154. Fisher DA, Nelson JC, Carlton EI, et al. Maturation of human hypothalamic-pituitary-thyroid function and control. *Thyroid.* 2000; 10:229-234.

155. Abuid J, Stinson DA, Larsen PR. Serum triiodothyronine and thyroxine in the neonate and the acute increases in these hormones following delivery. *J Clin Invest.* 1973;52:1195-1199.

156. de Jesus LA, Carvalho SD, Ribeiro MO, et al. The type 2 iodothyronine deiodinase is essential for adaptive thermogenesis in brown adipose tissue. *J Clin Invest.* 2001;108:1379-1385.

157. Fisher DA. Thyroid system immaturities in very low birth weight premature infants. *Semin Perinatol.* 2008;32:387-397.

158. Fisher DA. Thyroid function and dysfunction in premature infants. *Pediatr Endocrinol Rev.* 2007;4:317-328.

159. Shih JL, Agus MS. Thyroid function in the critically ill newborn and child. *Curr Opin Pediatr.* 2009;21:536-540.

160. Mariotti S, Franceschi C, Cossarizza A, et al. The aging thyroid. *Endocr Rev.* 1995;16:686-715.

161. Hershman JM, Pekary AE, Berg L, et al. Serum thyrotropin and thyroid hormone levels in elderly and middle-aged euthyroid persons. *J Am Geriatr Soc.* 1993;41:823-828.

162. Hoogendoorn EH, Hermus AR, de Vegt F, et al. Thyroid function and prevalence of anti-thyroperoxidase antibodies in a population with borderline sufficient iodine intake: influences of age and sex. *Clin Chem.* 2006;52:104-111.

163. Bowers J, Terrien J, Clerget-Froidevaux MS, et al. Thyroid hormone signaling and homeostasis during aging. *Endocr Rev.* 2013;34:556-589.

164. Chan JL, Bullen J, Stoyneva V, et al. Recombinant methionyl human leptin administration to achieve high physiologic or pharmacologic leptin levels does not alter circulating inflammatory marker levels in humans with leptin sufficiency or excess. *J Clin Endocrinol Metab.* 2005; 90:1618-1624.

165. Byerley LO, Heber D. Metabolic effects of triiodothyronine replacement during fasting in obese subjects. *J Clin Endocrinol Metab.* 1996;81:968-976.

166. Onur S, Haas V, Bosy-Westphal A, et al. L-tri-iodothyronine is a major determinant of resting energy expenditure in underweight patients with anorexia nervosa and during weight gain. *Eur J Endocrinol.* 2005; 152:179-184.

167. Danforth JE, Horton ES, O'Connell M, et al. Dietary-induced alterations in thyroid hormone metabolism during overnutrition. *J Clin Invest.* 1979;64:1336-1347.

168. Van den Berghe G. Novel insights into the neuroendocrinology of critical illness. *Eur J Endocrinol.* 2000;143:1-13.

169. Alkemade A, Friesema EC, Unmehopa UA, et al. Neuroanatomical pathways for thyroid hormone feedback in the human hypothalamus. *J Clin Endocrinol Metab.* 2005;90:4322-4334.

170. Fekete C, Sarkar S, Christoffolete MA, et al. Bacterial lipopolysaccharide (LPS)-induced type 2 iodothyronine deiodinase (D2) activation in the mediobasal hypothalamus (MBH) is independent of the LPS-induced fall in serum thyroid hormone levels. *Brain Res.* 2005;1056: 97-99.

171. Boelen A, Platvoet-Ter Schiphorst MC, Wiersinga WM. Association between serum interleukin-6 and serum 3,5,3′-triiodothyronine in nonthyroidal illness. *J Clin Endocrinol Metab.* 1993;77:1695-1699.

172. Vidart J, Magagnin Wajner S, Sarmento Leite R, et al. N-Acetylcysteine administration prevents nonthyroidal illness syndrome in patients with acute myocardial infarction: a randomized clinical trial. *J Clin Endocrinol Metab.* 2014;99(12):4537-4545.

173. Koenig RJ. Modeling the nonthyroidal illness syndrome. *Curr Opin Endocrinol Diabetes Obes.* 2008;15:466-469.

174. Peeters RP, Wouters PJ, Kaptein E, et al. Reduced activation and increased inactivation of thyroid hormone in tissues of critically ill patients. *J Clin Endocrinol Metab.* 2003;88:3202-3211.

175. Wadwekar D, Kabadi UM. Thyroid hormone indices during illness in six hypothyroid subjects rendered euthyroid with levothyroxine therapy. *Exp Clin Endocrinol Diabetes.* 2004;112:373-377.

176. Van den Berghe G, Wouters P, Weekers F, et al. Reactivation of pituitary hormone release and metabolic improvement by infusion of growth hormone-releasing peptide and thyrotropin-releasing hormone in patients with protracted critical illness. *J Clin Endocrinol Metab.* 1999; 84:1311-1323.

177. Hamblin PS, Dyer SA, Mohr VS, et al. Relationship between thyrotropin and thyroxine changes during recovery from severe hypothyroxinemia of critical illness. *J Clin Endocrinol Metab.* 1986;62: 717-722.

178. Brent GA, Hershman JM. Thyroxine therapy in patients with severe nonthyroidal illness and low serum thyroxine concentrations. *J Clin Endocrinol Metab.* 1986;63:1-8.

179. Bennett-Guerrero E, Jimenez JL, White WD, et al. Cardiovascular effects of intravenous triiodothyronine in patients undergoing coronary artery bypass graft surgery. A randomized, double-blind, placebo-controlled trial. Duke T3 study group. *JAMA.* 1996;275:687-692.

180. Klein I, Danzi S. Thyroid disease and the heart. *Circulation.* 2007; 116:1725-1735.

181. Novitzky D, Cooper DK. Thyroid hormone and the stunned myocardium. *J Endocrinol.* 2014;223:R1-R8.

182. Jackson IM. The thyroid axis and depression. *Thyroid.* 1998;8:951-956.

183. Topliss DJ, White EL, Stockigt JR. Significance of thyrotropin excess in untreated primary adrenal insufficiency. *J Clin Endocrinol Metab.* 1980; 50:52-56.

184. Ain KB, Mori Y, Refetoff S. Reduced clearance rate of thyroxine-binding globulin (TBG) with increased sialylation: a mechanism for estrogen-induced elevation of serum TBG concentration. *J Clin Endocrinol Metab.* 1987;65:689-696.

185. Marqusee E, Braverman LE, Lawrence JE, et al. The effect of droloxifene and estrogen on thyroid function in postmenopausal women. *J Clin Endocrinol Metab.* 2000;85:4407-4410.

186. Arafah BM. Decreased levothyroxine requirement in women with hypothyroidism during androgen therapy for breast cancer. *Ann Intern Med.* 1994;121:247-251.

187. Surks MI, Goswami G, Daniels GH. The thyrotropin reference range should remain unchanged. *J Clin Endocrinol Metab.* 2005;90: 5489-5496.

188. Wartofsky L, Dickey RA. The evidence for a narrower thyrotropin reference range is compelling. *J Clin Endocrinol Metab.* 2005;90:5483-5488.

189. Brucker-Davis F, Oldfield EH, Skarulis MC, et al. Thyrotropin-secreting pituitary tumors: diagnostic criteria, thyroid hormone sensitivity, and treatment outcome in 25 patients followed at the National Institutes of Health. *J Clin Endocrinol Metab.* 1999;84:476-486.

190. Kuzuya N, Kinji I, Ishibashi M. Endocrine and immunohistochemical studies on thyrotropin (TSH)-secreting pituitary adenomas: responses of TSH, α-subunit, and growth hormone to hypothalamic releasing hormones and their distribution in adenoma cells. *J Clin Endocrinol Metab.* 1990;71:1103-1111.

191. Wang R, Nelson JC, Weiss RM, et al. Accuracy of free thyroxine measurements across natural ranges of thyroxine binding to serum proteins. *Thyroid*. 2000;10:31-39.

192. Nelson JC, Weiss RM, Wilcox RB. Underestimates of serum free thyroxine (T_4) concentrations by free T_4 immunoassays. *J Clin Endocrinol Metab*. 1994;79:76-79.

193. Faix JD, Rosen HN, Velazquez FR. Indirect estimation of thyroid hormone-binding proteins to calculate free thyroxine index: comparison of nonisotopic methods that use labeled thyroxine ("T-uptake"). *Clin Chem*. 1995;41:41-47.

194. Nelson JC, Weiss RM. The effect of serum dilution on free thyroxine (T_4) concentrations in the low T_4 syndrome of nonthyroidal illness. *J Clin Endocrinol Metab*. 1985;61:239-246.

195. Demers LM, Spencer CA. Laboratory medicine practice guidelines: laboratory support for the diagnosis and monitoring of thyroid disease. *Clin Endocrinol (Oxf)*. 2003;58:138-140.

196. Afandi B, Vera R, Schussler GC, et al. Concordant decreases of thyroxine and thyroxine binding protein concentrations during sepsis. *Metabolism*. 2000;49:753-754.

197. Toft AD, Irvine WJ, Hunter WM, et al. Anomalous plasma TSH levels in patients developing hypothyroidism in the early months after ^{131}I therapy for thyrotoxicosis. *J Clin Endocrinol Metab*. 1974;39:607.

198. Rees-Jones RW, Larsen PR. Triiodothyronine and thyroxine content of desiccated thyroid tablets. *Metabolism*. 1977;26:1213-1218.

199. Kaptein EM. Thyroid hormone metabolism and thyroid diseases in chronic renal failure. *Endocr Rev*. 1996;17:45-63.

200. Bacci V, Schussler GC, Kaplan TB. The relationship between serum triiodothyronine and thyrotropin during systemic illness. *J Clin Endocrinol Metab*. 1982;54:1229.

201. Weiss RE, Refetoff S. Treatment of resistance to thyroid hormone—primum non nocere. *J Clin Endocrinol Metab*. 1999;84:401-404.

202. Refetoff S, Weiss RE, Usala SJ. The syndromes of resistance to thyroid hormone. *Endocr Rev*. 1993;14:348-399.

203. al-Adsani H, Hoffer LJ, Silva JE. Resting energy expenditure is sensitive to small dose changes in patients on chronic thyroid hormone replacement. *J Clin Endocrinol Metab*. 1997;82:1118-1125.

204. Becker C. Hypothyroidism and atherosclerotic heart disease: pathogenesis, medical management, and the role of coronary artery bypass surgery. *Endocr Rev*. 1985;6:432-440.

205. Mazzaferri EL, Robbins RJ, Spencer CA, et al. A consensus report of the role of serum thyroglobulin as a monitoring method for low-risk patients with papillary thyroid carcinoma. *J Clin Endocrinol Metab*. 2003;88:1433-1441.

206. Francis Z, Schlumberger M. Serum thyroglobulin determination in thyroid cancer patients. *Best Pract Res Clin Endocrinol Metab*. 2008;22:1039-1046.

207. Spencer CA, Lopresti JS. Measuring thyroglobulin and thyroglobulin autoantibody in patients with differentiated thyroid cancer. *Nat Clin Pract Endocrinol Metab*. 2008;4:223-233.

208. Schlumberger M, Hitzel A, Toubert ME, et al. Comparison of seven serum thyroglobulin assays in the follow-up of papillary and follicular thyroid cancer patients. *J Clin Endocrinol Metab*. 2007;92:2487-2495.

209. Snozek CL, Chambers EP, Reading CC, et al. Serum thyroglobulin, high-resolution ultrasound, and lymph node thyroglobulin in diagnosis of differentiated thyroid carcinoma nodal metastases. *J Clin Endocrinol Metab*. 2007;92:4278-4281.

210. Nascimento C, Borget I, Troalen F, et al. Ultrasensitive serum thyroglobulin measurement is useful for the follow-up of patients treated with total thyroidectomy without radioactive iodine ablation. *Eur J Endocrinol*. 2013;169:689-693.

211. Clarke NJ, Zhang Y, Reitz RE. A novel mass spectrometry-based assay for the accurate measurement of thyroglobulin from patient samples containing antithyroglobulin autoantibodies. *J Investig Med*. 2012;60:1157-1163.

212. Rapoport B, McLachlan SM. Thyroid autoimmunity. *J Clin Invest*. 2001;108:1253-1259.

213. Hollowell JG, Staehling NW, Flanders WD, et al. Serum TSH, T(4), and thyroid antibodies in the United States population (1988 to 1994): National Health and Nutrition Examination Survey (NHANES III). *J Clin Endocrinol Metab*. 2002;87:489-499.

214. Martin A, Barbesino G, Davies TF. T-cell receptors and autoimmune thyroid disease—signposts for T-cell-antigen driven diseases. *Int Rev Immunol*. 1999;18:111-140.

215. Latrofa F, Pichurin P, Guo J, et al. Thyroglobulin-thyroperoxidase autoantibodies are polyreactive, not bispecific: analysis using human monoclonal autoantibodies. *J Clin Endocrinol Metab*. 2003;88:371-378.

216. Guo J, Wang Y, Rapoport B, et al. Evidence for antigen presentation to sensitized T cells by thyroid peroxidase (TPO)-specific B cells in mice injected with fibroblasts co-expressing TPO and MHC class II. *Clin Exp Immunol*. 2000;119:38-46.

217. Stagnaro-Green A, Roman SH, Cobin RH, et al. Detection of at-risk pregnancy by means of highly sensitive assays for thyroid autoantibodies. *JAMA*. 1990;264:1422-1425.

218. Stagnaro-Green A, Glinoer D. Thyroid autoimmunity and the risk of miscarriage. *Best Pract Res Clin Endocrinol Metab*. 2004;18:167-181.

219. Thangaratinam S, Tan A, Knox E, et al. Association between thyroid autoantibodies and miscarriage and preterm birth: meta-analysis of evidence. *BMJ*. 2011;342:d2616.

220. Vanderpump MPJ, Tunbridge WMG, French JM, et al. The incidence of thyroid disorders in the community: a twenty-year follow-up of the Whickham survey. *Clin Endocrinol*. 1995;43:55-68.

221. Hayes AA, Akre CM, Gorman CA. Iodine-131 treatment of Graves' disease using modified early iodine-131 uptake measurements in therapy dose calculations. *J Nucl Med*. 1990;31:519-522.

222. Medeiros-Neto G, Kim PS, Vono J, et al. Congenital hypothyroid goiter with deficient thyroglobulin. *J Clin Invest*. 1996;98:2838-2844.

223. Mariotti S, Martino E, Cupini C, et al. Low serum thyroblobulin as a clue to the diagnosis of thyrotoxicosis factitia. *N Engl J Med*. 1982;307:410-412.

CHAPTER 12

Hyperthyroid Disorders

TERRY F. DAVIES • PETER LAURBERG • REBECCA S. BAHN

KEY POINTS

- Hyperthyroidism has a prevalence of 1% to 2% in women and 0.1% to 0.2% in men.
- The most common causes of an overactive thyroid are Graves disease and toxic multinodular goiter.
- Graves disease is caused by the development of unique human autoantibodies to the thyroid-stimulating hormone (thyrotropin, TSH) receptor; these autoantibodies act as TSH receptor agonists.
- Graves orbitopathy (GO) remains one of the most difficult endocrine diseases to treat and requires a multidisciplinary approach. It may occur before, during, or even long after resolution of the hyperthyroidism.
- Toxic thyroid nodules are caused by a constitutive activating mutation in the TSH receptor.
- Subacute thyroiditis secondary to infectious agents is usually painful, in marked contrast to the transient autoimmune thyroiditis seen in the postpartum period.
- The treatment of hyperthyroidism is best initiated with the antithyroid drug methimazole; propylthiouracil (PTU) is no longer recommended as first-line therapy because of its rare, but occasionally severe, hepatic toxicity. PTU may be useful in treating severe hyperthyroidism because of its capacity to block conversion of thyroxine (T_4) to triiodothyronine (T_3) by the type 1 deiodinase (D1) in liver, kidney, and Graves thyroid.
- Methimazole embryopathy is also rare. It may be avoided by the use of PTU in the first trimester as well as for women planning a pregnancy while under treatment for hyperthyroidism.
- Overtreatment of the pregnant hyperthyroid patient must be avoided because of the transplacental passage of both PTU and methimazole. Fetal hypothyroidism can impair cognitive development. Typically the TSH should remain suppressed and the free T_4 slightly above normal throughout pregnancy. If possible, the patient should be followed in concert with a high-risk obstetrician.

These days the terms *thyrotoxicosis* and *hyperthyroidism* are used interchangeably and refer to the classical or subtle physiologic manifestations of excessive quantities of the thyroid hormones, which are the characteristic of this condition (Table 12-1). In addition to overstimulation of the thyroid via the TSH receptor and true TSH receptor mutations, other common conditions causing hyperthyroidism include the passive release of thyroid hormones from damaged thyroid follicles; inflammation of the thyroid gland (called thyroiditis), which may be autoimmune, postviral, or drug induced; and extrathyroidal sources of thyroid hormone, most often iatrogenic or self-administered. For most patients with thyrotoxicosis, the symptoms and signs caused by an excess of the thyroid hormone, whatever the source, lead to medical attention. Others may have surprisingly few symptoms and are referred because of a suppressed TSH. This chapter begins with a brief review of the symptoms and signs of thyrotoxicosis and their pathophysiologic basis. The appropriate use of the laboratory tests already described in Chapter 11 is then presented to show how these results can focus the search for a diagnosis.

CLINICAL MANIFESTATIONS OF THYROTOXICOSIS

One very important clinical clue to the cause of the patient's thyrotoxicosis is the duration of the symptoms. Patients with hyperthyroidism have generally had manifestations for months before presentation but because the week-to-week increases in thyroid hormones are small, the effects of the disorder may become rather extreme, while going unnoticed by the patient. In addition, patients will often attribute the symptoms to other causes; for example, they may ascribe their fatigue to family or work responsibilities, heat intolerance to the weather, weight loss to an effective diet, and dyspnea and palpitations to a lack of regular exercise. On the other hand, patients with thyrotoxicosis due to thyroiditis can often date the onset of their symptoms precisely, usually to within a month or so of their seeking medical attention, as might be expected from the

TABLE 12-1

Causes of Hyperthyroidism

I. Excessive TSH-Receptor Stimulation

Graves disease (TRAbs)
Pregnancy-associated transient hyperthyroidism (hCG)
Trophoblastic disease (hCG)
Familial gestational hyperthyroidism (mutant TSH receptor)
TSH-producing pituitary adenoma

II. Autonomous Thyroid Hormone Secretion

Multinodular toxic goiter (somatic mutations)
Solitary toxic thyroid adenoma (somatic mutation)
Congenital activating TSH-receptor mutation (genomic mutation)

III. Destruction of Follicles With Release of Hormone

Subacute de Quervain thyroiditis (virus infection)
Painless thyroiditis/postpartum thyroiditis
    (hashitoxicosis—autoimmune)
Acute thyroiditis (bacterial infection)
Drug-induced thyroiditis (amiodarone, interferon-γ)

IV. Extrathyroidal Sources of Thyroid Hormone

Iatrogenic overreplacement with thyroid hormone
Excessive self-administered thyroid medication
Food and supplements containing excessive thyroid hormone
Functional thyroid cancer metastases
Struma ovarii

hCG, human chorionic gonadotropin; TRAbs, thyrotropin receptor antibodies; TSH, thyroid-stimulating hormone (thyrotropin).

effects of the release of the equivalent of 30 to 60 days' supply of thyroid hormone into the circulation over a few days to weeks. Thus, ascertaining the chronology as well as the spectrum of symptoms is a critical goal of the interview process.

Another general characteristic is that the symptoms and signs of thyrotoxicosis are more readily recognized in the younger than in the older patient. The term *masked* or *apathetic* thyrotoxicosis is used to describe the syndrome sometimes seen in the elderly, which may present as congestive heart failure with arrhythmia or as unexplained weight loss without the increased appetite and other typical symptoms and signs of the younger patient.

At present, the ready availability of sensitive serum TSH assays, a reliable indicator of excess thyroid hormone in the ambulatory patient (see Chapter 11), has made the more classical and severe manifestations of long-standing thyrotoxicosis less prevalent. In fact, a current area of controversy is how aggressively to treat the condition termed *subclinical* or *mild* hyperthyroidism, a biochemical diagnosis in which a subnormal serum TSH level is accompanied by normal free thyroid hormone concentrations. Nonetheless, the classical presentation is still common, serves to illustrate the pleiotropic physiologic effects of excess thyroid hormones, and, if not recognized, can progress to life-threatening severity despite the fact that hyperthyroidism is a benign condition (accelerated hyperthyroidism). The next sections review the pathophysiology of the most important manifestations of excess thyroid hormone.

Cardiovascular System

Alterations in cardiovascular function in the thyrotoxic patient are in part due to increased circulatory demands that result from the hypermetabolism and the need to dissipate the excess heat produced.[1] At rest, peripheral vascular resistance is decreased, and cardiac output is increased as a result of an increase first in heart rate and with more severe disease, in stroke volume. Thyroid hormones in

excess also have a direct ionotropic effect on cardiac contraction mediated by an increase in the ratio of α- to β-myosin heavy chain expression. Tachycardia is virtually always present and is due to a combination of increased sympathetic and decreased vagal tone.[2] Widening of the pulse pressure is due to the increase in systolic and decrease in diastolic pressure caused by reduced resistance.[3] The decreased resistance is due to increased nitric oxide production via the PI3K/AKT signaling pathway.[4] The increased systolic force is often felt by the patient as a palpitation and is evident on inspection or palpation of the precordium. Because of the diffuse and forceful nature of the apex beat, the heart may seem enlarged, and echocardiography may show an increased ventricular mass. In addition, the preejection period is shortened and the ratio of preejection period to left ventricular ejection time is decreased.[3,5] The heart sounds are enhanced, particularly S_1, and a scratchy systolic sound along the left sternal border, resembling a pleuropericardial friction rub (Means-Lerman scratch), may also be heard. These manifestations abate when a normal metabolic state is restored. Mitral valve prolapse occurs more frequently in Graves or Hashimoto disease than in the normal population[6] and has been suggested as autoimmune in origin.[7] Cardiac arrhythmias are almost invariably supraventricular, especially in younger patients. Between 2% and 20% of patients with thyrotoxicosis have atrial fibrillation, and about 15% of patients with otherwise unexplained atrial fibrillation are thyrotoxic,[1] which may be caused directly by the thyroid hormone excess or by activating autoantibodies to the β_1-adrenergic receptors.[8] In the Framingham cohort, individuals over age 60 with a suppressed TSH level had a 2.8-fold increased risk of developing atrial fibrillation compared to those with normal serum TSH values,[9] and such a finding has been widely confirmed.[10]

The increased cardiovascular cost of a standard workload or metabolic challenge is adequately met if the thyrotoxic patient is not, or has not previously been, in heart failure. Thus, in most patients without underlying heart disease, cardiac competence is maintained. Mild peripheral edema may occur in the absence of heart failure. Heart failure per se usually, but not always, occurs in patients with preexisting heart disease, and therefore is more typically seen in the elderly, but it may not be possible to determine whether underlying heart disease is present until after thyrotoxicosis is relieved. Atrial fibrillation decreases the efficiency of the cardiac response to any increased circulatory demand and may play a role in causing cardiac failure.[5] Attempts to convert or abate atrial fibrillation to sinus rhythm are not indicated while thyrotoxicosis is present, and about 60% of patients revert spontaneously to sinus rhythm after treatment, most within 4 months. For this reason and because thromboembolism is rare in patients under 50 with thyrotoxicosis, routine anticoagulation is not recommended for younger patients without a history of underlying heart disease or prior history of thrombotic disorder. Medical or electrical cardioversion of patients with thyrotoxicosis-induced atrial fibrillation is often successful even after a year has passed.[11]

Protein, Carbohydrate, and Lipid Metabolism

The stimulation of metabolism and heat production is reflected in increased appetite and heat intolerance but only rarely by elevated basal body temperature.[12] Despite an increased food intake, a state of chronic caloric and nutritional inadequacy often ensues, depending on the degree of increased metabolism. Both synthesis and degradation rates of proteins are increased, the latter to a greater extent than the former, with the result that in severe thyrotoxicosis there is a net decrease in tissue protein, as indicated by loss of weight, muscle wasting, proximal muscle weakness, and even mild hypoalbuminemia. Preexisting diabetes mellitus may be aggravated, one cause being accelerated turnover of insulin. Both lipogenesis and lipolysis are increased in thyrotoxicosis, but the net effect is lipolysis, as reflected by an increase in the plasma concentration of free fatty acids and glycerol and a decrease in serum cholesterol level; triglyceride levels are usually slightly decreased. The enhanced mobilization and oxidation of free fatty acids in response to fasting or catecholamines are due to enhancement of lipolytic pathways by thyroid hormones.[12]

Sympathetic Nervous System and Catecholamines

Many of the manifestations of thyrotoxicosis and of sympathetic nervous system activation are similar. Nonetheless, the plasma concentrations of epinephrine and norepinephrine, as well as their urinary excretion and that of their metabolites, are not increased in patients with thyrotoxicosis, and thyroid hormones exert effects separate from, but similar and additive to, those of the catecholamines. The improvement in cardiac function in patients with hyperthyroidism by β-adrenergic blockade has led to the concept that there is increased sympathetic tone or increased cardiac sensitivity to the sympathetic nervous system.[13] Support for the latter are the results in the transgenic mouse in which overexpression of type 2 deiodinase in the heart increases myocardial T_3 and the cyclic adenosine monophosphate (cAMP) response to norepinephrine in the cardiac myocytes due to alterations in G proteins.[14,15] In addition, adipocytes from thyrotoxic patients have threefold increases in norepinephrine-induced lipolysis, 15-fold increases in response to $β_2$-adrenergic receptor agonists, and threefold increases in response to forskolin or cAMP.[16-18] Thus, thyroid hormones increase sensitivity to catecholamines in both cardiomyocytes and adipocytes by a variety of mechanisms.

Nervous System

Alterations in the function of the nervous system in thyrotoxicosis are manifested by nervousness, emotional lability, and hyperkinesia. Fatigue may be due both to muscle weakness and to the insomnia that is commonly present. Emotional lability is common and in rare cases mental disturbance may be severe; manic depressive, schizoid, or paranoid reactions may emerge. The hyperkinesia of the thyrotoxic patient is characteristic and may manifest to such a point that the patient is almost levitating. During the interview the patient shifts positions frequently and movements are quick, jerky, exaggerated, and often purposeless. In children, in whom such manifestations tend to be more severe, inability to focus may lead to deterioration in school performance suggesting attention deficit hyperactivity disorder. There may be a fine tremor of the hands, tongue, or lightly closed eyelids. The electroencephalogram reveals an increase in fast wave activity, and in patients with convulsive disorders, the frequency of seizures is increased.

Muscle

Weakness and fatigability are usually not accompanied by objective evidence of muscle disease save for the generalized wasting associated with weight loss. The weakness is most prominent in the proximal muscles of the limbs, causing difficulty in climbing stairs or fatigue from minimal exertion such as using a blow dryer or lifting an infant. Proximal muscle wasting may be out of proportion to the overall loss of weight (often referred to as *thyrotoxic myopathy*). In the most severe forms, the myopathy may involve the more distal muscles of the extremities and the muscles of the trunk and face. Although myopathy of ocular muscles is unusual, the disorder may mimic myasthenia gravis or ophthalmic myasthenia.[18-22] Muscular strength returns to normal when a normal metabolic state is restored, but muscle mass takes longer to recover.

Graves disease occurs in about 3% to 5% of patients with myasthenia gravis, and about 1% of the patients with Graves disease develop myasthenia gravis. Antibodies and T cells specific for the TSH and acetylcholine receptors are involved in the pathogenesis of the two diseases.[23] Unlike thyrotoxic myopathy, the association of myasthenia gravis with Graves disease has a distinct female preponderance. The effect of both thyrotoxicosis and its alleviation on the course of myasthenia gravis is variable, but in the majority of instances, myasthenia is accentuated during the thyrotoxic state and improves when a normal metabolic state is restored. A form of myasthenia affecting mainly the orbital muscles may also occur more commonly in patients with Graves disease and needs to be distinguished from GO by the prominence of bilateral ptosis of a variable degree.[19]

Periodic paralysis of the hypokalemic type may occur together with thyrotoxicosis, and its severity is accentuated by the latter disorder. The coincidence of the two disorders is particularly common in Asian and Latino males.[24,25]

Eyes

Some retraction of the upper or lower eyelids, or both, evident as the presence of a rim of sclera between either lid and the limbus, may be seen in all forms of thyrotoxicosis, regardless of the underlying cause, and is responsible for the typical stare of the patient. Also common is either lid lag, a phenomenon in which the upper lid lags behind the globe when the patient is asked to shift the gaze slowly downward, or globe lag, which becomes evident when the eye lags behind the upper lid when the patient looks up. These ocular manifestations appear to be the result of increased adrenergic tone. It is important to differentiate these signs, which may occur in all forms of thyrotoxicosis, from those of infiltrative autoimmune orbitopathy, which are associated with Graves disease and are described later.

Skin and Hair

The most characteristic change in the patient with longstanding thyrotoxicosis is the warm, moist feel of the skin that results from cutaneous vasodilation and excessive sweating. The elbows may be smooth and pink; the complexion is rosy; and the patient blushes readily. Palmar erythema may resemble liver palms (palmar erythema), and telangiectasia may be present. The hair is fine and friable, and hair loss may increase. The nails are often soft and friable. A characteristic but uncommon finding is Plummer nails, onycholysis, typically involving the fourth and fifth fingers. Vitiligo, another autoimmune disease, is more common in patients with autoimmune thyroid disease.

Respiratory System

Dyspnea is common in severe thyrotoxicosis, and several factors may contribute to this condition. Vital capacity is commonly reduced, mainly from weakness of the respiratory muscles. During exercise, ventilation is increased out of proportion to the increase in oxygen uptake, but the diffusing capacity of the lung is normal. Because of the general increase in oxygen consumption associated with thyrotoxicosis, patients with chronic lung diseases may experience a rather severe worsening of the condition if they become thyrotoxic.

Alimentary System

An increase in appetite is common but is usually not seen in patients with mild disease. In more severe disease the increased intake of food is inadequate to meet the increased caloric requirements, and weight is lost at a variable rate. More often, the patient reports a gratifying success with a previously frustrated attempt at weight control. The frequency of bowel movements is increased, and diarrhea, although rare, can be a problem. The increased gastric emptying and intestinal motility in thyrotoxicosis appear to be responsible for slight malabsorption of fat, and these functions return to normal when a normal metabolic state has been restored. Celiac and Graves diseases coexist more commonly than once thought, and there is an increased prevalence of pernicious anemia.

Hepatic dysfunction occurs, particularly when thyrotoxicosis is severe; hypoproteinemia and increases in serum alanine aminotransferase (ALT) and bone or liver alkaline phosphatase levels may be elevated. Progressive hepatomegaly and jaundice was a cause of death prior to the development of successful treatment for Graves patients likely exacerbated by congestive heart failure.

Skeletal System: Calcium and Phosphorus Metabolism

Thyrotoxicosis is generally associated with increased excretion of calcium and phosphorus in urine and stool; with an increase in bone turnover and a net demineralization of bone, as demonstrated by routine bone densitometry; and occasionally with pathologic fractures, especially in elderly women.[16,20,26] In such instances the pathologic changes are variable and may include osteitis fibrosa, osteomalacia, or osteoporosis, most likely varying with vitamin D status. Urinary excretion of collagen breakdown products (teleopeptides) is increased in thyrotoxicosis. Kinetic studies indicate an increase in the exchangeable calcium pool and acceleration of both bone resorption and accretion, particularly the former. Thyroid hormone (T_3) has been shown to accelerate activity of the osteoclasts and helps explain these widespread changes.[17,18,21] Indeed, data indicate that TSH itself may have a local action, which may normally balance thyroid hormone action on osteoclasts and enhance osteoblast activity.[22,27,28] Such an action by TSH would be absent in hyperthyroidism, allowing accentuation of the thyroid hormone effects. These changes in hyperthyroidism lead to a decreased bone density in many patients. As the thyrotoxicosis is treated, bone density may normalize in many younger patients but not all.[29] Postmenopausal women, however, may have an accelerated reduction in bone density that requires treatment (see Chapter 29). Much controversy has existed over the induction of decreased bone density by TSH-suppression therapy in patients with thyroid cancer. Suffice it to say that postmenopausal, but not premenopausal, women given a TSH-suppressive dosage of thyroid hormones are at risk of osteopenia and require prophylaxis with calcium and vitamin D or more aggressive approaches.[30,31] The decision to relax TSH suppression in low-risk patients may be influenced by their bone status.

For all the same reasons, hypercalcemia may occur in patients with severe thyrotoxicosis. The total serum calcium concentration is increased in as many as 27% of patients, and the ionized serum calcium is elevated in 47%. The concentrations of heat labile serum alkaline phosphatase and osteocalcin are also frequently elevated. These findings resemble those of primary hyperparathyroidism, but the concentration of parathyroid hormone in serum is low normal in most. True primary hyperparathyroidism and thyrotoxicosis sometimes coexist. Plasma 25-hydroxycholecalciferol levels are decreased in thyrotoxic patients, and this alteration could contribute to the decreased intestinal absorption of calcium and osteomalacia noted in some.

Renal Function: Water and Electrolyte Metabolism

Thyrotoxicosis produces no symptoms referable to the urinary tract save for mild polyuria, which may lead to nocturia. Nevertheless renal blood flow, glomerular filtration, and tubular reabsorptive and secretory maxima are increased. Total exchangeable potassium is decreased, possibly due to a decrease in lean body mass, but electrolytes are normal except when hypokalemic periodic paralysis occurs.

Hematopoietic System

The red blood cells are usually normal, as judged by the usual indices, but red blood cell mass is increased. The increase in erythropoiesis is due both to the direct effect of thyroid hormones on the erythroid marrow and to increased production of erythropoietin. A parallel increase in plasma volume also occurs, with the result that the hematocrit is normal.

Approximately 3% of patients with Graves disease have pernicious anemia, and a further 3% have antibodies to intrinsic factor but normal absorption of vitamin B_{12}. Autoantibodies against gastric parietal cells may also be present in patients with Graves disease, and the requirements for vitamin B_{12} and folic acid appear to be increased. The total white blood cell count is often low because of a decrease in the number of neutrophils. The absolute lymphocyte count is normal or increased, leading to a relative lymphocytosis. The numbers of monocytes and eosinophils may also be increased. Splenic enlargement occurs in about 10% of the patients, and thymic enlargement is common in Graves disease.[32] The latter may present as a mediastinal mass. Thymic hyperplasia is also due to thyrotoxicosis because it is sometimes seen in patients receiving excess exogenous T_4 for TSH suppression.[33]

Platelet levels and the intrinsic clotting mechanism are normal, but the concentration of factor VIII is often increased and returns to normal when the thyrotoxicosis is treated. Despite this increase, there is an enhanced sensitivity to warfarin because of the accelerated clearance of the vitamin K–dependent clotting factors. Therefore, the dosage of warfarin needs to be reduced in thyrotoxic patients.[34] This must be kept in mind if initiating anticoagulant treatment for atrial fibrillation in older patients.[35] Coincidental autoimmune thrombocytopenia may also occur.

Pituitary and Adrenocortical Function

The thyrotoxic state imposes several challenges on pituitary and adrenocortical function. The hepatic inactivation of cortisol is accelerated, including enhanced

$5\alpha/5\beta$-reductases and 11β hydroxysteroid dehydrogenase. As a result of these changes, the disposal of cortisol is accelerated, but its rate of secretion is also increased, so the plasma cortisol concentration remains normal. The concentration of corticosteroid binding globulin in plasma is also normal. The urinary excretion of free cortisol is normal or slightly increased[36] (see Chapter 15).

Reproductive Function

Thyrotoxicosis in early life may cause delayed sexual maturation, although physical development is normal and skeletal growth may be accelerated. Thyrotoxicosis after puberty influences reproductive function, especially in women. The intermenstrual interval may be prolonged or shortened, and menstrual flow is initially diminished and ultimately ceases. Fertility may be reduced, and if conception takes place, there is an increased risk of miscarriage and other complications[37-39] In some patients, menstrual cycles are predominantly anovulatory with oligomenorrhea, but in most, ovulation occurs, as indicated by a secretory endometrium. In the former, a subnormal midcycle surge of luteinizing hormone (LH) may be responsible. In premenopausal women with thyrotoxicosis, basal plasma concentrations of LH and follicle-stimulating hormone (FSH) are reportedly normal but may display enhanced responsiveness to gonadotropin-releasing hormone (GnRH).

Thyrotoxicosis, whether spontaneous or induced by exogenous hormone, is accompanied by an increase in the concentration of sex hormone–binding globulin (SHBG) in plasma.[40] As a result the plasma concentrations of total testosterone, dihydrotestosterone, and estradiol are increased, but their unbound fractions are normal or transiently decreased. The increased binding in plasma may be responsible for the decreased metabolic clearance rate of testosterone and dihydrotestosterone. In the case of estradiol, however, the metabolic clearance rate is normal, suggesting that tissue metabolism of the hormone is increased. Conversion rates of androstenedione to testosterone, estrone, and estradiol and of testosterone to dihydrotestosterone are increased.[41] The increased rate of conversion of androgens to estrogenic byproducts may be the mechanism for gynecomastia and erectile dysfunction in some 10% of thyrotoxic men and one mechanism for menstrual irregularities in women. Another likely mechanism for menstrual changes is the disruption in amplitude and frequency of LH/FSH pulses due to thyroid hormone influences on GnRH signaling.

LABORATORY DIAGNOSIS

The effects of thyrotoxicosis on the major organ systems are the same regardless of the underlying cause. Their frequency and intensity and the other findings with which they are associated are influenced by the cause of the excess thyroid hormone. To a large extent, the same is true of laboratory test results. However, the patient with thyrotoxic symptoms will virtually always have a serum TSH concentration less than 0.1 mU/L and an elevated serum free T_4. In general, serum free T_3 is more elevated than is the free T_4, but free T_4 is relatively high if thyrotoxicosis is caused by thyroiditis or intake of levothyroxine.

If the possibility of exogenous thyroid hormone can be eliminated, the primary differential is between excess thyroid hormone production and excess thyroid hormone release from sick cells, as in thyroiditis (Fig. 12-1). Often this differentiation can be made on the basis of the history and physical. Laboratory tests, including an increased sedimentation rate and a high serum thyroglobulin (Tg) may favor thyroiditis, but the most critical differentiating test is the radioactive iodine uptake (RAIU), which is elevated or inappropriately high normal given the suppressed serum TSH level with excess thyroid hormone production and very low (<5%) in patients with thyroiditis. However, the RAIU may also be low in a hyperthyroid patient who has recently received an iodine load, usually iodinated contrast for a computed tomography (CT) scan or for angiography. A 24-hour urine iodine measurement can confirm this.

If the physical examination or thyroid ultrasonography indicates the presence of a nodular thyroid, thyroid scanning may confirm which nodules are hyperfunctioning. The association of thyrotoxicosis with an elevated TSH is rare and suggests a TSH-producing pituitary tumor (see Fig. 12-1). The possibility of an artifactually elevated TSH in a patient with Graves disease should be ruled out by repeating the assay by a different method in another laboratory (see Chapter 8). Exceptions to these general guidelines are discussed later within the appropriate subsection.

GRAVES DISEASE

Discovery

In the 19th century Caleb Hillier Parry,[42,43] Carl Adolph von Basedow,[44] and Robert James Graves[45] independently reported on a syndrome consisting of the three elements: (1) symptoms and signs of thyrotoxicosis, (2) swelling of the thyroid gland, and (3) protruding eyes. Internationally, the disease was named Graves disease, whereas it is called Basedow disease in German-speaking countries. A key element in the understanding of the nature of the disease was the discovery by Adams and Purves that the hyperthyroidism is caused by thyroid-stimulating autoantibodies.[46,47]

Our current understanding is that Graves disease is a common autoimmune disorder that may affect a number of organs and tissues and that the central element is autoimmunity against the TSH receptor (TSHR). In the majority of patients, circulating TSHR antibodies (TRAb) stimulate the thyroid after binding to the receptor, and hyperthyroidism is the most common manifestation of Graves disease. In populations with adequate iodine intake, Graves disease is the dominating cause of hyperthyroidism, representing around 80% of all cases of thyrotoxicosis.

Presentation

Graves disease may affect a number of organs and tissues (Table 12-2), and in each organ the disease may have

TABLE 12-2

Estimates for the Clinical Manifestations of Graves Disease

Manifestation	% Affected	Cases/Million/Year
All	100	350
Hyperthyroidism	90-95	325
Goiter	50	175
Orbitopathy	30	105
Severe orbitopathy	5	17
Hypothyroidism with orbitopathy	5	17
Dermopathy	0.5	4
Acropachy	0.1	0.5
Neonatal hyperthyroidism	0.2	1
Fetal hyperthyroidism	0.1	0.5

**Patient with symptoms and signs suggesting thyrotoxicosis, no amiodarone;
serum TSH <0.2 mU/L, free T₄ or T₃ elevated**

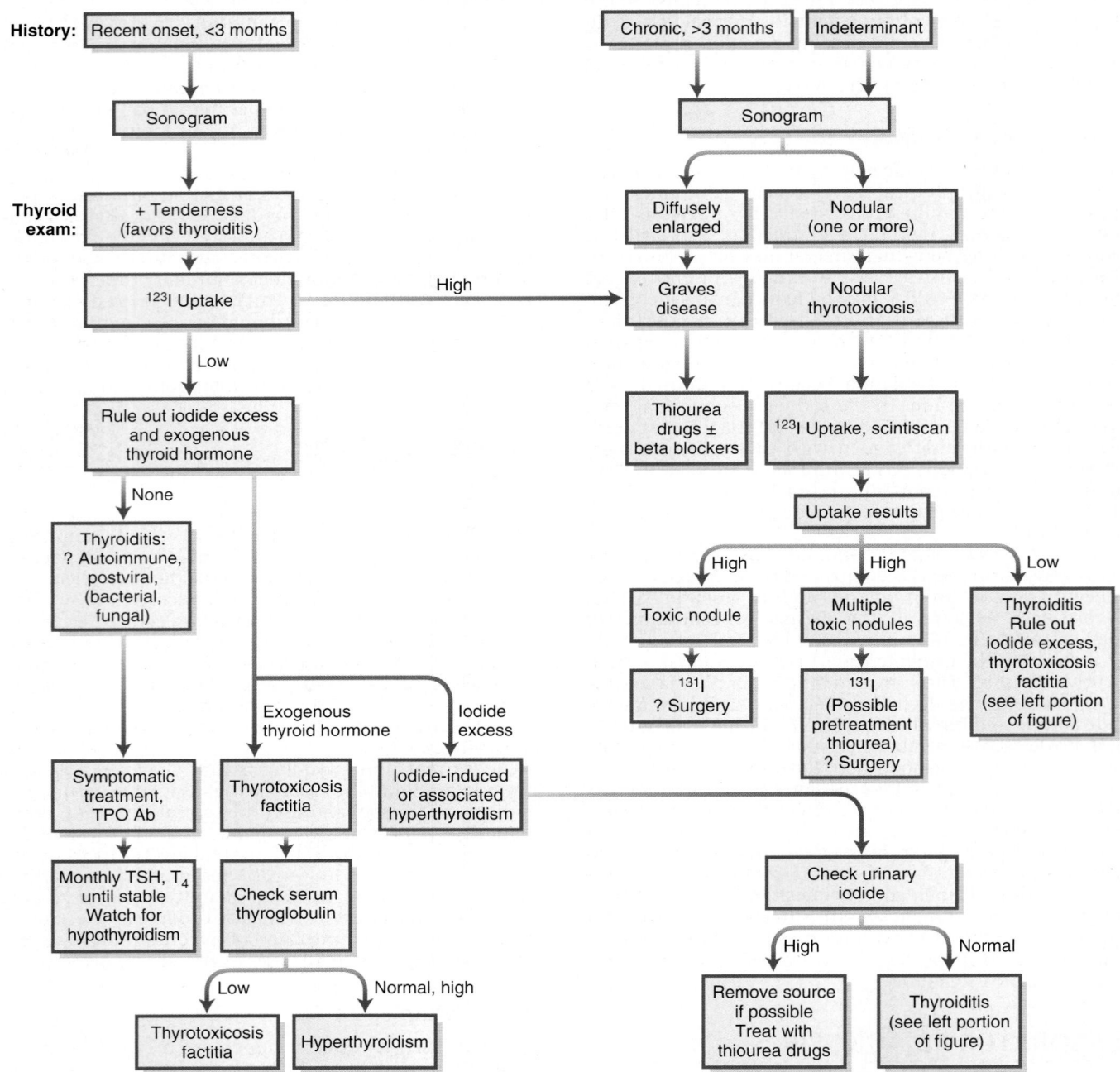

Figure 12-1 Algorithm for determining the cause of thyrotropin-independent thyrotoxicosis. T₃, triiodothyronine; T₄, thyroxine; TPO Ab, thyroid peroxidase antibody; TSH, thyroid-stimulating hormone (thyrotropin).

different presentations. The thyroid gland is affected in nearly all patients, and hyperthyroidism is the most common clinical manifestation. Around half of patients have enlarged thyroid by ultrasonography. The thyroid disease may be accompanied by an infiltrative orbitopathy and occasionally by infiltrative dermopathy. The presentation of the thyroid, eye, and skin signs is referred to as the *Graves triad*. In the individual patient, thyroid disease and the infiltrative phenomena may occur singly or together but run courses that may be largely independent. The

thyroid histologic appearance is distinct from autoimmune thyroiditis with the presence of a more sparse lymphocytic infiltrate. However, in Graves disease, hyperthyroidism occurs in the presence of some degree of autoimmune thyroiditis and may ultimately be replaced, in the long term, by thyroid hypofunction. Conversely, hyperthyroidism may occasionally supervene in patients with preexisting Hashimoto thyroiditis. Both of these diseases may occur within the same family, indicating their close interrelationship.

Autoimmune Characteristics

Autoimmune thyroid disease is characterized by the occurrence in the serum of antibodies against thyroid peroxidase (TPO), Tg, and the TSHR. T-cell–mediated autoimmunity can also be demonstrated against the three primary thyroid antigens, as judged by a variety of criteria, including the ability of the T cells to elaborate various cytokines and to exhibit a mitogenic response when exposed to thyroid antigens or to peptide sequences from the antigens. As mentioned earlier, autoimmune thyroid disease is also characterized by lymphocytic infiltration of the thyroid gland—intense in autoimmune thyroiditis and heterogeneous in Graves disease. In patients and their relatives, there is an increased frequency of other disorders of autoimmune origin, such as insulin-dependent diabetes mellitus, pernicious anemia, myasthenia gravis, Addison disease, Sjögren syndrome, lupus erythematosus, rheumatoid arthritis, and idiopathic thrombocytopenic purpura (see Chapter 40).

The circulating autoantibodies specific to Graves disease are directed against the TSHR and behave most often as thyroid-stimulating antibodies.[48] These antibodies can compete for the binding of TSH to its specific receptor site in the cell membrane and can activate multiple signaling pathways including adenylate cyclase.[49] Similar but distinct autoantibodies in the sera of some patients with autoimmune thyroiditis also compete for TSH binding but do not stimulate the thyroid cell very well and may block the ligand-binding site and act as TSH antagonists or weak agonists, whereas others are neutral in their influence on TSH binding and in the absence of cAMP generation are able to signal along cell destructive pathways (Fig. 12-2).

The thyroid gland itself is a major site of thyroid autoantibody secretion in autoimmune thyroid disease via the B cells that form part of the intrathyroidal infiltrate. Transplantation of Graves thyroid tissue into T cell–deficient and B cell–deficient mice with severe combined immunodeficiency (SCID mice) results in the appearance of human thyroid autoantibodies, including TRAbs, in the serum.[50] However, some patients show no loss of autoantibody secretion after thyroidectomy, which indicates the existence of extrathyroidal sources of continued production. The role of the TSHR expressed in extrathyroidal tissues, such as adipose tissue and bone cells, in perpetuating this response remains uncertain.

Autoimmune Thyroid Pathology

In patients with Graves disease, the thyroid gland is characterized by a nonhomogeneous lymphocytic infiltration with an absence of easily found follicular destruction, although areas of apoptosis can be discerned by specific staining (Fig. 12-3).[51] Antithyroid drug treatment may

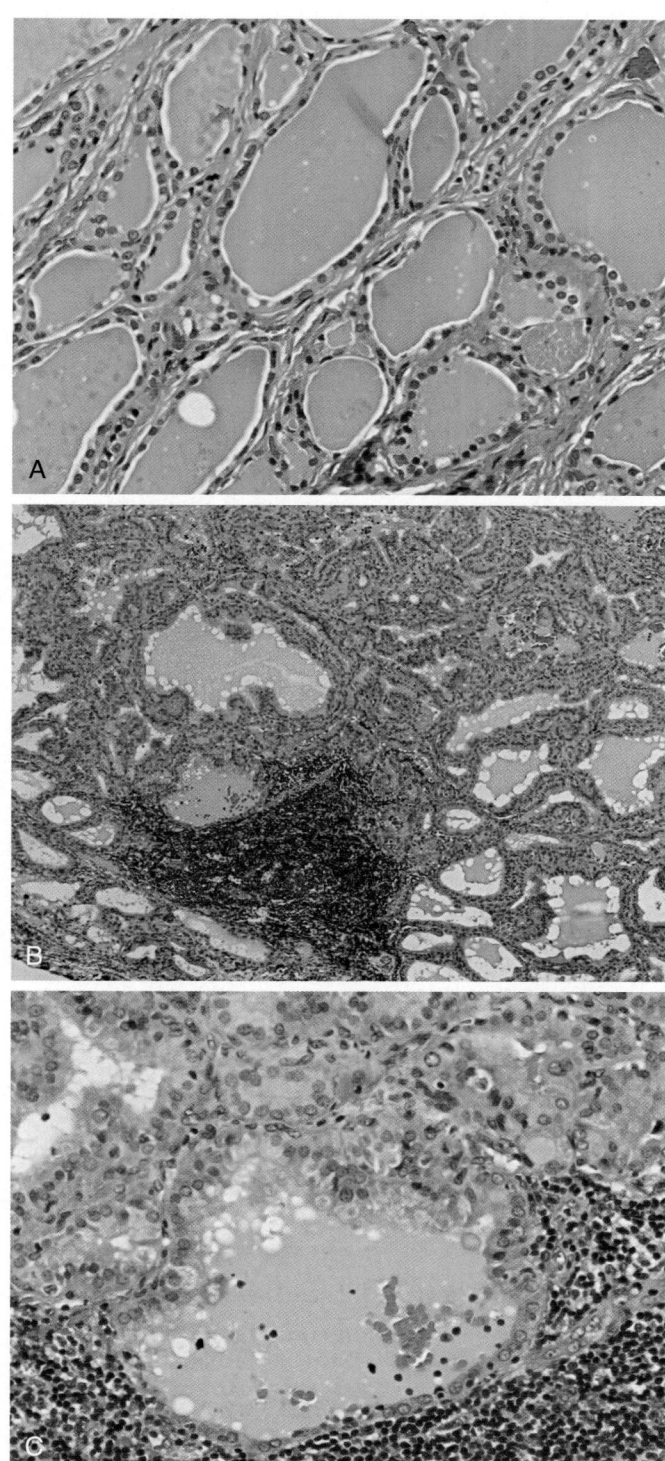

Figure 12-3 Histopathologic features of the thyroid gland in Graves disease. Sections of thyroid glands from normal tissue (**A**) and from a patient with Graves disease (**B** and **C**). (Courtesy of Dr. Pamela Unger, Mount Sinai School of Medicine, New York, NY.)

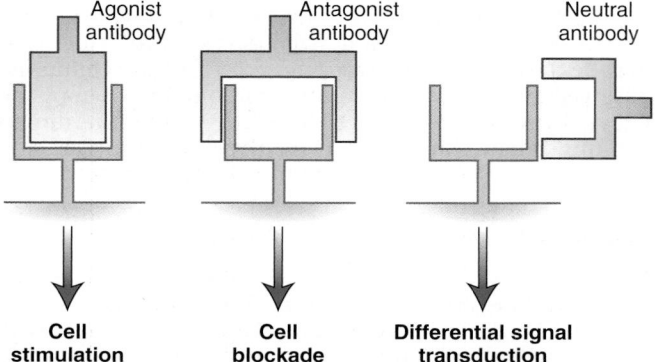

Figure 12-2 Schematic diagram of thyroid cell stimulation and blockade by antibodies to the thyroid-stimulating hormone receptor. Such autoantibodies may act as agonists or antagonists, or they may be neutral, depending on how they interact within the extracellular domain.

Agonist antibody — Cell stimulation

Antagonist antibody — Cell blockade

Neutral antibody — Differential signal transduction

reduce the degree of infiltration, influencing the observed histologic appearance in such patients. Although the intrathyroidal lymphocyte population is mixed, most are T lymphocytes (both Th1 and Th2 types along with CD25⁺ regulatory T cells), whereas B-cell germinal centers are much less common than in autoimmune thyroiditis. However, both intraepithelial T cells and plasma cells can be seen in peripolesis within the thyroid follicles. Follicular epithelial cell size correlates with the intensity of the local infiltrate, suggesting local thyroid cell stimulation by TRAbs. Memory T cells may predominate within the T-cell population, but this finding can vary from patient to patient. Activated B-cell and T-cell markers are more frequent in intrathyroidal lymphocyte cultures than in peripheral blood cultures.

Prevalence

The prevalence of hyperthyroidism varies with the degree of iodine sufficiency in the population under study. The National Health and Nutrition Examination Survey (NHANES III) data[52] from the United States and a detailed epidemiologic survey in the United Kingdom[53] demonstrate the female preponderance of thyroid patients and the lower prevalence of hyperthyroidism compared to hypothyroidism. Although relatively underpowered, these studies have indicated a prevalence of approximately 1% to 2% in women and about one tenth that frequency in men. Overall, in women the incidence was estimated to be 1 case per 1000 per year over a 20-year follow-up. Graves disease is uncommon in children. The incidence begins to increase around puberty and continues to rise until around 30 years of age. Therafter, the incidence is relatively stable. Graves disease is four to five times more common in women than in men.[54] The overall prevalence of autoimmune thyroid disease, comprising Graves disease and autoimmune thyroiditis, approaches or exceeds that of diabetes mellitus and when mild thyroid disease is included may be very much more.

Pathogenesis

The Major Antigen of Graves Disease— the Thyrotropin Receptor

The TSHR has seven transmembrane domains and employs multiple G proteins for signal transduction (Fig. 12-4). The human TSHR (hTSHR) is the primary autoantigen of Graves disease, as shown by the development of hyperthyroidism in mice and hamsters after exposure to normal hTSHR antigen.[55-58] It should be noted that expression of the TSHR in sites outside the thyroid gland has been reported in many tissues, including fibroblasts, fibrocytes, adipocytes, lymphocytes, osteoclasts and osteoblasts, and pituitary cells.[48] Although the physiologic role of TSHR in these sites is slowly being revealed, their role in autoimmune thyroid disease remains mostly unclear.

Molecular Structure of the Human Thyrotropin Receptor

The hTSHR gene is found on chromosome 14q31 and the crystallographic structure of the extracellular domain has been characterized[59] (see Fig. 12-4). Seven hydrophobic transmembrane spanning regions in the hTSHR indicate that it is a member of the G protein–coupled receptor gene superfamily, and those receptors with large extracellular domains have been designated subgroup B. The TSH holoreceptor consists of a 100-kDa, glycosylated, 744–amino acid sequence and a 20–amino acid signal peptide. The TSHR holoreceptor is cleaved into two subunits, α (or A)

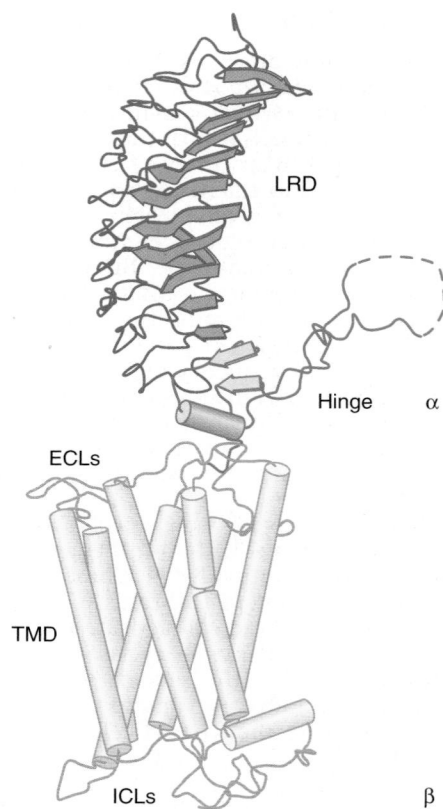

Figure 12-4 A model of the human thyroid-stimulating hormone receptor (TSHR) structure. The TSHR has seven transmembrane domains, a large extracellular domain, and a small intracellular domain. The receptor is cleaved, probably after activation, into α- (or A) and β- (or B) subunits. The α-subunit is thought to be shed from the cell surface. ECLs, extracellular loops; ICLs, intracellular loops; LRD, leucine-rich repeat domain; TMD, transmembrane domain.

and β (or B), which are linked by disulfide bonds to form the physiologic receptor. The 50-kDa α-subunit is water-soluble and has TSH-binding activity. TSH and TRAbs bind to the leucine-rich repeat (LRR) regions of the α-subunit.[59,60] The 30-kDa β-subunit is water-insoluble, contains the membrane-spanning domain with its three extracellular loops and three cytoplasmic loops, and is 70% to 75% homologous with the LH/human chorionic gonadotropin (hCG) receptor. Shedding of the α-subunit has been shown in vitro and has been suggested to also occur in vivo and may act as an important antigen in Graves disease. Enhanced subunit shedding from damaged follicular cells may be the cause for the worsening of TSHR autoimmunity observed in many patients after radioiodine therapy for Graves hyperthyroidism (see later). The TSHR forms dimers and multimeric complexes on the thyroid cell surface, and they appear to enhance the stability of the receptor.[48]

Autoantibodies to the Thyrotropin Receptor

In hyperthyroid Graves disease, TRAbs, discovered by Adams and Purves,[46,61] bind to the TSHR and may activate $G_s\alpha$ and G_q signaling complexes and induce thyroid growth, increase vascularity, and cause an increased rate of thyroid hormone production and secretion.[49] In contrast, receptor antibodies that act as TSH antagonists are referred to as *blocking TRAbs*, although they may still initiate some signaling, acting as weak agonists. In the same way, so-called neutral antibodies may also signal to varying degrees. These different types of TRAbs may be coincident with the stimulating type and may also predominate in certain patients after treatment with radioiodine, antithyroid drugs, or surgery (see Fig. 12-2).

TRAbs can also be found in approximately 15% of patients with autoimmune hypothyroidism. These TRAbs are usually of the blocking variety and may be more often found in the atrophic form of the disease.[62] TRAbs are not detectable in the normal population with the use of currently available methods and are highly specific markers for human autoimmune thyroid disease.

First Evidence for Bioactivity of Thyrotropin Receptor Autoantibodies

The self-infusion of sera from patients with Graves disease caused thyroid stimulation and was the first demonstration of the role of TRAbs in the induction of human hyperthyroidism.[63] Another example of the in vivo effects of TRAbs came from studies in neonates demonstrating the transplacental stimulation of the fetal thyroid in mothers with high titers of TRAbs.[64,65] TRAbs show light chain restriction in many patients with Graves disease, and TRAbs that exhibit TSH agonist bioactivity are in the immunoglobulin G1 (IgG1) subclass; both observations suggest oligoclonality,[66,67] indicating their primary role in disease causation.

Prevalence of Thyrotropin Receptor Autoantibodies in Graves Disease

The fact that TRAbs are detectable only in patients with autoimmune thyroid disease indicates that the autoantibodies are disease-specific, in contrast with the high prevalence of Tg antibodies and TPO antibodies in the population, and their measurement continues to be clinically useful. Furthermore, TRAbs are unique human autoantibodies and do not occur in natural animal disease. A total of 90% to 100% of untreated hyperthyroid patients with Graves disease have detectable TRAbs with thyroid-stimulating activity when using a sensitive assay.[68] The levels of TRAbs are decreased by treatment of the disease and, when they persist, may predict recurrence.[68-70] With time, TSHR-blocking autoantibodies may become the more prevalent type after treatment of patients with Graves disease and may be associated with hypothyroidism.

Intrathyroidal T Cells

In addition to the presence of TRAbs, some T cells in patients with autoimmune thyroid disease are highly reactive to thyroid antigens and to peptides derived from these antigens[71,72] and are also mostly oligoclonal.[73] About 10% of activated T cells infiltrating the thyroid gland in patients with autoimmune thyroid disease proliferate in response to thyroid cell antigens. Intrathyroidal T cells from patients with Graves disease exhibit characteristics of both the helper T-cell subset 1 (Th1) (which are recognized by their secretion of interleukin 2 [IL-2]) and interferon-γ and helper T-cell subset 2 (Th2) (which are recognized by their secretion of IL-4)[74] and include Treg cells.[75]

Regulation of the Immune Response in Autoimmune Thyroid Disease

Although thyroid hormone excess itself may give rise to changes in T-cell numbers and function, the immune system continues to exert its overall peripheral control. This is achieved by secretion of T-cell cytokines, by the suppressive influence of anergized T cells, and by the presence of regulatory cells, which are a subset of CD4+ T cells (D25+Fox3p+).[76,77] Considerable evidence now shows that Treg cells are deficient in Graves disease, and this change likely explains the propensity to autoimmune disease in such patients.[78,79] In addition to these potential regulatory influences, another important mechanism of control is central tolerance caused by positive and negative selection of T cells and B cells in the thymus, where thyroid antigens, including the TSHR, are expressed.[80,81] Regulation of thymic gene expression of the TSHR appears to be potentially important in susceptibility to Graves disease.[82]

Mechanisms in the Development of Autoimmune Thyroid Disease

The development of autoimmune thyroid disease depends on a combination of environmental and genetic factors. The human genome must harbor unique susceptibility genes because the disease has not been observed in any other species. Still, environmental factors acting through epigenetic pathways have strong influences and the disease appears to develop when a stochastic combination of genetic and environmental influences exceed a certain threshold. For example, release of thyroid antigens following an insult may be important as shown by the worsening of TSHR autoimmunity observed after radioiodine therapy or the direct insult caused by a virus or a drug such as interferon-α.[83]

The Consequences of an Insult

Initiation of autoimmune thyroid disease is thought to occur with an insult that leads to an immune response (Fig. 12-5). This may take the form of a direct insult to the thyroid gland by a viral infection[84] or another external influence, including trauma, leading to activation of T cells[85,86] presumed to be of the Th17 variety.[87] Alternatively, it may be initiated elsewhere in the body. In the latter case, the arrival of activated T cells in the thyroid gland would start the process. Such an arrival may be nonspecific

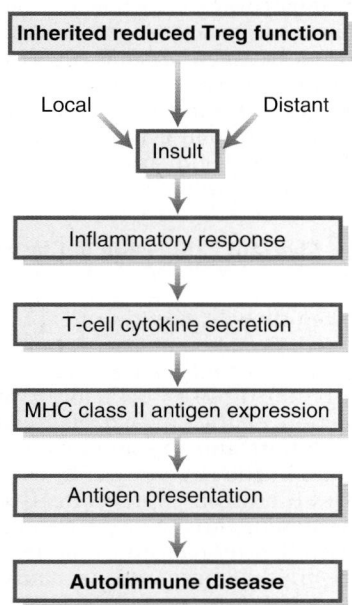

Figure 12-5 An overview of the most likely mechanisms involved in the cause and precipitation of Graves disease. MHC, major histocompatibility complex.

because the same T cells may arrive in many glands but the patient has a particular susceptibility to autoimmune thyroid disease. Initiation of disease may then be mediated by different mechanisms including bystander activation, molecular mimicry, or cryptic antigen presentation, as described later. The relative importance of these different mechanisms in Graves disease remains uncertain.

Mechanism #1—Bystander Activation

Evidence has mounted that bystander activation of local resident antigen-specific and nonspecific T cells may initiate autoimmunity. The presence of activated T cells within the thyroid gland following an insult may induce, via cytokine secretion, the activation of local thyroid-specific and non–thyroid-specific T cells as seen in animal models of thyroiditis.[88] This series of events can occur only in a susceptible individual with the right immune repertoire. Bystander activation would arise from any T cells within the thyroid gland, and these T cells may be activated by many different insults. The attractiveness of this model is that many different types of infections/insults would lead to the same clinical disease phenotype. There is much evidence for residual thyroid-resident T cells and dendritic cells in the glands of patients with Graves disease that could have been activated by this mechanism at the time of disease onset.[89]

Mechanism #2—Molecular Mimicry (Specificity Crossover)

In addition to the effects of the direct release of cytokines from T cells activated elsewhere via the bystander effect, intrathyroidal T cells may become activated in another nonspecific way. Structural or conformational similarity (i.e., sequence or shape or both) among different antigens can lead to specificity crossover (or molecular mimicry).[90] Antigenic similarity between bacteria and viruses and human proteins is common, and in one study 4% of monoclonal antibodies raised against a variety of viruses cross-reacted with antigens in tissues.[91] Furthermore, mice infected with reovirus type 1 developed an autoimmune polyendocrinopathy with autoantibodies directed against normal pancreas, pituitary, thyroid, and gastric mucosa, suggesting molecular mimicry between a reoviral antigen and a common tissue antigen.[92] Molecular mimicry has also been reported between *Yersinia enterocolitica* and the TSHR based on the observed cross-reaction between sera from patients with *Yersinia* infection and sera from patients with Graves disease.[93] Similar evidence has been presented on the basis of structural similarities between *Borrelia* and retroviral sequences and the TSHR.[94]

Mechanism #3—Aberrant Expression of Class II HLA Antigens

Normal thyroid epithelial cells do not express human leukocyte antigen (HLA) class II antigens, but they are markedly expressed in thyroid glands from patients with autoimmune thyroid disease.[95-98] A local insult, whether trauma or infection of the thyroid gland, may cause an inflammatory infiltrate and the production of interferons or other cytokines in the thyroid gland, which are able to induce HLA class II antigen expression. HLA class II antigens are used to present antigen to the immune system and overexpression on the thyroid cell would lead to enhanced presentation of thyroid autoantigens and activation of local autoreactive thyroid-specific T cells in a susceptible individual. Support for this concept comes from the in vivo induction of such molecules on mouse thyrocytes by

interferon-γ that also induced autoimmune thyroiditis[99] and the demonstration of the necessity for major histocompatibility complex (MHC) molecules on TSHR expressing fibroblasts used in the induction of Graves disease in mice.[55] A number of viruses may also induce thyroid cell expression of such antigens independent of immune cell cytokine secretion, including reovirus types 1 and 3 and cytomegalovirus.

Mechanism #4—Cryptic Antigens

T-cell tolerance depends on the visualization of self-antigens by the immune system in sufficient amounts to initiate continuous T-cell deletion, anergy induction, and regulatory T-cell activation. However, some antigens and antigenic epitopes are not seen in sufficient concentrations to cause the removal of T cells that may react to them. These molecules contain what are sometimes called *cryptic epitopes*.[100] Hence, T cells specific for these cryptic epitopes may be present in the immune repertoire. They may then induce autoaggressive T cells if such an epitope is uncovered or increased in concentration by a local insult. HLA class II antigen expression in a situation in which it normally does not occur, such as the thyroid epithelial cell, would then allow the presentation of these normally cryptic thyroid antigens to local autoreactive T cells if they are present. To date, however, such potential cryptic thyroid antigens have not been characterized.

Potential Risk Factors for Graves Disease

In addition to the possible mechanisms behind the pathogenesis of disease one has to consider the precipitating causes. Although disease causation may be stochastic, meaning a random occurrence of events, a number of specific factors have been shown to increase or decrease the risk of developing Graves disease. In addition to well-known associations such as family history of autoimmune thyroid disease and female sex, an increase in risk has been observed in people who smoke; Graves disease is also more common during the postpartum period and after radioiodine therapy for nontoxic goiter. Moreover, a number of immunomodulating drugs may increase the risk, and psychological stress may play a role. On the other hand, moderate alcohol consumption is associated with a severalfold decrease in risk compared with people who are abstainers,[101] and Graves disease tends to enter remission during the second half of pregnancy. We will discuss in more detail a number of these influences.

Risk Factor #1—Genetic Susceptibility

The development and the subsequent course of Graves disease are greatly influenced by heredity. The role of hereditary factors is evidenced by the increased incidence of other autoimmune disorders in members of patients' families, such as Hashimoto disease, insulin-dependent diabetes (type 1), celiac disease, Addison disease, and pernicious anemia.[102] Additionally, autoantibodies against endocrine tissues, especially thyroid antibodies, gastric parietal cell antibodies, and intrinsic factor in some families suggests a hereditary influence. The increased risk of a sibling being affected is shown by a high sibling recurrence risk (λs) of 11.6.[103] In addition, monozygotic twins have a higher concordance rate for Graves disease than do dizygotic twins,[104] despite the rearrangement of B-cell and T-cell V genes that cause the immune repertoires of identical twins to differ, thus implicating non-V genes in susceptibility. Indeed, there is also evidence that the propensity

TABLE 12-3
Confirmed Genes Associated With Graves Disease

Gene	Chromosome	SNPs	Odds Ratio
HLA	6p21		2.0-4.0
CTLA4	2q33	60	1.5-2.2
PTPN22	1p13	250	1.4-1.9
CD40	20q11	125	1.3-1.8
IL2RA	10p15	594	1.1-1.4
FCRL3	1q23	99	1.1-1.3
TG	8q24	1698	1.3-1.6
TSHR	14q31	984	1.4-2.6

CD40, cluster of differentiation 40; CTLA4, cytotoxic T-lymphocyte antigen 4; FCRL3, Fc receptor L3; HLA, human leukocyte antigen; IL2RA, interleukin 2 receptor-α; PTPN22, protein tyrosine phosphatase nonreceptor type 22; SNPs, single-nucleotide polymorphisms; TG, thyroglobulin; TSHR, thyroid-stimulating hormone receptor.

for the development of thyroid autoantibodies appears to be an autosomal dominant trait linked to the cytotoxic T-lymphocyte antigen 4 gene (CTLA4) that codes for a modulator of the second signal to T cells.[105] Because there are a large number of such genetic loci (Table 12-3) that may contribute to Graves disease susceptibility, it is referred to as a polygenic or complex genetic disorder. However, to date, these genes and gene regions only provide a small part of the calculated genetic susceptibility, so much more remains to be understood.

There is a long known and much investigated association with the HLA gene region (e.g., increased frequency of the HLA DR3 and DQA10501 haplotypes in Caucasians).[106] The HLA region provides approximately 5% of the genetic susceptibility to Graves disease and gives an increased risk of twofold to fourfold.[107,108] Additional nonspecific genetic susceptibility, after the HLA and CTLA4 contributions, includes the genes for lymphoid tyrosine phosphatase (PTPN22), the signaling molecule CD40, the IL-2 receptor-α, and the orphan Fc receptor L3, which may all be involved in providing a background autoimmunity susceptibility. In addition, a number of genome-wide association studies (GWAS) have also located additional sites, but many such observations have differed among studies and require further confirmation.[109,110] Of particular interest, however, has been the search for thyroid-specific genetic susceptibility that reveals small influences exerted by polymorphisms in the Tg gene and the TSHR gene, the latter being only associated with Graves disease.[111-113]

Epigenetics. As indicated by identical twin studies, the genetic contribution to Graves disease cannot explain all the disease susceptibility, and additional risk factors must be at work. A new major modifier of risk are the noncoding effects on gene expression and function referred to as *epigenetic influences*. These effects include DNA methylation, histone modifications, and RNA interference and can amplify a risk conferred by inherited polymorphism. Much more remains to be learned about how thyroid disease specificity is engineered into the genetic susceptibility to Graves disease, but the TSHR gene association has been neatly explained by such epigenetic changes influencing TSHR expression.[82] Because epigenetic changes can be influenced by infection and the environment, we need to learn more about such epigenetic-genetic interactions.

Risk Factor #2—Infection

Much has been written about the possible role of infection in the development of autoimmunity acting via bystander effects or molecular mimicry.[114,115] There is no evidence that a specific infection initiates Graves disease.[85] An identifiable agent should be present in most patients, and transfer of the agent to susceptible recipients should transfer the disease. As discussed earlier, it has been long suggested that Graves disease is associated with infectious agents (e.g., *Y. enterocolitica, Helicobacter pylori*), but no studies meet the necessary criteria to prove this even though molecular mimicry can be demonstrated in vitro.[93] Infections of the thyroid gland itself (e.g., subacute thyroiditis, congenital rubella, hepatitis C) may be associated with thyroid autoimmune phenomena but are not predictable initiators of Graves disease.[116] Reports of retroviral sequences in the thyroid glands of patients with Graves disease have failed to be reproduced. Hence, a causative role for infectious agents has not been definitively demonstrated in Graves disease. However, the potential influence of many different infections on the epigenetic characteristics of a variety of susceptibility genes remains a major hypothesis for the cause of Graves disease.

Risk Factor #3—Stress

As Parry first observed, Graves disease may become evident either after severe emotional stress, such as the actual or threatened separation from a loved one, or after an acute fright, such as an automobile accident.[117,118] Many clinical experiences and reports have associated major stress with the onset of Graves disease, including data on the high incidence of thyrotoxicosis among refugees from Nazi prison camps, although this may have been more directly related to replacement of iodine after their release. Some data suggest that stress induces an overall state of immune suppression by nonspecific mechanisms,[119-121] perhaps secondary to the effects of cortisol and corticotropin-releasing hormone action at the level of the immune cell. Following the acute immune suppression by stress, there is presumably an overcompensation by the immune system when the suppression is released. This reaction would then precipitate autoimmune thyroid disease, as seen after the release from the immunosuppression of pregnancy in the postpartum period when either thyroiditis or Graves disease may develop.[122] The rebound phenomenon would result in greater immune activity than normal and would initiate disease only if the individual were genetically susceptible.

Risk Factor #4—Gender

Graves disease is four to five times more common in women than in men (and it becomes more prevalent after puberty). The female preponderance and the fact that the disorder is uncommon before puberty have suggested that female sex steroids may be responsible for this difference.[123] Androgens may actually suppress autoimmune thyroiditis and favor the development of Th1 T cells and CD8+ T cells.[124,125] Estrogen and progesterone have also been shown to influence the immune system, particularly the B-cell repertoire, and have often been suggested as the reason for female susceptibility and having multiple effects favoring Th2 T cells and enhancing antigen presentation.[123] However, there is no fall in the incidence of Graves disease after menopause, and the disease is seen in many men. Such observations have suggested that perhaps it is the X chromosome rather than sex steroids that is the responsible element in female susceptibility. Women have two X chromosomes and, therefore, would receive twice any susceptibility gene dose. The forkhead box P3 gene (FOXP3) is a key gene in the development of regulatory T cells, is located within an X-chromosome locus (Xp11.23), and has been shown in some, but not all, studies to be linked with auto-immune thyroid diseases (AITDs).[126] The phenomenon of X-chromosome inactivation (XCI) has also been invoked in autoimmune disease.[127] Female cells may inactivate different X chromosomes to different degrees in different tissues leading to potentially differing immune responses. Evidence for XCI being important has been repeatedly described in Graves disease.[128,129]

Risk Factor #5—Pregnancy

Severe Graves disease is uncommon during pregnancy because hyperthyroidism is associated with reduced fertility. For those women with milder disease who successfully conceive, hyperthyroidism endows an increased risk of pregnancy loss and established pregnancy complications,[39,130-132] as exemplified by the influence of high thyroid hormone levels in normal pregnancy seen in thyroid hormone resistance.[133] Such data indicate that excess thyroid hormones themselves have a direct toxic effect on the fetus. However, pregnancy is a time of immunosuppression, so the disease tends to improve as pregnancy progresses. Both T-cell and B-cell functions are diminished as pregnancy progresses under the influence of both local placental factors and regulatory T cells (see later discussion).[123,134] Rebound from this immunosuppression after delivery may contribute to the development of postpartum thyroid disease.[135] In a retrospective Swedish study 30% of young women gave a history of pregnancy in the 12 months before the onset of Graves disease,[136] indicating that postpartum Graves disease is a surprisingly common presentation and that pregnancy is a major risk factor for development of the disease in susceptible women (see later section on Graves disease in pregnancy). Consistent with this observation is the higher rate of Graves disease relapse occurring in postpartum women who were previously in remission.[137]

Risk Factor #6—Drugs

Iodine and iodine-containing drugs, such as amiodarone, and iodine-containing contrast media may precipitate Graves disease or its recurrence in a susceptible individual.[138] Iodine is most likely to precipitate thyrotoxicosis in an iodine-deficient population simply by allowing TRAbs to effectively stimulate the formation of more thyroid hormone. Whether there is any other precipitating event is unclear, although iodine may also damage thyroid cells directly and release thyroid antigens to the immune system. Interferon-α has also been seen to precipitate not only a thyroiditis but also Graves disease.[116,139]

Risk Factor #7—Irradiation

There is no evidence that radiation exposure itself is a risk factor for Graves disease, although Graves disease is well known to be precipitated in some patients treated with radioactive iodine for multinodular goiter.[140,141] There is also evidence that thyroid autoantibodies are more prevalent in a radiation-exposed population, and claims of increased autoimmune thyroiditis in such populations have been made.[142-144] In addition, radioactive iodine treatment leads in the majority of patients to a steep increase in TRAb that returns to pretreatment level after 1 year.[145] Even 5 years after radioiodine therapy TRAb levels are considerably higher after radioiodine therapy than in patients treated with antithyroid drugs or surgery.[146] This flair in autoimmunity may be the cause for the onset or worsening of clinical ophthalmopathy in around 15% of patients. Fortunately, this is often transient (see later).[147]

Pathogenesis and Risk Factors for Graves Orbitopathy and Dermopathy

The pathogenesis of the orbitopathy and dermopathy is now better understood. The extraocular muscle and adipose tissue are swollen by the accumulation in the extracellular matrix of glycosaminoglycans (GAGs) and new fat cell development (adipogenesis) within the orbit. GAGs are secreted by fibroblasts under the influence of TRAbs and cytokines such as interferon-γ from local activated lymphocytes, and, therefore, orbital adipogenesis appears to also be enhanced by circulating TRAbs.[148] This accumulation of GAGs disrupts and impairs the function of the extraocular muscles. As the disease runs its course and inflammation decreases, the damaged muscles become fibrosed. Hence, histologic examination of the extraocular muscles shows disrupted muscle fibrils and a patchy lymphocytic infiltrate, predominantly of T cells, and some muscle cells exhibit HLA class II antigen as seen within the thyroid gland. Such T cells react in vitro with retroorbital tissue.[149,150] Transplantation of extraocular muscle into mice deficient in B cells and T cells (SCID/SCID mice) causes TRAbs to appear in the murine serum, showing accumulation of TSHR antibody-secreting B cells within the muscle samples.[151] Evidence of enhanced TSHR expression in retroorbital and pretibial tissues such as fibrocytes and adipocytes has strengthened the notion that it is the TSHR itself that is provoking the immune response.[148] Retroorbital fibrocytes may be derived from circulating marrow fibrocytes, and express more TSHR than is seen at other sites, which also supports the TSHRs as the primary antigen of GO.[152] The importance of the role of the insulin-like growth factor 1 (IGF-1) receptor as a retroorbital antigen and the role of serum IGF-1 and IGF-1 receptor antibodies acting synergistically with TSHR antibodies[153,154] remains unclear.[155,156]

High TSHR Antibodies and High Risk for Graves Orbitopathy

In keeping with the hypothesis that the TSHR is the primary antigen, patients with the most severe orbitopathy have the highest titers of TRAbs, and the level of TRAbs often correlates with the severity of the eye disease and is exemplified by patients with the Graves triad. It is likely that antigen-specific T cells play a major role in initiating the disorder and locally produced TRAbs effect many of the characteristic orbital tissue changes by providing additional signaling at the target cells. However, non–eye-specific antibodies may serve as markers of extraocular muscle inflammation including antibodies to the IGF-1 receptor.[157]

Specific Risk Factors for Graves Orbitopathy

Although there have been many claims, there is still no reproducible evidence that a separate and distinct genetic risk can be ascribed to severe ophthalmic Graves disease, suggesting that it is mainly environmental factors that lead to the enhanced retroorbital inflammation in some patients.[158,159] All of the same risk factors (e.g., infection, stress, gender, gonadal steroids, pregnancy, drugs, and irradiation) apply to the onset of both thyroid and eye involvement in Graves disease. There are, however, three additional distinct risk factors that deserve attention.

Smoking. The first risk factor is smoking, which has increased the risk for ophthalmic involvement in many studies, perhaps by causing tissue hypoxia or simply direct inflammation.[160,161]

Radioiodine. The second risk factor to consider is radioiodine, which in controlled clinical trials accentuates ophthalmic Graves disease.[147] This worsening may be related to the surge in thyroid autoimmunity seen after radioiodine therapy[145] and the severity of the baseline ophthalmopathy, which may be mild and transient and may be ameliorated with corticosteroid treatment for the subsequent 3 to 4 months. Many physicians are now reluctant to prescribe radioiodine to patients with moderate or severe eye disease unless the patients are receiving corticosteroids.

Trauma. Last, the role of trauma in the initiation and exacerbation of thyroid and retroorbital inflammation is well recognized.[81,86,158]

Natural History and Course of Graves Disease

The course of the thyrotoxic component of Graves disease is variable. In some patients, thyrotoxicosis persists, although it may vary in severity. In others, the course may be cyclic, exhibiting remissions of varying frequency, intensity, and duration. This cyclic feature has an important bearing on treatment. With the passage of months or years, thyrotoxicosis tends to give way to euthyroidism. In one study one third of patients actually became hypothyroid within 20 years of treatment with antithyroid agents,[162] echoing the hypothesis that Graves disease is usually accompanied by some degree of autoimmune thyroiditis.

The GO may or may not commence together with the thyrotoxic component. Thus, thyrotoxic patients may initially be free from eye disease but are affected by it months or years later or not at all. Conversely, orbitopathy may be the first manifestation of future Graves disease with the subsequent development of hyperthyroidism. In euthyroid patients with orbitopathy, evidence of a thyroid abnormality may only be manifest by the presence of TRAbs and other thyroid autoantibodies. As mentioned earlier, some such patients may become hypothyroid within a few years; others become hyperthyroid, and a few remain euthyroid. However, many such euthyroid patients do have evidence of autoimmune thyroiditis. The course of thyroid function in many of these patients is, therefore, unpredictable.

Histopathology of Graves Disease
Thyroid Gland

The older designation for Graves disease, *diffuse toxic goiter*, denoted that the gland was both enlarged and uniformly affected. The gland might vary in consistency from softer than normal to firm and rubbery, depending on the degree of thyroiditis, blood flow, and colloid content of follicles. The outer surface is usually smooth but may be somewhat lobular; less commonly, the gland is grossly nodular prior to treatment. The cut surface is red and glistening. Microscopically, the follicles are small and lined with hyperplastic columnar epithelium and contain scant colloid that displays much marginal scalloping and vacuolization (see Fig. 12-3). Nuclei are vesicular and basally located and exhibit occasional mitoses. Papillary projections of the hyperplastic epithelium extend into the lumina of the follicles. Vascularity is increased, and as described earlier, there is a varying heterogeneous infiltration by lymphocytes and plasma cells that collect in aggregates and may form infrequent germinal centers in contrast to their abundance in Hashimoto disease. In such regions, thyroid epithelial cells express HLA class II antigens, a phenomenon not seen in normal thyroid glands, and are large, perhaps due to local stimulation by TRAbs. When the patient is given iodine or antithyroid drugs, the thyroid gland may undergo involution as TRAbs decrease. Then hyperplasia and vascularity regress, papillary projections recede, and follicles enlarge and become filled with colloid once again.

Eyes

In patients with infiltrative orbitopathy, the volume of orbital contents is enlarged because of an increase both in retrobulbar connective tissue and adipose tissue and in the total extraocular muscle mass (Fig. 12-6). Some of the increase in muscle mass is due to edema resulting from accumulation of the ground substances of hyaluronic acid and chondroitin sulfates, which are hydrophilic, and are the result of cytokine action from activated lymphocytes. The extraocular muscles are swollen, and some fibers exhibit loss of striation, fragmentation, and lymphocytic infiltration. The lacrimal glands may also be involved. Ultimately, the tissues fibrose (see Fig. 12-6).

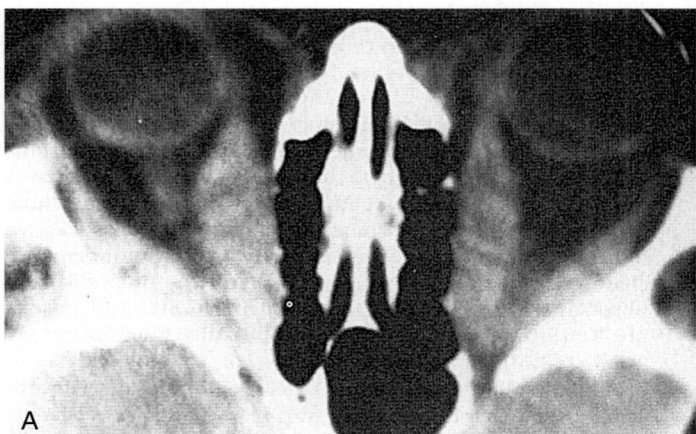
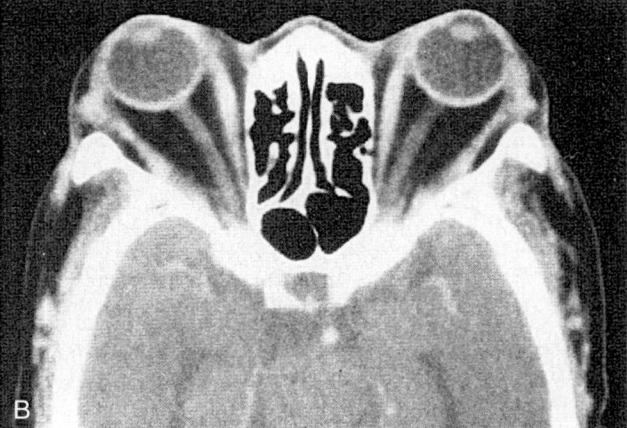

Figure 12-6 Computed tomographic scans of orbits in two patients with Graves orbitopathy. **A,** Notice the obviously grossly swollen medial rectus extraocular muscles in both orbits and the resulting proptosis. **B,** The patient shows considerable proptosis with only minimal muscle enlargement, suggesting the presence of a large amount of retroorbital fat. (Courtesy of Dr. Peter Som, Mount Sinai School of Medicine, New York, NY.)

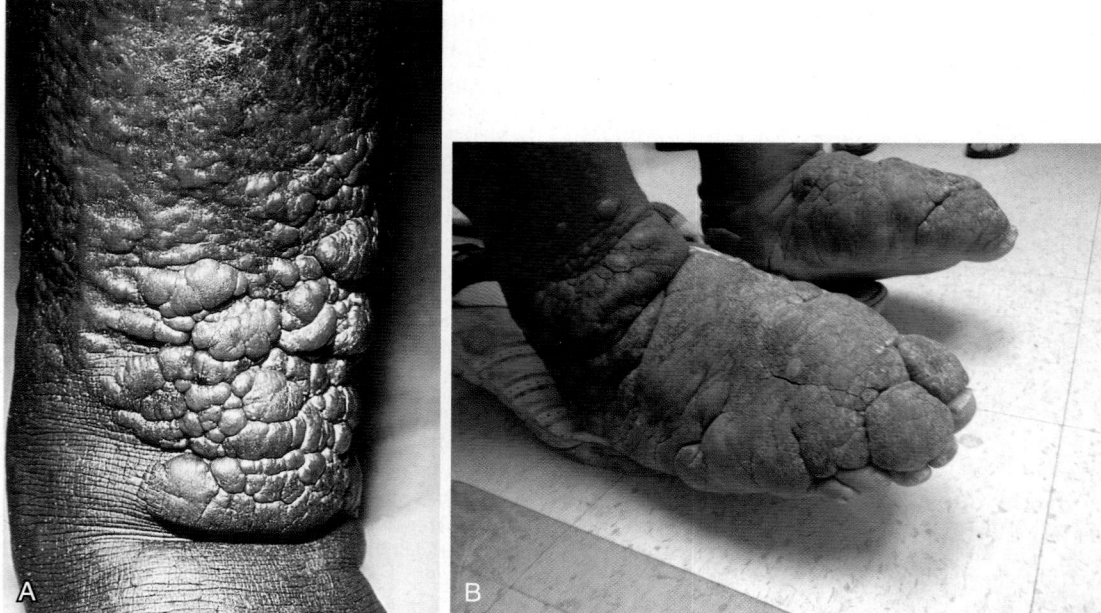

Figure 12-7 A, Chronic pretibial myxedema in a patient with Graves disease and orbitopathy. The lesions are firm and nonpitting, with a clear edge to feel. **B,** Here the chronic myxedma has continued to spread to the foot, causing severe disfiguration and immobility. (**A,** Courtesy of Dr. Andrew Werner, Mount Sinai School of Medicine, New York, NY.)

Skin

The dermopathy of Graves disease is the most uncommon manifestation of the Graves triad (also called the *Merseburg triad*, named after the city where von Basedow resided), which consisted of thyrotoxicosis and goiter, orbitopathy, and dermopathy (Fig. 12-7A and B). This dermopathy, often referred to as *pretibial myxedema* because of its most common site of development, is usually a late manifestation and 99% of patients with infiltrative dermopathy have clinical GO. The content of hyaluronic acid and chondroitin sulfates in the dermis is likely increased secondary to TRAb and cytokine activation of fibroblasts as seen behind the eye. This causes compression of the dermal lymphatics and nonpitting edema: the collagen fibers are separated and fragmented, and early lesions contain a lymphocytic infiltrate. As discussed earlier, TSHR expression can be demonstrated in fibroblasts and adipocytes,[148] and TRAb levels are usually extraordinarily high in such patients. Nodule and plaque formation may occur in chronic lesions, which can become large and disfiguring.

Thyroid Function

In Graves hyperthyroidism, normal pituitary regulatory mechanisms are overridden by the action of TRAbs of the stimulating variety. The resulting hyperfunction of the thyroid gland leads to suppression of TSH secretion that is reflected in undetectable serum TSH. In this context, the term *functional autonomy* may be misused when the intent is to imply that thyroid function is independent of TSH stimulation. True functional autonomy occurs when the thyroid gland is capable of functioning at a normal or an increased pace in the absence of both TSH and any other circulating thyroid stimulator (e.g., in congenital hyperthyroidism secondary to constitutively activated TSHRs). In Graves disease, the thyroid gland is controlled by an abnormal stimulator, the TRAbs (as in molar pregnancy, in which hCG is responsible). When that stimulator is withdrawn (i.e., when the disease enters remission), hyper-

function subsides, and the nonautonomous nature of thyroid function becomes evident in the reemergence of normal TSH secretion and control of thyroid function.

The molar ratio of T_3 to T_4 in Tg is about twice normal, reflective of chronic hyperstimulation of the gland that also leads to a high thyroidal activity of D1 with T_4 deiodination to T_3. The major product of glandular secretion is still T_4, but the ratio of T_3 to T_4 in the thyroid secretion is increased in proportion to the overproduction of T_3. In some instances, especially where there is iodine deficiency, T_3 appears to be the major secretory product, so the serum T_3 level is increased while serum T_4 concentration is within the normal range (T_3 thyrotoxicosis). The proportion of total plasma T_4 and T_3 in the free (or unbound) state is increased both because of a decrease in concentration of thyroxine-binding globulin (TBG) and because of the increase in the concentration of T_4.

Clinical Picture
The Thyroid Gland

The incidence of Graves disease is quite stable after 30 years of age. It is rare before age 10 years, and still occurs in the very old, sometimes in an apathetic form. The features include diffuse goiter, thyrotoxicosis, infiltrative orbitopathy, occasionally infiltrative dermopathy, and rarely achropachy with thickening of the terminal phalanges. Special manifestations to be discussed later are fetal and neonatal hyperthyroidism caused by transplacental passage of TRAbs. Because the orbitopathy and dermopathy may be independent of other manifestations, they are discussed separately. In other respects, the symptoms and signs of thyrotoxicosis are the same in Graves disease as in patients with other causes of hyperthyroidism.

In most patients, the thyroid gland is enlarged, but hyperthyroidism in Graves disease can also occur in a gland of normal size. In one study of 200 unselected patients only 50% had an enlarged thyroid by ultrasonography.[163] In patients with goiter, the size of the thyroid gland is most often two or three times normal but may be

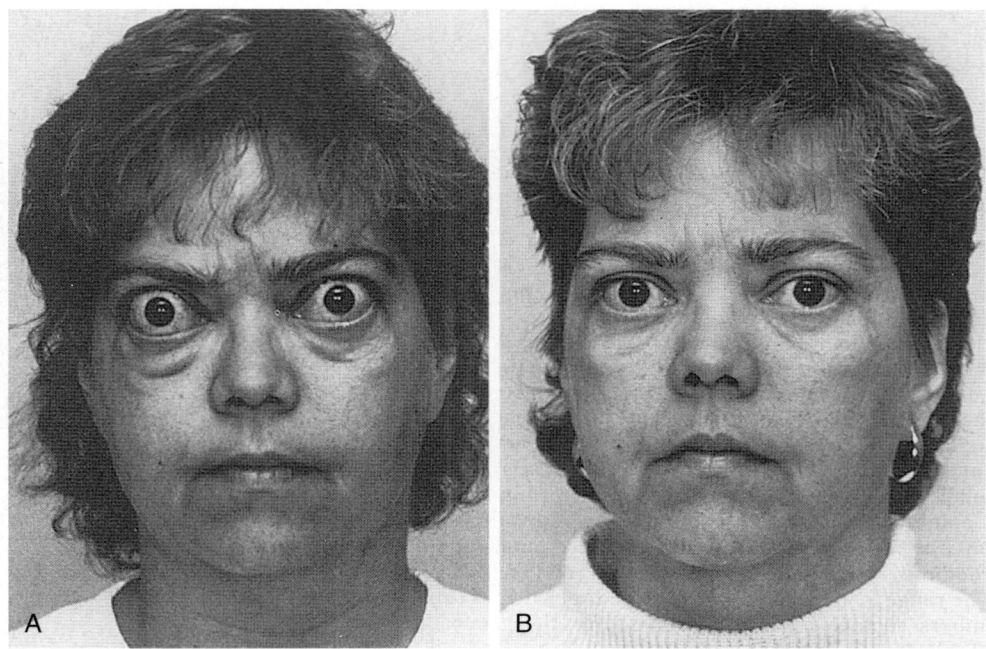

Figure 12-8 Characteristic signs of Graves orbitopathy (**A**) subsequently corrected by orbital decompression surgery (**B**). Note the thyroid stare, the asymmetry, the proptosis, and the periorbital edema prior to correction. (Courtesy of Dr. Jack Rootman, University of British Columbia, Vancouver, BC, Canada.)

massively enlarged. The consistency is usually soft but can range from soft to firm and rubbery usually because of associated autoimmune thyroiditis. The enlargement is usually symmetric. The surface is generally smooth but may feel lobular. In severe cases, a thrill may be felt, usually over the upper or lower poles where the superior and inferior thyroid arteries, respectively, enter the gland, and a thrill is always accompanied by an audible bruit. However, the bruit, which occurs in systole, may be difficult to auscultate if the patient is very tachycardic. The bruit should not be confused with a venous hum or murmur arising from the base of the heart. To differentiate a true bruit from a transmitted cardiac flow murmur, the auscultated bruit should be louder over the thyroid than in the upper left sternal area. In addition, mitral valve prolapse is more common than in the normal population[7] and may account for a cardiac murmur.

Graves Orbitopathy

Natural History. GO or ophthalmopathy is so named because the majority of cases of this ocular disorder occur in patients with active or past Graves hyperthyroidism. However, this entity is also termed *thyroid eye disease* or *thyroid-associated orbitopathy*, reflecting its association with both Graves disease and Hashimoto thyroiditis. The ocular manifestations of Graves disease follow an essentially independent course from the thyrotoxic manifestations but can be influenced by high or low thyroid hormone levels[164] and by the choice of therapy for hyperthyroidism.[165] As discussed earlier, the most important risk factors for the development of GO include smoking,[161] radioactive iodine therapy for Graves hyperthyroidism,[166] and high TRAb levels.[167,168] The natural history is characterized by rapid onset and deterioration followed by a plateau period that preceeds gradual improvement. The severity of the dynamic phase ranges from relatively mild to sight-threatening

disease, and its duration may span several months to 5 or more years.[165,169]

Infiltrative orbitopathy is clinically evident in about 25% to 50% of patients with Graves hyperthyroidism, depending on the diagnostic criteria.[165,170] However, ultrasonography, CT, or magnetic resonance imaging (MRI) of the orbits reveals changes, such as swelling of extraocular muscles and increased retroorbital fat volume, in a large majority of patients with Graves disease,[161] including those in whom the clinically apparent changes are minimal or absent.

Signs and Symptoms. Retraction of the eyelids leads to widening of the palpebral fissures so that the sclerae are exposed above the superior margin of the limbus (Fig. 12-8). When the patient looks downward, the upper lid lags behind the globe (lid lag), exposing more sclera. When the patient gazes upward, often with difficulty, the globe may lag behind the lid. Simple lid retraction and lid lag may be manifestations of the thyrotoxicosis per se and not indicative of GO. These manifestations will often abate when the thyrotoxicosis is relieved. In contrast, the early inflammatory signs and symptoms of bonafide GO include a sense of irritation in the eyes, resembling that caused by a foreign body, and excessive tearing that is often made worse by exposure to air or wind. In active disease, the conjunctivae and eyelids are generally injected and swollen, and the patient may complain of pain with eye motion.[171] Double vision can be intermittent, inconstant (at extremes of gaze only), or constant and may occur alone or in conjunction with other disease manifestations. Exophthalmos (proptosis), when present, is frequently asymmetric and associated with a feeling of pressure behind the globes. When exophthalmos is pronounced, the eyes may not close well during sleep, a condition termed *lagophthalmos* that may lead to corneal dryness. In severe cases, an exposed cornea may ulcerate or become infected. Subluxation, or anterior displacement of the globe out of the

TABLE 12-4

Clinical Assessment of the Patient With Graves Ophthalmopathy

Activity Measures*

Spontaneous retrobulbar pain
Pain on attempted up or down gaze
Redness of the eyelids
Redness of the conjunctivae
Swelling of the eyelids
Inflammation of the caruncle and/or plica
Conjunctival edema

Severity Measures

Lid aperture (distance between the lid margins in mm with the patient looking in the primary position, sitting relaxed, and with distant fixation)
Swelling of the eyelids (absent/equivocal, moderate, severe)
Redness of the eyelids (absent/present)
Redness of the conjunctivae (absent/present)
Conjunctival edema (absent, present)
Inflammation of the caruncle or plica (absent, present)
Exophthalmos (measured in millimeters using the same Hertel exophthalmometer and the same intercanthal distance for an individual patient)
Subjective diplopia score[†]
Eye muscle involvement (ductions in degrees)
Corneal involvement (absent/punctate keratopathy/ulcer)
Optic nerve involvement (best corrected visual acuity, color vision, optic disk, relative afferent pupillary defect (absent/present), plus visual fields if optic nerve compression is suspected

*Based on the classic features of inflammation in Graves ophthalmopathy. The clinical activity score (CAS) is the sum (one point each) of all items present; a CAS ≥ 3/7 indicates active ophthalmopathy.
[†]Subjective diplopia score: 0, no diplopia; 1, intermittent (i.e., diplopia in primary position of gaze, when tired or when first awakening); 2, inconstant (i.e., diplopia at extremes of gaze); 3, constant (i.e., continuous diplopia in primary or reading position).

orbit, is another manifestation of extreme proptosis that can be catastrophic if not promptly treated. Dysthyroid optic neuropathy is a sight-threatening condition that develops as the optic nerve is compressed by enlarged extraocular muscles at the orbital apex. This can occur with or without proptosis and may present as subtle changes in color vision or increased eye pressure symptoms.[172] If not properly treated, dysthyroid optic neuropathy can lead to decreased visual acuity and even sight loss.[173]

Objective Assessment of Eye Disease. The American Thyroid Association and the European Group on Graves Orbitopathy (EUGOGO) recommend that the inflammatory component of the eye changes of Graves disease be assessed using an overall activity score (Table 12-4).[174]

Thyroid Dermopathy

Dermopathy occurs in less than 5% of patients with Graves disease and is almost always accompanied by orbitopathy, usually of a severe degree.[175] These lesions cause hyperpigmented, nonpitting induration of the skin of the legs, commonly over the pretibial area (hence the name *pretibial myxedema*) and the dorsa of the feet, sometimes in the form of individual nodules and plaques or becoming confluent with a smooth characteristic edge or shoulder (see Fig. 12-7). Rarely, lesions develop on other areas of the body, such as the face, elbows, or dorsa of the hands, and are often associated with trauma to that area. The cause of the characteristic pretibial location of the dermopathy is unclear but may depend on impairment to venous flow in the lower extremities due to accumulation of glycosaminoglycans and edema or trauma to the exposed areas.[86]

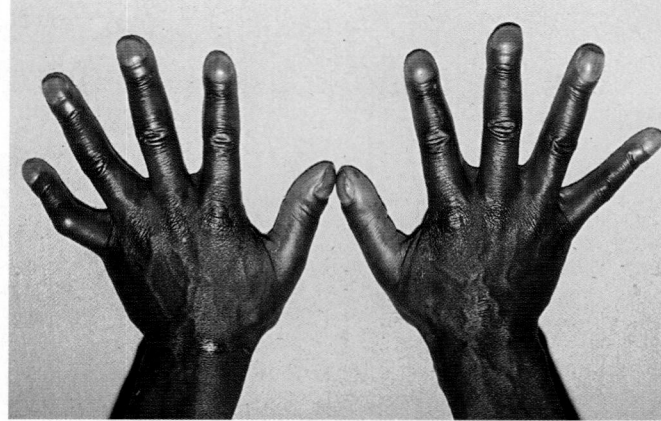

Figure 12-9 Rare thyroid acropachy in a patient with Graves disease. The hypermetabolic state leads to axial bone destruction, presumably secondary to enhanced osteoclast activity. Acropachy should not be confused with clubbing, which is usually painless. (Courtesy of Dr. Andrew Werner, Mount Sinai School of Medicine, New York, NY.)

Indeed, surgical trauma to such tissues aggravates the disease dramatically. Clubbing of the digits (thyroid acropachy) is also occasionally associated in such patients with long-standing Graves disease (Fig. 12-9).

Laboratory Tests for Graves Disease

In moderate or severe Graves disease, laboratory findings are consistent with the pathophysiology previously discussed. The serum TSH level, when measured by a sensitive immunoassay, is almost totally suppressed, and serum T_4 and T_3 levels are elevated (see Chapter 11 and Fig. 12-1). The free T_4 and T_3 are increased more than are the total T_4 and T_3 levels. The serum T_3 concentration is proportionally more elevated than the serum T_4 level. The increase in thyroid iodide uptake and clearance rate is often, but not always, reflected in the increased RAIU usually measured at 24 hours. The 24-hour RAIU may be inappropriately normal in a patient with milder disease given the suppressed serum TSH level, and also relatively low compared with the 24-hour uptake in patients with a very rapid iodine turnover in the hyperactive gland. In patients with severe accompanying illness, conversion of T_4 to T_3 may be impaired, permitting the return to normal of the free T_3 concentration but usually not the free T_4 (T_4 thyrotoxicosis). Occasionally, and usually in iodine deficiency, the discrepancy between T_4 and T_3 levels is exaggerated, the serum T_4 concentration being normal and the serum T_3 concentration alone being elevated (T_3 thyrotoxicosis).

Because there are other causes of suppressed serum TSH, such as depression and hypothalamic-pituitary disease, and to exclude the possibility that an increase in serum T_4 concentration is the result of an increase in hormone binding in the blood, the free T_4 concentration should also be measured. Determining the RAIU is not useful in the diagnosis when the clinical presentation is compatible with straightforward Graves disease or in a TRAb-positive thyrotoxic patient but may be appropriate in excluding thyrotoxicosis not caused by Graves disease. Very low values of the RAIU or absent thyroid uptake on a thyroid scan associated with thyrotoxicosis signal the presence of (1) thyroiditis (painless Hashimoto disease, subacute, acute, or drug induced); (2) factitious thyrotoxicosis; (3) ectopic thyroid tissue; or (4) iodine contamination by recent administration of iodinated radiographic contrast agent, such as for a CT scan examination or amiodarone administration (see Fig. 12-1). In some countries conventional thyroid scintigraphy is used to differentiate among different causes by showing diffuse uninodular or multinodular scans or no uptake at all.

Mild (Subclinical) Graves Disease

The term *mild disease* is used to refer to patients with a suppressed TSH but apparently normal T_4 and T_3 levels and is often referred to as subclinical disease (see later section). In clinical practice, a TSH concentration below 0.2 mU/L (normal range, 0.4 to 4.2 mU/L) may be associated with symptoms of an excessive thyroid hormone supply, but usually a value between 0.1 and 0.4 mU/L suggests a supranormal exposure to thyroid hormones but not a condition likely to be associated with the severe clinical manifestations seen in patients with almost completely suppressed TSH values.

Measuring TSH Receptor Autoantibodies

Two types of tests may be employed for the detection of TRAbs and both are available commercially. The first test assesses the capacity of patient serum or IgG to inhibit the binding of labeled TSH to solubilized TSHRs or to compete with a monoclonal antibody to the TSH binding site on the TSHR. These protein-binding inhibition assays are of low cost and good precision, and the frequency of positive results in patients with active and untreated disease has increased as the sensitivity of the assay has improved and is now greater than 95%.[68,176] The second type of test is a bioassay that assesses the capacity of the patient's serum or IgG to stimulate adenylate cyclase in thyroid epithelial cells or mammalian cells expressing recombinant TSHR. Tests of this type, which measure the biologic action of the antibodies, are much more expensive and have relatively poor precision but are also positive in the vast majority of the patients with active untreated Graves disease.[177] However, because the patient being assessed is already thyrotoxic there is usualy little need for a bioassay of the patient's antibody and a quantitative assessment is all that is necessary. Because of the proliferation of acronyms describing these antibodies, the authors encourage the designation of the specific assay used when providing the assay result.

Standardization. As with all autoantibody tests, it is important to use an internationally accepted standard to allow comparison of results from different laboratories. A TRAb standard from the Medical Research Council (MRC) is often employed and reported in MRC units. Alternatively, results have been reported in terms of equivalent TSH units. However, the TRAbs from different patients may not give parallel results with the MRC standards or TSH standards when measured in different dilutions; for this reason the conversion of TRAb data into MRC units or TSH units can be erroneous.

Indications for Measuring Thyrotropin Receptor Autoantibodies. Quantitation of TRAbs may be a useful indicator of the degree of disease activity in an individual patient and can confirm the clinical diagnosis of Graves disease in a scientific manner. Demonstration of TRAbs may also be of diagnostic value in the euthyroid patient with exophthalmos, especially when it is unilateral. High TRAb levels in a pregnant woman with Graves disease increase the likelihood that fetal or neonatal thyrotoxicosis will be present in her offspring, and in this situation a bioassay late in pregnancy can be helpful if the level of TRAb remains high. Another use of TRAb testing is in the prognosis of patients with Graves disease who are treated with antithyroid agents. A persisting high level of TRAbs is a useful predictor of relapse on cessation of the drug.[69,70,178] Unfortunately, in patients with low or negative titers, the test is less helpful because a minority of such patients may still experience a relapse of hyperthyroidism after drug withdrawal.

Differential Diagnosis

The patient with major manifestations of Graves disease (i.e., thyrotoxicosis, goiter with an accompanying bruit or thrill, and infiltrative orbitopathy) does not pose a diagnostic problem. In some patients, however, one of the major manifestations either dominates the clinical picture or is present alone, and the disorder may mimic another disease. All of these issues can be resolved by appropriate laboratory testing.

Thyroid Diseases

The diffuse goiter of Graves disease in a patient with severe hyperthyroidism may rarely be confused with that of other thyroid diseases. In subacute thyroiditis, asymmetry of the gland, tenderness on palpation, and systemic evidence of inflammation assist in the diagnosis. When Graves disease is in a latent or inactive phase and thyrotoxicosis is absent or in patients with extremely mild hyperthyroidism, the goiter may require differentiation from Hashimoto thyroiditis or simple nontoxic goiter as possible diagnoses. The goiter of Hashimoto disease is somewhat lobulated and firmer and more rubbery compared with that of Graves disease. Serum levels of TPO antibodies are generally higher in Hashimoto disease, and patients with Graves disease characteristically harbor TRAb, but diseases may overlap and measurement of antibodies may not always be helpful in distinguishing individual patients. The very low RAIU distinguishes thyrotoxicosis caused by painless or subacute thyroiditis from Graves disease in the absence of iodine excess (see Fig. 12-1).

Eye Diseases

The orbitopathy of Graves disease, if bilateral and associated with thyrotoxicosis past or present, does not require differentiation from exophthalmos of any other origin, such as that seen in morbid obesity. However, unilateral exophthalmos, even when associated with thyrotoxicosis, should alert the physician to the possibility of a local cause. Rare diseases that may produce either unilateral or bilateral exophthalmos include orbital neoplasms, carotid-cavernous sinus fistulas, cavernous sinus thrombosis, infiltrative disorders affecting the orbit, and pseudotumor of the orbit. Mild bilateral exophthalmos, without infiltrative signs, is seen commonly in morbid obesity and is occasionally present on a familial basis; it also sometimes occurs in patients with Cushing syndrome, cirrhosis, uremia, chronic obstructive pulmonary disease, and superior vena cava syndrome.

The eye motility decrease in GO is typically caused by restricted stiff extraocular muscles. Ophthalmoplegia as the sole manifestation of a suspected orbitopathy of Graves disease requires exclusion of diabetes mellitus and other disorders affecting the brainstem and its connections as well as myasthenia gravis. Demonstration of the characteristic swelling of the extraocular muscles (sparing of the muscle tendons with the lateral rectus least commonly affected) by orbital ultrasonography, CT scan, or MRI is diagnostic of GO if other causes of myositis or other infiltrative disorders can be excluded. The detection of TRAbs in serum or the demonstration of a suppressed TSH level is highly suggestive of the diagnosis.

Treatment

It is not possible to treat the basic pathogenetic factors in Graves disease in a risk-free way. Existing therapies for both the thyrotoxic and the ophthalmic manifestations all have significant side effects. The lack of general agreement as to which therapy is the best is due to the fact that none is ideal.[179] Because the therapeutic problems posed by thyrotoxicosis and orbitopathy differ, and because they run independent courses, their treatments are discussed separately.

Treatment of hyperthyroidism is designed to impose restraint on hormone secretion either by means of chemical agents that inhibit hormone synthesis or release or by reducing the quantity of thyroid tissue. There are three effective therapeutic options, and physician and patient preference often dictate the choice. Radioiodine is a more popular therapy in the United States when compared to Europe or Japan where the preference is for antithyroid drug therapy. Primary surgery is generally used much less often and dependent on the surgical expertise available.

Antithyroid Agents

Thionamides. The major agents for treating thyrotoxicosis are drugs of the thionamide class, most commonly methimazole, PTU, and carbimazole (10 mg of carbimazole is rapidly metabolized to approximately 6 mg of methimazole[180]). When this is taken into account the two drugs are interchangeable. Each of these agents inhibit the oxidation and organic binding of thyroid iodide and, therefore, produce intrathyroidal iodine deficiency that further increases the ratio of T_3 to T_4 in the thyroid secretion, as reflected in the high T_3/T_4 ratio in the serum. In addition, large doses of PTU (400 mg), but not methimazole, impair the conversion of T_4 to T_3 by D1 in the thyroid and peripheral tissues.[181] The PTU-sensitive D1 is the major source of peripheral T_3 production in the hyperthyroid patient.[182] Because of this additional action, large doses of PTU may provide more rapid alleviation of very severe thyrotoxicosis.[183]

The half-life in plasma of methimazole is about 6 hours, whereas that of PTU is about 1.5 hours, and both drugs are accumulated by the thyroid gland.[180] A single dose of methimazole may not exert an antithyroid effect for a full 24-hour period.[184] Thus, it may be more effective in patients with severe hyperthyroidism to split the dose of methimazole over the day. On the other hand, the partial block of a single daily dose of methimazole is normally sufficient to treat milder cases and during prolonged therapy when patients have become euthyroid. Single daily dosing improves compliance with therapy and should be used whenever possible. Both these drugs cross the placenta and can inhibit thyroid function in the fetus but both drugs have been used highly effectively in pregnancy (see later discussion of hyperthyroidism in pregnancy).

Action of Thionamides on the Immune System. Thionamide drugs may directly influence the immune response in patients with AITD.[185] This action may occur within the thyroid gland, where the drugs are concentrated. The action on the thyroid cells themselves decreases thyroid antigen expression and decreases prostaglandin and cytokine release from thyroid cells. Thionamides also inhibit the generation of oxygen radicals in T cells, B cells, and particularly antigen-presenting cells and hence may cause a further decline in antigen presentation. It has also been

TABLE 12-5
Incidence of Major Toxic Reactions to Antithyroid Drugs in Adults

Side Effect	Frequency (%)	Comments
Polyarthritis	1-2	—
ANCA+ vasculitis	Rare	Mostly PTU
Agranulocytosis	0.1-0.5	May be more common with PTU
Hepatitis	0.1-0.2	PTU only
Cholestasis	Rare	Methimazole only

ANCA+, antineutrophil cytoplasmic antibody–positive; PTU, propylthiouracil.
Adapted from Cooper DS. Antithyroid drugs. *N Engl J Med.* 2005;352: 905-917.

shown that methimazole induces the expression of Fas ligand on the thyroid epithelial cell, thus inducing apoptosis of infiltrating lymphocytes such as T cells that express Fas ligand and decreasing the lymphocytic infiltration.[186] The clinical importance of immunosuppression and induction of apoptosis compared with inhibition of thyroid hormone formation is unclear. Some investigators find that a more likely cause for the decrease in autoimmunity in patients treated with antithyroid drugs is that the patients become euthyroid. Thyroid hormones have multiple effects on the immune system, some of which appear to be non-genomic,[187] and the thyrotoxic state my worsen autoimmunity. The circle is broken when patients become euthyroid by drug therapy.

Adverse Actions of Thionamides. Adverse reactions occur in only a small number of patients taking thionamide drugs, although some may be very severe if left uncared for (Table 12-5). Mild side effects occur in up to 20% of patients and include skin reactions, arthralgias, GI symptoms, an abnormal sense of taste, and occasional sialadenitis. Other effects include thrombocytopenia, enlargement of lymph nodes or a lupus-like syndrome including the development of antineutrophil cytoplasmic antibody (ANCA)-positive vasculitis,[188] and toxic psychoses. The mechanisms underlying these reactions are not known, although some reactions disappear with discontinuance of treatment. Of the more serious side effects, the one most talked about is agranulocytosis, which occurs in 0.1% to 0.3% of the patients, generally within the first few weeks or months of treatment. Older patients and those taking higher antithyroid doses are at higher risk. It is accompanied by fever and sore throat.[180] When therapy with a thionamide is begun, the patient should be instructed to discontinue the drug and to notify the physician immediately should these symptoms develop. This precaution is more important than the frequent measurement of white blood cell counts because agranulocytosis may develop within a day or two. Because of the high frequency of lymphopenia in hyperthyroidism itself, a complete blood cell count with differential is recommended before antithyroid drug therapy is started. If the absolute neutrophil count falls below 1500 cells/µL, the drug should be withdrawn. Similarly, if agranulocytosis occurs, the drug should be discontinued immediately and the patient treated with antibiotics as appropriate. Granulocyte colony-stimulating factor may speed the recovery that invariably takes place. Lymphocytes of patients who have developed agranulocytosis while taking PTU undergo blast transformation when exposed in vitro to PTU or methimazole, and consequently, they should not be given a thionamide drug again. Granulocytopenia occurs during antithyroid therapy and is sometimes a forerunner of agranulocytosis, but as already mentioned, it can also be a manifestation of thyrotoxicosis itself. Granulocytopenia that develops during the first few weeks of therapy may be difficult to interpret. In this circumstance, serial measurements of the leukocyte count should be made. If they display a downward trend, the antithyroid drugs should be discontinued. When serial measurements of the white blood cell count remain constant or return to normal, treatment need not be interrupted.

No! to PTU. Although rare, PTU has been associated with fulminant hepatic necrosis, and it is the third most common cause of drug-related liver failure, accounting for 10% of all drug-related liver transplants. Children are at more risk than adults.[189] Fortunately, cessation of the treatment results in recovery in most cases. This PTU-associated liver failure may occur at any time during therapy, so routine monitoring of liver function may not be helpful.[190] Methimazole is associated with cholestasis rather than hepatic necrosis, and the risk is increased with higher doses administered in older patients.[191] There are no reported cases of liver transplantation attributed to methimazole toxicity. Because of this well-known rare but serious PTU side effect of hepatic failure, sometimes requiring liver transplantation, in June 2009 the Food and Drug Administration (FDA) finally issued an advisory that PTU should not be used as a first-line agent in hyperthyroidism in adults or children.[192] The use of PTU has remained recommended in the first trimester of pregnancy (see later) and in life-threatening thyrotoxicosis or thyroid storm to take advantage of its ability to inhibit peripheral conversion of T_4 to T_3 and for those who have experienced minor reactions to methimazole and are unable or unwilling to undergo ^{131}I therapy or thyroidectomy.[193]

For all patients initiating thioamide therapy, the 2010 American Thyroid Association Management Guidelines for Hyperthyroidism[194] recommend that patients should be informed about the possible side effects and must stop the medication and inform their physician if they develop pruritic rash, jaundice, acholic stools or dark urine, arthralgias, abdominal pain, nausea, fever, or pharyngitis. In addition, all patients should have both baseline complete blood counts with differential white blood cell count and liver function tests including transaminases, bilirubin, and alkaline phosphatase. We believe that the suspicion of any serious manifestation should be an indication for abandonment of antithyroid therapy and recourse to surgery or ^{131}I treatment.

Practical Use of Thionamides. Based on its half-life, methimazole can most often be prescribed on a once-daily basis. However, the initial dose of methimazole commonly employed in moderate thyrotoxicosis is 20 to 30 mg daily (or the equivalent of carbimazole) until the patient is euthyroid and then a maintenance dose of 5 to 10 mg daily can be employed. For significantly hyperthyroid patients, a randomized controlled trial reported that normalization of free T_4 at 3 months occurred in more patients on higher dose methimazole (30 mg daily) than in those with lower dose (15 mg daily).[195] In a large prospective multicenter study the time to normalization of T_4 depended on the dose of methimazole (40 vs. 10 mg/day), the size of the goiter, the initial biochemical abnormality, and the iodine intake of the patient.[196]

The therapeutic response to effective antithyroid therapy invariably occurs after a latent period because the agents inhibit the synthesis but not the release of hormone, and in very active disease the block of thyroid hormone production may not be complete; hence reduction in the supply of hormone to the tissues does not occur until glandular hormone stores are depleted. In a small percentage of patients the TRAb stimulation of the thyroid remains very active and the response to antithyroid drugs may be unsatisfactory with an increase in the size of a highly

vascular goiter, inappropriately high serum T_3 despite high doses of drugs, and an unstable clinical condition. After a time the best solution to this inappropriate response may be surgical thyroidectomy.

When using PTU it is important to remember that the biologic activity of PTU on a weight basis is around 1:20 that of methimazole.[195] Because PTU has a shorter duration of action, the dose should be split over the day; an equivalent initial PTU dose is 100 to 200 mg every 8 hours, depending upon the severity of hyperthyroidism. The dose can be reduced to a maintenance dose of 50 to 100 mg two to three times daily as hyperthyroidism ameliorates. When large amounts are required, PTU should be administered at 4- to 6-hour intervals. Although PTU differs from methimazole in having the additional effect of inhibiting the peripheral conversion of T_4 to T_3, there appears to be little difference in the duration of the latent period when either of these agents is employed alone in the usual dosage. This is because the thyroidal and extrathyroidal effect of PTU on conversion of T_4 to T_3 is more apparent at dosages greater than 600 mg/day. This effect may be an advantage in the acute treatment of severe hyperthyroidism.[181]

Generally, improvement within the first 2 to 4 weeks includes decreased nervousness and palpitations, increased strength, and weight gain. Usually, the metabolic state becomes normal within about 6 weeks. At this time, the dosage can often be reduced substantially to maintain a normal metabolic state. During treatment, the size of the thyroid gland generally decreases in one third to one half of the patients. In the remainder, it may remain unchanged or even enlarge. In the latter situation, the change signals either an intensification of the disease process, which often requires that the dosage of drug be increased, or the onset of hypothyroidism and increased TSH secretion as a result of excessive treatment. It is important to differentiate between these causes. Clinical criteria are not the main guidelines by which the adequacy of treatment is judged. Adequacy of therapy is assessed by measurement of free T_4 in the first several months when the serum TSH level usually remains suppressed and then subsequently by TSH assessment. Mild thyrotoxicosis may persist despite a serum T_4 concentration in the normal range because the serum T_3 concentration may still be elevated typically due to intrathyroidal iodine deficiency and the increased T_3/T_4 ratio in Graves Tg. The latter phenomenon may also account for maintenance of a normal metabolic state in the setting of a subnormal serum T_4 level. Importantly, the serum TSH concentration may remain subnormal for many months. An enlarging thyroid gland in a treated patient with Graves disease may also indicate the presence of a neoplasm and should be investigated appropriately.

Antithyroid agents can cause hypothyroidism if given in excessive amounts without proper biochemical control of thyroid function. The patient may develop signs and symptoms of hypothyroidism, and the thyroid gland may increase in size secondary to increased TSH. The hypothyroidism can be reversed by reducing the dosage of the antithyroid drug or by administering supplemental thyroid hormone.

Block-and-Replace Regimens. The logic behind prescribing a full dose of a thionamide drug and adding T_4 supplements to prevent the patient from becoming hypothyroid is twofold. First, a few patients are difficult to keep euthyroid with thionamide therapy alone, and a block-and-replace regimen can be helpful and requires fewer office visits. Second, it has been speculated that an immunosuppressive action of the thionamides may be helpful in attenuating the natural history of the AITDs directly. However, a series of controlled clinical trials have showed that doses of antithyroid drugs higher than necessary to make patients euthyroid do not improve the tendency to remission of the autoimmune abnormality and only increase the risk of side effects to the drugs. Therefore, block-and-replacement therapy with high-dose antithyroid drug is not generally recommended.[194]

Predicting the Response to Drug Withdrawal. A central question in the treatment of Graves disease patients with antithyroid drugs is how to determine the appropriate duration of antithyroid drug treatment. Remission after withdrawal of treatment will persist only if the disorder has entered an inactive phase. This latter transition and the natural decline in the levels of TRAbs are more likely to occur the longer the course of treatment. Accordingly, it has been shown that the risk of relapse is higher if drugs are withdrawn after 6 months rather than after 18 months of therapy. On the other hand, no further decrease in risk was observed after more prolonged therapy in the single study that has been performed. This is the basis for the recommendation of continuing antithyroid treatment for 12 to 18 months. A major advantage of a more prolonged therapy is that nearly all patients remain euthyroid as long as therapy is given, even if the dose of the drug is low.

Up to 50% of patients may go into remission after a course of antithyroid drugs.[197] Remission rates are reported to be lower in men, older patients, smokers, and those with more active Graves disease (including higher titer of TRAbs and larger goiters).[198] Factors preventing a recurrence also include (1) a change from stimulating TRAbs to blocking antibodies, which occurs rarely, (2) the progression of concomitant autoimmune thyroiditis, and (3) iodine deficiency itself. The persistence of high levels of circulating TRAbs during treatment of Graves disease portends recurrence after withdrawal of antithyroid drugs. Whether this is helpful in the management of the individual patient has been controversial because this may be unreliable in areas of iodine deficiency. However, most patients do not have persisting high levels of TRAb, and predicting their outcome is even more difficult. Genetic typing, for example, using HLA, is also not helpful in such predictions when examining the individual patient.

Antithyroid drug therapy should generally be continued for about 12 to 18 months and then withdrawn if the serum TSH returns to normal. Therapeutic durations longer than 18 months do not increase remission rates. The average rate of remission as defined by a normal serum TSH level after withdrawal of antithyroid therapy is 30% to 50%; hence about 50% of patients relapse or are unable to stop therapy.[180,197,199] About 75% of relapses occur in the first 3 months after withdrawal of therapy. Suppression of the TSH concentration below normal levels is the first signal of relapse even in the presence of a normal serum T_4 level. Nevertheless, about one third of patients experience a lasting remission. This fact alone indicates that antithyroid agents have a significant role as the sole therapy in the initial treatment of hyperthyroid Graves disease.

Iodide Transport Inhibitors. Both thiocyanate and perchlorate inhibit thyroid iodide transport and have been used to treat hyperthyroidism. Theoretical and practical disadvantages, such as frequent side effects, preclude their use except in special circumstances. Perchlorate has been used to treat patients with amiodarone-induced hyperthyroidism.[200]

Iodine and Iodine-Containing Agents. Iodine may be administered directly or may be contained in contrast media used therapeutically. However, iodine is now rarely used as a sole therapy. The mechanism of action of iodine in relieving thyrotoxicosis differs from that of the thionamides. Although quantities of iodine in excess of several milli-

grams can acutely inhibit organic binding (acute Wolff-Chaikoff effect), this transient phenomenon probably does not contribute to the therapeutic effect. Instead, the major action of iodine is to inhibit hormone release. Administration of iodine increases glandular stores of organic iodine, but the beneficial effect of iodine is evident more quickly than the effects of even large doses of agents that inhibit hormone synthesis. In patients with Graves disease, iodine acutely retards the rate of secretion of T_4, an effect that is rapidly lost when iodine is withdrawn. These features of iodine action provide both disadvantages and advantages. The enrichment of glandular organic iodine stores that occurs when this agent is given alone may retard the clinical response to subsequently administered thionamide, and the decrease in RAIU produced by iodine prevents the use of radioiodine as treatment for several weeks. Furthermore, if iodine is withdrawn, resumption of accelerated release of hormone from an enriched glandular hormone pool may exacerbate the disorder.

Another reason for not using iodine alone is that the therapeutic response on occasion is either incomplete or absent. Even if initially effective, iodine treatment may lose its effect with time. This phenomenon, which has been termed *iodine escape*, should not be confused with the escape from the acute Wolff-Chaikoff effect (see Chapter 11).[201] Nevertheless, the rapid slowing of hormone release by iodine makes it more effective than the thionamide drugs when prompt relief of thyrotoxicosis is mandatory. Therefore, aside from its use in preparation for thyroid surgery, iodine is useful mainly in patients with actual or impending thyrotoxic crisis, severe thyrocardiac disease, or acute surgical emergencies. If iodide is used in these circumstances, it should be administered with large doses of a thionamide.

The lowest dose of iodine required for control of thyrotoxicosis is approximately 6 mg daily, although a quantity much less than that is usually given. Six milligrams of iodine is present in one eighth of a drop of saturated solution of potassium iodide (SSKI) or approximately 1 drop of Lugol solution; many physicians, however, prescribe 5 to 10 drops of one of these agents three times daily. Although it is advisable to administer amounts larger than the suggested minimal effective dose, huge quantities of iodine are more likely to produce adverse reactions. We recommend the use of a maximum of 2 to 3 drops of SSKI twice daily.

In patients who are so ill that medications cannot be taken by mouth, antithyroid agents can be triturated and administered by stomach tube; iodine can be given by the same route or can be absorbed through the oral mucosa. When use of a stomach tube is contraindicated, thionamide drugs have been administerd rectally, but there are no parenteral preparations available. Here, iodine may be administered with high-dose corticosteroids. Iodine appears to be particularly effective after administration of a therapeutic dose of ^{131}I for the rapid alleviation of thyrotoxicosis.

Reactions to Iodine. Adverse reactions to iodine are unusual and are generally not serious but may include rash, which may be acneiform; drug fever; sialadenitis; conjunctivitis and rhinitis; vasculitis; and a leukemoid eosinophilic granulocytosis. Sialadenitis may respond to reduction of dosage and the addition of lemon/lime candies to increase salivary flow; in the case of the other reactions, iodine should be stopped.

Other Antithyroid Agents

Cholecystographic Agents. In doses of 1 g daily, the iodine-containing cholecystographic contrast agent sodium ipodate (or iopanoate) causes a prompt decrease in serum T_4 and serum T_3 concentrations in patients with hyperthyroidism. However, supplies of such agents are generally no longer available.

Cholestyramine. Cholestyramine also represents an effective and well-tolerated adjunctive therapy in patients with hyperthyroid Graves disease, and it can produce a rapid and complete decline in thyroid hormone levels.

Lithium. Lithium carbonate inhibits thyroid hormone secretion, but unlike iodine, it does not interfere with the accumulation of radioiodine. Lithium, 300 to 450 mg every 8 hours, is employed only to provide temporary control of thyrotoxicosis in patients who are allergic to both thionamide and iodide. This is because the blocking effect is often lost with time. The goal is to maintain a serum lithium concentration of 1 mEq/L. Another short-term use for lithium has been as an adjunct to radioiodine therapy because the drug slows the release of iodine from the thyroid.

Dexamethasone. Dexamethasone, 2 mg every 6 hours, inhibits the peripheral conversion of T_4 to T_3 and has well-known immunosuppressive effects. The inhibitory effect of dexamethasone on the conversion of T_4 to T_3 is additive to that of PTU, suggesting a different mechanism of action. Concurrent administration of PTU, SSKI, and dexamethasone to the patient with severe life-threatening thyrotoxicosis effects a rapid reduction in serum T_3 concentration, often to within the normal range in 24 to 48 hours.[202]

Beta-Blocking Agents. Drugs that block the response to catecholamines at the receptor site (e.g., propranolol) ameliorate some of the manifestations of thyrotoxicosis and are often used as adjuncts in management. Tremulousness, palpitations, excessive sweating, eyelid retraction, and heart rate decrease; effects are rapidly manifested and appear to be mediated largely through modulating the increased sensitivity to the sympathetic nervous system induced by excess thyroid hormone. Propranolol, but not other β-adrenergic blocking agents, may also weakly block the conversion of T_4 to T_3 via a mechanism independent of its effect on catecholamine signaling. Adrenergic antagonists are most useful in the interval before the response to thionamide or radioiodine therapy occurs. They are useful in patients with thyrotoxic symptoms and especially in those with impending or actual thyrotoxic crisis (see "Thyroid Storm"). Adrenergic antagonists are especially useful when tachycardia is contributing to cardiac insufficiency. However, the fact that β-adrenergic blockade can reduce cardiac output without altering oxygen consumption may have adverse effects in some organs, such as the liver, where the arteriovenous oxygen difference is already elevated in the hyperthyroid state.[203] Moreover, thyroid hormone also has a direct stimulatory effect on the myocardium independent of the adrenergic nervous system.

Propranolol has been the most widely used agent because it is relatively free from adverse effects and has a short half-life, allowing, in theory, easy control. It can be given orally in a dose of 10 to 60 mg every 6 or 8 hours. For intravenous use, a shorter-acting agent may be preferable (see "Thyroid Storm"). Propranolol may be contraindicated in patients with asthma or chronic obstructive pulmonary disease because it aggravates bronchospasm. Because of its myocardial depressant action, it is also contraindicated in patients with heart block and in patients with congestive failure, unless severe tachycardia is a contributory factor. Beta-blocking agents such as atenolol or metoprolol are longer-acting drugs that allow a once-a-day regimen much preferred by patients.

TABLE 12-6

Complications of Surgery in 322 Patients With Graves Hyperthyroidism in Experienced Hands (1986-1995)

Complication	%
Recurrent hyperthyroidism	2.0
Vocal cord paralysis	
Transient	2.5
Permanent	0.3
Prolonged postoperative hypocalcemia (>7 days)	3.7
Permanent hypoparathyroidism	0.6

Adapted from Werga-Kjellman P, Zedenius J, Tallstedt L, et al. Surgical treatment of hyperthyroidism: a ten-year experience. *Thyroid.* 2001;11: 187-192.

Surgery

Surgery was the original treatment for Graves disease before the advent of radioiodine and the thionamide drugs. Because of the occasional recurrence of hyperthyroidism after the popular technique of subtotal thyroidectomy, the surgical procedure of choice for the treatment of Graves disease has become a near total thyroidectomy.[194]

Complications of Surgery. The hazards of thyroidectomy are inversely related to the experience and skill of the surgical team.[204] Unless circumstances are otherwise compelling, thyroidectomy should not be performed by surgeons who do the operation only occasionally. In experienced hands, the frequency of complications such as permanent hypoparathyroidism and damage to the recurrent laryngeal nerve is quite low (Table 12-6). Bleeding into the operative site, the most serious postoperative complication, can rapidly produce death by asphyxia and requires immediate evacuation of the blood and ligation of the bleeding vessel. Even with subtotal surgery, the recurrent laryngeal nerve can be damaged. If such damage is unilateral, it causes dysphonia that usually improves in a few weeks but may leave the patient slightly hoarse, especially older patients. However, intraoperative recurrent laryngeal nerve monitoring does not necessarily improve long-term outcomes.[205] Hypoparathyroidism can be either transient or permanent. Transient hypoparathyroidism results from inadvertent removal of some parathyroids and impairment of blood supply to those that remain. Depending on the severity of these insults, symptoms and signs of hypocalcemia appear, usually within 1 to 7 days after surgery. Severe hypoparathyroidism should be treated with intravenous calcium gluconate. Milder cases can be treated with oral calcium carbonate and cholecalciferol in doses of 1 g of elemental calcium and 1000 U of vitamin D three times daily. However, the hypocalcemia that occurs immediately after surgery for thyrotoxicosis may not be due to transient hypoparathyroidism, because it occurs more frequently in the Graves patient than after surgery for other thyroid disorders. Instead, it may be due to "hungry bones" because of the demineralization of bone that occurs in hyperthyroidism. This begins to be reversed after cure of the hyperthyroid state and may contribute to the modest elevation in alkaline phosphatase during recovery unless the patients have been rendered euthyroid for some time prior to surgery. The treatment of hypoparathyroidism is discussed in Chapter 28, but many surgeons who fear that they have caused damage to the parathyroid glands at total thyroidectomy may reimplant the apparent parathyroid tissue into local muscles.

Preparation for Surgery. Preoperative use of antithyroid agents has greatly decreased the morbidity and mortality rates of surgery for Graves disease because these drugs deplete glandular hormone stores and restore the metabolic state to normal. However, these agents do not improve the hyperplasia and hypervascularity of the gland in the short term unless TRAb levels fall. Iodine, however, is reported to cause a decrease in height of the follicular cells, enlargement of follicles with retention of colloid, and reduction of hypervascularity. Hence, the aim of preoperative management is to restore the metabolic state to normal with antithyroid agents and then to induce involution of the gland with iodine.[206] Patients who are to undergo thyroidectomy are first given antithyroid therapy in the manner described earlier. Often, relatively large doses are given in order to hasten the clinical response and because surgical candidates are often patients with severe disease or large goiters. In addition, iodide (SSKI 2-3 drops twice daily) should be initiated at least 7 to 10 days before surgery to decrease thyroid blood flow and vascularity and hence intraoperative blood loss during thyroidectomy.[207] During this period, a preexisting bruit or thrill may decrease in intensity or disappear entirely, and the gland may become firm.

Several cautions should be observed: no date for surgery should be set until a normal metabolic state has been restored. Much too often, the operation is planned well in advance and the patient is given a standardized regimen independent of the clinical progress. Therapy with iodide should not be started until a normal metabolic state has been restored; iodine should not be relied on to complete an as yet incomplete response to antithyroid therapy because iodide will enrich glandular hormone stores if the antithyroid drug is not entirely effective. Antithyroid agents should not be withdrawn when iodine therapy is begun. Last, checking for vitamin D deficiency well before surgery will give enough time to replenish stores in deficient patients so that any postoperative hypocalcemia can be minimized.

Beta Blockade Alone Before Thyroid Surgery. Propranolol may be a useful adjunct in controlling signs and symptoms (see earlier) while the patient is being prepared for surgery. However, propranolol has been used alone in preoperative preparation of the patient in whom surgery is to be undertaken.[208] Although this mode of therapy is probably safe and effective in many patients with mild disease, thyroid crises can still occur when patients receive propranolol alone. Restoration of the patient to a eumetabolic state, as outlined earlier, is appropriate before subjecting the patient to the stress of surgery.

Radioiodine Therapy

Radioiodine produces thyroid ablation without the complications of surgery. There has been concern that this form of therapy might produce leukemia or an increase in thyroid cell mutation rates, and a hypothetical 0.8% lifetime cancer risk attributable to a 15-mCi ^{131}I dose at the age of 20 years has been calculated.[194] However, this is only a 3% increase in baseline cancer risk, and during the half-century in which radioiodine has been in use, most studies have found no significant increase in the prevalence of thyroid or other carcinomas in adults patients treated with radioiodine.[209] The prevalence of leukemia is also no greater, and the frequency of genetic damage in the offspring of patients treated earlier with radioiodine does not appear to be increased. As long as hypothyroidism is treated appropriately, there may be no increase in mortality rate or the rate may be similar to that seen after antithyroid drug treatment.[210] In view of the lack of evidence of serious toxicity from radioiodine in doses generally employed for treating adults with hyperthyroidism, as opposed to thyroid

cancer, the age limit for the use of radioiodine has been lowered progressively by some physicians from the initial lower limit of 40 years to age 10 or younger.[211] However, in a 5-year-old child the theoretical lifetime cancer risk after 15 mCi ^{131}I is 4%, so in childhood, antithyroid drugs should continue to be the first treatment of choice. The use of radioiodine in reproductive-age women also remains unpopular, and radioiodine is contraindicated during pregnancy. Fetuses exposed to ^{131}I after 10 weeks of gestation may be born athyreotic.[212] In addition, ^{131}I should not be administered for at least 8 weeks after cessation of lactation because it is concentrated in breast milk.

Preparation for Radioiodine Therapy. Antithyroid drugs are widely used before radioiodine treatment to theoretically decrease a posttreatment increase in thyroid hormone release. Such an increase is considered especially dangerous in older age groups with ischemic heart disease in whom cardiac deaths have been reported. Antithyroid drugs may also prevent the increase in thyroid autoantibodies that occurs after radioiodine therapy and may affect ophthalmopathy.[213] Normally, such drugs are withdrawn 3 to 7 days before treatment; if needed, they can then be reintroduced 7 days after treatment.

Radioiodine Dosing. National differences in radiation regulations have considerable impact on the way radioiodine therapy is given in different countries. Attempts have been made to standardize the radiation delivered to the thyroid gland by varying the dose of radioiodine according to the size of the gland, the uptake of ^{131}I, and its subsequent rate of release (so-called dosimetry). However, such calculations do not provide uniform results, especially because the true volume of the thyroid is difficult to calculate with accuracy. In general, therefore, it is difficult to make patients suffering from Graves disease euthyroid with radioiodine therapy. Either patients become hypothyroid or they remain hyperthyroid, perhaps even exacerbated by the radioiodine-induced increase in TRAbs. Thus, most clinics have redefined the goal of radioiodine therapy from making patients euthyroid to ablating the thyroid with a permanent need for thyroid hormone replacement.

A dose of 20 mCi alleviates hyperthyroidism in almost all patients and results in approximately 90% hypothyroidism.[214-219] Some physicians have settled on an arbitrary dose calculated to result in the delivery of 300 MBq (~8 mCi) of ^{131}I to the thyroid gland 24 hours after administration. Others aim to deliver 50 to 100 Gy (5000 to 10,000 rad) to the gland. No data support an advantage of dosimetry over a fixed-dose regimen. In addition, drug-induced radioresistance has been the subject of much discussion, particularly in relation to PTU, but it is not a major issue,[214] and a meta-analysis reported that methimazole therapy may also be associated with a similar small decrease in radioiodine efficacy of no practical import.[220] Because ^{131}I administration is contraindicated during pregnancy, a pregnancy test should be carried out in women of childbearing age before ^{131}I therapy is initiated.[221]

Treatment After Radioiodine Therapy. Treatment with antithyroid drugs after radioiodine therapy should be avoided for about 1 week because they may reduce the success of treatment, particularly if nonablative doses are used, via their acceleration of ^{131}I release.[222] Although exacerbation of thyrotoxicosis after radioiodine therapy is rare, methimazole use after radioiodine therapy should always be considered in patients with severe hyperthyroidism and other comorbid conditions. Clearly, it is important to monitor T_4 and T_3 levels in at-risk patients and to consider β-adrenergic blockade whether or not antithyroid drugs are used before or after radioiodine treatment. Patients are seen at 4-week intervals after ^{131}I administration, monitored by serum T_4

and TSH levels, and hypothyroidism is treated if it appears. Women planning to become pregnant are advised to wait for an arbitrary period of at least 6 months after ^{131}I therapy to allow for resolution of any transient effects of gonadal radiation and stabilization of thyroid function. If, after a period of 6 months, hyperthyroidism is still present and the patient is symptomatic, the treatment is repeated, generally with about 1.5 times the initial dose of ^{131}I or an ablative amount.

Complications of Radioiodine Therapy

#1—Thyroid Cancer From Low-Level Radiation Exposure. There is no increase in thyroid cancer or any other cancer following the diagnostic and therapeutic use of radioiodine in hyperthyroid adults.[209,223] There remain, however, concerns about a potential increased prevalence of thyroid carcinoma in patients treated with low amounts of radiation in childhood or adolescence as exemplified by the massive increase in childhood thyroid cancer in the United States after external neck radiation given for various benign disorders and the large increase in prevalence of thyroid cancer in children exposed to the Chernobyl radiation.[224,225] In Chernobyl the exposure for most of the children who developed thyroid carcinoma was to relatively low doses of radiation rather than the thyrodestructive doses prescribed in hyperthyroidism.[226] Nevertheless, many physicians think that the use of radioactivity in children should be avoided whenever possible.

#2—Mortality Rate After Radioiodine Therapy. Patients treated with radioiodine for hyperthyroidism had increased mortality rate versus age- and period-specific mortality rates.[227] This effect was not seen in patients rendered hypothyroid, and these findings further support the practice of treating hyperthyroidism with doses of radioiodine sufficient to induce overt hypothyroidism. An association was seen in this study with mortality rate from ischemic heart disease in patients with subclinical hypothyroidism, suggesting that T_4 replacement should be considered for this biochemical abnormality.[228]

#3—Hypothyroidism After Radioiodine Therapy. In theory, the therapeutic goal of ^{131}I administration is to induce euthyroidism so that Graves disease cannot recur. However, the incidence of hypothyroidism is significant during the first year or two after treatment with radioactive iodine, regardless of how the dose is calculated, and with ablative doses hypothyroidism normally occurs quite rapidly. Even with nonablative doses the rate of hypothyroidism continues to increase approximately 5% per year thereafter. The actual incidence depends upon the dose of radioiodine prescribed by the dosimetry or use of a standard dose.[229,230] When the dose delivered is an ablative dose, then permanent hypothyroidism will ensue in more than 80% of patients by 6 months. Many physicians prefer the certainty of induced hypothyroidism rather than the wait-and-see approach.

#4—Radiation Thyroiditis. The early induction of euthyroidism and later the development of hypothyroidism are both consequences of radiation-induced destruction of thyroid parenchyma. With the larger doses of radioactive iodine, a tender radiation thyroiditis may develop within the first week of treatment, as evidenced by epithelial swelling and necrosis, disruption of follicular architecture, edema, and infiltration with mononuclear cells. Resolution of the acute phase is followed by fibrosis, vascular narrowing, and further lymphocytic infiltration. Radiation thyroiditis may lead to an exacerbation of thyrotoxicosis 10 to 14 days after radioiodine is administered, with occasionally serious consequences, including precipitation of a thyrotoxic crisis and aggravation of patients with severe thyrotoxicosis or cardiac insufficiency. In thyrocardiac disease, therefore, antithyroid drugs should always be given for several months before radioiodine is given in order to deplete glandular hormone stores, and a β-adrenergic blocking regimen is initiated to limit any potential arrhythmias if appropriate. Antithyroid drugs prevent an outpouring of hormone if severe radiation thyroiditis should occur. The antithyroid agent should be withdrawn 3 to 7 days before administration of the radioiodine; if the clinical condition warrants, the agent can be started again 1 week later.

#5—Orbitopathy and Radioiodine Therapy. As discussed earlier, GO is probably the result of a crossover specificity between retroorbital and thyroid antigens, including the TSHR itself. Any worsening of the autoimmune thyroid response might therefore worsen the orbital immune response. Following radioiodine therapy, the levels of circulating TRAbs are elevated most strikingly,[231] perhaps secondary to impairment of immune restraint caused by the intrathyroidal irradiation that renders regulatory cells more sensitive. This change is in keeping with exacerbation of pretibial myxedema after radioiodine administration.[215] Similarly, carefully conducted studies indicate that significant eye disease worsens in about 10% of patients with GO who are treated with radioiodine (Fig. 12-10),[232,233] although this finding may not apply in mild disease.[234] Deterioration, if any, is usually mild and temporary but on occasion can involve a dramatic worsening. Hypothyroidism following radioiodine therapy increases the risk for development or worsening of orbitopathy.[235] Therefore, thyroid hormone levels are often initially measured 6 to 8 weeks following the treatment so that T_4 replacement can be started prior to the development of overt hypothyroidism.

Some physicians advocate the use of glucocorticoids at the time of radioiodine treatment to prevent such effects.[147,236] One regimen involves prednisone, 0.4 to 0.5 mg/kg 1 month before ^{131}I treatment, with a gradual tapering over 3 to 4 months. However, maneuvers such as careful control of thyroid function before and after therapy and cessation of smoking by the patient may also help minimize ocular changes. We do not advocate the use of radioiodine in patients with severe Graves ophthalmopathy unless steroid therapy is provided.

#6—Secondary Malignancies. The risk of long-term development of a malignancy after radiodine treatment has been found to be slightly increased in patients receiving large doses for thyroid cancer,[237] but a similar increased risk has not been reported in patients with Graves disease.

#7—Other Side Effects of Radioiodine. Additional hazards may attend the use of radioiodine, particularly in large doses. The parathyroid glands are exposed to radiation in patients treated with radioiodine. Although parathyroid reserve may be diminished in some patients, development of overt hypoparathyroidism is rare. The effect of radioiodine on other tissues that concentrate iodide (e.g., the salivary glands, the gastric glands, and the breasts) has often had attention but is not likely to be a problem with the relatively low doses prescribed for Graves disease when compared to the doses used for treatment of thyroid cancer.

Choice of Therapy

The choice of therapy for thyrotoxicosis is influenced by the experience of the treating clinician, emotional attitudes, economic considerations, and family and personal issues. Our choice of therapy takes into account the natural history of the disease, the advantages and disadvantages of the available therapies, and the features of the population group in which the patient falls. Apart from patients directly requesting surgery, this procedure is recommended only when the shortcomings of other modes of therapy are of particular importance (e.g., patients with antithyroid

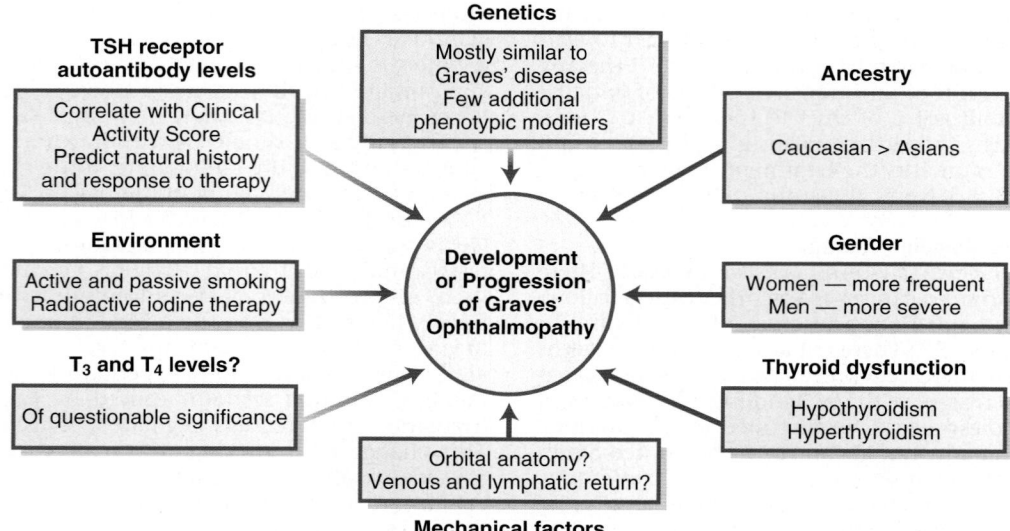

Figure 12-10 Probability of the development or worsening of orbitopathy in patients with Graves disease. T₃, triiodothyronine; T₄, thyroxine; TSH, thyroid-stimulating hormone. (From Stan MN, Bahn RS. Risk factors for development or deterioration of Graves' ophthalmopathy. *Thyroid.* 2010;20:777-783.)

drug allergy, a coincident cold nodule, patients with very large goiters, and patients with the need for a rapid return to normal). Occasionally, in young adults, it is necessary to remove a diffuse toxic goiter because of obstructive symptoms or cosmetic disfigurement. Nevertheless, only a small percentage of patients with Graves disease are now recommended for surgery in the United States. The choice, therefore, is among antithyroid drugs, radioiodine therapy, or a mixture of both.

In one common approach to therapy in adults, the physician initiates treatment with antithyroid drugs in all patients to produce a euthyroid state before reaching a final decision regarding a definitive therapeutic strategy. This step allows the patient to return to a euthyroid status as rapidly as possible and provides an estimate of the antithyroid drug dose requirement. The magnitude of the drug requirement and the size of the thyroid gland are two of a number of factors considered in the evaluation of the patient with regard to the likelihood of a remission. The options for treatment are explained to the patient during these first months of contact, and individual recommendations are then formulated. This approach allows the establishment of a workable physician-patient relationship, which is especially important in addressing anxieties about the use of radioiodine. Such concerns lead many patients, especially those younger than 50 years of age, to elect a prolonged trial of antithyroid drugs before definitive therapy with ¹³¹I.

Antithyroid drug therapy may be especially preferable in patients predicted to have a higher rate of remission. Patients with a large thyroid gland, a maintenance thionamide dose requirement of more than 10 mg of methimazole (or carbimazole equivalent), or high titers of TRAbs are likely to require prolonged antithyroid treatment and should be advised that the chance of spontaneous remission is a lot lower than 30%. A therapeutic trial is generally pursued for 12 months if long-term thionamide therapy is selected. One can, in theory, treat forever unless side effects occur.

When a decision in favor of radioiodine is made, ¹³¹I may be prescribed at a dose designed to result in the retention of about 300 MBq (8 mCi) ¹³¹I in the thyroid gland at 24 hours, or an ablative dose (20 mCi) may be prescribed. Radioiodine therapy may be used in young women desiring pregnancy but they should wait 6 months after ¹³¹I administration. Nevertheless, the long-term persistence of TRAbs after radioidine in many patients[146] raises the possibility of their transplacental passage, further complicating a pregnancy that already requires adjustment of levothyroxine dosages.

Hypothyroidism in the Recently Hyperthyroid Patient

The early onset of hypothyroidism may cause distinct symptoms in the previously thyrotoxic patient after ¹³¹I or surgical treatment or even with high doses of thionamide drugs. Such patients may develop severe muscle cramps, often in large muscle groups such as the trapezius or latissimus dorsi or the proximal muscles of the extremities. Such symptoms can develop even when the serum hormone levels are only low-normal or slightly decreased and before the serum TSH concentration has risen. It is possible to mistake a symptom such as back or hip pain for an unrelated illness and the patient should be warned in advance. It is also not unusual for patients to complain of hypothyroid symptoms when thyroid function test results return to within the normal range. Such patients appear to have trouble adjusting to the normal thyroid hormone levels after being exposed to excessive amounts for long periods. Weight gain is a frequent complaint after recovery from chronic thyrotoxicosis, and patients should be cautioned regarding their diet.[238]

Treatment of Graves Orbitopathy

GO varies in severity from the common mild form to a severe form that threatens vision. The latter type is rare and remains difficult to treat. The natural course of the disorder, which is variable and characterized by exacerbations and remissions, makes conclusions about the efficacy of any treatment difficult.[239] A further source of confusion is the variable terminology for describing the manifestations of orbitopathy and the lack of rigid criteria for defining their severity. Use of a clinical activity score to grade disease activity and quantitative measures of severity are strongly recommended for clinical practice (see Table 12-4).

Effect of Treatment of the Thyroid Gland on Orbitopathy. The first question that arises is whether different treatments for thyrotoxicosis affect the course of the eye disease differently. Subtotal or total thyroidectomy and thionamide drug therapy do not often influence orbitopathy unless they lead to the development of hypothyroidism,[240] although some experienced investigators have reported that total thyroidectomy followed by thyroid ablation of any remnant favors a better long-term outcome for this disorder.[241] However, both hypothyroidism and hyperthyroidism from any cause has an adverse effect on the disorder, and the patients should be promptly rendered euthyroid when it occurs. As discussed earlier, carefully controlled studies suggest that radioiodine treatment may lead to a slight but significant worsening of orbitopathy (see earlier discussion), and it may be best to avoid radioiodine in patients with active moderate to severe eye disease.[174] Alternatively, as mentioned earlier, coincidental glucocorticoid therapy may prevent deterioration of mild orbitopathy after radioiodine but may itself cause significant side effects.[236]

Symptomatic Treatment. With milder forms, little treatment other than symptomatic measures is required. The patient who experiences photophobia and sensitivity to wind or cold air can benefit from wearing dark glasses, which also afford protection from foreign bodies. Elevation of the head of the bed at night and use of ocular lubricants, such as 1% methylcellulose, may help when the eyelids do not close completely during sleep. Artificial tears can be used during the day. Because the ophthalmic manifestations tend to be self-limited and the progression to a more severe form is uncommon, such measures usually suffice to tide the patient over until the disorder regresses spontaneously.[165]

Glucocorticoids. The appearance of severe inflammatory manifestations, including conjunctival or periorbital erythema, chemosis, and eye pain with motion, warrants the use of more vigorous therapeutic measures.[242] Such changes, even when severe, may respond favorably and rapidly to glucocorticoids. Intravenous methylprednisolone pulse therapy (such as 500 mg initially and then 250 mg weekly for 6 weeks) has been shown to have fewer side effects than equivalent doses of oral prednisone and to have a more rapid onset of effectiveness.[1,243,244] Although liver necrosis has been reported in patients with orbitopathy given this treatment, total doses below 8 g total appear not to be hepatotoxic.[245] In the past decade, experience with intravenous methylprednisolone in both the United States and Europe has led to its becoming the initial therapy of choice for most patients with active moderate to severe orbitopathy[246] with the expectation that it will help at least 40% of these patients.[247]

External Radiation. The value of external radiation to the orbits has been established in some, but not all, clinical trials.[248-250] This treatment appears to be steroid-sparing rather than steroid-replacing therapy and is said by some to work best in combination, especially early in the onset of the disorder.[147,246] Side effects of orbital irradiation have included the development of blindness and retinal angiogenesis, and the presence of diabetes mellitus is a clear contraindication to this approach. The safe administration of highly collimated supervoltage radiation to the orbital space, therefore, requires experienced personnel.

Orbital Decompression. If glucocorticoid therapy or external radiation (or both) does not halt progression of the disease or if loss of vision is threatened either by ulceration or infection of the cornea or by changes in the retina or optic

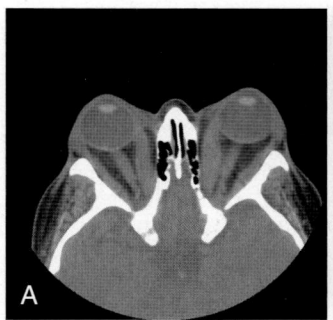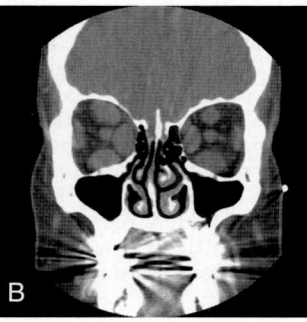

Figure 12-11 Axial (**A**) and coronal (**B**) computed tomographic scans of a patient with Graves orbitopathy demonstrating generalized enlargement of all extraocular muscles, expansion of the orbital fat, and marked bilateral proptosis.

nerve, orbital decompression can be performed by a variety of techniques.[251,252] In some patients, a desire for a nearly complete cosmetic correction may be such that decompression surgery is also the only satisfactory route. This procedure usually involves removal of either the lateral wall or the roof of the orbit or resection of the lateral wall of the ethmoid sinus and the roof of the maxillary sinus (Fig. 12-11). However, the operation often causes or worsens diplopia, and even in the best of hands corrective muscle surgery is necessary at a later stage. Overall, however, results are usually good in 95% of patients and up to a 5.0-mm reduction in proptosis can be achieved in experienced hands.

Newer Treatments for Graves Orbitopathy. The search for an immunosuppressive approach to GO has been long and tortuous. Without knowing the precise immunopathology such an approach cannot be disease specific. However, recent use of an anti–B cell monoclonal antibody (rituximab) has produced some beneficial results following single-dose treatments.[219] Unfortunately, side effects of this therapy may also occur, including the transient induction of dysthyroid optic neuropathy, which may threaten vision.[216] Carefully controlled trials now under way will decide whether this approach is suitable for general clinical use.[253]

An Approach to the Treatment of Orbitopathy. A trial of intravenous (or oral) glucocorticoid therapy for patients with active and severe or progressive orbitopathy is generally the initial approach to therapy. If a positive effect is not seen within a few weeks, a course of external radiation may be attempted in suitable patients if edema predominates and the expertise is available. Along with this treatment, local symptomatic measures should be employed. Ulceration and infection of the cornea should be promptly treated with antibiotics, lubricants, and protective shields. An attempt to close the eyelids by means of sutures (tarsorrhaphy) should be performed only by an experienced ophthalmologist because sutures may tear loose and cause scarring.

The management of severe orbitopathy should never be undertaken by the endocrinologist or by the ophthalmologist acting alone. Close, coordinated observation of the effects of medical therapy and the progress of the disease is necessary to determine whether and when surgery is appropriate.[171] Surgery or high-dose intravenous glucocorticoid therapy almost invariably will preserve vision if undertaken promptly when signs and symptoms of dysthyroid optic neuropathy appear. This decision is influenced by the ability of the available surgical team because the degree of success of such procedures is proportional to experience.

Treatment of Thyroid Dermopathy. Treatment of thyroid dermopathy is optimized only if initiated as soon as the condition is recognized. The application of a topical, high-potency glucocorticoid preparation with an occlusive dressing may cause regression or disappearance of the lesion.[217] Recently, rituximab has been observed to improve this condition in isolated case reports and requires further study for appropriate dosing[218,254,255] Unfortunately, many such lesions do not completely regress with treatment and can be troublesome for the long term. Long-standing untreated dermopathy is more resistant to treatment than new lesions (see Fig. 12-7).

Thyroid Storm (Accelerated Hyperthyroidism)

Thyroid storm, better called *accelerated hyperthyroidism*, is an extreme accentuation of thyrotoxicosis. It is an uncommon but serious complication, usually occurring in association with Graves disease but sometimes with toxic multinodular goiter in the elderly patient. It has a habit of causing panic in physicians because of its continuing high mortality rate.[256]

Presentation

Thyroid storm is usually of abrupt onset and occurs in patients in whom preexisting thyrotoxicosis has been treated incompletely or has not been treated at all. The condition is usually precipitated by infection, trauma, surgical emergencies, or operations and, less commonly, by radiation thyroiditis, diabetic ketoacidosis, toxemia of pregnancy, or parturition. The mechanism by which such factors worsen thyrotoxicosis may be related to cytokine release and acute immunologic disturbance caused by the precipitating condition. The serum thyroid hormone levels in crisis are not appreciably greater than those in severe uncomplicated thyrotoxicosis, but the patient can no longer adapt to the metabolic stress.

The clinical picture is one of severe hypermetabolism. Fever is almost invariable and may be severe; sweating is profuse. Marked tachycardia of sinus or ectopic origin and arrhythmias may be accompanied by pulmonary edema or congestive heart failure. Tremulousness and restlessness are present; delirium or frank psychosis may supervene. Nausea, vomiting, and abdominal pain may occur early in the course. As the disorder progresses, apathy, stupor, and coma may supervene, and hypotension can develop. If unrecognized, the condition may be fatal. This clinical picture in a patient with a history of preexisting thyrotoxicosis or with goiter or exophthalmos or both is sufficient to establish the diagnosis, and emergency treatment should not await laboratory confirmation. Thyroid storm in pregnancy is particularly treacherous for mother and child and must be taken most seriously. A clinical score (Table 12-7) can be used to help confirm the diagnosis.

Even with this approach, there are no foolproof criteria by which severe thyrotoxicosis complicated by some other serious disease can be distinguished from thyrotoxic crisis induced by that disease. In any event, the differentiation between these alternatives is of no great significance because treatment of the two is the same.

Treatment of Thyroid Storm

Treatment aims to correct both the severe thyrotoxicosis and the precipitating illness and to provide general support. There are no clinical trials of treatment for accelerated thyrotoxicosis, and opinions vary to some degree on the details, in particular the doses of antithyroid drugs that

TABLE 12-7
Diagnostic Criteria for Thyroid Storm

Diagnostic Parameter	Points*
Temperature (° F)	
99-99.9	5
100-100.9	10
101-101.9	15
102-102.9	20
103-103.9	25
≥104.0	30
Central Nervous System Effects	
Absent	0
Mild (agitation)	10
Moderate (delirium, psychosis, extreme lethargy)	20
Severe (seizures, coma)	30
Gastrointestinal-Hepatic Dysfunction	
Absent	0
Moderate (diarrhea, nausea/vomiting, abdominal pain)	10
Severe (unexplained jaundice)	20
Cardiovascular Dysfunction	
Tachycardia (beats/min)	
90-109	5
110-119	10
120-129	15
130-139	20
≥140	25
Congestive Heart Failure	
Absent	0
Mild (pedal edema)	5
Moderate (bibasilar rales)	10
Severe (pulmonary edema)	15
Atrial Fibrillation	
Absent	0
Present	10
Precipitating Event	
Absent	0
Present	10

*Scoring system: A score of 45 or greater is highly suggestive of thyroid storm; 25-44 is suggestive of impending storm, and <25 is unlikely to represent thyroid storm.
Adapted from Burch HB, Wartofsky L. Life-threatening thyrotoxicosis: thyroid storm. *Endocrinol Metab Clin North Am.* 1993;22:263-277.

should be used. However, all agree that the patient thought to have thyroid storm should be monitored in a medical intensive care unit during the initial phases of therapy. The therapy itself is designed to inhibit hormone synthesis and release and to antagonize the increased sensitivity to adrenergic stimulation mediated by severe thyrotoxicosis and to combat the hyperpyrexia.[202,257]

Large doses of an antithyroid agent (up to 400 mg of PTU every 4-6 hours) are given by mouth, by stomach tube, or, if necessary, per rectum. PTU is preferable to methimazole because it has the additional action of inhibiting the peripheral as well as the thyroidal generation of T_3 from T_4 by the type 1 iodothyronine deiodinase, which is the major source of the T_3.[181,182,258,259] Administration of PTU initiates therapy for the postcrisis period and prevents enrichment of glandular hormone stores by iodide, whose administration is of more immediate importance. The latter, administered either as SSKI (three drops twice daily) or the equivalent as Lugol solution (10 drops twice daily), acutely retards the release of preformed hormone from the thyroid gland.

Theoretically, PTU is administered before iodine to inhibit the synthesis of additional thyroid hormone from the administered iodine. Nonetheless, because iodide blocks its own organification through the Wolff-Chaikoff effect, its administration should not be delayed (until the availability of a thionamide) or omitted in the severely toxic patient in the absence of known allergy to iodide per se.

Large doses of dexamethasone (8 mg orally once daily) or hydrocortisone (150 mg every 8 hours) should be given to support the response to stress and inhibit both the release of hormone from the gland and possibly the peripheral generation of T_3 from T_4, synergizing with iodide and PTU, respectively, in these actions. Indeed, the combined use of PTU, iodide, and glucocorticoids can restore the concentration of T_3 to normal within 24 to 48 hours.[181] In the absence of cardiac insufficiency or asthma a β-adrenergic blocking agent should be given to ameliorate the hyperadrenergic state. Most experience has been with propranolol given at a dose of 40 to 80 mg orally every 6 hours, but a very short-acting β-adrenergic blocker such as labetalol or esmolol may be safer than propranolol in this situation. High-output congestive heart failure can develop in patients with severe thyrotoxicosis, and a β-adrenergic antagonist may further reduce cardiac output. If β-adrenergic blocking agents are contraindicated, a calcium channel blocker (diltiazem) may be used to slow the heart rate.

Supportive measures include correction of dehydration and hypernatremia, if present, and administration of glucose. Hyperpyrexia should be treated vigorously and the administration of a wide-spectrum antibiotic is appropriate after blood and urine cultures have been taken. In mild cases, acetaminophen may help, but a cold blanket or ice packs may be required. Salicylates should be avoided because they compete with T_3 and T_4 for binding to TBG and transthyretin (TTR) and therefore increase the free hormone levels. In addition, high doses of salicylates increase the metabolic rate. If heart failure or pulmonary congestion is present, appropriate diuretics are indicated. In patients with atrial fibrillation, the rapid ventricular response requires appropriate blockade of atrioventricular node conduction.

When treatment is successful, improvement is usually manifested within 1 or 2 days and recovery occurs within a week. At this time, the dexamethasone can be tapered and plans for long-term management made.

PREGNANCY AND THE THYROID

Human Chorionic Gonadotropin

hCG is a glycoprotein heterodimer composed of an α-subunit (identical to that of TSH, LH, and FSH) and a specific β-subunit, which has similarity to TSH. This glycoprotein binds and stimulates the hTSHR,[260-262] with an in vitro potency of about 1 U hCG = 0.7 µU of human TSH, depending on its carbohydrate content. In high concentrations hCG will cause hyperthyroidism characterized by a diffuse goiter, elevated free T_4, and suppressed TSH.

Transient Gestational Thyrotoxicosis

In the late first trimester of normal pregnancy there is often a physiologic mild transient gestational thyrotoxicosis (GTT) or hyperthyroidism. An exaggeration of this physiologic increase in thyroid stimulation in the first trimester may also be seen in some women and is associated with high levels of hCG (100,000-200,000 U/L), such as those found in twin pregnancies, and is often accompanied by hyperemesis.[263-265] In most patients, the condition is self-limited and the risk of birth defects warrants against the use of antithyroid drugs in early pregnancy, but in rare circumstances low doses of PTU (100-200 mg day or less) may be required for a few weeks until the hCG falls spontaneously. It may be difficult to separate this syndrome from early Graves disease, and a TRAb test may be helpful.[130]

Abnormal Responses to hCG

A few patients have been reported with an inherited variant of GTT in which a mutation in the TSHR gene resulted in a receptor protein with an increase in its responsiveness to hCG.[266] Such patients develop hyperthyroidism with each pregnancy because of even physiologic serum hCG concentrations. Similarly, the use of gonadotropins in in vitro fertilization and indirectly the use of GnRH agonists have all been associated with cases of thyroid dysfunction.[267]

Graves Disease During Pregnancy and the Postpartum Period

Although seen more regularly in clinical practice, a truly overactive thyroid gland is uncommon in established pregnancy, affecting approximately 0.2% of women. This low rate is because pregnancy tends to suppress autoimmune responses during pregnancy (Table 12-8), and Graves disease, an autoimmune disorder, is the most common cause of thyrotoxicosis in young women. Furthermore, although thyrotoxicosis has a variety of negative influences on fertility itself, it is also associated with increased pregnancy loss and serious medical complications for both the mother and the infant if it should persist.[38,39,134,268,269] More commonly, a woman under treatment for hyperthyroidism becomes pregnant. Whatever the sequence, pregnancy complicates the diagnosis and treatment of hyperthyroidism in Graves disease and influences its severity and course.

Influence of Pregnancy on the Immune System

The development of pregnancy and the growth of the placenta have profound influences on the immune system, as discussed earlier (see Risk Factor #5). The overall suppression of autoimmune responses, which occurs in pregnancy and is mediated by a variety of placental factors, is designed to allow the fetus with its 50% paternal antigens to survive immune assault[270,271] (see Table 12-8). These changes promote maternal-fetal tolerance, but the increased role of the regulatory T cells and their suppression of maternal responses to the fetus appears to be predominant

TABLE 12-8
Mechanisms of Immunosuppression in Pregnancy Leading to Immune Privilege

Maternal Peripheral Immune System

Regulatory T cells suppress fetal-reactive immune cells.
Sex steroids affect the immune system and negatively regulate B cells.

Maternal-Fetal Interface (Trophoblast–Immune Cell Interaction)

Apoptosis is induced in activated T cells by Fas expression on trophoblast cells.
T-cell proliferation is inhibited by local cytokines and chemokines.
Natural killer cells are inhibited by expression of human leukocyte antigen G (HLA-G).
Complement system is inactivated.

and long lived.[123,272] It has been shown that a major shift in such T-cell control reduces the effectiveness of all inflammatory T cells.

Fetal Microchimerism

In normal pregnancy, cells pass from mother to child and from child to mother. The presence of fetal microchimerism in parous women has been shown to persist for over 20 years,[273] indicating complete tolerance for the fetal cells. This exaggerated and long-lasting form of the immunosuppression of pregnancy, described earlier, is further exaggerated in patients with AITD.[274] Whether such cells can activate or reactivate an immune response as tolerance fades in the postpartum period has been the subject of much speculation, fueled by the apparent accumulation of fetal cells at sites of inflammation, including the thyroid, but the hypothesis remains unproved.[275,276] However, fetal microchimerism has also been associated with Graves disease–susceptible HLA haplotypes,[277] and a failure of fetal tolerance remains a possible contributing mechanism to postpartum thyroid disease.

Thyroid Antibodies in Pregnant Patients With Graves Disease

The hallmark of the immune effects initiated by the placenta is the fall in thyroid autoantibody secretion—TPO-Ab, Tg-Ab, and TRAbs—that is seen in almost all patients as pregnancy progresses.[278,279] This is now considered secondary to enhanced regulatory T-cell activity[280] and precedes a rapid increase in autoantibody levels after the immunosuppression is lost in the postpartum period. Assays for TRAbs in the serum of pregnant women with Graves disease may be of clinical value in selected cases because a failure of this immunosuppression may indicate potential fetal problems.[64,65] Because maternal antibodies cross the placenta, there is a correlation between the maternal level of stimulatory TRAbs and the development of fetal thyrotoxicosis. Fortunately, fetal and neonatal thyrotoxicosis occurs in only 1% of infants of mothers with Graves disease, and high levels of TRAbs, usually greater than three times the upper normal limit, are correlated with fetal thyroid stimulation.[132,281] Pregnant women at risk for failure to suppress thyroid autoantibodies include those with more severe hyperthyroidism and those with significant GO or infiltrative dermopathy. In addition, the prior treatment of the mother, especially with radioiodine, may not always be accompanied by a sufficient reduction in TRAbs. Thus, the fetus of a treated patient with Graves disease may still be at risk for development of fetal or neonatal thyrotoxicosis, and the mother may need antithyroid drug treatment and the fetus monitored by umbilical cord blood testing and ultrasonography.[282]

Differential Diagnosis

When mild thyrotoxicosis is present during early pregnancy, it may be due to GTT secondary to hCG stimulation of the thyroid gland (see later).[283,284] When it is more severe it is usually due to Graves disease because toxic multinodular goiters and hot nodules are uncommon in this age group.

Diagnosis

Pregnancy and hyperthyroidism are both accompanied by thyroid stimulation, a hyperdynamic circulation, and hypermetabolism. Note that amenorrhea may occur in thyrotoxicosis not associated with pregnancy. In pregnancy, serum TBG levels are increased by estrogen-induced changes in glycosylation, which increases TBG production and lengthens its half-life, and thus in both conditions, the total serum T_4 and T_3 levels are elevated so that the upper limit of the normal range during second and third trimesters of gestation is about 1.5 times the upper nonpregnant reference limit.[132] However, serum free T_4 levels, as measured by both analogue and equilibrium dialysis methodologies, may actually decrease as pregnancy progresses and the normal third trimester reference range for a given assay is significantly less than its nonpregnant reference range. Serum TSH levels also tend to decrease in early pregnancy, especially in women who already have a relatively low TSH, reaching a nadir between the 8th and 14th gestational weeks because of stimulation of the thyroid gland by hCG during this interval (GTT), as discussed earlier. The 95th percentile confidence interval lower limits for serum TSH levels are 0.06 mU/L, 0.3 mU/L, and 0.3 mU/L, respectively, for the first, second, and third trimesters. Nevertheless, each laboratory needs to establish its own normal ranges for thyroid testing in pregnancy.[285,286]

Biochemically, the diagnosis of thyrotoxicosis is confirmed when the serum TSH level is below the trimester specific lower limit and the total or free T_4 levels are above the normative range for pregnancy (Fig. 12-12). Detection of TRAbs can confirm the diagnosis of Graves disease, which may or may not be obvious from the clinical history and examination.

Treatment During Pregnancy

Hyperthyroidism in pregnancy is associated with a variety of complications for mother and child (Table 12-9). Although mild hyperthyroidism in pregnancy does not lead to a significant increase in risk for mother or fetus, severe thyrotoxicosis can lead to many complications and endanger the life of the mother and fetus. Furthermore, the management of hyperthyroidism during pregnancy can be an even greater problem than its diagnosis. Graves disease can worsen in the first trimester, but the subsequent trimesters have an attenuating influence on the hyperthyroid state because of the immunosuppression associated with pregnancy. Pregnancy is also one of the few clinical situations in which an assay of the biologic activity of the TRAbs is helpful in predicting its potential effect on the newborn. This assay is especially useful in pregnant women

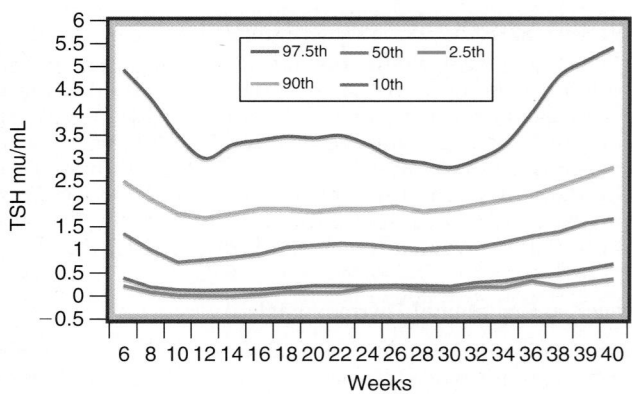

Figure 12-12 Gestation age-specific thyroid-stimulating hormone nomogram derived from 13,599 singleton and 132 twin pregnancies. Different percentiles are shown by colored lines. (From Dashe JS, Casey BM, Wells CE, et al. Thyroid-stimulating hormone in singleton and twin pregnancy: importance of gestational age-specific reference ranges. *Obstet Gynecol.* 2005;106:753-757.)

TABLE 12-9
Complications of Hyperthyroidism in Pregnancy

Increased and recurrent pregnancy loss
Preterm delivery
Preeclampsia
Fetal growth restriction
Fetal thyroid hyperfunction or hypofunction caused by TRAbs
Fetal goiter from excessive antithyroid drug treatment
Neonatal thyrotoxicosis
Increased perinatal and maternal mortality risk
Potential for decreased IQ of offspring because of excessive use of antithyroid drugs

IQ, intelligence quotient; TRAbs, thyrotropin receptor antibodies.

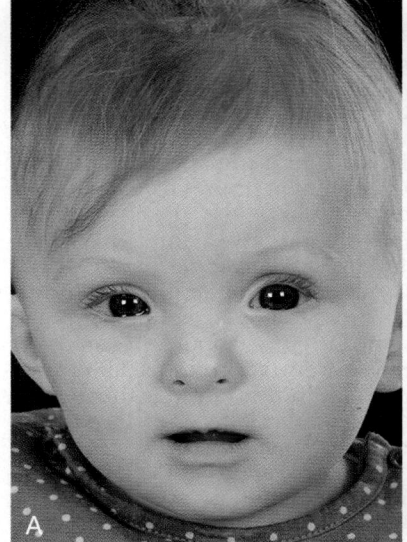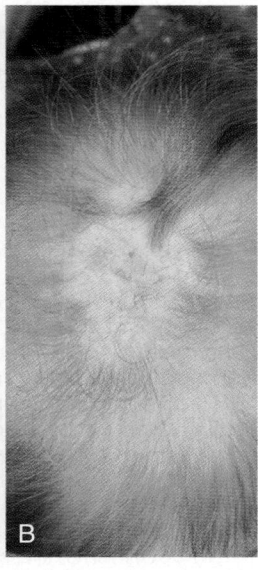

Figure 12-13 Examples of methimazole embryopathy: **A,** Dysmorphic astigmatism. **B,** Aplasia cutis. (From Bowman P, Osborne NJ, Sturley R, et al. Carbimazole embryopathy: implications for the choice of antithyroid drugs in pregnancy. *Q J Med.* 2012;105:189-193.)

who previously received ablative therapy for Graves hyperthyroidism and who still have high levels of TRAb.

Antithyroid Drugs in Pregnancy. Medical therapy is the method of choice in pregnancy. Because of the usual improvement in the disease, the dosage of antithyroid drug required to control the disease in the later phases of pregnancy is generally much less than that required in the same patient were she not pregnant. Overtreatment of the hyperthyroid pregnant woman remains a common but avoidable clinical problem with potentially severe consequences for the fetus. Thus, the clinician should prefer mild undertreatment to the risk of hypothyroidism.[282,287-289] Therefore, it is imperative for the clinician to understand the therapeutic targets for titrating antithyroid drug dosages during pregnancy.[290]

Certain aspects of placental physiology are relevant to the use of antithyroid drugs. PTU and methimazole readily and rapidly cross the placenta equally well and are concentrated in the fetal thyroid. In excess quantity these agents can cause goitrous hypothyroidism in the fetus.[291] Maternal T_4 crosses the placenta (as evidenced by infants born with significant circulating serum T_4 concentrations despite congenital hypothyroidism) and is the major source of fetal thyroid hormone prior to the complete functional development of the hypothalamic-pituitary axis in the fetus at around 20 weeks of gestation. Furthermore, the transplacental passage of maternal TRAbs in the latter half of pregnancy can result in fetal thyroid stimulation. Therefore, the fetal thyroid is subject to the same factors that influence maternal thyroid hormone production.

Until recently, the antithyroid drug of choice throughout pregnancy in the United States was PTU, but because of the rare yet serious side effect of PTU-induced hepatic failure (see Table 12-5), in June 2009 the FDA issued an advisory that PTU should be reserved for the first trimester of pregnancy while organogenesis is occurring[193] (see later). Subsequently, methimazole could be prescribed. One must keep in mind that the therapeutic antithyroid potency ratio of methimazole to PTU is around 20:1. Thus, a patient who requires only 50 mg of PTU in the first trimester may be given 2.5 mg methimazole, and she may not even require a thionamide during the later part of pregnancy. Of course, the best practice is to ensure definitive treatment prior to pregnancy so that antithyroid drugs are not needed at all.

Danger of Antithyroid Drugs in Pregnancy. The first report of birth defects after maternal use of antithyroid drugs was a brief letter reporting on congenital scalp skin defects after the use of methimazole.[292,293] Subsequently, several case reports confirmed the association and other types of defects were also described.[294] Such defects included a specific combination of facial features, and the condition was termed *methimazole/carbimazole embryopathy.* Because PTU was not at first associated with such birth defects, guidelines have been proposed that recommend the use of PTU in the first trimester and to consider shifting from methimazole to PTU in women planning a pregnancy.[295,296] Recent larger studies have since expanded our knowledge on methimazole-associated birth defects.[297,298] Apart from aplasia cutis, defects are seen in the abdominal wall (gastroschisis, omphalocele), gut (esophageal atresia), upper airways (choanal atresia), urinary system, heart (ventricular septal defect), and eye (Fig. 12-13). Around 1 in 30 women exposed to methimazole or carbimazole in early pregnancy will give birth to children with defects associated with this therapy. This is in addition to the 5% general population risk of giving birth to a child who has a birth defect diagnosed before the age of 2 years.[299] However, PTU is also teratogenic,[300,301] and the use of PTU is also associated with birth defects (estimated to be around 1 in 40 exposed).[298] These abnormalities tend to be milder than with methimazole-associated defects and include preauricular sinuses and cysts and urinary abnormalities.[302]

The period of risk when these drugs may be teratogenic is especially weeks 6 to 10 of pregnancy.[303] Accordingly, to reduce the risk of birth defects, withdrawal of antithyroid medication in patients who are considered in remission of Graves disease or an unavoidable shift from methimazole to PTU has to take place very early in pregnancy. The risk of birth defects has to be balanced against the risk of abnormal maternal thyroid function in early pregnancy. It is therefore wise to recommend to young women who receive antithyroid drugs for Graves disease that they test for pregnancy just a few days after a missing menstruation and immediately contact their physician to plan future therapy or withdrawal of medication. No firm international consensus has yet been reached on how to minimize the risk of birth defects from antithyroid drug use in early pregnancy.

Caring for the Pregnant Patient. The therapeutic target for a pregnant Graves patients is a healthy infant. In the second half of pregnancy both the untreated pregnant woman with hyperthyroidism caused by Graves disease and her fetus will be thyrotoxic, because TRAb passes the placenta and stimulates the fetal thyroid. Antithyroid drugs given to the mother also pass through the placenta and thus treat both the maternal and the fetal hyperthyroidism. However, the drugs may overtreat the fetus compared with the mother, and accordingly the aim of therapy is to keep the mother in a state of subclinical hyperthyroidism analogous to the normal gestational physiology of the first trimester.[290] This is associated with the lowest impact on fetal thyroid function and the highest rate of normal neonatal thyroid hormone levels.[304] The maternal serum free T_4 level should be maintained at or just above the upper normal *nonpregnant* range, and no attempt should be made to normalize the serum TSH concentration. Indeed a normal TSH during drug therapy is an indication that the dose of drug should be reduced. The clinical status of the patient is an important indication for treatment or increases in dosage. A modest tachycardia is a physiologic response to the increased metabolic demands of pregnancy; and pulse rates of 90 to 100 beats/minute are well tolerated without evidence of myocardial decompensation during delivery. The natural amelioration of Graves disease in the third trimester should be kept in mind, and repeated attempts should be made to reduce or discontinue the thionamide as the delivery date approaches to avoid TSH-induced fetal/newborn goiter, which may cause asphyxia (Fig. 12-14). The serum TSH concentration should be monitored monthly—more to avoid inadvertent overtreatment rather than as the target for normalization. Because thionamides, but not thyroid hormone given to the mother, pass the placenta rather freely, a *block and replace* strategy may induce severe fetal hypothyroidism and goiter, and it is in general not appropriate in the pregnant patient. The rare exception is a pregnant woman who was previously given ablative therapy for Graves disease but who still produces TRAb that leads to isolated fetal hyperthyroidism.

All pregnant patients with significant Graves disease should be managed in close cooperation with obstetricians experienced with modern techniques for monitoring the fetus for intrauterine thyroid dysfunction. These techniques normally include fetal heart rate monitoring and ultrasonographic assessment of fetal growth rate. With advanced ultrasonography it is usually possible to examine the fetus for the presence of goiter. Fetal goiter can develop both from the stimulatory effect of maternal TRAb passing through the placenta and secondary to antithyroid drugs given to the mother. Occasionally, cordocentesis with fetal thyroid function testing may be appropriate.

Iodide and Beta Blockers. Obviously, therapeutic radioiodine is contraindicated in pregnancy, although no harm has been found after diagnostic doses of [123]I.[216] Iodide itself should also not be used as therapy for more than 2 to 3 weeks in the pregnant woman because it readily crosses the placenta and can induce a large goiter that may cause airway obstruction in the newborn. Large amounts of iodide are contraindicated in the last month of pregnancy but can be used at earlier times in emergent situations. Whether propranolol or other beta blockers should be used in the pregnant woman with hyperthyroidism has been a matter of debate. In the experience of some, it can cause intrauterine growth retardation, delayed lung development, and neonatal hypoglycemia or depression,[305] but large studies have suggested that it can be employed with safety for short periods or at very low doses.[306,307]

Surgery. Surgery during the first and third trimesters is not desirable because of the possible induction of early pregnancy loss and later premature labor, respectively. Surgery may be successful during the second trimester, but it is best to avoid major surgery during pregnancy if possible. Nevertheless, if antithyroid drug requirements are very high or cannot be used, surgery may be indicated. Iodide can be given for 7 to 10 days to aid in patient preparation with large and highly vascular thyroid glands. Importantly, thyroid surgery may cure the hyperthyroidism of the mother, but TRAb will not disappear immediately. Thus, the fetal thyroid may still be stimulated, and withdrawal of antithyroid drugs from the pregnant woman may lead to isolated fetal hyperthyroidism.[308]

Consequences of Overtreatment. The influence of maternal hypothyroidism on fetal brain development and the subsequently reduced IQ of the children of hypothyroid mothers are discussed elsewhere (Chapter 13). Needless to say, the overuse of antithyroid drugs in pregnancy may lead to the same consequences. There is considerable evidence that many pregnant patients with Graves disease were overtreated in the past as far as the fetus is concerned, as evidenced by transiently elevated serum TSH levels on newborn screening tests.[309] This is another reason why one should accept patients being slightly hyperthyroid rather than slightly hypothyroid.

Graves Disease in the Postpartum Period

Changes in the Immune Response in the Postpartum Period. As discussed earlier, pregnancy induces a variety of immune changes that are responses to placental influences and the paternal foreign antigens and are designed to prevent rejection of the foreign fetus. These changes include enhanced regulatory T-cell influences and a T-cell shift from Th1 to Th2, resulting in an overall decrease in all autoimmune responses, as evidenced by marked decreases in thyroid autoantibodies.[279] Following delivery, these immune changes are slowly lost and a return to normal is observed but only after a period of exacerbated autoimmune reactivity in which large increases in T-cell and autoantibody activity occur. It is at this time—4 to 12 months post partum—that new-onset or recurrent thyrotoxicosis is seen. Such thyroid dysfunction may be transient or permanent.

Transient Postpartum Thyroiditis. Transient postpartum thyroiditis remains the most common form of hyperthyroidism in the postpartum period and precedes a period of

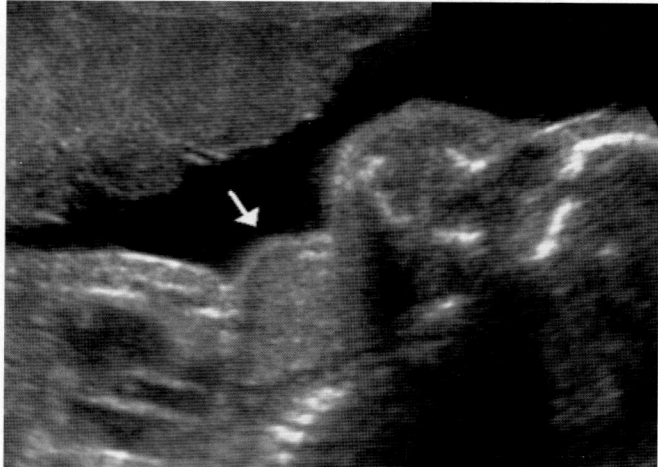

Figure 12-14 Sagittal view of a fetus at 23.9 weeks showing a large goiter *(arrow)* preventing neck flexion. (From Mayor-Lynn KA, Rohrs HJ 3rd, Cruz AC, et al. Antenatal diagnosis and treatment of a dyshormonogenetic fetal goiter. *J Ultrasound Med.* 2009;28[1]:67-71.)

hypothyroidism.[310] The transient thyrotoxicosis is due to thyroid cell destruction and may occur in approximately 5% to 10% of patients during the 4 to 12 months post partum.[311] However, the rapid return of true Graves hyperthyroidism is less common but is similarly dependent on the subsequent changes in the immune response.

Presentation of Postpartum Graves Disease. A high percentage of women with Graves disease in the 20- to 35-year-old age group give a history of pregnancy in the 12 months before the onset of Graves disease.[136,312] Pregnancy and the postpartum state also apparently influence the course of preexisting Graves disease. Patients in clinical remission during pregnancy are prone to postpartum relapse. In 41 pregnancies in 35 patients in remission, 78% were followed by development of thyrotoxicosis during the postpartum period. The patients with Graves disease and postpartum thyrotoxicosis were classified into three categories: some had persistent recurrent hyperthyroidism with an elevated RAIU (classic Graves disease). Some had a transient disorder associated with a normal or an elevated RAIU (transient Graves disease). Some patients, especially those with the highest titers of TPO antibodies, experienced the transient thyrotoxicosis with a decreased RAIU (the thyrotoxic phase of postpartum thyroiditis referred to earlier). This phase, in turn, may be followed by a hypothyroid phase.[122]

Preconception Counseling. A special problem related to hyperthyroidism and pregnancy is presented by the patient who wishes to conceive in the near future and is either in early remission after a course of antithyroid drug treatment or is being treated with antithyroid agents for active Graves disease.[313] For the first scenario, antithyroid drugs can be reluctantly reintroduced if required during pregnancy if symptomatic thyrotoxicosis recurs. In the second situation, definitive therapy (radioiodine therapy or surgery) should be considered to forestall the complexities of managing hyperthyroidism during pregnancy. As with the therapy of Graves disease in general, such decisions must involve education of the patient so that the risks and benefits of the various alternatives are clearly appreciated. Fertile women who receive antithyroid drugs should be educated to perform pregnancy testing already within the first days after a missed menstrual period if pregnancy is possible, and if the test is positive immediately contact the physician for further planning of therapy. The 1-year surge in TRAb after radioiodine therapy[145,146] may increase the risk of fetal exposure to high TRAb levels if the woman is treated with radioiodine shortly before she becomes pregnant.

Nursing and Antithyroid Drugs. Older studies suggested that relatively more methimazole than PTU appeared in breast milk of women receiving these drugs during lactation, but more recent evidence shows little difference between them.[291,314,315] It is occasionally recommended that women who take high doses of antithyroid drugs not nurse their infants because of the difficulty in monitoring thyroid function in infants. The drug doses transferred via breast milk are very small, and no drug side effects have been reported in neonates whose mothers were taking antithyroid drugs, although periodic tests of neonatal thyroid function may be appropriate in women taking very high doses.

INHERITED NONIMMUNE HYPERTHYROIDISM

Toxic diffuse thyroid hyperplasia without the pathologic characteristics of autoimmune disease has been reported in families and appears to be inherited as an autosomal dominant condition.[48,316,317] Polymorphic genomic mutations in the *TSHR* gene have been reported to cause constitutively activated TSHRs differing from family to family. Recessive mutations on both chromosomes have also been described as causing hyperthyroidism while the parents remained euthyroid. These gain of function mutations, mostly in the transmembrane regions of the TSHR, are similar to those somatic mutations seen in toxic adenomas but are in the germline.[318] A database for *TSHR* mutations is available from the University of Leipzig.[319] Treatment is by radioiodine ablation or thyroidectomy, depending on the age of the patient.

TOXIC MULTINODULAR GOITER

Toxic multinodular goiter is a disorder in which hyperthyroidism arises in a multinodular goiter, usually of long standing, and is the result of one of several pathogenetic factors.[320] Its incidence is highly dependent on the iodine intake of the population.

Pathogenesis

The pathogenesis of toxic multinodular goiter cannot be considered apart from that of its invariable forerunner, nontoxic multinodular goiter, from which it may slowly emerge. Two hallmarks of the disorder, structural and functional heterogeneity and functional autonomy, evolve over time; the increase in the extent of autonomous function causes the disease to move from the nontoxic to the toxic phase. Somatic mutations in the *TSHR* gene, first demonstrated in toxic adenomas,[48] have been demonstrated in toxic multinodular goiter, and the individual mutations appear to differ from nodule to nodule. However, only about 60% of toxic nodules have reported *TSHR* mutations, and only a very few have G protein mutations. Hence, there are many nodules with autonomy of undetermined cause[321] and that presumably involve mutations in additional parts of the signaling pathways.

Radioiodine scans show localization of isotope in one or more discrete nodules, whereas iodine accumulation in the remainder of the gland is usually suppressed because TSH is suppressed by the hyperthyroidism. However, the degree of hyperthyroidism can be variable and TSH may not be totally inhibited, so the background uptake of radioisotope may also be variable. Some clinicians refer to such nodules as *warm* rather than hot. Histopathologically, the functioning areas may resemble adenomas in being reasonably well demarcated from surrounding tissue. They generally consist of large follicles, sometimes with hyperplastic epithelium, but here, too, architecture correlates poorly with functional state. The remaining tissue appears inactive, and zones of degeneration are present in both functioning and nonfunctioning areas. Hence, from the pathophysiologic standpoint, these thyroids harbor multiple solitary hyperfunctioning and hypofunctioning adenomas interspersed by suppressed normal thyroid tissue.

Clinical Presentation

The overproduction of thyroid hormone in toxic multinodular goiter is usually less than that in Graves disease and the disease presentation milder (Fig. 12-15); in addition, toxic multinodular goiter usually occurs after the age of 50 in patients who have had nontoxic multinodular goiter for many years (Fig. 12-16). Like its forerunner, toxic multinodular goiter is more common in women than in men (6 : 1).[54] Sometimes, hyperthyroidism develops

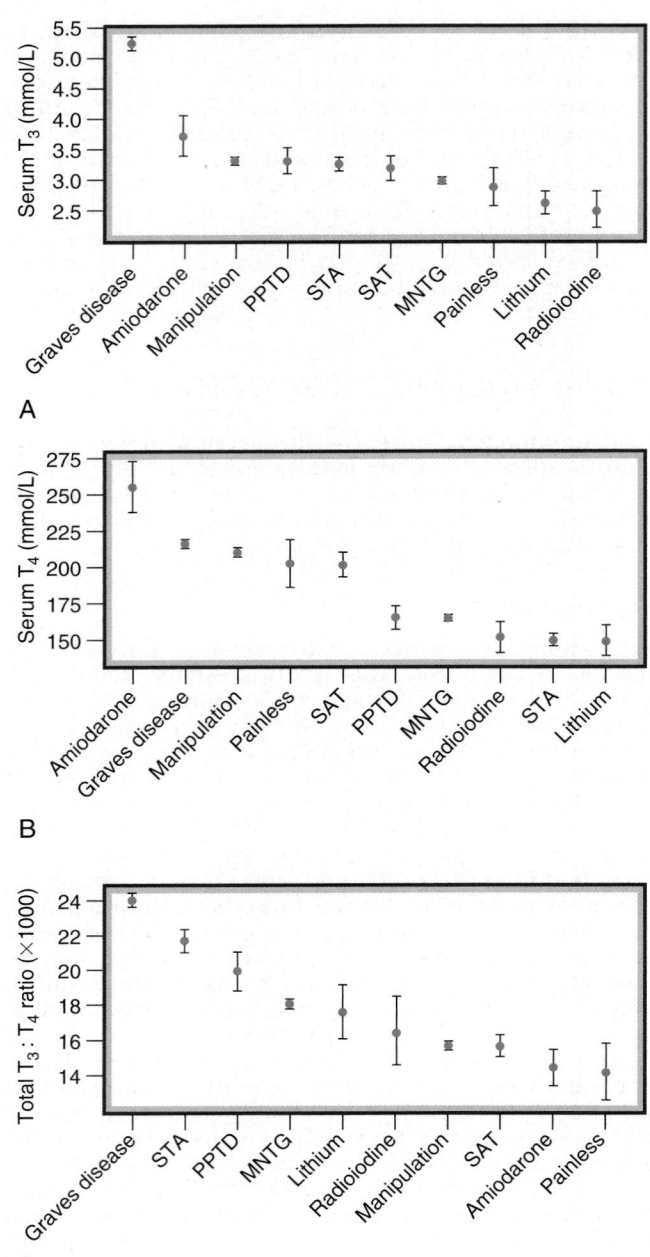

A

B

C

Figure 12-15 Serum T₃ (**A**), T₄ (**B**), and T₃:T₄ ratio (**C**) in 10 types of hyperthyroidism. Means (±SEM) are shown. MNTG, multinodular toxic goiter; PPTD, postpartum thyroid disease; SAT, subacute thyroiditis; SEM, standard error of the mean; STA, solitary toxic adenoma; T₃, triiodothyronine; T₄, thyroxine. (From Carlé A, Knudsen N, Pedersen IB, et al. Determinants of serum T4 and T3 at the time of diagnosis in nosological types of thyrotoxicosis: a population-based study. *Eur J Endocrinol.* 2013;169[5]: 537-545.)

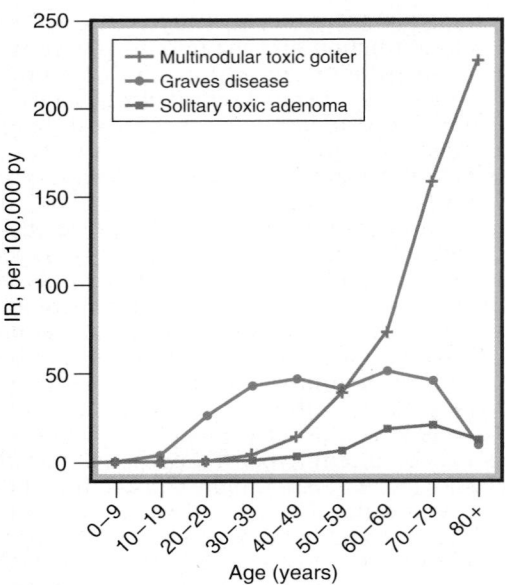

Figure 12-16 An example of age-specific incidence rates (IR) of the three most common types of hyperthyroidism. py, person-years. (From Carlé A, Pedersen IB, Knudsen N, et al. Epidemiology of subtypes of hyperthyroidism in Denmark: a population-based study. *Eur J Endocrinol.* 2011;164[5]:801-809.)

A toxic multinodular goiter may also be found as part of Graves disease as confirmed by the presence of TRAb of the stimulating variety.[322] Presumably this represents two separate diseases, although TRAbs have growth-stimulating activity but this should apply to all cells. Toxic multinodular goiter alone is not accompanied by infiltrative ophthalmopathy, and when the two coexist, it represents the emergence of Graves disease.

Cardiovascular manifestations often predominate, possibly because of the age of the patients, and include atrial fibrillation or tachycardia, with or without heart failure. Weakness and wasting of muscles are common, the so-called *apathetic* or *masked thyrotoxicosis*. The nervous manifestations are less prominent than in younger patients with thyrotoxicosis, but emotional lability may be pronounced and even osteoporosis may be the factor leading to thyroid function testing and diagnosis. Because of the physical characteristics of the thyroid gland and its frequent retrosternal extension, obstructive symptoms are more common than in Graves disease.

On palpation, the characteristics of the goiter are the same as those of the more common nontoxic multinodular goiter. In as many as 20% of elderly patients with thyrotoxicosis, the thyroid gland is firm and irregular but not distinctly enlarged. A thyroid scan and ultrasound examination will confirm the diagnosis as toxic multinodular goiter rather than a single toxic adenoma or Graves disease.

Laboratory Tests and Differential Diagnosis

All patients with a multinodular goiter should be screened annually with a serum TSH. If suppressed, the free T₄ (or if normal, the free T₃) should be determined. Serum TSH levels intermediate between 0.1 and 0.4 mU/L are not usually associated with significant symptoms. Such patients have thyroid autonomy but are not thyrotoxic (see "Mild (Subclinical) Hyperthyroidism"). For patients with established thyrotoxicosis, an RAIU with scan will help in

abruptly, often after exposure to increased quantities of iodine such as the contrast media for CT scanning, which permits autonomous foci to increase hormone secretion to excessive levels and which may simply exacerbate already established mild hyperthyroidism (see "Iodide-Induced Hyperthyroidism"). The serum T₄ and T₃ concentrations may be only marginally increased, and a suppressed TSH may be the major abnormality. The total RAIU is only slightly increased or within the normal range unless following iodine exposure.

gauging the dose of ^{131}I to be administered as well as identify the autonomously functioning nodules. The latter can then be followed by ^{131}I therapy.

Treatment

Radioiodine Therapy

Radioiodine may be the treatment of choice for patients with toxic multinodular goiter despite disagreement about the size and number of doses required to achieve a therapeutic response.[320,323] We attempt to deposit about 12 to 14 mCi into the gland at 24 hours based on a pretreatment RAIU test. In the United States, iodine intake is higher than in many regions in Europe so that 24-hour RAIU values of 20% to 30% are not unusual. Such patients will require 50 mCi or more radioiodine to restore a euthyroid state and may even require a second treatment.

Because a number of patients with this disorder have underlying heart disease, the administration of radioiodine should be preceded by a course of antithyroid therapy with methimazole until a near eumetabolic state is achieved, but still with a suppressed TSH to avoid iodine uptake in normal thyroid tissue. Medication is then discontinued for at least 4 to 7 days before radioiodine is administered. A week later the antithyroid drug may be reinstituted so that the thyrotoxicosis is controlled until radioiodine takes effect, which typically requires 3 to 4 months. A decrease in size of the hyperfunctioning nodules is a positive sign. At that time, the antithyroid drug can be tapered, but if the TSH level remains below 0.1 mU/L after 6 months, a second dose is usually given.

Surgery

Surgical therapy is often recommended after adequate preoperative preparation in patients with large goiters or obstructive manifestations. In these patients, a CT scan or MRI is recommended to define the extent of the goiter and the adequacy of the tracheal walls. Respiratory function studies may also be helpful in assessing the need for surgery. Patients with fixed, especially partially retrosternal, goiter should be considered for surgery because of the risk of more complete obstruction should hemorrhage into a nodule occur. However, when surgery is contraindicated, even significant obstructive symptoms can be relieved by adequate radioiodine therapy.[324] In elderly patients who are not candidates for either radioiodine therapy or surgery, lifelong low dose antithyroid drug therapy remains an option.

TOXIC ADENOMA

A third, less common form of hyperthyroidism (around 5% of cases)[54] is caused by one or more autonomous adenomas of the thyroid gland. As herein employed, the term *toxic adenoma* refers to a tumor in a thyroid that is otherwise intrinsically normal. The disorder is usually caused by a single adenoma that is either palpable or seen on ultrasound as a solitary nodule and hence is sometimes referred to as a *hyperfunctioning solitary nodule* or *toxic nodule*. Occasionally, two or three adenomas of similar character are present.

Pathogenesis

Toxic adenomas are true follicular adenomas (for histopathologic characteristics see Chapter 14). The basic pathogenesis of many toxic adenomas is one of several somatic

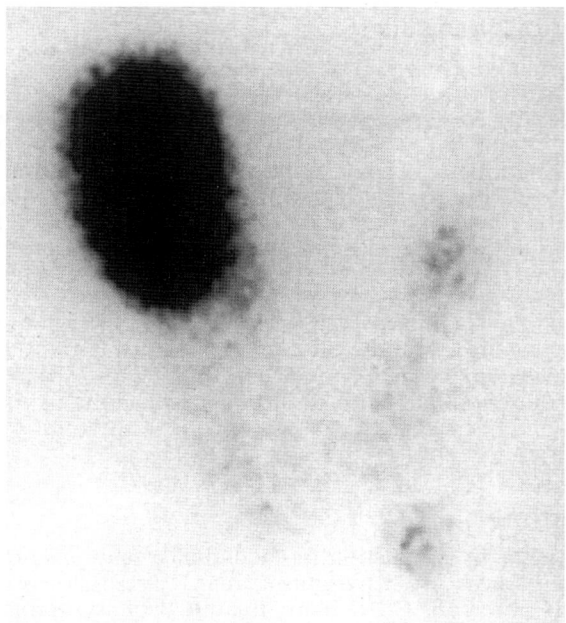

Figure 12-17 Radioiodine (^{123}I) thyroid scan shows a hyperfunctioning hot nodule corresponding to physical examination findings with a faint outline of the remaining suppressed gland. In this unusual case, Graves disease developed a few months later after an oral contrast agent load. (From Soule J, Mayfield R. Graves' disease after 131I therapy for toxic nodule. *Thyroid.* 2001;11:91-92.)

point mutations in the *TSHR* gene, commonly in the third transmembrane loop.[319] These single nucleotide substitutions cause amino acid changes that lead to constitutive activation of the TSHR in the absence of TSH.[325] It appears, therefore, that the TSHR is switched from an *off* state to an *on* state. Similarly, loss-of-function rather than gain-of-function mutations may also occur in the *TSHR* gene and cause hypothyroidism (see later). A small number of autonomous adenomas have mutations in the G protein genes that lead to a similar state of constitutive activation.[321]

Clinical Presentation

The toxic adenoma often presents as a nodule in a patient with a suppressed TSH; on ultrasound it appears as a single hypoechogenic nodule. A radioiodine thyroid scan shows a localized area of increased radioiodine accumulation (Fig. 12-17). This condition may occur at a younger age than toxic multinodular goiter and may be seen in patients in their 30s and 40s.

Frequently there is a history of a long-standing, slowly growing lump in the neck. It is unusual for adenomas to produce thyrotoxicosis until they have achieved a diameter of greater than 3 cm,[320] and up to that point, patients have subclinical hyperthyroidism. The adenoma can undergo central necrosis and hemorrhage spontaneously relieving the thyrotoxicosis, and the remainder of the thyroid may then resume its function. Calcification in the area of hemorrhage may take place and may be evident on sonogram examination. Such calcification is usually macroscopic and irregular and does not resemble the finely stippled calcification suggestive of papillary cancers. The peripheral clinical manifestations of a toxic adenoma are generally milder than those of Graves disease and are notable for the absence of infiltrative orbitopathy and myopathy, although cardiovascular manifestations may occur.

Laboratory Tests

The results of laboratory tests depend on the stage and function of the adenoma. At first, serum thyroid hormone concentrations are normal except for borderline suppression of the serum TSH. This, together with ultrasound examination to exclude multiple nodules, confirms the diagnosis. Later a thyroid scan may show localization of radioisotope in the palpated nodule, but this is not obvious until TSH secretion is suppressed. If the nodule continues to grow, frank hyperthyroidism is accompanied by elevation of serum thyroid hormone levels. Occasionally, the serum free T_4 concentration is normal, and only the serum T_3 level is increased (T_3 thyrotoxicosis). Incidental thyroid carcinoma may rarely coexist within a gland exhibiting a hyperfunctioning adenoma although autonomous malignant nodules causing functional hyperthyroidism are very rare.

Treatment

Although hyperfunctioning adenomas may eventually cause clinical hyperthyroidism, many do so slowly, and others not at all.[320] Therefore, treatment of asymptomatic patients with functional adenomas is decided on an individual basis. Clinically euthyroid subjects who wish to avoid both surgery and radioiodine can in theory be followed with annual assessments. However, suppression of TSH below normal, particularly to less than 0.1 mU/L, indicates hyperthyroidism, and therapy may be warranted. Two definitive therapies are available: radioiodine and surgery.

Radioiodine Therapy

In terms of the specificity of treatment, functioning thyroid nodules are candidates for radioiodine therapy. The radiation should, in theory, be directed almost exclusively to the diseased tissue. This is because TSH is suppressed and the normal thyroid tissue surrounding the nodule does not take up excess radioiodine. However, this suppression may be incomplete, and a significant fraction of patients receiving ^{131}I develop thyroid failure. For the patient over age 18 with a nodule 5 cm in diameter or smaller, ^{131}I is an appropriate treatment if the risk of eventual hypothyroidism is acceptable to the patient. For such lesions, doses of radioiodine are given sufficient to result in the presence of 300 to 370 MBq (8 to 10 mCi) in the nodule at 24 hours based on the uptake.[320] Recombinant TSH, used to enhance the RAIU in order to avoid a large treatment dose in nontoxic multinodular goiters, is not appropriate here because it will direct radioiodine into surrounding normal thyroid tissue. The potential for hypothyroidism also indicates the need for prolonged follow-up.

Surgery

Toxic nodules are readily treated by surgical excision. A hemithyroidectomy may avoid the long-term development of hypothyroidism and with modern surgical procedures can be performed on an outpatient basis or even under local anesthesia. Surgical excision is always preferable in patients younger than 18 years of age to avoid the long-term consequences of irradiation, including effects on perinodular tissue. The toxic adenoma is not diffusely hypervascular, and consequently preoperative preparation with iodine is not required. In the patient with overt thyrotoxicosis, however, a normal metabolic state should be restored with an antithyroid drug before surgery.

MILD (SUBCLINICAL) HYPERTHYROIDISM

Definition

The availability of sensitive assays for TSH allowed the recognition of mild hyperthyroidism, in which there are no signs or symptoms of thyrotoxicosis but the serum TSH is subnormal despite normal serum free thyroid hormone concentrations. The term *subclinical* is somewhat of a misnomer, because the condition is defined by biochemical characteristics, and it is preferable to use the term *mild thyroid dysfunction*.[326] Nonetheless, it is still not clear whether a patient is classified as having mild hyperthyroidism simply because our ability to detect physiologic evidence of excess thyroid hormone is less sensitive than our capacity to measure changes in TSH. This is further complicated by the fact that the hypothalamic-pituitary axis is sensitive to both serum free T_4 and T_3, whereas the peripheral tissues such as the heart primarily sense the free T_3 (see Chapter 11).[327,328] It is easy to assume, given the wide normal range for free thyroid hormone concentrations, that an individual with a low-normal free T_4 set-point for TSH secretion would have a reduced TSH if that concentration were increased by 50% but could still remain within the normal range. In fact, in patients with primary hypothyroidism, small additional quantities of levothyroxine given to patients with normal TSH will decrease TSH below normal without a supranormal free T_4.[327] On the other hand, in the now classic studies in the Framingham population over 60 years of age, the cumulative incidence of atrial fibrillation over 10 years was 28% in patients with a serum TSH concentration of 0.1 mU/L or less, whereas it was only 11% in those with serum TSH concentrations falling between 0.1 and 0.4 mU/L. The latter was only slightly higher than that in the normal population.[9,10] Nevertheless, heart failure is the leading cause of increased cardiovascular mortality rate in both overt and mild hyperthyroidism.[329]

Bone density is another end point for such studies because it is well known that thyroid hormone causes a net resorption of cortical bone[330] and that lack of TSH may contribute to this phenomenon.[28] Several studies demonstrate lower bone density in patients with mild thyrotoxicosis, although others do not.[31,331] This is a subject of considerable interest because the condition is much more common than overt thyrotoxicosis (0.7% of the population in NHANES III) and has broad implications with respect to the cost of diagnosis, treatment, and follow-up.[52] In general, normalization of thyroid function in postmenopausal women with subclinical hyperthyroidism seems to improve bone density and certain aspects of cardiac function.[332]

Overal, these data would generally favor treatment in the older population, but unfortunately, there are still no large, long-term randomized studies to allow evidence-based conclusions as to the risk/benefit ratio[333] (Table 12-10).

Diagnosis

The diagnosis of subclinical hyperthyroidism requires tests revealing several subnormal TSH concentration results spaced months apart in the presence of normal free T_3 and T_4 concentrations. Several studies show that suppressed TSH can normalize spontaneously over several years, particularly in patients without nodular goiter.[334,335] As with overt thyrotoxicosis, there are two sources of excess thyroid hormones, endogenous and exogenous. In a study of over

TABLE 12-10

Indications for Treatment of Persistent Subclinical Hyperthyroidism

Postmenopausal osteoporosis
Rheumatic valvular disease with left atrial enlargement or atrial fibrillation
Recent-onset atrial fibrillation or recurrent cardiac arrhythmias
Congestive heart failure
Angina pectoris
Infertility or menstrual disorders
Nonspecific symptoms such as fatigue, nervousness, depression, or gastrointestinal disorders, especially in patients older than 60 years of age (consider therapeutic trial)

25,000 individuals attending health fairs in Colorado, 58% of those with a TSH less than 0.3 mU/L were receiving thyroid hormones.[336] When this is not being done intentionally for the treatment of persistent thyroid carcinoma, it is easily treated by more careful monitoring of the levothyroxine dosage using serum TSH concentrations. Endogenous subclinical thyrotoxicosis has the same causes as overt thyrotoxicosis. In the population over 60, multinodular goiter is a more likely cause of hyperthyroidism than it is in younger individuals.

Treatment

There are insufficient data to conclude that individuals with serum TSH concentrations greater than 0.1 mU/L due to hyperthyroidism will benefit from treatment.[333] The decision for or against treatment of individuals with persistently subnormal TSH concentrations less than 0.1 mU/L (with normal free thyroid hormones) should be based on evaluation of the conditions that may benefit from treatment as well as determining the cause. In the elderly, postmenopausal osteoporosis and various cardiac diseases are the primary indications for which treatment should be considered. Infertility or menstrual disorders are important in young women.

Identifying the cause of the hyperthyroidism allows assessment of the potential risks of treatment. At one extreme, the treatment of mild Graves disease with radioiodine usually causes hypothyroidism, whereas this typically does not occur in patients with multinodular toxic goiter. Thus, in an asymptomatic patient with mild Graves disease, watchful waiting for several years, awaiting a possible spontaneous remission, may be the best course of action,[337] and if therapy is considered necessary the chance of prolonged remission after a course of antithyroid drug therapy is good. On the other hand, patients with subclinical hyperthyroidism due to toxic nodular goiter or a solitary hyperfunctioning adenoma can often be treated with a single dose of radioactive iodine with a relatively low risk of subsequent hypothyroidism. Thus, the threshold for treatment of such patients is lower. As always, the rationale for treatment, its risks, and its benefits should be carefully discussed with the patient, and one should be guided by common sense and not by the principle of simply treating an abnormal test result.[338]

IODIDE-INDUCED HYPERTHYROIDISM

In Iodine Deficiency

Administration of supplemental iodine to subjects with endemic iodine deficiency goiter can result in iodine-induced hyperthyroidism. This response, also termed the *Jod-Basedow effect*, occurs in only a small fraction of individuals at risk. The Jod-Basedow effect specifically refers to iodine-induced von Basedow (Graves) disease but is often used to refer to iodine-induced hyperthyroidism of any type. There are two major patterns of the underlying thyroid disorder.[339] The first, common in older individuals, is the development of a toxic nodular goiter with autonomous nodules, and TRAbs are not detectable in the blood. The second is the development of Graves disease, more common in younger individuals, with diffuse goiter in whom stimulating TRAbs are often present. These findings indicate that the Jod-Basedow effect occurs in thyroid glands in which thyroid function is independent of TSH stimulation. The occurrence of the Jod-Basedow effect is not a contraindication to treating endemic iodine deficiency. Apart from the many other benefits that accrue from iodine treatment and prophylaxis, over the long run the frequency of spontaneous hyperthyroidism due to toxic nodular goiter is diminished.[340,341]

In Iodine Sufficiency

Iodide-induced hyperthyroidism is also an important disorder in areas of the world in which dietary iodine intake is high.[342] In regions in which iodine intake is marginal but overt iodine deficiency is absent, moderate increments in iodine intake may induce hyperthyroidism in patients with autonomous thyroid nodules. Consequently the physician must be alert to the possibility of inducing hyperthyroidism when administering iodine in expectorants, x-ray and CT scan contrast media, medications containing iodine (e.g., amiodarone), povidone iodine, or any other form to patients with nodular goiter.[343,344] Nodular goiter is generally a disease of the elderly, so induction of the Jod-Basedow phenomenon can have serious consequences, because enrichment of the thyroid with iodine forestalls administration of ^{131}I and delays the response to antithyroid agents. Prevention of an acute exacerbation may be achieved by pretreatment of at-risk subjects with methimazole starting before exposure and for several weeks afterward.[345]

Amiodarone-Induced Hyperthyroidism

The most common drug associated with iodine-induced thyrotoxicosis is amiodarone. This iodine-rich drug is popular because of its effectiveness in combating severe cardiac arrhythmias. However, its use may be limited by toxicity due to its high fat solubility and high iodine content inducing thyroid disease and also by pulmonary fibrosis and liver disease. Amiodarone has complex effects on the thyroid, although the majority (~80%) of patients remain euthyroid.[346] Structurally, the drug resembles T_4 and contains 37% iodine by weight (Fig. 12-18).

About 6 mg of iodide are released per day of the 75 mg of iodine present in a 200-mg tablet compared with the typical daily iodine supply of about 150 to 200 µg in North America. Amiodarone has a half-life of 50 to 60 days and therefore remains available for a long period even after drug withdrawal. In addition to providing huge amounts of iodide, amiodarone inhibits the type 1 and probably the type 2 deiodinases and may compete with T_3 for binding to the thyroid hormone receptor. Amiodarone also has a direct cytotoxic effect on thyroid cells via induction of apoptosis.[347] In addition to the iodine load, the drug or its metabolites may precipitate AITD in susceptible individuals, most likely by increasing Tg iodination and enhancing its immunogenicity.

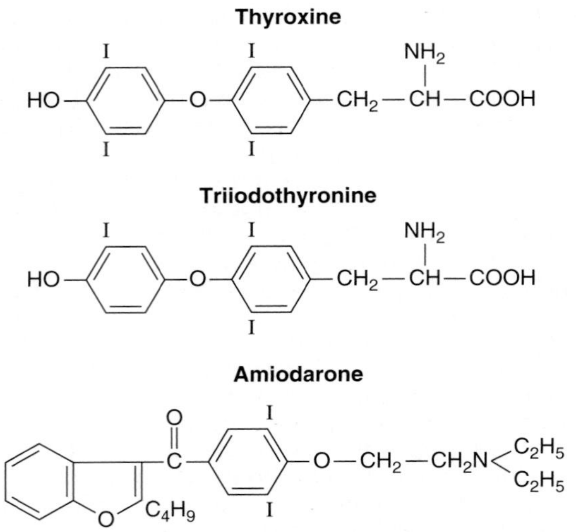

Thyroxine

Triiodothyronine

Amiodarone

Figure 12-18 The chemical structures of thyroxine (T_4), triiodothyronine (T_3), and amiodarone.

A new drug, dronedarone, is now available and is a benzofuran derivative related to amiodarone; in dronedarone, the iodine moieties were removed to reduce the toxic effects on the thyroid and other organs, and a methylsulfonamide group was added to reduce solubility in fats, although liver toxicity continues to be seen. Dronedarone displays amiodarone-like class III antiarrhythmic activity and is now in clinical practice.

Clinical Presentation

In all patients receiving amiodarone, its effects, particularly the inhibition of the deiodinases, cause a compensatory increase in TSH secretion. This increases serum free T_4 30% to 50% with the serum T_3 and TSH concentrations remaining normal after equilibrium occurs. The pathologic effects on the thyroid cell may result in iodide-induced thyroiditis and subsequent hypothyroidism (the most common thyroid complication in iodine-sufficient regions, see Chapter 13) or hyperthyroidism (more common in low iodine intake areas) in susceptible individuals due to either the Jod-Basedow effect in iodine-deficient regions or the development of Graves disease. The iodine-induced hyperthyroidism and thyroiditis-like syndromes have also been referred to as type I and type II amiodarone-induced thyrotoxicosis, respectively.[284,348]

Amiodarone-induced thyrotoxicosis, which is less common than the induction of hypothyroidism, may develop at the outset of exposure or not until after several years of treatment. It commonly presents as an exacerbation of the underlying cardiac disease that was the indication for its use in the first instance. This serious complication can sometimes be anticipated by its early recognition due to a progressive decrease in serum TSH. Monitoring of TSH throughout amiodarone treatment on a regular basis, such as every 6 months, should be undertaken by the supervising cardiologist or internist. This is especially important in areas of borderline or deficient iodine supply.

Diagnosis

All patients with amiodarone-induced thyrotoxicosis will have a suppressed TSH with the degree of suppression proportional to the clinical severity. Serum free T_4 will be elevated but the elevation in serum free T_3 will be less than

that in typical thyrotoxic states because of the blockade of T_4-to-T_3 conversion by the drug. Distinction between the two causes of thyrotoxicosis may not be possible, although many strategies have been suggested. In North America the cause of thyrotoxicosis is virtually always thyroiditis due to the lack of iodine deficiency, whereas a more evenly divided mix of the two causes occurs in Europe.[346,349,350] Doppler-flow ultrasonography showing hypervascularity accompanied by an enlarged gland favors iodine-induced hyperthyroidism, and a normal-sized gland and normal or reduced vascularity favors thyroiditis, but results can be equivocal.[346,349] RAIU values are virtually always low.

Treatment

If possible, amiodarone should be discontinued, but this is not absolutely necessary. In patients with thyroiditis, a spontaneous resolution may occur, but in most patients with amiodarone-associated hyperthyroidism a combination of methimazole or carbimazole (20 to 40 mg/day) and prednisolone/prednisone 20 to 40 mg/day is given to cover both diagnostic possibilities.[351,352] The latter may be tapered after 3 months to see if a remission has occurred. In patients with iodine-induced hyperthyroidism, perchlorate, 500 mg twice daily for 1 to 2 weeks, may accelerate the resolution of the condition, although this agent may have significant renal and bone marrow toxicities precluding the long-term use, but this is rare in the dose mentioned.[346,353] In patients who remain unstable or whose cardiac condition is likely to require lifelong amiodarone therapy, surgery is appropriate. Amiodarone has been restarted in patients who have recovered from thyroiditis, and these patients may remain euthyroid.[285,354]

HYPERTHYROIDISM DUE TO THYROTROPIN SECRETION

Pituitary Tumor

Excess TSH is an exceedingly rare cause of hyperthyroidism. However, pituitary thyrotroph tumors cause this condition and may present as a Graves-like syndrome with diffuse goiter and substantial thyrotoxicosis. Guidelines for the management of such patients have recently been released.[355] Laboratory studies demonstrating an inappropriately detectable or somewhat elevated TSH must first be confirmed by eliminating assay artifacts. This condition is discussed in depth in Chapter 9 and must be differentiated from the rare patient who has familial resistance to thyroid hormone (RTH).[356-358]

Thyroid Hormone Resistance

In some patients with familial thyroid hormone resistance due to mutations in the β-isoform of the thyroid hormone receptor, the hypothalamic-pituitary feedback mechanism is more resistant to the effects of thyroid hormone than are peripheral tissues such as the heart, which expresses the thyroid receptor α-isoform.[356-358] These patients may therefore present with a hyperthyroid appearance with tachycardia, nervousness, and goiter associated with an elevated free T_4. However, because the thyroid hormone hyperproduction is TSH-driven, serum TSH concentrations are detectable (>0.1 mU/L) or even elevated inappropriately for the high serum thyroid hormone levels. In general, the manifestations are due not to excessive but, rather, to an inadequate balance between activation of the different types of thyroid hormone receptors, and these individuals may require treatment with thyroid hormone or thyroid hormone analogues or β-adrenergic receptor blocking agents rather than antithyroid drugs (see Chapter 13 for a more extensive discussion of RTH). A critical historical point in such patients is a family history because RTH is inherited in an autosomal dominant pattern.

TUMOR CHORIONIC GONADOTROPIN-INDUCED HYPERTHYROIDISM

hCG exhibits specificity crossover with the TSHR (see earlier discussion under "Pregnancy and the Thyroid"). Thyroid hyperfunction may, therefore, accompany hydatidiform mole, choriocarcinoma, or metastatic embryonal carcinoma of the testis.[284] Such neoplasms, particularly hydatidiform mole, elaborate differentially glycosylated hCG molecules that exhibit crossover specificity for binding to the TSHR and can induce variable degrees of thyroid overactivity.[260,359] Some patients have clinically overt thyrotoxicosis; however, clinical manifestations are usually not prominent, and goiter is absent or minimal. The free T_4 and free T_3 levels are increased, and TSH values are suppressed. The possibility of a molar pregnancy should be considered in a young woman with hyperthyroidism and amenorrhea because the appropriate therapy is evacuation of the uterus.

TRANSIENT THYROTOXICOSIS

Overview

As mentioned at the outset of this chapter, transient thyrotoxicosis must be differentiated from the sustained hyperthyroidism of Graves disease and other causes of hyperthyroidism. Transient thyrotoxicosis is caused by thyroid cell breakdown, and the hyperthyroid symptoms are of abrupt onset and short duration. This process may be followed by recovery of thyroid function or the development of transient or permanent thyroid failure. The discussion in this chapter focuses on thyroiditis as the most common cause of transient thyrotoxicosis, and this disorder is covered more completely in Chapter 13 because Hashimoto disease most commonly causes hypothyroidism after the initial phase of transient hyperthyroidism. Unfortunately, transient thyrotoxicosis continues to have a confusing nomenclature, which can be clarified as follows:

1. Autoimmune thyroiditis: In the autoimmune forms (Hashimoto thyroiditis), there are typically no local symptoms of thyroid inflammation, leading to the terms *silent* or *painless thyroiditis*, also referred to as *lymphocytic thyroiditis* or *hashitoxicosis*. This condition may uncommonly present with thyroid tenderness if the thyroid has expanded rapidly, stretching the capsule.
2. Viral thyroiditis: In what is thought to be postviral thyroiditis (also termed *subacute, de Quervain,* or *granulomatous thyroiditis*), thyroid tenderness may be the most prominent symptom, and thyrotoxicosis is rare and typically self-limited, although this form may rarely also be painless.
3. Acute thyroiditis: Acute thyroiditis due to bacterial or fungal infections is only rarely accompanied by thyrotoxicosis and the local symptoms predominate (see Chapter 13).
4. Drug-induced thyroiditis: Thyroiditis may also be drug-induced, the principal offenders being amiodarone and lithium. Some of the new small molecule kinase inhibitors (such as sunitinib) may also cause this form of thyroiditis, resulting eventually in hypothyroidism.[360,361]

Transient Thyrotoxicosis Due to Autoimmune (Hashimoto) Thyroiditis

As described earlier, Hashimoto disease causes two different thyrotoxicosis-associated transient syndromes. The most common is the painless form in which the symptoms of thyrotoxicosis, usually mild, predominate; the much more uncommon form has a painful presentation probably secondary to a more acute onset. Histopathologic examination in such patients with thyroiditis shows diffuse or local lymphocytic infiltration, varying degrees of fibrosis, and disruption of the follicular architecture (Fig. 12-19).

Transient Thyrotoxicosis From Painless Autoimmune Thyroiditis

Painless autoimmune thyroiditis may occur post partum or spontaneously. Postpartum thyroiditis is the most common example, and its pathophysiology, postpartum enhancement of thyroid-directed autoimmunity (Hashimoto disease), is analogous to the postpartum exacerbation of Graves disease (see "Graves Disease in the Postpartum Period" earlier). The incidence of postpartum thyroiditis varies but may occur in as many as 10% of women and in more than 30% of those with positive TPO autoantibodies and even a larger fraction in patients with type 1 diabetes mellitus.[269,311] In women found to be TPO antibody positive prenatally, postpartum assessment of thyroid function is recommended at 3, 6, and 12 months. Thyrotoxicosis from spontaneous autoimmune thyroiditis has all the same characteristics as postpartum thyroiditis and is seen in patients early in their development of classic Hashimoto disease and before the onset of hypothyroidism.

Transient Thyrotoxicosis From Painful Autoimmune Thyroiditis

Although some patients may present with local thyroid tenderness, this occurrence is uncommon. Such tender

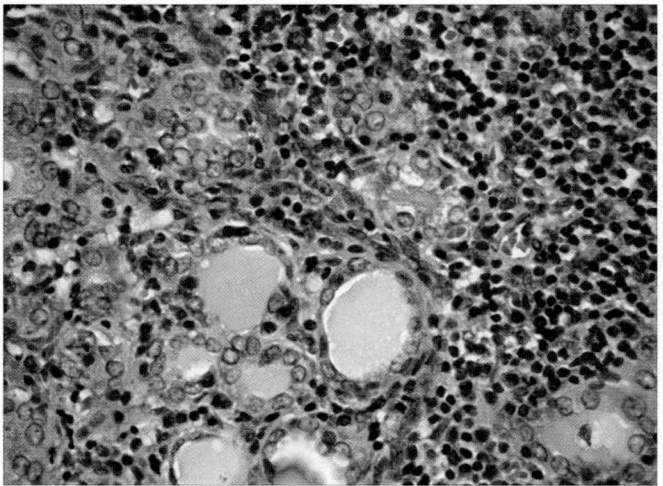

Figure 12-19 Lymphocytic thyroiditis in a patient with transient thyrotoxicosis (painless thyroiditis) secondary to autoimmune (Hashimoto) thyroiditis. Notice the diffuse lymphocytic invasion of the tissue, including the follicular epithelium, and the loss of follicles. Multinucleated giant cells may also be seen in the follicular lumen. (Courtesy of Dr. Vania Nosé, Brigham and Women's Hospital, Boston, MA.)

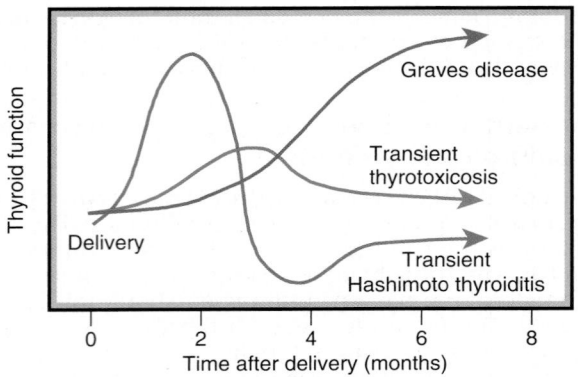

Figure 12-20 The postpartum thyroid syndromes. These potential patterns of thyroid dysfunction may be seen in the postpartum period.

episodes, which may be unilateral, may recur until the thyroid gland is completely destroyed by the disease process. Only rarely does the pain persist, sometimes requiring surgical intervention.

Clinical Presentation of Transient Autoimmune Thyrotoxicosis

More than 75% of patients are women who present with the acute onset of symptoms of thyrotoxicosis, usually nervousness, palpitations, and irritability; they can often pinpoint the time of recent onset. In the postpartum syndrome symptoms present 4 to 12 months after delivery but may be mild and overlooked in the myriad of events involved in the care of the newborn.[310] After 1 to 2 months the thyrotoxic symptoms fade but are often replaced by those suggesting hypothyroidism (Fig. 12-20).

In a significant number of postpartum patients, the thyrotoxic phase is too mild to be noticed and the patient presents somewhat later after delivery with hypothyroid symptoms. The physical examination shows mild signs of thyrotoxicosis, tachycardia being the most prominent, without the specific eye signs or dermopathy associated with Graves disease. The thyroid gland is normal in size but may be firm if the Hashimoto disease is chronic.

Diagnosis

Thyrotoxicosis is usually mild and is reflected in the degree of suppression of the serum TSH level and elevation of the serum free T_4. Significant elevation of the TPO antibodies is typical. Systemic manifestations of inflammation are lacking, and the erythrocyte sedimentation rate is normal or nearly normal but the ultrasound may indicate the heterogeneity of an inflamed gland. If true hyperthyroidism cannot be eliminated as a diagnosis on clinical grounds, TRAb should be measured or an RAIU test should be performed unless the patient is nursing. The classic decreased RAIU is due partly to feedback suppression of TSH secretion but also to thyroid follicular cell destruction. The tendency of the disorder to pass through a hypothyroid phase is not surprising in view of the extensive depletion of Tg, which is processed to T_4 and not replaced by the dysfunctional cells.

Natural History

The duration of the thyrotoxic phase, typically not severe enough to require treatment, averages about 1 to 2 months. About one half of the patients return to a euthyroid phase

and remain well in the short term. In the remaining half, a hypothyroid phase may follow and may last from 2 to 9 months. In most, there is eventual restoration of euthyroidism, but some develop permanent hypothyroidism years later.[362,363] About one third retain a goiter, usually with persistence of thyroid autoantibodies in the serum. The opposite sequela, recurrence of thyrotoxicosis, may also occur months or years after restoration of a euthyroid state or particularly after pregnancy.

Treatment

The thyrotoxic phase may require alleviation of the peripheral manifestations through the use of beta blockers. Prednisone (20 to 40 mg/day) may decrease the duration of the thyrotoxic phase but is typically not needed except when the painful form of the disease is present. If mild and brief, the hypothyroid phase may also not require treatment. When treatment with levothyroxine is required, it should be withdrawn slowly approximately 6 months later, because the hypothyroidism is often not permanent.

Subacute Thyroiditis

Subacute thyroiditis (also termed *granulomatous, giant cell,* or *de Quervain thyroiditis*) is thought to be caused directly or indirectly by a viral infection of the thyroid gland and often follows an upper respiratory illness. A tendency to appear in the spring in the Northern latitudes has been noted and again it predominates in the female. The mumps virus has been implicated in some cases, and coxsackievirus, influenza virus, echovirus, and adenoviruses may also be etiologic agents. Positive TPO antibodies are present transiently during the active phase of the disease, although some patients may retain evidence of thyroid autoimmunity for many years. A small number of patients eventually develop AITD.[364] Subacute thyroiditis is uncommon, but mild cases may be mistakenly diagnosed as pharyngitis.

Pathology

The histopathologic changes are different from those in Hashimoto disease. The lesions are patchy in distribution and vary in their stage of development from area to area. Affected follicles are infiltrated predominantly with mononuclear cells and show disruption of epithelium, partial or complete loss of colloid, and fragmentation and duplication of the basement membrane (Fig. 12-21). To this extent, the histopathologic appearance may resemble that in Hashimoto disease. A characteristic feature is the well-developed follicular lesion that consists of a central core of colloid surrounded by the multinucleated giant cells, from which stems the designation *giant cell thyroiditis*. Colloid may be found in the interstitium or within the giant cells. The follicular changes progress to form granulomas. Interfollicular fibrosis and an interstitial inflammatory reaction are present to varying degrees. When the disease subsides, an essentially normal histologic appearance is restored.

Pathophysiology

Apoptosis of follicular epithelium and loss of follicular integrity are the primary events in the pathophysiology. Tg, T_4, and iodinated Tg fragments are released into the circulation, often in quantities sufficient to elevate not just the serum Tg level but also the serum free T_4 level, producing clinical thyrotoxicosis and suppressing TSH secretion. As a result, the RAIU decreases to low levels, and hormone synthesis ceases. Later in the disease, when stores of preformed hormone are depleted, serum T_4 and T_3 concentrations decline, sometimes into the hypothyroid range, and the serum TSH level rises, often to elevated values exactly as occurs in silent thyroiditis (Fig. 12-22). As the disease becomes inactive, the RAIU may be greater than normal for a time as hormone stores are repleted. Ultimately, when hormone secretion resumes, serum T_4 and T_3 concentrations rise, and serum TSH concentration decreases to normal values.

Clinical Picture

The characteristic feature is the gradual or sudden appearance of pain in the region of the thyroid gland with or

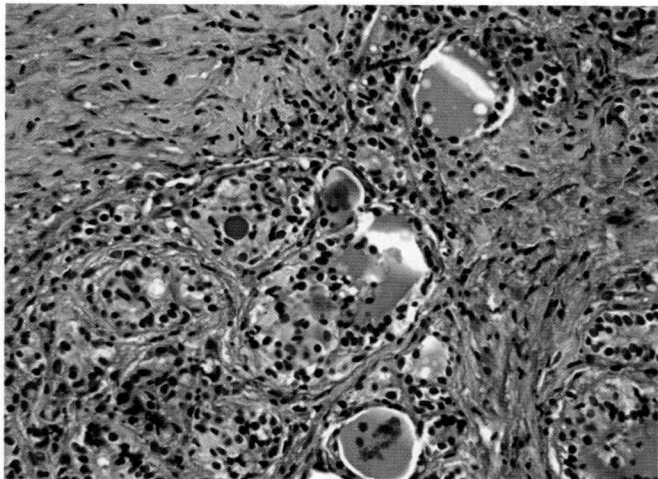

Figure 12-21 Subacute (viral or postviral) thyroiditis. Diffuse neutrophilic invasion with active destruction of follicles and a multinucleated giant cell. Fibrosis and near-complete loss of follicles have occurred. (Courtesy of Dr. Vania Nose, Brigham and Women's Hospital, Boston, MA.)

without fever. The pain, which is aggravated by turning the head or swallowing, characteristically radiates to the ear, jaw, or occiput and may mimic disorders arising in these areas. The absence of pain does not exclude the diagnosis, because biopsy-proven painless subacute thyroiditis occurs, but it must be distinguished from acute autoimmune thyroiditis. Hoarseness and dysphagia may be present; patients may complain of palpitation, nervousness, and lassitude. The latter symptoms can be extreme, considering the local nature of the disease, and suggest a systemic component. Although acute manifestations are present in severe cases, in milder disease, symptoms may be present for months yet are often overlooked.

On palpation at least part of the thyroid is slightly to moderately enlarged, firm, often nodular, and usually exquisitely tender, one lobe frequently being more severely affected than the other. Indeed the symptoms may be truly unilateral. The overlying skin may be warm and erythematous. Occasionally the locus of maximal involvement migrates over the course of a few weeks to other parts of the gland. The disease usually subsides within a few months, leaving no residual deficiency of thyroid function in 90% of patients. In rare patients the disease smolders, with repeated exacerbations over many months, hypothyroidism sometimes being the final result.

Diagnosis

The laboratory findings vary with the phase of the disease. During the active phase, the erythrocyte sedimentation rate is increased, often to a remarkable extent (>100 mm/hour). Indeed a diagnosis of active subacute thyroiditis is hardly tenable when the sedimentation rate is normal. The white blood cell count is normal or, at most, moderately increased. The serum Tg level is characteristically high, in keeping with the degree of thyroid destruction.

Subacute thyroiditis must be differentiated from acute hemorrhagic degeneration in a preexisting thyroid nodule,

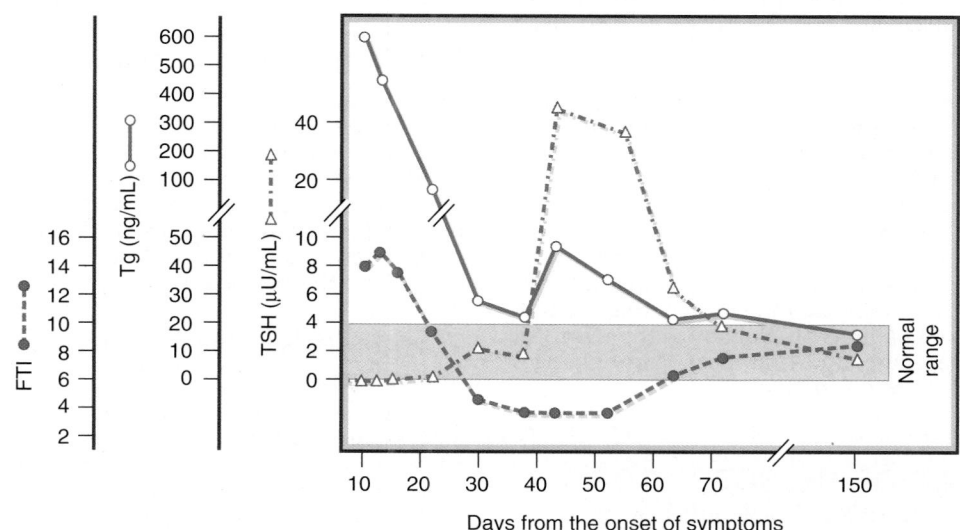

Days from the onset of symptoms

Figure 12-22 Thyroid function in a patient during the course of subacute (viral or postviral) thyroiditis. During the thyrotoxic phase (days 10 to 20), the serum thyroglobulin (Tg) concentration was greatly elevated, the free thyroxine index (FTI) was high, and the thyroid-stimulating hormone (TSH) was suppressed; the erythrocyte sedimentation rate was 86 mm/hour, and the thyroidal radioactive iodine uptake (RAIU) was 2%. The Tg level and the FTI declined in parallel. During the phase of hypothyroidism (days 30 to 63), when the FTI was below normal, a modest transient increase in serum Tg occurred in parallel with the increase in serum TSH. All parameters of thyroid function were normal by day 150, 5 months after the onset of symptoms. (From DeGroot LJ, Larsen PR, Hennemann G. Acute and subacute thyroiditis. In: DeGroot LJ, Larsen PR, Hennemann G, eds. *The Thyroid and Its Diseases*, 6th ed. New York, NY: Churchill Livingstone; 1996:705.)

Hashimoto disease with painful recurrence (see earlier), acute pyogenic thyroiditis or fungal infection, and rarely thyroid malignancy with painful nodules. Acute painful exacerbations of Hashimoto thyroiditis may be difficult to distinguish from subacute thyroiditis. Lack of elevation of the erythrocyte sedimentation rate and high titers of thyroid autoantibodies strongly suggest the former. Acute pyogenic thyroiditis is distinguished by the presence of a septic focus elsewhere by a greater inflammatory reaction in the tissues adjacent to the thyroid and by much greater leukocytic and febrile responses (see Chapter 13). The RAIU and thyroid function are usually preserved in acute pyogenic thyroiditis. Rarely, widespread infiltrating cancer of the thyroid can present with a clinical and laboratory picture almost indistinguishable from that of subacute thyroiditis. Ultrasound and fine-needle aspiration should be performed if this is a consideration.

Treatment

In mild cases, aspirin or nonsteroidal anti-inflammatory drugs or cyclooxygenase 2 (COX-2) inhibitors may control the symptoms. With more severe pain, glucocorticoids (e.g., prednisone up to 40 mg/day) are the only solution for the extreme discomfort. This drug may be required for several months and should then be withdrawn gradually. If the TSH is not suppressed, TSH-suppressive therapy with levothyroxine may decrease the size of the gland, relieving the pressure on the thyroid capsule. TSH is needed for thyroid cell regeneration, so such therapy should be decreased as the symptoms subside.

Drug-Associated Thyroiditis

Thyroiditis is an uncommon complication of pharmacotherapy. Amiodarone is an important exception and was discussed earlier. Most of the thyroiditis associated with various therapeutic agents appears to be due to drug-induced exacerbation of underlying autoimmune disease. This effect is understandable with agents that are specifically administered to modify the immune system. They include IL-2, interferon-α, and granulocyte/macrophage colony-stimulating factor (GM-CSF), all of which can precipitate silent thyroiditis.[115,365,366] This has also been described with lithium and the GnRH agonist leuprolide, but the pathophysiologic mechanism is obscure.[367-369]

Thyroiditis has been found in association with multitargeting kinase inhibitors such as sunitinib and sorafenib given for a variety of tumors including gastrointestinal stromal tumors, hepatocellular carcinoma, and renal cell carcinoma.[361,370] This may present as subacute thyroiditis with a suppressed TSH as the major manifestation of the early phase but then progress to destruction of the gland through an unclear mechanism. Although imatinib has been associated with an increase in levothyroxine requirements in hypothyroid patients (analogous to the effects of phenytoin, carbamazepine, and rifampin), those changes are independent of thyroid function.[371]

OTHER CAUSES OF THYROTOXICOSIS WITH A LOW RADIOIODINE UPTAKE

In addition to silent and subacute thyroiditis, several other entities should be considered in the patient with thyrotoxicosis in whom the thyroid gland is either not palpable or not enlarged and who has biochemical findings of thyrotoxicosis accompanied by a low RAIU.

Thyrotoxicosis Factitia

Thyrotoxicosis that arises from the ingestion, usually chronic, of excessive quantities of thyroid hormone usually occurs in individuals with a background of underlying psychiatric disease, especially in paramedical personnel who have access to thyroid hormone or in patients for whom thyroid hormone medication has been prescribed in the past. Generally the patient is aware of taking thyroid hormone but may adamantly deny it. In other instances, large doses of thyroid hormone or other thyroactive material may be given without the knowledge of the patient, usually as part of a regimen for weight reduction. Some "natural" products for weight reduction stated not to contain thyroid hormone nonetheless do. Symptoms are typical of thyrotoxicosis and may be severe.

In the absence of preexisting disease of the thyroid, the diagnosis is made from the combination of typical thyrotoxic manifestations, together with thyroid atrophy and hypofunction. Infiltrative ophthalmopathy never occurs, but lid lag, stare, and other thyrotoxic eye signs may be present; TSH levels are suppressed. Serum T_4 concentrations are increased unless the patient is taking T_3, in which case they will be subnormal. Serum T_3 concentrations are increased in either case. Hypofunction of the thyroid gland is evidenced by the subnormal values of RAIU. The presence of low, rather than elevated, values of serum Tg is a clear indication that the thyrotoxicosis results from exogenous hormone, rather than thyroid hyperfunction.

This disorder may be confused with other varieties of thyrotoxicosis associated with a subnormal RAIU and absence of goiter, including silent thyroiditis, ectopic thyroid tissue, and hyperfunctioning metastatic follicular carcinoma. Evidence for the two latter disorders can be obtained by demonstration of the ectopic focus or foci by external radioiodine scanning or the presence of normal to elevated serum Tg concentrations. Differentiation from silent thyroiditis may be difficult. The presence of TPO antibodies points to painless chronic autoimmune thyroiditis, whereas a firm thyroid and brief history suggest the painless variant of subacute thyroiditis. Treatment of thyrotoxicosis factitia consists of withdrawing the offending medication. Psychiatric consultation is often required.

Hamburger Thyrotoxicosis

An unusual form of exogenous thyrotoxicosis occurred in the midwestern portion of the United States in 1984 and 1985. The source was the inclusion of large quantities of bovine thyroid in ground beef preparations.[372] When the slaughtering practices were changed, this condition disappeared. Such a possibility, although remote, should be considered, especially if one is confronted with epidemic exogenous thyrotoxicosis.

Thyrotoxicosis Due to Extrathyroidal Tissue
Struma Ovarii

Thyroid tissue may be present in 5% to 10% of teratomas, and occasionally such foci are hyperfunctional.[373,374] About 5% to 10% of these tumors are bilateral. Although thyrotoxicosis is unusual, it may occur in as many as 8% to 10% of patients. Rarely, males with germ cell tumors may also develop hCG-induced hyperthyroidism.[375]

Clinical Presentation

Patients present with variable degrees of thyrotoxicosis but without goiter and generally have lower abdominal symptoms such as pain or a mass. Rarely ascites is present. Laboratory studies show reduced TSH and increased free T_4 of a variable degree, but the RAIU is low. The Tg may be elevated, particularly if the teratoma is malignant and has metastasized to the peritoneum. Abdominal CT scan or MRI shows a multilocular ovarian mass or masses.[376] Rarely a struma ovarii is accompanied by Graves disease.[377]

Treatment

The patient should be rendered euthyroid if thyrotoxicosis is significant followed by removal of the involved ovary or ovaries. Therapeutic radioiodine will be required for metastatic disease after ablation of the normal thyroid gland.

Thyrotoxicosis Due to Metastatic Thyroid Carcinoma

In general, thyroid carcinomas are made up of poorly functioning tissue. On occasion, follicular thyroid carcinomas will have sufficient function when combined with the total mass of the metastases to result in an elevation in serum free T_4 or T_3 and may even be seen in Graves disease with TRAbs activating the tissue.[378] Typically, such a course is a complication of a previously diagnosed lesion (see Chapter 14).[379] The symptoms of thyrotoxicosis will vary and the metastatic disease is usually obvious from radiologic studies. On occasion, the presentation may be confusing if the patient is receiving TSH-suppressive therapy, and diagnosis will require its discontinuation. In spite of that, TSH will remain suppressed and the serum free T_4 is elevated. Treatment of this condition is typical for that of thyroid carcinoma and is described in Chapter 14. In patients with thyrotoxicosis due to metastatic tumor, serum Tg is quite elevated, indicating that the thyrotoxicosis is caused by thyroidal tissue that is not located in the neck. An RAIU during the thyrotoxic phase will show no neck uptake due to TSH suppression even if the thyroid is still present.

REFERENCES

1. Kahaly GJ, Dillmann WH. Thyroid hormone action in the heart. *Endocr Rev.* 2005;26:704-728.
2. Burggraaf J, Tulen JH, Lalezari S, et al. Sympathovagal imbalance in hyperthyroidism. *Am J Physiol Endocrinol Metab.* 2001;281:E190-E195.
3. Fazio S, Palmieri EA, Lombardi G, Biondi B. Effects of thyroid hormone on the cardiovascular system. *Recent Prog Horm Res.* 2004;59:31-50.
4. Carrillo-Sepulveda MA, Ceravolo GS, Furstenau CR, et al. Emerging role of angiotensin type 2 receptor (AT2R)/Akt/NO pathway in vascular smooth muscle cell in the hyperthyroidism. *PLoS One.* 2013;8:e61982.
5. Grais IM, Sowers JR. Thyroid and the heart. *Am J Med.* 2014;127:691-698.
6. Brauman A, Rosenberg T, Gilboa Y, et al. Prevalence of mitral valve prolapse in chronic lymphocytic thyroiditis and nongoitrous hypothyroidism. *Cardiology.* 1988;75:269-273.
7. Evangelopoulos ME, Toumanidis S, Sotou D, et al. Mitral valve prolapse in young healthy individuals. An early index of autoimmunity? *Lupus.* 2009;18:436-440.
8. Stavrakis S, Yu X, Patterson E, et al. Activating autoantibodies to the beta-1 adrenergic and m2 muscarinic receptors facilitate atrial fibrillation in patients with Graves' hyperthyroidism. *J Am Coll Cardiol.* 2009;54:1309-1316.
9. Sawin CT, Geller A, Wolf PA, et al. Low serum thyrotropin concentrations as a risk factor for atrial fibrillation in older persons. *N Engl J Med.* 1994;331:1249-1252.
10. Cappola AR, Fried LP, Arnold AM, et al. Thyroid status, cardiovascular risk, and mortality in older adults. *JAMA.* 2006;295:1033-1041.
11. Nakazawa H, Lythall DA, Noh J, et al. Is there a place for the late cardioversion of atrial fibrillation? A long-term follow-up study of patients with post-thyrotoxic atrial fibrillation. *Eur Heart J.* 2000;21:327-333.
12. Silva JE. Thermogenic mechanisms and their hormonal regulation. *Physiol Rev.* 2006;86:435-464.
13. Palmieri EA, Fazio S, Palmieri V, et al. Myocardial contractility and total arterial stiffness in patients with overt hyperthyroidism: acute

14. Carvalho-Bianco SD, Kim B, Harney JW, et al. Chronic cardiac-specific thyrotoxicosis increases myocardial beta-adrenergic responsiveness. *Mol Endocrinol.* 2004;18:1840-1849.
15. Ojamaa K, Klein I, Sabet A, Steinberg SF. Changes in adenylyl cyclase isoforms as a mechanism for thyroid hormone modulation of cardiac beta-adrenergic receptor responsiveness. *Metabolism.* 2000;49:275-279.
16. Wakasugi M, Wakao R, Tawata M, et al. Change in bone mineral density in patients with hyperthyroidism after attainment of euthyroidism by dual energy X-ray absorptiometry. *Thyroid.* 1994;4:179-182.
17. Mundy GR, Shapiro JL, Bandelin JG, et al. Direct stimulation of bone resorption by thyroid hormones. *J Clin Invest.* 1976;58:529-534.
18. Williams GR. Thyroid hormone actions in cartilage and bone. *Eur Thyroid J.* 2013;2:3-13.
19. Marino M, Barbesino G, Pinchera A, et al. Increased frequency of euthyroid ophthalmopathy in patients with Graves' disease associated with myasthenia gravis. *Thyroid.* 2000;10:799-802.
20. Mohan HK, Groves AM, Fogelman I, Clarke SE. Thyroid hormone and parathyroid hormone competing to maintain calcium levels in the presence of vitamin D deficiency. *Thyroid.* 2004;14:789-791.
21. Wojcicka A, Bassett JH, Williams GR. Mechanisms of action of thyroid hormones in the skeleton. *Biochim Biophys Acta.* 2013;1830:3979-3986.
22. Zaidi M, Davies TF, Zallone A, et al. Thyroid-stimulating hormone, thyroid hormones, and bone loss. *Curr Osteoporos Rep.* 2009;7:47-52.
23. Yu Wai Man CY, Chinnery PF, Griffiths PG. Extraocular muscles have fundamentally distinct properties that make them selectively vulnerable to certain disorders. *Neuromuscul Disord.* 2005;15:17-23.
24. Kodali VR, Jeffcote B, Clague RB. Thyrotoxic periodic paralysis: a case report and review of the literature. *J Emerg Med.* 1999;17:43-45.
25. Dias Da Silva MR, Cerutti JM, Arnaldi LA, Maciel RM. A mutation in the KCNE3 potassium channel gene is associated with susceptibility to thyrotoxic hypokalemic periodic paralysis. *J Clin Endocrinol Metab.* 2002;87:4881-4884.
26. Wakasugi M, Wakao R, Tawata M, et al. Bone mineral density in patients with hyperthyroidism measured by dual energy X-ray absorptiometry. *Clin Endocrinol (Oxf).* 1993;38:283-286.
27. Abe E, Marians RC, Yu W, et al. TSH is a negative regulator of skeletal remodeling. *Cell.* 2003;115:151-162.
28. Baliram R, Sun L, Cao J, et al. Hyperthyroid-associated osteoporosis is exacerbated by the loss of TSH signaling. *J Clin Invest.* 2012;122:3737-3741.
29. Wejda B, Hintze G, Katschinski B, et al. Hip fractures and the thyroid: a case-control study. *J Intern Med.* 1995;237:241-247.
30. Faber J, Galloe AM. Changes in bone mass during prolonged subclinical hyperthyroidism due to L-thyroxine treatment: a meta-analysis. *Eur J Endocrinol.* 1994;130:350-356.
31. Bauer DC, Ettinger B, Nevitt MC, Stone KL. Risk for fracture in women with low serum levels of thyroid-stimulating hormone. *Ann Intern Med.* 2001;134:561-568.
32. Dalla Costa M, Mangano FA, Betterle C. Thymic hyperplasia in patients with Graves' disease. *J Endocrinol Invest.* [Epub 2014 Aug 23].
33. Godart V, Weynand B, Coche E, et al. Intense 18-fluorodeoxyglucose uptake by the thymus on PET scan does not necessarily herald recurrence of thyroid carcinoma. *J Endocrinol Invest.* 2005;28:1024-1028.
34. Erem C, Ersoz HO, Karti SS, et al. Blood coagulation and fibrinolysis in patients with hyperthyroidism. *J Endocrinol Invest.* 2002;25:345-350.
35. Kurnik D, Loebstein R, Farfel Z, et al. Complex drug-drug-disease interactions between amiodarone, warfarin, and the thyroid gland. *Medicine (Baltimore).* 2004;83:107-113.
36. Taniyama M, Honma K, Ban Y. Urinary cortisol metabolites in the assessment of peripheral thyroid hormone action: application for diagnosis of resistance to thyroid hormone. *Thyroid.* 1993;3:229-233.
37. Stagnaro-Green A, Roman SH, Cobin RH, et al. Detection of at-risk pregnancy by means of highly sensitive assays for thyroid autoantibodies. *JAMA.* 1990;264:1422-1425.
38. Stagnaro-Green A, Glinoer D. Thyroid autoimmunity and the risk of miscarriage. *Best Pract Res Clin Endocrinol Metab.* 2004;18:167-181.
39. Stagnaro-Green A, Pearce E. Thyroid disorders in pregnancy. *Nat Rev Endocrinol.* 2012;8:650-658.
40. Meikle AW. The interrelationships between thyroid dysfunction and hypogonadism in men and boys. *Thyroid.* 2004;14(Suppl 1):S17-S25.
41. Tagawa N, Takano T, Fukata S, et al. Serum concentration of androstenediol and androstenediol sulfate in patients with hyperthyroidism and hypothyroidism. *Endocr J.* 2001;48:345-354.
42. Parry CH. Disease of the heart: enlargement of the thyroid gland in connection with enlargement or palpitation of the heart. In: *Collections From the Unpublished Medical Writings of the Late Caleb Hillier Parry.* London: Underwoods, Fleet Street; 1825:111-125.
43. Weetman AP. Grave's disease 1835-2002. *Horm Res.* 2003;59(Suppl 1):114-118.
44. von Basedow CA. Exophthalmos durch Hypertrophie des Zellgewebes in der Augenhöhle. *Wochensch Ges Heilk.* 1840;6:197-204.
45. Graves RJ. *Clinical Lectures, Lecture XII.* Philadelphia: Barrington & Haswell; 1842.

46. Adams DD. The presence of an abnormal thyroid-stimulating hormone in the serum of some thyrotoxic patients. *J Clin Endocrinol Metab.* 1958;18:699-712.
47. Adams DD. The pathogenesis of thyrotoxicosis the discovery of LATS. *N Z Med J.* 1975;81:15-17.
48. Davies TF, Ando T, Lin RY, et al. Thyrotropin receptor-associated diseases: from adenomata to Graves disease. *J Clin Invest.* 2005;115: 1972-1983.
49. Morshed SA, Latif R, Davies TF. Characterization of thyrotropin receptor antibody-induced signaling cascades. *Endocrinology.* 2009;150: 519-529.
50. Martin A, Valentine M, Unger P, et al. Engraftment of human lymphocytes and thyroid tissue into Scid and Rag2-deficient mice: absent progression of lymphocytic infiltration. *J Clin Endocrinol Metab.* 1994; 79:716-723.
51. Hiromatsu Y, Hoshino T, Yagita H, et al. Functional Fas ligand expression in thyrocytes from patients with Graves' disease. *J Clin Endocrinol Metab.* 1999;84:2896-2902.
52. Hollowell JG, Staehling NW, Flanders WD, et al. Serum TSH, T(4), and thyroid antibodies in the United States population (1988 to 1994): National Health and Nutrition Examination Survey (NHANES III). *J Clin Endocrinol Metab.* 2002;87:489-499.
53. Vanderpump MPJ, Tunbridge WMG, French JM, et al. The incidence of thyroid disorders in the community: a twenty-year follow-up of the Whickham survey. *Clin Endocrinol (Oxf).* 1995;43:55-68.
54. Carle A, Pedersen IB, Knudsen N, et al. Epidemiology of subtypes of hyperthyroidism in Denmark: a population-based study. *Eur J Endocrinol.* 2011;164:801-809.
55. Shimojo N, Kohno Y, Yamaguchi K, et al. Induction of Graves-like disease in mice by immunization with fibroblasts transfected with the thyrotropin receptor and a class II molecule. *Proc Natl Acad Sci U S A.* 1996;93:11074-11079.
56. Kita M, Ahmad L, Marians RC, et al. Regulation and transfer of a murine model of thyrotropin receptor antibody mediated Graves' disease. *Endocrinology.* 1999;140:1392-1398.
57. Ando T, Imaizumi M, Graves P, et al. Induction of thyroid-stimulating hormone receptor autoimmunity in hamsters. *Endocrinology.* 2003;144: 671-680.
58. Nagayama Y, Kita-Furuyama M, Ando T, et al. A novel murine model of Graves' hyperthyroidism with intramuscular injection of adenovirus expressing the thyrotropin receptor. *J Immunol.* 2002;168: 2789-2794.
59. Sanders J, Chirgadze DY, Sanders P, et al. Crystal structure of the TSH receptor in complex with a thyroid-stimulating autoantibody. *Thyroid.* 2007;17:395-410.
60. Latif R, Teixeira A, Michalek K, et al. Antibody protection reveals extended epitopes on the human TSH receptor. *PLoS One.* 2012;7: e44669.
61. Adams DD, Purves HD. Abnormal responses in the assay of thyrotropin. *Proc Univ Otago Med Sch.* 1956;34:11-12.
62. Kraiem Z, Lahat N, Glaser B, et al. Thyrotropin receptor blocking antibodies: incidence, characterization and in-vitro synthesis. *Clin Endocrinol (Oxf).* 1987;27:409-421.
63. Adams DD, Fastier FN, Howie JB, et al. Stimulation of the human thyroid by infusions of plasma containing LATS protector. *J Clin Endocrinol Metab.* 1974;39:826-832.
64. Munro DS, Dirmikis SM, Humphries H, et al. The role of thyroid-stimulating immunoglobulins of Graves' disease in neonatal thyrotoxicosis. *Br J Obstet Gynaecol.* 1978;85:837-843.
65. Zakarija M, McKenzie JM. Pregnancy-associated changes in thyroid-stimulating antibody of Graves' disease and the relationship to neonatal hyperthyroidism. *J Clin Endocrinol Metab.* 1983;57:1036-1040.
66. Zakarija MJ. Immunochemical characterization of the thyroid-stimulating antibody (TSab) of Graves' disease: evidence for restricted heterogeneity. *J Clin Lab Immunol.* 1983;10:77-85.
67. Weetman AP, Yateman ME, Ealey PA, et al. Thyroid-stimulating antibody activity between different immunoglobulin G subclasses. *J Clin Invest.* 1990;86:723-727.
68. Tozzoli R, Bagnasco M, Giavarina D, Bizzaro N. TSH receptor autoantibody immunoassay in patients with Graves' disease: improvement of diagnostic accuracy over different generations of methods. Systematic review and meta-analysis. *Autoimmun Rev.* 2012;12:107-113.
69. Davies TF, Yeo PP, Evered DC, et al. Value of thyroid-stimulating-antibody determinations in predicting short-term thyrotoxic relapse in Graves' disease. *Lancet.* 1977;1:1181-1182.
70. Davies TF, Roti E, Braverman LE, DeGroot LJ. Thyroid controversy—stimulating antibodies. *J Clin Endocrinol Metab.* 1998;83(11):3777-3785.
71. Mackenzie WA, Schwartz AE, Friedman EW, Davies TF. Intrathyroidal T cell clones from patients with autoimmune thyroid disease. *J Clin Endocrinol Metab.* 1987;64:818-824.
72. Dayan CM, Londei M, Corcoran AE, et al. Autoantigen recognition by thyroid-infiltrating T cells in Graves disease. *Proc Natl Acad Sci U S A.* 1991;88:7415-7419.
73. Davies TF, Martin A, Concepcion ES, et al. Evidence of limited variability of antigen receptors on intrathyroidal T cells in autoimmune thyroid disease. *N Engl J Med.* 1991;325:238-244.
74. Grubeck Loebenstein B, Turner M, Pirich K, et al. CD4+ T-cell clones from autoimmune thyroid tissue cannot be classified according to their lymphokine production. *Scand J Immunol.* 1990;32: 433-440.
75. Zha B, Huang X, Lin J, et al. Distribution of lymphocyte subpopulations in thyroid glands of human autoimmune thyroid disease. *J Clin Lab Anal.* 2014;28:249-254.
76. Valmori D, Merlo A, Souleimanian NE, et al. A peripheral circulating compartment of natural naive CD4 Tregs. *J Clin Invest.* 2005;115: 1953-1962.
77. Wing JB, Sakaguchi S. Foxp3(+) T(reg) cells in humoral immunity. *Int Immunol.* 2014;26:61-69.
78. Glick AB, Wodzinski A, Fu P, et al. Impairment of regulatory T-cell function in autoimmune thyroid disease. *Thyroid.* 2013;23:871-878.
79. Morshed SA, Latif R, Davies TF. Delineating the autoimmune mechanisms in Graves' disease. *Immunol Res.* 2012;54:191-203.
80. Li HS, Carayanniotis G. Detection of thyroglobulin mRNA as truncated isoform(s) in mouse thymus. *Immunology.* 2005;115:85-89.
81. Murakami M, Hosoi Y, Negishi T, et al. Thymic hyperplasia in patients with Graves' disease. Identification of thyrotropin receptors in human thymus. *J Clin Invest.* 1996;98:2228-2234.
82. Stefan M, Wei C, Lombardi A, et al. Genetic-epigenetic dysregulation of thymic TSH receptor gene expression triggers thyroid autoimmunity. *Proc Natl Acad Sci U S A.* 2014;111:12562-12567.
83. Akeno N, Smith EP, Stefan M, et al. IFN-alpha mediates the development of autoimmunity both by direct tissue toxicity and through immune cell recruitment mechanisms. *J Immunol.* 2011;186: 4693-4706.
84. Blackard JT, Kong L, Huber AK, Tomer Y. Hepatitis C virus infection of a thyroid cell line: implications for pathogenesis of hepatitis C virus and thyroiditis. *Thyroid.* 2013;23:863-870.
85. Tomer Y, Davies TF. Infection, thyroid disease and autoimmunity. *Endocr Rev.* 1993;14:107-120.
86. Rapoport B, Aalsabeh R, Aftergood D, McLachlan S. Elephantiasic pretibial myxedema: insight into (and a hypothesis regarding) the pathogenesis of the extrathyroidal manifestations of Graves' disease. *Thyroid.* 2000;10:685-692.
87. Peng D, Xu B, Wang Y, et al. A high frequency of circulating th22 and th17 cells in patients with new onset Graves' disease. *PLoS One.* 2013;8:e68446.
88. Arata N, Ando T, Unger P, Davies TF. By-stander activation in autoimmune thyroiditis: studies on experimental autoimmune thyroiditis in the GFP+ fluorescent mouse. *Clin Immunol.* 2006;121:108-117.
89. De Riu A, Martin A, Valentine M, et al. Graves' disease thyroid transplants in Scid mice: persistent selectivity in hTcR V alpha gene family use. *Autoimmunity.* 1994;19:271-277.
90. Wickham S, Carr DJ. Molecular mimicry versus bystander activation: herpetic stromal keratitis. *Autoimmunity.* 2004;37:393-397.
91. Srinivasappa J, Saegusa J, Prabhakar BS, et al. Molecular mimicry: frequency of reactivity of monoclonal antiviral antibodies with normal tissues. *J Virol.* 1986;57:397-401.
92. Haspel MV, Onodrera T, Prabhakar BS, et al. Multiple organ-reactive monoclonal autoantibodies. *Nature.* 1983;304:73-76.
93. Hargreaves CE, Grasso M, Hampe CS, et al. *Yersinia enterocolitica* provides the link between thyroid-stimulating antibodies and their germline counterparts in Graves' disease. *J Immunol.* 2013;190: 5373-5381.
94. Benvenga S, Guarneri F, Vaccaro M, et al. Homologies between proteins of *Borrelia burgdorferi* and thyroid autoantigens. *Thyroid.* 2004;14: 964-966.
95. Mirakian R, Hammond LJ, Bottazzo GF. Pathogenesis of thyroid autoimmunity: the Bottazzo-Feldmann hypothesis. *Immunol Today.* 1998; 19:97-98.
96. Piccinini LA, Goldsmith NK, Schachter BS, Davies TF. Localization of HLA-DR alpha-chain messenger ribonucleic acid in normal and autoimmune human thyroid using in situ hybridization. *J Clin Endocrinol Metab.* 1988;66:1307-1315.
97. Pujol-Borrell R, Todd I, Londei M, et al. Inappropriate major histocompatibility complex class II expression by thyroid follicular cells in thyroid autoimmune disease and by pancreatic beta cells in type I diabetes. *Mol Biol Med.* 1986;3:159-165.
98. Yin X, Sachidanandam R, Morshed S, et al. mRNA-Seq reveals novel molecular mechanisms and a robust fingerprint in Graves' disease. *J Clin Endocrinol Metab.* 2014;99(10):E2076-E2083.
99. Kawakami Y, Kuzuya N, Watanabe T, et al. Induction of experimental thyroiditis in mice by recombinant interferon gamma administration. *Acta Endocrinol (Copenh).* 1990;122:41-48.
100. Moudgil KD, Sercarz EE. Understanding crypticity is the key to revealing the pathogenesis of autoimmunity. *Trends Immunol.* 2005;26: 355-359.
101. Carle A, Bulow Pedersen I, Knudsen N, et al. Graves' hyperthyroidism and moderate alcohol consumption: evidence for disease prevention. *Clin Endocrinol (Oxf).* 2013;79:111-119.
102. Weetman AP. Diseases associated with thyroid autoimmunity: explanations for the expanding spectrum. *Clin Endocrinol (Oxf).* 2011;74: 411-418.

103. Villanueva R, Greenberg DA, Davies TF, Tomer Y. Sibling recurrence risk in autoimmune thyroid disease. *Thyroid.* 2003;13:761-764.

104. Brix TH, Christensen K, Holm NV, et al. A population-based study of Graves' disease in Danish twins. *Clin Endocrinol (Oxf).* 1998;48:397-400.

105. Tomer Y, Greenberg DA, Barbesino G, et al. CTLA-4 and not CD28 is a susceptibility gene for thyroid autoantibody production. *J Clin Endocrinol Metab.* 2001;86:1687-1693.

106. Farid NR, Bear JC. The human major histocompatibility complex and endocrine disease. *Endocr Rev.* 1981;2:50-86.

107. Barbesino G, Tomer Y, Concepcion ES, et al. Linkage analysis of candidate genes in autoimmune thyroid disease: 1. Selected immunoregulatory genes. *J Clin Endocrinol Metab.* 1998;83:1580-1584.

108. Ban Y, Concepcion ES, Villanueva R, et al. Analysis of immune regulatory genes in familial and sporadic Graves' disease. *J Clin Endocrinol Metab.* 2004;89:4562-4568.

109. Chu X, Pan CM, Zhao SX, et al. A genome-wide association study identifies two new risk loci for Graves' disease. *Nat Genet.* 2011;43:897-901.

110. Zhao SX, Xue LQ, Liu W, et al. Robust evidence for five new Graves' disease risk loci from a staged genome-wide association analysis. *Hum Mol Genet.* 2013;22:3347-3362.

111. Tomer Y, Greenberg D. The thyroglobulin gene as the first thyroid-specific susceptibility gene for autoimmune thyroid disease. *Trends Mol Med.* 2004;10:306-308.

112. Yin X, Latif R, Bahn R, et al. Influence of the TSH receptor gene on susceptibility to Graves' disease and Graves' ophthalmopathy. *Thyroid.* 2008;18:1201-1206.

113. Brand OJ, Barrett JC, Simmonds MJ, et al. Association of the thyroid stimulating hormone receptor gene (TSHR) with Graves' disease. *Hum Mol Genet.* 2009;18:1704-1713.

114. Samarkos M, Vaiopoulos G. The role of infections in the pathogenesis of autoimmune diseases. *Curr Drug Targets Inflamm Allergy.* 2005;4:99-103.

115. Olson JK, Croxford JL, Miller SD. Virus-induced autoimmunity: potential role of viruses in initiation, perpetuation, and progression of T-cell-mediated autoimmune disease. *Viral Immunol.* 2001;14:227-250.

116. Menconi F, Hasham A, Tomer Y. Environmental triggers of thyroiditis: hepatitis C and interferon-alpha. *J Endocrinol Invest.* 2011;34:78-84.

117. Vita R, Lapa D, Trimarchi F, Benvenga S. Stress triggers the onset and the recurrences of hyperthyroidism in patients with Graves' disease. *Endocrine.* 2015;48(1):254-263.

118. Effraimidis G, Tijssen JG, Brosschot JF, Wiersinga WM. Involvement of stress in the pathogenesis of autoimmune thyroid disease: a prospective study. *Psychoneuroendocrinology.* 2012;37(8):1191-1198.

119. Irwin M. Stress-induced immune suppression: role of brain corticotropin releasing hormone and autonomic nervous system mechanisms. *Adv Neuroimmunol.* 1994;4:29-47.

120. Marshall GD. Neuroendocrine mechanisms of immune dysregulation: applications to allergy and asthma. *Ann Allergy Asthma Immunol.* 2004;93:S11-S17.

121. Falgarone G, Heshmati HM, Cohen R, Reach G. Mechanisms in endocrinology. Role of emotional stress in the pathophysiology of Graves' disease. *Eur J Endocrinol.* 2013;168:R13-R18.

122. Amino N, Tada H, Hidaka Y, et al. Therapeutic controversy: screening for postpartum thyroiditis. *J Clin Endocrinol Metab.* 1999;84:1813-1821.

123. Polese B, Gridelet V, Araklioti E, et al. The endocrine milieu and CD4 T-lymphocyte polarization during pregnancy. *Front Endocrinol (Lausanne).* 2014;5:106.

124. Ansar AS, Young PR, Penhale WJ. Beneficial effect of testosterone in the treatment of chronic autoimmune thyroiditis in rats. *J Immunol.* 1986;136:143-147.

125. Gleicher N, Barad DH. Gender as risk factor for autoimmune diseases. *J Autoimmun.* 2007;28:1-6.

126. Ban Y, Tozaki T, Tobe T, et al. The regulatory T cell gene FOXP3 and genetic susceptibility to thyroid autoimmunity: an association analysis in Caucasian and Japanese cohorts. *J Autoimmun.* 2007;28:201-207.

127. Chow JC, Yen Z, Ziesche SM, Brown CJ. Silencing of the mammalian X chromosome. *Annu Rev Genomics Hum Genet.* 2005;6:69-92.

128. Brix TH, Knudsen GP, Kristiansen M, et al. High frequency of skewed X-chromosome inactivation in females with autoimmune thyroid disease: a possible explanation for the female predisposition to thyroid autoimmunity. *J Clin Endocrinol Metab.* 2005;90:5949-5953.

129. Yin X, Latif R, Tomer Y, Davies TF. Thyroid epigenetics: X chromosome inactivation in patients with autoimmune thyroid disease. *Ann N Y Acad Sci.* 2007;1110:193-200.

130. Mestman JH. Hyperthyroidism in pregnancy. *Curr Opin Endocrinol Diabetes Obes.* 2012;19:394-401.

131. Mestman JH. Hyperthyroidism in pregnancy. *Endocrinol Metab Clin North Am.* 1998;27:127-149.

132. Chan GW, Mandel SJ. Therapy insight: management of Graves' disease during pregnancy. *Nat Clin Pract Endocrinol Metab.* 2007;3:470-478.

133. Anselmo J, Cao D, Karrison T, et al. Fetal loss associated with excess thyroid hormone exposure. *JAMA.* 2004;292:691-695.

134. Aluvihare VR, Kallikourdis M, Betz AG. Tolerance, suppression and the fetal allograft. *J Mol Med.* 2005;83:88-96.

135. Stagnaro-Green A, Roman SH, Cobin RH, et al. A prospective study of lymphocyte-initiated immunosuppression in normal pregnancy: evidence of a T-cell etiology for postpartum thyroid dysfunction. *J Clin Endocrinol Metab.* 1992;74:645-653.

136. Jansson R, Dahlberg PA, Winsa B, et al. The postpartum period constitutes an important risk for the development of clinical Graves' disease in young women. *Acta Endocrinol (Copenh).* 1987;116(3):321-325.

137. Rotondi M, Cappelli C, Pirali B, et al. The effect of pregnancy on subsequent relapse from Graves' disease after a successful course of antithyroid drug therapy. *J Clin Endocrinol Metab.* 2008;93:3985-3988.

138. Basaria S, Cooper DS. Amiodarone and the thyroid. *Am J Med.* 2005;118:706-714.

139. Tomer Y, Blackard JT, Akeno N. Interferon alpha treatment and thyroid dysfunction. *Endocrinol Metab Clin North Am.* 2007;36:x-xi, 1051-1066.

140. DeGroot L. Effects of irradiation on the thyroid gland. *Endocrinol Metab Clin North Am.* 1993;22:607-615.

141. Huysmans D, Hermus A, Edelbrook M, et al. Autoimmune hyperthyroidism occurring late after radioiodine treatment for volume reduction of large multinodular goiters. *Thyroid.* 1997;7:535-539.

142. Pacini F, Vorontsova T, Molinaro E, et al. Prevalence of thyroid autoantibodies in children and adolescents from Belarus exposed to the Chernobyl radioactive fallout. *Lancet.* 1998;352:763-766.

143. Vermiglio F, Castagna MG, Volnova E, et al. Post-Chernobyl increased prevalence of humoral thyroid autoimmunity in children and adolescents from a moderately iodine-deficient area in Russia. *Thyroid.* 1999;9:781-786.

144. Vykhovanets EV, Chernyshov VP, Slukvin I, et al. 131-I dose-dependent thyroid autoimmune disorders in children living around Chernobyl. *Clin Immunol Immunopathol.* 1997;84:251-259.

145. McGregor AM, Petersen MM, Capiffe120 R, et al. A prospective study of the effects of radioiodine therapy on thyroid-stimulating antibody synthesis in Grave's disease [proceedings]. *J Endocrinol.* 1979;81(2):114P-115P.

146. Laurberg P, Wallin G, Tallstedt L, et al. TSH-receptor autoimmunity in Graves' disease after therapy with anti-thyroid drugs, surgery, or radioiodine: a 5-year prospective randomized study. *Eur J Endocrinol.* 2008;158:69-75.

147. Bartalena L, Marcocci C, Tanda ML, et al. An update on medical management of Graves' ophthalmopathy. *J Endocrinol Invest.* 2005;28:469-478.

148. Prabhakar BS, Bahn RS, Smith TJ. Current perspective on the pathogenesis of Graves' disease and ophthalmopathy. *Endocr Rev.* 2003;24:802-835.

149. Feldon SE, Park DJ, O'Loughlin CW, et al. Autologous T-lymphocytes stimulate proliferation of orbital fibroblasts derived from patients with Graves' ophthalmopathy. *Invest Ophthalmol Vis Sci.* 2005;46:3913-3921.

150. Grubeck-Loebenstein B, Trieb K, Holter W, et al. Retrobulbar T cells from patients with Graves' ophthalmopathy are CD8+ and specifically autologous fibroblasts. *J Clin Invest.* 1993;93:2738-2743.

151. Mori S, Yoshikawa N, Tokoro T, et al. Studies of retroorbital tissue xenografts from patients with Graves' ophthalmopathy in severe combined immunodeficient (SCID) mice: detection of thyroid-stimulating antibody. *Thyroid.* 1996;6:275-281.

152. Douglas RS, Afifiyan NF, Hwang CJ, et al. Increased generation of fibrocytes in thyroid-associated ophthalmopathy. *J Clin Endocrinol Metab.* 2010;95(1):430-438.

153. Weightman DR, Perros P, Sherif IH, Kendall-Taylor P. Autoantibodies to IGF-1 binding sites in thyroid associated ophthalmopathy. *Autoimmunity.* 1993;16:251-257.

154. Smith TJ, Tsai CC, Shih MJ, et al. Unique attributes of orbital fibroblasts and global alterations in IGF-1 receptor signaling could explain thyroid-associated ophthalmopathy. *Thyroid.* 2008;18:983-988.

155. Minich WB, Dehina N, Welsink T, et al. Autoantibodies to the IGF1 receptor in Graves' orbitopathy. *J Clin Endocrinol Metab.* 2013;98:752-760.

156. Wiersinga WM. Autoimmunity in Graves' ophthalmopathy: the result of an unfortunate marriage between TSH receptors and IGF-1 receptors? *J Clin Endocrinol Metab.* 2011;96:2386-2394.

157. Gianoukakis AG, Douglas RS, King CS, et al. IgG from patients with Graves' disease induces IL-16 and RANTES expression in cultured human thyrocytes: a putative mechanism for T cell infiltration of the thyroid in autoimmune disease. *Endocrinology.* 2006;147(4):1941-1949.

158. Villanueva R, Inzerillo AM, Tomer Y, et al. Limited genetic susceptibility to severe Graves' ophthalmopathy: no role for CTLA-4 but evidence for an environmental etiology. *Thyroid.* 2000;10(9):791-798.

159. Yin X, Latif R, Bahn R, Davies TF. Genetic profiling in Graves' disease: further evidence for lack of a distinct genetic contribution to Graves' ophthalmopathy. *Thyroid.* 2012;22:730-736.

160. Shine B, Fells P, Edwards OM, Weetman AP. Association between Graves' ophthalmopathy and smoking. *Lancet.* 1990;335:1261-1263.

161. Wiersinga WM. Smoking and thyroid. *Clin Endocrinol (Oxf).* 2013;79:145-151.

162. Wood LC, Ingbar SH. Hypothyroidism as a late sequela in patients with Graves' disease treated with antithyroid agents. *J Clin Invest.* 1979; 64:1429-1436.

163. Laurberg P, Nygaard B, Andersen S, et al. Association between TSH-receptor autoimmunity, hyperthyroidism, goitre, and orbitopathy in 208 patients included in the remission induction and sustenance in Graves' disease study. *J Thyroid Res.* 2014;2014:165487.

164. Kung AW, Yau CC, Cheng A. The incidence of ophthalmopathy after radioiodine therapy for Graves' disease: prognostic factors and the role of methimazole. *J Clin Endocrinol Metab.* 1994;79:542-546.

165. Tanda ML, Piantanida E, Liparulo L, et al. Prevalence and natural history of Graves' orbitopathy in a large series of patients with newly diagnosed Graves' hyperthyroidism seen at a single center. *J Clin Endocrinol Metab.* 2013;98(4):1443-1449.

166. Traisk F, Tallstedt L, Abraham-Nordling M, et al. Thyroid-associated ophthalmopathy after treatment for Graves' hyperthyroidism with antithyroid drugs or iodine-131. *J Clin Endocrinol Metab.* 2009;94: 3700-3707.

167. Eckstein AK, Plicht M, Lax H, et al. Thyrotropin receptor autoantibodies are independent risk factors for Graves' ophthalmopathy and help to predict severity and outcome of the disease. *J Clin Endocrinol Metab.* 2006;91:3464-3470.

168. Stan MN, Bahn RS. Risk factors for development or deterioration of Graves' ophthalmopathy. *Thyroid.* 2010;20:777-783.

169. Rundle FF, Wilson CW. Development and course of exophthalmos and ophthalmoplegia in Graves' disease with special reference to the effect of thyroidectomy. *Clin Sci.* 1945;5:177-194.

170. Bahn RS. Graves' ophthalmopathy. *N Engl J Med.* 2010;362:726-738.

171. Stan MN, Garrity JA, Bahn RS. The evaluation and treatment of Graves ophthalmopathy. *Med Clin North Am.* 2012;96:311-328.

172. McKeag D, Lane C, Lazarus JH, et al. Clinical features of dysthyroid optic neuropathy: a European Group on Graves' Orbitopathy (EUGOGO) survey. *Br J Ophthalmol.* 2007;91:455-458.

173. Ben Simon GJ, Syed HM, Douglas R, et al. Clinical manifestations and treatment outcome of optic neuropathy in thyroid-related orbitopathy. *Ophthalmic Surg Lasers Imaging.* 2006;37(4):284-290.

174. Bartalena L, Baldeschi L, Dickinson A, et al. Consensus statement of the European Group on Graves' orbitopathy (EUGOGO) on management of GO. *Eur J Endocrinol.* 2008;158(3):273-285.

175. Fatourechi V. Thyroid dermopathy and acropachy. *Best Pract Res Clin Endocrinol Metab.* 2012;26:553-565.

176. Smith BR, Bolton J, Young S, et al. A new assay for thyrotropin receptor autoantibodies. *Thyroid.* 2004;14:830-835.

177. Leschik JJ, Diana T, Olivo PD, et al. Analytical performance and clinical utility of a bioassay for thyroid-stimulating immunoglobulins. *Am J Clin Pathol.* 2013;139:192-200.

178. Schott M, Minich WB, Willenberg HS, et al. Relevance of TSH receptor stimulating and blocking autoantibody measurement for the prediction of relapse in Graves' disease. *Horm Metab Res.* 2005;37:741-744.

179. Singer PA, Cooper DS, Levy E, et al. Treatment guidelines for patients with hyperthyroidism and hypothyroidism. *JAMA.* 1995;273: 808-812.

180. Cooper DS. Antithyroid drugs. *N Engl J Med.* 2005;352:905-917.

181. Abuid J, Larsen PR. Triiodothyronine and thyroxine in hyperthyroidism. Comparison of the acute changes during therapy with antithyroid agents. *J Clin Invest.* 1974;54:201-208.

182. Maia AL, Kim BW, Huang SA, et al. Type 2 iodothyronine deiodinase is the major source of plasma T3 in euthyroid humans. *J Clin Invest.* 2005;115:2524-2533.

183. Laurberg P, Vestergaard H, Nielsen S, et al. Sources of circulating 3,5,3'-triiodothyronine in hyperthyroidism estimated after blocking of type 1 and type 2 iodothyronine deiodinases. *J Clin Endocrinol Metab.* 2007;92:2149-2156.

184. Okamura Y, Shigemasa C, Tatsuhara T. Pharmacokinetics of methimazole in normal subjects and hyperthyroid patients. *Endocrinol Jpn.* 1986;33:605-615.

185. Weetman AP. The immunomodulatory effects of antithyroid drugs. *Thyroid.* 1994;4:145-146.

186. Stassi G, Zeuner A, Di Liberto D, et al. Fas-FasL in Hashimoto's thyroiditis. *J Clin Immunol.* 2001;21:19-23.

187. De Vito P, Incerpi S, Pedersen JZ, et al. Thyroid hormones as modulators of immune activities at the cellular level. *Thyroid.* 2011;21: 879-890.

188. Harper L, Chin L, Daykin J, et al. Propylthiouracil and carbimazole associated-antineutrophil cytoplasmic antibodies (ANCA) in patients with Graves' disease. *Clin Endocrinol (Oxf).* 2004;60:671-675.

189. Rivkees SA, Mattison DR. Propylthiouracil (PTU) hepatoxicity in children and recommendations for discontinuation of use. *Int J Pediatr Endocrinol.* 2009;2009:132041.

190. Cooper DS, Rivkees SA. Putting propylthiouracil in perspective. *J Clin Endocrinol Metab.* 2009;94:1881-1882.

191. Woeber KA. Methimazole-induced hepatotoxicity. *Endocr Pract.* 2002;8: 222-224.

192. Rivkees SA. 63 years and 715 days to the "boxed warning": unmasking of the propylthiouracil problem. *Int J Pediatr Endocrinol.* 2010;2010: 658267.

193. Bahn RS, Burch HS, Cooper DS, et al. The role of propylthiouracil in the management of Graves' disease in adults: report of a meeting jointly sponsored by the American Thyroid Association and the Food and Drug Administration. *Thyroid.* 2009;19:673-674.

194. Bahn Chair RS, Burch HB, Cooper DS, et al. Hyperthyroidism and other causes of thyrotoxicosis: management guidelines of the American Thyroid Association and American Association of Clinical Endocrinologists. *Thyroid.* 2011;21:593-646.

195. Nakamura H, Noh JY, Itoh K, et al. Comparison of methimazole and propylthiouracil in patients with hyperthyroidism caused by Graves' disease. *J Clin Endocrinol Metab.* 2007;92:2157-2162.

196. Benker G, Reinwein D, Kahaly G, et al. Is there a methimazole dose effect on remission rate in Graves' disease? Results from a long-term prospective study. The European Multicentre Trial Group of the Treatment of Hyperthyroidism with Antithyroid Drugs. *Clin Endocrinol (Oxf).* 1998;49:451-457.

197. Sundaresh V, Brito JP, Wang Z, et al. Comparative effectiveness of therapies for Graves' hyperthyroidism: a systematic review and network meta-analysis. *J Clin Endocrinol Metab.* 2013;98:3671-3677.

198. Allahabadia A, Daykin J, Holder RL, et al. Age and gender predict the outcome of treatment for Graves' hyperthyroidism. *J Clin Endocrinol Metab.* 2000;85:1038-1042.

199. Brent GA. Clinical practice. Graves' disease. *N Engl J Med.* 2008;358: 2594-2605.

200. Bogazzi F, Bartalena L, Tomisti L, et al. Potassium perchlorate only temporarily restores euthyroidism in patients with amiodarone-induced hypothyroidism who continue amiodarone therapy. *J Endocrinol Invest.* 2008;31:515-519.

201. Emerson CH, Anderson AJ, Howard WJ, Utiger RD. Serum thyroxine and triiodothyronine concentrations during iodide treatment of hyperthyroidism. *J Clin Endocrinol Metab.* 1975;40:33-36.

202. Chiha M, Samarasinghe S, Kabaker AS. Thyroid storm: an updated review. *J Intensive Care Med.* 2015;30(3):131-140.

203. Myers JD, Brannon ES, Holland BC. A correlative study of the cardiac output and the hepatic circulation in hyperthyroidism. *J Clin Invest.* 1950;29:1069-1077.

204. Sosa JA, Bowman HM, Tielsch JM, et al. The importance of surgeon experience for clinical and economic outcomes from thyroidectomy. *Ann Surg.* 1998;228:320-330.

205. Rulli F, Ambrogi V, Dionigi G, et al. Meta-analysis of recurrent laryngeal nerve injury in thyroid surgery with or without intraoperative nerve monitoring. *Acta Otorhinolaryngol Ital.* 2014;34:223-229.

206. Chang DC, Wheeler MH, Woodcock JP, et al. The effect of preoperative Lugol's iodine on thyroid blood flow in patients with Graves' hyperthyroidism. *Surgery.* 1987;102:1055-1061.

207. Erbil Y, Ozluk Y, Giris M, et al. Effect of lugol solution on thyroid gland blood flow and microvessel density in the patients with Graves' disease. *J Clin Endocrinol Metab.* 2007;92:2182-2189.

208. Toft AD, Irvine WJ, Sinclair I, et al. Thyroid function after surgical treatment of thyrotoxicosis. A report of 100 cases treated with propranolol before operation. *N Engl J Med.* 1978;298:643-647.

209. Franklyn JA, Maisonneuve P, Sheppard M, et al. Cancer incidence and mortality after radioiodine treatment for hyperthyroidism: a population-based cohort study. *Lancet.* 1999;353:2111-2115.

210. Boelaert K, Maisonneuve P, Torlinska B, Franklyn JA. Comparison of mortality in hyperthyroidism during periods of treatment with thionamides and after radioiodine. *J Clin Endocrinol Metab.* 2013;98: 1869-1882.

211. Cheetham TD, Wraight P, Hughes IA, Barnes ND. Radioiodine treatment of Graves' disease in young people. *Horm Res.* 1998;49: 258-262.

212. Berg GE, Nystrom EH, Jacobsson L, et al. Radioiodine treatment of hyperthyroidism in a pregnant women. *J Nucl Med.* 1998;39:357-361.

213. Nakazato N, Yoshida K, Mori K, et al. Antithyroid drugs inhibit radioiodine-induced increases in thyroid autoantibodies in hyperthyroid Graves' disease. *Thyroid.* 1999;9:775-779.

214. Razvi S, Basu A, McIntyre EA, et al. Low failure rate of fixed administered activity of 400 MBq 131I with pre-treatment with carbimazole for thyrotoxicosis: the Gateshead Protocol. *Nucl Med Commun.* 2004; 25:675-682.

215. Harvey RD, Metcalfe RA, Morteo C, et al. Acute pre-tibial myxedema following radioiodine therapy for thyrotoxic Graves' disease. *Clin Endocrinol (Oxf).* 1995;42:657-660.

216. Krassas GE, Stafilidou A, Boboridis KG. Failure of rituximab treatment in a case of severe thyroid ophthalmopathy unresponsive to steroids. *Clin Endocrinol (Oxf).* 2010;72:853-855.

217. Fatourechi V. Pretibial myxedema: pathophysiology and treatment options. *Am J Clin Dermatol.* 2005;6:295-309.

218. Heyes C, Nolan R, Leahy M, Gebauer K. Treatment-resistant elephantiasic thyroid dermopathy responding to rituximab and plasmapheresis. *Australas J Dermatol.* 2012;53:e1-e4.

219. Salvi M, Vannucchi G, Campi I, Beck-Peccoz P. Rituximab in the treatment of thyroid eye disease: science fiction? *Orbit.* 2009;28:251-255.

220. Walter MA, Briel M, Christ-Crain M, et al. Effects of antithyroid drugs on radioiodine treatment: systematic review and meta-analysis of randomised controlled trials. *BMJ.* 2007;334:514.

221. Gorman CA. Radioiodine and pregnancy. *Thyroid.* 1999;9:721-726.

222. Sabri O, Zimny M, Schreckenberger M, et al. Radioiodine therapy in Graves' disease patients with large diffuse goiters treated with or without carbimazole at the time of radioiodine therapy. *Thyroid.* 1999;9:1181-1188.

223. Dickman PW, Holm LE, Lundell G, et al. Thyroid cancer risk after thyroid examination with 131I: a population-based cohort study in Sweden. *Int J Cancer.* 2003;106:580-587.

224. Moysich KB, Menezes RJ, Michalek AM. Chernobyl-related ionising radiation exposure and cancer risk: an epidemiological review. *Lancet Oncol.* 2002;3:269-279.

225. Nikiforov Y, Heffess C, Korzenko A, et al. Characteristics of follicular tumors and nonneoplastic thyroid lesions in children and adolescents exposed to radiation as a result of the Chernobyl disaster. *Cancer.* 1995;76:900.

226. Gavrilin Y, Khrouch V, Shinkarev S, et al. Individual thyroid dose estimation for a case-control study of Chernobyl-related thyroid cancer among children of Belarus: part I. I-131, short-lived radioiodines (I-132, I-133, I-135), and short-lived radiotelluriums (Te-131M and Te-132). *Health Phys.* 2004;86:565-585.

227. Franklyn JA, Sheppard MC, Maisonneuve P. Thyroid function and mortality in patients treated for hyperthyroidism. *JAMA.* 2005;294: 71-80.

228. Collet TH, Gussekloo J, Bauer DC, et al. Subclinical hyperthyroidism and the risk of coronary heart disease and mortality. *Arch Intern Med.* 2012;172:799-809.

229. Leslie WD, Ward L, Salamon EA, et al. A randomized comparison of radioiodine doses in Graves' hyperthyroidism. *J Clin Endocrinol Metab.* 2003;88:978-983.

230. Metso S, Jaatinen P, Huhtala H, et al. Long-term follow-up study of radioiodine treatment of hyperthyroidism. *Clin Endocrinol (Oxf).* 2004;61:641-648.

231. McGregor AM, Petersen MM, Capiferri R, et al. Effects of radioiodine on thyrotrophin binding inhibiting immunoglobulins in Graves' disease. *Clin Endocrinol (Oxf).* 1979;11:437-444.

232. Bartalena L, Marcocci C, Bogazzi F, et al. Use of corticosteroids to prevent progression of Graves' ophthalmopathy after radioiodine therapy for hyperthyroidism. *N Engl J Med.* 1989;321:1349-1352.

233. Tallestedt L, Lundell G, Torring O, et al. Occurrence of ophthalmopathy after treatment for Graves' disease. *N Engl J Med.* 1992;326: 1733-1738.

234. Gorman CA. Therapeutic controversies. Radioiodine therapy does not aggravate Graves' ophthalmopathy. *J Clin Endocrinol Metab.* 1995;80: 340-342.

235. Stan MN, Durski JM, Brito JP, et al. Cohort study on radioactive iodine-induced hypothyroidism: implications for Graves' ophthalmopathy and optimal timing for thyroid hormone assessment. *Thyroid.* 2013;23:620-625.

236. Bartalena L. Steroid prophylaxis after radioiodine treatment for Graves' hyperthyroidism: selective or universal? *Thyroid.* 2014;24(10): 1441-1442.

237. Sawka AM, Thabane L, Parlea L, et al. Second primary malignancy risk after radioactive iodine treatment for thyroid cancer: a systematic review and meta-analysis. *Thyroid.* 2009;19:451-457.

238. Dale J, Daykin J, Holder R, et al. Weight gain following treatment of hyperthyroidism. *Clin Endocrinol (Oxf).* 2001;55:233-239.

239. Wiersinga WM, Prummel MF. Graves' ophthalmopathy: a rational approach to treatment. *Trends Endocrinol Metab.* 2002;13:280-287.

240. Jarhult J, Rudberg C, Larsson E, et al. Graves' disease with moderate-severe endocrine ophthalmopathy-long term results of a prospective, randomized study of total or subtotal thyroid resection. *Thyroid.* 2005;15:1157-1164.

241. Menconi F, Marino M, Pinchera A, et al. Effects of total thyroid ablation versus near-total thyroidectomy alone on mild to moderate Graves' orbitopathy treated with intravenous glucocorticoids. *J Clin Endocrinol Metab.* 2007;92:1653-1658.

242. Bartalena L, Tanda ML. Clinical practice. Graves' ophthalmopathy. *N Engl J Med.* 2009;360:994-1001.

243. Aktaran S, Akarsu E, Erbagci I, et al. Comparison of intravenous methylprednisolone therapy vs. oral methylprednisolone therapy in patients with Graves' ophthalmopathy. *Int J Clin Pract.* 2007;61:45-51.

244. Zang S, Ponto KA, Kahaly GJ. Clinical review: Intravenous glucocorticoids for Graves' orbitopathy: efficacy and morbidity. *J Clin Endocrinol Metab.* 2011;96:320-332.

245. Marino M, Morabito E, Brunetto MR, et al. Acute and severe liver damage associated with intravenous glucocorticoid pulse therapy in patients with Graves' ophthalmopathy. *Thyroid.* 2004;14:403-406.

246. Tanda ML, Piantanida E, Bartalena L. Treating Graves' orbitopathy: where are we? *Endocrine.* 2012;41:167-168.

247. Vannucchi G, Covelli D, Campi I, et al. The therapeutic outcome to intravenous steroid therapy for active Graves' orbitopathy is influenced by the time of response but not polymorphisms of the glucocorticoid receptor. *Eur J Endocrinol.* 2014;170:55-61.

248. Perros P, Krassas GE. Orbital irradiation for thyroid-associated orbitopathy: conventional dose, low dose or no dose? *Clin Endocrinol (Oxf).* 2002;56:689-691.

249. Gorman CA, Garrity JA, Fatourechi V, et al. A prospective, randomized, double-blind, placebo-controlled study of orbital radiotherapy for Graves' ophthalmopathy. *Ophthalmology.* 2001;108:1523-1534.

250. Prummel MF, Terwee CB, Gerding MN, et al. A randomized controlled trial of orbital radiotherapy versus sham irradiation in patients with mild Graves' ophthalmopathy. *J Clin Endocrinol Metab.* 2004;89: 15-20.

251. Boulos PR, Hardy I. Thyroid-associated orbitopathy: a clinicopathologic and therapeutic review. *Curr Opin Ophthalmol.* 2004;15: 389-400.

252. Mourits MP, Koornneef L, Wiersinga WM, et al. Orbital decompression for Graves' ophthalmopathy by inferomedial, by inferomedial plus lateral, and by coronal approach. *Ophthalmology.* 1990;97: 636-641.

253. Bartalena L. Commentary: rituximab, adalimumab, etanercept, tocilizumab—are biologics the future for Graves' orbitopathy? *Ophthal Plast Reconstr Surg.* 2014;30:420-423.

254. Mitchell AL, Gan EH, Morris M, et al. The effect of B cell depletion therapy on anti-TSH receptor antibodies and clinical outcome in glucocorticoid-refractory Graves' orbitopathy. *Clin Endocrinol (Oxf).* 2013;79:437-442.

255. Bartalena L, Fatourechi V. Extrathyroidal manifestations of Graves' disease: a 2014 update. *J Endocrinol Invest.* 2014;37(8):691-700.

256. Akamizu T, Satoh T, Isozaki O, et al. Diagnostic criteria, clinical features, and incidence of thyroid storm based on nationwide surveys. *Thyroid.* 2012;22:661-679.

257. Klubo-Gwiezdzinska J, Wartofsky L. Thyroid emergencies. *Med Clin North Am.* 2012;96:385-403.

258. Bianco AC, Salvatore D, Gereben B, et al. Biochemistry, cellular and molecular biology and physiological roles of the iodothyronine selenodeiodinases. *Endocr Rev.* 2002;23:38-89.

259. Laurberg P, Torring J, Weeke J. A comparison of the effects of propylthiouracil and methimazol on circulating thyroid hormones and various measures of peripheral thyroid hormone effects in thyrotoxic patients. *Acta Endocrinol (Copenh).* 1985;108:51-54.

260. Davies TF, Taliadouros GS, Catt KJ, Nisula BC. Assessment of urinary thyrotropin-competing activity in choriocarcinoma and thyroid disease: further evidence for human chorionic gonadotropin interacting at the thyroid cell membrane. *J Clin Endocrinol Metab.* 1979;49: 353-357.

261. Davies TF, Platzer M. hCG-induced TSH receptor activation and growth acceleration in FRTL-5 thyroid cells. *Endocrinology.* 1986;118: 2149-2151.

262. Tomer Y, Huber GK, Davies TF. Human chorionic gonadotropin (hCG) interacts directly with recombinant human TSH receptors. *J Clin Endocrinol Metab.* 1992;74:1477-1479.

263. Grun JP, Meuris S, De Nayer P, Glinoer D. The thyrotrophic role of human chorionic gonadotrophin (hCG) in the early stages of twin (versus single) pregnancies. *Clin Endocrinol (Oxf).* 1997;46:719-725.

264. Goodwin TM, Montoro M, Mestman JH, et al. The role of chorionic gonadotropin in transient hyperthyroidism of hyperemesis gravidarum. *J Clin Endocrinol Metab.* 1992;75:1333-1337.

265. Cooper DS, Laurberg P. Hyperthyroidism in pregnancy. *Lancet Diabetes Endocrinol.* 2013;1:238-249.

266. Rodien P, Bremont C, Sanson ML, et al. Familial gestational hyperthyroidism caused by a mutant thyrotropin receptor hypersensitive to human chorionic gonadotropin. *N Engl J Med.* 1998;339:1823-1826.

267. Han EJ, Song HD, Yang JH, et al. Thyroid dysfunction associated with administration of the long-acting gonadotropin-releasing hormone agonist. *Endocrinol Metab (Seoul).* 2013;28:221-225.

268. Galofre JC, Davies TF. Autoimmune thyroid disease in pregnancy: a review. *J Womens Health (Larchmt).* 2009;18:1847-1856.

269. Lazarus JH. Thyroid disease in pregnancy and childhood. *Minerva Endocrinol.* 2005;30:71-87.

270. Davies TF. The thyroid immunology of the postpartum period. *Thyroid.* 1999;9:675-684.

271. Weetman AP. Immunity, thyroid function and pregnancy: molecular mechanisms. *Nat Rev Endocrinol.* 2010;6:311-318.

272. Somerset DA, Zheng Y, Kilby MD, et al. Normal human pregnancy is associated with an elevation in the immune suppressive CD25+ CD4+ regulatory T-cell subset. *Immunology.* 2004;112:38-43.

273. Evans PC, Lambert N, Maloney S, et al. Long-term fetal microchimerism in peripheral blood mononuclear cell subsets in healthy women and women with scleroderma. *Blood.* 1999;93:2033-2037.

274. Lepez T, Vandewoestyne M, Hussain S, et al. Fetal microchimeric cells in blood of women with an autoimmune thyroid disease. *PLoS One.* 2011;6:e29646.

275. Ando T, Davies TF. Clinical review 160: Postpartum autoimmune thyroid disease: the potential role of fetal microchimerism. *J Clin Endocrinol Metab.* 2003;88:2965-2971.

276. Galofre JC. Microchimerism in Graves' disease. *J Thyroid Res.* 2012; 2012:724382.

277. Lambert NC, Evans PC, Hashizumi TL, et al. Cutting edge: persistent fetal microchimerism in T lymphocytes is associated with HLA-DQA1*0501: implications in autoimmunity. *J Immunol.* 2000;164: 5545-5548.

278. Amino N, Kuro R, Tanizawa O, et al. Changes of serum antithyroid antibodies during and after pregnancy in autoimmune thyroid diseases. *Clin Exp Immunol.* 1978;31:30-37.
279. Balucan FS, Morshed SA, Davies TF. Thyroid autoantibodies in pregnancy: their role, regulation and clinical relevance. *J Thyroid Res.* 2013;2013:182472.
280. Aluvihare VR, Kallikourdis M, Betz AG. Regulatory T cells mediate maternal tolerance to the fetus. *Nat Immunol.* 2004;5:266-271.
281. Abeillon-du Payrat J, Chikh K, Bossard N, et al. Predictive value of maternal second-generation thyroid-binding inhibitory immunoglobulin assay for neonatal autoimmune hyperthyroidism. *Eur J Endocrinol.* 2014;171:451-460.
282. Luton D, Le Gac I, Vuillard E, et al. Management of Graves' disease during pregnancy: the key role of fetal thyroid gland monitoring. *J Clin Endocrinol Metab.* 2005;90:6093-6098.
283. Amino N, Tanizawa O, Mori H, et al. Aggravation of thyrotoxicosis in early pregnancy and after delivery in Graves' disease. *J Clin Endocrinol Metab.* 1982;55:108-112.
284. Hershman JM. Human chorionic gonadotropin and the thyroid: hyperemesis gravidarum and trophoblastic tumors. *Thyroid.* 1999;9:653-657.
285. Springer D, Bartos V, Zima T. Reference intervals for thyroid markers in early pregnancy determined by 7 different analytical systems. *Scand J Clin Lab Invest.* 2014;74:95-101.
286. Khalid AS, Marchocki Z, Hayes K, et al. Establishing trimester-specific maternal thyroid function reference intervals. *Ann Clin Biochem.* 2014;51:277-283.
287. LeBeau SO, Mandel SJ. Thyroid disorders during pregnancy. *Endocrinol Metab Clin North Am.* 2006;35:117-136, vii.
288. Cheron RG, Kaplan M, Reed Larsen P, et al. Neonatal thyroid function after propylthiouracil therapy for maternal Graves' disease. *N Engl J Med.* 1981;304:525-528.
289. Stagnaro-Green A. Optimal care of the pregnant woman with thyroid disease. *J Clin Endocrinol Metab.* 2012;97:2619-2622.
290. Abalovich M, Amino N, Barbour LA, et al. Management of thyroid dysfunction during pregnancy and postpartum: an Endocrine Society Clinical Practice Guideline. *J Clin Endocrinol Metab.* 2007;92:S1-S47.
291. Mortimer RH, Cannell GR, Addison RS, et al. Methimazole and propylthiouracil equally cross the perfused human term placental lobule. *J Clin Endocrinol Metab.* 1997;82:3099-3102.
292. Milham S Jr, Elledge W. Maternal methimazole and congenital defects in children. *Teratology.* 1972;5:125-126.
293. Milham S Jr. Scalp defects in infants of mothers treated for hyperthyroidism with methimazole or carbimazole during pregnancy. *Teratology.* 1985;32:321.
294. Clementi M, Di Gianantonio E, Pelo E, et al. Methimazole embryopathy: delineation of the phenotype. *Am J Med Genet.* 1999;83:43-46.
295. Stagnaro-Green A, Abalovich M, Alexander E, et al. Guidelines of the American Thyroid Association for the diagnosis and management of thyroid disease during pregnancy and postpartum. *Thyroid.* 2011;21:1081-1125.
296. De Groot LJ, Mestman J. Detecting and treating thyroid nodules and cancer before, during, and after pregnancy: a patient's guide. *J Clin Endocrinol Metab.* 2012;97:37A-38A.
297. Yoshihara A, Noh J, Yamaguchi T, et al. Treatment of Graves' disease with antithyroid drugs in the first trimester of pregnancy and the prevalence of congenital malformation. *J Clin Endocrinol Metab.* 2012;97:2396-2403.
298. Andersen SL, Olsen J, Wu CS, Laurberg P. Birth defects after early pregnancy use of antithyroid drugs: a Danish nationwide study. *J Clin Endocrinol Metab.* 2013;98:4373-4381.
299. Moore KL, Persaud TVN, Torchia MG. Human birth defects. In: *The Developing Human: Clinically Oriented Embryology.* Philadelphia, PA: Saunders/Elsevier; 2013:471-501.
300. Benavides VC, Mallela MK, Booth CJ, et al. Propylthiouracil is teratogenic in murine embryos. *PLoS One.* 2012;7:e35213.
301. van Veenendaal NR, Ulmer B, Boskovski MT, et al. Embryonic exposure to propylthiouracil disrupts left-right patterning in *Xenopus* embryos. *FASEB J.* 2013;27:684-691.
302. Andersen SL, Olsen J, Wu CS, Laurberg P. Severity of birth defects after propylthiouracil exposure in early pregnancy. *Thyroid.* 2014;24(10):1522-1540.
303. Laurberg P, Andersen SL. Therapy of endocrine disease: antithyroid drug use in early pregnancy and birth defects: time windows of relative safety and high risk? *Eur J Endocrinol.* 2014;171:R13-R20.
304. Momotani N, Noh J, Oyanagi H, et al. Antithyroid drug therapy for Graves' disease during pregnancy: optimal regimen for fetal thyroid status. *N Engl J Med.* 1986;315:24-28.
305. Petit KP, Nielsen HC. Chronic in utero beta-blockade alters fetal lung development. *Dev Pharmacol Ther.* 1992;19:131-140.
306. Ray JG, Vermeulen MJ, Burrows EA, Burrows RF. Use of antihypertensive medications in pregnancy and the risk of adverse perinatal outcomes: McMaster Outcome Study of Hypertension In Pregnancy 2 (MOS HIP 2). *BMC Pregnancy Childbirth.* 2001;1:6.
307. Momotani N, Hisaoka T, Noh J, et al. Effects of iodine on thyroid status of fetus versus mother in treatment of Graves' disease complicated by pregnancy. *J Clin Endocrinol Metab.* 1992;75:738-744.
308. Laurberg P, Bournaud C, Karmisholt J, Orgiazzi J. Management of Graves' hyperthyroidism in pregnancy: focus on both maternal and foetal thyroid function, and caution against surgical thyroidectomy in pregnancy. *Eur J Endocrinol.* 2009;160:1-8.
309. Lamberg BA, Konen EI, Teramo K, et al. Treatment of maternal hyperthyroidism with antithyroid agents and changes in thyrotropin and thyroxine in the newborn. *Acta Endocrinol (Copenh).* 1981;97:186-195.
310. Amino N, Mori H, Iwatani Y, et al. High prevalence of transient postpartum thyrotoxicosis and hypothyroidism. *N Engl J Med.* 1982;306:849-852.
311. Stagnaro-Green A. Approach to the patient with postpartum thyroiditis. *J Clin Endocrinol Metab.* 2012;97:334-342.
312. Rochester DB, Davies TF. Increased risk of Graves' disease after pregnancy. *Thyroid.* 2005;15:1287-1290.
313. Lazarus JH. Pre-conception counselling in Graves' disease. *Eur Thyroid J.* 2012;1:24-29.
314. Mandel SJ, Cooper DS. The use of antithyroid drugs in pregnancy and lactation. *J Clin Endocrinol Metab.* 2001;86:2354-2359.
315. Karras S, Tzotzas T, Kaltsas T, Krassas GE. Pharmacological treatment of hyperthyroidism during lactation: review of the literature and novel data. *Pediatr Endocrinol Rev.* 2010;8:25-33.
316. Refetoff S. Resistance to thyrotropin. *J Endocrinol Invest.* 2003;26:770-779.
317. Duprez L, Parma J, Van Sande J, et al. Germline mutations in the thyrotropin receptor gene cause non-autoimmune autosomal dominant hyperthyroidism. *Nat Genet.* 1994;7:396-401.
318. Parma J, Duprez L, Van Sande J, et al. Somatic mutations of the thyrotropin receptor gene cause hyperfunctioning thyroid adenomas. *Nature.* 1993;365:649-651.
319. TSH Receptor Mutation Database. University of Leipzig, Leipzig, Germany, 2013. Available at: <http://endokrinologie.uniklinikum-leipzig.de/tsh/>.
320. Hegedus L, Bonnema SJ, Bennedbaek FN. Management of simple nodular goiter: current status and future perspectives. *Endocr Rev.* 2003;24:102-132.
321. Krohn K, Fuhrer D, Bayer Y, et al. Molecular pathogenesis of euthyroid and toxic multinodular goiter. *Endocr Rev.* 2005;26:504-524.
322. Kraiem Z, Glaser B, Yigla M, et al. Toxic multinodular goiter: a variant of autoimmune hyperthyroidism. *J Clin Endocrinol Metab.* 1987;65:659-664.
323. Nygaard B, Hegedus L, Nielsen KG, et al. Long-term effect of radioactive iodine on thyroid function and size in patients with solitary autonomously functioning toxic thyroid nodules. *Clin Endocrinol (Oxf).* 1999;50:197-202.
324. Huysmans DAKC, Hermus RMM, Corstens FHM, et al. Large, compressive, goiters treated with radioiodine. *Ann Intern Med.* 1994;121:757-762.
325. Tonacchera M, Agretti P, Rosellini V, et al. Sporadic nonautoimmune congenital hyperthyroidism due to a strong activating mutation of the thyrotropin receptor gene. *Thyroid.* 2000;10:859-863.
326. Evered D, Hall R. Hypothyroidism. *Br Med J.* 1972;1:290-293.
327. Carr K, Mcleod DT, Parry G, Thornes HM. Fine adjustment of thyroxine replacement dosage: comparison of the thyrotrophin releasing hormone tests using a sensitive thyrotrophin assay with measurement of free thyroid hormones and clinical assessment. *Clin Endocrinol (Oxf).* 1988;28:325-333.
328. Bell GM, Sawers JSA, Forfar JC, et al. The effect of minor increments in plasma thyroxine on heart rate and urinary sodium excretion. *Clin Endocrinol (Oxf).* 1983;18:511-516.
329. Selmer C, Olesen JB, Hansen ML, et al. Subclinical and overt thyroid dysfunction and risk of all-cause mortality and cardiovascular events: a large population study. *J Clin Endocrinol Metab.* 2014;99:2372-2382.
330. Nicholls JJ, Brassill MJ, Williams GR, Bassett JH. The skeletal consequences of thyrotoxicosis. *J Endocrinol.* 2012;213:209-221.
331. Garin MC, Arnold AM, Lee JS, et al. Subclinical thyroid dysfunction and hip fracture and bone mineral density in older adults: the cardiovascular health study. *J Clin Endocrinol Metab.* 2014;99:2657-2664.
332. Faber J, Wiinberg N, Schifter S, Mehlsen J. Haemodynamic changes following treatment of subclinical and overt hyperthyroidism. *Eur J Endocrinol.* 2001;145:391-396.
333. Surks MI, Ortiz E, Daniels GH, et al. Subclinical thyroid disease: scientific review and guidelines for diagnosis and management. *JAMA.* 2004;291:228-238.
334. Sawin CT, Geller A, Kaplan MM, et al. Low serum thyrotropin (thyroid-stimulating hormone) in older persons without hyperthyroidism. *Arch Intern Med.* 1991;151:165-168.
335. Meyerovitch J, Rotman-Pikielny P, Sherf M, et al. Serum thyrotropin measurements in the community: five-year follow-up in a large network of primary care physicians. *Arch Intern Med.* 2007;167:1533-1538.
336. Canaris GJ, Manowitz NR, Mayor G, Ridgway EC. The Colorado thyroid disease prevalence study. *Arch Intern Med.* 2000;160:526-534.

337. Woeber KA. Observations concerning the natural history of subclinical hyperthyroidism. *Thyroid.* 2005;15:687-691.

338. Col NF, Surks MI, Daniels GH. Subclinical thyroid disease: clinical applications. *JAMA.* 2004;291:239-243.

339. Roti E, Uberti ED. Iodine excess and hyperthyroidism. *Thyroid.* 2001;11:493-500.

340. Baltisberger BL, Minder CE, Burgi H. Decrease of incidence of toxic nodular goitre in a region of Switzerland after full correction of mild iodine deficiency. *Eur J Endocrinol.* 1995;132:546-549.

341. Taylor PN, Okosieme OE, Dayan CM, Lazarus JH. Therapy of endocrine disease: impact of iodine supplementation in mild-to-moderate iodine deficiency: systematic review and meta-analysis. *Eur J Endocrinol.* 2014;170:R1-R15.

342. Fradkin JE, Wolff J. Iodide-induced thyrotoxicosis. *Medicine.* 1983; 62:1-20.

343. Martin FIR, Tress BW, Colman PG, Deam DR. Iodine-induced hyperthyroidism due to nonionic contrast radiography in the elderly. *Am J Med.* 1993;95:78-82.

344. Conn JJ, Sebastian MJ, Deam D, et al. A prospective study of the effect of nonionic contrast media on thyroid function. *Thyroid.* 1996;6: 107-110.

345. Lawrence JE, Lamm SH, Braverman LE. The use of perchlorate for the prevention of thyrotoxicosis in patients given iodine rich contrast agents. *J Endocrinol Invest.* 1999;22:405-407.

346. Martino E, Bartalena L, Bogazzi F, Braverman LE. The effects of amiodarone on the thyroid. *Endocr Rev.* 2001;22:240-254.

347. Smyrk TC, Goellner JR, Brennan MD, Carney JA. Pathology of the thyroid in amiodarone-associated thyrotoxicosis. *Am J Surg Pathol.* 1987;11:197-204.

348. Cohen-Lehman J, Dahl P, Danzi S, Klein I. Effects of amiodarone therapy on thyroid function. *Nat Rev Endocrinol.* 2010;6:34-41.

349. Eaton SE, Euinton HA, Newman CM, et al. Clinical experience of amiodarone-induced thyrotoxicosis over a 3-year period: role of colour-flow Doppler sonography. *Clin Endocrinol (Oxf).* 2002;56: 33-38.

350. Osman F, Franklyn JA, Sheppard MC, Gammage MD. Successful treatment of amiodarone-induced thyrotoxicosis. *Circulation.* 2002;105: 1275-1277.

351. Pearce EN, Farwell AP, Braverman LE. Thyroiditis. *N Engl J Med.* 2003;348:2646-2655.

352. Bogazzi F, Tomisti L, Bartalena L, et al. Amiodarone and the thyroid: a 2012 update. *J Endocrinol Invest.* 2012;35:340-348.

353. Daniels GH. Amiodarone-induced thyrotoxicosis. *J Clin Endocrinol Metab.* 2001;86:3-8.

354. Ryan LE, Braverman LE, Cooper DS, et al. Can amiodarone be restarted after amiodarone-induced thyrotoxicosis? *Thyroid.* 2004;14:149-153.

355. Beck-Peccoz P, Lania A, Beckers A, et al. 2013 European thyroid association guidelines for the diagnosis and treatment of thyrotropin-secreting pituitary tumors. *Eur Thyroid J.* 2013;2:76-82.

356. Refetoff S, Weiss RE, Usala SJ. The syndromes of resistance to thyroid hormone. *Endocr Rev.* 1993;14:348-399.

357. Refetoff S, Weiss RE, Usala SJ, Hayashi Y. The syndromes of resistance to thyroid hormone: update 1994. *Endocr Rev.* 1994;3:336-342.

358. Beck-Peccoz P, Mannavola D, Persani L. Syndromes of thyroid hormone resistance. *Ann Endocrinol (Paris).* 2005;66:264-269.

359. Pekary AE, Jackson IM, Goodwin TM, et al. Increased in vitro thyrotropic activity of partially sialated human chorionic gonadotropin extracted from hydatidiform moles of patients with hyperthyroidism. *J Clin Endocrinol Metab.* 1993;76:70-74.

360. Desai J, Yassa L, Marqusee E, et al. Hypothyroidism after sunitinib treatment for patients with gastrointestinal stromal tumors. *Ann Intern Med.* 2006;145:660-664.

361. Illouz F, Braun D, Briet C, et al. Endocrine side-effects of anti-cancer drugs: thyroid effects of tyrosine kinase inhibitors. *Eur J Endocrinol.* 2014;171:R91-R99.

362. Sarvghadi F, Hedayati M, Mehrabi Y, Azizi F. Follow up of patients with postpartum thyroiditis: a population-based study. *Endocrine.* 2005;27: 279-282.

363. Stagnaro-Green A, Schwartz A, Gismondi R, et al. High rate of persistent hypothyroidism in a large-scale prospective study of postpartum thyroiditis in southern Italy. *J Clin Endocrinol Metab.* 2011;96: 652-657.

364. Weetman AP, Smallridge RC, Nutman TB, Burman KD. Persistent thyroid autoimmunity after subacute thyroiditis. *J Clin Lab Immunol.* 1987;23:1-6.

365. Koh LK, Greenspan FS, Yeo PP. Interferon-alpha induced thyroid dysfunction: three clinical presentations and a review of the literature. *Thyroid.* 1997;7:891-896.

366. Tomer Y. Hepatitis C and interferon induced thyroiditis. *J Autoimmun.* 2010;34(3):J322-J326.

367. Doi F, Kakizaki S, Takagi H, et al. Long-term outcome of interferon-alpha-induced autoimmune thyroid disorders in chronic hepatitis C. *Liver Int.* 2005;25:242-246.

368. Miller KK, Daniels GH. Association between lithium use and thyrotoxicosis caused by silent thyroiditis. *Clin Endocrinol (Oxf).* 2001;55: 501-508.

369. Baethge C, Blumentritt H, Berghofer A, et al. Long-term lithium treatment and thyroid antibodies: a controlled study. *J Psychiatry Neurosci.* 2005;30:423-427.

370. Hamnvik OP, Larsen PR, Marqusee E. Thyroid dysfunction from antineoplastic agents. *J Natl Cancer Inst.* 2011;103:1572-1587.

371. de Groot JW, Zonnenberg BA, Plukker JT, et al. Imatinib induces hypothyroidism in patients receiving levothyroxine. *Clin Pharmacol Ther.* 2005;78:433-438.

372. Hedberg CW, Fishbein DB, Janssen RS, et al. An outbreak of thyrotoxicosis caused by the consumption of bovine thyroid gland in ground beef. *N Engl J Med.* 1987;316(16):993-998.

373. DeSimone CP, Lele SM, Modesitt SC. Malignant struma ovarii: a case report and analysis of cases reported in the literature with focus on survival and I131 therapy. *Gynecol Oncol.* 2003;89:543-548.

374. Dunzendorfer T, deLas Morenas A, Kalir T, Levin RM. Struma ovarii and hyperthyroidism. *Thyroid.* 1999;9:499-502.

375. Giralt SA, Dexeus F, Amato R, et al. Hyperthyroidism in men with germ cell tumors and high levels of beta-human chorionic gonadotropin. *Cancer.* 1992;69:1286-1290.

376. Dujardin MI, Sekhri P, Turnbull LW. Struma ovarii: role of imaging? *Insights Imaging.* 2014;5(1):41-51.

377. Bayot MR, Chopra IJ. Coexistence of struma ovarii and Graves' disease. *Thyroid.* 1995;5:469-471.

378. Snow MH, Davies T, Smith BR, et al. Thyroid stimulating antibodies and metastatic thyroid carcinoma. *Clin Endocrinol (Oxf).* 1979;10:413-418.

379. Als C, Gedeon P, Rosler H, et al. Survival analysis of 19 patients with toxic thyroid carcinoma. *J Clin Endocrinol Metab.* 2002;87:4122-4127.

CHAPTER 13

Hypothyroidism and Thyroiditis

GREGORY A. BRENT • ANTHONY P. WEETMAN

KEY POINTS

- Autoimmunity is responsible for over 90% of noniatrogenic hypothyroidism in iodine-sufficient areas.
- A variety of genetic factors contribute to susceptibility in autoimmune thyroiditis, but epidemiologic data suggest a strong influence of environmental factors to explain the recent increase in prevalence.
- The risk of progression from *subclinical* to *overt* hypothyroidism is most closely related to the magnitude of serum thyrotropin (TSH, thyroid-stimulating hormone) elevation and the presence of anti-TPO (thyroid peroxidase) antibodies.
- In some patients with autoimmune hypothyroidism, a transient exacerbation of thyroiditis or a fluctuation in the balance between TSH receptor blocking and stimulating autoantibodies may result in episodes of thyrotoxicosis.
- Hypothyroidism due to direct thyroidal inflammation or activation of autoimmune destruction has been associated with a number of drugs, including tyrosine kinase inhibitors (TKIs).
- The quantity of levothyroxine required to normalize TSH in an athyreotic patient results in a slightly higher serum free thyroxine (T$_4$) concentration than is present in normal individuals.
- The current approach to thyroid replacement using levothyroxine alone, although not a perfect replication of normal physiology, is satisfactory for virtually all patients.
- Levothyroxine requirements are increased in malabsorption due to bowel diseases, as well as impaired gastric acid secretion, or adsorption of levothyroxine to coadministered medications.
- Athyreotic patients who are planning a pregnancy should be advised to increase the dose of levothyroxine by around 30% as soon as the diagnosis is confirmed; the increased dose requirement persists throughout pregnancy, but dosage can return to normal within a few weeks after delivery.

HYPOTHYROIDISM

Reduced production of thyroid hormone is the central feature of the clinical state termed *hypothyroidism*.[1,2] Permanent loss or destruction of the thyroid, through processes such as autoimmune destruction, referred to as Hashimoto disease,[3] or irradiation injury, is described as *primary hypothyroidism* (Table 13-1). Hypothyroidism due to transient or progressive impairment of hormone biosynthesis is typically associated with compensatory thyroid enlargement. Central or secondary hypothyroidism, due to insufficient stimulation of a normal gland, is the result of hypothalamic or pituitary disease or defects in the TSH molecule.[4] Transient or temporary hypothyroidism can be observed as a phase of subacute thyroiditis.[5] Primary hypothyroidism is the cause in approximately 99% of cases of hypothyroidism, with less than 1% being due to TSH deficiency or other causes. Central hypothyroidism is discussed in Chapter 11.

Reduced action of thyroid hormone at the tissue level, despite normal or increased thyroid hormone production from the thyroid gland, can also be associated with clinical hypothyroidism. Conditions associated with reduced thyroid hormone action are rare and include abnormalities of thyroid hormone metabolism and defects in nuclear signaling.[6] Consumptive hypothyroidism, identified in an increasing number of clinical settings, is the result of accelerated inactivation of thyroid hormone by the type 3 iodothyronine deiodinase (D3).[7] Defects of activation of the prohormone, T$_4$, to the active form, triiodothyronine (T$_3$), have also been identified.[8] Polymorphisms in genes regulating thyroid hormone production and activation may influence thyroid hormone action in some tissues.[9] Resistance to thyroid hormone (RTH), the result of defects in the thyroid hormone nuclear receptor (TR) or nuclear cofactors, is associated with elevated circulating levels of thyroid hormone. Some tissues, depending on the level of expression of the mutant receptor and other forms of local compensation, have evidence of reduced thyroid hormone action.[10]

Estimates of the incidence of hypothyroidism vary depending on the population studied.[11,12] In the United States, 0.3% have overt hypothyroidism, defined as an elevated serum TSH concentration and reduced free thyroxine concentration (fT$_4$), and 4.3% have what has been described as subclinical or mild hypothyroidism.[12] Although a number of clinical manifestations have been associated with this early or mild phase of hypothyroidism, we will use the term *subclinical* to describe this group, as is used in most clinical studies. Subclinical hypothyroidism is defined as an elevated serum TSH level with a normal serum fT$_4$ concentration.[13,14] Subclinical hypothyroidism can progress to overt hypothyroidism, as well as be associated with manifestations that, in some patients, may benefit from treatment.[15] The incidence of hypothyroidism is higher among women, in the elderly, and in some racial and ethnic groups.[16] Neonatal screening programs for congenital hypothyroidism identify hypothyroidism (almost all primary) in almost 1 in 3000 newborns.[17]

TABLE 13-1
Causes of Hypothyroidism

Primary Hypothyroidism

Acquired
Hashimoto thyroiditis
Iodine deficiency (endemic goiter)
Drugs blocking synthesis or release of T_4 (e.g., lithium, ethionamide, sulfonamides, iodide)
Goitrogens in foodstuffs or as endemic substances or pollutants
Cytokines (interferon-α, interleukin 2)
Thyroid infiltration (amyloidosis, hemochromatosis, sarcoidosis, Riedel struma, cystinosis, scleroderma)
Postablative thyroiditis due to ^{131}I, surgery, or therapeutic irradiation for nonthyroidal malignancy

Congenital
Iodide transport or utilization defect (NIS or pendrin mutations)
Iodotyrosine dehalogenase deficiency
Organification disorders (TPO deficiency or dysfunction)
Defects in thyroglobulin synthesis or processing
Thyroid agenesis or dysplasia
TSH receptor* defects
Thyroidal G_s protein abnormalities (pseudohypoparathyroidism type 1a)
Idiopathic TSH unresponsiveness

Transient (Post-thyroiditis) Hypothyroidism

Following painless (including postpartum thyroiditis) or painful subacute thyroiditis

Consumptive Hypothyroidism

Rapid destruction of thyroid hormone due to D3 expression in large hemangiomas or hemangioendotheliomas

Defects of Thyroxine to Triiodothyronine Conversion

Selenocysteine insertion sequence–binding protein 2 (SECISBP-2) defect

Drug-Induced Thyroid Destruction

Tyrosine kinase inhibitor (sunitinib)

Central Hypothyroidism

Acquired
Pituitary origin (secondary)
Hypothalamic disorders (tertiary)
Bexarotene (retinoid X receptor agonist)
Dopamine or severe illness

Congenital
TSH deficiency or structural abnormality
TSH receptor defect

Resistance to Thyroid Hormone

Generalized
"Pituitary" dominant

NIS, sodium-iodide symporter; TPO, thyroid peroxidase; TSH, thyroid-stimulating hormone (thyrotropin).

Clinical Presentation

Hypothyroidism can affect all organ systems, and these manifestations are largely independent of the underlying disorder but are a function of the degree of hormone deficiency. The following sections discuss the pathophysiology of each organ system at various levels of thyroid hormone deficiency, from mild to severe. The term *myxedema,* formerly used as a synonym for hypothyroidism, refers to the appearance of the skin and subcutaneous tissues in the patient in a severely hypothyroid state (Fig. 13-1). Hypothyroidism of this severity is rarely seen today, and the term should be reserved to describe the physical signs.

Skin and Appendages

Hypothyroidism causes an accumulation of hyaluronic acid that alters the composition of the ground substance in the dermis and other tissues.[18,19] This material is hygroscopic, producing the mucinous edema that is responsible for the thickened features and puffy appearance (myxedema) with full-blown hypothyroidism. Myxedematous tissue is characteristically boggy and nonpitting and is apparent around the eyes, on the dorsa of the hands and feet, and in the supraclavicular fossae (see Fig. 13-1). It causes enlargement of the tongue and thickening of the pharyngeal and laryngeal mucous membranes.

A clinically similar deposit may occur in patients with Graves disease, usually over the pretibial area (infiltrative dermopathy or pretibial myxedema), but it can be differentiated histologically.[20] In addition to having a puffy appearance, the skin is pale and cool as a result of cutaneous vasoconstriction. Anemia may contribute to the pallor; hypercarotenemia gives the skin a yellow tint but does not cause scleral icterus (see Fig. 13-1). The secretions of the sweat glands and sebaceous glands are reduced, leading to dryness and coarseness of the skin, which in extreme cases may resemble that seen in patients with ichthyosis.

Wounds of the skin tend to heal slowly. Easy bruising is due to an increase in capillary fragility. Head and body hair is dry and brittle, lacks luster, and tends to fall out. Hair may be lost from the temporal aspects of the eyebrows, although this is not specific for hypothyroidism (see Fig. 13-1B). Growth of hair is retarded so that haircuts and shaves are required less often. The nails are brittle and grow slowly. Topical T_3 has been shown to accelerate wound healing and stimulate hair growth in a euthyroid mouse model, demonstrating a role for thyroid hormone in these processes.[19]

Histopathologic examination of the skin reveals hyperkeratosis with plugging of hair follicles and sweat glands. The dermis is edematous, and the connective tissue fibers are separated by an increased amount of metachromatically staining, periodic acid–Schiff (PAS)–positive mucinous material. This material consists of protein complexed with two mucopolysaccharides: hyaluronic acid and chondroitin sulfate B. The hygroscopic glycosaminoglycans are mobilized early during treatment with thyroid hormone, leading to an increase in urinary excretion of nitrogen and hexosamine as well as tissue water.[18]

Patients with hypothyroidism due to Hashimoto thyroiditis may also have skin lesions with loss of pigmentation characteristic of the autoimmune skin condition vitiligo. This feature is not a manifestation of reduced thyroid hormone action, but reflects the common association of autoimmune endocrine disease and this skin condition, which is recognized as a component of autoimmune polyendocrine syndromes.[21]

Cardiovascular System

The cardiac output at rest is decreased because of reduction in both stroke volume and heart rate, reflecting loss of the inotropic and chronotropic effects of thyroid hormones. Peripheral vascular resistance at rest is increased, and blood volume is reduced. These hemodynamic alterations cause narrowing of pulse pressure, prolongation of circulation time, and decrease in blood flow to the tissues.[22,23] The reduction in cutaneous circulation is responsible for the coolness and pallor of the skin and the sensitivity to cold. In most tissues, the decrease in blood flow is proportional to the decrease in oxygen consumption, so the arteriovenous oxygen difference remains

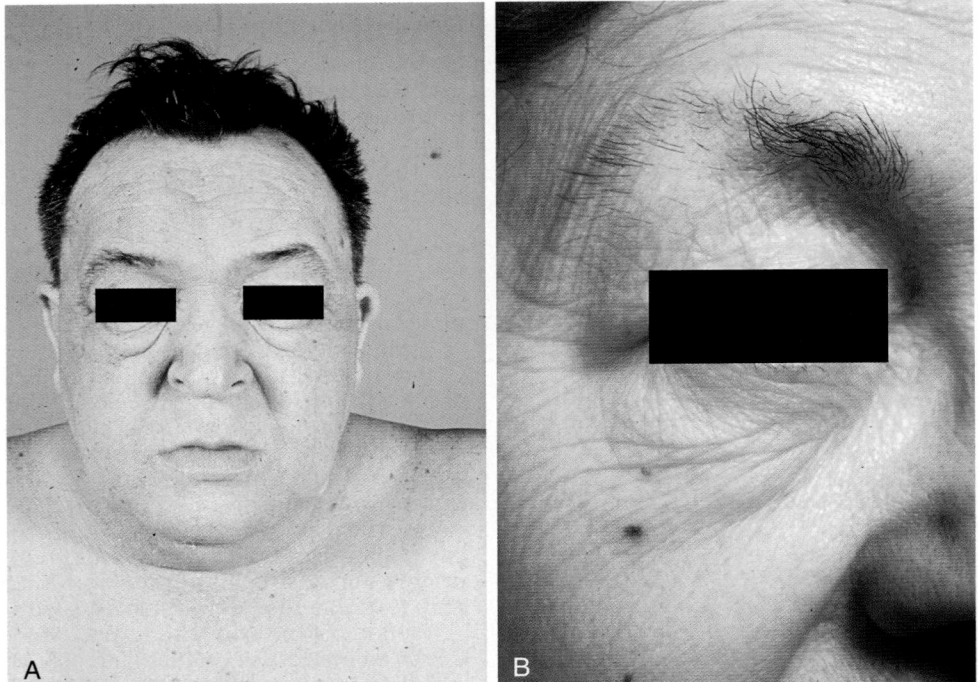

Figure 13-1 A and **B,** Typical appearance with moderately severe primary hypothyroidism or myxedema. Note dry skin and sallow complexion; the absence of scleral pigmentation differentiates the carotenemia from jaundice. Both individuals demonstrate periorbital myxedema. **B,** This patient illustrates the loss of the lateral aspect of the eyebrow, sometimes termed *Queen Anne's sign.* That finding is not unusual in the age group that is commonly affected by severe hypothyroidism and should not be considered to be a specific sign of the condition.

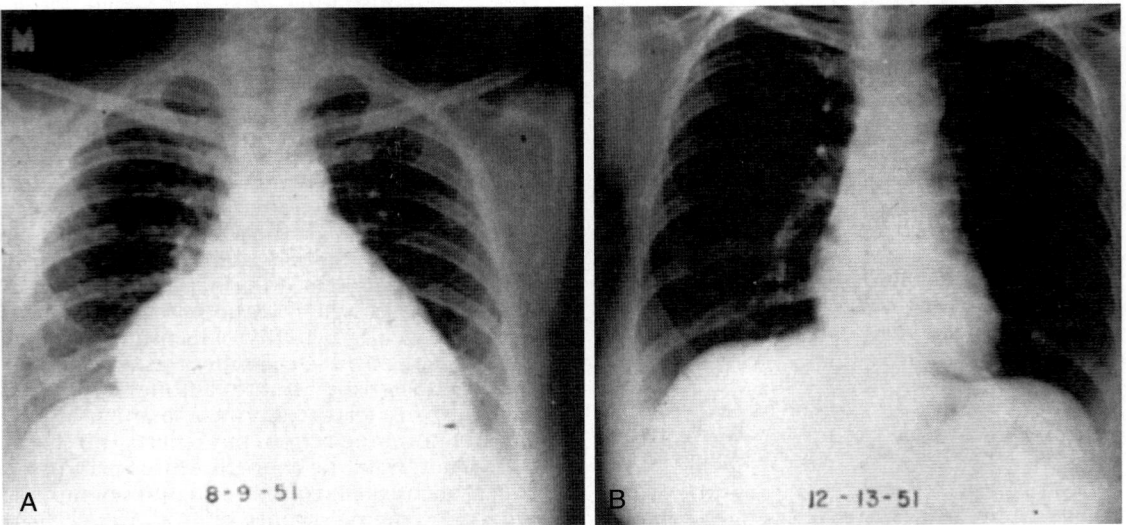

Figure 13-2 A and **B,** Chest roentgenograms in a patient with myxedema heart disease. The patient had signs of severe congestive heart failure and was given thyroid hormone alone. Within 4 months, the heart had returned to normal size (**B**) and there was no evidence of underlying heart disease.

normal. The hemodynamic alterations at rest resemble those of congestive heart failure. However, in hypothyroidism, cardiac output increases and peripheral vascular resistance decreases normally in response to exercise unless the hypothyroid state is severe and of long standing.

In severe primary hypothyroidism the cardiac silhouette is enlarged (Fig. 13-2), and the heart sounds are diminished in intensity.[24] These findings are the result largely of effusion into the pericardial sac of fluid rich in protein and glycosaminoglycans, but the myocardium may also be

dilated. Pericardial effusion is rarely of sufficient magnitude to cause tamponade.

Angina pectoris may first appear or worsen during treatment of the hypothyroid state with thyroid hormone, although most patients with hypothyroidism and coronary artery disease have no change, or improvement, in anginal symptoms with T_4 treatment.[25] Electrocardiographic changes include sinus bradycardia, prolongation of the PR interval, low amplitude of the P wave and QRS complex, alterations of the ST segment, and flattened or inverted T waves. Pericardial effusion is probably responsible for the low amplitude in severe hypothyroidism. Systolic time intervals are altered; the preejection period is prolonged, and the ratio of preejection period to left ventricular ejection time is increased. Echocardiographic studies have revealed resting left ventricular diastolic dysfunction in overt and, in some studies, subclinical hypothyroidism.[26] These findings normalize when the hypothyroidism is treated.

Serum levels of homocysteine, creatine kinase, aspartate aminotransferase, and lactate dehydrogenase may be increased in hypothyroidism.[23,27] Typically, the isoenzyme patterns suggest that the source of the increased creatine kinase and lactate dehydrogenase is skeletal, not cardiac, muscle. All levels return to normal with therapy. Sequential cardiac biopsies in a hypothyroid patient with heart failure showed that messenger RNA (mRNA) levels from genes regulated by thyroid hormone and important for the strength of myocardial contraction were normalized after T_4 treatment.[28]

The combination of large heart, hemodynamic and electrocardiographic alterations, and the serum enzyme changes has been termed *myxedema heart*. In the absence of coexisting organic heart disease, treatment with thyroid hormone corrects the hemodynamic, electrocardiographic, and serum enzyme alterations of myxedema heart and restores heart size to normal (see Fig. 13-2).

Hypothyroidism is consistently associated with elevations of total and low-density lipoprotein (LDL) cholesterol, which improve with T_4 replacement.[29] The higher the original serum TSH concentration and elevation of serum LDL, the greater the magnitude of reduction in LDL cholesterol after T_4 therapy. Lipoprotein fractionation has shown that the cholesterol elevation is predominantly due to the less atherogenic large LDL particles. A subset of younger (<50 years) male hypothyroid patients had elevated serum triglycerides and C-reactive protein that improved with T_4 treatment.[30] Most studies have shown that serum high-density lipoprotein (HDL) levels are not influenced by thyroid status.

Hypothyroidism has been shown to be a risk factor for atherosclerosis and cardiovascular disease by several studies, although others have not shown this association.[31] The Whickham Study showed no increase in cardiovascular mortality rate in patients with subclinical hypothyroidism followed for more than 20 years.[11] A prospective study in the United States, following men and women age 65 or older for more than 10 years, showed no influence of hypothyroidism (overt or subclinical) on cardiovascular outcome or mortality rate.[32] Cardiovascular outcome studies suggest that improvement from treatment of hypothyroidism, especially subclinical hypothyroidism, is primarily in those who are middle age and not older individuals (older than 65 years of age).[14,33,34]

Respiratory System

Hypothyroidism affects breathing by actions on the central regulation of respiration as well as the innervation and function of the respiratory muscles, upper airways, and tongue.[35] Pleural effusions usually are evident only on radiologic examination but in rare instances may cause dyspnea. Lung volumes are usually normal, but maximal breathing capacity and diffusing capacity are reduced. In severe hypothyroidism, myxedematous involvement of respiratory muscles and depression of both the hypoxic and the hypercapnic ventilatory drives may cause alveolar hypoventilation and carbon dioxide retention, which in turn can contribute to the development of myxedema

coma. An increased prevalence of obstructive sleep apnea is seen in hypothyroid patients, and it is usually reversed with restoration of a euthyroid state.[36]

Alimentary System

Although most patients experience a modest gain in weight, appetite is usually reduced. The weight gain that occurs is caused partly by retention of fluid by the hydrophilic glycoprotein deposits in the tissues, but generally does not exceed 10% of body weight. Peristaltic activity is decreased and, together with the decreased food intake, is responsible for the frequent complaint of constipation. The latter may lead to fecal impaction (myxedema megacolon). Gaseous distention of the abdomen (myxedema ileus), if accompanied by colicky pain and vomiting, may mimic mechanical ileus.[37]

Elevations in the serum levels of carcinoembryonic antigen, which may occur on the basis of hypothyroidism alone, add to the impression that an obstruction is present. Ascites in the absence of another cause is unusual in hypothyroidism, but it can occur, usually in association with pleural and pericardial effusions. Like pericardial and pleural effusions, the ascitic fluid is rich in protein and glycosaminoglycans.

Achlorhydria after maximal histamine stimulation may be present in patients with primary hypothyroidism. Circulating antibodies against gastric parietal cells have been found in about one third of patients with primary hypothyroidism and may be secondary to atrophy of the gastric mucosa. Hypothyroid patients with positive parietal cell antibodies have a higher T_4 requirement compared with antibody-negative patients.[38] Among Swedish celiac disease patients, there was a 4.4-fold increased risk for hypothyroidism, compared with the general population.[39] Overt pernicious anemia is reported in about 12% of patients with primary hypothyroidism. The coexistence of pernicious anemia and other autoimmune diseases with primary hypothyroidism reflects the fact that autoimmunity plays the central role in the pathogenesis of these diseases (see Chapter 40).[21]

Hypothyroidism has complex effects on intestinal absorption. Although the rates of absorption for many substances are decreased, the total amount absorbed may be normal or even increased because the decreased bowel motility may allow more time for absorption. Malabsorption is occasionally overt.

Liver function test results are usually normal, but levels of aminotransaminases may be elevated, probably because of impaired clearance.[40] The gallbladder contracts sluggishly and may be distended. In a population study of those without diagnosed thyroid disease, men, but not women, with an elevated TSH had a 3.8-fold increased risk of cholelithiasis.[41] Hypothyroidism is being recognized as a predisposing factor for nonalcoholic fatty liver disease.[42]

Atrophy of the gastric and intestinal mucosa and myxedematous infiltration of the bowel wall may be demonstrated on histologic examination. The colon may be greatly distended, and the volume of fluid in the peritoneal cavity is usually increased. The liver and pancreas are normal.

Central and Peripheral Nervous Systems

Thyroid hormone is essential for the development of the central nervous system.[17,43,44] Deficiency in fetal life or at birth impairs neurologic development, including hypoplasia of cortical neurons with poor development of cellular processes, retarded myelination, and reduced vascularity. If the deficiency is not corrected in early postnatal life, the damage is irreversible. Deficiency of thyroid hormone beginning in adult life causes less severe manifestations that usually respond to treatment with the hormone. Cerebral blood flow is reduced, but cerebral oxygen consumption is usually normal; this finding is in accord with the conclusion that the oxygen consumption of isolated brain tissue in vitro, unlike that of most other tissues, is not stimulated by administration of thyroid hormones. In severe cases, decreased cerebral blood flow may lead to cerebral hypoxia.

All intellectual functions, including speech, are slowed in thyroid hormone deficiency.[45] Loss of initiative is present and memory defects are common, lethargy and somnolence are prominent, and dementia in elderly patients may be mistaken for senile dementia.[46] Positron emission tomography (PET) brain scans of hypothyroid patients before and after T$_4$ therapy demonstrate reversible reduced glucose uptake in specific brain areas, such as the limbic system, which also correlates with behavioral and psychiatric symptoms.[47] Psychiatric disorders are common and are usually of the paranoid or depressive type and may induce agitation (myxedema madness).[46] Headaches are frequent. Cerebral hypoxia due to circulatory alterations may predispose to confusional attacks and syncope, which may be prolonged and lead to stupor or coma. Other factors predisposing to coma in hypothyroidism include exposure to severe cold, infection, trauma, hypoventilation with carbon dioxide retention, and depressant drugs.

Epileptic seizures have been reported and tend to occur in myxedema coma. Night blindness is due to deficient synthesis of the pigment required for dark adaptation. Hearing loss of the perceptive type is frequent due to myxedema of the eighth cranial nerve and serous otitis media. Perceptive deafness may also occur in association with a defect in the organic binding of thyroidal iodide (Pendred syndrome) (see Chapter 11), but in these instances it is not due to hypothyroidism per se.

Thick, slurred speech and hoarseness are due to myxedematous infiltration of the tongue and larynx, respectively.[44] Body movements are slow and clumsy, and cerebellar ataxia may occur. Numbness and tingling of the extremities are frequent; in the fingers these symptoms may be due to compression by glycosaminoglycan deposits in and around the median nerve in the carpal tunnel (carpal tunnel syndrome).[48] The tendon reflexes are slow, especially during the relaxation phase, producing the characteristic "hung-up reflexes"; this phenomenon is due to a decrease in the rate of muscle contraction and relaxation rather than a delay in nerve conduction.

The presence of extensor plantar responses or diminished vibration sense should alert the physician to the possibility of coexisting pernicious anemia with combined system disease. Electroencephalographic changes include slow alpha-wave activity and general loss of amplitude. The concentration of protein in the cerebrospinal fluid is often increased, but cerebrospinal fluid pressure is normal.

Histopathologic examination of the brain in patients with untreated hypothyroidism reveals that the nervous system is edematous with mucinous deposits in and around nerve fibers. In patients with cerebellar ataxia, neural myxedematous infiltrates of glycogen and mucinous material are present in the cerebellum. There may be foci of degeneration and an increase in glial tissue. The cerebral vessels show atherosclerosis, but this finding is much more common if the patient has had coexistent hypertension.

Hypothyroidism has been associated with several neurologic conditions, although a strong etiologic link has not been established. Epidemiologic studies have shown an association between Alzheimer disease and hypothyroidism.[49] It is difficult to convincingly demonstrate this association because the incidence of thyroid disease in the elderly population is high and, like dementia, increases with age. A mechanistic link is suggested by the observation of amyloid deposition in Down syndrome, a condition associated with an increased incidence of Hashimoto disease, and thyroid hormone regulates amyloid gene processing in a number of cellular and animal models. Subclinical hyperthyroidism, however, has also been associated with Alzheimer disease.[50] There is an increase in cerebrospinal fluid reverse T$_3$ levels in Alzheimer disease patients, all with normal circulating thyroid hormone levels, suggesting the potential for altered thyroid hormone metabolism in the brain.[51] The impact of normalizing T$_3$ levels in the brain, however, is not known. A corticosteroid-responsive encephalopathy is associated with chronic Hashimoto thyroiditis but may be linked to autoimmunity rather than a process mediated specifically by low thyroid hormone levels or thyroid autoantibodies.[52]

Muscular System

Stiffness and aching of muscles are common in hypothyroidism and are worsened by cold temperatures.[48] Delayed muscle contraction and relaxation cause slowness of movement and delayed tendon jerks.[44] Muscle mass may be reduced or enlarged due to interstitial myxedema. Muscle mass may be slightly increased, and the muscles tend to be firm. Rarely, a profound increase in muscle mass with slowness of muscular activity may be the predominant manifestation (the *Kocher-Debré-Sémélaigne*, or *Hoffmann*, syndrome). Myoclonus may be present. The electromyogram may be normal or may exhibit disordered discharge, hyperirritability, and polyphasic action potentials.

On histopathologic examination, the muscles appear pale and swollen. The muscle fibers may show swelling, loss of normal striations, and separation by mucinous deposits. Type I muscle fibers tend to predominate.

Skeletal System: Calcium and Phosphorus Metabolism

Thyroid hormone is essential for normal growth and maturation of the skeleton, and growth failure is due both to impaired general protein synthesis and to a reduction in growth hormone, but especially of insulin-like growth factor 1 (Fig. 13-3).[53,54] The thyroid hormone receptor isoforms α and β have specific roles in bone maturation. Before puberty, thyroid hormone plays a major role in the maturation of bone. Deficiency of thyroid hormone in early life leads to both a delay in development and an abnormal, stippled appearance of the epiphyseal centers of ossification (epiphyseal dysgenesis) (Fig. 13-4). Impairment of linear growth leads to dwarfism in which the limbs are disproportionately short in relation to the trunk but cartilage growth is unaffected (see Fig. 13-3). Children with prolonged hypothyroidism, even after adequate treatment, do not reach predicted height based on midparental height calculations.[55]

Urinary excretion of calcium is decreased, as is the glomerular filtration rate, whereas fecal excretion of calcium and both urinary and fecal excretion of phosphorus are variable. Calcium balance is also variable, and any changes are slight. The exchangeable pool of calcium and its rate of turnover are reduced, reflecting decreased bone formation and resorption. Because levels of parathyroid hormone are often slightly increased, some degree of resistance to its action may be present; levels of 1,25(OH)$_2$D (dihydroxyvitamin D) are also increased.

Levels of calcium and phosphorus in serum are usually normal, but calcium may be slightly elevated. The alkaline phosphatase level is usually below normal in infantile and juvenile hypothyroidism. Bone density may be increased. The radiologic appearance of the skeleton in cretinism and juvenile hypothyroidism is discussed subsequently.

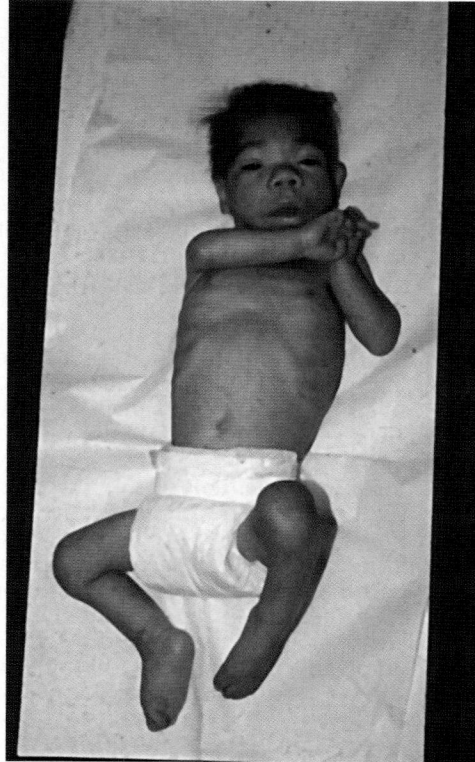

Figure 13-3 The consequences of untreated congenital hypothyroidism are demonstrated in this 17-year-old girl. Her condition had been diagnosed at birth but, through a series of misunderstandings, was not treated with thyroid hormone. Note her size, the poorly developed nasal bridge, the wide-set eyes, and the ears, which are larger than are appropriate for head size. Her tongue is enlarged, and her extremities are inappropriately short in relation to her trunk. (Courtesy of Dr. Ronald B. Stein.)

Renal Function: Water and Electrolyte Metabolism

Reversible reductions in renal blood flow, glomerular filtration rate, and tubular reabsorptive and secretory maxima are seen in hypothyroidism. Blood urea nitrogen and serum creatinine levels are normal, but uric acid levels may be increased. Urine flow is reduced, and delay in the excretion of a water load may result in reversal of the normal diurnal pattern of urine excretion. The delay in water excretion appears to be due to decreased volume delivery to the distal diluting segment of the nephron as a result of the diminished renal perfusion; evidence supporting inappropriate secretion of vasopressin (syndrome of inappropriate antidiuretic hormone [ADH] secretion) is less compelling.[56] There is a high prevalence of hypothyroidism in patients with chronic kidney disease, and improvement in renal function has been demonstrated with T$_4$ treatment.[57]

The impaired renal excretion of water and the retention of water by the hydrophilic deposits in the tissues result in an increase in total body water, even though plasma volume is reduced. This increase accounts for the hyponatremia occasionally noted because the level of exchangeable sodium is increased. The amount of exchangeable potassium is usually normal in relation to lean body mass. Serum magnesium concentration may be increased, but exchangeable magnesium levels and urinary magnesium excretion are decreased.

Hematopoietic System

In response to the diminished oxygen requirements and decreased production of erythropoietin, the red blood cell mass is decreased; this is evident in the mild normocytic, normochromic anemia that often occurs. Less commonly, the anemia is macrocytic, sometimes from deficiency of vitamin B$_{12}$. Reference has already been made to the high incidence of pernicious anemia (and of achlorhydria and vitamin B$_{12}$ deficiency without overt anemia) in primary hypothyroidism (see Chapter 40). Conversely, overt and subclinical hypothyroidism is present in 12% and 15% of patients, respectively, with pernicious anemia. Folate deficiency from malabsorption or dietary inadequacy may also cause macrocytic anemia. The frequent menorrhagia and

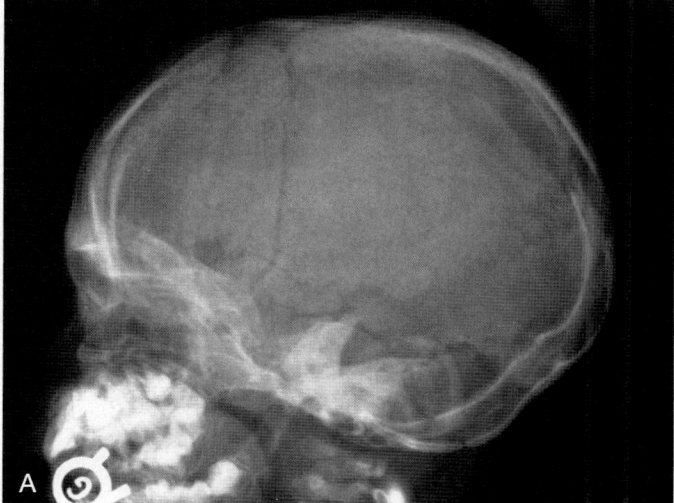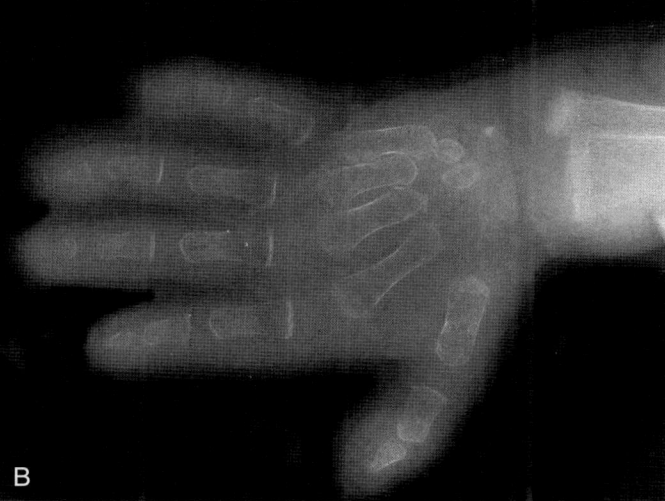

Figure 13-4 X-ray films of the skull and hand of the 17-year-old patient illustrated in Figure 13-3. **A,** Skull film shows that the posterior and anterior fontanels are open and that the sutures are not fused. The deciduous and permanent teeth are present. **B,** Radiograph of the wrist and hand shows the delayed appearance of the epiphyseal centers of the bones of the hand and the absence of the distal radial epiphysis. The estimated bone age is 9 months. (Courtesy of Dr. Ronald B. Stein.)

the defective absorption of iron resulting from achlorhydria may contribute to a microcytic, hypochromic anemia.

The total and differential white blood cell counts are usually normal, and platelets are adequate, although platelet adhesiveness may be impaired. If pernicious anemia or significant folate deficiency is present, the characteristic changes in peripheral blood and bone marrow will be found. The intrinsic clotting mechanism may be defective because of decreased concentrations in plasma of factors VIII and IX, which, together with an increase in capillary fragility and the decrease in platelet adhesiveness, may account for the bleeding tendency that sometimes occurs.[37,58,59]

Pituitary and Adrenocortical Function

In long-standing primary hypothyroidism, hyperplasia of the thyrotropes may cause the pituitary gland to be enlarged. This feature can be detected radiologically as an increase in the volume of the pituitary fossa.[60] Rarely, the pituitary enlargement compromises the function of other pituitary cells and causes pituitary insufficiency or visual field defects. Patients with severe hypothyroidism may have increased serum prolactin levels, stimulated by the elevation in thyrotropin-releasing hormone (TRH) and proportional to the level of serum TSH elevation, and galactorrhea may develop in some patients. Treatment with thyroid hormone normalizes the serum prolactin and TSH levels and causes disappearance of galactorrhea, if present.

In rodents, thyroid hormone directly regulates growth hormone synthesis. Growth hormone is not directly regulated by thyroid hormone in humans, but thyroid status influences the growth hormone axis.[61] Hypothyroid children have delayed growth and the response of growth hormone to provocative stimuli may be subnormal.

As a result of the decreased rate of turnover of cortisol due to decreased hepatic 11β-hydroxysteroid dehydrogenase type 1 (11β-HSD-1), the 24-hour urinary excretion of cortisol and 17-hydroxycorticosteroids is decreased but the plasma cortisol level is usually normal (see Chapter 15). The response of urinary 17-hydroxycorticosteroid to exogenous adrenocorticotropic hormone is usually normal but may be decreased. The response of plasma cortisol to insulin-induced hypoglycemia may be impaired.

In severe, long-standing primary hypothyroidism, pituitary and adrenal function may be secondarily decreased, and adrenal insufficiency may be precipitated by stress or by rapid replacement therapy with thyroid hormone.[61] The rate of turnover of aldosterone is decreased, but the plasma level is normal. Plasma renin activity is decreased, and sensitivity to angiotensin II is increased, which may contribute to the association of hypertension with hypothyroidism (see Chapter 16).[62,63]

Reproductive Function

In both sexes, thyroid hormones influence sexual development and reproductive function.[64] Infantile hypothyroidism, if untreated, leads to sexual immaturity, and juvenile hypothyroidism causes a delay in the onset of puberty followed by anovulatory cycles. Paradoxically, primary hypothyroidism may also rarely cause precocious sexual development and galactorrhea, presumably due to "spillover" of elevated TSH stimulating the luteinizing hormone (LH) receptor and elevated TRH initiating excess prolactin release.

In adult women, severe hypothyroidism may be associated with diminished libido and failure of ovulation. Secretion of progesterone is inadequate, and endometrial proliferation persists, resulting in excessive and irregular breakthrough menstrual bleeding. These changes may be due to deficient secretion of LH and pulse frequency and amplitude. Rarely, in primary hypothyroidism, secondary depression of pituitary function may lead to ovarian atrophy and amenorrhea. Fertility is reduced, and there is an increase in spontaneous abortion and preterm delivery, although many pregnancies are successful.[65] Pregnancy complications are associated with overt and subclinical hypothyroidism, although the impact has varied among different studies.[66-68] A randomized prospective study of levothyroxine treatment in pregnant women with thyroid peroxidase (TPO) antibody positivity but normal range TSH has shown that the increased incidence of preterm delivery and spontaneous abortions is reversed by treatment, although this result remains to be confirmed.[69] Primary ovarian failure can also be seen in patients with Hashimoto thyroiditis as part of an autoimmune polyendocrine syndrome.[21] Hypothyroidism in men may cause diminished libido, erectile dysfunction, and oligospermia. A significant fraction of men with both hypothyroidism and hyperthyroidism have moderate to severe erectile dysfunction, which improves with treatment of the thyroid disease.[70]

Values for plasma gonadotropins are usually in the normal range in primary hypothyroidism; in postmenopausal women, levels are usually somewhat lower than in euthyroid women of the same age but are nevertheless within the menopausal range. This feature provides a valuable means of differentiating primary from secondary hypothyroidism.

The metabolism of both androgens and estrogens is altered in hypothyroidism. Secretion of androgens is decreased, and the metabolism of testosterone is shifted toward etiocholanolone rather than androsterone. With respect to estradiol and estrone, hypothyroidism favors metabolism of these steroids via 16α-hydroxylation over that via 2-oxygenation, with the result that formation of estriol is increased and that of 2-hydroxyestrone and its derivative, 2-methoxyestrone, is decreased. The sex hormone–binding globulin in plasma is decreased, with the result that the plasma concentrations of both testosterone and estradiol are decreased, but the unbound fractions are increased. The alterations in steroid metabolism are corrected by restoration of the euthyroid state.[71]

Catecholamines

The plasma cyclic adenosine monophosphate (cAMP) response to epinephrine is decreased in hypothyroidism, suggesting a state of decreased adrenergic responsiveness. The fact that the responses of plasma cAMP to glucagon and parathyroid hormone are also decreased suggests that thyroid hormones have a general modulating influence on cAMP generation.[72] The reduced adrenergic responsiveness associated with hypothyroidism has been linked to all steps of catecholamine signaling, including receptor and postreceptor actions, resulting in an impaired cAMP response. Direct measurement of norepinephrine in abdominal fat of hypothyroid patients shows reduced levels, and there is reduced production of glycerol in response to adrenergic agonist stimulation.[73] Augmentation of α_2-receptor signaling has also been proposed as a factor reducing catecholamine responsiveness.

Energy Metabolism: Protein, Carbohydrate, and Lipid Metabolism

The decrease in energy metabolism and heat production is reflected in a low basal metabolic rate, decreased appetite, cold intolerance, and slightly low basal body temperature.[74-76] Both the synthesis and the degradation of protein are decreased, the latter especially so, with the result that nitrogen balance is usually slightly positive. The decrease in protein synthesis is reflected in retardation of both skeletal and soft tissue growth.

Permeability of capillaries to protein is increased, accounting for the high levels of protein in effusions and in cerebrospinal fluid. In addition, the albumin pool is increased because of the greater decrease in albumin degradation compared to albumin synthesis. A greater than normal fraction of exchangeable albumin is in the extravascular space. The total concentration of serum proteins may be increased.

Hypothyroidism is associated with a reduction in glucose disposal to skeletal muscle and adipose tissue.[77] Thyroid hormone has been shown to stimulate expression of the insulin-sensitive glucose transporter (GLUT4), and the levels of this transporter are reduced in hypothyroidism. Hypothyroidism is also, however, associated with reduced gluconeogenesis. The net effect of these influences is usually a minimal effect of hypothyroidism on serum glucose levels. Thyroid hormone downregulates expression of prohormone processing enzymes, which, therefore, have increased activity in hypothyroidism. Degradation of insulin, therefore, is slowed and the sensitivity to exogenous insulin may be increased. In a patient with preexisting diabetes mellitus who develops hypothyroidism, insulin requirements may be reduced. A further influence on glucose uptake may occur at the tissue level. Polymorphisms in the 5'-deiodinase type 2 (D2) gene, which may affect local T_3 production, have been shown to be associated with impaired glucose disposal.[78]

Both the synthesis and the degradation of lipid are depressed in hypothyroidism. Degradation, however, is reduced to a greater extent, with a net effect of accumulation of LDL and triglycerides.[29,74] The decrease in the lipid degradation rate may reflect the decrease in postheparin lipolytic activity, as well as reduced LDL receptors. Plasma free fatty acid levels are decreased, and the mobilization of free fatty acids in response to fasting, catecholamines, and growth hormone is impaired. Impaired lipolysis of white fat in hypothyroid patients at baseline and in response to catecholamine reflects impaired free fatty acid mobilization.[72,73] All of these abnormalities are relieved by treatment.

An elevation in serum LDL cholesterol has been associated, in most studies, with both overt and subclinical hypothyroidism.[29] According to most studies, serum HDL and triglyceride levels are not influenced by hypothyroidism.[74] The reduction in LDL with T_4 therapy is generally related to the original magnitude of LDL and TSH elevation; the higher the initial levels, the greater the reduction in LDL that is observed. A typical reduction in LDL is 5% to 10% of the original level.

The role of adipocytokines, such as leptin, adiponectin, and resistin, in metabolic regulation has been increasingly recognized as well as the potential for interaction with thyroid hormone.[76] Rodent studies have shown that leptin regulates central adaptation between the starved and fed state and that falling leptin levels, associated with starvation, lead to a suppression of the thyroid axis. Hypothyroidism in rodents is associated with reduced leptin and increased resistin levels. Leptin infusion into the cerebral ventricles reverses some of the metabolic changes seen with hypothyroidism, including improved glucose disposal and reduced skeletal muscle fat.[79] Human studies, however, have not shown consistent changes in adipocytokines in hypothyroidism.[80]

Current Clinical Picture

In the adult, the onset of hypothyroidism is usually so insidious that the typical manifestations may take months or years to appear and go unnoticed by family and friends. The gradual development of the hypothyroid state is due to slow progression both of thyroid hypofunction and of the clinical manifestations after thyroid failure is complete. This course is in contrast with the more rapid development of the hypothyroid state when replacement therapy is discontinued in a patient with treated primary hypothyroidism or when the thyroid gland of a normal subject is surgically removed. In such patients, manifestations of frank hypothyroidism are usually present by 6 weeks and myxedema appears by 3 months.

Hypothyroidism continues to be diagnosed at earlier stages.[1,2,81] Based on the most recent data, subclinical or early hypothyroidism is seen approximately 14 times more commonly than overt hypothyroidism. Early symptoms are variable and relatively nonspecific. The reason for the increased prevalence of hypothyroid patients presenting with minimal symptoms is largely the availability of sensitive and specific laboratory tests that allow recognition of the primary form of the disease long before severe symptoms have developed. There should, therefore, be a low threshold to test patients for suspected primary hypothyroidism with a serum TSH determination. Patients with significant biochemical abnormalities of hypothyroidism may not score high on indices of symptoms and signs.[82]

With respect to physical signs of hypothyroidism, the presence of coarse skin, periorbital puffiness that obscures the curve of the malar bone (see Fig. 13-1), cold skin, and delayed ankle reflex relaxation phase are all signs that should lead to appropriate diagnostic tests.

Acute hypothyroidism in the previously hyperthyroid patient seen after radioiodine therapy may also be characterized by painful cramping of large muscle groups, as is discussed under "Treatment of Graves Disease" in Chapter 12.

Hypothyroidism in Infants and Children

Severe hypothyroidism is seldom apparent at birth, perhaps due to the partial protection afforded by transplacental transfer of maternal thyroid hormones, hence the requirement for systematic screening for congenital hypothyroidism.[17] Congenital hypothyroidism can be due to complete thyroid agenesis, ectopic thyroid, or incomplete thyroid development. Mutations in genes important for thyroid development have been identified in a number of patients and in some cases may explain associated abnormalities in development of other structures, such as the heart, because of their spatial association during development. The age at which symptoms appear depends on the degree of impairment of thyroid function (see Figs. 13-3 and 13-4). Severe hypothyroidism in infancy is termed *cretinism*. As the age at onset increases, the clinical picture of cretinism merges imperceptibly with that of juvenile hypothyroidism. Retardation of mental development and growth, the hallmark of cretinism, becomes manifest only in later infancy, and the former is largely irreversible. Consequently, early recognition is crucial and has been achieved by universal population screening in the developed world by measuring serum T_4 or TSH concentrations routinely in filter paper blood spots from neonates. During the first few months of life, symptoms and signs of hypothyroidism include feeding problems, failure to thrive, constipation, a hoarse cry, somnolence, and jaundice. In succeeding months, especially in severe cases, protuberance of the abdomen, dry skin, poor growth of hair and nails, and delayed eruption of the deciduous teeth become evident. Retardation of mental and physical development is manifested by delay in reaching the normal milestones of development, such as holding up the head, sitting, walking, and talking.

Thyroid hormone plays a major role in bone development, and thyroid hormone receptors are expressed in osteoclasts and osteoblasts.[53,54] The primary targets of thyroid hormone have been identified in the epiphyseal plates. Impairment of linear growth in congenital hypothyroidism results in dwarfism, with the limbs disproportionately short in relation to the trunk (see Fig. 13-3). Delayed closure of the fontanels causes the head to be large in relation to the body. The naso-orbital configuration remains infantile. Maldevelopment of the femoral epiphyses results in a waddling gait. The teeth are malformed and susceptible to caries. The characteristic appearance includes a broad, flat nose; widely set eyes; periorbital puffiness; large protruding tongue; sparse hair; rough skin; short neck; and protuberant abdomen with an umbilical hernia. Mental deficiency is usually severe.

Radiologic examination of the skeleton is diagnostic. The skull shows a poorly developed base; delayed closure of the fontanels; widely set orbits; and a short, flat nasal bone. The pituitary fossa may be enlarged. Shedding of deciduous teeth and eruption of permanent teeth are delayed (see Fig. 13-4).

The radiologic picture of epiphyseal dysgenesis is virtually pathognomonic of hypothyroidism in infancy and childhood and may involve any center of endochondral ossification, depending on the age at onset of the hypothyroid state; it is usually best seen in the femoral and humeral heads and the navicular bone of the foot. The centers of ossification appear late, so bone age is retarded in relation to chronologic age, and when they eventually appear, instead of a single center, multiple small centers are scattered throughout a misshapen epiphysis (see Fig. 13-4). These small centers of ossification eventually coalesce and form a single center with an irregular outline and a stippled appearance (stippled epiphysis). Epiphyseal dysgenesis is evident only in centers that normally ossify at a time after the onset of the hypothyroidism. After a normal metabolic state is restored by treatment, centers destined to ossify at a later age develop normally.

Hypothyroidism that begins in childhood is usually Hashimoto disease and can be transient in this age group. Subclinical hypothyroidism is also seen in children and adolescents, and in one study those affected were more likely to be obese and have a family history of thyroid disease.[83] The clinical manifestations of hypothyroidism in children are intermediate, between those of infantile and those of adult hypothyroidism, in that the developmental retardation is not as severe as that of cretinism and the manifestations of full-blown adult myxedema are rarely seen. Growth and sexual development are affected predominantly. If left untreated, linear growth is severely retarded and sexual maturation and the onset of puberty are delayed.[53-55] On radiologic examination, epiphyseal dysgenesis may be present and epiphyseal union is always delayed, resulting in a bone age that is younger relative to chronologic age.

Laboratory Evaluation
Primary and Central Hypothyroidism

A decrease in secretion of the thyroid hormones is common to all varieties of hypothyroidism, except for disorders of thyroid hormone metabolism or action, such as *consumptive hypothyroidism* and *resistance to thyroid hormone* (see

TABLE 13-2
Laboratory Evaluation of Patients with Suspected Hypothyroidism or Thyroid Enlargement*

TSH, Free T_4	TPO-Ab	Diagnosis
TSH > 10 mU/L		
Low	+	Primary hypothyroidism due to autoimmune thyroid disease
Low normal	+	Primary "subclinical" hypothyroidism (autoimmune)
Low or low normal	–	Recovery from systemic illness
		External irradiation, drug-induced, congenital hypothyroidism
		Iodine deficiency
		Seronegative autoimmune thyroid disease
		Rare thyroid disorders (amyloidosis, sarcoidosis, etc.)
		Recovery from subacute granulomatous thyroiditis
Normal	+, –	Consider TSH or T_4 assay artifacts
Elevated	–	Thyroid hormone resistance
		Blockade of T_4 to T_3 conversion (amiodarone) or a congenital 5′-deiodinase deficiency
		Consider assay artifacts
TSH 5-10 mU/L		
Low, low normal	+	Early primary autoimmune hypothyroidism
Low, low normal	–	Milder forms of nonautoimmune hypothyroidism (see earlier)
		Central hypothyroidism with impaired TSH bioactivity
Elevated	– (+)	Consider thyroid hormone resistance
		T_4 to T_3 conversion blockade (e.g., amiodarone)
TSH 0.5-5 mU/L		
Low, low normal	– (+)	Central hypothyroidism
		Salicylate or phenytoin therapy
		Desiccated thyroid or T_3 replacement
TSH < 0.5 μU/L		
Low, low normal	– (+)	"Post-hyperthyroid" hypothyroidism (^{131}I or surgery)
		Central hypothyroidism
		T_3 or desiccated thyroid excess
		Following excess levothyroxine withdrawal

*Initial tests: serum TSH, serum free T_4, TPO, or Tg-Ab.
Tg-Ab, anti-thyroglobulin antibody; TPO-Ab, thyroid peroxidase autoantibody; TSH, thyroid-stimulating hormone (thyrotropin); +, present; –, not present.

later). In patients with primary thyroid disease, the cause of hypothyroidism in more than 99% of the patients, there is a significant increase in basal serum TSH concentration. A strategy for evaluating the patient suspected of hypothyroidism involves a TSH determination (Table 13-2). If the suspicion of hypothyroidism is strong, if a goiter is present, or if central hypothyroidism is part of the differential diagnosis, an fT$_4$ assay should be included (see Chapter 11). If hypothyroidism is thought to be unlikely but must be excluded, only a TSH determination is required because primary hypothyroidism is almost always the cause. If TSH is elevated, an fT$_4$ assay can be added to the same determination (Fig. 13-5). As hypothyroidism progresses, the serum TSH increases further, the serum fT$_4$ falls, and finally at the most severe stage, serum T$_3$ concentrations may become subnormal (see Table 13-2). The persistence of a normal serum T$_3$ is, in part, due to preferential synthesis and secretion of T$_3$ by residual functioning thyroid tissue under the influence of the increased plasma TSH. In addition, the efficiency of conversion of T$_4$ to T$_3$ by D2 is increased as

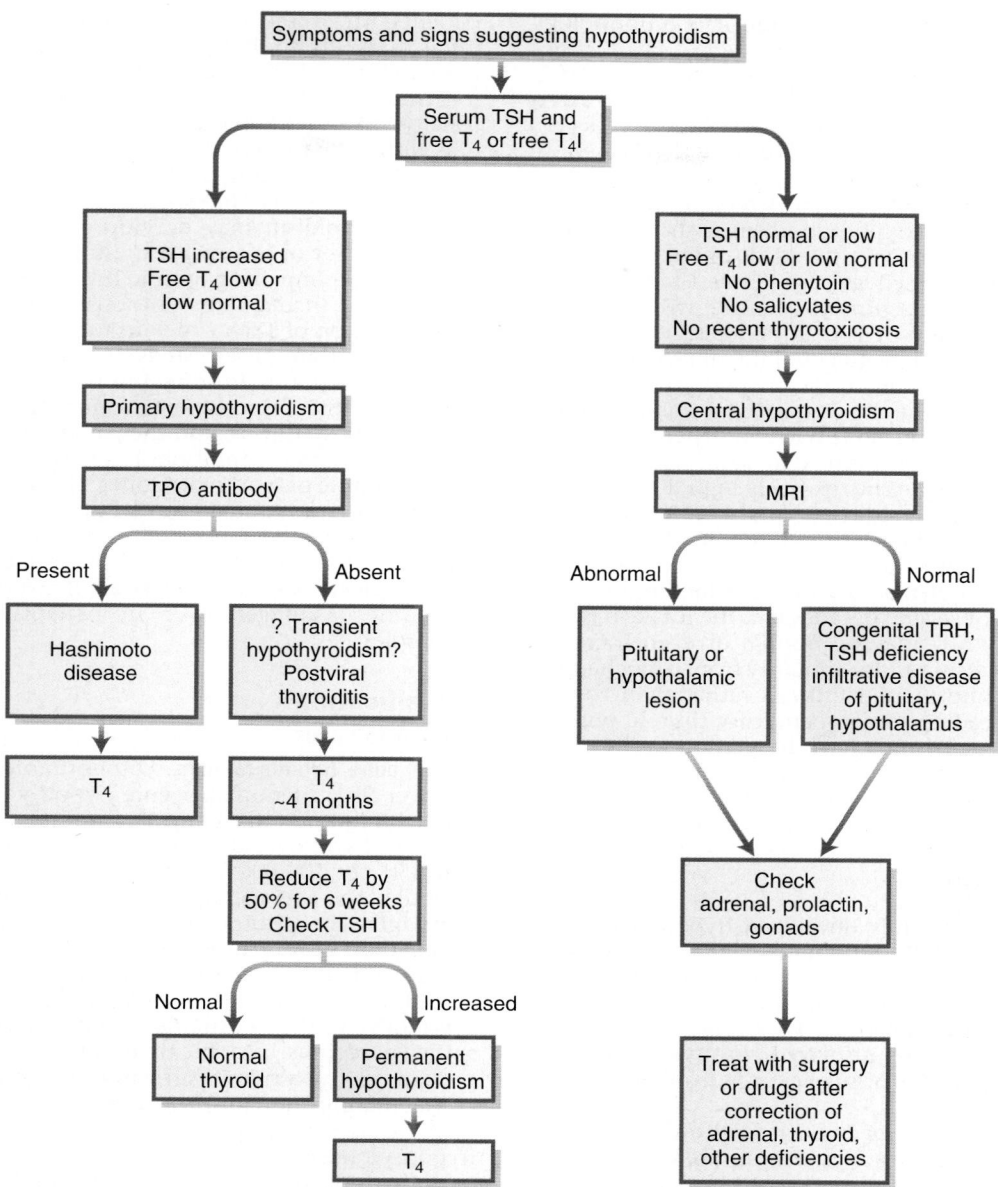

Figure 13-5 Strategy for the laboratory evaluation of patients with suspected hypothyroidism. The principal differential diagnosis is between primary and central hypothyroidism (see Chapter 9). The serum thyrotropin (TSH) concentration is the critical laboratory determination that, in general, allows recognition of the cause of the disease. An exception is the individual with a recent history of thyrotoxicosis (and suppressed TSH) in whom a low free thyroxine (T_4) level may be associated with a reduced TSH level for several months after relief of the thyrotoxicosis. In patients with primary hypothyroidism, the absence of thyroid peroxidase (TPO) antibodies raises a possible diagnosis of transient hypothyroidism following an undiagnosed episode of subacute or postviral thyroiditis. In such patients, a trial of levothyroxine in reduced dosage after 4 months may reveal recovery of thyroid function, thus avoiding permanent levothyroxine replacement. MRI, magnetic resonance imaging; TRH, thyrotropin-releasing hormone; T4I, thyroxine index.

the serum T_4 level falls.[84] Consequently, the serum T_3 concentration may remain within the normal range.

The principal differential diagnosis is between primary and central hypothyroidism (see Chapter 9).[85] The serum TSH concentration is the critical laboratory determination that, in general, allows recognition of the cause of the disease when the serum fT_4 is reduced. An exception is the individual with a recent history of thyrotoxicosis (and suppressed TSH) in whom a low fT_4 level may be associated with a reduced TSH level for several months after treatment of the thyrotoxicosis. In patients with primary hypothyroidism, the absence of TPO antibodies raises a possible diagnosis of transient hypothyroidism following an undiagnosed episode of painful subacute thyroiditis, also

referred to as postviral, de Quervain, granulomatous, or pseudotuberculous thyroiditis.

The differentiation of hypothyroidism due to intrinsic thyroid failure from hypothyroidism due to diminished TSH secretion from hypothalamic or pituitary disease (central or secondary hypothyroidism) is the most critical decision point in this pathway (see Fig. 13-5). A low thyroid hormone level with a normal or low TSH level should lead to an evaluation for the possibility of failure of other endocrine systems that require trophic pituitary hormones for normal function (see Table 13-1) (see Chapters 8 and 9). In some patients with central hypothyroidism, the basal serum TSH concentration (and the response to TRH) may even be somewhat elevated, but the TSH has reduced biologic potency even though it is immunologically reactive.[4]

In patients with an elevated TSH level and a reduced fT_4, the presence or absence of TPO antibodies should be ascertained (see Fig. 13-5). The presence of TPO antibodies generally points to autoimmune thyroid disease (Hashimoto disease) as the cause of the hypothyroidism. On the other hand, the absence of TPO antibodies requires a search for less common causes of hypothyroidism such as transient hypothyroidism, infiltrative thyroid disorders, and external irradiation, as discussed later (see Table 13-1), although rarely patients with Hashimoto disease will not have detectable thyroglobulin or TPO antibodies.

Measurement of radioactive iodine uptake (RAIU) is rarely required in the evaluation of hypothyroidism. Tests that employ radioiodine to assess the function of the thyroid gland display a variable pattern, depending on the underlying thyroid disorder. The diagnostic value of a low RAIU is limited because of the relatively high dietary iodine intake in North America, reducing uptake of the tracer dose of radioiodine, and variation in iodine intake from day to day in the same individual. National surveys of dietary iodine intake had shown a progressive reduction in iodine intake over the past several decades, but the intake has now stabilized.[86] The RAIU may be normal or even increased when hypothyroidism results primarily from a biochemical defect in thyroid hormone synthesis rather than thyroid cell destruction leading to compensatory thyroid enlargement. Specific functional patterns in relation to the causes of hypothyroidism are discussed later. Nonetheless, measurement of RAIU is almost never required in the diagnostic evaluation of the hypothyroid patient.

Differential Diagnosis

The clinical picture of fully developed hypothyroidism is quite characteristic, but the abnormalities can be overlooked, even by experienced clinicians, if the diagnosis is not considered. Despite the availability of inexpensive and specific tests, it is still surprising how often what is retrospectively obvious, severe, primary hypothyroidism is not recognized. A high index of suspicion is required to avoid this oversight.

For the milder forms of hypothyroidism, the clinical presentation overlaps to a significant extent with other conditions. The fact that these disorders often occur in older patients is partly responsible for the diagnostic uncertainty.[2] In some cases, slowing of mental and physical activity, dry skin, and loss of hair may mimic similar findings in hypothyroidism. Furthermore, older people often become hypothermic with cold exposure. In patients with chronic renal insufficiency, anorexia, torpor, periorbital puffiness, sallow complexion, and anemia (e.g., see Fig. 13-1) may suggest hypothyroidism and may call for specific testing. Distinguishing nephrotic states from hypothyroidism by clinical examination alone may be even more difficult. In this disorder, waxy pallor, edema, hypercholesterolemia, and hypometabolism may suggest hypothyroidism. In addition, the total serum T_4 concentration may be decreased if significant thyroid-binding globulin is lost in the urine but the fT_4 and TSH would be normal.

In patients with pernicious anemia, psychiatric abnormalities, pallor, and numbness and tingling of the extremities may mimic similar findings in hypothyroidism. Although there is a clinical and immunologic overlap between primary hypothyroidism and pernicious anemia, this association is not invariable (see Chapter 40). The presence of hypothyroidism is often suspected in patients who are severely ill, especially in the elderly.[34,87] In such patients, the total T_4 concentration may be decreased, often markedly so, but the fT_4 is generally normal unless the patient is severely ill (see Chapter 11). These features, together with the absence of an elevation of serum TSH, usually serve to differentiate the ill euthyroid patient from one with primary hypothyroidism. The serum TSH, however, can be transiently increased (up to 20 mU/L) during recovery from severe illness.

Hypothyroidism may develop either because of some extrinsic factor or acquired condition or because of a congenital defect impairing thyroid hormone biosynthesis (see Table 13-1). Inadequate synthesis of hormone leads to hypersecretion of TSH, which in turn produces both goiter and stimulation of all steps in hormone biosynthesis capable of response. In some instances, however, the compensatory TSH response overcomes the impairment in hormone biosynthesis, and the patient is euthyroid with a goiter. The latter condition is discussed in Chapter 14 under "Simple or Nontoxic Goiter." Less commonly, hypothyroidism is associated with an atrophic gland or, in the case of a congenital abnormality, one that never developed properly. Hypothyroidism occurs in about 20% of patients after surgical lobectomy, with an increased risk in areas of iodine insufficiency or in patients with anti-TPO antibodies.[88]

Classification
Acquired Causes
Autoimmune Hypothyroidism. Autoimmunity is responsible for over 90% of noniatrogenic hypothyroidism in countries with iodine sufficiency. The annual incidence of autoimmune hypothyroidism is around 80 per 100,000 men and 350 per 100,000 women.[89] All ages may be affected, although the average age of onset is between 40 and 60 years old. The disorder is more frequent in whites and Asians than in African Americans. The initial presentation depends on the stage of disease. Juvenile and adolescent autoimmune thyroiditis may be self-limiting. Hashimoto thyroiditis is the commonest cause of goiter in iodine-sufficient regions; atrophic thyroiditis (primary myxedema) presents as hypothyroidism without a goiter.

Circulating autoantibodies against thyroglobulin and TPO are present in almost all patients with autoimmune hypothyroidism. Up to 20% of patients with autoimmune hypothyroidism have TSH receptor antibodies that block the receptor, rather than stimulating it, as in Graves disease; in rare patients there may be switching from one type of antibody to the other, resulting in alternating hypothyroidism and hyperthyroidism.[90] Less commonly, patients produce autoantibodies against the sodium-iodide symporter (NIS), pendrin, and T_4 and T_3, but the functional relevance of these antibodies is not known.

Around 15% of women and 3% of men have positive thyroid autoantibodies but no other clinical features of thyroid disease; most of them, however, will have histologic evidence of focal thyroiditis. Longitudinal studies have shown that euthyroid women with high initial levels of autoantibodies against thyroglobulin or TPO and those whose TSH is within the upper half of the reference interval are the most likely to progress to overt hypothyroidism.[91]

Autoimmune hypothyroidism is commonly found in association with a range of autoimmune disorders, including pernicious anemia, systemic lupus erythematosus, Addison disease, celiac disease, and vitiligo.[92] A steroid-responsive encephalopathy (referred to as Hashimoto encephalopathy) has been reported in individuals with positive TPO antibodies, irrespective of thyroid dysfunction, but it is unclear whether there is a true causal

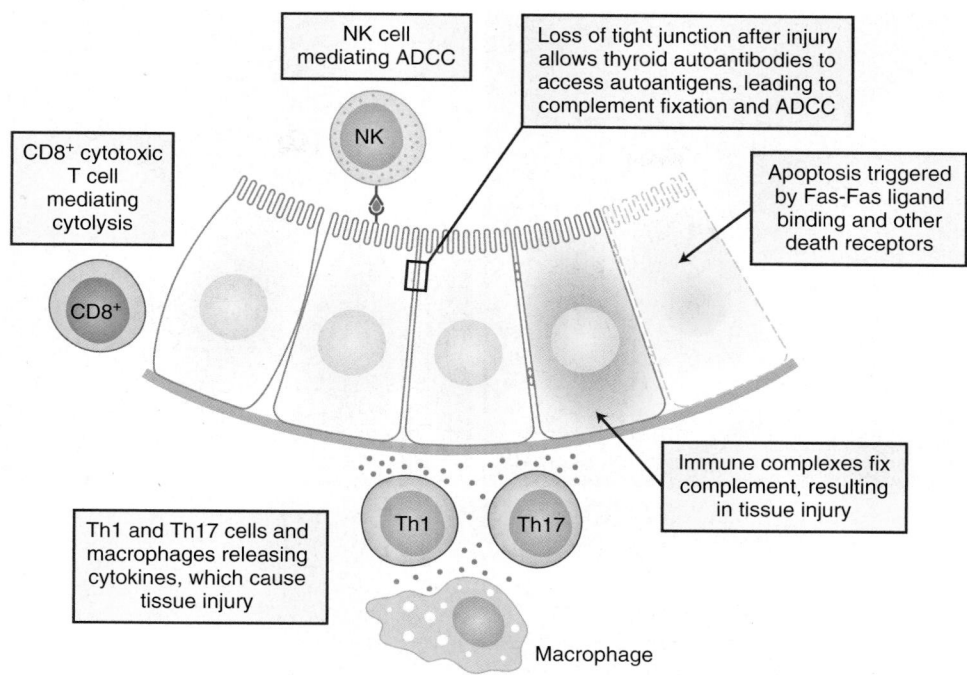

Figure 13-6 Summary of the main mechanisms involved in the pathogenesis of autoimmune hypothyroidism. ADCC, Antibody-dependent cell-mediated cytotoxicity; NK, natural killer.

relationship, for instance, through immunologic cross-reactivity with brain tissue.[52,93]

Pathophysiology. The current understanding of autoimmune mechanisms has been discussed in Chapter 12, and the main features associated with autoimmune hypothyroidism are summarized in Figure 13-6. T-cell–mediated tissue injury is believed to be the most important cause of autoimmune thyroid follicular cell destruction. Perforin-containing cytotoxic CD8+ T cells are abundant in the intrathyroidal lymphocytic infiltrate in Hashimoto thyroiditis. These T cells increase during the evolution of disease and recognize both thyroglobulin and TPO.[94] Apoptosis is an additional pathway for thyroid cell destruction. In Hashimoto thyroiditis, thyroid follicular cells express both Fas (CD95) and Fas ligand (CD95L) and may thus self-destruct when these molecules interact; it is now clear that other decoy death receptors and regulators of apoptosis signaling play an additional role.[95] There is also an increase in the number of intrathyroidal Th17 lymphocytes in Hashimoto thyroiditis, implying a pathogenic role for this proinflammatory T-cell subset.[96] The differentiation of Th17 cells may be enhanced by iodine. Cytokines released by T cells and other inflammatory cells cause Hürthle cell formation and thyroid dysfunction. The thyroid cells also respond to cytokines by expressing a number of proinflammatory molecules, such as chemokines and adhesion molecules, which increase the potential for T-cell binding and cytotoxicity.

Apart from the striking activity of TSH receptor blocking antibodies, which can induce temporary neonatal hypothyroidism following their transfer across the placenta,[97,98] the pathogenic role of antibodies in autoimmune hypothyroidism is unclear.[99] No neonatal disorders have been associated with the presence of high thyroglobulin or TPO autoantibodies in mothers, indicating that any role in tissue injury is likely to be secondary to an initial phase of T-cell–mediated damage, which allows the autoantibodies to access their target antigens. Such injury may be mediated through antibody-dependent cell-mediated cyto-

toxicity, involving natural killer (NK) cells, or through complement fixation in the case of TPO antibodies.[100]

Histopathology. The pathologic features of autoimmune hypothyroidism vary from mild focal thyroiditis to extensive lymphocytic infiltration and fibrosis. In classical Hashimoto thyroiditis (originally termed *struma lymphomatosa*), the thyroid gland may be diffusely enlarged or nodular; the tissue is pale and firm and has a rubbery texture (Fig. 13-7A). Typically, there is a diffuse lymphocytic infiltration with germinal center formation and obliteration of thyroid follicles, accompanied by a variable degree of fibrosis (see Fig. 13-7B). Destruction of thyroid epithelial cells occurs as disease progresses from euthyroidism to hypothyroidism; in some patients there is follicular cell metaplasia and the formation of Hürthle cells. Rarely, there are concurrent histologic changes of Graves disease, so-called hashitoxicosis. In the other broad type of autoimmune hypothyroidism, termed *atrophic thyroiditis* or *primary myxedema*, the gland is atrophied and consists of extensive fibrotic tissue, moderate lymphocytic infiltration, and widespread loss of thyroid follicles, but the fibrosis is not as extensive as in Riedel thyroiditis (see Fig. 13-7C). The histopathologic changes in painless thyroiditis resemble Hashimoto thyroiditis.

Although it is now generally thought that these variations represent a spectrum of disease arising from a common underlying autoimmune process, a distinct subset of patients with Hashimoto thyroiditis has been delineated recently in whom there are high circulating levels of IgG4 and increased numbers of IgG4-positive plasma cells in the thyroid. Such IgG4-related thyroiditis is characterized pathologically by a greater degree of stromal fibrosis, lymphoplasmacytic infiltration, and hypothyroidism.[101]

Risk Factors

Genetic Susceptibility. The importance of genetic factors in the cause of autoimmune hypothyroidism is indicated by the frequent presence of thyroid autoantibodies, thyroid disease, and other autoimmune disorders in family members and by twin studies, which show a high concordance

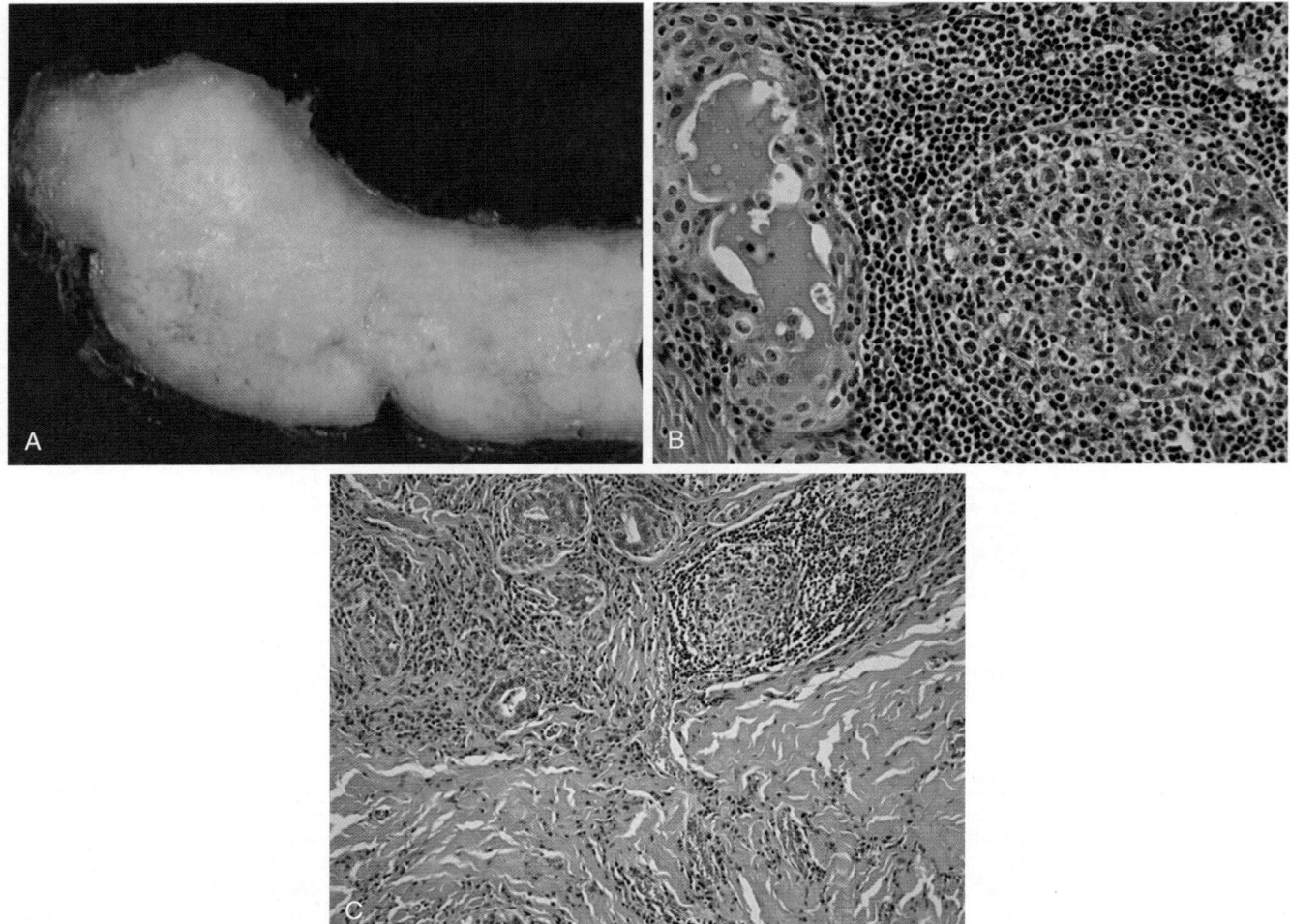

Figure 13-7 Hashimoto thyroiditis. **A,** Gross appearance of a cut section of the thyroid lobe demonstrating the pale color of the tissue due to lymphocytic infiltration, fibrosis, and loss of follicles. **B,** Typical histologic appearance illustrating a germinal center, heavy lymphocytic infiltration, and a partially disrupted thyroid follicle. **C,** Fibrous variant showing extensive fibrosis and loss of follicles. (**A** and **C,** Courtesy of Dr. Vania Nosé, Brigham and Women's Hospital, Boston, MA. **B,** From Nosé V, Asa SL, Erickson LA, et al: *Diagnostic Pathology:* Endocrine. Salt Lake City, Amirsys, 2012.)

rate (0.55) in monozygotic but not dizygotic twins.[102] As with all autoimmune endocrinopathies, human leukocyte antigen (HLA)-D region polymorphisms play a role in susceptibility, and Hashimoto thyroiditis is associated with HLA-DR3 and to a lesser extent HLA-DR4.[103] Polymorphisms in the *CTLA4* gene also confer susceptibility, with lesser contributions from polymorphisms in the *CD40* gene and the gene encoding thyroglobulin.[104,105] It is clear that new analytic approaches are likely to reveal many other genes, which make small etiologic contributions that account for the diversity of clinical presentation. For example, a combination of novel genetic markers have been described and are associated with an increased risk of progression from TPO antibody positivity to hypothyroidism, including polymorphism in the *MAGI3* gene.[106]

Shared genetic susceptibility accounts for the frequent occurrence of other autoimmune disorders in patients with autoimmune hypothyroidism. Around half of women with Turner syndrome are positive for thyroid autoantibodies and a third develop hypothyroidism.[107] There is also an increase in autoimmune hypothyroidism in children with Down syndrome, which may evolve into Graves disease in some cases.[108]

Nongenetic Risk Factors. Many of the factors that have been identified as increasing the risk for Graves disease (pregnancy, drugs, age, sex, iodine, and irradiation) apply equally to autoimmune thyroiditis. These factors are detailed in Chapter 12 and are briefly considered here. Epidemiologic data suggest a strong influence of environmental factors in Hashimoto thyroiditis, as this was a rare disease before the 1950s but it is now one of the most common autoimmune disorders.[109]

Sex and Pregnancy. The female preponderance of autoimmune hypothyroidism may be due to sex hormones; skewed X chromosome inactivation has also been proposed as an additional explanation. During pregnancy, fetal tolerance is maintained by changes in immunoregulation that have the coincidental effect of improving thyroid autoimmunity but then lead to postpartum exacerbation of the autoimmune process.[110] This phenomenon results in transient postpartum thyroiditis, a form of painless subacute thyroiditis (see Chapter 12), and in around 30% to 40% of these cases permanent hypothyroidism may appear over the next decade.[111] Those women with hypothyroidism and positive TPO antibodies during the phase of postpartum thyroiditis are most at risk of such an outcome.

Iodine and Selenium. An excessive intake of iodine can precipitate autoimmune thyroiditis in susceptible populations.[112,113] This form of hypothyroidism should be distinguished from direct blockade of a thyroid gland by iodine (the Wolff-Chaikoff effect).[114] Evidence accumulated in animal models suggests that increased iodination of thyroglobulin enhances its immunoreactivity, and iodine may also cause thyroid injury through the generation of reactive oxygen metabolites.[115] There are epidemiologic data to suggest that selenium deficiency exacerbates autoimmune thyroiditis, but trials of selenium supplementation have been inconclusive with regard to clinical benefit.[116]

Drugs and Smoking. Treatment of patients with cytokines may precipitate the appearance of autoimmune thyroid disease in the form of Hashimoto thyroiditis or Graves disease (see later).[117] A number of novel anticancer treatments, including tyrosine kinase inhibitors (TKIs), can also induce autoimmune thyroiditis.[118] There is a higher than expected prevalence of autoimmune hypothyroidism in patients treated with lithium. Anthracene derivatives and other chemicals produce autoimmune thyroiditis in animals, but the role of environmental toxins in human disease is poorly studied. Smoking is associated with a decreased risk of autoimmune thyroiditis, but the risk rises temporarily when smoking is stopped.[119] Moderate alcohol consumption is also protective.[120]

Irradiation. Radiation exposure has been shown to induce thyroid autoantibodies and autoimmune thyroid disease in a number of studies. These exposures include radiation from the atomic bomb detonation in Japan[121] and radioactive fallout from the Chernobyl disaster, which was followed by an increase in the prevalence of thyroid autoantibodies in exposed children, with a small overall increase in the prevalence of hypothyroidism 12 to 14 years later.[122] Hodgkin disease survivors have a 17-fold relative risk of developing hypothyroidism, but this may in part be a direct effect of irradiation.[123]

Age. Autoimmune hypothyroidism continues to occur throughout adult life (except in the very elderly whose longevity may be associated with superior immunoregulation) so that the prevalence of the disease increases markedly with age.[11,16,87] This feature is similar to other types of autoimmunity and may reflect an increasing loss of tolerance to self.

Infection. There is no direct evidence that infection causes autoimmune thyroiditis in humans, although there is some evidence that the hepatitis C virus may precipitate thyroid disease in susceptible patients.[117] In addition, there is follow-up evidence from patients with painful subacute thyroiditis, following a viral infection (see later), that long-term hypothyroidism occurs in around 15% of patients and some of these cases may have an autoimmune basis.

Clinical Picture. Goiter, the hallmark of classic Hashimoto disease, usually develops gradually and may be found during routine examination or by ultrasonography. On occasion, the thyroid gland enlarges rapidly and, when accompanied by pain and tenderness, may mimic painful subacute thyroiditis (see Chapter 12). Some patients are hypothyroid when first seen. The goiter is generally painless, moderate in size, and firm in consistency and moves freely on swallowing. The surface can be either smooth or nodular. Both lobes are enlarged, but the gland may be asymmetric. The pyramidal lobe may also be enlarged, and rarely, adjacent structures, such as the trachea, esophagus, and recurrent laryngeal nerves, may be compressed. Enlargement of regional lymph nodes is unusual.

Other patients with hypothyroidism present without a goiter (atrophic thyroiditis), which is thought to be the end result of autoimmune destruction of the thyroid, although the progression of goitrous Hashimoto thyroiditis to the atrophied state is not commonly seen in the individual patient. The atrophic thyroid is likely the reflection of rapid destruction early in the onset of autoimmune thyroiditis, combined in some patients with TSH receptor antibodies of the blocking variety, although such antibodies may also occur in those with a goiter. Generally, the disease tends to progress slowly with an increase in fibrous tissue and loss of thyroid follicular cells. A study of thyroid volume by ultrasound in patients with newly diagnosed autoimmune hypothyroidism found that there was a continuum of thyroid size, with atrophy and goiter representing extremes of the distribution, supporting the idea that these are not distinct entities but rather part of the same underlying autoimmune process.[124]

Clinically, the untreated goiter remains unchanged or enlarges gradually over many years. The manifestations of hypothyroidism vary and often develop over many years in patients who are initially euthyroid. Thyroid lymphoma occurs almost exclusively in patients with underlying Hashimoto thyroiditis and should be suspected if there is rapid and sometimes painful enlargement of the thyroid gland.[125] As mentioned earlier, the presence of coexistent Hashimoto thyroiditis may be a favorable prognostic factor in patients with papillary carcinoma, but the risk of papillary carcinoma is probably not increased in Hashimoto thyroiditis.[126]

Occasionally, hyperthyroidism due to Graves disease develops in patients with Hashimoto thyroiditis. In other patients with early autoimmune thyroiditis, transitory thyrotoxicosis (painless thyroiditis with thyrotoxicosis) occurs as the result of thyroid cell destruction. In such cases, evidence of ongoing thyroid hyperfunction is lacking because the thyroid RAIU is depressed. As described earlier, 50% of women with thyroid autoantibodies who are euthyroid in the first trimester of pregnancy develop postpartum thyroiditis, accompanied by transient thyrotoxicosis, hypothyroidism, or fluctuation from one state to the other.[127]

Laboratory Tests. The results of the common tests of thyroid function depend on the stage of the disease (see Table 13-2). Rarely, the tests may suggest thyrotoxicosis with a suppressed TSH and elevated serum T_4 and T_3 levels, due to either release of stored thyroid hormone as a result of rapid tissue destruction, or the relative overproduction of autoantibodies, which stimulate rather than block the TSH receptor (sometimes called hashitoxicosis). In the latter case, the RAIU may be increased, whereas it is decreased if there is tissue destruction. Typically, patients with Hashimoto thyroiditis present with a goiter and blood tests show a normal or slightly raised TSH, with normal serum T_4 and T_3 levels. As tissue destruction continues, the TSH level rises further, but the ability of the thyroid to respond to TSH diminishes, and the RAIU and serum T_4 level decline to subnormal values, resulting in overt hypothyroidism. This is the typical biochemical finding in atrophic thyroiditis, in which there is no goiter to alert the patient or physician to the underlying disorder. The serum T_3 level remains normal until late in the disease process, reflecting maximal stimulation of the failing thyroid by the increased serum TSH. The early phase of the foregoing sequence, when the serum TSH is increased but T_4 and T_3 are still normal, is termed *subclinical hypothyroidism* (see Table 13-2).

The diagnosis of autoimmune hypothyroidism is confirmed by the presence of thyroid autoantibodies in the serum, usually in high levels. TPO and thyroglobulin autoantibodies occur in roughly similar frequencies; the presence of both autoantibodies is twice as frequent as the isolated individual autoantibodies.[128] Thyroid autoantibodies may be absent in rare patients due to assay insensitivity or the occurrence of an entirely intrathyroidal autoimmune process. Sometimes part of a gland with autoimmune thyroiditis may look and feel like a firm thyroid nodule, and ultrasonography or even aspiration biopsy should be performed to confirm the diagnosis.

Differential Diagnosis. Differentiation of autoimmune hypothyroidism from other forms of hypothyroidism is facilitated by the demonstration that high levels of thyroid autoantibodies occur more commonly than in other thyroid disorders. The frequent coexistence of hypothyroidism and Hashimoto thyroiditis serves to distinguish this disease from nontoxic goiter and thyroid neoplasia.

Differentiation of a euthyroid Hashimoto goiter from a multinodular goiter is often difficult without ultrasonography, and diffuse nontoxic goiter tends to be softer than that of Hashimoto thyroiditis. Ultrasound examination typically reveals a diffuse and patchy heterogeneous echotexture or hypoechoic micronodules with echogenic septations in Hashimoto thyroiditis. In adolescents, differentiation of Hashimoto goiter from diffuse nontoxic goiter is even more difficult because in this age group Hashimoto thyroiditis may not be accompanied by such high levels of thyroid autoantibodies. The presence of well-defined nodules usually distinguishes nontoxic multinodular goiter from Hashimoto thyroiditis.

Differentiation between euthyroid Hashimoto thyroiditis and thyroid carcinoma can sometimes be made on clinical grounds, but an ultrasound examination and aspiration biopsy are necessary in any case in which there is uncertainty. Lymphoma must always be excluded if there is a sudden change in a known Hashimoto goiter; core needle biopsy or open surgical biopsy may be required for final diagnosis. Thyroid carcinoma usually occurs as a solitary nodule that is firm or hard, and the gland may be fixed to adjacent structures. Compression of the recurrent laryngeal nerve with hoarseness is virtually pathognomonic of thyroid carcinoma but occurs late in the cancer progression. A history of a recent enlargement of the goiter is more common in thyroid malignancies (either carcinoma or lymphoma) than in Hashimoto thyroiditis. Enlargement of regional lymph nodes also suggests thyroid malignancy but can rarely occur in autoimmune thyroiditis.

Treatment. In euthyroid patients with Hashimoto thyroiditis, no treatment is required because the goiter is usually asymptomatic. Levothyroxine treatment may be indicated in patients when the goiter presses on adjacent structures or is unsightly, and it is most effective in goiters of recent onset. The aim is to keep the TSH level in the lower half of the reference interval. In long-standing goiter, treatment with thyroid hormone is usually ineffective, possibly because of fibrosis. Rarely, the goiter may be painful and this symptom may respond to levothyroxine therapy; prednisolone is usually ineffective. Surgery may be justified if symptoms or unsightly enlargement persists after a trial of levothyroxine therapy.

Replacement doses of thyroid hormone should be given when hypothyroidism is present, appropriate to the degree of hormone deficiency (see later). There may be a spontaneous return to euthyroidism in up to 10% of patients after starting levothyroxine, associated in some cases with the disappearance of TSH receptor blocking antibodies. However, it has not been established that such remissions are durable and there is no need to routinely stop levothyroxine once it has been started. It has recently been suggested that prednisolone treatment can reverse the hypothyroidism of IgG4-related thyroiditis, but the long-term outcome in such cases is not yet known.[129]

Iodine Deficiency (Endemic Goiter). The term *endemic goiter* denotes any goiter occurring in a region where goiter is prevalent.[112] As mentioned, endemic goiter almost always occurs in areas of environmental iodine deficiency.[130]

Although this condition is estimated to affect more than 200 million people throughout the world and is of major public health significance, it is most common in mountainous areas, such as the Alps, Himalayas, and Andes, or in the Great Lakes and Mississippi Valley regions of the United States, owing to the depletion of iodine consequent to the persistent glacial run-off in these regions.

The causative role of iodine deficiency in the genesis of endemic goiter is supported by the inverse correlation between the iodine content of soil and water and the incidence of goiter, the kinetics of iodine metabolism in patients with the disorder, and a decrease in incidence after iodine prophylaxis. The latter accounts for its absence in the population residing in the Great Plains region of the United States.

The occurrence of endemic goiter can vary, even within an area of known iodine deficiency; the roles of dietary minerals or naturally occurring goitrogens and of pollution of water supplies have been suggested in instances of this type.[112] For example, in the Cauca Valley of Colombia, waterborne goitrogens have been implicated, and in many areas of endemic iodine deficiency, consumption of cassava meal, which gives rise to thiocyanate, aggravates the iodine-deficient state by inhibiting thyroid iodide transport. Familial clustering of goiters within iodine-insufficient areas, usually with an autosomal dominant inheritance, suggest an important genetic component.[131]

Most abnormalities in iodine metabolism in patients with endemic goiter are consistent with the expected effects of iodine deficiency (see Chapter 11, "Iodine Metabolism"). Thyroid iodide clearance rates and RAIU are increased in proportion to the decrease in the urinary excretion of stable iodine. The absolute iodine uptake is normal or low. In areas of moderate iodine deficiency, the serum T_4 concentration is usually in the lower range of normal; in areas of severe deficiency, however, values are decreased. Nevertheless, most patients in these areas do not appear to be in a hypothyroid state because of an increase in the synthesis of T_3 at the expense of T_4 and because of an increase in the activity of thyroidal D1 and D2.[84] TSH levels are typically in the upper range of normal.

The incidence and severity of endemic goiter and the metabolic state of the goitrous patient depend mainly on the degree of iodine deficiency. In the absence of hypothyroidism, the effects of the goiter are mainly cosmetic. When the goiter becomes nodular, however, hemorrhage into a nodule may cause acute pain and swelling, mimicking painful subacute thyroiditis or neoplasia. The goiter may also compress adjacent structures, such as the trachea, esophagus, and recurrent laryngeal nerves. The borderline nature of the iodine supply in many countries of Western Europe is exemplified by the development of compensatory maternal and fetal goiter during pregnancy due to the increased requirement for thyroid hormone during gestation.[112]

The incidence of endemic goiter has been greatly reduced in many areas by the introduction of iodized salt.[112] In the United States, table salt is enriched with potassium iodide to a concentration of 0.01%, which, if the intake of salt is average, would provide an iodine intake of approximately 150 to 300 μg/day, the desired amount in an adult (see Table 11-1). The use of iodine-containing flour in bread products and iodized salt in commercially produced food has been markedly reduced.[132] The iodine content of bread and infant formula is variable within a given product and often does not match the measured content.[132] As mentioned, iodine intake in the United States has been decreasing in recent decades, likely due to reduced iodine in commercial food products, although iodine intake has now stabilized. Pregnant women, however, remain a susceptible population because of their increased iodine requirements.[130] Most prescription prenatal vitamins do not contain iodine.[133] An annual injection of iodized oil is another effective means of administering iodine, and endemic goiter can be treated by the addition of iodine to communal drinking water.

Administration of iodine has little, if any, effect on a long-standing endemic goiter, but it causes the early endemic hyperplastic goiter of iodine deficiency to regress. Similarly, thyroid hormone usually has no effect on long-standing goiter or on established mental or skeletal changes, but it should be given in full-replacement doses if there is evidence of hypothyroidism. This is of paramount importance in pregnant women. Surgical treatment is indicated if the adjacent structures are compressed or if the goiter is either very large or is enlarging rapidly.

Endemic Cretinism. Endemic cretinism is a developmental disorder that occurs in regions of severe endemic goiter.[112] Both parents of an endemic cretin are usually goitrous, and in addition to the features of sporadic cretinism described earlier, endemic cretins often have deaf-mutism, spasticity, motor dysfunction, and abnormalities in the basal ganglia demonstrable by magnetic resonance imaging.

Three types of cretins can be discerned: (1) hypothyroid cretins, (2) neurologic cretins, and (3) cretins with combined features of the two. The pathogenesis of neurologic cretinism is obscure but may be due to severe thyroid hormone deficiency during a critical early phase of central nervous system development in utero.[43] Some cretins are goitrous, but the thyroid may also be atrophic, possibly as a consequence of exhaustion atrophy from continuous overstimulation or the lack of iodine.

Iodide Excess. Goiter and hypothyroidism, either alone or in combination, are sometimes induced by chronic administration of large doses of iodine in either organic or inorganic form (see Table 11-7).[112,134] Iodide-induced goiter was formerly seen in patients with chronic respiratory disease, who were given potassium iodide as an expectorant. The development of iodide goiter has also been reported after a single administration of radiographic contrast medium from which iodide is released slowly over a long period and may also occur during amiodarone administration. Iodide goiter without hypothyroidism may occur endemically, such as on the island of Hokkaido, Japan, where seaweed products are consumed in large quantities.

From an analysis of reported cases and from the fact that only a small percentage of patients who receive iodides chronically develop goiter, it appears that the disorder evolves on a background of underlying thyroid dysfunction.[134] Categories of susceptible individuals include the following: patients with Hashimoto disease; patients with Graves disease, especially after its treatment with radioiodine; and patients with cystic fibrosis.

Among these groups, many individuals display a positive iodide-perchlorate discharge test, indicating a defect in the thyroidal organic iodine-binding mechanism (see Chapter 11, "Iodine Metabolism"). However, intrinsic thyroid disease need not be present because a propensity to develop iodide goiter and hypothyroidism has also been demonstrated in patients who have undergone hemithyroidectomy for a solitary thyroid nodule in whom the remaining lobe was histologically normal.[88] In these patients, as in those with Hashimoto disease or Graves disease studied prospectively, individuals with the highest basal serum TSH concentrations, even within the normal range, were those who developed iodide goiter. Iodinated contrast material, amiodarone, and povidone-iodine are common sources.[134]

Goiter and hypothyroidism commonly occur in newborn infants born to women given large quantities of iodine during pregnancy, and death from neonatal asphyxia has been reported (see Fig. 11-11). In such cases, the mother is usually free from goiter. Pregnant women should not receive large doses of iodine (>1 mg/day) over prolonged periods (>10 days), especially near term. Maternal amiodarone therapy causes thyroidal dysfunction in up to 20% of newborns.[112] It is not known whether iodide goiter in newborns results from an inherent hypersensitivity of the fetal thyroid or from the fact that the placenta concentrates iodide several-fold, or both.

As discussed earlier (see Chapter 11, "Regulation of Thyroid Function"), large doses of iodine cause an acute inhibition of organic binding that abates in the normal individual, despite continued iodine administration (acute Wolff-Chaikoff effect and escape).[135] Iodide goiter appears to result from a more pronounced inhibition of organic binding and the failure of the escape phenomenon. As a consequence of decreased hormone synthesis and the consequent increase in TSH, iodide transport is enhanced. Because inhibition of organic binding is a function of the intrathyroidal concentration of iodide, a vicious circle, augmented by this increase in serum TSH, is set in motion.

The disorder usually appears as a goiter with or without hypothyroidism, although in rare instances iodine may produce hypothyroidism unaccompanied by goiter. Usually the thyroid gland is firm and diffusely enlarged, often greatly so. Histopathologic examination reveals intense hyperplasia. The fT_4 concentration is low, TSH concentration is increased, and the 24-hour urinary iodine excretion and the serum inorganic iodide concentration are increased. The disorder regresses after iodine is withdrawn. Thyroid hormone may also be given to relieve severe symptoms.

Drugs Blocking Thyroid Hormone Synthesis or Release, Causing Goiter Formation. Ingestion of compounds that block thyroid hormone synthesis or release may cause goiter with or without hypothyroidism. Apart from the agents used in the treatment of hyperthyroidism, antithyroid agents may be encountered either as drugs for the treatment of disorders unrelated to the thyroid gland or as natural agents in foodstuffs.

Goiter with or without hypothyroidism can occur in patients given lithium, usually for bipolar manic-depressive psychosis.[136] Like iodide, lithium inhibits thyroid hormone release, and in high concentrations it can inhibit organic binding reactions. At least acutely, iodide and lithium act synergistically in the latter respect. The mechanisms underlying the several effects of lithium are uncertain; what differentiates patients who develop thyroid disease during lithium therapy from those who do not is also unclear. A promoting effect on underlying autoimmune thyroiditis may be at least one factor because many patients with this combination have autoimmune thyroid disease.

Other drugs that occasionally produce goitrous hypothyroidism include para-aminosalicylic acid, phenylbutazone, aminoglutethimide, and ethionamide. Like the thionamides, these drugs interfere with both the organic binding of iodine and perhaps in later steps in hormone biosynthesis. Although soybean flour is not an antithyroid agent, soybean products in feeding formulas formerly resulted in goiter in infants by enhancing fecal loss of hormone, which, together with the low iodine content of soybean products, produced a state of iodine deficiency. Feeding formulas containing soybean products are now enriched with iodine.

Cigarette smoking reduces the hypothyroidism in patients with underlying autoimmune thyroid disease, although the risk is transiently increased if smoking is stopped.[119] Thiocyanate, hydroxypyridine, and benzopyrene derivatives found in cigarette smoke may also interfere with thyroid hormone action.[137]

Both the goiter and the hypothyroidism usually subside after the antithyroid agent is withdrawn. If continued administration of pharmacologic goitrogens is required, however, replacement therapy with thyroid hormone causes the goiter to regress.

Goitrogens in Foodstuffs or as Endemic Substances or Pollutants. Antithyroid agents also occur naturally in foods. They are widely distributed in the family Cruciferae or Brassicaceae, particularly in the genus *Brassica*, including cabbages, turnips, kale, kohlrabi, rutabaga, mustard, and various plants that are not eaten by humans but that serve as animal fodder. It is likely that some thiocyanate is present in such plants (particularly cabbage).[138] Cassava meal, a dietary staple in many regions of the world, contains linamarin, a cyanogenic glycoside, the preparation of which leads to the formation of thiocyanate. Ingestion of cassava can accentuate goiter formation in areas of endemic iodine deficiency. Except for thiocyanate, dietary goitrogens influence thyroid iodine metabolism in the same manner as do the thionamides, which they resemble chemically; their role in the induction of disease in humans is uncertain. Waterborne, sulfur-containing goitrogens of mineral origin are believed to contribute to the development of endemic goiter in certain areas of Colombia.

A number of synthetic chemical pollutants have been implicated as a cause of goitrous hypothyroidism, including polychlorinated biphenyls and resorcinol derivatives.[139] Perchlorate has also been noted in high concentrations in geographic regions in which explosives and rocket fuel were made. Perchlorate has been detected in water, food, and breast milk, although the amount does not appear to be sufficient to disrupt thyroid function. In an area of Chile with a high level of natural perchlorate contamination in the water, thyroid function in pregnant women was not different from that in a region with no perchlorate, although iodine intake is quite high in this area.[140]

Cytokines. Patients with chronic hepatitis C or various malignancies may be given interferon-α or interleukin 2.[117,141] Such patients may experience hypothyroidism, which is often a transient destructive thyroiditis and associated with an initial thyrotoxic phase but in other cases may persist. Graves disease with hyperthyroidism may also develop, and ablative therapy may be required to treat this condition. Women and those who have positive TPO antibodies prior to treatment are at higher risk for these complications and should be monitored especially carefully during and after a course of treatment with either of these cytokines.

Congenital Causes of Goiter. Inherited defects in hormone biosynthesis are rare causes of goitrous hypothyroidism and account for only about 10% to 15% of the 1 in 3000 newborns with congenital hypothyroidism.[17,142,143] In most instances, the defect appears to be transmitted as an autosomal recessive trait. Individuals with goitrous hypothyroidism are believed to be homozygous for the abnormal gene, whereas euthyroid relatives with slightly enlarged thyroids are presumably heterozygous. In the latter group, appropriate functional testing may disclose a mild abnormality of the same biosynthetic step that is defective in the homozygous individual. In contrast with nontoxic goiter, which is more common in females than in males, these defects, as a group, affect females only slightly more commonly than males.

Although goiter may be present at birth, it usually does not appear until several years later. Therefore, the absence of goiter in a child with functioning thyroid tissue does not exclude the presence of hypothyroidism. The goiter is initially diffusely hyperplastic, often intensely so, suggesting papillary carcinoma, but eventually it becomes nodular. In general, the more severe the biosynthetic defect, the earlier the goiter appears, the larger it is, and the greater the likelihood of early development of hypothyroidism or even cretinism.[142] Five specific defects in the pathways of hormone synthesis have been identified.

Iodide Transport Defect. An iodide transport defect, a result of impaired iodide transport by the NIS protein mechanism, is rare and is reflected in defective iodide transport in the thyroid, salivary gland, and gastric mucosa.[144,145] Some mutations in such patients produce reduced activity, and others completely inactivate NIS by preventing the protein from being transported and inserted into the membrane. With the milder NIS mutations, administration of iodide raises the plasma and intrathyroidal iodide concentration, permitting the synthesis of normal quantities of hormone.

Defects in Expression or Function of Thyroid Peroxidase. TPO is a protein that is required for normal synthesis of iodothyronines. Quantitative or qualitative abnormalities of TPO have been identified in 1 in 66,000 infants in the Netherlands. The most common of the 16 mutations identified in 35 families was a GGCC insertion in exon 8, leading to a premature stop codon.[146]

Pendred Syndrome. The most common presentation in patients with Pendred syndrome is a defect in iodine organification accompanied by sensory nerve deafness.[147] The abnormality is in the *PDS* gene encoding pendrin, which is involved in the apical secretion of iodide into the follicular lumen (see Fig. 11-2 and Chapter 11, "Iodine Metabolism"). Thyroid function is only mildly impaired in this disorder.

Defects in Thyroglobulin Synthesis. Defects in the synthesis of thyroglobulin due to genetic causes are rare, having been identified only in a small number of families with congenital hypothyroidism.[142] Some defects lead to premature termination of translation, whereas another defect causes deficiency in endoplasmic reticulum processing of the thyroglobulin molecule. The complex regulation and huge size of this gene makes screening for mutations a difficult task, and considerable work is still required to unravel the extent of the defects in this gene.

Iodotyrosine Dehalogenase Defect. The pathogenesis of goiter and hypothyroidism in the iodotyrosine dehalogenase defect is complex. The major abnormality is an impairment of both intrathyroidal and peripheral deiodination of iodotyrosines, presumably because of the dysfunction of the iodotyrosine *DEHAL1B* gene (see "Iodide Metabolism" in Chapter 11).[148,149]

As a consequence of intense thyroid stimulation and lack of intrathyroidal recycling of iodide derived from dehalogenation, iodide is rapidly accumulated by the thyroid gland and is rapidly released; monoiodotyrosine (MIT) and diiodotyrosine (DIT) are elevated in plasma and, together with their deaminated derivatives, in the urine. Hypothyroidism is presumed to result from the loss of large quantities of MIT and DIT in the urine and to secondary iodine deficiency. The goiter and hypothyroidism are relieved by administration of high doses of iodine.

Thyroid Infiltration Causing Hypothyroidism and Goiter. A number of infiltrative or fibrosing conditions may cause hypothyroidism. Some are often associated with goiter, such as Riedel struma (see later).[150] Others, such as amyloidosis,[151] hemochromatosis,[152] or scleroderma,[153] may not be. Although the other manifestations of these conditions are usually obvious and hypothyroidism is only a complication, the presence of significant hypothyroidism without evidence of autoimmune thyroiditis should lead to a consideration of these rare causes of this condition.

Postablative Hypothyroidism. Postablative hypothyroidism is a common cause of thyroid failure in adults. One type follows total thyroidectomy usually performed for thyroid carcinoma. Although functioning remnants may be present, as indicated by foci of radioiodine accumulation, hypothyroidism invariably develops. Another etiologic mechanism is subtotal resection of the diffuse goiter of Graves disease or multinodular goiter. Its frequency depends on the amount of tissue remaining, but continued autoimmune destruction of the thyroid remnant in patients with Graves disease may be a factor because some studies suggest a correlation between the presence of circulating thyroid autoantibodies in thyrotoxicosis and the development of hypothyroidism after surgery. Hypothyroidism can be manifested during the first year after surgery, but as with postradioiodine hypothyroidism, the incidence increases with time to approach 100%. In some patients, mild hypothyroidism appears during the early postoperative period and then may occasionally remit, as also occurs after radioiodine treatment.

Hypothyroidism after destruction of thyroid tissue with radioiodine is common and is the one established disadvantage of this form of treatment for hyperthyroidism in adults. Its frequency is determined, in large part, by the dose of radioiodine and radioiodine uptake, but it is also influenced by other factors including age, thyroid gland size, magnitude of thyroid hormone elevations, and use of antithyroid drugs.[154] The incidence of postradioiodine hypothyroidism increases with time, approaching 100%. Although the fT$_4$ is low in patients with postablative hypothyroidism, serum TSH levels may be anomalously low for several months after either surgical or ^{131}I-induced hypothyroidism if TSH synthesis has been suppressed for a long period prior to treatment.

Primary atrophic thyroid failure may also develop in patients with Hodgkin disease after treatment with mantle irradiation or after high-dose neck irradiation for other forms of lymphoma or carcinoma.[123] Surgical, radioiodine, or external beam therapy may also lead to a state of subclinical hypothyroidism (see Table 13-2).

Congenital Causes

Thyroid Agenesis or Dysplasia. Developmental defects of the thyroid are often responsible for the hypothyroidism that occurs in 1 in 3000 newborns.[17] These defects may take the form of complete absence of thyroid tissue or failure of the thyroid to descend properly during embryologic development. Thyroid tissue may then be found anywhere along its normal route of descent from the foramen cecum at the junction of the anterior two thirds and posterior third of the tongue (lingual thyroid) to the normal site or below. Absence of thyroid tissue or its ectopic location can be ascertained by scintiscanning.

As indicated, a number of proteins are known to be crucial for normal thyroid gland development.[17] These proteins include the thyroid-specific transcription factor PAX8, as well as thyroid transcription factors 1 and 2 (TTF-1 and TTF-2). It might be anticipated that defects in one or more of these proteins may explain abnormalities in thyroidal development. These abnormalities have been identified in several patients with *PAX8* mutations, and a mutation in the human *TTF2* gene was associated with thyroid agenesis, cleft palate, and choanal atresia. Despite a specific search, no mutations have been found in the *TTF1* gene in infants with congenital hypothyroidism.

Thyroid Aplasia Due to Thyrotropin Receptor Unresponsiveness. Several families exist in which thyroid hypoplasia, high

TSH concentrations, and a low fT$_4$ level are associated with loss-of-function mutations in the TSH receptor.[155] The thyroid gland of these patients was in the normal location but did not trap pertechnetate (TCO$_4^-$). Somewhat surprisingly, thyroglobulin levels were still detectable. The molecular details of these patients are still under study.

A second type of abnormality that may cause TSH unresponsiveness is a mutation in the G$_s$ protein that occurs in pseudohypoparathyroidism type 1A. These patients have inactivating mutations in the α-subunit of the G$_s$ protein and, consequently, mild hypothyroidism.[156] Other as yet unexplained patients with elevated TSH levels and hypothyroidism in which the molecular nature of the defect has not been defined have been reported.[157]

Transient Hypothyroidism. Transient hypothyroidism is defined as a period of reduced fT$_4$ with suppressed, normal, or elevated TSH levels that are eventually followed by a euthyroid state. This form of hypothyroidism usually occurs in the clinical context of a patient with painful or painless subacute thyroiditis.[127] These conditions are reviewed in detail in Chapter 12.

The patient reports mild to moderate symptoms of hypothyroidism of short duration, and serum TSH concentrations are typically elevated, although not greatly so. The patient often has a preceding episode of symptoms consistent with mild or moderate thyrotoxicosis. If these symptoms cannot be elucidated from the history, it may be difficult to distinguish such patients from those with a permanent form of hypothyroidism. In the early phases of post-thyroiditis hypothyroidism, TSH concentrations may still be suppressed even though the fT$_4$ is low because of the delayed recovery of pituitary TSH synthesis, such as in patients with Graves disease or with toxic nodules who have undergone surgery and who have experienced rapid relief of hypothyroidism (see Table 13-2). In that situation, the TSH response to hypothyroidism may be suppressed for many months; in post-thyroiditis hypothyroidism, this period is rarely longer than 3 to 4 weeks.

A significant fraction (50%) of women with autoimmune thyroiditis but normal thyroid function have episodes of hypothyroidism during the postpartum period.[127] In some, the preceding thyrotoxicosis is relatively asymptomatic, which can make an accurate clinical diagnosis difficult. Patients who have had an episode of typical painful subacute thyroiditis, with pain, tenderness, and thyrotoxicosis, are not difficult to recognize.

Diagnostic evaluation should include a determination of TSH, fT$_4$, and TPO antibodies. Negative or low antibodies argue strongly for a nonautoimmune cause. This is significant, in that it may be possible for the patient to be treated only temporarily for hypothyroidism. In such patients, a trial of a lower levothyroxine dosage after 3 to 6 months may reveal that thyroid function has recovered (see Fig. 13-5). This may also occur in patients with hypothyroidism that follows painless subacute thyroiditis (e.g., in the postpartum period), but it is somewhat less likely to occur because of the underlying progressive nature of the autoimmune thyroiditis.

In patients with hypothyroidism due to painful subacute thyroiditis, the thyroid gland is usually relatively small and atrophic. In patients with hypothyroidism that follows an episode of painless subacute thyroiditis, the gland is usually slightly enlarged and somewhat firm, reflecting the underlying scarring and infiltration associated with that condition.

Consumptive Hypothyroidism. *Consumptive hypothyroidism* is the term given to an unusual cause of hypothyroidism that has been identified in infants with visceral hemangiomas or related tumors.[7,158] The first patient reported with this syndrome presented with abdominal distention caused by a large hepatic hemangioma with respiratory compromise secondary to upward displacement of the diaphragm. However, clinical signs suggested hypothyroidism, which was confirmed by finding a markedly elevated TSH level and undetectable T_4 and T_3 levels. The infant's response to an initial intravenous infusion of liothyronine (T_3) was transient, leading to the decision to use parenteral thyroid hormone replacement to relieve the severe hypothyroidism. The accelerated degradation of thyroid hormone was apparent from the fact that 96 µg of liothyronine plus 50 µg of levothyroxine were required to normalize the TSH level. The equivalent dosage of levothyroxine alone is roughly nine times that ordinarily required for treatment of infants with congenital hypothyroidism. The infant succumbed to complications of the hemangioma, and a postmortem tumor biopsy showed D3 activity in the tumor at levels eightfold higher than those normally present in term placenta. The serum reverse T_3 was extremely elevated (400 ng/dL), and the serum thyroglobulin was greater than 1000 ng/mL, indicating the presence of a highly stimulated thyroid gland. Retrospective search revealed two other patients with similar pathophysiology in whom the cause of the hypothyroidism had not been recognized. Significant D3 expression has subsequently been noted in all proliferating cutaneous hemangiomas studied to date. The cutaneous hemangiomas of infancy, although they express D3, are not associated with hypothyroidism owing to their small size. Most infantile hemangiomas involute with propranolol therapy, but such patients must also receive adequate doses of thyroid hormone to prevent the permanent neurologic complications associated with untreated hypothyroidism during this critical phase of neurologic development.[159] Subsequent reports have identified a similar syndrome in adults, including a patient with an epithelioid hemangioendothelioma and an individual with a fibrous tumor as well as extensive gastrointestinal stromal tumors (GISTs).[160] Some of these tumors express D3 or this deiodinase may be induced during treatment with TKIs (see later).[161-164]

Defects in Conversion of Thyroxine to Triiodothyronine. The enzymes that convert the precursor T_4 to the active form, T_3, are 5′-deiodinase 1 (D1) and D2, both of which contain selenocysteine in their active site.[84] A stem loop structure in the 3′-untranslated region of the mRNA, termed a *SECIS element*, directs insertion of selenocysteine at the UGA codon, rather than allowing it to function as a stop codon. Defects in a SECIS-binding protein (selenocysteine insertion sequence–binding protein 2, SECISBP-2) were found in two families with an elevated fT_4, reduced T_3, and elevated TSH.[165] Affected individuals have growth retardation, compared with unaffected family members.

Polymorphisms in genes associated with thyroid hormone metabolism have been associated with patterns of thyroid function studies as well as obesity. The D2 polymorphism resulting in a change from threonine (Thr) to alanine (Ala) at codon 92 (Thr92Ala) has been associated with obesity, reduced glucose disposal, and lower D2 activity in skeletal muscle.[166] This polymorphism also has a higher frequency in groups with a high incidence of obesity and type 2 diabetes such as Mexican Americans and Pima Indians.[166]

Hypothyroidism Due to Drug-Induced Thyroid Destruction. Thyroid inflammation or activation of autoimmune thyroid destruction has been associated with a number of drugs.[116,141] The TKIs, such as sunitinib, have been associated with a high incidence of hypothyroidism due to thyroid destruction.[161,162] Sunitinib is used to treat renal cell carcinoma and GISTs and inhibits multiple cellular pathways including KIT, PDGF, VEGF, and RET. An abnormal TSH was found in 62% of patients receiving sunitinib who were followed for 37 weeks.[163] Patients studied by ultrasound demonstrated no thyroid tissue. Although 40% of hypothyroid patients initially had a suppressed TSH, suggesting thyroiditis, the long-term course was most consistent with sunitinib-induced follicular cell apoptosis. Thus, such patients require repeated thyroid function testing. These agents have now been shown to slow disease progression in advanced thyroid cancer unresponsive to radioiodine but may increase thyroid hormone requirements due to increased D3 expression.[167]

Central Hypothyroidism. Central hypothyroidism is due to TSH deficiency caused by either acquired or congenital hypothalamic or pituitary gland disorders (see Chapters 8 and 9). The causes of TSH deficiency may be classified as those of pituitary (*secondary* hypothyroidism) and hypothalamic (*tertiary* hypothyroidism) origins, but this distinction is not necessary in the initial separation of primary from central hypothyroidism.

In many cases, hyposecretion of TSH is accompanied by decreased secretion of other pituitary hormones, with the result that evidence of somatotroph, gonadotroph, and corticotroph failure is also present. Hyposecretion of TSH as the sole demonstrable abnormality (monotropic deficiency) is less common but does occur in both acquired and congenital forms. Hypothyroidism due to pituitary insufficiency varies in severity from instances in which it is mild and overshadowed by features of gonadal and adrenocortical failure to those in which the features of the hypothyroid state are predominant. Because a small but significant fraction of thyroid gland function is independent of TSH (~10% to 15%), hypothyroidism due to central causes is less severe than primary hypothyroidism.

The causes of central hypothyroidism are both acquired and congenital. The general subject is discussed in Chapters 8 and 9, and those causes with relatively specific thyroid-related deficiencies are mentioned here for completeness. In addition to pituitary tumors, hypothalamic disorders, and the like, an unusual cause of secondary hypothyroidism occurs in individuals given bexarotene (a retinoid X receptor [RXR] agonist) for T-cell lymphoma.[168,169] This drug suppresses the activity of the human TSH β-subunit promoter in vitro. Serum T_4 concentrations are reduced about 50%, and patients experience clinical benefit from thyroid hormone replacement. Dopamine, dobutamine, high-dose glucocorticoids, or severe illness may suppress TSH release transiently, leading to a pattern of thyroid hormone abnormalities suggesting central hypothyroidism.[169] As discussed earlier (see Chapter 11, "Changes in Thyroid Function During Severe Illness"), this severe state of hypothalamic-pituitary-thyroid suppression is a manifestation of stage 3 illness (see Table 11-10). Although these agents might be expected to have similar effects when given long term, they do not, nor does somatostatin have a similar effect when given for acromegaly, although it does block the response of TSH to TRH and it has been administered to patients with thyrotropin-secreting pituitary adenomas.[170]

Congenital defects in either the stimulation or the synthesis of TSH or in its structure have been identified as rare causes of congenital hypothyroidism[17] and include the consequences of defects in several of the homeobox genes, including *POU1F1* (formerly termed *Pit-1*), *PROP1,* and *HESX1.* The last gene encodes a factor necessary for the development of the hypothalamus, pituitary, and olfactory portions of the brain. Defects in *POU1F1* and *PROP1* cause hereditary hypothyroidism, usually accompanied by deficiencies in growth hormone and prolactin.[171] One patient has been identified with a familial defect in the TRH receptor gene.[172] All of these conditions are associated with the typical pattern of central hypothyroidism, a reduced fT_4, and inappropriately low TSH.

Structural defects in TSH have also been described. They include those with a mutation in the CAGYC peptide sequence of the β-subunit, thought to be necessary for its association with the α-subunit,[173] and defects that produce premature termination of the TSH β-subunit gene.[174] As mentioned, some of these abnormalities may be associated with elevations in TSH, suggesting the diagnosis of primary hypothyroidism, but the TSH molecule is immunologically, but not biologically, intact.

Resistance to Thyroid Hormone. The clinical manifestations of resistance to thyroid hormone (RTH) depend on the nature of the mutation.[6,10,175] The majority of patients with RTH have a mutation in the gene encoding the thyroid hormone receptor β (*TRβ* gene, *THRB*) that interferes with the capacity of that receptor to respond normally to T_3, usually by reducing its T_3-binding affinity (see Fig. 11-7 in Chapter 11). A small number of individuals have been identified with *TRα* gene (*THRA*) mutations, referred to as RTH-α1,[176] who differ in significant ways from patients with RTH due to *THRB* mutations.[177-179]

RTH is probably produced by the heterodimerization of the mutant *TRβ* with RXR or homodimerization with a normal *TRβ* or *TRα*. These mutant *TRβ*-containing dimers compete with wild-type TR-containing dimers for binding to the thyroid hormone response elements (TREs) of thyroid hormone–dependent genes (see Chapter 3).[175] Because these complexes bind corepressor molecules that cannot be released in the absence of T_3 binding, genes containing these TREs are more repressed than they would be normally at the prevailing concentrations of circulating thyroid hormones.[6] Receptors that contain mutations in the activation domain may have a combination of both decreased affinity for T_3 as well as impaired activating potential.

Thus, the mutant *TRβ* complex can interfere with the function of the wild-type TRs, producing a pattern termed *dominant negative inhibition* with an autosomal dominant pattern of inheritance. At least 400 families have been identified with this condition, and there are probably many more unreported cases. The gene frequency estimate is about 1:50,000 for mutations in *TRβ* and the study of the function of the mutant receptors in this disorder has provided valuable insights into the mechanism of thyroid hormone action.[175] The frequency of *TRα* mutations is probably much lower but undefined.

Patients with RTH usually are recognized because of thyroid enlargement, which is present in about two thirds of these individuals. Patients usually report a mixture of symptoms of hyperthyroidism and hypothyroidism. With respect to the heart, palpitations and tachycardia are more common than a reduced heart rate; however, patients may also demonstrate growth retardation and retarded skeletal maturation.[180] This has been attributed to the fact that thyroid hormone effects in the heart and bone appear to be primarily dependent on *TRα* rather than *TRβ*, whereas the hypothalamic-pituitary axis is primarily regulated through *TRβ*.

Abnormalities in neuropsychological development exist, with an increased prevalence of attention deficit hyperactivity disorder, which is found in approximately 10% of such individuals.[180] Other neuropsychological abnormalities have also been described. Deafness in patients with RTH reflects the important role of *TRβ* and thyroid hormone in the normal development of auditory function. The mixture of symptoms, some suggesting hypo-

thyroidism and others suggesting hyperthyroidism, may even differ in individuals within the same family, despite the identical mutation, thus confusing the clinical picture.

Because patients may present with symptoms suggesting hyperthyroidism, it is important to keep this diagnosis in mind in a patient with tachycardia, goiter, and elevated thyroid hormones. RTH is discussed here because a reduced response to thyroid hormone is the biochemical basis for the condition. However, the laboratory results may be the first clear evidence that a patient, otherwise thought to have hyperthyroidism, has RTH. These tests show the unusual combination of an increased fT_4 accompanied by normal or slightly increased TSH levels (see Table 13-2). Thus, the principal differential diagnosis is between a TSH-secreting pituitary tumor causing hyperthyroidism and RTH.[181]

Factors that may assist in the differential diagnosis are as follows: absence of a family history in patients with TSH-producing tumors, normal thyroid hormone levels in family members of individuals with TSH-induced hyperthyroidism due to pituitary tumor, and the presence of an elevated glycoprotein α-subunit in patients with pituitary tumor but not in those with RTH.

A definitive diagnosis requires sequencing of the *TRβ* gene demonstrating the abnormality. Mutations in the *TRβ* gene are found in about 90% of individuals with a clinical diagnosis. In a few individuals this is not the case, suggesting that there may be mutations in coactivator proteins or one of the RXR receptors, which can also present in a similar fashion.[182]

Treatment is difficult because thyroid hormone analogues designed to suppress TSH, thereby relieving the hyperthyroxinemia, may lead to worsening of the cardiovascular manifestations of the condition.[183] Therapy with 3,5,3'-triiodothyroacetic acid (TRIAC) has been used in several patients. The development of analogues of thyroid hormone with *TRβ*, as opposed to mixed or *TRα* preferential effects, as well as analogues that selectively bind mutant TRs, may eventually prove useful in treatment.

Individuals with RTH-α1 have more subtle changes in thyroid function studies, compared with RTH due to *TRβ* gene mutations, and a clinical phenotype consistent with hypothyroidism in tissue that predominantly expresses the *TRα* isoform β.[177,178] Because regulation of TSH is predominantly mediated by *TRβ*, these individuals have a normal serum TSH, but a reduced T_4/T_3 ratio and low concentration of serum reverse T_3, presumably due to reduced activity of the D3 enzyme. Common phenotypic features include growth failure, developmental delays, constipation, and delayed bone maturation, with some improvement associated with T_4 treatment.[179]

Treatment

Hypothyroidism, either primary or central, is gratifying to treat because of the ease and completeness with which it responds to thyroid hormone.[82,184] Treatment is nearly always with levothyroxine, and the proper use of this medication has been reviewed extensively.[81] A primary advantage of levothyroxine therapy is that the peripheral deiodination mechanisms can continue to produce the amount of T_3 required in tissues under the normal physiologic control.[84] If one accepts the principle that replicating the natural state is the goal of hormone replacement, it is logical to provide the "prohormone" and allow the peripheral tissues to activate it by physiologically regulated mechanisms. There is, however, significant interest in combined T_4 and T_3 therapy.[185,186]

Pharmacologic and Physiologic Considerations

Levothyroxine has a 7-day half-life; about 80% of the hormone is absorbed relatively slowly (over hours) and it equilibrates rapidly in its extracellular distribution volume, therefore avoiding large postabsorptive perturbations in fT_4 levels. With its long half-life, omission of a single day's tablet has no significant effect and the patient may safely take an omitted tablet the following day. In fact, the levothyroxine dosage can be calculated almost as satisfactorily on a weekly, as on a daily, basis. Although T_4 is well absorbed and does not require fasting, regular ingestion of levothyroxine on an empty stomach results in the least variation in serum TSH concentration.[187]

The Food and Drug Administration (FDA) has issued standards for single-dose bioequivalence studies in normal volunteers to assess and compare T_4 products in the United States.[188] The AUC (area under the curve) confidence interval must fall within 80% to 125% of the comparison product for a preparation to be considered equivalent. The desirability of a pharmacotherapeutic measurement, such as TSH level as an end point, has been suggested by many professional organizations.[188] The guidelines for measured T_4 content have narrowed from 90% to 110% to 95% to 105% of the stated tablet dose and require that content to be maintained for the entire shelf life.[189] The availability in many countries of a multiplicity of tablet strengths with content ranging from 25 to 300 µg allows precise titration of the daily levothyroxine dosage for most patients with a single daily tablet, improving compliance significantly.

The typical dose of levothyroxine, approximately 1.6 to 1.8 µg/kg ideal body weight per day (0.7 to 0.8 µg/pound), generally results in the prescription of between 75 and 125 µg/day for women and 125 to 200 µg/day for men. Replacement doses need not be adjusted upward in obese patients and should be based on lean body mass.[190] This dosage is about 20% greater than the T_4 production rate owing to incomplete absorption of the levothyroxine. In patients with primary hypothyroidism, these amounts usually result in serum TSH concentrations that are within the normal range. Because of the 7-day half-life, approximately 6 weeks are required before there is complete equilibration of the fT_4 and the biologic effects of levothyroxine. Accordingly, assessments of the adequacy of a given dose or the effects of a change in dosage, with rare exceptions such as pregnancy, should not be made until this interval has passed. This long half-life also means that it is safe for a patient to take any missed doses of T_4 for up to a week after missing tablets.

By and large, levothyroxine products are clinically equivalent, although problems do occur.[191] However, the variation permitted by the FDA in tablet content can result in slight variations in serum TSH in patients with primary hypothyroidism even when the same brand is used. Using levothyroxine from a single manufacturer reduces variability that may be relevant for patients, such as elderly, pregnant, and thyroid cancer patients, when close titration is required. Although the serum TSH level is an indirect reflection of the levothyroxine effect in patients with primary hypothyroidism, it is far superior to any other readily available method of assessing the adequacy of therapy. Return of the serum TSH level to normal is therefore the goal of levothyroxine therapy in the patient with primary hypothyroidism. Some patients may require slightly higher or lower doses than generally used, owing to individual variations in absorption, and a number of conditions or associated medications may change levothyroxine requirements in patients with established hypothyroidism (see later).

In decades past, desiccated thyroid was successfully employed for the treatment of hypothyroidism and still accounts for a small fraction of the prescriptions written for thyroid replacement in the United States. Although this approach was successful, desiccated thyroid preparations contain thyroid hormone derived from animal thyroids that have twofold to threefold higher ratios of T_3 to T_4 than the 1:15 value in normal human thyroglobulin.[192] Accordingly, these preparations may lead to superphysiologic levels of T_3 in the immediate postabsorptive period (2 to 4 hours) owing to the rapid release of T_3 from thyroglobulin, its immediate and nearly complete absorption, and the 1-day period required for T_3 to equilibrate with its 40-L volume of distribution (see Table 11-5).[193] A recent prospective double-blind randomized crossover study compared 4 months of levothyroxine monotherapy with desiccated thyroid preparations in the same hypothyroid patients.[194] There were no significant differences in outcomes, although among patients who had a preference, more preferred desiccated thyroid extract and these patients lost a modest amount of weight.

Mixtures of liothyronine and levothyroxine (liotrix) contain in a 1-grain (64-µg) equivalent tablet (Thyrolar-1 in the United States) the amounts of T_3 (12.5 µg) and T_4 (50 µg) present in the most popular desiccated thyroid tablet.[195] The levothyroxine equivalency of a 1-grain desiccated thyroid tablet or its liotrix equivalent can be estimated as follows. The 12.5 µg of liothyronine (T_3) is completely absorbed from desiccated thyroid or from liotrix tablets.[193] Levothyroxine is approximately 80% absorbed,[196] and about 36% of the 40 µg of levothyroxine absorbed is converted to T_3, with the molecular weight of T_3 (651) being 84% that of T_4 (777). Accordingly, a 1-grain tablet should provide about 25 µg of T_3, which would be approximately equivalent to that obtained from 100 µg of levothyroxine. This equivalency ratio can be used as an initial guide in switching patients from desiccated thyroid or liotrix to levothyroxine. Although levothyroxine is absorbed in the stomach and small intestine, normal gastric acid secretion is required for complete absorption.[197] Patients with impaired acid secretion on levothyroxine therapy require a 22% to 34% higher dose of levothyroxine to maintain the desired serum TSH. In those patients in whom acid secretion was normalized therapeutically, the levothyroxine dose returned to baseline.[197]

As indicated earlier, the use of levothyroxine as thyroid hormone replacement is a compromise with the normal pathway of T_3 production, in which about 80% of T_3 is derived from T_4 5′-monodeiodination and approximately 20% (~6 µg) is secreted directly from the thyroid gland.[84] Studies in thyroidectomized rats, for example, show that it is not possible to normalize T_3 simultaneously in all tissues by an intravenous infusion of T_4.[198] However, it should be recalled from the earlier discussion of T_4 deiodination that the ratio of T_3/T_4 in the human thyroid gland is about 0.09 but is 0.17 in the rat thyroid gland.[84] Thus, about 40% of the rat's daily T_3 production is derived from the thyroid versus about 20% in humans.[84] Accordingly, the demonstration that T_4 alone cannot provide normal levels of T_3 in all tissues in the rat is of interest but is not strictly applicable to thyroid hormone replacement in humans. Nonetheless, the ratio of T_3 to T_4 in the serum of a patient receiving levothyroxine as the only source of T_3 is about 20% lower than that in a normal individual.

Similarly, the quantity of levothyroxine required to normalize TSH in an athyreotic patient results in a slightly higher serum fT_4 concentration than is present in normal individuals. This has been shown in a comparison of thyroid function in the same patient before and after thyroidectomy.[199] Although serum T_3 was the same level in patients before or after thyroidectomy, a higher serum T_4 concentration was necessary when on T_4 replacement to maintain the same serum T_3.[199] T_4 has an independent mechanism for TSH suppression, owing to the intracellular generation of T_3 in the hypothalamic-pituitary-thyroid axis, resulting in a portion of the feedback TSH regulation being independent of the plasma T_3. A retrospective, cross-sectional study compared thyroid function studies in 1800 athyreotic thyroid cancer patients on levothyroxine monotherapy compared to control subjects.[200] In these patients, the serum fT_4 levels were significantly higher, and free T_3 levels significantly lower, than euthyroid control subjects. However, these patients came from a region of variable iodine intake, which makes interpretation of the control data difficult.

Although the concept of combined T_4/T_3 therapy has been recognized for many years, a positive study generated a great deal of interest in this approach.[201] Patients received 12.5 µg of T_3 as a substitution for 50 µg of their levothyroxine preparation and scored, on average, somewhat higher on tests of mood than when they were taking levothyroxine alone. The dosage of thyroid hormone used in these studies was excessive, as judged by the fact that 20% of the group had serum TSH values below normal on either regimen and the test period was only a few months. A large number of subsequent studies using a wide range of replacement strategies and relative T_4/T_3 content were performed in different populations, and none has shown an advantage of combination therapy over T_4 alone.[202] A study that compared T_4 monotherapy to T_4/T_3 combined therapy in hypothyroid patients evaluated the results based on the presence or absence of D2 gene polymorphisms.[203] The hypothyroid patients homozygous for the D2 polymorphism showed greater improvement in measures of well-being while on T_4/T_3 combination therapy compared to T_4 monotherapy. This study requires replication in a separate population but may indicate that T_4/T_3 combination therapy can be targeted to specific hypothyroid patients who will benefit based on a genetic profile of genes important for thyroid hormone metabolism and action.[186,204]

On the other hand, the fT_4 index correlated as closely with the resting energy expenditure, as did TSH levels, in a group of patients in whom small adjustments above or below their ideal replacement levothyroxine dosage were made.[205] The correlation with serum T_3 was not statistically significant, suggesting that in humans, perhaps as a result of differences in the peripheral metabolism of T_4 from that in rodents, the fT_4 concentration may be as accurate as the TSH value as an index of satisfactory thyroid hormone replacement. The practical difficulty with the design of tablets providing combinations of T_3 and T_4 is that the approximate dose of 6 µg of T_3 provided would need to be released in a sustained fashion over 24 hours, as well as replicating the diurnal rhythm of T_3,[206] which is quite different from the rapid absorption of T_3 with a peak at 2 to 4 hours when given in its conventional form. Thus, for the present, it appears that the current approach to thyroid replacement using levothyroxine alone, although not a perfect replication of normal physiology, is satisfactory for virtually all patients. A sustained-release T_3 preparation has been developed and produces more stable levels of serum T_3.[207] The clinical effects of this more "physiologic" replacement are not known.

Institution of Replacement Therapy

The initial dose of levothyroxine prescribed depends on the degree of hypothyroidism and the age and general health of the patient. Patients who are young or middle-aged and otherwise healthy with no associated cardiovascular or other abnormalities and mild to moderate hypothyroidism (TSH concentrations of 5 to 50 mU/L) can be given an initial complete replacement dose of about 1.7 µg/kg of ideal body weight. The resulting increase in serum T_4 concentration to normal requires 5 to 6 weeks, and the biologic effects of T_3 are sufficiently delayed that these patients do not experience adverse effects. At the other extreme, the elderly patient with heart disease, particularly angina pectoris, without reversible coronary lesions, should be given a small initial dose of levothyroxine (25 µg/day), and the dosage should be increased in 12.5-µg increments at 2- to 3-month intervals with careful clinical and laboratory evaluation.

The goal in the patient with primary hypothyroidism is to return serum TSH concentrations to normal, reflecting normalization of that patient's thyroid hormone supply. This usually results in a mid- to high-normal serum fT_4. The serum TSH should be evaluated 6 weeks after a theoretically complete replacement dose has been instituted to allow minor adjustments to optimize the individual dose.[208] In patients with central hypothyroidism, serum TSH is not a reliable index of adequate replacement, and the serum fT_4 should be restored to a concentration in the upper half of the normal range. T_4 dosing based on body weight and a serum fT_4 in the upper reference range improved markers of thyroid hormone action and was superior to replacement with a combination of T_4/T_3.[209] Patients with central hypothyroidism should also be evaluated and treated for glucocorticoid deficiency, if necessary, before institution of thyroid replacement (see Chapter 9).

Although the adverse effects of the rapid institution of therapy are unusual, pseudotumor cerebri has been reported in profoundly hypothyroid juveniles between ages 8 and 12 years who were given even modest initial levothyroxine replacement.[210] This complication appears 1 to 10 months after initiation of treatment and responds to acetazolamide and dexamethasone.

The interval between the initiation of treatment and the first evidence of improvement depends on the strength of dose given and the degree of the deficit. An early clinical response in moderate to severe hypothyroidism is a diuresis of 2 to 4 kg. The serum sodium (Na^+) level increases even sooner if hyponatremia was present initially. Thereafter, pulse rate and pulse pressure increase, appetite improves, and constipation may disappear. Later, psychomotor activity increases and the delay in the deep tendon reflex disappears. Hoarseness abates slowly, and changes in skin and hair do not disappear for several months. In individuals started on a complete replacement dose, the serum fT_4 level should normalize after 6 weeks; a somewhat longer period may be necessary for serum TSH levels to return to normal, perhaps up to 3 months.

In some cases (e.g., myxedema coma [see later]), it is clinically appropriate to alleviate hypothyroidism rapidly. For example, patients with severe hypothyroidism withstand acute infections or other serious illnesses poorly and myxedema coma may develop as a complication. In such circumstances, rapid near repletion of the peripheral hormone pool in the average adult can be accomplished by a single intravenous dose of 500 µg of levothyroxine. Alternatively, by virtue of its rapid onset of action, liothyronine (25 µg orally every 12 hours) can be administered if the patient can take medication by mouth. With both approaches, an initial biologic effect is achieved within 24 hours. Parenteral therapy with levothyroxine is then continued with a dose that is 80% of the appropriate oral dose but not in excess of 1.4 µg/kg of ideal body weight. Because of the possibility that rapid increases in metabolic rate will overtax the existing pituitary-adrenocortical reserve, supplemental glucocorticoid (intravenous hydrocortisone 5 mg/hour) should also be given to patients with severe hypothyroidism receiving high initial doses of thyroid hormones. Finally, in view of the tendency of hypothyroid patients to retain free water, intravenous fluids containing only dextrose should not be given.

When replacement therapy is withdrawn for short periods (4 to 6 weeks) for purposes of evaluating therapy for thyroid cancer, rapid reinstitution of levothyroxine using a loading dose of three times the daily replacement dose for 3 days can usually be given unless there are other complicating medical illnesses.

When hypothyroidism results from administration of iodine-containing or antithyroid drugs, withdrawal of the offending agent usually relieves both the hypothyroidism and the accompanying goiter, although it is appropriate to provide interim replacement until the gland recovers its function.[134,211] This is especially true for amiodarone, which may remain in tissues for up to a year.

Infants and Children. In infants with congenital hypothyroidism, the determining factor for eventual intellectual attainment is the age at which adequate treatment with thyroid hormone is begun.[17,212] The therapy for infants with congenital hypothyroidism should consist initially of raising the serum T_4 level to more than 130 nmol/L (10 µg/dL) as rapidly as possible and maintaining it at that level for the first 3 to 4 years of life. This is usually accomplished by administering an initial levothyroxine dose of 50 µg/day, which is higher than the adult dose on a weight basis and in keeping with the higher metabolic clearance of the hormone in the infant. The serum TSH concentration may not return to normal even with this high dose because of residual reset of the pituitary feedback mechanism. After 2 years of age, however, a TSH level in the normal range is an index of optimal therapy as it is in adults.[213]

Monitoring Replacement Therapy. Monitoring the adequacy of, and compliance with, thyroid hormone therapy in patients with primary hypothyroidism is easily done by measurement of serum TSH. This value should be within the normal range for an assay sufficiently sensitive to measure, with confidence, the lower limit of the normal range. The normal serum TSH concentration varies between 0.5 and 4.0 mU/L in most second-generation and third-generation assays, and results within this range are associated with the elimination of all clinical and biochemical manifestations of primary hypothyroidism, except in patients with RTH. Based on analysis of the NHANES III (National Health and Nutrition Examination Survey) reference group,[12] a reference TSH range with an upper limit of 2.5 mU/L has been suggested. This adjustment, however, would identify a large number of individuals as having abnormal thyroid function, without a clear indication of the clinical significance of TSH levels in this range. A more recent analysis, based on age-specific reference ranges, indicates that older adults, without thyroid autoantibodies, have an increased upper limit TSH (>4.5 mU/L) that is not associated with thyroid disease.[214] In related studies, this progressive shift with age to higher levels of TSH has been associated with extreme longevity in several populations.[215]

After the first 6 months of therapy, the dose should be reassessed because restoration of euthyroidism increases the metabolic clearance of T_4. A dose that was adequate during the early phases of therapy may not be so when the same patient is euthyroid owing to an acceleration in the clearance of thyroid hormone.

Under normal circumstances, the finding of a normal serum TSH level on an annual basis is adequate to ensure that the proper levothyroxine dose is being taken by the patient. If the serum TSH level is above the normal range and noncompliance is not the explanation, small adjustments, usually in 12-µg increments, can be made with reassessment of TSH concentrations after the 6 weeks required for full equilibration have passed. In North America, this strategy is simplified by the availability of multiple tablet strengths, many of which differ by only 12 µg. Most patients can receive the same dose until they reach their seventh or eighth decade, at which point a downward adjustment of 20% to 30% may be indicated because thyroid hormone clearance decreases in the elderly.

Thyroid hormone requirements may be altered in several situations (Table 13-3). A reduction in replacement dosage may be required in women who are receiving androgen therapy for adjuvant treatment of breast carcinoma.[216] Most other conditions or medications increase the levothyroxine requirement in patients receiving maintenance therapy. During pregnancy, the levothyroxine requirement is increased by 25% to 50% in most hypothyroid women,[217] and a prospective study demonstrated that the increased requirement occurs early in the first trimester.[67,68,218] The required increment is higher in athyreotic patients compared to those with autoimmune hypothyroidism.[219] Athyreotic patients who are planning a pregnancy should be advised to increase the dose by around 30% as soon as the diagnosis is confirmed because the change in requirement appears soon after implantation.

TABLE 13-3
Conditions That Alter Levothyroxine Requirements

Increased Levothyroxine Requirements

Pregnancy
Gastrointestinal Disorders
Mucosal diseases of the small bowel (e.g., sprue)
After jejunoileal bypass and small bowel resection
Impaired gastric acid secretion (e.g., atrophic gastritis)
Diabetic diarrhea

Therapy with Certain Pharmacologic Agents
Drugs That Interfere with Levothyroxine Absorption
Cholestyramine
Sucralfate
Aluminum hydroxide
Calcium carbonate
Ferrous sulfate

Drugs That Increase the Cytochrome P450 Enzyme (CYP3A4)
Rifampin
Carbamazepine
Estrogen
Phenytoin
Sertraline
? Statins

Drugs That Block T_4 to T_3 Conversion
Amiodarone

Conditions That May Block Deiodinase Synthesis
Selenium deficiency
Cirrhosis

Decreased Levothyroxine Requirements

Aging (65 years and older)
Androgen therapy in women

T_4, thyroxine; T_3, triiodothyronine.

The increased requirement is probably due to a combination of factors, including increases in T_4-binding globulin and the volume of distribution of T_4, an increase in body mass, and an increase in D3 in the placenta and uterus probably due to estradiol-induced increases in *Dio3* gene transcription.[84] The increased requirement persists throughout pregnancy but returns to normal within a few weeks after delivery. Therefore, the dose should be reduced to the original prepregnancy level at the time of delivery. Maternal T_4 is critically important to the athyreotic fetus and in the normal fetus in the first trimester before fetal thyroid function and feedback regulation mature.[220] Maternal hypothyroidism has been associated with fetal loss, preterm delivery, and intellectual deficit in the offspring.[67,68,127] These findings are not seen in hypothyroid women on T_4 replacement sufficient to normalize their TSH, suggesting that these associations are directly related to maternal thyroid hormone status. A randomized prospective study in pregnant women with anti-TPO antibodies and normal range TSH demonstrated the benefit of levothyroxine treatment to prevent these complications.[66]

Other conditions in which levothyroxine requirements are increased (see Table 13-3)[81,141] include malabsorption due to bowel diseases, impaired gastric acid secretion,[197] and adsorption of levothyroxine to coadministered medications such as sucralfate, aluminum hydroxide, calcium carbonate, ferrous sulfate, lovastatin, or various resins. Certain medications, notably rifampin, carbamazepine, phenytoin, and sertraline, increase the clearance of levothyroxine by inducing CYP3A4 in the liver. Estrogen given to postmenopausal women may act in the same way, although the increases in D3 also play a role.[221] Soy protein and soybean isoflavones have been proposed to interfere directly with thyroid hormone action as well as synthetic T_4 absorption.[222] There is no evidence that soy interferes with thyroid function in euthyroid individuals who are iodine sufficient, and the effect of soy on T_4 absorption in hypothyroid patients is modest.[222] Amiodarone increases levothyroxine requirements by blocking conversion of T_4 to T_3 and perhaps by interfering with T_3–thyroid hormone receptor binding.[223] Selenium deficiency is rare, but because it is rate limiting in the synthesis of D1 (see Fig. 11-6),[84] any significant deficiency, such as may occur in patients receiving diets restricted in protein, may increase levothyroxine requirements.

Occasionally, in patients who have been treated with radioactive iodine for Graves disease or toxic nodular goiter, some degree of thyroid hormone secretion persists and, although insufficient to sustain normal thyroid hormone levels, is autonomous. Such patients may have a suppressed TSH on what otherwise would be considered a replacement dose of levothyroxine. The levothyroxine dose in these individuals should be reduced until TSH levels rise to normal, keeping in mind that several months may be required before TSH secretion recovers after its prolonged suppression. Because of either the delayed effects of radioiodine or the natural history of Graves disease per se, this autonomous T_4 secretion may decrease with time, leading to an increase in levothyroxine requirements in subsequent years. Rarely, the opposite occurs; that is, a patient treated with radioiodine develops an increased TSH level, but after several months of therapy, the requirement for such replacement is either reduced or eliminated. This response may reflect transient impairment of thyroid function by a combination of preirradiation antithyroid drug therapy and immediate, but transient, effects of irradiation on the thyroid. In such patients, frequent monitoring of levothyroxine replacement is required to avoid overreplacement.

In North America, based on the recent previously discussed changes in assessment of levothyroxine bioequivalence, the possibility of a difference in tablet levothyroxine content should be considered if a new preparation changes the biologic or biochemical effects of the same dosage. Although the difference in preparation is unlikely to cause a significant difference in most patients, the change in manufacturer introduces another potential source of variability.

Adverse Effects of Levothyroxine Therapy

Although the administration of excessive doses of levothyroxine causes accelerated bone loss in postmenopausal patients, most authorities believe that returning thyroid status to normal does not have adverse effects on bone density.[224,225] Administration of excessive doses also increases cardiac wall thickness and contractility and, in elderly patients, increases the risk of atrial fibrillation.[15,23]

In some patients, TSH levels remain elevated despite the prescription of adequate replacement doses.[226] This response is most often a consequence of poor adherence. The combination of normal or even elevated serum fT_4 values and elevated TSH levels can occur if the patient does not take levothyroxine regularly but ingests several pills the day before testing. The integrated dose of levothyroxine over prior weeks is best reflected in the serum TSH level, and nonadherent patients require careful education as to the rationale for treatment. Subtle changes in dietary habits, such as increasing the ingestion of bran-containing products, soy, or calcium or proton pump inhibitors, may decrease levothyroxine absorption, and their recognition requires a careful history.[81,141,226]

Patients with Hypothyroid Symptoms Despite Restitution of Normal Thyroid Function

In patients taking levothyroxine replacement with a normal serum TSH concentration, symptoms consistent with hypothyroidism may persist. A survey of hypothyroid patients on levothyroxine with normal TSH and control patients included questions about symptoms that might be associated with thyroid hormone deficiency.[227] Although a significant fraction of both groups reported such symptoms, a greater fraction of patients on levothyroxine replacement had these symptoms. Such patients should be educated as to the relationship between symptoms of hypothyroidism and the role of thyroid hormone in relieving them, and other causes should be sought for the symptoms.

Special Aspects of Hypothyroidism
Subclinical Hypothyroidism

The term *subclinical hypothyroidism* was originally used to describe the patient with a low-normal fT_4 but a slightly elevated serum TSH level. Other terms for this condition are *mild hypothyroidism, early thyroid failure, preclinical hypothyroidism,* and *decreased thyroid reserve* (see Table 13-2). The TSH elevation in such patients is modest, with values typically between 5 and 15 mU/L, although patients with a TSH above 10 mU/L more often have a reduced fT_4 and may have true hypothyroid symptoms. The definition of this syndrome depends significantly on the reference range for a normal TSH concentration. This syndrome is most often seen in patients with early Hashimoto disease and is a common phenomenon, occurring in 7% to 10% of older women.[13-15]

A number of studies on the effects of thyroid hormone treatment in such patients have used physiologic end points (e.g., measurements of various serum enzymes, systolic time intervals, serum lipids, psychometric testing), and results have been variable.[13-15] In the most carefully controlled studies, one or another of the parameters has returned to normal in about 25% to 50% of patients. In general, fT_4 and TSH levels normalize, but free T_3, usually normal at the outset, does not change. Modest improvements in cardiac indices and lipid profiles have been noted in most, but not all, studies, although the benefit on cardiovascular risk is seen in middle-aged patients.[29,34] The association of mild hypothyroidism with an increase in risk for atherosclerotic heart disease has been shown by some studies, but not others.[13,15] The impact of treatment to reduce the risk of atherosclerotic heart disease, other than reduction in risk factors such as cholesterol and C-reactive protein, have not yet been studied.

One factor favoring a decision to recommend levothyroxine therapy is the likelihood of developing overt hypothyroidism. The risk of progression from *subclinical* to *overt* hypothyroidism (elevated serum TSH and reduced fT_4) is most closely related to the magnitude of serum TSH elevation and the presence of anti-TPO antibodies. Prospective studies of women with subclinical hypothyroidism have shown rates of progression from approximately 3% to 8% per year, with the higher rates seen in individuals with initial TSH concentration greater than 10 and those with positive anti-TPO antibodies.[228] Although most individuals progress slowly to overt hypothyroidism, rapid progression over weeks to months has been reported.[229] Factors that may predispose to rapid progression include increased age, high levels of TPO antibodies, intercurrent systemic infection or inflammation, iodine contrast agents, and medications such as amiodarone and lithium. The decision to treat with levothyroxine must also take into account the expense and inconvenience of a daily medication, not acceptable to some patients, and the possibility that unintended overdosage may exacerbate osteoporosis or cause cardiac arrhythmias. Ultimately, the decision to treat must depend on a careful consideration of the individual clinical situation and patient preference. If a therapeutic trial is performed, the TSH concentration should be monitored carefully and should not be reduced below normal. If no therapy is given, such patients should be monitored at intervals of 6 to 12 months both clinically and biochemically.

Metabolic Insufficiency

Nonspecific symptoms of true hypothyroidism include mild lassitude, fatigue, slight anemia, constipation, apathy, cold intolerance, menstrual irregularities, loss of hair, and weight gain. For this reason, some patients with such complaints but with normal laboratory results for thyroid function have been considered candidates for levothyroxine therapy. The response to thyroid hormone therapy is sometimes gratifying, at least initially, but symptomatic improvement usually disappears after a time unless the dose is increased. Eventually, even larger doses fail to alleviate the symptoms, confirming that they do not arise from a deficiency of thyroid hormone.

Thus, thyroid hormone therapy should be avoided in patients with no biochemical documentation of impaired thyroid function. Furthermore, even in patients with subclinical hypothyroidism, symptoms may be out of proportion to abnormalities in the fT_4. It is unwise to raise a patient's expectations that such symptoms will be relieved by correction of mild biochemical abnormalities.

Thyroid Function Testing in Patients Receiving Replacement Therapy for Unclear Reasons

Physicians are frequently confronted with patients receiving levothyroxine in whom the basis for the diagnosis cannot be established. It may be difficult to document previous clinical findings or laboratory data to determine whether thyroid hormone replacement is indicated. If serum TSH is in the normal range and primary hypothyroidism is suspected, a simple way of assessing the need for levothyroxine therapy is to switch levothyroxine to an every-other-day dosage or to reduce the daily dose by 50% and to reevaluate TSH and fT_4 after 4 weeks. If there is no significant increase in TSH concentration and fT_4 remains constant during that period, residual thyroid function is present, although it may still not be completely normal. To answer this question, levothyroxine can then be withdrawn and blood tests repeated 4 to 8 weeks later.

If the initial TSH level is suppressed, indicating overreplacement, the levothyroxine dose should be reduced until TSH becomes detectable before this trial is instituted. If central hypothyroidism is suspected, the fT_4 must be monitored.

Emergent Surgery in the Hypothyroid Patient

The perioperative course of patients with untreated hypothyroidism has been evaluated in several studies. In general, such patients were not recognized to be hypothyroid or did not require surgery despite the presence of significant hypothyroidism. Complications were uncommon. Perioperative hypotension, ileus, and central nervous system disturbances were more common in hypothyroid patients, and patients with major infections had fewer episodes of fever than did euthyroid control subjects.[230] Other complications were delayed recovery from anesthesia and abnormal hemostasis, possibly owing to an acquired form of von Willebrand disease.[59]

From these studies, one may conclude that emergent surgery should not be postponed in hypothyroid patients but that such patients should be rigorously monitored for evidence of carbon dioxide retention, bleeding, infection, and hyponatremia. These findings are also relevant to the treatment of hypothyroid individuals with symptomatic coronary artery disease. Considering the lack of significant increase in perioperative complications in the hypothyroid patient, the option of surgery for remediable coronary artery lesions is open to hypothyroid individuals without the risk of a myocardial infarction in association with restitution of the euthyroid state (see later).[231]

Heart Disease and Thyroid Hormone Therapy
Coexisting Coronary Artery Disease and Hypothyroidism

In many patients with coronary artery disease and primary hypothyroidism, cardiac function is improved in response to levothyroxine therapy because of a decrease in peripheral vascular resistance and improvement in myocardial function. However, patients with preexisting angina pectoris should be evaluated for correctable lesions of the coronary arteries and treated appropriately before levothyroxine is administered.[231,232] Retrospective studies indicate that this approach is safer than the institution of replacement therapy prior to angiography and angioplasty or even coronary artery bypass grafting (CABG).[231]

In a few patients, lesions may not be remediable or small-vessel disease is severe even after bypass grafting, so that complete replacement cannot be instituted. Such patients must receive optimal antianginal therapy combined with β-adrenergic receptor blockers in judicious quantities, and complete restitution of the euthyroid state may not be possible.

Thyroid Hormone for Compromised Cardiovascular Function

In addition to the issues raised in patients with combined hypothyroidism and coronary artery disease, there is interest in the potential therapeutic use of thyroid hormone in the treatment of patients with cardiomyopathy or those who have undergone CABG or other cardiac procedures.[23] As expected, T_3 levels are reduced in patients with advanced congestive heart failure, as with any illness. In one report, 23 patients with advanced heart failure (mean ejection fraction, 22%) were given up to 2.7 μg/kg of liothyronine over 6 hours with an increase in cardiac output and decrease in systemic vascular resistance but without increase in heart or metabolic rate.[233] Similar effects were seen with a dose of 110 μg liothyronine over 6 hours after CABG.[234]

Liothyronine has also been given postoperatively for congenital heart disease and, again, an improvement in cardiac output and decrease in vascular resistance occurred without adverse side effects.[200] These results suggest that, in certain selected circumstances, liothyronine may be useful as adjunctive therapy in patients with congestive heart failure because of its effect of relaxing vascular smooth muscle.

Although most therapeutic trials of thyroid hormone treatment have used T_3, thyroid hormone analogues have also been used.[23] The most extensively studied is 3,5-diiodothyropropionic acid (DITPA), an analogue that binds both $TR\alpha$ and $TR\beta$ with low affinity. A randomized study of DITPA in heart failure showed some improved cardiac performance,[235] but the study was terminated because of significant metabolic side effects including weight loss.[236]

Screening for Primary Hypothyroidism

The use of screening for hypothyroidism has been addressed by a number of studies but remains controversial.[184,237] The conclusions depend, to a great extent, on assumptions regarding the effectiveness and economic value of identifying and treating patients with subclinical hypothyroidism. An evidenced-based medicine review of the literature by an expert panel concluded that there was insufficient evidence to support population-based screening.[238] Aggressive "case finding," based on identification of risk factors such as family history, was advocated for pregnant women, women older than 60 years, and others at high risk. The fraction of patients with hypothyroidism missed when a "case finding" strategy is used, however, is not known. A report from the U.S. Preventive Services Task Force also concluded that population screening for hypothyroidism in nonpregnant adults was not justified.[237] Large, randomized, prospective studies of levothyroxine treatment in patients with subclinical hypothyroidism to establish benefit, however, have not yet been performed. Given the very high incidence of hypothyroidism in older women and the absence of robust clinical symptoms, an assessment of TSH levels at 5-year intervals in women older than age 50 years seems justified until more extensive studies have been performed.

A second complex issue involves whether women planning pregnancy should be screened for the presence of hypothyroidism as a routine part of a prenatal visit.[67,68] This question is raised because of increasing association of adverse outcomes in pregnancy, even with subclinical hypothyroidism including impairment of mental develop-ment in infants, fetal loss, and preterm delivery.[66,127] The prevalence of overt hypothyroidism during pregnancy is approximately 2%, and screening of all patients has been advocated by several professional organizations. Thyroid testing in high-risk patients, "case finding," has been advocated, although a prospective study showed that approximately a third of pregnant women with underlying thyroid disease are missed by this testing approach.[239]

Maternal fT_4 concentrations in the lowest 10% of the normal range, even with normal TSH levels, have also been suggested as a risk factor for impaired neuropsychological development of the fetus.[240] It is not clear why this is a risk factor for impaired fetal neuropsychological development, because such patients are not hypothyroid.

A number of questions are raised regarding the appropriate timing of testing, whether thyroid autoantibodies should be measured, the relative importance of TSH and fT_4, the influence of trimester on the normal ranges, and the threshold for intervention.[241] The association of maternal subclinical hypothyroidism and preterm delivery is a much more proximal and defined end point to study compared with intellectual performance in offspring. The morbidity and mortality rates from preterm delivery are significant for the newborn, and these findings are likely to allow for more focused intervention studies to determine the response to T_4 treatment.[65]

For the moment, it appears that any patient with a family history of autoimmune thyroid disease, with symptoms suggesting hypothyroidism, or with thyroid enlargement should be tested for thyroid dysfunction prior to pregnancy or as soon after conception as is feasible. Optimization of levothyroxine therapy for women known to have hypothyroidism prior to conception, when possible, may be the most effective intervention to prevent hypothyroid-related complications of pregnancy. Although the data do not yet reach the threshold to mandate universal screening, the ease of testing, associated adverse outcomes, and demonstrated benefit of intervention make thyroid testing of all pregnant women a reasonable choice.

Myxedema Coma

Myxedema coma is the ultimate stage of severe long-standing hypothyroidism.[242,243] This state, which almost invariably affects older patients, occurs most commonly during the winter months and is associated with a high mortality rate. It is usually accompanied by a subnormal temperature. Values as low as 23° C have been recorded. The external manifestations of severe myxedema, bradycardia, and severe hypotension are invariably present. The characteristic delay in deep tendon reflexes may be lacking if the patient is areflexic. Seizures may accompany the comatose state. Although the pathogenesis of myxedema coma is not clear, factors that predispose to its development include exposure to cold, infection, trauma, and central nervous system depressants or anesthetics. Alveolar hypoventilation, leading to carbon dioxide retention and narcosis, and dilutional hyponatremia resembling that seen with inappropriate ADH secretion may also contribute to the clinical state.

From the foregoing, it appears that myxedema coma should be readily recognized from its clinical signs, but this is not the case. Hypothermia of any cause, for example, to cold exposure, may cause changes suggestive of myxedema, including delayed relaxation of deep tendon reflexes. The importance of diagnosing myxedema coma is that a delay in therapy worsens the prognosis. Consequently, a rapid serum fT4 and TSH should be obtained whenever this diagnosis is being considered. Otherwise the diagnosis should be made on clinical grounds, and after serum has been sent for thyroid function tests, therapy should be initiated without awaiting the results of delayed confirmatory tests because the mortality rate may be 20% or higher.

Treatment consists of administration of thyroid hormone and correction of the associated physiologic disturbances.[242,243] Because of the sluggish circulation and severe hypometabolism, absorption of therapeutic agents from the gut or from subcutaneous or intramuscular sites is unpredictable, and medications should be administered intravenously if possible. Administration of levothyroxine as a single intravenous dose of 500 to 800 µg repletes the peripheral hormone pool and may cause improvement within hours. Daily doses of intravenous levothyroxine, 100 µg, are given thereafter. Hydrocortisone (5 to 10 mg/hour) should also be given because of the possibility of relative adrenocortical insufficiency as the metabolic rate increases.

Alternatively, intravenous liothyronine may be given at a dose of 25 µg every 12 hours. Others have used a combination of 200 to 300 µg T_4 and 25 µg T_3 intravenously as a single dose, followed by 25 µg T_3 and 100 µg T_4 24 hours later, and then 50 µg T_4 daily until the patient regains consciousness. *Hypotonic* fluids should not be given because of the danger of water intoxication owing to the reduced free water clearance of the hypothyroid patient. *Hypertonic* saline and glucose may be required to alleviate severe dilutional hyponatremia and the occasional hypoglycemia.

A critical element in therapy is support of respiratory function by means of assisted ventilation and controlled oxygen administration. Internal warming by gastric perfusion may be useful, but external warming should be avoided because it may lead to vascular collapse due to peripheral vasodilatation. Further heat loss can be prevented with blankets. An increase in temperature may be seen within 24 hours in response to levothyroxine. General measures applicable to the comatose patient should be undertaken, such as frequent turning, prevention of aspiration, and attention to fecal impaction and urinary retention.

Finally, the physician should assess the patient for the presence of coexisting disease, especially infection, cardiac disease, or cerebrovascular disease. The myxedematous patient may be afebrile despite a significant infection. As soon as the patient is able to take medication by mouth, treatment with oral levothyroxine should be instituted.

THYROIDITIS

Thyroiditis is a term indicating the presence of thyroid inflammation and thus comprises a large group of diverse inflammatory conditions. These conditions include the following: autoimmune or quasi-autoimmune causes and viral or postviral conditions and infections, including those of bacterial and fungal origins; a chronic sclerosing form of thyroiditis, termed *Riedel thyroiditis* (or struma); and miscellaneous causes of various types, including radiation-induced and granulomatous causes, such as sarcoidosis, as well as lithium.[5]

Not only are the causes of thyroiditis extremely varied, their clinical presentations may also be diverse and are difficult to categorize in a simple fashion (Table 13-4). Thus, as already discussed, autoimmune thyroiditis may present with hypothyroidism but often patients remain euthyroid for long periods after the disease begins. On the other hand, in a euthyroid patient with Hashimoto disease who becomes pregnant, the postpartum period is often complicated by an acute form of thyrotoxicosis due to the

TABLE 13-4
Causes of Thyroiditis
Autoimmune thyroiditis
Painless subacute thyroiditis, including postpartum thyroiditis (see Chapter 12)
Painful subacute thyroiditis (see Chapter 12)
Acute infectious thyroiditis
Riedel thyroiditis
Postirradiation (^{131}I or external-beam therapy)
Sarcoidosis

transient exacerbation of thyroiditis, often followed by a period of hypothyroidism (see Chapter 12).[127]

A similar syndrome has been observed in nonpregnant patients, called *painless subacute thyroiditis*. It is manifested primarily as thyrotoxicosis of sudden onset without localized pain and often without evidence of autoimmune disease. This condition may be viral in origin in some patients; however, the classic presentation of postviral thyroiditis, a condition referred to as painful subacute thyroidits, is characterized by extreme thyroid tenderness, with pain radiating to the oropharynx and ears, and must be differentiated from acute infectious thyroiditis caused by bacterial or fungal infection.[244]

Thus, inflammatory conditions of the thyroid present a didactic dilemma because one must decide whether to discuss these entities as a group with the common denominator of inflammation or to categorize them according to their principal clinical effects, namely, thyrotoxicosis or thyroid hormone deficiency. We have chosen the latter approach and have already discussed autoimmune thyroiditis, the major cause of thyroid gland failure (see Table 13-1). However, patients with acute autoimmune thyroiditis may also develop thyrotoxicosis, such as in postpartum painless thyroiditis (see Chapter 12, Autoimmune Thyroiditis). These patients must be differentiated from those with Graves disease. In addition, some patients with painful subacute thyroiditis have thyrotoxicosis as a major manifestation with varying degrees of neck discomfort. For that reason, this thyroiditis syndrome is also discussed in Chapter 12, even though the pain associated with the typical form of this condition makes the principal differential diagnosis lie between that and infectious thyroiditis. In that context, subacute thyroiditis is also mentioned later.

Acute Infectious Thyroiditis

Although the thyroid gland is remarkably resistant to infection, congenital abnormalities of the piriform sinus, underlying autoimmune disease, or immunocompromise of the host may lead to the development of an infectious disease of the thyroid gland, acute infectious thyroiditis.[244,245] The cause may be any bacterium, including *Staphylococcus*, *Pneumococcus*, *Salmonella*, or *Mycobacterium tuberculosis*. In addition, infections with certain fungi, including *Coccidioides immitis*, *Candida*, *Aspergillus*, and *Histoplasma*, have been reported.

The most common cause of repeated childhood infectious thyroiditis, particularly in the left lobe, is a consequence of an internal fistula extending from the piriform sinus to the thyroid.[245] This sinus is the residual connection following the path of migration of the ultimobranchial body from the fifth pharyngeal pouch to the thyroid gland. The predominance of thyroiditis of the left lobe is explained by the fact that the right ultimobranchial body is often atrophic, whereas this is not the case for the left side.

Nonetheless, a patient with a completely normal thyroid gland may develop bacterial thyroiditis. This is an extremely rare disease even as a complication of direct puncture of the thyroid gland, such as in fine-needle aspiration. In individuals with midline infections, persistence of the thyroglossal duct should be considered.

Incidence

Infectious thyroiditis is extremely rare, with no more than a few cases being seen in large tertiary care centers.

Clinical Manifestations

The clinical manifestations of infectious thyroiditis are dominated by local pain and tenderness in the affected lobe or entire gland. This is accompanied by painful swallowing and difficulty on swallowing. Because of the tendency for referral of pain to the pharynx or ear, the patient may not recognize the tenderness in the anterior neck. Depending on the virulence of the organism and the presence of septicemia, symptoms such as fever and chills may also accompany the condition.

The major differential diagnosis lies between an infectious form of thyroiditis and painful subacute thyroiditis. It is instructive to compare the principal features of these two diseases to arrive at an accurate diagnosis (Table 13-5). By and large, patients with acute infectious thyroiditis caused by a bacterium are much sicker than patients with painful subacute thyroiditis; they have more severe and localized tenderness and are less likely to have laboratory evidence of thyrotoxicosis, which is present in approximately 60% of patients with painful subacute thyroiditis. Ultrasonographic examination often reveals the abscess in the thyroid gland or evidence of swelling, and needle aspiration may help pinpoint the responsible organism. A gallium scan will be positive as a result of the diffuseness of the inflammation and, particularly in children with infectious thyroiditis of the left lobe, a barium swallow showing a fistula connecting the piriform sinus and left lobe of the thyroid is diagnostic.[245]

Occasionally, pertechnetate scanning is useful in showing normal function of one lobe of the thyroid gland, which is much less common in painful subacute thyroiditis (which more often affects the entire gland). Needle aspiration should be used to drain the affected lobe, although occasionally surgical drainage may be required. If a piriform sinus fistula can be demonstrated, it must be removed to prevent recurrence of the problem.

Antibiotics should be administered appropriate to the offending organism. Fungal infections should be treated appropriately, especially because many of these individuals are immunocompromised. Endemic organisms should be kept in mind as a cause, in that both *Echinococcus* and *Trypanosomiasis* infections of the thyroid gland have been reported.

The prognosis is excellent with preservation of thyroid function in general, although post-thyroiditis thyroid function tests should be monitored to ascertain that thyroid failure has not occurred.

Riedel Thyroiditis

Riedel chronic sclerosing thyroiditis is rare and occurs primarily in middle-age women.[150,246,247] The etiologic mechanism is uncertain, and any association with autoimmune thyroid disease is probably coincidental.[248] The morphologic similarities between the fibrosis of Riedel thyroiditis and IgG4-related sclerosing disease suggest that these enti-

TABLE 13-5

Features Useful in Differentiating Between Acute Infectious Thyroiditis and Subacute Thyroiditis

Characteristic	Acute Thyroiditis (% with Feature)	Subacute Thyroiditis (% with Feature)
History		
Preceding upper respiratory infection	88	17
Fever	100	54
Symptoms of thyrotoxicosis	Uncommon	47
Sore throat	90	36
Physical Examination of the Thyroid		
Painful thyroid swelling	100	77
Left side affected	85	Not specific
Migrating thyroid tenderness	Possible	27
Erythema of overlying skin	83	Not usually
Laboratory Findings		
Elevated white blood cell count	57	25-50
Elevated ESR (>30 mm/hr)	100	85
Abnormal thyroid hormone levels (elevated or depressed)	5-10	60
Alkaline phosphatase, transaminases increased	Rare	Common
Results of Needle Aspiration		
Purulent, bacteria or fungi present	~100	0
Lymphocytes, macrophages, some polyps, giant cells	0	~100
^{123}I uptake low	Uncommon	~100
Radiologic Findings		
Abnormal thyroid scan	92	—
Thyroid scan or ultrasound helpful in diagnosis	75	—
Gallium scan positive	~100	~100
Barium swallow showing fistula	Common	0
CT scan useful	Rarely	Not indicated
Clinical Course		
Clinical response to glucocorticoid treatment	Transient	100
Incision and drainage required	85	No
Recurrence following operative drainage	16	No
Piriform sinus fistula discovered	96	No

CT, computed tomography; ESR, erythrocyte sedimentation rate.
From DeGroot LJ, Larsen PR, Hennemann G. Acute and subacute thyroiditis. In: *The Thyroid and Its Diseases*, 6th ed. New York: Churchill Livingstone; 1996:700.

ties are closely related, with thyroiditis representing an initial manifestation of a more generalized process.[249] Retroperitoneal, orbital, and mediastinal fibrosis, as well as rarer fibrotic syndromes, are associated with Riedel thyroiditis.[250]

Symptoms develop insidiously and are related chiefly to compression of adjacent structures, including the trachea, esophagus, and recurrent laryngeal nerves. Systemic evidence of inflammation is uncommon. The thyroid gland is moderately enlarged, stony hard, and usually asymmetrical. The consistency of the gland and the invasion of adjacent structures suggest carcinoma, but there is no enlargement of regional lymph nodes. Temperature, pulse, and leukocyte count are normal. Severe hypothyroidism is unusual but does occur, as does loss of parathyroid function. The RAIU may be normal or low. Elevated circulating thyroid autoantibodies are much less common and are found in lower titers than in Hashimoto disease.

Tamoxifen, 10 to 20 mg/day (with or without corticosteroids), has been successful in many of these patients and is thought to suppress transforming growth factor beta (TGF-β).[150] Surgery may be required to preserve tracheal and esophageal function, although the response to tamoxifen will often preclude the necessity for this. Treatment with thyroid hormone relieves the hypothyroidism but has no effect on the primary process.

Miscellaneous Causes

Only a few causes of generalized inflammation of the thyroid gland have been reported. These include inflammation arising after ^{131}I treatment for Graves disease, a residual thyroid lobe in a patient with thyroid cancer of the contralateral lobe, and thyroiditis arising from external beam therapy for conditions such as Hodgkin or non-Hodgkin lymphoma, breast carcinoma, or other lesions of the oropharynx. Anaplastic thyroid carcinoma may rarely be associated with a diffuse thyroiditis and elevation of thyroid hormone levels.[251] In general, only radioiodine-induced thyroiditis is associated with pain, and glucocorticoid treatment may be useful in symptomatic therapy.

REFERENCES

1. Vaidya B, Pearce SH. Management of hypothyroidism in adults. BMJ. 2008;337:a801.
2. Almandoz JP, Gharib H. Hypothyroidism: etiology, diagnosis, and management. Med Clin North Am. 2012;96:203-221.
3. Caturegli P, De Remigis A, Rose NR. Hashimoto thyroiditis: clinical and diagnostic criteria. Autoimmun Rev. 2014;13:391-397.
4. Persani L. Clinical review: central hypothyroidism: pathogenic, diagnostic, and therapeutic challenges. J Clin Endocrinol Metab. 2012;97:3068-3078.
5. Samuels MH. Subacute, silent, and postpartum thyroiditis. Med Clin North Am. 2012;96:223-233.
6. Brent GA. Mechanisms of thyroid hormone action. J Clin Invest. 2012;122:3035-3043.
7. Luongo C, Trivisano L, Alfano F, Salvatore D. Type 3 deiodinase and consumptive hypothyroidism: a common mechanism for a rare disease. Front Endocrinol (Lausanne). 2013;4:115.
8. Arrojo EDR, Fonseca TL, Werneck-de-Castro JP, Bianco AC. Role of the type 2 iodothyronine deiodinase (D2) in the control of thyroid hormone signaling. Biochim Biophys Acta. 2013;1830:3956-3964.
9. Dayan CM, Panicker V. Novel insights into thyroid hormones from the study of common genetic variation. Nat Rev Endocrinol. 2009;5:211-218.
10. Visser WE, van Mullem AA, Visser TJ, Peeters RP. Different causes of reduced sensitivity to thyroid hormone: diagnosis and clinical management. Clin Endocrinol (Oxf). 2013;79(5):595-605.
11. Vanderpump MP, Tunbridge WM, French JM, et al. The incidence of thyroid disorders in the community: a twenty-year follow-up of the Whickham Survey. Clin Endocrinol (Oxf). 1995;43:55-68.
12. Hollowell JG, Staehling NW, Flanders WD, et al. Serum TSH, T(4), and thyroid antibodies in the United States population (1988 to 1994): National Health and Nutrition Examination Survey (NHANES III). J Clin Endocrinol Metab. 2002;87:489-499.
13. Cooper DS, Biondi B. Subclinical thyroid disease. Lancet. 2012;379:1142-1154.
14. Biondi B. Natural history, diagnosis and management of subclinical thyroid dysfunction. Best Pract Res Clin Endocrinol Metab. 2012;26:431-446.
15. Franklyn JA. The thyroid—too much and too little across the ages. The consequences of subclinical thyroid dysfunction. Clin Endocrinol (Oxf). 2013;78:1-8.
16. Boucai L, Hollowell JG, Surks MI. An approach for development of age-, gender-, and ethnicity-specific thyrotropin reference limits. Thyroid. 2011;21:5-11.
17. Gruters A, Krude H. Detection and treatment of congenital hypothyroidism. Nat Rev Endocrinol. 2012;8:104-113.
18. Smith TJ, Bahn RS, Gorman CA. Connective tissue, glycosaminoglycans, and diseases of the thyroid. Endocr Rev. 1989;10:366-391.
19. Safer JD. Thyroid hormone action on skin. Curr Opin Endocrinol Diabetes Obes. 2012;19:388-393.
20. Somach SC, Helm TN, Lawlor KB, et al. Pretibial mucin. Histologic patterns and clinical correlation. Arch Dermatol. 1993;129:1152-1156.
21. Wemeau JL, Proust-Lemoine E, Ryndak A, Vanhove L. Thyroid autoimmunity and polyglandular endocrine syndromes. Hormones (Athens). 2013;12:39-45.
22. Kahaly GJ, Dillmann WH. Thyroid hormone action in the heart. Endocr Rev. 2005;26:704-728.
23. Danzi S, Klein I. Thyroid hormone and the cardiovascular system. Med Clin North Am. 2012;96:257-268.
24. Hardisty CA, Naik DR, Munro DS. Pericardial effusion in hypothyroidism. Clin Endocrinol (Oxf). 1980;13:349-354.
25. Keating FR Jr, Parkin TW, Selby JB, Dickinson LS. Treatment of heart disease associated with myxedema. Prog Cardiovasc Dis. 1961;3:364-381.
26. Biondi B. Mechanisms in endocrinology: heart failure and thyroid dysfunction. Eur J Endocrinol. 2012;167:609-618.
27. Hussein WI, Green R, Jacobsen DW, Faiman C. Normalization of hyperhomocysteinemia with L-thyroxine in hypothyroidism. Ann Intern Med. 1999;131:348-351.
28. Ladenson PW, Sherman SI, Baughman KL, et al. Reversible alterations in myocardial gene expression in a young man with dilated cardiomyopathy and hypothyroidism. Proc Natl Acad Sci U S A. 1992;89:5251-5255.
29. Pearce EN. Update in lipid alterations in subclinical hypothyroidism. J Clin Endocrinol Metab. 2012;97:326-333.
30. Pearce EN, Wilson PW, Yang Q, et al. Thyroid function and lipid subparticle sizes in patients with short-term hypothyroidism and a population-based cohort. J Clin Endocrinol Metab. 2008;93:888-894.
31. Thvilum M, Brandt F, Brix TH, Hegedus L. A review of the evidence for and against increased mortality in hypothyroidism. Nat Rev Endocrinol. 2012;8:417-424.
32. Cappola AR, Fried LP, Arnold AM, et al. Thyroid status, cardiovascular risk, and mortality in older adults. JAMA. 2006;295:1033-1041.
33. Kvetny J, Heldgaard PE, Bladbjerg EM, Gram J. Subclinical hypothyroidism is associated with a low-grade inflammation, increased triglyceride levels and predicts cardiovascular disease in males below 50 years. Clin Endocrinol (Oxf). 2004;61:232-238.
34. Biondi B, Cooper DS. The clinical significance of subclinical thyroid dysfunction. Endocr Rev. 2008;29:76-131.
35. Schlenker EH. Effects of hypothyroidism on the respiratory system and control of breathing: human studies and animal models. Respir Physiol Neurobiol. 2012;181:123-131.
36. Attal P, Chanson P. Endocrine aspects of obstructive sleep apnea. J Clin Endocrinol Metab. 2010;95:483-495.
37. Tachman ML, Guthrie GP Jr. Hypothyroidism: diversity of presentation. Endocr Rev. 1984;5:456-465.
38. Checchi S, Montanaro A, Pasqui L, et al. L-thyroxine requirement in patients with autoimmune hypothyroidism and parietal cell antibodies. J Clin Endocrinol Metab. 2008;93:465-469.
39. Elfstrom P, Montgomery SM, Kampe O, et al. Risk of thyroid disease in individuals with celiac disease. J Clin Endocrinol Metab. 2008;93:3915-3921.
40. Burra P. Liver abnormalities and endocrine diseases. Best Pract Res Clin Gastroenterol. 2013;27:553-563.
41. Volzke H, Robinson DM, John U. Association between thyroid function and gallstone disease. World J Gastroenterol. 2005;11:5530-5534.
42. Hazlehurst JM, Tomlinson JW. Non-alcoholic fatty liver disease in common endocrine disorders. Eur J Endocrinol. 2013;169:R27-R37.
43. Williams GR. Neurodevelopmental and neurophysiological actions of thyroid hormone. J Neuroendocrinol. 2008;20:784-794.
44. Wood-Allum CA, Shaw PJ. Thyroid disease and the nervous system. Handb Clin Neurol. 2014;120:703-735.
45. Joffe RT, Pearce EN, Hennessey JV, et al. Subclinical hypothyroidism, mood, and cognition in older adults: a review. Int J Geriatr Psychiatry. 2013;28:111-118.
46. Bauer M, Goetz T, Glenn T, Whybrow PC. The thyroid-brain interaction in thyroid disorders and mood disorders. J Neuroendocrinol. 2008;20:1101-1114.
47. Bauer M, Silverman DH, Schlagenhauf F, et al. Brain glucose metabolism in hypothyroidism: a positron emission tomography study before and after thyroid hormone replacement therapy. J Clin Endocrinol Metab. 2009;94:2922-2929.
48. Tagoe CE, Zezon A, Khattri S. Rheumatic manifestations of autoimmune thyroid disease: the other autoimmune disease. J Rheumatol. 2012;39:1125-1129.
49. Tan ZS, Vasan RS. Thyroid function and Alzheimer's disease. J Alzheimers Dis. 2009;16:503-507.
50. Kalmijn S, Mehta KM, Pols HA, et al. Subclinical hyperthyroidism and the risk of dementia. The Rotterdam study. Clin Endocrinol (Oxf). 2000;53:733-737.
51. Sampaolo S, Campos-Barros A, Mazziotti G, et al. Increased cerebrospinal fluid levels of 3,3',5'-triiodothyronine in patients with Alzheimer's disease. J Clin Endocrinol Metab. 2005;90:198-202.
52. Schiess N, Pardo CA. Hashimoto's encephalopathy. Ann N Y Acad Sci. 2008;1142:254-265.
53. Combs CE, Nicholls JJ, Duncan Bassett JH, Williams GR. Thyroid hormones and bone development. Minerva Endocrinol. 2011;36:71-85.
54. Wojcicka A, Bassett JH, Williams GR. Mechanisms of action of thyroid hormones in the skeleton. Biochim Biophys Acta. 2013;1830:3979-3986.

55. Rivkees SA, Bode HH, Crawford JD. Long-term growth in juvenile acquired hypothyroidism: the failure to achieve normal adult stature. *N Engl J Med.* 1988;318:599-602.
56. Iwasaki Y, Oiso Y, Yamauchi K, et al. Osmoregulation of plasma vasopressin in myxedema. *J Clin Endocrinol Metab.* 1990;70:534-539.
57. Rhee CM, Brent GA, Kovesdy CP, et al. Thyroid functional disease: an under-recognized cardiovascular risk factor in kidney disease patients. *Nephrol Dial Transplant.* 2014. [Epub ahead of print].
58. Federici AB. Acquired von Willebrand syndrome associated with hypothyroidism: a mild bleeding disorder to be further investigated. *Semin Thromb Hemost.* 2011;37:35-40.
59. Squizzato A, Romualdi E, Buller HR, Gerdes VE. Clinical review: thyroid dysfunction and effects on coagulation and fibrinolysis: a systematic review. *J Clin Endocrinol Metab.* 2007;92:2415-2420.
60. Lecky BR, Williams TD, Lightman SL, et al. Myxoedema presenting with chiasmal compression: resolution after thyroxine replacement. *Lancet.* 1987;1:1347-1350.
61. Kamilaris TC, DeBold CR, Pavlou SN, et al. Effect of altered thyroid hormone levels on hypothalamic-pituitary-adrenal function. *J Clin Endocrinol Metab.* 1987;65:994-999.
62. Stabouli S, Papakatsika S, Kotsis V. Hypothyroidism and hypertension. *Expert Rev Cardiovasc Ther.* 2010;8:1559-1565.
63. Barreto-Chaves ML, Carrillo-Sepulveda MA, Carneiro-Ramos MS, et al. The crosstalk between thyroid hormones and the renin-angiotensin system. *Vascul Pharmacol.* 2010;52:166-170.
64. Mintziori G, Anagnostis P, Toulis KA, Goulis DG. Thyroid diseases and female reproduction. *Minerva Med.* 2012;103:47-62.
65. Stagnaro-Green A. Maternal thyroid disease and preterm delivery. *J Clin Endocrinol Metab.* 2009;94:21-25.
66. Negro R, Mestman JH. Thyroid disease in pregnancy. *Best Pract Res Clin Endocrinol Metab.* 2011;25:927-943.
67. Stagnaro-Green A, Abalovich M, Alexander E, et al. Guidelines of the American Thyroid Association for the diagnosis and management of thyroid disease during pregnancy and postpartum. *Thyroid.* 2011;21:1081-1125.
68. De Groot L, Abalovich M, Alexander EK, et al. Management of thyroid dysfunction during pregnancy and postpartum: an Endocrine Society clinical practice guideline. *J Clin Endocrinol Metab.* 2012;97:2543-2565.
69. Negro R, Formoso G, Mangieri T, et al. Levothyroxine treatment in euthyroid pregnant women with autoimmune thyroid disease: effects on obstetrical complications. *J Clin Endocrinol Metab.* 2006;91:2587-2591.
70. Krassas GE, Tziomalos K, Papadopoulou F, et al. Erectile dysfunction in patients with hyper- and hypothyroidism: how common and should we treat? *J Clin Endocrinol Metab.* 2008;93:1815-1819.
71. Brenta G, Schnitman M, Gurfinkiel M, et al. Variations of sex hormone-binding globulin in thyroid dysfunction. *Thyroid.* 1999;9:273-277.
72. Silva JE, Bianco SD. Thyroid-adrenergic interactions: physiological and clinical implications. *Thyroid.* 2008;18:157-165.
73. Haluzik M, Nedvidkova J, Bartak V, et al. Effects of hypo- and hyperthyroidism on noradrenergic activity and glycerol concentrations in human subcutaneous abdominal adipose tissue assessed with microdialysis. *J Clin Endocrinol Metab.* 2003;88:5605-5608.
74. Mullur R, Liu YY, Brent GA. Thyroid hormone regulation of metabolism. *Physiol Rev.* 2014;94:355-382.
75. Pearce EN. Thyroid hormone and obesity. *Curr Opin Endocrinol Diabetes Obes.* 2012;19:408-413.
76. Iwen KA, Schroder E, Brabant G. Thyroid hormones and the metabolic syndrome. *Eur Thyroid J.* 2013;2:83-92.
77. Crunkhorn S, Patti ME. Links between thyroid hormone action, oxidative metabolism, and diabetes risk? *Thyroid.* 2008;18:227-237.
78. Chidakel A, Mentuccia D, Celi FS. Peripheral metabolism of thyroid hormone and glucose homeostasis. *Thyroid.* 2005;15:899-903.
79. Vettor R. The metabolic actions of thyroid hormone and leptin: a mandatory interplay or not? *Diabetologia.* 2005;48:621-623.
80. Iglesias P, Alvarez Fidalgo P, Codoceo R, Diez JJ. Serum concentrations of adipocytokines in patients with hyperthyroidism and hypothyroidism before and after control of thyroid function. *Clin Endocrinol (Oxf).* 2003;59:621-629.
81. Biondi B, Wartofsky L. Treatment with thyroid hormone. *Endocr Rev.* 2014;35:433-512.
82. Zulewski H, Muller B, Exer P, et al. Estimation of tissue hypothyroidism by a new clinical score: evaluation of patients with various grades of hypothyroidism and controls. *J Clin Endocrinol Metab.* 1997;2:771-776.
83. Rapa A, Monzani A, Moia S, et al. Subclinical hypothyroidism in children and adolescents: a wide range of clinical, biochemical, and genetic factors involved. *J Clin Endocrinol Metab.* 2009;94:2414-2420.
84. Gereben B, Zavacki AM, Ribich S, et al. Cellular and molecular basis of deiodinase-regulated thyroid hormone signaling. *Endocr Rev.* 2008;29:898-938.
85. Yamada M, Mori M. Mechanisms related to the pathophysiology and management of central hypothyroidism. *Nat Clin Pract Endocrinol Metab.* 2008;4:683-694.
86. Caldwell KL, Jones R, Hollowell JG. Urinary iodine concentration: United States National Health and Nutrition Examination Survey 2001-2002. *Thyroid.* 2005;15:692-699.
87. Mariotti S, Franceschi C, Cossarizza A, Pinchera A. The aging thyroid. *Endocr Rev.* 1995;16:686-715.
88. Verloop H, Louwerens M, Schoones JW, et al. Risk of hypothyroidism following hemithyroidectomy: systematic review and meta-analysis of prognostic studies. *J Clin Endocrinol Metab.* 2012;97:2243-2255.
89. McGrogan A, Seaman HE, Wright JW, de Vries CS. The incidence of autoimmune thyroid disease: a systematic review of the literature. *Clin Endocrinol (Oxf).* 2008;69:687-696.
90. McLachlan SM, Rapoport B. Thyrotropin-blocking autoantibodies and thyroid-stimulating autoantibodies: potential mechanisms involved in the pendulum swinging from hypothyroidism to hyperthyroidism or vice versa. *Thyroid.* 2013;23:14-24.
91. Walsh JP, Bremner AP, Feddema P, et al. Thyrotropin and thyroid antibodies as predictors of hypothyroidism: a 13-year, longitudinal study of a community-based cohort using current immunoassay techniques. *J Clin Endocrinol Metab.* 2010;95:1095-1104.
92. Boelaert K, Newby PR, Simmonds MJ, et al. Prevalence and relative risk of other autoimmune diseases in subjects with autoimmune thyroid disease. *Am J Med.* 2010;123(183):e181-e189.
93. Blanchin S, Coffin C, Viader F, et al. Anti-thyroperoxidase antibodies from patients with Hashimoto's encephalopathy bind to cerebellar astrocytes. *J Neuroimmunol.* 2007;192:13-20.
94. Ehlers M, Thiel A, Bernecker C, et al. Evidence of a combined cytotoxic thyroglobulin and thyroperoxidase epitope-specific cellular immunity in Hashimoto's thyroiditis. *J Clin Endocrinol Metab.* 2012;97:1347-1354.
95. Wang SH, Baker JR. The role of apoptosis in thyroid autoimmunity. *Thyroid.* 2007;17:975-979.
96. Li D, Cai W, Gu R, et al. Th17 cell plays a role in the pathogenesis of Hashimoto's thyroiditis in patients. *Clin Immunol.* 2013;149:411-420.
97. Brown RS, Bellisario RL, Botero D, et al. Incidence of transient congenital hypothyroidism due to maternal thyrotropin receptor-blocking antibodies in over one million babies. *J Clin Endocrinol Metab.* 1996;81:1147-1151.
98. Leger J, Olivieri A, Donaldson M, et al. European Society for Paediatric Endocrinology consensus guidelines on screening, diagnosis, and management of congenital hypothyroidism. *J Clin Endocrinol Metab.* 2014;99:363-384.
99. Feingold SB, Smith J, Houtz J, et al. Prevalence and functional significance of thyrotropin receptor blocking antibodies in children and adolescents with chronic lymphocytic thyroiditis. *J Clin Endocrinol Metab.* 2009;94:4742-4748.
100. Rebuffat SA, Nguyen B, Robert B, et al. Antithyroperoxidase antibody-dependent cytotoxicity in autoimmune thyroid disease. *J Clin Endocrinol Metab.* 2008;93:929-934.
101. Li Y, Zhou G, Ozaki T, et al. Distinct histopathological features of Hashimoto's thyroiditis with respect to IgG4-related disease. *Mod Pathol.* 2012;25:1086-1097.
102. Brix TH, Kyvik KO, Hegedus L. A population-based study of chronic autoimmune hypothyroidism in Danish twins. *J Clin Endocrinol Metab.* 2000;85:536-539.
103. Jacobson EM, Huber A, Tomer Y. The HLA gene complex in thyroid autoimmunity: from epidemiology to etiology. *J Autoimmun.* 2008;30:58-62.
104. Simmonds MJ. GWAS in autoimmune thyroid disease: redefining our understanding of pathogenesis. *Nat Rev Endocrinol.* 2013;9:277-287.
105. Tomer Y. Mechanisms of autoimmune thyroid diseases: from genetics to epigenetics. *Annu Rev Pathol.* 2014;9:147-156.
106. Medici M, Porcu E, Pistis G, et al. Identification of novel genetic loci associated with thyroid peroxidase antibodies and clinical thyroid disease. *PLoS Genet.* 2014;10:e1004123.
107. Mortensen KH, Cleemann L, Hjerrild BE, et al. Increased prevalence of autoimmunity in Turner syndrome—influence of age. *Clin Exp Immunol.* 2009;156:205-210.
108. Aversa T, Lombardo F, Corrias A, et al. In young patients with Turner or Down syndrome, Graves' disease presentation is often preceded by Hashimoto's thyroiditis. *Thyroid.* 2014;24:744-747.
109. Caturegli P, De Remigis A, Chuang K, et al. Hashimoto's thyroiditis: celebrating the centennial through the lens of the Johns Hopkins hospital surgical pathology records. *Thyroid.* 2013;23:142-150.
110. Weetman AP. Immunity, thyroid function and pregnancy: molecular mechanisms. *Nat Rev Endocrinol.* 2010;6:311-318.
111. Stuckey BG, Kent GN, Ward LC, et al. Postpartum thyroid dysfunction and the long-term risk of hypothyroidism: results from a 12-year follow-up study of women with and without postpartum thyroid dysfunction. *Clin Endocrinol (Oxf).* 2010;73:389-395.
112. Zimmermann MB. Iodine deficiency. *Endocr Rev.* 2009;30:376-408.
113. Aghini Lombardi F, Fiore E, Tonacchera M, et al. The effect of voluntary iodine prophylaxis in a small rural community: the Pescopagano survey 15 years later. *J Clin Endocrinol Metab.* 2013;98:1031-1039.
114. Pramyothin P, Leung AM, Pearce EN, et al. Clinical problem-solving. A hidden solution. *N Engl J Med.* 2011;365:2123-2127.

115. Sundick RS, Herdegen DM, Brown TR, Bagchi N. The incorporation of dietary iodine into thyroglobulin increases its immunogenicity. *Endocrinology*. 1987;120:2078-2084.
116. Toulis KA, Anastasilakis AD, Tzellos TG, et al. Selenium supplementation in the treatment of Hashimoto's thyroiditis: a systematic review and a meta-analysis. *Thyroid*. 2010;20:1163-1173.
117. Tomer Y. Hepatitis C and interferon induced thyroiditis. *J Autoimmun*. 2010;34:J322-J326.
118. Torino F, Barnabei A, Paragliola R, et al. Thyroid dysfunction as an unintended side effect of anticancer drugs. *Thyroid*. 2013;23:1345-1366.
119. Wiersinga WM. Smoking and thyroid. *Clin Endocrinol (Oxf)*. 2013;79:145-151.
120. Carle A, Pedersen IB, Knudsen N, et al. Moderate alcohol consumption may protect against overt autoimmune hypothyroidism: a population-based case-control study. *Eur J Endocrinol*. 2012;167:483-490.
121. Imaizumi M, Usa T, Tominaga T, et al. Radiation dose-response relationships for thyroid nodules and autoimmune thyroid diseases in Hiroshima and Nagasaki atomic bomb survivors 55-58 years after radiation exposure. *JAMA*. 2006;295:1011-1022.
122. Ostroumova E, Brenner A, Oliynyk V, et al. Subclinical hypothyroidism after radioiodine exposure: Ukrainian-American cohort study of thyroid cancer and other thyroid diseases after the Chernobyl accident (1998-2000). *Environ Health Perspect*. 2009;117:745-750.
123. Sklar C, Whitton J, Mertens A, et al. Abnormalities of the thyroid in survivors of Hodgkin's disease: data from the Childhood Cancer Survivor Study. *J Clin Endocrinol Metab*. 2000;85:3227-3232.
124. Carle A, Pedersen IB, Knudsen N, et al. Thyroid volume in hypothyroidism due to autoimmune disease follows a unimodal distribution: evidence against primary thyroid atrophy and autoimmune thyroiditis being distinct diseases. *J Clin Endocrinol Metab*. 2009;94:833-839.
125. Graff-Baker A, Sosa JA, Roman SA. Primary thyroid lymphoma: a review of recent developments in diagnosis and histology-driven treatment. *Curr Opin Oncol*. 2010;22:17-22.
126. Jankovic B, Le KT, Hershman JM. Clinical review: Hashimoto's thyroiditis and papillary thyroid carcinoma: is there a correlation? *J Clin Endocrinol Metab*. 2013;98:474-482.
127. Stagnaro-Green A, Pearce E. Thyroid disorders in pregnancy. *Nat Rev Endocrinol*. 2012;8:650-658.
128. Unuane D, Velkeniers B, Anckaert E, et al. Thyroglobulin autoantibodies: is there any added value in the detection of thyroid autoimmunity in women consulting for fertility treatment? *Thyroid*. 2013;23:1022-1028.
129. Watanabe T, Maruyama M, Ito T, et al. Clinical features of a new disease concept, IgG4-related thyroiditis. *Scand J Rheumatol*. 2013;42:325-330.
130. Pearce EN, Andersson M, Zimmermann MB. Global iodine nutrition: where do we stand in 2013? *Thyroid*. 2013;23:523-528.
131. Bottcher Y, Eszlinger M, Tonjes A, Paschke R. The genetics of euthyroid familial goiter. *Trends Endocrinol Metab*. 2005;16:314-319.
132. Pearce EN, Pino S, He X, et al. Sources of dietary iodine: bread, cows' milk, and infant formula in the Boston area. *J Clin Endocrinol Metab*. 2004;89:3421-3424.
133. Leung AM, Pearce EN, Braverman LE. Iodine content of prenatal multivitamins in the United States. *N Engl J Med*. 2009;360:939-940.
134. Leung AM, Braverman LE. Iodine-induced thyroid dysfunction. *Curr Opin Endocrinol Diabetes Obes*. 2012;19:414-419.
135. Wolff J, Chaikoff IL. Plasma inorganic iodide as a homeostatic regulator of thyroid function. *J Biol Chem*. 1948;174:555-564.
136. Lazarus JH. Lithium and thyroid. *Best Pract Res Clin Endocrinol Metab*. 2009;23:723-733.
137. Muller B, Zulewski H, Huber P, et al. Impaired action of thyroid hormone associated with smoking in women with hypothyroidism. *N Engl J Med*. 1995;333:964-969.
138. Chu M, Seltzer TF. Myxedema coma induced by ingestion of raw bok choy. *N Engl J Med*. 2010;362:1945-1946.
139. Pearce EN, Braverman LE. Environmental pollutants and the thyroid. *Best Pract Res Clin Endocrinol Metab*. 2009;23:801-813.
140. Pearce EN, Spencer CA, Mestman JH, et al. Effect of environmental perchlorate on thyroid function in pregnant women from Cordoba, Argentina, and Los Angeles, California. *Endocr Pract*. 2011;17:412-417.
141. Barbesino G. Drugs affecting thyroid function. *Thyroid*. 2010;20:763-770.
142. Grasberger H, Refetoff S. Genetic causes of congenital hypothyroidism due to dyshormonogenesis. *Curr Opin Pediatr*. 2011;23:421-428.
143. Szinnai G. Genetics of normal and abnormal thyroid development in humans. *Best Pract Res Clin Endocrinol Metab*. 2014;28:133-150.
144. Portulano C, Paroder-Belenitsky M, Carrasco N. The Na+/I- symporter (NIS): mechanism and medical impact. *Endocr Rev*. 2014;35:106-149.
145. Kogai T, Brent GA. The sodium iodide symporter (NIS): regulation and approaches to targeting for cancer therapeutics. *Pharmacol Ther*. 2012;135:355-370.
146. Bakker B, Bikker H, Vulsma T, et al. Two decades of screening for congenital hypothyroidism in the Netherlands: TPO gene mutations in total iodide organification defects (an update). *J Clin Endocrinol Metab*. 2000;85:3708-3712.
147. Bizhanova A, Kopp P. Genetics and phenomics of Pendred syndrome. *Mol Cell Endocrinol*. 2010;322:83-90.
148. Iglesias A, Garcia-Nimo L, Cocho de Juan JA, Moreno JC. Towards the pre-clinical diagnosis of hypothyroidism caused by iodotyrosine deiodinase (DEHAL1) defects. *Best Pract Res Clin Endocrinol Metab*. 2014;28:151-159.
149. Moreno JC, Visser TJ. Genetics and phenomics of hypothyroidism and goiter due to iodotyrosine deiodinase (DEHAL1) gene mutations. *Mol Cell Endocrinol*. 2010;322:91-98.
150. Hennessey JV. Clinical review: Riedel's thyroiditis: a clinical review. *J Clin Endocrinol Metab*. 2011;96:3031-3041.
151. Ozdemir D, Dagdelen S, Erbas T. Endocrine involvement in systemic amyloidosis. *Endocr Pract*. 2010;16:1056-1063.
152. Oerter KE, Kamp GA, Munson PJ, et al. Multiple hormone deficiencies in children with hemochromatosis. *J Clin Endocrinol Metab*. 1993;76:357-361.
153. Shah AA, Wigley FM. Often forgotten manifestations of systemic sclerosis. *Rheum Dis Clin North Am*. 2008;34:221-238, ix.
154. Brent GA. Clinical practice. Graves' disease. *N Engl J Med*. 2008;358:2594-2605.
155. Biebermann H, Schoneberg T, Krude H, et al. Mutations of the human thyrotropin receptor gene causing thyroid hypoplasia and persistent congenital hypothyroidism. *J Clin Endocrinol Metab*. 1997;82:3471-3480.
156. Spiegel AM, Shenker A, Weinstein LS. Receptor-effector coupling by G proteins: implications for normal and abnormal signal transduction. *Endocr Rev*. 1992;13:536-565.
157. Xie J, Pannain S, Pohlenz J, et al. Resistance to thyrotropin (TSH) in three families is not associated with mutations in the TSH receptor or TSH. *J Clin Endocrinol Metab*. 1997;82:3933-3940.
158. Huang SA, Tu HM, Harney JW, et al. Severe hypothyroidism caused by type 3 iodothyronine deiodinase in infantile hemangiomas. *N Engl J Med*. 2000;343:185-189.
159. Puttgen KB. Diagnosis and management of infantile hemangiomas. *Pediatr Clin North Am*. 2014;61:383-402.
160. Huang SA, Fish SA, Dorfman DM, et al. A 21-year-old woman with consumptive hypothyroidism due to a vascular tumor expressing type 3 iodothyronine deiodinase. *J Clin Endocrinol Metab*. 2002;87:4457-4461.
161. Brown RL. Tyrosine kinase inhibitor-induced hypothyroidism: incidence, etiology, and management. *Target Onco*. 2011;6:217-226.
162. Makita N. Iiri T. Tyrosine kinase inhibitor-induced thyroid disorders: a review and hypothesis. *Thyroid*. 2013;23:151-159.
163. Desai J, Yassa L, Marqusee E, et al. Hypothyroidism after sunitinib treatment for patients with gastrointestinal stromal tumors. *Ann Intern Med*. 2006;145:660-664.
164. Maynard MA, Marino-Enriquez A, Fletcher JA, et al. Thyroid hormone inactivation in gastrointestinal stromal tumors. *N Engl J Med*. 2014;370:1327-1334.
165. Dumitrescu AM, Liao XH, Abdullah MS, et al. Mutations in SECISBP2 result in abnormal thyroid hormone metabolism. *Nat Genet*. 2005;37:1247-1252.
166. Canani LH, Capp C, Dora JM, et al. The type 2 deiodinase A/G (Thr92Ala) polymorphism is associated with decreased enzyme velocity and increased insulin resistance in patients with type 2 diabetes mellitus. *J Clin Endocrinol Metab*. 2005;90:3472-3478.
167. Haugen BR, Sherman SI. Evolving approaches to patients with advanced differentiated thyroid cancer. *Endocr Rev*. 2013;34:439-455.
168. Graeppi-Dulac J, Vlaeminck-Guillem V, Perier-Muzet M, et al. Endocrine side-effects of anti-cancer drugs: the impact of retinoids on the thyroid axis. *Eur J Endocrinol*. 2014;170:R253-R262.
169. Haugen BR. Drugs that suppress TSH or cause central hypothyroidism. *Best Pract Res Clin Endocrinol Metab*. 2009;23:793-800.
170. Comi RJ, Gesundheit N, Murray L, et al. Response of thyrotropin-secreting pituitary adenomas to a long-acting somatostatin analogue. *N Engl J Med*. 1987;317:12-17.
171. de Moraes DC, Vaisman M, Conceicao FL, Ortiga-Carvalho TM. Pituitary development: a complex, temporal regulated process dependent on specific transcriptional factors. *J Endocrinol*. 2012;215:239-245.
172. Collu R, Tang J, Castagne J, et al. A novel mechanism for isolated central hypothyroidism: inactivating mutations in the thyrotropin-releasing hormone receptor gene. *J Clin Endocrinol Metab*. 1997;82:1561-1565.
173. Hayashizaki Y, Hiraoka Y, Tatsumi K, et al. Deoxyribonucleic acid analyses of five families with familial inherited thyroid stimulating hormone deficiency. *J Clin Endocrinol Metab*. 1990;71:792-796.
174. Medeiros-Neto G, Herodotou DT, Rajan S, et al. A circulating, biologically inactive thyrotropin caused by a mutation in the beta subunit gene. *J Clin Invest*. 1996;97:1250-1256.
175. Refetoff S, Dumitrescu AM. Syndromes of reduced sensitivity to thyroid hormone: genetic defects in hormone receptors, cell transporters and deiodination. *Best Pract Res Clin Endocrinol Metab*. 2007;21:277-305.

176. Refetoff S, Bassett JH, Beck-Peccoz P, et al. Classification and proposed nomenclature for inherited defects of thyroid hormone action, cell transport, and metabolism. *J Clin Endocrinol Metab.* 2014;99:768-770.
177. Schoenmakers N, Moran C, Peeters RP, et al. Resistance to thyroid hormone mediated by defective thyroid hormone receptor alpha. *Biochim Biophys Acta.* 2013;1830:4004-4008.
178. Moran C, Agostini M, Visser WE, et al. Resistance to thyroid hormone caused by a mutation in thyroid hormone receptor (TR)α1 and TRα2: clinical, biochemical, and genetic analyses of three related patients. *Lancet Diabetes Endocrinol.* 2014;2(8):619-626.
179. van Mullem AA, Chrysis D, Eythimiadou A, et al. Clinical phenotype of a new type of thyroid hormone resistance caused by a mutation of the TRalpha1 receptor: consequences of LT4 treatment. *J Clin Endocrinol Metab.* 2013;98:3029-3038.
180. Weiss RE, Refetoff S. Effect of thyroid hormone on growth. Lessons from the syndrome of resistance to thyroid hormone. *Endocrinol Metab Clin North Am.* 1996;25:719-730.
181. Beck-Peccoz P, Persani L, Mannavola D, Campi I. Pituitary tumours: TSH-secreting adenomas. *Best Pract Res Clin Endocrinol Metab.* 2009;23:597-606.
182. Reutrakul S, Sadow PM, Pannain S, et al. Search for abnormalities of nuclear corepressors, coactivators, and a coregulator in families with resistance to thyroid hormone without mutations in thyroid hormone receptor beta or alpha genes. *J Clin Endocrinol Metab.* 2000;85:3609-3617.
183. Weiss RE, Refetoff S. Treatment of resistance to thyroid hormone—primum non nocere. *J Clin Endocrinol Metab.* 1999;84:401-404.
184. Garber JR, Cobin RH, Gharib H, et al. American Association of Clinical Endocrinologists and American Thyroid Association Taskforce on Hypothyroidism. Clinical practice guidelines for hypothyroidism in adults: cosponsored by the American Association of Clinical Endocrinologists and the American Thyroid Association. *Thyroid.* 2012;22:1200-1235.
185. Biondi B, Wartofsky L. Combination treatment with T4 and T3: toward personalized replacement therapy in hypothyroidism? *J Clin Endocrinol Metab.* 2012;97:2256-2271.
186. Wiersinga WM, Duntas L, Fadeyev V, et al. 2012 ETA guidelines: the use of L-T4 + L-T3 in the treatment of hypothyroidism. *Eur Thyroid J.* 2012;1:55-71.
187. Bach-Huynh TG, Nayak B, Loh J, et al. Timing of levothyroxine administration affects serum thyrotropin concentration. *J Clin Endocrinol Metab.* 2009;94:3905-3912.
188. Hennessey JV. Levothyroxine a new drug? Since when? How could that be? *Thyroid.* 2003;13:279-282.
189. Burman K, Hennessey J, McDermott M, et al. The FDA revises requirements for levothyroxine products. *Thyroid.* 2008;18:487-490.
190. Santini F, Pinchera A, Marsili A, et al. Lean body mass is a major determinant of levothyroxine dosage in the treatment of thyroid diseases. *J Clin Endocrinol Metab.* 2005;90:124-127.
191. Olveira G, Almaraz MC, Soriguer F, et al. Altered bioavailability due to changes in the formulation of a commercial preparation of levothyroxine in patients with differentiated thyroid carcinoma. *Clin Endocrinol (Oxf).* 1997;46:707-711.
192. Rees-Jones RW, Larsen PR. Triiodothyronine and thyroxine content of desiccated thyroid tablets. *Metabolism.* 1977;26:1213-1218.
193. LeBoff MS, Kaplan MM, Silva JE, Larsen PR. Bioavailability of thyroid hormones from oral replacement preparations. *Metabolism.* 1982;31:900-905.
194. Hoang TD, Olsen CH, Mai VQ, et al. Desiccated thyroid extract compared with levothyroxine in the treatment of hypothyroidism: a randomized, double-blind, crossover study. *J Clin Endocrinol Metab.* 2013;98:1982-1990.
195. Blumberg KR, Mayer WJ, Parikh DK, Schnell LA. Liothyronine and levothyroxine in Armour thyroid. *J Pharm Sci.* 1987;76:346-347.
196. Hays MT. Localization of human thyroxine absorption. *Thyroid.* 1991;1:241-248.
197. Centanni M, Gargano L, Canettieri G, et al. Thyroxine in goiter, *Helicobacter pylori* infection, and chronic gastritis. *N Engl J Med.* 2006;354:1787-1795.
198. Escobar-Morreale HF, Obregon MJ, Escobar del Rey F, Morreale de Escobar G. Replacement therapy for hypothyroidism with thyroxine alone does not ensure euthyroidism in all tissues, as studied in thyroidectomized rats. *J Clin Invest.* 1995;96:2828-2838.
199. Jonklaas J, Davidson B, Bhagat S, Soldin SJ. Triiodothyronine levels in athyreotic individuals during levothyroxine therapy. *JAMA.* 2008;299:769-777.
200. Gullo D, Latina A, Frasca F, et al. Levothyroxine monotherapy cannot guarantee euthyroidism in all athyreotic patients. *PLoS ONE.* 2011;6:e22552.
201. Bunevicius R, Kazanavicius G, Zalinkevicius R, Prange AJ Jr. Effects of thyroxine as compared with thyroxine plus triiodothyronine in patients with hypothyroidism. *N Engl J Med.* 1999;340:424-429.
202. Grozinsky-Glasberg S, Fraser A, Nahshoni E, et al. Thyroxine-triiodothyronine combination therapy versus thyroxine monotherapy for clinical hypothyroidism: meta-analysis of randomized controlled trials. *J Clin Endocrinol Metab.* 2006;91:2592-2599.
203. Panicker V, Saravanan P, Vaidya B, et al. Common variation in the DIO2 gene predicts baseline psychological well-being and response to combination thyroxine plus triiodothyronine therapy in hypothyroid patients. *J Clin Endocrinol Metab.* 2009;94:1623-1629.
204. Bianco AC, Casula S. Thyroid hormone replacement therapy: three "simple" questions, complex answers. *Eur Thyroid J.* 2012;1:88-98.
205. Al-Adsani H, Hoffer LJ, Silva JE. Resting energy expenditure is sensitive to small dose changes in patients on chronic thyroid hormone replacement. *J Clin Endocrinol Metab.* 1997;82:1118-1125.
206. Russell W, Harrison RF, Smith N, et al. Free triiodothyronine has a distinct circadian rhythm that is delayed but parallels thyrotropin levels. *J Clin Endocrinol Metab.* 2008;93:2300-2306.
207. Hennemann G, Docter R, Visser TJ, et al. Thyroxine plus low-dose, slow-release triiodothyronine replacement in hypothyroidism: proof of principle. *Thyroid.* 2004;14:271-275.
208. Carr D, McLeod DT, Parry G, Thornes HM. Fine adjustment of thyroxine replacement dosage: comparison of the thyrotrophin releasing hormone test using a sensitive thyrotrophin assay with measurement of free thyroid hormones and clinical assessment. *Clin Endocrinol (Oxf).* 1988;28:325-333.
209. Slawik M, Klawitter B, Meiser E, et al. Thyroid hormone replacement for central hypothyroidism: a randomized controlled trial comparing two doses of thyroxine (T4) with a combination of T4 and triiodothyronine. *J Clin Endocrinol Metab.* 2007;92:4115-4122.
210. Van Dop C, Conte FA, Koch TK, et al. Pseudotumor cerebri associated with initiation of levothyroxine therapy for juvenile hypothyroidism. *N Engl J Med.* 1983;308:1076-1080.
211. Bogazzi F, Tomisti L, Bartalena L, et al. Amiodarone and the thyroid: a 2012 update. *J Endocrinol Invest.* 2012;35:340-348.
212. LaFranchi SH, Austin J. How should we be treating children with congenital hypothyroidism? *J Pediatr Endocrinol Metab.* 2007;20:559-578.
213. Fisher DA, Schoen EJ, La Franchi S, et al. The hypothalamic-pituitary-thyroid negative feedback control axis in children with treated congenital hypothyroidism. *J Clin Endocrinol Metab.* 2000;85:2722-2727.
214. Surks MI, Boucai L. Age- and race-based serum thyrotropin reference limits. *J Clin Endocrinol Metab.* 2010;95:496-502.
215. Atzmon G, Barzilai N, Hollowell JG, et al. Extreme longevity is associated with increased serum thyrotropin. *J Clin Endocrinol Metab.* 2009;94:1251-1254.
216. Arafah BM. Decreased levothyroxine requirement in women with hypothyroidism during androgen therapy for breast cancer. *Ann Intern Med.* 1994;121:247-251.
217. Mandel SJ, Larsen PR, Seely EW, Brent GA. Increased need for thyroxine during pregnancy in women with primary hypothyroidism. *N Engl J Med.* 1990;323:91-96.
218. Alexander EK, Marqusee E, Lawrence J, et al. Timing and magnitude of increases in levothyroxine requirements during pregnancy in women with hypothyroidism. *N Engl J Med.* 2004;351:241-249.
219. Loh JA, Wartofsky L, Jonklaas J, Burman KD. The magnitude of increased levothyroxine requirements in hypothyroid pregnant women depends upon the etiology of the hypothyroidism. *Thyroid.* 2009;19:269-275.
220. Vulsma T, Gons MH, de Vijlder JJ. Maternal-fetal transfer of thyroxine in congenital hypothyroidism due to a total organification defect or thyroid agenesis. *N Engl J Med.* 1989;321:13-16.
221. Arafah BM. Increased need for thyroxine in women with hypothyroidism during estrogen therapy. *N Engl J Med.* 2001;344:1743-1749.
222. Messina M, Redmond G. Effects of soy protein and soybean isoflavones on thyroid function in healthy adults and hypothyroid patients: a review of the relevant literature. *Thyroid.* 2006;16:249-258.
223. Figge J, Dluhy RG. Amiodarone-induced elevation of thyroid stimulating hormone in patients receiving levothyroxine for primary hypothyroidism. *Ann Intern Med.* 1990;113:553-555.
224. Marcocci C, Golia F, Bruno-Bossio G, et al. Carefully monitored levothyroxine suppressive therapy is not associated with bone loss in premenopausal women. *J Clin Endocrinol Metab.* 1994;78:818-823.
225. Gogakos AI, Duncan Bassett JH, Williams GR. Thyroid and bone. *Arch Biochem Biophys.* 2010;503:129-136.
226. Benvenga S. When thyroid hormone replacement is ineffective? *Curr Opin Endocrinol Diabetes Obes.* 2013;20:467-477.
227. Saravanan P, Chau WF, Roberts N, et al. Psychological well-being in patients on "adequate" doses of L-thyroxine: results of a large, controlled community-based questionnaire study. *Clin Endocrinol (Oxf).* 2002;57:577-585.
228. Huber G, Staub JJ, Meier C, et al. Prospective study of the spontaneous course of subclinical hypothyroidism: prognostic value of thyrotropin, thyroid reserve, and thyroid antibodies. *J Clin Endocrinol Metab.* 2002;87:3221-3226.
229. Heymann R, Brent GA. Rapid progression from subclinical to symptomatic overt hypothyroidism. *Endocr Pract.* 2005;11:115-119.
230. Ladenson PW, Levin AA, Ridgway EC, Daniels GH. Complications of surgery in hypothyroid patients. *Am J Med.* 1984;77:261-266.
231. Sherman SI, Ladenson PW. Percutaneous transluminal coronary angioplasty in hypothyroidism. *Am J Med.* 1991;90:367-370.

232. Hay I, Duick DS, Vlietstra RE, et al. Thyroxine therapy in hypothyroid patients undergoing coronary revascularization: a retrospective analysis. *Ann Intern Med.* 1981;95:456-457.

233. Hamilton MA, Stevenson LW, Fonarow GC, et al. Safety and hemodynamic effects of intravenous triiodothyronine in advanced congestive heart failure. *Am J Cardiol.* 1998;81:443-447.

234. Klemperer JD, Klein I, Gomez M, et al. Thyroid hormone treatment after coronary-artery bypass surgery. *N Engl J Med.* 1995;333:1522-1527.

235. Goldman S, McCarren M, Morkin E, et al. DITPA (3,5-diiodothyropropionic acid), a thyroid hormone analog to treat heart failure: phase II trial Veterans Affairs cooperative study. *Circulation.* 2009;119:3093-3100.

236. Ladenson PW, McCarren M, Morkin E, et al. Effects of the thyromimetic agent diiodothyropropionic acid on body weight, body mass index, and serum lipoproteins: a pilot prospective, randomized, controlled study. *J Clin Endocrinol Metab.* 2010;95:1349-1354.

237. Helfand M. Screening for subclinical thyroid dysfunction in nonpregnant adults: a summary of the evidence for the U.S. Preventive Services Task Force. *Ann Intern Med.* 2004;140:128-141.

238. Surks MI, Ortiz E, Daniels GH, et al. Subclinical thyroid disease: scientific review and guidelines for diagnosis and management. *JAMA.* 2004;291:228-238.

239. Vaidya B, Anthony S, Bilous M, et al. Detection of thyroid dysfunction in early pregnancy: universal screening or targeted high-risk case finding? *J Clin Endocrinol Metab.* 2007;92:203-207.

240. Pop VJ, Kuijpens JL, van Baar AL, et al. Low maternal free thyroxine concentrations during early pregnancy are associated with impaired psychomotor development in infancy. *Clin Endocrinol (Oxf).* 1999;50:149-155.

241. Brent GA. Diagnosing thyroid dysfunction in pregnant women: is case finding enough? *J Clin Endocrinol Metab.* 2007;92:39-41.

242. Fliers E, Wiersinga WM. Myxedema coma. *Rev Endocr Metab Disord.* 2003;4:137-141.

243. Klubo-Gwiezdzinska J, Wartofsky L. Thyroid emergencies. *Med Clin North Am.* 2012;96:385-403.

244. Paes JE, Burman KD, Cohen J, et al. Acute bacterial suppurative thyroiditis: a clinical review and expert opinion. *Thyroid.* 2010;20:247-255.

245. Yolmo D, Madana J, Kalaiarasi R, et al. Retrospective case review of pyriform sinus fistulae of third branchial arch origin commonly presenting as acute suppurative thyroiditis in children. *J Laryngol Otol.* 2012;126:737-742.

246. Bartholomew LG, Cain JC, Woolner LB, et al. Sclerosing cholangitis: its possible association with Riedel's struma and fibrous retroperitonitis. Report of two cases. *N Engl J Med.* 1963;269:8-12.

247. Chopra D, Wool MS, Crosson A, Sawin CT. Riedel's struma associated with subacute thyroiditis, hypothyroidism, and hypoparathyroidism. *J Clin Endocrinol Metab.* 1978;46:869-871.

248. Papi G, LiVolsi VA. Current concepts on Riedel thyroiditis. *Am J Clin Pathol.* 2004;121(Suppl):S50-S63.

249. Pusztaszeri M, Triponez F, Pache JC, Bongiovanni M. Riedel's thyroiditis with increased IgG4 plasma cells: evidence for an underlying IgG4-related sclerosing disease? *Thyroid.* 2012;22:964-968.

250. Fatourechi MM, Hay ID, McIver B, et al. Invasive fibrous thyroiditis (Riedel thyroiditis): the Mayo Clinic experience, 1976-2008. *Thyroid.* 2011;21:765-772.

251. Heymann RS, Brent GA, Hershman JM. Anaplastic thyroid carcinoma with thyrotoxicosis and hypoparathyroidism. *Endocr Pract.* 2005;11:281-284.

CHAPTER 14

Nontoxic Diffuse Goiter, Nodular Thyroid Disorders, and Thyroid Malignancies

MARTIN-JEAN SCHLUMBERGER • SEBASTIANO FILETTI • ERIK K. ALEXANDER • IAN D. HAY

KEY POINTS

- Sonography is a noninvasive technique that has become an integral part of the clinical evaluation of a thyroid patient.
- Localization of functioning or nonfunctioning thyroid tissue in the area of the thyroid gland or elsewhere is made possible by techniques of external scintiscanning.
- Positron emission tomography (PET) scanners permit in vivo images related to regional glucose metabolism with high sensitivity and spatial resolution.
- Poorly differentiated thyroid carcinoma is rare, representing less than 5% of all thyroid cancers.
- For patients with locoregional recurrence of medullary thyroid carcinoma (MTC), a complete diagnostic workup should be obtained, principally to exclude distant metastases. Surgery is performed when feasible and is typically followed by external radiotherapy.

This chapter reviews the imaging techniques available for evaluating thyroid structural abnormalities; the units of measurement used in evaluation of the radiation dose and radioactivity are defined in Table 14-1.

Goiter resulting in thyrotoxicosis and other thyroid conditions arising from autoimmune thyroid disease are considered in Chapters 11 and 12. This chapter deals with all aspects of benign nontoxic goiter but concentrates on the increasingly recognized problem of nodular thyroid disease. Moreover, thyroid neoplasia, both benign and malignant, is discussed authoritatively. Appropriate histologic classification and staging of thyroid cancer are considered, and a management program for the most common thyroid cancer types is presented. The section on manage-ment of thyroid nodules and thyroid malignances is largely based on recently available consensus statements from the European Thyroid Association (ETA)[1,2] and guidelines from the American Thyroid Association (ATA).[3,4]

STRUCTURAL AND FUNCTIONAL IMAGING OF THE THYROID

Ultrasonography

Sonography is a noninvasive technique that has become an integral part of the clinical evaluation of a thyroid patient.[5] High-frequency sound waves are emitted by a transducer and reflected as they pass through the body, whereupon the returning echoes are received by the transducer, which also acts as a receiver. The amplitude of the reflected sound waves is influenced by differences in the acoustic impedance of tissues encountered by the sound; for example, *fluid-filled* structures reflect few echoes and therefore have no or few internal echoes and well-defined margins; *solid* structures reflect varying amounts of sound and thus have varying degrees of internal echoes and less well-defined margins; and *calcified* structures reflect virtually all incoming sound and yield pronounced echoes with an *acoustic shadow* posteriorly.

Thyroid parenchyma, surrounding anatomic structures, and thyroid nodules as small as 2 mm in diameter can be readily detected. Color flow Doppler ultrasonography allows visualization of vessels as well as permitting the assessment of nodular vascularity for the purposes of cancer risk assessment.

The thyroid gland must be examined thoroughly in transverse and longitudinal planes. Imaging of patients with thyroid nodules and during follow-up of thyroid cancer should also include the regional neck lymph node compartments, with the goal of identifying enlarged and pathologic nodes.[1,3,5-10]

The normal thyroid parenchyma has a characteristic homogeneous medium-level echogenicity, with little identifiable internal architecture (Fig. 14-1). The surrounding muscles have a hypoechoic appearance. The air-filled trachea in the midline gives a characteristic curvilinear reflecting surface with an associated reverberation artifact.

TABLE 14-1
Radiation Nomenclature: Traditional and International System (SI) Units

Absorbed Radiation Dose

Units:
Gy (gray) and rad (radiation absorbed dose)

Conversions:
1 Gy = 100 rad = absorption of 1 J/kg
1 rad = 0.01 Gy = 1 cGy

Dose Equivalent Radiation

Units:
Sv (sievert) and rem (roentgen equivalent in man)

Conversion:
1 Sv = 100 rem

Radioactivity (or Activity)

Units:
Bq (becquerel) and Ci (curie)

Conversions:
1 Bq = 1 disintegration per second = 27 pCi
1 mCi = 37 MBq
1 GBq = 10^3 MBq = 10^6 kBq = 10^9 Bq

Notes:
Because the becquerel is extremely small, commonly used multiples of the Bq unit are kBq (kilobecquerel), MBq (megabecquerel), and GBq (gigabecquerel).
A curie, however, is extremely large, so commonly used subunits are mCi (millicurie), μCi (microcurie), nCi (nanocurie), and pCi (picocurie).
Gy, Sv, and Bq are SI units; the rad, rem, and Ci are non-SI units.

TABLE 14-2
Clinical Utility of Neck Ultrasound

Map of the neck (thyroid and lymph node areas)
Thyroid gland: size, volume, characteristics
Nodules: number and characteristics of each nodule: diameters, shape, echogenicity, composition, limits, presence of calcifications, vascularization.
Lymph node compartments
Follow-up: numbers and diameters of nodules
Guidance for fine-needle aspiration biopsy
Follow-up of thyroid cancer: thyroid bed and regional lymph nodes
Guidance for radiofrequency and ethanol ablation

A diagrammatic representation of the neck showing the location or locations of any abnormal finding and their characteristics is a useful supplement to the routine film images recorded during an ultrasound examination. Such a cervical map with compartments[9] (Fig. 14-2) can help communicate the anatomic relationships of the disease more clearly to the referring clinician and serves as a reference for the sonographer on follow-up examinations.

Neck ultrasonography is clinically useful at each step of thyroid evaluation (Table 14-2). It confirms the presence or absence of a thyroid nodule when the findings on physical examination are equivocal and may reveal the presence of other nonpalpable nodules.

In patients with a thyroid nodule, gray-scale and color Doppler ultrasound are used to evaluate its sonographic features, including size, shape, echogenicity (hypoechoic or hyperechoic), margins, and composition (cystic, solid, or mixed) as well as the presence of coarse or fine calcifications, and internal blood flow. Such features are highly useful for initial cancer risk assessment. Ultrasound also permits a comprehensive evaluation of regional lymph node compartments. Elastography assesses tissue stiffness within an isolated, solid thyroid nodule and may prove useful as an indicator of malignancy risk. Early reports suggested very high specificity and sensitivity, independent of the nodule size. More recent reports suggest elastographic cancer risk assessment may be inferior to gray-scale ultrasound,[11] with positive predictive values of only 30% to 40%.[12] Although initially promising, these mixed data suggest that elastographic evaluation of thyroid nodules is highly user dependent. Furthermore, elastography can only be applied to solitary solid nodules using a special software package.

In patients with known thyroid cancer, sonography can be useful in evaluating the extent of disease, both preoperatively and postoperatively. Thus, in patients who present with cervical lymphadenopathy caused by papillary thyroid carcinoma (PTC) but in whom the gland is palpably normal, sonography may be used preoperatively to detect an occult, primary intrathyroid focus. A preoperative sonogram should be obtained in all patients with PTC or MTC in order to preoperatively identify the anatomic locations of any sonographically suspicious regional lymph nodes and thereby permit planning of nodal dissection.[1,3,4,13] Occasionally, impalpable residual cancer that had been identified by preoperative ultrasonography and proved to be cytologically positive by ultrasound-guided fine-needle aspiration biopsy (FNAB) can be identified intraoperatively by the use of a handheld ultrasound probe or by preoperative ultrasound-guided charcoal tattooing.[14]

After initial therapy for follicular cell–derived thyroid cancer (FCTC), sonography (together with measurement of serum thyroglobulin [Tg]) represents the most useful method for detecting residual, recurrent, or metastatic

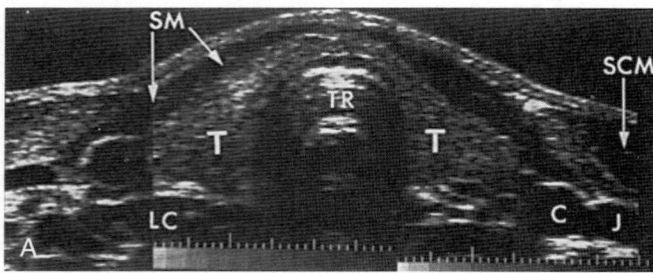

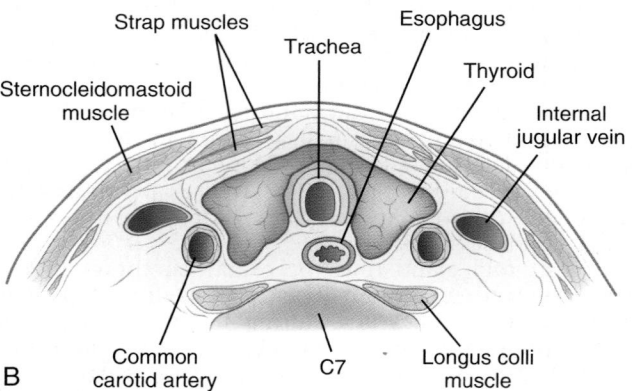

Figure 14-1 Transverse composite sonogram (**A**) and corresponding anatomic map (**B**) of the normal thyroid gland. C, common carotid artery; C7, seventh cervical vertebra; J, internal jugular vein; LC, longus colli muscle; SM, strap muscles; SCM, sternocleidomastoid muscle; T, thyroid; TR, trachea. (From Rifkin MD, Charboneau JW, Laing FC. Special course: ultrasound 1991. In: Reading CC, ed. *Syllabus: Thyroid, Parathyroid, and Cervical Lymph Nodes.* Oak Brook, IL: Radiological Society of North America; 1991:363-377.)

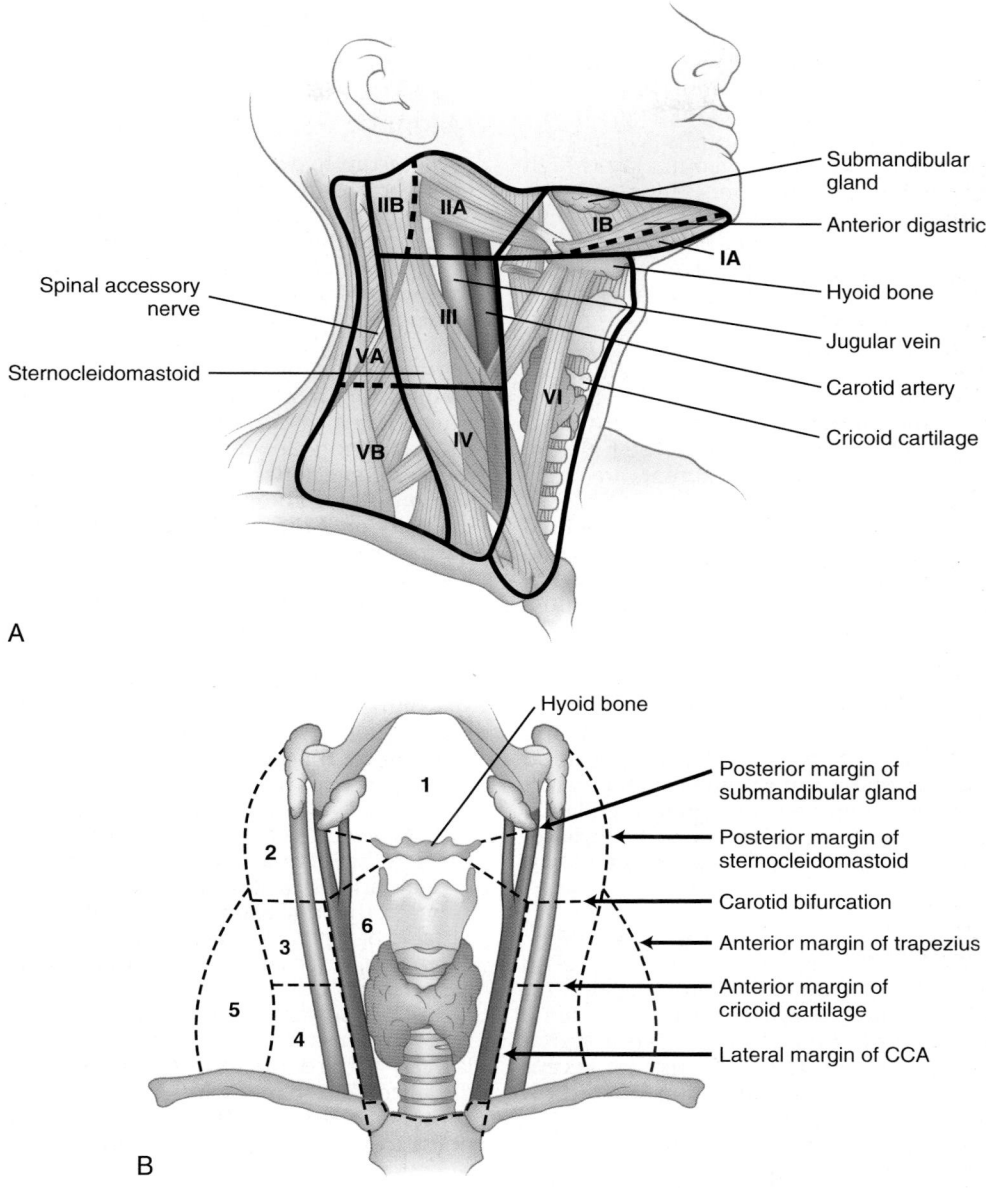

Figure 14-2 A, Anatomic scheme of the neck with compartments. **B,** Cervical map, derived from sonographic images, helps communicate anatomic relationships of disease to clinicians and serves as a reference for follow-up examinations; standard colors are used to characterize any finding. CCA, common carotid artery. (A from Cooper DS, Doherty GM, Haugen BR, et al. Revised management guidelines for patients with thyroid nodules and differentiated thyroid cancer. *Thyroid.* 2009;19:1167-1214, used with permission. B courtesy of J.W. Charboneau, Mayo Clinic, used with permission.)

disease in the neck.[6-8] In patients who have undergone less than a total thyroidectomy, the sonographic appearance of the remaining thyroid tissue may be an important factor in the decision whether to recommend completion thyroidectomy. Also, it is more sensitive than neck palpation in detecting recurrent disease within the thyroid bed and metastatic disease in cervical lymph nodes.

Sonography is also the standard modality for guiding FNAB of most thyroid nodules and cervical lymph nodes.[3,5]

External Scintiscanning

Localization of functioning or nonfunctioning thyroid tissue in the area of the thyroid gland or elsewhere is made

possible by techniques of external scintiscanning. The underlying principle is that isotopes that are selectively accumulated by thyroid tissue can be detected by a gamma camera and the data transformed into a visual display. Radioactivity in specific areas can be quantified.[15-17]

Several radioisotopes are employed in thyroid imaging. Technetium-99m (^{99m}Tc) pertechnetate is a monovalent anion that is actively concentrated by the thyroid gland but undergoes negligible organic binding and diffuses out of the thyroid gland as its concentration in the blood decreases. The short physical half-life of ^{99m}Tc (6 hours), its low fractional uptake, and its transient stay within the thyroid make the radiation delivered to the thyroid gland by a standard activity very low. Consequently, the intravenous administration of radioactivities greater than 37 MBq

(1 mCi) permits, about 30 minutes later, adequate imaging of the thyroid.

Two radioactive isotopes of iodine have been used in thyroid imaging. Iodine-131 (^{131}I) was commonly used in the past. Contrary to ^{99m}Tc, iodine isotopes undergo organic binding. However, ^{131}I is a beta emitter, its physical half-life is 8.1 days, and the energy of its main gamma ray is high and thus poorly adapted for its detection.[17] ^{123}I is, in many respects, an ideal isotope for thyroid imaging because of its short half-life (0.55 day) and the absence of beta radiation, but it is unfortunately much more expensive.[18]

The most important use of scintigraphic imaging of thyroid tissue is in defining areas of increased or decreased function (*hot* or *cold* areas, respectively) relative to the function of the remainder of the gland. Almost all malignant nodules are hypofunctioning, but more than 80% of benign nodules are also nonfunctioning. Conversely, functioning nodules (hot nodules), particularly if the function of the surrounding tissue is decreased or absent, are rarely malignant.

Scintiscanning with radioactive iodine can also be used to demonstrate that intrathoracic masses represent thyroid tissue and to detect ectopic thyroid tissue in the neck. In FCTC patients, total-body scanning is used to detect functioning metastases.[1,3] This scan is performed after the administration of larger activities of radioiodine, either for diagnosis (1-5 mCi of ^{131}I or 1-5 mCi ^{123}I) or therapy (30 mCi or more of ^{131}I) and following intense stimulation with TSH (thyroid-stimulating hormone, thyrotropin) and in the absence of iodine contamination. Superimposition of computed tomography (CT) and gamma camera images (single-photon emission computed tomography [SPECT]/CT) greatly improves both the sensitivity and specificity of the technique and the anatomic localization of any focus of uptake.[19-22]

Computed Tomography

The CT appearance of the anatomic structures depends on the attenuation of the tissue examined. The thyroid gland, because of its high concentration of iodine, has a higher attenuation than do the surrounding soft tissues. Recent advances with spiral CT and reconstruction algorithms have improved the performance of the method.[23,24]

CT scan does not distinguish benign from malignant nodules and does not assess functional status; however, it can define the anatomic extent of large goiters with great clarity. CT scanning can provide useful information regarding the presence and extent of intrathoracic (substernal) goiters. The CT findings of an intrathoracic mass in continuity with the thyroid gland, with high attenuation on non–contrast-enhanced images and marked enhancement after intravenous contrast material injection, all suggest intrathoracic goiter. Radioiodine scanning can also be performed in this clinical setting, but false-negative results can occur when little or no functional tissue is present in the intrathoracic goiter.

In aggressive pathologic processes, such as anaplastic thyroid carcinoma, CT with infusion of contrast medium is the most frequently recommended first-line technique to identify lymph node metastases and to define the tumor's relationships to surrounding structures, including vessels and the aerodigestive tract.[23,24] CT imaging is less sensitive than neck ultrasonography for the detection of lymph node metastases but may complement neck ultrasound for the detection of macrometastases in the central compartment, in the mediastinum and behind the trachea, and is the most sensitive tool for the detection of micrometastases in the lungs. Because of the necessity of infusing iodine-containing contrast agents for CT scanning of the neck and mediastinum, CT should be performed at least 4 weeks before any administration of radioiodine.[25]

Magnetic Resonance Imaging

Because the hydrogen atoms of different tissues have different relaxation times (termed *T1* and *T2*), a computer-assisted analysis of *T1*-weighted and *T2*-weighted signals is used to differentiate the thyroid gland from skeletal muscles, blood vessels, or regional lymph nodes. Normal thyroid tissue tends to be slightly more intense than muscles on a *T1*-weighted image, and tumors often appear more intense than normal thyroid tissue.

Magnetic resonance imaging (MRI) does not distinguish benign from malignant nodules and does not assess functional status. Recurrent neoplasms in the thyroid bed or regional lymph nodes can be detected with MRI. Recurrence is characterized by a mass with low to medium intensity on *T1*-weighted images and medium to high signal intensity on *T2*-weighted images. Conversely, scar tissue or fibrous tissue has low signal intensity on both *T1*-weighted and *T2*-weighted images.[23,24] Tumor invasion of adjacent skeletal muscle has high signal intensity on *T2*-weighted images. Edema or inflammation in the muscle can cause a similar appearance and can be difficult to differentiate from recurrent tumor.

Compared to CT scan, MRI may better delineate any involvement of the aerodigestive axis. It is often used as a second-line imaging technique in patients with demonstrated or suspicious lesions in the upper part of the neck on CT scan in order to better delineate these lesions from soft tissues. In the lower part of the neck, movements of the aerodigestive axis during the procedure that may last several minutes will decrease the quality of images. Endoscopy of the trachea and/or esophagus, with or without ultrasonography, looking for evidence of intraluminal extension, can also be helpful in cases of suspected aerodigestive tract invasion.

MRI is useful for assessment of the extent of bone involvement in cases of axial bone metastases from follicular cell–derived carcinomas and MTC, which are poorly visualized on bone scintigraphy.[26,27] For MTC patients, contrast-enhanced MRI is more sensitive than three-phase contrast-enhanced CT for the detection of liver metastases.[27]

Positron Emission Tomography

PET is both quantitative and tomographic. The radionuclide used emits a positron that is converted into a pair of photons after a short path of a few millimeters in the tissue. The coincident detection of the two photons, which travel on a line in opposite directions, permits the localization of the site of the radionuclide decay.

The agent most widely used with PET is [^{18}F]fluorodeoxyglucose (^{18}FDG). This agent is transported and phosphorylated as a glucose substitute but remains metabolically trapped inside tumor cells because of its inability to undergo glycolysis.

PET scanners permit in vivo images related to regional glucose metabolism, with high sensitivity and spatial resolution. Superimposition of CT and PET images greatly improves both the sensitivity and specificity of the technique and the anatomic localization of any focus of abnormal uptake. The uptake in any focus can be quantified, and the most frequently used parameter is the standardized uptake value (SUV). The sensitivity of ^{18}FDG-PET scanning may be improved with TSH stimulation.[28,29]

PET scanning should be performed in only selected patients with thyroid carcinoma. Low-risk patients are very unlikely to require [18]FDG-PET scanning as part of initial staging or follow-up. [18]FDG-PET scanning in thyroid cancer[3,28] may be used as follows:

- To localize disease in Tg-positive patients (having serum Tg levels > 10 ng/mL) with no other abnormality on diagnostic imaging; it is mostly useful for the detection of lymph node metastases in the posterior neck and mediastinum or distant metastases.
- For the initial staging and follow-up of patients with anaplastic, poorly differentiated, or Hürthle cell thyroid cancers in order to identify sites of disease that may be missed with conventional imaging; in these cancers, FDG uptake is usually high and ^{131}I uptake is either low or absent.
- In patients with known distant metastases in whom high FDG uptake in large metastases indicates a high risk for disease-specific fatality and poor response to ^{131}I therapy.[30,31]
- As a measurement of posttreatment response following local (external beam irradiation, surgical resection, thermal ablation, embolization) or systemic therapy.[32]

Inflammatory lymph nodes, suture granulomas, and increased muscle activity are common causes of false-positive [18]FDG-PET findings. Also, asymmetric laryngeal uptake is frequently observed in patients with vocal cord paralysis. Therefore, cytologic or histologic confirmation is required before one can be certain that an [18]FDG-positive lesion represents metastatic disease.

High uptake has also been observed in several thyroid diseases, such as thyroiditis, and PET cannot be used to differentiate benign from malignant thyroid nodules. The discovery of focal thyroid uptake on an FDG-PET scan performed for other reasons should lead to a complete workup, including FNA cytologic testing, because a third of these nodules may prove to be malignant.[33,34]

Delineation between lymph node metastases or local extension of the tumor and vessels or the aerodigestive axis is often not well visualized on FDG-PET/CT in the absence of contrast injection, and if necessary, other imaging techniques (CT and MRI with contrast medium) may be performed, especially for a preoperative workup.

In clinical research settings, PET scanning with [124]I has also been used for quantitation of uptake and for accurate dosimetry in distant metastases from thyroid cancer.[35] PET scanning with ^{18}F-labeled dihydroxyphenylalanine (^{18}F-DOPA) can be usefully employed to visualize neoplastic foci of MTC,[36,37] because the FDG uptake is usually low in MTC patients, and FDG-PET scan in that clinical setting is therefore rarely informative.[27,38]

NONTOXIC DIFFUSE GOITER AND NODULAR THYROID DISEASE

Nontoxic goiter may be defined as any thyroid enlargement that is characterized by uniform or selective (i.e., restricted to one or more areas) growth of thyroid tissue, is not associated with overt hyperthyroidism or hypothyroidism, and does not result from inflammation or neoplasia. A thyroid nodule is defined as a discrete lesion, within the thyroid gland, due to an abnormal, focal growth of thyroid cells.

Epidemiology

The prevalence of goiter, diffuse or nodular, differs widely, depending on the iodine intake by the population living in a given area. Thus, goiter may occur endemically, due mainly to iodine deficiency, or sporadically, depending on whether the goiter prevalence in children is more or less than 5%, respectively. In pregnancy, goitrous enlargement is physiologic and usually regresses post partum. In an adult nonpregnant population, the Framingham survey revealed a 4.6% prevalence, with a strong female predominance (6.4% in women and 1.5% in men), whereas the Wickham study displayed a 3.2% prevalence (6.6:1 hazard ratio of women to men).[39,40] However, different variables (regional variation in the iodine intake, smoking habits, age and sex distribution, and primarily the methodology [palpation vs. sonography] used to determine thyroid volume) may have influenced these data. Using sonography as the screening method, the prevalence rate of goiter in an unselected adult population has been reported to be as high as 30% to 50%. This prevalence is even higher in iodine-deficient areas and in older populations. Similarly, a prevalence of thyroid nodules nearing 50% has been described in adult and geriatric autopsy series[41] and up to 65% in healthy adults screened with sonography.[42]

Etiology and Pathophysiology

Goiter has been traditionally regarded as the adaptive response of the thyroid follicular cell to any factor that impairs thyroid hormone synthesis. This classic concept no longer appears to encompass the many aspects of goiters. Indeed, goiter is characterized by a variety of clinical, functional, and morphologic presentations, and whether this heterogeneity represents different entities remains to be clarified. Also, iodine deficiency as the sole factor responsible for goiter appears to be an oversimplification. Thus, not all inhabitants in an iodine-deficient region develop goiter; moreover, endemic goiter has been observed in countries with no iodine deficiency, and even in some regions with iodine excess, and has not been observed in some regions with severe iodine deficiency. These findings suggest that other factors, genetic, demographic, and environmental, may play a role in the genesis of diffuse and nodular goiter, and some of these factors may act synergistically.

The role of genetic factors is suggested by several lines of evidence,[43] such as (1) the clustering of goiters within families; (2) the higher concordance rate for goiters in monozygotic than in dizygotic twins; (3) the female-male ratio (1:1 in endemic vs. 7:1 to 9:1 in sporadic goiters); and (4) the persistence of goiters in areas where a widespread iodine prophylaxis program has been properly implemented.

By studying families affected by goiter, researchers have been able to detect several gene abnormalities involving proteins related to thyroid hormone synthesis, such as mutations in genes encoding Tg, sodium/iodide symporter (NIS), thyroid peroxidase (TPO), dual oxidase 2 (DUOX2), pendrin (Pendred syndrome [PDS]), and TSH receptor (TSHR). In addition, three loci for this disorder have been identified that map to chromosomes 14q, Xp22, and 3q26, respectively.[44,45] Although an autosomal dominant inheritance has been demonstrated in several families, multiple genes may be involved in other families, indicating a marked genetic background underlying the cause of the goiter. This complicated genetic pattern may explain why predisposing gene alterations remain unidentified in most patients with nontoxic goiter.

In addition to iodine deficiency and genetic susceptibility, the exposure to a variety of environmental factors has been linked to goiter generation.[46,47] Thus, endocrine disrupters, including perchlorate, thiocyanate, and nitrate; isoflavones; and organochlorines as well as drugs, smoking, selenium deficiency, insulin resistance, oral contraceptives, parity, and alcohol have been suggested to be involved in goiter development.[48,49]

TSH has long been considered the major stimulus for thyroid growth in response to any factor impairing thyroid hormone synthesis. Indeed, in the rare clinical setting of a functioning TSH-secreting pituitary adenoma, the increased serum TSH concentrations typically cause enlargement of the thyroid gland.[50] Similarly, goiter is also a typical feature of Graves disease, in which a stimulatory growth effect on thyroid tissue is induced by thyroid-stimulating antibody through TSHR activation.[51] Moreover, thyroid enlargement may appear during the course of Graves disease when increased TSH levels result from overtreatment with anti-thyroid drugs. In addition, toxic thyroid hyperplasia is usually present in nonautoimmune autosomal dominant hyperthyroidism, a disorder related to germline activating mutations of the *TSHR* gene.[52] This clinical condition further emphasizes the role of TSH-TSHR system activation in the genesis of thyroid hyperplasia.[43] Serum TSH concentration is normal in most patients with nontoxic goiter.[46] Experimentally, it has been demonstrated that in rats iodine depletion enhances the promotion of thyroid growth by normal levels of TSH.[53] Hence, any factor that impairs intrathyroidal iodine levels may lead to gradual development of goiter in response to normal concentrations of TSH.

More intriguing is the relationship between TSH levels and iodine supply. Indeed, even small differences in the level of iodine intake are correlated with significant differences in TSH levels; this change has been demonstrated after the 11-year follow-up in the longitudinal population-based Danish program monitoring the nationwide iodine fortification (DanThyr study).[54]

Indeed, a complex network of both TSH-dependent and TSH-independent pathways directs thyroid follicular cell growth and function and plays a role in the goitrogenic process. In particular, a variety of growth factors, derived either from the bloodstream or through autocrine or paracrine secretion, may serve to regulate thyroid cell proliferation and differentiation processes.[43]

Typically, early in the course of goiter formation, areas of microheterogeneity of structure and function are intermixed and include areas of functional autonomy and areas of focal hemorrhage.

Analysis of hyperplastic nodules by rigid criteria also indicated that morphologically indistinguishable hyperplastic thyroid nodules may be either monoclonal or polyclonal. Monoclonal adenomas within hyperplastic thyroid glands may reflect a stage in progression along the hyperplasia-neoplasia spectrum; accumulation of multiple somatic mutations may subsequently confer a selective growth advantage to this single-cell clone.[55]

Histologically, nodules contain irregularly enlarged, involuted follicles distended with colloid or clusters of smaller follicles lined by taller epithelium and containing small colloid droplets. The nodules tend to be incompletely encapsulated and are poorly demarcated from and merge with the internodular tissue, which also has an altered architecture. However, the nodules in some glands appear to be localized, with areas of apparently normal architecture elsewhere. Here, the distinction from a follicular adenoma may be difficult, and some pathologists apply terms such as *colloid* or *adenomatous* nodules to such lesions.

Natural History

Nontoxic goiter has a female preponderance. There appears to be no physiologic increase in thyroid volume during normal adolescence. Development of a goiter during adolescence, therefore, is a pathologic rather than a physiologic process.[56]

Iodine intake influences the natural history of nodular goiter disease. In the DanThyr follow-up study[49] it was demonstrated that 11 years after the iodization program one third of solitary thyroid nodules identified at baseline had disappeared; interestingly, one fifth of previous multinodular goiters turned out to be diffuse. This finding confirmed that the iodine intake is the main factor in determining the nodular thyroid disease appearance in a given area; furthermore, the survey demonstrated that the thyroid nodularity is a dynamic and not necessarily an irreversible process.

Therefore, the dissimilar iodine intake may account for the epidemiologic thyroid nodular disease differences between the United States, which carries an adequate iodine supply, and European as well other countries, which still display a severe to mild/moderate iodine deficiency.

Clinical Presentation

In an era when patients are advised on self-examination to detect cancer at an early stage, the finding of a palpable abnormality in such a superficial location as the thyroid gland can be disconcerting. The affected patient is likely to seek medical evaluation. At the end of an appropriate investigation, the clinician can usually reassure the patient that the goiter or the nodule is benign. Autonomous nodules or autonomous functional areas in the context of a multinodular goiter may result in an increased thyroid hormone secretion and subsequently a subclinical or overt thyrotoxicosis. This feature is, however, a rare event, especially in the United States, being mainly linked to the iodine deficiency. However, in general, thyroid nodules are usually not associated with abnormal thyroid hormone secretion. Therefore, affected patients do not exhibit clinical signs of thyroid dysfunction and are often asymptomatic. The only clinical features of nontoxic goiter may be those of thyroid enlargement. In a health care system in which the extent of cross-sectional imaging has increased, a large proportion of clinically relevant nodules are incidentally detected during carotid ultrasonography or CT and MRI studies of the chest, neck, or head. Such incidentally detected nodules carry the same risk of malignancy as do nodules identified on clinical examination.

Most thyroid nodules are asymptomatic. However, large nodules, which may displace or compress the trachea, esophagus, and neck vessels, can be rarely associated with symptoms and signs, including neck tightness, dysphagia, and a choking sensation. These obstructive symptoms may be accentuated by the so-called Pemberton maneuver (see Chapter 10). Invasion or compression of the recurrent laryngeal nerve, causing hoarseness, rarely occurs, though, when present, it suggests advanced thyroid carcinoma. More commonly, acute hemorrhage into a cystic nodule may produce acute, painful enlargement of the neck and can enhance or induce obstructive symptoms.[46]

Initial Investigation

Thyroid nodules are generally benign hyperplastic (or colloid) nodules or benign follicular adenomas. However, multiple retrospective studies confirm that about 5% to 15% of clinically relevant nodules prove cancerous.[57,58] The prevalence of thyroid cancer in the United States, as well as in most industrialized countries, has been steadily increasing.[59] This increase is mostly due to increased detection (and increased reporting) of small, indolent malignancies.[60,61] However, an increase in more advanced thyroid cancer has also been detected in some studies, raising questions that other factors beyond simply sampling bias may impact this finding. Regardless, the mortality rate attributable to thyroid cancer remains very low.[61]

Initial Clinical Evaluation

In the evaluation of a clinically relevant thyroid nodule, a thorough history and careful physical examination should be supplemented with laboratory testing, imaging procedures including neck ultrasonography, and most important, consideration of fine-needle aspiration (FNA). With this approach, an individualized assessment of malignant risk, as well as the specific morbidity and mortality risks attributable to such malignancy, can be made. This evaluation allows the health care worker to advise appropriate treatment in relation to the patient's other illnesses and desires.[46]

Historic features that suggest malignancy include young age (<20-30 years), male sex, a history of external neck radiation during childhood or adolescence, and rapid nodule growth or persistent changes in speaking, breathing, or swallowing. Rarely, a family history of multiple endocrine neoplasia (MEN) type 2 is detected, which should prompt evaluation.[46]

On physical examination, a large, fixed, and firm nodule is worrisome for malignancy, especially when suspicious regional lymphadenopathy is detected.[3,4] It should be noted, however, that most patients are asymptomatic at presentation, and physical examination simply detects a 1- to 3-cm nodule that is nontender and mobile with swallowing.

Many studies have shown that nodule size minimally impacts the risk of malignancy[62] and that the incidence of cancer in incidentally identified nodules is the same as in those with palpable nodules. However, in nodules larger than 4 cm in diameter, the incidence of carcinoma may be higher.[63] The presence of multiple nodules does not decrease the likelihood of thyroid cancer. In patients with multiple, clinically relevant nodules, the rate of malignancy per nodule decreases, but the decrease is approximately proportional to the number of detected nodules. Therefore, the overall cancer rate per patient is the same in those with multiple nodules as in those with a solitary nodule. Importantly, when multiple nodules are present, each must be separately evaluated because the dominant (largest) nodule is not solely representative of thyroid cancer risk.[64]

Initial Laboratory Evaluation

In all patients with suspected or known thyroid nodules, measurement of serum TSH is recommended. A low or undetectable serum TSH, even if associated with normal free thyroid hormone levels, should suggest the possibility of toxic, autonomously functioning nodules and prompt thyroid scintigraphy. Higher serum TSH concentrations, even within the normal reference range, may increase the risk that a thyroid nodule is cancerous.[65,66]

Measurement of serum anti-TPO antibody (TPO Ab) concentration may assist with the diagnosis of chronic lymphocytic thyroiditis (Hashimoto thyroiditis) if the serum TSH level is elevated. Hashimoto thyroiditis causes a heterogeneous parenchymal appearance on sonography that at times can mimic a pseudonodule. When an elevated TPO Ab and heterogeneous sonographic pattern are detected, a thyroid nodule must be sonographically discrete in three separate dimensions to warrant evaluation.

Hashimoto disease may also be associated with the presence of bilateral, enlarged, but benign-appearing lymphadenopathy. This feature is due to the immune nature of this disease and should not necessarily cause alarm. In some patients, an FNA (described later) will be required to help distinguish benign from suspicious disease.

FCTCs may release increased amounts of Tg into the bloodstream. Unfortunately, there is overlap of serum Tg levels in FCTCs and most benign conditions. Therefore, the measurement of serum Tg levels is not useful in the initial workup of nodular thyroid disease. Some investigators recommend routine measurement of serum calcitonin levels in all patients with nodular thyroid disease to screen for MTC.[67,68] However, because of the rarity of unsuspected MTC, the high frequency of false-positive results that often prompts further workup or thyroidectomy, and the unknown clinical relevance of medullary microcarcinomas (<1.0 cm), it is neither cost effective nor necessary to measure serum calcitonin levels in the initial evaluation of patients with nodular thyroid disease. In circumstances of greater suspicion (e.g., the presence of microcalcifications in the nodule), however, the measurement of serum calcitonin may prove useful.[3,46] If the unstimulated serum calcitonin determination is greater than 100 pg/mL, MTC is likely present.[68]

Imaging of the Thyroid

Ultrasonographic evaluation is the optimal means of evaluating the anatomic structure of the thyroid. Ultrasonography allows the health care provider to assess both the morphologic appearance and the size of the gland, while also assessing cancer risk in thyroid nodules.[1,3,5,46] Ultrasonography is capable of detecting even minute thyroid nodules. In fact, of 1000 normal control subjects, 65% had detectable nodularity on high-resolution sonography.[42] Numerous studies demonstrate that ultrasound can effectively stratify malignancy risk in thyroid nodules (Table 14-3). Such risk assessment then guides diagnostic and evaluative strategies for any given patient. For example, FNA of higher risk nodules is generally recommended when equal to or larger than 1 cm. In contrast, very low-risk nodules may not require FNA until growth beyond 2 cm is detected (ATA guidelines). Features with the highest specificity for thyroid cancer include the presence of microcalcifications, hypoechoic parenchyma, and infiltrative or irregular margins.[69-73] Such features are most predictive when present in combination. The presence of abnormal adenopathy, especially when unilateral and in the lower neck, also increases the risk of cancer when a thyroid nodule is confirmed. Macrocalcifications, however, do not predict malignancy, unless seen in combination with microcalcifications.[69,73] A taller-than-wider shape (i.e., the anteroposterior dimension is larger than transverse dimension on a transverse image) has been associated with increased malignancy risk in some studies, though this remains controversial, especially given the lack of a clear hypothesis suggesting why such a growth pattern would prove more malignant. In contrast, purely cystic nodules, a spongiform parenchyma, and homogeneously hyperechoic lesions carry the lowest risk of malignancy.[5,42,69,70,74]

Extensive published research confirming the utility of sonographic risk assessment, combined with substantial advances in ultrasound technology, has led experts to now routinely recommend a sonographic risk classification for all thyroid nodules (ATA guidelines, ETA, American Association of Clinical Endocrinologists [AACE]). Nodules should be classified into high-, intermediate-, low-, and

TABLE 14-3

Clinical and Sonographic Findings Distinguishing Benign From Malignant Thyroid Nodules

Clinical Features	Sonographic Risk Assessment
Historic Features	**Benign**
Young (<20-30 years old) age	Purely cystic nodules
Male sex	**Very Low Suspicion**
Neck irradiation during childhood or adolescence	Spongiform or partially cystic nodules *without* irregular margins, microcalcifications, or extrathyroidal extension
Rapid growth	
Recent, persistent changes in speaking, breathing, or swallowing	**Low Suspicion**
Family history of multiple endocrine neoplasia type 2	Solid, isoechoic or hyperechoic nodules *without* irregular margins, microcalcifications, or extrathyroidal extension
Physical Examination	Echo-free (cystic) lesion
	Spongiform appearance
Firm, fixed, and irregular consistency of nodule	Homogeneously hyperechoic lesions
Vocal cord paralysis or hoarseness	Hypoechoic halo
	Intermediate Suspicion
Persistent regional lymph adenopathy	Solid, hypoechoic nodule *without* irregular margins, microcalcifications, or extrathyroidal extension
	Hypoechoic lesions
	Presence of microcalcifications
	Irregular infiltrative margins
	Absence of halo
	A taller than wide shape measured in the transverse dimension
	Internal or central blood flow
	Suspicious cervical lymphadenopathy
	High Suspicion
	Solid, hypoechoic nodule *with* one or more features: irregular margins, microcalcifications, extrathyroidal extension

very low-suspicion categories, as this allows an evidenced-based strategy to support future intervention or conservative follow-up. High-risk nodules are solid and hypoechoic with additional findings of microcalcifications, or an irregular border. Cancer risk is estimated at 70% to 90% in such lesions. Intermediate- and low-risk nodules constitute the majority of nodules seen in clinical practice. Intermediate-risk nodules are solid and hypoechoic but without the additional concerning features listed for high-risk nodules. Low-risk nodules are solid, iso- or hyperechoic, or partially cystic, yet they also lack concerning features of microcalcifications, irregular margins, and abnormal adenopathy. Cancer risk in these two groups range from about 20% to 5% to 15%, respectively. Nodules at high or indeterminate risk are generally recommended for FNA if their maximal diameter exceeds 1 cm, whereas low-risk nodules can be followed until growth exceeds 1.5 cm. Very low-risk nodules are mostly cystic or spongiform, and risk of malignancy is very low. For this reason, growing consensus suggests that FNA should not be performed in such nodules unless the maximal nodule diameter exceeds 2 cm.[74-77] Importantly, purely cystic nodules are so rarely malignant that FNA is not indicated for diagnostic purposes. Such guidelines can provide a roadmap for clinicians to consider, though individual assessment is nonetheless required. Certain clinical factors, patient or physician concerns, or other findings may appropriately sway a practitioner to biopsy a low-risk nodule even when it is less than 1 cm, or conversely to choose to follow a high-risk nodule even without FNA. These are reasonable decisions, as the overall risk of thyroid cancer is considered in conjunction with the patient's comorbid illnesses, desires, and risks of intervention.

Ultrasound elastography (USE) is a technique that seeks to use pressure and ultrasound as a measurement of tissue stiffness. In general, the stiffer the nodule, the higher the risk of cancer. USE was initially reported as highly predictive of benign or malignant disease.[78] However, more recent trials indicate inferior performance of USE in comparison to ultrasound assessment.

CT and MRI studies of the neck have also been employed. Although such tests are highly useful to assess surrounding neck structures in preparation for surgery, their performance is generally inferior to that of thyroid ultrasound. Furthermore, cancer risk characteristics cannot be as readily defined (such as hypoechoic parenchyma or irregular margins) as with ultrasound.

Before the advent of ultrasound-guided FNA, thyroid scintigraphy using ^{131}I, ^{123}I, or ^{99m}Tc was used to image the gland. Most thyroid carcinomas are inefficient in trapping and organifying iodine and appear on scans as areas of diminished isotope uptake, referred to as a cold nodule. This feature reflects the early decrease of NIS expression during tumorigenesis.[79] Unfortunately, most benign nodules also do not concentrate iodine. Furthermore, not all nodules with normal or slightly increased ^{99m}Tc uptake are benign and some may appear cold on a thyroid scan with radioactive iodine.[15,16] This confirms the limited utility of thyroid scintigraphy. The only situation in which an iodine scan can exclude malignancy with reasonable certainty is in the case of a toxic (hot) adenoma. Such a nodule demonstrates focal ^{123}I uptake though markedly suppressed or absent uptake in the remainder of the gland. These lesions are typically associated with a suppressed serum TSH level. They account for fewer than 5% to 10% of thyroid nodules and are almost invariably benign.[46] Thyroid scintigraphy is employed much less often than previously, though it can still prove valuable in the assessment of a patient with multiple thyroid nodules or a borderline low serum TSH concentration. Scintigraphy in such cases allows the practitioner to initially target aspiration of the nonfunctional nodules. Finally, FDG-PET is increasingly performed during the evaluation of patients with various illnesses. Though not recommended for the routine evaluation of thyroid nodules, incidental PET-positive nodules have a cancer risk of 30% to 40%.[33,34,80-83] In such patients, FNA is warranted. Importantly, diffuse FDG-PET uptake most often is found in the setting of Hashimoto disease and should not be considered pathologic or malignant if ultrasound confirms the absence of any nodularity (Fig. 14-3).

Thyroid Nodule Fine-Needle Aspiration

FNA of thyroid nodules has eclipsed all other techniques for diagnosing thyroid cancer, with reported overall rates of sensitivity and specificity exceeding 90% in iodine-sufficient areas.[3,5,46,73,84,85] The technique is easy to perform and safe, with only a handful of complications having been reported in the literature,[86] and causes only mild discomfort. However, care must be taken to obtain an adequate specimen; most authors recommend 2 to 4 aspirations per nodule.[84,85] Routine use of ultrasound-guided biopsy even for clinically palpable solid nodules combined with on-site cytologic examination decreases the risk of inadequate sampling.[87-89] A satisfactory specimen must contain at least five groups of 10 to 15 well-preserved cells.

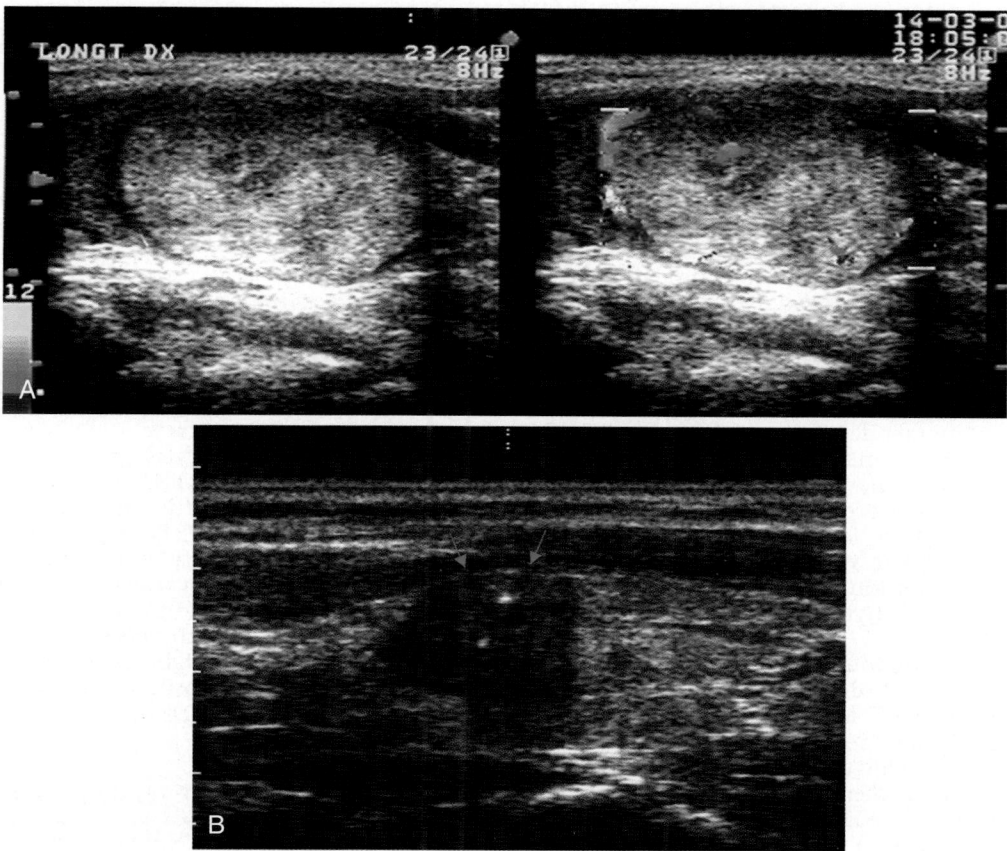

Figure 14-3 Conventional and color flow Doppler sonography. **A,** Benign lesion. Sonogram shows well-defined, oval, hyperechoic nodule with perinodular and slight intranodular blood flow. **B,** Malignant lesion. Sonogram shows a nodule with inhomogeneous hypoechoic aspect, microcalcifications, irregular borders, with invasion of the thyroid capsule *(arrows).*

Not all thyroid nodules require FNA, and many can be safely followed without intervention over time and pose minimal risk. A decision to consider thyroid nodule FNA should initially rest upon an assessment of whether cytologic interpretation would modify the clinical care ahead. If, for example, advancing patient age and comorbid conditions would render further surgical intervention unlikely, FNA may be unnecessary. For those in whom evaluation is warranted, however, recommendation for FNA is then based on nodule size and sonographic features. Although individual assessment is paramount, for those with high- or intermediate-risk features most nodules should generally be considered for FNA when larger than 1 cm. In contrast, low-suspicion and very low-suspicion nodules should be considered for FNA when larger than 1.5 cm and 2.0 cm, respectively. These guidelines were developed with hope of identifying clinically relevant thyroid cancer that benefits from therapeutic intervention while avoiding excessive diagnostic intervention, but prospective investigations of this approach are not yet available. Smaller nodules (generally <1 cm) can most often be conservatively followed with repeat sonographic assessment in 1 to 2 years unless unique circumstances or symptoms raise concern.

Thyroid nodule FNA cytologic findings should be reported using diagnostic categories outlined in the Bethesda System for Reporting Thyroid Cytopathology (Table 14-4).[90-95]

The diagnosis of PTC (Bethesda category: Malignant) by FNA on the basis of characteristic nuclear changes is both reliable and accurate, with sensitivity and specificity

TABLE 14-4

Probability of Malignancy Based on Fine-Needle Aspiration Cytologic Categorization[90-95]

Cytologic Appearance	% of Results	% of Malignancy, for Each Category
Insufficient/nondiagnostic	~5-10	<5% if cystic nodule; 10-20% in solid nodules
Benign	70 (53-90)	1-5%
Indeterminate	20 (5-23)	
Suspicious for papillary carcinoma		60-70%
Suspicious for a follicular neoplasm (SFN/FN)		15-30%
Atypia (follicular lesion) of undetermined significance (AUS/FLUS)		10-25%
Malignant	5 (1-10)	>97%

both approaching 100% provided that these changes are evaluated by an experienced cytopathologist. Similarly, a benign result should be viewed as highly accurate, as data confirm a low risk (~1-5%) of false-negative results, and negligible mortality risk from false-negative aspirates during an 8.5-year follow-up.[62] However, cytologically indeterminate nodules harbor malignant risk. Bethesda classification allows malignancy risk stratification within this category, ranging from those with highest indeterminate risk (SUSP [suspicious for papillary carcinoma]) to those with lower risk (SFN/FN [suspicious for a follicular neoplasm] or AUS/FLUS [atypia/follicular lesion of unde-termined significance]). Regardless, an indeterminate FNA cytologic finding implies concern that such a nodule may be a thyroid malignancy. Cytologic results should be com-bined with clinical and ultrasound characteristics, allowing further individual assessment. At times, such indetermi-nate cytologic findings—especially if SUSP, or combined with other clinical factors such as large nodule size, cos-metic concerns, or difficulty swallowing—may prove con-cerning enough to warrant a recommendation for surgical removal. This approach is very reasonable, though in every case therapy must be individualized.

However, low-risk indeterminate nodules (SFN/FN or AUS/FLUS) often harbor a relatively lower risk of malig-nancy. Furthermore, the interobserver reproducibiliy of these diagnoses is poor.[96] Historically, surgical intervention was commonly recommended for nodules with SFN/FN or AUS/FLUS cytologic findings, though the majority of patients would prove to have benign disease. For such patients, surgery was unnecessary yet exposed them to substantial morbidity, time lost for recovery, and excess health care cost. To address these issues, the field has witnessed a rapid expansion in the discovery, develop-ment, and validation of thyroid-specific molecular diag-nostic tests.

Historically, immunostaining for galectin-3 either alone or combined with TPO was suggested as a valuable adjunct to indeterminate nodules.[97] More recently, a series of 17 single gene oncogenic mutations or translocations in BRAF, RAS, RET/PTC, and PAX8/PPARγ demonstrated promise as an effective diagnostic marker for cytologically indetermi-nate thyroid nodules.[98-102] When detected, such mutations were initially felt to convey a very high positive predictive value and therefore hold promise as a "rule in" test. Although these data are validated when specific mutations in BRAF are detected, a recent blinded, multicenter pro-spective trial confirms worse test performance for the full 17-gene mutation panel than previously reported.[101] These data raise questions about the overall transferability of initial data into clinical practice, especially when applied to nodules with AUS/FLUS cytologic findings.[101] In general, the sensitivity and negative predictive value of the 17-gene mutation is not robust enough to warrant conservative management of indeterminate nodules with a negative (no mutations) result because many malignancies would be missed.[98,102]

A separate diagnostic molecular test has investigated the utility of an RNA gene expression classifier (GEC) using microarray technology. Through analysis of the expression patterns from 162 genes, a test was developed for use with nodules with SFN/FN and AUS/FLUS cytologic findings, with the goal of maximizing sensitivity and negative pre-dictive value. A prospective, blinded, multicenter valida-tion trial was performed enrolling nearly 4000 thyroid nodules with SFN/FN or AUS/FLUS cytologic findings.[103] A benign GEC test resulted in negative predictive values of 94% and 95%, respectively, which is similar to that of a benign FNA cytologic result itself. The positive predictive values were 37% and 38%, respectively. Further investiga-tions are under way to confirm these results and determine under what circumstances the expense of such testing is appropriately justified. Increasingly, molecular testing of cytologically indeterminate thyroid nodules is endorsed because of its ability to substantially improve preoperative cancer risk assessment and modify clinical care. For those in whom thyroid surgery is favored, use of the 17-gene mutation panel may prove most helpful, as its high specificity and positive predictive value will allow recom-mendations for partial versus near-total thyroidectomy.[102]

In contrast, for patients desiring nonoperative manage-ment, the GEC is favored because of its high sensitivity and negative predictive value. Furthermore, initial cost-effectiveness analyses have demonstrated a cost savings via this approach.[104]

MicroRNA testing has been proposed as a separate mo-lecular test for use in cytologically indeterminate nodules. Initial pilot data suggest potential for this approach, though no test is currently commercially available.[105] Further pro-spective validation is required.

The use of large-needle core biopsy in addition to stan-dard FNAB may improve diagnostic accuracy in difficult FNA cases, but the technique is associated with increased morbidity.[106] Particularly for cystic thyroid nodules, sam-pling from the margin of the nodule under ultrasound guidance, rather than from the cystic fluid and debris in the center, increases accuracy.

Initial nondiagnostic cytologic testing should prompt repeat ultrasound-guided FNA. If available, on-site cyto-logic evaluation will assist in ensuring an adequate speci-men for evaluation.[88,107-110] When the sonographic pattern of a nondiagnostic nodule is concerning, close observation or consideration for surgical excision should be given.[111] Although most nondiagnostic aspirates are due to cystic content, solid nodules with persistent nondiagnostic aspi-rates are associated with higher malignant risk. Repeat FNA of an initially nondiagnostic thyroid nodule yields ade-quate results in 60% to 80% of specimens.[109,112,113]

MANAGEMENT OF NONTOXIC DIFFUSE GOITER AND NODULAR THYROID DISEASE

Patients with small, asymptomatic, nontoxic goiters can be monitored by clinical examination and evaluated periodi-cally with ultrasound measurements. In fact, goiter growth can be variable, and some patients have stable goiters for many years. For more than a century, thyroid hormone supplementation was employed to reduce the size of non-toxic goiters. A 1953 report of Greer and Astwood, in which two thirds of patients' goiters regressed with thyroid therapy, led to widespread acceptance of suppressive therapy[114] despite some doubts about its value.[115] An over-view of studies performed from 1960 to 1992 suggested that 60% or more of sporadic nontoxic goiters responded to suppressive therapy.[115] In a prospective placebo-controlled, double-blind randomized clinical trial, 58% of the thyroxine-treated group had a significant response at 9 months, as measured by ultrasonography, in contrast with 5% after placebo.[116]

Patients with nodular thyroid disease appear to be less responsive to suppressive therapy than those with diffuse nontoxic goiters. A recent meta-analysis failed to demon-strate a significant benefit of thyroxine therapy, which was found to carry a relative risk of nodule shrinkage of only 1.9 (95% confidence interval, 0.95-3.81).[117] Statistical sig-nificance emerged from a multicenter, randomized, double-blind, placebo-controlled trial: after 18 months of follow-up the nodule shrinkage was significantly greater in the levo-thyroxine group than in the placebo group ($p = 0.01$), as well as the proportion of responders ($p = 0.04$).[118] It is likely that a subset of patients respond to thyroxine suppressive therapy, particularly younger patients with small or recently diagnosed nodules.[117] However, thyroid nodules rapidly return to the pretreatment size after discontinuation of therapy.[46] Therefore, maintainance of the size reduction may require continuous treatment.

A major concern in relation to long-term thyroxine suppression therapy is the possibility of detrimental effects on the skeleton and heart. It has been reported that TSH suppression therapy is associated with variable degrees of bone loss, particularly in postmenopausal women.[119,120] However, other studies did not demonstrate significant change in bone mass after long-term thyroxine therapy.[116] Furthermore, there is no evidence that levothyroxine per se is detrimental to the heart in young subjects when TSH is decreased to subnormal but still detectable values.[119,120]

Surgery for nontoxic goiter is physiologically unsound because it further restricts the ability of the thyroid to meet hormone requirements. Nevertheless, surgery may become necessary because of persistence of obstructive manifestations despite a trial of levothyroxine. Surgery should consist of a near-total or total thyroidectomy, but recurrence is seen in about 10% to 20% within 10 years.[121] Surgical complications have been reported in 7% to 10% of cases and are more common with large goiters and with reoperation.[122] Prophylactic treatment with levothyroxine after goiter resection probably does not prevent goiter recurrence.[123]

Traditionally, the role of ^{131}I therapy for nontoxic goiter was to reduce the size of a massive goiter in elderly patients who were poor candidates for surgery or to treat goiter that recurs after resection. However, several studies have demonstrated that primary treatment of nontoxic goiter with ^{131}I is followed by a reduction in thyroid volume.[124,125] In one study, thyroid volume (assessed by ultrasonography) was reduced by 40% after 1 year and 55% after 2 years with no further reduction thereafter, and 60% of the total reduction occurred within the first 3 months.[124]

Considering its effectiveness in reducing the size of the thyroid gland, ^{131}I therapy has also been used for the treatment of nonautonomous thyroid nodules: a significant shrinkage has been observed, ranging from 31% to 60%[126,127] (Fig. 14-4).

It was formerly argued that treatment of large goiters or goiters with substernal extension with ^{131}I should be avoided because of the risks of acute swelling of the gland and consequent tracheal compression. Ultrasonographic studies of thyroid volume after ^{131}I have failed to demonstrate significant early volume increase. Moreover, decreased tracheal deviation and increased tracheal lumen size were demonstrable by MRI in patients who had compression by nontoxic goiters with substernal extension.[124]

Therefore, it appears that ^{131}I treatment of nontoxic diffuse goiter or multinodular thyroid disease is effective and safe: hypothyroidism has been reported in 20% to 40%; transient thyrotoxicosis and mild pain can occur.[124] Regular follow-up, preferably by a systematic annual recall scheme, is necessary. The activities used are in the range of those used for ^{131}I treatment of hyperthyroidism, and thus radiation doses are comparable, and long-term thyroid and nonthyroidal cancer risk after ^{131}I treatment for hyperthyroidism is reassuring.[127,128] Stimulation with low doses of recombinant human TSH (rhTSH) (0.01 to 0.03 mg) increases the thyroid ^{131}I uptake and therefore may allow the administration of a lower dosage of ^{131}I, but rhTSH also increases thyroid hormone production, and overproduction of thyroid hormones should be excluded before its use.[129] Long-term randomized studies comparing the effects, side effects, and costs and benefits of surgery and ^{131}I treatment need to be performed.

Percutaneous ethanol injection (PEI) should be used only for recurrent symptomatic cystic nodules.[130] Laser ablation, cryoablation, and radiofrequency ablation are still generally experimental procedures and can be proposed, in experienced centers, for selected patients with symptomatic nodular goiters when surgery is not possible.[131]

MANAGEMENT OF MALIGNANT THYROID DISORDERS

Thyroid tumors are the most common endocrine neoplasms. The management of a patient with typical thyroid cancer is effective and usually consists of surgical resection, followed by medical therapy and regular surveillance.[1,3,4,132,133] Some degree of consensus has been achieved with regard to the initial management of differentiated thyroid cancer, but many important clinical and biologic questions remain unanswered. In the following discussion, a widely used scheme for classifying and staging tumors of the thyroid gland is presented. The distinguishing features of the principal types of benign and malignant thyroid neoplasms and the controversies in the management of differentiated thyroid carcinoma, based on recent consensus and guidelines, are also reviewed.[1,3,4]

Classification of Thyroid Tumors
Histologic Classification

Two monographs have had a major impact on the histologic classification of thyroid tumors. One is from the World Health Organization (WHO),[134] the other from the Armed Forces Institute of Pathology (AFIP).[135] The classification described in Table 14-5 is modified from the guidelines described by these organizations.

Lesions of follicular cell origin constitute more than 95% of the cases, and the remainder are largely made up of tumors exhibiting C-cell differentiation. Mixed medullary and follicular carcinomas, made up of cells with both C-cell and follicular differentiation, are rare and of uncertain histogenesis. Nonepithelial thyroid tumors mainly include malignant lymphomas, which may involve the thyroid gland as the only manifestation of the disease or as part of a systemic disease. True sarcomas and malignant hemangioendotheliomas are exceptional. Blood-borne metastases to the thyroid are not uncommon at autopsy in

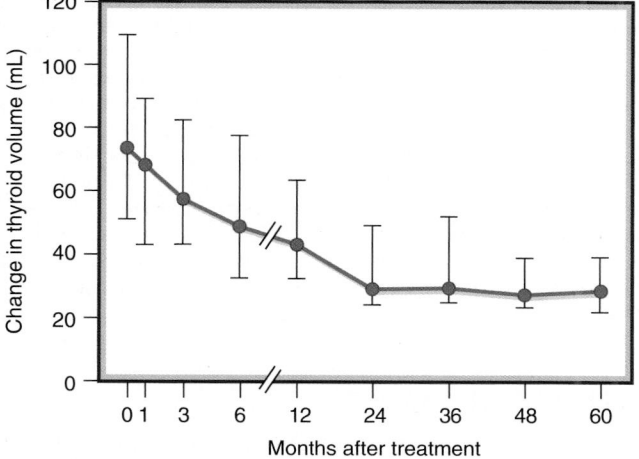

Figure 14-4 Median changes in thyroid volume alterations after ^{131}I treatment in 39 patients with nontoxic multinodular thyroid disease who remained euthyroid after a single dose. Vertical bars represent quartiles. (From Nygaard B, Hegedus L, Gervil M, et al. Radioiodine treatment of multinodular nontoxic goiter. *BMJ.* 1993;307: 828-832.)

TABLE 14-5

Classification of Thyroid Neoplasms

I. Primary Epithelial Tumors
  A. Tumors of Follicular Cells
    1. Benign: follicular adenoma
    2. Malignant: carcinoma
      a. Differentiated: papillary, follicular, poorly differentiated
      b. Undifferentiated (anaplastic)
  B. Tumors of C Cells
    1. Medullary carcinoma
  C. Tumors of Follicular and C Cells
    1. Mixed medullary-follicular carcinomas
II. Primary Nonepithelial Tumors
  A. Malignant Lymphomas
  B. Sarcomas
  C. Others
III. Secondary Tumors

patients with widespread malignancy but rarely cause clinically detectable thyroid enlargement.

Staging of Thyroid Carcinoma

In addition to the histologic classification of thyroid tumors developed by the WHO and AFIP groups, the International Union Against Cancer (UICC) and the American Joint Committee on Cancer (AJCC) have agreed on a staging system in thyroid cancer.[136-138] As stated by the AJCC, "The principal purpose served by international agreement on the classification of cancer cases by extent of disease was to provide a method of conveying clinical experience to others without ambiguity."[137]

The AJCC based its system of classification on the TNM (tumor-node-metastasis) system, which relies on assessing three components: (1) extent of the primary tumor (T), (2) absence or presence of regional lymph node metastases (N), and (3) absence or presence of distant metastases (M).

The TNM system allows a reasonably precise description and recording of the anatomic extent of disease. The classification may be either *clinical* (cTNM), based on evidence (including biopsy) acquired before treatment, or *pathologic* (pTNM), by which intraoperative and surgical pathologic data are available. Obviously, pTNM classification is preferable because a precise size can be assigned to the primary tumor, the histotype is identified, and extrathyroid invasion is demonstrated unequivocally.

Typically, in the earliest (1992) TNM classification,[136] the primary thyroid tumor (T) status was defined according to the size of the primary lesion: *T1*, greatest diameter 1 cm or smaller; *T2*, larger than 1 cm but not larger than 4 cm; T3, larger than 4 cm; and T4, direct (extrathyroidal) extension or invasion through the thyroid capsule. Therefore, a thyroid tumor with four degrees of T, two degrees of N, and two degrees of M could have 16 different TNM categories.

For purposes of tabulation and analysis, these categories were condensed into a convenient number of TNM stage groupings (Table 14-6). Whereas head and neck cancer was usually staged entirely on the basis of anatomic extent, in thyroid cancer staging both the histologic diagnosis and the age of the patient for PTC and follicular thyroid carcinoma (FTC) were included because of their importance in predicting the behavior and prognosis of thyroid cancer.

According to this staging scheme, first devised in 1992, all patients younger than age 45 years with PTC or FTC were considered to be stage I, unless they had distant metastases, in which case they would be in stage II. In young patients and especially in children, the risk of recurrence is high and may be underestimated by the TNM staging system.[139] Older patients (aged 45 years or older) with node-negative papillary or follicular microcarcinoma (*T1* N0 M0) were in stage I. Tumors between 1.1 and 4.0 cm were classified as stage II, and those with either nodal spread (N1) or extrathyroidal invasion (T4) are stage III.

The subsequent TNM classifications, published in 2002 and 2010, are more complicated, and the definition of minimal (T3) or more extensive (T4) thyroid tumor extension frequently may be difficult to define retrospectively.[137,138] Six lymph nodes, according to the newer TNM classifications, need to be examined at histologic diagnosis to qualify for the definition of N0. To date, prognostic differences and, especially, the differing risk of cause-specific mortality between central lymph node metastases (N1a) and other regional metastases (N1b) has yet to be widely validated; in fact, the risk of persistent/recurrent disease appears to be more related to the number and size of involved lymph nodes and the number of lymph nodes with extracapsular extension, but these characteristics are not taken into account in the current classification.[3,140,141] Another feature of the latest (7th edition) TNM classification was the introduction of a new definition of *T1* as tumors of up to 2-cm diameter, with subdivisions of T1a for tumors 1 cm or smaller and T1b for tumors from 1.1 cm up to 2 cm. Thus, what had been classically considered as a papillary thyroid microcarcinoma (PTM) would now be classified as a T1a tumor. Additionally, more complexity in the form of subclasses T3, T4a, and T4b was introduced to the extent of extrathyroidal invasion, as outlined in the accompanying Table 14-6.

For MTC, the scheme is similar, in that *T1* N0 M0 carcinoma is stage I, but *T2*-T3 N0 M0 is stage II and a *T1*-T3 N1a M0 tumor is stage III, underlying the prognostic impact of lymph node involvement. There is no age distinction for MTC, although age is a significant independent prognostic indicator in most multivariate analyses.[142-144]

All anaplastic carcinomas are considered T4 tumors. T4a describes tumors of any size limited to the thyroid, and T4b applies to a tumor of any size that extends beyond the thyroid capsule. All anaplastic carcinomas are staged IV, stage IVA being T4a, any N, M0; stage IVB being T4b, any N, M0; and stage IVC being any T, any N, and M1.

The UICC staging system predicts disease mortality risk but has also been used in practice to predict the risk of persistent/recurrent disease. Two other systems, more designed to predict postoperative tumor recurrence, have recently been established: the ATA initial risk stratification, based on clinical-pathologic features available after initial surgery, was introduced in the 2009 ATA guidelines and was refined in the 2014 ATA guidelines; it predicts the risk of structural persistent or recurrent disease. The ATA "response to therapy system" acknowledges that risk of recurrence and mortality risk change over time and that a reassessment of risk is required at each step of follow-up. The two latter systems are further discussed later in this chapter.

Follicular Adenoma

A follicular adenoma is a benign, encapsulated tumor with evidence of follicular cell differentiation.[134,135] It is the most common thyroid neoplasm and may be found in 4% to 20% of glands examined at autopsy.[145] The tumor has a well-defined fibrous capsule that is grossly and microscopically complete. There is a sharp demarcation and

TABLE 14-6

The Tumor-Node-Metastasis (TNM) Scoring System[136-138]

		Definition of TNM
1992 Version	**2002 Version**	**2010 Version**
Primary Tumor (T)		
T0:	No evidence of primary tumor	No evidence of primary tumor
T1:	Tumor ≤1 cm limited to the thyroid	Tumor ≤2 cm limited to the thyroid T1a: ≤1 cm T1b: >1 cm to 2 cm
T2:	Tumor >1 to ≤4 cm limited to the thyroid	Tumor >2 to ≤4 cm limited to the thyroid
T3:	Tumor >4 cm limited to the thyroid	Tumor >4 cm limited to the thyroid or any tumor with minimal extrathyroid extension (e.g., extension to sternothyroid muscle or perithyroid soft tissues)
T4:	Any size extending beyond the thyroid capsule	
T4a:		Tumor of any size with extension beyond the thyroid capsule and invades any of the following: subcutaneous soft tissues, larynx, trachea, esophagus, recurrent laryngeal nerve
T4b:		Tumor invades prevertebral fascia or mediastinal vessels or encases carotid artery
Regional Lymph Node (N)		
N0:	No regional lymph node metastasis	No regional lymph node metastasis*
N1:	Regional lymph node metastasis	Regional lymph node metastasis
N1a:		Metastases in pretracheal and paratracheal lymph nodes, including prelaryngeal and delphian lymph nodes
N1b:		Metastases in other unilateral, bilateral, or contralateral cervical or upper mediastinal lymph nodes
Distant Metastases (M)		
M0:	No distant metastasis	No distant metastasis
M1:	Distant metastasis	Distant metastasis
		TNM Staging†
1992 Version	**2002 Version**	**2010 Version**
Age <45 Years		
Stage I:	Any T, any N, M0	Any T, any N, M0
Stage II:	Any T, any N, M1	Any T, any N, M1
Stage III:	None	None
Stage IV:	None	None
Age ≥45 Years		
Stage I:	T1, N0, M0	T1, N0, M0
Stage II:	T2-T3, N0, M0	T2, N0, M0
Stage III:	T4, N0, M0 or any T, N1, M0	T3, N0, M0 or any T1-3, N1a, M0
Stage IV:	Any T, any N, M1	
Stage IVA		T1-3, N1b, M0 or T4a, any N, M0
Stage IVB		T4b, any N, M0
Stage IVC		Any T, any N, M1

*To classify as N0, at least six lymph nodes should be included at histologic examination. Otherwise, the disease is classified as Nx (2002) or N0 if the lymph nodes are negative but the number ordinarily examined is not met (2010).
†Stage grouping for papillary and follicular thyroid carcinomas.

distinct structural difference from the surrounding parenchyma. These adenomas vary in size, but most have a diameter of 1 to 3 cm at the time of excision. Degenerative changes, including necrosis, hemorrhage, edema, fibrosis, or calcification, are common features, particularly in larger tumors.

Follicular adenomas can be classified into subtypes according to the size or presence of follicles and degree of cellularity. Each adenoma tends to have a consistent architectural pattern. *Microfollicular, normofollicular,* and *macrofollicular* adenomas owe their names to the size of their follicles compared with follicles in the neighboring, nonneoplastic areas of the gland. *Trabecular adenomas* are cellular and consist of columns of cells arranged in compact cords. They show little follicle formation and rarely contain colloid. A variant, the *hyalinizing trabecular adenoma,* has unusually elongated cells and prominent hyaline changes in the extracellular space.[146]

The histologic differences among these subtypes are striking but of no clinical importance. The only practical value of the classification is that the more cellular a follicular nodule is, the more one should search for evidence of malignancy in the form of invasion of blood vessels and capsule, either singly or in combination.[134,135] Atypical adenomas are hypercellular or heterogeneous, or both, with gross and histologic appearances that suggest the possibility of malignancy but not invasion. Classification of these tumors is difficult and poorly reproducible among pathologists. They account for fewer than 3% of all follicular adenomas. Follow-up indicates that this lesion behaves in a benign fashion. However, the fact that the tumor does not recur or produce metastases after removal does not prove that it is actually benign; removal may have interrupted a natural history that would have culminated in invasion and metastases. For this reason they are classified as tumors of *undefined malignancy*.

The most important cytologic variant is the *oxyphilic* or *oncocytic (Hürthle cell) adenoma*, which is composed predominantly (at least 75%) or entirely of large cells with granular, eosinophilic cytoplasm.[147] Ultrastructurally, the cells are rich in mitochondria and may exhibit nuclear pleomorphism with distinct nucleoli. Although all such neoplasms are thought by some to be potentially malignant,[148] the biologic behavior and clinical course of oncocytic tumors correlate closely with the histologic appearance and the size of the initial lesion. The absence of invasion predicts a benign outcome,[147] but larger tumors may rarely be associated with later recurrence or metastases, even in the absence of obvious microscopic evidence of invasion; fortunately, such an occurrence is rare, and generally a diagnosis of benign Hürthle cell adenoma is reliable.[149,150]

Some normofollicular adenomas may contain pseudopapillary structures that can be confused with the papillae of papillary carcinoma. These structures are probably an expression of localized hyperactivity and are most common in adenomas that show autonomous function.

In the majority of hyperfunctioning follicular adenomas, activating point mutations have been identified in the TSHR or in the α-subunit of the stimulatory guanyl nucleotide protein ($G_s\alpha$) (Fig. 14-5).[52,151] Such mutations result in a constitutive hyperstimulation of the cells. Genetic abnormalities found in hypofunctioning adenomas are detailed later.

Papillary Thyroid Carcinoma

PTC has been defined as "a malignant epithelial tumor showing evidence of follicular cell differentiation, and characterized by the formation of papillae and/or a set of distinctive nuclear changes."[134,135] The most common thyroid malignancy, PTC constitutes 50% to 90% of differentiated FCTCs worldwide.[59,152]

PTM or pT1a is defined by WHO as a PTC 1.0 cm in diameter or smaller.[134,153,154] The incidence rate in the United States for clinically diagnosed PTM (approximately 1 per 100,000) is lower than that reported for tumors larger than 1 cm in diameter (approximately 5 per 100,000) and than the incidence of PTM in autopsy material from various continents (4-36%).[59,134,135] Screening is responsible for the increased detection of small PTCs that is currently observed in all industrialized countries.[59-61] Since the early 80s, the incidence of larger tumors has not increased significantly. Therefore, a large majority of thyroid cancers at diagnosis are currently small tumors with limited extension that carry an excellent prognosis and should not be overtreated. Protocols for initial treatment and follow-up should be modified accordingly.

PTCs appear as firm, unencapsulated or partially encapsulated tumors. PTCs may be partly necrotic and some are cystic. The presence of necrosis and a high mitotic rate are associated with an aggressive behavior similar to that of poorly differentiated thyroid cancer.[31,155] Typically, PTC shows a predominance of papillary structures, consisting of a fibrovascular core lined by a single layer of epithelial cells, but the papillae are usually admixed with neoplastic follicles having characteristic nuclear features.

The nuclei of PTC cells have a distinctive appearance that has a diagnostic significance comparable to that of the papillae. Indeed, the preoperative diagnosis of PTC can often be made on the basis of the characteristic nuclear changes seen in FNA material: nuclei are larger than in normal follicular cells and overlap; they may be fissured like coffee beans; chromatin is hypodense (ground-glass nuclei); limits are irregular; and they frequently contain an inclusion corresponding to a cytoplasmic invagination.

Psammoma bodies are often present in the core of papillae or in the tumor stroma; they are microscopic structures of calcified layers.

Several subtypes exist and account for about 20% of all PTCs: the tumor is designated a *follicular variant* of PTC when the lining cells of the neoplastic follicles have the same nuclear features as seen in typical PTC and the follicular predominance over the papillae is complete; the encapsulated follicular variant is associated with a favorable outcome.[134,135] The *diffuse sclerosing variant* is characterized by diffuse involvement of one or both thyroid lobes, widespread lymphatic permeation, prominent fibrosis, and lymphoid infiltration. The *tall cell variant* is characterized by well-formed papillae that are covered by cells twice as tall as they are wide. The *columnar cell variant* differs from other forms of PTC because of the presence of prominent nuclear stratification of elongated cells. The hobnail variant with *micropapillary pattern* is a recently recognized poor prognostic finding.[156] The tall cell and columnar cell variants are more aggressive, but controversy exists regarding outcome for the diffuse sclerosing variant.[133]

In children, PTCs represent the large majority of cases, and histologic subtypes include the classical PTC, the presence of solid trabecular features (of unknown prognostic significance), the follicular variant, and the diffuse sclerosing variant. Tumor extension is usually substantial at diagnosis: tumors are large, multifocal, unencapsulated, and invasive. Extension beyond the thyroid capsule, lymph node metastases, and lung metastases are frequently observed.[139,157,158]

Molecular Pathogenesis

The thyroid follicular cell may give rise to both benign and malignant tumors, and the malignancy can be of either papillary or follicular histotype. There is no evidence that human benign tumors ever undergo malignant transformation into classical PTC. Structural abnormalities of the chromosomes may occur in about 50% of PTCs, frequently involving the long arm of chromosome 10.[102,151,159-162] The *RET* proto-oncogene is located on chromosome 10q11-2. It encodes a transmembrane receptor with a tyrosine kinase

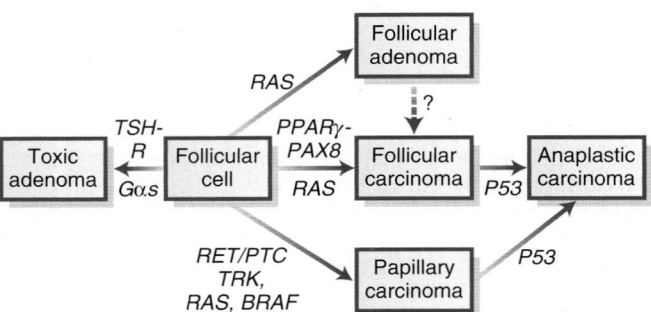

Figure 14-5 Genetic events in thyroid tumorigenesis. Activating point mutations of the *RAS* genes are found with a high frequency in both follicular adenomas and follicular carcinomas and are considered an early event in follicular tumorigenesis. The PPARγ-PAX8 rearrangement is found only in follicular tumors. Rearrangements of transmembrane receptors with tyrosine kinase activity (*RET/PTC*, *TRK* genes) and activating point mutation of the *BRAF* gene are found only in papillary thyroid carcinomas (PTCs). Inactivating point mutations of the *P53* gene are found only in poorly differentiated and anaplastic thyroid carcinomas. Activation of the cyclic adenosine monophosphate pathway, by point mutation of the thyrotropin receptor (TSH-R) or the α-subunit of the G protein genes, leads to the appearance of hyperfunctioning thyroid nodules. Gαs, α-subunit of stimulatory guanyl nucleotide protein; PPAR, peroxisome proliferator–activated receptor.

domain. Its ligands, such as the glial cell line–derived neutrophilic factor (GDNF), bind to the GDNF receptor (the GFRα-1) and induce RET protein dimerization. *RET* (REarranged during Transfection) activation was first demonstrated in transfection experiments and has been found only in PTC tumors. It was therefore called *RET/PTC*.[162,163]

All activated forms of the *RET* proto-oncogene are the consequence of oncogenic rearrangements fusing the tyrosine kinase domain of the *RET* gene with the 5′ domain of different genes. The foreign gene is constitutively expressed, and its 5′ domain acts as a promoter, resulting in permanent expression of the *RET* gene. Furthermore, these genes have domains that induce *RET* activation by permanent dimerization. Because of this fusion, the chimeric protein is localized in the cytoplasm and not in the plasma cell membrane.

Three major classes of *RET/PTC* have been identified: *RET/PTC1* is formed by an intrachromosomal rearrangement fusing the *RET* tyrosine kinase domain to a gene designated *H4 (CCDC6)*. *RET/PTC2* is formed by an interchromosomal rearrangement fusing the *RET* tyrosine kinase domain to a gene located on chromosome 17 encoding the RIα regulatory subunit of protein kinase A. *RET/PTC3* is formed by an intrachromosomal rearrangement fusing the *RET* tyrosine kinase domain to a gene designated RFG *(NCOA4)*. Several other variants of *RET/PTC* have been observed in post-Chernobyl thyroid tumors, including rearrangements formed by fusing the tyrosine kinase domain of the RET gene at other breakpoint sites or with other partners.

The frequency of *RET/PTC* rearrangements occurring in adult PTC patients without prior childhood neck irradiation varies widely among series (average less than 10%). In these tumors, the frequencies of *RET/PTC1* and *RET/PTC3* were similar and that of *RET/PTC2* was lower. The *RET/PTC* rearrangements were more frequently found (in 60-80% of cases) in PTC cases occurring either in children, even in the absence of radiation exposure, or in subjects of any age after radiation exposure during childhood, either external irradiation or contamination after the Chernobyl accident.[151,161] *RET/PTC3* was more frequently found in aggressive tumors that occurred early after the accident, and *RET/PTC1* in classic variant tumors that are less aggressive and occurred later. The finding of *RET/PTC* rearrangement in micropapillary thyroid carcinomas suggests that it constitutes an early event in thyroid carcinogenesis. On the other hand, *RET/PTC*-positive tumors lack evidence of progression to poorly or undifferentiated tumor phenotypes. Among thyroid cancer tissues from Ukraine, fusion oncogenes that arose primarily through intrachromosomal rearrangements and that aberrantly activate mitogen-activated protein kinase (MAPK) signaling were more frequently found in the tumors from patients who were younger than 10 years of age and living in contaminated areas during the time of the Chernobyl nuclear reactor accident than in tumors from children that had not been exposed to radiation.[164] An activating point mutation of the *RAS* genes is found in 10% to 20% of PTCs and mostly in the follicular variant.[165] A single activating point mutation of the *BRAF* gene at codon 600 (V600E) is found in 40% (range 29-69%) of PTCs occurring in adults.[166] Its presence did not overlap with *RET/PTC* or *RAS* mutation, and it was rarely found in PTC occurring in children or following neck exposure to radiation.[159] *BRAF* mutation is more frequently found in the tall cell variant and less frequently in the follicular variant; it has not been found in other thyroid tumor types.[166] Finally, an intrachromosomal rearrangement of the *BRAF* gene with the *AKAP9* gene has been found in PTCs occurring after the Chernobyl accident.[167]

Several additional oncogenes may occasionally be involved in PTC, including *NTRK1* (also named *TRKA*), which codes for a neural growth factor receptor with a tyrosine kinase domain and which is activated by rearrangement in less than 10% of PTCs.[168,169] Rearrangement of the anaplastic lymphoma kinase *(ALK)* gene has been found in few PTCs.[170] The receptor for hepatocyte growth factor is a transmembrane tyrosine kinase encoded by the *MET* oncogene; it is overexpressed in some patients with PTC, and low expression has been associated with the occurrence of distant metastases.[171]

Mutations in the promoter of the gene for telomerase reverse transcriptase (TERT) were found in 12% of PTCs, and more frequently in *BRAF* mutated PTCs; the tumor recurrence rate was 8.5-fold greater in patients who had both mutations compared with patients with neither mutation.[172]

Multiple other abnormalities have been found in follicular cell–derived tumors, including overexpression of vascular endothelial growth factor (VEGF) and of VEGF receptors (VEGFRs) and activation of other angiogenic pathways (fibroblast growth factor [FGF] and platelet-derived growth factor [PDGF] pathways), in line with the hypervascularization observed in these tumors.[173,174] These pathways may be targets for therapies.

In conclusion, the *RET/PTC, RAS, BRAF*, MAPK pathway is activated in at least 90% of sporadic or radiation-induced PTCs, and mutations affecting this pathway are considered as initiating events of PTC.[159] These data have been confirmed by the genome analysis of 496 PTC tumors, which also demonstrated that *BRAF* mutation is associated with a less differentiated phenotype although more heterogeneous than with *RAS* mutations.[175]

PTC has been associated with the deregulation of a specific set of microRNAs. Upregulation of miR-221, -222, -146b, and -181b was reported in several studies and may induce the loss of cell cycle control.[105]

A high incidence of PTC has been reported in patients with adenomatous polyposis coli who have a peculiar histologic appearance, with solid areas and elongated cells, and Cowden disease (the multiple hamartoma syndrome), suggesting that the predisposing genes may play a role in the occurrence of papillary carcinoma. The familial risk of thyroid cancer is higher than for other cancers, and about 3% to 10% of cases of PTC are familial[176]; their behavior is similar to or slightly more aggressive than that of nonfamilial cases.[177] At least five loci of predisposition have been individualized but they do not explain all hereditary cases[178-182]: the gene predisposing to familial thyroid tumors with cellular oxyphilia has been mapped to chromosome 19q13.2, and in a family with PTC and renal carcinoma a separate gene was mapped to chromosome 1p13.2.q22. Variants of two genes, *FOXE1* (TTF2) located at chromosomal locus at 9q22, and *NKX2-1* (TTF1) on 14q, both coding for thyroid-specific transcription factors, confer an increased risk of thyroid cancer.

The expression of thyroid-specific genes has been studied at the messenger ribonucleic acid (mRNA) and protein levels in large series of human thyroid tumors. Expression of *NIS* was profoundly decreased in both benign and malignant thyroid hypofunctioning nodules; moreover, in malignant nodules, low expression of TPO, PDS, and Tg was also found.[79] These abnormalities clearly explain many of the metabolic defects typically observed in thyroid cancer tissues: a low iodine concentration, a low rate of iodine organification, a low hormonal synthesis, and a short intrathyroidal half-life of iodine. NIS expression is heterogeneous among tumor cells.[79] However, Tg is expressed in variable amounts in almost all FCTCs and can be shown by immunohistochemistry, which can prove useful in cases with atypical histologic appearance. Also, TSHR is expressed in many FCTCs, and TSH may stimulate both their differentiation and growth.[79] Loss of differentiation is induced by *BRAF* mutation and by the activation of the MAPK pathway and can be reverted in experimental models and in humans by *BRAF* or MEK inhibitors.[183,184] In distant metastases from radioiodine refractory thyroid cancer, *BRAF* mutations are overrepresented, and the *RAS* and *BRAF* mutation spectrum was concordant with the primary tumor and between metastases; in contrast, *PIK3CA/AKT1* mutations may arise during progression.[185] *RAS* mutations are overrepresented in distant metastases with radioiodine uptake. Radioiodine therapy is ineffective in achieving cure in many patients with radioiodine avid metastatic disease, and recent evidence suggest that pretreatment with BRAF or MEK inhibitors enhances responses to ^{131}I, particularly in patients with *RAS*-mutant tumors.[184,186]

Presenting Features

Although PTCs can occur at any age, most occur in patients between 30 and 50 years of age (mean age, 45 years). Women are affected more frequently (female predominance, 60-80%). Most primary tumors are 1 to 4 cm, and in recent years the proportion of small tumors is increasing, largely due to detection of small PTCs by screening.[59,60,133,152,187] PTC is frequently multifocal when it occurs in a single lobe and is bilateral in 20% to 80% of cases, depending on whether or not the thyroid is meticulously examined. Some studies have suggested that contralateral PTCs may have independent clonal origins, but this idea remains controversial.[188] Extrathyroidal invasion of adjacent soft tissues is present in about 15% (range 5-34%) at primary surgery, and clinically evident lymphadenopathy at presentation is rarely associated with small thyroid tumors.[133,152] About 35% to 50% of excised neck nodes have histologic evidence of involvement, and in patients 17 years of age or younger nodal involvement may be present in up to 90%.[139,157,158,189] Only 1% to 7% of PTC patients have distant metastases at diagnosis.[133,152] Spread to superior mediastinal nodes is usually associated with extensive neck nodal involvement.

The TNM classification, as described earlier in this chapter, is a widely used system for tumor staging.[190] Most PTC patients presented with either stage I (60%) or stage II (22%), and in recent years the proportion of stage I tumors is increasing. Patients aged 45 years or older with either nodal metastases or extrathyroidal extension account for fewer than 20% of cases.[133,152] As already noted, few (1-7%) PTC patients present with distant metastases and have stage IV disease. Figure 14-6 (upper left) illustrates the distribution of pTNM stages in 2284 PTC cases seen at the Mayo Clinic, and Figure 14-7 demonstrates survival by TNM stage in this cohort of PTC patients treated from 1940 to 1997. In the figures shown in this chapter illustrating outcome results from the Mayo Clinic 1940-1997 cohort of PTC patients, the pTNM stages are derived from the older (2002) definition, in part, because of the challenges in defining from available records the N1a versus N1b status, and the exact location of the extrathyroidal extension necessary to ascribe T4a or T4b status to the tumor extent at surgery.

Recurrence and Mortality

Three types of tumor recurrences may occur with PTC: postoperative *nodal metastases* (NM), *local recurrence* (LR), and postoperative *distant metastases* (DM).

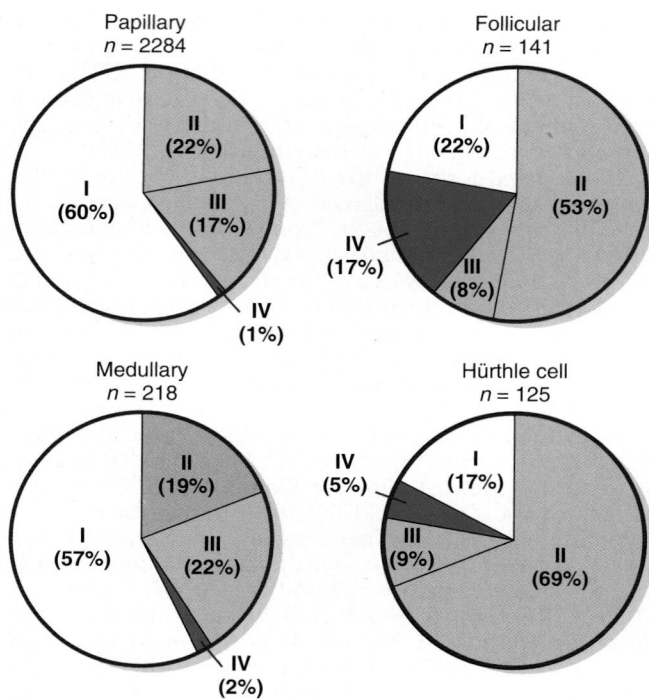

Figure 14-6 Distribution of pathologic tumor-node-metastasis (pTNM) stages in 2284 patients with papillary thyroid carcinoma *(upper left)*, 218 patients with medullary thyroid cancer *(lower left)*, 141 patients with follicular thyroid cancer *(upper right)*, and 125 patients with Hürthle cell cancer *(lower right)* undergoing primary surgical treatment at the Mayo Clinic from 1940 to 1997.

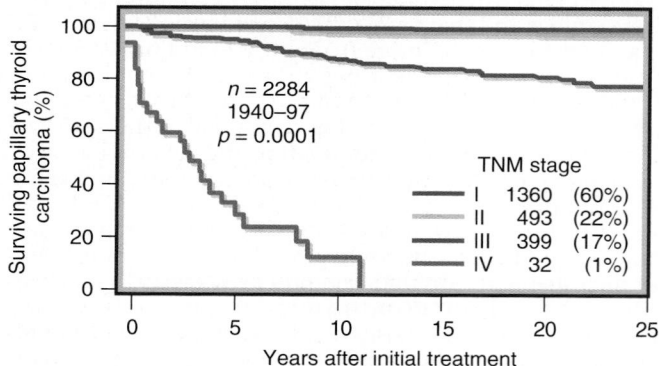

Figure 14-7 Cause-specific survival rate according to pathologic tumor-node-metastasis (pTNM) stage in a cohort of 2284 patients with papillary thyroid carcinoma treated at the Mayo Clinic from 1940 to 1997. The numbers in parentheses represent the percentages of patients in each pTNM stage grouping.

Local recurrence may be defined as "histologically confirmed tumor occurring in the resected thyroid bed, thyroid remnant, or other adjacent tissues of the neck (excluding lymph nodes)" after complete surgical removal of the primary tumor.[191] Nodal or distant spread may be considered postoperative if the metastases are discovered within 180 or 30 days, respectively.[133] Ideally, tumor recurrence should be considered only as it occurs in patients without initial distant metastases who had complete surgical resection of the primary tumors.

Figure 14-8 illustrates rates of PTC recurrence at local, nodal, and distant sites in 2150 patients with PTC treated at one institution from 1940 to 1997. After 20 years of follow-up, postoperative nodal metastases had been discovered in 9%, and local recurrence and distant metastases

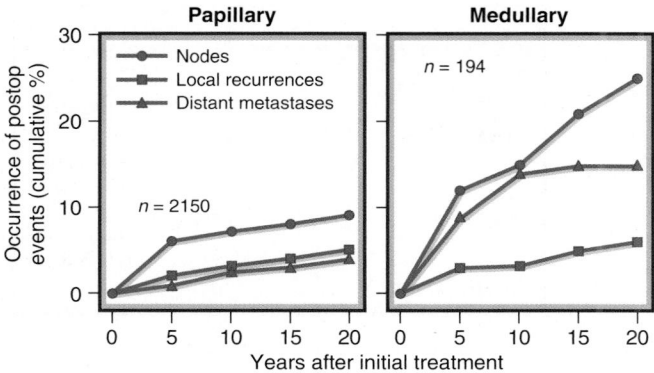

Figure 14-8 Development of neck nodal metastases, local recurrences, and distant metastases in the first 20 years after definitive surgery for papillary thyroid cancer (PTC) or medullary thyroid cancer (MTC) performed at the Mayo Clinic from 1940 to 1997. Based on 2150 consecutive PTC *(left)* and 194 MTC *(right)* patients who had complete surgical resection (i.e., had no gross residual disease) and were without distant metastases on initial examination. Postop, postoperative.

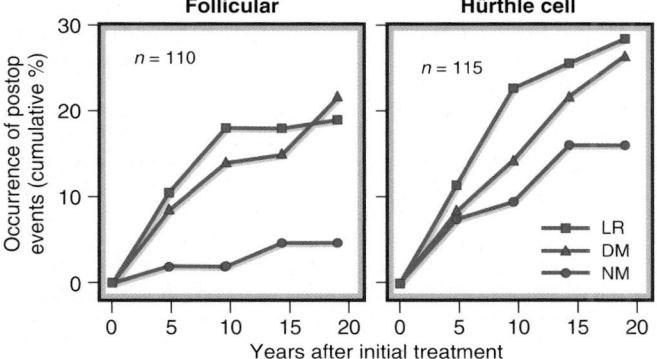

Figure 14-9 Development of neck nodal metastases (NM), local recurrences (LR), and distant metastases (DM) in the first 20 years after definitive surgery for follicular thyroid cancer (FTC) or Hürthle cell cancer (HCC) performed at the Mayo Clinic from 1940 to 1997. Based on 110 consecutive FTC patients *(left)* and 115 HCC patients *(right)* who had complete surgical resection and were without distant metastases on initial examination. Postop, postoperative.

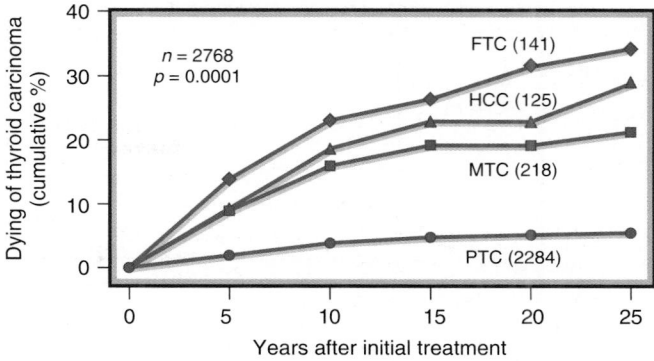

Figure 14-10 Cumulative cause-specific mortality rates for patients with differentiated thyroid carcinoma in the first 25 years after treatment with initial surgery performed at the Mayo Clinic from 1940 to 1997. Based on 2768 consecutively treated patients (2284 with papillary thyroid carcinoma [PTC], 141 with follicular thyroid cancer [FTC], 125 with Hürthle cell cancer [HCC], and 218 with medullary thyroid cancer [MTC]).

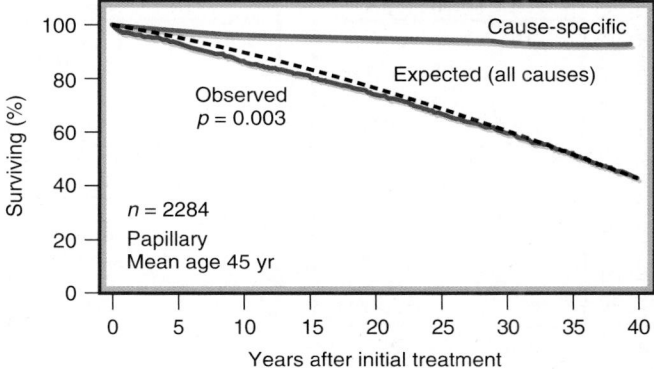

Figure 14-11 Survival to death from all causes and to death from thyroid cancer (cause-specific mortality) in 2284 consecutive patients with papillary thyroid carcinoma undergoing initial management at the Mayo Clinic from 1940 to 1997. Also plotted *(dashed line)* is the expected survival (all causes) of persons of the same age and sex and with the same date of treatment but living under mortality risk conditions of the northwest central United States.

occurred in 5% and 4%, respectively. Both local recurrence and distant metastases are less common in PTC than in FTC (Fig. 14-9). However, postoperative cases of nodal metastases were more frequent in PTC than in FTC.

Cause-specific mortality (CSM) rates for differentiated thyroid cancer are shown in Figure 14-10. CSM rates for PTC were 2% at 5 years, 4% at 10 years, and 5% at 20 years. Among those with lethal PTC, 20% of deaths occurred in the first year after diagnosis, and 80% of the deaths occurred within 10 years. The 25-year cause-specific survival rate of 95% for PTC was significantly higher than the 79%, 71%, and 66% rates seen with MTC, Hürthle cell cancer (HCC), and FTC, respectively.

Outcome Prediction

Only a fraction (~15-25%) of patients with PTC are likely to experience relapse of disease, and even fewer (~5%) have a lethal outcome. Exceptional patients, who have an aggressive course, tend to experience relapse early (Fig. 14-11), and the rare fatalities usually occur within 5 to 10 years of diagnosis.[133,152] Multivariate analyses have been used to identify variables predictive of CSM.[152,192-198] Increasing age of the patient and the presence of extrathyroidal invasion are independent prognostic factors in all studies.

The presence of initial distant metastases and large size of the primary tumor are also significant variables in most studies,[152,192-194,197] and some groups [133,152,193-196] have reported that histopathologic grade (degree of differentiation) is an independent variable. The completeness of initial tumor resection (postoperative status) is also a predictor of fatality.[133,193,197] The presence of initial neck nodal metastases, although relevant to future nodal recurrence, does not influence CSM rate (Fig. 14-12).[133,152,197]

Several scoring systems based on these significant prognostic indicators have been devised. Each system allows one to assign the majority of PTC patients (80% or more) to a low-risk group, in which the CSM rate at 25 years is less than 2%, and the others (a small minority) to a high-risk group, in which almost all cancer-related deaths are observed. In general, these systems provide prediction of postoperative events comparable to that of the internationally accepted TNM staging system.[198]

A scoring index devised to assign PTC patients to prognostic risk groups[192] was named the AGES scheme after the four independent variables: patient's *a*ge, tumor *g*rade, tumor *e*xtent (local invasion, distant metastases), and tumor *s*ize. With the use of such a scoring system, 86% of patients were in the minimal-risk group (AGES score <4) and they experienced a 20-year CSM rate of only 1%.[133] By

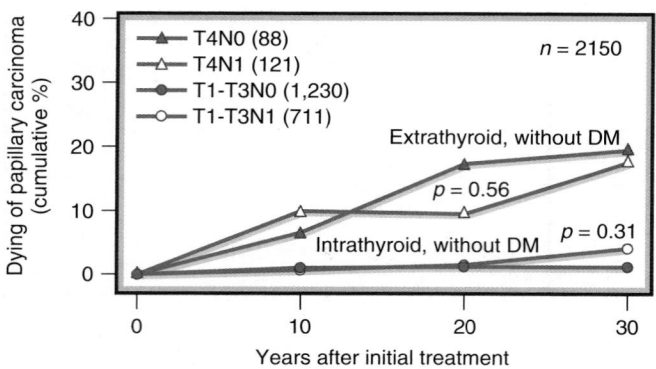

Figure 14-12 Lack of influence of nodal metastases at initial operation on cumulative mortality from papillary thyroid carcinoma in 1941 patients with pathologic T1 to T3 intrathyroidal tumors (completely confined to the thyroid gland) and 209 pathologic T4 patients with extrathyroidal (locally invasive) tumors. All patients had initial surgical treatment at the Mayo Clinic from 1940 to 1997. DM, distant metastases.

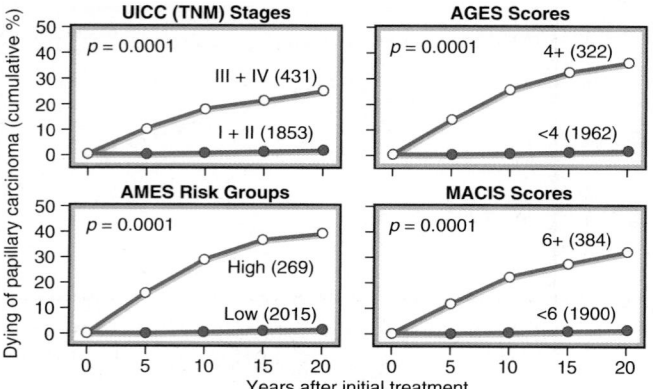

Figure 14-13 Cumulative mortality from papillary thyroid carcinoma in patients at either minimal risk or higher risk of cancer-related death as defined by International Union Against Cancer (UICC) pathologic tumor-node-metastasis (pTNM) stages *(upper left)*, AGES scores *(upper right)*, AMES risk groups *(lower left)*, and MACIS scores *(lower right)*. The minimal risk group constitutes 81% of the 2284 patients when defined by pTNM stages I and II, 86% as defined by AGES scores less than 4, 88% as defined by AMES low risk, and 83% when defined by a MACIS score less than 6. The cause-specific mortality (CSM) rates at 20 years were 25% for stages III and IV, 36% for AGES scores of 4+, 39% for AMES high risk, and 32% for patients with MACIS scores of 6+. The ratios between the CSM rates for high-risk versus low-risk groups at 20 years were 19 for pTNM, 36 for AGES, 35 for AMES, and 40 for MACIS. AGES, patient's *a*ge, tumor *g*rade, tumor *e*xtent (local invasion, distant metastases), and tumor *s*ize; AMES, *a*ge, *m*etastasis, *e*xtent, *s*ize; MACIS, *m*etastasis, *a*ge, *c*ompleteness of resection, *i*nvasion, and *s*ize.

contrast, patients with AGES scores of 4+ (high risk; 14% of the total) had a 20-year CSM rate of 36%.

Figure 14-13 compares the AGES scores with TNM stage and with two other subsequently introduced schemes designed to stratify PTC patients into groups at either minimal risk or high risk of cancer-related death. Such prognostic scoring systems make it possible to counsel patients and to aid in the planning of individualized postoperative management programs in PTC.[192,197]

Although the AGES scheme had the potential for universal application, some academic centers could not include the differentiation (G) variable because their surgical pathologists did not recognize higher-grade PTC tumors.[198] Accordingly, a prognostic scoring system for predicting PTC mortality rates was devised with the use of candidate variables that included completeness of primary tumor

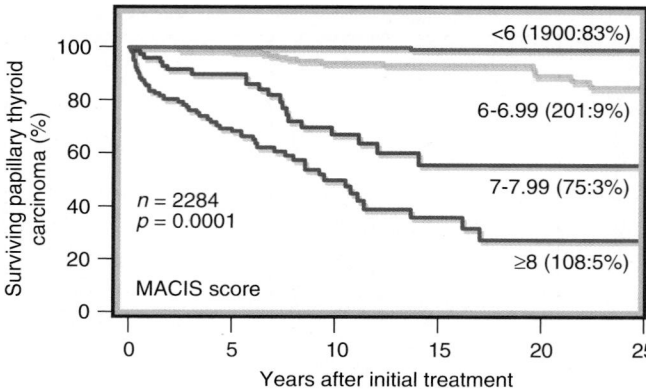

Figure 14-14 Cause-specific survival according to MACIS (*m*etastases, *a*ge, *c*ompleteness of resection, *i*nvasion, and *s*ize) scores of less than 6, 6 to 6.99, 7 to 7.99, and 8+ in a cohort of 2284 consecutive patients with papillary thyroid carcinoma (PTC) undergoing initial treatment at the Mayo Clinic from 1940 to 1997. The numbers in parentheses represent the numbers and percentages of PTC patients in each of the four risk groups.

resection but excluded histologic grade.[197] Cox model analysis and stepwise variable selection led to a final prognostic model that included five variables: *m*etastasis, *a*ge, *c*ompleteness of resection, *i*nvasion, and *s*ize (MACIS). The final score was defined as 3.1 (age 39 years or younger) or 0.08 × age (age 40 years or older) + 0.3 × tumor size (in centimeters) + 1 (if tumor not completely resected) + 1 (if locally invasive) + 3 (if distant metastases present).

As illustrated by Figure 14-14 , the MACIS scoring system permits identification of groups of patients with a broad range of risk of death from PTC. Twenty-year cause-specific survival rates for patients with MACIS scores of less than 6, 6 to 6.99, 7 to 7.99, and 8+ were 99%, 89%, 56%, and 27%, respectively ($p < 0.0001$). When the cumulative mortality rate from all causes of death was considered, approximately 85% of PTC patients with AGES scores below 4 or MACIS scores below 6 had no excess mortality rate over rates predicted for control subjects.[192,197]

It should be emphasized that the five variables in MACIS scoring are easy to define after primary operation; consequently, the system can be applied in any clinical setting. The MACIS system can be used for counseling individual PTC patients and can help guide decision making concerning the intensity of the postoperative tumor surveillance and the appropriateness of adjunctive radioiodine therapy. Because the CIS (*c*ompleteness of resection, *i*nvasion, and *s*ize) variables require information obtained at surgery, the system probably should not be used to decide the extent of primary surgery.[199,200]

The risk of thyroid cancer recurrence is higher than the risk of thyroid cancer–related death but is difficult to quantify because it needs active follow-up of all patients. Recently, the ATA proposed a stratification system for the risk of recurrence after initial treatment that could be taken into account for the indication of postoperative administration of radioiodine and for the subsequent follow-up strategy. The stratification is based on individual factors from various studies, and reports a continuous increasing risk of recurrence according to each factor, and no multivariate analysis is so far available. Of note, the age of the patient at the time of initial treatment is not taken into account for the risk of recurrence, but many other prognostic factors for thyroid cancer death are also prognostic for the risk of recurrence, such as some histologic characteristics, the size of the thyroid tumor, the extension of the tumor beyond the thyroid capsule, the presence of lymph node metastases, and the presence of residual disease due to either incomplete surgical resection or presence of distant metastases. The encapsulated follicular variant is associated with a low risk of recurrence; aggressive histologic subtypes, the presence of necrosis, a high mitotic count, and vascular invasion are in contrast associated with a higher risk. Indeed, the risk of recurrence is minimal (less than 2%) for unifocal micropapillary carcinoma, is higher for multifocal micropapillary carcinoma (around 4%), and increases with the size of the thyroid tumor but is still low (about 5%) in patients with an intrathyroid tumor of 3 to 4 cm without extension beyond the thyroid capsule.[201] The prognostic impact of the extension beyond the thyroid capsule is low in micropapillary carcinomas that are N0 and increases with the size of the thyroid tumor and with the extent of the extension.[202-204] Minimal lymph node involvement (less than three lymph node metastases of less than 2 mm each) is associated with a low risk of recurrence; the risk increases with the number of lymph node metastases, with the size of the lymph node metastases, and with the presence of extracapsular nodal extension.[140,141,205] Therefore, minimal lymph node involvement that is usually found at prophylactic lymph node dissection may have a minimal prognostic impact and may not change the indication for postoperative treatment with radioiodine. However, large lymph node metastases (>3 cm) that are usually palpable and easily visualized on neck ultrasonography and are frequently multiple and associated with extracapsular nodal extension have a major prognostic impact on recurrence that may occur in up to 40% of patients. The risk of recurrence is also associated with the genetic status, and the presence of *BRAF* mutation is associated with a higher risk of recurrence for most tumor stages[102,166,206]; the risk is even higher when both *BRAF* and *TERT* mutations are present in the tumor.[102,172] Each of these characteristics is associated with a risk of tumor recurrence that may range from less than 2% up to more than 40%. For practical purposes, three discrete groups have been individualized that may guide subsequent treatment and follow-up (see "Outcome Prediction" later in text and Table 14-7).

Follicular Thyroid Carcinoma

FTC is "a malignant epithelial tumor showing evidence of follicular cell differentiation but lacking the diagnostic features of papillary carcinoma."[134] Such a definition excludes the follicular variant of PTC, and it is also customary to exclude both the poorly differentiated carcinoma[207] and the rare mixed medullary and follicular carcinoma.[208] The correct classification of tumors with predominant oncocytic features (HCCs) is controversial.[147-149] The WHO committee has taken the stance that this tumor is an oxyphilic variant of FTC.[134] The AFIP monograph, by contrast, states that "the tumors made up of this cell type have gross, microscopic, behavioral, cytogenetic features that set them apart from all others and justify discussing them in a separate section."[135] The mutational, transcriptional, and copy number profiles of HCC were distinct from those of PTC and FTC, indicating HCC to be a unique type of thyroid malignancy. Molecular pathways that differentiate Hürthle cell adenoma from widely invasive HCC included the PIK3CA-Akt-mTOR (mammalian target of rapamycin) and Wnt/β-catenin pathways, potentially providing a rationale for new targets for this type of malignancy. Recent data have confirmed that molecular abnormalities are different from those found in follicular cancer.[209]

Thus categorized, FTC is a relatively rare neoplasm whose identification requires invasion of the capsule,

blood vessel, or adjacent thyroid. In epidemiologic surveys, FTC constituted from 5% to 50% of differentiated thyroid cancers and tended to be more common in areas with iodine deficiency.[210] Owing to a combination of changing diagnostic criteria and an increase in the incidence of PTC associated with dietary iodine supplementation, the diagnosis of FTC has decreased in frequency; in one North American experience, minimally invasive nonoxyphilic FTC made up fewer than 2% of thyroid malignancies.[211]

The microscopic appearance of FTC varies from well-formed follicles to a predominantly solid growth pattern.[134,135] Poorly formed follicles and atypical patterns (e.g., cribriform) may occur, and multiple architectural types may coexist. FTC is best divided into two categories on the basis of degree of invasiveness: (1) minimally invasive or encapsulated and (2) widely invasive. There is little overlap between these two types.

Minimally invasive FTC is an encapsulated tumor whose growth pattern resembles that of a trabecular or solid microfollicular or atypical adenoma. The diagnosis of malignancy depends on the demonstration of blood vessel or capsular invasion or both. The criteria for invasion must therefore be strict.[134,135] Blood vessel invasion is almost never seen grossly. Microscopically, the vessels "should be of venous caliber, be located in or immediately outside of the capsule and contain one or more clusters of tumor cells attached to the wall and protruding into the lumen."[134] Interruption of the capsule must involve the full thickness to qualify as capsular invasion. Penetration of only the inner half or the presence of tumor cells embedded in the capsule does not qualify for the diagnosis of FTC. Foci of capsular invasion must be distinguished from the capsular rupture that can result from FNA. The acronym WHAFFT (*worrisome histologic alterations following FNA of the thyroid*) is applied to such changes.[212] The diagnosis of malignancy of these tumors may be difficult and not reproducible among pathologists, and immunohistochemistry with markers such as TPO, galectin 3, or HMBE1 may help for this purpose,[97] but these techniques did not reliably improve the accuracy in case of suspicious findings.

Global gene expression studies with the microarray technology demonstrate and more recently the gene classifier or a panel of gene mutations may help to differentiate malignant from benign follicular tumors, but this needs confirmation.[213]

In contrast, the rare *widely invasive* form of FTC can be distinguished easily from benign lesions. Although the tumor may be partially encapsulated, the margins are infiltrative even on gross examination, and vascular invasion is often extensive. The structural features are variable, but a follicular element is always present. When follicular differentiation is poor or absent, or in the presence of trabecular, insular, or solid component, the tumor may be classified as a poorly differentiated carcinoma (see later).[135,214]

Focal or extensive clear-cell changes can occur. A rare clear-cell variant of FTC has been described in which glycogen accumulation or dilatation of the granular endoplasmic reticulum is responsible for the clear cells.[215] When more than 75% of cells in an FTC exhibit Hürthle cell (or oncocytic) features, the tumor is classified as a Hürthle cell or an oncocytic carcinoma[135,216] or an oxyphilic variant FTC.[134]

Molecular Pathogenesis

There is still no accepted paradigm for the pathogenesis of FTC. A multistep adenoma-to-carcinoma pathogenesis, similar to that for colon cancer and other adenocarcinomas, is not universally accepted because pathologists do not recognize follicular carcinoma in situ and documentation of the evolution of adenoma to carcinoma is rare. Nevertheless, several facts about the pathogenesis of FTC are firmly established.[102,151,161,165,217]

First, most follicular adenomas and all FTCs are probably of monoclonal origin. Second, oncogene activation, particularly by point mutation of the *RAS* oncogene, is common both in follicular adenomas (~20%) and in FTCs (~40%), supporting a role in early tumorigenesis.[165,218] The *RET* and *BRAF* oncogenes do not appear to be involved in follicular tumors.[102,151,217] Third, cytogenetic abnormalities and evidence of genetic loss are more common in FTC than in PTC and also occur in follicular adenomas.[161,217]

Of the cytogenetic abnormalities described in FTC, the most common are deletions, partial deletions, and deletion rearrangements involving the p arm of chromosome 3. Loss of heterozygosity (LOH) on chromosome 3p appears to be limited to FTC because no evidence for 3p LOH has been found in follicular adenomas or PTC. A translocation, t(2;3)(q13;p25), resulting in the fusion of the DNA binding domains of the thyroid transcription factor PAX-8 to domains of the peroxisome proliferator–activated receptor (PPAR)γ1, was detected in 30% (range 11-63%) of FTCs and in 10% of follicular adenomas, but not in PTCs or multinodular hyperplasia.[219-221] The chimeric protein may retard growth inhibition and follicular differentiation normally induced by PPARγ1.[220] The two main genetic alterations found in follicular carcinomas may act through distinct molecular pathways.[221]

Presenting Features

FTC tends to occur in older people, with the mean age in most studies being more than 50 years, about 10 years older than that for typical PTC.[210] The average median age of patients with oxyphilic FTC (HCC) is about 60 years.[210,216] As in most thyroid malignancies, women outnumber men by more than 2 to 1. Most patients with FTC present with a painless thyroid nodule, with or without background thyroid nodularity, and they rarely (4-6%) have clinically evident lymphadenopathy at presentation.[210] Lymph node metastases to the neck in FTC are so exceptional that "wherever they are observed, the alternative possibilities of follicular variant papillary carcinoma, oncocytic carcinoma, and poorly differentiated carcinoma should be considered."[135]

In most series in which tumor sizes were reported, the average tumor in FTC (oxyphilic or nonoxyphilic) was larger than those seen with PTC.[210,216] Direct extrathyroidal extension, by definition, does not occur with minimally invasive FTC but is common in the rare patients with widely invasive FTC. Between 5% and 20% of patients may have distant metastases at presentation.[210] The most common sites for distant metastases in FTC are lung and bone.[133,210] The bones most often involved are long bones (e.g., femur), flat bones (particularly the pelvis, sternum, and skull), and vertebrae. When a distant metastasis is the first manifestation of the disease, definitive proof of its thyroid origin should be obtained, usually by a biopsy of a metastasis, before performing any thyroid surgery. It is unusual for patients with FTC to have thyrotoxicosis caused by massive tumor burden.[222]

Most patients (53-69%) with FTC or HCC have pTNM stage II disease. Patients aged 45 years or older with nodal metastases or extrathyroidal extension (stage III) account for only 4% of FTCs and 9% of HCCs (see Fig. 14-6). About 5% of HCCs and 17% or more of nonoxyphilic FTCs have distant metastases at the time of diagnosis (stage IV).

Recurrence and Mortality

Nodal metastases are rare in typical FTC, and the nodal recurrence rate at 20 postoperative years is the lowest in differentiated thyroid carcinoma, being around 2% (see Fig. 14-9), and is higher (in about 17%) in HCC patients.[223] When recurrences at either neck or distant sites are taken into consideration, patients with HCC (Fig. 14-15) have the highest numbers of tumor recurrences after 10 to 20 years. As illustrated by Figure 14-9, local recurrences at 20 years have occurred in 20% of FTCs and 30% of HCCs. Comparable distant metastasis rates are 23% and 28%, respectively.

CSM rates vary with the presenting TNM stage in both FTC (Fig. 14-16) and HCC. The death rates tend to parallel the curves for development of distant metastases (see Fig. 14-9). In more than 5 decades of experience at the Mayo Clinic, the mortality rate for FTC initially exceeds that of HCC, but by 20 to 30 postoperative years there are no significant differences in cause-specific survival rates between FTC and HCC (Fig. 14-17), both being around 80% at 20 and 70% at 30 postoperative years.[210] Curves representing death from all causes differ in FTC and HCC.

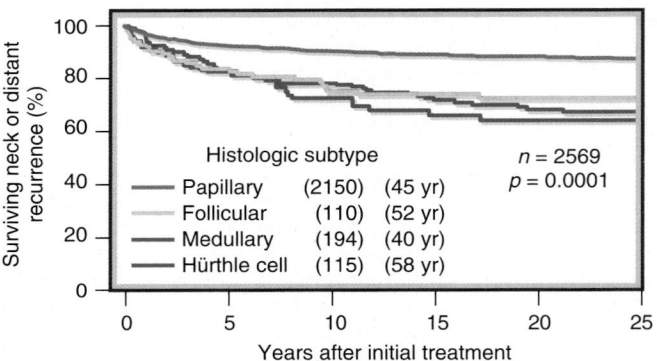

Figure 14-15 Postoperative recurrence (any site) in the first 20 years after definitive surgery for differentiated thyroid carcinoma performed at the Mayo Clinic from 1940 to 1997. Based on 2569 consecutive patients (2150 papillary thyroid carcinoma, 110 follicular thyroid carcinoma, 115 Hürthle cell carcinoma, and 194 medullary thyroid carcinoma) who had complete tumor resection and had no distant metastases at presentation. The ages in parentheses represent the median age at diagnosis for each of the four histologic subtypes.

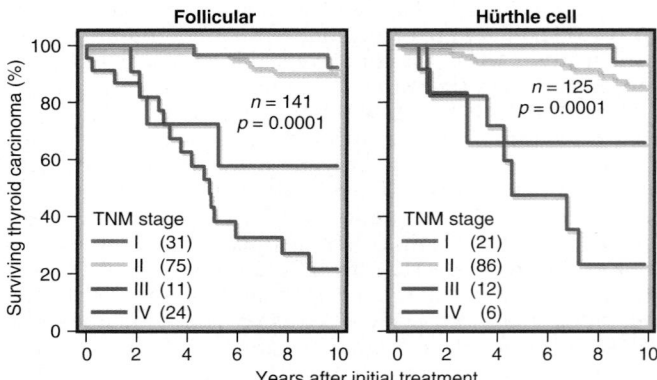

Figure 14-16 Cause-specific survival according to pathologic tumor-node-metastasis (pTNM) stages in a cohort of 141 patients with follicular thyroid carcinoma *(left panel)* and 125 patients with Hürthle cell carcinoma *(right panel)* treated at the Mayo Clinic from 1940 to 1997. Numbers in parentheses represent the number of patients in each pTNM stage grouping.

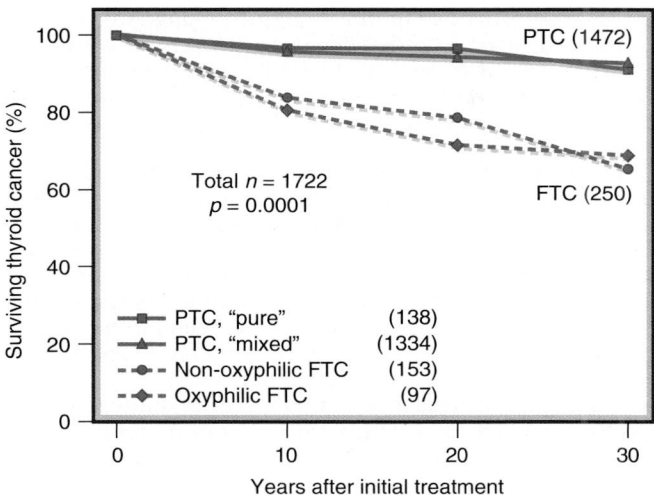

Figure 14-17 Comparison of cause-specific survival rates in 1472 papillary thyroid carcinoma (PTC) and 250 follicular thyroid carcinoma (FTC) patients treated at the Mayo Clinic from 1940 to 1990. Of the PTCs, 138 were "pure" papillary in histotype (no follicular elements); 97 of the FTC patients had predominantly oxyphilic tumors. There is a significant difference ($p = 0.0001$) between the PTC and the FTC survival curves. However, within either the PTC or FTC groups, the two survival curves are insignificantly different. (From Grebe SKG, Hay ID. Follicular thyroid cancer. *Endocrinol Metab Clin North Am.* 1995;24:761-801.)

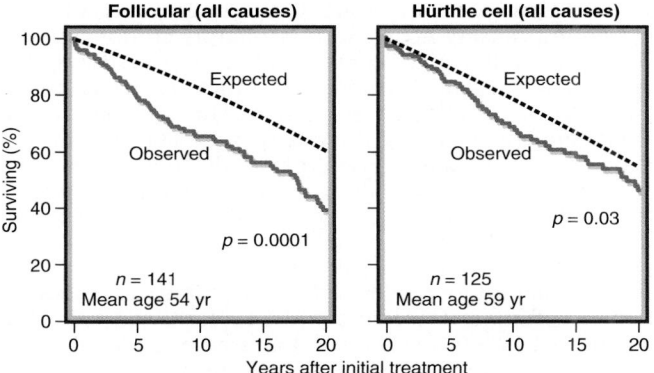

Figure 14-18 Survival to death from all causes in 141 consecutive patients with follicular thyroid carcinoma *(left)* and 125 patients with Hürthle cell cancer *(right)* undergoing initial management at the Mayo Clinic from 1940 to 1997. Also plotted *(dashed line)* is the expected survival (all causes) of persons of the same age and sex and with the same date of treatment but living under mortality risk conditions of the northwest central United States.

On average, patients with FTC are about 5 years younger, tend to die within the first 10 postoperative years, and have a high all-cause mortality rate for 10 to 30 postoperative years (Fig. 14-18). Deaths related to HCC occur gradually over the first 15 years; however, by 25 years, the average survivor of HCC is 84 years old, and by that time, almost 50% of the treated cohort would be predicted by the actuarial curve to have died from all causes.

Outcome Prediction

The risk factors that predict outcome in FTC are largely the same as in PTC[210,224-232]: distant metastases at presentation, increasing age of the patient, large tumor size, and the presence of local (extrathyroidal) invasion. To a lesser degree, increased mortality risk is associated with male sex and higher grade (less well differentiated) tumors. In

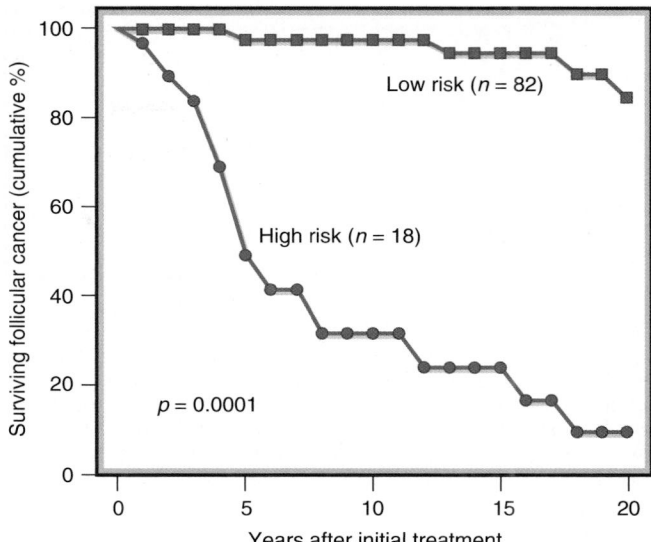

Figure 14-19 Cumulative cause-specific survival among 100 patients with nonoxyphilic follicular thyroid carcinoma treated at the Mayo Clinic from 1946 to 1970, plotted by high-risk and low-risk categories. *High-risk* means that two or more of the following factors were present: age older than 50 years, marked vascular invasion, and metastatic disease at time of initial diagnosis. (From Brennan MD, Bergstralh EJ, van Heerden JA, et al. Follicular thyroid cancer treated at the Mayo Clinic, 1946 through 1970: initial manifestations, pathologic findings, therapy, and outcome. *Mayo Clin Proc.* 1991;66:11-22.)

addition, vascular invasiveness, lymphatic involvement at presentation, DNA aneuploidy, and oxyphilic histologic findings are potential prognostic variables unique to FTC.[210] The importance of vascular invasion is underscored by a study showing that FTC patients with minimal capsular invasion and no evidence of vascular invasion had a 0% CSM rate at 10-year follow-up.[224] Indeed, the risk of recurrence and cancer-related death increases with the extent of vascular invasion and of capsular invasion.

Prognostic scoring systems for FTC[210,225] allow stratification of patients into high-risk and low-risk categories. A multivariate analysis at the Mayo Clinic found that distant metastases at presentation, patient's age greater than 50 years, and marked vascular invasion predict a poor outcome.[210] As illustrated by Figure 14-19, if two or more of these factors are present, the 5-year survival rate is only 47%, and 20-year survival rate is 8%. By contrast, if only one of these factors is present, 5-year survival rate is 99%, and 20-year survival rate is 86%.

Systems developed to predict outcome in either PTC or FTC have been applied to FTC patients. The pTNM as well as the AMES risk group categorization (*a*ge, *m*etastasis, *e*xtent, *s*ize) have proved to be useful in FTC.[226] Additionally, from a multivariate analysis of 228 patients with FTC treated at the Memorial Sloan Kettering Cancer Center, the independent adverse prognostic factors were identified as age older than 45 years, Hürthle cell histotype, extrathyroidal extension, tumor size exceeding 4 cm, and the presence of distant metastases.[227] The prognostic importance in FTC of histologic grade was also confirmed,[227] and this factor was included in assignment of risk groups to low, intermediate, or high categories (Fig. 14-20).

The AGES scheme, originally developed for PTC, has also been successfully applied to FTC.[228,229] Additionally, it has recently been demonstrated that, when compared to the TNM, AGES, and AMES prognostic schemes, the MACIS classification was the most accurate predictor of survival in

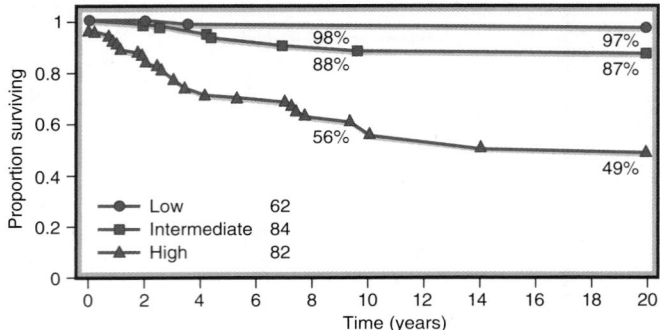

Figure 14-20 Survival differences in low-risk, intermediate-risk, and high-risk groups for 228 consecutive patients with follicular thyroid carcinoma who were seen and treated at the Memorial Sloan-Kettering Cancer Center during a period of 55 years from 1930 to 1985. (From Shaha AR, Loree TR, Shah JP. Prognostic factors and risk group analyses in follicular carcinoma of the thyroid. *Surgery.* 1995;118: 1131-1138.)

FTC.[230] It would therefore appear that scoring systems used in PTC may be cautiously applied to FTC as long as some of the unique features of this tumor, such as vascular invasiveness and the remarkable significance of DNA aneuploidy in HCC, are kept in mind.[210]

Poorly Differentiated Carcinoma

Poorly differentiated thyroid carcinoma is rare, representing less than 5% of all thyroid cancers. It has been defined as "a tumor of follicular cell origin with morphological and biologic attributes intermediate between differentiated and anaplastic carcinomas of the thyroid."[135] A recent study proposed new diagnostic criteria for poorly differentiated carcinoma: (1) solid, trabecular, and insular pattern of growth, (2) absence of the conventional nuclear features of papillary carcinomas, (3) presence of at least convoluted nuclei, mitotic activity greater than 3×10 high-power fields, and tumor necrosis.[214] Similarly, in well-differentiated cancer, necrosis, mitosis, and cellular atypia associated with vascular invasion are considered as features of poor prognosis and aggressiveness.[31,232] Most poorly differentiated tumors are larger than 5 cm in diameter at diagnosis, with extrathyroidal extension and blood vessel invasion.

RET rearrangements are rare and *BRAF* mutation is found in 15% of poorly differentiated carcinomas. *RAS* mutations are the most prevalent genetic lesion, which is identified in 44% of cases and predominantly affects NRAS codon 61.[233] Similar to anaplastic thyroid carcinoma, mutations have been found in several genes: p53 (15-30% of cases), PI3K and its downstream effector AKT, and ALK gene. The overexpression of the endothelial growth factor receptor is frequently observed.[170,185,234-236]

The mean age at diagnosis is about 55 years, and the female:male ratio is about 2:1. Poorly differentiated carcinoma is aggressive and often lethal. Radioiodine uptake is rarely present, FDG uptake on PET is frequently high; production of Tg in blood may be lower than in differentiated carcinomas. Metastases are common in regional nodes and distant sites (lung, bone, brain). In one series, 56% of patients died from their tumor within 8 years of initial therapy.[207,214,237]

Undifferentiated (Anaplastic) Carcinoma

Anaplastic carcinoma constitutes about 1% to 2% of all thyroid carcinomas, usually occurs after the age of 60 years, and is slightly more common in women (1.3:1 to

1.5:1).[238-240] This carcinoma is highly malignant, nonencapsulated, and extends widely. Evidence of invasion of adjacent structures, such as the skin, muscles, nerves, blood vessels, larynx, and esophagus, is common. Distant metastases occur early in the course of the disease in lungs, liver, bones, and brain.

On histopathologic examination, the lesion is composed of atypical cells that exhibit numerous mitoses and form a variety of patterns. Spindle-shaped cells, multinucleated giant cells, and squamoid cells usually predominate. Areas of necrosis and polymorphonuclear infiltration are common, and the presence of PTC or FTC suggests that they may be the precursors of anaplastic carcinoma. Immunohistochemistry revealed that a significant proportion of cells are tumor-associated macrophages.[241,242]

Mutations of the *p53* gene are present in many (60-80%) undifferentiated carcinomas but may not be found in the residual well-differentiated component, suggesting that these mutations occurred after the development of the original tumor and may have played a key role in tumor progression.[152,234] *BRAF* mutation is found mostly in anaplastic thyroid carcinoma with a papillary component, and *RAS* mutation is found in 20% or more anaplastic thyroid carcinoma; PI3KCA mutation is rare in differentiated thyroid cancer and was found in 23% of anaplastic thyroid carcinoma; finally, ALK rearrangement was found in about 10% of anaplastic thyroid carcinomas.[170]

The usual clinical complaint is of a rapid, often painful enlargement of a mass that may have been present in the thyroid gland for many years. The tumor invades adjacent structures, causing hoarseness, inspiratory stridor, and difficulty in swallowing. On examination, the overlying skin is often warm and discolored. The mass is tender and is often fixed to adjacent structures. The regional lymph nodes are enlarged, and there may be evidence of distant metastases. Anaplastic carcinomas do not accumulate iodine and do not typically produce Tg; high FDG uptake is usually found on PET, which is the best tool for tumor staging and for control of treatment efficacy.[243,244]

Treatment should be initiated rapidly to avoid death from locally infiltrative disease and possible suffocation. It consists of surgical resection of the tumor tissue present in the neck, when this is feasible, followed by a combination of external irradiation and chemotherapy, but despite aggressive treatment results are poor with a 1-year survival rate that does not exceed 20% to 30%.[238-240]

Chemotherapy is poorly effective in patients with distant metastases. Recently, the use of the *BRAF* inhibitor vemurafenib in a patient with a *BRAF* mutation, of the ALK inhibitor crizotinib in patients with an ALK rearrangement, or of everolimus in a patient with an activated PI3K-mTOR pathway produced tumor response in patients with advanced disease.[245-247]

Medullary Thyroid Carcinoma

MTC accounts for less than 5% of thyroid malignancies (see Chapter 39). It arises from the parafollicular or C cells of the thyroid gland, and the tumor cells typically produce an early biochemical signal (hypersecretion of calcitonin). MTC readily invades the intraglandular lymphatics and spreads to other parts of the gland, in addition to the pericapsular and regional lymph nodes. It also regularly spreads through the bloodstream to the lungs, bones, and liver.[2,4,142-144,248]

MTC tumors are firm and usually unencapsulated. On histopathologic examination, the tumor is composed of cells that vary in morphologic features and arrangement. Round, polyhedral, and spindle-shaped cells form a variety of patterns, which may vary from solid and trabecular to endocrine or glandular-like structures. An amyloid stroma is commonly present.[134,135] Gross or microscopic foci of carcinoma may be present in other parts of the gland, and blood vessels may be invaded. In all cases, the diagnosis can be confirmed by positive immunostaining of tumor tissue for calcitonin and carcinoembryonic antigen (CEA).

MTC first appears either as a hard nodule or mass in the thyroid gland or as an enlargement of the regional lymph nodes. Occasionally, a metastatic lesion in a distant site is found first. The neck masses are frequently painful; they are sometimes bilateral and are often localized to the upper two thirds of each lobe of the gland, which reflects the anatomic location of the parafollicular cells.

The tumor occurs in both sporadic and hereditary forms, the latter making up about 20% of the total. The hereditary variety arises as part of MEN syndrome type 2A or 2B. A germline activating *RET* point mutation is found in almost all hereditary cases, and *RET* proto-oncogene testing should be performed in all MTC patients. The finding of a germline *RET* mutation indicates a hereditary disease; the mutation should then be sought in all first-degree family members. The hereditary form is typically bilateral and is usually preceded by a premalignant C-cell hyperplasia. Total thyroidectomy at this premalignant stage can cure the disease in more than 95% of cases.[4,67,68,248-250]

There is a strong relationship between genotype and phenotype: most MEN2B are due to a codon 918 mutation in exon 16; the most frequent mutation found in patients with MEN2A is a codon 634 mutation in exon 11; the other mutations are located in exons 10, 13, 14, and 15 and are usually associated with less aggressive phenotypes. Somatic *RET* mutations are found in 40% of sporadic MTCs, the codon 918 mutation being the most frequent and associated with a more aggressive course.[251] In up to two thirds of tumors with no *RET* mutation, a *RAS* point mutation was found in most studies[252-254] but not in all.[255]

Early series of MTC mainly described sporadic cases, in which 80% of patients presented with TNM stage II or III. Patients with MEN2A are diagnosed earlier and have curable (stage I) disease.[248,249] Patients with MTC now have outcomes similar to or better than those of patients with nonpapillary FCTC (see Fig. 14-8). The cause-specific survival curves for 218 consecutive MTC cases treated from 1940 to 1997 at the Mayo Clinic, according to TNM stage, are presented in Figure 14-21.

In multivariate analysis, only the age of the patient at initial treatment and the stage of the disease remain significantly independent indicators of survival. This suggests that, in routine practice, clinicians attempting to predict outcome in MTC should take into account not only the presenting disease stage, as assessed by the pTNM system (see Fig. 14-21), but also the age of the patient at diagnosis.[142-144]

Cushing syndrome may occur at an advanced stage of the disease, because of secretion of corticotropin by the tumor. Prostaglandins, serotonin, kinins, and vasoactive intestinal peptide may also be secreted and are variously responsible for flushing and for the attacks of watery diarrhea that about one third of patients experience, usually at an advanced stage of the disease.[142-144,248] In MEN2A, hyperparathyroidism occurs late and is usually mild. Pheochromocytomas invariably occur later than MTC; they are often bilateral and may be clinically silent, and patients at risk should be screened with measurements of urinary metanephrine excretion. Familial MTC is a variant of MEN2A: MTC is transmitted as a single entity without any associated abnormality in the family and usually occurs later in life and is less aggressive than the MTC occurring in the context of other subgroups of MEN2A; pheochromocytoma should be screened even if its risk is low, because it cannot be totally excluded in any hereditary form. In MEN2B, MTC and pheochromocytomas are associated with multiple mucosal neuromas *(bumpy lip syndrome)*, a marfanoid habitus, and typical facies, but such patients do not have hyperparathyroidism.[4,248]

Differentiation of sporadic MTC from other types of thyroid nodules on clinical grounds alone may be difficult. In patients with a family history of thyroid cancer associated with hypertension or hyperparathyroidism, the MEN2A syndrome should be suspected. FNAB has made it possible to diagnose MTC before surgery. In some patients, however, cytologic findings may be misleading because the type of carcinoma is difficult to determine and HCC may occasionally be confused with MTC.[134,135] Positive immunocytochemical staining for calcitonin allows confirmation of the diagnosis. Basal plasma calcitonin levels are elevated in virtually all patients with clinical MTC, but it is still controversial whether it should be performed in all patients with thyroid nodules or only in those with suspicious or malignant cytologic findings.[67,68]

When the diagnosis of MTC is made from calcitonin measurements or FNAB, patients should be evaluated for hyperparathyroidism and for pheochromocytoma, unless a hereditary form of the disease has been excluded. If these diagnoses are satisfactorily excluded, a total thyroidectomy with removal of regional nodes can safely be performed.[4,249,250,256,257] In patients with MEN2, surgery should be performed for pheochromocytomas before surgery for MTC is performed. First-degree relatives of patients with MEN should undergo DNA testing for the presence of the mutant *RET* gene (see Chapter 41). Gene carriers should undergo a prophylactic total thyroidectomy at an age that depends on the mutation: within the first year of life for those with MEN2B and before they are 5 years old for those with the 634 *RET* mutation (the most frequent).[4,249,250] For carriers of other mutations, prophylactic total thyroidectomy may be delayed beyond age 5 years in the setting of a normal annual basal serum calcitonin, normal annual neck ultrasonography, less aggressive MTC family history, and family preference. Surgery is indicated if all of these features are not present and consists of a total thyroidectomy with lymph node dissection; lymph node dissection may be obviated when the thyroid nodule is smaller than 5 mm, when there is no lymph node abnormality at neck

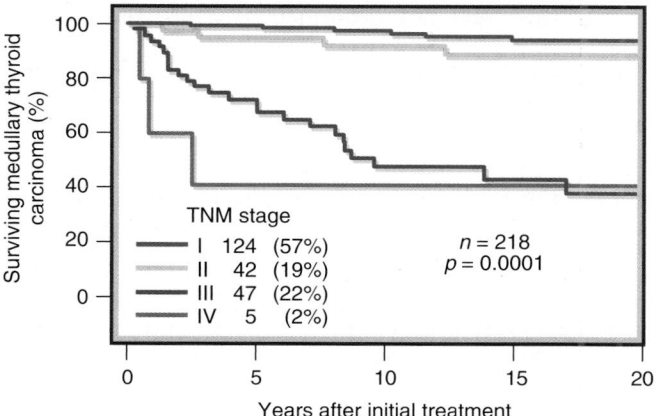

Figure 14-21 Cause-specific survival according to pathologic tumor-node-metastasis (pTNM) stage in a cohort of 218 patients with medullary thyroid carcinoma treated at the Mayo Clinic from 1940 to 1997. Numbers in parentheses represent the percentages of patients in each pTNM stage grouping.

ultrasonography, and when the plasma calcitonin level is less than 40 pg/mL.[4]

Primary Malignant Lymphoma

Primary thyroid lymphomas are rare tumors, accounting for 2.5% of all non-Hodgkin lymphomas and less than 2% of all malignant thyroid tumors. The peak incidence is during the seventh decade of life and the male-female ratio is 1:3.

Primary thyroid lymphoma almost always has a B-cell lineage.[258] The majority of thyroid malignant lymphomas are *mucosa-associated lymphoid tissue* (MALT) lymphomas that usually arise in a background of Hashimoto thyroiditis. These small cell lymphomas are characterized by a low grade of malignancy, a slow growth rate, and a tendency for recurrence at other MALT sites such as the gastrointestinal or respiratory tract, the thymus, or the salivary glands. At diagnosis, diffuse large cell lymphomas account for about 70% to 80% of tumors, and a substantial proportion of clinical cases arise from the transformation of low-grade MALT lymphoma to high-grade B-cell lymphoma. Other histologic findings are rare.

Clinical thyroid lymphomas almost invariably present as a rapidly enlarging, painless neck mass. One third of the patients have compressive symptoms. The mass is often fixed to surrounding tissues, and half of the patients have unilateral or bilateral cervical lymph node enlargement. Clinically evident distant disease is uncommon. About 20% of patients already have a long-standing goiter, and hypothyroidism is reported in up to 40% of cases. The palpated mass is solid and hypoechoic on ultrasonography, which often depicts a characteristic asymmetric pseudocystic pattern. Most patients have serum antiperoxidase and anti-Tg antibodies.

The diagnosis of lymphoma can often be established by FNA cytologic tests, particularly in diffuse large B-cell type. Large-bore needle biopsy or open surgical biopsy may be needed for immunohistochemical staining to diagnose small cell lymphomas and the frequently associated chronic autoimmune thyroiditis. Lymphocyte monoclonality for light chain immunoglobulin may be necessary to confirm malignant lymphoma.

Accurate staging is critical for treatment planning. Staging includes a physical examination; complete blood count; serum lactate dehydrogenase; liver function tests; bone marrow biopsy; CT scan or MRI of the neck; CT scan of the thorax, abdomen, and pelvis; and appropriate biopsies at other sites where tumor is suspected. Involvement of the Waldeyer ring and the gastrointestinal tract has been associated with thyroid lymphomas, and therefore, upper gastrointestinal tract radiographs or endoscopy should be performed.

Treatment is guided by the histologic subtype, the extent of the disease, and in case of diffuse large B-cell lymphoma, by the age-adjusted international prognostic index.[259,260] Surgical debulking of thyroid lymphomas is neither feasible nor necessary. Small tumors are often treated initially as primary thyroid carcinomas with surgery, and additional radiotherapy may be necessary in case of indolent lymphoma.

For high-grade B-cell lymphoma, chemotherapy combined with rituximab (chimeric human-mouse anti-CD20 monoclonal antibody) has become the standard treatment.[261] The chemotherapy prescribed should be an anthracycline-based regimen. It usually consists of 4 to 6 cycles of the CHOP regimen (cyclophosphamide 750 mg/m² on day 1, doxorubicin 50 mg/m² on day 1, vincristine 1.4 mg/m² on day 1, and prednisone 40 mg/m² per day on days 1-5) every 3 weeks. For localized aggressive lymphoma, the combination of chemotherapy and radiotherapy used before the era of rituximab reduced distant recurrence compared with radiotherapy alone that should be used only for elderly patients who cannot receive medical treatment, because a recurrence at distant sites will occur in one third of the patients and generally within the first year of treatment.

For MALT lymphomas, if disease is localized after accurate staging, total thyroidectomy (predicted overall survival rate and disease-free survival, 100% at 5 years) or involved-field radiation therapy alone, 2 Gy per fraction for 5 days per week up to a total dose of 30 to 40 Gy (5-year overall survival rate 90%) may be adequate.[262] For disseminated MALT lymphoma, chemotherapy alone with single agent such as chlorambucil or combined with local radiation therapy can be proposed.

SURGICAL TREATMENT OF THYROID CARCINOMA

Factors that influence the optimal extent of surgery include the histologic diagnosis, the size and the local extent of the original lesion, the presence of lymph node and distant metastases, and the patient's age, and these factors are taken into account in the risk group category.[1,3,4] Obviously, the surgeon must be appropriately skilled in thyroid surgery, and the goal of surgery should be to remove all the malignant neoplastic tissue present in the neck. Therefore, a preoperative ultrasound examination of the thyroid gland and of neck lymph node areas should be routinely performed and detected lesions adequately resected.[1,3,4]

CT scan of the neck and mediastinum with contrast medium and MRI as well as endoscopies may be performed in patients with extensive disease.

In the case of PTC and FTC, a near-total or total thyroidectomy is recommended for all patients.[1,3,132,133,190-192,263] Total thyroidectomy permits the eradication of bilateral disease and may reduce the recurrence rate, compared with more limited surgery, because many PTCs are both multifocal and bilateral. Removal of most, if not all, of the thyroid gland facilitates postoperative remnant ablation with ^{131}I and an easier detection of recurrence. However, most thyroid cancers are indolent tumors with an excellent prognosis, and total thyroidectomy is associated with a higher risk of morbidity but does not bring any benefit in terms of overall survival in low-risk patients, and its impact on survival[263] was not confirmed by a reanalysis of the data.[264]

For patients with unifocal intrathyroidal PTM, a lobectomy may be an appropriate primary surgical procedure.[1,3,153,154,265] A lobectomy may be also considered in patients with a pT1-2 tumor (<4 cm) and who have no extrathyroidal extension or clinical lymph node metastases and no abnormality in the contralateral lobe at neck ultrasonography and no high-risk histologic features, and in whom follow-up can be performed.[265] A completion thyroidectomy should be offered to the other patients who have undergone a unilateral lobectomy for a supposedly benign tumor that proves to be a cancer and for whom a total thyroidectomy would have been recommended had the diagnosis been available before the initial surgery.[3]

Surgery of lymph nodes is based on the preoperative workup, including neck ultrasound examination. In the presence of clinically involved lymph nodes, a therapeutic lymph node dissection is routinely performed.[3,13,205] In patients with central neck involvement, it includes dissection of the central compartment VI (paratracheal and tracheoesophageal areas) and may also include dissection of the ipsilateral supraclavicular area and the lower third of the jugulocarotid chain (compartments III and IV).[3,13,266] A modified ipsilateral neck dissection is performed if palpable lymph node metastases are present in the jugulocarotid chain or a preoperative ultrasound demonstrates biopsy-proven lateral neck nodal disease; in such cases, a compartment VI dissection is also performed. Compartment dissection is preferable to lymph node picking. In patients with PTC, in the absence of any evidence of lymph node involvement, a prophylactic central neck dissection is controversial and is performed either routinely or only for advanced primary tumors (T3 or T4).[3,13,267,268]

Although this type of lymph node dissection has not been shown to improve the recurrence and survival rates,[140,141,205,223,224] several arguments support its routine use in patients with papillary carcinomas: histologic evidence of lymph node metastases is present in up to two thirds of PTC patients, of whom more than 80% have involvement of the central compartment; metastases are difficult to detect by palpation in lymph nodes located behind the vessels or in the paratracheal groove; and finally, preoperative neck ultrasound detects only half of the involved lymph nodes.[140,269-271] The knowledge of initial lymph node status is a requisite for TNM classification, is useful for the indication of postsurgical radioiodine treatment,[266] and helps in the interpretation of any cervical abnormality identified during the subsequent postoperative follow-up.[1,3] The major drawbacks of lymph node dissection is that it may increase the morbidity rate and does not improve long-term outcomes, and for this reason it should be performed by a skilled surgeon. Finally, the negative prognostic impact of lymph node involvement increases with the number of N1, the size of N1, and the presence of extranodal extension. It is clear that the negative prognostic impact on recurrence of a few (<3-5) or very tiny/microscopic N1 (<2 mm) that are not detected on neck ultrasonography is much less important than that of clinical N1.[140,141,205]

In the case of FTC, lymph node metastases are less frequent, and a lymph node dissection should only be performed if involved lymph nodes are detected.[210]

MTC is treated by total thyroidectomy, with a dissection of the central compartment of the neck and the lower two thirds of the jugulocarotid chains. A modified neck dissection is performed either routinely or for MTC affecting the lateral neck nodes.[249,250,256,257]

Ideally, patients with anaplastic carcinoma should be treated with total thyroidectomy and lymph node dissection, but lesions are frequently too extensive for any procedure but palliative surgery.[238-240] In these cases, surgery may be performed later in the case of tumor regression after a combination of chemotherapy and external radiotherapy.

In recommending surgery, the endocrinologist should discuss potential operative complications with the patient. Unilateral lobectomy virtually never causes permanent hypocalcemia but can cause temporary vocal cord paralysis in as many as 3% of patients. Total thyroidectomy causes temporary hypocalcemia in 7% to 10% of patients and permanent hypocalcemia in 0.5% to 1%; permanent vocal cord paralysis occurs in less than 1%, and may benefit from specific treatments.[272] The risk of hypoparathyroidism is reduced by identifying parathyroid glands and, if viability is in doubt, by autotransplanting the parathyroid glands. The experience of the surgeon is important in terms of the finer technical points of thyroidectomy, including preservation of the external branch of the recurrent laryngeal nerve, which is important in the fine regulation of voice pitch. Intraoperative neural stimulation may facilitate nerve identification and confirm neural function.

A history of radiation in childhood increases the risk of both benign and malignant thyroid nodules in later life.[273] The risk increases with a younger age at exposure and larger radiation dose. Several issues are relevant for the thyroidologist. With respect to the extent of surgery, a near-total or total thyroidectomy should be performed in all patients with a history of radiation exposure to the neck with a thyroid carcinoma[273,274] and in those with benign lesions.

Indeed, one must weigh the relative risk of complications associated with a more extensive surgical procedure against the possibility of recurrence of thyroid nodules in the residual thyroid tissue. In one irradiated population, both benign and malignant nodules recurred after previous subtotal thyroidectomy. The overall risk of recurrence in this study was approximately 20% and was lower in those who had more thyroid tissue removed than in those who had less extensive procedures. In those patients, suppression of TSH by thyroid hormone led to a reduction in recurrence from 35% to approximately 8%, but TSH suppression had no influence on the occurrence of malignant nodules.[273] All irradiated patients who have had thyroid nodules removed should receive TSH-suppressive doses of levothyroxine regardless of the extent of surgery. The appearance of new thyroid nodules is, however, fairly common, and such patients should be monitored indefinitely for this possibility.

It is not clear whether this experience should be extrapolated to prescribe routine TSH suppression therapy for all irradiated patients, even if nodularity is not present, because its beneficial effects have not been quantified and the risks of long-term TSH suppression in women, especially vis-à-vis osteoporosis, have not been clearly defined and may be significant. At present, this approach cannot be recommended for all irradiated patients but can be recommended for patients at high risk of developing a thyroid nodule.[273]

POSTOPERATIVE MANAGEMENT

In view of the foregoing uncertainties and the different needs of individual patients, postoperative treatment of thyroid carcinoma cannot always accord with a rigid algorithm.[1,3] One must consider the extent of disease at surgery, the histotype and differentiation of the tumor, the age of the patient, the risk group category for tumor-related death and for recurrence, and the results of postoperative serum Tg determination and neck ultrasonography.

^{131}I Administration

^{131}I is an effective agent for delivering high radiation doses to the thyroid tissue with low spillover to other portions of the body. The radiation dose to the thyroid tissue is related to the tissue concentration, the ratio between the total tissue uptake and the volume of functional tissue, and the effective half-life of ^{131}I in the tissue.[79,275] Thyroid tissue is able to concentrate iodine only after TSH stimulation, but even after optimal TSH stimulation, iodine uptake in neoplastic tissue is always lower than in normal thyroid tissue and may not be detectable in about one third of cases.[79]

^{131}I therapy is given postoperatively for three reasons.[1,3] First, it destroys normal thyroid remnants (this is termed *ablation*), thereby increasing the sensitivity and the specificity of measurements of serum Tg for the detection of persistent or recurrent disease; ablation was mandatory for interpreting TSH-stimulated Tg determinations, because Tg may be produced by normal thyroid remnants and by neoplastic foci; during levothyroxine treatment, the production of Tg by normal thyroid cells may be low or suppressed and serum Tg can be used for the follow-up of these patients.[276] Second, it may destroy occult or known microscopic carcinoma, thereby potentially decreasing the long-term recurrence rate. Finally, it makes it possible to perform a postablative ^{131}I total-body scan (TBS), a sensitive tool for detecting persistent carcinoma.

It cannot be emphasized too strongly that postoperative ^{131}I therapy should be used *selectively* and that not all patients with a diagnosis of FCTC benefit from routine postoperative radioiodine ablative therapy.[1,3,133,277] In low-risk patients, the long-term prognosis after surgery alone is so favorable that ^{131}I ablation is not recommended.[1,3,278,279] However, patients who are at high risk of recurrence (Table 14-7) are routinely treated with ^{131}I because such therapy can potentially decrease both recurrence and death rates. Also, radioiodine is administered postoperatively when surgery has not been complete or its success is doubtful. Young children have traditionally been considered as candidates for postoperative radioiodine therapy because they may have extensive neck lymph node involvement and frequently harbor pulmonary metastases that may not be detectable even with CT imaging of the chest.[139,158,189] Finally, in the other patients, there is currently no evidence that radioiodine remnant ablation (RRA) may improve the long-term outcome, and prospective randomized trials are needed to validate its current indications.

The risk of persistent disease is low when postoperative serum Tg is undetectable, so that ^{131}I administration may not be justified.[280] This is particularly the case in N0 patients or those with minimal lymph node involvement.[281] On the contrary, the likelihood of identifying ^{131}I avid metastatic disease on the post-therapy ^{131}I TBS increases with postoperative Tg values greater than 5 to 10 ng/mL, suggesting that ^{131}I should be administered to such patients. Postoperative neck ultrasonography may also provide reassuring data or show abnormalities that should lead to ^{131}I administration.[282]

Usually, levothyroxine treatment is given soon after surgery, and both the indication and the protocol of stimulation and the ^{131}I activity to be administered are decided according to the ATA risk stratification and the data from postoperative serum Tg determination and neck ultrasonography. Pregnancy must be excluded in women of childbearing age.

In case of withdrawal, no levothyroxine treatment is given for 4 to 6 weeks, but liothyronine can be substituted for 3 to 4 weeks and then discontinued for 2 weeks before radioiodine studies. At that time, the serum TSH level should be greater than an empirically determined level of 25 to 30 mU/L. Intramuscular injections of rhTSH (0.9 mg for 2 consecutive days, with ^{131}I administered 1 day after the second injection) given on levothyroxine treatment may achieve an effective stimulation of radioiodine uptake by normal thyroid remnant, with ablation rates similar to those obtained with withdrawal, using either a high (100 mCi) or a low (30 mCi) activity.[283-285] Its use prevents hypothyroidism and maintains the quality of life, induces a lower radiation exposure to the body, and permits an earlier discharge from the hospital.[283-288] Similar outcomes were reported in intermediate- and in high-risk patients.[289-291] In addition, short-term recurrence rates have been found to be similar in patients prepared with thyroid hormone withdrawal or rhTSH, even in those with initial lymph node involvement.[292,293] A retrospective study reported a similar outcome at 10 years after ablation with a low activity in patients prepared with either withdrawal or rhTSH.[294] rhTSH is approved for RRA with 100 mCi (or more) or 30 mCi in the United States, Europe, and many other countries around the world.

In a patient who has undergone an incomplete thyroidectomy, neck uptake may be measured with a tracer activity of ^{131}I or ^{123}I; the activity used should be small enough to avoid stunning, that is, a decrease of thyroid uptake with the subsequent high activity of radioiodine.[295,296] High uptake (>10%) and high risk of persistent disease should lead to completion surgery. [131]I therapy can be administered to the other patients, with no pretherapy TBS because of its low impact on the decision to ablate.[297] A TBS is performed 3 to 7 days after the treatment activity and is highly informative in patients with a low uptake (<1%) in the thyroid bed. Additional metastatic foci have been reported in 10% to 26% of patients scanned following high-dose radioiodine treatment compared with the diagnostic scan.[298] [131]I SPECT/CT fusion imaging may provide superior lesion localization.[19-22]

After radioiodine therapy, levothyroxine therapy is then initiated or maintained. Total ablation (defined as no visible uptake) was verified in the past by an ^{131}I TBS 6 to 12 months later, typically with 2 to 5 mCi (74 to 185 MBq). However, a control ^{131}I TBS is no longer routinely performed when postablation scan has previously been informative, because it does not afford any further information.[299,300] Moreover, total ablation is currently defined by an undetectable serum Tg level following rhTSH stimulation in the absence of anti-Tg antibody (or a serum Tg level below 0.2-0.3 ng/mL on levothyroxine treatment when using a sensitive assay) and a normal neck ultrasonography.[1,3]

Total ablation (eradication of normal thyroid remnants) is achieved after administration of either 100 mCi (3700 MBq) or 30 mCi (1100 MBq) in more than 80% of

---

TABLE 14-7

Indications for Postoperative Administration of ^{131}I in Patients with Papillary, Follicular, or Hürthle Cell Thyroid Carcinoma After Initial Total Thyroidectomy*

Low Risk of Recurrence

T1a (≤1 cm, uni- or multifocal, intrathyroid), N0/Nx, M0/Mx: No benefits, no indication.

T1b-T2 (>1 cm to 4 cm), N0/Nx, M0/Mx: No demonstrated benefits. Not routine, but consider RAI if intermediate-risk features are present (vascular invasion, aggressive histology).

Intermediate Risk of Recurrence

T3 (>4 cm), N0/Nx, M0/Mx: Not routine. Consider if adverse features or older age.

T3 (microscopic extrathyroid extension): Consider RAI because of the higher risk of recurrence, but RAI is not routine for smaller tumors with no adverse features.

T1-T3, N1a, M0/Mx: Not routine for microscopic N1 without adverse features. Consider RAI for larger N1, multiple N1, extranodal extension or adverse features.

T1-T3, N1b, M0/Mx: Consider RAI for higher risk of recurrence, in particular if multiple N1, larger size, extranodal extension, or other adverse features.

High Risk of Recurrence

T4 any N, any M, M1, any T, any N, or any thyroid cancer patient with incompletely resected disease: RAI is recommended because it improves recurrence/mortality rates.

*According to the American Thyroid Association risk of recurrence.
pTNM, pathologic tumor-node-metastasis; RAI, radioactive iodine.

patients who had at least a near-total thyroidectomy, after preparation with either withdrawal or rhTSH.[283-285,301,302] After less extensive surgery, ablation is achieved in only two thirds of patients with 30 mCi (1100 MBq). Therefore, a total thyroidectomy should be performed in all patients who are to be treated with [131]I. Also, in low- or intermediate-risk patients levothyroxine treatment is initiated soon after surgery and 30 mCi (1100 MBq) is administered following injections of rhTSH, with the aim of irradiating normal thyroid remnants; in high-risk patients, a higher activity (100 mCi or more) is administered with the aims of both ablating normal thyroid remnants and irradiating residual neoplastic tissue; in patients with known distant metastases, ^{131}I is administered following thyroid hormone withdrawal, but in the low- or intermediate-risk patients rhTSH injections represents a valid alternative. High activities should be administered with caution to elderly patients.[303]

[131]I ablation therapy has no role in the management of patients with anaplastic thyroid cancer, MTC, or thyroid lymphoma.

External Radiotherapy

External radiotherapy to the neck and mediastinum is indicated only for older patients (>45 years) with extensive PTC in whom complete surgical excision is impossible and in whom the tumor tissue does not take up [131]I. Retrospective studies have shown that in these selected patients, external radiotherapy decreases the risk of neck recurrence.[304,305] The target volume encompasses the thyroid bed, bilateral neck lymph node areas, and the upper part of the mediastinum. Typically, 50 Gy (5000 rad) would be delivered in 25 fractions over 5 weeks, with a boost of 5 to 10 Gy on any residual macroscopic focus. The current approach with intensity-modulated radiation therapy permits the delivery of 63 to 66 Gy to gross disease and high-risk areas and 54 to 56 Gy in 30 to 33 fractions to cervical and mediastinal nodal regions. Its use may decrease late morbidity.

In patients with MTC, this protocol may be applied after incomplete resection of the tumor; after apparently complete surgery for extensive tumor involvement of the neck, when plasma calcitonin remains detectable in the absence of distant metastases, it may decrease the risk of neck recurrence by a factor of 2 to 4.[142,248]

In patients with anaplastic thyroid carcinoma, when the extent of disease is limited and surgery is feasible, accelerated external radiotherapy in combination with chemotherapy permits local control of the disease in two thirds of the patients and long-term survival in about 20%.[238-240]

Levothyroxine Treatment

The growth of thyroid tumor cells is controlled by TSH, and inhibition of TSH secretion with levothyroxine is thought to improve the recurrence and survival rates.[1,3,120] Therefore, levothyroxine should be given to all patients with FCTC, whatever the extent of thyroid surgery and other treatment. The initial effective dose is about 1.6 to 2.0 µg/Kg body weight in adults; children require a higher dose and elderly patients a lower dose. The adequacy of therapy is monitored by measuring serum TSH 3 months after it is begun, the initial goal being a serum TSH concentration below 0.1 mU/L for high-risk thyroid cancer patients, and maintenance of the TSH at or slightly below the lower limit of normal (0.1-0.5 mU/L) is appropriate for low-risk patients. Similar recommendations apply to low-risk patients who have not undergone remnant ablation (i.e., serum TSH 0.1-0.5 mU/L). The dose of levothyroxine

will be modified according to the initial response to therapy, and in patients with no evidence of disease, the dose of levothyroxine is decreased to maintain the serum TSH level within the normal range.

In patients with anaplastic thyroid carcinoma, MTC, or thyroid lymphoma, a replacement dose of levothyroxine is given with the aim of obtaining a serum TSH level in the normal range.

FOLLOW-UP

In patients with PTC or FTC, the goals of follow-up after initial therapy are to maintain adequate levothyroxine therapy and to detect persistent or recurrent thyroid carcinoma. Most recurrences appear during the first years of follow-up.

Detection of Recurrent Disease
Clinical and Ultrasonographic Examinations

Palpation of the thyroid bed and lymph node areas is routinely performed at all follow-up visits in patients with thyroid cancer. Ultrasonography is more sensitive and may detect lymph nodes as small as 2 to 3 mm in diameter.[5-8] Metastatic lymph nodes should be differentiated from frequent benign lymph node hyperplasia, and false-positive findings may have deleterious consequences. Lymph nodes that are small, thin, or oval and are found in the posterior neck chains, especially if they decrease in size after an interval of 3 months, are considered benign. By contrast, malignant lymph nodes are much more likely to occur in levels III, IV, and VI, and the feature with the highest sensitivity is absence of a hilus (100%), but this finding has a low specificity of only 29%; the most specific criteria are short axis greater than 5 mm, hyperechogenicity, presence of hyperechoic punctuations and of a cystic component, and peripheral hypervascularization.[271] These characteristics may be difficult to recognize in small lymph nodes, and in case of doubt such patients should be followed at short intervals. Serum Tg level on levothyroxine treatment is also indicative because less than 2% of patients with serum Tg level below 0.3 ng/mL and more than 25% of those with a level higher than 0.3 ng/mL will develop a recurrence.[306] However, using an assay with a functional sensitivity of 1 ng/mL, serum Tg is undetectable in more than 20% of patients receiving levothyroxine treatment who have isolated lymph node metastases.[132,276] Therefore, undetectable values do not exclude metastatic lymph node disease. Ultrasonographically suspicious lymph nodes greater than 8 mm in the smaller diameter should be biopsied for cytologic testing with Tg measurement in the needle washout fluid.[307]

Serum Thyroglobulin Determinations

Tg is a glycoprotein that is produced only by normal or neoplastic thyroid follicular cells. Methods used for serum Tg determination and serum interferences are detailed in Chapter 10.[308] Data have been obtained with assays with a sensitivity of 1 ng/mL, but functional sensitivity has now been improved to 0.1 ng/mL in many currently available assays. Serum Tg should not be detectable in patients who have had total thyroid ablation.[132,276] Serum Tg antibodies may induce falsely negative results and should be quantitatively assessed with every measurement of serum Tg.[1,3,308] In patients who are in complete remission after total thyroid ablation, serum Tg antibodies decline gradually to low or undetectable levels, with a median time of 3 years.[309]

Their persistence or their reappearance during follow-up should be considered suspicious for persistent or recurrent disease.

There is a close relationship between tumor burden and the Tg level, both during levothyroxine and following TSH stimulation[308,310]; this explains why serum Tg may be undetectable in patients with isolated lymph node metastases in the neck or with small lung metastases. The production of Tg by both normal and neoplastic thyroid tissue is in part TSH dependent. High serum TSH concentrations above an empirically determined value (>25 or 30 mU/L) can be achieved by withdrawing levothyroxine for 4 to 6 weeks. However, the resulting hypothyroidism is poorly tolerated by some patients. Intramuscular injections of rhTSH (0.9 mg for 2 consecutive days) are an alternative because levothyroxine treatment needs not be discontinued, there is no hypothyroidism, quality of life is maintained, and side effects are minimal. After rhTSH stimulation, the peak of serum Tg is usually obtained 3 days after the second injection.[288,311] Although the increase in serum Tg is frequently less impressive after stimulation with rhTSH compared to levothyroxine withdrawal, the diagnostic efficiency of rhTSH for stimulating Tg production in the serum is comparable to that of levothyroxine withdrawal in most patients.[276,311]

When serum Tg is detectable during levothyroxine treatment, it increases by 5- to 10-fold after TSH stimulation.[308,310] When the serum Tg is below 1 ng/mL during levothyroxine treatment in a blood test performed 3 months after initial treatment, it will increase 14% to 20% following TSH stimulation at 9 to 12 months.[276,299,300] At that time, the serum Tg concentration is an excellent prognostic indicator. Most patients with undetectable TSH-stimulated serum Tg concentrations remained free of relapse after more than 15 years of follow-up, and less than 2% had a neck lymph node recurrence that was detected usually by sonography.[276,299,300] Conversely, persistent or recurrent disease was found in one third of patients with detectable serum Tg concentrations and twice more frequently located in neck lymph nodes than at distant sites; in these patients serum Tg levels increased with time or remained elevated; in the other two thirds of patients with detectable stimulated Tg level, serum Tg obtained following TSH stimulation at subsequent blood tests performed some months or years later will decrease to low or undetectable levels, even in the absence of any further treatment; these patients can then also be considered cured.[276,300,312,313] Persistent thyroid cells may produce Tg for several months after ^{131}I treatment, and this may disappear during subsequent months. These data demonstrate that the trend in serum Tg level is more relevant than the actual serum Tg level by itself.

Modern Tg assays with a functional sensitivity of 0.1 ng/mL have an improved sensitivity for the detection of persistent disease during levothyroxine treatment.[306,314-318] In the large majority (>95%) of patients with serum Tg levels below 0.2 to 0.3 ng/mL on levothyroxine treatment, TSH-stimulated Tg will remain low (<1 ng/mL) or undetectable and, the negative predictive value being 99%, an rhTSH-stimulated Tg is usually not warranted.

[131]I Total-Body Scan

The results of a ^{131}I TBS depend on the ability of neoplastic thyroid tissue to take up ^{131}I in the presence of high serum TSH concentrations, which are achieved by either withdrawing levothyroxine, or administering intramuscular injections of rhTSH (0.9 mg for 2 consecutive days, with radioiodine administration on the day following the

TABLE 14-8
Nonthyroidal Conditions Associated With [131]I Accumulation

Contamination

Skin, hair, clothes

Physiologic Accumulations

Salivary glands (mouth, esophagus), nose
Stomach
Colon (if hypothyroidism)
Bladder
Breast in young women
Diffuse hepatic uptake (^{131}I-labeled iodoproteins)

Inflammatory Processes

Lung or bronchial, cutaneous, dental, sinusoidal

Various Other Conditions

Nonthyroidal neoplasms: salivary glands, stomach, lung, meningioma, hemangioma
Struma ovarii
Cysts: renal, pleuropericardial, hepatic, salivary, mammary, testicular hydrocele
Thymus: normal or hyperplastic
Ectasia of the common carotid artery with stasis
Esophagus: dilatation, hiatal hernia
Pericardial effusion, cardiac insufficiency

second injection).[288] When ^{131}I scanning is planned, patients should be instructed to avoid injection of contrast medium for 1 month,[25] iodine-containing medications, and iodine-rich foods, and urinary iodine should be measured in doubtful cases. Pregnancy must be excluded in women of childbearing age. For routine diagnostic scans, from 2 to 5 mCi (74 to 185 MBq) of ^{131}I is given; higher activities may reduce the uptake of a subsequent therapeutic activity of [131]I.[295,296] The scan is done and uptake, if any, is measured 48 to 72 hours after the activity, preferably using a SPECT/CT. False-positive results are rare and are usually easily recognized (Table 14-8). Assuming equivalent fractional uptake after administration of either a diagnostic or a therapeutic activity of ^{131}I, uptake too low to be detected with 2 to 5 mCi (74 to 185 MBq) may be detectable after the administration of 100 mCi (3700 MBq) or more. Thus, a TBS should be routinely performed 3 to 7 days after the administration of a high activity (Fig. 14-22).

Other Tests

These tests are performed only in selected cases and may include spiral CT with contrast medium or MRI of the neck and chest, bone scintigraphy, MRI of bones, and PET scanning using [18]FDG. FDG-PET scanning is performed both for diagnosing remote neoplastic foci and for prognostic assessment. The sensitivity of FDG-PET scan may be improved by TSH stimulation, obtained following levothyroxine withdrawal or injections of rhTSH.[28,29] The FDG-PET scan is particularly useful for the discovery of mediastinal and of posterior neck lymph node metastases (Fig. 14-23); a spiral CT scan is more sensitive for the discovery of small lung metastases. FDG uptake in metastases as quantified by SUV is closely related to clinical prognostic parameters: responses to radioiodine treatment are observed in metastases with radioiodine uptake and with no FDG uptake. Metastases with high SUVs are likely to progress rapidly and usually do not respond to therapy with radioiodine even when radioiodine uptake is present.[30,31]

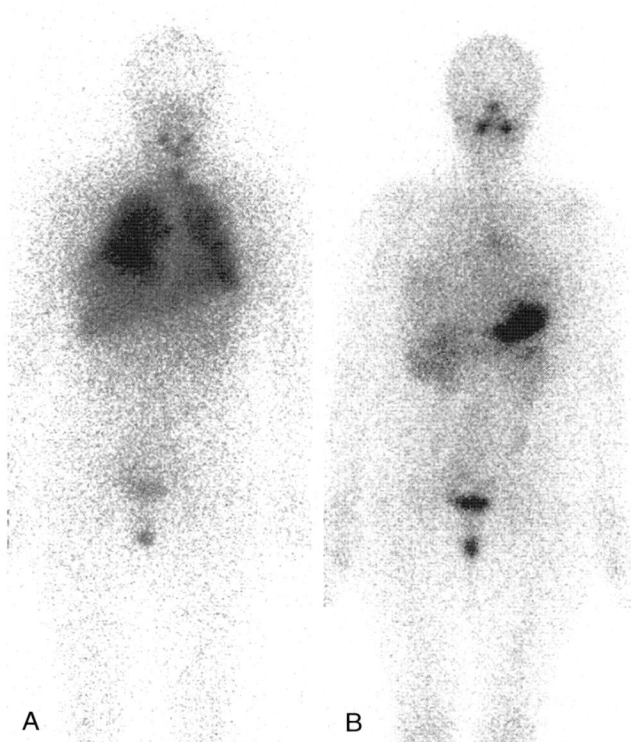

Figure 14-22 Total-body scans in an asymptomatic, 34-year-old patient who underwent surgery for a papillary thyroid carcinoma. The results of chest radiography were normal. **A,** This total-body scan was performed 4 days after postoperative administration of 100 mCi (3700 MBq) of radioactive iodine (^{131}I). Note the presence of diffuse uptake in the lungs and uptake in thyroid remnants and in the left supraclavicular lymph nodes. **B,** A total-body scan performed 6 months later, after the administration of a second treatment with 100 mCi of ^{131}I, demonstrated the disappearance of all foci of uptake. The thyroglobulin level became undetectable during levothyroxine therapy, and 6 years later the patient is still considered to be in complete remission.

Follow-up Strategy

Tests performed during follow-up permit a reassessment of initial prognostication.[319,320] According to the ATA guidelines, four responses to therapy may be observed:

1. *Excellent response* with no clinical, biologic, or imaging abnormality; the risk of recurrence is low.
2. *Biochemical incomplete response*, with elevated serum Tg level but no other evidence of disease; in many patients, the serum Tg will normalize with time in the absence of any subsequent treatment. Serum Tg may increase in some patients who will develop structural disease.
3. *Structural incomplete response*, with imaging evidence of disease; these patients require specific treatment modalities. Disease-specific mortality risk is observed only in this group of patients; morbidity may be significant.
4. *Indeterminate response*, which may be a low but detectable serum Tg, presence of anti-Tg antibodies, or small and avascular abnormalities in the thyroid bed[321] or small lymph nodes on neck ultrasonography; many of these patients will end up with no evidence of disease, but some may develop structural disease (Table 14-9).

TABLE 14-9

Sensitivity of Various Methods and of Their Combination for the Detection of Lymph Node Metastases*

Methods	Study Information N1/Patients		
	Pacini[7] 27/340	Frasoldati[6] 51/494	Torlontano[8] 38/456
Tg/TSH	85% (rhTSH)	57% (WD)	82% (WD)
^{131}I TBS	21%	45%	34%
Neck ultrasonography	70%	94%	100%
Tg/TSH + ultrasonography	96%	99.5%	100%

*Tg (serum thyroglobulin) and TBS (total body scan) were obtained either following withdrawal (WD) or recombinant human thyroid-stimulating hormone (rhTSH).

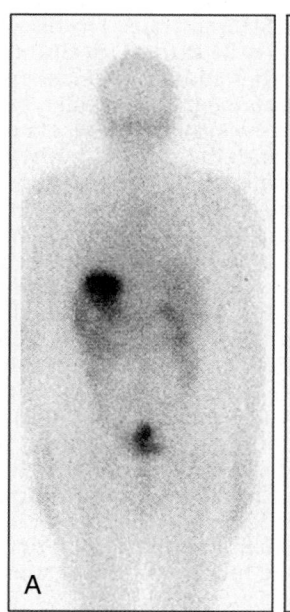
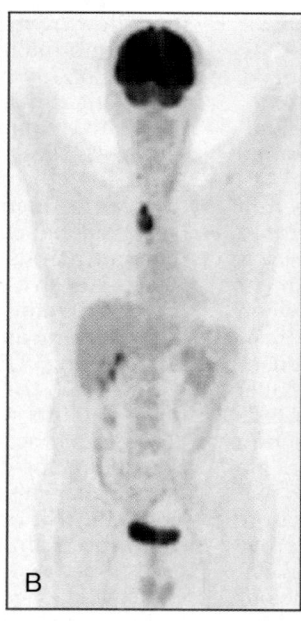
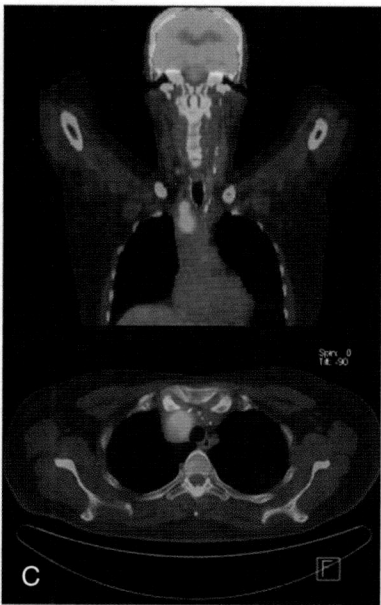

Figure 14-23 This patient was being monitored for a papillary thyroid carcinoma treated by total thyroidectomy and postoperative radioiodine. The serum thyroglobulin level was 45 ng/mL during levothyroxine suppressive treatment. **A,** Total-body scan performed 3 days after administration of 100 mCi (3.7 GBq); there is no visible uptake in the neck and thorax; note accumulation of radioiodine in the stomach, colon, and bladder (posterior view). **B,** Positron emission tomography (PET) scan using [^{18}F]-fluorodeoxyglucose (^{18}FDG) with maximal intensity projection demonstrating significant uptake in the upper mediastinum. **C,** Fusion images of ^{18}FDG-PET scan and computed tomography scan: axial and coronal slices localizing the FDG uptake in the right paratracheal mediastinum and corresponding to a lymph node metastasis that was subsequently excised. Serum thyroglobulin became undetectable during thyroid hormone treatment.

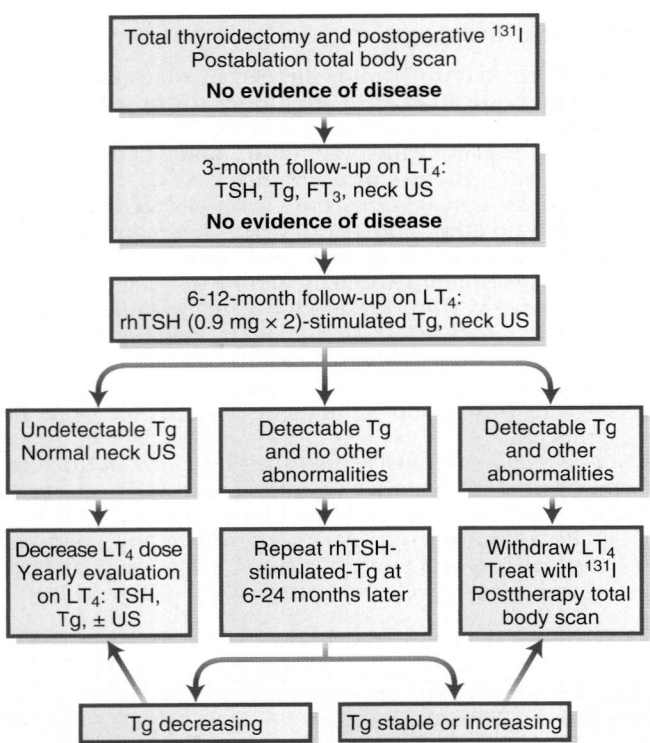

Total thyroidectomy and postoperative ^{131}I
Postablation total body scan
No evidence of disease

↓

3-month follow-up on LT$_4$:
TSH, Tg, FT$_3$, neck US
No evidence of disease

↓

6-12-month follow-up on LT$_4$:
rhTSH (0.9 mg × 2)-stimulated Tg, neck US

| Undetectable Tg Normal neck US | Detectable Tg and no other abnormalities | Detectable Tg and other abnormalities |

| Decrease LT$_4$ dose Yearly evaluation on LT$_4$: TSH, Tg, ± US | Repeat rhTSH-stimulated-Tg at 6-24 months later | Withdraw LT$_4$ Treat with ^{131}I Posttherapy total body scan |

Tg decreasing   Tg stable or increasing

Figure 14-24 Follow-up of patients with PTC or FTC after near-total thyroidectomy and radioactive iodine (^{131}I) ablation, based on serum thyroglobulin (Tg) measurements and neck ultrasonography (US). Undetectable Tg: Tg level below the detection limit of the assay; the institutional threshold should be determined by each institution for each assay used for serum Tg determination. FT$_3$, free T$_3$ (triiodothyronine); LT$_4$, levothyroxine; rhTSH, recombinant human thyroid-stimulating hormone; TSH, thyrotropin (thyroid-stimulating hormone). (From Pacini F, Schlumberger M, Dralle H, et al. European consensus for the management of patients with differentiated thyroid cancer of the follicular epithelium. *Eur J Endocrinol.* 2006;154:787-803, used with permission.)

If the TBS performed after administration of ^{131}I to destroy the thyroid remnants is informative (when uptake in normal thyroid remnants is low, <1%) and does not show any uptake outside the thyroid bed, physical examination is performed, and serum TSH and Tg are measured during levothyroxine treatment 3 months later (Fig. 14-24). A neck ultrasonography is performed and the serum Tg level is measured following rhTSH injections 6 to 12 months after initial treatment; when a sensitive assay is used, serum Tg is measured on levothyroxine treatment and is measured again after rhTSH stimulation only when it is higher than 0.2 to 0.3 ng/mL on levothyroxine treatment.[306,315-318] Suspicious lymph node abnormalities at neck ultrasonography greater than 8 to 10 mm in their smaller diameter should be submitted to FNAB for cytologic tests and Tg determination in the aspirate fluid, even if serum Tg remains undetectable.[307,315] Lymph node metastases are indeed treated, but currently there is no evidence that treatment at a very early stage (when lymph nodes measure less than 5-8 mm in their smaller diameter) may improve the outcome as compared to treatment at a stage when they measure 8 to 10 mm in diameter, and suspicious nonoperated lymph nodes may remain stable for long periods.[322] Abnormalities in the thyroid bed are frequently observed at neck ultrasonography and frequently correspond to sclerosis; they are usually followed up with repeated ultrasonography examinations.[321] A diagnostic ^{131}I TBS is no longer routinely performed in patients with undetectable serum Tg because the majority of patients with ^{131}I uptake in their metastases also have detectable serum Tg levels.[299,300] Also, visible low uptake in the thyroid bed should not be considered evidence of disease in the absence of any other abnormality. Successful remnant ablation is currently defined by two criteria: (1) an undetectable serum TSH-stimulated Tg or a serum Tg less than 0.2 to 0.3 ng/mL on levothyroxine treatment with a sensitive assay, in the absence of interfering anti-Tg antibodies, and (2) a neck ultrasonography that does not show any evidence of disease.[1,3] No other imaging studies are required in the majority of usual cases.

In patients with an excellent response to therapy, long-term risk of recurrence is low, being less than 2% in initially low- and intermediate-risk patients, and all recurrences occurred within 8 years after initial treatment.[299,300,323] The dose of levothyroxine is decreased to maintain a serum TSH concentration within the normal range (0.5-2.5 mU/L). Clinical and biochemical evaluations with serum TSH and Tg determination on levothyroxine treatment are performed annually; neck ultrasonography is performed in case of doubt, and any other testing is unnecessary as long as the patient's serum Tg concentration is undetectable and the patient does not produce an interfering anti-Tg autoantibody.[324,325]

In patients with biochemical or structural incomplete response to therapy, higher doses of levothyroxine are given, the goal being to maintain serum TSH concentration below 0.1 mU/L indefinitely in the absence of contraindication.[120,324]

At 9 to 12 months, serum Tg is higher than 0.2 to 0.3 ng/mL in a fourth of low-risk patients who are then submitted to rhTSH injections. Stimulated Tg obtained 3 days after the second injection will remain lower than 1.5 ng/mL in a third of these patients who had a low (<2%) risk of recurrence but will increase above this level in the other patients who had a higher (32%) risk of recurrence.[306] At that point, a higher percentage of initially intermediate- or high-risk patients may have a detectable serum Tg level on levothyroxine treatment that will increase above 1.5 ng/mL following rhTSH injections. The discovery of any structural abnormality will dictate specific treatments. In the absence of any other abnormalities, suppressive thyroxine treatment is maintained and another Tg determination is performed some months or years later, depending on serum Tg level and the clinical context. Serum Tg will decrease or become undetectable in the absence of any further treatment in two thirds of patients who then will be considered cured.[300,312,313] Serum Tg will increase in the remaining third of patients who should then be submitted to an extensive workup, which may include ultrasound of the neck; spiral CT with contrast medium of the neck, mediastinum, and lungs; bone scintigraphy; and FDG-PET/CT scanning. The administration of a large activity of ^{131}I with a TBS 3 to 5 days later is currently performed only in those patients with a negative FDG-PET/CT scan; in fact, FDG-PET/CT scanning is more sensitive than post-therapy ^{131}I TBS for the detection of neoplastic foci, and high FDG uptake characterizes radioresistant tumors.[326,327] In conclusion, the risk of recurrence should be reassessed at each follow-up examination, and examination findings may be used to decide the most appropriate subsequent follow-up strategy.

In low-risk PTC patients who have had a total thyroidectomy but who were not given ^{131}I postoperatively, the intensity of the follow-up strategy depends largely on the serum Tg level and on neck sonography. If the Tg is low or not detectable during levothyroxine treatment (with serum TSH maintained in the normal range) and a neck ultrasound is negative, ^{131}I TBS may be avoided; the Tg level will become undetectable with time in more than 95% of patients, or will fall below 0.5 ng/mL using a sensitive assay with the risk of recurrence being extremely low.[328-330] However, if the Tg is readily detectable, and more importantly, if it increases with time on levothyroxine treatment, administration of a high activity of ^{131}I may be indicated with a post-therapy scan some days later.[298] The follow-up protocol previously described is then applied on the basis of serum Tg determinations.

In low-risk PTC patients who have initially undergone only a unilateral lobectomy for PTM, yearly follow-up should consist of a careful neck examination and serum Tg determination during levothyroxine treatment (with serum TSH level maintained in the normal range). With time, ultrasonography is likely to show focal nodular abnormalities in the remaining lobe in most patients with detectable Tg concentrations. Usually, biopsies of these lesions can be performed under sonographic guidance, and most prove to be cytologically benign. However, if recurrent PTC is found on biopsy, a completion thyroidectomy should be performed.

For MTC patients, the tumor marker for follow-up is the plasma calcitonin level. In more than 90% of young patients whose disease is treated at a preclinical stage on the basis of a *RET* oncogene mutation, the postoperative basal calcitonin level is undetectable.[18,250,250,331,332] About 5% of them have subsequent biologic recurrence of the disease.[144]

In adults with sporadic MTC, who most often present with TNM stage III (node-positive) disease, postoperative basal calcitonin levels are rarely undetectable.[333,334] In general, calcitonin levels correlate with MTC tumor mass, and when it is below 150 pg/mL, the disease may be located in the neck and the risk of distant spread increases with higher calcitonin levels.[27] The localization of neoplastic foci may be difficult and may require multiple morphologic examinations, including neck and liver ultrasonography, CT scan with injection of the neck and chest, and MRI of bones and liver[26,27]; if those tests are negative, a venous sampling catheterization with selective calcitonin measurements may be indicated.[334,335] PET scanning with FDG is usually poorly sensitive[27,38] and with ^{18}F-DOPA seems more promising for localizing neoplastic MTC foci.[36,37] Reinterventions based on the results of selective venous sampling catheterization allow the removal of neoplastic foci in most patients, but they are not likely to improve the cure rate by more than 5% to 30%.[335-337] Such a situation may exist for several postoperative years, and slowly rising calcitonin levels may not necessarily imply a prognosis worse than that indicated by the presenting stage of disease.[334]

A second major tumor marker for MTC is CEA. In general, serum CEA levels are higher in more aggressive MTC, whereas the plasma calcitonin level is higher in those with better differentiated tumors. The doubling time of calcitonin and CEA levels represents a highly significant prognostic indicator for disease progression and for survival.[338,339]

Papillary and Follicular Thyroid Carcinoma
Locoregional Recurrences

Locoregional recurrences occur in 5% to 20% of patients with PTC and FTC. More than a third of reoperations for persistent or recurrent disease are related to inadequate initial thyroid surgery.[340] Small lymph node metastases may be treated with radioiodine, but their persistence after two or three treatments should lead to surgery.[341]

A recurrence larger than 8 to 10 mm in diameter should be excised.[341,342] Compartmental dissection of previously unexplored compartments with clinically significant persistent/recurrent disease while sparing vital structures is performed because microscopic lymph node metastases are commonly more extensive than would appear from imaging studies alone; this dissection provides a long-term local control of the disease in the majority of patients.[343] Conversely, compartmental surgical dissections may not be feasible in the setting of compartments that have been previously explored because of extensive scarring, and only a more limited or targeted lymph node resection may be possible.

Total excision may be facilitated by TBS 3 to 5 days after administration of 100 mCi (3700 MBq) of ^{131}I because additional tissue that should be excised may be identified. In some selected centers, surgery is performed 1 day after the TBS is done, typically using an intraoperative probe. The completeness of resection is verified 1 to 2 days after surgery by another TBS, and in one series total excision was achieved in 92% of cases.[342] Other methods may be used to facilitate the excision of small neoplastic foci located in scar tissue or in sites that are difficult to redissect, such as intraoperative ultrasound or preoperative ultrasound-guided charcoal tattooing.[14] External radiotherapy is indicated in FCTC patients with soft tissue recurrences that cannot be completely excised and that do not take up [131]I.

Recently, it has been reported that patients with PTC who were not eligible for further surgery or ^{131}I therapy have been treated for regional nodal recurrence with ultrasound-guided radiofrequency ablation or PEI.[344-346] For tumors that invade the upper aerodigestive tract, patient outcome is related to complete resection of all gross disease, with techniques ranging from shaving tumor off the trachea or esophagus for superficial invasion with the preservation of function to more aggressive techniques, including tracheal resection and anastomosis or laryngopharyngoesophagectomy.[347] Surgery is usually combined with ^{131}I and external beam radiation.

Distant Metastases

In a large group of patients with differentiated carcinoma (PTC, FTC, and HCC), only 9% developed distant metastases.[348] Mortality rates at 5 and 10 years after the diagnosis of metastasis were 65% and 75% for all patients with distant metastases, and nearly 80% of the deaths were due to thyroid cancer.[348-350] Of note, up to 20% of deaths were due to locoregional disease.[351] Thus, the development of distant metastases in FCTC portends an ominous prognosis. Lung metastases are more frequent in young patients with PTC, and the lung is almost the only site of distant spread in children. Bone metastases are more common in older patients and in those with FTC. Other less common sites are the brain, liver, and skin.[348-350]

Clinical symptoms of lung involvement are uncommon. By contrast, pain, swelling, or fracture occurs in more than 80% of patients with bone metastases. The pattern of lung involvement may vary from macronodular to diffuse infiltrates. The latter are usually diagnosed with ^{131}I TBS and may be confirmed by spiral CT; enlarged mediastinal lymph nodes are often present in patients with PTC, especially children. Bone metastases are osteolytic and are better visualized by CT scan or MRI. FDG-PET scanning is useful in these patients for both determining the extent of disease and for prognostic assessment.[3,28,30,31] Nearly all patients with distant metastases have high serum Tg concentrations unless the lung metastases are not visible on

CT scan, and two thirds of such patients have ^{131}I uptake in their sites of metastasis.[349]

Focal treatment of bone metastases includes either surgery after embolization, external beam radiation therapy, or thermal ablation (radiofrequency ablation or cryoablation) and cement injection. Focal treatment is indicated when there are neurologic or orthopedic complications or a high risk of such complications and when bone metastases are visible on CT scan or MRI, even in the presence of ^{131}I uptake, because radioiodine alone will not control the disease. In patients with a single or a few bone metastases, focal treatment may also be performed with a curative intent.[352] Surgery and stereotaxic radiation therapy may be indicated in patients with brain metastases. Thermal ablation or stereotaxic radiation therapy may be used in case of few lung metastases. Completenesss of thermal ablation and outcome of the treated lesions can be assessed with FDG-PET scanning.[32]

Patients with distant metastases that take up ^{131}I are treated with 100 to 200 mCi (3700 to 7400 MBq) every 4 to 6 months during the first 2 years and then at longer intervals. Between ^{131}I treatments, suppressive doses of levothyroxine are given to maintain the serum TSH level below 0.1 mUI/L. In one study, the radiation dose to the tumor tissue and outcome of ^{131}I therapy are correlated.[275] A radiation dose higher than 80 Gy (8000 rads) should be delivered to obtain cure; with radiation doses less than 35 Gy (3500 rads), there is little chance for success. This is the rationale for using higher activities of radioiodine either as standard activity or based on individual dosimetry but without demonstrated benefits for any of these techniques. In patients with functioning metastases, PET scanning with [124]I showed that in a given patient uptake may vary between metastases and also within a given metastasis.[35] Finally, uptake may be heterogeneous at the cellular level.[35,79] This heterogeneity in the dose distribution in neoplastic foci may explain the ineffectiveness of ^{131}I treatment, despite significant mean uptake on TBS. For treatment to be effective in this clinical setting, appropriate levels of TSH stimulation and absence of iodine contamination are essential. Excess iodine is eliminated 1 month after administration of an iodinated CT scan.[25] The urinary iodine excretion can be obtained to confirm clearance. Similar short-term survival rates were observed in patients with distant metastases after ^{131}I treatment prepared with either withdrawal or rhTSH.[353] However, most patients with ^{131}I uptake in their metastases are alive at 5 years, and there are no available data on long-term outcome after preparation with rhTSH. Prolonged withdrawal usually induces higher uptake in neoplastic foci than rhTSH and should be the preferred method of TSH stimulation in patients with metastatic disease.[354] rhTSH-mediated therapy may be indicated in selected patients with underlying comorbid conditions, making iatrogenic hypothyroidism potentially risky, and in patients with pituitary disease who are unable to raise their serum TSH.[288] Such patients should be given the same or higher activity that would have been given had they been prepared with hypothyroidism or a dosimetrically determined activity. Lower activities (1-2 mCi [37-74 MBq]/kg body weight) are given to children. There is no limit to the cumulative activity of ^{131}I that can be given to patients with distant metastases, although the risk of leukemia and of solid cancers rises significantly above a cumulative activity of 600 mCi (22,000 MBq); also, above this activity, further ^{131}I therapy may rarely provide a cure.[349]

Disappearance of imaging abnormalities have been obtained overall in about 45% of patients with distant metastases showing avidity for ^{131}I, and responses are more frequent in younger patients, those with small pulmonary metastases, those who had a well-differentiated cancer, and those who have no FDG uptake on PET scan; complete responses may be obtained several years after initiation of therapy.[348-350] When response was judged to have been complete after ^{131}I therapy, subsequent relapse rarely (<10%) occurred even though serum Tg levels were persistently detectable in some patients.[349]

Two thirds of distant metastases will become refractory to radioiodine, and treatment with ^{131}I will not provide any benefit. This group includes patients with metastatic disease that does not take up ^{131}I at the time of initial treatment or that loses the ability to take up ^{131}I after previous evidence of uptake, patients with ^{131}I uptake retained in some lesions but not in others, and patients with metastatic disease that progresses despite significant uptake of ^{131}I in the metastases.[355] Less clear is the situation for patients with persistent ^{131}I uptake in all lesions who are not cured despite several treatment courses (particularly after receiving more than 22,000 MBq [600 mCi] of ^{131}I) and whose disease does not progress according to RECIST (Response Evaluation Criteria in Solid Tumors) criteria.[349] The decision to continue ^{131}I treatment in such patients is generally based on their response to previous treatment courses, persistence of a significant level of ^{131}I uptake on the previous post-therapy TBS, low FDG uptake in tumor foci, and absence of side effects.[355] In patients with refractory disease, ^{131}I treatment should be abandoned, and follow-up is performed with imaging every 4 to 6 months on levothyroxine treatment that should maintain serum TSH below 0.1 mUI/L.[355,356] Focal treatment modalities are used as previously described. In patients with multiple lesions greater than 1 to 2 cm in diameter with documented progression on imaging within 12 months, a systemic treatment may be indicated.[355] Tyrosine kinase inhibitors with antiangiogenic effects are used as first-line treatment.[2-4] They provide significant rates of tumor responses, and one randomized phase II trial with vandetanib versus placebo[357] and two large phase III trials versus placebo have demonstrated that both sorafenib[358] and lenvatinib[359] significantly improve the progression-free survival. However, toxicities are significant and should be prevented and managed by dose reduction and symptomatic treatments. Of interest, a second-line treatment with another antiangiogenic drug may be beneficial.[360,361] Cytotoxic chemotherapy is considered poorly effective,[362] but newer cytotoxic drugs may be used in patients with rapidly progressive disease or who are resistant to tyrosine kinase inhibitors.[363]

Overall survival after the discovery of distant metastases is more favorable in young patients with well-differentiated tumors that take up ^{131}I and have metastases that are small when discovered. When the tumor mass is considered, the location of the distant metastases, be it in the lungs or bone, has no independent prognostic influence.[349] Small radio-avid bone metastases with no structural abnormalities respond to therapy and the poor prognosis of most patients with bone metastases is linked to the large size of their lesions.[348-350,364] Large distant metastases with high FDG uptake on PET scanning almost never respond to ^{131}I therapy and usually rapidly progress, confirming the clinical prognostic classification.[30,31]

Complications of Treatment with [131]I

Acute side effects (nausea, sialadenitis, lost of taste) after treatment with ^{131}I are common but are typically mild and resolve rapidly. Radiation thyroiditis is usually trivial, but if the thyroid remnant is large, the patient may have enough pain to warrant corticosteroid therapy for a few days. Tumor in certain locations, such as the brain, spinal cord, and paratracheal region, may swell in response to TSH stimulation or after ^{131}I therapy, causing compressive symptoms, and this problem should be prevented with corticosteroid therapy. Xerostomia and obstruction of lacrimal ducts may occur in 5% to 10% of patients treated with [131]I.[365,366] Radiation fibrosis may develop in patients with diffuse lung metastases and can eventually prove fatal if high activities (>150 mCi [5550 MBq]) are administered at short intervals (<3 months).[217]

Particular attention must be paid to avoid administration of ^{131}I to pregnant women. After ^{131}I treatment, spermatogenesis may be transiently depressed,[367] and women may have transient ovarian failure. Genetic damage induced by exposure to ^{131}I before conception has been a major subject of concern. However, no anomaly has been reported to date. Therefore, it is recommended that conception be postponed for 6 months after treatment with [131]I.[368] There is no evidence that pregnancy affects tumor growth in women receiving adequate levothyroxine therapy. In case of pregnancy in a patient treated with replacement dose of levothyroxine, the dose of levothyroxine is increased by 30% as soon as the pregnancy is confirmed and serum TSH level is measured every month during the first half of pregnancy.[369] In a patient treated with a suppressive dose of levothyroxine, serum TSH level is controlled every month, and the daily dose of levothyroxine is increased when serum TSH is increased.

Mild pancytopenia may occur after repeated ^{131}I therapy, especially in patients with bone metastases also treated with external radiotherapy. The overall relative risk of leukemia and of solid tumors was found to be increased in patients treated with a high cumulative activity of [131]I (>600 mCi [22,000 MBq]) or in association with external radiotherapy.[370]

Medullary Thyroid Carcinoma

For patients with locoregional recurrence of MTC, a complete diagnostic workup should be obtained, principally to exclude distant metastases. Surgery is performed when feasible and is typically followed by external radiotherapy.

Distant metastases are usually multifocal in each involved organ and frequently involve multiple organs, including liver, lungs, and bones.[2] They may progress slowly and may be compatible with decades of survival. Symptomatic treatments are given, in particular against diarrhea. Cytotoxic chemotherapy is poorly efficient and may be indicated only in cases of rapid tumor progression.[371] Chemoembolization with adriamycin of liver metastases provided a high response rate both on symptoms and on tumor masses.[372] Kinase inhibitors directed against tumor cells (RET and other kinases) and endothelial cells (VEGFR) provide a high response rate and should be used as first-line treatment.[373] Two phase III trials versus placebo have demonstrated that vandetanib[374] and cabozantinib[375] improve progression-free survival. However, toxicity was significant, and they should be proposed only to MTC patients with large tumor foci and progressive disease on imaging.

REFERENCES

1. Pacini F, Schlumberger M, Dralle H, et al. European consensus for the management of patients with differentiated thyroid cancer of the follicular epithelium. *Eur J Endocrinol.* 2006;154:787-803.
2. Schlumberger M, Bastholt L, Dralle H, et al; European Thyroid Association Task Force. 2012 European Thyroid Association guidelines for metastatic medullary thyroid cancer. *Eur Thyroid J.* 2012;1:5-14.
3. Cooper DS, Doherty GM, Haugen BR, et al. Revised management guidelines for patients with thyroid nodules and differentiated thyroid cancer. *Thyroid.* 2009;19:1167-1214.
4. Wells SA Jr, Asa SL, Dralle H, et al. Revised American Thyroid Association guidelines for the management of medullary thyroid carcinoma. *Thyroid.* 2015;25:567-610.
5. Frates MC, Benson CB, Charboneau JW, et al. Management of thyroid nodules detected at US: Society of Radiologists in Ultrasound consensus conference statement. *Radiology.* 2005;237:794-800.
6. Frasoldati A, Pesenti M, Gallo M, et al. Diagnosis of neck recurrences in patients with differentiated thyroid carcinoma. *Cancer.* 2003;97:90-96.
7. Pacini F, Molinaro E, Castagna MG, et al. Recombinant human thyrotropin-stimulated serum thyroglobulin combined with neck ultrasonography has the highest sensitivity in monitoring differentiated thyroid carcinoma. *J Clin Endocrinol Metab.* 2003;88:3668-3673.
8. Torlontano M, Attard M, Crocetti U, et al. Follow-up of low risk patients with papillary thyroid cancer: role of neck ultrasonography in detecting lymph node metastases. *J Clin Endocrinol Metab.* 2004;89:3402-3407.
9. Robbins KT, Shaha AR, Medina JE, et al; Committee for Neck Dissection Classification, American Head and Neck Society. Consensus statement on the classification and terminology of neck dissection. *Arch Otolaryngol Head Neck Surg.* 2008;134:536-538.
10. Rago T, Vitti P. Role of thyroid ultrasound in the diagnostic evaluation of thyroid nodules. *Best Pract Res Clin Endocrinol Metab.* 2008;22:913-928.
11. Moon HJ, Sung JM, Kim EK, et al. Diagnostic performance of gray-scale US and elastography in solid thyroid nodules. *Radiology.* 2012;262:1002-1013.
12. Azizi G, Keller J, Lewis M, et al. Performance of elastography for the evaluation of thyroid nodules: a prospective study. *Thyroid.* 2013;23:734-740.
13. Stulak JM, Grant CS, Farley DR, et al. Value of preoperative ultrasonography in the surgical management of initial and reoperative thyroid cancer. *Arch Surg.* 2005;141:489-496.
14. Hartl DM, Chami L, Ghuzlan AA, et al. Charcoal suspension tattoo localization for differentiated thyroid cancer recurrence. *Ann Surg Oncol.* 2009;16:2602-2608.
15. Price DC. Radioisotopic evaluation of the thyroid and the parathyroids. *Radiol Clin North Am.* 1993;31:991-1015.
16. Meller J, Becker W. The continuing importance of thyroid scintigraphy in the era of high-resolution ultrasound. *Eur J Nucl Med Mol Imaging.* 2002;29(Suppl 2):S425-S438.
17. Robbins RJ, Schlumberger MJ. The evolving role of ^{131}I for the treatment of differentiated thyroid carcinoma. *J Nucl Med.* 2005;46:28S-37S.
18. Loevinger R, Budinger TF, Watson EE. *MIRD Primer for Absorbed Dose Calculations.* New York, NY: The Society of Nuclear Medicine; 1988.
19. Wong KK, Zarzhevsky N, Cahill JM, et al. Incremental value of diagnostic ^{131}I SPECT/CT fusion imaging in the evaluation of differentiated thyroid carcinoma. *AJR Am J Roentgenol.* 2008;191:1785-1794.
20. Aide N, Heutte N, Rame JP, et al. Clinical relevance of single-photon emission computed tomography/computed tomography of the neck and thorax in postablation (131)I scintigraphy for thyroid cancer. *J Clin Endocrinol Metab.* 2009;94:2075-2084.
21. Avram AM. Radioiodine scintigraphy with SPECT/CT: an important diagnostic tool for thyroid cancer staging and risk stratification. *J Nucl Med.* 2012;53:754-764.
22. Grewal RK, Tuttle RM, Fox J, et al. The effect of posttherapy ^{131}I SPECT/CT on risk classification and management of patients with differentiated thyroid cancer. *J Nucl Med.* 2010;51:1361-1367.
23. Phan TT, Jager PL, van Tol KM, Links TP. Thyroid cancer imaging. *Cancer Treat Res.* 2004;122:317-343.
24. Alberico RA, Husain SH, Sirotkin I. Imaging in head and neck oncology. *Surg Oncol Clin North Am.* 2004;13:13-35.
25. Padovani RP, Kasamatsu TS, Nakabashi CC, et al. One month is sufficient for urinary iodine to return to its baseline value after the use of water-soluble iodinated contrast agents in post-thyroidectomy patients requiring radioiodine therapy. *Thyroid.* 2012;22:926-930.
26. Mirallie E, Vuillez JP, Bardet S, et al. High frequency of bone/bone marrow involvement in advanced medullary thyroid cancer. *J Clin Endocrinol Metab.* 2005;90:779-788.
27. Giraudet AL, Vanel D, Leboulleux S, et al. Imaging medullary thyroid carcinoma with persistent elevated calcitonin levels. *J Clin Endocrinol Metab.* 2007;92:4185-4190.
28. Leboulleux S, Schroeder PR, Schlumberger M, Ladenson PW. The role of PET in follow-up of patients treated for differentiated epithelial thyroid cancers. *Nat Clin Pract Endocrinol Metab.* 2007;3:112-121.
29. Leboulleux S, Schroeder PR, Busaidy NL, et al. Assessment of the incremental value of recombinant TSH stimulation before FDG PET/CT imaging to localize residual differentiated thyroid cancer. *J Clin Endocrinol Metab.* 2009;94:1310-1316.
30. Robbins RJ, Wan QW, Grewal RK, et al. Real-time prognosis for metastatic thyroid carcinoma based on 2-[18F] fluoro-2-deoxy-D-glucose positron emission tomography. *J Clin Endocrinol Metab.* 2006;91:498-505.

31. Deandreis D, Al Ghuzlan A, Leboulleux S, et al. Do histological, immunohistochemical and metabolic (radioiodine and fluorodeoxyglucose uptake) patterns of metastatic thyroid cancer correlate with patient outcome? *Endocr Relat Cancer.* 2011;18:159-169.

32. Deandreis D, Leboulleux S, Dromain C, et al. Role of FDG PET/CT and chest CT in the follow-up of lung lesions treated with radiofrequency ablation. *Radiology.* 2011;258:270-276.

33. Van den Bruel A, Maes A, De Potter T, et al. Clinical relevance of thyroid fluorodeoxyglucose-whole body positron emission tomography incidentaloma. *J Clin Endocrinol Metab.* 2002;87:1517-1520.

34. Kim JM, Ryu JS, Kim TY, et al. 18F-Fluorodeoxyglucose positron emission tomography does not predict malignancy in thyroid nodules cytologically diagnosed as follicular neoplasm. *J Clin Endocrinol Metab.* 2007;92:1630-1634.

35. Sgouros G, Kolbert KS, Sheikh A, et al. Patient specific dosimetry for ^{131}I thyroid cancer therapy using ^{124}I PET and 3-dimensional-internal dosimetry (3D-ID) software. *J Nucl Med.* 2004;45:1366-1372.

36. Gourgiotis L, Sarlis NJ, Reynolds JC, et al. Localization of medullary thyroid carcinoma metastasis in a multiple endocrine neoplasia type 2A patient by 6-(F-18)-fluorodopamine positron emission tomography. *J Clin Endocrinol Metab.* 2003;88:637-641.

37. Koopmans KP, de Groot JW, Plukker JT, et al. 18F-Dihydroxyphenylalanine PET in patients with biochemical evidence of medullary thyroid cancer: relation to tumor differentiation. *J Nucl Med.* 2008; 49:524-531.

38. Ong SC, Schoder H, Patel SG, et al. Diagnostic accuracy of 18F-FDG PET in restaging patients with medullary thyroid carcinoma and elevated calcitonin levels. *J Nucl Med.* 2007;48:501-507.

39. Vander JB, Gaston EA, Dawber TR. The significance of nontoxic thyroid nodules. Final report of a 15-year study of the incidence of thyroid malignancy. *Ann Intern Med.* 1968;69:537-540.

40. Tunbridge WM, Evered DC, Hall R, et al. The spectrum of thyroid disease in a community: the Whickham survey. *Clin Endocrinol (Oxf).* 1977;7:481-493.

41. Mortensen JD, Woolner LB, Bennett WA. Gross and microscopic findings in clinically normal thyroid glands. *J Clin Endocrinol Metab.* 1955; 15:1270-1280.

42. Tan GH, Gharib H. Thyroid incidentalomas: management approaches to nonpalpable nodules discovered incidentally on thyroid imaging. *Ann Intern Med.* 1997;126:226-231.

43. Krohn K, Fuhrer D, Bayer Y, et al. Molecular pathogenesis of euthyroid and toxic multinodular goiter. *Endocr Rev.* 2005;26:504-524.

44. Bignell GR, Canzian F, Shayeghi M, et al. Familial nontoxic multinodular thyroid goiter locus maps to chromosome 14q but does not account for familial nonmedullary thyroid cancer. *Am J Hum Genet.* 1997;61:1123-1130.

45. Capon F, Tacconelli A, Giardina E, et al. Mapping a dominant form of multinodular goiter to chromosome Xp22. *Am J Hum Genet.* 2000;67: 1004-1007.

46. Hegedus L, Bonnema SJ, Bennedbaek FN. Management of simple nodular goiter: current status and future perspectives. *Endocr Rev.* 2003;24:102-132.

47. Carlé A, Krejbjerg A, Laurberg P. Epidemiology of nodular goitre. Influence of iodine intake. *Best Pract Res Clin Endocrinol Metab.* 2014; 28:465-479.

48. Knudsen N, Brix TH. Genetic and non-iodine-related factors in the aetiology of nodular goiter. *Best Pract Res Clin Endocrinol Metab.* 2014; 28:495-506.

49. Krejbjerg A, Bjergved L, Pedersen IB, et al. Thyroid nodules in an 11-year DanThyr follow-up study. *J Clin Endocrinol Metab.* 2014;99:4749-4757.

50. Abs R, Stevenaert A, Beckers A. Autonomously functioning thyroid nodules in a patient with a thyrotropin-secreting pituitary adenoma: possible cause-effect relationship. *Eur J Endocrinol.* 1994;131:355-358.

51. Salvi M, Fukazawa H, Bernard N, et al. Role of autoantibodies in the pathogenesis and association of endocrine autoimmune disorders. *Endocr Rev.* 1988;9:450-466.

52. Van Sande J, Parma J, Tonacchera M, et al. Genetic basis of endocrine disease. Somatic and germline mutations of the TSH receptor gene in thyroid diseases. *J Clin Endocrinol Metab.* 1995;80:2577-2585.

53. Bray GA. Increased sensitivity of the thyroid in iodine-depleted rats to the goitrogenic effects of thyrotropin. *J Clin Invest.* 1968;47:1640-1647.

54. Bjergved L, Jørgensen T, Perrild H, et al. Predictors of change in serum TSH after iodine fortification: an 11-year follow-up to the DanThyr study. *J Clin Endocrinol Metab.* 2012;97:4022-4029.

55. Apel RL, Ezzat S, Bapat BV, et al. Clonality of thyroid nodules in sporadic goiter. *Diagn Mol Pathol.* 1995;4:113-121.

56. Foley TP. Goiter in adolescents. *Endocrinol Metab Clin North Am.* 1993;22:593-606.

57. Yassa L, Cibas ES, Benson CB, et al. Long-term assessment of a multidisciplinary approach to thyroid nodule diagnostic evaluation. *Cancer.* 2007;111:508-516.

58. Wang CC, Friedman L, Kennedy GC, et al. A large multicenter correlation study of thyroid nodule cytopathology and histopathology. *Thyroid.* 2011;21:243-251.

59. Davies L, Welch HG. Current thyroid cancer trends in the United States. *JAMA Otolaryngol Head Neck Surg.* 2014;140:317-322.

60. Ahn HS, Kim HJ, Welch HG. Korea's thyroid-cancer "epidemic"—screening and overdiagnosis. *N Engl J Med.* 2014;371:1765-1767.

61. Ito Y, Nikiforov Y, Schlumberger M, Vigneri R. Increasing incidence of thyroid cancer: controversies explored. *Nat Rev Endocrinol.* 2013;9: 178-184.

62. Nou E, Kwong N, Alexander LK, et al. Determination of the optimal time interval for repeat evaluation after a benign thyroid nodule aspiration. *J Clin Endocrinol Metab.* 2014;99:510-516.

63. McCoy KL, Jabbour N, Ogilvie JB, et al. The incidence of cancer and rate of false-negative cytology in thyroid nodules greater than or equal to 4 cm in size. *Surgery.* 2007;142:837-844.

64. Alexander EK, Hurwitz S, Heering JP, et al. Natural history of benign solid and cystic thyroid nodules. *Ann Intern Med.* 2003;138:315-318.

65. Boelaert K, Horacek J, Holder RL, et al. Serum thyrotropin concentration as a novel predictor of malignancy in thyroid nodules investigated by fine-needle aspiration. *J Clin Endocrinol Metab.* 2006;91: 4295-4301.

66. Haymart MR, Repplinger DJ, Leverson GE, et al. Higher serum thyroid stimulating hormone level in thyroid nodule patients is associated with greater risks of differentiated thyroid cancer and advanced tumor stage. *J Clin Endocrinol Metab.* 2008;93:809-814.

67. Elisei R, Bottici V, Luchetti F, et al. Impact of routine measurement of serum calcitonin on the diagnosis and outcome of medullary thyroid cancer: experience in 10,864 patients with nodular thyroid disorders. *J Clin Endocrinol Metab.* 2004;89:163-168.

68. Costante G, Durante C, Francis Z, et al. Clinical interest of calcitonin determination in C cell disease. *Nat Clin Pract Endocrinol Metab.* 2009; 5:35-44.

69. Kwak JY, Han KH, Yoon JH, et al. Thyroid imaging reporting and data system for US features of nodules: a step in establishing better stratification of cancer risk. *Radiology.* 2011;260:892-899.

70. Moon WJ, Jung SL, Lee JH, et al. Benign and malignant thyroid nodules: US differentiation—multicenter retrospective study. *Radiology.* 2008;247:762-770.

71. Moon HJ, Kwak JY, Kim MJ, et al. Can vascularity at power Doppler US help predict thyroid malignancy? *Radiology.* 2010;255:260-269.

72. Salmaslioglu A, Erbil Y, Dural C, et al. Predictive value of sonographic features in preoperative evaluation of malignant thyroid nodules in a multinodular goiter. *World J Surg.* 2008;32:1948-1954.

73. Papini E, Guglielmi R, Bianchini A, et al. Risk of malignancy in nonpalpable thyroid nodules: predictive value of ultrasound and color-Doppler features. *J Clin Endocrinol Metab.* 2002;87:1941-1946.

74. Brito JP, Gionfriddo MR, Al NA, et al. The accuracy of thyroid nodule ultrasound to predict thyroid cancer: systematic review and meta-analysis. *J Clin Endocrinol Metab.* 2014;99:1253-1263.

75. Horvath E, Majlis S, Rossi R, et al. An ultrasonogram reporting system for thyroid nodules stratifying cancer risk for clinical management. *J Clin Endocrinol Metab.* 2009;94:1748-1751.

76. Tae HJ, Lim DJ, Baek KH, et al. Diagnostic value of ultrasonography to distinguish between benign and malignant lesions in the management of thyroid nodules. *Thyroid.* 2007;17:461-466.

77. Shimura H, Haraguchi K, Hiejima Y, et al. Distinct diagnostic criteria for ultrasonographic examination of papillary thyroid carcinoma: a multicenter study. *Thyroid.* 2005;15:251-258.

78. Rago T, Santini F, Scutari M, et al. Elastography: new developments in ultrasound for predicting malignancy in thyroid nodules. *J Clin Endocrinol Metab.* 2007;92:2917-2922.

79. Schlumberger M, Lacroix L, Russo D, et al. Defects in iodide metabolism in thyroid cancer and implications for the follow-up and treatment of patients. *Nat Clin Pract Endocrinol Metab.* 2007;3:260-269.

80. Soelberg KK, Bonnema SJ, Brix TH, Hegedus L. Risk of malignancy in thyroid incidentalomas detected by 18F-fluorodeoxyglucose positron emission tomography: a systematic review. *Thyroid.* 2012;22:918-925.

81. Chen W, Parsons M, Torigian DA, et al. Evaluation of thyroid FDG uptake incidentally identified on FDG-PET/CT imaging. *Nucl Med Commun.* 2009;30:240-244.

82. Nishimori H, Tabah R, Hickeson M, How J. Incidental thyroid "PETomas": clinical significance and novel description of the self-resolving variant of focal FDG-PET thyroid uptake. *Can J Surg.* 2011; 54:83-88.

83. Deandreis D, Al Ghuzlan A, Auperin A, et al. Is 18F-fluorodeoxyglucose-PET/CT useful for the presurgical characterization of thyroid nodules with indeterminate fine needle aspiration cytology? *Thyroid.* 2012; 22:165-172.

84. Hamburger JI. Diagnosis of thyroid nodules by fine needle biopsy: use and abuse. *J Clin Endocrinol Metab.* 1994;79:335-339.

85. Gharib H. Changing concepts in the diagnosis and management of thyroid nodules. *Endocrinol Metab Clin North Am.* 1997;26:777-800.

86. Hales MS, Hsu FS. Needle tract implantation of papillary carcinoma of the thyroid following aspiration biopsy. *Acta Cytol.* 1990;34:801-804.

87. Mikosch P, Gallowitsch HJ, Kresnik E, et al. Value of ultrasound-guided fine-needle aspiration biopsy of thyroid nodules in an endemic goitre area. *Eur J Nucl Med.* 2000;27:62-69.

88. Baloch ZW, Tam D, Langer J, et al. Ultrasound-guided fine-needle aspiration biopsy of the thyroid: role of on-site assessment and multiple cytologic preparations. *Diagn Cytopathol.* 2000;23:425-429.

89. Danese D, Sciacchitano S, Farsetti A, et al. Diagnostic accuracy of conventional versus sonography-guided fine-needle aspiration biopsy of thyroid nodules. *Thyroid.* 1998;8:15-21.

90. Baloch ZW, LiVolsi VA, Asa SL, et al. Diagnostic terminology and morphologic criteria for cytologic diagnosis of thyroid lesions: a synopsis of the National Cancer Institute Thyroid Fine-Needle Aspiration State of the Science Conference. *Diagn Cytopathol.* 2008;36:425-437.

91. Crippa S, Mazzucchelli L, Cibas ES, Ali SZ. The Bethesda System for reporting thyroid fine-needle aspiration specimens. *Am J Clin Pathol.* 2010;134:343-344.

92. Theoharis CG, Schofield KM, Hammers L, et al. The Bethesda thyroid fine-needle aspiration classification system: year 1 at an academic institution. *Thyroid.* 2009;19:1215-1223.

93. Luu MH, Fischer AH, Pisharodi L, Owens CL. Improved preoperative definitive diagnosis of papillary thyroid carcinoma in FNAs prepared with both ThinPrep and conventional smears compared with FNAs prepared with ThinPrep alone. *Cancer Cytopathol.* 2011;119:68-73.

94. Bongiovanni M, Spitale A, Faquin WC, et al. The Bethesda System for reporting thyroid cytopathology: a meta-analysis. *Acta Cytol.* 2012;56:333-339.

95. Nayar R, Ivanovic M. The indeterminate thyroid fine-needle aspiration: experience from an academic center using terminology similar to that proposed in the 2007 National Cancer Institute Thyroid Fine Needle Aspiration State of the Science Conference. *Cancer.* 2009;117:195-202.

96. Cibas ES, Baloch ZW, Fellegara G, et al. A prospective assessment defining the limitations of thyroid nodule pathologic evaluation. *Ann Intern Med.* 2013;159:325-332.

97. Bartolazzi A, Orlandi F, Saggiorato E, et al. Galectin-3-expression analysis in the surgical selection of follicular thyroid nodules with indeterminate fine-needle aspiration cytology: a prospective multicentre study. *Lancet Oncol.* 2008;9:543-549.

98. Nikiforov YE, Ohori NP, Hodak SP, et al. Impact of mutational testing on the diagnosis and management of patients with cytologically indeterminate thyroid nodules: a prospective analysis of 1056 FNA samples. *J Clin Endocrinol Metab.* 2011;96:3390-3397.

99. Cantara S, Capezzone M, Marchisotta S, et al. Impact of proto-oncogene mutation detection in cytological specimens from thyroid nodules improves the diagnostic accuracy of cytology. *J Clin Endocrinol Metab.* 2010;95:1365-1369.

100. Moses W, Weng J, Sansano I, et al. Molecular testing for somatic mutations improves the accuracy of thyroid fine-needle aspiration biopsy. *World J Surg.* 2010;34:2589-2594.

101. Beaudenon-Huibregtse S, Alexander EK, Guttler RB, et al. Centralized molecular testing for oncogenic gene mutations complements the local cytopathologic diagnosis of thyroid nodules. *Thyroid.* 2014;24:1479-1487.

102. Xing M, Haugen BR, Schlumberger M. Progress in molecular-based management of differentiated thyroid cancer. *Lancet.* 2013;381:1058-1069.

103. Alexander EK, Kennedy GC, Baloch ZW, et al. Preoperative diagnosis of benign thyroid nodules with indeterminate cytology. *N Engl J Med.* 2012;367:705-715.

104. Li H, Robinson KA, Anton B, et al. Cost-effectiveness of a novel molecular test for cytologically indeterminate thyroid nodules. *J Clin Endocrinol Metab.* 2011;96:E1719-E1726.

105. Keutgen XM, Filicori F, Crowley MJ, et al. A panel of four miRNAs accurately differentiates malignant from benign indeterminate thyroid lesions on fine needle aspiration. *Clin Cancer Res.* 2012;18:2032-2038.

106. Carpi A, Nicolini A. The role of large-needle aspiration biopsy in the preoperative selection of palpable thyroid nodules: a summary of principal data. *Biomed Pharmacother.* 2000;54:350-353.

107. Braga M, Cavalcanti TC, Collaco LM, Graf H. Efficacy of ultrasound-guided fine-needle aspiration biopsy in the diagnosis of complex thyroid nodules. *J Clin Endocrinol Metab.* 2001;86:4089-4091.

108. Redman R, Zalaznick H, Mazzaferri EL, Massoll NA. The impact of assessing specimen adequacy and number of needle passes for fine-needle aspiration biopsy of thyroid nodules. *Thyroid.* 2006;16:55-60.

109. Orija IB, Pineyro M, Biscotti C, et al. Value of repeating a nondiagnostic thyroid fine-needle aspiration biopsy. *Endocr Pract.* 2007;13:735-742.

110. Wu HH, Rose C, Elsheikh TM. The Bethesda system for reporting thyroid cytopathology: an experience of 1,382 cases in a community practice setting with the implication for risk of neoplasm and risk of malignancy. *Diagn Cytopathol.* 2012;40:399-403.

111. Moon HJ, Kwak JY, Choi YS, Kim EK. How to manage thyroid nodules with two consecutive non-diagnostic results on ultrasonography-guided fine-needle aspiration. *World J Surg.* 2012;36:586-592.

112. Alexander EK, Heering JP, Benson CB, et al. Assessment of nondiagnostic ultrasound-guided fine needle aspirations of thyroid nodules. *J Clin Endocrinol Metab.* 2002;87:4924-4927.

113. Choi YS, Hong SW, Kwak JY, et al. Clinical and ultrasonographic findings affecting nondiagnostic results upon the second fine needle aspiration. *Ann Surg Oncol.* 2012;19:2304-2309.

114. Greer MA, Astwood EB. Treatment of simple goiter with thyroid. *J Clin Endocrinol.* 1953;13:1312-1331.

115. Ross DS. Thyroid hormone suppressive therapy of sporadic nontoxic goiter. *Thyroid.* 1992;2:263-269.

116. Berghout A, Wiersinga WM, Drexhage HA, et al. Comparison of placebo with L-thyroxine alone or with carbimazole for treatment of sporadic nontoxic goitre. *Lancet.* 1990;336:193-197.

117. Castro MR, Caraballo PJ, Morris JC. Effectiveness of thyroid hormone suppressive therapy in benign solitary thyroid nodules: a meta-analysis. *J Clin Endocrinol Metab.* 2002;87:4154-4159.

118. Wemeau JL, Caron P, Schvartz C, et al. Effects of thyroid-stimulating hormone suppression with levothyroxine in reducing the volume of solitary thyroid nodules and improving extranodular nonpalpable changes: a randomized, double-blind, placebo-controlled trial by the French Thyroid Research Group. *J Clin Endocrinol Metab.* 2002;87:4928-4934.

119. Surks MI, Ortiz E, Daniels GH, et al. Subclinical thyroid disease. Scientific review and guidelines for diagnosis and management. *JAMA.* 2004;291:228-238.

120. Biondi B, Wartofsky L. Treatment with thyroid hormone. *Endocr Rev.* 2014;35:433-512.

121. Berghout A, Wiersinga WM, Drexhage HA, et al. The long-term outcome of thyroidectomy for sporadic nontoxic goitre. *Clin Endocrinol (Oxf).* 1989;31:193-199.

122. Agerback H, Pilegaard HK, Watt-Boolsen S, et al. Complications of 2,028 operations for benign thyroid disease. *Ugeskr Laeger.* 1988;150:533-536.

123. Bistrup C, Nielsen JD, Gregersen G, et al. Preventive effect of levothyroxine in patients operated for nontoxic goitre: a randomized trial of one hundred patients with nine years follow-up. *Clin Endocrinol (Oxf).* 1994;40:323-327.

124. Bonnema SJ, Nielsen VE, Hegedus L. Long-term effects of radioiodine on thyroid function, size and patient satisfaction in non-toxic diffuse goitre. *Eur J Endocrinol.* 2004;150:439-445.

125. Wesche MFT, Tiel-V Buul MCC, Lips P, et al. A randomized trial comparing levothyroxine with radioactive iodine in the treatment of sporadic nontoxic goiter. *J Clin Endocrinol Metab.* 2001;86:998-1005.

126. Manders JMB, Corstens FHM. Radioiodine therapy of euthyroid multinodular goiters. *Eur J Nucl Med Mol Imaging.* 2002;29(Suppl 2):S466-S470.

127. Nygaard B, Faber J, Hegedus L. Acute changes in thyroid volume and function following ^{131}I therapy of multinodular goiter. *Clin Endocrinol (Oxf).* 1994;41:715-718.

128. Holm LE, Hall P, Wiklund K, et al. Cancer risk after iodine-131 therapy for hyperthyroidism. *J Natl Cancer Inst.* 1991;83:1072-1077.

129. Graf H, Fast S, Pacini F, et al. Modified-release recombinant human TSH (MRrhTSH) augments the effect of (131)I therapy in benign multinodular goiter: results from a multicenter international, randomized, placebo-controlled study. *J Clin Endocrinol Metab.* 2011;96:1368-1376.

130. Zingrillo M, Torlontano M, Chiarella R, et al. Percutaneous ethanol injection may be a definitive treatment for symptomatic thyroid cystic nodules not treatable by surgery: five-year follow-up study. *Thyroid.* 1999;9:763-767.

131. Papini E, Guglielmi R, Bizzarri G, et al. Ultrasound-guided laser thermal ablation for treatment of benign thyroid nodules. *Endocr Pract.* 2004;10:276-283.

132. Schlumberger MJ. Papillary and follicular thyroid carcinoma. *N Engl J Med.* 1998;338:297-306.

133. Hay ID. Papillary thyroid carcinoma. *Endocrinol Metab Clin North Am.* 1990;19:545-576.

134. Hedinger C, Williams ED, Sobin LH. *Histological Typing of Thyroid Tumours.* 2nd ed. Originally published by the World Health Organization as no. 11 in the International Histological Classification of Tumours series. New York, NY: Springer-Verlag; 1988:1-20.

135. Rosai J, Carganio ML, Delellis RA. *Tumors of the Thyroid Gland.* Washington, DC: Armed Forces Institute of Pathology; 1992.

136. Beahrs OH, Henson DE, Hutter RVP, et al. *Manual for Staging of Cancer.* Philadelphia, PA: JB Lippincott; 1992.

137. American Joint Committee on Cancer. Thyroid. In: Greene FL, Page DL, Fleming ID, et al, eds. *AJCC Cancer Staging Handbook.* 6th ed. New York, NY: Springer; 2002:89-98.

138. Sobin LH, Gospodarowicz MK, Wittekind CH, eds. *TNM Classification of Malignant Tumors.* 7th ed. New York, NY: International Union Against Cancer; 2010:58-62.

139. Schlumberger M, de Vathaire F, Travagli JP, et al. Differentiated thyroid carcinoma in childhood: long term follow-up of 72 patients. *J Clin Endocrinol Metab.* 1987;65:1088-1094.

140. Leboulleux S, Rubino C, Baudin E, et al. Prognostic factors for persistent or recurrent disease of papillary thyroid carcinoma with neck lymph node metastases and/or tumor extension beyond the thyroid capsule at initial diagnosis. *J Clin Endocrinol Metab.* 2005;90:5723-5729.

141. Bardet S, Ciappuccini R, Quak E, et al. Prognostic value of microscopic lymph node involvement in patients with papillary thyroid cancer. *J Clin Endocrinol Metab.* 2015;100:132-140.

142. Brierley J, Tsang R, Simpson WJ, et al. Medullary thyroid cancer: analyses of survival and prognostic factors and the role of radiation therapy in local control. *Thyroid.* 1996;6:305-310.

143. Kebebew E, Ituarte PH, Siperstein AE, et al. Medullary thyroid carcinoma: clinical characteristics, treatment, prognostic factors, and a comparison of staging systems. *Cancer.* 2000;88:1139-1148.

144. Modigliani E, Cohen R, Campos JM, et al. Prognostic factors for survival and for biochemical cure in medullary thyroid carcinoma: results in 899 patients. The GETC Study Group. Groupe d'étude des tumeurs à calcitonine. *Clin Endocrinol (Oxf).* 1998;48:265-273.

145. Bisi H, Fernandes VS, Asato de Camargo RY, et al. The prevalence of unsuspected thyroid pathology in 300 sequential autopsies, with special reference to the incidental carcinoma. *Cancer.* 1989;64:1888-1893.

146. Carney JA, Ryan J, Goellner JR. Hyalinizing trabecular adenoma of the thyroid gland. *Am J Surg Pathol.* 1987;11:583-592.

147. Carcangiu ML, Bianchi S, Savino D, et al. Follicular Hürthle cell neoplasms of the thyroid gland: a study of 153 cases. *Cancer.* 1991;68:1944-1953.

148. Gundry SR, Burney RE, Thompson NW, et al. Total thyroidectomy for Hürthle cell neoplasm of the thyroid. *Arch Surg.* 1983;118:529-532.

149. Grant CS, Barr D, Goellner JR, et al. Benign Hürthle cell tumors of the thyroid: a diagnosis to be trusted? *World J Surg.* 1988;12:488-494.

150. Chen H, Nicol TL, Zeiger MA, et al. Hürthle cell neoplasms of the thyroid: are there factors predictive of malignancy? *J Nucl Med.* 1998;34:1626-1631.

151. Xing M. Molecular pathogenesis and mechanisms of thyroid cancer. *Nat Rev Cancer.* 2013;13:184-199.

152. Hay ID, Thompson GB, Grant CS, et al. Papillary thyroid carcinoma managed at the Mayo Clinic during six decades (1940-1999): temporal trends in initial therapy and long-term outcome in 2444 consecutively treated patients. *World J Surg.* 2002;26:879-885.

153. Hay ID, Hutchinson ME, Gonzalez-Losada T, et al. Papillary thyroid microcarcinoma; a study of 900 cases observed in a 60-year period. *Surgery.* 2008;144:980-988.

154. Baudin E, Travagli J, Ropers J, et al. Microcarcinoma of the thyroid gland: the Gustave Roussy Institute experience. *Cancer.* 1998;83:553-559.

155. Hiltzik D, Carlson DL, Tuttle RM, et al. Poorly differentiated thyroid carcinomas defined on the basis of mitosis and necrosis: a clinicopathologic study of 58 patients. *Cancer.* 2006;106:1286-1295.

156. Motosugi U, Murata S, Nagata K, et al. Thyroid papillary carcinoma with micropapillary and hobnail growth pattern: a histological variant with intermediate malignancy? *Thyroid.* 2009;19:535-537.

157. Hay ID, Gonzalez-Losada T, Reinalda MS, et al. Long-term outcome in 215 children and adolescents with papillary thyroid cancer treated during 1940 through 2008. *World J Surg.* 2010;34:1192-1202.

158. Rivkees SA, Mazzaferri EL, Verburg FA, et al. The treatment of differentiated thyroid cancer in children: emphasis on surgical approach and radioactive iodine therapy. *Endocr Rev.* 2011;32:798-826.

159. Fagin JA. Challenging dogma in thyroid cancer molecular genetics. Role of RET/PTC and BRAF in tumor initiation. *J Clin Endocrinol Metab.* 2004;89:4264-4266.

160. Herrmann MA, Hay ID, Bartlet DH, et al. Cytogenetic and molecular genetic studies of follicular and papillary thyroid cancers. *J Clin Invest.* 1991;88:1596-1603.

161. Williams ED. Cancer after nuclear fallout: lessons from the Chernobyl accident. *Nature Rev.* 2002;2:543-549.

162. Grieco M, Santoro M, Berlingieri MT, et al. PTC is a novel rearranged form of the RET proto-oncogene and is frequently detected in vivo in human thyroid papillary carcinomas. *Cell.* 1990;60:557-563.

163. Santoro M, Dathan NA, Berlingieri MT, et al. Molecular characterization of RET/PTC3; a novel rearranged version of the RET proto-oncogene in a human thyroid papillary carcinoma. *Oncogene.* 1994;9:509-516.

164. Ricarte-Filho JC, Li S, Garcia-Rendueles ME, et al. Identification of kinase fusion oncogenes in post-Chernobyl radiation-induced thyroid cancers. *J Clin Invest.* 2013;123:4935-4944.

165. Vasko V, Ferrand M, Di Cristofaro J, et al. Specific pattern of RAS oncogene mutations in follicular thyroid tumors. *J Clin Endocrinol Metab.* 2003;88:2745-2752.

166. Xing M. BRAF mutation in papillary thyroid cancer: pathogenic role, molecular bases, and clinical implications. *Endocr Rev.* 2007;28:742-762.

167. Ciampi R, Knauf JA, Kerler R, et al. Oncogenic AKAP9-BRAF fusion is a novel mechanism of MAPK pathway activation in thyroid cancer. *J Clin Invest.* 2005;115:20-23.

168. Bongarzone I, Vigneri P, Mariani L, et al. RET/NTRK1 rearrangements in thyroid gland tumors of the papillary carcinoma family: correlation with clinicopathological features. *Clin Cancer Res.* 1998;4:223-228.

169. Leeman-Neill RJ, Kelly LM, Liu P, et al. 2014 ETV6–NTRK3 is a common chromosomal rearrangement in radiation associated thyroid cancer. *Cancer.* 2014;120:799-807.

170. Kelly LM, Barila G, Liu P, et al. Identification of the transforming STRN-ALK fusion as a potential therapeutic target in the aggressive forms of thyroid cancer. *Proc Natl Acad Sci U S A.* 2014;111:4233-4238.

171. Mineo R, Costantino A, Frasca F, et al. Activation of the hepatocyte growth factor (HGF)-Met system in papillary thyroid cancer: biological effects of HGF in thyroid cancer cells depend on Met expression levels. *Endocrinology.* 2004;145:4355-4365.

172. Xing M, Liu R, Liu X, et al. BRAF V600E and TERT promoter mutations cooperatively identify the most aggressive papillary thyroid cancer with highest recurrence. *J Clin Oncol.* 2014;32:2718-2726.

173. Mitchell JC, Parangi S. Angiogenesis in benign and malignant thyroid disease. *Thyroid.* 2005;15:494-510.

174. Guo M, Liu W, Serra S, et al. FGFR2 isoforms support epithelial-stromal interactions in thyroid cancer progression. *Cancer Res.* 2012;72:2017-2027.

175. Giordano TJ. The cancer genome atlas research network: a sight to behold. *Endocr Pathol.* 2014;25:362-365.

176. Goldgar DE, Easton DF, Cannon-Albright LA, Skolnick MH. Systematic population-based assessment of cancer risk in first-degree relatives of cancer probands. *J Natl Cancer Inst.* 1994;86:1600-1608.

177. Sturgeon C, Clark OH. Familial nonmedullary thyroid cancer. *Thyroid.* 2005;15:588-593.

178. Vriens MR, Suh I, Moses W, Kebebew E. Clinical features and genetic predisposition to hereditary nonmedullary thyroid cancer. *Thyroid.* 2009;19:1343-1349.

179. Gudmundsson J, Sulem P, Gudbjartsson DF, et al. Common variants on 9q22.33 and 14q13.3 predispose to thyroid cancer in European populations. *Nat Genet.* 2009;41:460-464.

180. Landa I, Ruiz-Llorente S, Montero-Conde C, et al. The variant rs1867277 in FOXE1 gene confers thyroid cancer susceptibility through the recruitment of USF1/USF2 transcription factors. *PLoS Genet.* 2009;5:e1000637.

181. Ngan ESW, Lang BHH, Liu T, et al. A germline mutation (A339V) in thyroid transcription factor-1 (TITF-1/NKX2.1) in patients with multinodular goiter and papillary thyroid carcinoma. *J Natl Cancer Inst.* 2009;101:162-175.

182. Tomaz RA, Sousa I, Silva JG, et al. FOXE1 polymorphisms are associated with familial and sporadic nonmedullary thyroid cancer susceptibility. *Clin Endocrinol (Oxf).* 2012;77:926-933.

183. Chakravarty D, Santos E, Ryder M, et al. Small-molecule MAPK inhibitors restore radioiodine incorporation in mouse thyroid cancers with conditional BRAF activation. *J Clin Invest.* 2011;121:4700-4711.

184. Ho AL, Grewal RK, Leboeuf R, et al. Selumetinib-enhanced radioiodine uptake in advanced thyroid cancer. *N Engl J Med.* 2013;368:623-632.

185. Ricarte-Filho JC, Ryder M, Chitale DA, et al. Mutational profile of advanced primary and metastatic radioactive iodine-refractory thyroid cancers reveals distinct pathogenetic roles for BRAF, PIK3CA, and AKT1. *Cancer Res.* 2009;69:4885-4893.

186. Sabra MM, Dominguez JM, Grewal RK, et al. Clinical outcomes and molecular profile of differentiated thyroid cancers with radioiodine-avid distant metastases. *J Clin Endocrinol Metab.* 2013;98:E829-E836.

187. Colonna M, Grosclaude P, Remontet L, et al. Incidence of thyroid cancer in adults recorded by French Cancer registries (1978-1997). *Eur J Cancer.* 2002;38:1762-1768.

188. Shattuck TM, Westra WH, Ladenson PW, et al. Independent clonal origins of distinct tumor foci in multifocal thyroid carcinoma. *N Engl J Med.* 2005;352:2406-2412.

189. Zimmerman D, Hay ID, Gough IR, et al. Papillary thyroid carcinoma in children and adults: long-term follow-up of 1,039 patients conservatively treated at one institution during three decades. *Surgery.* 1988;104:1157-1166.

190. Kukkonen ST, Haapiainen RK, Fransila KO, et al. Papillary thyroid carcinoma: the new, age-related TNM classification system in a retrospective analysis of 199 patients. *World J Surg.* 1990;14:837-842.

191. Grant CS, Hay ID, Gough IR, et al. Local recurrence in papillary thyroid carcinoma: is extent of surgical resection important? *Surgery.* 1988;104:954-962.

192. Hay ID, Grant CS, Taylor WF, et al. Ipsilateral lobectomy versus bilateral lobar resection in papillary thyroid carcinoma: a retrospective analysis of surgical outcome using a novel prognostic scoring system. *Surgery.* 1987;102:1088-1095.

193. Tsang RW, Brierley JD, Simpson WJ, et al. The effects of surgery, radioiodine, and external radiation therapy on the clinical outcome of patients with differentiated thyroid carcinoma. *Cancer.* 1998;82:375-388.

194. DeGroot LJ, Kaplan EL, McCormick M, et al. Natural history, treatment and course of papillary thyroid carcinoma. *J Clin Endocrinol Metab.* 1990;71:414-424.

195. Shah JP, Loree TR, Dharker D, et al. Prognostic factors in differentiated carcinoma of the thyroid gland. *Am J Surg.* 1992;164:658-661.

196. Akslen LA, LiVolsi VA. Prognostic significance of histologic grading compared with subclassification of papillary thyroid carcinoma. *Cancer.* 2000;88:1902-1908.

197. Hay ID, Bergstralh EJ, Goellner JR, et al. Predicting outcome in papillary thyroid carcinoma: development of a reliable prognostic scoring system in a cohort of 1,779 patients surgically treated at one institution during 1940 through 1989. *Surgery.* 1993;114:1050-1058.

198. Brierley JD, Panzarella T, Tsang RW, et al. A comparison of different staging systems predictability of patient outcome: thyroid carcinoma as an example. *Cancer.* 1997;79:2414-2423.

199. Hay ID. Management of patients with low-risk papillary thyroid carcinoma. *Endocr Pract.* 2007;13:521-533.

200. Pace-Asciak PZ, Payne RJ, Eski SJ, et al. Cost savings of patients with a MACIS score lower than 6 when radioactive iodine is not given. *Arch Otolaryngol Head Neck Surg.* 2007;133:870-873.

201. Rivera M, Ricarte-Filho J, Patel S, et al. Encapsulated thyroid tumors of follicular cell origin with high grade features (high mitotic rate/ tumor necrosis): a clinicopathologic and molecular study. *Hum Pathol.* 2010;41:172-180.

202. Chéreau N, Buffet C, Trésallet C, et al. Does extracapsular extension impact the prognosis of papillary thyroid microcarcinoma? *Ann Surg Oncol.* 2014;21:1659-1664.

203. Nixon IJ, Ganly I, Patel S, et al. The impact of microscopic extrathyroid extension on outcome in patients with clinical T1 and T2 well-differentiated thyroid cancer. *Surgery.* 2011;150:1242-1249.

204. Rivera M, Ricarte-Filho J, Tuttle RM, et al. Molecular, morphologic, and outcome analysis of thyroid carcinomas according to degree of extra-thyroid extension. *Thyroid.* 2010;20:1085-1093.

205. Randolph GW, Duh QY, Heller KS, et al; American Thyroid Association Surgical Affairs Committee's Taskforce on Thyroid Cancer Nodal Surgery. The prognostic significance of nodal metastases from papillary thyroid carcinoma can be stratified based on the size and number of metastatic lymph nodes, as well as the presence of extranodal extension. *Thyroid.* 2012;22:1144-1152.

206. Ricarte-Filho J, Ganly I, Rivera M, et al. Papillary thyroid carcinomas with cervical lymph node metastases can be stratified into clinically relevant prognostic categories using oncogenic BRAF, the number of nodal metastases, and extra-nodal extension. *Thyroid.* 2012;22:575-584.

207. Carcangiu MC, Zempi G, Rosai J. Poorly differentiated ("insular") thyroid carcinoma: a reinterpretation of Langhans "wuchernde" Struma. *Am J Surg Pathol.* 1984;8:655-668.

208. Sobrinho-Simoes M. Mixed medullary and follicular carcinoma of the thyroid. *Histopathology.* 1993;23:187-189.

209. Ganly I, Ricarte-Filho J, Eng S, et al. Genomic dissection of Hurthle cell carcinoma reveals a unique class of thyroid malignancy. *J Clin Endocrinol Metab.* 2013;98:E962-E972.

210. Grebe SKG, Hay ID. Follicular thyroid cancer. *Endocrinol Metab Clin North Am.* 1996;24:761-801.

211. LiVolsi VA, Asa SL. The demise of follicular carcinoma of the thyroid gland. *Thyroid.* 1994;4:233-236.

212. LiVolsi VA, Merino MJ. Worrisome histologic alterations following fine-needle aspiration of the thyroid. *Pathol Annu.* 1994;29:99-120.

213. Weber F, Shen L, Aldred MA, et al. Genetic classification of benign and malignant thyroid follicular neoplasia based on a three-gene combination. *J Clin Endocrinol Metab.* 2005;90:2512-2521.

214. Volante M, Collini P, Nikiforov YE, et al. Poorly differentiated thyroid carcinoma: the Turin proposal for the use of uniform diagnostic criteria and an algorithmic diagnostic approach. *Am J Surg Pathol.* 2007; 31:1256-1264.

215. Ishimaru Y, Fukuda S, Kurano R, et al. Follicular thyroid carcinoma with clear cell change showing unusual ultrastructural features. *Am J Surg Pathol.* 1988;12:240-246.

216. Watson RG, Brennan MD, Goellner JR, et al. Invasive Hürthle cell carcinoma of the thyroid: natural history and management. *Mayo Clin Proc.* 1984;59:851-855.

217. Pierotti MA, Bongarzone I, Borrello MG, et al. Cytogenetics and molecular genetics of carcinomas arising from thyroid epithelial follicular cells. *Genes Chromosomes Cancer.* 1996;16:1-14.

218. Challeton C, Bounacer A, Du Villard JA, et al. Pattern of ras and gsp oncogene mutations in radiation-associated human thyroid tumors. *Oncogene.* 1995;11:601-603.

219. Kroll TG, Sarraf P, Pecciarini L, et al. PAX8-PPARγ1 fusion oncogene in human thyroid carcinoma. *Science.* 2000;289:1357-1360.

220. Powell GJ, Wang X, Allard BL, et al. The PAX8/PPAR gamma fusion oncoprotein transforms immortalized human thyrocytes through a mechanism probably involving wild-type PPAR gamma inhibition. *Oncogene.* 2004;23:3634-3641.

221. Nikiforova MN, Lynch RA, Biddinger PW, et al. RAS point mutations and PAX8-PPAR gamma rearrangement in thyroid tumors: evidence for distinct molecular pathways in thyroid follicular carcinoma. *J Clin Endocrinol Metab.* 2003;88:2318-2326.

222. Paul SJ, Sisson JC. Thyrotoxicosis caused by thyroid cancer. *Endocrinol Metab Clin North Am.* 1990;19:593-612.

223. Grebe SKG, Hay ID. Thyroid cancer nodal metastases: biologic significance and therapeutic considerations. *Surg Oncol Clin North Am.* 1996;5:43-63.

224. van Heerden JA, Hay ID, Goellner JR, et al. Follicular thyroid carcinoma with capsular invasion alone: a non-threatening malignancy. *Surgery.* 1992;112:1130-1136.

225. Mueller-Gaertner HW, Brzac HT, Rehpenning W. Prognostic indices for tumor relapse and tumor mortality in follicular thyroid carcinoma. *Cancer.* 1991;67:1903-1908.

226. Cady R, Rossi R. An expanded view of risk-group definition in differentiated thyroid carcinoma. *Surgery.* 1985;98:1171-1176.

227. Shaha AR, Loree TR, Shah JP. Prognostic factors and risk group analysis in follicular carcinoma of the thyroid. *Surgery.* 1995;118:1131-1138.

228. Emerick GT, Duh QY, Siperstein AE, et al. Diagnosis, treatment, and outcome of follicular thyroid carcinoma. *Cancer.* 1993;72:3287-3294.

229. Davis NL, Bugis SD, McGregor GI, et al. An evaluation of prognostic scoring systems in patients with follicular thyroid cancer. *Am J Surg.* 1995;170:476-480.

230. Asari R, Koperek O, Scheuba C, et al. Follicular thyroid carcinoma in an iodine-replete endemic goiter region: a prospectively collected, retrospectively analyzed clinical trial. *Ann Surg.* 2009;249:1023-1031.

231. LiVolsi VA, Baloch ZW. Predicting prognosis in thyroid carcinoma: can histology do it? *Am J Surg Pathol.* 2002;26:1064-1065.

232. d'Avanzo A, Ituarte P, Treseler P, et al. Prognostic scoring systems in patients with follicular thyroid cancer: a comparison of different staging systems in predicting the patient outcome. *Thyroid.* 2004;14: 453-458.

233. Volante M, Rapa I, Gandhi M, et al. RAS mutations are the predominant molecular alteration in poorly differentiated thyroid carcinomas and bear prognostic impact. *J Clin Endocrinol Metab.* 2009;94: 4735-4741.

234. Fagin JA, Matsuo K, Karmakar A, et al. High prevalence of mutations of the p53 gene in poorly differentiated human thyroid carcinomas. *J Clin Invest.* 1993;91:179-184.

235. Elliott DD, Sherman SI, Busaidy NL, et al. Growth factor receptors expression in anaplastic thyroid carcinoma: potential markers for therapeutic stratification. *Hum Pathol.* 2008;39:15-20.

236. Saji M, Ringel MD. The PI3K-Akt-mTOR pathway in initiation and progression of thyroid tumors. *Mol Cell Endocrinol.* 2010;321:20-28.

237. Ibrahimpasic T, Ghossein R, Carlson DL, et al. Outcomes in patients with poorly differentiated thyroid carcinoma. *J Clin Endocrinol Metab.* 2014;99:1245-1252.

238. McIver B, Hay ID, Giuffrida DF, et al. Anaplastic thyroid carcinoma: a 50-year experience at a single institution. *Surgery.* 2001;130:1028-1034.

239. De Crevoisier R, Baudin E, Bachelot A, et al. Combined treatment of anaplastic thyroid carcinoma with surgery, chemotherapy, and hyper-fractionated accelerated external radiotherapy. *Int J Radiat Oncol Biol Phys.* 2004;60:1137-1143.

240. Smallridge RC. Approach to the patient with anaplastic thyroid carcinoma. *J Clin Endocrinol Metab.* 2012;97:2566-2572.

241. Ryder M, Ghossein RA, Ricarte-Filho JC, et al. Increased density of tumor-associated macrophages is associated with decreased survival in advanced thyroid cancer. *Endocr Relat Cancer.* 2008;15:1069-1074.

242. Caillou B, Talbot M, Weyemi U, et al. Tumor-associated macrophages (TAMs) form an interconnected cellular supportive network in anaplastic thyroid carcinoma. *PLoS ONE.* 2011;6:e22567.

243. Poisson T, Deandreis D, Leboulleux S, et al. 18F-fluorodeoxyglucose positron emission tomography and computerized tomography in anaplastic thyroid cancer. *Eur J Nucl Med.* 2010;37:2277-2285.

244. Bogsrud TV, Karantanis D, Nathan MA, et al. 18F-FDG PET in the management of patients with anaplastic thyroid carcinoma. *Thyroid.* 2008;18:713-719.

245. Rosove MH, Peddi PF, Glaspy JA. BRAF V600E inhibition in anaplastic thyroid cancer. *N Engl J Med.* 2013;368:684-685.

246. Godbert Y, Henriques de Figueiredo B, Bonichon F, et al. Remarkable response to crizotinib in woman with anaplastic lymphoma kinase-rearranged anaplastic thyroid carcinoma. *J Clin Oncol.* 2014;[Epub ahead of print].

247. Wagle N, Grabiner BC, Van Allen EM, et al. Response and acquired resistance to everolimus in anaplastic thyroid cancer. *N Engl J Med.* 2014;371:1426-1433.

248. Leboulleux S, Baudin E, Travagli JP, Schlumberger M. Medullary thyroid carcinoma. *Clin Endocrinol (Oxf).* 2004;61:299-310.

249. Machens A, Niccoli-Sire P, Hoegel J, et al. Early malignant progression of hereditary medullary thyroid cancer. *N Engl J Med.* 2003;349:1517-1525.

250. Skinner MA, Moley JA, Dilley WG, et al. Prophylactic thyroidectomy in multiple endocrine neoplasia type 2A. *N Engl J Med.* 2005;353: 1105-1113.

251. Elisei R, Cosci B, Romei C, et al. Prognostic significance of somatic RET oncogene mutations in sporadic medullary thyroid cancer: a 10-year follow-up study. *J Clin Endocrinol Metab.* 2008;93:682-687.

252. Boichard A, Al Ghuzlan A, Croux L, et al. H-RAS and K-RAS point mutations occur in a large proportion of sporadic RET-negative medullary thyroid carcinomas. *J Clin Endocrinol Metab.* 2012;97:2031-2035.

253. Moura MM, Cavaco BM, Pinto AE, Leite V. High prevalence of RAS mutations in RET-negative sporadic medullary thyroid carcinomas. *J Clin Endocrinol Metab.* 2011;96:E863-E868.

254. Agrawal N, Jiao Y, Sausen M, et al. Exomic sequencing of medullary thyroid cancer reveals dominant and mutually exclusive oncogenic mutations in RET and RAS. *J Clin Endocrinol Metab.* 2013;98:E364-E369.

255. Ciampi R, Mian C, Fugazzola L, et al. Evidence of a low prevalence of RAS mutations in a large medullary thyroid cancer series. *Thyroid.* 2013;23:50-57.

256. Moley JF, DeBenedetti MK. Patterns of nodal metastases in palpable medullary thyroid carcinoma. Recommendations for extent of node dissection. *Ann Surg.* 1999;6:880-888.

257. Scollo C, Baudin E, Travagli JP, et al. Rationale for central and bilateral lymph node dissection in sporadic and hereditary medullary thyroid cancer. *J Clin Endocrinol Metab.* 2003;88:2070-2075.

258. Thieblemont C, Mayer A, Dumontet C, et al. Primary thyroid lymphoma is a heterogeneous disease. *J Clin Endocrinol Metab.* 2002;87: 105-111.

259. Harris NL, Jaffe ES, Stein H, et al. A revised European-American classification of lymphoid neoplasms: a proposal from the International Lymphoma Study Group. *Blood.* 1994;84:1361-1392.

260. Shipp M. A predictive model for aggressive non-Hodgkin's lymphoma. The International Non-Hodgkin's Lymphoma Prognostic Factors Project. *N Engl J Med.* 1993;329:987-994.

261. Coiffier B, Lepage E, Briere J, et al. CHOP chemotherapy plus rituximab compared with CHOP alone in elderly patients with diffuse large-B-cell lymphoma. *N Eng J Med.* 2002;346:235-242.

262. Tsang RW, Gosodarowicz MK, Pintilie M, et al. Localized mucosa-associated lymphoid tissue lymphoma treated with radiation therapy has excellent clinical outcome. *J Clin Oncol.* 2003;21:4157-4164.

263. Bilimoria KY, Bentrem DJ, Ko CY, et al. Extent of surgery affects survival for papillary thyroid cancer. *Ann Surg.* 2007;246:375-384.

264. Adam MA, Pura J, Gu L, et al. Extent of surgery for papillary thyroid cancer is not associated with survival: an analysis of 61,775 patients. *Ann Surg.* 2014;260:601-605.

265. Nixon IJ, Ganly I, Patel SG, et al. Thyroid lobectomy for treatment of well differentiated intrathyroid malignancy. *Surgery.* 2012;151: 571-579.

266. Bonnet S, Hartl D, Leboulleux S, et al. Prophylactic lymph node dissection for papillary thyroid cancer less than 2 cm: implications for radioiodine treatment. *J Clin Endocrinol Metab.* 2009;94:1162-1167.

267. White MC, Gauger PG, Doherty GM. Central lymph node dissection in papillary thyroid carcinoma. *World J Surg.* 2007;31:895-904.

268. Mazzaferri EL, Doherty GM, Steward DL. The pros and cons of prophylactic central compartment lymph node dissection for papillary thyroid carcinoma. *Thyroid.* 2009;19:683-689.

269. Moreno MA, Edeiken-Monroe BS, Siegel ER, et al. In papillary thyroid cancer, preoperative central neck ultrasound detects only macroscopic surgical disease, but negative findings predict excellent long-term regional control and survival. *Thyroid.* 2012;22:347-355.

270. Hay ID, Bergstralh EJ, Grant CS, et al. Impact of primary surgery on outcome in 300 patients with pathologic tumor-node-metastasis stage III papillary thyroid carcinoma treated at one institution from 1940 through 1989. *Surgery.* 1999;126:1173-1181.

271. Leboulleux S, Girard E, Rose M, et al. Ultrasound criteria of malignancy for cervical lymph nodes in patients followed up for differentiated thyroid cancer. *J Clin Endocrinol Metab.* 2007;92:3590-3594.

272. Hartl DM, Travagli JP, Leboulleux S, et al. Current concepts in the management of unilateral recurrent laryngeal nerve paralysis after thyroid surgery. *J Clin Endocrinol Metab.* 2005;90:3084-3088.

273. Schneider AB, Sarne DH. Long-term risks for thyroid cancer and other neoplasm after exposure to radiation. *Nat Clin Pract Endocrinol Metab.* 2005;1:82-91.

274. Rubino C, Cailleux AF, Abbas M, et al. Characteristics of follicular cell-derived thyroid carcinomas occurring after external radiation exposure: results of a case control study nested in a cohort. *Thyroid.* 2002;12:299-304.

275. Maxon HR, Thomas SR, Hertzberg VS, et al. Relation between effective radiation dose and outcome of radioiodine therapy for thyroid cancer. *N Engl J Med.* 1983;309:937-941.

276. Eustatia-Rutten CFA, Smit JWA, Romijn JA, et al. Diagnostic value of serum thyroglobulin measurements in the follow-up of differentiated thyroid carcinoma, a structured meta-analysis. *Clin Endocrinol (Oxf).* 2004;61:61-74.

277. Jonklaas J, Cooper DS, Ain KB, et al; National Thyroid Cancer Treatment Cooperative Study Group. Radioiodine therapy in patients with stage I differentiated thyroid cancer. *Thyroid.* 2010;20:1423-1424.

278. Hay ID, McDougall IR, Sisson JC. Perspective: the case against radioiodine remnant ablation in patients with well-differentiated thyroid carcinoma. *J Nucl Med.* 2008;49:1395-1397.

279. Schvartz C, Bonnetain F, Dabakuyo S, et al. Impact on overall survival of radioactive iodine in low-risk differentiated thyroid cancer patients. *J Clin Endocrinol Metab.* 2012;97:1526-1535.

280. Ibrahimpasic T, Nixon IJ, Palmer FL, et al. Undetectable thyroglobulin after total thyroidectomy in patients with low- and intermediate-risk papillary thyroid cancer—is there a need for radioactive iodine therapy? *Surgery.* 2012;152:1096-1105.

281. Nascimento CL, Borget I, Al Ghuzlan A, et al. Persistent disease and recurrence in differentiated thyroid cancer patients with undetectable postoperative stimulated thyroglobulin level. *Endocr Relat Cancer.* 2011;18:29-40.

282. Lepoutre-Lussey C, Maddah D, Golmard JL, et al. Post-operative neck ultrasound and risk stratification in differentiated thyroid cancer patients with initial lymph node involvement. *Eur J Endocrinol.* 2014; 170:837-846.

283. Pacini F, Ladenson PW, Schlumberger M, et al. Radioiodine ablation of thyroid remnants after preparation with recombinant human thyrotropin in differentiated thyroid carcinoma: results of an international, randomized, controlled study. *J Clin Endocrinol Metab.* 2006;91: 926-932.

284. Schlumberger M, Catargi B, Borget I, et al. Tumeurs de la Thyroïde Refractaires Network for the Essai Stimulation Ablation Equivalence Trial. Strategies of radioiodine ablation in low-risk thyroid cancer patients. *N Engl J Med.* 2012;366:1663-1673.

285. Mallick U, Harmer C, Yap B, et al. Ablation with low-dose radioiodine and thyrotropin alfa in thyroid cancer. *N Engl J Med.* 2012;366: 1674-1685.

286. Hänscheid H, Lassmann M, Luster M, et al. Iodine biokinetics and dosimetry in radioiodine therapy of thyroid cancer: procedures and results of a prospective international controlled study of ablation after rhTSH or hormone withdrawal. *J Nucl Med.* 2006;47:648-654.

287. Rémy H, Borget I, Leboulleux S, et al. Iodine 131 effective half-life and dosimetry in thyroid cancer patients. *J Nucl Med.* 2008;49:1445-1450.

288. Schlumberger M, Ricard M, De Pouvourville G, Pacini F. How the availability of recombinant human TSH has changed the management of patients who have thyroid cancer. *Nat Clin Pract Endocrinol Metab.* 2007;3:641-650.

289. Castagna MG, Cevenini G, Theodoropoulou A, et al. Post-surgical thyroid ablation with low or high radioiodine activities results in similar outcomes in intermediate risk differentiated thyroid cancer patients. *Eur J Endocrinol.* 2013;169:23-29.

290. Rosário PW, Calsolari MR. Thyroid ablation with 1.1 GBq (30 mCi) iodine-131 in patients with papillary thyroid carcinoma at intermediate risk for recurrence. *Thyroid.* 2014;24:826-831.

291. Hugo J, Robenshtok E, Grewal R, et al. Recombinant human thyroid stimulating hormone-assisted radioactive iodine remnant ablation in thyroid cancer patients at intermediate to high risk of recurrence. *Thyroid.* 2012;22:1007-1015.

292. Tuttle RM, Brokhin M, Omry G, et al. RJ Recombinant human TSH-assisted radioactive iodine remnant ablation achieves short-term clinical recurrence rates similar to those of traditional thyroid hormone withdrawal. *J Nucl Med.* 2008;49:764-770.

293. Elisei R, Schlumberger M, Driedger A, et al. Follow-up of low-risk differentiated thyroid cancer patients who underwent radioiodine ablation of postsurgical thyroid remnants after either recombinant human thyrotropin or thyroid hormone withdrawal. *J Clin Endocrinol Metab.* 2009;94:4171-4179.

294. Molinaro E, Giani C, Agate L, et al. Patients with differentiated thyroid cancer who underwent radioiodine thyroid remnant ablation with low-activity ^{131}I after either recombinant human TSH or thyroid hormone therapy withdrawal showed the same outcome after a 10-year follow-up. *J Clin Endocrinol Metab.* 2013;98:2693-2700.

295. Lassmann M, Luster M, Hanscheid H, et al. The impact of I-131 diagnostic activities on the biokinetics of thyroid remnants. *J Nucl Med.* 2004;45:619-625.

296. Nordén MM, Larsson F, Tedelind S, et al. Down-regulation of the sodium/iodide symporter explains ^{131}I-induced thyroid stunning. *Cancer Res.* 2007;67:7512-7517.

297. Schlumberger M, Pacini F. The low utility of pretherapy scans in thyroid cancer patients. *Thyroid.* 2009;19:815-816.

298. Schlumberger M, Mancusi F, Baudin E, et al. [131]I therapy for elevated thyroglobulin levels. *Thyroid.* 1997;7:273-276.

299. Cailleux AF, Baudin E, Travagli JP, et al. Is diagnostic iodine-131 scanning useful after total thyroid ablation for differentiated thyroid cancer? *J Clin Endocrinol Metab.* 2000;85:175-178.

300. Pacini F, Capezzone M, Elisei R, et al. Diagnostic 131-iodine whole-body scan may be avoided in thyroid cancer patients who have undetectable stimulated serum Tg levels after initial treatment. *J Clin Endocrinol Metab.* 2002;87:1499-1501.

301. Bal CS, Kumar A, Pant GS. Radioiodine dose for remnant ablation in differentiated thyroid carcinoma: a randomized clinical trial in 509 patients. *J Clin Endocrinol Metab.* 2004;89:1666-1673.

302. Hackshaw A, Harmer C, Mallick U, et al. [131]I activity for remnant ablation in patients with differentiated thyroid cancer: a systematic review. *J Clin Endocrinol Metab.* 2007;92:28-38.

303. Tuttle RM, Leboeuf R, Robbins RJ, et al. Empiric radioactive iodine dosing regimens frequently exceed maximum tolerated activity levels in elderly patients with thyroid cancer. *J Nucl Med.* 2006;47: 1587-1591.

304. Farahati J, Reiners C, Stuschke M, et al. Differentiated thyroid cancer: impact of adjuvant external radiotherapy in patients with perithyroidal tumor infiltration (stage pT4). *Cancer.* 1996;77:172-180.

305. Romesser PB, Sherman EJ, Shaha AR, et al. External beam radiotherapy with or without concurrent chemotherapy in advanced or recurrent non-anaplastic non-medullary thyroid cancer. *J Surg Oncol.* 2014;110: 375-382. [Epub 2014 Jun 24].

306. Brassard M, Borget I, Edet-Sanson A, et al; THYRDIAG Working Group. Long-term follow-up of patients with papillary and follicular thyroid cancer: a prospective study on 715 patients. *J Clin Endocrinol Metab.* 2011;96:1352-1359.

307. Pacini F, Fugazzola L, Lippi F, et al. Detection of thyroglobulin in fine needle aspirates of nonthyroidal neck masses: a clue to the diagnosis of metastatic differentiated thyroid cancer. *J Clin Endocrinol Metab.* 1992;74:1401-1404.

308. Demers LM, Spencer CA. *Laboratory Support for the Diagnosis and Monitoring of Thyroid Disease.* NACB Laboratory Medicine Practice Guidelines. Washington, DC: American Association for Clinical Chemistry; 2003. Available at: <http://www.nacb.org/lmpg/thyroid/LMPH.stm>.

309. Chiovato L, Latrofa F, Braverman LE, et al. Disappearance of humoral thyroid autoimmunity after complete removal of thyroid antigens. *Ann Intern Med.* 2003;139:346-351.

310. Bachelot A, Cailleux AF, Klain M, et al. Relationship between tumor burden and serum thyroglobulin level in patients with papillary and follicular thyroid carcinoma. *Thyroid.* 2002;12:707-711.

311. Haugen BR, Pacini F, Reiners C, et al. A comparison of recombinant human thyrotropin and thyroid hormone withdrawal for the detection of thyroid remnant or cancer. *J Clin Endocrinol Metab.* 1999; 84:3877-3885.

312. Baudin E, Docao C, Cailleux AF, et al. Positive predictive value of serum thyroglobulin levels, measured during the first year of follow-up following thyroid hormone withdrawal, in thyroid cancer patients. *J Clin Endocrinol Metab.* 2003;88:1107-1111.

313. Padovani RP, Robenshtok E, Brokhin M, Tuttle RM. Even without additional therapy, serum thyroglobulin concentrations often decline for years after total thyroidectomy and radioactive remnant ablation in patients with differentiated thyroid cancer. *Thyroid.* 2012;22: 778-783.

314. Schlumberger M, Hitzel A, Toubert ME, et al. Comparison of seven serum thyroglobulin assays in the follow-up of papillary and follicular thyroid cancer patients. *J Clin Endocrinol Metab.* 2007;92:2487-2495.

315. Snozek CL, Chambers EP, Reading CC, et al. Serum thyroglobulin, high-resolution ultrasound, and lymph node thyroglobulin in diagnosis of differentiated thyroid carcinoma nodal metastases. *J Clin Endocrinol Metab.* 2007;92:4278-4281.

316. Spencer C, Fatemi S, Singer P, et al. Serum basal thyroglobulin measured by a second-generation assay correlates with the recombinant human thyrotropin-stimulated thyroglobulin response in patients treated for differentiated thyroid cancer. *Thyroid.* 2010;20:587-595.

317. Malandrino P, Latina A, Marescalco S, et al. Risk-adapted management of differentiated thyroid cancer assessed by a sensitive measurement of basal serum thyroglobulin. *J Clin Endocrinol Metab.* 2011;96: 1703-1709.

318. Chindris AM, Diehl NN, Crook JE, et al. Undetectable sensitive serum thyroglobulin (<0.1 ng/ml) in 163 patients with follicular cell-derived thyroid cancer: results of rhTSH stimulation and neck ultrasonography and long-term biochemical and clinical follow-up. *J Clin Endocrinol Metab.* 2012;97:2714-2723.

319. Castagna MG, Maino F, Cipri C, et al. Delayed risk stratification, to include the response to initial treatment (surgery and radioiodine ablation), has better outcome predictivity in differentiated thyroid cancer patients. *Eur J Endocrinol.* 2011;165:441-446.

320. Tuttle RM, Tala H, Shah J, et al. Estimating risk of recurrence in differentiated thyroid cancer after total thyroidectomy and radioactive iodine remnant ablation: using response to therapy variables to modify the initial risk estimates predicted by the new American Thyroid Association staging system. *Thyroid.* 2010;20:1341-1349.

321. Rondeau G, Fish S, Hann LE, et al. Ultrasonographically detected small thyroid bed nodules identified after total thyroidectomy for differentiated thyroid cancer seldom show clinically significant structural progression. *Thyroid.* 2011;21:845-853.

322. Robenshtok E, Fish S, Bach A, et al. Suspicious cervical lymph nodes detected after thyroidectomy for papillary thyroid cancer usually remain stable over years in properly selected patients. *J Clin Endocrinol Metab.* 2012;97:2706-2713.

323. Durante C, Montesano T, Torlontano M, et al; PTC Study Group. Papillary thyroid cancer: time course of recurrences during postsurgery surveillance. *J Clin Endocrinol Metab.* 2013;98:636-642.

324. Jonklaas J, Sarlis NJ, Litofsky D, et al. Outcomes of patients with differentiated thyroid carcinoma following initial therapy. *Thyroid.* 2006;16:1229-1242.

325. Castagna MG, Brilli L, Pilli T, et al. Limited value of repeat recombinant thyrotropin (rhTSH)-stimulated thyroglobulin testing in differentiated thyroid carcinoma patients with previous negative rhTSH-stimulated thyroglobulin and undetectable basal serum thyroglobulin levels. *J Clin Endocrinol Metab.* 2008;93:76-81.

326. Leboulleux S, El Bez I, Borget I, et al. Post-radioiodine treatment whole body scan in the era of fluorodesoxyglucose positron emission tomography for differentiated thyroid carcinoma with elevated serum thyroglobulin levels. *Thyroid.* 2012;22:832-838.

327. Rosario PW, Mourão GF, dos Santos JB, Calsolari MR. Is empirical radioactive iodine therapy still a valid approach to patients with thyroid cancer and elevated thyroglobulin? *Thyroid.* 2014;24: 533-536.

328. Durante C, Montesano T, Attard M, et al; PTC Study Group. Long-term surveillance of papillary thyroid cancer patients who do not undergo postoperative radioiodine remnant ablation: is there a role for serum thyroglobulin measurement? *J Clin Endocrinol Metab.* 2012;97: 2748-2753.

329. Nascimento C, Borget I, Troalen F, et al. Ultrasensitive serum thyroglobulin measurement is useful for the follow-up of patients treated with total thyroidectomy without RAI ablation. *Eur J Endocrinol.* 2013;169:689-693.

330. Angell TE, Spencer CA, Rubino BD, et al. In search of an unstimulated thyroglobulin baseline value in low-risk papillary thyroid carcinoma patients not receiving radioactive iodine ablation. *Thyroid.* 2014;24: 1127-1133.

331. Rohmer V, Vidal-Trecan G, Bourdelot A, et al. Prognostic factors of disease-free survival after thyroidectomy in 170 young patients 2 with a RET germline mutation. A multicenter study of the GTE (Groupe français d'Etude des Tumeurs Endocrines) for the Groupe Français des Tumeurs Endocrines. *J Clin Endocrinol Metab.* 2011;96:509-518.

332. Elisei R, Romei C, Renzini G, et al. The timing of total thyroidectomy in RET gene mutation carriers could be personalized and safely planned on the basis of serum calcitonin: 18 years experience at one single center. *J Clin Endocrinol Metab.* 2012;97:426-435.

333. Machens A, Lorenz K, Sekulla C, et al. Molecular epidemiology of multiple endocrine neoplasia 2: implications for RET screening in the new millennium. *Eur J Endocrinol.* 2013;168:307-314.

334. van Heerden JA, Grant CS, Gharib H, et al. Long-term course of patients with persistent hypercalcitoninemia after apparent curative primary surgery for medullary thyroid carcinoma. *Ann Surg.* 1990;212: 395-400.

335. Pellegriti G, Leboulleux S, Baudin E, et al. Long-term outcome of medullary thyroid carcinoma in patients with normal postoperative medical imaging. *Br J Cancer.* 2003;88:1537-1542.

336. Kebebew E, Kikuchi S, Duh QY, et al. Long-term results of reoperation and localizing studies in patients with persistent or recurrent medullary thyroid cancer. *Arch Surg.* 2000;135:895-901.

337. Fialkowski E, Debenedetti M, Moley J. Long-term outcome of re-operations for medullary thyroid carcinoma. *World J Surg.* 2008;32: 754-765.

338. Barbet J, Campion L, Kraeber-Bodéré F, et al. Prognostic impact of serum calcitonin and carcinoembryonic antigen doubling-times in patients with medullary thyroid carcinoma. *J Clin Endocrinol Metab.* 2005;90:6077-6084.

339. Giraudet AL, Al Ghuzlan A, Aupérin A, et al. Progression of medullary thyroid carcinoma: assessment with calcitonin and CEA doubling times. *Eur J Endocrinol.* 2008;158:239-246.

340. Kouvaraki MA, Lee JE, Shapiro SE, et al. Preventable reoperations for persistent and recurrent papillary thyroid carcinoma. *Surgery.* 2004;136: 1183-1191.

341. Pacini F, Cetani F, Miccoli P, et al. Outcome of 309 patients with metastatic differentiated thyroid carcinoma treated with radioiodine. *World J Surg.* 1994;18:600-604.

342. Travagli JP, Cailleux AF, Ricard M, et al. Combination of radioiodine (^{131}I) and probe-guided surgery for persistent or recurrent thyroid carcinoma. *J Clin Endocrinol Metab.* 1998;83:2675-2680.

343. Clayman GL, Agarwal G, Edeiken BS, et al. Long-term outcome of comprehensive central compartment dissection in patients with recurrent/persistent papillary thyroid carcinoma. *Thyroid.* 2011;21: 1309-1316.

344. Dupuy DE, Monchik JM, Decrea C, et al. Radiofrequency ablation of regional recurrence from well-differentiated thyroid malignancy. *Surgery.* 2001;130:971-977.

345. Hay ID, Lee RA, Davidge-Pitts C, et al. Long-term outcome of ultrasound-guided percutaneous ethanol ablation of selected "recurrent" neck nodal metastases in 25 patients with TNM stages III or IVA papillary thyroid carcinoma previously treated by surgery and ^{131}I therapy. *Surgery.* 2013;154:1448-1454.

346. Kim BM, Kim MJ, Kim EK, et al. Controlling recurrent papillary thyroid carcinoma in the neck by ultrasonographically-guided percutaneous ethanol injection. *Eur Radiol.* 2008;18:835-842.

347. Gaissert HA, Honings J, Grillo HC, et al. Segmental laryngotracheal and tracheal resection for invasive thyroid carcinoma. *Ann Thorac Surg.* 2007;83:1952-1959.

348. Ruegemer JJ, Hay ID, Bergstralh EJ, et al. Distant metastases in differentiated thyroid carcinoma: a multivariate analysis of prognostic variables. *J Clin Endocrinol Metab.* 1988;63:960-967.

349. Durante C, Haddy N, Baudin E, et al. Long term outcome of 444 patients with distant metastases from papillary and follicular thyroid carcinoma: benefits and limits of radioiodine therapy. *J Clin Endocrinol Metab.* 2006;92:450-455.

350. Casara D, Rubello D, Saladini G, et al. Different features of pulmonary metastases in differentiated thyroid cancer: natural history and multivariate statistical analysis of prognostic variables. *J Nucl Med.* 1993; 34:1626-1631.

351. Kitamura Y, Shimizu K, Nagahama M, et al. Immediate causes of death in thyroid carcinoma: clinicopathological analysis of 161 fatal cases. *J Clin Endocrinol Metab.* 1999;84:4043-4049.

352. Bernier MO, Leenhardt L, Hoang C, et al. Survival and therapeutic modalities in patients with bone metastases of differentiated thyroid carcinomas. *J Clin Endocrinol Metab.* 2001;86:1568-1573.

353. Tala H, Robbins R, Fagin JA, et al. Five-year survival is similar in thyroid cancer patients with distant metastases prepared for radioactive iodine therapy with either thyroid hormone withdrawal or recombinant human TSH. *J Clin Endocrinol Metab.* 2011;96:2105-2111.

354. Potzi C, Moameni A, Karanikas G, et al. Comparison of iodine uptake in tumour and nontumour tissue under thyroid hormone deprivation and with recombinant human thyrotropin in thyroid cancer patients. *Clin Endocrinol (Oxf).* 2006;65:519-523.

355. Schlumberger M, Brose M, Elisei R, et al. Definition and management of radioactive iodine-refractory differentiated thyroid cancer. *Lancet Diabetes Endocrinol.* 2014;2:356-358.

356. Sabra MM, Grewal RK, Tala H, et al. Clinical outcomes following empiric radioiodine therapy in patients with structurally identifiable metastatic follicular cell-derived thyroid carcinoma with negative diagnostic but positive post-therapy ^{131}I whole-body scans. *Thyroid.* 2012; 22:877-883.

357. Leboulleux S, Bastholt L, Krause T, et al. Vandetanib in locally advanced or metastatic differentiated thyroid cancer: a randomised, double-blind phase 2 trial. *Lancet Oncol.* 2012;13:897-905.

358. Brose MS, Nutting CM, Jarzab B, et al; DECISION investigators. Sorafenib in radioactive iodine-refractory, locally advanced or metastatic differentiated thyroid cancer: a randomised, double-blind, phase 3 trial. *Lancet.* 2014;384(9940):319-328.

359. Schlumberger M, Tahara M, Wirth LJ, et al. Lenvatinib versus placebo in ^{131}I-refractory differentiated thyroid cancer. *N Engl J Med.* 2015; 372:621-630.

360. Massicotte MH, Brassard M, Claude-Desroches M, et al. Tyrosine kinase inhibitor treatments in patients with metastatic thyroid carcinomas: a retrospective study of the TUTHYREF network. *Eur J Endocrinol.* 2014;170:575-582.

361. Dadu R, Devine C, Hernandez M, et al. Role of salvage targeted therapy in differentiated thyroid cancer patients who failed first-line sorafenib. *J Clin Endocrinol Metab.* 2014;99:2086-2094.

362. Shimaoka K, Schoenfeld DA, DeWys WD, et al. A randomized trial of doxorubicin versus doxorubicin plus cisplatin in patients with advanced thyroid carcinoma. *Cancer.* 1985;56:2155-2160.

363. Crouzeix G, Michels JJ, Sevin E, et al; French TUTHYREF network. Unusual short-term complete response to two regimens of cytotoxic chemotherapy in a patient with poorly differentiated thyroid carcinoma. *J Clin Endocrinol Metab.* 2012;97:3046-3050.

364. Robenshtok E, Farooki A, Grewal RK, Tuttle RM. Natural history of small radioiodine-avid bone metastases that have no structural correlate on imaging studies. *Endocrine.* 2014;47:266-272.

365. Kloos RT, Duvuuri V, Jhiang SM, et al. Nasolacrimal drainage system obstruction from radioactive iodine therapy for thyroid carcinoma. *J Clin Endocrinol Metab.* 2002;87:5817-5820.

366. Mandel SJ, Mandel L. Radioactive iodine and the salivary glands. *Thyroid.* 2003;13:265-271.

367. Pacini F, Gasperi M, Fugazzola L, et al. Testicular function in patients with differentiated thyroid carcinoma treated with radioiodine. *J Nucl Med.* 1994;35:1418-1422.

368. Garsi JP, Schlumberger M, Rubino C, et al. Therapeutic administration of ^{131}I for differentiated thyroid cancer, radiation dose to ovaries and outcome of pregnancies. *J Nucl Med.* 2008;49:845-852.

369. Alexander EK, Marqusee E, Lawrence J, et al. Timing and magnitude of increase in levothyroxine requirements during pregnancy in women with hypothyroidism. *N Engl J Med.* 2004;351:241-249.

370. Rubino C, De Vathaire F, Dottorini ME, et al. Second primary malignancies in thyroid cancer patients. *Br J Cancer.* 2003;89:1638-1644.

371. Nocera M, Baudin E, Pellegriti G, et al. Treatment of advanced medullary thyroid cancer with an alternating combination of doxorubicin-streptozocin and 5 FU-dacarbazine. Groupe d'Étude des Tumeurs a Calcitonine (GETC). *Br J Cancer.* 2000;83:715-718.

372. Fromigué J, De Baere T, Baudin E, et al. Chemoembolization for liver metastases from medullary thyroid carcinoma. *J Clin Endocrinol Metab.* 2006;91:2496-2499.

373. Schlumberger M, Carlomagno F, Baudin E, et al. New therapeutic approaches for medullary thyroid carcinoma. *Nat Clin Pract Endocrinol Metab.* 2008;4:22-32.

374. Wells SA, Robinson BG, Gagel RF, et al. Vandetanib in patients with locally advanced or metastatic medullary thyroid cancer: a randomized, double-blind phase III trial (ZETA). *J Clin Oncol.* 2012;30: 134-141.

375. Elisei R, Schlumberger MJ, Müller S, et al. Cabozantinib in progressive medullary thyroid cancer. *J Clin Oncol.* 2013;31:3639-3646.

Section IV

Adrenal Cortex and Endocrine Hypertension

CHAPTER 15

The Adrenal Cortex

PAUL M. STEWART • JOHN D. C. NEWELL-PRICE

KEY POINTS

- This chapter discusses mechanisms and regulation of adrenal steroid production, function of the hypothalamic-pituitary-adrenal axis, and negative regulation.
- The chapter goes on to describe the transactivating and transrepressive actions of glucocorticoids.
- Glucocorticoid excess and Cushing syndrome, adrenal insufficiency and Addison disease, and inherited disorders of the adrenal gland are also discussed.
- Optimizing corticosteroid replacement therapies is addressed.
- The chapter concludes with discussion of adrenal incidentalomas, adenomas, and carcinomas.

THE ADRENAL CORTEX—HISTORICAL MILESTONES

The anatomy of the adrenal glands was described almost 450 years ago by Bartholomeo Eustacius,[1] and the zonation of the gland and its distinction from the medulla were elucidated shortly thereafter. However, a functional role for the adrenal glands was not accurately defined until the pioneering work of Thomas Addison, who described the clinical and autopsy findings in 11 cases of Addison disease in his classic monograph in 1855.[2] Just a year later, Brown-Séquard demonstrated that the adrenal glands were "organs essential for life" by performing adrenalectomies in dogs, cats, and guinea pigs.[3] In 1896, William Osler first administered adrenal extract to a patient with Addison disease, a feat that was repeated by others in animal and human studies over the next 40 years. Between 1937 and 1955, the adrenocorticosteroid hormones were isolated, and their structures were defined and synthesized.[4] Notable breakthroughs included the discovery of cortisone and clinical evaluation of its anti-inflammatory effect in patients with rheumatoid arthritis[5] and the isolation of aldosterone.[6]

The control of adrenocortical function by a pituitary factor was demonstrated in the 1920s, and this led to the isolation of sheep adrenocorticotropic hormone (ACTH) by Li, Evans, and Simpson in 1943.[7] Such a concept was supported through clinical studies, notably by Harvey Cushing in 1932, who associated his original clinical observations of 1912 (a "polyglandular syndrome" caused by pituitary basophilism) with adrenal hyperactivity.[8] The neural control of pituitary ACTH secretion by corticotropin-releasing factor (later renamed corticotropin-releasing hormone, or CRH) was defined by Harris and other workers in the 1940s, but CRH was not characterized and synthesized until 1981 in the laboratory of Wylie Vale.[9] Jerome Conn described primary aldosteronism in 1955,[10] and the control of adrenal aldosterone secretion by angiotensin II was confirmed shortly afterward. Advances in radioimmunoassay, and particularly molecular biology, have facilitated an exponential increase in the understanding of adrenal physiology and pathophysiology (Table 15-1).

ANATOMY AND DEVELOPMENT

The cells forming the adrenal cortex originate from the intermediate mesoderm. These cells derive from the urogenital ridge and have a common embryologic origin with the gonad and the kidney. Early differentiation of the adrenogonadal primordium from the urogenital ridge requires signaling cascades and transcription factors GLI3, SALL1, FOXD2, WT1, PBX1, and WNT4, and the regulator of telomerase activity, ACD (Fig. 15-1). The adrenogonadal primordium can be seen as the medial part of the urogenital ridge at 4 weeks. Separation of the adrenogonadal primordium and formation of the adrenal primordium seem to depend on the actions of transcription factors SF1 (steroidogenic factor 1), DAX1, WNT4, and CITED2. The adrenocortical primordium develops at approximately 8 weeks of gestation and can be differentiated into two distinct layers, the inner fetal zone (FZ) and the outer definitive zone (DZ). At approximately 9 weeks, the adrenal blastema encapsulates and the adrenal medulla develops when neural crest cells migrate into the adrenal gland.[11] During the second trimester, the FZ enlarges, becomes larger than the fetal kidney, and secretes abundant amounts of dehydroepiandrosterone (DHEA) and dehydroepiandrosterone sulfate (DHEAS). Concentrations of these hormones abruptly decline postnatally, in parallel with the postnatal involution of the FZ. The neocortex develops over the subsequent years into the adult adrenal gland.

In fetal life and up to 12 months of age, two distinct zones are evident, an inner prominent FZ and an outer DZ that differentiates into the adult adrenal gland. After birth, the FZ regresses and the DZ, which contains an inner zona

TABLE 15-1	
History of the Adrenal Cortex: Important Milestones	
Year	**Event**
1563	Eustachius describes the adrenals (published by Lancisi in 1714).
1849	Thomas Addison, while searching for the cause of pernicious anemia, stumbles on a bronzed appearance associated with the adrenal glands—*melasma suprarenale.*
1855	Thomas Addison describes the clinical features and autopsy findings in 11 cases of diseases of the suprarenal capsules, at least 6 of which were tuberculous in origin.
1856	In adrenalectomy experiments, Brown-Séquard demonstrates that the adrenal glands are essential for life.
1896	William Osler prepares an oral glycerin extract derived from pig adrenals and demonstrates that it has clinical benefit in patients with Addison disease.
1905	Bulloch and Sequeira describe patients with congenital adrenal hyperplasia.
1929	Liquid extracts of cortical tissue are used to keep adrenalectomized cats alive indefinitely (Swingle and Pfiffner); subsequently, this extract was used successfully to treat a patient with Addison disease (Rowntree and Greene).
1932	Harvey Cushing associates the polyglandular syndrome of pituitary basophilism, which he first described in 1912, with hyperactivity of the pituitary-adrenal glands.
1936	The concept of stress and its effect on pituitary-adrenal function are described by Selye.
1937-1952	Isolation and structural characterization of adrenocortical hormones are reported by Kendall and Reichstein.
1943	Li and colleagues isolate pure adrenocorticotropic hormone from sheep pituitary.
1950	Hench, Kendall, and Reichstein share the Nobel Prize in Medicine for describing the anti-inflammatory effects of cortisone in patients with rheumatoid arthritis.
1953	Isolation and analysis of the structure of aldosterone are reported by Simpson and Tait.
1956	Conn describes primary aldosteronism.
1981	Characterization and synthesis of corticotropin-releasing hormone are reported by Vale.
1980-present	The *molecular era:* cloning and functional characterization of steroid receptors, steroidogenic enzymes, and adrenal transcription factors are reported, and the molecular basis for human adrenal diseases is defined.

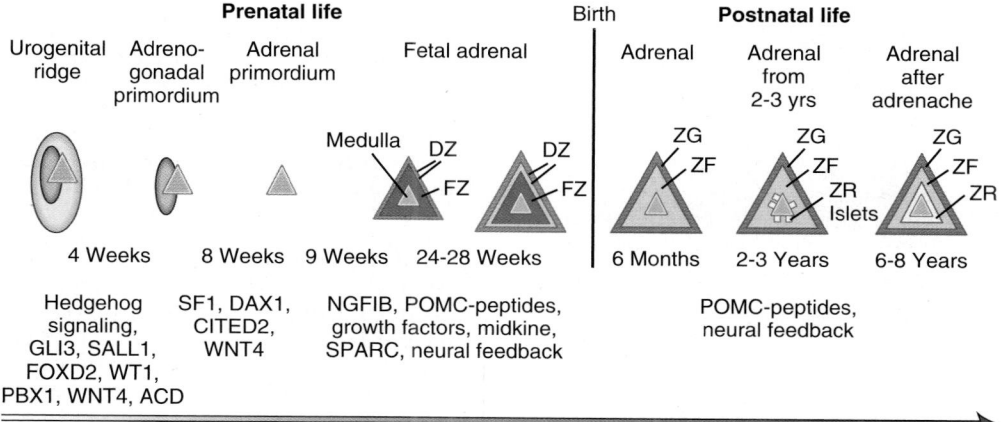

Figure 15-1 Schematic diagram of the development of the human adrenal cortex during prenatal and postnatal life showing transcription factors that are active at each stage (see text for details). DZ, definitive zone; FZ, fetal zone; POMC, pro-opiomelanocortin; SPARC, secreted protein, acidic, cysteine-rich (osteonectin); ZF, zona fasciculata; ZG, zona glomerulosa; ZR, zona reticularis.

fasciculata (ZF) and an outer zona glomerulosa (ZG), proliferates.[12,13] The innermost zone, the zona reticularis (ZR), is evident after 2 years of life. The differentiation of the adrenal cortex into distinct zones has important functional consequences and is thought to depend on the temporal expression of transcription factors including Pref-1/ZOG, inner zone antigen, and SF1.[14,15] In preadrenarchal children focal reticular zone islets can be found, but the ZG and ZF are clearly differentiated.[16] The occurrence of these ZR islets is consistent with the observation that DHEA and DHEAS concentrations gradually begin to rise from about 3 years of age.[17] At adrenarche, the inner zone (ZR) thickens, corresponding with increased production of DHEA and DHEAS. Concurrently, changes in zone-specific enzyme expression patterns, such as decreased 3β-hydroxysteroid dehydrogenase type 2 (HSD3B2) and increased cytochrome b_5 and sulfotransferase (SULT2A1) in the ZR, lead to increased flux toward DHEA. Clinically, adrenarche becomes apparent at 6 to 8 years of age. Adrenal androgen production peaks in the third decade and then declines at a variable rate. Mineralocorticoids and glucocorticoids show a less age-specific variation.

The adult adrenal gland is a pyramidal structure, approximately 4 g in weight, 2 cm wide, 5 cm long, and 1 cm thick, that lies immediately above the kidney on its posteromedial surface. Beneath the capsule, the ZG makes up approximately 15% of the cortex (depending on sodium intake) (Fig. 15-2). Cells are clustered in spherical nests and are small, with smaller nuclei in comparison with cells in other zones. The ZF makes up 75% of the cortex; cells are large and lipid-laden and form radial cords within the fibrovascular radial network. The innermost ZR is sharply demarcated from both the ZF and the adrenal medulla. Cells there are irregular with little lipid content. The maintenance of normal adrenal size appears to involve a progenitor cell population lying between the ZG and ZF; cell migration and differentiation occur within the fasciculata and senescence occurs within the ZR, but the factors regulating this important aspect of adrenal regeneration are unknown. ACTH administration results in glomerulosa

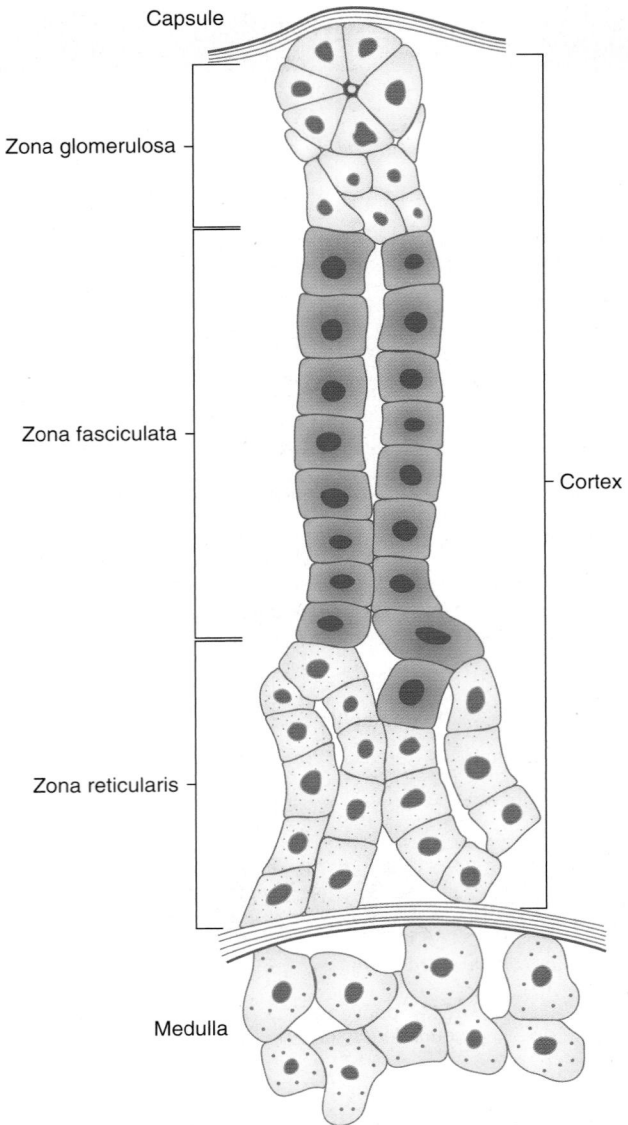

Figure 15-2 Schematic diagram of the structure of the human adrenal cortex, depicting the outer zona glomerulosa and inner zona fasciculata and zona reticularis.

TABLE 15-2

IUPAC and Trivial Names of Natural and Synthetic Steroids

Trivial Name	IUPAC Name
Aldosterone	4-Pregnen-11β,21-diol-3,18,20-trione
Androstenedione	4-Androsten-3,17-dione
Cortisol	4-Pregnen-11β,17α,21-triol-3,20-dione
Cortisone	4-Pregnen-17α,21-diol-3,11,20-trione
Dehydroepiandrosterone	5-Androsten-3β-ol-17-one
Deoxycorticosterone	4-Pregnen-21-ol-3,20-dione
Dexamethasone	1,4-Pregnadien-9α-fluoro-16α-methyl-11β,17α,21-triol-3,20-dione
Dihydrotestosterone	5α-Androstan-17β-ol-3-one
Estradiol	1,3,5(10)-Estratrien-3,17β-diol
Fludrocortisone	4-Pregnen-9α-fluoro-11β,17α,21-triol-3,20-dione
17-Hydroxyprogesterone	4-Pregnen-17α-ol-3,20-dione
Methylprednisolone	1,4-Pregnadien-6α-methyl-11β,17α,21-triol-3,20-dione
Prednisolone	1,4-Pregnadien-11β,17α,21-triol-3,20-dione
Prednisone	1,4-Pregnadien-17α,21-diol-3,11,20-trione
Pregnenolone	5-Pregnen-3β-ol-20-one
Progesterone	4-Pregnen-3,20-dione
Testosterone	4-Androsten-17β-ol-3-one
Triamcinolone	1,4-Pregnadien-9α-fluoro-11β,16α,17α,21-tetrol-3,20-dione

IUPAC, International Union of Pure and Applied Chemistry.

ocorticoids (aldosterone, deoxycorticosterone [DOC]), and sex steroids (mainly androgens). All steroid hormones are derived from the cyclopentanoperhydrophenanthrene structure, that is, three cyclohexane rings and a single cyclopentane ring (Fig. 15-3). Steroid nomenclature is defined in two ways: by trivial names (e.g., cortisol, aldosterone) or by the chemical structure as defined by the International Union of Pure and Applied Chemistry (IUPAC).[18] The IUPAC classification is inappropriate for clinical use but does provide an invaluable insight into steroid structure. The basic structure, trivial name, and IUPAC name of some common steroids are given in Figure 15-3 and Table 15-2. Estrogens have 18 carbon atoms (C18 steroids) and androgens have 19 carbon atoms (C19), whereas glucocorticoids and progestogens are C21-steroid derivatives.

Cholesterol is the precursor for adrenal steroidogenesis. It is provided principally from the circulation, in the form of low-density lipoprotein (LDL) cholesterol.[19] Uptake is by specific cell-surface LDL receptors present on adrenal tissue[20]; LDL is then internalized via receptor-mediated endocytosis,[21] the resulting vesicles fuse with lysozymes, and free cholesterol is produced after hydrolysis. However, it is clear that this cannot be the sole source of adrenal cholesterol, because patients with abetalipoproteinemia who have undetectable circulating LDL and patients with defective LDL receptors in the setting of familial hypercholesterolemia still have normal basal adrenal steroidogenesis. Cholesterol can be generated de novo within the adrenal cortex from acetyl coenzyme A (CoA). In addition, there is evidence that the adrenal gland can utilize high-density lipoprotein (HDL) cholesterol after uptake through the putative HDL receptor, SR-B1.[22]

The biochemical pathways involved in adrenal steroidogenesis are shown in Figure 15-4. The initial hormone-dependent, rate-limiting step is the transport of intracellular cholesterol from the outer to inner mitochondrial membrane for conversion to pregnenolone by cytochrome P450 side-chain cleavage enzyme (P450scc). Naturally occurring human mutations have confirmed the importance of a 30-kDa protein, steroidogenic acute regulatory protein

cells adopting a fasciculata phenotype, and in turn, the innermost fasciculata cells adopt a reticularis phenotype that is reversible on withdrawal of ACTH.

The vasculature of the adrenal cortex is complex. Arterial supply is conveyed by up to 12 small arteries from the aorta and the inferior phrenic, renal, and intercostal arteries. These arteries branch to form a subcapsular arteriolar plexus from which radial capillaries penetrate deeper into the cortex. In the ZR, a dense sinusoidal plexus is created, which empties into a central vein. The right adrenal vein is short, draining directly into the inferior vena cava, whereas the longer left adrenal vein usually drains into the left renal vein.

ADRENAL STEROIDS AND STEROIDOGENESIS

Three main types of hormones are produced by the adrenal cortex—glucocorticoids (cortisol, corticosterone), mineral-

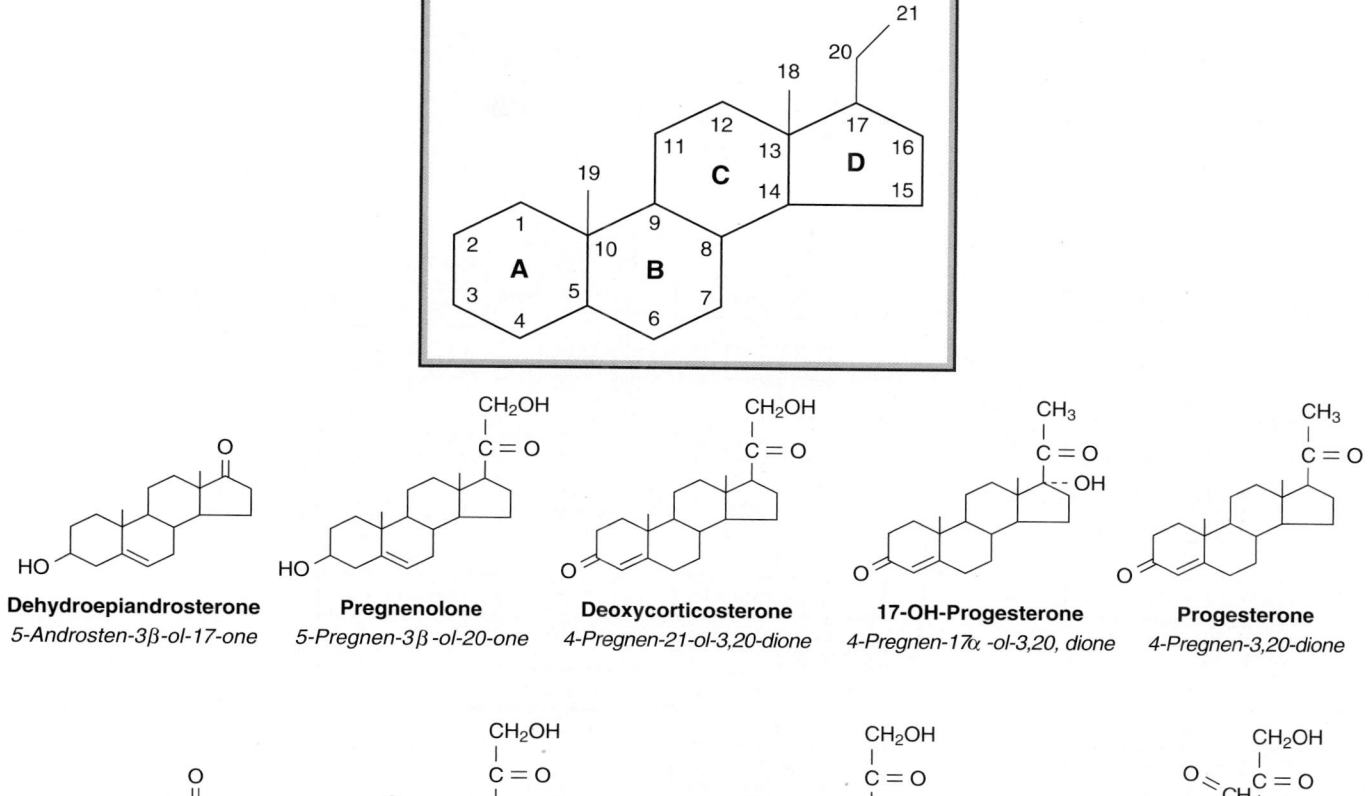

Figure 15-3 The cyclopentanoperhydrophenanthrene structure of corticosteroid hormones, highlighting the structure of some endogenous steroid hormones together with their nomenclature.

TABLE 15-3

Nomenclature for Adrenal Steroidogenic Enzymes and Their Genes

Enzyme Name	Enzyme Family	Gene	Chromosome
P450 Cholesterol side-chain cleavage (SCC) (desmolase)	Cytochrome P450 type I	CYP11A1	15q23-q24
3β-Hydroxysteroid dehydrogenase (3β-HSD) (type II isozyme)	Short-chain alcohol dehydrogenase reductase superfamily	HSD3B2	1p13.1
17α-Hydroxylase/17,20-lyase	Cytochrome P450 type II	CYP17A1	10q24.3
21-Hydroxylase	Cytochrome P450 type II	CYP21A2	6p21.3
11β-Hydroxylase	Cytochrome P450 type I	CYP11B1	8q24.3
Aldosterone synthase	Cytochrome P450 type I	CYP11B2	8q24.3

(StAR), in mediating this effect. StAR is induced by an increase in intracellular cyclic adenosine monophosphate (cAMP) after binding of ACTH to its cognate receptor, providing the first important rate-limiting step in adrenal steroidogenesis.[23] Other transporters, including the peripheral benzodiazepine-like receptor, may be involved.[24]

Steroidogenesis involves the concerted action of several enzymes, including a series of cytochrome P450 enzymes, all of which have been cloned and characterized (Table 15-3). Cytochrome P450 enzymes are classified into two types according to their subcellular localization and their specific electron shuttle system. Mitochondrial (type I)

cytochrome P450 enzymes such as CYP11A1 (P450scc), 11β-hydroxylase (CYP11B1, or P450c11b1), and aldosterone synthase (CYP11B2, or P450aldo) rely on electron transfer facilitated by adrenodoxin and adrenodoxin reductase.[25,26] Micrososomal (type II) cytochrome P450 enzymes localized to the endoplasmic reticulum include the steroidogenic enzymes 17α-hydroxylase (CYP17A1, or P450c17), 21-hydroxylase (CYP21A2, or P450c21), and P450 aromatase (CYP19A1, or P450aro). The functions of cytochrome P450 type II enzymes crucially depend on P450 oxidoreductase (POR), which provides electrons required for monooxygenase reaction catalyzed by the

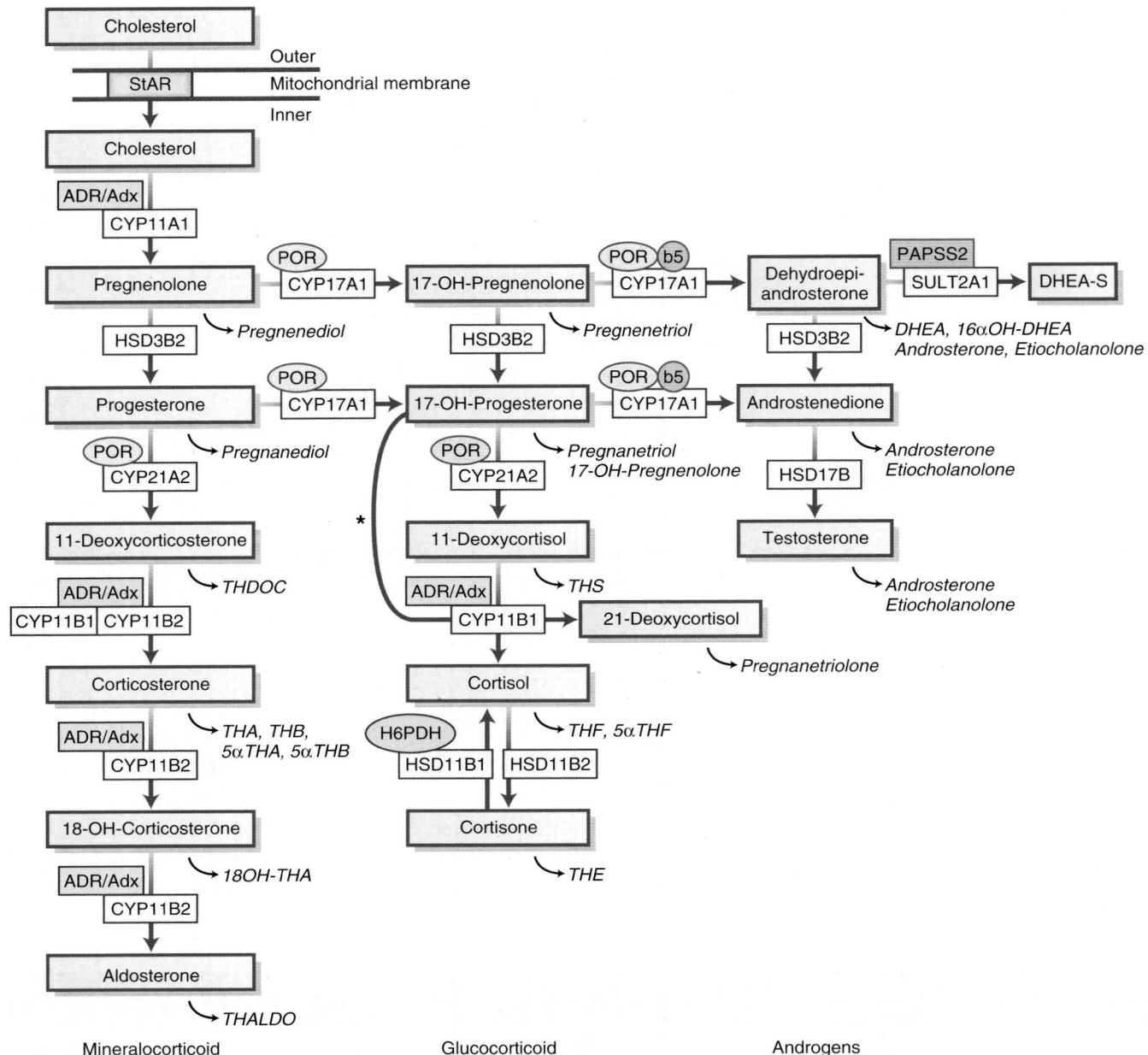

Figure 15-4 Adrenal steroidogenesis. After the steroidogenic acute regulatory (StAR) protein-mediated uptake of cholesterol into mitochondria within adrenocortical cells, aldosterone, cortisol, and adrenal androgens are synthesized through the coordinated action of a series of steroidogenic enzymes in a zone-specific fashion. The mitochondrial cytochrome P450 (CYP) type I enzymes (CYP11A1, CYP11B1, CYP11B2) requiring electron transfer via adrenodoxin reductase (ADR) and adrenodoxin (Adx) are marked with a box labeled ADR/Adx. The microsomal CYP type II enzymes (CYP17A1, CYP21A2) receive electrons from P450 oxidoreductase (circle labeled POR). The 17,20-lyase reaction catalyzed by CYP17A1 requires, in addition to POR, cytochrome b_5, indicated by a circle labeled b5. Urinary steroid hormone metabolites are given in italics below the plasma hormones. The asterisk (*) indicates 11-hydroxylation of 17-OH-progesterone to 21-deoxycortisol in cases of 21-hydroxylase deficiency. The adrenal conversion of androstenedione to testosterone is catalyzed by the aldo-keto reductase AKR1C3 (HSD17B5). CYP11A1, P450 side-chain cleavage enzyme; CYP11B1, 11β-hydroxylase; CYP11B2, aldosterone synthase; CYP17A1, 17α-hydroxylase; CYP21A2, 21-hydroxylase; DHEA, dehydroepiandrosterone; DHEA-S, dehydroepiandrosterone sulfate; H6PDH, hexose-6-phosphate dehydrogenase; HSD11B1, 11β-hydroxysteroid dehydrogenase 1; HSD11B2, 11β-hydroxysteroid dehydrogenase 2; HSD17B, 17β-hydroxysteroid dehydrogenase; HSD3B2, 3β-hydroxysteroid dehydrogenase type 2; 17-OH-progesterone, 17α-hydroxyprogesterone; PAPSS2, 3'-phosphoadenosine, 5'-phosphosulfate synthase 2; SULT2A1, sulfotransferase 2A1; THA, tetrahydro-11-dehydrocorticosterone; THB, tetrahydro-corticosterone; THALDO, tetrahydro-aldosterone; THDOC, tetrahydro-11-deoxycorticosterone; THF, tetrahydro-cortisol; THS, tetrahydro-11-deoxycortisol.

P450 enzyme.[26,27] This category also includes hepatic P450 enzymes involved in drug metabolism and enzymes involved in sterol and bile acid synthesis.[26,27] In addition, the 17,20-lyase activity of P450 CYP17A1 is dependent on a flavoprotein cytochrome b_5, which functions as an allosteric facilitator of CYP17A1, and POR interaction (Fig. 15-5; see also Fig. 15-4).[28]

Mutations in the genes encoding these enzymes result in human disease, so some understanding of the underlying pathways and steroid precursors is required.[29] After uptake of cholesterol to the mitochondrion, cholesterol is cleaved by the P450scc enzyme to form pregnenolone.[30] In the cytoplasm, pregnenolone is converted to progesterone by the type II isozyme 3β-HSD through a reaction

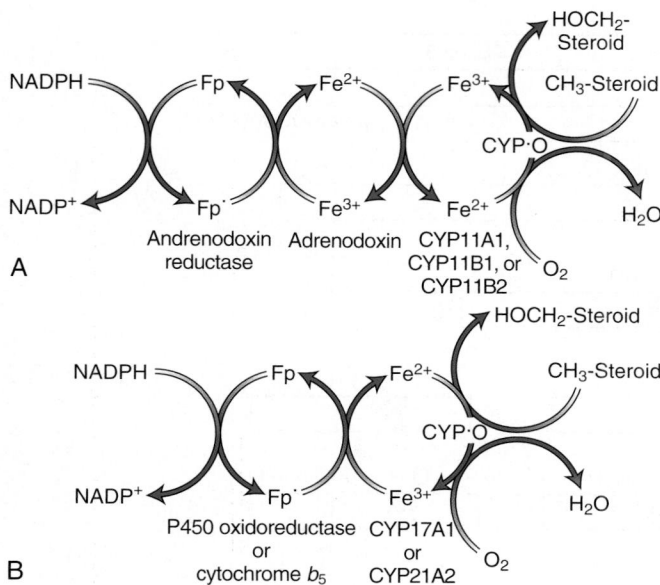

Figure 15-5 A, Electron shuttle system for the mitochondrial enzymes CYP11A1, CYP11B1, and CYP11B2. Adrenodoxin reductase receives electrons from reduced nicotinamide adenine dinucleotide phosphate (NADPH) and reduces adrenodoxin, which transfers reducing equivalents to the cytochrome P450 (CYP) enzyme. The enzyme then transfers electrons, by way of oxygen, to the steroid. **B,** Electron shuttle system for the microsomal enzymes CYP17A1 and CYP21A2. P450 oxidoreductase, a flavoprotein, accepts electrons from NADPH and transfers them to the NADPH-P450 enzyme. The enzyme then transfers electrons, by way of oxygen, to the steroid. A second reducing equivalent may be supplied to CYP17A1 by NADPH-P450 oxidoreductase or cytochrome b_5. Fp, flavoprotein; Fp•, reduced form of flavoprotein; NADP+, nicotinamide adenine dinucleotide phosphate.

involving dehydrogenation of the 3-hydroxyl group and isomerization of the double bond at C5.[31] Progesterone is hydroxylated to 17-hydroxyprogesterone (17-OHP) through the 17α-hydroxylase activity of CYP17A1. 17α-Hydroxylation is an essential prerequisite for glucocorticoid synthesis, and the ZG does not express 17α-hydroxylase. CYP17A1 also possesses 17,20-lyase activity, which results in production of the C19 adrenal androgens DHEA and androstenedione.[32] In humans, however, 17-OHP is not an efficient substrate for CYP17A1, and there is negligible conversion of 17-OHP to androstenedione. Adrenal androstenedione secretion is dependent on the conversion of DHEA to androstenedione by 3β-HSD. This enzyme also converts 17-hydroxypregnenolone to 17-OHP, but the preferred substrate is pregnenolone. The human adrenal gland is capable of synthesis of small but significant amounts of testosterone, which increases in clinical conditions associated with androgen excess. This conversion is facilitated by the enzyme 17β-HSD type 5 (HSD17B5), also called aldoketoreductase 1C3 (AKR1C3).[33] 21-Hydroxylation of either progesterone (in the ZG) or 17-OHP (in the ZF) is carried out by the product of the *CYP21A2* gene, 21-hydroxylase, to yield DOC or 11-deoxycortisol, respectively.[34] The final step in cortisol biosynthesis takes place in the mitochondria and involves the conversion of 11-deoxycortisol to cortisol by the enzyme CYP11B1 (11β-hydroxylase).[35] In the ZG, 11β-hydroxylase may also convert DOC to corticosterone. The enzyme CYP11B2 (aldosterone synthase) may also carry out this reaction; in addition, it is required for conversion of corticosterone to aldosterone via the intermediate 18-OH corticosterone; CYP11B1 lacks these two enzymatic activities.[36,37]

Therefore, CYP11B2 can carry out 11β-hydroxylation, 18-hydroxylation, and 18-methyloxidation to yield the characteristic C11-18 hemiacetyl structure of aldosterone.

Regulation of Adrenal Steroidogenesis: Functional Zonation of the Adrenal Cortex

Glucocorticoids are secreted in relatively high amounts (cortisol, 10 to 20 mg/day) from the ZF under the control of ACTH; mineralocorticoids are secreted in low amounts (aldosterone, 100 to 150 µg/day) from the ZG under the principal control of angiotensin II. As a class, adrenal androgens (DHEA, DHEAS, androstenedione) are the most abundant steroids secreted from the adult adrenal gland (>20 mg/day). In each case, secretion is facilitated through the expression of steroidogenic enzymes in a specific zonal manner. The ZG cannot synthesize cortisol because it does not express 17α-hydroxylase. In contrast, aldosterone secretion is confined to the outer ZG because of the restricted expression of CYP11B2. Although CYP11B1 and CYP11B2 share 95% homology, the 5′ promoter sequences differ, permitting regulation of the final steps in glucocorticoid and mineralocorticoid biosynthesis by ACTH and angiotensin II, respectively. In the ZR, high levels of cytochrome b_5 confer 17,20-lyase activity on CYP17A1 and androgen production. DHEA is sulfated in the ZR by the DHEA SULT2A1 to form DHEAS. This sulfonation reaction facilitated by SULT2A1 relies on the donor 3′-phosphoadenosine 5′-phosphosulfate (PAPS) to transfer a sulfonate group to an acceptor molecule. PAPS is synthesized by PAPS synthase, of which two isoenzymes exist (PAPSS1 and PAPSS2).[38]

In the fetal adrenal, steroidogenesis occurs primarily within the inner FZ. The FZ is a characteristic feature of higher primates, but the biologic role of fetal androgen production remains unclear. Because of a relative lack of 3β-HSD and high SULT2A1 activity, the principal steroidogenic products are DHEA and DHEAS, which are then aromatized by placental trophoblast to estrogens. Therefore, the majority of maternal estrogen across pregnancy is, indirectly, fetally derived.[39]

Classic endocrine feedback loops are in place to control the secretion of both hormones. Cortisol inhibits the secretion of CRH from the hypothalamus and ACTH from the pituitary, and aldosterone-induced sodium retention inhibits renal renin secretion.

Glucocorticoid Secretion: The Hypothalamic-Pituitary-Adrenal Axis

Pro-opiomelanocortin and ACTH

ACTH is the principal hormone stimulating adrenal glucocorticoid biosynthesis and secretion. ACTH has 39 amino acids but is synthesized within the anterior pituitary as part of a much larger, 241–amino acid precursor called *pro-opiomelanocortin* (POMC). A transcription factor, TPIT, appears to be essential for differentiation of POMC-expressing cells within the anterior pituitary.[40] POMC is cleaved in a tissue-specific fashion by prohormone convertases to yield smaller peptide hormones. In the anterior pituitary, this results in the secretion of β-lipoprotein (β-LPH) and pro-ACTH, the latter being further cleaved to an amino-terminal peptide, joining peptide, and ACTH itself (Fig. 15-6).[41,42] Postsecretion cleavage of the precursor to γ-melanocyte-stimulating hormone (pro-γ-MSH) by a serine protease (AsP) expressed in the outer adrenal cortex is thought to mediate the trophic action of ACTH on the adrenal cortex.[43] The first 24 amino acids of ACTH are common to all species, and a synthetic ACTH(1-24),

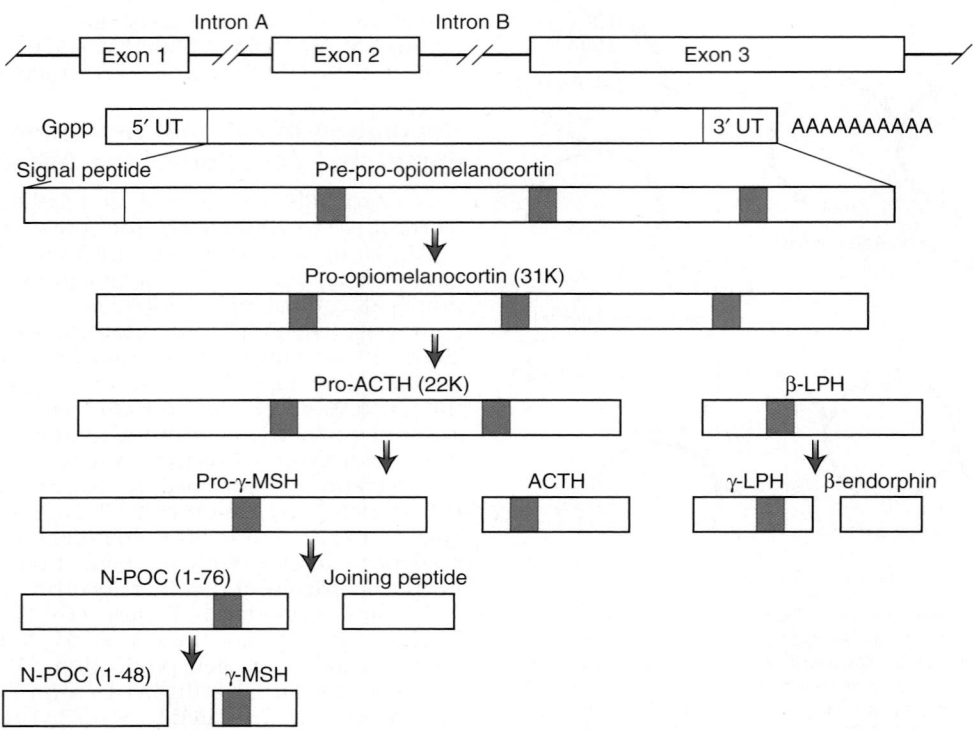

Figure 15-6 Synthesis and cleavage of pro-opiomelanocortin (POMC) within the human anterior pituitary gland. Prohormone convertase enzymes sequentially cleave POMC to adrenocorticotropic hormone (ACTH). Shaded areas represent melanocyte-stimulating hormone (MSH) structural units. β-LPH, β-lipoprotein; γ-LPH, γ-lipoprotein; N-POC, amino-terminal pro-opiomelanocortin.

Synacthen, is available commercially for clinical testing of the hypothalamic-pituitary-adrenal (HPA) axis and assessing adrenal glucocorticoid reserve. The hormones α-, β-, and γ-MSH are also cleaved products from POMC, but the increased pigmentation characteristic of Addison disease is thought to arise directly from increased ACTH concentrations binding to the melanocortin-1 receptor (MC1R) rather than from α-MSH secretion.[44]

POMC is also transcribed in many extrapituitary tissues, notably brain, liver, kidney, gonad, and placenta.[41,45,46] In these normal tissues, POMC messenger RNA (mRNA) is usually shorter (800nt) than the pituitary 1200nt transcript because of lack of exons 1 and 2 and the 5′ region of exon 3.[47] Because the POMC-like peptide product from this shorter transcript lacks a signal sequence needed to cross the endoplasmic reticulum, it is probable that it is neither secreted nor active in normal circumstances. However, in ectopic ACTH syndrome, additional POMC mRNA species are described that are longer than the normal pituitary POMC species (typically 1450nt) as a result of the use of alternative promoters in the 5′ region of the gene.[48,49] This may in part explain the resistance of POMC expression to glucocorticoid feedback in these tumors. Other factors, including interaction with tissue-specific transcription factors[50] and lack of *POMC* promoter methylation,[51] may explain the ectopic expression of ACTH in some malignant tissues. The cleavage of POMC is also tissue specific,[52] and it is possible, at least in some cases of ectopic ACTH syndrome, that circulating ACTH precursors (notably pro-ACTH) may cross-react in current ACTH radioimmunoassays.[53,54] The biologic activity of POMC itself on adrenal function is thought to be negligible.

POMC expression and processing within neurons in the hypothalamus, specifically the generation of α-MSH that interacts with melanocortin-4 receptors (MC4R), appears to be of crucial importance in appetite control and energy homeostasis (see later discussion).[55]

Corticotropin-Releasing Hormone and Arginine Vasopressin

POMC secretion is tightly controlled by numerous factors, notably CRH and arginine vasopressin (AVP) (Fig. 15-7).[56,57] Additional control is provided through an endogenous circadian rhythm and by stress and feedback inhibition by cortisol itself. CRH is a 41–amino acid peptide that is synthesized in neurons within the paraventricular nucleus of the hypothalamus.[9,58,59] Human and rat CRH are identical, but ovine CRH differs by 7 amino acids[60,61]; ovine-sequence CRH is slightly more potent than human-sequence CRH in stimulating ACTH secretion and has a longer half-life, but both are used diagnostically.

CRH is secreted into the hypophyseal portal blood, where it binds to specific type I CRH receptors on anterior pituitary corticotrophs[62] to stimulate *POMC* transcription through a process that includes activation of adenylate cyclase. It is unclear whether hypothalamic CRH contributes in any way to circulating levels; CRH is also synthesized in other tissues, and it is likely that circulating CRH reflects synthesis from testis, gastrointestinal tract, adrenal medulla, and particularly the placenta,[63] in which the increased secretion across pregnancy results in a threefold increase in circulating CRH levels.[64] In the circulation, CRH is bound to CRH-binding protein (CRH-BP); levels of CRH-BP also increase during pregnancy so that cortisol secretion is not markedly elevated.[65]

CRH is the principal stimulus for ACTH secretion,[66] but AVP is able to potentiate CRH-mediated secretion.[67] In this case, AVP acts through the V_{1b} receptor to activate protein kinase C. The peak response of ACTH to CRH does not differ across the day, but it is affected by endogenous

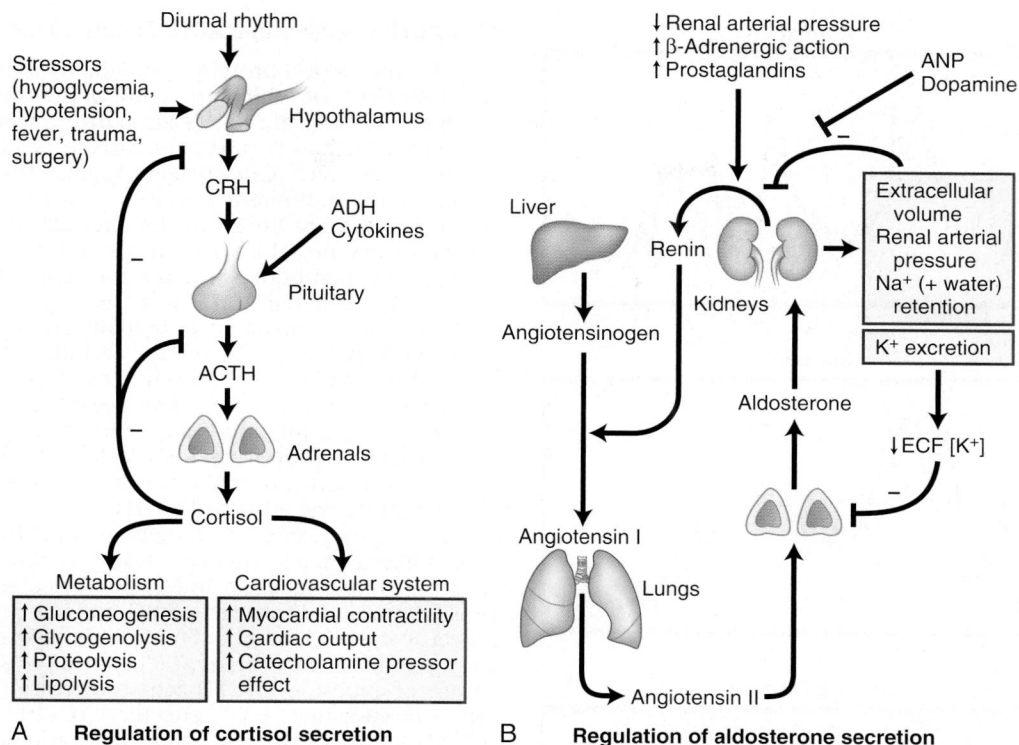

A   **Regulation of cortisol secretion**

B   **Regulation of aldosterone secretion**

Figure 15-7 Normal negative feedback regulation of cortisol and aldosterone secretion. **A,** Hypothalamic-pituitary-adrenal axis. Adrenocorticotropic hormone (ACTH) is secreted from the anterior pituitary under the influence of two principal secretagogues, corticotropin-releasing hormone (CRH) and arginine vasopressin; other factors, including cytokines, also play a role. CRH secretion is regulated by an inbuilt circadian rhythm and by additional stressors operating through the hypothalamus. Secretion of CRH and ACTH is inhibited by cortisol, highlighting the importance of negative feedback control. **B,** Renin-angiotensin-aldosterone system (RAAS). Renin is secreted from the juxtaglomerular cells in the kidney dependent on renal arterial blood pressure. Renin converts angiotensinogen to angiotensin I, which is converted in the lungs by angiotensin-converting enzyme (ACE) into angiotensin II. Angiotensin stimulates adrenal aldosterone synthesis. Extracellular fraction (ECF) of potassium has an important direct inhibitory influence on aldosterone secretion. ADH, antidiuretic hormone (arginine vasopressin); ANP, atrial natriuretic peptide.

function of the HPA axis in that responsiveness is reduced in subjects treated with corticosteroids but increased in subjects with Cushing disease. Other reported ACTH secretagogues, including angiotensin II, cholecystokinin, atrial natriuretic factor, and vasoactive peptides, probably act to modulate the CRH control of ACTH secretion.[68]

The Stress Response and Immune-Endocrine Axis. The proinflammatory cytokines, notably interleukin 1 (IL-1), IL-6, and tumor necrosis factor-α, also increase ACTH secretion, either directly or by augmenting the effect of CRH.[69,70] Leukemia inhibitory factor (LIF), a cytokine of the IL-6 family, is a further activator of the HPA axis.[71] This explains the response of the HPA axis to an inflammatory stimulus and is an important immune-endocrine interaction (see Chapter 7). Physical stresses increase ACTH and cortisol secretion, again through central actions mediated via CRH and AVP. Cortisol secretion rises in response to fever, surgery,[72] burn injury,[73] hypoglycemia,[74] hypotension, and exercise.[75] In all of these cases, this increased secretion can be viewed as a normal counterregulatory response to the insult. Acute psychological stress raises cortisol levels,[76] but secretion rates appear to be normal in patients with chronic anxiety states and underlying psychotic illness. However, depression is associated with high circulating cortisol concentrations, and this is an important consideration in the differential diagnosis of Cushing syndrome (see later discussion).

Circadian Rhythm. ACTH, and hence cortisol, is secreted in a pulsatile fashion with a circadian rhythm; levels are highest on wakening and decline throughout the day, reaching nadir values in the evening (Fig. 15-8).[77] The

average ACTH pulse frequency is higher in normal adult men compared with women (18 versus 10 pulses/24 hours, respectively). The circadian ACTH rhythm appears to be mediated principally by an increased ACTH pulse amplitude occurring between 5 and 9 AM but also by a reduction in ACTH pulse frequency occurring between 6 PM and midnight.[78,79] Food ingestion is a further stimulus to ACTH secretion. An ultradian rhythm overlies the circadian and appears to be driven by an oscillator created between the secretion of ACTH, the short delay in response at the adrenal, and the subsequent negative feedback by cortisol at the hypothalamus and pituitary.[80]

Circadian rhythm is dependent on both day-night[81] and sleep-wake[82] patterns and is disrupted by alternating day-night shift work and by long-distance travel across time zones.[83] It can take up to 2 weeks for the circadian rhythm to reset to an altered day-night cycle.

Negative Feedback. An important aspect of CRH and ACTH secretion is the negative feedback control exerted by glucocorticoids themselves. Glucocorticoids inhibit *POMC* transcription in the anterior pituitary[56] and CRH and AVP mRNA synthesis and secretion in the hypothalamus.[84,85] Annexin 1 (formerly called *lipocortin 1*) may also play a critical role in effecting the negative feedback of glucocorticoids on ACTH and CRH release.[86] The negative feedback effect depends on the dose, potency, half-life, and duration of administration of the glucocorticoid and has important physiologic and diagnostic consequences. Suppression of the HPA axis by pharmacologic corticosteroids may persist for many months after cessation of therapy, and adrenocortical insufficiency should be anticipated. Diagnostically,

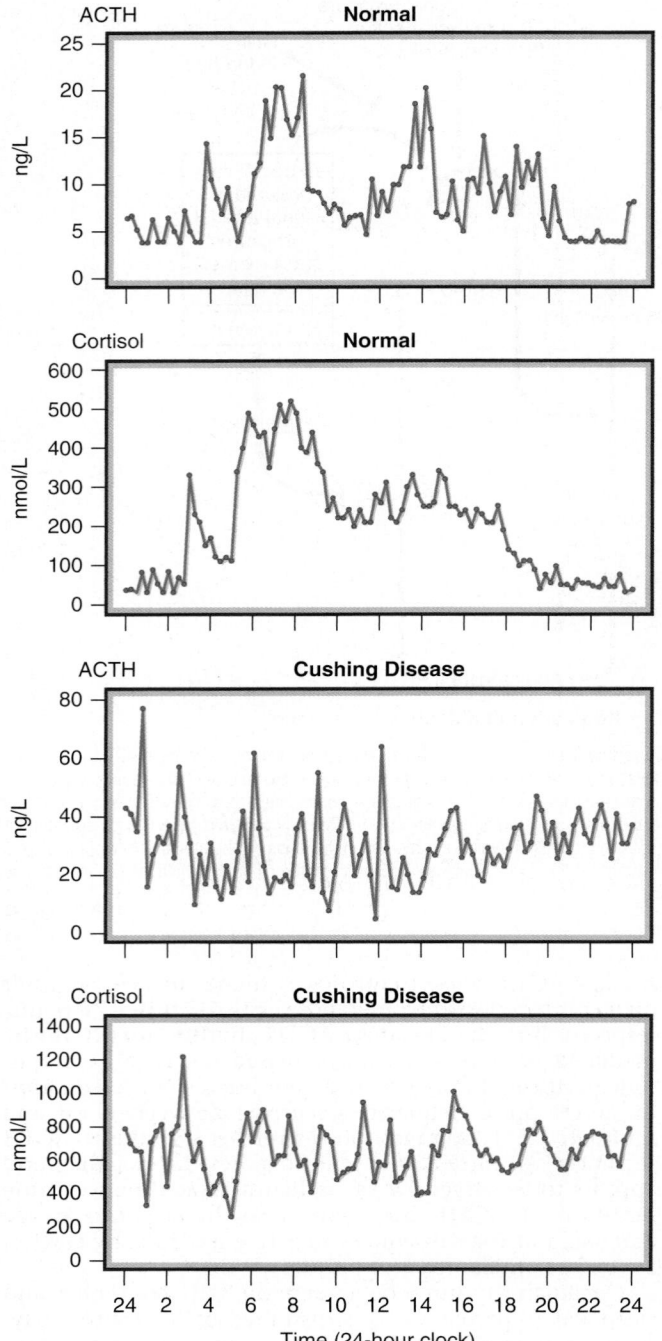

Figure 15-8 Circadian and pulsatile secretion of adrenocorticotropic hormone (ACTH) and cortisol in a normal subject (top two panels) and in a patient with Cushing disease. In a normal subject, secretion of ACTH and cortisol is highest in early morning and falls to a nadir at midnight. ACTH pulse frequency and pulse amplitude are increased in Cushing disease, and circadian rhythmic secretion is lost.

The ACTH Receptor and ACTH Effects on the Adrenal Gland

ACTH binds to a G protein–coupled, melanocortin-2 receptor (MC2R),[89] of which there are approximately 3500 on each adrenocortical cell. Melanocortin-2 receptor accessory protein (MRAP) is required for correct localization and signaling of MC2R.[90] Current data suggest that MRAP might promote three different activities: as a chaperone assisting correct folding of MC2R in the endoplasmic reticulum, as an accessory protein essential for trafficking of MC2R to the plasma membrane, and as a coreceptor enabling MC2R to bind or to signal ACTH response.[91] Downstream signal transduction is mediated principally through the stimulation of adenylate cyclase and intracellular cAMP,[92] although both extracellular and intracellular Ca^{2+} play a role.[93] Other factors synergize with or inhibit the effects of ACTH on the adrenal cortex, including angiotensin II, activin, inhibin, and cytokines (tumor necrosis factor-α and leptin).[94] Cell-to-cell communication via gap junctions is also important in mediating the effects of ACTH.[95]

ACTH produces both immediate and chronic effects on the adrenal gland; the end result is the stimulation of adrenal steroidogenesis and growth. Acutely, steroidogenesis is stimulated through a StAR-mediated increase in cholesterol delivery to the CYP11A1 enzyme in the inner mitochondrial membrane.[23] Chronically (within 24 to 26 hours of exposure), ACTH acts to increase the synthesis of all steroidogenic CYP enzymes (CYP11A1, CYP17A1, CYP21A2, CYP11B1) in addition to adrenodoxin,[96,97] the effects of which are mediated at the transcriptional level. ACTH increases synthesis of the LDL and HDL receptors and possibly also synthesis of 3-hydroxy-3-methylglutaryl (HMG)-CoA reductase, the rate-limiting step in cholesterol biosynthesis. ACTH increases adrenal weight by inducing both hyperplasia and hypertrophy. Adrenal atrophy is a feature of ACTH deficiency.

Mineralocorticoid Secretion: The Renin-Angiotensin-Aldosterone Axis

Aldosterone is secreted from the ZG under the control of three principal secretagogues: angiotensin II, potassium, and, to a lesser extent, ACTH (see Fig. 15-7). Other factors, notably somatostatin, heparin, atrial natriuretic factor, and dopamine, can directly inhibit aldosterone synthesis. The secretion of aldosterone and its intermediary 18-hydroxylated metabolites is restricted to the ZG because of the zone-specific expression of CYP11B2 (aldosterone synthase).[98] Corticosterone and DOC, synthesized in both the ZF and ZG, can act as mineralocorticoids, which becomes significant in some clinical diseases, notably some forms of congenital adrenal hyperplasia (CAH) and adrenal tumors. Similarly, it is now established that cortisol can act as a mineralocorticoid in the setting of impaired metabolism of cortisol to cortisone by the enzyme 11β-hydroxysteroid dehydrogenase type 2 (HSD11B2); this is important in patients with hypertension, ectopic ACTH syndrome, or renal disease. The renin-angiotensin system is described in detail in Chapter 16.

Angiotensin II and potassium stimulate aldosterone secretion principally by increasing the transcription of *CYP11B2* through common intracellular signaling pathways. cAMP response elements in the 5′ region of the *CYP11B2* gene are activated after an increase in intracellular Ca^{2+} and activation of calmodulin kinases. The potassium effect is mediated through membrane depolarization and opening of calcium channels and the angiotensin II effect after binding of angiotensin II to the surface AT_1 receptor and activation of phospholipase C.[98]

the feedback mechanism explains ACTH hypersecretion in Addison disease, as well as undetectable ACTH levels in patients with a cortisol-secreting adrenal adenoma. Feedback inhibition is principally mediated via the glucocorticoid receptor (GR); patients with glucocorticoid resistance resulting from mutations in the GR[87] and mice lacking the GR gene[88] have ACTH and cortisol hypersecretion due to perceived lack of negative feedback.

The effect of ACTH on aldosterone secretion is modest and differs in the acute and chronic situation (see Chapter 16). An acute bolus of ACTH will increase aldosterone secretion, principally by stimulating the early pathways of adrenal steroidogenesis (see earlier discussion), but circulating levels increase by no more than 10% to 20% above baseline values. ACTH has no effect on *CYP11B2* gene transcription or enzyme activity. Chronic continual ACTH stimulation has either no effect or an inhibitory effect on aldosterone production, possibly because of receptor down-regulation or suppression of angiotensin II–stimulated secretion because of a mineralocorticoid effect of cortisol, DOC, or corticosterone. Dopamine and atrial natriuretic peptide inhibit aldosterone secretion, as does heparin.

These separate lines of control—through the HPA axis for glucocorticoid biosynthesis and via the renin-angiotensin system for mineralocorticoid synthesis—have important clinical consequences. Patients with primary adrenal failure invariably have both cortisol and aldosterone deficiency, whereas patients with ACTH deficiency due to pituitary disease have glucocorticoid deficiency but normal aldosterone concentrations because the renin-angiotensin system is intact.

Adrenal Androgen Secretion

Adrenal androgens represent an important component (>50%) of circulating androgens in premenopausal women.[99] In men, this contribution is much smaller because of the testicular production of androgens, but adrenal androgen excess even in men may be of clinical significance, notably in patients with CAH, which results in a suppression of the hypothalamic-pituitary-gonadal axis. The adult adrenal secretes approximately 4 mg/day of DHEA, 7 to 15 mg/day of DHEAS, 1.5 mg of androstenedione, and 0.05 mg/day of testosterone.

DHEA is a crucial precursor of human sex steroid biosynthesis and exerts androgenic or estrogenic activity after conversion by the activities of the 3β-HSD superfamily (β-HSD isozymes and aromatase); these enzymes are expressed in peripheral target tissues, a fact that is of clinical importance in many diseases.[100] Some studies have postulated direct effects of DHEA acting as a classic hormone in peripheral tissues. Specific plasma membrane receptors have been identified but await full characterization.[101] Conventionally, desulfated DHEA is thought to be converted downstream to a biologically active hormone. Serum DHEAS was previously thought to represent a circulating storage pool for DHEA regeneration, but it was later suggested that conversion of DHEAS to DHEA by steroid sulfatase plays a minor role in adult physiology and that the equilibrium between serum DHEA and DHEAS is mainly regulated by SULT2A1 activity. This implies that serum DHEAS may not always appropriately reflect the active DHEA pool, particularly if SULT2A1 activity is impaired, as in the inflammatory stress response.[102]

DHEAS stimulates androgen secretion; DHEA (but not DHEAS because of its increased plasma half-life) and androstenedione demonstrate a circadian rhythm similar to that of cortisol.[103] However, there are many discrepancies between adrenal androgen and glucocorticoid secretion, leading to the suggestion of an additional cortical androgen-stimulating hormone (CASH). Many putative CASHs have been proposed, including POMC derivatives such as joining peptide, prolactin, and insulin-like growth factor type 1 (IGF-1), but conclusive proof is lacking. Efficient adrenal steroidogenesis toward androgen synthesis is crucially dependent on the relative activities of 3β-HSD and 17α-hydroxylase and, in particular, on the 17,20-lyase

activity of 17α-hydroxylase. Factors that determine whether the 17-hydroxylated substrates, 17-OH pregnenolone and 17-OHP, will undergo 21-hydroxylation to form glucocorticoid or side-chain cleavage by 17α-hydroxylase to form DHEA and androstenedione are unresolved and seem likely to be important in defining the activity of any putative CASH (Table 15-4).

TABLE 15-4
Dissociation of Adrenal Androgen and Glucocorticoid Secretion: Evidence for an Adrenal-Stimulating Hormone
Dexamethasone studies: Complete cortisol suppression with chronic high-dose dexamethasone; DHEA falls by only 20% (greater sensitivity of DHEA to acute low-dose dexamethasone administration).
Adrenarche: Clinically significant rise in circulating DHEA at 6 to 8 years of age; cortisol production unaltered.
Aging: Reduction in DHEA production; no change in cortisol.
Anorexia nervosa and illness: Fall in DHEA, no change (or increase) in cortisol.

DHEA, dehydroepiandrosterone.

CORTICOSTEROID HORMONE ACTION

Receptors and Gene Transcription

Both cortisol and aldosterone exert their effects after uptake of free hormone from the circulation and binding to intracellular receptors; these are termed, respectively, the *glucocorticoid receptor* (GR, encoded by *NR3C1*) and the *mineralocorticoid receptor* (MR, encoded by *NR3C2*).[104-106] These are members of the thyroid/steroid hormone receptor superfamily of transcription factors; they consist of a carboxy-terminal ligand-binding domain, a central DNA-binding domain that interacts with specific DNA sequences on target genes, and an amino-terminal hypervariable region. Although only single genes encode the GR and MR, splice variants have been described in both receptor types; this, together with tissue-specific post-translational modification (phosphorylation, sumoylation, and ubiquitination), is thought to account for many of the diverse actions of corticosteroids (Fig. 15-9).[107,108]

Glucocorticoid hormone action has been studied in more depth than mineralocorticoid action. The binding of steroid to the GRα in the cytosol results in activation of the steroid-receptor complex through a process that involves the dissociation of heat shock proteins (HSP90 and HSP70).[109] Following translocation to the nucleus, gene transcription is stimulated or repressed after binding of the dimerized GR-ligand complex to a specific DNA sequence in the promoter regions of target genes.[110] This sequence, known as the *glucocorticoid-response element* (GRE), is invariably a palindromic CGTACAnnnTGTACT sequence that binds with high affinity to two loops of DNA within the DNA-binding domain of the GR (zinc fingers). This stabilizes the RNA polymerase II complex, facilitating gene transcription. The GRβ variant may act as a dominant negative regulator of GRα transactivation.[107]

Naturally occurring mutations in the GR (as seen in patients with glucocorticoid resistance) and GR mutants generated in vitro have highlighted critical regions of the receptor that are responsible for binding and transactivation,[111] but numerous other factors are required (e.g., coactivators, corepressors[112]), and this may make responses tissue specific. This is a rapidly evolving field and beyond the scope of this chapter. However, the interaction between

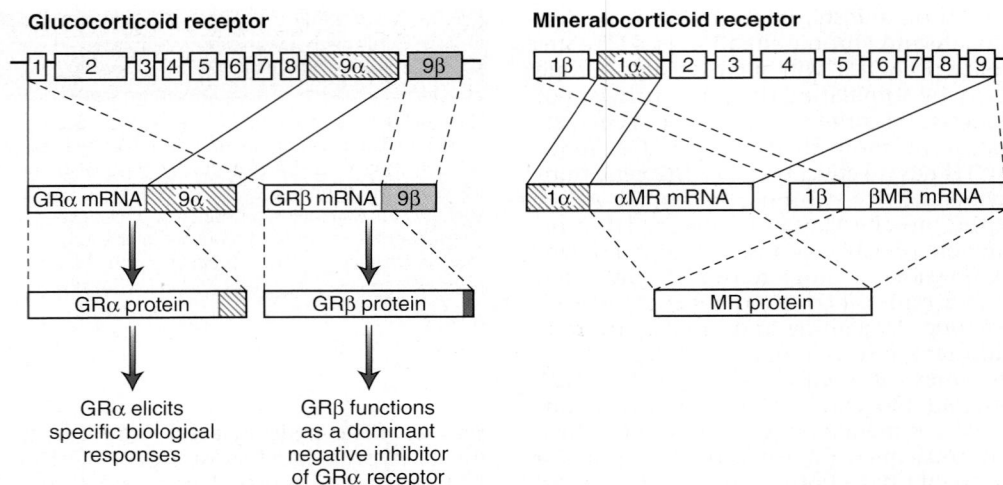

Figure 15-9 Schematic structure of the human genes encoding the glucocorticoid receptor (GR) and mineralocorticoid receptor (MR). In both cases, splice variants have been described. In the case of the GR, there is evidence that the GRβ isoform can act as a dominant negative inhibitor of GRα action. mRNA, messenger ribonucleic acid.

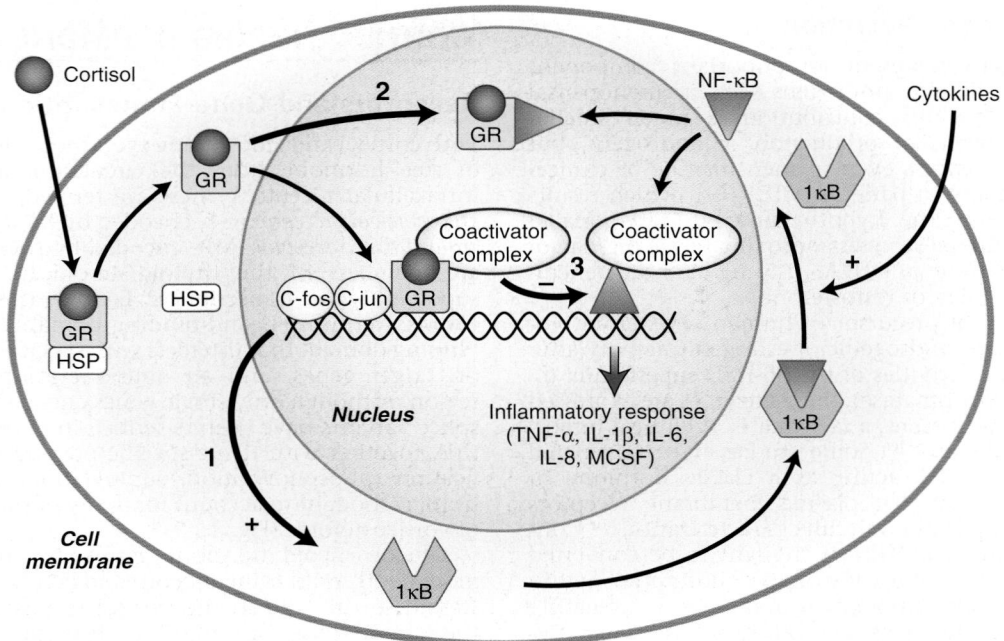

Figure 15-10 The anti-inflammatory action of glucocorticoids. Cortisol binds to the cytoplasmic glucocorticoid receptor (GR). Conformational changes in the receptor-ligand complex result in dissociation from heat shock proteins (HSP70 and HSP90) and migration to the nucleus. Binding occurs to specific DNA motifs—glucocorticoid response elements—in association with the activator protein 1 (AP1) comprising C-fos and C-jun. Glucocorticoids mediate their anti-inflammatory effects through several mechanisms: (1) the inhibitory protein 1κB, which binds and inactivates nuclear factor-κB (NF-κB), is induced; (2) the GR-cortisol complex is able to bind NF-κB and thereby prevent initiation of an inflammatory process; (3) GR and NF-κB compete for the limited availability of coactivators, which include cyclic adenosine monophosphate response element–binding protein (CREB) and steroid receptor coactivator-1. IL, interleukin; MCSF, macrophage colony-stimulating factor; TNF-α, tumor necrosis factor-α.

GR and two particular transcription factors are important in mediating the anti-inflammatory effects of glucocorticoids and explain the effect of glucocorticoids on genes that do not contain obvious GREs in their promoter regions.[113] Activator protein 1 (AP1) comprises Fos and Jun subunits and is a proinflammatory transcription factor induced by a series of cytokines and phorbol ester. The GR-ligand complex can bind to c-Jun and prevent interaction with the AP1 site, thereby mediating the so-called transrepressive effects of glucocorticoids.[114] Similarly, functional antagonism exists between the GR and

nuclear factor-κB (NF-κB), a ubiquitously expressed transcription factor that activates a series of genes involved in lymphocyte development, inflammatory response, host defense, and apoptosis (Fig. 15-10).[115] In keeping with the diverse array of actions of cortisol, many hundreds of glucocorticoid-responsive genes have been identified. Some glucocorticoid-induced genes and repressed genes are listed in Table 15-5.

In contrast to the diverse actions of glucocorticoids, mineralocorticoids have a more restricted role, principally stimulation of epithelial sodium transport in the distal

TABLE 15-5
Some of the Genes Regulated by Glucocorticoids or Glucocorticoid Receptors

Site of Action	Induced Genes	Repressed Genes
Immune system	IκB (nuclear factor-κB inhibitor)	Interleukins
	Haptoglobin	Tumor necrosis factor-α (TNF-α)
	T-cell receptor (TCR)-ζ	Interferon-γ
	p21, p27, and p57	E-selectin
	Lipocortin	Intercellular adhesion molecule-1
		Cyclooxygenase 2
		Inducible nitric oxide synthase (iNOS)
Metabolic	PPAR-γ	Tryptophan hydroxylase
	Tyrosine aminotransferase	Metalloprotease
	Glutamine synthase	
	Glycogen synthase	
	Glucose-6-phosphatase	
	PEPCK	
	Leptin	
	γ-Fibrinogen	
	Cholesterol 7α-hydroxylase	
	C/EBP/β	
Bone	Androgen receptor	Osteocalcin
	Calcitonin receptor	Collagenase
	Alkaline phosphatase	
	IGFBP6	
Channels and transporters	ENaC-α, -β, and -γ	
	SGK	
	Aquaporin 1	
Endocrine	Basic fibroblast growth factor (bFGF)	Glucocorticoid receptor
	Vasoactive intestinal peptide	Prolactin
	Endothelin	POMC/CRH
	Retinoid X receptor	PTHrP
	GHRH receptor	Vasopressin
	Natriuretic peptide receptors	
Growth and development	Surfactant proteins A, B, and C	Fibronectin
		α-Fetoprotein
		Nerve growth factor
		Erythropoietin
		G1 cyclins
		Cyclin-dependent kinases

CRH, corticotropin-releasing hormone; C/EBP/β, CAAT-enhancer binding protein-β; ENaC, epithelial sodium channel; GHRH, growth hormone–releasing hormone; IGFBP6, insulin-like growth factor–binding protein 6; PEPCK, phosphoenolpyruvate carboxykinase; POMC, pro-opiomelanocortin; PPAR, peroxisome proliferator-activated receptor; PTHrP, parathyroid hormone-related protein; SGK, serum- and glucocorticoid-induced kinase.
Modified from McKay LI, Cidlowski JA. Molecular control of immune/inflammatory responses: interactions between nuclear factor-κB and steroid receptor-signalling pathways. *Endocr Rev.* 1999;20:435-459.

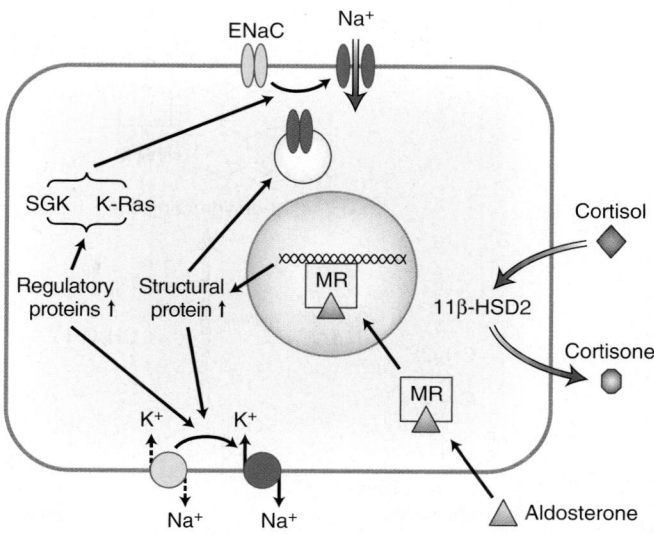

Figure 15-11 Mineralocorticoid hormone action. An epithelial cell in the distal nephron or distal colon is depicted. The much higher concentrations of cortisol are inactivated by the type 2 isozyme of 11β-hydroxysteroid dehydrogenase (11β-HSD2) to cortisone, permitting the endogenous ligand, aldosterone, to bind to the mineralocorticoid receptor (MR). Relatively few mineralocorticoid target genes have been identified, but they include serum- and glucocorticoid-induced kinase (SGK), subunits of the epithelial sodium channel (ENaC), and basolateral Na+/K+-adenosine triphosphatase.

The MR and GR share considerable homology—57% in the steroid-binding domain and 94% in the DNA-binding domain. It is perhaps not surprising, therefore, that there is promiscuity of ligand binding, with aldosterone (and the synthetic mineralocorticoid, fludrocortisone) binding to the GR and cortisol binding to the MR. For the MR, this is particularly impressive: in vitro, the MR has the same inherent affinity for aldosterone, corticosterone, or cortisol.[105] Specificity on the MR is conferred through the "pre-receptor" metabolism of cortisol via the enzyme HSD11B2, which converts cortisol and corticosterone to inactive 11-keto metabolites, enabling aldosterone to bind to the MR.[120,121] Mineralocorticoid hormone action was extended beyond this classic action in sodium-transporting epithelia with the demonstration that aldosterone can induce cardiac fibrosis and inflammatory changes in renal vasculature. The underlying signaling pathways remain to be fully clarified, but the effects are reversible with MR antagonists.[122]

Finally, for both glucocorticoids and mineralocorticoids, there is accumulating evidence for so-called nongenomic effects involving hormone response obviating the genomic GR or MR. A series of responses have been reported to occur within seconds or minutes after exposure to corticosteroids and are thought to be mediated by as yet uncharacterized membrane-coupled receptors.[123,124]

Cortisol-Binding Globulin and Corticosteroid Hormone Metabolism

More than 90% of circulating cortisol is bound predominantly to the α2-globulin, cortisol-binding globulin (CBG).[125] This 383–amino acid protein is synthesized in the liver and binds cortisol with high affinity. Affinity for synthetic corticosteroids is negligible except for prednisolone, which has an affinity for CBG approximately half that of cortisol. Circulating CBG concentrations are approximately 700 nmol/L. Levels are increased by estrogens and in some

nephron, distal colon, and salivary glands.[116] This action is mediated through induction of the apical sodium channel (comprising three subunits—α, β, and γ)[117] and the α1 and β1 subunits of the basolateral sodium-potassium adenosine triphosphatase pump (Na+/K+-ATPase)[118] through transcriptional regulation of serum- and glucocorticoid-induced kinase (SGK).[119] Aldosterone binds to the MR, principally in the cytosol (although there is evidence for expression of the unliganded MR in the nucleus), and the hormone-receptor complex is then translocated to the nucleus (Fig. 15-11).

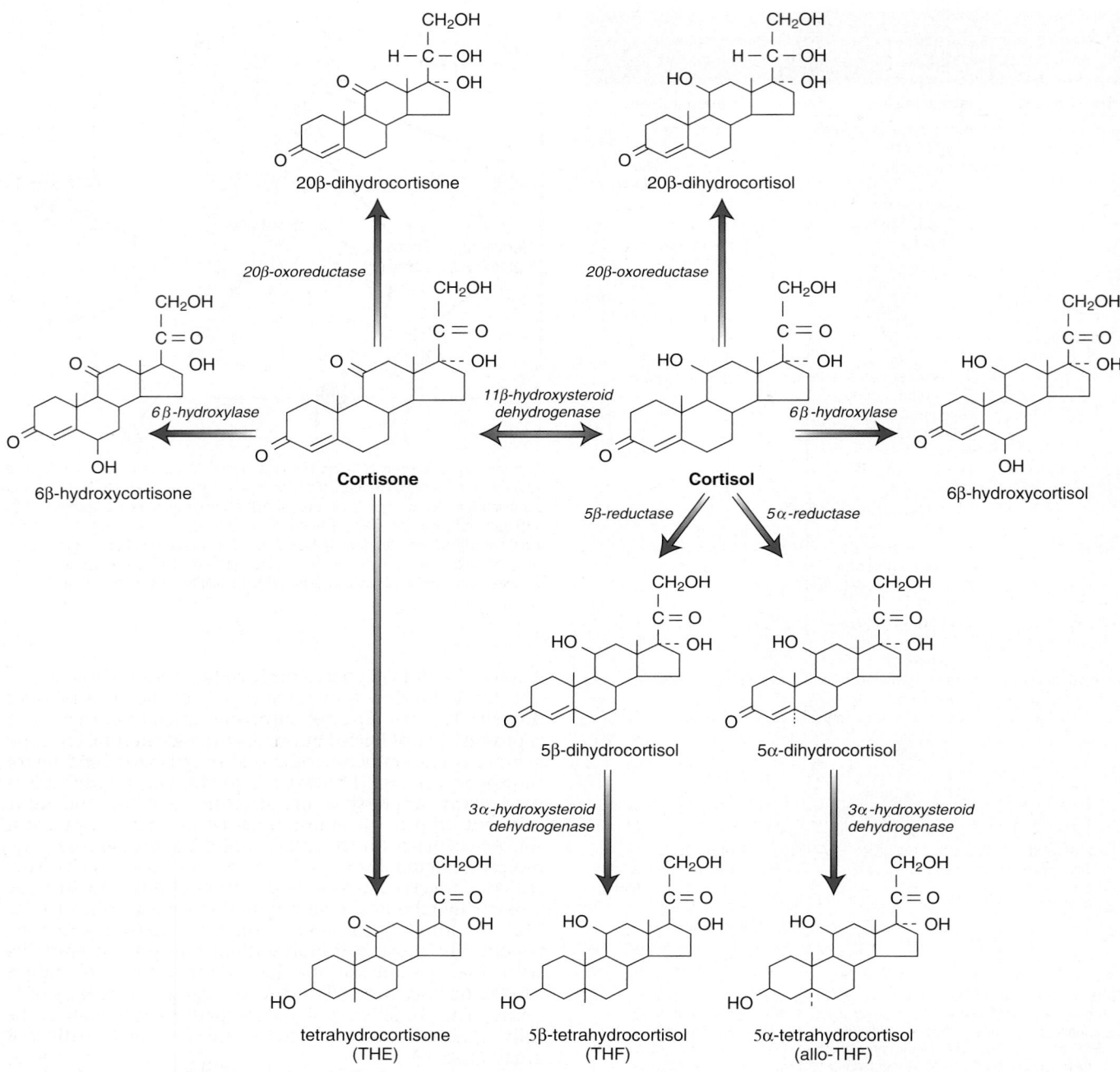

Figure 15-12 The principal pathways of cortisol metabolism. Interconversion of hormonally active cortisol to inactive cortisone is catalyzed by two isozymes of 11β-hydroxysteroid dehydrogenase (11β-HSD), with HSD11β1 principally converting cortisone to cortisol and HSD11β2 doing the reverse. Cortisol can be hydroxylated at the C6 and C20 positions. A ring reduction is undertaken by 5α-reductase or 5β-reductase and 3α-HSD.

patients with chronic active hepatitis; they are reduced by glucocorticoids and in patients with cirrhosis, nephrosis, and hyperthyroidism. The estrogen effect can be marked, with levels increasing twofold to threefold across pregnancy, a fact that should be taken into account when measuring plasma total cortisol in pregnancy and in women taking estrogens.

Inherited abnormalities in CBG synthesis are much rarer than those described for thyroxine-binding globulin but include cases of elevated CBG, partial or complete deficiency of CBG, and CBG variants with reduced affinity for cortisol.[126,127] In each case, alterations in CBG concentrations change the total circulating cortisol concentrations accordingly, but free cortisol concentrations are

normal. Only this free circulating fraction is available for transport into tissues for biologic activity. The excretion of free cortisol through the kidneys results in *urinary free cortisol*, which represents only 1% of the total cortisol secretion.

The circulating half-life of cortisol varies between 70 and 120 minutes. The major steps in cortisol metabolism are depicted in Figure 15-12[128] and can be summarized as follows:

• Interconversion of the 11-hydroxyl group (cortisol, Kendall's compound F) to the 11-oxo group (cortisone, compound E) through activity of the 11β-HSD system (EC 1.1.1.146).[129,130] The metabolism of cortisol and that of cortisone then follow similar pathways.

- Reduction of the C4-5 double bond to form dihydrocortisol or dihydrocortisone, followed by hydroxylation of the 3-oxo group to form tetrahydrocortisol (THF) or tetrahydrocortisone (THE). The reduction of the C4-5 double bond can be carried out by either 5β-reductase or 5α-reductase, yielding, respectively, 5β-THF (THF) and 5α-THF (allo-THF). In normal subjects, the ratio of THF to allo-THF is 2:1. THF, allo-THF, and THE are rapidly conjugated with glucuronic acid and excreted in the urine.
- Further reduction of the 20-oxo group by either 20α- or 20β-HSD to yield α- and β-cortols and cortolones from cortisol and cortisone, respectively. Reduction of the C20 position may also occur without A-ring reduction, giving rise to 20α- and 20β-hydroxycortisol.
- Hydroxylation at C6 to form 6β-hydroxycortisol.
- Cleavage of THF and THE to the C19 steroids, 11-hydroxy- or 11-oxo- androsterone, or etiocholanolone.
- Oxidation of the C21 position or cortols and cortolones to form the extremely polar metabolites, cortolic and cortolonic acids.

Approximately 50% of secreted cortisol appears in the urine as THF, allo-THF, and THE; 25% as cortols/cortolones; 10% as C19 steroids; and 10% as cortolic/cortolonic acids. The remaining metabolites are free unconjugated steroids (cortisol, cortisone, and their 6β-, and 20α/20β-metabolites).

The principal site of cortisol metabolism has been considered to be the liver, but many of the enzymes listed have been described in mammalian kidney, notably the interconversion of cortisol to cortisone by HSD11B2. Quantitatively, this is the most important pathway. Furthermore, the bioactivity of glucocorticoids is in part related to the hydroxyl group at C11; because cortisone with a C11-oxo group is an inactive steroid, expression of 11β-HSD in peripheral tissues plays a crucial role in regulating corticosteroid hormone action. Two distinct 11β-HSD isozymes have been reported: type 1, reduced nicotinamide adenine dinucleotide phosphate (NADPH)-dependent oxo-reductase expressed principally in the liver, which confers bioactivity on orally administered cortisone by converting it to cortisol,[130] and a type 2, nicotinamide adenine dinucleotide (NAD)-dependent dehydrogenase. It is the HSD11B2, coexpressed with the MR in the kidney, colon, and salivary gland, that inactivates cortisol to cortisone and permits aldosterone to bind to the MR in vivo. If this enzyme-protective mechanism is impaired, cortisol is able to act as a mineralocorticoid; this explains some forms of endocrine hypertension (apparent mineralocorticoid excess, licorice ingestion) and the mineralocorticoid excess state that characterizes the ectopic ACTH syndrome.[129,131]

Hyperthyroidism results in increased cortisol metabolism and clearance, and hypothyroidism produces the converse, principally because of an effect of thyroid hormone on hepatic HSD11B1 and 5α/5β-reductases.[130] IGF-1 increases cortisol clearance by inhibiting hepatic HSD11B1 (conversion of cortisone to cortisol).[132] 6β-Hydroxylation is normally a minor pathway, but cortisol itself induces 6β-hydroxylase so that 6β-hydroxycortisol excretion is markedly increased in patients with Cushing syndrome.[133] Some drugs, notably rifampicin and phenytoin, increase cortisol clearance through this pathway.[134] Patients with renal disease have impaired cortisol clearance because of reduced conversion of renal cortisol to cortisone.[135] These observations have clinical implications for patients with thyroid disease, acromegaly, or renal disease and for patients taking cortisol replacement therapy. Adrenal crisis has been reported in steroid-replaced addisonian patients

given rifampicin,[136] and hydrocortisone replacement therapy may need to be increased in treated patients who develop hyperthyroidism or reduced in patients with untreated growth hormone (GH) deficiency.

Aldosterone is also metabolized in the liver and kidneys. In the liver, it undergoes tetrahydro reduction and is excreted in the urine as a 3-glucuronide tetrahydroaldosterone derivative. However, glucuronide conjugation at the 18 position occurs directly in the kidney, as does 3α and 5α/5β metabolism of the free steroid.[137] Because of the aldehyde group at the C18 position, aldosterone is not metabolized by HSD11B2.[138] Hepatic aldosterone clearance is reduced in patients with cirrhosis, ascites, or severe congestive heart failure.

Effects of Glucocorticoids

The principal sites of action of glucocorticoids and some of the consequences of glucocorticoid excess are shown in Figure 15-13.

Carbohydrate, Protein, and Lipid Metabolism

Glucocorticoids increase blood glucose concentrations through their action on glycogen, protein, and lipid metabolism. In the liver, cortisol stimulates glycogen deposition by increasing glycogen synthase and inhibiting the glycogen-mobilizing enzyme, glycogen phosphorylase.[139] Hepatic glucose output increases through the activation of key enzymes involved in gluconeogenesis, principally glucose-6-phosphatase and phosphoenolpyruvate kinase (PEPCK).[140,141] In peripheral tissues (e.g., muscle, fat), cortisol inhibits glucose uptake and utilization.[142] In adipose tissue, lipolysis is activated, resulting in the release of free fatty acids into the circulation. An increase in total circulating cholesterol and triglycerides is observed, but HDL-cholesterol levels fall. Glucocorticoids also have a permissive effect on other hormones, including catecholamines and glucagon. The result is insulin resistance and an increase in blood glucose concentrations, at the expense of protein and lipid catabolism.

Glucocorticoids stimulate adipocyte differentiation, promoting adipogenesis through the transcriptional activation of key differentiation genes, including lipoprotein lipase, glycerol-3-phosphate dehydrogenase, and leptin.[143] Long-term effects of glucocorticoid excess on adipose tissue are more complex, at least in humans, in whom the deposition of visceral or central adipose tissue is stimulated,[144] providing a useful discriminatory sign for the diagnosis of Cushing syndrome. The predilection for visceral obesity may relate to the increased expression of the GR[145] and HSD11B1 in omental compared with subcutaneous adipose tissue.[146]

Skin, Muscle, and Connective Tissue

In addition to inducing insulin resistance in muscle tissue, glucocorticoids also cause catabolic changes in muscle, skin, and connective tissue. In the skin and connective tissue, glucocorticoids inhibit epidermal cell division and DNA synthesis and reduce synthesis and production of collagen.[147] In muscle, glucocorticoids cause atrophy (but not necrosis), which seems to be specific for type II (phasic) muscle fibers. Muscle protein synthesis is reduced.

Bone and Calcium Metabolism

Glucocorticoids inhibit osteoblast function, which is thought to account for the osteopenia and osteoporosis

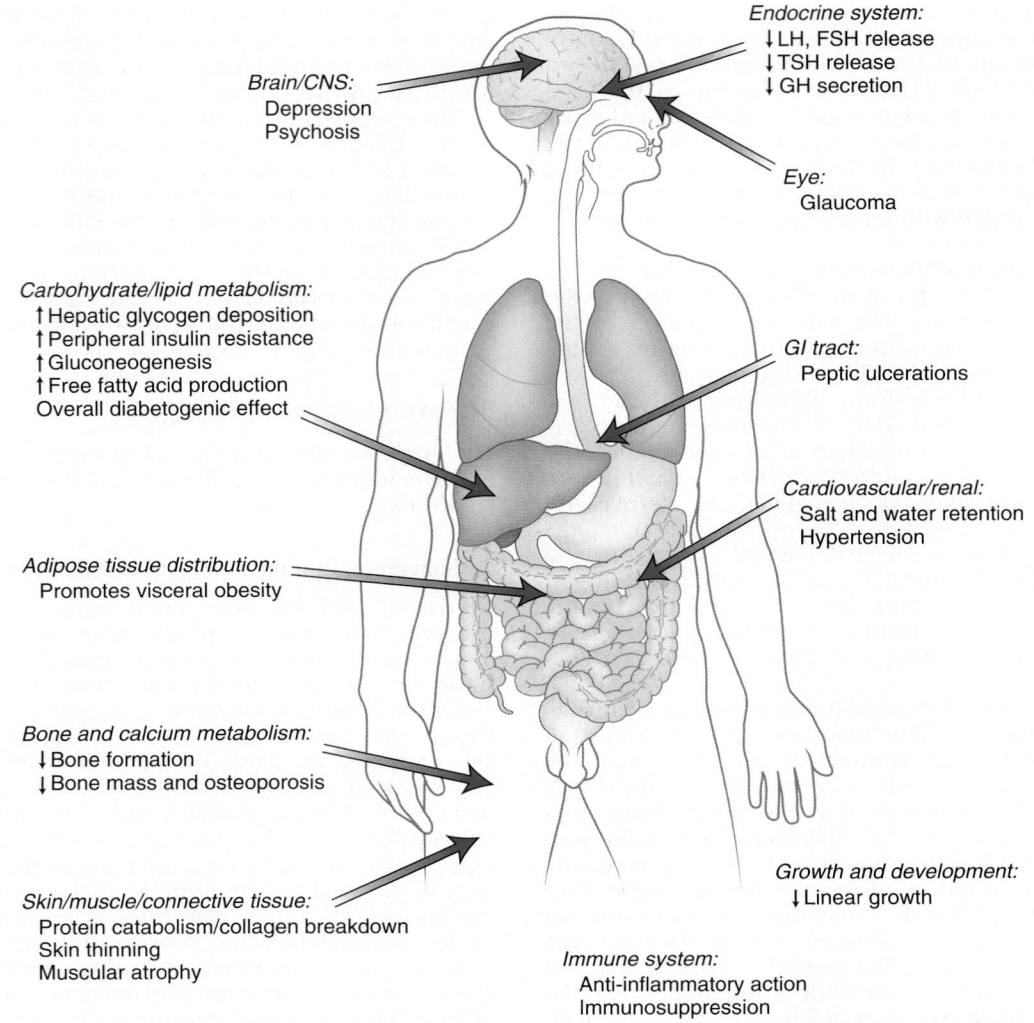

Endocrine system:
↓LH, FSH release
↓TSH release
↓GH secretion

Brain/CNS:
Depression
Psychosis

Eye:
Glaucoma

Carbohydrate/lipid metabolism:
↑Hepatic glycogen deposition
↑Peripheral insulin resistance
↑Gluconeogenesis
↑Free fatty acid production
Overall diabetogenic effect

GI tract:
Peptic ulcerations

Cardiovascular/renal:
Salt and water retention
Hypertension

Adipose tissue distribution:
Promotes visceral obesity

Bone and calcium metabolism:
↓Bone formation
↓Bone mass and osteoporosis

Growth and development:
↓Linear growth

Skin/muscle/connective tissue:
Protein catabolism/collagen breakdown
Skin thinning
Muscular atrophy

Immune system:
Anti-inflammatory action
Immunosuppression

Figure 15-13 The principal sites of action of glucocorticoids in humans, highlighting some of the consequences of glucocorticoid excess. CNS, central nervous system; FSH, follicle-stimulating hormone; GH, growth hormone; GI, gastrointestinal; LH, luteinizing hormone; TSH, thyroid-stimulating hormone.

that characterize glucocorticoid excess.[148] Up to 1% of Western populations are taking long-term glucocorticoid therapy,[149] and glucocorticoid-induced osteoporosis is becoming a prevalent health concern, affecting 50% of patients treated with corticosteroids for longer than 12 months. However, the complication perhaps most feared by physicians is osteonecrosis. Osteonecrosis (also termed *avascular necrosis*) produces rapid and focal deterioration of bone quality and primarily affects the femoral head, leading to pain and ultimately to collapse of the bone, often necessitating hip replacement. It can affect individuals of any age and may occur with relatively low doses of glucocorticoids (e.g., during corticosteroid replacement therapy for adrenal failure).[150] Importantly, defects may not be detectable on conventional radiographs but are readily seen on magnetic resonance imaging (MRI). Glucocorticoid-induced osteocyte apoptosis has been implicated in the pathogenesis of the condition,[151] and the lack of a direct role for an interrupted blood supply suggests that the term *osteonecrosis* is preferable to *avascular femoral necrosis.* However, there is still no explanation for individual susceptibility.

Glucocorticoids also induce negative calcium balance by inhibiting intestinal calcium absorption and increasing renal calcium excretion. As a consequence, parathyroid secretion is usually increased. In children, glucocorticoids suppress growth, but the increases in body mass index (BMI) are thought to offset a deleterious effect on bone mineral density.[152]

Salt and Water Homeostasis and Blood Pressure Control

Glucocorticoids increase blood pressure by a variety of mechanisms involving actions on the kidney and vasculature.[153] In vascular smooth muscle, they increase sensitivity to pressor agents such as catecholamines and angiotensin II while reducing nitric oxide–mediated endothelial dilatation. Angiotensinogen synthesis is increased by glucocorticoids.[154] In the kidney, depending on the activity of HSD11B2, cortisol can act on the distal nephron to cause sodium retention and potassium loss (mediated via the MR).[131] Elsewhere across the nephron, glucocorticoids increase the glomerular filtration rate, proximal tubular epithelial sodium transport, and free water clearance.[155] This last effect involves antagonism of the action of vasopressin and explains the dilutional hyponatremia seen in patients with glucocorticoid deficiency.[156]

Anti-inflammatory Actions and the Immune System

Glucocorticoids suppress immunologic responses, and this action has been the stimulus to develop a series of highly potent pharmacologic glucocorticoids to treat a variety of autoimmune and inflammatory conditions. The inhibitory effects are mediated at many levels. In the peripheral blood, glucocorticoids reduce lymphocyte counts acutely (T lymphocytes > B lymphocytes) by redistributing lymphocytes from the intravascular compartment to the spleen, lymph nodes, and bone marrow. Conversely, neutrophil counts increase after glucocorticoid administration. Eosinophil counts rapidly fall, an effect that was historically used as a bioassay for glucocorticoids. The immunologic actions of glucocorticoids involve direct actions on both T and B lymphocytes, including inhibition of immunoglobulin synthesis and stimulation of lymphocyte apoptosis. Inhibition of cytokine production from lymphocytes is mediated through inhibition of the action of NF-κB. NF-κB plays a crucial and generalized role in inducing cytokine gene transcription; glucocorticoids can bind directly to NF-κB to prevent nuclear translocation, and they induce NF-κB inhibitor, which sequesters NF-κB in the cytoplasm, thereby inactivating its effect.[115]

Additional anti-inflammatory effects involve the inhibition of monocyte differentiation into macrophages and macrophage phagocytosis and cytotoxic activity. Glucocorticoids reduce the local inflammatory response by preventing the actions of histamine and plasminogen activators. Prostaglandin synthesis is impaired through the induction of lipocortins, which inhibit phospholipase A2 activity.[157]

Central Nervous System and Mood

Clinical observations of patients with glucocorticoid excess and deficiency reveal that the brain is an important target tissue for glucocorticoids, with depression, euphoria, psychosis, apathy, and lethargy being important manifestations. Both GRs and MRs are expressed in discrete regions of the rodent brain, including hippocampus, hypothalamus, cerebellum, and cortex.[158] Glucocorticoids cause neuronal death, notably in the hippocampus[159]; this effect may underlie the interest in glucocorticoids in relation to cognitive function, memory, and neurodegenerative diseases such as Alzheimer disease.[160] Local blockade of cortisol generation by HSD11B1 has been shown to improve cognitive function.[161] DHEA has been shown to have neuroprotective effects in the hippocampus region.[162] CYP7B, an enzyme that metabolizes DHEA to its 7α-hydroxylated metabolite, is highly expressed in brain, but expression was decreased in dentate neurons in the hippocampus.[163]

Eye

In the eye, glucocorticoids act to raise intraocular pressure through an increase in aqueous humor production and deposition of matrix within the trabecular meshwork, which inhibits aqueous drainage. Steroid-induced glaucoma appears to have a genetic predisposition, but the underlying mechanisms are unknown.[164]

Gut

Long-term but not acute administration of glucocorticoids increases the risk of developing peptic ulcer disease.[165] Pancreatitis with fat necrosis is reported in patients with glucocorticoid excess. The GR is expressed throughout the gastrointestinal tract, and the MR is expressed in the distal colon; they mediate the corticosteroid control of epithelial ion transport.

Growth and Development

Although glucocorticoids stimulate transcription of the gene encoding GH in vitro, glucocorticoids in excess inhibit linear skeletal growth,[152,166] probably as a result of catabolic effects on connective tissue, muscle, and bone and through inhibition of the effects of IGF-1. The results of experiments on mice lacking the GR gene[88] have emphasized the role of glucocorticoids in normal fetal development. In particular, glucocorticoids stimulate lung maturation through the synthesis of surfactant proteins (SP-A, SP-B, and SP-C),[167] and mice lacking the GR die shortly after birth due to hypoxia from lung atelectasis. Glucocorticoids also stimulate the enzyme phenylethanolamine N-methyltransferase (PNMT), which converts noradrenaline to adrenaline in adrenal medulla and chromaffin tissue. Mice lacking the GR do not develop an adrenal medulla.[88]

Endocrine Effects

Glucocorticoids suppress the thyroid axis, probably through a direct action on the secretion of thyroid-stimulating hormone (TSH, thyrotropin). In addition, they inhibit 5′ deiodinase activity that mediates the conversion of thyroxine to active triiodothyronine.

Glucocorticoids also act centrally to inhibit gonadotropin-releasing hormone (GnRH) pulsatility and release of luteinizing hormone (LH) and follicle-stimulating hormone (FSH).

Therapeutic Corticosteroids

Since the dramatic anti-inflammatory effect of cortisone was first demonstrated in the 1950s, a series of synthetic corticosteroids have been developed for therapeutic purposes. These agents are used to treat a diverse variety of human diseases, principally relying on their anti-inflammatory and immunologic actions (Table 15-6). The main corticosteroids used in clinical practice, together with their relative glucocorticoid and mineralocorticoid potencies, are listed in Table 15-7.

The structures of common synthetic steroids are depicted in Figure 15-14. The biologic activity of a corticosteroid depends on a 4-3-keto, 11β-hydroxy, 17α,21-trihydroxyl configuration.[168] Conversion of the C11 hydroxyl group to a C11 keto group (i.e., cortisol to cortisone) inactivates the

TABLE 15-6

Therapeutic Use of Corticosteroids

Endocrine: Replacement therapy (Addison disease, pituitary disease, congenital adrenal hyperplasia), Graves ophthalmopathy
Skin: Dermatitis, pemphigus
Hematology: Leukemia, lymphoma, hemolytic anemia, idiopathic thrombocytopenic purpura
Gastrointestinal: Inflammatory bowel disease (ulcerative colitis, Crohn disease)
Liver: Chronic active hepatitis, transplantation, organ rejection
Renal: Nephrotic syndrome, vasculitides, transplantation, rejection
Central nervous system: Cerebral edema, raised intracranial pressure
Respiratory: Angioedema, anaphylaxis, asthma, sarcoidosis, tuberculosis, obstructive airway disease
Rheumatology: Systemic lupus erythematosus, polyarteritis, temporal arteritis, rheumatoid arthritis
Muscle: Polymyalgia rheumatica, myasthenia gravis

steroid. The addition of a 1,2 unsaturated bond to cortisol results in prednisolone, which is four times more potent than cortisol in classic glucocorticoid bioassays such as hepatic glycogen deposition, suppression of eosinophils, and anti-inflammatory actions. Prednisone, widely prescribed in the United States, is the cortisone equivalent of prednisolone and relies on conversion by HSD11B1 in the liver for bioactivity.[169] Potency is further increased by the addition of a 6α-methyl group to prednisolone (methylprednisolone).

Fludrocortisone is a synthetic mineralocorticoid having 125-fold greater potency than cortisol in stimulating sodium reabsorption. This effect is achieved through the addition of a 9α-fluoro group to cortisol. Fludrocortisone also has glucocorticoid potency (12-fold greater than cortisol). The addition of a 16α-methyl group and 1,2 saturated bond to fludrocortisone results in dexamethasone, a highly potent glucocorticoid (25-fold greater potency than cortisol) that has negligible mineralocorticoid activity.[168,170]

Administration

Widely used synthetic glucocorticoids in respiratory and nasal aerosol sprays are betamethasone, beclomethasone, and fluticasone. Betamethasone has the same structure as dexamethasone but with a 16β-methyl group. Beclomethasone has the same structure as betamethasone apart from the replacement of the 9α-fluoro group with a 9α-chloro group. Fluticasone has the same structure as dexamethasone with an additional 6α-fluoro group and a 5-fluoromethyl group replacing the hydroxymethyl group.

Corticosteroids are given orally, parenterally, and by numerous topical routes (e.g., eyes, skin, nose, inhalation, rectal suppositories).[170] Unlike hydrocortisone, which has a high affinity for CBG, most synthetic steroids have low affinity for this binding protein and circulate as free steroid (approximately 30%) or bound to albumin (approximately 70%). Circulating half-lives vary depending on individual variability and underlying disease, particularly renal and hepatic impairment. Cortisone acetate should not be used parenterally because it requires metabolism by the liver to active cortisol.

It is beyond the scope of this chapter to describe which steroid should be given and by which route for the non-endocrine conditions listed in Table 15-6. Acute and long-term corticosteroid therapy in patients with hypoadrenalism or CAH is discussed in later sections.

Long-Term Therapy

In addition to the undoubted benefit that corticosteroids provide, there is an increasing incidence of overuse,

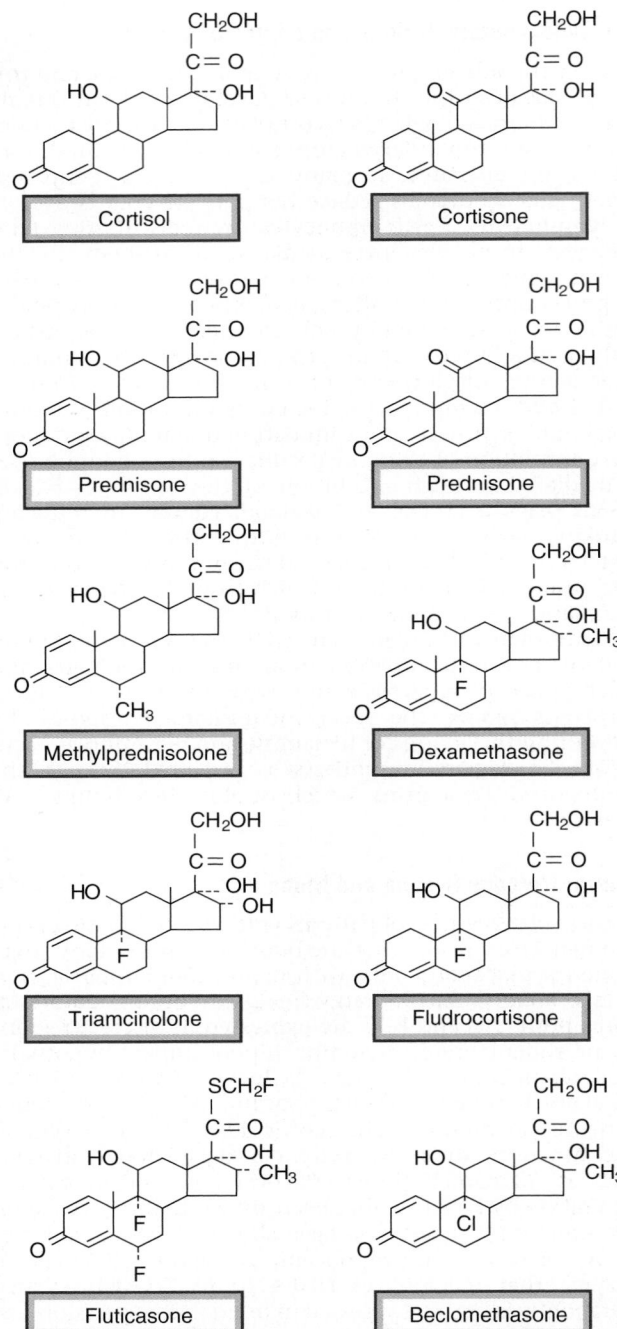

Figure 15-14 Structures of the natural glucocorticoid cortisol, some of the more commonly prescribed synthetic glucocorticoids, and the mineralocorticoid fludrocortisone. Triamcinolone is identical to dexamethasone except that a 16α-hydroxyl group is substituted for the 16α-methyl group. Betamethasone, another widely used glucocorticoid, has a 16β-methyl group. Beclomethasone is derived from betamethasone by replacement of the 9α-fluoro group with a chloro group. Fluticasone is identical to dexamethasone except that an additional 6α-fluoro group has been added, and the hydroxymethyl group at position 21 has been exchanged by a 5-fluoromethyl group.

particularly in patients with respiratory or rheumatologic disease, to such an extent that up to 1% of the population is now prescribed long-term corticosteroid therapy.[149] Because of their established euphoric effect, corticosteroids often make patients feel better but without any objective improvements in underlying disease parameters. In view of the long-term harm of chronic glucocorticoid excess,[171] decisions regarding treatment should be evidence based and subject to regular review based on efficacy and side effects. The endocrinologic consequences of chronic glucocorticoid excess, notably suppression of the HPA axis, are an important aspect of modern clinical practice and are described later (see "Primary and Central Hypoadrenalism"). Endocrinologists need to be aware of the effects of long-term therapy and of steroid withdrawal. Selective glucocorticoid receptor agonists (SEGRAs) are being developed with the aim of dissociating the transrepressive, anti-inflammatory actions of glucocorticoids from the transactivating effects that, by and large, mediate deleterious side effects.[172]

Adrenocortical Diseases

Adrenocortical diseases are relatively rare. Their importance lies in their high rates of morbidity and mortality if untreated, coupled with the relative ease of diagnosis and the availability of effective therapy. The diseases are most readily classified on the basis of hormone excess or deficiency (Table 15-8).

Glucocorticoid Excess
Cushing Syndrome

In 1912, Harvey Cushing first described a 23-year-old female with obesity, hirsutism, and amenorrhea, and 20 years later he postulated that this "polyglandular syndrome" was due to a primary pituitary abnormality causing adrenal hyperplasia.[8] Adrenal tumors were shown to cause the syndrome in some cases,[173] but ectopic ACTH production was not characterized until much later, in 1962.[174] The term *Cushing syndrome* is used to describe all causes, whereas *Cushing disease* is reserved for pituitary-dependent Cushing syndrome.

Cushing syndrome comprises the symptoms and signs associated with prolonged exposure to inappropriately elevated levels of free plasma glucocorticoids. The use of the term *glucocorticoid* in the definition covers excess from both endogenous (cortisol) and exogenous (e.g., predniso-

lone, dexamethasone) sources. Iatrogenic Cushing syndrome is common,[170,175] occurring to some degree in most patients taking long-term corticosteroid therapy. Endogenous causes of Cushing syndrome are rare and result in loss of the normal feedback mechanism of the HPA axis and the normal circadian rhythm of cortisol secretion.

The incidence of Cushing disease is estimated to be 2 to 3 cases per 1 million population per year. The incidence of ectopic ACTH syndrome parallels that of bronchogenic carcinoma, and although 0.5% of lung cancer patients have ectopic ACTH syndrome, rapid progression of the underlying disease often precludes an early diagnosis. Cushing disease and adrenal adenomas are four times more common in women, whereas ectopic ACTH syndrome is more common in men.

Clinical Features of Cushing Syndrome

The classic features of Cushing syndrome—centripetal obesity, moon face, hirsutism, and plethora—have been well known since Cushing's initial descriptions in 1912 and 1932 (Figs. 15-15 to 15-17). However, this gross clinical picture is not always present, and a high index of suspicion is required in many cases. Once the normal physiologic effects of glucocorticoids are appreciated (see Fig. 15-13), the clinical features of glucocorticoid excess are easier to define. They are summarized in Table 15-9 together with the most discriminatory features that will assist in distinguishing Cushing syndrome from simple obesity.[176,177]

Obesity. Weight gain and obesity are the most common signs of Cushing syndrome. At least in adults, this weight gain is invariably centripetal in nature.[144,178] In fact, generalized obesity is more common in the general population

TABLE 15-8
Adrenocortical Diseases
Glucocorticoid Excess
Cushing syndrome
Pseudo-Cushing syndromes
Glucocorticoid Resistance
Glucocorticoid Deficiency
Primary hypoadrenalism
Secondary hypoadrenalism
Postchronic corticosteroid replacement therapy
Congenital Adrenal Hyperplasia
Deficiencies of 21-hydroxylase, 3β-HSD, 17α-hydroxylase, 11β-hydroxylase, P450 oxidoreductase, P450 side chain cleavage, and StAR
Mineralocorticoid Excess
Mineralocorticoid Deficiency
Defects in aldosterone synthesis
Defects in aldosterone action
Hyporeninemic hypoaldosteronism
Adrenal Incidentalomas, Adenomas, and Carcinomas

HSD, hydroxysteroid dehydrogenase; StAR, steroidogenic acute regulatory (protein).

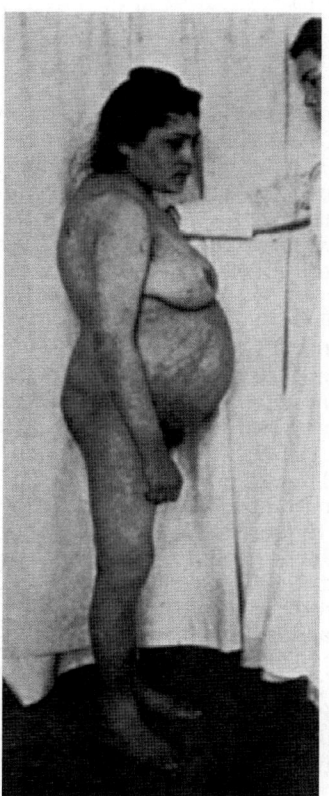

Figure 15-15 Minnie G., Cushing's index patient, at age 23 years. (From Cushing H. The basophil adenomas of the pituitary body and their clinical manifestations [pituitary basophilism]. *Bull Johns Hopkins Hosp.* 1932;50:137-195.)

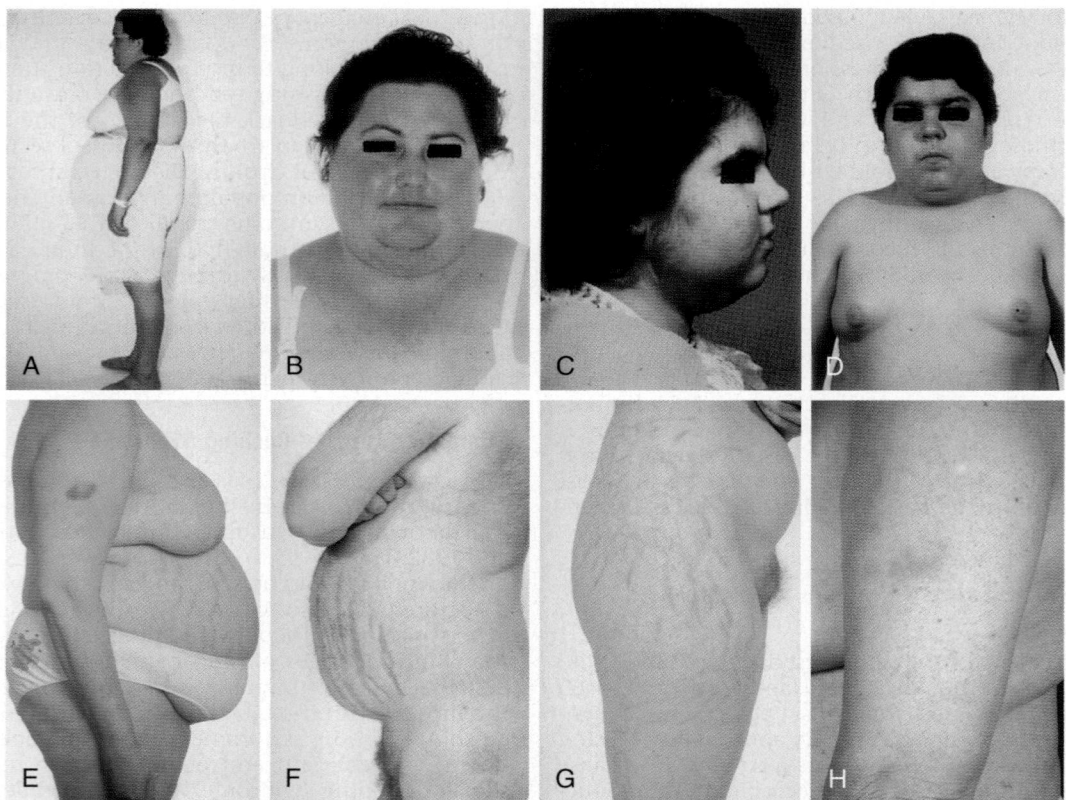

Figure 15-16 Clinical features of Cushing syndrome. **A,** Centripetal and some generalized obesity and dorsal kyphosis in a 30-year-old woman with Cushing disease. **B,** Same patient as in **A,** showing moon facies, plethora, hirsutism, and enlarged supraclavicular fat pads. **C,** Facial rounding, hirsutism, and acne in a 14-year-old girl with Cushing disease. **D,** Central and generalized obesity and moon facies in a 14-year-old boy with Cushing disease. **E** and **F,** Typical centripetal obesity with livid abdominal striae seen in a 41-year-old woman (**E**) and a 40-year-old man (**F**) with Cushing syndrome. **G,** Striae in a 24-year-old patient with congenital adrenal hyperplasia treated with excessive doses of dexamethasone as replacement therapy. **H,** Typical bruising and thin skin of a patient with Cushing syndrome. In this case, the bruising occurred without obvious injury.

than it is in patients with Cushing syndrome. One exception is seen in pediatric patients, in whom glucocorticoid excess may result in generalized obesity. In addition to centripetal obesity, patients develop fat depots over the thoracocervical spine (buffalo hump), in the supraclavicular region, and over the cheeks and temporal regions, giving rise to the rounded, moon-like facies. The epidural space, another site of abnormal fat deposition, may lead to neurologic deficits.

Reproductive Organs. Gonadal dysfunction is common, with menstrual irregularity in females and loss of libido in both sexes. Hirsutism is frequently found in female patients, as is acne. The most common form of hirsutism is vellus hypertrichosis on the face; this type should be distinguished from the darker, terminal differentiated hirsutism that may occur because of ACTH-mediated adrenal androgen excess. Hypogonadotropic hypogonadism occurs because of a direct inhibitory effect of cortisol on GnRH pulsatility and LH/FSH secretion, and it is reversible on correction of the hypercortisolism.[179,180]

Psychiatric Features. Psychiatric abnormalities occur in approximately 50% of patients with Cushing syndrome, regardless of cause.[181,182] Agitated depression and lethargy are among the most common problems, but paranoia and overt psychosis are also well recognized. Memory and cognitive function may also be affected, and increased irritability may be an early feature. Insomnia is common, and both rapid eye movement and delta-wave sleep patterns are reduced.[183] Lowering of plasma cortisol by medical or surgical therapy usually results in a rapid improvement in the psychiatric state. Overall quality of life is significantly reduced in patients with Cushing syndrome, particularly affecting physical health and functioning. Quality-of-life scores improve after treatment but do not return to normal.[184]

Bone. In childhood, the most common presentation is poor linear growth and weight gain[150]; as discussed earlier, glucocorticoids have profound effects on growth and development.[166] Many patients with long-standing Cushing syndrome have lost height because of osteoporotic vertebral collapse. This can be assessed by measuring the patient's sitting height or comparing the height with arm span; in normal subjects, height and arm span should be equal. Pathologic fractures, occurring spontaneously or after minor trauma, are not uncommon. Rib fractures, in contrast to those of the vertebrae, are often painless. The radiographic appearance is typical, with exuberant callus formation at the site of the healing fracture. In addition, osteonecrosis of the femoral and humeral heads is a recognized feature of endogenous Cushing syndrome (see Fig. 15-17). Hypercalciuria may lead to renal calculi, but hypercalcemia is not a feature.

Skin. Hypercortisolism results in thinning of the skin and separation and exposure of the subcutaneous vascular tissue. On examination, wrinkling of the skin on the dorsum of the hand may be seen, resulting in a "cigarette paper" appearance (Liddle sign). Minimal trauma may result in bruising, which frequently resembles the appearance of senile purpura. The plethoric appearance of the patient with Cushing syndrome is secondary to the

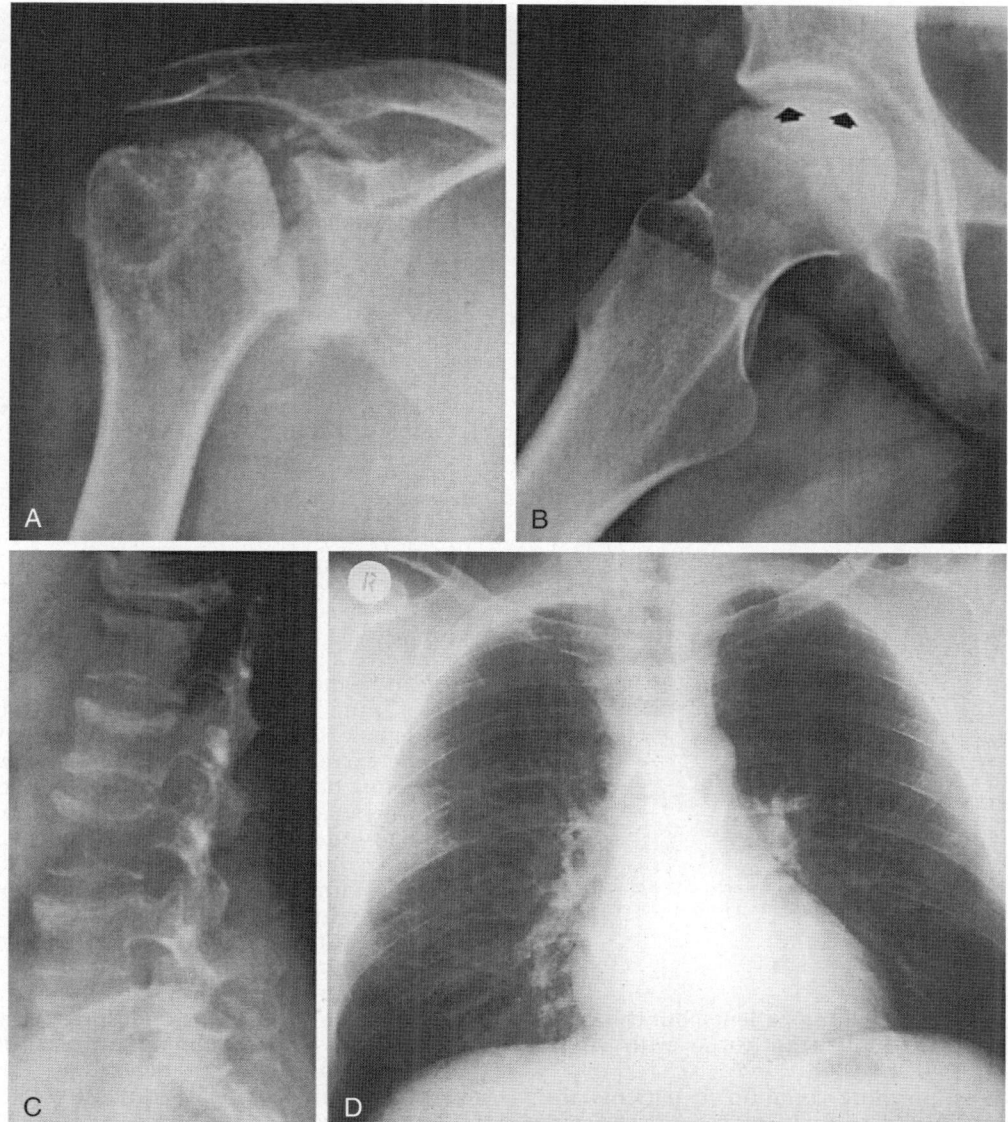

Figure 15-17 Bone abnormalities in Cushing disease. **A,** Aseptic necrosis of the right humeral head in a 43-year-old woman with Cushing disease of about 8 months' duration. **B,** Aseptic necrosis of the right femoral head in a 24-year-old woman with Cushing disease of about 4 ½ years' duration. The *arrows* indicate the crescent subchondral radiolucency, best seen in this lateral view. **C,** Diffuse osteoporosis, vertebral collapse, and subchondral sclerosis in the same patient shown in **A. D,** Rib fracture in a 38-year-old man with Cushing disease. (**A** through **C** from Phillips KA, Nance EP Jr, Rodriguez RM, et al. Avascular necrosis of bone: a manifestation of Cushing's disease. *South Med J.* 1986;79:825-829.)

thinning of the skin[185] combined with loss of facial subcutaneous fat and is not caused by true polycythemia. Acne and papular lesions may occur over the face, chest, and back.

The typical, almost pathognomonic, red-purple livid striae greater than 1 cm in width are most frequently found on the abdomen but may also be present on the upper thighs, breasts, and arms. They are very common in younger patients and less so in those older than 50 years of age. They must be differentiated from the paler, less pigmented striae that occur as a result of pregnancy (striae gravidarum) or in association with rapid weight loss.

Skin pigmentation is rare in Cushing disease but common in the ectopic ACTH syndrome. It arises because of overstimulation of melanocyte receptors by ACTH and possibly POMC-derived peptides.

Muscle. Myopathy and bruising are two of the most discriminatory features of the syndrome.[176] The myopathy of Cushing syndrome involves the proximal muscles of the lower limbs and the shoulder girdle.[186] Complaints of weakness, such as inability to climb stairs or get up from a deep chair, are relatively uncommon, but testing for proximal myopathy by asking the patient to rise from a crouching position often reveals the problem.

Cardiovascular Features. Hypertension is another prominent feature, occurring in up to 75% of cases. Even though epidemiologic data show a strong association between high blood pressure and obesity, hypertension is much more common in patients with Cushing syndrome than in those with simple obesity.[153] This, together with the established metabolic consequences of the disease (diabetes, hyperlipidemia), is thought to explain the increased cardiovascular mortality rate in untreated cases.[187-189] Cardiovascular events are also more common in patients with presumed iatrogenic Cushing syndrome resulting from prescribed corticosteroids.[171] In addition, thromboembolic events

TABLE 15-9

Prevalence of Symptoms and Signs in Cushing Syndrome and Discriminant Index Compared With Prevalence of Features in Patients With Simple Obesity

Findings	% of Patients	Discriminant Index
Symptoms		
Weight gain	91	
Menstrual irregularity	84	1.6
Hirsutism	81	2.8
Psychiatric dysfunction	62	
Backache	43	
Muscle weakness	29	8.0
Fractures	19	
Loss of scalp hair	13	
Signs		
Obesity	97	
Truncal	46	1.6
Generalized	55	0.8
Plethora	94	3.0
Moon facies	88	
Hypertension	74	4.4
Bruising	62	10.3
Red-purple striae	56	2.5
Muscle weakness	56	
Ankle edema	50	
Pigmentation	4	
Other Findings		
Hypertension	74	
Diabetes	50	
Overt	13	
Impaired glucose tolerance test	37	
Osteoporosis	50	
Renal calculi	15	

Data from Ross EJ, Linch DC. Cushing's syndrome-killing disease: discriminatory value of signs and symptoms aiding early diagnosis. *Lancet.* 1982;2:646-649.

may be more common in Cushing patients, but this development appears to be limited to those with ACTH-dependent disease.[190]

Infections. Infections are more common in patients with Cushing syndrome.[191,192] In many instances, infections are asymptomatic and occur because the normal inflammatory response is suppressed. Reactivation of tuberculosis has been reported[193] and has even been the presenting feature in some cases. Fungal infections of the skin (notably tinea versicolor) and nails may occur, as may opportunistic fungal infections. Bowel perforation is more common in patients with extreme hypercortisolism, and the hypercortisolism may mask the usual symptoms and signs of the condition. Wound infections are more common and contribute to poor wound healing.

Metabolic and Endocrine Features. Glucose intolerance occurs, and overt diabetes mellitus is present in up to one third of patients in some series. Hepatic lipoprotein synthesis is stimulated, and increases in circulating cholesterol and triglycerides may be found.[194] Hypokalemic alkalosis is found in 10% to 15% of patients with Cushing disease but in more than 95% of patients with ectopic ACTH syndrome. Several factors may contribute to this mineralocorticoid excess state, including corticosterone and DOC excess, but the principal culprit is thought to be cortisol itself. Depending on the prevailing cortisol production rate, cortisol swamps HSD11B2 in the kidney and acts as a mineralocorticoid. Hypokalemic alkalosis is more common in ectopic ACTH syndrome because cortisol production rates are higher than in patients with Cushing disease.[131]

TABLE 15-10

Classification of Causes of Cushing Syndrome

ACTH-Dependent Causes

Cushing disease (pituitary-dependent)
Ectopic ACTH syndrome
Ectopic CRH syndrome
Macronodular adrenal hyperplasia
Iatrogenic (treatment with 1-24 ACTH)

ACTH-Independent Causes

Adrenal adenoma and carcinoma
Primary pigmented nodular adrenal hyperplasia and Carney syndrome.
McCune-Albright syndrome
Aberrant receptor expression (gastric inhibitory polypeptide, interleukin-1β)
Iatrogenic (e.g., pharmacologic doses of prednisolone, dexamethasone)

Other Causes of Hypercortisolism

Alcoholism
Depression
Obesity
Pregnancy

ACTH, adrenocorticotropic hormone; CRH, corticotropin-releasing hormone.

This can be diagnosed by documenting an increase in the ratio of urinary cortisol to cortisone metabolites. In addition, hepatic 5α-reductase activity is inhibited, resulting in a greater excretion of 5α-cortisol metabolites.[195]

The functions of the pituitary-thyroid axis and the pituitary-gonadal axis are suppressed in patients with Cushing syndrome because of a direct effect of cortisol on TSH and gonadotropin secretion.[196,197] Cortisol causes a reversible form of hypogonadotropic hypogonadism but also directly inhibits Leydig cell function. GH secretion is reduced, possibly mediated through an increase in somatostatinergic tone.

Eye. Ocular effects include raised intraocular pressure[198] and exophthalmos[199] (in up to one third of patients in Cushing's original series), the latter occurring because of increased retro-orbital fat deposition. Cataracts, a well-recognized complication of corticosteroid therapy, seem to be uncommon,[200] except as a complication of diabetes. In our experience, chemosis is a sensitive and underreported feature of Cushing syndrome.

CLASSIFICATION AND PATHOPHYSIOLOGY OF CUSHING SYNDROME

Cushing syndrome is most readily classified into ACTH-dependent and ACTH-independent causes (Table 15-10).

ACTH-Dependent Causes

Cushing Disease

When iatrogenic causes are excluded, the most common cause of Cushing syndrome is Cushing disease, accounting for approximately 70% of cases. The adrenal glands in these patients show bilateral adrenocortical hyperplasia with widening of the ZF and ZR.[177]

Cushing himself raised the question as to whether this disease was a primary pituitary condition or secondary to an abnormality in the hypothalamus, and there has been an ongoing debate on this issue ever since.[201] The hypothalamic theory states that ACTH-secreting adenomas

TABLE 15-11

Etiology of Cushing Disease: Hypothalamic Theory Versus Pituitary Theory

Hypothalamic Theory	Pituitary Theory
Neuroendocrine abnormalities[202,203]	Lack of cure after pituitary stalk section
Loss of circadian rhythm, sleep disturbance, other hypothalamic defects (TSH, LH/FSH secretion)	Circulating and CSF CRH levels are suppressed[204]
Efficacy of centrally acting drugs[205,206] (bromocriptine, cyproheptadine, sodium valproate)	Reversal of hypothalamic defects on correction of hypercortisolism
Recurrences after pituitary surgery	High surgical cure rate (recurrences resulting from regrowth of inadequately resected tumor rather than real recurrence)[207,208]
Ectopic CRH-secreting tumors cause Cushing disease,[210] but pathologic examination shows basophil hyperplasia, not adenomas	Secondary hypoadrenalism after successful pituitary surgery (may be prolonged and associated with reduced ACTH expression in surrounding adjacent normal corticotrophs)[209]
	Pituitary ACTH-secreting adenoma in almost 90% of cases are monoclonal in origin[211,212]

Note: Superscript numbers indicate references listed at the end of the chapter.
ACTH, adrenocorticotropic hormone; CRH, corticotropin-releasing hormone; CSF, cerebrospinal fluid; FSH, follicle-stimulating hormone; LH, luteinizing hormone; TSH, thyroid-stimulating hormone.

arise because of dysfunctional regulation of corticotrophs through chronic stimulation by CRH (or AVP). Other studies provide data to support a primary pituitary defect as the cause of the condition (Table 15-11).

The hypothalamus may have an initiating role, but the overwhelming evidence is that, at presentation, the condition is pituitary-dependent. In 85% to 90% of cases, the disease is caused by a pituitary adenoma of monoclonal origin[213,214]; basophil hyperplasia alone is found in 9% to 33% of pathologic series.[201] The majority of tumors are small microadenomas (<1 cm), but larger macroadenomas occur in up to 10% of cases and usually signify a more invasive tumor.[215] Selective surgical removal of a causative corticotroph adenoma results in remission, but on very long-term follow-up, relapse may occur in up to 20% to 30% of micro- and macroadenoma patients.[215a] However, it is possible, particularly in cases with no identifiable pituitary adenoma, that Cushing disease is heterogeneous with different subtypes.

A key biochemical hallmark of the disease is a relative resistance of ACTH secretion to normal glucocorticoid feedback inhibition.[216] ACTH-secreting pituitary adenomas function at a higher than normal set-point for cortisol feedback. The predominant finding in Cushing disease is an increase in ACTH pulse amplitude with loss of normal circadian rhythm, but ACTH pulse frequency is also increased in some cases (see Fig. 15-8).[217]

Ectopic ACTH Syndrome

In 15% of cases, Cushing syndrome is associated with non-pituitary tumors secreting ACTH—the ectopic ACTH syndrome.[218] On clinical grounds, these tumors can be divided into two entities: highly malignant tumors such as small cell carcinoma of bronchus (Table 15-12) and highly proliferative neuroendocrine carcinoma (e.g., pancreas), and more indolent tumors occurring in patients with underlying neuroendocrine tumors such as bronchial carcinoids. In the former group, the clinical presentation is often that of a wasting syndrome with weakness and pigmentation. Circulating ACTH concentrations and cortisol secretion rates can be extremely high. As a result, duration of symptoms from onset to presentation is short (<3 months); patients are commonly pigmented, and the metabolic manifestations of glucocorticoid excess are often rapid and progressive. Weight loss, myopathy, and glucose intolerance are prominent symptoms and signs. The association of these features with hypokalemic alkalosis and peripheral edema should alert the clinician to the diagnosis.

Depending on local referral practice, approximately 20% of cases of ectopic ACTH syndrome are explained by

TABLE 15-12

Tumors Associated With the Ectopic Adrenocorticotropic Hormone Syndrome

Tumor Type	Approximate Incidence (%)
Small cell lung carcinoma	50
Non–small cell lung carcinoma	5
Pancreatic tumors (including carcinoids)	10
Thymic tumors (including carcinoids)	5
Lung carcinoids	10
Other carcinoids	2
Medullary carcinoma of thyroid	5
Pheochromocytoma and related tumors	3
Rare carcinomas of prostate, breast, ovary, gallbladder, colon	10

indolent tumors, such as benign bronchial carcinoids, that produce ACTH.[218,219] In these cases, symptoms and signs are commonly present for 18 months before clinical presentation. Such patients present with the typical features of Cushing syndrome and may be biochemically similar to patients with Cushing disease. Therefore, once a diagnosis of Cushing syndrome is established, the principal diagnostic dilemma is in the distinction of pituitary-dependent Cushing disease from these indolent causes of ectopic ACTH syndrome.

Tumors most commonly associated with ectopic ACTH syndrome arise from neuroendocrine tissues, the cells of which possess the ability to uptake and decarboxylate amine precursors (APUD cells). Although *POMC* transcripts of 1200-1450nt are frequently found in small cell lung cancer, only 0.5% to 1% of tumors are associated with ectopic ACTH syndrome, and the explanation for the development of ectopic ACTH secretion remains unclear. In contrast, *POMC* mRNA transcripts of the short 800nt length may be found in tumors not associated with ectopic ACTH syndrome. In addition to aberrant transcriptional regulation of the *POMC*, interaction with tissue-specific transcription factors or the promoter methylation status of *POMC* may be involved. Once translated, POMC is cleaved in the pituitary by specific serine endoproteases to produce ACTH precursors; in ectopic ACTH syndrome, aberrant peripheral processing of POMC may lead to increased concentrations of circulating ACTH precursors (pro-ACTH, N-POC) (see Fig. 15-6). In contrast to ACTH secretion from pituitary adenomas, ectopic POMC/ACTH production is not responsive to normal glucocorticoid feedback[220] because of the defective GR or GR-signaling mechanism.[221] However, this sensitivity to glucocorticoid feedback is far from clearcut, which is one reason why the differential diagnosis of ACTH-dependent Cushing syndrome can be challenging.[218]

Ectopic Corticotropin-Releasing Hormone Syndrome

Ectopic production of CRH is a very rare cause of pituitary-dependent Cushing disease. A number of cases have now been described in which a tumor (usually bronchial carcinoid, medullary thyroid, or prostate carcinoma) has been shown to secrete CRH alone or in combination with ACTH.[222-224] When available, pituitary histologic examination has revealed corticotroph hyperplasia but not adenoma formation. Biochemically, these patients, like those with ectopic ACTH syndrome, lose the normal negative glucocorticoid feedback mechanism—50% have resistance to high-dose dexamethasone therapy. Ectopic CRH production may explain the suppression of cortisol secretion after high-dose dexamethasone that is observed in some patients with the ectopic ACTH syndrome.

Macronodular Adrenal Hyperplasia

In 10% to 40% of patients with Cushing disease, there is bilateral adrenocortical hyperplasia associated with one or more nodules, which may be up to several centimeters in diameter.[225-228] Patients tend to be older and to have had symptoms for a longer time, but they otherwise present with the classic clinical features of Cushing syndrome. Pathologically, the nodules are lobulated and can be markedly enlarged, but internodular hyperplasia is invariably found. Macronodular adrenal hyperplasia (MAH) is thought to result from long-standing adrenal ACTH stimulation, which leads to autonomous adrenal adenoma formation. Therefore, as the adrenals in a patient with Cushing disease become more hyperplastic, they secrete more cortisol for a given ACTH level, which ultimately can lead to autosuppression. Individual clinical cases support this hypothesis, and MAH should be regarded as an ACTH-dependent form of Cushing syndrome, even though ACTH levels may be relatively low and dexamethasone suppressibility less marked than in other cases of Cushing disease.[229] These features can be a trap for the unwary because they may be mistaken for primary adrenal tumors, especially as up to 30% of patients with Cushing disease have asymmetric adrenal hyperplasia.

ACTH-Independent Causes
Cortisol-Secreting Adrenal Adenoma and Carcinoma

Excluding iatrogenic cases, adrenal adenomas are responsible for about 10% to 15% of Cushing syndrome cases, and carcinomas for less than 5%. By contrast, 65% of cases of Cushing syndrome in children have an adrenal cause (15% adenomas, 50% carcinomas).[227-229] Onset of clinical features is gradual in patients with adenomas, but it is often rapid in adrenal carcinoma. Mutations of PRKACA, which encodes the catalytic subunit of cAMP-dependent protein kinase A (PKA), at the hotspot L205R have been shown by several independent groups to be the cause of approximately 50% of adrenal adenomas causing Cushing syndrome.[230-233]

In addition to the features of hypercortisolism, patients may complain of loin or abdominal pain, and a tumor may be palpable. Adrenal carcinoma may secrete other steroids, such as androgens or mineralocorticoids, but this is very unusual in adenomas. Therefore, in females, there may be features of virilization, with hirsutism, clitoromegaly, breast atrophy, deepening of the voice, temporal recession, and severe acne. In pure cortisol-secreting adenomas,

hirsutism is uncommon. Subclinical Cushing syndrome has been reported in up to 10% of patients with adrenal incidentalomas (see later discussion).

Primary Pigmented Nodular Adrenal Hyperplasia and Carney Syndrome

About 100 cases of ACTH-independent Cushing syndrome have been reported in association with bilateral, small, pigmented adrenal nodules. Pathologically, these nodules are usually 2 to 4 mm in diameter (although they can be larger) and black or brown on cut section. Adjacent adrenal tissue is atrophic, distinguishing this primary pigmented nodular adrenal hyperplasia (PPNAD) from MAH. Presentation is with typical features of Cushing syndrome in persons younger than 30 years of age and, in 50% of cases, in persons younger than 15 years of age.[234] Cases of PPNAD have been reported without Cushing syndrome. Bilateral adrenalectomy is curative.

A familial autosomal dominant variant, called *Carney complex* (Table 15-13), comprises mesenchymal tumors (especially atrial myxomas), spotty skin pigmentation, peripheral nerve tumors, and various other tumors including breast lesions, testicular tumors, and GH-secreting pituitary tumors.[235] Mutations of the gene encoding the PKA regulatory subunit type IA *(PRKAR1A)* lead to abnormal PKA signaling and explain the phenotype in some cases.[236] Other cases have been mapped to chromosome 2p16, but the underlying genetic mutation is unknown.

McCune-Albright Syndrome

In McCune-Albright syndrome, fibrous dysplasia and cutaneous pigmentation may be associated with pituitary, thyroid, adrenal, and gonadal hyperfunction. The most common manifestation is with sexual precocity and GH excess, but Cushing syndrome has been reported.[237] The underlying abnormality is a somatic mutation in the α-subunit of the stimulatory G protein, which is linked to adenyl cyclase. The mutation results in constitutive activation of the G protein, mimicking constant ACTH stimulation at the level of the adrenal. ACTH levels are suppressed, and adrenal adenomas may occur.

Macronodular Hyperplasia

Although MAH commonly occurs in patients with ACTH-dependent Cushing syndrome, truly ACTH-independent

TABLE 15-13	
Clinical Features of Carney Complex	
Feature	**Prevalence (%)**
Skin lesions	80
Pigmented lesions	
Blue nevi	
Cutaneous myxomas	
Cardiac myxomas	72
Pigmented nodular adrenal hyperplasia	45
Breast lesions	
Bilateral fibroadenomas	45 (females only)
Testicular tumors	56 (males only)
Pituitary lesions, usually growth hormone secreting	10
Neural lesions (gastric schwannomas)	<5
Miscellaneous	
Thyroid cancers	Rare
Acoustic neuromas	Rare
Hepatomas	Rare

macronodular hyperplasia (AIMAH) is also recognized as a distinct entity.[238] The nodules are nonpigmented and greater than 5 mm in diameter; occasionally, the adrenals are massively enlarged. Most cases are explained on the basis of aberrant receptor expression within the adrenal cortex.[239] Food-induced hypercortisolism due to enhanced adrenal responsiveness to gastric inhibitory polypeptide (GIP) was the first cause of AIMAH described, due to expression of GIP receptors within the adrenal cortex, but aberrant expression of the vasopressin V_1, β-adrenergic, LH, serotonin, and angiotensin (AT_1) receptors have also been linked to AIMAH. Protocols have been suggested for the further investigation of AIMAH.[239]

Familial cases suggest a genetic cause for this condition in some patients, and inactivating mutations Armadillo repeat 5 (ARMC5) have been demonstrated as a cause.[240]

Iatrogenic Cushing Syndrome

A careful drug history is required to exclude iatrogenic Cushing syndrome. Development of the features of Cushing syndrome depends on the dose, duration, and potency of the corticosteroids used in clinical practice. ACTH is rarely prescribed, but long-term administration will also result in cushingoid features. Some features, such as an increase in intraocular pressure, cataracts, benign intracranial hypertension, aseptic necrosis of the femoral head, osteoporosis, and pancreatitis, are more common in iatrogenic than endogenous Cushing syndrome, whereas other features, notably hypertension, hirsutism, and oligomenorrhea/amenorrhea, are less prevalent.

Special Features of Cushing Syndrome
Cyclic Cushing Syndrome

Of particular clinical interest has been a group of patients with cyclic Cushing syndrome, characterized by periods of excess cortisol production interspersed with intervals of normal cortisol production (Fig. 15-18). Some of these patients demonstrate a paradoxical rise in plasma ACTH and cortisol when treated with dexamethasone, and occasionally a patient is benefited by dopamine agonist (bromocriptine or cabergoline) therapy. Most patients have been thought to have pituitary-dependent disease, and in many of these patients, basophil adenomas have been removed, with long-term cure in some cases. However, cortisol secretion may show some evidence of cyclicity in patients with an ectopic source of ACTH and in PPNAD.[241,242]

Cushing Syndrome in Children

Cushing syndrome can occur at any age, but the causes differ across age groups (Fig. 15-19). In children, adrenal causes account for 65% of all cases, and in addition to the previously mentioned features, growth arrest is almost invariable.[243] The dissociation between height and weight is obvious, with the height most commonly below the mean, whereas the BMI is almost always above the mean. If the height and weight are increasing along the same percentile line, then the diagnosis of Cushing syndrome is highly unlikely. Obesity in childhood Cushing syndrome tends to be generalized. Most patients have a delayed bone age that is negatively correlated with height standard deviation score (SDS), duration of symptoms, and age at diagnosis. The observed growth failure often precedes other manifestations such as weight gain, pubertal arrest, fatigue, depression, hypertension, and acne. Pubertal development can be advanced in patients with virilizing tumors causing precocious pseudopuberty. However, in patients with true

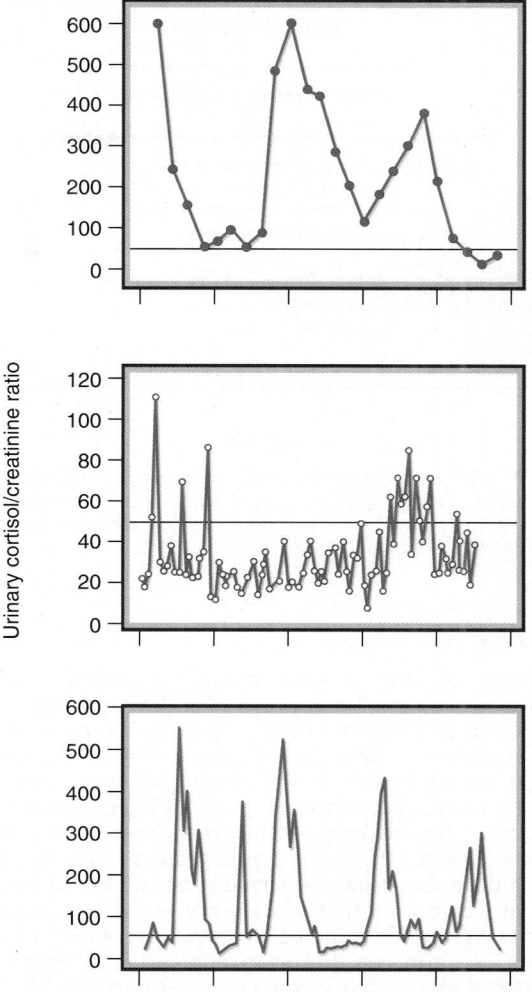

Figure 15-18 Patterns of cortisol secretion in three patients with cyclic Cushing syndrome. In each case, the ratio of early morning urinary cortisol (in nanomoles per liter) to creatinine (in millimoles per liter) are plotted against time. Variable periodicity in cortisol hypersecretion is shown. (From Atkinson AB, McCance DR, Kennedy L, et al. Cyclical Cushing's syndrome first diagnosed after pituitary surgery: a trap for the unwary. *Clin Endocrinol.* 1992;36:297-299.)

puberty, glucocorticoid-mediated suppression of gonadotropins may occur.[244]

Glucocorticoid excess influences not only the hypothalamic-pituitary-gonadal axis but also the GH/IGF-1 axis, leading to both reduction of spontaneous GH secretion and pharmacologic GH response. Furthermore, direct effects of glucocorticoids on epiphyseal chondrocytes, probably together with disturbance of microvascularization of the growth plate, result in a negative effect on growth. Poor catch-up has been reported in children after cure of Cushing disease, and evidence exists for GH inhibition by hypercortisolemia for 1 to 2 years after cure of Cushing disease. GH secretion should be assessed 3 months after treatment. If GH deficiency is demonstrated, GH in a replacement dose of 25 μg/kg per day should be given. Catch-up growth is observed in most patients and target adult height is achieved. However, many patients remain obese.

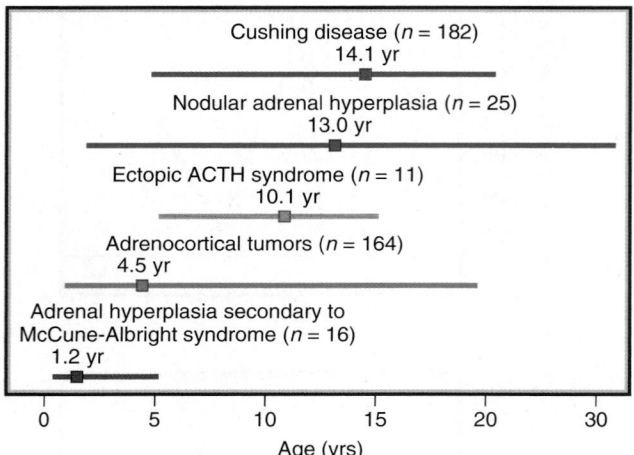

Figure 15-19 Etiology and age-dependency of pediatric Cushing syndrome. Note how the causes differ across age groups. (From Storr HL, Chan LF, Grossman AB, et al. Paediatric Cushing's syndrome: epidemiology, investigation and therapeutic advances. *Trends Endocrinol Metab.* 2007;18:167-174.)

Pregnancy

Pregnancy is rare in women with Cushing syndrome because of associated amenorrhea due to androgen excess or hypercortisolism. However, pregnancy has been reported in approximately 100 such women, 50% of whom had adrenal adenomas.[245] A few cases of true pregnancy-induced Cushing syndrome have been described, with regression after delivery.[246] In these cases, the cause is unknown. Establishing a diagnosis and a cause can be difficult. Clinically, striae, hypertension, and gestational diabetes are common features in normal pregnancies, yet hypertension and diabetes are also the most common signs of Cushing syndrome in a pregnant woman (70% and 30% of all cases, respectively). Furthermore, biochemically normal pregnancy is associated with a threefold increase in plasma cortisol due to increased production of cortisol and CBG. Urinary free cortisol also rises, and dexamethasone does not suppress plasma cortisol to the same degree as the nonpregnant state. Left untreated, the condition is associated with high rates of maternal and fetal morbidity and mortality. Any adrenal or pituitary adenomas should be excised. Metyrapone, which is not teratogenic, has been effective in many cases in controlling the hypercortisolism.

Other Syndromes of Hypercortisolemia

Other states occur when there are clinical and biochemical features of Cushing syndrome, but when hypercortisolemia is secondary to other factors it is often referred to as *pseudo-Cushing syndrome*. Resolution of the underlying cause results in disappearance of the cushingoid state. Several causes are described.

Alcohol

In the original description of alcohol-related pseudo-Cushing syndrome, urinary and plasma cortisol levels were elevated and failed to suppress with dexamethasone. Plasma ACTH has been found to be normal or suppressed. The condition is rare but should be suspected in a patient with an ongoing history of heavy alcohol intake and biochemical or clinical evidence of chronic liver disease.[247] The pathogenesis of this condition remains unknown, but

a two-hit hypothesis has been put forward. Chronic liver disease of any cause is associated with impaired cortisol metabolism, but in alcoholic patients there is an increased cortisol secretion rate, rather than concomitant suppression in the face of impaired metabolism.[248] In some studies, alcohol has directly stimulated cortisol secretion; alternatively, AVP levels are elevated in patients with decompensated liver disease and may stimulate the HPA axis. With abstinence from alcohol, the biochemical abnormalities revert to normal within days.

Depression

Although the cause is unknown, it is recognized that patients with depression may exhibit the hormonal abnormalities of patients with Cushing syndrome.[249] These abnormalities are reversible on correction of the psychiatric condition. Conversely, patients with Cushing syndrome are frequently depressed, and a careful clinical and endocrinologic assessment is required.

Obesity

Although one of the most common referrals to a clinical endocrinologist is for exclusion of an underlying endocrine cause in a patient with obesity, the diagnosis of Cushing syndrome in such patients should not cause difficulties. Patients with obesity have mildly increased cortisol secretion rates, and the data suggest that this is due to activation of the HPA axis.[250,251] However, circulating cortisol concentrations are invariably normal, and urinary free cortisol concentrations are either normal or only slightly elevated. The stimulus for the increased secretion of cortisol appears to be increased peripheral metabolism and clearance of cortisol—principally, reduced hepatic conversion of cortisone to cortisol by HSD11B1 and increased conversion of cortisol to 5α-reduced derivatives.[251]

Investigation of Patients With Suspected Cushing Syndrome

There are two stages in the investigation of suspected Cushing syndrome: (1) Does this patient have Cushing syndrome? and (2) If the answer is "yes," what is the cause? Unfortunately, many investigators fail to make this distinction and ill-advisedly use tests that are relevant to the second question in trying to answer the first question. In particular, it is essential that radiologic investigations not be undertaken until Cushing syndrome has been confirmed biochemically. The starting point should be to investigate patients in whom there is a high clinical index of suspicion for the diagnosis of Cushing syndrome, focusing on the features that are most discriminating for the condition (see Table 15-9). Widespread indiscriminate biochemical screening in obese, hypertensive, and diabetic populations is not recommended. Very few laboratories have developed methods for the measurement of free serum cortisol.[252] Because more than 90% of serum cortisol is protein bound, the results of the conventional assay are affected by drugs and by conditions that alter CBG levels. Estrogen therapy or pregnancy may elevate CBG and total serum cortisol, and estrogens should be stopped for 6 weeks prior to assessment by tests using serum cortisol. The major tests are listed in Table 15-14.[177,249,253,254]

Question 1: Does This Patient Have Cushing Syndrome?
Circadian Rhythm of Plasma Cortisol. In normal subjects, plasma cortisol levels are at their highest early in the

TABLE 15-14

Tests Used in the Diagnosis and Differential Diagnosis of Cushing Syndrome

Diagnosis—Does the Patient Have Cushing Syndrome?

Late night salivary cortisol/circadian rhythm of plasma cortisol
Urinary free cortisol excretion*
Low-dose dexamethasone suppression test*

Differential Diagnosis—What Is the Cause of the Cushing Syndrome?

Plasma ACTH
Plasma potassium, bicarbonate
High-dose dexamethasone suppression test
Corticotropin-releasing hormone
Inferior petrosal sinus sampling
CT, MRI scanning of pituitary, adrenals
Scintigraphy
Tumor markers

*Valuable outpatient screening tests (see text discussion).
ACTH, adrenocorticotropic hormone; CT, computed tomography; MRI, magnetic resonance imaging.

morning and reach a nadir (<50 nmol/L [<2 µg/dL] in a nonstressed subject) at about midnight.[255] This circadian rhythm is lost in patients with Cushing syndrome; in the majority, the 9 AM plasma cortisol is normal but nocturnal levels are raised. Random morning plasma cortisol levels are therefore of little value in making the diagnosis, whereas a midnight cortisol level greater than 200 nmol/L (>7.5 µg/dL) indicates Cushing syndrome. However, various factors such as stress of venipuncture, intercurrent illness, and admission to hospital may lead to false-positive results. Conversely, if a serum cortisol value is less than 50 nmol/L at midnight, Cushing syndrome is excluded at that time. Ideally, patients should be hospitalized for 24 to 48 hours before the midnight cortisol level is measured, but some centers have reported discriminant results for midnight levels measured in outpatients. Nevertheless, this is a cumbersome test and has been largely supplanted by measurement of salivary cortisol (see next).

Salivary Cortisol. CBG is absent from saliva, and the use of salivary cortisol measurements offers a sensible alternative in that the test does not require hospitalization. The diagnostic accuracy of a single midnight salivary cortisol level has been established in several studies. The cutoff points that define disease vary depending on the assay used. In one study, a cortisol value greater than 2.0 ng/mL (5.5 nmol/L) had a 100% sensitivity and a 96% specificity for diagnosis of Cushing syndrome.[253,256,257] It is important to note, however, that late-night salivary cortisol tends to increase with age and cardiovascular comorbid conditions such as hypertension and diabetes, and thus the discriminating power diminishes in the elderly population.[258]

Urinary Free Cortisol Excretion. For many years, the diagnosis of Cushing syndrome was based on the measurement of urinary metabolites of cortisol (24-hour urinary 17-hydroxycorticosteroid or 17-oxogenic steroid excretion, depending on the method used). However, the sensitivity and specificity of these methods are poor, and most centers have replaced these assays with the more sensitive measurement of urinary free cortisol. This is an integrated measure of plasma free cortisol: as cortisol secretion increases, the binding capacity of CBG is exceeded, resulting in a disproportionate rise in urinary free cortisol. Normal values depend on the assay used and tend to be lower when analyzed by liquid chromatography and tandem mass spectrometry. Although in widespread use, urinary free cortisol is less sensitive that salivary cortisol

and dexamethasone suppression testing. Patients should make two or three complete consecutive collections to account for patient error in collecting samples and for episodic cortisol secretion, notably from adrenal adenomas. Simultaneous creatinine excretion (which differs by no more than 10% from day to day) may be used to ensure adequacy of collection. Urinary free cortisol is a useful screening test, although it is accepted that the value can be normal in up to 8% to 15% of patients with Cushing syndrome.[253,254,259] Conversely, moderately elevated results should always be verified by further testing before a diagnosis of Cushing syndrome is made. In addition, variations in levels of up to 50% have been observed in patients with proven Cushing disease, reinforcing the need for multiple collections.[260]

Measurement of the cortisol-to-creatinine ratio in the first urine specimen passed on waking obviates the need for a timed collection and has been used as a screening test, particularly when cyclic Cushing syndrome is suspected.[261] Urine aliquots may be sent to the local endocrinology laboratory, with cortisol-to-creatinine ratios greater than 25 nmol/mmol on repeated measurement being indicative of hypercortisolism.

Low-Dose Overnight Dexamethasone Suppression Tests. In normal subjects, the administration of a supraphysiologic dose of glucocorticoid results in suppression of ACTH and cortisol secretion. In Cushing syndrome of whatever cause, there is a failure of this suppression when low doses of the synthetic glucocorticoid dexamethasone are given.[216]

The overnight test is a useful outpatient screening test,[249,253,262] in which 1 mg of dexamethasone is given at 11 PM. A normal response is a plasma cortisol level of less than 50 nmol/L (<1.8 µg/dL) between 8 and 9 AM the following morning. The outpatient overnight test has high sensitivity (95%) but lower specificity, and further investigation is often required.[263,264]

In the 48-hour low-dose dexamethasone test, plasma cortisol is measured at 9 AM on day 0 and again 48 hours later, after administration of dexamethasone 0.5 mg every 6 hours for 48 hours. Using a postdexamethasone plasma cortisol concentration of less than 50 nmol/L (<1.8 µg/dL) as the cutoff point, this test is reported to have a 97% to 100% true-positive rate and a false-positive rate of less than 1%.[249,263]

Certain drugs (e.g., phenytoin, rifampicin) may increase the metabolic clearance rate of dexamethasone, leading to false-positive results. Simultaneous measurement of plasma dexamethasone may be useful in such cases and will also detect whether patients failed to take the drug, but the values of plasma dexamethasone that predict suppression of serum cortisol are not fully defined.[264]

Other Causes of Hypercortisolemia: Pseudo-Cushing or True Cushing Syndrome? In patients with depression, urinary free cortisol concentrations may be elevated and may overlap with those seen in patients with true Cushing syndrome. Compared with patients with Cushing disease, depressed patients have greater suppressibility after dexamethasone and reduced response to CRH, but neither test is diagnostic.[249,265] The dexamethasone-suppressed CRH test has been proposed as a tool to discriminate between true Cushing syndrome and other states but has been shown to have no advantage over the standard low-dose dexamethasone suppression test. In normal subjects and in patients with endogenous depression, insulin-induced hypoglycemia results in a rise in ACTH and cortisol levels, a response that usually is not seen in patients with Cushing syndrome, but this test has largely been abandoned for this purpose.[249]

Diagnostic Guidelines. The Endocrine Society, in collaboration with the European Society for Endocrinology, has

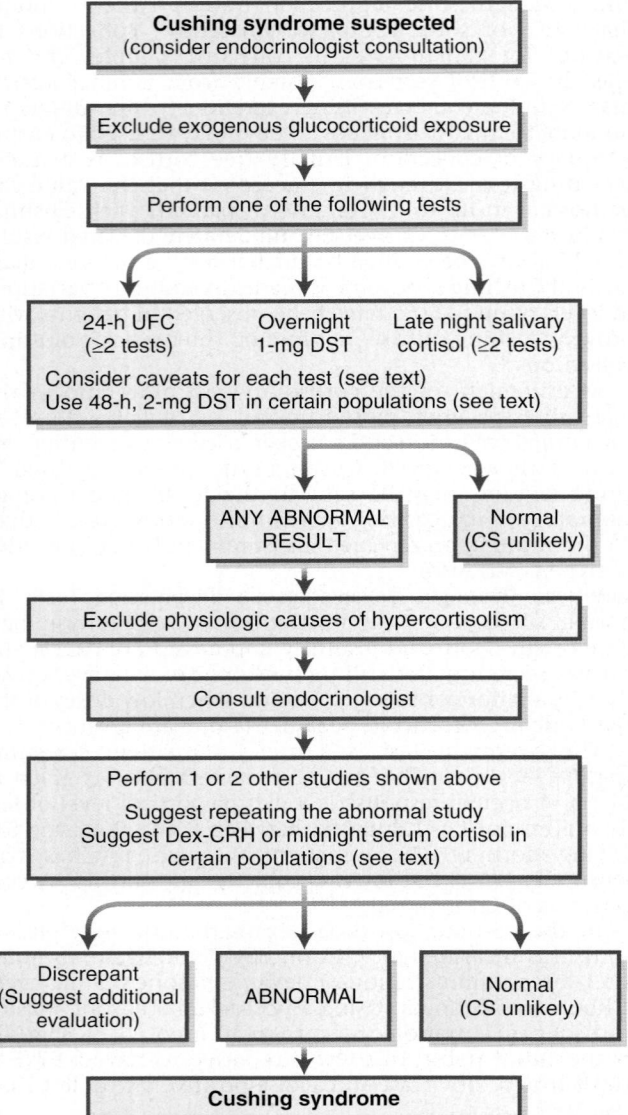

Figure 15-20 Algorithm for testing patients with suspected Cushing syndrome (CS) according to the 2008 Endocrine Society clinical practice guideline. All statements are recommendations except for those prefaced by the word *Suggest*. Diagnostic criteria that point to Cushing syndrome are a urinary free cortisol (UFC) value greater than the normal range for the assay, a serum cortisol level greater than 1.8 µg/dL (>50 nmol/L) after administration of 1 mg dexamethasone (1-mg DST), and a late-night salivary cortisol concentration greater than 145 ng/dL (>4 nmol/L). CRH, corticotropin-releasing hormone; Dex, dexamethasone; DST, dexamethasone suppression test. (From Nieman LK, Biller BM, Findling JW, et al. The diagnosis of Cushing's syndrome: an Endocrine Society Clinical Practice Guideline. *J Clin Endocrinol Metab.* 2008;93:1526-1540.)

issued evidence-based guidelines for the diagnosis of Cushing syndrome.[266] Recommendations are to proceed initially with one of four highly sensitive screening tests: urinary free cortisol, late-night salivary cortisol, long overnight dexamethasone, or the 2-mg/48-hour dexamethasone screening test. Abnormality detected by of any of these tests in a patient with clinically suspected Cushing syndrome should be confirmed with one of the additional tests; if both test results are abnormal, patients should then undergo testing for the cause of the Cushing syndrome (Fig. 15-20).

Question 2: What Is the Cause of Cushing Syndrome in This Patient?

Having confirmed Cushing syndrome clinically and biochemically, the clinician's next step is to determine the cause (Fig. 15-21).

Morning Plasma ACTH. Ideally, ACTH should be measured with the use of a modern, two-site immunoradiometric assay. Such a test differentiates ACTH-dependent from ACTH-independent causes. The samples should be taken in ice cold tubes and immediately separated ahead of storage at −40° C ahead of analysis to prevent inadvertent degradation. In Cushing disease, 50% of patients have a 9 AM ACTH level within the normal reference range (2 to 11 pmol/L [9 to 52 pg/mL]); in the remainder, it is modestly elevated. Occasionally, due to episodic secretion, levels may be very low, and thus measurement of at least two values is recommended to avoid misclassification of mild Cushing disease as ACTH-independent. ACTH levels in the ectopic ACTH syndrome are high (usually >20 pmol/L [>90 pg/mL]); nevertheless, overlap values are seen in Cushing disease in 30% of cases.[267] Therefore, this test cannot be used to differentiate the two conditions (Fig. 15-22). The measurement of ACTH precursors (pro-ACTH, POMC) has been suggested, but it is not routinely available and has not been proved to detect an ectopic source of ACTH.

In patients with adrenal tumors, plasma ACTH is invariably undetectable (<1 pmol/L). The presence of plasma ACTH levels that are low-normal or intermittently detectable, which may occur in MAH, is problematic. The danger is that in some patients the asymmetry of the nodular hyperplasia may lead to a diagnosis of adrenal adenoma, the plasma ACTH is ignored, and an inappropriate adrenalectomy is performed. Conversely, in some patients with this syndrome, an autonomous adrenal tumor develops, and unilateral adrenalectomy is required despite the detectable ACTH.

Plasma Potassium. Hypokalemic alkalosis is present in more than 95% of patients with the ectopic ACTH syndrome but in fewer than 10% of those with Cushing disease. The cause of this mineralocorticoid excess state is now established. Patients with the ectopic syndrome usually have higher rates of cortisol secretion. Cortisol saturates the renal-protective HSD11B2 enzyme, resulting in cortisol-induced mineralocorticoid hypertension (see Chapter 16).[131] In addition, these patients have higher levels of the ACTH-dependent mineralocorticoid, DOC.

High-Dose Dexamethasone Suppression Test. The rationale for the high-dose dexamethasone suppression test is that in Cushing disease the negative feedback control of ACTH is reset to a higher level than normal. Therefore, cortisol levels do not suppress with low-dose dexamethasone but do so after high doses. The original test introduced by Liddle was based on giving 2 mg dexamethasone every 6 hours for 48 hours and demonstrating a fall of greater than 50% in urinary 17-hydroxycorticosteroids.[216] In the modern test, the plasma or urinary free cortisol (or both) is measured at 0 and +48 hours, and a greater than 50% suppression of plasma cortisol from the basal value has been used to define a positive response. In all cases, the response is graded and is dependent on the original cortisol secretion rate: greater suppression is often observed in patients with lower basal cortisol values. In women with ACTH-dependent Cushing syndrome, in whom the *a priori* likelihood of Cushing disease is 90%, the sensitivity of this test for the Cushing disease is 80%, lower than the pretest probability. Because of this there is little logic to the continued use of this test when inferior petrosal sinus sampling (IPSS)

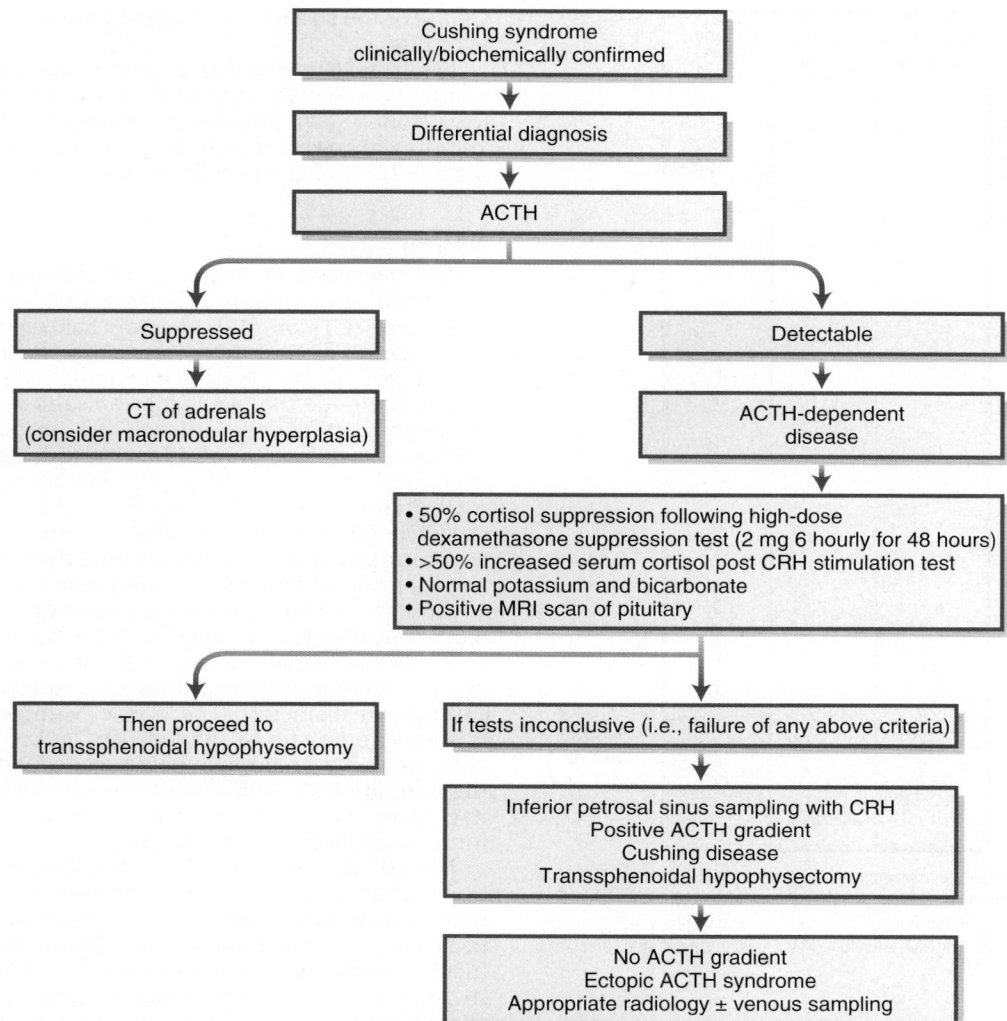

Figure 15-21 The tests to uncover the cause of Cushing syndrome are debatable and differ in any given center depending on many factors, including familiarity and turnaround time of hormone assays and local expertise in techniques such as inferior petrosal sinus sampling. Depicted here is an algorithm in use within many endocrine units based on the reported sensitivity and specificity of each endocrine test. ACTH, adrenocorticotropic hormone; CRH, corticotropin-releasing hormone; CT, computed tomography; MRI, magnetic resonance imaging.

is available (see later). Moreover, if the low-dose dexamethasone suppression test has been used in the diagnosis of Cushing syndrome and a greater than 50% fall in cortisol is observed, there is no added value in the high-dose dexamethasone suppression test.[263]

Corticotropin-Releasing Hormone Test. CRH is a 41–amino acid peptide that was identified by Vale in 1981 from ovine hypothalami. The ovine sequence differs by seven amino acid residues from that of the human hormone but is slightly more effective in stimulating the release of ACTH in humans.[268] The test involves the intravenous injection of either ovine or human sequence CRH in a dose of 1 μg/kg body weight or a single dose of 100 μg (Fig. 15-23). The test can be performed in the morning or afternoon. After basal sampling, CRH is administered and blood samples for ACTH and cortisol are then taken every 15 minutes for 1 to 2 hours.[261,263,269,270]

In normal subjects, CRH produces a rise in ACTH and cortisol of 15% to 20%. This response is exaggerated in Cushing disease, in which typically an ACTH increase greater than 50% and a cortisol rise greater than 20% over baseline values are seen. Responses are seldom seen in the

ectopic ACTH syndrome, but false-positive results have been reported. In distinguishing pituitary-dependent Cushing disease from the ectopic ACTH syndrome, the response of ACTH and cortisol to CRH has a specificity and a sensitivity of approximately 90%. However, a positive response defined as an ACTH increase of 100% or a cortisol rise of 50% over baseline values effectively eliminates a diagnosis of ectopic ACTH syndrome, which is the real benefit of this test. Up to 10% of patients with Cushing disease do not respond to CRH.

Inferior Petrosal Sinus Sampling and Selective Venous Catheterization. The most robust test to distinguish Cushing disease from the ectopic ACTH syndrome is IPSS.[177] Because blood from each half of the pituitary drains into the ipsilateral inferior petrosal sinus, catheterization and venous sampling of both sinuses simultaneously can distinguish a pituitary from an ectopic source of ACTH (Fig. 15-24).[271,272] In virtually all patients with the ectopic ACTH syndrome, the ratio of the ACTH concentration in the inferior petrosal sinus and that in simultaneously drawn peripheral venous blood is less than 1.4:1. In contrast, the ratio is elevated to greater than 2.0 in Cushing disease. However, because

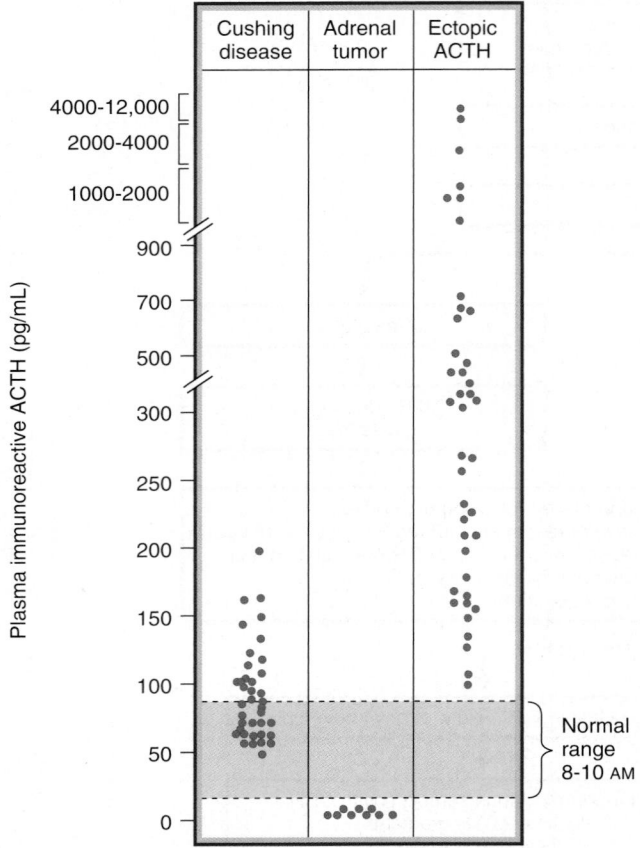

Figure 15-22 Plasma adrenocorticotropic hormone (ACTH) concentrations in patients with Cushing disease, Cushing syndrome associated with adrenocortical tumors, or the ectopic ACTH syndrome. To convert values to picomoles per liter, multiply by 0.2202. (From Besser GM, Edwards CRW. Cushing's syndrome. *Clin Endocrinol Metab.* 1972;1:451-490.)

sponse or the absence of a macroadenoma on pituitary MRI scanning).

Rarely, selective catheterization of vascular beds may be required to identify the source of ectopic ACTH secretion (e.g., from a small pulmonary carcinoid or thymic tumor). Tumors causing ectopic ACTH syndrome may also produce peptide hormones other than ACTH or its precursors.

Imaging

CT/MRI Scanning of Pituitary and Adrenal Glands. High-resolution, thin-section, contrast-enhanced computed tomography (CT) or MRI imaging has revolutionized the investigation of Cushing syndrome.[271,272] However, it is essential that the results of any imaging technique be interpreted alongside the biochemical results if mistakes are to be avoided. When the adrenals are imaged, asymmetric nodular hyperplasia may lead to a false diagnosis of adrenal adenoma. In the general population there is an approximately 10% rate of small abnormalities on pituitary MRI, so-called pituitary incidentalomas, which may mimic a corticotrope adenoma to the unwary, thus emphasizing the need for careful biochemical assessment.[276]

Pituitary MRI is the investigation of choice once the biochemical tests have suggested Cushing disease, with a sensitivity of 60% and specificity of 87%. About 90% of ACTH-secreting pituitary tumors are microadenomas (i.e., <10 mm in diameter). The classic features of a pituitary microadenoma are a hypodense lesion after contrast enhancement, which may be associated with deviation of the pituitary stalk, and a convex upper surface of the pituitary gland (Fig. 15-25). CT scanning is no longer indicated for investigation of Cushing disease.

For adrenal imaging, CT offers better spatial resolution[277] (Fig. 15-26) and is the procedure of choice, but MRI may provide diagnostic information in patients with suspected adrenal carcinoma. Once again, so-called adrenal incidentalomas are present in up to 5% of normal subjects, so adrenal imaging should not be performed unless biochemical investigation has suggested a primary adrenal cause (i.e., undetectable ACTH concentrations). Adrenal carcinomas are usually large and are often associated with metastatic spread at presentation (Fig. 15-27).

In patients with occult ectopic ACTH syndrome, high-definition CT/MRI scanning of thorax, abdomen, and pelvis with images obtained every 0.1-0.5 cm may be required to detect small ACTH-secreting carcinoid tumors (Fig. 15-28).

Scintigraphy Studies. Scintigraphy is of value in certain patients with primary adrenal disease. The most commonly used agent is ^{131}I-labeled 6β-iodomethyl-19-norcholesterol,[278] a marker of adrenocortical cholesterol uptake. In patients with adrenal adenomas, the isotope is taken up by the adenoma but not by the contralateral suppressed adrenal gland. Adrenal scintigraphy is useful in patients with suspected adrenocortical macronodular hyperplasia, although it is not in widespread use; CT scanning may misleadingly suggest unilateral disease, whereas isotope scanning identifies the bilateral adrenal involvement.

Many neuroendocrine tumors giving rise to the ectopic ACTH syndrome express somatostatin receptors and can be imaged by administering radiolabeled analogues of somatostatin (most commonly ^{111}In-labeled octreotide). This technique can detect tumors as small as a few millimeters in diameter and should be considered for patients with ACTH-dependent Cushing syndrome in whom pituitary disease has been excluded, although discovery of a lesion that has not been seen on axial imaging is rare.[279]

of the problem of intermittent ACTH secretion, it is useful to take measurements before and at intervals (e.g., 2, 5, and 15 minutes) after intravenous injection of 100 μg synthetic ovine or human CRH.[273,274] Using this approach, an ACTH petrosal sinus/peripheral ratio greater than 3.0 after CRH administration has a sensitivity of 95% and specificity of nearly 100% for diagnosing Cushing disease.[274] When CRH is not available some centers use desmopressin as a secretagogue, but central to peripheral gradients have been observed in some patients with ectopic ACTH when using this peptide. When a negative gradient is found and venograms confirm correct catheter placement, measurement of prolactin in the samples and correction of the ACTH values can reduce the false-negative rate in Cushing disease.[275]

IPSS may also be of value in lateralizing a pituitary tumor in a patient in whom imaging techniques have failed to demonstrate a microadenoma; however, some centers have found this procedure to be of little value in predicting tumor location. Because many tumors are central and drain into both sinuses, current evidence suggests that it is unwise to base the surgical procedure on the results of IPSS studies alone.

IPSS is technically demanding; it has been associated with complications (referred aural pain, thrombosis) and should be performed only in an experienced tertiary referral center. In some centers, a clinical diagnostic algorithm is used (see Fig. 15-21), and IPSS is performed if the differential diagnosis remains in doubt (i.e., lack of adequate suppression after high-dose dexamethasone or CRH re-

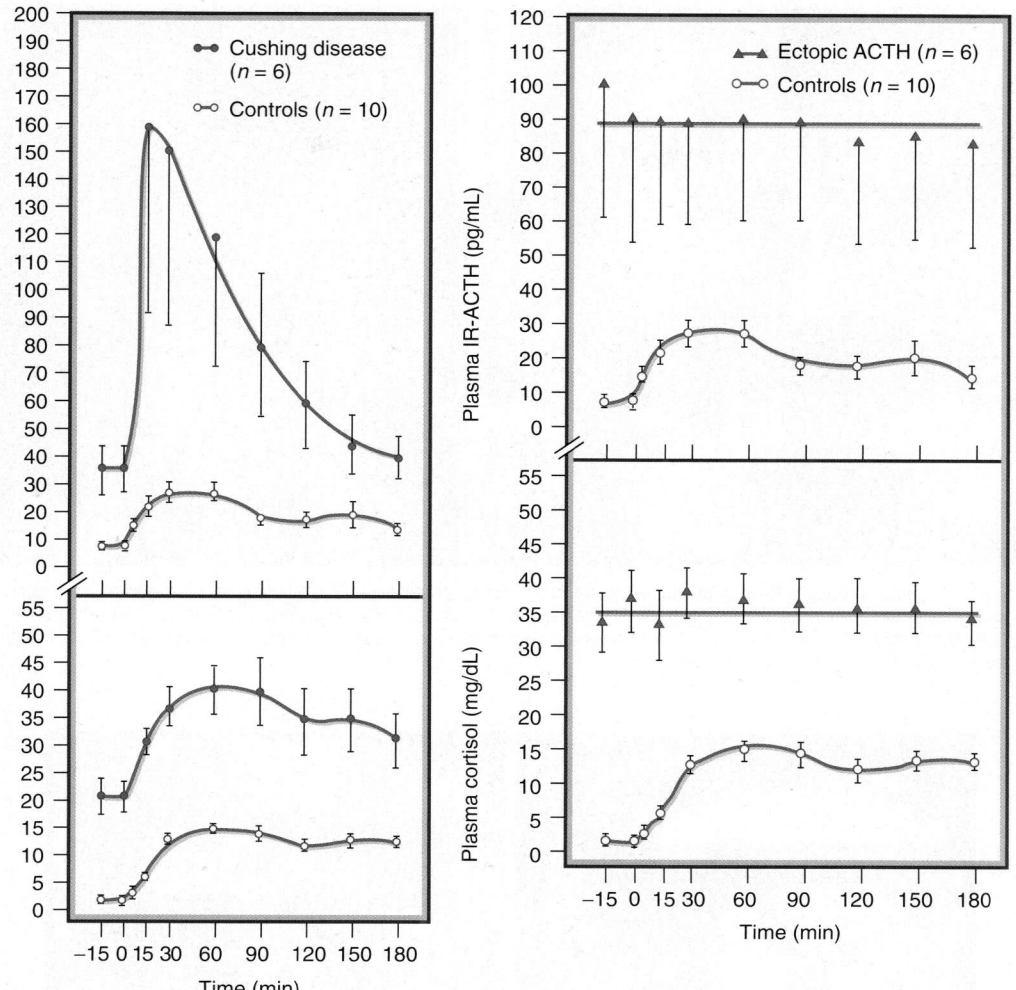

Figure 15-23 Comparison of cortisol and adrenocorticotropic hormone (ACTH) responses to an intravenous injection of ovine corticotropin-releasing hormone (1 µg/kg) in normal subjects, patients with Cushing disease, and patients with the ectopic ACTH syndrome. IR, immunoreactive. (From Chrousos GP, Schulte HM, Oldfield EH, et al. The corticotropin-releasing factor stimulation test: an aid in the evaluation of patients with Cushing's syndrome. *N Engl J Med.* 1984;310:622-626.)

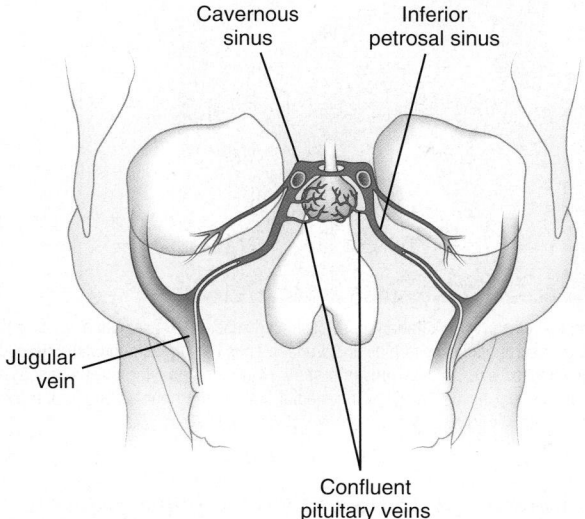

Figure 15-24 Anatomy of the venous drainage of the pituitary gland through the inferior petrosal venous sinuses. (From Oldfield EH, Chrousos GP, Schulte HM, et al. Preoperative lateralization of ACTH-secreting pituitary microadenomas by bilateral and simultaneous inferior petrosal sinus sampling. *N Engl J Med.* 1985;312: 100-103.)

Treatment of Cushing Syndrome
Adrenal Causes

Unilateral adrenal adenomas should be removed by adrenalectomy; the cure rate is 100%, with serum cortisol values that are less than 50 nmol/L at 9 AM, or even lower in many modern assays.[280] With the increasing experience of laparoscopic adrenalectomy in most tertiary centers, this procedure has now become the surgical treatment of choice for unilateral tumors, offering reduced surgical morbidity and postoperative hospital stay compared with traditional open approaches.[281] After surgery, it may take many months or even years for the contralateral suppressed adrenal to recover. Glucocorticoid replacement regimens vary, but many centers use low doses (15-20 mg) of hydrocortisone, and withdrawal regimens differ. One practical approach is to measure the morning plasma cortisol having omitted the dose of hydrocortisone in the morning at 3-month intervals. Patients with serum cortisol values less than 200 nmol/L (7.0 µg/dL) should continue glucocorticoid replacement, whereas in patients with values above 500 nmol/L (18.3 µg/dL) this replacement can be stopped. In patients with values between 200 and 500 nmol/L, ACTH(1-24) testing can be used to assess whether there is sufficient response to stress, although insulin tolerance

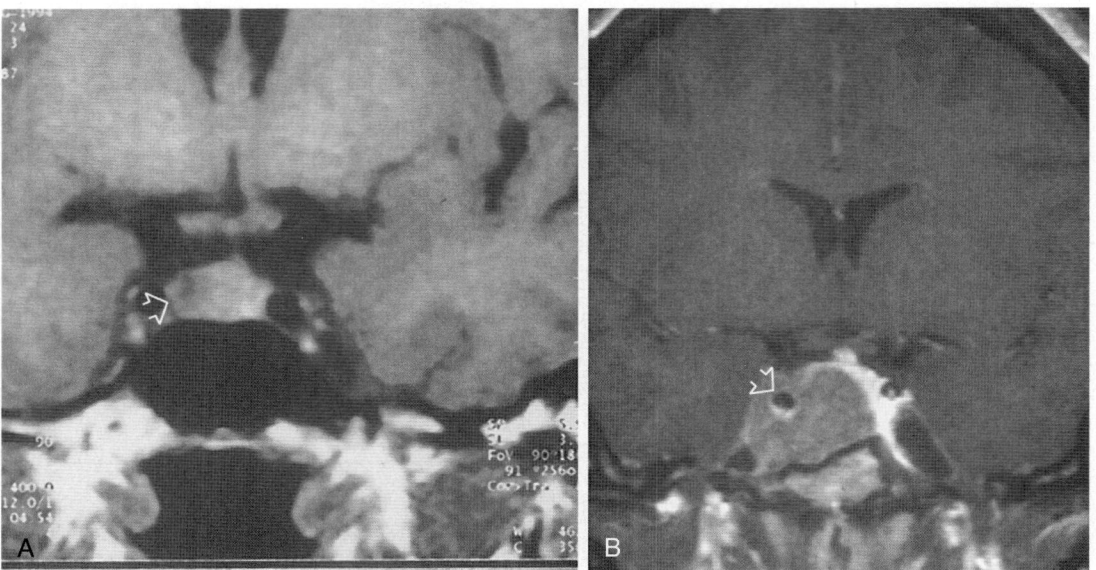

Figure 15-25 A, Magnetic resonance imaging (MRI) scan of pituitary demonstrates the typical appearance of a pituitary microadenoma. A hypodense lesion is seen in the right side of the gland *(arrow)*, with deviation of the pituitary stalk away from the lesion. After a biochemical diagnosis of Cushing disease, this patient was cured by trans-sphenoidal hypophysectomy. **B,** MRI scan of the pituitary gland demonstrates a large macroadenoma *(arrow)* in a patient with Cushing disease. In contrast to smaller tumors, large macroadenomas are invariably invasive and recur after surgery.

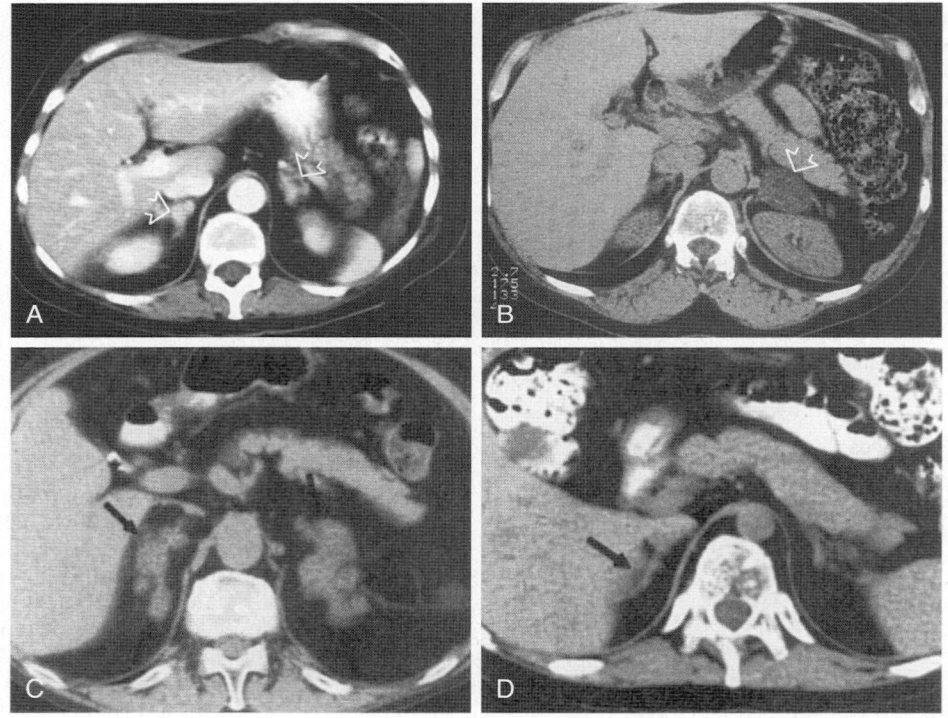

Figure 15-26 A, Adrenal computed tomographic (CT) scan demonstrates bilateral adrenal hyperplasia *(arrows)* in a patient with Cushing disease. **B,** CT scan of a typical solitary left adrenal adenoma *(arrow)* causing Cushing syndrome. **C,** Cushing syndrome caused by massive macronodular hyperplasia. Adrenal glands are replaced by multiple nodules *(arrows)*. The combined weight of the adrenal glands was more than 100 g. **D,** Cushing syndrome caused by surgically proven primary pigmented nodular adrenal disease in a 21-year-old patient. Notice the multiple small nodules with relatively atrophic internodular adrenocortical tissue involving the medial limb of the right adrenal gland *(arrow)*. (**C** and **D,** From Findling JW, Doppman JL. Biochemical and radiologic diagnosis of Cushing's syndrome. *Endocrinol Metab Clin North Am.* 1994;23:511-537.)

testing may be used in some centers. In the interim, all patients should carry a steroid alert card and increase their dose of replacement therapy in the event of an intercurrent illness.

Adrenal carcinomas have had a very poor prognosis, and most patients have died within 2 years of diagnosis.[282] It is

usual practice to try to remove the primary tumor, even though metastases may be present, so as to enhance the response to the adrenolytic agent *o,p´*-DDD[283] (mitotane). Radiotherapy to the tumor bed and to some metastases, such as those in the spine, may be of limited value. However, in recent years significant progress has been

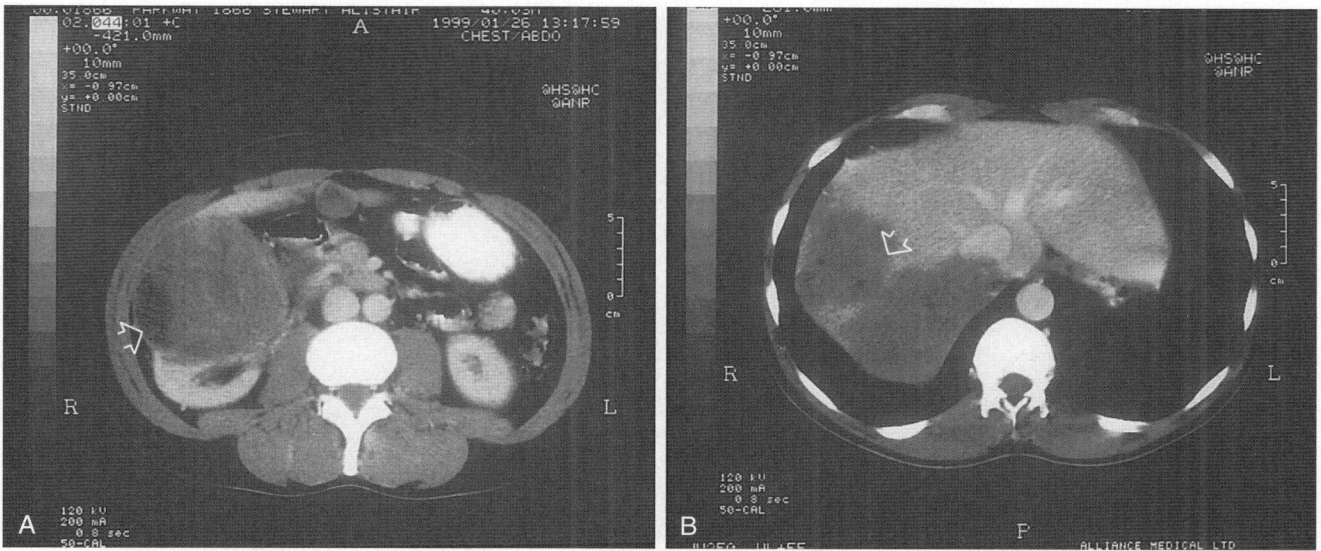

Figure 15-27 Computed tomographic scan of a patient with rapidly progressing Cushing syndrome caused by an adrenal carcinoma. An irregular right adrenal mass is shown in **A,** and a large liver metastasis is seen in **B.**

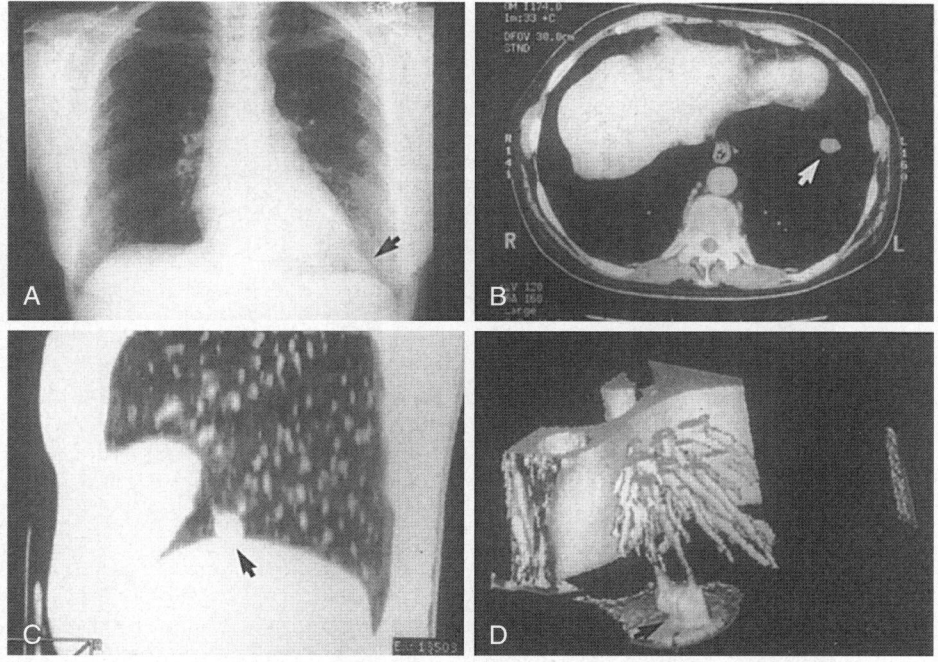

Figure 15-28 Imaging of the thorax in a patient with the ectopic adrenocorticotropic hormone (ACTH) syndrome. **A,** Plain chest radiograph demonstrates a suspicious lesion behind the left heart border *(arrow).* **B** and **C,** Axial and sagittal computed tomographic images demonstrate a bronchial carcinoid tumor *(arrow)* abutting the diaphragm. **D,** Three-dimensional reconstruction illustrates adherence of the tumor to the diaphragm *(arrow),* which was confirmed at surgery. (From Newell-Prince J, Trainer P, Besser M, et al. The diagnosis and differential diagnosis of Cushing's syndrome and pseudo-Cushing's states. *Endocr Rev.* 1998;19:647-672.)

made by implementing collaborative multicenter studies. Phase III trials of mitotane therapy achieving therapeutic plasma mitotane levels have shown significant benefit[284]; drug combinations include etoposide, doxorubicine, and cisplatin plus mitotane or streptozotocin plus mitotane. Several targeted therapies, including IGF-1 inhibitors, sunitinib, and sorafenib, may be of value in cases of mitotane failure. The 10-year survival rate for patients with T1 N0 M0 disease is about 80% but is significantly impaired with increased tumor mass, positive lymph nodes, and distant metastases, reaching less than 20% for patients with T1-4 N0-1 M1.[285]

Pituitary-Dependent Cushing Syndrome

The treatment of Cushing disease has been significantly enhanced with transsphenoidal surgery conducted by an experienced surgeon.[286] Before the capability of selective removal of a pituitary microadenoma was developed, the treatment of choice was bilateral adrenalectomy, which had an appreciable mortality rate even in the best centers (up to 4%) and a significant morbidity rate. The major risk was the subsequent development of Nelson syndrome (postadrenalectomy hyperpigmentation with a locally aggressive pituitary tumor) (Fig. 15-29), which was

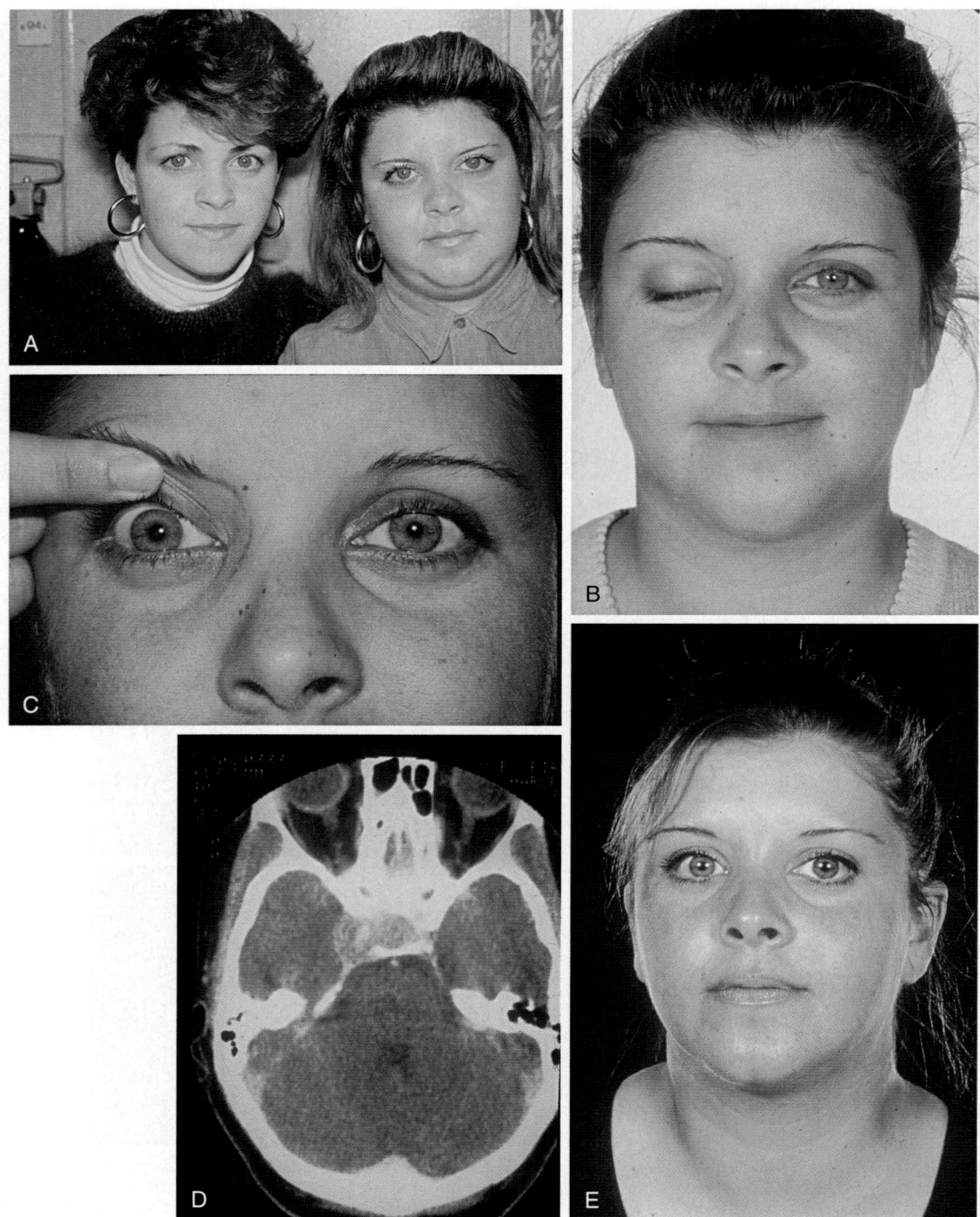

Figure 15-29 A young woman with Cushing disease, photographed initially beside her identical twin sister (**A**). In this case, treatment with bilateral adrenalectomy was undertaken. Several years later, the patient presented with Nelson syndrome and a right third cranial nerve palsy (**B** and **C**) related to cavernous sinus infiltration from a locally invasive corticotropinoma (**D**). Hypophysectomy and radiotherapy were performed with reversal of the third cranial nerve palsy (**E**). Note the advancing skin pigmentation of Nelson syndrome.

attributed to loss of any negative feedback after adrenalectomy but is more likely to be due to an aggressive pituitary tumor from the outset.[287] In an attempt to avoid this complication, pituitary irradiation was often carried out at the time of bilateral adrenalectomy.[288] In addition, these patients required lifelong replacement therapy with hydrocortisone and fludrocortisone. Currently, bilateral adrenalectomy is rarely indicated for patients with Cushing disease

but may be performed if pituitary surgery has failed or the condition has recurred.

The surgical outcome for transsphenoidal hypophysectomy varies from center to center and with surgical expertise.[210] Because of the hazards of untreated Cushing disease and the potential complications of surgery, the endocrinologist should refer patients only to a recognized surgical specialist at a center in which outcome data have been

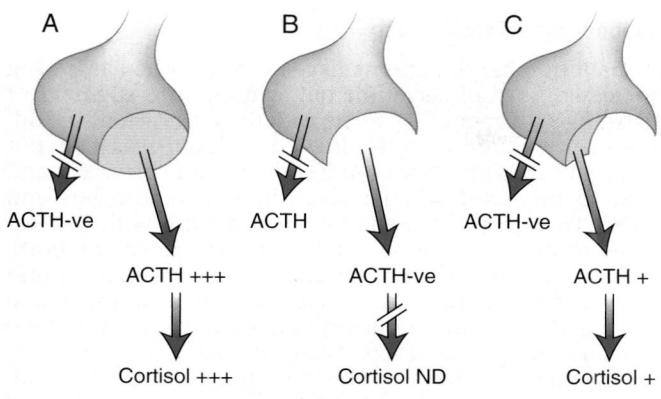

+++ Secretion above normal
+ Secretion is detectable
-ve Secretion suppressed
▢ ACTH secreting tumor

Figure 15-30 Selective removal of a microadenoma and its effect on the hypothalamic-pituitary-adrenal axis. **A,** Before treatment. **B,** After total removal of adenoma. **C,** After incomplete excision. Because the surrounding normal pituitary corticotrophs are suppressed in a patient with an adrenocorticotropic hormone (ACTH)-secreting pituitary adenoma, successful removal of the tumor results in ACTH, and hence adrenocortical, deficiency, with an undetectable (<50 nmol/L [2 µg/dL]) plasma cortisol level. A postoperative plasma cortisol level higher than 50 nmol/L (2 µg/dL) implies that the patient is not cured. (Courtesy of Professor Peter Trainer.)

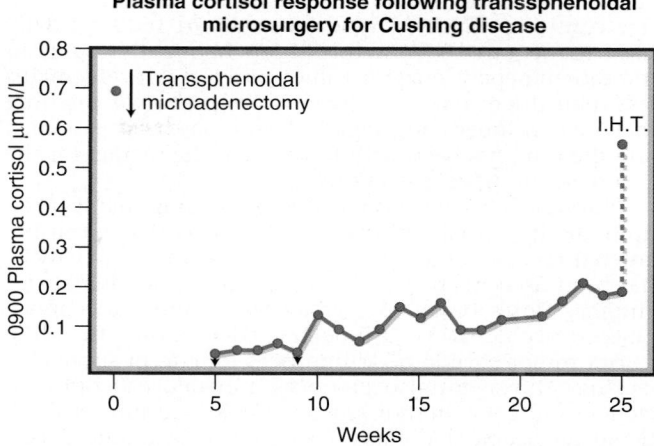

Figure 15-31 Gradual recovery of function of the hypothalamic-pituitary-adrenal axis in a patient after removal of a pituitary adrenocorticotropic hormone-secreting microadenoma. Morning (9 AM) plasma cortisol levels were measured. The insulin hypoglycemia test (I.H.T.) eventually demonstrated the return of a normal stress response.

established. In optimal centers, remission rates are 70% to 90% for microadenomas and 50% for macroadenomas.[202] Rates for postoperative hypopituitarism and permanent diabetes insipidus depend on how aggressive the surgeon was in removing pituitary tissue. The ideal outcome is a cured patient with intact pituitary function, but this result may not be possible for a patient with Cushing disease in whom a pituitary adenoma was not identified preoperatively or during the operation itself.

In centers that lack facilities for frequent monitoring of cortisol levels, perioperative and postoperative hydrocortisone cover is advised; this can be reduced to maintenance replacement doses usually within 3 to 7 days. On days 2 to 5 postoperatively, a 9 AM plasma cortisol level should be measured with the patient having omitted hydrocortisone for 24 hours. After selective removal of a microadenoma, the surrounding corticotrophs are usually suppressed (Fig. 15-30). As a result, plasma cortisol levels are less than 30 nmol/L (<1 µg/dL) postoperatively, and ongoing glucocorticoid replacement therapy is required. The HPA axis usually (but not invariably) exhibits gradual recovery, and glucocorticoid therapy is needed until this occurs (Fig. 15-31). A nonsuppressed plasma cortisol postoperatively suggests that the patient is not in remission even though cortisol secretion may have fallen to normal or subnormal values.[203,204] The recurrence rate in patients with an established remission after pituitary surgery is 2%, but this value is higher in children (up to 40%).[205,206] A detailed assessment of residual pituitary function is required in each patient, and close follow-up of such individuals is warranted.

In the past, pituitary irradiation was often used in the treatment of Cushing disease. However, because of the improvements in pituitary surgery, far fewer patients are so treated. In children, pituitary irradiation appears to be more effective.[207] Radiotherapy is not recommended as a primary treatment but is reserved for patients not responding to pituitary microsurgery, those who have undergone

bilateral adrenalectomy, and patients with established Nelson syndrome.

The management of recurrent Cushing disease involves a consideration of repeat surgery, gamma knife radiosurgery, and medical therapies.[286,289]

Ectopic ACTH Syndrome

Treatment of the ectopic ACTH syndrome depends on the cause. If the tumor can be found and has not spread, then its removal can lead to cure (e.g., bronchial carcinoid, thymoma). However, the prognosis for small cell lung cancer associated with the ectopic ACTH syndrome is poor. The cortisol excess and associated hypokalemic alkalosis and diabetes mellitus can be ameliorated by medical therapy. Treatment of the small cell tumor itself will also, at least initially, produce improvement. Sometimes, if the ectopic source of ACTH cannot be found, it may be necessary to perform bilateral adrenalectomy and then monitor the patient carefully (sometimes for several years) before the primary tumor becomes apparent.

Medical Treatment of Cushing Syndrome

Several drugs have been used in the treatment of Cushing syndrome.[286] Metyrapone inhibits 11β-hydroxylase and has been the most commonly given agent, often with a goal of lowering cortisol concentrations before definitive therapy or while awaiting benefit from pituitary irradiation. The daily dose must be determined by measurements of plasma or urinary free cortisol. The aim should be to achieve a mean plasma cortisol concentration of about 300 nmol/L (11 µg/dL) during the day or a normal urinary free cortisol level. The drug is usually given in doses ranging from 250 mg twice daily to 1.5 g every 6 hours, with lower doses for adrenal adenoma and higher for ectopic ACTH. Nausea is a side effect that can be helped (if it is not caused by adrenal insufficiency) by giving the drug with milk.[208]

Ketoconazole is an imidazole that has been widely used as an antifungal agent but causes abnormal liver function tests in about 15% of patients. Ketoconazole blocks a variety of steroidogenic cytochrome P450–dependent enzymes and thus lowers plasma cortisol levels. For effective control of Cushing syndrome, 400 to 1600 mg daily has been required.[212,290] Ketoconazole frequently causes an increase in hepatic enzyme values, and if this level remains less than three times the upper limit of normal the drug may be continued, but hepatic failure has been described and the drug has been withdrawn from the market for the treatment of fungal infections.

Mitotane (o,p′-DDD) is an adrenolytic drug that is taken up by both normal and malignant adrenal tissue, causing adrenal atrophy and necrosis.[283] Because of its toxicity, it has been used mainly in the management of adrenal carcinoma. Doses of up to 5 g/day are required to control glucocorticoid excess, although evidence that the drug causes tumor shrinkage or improves long-term survival is lacking. This agent also produces mineralocorticoid deficiency, and concomitant glucocorticoid and mineralocorticoid replacement therapy may be required. Side effects are common and include fatigue, skin rashes, neurotoxicity, and gastrointestinal disturbance. It has also been used at lower doses in Cushing disease.[291]

Somatostatin analogues such as octreotide and lanreotide are generally ineffective in Cushing disease. However, the multireceptor somatostatin analogue, pasireotide, which demonstrates high-affinity binding to somatostatin receptor subtypes 1, 2, 3, and 5, normalizes urinary free cortisol in 17% of patients with Cushing disease, with hyperglycemia being a common side effect.[292] The GR antagonist mifepristone has been shown to improve diabetes in patients with Cushing syndrome, but biochemical monitoring is not possible when using this drug.[293]

Prognosis of Cushing Syndrome

Studies performed before the introduction of effective therapy revealed that 50% of patients with untreated Cushing syndrome died within 5 years, principally from vascular disease.[187] Even with modern management, an increased prevalence of cardiovascular risk factors persists for many years after an apparent remission.[188,189] Paradoxically, on correction of the hypercortisolism, patients often feel worse. Skin desquamation, steroid-withdrawal arthropathy, profound lethargy, and mood changes may occur and can take several weeks or months to resolve.[294] In our experience, these features, together with postural hypotension, are particularly severe in patients in remission who are also rendered vasopressin deficient. They can usually be ameliorated by a transient increase in glucocorticoid replacement therapy. Patients are invariably GH deficient, and GH replacement therapy may produce clinical benefit.

Features of Cushing syndrome disappear over a period of 2 to 12 months after treatment. Hypertension and diabetes mellitus improve, but as with other secondary causes, they may not resolve completely. The osteopenia of Cushing syndrome improves rapidly during the first 2 years after treatment but resolves more slowly thereafter.[295] Vertebral fractures and osteonecrosis are irreversible, and permanent deformity results. Visceral obesity and myopathy are both reversible features. Reproductive and sexual function return to normal within 6 months, provided that anterior pituitary function was not compromised. Long-term health-related quality of life in adults significantly improves after treatment, but quality-of-life scores do not return to normal levels.[184] Similar observations have been made in pediatric patients, in whom significant improvement was noted before and after treatment but residual impairment of health-related quality of life persisted 1 year after cure.[296]

Glucocorticoid Resistance

A small number of patients have been described as having increased cortisol secretion but without the stigmata of Cushing syndrome.[87,297] These patients are resistant to suppression of cortisol with low-dose dexamethasone but respond to high doses. ACTH levels are elevated and lead to increased adrenal production of androgens and DOC. Therefore, these patients may present with the features of androgen or mineralocorticoid excess, or both. Treatment with a dose of dexamethasone (usually >3 mg/ day) adequate to suppress ACTH results in a fall in adrenal androgens and often returns plasma potassium and blood pressure to normal levels. Many of these patients have been found to have point mutations in the steroid-binding domain of the GR, with consequent reduction of glucocorticoid-binding affinity, but this finding is not invariable. A useful clinical discriminatory test to differentiate this condition from Cushing syndrome is to measure bone mineral density: it is preserved in patients with glucocorticoid resistance or even increased in females because of the androgen excess. In addition, the circadian rhythm for ACTH and cortisol is preserved in patients with glucocorticoid resistance.

GLUCOCORTICOID DEFICIENCY

Primary and Central Hypoadrenalism

Primary hypoadrenalism refers to glucocorticoid deficiency occurring in the setting of adrenal disease, whereas central hypoadrenalism arises because of deficiency of ACTH (Table 15-15). A major distinction between these forms of hypoadrenalism is that mineralocorticoid deficiency invariably accompanies primary hypoadrenalism, but this does not occur in central hypoadrenalism: here only ACTH is deficient, and the renin-angiotensin-aldosterone (RAA) axis is intact. A further important cause of adrenal insufficiency in which there may be dissociation of glucocorticoid and mineralocorticoid secretion is CAH.

Primary Hypoadrenalism
Addison Disease

Thomas Addison described the condition now known as *primary hypoadrenalism* in his classic monograph published in 1855.[2] Addison disease is a rare condition with an estimated incidence in the developed world of 0.8 cases per 100,000 and a prevalence of 4 to 11 cases per 100,000 population. Nevertheless, it is associated with significant morbidity and mortality rates, but once the diagnosis is made it can be easily treated.[298,299] Causes of Addison disease are listed in Table 15-15.

Autoimmune Adrenalitis. In the Western world, autoimmune adrenalitis accounts for more than 70% of all cases of primary hypoadrenalism.[300] Pathologically, the adrenal glands are atrophic with loss of most of the cortical cells, but the medulla is usually intact. In 75% of cases, adrenal autoantibodies can be detected.[301] Fifty percent of patients with this form of Addison disease have an associated autoimmune disease (Table 15-16), thyroid disease being the most common. Conversely, only 1% to 2% of patients with more common autoimmune diseases such as insulin-dependent diabetes mellitus or thyrotoxicosis have antiadrenal autoantibodies and develop adrenal disease, although the figure is higher in patients with autoimmune hypoparathyroidism (16%). These autoimmune polyglandular syndromes (APSs) have been

TABLE 15-15

Etiology of Adrenocortical Insufficiency (Excluding Congenital Adrenal Hyperplasia)

Primary Causes: Addison Disease

Autoimmune
  Sporadic
  Autoimmune polyendocrine syndrome type I (Addison disease, chronic mucocutaneous candidiasis, hypoparathyroidism, dental enamel hypoplasia, alopecia, primary gonadal failure—see Chapter 40)
  Autoimmune polyendocrine syndrome type II (Schmidt syndrome) (Addison disease, primary hypothyroidism, primary hypogonadism, insulin-dependent diabetes, pernicious anemia, vitiligo—Chapter 40)
Infections
  Tuberculosis
  Fungal infections
  Cytomegalovirus
  HIV
Metastatic tumor
Infiltrations
  Amyloid
  Hemochromatosis
Intra-adrenal hemorrhage (Waterhouse-Friderichsen syndrome) after meningococcal septicemia
Adrenoleukodystrophies
Congenital adrenal hypoplasia
  DAX1 (NR0B1) mutations
  SF1 mutations
ACTH resistance syndromes
  MC2R gene mutations
  MRAP gene mutations
  AAAS (ALADIN) gene mutations (triple-A syndrome)
Bilateral adrenalectomy

Secondary Causes: Central Hypoadrenalism

Exogenous glucocorticoid therapy
Hypopituitarism
Selective removal of ACTH-secreting pituitary adenoma
Pituitary tumors and pituitary surgery, craniopharyngiomas
Pituitary apoplexy
Granulomatous disease (tuberculosis, sarcoid, eosinophilic granuloma)
Secondary tumor deposits (breast, bronchus)
Postpartum pituitary infarction (Sheehan syndrome)
Pituitary irradiation (effect usually delayed for several years)
Isolated ACTH deficiency
  Idiopathic
  Lymphocytic hypophysitis
  TPIT (TBX19) gene mutations
  PCSK1 gene mutation (POMC processing defect)
  POMC gene mutations
Multiple pituitary hormone deficiencies
  HESX1 gene mutations
  LHX4 gene mutations
  SOX3 gene mutations
  PROP1 gene mutations

ACTH, adrenocorticotropic hormone; HIV, human immunodeficiency virus; POMC, pro-opiomelanocortin.

TABLE 15-16

Incidence of Other Endocrine and Autoimmune Diseases in Patients With Autoimmune Adrenal Insufficiency

Disease	Incidence (%)
Thyroid disease	
Hypothyroidism	8
Nontoxic goiter	7
Thyrotoxicosis	7
Gonadal failure	
Ovarian	20
Testicular	2
Insulin-dependent diabetes mellitus	11
Hypoparathyroidism	10
Pernicious anemia	5
None	53

Infections. Worldwide, infectious diseases are the most common cause of primary adrenal insufficiency. These diseases include tuberculosis, fungal infections (histoplasmosis, cryptococcosis), and cytomegalovirus infection. Adrenal failure may also occur in the acquired immunodeficiency syndrome (AIDS).[302]

Tuberculous Addison disease results from hematogenous spread of the infection from elsewhere in the body; extraadrenal disease is usually evident. The adrenals are initially enlarged, with extensive epithelioid granulomas and caseation, and both the cortex and the medulla are affected. Fibrosis ensues, and the adrenals become normal in size or smaller, with calcification evident in 50% of cases.

The adrenals are frequently involved in patients with AIDS[302,303]; adrenalitis may occur after infection with cytomegalovirus or atypical mycobacteria, and Kaposi sarcoma may result in adrenal replacement. Onset is often insidious, but if tested, more than 10% of patients with AIDS will demonstrate a subnormal cortisol response to a short Synacthen test. Adrenal insufficiency may be precipitated through the concomitant administration of appropriate anti-infectives such as ketoconazole (which inhibits cortisol synthesis) or rifampicin (which increases cortisol metabolism). Rarely, patients with AIDS and features of adrenal insufficiency are found to have elevated circulating ACTH and cortisol concentrations that fail to suppress normally after low-dose dexamethasone administration. This is thought to reflect an acquired form of glucocorticoid resistance resulting from reduced GR affinity, but the underlying cause remains unknown.[304]

Acquired Primary Adrenal Insufficiency

With the exception of tuberculosis and autoimmune adrenal failure, other causes of Addison disease are rare (see Table 15-15). Adrenal metastases (most commonly from primary tumors in the lung or breast) are often found at postmortem examinations, but they uncommonly cause adrenal insufficiency,[305] perhaps because more than 90% of the adrenal cortex must be compromised before symptoms and signs become apparent. Necrosis of the adrenals due to intra-adrenal hemorrhage should be considered in any severely sick patient, particularly a patient with underlying infection, trauma, or coagulopathy.[306] Intra-adrenal bleeding may be found in patients with severe septicemia of any cause, particularly in children, in whom a common cause is infection with *Pseudomonas aeruginosa*. When caused by meningococci, the association with adrenal insufficiency is known as the Waterhouse-Friderichsen syndrome. Adrenal replacement may also occur with amyloidosis and hemochromatosis.

classified into two distinct variants.[301] APS type I, or autoimmune polyendocrinopathy-candidiasis-ectodermal dysplasia (APECED), is a rare autosomal recessive condition comprising Addison disease, chronic mucocutaneous candidiasis, and hypoparathyroidism. The more common APS type II comprises Addison disease, autoimmune thyroid disease, diabetes mellitus, and hypogonadism. Here, autoantibodies to 21-hydroxylase are usually present and are predictive for the development of adrenal destruction.[301] Polyglandular autoimmune syndromes are discussed in greater detail in Chapter 40.

Inherited Primary Adrenal Insufficiency

Adrenal hypoplasia congenita (AHC) is an X-linked disorder comprising congenital adrenal insufficiency and combined primary and central hypogonadotropic hypogonadism. The condition is caused by mutations in the *DAX1 (NROB1)* gene, a member of a nuclear receptor family that is expressed in the adrenal cortex, gonads, and hypothalamus.[307,308] Depending on the molecular defect, the clinical presentation can be highly variable. Severe cases often manifest with mineralocorticoid deficiency and gradually develop glucocorticoid deficiency. Hypogonadism is combined with primary testicular abnormalities and low gonadotropin levels. However, the so-called minipuberty of infancy can be normal.[309,310] Patients presenting with late-onset adrenal failure have also been described.[311]

Mutations in another transcription factor, SF1, may also result in adrenal insufficiency due to lack of development of a functional adrenal cortex. The transcriptional regulation of many P450 steroidogenic enzymes is dependent on SF1.[15] When it was first described, SF1 mutation was associated with complete sex reversal causing 46,XY disorder of sex development (DSD).[312] However, novel clinical phenotypes in SF1-deficient patients are now emerging; they range from isolated adrenal failure[313] to isolated gonadal failure[314] and ovarian insufficiency.[315] AHC may also occur in association with glycerol kinase deficiency and muscular dystrophy caused by gene deletion, including the *DAX1* gene.[316]

Adrenoleukodystrophy has a prevalence rate of 1:20,000 and is a cause of adrenal insufficiency in association with demyelination within the nervous system; demyelination results from a failure of β-oxidation of fatty acids within peroxisomes owing to reduced activity of very long chain acyl-CoA synthetase.[317] Increased accumulation of very long chain fatty acids (VLCFAs) occurs in many tissues, and serum assays can be used diagnostically. Only males have the fully expressed condition, and carrier females are usually normal. Several forms are recognized: a childhood cerebral form (30% to 40% of cases), adult adrenomyeloneuropathy (40%), and Addison disease (7%). The childhood-onset form manifests at 5 to 10 years of age with progression eventually to a blind, mute, and severely spastic tetraplegic state. Adrenal insufficiency is usually present but does not appear to correlate with the neurologic deficit. Nevertheless, this is the most common form of adrenal insufficiency in a child younger than 7 years of age.[318] Adrenomyeloneuropathy, by contrast, manifests later in life with the gradual development of spastic paresis and peripheral neuropathy. Both the childhood and the adult condition result from mutations in the *ABCD1* gene on chromosome Xq28, which encodes for an ABC peroxisomal membrane protein involved in the import of VLCFA into the peroxisome.[319] So far, more than 400 mutations have been reported in the *ABCD1* gene with no relationship between genotype and phenotype.[320,321] Treatment options are few. Monounsaturated fatty acids, which block the synthesis of the saturated VLCFA, have been used; a combination of erucic acid and oleic acid (Lorenzo's oil) has led to normal levels of VLCFA. Treatment does not alter the rate of neurologic deterioration but may prevent new neurologic damage in asymptomatic cases.[321] Bone marrow transplantation is a further possibility.

Familial glucocorticoid deficiency (FGD), or inherited unresponsiveness to ACTH, is a rare autosomal recessive cause of hypoadrenalism that usually manifests in childhood. Most patients present with neonatal hypoglycemia or later in life with increasing pigmentation, and they often have enhanced growth velocity. Primary adrenal failure in a child with normal activity of the RAA system is highly suggestive of FGD. The diagnosis can be confirmed by demonstrating low cortisol in combination with increased ACTH concentrations and normal plasma renin and aldosterone measurements.[91] The type 1 variant accounts for approximately 25% of all cases and is explained by inactivating mutations in the ACTH-binding receptor, MC2R.[322-324] The FGD type 2 variant is caused by mutations in the *MRAP* gene, which is thought to mediate intracellular trafficking of the *MC2R*, has been reported in some families.[90] However, 50% of patients with FGD do not have mutations in either *MC2R* or *MRAP*; other loci are being defined.

A variant called the *triple A syndrome* or *Allgrove syndrome* refers to the triad of adrenal insufficiency due to ACTH resistance, achalasia, and alacrima. It is caused by mutations in the *AAAS* gene, which encodes ALADIN, a tryptophan/aspartate WD-repeat–containing protein of the nuclear pore complex.[325,326] The exact function of ALADIN is unknown, but its interaction with other proteins of the nuclear pore complex suggest that it is part of a structural scaffold.

Several syndromic disorders are associated with adrenal insufficiency for which the underlying molecular genetic defect remains to be elucidated.[11]

Secondary Hypoadrenalism
Inherited Central Hypoadrenalism

Central hypoadrenalism may be defined as hypocortisolemia secondary to a deficiency in ACTH. The prevalence of central hypoadrenalism is 125 to 280 per million,[1,326a] which is likely to be an underestimate considering the use of therapeutic corticosteroids in the general population. It occurs in up to one third of patients with pituitary disease.[3,326b] ACTH deficiency is an important diagnosis to make; in subjects with tumoral and posttraumatic hypopituitarism, central hypoadrenalism is associated with increased mortality rates.[4-6,326c-326e] The causes of central hypoadrenalism are outlined in Table 15-15; the most common reason is ACTH suppression by exogenous glucocorticoid treatment.[7,178]

When caused by pituitary disease, other pituitary hormones are often deficient, so the patient presents with partial or complete hypopituitarism. The clinical features of hypopituitarism make this a relatively easy diagnosis. By contrast, isolated ACTH deficiency is rare, and the diagnosis is difficult to make. It may occur in patients with lymphocytic hypophysitis. Mutations in the *TBX19* gene, the product of which (TPIT) regulates *POMC* expression, have been reported in a few cases of isolated ACTH deficiency occurring in neonatal life.[327] A rare but fascinating cause relates to a defect in the normal post-translational processing of POMC to ACTH by the prohormone convertase enzymes (PC1 and PC2).[328] Such patients may have more generalized defects in peptide processing (e.g., cleavage of proinsulin to insulin) giving rise to diabetes mellitus.

Some patients have mutations in the *POMC* gene that interrupt the synthesis of ACTH and cause ACTH deficiency. Elucidation of the phenotype of these patients has uncovered a novel role for POMC peptides in regulating appetite and hair color: in addition to adrenal insufficiency, *POMC* mutations result in severe obesity and red hair pigmentation.[329] A central role for α-MSH in regulating food intake via the hypothalamic MC4R has been established,[55] and in recombinant mice lacking the POMC gene, the obese phenotype can be reversed by giving an α-MSH agonist peripherally.[330]

Other rare inborn causes of secondary insufficiency are the result of mutations in genes involved in pituitary development, such as *HESX1*,[331] *LHX4*,[332] *SOX3*,[333] and *PROP1*.[334] These defects result in congenital hypopituitarism with multiple pituitary hormone deficiencies: ACTH deficiency may not be present at the time of diagnosis, it but develops progressively over time.

Secondary hypoadrenalism is also observed in patients with Cushing disease after successful and selective removal of the ACTH-secreting pituitary adenoma. The function of adjacent normal pituitary corticotrophs is suppressed and may remain so for many months after curative surgery.[203-205]

ACTH Suppression by Exogenous Glucocorticoids

The ability of exogenously administered corticosteroids to cause adrenal atrophy has been appreciated since their discovery in the 1940s. HPA axis suppression by exogenous glucocorticoid is not trivial and has been described with intra-articular, topical, ocular, rectal, and inhaled, as well as systemic, therapy.[334a,334b,337]

There is considerable interindividual variability in response to glucocorticoids; there are no absolute cutoff values for the type of steroid taken, dose, route of administration, duration of treatment, or time since steroid withdrawal that predict adrenal suppression. However, there are some generic issues that can guide diagnosis and therapy. Relative steroid potencies in their affinity/transactivation of the GR have been described based on suppression of corticosterone production, in vitro binding to the glucocorticoid (GR), and by functional changes in GC target tissues by individual steroids[334c]; these suggest that oral doses of 20 mg hydrocortisone, 5 mg of prednisolone, and 0.75 mg of dexamethasone are bioequivalent. Dexamethasone has a longer half-life and higher affinity for the GR than hydrocortisone and exerts a more sustained suppressive effect on the HPA axis. Similarly, it is unclear how the potency of oral hydrocortisone compares to that of glucocorticoids taken by other routes. Budesonide has more potent action at the GR than dexamethasone or prednisolone,[334d] but its effect on adrenal suppression is dependent on systemic absorption of the inhaled compound. Comparison of inhaled fluticasone with inhaled steroids such as budesonide or beclomethasone indicated that fluticasone was more frequently associated with suppression of the HPA axis and that adults using over 1000 µg of inhaled fluticasone for over a year were at risk of adrenal suppression.[175]

Concomitant therapies can augment potency and adrenal suppression. The coadministration of inhaled fluticasone with one of the many medications that suppress its clearance by inhibition of CYP3A4 is associated with adrenal suppression (see Table 15-2).[334f] Co-prescriptions of agents that do not affect glucocorticoid clearance but have affinity for the GR are also associated with adrenal suppression, the most notorious example being progesterone derivatives such as medroxyprogesterone acetate given in high dose to oncology patients.[172]

In terms of dose and duration adrenal atrophy and subsequent deficiency should be anticipated in any subject who has taken more than the equivalent of 30 mg hydrocortisone per day orally (>7.5 mg/day prednisolone or >0.75 mg/day dexamethasone) for longer than 3 weeks. In addition to the magnitude of the dose of glucocorticoid, the timing of administration may affect the degree of adrenal suppression. If prednisolone is given as 5 mg at night and 2.5 mg in the morning, there will be more marked suppression of the HPA axis compared with 2.5 mg at night and 5 mg in the morning, because the larger evening dose blocks the early morning surge of ACTH. LaRochelle and colleagues reported that adrenal function recovered if patients' steroid doses could be tapered to 5 mg of prednisone daily.[335] This report has formed the basis of the practice of assessing HPA axis function in patients who have been on more than 5 mg of prednisolone or equivalent for more than 3 months. Recently, lower doses of glucocorticoid have been shown to suppress cortisol production; in one study, more than 60% of subjects on a glucocorticoid dose equivalent of less than 5 mg of prednisolone per day had a subnormal ACTH or cortisol response to CRF.[335a] In patients on long-term tapering of prednisolone who were considered for steroid withdrawal once they had reached a dose of 7 mg/day, 48% had adrenal insufficiency defined by basal cortisol (<100 nmol/L) or response to 250 µg synthetic ACTH (<550 nmol/L); a longer duration of prednisolone therapy (13.7 years) was seen in the hypoadrenal group defined by a low baseline cortisol but not in the group defined by cortisol response to 250 µg synthetic ACTH (6.1 years).[335b] Dynamic testing of adrenal function, such as the Synacthen stimulation test (SST) and CRF tests, suggests that cortisol production recovers after withdrawal of long-term glucocorticoids; in a meta-analysis of patients receiving glucocorticoid therapy, 46% to 100% had insufficient cortisol response 1 day after withdrawal, which improved to 26% to 49% in patients at assessment 1 week later.[36] Up to 10% of patients still have biochemical evidence of hypoadrenalism between 6 and 20 months after withdrawal of glucocorticoids.[335c]

All patients receiving long-term therapy with corticosteroids should be treated in a similar fashion to patients with chronic ACTH deficiency; they should carry steroid cards and be offered steroid alert bracelets or necklaces. In the event of an intercurrent stress (e.g., infection, surgery), supplemental steroid cover should be given. If the patient is unable to take drugs orally, parenteral therapy is required.

During recovery from suppression and without replacement therapy, patients may experience symptoms of glucocorticoid deficiency, including anorexia, nausea, weight loss, arthralgia, lethargy, skin desquamation, and postural dizziness (see the later discussions of adrenal insufficiency).[336] To avoid these symptoms, steroids should be cautiously withdrawn over a period of months.[175] Assuming that the underlying disease permits steroid reduction, doses should be reduced from pharmacologic levels to physiologic levels (equivalent to 7.5 mg/day prednisolone) over a few weeks. Thereafter, doses should be reduced by 1 mg/day of prednisolone every 2 to 4 weeks depending on patient well-being. An alternative approach is to switch the patient to hydrocortisone 20 mg/day and reduce the daily dose by 2.5 mg/day every week to a level of 10 mg/day. After 2 to 3 months on reduced doses, endogenous function of the HPA axis can be assessed by a corticotropin (ACTH-Synacthen) stimulation test or an insulin-induced hypoglycemia test. A "pass" response to these tests indicates adequate function of the HPA axis, and corticosteroid therapy can be safely withdrawn. In those patients who are taking physiologic doses of prednisolone (less than 5 to 7.5 mg/day) or equivalent corticosteroid, an SST given 12 to 24 hours after omitted steroid therapy will provide an immediate answer as to whether sudden or gradual withdrawal of steroid therapy is indicated (Table 15-17).[337]

Iatrogenic-induced Cushing syndrome occurs in patients who take suppressive doses of corticosteroids for longer than 3 weeks.[175] The rapidity of onset of clinical features depends on the administered dose but can occur within 1 month of therapy.

Hypoadrenalism During Critical Illness

Hypoadrenalism may also complicate critical illness, even in individuals with a previously intact HPA axis.[338] This has

TABLE 15-17

Suggested Plan for Steroid Replacement in Patients Withdrawing From Chronic Corticosteroid Therapy

	Duration of Glucocorticoid Treatment			
Pred Dose (mg/day)	**≤3 wk***	**>3 wk**		
≥7.5	Can stop	↓ rapidly (e.g., 2.5 mg q3-4d) THEN		
5-7.5	Can stop	↓ 1 mg q2-4 wk THEN	OR	Convert 5 mg pred to 20 mg HC, then ↓ 2.5 mg/wk to 10 mg/day THEN
<5	Can stop	↓ 1 mg q2-4 wk		After 2-3 mo HC 10 mg/day, administer SST/ITT: Pass → Withdraw Fail → Continue

*Beware of frequent steroid courses (e.g., in asthma).
HC, hydrocortisone; ITT, insulin tolerance test; pred, prednisolone; SST, short Synacthen test.

been termed *functional adrenal insufficiency* to reflect the notion that hypoadrenalism is transient and is not caused by a structural lesion. Functional adrenal insufficiency has been difficult to define biochemically and is of uncertain cause. Inability to mount an adequate and appropriate cortisol response to overwhelming stress or sepsis is frequently encountered in intensive care units and substantially increases the risk of death during acute illness.[339] This has stimulated attempts to define functional adrenal insufficiency quantitatively and to treat it with supplemental corticosteroids. Although this diagnosis remains highly contentious, if a suboptimal cortisol response is suspected, the current recommendations suggest (1) treatment with hydrocortisone, 200 mg/day in four divided doses or, preferably, 10 mg/hour as a continuous infusion, for patients with septic shock and (2) treatment with methylprednisolone, 1 mg/kg per day, for patients with severe early acute respiratory distress syndrome. Glucocorticoid treatment should be tapered off rather than stopped abruptly. Treatment of critical illness–related adrenal insufficiency with dexamethasone is not recommended.[340]

Clinical Features of Adrenal Insufficiency

Patients with primary adrenal failure usually have both glucocorticoid and mineralocorticoid deficiency. In contrast, those with secondary adrenal insufficiency have an intact RAA system. This accounts for differences in salt and water balance in the two groups of patients, which in turn result in different clinical presentations. The most obvious feature that differentiates primary from secondary hypoadrenalism is skin pigmentation (Table 15-18), which is almost always present in cases of primary adrenal insufficiency (unless of short duration) and absent in secondary insufficiency. The pigmentation is seen in sun-exposed areas, recent rather than old scars, axillae, nipples, palmar creases, pressure points, and mucous membranes (buccal, vaginal, vulval, anal). The cause of the pigmentation has long been debated but is thought to reflect increased stimulation of the MC1R by ACTH itself. In autoimmune Addison disease, there may be associated vitiligo (Fig. 15-32).

The clinical features relate to the rate of onset and the severity of adrenal deficiency.[298] In many cases, the disease has an insidious onset and a diagnosis is made only when the patient presents with an acute crisis during an intercurrent illness. Acute adrenal insufficiency, termed an *adrenal crisis* or *addisonian crisis,* is a medical emergency manifesting as hypotension and acute circulatory failure (Table 15-19). Anorexia may be an early feature; it progresses to nausea, vomiting, diarrhea, and sometimes abdominal pain. Fever may be present, and hypoglycemia may occur. Patients presenting acutely with adrenal hemorrhage have

TABLE 15-18

Clinical Features of Primary Adrenal Insufficiency

Feature	Frequency (%)
Symptoms	
Weakness, tiredness, fatigue	100
Anorexia	100
Gastrointestinal symptoms	92
Nausea	86
Vomiting	75
Constipation	33
Abdominal pain	31
Diarrhea	16
Salt craving	16
Postural dizziness	12
Muscle or joint pains	13
Signs	
Weight loss	100
Hyperpigmentation	94
Hypotension (<110 mm Hg systolic)	88-94
Vitiligo	10-20
Auricular calcification	5
Laboratory Findings	
Electrolyte disturbances	92
Hyponatremia	88
Hyperkalemia	64
Hypercalcemia	6
Azotemia	55
Anemia	40
Eosinophilia	17

hypotension; abdominal, flank, or lower chest pain; anorexia; and vomiting. The condition is difficult to diagnose, but evidence of occult hemorrhage (rapidly falling hemoglobin), progressive hyperkalemia, and shock should alert the clinician to the diagnosis.

Alternatively, the patient may present with vague features of chronic adrenal insufficiency—weakness, tiredness, weight loss, nausea, intermittent vomiting, abdominal pain, diarrhea or constipation, general malaise, muscle cramps, arthralgia, and symptoms suggestive of postural hypotension (see Table 15-18). Salt craving may be a feature, and a low-grade fever may be present. Supine blood pressure is usually normal, but almost invariably there is a fall in blood pressure on standing. Adrenal androgen secretion is lost; this is clinically more apparent in women, who may complain of loss of axillary and pubic hair and frequently have dry and itchy skin. Psychiatric symptoms may occur in long-standing cases and include memory impairment, depression, and psychosis. Formal

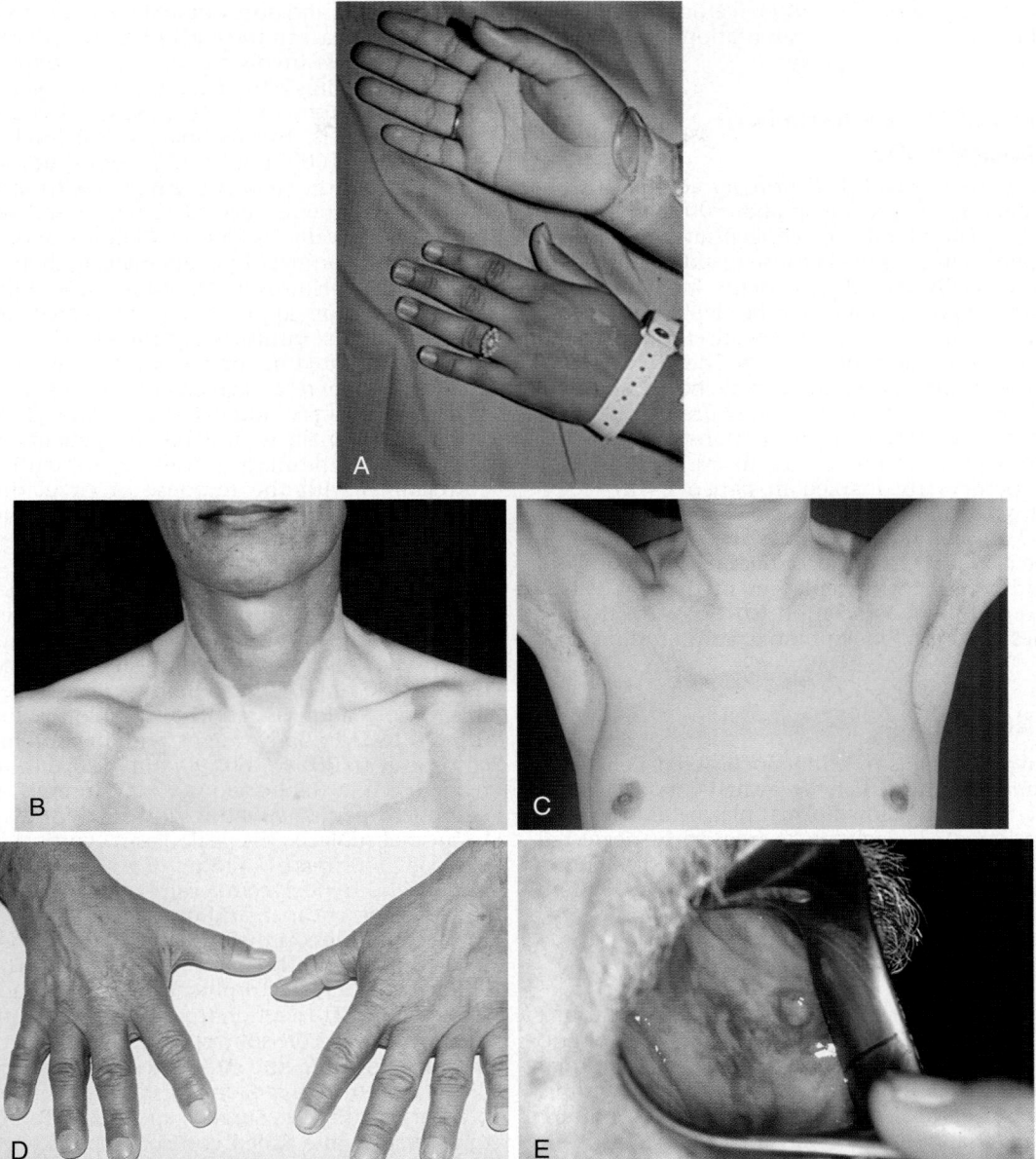

Figure 15-32 Pigmentation in Addison disease. **A,** Hands of an 18-year-old woman with autoimmune polyendocrine syndrome and Addison disease. Pigmentation in a patient with Addison disease before (**B**) and after (**C**) treatment with hydrocortisone and fludrocortisone. Notice the additional presence of vitiligo. **D,** Similar changes in a 60-year-old man with tuberculous Addison disease before *(left)* and after *(right)* corticosteroid therapy. **E,** Buccal pigmentation in the same patient as in **D**. (**B** and **C**, Courtesy of Professor C.R.W. Edwards.)

TABLE 15-19
Clinical and Laboratory Features of an Adrenal Crisis

Dehydration, hypotension, or shock out of proportion to severity of current illness
Nausea and vomiting with a history of weight loss and anorexia
Abdominal pain, so-called acute abdomen
Unexplained hypoglycemia
Unexplained fever
Hyponatremia, hyperkalemia, azotemia, hypercalcemia, or eosinophilia
Hyperpigmentation or vitiligo
Other autoimmune endocrine deficiencies, such as hypothyroidism or gonadal failure

quality-of-life measures indicate significant impairment in patients with primary or secondary adrenal insufficiency.[341] Tiredness is often profound, and patients may be inappropriately diagnosed with chronic fatigue syndrome or anorexia nervosa.

In secondary adrenal insufficiency due to hypopituitarism, the presentation may relate to deficiency of hormones other than ACTH, notably LH/FSH (infertility, oligorrhea/amenorrhea, poor libido) and TSH (weight gain, cold intolerance). Fasting hypoglycemia occurs because of loss of the gluconeogenic effects of cortisol. It is rare in adults unless there is concomitant alcohol abuse or additional GH deficiency. However, hypoglycemia is a common presenting feature of ACTH/adrenal insufficiency in childhood.[342] In addition, patients with ACTH deficiency present with malaise, weight loss, and other features of chronic adrenal insufficiency. Rarely, the presentation is more acute in patients with pituitary apoplexy.

Investigation of Hypoadrenalism

Routine Biochemical Profile

Among patients with established primary adrenal insufficiency, hyponatremia is present in about 90% and hyperkalemia in 65%. The blood urea concentration is usually elevated. Hyperkalemia occurs because of aldosterone deficiency, so it is usually absent in patients with secondary adrenal failure. Hyponatremia may be depletional in an addisonian crisis, but vasopressin levels are elevated, resulting in increased free water retention.[343] Therefore, in secondary adrenal insufficiency, there may be a dilutional hyponatremia with normal or low blood urea.

Reversible abnormalities in liver transaminases frequently occur. Hypercalcemia occurs in 6% of all cases[344] and may be particularly marked in patients with coexisting thyrotoxicosis. Free thyroxine concentrations are usually low or normal, but TSH values are frequently moderately elevated.[345] This is a direct effect of glucocorticoid deficiency and reverses with replacement therapy. Persistent elevation of TSH in association with positive thyroid autoantibodies suggests concomitant autoimmune thyroid disease.

Mineralocorticoid Status

In primary hypoadrenalism, mineralocorticoid deficiency usually occurs, manifested by elevated plasma renin activity and either low or low-normal plasma aldosterone. The investigation of ZG activity is frequently neglected in Addison disease, compared with assessment of ZF function. In secondary adrenal insufficiency, the RAA system is intact.

Assessing Adequacy of Function of the HPA Axis

Clinical suspicion of the diagnosis should be confirmed with definitive diagnostic tests. Basal plasma cortisol and urinary free cortisol levels are often in the low-normal range and cannot be used to exclude the diagnosis. However, a basal cortisol value greater than 400 nmol/L (14.5 μg/dL) invariably indicates an intact HPA axis.[346] In practice, rather than wait for results of insensitive basal tests, all patients with suspected adrenal insufficiency should have an ACTH stimulation test; in patients with an addisonian crisis, however, treatment should be instigated immediately and stimulation tests conducted at a later stage.

The ACTH stimulation test or SST involves intramuscular or intravenous administration of 250 μg tetracosactin, a synthetic ACTH(1-24) comprising the first 24 amino acids of normally secreted ACTH(1-39).[347] Plasma cortisol levels are measured at 0 and 30 minutes after ACTH administration, and a normal response is defined by a peak plasma cortisol level greater than 550 nmol/L (>20 μg/dL).[348] This value equates to the 5th percentile response in normal subjects but is very much assay-dependent, with different cortisol radioimmunoassays giving different results. Incremental responses (i.e., the difference between peak and basal values) are of no value in defining a "pass" response, with the possible exception of diagnosing relative adrenal insufficiency in patients with critical illness. Response is unaffected by the time of day of the test, and the test can be performed in patients who have commenced corticosteroid replacement therapy, as long as this therapy is of

short duration and does not include hydrocortisone (which would cross-react in the cortisol assay). A prolonged ACTH stimulation test involving the administration of depot or intravenous infusions of tetracosactin for 24 to 48 hours differentiates primary from secondary hypoadrenalism. In normal subjects, the plasma cortisol level at 4 hours is greater than 1000 nmol/L (36 μg/dL); beyond that time, there is no further increase. Patients with secondary hypoadrenalism show a delayed response and usually have a much higher value at 24 and 48 hours than at 4 hours. In patients with primary hypoadrenalism, there is no response at either time. However, the test is rarely required if plasma ACTH has been appropriately measured at baseline. In primary adrenal insufficiency, the ACTH level is disproportionately elevated in comparison to plasma cortisol.[349]

Whereas there is agreement on the investigation of suspected primary adrenal failure, the diagnosis of central hypoadrenalism, notably in patients with existing hypothalamic/pituitary disease, is contentious. Based on correlations with the response of circulating cortisol to surgery, the insulin-induced hypoglycemia test or insulin tolerance test (ITT) was introduced more than 40 years ago as a laboratory test to assess integrity of the HPA axis, and it should be considered the gold standard in this regard.[350] It should not be performed in patients with ischemic heart disease (always check an electrocardiogram before the test), epilepsy, or severe hypopituitarism (i.e., 9 AM plasma cortisol < 180 nmol/L [<6.5 μg/dL]). The test involves the intravenous administration of soluble insulin in a dose of 0.1 to 0.15 U/kg body weight, with measurement of plasma cortisol at 0, 30, 45, 60, 90, and 120 minutes. Adequate hypoglycemia (blood glucose <2.2 mmol/L with signs of neuroglycopenia—sweating and tachycardia) is essential. In normal subjects, the peak plasma cortisol concentration exceeds 500 nmol/L (18 μg/dL). However, the cortisol response to hypoglycemia can be reliably predicted by the SST—a safer, cheaper, and quicker test.[347,351]

The SST relies on the principle that the cortisol response to an exogenous bolus of ACTH is determined by the endogenous ACTH trophic drive to the adrenal cortex; impaired ACTH secretion from the anterior pituitary results in an impaired cortisol response after Synacthen administration. However, the ACTH test should not be used to diagnose central hypoadrenalism in patients with a recent pituitary insult (e.g., surgery, apoplexy). Total hypophysectomy results in a failed cortisol response to ITT immediately thereafter, but it takes 2 to 3 weeks for the adrenal cortex to readjust to the reduced level of ACTH secretion; in the interim, a false-positive cortisol response is seen. The SST should also be avoided in patients with a primary diagnosis of Cushing disease, in whom an exaggerated cortisol response to ACTH may persist.

In clinical practice, if the ACTH test is normal, insulin hypoglycemia testing is not necessary in most cases unless there is also a need to document endogenous GH reserve in a patient with pituitary disease. In our practice, an ITT is performed in a patient with suspected hypopituitarism if there is a subnormal response to ACTH. Some patients have an inadequate response to ACTH but then respond normally to hypoglycemia[351]; they do not require corticosteroid replacement therapy. This approach is open to debate, and even taking into account the caveats listed, false-positive results have been reported for the SST.[352] Although these are rare (<2%), the possibility should be noted, particularly in patients with ongoing symptoms and signs indicative of hypoadrenalism.

A low-dose SST giving only 1 μg ACTH has been proposed as a screen for adequacy of function of the HPA axis, with the suggestion that it may be more sensitive than the conventional 250-μg test.[353-355] Other researchers dispute this suggestion,[356,357] and further validation of this test is required to support such a concept.

Two other tests have been advocated to assess adequacy of function of the HPA axis, but their use in modern clinical practice should be restricted to difficult diagnostic cases. In the overnight metyrapone test, 30 mg/kg (maximum, 3 g) metyrapone is given at midnight, and plasma cortisol and 11-deoxycortisol are measured at 8 AM the following morning. In patients with an intact axis, ACTH levels rise after the blockade of cortisol synthesis by metyrapone, and a normal result is signified by a peak 11-deoxycortisol value greater than 7 μg/dL.[358] The CRH stimulation test has been used to diagnose adrenal insufficiency; unlike the metyrapone test, it differentiates primary from secondary causes. Patients with primary adrenal failure have high ACTH levels that rise further after CRH stimulation. Patients with secondary adrenal failure have low ACTH levels that fail to respond to CRH. Patients with hypothalamic disease show a steady rise in ACTH levels after CRH administration.[359]

Testing the HPA Axis During Critical Illness. Many factors complicate investigation of the HPA axis during critical illness. Cortisol levels vary broadly with disease severity, making it difficult to define appropriate responses. Additionally, CBG levels decrease substantially, leading to increases in the ratio of free to bound serum cortisol; for this reason, tests that assess the whole axis (e.g., ITT) are not appropriate in the critical care setting. Investigations are therefore limited to basal cortisol levels or values measured after the SST.

Recent guidance has indicated that a random cortisol value of less than 400 nmol/L (<15 μg/dL) suggests corticosteroid insufficiency, whereas a level greater than 900 nmol/L (>33 μg/dL) is unlikely to occur in patients with compromised HPA axis function. For individuals with intermediate cortisol levels, an SST should be performed; a cortisol increment of less than 250 nmol/L (<9 μg/dL) is an independent prognostic marker for death in critically ill patients.[339]

An initial multicenter randomized trial of patients with septic shock showed that those with an increment less than 250 nmol/L across an SST had a significant improvement in survival when given replacement corticosteroids.[360] However, in a more recent study hydrocortisone treatment hastened reversal of shock but did not improve overall survival in patients with septic shock.[361] The SST was not useful in predicting benefit from glucocorticoids. It is possible that differences in results between these two trials were due to differences in patient selection (e.g., severity of sepsis) and the speed of administration of glucocorticoids.

In light of this uncertainty, recent recommendations continue to suggest hydrocortisone treatment for septic shock and methylprednisolone for patients with severe early acute respiratory distress syndrome, particularly those with poor response to fluid resuscitation and vasopressor agents.[340] The role of glucocorticoids in the management of critically ill patients with other conditions requires further research.

Other Tests. Radioimmunoassays to detect autoantibodies such as those against the 21-hydroxylase antigen are now available and should be analyzed in patients with primary adrenal failure. In autoimmune Addison disease, it is also important to look for evidence of other organ-specific autoimmune disease. A CT scan may reveal enlarged or calcified adrenals, suggesting an infective, hemorrhagic, or malignant diagnosis (Fig. 15-33). Chest radiography, tuberculin testing, and early morning urine samples cultured for

Mycobacterium tuberculosis should be performed if tuberculosis is suspected. CT-guided adrenal biopsy may reveal an underlying diagnosis in patients with suspected malignant deposits in the adrenal gland. Adrenoleukodystrophy can be diagnosed by measuring circulating levels of VLCFA. Finally, appropriate investigations, including pituitary MRI scans and an assessment of anterior function, are required for patients with suspected secondary hypoadrenalism who are not taking corticosteroid therapy.

Treatment of Acute Adrenal Insufficiency

Acute adrenal insufficiency is a life-threatening emergency, and treatment should not be delayed while waiting for definitive proof of diagnosis (Table 15-20). However, in addition to measurement of plasma electrolytes and blood glucose, appropriate samples for ACTH and cortisol should be taken before corticosteroid therapy is given. If the patient is not critically ill, an acute ACTH stimulation test can be performed.

In adults, intravenous hydrocortisone should be given in a dose of 100 mg every 6 to 8 hours. If this is not possible, then the intramuscular route should be used. In the patient with shock, 1 L of normal saline should be given intravenously over the first hour. Because of possible hypoglycemia, it is normal to give 5% dextrose in saline. Subsequent saline and dextrose therapy will depend on biochemical monitoring and the patient's condition. Clinical improvement, especially in the blood pressure, should be seen within 4 to 6 hours if the diagnosis is correct. It is important to recognize and treat any associated condition (e.g., infection) that may have precipitated the acute adrenal crisis.

After the first 24 hours, the dose of hydrocortisone can be reduced, usually to 50 mg intramuscularly every 6 hours

TABLE 15-20
Treatment of Acute Adrenal Insufficiency (Adrenal Crisis) in Adults

Emergency Measures

1. Establish intravenous access with a large-gauge needle.
2. Draw blood for immediate serum electrolytes and glucose and routine measurement of plasma cortisol and ACTH. Do not wait for laboratory results.
3. Infuse 2-3 L of 154 mmol/L NaCl (0.9% saline) solution, or 50 g/L (5%) dextrose in 154 mmol/L NaCl (0.9% saline) solution, as quickly as possible. Monitor for signs of fluid overload by measuring central or peripheral venous pressure and listening for pulmonary rales. Reduce infusion rate if indicated.
4. Inject intravenous hydrocortisone (100 mg immediately and every 6 hr).
5. Use supportive measures as needed.

Subacute Measures After Stabilization of the Patient

1. Continue intravenous 154 mmol/L NaCl (0.9% saline) solution at a slower rate for next 24-48 hr.
2. Search for and treat possible infectious precipitating causes of the adrenal crisis.
3. Perform a short ACTH stimulation test to confirm the diagnosis of adrenal insufficiency (if patient does not have known adrenal insufficiency).
4. Determine the type of adrenal insufficiency and its cause, if not already known.
5. Taper glucocorticoids to maintenance dosage over 1-3 days, if precipitating or complicating illness permits.
6. Begin mineralocorticoid replacement with fludrocortisone (0.1 mg by mouth daily) when saline infusion is stopped.

ACTH, adrenocorticotropic hormone.

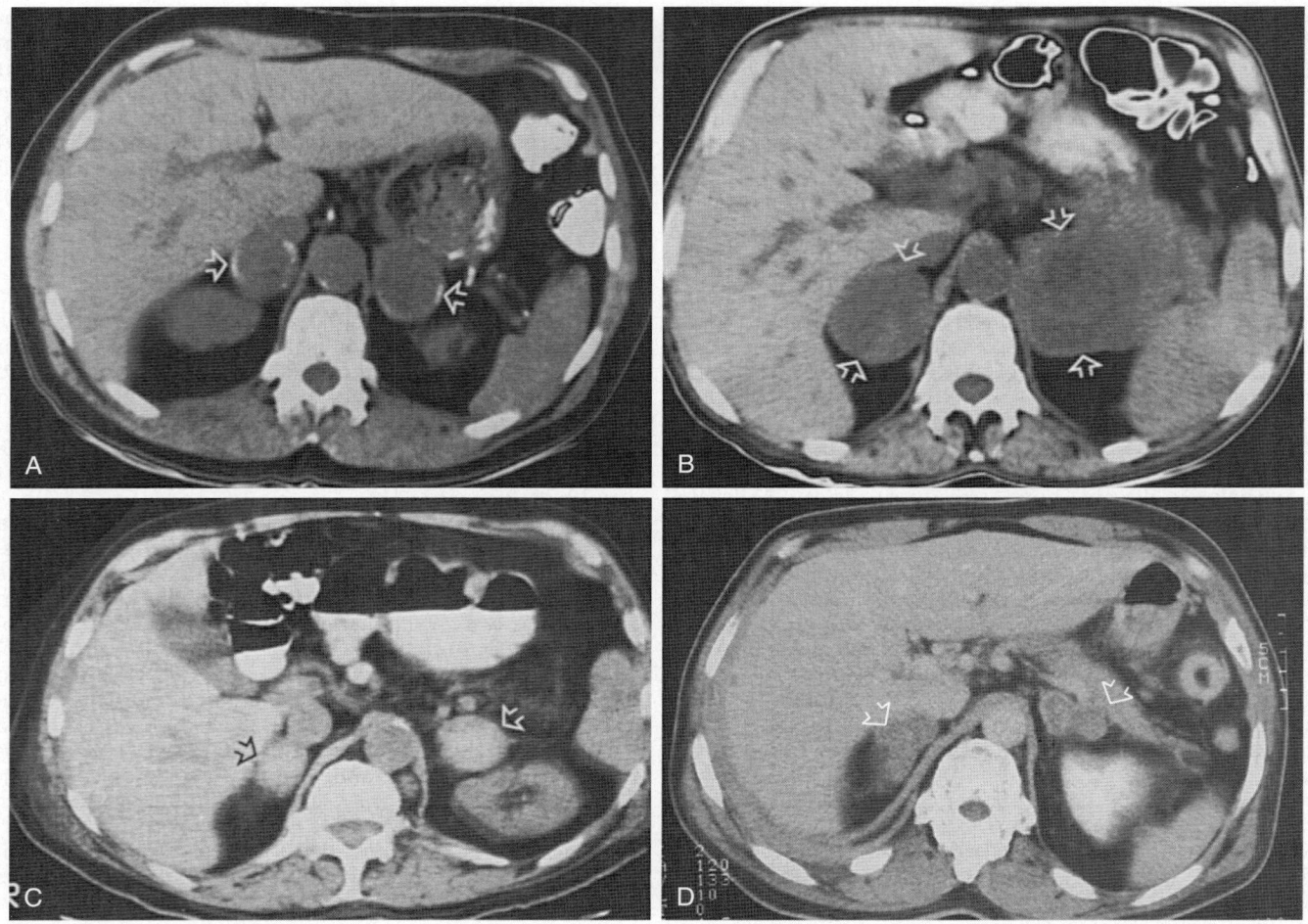

Figure 15-33 Computed tomographic (CT) scans of patients with primary adrenal insufficiency. The affected adrenal glands are indicated by arrows. **A,** CT scan of a 59-year-old man with histoplasmosis. Notice the subcapsular calcium in both glands. **B,** CT scan of a 59-year-old man with metastatic melanoma. **C,** CT scan of an 80-year-old man with bilateral adrenal hemorrhage resulting from anticoagulation for pulmonary emboli. **D,** Bilateral adrenal tuberculomas in a 79-year-old man with tuberculosis affecting the urogenital tract. (**A** and **B,** Courtesy of Dr. William D. Salmon, Jr.; **C,** Courtesy of Dr. Craig R. Sussman.)

and then to oral hydrocortisone, 40 mg in the morning and 20 mg at 6 PM. This dose can then be rapidly reduced to a more standard replacement dose of 20 mg on awakening and 10 mg at 6 PM.

Long-Term Replacement Therapy

The aim of long-term therapy is to give replacement doses of hydrocortisone to mimic the normal cortisol secretion rate (Table 15-21). In the past, this rate was thought to be approximately 25 to 30 mg/day, but stable isotope studies have indicated lower normal cortisol production rates of 8 to 15 mg/day.[362] Most patients can cope with less than 30 mg/day (usually 15 to 25 mg/day in divided doses). Doses are usually given on awakening, with a smaller dose at 6 PM, but some patients feel better with three-times-a-day dosing. In cases of primary adrenal failure, cortisol day curves with simultaneous ACTH measurements are advocated to provide some insight into the adequacy of replacement therapy.[363] There are no good biomarkers of glucocorticoid adequacy in patients with central hypoadrenalism. Decisions regarding doses of replacement therapy are largely based on crude yet important end points such as weight, well-being, and blood pressure.[364] Bone mineral density is moderately reduced in a dose-dependent manner in patients treated with more than 25 mg/day of

hydrocortisone,[365] highlighting the need to strive for minimally effective but safe doses.[366,367] Possibly because of the known action of IGF-1 to increase cortisol clearance,[132] it is our experience that glucocorticoid requirements are slightly lower in hypopituitary, GH-deficient subjects than in patients with primary adrenal insufficiency.

In primary adrenal failure, mineralocorticoid replacement is usually also required in the form of fludrocortisone (or 9α-fluorinated hydrocortisone), 0.05 to 0.2 mg/day. The mineralocorticoid activity of this is about 125 times that of hydrocortisone. After the acute phase has passed, the adequacy of mineralocorticoid replacement should be assessed by measuring electrolytes, supine and erect blood pressures, and plasma renin activity.[368] Too little fludrocortisone may cause postural hypotension with elevated plasma renin activity, whereas too much causes the converse. Mineralocorticoid replacement therapy is all too frequently neglected in patients with adrenal failure.

Patients on glucocorticoid replacement therapy should be advised to double their daily dose in the event of intercurrent febrile illness, accident, or mental stress such as an important examination. If the patient is vomiting and cannot take medication by mouth, parenteral hydrocortisone must be given urgently. For minor surgery, 50 to 100 mg hydrocortisone hemisuccinate is given with the premedication. For major operations, this pretreatment is

TABLE 15-21
Treatment of Chronic Primary Adrenal Insufficiency in Adults

Maintenance Therapy

Glucocorticoid Replacement
- Hydrocortisone 15-20 mg on awakening and 5-10 mg in early afternoon
- Monitor clinical symptoms and morning plasma ACTH.

Mineralocorticoid Replacement
- Fludrocortisone 0.1 (0.05-0.2) mg orally
- Liberal salt intake
- Monitor lying and standing blood pressure and pulse, edema, serum potassium, and plasma renin activity.
- Educate patient about the disease, how to manage minor illnesses and major stresses, and how to inject steroid intramuscularly.
- Obtain MedicAlert bracelet/necklace, Emergency Medical Information card.

Treatment of Minor Febrile Illness or Stress

- Increase glucocorticoid dose twofold to threefold for the few days of illness; do not change mineralocorticoid dose.
- Contact physician if illness worsens or persists for more than 3 days or if vomiting develops.
- No extra supplementation is needed for most uncomplicated, outpatient dental procedures with local anesthesia. General anesthesia or intravenous sedation should not be used in the office.

Emergency Treatment of Severe Stress or Trauma

- Inject contents of prefilled dexamethasone (4-mg) syringe intramuscularly.
- Get to physician as quickly as possible.

Steroid Coverage for Illness or Surgery in Hospital

- For moderate illness, give hydrocortisone 50 mg bid PO or IV. Taper rapidly to maintenance dose as patient recovers.
- For severe illness, give hydrocortisone 100 mg IV q8h. Taper to maintenance level by decreasing by half every day. Adjust dose according to course of illness.
- For minor procedures under local anesthesia and most radiologic studies, no extra supplementation is needed.
- For moderately stressful procedures such as barium enema, endoscopy, or arteriography, give a single 100-mg IV dose of hydrocortisone just before the procedure.
- For major surgery, give hydrocortisone 100 mg IV just before induction of anesthesia and continue q8h for first 24 hr. Taper dose rapidly, decreasing by half per day, to maintenance level.

ACTH, adrenocorticotropic hormone; bid, twice a day; IV, intravenous; PO, orally; q, every.

followed by the same regimen as for acute adrenal insufficiency (see Table 15-21). Pregnancy proceeds normally in patients taking replacement therapy, but daily doses of hydrocortisone are usually increased modestly (5 to 10 mg/day) in the last trimester. Progesterone is a mineralocorticoid antagonist, and the rising levels across pregnancy may necessitate an increased dose of fludrocortisone. During labor, patients should be well hydrated with a saline drip and should receive hydrocortisone 50 mg intramuscularly every 6 hours until delivery. Thereafter, doses can be rapidly tapered to prepregnancy levels.

Every patient on glucocorticoid therapy should be advised to register for a medical alert bracelet or necklace and to carry a steroid card. Patients should receive regular education regarding the requirements of stress-related glucocorticoid dose adjustment, which should involve the patient's partner and family as well. Parenteral preparations of hydrocortisone for self-administration may be required for patients living far from hospitals and those planning vacations.

For patients with both primary and secondary adrenal failure, beneficial effects of adrenal androgen replacement therapy with 25 to 50 mg/day of DHEA have been reported. To date, reported benefit is principally confined to female patients and includes improvement in sexual function and well-being.[369] However, patients with adrenal insufficiency on current steroid replacement regimens have significantly impaired health-related subjective health status irrespective of the origin of disease or concomitant disease.[341] Delayed-release hydrocortisone preparations, such as Plenadren, that more closely replicate normal circadian cortisol concentrations, have recently been licensed and approved; early clinical trials show improved quality of life in both primary and central hypoadrenalism compared to conventional twice- or thrice-daily hydrocortisone administration.[369a]

CONGENITAL ADRENAL HYPERPLASIA

CAH comprises a group of autosomal recessive disorders caused by deficient adrenal corticosteroid biosynthesis.[370,371] It results from defects in one of the steroidogenic enzymes involved in cortisol biosynthesis or in the electron-providing factor, POR. Congenital lipoid adrenal hyperplasia, caused by StAR deficiency affecting mitochondrial cholesterol uptake, is a subform of this disease complex with the unique feature of lipid accumulation leading to cell destruction. In each case, there is reduced negative feedback inhibition of cortisol and, depending on the steroidogenic pathway involved, alteration in adrenal mineralocorticoid and androgen secretion (Table 15-22).

Aldosterone synthase deficiency does not affect glucocorticoid biosynthesis and does not lead to adrenal hyperplasia, but it has been historically grouped into this disease complex. All forms of CAH together represent a disease continuum, ranging from severe forms caused by complete loss-of-function defects to milder forms in which the defective proteins have partial residual activity.

21-Hydroxylase Deficiency

Between 90% and 95% of cases of CAH are caused by 21-hydroxylase deficiency.[370] In Western societies, the incidence varies from 1 in 10,000 to 1 in 15,000 live births, but in isolated communities the incidence may be much higher (e.g., 1:300 in Alaskan Inuit populations). Nonclassic CAH is more common, with an incidence of about 1 in 500 to 1 in 1000 live births. The condition arises because of defective conversion of 17α-OHP to 11-deoxycortisol. Reduced cortisol biosynthesis results in reduced negative feedback drive and increased ACTH secretion; as a consequence, adrenal androgens are produced in excess (Fig. 15-34). Seventy-five percent of patients have clinically manifest mineralocorticoid deficiency because of failure to convert sufficient progesterone to DOC in the ZG. Clinically, several distinct variants of 21-hydroxylase deficiency have been recognized (Table 15-23).

Simple Virilizing Form

In the simple virilizing form of 21-hydroxylase deficiency, the enhanced ACTH drive to adrenal androgen secretion in utero leads to virilization of an affected female fetus. Depending on the severity, clitoral enlargement, labial fusion, and development of a urogenital sinus may occur, leading to sexual ambiguity at birth and even inappropriate sex assignment. Males are phenotypically normal at birth and are at risk of not being diagnosed; this explains

TABLE 15-22
Congenital Adrenal Hyperplasia: Features for Each Enzyme Defect

Deficiency	21-Hydroxylase	11β-Hydroxylase	17α-Hydroxylase	3β-HSD Type 2	P450 Oxidoreductase	Lipoid Adrenal Hyperplasia	P450 Side-Chain Cleavage	Aldosterone Synthase	Apparent Cortisone Reductase
OMIM No. / Gene/Protein / Alias	+201910 CYP21A2 P450c21	#202010 CYP11B1 P450c11	#202110 CYP17A1 P450c17	+201810 HSD3B2 3β-HSD	#201750 POR CPR, CYPOR	*600617 StAR	+118485 CYP11A1 P450scc	*124080 CYP11B2 P450aldo	*138090 H6PDH
Incidence	Classic: 1:10,000 to 1:15,000 Nonclassic: 1:500 to 1:1000	1:100,000 to 1:200,000	Rare	Rare	Unknown	Rare	Rare	Rare	Rare
DSD	Classic: 46,XX Nonclassic: No	46,XX	46,XY	46,XY*	46,XX + 46,XY†	46,XY	46,XY	No	No
Primary affected organ	Adrenal	Adrenal	Adrenal, gonads	Adrenal, gonads	Adrenal, gonads, liver, all CYP type 2-expressing tissues	Adrenal, gonads	Adrenal, gonads	Adrenal	Liver, adrenal, all H6PDH/HSD11B1-expressing tissues
Glucocorticoids	Classic: Reduced Nonclassic: Normal	Reduced	Reduced	Reduced	Reduced to normal, impaired stress response	Reduced	Reduced	Normal	Normal, but reduced tissue levels due to increased cortisol clearance
Mineralocorticoids	Classic: Reduced in SW Nonclassic: Normal	Increased, mainly precursors	Increased	Reduced often	Reduced to increased	Reduced	Reduced	Reduced	Normal
Sex hormones	Increased	Increased	Reduced	Reduced in males, increased in females‡	Reduced	Reduced	Reduced	Normal	Increased
Increased marker metabolites in plasma	17-OHP, 21-DOF	DOC, S	Pregnenolone, progesterone, DOC, S	17-OH, pregnenolone, DHEA	Pregnenolone, progesterone, 17-OHP			DOC, B, 18-OHB	
Increased marker metabolites in urine	Pregnanetriol, 17-OH pregnenolone, pregnanetriolone	THDOC, THS	THDOC, THB, pregnenediol, pregnanediol	Pregnanetriol	Pregnanediol, pregnanediol, pregnanetriol, 17-OH pregnanolone				
PRA	Classic: Increased Nonclassic: Normal to mildly increased	Reduced	Reduced	Increased	Reduced	Increased	Increased	Increased	Normal
Hypertension	No	Yes	Yes	No	No or mild	No	No	No	Normal
Plasma sodium	Classic: Reduced in SW Nonclassic: Normal	Increased	Increased	Reduced in SW	Normal	Reduced	Reduced	Reduced	Normal
Plasma potassium	Classic: Increased in SW Nonclassic: Normal	Reduced	Reduced	Increased in SW	Normal	Increased	Increased	Increased	Normal
Urinary salt loss	Classic: Yes Nonclassic: No	No	No	Yes	No	Yes	Yes	Yes	No
Skeletal malformation	No	No	No	No	Yes§	No	No	No	No

*Masculinization of the external genitalia in females at birth is rare and usually mild; signs of increased androgens usually manifest later.
†DSD is observed in both sexes, and normal sex-specific development is also reported.
‡Steroid hormone conversion by HSD3B1 in peripheral tissues.
§In most cases published thus far, however, absence of skeletal malformations does not rule out POR deficiency.

B, corticosterone; CYP, cytochrome P450; DHEA, dehydroepiandrosterone; DOC, 11-deoxycorticosterone; 21-DOF, 21-deoxycortisol; DSD, disorder of sex development; H6PDH, hexose-6-phosphate dehydrogenase; HSD, hydroxysteroid dehydrogenase; OMIM, Online Mendelian Inheritance in Man; 18-OHB, 18-hydroxycorticosterone; 17-OHP, 17-hydroxyprogesterone; POR, P450 oxidoreductase; PRA, plasma renin activity; S, 11-deoxycortisol; StAR, steroidogenic acute regulatory protein; SW, salt wasting; THB, tetrahydro-corticosterone; THS, tetrahydro-11-deoxycortisol; THDOC, tetrahydro-11-deoxycorticosterone.

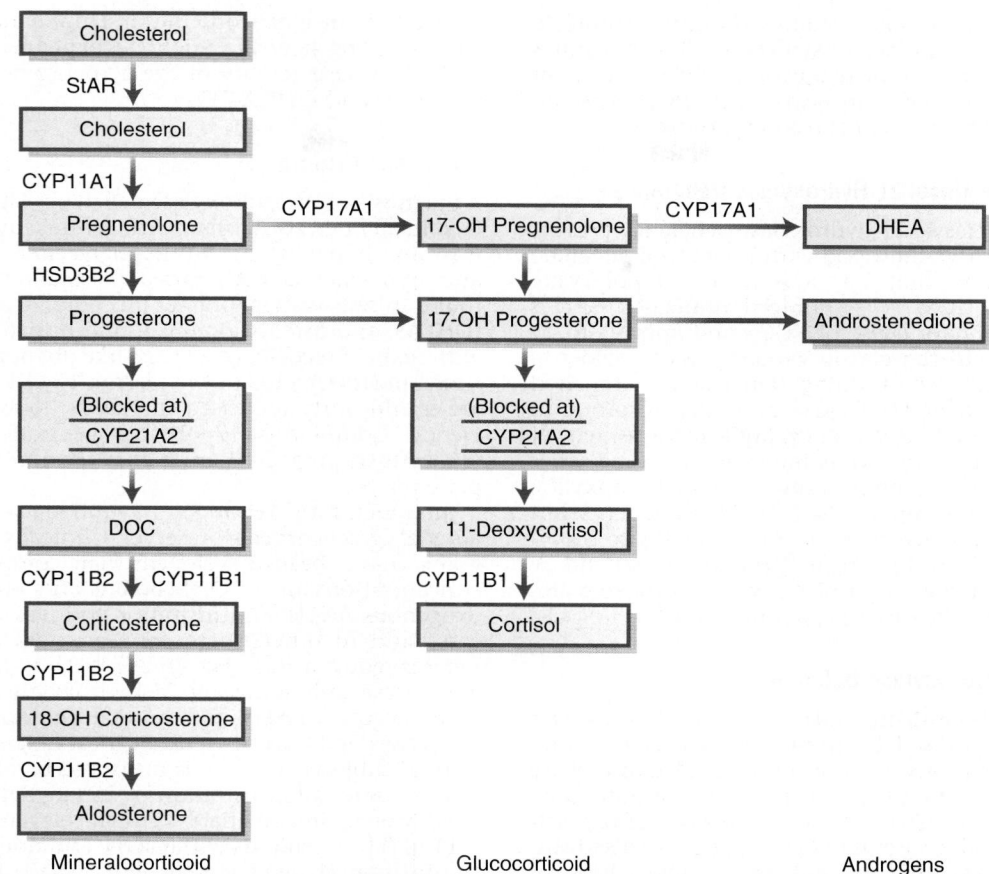

Figure 15-34 Congenital adrenal hyperplasia related to 21-hydroxylase deficiency. The normal synthesis of cortisol is impaired, and adrenocorticotropic hormone (ACTH) levels increase because of loss of normal negative feedback inhibition, resulting in an increase in adrenal steroid precursors proximal to the block. The results are cortisol deficiency, variable mineralocorticoid deficiency, and excessive secretion of adrenal androgens. CYP, cytochrome P450; DHEA, dehydroepiandrosterone; DOC, deoxycorticosterone; HSD, hydroxysteroid dehydrogenase; StAR, steroidogenic acute regulatory protein.

TABLE 15-23

Forms of 21-Hydroxylase Deficiency

Phenotype	Classic Salt Wasting	Simple Virilizing	Nonclassic
Age at diagnosis	Newborn to 6 mo	*Female:* Newborn to 2 yr *Male:* 2-4 yr	Child to adult
Genitalia	*Female:* Ambiguous *Male:* Normal	*Female:* Ambiguous *Male:* Normal	*Female:* Virilized *Male:* Normal
Incidence	1:20,000	1:60,000	1:1000
Hormones			
Aldosterone	Reduced	Normal	Normal
Renin	Increased	Normal or increased	Normal
Cortisol	Reduced	Reduced	Normal
17-OHP	>5000 ng/dL	2500-5000 ng/dL	500-2500 ng/dL (ACTH stimulation)
Testosterone	Increased	Increased	Variable, increased
Growth	−2 to −3 SD	−1 to −2 SD	Probably normal
21-Hydroxylase activity (% of wild type)	0	1-5	20-50
Typical *CYP21A2* mutations	Deletions, conversions, nt656g G110Δ8nt, R356W I236N, V237E, M239K, Q318X	I172N Intron 2 splice site (nt656g)	V281L P30L

ACTH, adrenocorticotropic hormone; 17-OHP, 17-hydroxyprogesterone; SD, standard deviation.

the skewed female-to-male ratio of simple virilizing CAH diagnosed in the preneonatal screening era. Such patients may present in early childhood with signs of precocious pseudopuberty such as sexual precocity, pubic hair development, or growth acceleration due to premature androgen excess. If left untreated, this stimulates premature epiphyseal closure, and final adult height is invariably diminished.[372,373]

Salt-Wasting Form

Seventy-five percent of patients of both sexes who have the salt-wasting form of 21-hydroxylase deficiency also have concomitant, clinically manifested aldosterone deficiency. In addition to the described features, neonates commonly present after the first 2 weeks of life with a salt-wasting crisis and hypotension. The clinical signs and symptoms of salt wasting include poor feeding, vomiting, failure to thrive, lethargy, and sepsis-like symptoms. These features may alert the clinician to the diagnosis in a male baby, but the diagnosis is still delayed in many cases, and the condition carries a significant neonatal mortality rate.

Nonclassic or Late-Onset 21-Hydroxylase Deficiency

Patients with nonclassic 21-hydroxylase deficiency present in childhood or early adulthood with premature pubarche or with a phenotype that may masquerade as polycystic ovary syndrome (PCOS).[370,374,375] Indeed, nonclassic CAH is a recognized secondary cause of PCOS and appears to be more common than the classic variant. Recent evidence suggests that at least 30% of adult patients have an impaired cortisol response to ACTH(1-24)[376] and may be prone to stress-induced adrenal insufficiency. Routine assessment of adrenal glucocorticoid reserve is indicated. In some series from tertiary referral centers, nonclassic 21-hydroxylase deficiency accounts for up to 12% of all PCOS patients, but more realistic prevalence rates are probably 1% to 3%.[377] Females present with hirsutism, primary or secondary amenorrhea, or anovulatory infertility.[374] Androgenic alopecia and acne may be other presenting features.

Heterozygote 21-Hydroxylase Deficiency

Salt wasting, simple virilizing, and late-onset 21-hydroxylase deficiency are all caused by homozygous or compound heterozygote mutations in the human 21-hydroxylase gene *(CYP21A2)*. In the carrier or heterozygote state, only one allele is mutated. The clinical significance of the heterozygote state is uncertain; it does not appear to disadvantage reproductive capability but may cause signs of hyperandrogenism in adult women.[370]

Molecular Genetics

21-Hydroxylase deficiency is inherited as an autosomal recessive trait, and the higher incidence of the condition in some ethnic communities almost certainly relates to consanguinity. The *CYP21A2* gene and its highly homologous pseudogene *(CYP21A1P)* are located on the short arm of chromosome 6 (6p21.3). Because of the genomic localization within the human leukocyte antigen (HLA) locus, a region with a high frequency of genomic recombinations, most of the mutations causing 21-hydroxylase deficiency are generated by gene conversion events. Complete gene deletions or conversions of the *CYP21A2* gene, eight pseudogene-derived point mutations, and an 8–base pair deletion are found in more than 95% of cases. Other rare pseudogene-independent *CYP21A2*-inactivating mutations have been reported in single families or small populations. Approximately 65% to 75% of CAH patients are compound heterozygous for the disease-causing mutations.[378]

The genotype-phenotype correlation in CAH due to the 21-hydroxylase deficiency is well established. The clinical phenotype correlates with the less severely mutated allele and, consequently, with the residual 21-hydroxylase activity (Fig. 15-35).[379,380] This correlation appears to be high, although divergence between genotype and phenotype has been observed.[381] The 21-hydroxylase activity measured by in vitro analysis provides a possibility for estimating disease severity, although some phenotypic variability (e.g., salt wasting, age at onset) seems likely to depend on other interacting genes and maturation processes rather than *CYP21A2* itself. One such factor might be the length of the CAG repeats in the androgen receptor modulating androgen action.[382] Potential variations in the degree of

recovery from glucocorticoid and mineralocorticoid deficiency during later life might be explained by significant 21-hydroxylase activity of the cytochrome P450 enzymes CYP2C19 and CYP3A4.[383]

Diagnostic Criteria

A diagnosis of 21-hydroxylase deficiency should be considered in any newborn infant with genital ambiguity and salt wasting, hypotension, or hypoglycemia. Hyponatremia and hypokalemia with raised plasma renin activity are found in salt-wasters. In later life, adrenal androgen excess (DHEAS, androstenedione) is found in patients presenting with sexual precocity or a PCOS-like phenotype. Randomly timed measurements of the plasma 17-OHP concentration are significantly increased in classic 21-hydroxylase deficiency. Commonly, 17-OHP concentrations in patients with salt-wasting CAH are higher than in non–salt-losing patients.

In nonclassic CAH, an SST is required to establish normal adrenal glucocorticoid reserve. Clinically useful nomograms have been developed that compare circulating concentrations of 17-OHP before and 60 minutes after exogenous ACTH administration to investigate borderline cases and to differentiate between nonclassic CAH and heterozygous carriers (Fig. 15-36).[384] This separates patients with classic and nonclassic 21-hydroxylase deficiency from heterozygote carriers and normal subjects, but there is some overlap between values seen in heterozygotes and in normal subjects. 17-OHP is measured basally and then 60 minutes after administration of 250 µg Synacthen. Stimulated values are invariably grossly elevated (>35 nmol/L [>11 µg/L]) in patients with classic and nonclassic forms of the disorder. Heterozygote patients usually have stimulated values between 10 and 30 nmol/L (330 and 1000 ng/dL) (see Fig. 15-36). Stimulation tests are not always required to make a diagnosis; for example, a basal 17-OHP concentration of less than 5 nmol/L (<150 ng/dL) in the follicular phase of the menstrual cycle effectively excludes late-onset 21-hydroxylase deficiency.[374] *CYP21A2* genotyping to confirm the clinical and biochemical diagnosis is a useful adjunct to hormonal measurements. Androgen excess in 21-hydroxylase deficiency is readily suppressed after glucocorticoid administration.

Prenatal diagnosis of 21-hydroxylase deficiency has been advocated, because treatment of an affected female may prevent masculinization in utero.[385] 17-OHP can be assayed in amniotic fluid, but the most robust approach is the rapid genotyping of fetal cells obtained by chorionic villous sampling in early gestation. In patients with known 21-hydroxylase deficiency (male or female) seeking fertility, determination of 17-OHP levels across an SST in the partner before conception will uncover nonclassic or heterozygote cases and provide the endocrinologist/geneticist with some assignment of risk before pregnancy.

Treatment

The objectives for treatment of 21-hydroxylase deficiency differ with age, but at all ages treatment and overall patient management can be fraught with difficulties. In childhood, the overall goal is to replace glucocorticoid and mineralocorticoid, thereby preventing further salt-wasting crises, but also to normalize adrenal androgen secretion so that normal growth and skeletal maturation can proceed. Accurate replacement is essential; in excess, glucocorticoids will suppress growth, whereas inadequate replacement will result initially in accelerated linear growth and ultimately in short stature due to premature epiphyseal closure.[370]

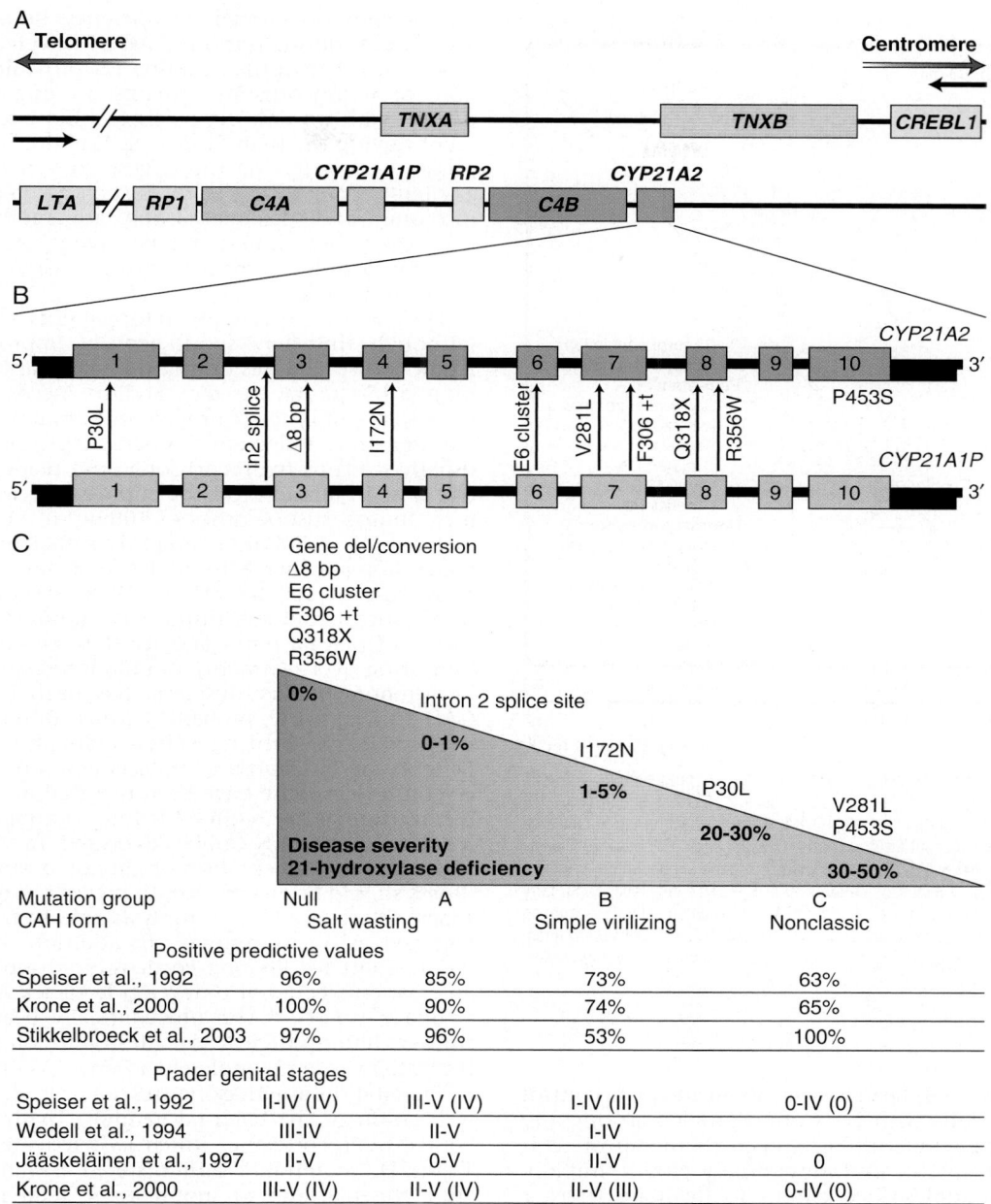

Figure 15-35 Genetics of 21-hydroxylase deficiency. **A,** Genomic organization of the functional *CYP21A2* gene and its nonfunctional *CYP21A1P* pseudogene. **B,** Nine out of 10 common mutations are transferred by microconversions from the *CYP21A1P* pseudogene into the *CYP21A2* gene. **C,** Genotype-phenotype correlation in 21-hydroxylase deficiency is well established. Based on the in vitro enzyme activity, the *CYP21A2* gene-inactivating mutations can be categorized into four major mutation groups. Although variation has been reported for the milder mutations, the overall correlation is high regarding expression of the adrenal phenotype. Considerable variability exists for the correlation with genital virilization. CAH, congenital adrenal hyperplasia.

Response is best monitored through growth velocity and bone age, with biochemical markers from blood (17-OHP, androstenedione, testosterone), urine, and saliva (17-OHP, androstenedione, testosterone) being useful adjuncts. In difficult cases, a day curve study, as described for patients with primary adrenal failure but measuring the ACTH and 17-OHP response before and after corticosteroid replacement, may confirm overreplacement or underreplacement. The optimal glucocorticoid dose fails to suppress 17-OHP and its metabolites and maintains sex hormone concentrations in the middle of the age- and sex-specific normal range. Ideally, the biochemical investigations will indicate the need for dose adjustments before physical changes,

growth, and skeletal maturation indicate inadequate or excessive glucocorticoid treatment.[386]

Corrective surgery (e.g., clitoral reduction, vaginoplasty) is frequently required during childhood. The method of choice should be a one-stage complete repair using the newest techniques of vaginoplasty, clitoral, and labial surgery.[386]

In late childhood and adolescence, appropriate replacement therapy is equally important. Overtreatment may result in obesity and delayed menarche/puberty with sexual infantilism, whereas underreplacement will result in sexual precocity. Compliance with regular medication is often an issue throughout adolescence.

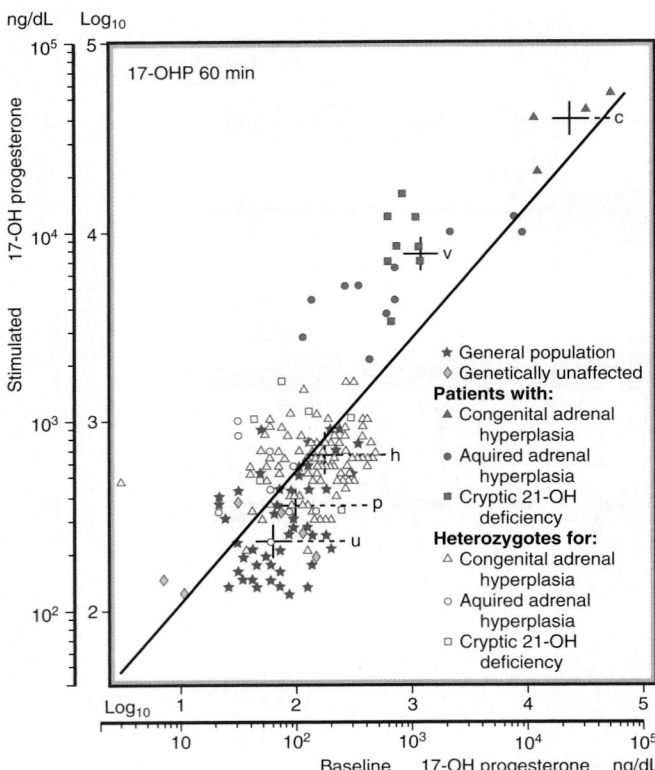

Figure 15-36 Basal and stimulated plasma 17α-hydroxyprogesterone (17-OHP) concentrations in patients with 21-hydroxylase (21-OH, CYP21A2) deficiency. To convert values to nmol/L, multiply by 0.0303. The mean for each group is indicated by a large cross and an adjacent letter: *c*, patients with classic CYP21A2 deficiency; *h*, heterozygotes for all forms of CYP21A2 deficiency; *p*, general population; *u*, known unaffected persons (e.g., siblings of patients with CYP21A2 deficiency who carry neither affected parental haplotype as determined by human leukocyte antigen typing); *v*, patients with nonclassic (acquired and cryptic) CYP21A2 deficiency. (From White PC, New MI, Dupont B. Congenital adrenal hyperplasia: part 1. *N Engl J Med.* 1987;316:1519-1524.)

Although much has been written about adequate control in childhood, adults with CAH often provide an ongoing dilemma for the endocrinologist. The follow-up of such patients should involve multidisciplinary clinics, initially with transition adolescence clinics to facilitate transfer from pediatric to adult care. Problems in adulthood relate to fertility concerns, hirsutism, and menstrual irregularity in women; obesity, metabolic consequences, and impact of short stature; probable increased cardiovascular risk; sexual dysfunction; and psychological problems.[370,387,388] Counseling is often required in addition to endocrine support. Males may develop enlargement of the testes due to so-called testicular adrenal rest tumors—that is, ectopic adrenal tissue, which may regress after glucocorticoid suppression. These patients need adequate endocrine therapy rather than urologic referral with ensuing risk of removal of testis mistaken for a tumor.[389]

In the absence of any evidence-based data, there are no prescriptive steroid regimens to treat patients with CAH at any age, and as a result, many individualized regimens are used in clinical practice. Hydrocortisone is recommended for replacement therapy from the newborn period to adolescence.[386] Usual starting doses of hydrocortisone in childhood are 10 to 15 mg/m² per day in three divided doses, with up to 25 mg/m² in infancy only seldom required. These doses are higher than those employed for replacement of adrenal insufficiency because treatment also aims at normalization of ACTH-driven adrenal androgen excess. The optimal timing for providing the highest dose of hydrocortisone remains an ongoing matter of debate, with no data supporting either circadian replacement (giving the highest dose in the morning) or reverse-phase therapy (giving the largest dose of hydrocortisone at night). Long-acting steroids such as prednisone, prednisolone, and dexamethasone are more effective in this regard but should not be given before the end of puberty in order to avoid oversuppression and reduction in linear growth.

Fludrocortisone is required for patients with salt wasting (although this may spontaneously improve with age). Fludrocortisone doses during the first year of life are commonly 150 µg/m² per day. Sodium needs to be supplemented, as milk feeds provide only maintenance sodium requirements. Adequate mineralocorticoid replacement usually leads to hydrocortisone dose reduction. The relative dose in relation to body surface decreases throughout life. Fludrocortisone doses of 100 µg/m² per day after the first 2 years of life are commonly sufficient. This requirement drops further with adolescence and adulthood to a daily dose of 100 to 200 µg (50 to 100 µg/m² per day). Mineralocorticoid substitution is monitored by measurements of plasma renin activity (low or suppressed levels indicating overtreatment) and blood pressure.[390]

Adrenomedullary dysplasia has been reported in the CAH adrenal gland, probably because of relative glucocorticoid deficiency, which results in epinephrine deficiency.[391] Benefits of epinephrine replacement on the metabolic response to exercise have been reported in children,[392] but further studies are required before routine catecholamine replacement therapy can be advocated. In clinical practice, sufficient supplementation of glucose during exercise and illness should be guaranteed, to prevent hypoglycemic episodes. Bilateral adrenalectomy is effective but should be regarded as a last resort[393]; in addition, because of the requirement for lifelong corticosteroid replacement therapy, patients could also develop feedback ACTH-secreting pituitary tumors.[394] This procedure also bears a number of risks, including surgical and anesthetic complications, and the patient is left completely adrenal insufficient.

Prenatal dexamethasone treatment is effective to avoid virilization of the external genitalia in the female fetus. Unlike hydrocortisone, which is inactivated by placental 11β-HSD, maternally administered dexamethasone can cross the placenta to suppress the fetal HPA axis. One approach is to advocate use of dexamethasone therapy as soon as pregnancy is confirmed in high-risk cases and to continue this therapy until the diagnosis is excluded in the female fetus. If the fetus is affected, only those of female sex require dexamethasone therapy across gestation. Therapy must be instigated at 6 to 7 weeks of gestation to be effective. The suggested dexamethasone dose is 20 to 25 µg/kg in three divided doses per day (total maximum dose, 1.5 mg/day).[370] However, because only one in eight pregnancies treated in this way will result in an affected female fetus, the use of steroid therapy in this setting has been questioned.[395] The fetal sex can be determined as early as week 6 of gestation with the use of novel molecular diagnostic methods that analyze free fetal DNA from maternal blood using real-time polymerase chain reaction. In this way, the number of unnecessarily treated cases can be reduced to three out of eight. Dexamethasone can lead to maternal cushingoid effects in pregnancy[396] and may in turn have long-term, deleterious effects on the fetus, including metabolic, psychological, and intellectual consequences. Prenatal treatment is controversial and has to be regarded as experimental; patients treated should be included in ongoing multicenter studies.[397]

In adult women with hyperandrogenism and untreated nonclassic CAH, there is no evidence that final height is affected. In this setting, glucocorticoid suppression in isolation rarely controls hirsutism, and additional antiandrogen therapy is often required (e.g., cyproterone acetate, spironolactone, flutamide together with an oral estrogen contraceptive pill). However, ovulation induction rates with gonadotropin therapy are improved after suppression of nocturnal ACTH levels with 0.25 to 0.5 mg dexamethasone. Hypogonadotropic hypogonadism in male patients is a consequence of increased aromatization of adrenal androgens, in particular androstenedione to estrone, resulting in suppression of pituitary LH and FSH secretion. The condition is reversible after optimization of glucocorticoid therapy. However, overreplacement in men or women may also lead to hypogonadotropic hypogonadism due to glucocorticoid-mediated suppression of GnRH secretion.

Long-Term Complications and Comorbid Conditions

Outcome assessed by final height is not optimal in many patients treated for 21-hydroxylase deficiency. In a meta-analysis including 18 studies published between 1977 and 2001, the mean adult height of patients with classic CAH was 10 cm (−1.4 SDS) below the population mean and −1.2 SDS calculated for target height. The pubertal growth spurt occurs earlier and is less pronounced than normal. An often overlooked problem is glucocorticoid overtreatment during the first 2 years of life; overtreatment suppresses the infant growth spurt, which is characterized by the highest postnatal growth velocity. Therefore, the lowest optimal dose of glucocorticoid replacement should be established as early in life as possible.

Increased fat mass and obesity are common among children and adolescents with CAH.[398-400] Glucocorticoid dose, chronologic age, advanced bone age maturation, and parental obesity all contribute to elevated BMI SDS.[399]

Increased fat mass and higher insulin levels have been described in women older than 30 years of age with CAH. However, clear evidence of cardiovascular risk factors had not been shown. Women with CAH do have a significantly higher rate of gestational diabetes, a possible forerunner for the development of type 2 diabetes,[401] and women with nonclassic CAH[402] and young adult CAH patients[403] have reduced insulin sensitivity. Increased intima media thickness as a marker of atherosclerosis has been detected.[403]

Daytime systolic blood pressure in children and adolescents with CAH is elevated, and the physiologic nocturnal dip in blood pressure is absent.[404] Elevated systolic blood pressure correlates with the degree of overweight and obesity.[405] There are no long-term outcome data on adults.

11β-Hydroxylase Deficiency

11β-Hydroxylase deficiency accounts for 7% of all cases of CAH, with an incidence of 1 in 100,000 live births.[406] The condition arises because of mutations in the 11β-hydroxylase (CYP11B1) gene that result in loss of enzyme activity and a block in the conversion of 11-deoxycortisol to cortisol. The CYP11B1 gene is located on chromosome 8q24.3, approximately 40 kilobases from the highly homologous aldosterone synthase gene (CYP11B2).[406] CYP11B1-inactivating mutations have been shown to be distributed over the entire coding region consisting of nine exons. Although mutation clusters are reported in exons 2, 6, 7, and 8,[378,406] real hot spots, as seen in 21-hydroxylase deficiency, do not exist. Most of the reported mutations lead to absent or almost absent 11β-hydroxylase enzyme activity, with only some cases of mild or nonclassic 11-hydroxylase deficiency reported.[407,408]

Loss of negative cortisol feedback and enhanced ACTH-mediated adrenal androgen excess occur in 11β-hydroxylase deficiency (Fig. 15-37). Clinical features therefore are very similar to those reported in the simple virilizing form of CAH (46,XX DSD including virilization of the external genitalia and sexual ambiguity); and again, milder cases can manifest later in childhood or even young adulthood. The principal difference from 21-hydroxylase deficiency is hypertension, which is thought to be secondary to the mineralocorticoid effect of DOC excess. However, there is a poor correlation between DOC secretion and the presence of hypertension, and unexplained salt wasting has been reported in few patients during early life. On this clinical background, the diagnosis can be made by measuring a plasma ACTH–stimulated 11-deoxycortisol value, which will be higher than three times the 95th percentile for an age-matched normal group. Basal concentrations of 17-OHP are commonly increased but may be normal even during the first weeks of life.[409]

Although established heterozygotes may not demonstrate an increase in 11-deoxycortisol above normal values after Synacthen stimulation[410] (unlike the 17-OHP response observed in heterozygote patients with 21-hydroxylase deficiency), exaggerated ACTH-stimulated responses have been observed in patients with hirsutism[411] and in patients with essential hypertension,[412] suggesting partial defects in 11β-hydroxylase activity.

Treatment is with replacement glucocorticoid therapy; with suppression of DOC secretion, the plasma renin activity, which is suppressed at baseline, increases into the normal range. In general, higher glucocorticoid doses are needed to suppress hyperandrogenism compared with the situation in 21-hydroxylase deficiency, and add-on antihypertensive therapy may be necessary in some cases. Antihypertensive treatment should be commenced at an early stage to avoid excessive glucocorticoid exposure.

17α-Hydroxylase Deficiency

Approximately 150 cases of 17α-hydroxylase deficiency have been reported.[413-415] Mutations within the CYP17A1 gene result in failure to synthesize cortisol (17α-hydroxylase activity), adrenal androgens (17,20-lyase activity), and gonadal steroids (Fig. 15-38). Therefore, in contrast to 21- and 11β-hydroxylase deficiencies, 17α-hydroxylase deficiency results in adrenal and gonadal insufficiency and causes 46,XY DSD. A single enzyme is expressed in the adrenal and the gonads and possesses both 17α-hydroxylation and 17,20-lyase activities, but rare patients with isolated deficiency in the hydroxylation of 17-OHP or 17,20-lyase deficiency have been reported.[414] Loss of negative feedback results in increased secretion of steroids proximal to the block, and mineralocorticoid synthesis is enhanced. Corticosterone has weaker glucocorticoid activity than cortisol, but corticosterone excess generally prevents adrenal crises. Accumulation of corticosterone and DOC results in severe hypokalemic hypertension. Sex steroid deficiency caused by loss of 17,20-lyase activity results in 46,XY DSD; this manifests as undervirilization in male newborns and primary amenorrhea in 46,XX individuals. There is lack of pubertal development due to hypergonadotropic hypogonadism in both sexes.[415]

The 17α-hydroxylase enzyme is a microsomal cytochrome P450 type II enzyme that requires electron transfer from NADPH via POR for catalytic activity.[26] For efficient catalysis of the 17,20-lyase reaction, the CYP17A1-POR

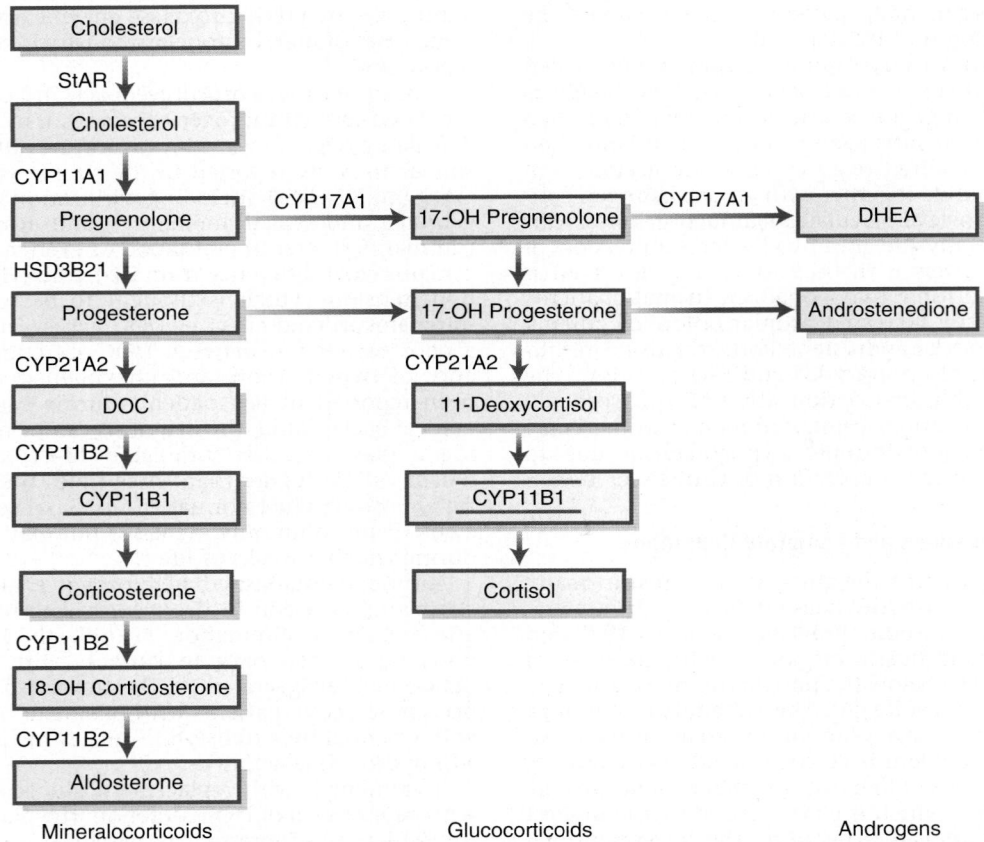

Figure 15-37 Congenital adrenal hyperplasia related to 11β-hydroxylase deficiency. The normal synthesis of cortisol is impaired, and adrenocorticotropic hormone (ACTH) levels increase because of the loss of normal negative feedback inhibition, which results in an increase in adrenal steroid precursors proximal to the block. The results are cortisol deficiency, mineralocorticoid excess related to excessive deoxycorticosterone (DOC) secretion, and excessive secretion of adrenal androgens. CYP, cytochrome P450; DHEA, dehydroepiandrosterone; HSD, hydroxysteroid dehydrogenase; StAR, steroidogenic acute regulatory protein.

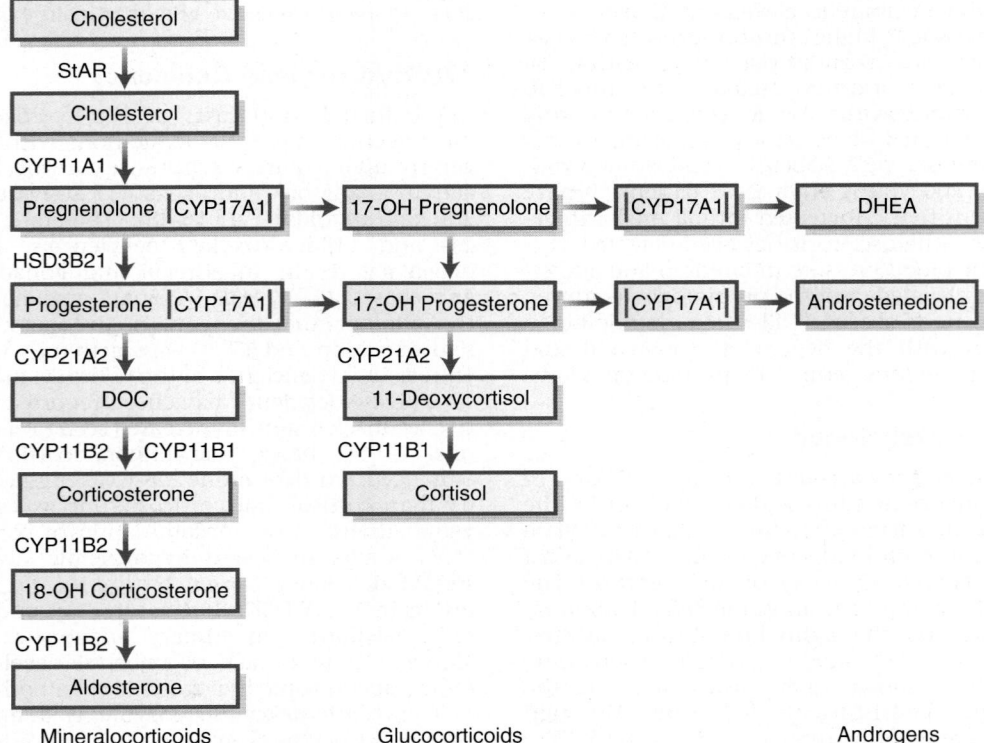

Figure 15-38 Congenital adrenal hyperplasia related to 17α-hydroxylase deficiency. The normal synthesis of cortisol is impaired, and adrenocorticotropic hormone (ACTH) levels increase because of loss of normal negative feedback inhibition resulting in an increase in adrenal steroid precursors proximal to the block. The result is cortisol deficiency and mineralocorticoid excess usually related to deoxycorticosterone (DOC) excess. Because gonadal 17α-hydroxylase activity is also absent, sex steroid secretion in addition to adrenal androgen secretion is severely impaired, resulting in hypogonadism. CYP, cytochrome P450; DHEA, dehydroepiandrosterone; HSD, hydroxysteroid dehydrogenase; StAR, steroidogenic acute regulatory protein.

complex requires additional allosteric interaction with cytochrome b_5.[416,417] The *CYP17A1* gene consists of eight exons and is located on chromosome 10q24.3. A variety of different mutations have been described, without evidence of a hot spot.[378,418] Relative hydroxylase/lyase activities of CYP17A1 mutants have been shown to vary in in vitro functional assays, but correlations with clinical phenotype are lacking. Patients with clinically pure 17,20-lyase deficiency have CYP17A1 mutations that selectively compromise 17,20-lyase activity.[416,419,420] Mutations underlying isolated 17,20-lyase deficiency are located within the area of the CYP17A1 molecule that is thought to interact with the cofactor cytochrome b_5, thereby disrupting the electron transfer from POR to CYP17A1, specifically for the conversion of 17-hydroxypregnenolone to DHEA.[416,419]

The diagnosis is usually made at the time of puberty when patients present with hypertension, hypokalemia, and hypergonadotropic hypogonadism, the last occurring because of lack of CYP17A1 expression within the gonad and impaired gonadal steroidogenesis. As a result, LH and FSH levels are elevated. Female patients (XX) have primary amenorrhea with absent sexual characteristics, whereas 46,XY individuals present with 46,XY DSD with female external genitalia but absent uterus and fallopian tubes. The intra-abdominal testes should be removed, and such patients are usually reared as females.

Glucocorticoid replacement reverses the DOC-induced suppression of the renin-angiotensin system and lowers blood pressure. Additional sex steroid replacement is required from puberty onward.

P450 Oxidoreductase Deficiency: Apparent Combined 17α-Hydroxylase and 21-Hydroxylase Deficiencies

Patients have been described with biochemical evidence of apparent combined 17α-hydroxylase and 21-hydroxylase deficiencies.[421] Urinary gas chromatography/mass spectrometry analysis reveals a typical pattern comprising increased pregnenolone and progesterone metabolites, slightly increased corticosterone metabolites, increased pregnanetriolone excretion, and low androgen metabolites (see Fig. 15-4). Mothers pregnant with an affected child present with low serum estriol and a characteristic urinary steroid profile, allowing for prenatal biochemical diagnosis.[422,423] The analysis of serum steroids only may lead to misdiagnosis.[424] Cortisol baseline secretion may be normal, but most, if not all, patients show an insufficient cortisol response to ACTH stimulation and therefore require glucocorticoid replacement. Impaired 17,20-lyase activity results in deficient androgen synthesis, and affected boys are often born undervirilized. Most of the affected girls are born with virilized genitalia. Therefore, patients can present with 46,XY or 46,XX DSD or with appropriate development of the external genitalia in both sexes. After birth, virilization does not progress, and circulating androgen concentrations are typically low. Some mothers develop signs of virilization during midpregnancy with an affected child; this commonly resolves soon after birth, further indicating intrauterine androgen excess.[422] In addition to these features of CAH, affected children may also present with bone malformations, including midface hypoplasia, craniosynostosis, and radiohumeral synostosis, in some cases resembling the Antley-Bixler congenital malformation syndrome.[425,426] The bone phenotype in affected patients with POR deficiency is most likely caused by an impairment of sterol biosynthesis, specifically POR-dependent 14α-lanosterol demethylase (CYP51A1).

The paradox of fetal virilization but sex hormone deficiency in postnatal life might be mediated by a newly discovered "backdoor" pathway of androgen synthesis in fetal life that relies on neither androstenedione nor testosterone as an intermediate.[426-428] Pubertal development in POR deficiency appears to be dominated by the consequences of sex steroid deficiency,[428] and most patients require sex hormone substitution. The overall incidence of POR deficiency has not been established. However, a relatively large number of patients with POR deficiency were reported within a short period after the initial description of the molecular cause of the disease.[428,429]

The *POR* gene is located on chromosome 7q11.2 and consists of 15 translated exons spanning 32.9 kilobytes and encoding a protein of 680 amino acids. A variety of POR-inactivating mutations have been reported, including missense, frameshift, and splice site mutations. A287P is the most common mutation in Caucasians, whereas R457H is the most frequent founder mutation in the Japanese population. All patients carry POR mutations that are either partially inactivating or, in case of major loss-of-function mutations, manifest only in the compound heterozygous state. Homozygous mutations with total loss of function are most likely not viable—a view supported by the nonviability of complete POR gene deletion in the murine model.[430]

3β-Hydroxysteroid Dehydrogenase Deficiency

In this rare form of CAH, the secretion of all classes of adrenal and ovarian steroids is impaired due to mutations within the *HSD3B2* gene encoding 3β-HSD type 2.[431,432] There are two isoforms of 3β-HSD, encoded by *HSD3B1* and *HSD3B2*, respectively. The *HSD3B2* gene is located on chromosome 1p13.1 and consists of four exons. HSD3B2 is expressed mainly in the adrenal and the gonad, whereas HSD3B1 is expressed in the placenta and almost ubiquitously in peripheral target tissues.[27,432] The enzyme HSD3B2 catalyzes three key reactions in adrenal steroidogenesis: the conversion of the Δ^5 steroids pregnenolone, 17-hydroxypregnenolone, and DHEA to the Δ^4 steroids progesterone, 17-OHP, and androstenedione, respectively. 3β-HSDII deficiency affects all three steroid hormone pathways (i.e., mineralocorticoids, glucocorticoids, and sex steroids).

The clinical spectrum shows a wide variety of disease expression. Patients usually present in early infancy with adrenal insufficiency. Loss of mineralocorticoid secretion results in salt wasting, although this is absent in 30% to 40% of cases (Fig. 15-39). As with 21-hydroxylase deficiency, absence of salt wasting may delay the presentation into childhood or puberty, ranging from a severe salt-wasting form with or without ambiguous genitalia in affected male neonates to isolated premature pubarche in infants and children of both sexes and a late-onset variant manifesting with hirsutism and menstrual irregularities. In general, the functional and biochemical data are in close agreement with the expressed phenotype in patients with the non–salt-wasting form of HSD3B2 deficiency. However, some variability exists, and identical mutations have been found in the *HSD3B2* gene in both salt-wasters and non–salt-wasters.[431,432] The correlation between the impairment in male sexual differentiation and salt wasting is poor. The spectrum of genital development is variable in both sexes. In males, because the HSD3B2 enzyme is also expressed within the gonad, 46,XY DSD may occur, resulting in female external genitalia. However, most patients present with hypospadias, and even normal male genitalia may be found. In females, genital development can be normal, but

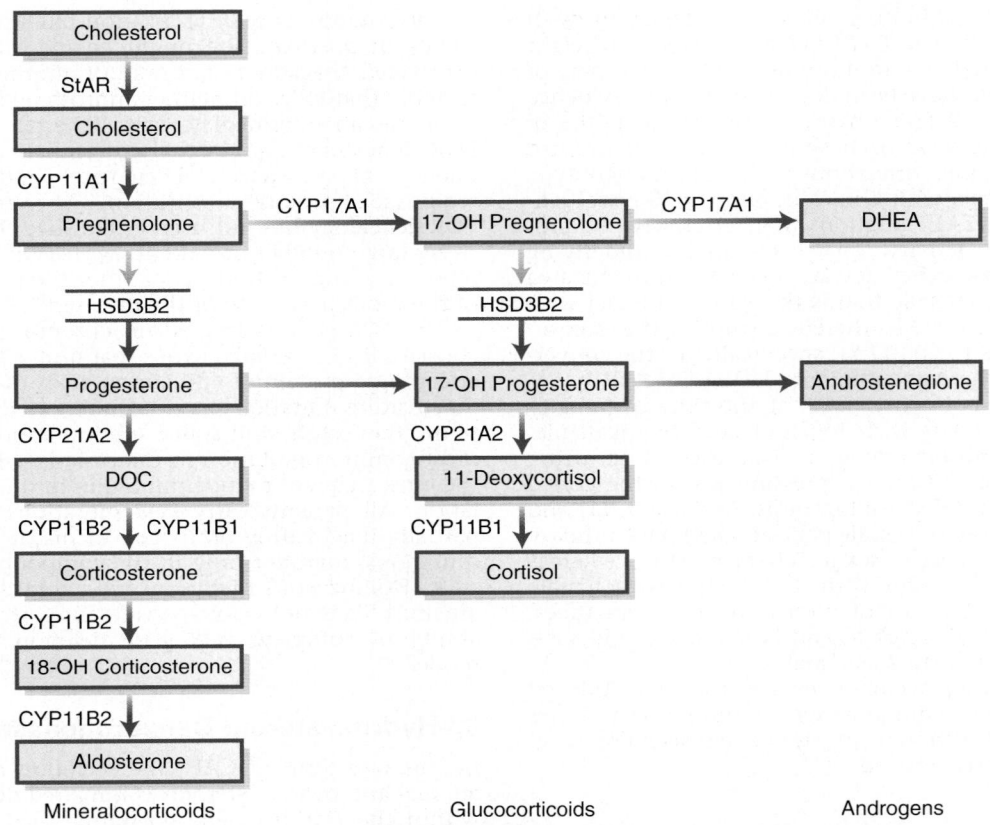

Figure 15-39 Congenital adrenal hyperplasia related to 3β-hydroxysteroid dehydrogenase (3β-HSD) type 2 deficiency resulting in cortisol deficiency and variable mineralo-corticoid deficiency. Gonadal 3β-HSD type 2 activity is also absent, resulting in 46,XY DSD and hypogonadism or primary amenorrhea in females. Virilization in females can occur due to 3β-hydroxysteroid dehydrogenase type 1 activity. DOC, deoxycorticosterone; DHEA, dehydroepiandrosterone; DSD, disorder of sex development; StAR, steroidogenic acute regulatory protein.

usually there is evidence of mild virilization, presumably because of enhanced adrenal DHEA secretion, which is converted peripherally to testosterone. A late-onset form has been described in patients with premature pubarche[433] and a PCOS-like phenotype (i.e., hirsutism, oligorrhea/amenorrhea).[434]

Because activity of the HSD3B1 enzyme, present in peripheral tissues, is intact, levels of circulating Δ⁴ steroids (progesterone, 17-OHP, androstenedione) may be normal (or even increased). However, a diagnosis is established by demonstration of an increased ratio of Δ⁵ steroids (pregnenolone, 17-hydroxypregnenolone, DHEA) to Δ⁴ steroids in plasma or urine. Hormonal criteria have been refined for the diagnosis of HSD3B2 deficiency based on genotyping of the *HSD3B2* gene. The 17-hydroxypregnenolone concentrations and the ratios of 17-hydroxypregnenolone to cortisol at baseline and after ACTH stimulation are of the highest discriminatory value in differentiating between patients affected by HSD3B2 deficiency and those with milder biochemical abnormalities, who are commonly negative for *HSD3B2* mutations.[435,436] Treatment is with replacement glucocorticoids, fludrocortisone (if indicated), and sex steroids from puberty onward.

StAR Deficiency: Congenital Lipoid Adrenal Hyperplasia

Mutations in the gene encoding StAR results in a failure of transport of cholesterol from the outer to the inner mitochondrial membrane in steroidogenic tissues. StAR-independent cholesterol transport occurs only at a low rate. As a result, there is deficiency of all adrenal and gonadal steroid hormones.[23,437] The adrenal glands are often massively enlarged and full of lipid; before the characterization of StAR, the condition was termed *congenital lipoid adrenal hyperplasia*.[437] StAR deficiency severely but incompletely abolishes pregnenolone synthesis. Cholesterol esters accumulate under the increased tone of ACTH stimulation. Consequently, the lipid accumulation worsens the dysfunction and leads to adrenal cell destruction. Presentation is with acute adrenal insufficiency in the neonatal period, and males exhibit 46,XY DSD due to absent gonadal steroids.

The most severe form of this disorder manifests with 46,XY DSD and combined adrenal insufficiency. Salt wasting typically develops in the neonatal period or after a few weeks of life, but later onset may also occur. Females can show spontaneous pubertal development. A milder form of StAR deficiency has also been described in normally virilized 46,XY individuals who present with adrenal failure during early childhood.[438] Treatment consists of glucocorticoid and mineralocorticoid replacement and substitution of sex hormones in later life.

P450 Side-Chain Cleavage Deficiency

Deficiency of P450scc (CYP11A1) enzyme is a rare inborn error of steroidogenesis, with only seven cases reported. It was previously thought that such mutations would not be viable, because the maintenance of human pregnancy relies on placentally produced progesterone. The production is facilitated by the fetal part of the placenta from the second trimester onward. P450scc deficiency manifests clinically and biochemically with similar signs and symptoms as StAR deficiency, but patients do not have enlarged adrenals.[439-441] Depending on the impairment of CYP11A1 function, a spectrum of clinical presentation ranges from 46,XY DSD with severe adrenal insufficiency in the newborn period to hypospadias and cryptorchidism and later manifestation of adrenal insufficiency during childhood.[442] Concentrations of all steroid hormones are decreased, in keeping with impaired conversion of cholesterol to pregnenolone. Treatment with glucocorticoid, mineralocorticoid, and sex steroid replacement is required.

Cortisone Reductase Deficiency

In cortisone reductase deficiency, adrenal glands become hyperplastic because of ACTH stimulation due to a defect in cortisol metabolism rather than an inherent defect within the gland itself.[130,443,444] Patients with this condition have a defect in the conversion of cortisone to cortisol, suggesting inhibition of 11-oxo-reductase activity and, by implication, inhibition of HSD11B1 (see Fig. 15-12). Cortisol clearance is increased, and as a consequence, ACTH secretion is elevated to maintain normal circulating cortisol concentrations but at the expense of adrenal androgen excess. Female patients present with hirsutism, menstrual irregularity, androgenic alopecia, or some combination of these features. Males may present with premature pubarche. Dexamethasone treatment to suppress ACTH has been used with some success to control the hyperandrogenism in these cases. Urinary tetrahydrometabolites of cortisol and cortisone show almost exclusively THE with little or no detectable THF or allo-THF; the ratio of THF+allo-THF to THE is less than 0.05 (reference range, 0.8 to 1.3). The molecular bases for cortisone reductase deficiency are inactivating mutations in hexose-6-phosphate dehydrogenase (H6PDH).[444] H6PDH, located in the endoplasmic reticulum, catalyzes the conversion of glucose 6-phosphate to glucose 6-phosphogluconate, thereby generating NADPH, which is crucial in conveying oxo-reductase activity on HSD11B1.

Patients with PCOS share many of the same clinical characteristics as those with cortisone reductase deficiency. Whereas there is evidence to support increased cortisol secretion rates in PCOS, perhaps indicating a defect in the conversion of cortisone to cortisol, a consensus with respect to THF+allo-THF:THE ratios is still lacking.[445] Association studies using single-nucleotide polymorphic markers in the HSD11B1 and H6PDH genes have largely been negative.

Mineralocorticoid Deficiency

The mineralocorticoid deficiency syndromes are listed in Table 15-24. They can be divided into congenital and acquired syndromes. Mineralocorticoid deficiency may occur in some forms of CAH and with other causes of adrenal insufficiency (e.g., Addison disease, CAH).

TABLE 15-24

Causes of Mineralocorticoid Deficiency

Addison disease
Adrenal hypoplasia
Congenital adrenal hyperplasia (21-hydroxylase and 3β-hydroxysteroid
    dehydrogenase deficiencies)
Pseudohypoaldosteronism types I and II
Hyporeninemic hypoaldosteronism
Aldosterone biosynthetic defects
Drug induced

Primary Defects in Aldosterone Biosynthesis: Aldosterone Synthase Deficiency

Before the characterization of the CYP11B2 gene, two diseases were recognized: *corticosterone methyl oxidase type I (CMO I) deficiency* and *corticosterone methyl oxidase type II (CMO II) deficiency*.[446] Subsequently, both variants were shown to be secondary to mutations in aldosterone synthase (CYP11B2), and they are now termed *aldosterone synthase deficiency, types I and II*.[447] Aldosterone synthase catalyzes the three terminal steps of aldosterone biosynthesis, 11β-hydroxylation of DOC to corticosterone, 18-hydroxylation to 18-hydroxycorticosterone, and 18-oxidation to aldosterone. Patients with type I aldosterone synthase deficiency have low to normal levels of 18-hydroxycorticosterone but undetectable levels of aldosterone (or urinary tetrahydroaldosterone), whereas patients with the type II variant have high levels of 18-hydroxycorticosterone and only subnormal or even normal levels of aldosterone. This suggests blockade of only the terminal 18-oxidation step, with some residual aldosterone synthase activity remaining. The explanation for the variable biochemical phenotype is unknown, particularly now that the same mutation in aldosterone synthase has been uncovered in both variants. It is possible that the phenotypic variation may reflect polymorphic variants in the residual and normal product of the CYP11B1 gene, 11β-hydroxylase.

Both variants are rare and are inherited as autosomal recessive traits.[447] Patients usually present in neonatal life with a salt-wasting crisis involving severe dehydration, vomiting, and failure to grow and thrive. Hyperkalemia, metabolic acidosis, dehydration, and hyponatremia are found. The plasma renin activity is elevated, and plasma aldosterone levels are low. Plasma 18-hydroxycorticosterone levels, the ratio of plasma 18-hydroxycorticosterone to aldosterone, and the levels of their urinary metabolites are used to differentiate the type I and II variants. In most infants, the disorders become less severe as the child ages; indeed, in older children, adolescents, and adults, the abnormal steroid pattern described may be present and may persist throughout life without clinical manifestations.

Patients with CYP11B2 deficiency typically respond well to 9α-fludrocortisone (starting dose, 150 µg/m² per day in neonates and infants) and may also benefit from salt supplementation. Patients with failure to grow and thrive usually show a good catch-up growth. Electrolytes often tend to normalize spontaneously between 3 and 4 years of age. However, untreated patients are at significant risk for being growth retarded, although spontaneous normalization of growth can occur. Adults are usually asymptomatic but are more susceptible to salt loss. Rarely, presentation is in adulthood.[448] Mineralocorticoid treatment in later life has to be established on an individual basis.

Postadrenalectomy Hypoaldosteronism

In a patient with a unilateral aldosteronoma (Conn syndrome), the contralateral ZG is frequently suppressed. Without reversal of the chronic volume expansion preoperatively, patients may develop severe hyperkalemia and hypotension lasting several days to several weeks after adrenalectomy. This effect may be exacerbated by the use of spironolactone preoperatively. Spironolactone has a long half-life and should be discontinued 2 to 3 days before surgery to minimize the risk of postoperative mineralocorticoid deficiency.

Defects in Aldosterone Action: Pseudohypoaldosteronism

Pseudohypoaldosteronism (PHA) is a rare, inherited salt-wasting disorder that was first described by Cheek and Perry in 1958 as a defective renal tubular response to mineralocorticoid in infancy. Patients present in the neonatal period with dehydration, hyponatremia, hypokalemia, metabolic acidosis, and failure to thrive despite normal glomerular filtration and normal renal and adrenal function.[449] Renin levels and plasma aldosterone are grossly elevated. When patients fail to respond to mineralocorticoid therapy, PHA is suspected as the underlying disorder.

PHA type I can be divided into two distinct disorders based on unique physiologic and genetic characteristics: the renal form of PHA, which is inherited as an autosomal dominant trait, and a generalized autosomal recessive form of PHA. The autosomal dominant form is usually less severe; the patient's condition often improves spontaneously within the first several years of life, allowing discontinuation of therapy. By contrast, the autosomal recessive form produces a multiorgan disorder, with mineralocorticoid resistance seen in the kidney, sweat and salivary glands, and the colonic mucosa. The condition does not spontaneously improve with age and is generally more severe than the autosomal dominant form.

The underlying basis for the autosomal dominant form of PHA is explained on the basis of inactivating mutations in the MR (hMR, NR3C2).[449,450] By contrast, inactivating mutations in the α-subunit and, to a lesser extent, in the β- and γ-subunits of the epithelial sodium channel (ENaC) account for the generalized autosomal recessive form of mineralocorticoid resistance.[451,452] (In effect, this represents the opposite of Liddle syndrome—see Chapter 16.) Generalized loss of ENaC activity leads to renal salt wasting (as seen in the renal form) in addition to recurrent respiratory infections and neonatal respiratory distress, cholelithiasis, and polyhydramnios.

PHA type I is resistant to mineralocorticoid therapy, so standard treatment involves supplementation with salt (2 to 8 g/day) in the form of sodium chloride and sodium bicarbonate as well as cation exchange resins. This supplementation usually corrects the patient's biochemical imbalance. However, if a patient shows signs of severe hyperkalemia, peritoneal dialysis may be necessary. Hypercalciuria has been reported in some cases of PHA-I. The recommended course of treatment for these patients usually involves indomethacin or hydrochlorothiazide. Indomethacin is thought to act by causing a reduction in the glomerular filtration rate or an inhibition of the effect of prostaglandin E_2 on renal tubules. Indomethacin has been shown to reduce polyuria, sodium loss, and hypercalciuria. Hydrochlorothiazide has been used to diminish hyperkalemia and reduce hypercalciuria in patients with PHA-I.

In patients with the autosomal dominant or renal form of PHA-I, the signs and symptoms of PHA decrease with age; nevertheless, these patients usually require salt supplementation for the first 2 to 3 years of life. In patients with the autosomal recessive or multiorgan type of PHA-I, resistance to therapy with sodium chloride or drugs that decrease serum potassium concentrations often occurs and may even lead to death in infancy from hyperkalemia. PHA-I patients with multiorgan involvement often require very high amounts of salt in their diet (up to 45 g NaCl per day). Carbenoxolone, a derivative of glycyrrhetinic acid in licorice, has been used with moderate success in helping to reduce the high levels of dietary salt needed by renal PHA-I patients. Carbenoxolone acts by inhibiting

HSD11B2 activity and allows unmetabolized cortisol to bind to and activate MRs in a manner similar to that of aldosterone.[453] It was found to be ineffective in patients with multiorgan PHA-I.

Two other variants of PHA have been described—types II and III. Type II PHA, or Gordon syndrome, is in retrospect a misnomer. Patients with Gordon syndrome share some of the features of patients with PHA-I, notably hyperkalemia and metabolic acidosis, but they exhibit salt retention with mild hypertension and suppressed plasma renin activity rather than salt wasting. The condition is explained by mutations in a serine threonine kinase family (WNK1 and WNK4) that result in increased expression of these proteins with activation of the thiazide-sensitive sodium chloride cotransporter in the cortical and medullary collecting ducts.[454] The condition represents the exact opposite of Gitelman syndrome but is not a true form of PHA.

Type III PHA is an acquired and usually transient form of mineralocorticoid resistance seen in patients with underlying renal diseases including obstruction and infection and in patients with excessive loss of salt through the gut or skin. Reduced glomerular filtration rate is a hallmark of the condition. The cause is unknown, although increased transforming growth factor-β–mediated aldosterone resistance has been suggested to be an underlying factor.

Hyporeninemic Hypoaldosteronism

Angiotensin II is a key stimulus to aldosterone secretion, and damage or blockade of the renin-angiotensin system may result in mineralocorticoid deficiency. Various renal diseases have been associated with damage to the juxtaglomerular apparatus and subsequent renin deficiency. These include systemic lupus erythematosus, myeloma, amyloid, AIDS, and damage related to use of nonsteroidal anti-inflammatory drugs, but the most common (>75% of cases) is diabetic nephropathy.[455,456]

The usual picture is that of an elderly patient with hyperkalemia, acidosis, and mild to moderate impairment of renal function. Plasma renin activity and aldosterone levels are low and fail to respond to sodium depletion, erect posture, or furosemide administration. In contrast to adrenal insufficiency, patients have normal or elevated blood pressure and no postural hypotension. Muscle weakness and cardiac arrhythmias may also occur. Other factors may contribute to the hyperkalemia, including the use of potassium-sparing diuretics, potassium supplementation, insulin deficiency, and use of β-adrenoceptor blocking drugs or prostaglandin synthetase inhibitors, which inhibit renin release.

Treatment of primary renin deficiency is with fludrocortisone in the first instance together with dietary potassium restriction. However, these patients are not salt depleted and may become hypertensive with fludrocortisone. In such a scenario, the addition of a loop-acting diuretic such as furosemide is appropriate. This will increase acid excretion and improve the metabolic acidosis.

ADRENAL ADENOMAS, INCIDENTALOMAS, AND CARCINOMAS

Adenomas

Cortisol-secreting adrenal adenomas were discussed earlier, and aldosterone-secreting adenomas (Conn syndrome) are discussed in Chapter 16. Pure virilizing benign adrenal adenomas are rare, with approximately 50 cases reported in the literature. Most cases occur in women; in males, the disorder is restricted to childhood, when presentation is with sexual precocity and accelerated bone age. Such tumors have to be considered in the differential diagnosis of CAH in patients presenting during childhood. In females, most patients present before menopause with marked hirsutism, deepening of the voice, and amenorrhea. Clitoromegaly is found in 80% of cases. Testosterone is usually strikingly elevated, but gonadotropin levels may not be suppressed. By definition, urinary free cortisol is normal. Tumors vary in size and should be treated surgically. Postoperatively, clinical features invariably improve, and normal menses return.[457]

Incidentalomas

Autopsy series had defined the prevalence of adrenal adenomas greater than 1 cm in diameter to be between 1.5% and 7% before the advent of high-resolution imaging procedures such as CT and MRI; since that time, incidentally discovered adrenal masses have become a common clinical problem. An adrenal mass is uncovered in up to 4% of patients imaged for nonadrenal disease.[458] Incidentalomas are uncommon in patients younger than 30 years of age but increase in frequency with age; they occur equally in males and females, most commonly in the sixth and seventh decades. Clinically, two issues arise: whether the lesion is functional (i.e., secreting hormones) and whether it is malignant. Most incidentalomas are adrenocortical adenomas, but occasionally they represent myelolipomas, hamartomas, or granulomatous infiltrations of the adrenal gland and result in a characteristic CT/MRI appearance (Fig. 15-40). Functioning tumors (pheochromocytomas and those secreting cortisol, aldosterone, or sex steroids) and carcinomas account for around 4% of all incidentalomas. In addition, it is established that some incidentalomas cause abnormal hormone secretion without obvious clinical manifestations of a hormone excess state. The best example is so-called subclinical Cushing syndrome, which occurs in up to 20% to 30% of all cases.[458-460] There is debate as to the best means to biochemically define this phenomenon, but serum cortisol after dexamethasone testing has the widest acceptance, although cutoff values vary. When there is evidence of low-grade excess biochemical hypercortisolism there is an associated increase in the prevalence of diabetes, obesity, hypertension, new cardiovascular

events, osteoporosis, and fatality. However, no prospective study has proved that the adrenal adenoma is the cause of the observed complications, as these are highly prevalent in the population at this age. Intervention by adrenalectomy has shown some benefit, but the studies performed have been retrospective and highly selected, and hence the approach to each patient needs individualization with most being observed in current clinical practice.

As a result, all patients with incidentally discovered adrenal masses should undergo appropriate endocrine screening tests. This testing should comprise 24-hour urinary catecholamine collection or measurement of plasma metanephrines, 24-hour urinary free cortisol (or a midnight salivary cortisol level), and overnight dexamethasone suppression tests. Because of the reported poor sensitivity of serum potassium measurements in detecting primary aldosteronism, circulating levels of plasma renin activity and aldosterone are required in hypertensive patients. DHEAS should be measured as a marker of adrenal androgen secretion. Low levels may occur in patients with suppressed ACTH concentrations due to autonomous cortisol secretion from the adenoma.[461] Some studies have also documented high levels of 17-OHP after ACTH stimulation tests, suggesting partial defects in 21-hydroxylase in some tumors.

The possibility of malignancy should be considered in each case. In patients with a known extra-adrenal primary tumor, the incidence of malignancy is obviously much higher; for example, up to 20% of patients with lung cancer have adrenal metastases on CT scanning. In those with no evidence of malignancy, adrenal carcinoma is rare; in one study, only 26 of 630 incidentalomas were found to be adrenal carcinomas.[458] Many studies contain a positive bias, and true risk of malignancy may be much lower.[462] In true incidentalomas, size appears to be predictive of malignancy: fewer than 2% of incidentalomas smaller than 4 cm but 25% of those larger than 6 cm in diameter are malignant (Fig. 15-41).[463] Smooth, homogeneous adenomas on an enhanced adrenal scan with a Hounsfield unit score (a marker of radiodensity) less than 10 HU are invariably benign; malignancy is suspected in irregular, inhomogeneous adenomas with a score greater than 20 HU. On this background, adrenalectomy is indicated for functional tumors and for tumors larger than 4 cm in diameter. Repeat CT scanning in patients with smaller tumors can be used to guide management, but development of functional

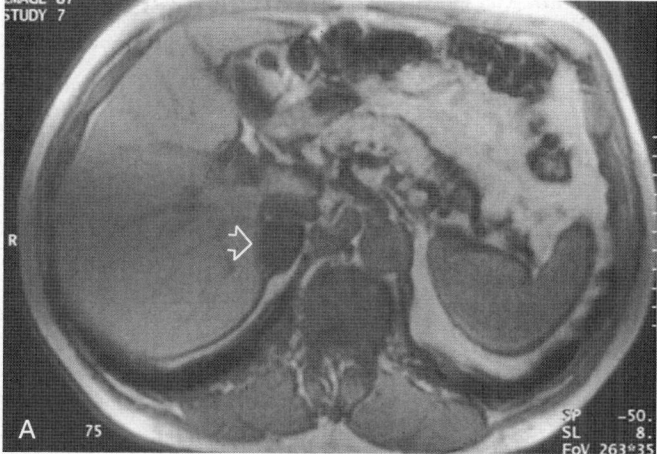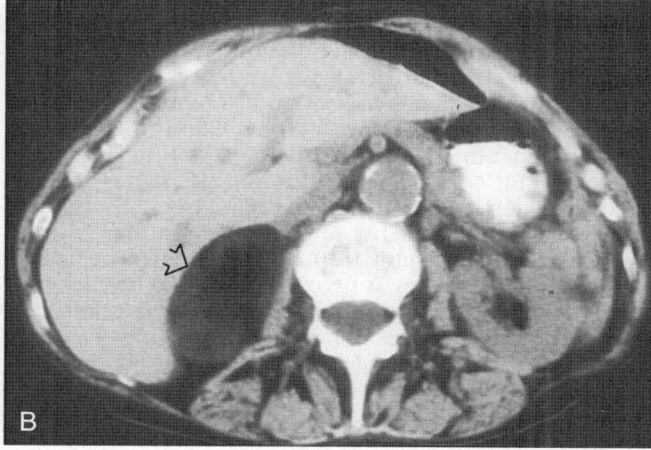

Figure 15-40 A, Adrenal incidentaloma *(arrow)* discovered in a woman undergoing investigation for abdominal pain. **B,** Incidentally discovered right adrenal myelolipoma *(arrow).*

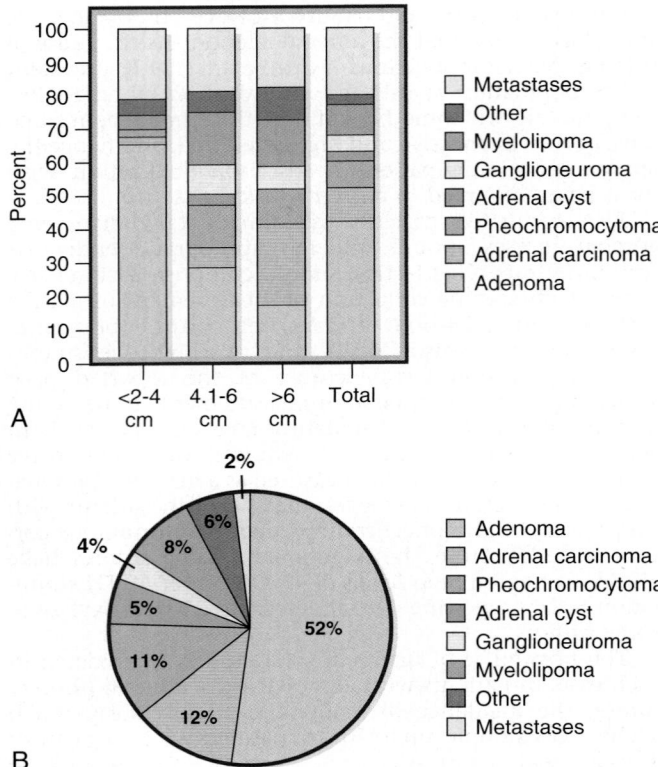

Figure 15-41 Distribution of diagnosis of adrenal incidentalomas. **A,** Data from eight studies with histologically determined diagnoses (*n* = 103) relating to tumor size. **B,** Distribution of 380 incidental adrenal masses by histologic diagnosis. (From Mansmann G, Lau L, Balk E, et al. The clinically inapparent adrenal mass: update in diagnosis and management. *Endocr Rev.* 2004;25:309-340.)

autonomy is very rare, and patients may be discharged if tumors are static. Laparoscopic adrenalectomy is the treatment of choice, offering shorter hospital stays and reduced operative complications (e.g., blood loss, morbidity) compared with open adrenalectomy. The possible exception is the patient with highly suggestive adrenal carcinoma, because breach of the tumor capsule is associated with a poorer outcome. Adequate preparation and close endocrine supervision perioperatively and postoperatively are required for functional tumors.

Carcinomas

Primary adrenal carcinoma is very rare, with an annual incidence of 1 per 1 million population. Women are more commonly affected than men, with a ratio of 2.5:1. The mean age at onset is between 40 and 50 years, although men tend to be older at presentation. Eighty percent of tumors are functional, most commonly secreting glucocorticoids alone (45%), glucocorticoids and androgens (45%), or androgens alone (10%). Fewer than 1% of all tumors secrete aldosterone. Patients present with features of the hormone excess state (glucocorticoid, androgen, or both) but abdominal pain, weight loss, anorexia, and fever occur in 25% of cases. An abdominal mass may be palpable. Current treatment choices for what is often an aggressive tumor are poor. Surgery offers the only chance of cure for patients with local disease, but metastatic spread is evident in 75% of cases at presentation. Radiotherapy is ineffective, as are most chemotherapeutic regimens. Mitotane in high doses offers benefit in reducing tumor growth[284] and in controlling hormonal hypersecretion in 75% of cases.[283]

Overall, the prognosis is poor, with 5-year survival rates of less than 20%. Newer chemotherapies are being evaluated.[285]

Etiology of Adrenal Tumors

Other than the factors discussed under adrenal Cushing syndrome, the underlying basis for adrenal tumorigenesis is unknown. Clonal analysis suggests progression from a normal to an adenomatous to a carcinomatous lesion, but the molecular pathways involved remain obscure. Several factors have been associated with malignant transformation, including the genes encoding p53, p57 cyclin-dependent kinase, menin, IGF-2, MC2R, and inhibin-α.[464] Mice lacking the inhibin-α gene develop adrenal tumors through a process that is also gonadotropin dependent.[465]

ACKNOWLEDGMENTS

Acknowledgment is given to Professor W. Arlt, Dr. M.S. Cooper, Dr. J.W. Tomlinson, and Dr. W. Young for assistance with parts of this chapter.

REFERENCES

1. Eustachius B. *Tabulae Anatomicae*. In: Lancisi JM, ed. Amsterdam: R. & G. Wetstenios; 1774.
2. Addison T. *On the Constitutional and Local Effects of Disease of the Supra-Renal Capsules*. London: Highley; 1866.
3. Brown-Sequard CE. Recherches experimentales sur la physiologie et la pathologie des capsules surrenales. *Arch Gen Med.* 1856;5:385-401.
4. Medvei VC. *A History of Clinical Endocrinology*. Pearl River, NY: Parthenon; 1993.
5. Hench PS, Kendall EC, Slocumb CH, et al. The effect of a hormone of the adrenal cortex (17-hydroxy-11-dehydrocorticosterone; compound E) and of pituitary adrenocorticotropic hormone on rheumatoid arthritis. *Mayo Clin Proc.* 1949;24:181-197.
6. Simpson SA, Tait JF. Recent progress in methods of isolation, chemistry, and physiology of aldosterone. *Recent Prog Horm Res.* 1955;11:183-210.
7. Li CH, Evans HM, Simpson ME. Adrenocorticotrophic hormone. *J Biol Chem.* 1943;149:413-424.
8. Cushing H. The basophil adenomas of the pituitary body and their clinical manifestations (pituitary basophilism). *Bull Johns Hopkins Hosp.* 1932;50:137-195.
9. Vale W, Spiess J, Rivier C, et al. Characterization of a 41-residue ovine hypothalamic peptide that stimulates secretion of corticotropin and β-endorphin. *Science.* 1981;213:1394-1397.
10. Conn JW. Primary aldosteronism, a new clinical syndrome. *J Lab Clin Med.* 1955;45:3-17.
11. Else T, Hammer GD. Genetic analysis of adrenal absence: agenesis and aplasia. *Trends Endocrinol Metab.* 2005;16:458.
12. Mesiano S, Jaffe RB. Developmental and functional biology of the primate fetal adrenal cortex. *Endocr Rev.* 1997;18:378-403.
13. Jaffe RB, Mesiano S, Smith R, et al. The regulation and role of fetal adrenal development in human pregnancy. *Endocr Res.* 1998;24:919-926.
14. Okamoto M, Takemori H. Differentiation and zonation of the adrenal cortex. *Curr Opin Endocrinol Diab.* 2000;7:122-127.
15. Luo X, Ikeda Y, Parker KL. A cell-specific nuclear receptor is essential for adrenal and gonadal development and sexual differentiation. *Cell.* 1994;77:481-490.
16. Havelock JC, Auchus RJ, Rainey WE. The rise in adrenal androgen biosynthesis: adrenarche. *Semin Reprod Med.* 2004;22:337-347.
17. Remer T, Boye KR, Hartmann MF, et al. Urinary markers of adrenarche: reference values in healthy subjects, aged 3-18 years. *J Clin Endocrinol Metab.* 2005;90:2015-2021.
18. IUPAC Commission on the Nomenclature of Organic Chemistry (CNOC) and IUPAC-IUB Commission on Biochemical Nomenclature (CBN). Definitive rules for the nomenclature of steroids. *Pure Appl Chem.* 1972;31:285-322.
19. Gwynne JT, Strauss JF 3rd. The role of lipoproteins in steroidogenesis and cholesterol metabolism in steroidogenic glands. *Endocr Rev.* 1982;3:299-329.
20. Faust JR, Goldstein JL, Brown MS. Receptor-mediated uptake of low density lipoprotein and utilization of its cholesterol for steroid synthesis in cultured mouse adrenal cells. *J Biol Chem.* 1977;252:4861-4871.

21. Goldstein JL, Anderson RG, Brown MS. Coated pits, coated vesicles, and receptor-mediated endocytosis. *Nature.* 1979;279:679-685.

22. Landschulz KT, Pathak RK, Rigotti A, et al. Regulation of scavenger receptor, class B, type I, a high density lipoprotein receptor, in liver and steroidogenic tissues of the rat. *J Clin Invest.* 1996;98:984-995.

23. Stocco DM, Clark BJ. Regulation of the acute production of steroids in steroidogenic cells. *Endocr Rev.* 1996;17:221-244.

24. Amri H, Li H, Culty M, et al. The peripheral-type benzodiazepine receptor and adrenal steroidogenesis. *Curr Opin Endocrinol Diabetes.* 1999;6:179-184.

25. Bernhardt R. The role of adrenodoxin in adrenal steroidogenesis. *Curr Opin Endocrinol Diabetes.* 2000;7:109-115.

26. Miller WL. Minireview: regulation of steroidogenesis by electron transfer. *Endocrinology.* 2005;146:2544-2550.

27. Payne AH, Hales DB. Overview of steroidogenic enzymes in the pathway from cholesterol to active steroid hormones. *Endocr Rev.* 2004;25:947-970.

28. Onoda M, Hall PF. Cytochrome b5 stimulates purified testicular microsomal cytochrome P-450 (C21 side-chain cleavage). *Biochem Biophys Res Commun.* 1982;108:454-460.

29. Miller WL. Molecular biology of steroid hormone synthesis. *Endocr Rev.* 1988;9:295-318.

30. John ME, John MC, Ashley P, et al. Identification and characterization of cDNA clones specific for cholesterol side-chain cleavage cytochrome P-450. *Proc Natl Acad Sci U S A.* 1984;81:5628-5632.

31. Lorence MC, Murry BA, Trant JM, et al. Human 3 β-hydroxysteroid dehydrogenase/delta 5-4 isomerase from placenta: expression in nonsteroidogenic cells of a protein that catalyzes the dehydrogenation/isomerization of C21 and C19 steroids. *Endocrinology.* 1990;126:2493-2498.

32. Bradshaw KD, Waterman MR, Couch RT, et al. Characterization of complementary deoxyribonucleic acid for human adrenocortical 17 alpha-hydroxylase: a probe for analysis of 17 alpha-hydroxylase deficiency. *Mol Endocrinol.* 1987;1:348-354.

33. Nakamura Y, Hornsby PJ, Casson P, et al. Type 5 17β-hydroxysteroid dehydrogenase (AKR1C3) contributes to testosterone production in the adrenal reticularis. *J Clin Endocrinol Metab.* 2009;94:2192-2198.

34. White PC, New MI, Dupont B. Cloning and expression of cDNA encoding a bovine adrenal cytochrome P-450 specific for steroid 21-hydroxylation. *Proc Natl Acad Sci U S A.* 1984;81:1986-1990.

35. Chua SC, Szabo P, Vitek A, et al. Cloning of cDNA encoding steroid 11 β-hydroxylase (P450c11). *Proc Natl Acad Sci U S A.* 1987;84:7193-7197.

36. Mornet E, Dupont J, Vitek A, et al. Characterization of two genes encoding human steroid 11 β-hydroxylase (P-450(11) β). *J Biol Chem.* 1989;264:20961-20967.

37. Curnow KM, Tusie-Luna MT, Pascoe L, et al. The product of the CYP11B2 gene is required for aldosterone biosynthesis in the human adrenal cortex. *Mol Endocrinol.* 1991;5:1513-1522.

38. Strott CA. Sulfonation and molecular action. *Endocr Rev.* 2002;23:703-732.

39. Siiteri PK, MacDonald PC. The utilization of dehydroisoandrosterone sulphate for estrogen synthesis during human pregnancy. *Steroids.* 1963;2:713-730.

40. Lamolet B, Pulichino AM, Lamonerie T, et al. A pituitary cell-restricted T box factor, Tpit, activates POMC transcription in cooperation with Pitx homeoproteins. *Cell.* 2001;104:849-859.

41. Smith AI, Funder JW. Proopiomelanocortin processing in the pituitary, central nervous system, and peripheral tissues. *Endocr Rev.* 1988;9:159-179.

42. Donald RA. ACTH and related peptides. *Clin Endocrinol (Oxf).* 1980;12:491-524.

43. Bicknell AB, Lomthaisong K, Woods RJ, et al. Characterization of a serine protease that cleaves pro-gamma-melanotropin at the adrenal to stimulate growth. *Cell.* 2001;105:903-912.

44. Suzuki I, Cone RD, Im S, et al. Binding of melanotropic hormones to the melanocortin receptor MC1R on human melanocytes stimulates proliferation and melanogenesis. *Endocrinology.* 1996;137:1627-1633.

45. DeBold CR, Nicholson WE, Orth DN. Immunoreactive proopiomelanocortin (POMC) peptides and POMC-like messenger ribonucleic acid are present in many rat nonpituitary tissues. *Endocrinology.* 1988;122:2648-2657.

46. de Keyzer Y, Lenne F, Massias JF, et al. Pituitary-like proopiomelanocortin transcripts in human Leydig cell tumors. *J Clin Invest.* 1990;86:871-877.

47. Clark AJ, Lavender PM, Coates P, et al. In vitro and in vivo analysis of the processing and fate of the peptide products of the short proopiomelanocortin mRNA. *Mol Endocrinol.* 1990;4:1737-1743.

48. de Keyzer Y, Bertagna X, Luton JP, et al. Variable modes of proopiomelanocortin gene transcription in human tumors. *Mol Endocrinol.* 1989;3:215-223.

49. Clark AJ, Lavender PM, Besser GM, et al. Pro-opiomelanocortin mRNA size heterogeneity in ACTH-dependent Cushing's syndrome. *J Mol Endocrinol.* 1989;2:3-9.

50. Picon A, Bertagna X, de Keyzer Y. Analysis of the human proopiomelanocortin gene promoter in a small cell lung carcinoma cell line reveals an unusual role for E2F transcription factors. *Oncogene.* 1999;18:2627-2633.

51. Newell-Price J, King P, Clark AJ. The CpG island promoter of the human proopiomelanocortin gene is methylated in nonexpressing normal tissue and tumors and represses expression. *Mol Endocrinol.* 2001;15:338-348.

52. Zhou A, Bloomquist BT, Mains RE. The prohormone convertases PC1 and PC2 mediate distinct endoproteolytic cleavages in a strict temporal order during proopiomelanocortin biosynthetic processing. *J Biol Chem.* 1993;268:1763-1769.

53. Stewart PM, Gibson S, Crosby SR, et al. ACTH precursors characterize the ectopic ACTH syndrome. *Clin Endocrinol (Oxf).* 1994;40:199-204.

54. Oliver RL, Davis JR, White A. Characterisation of ACTH related peptides in ectopic Cushing's syndrome. *Pituitary.* 2003;6:119-126.

55. Coll AP, Farooqi IS, Challis BG, et al. Proopiomelanocortin and energy balance: insights from human and murine genetics. *J Clin Endocrinol Metab.* 2004;89:2557-2562.

56. Lundblad JR, Roberts JL. Regulation of proopiomelanocortin gene expression in pituitary. *Endocr Rev.* 1988;9:135-158.

57. Orth DN. Corticotropin-releasing hormone in humans. *Endocr Rev.* 1992;13:164-191.

58. Taylor AL, Fishman LM. Corticotropin-releasing hormone. *N Engl J Med.* 1988;319:213-222.

59. Antoni FA. Hypothalamic control of adrenocorticotropin secretion: advances since the discovery of 41-residue corticotropin-releasing factor. *Endocr Rev.* 1986;7:351-378.

60. Shibahara S, Morimoto Y, Furutani Y, et al. Isolation and sequence analysis of the human corticotropin-releasing factor precursor gene. *EMBO J.* 1983;2:775-779.

61. Furutani Y, Morimoto Y, Shibahara S, et al. Cloning and sequence analysis of cDNA for ovine corticotropin-releasing factor precursor. *Nature.* 1983;301:537-540.

62. Chen R, Lewis KA, Perrin MH, et al. Expression cloning of a human corticotropin-releasing-factor receptor. *Proc Natl Acad Sci U S A.* 1993;90:8967-8971.

63. Sasaki A, Sato S, Murakami O, et al. Immunoreactive corticotropin-releasing hormone present in human plasma may be derived from both hypothalamic and extrahypothalamic sources. *J Clin Endocrinol Metab.* 1987;65:176-182.

64. Campbell EA, Linton EA, Wolfe CD, et al. Plasma corticotropin-releasing hormone concentrations during pregnancy and parturition. *J Clin Endocrinol Metab.* 1987;64:1054-1059.

65. Linton EA, Wolfe CD, Behan DP, et al. A specific carrier substance for human corticotrophin releasing factor in late gestational maternal plasma which could mask the ACTH-releasing activity. *Clin Endocrinol (Oxf).* 1988;28:315-324.

66. Rivier C, Rivier J, Vale W. Inhibition of adrenocorticotropic hormone secretion in the rat by immunoneutralization of corticotropin-releasing factor. *Science.* 1982;218:377-379.

67. Hauger RL, Aguilera G. Regulation of pituitary corticotropin releasing hormone (CRH) receptors by CRH: interaction with vasopressin. *Endocrinology.* 1993;133:1708-1714.

68. Watanabe T, Oki Y, Orth DN. Kinetic actions and interactions of arginine vasopressin, angiotensin-II, and oxytocin on adrenocorticotropin secretion by rat anterior pituitary cells in the microperifusion system. *Endocrinology.* 1989;125:1921-1931.

69. Bateman A, Singh A, Kral T, et al. The immune-hypothalamic-pituitary-adrenal axis. *Endocr Rev.* 1989;10:92-112.

70. Chrousos GP. The hypothalamic-pituitary-adrenal axis and immune-mediated inflammation. *N Engl J Med.* 1995;332:1351-1362.

71. Ray DW, Ren SG, Melmed S. Leukemia inhibitory factor (LIF) stimulates proopiomelanocortin (POMC) expression in a corticotroph cell line: role of STAT pathway. *J Clin Invest.* 1996;97:1852-1859.

72. Udelsman R, Norton JA, Jelenich SE, et al. Responses of the hypothalamic-pituitary-adrenal and renin-angiotensin axes and the sympathetic system during controlled surgical and anesthetic stress. *J Clin Endocrinol Metab.* 1987;64:986-994.

73. Vaughan GM, Becker RA, Allen JP, et al. Cortisol and corticotrophin in burned patients. *J Trauma.* 1982;22:263-273.

74. Fish HR, Chernow B, O'Brian JT. Endocrine and neurophysiologic responses of the pituitary to insulin-induced hypoglycemia: a review. *Metabolism.* 1986;35:763-780.

75. Luger A, Deuster PA, Kyle SB, et al. Acute hypothalamic-pituitary-adrenal responses to the stress of treadmill exercise: physiologic adaptations to physical training. *N Engl J Med.* 1987;316:1309-1315.

76. Aguilera G. Regulation of pituitary ACTH secretion during chronic stress. *Front Neuroendocrinol.* 1994;15:321-350.

77. Weitzman ED, Fukushima D, Nogeire C, et al. Twenty-four hour pattern of the episodic secretion of cortisol in normal subjects. *J Clin Endocrinol Metab.* 1971;33:14-22.

78. Veldhuis JD, Iranmanesh A, Johnson ML, et al. Amplitude, but not frequency, modulation of adrenocorticotropin secretory bursts gives rise to the nyctohemeral rhythm of the corticotropic axis in man. *J Clin Endocrinol Metab.* 1990;71:452-463.

79. Horrocks PM, Jones AF, Ratcliffe WA, et al. Patterns of ACTH and cortisol pulsatility over twenty-four hours in normal males and females. *Clin Endocrinol (Oxf).* 1990;32:127-134.
80. Walker JJ, Spiga F, Waite E, et al. The origin of glucocorticoid hormone oscillations. *PLoS Biol.* 2012;10(6):e1001341.
81. Boivin DB, Duffy JF, Kronauer RE, et al. Dose-response relationships for resetting of human circadian clock by light. *Nature.* 1996;379:540-542.
82. Czeisler CA, Dumont M, Duffy JF, et al. Association of sleep-wake habits in older people with changes in output of circadian pacemaker. *Lancet.* 1992;340:933-936.
83. Desir D, Van Cauter E, Fang VS, et al. Effects of "jet lag" on hormonal patterns: I. Procedures, variations in total plasma proteins, and disruption of adrenocorticotropin-cortisol periodicity. *J Clin Endocrinol Metab.* 1981;52:628-641.
84. Davis LG, Arentzen R, Reid JM, et al. Glucocorticoid sensitivity of vasopressin mRNA levels in the paraventricular nucleus of the rat. *Proc Natl Acad Sci U S A.* 1986;83:1145-1149.
85. Keller-Wood ME, Dallman MF. Corticosteroid inhibition of ACTH secretion. *Endocr Rev.* 1984;5:1-24.
86. Buckingham JC, John CD, Solito E, et al. Annexin 1, glucocorticoids, and the neuroendocrine-immune interface. *Ann N Y Acad Sci.* 2006;1088:396-409.
87. Lamberts SW, Koper JW, Biemond P, et al. Cortisol receptor resistance: the variability of its clinical presentation and response to treatment. *J Clin Endocrinol Metab.* 1992;74:313-321.
88. Cole TJ, Blendy JA, Monaghan AP, et al. Targeted disruption of the glucocorticoid receptor gene blocks adrenergic chromaffin cell development and severely retards lung maturation. *Genes Dev.* 1995;9:1608-1621.
89. Mountjoy KG, Robbins LS, Mortrud MT, et al. The cloning of a family of genes that encode the melanocortin receptors. *Science.* 1992;257:1248-1251.
90. Metherell LA, Chapple JP, Cooray S, et al. Mutations in MRAP, encoding a new interacting partner of the ACTH receptor, cause familial glucocorticoid deficiency type 2. *Nat Genet.* 2005;37:166-170.
91. Clark AJ, Chan LF, Chung TT, et al. The genetics of familial glucocorticoid deficiency. *Best Pract Res Clin Endocrinol Metab.* 2009;23:159-165.
92. Cooke BA. Signal transduction involving cyclic AMP-dependent and cyclic AMP-independent mechanisms in the control of steroidogenesis. *Mol Cell Endocrinol.* 1999;151:25-35.
93. Enyeart JJ, Mlinar B, Enyeart JA. T-type Ca^{2+} channels are required for adrenocorticotropin-stimulated cortisol production by bovine adrenal zona fasciculata cells. *Mol Endocrinol.* 1993;7:1031-1040.
94. Ehrhart-Bornstein M, Hinson JP, Bornstein SR, et al. Intraadrenal interactions in the regulation of adrenocortical steroidogenesis. *Endocr Rev.* 1998;19:101-143.
95. Munari-Silem Y, Lebrethon MC, Morand I, et al. Gap junction-mediated cell-to-cell communication in bovine and human adrenal cells. A process whereby cells increase their responsiveness to physiological corticotropin concentrations. *J Clin Invest.* 1995;95:1429-1439.
96. Simpson ER, Waterman MR. Regulation of the synthesis of steroidogenic enzymes in adrenal cortical cells by ACTH. *Annu Rev Physiol.* 1988;50:427-440.
97. Waterman MR, Bischof LJ. Cytochromes P450 12: diversity of ACTH (cAMP)-dependent transcription of bovine steroid hydroxylase genes. *FASEB J.* 1997;11:419-427.
98. Rainey WE. Adrenal zonation: clues from 11β-hydroxylase and aldosterone synthase. *Mol Cell Endocrinol.* 1999;151:151-160.
99. Longcope C. Adrenal and gonadal androgen secretion in normal females. *Clin Endocrinol Metab.* 1986;15:213-228.
100. Labrie F, Belanger A, Simard J, et al. DHEA and peripheral androgen and estrogen formation: intracinology. *Ann N Y Acad Sci.* 1995;774:16-28.
101. Liu D, Dillon JS. Dehydroepiandrosterone activates endothelial cell nitric-oxide synthase by a specific plasma membrane receptor coupled to Galpha(i2,3). *J Biol Chem.* 2002;277:21379-21388.
102. Hammer F, Subtil S, Lux P, et al. No evidence for hepatic conversion of dehydroepiandrosterone (DHEA) sulfate to DHEA: in vivo and in vitro studies. *J Clin Endocrinol Metab.* 2005;90:3600-3605.
103. McKenna TJ, Fearon U, Clarke D, et al. A critical review of the origin and control of adrenal androgens. *Baillieres Clin Obstet Gynaecol.* 1997;11:229-248.
104. Weinberger C, Hollenberg SM, Rosenfeld MG, et al. Domain structure of human glucocorticoid receptor and its relationship to the v-erb-A oncogene product. *Nature.* 1985;318:670-672.
105. Arriza JL, Weinberger C, Cerelli G, et al. Cloning of human mineralocorticoid receptor complementary DNA: structural and functional kinship with the glucocorticoid receptor. *Science.* 1987;237:268-275.
106. Gustafsson JA, Carlstedt-Duke J, Poellinger L, et al. Biochemistry, molecular biology, and physiology of the glucocorticoid receptor. *Endocr Rev.* 1987;8:185-234.
107. Zhou J, Cidlowski JA. The human glucocorticoid receptor: one gene, multiple proteins and diverse responses. *Steroids.* 2005;70:407-417.
108. Pascual-Le Tallec L, Lombes M. The mineralocorticoid receptor: a journey exploring its diversity and specificity of action. *Mol Endocrinol.* 2005;19:2211-2221.
109. Pratt WB. The role of heat shock proteins in regulating the function, folding, and trafficking of the glucocorticoid receptor. *J Biol Chem.* 1993;268:21455-21458.
110. Beato M, Sanchez-Pacheco A. Interaction of steroid hormone receptors with the transcription initiation complex. *Endocr Rev.* 1996;17:587-609.
111. Bamberger CM, Schulte HM, Chrousos GP. Molecular determinants of glucocorticoid receptor function and tissue sensitivity to glucocorticoids. *Endocr Rev.* 1996;17:245-261.
112. McKenna NJ, Lanz RB, O'Malley BW. Nuclear receptor coregulators: cellular and molecular biology. *Endocr Rev.* 1999;20:321-344.
113. Rhen T, Cidlowski JA. Antiinflammatory action of glucocorticoids: new mechanisms for old drugs. *N Engl J Med.* 2005;353:1711-1723.
114. Schule R, Rangarajan P, Kliewer S, et al. Functional antagonism between oncoprotein c-Jun and the glucocorticoid receptor. *Cell.* 1990;62:1217-1226.
115. McKay LI, Cidlowski JA. Molecular control of immune/inflammatory responses: interactions between nuclear factor-kappa B and steroid receptor-signaling pathways. *Endocr Rev.* 1999;20:435-459.
116. Funder JW. Aldosterone action. *Annu Rev Physiol.* 1993;55:115-130.
117. Rossier BC, Alpern RJ. Cell and molecular biology of epithelial transport. *Curr Opin Nephrol Hypertens.* 1999;8:579-580.
118. Verrey F, Kraehenbuhl JP, Rossier BC. Aldosterone induces a rapid increase in the rate of Na,K-ATPase gene transcription in cultured kidney cells. *Mol Endocrinol.* 1989;3:1369-1376.
119. Chen SY, Bhargava A, Mastroberardino L, et al. Epithelial sodium channel regulated by aldosterone-induced protein sgk. *Proc Natl Acad Sci U S A.* 1999;96:2514-2519.
120. Edwards CR, Stewart PM, Burt D, et al. Localisation of 11 β-hydroxysteroid dehydrogenase: tissue specific protector of the mineralocorticoid receptor. *Lancet.* 1988;2:986-989.
121. Funder JW, Pearce PT, Smith R, et al. Mineralocorticoid action: target tissue specificity is enzyme, not receptor, mediated. *Science.* 1988;242:583-585.
122. Funder JW. New biology of aldosterone, and experimental studies on the selective aldosterone blocker eplerenone. *Am Heart J.* 2002;144:S8-S11.
123. Iwasaki Y, Aoki Y, Katahira M, et al. Non-genomic mechanisms of glucocorticoid inhibition of adrenocorticotropin secretion: possible involvement of GTP-binding protein. *Biochem Biophys Res Commun.* 1997;235:295-299.
124. Funder JW. The nongenomic actions of aldosterone. *Endocr Rev.* 2005;26:313-321.
125. Hammond GL. Molecular properties of corticosteroid binding globulin and the sex-steroid binding proteins. *Endocr Rev.* 1990;11:65-79.
126. Roitman A, Bruchis S, Bauman B, et al. Total deficiency of corticosteroid-binding globulin. *Clin Endocrinol (Oxf).* 1984;21:541-548.
127. Smith CL, Power SG, Hammond GL. A Leu-His substitution at residue 93 in human corticosteroid binding globulin results in reduced affinity for cortisol. *J Steroid Biochem Mol Biol.* 1992;42:671-676.
128. Fukushima DK, Bradlow HL, Hellman L, et al. Metabolic transformation of hydrocortisone-4-C14 in normal men. *J Biol Chem.* 1960;235:2246-2252.
129. White PC, Mune T, Agarwal AK. 11β-Hydroxysteroid dehydrogenase and the syndrome of apparent mineralocorticoid excess. *Endocr Rev.* 1997;18:135-156.
130. Tomlinson JW, Walker EA, Bujalska IJ, et al. 11β-Hydroxysteroid dehydrogenase type 1: a tissue-specific regulator of glucocorticoid response. *Endocr Rev.* 2004;25:831-866.
131. Quinkler M, Stewart PM. Hypertension and the cortisol-cortisone shuttle. *J Clin Endocrinol Metab.* 2003;88:2384-2392.
132. Moore JS, Monson JP, Kaltsas G, et al. Modulation of 11β-hydroxysteroid dehydrogenase isozymes by growth hormone and insulin-like growth factor: in vivo and in vitro studies. *J Clin Endocrinol Metab.* 1999;84:4172-4177.
133. Voccia E, Saenger P, Peterson RE, et al. 6β-Hydroxycortisol excretion in hypercortisolemic states. *J Clin Endocrinol Metab.* 1979;48:467-471.
134. Yamada S, Iwai K. Induction of hepatic cortisol-6-hydroxylase by rifampicin (Letter). *Lancet.* 1976;2:366-367.
135. Whitworth JA, Stewart PM, Burt D, et al. The kidney is the major site of cortisone production in man. *Clin Endocrinol (Oxf).* 1989;31:355-361.
136. Kyriazopoulou V, Parparousi O, Vagenakis AG. Rifampicin-induced adrenal crisis in addisonian patients receiving corticosteroid replacement therapy. *J Clin Endocrinol Metab.* 1984;59:1204-1206.
137. Morris DJ, Brem AS. Metabolic derivatives of aldosterone. *Am J Physiol.* 1987;252:F365-F373.
138. Edwards C, Hayman A. Enzyme protection of the mineralocorticoid receptor: evidence in favour of the hemi-acetal structure of aldosterone. In: Bonvalet JP, Farman N, Lombès M, et al., eds. *Aldosterone Fundamental Aspects.* London: Colloque INSERM/John Libbey Eurotext; 1991:67-76.

139. Stalmans W, Laloux M. Glucocorticoids and hepatic glycogen metabolism. In: Baxter JD, Rousseau GG, eds. *Glucocorticoid Hormone Action.* New York, NY: Springer-Verlag; 1979:518-533.
140. Watts LM, Manchem VP, Leedom TA, et al. Reduction of hepatic and adipose tissue glucocorticoid receptor expression with antisense oligonucleotides improves hyperglycemia and hyperlipidemia in diabetic rodents without causing systemic glucocorticoid antagonism. *Diabetes.* 2005;54:1846-1853.
141. Chakravarty K, Cassuto H, Reshef L, et al. Factors that control the tissue-specific transcription of the gene for phosphoenolpyruvate carboxykinase-C. *Crit Rev Biochem Mol Biol.* 2005;40:129-154.
142. Olefsky JM. Effect of dexamethasone on insulin binding, glucose transport, and glucose oxidation of isolated rat adipocytes. *J Clin Invest.* 1975;56:1499-1508.
143. Hauner H, Entenmann G, Wabitsch M, et al. Promoting effect of glucocorticoids on the differentiation of human adipocyte precursor cells cultured in a chemically defined medium. *J Clin Invest.* 1989;84:1663-1670.
144. Rebuffe-Scrive M, Krotkiewski M, Elfverson J, et al. Muscle and adipose tissue morphology and metabolism in Cushing's syndrome. *J Clin Endocrinol Metab.* 1988;67:1122-1128.
145. Bronnegard M, Arner P, Hellstrom L, et al. Glucocorticoid receptor messenger ribonucleic acid in different regions of human adipose tissue. *Endocrinology.* 1990;127:1689-1696.
146. Bujalska IJ, Kumar S, Stewart PM. Does central obesity reflect "Cushing's disease of the omentum"? *Lancet.* 1997;349:1210-1213.
147. Leibovich SJ, Ross R. The role of the macrophage in wound repair: a study with hydrocortisone and antimacrophage serum. *Am J Pathol.* 1975;78:71-100.
148. Canalis E. Mechanisms of glucocorticoid action in bone: implications to glucocorticoid-induced osteoporosis. Clinical Review 83. *J Clin Endocrinol Metab.* 1996;81:3441-3447.
149. van Staa TP, Leufkens HG, Abenhaim L, et al. Use of oral corticosteroids in the United Kingdom. *Q J Med.* 2000;93:105-111.
150. Williams PL, Corbett M. Avascular necrosis of bone complicating corticosteroid replacement therapy. *Ann Rheum Dis.* 1983;42:276-279.
151. Weinstein RS, Nicholas RW, Manolagas SC. Apoptosis of osteocytes in glucocorticoid-induced osteonecrosis of the hip. *J Clin Endocrinol Metab.* 2000;85:2907-2912.
152. Leonard MB, Feldman HI, Shults J, et al. Long-term, high-dose glucocorticoids and bone mineral content in childhood glucocorticoid-sensitive nephrotic syndrome. *N Engl J Med.* 2004;351:868-875.
153. Fraser R, Davies DL, Connell JM. Hormones and hypertension. *Clin Endocrinol (Oxf).* 1989;31:701-746.
154. Saruta T, Suzuki H, Handa M, et al. Multiple factors contribute to the pathogenesis of hypertension in Cushing's syndrome. *J Clin Endocrinol Metab.* 1986;62:275-279.
155. Marver D. Evidence of corticosteroid action along the nephron. *Am J Physiol.* 1984;246:F111-F123.
156. Raff H. Glucocorticoid inhibition of neurohypophysial vasopressin secretion. *Am J Physiol.* 1987;252:R635-R644.
157. Peers SH, Flower RJ. The role of lipocortin in corticosteroid actions. *Am Rev Respir Dis.* 1990;141:S18-S21.
158. McEwen BS, De Kloet ER, Rostene W. Adrenal steroid receptors and actions in the nervous system. *Physiol Rev.* 1986;66:1121-1188.
159. Sapolsky RM, Krey LC, McEwen BS. Prolonged glucocorticoid exposure reduces hippocampal neuron number: implications for aging. *J Neurosci.* 1985;5:1222-1227.
160. Lupien SJ, de Leon M, de Santi S, et al. Cortisol levels during human aging predict hippocampal atrophy and memory deficits. *Nat Neurosci.* 1998;1:69-73.
161. Sandeep TC, Yau JL, MacLullich AM, et al. 11β-Hydroxysteroid dehydrogenase inhibition improves cognitive function in healthy elderly men and type 2 diabetics. *Proc Natl Acad Sci U S A.* 2004;101:6734-6739.
162. Hajszan T, MacLusky NJ, Leranth C. Dehydroepiandrosterone increases hippocampal spine density in ovariectomized female rats. *Endocrinology.* 2004;145:1042-1045.
163. Yau JL, Rasmuson S, Andrew R, et al. Dehydroepiandrosterone 7-hydroxylase CYP7B: predominant expression in primate hippocampus and reduced expression in Alzheimer's disease. *Neuroscience.* 2003;121:307-314.
164. Clark AF. Steroids, ocular hypertension, and glaucoma. *J Glaucoma.* 1995;4:354-369.
165. Messer J, Reitman D, Sacks HS, et al. Association of adrenocorticosteroid therapy and peptic-ulcer disease. *N Engl J Med.* 1983;309:21-24.
166. Strickland AL, Underwood LE, Voina SJ, et al. Growth retardation in Cushing's syndrome. *Am J Dis Child.* 1972;123:207-213.
167. Ballard PL, Ertsey R, Gonzales LW, et al. Transcriptional regulation of human pulmonary surfactant proteins SP-B and SP-C by glucocorticoids. *Am J Respir Cell Mol Biol.* 1996;14:599-607.
168. Dluhy RG, Newmark SR, Lauler DP, et al. Pharmacology and chemistry of adrenal glucocorticoids. In: Azarnoff DL, ed. *Steroid Therapy.* Philadelphia, PA: Saunders; 1975:1-14.
169. Meikle AW, Weed JA, Tyler FH. Kinetics and interconversion of prednisolone and prednisone studied with new radioimmunoassays. *J Clin Endocrinol Metab.* 1975;41:717-721.
170. Axelrod L. Glucocorticoid therapy. *Medicine (Baltimore).* 1976;55:39-65.
171. Wei L, MacDonald TM, Walker BR. Taking glucocorticoids by prescription is associated with subsequent cardiovascular disease. *Ann Intern Med.* 2004;141:764-770.
172. Schacke H, Schottelius A, Docke WD, et al. Dissociation of transactivation from transrepression by a selective glucocorticoid receptor agonist leads to separation of therapeutic effects from side effects. *Proc Natl Acad Sci U S A.* 2004;101:227-232.
173. Walters W, Wilder RM, Kepler EJ. The suprarenal cortical syndrome with presentation of ten cases. *Ann Surg.* 1934;100:670-688.
174. Meador CK, Liddle GW, Island DP, et al. Cause of Cushing's syndrome in patients with tumors arising from "nonendocrine" tissue. *J Clin Endocrinol Metab.* 1962;22:693-703.
175. Hopkins RL, Leinung MC. Exogenous Cushing's syndrome and glucocorticoid withdrawal. *Endocrinol Metab Clin North Am.* 2005;34:371-384, ix.
176. Ross EJ, Linch DC. Cushing's syndrome—killing disease: discriminatory value of signs and symptoms aiding early diagnosis. *Lancet.* 1982;2:646-649.
177. Newell-Price J, Bertagna X, Grossman AB, et al. Cushing's syndrome. *Lancet.* 2006;367:1605-1617.
178. Wajchenberg BL, Bosco A, Marone MM, et al. Estimation of body fat and lean tissue distribution by dual energy x-ray absorptiometry and abdominal body fat evaluation by computed tomography in Cushing's disease. *J Clin Endocrinol Metab.* 1995;80:2791-2794.
179. Luton JP, Thieblot P, Valcke JC, et al. Reversible gonadotropin deficiency in male Cushing's disease. *J Clin Endocrinol Metab.* 1977;45:488-495.
180. Lado-Abeal J, Rodriguez-Arnao J, Newell-Price JD, et al. Menstrual abnormalities in women with Cushing's disease are correlated with hypercortisolemia rather than raised circulating androgen levels. *J Clin Endocrinol Metab.* 1998;83:3083-3088.
181. Jeffcoate WJ, Silverstone JT, Edwards CR, et al. Psychiatric manifestations of Cushing's syndrome: response to lowering of plasma cortisol. *Q J Med.* 1979;48:465-472.
182. Dorn LD, Burgess ES, Dubbert B, et al. Psychopathology in patients with endogenous Cushing's syndrome: "atypical" or melancholic features. *Clin Endocrinol (Oxf).* 1995;43:433-442.
183. Friess E, Wiedemann K, Steiger A, et al. The hypothalamic-pituitary-adrenocortical system and sleep in man. *Adv Neuroimmunol.* 1995;5:111-125.
184. Lindsay JR, Nansel T, Baid S, et al. Long-term impaired quality of life in Cushing's syndrome despite initial improvement after surgical remission. *J Clin Endocrinol Metab.* 2006;91:447-453.
185. Ferguson JK, Donald RA, Weston TS, et al. Skin thickness in patients with acromegaly and Cushing's syndrome and response to treatment. *Clin Endocrinol (Oxf).* 1983;18:347-353.
186. Pleasure DE, Walsh GO, Engel WK. Atrophy of skeletal muscle in patients with Cushing's syndrome. *Arch Neurol.* 1970;22:118-125.
187. Plotz CM, Knowlton AI, Ragan C. The natural history of Cushing's syndrome. *Am J Med.* 1952;13:597-614.
188. Etxabe J, Vazquez JA. Morbidity and mortality in Cushing's disease: an epidemiological approach. *Clin Endocrinol (Oxf).* 1994;40:479-484.
189. Colao A, Pivonello R, Spiezia S, et al. Persistence of increased cardiovascular risk in patients with Cushing's disease after five years of successful cure. *J Clin Endocrinol Metab.* 1999;84:2664-2672.
190. Stuijver DJ, van Zaane B, Feelders RA, et al. Incidence of venous thromboembolism in patients with Cushing's syndrome: a multicenter cohort study. *J Clin Endocrinol Metab.* 2011;96(11):3525-3532.
191. Dale DC, Petersdorf RG. Corticosteroids and infectious diseases. *Med Clin North Am.* 1973;57:1277-1287.
192. Graham BS, Tucker WS Jr. Opportunistic infections in endogenous Cushing's syndrome. *Ann Intern Med.* 1984;101:334-338.
193. Hill AT, Stewart PM, Hughes EA, et al. Cushing's disease and tuberculosis. *Respir Med.* 1998;92:604-606.
194. Taskinen MR, Nikkila EA, Pelkonen R, et al. Plasma lipoproteins, lipolytic enzymes, and very low density lipoprotein triglyceride turnover in Cushing's syndrome. *J Clin Endocrinol Metab.* 1983;57:619-626.
195. Stewart PM, Walker BR, Holder G, et al. 11β-Hydroxysteroid dehydrogenase activity in Cushing's syndrome: explaining the mineralocorticoid excess state of the ectopic adrenocorticotropin syndrome. *J Clin Endocrinol Metab.* 1995;80:3617-3620.
196. Benker G, Raida M, Olbricht T, et al. TSH secretion in Cushing's syndrome: relation to glucocorticoid excess, diabetes, goitre, and the "sick euthyroid syndrome." *Clin Endocrinol (Oxf).* 1990;33:777-786.
197. Saketos M, Sharma N, Santoro NF. Suppression of the hypothalamic-pituitary-ovarian axis in normal women by glucocorticoids. *Biol Reprod.* 1993;49:1270-1276.
198. Sayegh F, Weigelin E. Intraocular pressure in Cushing's syndrome. *Ophthalmic Res.* 1975;7:390-394.
199. Kelly W. Exophthalmos in Cushing's syndrome. *Clin Endocrinol (Oxf).* 1996;45:167-170.

200. Bouzas EA, Mastorakos G, Friedman TC, et al. Posterior subcapsular cataract in endogenous Cushing syndrome: an uncommon manifestation. *Invest Ophthalmol Vis Sci.* 1993;34:3497-3500.
201. Biller BM. Pathogenesis of pituitary Cushing's syndrome: pituitary versus hypothalamic. *Endocrinol Metab Clin North Am.* 1994;23:547-554.
202. Utz AL, Swearingen B, Biller BM. Pituitary surgery and postoperative management in Cushing's disease. *Endocrinol Metab Clin North Am.* 2005;34:459-478, xi.
203. Trainer PJ, Lawrie HS, Verhelst J, et al. Transsphenoidal resection in Cushing's disease: undetectable serum cortisol as the definition of successful treatment. *Clin Endocrinol (Oxf).* 1993;38:73-78.
204. McCance DR, Besser M, Atkinson AB. Assessment of cure after transsphenoidal surgery for Cushing's disease. *Clin Endocrinol (Oxf).* 1996; 44:1-6.
205. Leinung MC, Kane LA, Scheithauer BW, et al. Long term follow-up of transsphenoidal surgery for the treatment of Cushing's disease in childhood. *J Clin Endocrinol Metab.* 1995;80:2475-2479.
206. Joshi SM, Hewitt RJ, Storr HL, et al. Cushing's disease in children and adolescents: 20 years of experience in a single neurosurgical center. *Neurosurgery.* 2005;57:281-285, discussion 281-285.
207. Storr HL, Plowman PN, Carroll PV, et al. Clinical and endocrine responses to pituitary radiotherapy in pediatric Cushing's disease: an effective second-line treatment. *J Clin Endocrinol Metab.* 2003;88: 34-37.
208. Verhelst JA, Trainer PJ, Howlett TA, et al. Short and long-term responses to metyrapone in the medical management of 91 patients with Cushing's syndrome. *Clin Endocrinol (Oxf).* 1991;35:169-178.
209. Child DF, Burke CW, Burley DM, et al. Drug controlled of Cushing's syndrome; combined aminoglutethimide and metyrapone therapy. *Acta Endocrinol (Copenh).* 1976;82:330-341.
210. Burch W. A survey of results with transsphenoidal surgery in Cushing's disease. *N Engl J Med.* 1983;308:103-104.
211. Semple CG, Beastall GH, Gray CE, et al. Trilostane in the management of Cushing's syndrome. *Acta Endocrinol (Copenh).* 1983;102:107-110.
212. McCance DR, Hadden DR, Kennedy L, et al. Clinical experience with ketoconazole as a therapy for patients with Cushing's syndrome. *Clin Endocrinol (Oxf).* 1987;27:593-599.
213. Gicquel C, Le Bouc Y, Luton JP, et al. Monoclonality of corticotroph macroadenomas in Cushing's disease. *J Clin Endocrinol Metab.* 1992; 75:472-475.
214. Biller BM, Alexander JM, Zervas NT, et al. Clonal origins of adrenocorticotropin-secreting pituitary tissue in Cushing's disease. *J Clin Endocrinol Metab.* 1992;75:1303-1309.
215. Woo YS, Isidori AM, Wat WZ, et al. Clinical and biochemical characteristics of adrenocorticotropin-secreting macroadenomas. *J Clin Endocrinol Metab.* 2005;90:4963-4969.
215a. Alexandraki KI, Kaltsas GA, Isidori AM, et al. Long-term remission and recurrence rates in Cushing's disease: predictive factors in a single-centre study. *Eur J Endocrinol.* 2013;168(4):639-648.
216. Liddle GW. Tests of pituitary-adrenal suppressibility in the diagnosis of Cushing's syndrome. *J Clin Endocrinol Metab.* 1960;20:1539-1560.
217. Stewart PM, Penn R, Gibson R, et al. Hypothalamic abnormalities in patients with pituitary-dependent Cushing's syndrome. *Clin Endocrinol (Oxf).* 1992;36:453-458.
218. Isidori AM, Kaltsas GA, Pozza C, et al. The ectopic adrenocorticotropin syndrome: clinical features, diagnosis, management, and long-term follow-up. *J Clin Endocrinol Metab.* 2006;91(2):371-377.
219. Limper AH, Carpenter PC, Scheithauer B, et al. The Cushing syndrome induced by bronchial carcinoid tumors. *Ann Intern Med.* 1992; 117:209-214.
220. Odell WD. Ectopic ACTH secretion: a misnomer. *Endocrinol Metab Clin North Am.* 1991;20:371-379.
221. Ray DW, Littlewood AC, Clark AJ, et al. Human small cell lung cancer cell lines expressing the proopiomelanocortin gene have aberrant glucocorticoid receptor function. *J Clin Invest.* 1994;93:1625-1630.
222. Carey RM, Varma SK, Drake CR Jr, et al. Ectopic secretion of corticotropin-releasing factor as a cause of Cushing's syndrome: a clinical, morphologic, and biochemical study. *N Engl J Med.* 1984; 311:13-20.
223. Muller OA, von Werder K. Ectopic production of ACTH and corticotropin-releasing hormone (CRH). *J Steroid Biochem Mol Biol.* 1992;43:403-408.
224. Preeyasombat C, Sirikulchayanonta V, Mahachokelertwattana P, et al. Cushing's syndrome caused by Ewing's sarcoma secreting corticotropin releasing factor-like peptide. *Am J Dis Child.* 1992;146: 1103-1105.
225. Aron DC, Findling JW, Fitzgerald PA, et al. Pituitary ACTH dependency of nodular adrenal hyperplasia in Cushing's syndrome: report of two cases and review of the literature. *Am J Med.* 1981;71:302-306.
226. Doppman JL, Nieman LK, Travis WD, et al. CT and MR imaging of massive macronodular adrenocortical disease: a rare cause of autonomous primary adrenal hypercortisolism. *J Comput Assist Tomogr.* 1991;15:773-779.
227. Samuels MH, Loriaux DL. Cushing's syndrome and the nodular adrenal gland. *Endocrinol Metab Clin North Am.* 1994;23:555-569.
228. Sturrock ND, Morgan L, Jeffcoate WJ. Autonomous nodular hyperplasia of the adrenal cortex: tertiary hypercortisolism? *Clin Endocrinol (Oxf).* 1995;43:753-758.
229. Hermus AR, Pieters GF, Smals AG, et al. Transition from pituitary-dependent to adrenal-dependent Cushing's syndrome. *N Engl J Med.* 1988;318:966-970.
230. Beuschlein F, Fassnacht M, Assié G, et al. Constitutive activation of PKA catalytic subunit in adrenal Cushing's syndrome. *N Engl J Med.* 2014;370(11):1019-1028.
231. Cao Y, He M, Gao Z, et al. Activating hotspot L205R mutation in PRKACA and adrenal Cushing's syndrome. *Science.* 2014;344(6186): 913-917.
232. Goh G, Scholl UI, Healy JM, et al. Recurrent activating mutation in PRKACA in cortisol-producing adrenal tumors. *Nat Genet.* 2014; 46(6):613-617. [Erratum in: *Nat Genet.* 2014;46(7):759.]
233. Sato Y, Maekawa S, Ishii R, et al. Recurrent somatic mutations underlie corticotropin-independent Cushing's syndrome. *Science.* 2014; 344(6186):917-920.
234. Young WF Jr, Carney JA, Musa BU, et al. Familial Cushing's syndrome due to primary pigmented nodular adrenocortical disease: reinvestigation 50 years later. *N Engl J Med.* 1989;321:1659-1664.
235. Stratakis CA, Kirschner LS, Carney JA. Clinical and molecular features of the Carney complex: diagnostic criteria and recommendations for patient evaluation. *J Clin Endocrinol Metab.* 2001;86: 4041-4046.
236. Kirschner LS, Carney JA, Pack SD, et al. Mutations of the gene encoding the protein kinase A type I-alpha regulatory subunit in patients with the Carney complex. *Nat Genet.* 2000;26:89-92.
237. Kirk JM, Brain CE, Carson DJ, et al. Cushing's syndrome caused by nodular adrenal hyperplasia in children with McCune-Albright syndrome. *J Pediatr.* 1999;134:789-792.
238. Malchoff CD, MacGillivray D, Malchoff DM. Adrenocorticotropic hormone-independent adrenal hyperplasia. *Endocrinologist.* 1996;6: 79-85.
239. Christopoulos S, Bourdeau I, Lacroix A. Aberrant expression of hormone receptors in adrenal Cushing's syndrome. *Pituitary.* 2004; 7:225-235.
240. Assié G, Libé R, Espiard S, et al. ARMC5 mutations in macronodular adrenal hyperplasia with Cushing's syndrome. *N Engl J Med.* 2013; 369(22):2105-2114.
241. Atkinson AB, Kennedy AL, Carson DJ, et al. Five cases of cyclical Cushing's syndrome. *Br Med J (Clin Res Ed).* 1985;291:1453-1457.
242. Mantero F, Scaroni CM, Albiger NM. Cyclic Cushing's syndrome: an overview. *Pituitary.* 2004;7:203-207.
243. Leinung MC, Zimmerman D. Cushing's disease in children. *Endocrinol Metab Clin North Am.* 1994;23:629-639.
244. Storr HL, Chan LF, Grossman AB, et al. Paediatric Cushing's syndrome: epidemiology, investigation and therapeutic advances. *Trends Endocrinol Metab.* 2007;18:167-174.
245. Lindsay JR, Jonklaas J, Oldfield EH, et al. Cushing's syndrome during pregnancy: personal experience and review of the literature. *J Clin Endocrinol Metab.* 2005;90:3077-3083.
246. Wallace C, Toth EL, Lewanczuk RZ, et al. Pregnancy-induced Cushing's syndrome in multiple pregnancies. *J Clin Endocrinol Metab.* 1996; 81:15-21.
247. Kirkman S, Nelson DH. Alcohol-induced pseudo-Cushing's disease: a study of prevalence with review of the literature. *Metabolism.* 1988; 37:390-394.
248. Stewart PM, Burra P, Shackleton CH, et al. 11β-Hydroxysteroid dehydrogenase deficiency and glucocorticoid status in patients with alcoholic and non-alcoholic chronic liver disease. *J Clin Endocrinol Metab.* 1993;76:748-751.
249. Newell-Price J, Trainer P, Besser M, et al. The diagnosis and differential diagnosis of Cushing's syndrome and pseudo-Cushing's states. *Endocr Rev.* 1998;19:647-672.
250. Glass AR, Burman KD, Dahms WT, et al. Endocrine function in human obesity. *Metabolism.* 1981;30:89-104.
251. Stewart PM, Boulton A, Kumar S, et al. Cortisol metabolism in human obesity: impaired cortisone → cortisol conversion in subjects with central adiposity. *J Clin Endocrinol Metab.* 1999;84:1022-1027.
252. Hamrahian AH, Oseni TS, Arafah BM. Measurements of serum free cortisol in critically ill patients. *N Engl J Med.* 2004;350:1629-1638.
253. Arnaldi G, Angeli A, Atkinson AB, et al. Diagnosis and complications of Cushing's syndrome: a consensus statement. *J Clin Endocrinol Metab.* 2003;88:5593-5602.
254. Findling JW, Raff H. Screening and diagnosis of Cushing's syndrome. *Endocrinol Metab Clin North Am.* 2005;34:385-402, ix-x.
255. Newell-Price J, Trainer P, Perry L, et al. A single sleeping midnight cortisol has 100% sensitivity for the diagnosis of Cushing's syndrome. *Clin Endocrinol (Oxf).* 1995;43:545-550.
256. Raff H, Raff JL, Findling JW. Late-night salivary cortisol as a screening test for Cushing's syndrome. *J Clin Endocrinol Metab.* 1998;83:2681-2686.
257. Yaneva M, Mosnier-Pudar H, Dugue MA, et al. Midnight salivary cortisol for the initial diagnosis of Cushing's syndrome of various causes. *J Clin Endocrinol Metab.* 2004;89:3345-3351.

258. Liu H, Bravata DM, Cabaccan J, et al. Elevated late-night salivary cortisol levels in elderly male type 2 diabetic veterans. *Clin Endocrinol (Oxf)*. 2005;63(6):642.
259. Invitti C, Pecori Giraldi F, de Martin M, et al. Diagnosis and management of Cushing's syndrome: results of an Italian multicentre study. Study Group of the Italian Society of Endocrinology on the Pathophysiology of the Hypothalamic-Pituitary-Adrenal Axis. *J Clin Endocrinol Metab*. 1999;84:440-448.
260. Petersenn S, Newell-Price J, Findling JW, et al. Pasireotide B2305 Study Group. High variability in baseline urinary free cortisol values in patients with Cushing's disease. *Clin Endocrinol (Oxf)*. 2014;80(2):261.
261. Corcuff JB, Tabarin A, Rashedi M, et al. Overnight urinary free cortisol determination: a screening test for the diagnosis of Cushing's syndrome. *Clin Endocrinol (Oxf)*. 1998;48:503-508.
262. Cronin C, Igoe D, Duffy MJ, et al. The overnight dexamethasone test is a worthwhile screening procedure. *Clin Endocrinol (Oxf)*. 1990;33:27-33.
263. Isidori AM, Kaltsas GA, Mohammed S, et al. Discriminatory value of the low-dose dexamethasone suppression test in establishing the diagnosis and differential diagnosis of Cushing's syndrome. *J Clin Endocrinol Metab*. 2003;88(11):5299-5306.
264. Meikle AW. Dexamethasone suppression tests: usefulness of simultaneous measurement of plasma cortisol and dexamethasone. *Clin Endocrinol (Oxf)*. 1982;16:401-408.
265. Yanovski JA, Cutler GB Jr, Chrousos GP, et al. Corticotropin-releasing hormone stimulation following low-dose dexamethasone administration. A new test to distinguish Cushing's syndrome from pseudo-Cushing's states. *JAMA*. 1993;269:2232-2238.
266. Nieman LK, Biller BM, Findling JW, et al. The diagnosis of Cushing's syndrome: an Endocrine Society Clinical Practice Guideline. *J Clin Endocrinol Metab*. 2008;93:1526-1540.
267. Findling JW. Clinical application of a new immunoradiometric assay for ACTH. *Endocrinologist*. 1992;2:360-365.
268. Trainer PJ, Faria M, Newell-Price J, et al. A comparison of the effects of human and ovine corticotropin-releasing hormone on the pituitary-adrenal axis. *J Clin Endocrinol Metab*. 1995;80:412-417.
269. Chrousos GP, Schulte HM, Oldfield EH. The corticotropin-releasing factor stimulation test: an aid in the evaluation of patients with Cushing's syndrome. *N Engl J Med*. 1984;310:622-626.
270. Nieman LK, Oldfield EH, Wesley R, et al. A simplified morning ovine corticotropin-releasing hormone stimulation test for the differential diagnosis of adrenocorticotropin-dependent Cushing's syndrome. *J Clin Endocrinol Metab*. 1993;77:1308-1312.
271. Findling JW, Doppman JL. Biochemical and radiologic diagnosis of Cushing's syndrome. *Endocrinol Metab Clin North Am*. 1994;23:511-537.
272. Lindsay JR, Nieman LK. Differential diagnosis and imaging in Cushing's syndrome. *Endocrinol Metab Clin North Am*. 2005;34:403-421.
273. Oldfield EH, Doppman JL, Nieman LK, et al. Petrosal sinus sampling with and without corticotropin-releasing hormone for the differential diagnosis of Cushing's syndrome. *N Engl J Med*. 1991;325:897-905.
274. Kaltsas GA, Giannulis MG, Newell-Price JD, et al. A critical analysis of the value of simultaneous inferior petrosal sinus sampling in Cushing's disease and the occult ectopic adrenocorticotropin syndrome. *J Clin Endocrinol Metab*. 1999;84:487-492.
275. Sharma ST, Nieman LK. Is prolactin measurement of value during inferior petrosal sinus sampling in patients with adrenocorticotropic hormone-dependent Cushing's syndrome? *J Endocrinol Invest*. 2013;36(11):1112-1116.
276. Hall WA, Luciano MG, Doppman JL, et al. Pituitary magnetic resonance imaging in normal human volunteers: occult adenomas in the general population. *Ann Intern Med*. 1994;120:817-820.
277. Korobkin M, Francis IR. Adrenal imaging. *Semin Ultrasound CT MR*. 1995;16(4):317-330.
278. Miles JM, Wahner HW, Carpenter PC, et al. Adrenal scintiscanning with NP-59, a new radioiodinated cholesterol agent. *Mayo Clin Proc*. 1979;54:321-327.
279. de Herder WW, Krenning EP, Malchoff CD, et al. Somatostatin receptor scintigraphy: its value in tumor localization in patients with Cushing's syndrome caused by ectopic corticotropin or corticotropin-releasing hormone secretion. *Am J Med*. 1994;96:305-312.
280. Valimaki M, Pelkonen R, Porkka L, et al. Long-term results of adrenal surgery in patients with Cushing's syndrome due to adrenocortical adenoma. *Clin Endocrinol (Oxf)*. 1984;20:229-236.
281. Young WF Jr, Thompson GB. Laparoscopic adrenalectomy for patients who have Cushing's syndrome. *Endocrinol Metab Clin North Am*. 2005;34:489-499, xi.
282. Kasperlik-Zaluska AA, Migdalska BM, Zgliczynski S, et al. Adrenocortical carcinoma: a clinical study and treatment results of 52 patients. *Cancer*. 1995;75:2587-2591.
283. Allolio B, Hahner S, Weismann D, et al. Management of adrenocortical carcinoma. *Clin Endocrinol (Oxf)*. 2004;60:273-287.
284. Terzolo M, Angeli A, Fassnacht M, et al. Adjuvant mitotane treatment for adrenocortical carcinoma. *N Engl J Med*. 2007;356:2372-2380.
285. Fassnacht M, Allolio B. Clinical management of adrenocortical carcinoma. *Best Pract Res Clin Endocrinol Metab*. 2009;23:273-289.
286. Biller BM, Grossman AB, Stewart PM, et al. Treatment of adrenocorticotropin-dependent Cushing's syndrome: a consensus statement. *J Clin Endocrinol Metab*. 2008;93:2454-2462.
287. Assie G, Bahurel H, Coste J, et al. Corticotroph tumor progression after adrenalectomy in Cushing's disease: a reappraisal of Nelson's syndrome. *J Clin Endocrinol Metab*. 2007;92:172-179.
288. Jenkins PJ, Trainer PJ, Plowman PN, et al. The long-term outcome after adrenalectomy and prophylactic pituitary radiotherapy in adrenocorticotropin-dependent Cushing's syndrome. *J Clin Endocrinol Metab*. 1995;80:165-171.
289. Aghi MK. Management of recurrent and refractory Cushing disease. *Nat Clin Pract Endocrinol Metab*. 2008;4:560-568.
290. Castinetti F, Guignat L, Giraud P, et al. Ketoconazole in Cushing's disease: is it worth a try? *J Clin Endocrinol Metab*. 2014;99(5):1623-1630.
291. Baudry C, Coste J, Bou Khalil R, et al. Efficiency and tolerance of mitotane in Cushing's disease in 76 patients from a single center. *Eur J Endocrinol*. 2012;167(4):473-478.
292. Colao A, Petersenn S, Newell-Price J, et al. Pasireotide B2305 Study Group. A 12-month phase 3 study of pasireotide in Cushing's disease. *N Engl J Med*. 2012;366(10):914-924.
293. Fleseriu M, Biller BM, Findling JW, et al. SEISMIC Study Investigators. Mifepristone, a glucocorticoid receptor antagonist, produces clinical and metabolic benefits in patients with Cushing's syndrome. *J Clin Endocrinol Metab*. 2012;97(6):2039-2049.
294. Bhattacharyya A, Kaushal K, Tymms DJ, et al. Steroid withdrawal syndrome after successful treatment of Cushing's syndrome: a reminder. *Eur J Endocrinol*. 2005;153:207-210.
295. Hermus AR, Smals AG, Swinkels LM, et al. Bone mineral density and bone turnover before and after surgical cure of Cushing's syndrome. *J Clin Endocrinol Metab*. 1995;80:2859-2865.
296. Keil MF, Merke DP, Gandhi R, et al. Quality of life in children and adolescents 1 year after cure of Cushing syndrome: a prospective study. *Clin Endocrinol (Oxf)*. 2009;71:326-333.
297. Charmandari E, Kino T, Souvatzoglou E, et al. Natural glucocorticoid receptor mutants causing generalized glucocorticoid resistance: molecular genotype, genetic transmission, and clinical phenotype. *J Clin Endocrinol Metab*. 2004;89:1939-1949.
298. Oelkers W. Adrenal insufficiency. *N Engl J Med*. 1996;335:1206-1212.
299. Arlt W, Allolio B. Adrenal insufficiency. *Lancet*. 2003;361:1881-1893.
300. Carey RM. The changing clinical spectrum of adrenal insufficiency. *Ann Intern Med*. 1997;127:1103-1105.
301. Betterle C, Dal Pra C, Mantero F, et al. Autoimmune adrenal insufficiency and autoimmune polyendocrine syndromes: autoantibodies, autoantigens, and their applicability in diagnosis and disease prediction. *Endocr Rev*. 2002;23:327-364.
302. Piedrola G, Casado JL, Lopez E, et al. Clinical features of adrenal insufficiency in patients with acquired immunodeficiency syndrome. *Clin Endocrinol (Oxf)*. 1996;45:97-101.
303. Freda PU, Bilezikian JP. The hypothalamus-pituitary-adrenal axis in HIV disease. *AIDS Read*. 1999;9(1):43-50.
304. Norbiato G, Galli M, Righini V, et al. The syndrome of acquired glucocorticoid resistance in HIV infection. *Baillieres Clin Endocrinol Metab*. 1994;8:777-787.
305. Seidenwurm DJ, Elmer EB, Kaplan LM, et al. Metastases to the adrenal glands and the development of Addison's disease. *Cancer*. 1984;54:552-557.
306. Xarli VP, Steele AA, Davis PJ, et al. Adrenal hemorrhage in the adult. *Medicine (Baltimore)*. 1978;57:211-221.
307. Lalli E, Sassone-Corsi P. DAX-1 and the adrenal cortex. *Curr Opin Endocrinol Metab*. 1999;6:185-190.
308. Tabarin A, Achermann JC, Recan D, et al. A novel mutation in DAX1 causes delayed-onset adrenal insufficiency and incomplete hypogonadotropic hypogonadism. *J Clin Invest*. 2000;105:321-328.
309. Takahashi T, Shoji Y, Shoji Y, et al. Active hypothalamic-pituitary-gonadal axis in an infant with X-linked adrenal hypoplasia congenita. *J Pediatr*. 1997;130:485-488.
310. Kaiserman KB, Nakamoto JM, Geffner ME, et al. Minipuberty of infancy and adolescent pubertal function in adrenal hypoplasia congenita. *J Pediatr*. 1998;133:300-302.
311. Ozisik G, Mantovani G, Achermann JC, et al. An alternate translation initiation site circumvents an amino-terminal DAX1 nonsense mutation leading to a mild form of X-linked adrenal hypoplasia congenita. *J Clin Endocrinol Metab*. 2003;88:417-423.
312. Achermann JC, Ito M, Ito M, et al. A mutation in the gene encoding steroidogenic factor-1 causes XY sex reversal and adrenal failure in humans. *Nat Genet*. 1999;22:125-126.
313. Biason-Lauber A, Schoenle EJ. Apparently normal ovarian differentiation in a prepubertal girl with transcriptionally inactive steroidogenic factor 1 (NR5A1/SF-1) and adrenocortical insufficiency. *Am J Hum Genet*. 2000;67:1563-1568.
314. Lin L, Philibert P, Ferraz-de-Souza B, et al. Heterozygous missense mutations in steroidogenic factor 1 (SF1/Ad4BP, NR5A1) are associated with 46,XY disorders of sex development with normal adrenal function. *J Clin Endocrinol Metab*. 2007;92:991-999.
315. Lourenco D, Brauner R, Lin L, et al. Mutations in NR5A1 associated with ovarian insufficiency. *N Engl J Med*. 2009;360:1200-1210.

316. Scheuerle A, Greenberg F, McCabe ER. Dysmorphic features in patients with complex glycerol kinase deficiency. *J Pediatr.* 1995;126:764-767.

317. Moser HW, Moser AE, Singh I, et al. Adrenoleukodystrophy—survey of 303 cases: biochemistry, diagnosis, and therapy. *Ann Neurol.* 1984;16:628-641.

318. Laureti S, Casucci G, Santeusanio F, et al. X-linked adrenoleukodystrophy is a frequent cause of idiopathic Addison's disease in young adult male patients. *J Clin Endocrinol Metab.* 1996;81:470-474.

319. Mosser J, Douar AM, Sarde CO, et al. Putative X-linked adrenoleukodystrophy gene shares unexpected homology with ABC transporters. *Nature.* 1993;361:726-730.

320. Kemp S, Pujol A, Waterham HR, et al. ABCD1 mutations and the X-linked adrenoleukodystrophy mutation database: role in diagnosis and clinical correlations. *Hum Mutat.* 2001;18:499-515.

321. Moser HW, Raymond GV, Lu SE, et al. Follow-up of 89 asymptomatic patients with adrenoleukodystrophy treated with Lorenzo's oil. *Arch Neurol.* 2005;62:1073-1080.

322. Clark AJ, McLoughlin L, Grossman A. Familial glucocorticoid deficiency associated with point mutation in the adrenocorticotropin receptor. *Lancet.* 1993;341:461-462.

323. Tsigos C, Arai K, Hung W, et al. Hereditary isolated glucocorticoid deficiency is associated with abnormalities of the adrenocorticotropin receptor gene. *J Clin Invest.* 1993;92:2458-2461.

324. Huebner A, Elias LL, Clark AJ. ACTH resistance syndromes. *J Pediatr Endocrinol Metab.* 1999;12(Suppl 1):277-293.

325. Tullio-Pelet A, Salomon R, Hadj-Rabia S, et al. Mutant WD-repeat protein in triple-A syndrome. *Nat Genet.* 2000;26:332-335.

326. Handschug K, Sperling S, Yoon SJ, et al. Triple A syndrome is caused by mutations in AAAS, a new WD-repeat protein gene. *Hum Mol Genet.* 2001;10:283-290.

326a. Crowley RK, Argese N, Tomlinson JW, Stewart PM. Central hypoadrenalism. *J Clin Endocrinol Metab.* 2014;99(11):4027-4036. doi: 10.1210/jc.2014-2476; [Epub 2014 Aug 20].

326b. Clark PM, Neylon I, Raggatt PR, et al. Defining the normal cortisol response to the short Synacthen test: implications for the investigation of hypothalamic-pituitary disorders. *Clin Endocrinol (Oxf).* 1998;49(3):287-292.

326c. Sherlock M, Reulen RC, Alonso AA, et al. ACTH deficiency, higher doses of hydrocortisone replacement, and radiotherapy are independent predictors of mortality in patients with acromegaly. *J Clin Endocrinol Metab.* 2009;94(11):4216-4223. doi: 10.1210/jc.2009-1097; [Epub 2009 Oct 6].

326d. Hannon MJ, Crowley RK, Behan LA, et al. Acute glucocorticoid deficiency and diabetes insipidus are common after acute traumatic brain injury and predict mortality. *J Clin Endocrinol Metab.* 2013;98(8):3229-3237. doi: 10.1210/jc.2013-1555; [Epub 2013 May 20].

326e. Zueger T, Kirchner P, Herren C, et al. Glucocorticoid replacement and mortality in patients with nonfunctioning pituitary adenoma. *J Clin Endocrinol Metab.* 2012;97(10):E1938-E1942. doi: 10.1210/jc.2012-2432; [Epub 2012 Aug 7].

327. Pulichino AM, Vallette-Kasic S, Couture C, et al. Human and mouse TPIT gene mutations cause early onset pituitary ACTH deficiency. *Genes Dev.* 2003;17:711-716.

328. O'Rahilly S, Gray H, Humphreys PJ, et al. Brief report: impaired processing of prohormones associated with abnormalities of glucose homeostasis and adrenal function. *N Engl J Med.* 1995;333:1386-1390.

329. Krude H, Biebermann H, Luck W, et al. Severe early-onset obesity, adrenal insufficiency and red hair pigmentation caused by POMC mutations in humans. *Nat Genet.* 1998;19:155-157.

330. Yaswen L, Diehl N, Brennan MB, et al. Obesity in the mouse model of pro-opiomelanocortin deficiency responds to peripheral melanocortin. *Nat Med.* 1999;5:1066-1070.

331. Dattani MT, Martinez-Barbera JP, Thomas PQ, et al. Mutations in the homeobox gene HESX1/Hesx1 associated with septo-optic dysplasia in human and mouse. *Nat Genet.* 1998;19:125-133.

332. Machinis K, Pantel J, Netchine I, et al. Syndromic short stature in patients with a germline mutation in the LIM homeobox LHX4. *Am J Hum Genet.* 2001;69:961-968.

333. Lagerstrom-Fermer M, Sundvall M, Johnsen E, et al. X-linked recessive panhypopituitarism associated with a regional duplication in Xq25-q26. *Am J Hum Genet.* 1997;60:910-916.

334. Wu W, Cogan JD, Pfaffle RW, et al. Mutations in PROP1 cause familial combined pituitary hormone deficiency. *Nat Genet.* 1998;18:147-149.

334a. Mader R, Lavi I, Luboshitzky R. Evaluation of the pituitary-adrenal axis function following single intraarticular injection of methylprednisolone. *Arthritis Rheum.* 2005;52(3):924-928.

334b. van Velsen SG, De Roos MP, Haeck IM, et al. The potency of clobetasol propionate: serum levels of clobetasol propionate and adrenal function during therapy with 0.05% clobetasol propionate in patients with severe atopic dermatitis. *J Dermatolog Treat.* 2012;23(1):16-20. doi: 10.3109/09546634.2010.534127; [Epub 2011 Jan 22].

334c. Meikle AW, Tyler FH. Potency and duration of action of glucocorticoids. Effects of hydrocortisone, prednisone and dexamethasone on human pituitary-adrenal function. *Am J Med.* 1977;63(2):200-207.

334d. Grossmann C, Scholz T, Rochel M, et al. Transactivation via the human glucocorticoid and mineralocorticoid receptor by therapeutically used steroids in CV-1 cells: a comparison of their glucocorticoid and mineralocorticoid properties. *Eur J Endocrinol.* 2004;151(3):397-406.

334f. Foisy MM, Yakiwchuk EM, Chiu I, Singh AE. Adrenal suppression and Cushing's syndrome secondary to an interaction between ritonavir and fluticasone: a review of the literature. *HIV Med.* 2008;9(6):389-396. doi: 10.1111/j.1468-1293.2008.00579.x; [Epub 2008 May 4].

335. LaRochelle GE Jr, LaRochelle AG, Ratner RE, Borenstein DG. Recovery of the hypothalamic-pituitary-adrenal (HPA) axis in patients with rheumatic diseases receiving low-dose prednisone. *Am J Med.* 1993;95:258-264.

335a. Schlaghecke R, Kornely E, Santen RT, Ridderskamp P. The effect of long-term glucocorticoid therapy on pituitary-adrenal responses to exogenous corticotropin-releasing hormone. *N Engl J Med.* 1992;326(4):226-230.

335b. Sacre K, Dehoux M, Chauveheid MP, et al. Pituitary-adrenal function after prolonged glucocorticoid therapy for systemic inflammatory disorders: an observational study. *J Clin Endocrinol Metab.* 2013;98(8):3199-3205. doi: 10.1210/jc.2013-1394; [Epub 2013 Jun 12].

335c. Henzen C, Suter A, Lerch E, et al. Supression and recovery of adrenal response after short-term, high-dose glucocorticoid treatment. *Lancet.* 2000;355(9203):542-545.

336. Dixon RB, Christy NP. On the various forms of corticosteroid withdrawal syndrome. *Am J Med.* 1980;68:224-230.

337. Holme J, Tomlinson JW, Stockley RA, et al. Adrenal suppression in bronchiectasis and the impact of inhaled corticosteroids. *Eur Respir J.* 2008;32:1047-1052.

338. Cooper MS, Stewart PM. Corticosteroid insufficiency in acutely ill patients. *N Engl J Med.* 2003;348:727-734.

339. Annane D, Sebille V, Troche G, et al. A 3-level prognostic classification in septic shock based on cortisol levels and cortisol response to corticotropin. *JAMA.* 2000;283:1038-1045.

340. Marik PE, Pastores SM, Annane D, et al. Recommendations for the diagnosis and management of corticosteroid insufficiency in critically ill adult patients: consensus statements from an international task force by the American College of Critical Care Medicine. *Crit Care Med.* 2008;36:1937-1949.

341. Hahner S, Loeffler M, Fassnacht M, et al. Impaired subjective health status in 256 patients with adrenal insufficiency on standard therapy based on cross-sectional analysis. *J Clin Endocrinol Metab.* 2007;92:3912-3922.

342. Artavia-Loria E, Chaussain JL, Bougneres PF, et al. Frequency of hypoglycemia in children with adrenal insufficiency. *Acta Endocrinol Suppl (Copenh).* 1986;279:275-278.

343. Laczi F, Janaky T, Ivanyi T, et al. Osmoregulation of arginine-8-vasopressin secretion in primary hypothyroidism and in Addison's disease. *Acta Endocrinol (Copenh).* 1987;114:389-395.

344. Muls E, Bouillon R, Boelaert J, et al. Etiology of hypercalcemia in a patient with Addison's disease. *Calcif Tissue Int.* 1982;34:523-526.

345. Topliss DJ, White EL, Stockigt JR. Significance of thyrotropin excess in untreated primary adrenal insufficiency. *J Clin Endocrinol Metab.* 1980;50:52-56.

346. Hagg E, Asplund K, Lithner F. Value of basal plasma cortisol assays in the assessment of pituitary-adrenal insufficiency. *Clin Endocrinol (Oxf).* 1987;26:221-226.

347. Lindholm J, Kehlet H. Re-evaluation of the clinical value of the 30 min ACTH test in assessing the hypothalamic-pituitary-adrenocortical function. *Clin Endocrinol (Oxf).* 1987;26:53-59.

348. Clark PM, Neylon I, Raggatt PR, et al. Defining the normal cortisol response to the short Synacthen test: implications for the investigation of hypothalamic-pituitary disorders. *Clin Endocrinol (Oxf).* 1998;49:287-292.

349. Oelkers W, Diederich S, Bahr V. Diagnosis and therapy surveillance in Addison's disease: rapid adrenocorticotropin (ACTH) test and measurement of plasma ACTH, renin activity, and aldosterone. *J Clin Endocrinol Metab.* 1992;75:259-264.

350. Erturk E, Jaffe CA, Barkan AL. Evaluation of the integrity of the hypothalamic-pituitary-adrenal axis by insulin hypoglycemia test. *J Clin Endocrinol Metab.* 1998;83:2350-2354.

351. Stewart PM, Corrie J, Seckl JR, et al. A rational approach for assessing the hypothalamo-pituitary-adrenal axis. *Lancet.* 1988;1:1208-1210.

352. Streeten DH, Anderson GH Jr, Bonaventura MM. The potential for serious consequences from misinterpreting normal responses to the rapid adrenocorticotropin test. *J Clin Endocrinol Metab.* 1996;81:285-290.

353. Oelkers W. Dose-response aspects in the clinical assessment of the hypothalamo-pituitary-adrenal axis, and the low-dose adrenocorticotropin test. *Eur J Endocrinol.* 1996;135:27-33.

354. Abdu TA, Elhadd TA, Neary R, et al. Comparison of the low dose short synacthen test (1 microg), the conventional dose short synacthen test (250 microg), and the insulin tolerance test for assessment of the hypothalamo-pituitary-adrenal axis in patients with pituitary disease. *J Clin Endocrinol Metab.* 1999;84:838-843.

355. Kazlauskaite R, Evans AT, Villabona CV, et al. Corticotropin tests for hypothalamic-pituitary-adrenal insufficiency: a metaanalysis. *J Clin Endocrinol Metab*. 2008;93:4245-4253.

356. Suliman AM, Smith TP, Labib M, et al. The low-dose ACTH test does not provide a useful assessment of the hypothalamic-pituitary-adrenal axis in secondary adrenal insufficiency. *Clin Endocrinol (Oxf)*. 2002; 56:533-539.

357. Stewart PM, Clark PM. The low-dose corticotropin-stimulation test revisited: the less, the better? *Nat Clin Pract Endocrinol Metab*. 2009; 5:68-69.

358. Fiad TM, Kirby JM, Cunningham SK, et al. The overnight single-dose metyrapone test is a simple and reliable index of the hypothalamic-pituitary-adrenal axis. *Clin Endocrinol (Oxf)*. 1994;40:603-609.

359. Schlaghecke R, Kornely E, Santen RT, et al. The effect of long-term glucocorticoid therapy on pituitary-adrenal responses to exogenous corticotropin-releasing hormone. *N Engl J Med*. 1992;326: 226-230.

360. Annane D, Sebille V, Charpentier C, et al. Effect of treatment with low doses of hydrocortisone and fludrocortisone on mortality in patients with septic shock. *JAMA*. 2002;288:862-871.

361. Sprung CL, Annane D, Keh D, et al. Hydrocortisone therapy for patients with septic shock. *N Engl J Med*. 2008;358:111-124.

362. Esteban NV, Loughlin T, Yergey AL, et al. Daily cortisol production rate in man determined by stable isotope dilution/mass spectrometry. *J Clin Endocrinol Metab*. 1991;72:39-45.

363. Feek CM, Ratcliffe JG, Seth J, et al. Patterns of plasma cortisol and ACTH concentrations in patients with Addison's disease treated with conventional corticosteroid replacement. *Clin Endocrinol (Oxf)*. 1981; 14:451-458.

364. Arlt W, Rosenthal C, Hahner S, et al. Quality of glucocorticoid replacement in adrenal insufficiency: clinical assessment vs. timed serum cortisol measurements. *Clin Endocrinol (Oxf)*. 2006;64:384-389.

365. Lovas K, Gjesdal CG, Christensen M, et al. Glucocorticoid replacement therapy and pharmacogenetics in Addison's disease: effects on bone. *Eur J Endocrinol*. 2009;160:993-1002.

366. Peacey SR, Guo CY, Robinson AM, et al. Glucocorticoid replacement therapy: are patients over treated and does it matter? *Clin Endocrinol (Oxf)*. 1997;46:255-261.

367. Howlett TA. An assessment of optimal hydrocortisone replacement therapy. *Clin Endocrinol (Oxf)*. 1997;46:263-268.

368. Fiad TM, Conway JD, Cunningham SK, et al. The role of plasma renin activity in evaluating the adequacy of mineralocorticoid replacement in primary adrenal insufficiency. *Clin Endocrinol (Oxf)*. 1996;45: 529-534.

369. Arlt W, Callies F, van Vlijmen JC, et al. Dehydroepiandrosterone replacement in women with adrenal insufficiency. *N Engl J Med*. 1999; 341:1013-1020.

369a. Johannsson G, Falorni A, Skrtic S, et al. Adrenal insufficiency: review of clinical outcomes with current glucocorticoid replacement therapy. *Clin Endocrinol (Oxf)*. 2015;82(1):2-11. doi: 10.1111/cen.12603; [Epub 2014 Oct 10].

370. White PC, Speiser PW. Congenital adrenal hyperplasia due to 21-hydroxylase deficiency. *Endocr Rev*. 2000;21:245-291.

371. Merke DP, Bornstein SR. Congenital adrenal hyperplasia. *Lancet*. 2005;365:2125-2136.

372. Eugster EA, Dimeglio LA, Wright JC, et al. Height outcome in congenital adrenal hyperplasia caused by 21-hydroxylase deficiency: a meta-analysis. *J Pediatr*. 2001;138:26-32.

373. Cabrera MS, Vogiatzi MG. New MI. Long term outcome in adult males with classic congenital adrenal hyperplasia. *J Clin Endocrinol Metab*. 2001;86:3070-3078.

374. Azziz R, Dewailly D, Owerbach D. Nonclassic adrenal hyperplasia: current concepts. Clinical Review 56. *J Clin Endocrinol Metab*. 1994; 78:810-815.

375. New MI. Extensive clinical experience: nonclassical 21-hydroxylase deficiency. *J Clin Endocrinol Metab*. 2006;91:4205-4214.

376. Bidet M, Bellanne-Chantelot C, Galand-Portier M-B, et al. Clinical and molecular characterization of a cohort of 161 unrelated women with nonclassical congenital adrenal hyperplasia due to 21-hydroxylase deficiency and 330 family members. *J Clin Endocrinol Metab*. 2009; 94:1570-1578.

377. Azziz R, Sanchez LA, Knochenhauer ES, et al. Androgen excess in women: experience with over 1000 consecutive patients. *J Clin Endocrinol Metab*. 2004;89:453-462.

378. Krone N, Arlt W. Genetics of congenital adrenal hyperplasia. *Best Pract Res Clin Endocrinol Metab*. 2009;23:181-192.

379. Speiser PW, Dupont J, Zhu D, et al. Disease expression and molecular genotype in congenital adrenal hyperplasia due to 21-hydroxylase deficiency. *J Clin Invest*. 1992;90:584-595.

380. Krone N, Braun A, Roscher AA, et al. Predicting phenotype in steroid 21-hydroxylase deficiency? Comprehensive genotyping in 155 unrelated, well defined patients from southern Germany. *J Clin Endocrinol Metab*. 2000;85:1059-1065.

381. Wilson RC, Mercado AB, Cheng KC, et al. Steroid 21-hydroxylase deficiency: genotype may not predict phenotype. *J Clin Endocrinol Metab*. 1995;80:2322-2329.

382. Rocha RO, Billerbeck AE, Pinto EM, et al. The degree of external genitalia virilization in girls with 21-hydroxylase deficiency appears to be influenced by the CAG repeats in the androgen receptor gene. *Clin Endocrinol (Oxf)*. 2008;68:226-232.

383. Gomes LG, Huang N, Agrawal V, et al. Extraadrenal 21-hydroxylation by CYP2C19 and CYP3A4: effect on 21-hydroxylase deficiency. *J Clin Endocrinol Metab*. 2009;94:89-95.

384. New MI, Lorenzen F, Lerner AJ, et al. Genotyping steroid 21-hydroxylase deficiency: hormonal reference data. *J Clin Endocrinol Metab*. 1983;57: 320-326.

385. Forest MG, Betuel H, David M. Prenatal treatment in congenital adrenal hyperplasia due to 21-hydroxylase deficiency: up-date 88 of the French multicentric study. *Endocr Res*. 1989;15:277-301.

385a. Wedell A, Thilén A, Ritzén EM, et al. Mutational spectrum of the steroid 21-hydroxylase gene in Sweden: implications for genetic diagnosis and association with disease manifestation. *J Clin Endocrinol Metab*. 1994;78(5):1145-1152.

385b. Jääskeläinen J, Levo A, Voutilainen R, Partanen J. Population-wide evaluation of disease manifestation in relation to molecular genotype in steroid 21-hydroxylase (CYP21) deficiency: good correlation in a well defined population. *J Clin Endocrinol Metab*. 1997;82(10): 3293-3297.

386. Joint LWPES/ESPE CAH Working Group. Consensus statement on 21-hydroxylase deficiency from the Lawson Wilkins Pediatric Endocrine Society and the European Society for Paediatric Endocrinology. *J Clin Endocrinol Metab*. 2002;87(9):4048-4053.

387. Meyer-Bahlburg HF. What causes low rates of child-bearing in congenital adrenal hyperplasia? *J Clin Endocrinol Metab*. 1999;84:1844-1847.

388. Morgan JF, Murphy H, Lacey JH, et al. Long term psychological outcome for women with congenital adrenal hyperplasia: cross sectional survey. *BMJ*. 2005;330:340-341, discussion 341.

389. Claahsen-van der Grinten HL, Otten BJ, Stikkelbroeck MM, et al. Testicular adrenal rest tumours in congenital adrenal hyperplasia. *Best Pract Res Clin Endocrinol Metab*. 2009;23:209-220.

390. Hindmarsh PC. Management of the child with congenital adrenal hyperplasia. *Best Pract Res Clin Endocrinol Metab*. 2009;23:193-208.

391. Merke DP, Chrousos GP, Eisenhofer G, et al. Adrenomedullary dysplasia and hypofunction in patients with classic 21-hydroxylase deficiency. *N Engl J Med*. 2000;343:1362-1368.

392. Weise M, Mehlinger SL, Drinkard B, et al. Patients with classic congenital adrenal hyperplasia have decreased epinephrine reserve and defective glucose elevation in response to high-intensity exercise. *J Clin Endocrinol Metab*. 2004;89:591-597.

393. Van Wyk JJ, Ritzen EM. The role of bilateral adrenalectomy in the treatment of congenital adrenal hyperplasia. *J Clin Endocrinol Metab*. 2003;88:2993-2998.

394. Charmandari E, Chrousos GP, Merke DP. Adrenocorticotropin hypersecretion and pituitary microadenoma following bilateral adrenalectomy in a patient with classic 21-hydroxylase deficiency. *J Pediatr Endocrinol Metab*. 2005;18:97-101.

395. Seckl JR, Miller WL. How safe is long-term prenatal glucocorticoid treatment? *JAMA*. 1997;277:1077-1079.

396. Pang S, Clark AT, Freeman LC, et al. Maternal side effects of prenatal dexamethasone therapy for fetal congenital adrenal hyperplasia. *J Clin Endocrinol Metab*. 1992;75:249-253.

397. Lajic S, Nordenstrom A, Hirvikoski T. Long-term outcome of prenatal treatment of congenital adrenal hyperplasia. *Endocr Dev*. 2008;13: 82-98.

398. Cornean RE, Hindmarsh PC, Brook CG. Obesity in 21-hydroxylase deficient patients. *Arch Dis Child*. 1998;78:261-263.

399. Volkl TM, Simm D, Beier C, et al. Obesity among children and adolescents with classic congenital adrenal hyperplasia due to 21-hydroxylase deficiency. *Pediatrics*. 2006;117:e98-e105.

400. Stikkelbroeck NM, Oyen WJ, van der Wilt GJ, et al. Normal bone mineral density and lean body mass, but increased fat mass, in young adult patients with congenital adrenal hyperplasia. *J Clin Endocrinol Metab*. 2003;88:1036-1042.

401. Falhammar H, Filipsson H, Holmdahl G, et al. Metabolic profile and body composition in adult women with congenital adrenal hyperplasia due to 21-hydroxylase deficiency. *J Clin Endocrinol Metab*. 2007; 92:110-116.

402. Speiser PW, Serrat J, New MI, et al. Insulin insensitivity in adrenal hyperplasia due to nonclassical steroid 21-hydroxylase deficiency. *J Clin Endocrinol Metab*. 1992;75:1421-1424.

403. Sartorato P, Zulian E, Benedini S, et al. Cardiovascular risk factors and ultrasound evaluation of intima-media thickness at common carotids, carotid bulbs, and femoral and abdominal aorta arteries in patients with classic congenital adrenal hyperplasia due to 21-hydroxylase deficiency. *J Clin Endocrinol Metab*. 2007;92:1015-1018.

404. Roche EF, Charmandari E, Dattani MT, et al. Blood pressure in children and adolescents with congenital adrenal hyperplasia (21-hydroxylase deficiency): a preliminary report. *Clin Endocrinol*. 2003;58:589-596.

405. Volkl TMK, Simm D, Dotsch J, et al. Altered 24-hour blood pressure profiles in children and adolescents with classical congenital adrenal hyperplasia due to 21-hydroxylase deficiency. *J Clin Endocrinol Metab*. 2006;91:4888-4895.

406. White PC, Curnow KM, Pascoe L. Disorders of steroid 11 β-hydroxylase isozymes. *Endocr Rev.* 1994;15:421-438.
407. Joehrer K, Geley S, Strasser-Wozak EM, et al. CYP11B1 mutations causing non-classic adrenal hyperplasia due to 11β-hydroxylase deficiency. *Hum Mol Genet.* 1997;6:1829-1834.
408. Peters CJ, Nugent T, Perry LA, et al. Cosegregation of a novel homozygous CYP11B1 mutation with the phenotype of non-classical congenital adrenal hyperplasia in a consanguineous family. *Horm Res.* 2007;67:189-193.
409. Peter M, Janzen N, Sander S, et al. A case of 11β-hydroxylase deficiency detected in a newborn screening program by second-tier LC-MS/MS. *Horm Res.* 2008;69:253-256.
410. Pang S, Levine LS, Lorenzen F, et al. Hormonal studies in obligate heterozygotes and siblings of patients with 11β-hydroxylase deficiency congenital adrenal hyperplasia. *J Clin Endocrinol Metab.* 1980;50:586-589.
411. Gabrilove JL, Sharma DC, Dorfman RI. Adrenocortical 11-β-hydroxylase deficiency and virilism first manifest in the adult women. *N Engl J Med.* 1965;272:1189-1194.
412. de Simone G, Tommaselli AP, Rossi R, et al. Partial deficiency of adrenal 11-hydroxylase: a possible cause of primary hypertension. *Hypertension.* 1985;7:204-210.
413. Biglieri EG. 17 Alpha-hydroxylase deficiency: 1963-1966. *J Clin Endocrinol Metab.* 1997;82:48-50.
414. Zachmann M, Werder EA, Prader A. Two types of male pseudohermaphroditism due to 17,20-desmolase deficiency. *J Clin Endocrinol Metab.* 1982;55:487-490.
415. Auchus RJ. The genetics, pathophysiology, and management of human deficiencies of P450c17. *Endocrinol Metab Clin North Am.* 2001;30:101-119, vii.
416. Geller DH, Auchus RJ, Miller WL. P450c17 mutations R347H and R358Q selectively disrupt 17,20-lyase activity by disrupting interactions with P450 oxidoreductase and cytochrome b5. *Mol Endocrinol.* 1999;13:167-175.
417. Auchus RJ, Lee TC, Miller WL. Cytochrome b5 augments the 17,20-lyase activity of human P450c17 without direct electron transfer. *J Biol Chem.* 1998;273:3158-3165.
418. Yanase T, Simpson ER, Waterman MR. 17 Alpha-hydroxylase/17,20-lyase deficiency: from clinical investigation to molecular definition. *Endocr Rev.* 1991;12:91-108.
419. Geller DH, Auchus RJ, Mendonca BB, et al. The genetic and functional basis of isolated 17,20/lyase deficiency. *Nat Genet.* 1997;17:201-205.
420. Sherbet DP, Tiosano D, Kwist KM, et al. CYP17 mutation E305G causes isolated 17,20-lyase deficiency by selectively altering substrate binding. *J Biol Chem.* 2003;278:48563-48569.
421. Peterson RE, Imperato-McGinley J, Gautier T, et al. Male pseudohermaphroditism due to multiple defects in steroid-biosynthetic microsomal mixed-function oxidases: a new variant of congenital adrenal hyperplasia. *N Engl J Med.* 1985;313:1182-1191.
422. Shackleton C, Marcos J, Arlt W, et al. Prenatal diagnosis of P450 oxidoreductase deficiency (ORD): a disorder causing low pregnancy estriol, maternal and fetal virilization, and the Antley-Bixler syndrome phenotype. *Am J Med Genet.* 2004;129A:105-112.
423. Cragun DL, Trumpy SK, Shackleton CH, et al. Undetectable maternal serum uE3 and postnatal abnormal sterol and steroid metabolism in Antley-Bixler syndrome. *Am J Med Genet.* 2004;129A:1-7.
424. Fukami M, Hasegawa T, Horikawa R, et al. Cytochrome P450 oxidoreductase deficiency in three patients initially regarded as having 21-hydroxylase deficiency and/or aromatase deficiency: diagnostic value of urine steroid hormone analysis. *Pediatr Res.* 2006;59:276-280.
425. Fluck CE, Tajima T, Pandey AV, et al. Mutant P450 oxidoreductase causes disordered steroidogenesis with and without Antley-Bixler syndrome. *Nat Genet.* 2004;36:228-230.
426. Arlt W, Walker EA, Draper N, et al. Congenital adrenal hyperplasia caused by mutant P450 oxidoreductase and human androgen synthesis: analytical study. *Lancet.* 2004;363:2128-2135.
427. Homma K, Hasegawa T, Nagai T, et al. Urine steroid hormone profile analysis in cytochrome P450 oxidoreductase deficiency: implication for the backdoor pathway to dihydrotestosterone. *J Clin Endocrinol Metab.* 2006;91:2643-2649.
428. Fukami M, Nishimura G, Homma K, et al. Cytochrome P450 oxidoreductase deficiency: identification and characterization of biallelic mutations and genotype-phenotype correlations in 35 Japanese patients. *J Clin Endocrinol Metab.* 2009;94:1723-1731.
429. Huang N, Pandey AV, Agrawal V, et al. Diversity and function of mutations in p450 oxidoreductase in patients with Antley-Bixler syndrome and disordered steroidogenesis. *Am J Hum Genet.* 2005;76:729-749.
430. Otto DM, Henderson CJ, Carrie D, et al. Identification of novel roles of the cytochrome p450 system in early embryogenesis: effects on vasculogenesis and retinoic acid homeostasis. *Mol Cell Biol.* 2003;23:6103-6116.
431. Rheaume E, Simard J, Morel Y, et al. Congenital adrenal hyperplasia due to point mutations in the type II 3β-hydroxysteroid dehydrogenase gene. *Nat Genet.* 1992;1:239-245.
432. Simard J, Ricketts M-L, Gingras S, et al. Molecular biology of the 3β-hydroxysteroid dehydrogenase/δ5-δ4 isomerase gene family. *Endocr Rev.* 2005;26:525-582.
433. Marui S, Castro M, Latronico AC, et al. Mutations in the type II 3β-hydroxysteroid dehydrogenase (HSD3B2) gene can cause premature pubarche in girls. *Clin Endocrinol (Oxf).* 2000;52:67-75.
434. Pang SY, Lerner AJ, Stoner E, et al. Late-onset adrenal steroid 3β-hydroxysteroid dehydrogenase deficiency: I. A cause of hirsutism in pubertal and postpubertal women. *J Clin Endocrinol Metab.* 1985;60:428-439.
435. Lutfallah C, Wang W, Mason JI, et al. Newly proposed hormonal criteria via genotypic proof for type II 3β-hydroxysteroid dehydrogenase deficiency. *J Clin Endocrinol Metab.* 2002;87:2611-2622.
436. Mermejo LM, Elias LLK, Marui S, et al. Refining hormonal diagnosis of type II 3β-hydroxysteroid dehydrogenase deficiency in patients with premature pubarche and hirsutism based on HSD3B2 genotyping. *J Clin Endocrinol Metab.* 2005;90:1287-1293.
437. Bose HS, Sugawara T, Strauss JF 3rd, et al. The pathophysiology and genetics of congenital lipoid adrenal hyperplasia. International Congenital Lipoid Adrenal Hyperplasia Consortium. *N Engl J Med.* 1996;335:1870-1878.
438. Baker BY, Lin L, Kim CJ, et al. Nonclassic congenital lipoid adrenal hyperplasia: a new disorder of the steroidogenic acute regulatory protein with very late presentation and normal male genitalia. *J Clin Endocrinol Metab.* 2006;91:4781-4785.
439. Tajima T, Fujieda K, Kouda N, et al. Heterozygous mutation in the cholesterol side chain cleavage enzyme (p450scc) gene in a patient with 46,XY sex reversal and adrenal insufficiency. *J Clin Endocrinol Metab.* 2001;86:3820-3825.
440. Hiort O, Holterhus PM, Werner R, et al. Heterozygous mutation in the cholesterol side chain cleavage enzyme (p450scc) gene in a patient with 46,XY sex. *J Clin Endocrinol Metab.* 2005;90:538-541.
441. Kim CJ, Lin L, Huang N, et al. Severe combined adrenal and gonadal deficiency caused by novel mutations in the cholesterol side chain cleavage enzyme, P450scc. *J Clin Endocrinol Metab.* 2008;93:696-702.
442. Rubtsov P, Karmanov M, Sverdlova P, et al. A novel homozygous mutation in CYP11A1 gene is associated with late-onset adrenal insufficiency and hypospadias in a 46,XY patient. *J Clin Endocrinol Metab.* 2009;94:936-939.
443. Jamieson A, Wallace AM, Andrew R, et al. Apparent cortisone reductase deficiency: a functional defect in 11β-hydroxysteroid dehydrogenase type 1. *J Clin Endocrinol Metab.* 1999;84:3570-3574.
444. Lavery GG, Walker EA, Tiganescu A, et al. Steroid biomarkers and genetic studies reveal inactivating mutations in hexose-6-phosphate dehydrogenase in patients with cortisone reductase deficiency. *J Clin Endocrinol Metab.* 2008;93:3827-3832.
445. Vassiliadi DA, Barber TM, Hughes BA, et al. Increased 5 alpha-reductase activity and adrenocortical drive in women with polycystic ovary syndrome. *J Clin Endocrinol Metab.* 2009;94:3558-3566.
446. Veldhuis JD, Melby JC. Isolated aldosterone deficiency in man: acquired and inborn errors in the biosynthesis or action of aldosterone. *Endocr Rev.* 1981;2:495-517.
447. White PC. Aldosterone synthase deficiency and related disorders. *Mol Cell Endocrinol.* 2004;217:81-87.
448. Kayes-Wandover KM, Schindler RE, Taylor HC, et al. Type 1 aldosterone synthase deficiency presenting in a middle-aged man. *J Clin Endocrinol Metab.* 2001;86:1008-1012.
449. Zennaro MC, Lombes M. Mineralocorticoid resistance. *Trends Endocrinol Metab.* 2004;15:264-270.
450. Geller DS, Rodriguez-Soriano J, Vallo Boado A, et al. Mutations in the mineralocorticoid receptor gene cause autosomal dominant pseudohypoaldosteronism type I. *Nat Genet.* 1998;19:279-281.
451. Chang SS, Grunder S, Hanukoglu A, et al. Mutations in subunits of the epithelial sodium channel cause salt wasting with hyperkalaemic acidosis, pseudohypoaldosteronism type 1. *Nat Genet.* 1996;12:248-253.
452. Strautnieks SS, Thompson RJ, Gardiner RM, et al. A novel splice-site mutation in the gamma subunit of the epithelial sodium channel gene in three pseudohypoaldosteronism type 1 families. *Nat Genet.* 1996;13:248-250.
453. Hanukoglu A, Joy O, Steinitz M, et al. Pseudohypoaldosteronism due to renal and multisystem resistance to mineralocorticoids respond differently to carbenoxolone. *J Steroid Biochem Mol Biol.* 1997;60:105-112.
454. Wilson FH, Disse-Nicodeme S, Choate KA, et al. Human hypertension caused by mutations in WNK kinases. *Science.* 2001;293:1107-1112.
455. DeFronzo RA. Hyperkalemia and hyporeninemic hypoaldosteronism. *Kidney Int.* 1980;17:118-134.
456. Sunderlin FS Jr, Anderson GH Jr, Streeten DH, et al. The renin-angiotensin-aldosterone system in diabetic patients with hyperkalemia. *Diabetes.* 1981;30:335-340.
457. Gabrilove JL, Seman AT, Sabet R, et al. Virilizing adrenal adenoma with studies on the steroid content of the adrenal venous effluent and a review of the literature. *Endocr Rev.* 1981;2:462-470.
458. Kloos RT, Gross MD, Francis IR, et al. Incidentally discovered adrenal masses. *Endocr Rev.* 1995;16:460-484.

459. Terzolo M, Bovio S, Reimondo G, et al. Subclinical Cushing's syndrome in adrenal incidentalomas. *Endocrinol Metab Clin North Am.* 2005;34:423-439, x.

460. Catargi B, Rigalleau V, Poussin A, et al. Occult Cushing's syndrome in type-2 diabetes. *J Clin Endocrinol Metab.* 2003;88:5808-5813.

461. Flecchia D, Mazza E, Carlini M, et al. Reduced serum levels of dehydroepiandrosterone sulphate in adrenal incidentalomas: a marker of adrenocortical tumour. *Clin Endocrinol (Oxf).* 1995;42:129-134.

462. Cawood TJ, Hunt PJ, O'Shea D, et al. Recommended evaluation of adrenal incidentalomas is costly, has high false-positive rates and confers a risk of fatal cancer that is similar to the risk of the adrenal lesion becoming malignant: time for a rethink? *Eur J Endocrinol.* 2009; 161:513-527.

463. Mansmann G, Lau J, Balk E, et al. The clinically inapparent adrenal mass: update in diagnosis and management. *Endocr Rev.* 2004;25: 309-340.

464. Gicquel C, Le Bouc Y, Luton JP, et al. Pathogenesis and treatment of adrenocortical carcinoma. *Curr Opin Endocrinol Diab.* 1998;5:189-196.

465. Matzuk MM, Finegold MJ, Mather JP, et al. Development of cancer cachexia-like syndrome and adrenal tumors in inhibin-deficient mice. *Proc Natl Acad Sci U S A.* 1994;91:8817-8821.

Endocrine Hypertension

WILLIAM F. YOUNG, JR.

KEY POINTS

- There are at least 14 endocrine disorders for which hypertension may be the initial clinical presentation. An accurate diagnosis of endocrine hypertension provides the clinician with a unique treatment opportunity: to render a surgical cure or to achieve a dramatic response with pharmacologic therapy.
- Catecholamines affect many cardiovascular and metabolic processes—they increase heart rate, blood pressure, myocardial contractility, and cardiac conduction velocity. The identification of three types of adrenergic receptors (α, β, and dopaminergic receptors) and their subtypes (α_1, α_2, β_1, β_2, β_3, D_1, and D_2) has led to understanding of the physiologic responses to endogenous and exogenous administration of catecholamines.
- Catecholamine-secreting tumors are rare, with an annual incidence of 2 to 8 cases per 1 million people. Nevertheless, it is important to suspect, confirm, localize, and resect these tumors because (1) the associated hypertension is curable with surgical removal of the tumor, (2) a risk of lethal paroxysm exists, (3) at least 10% of the tumors are malignant, and (4) 40% of these tumors are familial and their detection in the proband may result in early diagnosis in other family members.
- Germline mutations are responsible for approximately 40% of all catecholamine-secreting tumors. Mutations contributing to pheochromocytoma and paraganglioma have two general transcription signatures: cluster 1—genes encoding proteins that function in the cellular response to hypoxia, and cluster 2—genes encoding proteins that activate kinase signaling.
- Pheochromocytoma/paraganglioma must be confirmed biochemically by the presence of increased concentrations of fractionated metanephrines and catecholamines in urine or plasma. Then the tumor should be localized with computed tomography (CT) of the abdomen and pelvis. Approximately 85% of these tumors are found in the adrenal glands, and 95% are found in the abdomen and pelvis.
- Some form of preoperative pharmacologic preparation is indicated for all patients with catecholamine-secreting neoplasms, including those who are asymptomatic and normotensive. Surgical resection of a catecholamine-secreting tumor is a high-risk surgical procedure, and an experienced surgeon-anesthesiologist team is required.
- Hypertension, suppressed plasma renin activity, and increased aldosterone excretion characterize the syndrome of primary aldosteronism, which was first described in 1955.
- Aldosterone-producing adenoma and bilateral idiopathic hyperaldosteronism are the most common subtypes of primary aldosteronism. Somatic mutations account for about half of aldosterone-producing adenomas and include mutations in genes encoding components of the potassium channel (KCNJ5); the sodium/potassium and calcium adenosine triphosphatases (ATPases) (ATP1A1 and ATP2B3); and a voltage-dependent C-type calcium channel (CACNA1D).
- Use of the plasma aldosterone to plasma renin activity ratio as a case-detection test, followed by aldosterone suppression for confirmatory testing, has resulted in much higher prevalence estimates for primary aldosteronism—5% to 10% of all patients with hypertension.
- The treatment goal in patients with primary aldosteronism is to prevent the morbidity and fatality associated with hypertension, hypokalemia, and cardiovascular damage. Knowing the cause of the primary aldosteronism helps to determine the appropriate treatment. Normalization of blood pressure should not be the only goal—normalization of circulating aldosterone or mineralocorticoid receptor blockade should be part of the management plan for all patients with primary aldosteronism.

An estimated 68 million people in the United States are hypertensive.[1,2] In most, hypertension is *primary* (i.e., *essential* or *idiopathic*), but a subgroup of approximately 15% have *secondary* hypertension. The secondary causes of hypertension can be divided into renal causes, such as renal parenchymal or renovascular disease, and endocrine causes. There are at least 14 endocrine disorders for which hypertension may be the initial clinical presentation (Table 16-1). An accurate diagnosis of endocrine hypertension provides the clinician with a unique treatment opportunity: to render a surgical cure or to achieve a dramatic response with pharmacologic therapy. The diagnostic and therapeutic approaches to endocrine hypertension—ranging from the classic adrenal causes of hypertension (e.g., pheochromocytoma, primary aldosteronism) to pituitary-dependent hypertension (e.g., Cushing syndrome, acromegaly)—are reviewed in this chapter.

ADRENAL MEDULLA AND CATECHOLAMINES

The adrenal medulla occupies the central portion of the adrenal gland and accounts for 10% of total adrenal gland volume. There is no clear demarcation between the adrenal cortex and adrenal medulla. The adrenal glands derive blood supply from the superior, middle, and inferior branches of the inferior phrenic artery, from the renal arteries, and directly from the aorta. The adrenal arteries branch and form a plexus under the capsule. This plexus supplies the cortex. Some of the plexus arteries penetrate the cortex and supply the medulla, as do capillaries drain-

TABLE 16-1

Endocrine Causes of Hypertension

Adrenal-Dependent Causes

Pheochromocytoma
Primary aldosteronism
Hyperdeoxycorticosteronism
   Congenital adrenal hyperplasia
      11β-Hydroxylase deficiency
      17α-Hydroxylase deficiency
   Deoxycorticosterone-producing tumor
Primary cortisol resistance
Cushing syndrome

AME/11β-HSD Deficiency

Genetic
   Type 1 AME
   Type 2 AME
Acquired
   Licorice or carbenoxolone ingestion (type 1 AME)
   Cushing syndrome (type 2 AME)

Thyroid-Dependent Causes

Hypothyroidism
Hyperthyroidism

Calcium/Parathyroid-Dependent Causes

Hyperparathyroidism

Pituitary-Dependent Causes

Acromegaly
Cushing syndrome

AME, apparent mineralocorticoid excess; HSD, hydroxysteroid dehydrogenase.

ing the cortical cells, forming the corticomedullary portal system. The right adrenal vein is short and drains directly into the inferior vena cava (IVC). The left adrenal vein merges with the inferior phrenic vein, and this larger vein (the common phrenic vein) drains into the left renal vein.

Adrenomedullary cells are called *chromaffin cells* (stain brown with chromium salts) or *pheochromocytes*. Cytoplasmic granules turn dark when stained with chromic acid because of the oxidation of epinephrine and norepinephrine to melanin. Chromaffin cells differentiate in the center of the adrenal gland in response to cortisol; some chromaffin cells also migrate to form paraganglia, collections of chromaffin cells located on both sides of the aorta. The largest cluster of chromaffin cells outside the adrenal medulla is located near the level of the inferior mesenteric artery and is referred to as the *organ of Zuckerkandl*; it is quite prominent in the fetus and is a major source of catecholamines during the first year of life. The preganglionic sympathetic neurons receive synaptic input from neurons within the pons, medulla, and hypothalamus, providing regulation of sympathetic activity by the brain. Axons from the lower thoracic and lumbar preganglionic neurons, via splanchnic nerves, directly innervate the cells of the adrenal medulla.

The term *catecholamine* refers to substances that contain catechol (ortho-dihydroxybenzene) and a side chain with an amino group—the catechol nucleus (Fig. 16-1).[3] Epinephrine is synthesized and stored in the adrenal medulla and released into the systemic circulation. Norepinephrine is synthesized and stored not only in the adrenal medulla but also in the peripheral sympathetic nerves. Dopamine, the precursor of norepinephrine, is found in the adrenal medulla and peripheral sympathetic nerves and acts primarily as a neurotransmitter in the central nervous system.

Catecholamines affect many cardiovascular and metabolic processes. They increase the heart rate, blood pressure, myocardial contractility, and cardiac conduction velocity. Activation of G protein–coupled receptors mediates the biologic actions of catecholamines. The identification of three types of adrenergic receptors (α, β, and dopaminergic receptors) and their subtypes (α_1, α_2, β_1, β_2, β_3, D_1, and D_2) has led to understanding of the physiologic responses to endogenous and exogenous administration of catecholamines.[4] The 2012 Nobel Prize in Chemistry was awarded to Brian K. Kobilka and Robert J. Lefkowitz for their studies of G protein–coupled receptors.[5] The α_1 subtype is a postsynaptic receptor that mediates vascular and smooth muscle contraction; stimulation causes vasoconstriction and increases blood pressure. The α_2 receptors

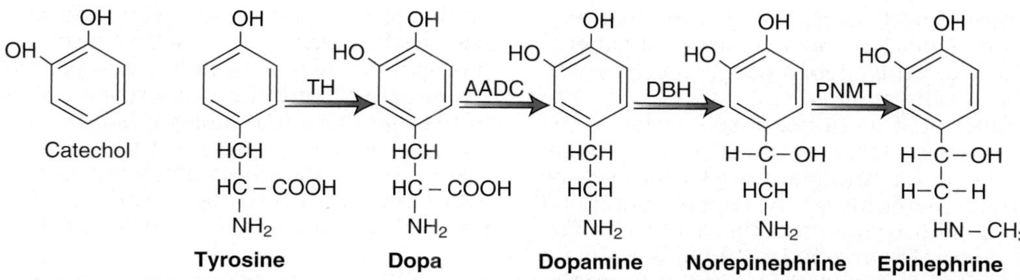

Figure 16-1 Biosynthetic pathway for catecholamines. The term *catecholamine* comes from the catechol (ortho-dihydroxybenzene) structure and a side chain with an amino group—the catechol nucleus (shown on left). Tyrosine is converted to 3,4-dihydroxyphenylalanine (dopa) by tyrosine hydroxylase (TH); this rate-limiting step provides the clinician with the option to treat pheochromocytoma with a TH inhibitor, α-methyl-paratyrosine (metyrosine). Aromatic L-amino acid decarboxylase (AADC) converts dopa to dopamine. Dopamine is hydroxylated to norepinephrine by dopamine β-hydroxylase (DBH). Norepinephrine is converted to epinephrine by phenylethanolamine *N*-methyltransferase (PNMT). Cortisol serves as a cofactor for PNMT, which explains why epinephrine-secreting neoplasms are almost exclusively localized to the adrenal medulla. (Modified and redrawn from Dluhy RG, Lawrence JE, Williams GH. Endocrine hypertension. In: Larsen PR, Kronenberg HM, Melmed S, et al, eds. *Williams Textbook of Endocrinology*, 10th ed. Philadelphia, PA: Saunders; 2003:555.)

are located on presynaptic sympathetic nerve endings; when activated, they inhibit release of norepinephrine. Stimulation causes suppression of central sympathetic outflow and decreased blood pressure.

There are three major β-receptor subtypes. The β_1 receptor mediates cardiac effects and is more responsive to isoproterenol than to epinephrine or norepinephrine. Stimulation causes positive inotropic and chronotropic effects on the heart, increased renin secretion in the kidney, and lipolysis in adipocytes. The β_2 receptor mediates bronchial, vascular, and uterine smooth muscle relaxation. Stimulation causes bronchodilation, vasodilatation in skeletal muscle, glycogenolysis, and increased release of norepinephrine from sympathetic nerve terminals. The β_3 receptor regulates energy expenditure and lipolysis.

D_1 receptors are localized to the cerebral, renal, mesenteric, and coronary vasculatures; stimulation causes vasodilation in these vascular beds. D_2 receptors are presynaptic; they are localized to sympathetic nerve endings, sympathetic ganglia, and brain. Stimulation of D_2 receptors in these locations inhibits the release of norepinephrine, inhibits ganglionic transmission, and inhibits prolactin release, respectively.

Most cells in the body have adrenergic receptors. The pharmacologic development of selective α- and β-adrenergic agonists and antagonists has advanced pharmacotherapy for various clinical disorders. For example, β_1 antagonists (e.g., atenolol, metoprolol) are now considered standard therapies for angina pectoris, hypertension, and cardiac arrhythmias.[6] Administration of β_2 agonists (e.g., terbutaline, albuterol) causes bronchial smooth muscle relaxation; these agents are commonly prescribed in inhaled formulations for the treatment of asthma.[7]

Catecholamine Synthesis

Catecholamines are synthesized from tyrosine by a process of hydroxylation and decarboxylation (see Fig. 16-1). Tyrosine is derived from ingested food or synthesized from phenylalanine in the liver, and it enters neurons and chromaffin cells by active transport. Tyrosine is converted to 3,4-dihydroxyphenylalanine (dopa) by tyrosine hydroxylase, the rate-limiting step in catecholamine synthesis. Increased intracellular levels of catechols downregulate the activity of tyrosine hydroxylase; as catecholamines are released from secretory granules in response to a stimulus, cytoplasmic catecholamines are depleted and the feedback inhibition of tyrosine hydroxylase is released. Transcription of tyrosine hydroxylase is stimulated by glucocorticoids, cyclic adenosine monophosphate (cAMP)–dependent protein kinases, calcium/phospholipid-dependent protein kinase, and calcium/calmodulin-dependent protein kinase. α-Methyl-paratyrosine (metyrosine) is a tyrosine hydroxylase inhibitor that may be used therapeutically in patients with catecholamine-secreting neoplasms to decrease tumoral synthesis of catecholamines.[8]

Aromatic L-amino acid decarboxylase catalyzes the decarboxylation of dopa to dopamine (see Fig. 16-1). Dopamine is actively transported into granulated vesicles to be hydroxylated to norepinephrine by the copper-containing enzyme dopamine β-hydroxylase. Ascorbic acid is a cofactor and hydrogen donor. The enzyme is structurally similar to tyrosine hydroxylase and may share similar transcriptional regulatory elements, and both are stimulated by glucocorticoids and cAMP-dependent kinases. These reactions occur in the synaptic vesicle of adrenergic neurons in the central nervous system, the peripheral nervous system, and the chromaffin cells of the adrenal medulla. The major constituents of the granulated vesicle are dopamine β-hydroxylase, ascorbic acid, chromogranin A, and adenosine triphosphate (ATP).

In the adrenal medulla, norepinephrine is released from the granule into the cytoplasm, where the cytosolic enzyme phenylethanolamine N-methyltransferase (PNMT) converts it to epinephrine (see Fig. 16-1). Epinephrine is then transported back into another storage vesicle. The N-methylation reaction by PNMT involves S-adenosylmethionine as the methyl donor as well as oxygen and magnesium. PNMT expression is regulated by the presence of glucocorticoids, which are in high concentration in the adrenal medulla through the corticomedullary portal system. Therefore, catecholamine-secreting tumors that secrete primarily epinephrine are localized to the adrenal medulla. In normal adrenal medullary tissue, approximately 80% of the catecholamines released are epinephrine.

Catecholamine Storage and Secretion

Catecholamines are found in the adrenal medulla and in sympathetically innervated organs. Catecholamines are stored in electron-dense granules that also contain ATP, neuropeptides (e.g., adrenomedullin, corticotropin [ACTH, adrenocorticotropic hormone], vasoactive intestinal polypeptide), calcium, magnesium, and chromogranins. Uptake into the storage vesicles is facilitated by active transport by vesicular monoamine transporters (VMAT).[9] The VMAT ATP-driven pump maintains a steep electrical gradient. For every monoamine transported, ATP is hydrolyzed and two hydrogen ions are transported from the vesicle into the cytosol. Iodine-123 (^{123}I) and ^{131}I-labeled metaiodobenzylguanidine (MIBG) are imported by VMAT into the storage vesicles in the adrenal medulla, which makes ^{123}I-MIBG useful for imaging localization of catecholamine-secreting tumors and ^{131}I-MIBG potentially useful in treating malignant catecholamine-secreting tumors.[10-12] Catecholamine uptake, as well as that of MIBG, is inhibited by reserpine.[13] The catecholamine stores are dynamic, with constant leakage and reuptake.[9]

Stressful stimuli (e.g., myocardial infarction, anesthesia, hypoglycemia) trigger adrenal medullary catecholamine secretion. Acetylcholine from preganglionic sympathetic fibers stimulates nicotinic cholinergic receptors and causes depolarization of adrenomedullary chromaffin cells. Depolarization leads to activation of voltage-gated calcium channels, which results in exocytosis of secretory vesicle contents. A calcium-sensing receptor appears to be involved in the process of exocytosis. During exocytosis, all the granular contents are released into the extracellular space. Norepinephrine modulates its own release by activating the α_2 receptors on the presynaptic membrane. Stimulation of the presynaptic α_2 receptors inhibits norepinephrine release (the mechanism of action of some antihypertensive medications such as clonidine and guanfacine). Catecholamines are among the shortest lived signaling molecules in plasma; the initial biologic half-life of circulating catecholamines is between 10 and 100 seconds. Approximately one half of the catecholamines circulate in plasma in loose association with albumin. Therefore, plasma concentrations of catecholamines fluctuate widely.

Catecholamine Metabolism and Inactivation

Catecholamines are removed from the circulation either by reuptake in sympathetic nerve terminals or by metabolism through two enzyme pathways (Fig. 16-2), followed by sulfate conjugation and renal excretion. Most of the metabolism of catecholamines occurs in the same cell in

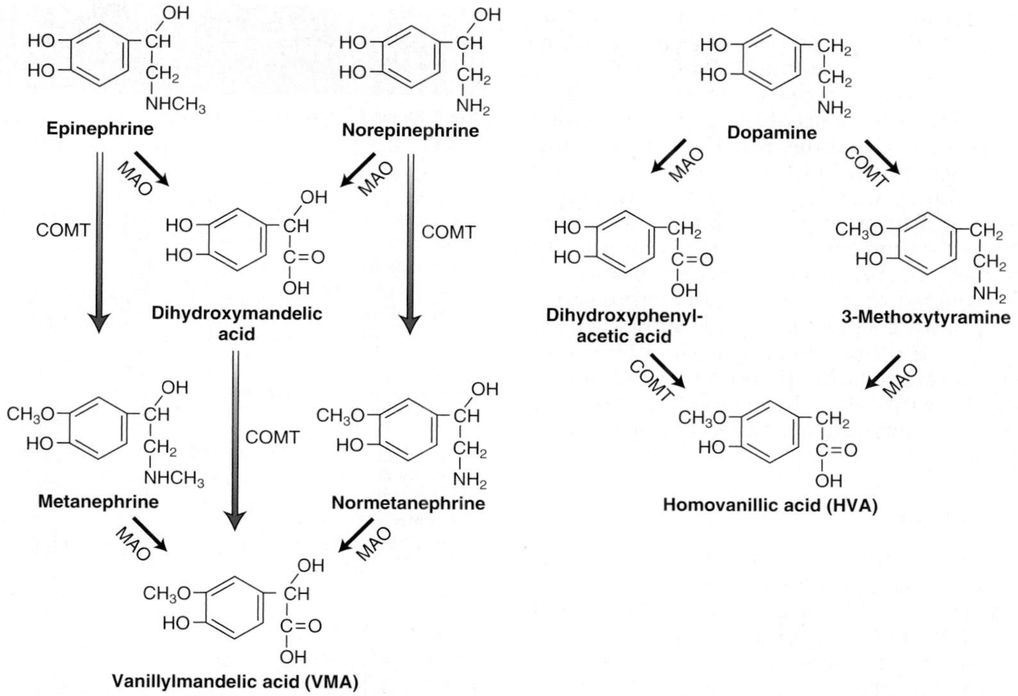

Figure 16-2 Catecholamine metabolism. Metabolism of catecholamines occurs through two enzymatic pathways. Catechol-*O*-methyltransferase (COMT) converts epinephrine to metanephrine and converts norepinephrine to normetanephrine through meta-*O*-methylation. Metanephrine and normetanephrine are oxidized by monoamine oxidase (MAO) to vanillylmandelic acid (VMA) by oxidative deamination. MAO also may oxidize epinephrine and norepinephrine to dihydroxymandelic acid, which is then converted by COMT to VMA. Dopamine is also metabolized by MAO and COMT to the final metabolite, homovanillic acid (HVA). (Modified and redrawn from Dluhy RG, Lawrence JE, Williams GH. Endocrine hypertension. In Larsen PR, Kronenberg HM, Melmed S, et al, eds. *Williams Textbook of Endocrinology*, 10th ed. Philadelphia, PA: Saunders; 2003:556.)

which they are synthesized.[9] Almost 90% of catecholamines released at sympathetic synapses are taken up locally by the nerve endings, termed *uptake 1*. Uptake 1 can be blocked by cocaine, tricyclic antidepressants, and phenothiazines. Extraneuronal tissues also take up catecholamines, and this is termed *uptake 2*. Most of these catecholamines are metabolized by catechol-*O*-methyltransferase (COMT).

Although COMT is found primarily outside neural tissue, *O*-methylation in the adrenal medulla is the predominant source of metanephrine (COMT converts epinephrine to metanephrine) and a major source of normetanephrine (COMT converts norepinephrine to normetanephrine) through methylation of the 3-hydroxy group.[9] *S*-Adenosylmethionine is used as the methyl donor, and calcium is required for this enzymatic step. Metanephrine and normetanephrine are oxidized by monoamine oxidase (MAO) to vanillylmandelic acid (VMA) by oxidative deamination. MAO may also oxidize epinephrine and norepinephrine to 3,4-dihydroxymandelic acid, which is then converted by COMT to VMA. MAO is located on the outer membrane of mitochondria. In the storage vesicle, norepinephrine is protected from metabolism by MAO. MAO and COMT metabolize dopamine to homovanillic acid (see Fig. 16-2).

PHEOCHROMOCYTOMA AND PARAGANGLIOMA

Catecholamine-secreting tumors that arise from chromaffin cells of the adrenal medulla and the sympathetic ganglia are referred to as *pheochromocytomas* and *catecholamine-*

secreting paragangliomas, respectively.[14] Because the tumors have similar clinical presentations and are treated with similar approaches, many clinicians use the term *pheochromocytoma* to refer to both adrenal pheochromocytomas and extra-adrenal catecholamine-secreting paragangliomas. However, the distinction between pheochromocytoma and paraganglioma is an important one because of implications for associated neoplasms, risk for malignancy, and genetic testing. Catecholamine-secreting tumors are rare, with an annual incidence of 2 to 8 cases per 1 million people.[15] Based on screening studies for secondary causes of hypertension in outpatients, the prevalence of pheochromocytoma has been estimated at 0.1% to 0.6%.[16,17] Nevertheless, it is important to suspect, confirm, localize, and resect these tumors because (1) the associated hypertension is curable with surgical removal of the tumor, (2) a risk of lethal paroxysm exists, (3) at least 10% of the tumors are malignant, and (4) 40% of these tumors are familial and their detection in the proband may result in early diagnosis in other family members.

History

The association between adrenal medullary tumors and symptoms was first recognized by Fränkel in 1886.[18] He described Fraulein Minna Roll, age 18 years, who had intermittent attacks of palpitation, anxiety, vertigo, headache, chest pain, cold sweats, and vomiting. She had a hard, noncompressible pulse and retinitis. Despite champagne therapy and injections of ether, she died. At autopsy, bilateral adrenal tumors were initially thought to be angiosarcomas, but later a positive chromaffin reaction confirmed pheochromocytoma. A subsequent study published in 2007 documented the presence of a germline *RET* proto-oncogene mutation in four living relatives of Frau-lein Roll—proving that the original patient and her family had multiple endocrine neoplasia type 2 (MEN2).[19]

The term *pheochromocytoma*, proposed by Pick in 1912,[20] comes from the Greek words *phaios* (dusky), *chroma* (color), and *cytoma* (tumor)—words that describe the dark staining reaction that is caused by the oxidation of intracellular catecholamines when they are exposed to dichromate salts. In 1926, César Roux in Lausanne, Switzerland, and Charles Mayo in Rochester, Minnesota, successfully surgically removed abdominal catecholamine-secreting tumors.[21,22] In 1929, it was discovered that a pheochromocytoma contained an excess amount of a pressor agent.[23] Subsequently, epinephrine (in 1936) and norepinephrine (in 1949) were isolated from pheochromocytoma tissue.[23] In 1950, it was found that patients with pheochromocytoma excreted increased amounts of epinephrine, norepinephrine, and dopamine in the urine.[24]

Clinical Presentation

Catecholamine-secreting tumors occur with equal frequency in men and women, primarily in the third, fourth, and fifth decades. These tumors are rare in children, and when discovered, they may be multifocal and associated with a hereditary syndrome. The symptoms, listed in Table 16-2, are caused by the pharmacologic effects of excess concentrations of circulating catecholamines.[25] The associated hypertension may be sustained or paroxysmal, and patients whose pheochromocytoma is diagnosed in the presymptomatic stage may have normal blood pressure. The lability in blood pressure can be attributed to episodic release of catecholamines, chronic volume depletion, and impaired sympathetic reflexes. In addition to volume depletion, altered sympathetic vascular regulation may have a role in orthostasis, which may be observed in patients with pheochromocytoma.[26] Symptoms of orthostatic hypotension (e.g., lightheadedness, presyncope, syncope) may dominate the presentation, especially in patients with epinephrine- or dopamine-predominant tumors.[27]

Episodic symptoms may occur in spells, or paroxysms, that can be extremely variable in presentation but typically include forceful heartbeat, pallor, tremor, headache, and diaphoresis.[28] The spell may start with a sensation of a "rush" in the chest and a sense of shortness of breath, followed by a forceful heartbeat and a throbbing headache. Peripheral vasoconstriction associated with a spell results in cool or cold hands and feet and facial pallor. Increased sense of body heat and sweating are common symptoms that occur toward the end of the spell. Spells may be either spontaneous or precipitated by postural change, anxiety, medications (e.g., β-adrenergic antagonists, metoclopramide, anesthetic agents), exercise, or maneuvers that increase intra-abdominal pressure (e.g., change in position, lifting, defecation, exercise, colonoscopy, pregnancy, trauma). Although the types of spells experienced across the patient population are highly variable, spells tend to be stereotypical for each patient. Spells may occur multiple times daily or as infrequently as once monthly. The typical duration of a pheochromocytoma spell is 15 to 20 minutes, but it may be much shorter or last several hours. However, the clinician must recognize that most patients with spells do not have a pheochromocytoma (Table 16-3).[29]

Additional clinical signs of pheochromocytoma include hypertensive retinopathy, orthostatic hypotension, angina, nausea, constipation (megacolon may be the presenting symptom), hyperglycemia, diabetes mellitus, hypercalcemia, Raynaud phenomenon, livedo reticularis, erythrocy-

TABLE 16-2

Signs and Symptoms Associated With Catecholamine-Secreting Tumors

Spell-Related Signs and Symptoms

Anxiety and fear of impending death
Diaphoresis
Dyspnea
Epigastric and chest pain
Headache
Hypertension
Nausea and vomiting
Pallor
Palpitation (forceful heartbeat)
Tremor

Chronic Signs and Symptoms

Cold hands and feet
Congestive heart failure—dilated or hypertrophic cardiomyopathy
Constipation
Diaphoresis
Dyspnea
Ectopic hormone secretion–dependent symptoms (e.g., CRH/ACTH, GHRH, PTHrP, VIP)
Epigastric and chest pain
Fatigue
Fever
General increase in sweating
Grade II to IV hypertensive retinopathy
Headache
Hyperglycemia
Hypertension
Nausea and vomiting
Orthostatic hypotension
Painless hematuria (associated with urinary bladder paraganglioma)
Pallor
Palpitation (forceful heartbeat)
Tremor
Weight loss

Not Typical of Pheochromocytoma

Flushing

ACTH, adrenocorticotropic hormone; CRH, corticotropin–releasing hormone; GHRH, growth hormone–releasing hormone; PTHrP, parathyroid hormone–related peptide; VIP, vasoactive intestinal polypeptide.
Adapted from Young WF Jr. Pheochromocytoma, 1926-1993. *Trends Endocrinol Metab.* 1993;4:122-127.

tosis, and mass effects from the tumor. Although hypercalcemia may be a sign of primary hyperparathyroidism in patients with MEN2A, in most patients with pheochromocytoma it is an isolated finding and resolves with resection of the catecholamine-secreting tumor. In addition, calcitonin secretion is in part a catecholamine-dependent process; serum calcitonin concentrations are frequently mildly elevated in patients with pheochromocytoma, usually unrelated to MEN2. Fasting hyperglycemia and diabetes mellitus are caused in part by the α-adrenergic inhibition of insulin release. Painless hematuria and paroxysmal attacks induced by micturition and defecation are associated with urinary bladder paragangliomas.

Some of the cosecreted hormones that may dominate the clinical presentation include ACTH (Cushing syndrome), parathyroid hormone–related peptide (hypercalcemia), vasopressin (syndrome of inappropriate antidiuretic hormone secretion), vasoactive intestinal peptide (watery diarrhea), and growth hormone–releasing hormone (acromegaly).[30-33] Cardiomyopathy and congestive heart failure are the symptomatic presentations caused by pheochromocytoma that are most frequently unrecognized by clinicians.[34] The cardiomyopathy, whether dilated or

TABLE 16-3
Differential Diagnosis of Pheochromocytoma-Type Spells

Endocrine Causes

Carbohydrate intolerance
Hyperadrenergic spells
Hypoglycemia
Pancreatic tumors (e.g., insulinoma)
Pheochromocytoma
Primary hypogonadism (menopausal syndrome)
Thyrotoxicosis

Cardiovascular Causes

Angina
Cardiovascular deconditioning
Labile essential hypertension
Orthostatic hypotension
Paroxysmal cardiac arrhythmia
Pulmonary edema
Renovascular disease
Syncope (e.g., vasovagal reaction)

Psychological Causes

Factitious (e.g., drugs, Valsalva maneuver)
Hyperventilation
Severe anxiety and panic disorders
Somatization disorder

Pharmacologic Causes

Chlorpropamide-alcohol flush
Combination of a monoamine oxidase inhibitor and a decongestant
Illegal drug ingestion (cocaine, phencyclidine, lysergic acid diethylamide)
Sympathomimetic drug ingestion
Vancomycin (red man syndrome)
Withdrawal of adrenergic-inhibitor

Neurologic Causes

Autonomic neuropathy
Cerebrovascular insufficiency
Diencephalic epilepsy (autonomic seizures)
Migraine headache
Postural orthostatic tachycardia syndrome
Stroke

Other Causes

Carcinoid syndrome
Mast cell disease
Recurrent idiopathic anaphylaxis
Unexplained flushing spells

hypertrophic, may be totally reversible with tumor resection.[35] Myocarditis and myocardial infarction with normal coronary arteries seen on angiography are cardiac-based presentations that may not be recognized as pheochromocytoma. The myocarditis is characterized by infiltration of inflammatory cells and focal contraction-band necrosis. Many physical examination findings can be associated with genetic syndromes that predispose to pheochromocytoma; these findings include retinal angiomas, iris hamartomas, marfanoid body habitus, café au lait spots, axillary freckling, subcutaneous neurofibromas, and mucosal neuromas on the eyelids and tongue. Some patients with pheochromocytoma are asymptomatic despite high circulating levels of catecholamines; this type most likely reflects adrenergic receptor desensitization related to chronic stimulation.

Because of the increased and widespread use of CT and magnetic resonance imaging (MRI) in patients with abdominal symptoms, pheochromocytoma and abdominal paraganglioma may be detected as an incidental adrenal mass in many patients before any symptoms develop.[36] In recent studies, approximately 50% of adrenal pheochromocytoma patients had their adrenal tumors discovered incidentally on imaging performed for other reasons.[37-40] Although typically these incidentally discovered tumors in asymptomatic patients are small (<3 cm), they may be up to 10 cm in largest diameter.

At the time of symptom-based detection, pheochromocytomas have an average diameter of 4.5 cm (Fig. 16-3).[41] Paragangliomas are found where there is chromaffin tissue: along the para-aortic sympathetic chain, within the organ of Zuckerkandl (at the origin of the inferior mesenteric artery), in the wall of the urinary bladder, and along the sympathetic chain in the neck or mediastinum.[42] During early postnatal life, the extra-adrenal sympathetic paraganglionic tissues are prominent; later they degenerate, leaving residual foci associated with the vagus nerves, carotid vessels, aortic arch, pulmonary vessels, and mesenteric arteries. Odd locations for paragangliomas include the neck, intra-atrial cardiac septum, spermatic cord, vagina, scrotum, and sacrococcygeal region. Paragangliomas in the head and neck region (e.g., carotid body tumors, glomus tumors, chemodectomas) usually arise from parasympathetic tissue and typically do not hypersecrete catecholamines and metanephrines. Paragangliomas in the mediastinum, abdomen, and pelvis usually arise from

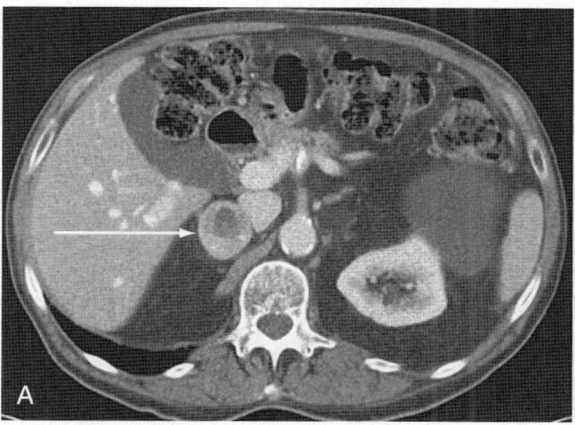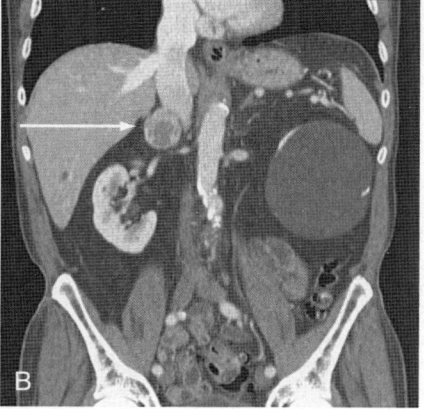

Figure 16-3 A computed tomographic (CT) scan of the abdomen with intravenous contrast in a 71-year-old man with an incidentally discovered right adrenal mass. The concentrations of plasma fractionated free metanephrines were abnormal: metanephrine, 0.34 nmol/L (normal, <0.5 nmol/L) and normetanephrine, 8.59 nmol/L (normal, <0.9 nmol/L). The 24-hour urine studies were abnormal: norepinephrine, 455 μg (normal, <170 μg); epinephrine, 7.2 μg (normal, <35 μg); dopamine, 160 μg (normal, <700 μg); metanephrine, 173 μg (normal, <400 μg); and normetanephrine, 3147 μg (normal, <900 μg). **A,** The axial CT image shows a typical 3.8-cm heterogeneously enhancing right adrenal mass just lateral to the inferior vena cava and consistent with pheochromocytoma *(arrow).* **B,** Coronal view shows the location *(arrow)* of the mass superior to the right kidney and inferior and medial to the liver. After α- and β-adrenergic blockade, a 20-g (2.5 × 1.5 × 1.5 cm) pheochromocytoma was removed laparoscopically.

sympathetic chromaffin tissue and usually do hypersecrete catecholamines and metanephrines.

Syndromic Forms of Pheochromocytoma and Paraganglioma

Multiple Endocrine Neoplasia Type 2A

MEN2A (previously known as Sipple syndrome) is an autosomal dominant disorder with age-related penetrance.[43] MEN2A is characterized by medullary thyroid cancer (MTC) in all patients, adrenergic (epinephrine and metanephrines are predominant) pheochromocytoma in 50% (usually bilateral and frequently asynchronous), primary hyperparathyroidism in 20%, cutaneous lichen amyloidosis in 5%, and very rarely Hirschsprung disease. Cutaneous lichen amyloidosis is a pruritic, papular, scaly, and pigmented skin lesion that is typically located in the interscapular region or on the extensor surfaces of the extremities.

MTC is usually detected before the pheochromocytoma is diagnosed. The prevalence of MEN2A is approximately 1 in 200,000 live births. Numerous activating mutations throughout the *RET* (REarranged during Transfection) proto-oncogene have been documented in persons with MEN2A. *RET*, located on chromosome 10q11.2, encodes a transmembrane receptor tyrosine kinase that is involved in the regulation of cell proliferation and apoptosis by activation of the PI3K/AKT (phosphoinositide 3-kinase) and MAPK/ERK (mitogen-activated protein kinase/extracellular signal-regulated kinase) signaling pathways. *RET* can be constitutively activated by gain-of-function mutations in seven specific exons of the *RET* gene (exons 8, 10, 11, 13, 14, 15, or 16). Most mutations in MEN2A kindreds (>90%) involve *RET* exons 10 (codons 609, 611, 618, and 620) or 11 (codons 630 or 634). Eighty-five percent of individuals with MEN2A have a mutation in codon 634, particularly p.Cys634Arg (c.1900C>T).

Hirschsprung disease is characterized by the absence of autonomic ganglion cells within the distal colon parasympathetic plexus, which results in constipation, megacolon, or obstipation. Hirschsprung disease may occur in patients with MEN2A who have a Janus mutation—a mutation that acts simultaneously as both a gain-in-function and a loss-of-function mutation—in the *RET* proto-oncogene (exon 10: codons 609, 611, 618, 620).[44] It is important to distinguish the constipation/obstipation due to Hirschsprung disease in patients with MEN2A from that due to ganglioneuromatosis of MEN2B or from the colonic paralytic effects seen in patients with massive elevations in catecholamines (most commonly seen in patients with widespread metastatic paraganglioma or pheochromocytoma).

Multiple Endocrine Neoplasia Type 2B

MEN2B (previously known as Gorlin syndrome) is also an autosomal dominant disorder with age-related penetrance, and it represents approximately 5% of all MEN2 cases.[43] MEN2B is characterized by MTC in all patients, adrenergic (epinephrine and metanephrines predominant) pheochromocytoma in 50%, mucocutaneous neuromas (typically involving the tongue, lips, and eyelids) in most patients, and by skeletal deformities (e.g., kyphoscoliosis, lordosis), joint laxity, myelinated corneal nerves, and intestinal ganglioneuromas.

MEN2B-associated tumors are caused by mutations in the *RET* protein's intracellular domain. A single methionine-to-threonine missense mutation in exon 16 (p.Met918Thr; c.2753T>C) is responsible for more than 95% of MEN2B cases. Another mutation, alanine to phenylalanine at codon 883 in exon 15, has been found in 4% of MEN2B kindreds.

More than 95% of patients with MEN2A and more than 98% of those with MEN2B have an identifiable mutation in the *RET* proto-oncogene. Pheochromocytoma in MEN2 has an adrenergic (epinephrine and metanephrines are predominant) biochemical phenotype, and this knowledge directs genetic testing. Genetic testing for mutations in the *RET* proto-oncogene should be considered for patients with co-phenotype disorders (e.g., medullary thyroid carcinoma) or adrenergic biochemical phenotype pheochromocytoma (unilateral or bilateral). In a family with MEN2, a family member with a clinical diagnosis of MEN2 should be tested first. If a *RET* mutation is found, all family members of unknown status should be offered genotyping. Genetic counseling consultation should be considered before genetic testing is performed. In families with known MEN2, genetic testing shortly after birth facilitates prompt surgical management of the thyroid gland (see Chapter 39 for further discussion of MEN2).

von Hippel-Lindau Disease

von Hippel-Lindau (VHL) syndrome is an autosomal dominant disorder that may manifest with a variety of benign and malignant neoplasms: noradrenergic (norepinephrine and normetanephrine are predominant) pheochromocytoma or paraganglioma (mediastinal, abdominal, pelvic), hemangioblastoma (involving the cerebellum, spinal cord, or brainstem), retinal angioma, clear cell renal cell carcinoma, pancreatic neuroendocrine tumors, endolymphatic sac tumors of the middle ear, serous cystadenomas of the pancreas, and papillary cystadenomas of the epididymis and broad ligament.[45] The appearance of these VHL-related neoplasms in mutation-positive individuals is close to 100% by age 65 years. The average age of detection of pheochromocytoma is 20 to 29 years of age.[45]

The prevalence of VHL syndrome is between 1 in 35,000 and 1 in 91,000 people.[46,47] The *VHL* tumor suppressor gene, located on chromosome 3p25-26, encodes a protein that regulates ubiquitination and proteosomal degradation of hypoxia-inducible factor (HIF). Loss-of-function mutations in VHL lead to the inappropriate activation of the hypoxic response—promoting glycolysis, angiogenesis, and proliferation. Genotype-phenotype correlations may be used to divide patients into two groups: type 1 and type 2. Patients from kindreds with the type 1 syndrome have mutations that lead to total loss of biologic activity of the VHL protein and are at very low risk to develop pheochromocytoma; whereas those from kindreds with the type 2 syndrome have missense mutations that allow residual activity of the VHL protein and are at high risk for developing pheochromocytoma. In addition, kindreds with type 2 VHL syndrome are subdivided into type 2A (low risk for renal cell carcinoma), type 2B (high risk for renal cell carcinoma), and type 2C (pheochromocytomas only).

Genetic testing for VHL syndrome should be considered for patients with bilateral noradrenergic (norepinephrine and normetanephrine predominant) pheochromocytoma, diagnosis of unilateral noradrenergic pheochromocytoma at a young age (e.g., ≤45 years), or pheochromocytoma/paraganglioma patients with co-phenotype disorders (e.g., retinal angioma).

Pheochromocytomas occurring in patients with MEN2 produce predominantly epinephrine and its major metabolite, metanephrine, whereas those occurring in patients with VHL syndrome produce predominantly norepinephrine and its major metabolite, normetanephrine. These biochemical phenotypes result from mutation-specific differential gene expression. PNMT is overexpressed in MEN2-associated tumors (epinephrine and metanephrine profile) and underexpressed in VHL-associated tumors (norepinephrine and normetanephrine profile).[48,49] In addition, pheochromocytomas occurring in patients with MEN2 have increased tyrosine hydroxylase activity compared with those occurring in patients with VHL; this difference accounts for higher levels of catecholamines and metabolites in patients with MEN2.

Neurofibromatosis Type 1

Neurofibromatosis 1 (NF1), previously known as von Recklinghausen disease, is one of the most common genetic syndromes, with a prevalence of 1 in 2000 to 1 in 5000 persons.[50] NF1 is an autosomal dominant disorder with 100% penetrance and is characterized by neurofibromas, multiple café au lait spots, axillary and inguinal freckling, iris hamartomas (Lisch nodules), bony abnormalities, central nervous system gliomas, pheochromocytoma and paraganglioma, macrocephaly, and cognitive deficits. Although penetrance is 100%, the expression of NF1 features is variable. Approximately 2% of patients with NF1 develop catecholamine-secreting tumors.[51-53] In these patients, the catecholamine-secreting tumor is usually a solitary, benign adrenal pheochromocytoma, occasionally a bilateral adrenal pheochromocytoma, and rarely an abdominal periadrenal paraganglioma.[53] Frequently the adrenal pheochromocytoma is detected as an incidental adrenal mass on imaging performed for other reasons.[54]

The NF1 tumor suppressor gene, located on chromosome 17q11.2, encodes neurofibromin, which downregulates RAS proteins and the downstream RAS-RAF-MAPK signaling cascade. Inactivating NF1 mutations cause the disorder. Unless a patient with pheochromocytoma presents with additional clinical characteristics consistent with an NF1 diagnosis, genetic testing of the NF1 gene is not recommended.

Carney Triad or Syndrome

The Carney triad (gastrointestinal stromal tumor, pulmonary chondroma, and catecholamine-secreting paraganglioma; less frequent neoplasms include esophageal leiomyoma and adrenal adenoma) is another syndrome associated with catecholamine-secreting tumors.[55] This syndrome is a rare (approximately 150 patients have been reported) disorder of unknown cause that primarily affects young women.[56] The gastric stromal tumors are frequently multicentric and associated with early liver metastases; however, most affected patients have a very indolent course.[57] The pulmonary chondromas are benign and, if asymptomatic, require no specific therapy. The paragangliomas secrete catecholamines and should be resected when discovered. Additional features of the Carney triad include esophageal leiomyomas and adrenocortical adenomas. The esophageal leiomyomas are benign and usually asymptomatic. The adrenocortical adenomas may be nonfunctioning or may secrete cortisol autonomously.[58]

Other Genetic Forms of Pheochromocytoma and Paraganglioma

Mutations contributing to pheochromocytoma and paraganglioma have two general transcription signatures: cluster 1—genes encoding proteins that function in the cellular response to hypoxia, and cluster 2—genes encoding proteins that activate kinase signaling (Table 16-4).

TABLE 16-4		
Germline Mutations Associated With Pheochromocytoma and Paraganglioma		
Syndrome/Name	**Gene**	**Typical Tumor Location and Other Associations**
Hypoxic Pathway: Cluster 1*		
SDHD mutation (familial paraganglioma type 1)[†]	SDHD	Primarily skull base and neck; occasionally adrenal medulla, mediastinum, abdomen, pelvis; GIST; possible pituitary adenoma
SDHAF2 mutation (familial paraganglioma type 2)[†]	SDHAF2	Primarily skull base and neck; occasionally abdomen and pelvis
SDHC mutation (familial paraganglioma type 3)	SDHC	Primarily skull base and neck; occasionally abdomen, pelvis, or chest; GIST; possible pituitary adenoma
SDHB mutation (familial paraganglioma type 4)	SDHB	Abdomen, pelvis, and mediastinum; rarely adrenal medulla, skull base, and neck; GIST; possible pituitary adenoma
SDHA mutation	SDHA	Primarily skull base and neck; occasionally abdomen and pelvis; GIST; possible pituitary adenoma
von Hippel-Lindau (VHL) disease	VHL	Adrenal medulla, frequently bilateral; occasionally paraganglioma that may be localized from skull base to pelvis; see text for VHL-associated findings
Hereditary leiomyomatosis and renal cell carcinoma (Reed syndrome)—fumarate hydratase mutation	FH	Multifocal and metastatic; associated with hereditary leiomyomatosis, uterine fibroids, and renal cell cancer
Hypoxia-inducible factor (HIF) 2α	HIF2A	Paraganglioma, polycythemia, and rarely somatostatinoma
Familial erythrocytosis associated with mutation in prolyl hydroxylase isoform 1 (PDH1)	EGLN2	Polycythemia associated with pheochromocytoma and paraganglioma
Familial erythrocytosis associated with mutation in prolyl hydroxylase isoform 2 (PDH2)	EGLN1	Polycythemia associated with pheochromocytoma and paraganglioma
KIF1B	KIF1B	Neuroblastoma
Kinase Signaling Pathway: Cluster 2[‡]		
MEN2A and MEN2B	RET	Adrenal medulla, frequently bilateral; see text for MEN2A and MEN2B associated findings
Neurofibromatosis type 1 (NF1)	NF1	Adrenal or periadrenal; see text for NF1-associated findings
MAX[†]	MAX	Adrenal medulla
Familial pheochromocytoma	TMEM127	Adrenal medulla; possible renal cell carcinoma

*Cluster 1 tumors are mostly extra-adrenal paragangliomas (except in VHL where most tumors are localized to the adrenal) and nearly all have a noradrenergic biochemical phenotype.
[†]Associated with maternal imprinting—see text.
[‡]Cluster 2 tumors are usually adrenal pheochromocytomas with an adrenergic biochemical phenotype.
GIST, gastrointestinal stromal tumor; MEN, multiple endocrine neoplasia; SDH, succinate dehydrogenase.

Cluster 1 tumors are mostly extra-adrenal paragangliomas (except in VHL, in which most tumors are localized to the adrenal gland) and nearly all have a noradrenergic biochemical phenotype. Cluster 2 tumors are usually adrenal pheochromocytomas with an adrenergic biochemical phenotype (see Table 16-4). Since 1990, 16 pheochromocytoma/paraganglioma susceptibility genes have been reported: *NF1, RET, VHL, SDHD, SDHC, SDHB, EGLN1 (PHD2), EGLN2 (PDH1), KIF1B, SDHAF2, IDH1, TMEM127, SDHA, MAX, HIF2A,* and *FH.*[59]

Succinate Dehydrogenase Gene Mutations

Most cases of familial paraganglioma are caused by mutations in the succinate dehydrogenase (SDH; succinate:ubiquinone oxidoreductase) subunit genes (*SDHB, SDHC, SDHD, SHDA,* and *SDHAF2*), which make up portions of mitochondrial complex II.[60,61] The SDH genes are considered tumor suppressor genes and encode the proteins that form the mitochondrial complex II, a crucial link between the Krebs cycle and mitochondrial electron transport chain. SDH is a heterotetramer protein complex consisting of four subunits encoded by nuclear genes. *SDHA* and *SDHB* form the catalytic domain and *SDHC* and *SDHD* anchor the complex to the inner mitochondrial membrane. The assembly factors, *SDHAF1* and *SDHAF2,* are needed for functional and structural integrity of the complex. Defects in the *SDH* genes result in succinate accumulation, which is a competitive inhibitor of the 2-oxoglutarate-dependent dioxygenases (e.g., HIF prolyl hydroxylases and histone or DNA demethylases), which leads to the stabilization of HIF-α and the activation of hypoxic signaling and to epigenetic modifications.

As of 2014, a total of 403 different germline mutations in the *SDH* genes associated with pheochromocytoma/paraganglioma were reported in the literature;[62] 52% in *SDHB,* 35% in *SDHD,* 10% in *SDHC,* 2% in *SDHA,* and 1% in *SDHAF2.* Missense mutations occurred most frequently except for *SDHD,* in which more frameshift mutations were observed. Seventy-eight mutations were found in malignant tumors: 76% in *SDHB,* 19% in *SDHD,* and 5% in *SDHC.*[62]

In patients with *SDHD* or *SDHAF2* mutations, penetrance depends on the mutation's parent of origin. With rare exceptions,[63,64] the disease is not manifested when the mutation is inherited from the mother but is highly penetrant when inherited from the father.[65] This phenomenon is known as *maternal imprinting.*[66]

TMEM127 Mutations

TMEM127 is a negative regulator of mammalian target of rapamycin (mTOR) effector proteins. In a study of 990 individuals with pheochromocytoma or paraganglioma, germline mutations in *TMEM127* were identified in 20 individuals with adrenal tumors, 5 of whom had a family history of pheochromocytoma.[67] Among 547 patients who presented with sporadic pheochromocytoma (unilateral adrenal tumor with negative family history), 11 (2%) had *TMEM127* mutations.

MAX Mutations

In 2011, loss-of-function mutations in the MYC-associated factor X *(MAX)* gene were identified in patients with familial pheochromocytoma.[68] In an initial study of three individuals with familial pheochromocytoma (who did not have mutations in any of the nine previously described susceptibility genes), *MAX* germline mutations were found. *MAX* is a component of the MYC-MAX-MXD1 transcription factors that regulate cell proliferation, differentiation, and apoptosis. In an extension of this study, *MAX* mutations were found in 5 of 59 patients (8.5%) with suspected familial pheochromocytoma (based on age of onset <30 years, bilateral pheochromocytoma, or positive family history).[68]

FH Mutations

In 2014, 598 patients with pheochromocytoma/paraganglioma without mutations in known susceptibility gene mutations were screened for germline mutations in the *FH* gene encoding fumarate hydratase.[69] Five patients (1%) were found to have pathogenic germline *FH* mutations. Clinically, a metastatic phenotype and multiple tumors were significantly more frequent in patients with *FH* mutations than those without such mutations.

Genetic Testing

Genetic testing should be considered if a patient has one or more of the following: (1) paraganglioma, (2) bilateral adrenal pheochromocytoma, (3) unilateral adrenal pheochromocytoma and a family history of pheochromocytoma/paraganglioma, (4) unilateral adrenal pheochromocytoma with onset at a young age (<45 years), or (5) other clinical findings suggestive of one of the previously discussed syndromic disorders. An asymptomatic person at risk for disease on the basis of family history of pheochromocytoma/paraganglioma should have genetic testing only if an affected family member has a known mutation. Genetic testing can be complex, and testing of one family member has implications for related individuals. Genetic counseling is recommended to help families understand the implications of genetic test results, to coordinate testing of at-risk individuals, and to help families work through the psychosocial issues that may arise before, during, or after the testing process.

The clinician may obtain a list of clinically approved molecular genetic diagnostic laboratories.[70] A sequential genetic testing algorithm, based on biochemical phenotype, age, and tumor has been proposed.[28] However, the field of genetic testing is rapidly evolving, and at many clinical laboratories sequential genetic testing is no longer done as it is less expensive to utilize next generation sequencing technology for all clinically available mutations as a package.

Evaluation and Monitoring of Carriers of Succinate Dehydrogenase Mutations

If an SDHx mutation is identified in a relative of a proband, annual clinical assessment including blood pressure check and biochemical testing is indicated for early detection of pheochromocytoma/paraganglioma. Prospective studies to guide the clinician in the frequency, age to start, and type of testing are lacking. Biochemical testing for fractionated metanephrines in plasma or in a 24-hour urine collection for fractionated metanephrines and catecholamines should be performed annually in all carriers of an SDHx mutation starting around age 10 years. Because paragangliomas may be nonfunctioning or may be detected before catecholamine-secretory autonomy is evident, periodic imaging studies are advised. For example, at-risk SDHx (e.g., paternally inherited for *SDHD* and *SDHAF2*) mutation carriers should have MRI of the abdomen, pelvis, chest, and neck every 2 to 3 years; ^{123}I-MIBG scintigraphy should be performed every 5 years. In addition, as new tumor associations are identified, additional surveillance testing will be indicated. For example, several reports have

TABLE 16-5

Medications That May Increase Measured Levels of Fractionated Catecholamines and Metanephrines

Tricyclic antidepressants (including cyclobenzaprine)
Levodopa
Drugs containing adrenergic receptor agonists (e.g., decongestants)
Amphetamines
Buspirone and antipsychotic agents
Prochlorperazine
Reserpine
Withdrawal from clonidine and other drugs (e.g., illicit drugs)
Illicit drugs (e.g., cocaine, heroin)
Ethanol

identified an association between SDHx mutations and pituitary tumor risk.[59] If this risk proves to be real and clinically important, then pituitary-directed MRI may become part of the surveillance program.

Diagnostic Investigation

Differential Diagnosis

Numerous disorders can cause signs and symptoms that may prompt the clinician to test for pheochromocytoma (see Table 16-3). The disorders span much of medicine and include endocrine disorders (e.g., primary hypogonadism), cardiovascular disorders (e.g., idiopathic orthostatic hypotension), psychological disorders (e.g., panic disorder), pharmacologic causes (e.g., withdrawal from an adrenergic inhibitor), neurologic disorders (e.g., postural orthostatic tachycardia syndrome), and miscellaneous disorders (e.g., mast cell disease). Indeed, most patients tested for pheochromocytoma do not have it. In addition, levels of fractionated catecholamines and metanephrines may be elevated in several clinical scenarios, including withdrawal from medications or drugs (e.g., clonidine, alcohol), any acute illness (e.g., subarachnoid hemorrhage, migraine headache, preeclampsia), and administration of many drugs and medications (e.g., tricyclic antidepressants, levodopa, buspirone, antipsychotic agents, cocaine, phencyclidine, amphetamines, ephedrine, pseudoephedrine, phenylpropanolamine, isoproterenol) (Table 16-5).[28]

Case Detection

Pheochromocytoma should be suspected in patients who have one or more of the following:
- Hyperadrenergic spells (e.g., self-limited episodes of nonexertional forceful palpitations, diaphoresis, headache, tremor, or pallor)[29]
- Resistant hypertension
- A familial syndrome that predisposes to catecholamine-secreting tumors (e.g., MEN2, NF1, VHL, Carney triad)
- A family history of pheochromocytoma
- An incidentally discovered adrenal mass with imaging characteristics consistent with pheochromocytoma[36,40]
- Pressor response during anesthesia, surgery, or angiography
- Onset of hypertension at a young age (<20 years)
- Idiopathic dilated cardiomyopathy[71]

Measurement of Fractionated Metanephrines and Catecholamines in Urine and Blood. The diagnosis must be confirmed biochemically by the presence of increased concentrations of fractionated metanephrines and catecholamines in urine or plasma (Fig. 16-4).[28,72,73] The metabolism of catecholamines is primarily intratumoral, with formation of metanephrine from epinephrine and normetanephrine

from norepinephrine.[9] Most laboratories now measure fractionated catecholamines (dopamine, norepinephrine, and epinephrine) and fractionated metanephrines (metanephrine and normetanephrine) by high-performance liquid chromatography with electrochemical detection or tandem mass spectrometry.[74] These techniques have overcome the problems with fluorometric analysis, which include false-positive results caused by α-methyldopa, labetalol, sotalol, and imaging contrast agents.

At Mayo Clinic, the most reliable case-detection strategy is measurement of fractionated metanephrines and catecholamines in a 24-hour urine collection (sensitivity, 98%; specificity, 98%).[72,75] Because of the higher false-positive rate with plasma fractionated metanephrines, they should be reserved for high clinical suspicion cases. The index of suspicion for pheochromocytoma should be high in the following scenarios: resistant hypertension; spells with associated pallor; a family history of pheochromocytoma; a genetic syndrome that predisposes to pheochromocytoma (e.g., MEN2); a past history of resected pheochromocytoma and present history of recurrent hypertension or spells; and an incidentally discovered adrenal mass that has imaging characteristics consistent with pheochromocytoma (Table 16-6).[36] In addition, measurement of plasma fractionated metanephrines is a good first-line test for children, because obtaining a complete 24-hour urine collection is difficult in pediatric patients. Measurement of urinary dopamine or plasma methoxytyramine can be very useful in detecting the rare tumor with selective dopamine hypersecretion, because plasma metanephrine fractions are not direct metabolites of dopamine and may be normal in the setting of a dopamine-secreting tumor.[27,75,76]

The 24-hour urine collection for fractionated metanephrines and catecholamines should include measurement of urinary creatinine to verify an adequate collection. The diagnostic cutoffs for most 24-hour urinary fractionated metanephrine assays are based on normal ranges derived from normotensive volunteer reference groups, and this can result in excessive false-positive test results. For example, in normotensive laboratory volunteers, the 95th percentiles are 428 μg for normetanephrine and 200 μg for metanephrine, whereas the corresponding values in individuals who are being tested for pheochromocytoma as part of routine clinical practice but who do not have the neoplasm are, respectively, 71% and 51% higher than those of the normal volunteers (<900 μg for normetanephrine and <400 μg for metanephrine).[73]

Although it is preferred that patients not receive any medication during the diagnostic evaluation, treatment with most medications may be continued. Tricyclic antidepressants are the drugs that interfere most frequently with the interpretation of 24-hour urinary catecholamines and metabolites. To effectively screen for catecholamine-secreting tumors, treatment with tricyclic antidepressants and other psychoactive agents listed in Table 16-5 should be tapered and discontinued at least 2 weeks before any hormonal assessments. In some clinical situations it is contraindicated to discontinue certain medications (e.g., antipsychotics), and if case-detection testing is positive, then CT or MRI would be needed to exclude a catecholamine-secreting tumor. Furthermore, catecholamine secretion may be appropriately increased in situations of physical stress or illness (e.g., stroke, myocardial infarction, congestive heart failure, obstructive sleep apnea). There are no reliable references ranges for fractionated metanephrines or catecholamines in patients requiring intensive care unit hospitalization. Therefore, the clinical circumstances under which catecholamines and metanephrines are measured must be assessed in each case.

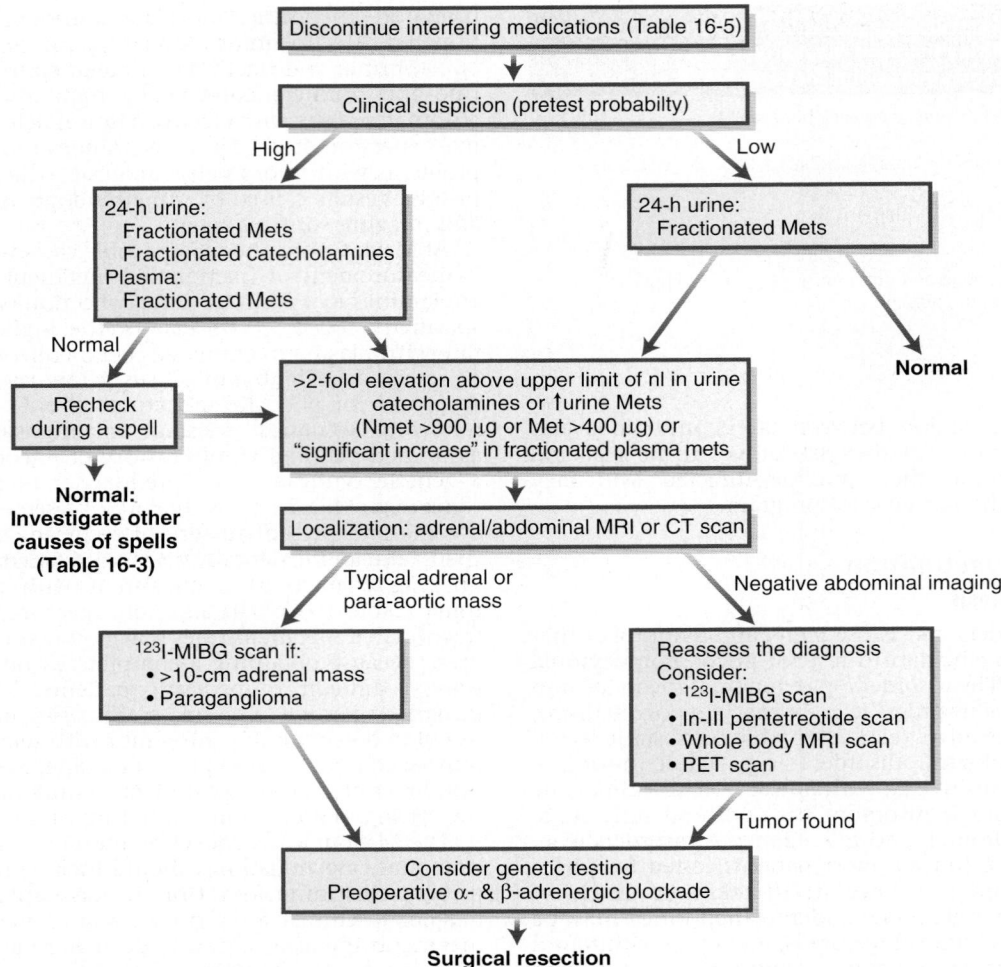

Figure 16-4 Evaluation and treatment of catecholamine-secreting tumors. Clinical suspicion is triggered by paroxysmal symptoms (especially hypertension); hypertension that is intermittent, unusually labile, or resistant to treatment; a family history of pheochromocytoma or associated conditions; or an incidentally discovered adrenal mass (see text for details). CT, computed tomography; In-111, indium-111; ^{123}I-MIBG, iodine-123–labeled metaiodobenzylguanidine; Mets, metanephrines; MRI, magnetic resonance imaging; nl, normal; Nmet, normetanephrine; PET, positron emission tomography. (Modified from Young WF Jr. Pheochromocytoma, 1926-1993. *Trends Endocrinol Metab.* 1993;4:122-127, used with permission.)

TABLE 16-6
Typical Imaging Phenotypes of Adrenal Masses

Tumor Type	Size (cm)	Shape	Texture	Laterality	Contrast Enhancement	CT*	MRI[†]	Necrosis, Hemorrhage, or Calcifications	Growth
Cortical adenoma	≤3	Round to oval with smooth margins	Homogeneous	Usually unilateral	Limited	<10 HU; >50% washout	Isointense	Rare	Slow
Cortical carcinoma	>4	Irregular with unclear margins	Inhomogeneous	Usually unilateral	Marked	>10 HU; <50% washout	Hyperintense	Common	Rapid
Pheochromocytoma	>3	Round to oval with smooth margins	Inhomogeneous with areas of cystic degeneration	Usually solitary and unilateral	Marked	>10 HU; <50% washout	Hyperintense	Common	1 cm/yr
Metastasis	Variable	Oval to irregular with unclear margins	Inhomogeneous	Often bilateral	Marked	>10 HU; <50% washout	Hyperintense	Common	Variable

*Precontrast radiodensity (HU) and percentage of contrast medium washout at 10 min.
[†]Relative intensity compared with liver on T2-weighted images.
CT, computed tomography; HU, Hounsfield unit; MRI, magnetic resonance imaging.

Other Tests That Have Been Used to Assess for Pheochromocytoma. Because of poor overall accuracy in testing for pheochromocytoma, measurement of plasma catecholamines no longer has a role except to detect dopamine-secreting paragangliomas.[77] Chromogranin A is stored and released from dense-core secretory granules of neuroendocrine cells and is increased in 80% of patients with pheochromocytoma.[78] Chromogranin A is not specific for pheochromocytoma, and elevations may be seen with other neuroendocrine tumors.[79] The 24-hour urinary VMA excretion has poor diagnostic sensitivity and specificity compared with fractionated 24-hour urinary metanephrines.

Clonidine Suppression Test. The high false-positive rate for plasma fractionated catecholamines and fractionated metanephrines triggered the development of a confirmatory test, the clonidine suppression test.[80] This test is intended to distinguish between pheochromocytoma and false-positive increases in plasma fractionated catecholamines and metanephrines. Clonidine is a centrally acting α_2-adrenergic receptor agonist that normally suppresses the release of catecholamines from neurons but does not affect the catecholamine secretion from a pheochromocytoma. Clonidine (0.3 mg) is administered orally, and plasma fractionated catecholamines or metanephrines are measured before and 3 hours after the dose.[81] In patients with essential hypertension, plasma catecholamine concentrations decrease (norepinephrine + epinephrine <500 pg/mL or >50% decrease in norepinephrine), as do plasma normetanephrine concentrations (into the normal range or >40% decrease).[82] However, these concentrations remain increased in patients with pheochromocytoma.

Provocative Testing and Suppression Testing. Because of advances in the methodology for measuring catecholamines and metanephrines, phentolamine, glucagon, histamine, metoclopramide, and tyramine tests are rarely needed. From 1975 to 1994 at Mayo Clinic, we performed histamine and glucagon stimulation testing in 542 patients in whom pheochromocytoma was highly suspected despite normal 24-hour urinary excretion of total metanephrines or catecholamines; not one patient had a positive stimulation test in this setting.[83]

Renal Failure. Measurements of urinary catecholamines and metabolites may be invalid if the patient has advanced renal insufficiency.[84] Serum chromogranin A levels have poor diagnostic specificity in these patients.[85] In patients without pheochromocytoma who are receiving hemodialysis, plasma norepinephrine and dopamine concentrations are increased, respectively, threefold and twofold above the upper limit of normal.[86] However, standard normal ranges can be used for interpreting plasma epinephrine concentrations.[87] Therefore, when patients with renal failure have plasma norepinephrine concentrations more than three times above the upper normal limit or epinephrine concentrations greater than the upper normal limit, pheochromocytoma should be suspected. The findings of one study suggested that plasma concentrations of fractionated metanephrines are increased approximately twofold in patients with renal failure and may be useful in the biochemical evaluation of patients with marked renal insufficiency or renal failure.[88] However, the results of an earlier study suggested that concentrations of plasma fractionated metanephrines could not distinguish between 10 patients with pheochromocytoma and 11 patients with end-stage renal disease who required long-term hemodialysis.[89]

Factitious Pheochromocytoma. As with other similar disorders, factitious pheochromocytoma can be very difficult to confirm.[90] The patient usually has a medical background. The patient may "spike" the 24-hour urine container, or the catecholamines may be administered systemically.

Localization

Localization studies should not be initiated until biochemical studies have confirmed the diagnosis of a catecholamine-secreting tumor (see Fig. 16-4). CT or MRI of the abdomen and pelvis should be the first localization test (sensitivity, >95%; specificity, >65%).[28,91] Approximately 85% of these tumors are found in the adrenal glands, and 95% are found in the abdomen and pelvis. The most common locations of catecholamine-secreting paragangliomas include superior abdominal para-aortic region, 46%; inferior abdominal para-aortic region, 29%; urinary bladder, 10%; mediastinum, 10%; head and neck, 3%; and pelvis, 2%.[42]

Imaging Phenotype. The term *imaging phenotype* refers to the characteristics of the mass on CT or MRI (see Table 16-6).[36] The lipid-rich nature of cortical adenomas is helpful in distinguishing these benign neoplasms from pheochromocytoma. On CT scans, the density of the image (with darker tissues being less dense) is attributed to x-ray attenuation. At the extremes of the CT density spectrum are air (black) and bone (white). The Hounsfield scale is a semiquantitative method of measuring x-ray attenuation. Typical Hounsfield unit (HU) values are −20 to −150 HU for adipose tissue and 20 to 50 HU for kidney. If an adrenal mass is less than 0 HU on unenhanced CT, it is almost certainly a benign adenoma.[92] Adrenal adenomas show a much earlier washout of contrast enhancement than do nonadenomas.[93] For example, Korobkin and colleagues[93] found that the mean percentage washout for adenomas was 51% at 5 minutes and 70% at 15 minutes, compared with 8% and 20%, respectively, for nonadenomas.

Although CT is still the primary adrenal imaging modality, MRI has advantages in certain clinical situations.[94] Several different MRI techniques have been used to characterize adrenal masses. Conventional spin-echo MRI was the first and is still the most frequently used technique. Early in the history of abdominal MRI, it became clear that with low- or midfield-strength magnets, T1- and T2-weighted imaging could be used to differentiate pheochromocytoma and malignancies from benign adenomas. On gadolinium-diethylenetriaminepenta-acetic acid (DPTA)-enhanced MRI, pheochromocytomas and malignant lesions show rapid and marked enhancement and a slower washout pattern, whereas adenomas demonstrate mild enhancement and a rapid washout of contrast agent.[93] Similar findings are made with CT.

Chemical shift MRI is a form of lipid-sensitive imaging. Chemical shift MRI is based on the principle that the hydrogen protons in water and lipid molecules resonate at different frequencies. Benign cortical adenomas contain approximately equal amounts of lipid and water, whereas the lipid content of pheochromocytomas is usually low.[95] When the protons of water and lipid are aligned, they are said to be in phase, and when opposite each other, they are out of phase. When fat and water are in phase on MRI, the signal intensity is maximized; when they are out of phase, the signal intensity is reduced. This in-phase and out-of-phase process is the chemical shift technique. Benign adrenal cortical adenomas lose signal on out-of-phase images but appear relatively bright on in-phase images.[95] A modification of the chemical shift MRI technique uses gradient echo pulse sequences to produce a similar effect.

Imaging characteristics consistent with a benign cortical adenoma include round and homogeneous density, smooth contour with sharp margination, diameter usually less than 3 cm, unilateral location, low unenhanced CT attenuation values (<10 HU) with rapid contrast medium washout at 10 minutes after administration of contrast medium,[93,96] isointensity with liver on both T1- and T2-weighted MRI sequences, and chemical shift evidence of lipid on MRI (see Table 16-6). The imaging phenotype consistent with pheochromocytoma includes enhancement with intravenous contrast medium on CT (see Fig. 16-3), high signal intensity on T2-weighted MRI (Fig. 16-5), cystic and hemorrhagic changes, and variable size; also, the tumor may be bilateral. Although it has been suggested that patients with apparent simple adrenal cysts do not require hormonal evaluation, pheochromocytoma can mimic an adrenal cyst.

^{123}I-MIBG Scintigraphy. If the results of abdominal imaging are negative, scintigraphic localization with ^{123}I-MIBG is indicated (Fig. 16-6). This radiopharmaceutical agent accumulates preferentially in catecholamine-producing tumors; however, this procedure is not as sensitive as was initially hoped (sensitivity, 80%; specificity, 99%).[11,94] ^{123}I-MIBG is superior to ^{131}I-MIBG because the photon energy allows single-photon emission computed tomographic (SPECT)

images.[11] Thyroid uptake of ^{123}I should be blocked with the administration of an iodide preparation (e.g., Lugol solution). In a study of 282 patients with catecholamine-secreting tumors that were surgically confirmed, the overall sensitivity was 89% for CT, 98% for MRI, and 81% for ^{131}I-MIBG.[11] If a typical (<10 cm) unilateral adrenal pheochromocytoma is found on CT or MRI, ^{123}I-MIBG scintigraphy is superfluous and the results may even confuse the clinician.[97-99] On the other hand, if the adrenal pheochromocytoma is more than 10 cm in diameter or if a paraganglioma is identified on CT or MRI, then ^{123}I-MIBG scintigraphy is indicated, because the patient has increased risk of malignant disease and additional paragangliomas. It is important for the clinician to recognize the medications that may interfere with ^{123}I-MIBG uptake (e.g., tricyclic antidepressants, labetalol, calcium channel blockers) and have the patient discontinue them before imaging is performed (Table 16-7).[100]

Other Localizing Procedures. Localizing procedures that also can be used, but are rarely required, include computer-assisted imaging of the chest, neck, and skull base. Other localizing studies, such as somatostatin receptor imaging with ^{111}In-DTPA-pentetreotide, may also be considered. Although somatostatin receptors are usually expressed in pheochromocytomas and paragangliomas, the sensitivity of somatostatin receptor imaging with ^{111}In-DTPA-pentetreotide is low.[28] Although positron emission tomography (PET) scanning with ^{18}F-fluorodeoxyglucose (FDG) or ^{11}C-hydroxyephedrine or 6-[^{18}F]fluorodopamine can identify paragangliomas, these expensive techniques probably should be reserved for identifying sites of metastatic disease in patients with negative ^{123}I-MIBG scintigraphic results.[101] Because of activation of aerobic glycolysis in patients with pheochromocytoma or paraganglioma associated with SDHx mutations, FDG-PET is the ideal imaging technique for localization of primary and metastatic tumors.[102,103] There has been recent development of the somatostatin analogue ^{68}Ga-DOTA-Tyr3-octreotide (DOTA-TOC). DOTA-TOC for PET-CT and initial studies appears promising.[104]

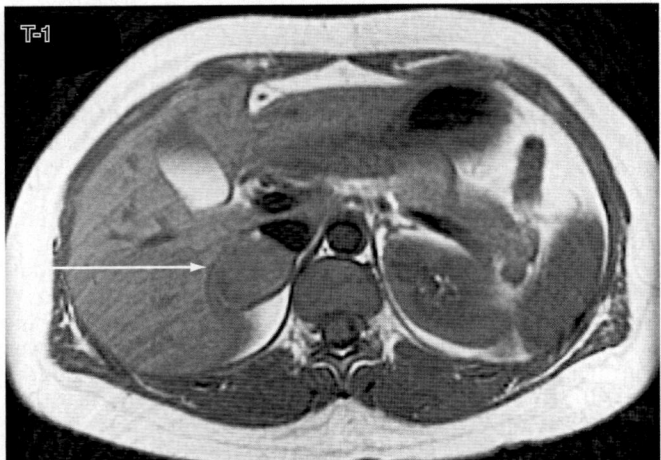

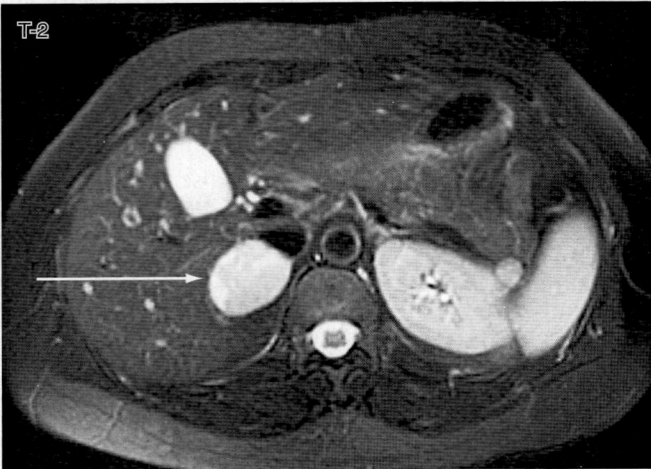

Figure 16-5 Magnetic resonance images of the abdomen of a 34-year-old woman with a recent onset of palpitations and hypertension. She presented with acute left ventricular failure after a single dose of a β-adrenergic blocker. The 24-hour urine test for total metanephrines and catecholamines showed the following: total metanephrines, 3800 μg (normal, <1000 μg); norepinephrine, 37 μg (normal, <170 μg); epinephrine, 7.7 μg (normal, <35 μg); and dopamine, 147 μg (normal, <700 μg). The images show a slightly heterogeneous, right adrenal mass (3.3 × 3.5 × 4.5 cm) consistent with pheochromocytoma *(arrows)* that has increased signal intensity on T2-weighted images *(lower panel)*. After α-adrenergic blockade and restoration of normal left ventricular function, the patient had a laparoscopic adrenalectomy to remove a 5 cm × 4 cm × 3 cm, 33-g pheochromocytoma. Postoperatively, the 24-hour urinary excretion of total metanephrines normalized.

TABLE 16-7
Drugs That May Interfere With Metaiodobenzylguanidine (MIBG) Uptake

Uptake-1 Inhibition*

Antiemetics (e.g., prochlorperazine)
Antipsychotics (e.g., chlorpromazine, haloperidol)
Cocaine
Labetalol
Phenylpropanolamine
Tricyclic antidepressants (e.g., amitriptyline, amoxapine, desipramine, doxepin, imipramine, nortriptyline)

Depletion of Storage Vesicle Contents†

Amphetamines (e.g., dextroamphetamine, fenfluramine, phentermine)
Dopamine
Labetalol
Reserpine
Sympathomimetics (e.g., ephedrine, phenylephrine, pseudoephedrine, salbutamol, terbutaline)

Inhibition of Vesicular Monoamine Transporters†

Reserpine

Unknown Mechanism*

Calcium channel blockers (e.g., diltiazem, nicardipine, nifedipine, nimodipine, verapamil)

*Should be stopped at least 48 hr before MIBG administration.
†Should be stopped at least 72 hr before MIBG administration.

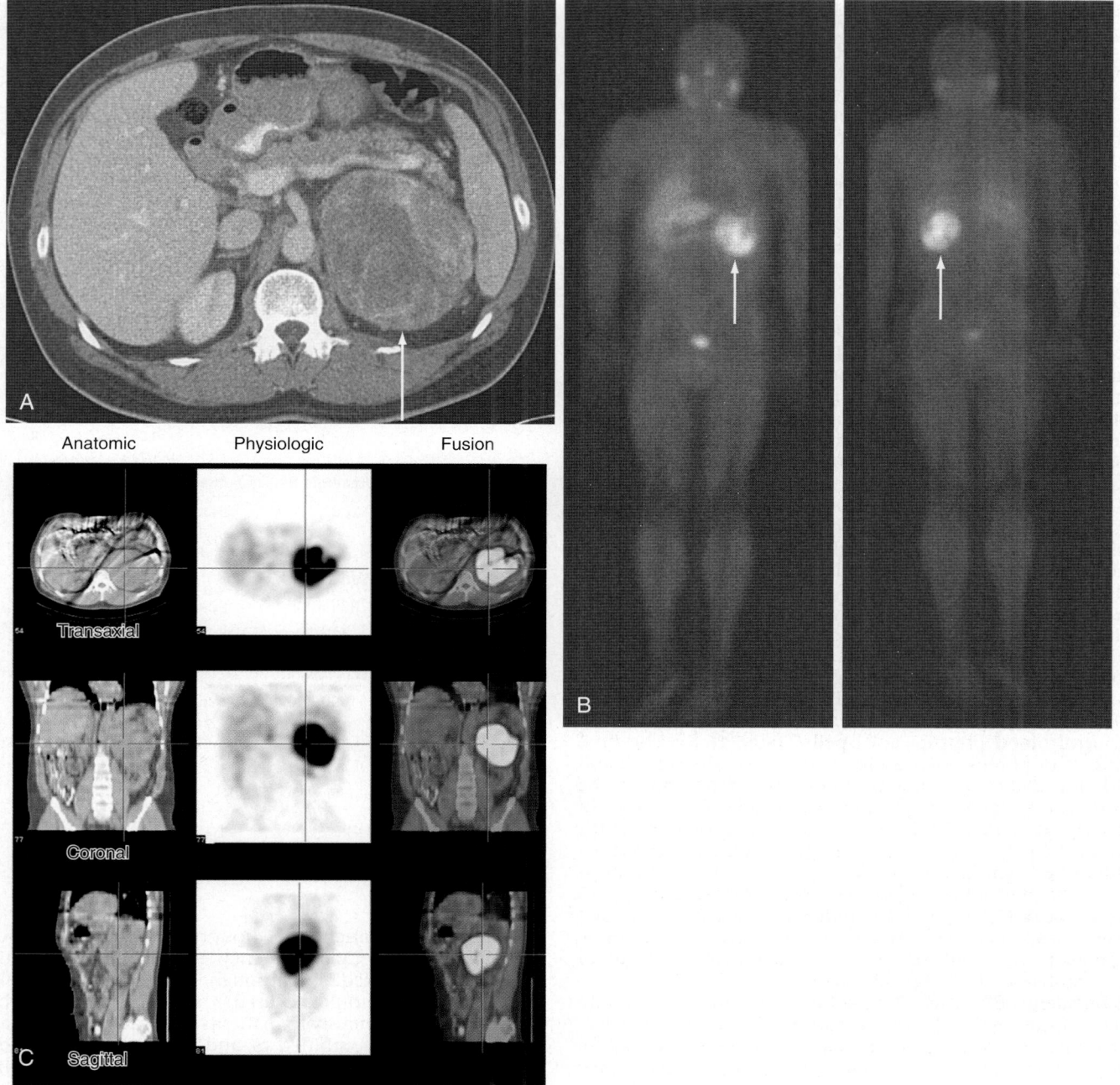

Figure 16-6 Computed tomography (CT) and ^{123}I-metaiodobenzylguanidine (^{123}I-MIBG) imaging from a 44-year-old man. He presented with a 9-year history of hypertension and recent onset of head throbbing, chest pressure, and abdominal pain. The 24-hour urine studies were abnormal: norepinephrine, 900 μg (normal, <170 μg); epinephrine, 28 μg (normal, <35 μg); dopamine, 468 μg (normal, <700 μg); and total metanephrines, 17,958 μg (normal, <1000 μg). **A,** Axial CT image with contrast shows a large, partially vascular and partially necrotic left adrenal tumor *(arrow).* **B,** ^{123}I-MIBG whole-body scan shows a large focus of increased radiotracer uptake in the left upper abdomen *(arrow)* that corresponds to the mass seen on the CT image; no other abnormal uptake is seen. **C,** ^{123}I-MIBG and single-photon emission computed tomography (SPECT) fusion CT images correlate with the images seen on CT (anatomic) with those seen on ^{123}I-MIBG (physiologic) in the axial, coronal, and sagittal planes. After α- and β-adrenergic blockade, a 680-g pheochromocytoma (13.5 × 12 × 9 cm) was removed.

Selective adrenal venous sampling (AVS) for catecholamines is usually misleading and should be avoided.[105]

Treatment

The treatment of choice for pheochromocytoma is complete surgical resection. Surgical survival rates are 98% to 100% and are highly dependent on the skill of the endocrinologist, endocrine surgeon, and anesthesiologist team.[28,41,106] The most common adverse event after surgery

is sustained hypertension. Careful preoperative pharmacologic preparation is crucial for successful treatment.[28,107,108] Most catecholamine-secreting tumors are benign and can be totally excised. Tumor excision usually cures hypertension.

Preoperative Management

Some form of preoperative pharmacologic preparation is indicated for all patients with catecholamine-secreting neoplasms, including those who are asymptomatic and normotensive.[28,108,109] However, no randomized controlled trials have compared the different approaches.[110] Combined α- and β-adrenergic blockade is one approach to control blood pressure and prevent intraoperative hypertensive crises.[25] α-Adrenergic blockade should be started 7 to 10 days preoperatively to normalize blood pressure and expand the contracted blood volume. A longer duration of preoperative α-adrenergic blockade is indicated for patients with recent myocardial infarction, catecholamine cardiomyopathy, or catecholamine-induced vasculitis. Blood pressure should be monitored with the patient in the seated and standing positions twice daily. Target blood pressure is low-normal blood pressure for age (e.g., <120/80 mm Hg in the seated position), with systolic blood pressure greater than 90 mm Hg (standing); both targets should be modified on the basis of the patient's age and comorbid disease. Orthostasis is not a goal of treatment but rather a side effect. Therefore, on the second or third day of α-adrenergic blockade, patients are encouraged to start a diet high in sodium content (≥5000 mg/day) because of the catecholamine-induced volume contraction and the orthostasis associated with α-adrenergic blockade. This degree of volume expansion may be contraindicated in patients with congestive heart failure or renal insufficiency. After adequate α-adrenergic blockade has been achieved, β-adrenergic blockade is initiated, typically 2 to 3 days preoperatively.

α-Adrenergic Blockade. Phenoxybenzamine is the preferred drug for preoperative preparation to control blood pressure and arrhythmia. It is an irreversible, long-acting, nonspecific α-adrenergic blocking agent. The initial dosage is 10 mg once or twice daily, and the dose is increased by 10 to 20 mg in divided doses every 2 to 3 days as needed to control blood pressure and spells (Table 16-8). The final dosage of phenoxybenzamine is typically between 20 and 100 mg daily. The patient should be warned about the orthostasis, nasal congestion, retrograde ejaculation in men, and marked fatigue that occur in almost all patients. With their more favorable side effect profiles, selective α₁-adrenergic blocking agents (e.g., prazosin, terazosin, doxazosin) are preferable to phenoxybenzamine when long-term pharmacologic treatment is indicated (e.g., for metastatic pheochromocytoma). However, treatment with these agents is not routinely used preoperatively because of incomplete α-adrenergic blockade.[111]

β-Adrenergic Blockade. The β-adrenergic antagonist should be administered only after α-adrenergic blockade is effective because with β-adrenergic blockade alone, severe hypertension or cardiopulmonary decompensation may occur as a result of the unopposed α-adrenergic stimulation.[112] Preoperative α-adrenergic blockade is indicated to control the tachycardia associated with both the high concentrations of circulating catecholamines and the α-adrenergic blockade. The clinician should exercise caution if the patient is asthmatic or has congestive heart failure. Chronic catecholamine excess can produce a myocardiopathy that may become evident with the initiation of β-adrenergic blockade, resulting in acute pulmonary edema.[112] Therefore, when the β-adrenergic blocker is administered, it should be used cautiously and at a low dose. For example, a patient is usually given 10 mg of propranolol every 6 hours to start. On the second day of treatment, the β-adrenergic blockade (assuming the patient tolerates the drug) is converted to a single long-acting dose. The dose is then increased as necessary to control the tachycardia (goal heart rate is 60-80 beats per minute).

Catecholamine Synthesis Inhibitor. Metyrosine should be used with caution and only after other agents have been

TABLE 16-8

Orally Administered Drugs Used to Treat Pheochromocytoma

Drug	Initial Dosage, mg/day* (Maximum)	Side Effects
α-Adrenergic Blocking Agents		
Phenoxybenzamine	10[†] (100)[†]	Postural hypotension, tachycardia, miosis, nasal congestion, diarrhea, retrograde ejaculation, fatigue
Prazosin	1 (20)[‡]	First-dose effect, dizziness, drowsiness, headache, fatigue, palpitations, nausea
Terazosin	1 (20)[†]	First-dose effect, asthenia, blurred vision, dizziness, nasal congestion, nausea, peripheral edema, palpitations, somnolence
Doxazosin	1 (20)	First-dose effect, orthostasis, peripheral edema, fatigue, somnolence
Combined α- and β-Adrenergic Blocking Agent		
Labetalol	200[†] (1200)[†]	Dizziness, fatigue, nausea, nasal congestion, impotence
Calcium Channel Blocker		
Nicardipine sustained-release	30[†] (120)[†]	Edema, dizziness, headache, flushing, nausea, dyspepsia
Catecholamine Synthesis Inhibitor		
α-Methyl-ρ-L-tyrosine (metyrosine)	1000[‡] (4000)[‡]	Sedation, diarrhea, anxiety, nightmares, crystalluria, galactorrhea, extrapyramidal symptoms

*Given once daily unless otherwise indicated.
[†]Given in two doses daily.
[‡]Given in three or four doses daily.

ineffective or in patients in whom tumor manipulation or destruction (e.g., radiofrequency ablation of metastatic sites) will be marked.[8,113] Although some centers advocate that this agent should be used routinely preoperatively, most reserve it primarily for patients who cannot be treated with the typical combined α- and β-adrenergic blockade protocol for cardiopulmonary reasons. Metyrosine inhibits catecholamine synthesis by blocking the enzyme tyrosine hydroxylase.[113] The side effects of metyrosine can be disabling; with long-term therapy, they include sedation, depression, diarrhea, anxiety, nightmares, crystalluria and urolithiasis, galactorrhea, and extrapyramidal signs. Metyrosine may be added to α- and β-adrenergic blockade if the resection will be difficult (e.g., malignant paraganglioma) or if destructive therapy is planned (e.g., radiofrequency ablation of hepatic metastases). Our typical protocol with short-term preprocedure preparation is to start with metyrosine 250 mg every 6 hours on day 1, 500 mg every 6 hours on day 2, 750 mg every 6 hours on day 3, and 1000 mg every 6 hours on the day before the procedure, with the last dose (1000 mg) given on the morning of the procedure. With this short-course therapy, the main side effect is hypersomnolence.

Calcium Channel Blockers. Calcium channel blockers, which block norepinephrine-mediated calcium transport into vascular smooth muscle, have been used successfully at several

TABLE 16-9
Intravenously Administered Drugs Used to Treat Pheochromocytoma

Agent	Dosage Range
For Hypertension	
Phentolamine	Administer a 1-mg IV test dose, then 2- to 5-mg IV boluses as needed or continuous infusion.
Nitroprusside	IV infusion rates of 2 µg/kg of body weight per minute are suggested as safe. Rates >4 µg/kg per minute may lead to cyanide toxicity within 3 hr. Doses >10 µg/kg per minute are rarely required, and the maximal dose should not exceed 800 µg/min.
Nicardipine	Initiate therapy at 5.0 mg/hr; the IV infusion rate may be increased by 2.5 mg/hr q15min up to a maximum of 15.0 mg/hr.
For Cardiac Arrhythmia	
Lidocaine	Initiate therapy with an IV bolus of 1-1.5 mg/kg (75-100 mg); additional boluses of 0.5-0.75 mg/kg (25-50 mg) can be given q5-10min if needed up to a maximum of 3 mg/kg. Loading is followed by maintenance IV infusion of 2-4 mg/min (30-50 µg/kg per minute) adjusted for effect and settings of altered metabolism (e.g., heart failure, liver congestion) and as guided by blood level monitoring.
Esmolol	An initial IV loading dose of 0.5 mg/kg is infused over 1 min, followed by a maintenance infusion of 0.05 mg/kg per minute for the next 4 min. Depending on the desired ventricular response, the maintenance infusion may then be continued at 0.05 mg/kg per minute or increased stepwise (e.g., by 0.1 mg/kg per minute increments to a maximum of 0.2 mg/kg per minute), with each step being maintained for ≥4 min.

IV, intravenous; q, every.

medical centers to preoperatively prepare patients with pheochromocytoma.[114] Nicardipine is the most commonly used calcium channel blocker in this setting; the starting dose is 30 mg twice daily of the sustained-release preparation (see Table 16-8).[115,116] Nicardipine is given orally to control blood pressure preoperatively and if needed is given as an intravenous infusion intraoperatively (Table 16-9). Although there is less collective experience with calcium channel blockers than with α- and β-adrenergic blockers, when calcium channel blockers are used as the primary mode of antihypertensive therapy, they may be just as effective.[116,117] Clearly, the exclusive use of calcium channel blockers for the perioperative management of patients with catecholamine-secreting tumors does not prevent all hemodynamic changes; however, its use has been associated with low morbidity and mortality rates.[117] The main role for this class of drugs may be either to supplement the combined α- and β-adrenergic blockade protocol when blood pressure control is inadequate or to replace the adrenergic blockade protocol in patients with intolerable side effects.

Acute Hypertensive Crises

Acute hypertensive crises may occur before or during an operation, and they should be treated with intravenously administered sodium nitroprusside, phentolamine, or nicardipine (see Table 16-9). Sodium nitroprusside is an ideal vasodilator for intraoperative management of hypertensive episodes because of its rapid onset of action and short duration of effect. It is administered as an intravenous infusion at 0.5 to 5.0 µg/kg of body weight per minute and adjusted every few minutes for target blood pressure response; to keep the steady-state thiocyanate concentration below 1 mmol/L, the rate of a prolonged infusion should be no more than 3 µg/kg per minute. Phentolamine is a short-acting, nonselective α-adrenergic blocker that is available in lyophilized form in 5-mg vials. An initial test dose of 1 mg is administered and is followed, if necessary, by repeat 5-mg boluses or continuous infusion. The response to phentolamine is maximal 2 to 3 minutes after a bolus injection and lasts 10 to 15 minutes. Nicardipine can be started at an infusion rate of 5 mg/hour and titrated for blood pressure control (the infusion rate may be increased by 2.5 mg/hour every 15 minutes up to a maximum of 15.0 mg/hour) (see Table 16-9).

Anesthesia and Surgery

Surgical resection of a catecholamine-secreting tumor is a high-risk surgical procedure, and an experienced surgeon-anesthesiologist team is required. The last oral doses of α- and β-adrenergic blockers can be administered early in the morning on the day of the operation. Fentanyl, ketamine, and morphine should be avoided, because they potentially can stimulate catecholamine release from a pheochromocytoma.[118] Also, parasympathetic nervous system blockade with atropine should be avoided because of the associated tachycardia. Anesthesia may be induced with intravenous injection of propofol, etomidate, or barbiturates in combination with synthetic opioids.[118] Most anesthetic gases can be used, but halothane and desflurane should be avoided. Cardiovascular and hemodynamic variables must be monitored closely. Continuous measurement of intra-arterial pressure and heart rhythm is required. If the patient has congestive heart failure or decreased cardiac reserve, monitoring of pulmonary capillary wedge pressure is indicated. The preoperative and perioperative treatment approach outlined here is the same for adults and children.[119,120]

In the past, an anterior midline abdominal surgical approach was typically used for resecting adrenal pheochromocytoma. However, the laparoscopic approach to the adrenal gland is currently the procedure of choice for patients with solitary intra-adrenal pheochromocytomas smaller than 8 cm in diameter.[121-123] If the pheochromocytoma is in the adrenal gland, the entire gland should be removed. Laparoscopic adrenalectomy for pheochromocytoma should be converted to open adrenalectomy in cases of difficult dissection, invasion, adhesions, or surgeon inexperience.[124] Great care should be taken to avoid tumor capsule rupture—this can transform a benign pheochromocytoma to an incurable one with diffuse peritoneal disease.[125] If the tumor is malignant, as much of the tumor should be removed as possible. If a bilateral adrenalectomy is planned preoperatively, the patient should receive glucocorticoid stress coverage while awaiting transfer to the operating room. In addition, glucocorticoid coverage should be initiated in the operating room if unexpected bilateral adrenalectomy is necessary. Cortical-sparing bilateral adrenalectomies have been used to treat patients with VHL disease.[126,127]

An anterior midline abdominal surgical approach is indicated for abdominal paragangliomas. The midline abdomen should be inspected carefully. Paragangliomas of the neck, chest, and urinary bladder require specialized approaches. Unresectable cardiac pheochromocytomas may require cardiac transplantation.[128]

Hypotension may occur during and after surgical resection of the pheochromocytoma, and it should be treated with fluids and colloids and then intravenous pressor agents if necessary. Postoperative hypotension occurs less frequently in patients who have had adequate preoperative α-adrenergic blockade and volume expansion. If both adrenal glands were manipulated during surgery, adrenocortical insufficiency should be considered as a potential cause of postoperative hypotension. Because hypoglycemia can occur in the immediate postoperative period, blood glucose levels should be monitored, and fluid given intravenously should contain 5% dextrose. Blood pressure is usually normal by the time of hospital discharge. Longstanding, persistent hypertension does occur and may be related to resection-related renal injury, resetting of baroreceptors, hemodynamic changes, structural changes of the blood vessels, altered sensitivity of the vessels to pressor substances, functional or structural renal changes, or coincident primary hypertension.

Long-Term Postoperative Follow-Up

Approximately 1 to 2 weeks after surgery, 24-hour urinary fractionated catecholamines and metanephrines should be measured. If the levels are normal, the resection of the pheochromocytoma should be considered complete. The survival rate after removal of a benign pheochromocytoma is almost equal to that of age- and sex-matched normal control subjects. Increased levels of fractionated catecholamines and metanephrines detected postoperatively are consistent with residual tumor (i.e., a second primary lesion or occult metastases). If bilateral adrenalectomy was performed, lifelong glucocorticoid and mineralocorticoid replacement therapy is prescribed.

The risk for recurrent disease (usually metastatic) in patients with apparent benign pheochromocytoma or paraganglioma is approximately 15% on long-term follow-up.[129] The 24-hour urinary excretion of fractionated catecholamines and metanephrines or plasma fractionated metanephrines should be checked annually for life.[28] Annual biochemical testing assesses for metastatic disease, tumor recurrence in the adrenal bed, and delayed appearance of multiple primary tumors. Recurrence rates are highest for patients with familial disease, large tumor size (>5 cm), or paraganglioma.[130] Follow-up CT or MRI is not needed unless metanephrine or catecholamine levels become elevated or the original tumor was associated with minimal catecholamine excess.

Genetic testing should be considered for patients younger than 45 years of age or those with one or more of the following: a family history of pheochromocytoma; paraganglioma; and any sign that suggests a genetic cause, such as retinal angiomas, axillary freckling, café au lait spots, cerebellar tumor, MTC, or hyperparathyroidism. In addition, all first-degree relatives of a patient with pheochromocytoma or paraganglioma should have biochemical testing (e.g., 24-hour urine collection for fractionated metanephrines and catecholamines). If mutation testing in a patient is positive, the patient's parents and children should be offered genetic testing.

Malignant Pheochromocytoma and Paraganglioma

Distinguishing between benign and malignant catecholamine-secreting tumors is difficult on the basis of clinical, biochemical, or histopathologic characteristics. Malignancy is rare in patients with MEN2 or VHL syndrome, but it is common in those with familial paraganglioma caused by mutations in *SDHB*.[131,132] Patients with *SDHB* mutations are more likely to develop malignant disease and nonpara-

ganglioma neoplasms (e.g., renal cell carcinoma).[62,133] Although the 5-year survival rate for patients with malignant pheochromocytoma is less than 50%, the prognosis is variable: approximately 50% of patients have an indolent form of the disease, with a life expectancy of more than 20 years, and the other half have rapidly progressive disease, with death occurring within 1 to 3 years after diagnosis. The clinician should first assess the pace of the malignant disease and then target the level of therapy to the aggressiveness of tumor behavior. A multimodality, multidisciplinary, individualized approach is indicated to control catecholamine-dependent symptoms, local mass effect symptoms from the tumor, and overall tumor burden. Long-term pharmacologic therapy for the patient with metastatic pheochromocytoma is similar to that outlined for preoperative preparation in a patient with a catecholamine-secreting tumor.

Metastatic sites include local tissue invasion, liver, bone, lung, omentum, and lymph nodes. Metastatic lesions should be resected, if possible, to decrease tumor burden. Skeletal metastatic lesions that are painful or threaten structural function can be treated with external radiotherapy or cryoablation or approached surgically.[8] Thrombotic therapy for large, unresectable liver metastases and radiofrequency ablation for small liver metastases are options to be considered.[8] In selected cases, long-acting octreotide has been beneficial.[134] Because of the risk of massive catecholamine release, ablative therapy should be performed with great caution and only at centers with experience with these techniques; in addition to α- and β-adrenergic blockade, these patients are usually treated with metyrosine before the procedure.[8] External radiotherapy can also be used to treat unresectable soft tissue lesions.[135]

Local tumor irradiation with therapeutic doses of ^{131}I-MIBG has produced partial and temporary responses in approximately one third of patients.[12] If the tumor is considered aggressive and the patient's quality of life is affected, combination chemotherapy can provide disease stabilization.[136,137] In a nonrandomized, single-arm trial, the efficacy of chemotherapy with a combination CVD protocol (cyclophosphamide 750 mg/m^2 body surface area on day 1; vincristine 1.4 mg/m^2 on day 1; and dacarbazine 600 mg/m^2 on days 1 and 2; repeated every 21 days) was studied in 14 patients with malignant pheochromocytoma.[138,139] This protocol produced a complete and partial response rate of 57% (median duration, 21 months; range, 7 to >34 months). Complete and partial biochemical responses were seen in 79% of patients (median duration, >22 months; range, 6 to >35 months). All responding patients had objective improvement in performance status and blood pressure.[138,139] CVD chemotherapy can be continued until the patient develops new lesions or there is a significant (e.g., >25%) increase in size of known tumor sites. Because CVD chemotherapy may induce massive catecholamine release, it is important that the patient be optimally α- and β-blocked, just as for surgery. In addition, the first cycle of CVD should be completed in the hospital and with close medical observation. Management of malignant pheochromocytoma can be frustrating because curative options are limited. Recent studies suggest that tyrosine kinase inhibitors (e.g., sunitinib) may have a role in the treatment of metastatic pheochromocytoma; however, they are not curative.[140]

Pheochromocytoma in Pregnancy

Pheochromocytoma in pregnancy can cause the death of both the fetus and the mother.[141,142] The approach to the biochemical diagnosis is the same as that for the nonpregnant patient. MRI (without gadolinium enhancement) is the preferred imaging modality, and ¹²³I-MIBG is contraindicated. The treatment of hypertensive crises is the same as for nonpregnant patients except that use of nitroprusside should be avoided. Although the most appropriate management is debated, adrenal pheochromocytomas should be removed promptly if diagnosed during the first or second trimester of pregnancy. The preoperative preparation is the same as for a nonpregnant patient. If the pregnancy is already in the third trimester, a single operation is recommended, to perform a cesarean section and remove the adrenal pheochromocytoma at the same time. Spontaneous labor and delivery should be avoided. The management of catecholamine-secreting paragangliomas in pregnancy may require modification of these guidelines depending on tumor location.

RENIN-ANGIOTENSIN-ALDOSTERONE SYSTEM

The components of the renin-angiotensin-aldosterone (RAA) system are shown in Figure 16-7.[143] Aldosterone is secreted from the zona glomerulosa under the control of three primary factors: angiotensin II, potassium, and ACTH. The secretion of aldosterone is restricted to the zona glomerulosa because of zone-specific expression of aldosterone synthase (CYP11B2) (see Chapter 15). Dopamine, atrial natriuretic peptide, and heparin inhibit aldosterone secretion.

Renin and Angiotensin

Renin is an enzyme that is produced primarily in the juxtaglomerular apparatus of the kidney; it is stored in granules and released in response to specific secretagogues. The protein consists of 340 amino acids, of which the first 43 are a prosegment that is cleaved to produce the active

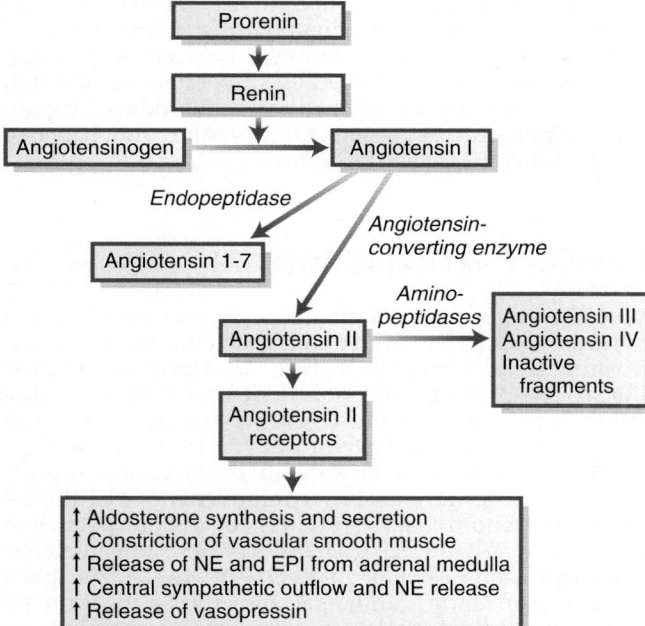

Figure 16-7 Components of the renin-angiotensin system. EPI, epinephrine; NE, norepinephrine. (Adapted and redrawn from Williams GH, Chao J, Chao L. Kidney hormones. In: Conn PM, Melmed S, eds. *Endocrinology: Basic and Clinical Principles.* Totowa, NJ: Humana Press; 1997:393-404.)

enzyme. The release of renin into the circulation is the rate-limiting step in the RAA system. Renal renin release is controlled by four factors:
1. The macula densa, a specialized group of convoluted distal tubular cells that function as chemoreceptors for monitoring the sodium and chloride loads present in the distal tubule
2. Juxtaglomerular cells acting as pressure transducers that sense stretch of the afferent arteriolar wall and thus renal perfusion pressure
3. The sympathetic nervous system, which modifies the release of renin, particularly in response to upright posture
4. Humoral factors, including potassium, angiotensin II, and atrial natriuretic peptides

Renin release is maximized in conditions of low renal perfusion pressure or low tubular sodium content (e.g., renal artery stenosis, hemorrhage, dehydration). Renin release is suppressed by elevated perfusion pressure at the kidney (e.g., hypertension) and a high-sodium diet. Renin release is increased directly by hypokalemia and decreased by hyperkalemia.

Angiotensinogen, an α₂-globulin synthesized in the liver, is the only known substrate for renin and is broken down into the angiotensin peptides. The protein consists of 485 amino acids, 33 of which constitute a presegment that is cleaved after secretion. The action of renin on angiotensinogen produces angiotensin I. Angiotensin I comprises the first 10–amino acid sequence after the presegment and does not appear to have biologic activity. Angiotensin II, the main biologically active angiotensin, is created by cleavage of the two carboxy-terminal peptides of angiotensin I by angiotensin-converting enzyme (ACE) (see Fig. 16-7). ACE is localized to cell membranes in the lung and intracellular granules in certain tissues that produce angiotensin II. Amino peptidase A can remove the amino-terminal aspartic acid to produce the heptapeptide, angiotensin III. Angiotensin II and angiotensin III have equivalent efficacy in promoting aldosterone secretion and modifying renal blood flow. The half-life in the circulation of angiotensin II is short (<60 seconds). Elements of the RAA system are present in the adrenals, kidneys, heart, and brain. For example, the adrenal glomerulosa cells contain the proteins needed to produce and secrete angiotensin II. Other tissues contain one or more components of the system but require other cells or circulating components, or both, to generate angiotensin II.

Angiotensin II functions through the angiotensin receptor to maintain normal extracellular volume and blood pressure by (1) increasing aldosterone secretion from the zona glomerulosa via increased transcription of CYP11B2; (2) constricting vascular smooth muscle, thereby increasing blood pressure and reducing renal blood flow; (3) releasing norepinephrine and epinephrine from the adrenal medulla; (4) enhancing the activity of the sympathetic nervous system by increasing central sympathetic outflow, thereby increasing norepinephrine discharge from sympathetic nerve terminals; and (5) promoting the release of vasopressin.

Aldosterone

Approximately 50% to 70% of aldosterone circulates bound to albumin or weakly bound to corticosteroid-binding globulin; 30% to 50% of total plasma aldosterone is free. The half-life is relatively short at 15 to 20 minutes. In the liver, aldosterone is rapidly inactivated to tetrahydroaldosterone. The classic functions of aldosterone are regulation of extracellular volume and control of potassium

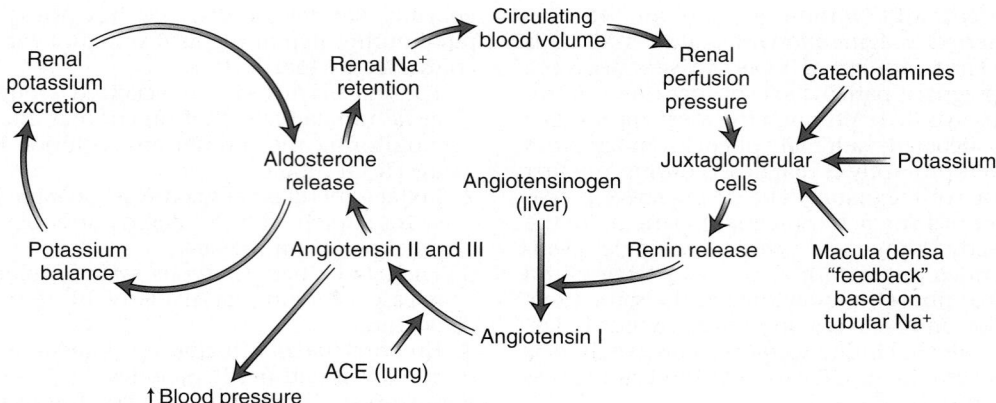

Figure 16-8 Renin-angiotensin-aldosterone and potassium-aldosterone negative feedback loops. Aldosterone production is determined by input from each loop. ACE, angiotensin-converting enzyme; Na+, sodium. (Adapted and redrawn from Williams GH, Dluhy RG. Diseases of the adrenal cortex. In: Braunwald E, Fauci AD, Kasper D, et al, eds. *Harrison's Principles of Internal Medicine*, 15th ed. New York, NY: McGraw-Hill; 2001:2087.)

homeostasis. These effects are mediated by the binding of free aldosterone to the mineralocorticoid receptor in the cytosol of epithelial cells, principally in the kidney.

Mineralocorticoid receptors have tissue-specific expression. For example, the tissues with the highest concentrations of these receptors are the distal nephron, colon, and hippocampus. Lower levels of mineralocorticoid receptors are found in the rest of the gastrointestinal tract and heart. Transport to the nucleus and binding to specific binding domains on targeted genes leads to their increased expression. Aldosterone-regulated kinase appears to be a key intermediary, and its increased expression leads to modification of the apical sodium channel, resulting in increased sodium ion transport across the cell membrane (see Chapter 15). The increased luminal negativity augments tubular secretion of potassium by the tubular cells and of hydrogen ion by the interstitial cells.

Glucocorticoids and mineralocorticoids bind equally to the mineralocorticoid receptor. Specificity of action is provided in many tissues by the presence of a glucocorticoid-inactivating enzyme, 11β-hydroxysteroid dehydrogenase, which prevents glucocorticoids from interacting with the receptor (see Chapter 15). Mineralocorticoid escape refers to the counterregulatory mechanisms that are manifested after 3 to 5 days of excessive mineralocorticoid administration. Several mechanisms contribute to this escape, including renal hemodynamic factors and increased levels of atrial natriuretic peptide.

In addition to the classic genomic actions mediated by aldosterone binding to cytosolic receptors, mineralocorticoids have acute, nongenomic actions resulting from activation of an unidentified cell surface receptor. This action involves a G protein signaling pathway and probably a modification of the sodium-hydrogen exchange activity. This effect has been demonstrated in both epithelial and nonepithelial cells.[144]

Aldosterone has additional, nonclassic effects primarily on nonepithelial cells.[145] These actions, although probably genomic and therefore mediated by activation of the cytosolic mineralocorticoid receptor, do not include modification of sodium-potassium balance. Aldosterone-mediated actions include the expression of several collagen genes; genes controlling tissue growth factors (e.g., transforming growth factor-β, plasminogen activator inhibitor type 1); and genes mediating inflammation.[146] The resultant actions lead to microangiopathy, necrosis (acutely), and fibrosis in various tissues such as the heart, the vasculature, and the kidney.[145] Increased levels of aldosterone are not necessary

to cause this damage; an imbalance between the volume or sodium balance state and the level of aldosterone appears to be the critical factor.[145]

The action of angiotensin II on aldosterone involves a negative feedback loop that also includes extracellular fluid volume (Fig. 16-8).[147] The major function of this feedback loop is to modify sodium homeostasis and, secondarily, to regulate blood pressure. Sodium restriction activates the RAA axis. The effects of angiotensin II on both the adrenal cortex and the renal vasculature promote renal sodium conservation. On the other hand, with suppression of renin release and suppression of the level of circulating angiotensin, aldosterone secretion is reduced and renal blood flow is increased, promoting sodium loss. The RAA loop is very sensitive to dietary sodium intake. Sodium excess enhances the responsiveness of the renal and peripheral vasculature and reduces the adrenal responsiveness to angiotensin II. Sodium restriction has the opposite effect. Therefore, sodium intake modifies target tissue responsiveness to angiotensin II, a fine-tuning mechanism that appears to be critical to maintaining normal sodium homeostasis without a chronic effect on blood pressure. Excess aldosterone secretion causes hypertension through two main mechanisms: mineralocorticoid-induced expansion of plasma and extracellular fluid volume and increased total peripheral vascular resistance.

PRIMARY ALDOSTERONISM

Hypertension, suppressed plasma renin activity (PRA), and increased aldosterone excretion characterize the syndrome of primary aldosteronism, first described in 1955.[148] Aldosterone-producing adenoma (APA) and bilateral idiopathic hyperaldosteronism (IHA) are the most common subtypes of primary aldosteronism (Table 16-10). Somatic mutations account for about half of APAs and include mutations in genes encoding components of the Kir 3.4 (GIRK4) potassium channel (KCNJ5); the sodium/potassium and calcium ATPases (ATP1A1 and ATP2B3); and a voltage-dependent C-type calcium channel (CACNA1D).[149] A much less common form, unilateral hyperplasia or primary adrenal hyperplasia (PAH), is caused by micronodular or macronodular hyperplasia of the zona glomerulosa of predominantly one adrenal gland. Familial hyperaldosteronism (FH) is also rare, and three types have been described (see later discussion).[149]

TABLE 16-10
Adrenocortical Causes of Hypertension

Low Renin and High Aldosterone

Primary Aldosteronism
Aldosterone-producing adenoma (APA)—30% of cases
Bilateral idiopathic hyperplasia (IHA)—60% of cases
Primary (unilateral) adrenal hyperplasia—2% of cases
Aldosterone-producing adrenocortical carcinoma—<1% of cases
Familial hyperaldosteronism (FH)
    Glucocorticoid-remediable aldosteronism (FH type 1)—<1% of cases
    FH type 2 (APA or IHA)—<6% of cases
    FH type 3 (germline KCNJ5 mutations)—<1% of cases
Ectopic aldosterone-producing adenoma or carcinoma—<0.1% of cases

Low Renin and Low Aldosterone

Hyperdeoxycorticosteronism
Congenital adrenal hyperplasia
    11β-Hydroxylase deficiency
    17α-Hydroxylase deficiency
Deoxycorticosterone-producing tumor
Primary cortisol resistance
Apparent mineralocorticoid excess (AME)/11β-HSD deficiency
    Genetic
        Type 1 AME
    Acquired
        Licorice or carbenoxolone ingestion (type 1 AME)
        Cushing syndrome (type 2 AME)

Cushing Syndrome
Exogenous glucocorticoid administration—most common cause
Endogenous
    ACTH-dependent—85% of cases
        Pituitary
        Ectopic
    ACTH-independent—15% of cases
        Unilateral adrenal disease (adenoma or carcinoma)
        Bilateral adrenal disease
            Massive macronodular hyperplasia (rare)
            Primary pigmented nodular adrenal disease (rare)

ACTH, corticotropin; HSD, hydroxysteroid dehydrogenase.

History

In his presidential address at the annual meeting of the Central Society for Clinical Research, Chicago, Illinois, October 29, 1954, Dr. Jerome W. Conn stated[148]: "I have prepared no comprehensive review of my personal philosophy of clinical investigation. Instead, I plan to make a scientific report to you about a clinical syndrome, the investigation of which has been most exciting to me since I initiated it in April of this year." Conn, a professor of Medicine at the University of Michigan, had been active in government-funded research on the mechanisms of human acclimatization to humid heat. He established that the body's acclimatization response was to rapidly diminish renal salt and water loss and to abruptly curtail the salt content of body sweat and saliva. He suggested that these responses were the result of increased adrenocortical function with elaboration of salt-retaining steroids. He also showed that intramuscular administration of deoxycorticosterone acetate (DOCA) produced similar changes in the electrolyte composition of urine, sweat, and saliva.

In April 1954, Professor Conn was asked to see M.W., a 34-year-old woman with a 7-year history of muscle spasms, temporary paralysis, tetany, and weakness and a 4-year history of hypertension. She was found to have a blood pressure of 176/104 mm Hg, severe hypokalemia (1.6 to 2.5 mEq/L), mild hypernatremia (146 to 151 mEq/L), and alkalosis (serum pH 7.62). Because there were no signs or symptoms of glucocorticoid or androgen excess, Conn suspected, based on his past research, that M.W.'s clinical presentation could result from excess secretion of the adrenal salt-retaining corticoid. Conn studied M.W. in the Metabolism Research Unit for 227 days. Streeten's bioassay technique developed to measure sodium retention in adrenalectomized rats after intraperitoneal injection of human urine was used, and M.W. averaged 1333 µg DOCA equivalent per day, compared with normotensive control subjects at 61.4 µg/day. In his presidential address, Conn stated: "It is believed that these studies delineate a new clinical syndrome which is designated temporarily as primary aldosteronism."[148] (Note: The word *temporarily* was used because aldosterone was yet to be measured in any human bodily fluid.)

Conn planned for a bilateral adrenalectomy for his patient on December 10, 1954. In 1995, Gittler and Fajans described the surgical scene: "To the immense delight of Conn and those in the operating room, the surgeon, Dr. William Baum, encountered a right 13-g adrenal tumor which was removed while leaving the contralateral gland intact. The patient's postoperative studies showed an almost total reversal of the preoperative metabolic and clinical abnormalities. Conn had achieved irrefutable proof of the validity of his investigative conclusions and established for the first time the relationship among adrenal aldosterone-producing tumors, hypertension, and hypokalemia. A new era had arrived in the study of hypertension and adrenal mineralocorticoids."[150]

By 1964, Conn had collected 145 cases,[151] and he suggested that up to 20% of patients with essential hypertension might have primary aldosteronism.[152] This suggestion was downplayed by most as a gross overestimate.[153,154] Later, Conn decreased his predicted prevalence of primary aldosteronism to 10% of hypertensives,[155] a prediction that was substantiated nearly 40 years later.

Prevalence

In the past, clinicians would not consider the diagnosis of primary aldosteronism unless the patient presented with spontaneous hypokalemia, and then the diagnostic evaluation would require discontinuation of antihypertensive medications for at least 2 weeks. This diagnostic approach resulted in predicted prevalence rates of less than 0.5% of hypertensive patients.[16,153,154,156-159] However, it is now recognized that most patients with primary aldosteronism are not hypokalemic[160-162] and that screening can be completed while the patient is taking antihypertensive drugs with a simple blood test that yields the ratio of plasma aldosterone concentration (PAC) to PRA.[161] Use of the PAC/PRA ratio as a case-detection test, followed by aldosterone suppression for confirmatory testing, has resulted in much higher prevalence estimates for primary aldosteronism—5% to 10% of all patients with hypertension.[161-164]

Clinical Presentation

The diagnosis of primary aldosteronism is usually made in patients who are in the third to sixth decades of life. Few symptoms are specific to the syndrome. Patients with marked hypokalemia may have muscle weakness and cramping, headaches, palpitations, polydipsia, polyuria, nocturia, or a combination of these.[160] Periodic paralysis is a very rare presentation in Caucasians, but it is not an infrequent presentation in patients of Asian descent.[165] For example, in a series of 50 patients with APA reported from Hong Kong, 21 (42%) presented with periodic paralysis.[165]

Another rare presentation is tetany associated with the decrease in ionized calcium with marked hypokalemic alkalosis. The polyuria and nocturia are a result of hypokalemia-induced renal concentrating defect, and the presentation is frequently mistaken for prostatism in men. There are no specific physical findings. Edema is not a common finding because of the phenomenon of mineralocorticoid escape, described earlier. The degree of hypertension is typically moderate to severe and may be resistant to the usual pharmacologic treatments.[160,166] In the first 262 cases of primary aldosteronism diagnosed at Mayo Clinic (1957-1986), the highest blood pressure was 260/155 mm Hg; the mean (± SD [standard deviation]) was 184/112 ± 28/16 mm Hg.[166] Patients with APA tend to have higher blood pressures than those with IHA.

Hypokalemia is frequently absent, so all patients with hypertension are candidates for this disorder. In other patients, the hypokalemia becomes evident only with the addition of a potassium-wasting diuretic (e.g., hydrochlorothiazide, furosemide). Deep-seated renal cysts are found in up to 60% of patients with chronic hypokalemia.[167] Because of a reset osmostat, the serum sodium concentration tends to be high-normal or slightly above the upper limit of normal. This clinical clue is very useful in the initial assessment for potential primary aldosteronism.

Several studies have shown that patients with primary aldosteronism are at higher risk than other patients with hypertension for target-organ damage of the heart and kidney.[168,169] Chronic kidney disease is common in patients with long-standing primary aldosteronism.[170] When matched for age, blood pressure, and duration of hypertension, patients with primary aldosteronism have greater left ventricular mass measurements than patients with other types of hypertension (e.g., pheochromocytoma, Cushing syndrome, essential hypertension).[171] In patients with APA, the left ventricular wall thickness and mass were markedly decreased 1 year after adrenalectomy.[172] A case-control study of 124 patients with primary aldosteronism and 465 patients with essential hypertension (matched for age, sex, and systolic and diastolic blood pressure) found that patients presenting with either APA or IHA had a significantly higher rate of cardiovascular events (e.g., stroke, atrial fibrillation, myocardial infarction) than the matched patients with essential hypertension.[169] A negative effect of circulating aldosterone on cardiac function was found in young nonhypertensive subjects with glucocorticoid-remediable aldosteronism (GRA) who had increased left ventricular wall thickness and reduced diastolic function compared with age- and sex-matched control subjects.[168]

Diagnosis

The diagnostic approach to primary aldosteronism can be considered in three phases: case-detection tests, confirmatory tests, and subtype evaluation tests.

Case-Detection Tests

Spontaneous hypokalemia is uncommon in patients with uncomplicated hypertension; when present, it strongly suggests associated mineralocorticoid excess. However, several studies have shown that most patients with primary aldosteronism have baseline serum levels of potassium in the normal range.[161,163] Therefore, hypokalemia should not be the major criterion used to trigger case-detection testing for primary aldosteronism. Patients with hypertension and hypokalemia (regardless of presumed cause), treatment-resistant hypertension (poor control on three antihyper-

When to consider testing for primary aldosteronism:
- Hypertension and hypokalemia
- Resistant hypertension
- Adrenal incidentaloma and hypertension
- Onset of hypertension at a young age (<20 y)
- Severe hypertension (≥160 mm Hg systolic or ≥100 mm Hg diastolic)
- Whenever considering secondary hypertension

Morning blood sample in seated ambulant patient
- Plasma aldosterone concentration (PAC)
- Plasma renin activity (PRA) or PRC

↑PAC (≥15 ng/dL)
↓PRA (<1.0 ng/mL per hour) or
↓PRC (<lower limit of detection for the assay)
and
PAC/PRA ratio ≥20 ng/dL per ng/mL per hour

Investigate for primary aldosteronism

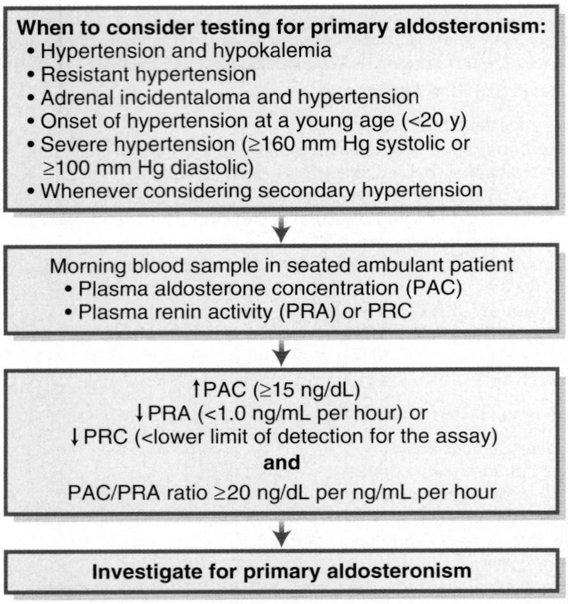

Figure 16-9 This algorithm provides guidance on when to consider testing for primary aldosteronism and use of the ratio of plasma aldosterone concentration (PAC) to plasma renin activity (PRA) as a case-detection tool. PRC, plasma renin concentration.

tensive drugs), severe hypertension (≥160 mm Hg systolic or ≥100 mm Hg diastolic), hypertension and an incidental adrenal mass, or onset of hypertension at a young age should undergo screening for primary aldosteronism (Fig. 16-9).[160,161]

In patients with suspected primary aldosteronism, screening can be accomplished (see Fig. 16-9) by paired measurements of PAC and PRA in a random morning ambulatory blood sample (preferably obtained between 8 and 10 AM). This test may be performed while the patient is taking antihypertensive medications (with some exceptions, discussed later) and without posture stimulation.[160] Hypokalemia reduces the secretion of aldosterone, and it is optimal to restore the serum level of potassium to normal before performing diagnostic studies.

It may be difficult to interpret data obtained from patients treated with a mineralocorticoid receptor antagonist (spironolactone and eplerenone). These drugs prevent aldosterone from activating the receptor, resulting sequentially in sodium loss, a decrease in plasma volume, and an elevation in PRA, which will reduce the utility of the PAC/PRA ratio. For this reason, spironolactone and eplerenone should not be initiated until the evaluation is completed and the final decisions about treatment are made. However, there are rare exceptions to this rule. For example, if the patient is hypokalemic despite treatment with spironolactone or eplerenone, then the mineralocorticoid receptors are not fully blocked and PRA or PRC should be suppressed in such a patient with primary aldosteronism. In this unique circumstance, the evaluation for primary aldosteronism can proceed despite treatment with mineralocorticoid receptor antagonists. However, in most patients already receiving spironolactone, therapy should be discontinued for at least 6 weeks. Other potassium-sparing diuretics, such as amiloride and triamterene, usually do not interfere with testing unless the patient is on high doses.

ACE inhibitors and angiotensin receptor blockers (ARBs) have the potential to falsely elevate the PRA. Therefore, the finding of a detectable PRA level or a low PAC/PRA ratio in a patient taking one of these drugs does not exclude the diagnosis of primary aldosteronism. However, an undetectably low PRA level in a patient taking an ACE inhibitor or ARB makes primary aldosteronism likely, and the PRA is suppressed (<1.0 ng/mL per hour) in almost all patients with primary aldosteronism.

The PAC/PRA ratio, first proposed as a case-detection test for primary aldosteronism in 1981,[173] is based on the concept of paired hormone measurements. The PAC is measured in nanograms per deciliter, and the PRA in nanograms per milliliter per hour. In a hypertensive hypokalemic patient, secondary hyperaldosteronism should be considered if both PRA and PAC are increased and the PAC/PRA ratio is less than 10 (e.g., renovascular disease). An alternative source of mineralocorticoid receptor agonism should be considered if both PRA and PAC are suppressed (e.g., hypercortisolism). Primary aldosteronism should be suspected if the PRA is suppressed (<1.0 ng/mL per hour) and the PAC is increased. At least 14 prospective studies have been published on the use of the PAC/PRA ratio in detecting primary aldosteronism.[174] Although there is some uncertainty about test characteristics and lack of standardization (see later discussion), the PAC/PRA ratio is widely accepted as the case-detection test of choice for primary aldosteronism.[161]

It is important to understand that the lower limit of detection varies among different PRA assays and can have a dramatic effect on the PAC/PRA ratio. As an example, if the lower limit of detection for PRA is <0.6 ng/mL per hour and the PAC is 16 ng/dL, then the PAC/PRA ratio with an "undetectable" PRA would be 27; however, if the lower limit of detection for PRA is 0.1 ng/mL per hour, the same PAC level would yield a PAC/PRA ratio of 160. Thus, the cutoff for a high PAC/PRA ratio is laboratory dependent and, more specifically, PRA assay dependent. In a retrospective study, the combination of a PAC/PRA ratio greater than 30 and a PAC level greater than 20 ng/dL had a sensitivity of 90% and a specificity of 91% for APA.[175] At Mayo Clinic, the combination of a PAC/PRA ratio of 20 or higher and a PAC level of at least 15 ng/dL is found in more than 90% of patients with surgically confirmed APA. In patients without primary aldosteronism, most of the variation occurs within the normal range.[176] A high PAC/PRA ratio is a positive screening test result, a finding that warrants further testing.[161]

It is critical for the clinician to recognize that the PAC/PRA ratio is only a case-detection tool, and all positive results should be followed by a confirmatory aldosterone suppression test to verify autonomous aldosterone production before treatment is initiated.[161] In a systematic review of 16 studies with 3136 participants, the PAC/PRA cutoff levels used varied between 7.2 and 100.[174] The sensitivity for APA varied between 64% and 100%, and the specificity ranged between 87% and 100%. However, the description of the reference standard and the attribution of diagnosis at the end of the studies were incomplete, and there was a lack of standardization concerning the origin of the study cohort, ongoing antihypertensive medications, use of high-salt versus low-salt diet, and circumstances during blood sampling. The authors concluded that none of the studies provided any valid estimates of test characteristics (sensitivity, specificity, and likelihood ratio at various cutoff levels).[174] In a study of 118 subjects with essential hypertension, neither antihypertensive medications nor acute variation of dietary sodium affected the accuracy of the PAC/PRA ratio adversely; the sensitivities on and off therapy were 73% and 87%, respectively, and the specificities were 74% and 75%, respectively.[177] In a study of African American and Caucasian subjects with resistant hyperten-

sion, the PAC/PRA ratio was elevated (>20) in 45 of 58 subjects with primary aldosteronism and in 35 of 207 patients without primary aldosteronism (sensitivity, 78%; specificity, 83%).[178]

The measurement of PRA is time-consuming, shows high interlaboratory variability, and requires special preanalytic prerequisites. To overcome these disadvantages, a monoclonal antibody against active renin is being used by several reference laboratories to measure the plasma renin concentration (PRC) instead of PRA. However, few studies have compared the different methods of testing for primary aldosteronism, and these studies lack confirmatory testing. It is reasonable to consider a positive PAC/PRC test if the PAC is greater than 15 ng/dL and the PRC is below the lower limit of detection for the assay (see Fig. 16-9).

Confirmatory Tests

An increased PAC/PRA ratio is not diagnostic by itself, and primary aldosteronism must be confirmed by demonstration of inappropriate aldosterone secretion.[162] The list of drugs and hormones capable of affecting the RAA axis is extensive, and a medication-contaminated evaluation is frequently unavoidable in patients with poorly controlled hypertension despite a three-drug program. Calcium channel blockers and α_1-adrenergic receptor blockers do not affect the diagnostic accuracy in most cases.[161] It is impossible to interpret data obtained from patients receiving treatment with mineralocorticoid receptor antagonists (e.g., spironolactone, eplerenone) when the PRA is not suppressed (see earlier). Therefore, treatment with a mineralocorticoid receptor antagonist should not be initiated until the evaluation has been completed and the final decisions about treatment have been made. Aldosterone suppression testing can be performed with orally administered sodium chloride and measurement of urinary aldosterone or with intravenous sodium chloride loading and measurement of PAC.[160,161]

Oral Sodium Loading Test. After hypertension and hypokalemia have been controlled, patients should receive a high-sodium diet (supplemented with sodium chloride tablets if needed) for 3 days, with a goal sodium intake of 5000 mg (equivalent to 218 mEq of sodium or 12.8 g sodium chloride).[166] The risk of increasing dietary sodium in patients with severe hypertension must be assessed in each case.[179] Because the high-salt diet can increase kaliuresis and hypokalemia, vigorous replacement of potassium chloride may be needed, and the serum level of potassium should be monitored daily. On the third day of the high-sodium diet, a 24-hour urine specimen is collected for measurement of aldosterone, sodium, and creatinine. To document adequate sodium repletion, the 24-hour urinary sodium excretion should exceed 200 mEq. Urinary aldosterone excretion of more than 12 μg/24 hours in this setting is consistent with autonomous aldosterone secretion.[166] The sensitivity and specificity of the oral sodium loading test are 96% and 93%, respectively.[180]

Intravenous Saline Infusion Test. The intravenous saline infusion test has also been used widely for the diagnosis of primary aldosteronism.[161,162] Normal subjects show suppression of PAC after volume expansion with isotonic saline; subjects with primary aldosteronism do not show this suppression. The test is done after an overnight fast. Two liters of 0.9% sodium chloride solution is infused intravenously with an infusion pump over 4 hours with the patient recumbent. Blood pressure and heart rate are monitored during the infusion. At the completion of the infusion, blood is drawn for measurement of PAC. PAC levels in normal subjects decrease to less than 5 ng/dL, whereas most patients with primary aldosteronism do not suppress to less than 10 ng/dL. Postinfusion PAC values between 5 and 10 ng/dL are indeterminate and may be seen in patients with IHA. Historically the saline infusion test has been performed in the supine position and the false-negative rate has been excessive; preliminary data suggest that if the saline infusion test is performed in the seated position the accuracy is improved.[181]

Fludrocortisone Suppression Test. In the fludrocortisone suppression test, fludrocortisone acetate is administered for 4 days (0.1 mg every 6 hours) in combination with sodium chloride tablets (2 g three times daily with food). Blood pressure and serum potassium levels must be monitored daily. In the setting of low PRA, failure to suppress the upright 10 AM PAC to less than 6 ng/dL on day 4 is diagnostic of primary aldosteronism.[182] Increased QT interval dispersion and deterioration of left ventricular function have been reported during fludrocortisone suppression tests.[179] Most centers no longer use this test.

Subtype Studies

After case-detection and confirmatory testing, the third management issue guides the therapeutic approach by distinguishing APA and PAH from IHA and GRA. Unilateral adrenalectomy in patients with APA or PAH results in normalization of hypokalemia in all cases; hypertension is improved in all cases and is cured in 30% to 60%.[183-185] In IHA and GRA, unilateral or bilateral adrenalectomy seldom corrects the hypertension.[166] IHA and GRA should be treated medically. APA is found in approximately 35% of cases and bilateral IHA in approximately 60% (see Table 16-10). APAs are usually small hypodense adrenal nodules (<2 cm in diameter) on CT and are golden yellow in color when resected. IHA adrenal glands may be normal on CT or may show nodular changes. Aldosterone-producing adrenal carcinomas are almost always larger than 4 cm in diameter and have an inhomogeneous phenotype on CT (see Table 16-6).

Computed Tomography of the Adrenal Glands. Primary aldosteronism subtype evaluation may require one or more tests, the first of which is imaging of the adrenal glands with CT (Fig. 16-10). If a solitary unilateral hypodense (HU < 10) macroadenoma (>1 cm) and normal contralateral adrenal morphologic appearance are found on CT in a young patient (<35 years) with severe primary aldosteronism, unilateral adrenalectomy is a reasonable therapeutic option (see Fig. 16-10).[186] However, in many cases, CT shows normal-appearing adrenals, minimal unilateral adrenal limb thickening, unilateral microadenomas (≤1 cm), or bilateral macroadenomas (Fig. 16-11). In these cases, additional testing is required to determine the source of excess aldosterone secretion.

Small APAs may be labeled incorrectly as IHA on the basis of CT findings of bilateral nodularity or normal-appearing adrenals. Also, apparent adrenal microadenomas may actually represent areas of hyperplasia, and unilateral adrenalectomy would be inappropriate. In addition, nonfunctioning unilateral adrenal macroadenomas are not uncommon, especially in older patients (>40 years).[187] Unilateral PAH may be visible on CT, or the PAH may appear normal on CT. In general, patients with APAs have more severe hypertension, more frequent hypokalemia, higher levels of plasma aldosterone (>25 ng/dL) and urinary aldosterone (>30 µg/24 hours), and are younger (<50 years), compared with those who have IHA.[166] Patients fitting these descriptors are considered to have a high probability of APA regardless of the CT findings (see Fig. 16-10), and 41% of patients with a high probability of APA and a

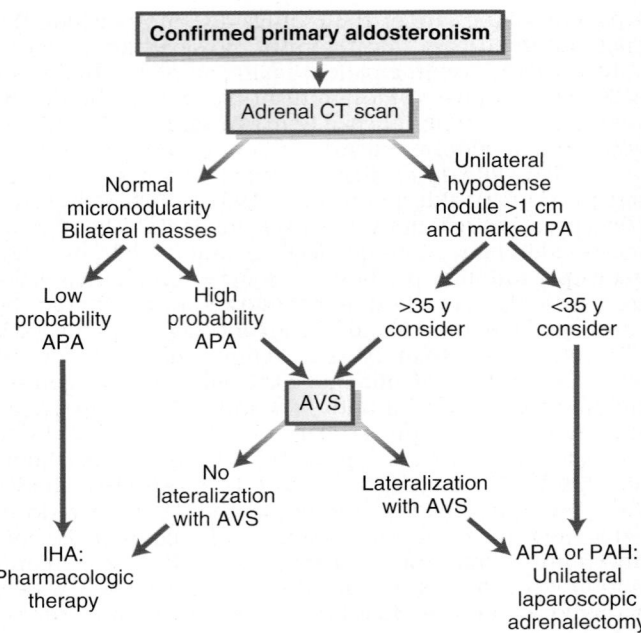

Figure 16-10 Subtype evaluation of primary aldosteronism. For patients who want to pursue a surgical treatment for their hypertension, adrenal venous sampling is frequently a key diagnostic step (see text for details). APA, aldosterone-producing adenoma; AVS, adrenal venous sampling; CT, computed tomography; IHA, idiopathic hyperaldosteronism; PA, primary aldosteronism; PAH, primary adrenal hyperplasia. (Modified from Young WF Jr, Hogan MJ. Renin-independent hypermineralocorticoidism. *Trends Endocrinol Metab.* 1994;5:97-106.)

normal adrenal CT scan prove to have unilateral aldosterone hypersecretion.[188]

Adrenal CT is not accurate in distinguishing between APA and IHA.[186,188,189] In one study of 203 patients with primary aldosteronism who were evaluated with both CT and AVS, CT was accurate in only 53% of patients; based on the CT findings, 42 patients (22%) would have been incorrectly excluded as candidates for adrenalectomy, and 48 (25%) might have had unnecessary or inappropriate surgery.[188] In a systematic review of 38 studies involving 950 patients with primary aldosteronism, adrenal CT/MRI results did not agree with the findings from AVS in 359 patients (38%); based on CT/MRI, 19% of the 950 patients would have undergone noncurative surgery, and 19% would have been offered medical therapy instead of curative adrenalectomy.[189] Therefore, AVS is essential to direct appropriate therapy in patients with primary aldosteronism who have a high probability of APA and are seeking a potential surgical cure.

Adrenal Venous Sampling. AVS is the criterion standard test to distinguish between unilateral and bilateral disease in patients with primary aldosteronism.[161,186,189] AVS is an intricate procedure because the right adrenal vein is small and may be difficult to locate and cannulate; the success rate depends on the proficiency of the angiographer.[190] A review of 47 reports found that the success rate for cannulation of the right adrenal vein in 384 patients was 74%.[166] With experience and focusing the expertise to one or two radiologists at a referral center, the AVS success rate can be as high as 96%.[188,191,192]

The five keys to a successful AVS program are (1) appropriate patient selection, (2) careful patient preparation, (3) focused technical expertise, (4) defined protocol, and (5) accurate data interpretation.[190] A center-specific written protocol is mandatory. The protocol should be developed

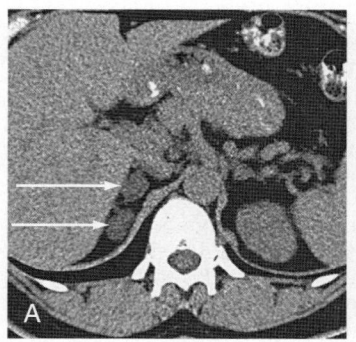 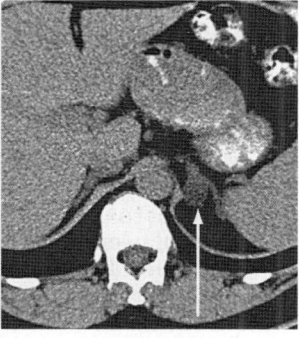

Results of bilateral adrenal venous sampling

Vein	Aldosterone (A), ng/dL	Cortisol (C), μg/dL	A/C ratio	Aldosterone ratio*
R adrenal vein	29,338	668	43.9	62.7
L adrenal vein	363	540	0.7	
Inferior vena cava	259	31	8.4	

*R adrenal vein A/C ratio divided by L adrenal vein A/C ratio.

B

Figure 16-11 A 43-year-old woman had a 2-year history of hypertension and hypokalemia. The screening test for primary aldosteronism was positive, with a plasma aldosterone concentration (PAC) of 37 ng/dL and low plasma renin activity (PRA) at less than 0.6 ng/mL per hour (PAC/PRA ratio > 61). The confirmatory test for primary aldosteronism was also positive, with the 24-hour urinary excretion of aldosterone measured at 53 μg on a high-sodium diet (urinary sodium, 196 mEq/24 hours). **A,** Adrenal computed tomography shows a 12-mm, low-density mass *(arrow, right panel)* in the medial limb of the left adrenal and two low-density, 10-mm nodules *(arrows, left panel)* within the right adrenal gland. **B,** Adrenal venous sampling lateralized aldosterone secretion to the right, and two cortical adenomas (1.8 × 1.2 × 0.8 cm and 2.5 × 1.5 × 1.2 cm) were found at laparoscopic right adrenalectomy. The postoperative plasma aldosterone concentration was less than 1.0 ng/dL. Hypokalemia was cured and blood pressure was normal without the aid of antihypertensive medications.

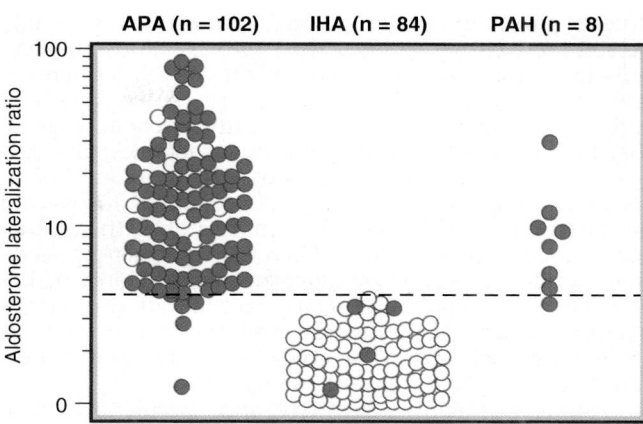

Figure 16-12 Adrenal vein aldosterone lateralization ratios for patients with unilateral aldosterone-producing adenomas (APA), bilateral idiopathic hyperplasia (IHA), and unilateral primary adrenal hyperplasia (PAH). Shaded symbols indicate that the diagnosis was confirmed surgically. The sensitivity and specificity of a cortisol-corrected plasma aldosterone concentration lateralization ratio greater than 4.0 for unilateral disease are 95.2% and 100%, respectively. (From Young WF Jr, Stanson AW, Thompson GB, et al. Role for adrenal venous sampling in primary aldosteronism. *Surgery.* 2004;136:1227-1235; used with permission.)

by an interested group of endocrinologists, hypertension specialists, internists, radiologists, and laboratory personnel. Safeguards should be in place to prevent mislabeling of the blood tubes in the radiology suite and to prevent sample mixup in the laboratory.[190]

At Mayo Clinic, we use continuous cosyntropin infusion during AVS (50 μg/hour starting 30 minutes before sampling and continuing throughout the procedure) for the following reasons: (1) to minimize stress-induced fluctuations in aldosterone secretion during nonsimultaneous AVS; (2) to maximize the gradient in cortisol from adrenal vein to IVC and thus confirm successful sampling of the adrenal veins; and (3) to maximize the secretion of aldosterone from an APA.[188,190] The adrenal veins are catheterized through the percutaneous femoral vein approach, and the position of the catheter tip is verified by gentle injection of a small amount of nonionic contrast medium and radiographic documentation. Blood is obtained from both adrenal veins and from the IVC below the renal veins and assayed for aldosterone and cortisol concentrations. To be sure that there is no cross-contamination, the IVC sample should be obtained from the external iliac vein. The venous sample from the left side typically is obtained from the common phrenic vein immediately adjacent to the entrance of the adrenal vein. The cortisol concentrations from the adrenal veins and IVC are used to confirm successful catheterization; the adrenal vein/IVC cortisol ratio is typically greater than 10:1.

Dividing the right and left adrenal vein PAC values by their respective cortisol concentrations corrects for the dilutional effect of the inferior phenic vein flow into the left adrenal vein; these are termed *cortisol-corrected ratios* (Fig. 16-12). In patients with APA, the mean cortisol-corrected aldosterone ratio (i.e., the ratio of PAC/cortisol from the APA side to that from the normal side) is 18.0:1.[188] A cutoff point of 4.0:1 for this ratio is used to indicate unilateral aldosterone excess (see Fig. 16-12). In patients with IHA, the mean cortisol-corrected aldosterone ratio is 1.8:1 (high side to low side), and a ratio of less than 3.0:1 suggests bilateral aldosterone hypersecretion (see Fig. 16-12).[188] Therefore, most patients with a unilateral source of aldosterone have cortisol-corrected aldosterone lateralization ratios greater than 4.0, and ratios greater than 3.0 but less than 4.0 represent a zone of overlap. Ratios no higher than 3.0 are consistent with bilateral aldosterone secretion. The test characteristics of adrenal vein sampling for detection of unilateral aldosterone hypersecretion (APA or PAH) are 95% sensitivity and 100% specificity.[188] At centers with experience with AVS, the complication rate is 2.5% or less.[188,191] Complications can include symptomatic groin hematoma, adrenal hemorrhage, and dissection of an adrenal vein.

Some centers and clinical practice guidelines recommend that AVS should be performed in all patients who have the diagnosis of primary aldosteronism.[161] The use of AVS should be based on patient preference, patient age, clinical comorbid conditions, and the clinical probability of finding an APA. A more practical approach is the selective use of AVS as outlined in Figure 16-10.[193]

Familial Hyperaldosteronism

Glucocorticoid-Remediable Aldosteronism: Familial Hyperaldosteronism Type I.
GRA (FH type I) was first described in a single family in 1966.[194] Twenty-six years later the causative *CYP11B1/CYP11B2* chimeric gene was discovered.[195] GRA is a form of hyperaldosteronism in which the hypersecretion of aldosterone can be reversed with physiologic

doses of glucocorticoid.[196] It is rare, as illustrated by a study of 300 consecutive patients with primary aldosteronism; only two patients were diagnosed with GRA (prevalence = 0.66%) (see Table 16-10).[197] GRA is characterized by early-onset hypertension that is usually severe and refractory to conventional antihypertensive therapies, aldosterone excess, suppressed PRA, and excess production of 18-hydroxycortisol and 18-oxycortisol. Mineralocorticoid production is regulated by ACTH instead of by the normal secretagogue, angiotensin II. Therefore, aldosterone secretion can be suppressed by glucocorticoid therapy. In the absence of glucocorticoid therapy, this mutation results in overproduction of aldosterone and the hybrid steroids 18-hydroxycortisol and 18-oxycortisol, which can be measured in the urine to make the diagnosis.

Genetic testing is a sensitive and specific means of diagnosing GRA and obviates the need to measure the urinary levels of 18-oxycortisol and 18-hydroxycortisol or to perform dexamethasone suppression testing. Genetic testing for GRA should be considered for patients with primary aldosteronism who have a family history of primary aldosteronism, onset of primary aldosteronism at a young age (<20 years), or family history of strokes at a young age.

Familial Hyperaldosteronism Type II. FH type II is autosomal dominant and may be monogenic.[149,198,199] The hyperaldosteronism in FH type II does not suppress with dexamethasone, and GRA mutation testing is negative. FH type II is more common than FH type I, but it still accounts for fewer than 6% of all patients with primary aldosteronism.[197] The molecular basis for FH type II is unclear, although a recent linkage analysis study showed an association with chromosomal region 7p22.[198,199]

Familial Hyperaldosteronism Type III. FH type III was first described in a single family in 2008.[200] This initial report included a father and two daughters who all presented with refractory hypertension before age 7 years, and all three were treated with bilateral adrenalectomy. The adrenal glands showed massive hyperplasia. Three years later the causative germline mutation in this family was discovered: a point mutation in and near the selectivity filter of the potassium channel KCNJ5.[201] This KCNJ5 mutation produces increased sodium conductance and cell depolarization, triggering calcium entry into glomerulosa cells, the signal for aldosterone production and cell proliferation. Other families with early-onset hyperaldosteronism have also been identified to have germline point mutations in the KCNJ5 gene.[202,203] In families in Europe with FH (GRA excluded), a new germline G151E KCNJ5 mutation was found in two patients with primary aldosteronism from Italy, and they presented a remarkably milder clinical and biochemical phenotype.[204] In four families with early-onset primary aldosteronism, germline G151R KCNJ5 mutations were found in two with severe hyperplasia requiring surgery; two kindreds had G151E mutations and mild primary aldosteronism.[205]

Somatic Mutations in *KCNJ5, ATP1A1, ATP2B3,* and *CACNA1D* Genes. In a multicenter study of 351 APAs from patients with primary aldosteronism and 130 other adrenocortical lesions, two somatic mutations in *KCNJ5* (G151R or L168R) were identified in 47% of APAs.[206] Somatic *KCNJ5* mutations were absent in patients with primary aldosteronism due to unilateral hyperplasia and in 130 nonaldosterone-secreting adrenal lesions. *KCNJ5* mutations were overrepresented in APAs from women compared with men (63% vs. 24%) and APAs with *KCNJ5* mutations were larger than those without (2.7 cm vs. 1.7 cm).

In a separate multicenter study, *KCNJ5* sequencing was performed on somatic (APA, *n* = 380) and peripheral (APA,

n = 344; bilateral IHA, *n* = 174) DNA of patients with primary aldosteronism.[207] Somatic *KCNJ5* mutations (G151R or L168R) were found in 34% of APAs; they were more prevalent in women (49%) than men (19%) (*p* < 0.001) and associated with higher preoperative aldosterone levels but not with therapeutic outcome after surgery. In this study, no germline *KCNJ5* mutations were found in patients with APA or IHA.[207]

Additional somatic APA mutations have been identified in three other genes: *ATP1A1* and *ATP2B3*, encoding Na+/K+-ATPase 1 and Ca2+-ATPase 3, respectively; and *CACNA1D*, encoding a voltage-gated calcium channel.[208,209] In a subsequent study, somatic APA mutations in *ATP1A1, ATP2B3,* and *KCNJ5* were present in 6.3%, 0.9%, and 39.3% of 112 APAs, respectively.[210] In addition, germline mutations in *CACNA1D* have now been reported in two children with primary aldosteronism.[211]

Principles of Treatment

The treatment goal is to prevent the morbidity and fatality associated with hypertension, hypokalemia, and cardiovascular damage. Knowing the cause of the primary aldosteronism helps to determine the appropriate treatment. Normalization of blood pressure should not be the only goal. In addition to the kidney and colon, mineralocorticoid receptors are present in the heart, brain, and blood vessels. Excessive secretion of aldosterone is associated with increased risk of cardiovascular disease and morbidity. Therefore, normalization of circulating aldosterone or mineralocorticoid receptor blockade should be part of the management plan for all patients with primary aldosteronism. However, clinicians must understand that most patients with long-standing primary aldosteronism have some degree of renal insufficiency that is masked by the glomerular hyperfiltration associated with aldosterone excess.[212,213] The true degree of renal insufficiency may become evident only after effective pharmacologic or surgical therapy.[212,213]

Surgical Treatment of Aldosterone-Producing Adenoma and Unilateral Hyperplasia

Unilateral laparoscopic adrenalectomy is an excellent treatment option for patients with APA or unilateral hyperplasia.[121] Although blood pressure control improves in almost 100% of patients postoperatively, average long-term cure rates of hypertension after unilateral adrenalectomy for APA range from 30% to 60%.[183,186] Persistent hypertension after adrenalectomy is correlated directly with having more than one first-degree relative with hypertension, use of more than two antihypertensive agents preoperatively, older age, increased serum creatinine level, and duration of hypertension and is most likely caused by coexistent primary hypertension.[183,214]

Laparoscopic adrenalectomy is the preferred surgical approach and is associated with shorter hospital stays and less long-term morbidity than the open approach. Because APAs are small and may be multiple, the entire adrenal gland should be removed.[215] To decrease the surgical risk, hypokalemia should be corrected with potassium supplements or a mineralocorticoid receptor antagonist, or both, preoperatively. These medications should be discontinued postoperatively. PAC should be measured 1 to 2 days after the operation to confirm a biochemical cure.[186] Serum potassium levels should be monitored weekly for 4 weeks after surgery, and a generous sodium diet should be followed to avoid the hyperkalemia of hypoaldosteronism that may occur because of the chronic suppression of the

RAA axis.[216] Clinically significant hyperkalemia develops after surgery in approximately 5% of APA patients, and short-term fludrocortisone supplementation may be required. Typically, the hypertension that was associated with aldosterone excess resolves in 1 to 3 months after the surgery. It has been found that adrenalectomy for APA is significantly less expensive than long-term medical therapy.[217]

Pharmacologic Treatment

IHA and GRA should be treated medically. In addition, APA may be treated medically if the medical treatment includes mineralocorticoid receptor blockade.[218] A sodium-restricted diet (<100 mEq of sodium per day), maintenance of ideal body weight, tobacco avoidance, and regular aerobic exercise contribute significantly to the success of pharmacologic treatment. No placebo-controlled, randomized trials have evaluated the relative efficacy of drugs in the treatment of primary aldosteronism.[219]

Spironolactone has been the drug of choice to treat primary aldosteronism for more than 4 decades. It is available as 25-, 50-, and 100-mg tablets. The dosage is 12.5 to 25 mg/day initially and can be increased to 400 mg/day if necessary to achieve a high-normal serum potassium concentration without the aid of oral potassium chloride supplementation. Hypokalemia responds promptly, but hypertension can take as long as 4 to 8 weeks to be corrected. After several months of therapy, the dosage of spironolactone often can be decreased to as little as 25 to 50 mg/day; dosage titration is based on a goal serum potassium level in the high-normal range. Serum potassium and creatinine should be monitored frequently during the first 4 to 6 weeks of therapy (especially in patients with renal insufficiency or diabetes mellitus). Spironolactone increases the half-life of digoxin, and the digoxin dosage may need to be adjusted when treatment with spironolactone is started. Concomitant therapy with salicylates should be avoided because they interfere with the tubular secretion of an active metabolite and decrease the effectiveness of spironolactone. However, spironolactone is not selective for the mineralocorticoid receptor. For example, antagonism at the testosterone receptor may result in painful gynecomastia, erectile dysfunction, and decreased libido in men, and agonist activity at the progesterone receptor results in menstrual irregularity in women.[220]

Eplerenone is a steroid-based antimineralocorticoid that acts as a competitive and selective mineralocorticoid receptor antagonist and was approved by the U.S. Food and Drug Administration (FDA) for the treatment of uncomplicated essential hypertension in 2003. The 9,11-epoxide group in eplerenone results in a marked reduction of the molecule's progestational and antiandrogenic actions; compared with spironolactone, eplerenone has 0.1% of the binding affinity to androgen receptors and less than 1% of the binding affinity to progesterone receptors. In a randomized, double-blind trial comparing the efficacy, safety, and tolerability of eplerenone to that of spironolactone (100-300 mg vs. 75-225 mg, respectively) in patients with primary aldosteronism found spironolactone to be superior in terms of blood pressure lowering but to be associated with higher rates of male gynecomastia (21% vs. 5% for eplerenone) and female mastodynia (21% vs. 0%).[221] Eplerenone is available as 25- and 50-mg tablets. For primary aldosteronism, it is reasonable to start with a dose of 25 mg twice daily (twice daily because of the shorter half-life of eplerenone compared with spironolactone) and titrated upward; the target is a high-normal serum potassium concentration without the aid of potassium supplements. The maximum dose approved by the FDA for hypertension is 100 mg/day. Potency studies with eplerenone show 25% to 50% less milligram-per-milligram potency compared with spironolactone. As with spironolactone, it is important to monitor blood pressure, serum potassium, and serum creatinine levels closely. Side effects include dizziness, headache, fatigue, diarrhea, hypertriglyceridemia, and elevated liver enzymes.

Patients with IHA frequently require a second antihypertensive agent to achieve good blood pressure control. Hypervolemia is a major reason for resistance to drug therapy, and low doses of a thiazide (e.g., 12.5 to 50 mg of hydrochlorothiazide daily) or a related sulfonamide diuretic are effective in combination with the mineralocorticoid receptor antagonist. Because these agents often lead to further hypokalemia, serum potassium levels should be monitored.

Before treatment for GRA is initiated, the diagnosis of GRA should be confirmed with genetic testing. In the GRA patient, chronic treatment with physiologic doses of a glucocorticoid normalizes blood pressure and corrects hypokalemia. The clinician should be cautious about iatrogenic Cushing syndrome with excessive doses of glucocorticoids, especially when dexamethasone is used in children. Shorter-acting agents such as prednisone or hydrocortisone should be prescribed, using the smallest effective dose in relation to body surface area (e.g., hydrocortisone, 10 to 12 mg/m^2 per day). Target blood pressure in children should be guided by age-specific blood pressure percentiles. Children should be monitored by pediatricians with expertise in glucocorticoid therapy, with careful attention paid to preventing retardation of linear growth due to overtreatment. Treatment with mineralocorticoid receptor antagonists in these patients may be just as effective as glucocorticoids and avoids the potential disruption of the hypothalamic-pituitary-adrenal axis and risk of iatrogenic side effects. In addition, glucocorticoid therapy or mineralocorticoid receptor blockade may even have a role in normotensive GRA patients.[168]

OTHER FORMS OF MINERALOCORTICOID EXCESS OR EFFECT

The medical disorders associated with excess mineralocorticoid effect from 11-deoxycorticosterone (DOC) and cortisol are listed in Table 16-10. These diagnoses should be considered if PAC and PRA are low in a patient with hypertension and hypokalemia.

Hyperdeoxycorticosteronism

Congenital Adrenal Hyperplasia

Congenital adrenal hyperplasia (CAH) is group of autosomal recessive disorders caused by enzymatic defects in adrenal steroidogenesis that result in deficient secretion of cortisol (see Chapter 15).[222,223] Approximately 90% of CAH cases are caused by 21-hydroxylase deficiency, which does not result in hypertension.[224] Deficiencies of 11β-hydroxylase (CYP11B1, P450c11) or 17α-hydroxylase (CYP17, P450c17) cause hypertension and hypokalemia because of hypersecretion of the mineralocorticoid DOC. The mineralocorticoid effect of increased circulating levels of DOC also decreases renin and aldosterone secretion. These mutations are autosomal recessive in inheritance and typically are diagnosed in childhood. However, partial enzymatic defects have been shown to cause hypertension in adults.

11β-Hydroxylase Deficiency. Approximately 5% of all cases of CAH are caused by 11β-hydroxylase deficiency; the prevalence in Caucasians is 1 in 100,000.[225] More than 40 mutations have been described in *CYP11B1*, the gene encoding 11β-hydroxylase.[226] There is an increased prevalence among Sephardic Jews from Morocco, suggestive of a founder effect. The impaired conversion of DOC to corticosterone results in high levels of DOC and 11-deoxycortisol; the substrate mass effect results in increased levels of adrenal androgens. Girls present in infancy or childhood with hypertension, hypokalemia, acne, hirsutism, and virilization. Boys with CAH due to 11β-hydroxylase deficiency present with hypertension, hypokalemia, and pseudoprecocious puberty. Approximately two thirds of patients have mild to moderate hypertension. The initial screening tests include measurement of blood levels of DOC, 11-deoxycortisol, androstenedione, testosterone, and dehydroepiandrosterone sulfate (DHEAS)—all of which should be increased above the upper limit of the respective reference ranges. Confirmatory testing includes germline mutation testing.[70]

17α-Hydroxylase Deficiency. 17α-Hydroxylase deficiency is a very rare cause of CAH and good prevalence data are not available, but the prevalence is likely less than 1 in 1 million live births.[227] 17α-Hydroxylase is essential for the synthesis of cortisol and gonadal hormones, and deficiency results in decreased production of cortisol and sex steroids. Genetic 46,XY males present with either pseudohermaphroditism or as phenotypic females, and 46,XX females present with primary amenorrhea. Therefore, a person with this form of CAH may not come to medical attention until puberty. Children, adolescents, and young adults present with hypertension and spontaneous hypokalemia and low levels of aldosterone and renin. Although very rare, there is an increased prevalence of 17α-hydroxylase deficiency among Dutch Mennonites. The initial screening tests include measurement of blood levels of adrostenedione, testosterone, DHEAS, 17-hydroxyprogesterone, aldosterone, and cortisol—all of which should be either low or at the lower quartile of the respective references ranges. The plasma concentrations of DOC and corticosterone should be above the upper limit of the respective reference ranges. Confirmatory testing includes germline mutation testing.[70]

Deoxycorticosterone-Producing Tumor

Pure DOC-producing adrenal tumors are very rare and usually large and malignant.[228] Some patients have been documented to have benign DOC-producing adrenocortical adenomas.[229] Some of these adrenal neoplasms cosecrete androgens and estrogens in addition to DOC, which may cause virilization in women or feminization in men. The typical clinical presentation would be that of relatively rapid onset of marked hypertension associated with hypokalemia and low blood levels of aldosterone and renin. A high level of plasma DOC or urinary tetrahydrodeoxycorticosterone and a large adrenal tumor seen on CT confirm the diagnosis. Aldosterone secretion in these patients is typically suppressed.

Primary Cortisol Resistance

Increased cortisol secretion and plasma cortisol concentrations without evidence of Cushing syndrome are found in patients with primary cortisol resistance (or glucocorticoid resistance), a rare familial syndrome.[230,231] Primary cortisol resistance is caused by genetic defects in the glucocorticoid receptor and the steroid-receptor complex. The syndrome is characterized by hypokalemic alkalosis, hypertension,

increased plasma concentrations of DOC, and increased adrenal androgen secretion. The hypertension and hypokalemia result from the combined effects of excess DOC and increased cortisol access to the mineralocorticoid receptor, resulting in high rates of cortisol production that overwhelm 11β-hydroxysteroid dehydrogenase type 2 (HSD11B2) activity. Most affected individuals present in childhood with hypertension and spontaneous hypokalemia and low levels of aldosterone and renin. The initial screening tests include measurement of blood levels of cortisol, DOC, 11-deoxycortisol, androstenedione, testosterone, and DHEAS—all of which should be increased above the upper limit of the respective reference ranges. In addition, 24-hour urinary cortisol excretion is above the upper limit of the reference range, and serum ACTH is not suppressed. Confirmatory testing includes germline mutation testing.[70]

Apparent Mineralocorticoid Excess Syndrome

Apparent mineralocorticoid excess is the result of impaired activity of the microsomal enzyme HSD11B2, which normally inactivates cortisol in the kidney by converting it to the inactive 11-keto compound, cortisone.[232] Cortisol can be a potent mineralocorticoid, and when HSD11B2 is genetically deficient or its activity blocked, high levels of cortisol accumulate in the kidney. Decreased HSD11B2 activity may be hereditary, or it may be secondary to pharmacologic inhibition of enzyme activity by glycyrrhizic acid, the active principle of licorice root (*Glycyrrhiza glabra*).[233] The congenital forms are rare autosomal recessive disorders; fewer than 50 patients have been identified worldwide.[234] Congenital apparent mineralocorticoid excess typically presents in childhood with hypertension, hypokalemia, low birth weight, failure to thrive, hypertension, polyuria and polydipsia, and poor growth.[226] Acquired apparent mineralocorticoid excess due to licorice root ingestion presents with hypertension and hypokalemia—the cause becomes evident when a good medical history is obtained. In addition, when HSD11B2 is overwhelmed by massive cortisol hypersecretion associated with Cushing syndrome due to ectopic ACTH syndrome, hypokalemic hypertension may be one of the outcomes.[235] The clinical phenotype of patients with apparent mineralocorticoid excess due to congenital deficiency of or inhibition of HSD11B2 includes hypertension, hypokalemia, metabolic alkalosis, low renin, low aldosterone, and normal plasma cortisol levels. The diagnosis of apparent mineralocorticoid excess is confirmed by demonstration of an abnormal (high) ratio of cortisol to cortisone in a 24-hour urine collection. The characteristic abnormal urinary cortisol-cortisone metabolite profile reflects decreased HSD11B2 activity; the ratio of cortisol to cortisone is typically increased 10-fold above the normal value.[232] DOC levels may also be increased in severe ACTH-dependent Cushing syndrome and contribute to the hypertension and hypokalemia in this disorder.

Liddle Syndrome: Abnormal Renal Tubular Ionic Transport

In 1963, Grant Liddle described an autosomal dominant renal disorder with a presentation similar to primary aldosteronism with hypertension, hypokalemia, and inappropriate kaliuresis.[236] However, blood levels of aldosterone and renin were very low so the disorder was termed *pseudoaldosteronism*. Liddle syndrome is caused by autosomal dominant mutations in the β- or γ-subunit of the amiloride-sensitive epithelial sodium channel.[226] It is extremely rare, with fewer than 30 families reported worldwide.[237] This mutation results in enhanced activity of the epithelial sodium channel, and patients present with increased renal sodium reabsorption, potassium wasting, hypertension, and hypokalemia. However, as mentioned earlier, blood levels of aldosterone and renin are low. Affected individuals usually present as children or young adults with hypertension and spontaneous hypokalemia and low levels of aldosterone and renin. A family history of hypertension associated with hypokalemia makes Liddle syndrome more likely. The finding of low aldosterone and renin levels in the hypokalemic hypertensive patient should raise the possibility of Liddle syndrome. When the other causes of this presentation have been excluded, then a treatment trial with amiloride or triamterene should be considered. Liddle syndrome can easily be distinguished from apparent mineralocorticoid excess based on the good clinical response to amiloride or triamterene combined with a sodium-restricted diet, lack of efficacy of spironolactone and dexamethasone, and normal 24-hour urine cortisone/cortisol ratio. Clinical genetic testing is available.[70]

OTHER ENDOCRINE DISORDERS ASSOCIATED WITH HYPERTENSION

Cushing Syndrome

Iatrogenic Cushing syndrome is relatively common. However, endogenous Cushing disease is rare, with an incidence of less than 1 case per 1 million people per year.[238] Hypertension occurs in 75% to 80% of patients with Cushing syndrome (see Chapter 15).[239,240] The mechanisms of hypertension include increased production of DOC, enhanced pressor sensitivity to endogenous vasoconstrictors (e.g., epinephrine, angiotensin II), increased cardiac output, activation of the RAA system by increased hepatic production of angiotensinogen, and cortisol activation of the mineralocorticoid receptor.

Thyroid Dysfunction
Hyperthyroidism

When excessive amounts of circulating thyroid hormones interact with thyroid hormone receptors on peripheral tissues, both metabolic activity and sensitivity to circulating catecholamines increase. Thyrotoxic patients usually have tachycardia, high cardiac output, increased stroke volume, decreased peripheral vascular resistance, and increased systolic blood pressure.[241] The initial management in patients with hypertension and hyperthyroidism includes use of a β-adrenergic blocker to treat hypertension, tachycardia, and tremor. The definitive treatment of hyperthyroidism is cause-specific (see Chapter 12).[242]

Hypothyroidism

The frequency of hypertension (usually diastolic) is increased threefold in hypothyroid patients and may account for as many as 1% of cases of diastolic hypertension in the general population.[243,244] The mechanisms for the elevation in blood pressure include increased systemic vascular resistance and extracellular volume expansion. Treatment of thyroid hormone deficiency decreases blood pressure in most patients with hypertension and normalizes blood pressure in one third of them. Synthetic levothyroxine is the treatment of choice for hypothyroidism (see Chapter 13).[245]

Hypercalcemia and Primary Hyperparathyroidism

Hypercalcemia is associated with an increased frequency of hypertension (see Chapter 28).[246] The frequency of hypertension in patients with primary hyperparathyroidism varies from 10% to 60%.[247] The mechanisms of hypertension are unclear because there is no direct correlation with the elevated parathyroid hormone or calcium levels. The hypertension associated with hyperparathyroidism can also occur as a complication of hypercalcemia-induced renal impairment. The treatment of hyperparathyroidism is surgical; hypertension may or may not remit after successful parathyroidectomy.[248,249]

Acromegaly

Hypertension occurs in 20% to 40% of the patients with acromegaly and is associated with sodium retention and extracellular volume expansion (see Chapter 9).[250,251] The hypertension of acromegaly is treated most effectively by curing the excess of growth hormone.[251] If a surgical cure is not possible, the hypertension usually responds well to diuretic therapy.

REFERENCES

1. Yoon SS, Ostchega Y, Louis T. Recent trends in the prevalence of high blood pressure and its treatment and control, 1999-2008. *NCHS Data Brief*. 2010;(48):1-8.
2. Hajjar I, Kotchen TA. Trends in prevalence, awareness, treatment, and control of hypertension in the United States, 1988-2000. *JAMA*. 2003; 290:199-206.
3. Dluhy RG, Lawerence JE, Williams GH. Endocrine hypertension. In: Larsen PR, Kronenberg HM, Melmed S, eds. *Williams Textbook of Endocrinology*. 10th ed. Philadelphia, PA: Saunders; 2003:555.
4. Lefkowitz RJ. A brief history of G-protein coupled receptors (Nobel Lecture). *Angew Chem Int Ed Engl*. 2013;52:6366-6378.
5. Benovic JL. G-protein-coupled receptors signal victory. *Cell*. 2012;151: 1148-1150.
6. James PA, Oparil S, Carter BL, et al. 2014 evidence-based guideline for the management of high blood pressure in adults: report from the panel members appointed to the Eighth Joint National Committee (JNC 8). *JAMA*. 2014;311:507-520.
7. Penn RB, Bond RA, Walker JK. GPCRs and arrestins in airways: implications for asthma. *Handb Exp Pharmacol*. 2014;219:387-403.
8. McBride JF, Atwell TD, Charboneau WJ, et al. Minimally invasive treatment of metastatic pheochromocytoma and paraganglioma: efficacy and safety of radiofrequency ablation and cryoablation therapy. *J Vasc Interv Radiol*. 2011;22(9):1263-1270.
9. Eisenhofer G, Kopin IJ, Goldstein DS. Catecholamine metabolism: a contemporary view with implications for physiology and medicine. *Pharmacol Rev*. 2004;56:331-349.
10. van Hulsteijn LT, Niemeijer ND, Dekkers OM, Corssmit EP. (131) I-MIBG therapy for malignant paraganglioma and phaeochromocytoma: systematic review and meta-analysis. *Clin Endocrinol (Oxf)*. 2014; 80:487-501.
11. Wiseman GA, Pacak K, O'Dorisio MS, et al. Usefulness of ^{123}I-MIBG scintigraphy in the evaluation of patients with known or suspected primary or metastatic pheochromocytoma or paraganglioma: results from a prospective multicenter trial. *J Nucl Med*. 2009;50:1448-1454.
12. Rutherford MA, Rankin AJ, Yates TM, et al. Management of metastatic phaeochromocytoma and paraganglioma: use of iodine-131-metaiodobenzylguanidine therapy in a tertiary referral centre. *QJM*. [Epub 2014 Sep 29].
13. Rose B, Matthay KK, Price D, et al. High-dose ^{131}I-metaiodobenzylguanidine therapy for 12 patients with malignant pheochromocytoma. *Cancer*. 2003;98:239-248.
14. DeLellis R, Lloyd R, Heitz P, Eng C. *Pathology and Genetics of Tumours of Endocrine Organs*. Lyon, France: IARC Press; 2004.
15. Stenstrom G, Svardsudd K. Pheochromocytoma in Sweden 1958-1981. An analysis of the National Cancer Registry Data. *Acta Med Scand*. 1986;220:225-232.
16. Sinclair AM, Isles CG, Brown I, et al. Secondary hypertension in a blood pressure clinic. *Arch Intern Med*. 1987;147:1289-1293.
17. Omura M, Saito J, Yamaguchi K, et al. Prospective study on the prevalence of secondary hypertension among hypertensive patients visiting a general outpatient clinic in Japan. *Hypertens Res*. 2004; 27:193-202.

18. Felix Fränkel. [Classics in oncology. A case of bilateral completely latent adrenal tumor and concurrent nephritis with changes in the circulatory system and retinitis: Felix Fränkel, 1886]. *CA Cancer J Clin.* 1984;34:93-106.

19. Neumann HP, Vortmeyer A, Schmidt D, et al. Evidence of MEN-2 in the original description of classic pheochromocytoma. *N Engl J Med.* 2007;357:1311-1315.

20. Pick L. Das Ganglioma embryonale sympathicum (sympathoma embryonale), eine typische bösartige geschwuestform des sympathischen nervensystems. *Berl Klin Wochenschr.* 1912;49:16-22.

21. Welbourn RB. Early surgical history of phaeochromocytoma. *Br J Surg.* 1987;74:594-596.

22. Young WF Jr. Endocrine hypertension: then and now. *Endocr Pract.* 2010;16:888-902.

23. Manger WM, Gifford RW. Background and importance and diagnosis. In: Manger WM, Gifford RW, eds. *Clinical and Experimental Pheochromocytoma.* 2nd ed. Cambridge, MA: Blackwell Science; 1996:1-7.

24. Engel A, von Euler US. Diagnostic value of increased urinary output of noradrenaline and adrenaline in pheochromocytoma. *Lancet.* 1950;2:387.

25. Young WF Jr. Pheochromocytoma: 1926-1993. *Trends Endocrinol Metab.* 1993;4:122-127.

26. Bortnik M, Occhetta E, Marino P. Orthostatic hypotension as an unusual clinical manifestation of pheochromocytoma: a case report. *J Cardiovasc Med (Hagerstown).* 2008;9(8):839-841.

27. Eisenhofer G, Goldstein DS, Sullivan P, et al. Biochemical and clinical manifestations of dopamine-producing paragangliomas: utility of plasma methoxytyramine. *J Clin Endocrinol Metab.* 2005;90:2068-2075.

28. Lenders JW, Duh QY, Eisenhofer G, et al. Pheochromocytoma and paraganglioma: an Endocrine Society clinical practice guideline. *J Clin Endocrinol Metab.* 2014;99:1915-1942.

29. Young WF Jr, Maddox DE. Spells: in search of a cause. *Mayo Clin Proc.* 1995;70:757-765.

30. Folkestad L, Andersen MS, Nielsen AL, Glintborg D. A rare cause of Cushing's syndrome: an ACTH-secreting phaeochromocytoma. *BMJ Case Rep.* 2014.

31. Lebowitz-Amit R, Mete O, Asa SL, et al. Malignant pheochromocytoma secreting vasoactive intestinal peptide and response to sunitinib: a case report and literature review. *Endocr Pract.* 2014;20:e145-e150.

32. Takeda K, Hara N, Kawaguchi M, et al. Parathyroid hormone-related peptide-producing non-familial pheochromocytoma in a child. *Int J Urol.* 2010;17:673-676.

33. Mumby C, Davis JR, Trouillas J, Higham CE. Phaeochromocytoma and acromegaly: a unifying diagnosis. *Endocrinol Diabetes Metab Case Rep.* 2014;2014:140036.

34. Dalby MC, Burke M, Radley-Smith R, Banner NR. Pheochromocytoma presenting after cardiac transplantation for dilated cardiomyopathy. *J Heart Lung Transplant.* 2001;20:773-775.

35. Giavarini A, Chedid A, Bobrie G, et al. Acute catecholamine cardiomyopathy in patients with phaeochromocytoma or functional paraganglioma. *Heart.* 2013;99:1438-1444.

36. Young WF Jr. Clinical practice. The incidentally discovered adrenal mass. *N Engl J Med.* 2007;356:601-610.

37. Oshmyansky AR, Mahammedi A, Dackiw A, et al. Serendipity in the diagnosis of pheochromocytoma. *J Comput Assist Tomogr.* 2013;37:820-823.

38. Kopetschke R, Slisko M, Kilisli A, et al. Frequent incidental discovery of phaeochromocytoma: data from a German cohort of 201 phaeochromocytoma. *Eur J Endocrinol.* 2009;161:355-361.

39. Motta-Ramirez GA, Remer EM, Herts BR, et al. Comparison of CT findings in symptomatic and incidentally discovered pheochromocytomas. *AJR Am J Roentgenol.* 2005;185:684-688.

40. Wachtel H, Cerullo I, Bartlett EK, et al. Clinicopathologic characteristics of incidentally identified pheochromocytoma. *Ann Surg Oncol.* 2015;22:132-138.

41. Kinney MA, Warner ME, vanHeerden JA, et al. Perianesthetic risks and outcomes of pheochromocytoma and paraganglioma resection. *Anesth Analg.* 2000;91:1118-1123.

42. Erickson D, Kudva YC, Ebersold MJ, et al. Benign paragangliomas: clinical presentation and treatment outcomes in 236 patients. *J Clin Endocrinol Metab.* 2001;86:5210-5216.

43. Taieb D, Kebebew E, Castinetti F, et al. Diagnosis and preoperative imaging of multiple endocrine neoplasia type 2: current status and future directions. *Clin Endocrinol (Oxf).* 2014;81:317-328.

44. Coyle D, Friedmacher F, Puri P. The association between Hirschsprung's disease and multiple endocrine neoplasia type 2a: a systematic review. *Pediatr Surg Int.* 2014;30:751-756.

45. Binderup ML, Bisgaard ML, Harbud V, et al. Von Hippel-Lindau disease (vHL). National clinical guideline for diagnosis and surveillance in Denmark. 3rd edition. *Dan Med J.* 2013;60:B4763.

46. Maddock IR, Moran A, Maher ER, et al. A genetic register for von Hippel-Lindau disease. *J Med Genet.* 1996;33:120-127.

47. Evans DG, Howard E, Giblin C, et al. Birth incidence and prevalence of tumor-prone syndromes: estimates from a UK family genetic register service. *Am J Med Genet A.* 2010;152A:327-332.

48. Eisenhofer G, Walther MM, Huynh TT, et al. Pheochromocytomas in von Hippel-Lindau syndrome and multiple endocrine neoplasia type 2 display distinct biochemical and clinical phenotypes. *J Clin Endocrinol Metab.* 2001;86:1999-2008.

49. Eisenhofer G, Pacak K, Huynh TT, et al. Catecholamine metabolomic and secretory phenotypes in phaeochromocytoma. *Endocr Relat Cancer.* 2011;18:97-111.

50. Rasmussen SA, Friedman JM. NF1 gene and neurofibromatosis 1. *Am J Epidemiol.* 2000;151:33-40.

51. Bausch B, Borozdin W, Mautner VF, et al. Germline NF1 mutational spectra and loss-of-heterozygosity analyses in patients with pheochromocytoma and neurofibromatosis type 1. *J Clin Endocrinol Metab.* 2007;92:2784-2792.

52. Patil S, Chamberlain RS. Neoplasms associated with germline and somatic NF1 gene mutations. *Oncologist.* 2012;17(1):101-116.

53. Walther MM, Herring J, Enquist E, et al. von Recklinghausen's disease and pheochromocytomas. *J Urol.* 1999;162:1582-1586.

54. Shinall MC, Solorzano CC. Pheochromocytoma in neurofibromatosis type 1: when should it be suspected? *Endocr Pract.* 2014;20:792-796.

55. Carney JA. Carney triad: a syndrome featuring paraganglionic, adrenocortical, and possibly other endocrine tumors. *J Clin Endocrinol Metab.* 2009;94:3656-3662.

56. Carney JA. Carney triad. *Front Horm Res.* 2013;41:92-110.

57. Zhang L, Smyrk TC, Young WF Jr, et al. Gastric stromal tumors in Carney triad are different clinically, pathologically, and behaviorally from sporadic gastric gastrointestinal stromal tumors: findings in 104 cases. *Am J Surg Pathol.* 2010;34:53-64.

58. Carney JA, Stratakis CA, Young WF Jr. Adrenal cortical adenoma: the fourth component of the Carney triad and an association with subclinical Cushing syndrome. *Am J Surg Pathol.* 2013;37:1140-1149.

59. Kirmani S, Young WF, et al. Hereditary paraganglioma-pheochromocytoma syndromes. In: Pagon RA, Adam MP, Ardinger HH, eds. *GeneReviews(R).* Seattle, WA: 1993.

60. Baysal BE, Ferrell RE, Willett-Brozick JE, et al. Mutations in SDHD, a mitochondrial complex II gene, in hereditary paraganglioma. *Science.* 2000;287:848-851.

61. Bayley JP, Devilee P, Taschner PE. The SDH mutation database: an online resource for succinate dehydrogenase sequence variants involved in pheochromocytoma, paraganglioma and mitochondrial complex II deficiency. *BMC Med Genet.* 2005;6:39.

62. Evenepoel L, Papathomas TG, Krol N, et al. Toward an improved definition of the genetic and tumor spectrum associated with SDH germline mutations. *Genet Med.* 2015;17:610-620.

63. Pigny P, Vincent A, Cardot Bauters C, et al. Paraganglioma after maternal transmission of a succinate dehydrogenase gene mutation. *J Clin Endocrinol Metab.* 2008;93:1609-1615.

64. Yeap PM, Tobias ES, Mavraki E, et al. Molecular analysis of pheochromocytoma after maternal transmission of SDHD mutation elucidates mechanism of parent-of-origin effect. *J Clin Endocrinol Metab.* 2011;96:E2009-E2013.

65. Astuti D, Douglas F, Lennard TW, et al. Germline SDHD mutation in familial phaeochromocytoma. *Lancet.* 2001;357:1181-1182.

66. Baysal BE. Mitochondrial complex II and genomic imprinting in inheritance of paraganglioma tumors. *Biochim Biophys Acta.* 2013;1827:573-577.

67. Yao L, Schiavi F, Cascon A, et al. Spectrum and prevalence of FP/TMEM127 gene mutations in pheochromocytomas and paragangliomas. *JAMA.* 2010;304:2611-2619.

68. Comino-Mendez I, Gracia-Aznarez FJ, Schiavi F, et al. Exome sequencing identifies MAX mutations as a cause of hereditary pheochromocytoma. *Nat Genet.* 2011;43:663-667.

69. Castro-Vega LJ, Buffet A, De Cubas AA, et al. Germline mutations in FH confer predisposition to malignant pheochromocytomas and paragangliomas. *Hum Mol Genet.* 2014;23:2440-2446.

70. GeneTests website. 2015. Accessed at <www.genetests.org>.

71. Brilakis ES, Young WF Jr, Wilson JW, et al. Reversible catecholamine-induced cardiomyopathy in a heart transplant candidate without persistent or paroxysmal hypertension. *J Heart Lung Transplant.* 1999;18:376-380.

72. Kudva YC, Sawka AM, Young WF Jr. Clinical review 164: the laboratory diagnosis of adrenal pheochromocytoma: the Mayo Clinic experience. *J Clin Endocrinol Metab.* 2003;88:4533-4539.

73. Perry CG, Sawka AM, Singh R, et al. The diagnostic efficacy of urinary fractionated metanephrines measured by tandem mass spectrometry in detection of pheochromocytoma. *Clin Endocrinol (Oxf).* 2007;66:703-708.

74. Taylor RL, Singh RJ. Validation of liquid chromatography-tandem mass spectrometry method for analysis of urinary conjugated metanephrine and normetanephrine for screening of pheochromocytoma. *Clin Chem.* 2002;48:533-539.

75. Sawka AM, Jaeschke R, Singh RJ, Young WF Jr. A comparison of biochemical tests for pheochromocytoma: measurement of fractionated plasma metanephrines compared with the combination of 24-hour urinary metanephrines and catecholamines. *J Clin Endocrinol Metab.* 2003;88:553-558.

76. Peitzsch M, Prejbisz A, Kroiss M, et al. Analysis of plasma 3-methoxytyramine, normetanephrine and metanephrine by ultraperformance liquid chromatography-tandem mass spectrometry: utility for diagnosis of dopamine-producing metastatic phaeochromocytoma. *Ann Clin Biochem*. 2013;50:147-155.

77. Lenders JW, Keiser HR, Goldstein DS, et al. Plasma metanephrines in the diagnosis of pheochromocytoma. *Ann Intern Med*. 1995;123: 101-109.

78. Algeciras-Schimnich A, Preissner CM, Young WF Jr, et al. Plasma chromogranin A or urine fractionated metanephrines follow-up testing improves the diagnostic accuracy of plasma fractionated metanephrines for pheochromocytoma. *J Clin Endocrinol Metab*. 2008;93:91-95.

79. Wang YH, Yang QC, Lin Y, et al. Chromogranin a as a marker for diagnosis, treatment, and survival in patients with gastroenteropancreatic neuroendocrine neoplasm. *Medicine (Baltimore)*. 2014;93:e247.

80. Bravo EL, Tarazi RC, Fouad FM, et al. Clonidine-suppression test: a useful aid in the diagnosis of pheochromocytoma. *N Engl J Med*. 1981;305:623-626.

81. Sjoberg RJ, Simcic KJ, Kidd GS. The clonidine suppression test for pheochromocytoma. A review of its utility and pitfalls. *Arch Intern Med*. 1992;152:1193-1197.

82. Eisenhofer G, Goldstein DS, Walther MM, et al. Biochemical diagnosis of pheochromocytoma: how to distinguish true- from false-positive test results. *J Clin Endocrinol Metab*. 2003;88:2656-2666.

83. Young WF Jr. Phaeochromocytoma: how to catch a moonbeam in your hand. *Eur J Endocrinol*. 1997;136:28-29.

84. Godfrey JA, Rickman OB, Williams AW, et al. Pheochromocytoma in a patient with end-stage renal disease. *Mayo Clin Proc*. 2001;76: 953-957.

85. Bech PR, Ramachandran R, Dhillo WS, et al. Quantifying the effects of renal impairment on plasma concentrations of the neuroendocrine neoplasia biomarkers chromogranin A, chromogranin B, and cocaine- and amphetamine-regulated transcript. *Clin Chem*. 2012;58:941-943.

86. Stumvoll M, Radjaipour M, Seif F. Diagnostic considerations in pheochromocytoma and chronic hemodialysis: case report and review of the literature. *Am J Nephrol*. 1995;15:147-151.

87. Morioka M, Yuihama S, Nakajima T, et al. Incidentally discovered pheochromocytoma in long-term hemodialysis patients. *Int J Urol*. 2002;9:700-703.

88. Eisenhofer G, Huysmans F, Pacak K, et al. Plasma metanephrines in renal failure. *Kidney Int*. 2005;67:668-677.

89. Marini M, Fathi M, Vallotton M. [Determination of serum metanephrines in the diagnosis of pheochromocytoma]. *Ann Endocrinol (Paris)*. 1994;54(5):337-342.

90. Stern TA, Cremens CM. Factitious pheochromocytoma. One patient history and literature review. *Psychosomatics*. 1998;39:283-287.

91. Jalil ND, Pattou FN, Combemale F, et al. Effectiveness and limits of preoperative imaging studies for the localisation of pheochromocytomas and paragangliomas: a review of 282 cases. French Association of Surgery (AFC) and French Association of Endocrine Surgeons (AFCE). *Eur J Surg*. 1998;164:23-28.

92. Boland GW, Lee MJ, Gazelle GS, et al. Characterization of adrenal masses using unenhanced CT: an analysis of the CT literature. *AJR Am J Roentgenol*. 1998;171:201-204.

93. Korobkin M, Brodeur FJ, Francis IR, et al. CT time-attenuation washout curves of adrenal adenomas and nonadenomas. *AJR Am J Roentgenol*. 1998;170:747-752.

94. Brink I, Hoegerle S, Klisch J, Bley TA. Imaging of pheochromocytoma and paraganglioma. *Fam Cancer*. 2005;4:61-68.

95. Schieda N, Al Dandan O, Kielar AZ, et al. Pitfalls of adrenal imaging with chemical shift MRI. *Clin Radiol*. 2014;69:1186-1197.

96. Szolar DH, Korobkin M, Reittner P, et al. Adrenocortical carcinomas and adrenal pheochromocytomas: mass and enhancement loss evaluation at delayed contrast-enhanced CT. *Radiology*. 2005;234:479-485.

97. Miskulin J, Shulkin BL, Doherty GM, et al. Is preoperative iodine 123 meta-iodobenzylguanidine scintigraphy routinely necessary before initial adrenalectomy for pheochromocytoma? *Surgery*. 2003;134:918-922, discussion 922-913.

98. Mihai R, Gleeson F, Roskell D, et al. Routine preoperative (123)I-MIBG scintigraphy for patients with phaeochromocytoma is not necessary. *Langenbecks Arch Surg*. 2008;393:725-727.

99. van Berkel A, Pacak K, Lenders JW. Should every patient diagnosed with a phaeochromocytoma have a (1)(2)(3) I-MIBG scintigraphy? *Clin Endocrinol (Oxf)*. 2014;81:329-333.

100. Solanki KK, Bomanji J, Moyes J, et al. A pharmacological guide to medicines which interfere with the biodistribution of radiolabelled meta-iodobenzylguanidine (MIBG). *Nucl Med Commun*. 1992;13: 513-521.

101. Rufini V, Treglia G, Castaldi P, et al. Comparison of metaiodobenzylguanidine scintigraphy with positron emission tomography in the diagnostic work-up of pheochromocytoma and paraganglioma: a systematic review. *Q J Nucl Med Mol Imaging*. 2013;57:122-133.

102. van Berkel A, Rao JU, Kusters B, et al. Correlation between in vivo 18F-FDG PET and immunohistochemical markers of glucose uptake and metabolism in pheochromocytoma and paraganglioma. *J Nucl Med*. 2014;55:1253-1259.

103. Fikri AS, Kroiss A, Ahmad AZ, et al. Localization and prediction of malignant potential in recurrent pheochromocytoma/paraganglioma (PCC/PGL) using 18F-FDG PET/CT. *Acta Radiol*. 2014;55:631-640.

104. Kroiss A, Putzer D, Decristoforo C, et al. 68Ga-DOTA-TOC uptake in neuroendocrine tumour and healthy tissue: differentiation of physiological uptake and pathological processes in PET/CT. *Eur J Nucl Med Mol Imaging*. 2013;40:514-523.

105. Freel EM, Stanson AW, Thompson GB, et al. Adrenal venous sampling for catecholamines: a normal value study. *J Clin Endocrinol Metab*. 2010;95:1328-1332.

106. Plouin PF, Duclos JM, Soppelsa F, et al. Factors associated with perioperative morbidity and mortality in patients with pheochromocytoma: analysis of 165 operations at a single center. *J Clin Endocrinol Metab*. 2001;86:1480-1486.

107. Pacak K. Preoperative management of the pheochromocytoma patient. *J Clin Endocrinol Metab*. 2007;92:4069-4079.

108. Hariskov S, Schumann R. Intraoperative management of patients with incidental catecholamine producing tumors: a literature review and analysis. *J Anaesthesiol Clin Pharmacol*. 2013;29:41-46.

109. Lafont M, Fagour C, Haissaguerre M, et al. Per-operative hemodynamic instability in normotensive patients with incidentally discovered pheochromocytomas. *J Clin Endocrinol Metab*. 2015;100(2):417-421.

110. van der Zee PA, de Boer A. Pheochromocytoma: a review on preoperative treatment with phenoxybenzamine or doxazosin. *Neth J Med*. 2014;72:190-201.

111. Kiernan CM, Du L, Chen X, et al. Predictors of hemodynamic instability during surgery for pheochromocytoma. *Ann Surg Oncol*. 2014;21: 3865-3871.

112. Sibal L, Jovanovic A, Agarwal SC, et al. Phaeochromocytomas presenting as acute crises after beta blockade therapy. *Clin Endocrinol (Oxf)*. 2006;65:186-190.

113. Steinsapir J, Carr AA, Prisant LM, Bransome ED Jr. Metyrosine and pheochromocytoma. *Arch Intern Med*. 1997;157:901-906.

114. Brunaud L, Boutami M, Nguyen-Thi PL, et al. Both preoperative alpha and calcium channel blockade impact intraoperative hemodynamic stability similarly in the management of pheochromocytoma. *Surgery*. 2014;156:1410-1418.

115. Siddiqi HK, Yang HY, Laird AM, et al. Utility of oral nicardipine and magnesium sulfate infusion during preparation and resection of pheochromocytomas. *Surgery*. 2012;152:1027-1036.

116. Combemale F, Carnaille B, Tavernier B, et al. [Exclusive use of calcium channel blockers and cardioselective beta-blockers in the pre- and peri-operative management of pheochromocytomas. 70 cases]. *Ann Chir*. 1998;52(4):341-345.

117. Lebuffe G, Dosseh ED, Tek G, et al. The effect of calcium channel blockers on outcome following the surgical treatment of phaeochromocytomas and paragangliomas. *Anaesthesia*. 2005;60:439-444.

118. Jugovac I, Antapli M, Markan S. Anesthesia and pheochromocytoma. *Int Anesthesiol Clin*. 2011;49:57-61.

119. Hack HA. The perioperative management of children with phaeochromocytoma. *Paediatr Anaesth*. 2000;10:463-476.

120. Reddy VS, O'Neill JA Jr, Holcomb GW 3rd, et al. Twenty-five-year surgical experience with pheochromocytoma in children. *Am Surg*. 2000;66:1085-1091, discussion 1092.

121. Assalia A, Gagner M. Laparoscopic adrenalectomy. *Br J Surg*. 2004;91: 1259-1274.

122. Bittner JG, Gershuni VM, Matthews BD, et al. Risk factors affecting operative approach, conversion, and morbidity for adrenalectomy: a single-institution series of 402 patients. *Surg Endosc*. 2013;27(7): 2342-2350.

123. Agarwal G, Sadacharan D, Aggarwal V, et al. Surgical management of organ-contained unilateral pheochromocytoma: comparative outcomes of laparoscopic and conventional open surgical procedures in a large single-institution series. *Langenbecks Arch Surg*. 2012;397: 1109-1116.

124. Shen WT, Sturgeon C, Clark OH, et al. Should pheochromocytoma size influence surgical approach? A comparison of 90 malignant and 60 benign pheochromocytomas. *Surgery*. 2004;136:1129-1137.

125. Rafat C, Zinzindohoue F, Hernigou A, et al. Peritoneal implantation of pheochromocytoma following tumor capsule rupture during surgery. *J Clin Endocrinol Metab*. 2014;99:E2681-E2685.

126. Baghai M, Thompson GB, Young WF Jr, et al. Pheochromocytomas and paragangliomas in von Hippel-Lindau disease: a role for laparoscopic and cortical-sparing surgery. *Arch Surg*. 2002;137:682-688, discussion 688-689.

127. Yip L, Lee JE, Shapiro SE, et al. Surgical management of hereditary pheochromocytoma. *J Am Coll Surg*. 2004;198:525-534, discussion 534-525.

128. Ramlawi B, David EA, Kim MP, et al. Contemporary surgical management of cardiac paragangliomas. *Ann Thorac Surg*. 2012;93: 1972-1976.

129. Amar L, Fassnacht M, Gimenez-Roqueplo AP, et al. Long-term postoperative follow-up in patients with apparently benign pheochromocytoma and paraganglioma. *Horm Metab Res*. 2012;44:385-389.

130. Press D, Akyuz M, Dural C, et al. Predictors of recurrence in pheochromocytoma. *Surgery*. 2014;156:1523-1528.

131. Young AL, Baysal BE, Deb A, Young WF Jr. Familial malignant catecholamine-secreting paraganglioma with prolonged survival associated with mutation in the succinate dehydrogenase B gene. *J Clin Endocrinol Metab*. 2002;87:4101-4105.

132. Ricketts CJ, Forman JR, Rattenberry E, et al. Tumor risks and genotype-phenotype-proteotype analysis in 358 patients with germline mutations in SDHB and SDHD. *Hum Mutat*. 2010;31:41-51.

133. Williamson SR, Eble JN, Amin MB, et al. Succinate dehydrogenase-deficient renal cell carcinoma: detailed characterization of 11 tumors defining a unique subtype of renal cell carcinoma. *Mod Pathol*. 2015; 28:80-94.

134. Elshafie O, Al Badaai Y, Alwahaibi K, et al. Catecholamine-secreting carotid body paraganglioma: successful preoperative control of hypertension and clinical symptoms using high-dose long-acting octreotide. *Endocrinol Diabetes Metab Case Rep*. 2014;2014:140051.

135. Vogel J, Atanacio AS, Prodanov T, et al. External beam radiation therapy in treatment of malignant pheochromocytoma and paraganglioma. *Front Oncol*. 2014;4:166.

136. Deutschbein T, Fassnacht M, Weismann D, et al. Treatment of malignant phaeochromocytoma with a combination of cyclophosphamide, vincristine and dacarbazine: own experience and overview of the contemporary literature. *Clin Endocrinol (Oxf)*. 2015;82:84-90.

137. Niemeijer ND, Alblas G, van Hulsteijn LT, et al. Chemotherapy with cyclophosphamide, vincristine and dacarbazine for malignant paraganglioma and pheochromocytoma: systematic review and meta-analysis. *Clin Endocrinol (Oxf)*. 2014;81(5):642-651.

138. Averbuch SD, Steakley CS, Young RC, et al. Malignant pheochromocytoma: effective treatment with a combination of cyclophosphamide, vincristine, and dacarbazine. *Ann Intern Med*. 1988;109:267-273.

139. Huang H, Abraham J, Hung E, et al. Treatment of malignant pheochromocytoma/paraganglioma with cyclophosphamide, vincristine, and dacarbazine: recommendation from a 22-year follow-up of 18 patients. *Cancer*. 2008;113:2020-2028.

140. Ayala-Ramirez M, Chougnet CN, Habra MA, et al. Treatment with sunitinib for patients with progressive metastatic pheochromocytomas and sympathetic paragangliomas. *J Clin Endocrinol Metab*. 2012;97: 4040-4050.

141. Salazar-Vega JL, Levin G, Sanso G, et al. Pheochromocytoma associated with pregnancy: unexpected favourable outcome in patients diagnosed after delivery. *J Hypertens*. 2014;32:1458-1463, discussion 1463.

142. Biggar MA, Lennard TW. Systematic review of phaeochromocytoma in pregnancy. *Br J Surg*. 2013;100:182-190.

143. Williams GH, Chao J, Chao L. Kidney hormones: the kallikrein kinin and renin-angiotensin systems. In: Conn PM, Melmed S, eds. *Endocrinology: Basic and Clinical Principles*. Totowa, NJ: Humana Press; 1997:393-404.

144. Mihailidou AS, Funder JW. Nongenomic effects of mineralocorticoid receptor activation in the cardiovascular system. *Steroids*. 2005;70: 347-351.

145. Funder JW. The nongenomic actions of aldosterone. *Endocr Rev*. 2005;26:313-321.

146. Brown NJ. Aldosterone and end-organ damage. *Curr Opin Nephrol Hypertens*. 2005;14:235-241.

147. Williams GH, Dluhy RG, et al. Diseases of the adrenal cortex. In: Braunwald E, Fauci AD, Kasper D, eds. *Harrison's Principles of Internal Medicine*. New York, NY: McGraw-Hill; 2001:2087.

148. Conn JW. Presidential address. I. Painting background. II. Primary aldosteronism, a new clinical syndrome. *J Lab Clin Med*. 1955;45:3-17.

149. Funder JW. Genetics of primary aldosteronism. *Front Horm Res*. 2014; 43:70-78.

150. Gittler RD, Fajans SS. Primary aldosteronism (Conn's syndrome). *J Clin Endocrinol Metab*. 1995;80:3438-3441.

151. Conn JW, Knopf RF, Nesbit RM. Clinical characteristics of primary aldosteronism from an analysis of 145 cases. *Am J Surg*. 1964; 107:159-172.

152. Conn JW. Plasma renin activity in primary aldosteronism. Importance in differential diagnosis and in research of essential hypertension. *JAMA*. 1964;190:222-225.

153. Fishman LM, Kuchel O, Liddle GW, et al. Incidence of primary aldosteronism uncomplicated "essential" hypertension. A prospective study with elevated aldosterone secretion and suppressed plasma renin activity used as diagnostic criteria. *JAMA*. 1968;205:497-502.

154. Kaplan NM. Hypokalemia in the hypertensive patient, with observations on the incidence of primary aldosteronism. *Ann Intern Med*. 1967;66:1079-1090.

155. Conn JW. The evolution of primary aldosteronism: 1954-1967. *Harvey Lect*. 1966;62:257-291.

156. Andersen GS, Toftdahl DB, Lund JO, et al. The incidence rate of phaeochromocytoma and Conn's syndrome in Denmark, 1977-1981. *J Hum Hypertens*. 1988;2:187-189.

157. Berglund G, Andersson O, Wilhelmsen L. Prevalence of primary and secondary hypertension: studies in a random population sample. *Br Med J*. 1976;2:554-556.

158. Streeten DH, Tomycz N, Anderson GH. Reliability of screening methods for the diagnosis of primary aldosteronism. *Am J Med*. 1979; 67:403-413.

159. Tucker RM, Labarthe DR. Frequency of surgical treatment for hypertension in adults at the Mayo Clinic from 1973 through 1975. *Mayo Clin Proc*. 1977;52:549-555.

160. Young WF. Primary aldosteronism: renaissance of a syndrome. *Clin Endocrinol (Oxf)*. 2007;66:607-618.

161. Funder JW, Carey RM, Fardella C, et al. Case detection, diagnosis, and treatment of patients with primary aldosteronism: an Endocrine Society clinical practice guideline. *J Clin Endocrinol Metab*. 2008;93: 3266-3281.

162. Stowasser M. Update in primary aldosteronism. *J Clin Endocrinol Metab*. 2015;100:1-10.

163. Mulatero P, Stowasser M, Loh KC, et al. Increased diagnosis of primary aldosteronism, including surgically correctable forms, in centers from five continents. *J Clin Endocrinol Metab*. 2004;89:1045-1050.

164. Piaditis G, Markou A, Papanastasiou L, et al. Progress in primary aldosteronism: a review of the prevalence of primary aldosteronism in pre-hypertension and hypertension. *Eur J Endocrinol*. 2015;172(5): R191-R203.

165. Ma JT, Wang C, Lam KS, et al. Fifty cases of primary hyperaldosteronism in Hong Kong Chinese with a high frequency of periodic paralysis. Evaluation of techniques for tumour localisation. *Q J Med*. 1986;61: 1021-1037.

166. Young WF Jr, Klee GG. Primary aldosteronism. Diagnostic evaluation. *Endocrinol Metab Clin North Am*. 1988;17:367-395.

167. Torres VE, Young WF Jr, Offord KP, Hattery RR. Association of hypokalemia, aldosterone, and renal cysts. *N Engl J Med*. 1990;322: 345-351.

168. Stowasser M, Sharman J, Leano R, et al. Evidence for abnormal left ventricular structure and function in normotensive individuals with familial hyperaldosteronism type I. *J Clin Endocrinol Metab*. 2005;90: 5070-5076.

169. Milliez P, Girerd X, Plouin PF, et al. Evidence for an increased rate of cardiovascular events in patients with primary aldosteronism. *J Am Coll Cardiol*. 2005;45:1243-1248.

170. Iwakura Y, Morimoto R, Kudo M, et al. Predictors of decreasing glomerular filtration rate and prevalence of chronic kidney disease after treatment of primary aldosteronism: renal outcome of 213 cases. *J Clin Endocrinol Metab*. 2014;99:1593-1598.

171. Tanabe A, Naruse M, Naruse K, et al. Left ventricular hypertrophy is more prominent in patients with primary aldosteronism than in patients with other types of secondary hypertension. *Hypertens Res*. 1997;20:85-90.

172. Rossi GP, Sacchetto A, Visentin P, et al. Changes in left ventricular anatomy and function in hypertension and primary aldosteronism. *Hypertension*. 1996;27:1039-1045.

173. Hiramatsu K, Yamada T, Yukimura Y, et al. A screening test to identify aldosterone-producing adenoma by measuring plasma renin activity. Results in hypertensive patients. *Arch Intern Med*. 1981;141: 1589-1593.

174. Montori VM, Young WF Jr. Use of plasma aldosterone concentration-to-plasma renin activity ratio as a screening test for primary aldosteronism. A systematic review of the literature. *Endocrinol Metab Clin North Am*. 2002;31:619-632, xi.

175. Weinberger MH, Fineberg NS. The diagnosis of primary aldosteronism and separation of two major subtypes. *Arch Intern Med*. 1993;153: 2125-2129.

176. Young WF Jr. Primary aldosteronism: diagnosis. In: Mansoor GA, ed. *Secondary Hypertension: Clinical Presentation, Diagnosis, and Treatment*. Totowa, NJ: Humana Press; 2004:119-137.

177. Schwartz GL, Turner ST. Screening for primary aldosteronism in essential hypertension: diagnostic accuracy of the ratio of plasma aldosterone concentration to plasma renin activity. *Clin Chem*. 2005;51: 386-394.

178. Nishizaka MK, Pratt-Ubunama M, Zaman MA, et al. Validity of plasma aldosterone-to-renin activity ratio in African American and white subjects with resistant hypertension. *Am J Hypertens*. 2005;18:805-812.

179. Lim PO, Farquharson CA, Shiels P, et al. Adverse cardiac effects of salt with fludrocortisone in hypertension. *Hypertension*. 2001;37:856-861.

180. Bravo EL, Tarazi RC, Dustan HP, et al. The changing clinical spectrum of primary aldosteronism. *Am J Med*. 1983;74:641-651.

181. Ahmed AH, Cowley D, Wolley M, et al. Seated saline suppression testing for the diagnosis of primary aldosteronism: a preliminary study. *J Clin Endocrinol Metab*. 2014;99:2745-2753.

182. Stowasser M, Gordon RD. Primary aldosteronism—careful investigation is essential and rewarding. *Mol Cell Endocrinol*. 2004;217:33-39.

183. Sawka AM, Young WF, Thompson GB, et al. Primary aldosteronism: factors associated with normalization of blood pressure after surgery. *Ann Intern Med*. 2001;135:258-261.

184. Citton M, Viel G, Rossi GP, et al. Outcome of surgical treatment of primary aldosteronism. *Langenbecks Arch Surg*. [Epub 2015 Jan 8].

185. Wachtel H, Cerullo I, Bartlett EK, et al. Long-term blood pressure control in patients undergoing adrenalectomy for primary hyperaldosteronism. *Surgery*. 2014;156:1394-1403.

186. Lim V, Guo Q, Grant CS, et al. Accuracy of adrenal imaging and adrenal venous sampling in predicting surgical cure of primary aldosteronism. *J Clin Endocrinol Metab*. 2014;99:2712-2719.

187. Kloos RT, Gross MD, Francis IR, et al. Incidentally discovered adrenal masses. *Endocr Rev.* 1995;16:460-484.

188. Young WF, Stanson AW, Thompson GB, et al. Role for adrenal venous sampling in primary aldosteronism. *Surgery.* 2004;136:1227-1235.

189. Kempers MJ, Lenders JW, van Outheusden L, et al. Systematic review: diagnostic procedures to differentiate unilateral from bilateral adrenal abnormality in primary aldosteronism. *Ann Intern Med.* 2009;151: 329-337.

190. Young WF, Stanson AW. What are the keys to successful adrenal venous sampling (AVS) in patients with primary aldosteronism? *Clin Endocrinol (Oxf).* 2009;70:14-17.

191. Daunt N. Adrenal vein sampling: how to make it quick, easy, and successful. *Radiographics.* 2005;25(Suppl 1):S143-S158.

192. Rossi GP, Auchus RJ, Brown M, et al. An expert consensus statement on use of adrenal vein sampling for the subtyping of primary aldosteronism. *Hypertension.* 2014;63:151-160.

193. Young WF Jr, Hogan MJ. Renin-Independent hypermineralocorticoidism. *Trends Endocrinol Metab.* 1994;5:97-106.

194. Sutherland DJ, Ruse JL, Laidlaw JC. Hypertension, increased aldosterone secretion and low plasma renin activity relieved by dexamethasone. *Can Med Assoc J.* 1966;95:1109-1119.

195. Lifton RP, Dluhy RG, Powers M, et al. A chimaeric 11 beta-hydroxylase/aldosterone synthase gene causes glucocorticoid-remediable aldosteronism and human hypertension. *Nature.* 1992;355:262-265.

196. Rich GM, Ulick S, Cook S, et al. Glucocorticoid-remediable aldosteronism in a large kindred: clinical spectrum and diagnosis using a characteristic biochemical phenotype. *Ann Intern Med.* 1992;116:813-820.

197. Mulatero P, Tizzani D, Viola A, et al. Prevalence and characteristics of familial hyperaldosteronism: the PATOGEN study (Primary Aldosteronism in TOrino-GENetic forms). *Hypertension.* 2011;58:797-803.

198. Sukor N, Mulatero P, Gordon RD, et al. Further evidence for linkage of familial hyperaldosteronism type II at chromosome 7p22 in Italian as well as Australian and South American families. *J Hypertens.* 2008; 26:1577-1582.

199. Carss KJ, Stowasser M, Gordon RD, O'Shaughnessy KM. Further study of chromosome 7p22 to identify the molecular basis of familial hyperaldosteronism type II. *J Hum Hypertens.* 2011;25:560-564.

200. Geller DS, Zhang J, Wisgerhof MV, et al. A novel form of human mendelian hypertension featuring nonglucocorticoid-remediable aldosteronism. *J Clin Endocrinol Metab.* 2008;93:3117-3123.

201. Choi M, Scholl UI, Yue P, et al. K+ channel mutations in adrenal aldosterone-producing adenomas and hereditary hypertension. *Science.* 2011;331:768-772.

202. Mussa A, Camilla R, Monticone S, et al. Polyuric-polydipsic syndrome in a pediatric case of non-glucocorticoid remediable familial hyperaldosteronism. *Endocr J.* 2012;59:497-502.

203. Charmandari E, Sertedaki A, Kino T, et al. A novel point mutation in the KCNJ5 gene causing primary hyperaldosteronism and early-onset autosomal dominant hypertension. *J Clin Endocrinol Metab.* 2012;97: E1532-E1539.

204. Mulatero P, Tauber P, Zennaro MC, et al. KCNJ5 mutations in European families with nonglucocorticoid remediable familial hyperaldosteronism. *Hypertension.* 2012;59:235-240.

205. Scholl UI, Nelson-Williams C, Yue P, et al. Hypertension with or without adrenal hyperplasia due to different inherited mutations in the potassium channel KCNJ5. *Proc Natl Acad Sci U S A.* 2012;109: 2533-2538.

206. Akerstrom T, Crona J, Delgado Verdugo A, et al. Comprehensive re-sequencing of adrenal aldosterone producing lesions reveal three somatic mutations near the KCNJ5 potassium channel selectivity filter. *PLoS One.* 2012;7:e41926.

207. Boulkroun S, Beuschlein F, Rossi GP, et al. Prevalence, clinical, and molecular correlates of KCNJ5 mutations in primary aldosteronism. *Hypertension.* 2012;59:592-598.

208. Beuschlein F, Boulkroun S, Osswald A, et al. Somatic mutations in ATP1A1 and ATP2B3 lead to aldosterone-producing adenomas and secondary hypertension. *Nat Genet.* 2013;45(4):440-444, 444e1-444e2.

209. Azizan EA, Poulsen H, Tuluc P, et al. Somatic mutations in ATP1A1 and CACNA1D underlie a common subtype of adrenal hypertension. *Nat Genet.* 2013;45:1055-1060.

210. Williams TA, Monticone S, Schack VR, et al. Somatic ATP1A1, ATP2B3, and KCNJ5 mutations in aldosterone-producing adenomas. *Hypertension.* 2014;63:188-195.

211. Scholl UI, Goh G, Stolting G, et al. Somatic and germline CACNA1D calcium channel mutations in aldosterone-producing adenomas and primary aldosteronism. *Nat Genet.* 2013;45:1050-1054.

212. Sechi LA, Di Fabio A, Bazzocchi M, et al. Intrarenal hemodynamics in primary aldosteronism before and after treatment. *J Clin Endocrinol Metab.* 2009;94:1191-1197.

213. Reincke M, Rump LC, Quinkler M, et al. Risk factors associated with a low glomerular filtration rate in primary aldosteronism. *J Clin Endocrinol Metab.* 2009;94:869-875.

214. Celen O, O'Brien MJ, Melby JC, Beazley RM. Factors influencing outcome of surgery for primary aldosteronism. *Arch Surg.* 1996;131: 646-650.

215. Ishidoya S, Ito A, Sakai K, et al. Laparoscopic partial versus total adrenalectomy for aldosterone producing adenoma. *J Urol.* 2005;174:40-43.

216. Chiang WF, Cheng CJ, Wu ST, et al. Incidence and factors of post-adrenalectomy hyperkalemia in patients with aldosterone producing adenoma. *Clin Chim Acta.* 2013;424:114-118.

217. Sywak M, Pasieka JL. Long-term follow-up and cost benefit of adrenalectomy in patients with primary hyperaldosteronism. *Br J Surg.* 2002; 89:1587-1593.

218. Ghose RP, Hall PM, Bravo EL. Medical management of aldosterone-producing adenomas. *Ann Intern Med.* 1999;131:105-108.

219. Lim PO, Young WF, MacDonald TM. A review of the medical treatment of primary aldosteronism. *J Hypertens.* 2001;19:353-361.

220. Jeunemaitre X, Chatellier G, Kreft-Jais C, et al. Efficacy and tolerance of spironolactone in essential hypertension. *Am J Cardiol.* 1987;60: 820-825.

221. Parthasarathy HK, Menard J, White WB, et al. A double-blind, randomized study comparing the antihypertensive effect of eplerenone and spironolactone in patients with hypertension and evidence of primary aldosteronism. *J Hypertens.* 2011;29:980-990.

222. Speiser PW, Azziz R, Baskin LS, et al. Congenital adrenal hyperplasia due to steroid 21-hydroxylase deficiency: an Endocrine Society clinical practice guideline. *J Clin Endocrinol Metab.* 2010;95:4133-4160.

223. Krone N, Arlt W. Genetics of congenital adrenal hyperplasia. *Best Pract Res Clin Endocrinol Metab.* 2009;23:181-192.

224. White PC, Dupont J, New MI, et al. A mutation in CYP11B1 (Arg-448—His) associated with steroid 11 beta-hydroxylase deficiency in Jews of Moroccan origin. *J Clin Invest.* 1991;87(5):1664-1667.

225. Merke DP, Bornstein SR. Congenital adrenal hyperplasia. *Lancet.* 2005;365:2125-2136.

226. New MI, Geller DS, Fallo F, Wilson RC. Monogenic low renin hypertension. *Trends Endocrinol Metab.* 2005;16:92-97.

227. Kim YM, Kang M, Choi JH, et al. A review of the literature on common CYP17A1 mutations in adults with 17-hydroxylase/17,20-lyase deficiency, a case series of such mutations among Koreans and functional characteristics of a novel mutation. *Metabolism.* 2014;63:42-49.

228. Mussig K, Wehrmann M, Horger M, et al. Adrenocortical carcinoma producing 11-deoxycorticosterone: a rare cause of mineralocorticoid hypertension. *J Endocrinol Invest.* 2005;28:61-65.

229. Ishikawa SE, Saito T, Kaneko K, et al. Hypermineralocorticism without elevation of plasma aldosterone: deoxycorticosterone-producing adrenal adenoma and hyperplasia. *Clin Endocrinol (Oxf).* 1988;29: 367-375.

230. Nicolaides NC, Roberts ML, Kino T, et al. A novel point mutation of the human glucocorticoid receptor gene causes primary generalized glucocorticoid resistance through impaired interaction with the LXXLL motif of the p160 coactivators: dissociation of the transactivating and transrepressive activities. *J Clin Endocrinol Metab.* 2014;99: E902-E907.

231. Charmandari E, Kino T, Chrousos GP. Primary generalized familial and sporadic glucocorticoid resistance (Chrousos syndrome) and hypersensitivity. *Endocr Dev.* 2013;24:67-85.

232. Chapman K, Holmes M, Seckl J. 11beta-hydroxysteroid dehydrogenases: intracellular gate-keepers of tissue glucocorticoid action. *Physiol Rev.* 2013;93:1139-1206.

233. Robles BJ, Sandoval AR, Dardon JD, Blas CA. Lethal liquorice lollies (liquorice abuse causing pseudohyperaldosteronism). *BMJ Case Rep.* 2013;2013.

234. Stewart PM, Krozowski ZS, Gupta A, et al. Hypertension in the syndrome of apparent mineralocorticoid excess due to mutation of the 11 beta-hydroxysteroid dehydrogenase type 2 gene. *Lancet.* 1996;347: 88-91.

235. Nieman LK, Biller BM, Findling JW, et al. The diagnosis of Cushing's syndrome: an Endocrine Society clinical practice guideline. *J Clin Endocrinol Metab.* 2008;93:1526-1540.

236. Liddle GW. A familial renal disorder simulating primary aldosteronism but with negligible aldosterone secretion. *Trans Assoc Am Physicians.* 1963;76:199-213.

237. Rossier BC, Schild L. Epithelial sodium channel: mendelian versus essential hypertension. *Hypertension.* 2008;52:595-600.

238. Lindholm J, Juul S, Jorgensen JO, et al. Incidence and late prognosis of Cushing's syndrome: a population-based study. *J Clin Endocrinol Metab.* 2001;86:117-123.

239. Sacerdote A, Weiss K, Tran T, et al. Hypertension in patients with Cushing's disease: pathophysiology, diagnosis, and management. *Curr Hypertens Rep.* 2005;7:212-218.

240. Baid S, Nieman LK. Glucocorticoid excess and hypertension. *Curr Hypertens Rep.* 2004;6:493-499.

241. Danzi S, Klein I. Thyroid hormone and blood pressure regulation. *Curr Hypertens Rep.* 2003;5:513-520.

242. Bahn RS, Burch HB, Cooper DS, et al. Hyperthyroidism and other causes of thyrotoxicosis: management guidelines of the American Thyroid Association and American Association of Clinical Endocrinologists. *Endocr Pract.* 2011;17:456-520.

243. Streeten DH, Anderson GH Jr, Howland T, et al. Effects of thyroid function on blood pressure. Recognition of hypothyroid hypertension. *Hypertension.* 1988;11:78-83.

244. Jian WX, Jin J, Qin L, et al. Relationship between thyroid-stimulating hormone and blood pressure in the middle-aged and elderly population. *Singapore Med J.* 2013;54:401-405.

245. Garber JR, Cobin RH, Gharib H, et al. Clinical practice guidelines for hypothyroidism in adults: cosponsored by the American Association of Clinical Endocrinologists and the American Thyroid Association. *Thyroid.* 2012;22:1200-1235.

246. Han D, Trooskin S, Wang X. Prevalence of cardiovascular risk factors in male and female patients with primary hyperparathyroidism. *J Endocrinol Invest.* 2012;35:548-552.

247. Richards AM, Espiner EA, Nicholls MG, et al. Hormone, calcium and blood pressure relationships in primary hyperparathyroidism. *J Hypertens.* 1988;6:747-752.

248. Heyliger A, Tangpricha V, Weber C, Sharma J. Parathyroidectomy decreases systolic and diastolic blood pressure in hypertensive patients with primary hyperparathyroidism. *Surgery.* 2009;146:1042-1047.

249. Rydberg E, Birgander M, Bondeson AG, et al. Effect of successful parathyroidectomy on 24-hour ambulatory blood pressure in patients with primary hyperparathyroidism. *Int J Cardiol.* 2010;142:15-21.

250. Terzolo M, Matrella C, Boccuzzi A, et al. Twenty-four hour profile of blood pressure in patients with acromegaly. Correlation with demographic, clinical and hormonal features. *J Endocrinol Invest.* 1999;22: 48-54.

251. Berg C, Petersenn S, Lahner H, et al. Cardiovascular risk factors in patients with uncontrolled and long-term acromegaly: comparison with matched data from the general population and the effect of disease control. *J Clin Endocrinol Metab.* 2010;95:3648-3656.

Section V

Reproduction

CHAPTER 17

Physiology and Pathology of the Female Reproductive Axis

SERDAR E. BULUN

KEY POINTS

- Ovulation and the preparation of the uterus for pregnancy are extremely delicate and parallel physiologic processes that are tightly regulated by a number of hormones released primarily by the hypothalamus, pituitary, and ovary.
- In women, the biologically active steroids—testosterone, dihydrotestosterone (DHT), and estradiol—are formed in the ovary, peripheral tissues, and locally in androgen or estrogen target tissues. Additionally, the adrenal gland and ovary secrete androgen and estrogen precursors that are converted to biologically active steroids in the peripheral tissues.
- A premenopausal woman often seeks medical help because of disorders that disrupt or complicate ovulation, normal menses, or fertility; these disorders include hypothalamic anovulation, hyperprolactinemia, polycystic ovary syndrome, ovarian insufficiency, endometriosis, and uterine fibroids.
- Combination oral contraceptives are commonly prescribed to suppress ovarian activity for the management of various benign causes of anovulatory uterine bleeding or androgen excess, such as polycystic ovary syndrome, and for the management of cyclic or chronic pelvic pain associated with endometriosis.
- Menopause is the depletion of all ovarian follicles; it effectively stops secretion of estradiol and progesterone. The management of postmenopausal ovarian deficiency, characterized thus by vasomotor symptoms, bone loss, and vaginal atrophy, is challenging and still highly debated in regard to the effectiveness and the side effects of existing treatment regimens.

REPRODUCTIVE PHYSIOLOGY

Tightly coordinated functions of the hypothalamus, pituitary, ovaries, and endometrium give rise to cyclic, predictable menses that indicate regular ovulation. Regular ovulation requires normal functioning of other endocrine glands, such as the thyroid and adrenals, and patients with hypothyroidism, hyperthyroidism, Cushing syndrome, or glucocorticoid resistance may present with anovulation. Clinicians need a thorough knowledge of the functions and interactions of the hypothalamus, pituitary, ovaries, and uterus with other systems to correctly diagnose reproductive disorders and design treatment strategies.

A prominent reproductive function of the hypothalamus is pulsatile secretion of gonadotropin-releasing hormone (GnRH). Negative feedback effects of several factors, including ovarian steroids, regulate hypothalamic GnRH secretion into the portal vessels. Dopamine, norepinephrine, serotonin, and opioids produced in the brain may mediate the regulation of GnRH secretion by ovarian hormones or other stimuli. In response to GnRH, the anterior pituitary cells secrete follicle-stimulating hormone (FSH) and luteinizing hormone (LH). Steroids (e.g., estradiol, progesterone) and peptides (e.g., inhibin) of ovarian origin and activin and follistatin of pituitary origin modify secretion of FSH and LH. LH stimulates androstenedione production in theca cells of the ovary; FSH regulates estradiol and inhibin B production in the granulosa cells and follicular growth. Release of an egg from the mature follicle depends on a sudden rise in LH levels in midcycle. After ovulation, the follicle transforms into a corpus luteum that secretes estradiol and progesterone under the control of FSH and LH. LH also stimulates granulosa-lutein cells of the corpus luteum to secrete inhibin A (Fig. 17-1A).

The endocrine effects of FSH, LH, estradiol, progesterone, inhibin A, and inhibin B have been deduced from changes in their serum levels throughout the menstrual cycle (see Fig. 17-1A). The postulated endocrine effects were then demonstrated in cell-based and in vivo studies (see Fig. 17-1B). Activin and follistatin are produced in the ovary and the pituitary. They appear to regulate FSH release

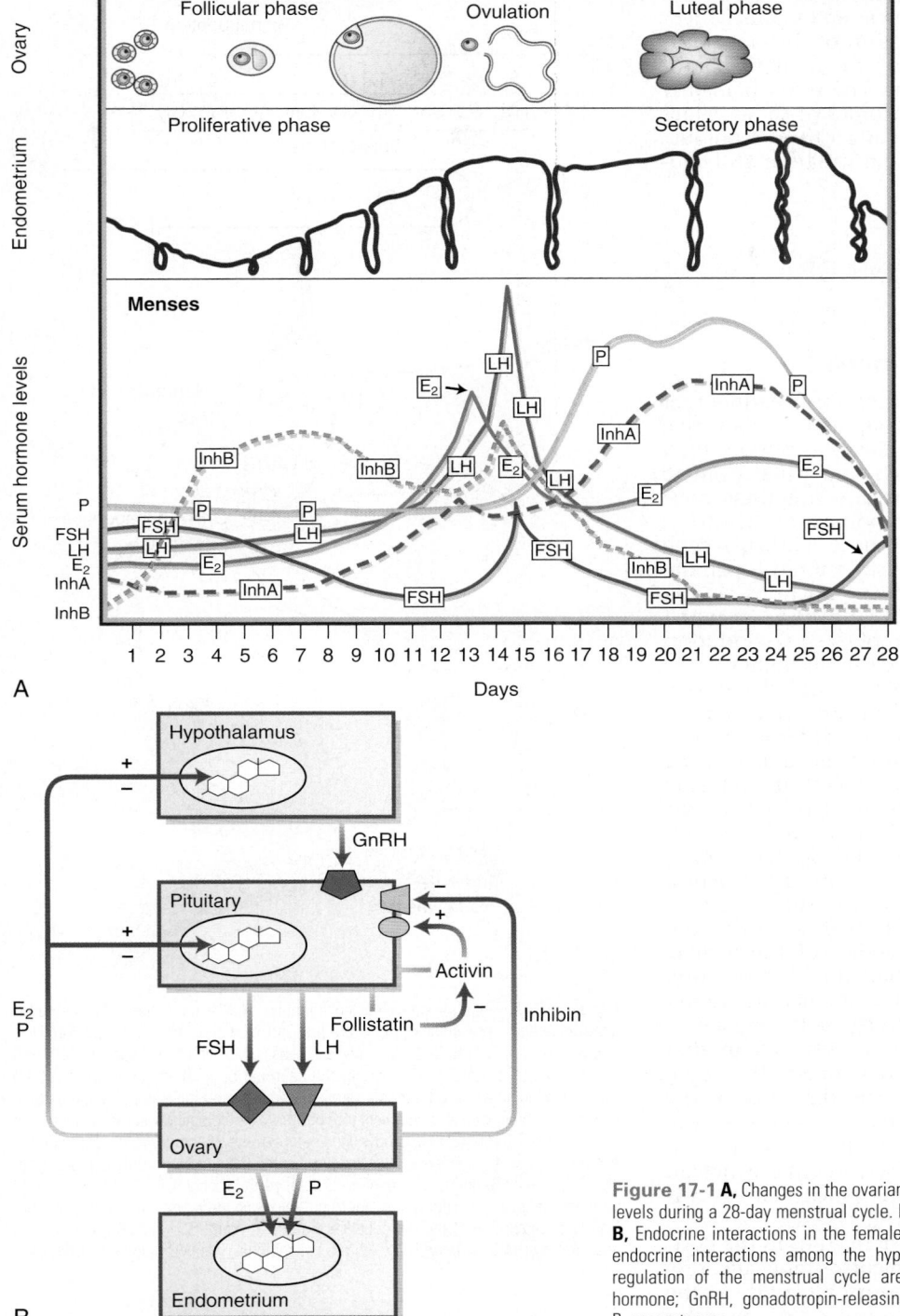

Figure 17-1 A, Changes in the ovarian follicle, endometrial thickness, and serum hormone levels during a 28-day menstrual cycle. Menses occur during the first few days of the cycle. **B,** Endocrine interactions in the female reproductive axis. Some of the well-characterized endocrine interactions among the hypothalamus, pituitary, ovary, and endometrium for regulation of the menstrual cycle are depicted. E_2, estradiol; FSH, follicle-stimulating hormone; GnRH, gonadotropin-releasing hormone; Inh, inhibin; LH, luteinizing hormone; P, progesterone.

from the pituitary via autocrine or paracrine but not endocrine pathways. Activin stimulates FSH production, whereas follistatin suppresses this action of activin.

Endometrium, the mucosal lining of the uterine cavity, has extremely high concentrations of nuclear receptors for estrogen and progesterone and is highly sensitive to these hormones. The biologically active estrogen, estradiol, induces the growth of endometrium; progesterone limits this estrogenic effect and enhances differentiation. Sloughing off the functional layer (stratum functionalis) of the endometrium follows withdrawal of estrogen or progester-

one. The remaining basal layer (stratum basalis) is capable of full regeneration in response to estrogen.

Ovaries remain quiescent until puberty because the GnRH-releasing system in the hypothalamus is immature in prepubertal children associated with very low circulating FSH and LH. The entire reproductive function and most of the endocrine function of the ovaries cease after menopause because ovaries are depleted of all oocytes and surrounding steroidogenic cells by this time. These prepubertal and postmenopausal states, characterized by the absence of ovarian function, are associated with the lack of menses.

In summary, the female reproductive function from puberty to menopause can be viewed as an extremely delicate ticking clock. The normal function of this apparatus depends on coordinated actions of the hypothalamus, pituitary, ovaries, and endometrium. The result is regular menses every 24 to 35 days. Any disorder of these tissues or dysfunction of other systems that affect these reproductive units secondarily may result in anovulation and consequent irregular uterine bleeding.

REPRODUCTIVE FUNCTIONS OF THE HYPOTHALAMUS

Gonadotropin-Releasing Hormone

GnRH and its analogues are used for the treatment of hormone-dependent disorders and assisted reproductive technologies such as in vitro fertilization (IVF).[1] In a number of vertebrates, three GnRHs and three cognate receptors with distinct distributions and functions have been identified. In humans, the hypothalamic GnRH is primarily encoded by the GnRH type I (GnRH-I) gene *(GNRH1)* and regulates gonadotropin secretion through the pituitary GnRH type I receptor, which functions as a G protein–coupled receptor. Binding of GnRH-I to its type I receptor leads primarily to activation of G_q. A second form of GnRH, called *GnRH-II*, is conserved in all higher vertebrates, including humans.[1] In contrast to GnRH-I, GnRH-II is expressed at the highest levels outside the brain. A cognate receptor for GnRH-II has been cloned from various vertebrate species, including primates.[1] The human gene homologue of this receptor has a frameshift and stop codon, and it appears that GnRH-II signaling occurs through the type I GnRH receptor. There seems to be considerable plasticity in the use of different GnRHs, receptors, and signaling pathways for diverse functions.[1] For practical purposes, GnRH-I is referred to as *GnRH* in this chapter.

GnRH is a 10–amino acid peptide that is synthesized primarily in specialized neuronal bodies of the arcuate nucleus of the medial basal hypothalamus.[1] Axons from GnRH neurons project to the median eminence and terminate in the capillaries that drain into the portal vessels.

The portal vein is a low-flow transport system that descends along the pituitary stalk and connects the hypothalamus to the anterior pituitary. The direction of the blood flow in this hypophyseal portal circulation is from the hypothalamus to the pituitary. GnRH originating in the neurons of the arcuate nucleus is secreted at the median eminence into the portal circulation, which delivers this hormone to the anterior pituitary (Fig. 17-2).

The mature decapeptide GnRH is derived from the posttranslational processing of a large precursor molecule, pre-pro-GnRH (see Fig. 17-2).[2] This precursor peptide is the product of the GnRH gene.[1] The pre-pro-GnRH consists of 92 amino acids and contains four parts (from aminoterminal to carboxyl-terminal): a 23–amino acid signal domain, the GnRH decapeptide, a 3–amino acid proteolytic processing site, and a 56–amino acid domain called *GnRH-associated peptide*.[3] The cleavage products of this precursor, GnRH and gonadotropin-releasing hormone–associated peptide (GAP), are transported to the nerve terminals and secreted into the portal circulation (see Fig. 17-2).[2,4] A physiologic role for GAP has not been established.[4]

In humans, GnRH neurons are located primarily in the arcuate nucleus of the medial basal hypothalamus and the preoptic area of the anterior hypothalamus.[5] The popula-

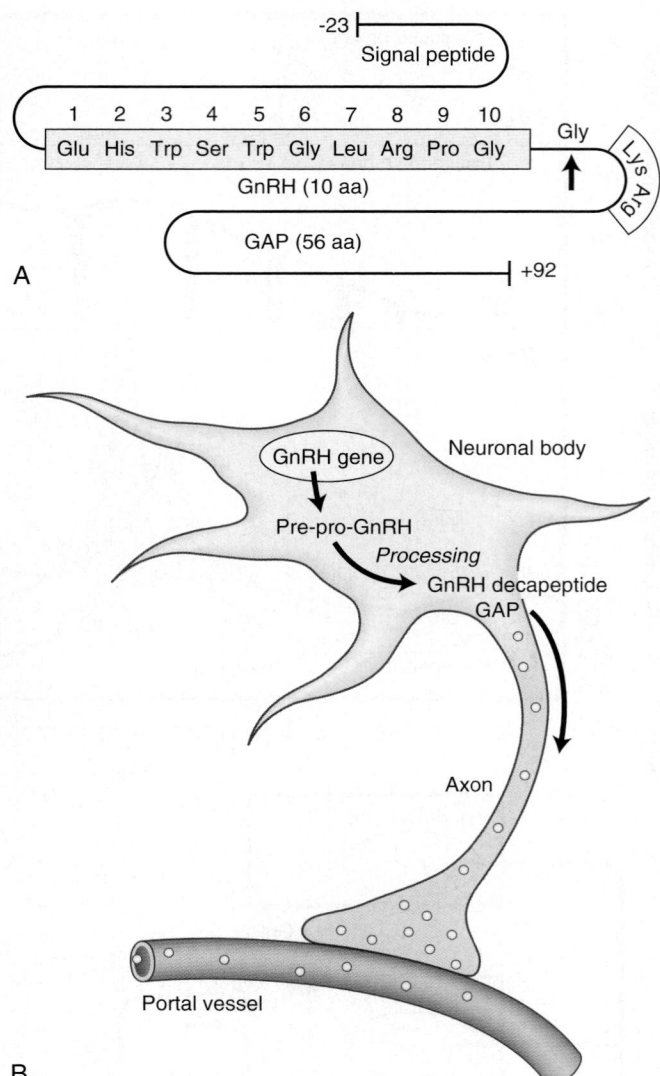

Figure 17-2 Gonadotropin-releasing hormone (GnRH) production. **A,** The GnRH gene encodes a precursor protein, pre-pro-GnRH, in the neuronal body. GnRH is released from this protein by proteolytic processing, which gives rise to GnRH and GnRH-associated protein (GAP) within the neuronal body. Both GnRH and GAP are transported in an axon to the nerve terminal and secreted into the portal circulation. **B,** Pre-pro-GnRH is a 92–amino acid (aa) protein. The biologically active decapeptide (amino acids 1 through 10) is sandwiched between the 23–amino acid signal peptide and the Gly-Lys-Arg sequence. The *arrow* indicates the site of proteolytic processing. The C-terminal 56–amino acid peptide is cleaved to produce GAP. LHRH, luteinizing hormone–releasing hormone (gonadotropin-releasing hormone 1). (From Yen SSC. Endocrine regulation of the reproductive system. In: Yen SSC, Jaffe RB, Barbieri RL, eds. *Reproductive Endocrinology*, 4th ed. Philadelphia, PA: WB Saunders; 1999:44.)

tion of GnRH-producing neurons is relatively limited and is in the range of 1000 to 2000. The neurons that produce GnRH originate from the olfactory area during embryogenesis.[5] GnRH and olfactory neurons migrate together along cranial nerves connecting the nose and forebrain to the hypothalamus during embryologic development, and disruption of this process causes idiopathic hypogonadotropic hypogonadism with anosmia, or Kallmann syndrome.[5] Individuals with Kallmann syndrome usually have lack of pubertal development and subsequent infertility due to deficient GnRH and pituitary gonadotropins. The neuronal proteins anosmin 1 (encoded by the *KAL1* gene) and fibroblast growth factor receptor type 1 (encoded by the *FGFR1*

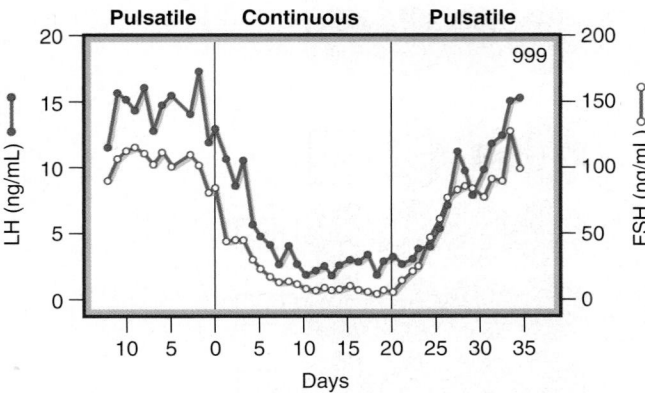

Figure 17-3 Effect of pulsatile or continuous administration of gonadotropin-releasing hormone (GnRH) to ovariectomized monkeys previously rendered GnRH deficient by placement of a lesion in the hypothalamus. Release of luteinizing hormone (LH) and follicle-stimulating hormone (FSH) was restored by hourly GnRH infusion, inhibited during a continuous infusion, and again restored after reinstitution of pulsatile GnRH administration. (Adapted from Belchetz PE, Plant TM, Nakai Y, et al. Hypophysial responses to continuous and intermittent delivery of hypothalamic gonadotropin releasing hormone. *Science*. 1978;202:631-633. Copyright © 1978 by American Association for the Advancement of Science.)

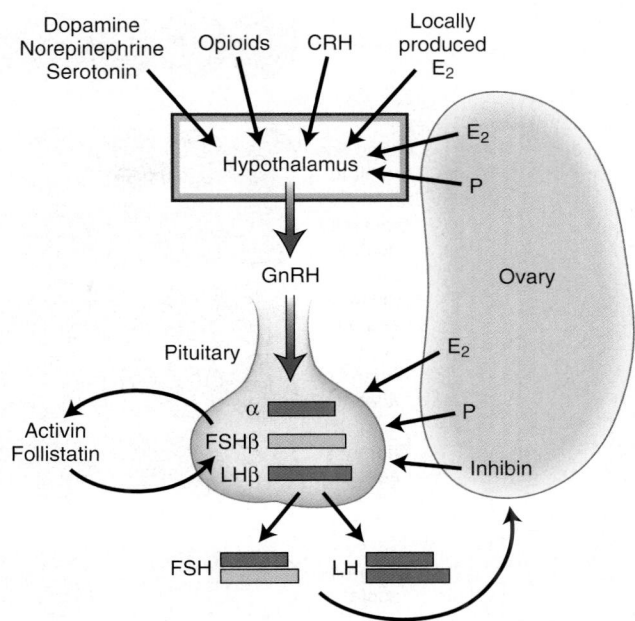

Figure 17-4 Regulation of gonadotropin-releasing hormone (GnRH), luteinizing hormone (LH), and follicle-stimulating hormone (FSH) secretion. Locally synthesized and systemic hormones regulate the pulsatile secretion of GnRH from the hypothalamus into the portal circulation. GnRH and a number of steroid and peptide hormones regulate the synthesis of gonadotropin subunits, including the common α-subunit and specific β-subunits for LH and FSH, and the formation and secretion of FSH and LH. CRH, corticotropin-releasing hormone; E_2, estradiol; P, progesterone.

gene) affect olfactory and GnRH neuron migration. Mutations in these genes cause Kallmann syndrome.[5] Data suggest that mutations of the genes for nasal embryonic luteinizing hormone–releasing hormone factor *(NELF)* and chromodomain helicase DNA-binding protein 7 *(CHD7)* may cause Kallmann syndrome, but this correlation is not as conclusively established as it is for *KAL1* and *FGFR1*.[5] Selective clinical phenotypes in men and women are highly associated with genetic causes of Kallman syndrome. Synkinesia *(KAL1)*, dental agenesis *(FGF8/FGFR1)*, digital bony abnormalities *(FGF8/FGFR1)*, and hearing loss *(CHD7)* may be useful for prioritizing genetic testing.[6]

Knobil demonstrated in a pioneering series of experiments that normal gonadotropin secretion requires pulsatile GnRH discharge within a critical frequency and amplitude.[7] The periodicity and amplitude of the pulsatile rhythm of GnRH and gonadotropin secretion are crucial in regulating gonadal activity and therefore the entire reproductive axis (Fig. 17-3). The self-priming effect of GnRH in upregulating its receptors on pituitary gonadotropin-producing cells manifests only at the physiologic periodicity of 60 to 90 minutes.[8,9] Slower frequency causes anovulation and amenorrhea because of inadequate stimulation. Higher frequency or constant exposure to GnRH also gives rise to anovulation by downregulating expression of GnRH receptors, thereby abolishing gonadotropin responses.

The activation of gene expression for gonadotropin subunits, including the common α-subunit and specific β-subunits for LH and FSH, dimerization of αβ subunits, and glycosylation appear to be governed by intermittency of GnRH inputs to pituitary gonadotrophs.[10] In humans, measurement of LH pulses is commonly used as an indication of GnRH pulsatile secretion.[11] The LH pulse frequency is approximately 90 minutes during the early follicular phase, 60 to 70 minutes during the late follicular phase, 100 minutes during the early luteal phase, and 200 minutes during the late luteal phase.[12] This variation is accompanied by predictable changes in FSH and LH levels and ovarian steroid release during these phases of the menstrual cycle. More rapid pulse frequencies favor LH secretion, whereas slower pulse frequencies favor FSH. It appears

that variations in GnRH pulse frequency markedly influence both the absolute levels and the ratio of LH and FSH release.

Regulation of Gonadotropin-Releasing Hormone Secretion

Cyclic, predictable menses require the pulsatile release of GnRH within a critical range of frequencies. Pulsatile, rhythmic activity is an intrinsic property of GnRH neurons, and various hormones and neurotransmitters modulate this rhythm (Fig. 17-4).

The variations in GnRH pulse frequency are achieved, in part, by gonadal steroid feedback. Estradiol increases GnRH pulse frequency, and elevated progesterone levels decrease GnRH pulsatility.[10] Increased progesterone levels may decrease GnRH pulse frequency and thereby lead to preferential biosynthesis and secretion of FSH, as observed in the late luteal phase.[10]

GnRH pulsatility is also modulated by the actions of locally released neurotransmitters. Norepinephrine stimulates GnRH release, whereas dopamine exerts an inhibitory effect (see Fig. 17-4).[13] β-Endorphin and other opioids may suppress the hypothalamic release of GnRH.[14,15] It was proposed that sex steroids enhance the activity of endogenous opioids that exert an inhibitory effect on GnRH secretion.[12] The negative effect of opioids on GnRH secretion is clinically explicable because the reduced GnRH secretion associated with hypothalamic amenorrhea may be mediated by an increase in endogenous opioid inhibitory tone.[16]

Estrogen signaling to GnRH neurons appears to be critical for suppressing FSH and LH and for coordinating the preovulatory surge release of LH. The precise roles of estrogen receptors α and β (ERα and ERβ, respectively) within the GnRH neurons or estradiol-sensitive afferent neurons

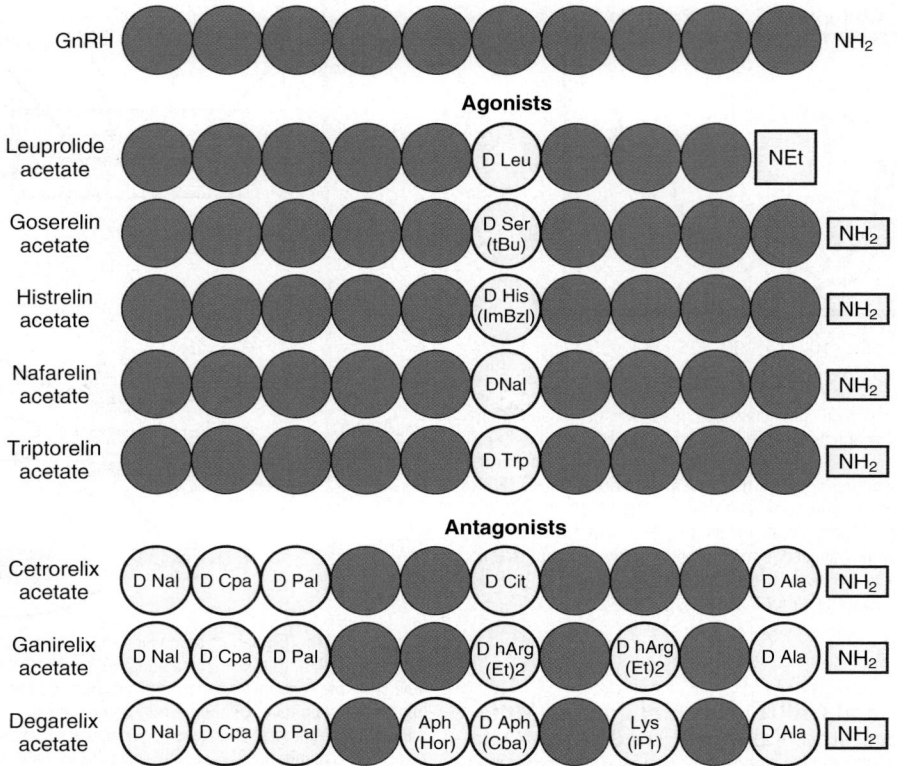

Figure 17-5 Gonadotropin-releasing hormone (GnRH) agonist and antagonist analogues in clinical practice. *Purple circles* indicate amino acids in the wild-type GnRH deca-peptide, and *white circles* are labeled with the changes made to the analogues. (Modified from Millar RP, Lu Z, Pawson AJ, et al. Gonadotropin-releasing hormone receptors. *Endocr Rev.* 2004;25:235-275. Copyright © 2004 by the Endocrine Society.)

in these negative and positive feedback effects of estrogen are not well understood.[17] Stimulation of FSH release after treatment of premenopausal women with an aromatase inhibitor and in vitro studies suggest that estrogen locally produced by aromatase activity in hypothalamic neurons may regulate gonadotropin secretion.[18,19]

Binding of the peptide kisspeptin to its G protein–coupled receptor KISS1R (previously known as GPR54), which is expressed in GnRH neurons, stimulates GnRH release in the hypothalamus.[20,21] Kisspeptin neurons contact GnRH neurons and act at the cell body and the nerve terminals. Kisspeptin can act directly on GnRH neurons or indirectly through synaptic input from other neurons to inhibit inwardly rectifying potassium channels and activate nonspecific cation channels, producing long-lasting depolarization and an increased action potential firing rate.[22] Mutations or knockout of KISS1R produces isolated hypogonadotropic hypogonadism in humans and mice, indicating that signaling through this receptor is essential for sexual development and function.[20,21] Moreover, kisspeptin- and KISS1R-expressing neurons may be critical targets for the negative and positive feedback actions of estrogen and progesterone.[23]

Gonadotropin-Releasing Hormone Analogues

The half-life of GnRH is short (2 to 4 minutes) because it is degraded rapidly by peptidases in the hypothalamus and pituitary gland.[24] These peptidases cleave the bonds between amino acids 5 and 6, 6 and 7, and 9 and 10. Analogues of GnRH with different properties have been synthesized by alteration of amino acids at these positions. Many agonistic and antagonistic GnRH analogues with various biologic effects have been produced.

Peptide Gonadotropin-Releasing Hormone Agonists

Several GnRH agonist peptides are generated by substitution of amino acids at the 6 or 10 position (Fig. 17-5). The increased biologic activity of agonistic peptides has been attributed to their high binding affinity to GnRH receptors and their reduced susceptibility to enzymatic degradation. An amino acid substitution at position 6 gives rise to metabolic stability, whereas replacement of the carboxy-terminal glycinamide residue by an ethylamide group increases strikingly the affinity for the receptors.[24,25] Peptide GnRH agonists are administered subcutaneously, intranasally, or intramuscularly. An initial agonistic action (i.e., flare effect) is associated with an increase in the circulating levels of LH and FSH. The most prominent agonistic response is observed during the early follicular phase, when the combined effects of GnRH agonist and elevated levels of estradiol create a large reserve pool of gonadotropins.[26]

Administration of a long-acting depot formulation of a GnRH agonist gives rise to an initial flare followed by downregulation of the gonadotropin-gonadal axis within 1 to 3 weeks. The initial downregulation effect is caused by desensitization, whereas the sustained response results from loss of receptors and the uncoupling of the receptor from its effector system.

The U.S. Food and Drug Administration (FDA) approved the use of these agonists for the treatment of GnRH-dependent precocious puberty, endometriosis, and prostate cancer. Another indication is preoperative hematologic improvement of patients with anemia caused by uterine leiomyomas. Off-label indications for GnRH agonists include downregulation of the pituitary during ovulation induction, induction of endometrial atrophy before endometrial ablation surgery, and prevention of menstrual bleeding in patients with coagulation defects. GnRH agonists have also been used to suppress ovarian steroidogenesis in hirsute patients.[27]

The most prominent side effects of long-term use of depot GnRH agonist formulations are caused by estrogen deficiency. Depot GnRH agonists induce a menopause-like state characterized by hot flashes, vaginal dryness, bone resorption, and osteopenia. Osteopenia is reversible in young women if treatment is maintained for no more than 6 months.[28,29] The risk/benefit ratio must be considered carefully before GnRH agonist treatment is extended for longer periods. Add-back regimens employing low-dose estrogens or progestins, or both, administered along with GnRH agonists have provided a means to overcome these side effects and to extend the length of agonist therapy.[30]

Peptide Gonadotropin-Releasing Hormone Antagonists

Inhibition of a premature LH rise by GnRH agonists requires at least 7 days, because it is accompanied by an initial stimulation of GnRH receptors before gonadotroph desensitization is achieved. In contrast, GnRH antagonists compete directly with endogenous GnRH for receptor binding and therefore rapidly inhibit secretion of gonadotropin and steroid hormones (see Fig. 17-5).[31-34] This property conveys a potential advantage over GnRH agonists in the management of ovarian stimulation. However, because of the constant need to block endogenous GnRH, much higher doses of antagonists are required. The GnRH antagonists incorporate a number of amino acid substitutions in the amino-terminal domain (involved in receptor activation) combined with a D-amino acid substitution for Gly6, which enhances the βII-type bend necessary for receptor binding.[1] GnRH antagonists have the advantage of inducing an immediate decrease in circulating gonadotropin levels with rapid reversal.[31-34] GnRH antagonists are alternative drugs to GnRH agonists for the prevention of a natural LH surge during ovulation induction by injectable FSH.[35] Use of GnRH antagonists has become popular in ovulation induction protocols for IVF (see Fig. 17-5).[35]

Nonpeptide Gonadotropin-Releasing Hormone Antagonists

Small molecular compound collections have been screened using mammalian cells that ectopically expressed human GnRH type I receptor. These studies led to the identification of synthetic compounds that bind to the GnRH type I receptor and block it. Several companies have manufactured orally administered GnRH antagonists intended for various indications, including endometriosis. None of these medications has yet reached the market.[1]

REPRODUCTIVE FUNCTIONS OF THE ANTERIOR PITUITARY

Gonadotrophs

Gonadotrophs are specialized cell types of the anterior pituitary that synthesize and secrete LH and FSH. These cells constitute 7% to 15% of the total number of anterior pituitary cells and are detected in this location from early fetal life.[36] Most gonadotrophs are capable of synthesizing both LH and FSH.[36,37] LH and FSH are each composed of two distinct, noncovalently associated protein subunits called α and β (see Fig. 17-4). In the gonadotroph, the subunit genes encode the subunit precursors. Gonadotrophs contain cell-surface GnRH type I receptors that

mediate the action of GnRH. These receptors belong to the seven-transmembrane domain and G protein–coupled receptor family.

Gonadotropin-Releasing Hormone Receptor

In humans, hypothalamic GnRH regulates gonadotropin secretion through the pituitary GnRH type I receptor by activation of $G_{q/11}$.[38] Although the predominant coupling of the type I GnRH receptor in the gonadotroph is through $G_{q/11}$ stimulation, signal transduction can occur through other G proteins and potentially by G protein–independent means.[1,38] A number of downstream cascades include protein kinase C (PKC)–, Ca^{2+}-, and tyrosine kinase–dependent pathways.[1] In mouse pituitary gonadotrophs, the GnRH receptor activates several mitogen-activated protein (MAP) kinase cascades, including the ERK1/2, the JUN amino-terminal kinase (JNK), the p38 MAP kinase, and the big MAP kinase (BMK1/ERK5).[1] The cross-talk between these pathways remains to be clarified.

Luteinizing Hormone and Follicle-Stimulating Hormone

LH and FSH are made of two peptide subunits called α and β, which are associated with noncovalent bonds. The α-subunits of human LH, FSH, thyroid-stimulating hormone (TSH), and human chorionic gonadotropin (hCG) have an identical polypeptide structure. In contrast, the β-subunit of each hormone has a unique amino acid sequence and confers the specific activity of the αβ-heterodimer. Each subunit is rich in cysteine and contains multiple disulfide linkages. Each subunit also contains multiple carbohydrate moieties that play important roles in the biologic activity and metabolism of these hormones.

The human common α-subunit gene encodes a precursor polypeptide with a 24–amino acid leader sequence that is cleaved post-translationally to produce the mature 92–amino acid α-subunit. The β-subunits of human FSH, LH, and hCG contain 117, 121, and 145 amino acids, respectively.[39-42] On binding of GnRH to its receptor, the biosynthesis of the gonadotropins proceeds by transcription of the subunit genes, translation of the subunit messenger ribonucleic acids (mRNAs), post-translational modifications of the precursor subunits and subunit folding and combination, mature hormone packaging, and secretion (see Fig. 17-4).

The human LH and hCG β-subunit genes are located on chromosome 19q13.3, which contains a cluster of seven β-subunit–like genes.[40] Five of these sequences are noncoding pseudogenes arranged in groups of tandem and inverted pairs. Only LH and hCG β-subunit genes give rise to two distinct and functional mRNA species. The LH β-subunit mRNA encodes a 145–amino acid precursor protein that is later cleaved to produce a 24–amino acid leader peptide and a 121–amino acid, biologically active, mature peptide. The hCG β-subunit mRNA also encodes a 145–amino acid protein. This protein, however, is not processed post-translationally and functions as the biologically active hCG β-subunit. The amino acid sequences of the human LH and hCG β-subunits are 82% homologous. These two β-subunits confer identical biologic activities when associated with the α-subunit.[40-42]

A single gene encodes the FSH β-subunit.[43] Complementary DNA encoding human FSH-β, LH-β, or hCG-β in combination with the complementary DNA of the α-subunit is expressed in mammalian cells in culture. These cells can synthesize these proteins, modify them after translation, glycosylate and combine the subunits, and secrete them as intact FSH, LH, or hCG.[44] Recombinant gonadotropins are used clinically to stimulate gonadal function.[45]

Regulation of Circulating Levels of Follicle-Stimulating Hormone and Luteinizing Hormone

The molecular mechanisms responsible for formation and combination of the α- and β-subunits of FSH and LH are not completely understood. Production rates of α- and β-subunits are regulated in part by negative feedback by estrogen, which regulates the pulsatile release of GnRH from the hypothalamus.[44,46] The pituitary contains more α-subunit than β-subunit mRNA, and readily detectable levels of free α-subunit are present in serum. The free β-subunit is present at relatively low levels in the pituitary and is rarely found in serum or urine. The specific β-subunit may be the rate-limiting factor in the synthesis of these glycoprotein hormones.

Inhibin, activin, and follistatin were first identified as gonadal hormones that exerted selective effects on FSH secretion.[47] Although the primary source of inhibin remains the ovary, activin and follistatin are produced in extragonadal tissues and can exert effects on FSH through an autocrine-paracrine mechanism. Inhibin B is secreted by ovarian granulosa cells during the follicular phase (under the control of FSH) and inhibin A by the corpus luteum in the luteal phase (under the control of LH). Inhibins act synergistically with estradiol to inhibit FSH secretion. Activin can directly stimulate FSH biosynthesis and release from the gonadotroph cells of the pituitary gland.[47] Follistatin can negatively regulate biologic functions of activin via binding and preventing it from interacting with the activin receptor at the cell membrane.[48]

Serum levels of gonadotropins are proportional to their secretion rates and serum half-lives, which are regulated by the number of carbohydrate residues. The sialic acid content of gonadotropic hormones and other glycoproteins has a marked effect on their rate of clearance and influences their apparent molecular size.[49] The higher content of sialic acid in FSH compared with LH is responsible for slower clearance of FSH, which has a half-life of 3 to 4 hours. LH, which has a half-life of 20 minutes, has the most rapid clearance rate. The hCG is highly sialylated and has the longest half-life (24 hours).

OVARY

The ovary is essential for periodic release of oocytes and production of the steroid hormones, estradiol and progesterone. These activities are integrated into the cyclic repetitive process of follicular maturation, ovulation, and formation and regression of the corpus luteum. The ovary fulfills two major objectives: generation of a fertilizable ovum and preparation of the endometrium for implantation through the sequential secretion of estradiol and progesterone.[45] The ovarian follicle comprising the egg and surrounding granulosa and theca cells constitutes the fundamental functional unit of the ovary.

Adult human ovaries are oval bodies with a length of 2 to 5 cm, a width of 1.5 to 3 cm, and a thickness of 0.5 to 1.5 cm. The ovaries lie near the posterior and lateral pelvic wall and are attached to the posterior surface of the broad ligament by the peritoneal fold, called the *mesovarium*.

The ovary consists of three structurally distinct regions: an outer cortex containing the surface germinal epithelium and the follicles; a central medulla consisting of stroma; and a hilum around the area of attachment of the ovary to the mesovarium (Fig. 17-6). The hilum is the point of attachment of the ovary to the mesovarium. It contains nerves, blood vessels, and hilus cells, which have the

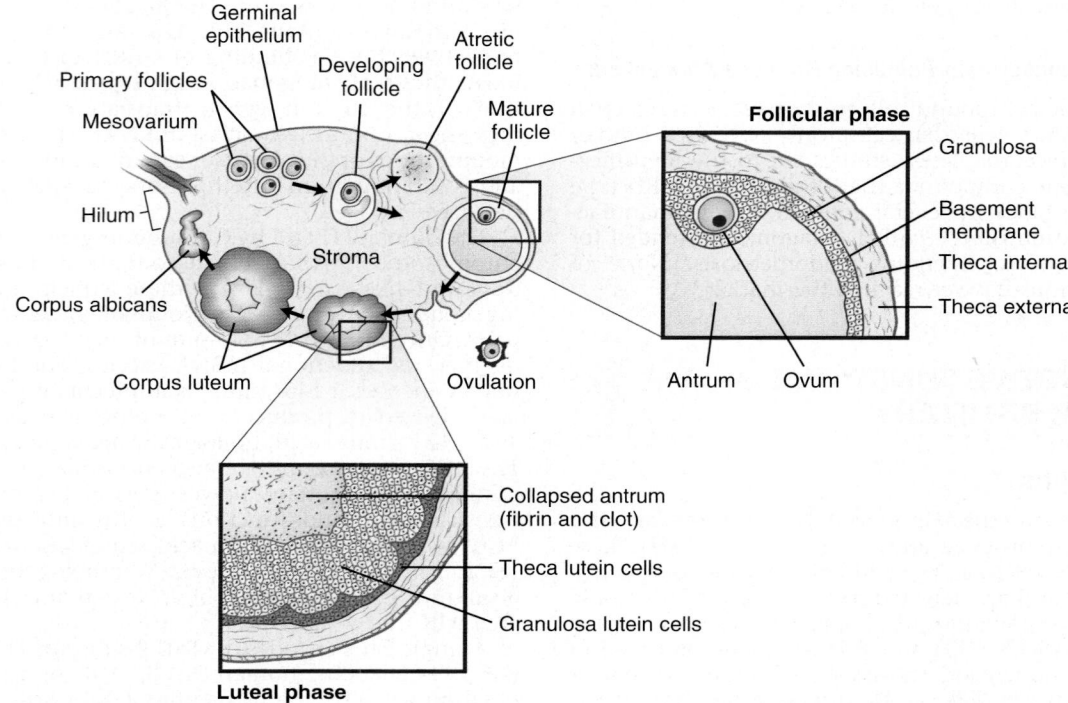

Figure 17-6 Functional anatomy and changes in the adult ovary during an ovarian cycle. (From Carr BR, Wilson JD. Disorders of the ovary and female reproductive tract. In: Braunwald E, Isselbacher KJ, Petersdorf RG, et al, eds. *Harrison's Principles of Internal Medicine*, 11th ed. New York, NY: McGraw-Hill; 1987:1818-1837.)

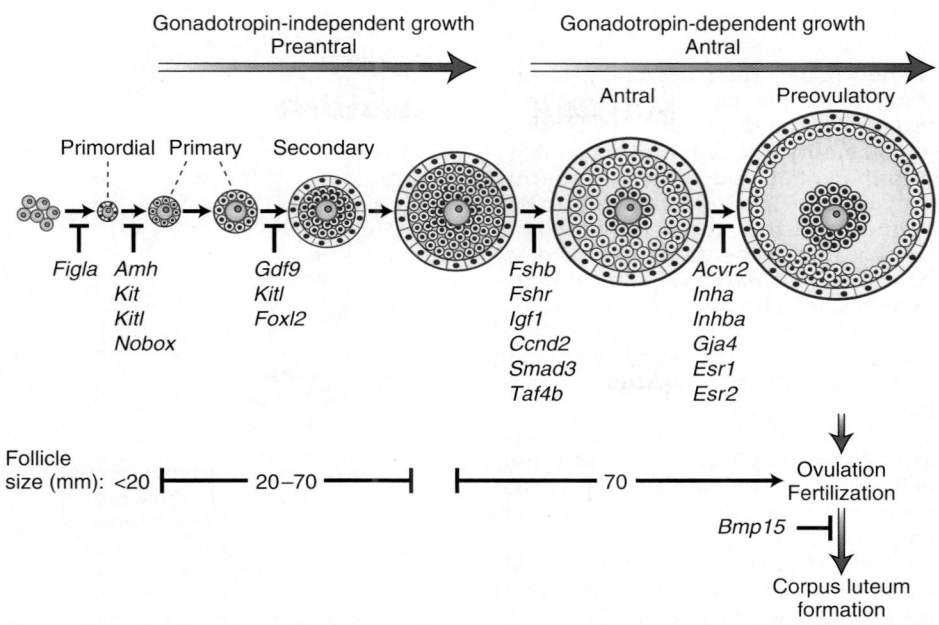

Figure 17-7 Developmental stages at which certain murine genes affect oogenesis. Data from transgenic mice with disruption of various genes have delineated critical roles of several genes during various phases of the follicular development. Preantral follicular growth is thought to be gonadotropin independent, whereas antrum formation and follicular maturation require the action of follicle-stimulating hormone (FSH). Acvr2, activin type II receptor; Amh, antimüllerian hormone; Bmp15, bone morphogenetic protein-15; Ccnd2, cyclin d2; Esr1, estrogen receptor-α; Esr2, estrogen receptor-β; Figla, factor in the germline-α; Foxl2, forkhead box L2; Fshb, FSH β-subunit; Fshr, FSH receptor; GDF-9, growth differentiation factor 9; Gja4, gap junction protein connexin 37; Igf1, insulin-like growth factor 1; Inha, inhibin α-subunit; Inhba, activin βA-subunit; Kit, kit receptor; Kitl, kit-ligand; Nobox, newborn oogenesis homeobox gene; Smad3, Sma mothers against decapentaplegic-3; Taf4b, TATA-box-binding protein-associated factor-4b. (Modified from Simpson JL, Rajkovic A. Ovarian differentiation and gonadal failure. *Am J Med Genet.* 1999;89:186-2000; and Choi Y, Rajkovic A. Genetics of mammalian folliculogenesis. *Cell Mol Life Sci.* 2006;63:579-590.)

potential to become active in steroidogenesis or to form androgen-secreting tumors. These cells are similar to the testosterone-producing Leydig cells of the testes.

The outermost portion of the cortex, called the *tunica albuginea*, is covered by a single layer of surface cuboidal epithelium called the *germinal epithelium*. The oocytes, enclosed in complexes called *follicles*, are in the inner part of the cortex, embedded in stromal tissue. One dominant follicle is recruited for ovulation during each cycle (see Fig. 17-6). The preovulatory follicle transforms into a corpus luteum after ovulation. In the absence of pregnancy, the corpus luteum regresses to become the corpus albicans (see Fig. 17-6). The stromal tissue is composed of connective tissue and interstitial cells, which are derived from mesenchymal cells and are presumed to have the ability to respond to LH or hCG with the production of androstenedione. The central medullary area of the ovary is derived largely from mesonephric cells.

Genetic Determinants of Ovarian Differentiation and Folliculogenesis

Nascent components of the human ovary develop long before a distinct ovary-like organ can be discerned. The female germ cells are formed during embryogenesis when the precursors of primordial germ cells differentiate from somatic lineages of the embryo and take a unique route from the base of the yolk sac along the hindgut to reach the genital ridge. This starts the differentiation of female gonads (ovaries) at the genital ridge. The originally undifferentiated gonad differentiates along a female pathway, and the newly formed oocytes proliferate and subsequently enter meiosis.[45]

Ovarian differentiation and folliculogenesis depend on coordinated expression and interaction of a multitude of genes.[50] Targeted gene disruption or insertion in mice has made it possible to inquire about the function of specific genes in ovarian differentiation and folliculogenesis. Figure 17-7 summarizes the biologic roles of some of these genes.[50] Genetically altered mice represent a first step in attempts to understand in vivo the various gene interactions that result in a functional ovary. Ovarian pathologic conditions in transgenic mice closely resemble disorders observed in mutant human homologues, as exemplified in cases involving the FSH β-subunit and FSH receptor. Many mouse models of ovarian pathologic conditions are available.[45,50] They can be divided into mice that have prenatal ovarian insufficiency with disordered gonad formation and diminished number of germ cells or absent germ cells and mice that have postnatal ovarian insufficiency as a result of defects at various stages of folliculogenesis (see Fig. 17-7).[50] These models should lead to the identification of genetic and molecular mechanisms responsible for the development and function of the human ovary.

In humans, certain gene defects give rise to specific defects in folliculogenesis. This was demonstrated by the discovery of a heterozygous mutation in the bone morphogenetic protein 15 gene *(BMP15)* that caused ovarian dysgenesis. BMP15 is a growth and differentiation factor that is primarily expressed in the oocyte and stimulates folliculogenesis and granulosa cell growth. In vitro, mutant BMP15 reduced granulosa cell growth and antagonized the stimulatory activity of wild-type protein on granulosa cell proliferation. In vivo, this mutation was associated with familial ovarian dysgenesis, indicating that the action of BMP15 is required for progression of human folliculogenesis.[51] A comprehensive discussion of genes responsible for ovarian development, folliculogenesis, and ovulation is provided in an excellent review article by Edson and colleagues.[45]

Oocytes

The fertilization of an oocyte by a spermatozoon gives rise to a zygote that starts to divide rapidly. An eight-cell embryo is formed usually on the third day after fertilization. Up to that point, all embryonic cells are morphologically identical, truly totipotential, and capable of starting a new individual or any lineage. The formation of a 16-cell morula marks the beginning of the process of differentiation, with cells being allocated to the inside or outside of the embryo. At the next stage, the blastocyst, three lineages are defined: trophectoderm, which is the precursor of the placenta; epiblast, which gives rise to the somatic cells of the embryo; and primitive endoderm, which eventually forms the yolk sac. After the embryo implants, a group of cells within the epiblast form the precursors of the primordial germ cells, the first cells of the future ovary to be defined.[45] The extraembryonic trophectoderm and primitive endoderm, which surround the epiblast cells of the postimplantation egg cylinder, are the sources of signals that instruct this small number of epiblast cells to become primordial germ cells; the rest of the cells commence differentiation into somatic tissues. The first primordial germ cell precursors express a key protein named PRDM1 (PRDI-BF1-RIZ domain containing 1, formerly called BLIMP1); these precursor cells represent the first cells of the mammalian embryo with committed cell fates.[45]

The primordial germ cells first become recognizable as a cluster of cells that stain intensely for alkaline phosphatase activity; these epiblast cells are observed at the base of the yolk sac before formation of the allantois.[45] Studies have confirmed that these cells are the only primordial germ cells, because their ablation results in embryos without germ cells, whereas transplantation of these cells leads to their proliferation followed by migration to the genital ridge.[45]

With the use of alkaline phosphatase as a marker, migration of these primordial germ cells from the yolk sac–epiblast junction to the indifferent gonad can be tracked; eventually, the ovary forms and permits the primordial germ cells to differentiate into oocytes. The oocytes enter meiosis and subsequently arrest. Entry into meiosis marks the developmental stage at which any progenitor cells that are capable of differentiating to oocytes disappear. The meiotically arrested oocytes eventually become surrounded by pre-granulosa cells and form individual primordial follicles, the resting pool of oocytes that have the potential to be recruited into the growing follicle pool during the postpubertal stage to be fertilized and to contribute to the next generation. These phenomena have been primarily observed in mice and are thought to be applicable to humans.[45]

Primordial germ cells of epiblast origin migrate to cross a remarkably long distance from the base of the yolk sac to the genital ridge in the fetus by ameboid movements with the aid of pseudopodia.[52] This long route of migration along the dorsal mesentery of the hindgut is interrupted only by the required lateral crossing of the coelomic angle at the level of the genital ridge (Fig. 17-8). The triggers that initiate primordial germ cell migration and the chemoattractants required for directional movement toward the genital ridge are beginning to be uncovered. A critical trigger may be expression of a key receptor on the primordial germ cell and expression of the secreted chemoattractants from the genital ridge. For example, suppression of transforming growth factor-β (TGF-β) signaling leads to enhanced migration due to reduction in the levels of TGF-β–induced collagen type 1 in the extracellular matrix.[53] An extracellular matrix gradient along the path of migra-

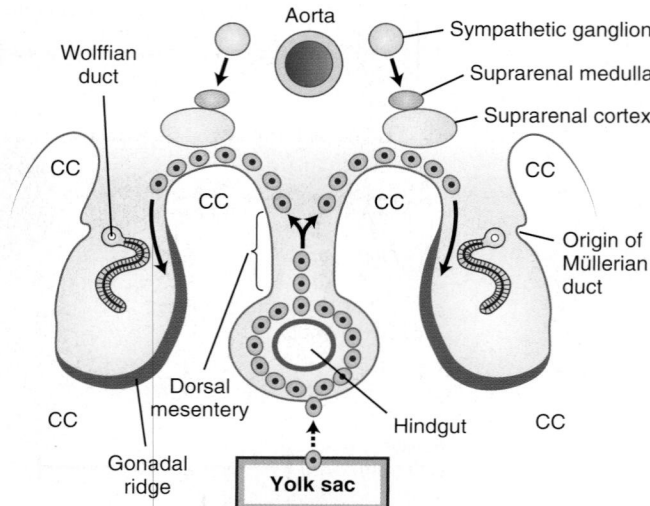

Figure 17-8 Transverse section of the caudal region of a 5-week embryo shows the location of gonadal ridges, the primordium of the adrenal glands, and the migration path of primordial germ cells. From the third week on, germ cells of epiblast origin located at the base of the yolk sac cross the dorsal mesentery of the hindgut and migrate to the gonadal ridges. By the end of the fifth week, rapid division of primordial germ cells, gonadal epithelium, and mesenchyme starts the early gonad that differentiates subsequently into the ovary in a 46,XX fetus. CC, coelomic cavity. (Modified from Moore K. *The Developing Human.* Philadelphia, PA: WB Saunders; 1983.)

tion is important, and if too much matrix is laid down, germ cells show reduced migration. The KIT ligand (KITLG) may function as an effective chemoattractant for the primordial germ cells. The phosphatidylinositol 3-kinase (PI3K)/AKT and SRC kinase pathways are involved downstream of KIT in the primordial germ cell.[54]

Germ cells appear to be unable to persist outside the genital ridge, which may be viewed as the only region competent to sustain gonadal development. By the same token, germ cells play an indispensable role in the induction of gonadal development. No functional gonad can form in the absence of germ cells.

On arrival at the genital ridge by the fifth week of gestation, the premeiotic germ cells are referred to as *oogonia.*[55] During the subsequent 2 weeks of intrauterine life (weeks 5 to 7 of gestation, or the *indifferent stage*), the primordial gonadal structure constitutes no more than a bulge on the medial aspect of the urogenital ridge (see Fig. 17-8). This protuberance is created by proliferation of surface (coelomic) germinal epithelium, by growth of the underlying mesenchyme, and by oogonial multiplication. The oogonia total 10,000 by about 6 to 7 weeks of intrauterine life.[55] Because meiosis and oogonial atresia are not occurring, the actual number of germ cells is dictated by mitotic division at this time.[55]

During the indifferent phase, the gonadal cortex and medulla are first delineated. However, short of cytogenetic evidence, the precise sexual identity of the gonadal ridge cannot be ascertained at this point. Nevertheless, the absence of testicular development beyond 7 weeks' gestation is considered presumptive evidence of formation of the ovary. Additional clues to the sexual identity of the gonad can be derived from the detection of oogonial meiosis at about 8 weeks' gestation, because no comparable process is observed in the testis until puberty. The sexual identity of the gonadal ridge is histologically clear by 16 weeks' gestation, when the first primordial follicles can be visualized.

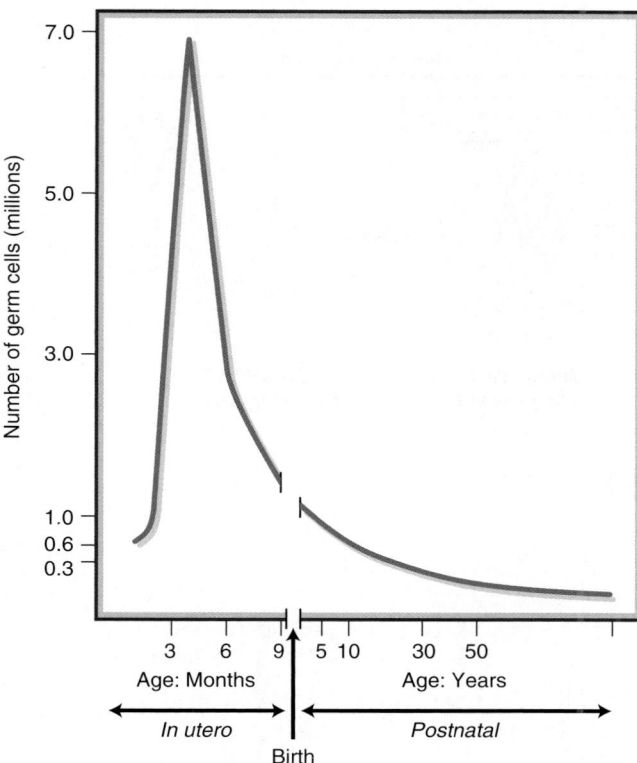

Figure 17-9 Age-dependent changes in germ cell number in the human ovary. The highest number of oocytes is found in the ovaries of a human fetus at midgestation. This number decreases sharply during the third trimester. After birth, the progressive decline in the number of ovarian follicles containing oocytes continues until complete depletion at menopause. (From Baker TG. A quantitative and cytological study of germ cells in the human ovaries. *Proc R Soc Biol Sci.* 1963;158:417-433.)

By about 8 weeks of intrauterine life, persistent mitosis increases the total number of oogonia to 600,000 (Fig. 17-9). From this point on, the oogonial endowment is subject to three simultaneous processes: mitosis, meiosis, and oogonial atresia. Stated differently, the onset of oogonial meiosis and oogonial atresia is superimposed on oogonial mitosis. As a result of the combined impact of these processes, the number of germ cells peaks at 6 to 7×10^6 by 20 weeks' gestation (see Fig. 17-9). At this time, two thirds of the total germ cells are intrameiotic primary oocytes; the remaining third can still be viewed as oogonial. The midgestational peak and the postpeak decline are accounted for in part by the progressively decreasing rate of oogonial mitosis, a process destined to end entirely by about the seventh month of intrauterine life. Equally relevant is the increasing rate of oogonial atresia, which peaks at 5 months' gestation. During this period, regulation of the ovarian developmental process is complex and probably involves a diverse group of genes (see Fig. 17-7).

From midgestation onward, relentless and irreversible attrition progressively diminishes the germ cell endowment of the gonad.[56] About 50 years later, it is exhausted. For the most part, this is accomplished through follicular atresia rather than oogonial atresia, begins at about month 6 of gestation, and continues throughout life (see Fig. 17-9). In contrast, oogonial atresia is destined to end at 7 months of intrauterine life as follicular atresia sets in. Follicular atresia has a profound effect on germ cell endowment, because only 1 to 2×10^6 germ cells are present at birth (see Fig. 17-9).[56] Remarkably, this dramatic depletion of the germ cell mass occurs during a period as short as 20

weeks. No similar rate of depletion occurs earlier or subsequently. Consequently, newborn girls enter life still far from realizing their reproductive potential but having lost as much as 80% of their germ cell endowment. The germ cell mass decreases further to approximately 300,000 by the onset of puberty. Of these follicles, only 400 to 500 (<1% of the total) are recruited for ovulation in the course of a reproductive life span.

Between weeks 8 and 13 of fetal life, some of the oogonia depart from the mitotic cycle to enter the prophase of the first meiotic division. This change marks the conversion of these cells to primary oocytes well before actual follicle formation. Meiosis (beginning at about 8 weeks' gestation) provides temporary protection from oogonial atresia, allowing the germ cells to invest themselves with granulosa cells and to form primordial follicles. Oogonia that persist beyond the seventh month of gestation and have not entered meiosis are subject to oogonial atresia; consequently, no oogonia are usually present at birth.

Once formed, the primary oocyte persists in prophase of the first meiotic division until the time of ovulation, when meiosis is resumed and the first polar body is formed and extruded (Fig. 17-10). Although the exact cellular mechanisms responsible for this meiotic arrest remain uncertain, it is presumed that a granulosa cell–derived meiosis inhibitor is in play. This hypothesis is based on the observation that denuded (granulosa-free) oocytes are capable of spontaneously completing meiotic maturation in vitro.

The primary oocyte is converted into a secondary oocyte by completion of the first meiotic metaphase and formation of the first polar body, which occurs before ovulation but after the LH surge. At ovulation, the secondary oocyte and the surrounding granulosa cells (cumulus oophorus) are extruded and enter the fallopian tube. If sperm penetration occurs, the secondary oocyte undergoes a second meiotic division, after which the second polar body is eliminated (see Fig. 17-10).

Granulosa Cell Layer

In the developing ovaries of a human female fetus, oocytes initially exist as germ cell clusters before an ovarian follicle is formed. During the second half of in utero life, these germ cell clusters break down, and the surviving oocytes become individually surrounded with squamous pregranulosa cells to give rise to primordial follicles. The transition from primordial to primary follicle is marked histologically by a morphologic change in granulosa cells from squamous to cuboidal. By the secondary stage, there are at least two layers of cuboidal granulosa cells and an additional layer of somatic cells, the theca, which forms outside the basement membrane of the follicle (Fig. 17-11).[45] At puberty, FSH secreted by the pituitary promotes further granulosa cell proliferation and survival.

A basement lamina separates the oocyte and granulosa cells from the surrounding stromal cells.[55] The granulosa cells do not have direct access to the circulation before ovulation (Fig. 17-12).

The avascular nature of the granulosa cell compartment necessitates contact between neighboring cells. The granulosa cells are interconnected by extensive intercellular gap junctions, which result in their coupling to yield an expanded, integrated, and functional syncytium (Fig. 17-13).[57] Gap junctions are composed of proteins called *connexins*. Connexin 37 and other connexins have been demonstrated in gap junctions in follicles. Gap junction protein connexin 37 (GJA4)–deficient mice lack graafian follicles, fail to ovulate, and develop inappropriate corpora

Meiosis I

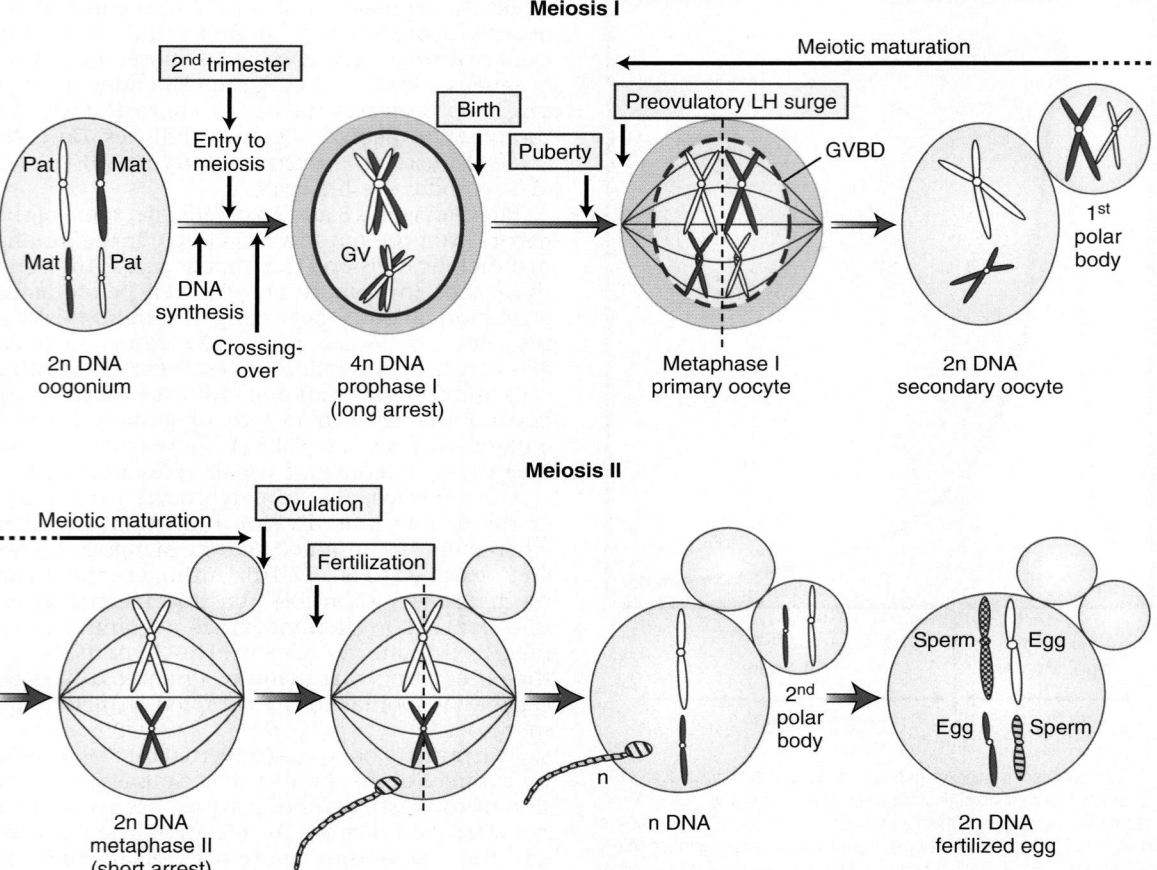

Figure 17-10 Meiotic cell division. During meiosis, the chromosomes that were inherited from the parents of the individual and stored in gonads are processed to prepare their genetic material for transmission to the offspring. Meiosis occurs exclusively in germ cells and serves two critical purposes: generation of germ cells genetically distinct from the somatic cells and generation of a mature egg (or sperm) with a reduction in the number of chromosomes from 46 to 23. Genetic recombination through crossover of genes between homologous chromosomes and random assortment of (grand-) maternal and (grand-) paternal chromosomes into daughter cells during the first meiotic division are responsible for the first function of meiosis, maintenance of genetic diversity. The second function is provided by a reduction in the number of chromosomes so that each daughter cell, or ovum, receives randomly one chromosome from each of the 23 pairs. During fertilization, the fusion of ovum and sperm, each of which contributes 23 chromosomes, produces a genetically novel individual with 46 chromosomes. The chromosome marked as *white* in the oogonium *(upper left corner)* originates from the father of the female fetus, whereas the *blue* chromosome comes from the mother of the fetus. The random exchange of genes (alleles) between homologous chromosomes (crossover) takes place before the meiotic arrest in the prophase I stage before birth. After birth, the oocytes of this child remain in meiotic arrest until puberty. In the developing oocyte in the graafian follicle, meiosis I is resumed immediately after the preovulatory luteinizing hormone (LH) surge during each ovulatory cycle. Meiotic maturation is defined as the period from the breakdown of the oocyte's nucleus (germinal vesicle [GV]) until the oocyte reaches metaphase II (i.e., transition from oocyte to egg). A second and short meiotic arrest occurs at metaphase II until the oocyte is fertilized by a sperm. DNA, deoxyribonucleic acid; GVBD, germinal vesicle breakdown; Mat, maternal; n, amount of DNA material in the haploid number (23) of chromosomes; Pat, paternal.

lutea.[57] These specialized cell junctions may be important in metabolic exchange and in the transport of small molecules between neighboring granulosa cells. Moreover, the granulosa cells extend cytoplasmic processes that penetrate the zona pellucida to form gap junctions with the plasma membrane of the oocyte (see Fig. 17-13). In the GJA4-deficient mice, oocyte development is arrested before meiotic competence.[58] Gap junctions represent a crucial communication system that is needed for the tight control exerted by the cumulus granulosa cells on the resumption of meiosis by the enclosed primary oocyte.

Several gene products regulate the transition from primordial to primary follicle, which is marked by a change in the morphologic appearance of granulosa cells from squamous to cuboidal, followed by an increase in granulosa cell layers in the secondary follicle.[45] These genes are expressed in the oocyte or granulosa cells, emphasizing the active role of the oocyte in granulosa cell differentiation. Newborn oogenesis homeobox (NOBOX), spermatogenesis and oogenesis helix-loop-helix 1 (SOHLH1), and SOHLH2

are critical transcription factors during the transition from primordial to primary follicles.[45] Interactions between KITLG expressed in granulosa cells and the KIT tyrosine kinase receptor expressed in oocytes also appear to be critical in early folliculogenesis. The KITLG/KIT pathway induces the PI3K/AKT pathway, leading to phosphorylation and inactivation of forkhead box O3 (FOXO3), an inhibitor of primordial follicle activation.[45] These genetic studies supported a critical role of the PI3K/AKT/FOXO3 pathway in early follicle development and granulosa cell differentiation. Whereas FOXO3 is the key oocyte factor critical for suppressing primordial follicle activation, another forkhead domain transcription factor, forkhead box L2 (FOXL2), is crucial in the transition from squamous to cuboidal granulosa cells.[45]

Antimüllerian hormone (AMH) produced by the granulosa cells of growing follicles appears to inhibit the growth of primordial follicles, and in its absence, there is a faster depletion of growing follicles, although it is unknown whether this is a direct or indirect effect of AMH.[45]

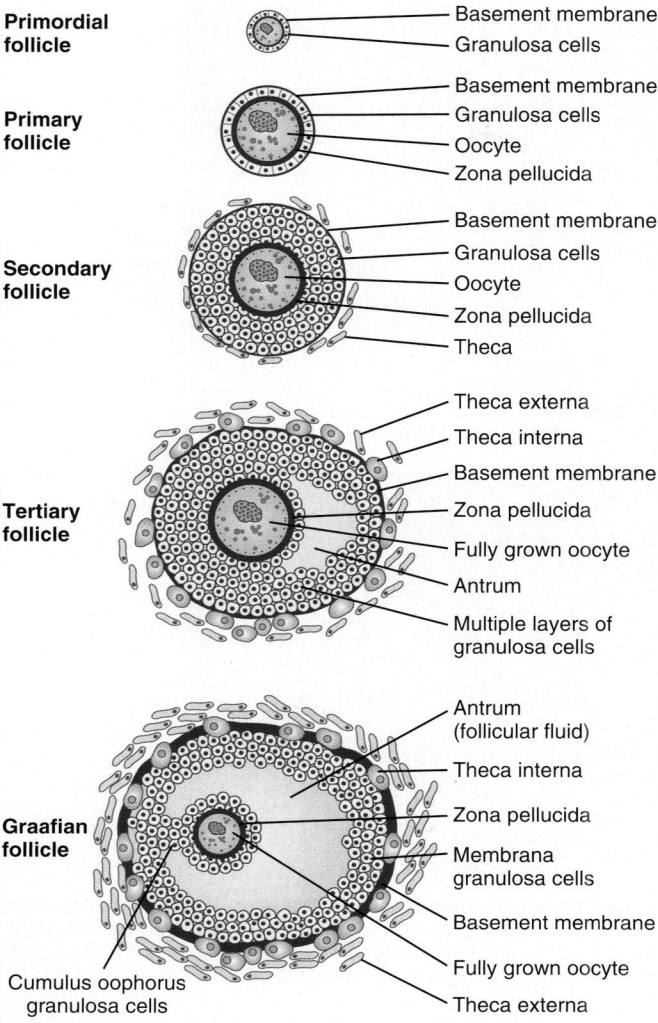

Primordial follicle
— Basement membrane
— Granulosa cells

Primary follicle
— Basement membrane
— Granulosa cells
— Oocyte
— Zona pellucida

Secondary follicle
— Basement membrane
— Granulosa cells
— Oocyte
— Zona pellucida
— Theca

Tertiary follicle
— Theca externa
— Theca interna
— Basement membrane
— Zona pellucida
— Fully grown oocyte
— Antrum
— Multiple layers of granulosa cells

Graafian follicle
— Antrum (follicular fluid)
— Theca interna
— Zona pellucida
— Membrana granulosa cells
— Basement membrane
— Fully grown oocyte
— Theca externa

Cumulus oophorus granulosa cells

Figure 17-11 Developmental stages of the ovarian follicle. The primordial follicle is composed of a single layer of granulosa cells and a single immature oocyte arrested in the diplotene stage of the first meiotic division. The primordial follicle is separated from the surrounding stroma by a thin basal lamina (i.e., basement membrane). The oocyte and granulosa cells do not have a direct blood supply. The first sign of follicular recruitment is cuboidal differentiation in the spindle-shaped cells inside the basal lamina, which thereafter undergo successive mitotic divisions to form a multilayered granulosa cell zone. The oocyte enlarges and secretes a glycoprotein-containing mucoid substance called the zona pellucida, which surrounds the oocyte and separates the granulosa cells from the oocyte. This structure is a primary follicle. The secondary follicle is formed by further proliferation of granulosa cells and by the final phase of oocyte growth, in which the oocyte reaches 120 μm in diameter, coincident with proliferation of layers of cells immediately outside the basal lamina to constitute the theca. The portion of the theca adjacent to the basal lamina is called the *theca interna*. Theca cells that merge with the surrounding stroma are designated the *theca externa*. The secondary follicle acquires an independent blood supply consisting of one or more arterioles that terminate in a capillary bed at the basal lamina. Capillaries do not penetrate the basement membrane, and the granulosa and oocyte remain avascular. The tertiary follicle is characterized by further hypertrophy of the theca and the appearance of a fluid-filled space among the granulosa cells, called the *antrum*. The fluid in the antrum consists of a plasma transudate and secretory products of granulosa cells, some of which (estrogens) are found there in strikingly higher concentrations than in peripheral blood. The follicle rapidly increases in size under the influence of gonadotropins to form the mature or graafian follicle. In the graafian follicle, the granulosa and oocyte remain encased by the basal lamina and are devoid of direct vascularization. The antral fluid increases in volume, and the oocyte, surrounded by an accumulation of granulosa cells (i.e., cumulus oophorus), occupies a polar, eccentric position within the follicle. The mature graafian follicle is then ready to release the ovum by the process of ovulation. (Adapted from Erickson GF, Magoffin DA, Dyer CA. The ovarian androgen producing cells: a review of structure-function relations. *Endocr Rev.* 1985;6:371-379. Copyright © 1985 by The Endocrine Society.)

Clinically, serum AMH may be a useful biomarker of ovarian reserve. In humans and mice, serum AMH declines with increasing age. Although it is difficult to establish a direct link between serum AMH and the primordial follicle pool in humans, antral follicle number is positively correlated with AMH levels.[45] More detailed information has been reviewed by Edson and colleagues.[45]

The granulosa cells in the fully developed graafian follicle shortly before ovulation are stratified in a manner that allows the distinction of a number of populations of cells.[59] Distinct populations of granulosa cells exhibit specific, specialized functions.[59,60] Mural granulosa cells within the outermost layer adjacent to the basement layer contain high levels of gonadotropin hormone receptors and steroidogenic enzymes and account for most of the steroidogenesis in the follicle.[59,60] The *cumulus oophorus* contains the egg and a surrounding mass of granulosa cells that have cell-cell interactions with the egg and seem to have critical roles in oocyte development (see Figs. 17-12 and 17-13).[59,60]

Mural and cumulus granulosa cells also exhibit distinct patterns of gene expression. For example, the tumor suppressor BRCA1 is highly expressed in ovarian granulosa cells of developing follicles.[61] However, in large antral or preovulatory follicles, BRCA1 expression significantly decreases in mural granulosa cells and becomes restricted to cumulus granulosa cells; these cells, unlike the mural ones, do not contain abundant aromatase, so this development gives rise to an intriguing inverse correlation of BRCA1 with aromatase mRNA and protein levels.[61] Stimulation of an FSH-dependent signaling pathway greatly induces aromatase but suppresses BRCA1 expression in granulosa cells. Moreover, BRCA1 binds to the aromatase promoter and inhibits its activity.[62] Therefore, BRCA1 may exert its tumor suppressor activity, in part, by limiting excessive estrogen formation in the ovary. A summary of ovarian follicle development is presented in Figure 17-11.

Theca Cell Layer

After the follicle achieves two layers of granulosa cells, another morphologically distinct layer of somatic cells, the theca, differentiates from ovarian stroma (see Figs. 17-11 to 17-13).[45] The cells making up the theca-interstitial compartment are heterogeneous in nature.[63] Cells of the theca interna layer, which forms just outside the basement membrane surrounding the granulosa cells, show typical steroidogenic features, including mitochondria with tubular cristae, smooth endoplasmic reticulum, and abundant lipid vesicles (see Figs. 17-11 and 17-12). Theca interna cells are responsible for producing the C19 steroids that diffuse into the neighboring granulosa cells and serve as substrates for estrogen production. Theca externa is the outermost layer of the follicle and is composed of fibroblasts, smooth muscle–like cells, and macrophages (see Figs. 17-11 and 17-12). The theca externa is thought to have an important function during ovulation. Cells that contribute to the theca differentiate from mesenchymal precursor cells present in the ovarian stroma, adjacent to developing follicles. Like preantral folliculogenesis, theca formation is gonadotropin-independent. Thecal precursor cells lack LH receptors, and the theca layer still forms in the ovaries of FSH-deficient mice.[45] After a discernible theca interna layer has developed, theca cell C19 steroid production is regulated primarily by LH.

The differentiated state of theca interna cells is marked by expression of a number of steroidogenic genes, including those that encode the LH receptor *(LHCGR)*; steroidogenic acute regulatory protein *(STAR)*; side-chain cleavage enzyme *(CYP11A1)*; 3β-hydroxysteroid dehydrogenase-Δ[5,4]

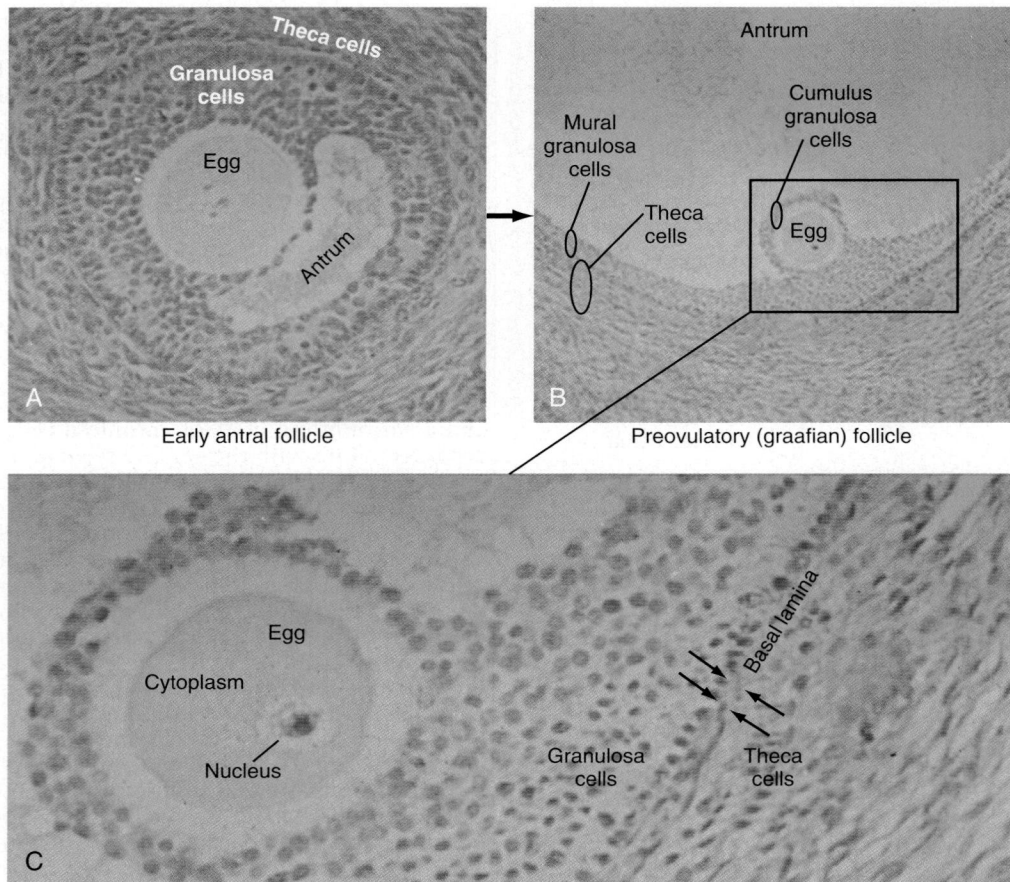

Figure 17-12 Histology of gonadotropin-dependent ovarian follicle development. **A,** Development of an antrum marks gonadotropin dependency. Multiple layers of granulosa and theca cells are present. **B,** The follicle destined to ovulate distinguishes itself from the rest of the cohort through accumulation of large quantities of antral fluid. The granulosa cells, which accumulate around the oocyte, are called *cumulus granulosa cells* and primarily function to support egg development. The mural granulosa cells in the periphery primarily serve as steroidogenic cells. **C,** A membrane called the *basal lamina (arrows),* which has been formed at the primary stage, separates the granulosa cells from the theca component of the follicle.

isomerase type 2 *(HSD3B2)*; and 17-hydroxylase/17,20-lyase *(CYP17A1)* in the human. Granulosa cells of the developing follicles appear to secrete factors that regulate theca cell differentiation. Candidate factors that may contribute to theca cell differentiation include insulin-like growth factor (IGF), KITLG, and growth differentiation factor 9 (GDF9). IGF-1 induces expression of *Lhcgr, Cyp11a1,* and *Hsd3b1* (counterpart of human *HDS3B2*), whereas KITLG stimulates *Star* and *Cyp17a1* expression in rat theca cells.[45] In mice lacking the *Gdf9* gene, a theca layer fails to form in the ovary. Whether *GDF9* regulates theca cell recruitment or differentiation directly or indirectly through regulation of preantral granulosa cell development is unknown.[45]

Follicles

The follicle represents the key functional unit in the ovary with respect to germ cell development and steroid production. The follicles are embedded in loose connective tissue of the ovarian cortex and can be subdivided into two functional types: nongrowing (primordial) and growing. Between 90% and 95% of follicles are nongrowing throughout reproductive life. Recruitment of a primordial follicle initiates dramatic changes in growth, structure, and function. The growing follicles are divided into four stages: primary, secondary, tertiary, and graafian (see Figs. 17-7

and 17-11). The first three stages of growth can occur in the absence of the pituitary and therefore appear to be controlled by intraovarian mechanisms (see Figs. 17-7 and 17-11). The follicle destined to ovulate is recruited during the first few days of the current cycle.[64]

The early growth of follicles occurs over several menstrual cycles, but the ovulatory follicle is one of a cohort recruited at the time of transition from the previous cycle's luteal phase to the current cycle's follicular phase.[64] The total time to achieve preovulatory status is approximately 85 days.[64] Most of this developmental period is FSH-independent. Eventually, this cohort of follicles reaches a stage at which, unless recruited by FSH, the next step is atresia. A cohort of follicles measuring 2 to 5 mm in diameter is continuously available for a response to FSH. The late luteal increase in FSH is the critical feature in rescuing this cohort of follicles from atresia; it allows a dominant follicle to emerge and pursue a path to ovulation. The increase in the FSH level must be maintained for a critical period (see Fig. 17-1).[65]

Recruited primordial follicles either develop into dominant, mature graafian follicles destined to ovulate or degenerate as a result of atresia.[66] The average time for development of a selected follicle to the point of ovulation is 10 to 14 days. If a follicle is not recruited, it goes through a process called *atresia*, during which the oocyte and granulosa cells within the basal lamina die and are replaced by

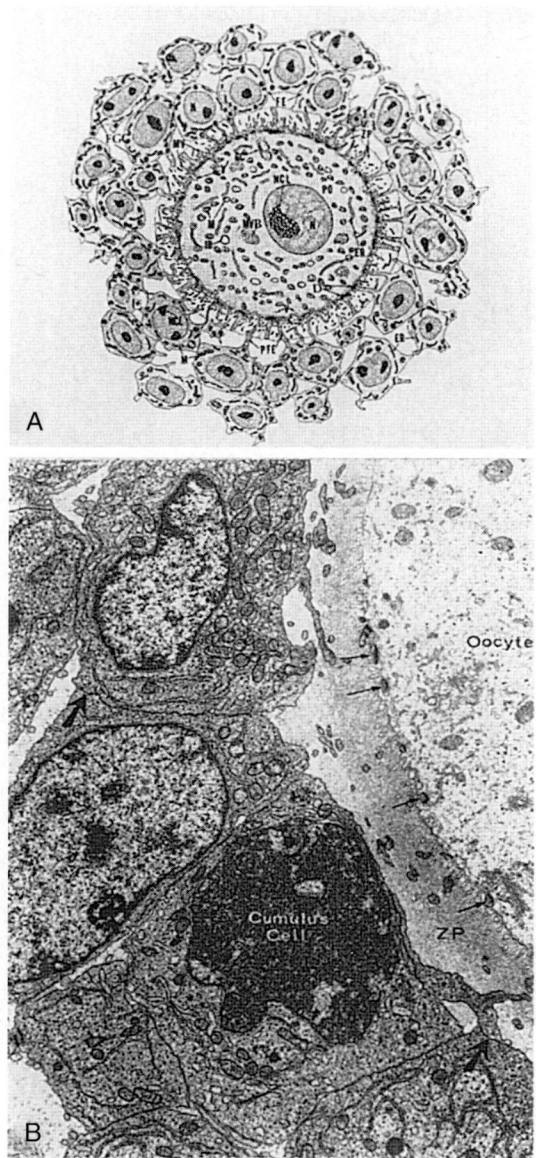

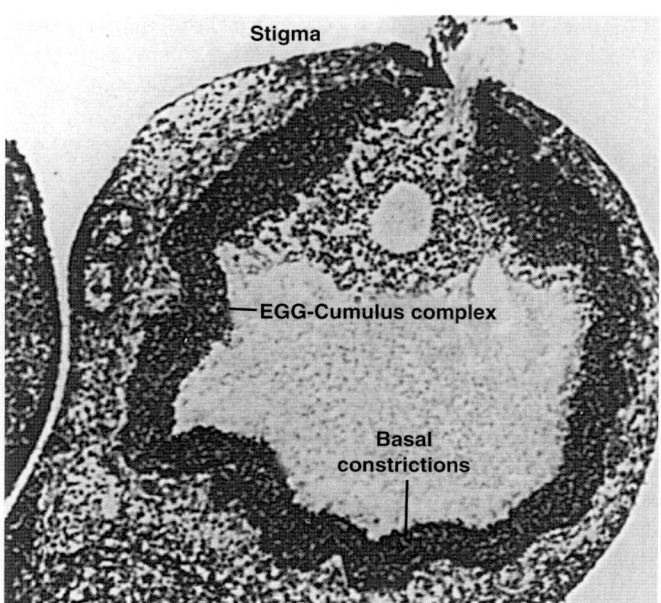

Figure 17-14 Ovulation of the cumulus-oocyte complex through the stigma. (From Erickson GF. An analysis of follicle development and ovum maturation. *Semin Reprod Endocrinol.* 1986;4:233, used with permission of Thieme Medical Publishers, New York.)

Figure 17-13 Structural relationship between the cumulus granulosa cell and the oocyte. **A,** Microvilli of an oocyte interdigitate with cytoplasmic extensions of granulosa cells, penetrating the zona pellucida. **B,** Notice the penetration of the zona pellucida (ZP) by cytoplasmic processes of the granulosa cells. Small gap junctions *(thin arrows)* are observed between processes of the granulosa cell and the oocyte membrane. The *thick arrows* indicate a gap junction between granulosa cells. (From Erickson GF. An analysis of follicle development and ovum maturation. *Semin Reprod Endocrinol.* 1986;4:233, used with permission of Thieme Medical Publishers, New York.)

fibrous tissue. There is general agreement that atresia of follicles occurs through apoptosis.[67]

Ovulation

There is a dramatic rise in circulating estradiol level as midcycle approaches. This is followed by a striking LH surge and, to a lesser extent, an FSH surge, which trigger the dominant follicle to ovulate. During each menstrual cycle, usually one follicle ovulates and gives rise to a corpus luteum. In women, LH or its surrogate, hCG, is essential to stimulate rupture of the mature follicle. It has been proposed that increased local prostaglandin biosynthesis in the follicle mediates the ovulatory effect of LH.[68,69]

Ovulation consists of rapid follicular enlargement followed by protrusion of the follicle from the surface of the ovarian cortex. This is followed by the rupture of the follicle and extrusion of an egg-cumulus complex into the peritoneal cavity (Fig. 17-14). Follicular rupture or ovulation occurs predictably 34 to 36 hours after the start of the LH surge. Elevation of a conical *stigma* on the surface of the protruding follicle precedes rupture (see Fig. 17-14). Rupture of this stigma is accompanied by a gentle rather than explosive expulsion of the ovum and antral fluid. A number of transcriptional regulators downstream of the LH receptor are required for ovulation. After the LH surge, progesterone receptor (PR) levels rapidly increase in the mural granulosa cells of the preovulatory follicle.[45] LH- or PR-dependent production of proteases acting locally on protein substrates in the basal lamina may play an important role in stigma formation and follicular rupture.[58,70] In particular, levels of plasminogen activator increase in the follicle before rupture.[71] Plasminogen activator–mediated conversion of plasminogen to plasmin may contribute to the proteolytic digestion of the follicular wall, which is a prerequisite for follicular rupture. Gene knockout studies in mice suggest that other factors important for ovulation or follicular rupture include endothelin 2, peroxisome proliferator-activated receptor-γ (PPARγ), CCAAT/enhancer-binding protein-β, liver receptor homologue 1 (LRH1), steroidogenic factor 1 (SF1), and nuclear receptor–interacting protein 1.[45]

Corpus Luteum

After ovulation, the dominant follicle reorganizes to become the corpus luteum (Fig. 17-15). After rupture of the follicle, capillaries and fibroblasts from the surrounding stroma proliferate and penetrate the basal lamina (see Fig. 17-11). This rapid vascularization of the corpus luteum may be guided by angiogenic factors, some of which are

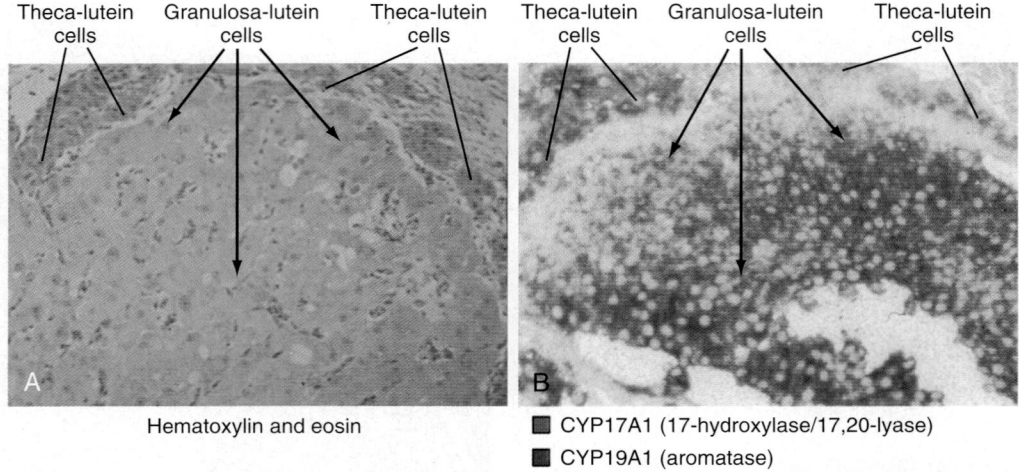

Figure 17-15 Corpus luteum. **A,** Hematoxylin and eosin stain shows the large granulosa-lutein cells occupying the center and smaller theca-lutein cells in the periphery. **B,** Immunoreactive aromatase, the product of the *CYP19A1* gene (brown stain), is the hallmark of granulosa-lutein cells, whereas immunoreactive 17-hydroxylase/17,20-lyase, the product of the *CYP17A1* gene (purple stain), is selectively localized to theca-lutein cells. (Courtesy of Dr. Hironobu Sasano, Tohoku University, Sendai, Japan.)

detected in the follicular fluid.[72] Vascular endothelial growth factor has been isolated from corpora lutea and has been postulated, along with basic fibroblast growth factor, to be a potential angiogenic agent in corpora lutea.[73] Concurrently, the granulosa and theca cells undergo morphologic changes collectively referred to as *luteinization*. The granulosa cells become granulosa-lutein cells (large cells), and the theca cells are transformed into theca-lutein cells (small cells) (see Fig. 17-15).[74] The so-called K cells, scattered throughout the corpus luteum, are believed to be macrophages.

The corpus luteum is the major source of sex steroid hormones secreted by the postovulatory ovary. The human corpus luteum secretes as much as 40 mg of progesterone per day during the midluteal phase of the ovarian cycle.[75] In view of the small size of the corpus luteum, it is the most active steroidogenic tissue in humans. An important aspect of corpus luteum formation is the penetration of the follicle basement membrane by blood vessels. This vascularization provides the granulosa-lutein cells with low-density lipoprotein (LDL) cholesterol.[72] LDL cholesterol serves as the primary substrate for corpus luteum progesterone production.

A key regulator of steroidogenesis in the corpus luteum is LH. In humans, the LH receptor is maintained throughout the functional life span of the corpus luteum and is not downregulated during the maternal recognition of pregnancy.[76] The rate-limiting step in LH-mediated progesterone formation in luteinized granulosa cells is the entry of cholesterol into the mitochondria, which is regulated by the STAR protein.[77] The availability of LDL cholesterol and the STAR-mediated mitochondrial entry of cholesterol into the mitochondria seem to be the two critical factors that account for the production of large amounts of progesterone in the corpus luteum.

Unless pregnancy occurs, the functional life span of the corpus luteum is normally 14 ± 2 days, after which it spontaneously regresses and is replaced by an avascular scar named the *corpus albicans*. There is little doubt about the central role of LH or hCG in the maintenance of corpus luteum function. Withdrawal of LH support in a variety of experimental circumstances has almost invariably resulted in luteal regression.[78] In pregnancy, however, the LH surrogate, hCG, secreted by the gestational trophoblast, maintains the ability of the corpus luteum to elaborate progesterone; this stimulus helps to maintain the early gestation until the luteoplacental shift.[78] The corpus luteum doubles in size (compared with the prepregnancy size) during the first 6 weeks of gestation because of hypertrophy of the luteinized granulosa and theca cells (see Fig. 17-15). This early hypertrophy is followed by regression. The corpus luteum at term is only one half of its size during the menstrual cycle.

Hormones such as estrogens and prostaglandins have been suggested to be important factors in the promotion of luteal demise.[79,80] Immune factors may influence luteal life span because corpus luteal regression is associated with a progressive infiltration of lymphocytes and macrophages. In the absence of LH or hCG, apoptosis is a critical end-point mechanism by which human corpora lutea are deleted.[81]

Ovarian Follicle-Stimulating Hormone and Luteinizing Hormone Receptors

The FSH receptor is expressed exclusively by granulosa cells. The LH or hCG receptor (LHCGR) is expressed primarily by the theca-interstitial cells of all follicles and by granulosa cells of large preovulatory follicles.

Granulosa cells in primary or secondary follicles that are in the early developmental stages before antrum formation primarily bind FSH but not LH. In these preantral follicles, the binding of LH or hCG is confined to theca-interstitial cells.[82] Granulosa cells in more mature tertiary follicles with an antrum appear capable of binding both LH and FSH. The FSH receptors are found in granulosa cells from follicles of all sizes, but LH receptors are found only in granulosa cells of large preovulatory follicles.[83,84] These observations are consistent with the concept that the acquisition of LH receptors on granulosa cells is under the influence of FSH.[85]

The receptors for the glycoprotein hormones have related structures (see Fig. 17-17 later). The receptors belong to the large family of G protein–coupled receptors, whose members all have a transmembrane domain that consists of seven membrane–traversing α-helices connected by three extracellular and three intracellular loops. The glycoprotein hormone receptors form a separate subgroup within this large family by virtue of their large extracellular hormone-binding domain at the amino-terminus. FSH binds to the FSH receptor, and LH and hCG bind to the same LH receptor. The LH and FSH receptor genes are located on chromosome 2 in the p21 region.[43] The carboxy-terminal half of the receptor is encoded by a single last exon and contains the seven transmembrane segments and the G protein–coupling domain. The unusually large extra-cellular domain of the glycoprotein hormone receptors, on the other hand, is encoded by the first 9 or 10 exons.

Role of Follicle-Stimulating Hormone in Ovarian Function. FSH is the main promoter of follicular maturation. Given that FSH receptors have been exclusively localized to granulosa cells, it is presumed that FSH action in the ovary involves the granulosa cells. The ability of FSH to orchestrate follicular growth and differentiation depends on its ability to exert multiple actions concurrently.

Phenotypes of women with mutations that disrupt the function of the FSH β-subunit gene are in good agreement and demonstrate that FSH is necessary for normal follicular development, ovulation, and fertility. Pubertal development is hampered in the absence of sufficient numbers of later-stage follicles with the granulosa cells needed for adequate estrogen production. Treatment of affected patients with exogenous FSH has resulted in follicular maturation, ovulation, and normal pregnancy.[43] The presenting phenotype of FSH β-subunit deficiency is practically identical to that caused by inactivating mutations of the FSH receptor.[43]

Women with FSH receptor mutations are clinically similar to patients with gonadal dysgenesis; they have absent or poorly developed secondary sexual characteristics and high serum levels of FSH and LH. The notable difference is the presence of ovarian follicles in women with mutated FSH receptors, consistent with the FSH independence of primordial follicle recruitment and early follicular growth and development. Total absence of any follicles, including those in the primordial stage, occurs in women in whom FSH receptor mutations cannot be demonstrated.[43] The ovarian phenotype of FSH receptor deficiency is distinct from the common form of gonadal dysgenesis (Turner syndrome), which is characterized by streak gonads and an absence of growing follicles.[43]

In vivo rodent studies suggest that FSH is capable of increasing the number of its own receptors in the granulosa cell. Whereas estradiol by itself may be without effect on the distribution, number, or affinity of granulosa cell FSH receptors, estrogens synergize with FSH to enhance the overall number of granulosa cell FSH receptors.[86] Changes in the production of estradiol by preantral follicles can increase their response to FSH through regulation of granulosa cell surface FSH receptors. This interaction between FSH and estradiol in follicular development has been well established in rodents. It appears that ERα and ERβ mediate the estrogenic effect on ovarian development and follicular maturation in mice.[87] However, it is not clear whether a similar relationship exists in the human ovary. ERα is not detected in the human ovary in significant quantities. Nevertheless, the demonstration of ERβ in the human ovary suggests an interaction between FSH and estrogen in the regulation of normal follicle development and ovulation in women.[88]

One of the major actions of FSH is induction of granulosa cell aromatase activity.[89] Little or no estrogen can be produced by FSH-unprimed granulosa cells even if they are supplied with aromatizable androgen precursors. Treatment with FSH enhances the aromatization capability of granulosa cells, an effect related to enhancement of the granulosa cell aromatase content.[89]

Treatment with FSH has also been shown to induce LH receptors in granulosa cells. The ability of FSH to induce LH receptors is augmented by the concomitant presence of estrogens.[90] Progestins, androgens, and LH itself may also induce LH receptors. After induction, the granulosa cell LH receptor requires the continued presence of FSH for its maintenance.

Circumstantial evidence, deduced from studies of women with disrupting mutations of the genes that encode FSH and LH receptors and aromatase (CYP19A1), indicates that FSH action, but not estrogen or LH action, is essential for follicular growth in humans.[43,90] Follicular growth and development up to the antral stage were observed in women with deficient LH action or estrogen biosynthesis, although these individuals were anovulatory.[43,90] Women with mutations of the FSH β-subunit or FSH receptor have only primordial follicles in their ovaries.[43] These data indicate that estrogen and LH are not critical for follicular development at least until the tertiary stage (see Figs. 17-11 and 17-12). However, FSH by itself is not sufficient to achieve normal follicular development and ovulation.

Role of Luteinizing Hormone in Ovarian Function. LH is essential for ovulation (follicular rupture) and the sustenance of corpus luteum function; in addition, it plays other important roles in follicular function.[90] First, LH probably plays a major role in the promotion of theca-interstitial cell androgen production. Second, LH may well synergize with FSH in the more advanced phases of follicular development. Third, small and sustained increments in the circulating levels of LH are necessary and sufficient to cause small antral follicles to grow and develop to the preovulatory stage.[90]

It is presumed that LH acts on the theca-interstitial cells of small follicles, where it promotes the biosynthesis of C19 steroids.[90] The consequent increase in estrogen production is presumed to contribute to the growth and development of the follicles. Treatment with small doses of LH also results in an increase in LH receptor content and in induction of the key steroidogenic proteins, such as STAR, CYP11A1, HSD3B2, and CYP17A1.[90]

The role of LH action in human ovarian physiology was exemplified by the phenotype of a woman with a disrupting mutation of the LH receptor gene.[43] She presented with amenorrhea, normally developed secondary sexual characteristics, increased circulating FSH and LH levels, and low levels of estradiol and progesterone that were unresponsive to hCG treatment.[43] The ovary contained follicles that developed up to antral stage with a well-developed theca layer but no preovulatory follicles or corpora lutea. These observations collectively support the view that LH is essential for ovulation and sufficient estrogen production, whereas follicular development is initially autonomous but at later stages depends on intact FSH action.[43]

Ovarian Steroidogenesis

The steroid hormone contents of the ovarian vein effluents and peripheral venous blood were compared to distinguish steroids secreted by the ovary from those secreted by the adrenal or produced by peripheral conversion of precursors.[91] These studies revealed that the ovaries secrete pregnenolone, progesterone, 17α-hydroxyprogesterone, dehydroepiandrosterone (DHEA), androstenedione, testosterone, estrone, and estradiol.[92] Although such measurements provide insights into the steroidogenic pathways under study, they do not identify the specific ovarian cells involved. Studies using microdissected preovulatory follicles identified estrone and estradiol as the major steroid products (Fig. 17-16). Progesterone and 17α-hydroxyprogesterone proved to be the major products of the corpus luteum (see Fig. 17-16).

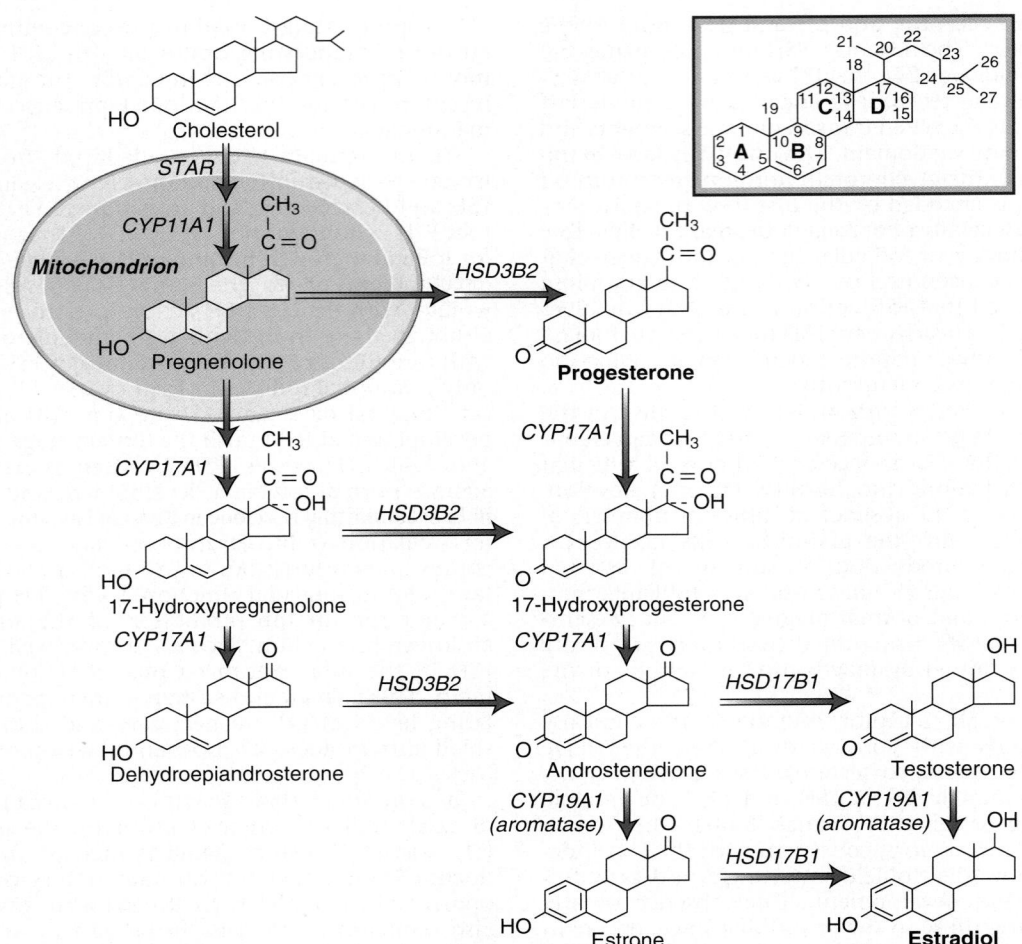

Figure 17-16 Steroidogenic pathway in the human ovary. The biologically active steroids progesterone and estradiol are produced primarily in the ovary of a woman of reproductive age. Estradiol production requires the activity of six steroidogenic proteins, including STAR, and six enzymatic steps. 17-Hydroxylase/17,20-lyase, the product of the *CYP17A1* gene, catalyzes two enzymatic reactions. The four rings of the cholesterol molecule and its derivative steroids are identified by the first four letters in the alphabet, and the carbons are numbered in the sequence shown in the insert. CYP17A1, 17-hydroxylase/17,20-lyase; CYP19A1, aromatase; HSD17B1, 17β-hydroxysteroid dehydrogenase type 1; HSD3B2, 3β-hydroxysteroid dehydrogenase-$\Delta^{5,4}$ isomerase type 2; STAR, steroidogenic acute regulatory protein.

The general steroidogenic pathway for the production of estrogens and androgens is depicted in Figure 17-16. The biologically active ovarian steroids are estradiol and progesterone. The major C19 steroid product of the ovary, androstenedione, is not biologically active. However, it acts as a dual precursor and contributes to circulating levels of estrone and testosterone through conversion in extraglandular tissues such as adipose tissue and skin (discussed later).[93] It is likely that estrogenically weak estrone is further converted to the potent estrogen estradiol and androgenically weak testosterone is converted to the potent androgen dihydrotestosterone (DHT) locally in target tissues such as brain, breast, prostate, and genital skin and subsequently exert potent biologic effects. This notion is supported by the presence in many human tissues of multiple proteins with overlapping enzymatic activities that catalyze these conversions (e.g., reductive 17β-HSD and 5α-reductase).[94]

The preovulatory follicle secretes estradiol during the first half of the menstrual cycle, and the corpus luteum secretes estradiol and progesterone during the second half of the cycle. The production of these two biologically active steroids is orchestrated in the follicle and corpus luteum in a cell-specific manner that is under the control of LH and FSH.

Steroids formed by the ovary and other steroid-producing organs are derived from cholesterol (see Fig. 17-16). Several sources of cholesterol can provide the ovary with substrate for steroidogenesis, including plasma lipoprotein cholesterol, cholesterol synthesized de novo within the ovary, and cholesterol from intracellular stores of cholesterol esters within lipid droplets. In the human ovary, LDL cholesterol is an important source of cholesterol used for steroidogenesis.[75] LH stimulates the activity of adenylate cyclase, increasing production of cyclic adenosine monophosphate (cAMP), which serves as a second messenger to increase LDL receptor mRNA, binding and uptake of LDL cholesterol, and the formation of cholesterol esters.[74,75] LDL-derived cholesterol is particularly essential for normal levels of progesterone production in the granulosa-lutein cells of the corpus luteum.[75]

Steroidogenic Genes and Their Functions in the Ovary

The ovarian granulosa, theca, and corpus luteum cells possess STAR plus five distinct proteins with specific enzyme activities for steroid hormone formation. These steroidogenic enzymes are CYP11A1 (side-chain cleavage of P450), HSD3B2 (3β-hydroxysteroid dehydrogenase-$\Delta^{5,4}$ isomerase type 2), CYP17A1 (17-hydroxylase/17,20-lyase),

CYP19A1 (aromatase), and HSD17B1 (17β-hydroxysteroid dehydrogenase type 1).[89] These enzymes are responsible for the conversion of cholesterol to the two major biologically active products: estradiol and progesterone.[89,93]

The first and rate-limiting step in the synthesis of all ovarian steroid hormones is the movement of cholesterol into the mitochondrion, which is regulated by a mitochondrial membrane protein encoded by the *STAR* gene (see Fig. 17-16).[95] This movement is followed by conversion of cholesterol to pregnenolone, which is catalyzed by the mitochondrial side-chain cleavage enzyme complex consisting of CYP11A1, adrenodoxin, and flavoprotein. LH induces steroidogenesis by increasing the conversion of cholesterol to pregnenolone in two distinct ways: acute regulation, which occurs over minutes through phosphorylation of preexisting STAR and rapid synthesis of new STAR, and chronic stimulation, which occurs within hours to days through the induction of CYP11A1 expression and consequent increased steroidogenesis (Fig. 17-17). STAR increases the flow of cholesterol to mitochondria, regulating substrate availability to CYP11A1 on the inner mitochondrial membrane.[95] In the absence of STAR, only 14% of the maximal STAR-induced level of steroidogenesis persists.[95]

STAR expression in the preovulatory graafian follicle is limited primarily to the theca cells (see Fig. 17-17).[96] The most important product of the theca cell during the follicular phase is the estrogen precursor androstenedione, and its production is controlled primarily by STAR. The biologically active steroid product of the ovary during the follicular phase is estradiol, which arises from the granulosa cells located adjacent to theca cells. The rate-limiting step for granulosa cell estradiol production is regulated by the FSH-dependent activity of the aromatase enzyme in a cyclic fashion.[89] During the luteal phase, cells of the corpus luteum, including granulosa-lutein cells, also show intense STAR immunoreactivity with a patchy distribution.[77,96] The delivery of cholesterol to the mitochondrial side-chain cleavage enzyme system in the corpus luteum is the rate-limiting step for progesterone biosynthesis and is regulated by STAR.[77] Thus, estradiol production seems to be regulated primarily by STAR and aromatase, whereas progesterone biosynthesis may be primarily under the control of STAR.

Steroidogenesis that depends on LH and FSH in theca and granulosa cells is mediated by common signaling molecules, including cAMP and the specific transcription factors SF1, product of the *NR5A1* gene, and LRH1, product of the *NR5A2* gene, which belong to the nuclear receptor family (see Fig. 17-17).[97,98] SF1 and LRH1 regulate the expression of genes that encode STAR, CYP11A1, HSD3B2, CYP17A1, and CYP19A1 (see Fig. 17-17). SF1 and possibly LRH1 can be regarded as downstream master switches that orchestrate ovarian steroidogenesis.[98]

All steroid hormones are derived from cholesterol. C27 cholesterol is converted to the 18-, 19-, and 21-carbon steroid hormones that are secreted by the ovary (see Fig. 17-16).

C21 Steroids. The principal progestogens are C21 steroids and include pregnenolone, progesterone, and 17- hydroxyprogesterone (see Fig. 17-16). Pregnenolone is of primary importance in the ovary because of its key position as a precursor of all steroid hormones.[99] Progesterone, the principal secretory product of the corpus luteum, is responsible for the progestational effects (i.e., cell differentiation and induction of secretory activity in the endometrium of the estrogen-primed uterus).[99] Progesterone is essential for implantation of the fertilized ovum and maintenance of pregnancy. It also induces decidualization of the endometrium, inhibits uterine contractions, increases the vis-

cosity of cervical mucus, promotes lateral (alveolar) development of the breast glands, and increases basal body temperature.[99]

C19 Steroids. The ovary secretes a variety of C19 steroids, including DHEA, androstenedione, and testosterone, all of which primarily serve as distant or immediate precursors for the potent androgen, DHT, or potent estrogen, estradiol (see Fig. 17-16; also see Fig. 17-26).[93] C19 steroids are produced by the theca cells and, possibly, to a lesser degree by the ovarian stroma. The major C19 steroid is androstenedione, part of which is secreted directly into plasma, with the remainder converted to estrogen by the granulosa cells.[89] DHEA and androstenedione do not appear to have major androgenic actions. In the ovary and in peripheral tissues, DHEA is converted to androstenedione, which can be converted to estrone or testosterone.[93] Testosterone is converted locally to DHT at target tissues for full androgenic action or estradiol for estrogenic activity.

C18 Steroids. Estrogen regulates gonadotropin secretion, development of the secondary sexual characteristics of women, uterine growth, thickening of the vaginal mucosa, thinning of the cervical mucus, linear growth of the ductal system of the breast, growth spurt, epiphyseal closure, and bone mineralization.[100] The naturally occurring estrogens are C18 steroids characterized by the presence of an aromatic A ring, a phenolic hydroxyl group at C3, and a hydroxyl group (estradiol) or a ketone group (estrone) at C17.[89,93] Aromatase is the key enzyme for estrogen production in the ovary (see Fig. 17-16).[89] The protein aromatase, encoded by the *CYP19A1* gene, confers the specific activity of the aromatase enzyme complex.

Aromatase mRNA and protein expression and its enzyme activity in the ovarian granulosa cell are regulated primarily by FSH.[89,93] The principal and most potent estrogen secreted by the ovary is estradiol. Although estrone is also secreted by the ovary, another important source of estrone is extraglandular conversion of androstenedione in peripheral tissues.[93] Estriol (16-hydroxyestradiol) is the most abundant estrogen in urine and is produced by metabolism of estrone and estradiol in extraovarian tissues. All C18 steroids, including estrone, estradiol, and estriol, are commonly referred to as estrogens. However, estrone and estriol are only weakly estrogenic and must be converted to estradiol to show full estrogenic action. At least seven enzymes with overlapping activities are capable of converting estrone to estradiol in the ovary and extraovarian tissues.[101]

Catechol estrogens are formed by hydroxylation of estrogens at the C2 or C4 position. The physiologic role of catechol estrogen is unclear. Estrone sulfate, formed by peripheral conversion of estradiol and estrone, is the most abundant estrogen in blood, but it is not physiologically active. Estrone sulfate is presumed to serve as a reservoir for estrone and eventually estradiol formation in a number of tissues, including those that are targets of estrogen.[93]

Two-Cell Theory for Ovarian Steroidogenesis

The classic two-cell theory is supported by molecular findings. Ovarian steroidogenesis in the preovulatory follicle takes place through LH receptors on theca cells and FSH (possibly also LH) receptors on granulosa cells (see Fig. 17-17). cAMP production and increased SF1 (product of the *NR5A1* gene) binding to multiple steroidogenic promoters mediate LH action in theca cells.[102] The STAR protein is the primary regulator of production of androstenedione, which subsequently diffuses into granulosa cells to serve as the estrogen precursor.[93] In the preovulatory follicle, cholesterol in theca cells arises from circulating lipoproteins and de novo biosynthesis. FSH is responsible for follicular

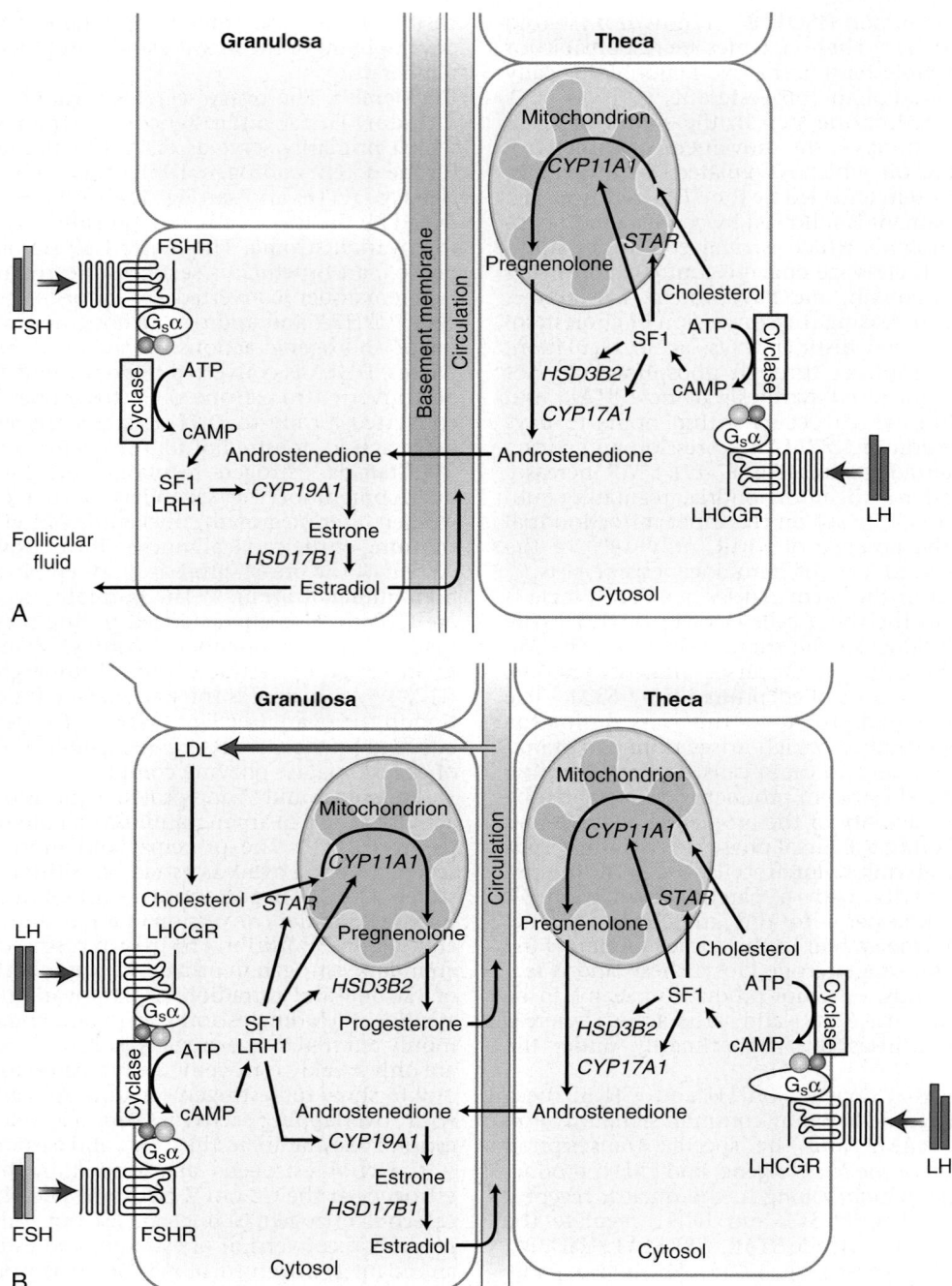

Figure 17-17 Two-cell hypothesis for ovarian steroidogenesis. **A,** The preovulatory follicle produces estradiol through a paracrine interaction between theca and granulosa cells. In response to stimulation with a gonadotropin, steroidogenic factor 1 (SF1, encoded by NR5A1, a member of the nuclear receptor family) acts as a master switch to initiate transcription of a series of steroidogenic genes in theca cells. In follicular granulosa cells, another nuclear receptor, liver homologue receptor 1 (LRH1, encoded by NR5A2), seems to primarily mediate the downstream effects of follicle-stimulating hormone (FSH) in the rodent ovary. In humans, the roles of SF1 and LRH1 in steroidogenesis in pre-ovulatory granulosa cells are not well understood. Because granulosa cells do not have a direct connection to the circulation, CYP19A1 (aromatase) in granulosa cells depends for substrate on androstenedione that diffuses from theca cells. Two critical steps in estradiol formation are the entry of cholesterol into mitochondria facilitated by steroidogenic acute regulatory protein (STAR) in theca cells and the conversion of androstenedione to estrone catalyzed by CYP19A1 in granulosa cells. **B,** In the corpus luteum, granulosa-lutein cells are heavily vascularized, a condition that is critical for entry of abundant quantities of cholesterol into this cell type through primarily low-density lipoprotein (LDL)-cholesterol receptors and for secretion of large amounts of progesterone into the circulation. The entry of cholesterol into mitochondria (mediated by STAR) is probably the most critical steroidogenic step for progesterone formation in granulosa-lutein cells. Androstenedione produced in theca-lutein cells serves as a substrate for estrone, which is further converted to estradiol in granulosa-lutein cells. Human data suggest that LRH1 may mediate at least a portion of gonadotropin-dependent steroidogenesis in the corpus luteum. Gonadotropins, SF1, and possibly LRH1 play key roles for important steroidogenic steps in the ovary. ATP, adenosine triphosphate; cAMP, cyclic adenosine monophosphate; FSHR, FSH receptor; HSD, hydroxysteroid dehydrogenase; LHCGR, LH receptor.

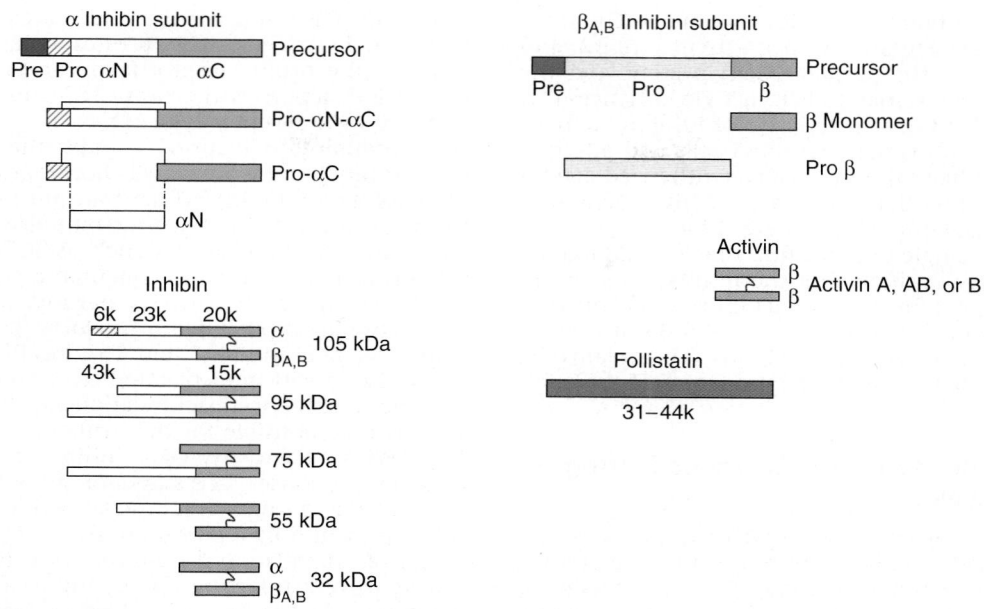

Figure 17-18 Structures of inhibin subunit precursors and processed forms in serum, the activins and the follistatins. The precise contribution of each molecular-weight form of inhibin to the biologic activity in serum is not known, but it has been established that the 55-kDa and 32-kDa forms are biologically active. αN, amino region of alpha-inhibin; αC, carboxy region of alpha-inhibin. (Modified from Burger H. Inhibin, activin and neoplasia. In: Yen SC, Jaffe RB, Barbieri RL, eds. *Reproductive Endocrinology*, 4th ed. Philadelphia, PA: Saunders; 1999:669-675.)

growth and estrogen formation. FSH induces cAMP formation, activation of protein kinase A and certain MAP kinases, and increased binding activity of LRH1 or SF1 to the *CYP191A1* promoter in preovulatory granulosa cells to form estrone and then estradiol primarily through aromatization of androstenedione (see Fig. 17-17). The relative roles of SF1 and LRH1 in estrogen formation in human ovarian granulosa cells are not well understood.[102]

In the corpus luteum, large deposits of cholesterol (which provide the yellow color) arise primarily from circulating lipoproteins to support the production of extremely high quantities of progesterone.[103] Other key anatomic events in formation of the corpus luteum are the disruption of the basement membrane between the granulosa and theca cells and strikingly increased vascularization of granulosa-lutein cells (see Fig. 17-15). Theca-lutein cells possess LH receptors and produce androstenedione. cAMP, SF1, and STAR induced by LH remain as the key regulators for biosynthesis of androstenedione, which serves as the estrogen precursor in neighboring granulosa-lutein cells (see Fig. 17-17).

The granulosa-lutein cell of the corpus luteum is anatomically and functionally different from its counterpart in the preovulatory follicle in several ways. First, these cells are characterized by large and granular cytoplasms, are heavily vascularized, and contain large quantities of cholesterol. Second, granulosa-lutein cells contain high levels of LH receptors in addition to FSH receptors. Third, they produce large quantities of progesterone; this function is regulated primarily by LH and STAR. Granulosa-lutein cells also aromatize androstenedione of thecal origin and eventually give rise to estradiol formation through FSH action and CYP19A1. The known mediators of LH and FSH in human granulosa-lutein cells are cAMP and increased LRH1 levels.[102,103] The relative roles of LRH1 and SF1 for progesterone and estradiol production in granulosa-lutein cells are not clear. Specific functions of the two gonadotropins (i.e., differentiation, growth, and progesterone versus estradiol formation) are probably determined by numerous modifying factors (see Fig. 17-17).

Peptide Hormones Produced by the Ovary

The ovary produces a large number of peptides that can act in an intracrine, autocrine, paracrine, or endocrine fashion.[102,104,105] They include numerous growth factors (e.g., IGFs) and cytokines (e.g., interleukin 1β). IGFs crosstalk with the FSH-dependent signaling cascade to augment the effects of FSH in granulosa cells.[104,105]

Inhibin, activin, and follistatin are produced in ovarian granulosa cells under the control of FSH and LH (Fig. 17-18).[102] Production of inhibin and activin is not limited to the ovary; a number of other tissues, including adrenal, pituitary, and placenta, synthesize these members of the broader TGF-β family of paracrine/endocrine factors. Two isoforms of inhibin have been isolated: inhibin A and inhibin B.[102] They contain an identical α-subunit but distinct β-subunits (βA and βB), encoded by separate genes. The heterodimers of inhibin, αβA and αβB, are called inhibin A and inhibin B, respectively (see Fig. 17-18). Although inhibin is produced by a number of tissues in the body, most of it is derived from the gonads. In the ovary, the source of inhibin is granulosa cells. The main role of inhibin is to suppress FSH production in the pituitary.[102]

Although both inhibin isoforms seem to have similar biologic properties, their synthesis is regulated differently during the follicular and luteal phases (see Fig. 17-1A). Under the influence of FSH, inhibin B is secreted mainly during the early follicular phase, with levels decreasing in midfollicular phase and becoming undetectable after the LH surge.[102] LH-induced inhibin A levels are low during the first half of the follicular phase but increase gradually during the midfollicular phase and peak during the luteal phase. All three subunits are detected in small antral follicles by immunohistochemistry and in situ hybridization.[102] The α- and βA-subunits are found in the dominant follicle and in the corpus luteum. All three subunits are expressed in response to gonadotropins or factors that increase intracellular cAMP.[102]

Activin is structurally related to inhibin but exerts opposite actions.[102] Activin contains two subunits that are identical to the β-subunits of inhibins A and B. The three activin isoforms are activin A ($\beta_A\beta_A$), activin B ($\beta_B\beta_B$), and activin AB ($\beta_A\beta_B$). In the pituitary, activin stimulates the release of FSH. In the ovarian follicle, activin enhances FSH action (see Fig. 17-18). As in the case of inhibin, activins are also produced in ovarian granulosa cells and pituitary gonadotrophs. Unlike inhibin, locally synthesized activin in the pituitary, rather than the ovarian-derived activin, is responsible for regulating FSH (see Fig. 17-4).[102]

Follistatin is a single-unit peptide that is produced in several human tissues, including the pituitary and ovary (see Fig. 17-18).[102] It binds and neutralizes the biologic functions of activin. It appears that local follistatin levels in tissues modulate the effects of activin. This explains the inhibitory effect of follistatin on pituitary FSH secretion (see Fig. 17-4).[102]

Overview of the Hormonal Changes During the Ovarian Cycle

FSH secretion is suppressed by negative feedback of the ovarian hormones estradiol, inhibin, and progesterone during the early and midluteal phase. The sharp decline of these hormones upon regression of the corpus luteum during the late luteal phase abolishes this negative feedback (see Fig. 17-1A). This permits increased secretion of FSH just before and during menses. This initial increase in FSH is essential for follicle recruitment and growth and steroidogenesis. With continued growth of the follicle, autocrine and paracrine factors produced within the follicle maintain follicular sensitivity to FSH. Continuing and combined action of FSH and activin leads to the appearance of LH receptors on the granulosa cells, a prerequisite for ovulation and luteinization.

Ovulation is triggered by the rapid rise in circulating levels of estradiol. A positive feedback response at the level of the anterior pituitary and possibly at the hypothalamus results in the midcycle surge of LH that is necessary for expulsion of the egg and formation of the corpus luteum (see Fig. 17-1A). A rise in the progesterone level follows ovulation, along with a second rise in the estradiol level, producing the 14-day luteal phase characterized by low FSH and LH levels. Demise of the corpus luteum concomitant with a fall in hormone (progesterone, estradiol, and inhibin A) levels allows FSH to increase again toward the end of the luteal phase, initiating a new cycle. If pregnancy is established by implantation of a blastocyst, the structural integrity and function (i.e., progesterone and estradiol production) of the corpus luteum are maintained by hCG secreted from the trophoblast. The hCG acts as a surrogate for LH on the corpus luteum.

In addition to FSH and LH, local factors (e.g., activin, inhibin) regulate follicular development and steroidogenesis. In the early follicular phase, activin produced by granulosa cells in immature follicles enhances the action of FSH on aromatase activity and FSH and LH receptor formation while simultaneously suppressing C19 steroid formation in theca cells. In the late follicular phase, increased production of inhibin by the granulosa cells and decreased activin levels promote the synthesis of C19 steroids in the theca layer in response to LH and local growth factors and cytokines; this provides larger amounts of the precursor androstenedione for production of estrone and ultimately of estradiol in the granulosa cells.[106]

LH-mediated androstenedione production in theca cells and FSH-mediated estradiol production in granulosa cells are potentiated by IGFs.[104] The major endogenous IGF produced in the human ovarian follicle is IGF-2 (rather than IGF-1), which is produced by granulosa and theca cells. The actions of IGF-1 and IGF-2 are mediated by IGF receptor type I in both cells. IGF receptor type I is structurally similar to the insulin receptor. It appears that gonadotropin-related IGF action in the ovary is regulated primarily by IGF-2 and IGF receptor type I.[104,105]

In summary, ovulation is under the control of substances functioning as classic hormones (i.e., FSH, LH, estradiol, and inhibin), which transmit messages between the ovary and the hypothalamic-pituitary axis and of paracrine and autocrine factors such as IGF-2, inhibin, and activin, which coordinate sequential activities within the follicle destined to ovulate. The negative feedback relationship between corpus luteum products (i.e., estradiol, progesterone, and inhibin) and FSH results in the critical initial rise in FSH immediately before and during menses, and the positive feedback relationship between estradiol and LH is responsible for the ovulatory stimulus (see Fig. 17-1). Within the ovary, IGF-2, inhibin, and activin modify follicular responses necessary for growth and function. These endocrine, paracrine, and autocrine factors undoubtedly represent only a portion of the complete picture. The causes of anovulation are diverse and may be related to defects in cell-surface receptors, intracellular elements of signal transduction, or cell-cell interactions.[107,108]

Extraovarian Steroidogenesis

Estradiol formation takes place in several tissues in the woman of reproductive age, including the ovary, peripheral tissues such as subcutaneous fat and skin, and physiologic and pathologic target sites such as the hypothalamus, breast cancer cells, and the cells of endometriosis (Fig. 17-19).[93] The latter two sources of estrogen are particularly critical in anovulatory premenopausal and postmenopausal women. Although only small quantities of estrogen are produced by an individual adipocyte or skin fibroblast in a continuous fashion, these cell types contribute to circulating estradiol levels because of their relative abundance.[93] This effect is more pronounced in obese women because of increased mass of the adipose tissue and skin.[93]

Aromatase (CYP19A1) in adipocytes and skin fibroblasts is responsible for peripheral aromatization of androstenedione that arises from the ovary and the adrenal gland in premenopausal women and primarily from the adrenal in postmenopausal women (see Fig. 17-19).[93] However, the product of this reaction, estrone, is only weakly estrogenic. Estrone is further converted to estrone sulfate, which serves as a reservoir for estrone in blood and other tissues. Estrone (arising from androstenedione and estrone sulfate) is further converted to the biologically active estradiol in target tissues such as the endometrium and breast by a number of enzymatic proteins with overlapping reductive 17β-HSD activity (see Fig. 17-19).[93,101] It is likely that local CYP19A1 expression in hypothalamus is critical for the regulation of gonadotropin secretion.[18,109] Estrogen-dependent pathologic tissues such as those in breast cancer and endometriosis contain extremely high levels of CYP19A1 that enhances tissue growth by increasing local estradiol concentrations (see Fig. 17-19).[93] Circulating androstenedione is the major substrate for aromatase activity in these physiologic and pathologic target tissues.[93]

Significant quantities of circulating androstenedione can also be converted to testosterone in peripheral tissues (discussed later). This is probably accomplished by the presence of multiple 17β-HSDs with overlapping reductive activities in peripheral tissues.[101] Androgenic action of testosterone is strikingly amplified by its conversion to DHT in peripheral and target tissues (e.g., skin, prostate). At least

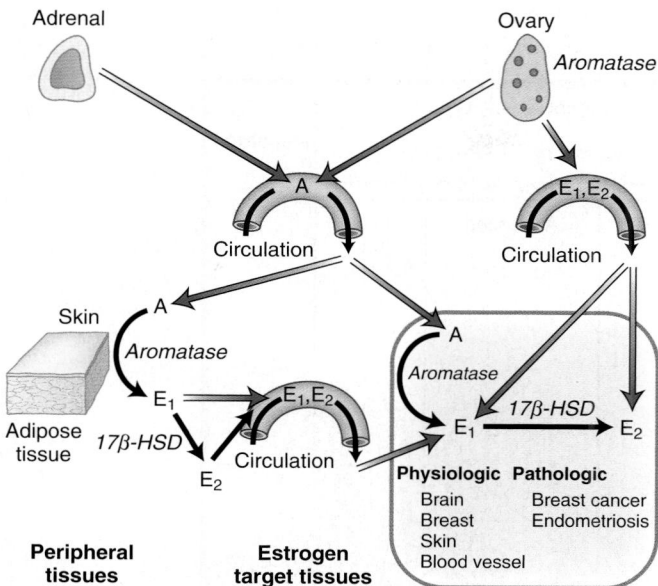

Figure 17-19 Estrogen biosynthesis in women. The biologically active estrogen, estradiol (E$_2$), is produced in at least three major sites: (1) by direct secretion from the ovary in reproductive-age women; (2) by conversion of circulating androstenedione (A), originating from the adrenal or ovary or both, to estrone (E$_1$) in peripheral tissues; and (3) by conversion of A to E$_1$ in estrogen target tissues. In the latter two instances, estrogenically weak estrone (E$_1$) is converted to E$_2$ within the same tissue. The expression of genes that encode the enzymes aromatase and reductive 17β-hydroxysteroid dehydrogenases (17β-HSD) is critical for E$_2$ formation at these sites. Reductive 17β-HSD activity in peripheral tissues may be conferred by protein products of several genes with overlapping functions. HSD17B1 is a distinct reductive 17β-HSD enzyme that is encoded by a specific gene expressed primarily in the ovary. Aromatase is encoded by a single gene *(CYP19A1)*. E$_2$ formation by peripheral and local conversion is particularly important in postmenopausal women and in those with estrogen-dependent diseases such as breast cancer, endometriosis, or endometrial cancer.

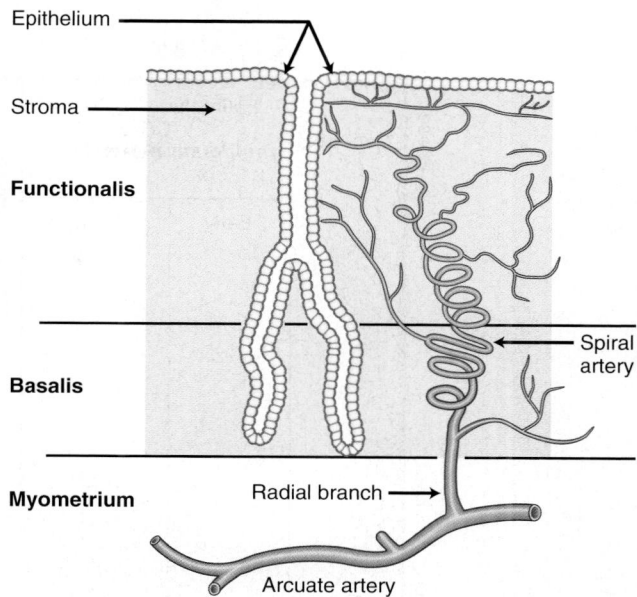

Figure 17-20 Functional anatomy of the endometrium. Endometrium is a multilayered mucosa specialized for implantation and support of pregnancy. A single, continuous layer of epithelial cells lines the surface of the stroma and penetrates the stroma with deep invaginations almost all the way down to the myometrium-endometrium junction. The entire thickness of the endometrium is penetrated by the spiral arteries and their capillaries. Spiral arteries originate from the radial branches of arcuate arteries, which arise from uterine arteries. The superficial layer (functionalis) is shed during menstruation, whereas the permanent bottom layer (basalis) gives rise to the regeneration of endometrium after each menstruation. The striking changes in the spiral arteries (i.e., coiling, stasis, and vasodilatation followed by intense vasoconstriction) are consistently observed before the onset of every menstruation episode. (Courtesy of Dr. Kristof Chwalisz, AbbVie, Inc., North Chicago, IL.)

two distinct proteins encoded by two separate genes, 5α-reductase type 1 and type 2, catalyze the conversion of testosterone to DHT in liver, prostate, and skin.[94] Local production of DHT in genital skin fibroblasts is critical for normal masculinization of external genitalia of male fetuses in utero.[110] DHT formation in the skin is an important cause of hirsutism.[111]

ENDOMETRIUM

The endometrium is the mucosal lining of the uterine cavity. The decidua is the highly modified and specialized endometrium of pregnancy. From an evolutionary perspective, the human endometrium is highly developed to accommodate the hemochorioendothelial type of placentation, which requires the presence of spiral arteries (Fig. 17-20). Trophoblasts of the blastocyst invade spiral arteries during implantation and placentation in the establishment of uteroplacental vessels.

Spiral arteries of the human endometrium confer another unique process, *menstruation.* Menstruation is shedding of endometrial tissue with hemorrhage that depends on sex steroid hormone–directed changes in blood flow in the spiral arteries. Spiral arteries are essential for menstruation; only humans and a few other primates that have endometrial spiral arteries experience menstruation. With nonfertile but ovulatory ovarian cycles, menstruation effects desquamation of the endometrium. New endometrial growth and development must be initiated with each ovarian cycle, so endometrial maturation corresponds with the next opportunity for pregnancy. There seems to be a

narrow window of endometrial receptivity to blastocyst implantation, comprising the period between days 20 and 24 during a 28-day menstrual cycle.[112]

Functional Anatomy of the Endometrium

The endometrium can be divided morphologically into an upper two-thirds *functionalis* layer and a lower one-third *basalis* layer (see Fig. 17-20). The purpose of the functionalis layer is to prepare for the implantation of the blastocyst; it is the site of proliferation, secretion, and degeneration. The purpose of the basalis layer is to provide the regenerative endometrium after menstrual loss of the functionalis.[113] Major histologic components of the endometrium include stromal cells, which constitute the skeleton of the tissue; a single layer of epithelial cells, which lines the lumen of the endometrial cavity and invaginations of the stroma; blood vessels; and resident immune cells. The epithelial cells that line the rather deep invaginations of the stroma are also referred to as *glandular cells.* However, these deep crypts represent extensions of the intracavitary lumen and are not true glands. These invaginations lined by epithelial cells extend from the surface of the functionalis layer (i.e., luminal epithelium) deep into the basalis level (i.e., glandular epithelium). After the functionalis layer is shed at the time of menstruation, the tissue stem cells in the basalis layer respond rapidly to estrogen and give rise to a new functionalis layer for the upcoming cycle (Fig. 17-21).[114] In humans and some other primates, the cellular components of the functionalis layer undergo a striking progression during the menstrual cycle, whereas the basalis layer shows only modest alterations.[113,115,116]

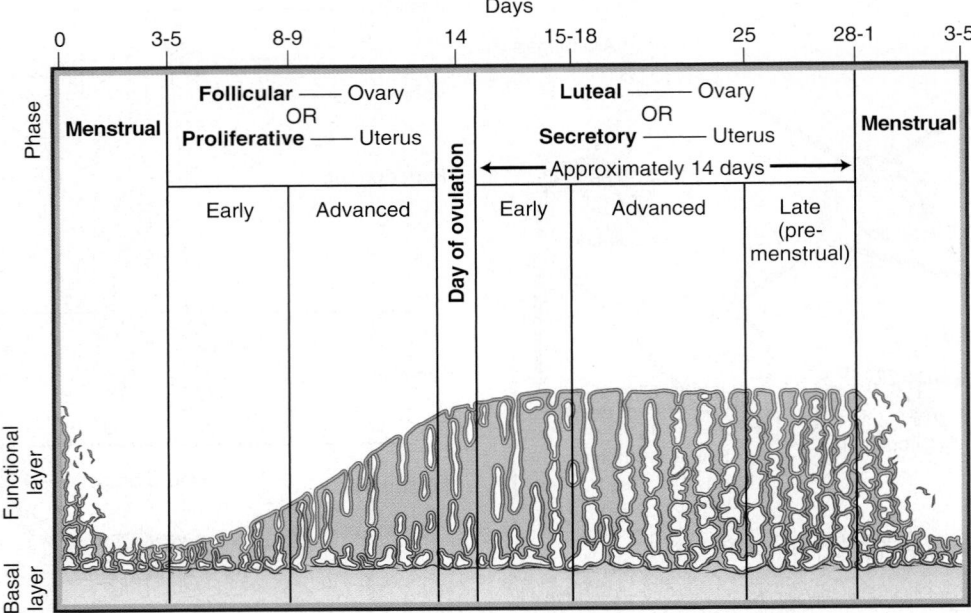

Figure 17-21 Cyclic changes in thickness and morphologic changes of endometrium and the relationship of these changes to those of the ovarian cycle. (From Cunningham FG, MacDonald PC, Gant NF, et al. The endometrium and decidua: menstruation and pregnancy. In: Cunningham FG, ed. *Williams Obstetrics*, 19th ed. Stamford, CT: Appleton & Lange; 1993:81-109.)

Hormone-Induced Morphologic Changes of the Endometrium

The cyclic changes in endometrial histology are faithfully reproduced during each ovulatory ovarian cycle (see Fig. 17-21). First, during the preovulatory, or follicular, phase of the cycle, estradiol is secreted (principally by a single dominant follicle of one ovary) in increasing quantities until just before ovulation. Second, during the postovulatory, or luteal, phase of the cycle, progesterone is secreted by the corpus luteum in increasing amounts (up to 40 to 50 mg/day) until the midluteal phase. Third, beginning about 7 to 8 days after ovulation, the rates of progesterone and estradiol secretion by the corpus luteum begin to decline and then diminish progressively before menstruation (see Fig. 17-1).

In response to these cyclic changes in the rates of ovarian sex steroid hormone secretion, there are five main stages of the corresponding endometrial cycle: (1) menstrual-postmenstrual *reepithelialization*; (2) *endometrial proliferation* in response to stimulation by estradiol; (3) abundant *epithelial secretion*, occurring in response to the combined action of estradiol and progesterone; (4) *premenstrual ischemia*, the result of endometrial tissue volume involution, which causes stasis of blood in the spiral arteries; and (5) *menstruation*, which is preceded and accompanied by severe vasoconstriction of the endometrial spiral arteries and collapse and desquamation of all but the deepest layer of the endometrium. In the final analysis, menstruation is the consequence of the withdrawal of factors that maintain endometrial growth and differentiation (see Fig. 17-21).

Commonly, the initiation of menstruation is attributed to progesterone withdrawal. This concept was developed because the administration of estrogen to postmenopausal women and treatment with and then withdrawal of a progestin causes menstruation, even with continued estrogen treatment. Moreover, progesterone facilitates decidualiza-

tion of the endometrium and the maintenance of pregnancy, whereas progesterone withdrawal favors the initiation of menstruation, lactation, and parturition.

The preovulatory (follicular or proliferative) phase and the postovulatory (luteal or secretory) phase of the ovarian-endometrial cycles are customarily divided into early and late stages (see Fig. 17-21). The normal secretory phase of the menstrual cycle can be subdivided almost daily by histologic criteria, from shortly after ovulation until the onset of menstruation.[117] Some gynecologists use histologic dating of endometrial biopsies obtained during the luteal phase to evaluate ovulation, progesterone production, or the degree of biologic response of the endometrium to progesterone.[117]

Effects of Ovarian Steroids on Endometrium

The exogenous administration of only estradiol and progesterone is sufficient to prepare the endometrium for implantation in the absence of ovarian function.[118,119] This observation underscores the essential roles of these steroids in uterine physiology. Estradiol or synthetic estrogens such as ethinyl estradiol cause a striking thickening of endometrial tissue. Stromal and epithelial cells of the endometrium proliferate rapidly under the influence of estradiol. Estradiol greatly increases mitotic activity and DNA synthesis in both cell types (Fig. 17-22). While promoting growth, estradiol also renders endometrial tissue responsive to progesterone by inducing the expression of PRs; progesterone action depends on previous or concurrent estrogen exposure of the endometrium.[120]

In contrast to the proliferative effects of estrogen, progesterone action primarily enables differentiation of the endometrium. Progesterone can inhibit and even reverse the proliferative action of estrogen on the functionalis layer (see Fig. 17-22). Moreover, progesterone action prepares the endometrium for implantation of the embryo through differentiation of stromal and epithelial cells.

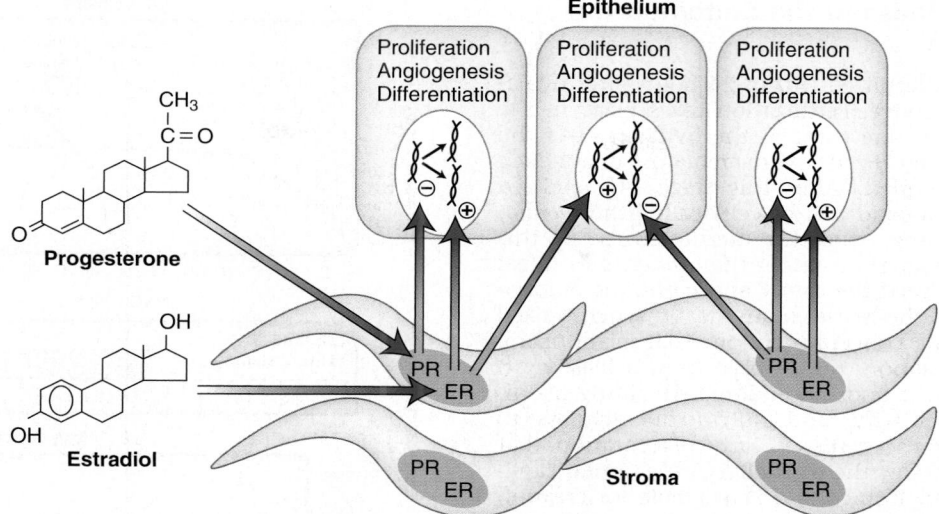

Figure 17-22 Critical epithelial effects of estrogen (i.e., deoxyribonucleic acid [DNA] synthesis, proliferation, and gene expression) are mediated primarily by estrogen receptor-α (ER) in stromal cells in a paracrine manner in the endometrium. This was demonstrated in mice. It was also shown in mice and humans that the antiestrogenic effects of progesterone on epithelial cells (e.g., decreased proliferation, enhanced differentiation) are mediated primarily by progesterone receptors (PRs) in stromal cells.

Progesterone induces the production and secretion of a glycogen-rich substance from the epithelial cells. Progesterone also causes an increase in stromal cell cytoplasm, a process called *pseudodecidualization*. The term *decidualization* is reserved for stroma differentiated under the combined influence of progesterone and hCG of placental origin during pregnancy.

Blood vessels that carry estrogen or progesterone come first in contact with endometrial stromal cells. These steroid ligands interact with their nuclear receptors in endometrial stromal cells, which in turn send paracrine signals to neighboring epithelial cells to regulate their functions.[99,120]

Estrogen Action

Estradiol enters endometrial cells from blood by simple diffusion and binds ERs, proteins with a high affinity for estradiol and biologically active synthetic estrogens. Although both ERα and ERβ are present in the endometrium, ERα is the primary mediator of the estrogenic action in that tissue.[121,122] The estradiol-ERα complex is a transcriptional factor that becomes associated with chromatin.[123] Estradiol-ERα complexes bind thousands of DNA sites across the entire genome and regulate the transcription of hundreds of genes at one time.[123] Most ERα binding sites are outside basal promoters and interact with the transcriptional start sites through DNA looping.[110,123] This interaction brings about ER-specific initiation of gene transcription, which promotes the synthesis of specific mRNAs and, thereafter, specific proteins.[110,123] Estradiol acts in the endometrium and in other estrogen-responsive tissues to promote the responsiveness of that tissue to progesterone via inducing PR expression.[99]

The endometrial epithelial cells are estrogen-responsive but probably do not replicate as a result of direct action of estradiol on them. Replication of human endometrial epithelial cells in culture is not increased appreciably, if at all, when estrogen is added to the medium. Estrogen acts on mouse uterine stromal cells to promote the synthesis of growth factors that act on epithelial cells (see Fig. 17-22).[120] These growth factors operate in a paracrine manner to cause increased DNA synthesis and replication in the adjacent epithelial cells.

Progesterone Action

Progesterone enters cells by diffusion and binds to its nuclear receptor (PR). Two PR isoforms, PR-A and PR-B, are present in the human endometrium.[124] Because PR-B but not PR-A levels in the endometrium are tightly regulated during the human menstrual cycle, PR-B is presumed to play a more important biologic role.[124] The cellular content of PRs typically depends on previous estrogen action.

The progesterone-PR complex regulates gene transcription, but the response to progesterone is strikingly different from that evoked by the estradiol-ER complex. Similar to ERα, PR binding sites are also widely distributed across the genome, lie frequently outside basal promoters, and do not involve classically defined progesterone response elements.[125] Interaction of PR binding sites with basal promoters possibly requires DNA looping.[125]

Progesterone acts as an antiestrogen by reducing ERα expression, by decreasing the tissue levels of estradiol through its conversion to estrone via inducing the HSD17B2 enzyme, and by enhancing estrogen inactivation through sulfation.[126-128] Tissue recombination experiments using uteri of PR knockout and normal mice have demonstrated that many effects of progesterone on epithelial cells are also mediated in a paracrine fashion by PRs in stromal cells but not by those in epithelial cells (see Fig. 17-22).[99,128]

The most striking consequences of progesterone action, stromal predecidualization and epithelial secretion, parallel increased levels of circulating progesterone during the luteal phase. The PR content of human endometrial tissue peaks during the late proliferative phase, just before ovulation, and declines sharply before circulating progesterone levels increase during the luteal phase.[124] This dyssynchrony between endometrial PR expression and circulating progesterone is not well understood. Molecular correlates of progesterone action with respect to differentiation include increased production of lactoferrin and glycodelin in epithelial cells and of prolactin and IGF-binding protein 1 in stromal cells of the endometrium.[99]

The Receptive Phase of the Endometrium for Implantation

Unless the ovum is fertilized within 24 hours after ovulation, it does not survive. Fertilization takes place in the ampullary, the distal one third of the oviduct. Over the next 2 days, the fertilized ovum remains unattached within the tubal lumen. After this stage, the embryo (which consists of a solid ball of cells called the *morula*) leaves the oviduct and enters the uterine cavity. By this time, endometrial secretions under the influence of luteal progesterone have filled the cavity and bathe the embryo in nutrients. This is the first of many neatly synchronized events that mark the conceptus-endometrial relationship. By 6 days after ovulation, the embryo (now a blastocyst) is ready to implant. It finds an endometrial lining of sufficient depth, vascularity, and nutritional richness to sustain the important events of early placentation that are to follow. Just below the epithelial lining, a rich capillary plexus has been formed and is available for creation of the trophoblast-maternal blood interface. Later, the surrounding superficial portion of the functionalis zone, now occupying more and more of the endometrial cavity, provides a sturdy splint to retain endometrial architecture despite the invasive inroads of the burgeoning trophoblast.

Progesterone is essential for the maintenance of pregnancy. The blastocyst depends on progesterone produced by the corpus luteum at this time. The hCG secreted by the trophoblast acts as a surrogate LH and prevents regression of the corpus luteum that provides a continuous supply of progesterone until the placental tissue starts to produce sufficient quantities of progesterone (6 to 7 weeks after fertilization).

The receptive phase of the endometrium is the temporal window of endometrial maturation during which the trophectoderm of the blastocyst can attach to the endometrial epithelial cells and proceed to invade the endometrial stroma. The window of uterine receptivity can be inferred from what has been learned from transfer of embryos to uteri of women primed with exogenous estrogen and progesterone preparations (Fig. 17-23). There is a distinct window for embryo transfer leading to implantation, which spans endometrial cycle days 16 to 20. The actual window of implantation follows this window of transfer, because embryos need to develop further, from the four-cell to eight-cell stage to the blastocyst stage, before initiation of attachment and frank invasion can occur. Based on serial measurements of serum hCG as a marker of initial embryonic-maternal interaction, the window of implantation in humans is estimated to be between days 20 and 24 of the cycle.[129] This relatively wide window agrees with the earlier morphologic data.[130]

Control of Endometrial Function With the Use of Exogenous Hormones

The fertility potential of a woman is primarily determined by the biologic quality of her oocytes, reflected in part by the capacity of the fertilized ovum to divide at an optimal rate and contain a normal chromosomal complement. This biologic quality declines sharply after the age of 35 years. However, the biologic potential of the endometrium for successful implantation remains intact even at advanced ages.[118] Oocyte donation from a fertile woman and fertilization of the donor eggs in vitro with the recipient's male partner's sperm, followed by embryo transfer into the uterine cavity of the recipient woman with nonfunction-

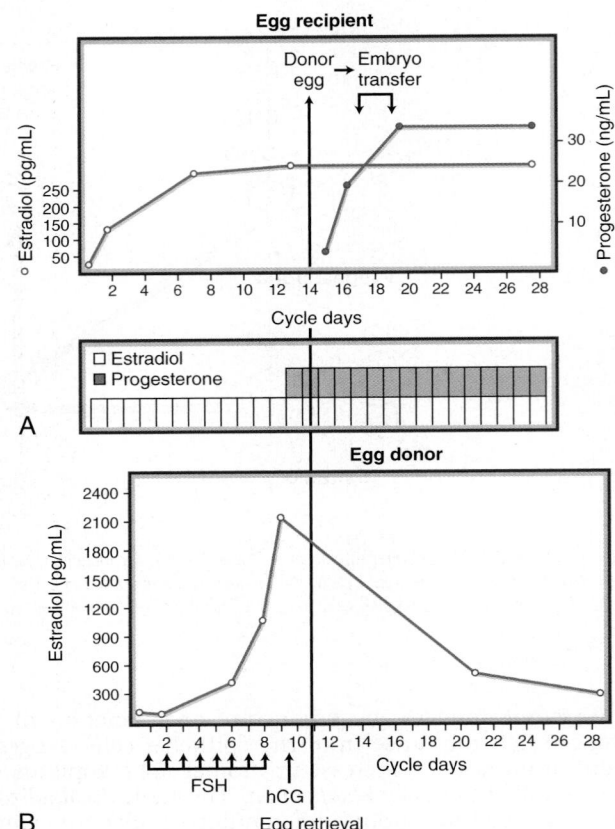

Figure 17-23 Donation of oocytes by a woman undergoing egg retrieval to a woman with ovarian insufficiency treated with exogenous estrogen and progesterone. The window of implantation in both women is synchronized by different but comparable hormonal treatments **A,** Woman with ovarian insufficiency is initially treated with oral micronized estradiol during days 1 through 14 of the cycle. Exogenous intramuscular progesterone is added to the estradiol treatment on days 15 through 28 and continued if pregnancy is diagnosed. Several donor eggs are fertilized with sperm from the recipient's husband, and one or two embryos are transferred to the uterus on day 16 to 19, depending on the stage of embryo development. These embryos are expected to implant between days 20 and 24. **B,** The egg donor is simultaneously treated with human recombinant follicle-stimulating hormone (FSH) with or without menopausal gonadotropin until cycle day 8 to 12, when human chorionic gonadotropin (hCG) is given to induce ovulation, and oocytes are harvested 32 to 36 hours later. One or two fertilized eggs are transferred to the uterus of the recipient. Progesterone supplement to the recipient is started before the embryo transfer. Serum levels of estradiol and progesterone in both women are shown. To convert estradiol values to picomoles per liter, multiply by 3.671. To convert progesterone values to nanomoles per liter, multiply by 3.180.

ing ovaries (e.g., premature ovarian insufficiency [POI]), have been used successfully as a therapeutic strategy to treat infertility (see Fig. 17-23).[118,119] This clinical application has provided unique opportunities to examine the hormonal therapy for endometrial maturation. The success of these procedures (i.e., pregnancy rate) has averaged higher than in conventional IVF.[119]

The follicular phase is mimicked by administration of oral micronized estradiol in daily doses of up to 8 mg for about 10 days. Serum estradiol during the replacement follicular phase reaches sufficiently high levels to stimulate endometrial growth. This is followed by up to 8 mg/day of oral estradiol combined with daily intramuscular (50 mg) or vaginal (200-400 mg) progesterone to promote the secretory transformation. Progesterone supplementation is ordinarily continued until 8 to 10 weeks of gestation.

Mechanism of Menstruation

In the absence of pregnancy, failure of the appearance of hCG despite otherwise appropriate tissue reactions leads to the vasomotor changes associated with estrogen-progesterone withdrawal and menstrual desquamation. A program of endometrial remodeling is initiated; alterations in the extracellular matrix and infiltration of leukocytes lead to hypoxia-reperfusion injury and sloughing of the functionalis, followed by activation of hemostatic and regenerative processes. The main histologic features of the premenstrual phase are degradation of the stromal reticular network, stromal infiltration by polymorphonuclear and mononuclear leukocytes, and secretory exhaustion of the endometrial glands, whose epithelial cells now have basal nuclei. The endometrium shrinks preceding menstruation in part as a result of diminished secretory activity and the catabolism of extracellular matrix.

An ischemic phase caused by vasoconstriction of the arterioles and coiled arteries precedes the onset of menstrual bleeding by 4 to 24 hours.[115] Bleeding occurs after the arterioles and arteries relax, leading to hypoxia-reperfusion injury. The superficial endometrial layers are distended by the formation of hematomas, and fissures develop, leading to the detachment of tissue fragments. Lysis and fragmentation of cells and apoptosis are evident. The menstrual efflux is composed of shed fragments of endometrium mixed with blood and liquefied by the fibrinolytic activity of the cellular debris (see Fig. 17-21). Clots of various sizes may be present if blood flow is excessive. Myometrium contracts to mechanically stop bleeding from the spiral arteries and other endometrial vessels.

APPROACH TO THE WOMAN WITH REPRODUCTIVE DYSFUNCTION

Reproductive dysfunction in an adult woman is most often manifested by disruption of cyclic, predictable menses. Efficient diagnosis of the underlying disorder requires a thorough understanding of female reproductive physiology and pathologic conditions and an accurate history and physical examination. Without a critical analysis of clinical findings based on thorough knowledge of normal and abnormal reproductive function, the application of predetermined algorithms of laboratory testing causes unnecessary use of hormone measurements or imaging studies and delays diagnosis.

History

An essential tool for the evaluation of a woman with a reproductive disorder is a carefully recorded history. The history should be obtained from the patient with the aim of assessing the biologic effects of each of the various hormones. Recording the details of pubertal development as a reference for the onset of particular symptoms provides critical clues to the cause of certain reproductive disorders. For example, anovulation manifested by irregular uterine bleeding associated with the polycystic ovary syndrome (PCOS) most often begins during the pubertal years. The onset of gradually progressing hirsutism at about the time of puberty suggests nonclassic adrenal hyperplasia or PCOS. In these cases, measurement of serum 17-hydroxyprogesterone may help to differentiate nonclassic adrenal hyperplasia from PCOS. The appearance of hirsutism before puberty or several years after normal pubertal development should alert the clinician to the possibility of

ovarian or adrenal neoplasms. Sudden onset of hirsutism at any age or the presence of virilization should prompt the physician to rule out steroid-secreting ovarian or adrenal tumors. Most women with symptomatic endometriosis suffer from severe episodes of painful menses (i.e., dysmenorrhea) that start during pubertal years.

Evaluation of female reproductive function depends on a detailed history of the menses. For example, PCOS is unlikely without a long-standing history of irregular periods since the menarche. A history of a period of cyclic, predictable menses before the onset of menstrual irregularities should draw attention to hypothalamic or other causes of anovulation. The current frequency, regularity, length, and quantity of uterine bleeding should be carefully recorded for several reasons. First, this information reflects tightly regulated interactions of several tissues, including the hypothalamus, pituitary, ovaries, and endometrium. Second, regular, predictable menses imply ovulation. Third, defining the type of menstrual irregularity may help with diagnosis of the underlying cause. For example, prolonged amenorrhea in a thin and estrogen-deficient woman suggests anovulation of hypothalamic origin. Infrequent periods of varying duration and with a varying amount of blood loss in a well-estrogenized, overweight woman suggest a primary ovarian dysfunction such as PCOS. Anovulation in a thin but well-estrogenized woman may also be caused by PCOS. Regular but heavy and prolonged menses with intermittent spotting may result from uterine anatomic disorders such as adenomyosis or leiomyomas. Fourth, neoplastic disorders of the endometrium, including endometrial polyps, hyperplasia, or malignancies, may be manifested by any pattern of irregular bleeding. The combination of vaginal ultrasonography and endometrial biopsy is helpful for the diagnosis of endometrial neoplasia.[131]

Disruption of cyclic and predictable menses is a common and alarming symptom that initially brings the patient to the clinician. After a careful evaluation of the menstrual symptoms, the clinician should identify other obvious symptoms of the endocrine disorder underlying the irregular periods. Pregnancy is the most common cause of amenorrhea (and other menstrual irregularities) in a woman of reproductive age. In a woman presenting with amenorrhea or any other menstrual irregularity, normal pregnancy, ectopic pregnancy, or gestational trophoblastic disease must be excluded at the onset. Careful evaluation of past reproductive history and the patient's sexual activity and contraceptive practices can provide useful indications of the likelihood of pregnancy. The reproductive history may suggest the possibility of Sheehan syndrome of postpartum pituitary necrosis if menses did not resume after a delivery complicated by significant hemorrhage.[132] In such instances, evidence of adrenal and thyroid insufficiency should be sought. A classic symptom of Sheehan syndrome is the absence of postpartum lactation, which is related to prolactin deficiency.

Amenorrhea is traditionally categorized as primary (no history of menstruation) or secondary (cessation of menses after a variable time). The diverse causes of primary amenorrhea are discussed extensively in Chapters 23 and 25. Although the distinction between primary and secondary amenorrhea may be useful for identifying the mechanism of disease and the differential diagnosis, the clinician should be aware that a disorder can initially manifest with either primary or secondary amenorrhea. For example, most women with gonadal dysgenesis have primary amenorrhea, but some patients have residual follicles and ovulate, and in these women with partial gonadal dysgenesis, some menstruation and rare pregnancies may occur before the cessation of ovarian function.[133,134] Patients with PCOS usually have secondary amenorrhea but occasionally have primary amenorrhea. Rarely, pregnancy may manifest as primary amenorrhea.

After pregnancy is ruled out, secondary amenorrhea is most often caused by chronic anovulation, which can be broadly categorized as hypothalamic dysfunction, hyperprolactinemia-associated anovulation, ovarian insufficiency, androgen excess, or chronic illness or primary uterine disease (e.g., intrauterine adhesion formation after a postpartum curettage). Establishing any association of secondary amenorrhea with life events is extremely useful. Strenuous exercise is often associated with amenorrhea. Weight loss often precedes or accompanies secondary amenorrhea and has been suggested as evidence of hypothalamic dysfunction. An unusual dietary history may suggest bulimia or anorexia nervosa. The presence of any signs or symptoms of estrogen deficiency, including painful intercourse, atrophic vagina, emotional lability, and vasomotor instability, suggests anovulation of a central nature with low concentrations of circulating gonadotropins (i.e., hypogonadotropic hypogonadism) or ovarian insufficiency with elevated gonadotropins (i.e., hypergonadotropic hypogonadism).

Galactorrhea in the absence of a recent history of pregnancy suggests a host of diagnostic possibilities and is frequently a manifestation of excessive prolactin secretion, although it may result from increased sensitivity of breast tissue to the hormones necessary for milk production. This history frequently reveals drug ingestion as the cause. Various drugs, including several psychotropic agents, antihypertensive agents, and oral contraceptives, have been implicated. Primary hypothyroidism may be associated with precocious puberty with galactorrhea in the child and with amenorrhea or galactorrhea, or both, in the adult woman. A history of excessive nipple manipulation or chest wall disease should be elicited because it may be the cause of galactorrhea. Prolactinomas, the prolactin-secreting adenomas of the pituitary, are a common cause of galactorrhea related to abnormally high serum levels of prolactin. A history of dilatation and curettage, postpartum endometritis, or disseminated tuberculosis with absent to scant menses suggests the possibility of intrauterine adhesion.[135]

Physical Examination

The quantity and distribution of excessive hair growth should be considered in light of the familial history. Hypertrichosis—excessive growth of hair on the extremities, the head, and the back—must be distinguished from true hirsutism, which is the development of facial hair, chest hair, and a male escutcheon with or without signs of virilization in response to increased production of or sensitivity to biologically active androgens. Some degree of hypertrichosis is not uncommon in women of Mediterranean descent, whereas the occurrence of any facial hirsutism in the relatively hairless Asian woman may require thorough investigation. Hirsutism is best documented and quantified with the help of photographs. Virilization is characterized as thickening of the voice, severe cystic acne, hair loss, increased muscle mass, and clitoromegaly and implies a more severe degree of androgen excess than that found with hirsutism. The syndrome of complete androgen insensitivity is characterized by sparse to absent pubic and axillary hair due to resistance to androgen.

A careful inspection of the breasts is essential for a thorough physical examination. Classification of the stage of breast development according to the method of Marshall and Tanner[136] is a convenient and valuable adjunct. The physician should assess whether the breasts appear to have decreased in size recently (e.g., severe androgen excess), whether the areolae are well formed and pigmented (as they are in pregnancy), and whether a discharge (e.g., galactorrhea) can be expressed.

A woman with PCOS who has never ovulated or taken a progestin-containing medication may have Tanner stage 4 breast development related to adequate estrogen production, whereas the progression to Tanner stage 5 requires exposure to progesterone through ovulation, ingestion of a progestin (e.g., administration of oral contraceptives), or pregnancy. Chapter 25 discusses Tanner staging of breast development.

The vulva, vagina, and cervix also represent sensitive indicators of gonadal steroid action. Because sensitivity of the genital skin and mucosa to androgen decreases with time from the early stages of fetal development to adulthood, the extent of any virilization can be helpful in suggesting the timing of androgen exposure. The most profound androgenic effects, such as posterior labial fusion with or without formation of a penile urethra, usually are observed in 46,XX fetuses exposed to androgens during the first 8 to 10 weeks of pregnancy. Similar findings have been described in patients with virilizing congenital adrenal hyperplasia, true hermaphroditism, and drug-induced virilization. Postnatal development of significant clitoromegaly in a 46,XX infant requires marked hormonal stimulation and, in the absence of significant exogenous steroids, strongly implicates an androgen-secreting tumor. The size of the glans clitoris can be quantified by determining the clitoral index, which is the product of the sagittal and transverse diameters of the glans. Ninety-five percent of normal women have a clitoral index less than 35 mm².

The vagina and uterine cervix are the most sensitive indicators of estrogen action. Under the influence of estrogen, the vaginal mucosa progresses during sexual maturation from a tissue with a shiny, bright red appearance with sparse, thin secretions to a tissue with a dull, gray-pink, rugated surface with copious, thick secretions. Well-estrogenized vaginal mucosa with stretchable cervical mucus (i.e., *spinnbarkeit*) may indicate the proliferative phase of the menstrual cycle in an ovulatory woman or extraovarian estrogen formation in an anovulatory woman with PCOS. The biologic activity of estrogen can also be quantified by vaginal cytologic examination.

To summarize, irregular uterine bleeding is a common symptom that brings the woman with reproductive dysfunction to the physician's office. Various disorders of the hypothalamus, pituitary, ovaries, or uterus or other tissues that affect reproductive function may be responsible for this alarming symptom. After pregnancy is ruled out, a detailed history and physical examination should be carefully recorded. In particular, the physician should pay attention to the salient features in the history and the biologic indicators of hormone action at target tissues during the physical examination. An analysis of these findings most often leads to a tentative diagnosis, which may be confirmed by laboratory testing.

DISORDERS OF THE FEMALE REPRODUCTIVE SYSTEM

Chronic Anovulation

Chronic anovulation is one of the most common gynecologic problems encountered by the practitioner. Patients may present with secondary amenorrhea, infrequent uterine bleeding (i.e., oligomenorrhea), or irregular episodes of excessive uterine bleeding. Infertility is an obvious consequence of chronic anovulation. Pregnancy, end-organ defects (e.g., intrauterine adhesions, müllerian agenesis), amenorrhea associated with genital ambiguity at birth (e.g., male or female pseudohermaphroditism, true hermaphroditism), or sexual infantilism due to gonadal dysgenesis should initially be ruled out.

For practical purposes, most of the etiologic factors giving rise to chronic anovulation in a woman of reproductive age fall into five broad categories: hypothalamic anovulation, hyperprolactinemia, androgen excess, POI, and chronic illness (e.g., hepatic or renal insufficiency, acquired immunodeficiency syndrome [AIDS]). Salient features of the history and physical examination help to place a woman with anovulation in one or more of these categories.

One group of anovulatory patients is estrogen deficient. Common disorders in this group include hypothalamic anovulation, galactorrhea-hyperprolactinemia (e.g., hypothyroidism, prolactinoma, nonfunctioning pituitary tumor), and POI in a woman of reproductive age. These patients are usually amenorrheic. All patients present with signs of estrogen deficiency (e.g., vaginal atrophy). Patients with hypothalamic anovulation or galactorrhea-hyperprolactinemia usually do not complain of hot flashes, whereas women with POI present with vasomotor symptoms. One serious consequence of estrogen deficiency is bone loss, giving rise to osteopenia and osteoporosis. If possible, the underlying cause should be corrected. Hormone therapy should be provided if ovulation cannot be restored.

Women with androgen excess constitute the second major group of anovulatory patients. A serious consequence of anovulation in this group is the greater risk for carcinoma of the endometrium because of unopposed action of estrogen formed continuously in extraovarian tissues. The most common disorder of the ovary associated with androgen excess and anovulation is PCOS. Insulin resistance plays a significant role in this condition and, along with hyperandrogenism, increases the risk of developing cardiovascular disease (CVD), diabetes mellitus, or both.[107] The clinician must recognize the long-term impact of PCOS and undertake therapeutic management of these anovulatory patients to avoid unwanted consequences. The clinician should also develop a plan with the patient to address long-term complications of unopposed estrogen formation associated with PCOS (e.g., endometrial neoplasia). Oral contraceptives or periodic progestin supplementation may be provided to prevent endometrial hyperplasia and cancer.

Many mechanisms may be responsible for anovulation in chronic illness. Effective treatment of the primary illness may restore normal menses. Alternatively, anovulatory bleeding may be managed with the use of exogenous hormones in these chronically ill patients (discussed later).

Measurements of FSH and prolactin help to categorize anovulatory patients. An undetectable or low-normal FSH level is consistent with hypothalamic amenorrhea, PCOS, or hyperprolactinemia, whereas high FSH levels suggest ovarian insufficiency. High prolactin levels may indicate a pituitary prolactinoma or hypothyroidism. The following sections describe specific disorders that cause chronic anovulation in women of reproductive age.

Hypothalamic Anovulation

Anovulation of hypothalamic origin usually manifests as amenorrhea. The terms *hypothalamic anovulation* and *hypo-thalamic amenorrhea* are used interchangeably in this chapter. A reduction in GnRH pulse frequency from the characteristic 60 to 120 minutes to intervals longer than 180 minutes leads to lower levels of LH and FSH secretion by the pituitary gland.[10,137] This functional gonadotropin deficiency fails to provide adequate stimulation to the ovarian follicles, and the normal sequence of follicular growth, maturation, follicular selection, and ovulation becomes attenuated. Downstream ovarian estradiol production remains low, and endometrial growth is reduced or arrested, resulting in a prolonged interval of amenorrhea. The transition from normal menstrual cyclicity to anovulation and amenorrhea can take place gradually and may be characterized by inadequate luteal phases, irregular menstrual bleeding, and amenorrhea. Patients with hypothalamic amenorrhea do not complain of hot flashes, even though circulating levels of estradiol are within the menopausal range. This suggests a significant role for GnRH or gonadotropins in the cause of hot flashes.

Any disorder of the central nervous system that interferes with normal GnRH pulse frequency can cause anovulation. Some of these disorders may be defined genetic or anatomic evidence such as isolated gonadotropin deficiency (with or without anosmia), infection, suprasellar tumors (e.g., pituitary adenomas, craniopharyngioma), and head trauma.[7] These genetic and anatomic disorders affect the function of the hypothalamus, and some of them may be ruled out by the medical history, physical examination, and imaging of the head (Table 17-1).

The most commonly observed form of hypothalamic anovulation is not associated with a demonstrable neuroanatomic finding.[138] This common form is called *functional hypothalamic amenorrhea* because it is presumed to involve aberrant but reversible regulation of otherwise normal neuroendocrine pathways. Other causes of hypothalamic anovulation demonstrable by neuroanatomic or genetic evidence are uncommon (see Table 17-1).

Functional Hypothalamic Amenorrhea

Anovulation resulting from stress-associated changes is viewed as a functional disorder in which no anatomic or organic abnormalities of the hypothalamic-pituitary-ovarian axis can be identified. This condition typically manifests as amenorrhea of 6 months' duration and has also been called *functional hypothalamic amenorrhea*. The overall prevalence of functional hypothalamic amenorrhea among all amenorrhea disorders ranges from 15% to 48%.[138]

Anovulation of hypothalamic origin is characterized by estrogen deficiency and low levels of gonadotropins. No genetic or anatomic disorders are identified in most patients. The concept of functional hypothalamic anovulation (i.e., amenorrhea) was first postulated in the 1940s as the failure of the hypothalamic-pituitary pathways to release gonadotropins from the anterior pituitary.[139] Since then, clinical studies have supported this common mechanism associated with an alteration in the pulsatile secretion of GnRH.[11] Diverse etiologic factors such as malnutrition or caloric restriction, depression, psychogenic stress, excessive energy expenditure related to exercise, or combinations of these disorders precede the onset of functional hypothalamic anovulation. Heightened awareness of diet or exercise and unrealistic expectations with respect to body image most likely contributed to the epidemic of this anovulatory disorder.

Diagnosis of Functional Hypothalamic Amenorrhea. Patients most commonly present with secondary amenorrhea characterized by absence of menstrual cycles for longer than 6 months without evidence of an organic disorder. The

TABLE 17-1

Classification of Anovulation Caused by Disorders of the Hypothalamic-Pituitary Unit

Functional Hypothalamic Anovulation (Amenorrhea)

Stress (psychogenic or physical)
Dieting
Vigorous exercise
Chronic illness (e.g., chronic liver or renal insufficiency, AIDS)

Psychiatric-Medical Emergencies

Anorexia nervosa

Medications

Antipsychotics (e.g., olanzapine, risperidone, amisulpride, clozapine)
Opiates

Hypothyroidism

Anatomically or Genetically Defined Pathologic Conditions of the Hypothalamic-Pituitary Unit

Pituitary tumors
Prolactinoma
Clinically nonfunctioning adenoma
GH-secreting adenoma (acromegaly)
ACTH-secreting adenoma (Cushing disease)
Other pituitary tumors (e.g., metastasis, meningioma)
Pituitary stalk section
Hemorrhagic pituitary destruction, including pituitary apoplexy and Sheehan syndrome
Pituitary aneurysm
Infiltrative disease of the pituitary (e.g., lymphocytic hypophysitis, sarcoidosis, histiocytosis X, tuberculosis)
Empty sella syndrome
Tumors that affect hypothalamic function (e.g., metastasis, craniopharyngioma)
Infiltrative granulomatous disease of the hypothalamus (e.g., sarcoidosis, histiocytosis X, tuberculosis)
Head trauma
Irradiation to the head
CNS infection
Isolated gonadotropin deficiency (including Kallmann syndrome)
Other

ACTH, adrenocorticotropic hormone; AIDS, acquired immunodeficiency syndrome; CNS, central nervous system; GH, growth hormone.

diagnosis of is one of exclusion. There are many neuroanatomic or genetic disorders that can mimic functional hypothalamic anovulation (see Table 17-1), and a careful and complete evaluation is essential to make this diagnosis.

Women with functional hypothalamic amenorrhea usually present with a history of regular menses for some period after menarche. This period of normal ovulatory function (determined by history) is interrupted by anovulation that usually manifests as secondary amenorrhea. Women with functional hypothalamic anovulation may occasionally present with primary amenorrhea.

Women with functional hypothalamic amenorrhea typically have a normal body weight or are thin. They may be highly driven for success and involved in high-stress occupations. The occupation of the patient (e.g., ballerina, competitive athlete) may be an important clue. A detailed interview may also reveal a variety of emotional crises or stressful events (e.g., divorce, death of a friend) preceding the onset of amenorrhea. During the interview, additional environmental and interpersonal factors may become evident, such as academic pressure, social maladjustment, or psychosexual problems.

When evaluating the patient, the physician should take note of the current diet regimen, the use of any sedatives or hypnotics, and the nature and extent of the patient's exercise habits. Despite a careful interview, a history of stress, excessive physical exercise, or an eating disorder may not be readily revealed by some women with functional hypothalamic anovulation. These women do not complain of hot flashes, in contrast to women with ovarian insufficiency.

These women usually have normal secondary sexual characteristics. The pelvic examination usually shows a thinning vaginal mucosa accompanied by scant to absent cervical mucus with a normal to small uterus, which are all evidence of estrogen deficiency. Signs of a well-estrogenized vagina and cervix observed during the physical examination make the diagnosis of hypothalamic amenorrhea unlikely. The physician should exclude a possible hyperprolactinemic cause (e.g., prolactinoma, hypothyroidism) and evidence of androgen excess (e.g., PCOS).

Laboratory tests are obtained to exclude other causes of anovulation and secondary amenorrhea. LH and FSH levels are usually lower than the normal values ordinarily found in the early follicular phase. TSH and prolactin levels are obtained to rule out hypothyroidism and hyperprolactinemia. The progestin challenge test (medroxyprogesterone acetate [MPA] at 5 mg/day for 10 days) elicits either a small spotting episode or an absence of withdrawal uterine bleeding in most patients. The administration of combined estrogen (2 mg/day of oral micronized estradiol) with progestin (5 mg/day of MPA for 10 days) will result in endometrial growth followed by vaginal bleeding because the uterine compartment remains functionally normal.

These results suggest that there is a scant or absent estrogenic effect on the endometrium, because circulating estradiol levels are typically in the low or early follicular phase range. Measurement of the serum estradiol level is not necessary. Because a suprasellar or large pituitary tumor is in the differential diagnosis, magnetic resonance imaging (MRI) of the head is necessary to rule out these possibilities. Imaging of the head is especially important if amenorrhea develops suddenly or is associated with a neurologic sign, both of which make the presence of a tumor more likely.

Pathophysiology of Functional Hypothalamic Anovulation. A critical defect in hypothalamic amenorrhea is the reduction in GnRH release from the medial basal hypothalamus, which leads to a reduction in GnRH pulse frequency.[11,140] LH pulse frequency is used as a surrogate measure to evaluate GnRH secretion because each GnRH pulse is accompanied by a concomitant LH pulse.[138] A key observation in functional hypothalamic anovulation is the absence of increased gonadotropin secretion despite the lack of inhibitory factors of ovarian origin, such as estradiol and inhibin.

There is considerable variability in the amplitude and frequency of the pulsatile LH secretion in women with functional hypothalamic amenorrhea. When the LH secretory patterns are compared with those of the follicular phase of the menstrual cycle, a characteristic abnormality in LH pulse frequency and amplitude is seen, and occasionally, regression to a pronounced variability similar to what is seen in the prepubertal pattern is observed.[11,138,140] In severe cases, the frequency and amplitude of LH pulses are markedly reduced. These LH patterns also suggest that GnRH pulsatile secretion is not altered to the same degree in every patient. During the recovery phase of hypothalamic amenorrhea, reversal to a pattern of LH secretion seen early in puberty often occurs, and it is characterized by a sleep-associated increase in LH amplitude.[138]

The response of the pituitary gland to GnRH with respect to production and release of gonadotropins is not impaired in functional hypothalamic anovulation. Intravenous pulsatile GnRH administration can restore normal levels of LH and FSH.[141]

Norepinephrine, dopamine, and serotonin produced in the brain have been shown to modulate GnRH or LH release in animal studies.[142] Patients receiving medication that alters these neurotransmitters (e.g., sedatives, antidepressants, stimulants, antipsychotics) have presented with abnormalities in their menstrual cycles. These responses to medications provide circumstantial evidence that disruptions of neural pathways can alter GnRH release in humans. It appears that activation of the noradrenergic neurons principally stimulates release of GnRH, whereas dopaminergic and serotoninergic neurons can stimulate or inhibit GnRH-LH secretion.[142]

Another group of substances that have inhibitory influences on GnRH secretion are endogenous opioid peptides.[143,144] Blockade of endogenous opiate receptors by the administration of naloxone, an opiate antagonist, causes an increase in the frequency and amplitude of pulsatile LH release in the majority of women with hypothalamic amenorrhea.[140] Gonadotropin secretion resumes if the activity of the opiate receptor is blocked by long-term naloxone use, and ovulatory function may be regained in some cases.[145] These studies suggest that there is an overall increase in endogenous opiate activity, which can reduce pulsatile GnRH secretion in some cases of functional hypothalamic amenorrhea.

The hypothalamic-pituitary-adrenal axis is dysfunctional in many women with functional hypothalamic amenorrhea, with increased secretion of corticotropin-releasing hormone (CRH), adrenocorticotropic hormone (ACTH), and cortisol. Activation of the pituitary-adrenocortical system is a common response in patients with chronic stress.[146] In functional hypothalamic amenorrhea, stressors such as exercise or emotional distress can chronically activate the hypothalamic-pituitary-adrenal axis and disrupt reproductive function.

Studies have demonstrated an increase in pulsatile ACTH secretion, increased adrenal sensitivity to ACTH, and increased cortisol secretion with a normal diurnal rhythm.[138] Daytime cortisol levels are markedly elevated, and the pituitary response to CRH is blunted.[147] In an animal model, CRH seems to be an important factor in the inhibition of GnRH pulsatility.[148,149] This inhibitory effect can be prevented by coadministration of a CRH antagonist or reversed by the opiate antagonist naloxone, suggesting that cross-talk occurs between the action of CRH and activation of the opioidergic system. Moreover, ACTH administration blocks the pituitary response to GnRH at the pituitary level.[150,151] In summary, overproduction of CRH and other stress-related hormones in the brain and activation of the pituitary-adrenocortical system by chronic stress seem to play causative roles in the inhibition of gonadotropin secretion in functional hypothalamic anovulation.

The roles of energy balance–regulating peptides such as leptin and ghrelin were investigated in the mechanism of hypothalamic amenorrhea.[138] Leptin is a cytokine produced by the adipocytes and is considered to be an appetite-suppressor peptide. Leptin is secreted in a pulsatile manner with a diurnal rhythm. A decrease in total circulating leptin with loss of the normal diurnal rhythm was reported in women with hypothalamic amenorrhea.[152] This relative hypoleptinemia is a common characteristic of several energy-deficient conditions and is associated with slowing of the LH pulse frequency.[152] Leptin administration to correct the relative leptin deficiency in women with hypothalamic amenorrhea was shown to improve reproductive, thyroid, and growth hormone axes and markers of bone formation, suggesting that leptin, a peripheral signal reflecting the adequacy of energy stores, is required for normal reproductive and neuroendocrine function.[152] In contrast to leptin, ghrelin is an appetite-inducing peptide secreted from the stomach. During the fasting state, ghrelin serves as the hunger signal from the periphery to the hypothalamic arcuate nucleus, a region that is known to control food intake. Ghrelin levels are reported to be elevated in women with hypothalamic amenorrhea.[153]

Hypothalamic Anovulation and Exercise. Regular vigorous exercise can lead to menstrual disturbances, a delay in menarche, luteal phase dysfunction, and secondary amenorrhea. Thirty percent of adolescent ballet dancers have problems with the progression of puberty. The mean age at menarche is delayed until the age of 15 years. Advancement of pubertal stages seems to coincide with times of prolonged rest or after recovery from an injury.[154-157] The intensity, length, and type of the sport determine the severity of the disease. Activities associated with an increased frequency of reproductive dysfunction are those that favor a lower body weight and include middle-distance and long-distance running, competitive swimming, gymnastics, and ballet dancing.

Competitive athletes show endocrine abnormalities in the central nervous system consistent with those in other forms of functional hypothalamic anovulation. Abnormalities include elevations of central CRH and β-endorphin levels.

The management of exercise-related anovulation depends on the patient's choices and expectations. Side effects such as osteoporosis and delay of puberty must be discussed thoroughly with the patient.[158] Decrease in exercise level and behavioral modification may be sufficient for the return of ovulatory function. Hormone therapy should be provided if sufficient results are not achieved. A low-dose oral contraceptive is a suitable option for women younger than 35 years of age.

Hypothalamic Anovulation Associated with Eating Disorders. Two common eating disorders associated with hypothalamic dysfunction are anorexia nervosa and bulimia. Patients with anorexia nervosa have extreme weight loss (>25% of original body weight) and a distorted body image accompanied by a striking fear of obesity. Bulimia is a related disorder characterized by alternating episodes of binge eating followed by periods of food restriction, self-induced vomiting, or excessive use of laxatives or diuretics. About 90% to 95% of these patients are women. The incidence of classic anorexia nervosa is about 1 case per 100,000 people in the general population.[159] Among female high school and college students, bulimia is fairly common. The incidence of anorexia nervosa peaks twice during the teen years, at ages 13 and 17. Bulimia usually begins at a later age, between 17 and 25 years. Anorexia nervosa has an extremely high mortality rate of 9% and is a true medical emergency. Death may result from cardiac arrhythmia, which may be precipitated by diminished heart muscle mass and associated electrolyte abnormalities.[160] These patients are also at increased risk for suicide.[161]

Gonadotropin secretion in anorexic women exhibits a prepubertal pattern that is similar to that observed in other forms of hypothalamic anovulation. Transitional patterns of LH secretion are seen with moderate degrees of weight recovery, and there is a normal or supranormal response to GnRH. Anovulation can persist in up to 50% of anorexic patients, even after normal weight is achieved. Anorexic and bulimic patients exhibit hyperactivation of the hypothalamus-pituitary-adrenal system. Although the diurnal variation is maintained, persistent hypersecretion of cortisol occurs throughout the day.[162] Cushingoid features are not present, in part because of mild hypercortisolemia and a reduction of peripheral glucocorticoid receptors. Levels of CRH and β-endorphin are increased in the central nervous system.[163,164]

In anorexia nervosa, basal metabolism is decreased because peripheral conversion of thyroxine (T_4) to biologically potent triiodothyronine (T_3) is decreased. Instead, T_4 is converted to reverse T_3, an inactive isoform. This alteration is also observed in severely ill patients and during starvation.[165] Anorexics have partial diabetes insipidus and are unable to concentrate urine appropriately because of the impaired secretion of vasopressin.[166]

Anorexia nervosa and bulimia are extremely difficult to treat. The most accepted approaches include individual psychotherapy, group therapy, and behavior modification. Patients with eating disorders should have psychiatric consultation and follow-up. This helps with the diagnosis and treatment. For patients who weigh less than 75% of their ideal body weight, immediate hospitalization and aggressive treatment are recommended. Complications of anorexia nervosa include osteoporosis, estrogen deficiency, and generalized effects of malnutrition.[155] Hormone therapy in the form of a low-dose oral contraceptive should be provided until ovulatory function is achieved.

Treatment and Management of Functional Hypothalamic Anovulation. Treatment of chronic anovulation resulting from central nervous system–hypothalamic disorders should be directed at reversal of the primary cause (e.g., stress management, reduction of exercise, correction of weight loss). The importance of successful treatment of this disease state is underscored because these women are prone to the development of osteoporosis. For a considerable number of patients, spontaneous recovery of menstrual function takes place after a modification of lifestyle, psychological guidance, or accommodation to environmental stress. The initial treatment should be directed to a change in lifestyle and tailored to the individual patient. For individuals who remain amenorrheic, periodic assessment of reproductive status (every 4 to 6 months) is prudent.

Modification of the stress response through cognitive-behavioral therapy is a logical approach to lowering the endogenous stress levels in women with hypothalamic amenorrhea. This approach was explored in 16 subjects with hypothalamic amenorrhea randomized to cognitive-behavioral therapy or observation for a 20-week period.[167] The therapy design focused on attitudes and habits concerning eating, exercise, body image, problem-solving skills, and stress reduction. The results are encouraging. About 88% of those who underwent cognitive-behavioral therapy had evidence of ovulation, compared with only 25% of those who were observed.[167] These results suggest that endogenous stress is a major factor in the development and maintenance of hypothalamic amenorrhea and that modification of this stress response can restore normal menses.

If anovulation persists for longer than 6 months or if reversal of the primary cause is not practical (e.g., professional athletes, ballerinas), a major concern is the long-term effect of hypoestrogenism, especially on bone metabolism. In addition to estrogen deficiency, IGF-1 deficiency, hypercortisolism, and nutritional factors may contribute to bone loss in this disorder.[168] However, epidemiologic data on the risk of fractures and the benefits of hormone therapy are scant.[158,168] On the basis of studies of reproductive-age women who were ovariectomized or underwent treatment with GnRH agonist for endometriosis, bone density is expected to decrease significantly, even within the first 6 months of amenorrhea. Because these patients are often reluctant to take medications, serial bone density studies of the lumbar spine and femur may be necessary to convince them of the necessity to begin

estrogen replacement therapy. If the patient is not at risk for thromboembolism and does not smoke cigarettes, a low-dose combination oral contraceptive is a reasonable replacement option. Alternatively, a combination of conjugated equine estrogens (0.625 mg) and MPA (2.5 mg) daily may be administered to provide estrogenic support. The progestin (MPA) is added solely to prevent endometrial hyperplasia.

If the patient desires ovulation to achieve pregnancy, the most physiologic approach is ovulation induction with pulsatile GnRH. This is the best physiologic means of induction because the cause of the anovulatory state is decreased endogenous GnRH secretion. Pulsatile intravenous GnRH (5 μg every 90 minutes) was shown to be effective.[169] Monitoring of serum estradiol levels or follicular development can be minimized because the ovarian follicular response and gonadotropin output mimic the natural menstrual cycle. In these patients, continuation of pulsatile GnRH or hCG (1500 units administered intramuscularly every 3 days for a total of four doses) can support the function of the corpus luteum. Intravenous GnRH treatment results in ovulation rates of approximately 90%, pregnancy rates of up to 30%, and hyperstimulation rates of less than 1% per treatment cycle. Because the intravenous GnRH pump is not a practical choice for many women, an alternative strategy is the use of subcutaneous recombinant FSH for the development of one to three follicles and the induction of ovulation with intramuscular hCG followed by luteal support using intramuscular hCG or progesterone in oil.

Chronic Anovulation Associated With Pituitary Disorders

The most common pituitary-related causes of anovulation are associated with hyperprolactinemia caused by prolactinomas or other functional or anatomic disorders of the pituitary. These disorders are frequently associated with dysregulation of gonadotropin secretion. Hyperprolactinemia and other pituitary disorders and their relation to reproduction are discussed in Chapter 9.

Chronic Anovulation Associated With Androgen Excess

The most common ovary-related disorder of chronic anovulation is PCOS. Irregular periods or amenorrhea and androgen excess are the most commonly observed features of PCOS. Other causes of ovary-related anovulation include steroid-secreting ovarian tumors and POI. Androgen excess arising from extraovarian sources (e.g., adrenal disorders) is also associated with anovulation.

Approach to the Patient With Androgen Excess

Two natural androgens are testosterone, which is transported to target tissue by the circulation, and DHT, which is produced primarily by target tissues. Increased levels of these androgens can lead to hirsutism, which is excessive androgenic hair growth, or to virilization, a more severe form of androgen excess. Hirsutism is defined as the presence of terminal (coarse) hair in locations at which hair is not commonly found in women, including facial hair on the cheek, above the upper lip, and on the chin (Fig. 17-24A and B). The presence of midline chest hair is also significant (see Fig. 17-24C). A male escutcheon, hair on the inner aspects of the thighs, and midline lower back hair entering the intergluteal area are hair growth patterns compatible with androgen excess. A moderate amount of hair

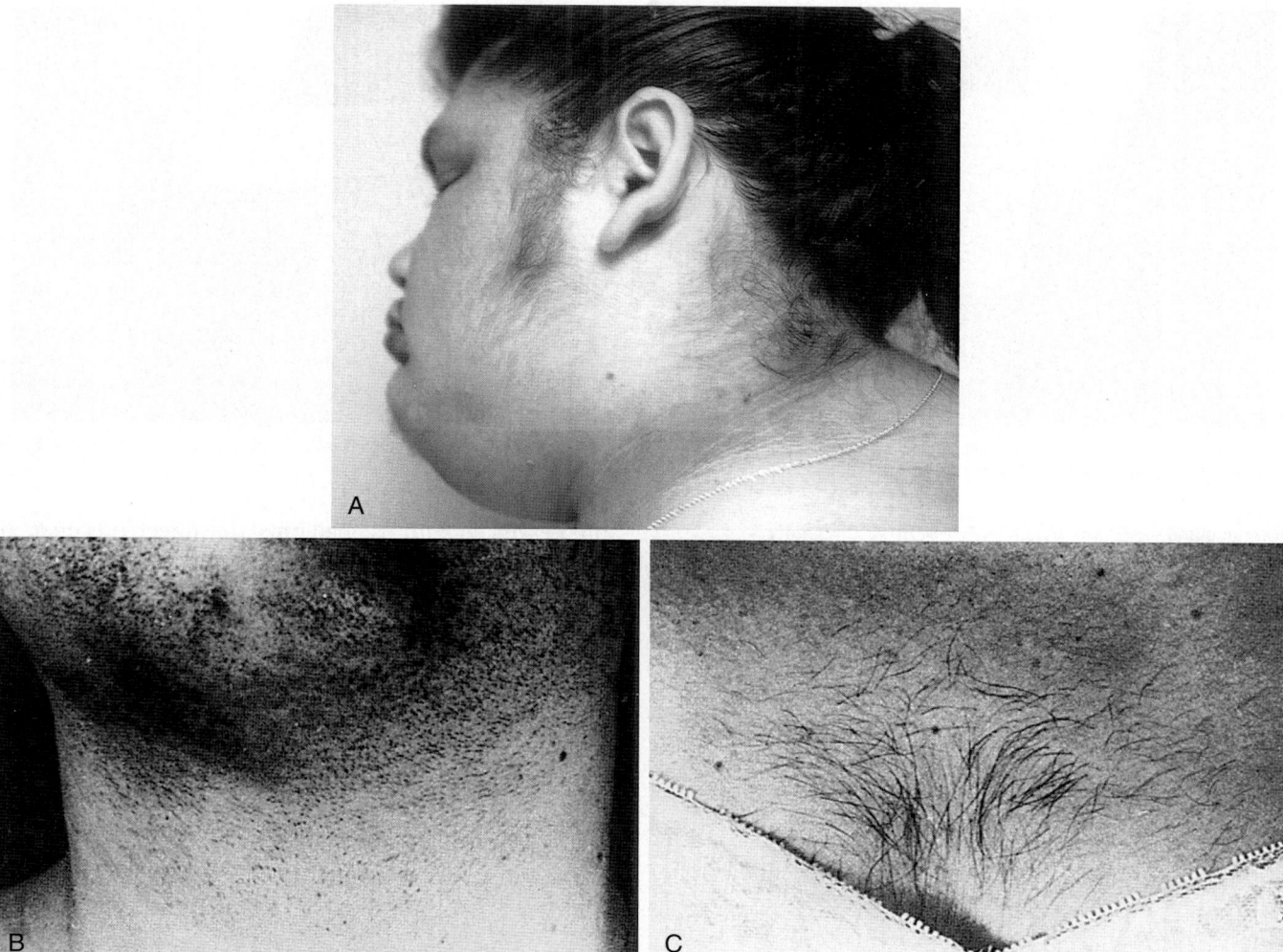

Figure 17-24 Hirsutism. **A,** Mild facial hirsutism. **B,** Severe facial hirsutism (chin), which requires regular shaving. **C,** Severe hirsutism on chest. (B and C from Dunaif A, Hoffman AR, Scully RE, et al. The clinical, biochemical and ovarian morphologic features in women with acanthosis nigricans and masculinization. *Obstet Gynecol.* 1985;66:545-552.)

on the forearms and lower legs by itself may not be abnormal, although it may be viewed by the patient as undesirable and may be mistaken for hirsutism. Numerous scoring systems are available for quantifying hirsutism. One of the most detailed scales was proposed by Ferriman and Gallwey.[170] A practical and clinically useful means of quantifying hirsutism is recording the hair growth in detail using simple drawings and photographs. In particular, photographs are invaluable for documenting hirsutism accurately.

Compared with hirsutism, virilization is a more severe form of androgen excess and implies significantly higher rates of testosterone production. Its manifestations include temporal balding, deepening of voice, decreased breast size, increased muscle mass, loss of female body contours, and clitoral enlargement (Fig. 17-25). Even if testosterone levels are moderately increased (<1.5 ng/mL), temporal balding and clitoromegaly may be observed after a long period (>1 year) in the presence of persistent androgen excess. A marked increase in androgen secretion, such as that may occur from production by neoplasms, leads to a more full-blown picture of virilization in less than a few months (see Fig. 17-25).

Measurements of an enlarged clitoris may be used for the quantification of virilization. A clitoral length greater than 10 mm is considered abnormal (see Fig. 17-25). Clitoral length is quite variable, however. An increase in clitoral diameter is a much more sensitive indicator of androgen action. Normal values for clitoral diameter are less than 7 mm at the base of the glans (see Fig. 17-25). The most accurate definition of clitoromegaly involves use of the clitoral index (the product of the sagittal and transverse diameters of the glans clitoris). A clitoral index greater than 35 mm² is abnormal and correlates statistically with androgen excess.[171]

Origins of Androgens

Among the natural C19 steroids, DHT is a biologically potent androgen that is capable of acting through androgen receptors on target cells. Almost all testosterone target tissues contain 5α-reductase activity, which converts testosterone to DHT, or aromatase activity, which produces estradiol in an intracrine fashion. It is not clear whether testosterone has any direct biologic effects independent of DHT or estradiol produced locally. There is no convincing

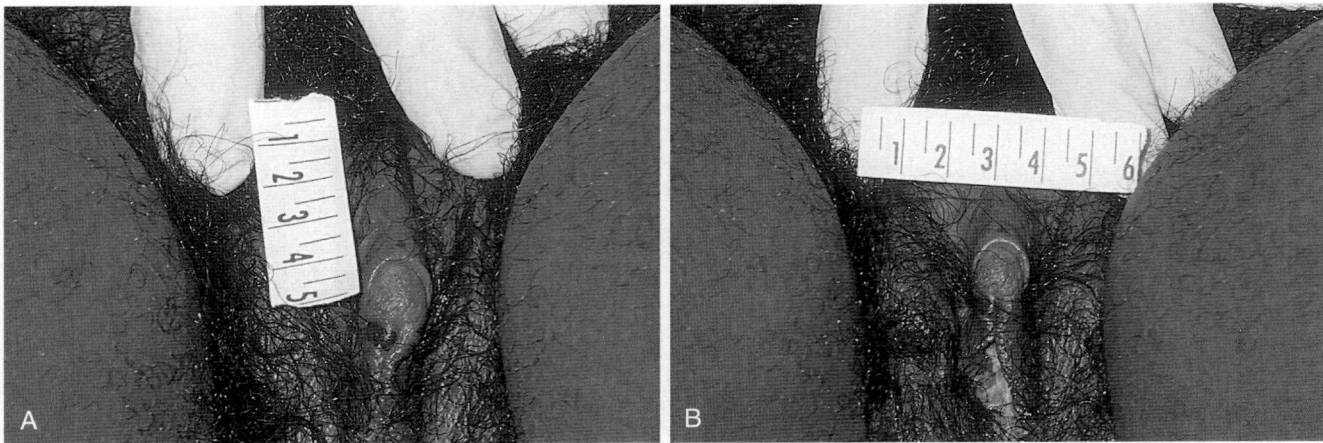

Figure 17-25 Severe clitoromegaly resulting from a testosterone-secreting ovarian tumor. **A,** The entire length of the clitoris is approximately 4 cm (normal, <1 cm). **B,** The transverse diameter of the clitoris measures 1.5 cm (normal, <0.7 cm).

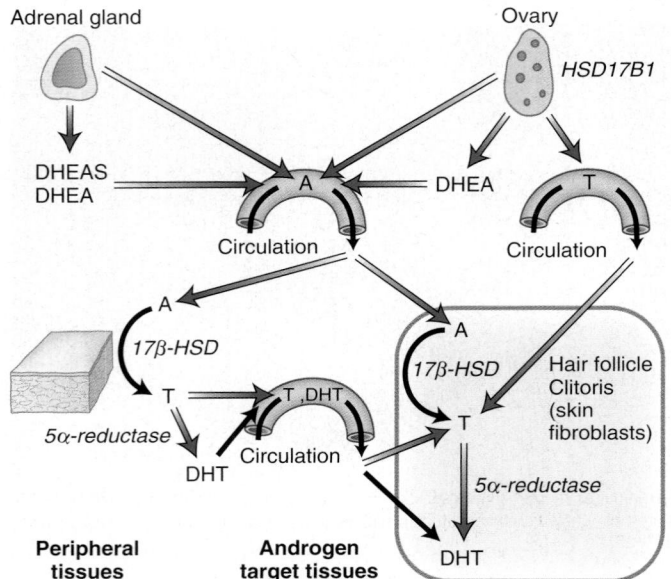

Figure 17-26 Androgen biosynthesis in women. Depending on the menstrual cycle phase or postmenopausal status, 20% to 30% of testosterone (T) is secreted by the ovary. The rest is accounted for by the conversion of circulating androstenedione (A) to T in various peripheral tissues. Both the adrenal gland and the ovary contribute to circulating A directly or indirectly, depending on the cycle phase or postmenopausal status and chronologic age. T may also be formed locally in androgen target tissues. T is converted to the biologically potent androgen dihydrotestosterone (DHT) within the target tissues and cells. For example, local conversion of T to DHT by 5α-reductase activity, which is conferred by products of at least two genes, in sex skin fibroblasts and hair follicles plays a key role in clitoral enlargement and hirsutism. The enzyme activity of 17β-HSD in peripheral tissues may be conferred by protein products of several genes with overlapping functions; HSD17B1, a distinct reductive 17β-HSD enzyme, is encoded by a specific gene expressed primarily in the ovary. DHEAS, dehydroepiandrosterone sulfate; 17β-HSD, reductive 17β-hydroxysteroid dehydrogenase.

evidence that the other C19 steroids, including androstenedione, DHEA, and dehydroepiandrosterone sulfate (DHEAS), are biologically active.

Testosterone in reproductive-age women is produced by two major mechanisms: direct secretion by the ovary, which accounts for roughly one third of testosterone production, and conversion of the precursor, androstenedione, to testosterone in the peripheral (extragonadal) tissues, which accounts for two thirds of testosterone production (Fig. 17-26).[172] These peripheral tissues include the skin and

adipose tissue. Androstenedione, the direct precursor of testosterone, is produced in the ovary and the adrenal gland. The C19 steroids DHEAS and DHEA of adrenal origin and DHEA of ovarian origin indirectly contribute to testosterone formation by first being converted to androstenedione, which is subsequently converted to testosterone (see Fig. 17-26). Only androstenedione can be converted directly to testosterone. The conversion rate of circulating androstenedione to testosterone in extragonadal tissues is about 5% in both men and women.

Testosterone is converted to a potent steroid, DHT, to exert full androgenic effects on certain target tissues such as hair follicles and external genitalia.[94,111] This conversion is catalyzed by the enzyme 5α-reductase and takes place in the liver for systemic DHT production and within androgen target cells such as sex skin fibroblasts for an intracrine effect.[94]

The androgenic effects of testosterone in target tissues are determined by the level of local 5α-reductase activity and the androgen receptor content (see Fig. 17-26). Androgen receptors mediate androgenic action in critical target tissues.[111,173] Other local enzymes at target tissues (e.g., aromatase, oxidative 17β-HSD) also regulate hormone action by metabolizing testosterone to the androgenically inactive androstenedione or to estradiol, a potent estrogen. There appears to be a balance between potent androgen action when DHT is formed and reduction of androgenicity when inactive C19 steroids or estradiol is formed from testosterone in target tissues and other extragonadal tissues. This may be particularly relevant for androgen-dependent disorders (e.g., hirsutism, virilization) and estrogen-dependent disorders such as malignancies of breast and endometrium (see Figs. 17-19 and 17-26).

Laboratory Evaluation of Androgen Action

Testosterone circulates in three forms: that which is bound to sex hormone–binding globulin (SHBG), the portion not bound to SHBG but loosely associated with albumin, and the fraction not bound by SHBG or albumin (i.e., free or dialyzable testosterone). The blood testosterone that is available to diffuse into target tissues includes the free and albumin-bound fractions and is referred to as bioavailable or non–SHBG-bound testosterone. The remainder is tightly bound to the protein SHBG.

SHBG is one of the primary regulators that determine the amounts of circulating bound and bioavailable testosterone available to act on target tissues. Conditions that decrease SHBG binding (e.g., androgen excess, obesity, acromegaly, hypothyroidism, liver disease) also increase bioavailable testosterone, augmenting the effect of testosterone. SHBG also regulates the circulating amounts of bioavailable estradiol by binding a significant fraction of circulating estradiol. Conditions that decrease SHBG levels give rise to increased bioavailable (non–SHBG-bound) estradiol.

The measurement of non–SHBG-bound (bioavailable) forms of testosterone has been advocated for states of androgen excess to detect more accurately subtle forms of hirsutism. Although the diagnostic yield of this measurement is superior to that of total serum testosterone, the correlation between total and non–SHBG-bound testosterone is excellent, so that bioavailable testosterone can usually be predicted from the total testosterone level.[174] The purpose of measuring serum testosterone is to establish the presence of circulating androgen excess and to detect extremely high values that may originate from an androgen-secreting neoplasm.

The normal serum levels of androgens, especially free testosterone determined by radioimmunoassay (RIA) or other direct methods, vary from laboratory to laboratory. A group of investigators compared serum free testosterone levels measured by equilibrium dialysis with those measured by direct RIA and with those calculated from the free androgen index (100 × testosterone/SHBG), a simple index that correlates with the free testosterone level.[175] Calculated values for free testosterone using the free androgen index correlated well with those obtained from equilibrium dialysis. In contrast, the direct free testosterone measurements had unacceptably high systematic bias and random variability and did not correlate as well with equilibrium dialysis values. Moreover, the lower limit of detection was higher for the direct RIA than for equilibrium dialysis or calculated free testosterone.[175] The clinician should be aware of the limitations of direct free testosterone measurements performed without rigorous quality control.

Measuring the levels of all C19 steroids is not clinically necessary for most patients presenting with androgen excess. The most useful initial test is a serum total testosterone level. An abnormal level in the presence of hirsutism or virilization may be associated with PCOS, hyperthecosis, nonclassic adrenal hyperplasia, or an androgen-secreting neoplasm. Most androgen-secreting tumors are of ovarian origin. The likelihood of a neoplasm correlates roughly with increasing testosterone levels. The following tests may be added on the basis of the clinical presentation: serum 17-hydroxyprogesterone (i.e., nonclassic adrenal hyperplasia), serum prolactin and TSH (i.e., mild androgen excess associated with hyperprolactinemia), serum FSH and LH (i.e., elevated LH/FSH ratio in PCOS), serum DHEAS (i.e., adrenal tumors), and imaging of ovaries and adrenals (i.e., PCOS and steroid-secreting tumors).

Causes of Androgen Excess

Several disorders give rise to androgen excess. They include unusual causes such as iatrogenic or drug-induced androgen excess, congenital genital ambiguity (e.g., excessive in utero androgen formation in female pseudohermaphroditism), and conditions unique to pregnancy (e.g., luteoma of pregnancy, hyperreactio luteinalis). These uncommon causes and relatively more prevalent disorders associated with androgen excess are listed in Table 17-2. The term *extraovarian steroid formation* is used synonymously with *extraglandular*, *extragonadal*, or *peripheral steroid formation* in this text.

TABLE 17-2
Causes of Androgen Excess in Women of Reproductive Age
Ovarian
Polycystic ovary syndrome (PCOS) Hyperthecosis (a severe PCOS variant) Ovarian tumor (e.g., Sertoli-Leydig cell tumor)
Adrenal
Nonclassic adrenal hyperplasia Cushing syndrome Glucocorticoid resistance Adrenal tumor (e.g., adenoma, carcinoma)
Specific Conditions of Pregnancy
Luteoma of pregnancy Hyperreactio luteinalis Aromatase deficiency in fetus
Other Causes
Hyperprolactinemia, hypothyroidism Medications (danazol, testosterone, anabolizing agents) Idiopathic hirsutism (normal serum testosterone in an ovulatory woman) Idiopathic hyperandrogenism (patients who do not fall into any of the other categories listed)

Overall, the prevalence of androgen-excess disorders was found to be as follows: 72.1% for PCOS (anovulatory patients, 56.6%; mildly affected ovulatory patients, 15.5%); 15.8% for idiopathic hyperandrogenism; 7.6% for idiopathic hirsutism; 4.3% for 21-hydroxylase-deficient nonclassic adrenal hyperplasia; and 0.2% for androgen-secreting tumors.[176]

In most hyperandrogenic disorders, androgen originates from more than one source (see Fig. 17-26). For example, testosterone secretion is somewhat increased from the ovary in PCOS, but the bulk of testosterone comes from extraovarian conversion of significantly elevated circulating androstenedione of ovarian origin to testosterone. Patients with PCOS also show increased adrenal output of DHEAS, which (after peripheral conversion to DHEA that is further converted to androstenedione) contributes indirectly to extraovarian testosterone formation.

If androgen excess is associated with primary amenorrhea, abnormal in utero sexual differentiation should be strongly suspected. These disorders are discussed in Chapter 23. Before embarking on a major workup for hirsutism or virilization, the physician is well advised to rule out exogenous androgen use. It is best to ask the patient to list all prescriptions and over-the-counter medications that she takes on her own, including injections. This is usually more rewarding than asking the patient whether she takes any androgens. Medications that can cause hirsutism or virilization are related to testosterone and include anabolic steroids and similar compounds.

The most common identifiable cause of androgen excess is PCOS, which is discussed elsewhere in this chapter. In this section, we first define some of the other disorders associated with hirsutism or virilization. This is followed by a simplified treatment strategy that may be applied to most hirsute patients within the categories of PCOS, nonclassic adrenal hyperplasia, and idiopathic hirsutism.

Idiopathic Hirsutism

Hirsutism is defined subjectively as the presence in a woman of terminal hair growth in a male-distribution pattern that affects quality of life sufficiently to prompt her to seek medical advice. Hirsutism should be distinguished from hypertrichosis, in which the excessive hair growth is not restricted to androgen-dependent areas and comprises vellus or lanugo-type hair. Hypertricosis is considered to be a phenotype not associated with male pattern hair growth and is unlikely to be modified by the known treatments of hirsutism.

Idiopathic (constitutional) hirsutism is characterized by excessive hair growth in the absence of elevated circulating androgen levels in ovulatory women, and it occurs more frequently in certain ethnic populations, particularly in women of Mediterranean ancestry.[111] It is defined as hirsutism in conjunction with regular menstrual cycles and normal levels of serum testosterone. Idiopathic hirsutism is not associated with any signs of virilization. Its cause is not understood completely. It has been proposed that women with idiopathic hirsutism have significantly increased cutaneous 5α-reductase activity,[177] but this association has not been confirmed. It is also unclear whether a certain 5α-reductase isoenzyme (type 1 or 2) is involved in the development of idiopathic hirsutism.[111]

Idiopathic hirsutism is diagnosed in women who have hirsutism,[111] normal ovulatory function, and normal total or free testosterone levels. Cyclic predictable menses are usually indicative of regular ovulation. If in doubt, ovulatory function may be verified by a luteal phase day 7 progesterone level, which should be at least 5 ng/mL. Luteal phase day 7 corresponds to cycle day 17 for 24-day intervals, cycle day 21 for 28-day intervals, and cycle day 28 for 35-day intervals. The presence of oligo-ovulation or anovulation in hirsute women after exclusion of related disorders (e.g., hypothyroidism, hyperprolactinemia, nonclassic adrenal hyperplasia) is consistent with the diagnosis of PCOS.[111] Thyroid dysfunction or hyperprolactinemia should be excluded by the measurements of TSH and prolactin. The follicular-phase basal 17-hydroxyprogesterone level should be measured to exclude 21-hydroxylase–deficient, nonclassic adrenal hyperplasia. The use of exogenous androgens should also be excluded. In summary, the diagnosis of idiopathic hirsutism is one of exclusion in which ovulatory dysfunction, elevated circulating testosterone levels, and other causes of androgen excess are ruled out.

Androgen-Secreting Tumors of the Ovary and Adrenal

Most androgen-secreting tumors arise from the ovary and secrete large quantities of testosterone or its precursor, androstenedione. These include Sertoli-Leydig cell tumors, hilus cell tumors, lipoid cell tumors, and infrequently, granulosa-theca tumors. Steroidogenically inert ovarian neoplasms such as epithelial cystadenomas or cystadenocarcinomas may produce factors that stimulate steroidogenesis in adjacent non-neoplastic ovarian stroma and induce production of sufficient amounts of androgen precursors such as androstenedione to give rise to clinically detectable androgen excess. Approximately 5% of androstenedione is converted to testosterone in extraovarian tissues, ultimately producing androgen excess (see Fig. 17-26).

Sertoli-Leydig cell tumors, which account for fewer than 1% of all solid ovarian tumors, tend to occur during the second to fourth decades of life, whereas hilus cell tumors occur more frequently in postmenopausal women. By the time the signs and symptoms of androgen excess cause the patient to seek medical assistance, Sertoli-Leydig cell tumors are usually so large that they are readily palpable on pelvic examination, whereas hilus cell tumors are still small. In women with either type of tumor, the serum testosterone level is markedly elevated. Granulosa-theca tumors primarily produce estradiol but may occasionally produce testosterone.

Rapidly progressing symptoms of androgen excess suggest the presence of an androgen-producing tumor unless proved otherwise. This rapid progression is typical of both ovarian and adrenal androgen-producing tumors. Progression is usually associated with defeminizing signs, such as loss of female body contour, increased muscle mass, and decreased breast size. As the tumor continues to grow, more and more testosterone is produced, resulting in rapidly worsening hirsutism and progressive virilization. Elevated serum testosterone levels are characteristically associated with ovarian tumors. This change may be mediated by production and secretion of testosterone directly by the tumor or by secretion of large quantities of androstenedione that are converted to testosterone in extragonadal tissues. The testosterone levels produced by certain ovarian tumors (e.g., Sertoli-Leydig cell tumors) may be suppressed by GnRH agonists,[178] so use of a GnRH agonist cannot be relied on to differentiate a neoplasm from another functional state.

In interpreting testosterone levels, the clinician should be familiar with the normal ranges of the clinical laboratory used. A value of three times the upper-normal range (or >2 ng/mL) suggests a neoplasm, particularly if the clinical history supports this diagnosis. Lower serum testosterone levels occasionally may be associated with virilizing ovarian tumors. If an androgen-secreting tumor is suspected, measurement of androstenedione is clinically useful. A severely elevated level of androstenedione is consistent with an ovarian or adrenal tumor. When an elevated level of testosterone is associated with suggestive clinical history, meticulously performed transvaginal ultrasonography is the most sensitive method to detect an ovarian tumor.

In contrast to testosterone-secreting tumors of the ovary, testosterone-secreting tumors of the adrenal are rare. The cells of some testosterone-producing adrenal tumors may resemble ovarian hilus cells, which are analogous to Leydig cells. These tumor cells produce testosterone and may be stimulated by LH or hCG. In patients with testosterone-producing adrenal adenomas, testosterone secretion usually decreases after LH suppression and increases after hCG stimulation. Testosterone-secreting adrenal carcinomas also have been reported.[179]

Virilizing adrenal tumors commonly secrete large quantities of DHEAS, DHEA, and androstenedione, and testosterone is usually produced by extraovarian conversion of these precursors. Levels of serum DHEAS are highly elevated in most patients with virilizing adrenal tumors.[180] If DHEAS levels exceed 8 μg/mL, adrenal imaging by computed tomography (CT) or MRI should be ordered. Occasionally, such high levels of DHEAS are associated with a functional abnormality such as congenital adrenal hyperplasia caused by an enzymatic defect or an unexplained hyperfunctional adrenal state that is commonly associated with PCOS. These circumstances may explain a negative CT or MRI result, which warrants further investigation.

Levels of a variety of adrenal steroids, including corticosteroids, may be elevated in various combinations in the presence of an adrenal tumor. It is not possible to describe a particular pattern of hormones that defines an adrenal tumor.[180] Very high levels of serum DHEAS (>8 μg/mL) suggest an adrenal tumor. Virilizing ovarian tumors are encountered much more frequently than those of adrenal origin. If the presentation is compatible with an androgen-secreting tumor and the ovaries are normal by transvaginal ultrasonography, the adrenals should be evaluated next by imaging.

Testosterone levels three times the upper-normal range (i.e., >2 ng/mL) and DHEAS levels higher than 8 µg/mL have been used traditionally as guidelines to investigate further whether neoplasms of the ovary or adrenal are the sources of androgen excess. These numbers are provided only as guidelines, not as rules, and there are exceptions. First, because tumors secrete androgens episodically, more than one measurement may be required to detect a significantly elevated level.[181] Second, other precursor steroids are often elevated as well (particularly androstenedione), and their measurement should be considered. Third, some tumors may give rise to milder elevations of DHEAS and testosterone levels. Even mild elevations in a postmenopausal woman are highly suspicious for an androgen-secreting tumor. By the same token, greatly elevated serum testosterone levels may be observed in women with severe ovarian hyperthecosis (a severe variant of PCOS) in the absence of a tumor.

Virilization of recent onset and short duration warrants immediate investigation, even if testosterone and DHEAS levels are mildly elevated. With improvements in scanning techniques—vaginal ultrasonography for the ovary; abdominal ultrasonography, CT, and MRI for the adrenal glands—the diagnosis of even a small ovarian or adrenal tumor may be made. If no neoplasm can be localized, imaging of the ovary or adrenal after intravenous administration of radiolabeled iodomethylnorcholesterol (NP-59), which detects active steroid-producing tumors, has proved useful.[182] These diagnostic studies should be pursued aggressively before surgical exploration of a suspected tumor.

The clinician should question whether an ovarian or adrenal tumor detected by imaging is the actual source of androgen excess before resorting to its surgical resection. Occasionally, a hemorrhagic corpus luteum cyst of the ovary may mimic an androgen-secreting tumor, or a woman with androgen excess may have an adrenal incidentaloma, which does not secrete androgen. Intraoperative selective ovarian or adrenal vein catheterization may be considered as a last resort to demonstrate significant steroid gradients before surgical exploration of an adrenal or ovary for a small tumor is undertaken, especially if the clinical picture is not certain.[183]

Non-neoplastic Adrenal Disorders and Androgen Excess

Adrenal disorders such as classic congenital adrenal hyperplasia, Cushing syndrome, and glucocorticoid resistance give rise to androgen excess related to overproduction of testosterone precursors from the adrenal gland. These disorders are discussed elsewhere in this text. In this chapter, we discuss nonclassic adrenal hyperplasia.

The diagnosis and prevalence of nonclassic adrenal hyperplasia continue to be debated, although the disorder clearly exists. Other terms that have been used to describe this syndrome include late-onset, adult-onset, attenuated, incomplete, and cryptic adrenal hyperplasia. This form of adrenal hyperplasia is caused by a partial deficiency in 21-hydroxylase activity. Although deficiencies in 11β-hydroxylase and 3β-HSD may result in the disorder, defects in 21-hydroxylase account for more than 90% of cases.[184]

The clinical presentation is almost identical to that of patients with PCOS. The prevalence of this disorder varies according to ethnic background, and the prevalence reported by different investigators has varied widely. The characteristic presentation consists of anovulatory uterine bleeding and progressive hirsutism of pubertal onset. These individuals are born with normal genitalia, do not exhibit

salt wasting, and are symptom-free until puberty. Patients of northern European ancestry have a low frequency of this disorder, whereas Ashkenazi Jews, Hispanics, and patients of central European ancestry have a much higher prevalence.[185] The patient with androgen excess from a high-risk ethnic group should be screened.

Screening may first be carried out by obtaining an 8 AM serum level of 17-hydroxyprogesterone in an anovulatory patient on any day. Although most women with nonclassic adrenal hyperplasia are anovulatory, some women with this disorder present with regular periods and hirsutism of pubertal onset or with only unexplained infertility.[184] If nonclassic adrenal hyperplasia is suspected in an ovulatory patient on the basis of clinical presentation, an 8 AM serum level of 17-hydroxyprogesterone should be obtained during the follicular phase, because 17-hydroxyprogesterone levels are higher in the luteal phase in ovulatory women.[184] A level of less than 2 ng/mL effectively rules out this diagnosis.[184]

The diagnosis of nonclassic adrenal hyperplasia can be made if the basal 17-hydroxyprogesterone level is higher than 8 ng/mL. No further testing is required in these cases. Values between 2 and 8 ng/mL are considered increased but not diagnostic of nonclassic adrenal hyperplasia. For example, disease-free women and patients with PCOS may also have basal levels of 17-hydroxyprogesterone in this indeterminate range.[184] In these circumstances, an ACTH stimulation test should be used to distinguish nonclassic adrenal hyperplasia from PCOS.[184] A rise of the 17-hydroxyprogesterone level to at least 10 ng/mL 60 minutes after intravenous injection of ACTH is considered diagnostic of nonclassic adrenal hyperplasia.[186] A higher basal level of 17-hydroxprogesterone within the 2-to 8-ng/mL range is associated with a higher likelihood of nonclassic adrenal hyperplasia. For example, an 8 AM 17-hydroxyprogesterone level higher than 4 ng/mL had a sensitivity of 90% for the diagnosis of nonclassic adrenal hyperplasia.[184]

In an androgen excess patient from a high-risk ethnic group, a baseline level of 17-hydroxyprogesterone should be measured at 8 AM. A screening baseline level of 17-hydroxyprogesterone should be obtained for patients with premature pubarche, those with androgen excess of early pubertal onset, women with progressive hirsutism or virilization, and patients with strong family histories of severe androgen excess.

Laboratory Testing to Aid the Differential Diagnosis of Androgen Excess

Algorithms exist for the differential diagnosis of anovulation associated with hirsutism or virilization or both. Salient clinical features are of paramount importance to guide laboratory testing. The most important features are the onset and severity of the signs and the rapidity with which they progress. Rapidly progressing severe androgen excess implies an androgen-secreting tumor until proved otherwise. The possibility of a tumor is further underscored in a postmenopausal woman or in a reproductive-age woman with a recent history of cyclic, predictable periods. Ovarian hyperthecosis, a severe variant of PCOS, also gives rise to severe androgen excess that may progress rapidly, especially at the time of expected puberty. Androgen excess emerging at the time of puberty may be indicative of PCOS or nonclassic adrenal hyperplasia.

The most useful initial test to evaluate androgen excess is the serum level of total testosterone (Table 17-3). Testosterone levels in most normal ovulatory women are lower than 0.6 ng/mL, although the value may vary from laboratory to laboratory. Women with idiopathic hirsutism have

TABLE 17-3

Laboratory Tests for the Differential Diagnosis of Androgen Excess

Initial Testing

Total testosterone
Prolactin
Thyroid-stimulating hormone

Further Testing Based on Clinical Presentation*

17-Hydroxyprogesterone (8 AM)
17-Hydroxyprogesterone 60 min after intravenous ACTH
Cortisol (8 AM) after 1 mg dexamethasone at midnight
DHEAS
Androstenedione
Imaging of ovaries (transvaginal ultrasonography)
Imaging of adrenal glands (abdominal ultrasonography, CT, MRI)
Nuclear imaging after intravenous administration of radiolabeled cholesterol

*See text.
ACTH, adrenocorticotropic hormone; CT, computed tomography; DHEAS, dehydroepiandrosterone sulfate; MRI, magnetic resonance imaging.

cyclic menses and normal testosterone levels. No further testing for androgen excess is required in this group.

If the testosterone level is elevated in an anovulatory woman, serum levels of TSH and prolactin should be obtained to rule out anovulation associated with hyperprolactinemia. Ultrasonography of the ovaries also can help to identify an ovarian tumor or polycystic ovaries. If the ethnic background of the patient (i.e., Ashkenazi Jews, Hispanics, and those of central European ancestry), onset of hirsutism (i.e., puberty), or family history suggests nonclassic adrenal hyperplasia, a baseline serum level of 17-hydroxyprogesterone should be obtained at 8 AM. Rare causes of androgen excess include an adrenal tumor, Cushing syndrome, and glucocorticoid resistance. A serum level of DHEAS and adrenal imaging are required to assess the presence or absence of an adrenal tumor. CT, MRI, or abdominal ultrasonography may be used to assess the adrenals, depending on the expertise of the local radiology laboratory. A screening test for Cushing syndrome and glucocorticoid resistance may be performed to explore rare adrenal causes of androgen excess (see Chapter 15).[187]

Most women with chronic anovulation and mild to moderate hirsutism of pubertal onset fall into the category of PCOS. These women have high-normal or elevated testosterone levels and no other laboratory abnormalities. After other diagnoses are ruled out by laboratory testing or on clinical grounds, a diagnosis of PCOS can be made.

Treatment of Hirsutism

Therapy for androgen excess should be directed toward its specific cause and suppression of abnormal androgen secretion. Neoplasms warrant surgical intervention and are not discussed in greater detail here. Suppression with a GnRH analogue may be tried initially for ovarian hyperthecosis. However, bilateral oophorectomy may become necessary to control androgen excess arising from hyperthecosis (see later discussion). Patients with adrenal disease are treated specifically. For Cushing syndrome, treatment correlates with the source of hypercortisolism. When treating androgen excess associated with nonclassic adrenal hyperplasia, an antiandrogen (e.g., spironolactone) in combination with an oral contraceptive is used. Although a glucocorticoid may be considered, the doses of glucocorticoids needed to suppress the adrenal can often cause symptoms and signs of glucocorticoid excess during long-term treatment. Thus, a combination oral contraceptive plus spironolactone is favored to treat androgen excess if the patient responds to this treatment with decreased hirsutism. Several classes of medications are reviewed in detail below for the treatment of androgen excess and hirsutism.

Oral Contraceptives. Oral contraceptives reduce circulating testosterone and androgen precursors by suppression of LH and stimulation of SHBG levels, thereby reducing hirsutism in hyperandrogenic patients.[111] Oral contraceptives decrease circulating androgen in patients with PCOS and synergize with the effects of antiandrogens. Oral contraceptives may further improve the results of antiandrogen therapy in patients with idiopathic hirsutism or nonclassic adrenal hyperplasia. It is advisable to use an oral contraceptive containing 30 or 35 µg of ethinyl estradiol to achieve effective suppression of LH.[111] A meta-analysis showed that treatment with oral contraceptives for 6 months reduced Ferriman-Gallwey scores of hirsutism by an average of 27%.[188]

Spironolactone. The most commonly used androgen blocker for the treatment of hirsutism in the United States is spironolactone, an aldosterone antagonist structurally related to progestins. Spironolactone is effective for abnormal hair growth associated with PCOS, nonclassic adrenal hyperplasia, or idiopathic hirsutism. Treatment with spironolactone for 6 months reduces Ferriman-Gallwey scores of hirsutism by an average of 38.4%.

Because spironolactone acts through mechanisms different from those of oral contraceptives, overall effectiveness is improved by combining these two medications in patients with hirsutism, including those with PCOS, idiopathic hirsutism, or nonclassic adrenal hyperplasia. Apart from inhibiting steroidogenesis and acting as an androgen antagonist, spironolactone has a significant effect in inhibiting 5α-reductase activity.[111,189] Basic experimental and several clinical studies have confirmed the efficacy of spironolactone for hyperandrogenism and suggest that the principal effect is related to its ability to block peripheral androgen production and action.[111]

Doses of spironolactone used in clinical studies have varied from 50 to 400 mg daily. Although doses of 100 mg/day usually are effective for the treatment of hirsutism, higher doses (200 to 300 mg/day) may be preferable in extremely hirsute or markedly obese women.[111,189] The initial recommended dosage is 100 mg/day, which is gradually increased by increments of 25 mg/day every 3 months up to 200 mg/day on the basis of the response. This approach may be helpful to minimize side effects such as gastritis, dry skin, and anovulation. In patients with normal renal function, hyperkalemia is almost never seen. Hypotension is rare except in older women. Monitoring for electrolytes and blood pressure is imperative within the first 2 weeks at each dose level. Adjustments in dose should be made only after 3 to 6 months, as with other antiandrogens, to account for the slow changes in the hair cycle.

Patients usually notice an initial transient diuretic effect. Some women with normal cycles complain of menstrual irregularity with spironolactone; this is remedied by a downward dose adjustment or the addition of an oral contraceptive. The mechanism for abnormal bleeding is unclear. In women with oligomenorrhea, such as those with PCOS, resumption of normal menses may occur. This change may be caused in part by an alteration in levels of circulating androgens; LH levels have only occasionally been reported to decrease.[190] Another important consideration is the potential in utero feminizing effect of this antiandrogen on the genitalia of a 46,XY fetus. Effective contraception should always be provided in women taking spironolactone.

Cyproterone Acetate. Cyproterone acetate is a 17-hydroxy-progesterone acetate derivative with strong progestagenic properties. Cyproterone acetate acts as an antiandrogen by competing with DHT and testosterone for binding to the androgen receptor. There is also some evidence that cyproterone acetate and ethinyl estradiol in combination can inhibit 5α-reductase activity in skin.[191] Cyproterone acetate is not available in the United States but has been used in other countries. The drug usually is administered daily in doses of 50 to 100 mg on days 5 through 15 of the treatment cycle. Because of its slow metabolism, it is administered early in the treatment cycle; when ethinyl estradiol is added, it is usually administered in 50-μg doses on days 5 through 26. This regimen is needed for menstrual control and is usually referred to as the *reverse sequential regimen*. Cyproterone acetate in doses of 50 to 100 mg/day, combined with ethinyl estradiol at 30 to 35 μg/day, is as effective as the combination of spironolactone (100 mg/day) and an oral contraceptive in the treatment of hirsutism.[111] In smaller doses (2 mg), cyproterone acetate has been administered as an oral contraceptive in daily combination with 50 or 35 μg of ethinyl estradiol. This regimen is primarily suited for individuals with a milder form of hyperandrogenism.[111]

Finasteride. Finasteride inhibits 5α-reductase activity and has been used primarily for the treatment of prostatic hyperplasia. It can also be used in the treatment of hirsutism.[192,193] At a dose of 5 mg/day, a significant improvement of hirsutism is observed after 6 months of therapy, without significant side effects. In hirsute women, the decline in circulating DHT levels is small and cannot be used to monitor therapy. Although this treatment regimen increases testosterone levels, SHBG levels remain unaffected.[192] A meta-analysis showed that finasteride treatment for 6 months reduced Ferriman-Gallwey scores of hirsutism by an average of 20.3%.[188]

Finasteride primarily inhibits 5α-reductase type 2. Because hirsutism results from the combined effects of type 1 and type 2, this agent is only partially effective. Although prolonged experience with finasteride is lacking, one of the potential advantages of this agent is its benign side effect profile. One study showed efficacy with 1 year of hirsutism treatment.[194] It was also reported that finasteride is less effective than spironolactone with respect to the reduction of hirsutism in women.[111] Nevertheless, finasteride at a dose of 5 mg/day for prolonged periods represents a useful option because of its benign side effect profile and good tolerance by patients. Like spironolactone, finasteride may cause congenital genital ambiguity in a 46,XY fetus, and effective contraception should be provided during its use.

Flutamide. Flutamide is a potent antiandrogen used in the treatment of prostate cancer. It has been shown to be effective in the treatment of hirsutism.[195,196] The mean Ferriman-Gallwey score is reduced by 41.3%.[188] Nevertheless, occasional severe hepatotoxicity makes this drug unsuitable for the indication of hirsutism.[197]

Metformin and Thiazolidinediones. Because PCOS is often associated with insulin resistance, drugs that mitigate insulin resistance have been used in this disorder.[106] Metformin (1500 to 2700 mg/day) for 6 months significantly reduces hirsutism by 19.1% as assessed by the Ferriman-Gallwey scoring system.[188] In obese adolescent women with PCOS, metformin in combination with lifestyle modification (i.e., diet with a 500-kcal/day deficit and exercise 30 minute/day) and oral contraceptives reduced the total testosterone level and waist circumference.[198] The thiazoli-

dinediones (4 mg/day of rosiglitazone or 30 mg/day of pioglitazone) also reduced Ferriman-Gallwey scores significantly.[188] These studies suggested that insulin-sensitizing agents may be used in the treatment of hirsutism of PCOS, especially for women who do not wish to use other oral agents.

Lifestyle Modification. In obese adolescent women with PCOS, lifestyle modification (i.e., diet with a 500-kcal/day deficit and exercise 30 minute/day) alone resulted in a 59% reduction in the testosterone/SHBG ratio, with a 122% increase in SHBG.[198] A moderate diet and exercise program should be recommended as part of hirsutism management, particularly for obese women.

A Comprehensive Treatment Strategy for Hirsutism. The medications described in the previous paragraphs may be effective when administered as individual treatments. Patients with the most common form of hirsutism (i.e., PCOS, nonclassic adrenal hyperplasia, or idiopathic hirsutism) are often initially treated with a combination of two agents, one that suppresses the ovary (e.g., an oral contraceptive) and another that suppresses the extraovarian (peripheral) action of androgens (e.g., spironolactone). An oral contraceptive containing 30 to 35 μg of ethinyl estradiol combined with spironolactone (100 mg/day) is the initial treatment of choice. Even in women with idiopathic hirsutism, the addition of an oral contraceptive to the antiandrogen spironolactone can improve efficacy and prevent abnormal bleeding. For women with only minor complaints of hirsutism, the use of an oral contraceptive alone may be an appropriate first approach. Moderate lifestyle modification (i.e., diet with a 500-kcal/day deficit and 30 minute/day of exercise) should be a part of hirsutism management in obese patients.

Because the growth phase of body hairs lasts 3 to 6 months, a response should not be expected before 6 months after onset of treatment. Objective means should be used to assess changes in hair growth. Scoring systems and evaluation of anagen hair shafts are difficult; taking photographs is the simplest and most objective tool. Patients are often unaware that change is taking place unless there is some objective measurement. Pictures of the face and selected midline body areas before and during therapy are especially useful for the encouragement of the patient and compliance with the treatment.

Suppression of androgen production and action inhibits only new hair growth. Existing coarse hair should be removed mechanically. Plucking, waxing, and shaving are ineffective for hair removal and cause irritation, folliculitis, and ingrown hairs. Electrolysis is still the method of choice. Laser epilation is relatively new and needs further evaluation.[111]

Most patients with PCOS, nonclassic adrenal hyperplasia, or idiopathic hirsutism respond to this strategy within 1 year. Patients should be encouraged to continue treatment for at least 2 years. Then, depending on the wishes and clinical responses of patients, therapy can be stopped and the patient reevaluated. Many patients require continuous treatment for suppression of hirsutism. Patients with clitoromegaly may be referred to a urologist for clitoral reduction surgery after the source of virilization has been effectively eliminated.

Polycystic Ovary Syndrome

PCOS is the most common form of chronic anovulation associated with androgen excess; it occurs in perhaps 5% to 10% of reproductive-age women.[107] The diagnosis of PCOS is made by excluding other hyperandrogenic disorders (e.g., nonclassic adrenal hyperplasia, androgen-secreting tumors, hyperprolactinemia) in women with chronic anovulation and androgen excess.

During the reproductive years, PCOS is associated with important reproductive morbidity, including infertility, irregular uterine bleeding, and increased pregnancy loss. The endometrium of the patient with PCOS must be evaluated by biopsy, because long-term unopposed estrogen stimulation leaves these patients at increased risk for endometrial cancer. PCOS is also associated with increased metabolic and cardiovascular risk factors.[199] These risks are linked to insulin resistance and are compounded by the common occurrence of obesity, although insulin resistance also occurs in nonobese women with PCOS.[107]

PCOS is considered to be a heterogeneous disorder with multifactorial causes. PCOS risk is significantly increased with a positive family history of chronic anovulation and androgen excess, and this complex disorder may be inherited in a polygenic fashion.[200,201]

Historical Perspective

In their pioneering studies, Stein and Leventhal described an association between the presence of bilateral polycystic ovaries and signs of amenorrhea, oligomenorrhea, hirsutism, and obesity (Fig. 17-27).[202] At the time, these signs

were strictly adhered to in the diagnosis of what was then known as *Stein-Leventhal syndrome*. These investigators also reported the results of bilateral wedge resection of the ovaries, in which at least half of each ovary was removed as a therapy for PCOS; most of their patients resumed menses and achieved pregnancy after ovarian wedge resection. The exact mechanism responsible for the therapeutic effect of removal or destruction of part of the ovarian tissue is still not well understood.

On the basis of Stein and Leventhal's original work, a primary ovarian defect was inferred. Subsequent clinical, morphologic, hormonal, and metabolic studies uncovered multiple underlying pathologies, and the term *polycystic ovary syndrome* was introduced to reflect the heterogeneity of this disorder. One of the most significant discoveries regarding the pathophysiology of PCOS was the demonstration of a unique form of insulin resistance and associated hyperinsulinemia.[107,202]

Diagnosis of Polycystic Ovary Syndrome and Laboratory Testing

One of the most prominent features of PCOS is the history of ovulatory dysfunction (i.e., amenorrhea, oligomenorrhea, or other forms of irregular uterine bleeding) of

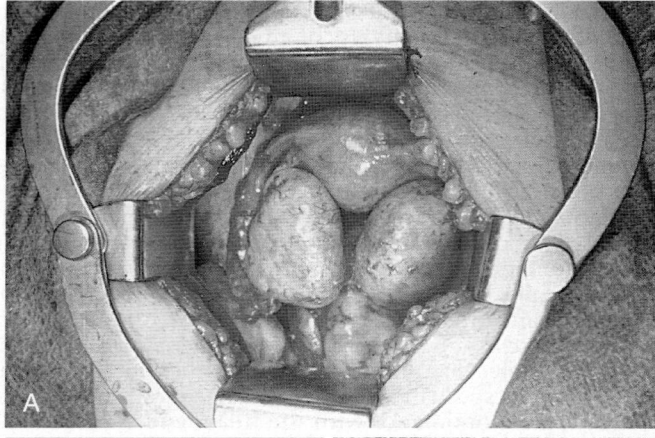
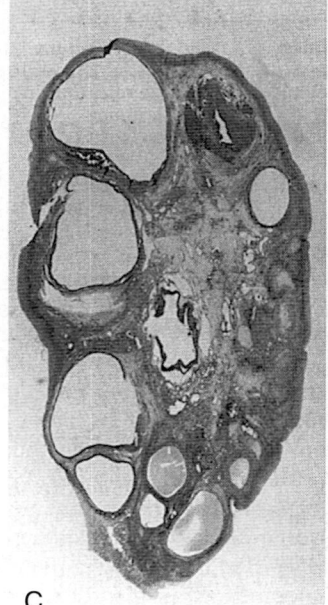
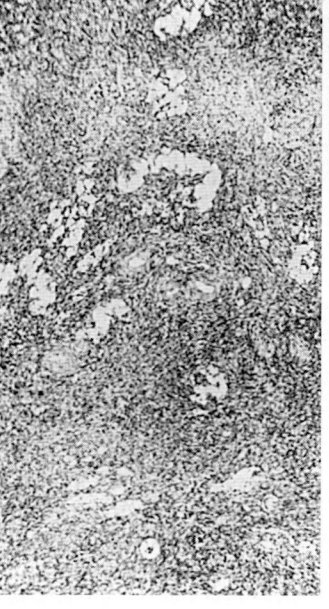
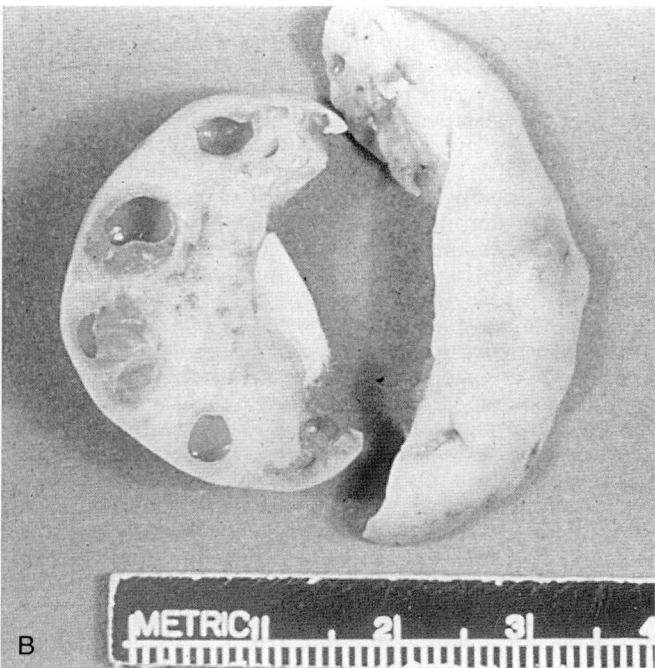

Figure 17-27 Polycystic ovaries. **A,** Operative findings of classic enlarged polycystic ovaries. The uterus is located adjacent to the two enlarged ovaries. **B,** Sectioned polycystic ovary with numerous follicles. **C,** Histologic section of a polycystic ovary with multiple subcapsular follicular cysts and stromal hypertrophy at low power *(left)*. At higher power (×100), islands of luteinized theca cells are visible in the stroma *(right)*. This morphologic change is called *stromal hyperthecosis*, and it appears to correlate directly with circulating insulin levels. (C from Dunaif A. Insulin resistance and the polycystic ovary syndrome: mechanism and implications for pathogenesis. *Endocr Rev.* 1997;18:774-800. Copyright © 1997 by The Endocrine Society.)

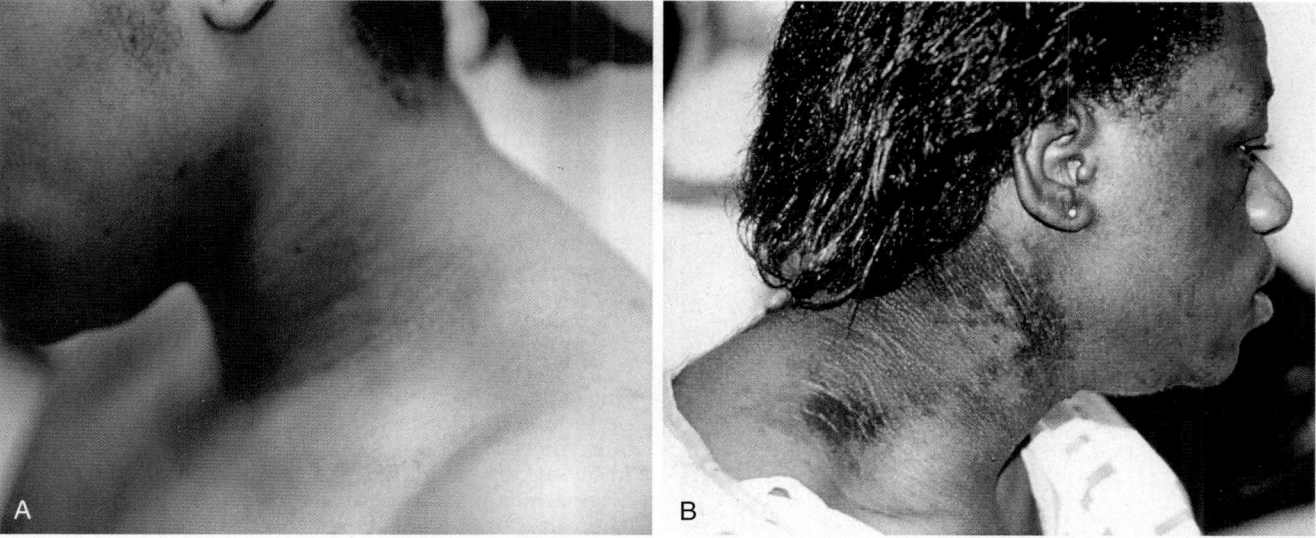

Figure 17-28 Acanthosis nigricans. **A,** Moderate acanthosis nigricans (i.e., darkening and thickening of skin) at the lateral lower fold of the neck. Notice facial hirsutism (sideburns) in the same patient. **B,** Severe acanthosis nigricans in another patient with severe insulin resistance. (B courtesy of Dr. R. Ann Word, UT Southwestern Medical Center, Dallas, TX.)

TABLE 17-4

Differential Diagnosis of Polycystic Ovary Syndrome

Idiopathic hirsutism
Hyperprolactinemia, hypothyroidism
Nonclassic adrenal hyperplasia
Ovarian tumors
Adrenal tumors
Cushing syndrome
Glucocorticoid resistance
Other rare causes of androgen excess

TABLE 17-5

Criteria for the Definition of Polycystic Ovary Syndrome (PCOS)

NIH Statement (1990)[204]

To include all of the following:
1. Hyperandrogenism and/or hyperandrogenemia
2. Oligo-ovulation
3. Exclusion of related disorders*

ESHRE/ASRM Statement (Rotterdam, 2003)[205]

To include two of the following, in addition to exclusion of related disorders*:
1. Oligo-ovulation or anovulation (e.g., amenorrhea, irregular uterine bleeding)
2. Clinical and/or biochemical signs of hyperandrogenism (e.g., hirsutism, elevated serum total or free testosterone)
3. Polycystic ovaries (by ultrasonography)

AES Suggested Criteria for the Diagnosis of PCOS (2006)[206]

To include all of the following:
1. Hyperandrogenism: hirsutism and/or hyperandrogenemia
2. Ovarian dysfunction: oligo-anovulation and/or polycystic ovaries
3. Exclusion of other androgen excess or related disorders*

*Including but not limited to 21-hydroxylase-deficient nonclassic adrenal hyperplasia, thyroid dysfunction, hyperprolactinemia, neoplastic androgen secretion, drug-induced androgen excess, the syndromes of severe insulin resistance, Cushing syndrome, and glucocorticoid resistance.
Superscript numbers in table indicate references at the end of the chapter.
AES; Androgen Excess Society, ASRM, American Society for Reproductive Medicine; ESHRE, European Society for Human Reproduction and Embryology; NIH, National Institutes of Health.

---

pubertal onset. A clear history of cyclic predictable menses of menarchal onset makes the diagnosis of PCOS unlikely. Acquired insulin resistance associated with significant weight gain or an unknown cause may induce the clinical picture of PCOS in a woman with a history of previously normal ovulatory function. Hirsutism may develop prepubertally or during adolescence, or it may be absent until the third decade of life. Seborrhea, acne, and alopecia are other common clinical signs of androgen excess. In extreme cases of ovarian hyperthecosis (a severe variant of PCOS), clitoromegaly may be observed. Nonetheless, a history of rapid progression of androgenic symptoms and virilization is unusual. Some women may never have signs of androgen excess because of hereditary differences in target tissue sensitivity to androgens.[111] Infertility related to the anovulation may be the only presenting symptom.

During the physical examination, it is essential to search for and document signs of androgen excess (hirsutism, virilization, or both), insulin resistance (acanthosis nigricans, Fig. 17-28), and the presence of unopposed estrogen action (well-rugated vagina and stretchable, clear cervical mucus) to support the diagnosis of PCOS. None of these signs is specific for PCOS, and each may be associated with any of the conditions listed in the differential diagnosis of PCOS (Table 17-4).

PCOS was previously defined according to the proceedings of an expert conference sponsored by the National Institutes of Health (NIH) in 1990, which described the disorder as including hyperandrogenism or hyperandrogenemia (or both), oligo-ovulation, and exclusion of known disorders of androgen excess and anovulation (Table 17-5).[203,204] Another expert conference held in Rotterdam in 2003 defined PCOS, after the exclusion of related disorders, by the presence of two of the following three features: oligo-ovulation or anovulation, clinical or biochemical signs of hyperandrogenism (or both), and polycystic ovaries (Fig. 17-29).[205] In essence, the Rotterdam 2003 criteria expanded the NIH 1990 definition by creating two new phenotypes: ovulatory women with polycystic ovaries plus hyperandrogenism and oligo-anovulatory women with polycystic ovaries but without hyperandrogenism. The clinical usefulness of including these new

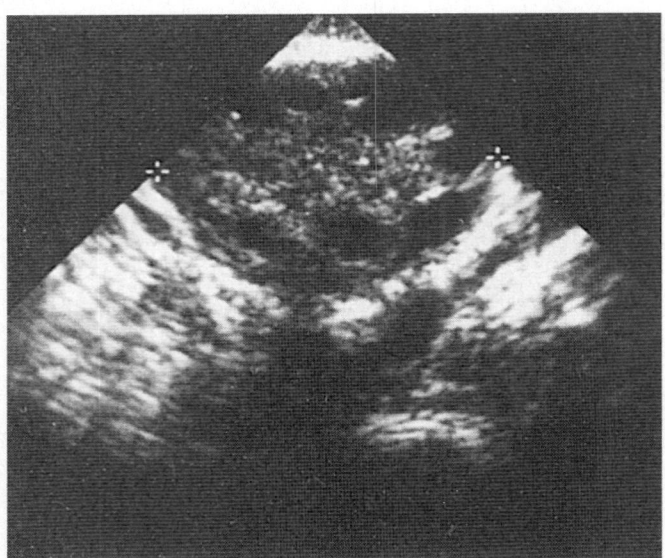

Figure 17-29 Transvaginal ultrasound image of a polycystic ovary. Notice the multiple, midsized follicles in the periphery and the increased solid area in the middle. (From Franks S. Medical progress: polycystic ovary syndrome. *N Engl J Med.* 1995;333:853-861.)

groups with respect to increased risk of infertility, insulin resistance, and long-term metabolic complications is not clear at this time.[206] More recently, the Androgen Excess Society published a broad consensus statement that included discussions of the merits and disadvantages of the NIH and Rotterdam criteria and suggested a practical definition that integrates both sets of diagnostic criteria (see Table 17-5).[205]

The exclusion of hyperprolactinemia, hypothyroidism, nonclassic adrenal hyperplasia, and tumors requires a careful history, physical examination, and laboratory testing, as detailed previously (see Table 17-4). Cushing syndrome and glucocorticoid resistance may give rise to androgen excess and anovulation after a period of normal ovulatory function in teens. An 8 AM cortisol level after dexamethasone (1 mg) administration at midnight is a useful screening test for both conditions. Cushing syndrome may be recognized by its typical signs, whereas 8 AM and 4 PM cortisol levels are essential to confirm the diagnosis of glucocorticoid resistance.[187] Glucocorticoid resistance is characterized by preserved diurnal rhythm despite significantly elevated cortisol, ACTH, and adrenal C19 steroid levels and absence of cushingoid symptoms and signs.[187]

Elevated total testosterone is the most direct evidence for androgen excess. Various levels of testosterone are found in women with PCOS. Rarely, serum testosterone levels higher than 2 ng/mL may be encountered in association with the most severe form of PCOS, ovarian hyperthecosis. Overall, it is much more common to observe high-normal levels or borderline elevations of testosterone in women with PCOS.

Prolactin and TSH concentrations should be measured routinely to rule out mild androgen excess and anovulation that may be associated with hyperprolactinemia. If basal LH levels are used as a marker for PCOS, a significant number of patients will slip through the cracks because they do not manifest elevated LH levels or increased LH/FSH ratios. The NIH-sponsored consensus conference on diagnostic criteria for PCOS in 1990 recommended that LH

and the LH/FSH ratio are not required for the diagnosis of PCOS.[204,207] The heterogeneity of LH values in PCOS may be caused by the pulsatile nature of LH secretion and negative effects of obesity on LH levels. An elevated LH/FSH ratio supports the diagnosis of PCOS and may be useful in differentiating mild cases of nonobese PCOS without prominent androgen excess from hypothalamic anovulation. However, failure to exhibit an elevated LH level is of no diagnostic value. By definition, nonclassic adrenal hyperplasia does not manifest as congenital virilization of external genitalia. Hyperandrogenic symptoms most commonly appear peripubertally or postpubertally. The clinical evaluation and laboratory-based diagnosis of nonclassic adrenal hyperplasia was discussed earlier. Chapter 15 describes the ACTH stimulation test. A screening test for Cushing syndrome or glucocorticoid resistance should be performed as clinically indicated (see Chapter 15).

Serum DHEAS levels may be increased (up to 8 µg/mL) in about 50% of anovulatory women with PCOS. DHEAS originates almost exclusively from the adrenal gland.[208] The cause of adrenal hyperactivity in PCOS is unknown. Obtaining a DHEAS level routinely in a patient with PCOS is not recommended because it does not change the diagnosis or management. If an adrenal tumor is suspected, a DHEAS level should be obtained. DHEAS levels higher than 8 µg/mL may be associated with steroidogenically active adrenal tumors, and imaging is then indicated.

The Rotterdam 2003 criteria include the use of ultrasound as a diagnostic tool. The use of ultrasonography in the diagnosis of PCOS must be tempered by an awareness of the broad spectrum of women with ultrasonographic findings characteristic of polycystic ovaries. The typical polycystic-appearing ovary may emerge in a nonspecific fashion when a state of anovulation of any cause persists for any length of time (see Fig. 17-29).[209] Thus, the polycystic-appearing ovary is the result of a functional derangement but not a specific central or local defect.

Biochemical evidence of insulin resistance or glucose intolerance is not necessary for the diagnosis of PCOS. Nonetheless, glucose intolerance should be investigated. Plasma glucose levels should be measured after a 75-g glucose load as a screen for glucose intolerance.

Women with PCOS commonly present with irregular uterine bleeding in the form of infrequent periods (i.e., oligomenorrhea) or amenorrhea. It is not necessary to document anovulation by ultrasonography, progesterone levels, or otherwise, especially if menstrual cycles are irregular with periods of amenorrhea. To confirm the diagnosis of chronic anovulation and unopposed estrogen exposure, most clinicians perform a progestin challenge test after a negative urine pregnancy test. Because endometrium is exposed to estradiol chronically in PCOS, these women respond to a challenge with a progestin (e.g., 5 mg/day of MPA given orally for 10 days) by uterine bleeding within a few days after the last pill of progestin. Reasons for lack of uterine bleeding after a progestin challenge include pregnancy, insufficient prior estrogen exposure of the endometrium, or an anatomic defect. If uterine bleeding does not follow progestin challenge, pregnancy should be ruled out again, along with other causes of chronic anovulation, as described in this chapter. An anatomic defect such as intrauterine adhesions may be ruled out with a hysterosalpingogram or hysteroscopy.

During the initial workup, an endometrial biopsy specimen should be obtained with the use of a plastic minisuction cannula (e.g., Pipelle) in the physician's office. If chronic anovulation persists, endometrial biopsies should be repeated periodically. Pregnancy should be ruled out by a urine or serum pregnancy test before each biopsy.

Response to oral contraceptives or periodic progestin treatment with predictable withdrawal bleeding episodes is reassuring, and patients with predictable bleeding patterns do not need endometrial sampling during these treatments. In untreated patients, the risk of endometrial hyperplasia and malignancy is significantly increased even in young women with PCOS because of unopposed estrogen exposure.

Gonadotropin Production in Polycystic Ovary Syndrome

Women with PCOS have higher mean concentrations of LH but low or low-normal levels of FSH compared with levels found in normal women in the early follicular phase.[210] The elevated LH levels in PCOS are presumed to be primarily caused by accelerated GnRH-LH pulsatile activity (Fig. 17-30).[211-213] Central opioid tone appears to be suppressed because the pattern of LH secretion does not change in response to naloxone.[214] The enhanced pulsatile secretion of GnRH has been attributed to a reduction in hypothalamic opioid inhibition caused by the chronic absence of progesterone.[183] An increase in amplitude and frequency of LH secretion also correlates with steady-state levels of circulating estrogen.

In obese women with PCOS, LH levels may not be increased. The increase in LH pulse frequency is characteristic of the anovulatory state regardless of body fat content.[215] LH pulse amplitude, however, is comparatively normal in overweight women with PCOS, whereas it is increased in nonobese women with PCOS.[216] The overall LH reduction in obese women with PCOS may result from factors other than changes in LH pulse amplitude.[217] A low LH value does not rule out the diagnosis of PCOS, whereas a high LH/FSH ratio supports this diagnosis in an anovulatory woman.

Insulin has been implicated as a potential regulator of LH secretion in PCOS. Insulin enhances the transcription of the LH-β gene *(LHB)*.[218,219] This laboratory observation was supported by an in vivo human study showing that insulin infusion suppresses pituitary response to GnRH in normal women and in women with PCOS.[220] These studies support the concept that insulin resistance or hyperinsulinemia may be responsible for abnormal gonadotropin release (see Fig. 17-30).

Steroid Production in Polycystic Ovary Syndrome

Ovulatory cycles are characterized by cyclic fluctuating hormone levels that regulate ovulation and menses (see Fig. 17-1A). Anovulation in women with PCOS is associated with steady-state levels of gonadotropins and ovarian steroids. In patients with persistent anovulation, the average daily production of estrogen and androgens is increased and depends on LH stimulation (see Fig. 17-30).[221] This is reflected in higher circulating levels of testosterone, androstenedione, DHEA, DHEAS, 17-hydroxyprogesterone, and estrone.[222] Testosterone, androstenedione, and DHEA are secreted directly by the ovary, whereas DHEAS, which is elevated in about 50% of anovulatory women with PCOS, is almost exclusively an adrenal contribution.[208] Circulating levels of androstenedione, secreted by polycystic ovaries, are particularly high.

Local conversion of steroid precursors to estradiol is an important physiologic process for certain estrogen target tissues, such as disease-free breast and genital skin, and can also promote the growth of pathologic estrogen-dependent tissues, such as endometrial or breast cancer (Fig. 17-31).[93,101,222-224] Androstenedione of ovarian origin is the most strikingly elevated steroid in PCOS. Androstenedione is not biologically active but serves as a dual precursor for

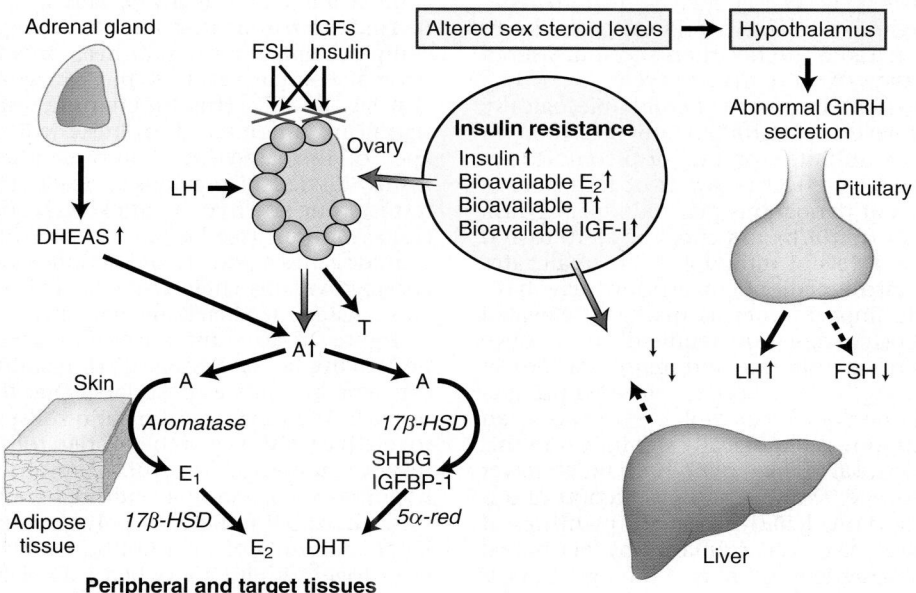

Peripheral and target tissues

Figure 17-30 Pathologic mechanisms in polycystic ovary syndrome (PCOS). A deficient in vivo response of the ovarian follicle to physiologic quantities of follicle-stimulating hormone (FSH), possibly because of an impaired interaction between signaling pathways associated with FSH and insulin-like growth factors (IGFs) or insulin, may be an important defect responsible for anovulation in PCOS. Insulin resistance associated with increased circulating and tissue levels of insulin and bioavailable estradiol (E_2), testosterone (T), and IGF-I gives rise to abnormal hormone production in a number of tissues. Oversecretion of luteinizing hormone (LH) and decreased output of FSH by the pituitary, decreased production of sex hormone–binding globulin (SHBG) and IGF-binding protein 1 (IGFBP-1) in the liver, increased adrenal secretion of dehydroepiandrosterone sulfate (DHEAS), and increased ovarian secretion of androstenedione (A) all contribute to the feed-forward cycle that maintains anovulation and androgen excess in PCOS. Excessive amounts of E_2 and T arise primarily from the conversion of A in peripheral and target tissues. T is converted to the potent steroids estradiol or DHT (dihydrotestosterone). Reductive 17β-hydroxysteroid dehydrogenase (17β-HSD) enzyme activity may be conferred by protein products of several genes with overlapping functions; 5α-reductase (5α-red) is encoded by at least two genes, and aromatase is encoded by a single gene. GnRH, gonadotropin-releasing hormone.

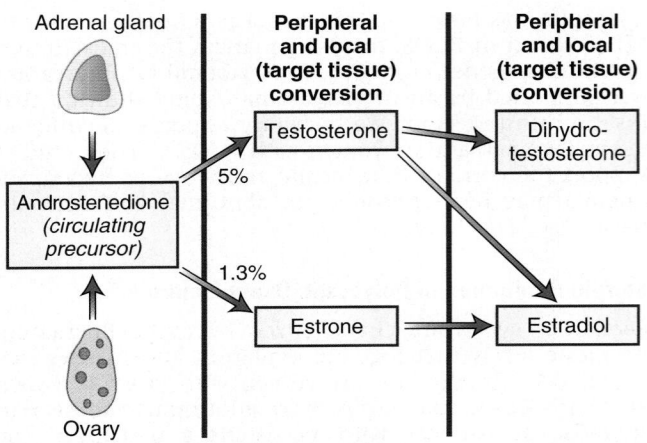

Figure 17-31 Extraovarian conversion of androstenedione to androgen and estrogen. Androstenedione of adrenal or ovarian origin, or both, acts as a dual precursor for androgen and estrogen. Approximately 5% of circulating androstenedione is converted to circulating testosterone, and approximately 1.3% of circulating androstenedione is converted to circulating estrone in peripheral tissues. Testosterone and estrone are further converted to biologically potent steroids, dihydrotestosterone and estradiol, in peripheral and target tissues. Biologically active amounts of estradiol in serum are measured in picograms or picomoles per milliliter (pg/mL or pmol/L), whereas biologically active levels of testosterone in serum are measured in nanograms or nanomoles per milliliter (ng/mL or nmol/L). The 1.3% conversion of normal quantities of androstenedione to estrone may have a critical biologic impact in settings such as postmenopausal endometrial or breast cancer. Significant androgen excess is observed in conditions with abnormally increased androstenedione formation (e.g., polycystic ovary syndrome).

androgen (i.e., testosterone that is further converted to the biologically far stronger androgen DHT) and estrogen (i.e., estrone that is further converted to biologically active estradiol in target tissues; Fig. 17-31). Increased androstenedione of ovarian origin in women with PCOS gives rise to circulating levels of estradiol higher than those measured during the first few days of an ovulatory cycle.

Estradiol is an extremely potent steroid. Biologically effective circulating levels of estradiol are measured in units of picograms per milliliter (pg/mL) or picomoles per liter (pmol/L); biologically effective levels of testosterone are measured in units of nanograms per milliliter (ng/mL) or nanomoles per liter (nmol/L) and circulate at 10 to 100 times the physiologic levels of estradiol. Even small rates of conversion of androstenedione to estrone may have a significant biologic impact, whereas markedly elevated production of androstenedione is required to produce significant amounts of testosterone and manifestations of androgen excess (see Fig. 17-31). Because elevated production of androstenedione does occur in PCOS, extraovarian production of testosterone is biologically significant in this disease. In postmenopausal women, who have much lower levels of androstenedione, extraovarian production of testosterone is less important. Relatively small quantities of estrone (and estradiol) produced primarily by peripheral aromatization of androstenedione have a biologic impact in men and postmenopausal women.

Production of Sex Hormone–Binding Globulin in Polycystic Ovary Syndrome

SHBG binds testosterone and estradiol and decreases their biologic activities. In PCOS, the net production of androgen and estrogen is increased. Amplified estrogenic and androgenic effects in PCOS also are caused by a decreased

SHBG concentration, giving rise to increased free or biologically active circulating levels of estradiol and testosterone (see Fig. 17-30). The levels of SHBG are controlled by a balance of hormonal influences on its synthesis in the liver. Testosterone and insulin inhibit and estrogen and thyroid hormone stimulate SHBG formation.[225] In anovulatory women with PCOS, circulating levels of SHBG are reduced by approximately 50%; this effect may be a hepatic response to increased circulating levels of testosterone and insulin (see Fig. 17-30).[225]

Testosterone decreases serum SHBG levels, giving rise to a vicious feedback circle favoring low SHBG and high bioavailable testosterone levels (see Fig. 17-30). Insulin directly decreases serum SHBG concentrations in women with PCOS independent of any action of sex steroids.[225] Insulin increases free testosterone levels in PCOS by two mechanisms: increasing ovarian secretion of testosterone precursors (e.g., androstenedione) and suppressing SHBG.[225]

Follicular Fate in Polycystic Ovary Syndrome

Under the influence of relatively low but constant levels of FSH, follicular growth is continuously stimulated, although not to the point of full maturation and ovulation.[226] Although full growth potential is not realized, the follicular life span may be extended by several months in the form of multiple follicular cysts. Most of these follicles in polycystic ovaries are 2 to 10 mm in diameter, and some can be as large as 20 mm. Hyperplastic theca cells, often luteinized in response to the high LH levels, surround these follicles (see Fig. 17-27). The accumulation of follicles arrested at various stages of development allows increased and relatively constant production of steroids in response to steady-state levels of gonadotropins.

These follicles are subject to atresia and are replaced by new follicles of similar limited growth potential. Steady-state turnover of stromal cells contributes to the stromal compartment of the ovary, and it is sustained by tissue derived from follicular atresia. A degenerating granulosa compartment, leaving the theca cells to contribute to the stromal compartment of the ovary, accompanies atresia (see Fig. 17-27). This functioning stromal tissue secretes significant amounts of androstenedione under the influence of increased LH. Androstenedione, by the mechanisms discussed previously, leads to increases in free testosterone and free estradiol levels and decreases in SHBG concentrations (see Fig. 17-30). From the point of view of steroidogenesis and steroid action, PCOS is the result of a complex vicious circle that includes a number of positive and negative feedback mechanisms.

Figure 17-30 summarizes the postulated mechanisms underlying PCOS. Because FSH, insulin, and IGF pathways can synergize, it was postulated that this synergy does not occur in the presence of insulin resistance and might lead to relative resistance of the ovarian follicle to FSH. However, in vitro studies provide mixed results with respect to this hypothesis. For example, cultured granulosa cells obtained from the small follicles of polycystic ovaries produce negligible amounts of estradiol but show a dramatic increase in estrogen production when FSH or IGF-I is added to the culture medium. When FSH and IGF-I were added together in vitro, they synergized to increase estrogen biosynthesis in granulosa cells from polycystic ovaries.[227]

Induction of ovulation in PCOS is achieved by increasing FSH levels that are hypothesized to overcome this postulated in vivo block to FSH at the granulosa cell level. Two popular treatments, oral clomiphene citrate and injectable recombinant FSH, can provide increased levels of endogenous or exogenous FSH that may lead to ovulation at various doses. Some PCOS patients require large doses of clomiphene citrate or FSH to achieve ovulation. Paradoxically, the polycystic ovary may overreact to pharmacologic levels of FSH by recruiting a large number of developing follicles at once; this occasionally gives rise to the ovarian hyperstimulation syndrome (OHSS) (discussed later).[228] The therapeutic window between ovarian nonresponsiveness and hyperreactivity is usually narrow. There are significant gaps of knowledge that do not permit reconciliation of clinical postulates derived from in vitro or in vivo studies of PCOS.

Ovarian Hyperthecosis

Ovarian hyperthecosis is a severe variant of PCOS. The term refers to significantly increased stromal tissue with luteinized theca-like cells scattered throughout large sheets of fibroblast-like cells. The clinical and histologic findings and pathophysiology represent an exaggerated version of PCOS.[229] This diagnosis can be made on clinical grounds; an ovarian biopsy is not necessary except to rule out an ovarian tumor.

Increased androgen production leads to the clinical picture of more intense androgenization. The higher testosterone levels may also lower LH levels by blocking estrogen action at the hypothalamic-pituitary level.[217] The severity of hyperthecosis correlates with the degree of insulin resistance.[217] Because insulin and IGF-1 stimulate proliferation of thecal interstitial cells, hyperinsulinemia may be an important pathophysiologic factor in the cause of hyperthecosis.

It is not uncommon to encounter markedly high levels of testosterone, even above 2 ng/mL, in patients with ovarian hyperthecosis. Virilization is common. These patients usually do not ovulate in response to clomiphene or recombinant FSH. It is usually difficult to suppress testosterone production, even using a GnRH analogue. Bilateral oophorectomy should be a last resort, but it may be necessary to control testosterone production in some of these patients.

Genetics of Polycystic Ovary Syndrome

The strong trend of PCOS to aggregate in families suggests an underlying genetic basis.[230,231] Some key clinical features of PCOS are genetically transmitted. In particular, there is familial aggregation of hyperandrogenemia (with or without oligomenorrhea) in PCOS kindreds, suggesting that it is a genetic trait.[201] Another study showed that hyperinsulinism may be a familial characteristic in daughters of women with PCOS.[232]

The PCOS phenotype is a consequence of genes and environment. For example, obesity associated with unhealthy lifestyle choices aggravates the PCOS phenotype in genetically susceptible women. The lack of a clearcut phenotype adds further challenge to genetic studies of PCOS. Several genomic loci have been proposed to account for the PCOS phenotype. These include *CYP11A1*, the insulin gene, and the follistatin gene; however, no convincing evidence regarding any of these loci has been published.[233] Although independent studies identified a dinucleotide repeat marker near the insulin receptor gene that maps to chromosome 19p13.2, the particular PCOS gene in this locus has not been isolated.[234] Recently, in the Han Chinese population, genome-wide PCOS association signals showed evidence of enrichment for candidate genes related to insulin signaling *(INSR)*, gonadotropin receptors *(FSHR, LHCGR)*, and type 2 diabetes *(HMGA2, THADA)*.[235]

Insulin Resistance and Polycystic Ovary Syndrome

Insulin resistance is a major factor in the pathogenesis of non–insulin-dependent diabetes mellitus (NIDDM). The term *insulin resistance* can be defined as impaired wholebody insulin-mediated glucose disposal, as determined with the use of techniques such as the hyperinsulinemic glucose clamp technique.[107] Insulin resistance is defined clinically as the inability of a known quantity of exogenous or endogenous insulin to increase glucose uptake and use in an affected individual as much as it does in a normal person. Insulin resistance is frequently observed in lean and obese women with PCOS. More severe degrees of insulin resistance or impaired glucose tolerance are more common in obese women with PCOS.[107]

Androgen excess and insulin resistance are often associated with acanthosis nigricans. Acanthosis nigricans is a gray-brown, velvety discoloration and increased thickness of the skin, usually seen at the neck, groin, and axillae and under the breasts; it is a marker for insulin resistance (see Fig. 17-28). Hyperkeratosis and papillomatosis are the histologic characteristics of acanthosis nigricans. Acanthosis nigricans in hyperandrogenic women depends on the presence and severity of hyperinsulinemia and insulin resistance.[236] The mechanism responsible for the development of acanthosis nigricans is uncertain. This abnormal growth response of the skin may be mediated through receptors for various growth factors, including those for insulin and IGF-1. Acanthosis nigricans can also be observed in the absence of insulin resistance or androgen excess.

Insulin resistance is characterized by an impaired glucose response to a specific amount of insulin. In many of these patients, normal glucose levels are maintained at the expense of increased circulating insulin to overcome the underlying defect. More severe forms of insulin resistance in PCOS range from impaired glucose tolerance to frank NIDDM. Resistance to insulin-stimulated glucose uptake is a relatively common phenomenon in the general population and is sometimes referred to as *syndrome X* or *metabolic syndrome*. The fundamental abnormality leading to the manifestations that make up the metabolic syndrome is resistance to insulin-mediated glucose uptake in muscle and increased lipolysis, which produces elevated levels of circulating free fatty acids.[237] These individuals also have dyslipidemia, hypertension, and increased risk of developing CVD. Not surprisingly, the incidences of dyslipidemia and cardiovascular risk are increased significantly in women with PCOS.[238,239] The incidence of hypertension increases significantly after menopause in women with a history of PCOS.[107] There is a significant clinical and pathologic overlap between the metabolic syndrome and PCOS.[240]

The clinical presentation of patients with insulin resistance depends on the ability of the pancreas to compensate for the target tissue resistance to insulin. During the first stages of this condition, compensation is effective, and the only metabolic abnormality is hyperinsulinemia. In many patients, the beta cells of the pancreas eventually fail to meet the challenge, and declining insulin levels lead to impaired glucose tolerance and eventually to frank diabetes mellitus. Beta-cell dysfunction is demonstrable in women with PCOS before the onset of glucose intolerance.[241]

Studies of well-characterized causes of hyperinsulinemia and androgen excess have illuminated various mechanisms of insulin resistance. Factors such as a decrease in insulin binding related to autoantibodies to insulin receptors, postreceptor defects, and a decrease in insulin receptor sites in target tissues are all involved in insulin resistance.[242] These rare syndromes are found in an extremely small portion of women with anovulation, androgen excess, and insulin resistance, leaving most PCOS patients without any demonstrable abnormalities in the number or quality of receptors or in antibody formation. The exact nature of insulin resistance in most women with PCOS is not well understood.

To understand the molecular defect underlying insulin resistance in PCOS, Dunaif and coworkers studied the differences between skin fibroblasts from women with and without PCOS with respect to insulin-dependent signal transduction.[107] The fibroblasts of women with PCOS showed no change in insulin binding or receptor affinity, but a postreceptor defect was observed in one half of the women with PCOS.[107] This defect is characterized by increased basal insulin receptor serine phosphorylation and decreased insulin-dependent tyrosine phosphorylation of the insulin receptor.[107] At about the same time, Miller and coworkers evaluated whether post-translational modification of the product of the CYP17A1 gene alters the ratio of its hydroxylase to lyase activity; they found that serine phosphorylation of CYP17A1 dramatically increases the enzyme's 17,20-lyase but not its 17α-hydroxylase activity. These observations led the investigators to hypothesize that a dominantly inherited aberrant kinase activity phosphorylates serine residues at the insulin receptor-β and CYP17A1 product, leading to insulin resistance and increased androgen production, respectively. The cause of this abnormal phosphorylation pattern and consequences for insulin action and androgen production are important topics for further study.[243]

Within the context of a unified hypothesis, insulin resistance seems to be a critical defect that explains most of the endocrine abnormalities observed in PCOS (see Fig. 17-30). Insulin resistance is associated with abnormal responses of the ovarian follicle to FSH, which lead to anovulation and androgen secretion. This results in noncyclic formation of estrogen from androgens in peripheral tissues. Estradiol together with elevated androgen and insulin levels gives rise to abnormal gonadotropin secretion. This creates an anovulatory state favoring continuous excess of LH, steroid precursors, androgen, and estrogen (see Fig. 17-30).

Role of Obesity in Insulin Resistance and Anovulation. Increased waist-to-hip ratio compounded by significantly increased body mass index is called *android obesity* because this type of adipose tissue distribution is observed more commonly in men. Overweight women with anovulatory androgen excess commonly have this particular body fat distribution.[244] Android obesity is the result of fat deposition in the abdominal wall and in visceral mesenteric locations. This fat is more sensitive to catecholamines, less sensitive to insulin, and more active metabolically. Android obesity is associated with insulin resistance, glucose intolerance, diabetes mellitus, and an increase in androgen production rate and results in decreased levels of SHBG and increased levels of free testosterone and estradiol.[244] Android obesity is associated significantly with cardiovascular risk factors, including hypertension and dyslipidemia, and it has been tied to a notable increase in the risk of poor-prognosis breast cancer.[245,246] However, no direct association has been reported between PCOS and breast cancer risk.[247]

Although the combination of insulin resistance and androgen excess is often observed in obese women overall, women with android-type obesity appear to be at a significantly higher risk for insulin resistance and androgen excess. However, insulin resistance and androgen excess are not confined to obese anovulatory women but also occur in nonobese anovulatory women.[215] Although obesity by itself causes insulin resistance, the combination of insulin resistance and androgen excess is a specific feature of PCOS. Not surprisingly, the combination of obesity and PCOS is associated with more severe degrees of insulin resistance than those found in nonobese women with PCOS.[215,248] Android-type obesity, in contrast to general obesity, is a more specific risk factor for PCOS.

Laboratory Evaluation of Metabolic Syndrome in PCOS. In everyday clinical practice, the criteria for diagnosing insulin resistance in an individual patient have not been standardized and present extremely complex issues. One fourth of the normal population has fasting and glucose-stimulated insulin levels that overlap with those of insulin-resistant individuals because of the great variability of insulin sensitivity in normal subjects.[107] Clinically available measures of insulin action, such as fasting or glucose-stimulated insulin levels, do not correlate well with more detailed measurements of insulin sensitivity in research settings.

In view of these constraints, it is reasonable to consider all women with PCOS at risk for insulin resistance and the associated abnormalities of the metabolic syndrome—dyslipidemia, hypertension, and CVD.[240] A lipid profile should be obtained in all cases of PCOS. Especially for obese women with PCOS, fasting glucose levels and glucose levels 2 hours after a 75-g glucose load should be obtained as a screen for glucose intolerance. The clinician should encourage the patient to take every possible measure (e.g., weight reduction, exercise) to reduce insulin resistance.

Use of Antidiabetic Drugs to Treat Anovulation and Androgen Excess. A logical approach to the management of PCOS includes using medications that improve insulin sensitivity in target tissues, achieving reductions in insulin secretion, and stabilizing glucose tolerance. Antidiabetic medications in the classes of biguanides (metformin) and thiazolidinediones (pioglitazone and rosiglitazone) have been used to reduce insulin resistance. Although metformin appears to influence ovarian steroidogenesis directly, this effect does not appear to be primarily responsible for the attenuation of ovarian androgen production in women with PCOS. Rather, metformin inhibits the output of hepatic glucose, necessitating a lower insulin concentration and thereby probably reducing androgen production by theca cells.[249]

Metformin at a dose of 500 mg three times daily reduced hyperinsulinemia, basal and stimulated levels of LH, and free testosterone concentrations in overweight women with PCOS.[250,251] Some anovulatory women ovulated and achieved pregnancy; however, clomiphene is superior to metformin in achieving live births in infertile women with PCOS.[252-254] Among published studies of metformin use in women with PCOS, subject characteristics and control measures for effects of weight change, dose of metformin, and outcome vary widely. A meta-analysis of 13 studies in which metformin was administered to 543 participants reported that patients taking metformin had an odds ratio for ovulation of 3.88 (95% confidence interval [CI], 2.25 to 6.69) compared with placebo and an odds ratio for ovulation of 4.41 (95% CI, 2.37 to 8.22) for metformin plus clomiphene compared with clomiphene alone.[255] Although the addition of metformin to clomiphene seems to increase the ovulation rate, it does not result in a higher rate of live births.[253] Metformin also improved fasting insulin levels, blood pressure, and levels of LDL cholesterol. These effects were judged to be independent of any changes in weight that were associated with metformin treatment, but controversy persists about whether the beneficial effects of metformin are entirely independent of the weight loss that is typically seen early in the course of therapy.[254,255]

The thiazolidinediones are pharmacologic ligands for the nuclear receptor PPARγ. They improve the action of insulin in the liver, skeletal muscle, and adipose tissue and have only a modest effect on hepatic glucose output. As with metformin, the thiazolidinediones are reported to affect ovarian steroid synthesis directly, although most evidence indicates that the reduction in insulin levels is responsible for decreased concentrations of circulating androgen.[249]

Women with PCOS who took troglitazone had consistent improvements in insulin resistance, pancreatic beta-cell function, hyperandrogenemia, and glucose tolerance.[256,257] In a double-blind, randomized, placebo-controlled study, ovulation was significantly greater for women with PCOS who received troglitazone than for those who received placebo; free testosterone levels decreased, and levels of SHBG increased in a dose-dependent fashion.[258] Although troglitazone is no longer available because of its hepatotoxicity, subsequent studies using rosiglitazone and pioglitazone had similar results.[259-261] Because of concern about the use of thiazolidinediones in pregnancy and recent evidence linking these drugs to serious side effects such as heart failure and stroke, they have been less readily adopted for routine treatment of PCOS. The success of the strategy of reversing insulin resistance as a way to correct the critical abnormalities in PCOS argues for this defect as central to the pathogenesis of the disorder.

Management of Long-Term Deleterious Effects of Polycystic Ovary Syndrome

The long-term consequences of PCOS include irregular uterine bleeding, anovulatory infertility, androgen excess, chronically elevated levels of free estrogen associated with an increased risk of endometrial cancer, and insulin resistance associated with an increased risk of CVD and diabetes mellitus. Treatment must aid in achieving a healthy lifestyle and normal body weight, protect the endometrium from the effects of unopposed estrogen, and reduce testosterone levels.

Any woman with PCOS should be counseled to maintain a healthy lifestyle. In obese PCOS women, permanent lifestyle modification should be emphasized as the primary preventive measure to minimize short-term and long-term deleterious effects. Simple measures such as decreasing daily food intake by 500 kcal and introducing any type of moderate exercise for 30 minutes daily for 6 months can decrease hyperandrogenemia and diastolic blood pressure.[198] Because insulin resistance contributes to the abnormal lipid profile and increased cardiovascular risk in women with PCOS, weight loss is a high priority for patients who are overweight.[262] Insulin resistance and androgen excess can be reduced with a weight reduction of at least 5%.[263,264] Significant weight loss has also resulted in ovulation and pregnancy in a number of patients with PCOS.[265] Nutritional counseling and an emphasis on lifestyle changes are essential components of the long-term management of PCOS.

If the patient does not wish to become pregnant, medical therapy is directed toward the interruption of the effect of unopposed estrogen on the endometrium. Nonfluctuating levels of unopposed estradiol in the absence of progesterone cause irregular uterine bleeding, amenorrhea, and infertility and increase the risk of endometrial cancer. Anovulatory women with PCOS may have endometrial cancer even in their early 20s.[266] Endometrial biopsy should be performed periodically in untreated women with PCOS regardless of age. Pregnancy should be ruled out before each endometrial biopsy. The uterine bleeding pattern should not influence the decision to perform an endometrial biopsy. The presence of amenorrhea does not rule out

endometrial hyperplasia. The critical factor that determines the risk of endometrial neoplasia is the duration of anovulation and exposure to unopposed estradiol. Long-term treatment with a progestin or oral contraceptive significantly decreases the risk of endometrial cancer.

One of the simplest and most effective ways to administer a progestin in the long term is to use an oral contraceptive. Oral contraceptives provide two additional benefits: reduction of androgen excess and contraception. Oral contraceptive pills reduce circulating androgen levels through suppression of circulating LH and stimulation of SHBG levels, and they have been shown to reduce hirsutism.[148] Oral contraceptive treatment for anovulation and hyperinsulinemia in women with androgen excess does not increase cardiovascular risk.[267]

For the patient who does not complain of hirsutism but is anovulatory and has irregular bleeding, treatment with a single progestin may be attempted as an alternative to oral contraceptive use. Progestin therapy is directed toward interruption of the chronic exposure of endometrium to unopposed effects of estrogen. MPA may be administered intermittently (e.g., 5 mg daily for the first 10 days of every other month) to ensure withdrawal bleeding and prevent endometrial hyperplasia. This treatment does not decrease androgen excess, nor does it provide contraception. Because an oral contraceptive with an ethinyl estradiol content of 30 μg or less can suppress androgen excess of ovarian origin, provide contraception, and protect the endometrium and does not increase insulin resistance, a low-dose oral contraceptive is the treatment of choice for nonsmokers with PCOS. An oral contraceptive together with the antiandrogen spironolactone (100 mg/day) is the recommended starting treatment for a hirsute woman with PCOS. The dose of spironolactone can be increased in increments to suppress hair growth, as described earlier.

Treatment with an oral contraceptive, with or without spironolactone, may not be effective in androgen suppression in severe cases of PCOS. In patients resistant to oral contraceptives, suppression of the ovary using a depot GnRH agonist may be required. Because glucocorticoids increase insulin resistance, they should be used with caution in patients with hyperinsulinemia. Spironolactone does not affect insulin sensitivity in anovulatory women and can be used safely without causing adverse effects on carbohydrate or lipid metabolism.[268]

The clinician must counsel women with PCOS regarding their increased risk of future diabetes mellitus. The age at onset of NIDDM is significantly earlier in these women than in the general population.[199] Women with PCOS are more likely to experience gestational diabetes.[269] Long-term follow-up studies have shown a significantly increased risk for frank diabetes mellitus in anovulatory patients with PCOS.[107] It is therefore important to monitor glucose tolerance with periodic measurements of glucose levels after fasting and after a 75-g glucose load. The place of metformin in the long-term treatment of PCOS remains to be determined.[254,270]

The physician should alert the patient with PCOS that up to one half of first-degree relatives and sisters may be affected by PCOS or at least by androgen excess in the presence of regular menses.[201] These individuals may be at higher than average risk for CVD and may benefit from preventive measures that reduce this risk.

Ovulation Induction in Polycystic Ovary Syndrome

When pregnancy is achieved, patients with PCOS appear to have an increased risk of spontaneous miscarriage.[271] This increased risk may be related to elevated levels of LH that may produce an adverse environment for the oocyte and the endometrium. LH levels should be suppressed with oral contraceptives before ovulation is induced. Suppression can be achieved in most patients with PCOS by the use of an oral contraceptive for 4 to 6 weeks before ovulation induction with clomiphene citrate, an aromatase inhibitor or recombinant FSH.

To induce ovulation in women with PCOS, FSH levels may be increased by oral administration of an antiestrogen (clomiphene citrate) or an aromatase inhibitor (letrozole, anastrozole) or by subcutaneous injection of recombinant FSH. Presumably, pharmacologic levels of FSH overcome the ovarian defect that is responsible for anovulation in PCOS.

Clomiphene Citrate. Clomiphene citrate is a nonsteroidal, ovulation-inducing ER ligand with mixed agonistic-antagonistic properties.[272] Acting as an antiestrogen, clomiphene citrate is thought to displace endogenous estrogen from hypothalamic ERs, thereby removing the negative feedback effect exerted by endogenous estrogens. The resultant change in pulsatile GnRH release is thought to normalize the release of pituitary FSH and LH, which is followed by follicular recruitment and selection, assertion of dominance, and ovulation.[272]

Clomiphene citrate treatment can be started at any time to induce ovulation in an amenorrheic and anovulatory patient provided that a pregnancy test is performed beforehand (Fig. 17-32). Alternatively, uterine bleeding may be induced after a 10-day treatment with a combination oral contraceptive or MPA (5 mg/day). On cycle day 2 or 3 (day 1 is the first day of uterine bleeding), a baseline ultrasound study is performed to rule out any ovarian follicular cyst of more than 25-mm average diameter. If one or more large cysts are seen, ovulation induction should be delayed until after gonadotropin suppression by continuous oral contraception treatment for 4 to 6 weeks to eliminate these cysts or decrease their size. Clomiphene citrate is started at 50 mg/day orally on day 3 of the cycle and continued for 5 days. Ultrasonography is performed on cycle day 13 or 14 to ensure follicular development (i.e., at least one new follicle measuring at least 16 mm in diameter). The patient should be encouraged to have intercourse every other day during the 10-day period following the last clomiphene citrate dose. Alternatively, measurement of urinary LH to detect an LH surge can be used to time intercourse. Intercourse is recommended on the day of a positive urinary LH peak and on the next day. If an hCG injection is used to induce ovulation, intercourse is recommended within 24 to 34 hours after the injection.

If follicular development does not occur after the first course of therapy with clomiphene citrate at 50 mg/day, a second course of 100 mg daily for 5 days may be started. Lack of response at doses of 150 to 200 mg daily for 5 days should be an indication for a change of treatment. Most patients destined to conceive do so with the starting dose of clomiphene citrate (50 mg/day for 5 days). Most clomiphene citrate–initiated conceptions occur within the first 6 ovulatory cycles.[272] The incidence rate for multiple gestation in clomiphene citrate–induced pregnancies is 6% (4% for twins and 2% for triplets).[253] Failure to achieve pregnancy after three clomiphene cycles despite sonographic evidence of follicular development should prompt the clinician to perform a comprehensive infertility workup, including a semen analysis and evaluation of the uterine cavity and tubal patency.

Aromatase Inhibitors. Via decreasing aromatization of the estrogen precursor steroids in the brain, aromatase inhibitors reduce hypothalamic-pituitary estrogen feedback, and this leads to increased GnRH secretion, concomitant elevations in LH and FSH, and increased ovarian follicular development in premenopausal women.[100,273] The gonadotropin-stimulating aromatase inhibitors letrozole and anastrozole have been used off-label in the treatment of patients with ovulatory dysfunction, such as PCOS, and for increasing the number of ovarian follicles recruited for ovulation in women who are already ovulatory.[274] Oral administration of letrozole (2.5 or 5 mg/day) or anastrozole (1 mg/day) on days 3 to 7 after uterine bleeding is effective for ovulation induction in women with anovulatory infertility (see Fig. 17-32).[274,275] In a randomized study, as compared with clomiphene (50 mg/day), letrozole (2.5 mg/day) was associated with higher live-birth and ovulation rates among infertile women with PCOS.[275] A retrospective study did not show any difference in the overall rates of major and minor congenital malformations among newborns from mothers who conceived after letrozole or clomiphene treatment.[276]

Metformin. Head-to-head randomized trials showed that clomiphene alone is clearly superior to metformin only with respect to achieving ovulation and live births in women with PCOS.[253] However, the ovulatory response to clomiphene was increased in obese women with PCOS by decreasing insulin secretion with the addition of metformin.[270] Another randomized study showed that the higher rate of ovulation in the users of clomiphene plus metformin seemed to be offset by a higher rate of pregnancy losses, producing similar live-birth rates in clomiphene-only and clomiphene plus metformin groups.[253] The benefit of the addition of metformin to clomiphene in obese clomiphene-nonresponders with PCOS needs to be assessed further.

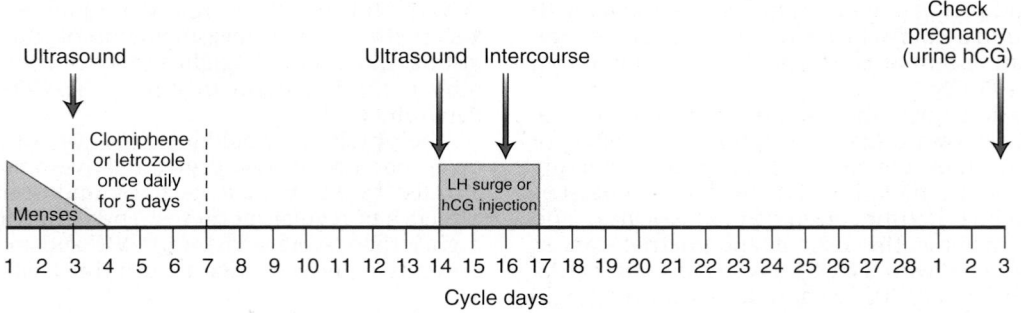

Figure 17-32 Monitoring of clomiphene citrate or letrozole-initiated ovulation. On cycle day 2 or 3, a baseline ultrasound examination is performed to rule out any large ovarian follicular cyst. Oral administration of clomiphene citrate or letrozole is started on day 3 of the cycle and continued for 5 days. Ultrasonography is performed on cycle day 13 or 14 to ensure follicular development. Upon observing at least one mature follicle by ultrasound, ovulation may be triggered by an hCG (human chorionic gonadotropin) injection followed by intercourse in 24 to 34 hours. Alternatively, the patient may be encouraged to have intercourse every other day during the 12-day period after the last clomiphene citrate or letrozole dose. Urinary hCG levels are checked to determine whether pregnancy has occurred. LH, luteinizing hormone.

Low-Dose Gonadotropin Therapy. For women who do not ovulate in response to clomiphene citrate or letrozole, FSH injections are started on day 3 of spontaneous or progestin-induced uterine bleeding. Recombinant FSH is administered subcutaneously starting with a daily dose of 75 IU for up to 10 days, if necessary, and using small incremental dose increases (12.5 to 37.5 IU) from then on at 3- to 7-day intervals until serum estradiol concentrations begin to increase. The dose is then maintained until follicular rupture, which is induced by subcutaneous injection of recombinant hCG (250 µg). Follicular growth is monitored by transvaginal ultrasonography and blood estradiol levels, which serve as biochemical markers for the granulosa cell mass in the growing follicle.[228] This regimen induces development of a single follicle in most cycles and has succeeded in reducing the rate of multiple pregnancies to as low as 6% in some series.[228] The low-dose regimen also practically eliminated the complication of severe OHSS.[228] Conception rates are comparable to those achieved with conventional therapy. The miscarriage rate remains somewhat higher than that after spontaneous conceptions (20% to 25%).

Conventional-dose gonadotropin therapy (starting FSH dose, 150 IU daily) should not be used as first-line treatment in patients with PCOS because it causes an alarming number of multiple pregnancies (14% to 50% of treatment cycles) and a significantly increased risk of OHSS (1.3% to 9.4% of treatment cycles).[277] OHSS is a more common complication of conventional-dose gonadotropin treatment. Milder forms are relatively common and are characterized by weight gain, abdominal discomfort, and enlarged ovaries. Home bed rest and increased oral intake of fluids are sufficient to manage this form. Severe OHSS occurs in 0.1% to 0.2% of stimulation attempts and is accompanied by severe ascites, pleural effusion, electrolyte imbalance, and hypovolemia with oliguria. The most dreaded complication is deep venous thrombosis and embolism. Its cause is poorly understood. Large numbers of follicles, peak estradiol levels greater than 2000 pg/mL, and pregnancy are associated with a higher likelihood of OHSS. Prevention includes withholding of the hCG injection and intrauterine insemination. Treatment of severe OHSS includes hospitalization, maintenance of fluid and electrolyte balance, prophylaxis for thromboembolism by heparin, and drainage of severe ascites or pleural effusions. Frequently, supportive measures are sufficient to manage this self-limited condition.

Premature Ovarian Insufficiency

On average, menopause occurs at the age of 50 years, with 1% of women continuing to menstruate beyond the age of 60 years and another 1% whose menopause occurs before age 40 years. Premature menopause or ovarian insufficiency has been arbitrarily defined as the cessation of menses before 40 years of age.[278]

POI, which is defined as early depletion of ovarian follicles (before the age of 40 years), is a state of hypergonadotropic hypogonadism. These patients go through a normal puberty and a variable period of cyclic menses followed by oligomenorrhea or amenorrhea accompanied by hot flashes and urogenital atrophy. POI should always be included in the differential diagnosis of chronic anovulation. History and physical examination may reveal menstrual irregularity or secondary amenorrhea accompanied by symptoms and signs of estrogen deficiency, such as hot flashes and urogenital atrophy.[279]

The cause or genetic basis of POI is not well understood. Two genetic syndromes associated with POI are gonadal dysgenesis with primarily mosaic X-chromosome defects and *FMR1* gene premutation, a variant of fragile X syndrome.[280] Syndromes resulting from single-gene mutations (e.g., blepharophimosis-ptosis-epicanthus inversus syndrome [*FOXL2* mutation], galactosemia [*GALT* mutation]) may be associated with POI.[280] However, the cause of POI remains unknown in most cases.

The underlying ovarian defect may manifest at various ages, depending on the number of functional follicles left in the ovaries. If loss of follicles occurs rapidly before puberty, primary amenorrhea and lack of secondary sexual development ensue. The degree to which the adult phenotype develops and the age at which secondary amenorrhea actually occurs depend on whether follicle loss took place during or after puberty. In cases of primary amenorrhea associated with sexual infantilism, the ovarian remnants exist as streaks, and transvaginal ultrasonography usually cannot detect any ovaries. Many gene defects (e.g., *FSHR*, *CYP17A1*, *CYP19A1*) involve ovarian failure at the expected time of puberty, and the phenotypes manifest with primary amenorrhea and lack of secondary sexual development (see Chapter 25).[280]

POI can also result from an autoimmune process and may be associated with an autoimmune polyendocrine syndrome.[281] Other causes of premature insufficiency can be related to the sudden destruction of follicles by chemotherapy, irradiation, or infections such as mumps oophoritis. The effect of irradiation depends on the patient's age and the x-ray dose.[282] Steroid levels begin to fall and gonadotropins rise within 2 weeks after irradiation of the ovaries. Younger women exposed to radiation are less likely to have permanent ovarian insufficiency because of the higher number of oocytes present at earlier ages. When the radiation field excludes the pelvis or the ovaries are transposed out of the pelvis by laparoscopic surgery before irradiation, the risk for POI is minimized.[283] Most chemotherapeutic agents used for eradication of malignancies are toxic to the ovaries and cause ovarian insufficiency.[284] Resumption of menses and pregnancy have been reported after radiotherapy or chemotherapy,[285] but POI may occur years after these therapies.[265]

Diagnosis and Management of Premature Ovarian Insufficiency

POI should be suspected in a woman younger than 40 years of age who presents with amenorrhea, oligomenorrhea, or another form of menstrual irregularity accompanied by hot flashes. Menopausal serum FSH levels (40 IU/L) on at least two occasions are sufficient for the diagnosis of POI.

Case reports of pregnancies in affected women occurring during hormone replacement therapy have been published.[286,287] In particular, young women with POI may experience intermittent periods of ovarian function, with antral follicles present at ovarian ultrasonography and ovulation described in cases that followed up with regular endocrine assessments. A randomized trial of hormone therapy in this setting showed that folliculogenesis occurred often but was less frequently followed by ovulation and even less frequently by pregnancy (up to 14%); conventional-dose estrogen therapy did not improve the rate of folliculogenesis, ovulation, or pregnancy.[279] Later pilot studies or case reports suggested that lowering FSH levels to less than 15 IU/L by use of high-dose estrogen or a GnRH antagonist in young women with POI may trigger ovulation or permit ovulation induction and pregnancy in a small number of patients.[288,289]

The clinician should inform patients diagnosed with POI that there is a small but significant likelihood of spontaneous pregnancy or pregnancy after ovulation induction. Women who desire pregnancy are still best served by assisted reproductive technology employing donor oocytes, because the probability of pregnancy with an autologous egg is low. Use of donor oocytes followed by IVF with the partner's sperm and intrauterine embryo transfer after synchronization of the recipient patient's endometrium with the donor's cycle using exogenous estrogen and progesterone is offered to the patient who wishes to carry a pregnancy in her uterus (see Fig. 17-23). This approach offers an excellent chance of achieving live birth (>50% per donor oocyte IVF cycle).

Patients with POI have an increased incidence of an abnormal complement of chromosomes.[290] The risk of having an abnormal karyotype increases with decreasing age at onset of the POI. A chromosomal analysis is recommended for the POI patients younger than 30 years of age because of the increased risk of a gonadal tumor associated with the presence of a Y chromosome.[291] It is extremely rare to encounter a gonadal tumor in patients with POI after the age of 30 years.[292]

Mosaicism that includes a Y chromosome has been associated with a high incidence of gonadal tumors.[291] These malignant tumors arise from germ cells and include gonadoblastomas, dysgerminomas, yolk sac tumors, and choriocarcinoma. Secondary virilization in patients with karyotypic abnormalities and POI is associated with a significantly increased risk of a gonadal tumor. The precise risk of a tumor in various subsets of these patients is not well known because a significant number of women carrying a Y chromosome do not have symptoms of virilization. The frequency of Y chromosomal material determined by polymerase chain reaction is high in those with Turner syndrome (12.2%), but the occurrence of a gonadal tumor among these Y-positive patients is about 7% to 10%.[293]

Fragile X–associated disorders are caused by a CGG trinucleotide repeat expansion in the promoter region of the *FMR1* gene. Expansion of the CGG trinucleotide repeats to more than 200 copies induces methylation of the *FMR1* gene, with an outcome of transcriptional silencing.[294] This so-called full mutation was linked to mental retardation or autism. Individuals who carried the premutation (defined as >55 but <200 CGG repeats) have increased *FMR1* mRNA levels with decreased levels of fragile X mental retardation protein (FMRP). Convincing evidence relates the *FMR1* premutation to altered ovarian function and loss of fertility.[295] The natural history of the altered ovarian function in women who carry the *FMR1* premutation is still not well understood. Women with POI are at increased risk for an *FMR1* premutation and should be informed of the availability of fragile X testing.

POI usually occurs as an isolated autoimmune disorder. Rarely, it may be associated with hypothyroidism, diabetes mellitus, hypoadrenalism, hypoparathyroidism, or systemic lupus erythematosus.[296] It can be part of an autoimmune polyendocrine syndrome.[281] Thyroid insufficiency, adrenal insufficiency, and diabetes mellitus are the endocrine disorders most frequently associated with POI.[297] Periodic endocrine testing for glucose intolerance, adrenal or parathyroid function, and autoimmune disease (e.g., systemic lupus erythematosus) should be considered based on the clinical presentation (Table 17-6). Because hypothyroidism is more commonly found than other endocrine disorders associated with POI, this author prefers to check a TSH level during the initial evaluation (see Table 17-6).

Treatment of POI should be directed toward its specific cause. In most cases, however, it is not possible to identify a specific cause if there are no karyotypic anomalies. Besides infertility, long-term ovarian steroid deficiency has far-

---

TABLE 17-6

Laboratory Evaluation of Premature Ovarian Insufficiency

Follicle-stimulating hormone (to establish the diagnosis of premature ovarian insufficiency)
Karyotype (<30 yr of age or sexual infantilism)
Testing for *FMR1* gene premutation carrier state
Thyroid-stimulating hormone (hypothyroidism)

FMR1, fragile X mental retardation 1.

---

reaching health implications. Early menopause has been associated with increased cardiovascular mortality and stroke, bone fracture, and colorectal cancer risks.[230] Despite reduced risks for development of breast cancer, overall quality of life and life expectancy decline with early menopause.[280] Hormone therapy, using combined estrogen and progestin or a low-dose oral contraceptive, is the cornerstone of the management for these women. The added value of androgen replacement remains uncertain.[280]

DIAGNOSIS AND MANAGEMENT OF ANOVULATORY UTERINE BLEEDING

Acyclic production of estrogen during anovulatory cycles gives rise to irregular shedding of the endometrium. These bleeding manifestations of anovulatory cycles in the absence of uterine pathology or systemic illness are commonly referred to as *dysfunctional uterine bleeding*. Anovulatory uterine bleeding, which is the most common cause of chronic menstrual irregularities, is a diagnosis of exclusion. Pregnancy, uterine leiomyomas, endometrial polyps, and adenomyosis should be ruled out as anatomic causes of irregular or excessive uterine bleeding. Malignancies of the vagina, cervix, endometrium, myometrium, fallopian tubes, and ovaries or coagulation abnormalities should also be ruled out before a diagnosis of anovulatory uterine bleeding is made.

Anovulatory uterine bleeding can be managed without surgical intervention by either restoring ovulation or mimicking the ovulatory hormonal profile by providing exogenous steroids. The rationale for use of exogenous steroids is based on the knowledge of predictable responses of the endometrium to estrogen and progesterone. Physiologic responses of the endometrium to natural ovarian steroids have been uncovered by observation of the gross and microscopic changes occurring in the endometrium during thousands of normal ovulatory cycles in humans and other primates.[115,116,298] The pharmacologic application of exogenous estrogens and progestins in women with anovulatory bleeding aims to correct the production of local tissue factors that mediate physiologic steroid action and reverse the excessive and prolonged flow typical of anovulatory cycles.

Clinical management of irregular uterine bleeding with exogenous hormones is a time-honored method, and it has diagnostic value. Failure to control vaginal bleeding with hormonal therapy, despite appropriate application and use, makes the diagnosis of anovulatory uterine bleeding considerably less likely. In such cases, attention is directed to an anatomic pathologic entity within the reproductive axis as the cause of abnormal bleeding.

Heavy but regular menstrual bleeding (i.e., hypermenorrhea) can be encountered in ovulatory women. It may have an anatomic cause, such as a leiomyoma impinging on the endometrial cavity or the diffuse and pathologic presence of benign endometrial glands in the myometrium (i.e., adenomyosis). In the absence of a specific pathologic cause, it is presumed that hypermenorrhea reflects subtle disturbances in the endometrial tissue mechanism. In essentially all cases, evaluation and treatment are identical to the approach detailed in this section.

Characteristics of Normal Menses

Normal menstruation takes place about 14 days after each ovulation episode as a consequence of postovulatory estrogen-progesterone withdrawal. The quantity and duration of bleeding are quite reproducible. This predictability leads many women to expect a certain characteristic flow pattern. Any slight deviations, such as plus or minus 1 day in duration or minor deviation from expected tampon use, are causes for major concern in the patient. Most women of reproductive age can predict the timing of their flows so accurately that even minor variability may require reassurance by the clinician. Although variability of menstrual cycles is a common feature during the teenage years and perimenopausal transition, the characteristics of menstrual bleeding do not undergo appreciable change between ages 20 and 40.[299]

For ovulatory women, the changes in the length of the menstrual cycle over the period of reproductive age are predictable. Between menarche and age 20, the cycle length for most ovulatory women is relatively longer. Between 20 and 40 years, there is increased regularity as cycles shorten. In the 40s, cycles begin to lengthen again. The highest incidence of anovulatory cycles occurs before age 20 and after age 40.[300] In these age groups, the average length of a cycle is between 25 and 28 days. Among ovulatory women, the frequency of a cycle of less than 21 days or more than 35 days is rare (<2%).[301] Overall, most women have cycles that last 24 to 35 days (Fig. 17-33).[299] Between ages 40 and 50, menstrual cycle length increases and anovulation becomes more prevalent.[302]

The average postovulatory bleeding lasts from 4 to 6 days. The normal volume of menstrual blood loss is 30 mL. More than 80 mL is considered abnormal. Most of the

blood loss occurs during the first 3 days of a period, so excessive flow may exist without prolongation of flow.[303,304]

During an ovulatory cycle, the duration from ovulation to menses is relatively constant and averages 14 days (see Fig. 17-1A). Greater variability in the length of the proliferative phase, however, produces a distribution in the duration of the menstrual cycle. Menstrual bleeding more often than every 24 days or less often than every 35 days requires evaluation.[299,302] Flow that lasts 7 or more days also requires evaluation. A flow that totals more than 80 mL per month usually leads to anemia and should be treated.[305] In clinical practice, however, it is difficult to quantify menstrual flow because evaluation and treatment are based solely on the patient's perceptions regarding the duration, amount, and timing of her menstrual bleeding. Despite this difficulty in quantifying menstrual blood loss, the clinician should evaluate the cause of excessive uterine bleeding. Anemia should be ruled out by a complete blood cell count.[306] A low hemoglobin value accompanied by microcytic and hypochromic red blood cells suggests excessive blood loss during menses. These patients should be provided with iron supplementation. The likely presence of coagulation defects, uterine leiomyomas, or adenomyosis underlying prolonged menses should be evaluated in anemic patients through a meticulous history and physical examination followed by relevant laboratory tests.

Terminology Describing Abnormal Uterine Bleeding

Oligomenorrhea is defined as intervals between episodes of uterine bleeding longer than 35 days, and the term *polymenorrhea* is used to describe intervals shorter than 24 days. *Hypermenorrhea* refers to regular intervals (24 to 35 days) but excessive flow or duration of bleeding, or both. *Hypomenorrhea* refers to diminution of the flow or shortening of the duration of regular menses, or both.

Uterine Bleeding in Response to Steroid Hormones

Estrogen Withdrawal Bleeding

Uterine bleeding follows acute cessation of estrogen support to the endometrium. This type of uterine bleeding can occur after bilateral oophorectomy, irradiation of mature follicles, or administration of estrogen to a woman, who previously underwent removal of both of her ovaries, followed by discontinuation of therapy. Similarly, the bleeding that occurs after bilateral removal of ovaries can be delayed by concomitant estrogen therapy. Flow occurs on discontinuation of exogenous estrogen. Estrogen withdrawal by itself (in the absence of progesterone) almost invariably causes uterine bleeding.

Estrogen Breakthrough Bleeding

Chronic exposure to various quantities of estrogen stimulates the growth of endometrium continuously in the absence of progesterone, as in the case of excessive extragonadal estrogen production in PCOS. After a certain point, the amount of estrogen produced in extraovarian tissue remains insufficient to maintain structural support for the endometrium. This gives rise to unpredictable episodes of shedding of the surface endometrium. Relatively low doses of estrogen yield intermittent spotting that may be prolonged, but the quantity is light. High levels of estrogen and sustained availability lead to prolonged periods of amenorrhea followed by acute, often profuse episodes of bleeding with excessive loss of blood.

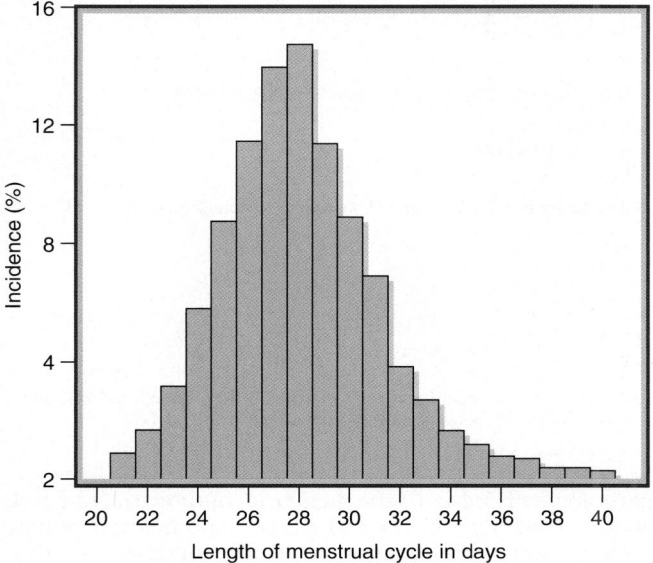

Figure 17-33 Variation of the duration of the menstrual cycle in women with regular cycles. (From Cunningham FG, MacDonald PC, Gant NF, et al. The endometrium and decidua: menstruation and pregnancy. In: Cunningham FG, ed. *Williams Obstetrics*, 19th ed. Stamford, CT: Appleton & Lange; 1993:81-109.)

Progesterone Withdrawal Bleeding

Typical progesterone withdrawal bleeding occurs after ovulation in the absence of pregnancy. Removal of the corpus luteum also leads to endometrial desquamation. Pharmacologically, a similar event can be achieved by administration and then discontinuation of progesterone or a synthetic progestin. Progesterone withdrawal bleeding occurs only if the endometrium is initially primed by endogenous or exogenous estrogen. If estrogen therapy is continued as progesterone is withdrawn, the progesterone withdrawal bleeding still occurs. Only when estrogen levels are increased markedly is progesterone withdrawal bleeding delayed.[307] Progesterone withdrawal bleeding is quite predictable in the presence of previous or concomitant estrogen exposure.

Progestin Breakthrough Bleeding

The pharmacologic phenomenon of breakthrough bleeding occurs in the setting of an unfavorably high ratio of progestin to estrogen. In the absence of sufficient estrogen, continuous progestin therapy leads to intermittent bleeding of variable duration, similar to the low-dose estrogen breakthrough bleeding described previously. This type of bleeding is associated with combination oral contraceptives that contain low-dose estrogen and the long-acting, progestin-only contraceptive methods such as Norplant and Depo-Provera.[308] Progestin breakthrough bleeding is highly unpredictable and is characterized by extensive variability among women.

Causes of Irregular Uterine Bleeding

The most common cause of disruption of a normal menstrual pattern is pregnancy or a complication of pregnancy. Pregnancy and pregnancy-related problems such as ectopic pregnancy or spontaneous miscarriage are extremely common causes of abnormal uterine bleeding (Table 17-7). Pregnancy should be ruled out by a urine test in any woman of reproductive age who presents with irregular bleeding (Table 17-8).

Anovulatory uterine bleeding is a diagnosis of exclusion for several reasons. Vulvar, vaginal, or uterine malignancies or an estrogen- or androgen-secreting ovarian tumor may cause abnormal uterine bleeding (see Table 17-7). Anovulatory uterine bleeding arising from responses of the endometrium to inappropriate production of ovarian steroids has also been called *dysfunctional uterine bleeding* because treatments that restore ovulatory function potentially reverse the irregular bleeding pattern. Common examples of anovulatory bleeding include those associated with exercise-related anovulation, hyperprolactinemia, hypothyroidism, or PCOS.[309] In these cases, restoration of ovulatory menses by correction of the underlying disorder or use of exogenous hormones can achieve predictable uterine bleeding.

Another common cause of irregular uterine bleeding is observed in oral contraceptive users in the form of progestin breakthrough bleeding. Progestin breakthrough bleeding during postmenopausal hormone therapy is also common. Patients may be unknowingly using other hormonal medications with an impact on the endometrium. For example, the use of ginseng, an herbal root, has been associated with estrogenic activity and abnormal bleeding.[310] Although uterine bleeding is a common benign side effect of various long-term hormone treatments, the clinician should always be convinced first that no other pathologic condition is present. Anatomically demonstrable

TABLE 17-7
Causes of Irregular Uterine Bleeding

Complications of Pregnancy

Threatened miscarriage
Incomplete miscarriage
Ectopic pregnancy

Anovulation

Physiologic
    Uncomplicated pregnancy (amenorrhea)
    Pubertal (postmenarchal) anovulation
    Anovulation immediately before menopause
Medications (e.g., oral contraceptives, GnRH agonists, danazol)
Hypothalamic (frequently presents as amenorrhea)
    Functional (e.g., diet, exercise, stress)
    Anatomic (e.g., tumor, granulomatous disease, infection)
Hyperprolactinemia, other pituitary disorders
    Prolactinoma
    Other pituitary tumors, granulomatous disease
    Hypothyroidism
    Medications
    Other
Androgen excess
    PCOS, hyperthecosis
    Ovarian tumor (e.g., Sertoli-Leydig cell tumor)
    Nonclassic adrenal hyperplasia
    Cushing syndrome
    Glucocorticoid resistance
    Adrenal tumor (e.g., adenoma, carcinoma)
    Medications (e.g., testosterone, danazol)
    Other
Premature ovarian insufficiency (frequently presents as amenorrhea)
Chronic illness
    Liver insufficiency
    Renal insufficiency
    AIDS
Other

Anatomic Defects Affecting the Uterus

Uterine leiomyomas
Endometrial polyps
Adenomyosis (usually manifests as hypermenorrhea)
Intrauterine adhesions (usually manifests as amenorrhea)
Endometritis
Endometrial hyperplasia, cancer
Chronic estrogen exposure (e.g., PCOS, medication, liver insufficiency)
Estrogen-secreting ovarian tumor (e.g., granulosa cell tumor)
Advanced cervical cancer
Other

Coagulation Defects (Usually Manifest as Hypermenorrhea)

Von Willebrand disease
Factor XI deficiency
Other

Extrauterine Genital Bleeding (May Mimic Uterine Bleeding)

Vaginitis
Genital trauma
Foreign body
Vaginal neoplasia
Vulvar neoplasia
Other

AIDS, acquired immunodeficiency syndrome; GnRH, gonadotropin-releasing hormone; PCOS, polycystic ovary syndrome.

pathologic disorders of the menstrual outflow tract include endometrial hyperplasia and cancer, endometrial polyps, uterine leiomyomas, adenomyosis, and endometritis. Irregular uterine bleeding may be associated with chronic illness, such as renal insufficiency, liver insufficiency, or AIDS. Careful examination may discover genital injury or a foreign object (see Table 17-7).

TABLE 17-8
Diagnostic Tests to Evaluate Irregular Uterine Bleeding

Commonly Used Tests

Urine hCG test
Serum hCG level (incomplete miscarriage, ectopic pregnancy)
Transvaginal pelvic ultrasonography (intrauterine or ectopic pregnancy, uterine leiomyoma, endometrial polyp or neoplasia, ovarian tumor)
Serum FSH, LH (anovulation; ovarian insufficiency)
Serum prolactin, TSH (anovulation; hyperprolactinemia)
Complete blood count, PT, PTT (evaluation for anemia, coagulation defect)
Liver and renal functions, HIV (anovulation; chronic disease)
Endometrial biopsy (endometrial disease; polyp, neoplasia, endometritis)

Less Commonly Used Tests

Evaluation for PCOS, ovarian or adrenal tumor, nonclassic adrenal hyperplasia, Cushing syndrome, and glucocorticoid resistance (androgen excess)
Head CT or MRI scan (hypothalamic anovulation, hyperprolactinemia)
Pelvic MRI scan (adenomyosis, uterine leiomyoma)
Hysterosonography with intrauterine saline instillation (endometrial polyp, uterine leiomyoma)
Hysteroscopy (endometrial polyp, uterine leiomyoma)
Dilatation and curettage (endometrial disease not diagnosed by ultrasonography or biopsy)

CT, computed tomography; FSH, follicle-stimulating hormone; hCG, human chorionic gonadotropin; HIV, human immunodeficiency virus; LH, luteinizing hormone; MRI, magnetic resonance imaging; PCOS, polycystic ovary syndrome; PT, prothrombin time; PTT, partial thromboplastin time; TSH, thyroid-stimulating hormone.

At puberty, the most common cause of irregular uterine bleeding is anovulation. Approximately 20% of adolescents with excessive irregular uterine bleeding have a coagulation defect.[311,312] Among all women of reproductive age with hypermenorrhea, the prevalence of a coagulation disorder is 17%; von Willebrand disease is the most common defect, and factor XI deficiency is the second common diagnosis. Bleeding because of a coagulation defect usually consists of a heavy flow with regular, cyclic menses (i.e., hypermenorrhea), and the same pattern can be seen in patients being treated with anticoagulants.[313] Bleeding disorders are usually associated with hypermenorrhea since menarche and a history of bleeding with surgery or trauma. Hypermenorrhea may be the only sign of an inherited bleeding disorder.[314]

Early pregnancy or its complications should always be ruled out first by a sensitive urine hCG measurement in any reproductive-age woman presenting with irregular bleeding. Other tests should be ordered on the basis of the initial clinical evaluation, including tests to evaluate anovulatory disorders of various causes (see Table 17-8). In patients with a history of prolonged heavy menses (i.e., hypermenorrhea) of pubertal origin, coagulation studies (e.g., prothrombin time, partial thromboplastin time, bleeding time) and a complete blood cell count should be obtained.

Pelvic ultrasonography through a vaginal probe is an extremely useful test for the evaluation of normal or abnormal pregnancy, uterine leiomyomas, endometrial neoplasia, and ovarian tumors (see Table 17-8). Other imaging studies may be used judiciously to rule out pathologic involvement of the hypothalamus, pituitary, and adrenal (discussed earlier). Pelvic MRI or ultrasound is used to assess adenomyosis, a uterine disorder characterized by the abnormal presence of diffuse endometrial tissue in the myometrial layer. Advanced adenomyosis is associated with diffuse enlargement of the uterus, hypermenorrhea, and anemia.

Endometrial histologic evaluation should be determined by an endometrial biopsy performed in the physician's office in patients at risk for endometrial hyperplasia or cancer (e.g., PCOS, liver insufficiency, obesity, diabetes mellitus, hormone therapy). A benign endometrial polyp or a uterine leiomyoma protruding into the uterine cavity can be diagnosed by hysterosonography using intrauterine saline installation or by hysteroscopy. Hysterosonography and hysteroscopy are not appropriate tests to evaluate endometrial hyperplasia or cancer because these procedures may cause dissemination of malignant cells. If malignancy is suspected, it should be ruled out by an office endometrial biopsy (see Table 17-8). Occasionally, an office endometrial biopsy cannot be performed or is not diagnostic of endometrial neoplasia. In these rare instances, endometrial curettage under anesthesia is performed for a reliable tissue diagnosis.

A careful history and physical examination may eliminate the need for most of these diagnostic tests. Before ordering a certain diagnostic study, it is useful to consider whether a particular test result would alter the ultimate clinical management.

Management of Anovulatory Uterine Bleeding

If ovulatory function can be restored, anovulatory bleeding usually gives way to predictable cyclic periods. Because restoration of ovulatory function may not be possible or practical in many of these women, exogenous estrogen and progestin are administered for several purposes. The indications for hormonal treatment of uterine bleeding include the need to stop acute uterine bleeding, to maintain predictable bleeding episodes, or to prevent endometrial hyperplasia.

Anovulatory uterine bleeding is a diagnosis of exclusion. Various anatomically demonstrable pathologic involvement of the genital tract (see Table 17-7) should be ruled out before administration of estrogen, progestin, or GnRH analogues.

Oral Contraceptives

Use of combination oral contraceptives in an acute or chronic fashion is the most common treatment for irregular uterine bleeding. The estrogen component of the combination pill stabilizes the endometrial tissue and stops shedding within hours; it decreases ovarian secretion of sex steroids by suppression of gonadotropins within several days. The progestin component of the pill directly affects endometrial tissue to decrease shedding over days and potentiates ovarian suppression induced by estrogen. The progestin (in the presence of estrogen) induces differentiation of the endometrial tissue into a stable form called *pseudodecidua*. Typically, a monophasic oral contraceptive preparation that contains 30 or 35 µg of ethinyl estradiol is preferred. Triphasic oral contraceptives and those with less than 30 µg of ethinyl estradiol are not suitable for the treatment of excessive anovulatory uterine bleeding. A combination oral contraceptive in high doses (two or three pills per day) can be used for short intervals (i.e., weeks) to treat an acute episode of excessive uterine bleeding. The usual dose of one pill per day may be administered for years to manage chronic anovulatory bleeding associated with PCOS or hyperprolactinemia.

Oral Contraceptives and Acute Excessive Uterine Bleeding Associated With Anemia. Unopposed estrogen exposure in women with anovulatory uterine bleeding is commonly associated with chronic endometrial buildup and heavy bleeding episodes. Therapy is administered as one combination oral contraceptive pill twice daily for 1 week. In obese women, the oral contraceptive may be given three times daily. This therapy is maintained despite cessation of flow within 2 days. If flow does not abate, other diagnostic possibilities (e.g., previously missed diagnosis of polyps, incomplete abortion, or neoplasia) should be reevaluated. In case of anovulatory bleeding, the flow does diminish rapidly within 2 days after the beginning of high-dose oral contraceptive treatment (i.e., one pill two or three times daily). Specific causes of anovulation and possible coagulation disorders should be evaluated during the next few days. The physician also should consider whether blood replacement or initiation of iron therapy is necessary. The patient should also be warned of possible nausea that may be caused by high-dose oral contraceptive treatment.

At the end of a week of high-dose oral contraceptive treatment, the pill is stopped temporarily. A heavy flow usually starts within a few days. On the third day of this withdrawal bleeding, a regular dose of combination oral contraceptive medication (one pill/day) is started. This is repeated for several 3-week treatments interrupted by 1-week withdrawal intervals. A decrease in volume with each successive cycle is expected. Oral contraceptives reduce menstrual flow by more than one half in most women.[315]

Because oral contraceptive use does not treat the underlying cause of anovulation but provides symptomatic relief by directly affecting the endometrium, its cessation results in the return of erratic uterine bleeding. Regardless of the requirement for contraception, use of oral contraceptives represents the best choice for hormonal management of heavy anovulatory bleeding and should be offered as long-term management.

Oral Contraceptives and Chronic Irregular Uterine Bleeding. PCOS is a common form of anovulation associated with chronic steady-state levels of unopposed estrogen that may give rise to endometrial hyperplasia and cancer (discussed earlier). Hypothalamic anovulation and hyperprolactinemia are associated with low estrogen levels that are insufficient to prevent bone loss. A combination oral contraceptive is a suitable long-term treatment for both forms of chronic anovulation.

Before the administration of an oral contraceptive, pregnancy should be ruled out. One pill per day is ordinarily administered for 3-week periods interrupted by 1-week hormone-free intervals. Withdrawal bleeding is expected during the hormone-free interval. The progestin component serves to prevent endometrial hyperplasia associated with steady-state unopposed estrogen exposure in PCOS. In cases of anovulation associated with hypoestrogenism (e.g., hypothalamic anovulation, hyperprolactinemia), the estrogen component of the pill provides sufficient replacement to prevent bone loss. The risk of thromboembolism, stroke, or myocardial infarction associated with long-term administration is extremely low in current nonsmokers and in the absence of a history of thromboembolism. Provided that the oral contraceptive controls the abnormal uterine bleeding effectively, a chronically anovulatory woman can continue this regimen until menopause.

Synthetic Progestins

Synthetic progestins enhance endometrial differentiation and antagonize the proliferative effects of estrogen on the endometrium (see Fig. 17-22).[126,316] The effects of progestins or natural progesterone include limitation of estrogen-induced endometrial growth and prevention of endometrial hyperplasia. The absence of naturally synthesized proges-

terone in anovulatory states is the rationale for administering a progestin.

The most common indication for long-term cyclic progestin administration is to prevent endometrial malignancy in a patient with PCOS and unopposed chronic estrogen exposure of the endometrium. A combination oral contraceptive is the treatment of choice in these cases. If the patient cannot use an oral contraceptive for some reason (e.g., history of thromboembolism), a progestin may be administered in a cyclic fashion to prevent endometrial hyperplasia. Before the administration of a progestin (or oral contraceptive), pregnancy should be ruled out. In the treatment of oligomenorrhea associated with PCOS, orderly, limited withdrawal bleeding can be accomplished by administration of a progestin such as MPA (5 mg/day) for at least 10 days every 2 months. Alternatively, norethindrone acetate at 5 mg/day or megestrol acetate at 20 mg/day may be administered for 10 days every 2 months. Absence of withdrawal bleeding requires further workup.

In the treatment of excessive uterine bleeding (i.e., hypermenorrhea or polymenorrhea), these progestins at higher daily doses (20 mg/day of MPA, 10 mg/day of norethindrone acetate, or 40 mg/day of megestrol acetate) are prescribed for 2 weeks to induce predecidual stromal changes in the endometrium. A heavy progestin withdrawal flow usually follows within 3 days after the last dose is administered. Thereafter, repeated progestin treatment (5 mg/day of MPA, 5 mg/day of norethindrone acetate, or 20 mg/day of megestrol acetate) is offered cyclically for at least the first 10 days of every other month to ensure therapeutic effect. Failure of progestin to correct irregular bleeding requires diagnostic reevaluation such as endometrial biopsy. Predictable withdrawal bleeding within several days after each cycle of progestin administration suggests the absence of endometrial malignancy.

High-Dose Estrogen for Acute Excessive Uterine Bleeding

An oral contraceptive given two or three times daily is the treatment of choice to stop heavy anovulatory bleeding. A high-dose oral contraceptive regimen should be offered to women with heavy uterine bleeding with or without asymptomatic anemia after anatomically demonstrable pathology of the genital tract has been ruled out (see Table 17-7). A patient with acute and severe anovulatory bleeding accompanied by symptomatic anemia represents a medical emergency. These patients should be hospitalized immediately and offered a blood transfusion. After genital tract disease has been ruled out by history, physical examination, and pelvic ultrasonography, intravenously administered high-dose estrogen is the treatment of choice to stop life-threatening bleeding. A well-established regimen is to administer 25 mg of conjugated estrogen intravenously every 4 hours until bleeding markedly slows down or for at least 24 hours.[317] Estrogen most likely acts on the capillaries to induce clotting.[318] Before intravenous estrogen treatment is discontinued, an oral contraceptive pill is started three times daily. Oral contraceptive treatment is then continued as described previously.

Because high-dose estrogen is a risk factor for thromboembolism, taking two or three oral contraceptive pills per day for a week or large doses of intravenous conjugated equine estrogens for 24 hours should be regarded as presenting a significant risk. However, no data are available to evaluate any risk associated with this type of acute use of hormonal therapy for such short intervals. The physician and patient should make a decision regarding high-dose hormone therapy after considering its risks and benefits. Alternative treatment options may be offered to patients with significant risk factors. Exposure to high doses of estrogen should be avoided in women with a past episode or a strong family history of idiopathic venous thromboembolism. High-dose hormone treatment should also be avoided in women with severe chronic illness such as liver insufficiency or renal insufficiency. One alternative for these patients is dilatation and curettage, followed by treatment with an oral contraceptive (one pill per day) until the uterine bleeding is under control.

Gonadotropin-Releasing Hormone Analogues for Excessive Anovulatory Uterine Bleeding

A GnRH analogue may be given to women with excessive anovulatory bleeding or hypermenorrhea related to severe chronic illness such as liver insufficiency or coagulation disorders. Monthly depot injections of GnRH agonists are not effective for acute excessive uterine bleeding and may increase uterine bleeding for the first 2 weeks. GnRH antagonists downregulate FSH and LH without a delay and achieve amenorrhea more rapidly. The GnRH agonist leuprolide acetate depot (3.75 mg/month intramuscularly) may be administered for 6 months or longer to control uterine bleeding due to chronic illness. GnRH antagonists can probably be used to halt acute or chronic anovulatory bleeding; however, insufficient published data are available to provide dose recommendations. Long-term side effects of GnRH analogues, including osteoporosis, make this an undesirable choice for long-term therapy. If long-term treatment with GnRH analogues is chosen, norethindrone acetate (2.5 mg daily) should be added back. This add-back regimen is usually sufficient to prevent osteoporosis and does not ordinarily worsen the uterine bleeding.

HORMONE-DEPENDENT BENIGN GYNECOLOGIC DISORDERS

Endometriosis

Endometriosis is defined as the presence of endometrium-like tissue in ectopic sites outside the uterine cavity, primarily on pelvic peritoneum and ovaries, and it is associated with chronic pelvic pain, pain during intercourse, and infertility.[319] This estrogen-dependent inflammatory disease affects 5% to 10% of U.S. women of reproductive age.[319] This classic presentation may represent a common phenotype resulting from diverse anatomic or biochemical aberrations of uterine function. As cellular and molecular mechanisms in endometriosis are uncovered, this condition is coming to be viewed as a systemic and chronic complex disease, much like diabetes mellitus or asthma.[320] Endometriosis may be inherited in a polygenic manner, because its incidence is increased by up to sevenfold in relatives of women with endometriosis.[321]

Pathology

There are three clinically distinct forms of endometriosis: endometriotic implants on the surface of pelvic peritoneum and ovaries (i.e., peritoneal endometriosis), ovarian cysts lined by endometrioid mucosa (i.e., endometriomas), and a complex, solid mass composed of endometriotic tissue blended with adipose and fibromuscular tissue and residing between rectum and vagina (i.e., rectovaginal nodule). These three types of lesions may be variant phenotypes of the same pathologic process, or they may be caused by different mechanisms.[322,323] Their common histologic characteristic is the presence of endometrial stromal or epithelial cells, along with chronic bleeding and inflammatory changes. These lesions may occur singly or in combination and are associated with significantly increased risk of infertility and chronic pelvic pain.[322,323] The inflammatory process in endometriosis may stimulate nerve endings in the pelvis to cause pain, impair the function of the uterine tubes, decrease receptivity of the endometrium, and negatively affect development of the oocyte and embryo. Endometriosis may also cause infertility by physically blocking the tubes. An ovarian endometrioma may decrease the quality of the eggs or become sufficiently large to interefere with the ovulation process.

Clinical evidence points to a deleterious effect of uninterrupted ovulatory cycles on the development and persistence of endometriosis.[320] First, symptoms of endometriosis usually appear after menarche and vanish after menopause. Occasionally, a rectovaginal nodule remains symptomatic in a postmenopausal woman, suggesting that its persistence is independent of ovarian estrogen. Second, multiparity is associated with a decreased risk of endometriosis. Third, disruption of ovulation by GnRH analogues, oral contraceptives, or progestins reduces pelvic disease and associated pain. In line with these observations, basic and clinical research findings indicate major roles of the ovarian steroids estrogen and progesterone in the pathologic development of endometriosis. In humans and primate models, estrogen stimulates the growth of endometriotic tissue, whereas aromatase inhibitors that block estrogen formation and antiprogestins are therapeutic.[320] Levels of nuclear receptors for estrogen and progesterone in endometriotic tissue are strikingly different from those in normal endometrium.[320] Fourth, biologically significant quantities of progesterone and estrogen are produced locally by an abnormally active steroidogenic cascade that includes aromatase.[320]

Mechanism of Disease

A number of hypotheses have been proposed regarding the histologic origin of endometriosis. Sampson suggested that fragments of menstrual endometrium pass retrograde through the tubes and then implant and persist on peritoneal surfaces.[324] This mechanism has been demonstrated in primate models and observed naturally in human disease, and it is supported by the observation that spontaneous endometriosis occurs exclusively in species that menstruate. Alternatively, the coelomic-metaplasia hypothesis describes the genesis of endometriotic lesions within the peritoneal cavity by differentiation of mesothelial cells into endometrium-like tissue. A third hypothesis argues that menstrual tissue from the endometrial cavity reaches other body sites through veins or lymphatic vessels.[320] Finally, it has been proposed that circulating blood cells originating from bone marrow differentiate into endometriotic tissue at various body sites.[325] Sampson's implantation hypothesis offers a plausible mechanism for most endometriotic lesions but does not explain why only some women develop endometriosis. Although most women of reproductive age have reflux menstruation into the peritoneal cavity, endometriosis is encountered in only 5% to 10% of this population.

Two possible mechanisms may explain the successful implantation of refluxed endometrium on the peritoneal surface or in a hemorrhagic corpus luteum cyst of the ovary. First, the eutopic endometrium of women with endometriosis exhibits multiple subtle but significant molecular abnormalities, including activation of oncogenic pathways or biosynthetic cascades favoring increased production of estrogen, cytokines, prostaglandins, and metalloproteinases.[320] When this biologically distinct tissue attaches to mesothelial cells, the magnitude of these abnormalities is amplified dramatically to enhance implant survival.[320] A second mechanism suggests that a defective immune system fails to clear implants off the peritoneal surface.[320] It is possible that both mechanisms may contribute to the same phenotype.

Clear molecular distinctions, such as overproduction of estrogen, prostaglandins, and cytokines, are observed between endometriotic tissue and endometrium (Fig. 17-34).[320] Subtler forms of these abnormalities are also observed in endometrium from a patient with endometriosis compared with endometrium from a disease-free woman. Inflammation is a hallmark of endometriotic tissue that overproduces prostaglandins, metalloproteinases, cytokines, and chemokines.[320] Increased levels of

acute inflammatory cytokines such as interleukin 1β (IL-1β), IL-6, and tumor necrosis factor (TNF) likely enhance adhesion of shed endometrial tissue fragments on peritoneal surfaces, and proteolytic membrane metalloproteinases may further promote their implantation.[320] Monocyte chemoattractant protein 1, IL-8, and RANTES (i.e., regulated on activation, normal T cell expressed and secreted) attract the granulocytes, natural killer cells, and macrophages typically observed in endometriosis.[326] Autoregulatory positive feedback loops ensure further accumulation of these immune cells, cytokines, and chemokines in established lesions.

Basic biologic functions such as inflammation, immune response, angiogenesis, and apoptosis are altered in favor of survival and replenishment of endometriotic tissue.[320] These functions depend in part on estrogen or progesterone action. Excessive formation of estrogen and

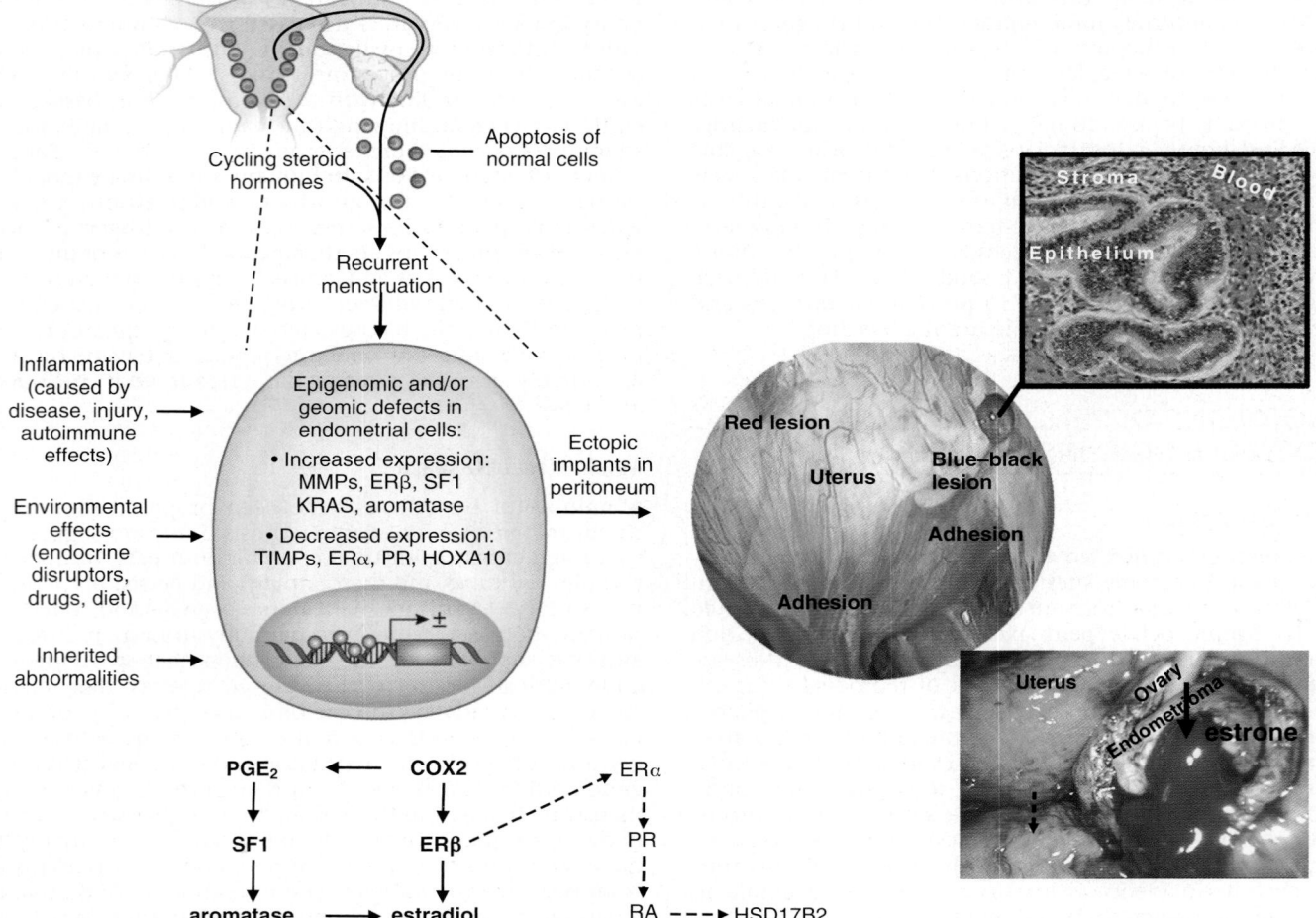

Figure 17-34 Molecular mechanisms in endometriosis. Endometriosis is defined as the presence of endometrium-like tissue on the pelvic peritoneum (red and blue-black lesions) or in the ovary (blood-filled cyst, i.e., endometrioma). These lesions are thought to originate from abnormal endometrial tissue stem cells (colored blue), which have migrated retrograde during menstruation. Normal endometrial cells (colored red) without such survival capabilities are thought to go through apoptosis in the peritoneal or ovarian environments. It is possible that women with endometriosis have higher numbers of the abnormal cells in their eutopic endometrial tissues. Thus, recurrent menstruation seems to be a significant risk factor for developing endometriosis. These abnormal cells (blue) contain genome-wide epigenetic abnormalities, such as DNA methylation, that affect the expression of a wide variety of genes. These epigenetic abnormalities may be inherited or caused by environmental influences such as inflammation and endocrine disruptors. Two nuclear receptors, steroidogenic factor 1 (SF1) and estrogen receptor-β (ERβ), play significant roles in the pathology of endometriosis. In normal endometrial stromal cells, cytosine-phosphate-guanine islands located at the SF1 and ERβ promoters are robustly methylated and silenced. A lack of promoter methylation is associated with promoter activation and the presence of extraordinarily large quantities of these nuclear receptors in endometriotic stromal cells. Prostaglandin E_2 (PGE$_2$) induces multiple steroidogenic genes, including aromatase, and formation of estradiol from cholesterol. SF1 mediates this steroidogenic action of PGE$_2$. ERβ suppresses ERα and progesterone receptors (PR). This results in defective retinoic acid (RA) production and action, leading to 17β-hydroxysteroid dehydrogenase 2 (HSD17B2) deficiency and failure to metabolize estradiol. ERβ also induces cyclooxygenase 2 (COX2) and formation of PGE$_2$. Estradiol and PGE$_2$ are produced in large quantities and enhance cell survival and inflammation in endometriotic tissue. MMPs, matrix metalloproteinases; KRAS, V-Ki-ras2 Kirsten rat sarcoma viral oncogene homologue; TIMPs, tissue inhibitors of metalloproteinases; HOXA10, homeobox A10.

prostaglandin and development of progesterone resistance have emerged as clinically useful concepts, because targeting of aromatase in the estrogen biosynthetic pathway, cyclooxygenase 2 (COX2) in the prostaglandin pathway, or the PR significantly reduces laparoscopically visible endometriosis and pelvic pain (see Fig. 17-34).[320] These three critical mechanisms have been linked by specific epigenetic (hypomethylation) defects that cause overexpression of the nuclear receptors SF1 and ERβ.[320] The genome-wide unique epigenetic fingerprint in endometriosis suggests DNA methylation is an integral component of the disease and identifies a novel role for the GATA family as key regulators of uterine physiology; aberrant DNA methylation in endometriotic cells correlates with a shift in GATA isoform expression that facilitates progesterone resistance and disease progression.[327]

Diagnosis

A history of severely painful menses during the teenage years, which eventually progressed into chronic pelvic pain experienced both during and between periods, is suggestive of endometriosis. Reliable diagnosis of peritoneal endometriosis can be made only by direct visualization of these lesions by laparoscopy or laparotomy. Ovarian endometriotic cysts filled with a thick, bloody fluid (i.e., endometriomas) can be diagnosed accurately by vaginal ultrasonography.

Treatment

Treatment of infertility caused by endometriosis consists of surgical removal with or without assisted reproductive technology, whereas pain is usually treated with a combination of medical suppression of ovulation and surgery. Peritoneal implants are resected or vaporized by electric current or laser. Ovarian endometriomas and rectovaginal endometriotic nodules may be effectively removed only by full dissection. Epidemiologic and laboratory data suggest a link between ovarian endometriosis and distinct types of ovarian cancers.[320]

Although current hormonal therapy for infertility associated with endometriosis is not of proven value, it is somewhat successful for pelvic pain associated with endometriosis. Various agents used are comparable in terms of efficacy. Most of the current medical treatments were designed to suppress ovulation (e.g., GnRH agonists, oral contraceptives, danazol, progestins). A possible alternative mechanism of action of the androgenic steroid danazol or a progestin is a direct growth-suppressive effect on endometriotic tissue.

Many patients and physicians do not favor danazol because of its anabolic and androgenic side effects of weight gain and muscle cramps and occasional irreversible virilization (e.g., clitoromegaly, voice changes).[328] Up to 50% of patients with endometriosis fail to complete 6 months of treatment with danazol.[329] The rest of the hormonal agents—oral contraceptives, progestins, and GnRH agonists—show comparable efficacy for control of endometriosis-associated pain.[330-332] A 6-month course using any one of these agents results in a significant reduction of pain in more than 50% of patients.[330-332] Induction of pain relief with a continuously administered oral contraceptive or progestin takes longer than with a GnRH agonist.

There is a high incidence of recurrence or persistence of the disease and pain after all of these medical therapies.[333] Thus, successful medical management of pain requires long-term ovarian suppression for years. Because it is not practical to maintain these patients on a depot GnRH agonist regimen for more than 6 months, treatment with a combination oral contraceptive is the most suitable long-term management option.[30]

We are still far from the cure of endometriosis, and current treatments are not satisfactory for effective control of pain. The radical treatment is removal of both ovaries, and even this was not found to be effective in a number of cases of postmenopausal endometriosis.[334] New alternative strategies are needed to offer women with endometriosis a reasonable chance to live without suffering from chronic pelvic pain for decades.

There are two important caveats about ovulation suppression–based treatments. First, large quantities of estrogen can be produced locally within the endometriotic cells. This represents an intracrine mechanism of estrogen action, in contrast to ovarian secretion, which is an endocrine means of supplying this steroid to target tissues (see Fig. 17-19).[93,331] Second, estradiol produced in peripheral tissue sites (e.g., adipose tissue, skin fibroblasts) may give rise to pathologically significant circulating levels of estradiol in a subset of women.[93] GnRH agonists do not inhibit peripheral estrogen formation or local estrogen production within the estrogen-responsive lesion. Moreover, endometriosis is resistant to selective effects of progesterone and progestins.[320]

Aromatase inhibitors and selective progesterone response modulators are candidate therapeutic agents for endometriosis refractory to existing treatment options. Aromatase expression and local estrogen biosynthesis in endometriotic implants prompted pilot studies to target aromatase in endometriosis using its third-generation inhibitors. Among these inhibitors, anastrozole and letrozole were used successfully to treat endometriosis in postmenopausal and premenopausal women.[329,335-338] An aromatase inhibitor is the medical treatment of choice for persistent postmenopausal endometriosis. Use of aromatase inhibitors in premenopausal women with endometriosis requires concomitant ovarian suppression by the addition of a GnRH analogue, progestin, or combination oral contraceptive.

For the medical management of pain in premenopausal women with endometriosis, this author favors the following simple algorithm. Unless contraindicated, the continuous use of a combination oral contraceptive is the initial treatment of choice. The patient is reassured that the majority of women will have minimal or no breakthrough bleeding after 6 months of continuous oral contraceptive treatment. If pain relief is adequate, the patient can remain on this regimen for years. If adequate pain relief is not achieved after 6 months of use, a daily oral aromatase inhibitor (anastrozole, 1 mg/day or letrozole 2.5 mg/day) is added to the continuous oral contraceptive regimen. This combination may be maintained for at least a year. If pain relief is still not satisfactory, conservative laparoscopic surgery is considered.

Uterine Leiomyomas

Uterine fibroids (leiomyomas) represent the most common tumor in women.[339] These lesions disrupt the functions of the uterus and cause excessive uterine bleeding, anemia, defective implantation of an embryo, recurrent pregnancy loss, preterm labor, obstruction of labor, pelvic discomfort, and urinary incontinence and may mimic or mask malignant tumors. By the time they reach 50 years of age, nearly 70% of white women and more than 80% of black women will have had at least one fibroid; severe symptoms develop in 15% to 30% of these women. Uterine fibroids in black women are significantly larger at diagnosis than those in white women, are diagnosed at an earlier age, and are characterized by more severe symptoms and a longer period of sustained growth. Approximately 200,000 hysterectomies, 30,000 myomectomies, and thousands of selective uterine-artery embolizations and high-intensity focused ultrasound procedures are performed annually in the United States to remove or destroy uterine fibroids.[339]

Each fibroid seems to originate from the transformation and monoclonal expansion of a single somatic stem cell of the myometrium under the influence of ovarian hormones. Human uterine fibroid tissue contains fewer stem cells than normal myometrium. However, stem cells derived from fibroid tissue—not the myometrium—carry *MED12* mutations, which suggests that at least one genetic hit initially transforms a myometrial stem cell, which subsequently interacts with the surrounding myometrial tissue to give rise to a fibroid tumor.[339]

Estrogen stimulates the growth of uterine fibroids through its receptor ERα. The primary roles of estrogen and ERα in fibroid growth are permissive in that they enable tissue to respond to progesterone by inducing the expression of PR, which is essential and sufficient for tumor growth, as indicated by the stimulation of cell proliferation, the accumulation of extracellular matrix, and cellular hypertrophy.[339] Since the stem cell population expresses much lower levels of PR than the population of mature cells but serves as the key source of tissue growth, a paracrine signal originating from PR-rich differentiated cells may mediate the proliferative effects of progesterone on fibroid stem cells.[339]

Diagnosis can be made by abdominal or transvaginal ultrasonography. Transvaginal ultrasonography is a sensitive method for determining the size, number, and location of uterine leiomyomas.

The therapeutic choices depend on the goals of therapy, with hysterectomy most often used for definitive treatment and myomectomy used when preservation of childbearing capability is desired. Intracavitary and submucous leiomyomas can be removed by hysteroscopic resection. Laparoscopic myomectomy is technically possible but involves an increased risk of uterine rupture during pregnancy. The overall recurrence rate after myomectomy varies widely, from 10% to 50%. Other FDA-approved treatment options include selective uterine artery embolization and extracorporeal ablation of uterine fibroids with MRI-guided, high-intensity, focused ultrasound.[340]

Although GnRH agonist–induced hypogonadism can reduce the overall volume of the uterus containing leiomyomas and tumor vascularity, the severe side effects and prompt recurrences make GnRH agonists useful only for short-term goals such as reducing anemia related to uterine bleeding or decreasing tumor vascularity before hysteroscopic resection. Trials have consistently demonstrated that treatment with an antiprogestin such as mifepristone or ulipristal acetate reduces fibroid size.[339] This observation underscores the role of progesterone in the cause of uterine fibroids and opens a new area of therapeutic investigation.[339]

MANAGEMENT OF MENOPAUSE

Consequences of Menopause

Perimenopause Stage

Menopause is the permanent cessation of menses as a result of the irreversible loss of a number of ovarian functions, including ovulation and estrogen production. Perimenopause is a critical period of life during which striking endocrinologic, somatic, and psychological alterations occur in the transition to menopause. Perimenopause encompasses the change from ovulatory cycles to cessation of menses and is marked by irregularity of menstrual bleeding.

The most sensitive clinical indication of perimenopause is the progressively increasing occurrence of menstrual irregularities. The menstrual cycle for most ovulatory women lasts 24 to 35 days, and approximately 20% of all reproductive-age women experience irregular cycles.[299] When women are in their 40s, anovulation becomes more prevalent and the menstrual cycle length increases, beginning several years before menopause.[302] The median age at the onset of perimenopause is 47.5 years.[341] Regardless of the age at onset, menopause (i.e., cessation of menses) is consistently preceded by a period of prolonged cycle intervals.[342] Elevated circulating levels of FSH mark this menstrual cycle change before menopause and are accompanied by decreased inhibin levels, normal levels of LH, and slightly elevated levels of estradiol.[343] These changes in serum hormone levels reflect a decreasing ovarian follicular reserve and can be detected most reliably on day 2 or 3 of the menstrual cycle.

Serum estradiol levels do not begin to decline until less than a year before menopause. The average circulating estradiol levels in perimenopausal women are estimated to be somewhat higher than those in younger women because of an increased follicular response to elevated FSH levels.[344] The decline in inhibin production by the follicle, which allows a rise in FSH levels, in the later reproductive years reflects diminishing follicular reserve and competence. Ovarian follicular output of inhibin begins to decrease after 30 years of age, and this decline becomes much more pronounced after age 40. These hormonal changes parallel a sharp decline in fecundity, which starts at age 35.

Perimenopause is a transitional period during which postmenopausal levels of FSH can be observed despite continued menses; LH levels remain in the normal range. Pregnancy is still possible in the perimenopausal woman, because occasional ovulation and functional corpus luteum formation can occur. Until complete cessation of menses is observed or FSH levels higher than 40 IU/L are measured on two separate occasions, some form of contraception should be recommended to prevent unwanted pregnancy.

Perimenopause represents an optimal period in which to evaluate the general health of the mature woman and introduce measures to prepare her for the striking physiologic changes that come with menopause. The patient and her clinician should attempt to achieve several important aims during perimenopause. The long-term goal is to maintain an optimal quality of physical and social life. Another immediate objective is the detection of any major chronic disorders that occur with aging. The benefits and risks of hormone therapy should be discussed thoroughly at this time.

Menopause Features

The median age at menopause is approximately 51 years.[345] The age at menopause is probably determined in part by genetic factors, because mothers and daughters tend to experience menopause at about the same age.[346-348] Environmental factors may modify the age at menopause. For example, current smoking is associated with an earlier menopause, whereas alcohol consumption delays menopause.[345] Oral contraceptive use does not affect the age at which menopause begins.

The symptoms frequently seen and related to decreased estrogen production in menopause include irregular frequency of menses followed by amenorrhea, vasomotor instability manifested as hot flashes and sweats, urogenital atrophy giving rise to pain during intercourse and a variety of urinary symptoms, and consequences of osteoporosis and CVD. The combination and extent of these symptoms vary widely for each patient. Some patients experience multiple severe symptoms that may be disabling, whereas others have no symptoms or only mild discomfort associated with perimenopause.

Biosynthesis of Estrogen and Other Steroids in the Postmenopausal Woman

No follicular units can be detected histologically in the ovaries after menopause. In reproductive-age women, the granulosa cell of the ovulatory follicle is the major source of inhibin and estradiol. In the absence of these factors that inhibit gonadotropin secretion, FSH and LH levels increase sharply after menopause. These levels peak a few years after menopause and decrease gradually and slightly thereafter.[349] The postmenopausal serum level of either gonadotropin may be more than 100 IU/L. FSH levels are usually higher than LH levels because LH is cleared from the blood much more quickly and possibly because the low levels of inhibin in menopause selectively lead to increased FSH secretion. Nevertheless, increased LH is a major factor that maintains significant quantities of androstenedione and testosterone secretion from the ovary, although the total production rates of both steroids decline after menopause.

The primary steroid products of the postmenopausal ovary are androstenedione and testosterone.[93] The average premenopausal rate of production of androstenedione of 3 mg/day is decreased by one half to approximately 1.5 mg/day.[93] The decrease primarily results from a substantial reduction in the ovarian contribution to the circulating androstenedione pool. Adrenal secretion accounts for most of the androstenedione production in the postmenopausal woman, with only a small amount secreted from the ovary.[93] DHEA and DHEAS originate almost exclusively from the adrenal gland and decline steadily with advancing age independent of menopause. The serum levels of DHEA and DHEAS after menopause are about one fourth of those in young adult women.[350]

Testosterone production is decreased by approximately one third after menopause.[93] Total testosterone production can be approximated by the sum of ovarian secretion and peripheral formation from androstenedione (see Fig. 17-26). In the premenopausal woman, significant amounts of testosterone are produced by conversion of androstenedione in extraovarian tissues. Because ovarian androstenedione secretion is substantially decreased after menopause, the decrease in postmenopausal testosterone production is accounted for in large measure by a decrease in the relative contribution of extraovarian sources.[93] With the disappearance of follicles and decreased estrogen, the elevated gonadotropins drive the remaining stromal tissue in the ovary to maintain testosterone secretion at levels observed during the premenopausal years. The contribution of the postmenopausal ovary to the total testosterone production is increased in the presence of seemingly unaltered ovarian secretion.

The most dramatic endocrine alteration of perimenopause involves the decline in the circulating level and production rate of estradiol. The average menopausal level of circulating estradiol is less than 20 pg/mL. The estradiol and estrone levels in postmenopausal women are usually slightly less than those in adult men. Circulating estradiol in postmenopausal women (and men) is derived from the peripheral conversion of androstenedione to estrone, which is converted peripherally to estradiol (see Fig. 17-19).[93] The mean circulating level of estrone in postmenopausal women (37 pg/mL) is higher than that of estradiol. The average postmenopausal production rate of estrone is approximately 42 µg/24 hours. After menopause, almost all estrone and estradiol is derived from the peripheral aromatization of androstenedione. There is a dramatic change in the androgen-to-estrogen ratio because of the sharp decrease in estradiol level and the only slightly reduced testosterone. The frequent onset of mild hirsutism after menopause reflects this striking shift in the hormone ratio. During the postmenopausal years, DHEAS and DHEA levels continue to decline steadily with advancing age, whereas serum androstenedione, testosterone, estrone, and estradiol levels do not change significantly.[349]

The aromatization of androstenedione to estrone in extraovarian tissues correlates positively with weight and advancing age (see Figs. 17-19 and 17-31).[93] Body weight correlates positively with the circulating levels of estrone and estradiol. Because aromatase enzyme activity is present in significant quantities in adipose tissue, increased aromatization of androstenedione in overweight individuals may reflect the increased bulk of tissue containing the enzyme.[93] There is a two- to fourfold increase in the specific activity of aromatase per cell with advancing age.[93] An increased overall number of adipose fibroblasts with aromatase activity and a decrease in the levels of SHBG increase the free estradiol level and contribute to the increased risk of endometrial cancer in obese women.[93]

In postmenopausal women, estrogen produced from androstenedione peripherally in fat and skin and locally in breast cancer tissue promotes the growth of this malignancy (Fig. 17-35).[93] The clinical relevance of extraovarian estrogen formation is exemplified by the successful use of aromatase inhibitors as the current endocrine treatment for postmenopausal breast cancer.[93]

Postmenopausal Uterine Bleeding

Perimenopausal or postmenopausal bleeding can be caused by hormone administration or excessive extraovarian estrogen formation. Irregular uterine bleeding is commonly observed during the perimenopausal transition as anovulatory cycles alternate with ovulatory cycles. Uterine bleeding after menopause is less common if the patient is not receiving hormone therapy. Obese women are more likely to experience postmenopausal bleeding because of increased peripheral aromatization of adrenal androstenedione. Patients receiving a continuous combination regimen of hormone therapy may experience unpredictable uterine bleeding. The major objective in these circumstances is to rule out endometrial malignancy. This can be best achieved by tissue diagnosis through an office endometrial biopsy using a plastic cannula. Transvaginal ultrasonographic measurement of endometrial thickness may be used in postmenopausal women to avoid unnecessary biopsies.[131] A biopsy is required if an endometrial thickness of 5 mm or greater is observed.

Unpredictable irregular uterine bleeding is observed in approximately 20% of postmenopausal women receiving a long-term (>1 year) continuous estrogen-progestin combination. Before employing ultrasonography and endometrial biopsy to explore the cause of bleeding that is assumed to arise from the intrauterine cavity, the clinician should

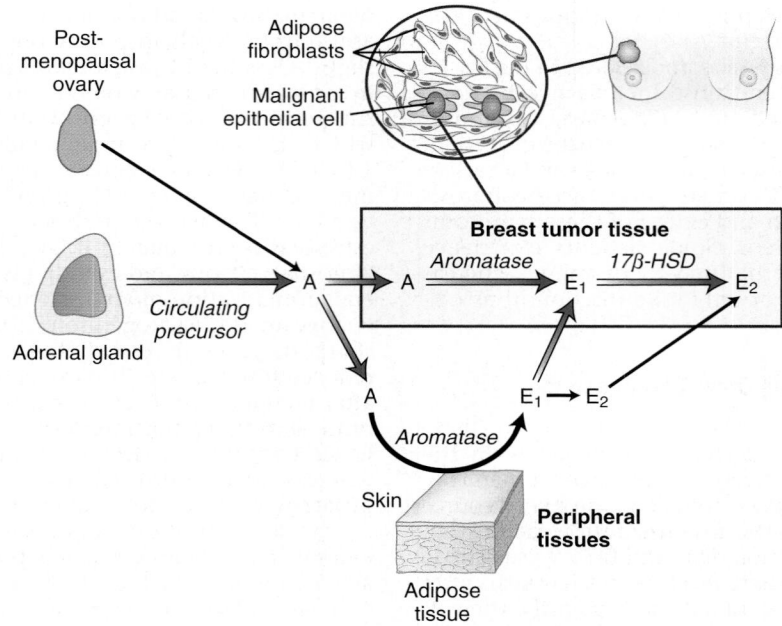

Figure 17-35 Tissue sources of estrogen in postmenopausal breast cancer. The important pathologic roles of extraovarian (peripheral) and local estrogen biosynthesis are shown for an estrogen-dependent disease in postmenopausal women. The estrogen precursor androstenedione (A) originates primarily from the adrenal gland in the postmenopausal woman. Aromatase expression and enzyme activity in extraovarian tissues such as fat increase with advancing age. The aromatase activity in skin and subcutaneous adipose fibroblasts gives rise to formation of systemically available estrone (E_1) and, to a smaller extent, estradiol (E_2). The conversion of circulating A to E_1 in undifferentiated breast adipose fibroblasts compacted around malignant epithelial cells and subsequent conversion of E_1 to E_2 in malignant epithelial cells provide high tissue concentrations of E_2 for tumor growth. The clinical relevance of these findings is exemplified by the successful use of aromatase inhibitors to treat breast cancer in postmenopausal women. 17β-HSD, reductive-type 17β-hydroxysteroid dehydrogenase.

rule out diseases of the vulva, vagina, and cervix.[131] Careful inspection of these organs along with a normal cervical Papanicolaou (Pap) smear within the past year is sufficient to rule out the vulva, vagina, and cervix as potential sources of bleeding. The causes of postmenopausal uterine bleeding are benign most of the time. Endometrial malignancy is encountered in patients with bleeding in only about 1% to 2% of postmenopausal endometrial biopsies.[351] Approximately three fourths of endometrial biopsies from postmenopausal women reveal no pathologic change or an atrophic endometrium. Other histologic findings include hyperplasia (15%) and endometrial polyps (3%). Persistent unexplained uterine bleeding requires repeated evaluation, biopsy, hysteroscopy, or dilatation and curettage.

Hot Flashes

The most frequent and striking symptom during perimenopause is the hot flash. It typically occurs during the transition from perimenopause to postmenopause. The flash is also a major symptom of postmenopause, and it can occur up to 5 years after menopause.[352] More than four fifths of postmenopausal women experience hot flashes within 3 months after the cessation of ovarian function, whether natural or surgical in origin. Of these women, more than three fourths have hot flashes for more than 1 year, and approximately one half have them for up to 5 years.[352] Hot flashes lessen in frequency and intensity with advancing age, unlike other sequelae of menopause, which progress with time.

A hot flash is a subjective sensation of intense warmth of the upper body, which typically lasts for approximately 4 minutes but may range in duration from 30 seconds to 5 minutes. It can follow a prodrome of palpitations or headache and is frequently accompanied by weakness,

faintness, or vertigo. The episode usually ends in profuse sweating and a cold sensation. Hot flashes may occur rarely or recur every few minutes. At night, hot flashes are more frequent and can be severe enough to awaken a woman from sleep. They are also more intense during times of stress. In a cool environment, hot flashes are fewer, less intense, and shorter in duration than in a warm environment.[353]

The hot flash results from a sudden reduction of estrogen levels rather than from hypoestrogenism itself. Regardless of the cause of menopause—natural, surgical, or estrogen withdrawal caused by a GnRH agonist—hot flashes are associated with an acute and significant drop in estrogen level. The consistent association between the onset of flashes and acute estrogen withdrawal is supported by the effectiveness of estrogen therapy and the absence of flashes in prolonged hypoestrogenic states, such as gonadal dysgenesis or hypothalamic amenorrhea. Hypogonadal women experience hot flashes only after estrogen is administered and withdrawn.[354] Higher body mass index, and body fat in particular, is associated with greater vasomotor symptom reporting, primarily hot flashes.[355]

Not all hot flashes are caused by menopause. Sudden episodes of sweating and flashes may be caused by catecholamine- or histamine-secreting tumors (e.g., pheochromocytoma, carcinoid), hyperthyroidism, or chronic infection (e.g., tuberculosis). The hot flash may also be psychosomatic in origin. In these circumstances, the clinician should obtain a serum FSH level to confirm perimenopause or menopause before initiating hormone therapy.

Urogenital Atrophy

The urogenital sinus gives rise to development of the lower vagina, vulva, and urethra during embryonic development, and these tissues are estrogen dependent. The decrease in estrogen at menopause causes the vaginal walls to become pale because of diminished vascularity and to thin down to only three or four squamous epithelial cell layers. Loss of this protective mechanism leaves the thin, friable tissue vulnerable to infection and ulceration. The vagina also loses its rugae and becomes shorter and inelastic. Postmenopausal women may complain of symptoms caused by vaginal dryness, such as pain during intercourse, vaginal discharge, burning, itching, or bleeding. Genitourinary atrophy leads to a variety of symptoms that affect the ease and quality of living.

Urethritis with dysuria, stress urinary incontinence, urinary frequency, and dyspareunia are further results of mucosal thinning of the urethra and bladder. Intravaginal estrogen treatment can effectively alleviate recurrent urinary tract infections and vaginal symptoms in the postmenopausal patient.[356]

Postmenopausal Osteoporosis

Osteoporosis is a disorder characterized by low bone mass and microarchitectural deterioration of bone tissue, leading to enhanced bone fragility and a consequent increase in fracture risk. The standard criterion for defining and diagnosing osteoporosis and applying the ICD-9 code 733.0 is the finding of a T-score of −2.5 or lower at the lumbar spine, femur neck, or total hip by bone mineral density (BMD) testing.[357] Osteoporosis is a public health concern that is associated with over 2 million fractures per year in the United States.[357] The most frequent sites of fracture are the vertebral bodies, distal radius, and femoral neck. Most osteoporotic patients are postmenopausal women.

Osteoporosis in postmenopausal women is a function of advancing age and estrogen deficiency. Seventy-five percent or more of the bone loss in women during the first 15 years after menopause is attributed to estrogen deficiency rather than to aging.[358,359] For the first 20 years after the cessation of ovarian estrogen secretion, postmenopausal osteoporosis accounts for a 50% reduction in trabecular bone and 30% loss of cortical bone.[358,359] Vertebral bone is especially vulnerable because the trabecular portion of the vertebral bodies is metabolically very active and decreases dramatically in amount in response to estrogen deficiency. Vertebral bone mass is already significantly decreased in perimenopausal and early postmenopausal women who have rising FSH and decreasing estrogen levels, whereas bone loss from the radius is not detected until at least 1 year after menopause.[359]

The risk of fracture depends on two factors: the peak bone mass achieved at maturity (at approximately age 30) and the subsequent rate of bone loss. An accelerated rate of bone loss after menopause strongly predicts an increased risk of fracture. The unfavorable effects of low premenopausal bone mass and accelerated loss of bone after menopause are additive, and these individuals are at the highest risk for fracture. An increased rate of average bone loss during menopause is an indicator of lower endogenous estrogen levels, possibly because postmenopausal bone loss is considerably slower in women with increased adipose tissue mass and consequent increased peripheral estrogen formation.[223]

Numerous studies showed that hormone therapy started at perimenopause prevents postmenopausal bone loss.[360] Hormone therapy started at any age in a postmenopausal woman prevents additional bone loss. The Women's Health Initiative (WHI) trial results revealed the most conclusive evidence for a decreased number of vertebral and hip fractures in the group of postmenopausal women receiving estrogen plus progestin (E+P) or estrogen (E) only.[361] The risk reductions were attenuated in both trials after intervention; however, a significant hip fracture benefit persisted over 13 years for women assigned to conjugated equine estrogens (CEEs) plus MPA.[361]

POSTMENOPAUSAL HORMONE THERAPY

A key and complex decision facing postmenopausal women is whether to use menopausal hormone therapy (HT). HT is very effective for managing vasomotor symptoms of the menopause. Postmenopausal women who have undergone a hysterectomy ordinarily receive HT with estrogen only (HT-E). A progestin is added to estrogen (HT-EP) in the postmenopausal woman with a uterus to prevent endometrial hyperplasia and cancer. Although either form of HT was originally prescribed primarily to treat vasomotor symptoms, starting from the 1950s, HT-E and later HT-EP had been increasingly viewed as a way to forestall many chronic diseases of aging, including CVD, cognitive impairment, and osteoporotic fractures. Approximately 40% of postmenopausal women in the United States were using HT shortly before the publication of the initial findings from the WHI.[361,362] A number of observational studies had suggested benefits of HT for CVD including coronary heart disease (CHD) and all-cause mortality, and an overall favorable benefit-risk profile.[363] There had been, however, no large-scale randomized prevention trials to address the balance of risks and benefits of HT. In these observational studies, the apparent benefits of HT may result in part from differences between women who choose to take postmenopausal HT and women who do not; HT users tend to be healthier and have better access to medical care.[364]

Until the late 1990s, the most common practice was to treat all women disturbed by the symptoms of hormone deprivation (e.g., hot flashes) with HT and to use long-term hormonal prophylaxis against osteoporosis. The assumption that HT was cardioprotective played an important role in encouraging postmenopausal women to stay on this regimen indefinitely.[365] This trend changed dramatically in the early 2000s, after publication of the principal results of two large randomized trials, the Heart and Estrogen/Progestin Replacement Study (HERS) in 1998 and the WHI trial in 2002.[366-368] The WHI results constituted the direct cause of discontinuation of HT in approximately 30% of postmenopausal women.[368] Debate continues regarding the applicability of the WHI results to all or various subsets of postmenopausal women.[365] Although the use of HT has dramatically decreased, the WHI trials raised a number of important issues that require further studies to address.[365,369]

The WHI investigators sought to determine the benefits and risks of HT taken for chronic disease prevention in predominantly healthy postmenopausal women aged 50 to 79 years at enrollment.[361,362] The WHI trials elected to include the most popular HT formulations in the United States at that time, which were CEEs (0.625 mg/day) plus MPA (2.5 mg/day) and CEEs (0.625 mg/day) alone.[361,362] Starting from 2002, a large number of original and review articles came from the WHI trials. Most recently, a comprehensive integrated overview of findings from the two WHI HT trials with extended postintervention follow-up for a median of 13 years was published.[361] Here the WHI investigators reported the key outcomes and stratified results by age and by time since menopause onset.[361] A discussion of the WHI trials and how they changed HT practices is provided next.

The Fundamental Findings of the WHI Trials

Results from the WHI and other randomized clinical trials provided a clearer picture regarding the benefits and risks of HT and have provided insights to improve decision making in HT practices.[361,362,365-368] A number of clinical characteristics are useful in identifying postmenopausal women for whom benefits of HT are likely to outweigh the risks.[361] Age and time since menopause are strong predictors of risks of HT.[361] The role of age was particularly prominent in the HT-E (estrogen only, for women without uteri) trial.[361] Younger women (50-59 years) taking HT-E had more favorable results for all-cause mortality, myocardial infarction, and the global index but not for stroke and venous thrombosis.[361] The influence of age was less clear for HT-EP (women with intact uteri, taking estrogen/ progestin), owing to increased risks of breast cancer, stroke, and venous thrombosis in all age groups. Overall, risks of adverse events were lower in younger than in older women among both HT-E and HT-EP users.[361]

The most recent and comprehensive results of the two WHI trials (HT-EP and HT-E) are summarized in Table 17-9, showing intervention-phase findings such as absolute risks per 10,000 women per year, rate differences, and relative risks for a wide range of chronic disease outcomes. Among the HT-EP users, the hazard ratio (HR) for CHD during the intervention phase was 1.18 (95% CI 0.95-1.45), and the risks of invasive breast cancer, stroke,

pulmonary embolism, and the global index increased (see Table 17-9).[361,362] Other risks included an increased rate of dementia (in women ≥65 years), gallbladder disease, and urinary incontinence.[361,362] On the other hand, the benefits included decreased risk of hip fractures, diabetes, and vasomotor symptoms.[361,362] Overall, the risks of HT-EP outweighed the benefits. After the intervention ended, most risks and benefits diminished or disappeared, although some elevation in breast cancer risk persisted (cumulative HR 1.28, 95% CI 1.11-1.48) among the HT-EP users.[361,362] At the time of treatment with HT-E, risks and benefits were more balanced, with an HR for CHD of 0.94 (95% CI 0.78-1.14), significantly elevated risks of stroke and venous thrombosis, significantly decreased risks of hip fractures and diabetes, and over cumulative follow-up, decreased risk of breast cancer (HR 0.79, 95% CI 0.65-0.97; see Nilas and Christiansen[359]).[361,362] Neither HT modality altered the mortality rate. Interestingly, breast cancer findings were divergent between the two trials, and for both cancer and CVD outcomes, results tended to be more adverse for HT-EP than for HT-E.[361,362] There was a clear and sizable benefit for reducing vasomotor symptoms; the results for other quality of life measures, however, varied widely.[361,362]

The age of the woman and time since menopause seemed to be the key modifiers of most of the WHI results.[361,362] In the HT-E trial, younger women 50 to 59 years of age had more favorable results for all-cause

TABLE 17-9
Results of the Women's Health Initiative (WHI) Estrogen-Progestin (E + P) and Estrogen-Alone (EA) Trials During the Intervention Phases[a]

Outcome	E + P Trial (*n* = 16,608)[b]				EA Trial (*n* = 10,739)[c]			
	E + P	Placebo	Difference[d]	RR (95% CI)[d]	EA	Placebo	Difference[d]	RR (95% CI)[d]
Benefits (in Addition to Menopausal Symptom Management)								
Hip fracture	11	17	−6	0.67 (0.47-0.95)	13	19	−6	0.67 (0.46-0.96)
Type 2 diabetes	72	88	−16	0.81 (0.70-0.94)	134	155	−21	0.86 (0.76-0.98)
Risks								
Stroke	33	24	+8	1.37 (1.07-1.76)	45	34	+11	1.35 (1.07-1.70)
Pulmonary embolism	18	9	+9	1.98 (1.36-2.87)	14	10	+4	1.35 (0.89-2.05)
Deep vein thrombosis	25	14	+11	1.87 (1.37-2.54)	23	15	+8	1.48 (1.06-2.07)
Breast cancer[e]	43	35	+8	1.24 (1.01-1.53)	28	35	−7	0.79 (0.61-1.02)
Gallbladder disease	131	84	+47	1.57 (1.36-1.80)	164	106	+58	1.55 (1.34-1.79)
Neutral or Uncertain Risks and Benefits[f]								
Coronary heart disease[g]	41	35	+6	1.18 (0.95-1.45)	55	58	−3	0.94 (0.78-1.14)
Myocardial infarction	35	29	+6	1.24 (0.98-1.56)	44	45	−1	0.97 (0.79-1.21)
Ovarian cancer	5	4	+1	1.41 (0.75-2.66)	—	—	—	Not available
Colorectal cancer	10	17	−7	0.62 (0.43-0.89)	17	15	+2	1.15 (0.81-1.64)
Dementia (age ≥ 65 y)	46	23	+23	2.01 (1.19-3.42)	44	29	+15	1.47 (0.85-2.52)
Total mortality	52	53	−1	0.97 (0.81-1.16)	80	77	+3	1.03 (0.88-1.21)
Global index[f,h]	189	168	+21	1.12 (1.02-1.24)	208	204	+4	1.03 (0.93-1.13)

[a]Benefits and risks (absolute risks per 10,000 women per year, rate differences, and relative risks) of menopausal hormone therapy on chronic disease outcomes in the overall study population of women aged 50-79 years.
[b]The E + P arm of the WHI assessed a median of 5.6 years of conjugated equine estrogens (0.625 mg/day) plus medroxyprogesterone acetate (2.5 mg/day) versus placebo.
[c]The estrogen-alone arm of the WHI assessed a median of 7.2 years of conjugated equine estrogens (0.625 mg/day) versus placebo.
[d]Rate difference is rate in the hormone arm minus rate in the placebo arm.
[e]Divergent results for the two interventions.
[f]Also includes outcomes with divergent results for the two interventions.
[g]Coronary heart disease is defined as nonfatal myocardial infarction or coronary death.
[h]The global index is a composite representing the first event for each participant from among the following: coronary heart disease, stroke, pulmonary embolism, breast cancer, colorectal cancer, endometrial cancer (E + P trial only), hip fracture, and death. Because participants can experience more than one type of event, the global index cannot be derived by a simple summing of the component events.
RR, relative risk; CI, confidence interval.
From Manson JE, Chlebowski RT, Stefanick ML, et al. Menopausal hormone therapy and health outcomes during the intervention and extended poststopping phases of the Women's Health Initiative randomized trials. *JAMA.* 2013;310:1353-1368.
Modified from Manson JE. Current recommendations: what is the clinician to do? *Fertil Steril.* 2014;101:916-921. ©2014 by American Society for Reproductive Medicine.

mortality, myocardial infarction, colorectal cancer, and the global index.[361] Age, however, did not affect increased risks of stroke, venous thrombosis, gallbladder disease, or urinary incontinence associated with both HT regimens. Among HT-EP users, breast cancer was an additional adverse effect. Although risk of myocardial infarction varied by time since menopause, the overall risks of chronic disease events outweighed benefits across all age groups for HT-EP.[361] In general, variations in hazard ratios by age were more apparent among the HT-E users than in the HT-EP users.[361,362] However, risks of unfavorable outcomes were much lower in younger women than in older women in both HT-E and HT-EP trials. Absolute risks measured by the global index per 10,000 women per year on HT-EP varied from 12 excess cases for ages 50 to 59 years to 38 excess cases for ages 70 to 79 years and, for HT-E, from 19 fewer cases for ages 50 to 59 years to 51 excess cases for the 70- to 79-year-old age group.[362] Overall, findings from both WHI trials suggest that HT has a harmful effect on CHD risk in older women and those at higher baseline risk of CVD, whereas the results in younger and low-risk women tend to be neutral for HT-EP and in a favorable direction for HT-E.[362] HT use had a negative impact on cognitive function among women older than 65 years, whereas HT effect was neutral for women younger than 55 years of age.[362,370]

Risks and Contraindications of Hormone Therapy

Coronary Heart Disease

Data suggest that initiation of HT many years after menopause is associated with excess CHD risk, whereas HT given for a limited period soon after menopause is not. HT-EP or HT-E does not prevent CHD as was previously proposed. To the contrary, there may be a small but significant increase in the rate of CHD among HT-EP users; these women with preexisting CHD and healthy women are at risk.[361,371] HT-E, on the other hand, does not increase the risk for CHD in healthy women.[361]

Stroke

Another outcome that was consistent across the two WHI trials and HERS is the increased risk of stroke among women assigned to HT-E or HT-EP. Increased stroke risk may be attributable to the estrogen component of the hormone regimen because its increase is statistically significant among both HT-E and HT-EP users.[361,362,371]

Pulmonary Embolism

A pattern of increased pulmonary embolism was observed in all randomized studies, although the risk was attenuated and was not statistically significant in the WHI HT-E trial.[361,362,371]

Breast Cancer

Findings of the WHI HT-E trial were markedly different from those of the HERS and WHI HT-EP trials with respect to breast cancer risk.[362] The WHI HT-E trial indicated a trend, albeit statistically not significant, toward a lower breast cancer risk during the intervention phase. This protective effect was statistically significant during cumulative (intervention plus postintervention) follow-up (HR 0.79, CI 0.65-0.97).[361] This result was in contrast to findings of an observational literature that mostly reports a moderate increase in risk with estrogen-alone preparations.[372] However, after control for prior use of postmenopausal HT

and additional control for time from menopause to first use of postmenopausal HT, the hazard ratios agreed closely between the observational and randomized trial data.[372] Nonetheless, the higher risk for breast cancer observed in the HT-EP trials probably represents a harmful additional effect of MPA, the progestin used in these studies.[361] The increased breast cancer risk was statistically significant in the WHI HT-EP trial, which demonstrated an attributable risk of 9 cases per 10,000 person-years during the 5.6-year intervention phase.[361] This risk persisted and remained significant during the postintervention phase, giving rise to an overall risk of 9 cases per 10,000 person-years during the 13 years of cumulative follow-up.[361] This result was matched by a trend of the same magnitude in the HERS study and was supported by evidence from large observational studies suggesting that the addition of MPA or another progestin to estrogen may significantly increase the risk for breast cancer (see Table 17-9).[373]

Ovarian Cancer

A retrospective 1979-1998 cohort study of 44,241 postmenopausal women revealed that HT-E, particularly when taken for 10 or more years, significantly increases the risk of ovarian cancer. The relative risks for 10 to 19 years and for 20 or more years were 1.8 (95% CI, 1.1 to 3.0) and 3.2 (95% CI, 1.7 to 5.7), respectively (p value for trend < 0.001). This study did not show an increased risk among women who used short-term HT-EP, but the investigators suggested that the risk associated with longer-term HT-EP use warrants further investigation.[374] The WHI HT-E data for ovarian cancer risk were not reported because of small numbers.[361] The WHI HT-EP trial found a trend for slightly increased ovarian cancer risk that was not significant.[361]

Dementia

In postmenopausal women 65 years of age or older, HT-EP significantly increased risk and resulted in an additional 23 cases of probable dementia per 10,000 women per year.[375] Alzheimer disease was the most common classification of dementia. A similar trend was observed for HT-E but did not reach statistical significance.[375] When the data were pooled, HT significantly increased probable dementia risk.[375]

Hyperlipidemia

Hyperlipidemia is a rare side effect observed in patients with severe familial hypertriglyceridemia. An oral estrogen regimen can hasten development of severe hypertriglyceridemia or pancreatitis in women with severely elevated triglyceride levels.[376] Estrogen replacement is relatively contraindicated in women with substantially increased triglyceride levels.

Gallbladder Disease

Both WHI trials (HT-E and HT-EP) showed substantially greater risk for any gallbladder disease or surgery with estrogen.[377] Both trials indicated a higher risk for cholecystitis and for cholelithiasis. Women on either HT regimen were more likely to undergo cholecystectomy.[361,362] These data suggest an increase in risk of biliary tract disease among postmenopausal women using estrogen therapy. The morbidity and cost associated with these outcomes may need to be considered in decisions regarding the use of estrogen therapy. Preexisting gallbladder disease is a relative contraindication for estrogen replacement.

Indications for Hormone Therapy

Hot Flashes

HT-E or HT-EP reliably treats hot flashes in most women.[378] Currently, hot flashes constitute the most common indication for a short course of HT (<5 years).

Fractures

HT-EP or HT-E significantly decreased the incidence of hip, vertebral, and other osteoporotic fractures.[361] In this case, the results of observational studies of estrogen and fracture risk and of trials using a surrogate end point (i.e., BMD) agree with the results of clinical trials of fracture prevention.

Colon Cancer

Colon cancer was significantly less common with HT-EP in the WHI study but not with HT-E, for reasons that are not clear.[361,362] It is possible that progestin is the protective hormone in this case.

Post-WHI Recommendations for Hormone Therapy

A number of publications with flow charts are available to clinicians for decision making about HT use.[362] Here, a number of useful principles are offered to guide the clinician and the patient for an optimal plan that suits her short-term and long-term needs and expectations. Decision making for women interested in HT involves balancing the potential benefits of HT against the potential risks.[362,379] HT is extremely effective for treatment of hot flashes, and for this indication women with intact uteri should receive HT-EP, whereas women without uteri should be prescribed HT-E because the only known benefit of adding a progestin is to prevent endometrial cancer. HT-E seems to be associated with less risk than HT-EP.[378] Nonetheless, HT-E also has adverse effects, and it is prudent to keep the dose low and the duration of treatment short for all HT regimens.[378]

Many clinicians and epidemiologists agree that short-term estrogen therapy using the lowest effective estrogen dose is a reasonable option for recently menopausal women who have moderate to severe symptoms and no previous history or elevated risk of CHD, stroke, breast cancer, or venous thromboembolism.[362,379] HT usually lasts for 2 to 3 years but rarely more than 5 years, because menopausal symptoms diminish after several years, whereas the risk of breast cancer increases with longer duration of HT.[378]

A small group of women may need long-term therapy for severe, persistent symptoms after stopping HT. These few women may be encouraged to first try nonhormonal options such as selective serotonin reuptake inhibitors (SSRIs); estrogen treatment should be resumed only if these alternatives are not helpful.[378] For isolated symptoms of genitourinary atrophy, low-dose vaginal estrogens with minimal systemic absorption and endometrial effects are highly beneficial.[379]

In the absence of evidence for an overall net benefit of postmenopausal treatment with HT-E and with the evidence that HT-EP is harmful, neither therapy should be used for preventing CHD or improving mental function.

Target Groups for Hormone Therapy

In women with gonadal dysgenesis and surgical menopause, the duration of estrogen deprivation is prolonged. Estrogen replacement is recommended for these patients for reduction of hot flashes and for long-term prophylaxis against osteoporosis and target organ atrophy. A low-dose contraceptive may be offered to nonsmoking women until the age of 45 years. After that point, doses of estrogen equivalent to 0.625 mg of conjugated equine estrogens may be more appropriate because of a sharp age-related increase in risk for thromboembolic events. The physician should recommend a continuous estrogen-progestin combination to those women with a uterus and an estrogen-only regimen to women without a uterus.

During perimenopause, hot flashes can be suppressed with an estrogen-progestin combination. Because bone loss related to estrogen deprivation also begins during this period, a benefit for women who take HT to prevent hot flashes is that bone loss will not start for the few years of therapy.[380] In perimenopausal women, unexplained uterine bleeding should be evaluated with an endometrial biopsy before the start of HT.

Estrogen Preparations and Beneficial Dose of Estrogen

Oral Estrogens: Combined Conjugated Equine Estrogens

The amount of estrogen that provides effective treatment for hot flashes varies. For this purpose, it is reasonable to start with CEEs at 0.3 mg/day (or micronized estradiol at 0.5 mg/day) and gradually increase this dose to CEEs at 0.625 mg/day (equivalent to micronized estradiol at 1 mg/day) and 1.25 mg/day (equivalent to micronized estradiol at 2 mg/day). If hot flashes in a postmenopausal woman are not alleviated by 1.25 mg/day of CEEs or an equivalent transdermal estradiol dose, it is unlikely that higher doses will be effective. In this case, alternative diagnoses (e.g., tuberculosis, depression, thyroid disease) should be ruled out.

Low-dose estrogen (0.3 mg/day of CEEs or 0.5 mg/day of micronized estradiol) maintains blood estradiol levels between 17 to 32 pg/mL (average, 22 pg/mL) and may be sufficient for preserving bone density and for alleviating menopausal symptoms in early postmenopausal women.[381] Osteoporosis and fracture risk should be assessed via periodic DXA (dual-energy x-ray absorptiometry) scans, especially because low-dose estrogen preparations may not prevent bone loss. The effect of estrogen on arterial thrombosis is probably dose related.[381] For example, oral contraceptives with higher doses of estrogen are more likely to be associated with increased risks of myocardial infarction and stroke, especially in smokers. When choosing a dose for HT, it is imperative to achieve and maintain the lowest beneficial levels of circulating estradiol and to avoid higher levels in order to minimize the risk of thrombosis.

The addition of a progestin, either cyclically or continuously, to concomitant estrogen replacement reduces the risk of estrogen-induced endometrial hyperplasia or carcinoma but poses additional problems,[382] which include regular withdrawal bleeding in up to 90% of women treated with cyclic therapy and irregular spotting in 20% of women treated with continuous estrogen plus progestin. Progestins appear to reduce the beneficial effects of estrogen on high-density lipoprotein (HDL) and LDL cholesterol and to increase the risks of pulmonary embolism, CHD, and breast cancer.[361,362,371]

A time-honored sequential regimen involves oral administration of 0.625 mg of CEEs or the equivalent dose of a variety of available products on days 1 through 25 of each month (Fig. 17-36). A daily dose of 5 mg of MPA is added on days 12 through 25 or on days 16 through 25.

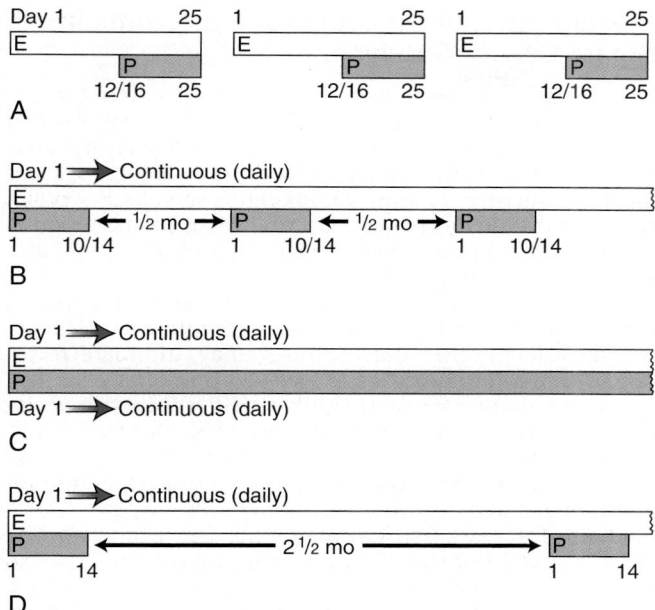

Figure 17-36 Regimens of hormone therapy. Estrogen (E) is replaced in a post-menopausal woman to prevent osteoporosis, urogenital atrophy, and hot flashes. In the postmenopausal woman with a uterus, a progestin (P) should be added to estrogen to prevent endometrial hyperplasia and cancer. E and P can be administered in several ways. **A** and **B**, Postmenopausal women receiving hormone therapy have predictable withdrawal bleeding episodes after each P course. **C**, E and P are administered together. After a year of continuous combination therapy, the rate of unpredictable breakthrough spotting is 20%. **D**, This relatively new regimen was introduced to minimize the harmful effects of a progestin. Its long-term safety for endometrial hyperplasia or cancer risk is unknown. Predictable bleeding after each P course every 3 months is presumed to be reassuring.

Withdrawal bleeding is expected on or after day 26 of each month. Another common cyclic regimen involves continuous oral administration of 0.625 mg of CEEs or the equivalent daily dose (see Fig. 17-36). A daily dose of 5 mg of MPA is added for the first 10 to 14 days of every month. One-year randomized trial data indicate that the 5-mg dose protects the endometrium as well as the 10-mg dose does.[383] Progestin withdrawal bleeding occurs in 90% of women with a sequential or cyclic regimen.[384,385] These regimens can also cause adverse symptoms related to the relatively high daily doses of progestin, including breast tenderness, bloating, fluid retention, and depression. The lowest possible dose of a progestin is recommended.

The continuous combined method of treatment has the potential benefit of reduced bleeding and amenorrhea, but it is occasionally complicated by breakthrough bleeding (see Fig. 17-36).[384,385] In this regimen, a combination of 0.625 mg of CEEs and 2.5 mg of MPA is given orally every day. The continuous combination regimen is simple and convenient, and it is associated with an incidence of amenorrhea in 80% of patients after at least 6 months of use. The other 20% of patients continue to experience some degree of unpredictable spotting. Overall compliance is much better in users of the continuous combination regimen. Moreover, the lower daily dose of MPA is associated with a lower incidence of breast tenderness with this regimen. Other estrogen-progestin combinations are also available for similar continuous use.

Cyclic progestin has also been used at less frequent intervals, such as every 3 to 6 months. When added to

standard-dosage estrogen, 10 mg of MPA every 3 months for 14 days produced a 1.5% rate of hyperplasia (a rate low enough to be interpreted as endometrial protection), and long-term use of MPA at 6-month intervals was associated with a low rate of endometrial cancer.[386,387] However, clinicians have not determined the optimal progestin dosage and schedule to use with low-dosage estrogen. Low-dosage estrogen use can reasonably be assumed to require less progestin for protection of the endometrium.

Most postmenopausal women can switch their HT regimen from standard-dosage HT to low-dosage estrogen opposed by MPA at 3-month intervals or start HT at this low dose.[381] Although its long-term safety has not been proved with respect to endometrial hyperplasia, the following regimen appears to be a reasonable compromise for treating hot flashes and preventing osteoporosis while minimizing the harmful effects of progestins and high-dose estrogen[381]: 0.3 mg/day of CEEs or 0.025 mg of transdermal estradiol is administered continuously. Every 3 months, a 14-day course of 5 mg of MPA is added (see Fig. 17-36D). Endometrial biopsy is not required in the presence of withdrawal bleeding after each periodic progestin intake and in the absence of irregular bleeding. This regimen may be continued for up to 5 years. After discontinuation of HT, the postmenopausal woman can be switched to a bisphosphonate or a selective estrogen receptor modulator (SERM) for bone protection if needed.

Transdermal Estrogen

Transdermal estrogen preparations appear to be as effective as oral estrogens for treating hot flashes and maintaining BMD, but they have different metabolic profiles. Oral estrogens are easier to administer and seem to have favorable effects on lipoprotein profiles. However, oral estrogens are associated with several disadvantages, including unfavorable changes in serum levels of triglycerides, C-reactive protein, fibrinogen, factor VII, and plasminogen activator inhibitor type 1.[379] A meta-analysis of clinical trials suggested a higher risk of venous thromboembolic events among oral HT users compared with transdermal estrogen users.[379] Clinical trial data that address the effect of transdermal estrogen on CHD and stroke risk are limited.[379]

A daily dose of 0.05 mg of transdermal estradiol is equivalent to 0.625 mg of oral CEEs or 1 mg of oral micronized estradiol. A lower-dose transdermal preparation includes 0.025 mg of estradiol (equivalent to 0.3 mg of oral CEEs). An ultralow-dose transdermal estradiol preparation (0.014 mg) is also available. In women with symptoms not responding to smaller doses, high-dose transdermal estradiol at 0.1 mg/day (equivalent to CEEs at 1.25 mg/day) may be used. For the average menopausal woman with hot flashes, it is reasonable to start with a daily dose of 0.025 mg, which should be accompanied by a progestin in a woman with a uterus.

Vaginal Estrogen

Vaginal estrogen formulations are the first choice for the initial management of menopause-related vaginal atrophy symptoms. Low-dose vaginal tablets, rings, and creams administered via the vagina are equally effective when used for relief of vulvovaginal symptoms. A usual starting dose is 0.625 mg CEEs (in 1 g cream) applied vaginally daily for 1 week; the following maintenance dose is twice weekly. A 12-week study designed to elucidate the lowest effective dose of estradiol cream for relieving vaginal symptoms reported that 100% of women responded to the lowest dose tested (10 μg daily). Circulating estradiol levels remained in the postmenopausal range (3-10 pg/mL, 13.6-36.7 pmol/L) using a highly sensitive assay, and improvements in vaginal cytologic features and decreases in vaginal pH were significant. No endometrial hyperplasia was noted during the course of the study.[388]

Management of Breakthrough Bleeding During Postmenopausal Hormone Therapy

Approximately 90% of women receiving estrogen plus cyclic administration of a progestin have monthly progestin withdrawal bleeding in a predictable fashion. Continuous combined estrogen-progestin therapy causes breakthrough bleeding in approximately 40% of women during the first 6 months, with the remaining 60% being amenorrheic. The pattern of vaginal bleeding in women taking the continuous combined regimen is unpredictable and causes anxiety in most patients, but the incidence of breakthrough bleeding decreases to 20% after 1 year of treatment.[384,385,389] Nevertheless, breakthrough bleeding remains the most important reason for discontinuance of this therapy. Most patients find it unacceptable and prefer to switch to a cyclic progestin regimen or to discontinue HT altogether. There is no effective pharmacologic method to manage the breakthrough bleeding associated with continuous combined estrogen-progestin regimens. The physician can only reassure the patient that the bleeding is likely to subside within 1 year from the start of HT. If breakthrough bleeding continues beyond 1 year, the regimen should be changed to daily estrogen plus cyclic progestin.

HT can be started in the amenorrheic postmenopausal patient at any time. Perimenopausal women with oligomenorrhea, hot flashes, or other associated symptoms can also be treated with HT. In the oligomenorrheic patient, an HT regimen may be initiated on day 3 of one of the infrequent menses. If the candidate for HT does not have irregular uterine bleeding, it is not essential to perform endometrial biopsies routinely before beginning treatment. Studies indicate that asymptomatic postmenopausal women rarely have endometrial abnormalities.[334,389,390] Pretreatment biopsies using a thin plastic biopsy cannula in the office may be limited to patients who are at higher risk for endometrial hyperplasia (e.g., unpredictable uterine bleeding, history of PCOS or chronic anovulation, obesity, liver disease, diabetes mellitus).

Prescribing a combined estrogen-progestin regimen does not preclude the development of endometrial cancer.[391] Therefore, it is necessary to rule out endometrial malignancy in women receiving HT who are experiencing irregular uterine bleeding. The important task is to differentiate breakthrough bleeding from bleeding induced by hyperplasia or cancer. Because breakthrough bleeding is extremely common, many biopsies must be performed to detect a rare case of endometrial abnormality during HT. To decrease the number of endometrial biopsies, a screening method using transvaginal ultrasonography has been introduced.[131] The thickness of the postmenopausal endometrium as measured by transvaginal ultrasonography in postmenopausal women correlates with the presence or absence of pathologic changes.[131] Patients receiving a cyclic or daily combination HT regimen who have an endometrial thickness of less than 5 mm can be managed conservatively.[392-394] An endometrial thickness equal to or greater than 5 mm requires biopsy. Based on this algorithm, it is estimated that 50% to 75% of bleeding patients receiving HT and evaluated by ultrasonography require biopsy.[131]

Management of Menopausal Symptoms in Breast Cancer Survivors

Vasomotor symptoms constitute a major problem for survivors of breast cancer. Approximately 65% of women become symptomatic with hot flashes (mostly severe) after treatment for breast cancer.[395] Hot flashes are encountered more frequently among tamoxifen users and women treated with chemotherapy. Up to 90% of premenopausal women who receive chemotherapy and tamoxifen have vasomotor symptoms.[395]

Breast cancer survivors often seek relief from hot flashes. HT is typically withheld from women with breast cancer because of concerns that estrogen may stimulate recurrence. One randomized study showed that after extended follow-up, there was a statistically significant increased risk of a new breast cancer event in survivors who took HT.[396] In this randomized, non–placebo-controlled study, 442 women assigned to receive HT-EP/HT-E or best symptomatic management without hormones were followed for a median of 4 years. Thirty-nine of the 221 women in the HT arm and 17 of the 221 women in the control arm had a new breast cancer diagnosed (hazard ratio, 2.4; 95% CI, 1.3 to 4.2). Cumulative breast cancer incidences at 5 years were 22.2% in the HT arm and 8.0% in the control arm. No difference in mortality rate from breast cancer was found.[396]

Because of higher breast cancer recurrence associated with HT, many breast cancer survivors have sought nonhormonal alternatives, including other pharmaceutical agents, herbal or dietary remedies, and mind-body or behavioral therapies.[395] Mind-body or behavioral treatments for hot flashes are particularly attractive to survivors of breast cancer because they do not have the side effects caused by pharmaceutical agents, but it is not yet known whether they are effective.[378,395]

Several nonhormonal pharmaceutical agents have been used off-label for women who cannot take or elect not to take HT. Among the non-HT treatments, SSRIs, serotonin-norepinephrine reuptake inhibitors (SNRIs), clonidine, and gabapentin were found to be more effective than placebo.[379] Although all of these nonsteroidal medications could reduce the number of hot flashes per day, their beneficial effects were far less than what has been observed with estrogen, and these drugs are all associated with significant side effects that can limit their use in some women. Extracts of black cohosh or red clover were found to be ineffective, and the results for soy isoflavone extracts were mixed.[379] The beneficial doses for hot flashes include paroxetine (an SSRI) at 10 to 20 mg/day, paroxetine controlled release at 12.5 to 25 mg/day, venlafaxine (an SNRI) at 75 mg/day, desvenlafaxine (an SNRI) at 100 mg/day, and gabapentin at 900 mg/day.[378] Gabapentin should be started with a smaller dose given at bedtime, and the dose should be gradually increased. Paroxetine reduces the metabolism of tamoxifen to its most active metabolite, endoxifen, and should be avoided in women with breast cancer who are receiving tamoxifen.[379]

For long-term prophylaxis against osteoporosis in breast cancer survivors, tamoxifen, raloxifene, or a bisphosphonate are viable options. However, tamoxifen and raloxifene intensify hot flashes.

Selective Estrogen Receptor Modulators and Bisphosphonates for Osteoporosis Prevention

Postmenopausal women who are at risk for osteoporosis should be screened at least once for osteoporosis by DXA scan. Based on the initial results and other risk factors,

DXA should be repeated periodically, preferably annually or every other year, to monitor the effectiveness of osteoporosis treatment and prevention.[397]

SERMs are compounds that act like estrogen in some target tissues but antagonize estrogenic effects in others (see Chapter 29).[398] One of the first SERMs was tamoxifen, for which estrogen-like agonist activity on bone was observed to occur simultaneously with estrogen antagonist activity on the breast.[398] Tamoxifen had been approved initially for treatment and prevention of breast cancer. An unwanted effect of tamoxifen is its estrogen-like action on the endometrium. Second-generation compounds have since been developed, most notably raloxifene, which has estrogen-like actions on bone, lipids, and the coagulation system; estrogen antagonist effects on the breast; and no detectable action in the endometrium.[399] In 2007, the FDA approved raloxifene for reducing the risk of invasive breast cancer in postmenopausal women with osteoporosis and in postmenopausal women who are at high risk for invasive breast cancer. Raloxifene is most often used to prevent and treat osteoporosis in postmenopausal women.

In placebo-controlled trials, raloxifene reduced vertebral fractures, whereas tamoxifen reduced nonvertebral fractures.[399] Tamoxifen and raloxifene had similar effects on fractures at multiple sites in a randomized, head-to-head trial.[399] Neither drug has been shown to prevent hip fractures, however. Tamoxifen or raloxifene reduced risk for invasive breast cancer compared with placebo by approximately 7 to 10 cases per 1000 women per year.[399] Tamoxifen and raloxifene reduced ER-positive breast cancer but not ER-negative breast cancer, noninvasive breast cancer, or mortality rate.[399] Tamoxifen and raloxifene increase thromboembolic events by 4 to 7 cases per 1000 women per year; raloxifene causes fewer events than tamoxifen. Tamoxifen increases risk for endometrial cancer compared with placebo by 4 cases per 1000 women per year and causes cataracts.[399] Raloxifene use is not associated with endometrial cancer or cataract risk.[399] The most common side effects for tamoxifen are hot flashes and other vasomotor symptoms and vaginal discharge, itching, or dryness. For raloxifene, vasomotor symptoms and leg cramps are most common. In a head-to-head trial, raloxifene users reported more musculoskeletal problems, dyspareunia, and weight gain, whereas tamoxifen users had more gynecologic problems, vasomotor symptoms, and bladder control symptoms.[399] Tamoxifen and raloxifene may be used to reduce the incidence of vertebral fractures and invasive breast cancer in postmenopausal women. The major drawbacks include hot flashes and increased thromboembolic events for both drugs and endometrial cancer for tamoxifen.

SERMs are effective for managing certain aspects of estrogen deficiency in postmenopausal women, but recent data suggest that pairing a SERM with estrogens may provide a more optimal therapeutic profile for women with a uterus. The drug combination bazedoxifene/CEE is a medication approved by the FDA in 2013 for the treatment of menopause symptoms and postmenopausal osteoporosis. It is a fixed-dose combination drug containing the SERM bazedoxifene and CEE.[400] This new agent demonstrated efficacy in postmenopausal women with a uterus, while allowing these women to avoid progestins and their possible adverse effects.[400]

The major treatment goal in postmenopausal osteoporosis is to prevent fractures by maintaining or increasing BMD and reducing excessive bone turnover.[401] Bisphosphonates suppress resorption by inhibiting the attachment of osteoclasts to bone matrix and enhancing programmed

cell death in osteoclasts. They have increased BMD and reduced the risk for osteoporotic fractures in numerous clinical trials.[401] The FDA has approved a number of bisphosphonates for treatment. Oral alendronate and oral risedronate were approved in 1995 and 2000, respectively. In 2003, oral ibandronate was approved, followed by intravenous ibandronate in 2006. Intravenous zoledronic acid was approved in 2007. A 5-mg dose of zoledronic acid is infused over 15 minutes once each year. Alendronate is given as a once-weekly 35- or 70-mg tablet or a once-daily 5- or 10-mg tablet; risedronate is given as a once-daily 5-mg tablet, a once-weekly 35-mg tablet, or a once-monthly 150-mg tablet, and ibandronate is given as a once-monthly 150-mg tablet or as 3 mg intravenously every 3 months.[402]

Compared with placebo control subjects, all approved bisphosphonates reduce the relative risk of new vertebral fractures by on average 50% in women with postmenopausal osteoporosis.[402,403] Alendronate, risedronate, and zoledronic acid reduce the relative risk of new nonvertebral and hip fractures.[401] Clinical trial extensions of up to 10 years with alendronate and 7 years with risedronate have shown that efficacy is maintained during long-term treatment.[401] Moreover, discontinuation of long-term (≥5 years) alendronate therapy results in minimal bone loss over the ensuing 3 to 5 years.[404] As in the case of SERMs, definitive data are lacking on optimal doses, duration, timing, long-term effects, and effects in nonwhite women. Once-yearly zoledronic acid infusions appear to be an attractive choice because of better compliance and lack of esophagitis, a side effect associated with oral bisphosphonates.

Osteonecrosis of the jaw is a rare but serious side effect of bisphosphonate therapies. Bisphosphonate users who plan to undergo tooth extraction should discuss this side effect to their dental surgeons, because tooth extraction may predispose them to osteonecrosis of the jaw.[405] In premenopausal patients with estrogen-responsive early breast cancer, the addition of zoledronic acid to adjuvant endocrine therapy reduced disease recurrence in all body sites and improved disease-free survival.[406] Further studies are required to explore the potential of bisphosphonates in preventing breast cancer in postmenopausal women with no previous history of breast cancer.

A number of case reports and a recent retrospective study suggested that the risk of esophageal cancer increased with oral bisphosphonate use over about a 5-year period. In Western countries, the incidence of esophageal cancer in patients over the age of 60 is estimated to increase from 1 to 2 per 1000 population with 5 years' use of an oral bisphosphonate.[407,408] Another retrospective study, however, did not find such a link.[409] Until more accurate data are available, health care providers should avoid prescribing oral bisphosphonates to patients with Barrett esophagus, a known risk factor for esophageal cancer.[407]

Tibolone for Osteoporosis Prevention

Tibolone, a synthetic steroid with estrogenic, androgenic, and progestagenic properties, is approved in many countries for treatment of menopausal symptoms and prevention of osteoporosis. Tibolone preserves BMD, reduces hot flashes, and may increase libido and vaginal lubrication in postmenopausal women.[410] A randomized study showed that tibolone reduced the risks of fracture and breast cancer and possibly colon cancer but increased the risk of stroke in older women with osteoporosis.[410] Tibolone should not be used in breast cancer survivors, as it increases breast cancer recurrence.[411] Tibolone is not available in the United States.

REFERENCES

1. Cheng CK, Leung PC. Molecular biology of gonadotropin-releasing hormone (GnRH)-I, GnRH-II, and their receptors in humans. *Endocr Rev.* 2005;26:283-306.
2. Seeburg PH, Mason AJ, Stewart TA, Nikolics K. The mammalian GnRH gene and its pivotal role in reproduction. *Recent Prog Horm Res.* 1987;43:69-98.
3. Nikolics K, Mason AJ, Szonyi E, et al. A prolactin-inhibiting factor within the precursor for human gonadotropin-releasing hormone. *Nature.* 1985;316:511-517.
4. Ackland J, Nikolics K, Seeburg P, et al. Molecular forms of gonadotropin-releasing hormone associated peptide (GAP): changes within the rat hypothalamus and release from hypothalamic cells in vitro. *Neuroendocrinology.* 1988;48:376-386.
5. Kim HG, Bhagavath B, Layman LC. Clinical manifestations of impaired GnRH neuron development and function. *Neurosignals.* 2008;16:165-182.
6. Costa-Barbosa FA, Balasubramanian R, Keefe KW, et al. Prioritizing genetic testing in patients with Kallmann syndrome using clinical phenotypes. *J Clin Endocrinol Metab.* 2013;98:E943-E953.
7. Knobil E. The neuroendocrine control of the menstrual cycle. *Recent Prog Horm Res.* 1980;36:53-88.
8. Van Vugt DA, Diefenbach WD, Alston E, Ferin M. Gonadotropin-releasing hormone pulses in third ventricular cerebrospinal fluid of ovariectomized rhesus monkeys: correlation with luteinizing hormone pulses. *Endocrinology.* 1985;117:1550-1558.
9. Gross KM, Matsumoto AM, Southworth MB, Bremner WJ. Evidence for decreased luteinizing hormone-releasing hormone pulse frequency in men with selective elevations of follicle-stimulating hormone. *J Clin Endocrinol Metab.* 1985;60:197-202.
10. Haisenleder DJ, Dalkin AC, Ortolano GA, et al. A pulsatile gonadotropin-releasing hormone stimulus is required to increase transcription of the gonadotropin subunit genes: evidence for differential regulation of transcription by pulse frequency in vivo. *Endocrinology.* 1991;128:509-517.
11. Reame N, Sauder S, Case G, et al. Pulsatile gonadotropin secretion in women with hypothalamic amenorrhea: evidence that reduced frequency of gonadotropin secretion is the mechanism of persistent anovulation. *J Clin Endocrinol Metab.* 1985;61:851-858.
12. Goodman RL, Parfitt DB, Evans NP, et al. Endogenous opioid peptides control the amplitude and shape of gonadotropin-releasing hormone pulses in the ewe. *Endocrinology.* 1995;136:2412-2420.
13. Herbison AE. Noradrenergic regulation of cyclic GnRH secretion. *Rev Reprod.* 1997;2:1-6.
14. Gindoff PR, Ferin M. Endogenous opioid peptides modulate the effect of corticotropin-releasing factor on gonadotropin release in the primate. *Endocrinology.* 1987;121:837-842.
15. Rabinovici J, Rothman P, Monroe S, et al. Endocrine effects and pharmacokinetic characteristics of a potent new gonadotropin-releasing hormone antagonist (Ganirelix) with minimal histamine-releasing properties: studies in postmenopausal women. *J Clin Endocrinol Metab.* 1992;75:1220-1225.
16. Wildt L, Leyendecker G, Sir-Petermann T, Waibel-Treber S. Treatment with naltrexone in hypothalamic ovarian failure: induction of ovulation and pregnancy. *Hum Reprod.* 1993;8:350-358.
17. Petersen SL, Ottem EN, Carpenter CD. Direct and indirect regulation of gonadotropin-releasing hormone neurons by estradiol. *Biol Reprod.* 2003;69:1771-1778.
18. Yilmaz MB, Wolfe A, Cheng YH, et al. Aromatase promoter I.f is regulated by estrogen receptor alpha (ESR1) in mouse hypothalamic neuronal cell lines. *Biol Reprod.* 2009;81:956-965.
19. Casper RF. Aromatase inhibitors in ovarian stimulation. *J Steroid Biochem Mol Biol.* 2007;106:71-75.
20. Seminara SB, Messager S, Chatzidaki EE, et al. The GPR54 gene as a regulator of puberty. *N Engl J Med.* 2003;349:1614-1627.
21. de Roux N, Genin E, Carel JC, et al. Hypogonadotropic hypogonadism due to loss of function of the KiSS1-derived peptide receptor GPR54. *Proc Natl Acad Sci U S A.* 2003;100:10972-10976.
22. Colledge WH. Kisspeptins and GnRH neuronal signalling. *Trends Endocrinol Metab.* 2009;20:115-121.
23. Popa SM, Clifton DK, Steiner RA. The role of kisspeptins and GPR54 in the neuroendocrine regulation of reproduction. *Annu Rev Physiol.* 2008;70:213-238.
24. Handelsman DJ, Swerdloff RS. Pharmacokinetics of gonadotropin-releasing hormone and its analogs. *Endocr Rev.* 1986;7:95-105.
25. Karten MJ, Rivier JE. Gonadotropin-releasing hormone analog design. Structure-function studies toward the development of agonists and antagonists: rationale and perspective. *Endocr Rev.* 1986;7:44-66.
26. Lemay A, Maheux R, Faure N, et al. Reversible hypogonadism induced by a luteinizing hormone-releasing hormone (LH-RH) agonist (buserelin) as a new therapeutic approach for endometriosis. *Fertil Steril.* 1984;41:863-871.
27. Carr BR, Breslau NA, Givens C, et al. Oral contraceptive pills, gonadotropin-releasing hormone agonists, or use in combination for treatment of hirsutism: a clinical research center study. *J Clin Endocrinol Metab.* 1995;80:1169-1178.
28. Cann C, Martin M, Genant H, Jaffe R. Decreased spinal mineral content in amenorrheic women. *JAMA.* 1984;251:626-629.
29. Matta WH, Shaw RW, Hesp R, Evans R. Reversible trabecular bone density loss following induced hypo-oestrogenism with the GnRH analogue buserelin in premenopausal women. *Clin Endocrinol (Oxf).* 1988;29:45-51.
30. Surrey E. Add-back therapy and gonadotropin-releasing hormone agonists in the treatment of patients with endometriosis: can a consensus be reached? Add-Back Consensus Working Group. *Fertil Steril.* 1999;71:420-424.
31. Pavlou S, Debold C, Island D, et al. Single subcutaneous doses of a luteinizing hormone-releasing hormone antagonist suppress serum gonadotropin and testosterone levels in normal men. *J Clin Endocrinol Metab.* 1986;63:303-308.
32. Pavlou SN, Wakefield G, Schlechter NL, et al. Mode of suppression of pituitary and gonadal function after acute or prolonged administration of a luteinizing hormone-releasing hormone antagonist in normal men. *J Clin Endocrinol Metab.* 1989;68:446-454.
33. Edelstein MC, Gordon K, Williams RF, et al. Single dose long-term suppression of testosterone secretion by a gonadotropin-releasing hormone antagonist (Antide) in male monkeys. *Contraception.* 1990;42:209-214.
34. Behre HM, Kliesch S, Puhse G, et al. High loading and low maintenance doses of a gonadotropin-releasing hormone antagonist effectively suppress serum luteinizing hormone, follicle-stimulating hormone, and testosterone in normal men. *J Clin Endocrinol Metab.* 1997;82:1403-1408.
35. Al-Inany HG, Youssef MA, Aboulghar M, et al. Gonadotrophin-releasing hormone antagonists for assisted reproductive technology. *Cochrane Database Syst Rev.* 2011;(5):CD001750.
36. Childs GV, Hyde C, Naor Z, Catt K. Heterogeneous luteinizing hormone and follicle-stimulating hormone storage patterns in subtypes of gonadotropes separated by centrifugal elutriation. *Endocrinology.* 1983;113:2120-2128.
37. Childs GV. Functional ultrastructure of gonadotropes: a review. *Curr Top Neuroendocrinol.* 1986;7:49-97.
38. Millar RP, Lu ZL, Pawson AJ, et al. Gonadotropin-releasing hormone receptors. *Endocr Rev.* 2004;25:235-275.
39. Gharib SD, Wierman ME, Shupnik MA, Chin WW. Molecular biology of the pituitary gonadotropins. *Endocr Rev.* 1990;11:177-199.
40. Talmadge K, Vamvakopoulos NC, Fiddes JC. Evolution of the genes for the beta subunits of human chorionic gonadotropin and luteinizing hormone. *Nature.* 1984;307:37-40.
41. Jameson JL, Becker CB, Lindell CM, Habener JF. Human follicle-stimulating hormone beta-subunit gene encodes multiple messenger ribonucleic acids. *Mol Endocrinol.* 1988;2:806-815.
42. Jameson L, Chin WW, Hollenberg AN, et al. The gene encoding the beta-subunit of rat luteinizing hormone. Analysis of gene structure and evolution of nucleotide sequence. *J Biol Chem.* 1984;259:15474-15480.
43. Themmen APN, Huhtaniemi IT. Mutations of gonadotropins and gonadotropin receptors: elucidating the physiology and pathophysiology of pituitary-gonadal function. *Endocr Rev.* 2000;21:551-583.
44. Shupnik M. Gonadotropin gene modulation by steroids and gonadotropin-releasing hormone. *Biol Reprod.* 1996;54:279-286.
45. Edson MA, Nagaraja AK, Matzuk MM. The mammalian ovary from genesis to revelation. *Endocr Rev.* 2009;30:624-712.
46. Abbud RA, Ameduri RK, Rao JS, et al. Chronic hypersecretion of luteinizing hormone in transgenic mice selectively alters responsiveness of the alpha-subunit gene to gonadotropin-releasing hormone and estrogens. *Mol Endocrinol.* 1999;13:1449-1459.
47. Thackray VG, Mellon PL, Coss D. Hormones in synergy: regulation of the pituitary gonadotropin genes. *Mol Cell Endocrinol.* 2009;314:192-203.
48. Bernard DJ, Fortin J, Wang Y, Lamba P. Mechanisms of FSH synthesis: what we know, what we don't, and why you should care. *Fertil Steril.* 2010;93:2465-2485.
49. de Leeuw R, Mulders J, Voortman G, et al. Structure-function relationship of recombinant follicle stimulating hormone (Puregon). *Mol Hum Reprod.* 1996;2:361-369.
50. Choi Y, Rajkovic A. Genetics of early mammalian folliculogenesis. *Cell Mol Life Sci.* 2006;63:579-590.
51. Di Pasquale E, Beck-Peccoz P, Persani L. Hypergonadotropic ovarian failure associated with an inherited mutation of human bone morphogenetic protein-15 (BMP15) gene. *Am J Hum Genet.* 2004;75:106-111.
52. Witschi E. Migration of the germ cells of human embryos from the yolk sac to the primitive gonadal folds. *Contrib Embryol.* 1948;32:67.
53. Chuva S, van den Driesche S, Carvalho S, et al. Altered primordial germ cell migration in the absence of transforming growth factor β signaling via ALK5. *Dev Biol.* 2005;284(1):194-203.
54. Farini D, La Sala G, Tedesco M, De Felici M. Chemoattractant action and molecular signaling pathways of Kit ligand on mouse primordial germ cells. *Dev Biol.* 2007;306(2):572-583.
55. Oktem O, Oktay K. The ovary: anatomy and function throughout human life. *Ann N Y Acad Sci.* 2008;1127:1-9.

56. Himelstein-Braw R, Byskov AG, Peters H, Faber M. Follicular atresia in the infant human ovary. *J Reprod Fertil.* 1976;46:55-59.

57. Simon AM, Goodenough DA, Li E, Paul DL. Female infertility in mice lacking connexin 37. *Nature.* 1997;385:525-529.

58. Espey L. Ovarian proteolytic enzymes and ovulation. *Biol Reprod.* 1974;10:216-235.

59. Zoller LC, Weisz J. A quantitative cytochemical study of glucose-6-phosphate dehydrogenase and delta 5-3 beta-hydroxysteroid dehydrogenase activity in the membrana granulosa of the ovulable type of follicle of the rat. *Histochemistry.* 1979;62:125-135.

60. Magnusson C, Billig H, Eneroth P, et al. Comparison between the progestin secretion responsiveness to gonadotrophins of rat cumulus and mural granulosa cells in vitro. *Acta Endocrinol (Copenh).* 1982;101:611-616.

61. Hu Y, Ghosh S, Amleh A, et al. Modulation of aromatase expression by BRCA1: a possible link to tissue-specific tumor suppression. *Oncogene.* 2005;24:8343-8348.

62. Lu M, Chen D, Lin Z, et al. BRCA1 negatively regulates the cancer-associated aromatase promoters I.3 and II in breast adipose fibroblasts and malignant epithelial cells. *J Clin Endocrinol Metab.* 2006;91:4514-4519.

63. Erickson G, Magoffin D, Dyer C, Hofeditz C. The ovarian androgen producing cells: a review of structure/function relationships. *Endocr Rev.* 1985;6:371-399.

64. Gougeon A. Regulation of ovarian follicular development in primates: facts and hypotheses. *Endocr Rev.* 1996;17:121-155.

65. Schipper I, Hop W, Fauser B. The follicle-stimulating hormone (FSH) threshold/window concept examined by different interventions with exogenous FSH during the follicular phase of the normal menstrual cycle: duration, rather than magnitude, of FSH increase affects follicle development. *J Clin Endocrinol Metab.* 1998;83:1292-1298.

66. Peters H, McNatty KP. *The Ovary: A Correlation of Structure and Function in Mammals.* Berkeley, CA: University of California Press; 1980:12-34.

67. Tilly JL, Kowalski KI, Johnson AL, Hsueh AJ. Involvement of apoptosis in ovarian follicular atresia and postovulatory regression. *Endocrinology.* 1991;129:2799-2801.

68. Bauminger S, Lindner H. Periovulatory changes in ovarian prostaglandin formation and their hormonal control in the rat. *Prostaglandins.* 1975;9:737-751.

69. Tsafriri A, Lindner HR, Zor U, Lamprecht SA. Physiological role of prostaglandins in the induction of ovulation. *Prostaglandins.* 1972;2:1-10.

70. Bjersing L, Cajander S. Ovulation and the mechanism of follicle rupture. IV. Ultrastructure of membrana granulosa of rabbit graafian follicles prior to induced ovulation. *Cell Tissue Res.* 1974;153:1-14.

71. Beers WH, Strickland S, Reich E. Ovarian plasminogen activator: relationship to ovulation and hormonal regulation. *Cell.* 1975;6:387-394.

72. Frederick JL, Shimanuki T, diZerega GS. Initiation of angiogenesis by human follicular fluid. *Science.* 1984;224:389-390.

73. Kamat BR, Brown LF, Manseau EJ, et al. Expression of vascular permeability factor/vascular endothelial growth factor by human granulosa and theca lutein cells. Role in corpus luteum development. *Am J Pathol.* 1995;146:157-165.

74. Ohara A, Mori T, Taii S, et al. Functional differentiation in steroidogenesis of two types of luteal cells isolated from mature human corpora lutea of menstrual cycle. *J Clin Endocrinol Metab.* 1965;65:1192-1200.

75. Carr B, MacDonald P, Simpson E. The role of lipoproteins in the regulation of progesterone secretion by the human corpus luteum. *Fertil Steril.* 1982;38:303-311.

76. Duncan WC, McNeilly AS, Fraser HM, Illingworth PJ. Luteinizing hormone receptor in the human corpus luteum: lack of downregulation during maternal recognition of pregnancy. *Hum Reprod.* 1996;11:2291-2297.

77. Strauss JF 3rd, Christenson LK, Devoto L, Martinez F. Providing progesterone for pregnancy: control of cholesterol flux to the side-chain cleavage system. *J Reprod Fertil Suppl.* 2000;55:3-12.

78. Casper R, Yen S. Induction of luteolysis in the human with a long acting analog of luteinizing hormone-releasing factor. *Science.* 1979;205:408-410.

79. Schoonmaker JN, Victery W, Karsch FJ. A receptive period for estradiol-induced luteolysis in the rhesus monkey. *Endocrinology.* 1981;108:1874-1877.

80. O'Grady JP, Kohorn EI, Glass RH, et al. Inhibition of progesterone synthesis in vitro by prostaglandin F2. *J Reprod Fertil.* 1972;30:153-156.

81. Shikone T, Yamoto M, Kokawa K, et al. Apoptosis of human corpora lutea during cyclic luteal regression and early pregnancy. *J Clin Endocrinol Metab.* 1996;81:2376-2380.

82. Bortolussi M, Marini G, Dal Lago A. Autoradiographic study of the distribution of LH (hCG) receptors in the ovary of untreated and gonadotrophin-primed immature rats. *Cell Tissue Res.* 1977;183:329-342.

83. Nimrod A, Erickson GF, Ryan KJ. A specific FSH receptor in rat granulosa cells: properties of binding in vitro. *Endocrinology.* 1976;98:56-64.

84. Nimrod A, Bedrak E, Lamprecht SA. Appearance of LH-receptors and LH-stimulable cyclic AMP accumulation in granulosa cells during follicular maturation in the rat ovary. *Biochem Biophys Res Commun.* 1977;78:977-984.

85. Zeleznik AJ, Midgley AR Jr, Reichert LE Jr. Granulosa cell maturation in the rat: increased binding of human chorionic gonadotropin following treatment with follicle-stimulating hormone in vivo. *Endocrinology.* 1974;95:818-825.

86. Richards J, Ireland J, Rao M, et al. Ovarian follicular development in the rat: hormone receptor regulation by estradiol, follicle-stimulating hormone and luteinizng hormone. *Endocrinology.* 1976;99:1562-1570.

87. Couse JF, Korach KS. Estrogen receptor null mice: what have we learned and where will they lead us? *Endocr Rev.* 1999;20:358-417.

88. Brandenberger AW, Tee MK, Jaffe RB. Estrogen receptor alpha (ER-alpha) and beta (ER-beta) mRNAs in normal ovary, ovarian serous cystadeno-carcinoma and ovarian cancer cell lines: down-regulation of ER-beta in neoplastic tissues. *J Clin Endocrinol Metab.* 1998;83:1025-1028.

89. Simpson ER, Mahendroo MS, Means GD, et al. Aromatase cytochrome P450, the enzyme responsible for estrogen biosynthesis. *Endocr Rev.* 1994;15:342-355.

90. Richards JS, Pangas SA. The ovary: basic biology and clinical implications. *J Clin Invest.* 2010;120:963-972.

91. Barlow JJ, Emerson K Jr, Saxena BN. Estradiol production after ovariectomy for carcinoma of the breast. *N Engl J Med.* 1969;280:633-637.

92. Baird DT, Fraser IS. Concentrations of oestrone and oestradiol in follicular fluid and ovarian venous blood of women. *Clin Endocrinol.* 1975;4:259-266.

93. Bulun SE, Lin Z, Imir G, et al. Regulation of aromatase expression in estrogen-responsive breast and uterine disease: from bench to treatment. *Pharmacol Rev.* 2005;57:359-383.

94. Mahendroo M, Russell D. Male and female isoenzymes of steroid 5alpha-reductase. *Rev Reprod.* 1999;4:179-183.

95. Miller WL, Strauss JF 3rd. Molecular pathology and mechanism of action of the steroidogenic acute regulatory protein, StAR. *J Steroid Biochem Mol Biol.* 1999;69:131-141.

96. Pollack SE, Furth EE, Kallen CB, et al. Localization of the steroidogenic acute regulatory protein in human tissues. *J Clin Endocrinol Metab.* 1997;82:4243-4251.

97. Leers-Sucheta S, Morohashi K, Mason JI, Melner MH. Synergistic activation of the human type II 3beta-hydroxysteroid dehydrogenase/delta5-delta4 isomerase promoter by the transcription factor steroidogenic factor-1/adrenal 4-binding protein and phorbol ester. *J Biol Chem.* 1997;272:7960-7967.

98. Hanley NA, Ikeda Y, Luo X, Parker KL. Steroidogenic factor 1 (SF-1) is essential for ovarian development and function. *Mol Cell Endocrinol.* 2000;163:27-32.

99. Kim JJ, Kurita T, Bulun SE. Progesterone action in endometrial cancer, endometriosis, uterine fibroids, and breast cancer. *Endocr Rev.* 2013;34:130-162.

100. Bulun SE. Aromatase and estrogen receptor alpha deficiency. *Fertil Steril.* 2014;101:323-329.

101. Peltoketo H, Luu-The V, Simard J, Adamski J. 17Beta-hydroxysteroid dehydrogenase (HSD)/17-ketosteroid reductase (KSR) family; nomenclature and main characteristics of the 17HSD/KSR enzymes. *J Mol Endocrinol.* 1999;23:1-11.

102. Makanji Y, Zhu J, Mishra R, et al. Inhibin at 90: from discovery to clinical application, a historical review. *Endocr Rev.* 2014;35(5):747-794.

103. Peng N, Kim JW, Rainey WE, et al. The role of the orphan nuclear receptor, liver receptor homologue-1, in the regulation of human corpus luteum 3beta-hydroxysteroid dehydrogenase type II. *J Clin Endocrinol Metab.* 2003;88:6020-6028.

104. Adashi EY, Resnick CE, D'Ercole AJ, et al. Insulin-like growth factors as intraovarian regulators of granulosa cell growth and function. *Endocr Rev.* 1985;6:400-420.

105. Kwintkiewicz J, Giudice LC. The interplay of insulin-like growth factors, gonadotropins, and endocrine disruptors in ovarian follicular development and function. *Semin Reprod Med.* 2009;27:43-51.

106. Groome NP, Illingworth PJ, O'Brien M, et al. Measurement of dimeric inhibin B throughout the human menstrual cycle. *J Clin Endocrinol Metab.* 1996;81:1401-1405.

107. Dunaif A. Insulin resistance and the polycystic ovary syndrome: mechanism and implications for pathogenesis. *Endocr Rev.* 1997;18:774-800.

108. Franks S, Stark J, Hardy K. Follicle dynamics and anovulation in polycystic ovary syndrome. *Hum Reprod Update.* 2008;14:367-378.

109. Konkle AT, McCarthy MM. Developmental time course of estradiol, testosterone, and dihydrotestosterone levels in discrete regions of male and female rat brain. *Endocrinology.* 2011;152:223-235.

110. Lin Z, Reierstad S, Huang CC, Bulun SE. Novel estrogen receptor-alpha binding sites and estradiol target genes identified by chromatin immunoprecipitation cloning in breast cancer. *Cancer Res.* 2007;67:5017-5024.

111. Azziz R, Carmina E, Sawaya ME. Idiopathic hirsutism. *Endocr Rev.* 2000;21:347-362.

112. Diedrich K, Fauser BC, Devroey P, et al. The role of the endometrium and embryo in human implantation. *Hum Reprod Update*. 2007;13: 365-377.

113. Dallenbach-Hellweg G. Normal endometrium. In: Dallenbach-Hellweg G, ed. *Atlas of Histopathology*. Berlin, Germany: Springer-Verlag; 2010.

114. Gargett CE, Schwab KE, Zillwood RM, et al. Isolation and culture of epithelial progenitors and mesenchymal stem cells from human endometrium. *Biol Reprod*. 2009;80:1136-1145.

115. Markee J. Menstruation in intraocular endometrial transplants in the rhesus monkey. *Contrib Embryol*. 1940;28:219.

116. Markee J. Morphological basis for menstrual bleeding: relation of regression to the initiation of bleeding. *Bull N Y Acad Med*. 1948;36:153.

117. Noyes RW, Hertig AT, Rock J. Dating the endometrial biopsy. *Fertil Steril*. 1950;1:3-25.

118. Sauer M, Paulson R, Lobo R. Reversing the natural decline in human fertility. An extended clinical trial of oocyte donation to women of advanced reproductive age. *JAMA*. 1992;268:1275-1279.

119. Rosenwaks Z. Donor eggs: their application in modern reproductive technologies. *Fertil Steril*. 1987;47:895-909.

120. Cooke PS, Buchanan DL, Young P, et al. Stromal estrogen receptors mediate mitogenic effects of estradiol on uterine epithelium. *Proc Natl Acad Sci U S A*. 1997;94:6535-6540.

121. Matsuzaki S, Fukaya T, Suzuki T, et al. Oestrogen receptor alpha and beta mRNA expression in human endometrium throughout the menstrual cycle. *Mol Hum Reprod*. 1999;559-564.

122. Cooke P, Buchanan D, Lubahn D, Cunha G. Mechanism of estrogen action: lessons from the estrogen receptor-alpha knockout mouse. *Biol Reprod*. 1998;59:470-475.

123. Carroll JS, Liu XS, Brodsky AS, et al. Chromosome-wide mapping of estrogen receptor binding reveals long-range regulation requiring the forkhead protein FoxA1. *Cell*. 2005;122(1):33-43.

124. Attia GR, Zeitoun K, Edwards D, et al. Progesterone receptor isoform A but not B is expressed in endometriosis. *J Clin Endocrinol Metab*. 2000;85:2897-2902.

125. Yin P, Roqueiro D, Huang L, et al. Genome-wide progesterone receptor binding: cell type-specific and shared mechanisms in T47D breast cancer cells and primary leiomyoma cells. *PLoS ONE*. 2012;7:e29021.

126. Tseng L, Gurpide E. Effects of progestins on estradiol receptor levels in human endometrium. *J Clin Endocrinol Metab*. 1975;41:402-404.

127. Tseng L, Liu H. Stimulation of acylsulfotransferase activity by progestin in human endometrium in vitro. *J Clin Endocrinol Metab*. 1981; 53:418-421.

128. Yang S, Fang Z, Gurates B, et al. Stromal progesterone receptors mediate induction of 17beta-hydroxysteroid dehydrogenase type 2 expression in human endometrial epithelium: a paracrine mechanism for inactivation of estradiol. *Mol Endocrinol*. 2001;15:2093-2105.

129. Bergh PA, Navot D. The impact of embryonic development and endometrial maturity on the timing of implantation. *Fertil Steril*. 1992; 58:537-542.

130. Hertig A, Rock J, Adams E. A description of 34 human ova within the first 17 days of development. *Am J Anat*. 1956;98:435.

131. Langer RD, Pierce JJ, O'Hanlan KA, et al. Transvaginal ultrasonography compared with endometrial biopsy for the detection of endometrial disease. Postmenopausal Estrogen/Progestin Interventions Trial. *N Engl J Med*. 1997;337:1792-1798.

132. Sheehan HL. The recognition of chronic hypopituitarism resulting from postpartum pituitary necrosis. *Am J Obstet Gynecol*. 1971;111: 852-854.

133. Simpson J, Christakos A, Horwith M, et al. Gonadal dysgenesis in individuals with apparently normal chromosomal complements: tabulation of cases and compilation of genetic data. *Birth Defects Orig Artic Ser*. 1971;7(6):215-228.

134. Hague WM, Adams J, Reeders ST, Jacobs HS. 45 X Turner's syndrome in association with polycystic ovaries. Case report. *Br J Obstet Gynaecol*. 1989;96:613-618.

135. Asherman JG. Amenorrhoea traumatica (atretica). *J Obstet Gynaecol Br Emp*. 1948;55:23-30.

136. Marshall W, Tanner JM. Variations in patterns of pubertal changes in girls. *Arch Dis Child*. 1969;44:291-303.

137. Filicori M, Santoro N, Merriam GR, Crowley WF Jr. Characterization of the physiological pattern of episodic gonadotropin secretion throughout the human menstrual cycle. *J Clin Endocrinol Metab*. 1986;62:1136-1144.

138. Liu JH, Bill AH. Stress-associated or functional hypothalamic amenorrhea in the adolescent. *Ann N Y Acad Sci*. 2008;1135:179-184.

139. Klinefelter HJ, Albrigh F, Griswold GC. Experience with a quantitative test for normal or decreased amounts of follicle-stimulating hormone in urine in endocrinological diagnosis. *J Clin Endocrinol Metab*. 1943;3: 529-544.

140. Khoury SA, Reame NE, Kelch RP, Marshall JC. Diurnal patterns of pulsatile luteinizing hormone secretion in hypothalamic amenorrhea: reproducibility and responses to opiate blockade and an alpha 2-adrenergic agonist. *J Clin Endocrinol Metab*. 1987;64:755-762.

141. Yen S, Rebar R, Vandenberg G. Hypothalamic amenorrhea and hypogonadotropism: responses to synthetic LRF. *J Clin Endocrinol Metab*. 1973;36:811.

142. Han SK, Herbison AE. Norepinephrine suppresses gonadotropin-releasing hormone neuron excitability in the adult mouse. *Endocrinology*. 2008;149:1129-1135.

143. Grachev P, Li XF, Kinsey-Jones JS, et al. Suppression of the GnRH pulse generator by neurokinin B involves a kappa-opioid receptor-dependent mechanism. *Endocrinology*. 2012;153:4894-4904.

144. Ropert J, Quigley M, Yen S. Endogenous opiates modulate pulsatile luteinizing hormone release in humans. *J Clin Endocrinol Metab*. 1981; 52:583-585.

145. Genazzani AD, Petraglia F, Gastaldi M, et al. Naltrexone treatment restores menstrual cycles in patients with weight loss-related amenorrhea. *Fertil Steril*. 1995;64:951-956.

146. Selye H. The stress syndrome. *Nature*. 1936;138:32.

147. Suh BY, Liu JH, Berga SL, et al. Hypercortisolism in patients with functional hypothalamic-amenorrhea. *J Clin Endocrinol Metab*. 1988;66: 733-739.

148. Xiao E, Luckhaus J, Niemann W, Ferin M. Acute inhibition of gonadotropin secretion by corticotropin-releasing hormone in the primate: are the adrenal glands involved? *Endocrinology*. 1989;124: 1632-1637.

149. Rivier C, Vale W. Influence of corticotropin-releasing factor on reproductive functions in the rat. *Endocrinology*. 1984;114:914-921.

150. Matteri R, Moberg G, Watson J. Adrenocorticotropin-induced changes in ovine pituitary gonadotropin secretion in vitro. *Endocrinology*. 1986;118:2091-2096.

151. Kamel F, Kubajak CL. Modulation of gonadotropin secretion by corticosterone: interaction with gonadal steroids and mechanism of action. *Endocrinology*. 1987;121:561-568.

152. Welt CK, Chan JL, Bullen J, et al. Recombinant human leptin in women with hypothalamic amenorrhea. *N Engl J Med*. 2004;351: 987-997.

153. Schneider LF, Monaco SE, Warren MP. Elevated ghrelin level in women of normal weight with amenorrhea is related to disordered eating. *Fertil Steril*. 2008;90:121-128.

154. Morley JE, Levine AS. Stress-induced eating is mediated through endogenous opiates. *Science*. 1980;209:1259-1261.

155. Rigotti NA, Neer RM, Skates SJ, et al. The clinical course of osteoporosis in anorexia nervosa. A longitudinal study of cortical bone mass. *JAMA*. 1991;265:1133-1138.

156. Frisch RE, Wyshak G, Vincent L. Delayed menarche and amenorrhea in ballet dancers. *N Engl J Med*. 1980;303:17-19.

157. Frisch RE, Gotz-Welbergen AV, McArthur JW, et al. Delayed menarche and amenorrhea of college athletes in relation to age of onset of training. *JAMA*. 1981;246:1559-1563.

158. Drinkwater BL, Nilson K, Chesnut CH 3rd, et al. Bone mineral content of amenorrheic and eumenorrheic athletes. *N Engl J Med*. 1984;311: 277-281.

159. Willi J, Grossmann S. Epidemiology of anorexia nervosa in a defined region of Switzerland. *Am J Psychiatry*. 1983;140:564-567.

160. Schwartz DM, Thompson MG. Do anorectics get well? Current research and future needs. *Am J Psychiatry*. 1981;138:319-323.

161. Swift WJ. The long-term outcome of early onset anorexia nervosa. A critical review. *J Am Acad Child Psychiatry*. 1982;21:38-46.

162. Boyar RM, Hellman LD, Roffwarg H, et al. Cortisol secretion and metabolism in anorexia nervosa. *N Engl J Med*. 1977;296:190-193.

163. Gold PW, Gwirtsman H, Avgerinos PC, et al. Abnormal hypothalamic-pituitary-adrenal function in anorexia nervosa. Pathophysiologic mechanisms in underweight and weight-corrected patients. *N Engl J Med*. 1986;314:1335-1342.

164. Kaye WH, Gwirtsman HE, George DT, et al. Elevated cerebrospinal fluid levels of immunoreactive corticotropin-releasing hormone in anorexia nervosa: relation to state of nutrition, adrenal function, and intensity of depression. *J Clin Endocrinol Metab*. 1987;64:203-208.

165. Moshang T Jr, Utinger RD. Low triiodothyronine euthyroidism in anorexia nervosa. In: Vigersky RS, ed. *Anorexia Nervosa*. New York, NY: Raven Press; 1977:263-270.

166. Gold PW, Kaye W, Robertson GL, Ebert M. Abnormalities in plasma and cerebrospinal-fluid arginine vasopressin in patients with anorexia nervosa. *N Engl J Med*. 1983;308:1117-1123.

167. Berga SL, Loucks TL. Use of cognitive behavior therapy for functional hypothalamic amenorrhea. *Ann N Y Acad Sci*. 2006;1092:114-129.

168. Soyka LA, Grinspoon S, Levitsky LL, et al. The effects of anorexia nervosa on bone metabolism in female adolescents. *J Clin Endocrinol Metab*. 1999;84:4489-4496.

169. Liu JH, Yen SS. The use of gonadotropin-releasing hormone for the induction of ovulation. *Clin Obstet Gynecol*. 1984;27:975-982.

170. Ferriman D, Gallwey JD. Clinical assessment of body hair growth in women. *J Clin Endocrinol Metab*. 1961;21:1440-1447.

171. Tagatz GE, Kopher RA, Nagel TC, Okagaki T. The clitoral index: a bioassay of androgenic stimulation. *Obstet Gynecol*. 1979;54:562-564.

172. Bardin CW, Lipsett MB. Testosterone and androstenedione blood production rates in normal women and women with idiopathic hirsutism or polycystic ovaries. *J Clin Invest*. 1967;46:891-902.

173. Mowszowicz I, Melanitou E, Doukani A, et al. Androgen binding capacity and 5 alpha-reductase activity in pubic skin fibroblasts from hirsute patients. *J Clin Endocrinol Metab*. 1983;56:1209-1213.

174. Schwartz U, Moltz L, Brotherton J, Hammerstein J. The diagnostic value of plasma free testosterone in non-tumorous and tumorous hyperandrogenism. *Fertil Steril*. 1983;40:66-72.

175. Miller KK, Rosner W, Lee H, et al. Measurement of free testosterone in normal women and women with androgen deficiency: comparison of methods. *J Clin Endocrinol Metab*. 2004;89:525-533.

176. Carmine E, Rosato F, Janni A, et al. Extensive clinical experience: relative prevalence of different androgen excess disorders in 950 women referred because of clinical hyperandrogenism. *J Clin Endocrinol Metab*. 2006;91:2-6.

177. Paulson RJ, Serafini PC, Catalino JA, Lobo RA. Measurements of 3 alpha,17 beta-androstanediol glucuronide in serum and urine and the correlation with skin 5 alpha-reductase activity. *Fertil Steril*. 1986;46: 222-226.

178. Kennedy L, Traub AI, Atkinson AB, Sheridan B. Short term administration of gonadotropin-releasing hormone analog to a patient with a testosterone-secreting ovarian tumor. *J Clin Endocrinol Metab*. 1987;64: 1320-1322.

179. Bavdekar SB, Kasla RR, Parmar RC, Hathi GS. Selective testosterone secreting adrenocortical carcinoma in an infant. *Indian J Pediatr*. 2001;68:95-97.

180. Derksen J, Nagesser SK, Meinders AE, et al. Identification of virilizing adrenal tumors in hirsute women. *N Engl J Med*. 1994;331:968-973.

181. Friedman CI, Schmidt GE, Kim MH, Powell J. Serum testosterone concentrations in the evaluation of androgen-producing tumors. *Am J Obstet Gynecol*. 1985;153:44-49.

182. Taylor L, Ayers JW, Gross MD, et al. Diagnostic considerations in virilization: iodomethyl-norcholesterol scanning in the localization of androgen secreting tumors. *Fertil Steril*. 1986;46:1005-1010.

183. Bricaire C, Raynaud A, Benotmane A, et al. Selective venous catheterization in the evaluation of hyperandrogenism. *J Endocrinol Invest*. 1991;14:949-956.

184. Azziz R, Hincapie LA, Knochenhauer ES, et al. Screening for 21-hydroxylase-deficient nonclassic adrenal hyperplasia among hyperandrogenic women: a prospective study. *Fertil Steril*. 1999;72:915-925.

185. Speiser PW, Dupont B, Rubinstein P, et al. High frequency of nonclassical steroid 21-hydroxylase deficiency. *Am J Hum Genet*. 1985;37: 650-667.

186. New MI, Lorenzen F, Lerner AJ, et al. Genotyping steroid 21-hydroxylase deficiency: hormonal reference data. *J Clin Endocrinol Metab*. 1983;57: 320-326.

187. Stratakis CA, Karl M, Schulte HM, Chrousos GP. Glucocorticosteroid resistance in humans. Elucidation of the molecular mechanisms and implications for pathophysiology. *Ann N Y Acad Sci*. 1994;746:362-374, discussion 374-376.

188. Koulouri O, Conway GS. A systematic review of commonly used medical treatments for hirsutism in women. *Clin Endocrinol (Oxf)*. 2008;68:800-805.

189. Lobo RA, Shoupe D, Serafini P, et al. The effects of two doses of spironolactone on serum androgens and anagen hair in hirsute women. *Fertil Steril*. 1985;43:200-205.

190. Evron S, Shapiro G, Diamant YZ. Induction of ovulation with spironolactone (Aldactone) in anovulatory oligomenorrheic and hyperandrogenic women. *Fertil Steril*. 1981;36:468-471.

191. Mowszowicz I, Wright F, Vincens M, et al. Androgen metabolism in hirsute patients treated with cyproterone acetate. *J Steroid Biochem*. 1984;20:757-761.

192. Rittmaster RS. Finasteride. *N Engl J Med*. 1994;330:120-125.

193. Wong IL, Morris RS, Chang L, et al. A prospective randomized trial comparing finasteride to spironolactone in the treatment of hirsute women. *J Clin Endocrinol Metab*. 1995;80:233-238.

194. Castello R, Tosi F, Perrone F, et al. Outcome of long-term treatment with the 5 alpha-reductase inhibitor finasteride in idiopathic hirsutism: clinical and hormonal effects during a 1-year course of therapy and 1-year follow-up. *Fertil Steril*. 1996;66:734-740.

195. Diamanti-Kandarakis E, Mitrakou A, Raptis S, et al. The effect of a pure antiandrogen receptor blocker, flutamide, on the lipid profile in the polycystic ovary syndrome. *J Clin Endocrinol Metab*. 1998;83: 2699-2705.

196. Moghetti P, Castello R, Negri C, et al. Flutamide in the treatment of hirsutism: long-term clinical effects, endocrine changes, and androgen receptor behavior. *Fertil Steril*. 1995;64:511-517.

197. Wysowski DK, Freiman JP, Tourtelot JB, Horton ML 3rd. Fatal and nonfatal hepatotoxicity associated with flutamide. *Ann Intern Med*. 1993;118:860-864.

198. Hoeger K, Davidson K, Kochman L, et al. The impact of metformin, oral contraceptives, and lifestyle modification on polycystic ovary syndrome in obese adolescent women in two randomized, placebo-controlled clinical trials. *J Clin Endocrinol Metab*. 2008;93:4299-4306.

199. Legro RS, Kunselman AR, Dodson WC, Dunaif A. Prevalence and predictors of risk for type 2 diabetes mellitus and impaired glucose tolerance in polycystic ovary syndrome: a prospective, controlled study in 254 affected women. *J Clin Endocrinol Metab*. 1999;84:165-169.

200. Urbanek M, Legro RS, Driscoll DA, et al. Thirty-seven candidate genes for polycystic ovary syndrome: strongest evidence for linkage is with follistatin. *Proc Natl Acad Sci U S A*. 1999;96:8573-8578.

201. Legro RS, Driscoll D, Strauss JF 3rd, et al. Evidence for a genetic basis for hyperandrogenemia in polycystic ovary syndrome. *Proc Natl Acad Sci U S A*. 1998;95:14956-14960.

202. Stein I, Leventhal M. Amenorrhea associated with bilateral polycystic ovaries. *Am J Obstet Gynecol*. 1935;29:181-191.

203. Tamura M, Deb S, Sebastian S, et al. Estrogen up-regulates cyclooxygenase-2 via estrogen receptor in human uterine microvascular endothelial cells. *Fertil Steril*. 2004;81:1351-1356.

204. Zawadzki JK, Dunaif A. Diagnostic criteria for polycystic ovary syndrome: towards a rational approach. In: Dunaif A, Givens JR, Haseltine FP, Merriam GR, eds. *Polycystic Ovary Syndrome*. Boston: Blackwell Scientific Publications; 1992:377-384.

205. Rotterdam ESHRE/ASRM-Sponsored PCOS Consensus Workshop Group. Revised 2003 consensus on diagnostic criteria and long-term health risks related to polycystic ovary syndrome. *Fertil Steril*. 2004;81: 19-25.

206. Azziz R. Controversy in clinical endocrinology: diagnosis of polycystic ovarian syndrome: the Rotterdam criteria are premature. *J Clin Endocrinol Metab*. 2006;91:781-785.

207. Dunaif A. Insulin resistance in polycystic ovarian syndrome. *Ann N Y Acad Sci*. 1993;687:60-64.

208. Hoffman D, Klove K, Lobo R. The prevalence and significance of elevated dehydroepiandrosterone sulfate levels in anovulatory women. *Fertil Steril*. 1980;42:853-861.

209. Franks S. Polycystic ovary syndrome. *N Engl J Med*. 1995;333: 853-861.

210. Kletzky OA, Davajan V, Nakamura RM, et al. Clinical categorization of patients with secondary amenorrhea using progesterone-induced uterine bleeding and measurement of serum gonadotropin levels. *Am J Obstet Gynecol*. 1975;121:695-703.

211. Venturoli S, Porcu E, Fabbri R, et al. Episodic pulsatile secretion of FSH, LH, prolactin, oestradiol, oestrone, and LH circadian variations in polycystic ovary syndrome. *Clin Endocrinol (Oxf)*. 1988;28:93-107.

212. Imse V, Holzapfel G, Hinney B, et al. Comparison of luteinizing hormone pulsatility in the serum of women suffering from polycystic ovarian disease using a bioassay and five different immunoassays. *J Clin Endocrinol Metab*. 1992;74:1053-1061.

213. Hayes FJ, Taylor AE, Martin KA, Hall JE. Use of a gonadotropin-releasing hormone antagonist as a physiologic probe in polycystic ovary syndrome: assessment of neuroendocrine and androgen dynamics. *J Clin Endocrinol Metab*. 1998;83:2343-2349.

214. Barnes RB, Lobo RA. Central opioid activity in polycystic ovary syndrome with and without dopaminergic modulation. *J Clin Endocrinol Metab*. 1985;61:779-782.

215. Morales AJ, Laughlin GA, Butzow T, et al. Insulin, somatotropic, and luteinizing hormone axes in lean and obese women with polycystic ovary syndrome: common and distinct features. *J Clin Endocrinol Metab*. 1996;81:2854-2864.

216. Taylor AE, McCourt B, Martin KA, et al. Determinants of abnormal gonadotropin secretion in clinically defined women with polycystic ovary syndrome. *J Clin Endocrinol Metab*. 1997;82:2248-2256.

217. Nagamani M, Van Dinh T, Kelver ME. Hyperinsulinemia in hyperthecosis of the ovaries. *Am J Obstet Gynecol*. 1986;154:384-389.

218. Dorn C, Mouillet JF, Yan X, et al. Insulin enhances the transcription of luteinizing hormone-beta gene. *Am J Obstet Gynecol*. 2004;191: 132-137.

219. Adashi EY, Hsueh AJ, Yen SS. Insulin enhancement of luteinizing hormone and follicle-stimulating hormone release by cultured pituitary cells. *Endocrinology*. 1981;108:1441-1449.

220. Lawson MA, Jain S, Sun S, et al. Evidence for insulin suppression of baseline luteinizing hormone in women with polycystic ovarian syndrome and normal women. *J Clin Endocrinol Metab*. 2008;93: 2089-2096.

221. Chang RJ. Ovarian steroid secretion in polycystic ovarian disease. *Semin Reprod Endocrinol*. 1984;2:244.

222. Wajchenberg BL, Achando SS, Mathor MM, et al. The source(s) of estrogen production in hirsute women with polycystic ovarian disease as determined by simultaneous adrenal and ovarian venous catheterization. *Fertil Steril*. 1988;49:56-61.

223. Chen D, Reierstad S, Lu M, et al. Regulation of breast cancer-associated aromatase promoters. *Cancer Lett*. 2009;273:15-27.

224. Reed MJ, Singh A, Ghilchik MW, et al. Regulation of oestradiol 17 beta hydroxysteroid dehydrogenase in breast tissues: the role of growth factors. *J Steroid Biochem Mol Biol*. 1991;39:791-798.

225. Nestler JE. Obesity, insulin, sex steroids and ovulation. *Int J Obes Relat Metab Disord*. 2000;24(Suppl 2):S71-S73.

226. Fauser BC. Observations in favor of normal early follicle development and disturbed dominant follicle selection in polycystic ovary syndrome. *Gynecol Endocrinol*. 1994;8:75-82.

227. Mason HD, Margara R, Winston RM, et al. Insulin-like growth factor-I (IGF-I) inhibits production of IGF-binding protein-1 while stimulating estradiol secretion in granulosa cells from normal and polycystic human ovaries. *J Clin Endocrinol Metab*. 1993;76:1275-1279.

228. Homburg R, Howles CM. Low-dose FSH therapy for anovulatory infertility associated with polycystic ovary syndrome: rationale, results, reflections and refinements. *Hum Reprod Update*. 1999;5:493-499.

229. Judd HL, Scully RE, Herbst AL, et al. Familial hyperthecosis: comparison of endocrinologic and histologic findings with polycystic ovarian disease. *Am J Obstet Gynecol.* 1973;117:976-982.

230. Cooper HE, Spellacy WN, Prem KA, Cohen WD. Hereditary factors in the Stein-Leventhal syndrome. *Am J Obstet Gynecol.* 1968;100:371-387.

231. Ferriman D, Purdie AW. The inheritance of polycystic ovarian disease and a possible relationship to premature balding. *Clin Endocrinol (Oxf).* 1979;11:291-300.

232. Kent SC, Gnatuk CL, Kunselman AR, et al. Hyperandrogenism and hyperinsulinism in children of women with polycystic ovary syndrome: a controlled study. *J Clin Endocrinol Metab.* 2008;93:1662-1669.

233. Diamanti-Kandarakis E, Kandarakis H, Legro RS. The role of genes and environment in the etiology of PCOS. *Endocrine.* 2006;30:19-26.

234. Urbanek M. The genetics of the polycystic ovary syndrome. *Nat Clin Pract Endocrinol Metab.* 2007;3:103-111.

235. Shi Y, Zhao H, Shi Y, et al. Genome-wide association study identifies eight new risk loci for polycystic ovary syndrome. *Nat Genet.* 2012;44:1020-1025.

236. Dunaif A, Green G, Phelps RG, et al. Acanthosis nigricans, insulin action, and hyperandrogenism: clinical, histological, and biochemical findings. *J Clin Endocrinol Metab.* 1991;73:590-595.

237. Reaven GM, Lithell H, Landsberg L. Hypertension and associated metabolic abnormalities: the role of insulin resistance and the sympathoadrenal system. *N Engl J Med.* 1996;334:374-381.

238. Mather KJ, Kwan F, Corenblum B. Hyperinsulinemia in polycystic ovary syndrome correlates with increased cardiovascular risk independent of obesity. *Fertil Steril.* 2000;73:150-156.

239. Talbott E, Guzick D, Clerici A, et al. Coronary heart disease risk factors in women with polycystic ovary syndrome. *Arterioscler Thromb Vasc Biol.* 1995;15:821-826.

240. Ehrmann DA, Liljenquist DR, Kasza K, et al. Prevalence and predictors of the metabolic syndrome in women with polycystic ovary syndrome. *J Clin Endocrinol Metab.* 2006;91:48-53.

241. Dunaif A, Finegood DT. Beta-cell dysfunction independent of obesity and glucose intolerance in the polycystic ovary syndrome. *J Clin Endocrinol Metab.* 1996;81:942-947.

242. Reddy SS, Kahn CR. Epidermal growth factor receptor defects in leprechaunism. A multiple growth factor-resistant syndrome. *J Clin Invest.* 1989;84:1569-1576.

243. Bremer AA, Miller WL. The serine phosphorylation hypothesis of polycystic ovary syndrome: a unifying mechanism for hyperandrogenemia and insulin resistance. *Fertil Steril.* 2008;89:1039-1048.

244. Kirschner MA, Samojlik E, Drejka M, et al. Androgen-estrogen metabolism in women with upper body versus lower body obesity. *J Clin Endocrinol Metab.* 1990;70:473-479.

245. Schapira DV, Kumar NB, Lyman GH, Cox CE. Abdominal obesity and breast cancer risk. *Ann Intern Med.* 1990;112:182-186.

246. Kumar N, Cantor A, Allen K, Cox C. Android obesity at diagnosis and breast carcinoma survival: evaluation of the effects of anthropometric variables at diagnosis, including body composition and body fat distribution and weight gain during life span, and survival from breast carcinoma. *Cancer.* 2000;88:2751-2757.

247. Anderson KE, Sellers TA, Chen PL, et al. Association of Stein-Leventhal syndrome with the incidence of postmenopausal breast carcinoma in a large prospective study of women in Iowa. *Cancer.* 1997;79:494-499.

248. Campbell PJ, Gerich JE. Impact of obesity on insulin action in volunteers with normal glucose tolerance: demonstration of a threshold for the adverse effect of obesity. *J Clin Endocrinol Metab.* 1990;70:1114-1118.

249. Ehrmann DA. Polycystic ovary syndrome. *N Engl J Med.* 2005;352:1223-1236.

250. Velazquez EM, Mendoza S, Hamer T, et al. Metformin therapy in polycystic ovary syndrome reduces hyperinsulinemia, insulin resistance, hyperandrogenemia, and systolic blood pressure, while facilitating normal menses and pregnancy. *Metabolism.* 1994;43:647-654.

251. Nestler J, Jakubowicz D. Decreases in ovarian cytochrome P450c 17 alpha activity and serum free testosterone after reduction of insulin secretion in polycystic ovary syndrome. *N Engl J Med.* 1996;335:617-623.

252. Velazquez E, Acosta A, Mendoza SG. Menstrual cyclicity after metformin therapy in polycystic ovary syndrome. *Obstet Gynecol.* 1997;90:392-395.

253. Legro RS, Barnhart HX, Schlaff WD, et al. Clomiphene, metformin, or both for infertility in the polycystic ovary syndrome. *N Engl J Med.* 2007;356:551-566.

254. Palomba S, Falbo A, Zullo F, Orio F Jr. Evidence-based and potential benefits of metformin in the polycystic ovary syndrome: a comprehensive review. *Endocr Rev.* 2009;30:1-50.

255. Tang T, Lord JM, Norman RJ, et al. Insulin-sensitising drugs (metformin, rosiglitazone, pioglitazone, D-chiro-inositol) for women with polycystic ovary syndrome, oligo amenorrhoea and subfertility. *Cochrane Database Syst Rev.* 2010;(1):CD003053.

256. Dunaif A, Scott D, Finegood D, et al. The insulin-sensitizing agent troglitazone improves metabolic and reproductive abnormalities in the polycystic ovary syndrome. *J Clin Endocrinol Metab.* 1996;81:3299-3306.

257. Ehrmann DA, Schneider DJ, Sobel BE, et al. Troglitazone improves defects in insulin action, insulin secretion, ovarian steroidogenesis, and fibrinolysis in women with polycystic ovary syndrome. *J Clin Endocrinol Metab.* 1997;82:2108-2116.

258. Azziz R, Ehrmann D, Legro RS, et al. Troglitazone improves ovulation and hirsutism in the polycystic ovary syndrome: a multicenter, double blind, placebo-controlled trial. *J Clin Endocrinol Metab.* 2001;86:1626-1632.

259. Ghazeeri G, Kutteh WH, Bryer-Ash M, et al. Effect of rosiglitazone on spontaneous and clomiphene citrate-induced ovulation in women with polycystic ovary syndrome. *Fertil Steril.* 2003;79:562-566.

260. Belli SH, Graffigna MN, Oneto A, et al. Effect of rosiglitazone on insulin resistance, growth factors, and reproductive disturbances in women with polycystic ovary syndrome. *Fertil Steril.* 2004;81:624-629.

261. Romualdi D, Guido M, Ciampelli M, et al. Selective effects of pioglitazone on insulin and androgen abnormalities in normo- and hyperinsulinaemic obese patients with polycystic ovary syndrome. *Hum Reprod.* 2003;18:1210-1218.

262. Wild RA, Alaupovic P, Parker IJ. Lipid and apolipoprotein abnormalities in hirsute women. I. The association with insulin resistance. *Am J Obstet Gynecol.* 1992;166:1191-1196, discussion 1196-1197.

263. Kiddy DS, Hamilton-Fairley D, Bush A, et al. Improvement in endocrine and ovarian function during dietary treatment of obese women with polycystic ovary syndrome. *Clin Endocrinol (Oxf).* 1992;36:105-111.

264. Guzick DS, Wing R, Smith D, et al. Endocrine consequences of weight loss in obese, hyperandrogenic, anovulatory women. *Fertil Steril.* 1994;61:598-604.

265. Clark AM, Ledger W, Galletly C, et al. Weight loss results in significant improvement in pregnancy and ovulation rates in anovulatory obese women. *Hum Reprod.* 1995;10:2705-2712.

266. Gitsch G, Hanzal E, Jensen D, Hacker NF. Endometrial cancer in premenopausal women 45 years and younger. *Obstet Gynecol.* 1995;85:504-508.

267. Kjos SL, Peters RK, Xiang A, et al. Contraception and the risk of type 2 diabetes mellitus in Latina women with prior gestational diabetes mellitus. *JAMA.* 1998;280:533-538.

268. Diamanti-Kandarakis E, Mitrakou A, Hennes MM, et al. Insulin sensitivity and antiandrogenic therapy in women with polycystic ovary syndrome. *Metabolism.* 1995;44:525-531.

269. Lanzone A, Fulghesu AM, Cucinelli F, et al. Preconceptional and gestational evaluation of insulin secretion in patients with polycystic ovary syndrome. *Hum Reprod.* 1996;11:2382-2386.

270. Nestler JE, Jakubowicz DJ, Evans WS, Pasquali R. Effects of metformin on spontaneous and clomiphene-induced ovulation in the polycystic ovary syndrome. *N Engl J Med.* 1998;338:1876-1880.

271. Regan L, Owen EJ, Jacobs HS. Hypersecretion of luteinising hormone, infertility, and miscarriage. *Lancet.* 1990;336:1141-1144.

272. Adashi EY. Clomiphene citrate-initiated ovulation: a clinical update. *Semin Reprod Endocrinol.* 1986;4:225-276.

273. Mitwally MF, Casper RF. Use of an aromatase inhibitor for induction of ovulation in patients with an inadequate response to clomiphene citrate. *Fertil Steril.* 2001;75:305-309.

274. Badawy A, Mosbah A, Shady M. Anastrozole or letrozole for ovulation induction in clomiphene-resistant women with polycystic ovarian syndrome: a prospective randomized trial. *Fertil Steril.* 2008;89:1209-1212.

275. Legro RS, Brzyski RG, Diamond MP, et al. Letrozole versus clomiphene for infertility in the polycystic ovary syndrome. *N Engl J Med.* 2014;371:119-129.

276. Tulandi T, Martin J, Al-Fadhli R, et al. Congenital malformations among 911 newborns conceived after infertility treatment with letrozole or clomiphene citrate. *Fertil Steril.* 2006;85:1761-1765.

277. Hamilton-Fairley D, Franks S. Common problems in induction of ovulation. *Baillieres Clin Obstet Gynaecol.* 1990;4:609-625.

278. Conway GS. Premature ovarian failure. *Br Med Bull.* 2000;56:643-649.

279. Taylor AE, Adams JM, Mulder JE, et al. A randomized, controlled trial of estradiol replacement therapy in women with hypergonadotropic amenorrhea. *J Clin Endocrinol Metab.* 1996;81:3615-3621.

280. Broekmans FJ, Soules MR, Fauser BC. Ovarian aging: mechanisms and clinical consequences. *Endocr Rev.* 2009;30:465-493.

281. Myhre AG, Halonen M, Eskelin P, et al. Autoimmune polyendocrine syndrome type 1 (APS I) in Norway. *Clin Endocrinol (Oxf).* 2001;54:211-217.

282. Wallace WH, Shalet SM, Crowne EC, et al. Ovarian failure following abdominal irradiation in childhood: natural history and prognosis. *Clin Oncol (R Coll Radiol).* 1989;1(2):75-79.

283. Morice P, Thiam-Ba R, Castaigne D, et al. Fertility results after ovarian transposition for pelvic malignancies treated by external irradiation or brachytherapy. *Hum Reprod.* 1998;13:660-663.

284. Bines J, Oleske DM, Cobleigh MA. Ovarian function in premenopausal women treated with adjuvant chemotherapy for breast cancer. *J Clin Oncol.* 1996;14:1718-1729.

285. Byrne J, Mulvihill JJ, Myers MH, et al. Effects of treatment on fertility in long-term survivors of childhood or adolescent cancer. *N Engl J Med.* 1987;317:1315-1321.

286. Rebar RW, Connolly HV. Clinical features of young women with hypergonadotropic amenorrhea. *Fertil Steril.* 1990;53:804-810.

287. Nelson LM, Anasti JN, Kimzey LM, et al. Development of luteinized graafian follicles in patients with karyotypically normal spontaneous premature ovarian failure. *J Clin Endocrinol Metab.* 1994;79: 1470-1475.

288. Check JH, Katsoff B. Ovulation induction and pregnancy in a woman with premature menopause following gonadotropin suppression with the gonadotropin releasing hormone antagonist, cetrorelix: a case report. *Clin Exp Obstet Gynecol.* 2008;35:10-12.

289. Tartagni M, Cicinelli E, De Pergola G, et al. Effects of pretreatment with estrogens on ovarian stimulation with gonadotropins in women with premature ovarian failure: a randomized, placebo-controlled trial. *Fertil Steril.* 2007;87:858-861.

290. Dewald G, Spurbeck J. Sex chromosome anomalies associated with premature gonadal failure. *Semin Reprod Endocrinol.* 1983;1:79-92.

291. Giltay JC, Ausems MG, van Seumeren I, et al. Short stature as the only presenting feature in a patient with an isodicentric (Y)(q11.23) and gonadoblastoma. A clinical and molecular cytogenetic study. *Eur J Pediatr.* 2001;160:154-158.

292. Manuel M, Katayama PK, Jones HW Jr. The age of occurrence of gonadal tumors in intersex patients with a Y chromosome. *Am J Obstet Gynecol.* 1976;124:293-300.

293. Gravholt CH, Fedder J, Naeraa RW, Muller J. Occurrence of gonadoblastoma in females with Turner syndrome and Y chromosome material: a population study. *J Clin Endocrinol Metab.* 2000;85:3199-3202.

294. Peprah E, He W, Allen E, et al. Examination of FMR1 transcript and protein levels among 74 premutation carriers. *J Hum Genet.* 2010;55: 66-68.

295. Wittenberger MD, Hagerman RJ, Sherman SL, et al. The FMR1 premutation and reproduction. *Fertil Steril.* 2007;87:456-465.

296. Nelson LM. Autoimmune ovarian failure: comparing the mouse model and the human disease. *J Soc Gynecol Investig.* 2001;8:S55-S57.

297. Wheatcroft NJ, Salt C, Milford-Ward A, et al. Identification of ovarian antibodies by immunofluorescence, enzyme-linked immunosorbent assay or immunoblotting in premature ovarian failure. *Hum Reprod.* 1997;12:2617-2622.

298. Ramathal CY, Bagchi IC, Taylor RN, Bagchi MK. Endometrial decidualization: of mice and men. *Semin Reprod Med.* 2010;28:17-26.

299. Belsey EM, Pinol AP. Menstrual bleeding patterns in untreated women. Task Force on Long-Acting Systemic Agents for Fertility Regulation. *Contraception.* 1997;55:57-65.

300. Chiazze L Jr, Brayer FT, Macisco JJ Jr, et al. The length and variability of the human menstrual cycle. *JAMA.* 1968;203:377-380.

301. Munster K, Schmidt L, Helm P. Length and variation in the menstrual cycle: a cross-sectional study from a Danish county. *Br J Obstet Gynaecol.* 1992;99:422-429.

302. Treloar AE, Boynton RE, Behn BG, Brown BW. Variation of the human menstrual cycle through reproductive life. *Int J Fertil.* 1967;12: 77-126.

303. Rybo G. Menstrual blood loss in relation to parity and menstrual pattern. *Acta Obstet Gynecol Scand.* 1966;45(Suppl 7):25-45.

304. Haynes PJ, Hodgson H, Anderson AB, Turnbull AC. Measurement of menstrual blood loss in patients complaining of menorrhagia. *Br J Obstet Gynaecol.* 1977;84:763-768.

305. Higham JM, O'Brien PM, Shaw RW. Assessment of menstrual blood loss using a pictorial chart. *Br J Obstet Gynaecol.* 1990;97:734-739.

306. Fraser IS, McCarron G, Markham R. A preliminary study of factors influencing perception of menstrual blood loss volume. *Am J Obstet Gynecol.* 1984;149:788-793.

307. de Ziegler D, Bergeron C, Cornel C, et al. Effects of luteal estradiol on the secretory transformation of human endometrium and plasma gonadotropins. *J Clin Endocrinol Metab.* 1992;74:322-331.

308. Belsey EM. Vaginal bleeding patterns among women using one natural and eight hormonal methods of contraception. *Contraception.* 1988;38: 181-206.

309. Wilansky DL, Greisman B. Early hypothyroidism in patients with menorrhagia. *Am J Obstet Gynecol.* 1989;160:673-677.

310. Hopkins MP, Androff L, Benninghoff AS. Ginseng face cream and unexplained vaginal bleeding. *Am J Obstet Gynecol.* 1988;159: 1121-1122.

311. Claessens EA, Cowell CA. Acute adolescent menorrhagia. *Am J Obstet Gynecol.* 1981;139:277-280.

312. Smith YR, Quint EH, Hertzberg RB. Menorrhagia in adolescents requiring hospitalization. *J Pediatr Adolesc Gynecol.* 1998;11:13-15.

313. van Eijkeren MA, Christiaens GC, Haspels AA, Sixma JJ. Measured menstrual blood loss in women with a bleeding disorder or using oral anticoagulant therapy. *Am J Obstet Gynecol.* 1990;162:1261-1263.

314. Edlund M, Blomback M, von Schoultz B, Andersson O. On the value of menorrhagia as a predictor for coagulation disorders. *Am J Hematol.* 1996;53:234-238.

315. Nilsson L, Rybo G. Treatment of menorrhagia. *Am J Obstet Gynecol.* 1971;110:713-720.

316. Kirkland JL, Murthy L, Stancel GM. Progesterone inhibits the estrogen-induced expression of c-fos messenger ribonucleic acid in the uterus. *Endocrinology.* 1992;130:3223-3230.

317. DeVore GR, Owens O, Kase N. Use of intravenous Premarin in the treatment of dysfunctional uterine bleeding: a double-blind randomized control study. *Obstet Gynecol.* 1982;59:285-291.

318. Livio M, Mannucci PM, Vigano G, et al. Conjugated estrogens for the management of bleeding associated with renal failure. *N Engl J Med.* 1986;315:731-735.

319. Giudice LC, Kao LC. Endometriosis. *Lancet.* 2004;364:1789-1799.

320. Bulun SE. Endometriosis. *N Engl J Med.* 2009;360:268-279.

321. Simpson JL, Elias S, Malinak LR, Buttram VC Jr. Heritable aspects of endometriosis. I. Genetic studies. *Am J Obstet Gynecol.* 1980;137: 327-331.

322. Garry R. Is insulin resistance an essential component of PCOS? The endometriosis syndromes: a clinical classification in the presence of aetiological confusion and therapeutic anarchy. *Hum Reprod.* 2004; 19(4):760-768.

323. Brosens I. Endometriosis rediscovered? *Hum Reprod.* 2004;19:1679-1680, author reply 1680-1681.

324. Sampson J. Peritoneal endometriosis due to the menstrual dissemination of endometrial tissue into the peritoneal cavity. *Am J Obstet Gynecol.* 1927;14:422-469.

325. Sasson IE, Taylor HS. Stem cells and the pathogenesis of endometriosis. *Ann N Y Acad Sci.* 2008;1127:106-115.

326. Hornung D, Ryan IP, Chao VA, et al. Immunolocalization and regulation of the chemokine RANTES in human endometrial and endometriosis tissues and cells. *J Clin Endocrinol Metab.* 1997;82:1621-1628.

327. Dyson MT, Roqueiro D, Monsivais D, et al. Genome-wide DNA methylation analysis predicts an epigenetic switch for GATA factor expression in endometriosis. *PLoS Genet.* 2014;10(3):e1004158.

328. Shaw RW. An open randomized comparative study of the effect of goserelin depot and danazol in the treatment of endometriosis. Zoladex Endometriosis Study Team. *Fertil Steril.* 1992;58:265-272.

329. A decision tree for the use of estrogen replacement therapy or hormone replacement therapy in postmenopausal women: consensus opinion of the North American Menopause Society. *Menopause.* 2000;7: 76-86.

330. Vercellini P, Cortesi I, Crosignani PG. Progestins for symptomatic endometriosis: a critical analysis of the evidence. *Fertil Steril.* 1997; 68:393-401.

331. Takayama K, Zeitoun K, Gunby RT, et al. Treatment of severe postmenopausal endometriosis with an aromatase inhibitor. *Fertil Steril.* 1998;69:709-713.

332. Vercellini P, Trespidi L, Colombo A, et al. A gonadotropin-releasing hormone agonist versus a low-dose oral contraceptive for pelvic pain associated with endometriosis. *Fertil Steril.* 1993;60:75-79.

333. Waller KG, Shaw RW. Gonadotropin-releasing hormone analogues for the treatment of endometriosis: long-term follow-up. *Fertil Steril.* 1993;59:511-515.

334. Archer DF, McIntyre-Seltman K, Wilborn WW Jr, et al. Endometrial morphology in asymptomatic postmenopausal women. *Am J Obstet Gynecol.* 1991;165:317-320, discussion 320-322.

335. Amsterdam A, Knecht M, Catt K. Hormonal regulation of cytodifferentiation and intercellular communication in cultured granulosa cells. *Proc Natl Acad Sci U S A.* 1981;78:3000-3004.

336. Ailawadi RK, Jobanputra S, Kataria M, et al. Treatment of endometriosis and chronic pelvic pain with letrozole and norethindrone acetate: a pilot study. *Fertil Steril.* 2004;81:290-296.

337. Soysal S, Soysal ME, Ozer S, et al. The effects of post-surgical administration of goserelin plus anastrozole compared to goserelin alone in patients with severe endometriosis: a prospective randomized trial. *Hum Reprod.* 2004;19:160-167.

338. Attar E, Bulun SE. Aromatase inhibitors: the next generation of therapeutics for endometriosis? *Fertil Steril.* 2006;85:1307-1318.

339. Bulun SE. Uterine fibroids. *N Engl J Med.* 2013;369:1344-1355.

340. Bouwsma EV, Hesley GK, Woodrum DA, et al. Comparing focused ultrasound and uterine artery embolization for uterine fibroids-rationale and design of the Fibroid Interventions: Reducing Symptoms Today and Tomorrow (FIRSTT) trial. *Fertil Steril.* 2011;96:704-710.

341. McKinlay SM, Brambilla DJ, Posner JG. The normal menopause transition. *Maturitas.* 1992;14:103-115.

342. den Tonkelaar I, te Velde ER, Looman CW. Menstrual cycle length preceding menopause in relation to age at menopause. *Maturitas.* 1998;29:115-123.

343. Buckler HM, Evans CA, Mamtora H, et al. Gonadotropin, steroid, and inhibin levels in women with incipient ovarian failure during anovulatory and ovulatory rebound cycles. *J Clin Endocrinol Metab.* 1991;72: 116-124.

344. Santoro N, Brown JR, Adel T, Skurnick JH. Characterization of reproductive hormonal dynamics in the perimenopause. *J Clin Endocrinol Metab.* 1996;81:1495-1501.

345. McKinlay SM, Bifano NL, McKinlay JB. Smoking and age at menopause in women. *Ann Intern Med.* 1985;103:350-356.

346. Torgerson DJ, Avenell A, Russell IT, Reid DM. Factors associated with onset of menopause in women aged 45-49. *Maturitas.* 1994;19:83-92.

347. Torgerson DJ, Thomas RE, Campbell MK, Reid DM. Alcohol consumption and age of maternal menopause are associated with menopause onset. *Maturitas.* 1997;26:21-25.

348. Cramer DW, Xu H, Harlow BL. Family history as a predictor of early menopause. *Fertil Steril.* 1995;64:740-745.

349. Jiroutek MR, Chen MH, Johnston CC, Longcope C. Changes in reproductive hormones and sex hormone-binding globulin in a group of postmenopausal women measured over 10 years. *Menopause.* 1998;5:90-94.

350. Labrie F, Belanger A, Cusan L, et al. Marked decline in serum concentrations of adrenal C19 sex steroid precursors and conjugated androgen metabolites during aging. *J Clin Endocrinol Metab.* 1997;82:2396-2402.

351. Feldman S, Shapter A, Welch WR, Berkowitz RS. Two-year follow-up of 263 patients with post/perimenopausal vaginal bleeding and negative initial biopsy. *Gynecol Oncol.* 1994;55:56-59.

352. Oldenhave A, Jaszmann LJ, Haspels AA, Everaerd WT. Impact of climacteric on well-being. A survey based on 5213 women 39 to 60 years old. *Am J Obstet Gynecol.* 1993;168:772-780.

353. Kronenberg F, Barnard R. Modulation of menopausal hot flashes by ambient temperature. *J Therm Biol.* 1992;17:43-49.

354. Yen SS. The biology of menopause. *J Reprod Med.* 1977;18:287-296.

355. Thurston RC, Sowers MR, Sternfeld B, et al. Gains in body fat and vasomotor symptom reporting over the menopausal transition: the study of women's health across the nation. *Am J Epidemiol.* 2009;170:766-774.

356. Raz R, Stamm WE. A controlled trial of intravaginal estriol in postmenopausal women with recurrent urinary tract infections. *N Engl J Med.* 1993;329:753-756.

357. Siris ES, Adler R, Bilezikian J, et al. The clinical diagnosis of osteoporosis: a position statement from the National Bone Health Alliance Working Group. *Osteoporos Int.* 2014;25:1439-1443.

358. Richelson LS, Wahner HW, Melton LJ 3rd, Riggs BL. Relative contributions of aging and estrogen deficiency to postmenopausal bone loss. *N Engl J Med.* 1984;311:1273-1275.

359. Nilas L, Christiansen C. Bone mass and its relationship to age and the menopause. *J Clin Endocrinol Metab.* 1987;65:697-702.

360. Christiansen C. Hormone replacement therapy and osteoporosis. *Maturitas.* 1996;23(Suppl):S71-S76.

361. Manson JE, Chlebowski RT, Stefanick ML, et al. Menopausal hormone therapy and health outcomes during the intervention and extended poststopping phases of the Women's Health Initiative randomized trials. *JAMA.* 2013;310:1353-1368.

362. Manson JE. Current recommendations: what is the clinician to do? *Fertil Steril.* 2014;101:916-921.

363. Nicholson WK, Brown AF, Gathe J, et al. Hormone replacement therapy for African American women: missed opportunities for effective intervention. *Menopause.* 1999;6:147-155.

364. Prentice RL, Anderson GL. The women's health initiative: lessons learned. *Annu Rev Public Health.* 2008;29:131-150.

365. American College of Obstetrics and Gynecology. ACOG Committee Opinion No. 420, November 2008: hormone therapy and heart disease. *Obstet Gynecol.* 2008;112:1189-1192.

366. Ness J, Aronow WS, Newkirk E, McDaniel D. Use of hormone replacement therapy by postmenopausal women after publication of the Women's Health Initiative Trial. *J Gerontol A Biol Sci Med Sci.* 2005;60:460-462.

367. Hoffmann M, Hammar M, Kjellgren KI, et al. Changes in women's attitudes towards and use of hormone therapy after HERS and WHI. *Maturitas.* 2005;52:11-17.

368. Thunell L, Milsom I, Schmidt J, Mattsson LA. Scientific evidence changes prescribing practice: a comparison of the management of the climacteric and use of hormone replacement therapy among Swedish gynaecologists in 1996 and 2003. *BJOG.* 2006;113:15-20.

369. Miller VM, Black DM, Brinton EA, et al. Using basic science to design a clinical trial: baseline characteristics of women enrolled in the Kronos Early Estrogen Prevention Study (KEEPS). *J Cardiovasc Transl Res.* 2009;2:228-239.

370. Shumaker SA, Legault C, Rapp SR, et al. Estrogen plus progestin and the incidence of dementia and mild cognitive impairment in postmenopausal women: the Women's Health Initiative Memory Study: a randomized controlled trial. *JAMA.* 2003;289:2651-2662.

371. Hulley S, Grady D, Bush T, et al. Randomized trial of estrogen plus progestin for secondary prevention of coronary heart disease in postmenopausal women. Heart and Estrogen/progestin Replacement Study (HERS) Research Group. *JAMA.* 1998;280:605-613.

372. Prentice RL, Chlebowski RT, Stefanick ML, et al. Estrogen plus progestin therapy and breast cancer in recently postmenopausal women. *Am J Epidemiol.* 2008;167:1207-1216.

373. Vandenbroucke JP. The HRT controversy: observational studies and RCTs fall in line. *Lancet.* 2009;373:1233-1235.

374. Lacey JV Jr, Mink PJ, Lubin JH, et al. Menopausal hormone replacement therapy and risk of ovarian cancer. *JAMA.* 2002;288:334-341.

375. Shumaker SA, Legault C, Kuller L, et al. Conjugated equine estrogens and incidence of probable dementia and mild cognitive impairment in postmenopausal women: Women's Health Initiative Memory Study. *JAMA.* 2004;291:2947-2958.

376. Glueck CJ, Lang J, Hamer T, Tracy T. Severe hypertriglyceridemia and pancreatitis when estrogen replacement therapy is given to hypertriglyceridemic women. *J Lab Clin Med.* 1994;123:59-64.

377. Cirillo DJ, Wallace RB, Rodabough RJ, et al. Effect of estrogen therapy on gallbladder disease. *JAMA.* 2005;293:330-339.

378. Chlebowski RT, Schwartz AG, Wakelee H, et al. Oestrogen plus progestin and lung cancer in postmenopausal women (Women's Health Initiative trial): a post-hoc analysis of a randomised controlled trial. *Lancet.* 2009;374:1243-1251.

379. Martin KA, Manson JE. Approach to the patient with menopausal symptoms. *J Clin Endocrinol Metab.* 2008;93:4567-4575.

380. Riis BJ, Hansen MA, Jensen AM, et al. Low bone mass and fast rate of bone loss at menopause: equal risk factors for future fracture: a 15-year follow-up study. *Bone.* 1996;19:9-12.

381. Ettinger B, Pressman A, Van Gessel A. Low-dosage esterified estrogens opposed by progestin at 6-month intervals. *Obstet Gynecol.* 2001;98:205-211.

382. Lindheim SR, Presser SC, Ditkoff EC, et al. A possible bimodal effect of estrogen on insulin sensitivity in postmenopausal women and the attenuating effect of added progestin. *Fertil Steril.* 1993;60:664-667.

383. Woodruff JD, Pickar JH. Incidence of endometrial hyperplasia in postmenopausal women taking conjugated estrogens (Premarin) with medroxyprogesterone acetate or conjugated estrogens alone. The Menopause Study Group. *Am J Obstet Gynecol.* 1994;170:1213-1223.

384. Archer DF, Pickar JH, Bottiglioni F. Bleeding patterns in postmenopausal women taking continuous combined or sequential regimens of conjugated estrogens with medroxyprogesterone acetate. Menopause Study Group. *Obstet Gynecol.* 1994;83:686-692.

385. The Writing Group for the PEPI Trial. Effects of estrogen or estrogen/progestin regimens on heart disease risk factors in postmenopausal women. The Postmenopausal Estrogen/Progestin Interventions (PEPI) Trial. *JAMA.* 1995;273:199-208.

386. Reed SD, Newton KM, Lacroix AZ. Indications for hormone therapy: the post-Women's Health Initiative era. *Endocrinol Metab Clin North Am.* 2004;33:691-715.

387. Harman SM, Naftolin F, Brinton EA, Judelson DR. Is the estrogen controversy over? Deconstructing the Women's Health Initiative study: a critical evaluation of the evidence. *Ann N Y Acad Sci.* 2005;1052:43-56.

388. Espeland MA, Rapp SR, Shumaker SA, et al. Conjugated equine estrogens and global cognitive function in postmenopausal women: Women's Health Initiative Memory Study. *JAMA.* 2004;291:2959-2968.

389. Nand SL, Webster MA, Baber R, O'Connor V. Bleeding pattern and endometrial changes during continuous combined hormone replacement therapy. The Ogen/Provera Study Group. *Obstet Gynecol.* 1998;91:678-684.

390. Korhonen MO, Symons JP, Hyde BM, et al. Histologic classification and pathologic findings for endometrial biopsy specimens obtained from 2964 perimenopausal and postmenopausal women undergoing screening for continuous hormones as replacement therapy (CHART 2 Study). *Am J Obstet Gynecol.* 1997;176:377-380.

391. McGonigle KF, Karlan BY, Barbuto DA, et al. Development of endometrial cancer in women on estrogen and progestin hormone replacement therapy. *Gynecol Oncol.* 1994;55:126-132.

392. Karlsson B, Granberg S, Wikland M, et al. Transvaginal ultrasonography of the endometrium in women with postmenopausal bleeding: a Nordic multicenter study. *Am J Obstet Gynecol.* 1995;172:1488-1494.

393. Bakos O, Smith P, Heimer G. Transvaginal ultrasonography for identifying endometrial pathology in postmenopausal women. *Maturitas.* 1994;20:181-189.

394. Granberg S, Ylostalo P, Wikland M, Karlsson B. Endometrial sonographic and histologic findings in women with and without hormonal replacement therapy suffering from postmenopausal bleeding. *Maturitas.* 1997;27:35-40.

395. Avis NE. Breast cancer survivors and hot flashes: the search for nonhormonal treatments. *J Clin Oncol.* 2008;26:5008-5010.

396. Holmberg L, Iversen OE, Rudenstam CM, et al. Increased risk of recurrence after hormone replacement therapy in breast cancer survivors. *J Natl Cancer Inst.* 2008;100:475-482.

397. Brunner RL, Gass M, Aragaki A, et al. Effects of conjugated equine estrogen on health-related quality of life in postmenopausal women with hysterectomy: results from the Women's Health Initiative Randomized Clinical Trial. *Arch Intern Med.* 2005;165:1976-1986.

398. Jordan VC, O'Malley BW. Selective estrogen-receptor modulators and antihormonal resistance in breast cancer. *J Clin Oncol.* 2007;25:5815-5824.

399. Nelson HD, Fu R, Griffin JC, et al. Systematic review: comparative effectiveness of medications to reduce risk for primary breast cancer. *Ann Intern Med.* 2009;151:703-715, W-226-235.

400. Rapp SR, Espeland MA, Shumaker SA, et al. Effect of estrogen plus progestin on global cognitive function in postmenopausal women: the Women's Health Initiative Memory Study: a randomized controlled trial. *JAMA.* 2003;289:2663-2672.

401. Bilezikian JP. Efficacy of bisphosphonates in reducing fracture risk in postmenopausal osteoporosis. *Am J Med.* 2009;122:S14-S21.

402. Jansen JP, Bergman GJ, Huels J, Olson M. Prevention of vertebral fractures in osteoporosis: mixed treatment comparison of bisphosphonate therapies. *Curr Med Res Opin.* 2009;25:1861-1868.

403. Bianchi G, Sambrook P. Oral nitrogen-containing bisphosphonates: a systematic review of randomized clinical trials and vertebral fractures. *Curr Med Res Opin.* 2008;24:2669-2677.

404. Bonnick S, Saag KG, Kiel DP, et al. Comparison of weekly treatment of postmenopausal osteoporosis with alendronate versus risedronate over two years. *J Clin Endocrinol Metab.* 2006;91:2631-2637.

405. Lodi G, Sardella A, Salis A, et al. Tooth extraction in patients taking intravenous bisphosphonates: a preventive protocol and case series. *J Oral Maxillofac Surg.* 2010;68:107-110.

406. Gnant M, Mlineritsch B, Schippinger W, et al. Endocrine therapy plus zoledronic acid in premenopausal breast cancer. *N Engl J Med.* 2009;360:679-691.

407. Wysowski DK. Reports of esophageal cancer with oral bisphosphonate use. *N Engl J Med.* 2009;360:89-90.

408. Green J, Czanner G, Reeves G, et al. Oral bisphosphonates and risk of cancer of oesophagus, stomach, and colorectum: case-control analysis within a UK primary care cohort. *BMJ.* 2010;341:c4444.

409. Cardwell CR, Abnet CC, Cantwell MM, Murray LJ. Exposure to oral bisphosphonates and risk of esophageal cancer. *JAMA.* 2010;304:657-663.

410. Cummings SR, Ettinger B, Delmas PD, et al. The effects of tibolone in older postmenopausal women. *N Engl J Med.* 2008;359:697-708.

411. Bundred NJ, Kenemans P, Yip CH, et al. Tibolone increases bone mineral density but also relapse in breast cancer survivors: LIBERATE trial bone substudy. *Breast Cancer Res.* 2012;14:R13.

CHAPTER 18

Hormonal Contraception

REBECCA H. ALLEN • ANDREW M. KAUNITZ • MARTHA HICKEY

KEY POINTS

- Because pregnancy in women with underlying medical conditions is associated with higher risks of maternal and perinatal morbidity and mortality, achieving effective preconception and family planning care is particularly important in this setting. Health care providers should consult the U.S. Medical Eligibility Criteria for Contraceptive Use (USMEC) from the Centers for Disease Control and Prevention (CDC) when caring for these women.
- Reducing health care system barriers to contraceptive initiation and continuation is important to reduce unintended pregnancy rates. Such barriers include requiring unnecessary health screenings, waiting until menstruation to begin methods, inappropriate contraindications, and failure to provide adequate refills for prescription-based methods. The Selected Practice Recommendations for Contraceptive Use from the CDC offers evidence-based guidelines to assist providers in caring for women who need contraception.
- Long-acting reversible contraceptive methods, which include the copper intrauterine device (IUD), the two levonorgestrel intrauterine systems, and the etonogestrel subdermal implant, provide superior contraceptive effectiveness, equivalent to sterilization, and higher continuation and satisfaction rates compared with shorter-acting methods. These methods should be offered preferentially to all women, including adolescents.
- Emergency contraception should be readily available to all women at risk for unplanned pregnancy. The copper IUD is the most effective emergency contraceptive, followed by ulipristal acetate and levonorgestrel.
- Besides offering highly effective contraception, the higher dose levonorgestrel intrauterine system is a first-line treatment for heavy menstrual bleeding and an effective alternative to endometrial ablation and hysterectomy.

Prevention of unplanned pregnancy continues to challenge clinicians and consumers in developed and developing countries. Pregnancies that are unintended or too closely spaced can lead to adverse maternal and child health outcomes.[1] Most women in the United States and other developed countries desire to have two children.[2] Therefore, on average, sexually active women devote more than 3 decades of their lives to avoiding unintended pregnancy. However, over half (51%) of all pregnancies in the United States are unintended.[3] Women who use contraception consistently and correctly account for only 5% of unintended pregnancies, but women who use contraception inconsistently or incorrectly account for 43%, and women who do not use contraception account for 52% of unintended pregnancies.[2] In developing countries, childbirth and unsafe abortion are important causes of maternal death and morbidity, and the unintended pregnancy rate is estimated at 40%.[4] For all couples, access to contraception is critical to be able to plan the timing and spacing of their childbearing for social, economic, and health reasons.[5]

Contraceptive advice and provision should start before the commencement of sexual activity and continue through the reproductive years. Although on the decline, the United States still has one of the highest teenage pregnancy rates in the developed world.[6] Teenaged parenting commonly has adverse consequences for the adolescent, her children, and her family.[7] Programs to prevent unplanned pregnancy by promoting abstinence have largely been ineffective. Nonhormonal contraceptives, such as male condoms, may offer benefits in terms of protection against sexually transmitted infection (STI) but are highly user-dependent and do not reliably prevent unplanned pregnancy in many populations. Female hormonal contraception, along with the copper IUD, represents the most effective and acceptable reversible contraceptive option; male hormonal contraception has not achieved this goal. The ideal contraceptive would be safe, highly effective, discreet, inexpensive, long acting, easily reversible, and under the woman's control. It would not need to be activated at or around the time of intercourse and would not disrupt vaginal bleeding patterns. The ideal contraceptive would also protect against STIs. Because an ideal contraceptive does not exist, the challenge for clinicians is to tailor the available methods to the medical, personal, and social needs of the woman and her partner as these needs evolve throughout her reproductive life span. The clinician must also learn to recognize and address barriers to the safe and effective implementation of the selected methods. Hormonal contraceptives are most effectively used by women who are well informed about the advantages and likely side effects of the method and who have actively participated in selecting the method. Guidance on medical eligibility for contraceptives can be found in two companion documents from the CDC, entitled "U.S. Medical Eligibility Criteria for Contraceptive Use, 2010" and "U.S. Selected Practice Recommendations for Contraceptive Use, 2013."[8,9]

In addition to enhancing quality of life by allowing couples to choose whether and when they wish to bear children, effective contraception lowers health care costs.[10] Male and female sterilization and long-acting reversible methods (e.g., IUDs, subdermal implants) constitute the most cost-effective contraceptive options, followed by other hormonal methods (e.g., oral contraceptives). Depot medroxyprogesterone acetate (DMPA) injection is more cost-effective than oral contraception. Barrier and behavioral methods (i.e., male condom and withdrawal, respectively) are the least cost-effective compared with other contraceptive options. Nevertheless, when compared with no method, they still prevent a large number of unintended pregnancies, leading to important cost savings.

COMBINED ESTROGEN AND PROGESTIN CONTRACEPTIVES

Methods that combine estrogen and progestin offer the advantage of relatively regular bleeding patterns and high efficacy if used consistently. These combined methods are available in oral, transdermal, and transvaginal preparations that thereby provide increased flexibility in choice of delivery system.

The Combined Oral Contraceptive Pill

Combined oral contraceptives (COCs) offer safe, reversible, and convenient birth control that is highly effective for those who take pills correctly. In many settings, oral contraception provides important noncontraceptive benefits that should be discussed during counseling.[11] By individualizing counseling and follow-up strategies based on relevant behavioral and medical considerations, clinicians can maximize their patients' success with COCs. The effectiveness of COCs is closely linked with correct and consistent use. Women who consistently take pills correctly have one or two pregnancies per 100 woman-years. However, with typical use, the failure rate is 9 pregnancies per 100 women-years.[12] Unscheduled spotting and bleeding occur in about 30% to 50% of women during the first 3 months of use but become much less common with ongoing use.[13] Counseling patients to anticipate early breakthrough bleeding and reassuring those who experience this side effect may improve continuation rates. Women who are bothered by hormone withdrawal symptoms during the hormone-free interval (HFI) or who may benefit from less frequent withdrawal bleeding may benefit from the newer formulations of oral contraceptives that shorten or eliminate the HFI.[14] Perimenopausal women may benefit from the regularity of bleeding, relief from vasomotor symptoms, and positive impact on bone mineral density (BMD) offered by combination oral contraception.[15] COCs have been available for more than 50 years and have gradually been refined to improve safety, efficacy, and acceptability. COCs are used by more than 10 million U.S. women, making them the most widely used hormonal contraceptive method.[16] Currently used methods contain estrogen, usually as ethinyl estradiol, at doses of 10 to 35 μg/day and a range of progestins. This section describes COCs available in the United States, focusing on education, counseling, and management measures to maximize contraceptive efficacy.

Composition and Formulations

Over time, the dose of estrogen and progestin in COCs has gradually decreased, and the types of progestins have changed. Currently, the highest-dose formulations marketed in the United States contain 50 μg of estrogen, and most COCs prescribed contain 35 μg or less. The vast majority modern COCs formulated with 35 μg of estrogen or less use ethinyl estradiol, which is a potent synthetic estrogen with similar metabolic effects (e.g., liver protein production) regardless of the route of administration because of its long half-life and slow metabolism.[17] Estradiol valerate has been released as a component of one newer COC, Natazia (Bayer Healthcare Pharmaceuticals). Estradiol valerate is a synthetic hormone that is extensively metabolized to estradiol and valeric acid before reaching the systemic circulation. A daily dose of 2 mg of estradiol valerate has biologic effects on the uterus, ovary, and hypothalamic-pituitary-ovarian axis similar to those of a 20-μg dose of ethinyl estradiol.[18] A COC formulated with 1.5 mg of micronized estradiol and the progestin nomegestrol acetate has been approved for use in some European countries but is not currently marketed in the United States.[19] Older COC preparations marketed in the United States contain one of five progestins: norethindrone, norethindrone acetate, ethynodiol diacetate, norgestrel, or levonorgestrel. Newer formulations contain the more potent progestins norgestimate, desogestrel, drospirenone, and dienogest.

Many COC formulations are marketed in the United States (Table 18-1). These products do not appear to be different in terms of safety or efficacy if used correctly.[13] COCs were originally formulated to mimic the normal menstrual cycle by providing 21 days of combined estrogen and progestin, followed by a 7-day pill-free week when withdrawal bleeding occurred. Most modern COCs mainly continue to follow this regimen and contain active pills for 21 to 24 days, although there is no evidence that an HFI provides any health benefits. COCs typically come in 28-day packages designed to be simple to use. Pills are still taken during the HFI, but they do not contain sex steroids.

Hormone-withdrawal symptoms, including pelvic pain, breast tenderness, and mood symptoms, may occur during the HFI.[20,21] A 4-day HFI has been shown to reduce these hormone withdrawal symptoms compared to a 7-day interval. In addition, less pituitary-ovarian activity during the HFI is noted in the 24/4 regimen compared to the 21/7 regimen.[22,23] Some women may ovulate if the HFI is extended beyond 7 days. There is less opportunity for follicle development and possible ovulation during shorter HFIs.[24] This may potentially increase efficacy.[25] COC regimens differ in whether the dose of ethinyl estradiol and progestin is the same throughout the 21 days of use or the doses vary. Monophasic preparations have a constant dose of estrogen and progestin in each of the 21 or 24 active hormone tables in each cycle pack. Phasic preparations alter the dose of the progestin and, in some formulations, the estrogen component among the active tablets in each pack. There is no evidence that phasic preparations are superior to monophasic formulations in terms of efficacy or bleeding patterns.[26]

The HFI can be modified or eliminated in order to improve contraceptive success; reduce the hormone-withdrawal symptoms; improve treatment of problems such as dysmenorrhea, pelvic pain, and anemia; and be more convenient for some women.[27] Newer oral contraception pills offer extended-cycle regimens of 84 pills, followed by 7 days of inert tablets or tablets containing 10 μg of ethinyl estradiol in place of the conventional HFI. These formulations offer only four scheduled withdrawal bleeds per year. In addition, a continuous COC with no HFI is available.

TABLE 18-1

Oral Contraceptive Formulations Available in the United States

Description	Name	Estrogen	Progestin	Progestin Dose (mg)
EE, 50 µg monophasic	Ovcon 50	EE	Norethindrone	1
	Ogestrel 0.5/50	EE	Norgestrel	0.5
	Zovia 1/50	EE	Ethynodiol diacetate	1
	Norinyl 1 + 50*	Mestranol	Norethindrone	1
EE, 35 µg monophasic	Femcon Fe chewable	EE	Norethindrone	0.4
	Modicon*	EE	Norethindrone	0.5
	Brevicon*	EE	Norethindrone	0.5
	Ovcon 35*	EE	Norethindrone	0.4
	Ortho-Cyclen*	EE	Norgestimate	0.25
	Zovia 1/35*	EE	Ethynodiol diacetate	1
	Ortho-Novum 1/35*	EE	Norethindrone	1
	Norinyl 1 + 35*	EE	Norethindrone	1
EE, 35 µg biphasic	Ortho-Novum 10/11*	EE	Norethindrone	0.5/1
EE, 35 µg triphasic	Ortho-Novum 7/7/7*	EE	Norethindrone	0.5/0.75/1
	Ortho Tri-Cyclen*†	EE	Norgestimate	0.18/0.215/0.25
	Tri-Norinyl*	EE	Norethindrone	0.5/1.0/0.5
	Estrostep*†	EE (µg) (20/30/35)	Norethindrone acetate	1
EE, 30 µg monophasic	Loestrin 1.5/30*	EE	Norethindrone acetate	1.5
	Ortho-Cept*	EE	Desogestrel	0.15
	Desogen*	EE	Desogestrel	0.15
	Lo-Ovral*	EE	Norgestrel	0.3
	Nordette*	EE	Levonorgestrel	0.15
	Levora*	EE	Levonorgestrel	0.15
	Yasmin*	EE	Drosperinone	3.0
EE, 30 µg triphasic	Triphasil*	EE (µg) (30/40/30)	Levonorgestrel	0.05/0.075/0.125
	Trivora*	EE (µg) (30/40/30)	Levonorgestrel	0.05/0.075/0.125
EE, 30 µg extended cycle (84 estrogen/progestin tablets)	Seasonale*	EE	Levonorgestrel	0.15
EE, 30 µg extended cycle (84 estrogen/progestin tablets, 7 tablets 10 µg EE)	Seasonique*	EE	Levonorgestrel	0.15
EE, 30 µg extended cycle triphasic (84 estrogen/progestin tablets, 7 tablets 10 µg EE)	Quartette	EE (µg) (20/25/30)	Levonorgestrel	0.15
EE, 25 µg monophasic	Generess Fe chewable	EE	Norethindrone	0.8
EE, 25 µg triphasic	Cyclessa*	EE	Desogestrel	0.10/0.125/0.15
	Ortho Tri-Cyclen Lo*	EE	Norgestimate	0.18/0.215/0.25
EE, 20 µg monophasic	Loestrin 1/20*	EE	Norethindrone acetate	1
	Lutera*	EE	Levonorgestrel	0.1
EE, 20 µg biphasic	Mircette*	EE (µg) (20/10)	Desogestrel	0.15
EE, 20 µg 24/4 (24 estrogen/progestin tablets)	Yaz*†‡	EE	Drosperinone	3.0
	Minastrin 24 Fe chewable	EE	Norethindrone acetate	1
EE, 20 µg extended cycle (84 estrogen/progestin tablets, 7 tablets 10 µg EE)	LoSeasonique*	EE	Levonorgestrel	0.1
EE, 20 µg extended cycle (all estrogen/progestin tablets)	Amethyst	EE	Levonorgestrel	0.09
EE, 10 µg 24/4 (24 estrogen/progestin tablets, 2 tablets 10 µg EE)	Lo Loestrin Fe	EE	Norethindrone	1
Estradiol valerate, quadriphasic	Natazia§	EV (mg) (3/2/2/1)	Dienogest	2/3
Progestin-only	Micronor*	N/A	Norethindrone	0.35

*Generic versions available.
†Indicated for the treatment of acne in women desiring to use oral contraception.
‡Indicated for the treatment of premenstrual dysphoric disorder in women desiring to use oral contraception.
§Indicated for the treatment of heavy menstrual bleeding in women desiring to use oral contraception.
EE, ethinyl estradiol; EV, estradiol valerate.

Mechanism of Action, Efficacy, Administration, and Effect on Pregnancy

Administration of COCs prevents ovulation by inhibiting gonadotropin secretion through the effect of estrogen and progestin on the pituitary and hypothalamus. Both steroids in COCs contribute to the suppression of ovulation.

Because the contraceptive efficacy of COCs relies on daily use, failure rates are largely attributable to poor adherence. Failure rates range from less than 1 per 100 woman-years (Pearl index) with excellent adherence to more than 15 pregnancies per 100 woman-years with low adherence. Typical first-year combination oral contraception failure rates are estimated at 9 per 100 women.[12]

Traditionally, COCs have been started on the first day of menses, but the pills can be safely started at any time if pregnancy has been excluded (quick start method).[28] This approach may reduce unplanned pregnancies occurring while women are waiting until menses to start the pills. If the COCs are inadvertently taken during pregnancy, they do not appear to increase the rate of miscarriage or adversely affect the developing fetus.[29]

Because daily use is critical to ensure contraceptive efficacy, some women prefer to link pill taking with a daily ritual (e.g., tooth brushing) or to use daily reminders through e-mail or text-messaging. Clear instructions for managing missed pills are an essential component of COC counseling. If a woman misses one tablet, she should take the missed pill as soon as possible even if it means taking two pills on the same day. She should then continue to take one tablet daily and no additional contraceptive protection is needed.[9] If she has missed two or more consecutive tablets, she should take the most recent pill and continue taking the remaining pills at the usual time, even if it means taking two pills on the same day. In this instance, she should use an additional form of contraception (e.g., condoms) for 7 days. If two or more pills were missed in the third week of the 28-day pack, she can omit the HFI in the current pack and start a new pack.[9] Emergency contraception can also be considered in these cases. COCs are not suitable for women who consistently miss pills, because this undermines contraceptive efficacy. In these cases, a method that does not require daily adherence (e.g., contraceptive rings; patches; an injectable, intrauterine, or implantable method) should be considered.

After discontinuation of COCs, most women rapidly resume ovulation. Some women may ovulate if the HFI is extended beyond 7 days. In some women, ovulation may be temporarily delayed for several months after discontinuing oral contraception; however, 12-month conception rates are no different in former pill users compared to women who discontinue other contraceptive methods.[30]

Noncontraceptive Health Benefits

For many users, COCs offer substantial noncontraceptive health benefits. These advantages include reductions in dysmenorrhea and symptoms of premenstrual syndrome, creating predictable withdrawal bleeding in women with abnormal uterine bleeding, reducing the daily intensity and duration of menstrual flow, improving anemia, and markedly reducing the risk of ovarian and endometrial cancer.[11] Educating COC candidates and users regarding these noncontraceptive benefits can assist the patient in making a choice and can increase oral contraception adherence and continuation.

Benign breast diseases, including fibroadenoma and cystic changes, occur less commonly in COC users. Functional follicular ovarian cysts are not reliably suppressed by modern COC formulations containing 35 μg of estradiol or less; however, postovulatory ovarian cysts (corpus luteum cysts) are reduced. COC use reduces the incidence of ectopic pregnancy, a common and potentially life-threatening condition.[31] The perimenopausal transition is a time of accelerated loss of BMD. In perimenopausal women, COCs can maintain BMD, improve reduced BMD, and possibly reduce the risk of postmenopausal fracture. Skeletal health benefits associated with COC use may also apply to women who have been hypoestrogenic and those with hypothalamic amenorrhea.[32]

Reducing the risk of epithelial ovarian and endometrial cancer is perhaps the most important noncontraceptive benefit of COC use. Although the incidence is low, epithelial ovarian cancer is the most common cause of death from gynecologic malignancy in the United States. The reduction in borderline and invasive ovarian cancer risk with COC use is consistently about 40% among short-term users and as much as 80% among women who have taken COCs for more than 10 years; risk reduction persists for more than 15 years after discontinuation of oral contraception.[33] A woman in her late 30s or 40s taking COCs reduces her risk of ovarian cancer during the peak presentation of this disease (i.e., age of 50 to 60 years). Worldwide, an estimated 100,000 deaths from epithelial ovarian cancer have been prevented since COCs first became available in the 1960s; current COC use is estimated to prevent an additional 30,000 such deaths each year.[33] There is also some evidence that women with an inherited increased risk of ovarian cancer due to *BRCA1* or *BRCA2* mutations may have a reduced risk of ovarian cancer when using COCs.[34,35] Although only limited data address this issue and study findings have not been consistent, use of COCs does not appear to increase breast cancer risk in *BRCA* mutation carriers.[36] Accordingly, although it is reasonable for women with *BRCA1* or *BRCA2* mutations to use COCs, the risks and benefits should be weighed by each woman and her clinician.[37,38]

Endometrial adenocarcinoma is the most common gynecologic cancer in U.S. women, and rising obesity rates put more women at risk. The risk of endometrial adenocarcinoma is reduced by 40% with 12 months of COC use and by 80% with 10 years of COC use,[39] and the protection persists for at least 20 years after oral contraception discontinuation.[40] All COC formulations appear to treat acne.[41] Selected COC formulations are approved by the U.S. Food and Drug Administration (FDA) for the treatment of acne (i.e., ethinyl estradiol/triphasic norgestimate, estrophasic norethindrone acetate, and ethinyl estradiol/drospirenone), for premenstrual dysphoric disorder (24/4 20-μg ethinyl estradiol/3-mg drospirenone) and for heavy menstrual bleeding (estradiol valerate/dienogest).

Side Effects

Contrary to popular perception, randomized, placebo-controlled trials have not shown that COCs cause weight gain, headaches, nausea, breast tenderness, or mood changes.[42,43] Therefore, COCs are well tolerated by most users. Nevertheless, some individuals report side effects that they attribute to COCs that may affect quality of life, contraceptive continuation, and patient satisfaction. Therefore, counseling about side effects or lack thereof is an important aspect of contraceptive care and may improve patient tolerance and adherence to COCs when they occur.[44]

The side effect of unscheduled vaginal bleeding, however, is common and attributable to COCs. Unscheduled bleeding affects about 30% to 50% of COC users during the initial 3 months of use, but the incidence declines with ongoing use. Unscheduled bleeding is more common with lower-dose (20 μg) than standard-dose (30 or 35 μg) ethinyl estradiol preparations.[45] In addition, unscheduled bleeding is more common in women using extended COC formulations in the early cycles, but this bleeding will lessen over time. If unscheduled bleeding during extended COC use is bothersome, women may opt to stop active tablets for 3 days, thereby inducing withdrawal bleeding, and then continue with active pills. This strategy has been shown to reduce subsequent unscheduled bleeding in this setting.[46]

Because irregular bleeding may be a manifestation of pregnancy or disease such as cervical or endometrial infection, polyps, or neoplasia, persistent or new-onset bleeding should be investigated. There are no FDA-approved treatments for unscheduled bleeding associated with hormonal contraception. Amenorrhea may occur with long-term COC use, and it is variably tolerated by patients. It may be more acceptable with counseling that provides appropriate reassurance.[44] Women who experience absence of withdrawal bleeding or who for other reasons suspect they could be pregnant should use a urine pregnancy test.

Headaches are common, but for most women, there is no evidence that COC use contributes to headaches.[47] Nevertheless, any new-onset or worsening headache with COC use must be evaluated. A history of migraine plus aura is a contraindication for use of COCs because of the increased risk of stroke.[8] For women 35 years of age or older, combination estrogen-progestin contraceptives should be avoided by all with migraines. Similarly, any COC users who experience increased frequency or intensity of any type of migraine headache should discontinue estrogen-containing contraceptives. If migraine headaches occur only during withdrawal bleeding, elimination of the HFI may be therapeutic.[47]

Health Risks

Extensive studies in large populations have established the risks and benefits of COCs for most women.[48] Results indicate that for most women, use of COCs represents a safe contraceptive choice. However, clinicians should be aware of circumstances in which the COC may pose health risks. The U.S. Medical Eligibility Criteria (USMEC), released in 2010 from the CDC, were adapted from the World Health Organization (WHO) document Medical Eligibility Criteria for Contraceptive Use, 4th edition (Tables 18-2 and 18-3).[8] The guidelines provide evidence-based advice on eligibility for use of hormonal contraceptives. The guidelines will be updated every 3 to 4 years as new evidence emerges. Although the WHO document covered many conditions such as postpartum status, breastfeeding, smoking, obesity, cardiovascular disease, diabetes, and cancer, the USMEC added new categories: endometrial hyperplasia, rheumatoid arthritis, solid organ transplantation, inflammatory bowel disease, bariatric surgery, and peripartum cardiomyopathy. The USMEC assists providers in deciding what contraceptive methods are appropriate for their patients. This guidance will likely improve access to contraception, especially among women with medical problems for which providers may have been hesitant to prescribe contraception in the past.[8,49] The safety of contraception in the USMEC is considered in four categories:

1. Conditions with no restriction on the use of the contraceptive method.
2. Conditions in which the advantages of the method usually outweigh the theoretical or proven risks. The method can generally be used, but careful follow-up may be required.
3. Conditions in which the theoretical or proven risks usually outweigh the advantages; examples include current gallbladder disease, diabetes with end-organ damage, controlled hypertension, and taking medications that may interfere with COC efficacy. The method is generally not recommended unless other more appropriate methods are not available or acceptable.
4. Conditions that present an unacceptable health risk if the contraceptive method is used; examples include delivery during the past 21 days, a personal history of deep venous thrombosis or pulmonary embolism, cardiovascular accident, known thrombogenic mutations, and migraine headaches with aura or other neurologic signs.

TABLE 18-2

U.S. Medical Eligibility Criteria for Contraceptive Use Categories for the Use of Estrogen-Containing Contraception According to Medical Condition

Condition	USMEC
Smoking age ≥ 35	
<15 cigarettes/day	Risks outweigh benefits
≥15 cigarettes/day	Unacceptable risk
Obesity (body mass index ≥ 30)	Benefits outweigh risks
Hypertension	
Controlled hypertension	Risks outweigh benefits
Elevated blood pressure	
Systolic 140-159 mm Hg or diastolic 90-99 mm Hg	Risks outweigh benefits
Systolic ≥ 160 mm Hg or diastolic ≥ 100 mm Hg	Unacceptable risk
Vascular disease	Unacceptable risk
Diabetes	
No vascular disease	Benefits outweigh risks
Vascular disease or > 20 years' duration	Either risks outweigh benefits or unacceptable risk (based on severity of condition)
Stroke	Unacceptable risk
Current or history of ischemic heart disease	Unacceptable risk
Multiple risk factors for cardiovascular disease (older age, smoking, obesity, diabetes, hypertension)	Either risks outweigh benefits or unacceptable risk (based on severity of condition)
Breast cancer	
Current	Unacceptable risk
Past and no evidence of disease for 5 years	Risks outweigh benefits
Migraines	
Without aura	
Age < 35 years	Benefits outweigh risks
Age ≥ 35 years	Risks outweigh benefits
With aura	Unacceptable risk

Thromboembolic Disease. The established increased risk of venous thromboembolism (VTE) is related to the estrogenic component.[50] Modern low-dose preparations (≤35 µg) carry a lower risk than the original oral contraceptives, but the incidence of VTE is still increased. No differences in VTE risk between 35- and 20- or 10-µg preparations have been established. Furthermore, there is no convincing evidence that VTE risk varies by type of progestin.[33,51,52] Other risk factors for VTE include, but are not limited to, age, obesity, smoking, and thrombogenic mutations.[52-54] In otherwise healthy reproductive age women, the risk of VTE ranges from 1 to 5 per 10,000 woman-years.[55] In women taking COCs, the absolute risk of VTE remains small, ranging from 3 to 9 cases per 10,000 woman-years (Fig. 18-1).[56] The VTE risk for COC use is significantly lower than that for women who are pregnant (5 to 20 per 10,000 woman-years) or post partum (40 to 65 per 10,000 woman-years).[57]

National guidelines recommend that the use of COC is contraindicated for those at increased risk for VTE: these high-risk women include those with a personal history of VTE, women immediately after delivery, women undergoing surgery with prolonged immobilization, and those with known inherited thrombophilic conditions.[8] Nonetheless, for the individual woman, a clinician may need to take into account her VTE risk based on the type of thrombophilia present and its association with risk factors, such as the coexistence of multiple thrombophilias, obesity, age, and any VTE events during prior periods of hormonal exposure, such as pregnancy and

TABLE 18-3

U.S. Medical Eligibility Criteria for Contraceptive Use Categories for the Use of Progestin-Only Methods of Contraception According to Medical Condition

Condition	POP	DMPA	Implant	Levonorgestrel IUD
Smoking age ≥ 35	No restriction	No restriction	No restriction	No restriction
Obesity ≥ 30 BMI	No restriction	No restriction	No restriction	No restriction
Menarche to age 18 and ≥ 30 BMI	No restriction	Benefits outweigh risks	No restriction	No restriction
Hypertension				
Controlled hypertension Elevated BP	No restriction	Benefits outweigh risks	No restriction	No restriction
Systolic 140-159 mm Hg or diastolic 90-99 mm Hg	No restriction	Benefits outweigh risks	No restriction	No restriction
Systolic ≥ 160 mm Hg or diastolic ≥ 100 mm Hg	Benefits outweigh risks	Risks outweigh benefits	Benefits outweigh risks	Benefits outweigh risks
Vascular disease	Benefits outweigh risks	Risks outweigh benefits	Benefits outweigh risks	Benefits outweigh risks
Diabetes				
No vascular disease	Benefits outweigh risks	Benefits outweigh risks	Benefits outweigh risks	Benefits outweigh risks
Vascular disease or > 20 years' duration	Benefits outweigh risks	Risks outweigh benefits	Benefits outweigh risks	Benefits outweigh risks
Stroke	I: Benefits outweigh risks C: Risks outweigh benefits	Risks outweigh benefits	I: Benefits outweigh risks C: Risks outweigh benefits	Benefits outweigh risks
Current or history of ischemic heart disease	I: Benefits outweigh risks C: Risks outweigh benefits	Risks outweigh benefits	I: Benefits outweigh risks C: Risks outweigh benefits	I: Benefits outweigh risks C: Risks outweigh benefits
Multiple risk factors for cardiovascular disease (older age, smoking, obesity, diabetes, hypertension)	Benefits outweigh risks	Risks outweigh benefits	Benefits outweigh risks	Benefits outweigh risks
Breast cancer				
Current	Contraindicated	Contraindicated	Contraindicated	Contraindicated
Past and no evidence of disease for 5 years	Risks outweigh benefits	Risks outweigh benefits	Risks outweigh benefits	Risks outweigh benefits
Migraines				
Without aura				
Age < 35 years	No restrictions	Benefits outweigh risks	Benefits outweigh risks	Benefits outweigh risks
Age ≥ 35 years	No restrictions	Benefits outweigh risks	Benefits outweigh risks	Benefits outweigh risks
With aura	Benefits outweigh risks	Benefits outweigh risks	Benefits outweigh risks	Benefits outweigh risks

BMI, body mass index; BP, blood pressure; C, continuation; DMPA, depot medroxyprogesterone acetate; I, initiation; IUD, intrauterine device; POP, progestin-only pill.

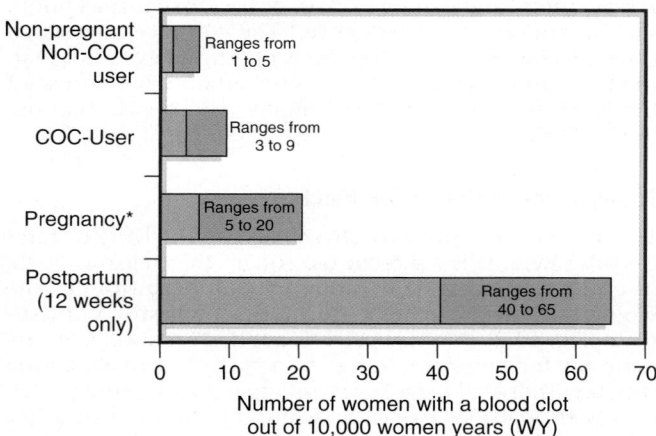

*Pregnancy data based on actual duration of pregnancy in the reference studies. Based on a model assumption that pregnancy duration is 9 months, the rate is 7 to 27 per 10,000 WY.

Figure 18-1 Venous thromboembolism risk among women of reproductive age by various conditions. COC, combined oral contraceptives. (From U.S. Food and Drug Administration. FDA Drug Safety Communication: Updated information about the risk of blood clots in women taking birth control pills containing drospirenone. Available at http://www.fda.gov/Drugs/DrugSafety/ucm299305.)

estrogen-containing contraceptives, in order to balance the risks and benefits of estrogen use. It is accepted, however, that routine screening of the general population for familial thrombophilic markers is not recommended before initiating COC use.[58]

Myocardial Infarction and Thrombotic and Hemorrhagic Stroke. Although arterial events are less common than VTE in reproductive-aged women, the sequelae of strokes and myocardial infarctions are more devastating than those of VTE. Myocardial infarction occurs rarely in COC users and is largely confined to thrombotic events in smokers.[29] Because cigarette smoking and COCs may act synergistically to increase the risk of myocardial infarction, and the absolute risk of myocardial infarction and stroke increases with age, COCs are generally contraindicated in smokers older than 35 years.[8] In a large Danish retrospective cohort study, the absolute risks of thrombotic stroke and myocardial infarction associated with COC use were low, but the risk was increased by a factor of 0.9 to 1.7 with COCs containing ethinyl estradiol at a dose of 20 μg and by a factor of 1.3 to 2.3 with those containing ethinyl estradiol at a dose of 30 to 40 μg. Risks were not increased with past use.[59] Among women with risk factors for myocardial infarction or stroke, including smoking, hypertension, diabetes, and migraine headache, COCs should be avoided by those older than 35 years.[8] Because COCs containing estradiol valerate are relatively new, there is limited data on their effects on the risk of VTE.

Breast Cancer. The association between use of menopausal estrogen-progestin therapy and breast cancer has led many to assume that COC use is associated with an increased risk of breast cancer. However, findings from a large, long-term cohort study in Britain and large case-control studies in the United States found that regardless of duration of use, neither current nor prior use of COC is associated with an increased risk of invasive or in situ breast cancer or death from breast cancer.[60,61] There is some evidence that women currently using COCs may be more likely to be diagnosed with breast cancer, but it is unknown if that is due to detection bias or promotion of an already existing cancer.[62] Although many women at elevated risk for breast cancer due to affected family members are concerned that use of COC is unsafe, a large Canadian prospective study of women with a family history of breast cancer found that neither current nor prior use of COC was associated with an elevated risk of breast cancer.[63] Studies of women with known *BRCA* gene mutations have yielded mixed results with respect to the impact of COC use on breast cancer risk.[36,37]

Cervical Cancer. Pooled data from 24 studies including more than 16,000 women with cervical cancer and 35,000 without cervical cancer found that for current COC users, the risk of invasive cervical cancer increased with increasing duration of use (relative risk for ≥5 years' use versus never use = 1.90; 95% confidence interval [CI], 1.69 to 2.13). The risk declined after use ceased, and after 10 or more years, it returned to the risk level of never users. A similar pattern of risk was seen for invasive and in situ cancer and for women who tested positive for high-risk human papillomavirus (HPV) strains. However, 10 years' use of oral contraceptives from about age 20 to 30 years is estimated to increase the cumulative incidence of invasive cervical cancer by age 50 from only 7.3 to 8.3 cases per 1000 women in less developed countries and from 3.8 to 4.5 cases per 1000 women in more developed countries.[64] Regular cervical cancer screening according to national protocols is advised for all sexually active women, regardless of contraceptive use. A history of cervical intraepithelial neoplasia or genital HPV infection is not a contraindication for COC use.[8]

Use of Combined Oral Contraceptive Pills After Pregnancy

COCs may be initiated immediately after induced or spontaneous termination of a first- or second-trimester pregnancy but not immediately after term delivery because the risk of VTE is elevated during the puerperium.[57,65] Because estrogens may reduce milk production, some experts do not think they represent an optimal contraceptive choice in lactating women.[66] However, ovulation may occur as early as 3 weeks after delivery in nonbreastfeeding women, and this consideration may be foremost for women wishing to initiate use of COCs.[49] The use of progestin-only contraceptives in postpartum and lactating women is addressed later in this chapter.

Use of Concomitant Medications With Combined Oral Contraceptive Pills

Certain anticonvulsants (phenytoin, carbamazepine, barbiturates, primidone, topiramate, and oxcarbazepine) that induce hepatic enzymes may reduce the contraceptive efficacy of COCs.[8] The antibiotic rifampicin/rifabutin can also interact with contraceptive hormones and reduce the efficacy of the contraceptive during and up to 4 weeks after use. In addition, antiretrovirals can reduce the efficacy of hormonal contraception including some nonnucleoside reverse transcriptase inhibitors (efavirenz and nevirapine) and some ritonavir-boosted (/r) protease inhibitors (darunavir/r, fosamprenavir/r, lopinavir/r, saquinavir/r, and tipranavir/r).[67] If oral contraceptives are used with these medications, a formulation containing at least 30 µg of ethinyl estradiol and backup contraception in the form of condoms should be used.[8] Alternatively, high-dose progestin-only methods such as DMPA or intrauterine contraceptives may be preferable because their efficacy is not reduced by medications that induce liver enzymes.

Contraceptive Vaginal Ring and Contraceptive Patch

The transdermal and transvaginal routes are safe and acceptable alternatives to COCs to deliver combined estrogen-progestin contraception. The contraceptive patch (Ortho Evra, Janssen Pharmaceuticals) and the contraceptive vaginal ring (NuvaRing, Merck) offer women combination estrogen-progestin contraception without the need to take pills daily. In consistent users, the contraceptive failure rates with the patch and ring are similar to those for oral contraceptives at 9%.[12] Contraceptive efficacy may be slightly reduced in patch users weighing more than 90 kg,[68] but the patch is still a contraceptive option for those women.[8] It is important to note that the use of nonoral combined hormonal contraceptives is not necessarily "safer" than oral contraceptives in terms of VTE risk because ethinyl estradiol activates clotting factors regardless of whether the route of administration is oral, vaginal, or transdermal.[69] Contraindications to the patch and the vaginal ring are the same as those for COCs. In the absence of adequate evidence to determine how the risks and noncontraceptive benefits of the patch and the ring compare with those of the COC, they are usually considered to be equivalent.

The contraceptive patch and vaginal ring act primarily by suppression of ovulation. The patch and ring are immediately effective if commenced within the first 5 days of the onset of menstruation, but because therapeutic steroid levels are achieved over the course of several days, starting at any other time requires 7 days of backup contraception, such as condoms or abstinence.[9] The contraceptive patch generates higher circulating levels of ethinyl estradiol than the COC and vaginal ring.[70] It is uncertain whether use of the patch is associated with a higher risk of VTE than use of the COC.[71,72]

Transdermal Contraceptive Patch

The only contraceptive patch available in the United States is Ortho Evra. It is a 4.5-cm tan square that releases 20 µg of ethinyl estradiol daily along with norelgestromin, the biologically active metabolite of the progestin norgestimate (Fig. 18-2).[73] A new patch is applied each week on the same day for 3 weeks, followed by a patch-free week, during which withdrawal bleeding is anticipated. Sweating associated with vigorous exercise, swimming, and use of a hot tub or sauna should not result in patch detachment. Unscheduled bleeding in patch users is similar to that seen with COCs.[74] Although patch users are more compliant than pill users, they are more likely to report breast discomfort, dysmenorrhea, nausea, and vomiting.[75] Mild local skin reactions are common. A contraceptive patch that releases less ethinyl estradiol than the Ortho Evra transdermal contraceptive has been developed but is not currently approved.[76]

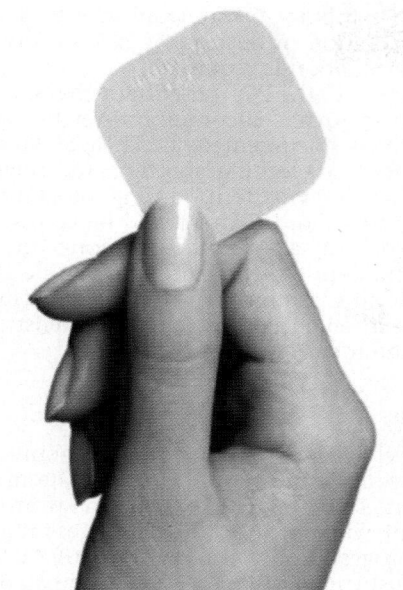

Figure 18-2 The contraceptive patch, Ortho Evra.

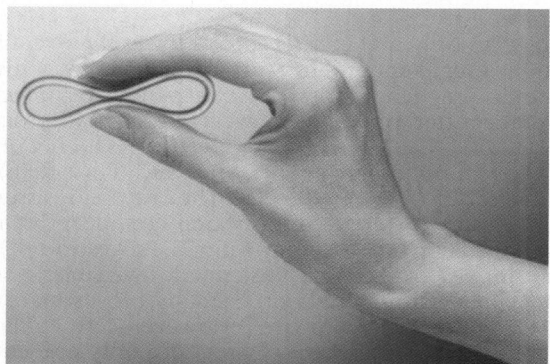

Figure 18-3 The contraceptive vaginal ring, NuvaRing.

Contraceptive Vaginal Ring

The vaginal mucosa offers excellent absorption of sex steroids. The only contraceptive vaginal ring available in the United States is the NuvaRing, a flexible plastic ring that is 4 mm thick and has an outside diameter of 54 mm.[77] The ring releases 15 µg daily of ethinyl estradiol along with etonogestrel, the biologically active metabolite of the progestin desogestrel (Fig. 18-3). The ring does not require individual fitting; as long as it remains in the vagina, appropriate absorption of steroids occurs. Expulsion is uncommon. Women's interest in using a contraceptive vaginal ring varies; some women are highly motivated and comfortable with this method. Some users keep the ring in place during sexual relations; in this setting, male discomfort is not common. Other users prefer to remove the ring before intercourse, and removal for less than 48 hours does not appear to impair efficacy.[9] Backup contraception is required for 7 days if the ring is removed for 48 hours or longer.

Like the traditional COC regimen, the contraceptive vaginal ring is inserted in the vagina for 3 weeks and then withdrawn for 1 week, during which withdrawal bleeding is anticipated. A new ring is required every 4 weeks. Rates of unscheduled (breakthrough) bleeding and spotting are lower with the ring than with COCs.[74] The ring is well tolerated, with increased physiologic vaginal discharge being the main bothersome side effect.[75]

PROGESTIN-ONLY CONTRACEPTIVE METHODS

Progestin-only contraceptives offer many advantages over estrogen-containing methods. There are fewer contraindications to progestin-only contraception (see Table 18-3). Progestin-only contraceptives may be appropriate for many women with contraindications to contraceptive doses of estrogen, including women age 35 or older who smoke, who have hypertension, or who have diabetes. In addition, they can be used immediately after delivery and in women at elevated risk for VTE. Unfortunately, package labeling for some progestin-only contraceptives does not reflect this distinction. For example, package labeling for DMPA inappropriately lists a history of VTE as a contraindication.[78] In these circumstances, clinicians may follow the recommendations of the USMEC, which indicate that in women with a history of VTE, the benefits of DMPA use outweigh the risks.[8]

Progestin-only contraceptives are formulated in long-acting preparations that provide a high level of contraceptive efficacy and acceptability. The main disadvantage of the progestin-only contraceptives is changes in vaginal bleeding patterns. This is common in progestin-only oral contraceptive users and represents the most frequent cause for contraceptive discontinuation. Types of progestin-only contraceptives include the following:

- Oral progestin-only contraception (progestin-only pill [POP], minipills)
- Progestin implants (Nexplanon)
- Intrauterine contraception (Mirena/Skyla)
- Injectable contraception (DMPA, Depo-Provera)

Oral Progestin-Only Contraception

Only one POP formulation is marketed in the United States: norethindrone in 0.35-mg tablets (e.g., Micronor, Nor-QD, and generics). The progestin dose is lower than the dose in any combination oral contraceptive. Due to the short half-life of POPs, serum steroid levels are near baseline as quickly as 24 hours after administration.[9] It is dispensed in packs of 28 active pills, which are taken continuously (i.e., no HFI) (Table 18-4). Contraindications to POPs are few (see Table 18-3).

Mechanism of Action

The mechanism of action of progestin-only oral contraceptives varies among patients and may include suppression of ovulation, thickening of cervical mucus, and induction of endometrial atrophy. Unlike with COCs, ovulation is not consistently suppressed with the 0.35-mg norethindrone progestin-only oral contraceptive, and the progestin effects on cervical mucus and the endometrium are critical factors in preventing conception. Within hours of administration, progestin-only oral contraceptives thicken cervical mucus that acts as a barrier to stop sperm at the cervical canal; 48 hours of norethindrone POP use is necessary to achieve the full contraceptive effects on cervical mucus.[9] In European countries, a POP containing 75 µg desogestrel is available.[79] In contrast with the norethindrone POP available in the United States, the desogestrel POP inhibits ovulation, and contraceptive efficacy is as high as that with COCs.[80]

TABLE 18-4

Summary and Recommendations for Progestin-Only Oral Contraceptive Use

1. Progestin-only contraception is an option for women in whom an estrogen-containing contraceptive is either contraindicated or causes additional health concerns.
2. Ovulation is not consistently suppressed; the main contraceptive actions of progestin-only oral contraception are effects on cervical mucus and the endometrium.
3. The typical user failure rate with progestin-only oral contraception is estimated to be more than 9%. Women choosing progestin-only oral contraception are often subfertile as a result of breastfeeding or older reproductive age, so the failure rate in these populations may be lower than in more fertile populations.
4. It is essential that the pill be taken at the same time each day to maximize contraceptive efficacy.
5. Menstrual irregularities are common in users of progestin-only oral contraception and represent the most frequent cause for contraceptive discontinuation.

Efficacy

The efficacy of progestin-only oral contraceptives is not well established.[81] National survey data used to estimate contraceptive failure rates with typical use have failed to distinguish between COCs (the larger group) and POPs. A potential confounding factor is that the women using progestin-only oral contraceptives may have reduced fertility as a result of breastfeeding or older reproductive age. It is thought that the typical first-year failure rates with progestin-only oral contraceptives are higher than those seen with COCs (9%).[12] In general, POPs are not a first-line contraceptive except in women who cannot or do not wish to use estrogen.

Starting the Progestin-Only Pill

Progestin-only oral contraceptives can be initiated within the first 5 days of menses, without the need for backup contraception.[9] Some clinicians initiate progestin-only oral contraceptives at any time in the cycle, as long as the clinician is reasonably certain that the patient is not pregnant. With this strategy, backup contraception should be used for the first 2 days of use. Because of the short duration of action and the short half-life of POPs, the pill must be taken at the same time each day to maximize contraceptive efficacy. A backup contraceptive (e.g., condoms) should be used for at least 2 days if the progestin-only oral contraceptive is taken more than 3 hours late or forgotten on any day.[9] The patient should also resume taking daily progestin-only oral contraceptives as soon as possible. Progestin-only oral contraceptives may be initiated immediately or within 7 days after induced or spontaneous abortion. If not administered immediately after abortion, the woman must use alternative contraception or abstinence for 2 days. After delivery, POPs can be started at any time, including immediately post partum in breastfeeding and nonbreastfeeding women.[8] If the woman is more than 21 days post partum and is not using POPs to augment lactational amenorrhea, then backup contraception should be used for 2 days.[9]

Side Effects of the Progestin-Only Oral Contraceptives

Sonographic studies have shown that follicular cysts are more common among progestin-only oral contraceptive users than among other women, but they may come and go over time.[82] No intervention is required in asymptomatic women, other than reassurance and sonographic follow-up. If a follow-up sonogram in 6 to 8 weeks demonstrates resolution or decrease in size of follicular cysts, no further evaluation is required.

Side effects with the POP other than changes in bleeding patterns are relatively uncommon. Weight gain has not been objectively documented, and headaches are uncommon. Unscheduled bleeding, spotting, and amenorrhea are common menstrual patterns during progestin-only oral contraceptive use, and users should be counseled accordingly. Interpreting signs and symptoms of pregnancy, whether intrauterine or extrauterine, can be challenging. Pregnancy testing is appropriate for POP users experiencing nausea, breast tenderness, a change in menstrual pattern, or lower abdominal pain (see Table 18-2).

Other Effects

Most studies have reported that progestin-only oral contraceptives have little impact on carbohydrate metabolism.[83] However, one study conducted in Latina women observed that lactating women with a history of gestational diabetes who used progestin-only oral contraceptives after delivery had an almost tripled risk of diabetes compared with those who used low-dose COCs.[84] All women with gestational diabetes, regardless of contraceptive used, should be screened for diabetes post partum with a 2-hour glucose tolerance test.[85]

Progestin-only oral contraceptives lower the overall risk of ectopic pregnancy and intrauterine pregnancy. A history of ectopic pregnancy does not contraindicate progestin-only oral contraceptive use. However, if pregnancy occurs, the likelihood that the pregnancy is ectopic is higher in POP users than in nonusers of contraceptives.[86] Bone density is not adversely affected by the POP. The only study assessing skeletal health in progestin-only oral contraceptive users was conducted in breastfeeding women. Progestin-only oral contraceptives protected against small, reversible losses in BMD occurring during lactation.[87] Finally, progestins usually suppress endometrial growth.[82] However, few epidemiologic data address the effect of progestin-only oral contraceptives on endometrial cancer risk or on any cancer risk.

Progestin-Only Oral Contraceptives During Lactation

The progestin-only oral contraceptive does not interfere with the quality or quantity of breast milk.[88] Very little progestin is passed from nursing mothers into their breast milk, and no adverse impact on infant growth has been observed. Package labeling advises delaying administration in lactating women until 6 weeks after delivery. Based on the absence of data suggesting harm to the infant or mother and the contraceptive benefits of early initiation, some experts recommend initiation of POPs before hospital discharge and no later than the third postpartum week, regardless of lactation status.[49]

Depot Medroxyprogesterone Acetate for Contraception

DMPA is an injectable, progestin-only contraceptive that provides effective, private, and reversible contraception. It avoids the need for user action daily or near the time of sexual intercourse and the need for partner cooperation (Table 18-5).

Formulations and Pharmacology

DMPA is available in two formulations: 150 mg/1 mL for intramuscular injection and 104 mg/0.65 mL for

TABLE 18-5

Summary and Recommendations for Depot Medroxyprogesterone Acetate Use

1. DMPA is an excellent method of contraception for women who desire a long-term, reversible contraceptive method.
2. DMPA primarily acts by inhibiting follicular maturation and ovulation through inhibition of gonadotropin secretion; it also affects cervical mucus.
3. DMPA is available in two formulations: 150 mg/1 mL for IM injection and 104 mg/0.65 mL for SC injection.
4. The ideal time to initiate DMPA is within 7 days of the onset of menses so as to ensure absence of pregnancy. The dose is repeated every 3 months (13 weeks), with a 2-week grace period.
5. Although DMPA does not permanently affect endocrine function, return of fertility may be delayed.
6. Thorough, candid counseling about side effects is important. Women who are well informed when they choose this method of contraception are much more likely to become highly satisfied users with high continuation rates.
7. Menstrual changes occur in all women using DMPA and are the most frequent cause for discontinuation.
8. Because DMPA induces amenorrhea, it can be used for managing a variety of gynecologic and nongynecologic disorders, such as heavy menstrual bleeding, dysmenorrhea, and iron deficiency anemia.
9. There is no high-quality evidence that use of DMPA increases the risk of developing cancer, cardiovascular disease, or sexually transmitted infection. DMPA use significantly reduces the risk of developing endometrial cancer.
10. There is an association between current DMPA use and decreased bone mineral density; losses in bone mineral density are temporary, reverse after discontinuation of DMPA, and have not been linked to postmenopausal osteoporosis or fractures.

DMPA, depot medroxyprogesterone acetate; IM, intramuscular; SC, subcutaneous.

subcutaneous injection. The newer subcutaneous injection may be less painful and is available in a prefilled syringe, offering the potential for self-administration.[89] The injections can be given every 3 months because low solubility of the microcrystals at the injection site allows pharmacologically active drug levels to persist for several months. Intramuscular DMPA is available as a generic formulation, which is less costly than subcutaneous DMPA. Otherwise, the benefits and risks are similar for intramuscular and subcutaneous administration.[90]

DMPA primarily acts by inhibiting follicular maturation and ovulation through inhibition of gonadotropin secretion. Unlike other progestin-only contraceptives, mean estradiol levels may be lower than normal for cycling premenopausal women.[91] Although some women may be hypoestrogenic, vasomotor symptoms and vaginal atrophy are uncommon. Because of its progestin effect, it also causes changes in cervical mucus that are hostile to sperm migration and endometrial atrophy.

DMPA is an effective contraceptive. Following a 150-mg intramuscular injection, failure rates in clinical trials have ranged from 0.0 to 0.7 per 100 woman-years. The typical-user failure rate is 6 failures per 100 woman-years, reflecting the fact that some users do not return for their injections as scheduled.[12] Because progestin levels are high, efficacy has not been reduced by obesity or use of concurrent medications such as anticonvulsants. For the 104-mg subcutaneous injection, no contraceptive failures were reported in phase III clinical trials.[92] This formulation is relatively new, so typical-user failure rates are not available, but they are expected to be similar to those for the intramuscular preparation.

Administration of Depot Medroxyprogesterone Acetate

Starting Injections. The ideal time to initiate DMPA is within 7 days of the onset of menses.[9] This approach ensures that the patient is not pregnant at the time of injection and prevents ovulation during the first month of use, so that backup contraception is unnecessary. Most women have pharmacologically active drug levels and a poor cervical mucus score within 24 hours after injection.[91] The "same-day," "quick-start," or "Depo-now" approach when a pregnancy test result is negative facilitates DMPA initiation for many users, and it may prevent some pregnancies.[93] However, there is a small possibility of undiagnosed pregnancy despite a negative pregnancy test result. When the quick-start approach is used for initiating DMPA, backup contraception or abstinence should be used for 7 days and a repeat pregnancy test should be performed in 2 to 4 weeks. Nevertheless, DMPA given inadvertently during pregnancy does not appear to be teratogenic.[94] DMPA may be initiated immediately after spontaneous or induced abortion or within the first 7 days. If given in the first 7 days after the event, then backup contraception should be used. After delivery, DMPA can be started at any time, including immediately post partum in breastfeeding and nonbreastfeeding women.[8,95] If the woman is more than 21 days post partum and not breastfeeding exclusively, then backup contraception should be used for 7 days after the first DMPA injection.[9]

Repeat Injections. Repeat injections of DMPA should be scheduled every 3 months (13 weeks). After a 150-mg injection, ovulation does not occur for at least 14 weeks. A 2-week grace period (repeat injection without pregnancy testing, up to 15 weeks following the prior injection) is appropriate for women receiving injections every 3 months.[9] In women more than 2 weeks late for an injection, a urine pregnancy test should be performed before administering further DMPA and backup contraception for 7 days is advised.

Side Effects of Depot Medroxyprogesterone Acetate

Candid counseling regarding the side effects of DMPA and the need for timed injections should be provided. Women who are well informed when they choose this method of contraception are more likely to become satisfied users with high continuation rates.[96] Menstrual changes occur in almost all women using DMPA and are the most frequent cause for discontinuation of injectable and all other progestin-only contraceptives.[97] Proactive patient education before initiation of DMPA and supportive follow-up can improve tolerance of menstrual changes. During the first months of use, episodes of unpredictable bleeding and spotting lasting 7 days or longer are common. Bleeding decreases with use, and at 1 year, 50% of women experience amenorrhea; this rate increases to 75% with long-term use.[91] Similar bleeding patterns are reported with the subcutaneous preparation.[98] Some women may view amenorrhea (along with a reduction or elimination of menstrual cramps) as one of the advantages of using this method.

There are no established methods for predicting, preventing, or treating unscheduled bleeding in DMPA users. Small studies have shown that estrogen supplements (e.g., 1.25 mg of oral conjugated estrogen, 1 to 2 mg of oral micronized estradiol, or 0.1-mg estradiol patches for 10 to 20 days) may terminate a bleeding episode.[9] Another treatment option endorsed by the U.S. Selected Practice Recommendations (USSPR) is nonsteroidal anti-inflammatory drugs (NSAIDs) for 5 to 7 days. However, a systematic review concluded that there is a lack of high-quality data to support routine clinical use of any interventions to treat persistent unscheduled bleeding with progestin-only contraceptives.[97]

Observational studies have not reported any consistent effects of DMPA on mood. Some evidence indicates that progestins may cause or exacerbate depressive symptoms in certain subpopulations of women, including those with a history of premenstrual syndrome or mood disorders. However, depression is not a contraindication to DMPA use.[8]

The impact of DMPA on weight has been controversial.[99] Randomized controlled trials, though limited, have failed to show that DMPA causes weight gain.[91,100] Observational studies are difficult to interpret given that individuals tend to gain weight over time irrespective of contraceptive use. On average, the weight gain with DMPA use is small (2 kg); however, there is marked individual variation. Weight gain with the use of DMPA may be associated with user subgroups at particular risk for obesity, including adolescents and ethnic minorities.[101] However, it is reasonable to monitor weight over time in women using DMPA.[9]

Risks and Benefits of Depot Medroxyprogesterone Acetate

DMPA has been used to manage a variety of gynecologic and nongynecologic disorders. The tendency of DMPA to cause amenorrhea makes it a particularly appropriate contraceptive choice for women with heavy menstrual bleeding, dysmenorrhea, or iron-deficiency anemia. DMPA is a useful means of suppressing menstrual bleeding and managing menstrual hygiene in individuals with special needs (e.g., cognitive impairment, military personnel).[91]

Progestins inhibit endometriotic tissue growth by directly causing initial decidualization and eventual atrophy and by inhibiting pituitary gonadotropin secretion and ovarian estrogen production. Randomized trials have shown that DMPA is more effective than oral contraceptives and danazol and as effective as leuprolide injections for treatment of pain associated with endometriosis.[100,102] In the United States, subcutaneous DMPA is approved for the treatment of pain associated with endometriosis.

Effect on Cancer Risk. Large case-control studies conducted by the WHO have shown that use of DMPA is associated with an 80% reduced risk of endometrial cancer and does not affect the incidence of ovarian or cervical cancer.[103-105] Multicountry data from the WHO and data from the United States, South Africa, and New Zealand provide reassurance that use of DMPA is not associated with an increased risk of breast cancer.[106]

Effect on Cardiovascular Risk. DMPA has an adverse effect on circulating lipids but does not increase production of coagulation factors and has no adverse effect on blood pressure. No adverse clinical effects on cardiovascular disease have been observed.[91] Based on these findings, the USMEC allows DMPA and other progestin-only contraceptives for use in women with a history of VTE and those in whom use of combination estrogen-progestin contraceptive is contraindicated.[8] This recommendation is different from package labeling for DMPA (written in the 1960s), which indicates that a prior history of VTE is a contraindication to DMPA use. In women with multiple risk factors for cardiovascular disease (e.g., smoking, older age, hypertension, diabetes), the USMEC classifies DMPA as category 3 (see Table 18-3), indicating that the risks of use may exceed the benefits. The basis for this caution seems to be the hypoestrogenic effects of DMPA and reduced high-density lipoprotein (HDL) levels. In addition, the effects of DMPA might persist for some time after discontinuation, so it would not be immediately reversible if there were an adverse event.

Effect on Skeletal Health. DMPA's impact on BMD has generated much controversy. In suppressing gonadotropin production and ovulation, DMPA also suppresses ovarian production of estradiol.[107] The resulting hypoestrogenemia causes a decline in BMD in current DMPA users.[108] Compared with nonusers, BMD at the hip and spine of DMPA users decreases by 0.5% to 3.5% after 1 year of use and by 5.7% to 7.5% after 2 years of use. The rate of loss is greatest during the first 1 to 2 years of use.[109] The intramuscular and subcutaneous formulations of DMPA have similar effects on BMD.[90] Because of this finding, the FDA added a black box warning to DMPA package labeling in 2004 stating, "DMPA should be used as a long-term birth control method (e.g., longer than 2 years) only if other birth control methods are inadequate." Nonetheless, although it is well established that DMPA leads to BMD declines in current users, the long-term impact of injectable contraception on skeletal health, if any, is uncertain.[110]

Published data do not suggest that DMPA use reduces peak bone mass or increases the risk of postmenopausal osteoporotic fractures.[111,112] Studies involving premenopausal women and adolescents treated with DMPA for up to 5 years indicate that the decline in BMD associated with injectable contraception is largely reversed after discontinuation.[100,111,113-115] The true association between fracture and DMPA use in the general population is difficult to elucidate. Further analyses of case-control studies showing a positive association have demonstrated that either DMPA users have an increased risk of fracture at baseline compared to non-DMPA users or baseline risk factors such as smoking or body mass index (BMI) were not assessed.[116,117] These analyses suggest that women who choose DMPA may be behaviorally different from women who choose other methods of contraception. To our knowledge, no prospective study has assessed the impact of DMPA contraceptive use on subsequent fracture risk in postmenopausal women.

To summarize, current use of DMPA is associated with BMD declines, but a significant increase in risk of fractures in DMPA users has not been demonstrated.[112] Professional organizations state that the advantages of DMPA use as a contraceptive outweigh the theoretical concerns regarding skeletal harm.[8,108,118] Skeletal health concerns should not restrict initiation or continuation of DMPA in reproductive-age women, including teens and women older than 35 years.[110] Likewise, published evidence does not support limiting the duration of DMPA therapy. The effect of DMPA on BMD is similar to that with pregnancy (decrease in BMD of 0% to 5%) or lactation (decrease in BMD of 5% to 10%).[119] Use of DMPA is not an indication for BMD testing before, during, or as follow-up of administration. Likewise, antiresorptive agents, including bisphosphonates, are not appropriate to prevent bone loss in women using injectable contraception.[108] As with all reproductive-age patients, clinicians should encourage DMPA users to consume adequate amounts of calcium and vitamin D, to perform weight-bearing exercise, and to quit smoking. Clinical judgment is called for when helping women with risk factors for osteoporosis make sound choices regarding DMPA and alternative contraceptives.

Effect on Sexually Transmitted Infections. The association between use of DMPA and risk of STI is uncertain. Some studies have shown an increased risk of STI in DMPA users, but it is unclear whether this reflects differences in sexual practices, such as a condom use, in DMPA users.[120] The relationship between DMPA use and human immunodeficiency virus (HIV) acquisition and transmission is also unclear, but several clinical trials have shown an increased risk.[121-125] Of particular concern is that DMPA is widely used in the areas of high HIV prevalence where there are limited alternative contraceptive options. There are a number of mechanisms through which DMPA may increase the risk of HIV transmission.[126] The USMEC currently places no restrictions (category 1) on hormonal contraceptive use in women at high risk for acquiring STIs or HIV or in women who are HIV-positive.[8] However, the USMEC recommends that because of the unclear information, women with HIV or those at risk for HIV should always use condoms to prevent HIV and other STI transmission.[127]

Effect on Return of Fertility. Although DMPA does not permanently impact endocrine function, return of fertility may be delayed after stopping DMPA use. Within 10 months of the last injection, 50% of women who discontinue DMPA to become pregnant will conceive. However, in some women, fertility is not reestablished until up to 18 months after the last injection.[91] The persistence of ovulation suppression after DMPA discontinuation is not related to the duration of use, but it is related to weight, as clearance is slower in heavier women.[128] Before initiating DMPA contraception, clinicians should counsel candidates about the possible prolonged duration of action. Women who may want to become pregnant within the next 1 or 2 years should choose an alternative contraceptive.

Intrauterine Progestins

The levonorgestrel-releasing intrauterine system (LNG-IUS) is an effective, safe, and convenient form of long-term, reversible contraception.[129] Intrauterine contraception use in the United States fell dramatically after earlier flawed studies reported an association between intrauterine contraception use and later tubal infertility. It is now acknowledged, however, that modern intrauterine contraception is not only highly effective but also safe for most women to use.[130] The addition of progestin to the IUD increases contraceptive efficacy and the 52-mg LNG-IUS is approved in the United States for contraception and for treatment of heavy menstrual bleeding. The LNG-IUS provides other off-label therapeutic benefits, including treatment of pain associated with endometriosis; treatment of symptoms associated with uterine adenomyosis, endometrial hyperplasia, or carcinoma; and protection of the endometrium in women during use of menopausal estrogen therapy.

Contraceptive Uses

Mirena and Skyla (Bayer Healthcare Pharmaceuticals, Wayne, NJ) are the two levonorgestrel-releasing IUDs approved in the United States. Mirena or the high-dose LNG-IUS is a T-shaped device with a reservoir containing 52 mg of levonorgestrel. It delivers 20 μg of levonorgestrel per day and maintains its contraceptive efficacy for at least 5 years.[131] The maximum plasma levonorgestrel levels are reached within a few hours, and they plateau between 100 and 200 pg/mL, levels that are lower than those with implants or oral contraceptives. Skyla is a new smaller and lower-dose LNG-IUS containing 13.5 mg of levonorgestrel, releasing 14 μg/day and declining to 5 μg/day after 3 years. The low-dose LNG-IUS is approved for use for 3 years and is distinguished from Mirena by its smaller size (30 mm × 28 mm compared to 32 mm × 32 mm) and a silver ring at the top of the vertical stem (visible with ultrasound). The inserter diameter is also narrower than Mirena (3.8 mm vs. 4.5 mm). The smaller dimensions of the Skyla device make it particularly suitable for women with smaller uterine cavities or tight cervices.

Data from large international studies confirm extremely low pregnancy rates with the LNG-IUS, ranging between 0.1 and 0.3 per 100 woman-years.[12,131,132] Despite endometrial suppression, fertility resumes rapidly after contraceptive removal.[133] The mechanism of action of the contraceptive effects of LNG-IUS is by thickening cervical mucus and profound endometrial suppression. Most LNG-IUS users continue to ovulate, even when there is amenorrhea.[131] There are few contraindications to IUDs, and most women are appropriate candidates including adolescents and nulliparous women.[129] Contraindications to IUD use are pregnancy, active cervicitis or uterine infection, malignancy in the uterus or cervix, a distorted uterine cavity, unexplained abnormal bleeding, and adverse reaction to product ingredients.[134] Although systemic concentrations of levonorgestrel are very low in LNG-IUS users, all hormonal contraceptives are generally avoided after breast cancer.

Expanding the Use of Intrauterine Devices

There is growing consensus that women in the United States will benefit from broader use of IUDs, including the LNG-IUS.[129] The Contraceptive CHOICE Project in St. Louis, Missouri, provides women ($n = 5000$) who do not desire pregnancy for at least 1 year with free contraception for up to 3 years. This project has shown that with standardized counseling, the majority of women (68%) will choose long-acting reversible contraceptive methods (45% levonorgestrel IUD, 10% copper IUD, and 13% etonogestrel implant).[135] Continuation rates at 12 and 24 months were 88% and 79% for the levonorgestrel IUD, 84% and 77% for the copper IUD, and 83% and 69% for the etonogestrel implant, respectively.[136] Satisfaction rates were also higher for long-acting reversible methods compared to other methods of contraception such as oral contraceptives and the injectable DMPA. In addition, among women participating in the Contraceptive CHOICE Project, rates of unintended pregnancy, birth, and abortion were substantially lower than for other women in St. Louis and compared to U.S. women overall.[137]

Adolescents in this study also frequently chose both IUDs and implants.[138] With appropriate counseling regarding STI prevention and anticipated side effects and their management, it is now accepted that the IUD can be used safely and effectively in adolescents.[8,139] Adolescents and young women have higher continuation rates and lower repeat unintended pregnancy rates when using a method that does not require ongoing adherence.[140] Additionally, the use of long-acting reversible contraception immediately after abortion has been shown to decrease repeat abortion rates.[141,142]

Abnormal Bleeding, Expulsion, and Uterine Perforation

As with DMPA and other progestin-only contraceptives, unpredictable uterine bleeding is the most common reason for discontinuation of the LNG-IUS.[143] Unscheduled bleeding is most common during the early months of LNG-IUS use and tends to resolve with time. By 12 months, up to 50% of women have amenorrhea or infrequent bleeding. With the 13.5-mg LNG-IUS, by 12 months approximately 26% of women have amenorrhea or infrequent bleeding.[144] Addressing patient preferences and assessing acceptance of menstrual disturbances are integral to efforts aimed at reducing early discontinuation rates. Adequate and specific counseling about likely changes in bleeding patterns before placement is essential for increasing patient acceptability.

Expulsion, the most common cause of IUD failure, occurs in about 2% to 4% of users. Those at increased risk for expulsion include nulliparous women, women with severe dysmenorrhea or uterine adenomyosis, those with uterine cavity abnormalities, and women with insertions immediately after delivery.[129,145] The USMEC recommends immediate insertion after first-trimester (category 1) and second-trimester (category 2) abortions.[8] Postpartum insertion is recommended after a 4-week interval (category 1). Immediate postpartum insertion is also an option (category 2) within 10 minutes of placental delivery as long as there is no evidence of puerperal sepsis. Expulsion rates with immediate postpartum insertion range from 10% to 20%, with lower rates seen after cesarean delivery. Because expulsion usually occurs within the first few months, women are encouraged to follow up with their care provider within 12 weeks of insertion.

Uterine perforation is an uncommon but potentially serious complication of LNG-IUS placement. Perforation rates are approximately 1 case per 1000 IUD insertions. The risk is increased sixfold for lactating women, but the absolute risk is still very low.[146]

Upper Genital Tract Infection and Infertility

The use of intrauterine contraception does not increase the risk of pelvic infection.[147] The insertion of the device results in a small transient risk of infection limited to the first 20 days after placement.[148] Similarly there is no evidence that intrauterine contraception increases the risk of subsequent infertility.[149] Intrauterine methods are suitable for nulliparous and adolescent women.[8]

Prophylactic antibiotics are not recommended for IUD insertion. A clinical history (including sexual history) should be taken as part of the routine assessment for intrauterine contraception to identify women at high risk for STIs; testing before insertion should be performed selectively, not routinely. Even among high-risk women, testing on the same day of insertion was found to be as safe as testing prior to insertion in terms of subsequent pelvic inflammatory disease (PID) risk.[150] An IUD should not be inserted in women with current PID, purulent cervicitis, or current chlamydial or gonorrheal infection.[8] Cervical or vaginal infection is not an indication to remove an IUD.[9] If a woman develops PID with an LNG-IUS in place, treatment follows the CDC Sexually Transmitted Diseases Treatment guidelines, and if the patient responds to therapy, the IUD can remain in place.[9]

Metabolic and Systemic Effects

Low but detectable circulating levels of progestin in LNG-IUS users have raised concerns that glucose control, lipid profile, and blood pressure may be negatively affected. However, these concerns have not been substantiated in high-quality clinical trials.[131] The data suggest that the LNG-IUS is safe to use in patients with diabetes, hypertension, or hyperlipidemia.[8] Progestins are not thought to increase the risk of thromboembolic disease, and the LNG-IUS has not been shown to be associated with venous or arterial events.[151]

Noncontraceptive Uses of the Levonorgestrel-Releasing Intrauterine System

Heavy Menstrual Bleeding. The high-dose LNG-IUS is a well-established and highly effective treatment intervention for heavy menstrual bleeding. In comparative studies, it offers efficacy equal to or greater than other surgical uterine-conserving treatments (e.g., global endometrial ablation, transcervical endometrial resection), is an acceptable alternative to hysterectomy for many women, and offers comparable improvement in health-related quality of life for menstrual disorders.[145,152,153] Although up to 43% of women using the LNG-IUS to treat abnormal uterine bleeding will eventually undergo hysterectomy, the system still offers lower direct and indirect healthcare costs at 5 years compared to immediate hysterectomy.[152,154]

Symptomatic Fibroids and Uterine Adenomyosis. Data suggest that the LNG-IUS is also an effective treatment for heavy menstrual bleeding associated with uterine fibroids.[155,156] However, submucous fibroids may be more likely to cause heavy bleeding and are more likely to lead to LNG-IUS expulsion because they distort the uterine cavity.[157] Therefore, the effectiveness of the LNG-IUS likely depends on fibroid number, size, and location in the uterus.

Uterine adenomyosis also is a common, benign condition that may be associated with heavy menstrual bleeding and pelvic pain. Limited data suggest that the LNG-IUS reduces bleeding and pain in women with this condition.[158,159]

Endometriosis. Results of small, prospective studies using the 52-mg LNG-IUS as a treatment for pelvic pain and dysmenorrhea associated with endometriosis are encouraging. The system may offer effective symptom relief, at least in the short term and is useful after the surgical treatment of endometriosis. However, these studies are limited by small sample sizes and vary significantly with regard to enrollment criteria and by stage and location of disease.[160] A short-term randomized trial found that the LNG-IUS was as effective as a gonadotropin-releasing hormone agonist in reducing pain in women with endometriosis.[161] Advantages of the LNG-IUS in this setting include the absence of hypoestrogenic effects associated with the use of gonadotropin-releasing hormone agonists as well as lower medication costs. Follow-up of these women for 3 years showed no further improvement in pelvic pain after 12 months of use.[162] Additional studies are needed to confirm the original findings and to determine how to best integrate use of LNG-IUS into current clinical protocols. As expected, all studies also reported increased menstrual disturbances in the LNG-IUS groups.

Endometrial Protection With Estrogen Replacement Therapy. Good-quality evidence supports the long-term use of LNG-IUS for endometrial suppression during estrogen replacement therapy and it is approved for this indication in other countries.[163] However, the 52-mg LNG-IUS is relatively large and may be difficult to insert into a postmenopausal woman's uterus. The smaller 13.5-mg LNG-IUS may be a better choice in menopausal women. Acceptability studies are needed, and more studies are necessary to determine the lowest effective dose of levonorgestrel required to achieve effective endometrial suppression.[164]

Endometrial Protection With Tamoxifen Use. Tamoxifen is commonly used as adjuvant endocrine therapy in the treatment of estrogen receptor–positive breast cancer in premenopausal women and in selected postmenopausal women. In postmenopausal women, tamoxifen increases the risk of endometrial polyps, hyperplasia, and cancer. A systematic review of the 52-mg LNG-IUS in the prevention of endometrial disease in tamoxifen users concluded that the device reduced the risk of endometrial polyps, but it is not known whether LNG-IUS reduces the risk of endometrial hyperplasia or cancer.[165] LNG-IUS users had a higher incidence of unscheduled bleeding, which may increase the need for diagnostic intervention in this high-risk group. The FDA lists a personal history of breast cancer as a contraindication to use of all progestational medications, including the LNG-IUS. Reflecting the uncertain safety of LNG-IUS use in women with breast cancer, guidance released in 2014 from the American College of

Obstetricians and Gynecologists suggests that this intra-uterine system not be used in this patient population.[166] **Treatment for Endometrial Hyperplasia or Carcinoma.** The efficacy of the LNG-IUS for endometrial hyperplasia is still uncertain.[167] Small, prospective studies, and one randomized controlled trial, have shown that the LNG-IUS is an effective and safe alternative in the treatment of perimenopausal and postmenopausal women with endometrial hyperplasia without atypia.[168,169] When atypia is present, the device may be less effective in achieving regression but no less so than oral progestins.[168,170] Although hysterectomy represents the best treatment for early endometrial cancer, progestins are sometimes used to treat endometrial hyperplasia with atypia or early endometrial cancer in women who wish to preserve future fertility. Small studies of selected patients suggest that intrauterine progestin in surgical high-risk candidates with endometrial cancer may be an alternative management option.[171] Larger studies are needed to better determine the value of LNG-IUS in this context.

Contraceptive Implants

Contraceptive implants provide long-acting, highly effective, convenient, and reversible contraception. All subdermal implants for clinical use in humans employ progestins. These methods offer an excellent contraceptive option for women who have contraindications to combined hormonal methods and an option for any woman who desires long-term protection against pregnancy that is rapidly reversible. The only subdermal implant available to women in the United States is Nexplanon (Merck & Co., Whitehouse Station, NJ) (Fig. 18-4), released in 2006. In 2011 Nexplanon replaced Implanon, which was the first version of the etonogestrel implant, and the device is now radiopaque.

Nexplanon contains 68 mg of etonogestrel as a single-rod subdermal implant.[172] Nexplanon is approved for 3 years of use, provides excellent efficacy throughout its use, and is easy to insert and remove. Nexplanon can be used during lactation; may improve dysmenorrhea; does not significantly affect weight, acne, lipids, or liver enzymes; and has only modest effects on BMD.[173] Like other

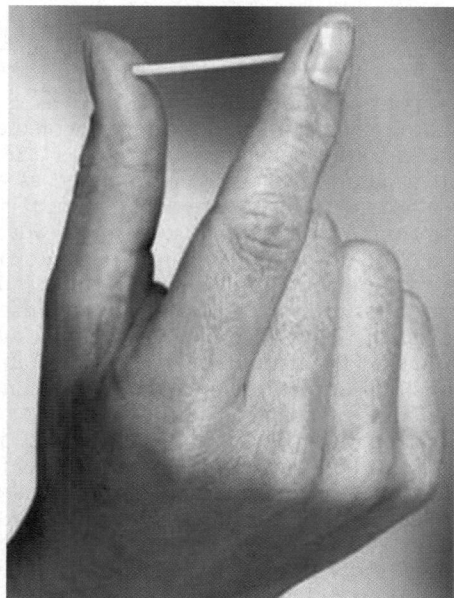

Figure 18-4 Nexplanon.

progestin-only contraceptives, the etonogestrel implant commonly causes irregular vaginal bleeding.

Description and Pharmacology

The Nexplanon rod releases the gonane progestin etonogestrel, formerly known as 3-ketodesogestrel, the biologically active metabolite of desogestrel.[173] Etonogestrel is the same progestin used in the contraceptive vaginal ring. The implant is 4 cm long and 2 mm in diameter, is radiopaque, and has a core made from a nonbiodegradable solid composed of ethylene vinyl acetate impregnated with 68 mg of etonogestrel (see Fig. 18-4). The ethylene vinyl acetate copolymer of Nexplanon allows controlled release of hormone over 3 years of use. Each implant is provided in a disposable sterile inserter for subdermal application. Maximum serum concentrations of etonogestrel are usually seen by day 4 after implant insertion. Etonogestrel levels decrease slightly by 1 year and further by 3 years but remain above the threshold needed to suppress ovulation.[172] After removal, serum levels are undetectable by 1 week in most users, who resume ovulation within 6 weeks of implant removal. Despite effective suppression of ovulation, estradiol levels only fall into the early follicular level range, and the implant does not cause hypoestrogenism. Consistent with that observation, based on limited data from clinical trials, there does not appear to be a clinically significant adverse effect of the etonogestrel implant on BMD.[173]

Mechanism of Action and Efficacy

The contraceptive action of Nexplanon is primarily inhibition of ovulation, although some thickening of cervical mucus may also occur.[174] The etonogestrel implant provides highly effective contraception. In an integrated analysis of 11 international clinical trials that included more than 900 healthy women between 18 and 40 years old, no pregnancies were reported while the etonogestrel implants were in place. Six pregnancies occurred during the first 14 days after etonogestrel implant removal. Including these six pregnancies, the cumulative Pearl index (number of pregnancies per 100 woman-years) was 0.38 (year 1 and 2 Pearl indices were 0.27 and 0.30, respectively).[174] After the implant has been removed, normal ovulation and fertility rapidly return.

Reported pregnancies among implant users have primarily been due to unrecognized pregnancies at the time of insertion and failure to insert the device. Postmarketing data of the etonogestrel implant from Australia show a real-world failure rate of 1.07 per 1000 insertions.[175] Of the 218 pregnancies identified in the Australian study, data were insufficient to assess the reason for contraceptive failure in 45 women, and 46 women were determined to have been already pregnant prior to implant insertion. Of the remaining 127 cases, failure to insert the implant caused pregnancies in 84 women. Other reasons included incorrect timing of insertion (19 cases), expulsion of the implant out of the insertion site (3 cases), and interaction with hepatic enzyme-inducing medicines (8 cases). The remaining 13 cases were classified as product failures. However, even when these method failures are accounted for, Nexplanon continues to have one of the highest efficacies of any method available.

There are reports of implant failure in women using anticonvulsants, particularly carbamazepine,[175] and contraceptive implants are not recommended in women taking anticonvulsants or other medications that induce hepatic enzymes.[8] Overweight and obese women were not included in the trials for approval of the etonogestrel implant. However, a prospective cohort study that examined 1168 women (28% overweight and 35% obese) found that failure rates were not impacted by BMI.[176]

Safety and Side Effect Profile

Nexplanon users commonly experience irregular and unpredictable bleeding patterns, similar to the experience of users of other continuous progestin-only contraceptives. Combined data from 11 clinical trials showed that the most common bleeding patterns with the etonogestrel implant were amenorrhea (22%), infrequent bleeding (34%), frequent bleeding (7%), and frequent or prolonged bleeding, or both (18%).[174] The number of bleeding days usually was not increased, but the pattern was unpredictable. Of clinical relevance is that bleeding patterns experienced during the initial 3 months predicted future patterns for most women.[177] The group of women with favorable bleeding patterns during the first 3 months tended to continue with this pattern throughout the first 2 years of use, whereas the group with unfavorable initial patterns had at least a 50% chance that the pattern would improve. Only 11.3% of patients discontinued use because of bleeding irregularities, mainly because of prolonged flow and frequent irregular bleeding.[177] Most women (77%) who had baseline dysmenorrhea experienced complete resolution of symptoms due to ovulation suppression. Effective preinsertion counseling on the possible changes in bleeding patterns may improve continuation rates.[178] Despite extensive clinical trials of agents to improve bleeding patterns with long-acting progestin-only contraceptives, there are no reliable treatment methods.[178] If a patient desires treatment to shorten a bleeding episode, the USSPR recommends two options: (1) NSAIDs for 5 to 7 days or (2) low-dose COCs or estrogen for 10 to 20 days.[9] These treatments may shorten bleeding episodes and offer temporary relief but do not change long-term bleeding patterns.

Several studies have observed a small (<1 kg) weight increase in etonogestrel implant users.[174] However, only 3% to 7% of women chose to remove the implant because of weight changes. Similar to the effect seen in women using POPs, ovarian cysts occur in up to 15% of users. Most cysts regress spontaneously and do not need additional treatment.[179] Nexplanon does not appear to change the content of breast milk and does not influence infant growth up to 3 years. Limited data show that the etonogestrel implant is safe for use during lactation.[180] Lipid measurements reveal an overall decrease in serum total cholesterol, HDL cholesterol, and low-density lipoprotein (LDL) cholesterol. Some studies have also shown a decrease in triglyceride levels. Minor reductions in the HDL/LDL ratio have been observed, although not into ranges thought to be clinically significant. Etonogestrel implant use does not significantly increase the risk of cardiovascular disease.[181]

Patient Selection

Before recommending the contraceptive implant, providers should review the indications and contraindications for its use. Contraindications to etonogestrel implant use are few and include breast cancer, use of hepatic enzyme–inducing drugs, unexplained and unevaluated abnormal vaginal bleeding, severe cirrhosis, systemic lupus erythematosus (SLE) with positive or unknown antiphospholipid antibodies, and liver tumors.[8] There is also one case report describing etonogestrel implant failure in a woman taking the antiretroviral drug efavirenz.[182] When explaining the etonogestrel implant, the clinician needs to address any

concerns and fears a woman may have about this method of contraception. In particular, women may have concerns about implant removal, although removal problems with single-rod devices such as Nexplanon are uncommon. Side effects (particularly irregular bleeding) should be discussed in advance, because an unexpected side effect may cause women to request early removal of the implant. The implant does not provide protection against STIs. Accordingly, and as is appropriate for all sexually active women, implant users should be reminded about safe sexual practices. Appropriate candidates for implantable contraception are women who desire long-term reversible birth control, have no contraindications to etonogestrel implant use, accept implant insertion and removal, and are ready to accept a change in menstrual bleeding patterns.

Insertion and Removal

Proper insertion and removal techniques are essential for clinical efficacy and for the prevention of complications. Timing of insertion depends on the patient's prior use of contraception and the clinician's evaluation of the appropriateness for the individual.[9] In the United States, Nexplanon has been made available only to clinicians who have completed insertion and removal training provided by the manufacturer. Proper training of clinicians appears to reduce the incidence of complications at insertion and removal. Complications of Nexplanon insertion are rare (<2%) but may include local pain, infection, and bleeding.[173] There is no indication for routine postinsertion follow-up.[9]

Nexplanon is licensed for 3 years of use and should then be removed. Prolonged use beyond 3 years has not been associated with any specific nonpregnancy complications. Before removal, the clinician needs to palpate the implant. Under sterile conditions, a 2- to 3-mm incision is made vertically over the implant. The rod is then removed using the pop-out technique described by Pymar and associates for Norplant System removal.[183] If inserted correctly, removal is usually simple and should take less than 5 minutes. The most common reason for difficulty in removal is placement of the implant too deeply. If the clinician cannot palpate the implant, imaging techniques may be necessary before proceeding.

EMERGENCY CONTRACEPTION

Emergency contraception (EC) is defined as a drug or device used to prevent pregnancy after unprotected sexual intercourse (including sexual assault) or after a recognized contraceptive failure.[184] Oral EC is intended as a backup method for occasional use, rather than a regular method of contraception. Although EC is sometimes called postcoital contraception or the morning-after pill, these labels are confusing, because they imply that EC can be taken only the morning after unprotected sexual intercourse. EC can reduce the risk of unintended pregnancy up to 5 days after unprotected sex. EC should be readily available to all women at risk for unplanned pregnancy, including adolescents and victims of sexual assault.

Research has shown that increased access to EC improves use, but it is not yet clear whether this access translates into a reduction in unintended pregnancy or abortion.[185] Although access is an important factor, how women use EC may be a stronger determinant of its ultimate effect. Studies show that even when women have EC at home, they often fail to use it after unprotected sexual intercourse. The most common reason for this is a lack of recognition of the risk of pregnancy or neglect of the perceived risk.[186] Although increasing knowledge of and access to EC is a public health priority, the use of regular, ongoing contraception is a more effective way to reduce unplanned pregnancy and abortion.

Emergency Contraception Regimens

Currently in the United States, 1.5 mg of levonorgestrel (Plan B One-Step, Next Choice), 30 mg of ulipristal acetate (UPA), and the copper T 380A IUD (Paragard) are the emergency contraceptives available to women. In 2006, Plan B (generic, Next Choice, Watson Pharmaceuticals) was released as two 0.75-mg levonorgestrel tablets to be taken as soon as possible and within 72 hours of unprotected intercourse, although clinical guidelines allowed its use up to 120 hours.[184] This progestin-only oral EC regimen was better tolerated compared to the older Yuzpe method of EC that used high doses of COCs. This was followed by the release of Plan B One-Step (Teva Women's Health, Inc.) in 2009, a combined 1.5-mg levonorgestrel tablet to be taken as one dose. After much political debate in the United States, the levonorgestrel products are now available in pharmacies over the counter for women aged 17 and older and by prescription for women under age 17.[187,188] Efforts to remove the age restriction for over-the-counter status failed in 2011.[189] UPA was approved in 2010 for EC in the United States and is marketed as Ella (HRA Pharma, Paris, France).[190] UPA is approved for use as soon as possible and up to 5 days after unprotected intercourse and is available by prescription only. UPA is a progesterone receptor modulator in the same class as mifepristone and is more effective than levonorgestrel EC.[191] The only contraindications to the oral EC regimens are allergy to the active substance or pregnancy. Of note, breastfeeding should be avoided for 36 hours after using UPA.

The copper T 380A IUD is also available for EC in women for up to 5 days after unprotected intercourse who desire to continue the device for their long-acting contraceptive method. The logistics of obtaining the copper T IUD for EC in the United States are more difficult than those for the oral regimens. Nevertheless, there is growing interest among U.S. women for this option, and it has the advantage of providing long-term contraception and decreasing the subsequent risk of unintended pregnancy.[192,193]

Mechanism of Action

The mode of action of hormonal EC is multifactorial and not completely understood. Because sperm are viable in the female reproductive tract for up to 5 days but eggs can be fertilized only within 1 day of ovulation, the mechanism of action most likely depends on when the oral EC regimen is given in relation to the time of intercourse and time of ovulation. No evidence supports the theory that hormonal EC interferes with postfertilization events, and most evidence suggests that it prevents pregnancy by preventing conception.[194] Because oral EC does not interrupt an established pregnancy, defined as beginning with implantation, hormonal EC is not considered an abortifacient.[195] The copper IUD works primarily by preventing fertilization because the copper ions are toxic to sperm and ova.[196] However, given its high efficacy, a secondary mechanism of preventing implantation cannot be ruled out.[194]

Efficacy

The effectiveness of EC depends on the mechanism of action of the method and when the method is used after unprotected intercourse. The probability of pregnancy after a single act of unprotected intercourse varies (3% to 8%) according to the day of the menstrual cycle and the couple's fertility status.[197] Calculating the efficacy of EC is complex because it is impossible to know how many pregnancies would otherwise have occurred. It is known, however, that the use of levonorgestrel-only EC is more effective than no treatment at all after a single episode of unprotected intercourse.[198] Plan B labeling cites an average preventive action of 89%. If 100 women had unprotected intercourse once during the second or third week of the cycle and were not treated with EC, about 8 would become pregnant, but after treatment with EC, typically only 1 woman would become pregnant. Taking a total of 1.5 mg of levonorgestrel in a single dose is as effective as the 0.75-mg split dose and single-dosing is more user-friendly.[199] The timing of levonorgestrel EC influences its effectiveness significantly. Waiting 12 hours to initiate treatment after unprotected intercourse increases the odds of pregnancy by almost 50%, and its efficacy decreases linearly with time.[200]

UPA is more effective than levonorgestrel EC when used within 24 hours and up to 5 days after unprotected sexual intercourse or suspected failure of a contraceptive method.[201] Unlike levonorgestrel, UPA prevents follicle rupture after the luteinizing hormone surge and therefore is superior at preventing ovulation.[202,203] Combining data from two studies allowed analysis of a sample sufficiently large to demonstrate that UPA almost halved the risk of pregnancy compared with levonorgestrel in women who received EC within 120 hours after sexual intercourse (odds ratio [OR], 0.55; 95% CI, 0.32-0.93).[201] When EC was used within 24 hours of unprotected sex, the risk of pregnancy was reduced by almost two thirds compared with levonorgestrel (OR, 0.35; 95% CI, 0.11-0.93).

Risk factors for failure of oral EC are body weight, intercourse during the fertile time of the cycle, and repeated acts of unprotected intercourse in the same cycle.[204] Preliminary data generate concern regarding the efficacy of oral EC in overweight and obese women. One study found that obese women have a three times greater risk of pregnancy following use of oral EC compared to normal-weight women (OR, 3.60; 95% CI, 1.96-6.53, $p < 0.001$).[204] Levonorgestrel performs worse than UPA in overweight and obese women, losing efficacy when BMI exceeds 26 kg/m^2, and UPA appears to retain effectiveness up to a BMI of 34 kg/m^2.[205] Of course, the most effective method of EC is the copper T 380A IUD, which has failure rates of less than 1 per 1000 and is not affected by body weight.[196]

Indications

EC is indicated for any woman at risk for unintended pregnancy from an episode of contraceptive failure or unprotected intercourse. Experts recommend the advance provision of EC to women.[206] However, surveys have found that the level of knowledge and use of EC in the United States by women and their health care providers is low.[184,207] Relatively few women presenting for termination of pregnancy or antenatal care were aware of EC.

No clinical examination or pregnancy testing is required before using oral hormonal EC.[9] There are no medical contraindications to the use of oral EC regimens because of their short duration of use.[8] Pregnancy is a relative contraindication because EC is ineffective if a pregnancy is already established. There is no evidence of teratogenicity. USMEC recommendations state that women with previous ectopic pregnancy, cardiovascular disease, migraines, or liver disease and women who are breastfeeding can use

EC.[8] There may be reduced efficacy of oral EC in women with severe malabsorption syndromes and those taking hepatic enzyme–inducing drugs and certain antiretroviral drugs. Contraindications for the copper IUD for EC are the same as those for regular contraceptive use.

Side Effects

The FDA has determined that levonorgestrel EC is safe enough to be available as an over-the-counter preparation only for women at least 17 years old. Women 16 years old or younger must obtain levonorgestrel EC with a prescription or without a prescription in states with direct pharmacy access. Not all pharmacies stock Plan B or participate in this program, but lists of participating pharmacies are available.[208] Although UPA is available by prescription only, this approach to EC has an excellent safety profile.[199] The side effects of the copper IUD for EC are the same as those for its use for long-term contraception.

There have been no deaths or serious complications directly linked to EC. The most common short-term side effects of oral EC include nausea, vomiting, and irregular bleeding, which affect up to 20% of users. Other minor adverse effects reported by women in clinical trials included dizziness, fatigue, breast tenderness, headache, and abdominal pain.[199] If vomiting occurs within 3 hours of taking oral EC, most experts recommend that the dose be repeated.[9]

Irregular bleeding caused by hormonal EC typically resolves by the next menstrual cycle. There is a low incidence of intermenstrual spotting after using hormonal EC, ranging from 3% to 37% in trials. After hormonal EC is taken, menses usually occurs within 1 week before or after the expected time. If the delay in the onset of menses is greater than 1 week or if the expected menses is lighter than usual, a pregnancy test should be performed. Because hormonal EC can postpone ovulation, making a woman vulnerable to pregnancy later in the cycle, women should be counseled to begin a regular method of contraception *immediately* after using EC.[9] A woman should also be advised to seek medical attention for continued irregular bleeding or abdominal pain, because these symptoms may be a sign of a spontaneous abortion or ectopic pregnancy.

CLINICAL CHALLENGES IN CONTRACEPTIVE CARE

Hormonal Contraception for Adolescents

Although on the decline, rates of teenage pregnancy are higher in the United States than in other Western industrialized countries.[6] Approximately 80% of these pregnancies are unplanned, of which about 26% end in induced abortion, 60% in live births, and 15% in miscarriage. Teenage pregnancy and parenting are precursors of poor medical, educational, and psychosocial outcomes for mother and child.[7] Children of teenage mothers are at greater risk for preterm birth, low birth weight, neonatal death, and later behavioral problems and poor academic performance. Teenage parenting contributes to the intergenerational transmission of poverty.[209] Studies show that sexually active adolescents will also be more motivated to use contraception if they are academically successful, believe pregnancy would be an impediment to their goals, and are involved in a stable relationship with a sexual partner.[7,210]

Considerations for clinicians advising adolescents about contraception should include the potentially high fertility rates in these young women, their high rates of unprotected intercourse, elevated risk of sexual assault, and increased risk of STIs.[211] Consistent and correct use of contraceptive methods can be challenging for adolescents and long-acting methods increase efficacy.[212] These methods, including DMPA injection, contraceptive implants, and IUDs, should be made available to teens.[213,214] With proper patient selection and counseling, IUDs and implants can be successful contraceptive options for adolescents.[215] Clinicians should also be aware of the legal conditions surrounding prescribing contraception to minors in the state in which they are practicing.[216]

Sexually active adolescents benefit from health guidance annually regarding responsible health behaviors, including abstinence, latex condoms to prevent STIs, and appropriate methods of birth control, along with instructions on ways to use them effectively.[209] Adolescents should also be counseled in a nonjudgmental manner about the need to use condoms during anal and oral intercourse. Barriers to effective contraception use by adolescents include lack of forward planning, nonconsensual intercourse, lack of confidential care, fear of disapproval by parents and doctors, absence of adolescent-friendly services, language and cultural barriers, fear of pelvic examination, and cost.[217] Misconceptions about contraception, including effects on weight gain, future fertility, acne, and risk of cancer, may also prevent adolescents from using effective contraception and should be addressed in counseling. The National Campaign to Prevent Teen and Unplanned Pregnancy operates a website that provides excellent information, decision tools, and reminders specifically designed for young women.[218]

Combined Hormonal Contraceptives in Adolescents

Although COCs, the patch, and the ring represent safe and effective methods for adolescents, many young women are not effectively educated about correct use and potential unwanted effects. They may use these short-acting hormonal contraceptives inconsistently, which will lead to very high pregnancy rates.[217] During counseling it is important to provide clear oral and written instructions about initiating these methods, ways to ensure correct use, and what to do if one or more pills are missed or if the patch or ring is not used correctly. By the same token, POPs are not favored for adolescents because they require stricter adherence for efficacy.

Initiating or continuing hormonal contraception does not require pelvic examination, cervical cancer screening, or sexually transmitted disease screening in adolescents or older reproductive-age women.[9] A history excluding contraindications, blood pressure measurement, and a negative urinary pregnancy test result are sufficient before initiating hormonal contraception.[219] Before beginning COCs, education about appropriate use, missed pills, and adverse effects is appropriate. Age-appropriate screening for STIs or cervical cancer should be considered regardless of contraceptive use. Screening for chlamydial infection and gonorrhea, as recommended by the CDC for women under the age of 26, can be accomplished through urine tests or a vaginal swab without a speculum.[220] The use of condoms should be encouraged in conjunction with the use of hormonal contraceptives to prevent STIs.

Initial follow-up should be at 8 to 12 weeks after commencing the COCs to monitor correct use and adverse events and should be done thereafter at 6- to 12-month intervals. Education and ongoing counseling are essential to ensure correct usage. Many adolescents are concerned that the COCs will cause weight gain or acne, and these issues should be directly addressed.[217] Chewable pills are available and may be more acceptable to young women who find it difficult to swallow pills. Unscheduled bleeding may be less acceptable to adolescents compared with adult women. Clinicians must consider the possibility that unscheduled bleeding represents cervicovaginal infection in this high-risk population and investigate and treat it accordingly.

Injectable Contraceptives in Adolescents

Discontinuation rates for DMPA in adolescents are high, with half of adolescents discontinuing the method by 12 months.[221] However, because DMPA suppresses ovulation for an extended period of time, prior use of DMPA protects many adolescents from unintended pregnancy despite inconsistent use. Weight gain is the most commonly cited reason for adolescents to discontinue DMPA, and it may be more common in African-American adolescents.[110] Although loss of bone density has been a concern in adolescents using DMPA, the position statement of the Society for Adolescent Medicine is that DMPA represents an extremely effective contraceptive and that clinical concerns about loss of BMD must be placed within the context of likely bone recovery on discontinuation, low risk of fractures, and benefits of preventing unintended pregnancy among adolescents.[118]

Hormonal Contraception in Postpartum and Lactating Women

The postpartum period is a critical time period for initiating contraception that helps women achieve optimal interpregnancy intervals.[222] The immediate postpartum period offers an ideal time for women to initiate contraception because of patient access and convenience. Delaying initiation of contraception until the standard 6-week postpartum visit places many women at risk for unintended pregnancy. By 6 weeks post partum, up to 40% of women will have had unprotected intercourse and nearly 50% will have ovulated.[223,224] Furthermore, not all women seek postpartum medical care, resulting in a large proportion with unmet contraceptive needs.[225] Therefore, evidence-based guidelines on the use of contraception in the postpartum period are essential.

Postpartum women remain in a hypercoagulable state for weeks after childbirth.[57] The USMEC recommends deferring use of estrogen-containing methods (category 4) until 3 weeks after delivery in all women. The guidelines further state that the benefits of estrogen-containing methods outweigh the risks (category 3) in breastfeeding women until 4 weeks after delivery; and depending on the risk factor, estrogen-containing methods outweigh the risk (category 3) or are contraindicated (category 4) in those with risk factors for VTE (such as age ≥ 35 years, previous VTE, thrombophilia, immobility, transfusion at delivery, BMI ≥ 30, postpartum hemorrhage, cesarean delivery, preeclampsia, and smoking) up to 6 weeks post partum or further.[49] Progestin-only methods are not restricted post partum for hypercoagulable or breastfeeding reasons.

Traditionally, combined hormonal contraception has not been recommended as the first choice for breastfeeding mothers because of concerns that the estrogenic component can reduce the volume of milk production and the caloric and mineral content of breast milk in lactating women. However, use of COCs by well-nourished breastfeeding women does not appear to result in problems with infant development. A systematic review of randomized, controlled trials concluded that existing data are of poor quality and insufficient to establish an effect of hormonal contraception on lactation.[226] Use of combination hormonal contraceptives can be considered after milk flow is well established. The USMEC allows the use of estrogen-containing methods after 30 days post partum in breastfeeding women without risk factors for VTE.[49]

Evidence from limited studies suggests that progestin-only contraception does not interfere with lactation or infant development and does not increase the risk of thromboembolic disease.[226] It appears reasonable to initiate progestin-only contraception, including DMPA, POPs, and implants, immediately after delivery, regardless of whether mothers are nursing their infants.[95] In addition, the insertion of IUDs immediately after the delivery of the placenta or as early as 4 weeks post partum is an option for women unless there is evidence of puerperal sepsis.[49,214]

Hormonal Contraception in Women Older Than 35 Years

No contraceptive methods are contraindicated based on age alone.[8] However, risks associated with the use of some methods may increase with age and additional comorbid conditions. For example, although the incidence of VTE, myocardial infarction, and stroke is low, these risks increase with age, obesity, smoking, and hypertension. However, because lean, healthy, nonsmoking women are at low risk for these rare events, they can use any method, including combined (estrogen-progestin pills, patch, and vaginal ring) methods, until menopause.[15] Large U.S. population-based case-control studies have found no increased risk of myocardial infarction or stroke among healthy, nonsmoking women older than 35 years who use COCs formulated with less than 50 μg of estrogen.[227,228]

The most effective reversible methods of contraception are long-acting reversible methods: the copper and progestin IUDs and the progestin implant. Because the copper IUD is nonhormonal and the hormonal IUD and implant do not contain estrogen, their use is not associated with an increased risk of cardiovascular events. In large prospective trials of users of progestin-only methods—pills, injections, implants, or IUDs—no substantial increase in the overall incidence of VTE, myocardial infarction, or cerebrovascular accidents has been noted.[229-231] Therefore, safe, effective options are available for the high-risk woman over 35.

Approximately 4 to 6 years prior to menopause, women will enter the menopausal transition and will likely experience changes in menstrual bleeding, including excessive or irregular menstruation, and vasomotor symptoms such as hot flashes and night sweats.[232] In healthy nonsmoking perimenopausal women, hormonal contraceptives represent appropriate treatment options for these symptoms, whether or not contraception is needed. Use of COCs and DMPA may reduce vasomotor symptoms in perimenopausal women, and most hormonal contraceptives will effectively treat abnormal uterine bleeding and prevent endometrial hyperplasia.[15] The reduced risk of endometrial and ovarian cancers associated with hormonal contraception use is of particular importance to older women of reproductive age.

Discontinuation of Hormonal Contraception at Menopause

The median age of menopause in North America is 51 years and, although pregnancy is uncommon after age 44,

TABLE 18-6

When to Discontinue Contraception

Contraceptive Method	Advice on Stopping Contraception	
	Age < 50 Years	Age ≥ 50 Years
Nonhormonal	May stop contraception after 2 years of amenorrhea	May stop contraception after 1 year of amenorrhea
Progestin-only methods: IUD, implant, injection, pill	Can be continued to age 55 years	Can be continued to age 55 years OR switch to nonhormonal method and stop after 1 year of amenorrhea
Estrogen-containing methods: ring, patch, pill	Can be continued to age 50 years or longer if no cardiovascular risk factors	Can be continued to age 55 years if no cardiovascular risk factors OR switch to nonhormonal method and stop after 1 year of amenorrhea

IUD, intrauterine device.

TABLE 18-7

Conditions Associated With Increased Risk for Adverse Health Events as a Result of Unintended Pregnancy

- Breast cancer
- Complicated valvular heart disease
- Diabetes: insulin-dependent; with nephropathy/retinopathy/neuropathy or other vascular disease; or of >20 years' duration
- Endometrial or ovarian cancer
- Epilepsy
- Hypertension (systolic > 160 mm Hg or diastolic > 100 mm Hg)
- History of bariatric surgery in the past 2 years
- HIV/AIDS
- Ischemic heart disease
- Malignant gestational trophoblastic disease
- Malignant liver tumors (hepatoma) and hepatocellular carcinoma of the liver
- Peripartum cardiomyopathy
- Schistosomiasis with fibrosis of the liver
- Severe (decompensated) cirrhosis
- Sickle cell disease
- Solid organ transplantation within the past 2 years
- Stroke
- Systemic lupus erythematosus
- Thrombogenic mutations
- Tuberculosis

AIDS, acquired immunodeficiency syndrome; HIV, human immunodeficiency virus.

From Centers for Disease Control and Prevention. U.S. Medical Eligibility Criteria for Contraceptive Use, 2010. *MMWR Morb Mortal Wkly Rep.* 2010;59:1-86.

spontaneous conception can occur. Assessment of follicle-stimulating hormone levels to determine when a woman is menopausal is often inaccurate. Therefore, it is recommended that women continue to use contraception until menopause or age 50 to 55 years.[9] Most women will be able to use contraception safely until they are assured of menopause. The decision of when to stop a contraception method must involve evaluation of the benefits of the method, health risks resulting from its use as age increases, diminishing risk of pregnancy, and availability of alternative methods (Table 18-6).[15] The use of the copper IUD is safe up to and into menopause unless bleeding abnormalities develop. For progestin-only methods, the potential benefits of decreased bleeding and endometrial protection outweigh risks of continuing use because arterial and venous cardiovascular events are not increased.[9] Healthy, lean, nonsmoking women can generally use combined methods until menopause; however, if new cardiovascular risk factors develop, reevaluation of contraceptive choice is appropriate.

Contraception in Women With Underlying Medical Conditions

Because pregnancy in women with underlying medical conditions is associated with higher risks of maternal and perinatal morbidity and mortality, achieving effective contraception is particularly important in this setting (Table 18-7). Providers should remember that the risk of using a contraceptive must be balanced with the risk of pregnancy in these patients. Although numerous studies have addressed the safety and effectiveness of hormonal contraceptive use in healthy women, data unfortunately are far less complete for women with underlying medical problems or other special circumstances. Using the best available scientific evidence, this chapter provides information to help clinicians and women with coexisting medical conditions make sound decisions regarding the selection and appropriateness of various hormonal contraceptives, including the levonorgestrel IUD. Guidelines from the CDC (USMEC, 2010) provide an important evidence-based resource for clinicians.[8]

Decisions regarding contraception for women with coexisting medical problems may be complicated. In some cases, medications taken for certain chronic conditions may alter the effectiveness of hormonal contraception, and pregnancy in these cases may pose substantial risks to the mother and her fetus. Differences in content and delivery methods of hormonal contraceptives may affect patients with certain conditions differently. Because transdermal and vaginal ring contraception is relatively new, few data address its use in women with medical concerns. In the absence of more extensive data, contraindications to the use of estrogen-progestin COCs should also be considered as contraindications to the use of transdermal and vaginal ring contraception. Practitioners should recognize that the use of nonhormonal forms of contraception, such as the copper IUD, remains a safe, effective choice for many women with medical conditions.

Hormonal Contraception in Obese Women

The proportion of Americans who are obese (BMI ≥ 30) is rising.[233] Concerns about obesity and contraception include possible complications such as VTE or reduced efficacy and the increased risk of pregnancy associated with obesity. The prospect of effective contraception with weight loss may also provide a window of opportunity for obese women to achieve a normal BMI, increase their chances of successful pregnancy, and reduce pregnancy complications.[234] Because pregnancy confers increased risks to mother and child in these pregnancies, the clinician must ensure that safe and effective contraception is provided when pregnancy is not planned.

More data are needed to determine whether the efficacy of combined hormonal contraception is decreased in obese women.[235] The true rate of contraceptive failure in overweight and obese women is unknown, because past clinical trials of efficacy routinely excluded women who weighed more than 90 kg. Observational studies have reported conflicting results, and most large studies did not control for compliance with the medication.[25,236] The efficacy of COCs, contraceptive rings, and transdermal patches primarily reflects the suppression of ovulation that results from the dose of progestin. Time to reach steady-state levels of levonorgestrel after ingestion appears to be twice as long among obese women compared with women of normal weight; the interval until hypothalamic-pituitary-ovarian activity is suppressed may be lengthened, placing obese women at higher risk for ovulation.[237] Therefore, the traditional 7-day HFI may increase the risk of failure, and it may be that obese women would have higher efficacy with 24/4 or continuous formulations of COCs.[238] All in all, the failure rate among obese COC users is estimated to be between 60% and 120% greater than among those with a normal BMI.[237] Despite this observation, COCs are more effective than barrier methods in obese women.

In clinical trials of the marketed transdermal patch, women in the highest weight decile (≥90 kg) had a substantially higher contraceptive failure rate.[68] However, in a phase 3 trial of an investigational low-dose estrogen-progestin contraceptive patch in which approximately 30% of participants were obese, the rate of contraceptive failure was similar among obese and nonobese women.[76] The incrementally higher rates in this setting with oral and transdermal methods should not exclude their use in overweight women motivated to use these methods in preference to less effective methods. There is very little information on the efficacy of the vaginal ring in obese women.

Obese women who are concerned about the possibility of decreased efficacy with COCs can consider using an IUD or implant as highly effective alternatives, especially because many obese women have hypertension and other risk factors for vascular disease that may be exacerbated by exogenous estrogen.[176] Because obese women have an elevated risk for abnormal uterine bleeding and endometrial neoplasia, use of the LNG-IUS may represent a particularly sound choice.

There is relatively little high-quality information regarding the efficacy of DMPA in obese women, but in overweight women, higher pregnancy rates have not been observed with use of the 150-mg intramuscular formulation or 106-mg subcutaneous formulation of DMPA.[92] Although DMPA does not appear to increase BMI in women overall, adolescents who are already obese may gain more weight when using DMPA compared with other methods.[110]

The health risks associated with use of estrogen-containing contraceptives may be increased in obese women. Exogenous estrogen and obesity are independent risk factors for VTE.[69] Case-control studies suggest that higher BMI values (>25) may increase the risk of VTE by up to 10-fold in COC users.[239] However, obese women are also at higher risk for VTE in pregnancy compared to normal-weight women, and pregnancy may pose a greater risk than combined hormonal contraception use.[240] In helping overweight women make sound contraceptive choices, practitioners should incorporate these observations in discussions with patients. It is important to remember that no contraceptive method is contraindicated based on weight alone.[8]

Hormonal Contraception in Women Taking Antiepileptic Drugs

Effective contraception is a critical component of the management of the female patient with epilepsy because of the increased risk of seizures in pregnancy, the teratogenic effect of some antiepileptic drugs (AEDs), and the multitude of interactions between AEDs and hormonal contraception. Steroid hormones and many of the AEDs are substrates for the cytochrome P450 enzyme system, in particular, the CYP3A4 isoenzyme. Concomitant use of hormonal contraceptives and AEDs may pose a risk of unexpected pregnancy, seizures, and drug-related adverse effects.[241] The risk of COC failure is slightly increased in the presence of CYP3A4 enzyme-inducing AEDs. Enzyme-inducing AEDs include carbamazepine, felbamate, lamotrigine, phenobarbital, phenytoin, oxcarbazepine, primidone, topiramate, and rufinamide.[8] Several AEDs also induce the production of sex hormone–binding globulin (SHBG) to which the progestins are tightly bound, resulting in lower concentrations of free progestin that may also lead to COC failure. There is no increase in the risk of COC failure in women taking non–enzyme-inducing AEDs. In addition, oral contraceptives significantly increase the metabolism of lamotrigine, posing a risk of seizures when hormonal agents are initiated and of toxicity during pill-free weeks.[241] There is no evidence that COCs increase seizures in women with epilepsy. The USMEC recommends that when a COC is chosen, a preparation containing a minimum of 30 µg of ethinyl estradiol should be used. POPs are subject to the same limitations as COCs in the setting of enzyme-inducing AEDs. There are few data regarding the contraceptive patch and vaginal ring. Contraceptive failures have also been reported in women taking enzyme-inducing AEDs and using the etonogestrel implant system (Nexplanon).[175] Although higher-dose COCs are one contraceptive option for women on enzyme-inducing AEDs, a variety of other options are available. Injectable contraception (DMPA) appears effective with concomitant AED use, and IUDs are highly effective in women taking anticonvulsants.[8]

Hormonal Contraception in Women Taking Antibiotics

Although there have been many retrospective case series and anecdotal reports of COC failure in women taking concomitant antibiotics, pharmacokinetic evidence of lower serum steroid levels exists only for rifampin. Women taking rifampin should not rely on oral, transdermal, vaginal ring, or implantable contraception alone for protection.[8] In contrast to rifampin, use of ampicillin, doxycycline, fluconazole, metronidazole, miconazole, quinalones, and tetracycline have not lowered steroid levels in women using COCs. The use of combined hormonal methods is not restricted among women taking broad-spectrum antibiotics, antifungals, or antiparasitics.[8] It is possible, however, that individual differences in pharmacokinetic responses to antibiotics can cause contraceptive failures.[242] For women who are concerned about the small possibility of a drug interaction, backup condoms or abstinence can be used while on the antibiotic.

Hormonal Contraception in HIV-Positive Women

More than 17 million women, many of reproductive age, are infected with HIV.[243] HIV transmission increasingly is linked to heterosexual intercourse. The role of hormonal contraception in HIV-positive women has been controversial. There may be an increased risk for acquiring or transmitting HIV in DMPA users, but DMPA is a needed contraceptive in areas of high HIV prevalence (sub-Saharan Africa) where there are limited alternative contraceptive options.[121] After reviewing the evidence, the WHO and CDC recently concluded that the use of hormonal contraceptives, including combined hormonal contraceptives, POPs, DMPA, and implants, is safe (category 1) for women at high risk for HIV infection or infected with HIV.[127] However, for women using DMPA who are at high risk for HIV infection, condom use is even more strongly encouraged, given the inconclusive nature of the evidence regarding an increased risk for HIV acquisition with injectables. Hormonal contraceptives, including DMPA, do not appear to have an impact on HIV disease progression.[244] For women on antiretroviral therapy, it is important to note there are several drug-drug interactions with hormonal contraceptives (particularly some non-nucleoside reverse transcriptase inhibitors and ritonavir-boosted protease inhibitors). These interactions might alter the safety and efficacy of both the hormonal contraceptive and the antiretroviral drug.[127] Case reports suggest that the antiretroviral drug efavirenz reduces contraceptive implant protection; IUDs and DMPA represent preferable contraceptive choices for women taking this medication or others that induce hepatic enzymes.[182]

IUDs are allowed by the USMEC for women with HIV (category 2) as there is no evidence that they are at higher risk for infectious complications compared to HIV-uninfected women.[245] The IUD has not been shown to affect disease progression or increase risk of transmission to sex partners. For women with AIDS, IUDs can be used if they are clinically well on antiretroviral therapy (category 2) and generally are not recommended (category 3) if not.[8] All IUD users with AIDS should be closely monitored for pelvic infection.

Hormonal Contraception and Chronic Hypertension

All women should have their blood pressure measured prior to initiating combined hormonal contraception.[9] Modern low-dose COCs may increase systolic and diastolic blood pressure, on average, by 8 and 6 mm Hg, respectively.[246] Nevertheless, a systematic review of the literature found that only a small percentage of women developed incident hypertension in up to 2 years of follow-up after starting a COC.[247] For women with preexisting hypertension, the concern with combined hormonal methods is the increased risk of arterial thrombosis leading to myocardial infarction and stroke.[248] Although the absolute risk of these events is low, the decision to use combined contraception in hypertensive women should be balanced against the higher risks of pregnancy. The USMEC rates combined hormonal contraception as contraindicated (category 4) for women with blood pressures higher than 160/100 mm Hg.[8] For women with blood pressures in the range of 140-159/90-99 mm Hg or women with adequately treated hypertension, the USMEC rates combined methods as category 3, in which the method is generally not recommended unless other more appropriate methods are not available or acceptable (see Table 18-2). As such, progestin-only methods and IUDs are a safer option for hypertensive women. Among these options, for women with controlled hypertension, or hypertension less than 160/100 mm Hg, the USMEC rates progestin-only methods as category 1 or 2. For women with severe hypertension at 160/100 mm Hg or higher, only DMPA is given a rating of category 3, perhaps because it cannot be discontinued easily once the injection is given. The only study to examine the risks of cardiovascular disease among women with hypertension using progestin-only methods showed that women on POPs or DMPA had only a slightly increased risk of cardiovascular events.[231] There are no studies evaluating the use of the levonorgestrel IUD or etonogestrel implant in women with hypertension.

Hormonal Contraception in Women with Lipid Disorders

The term *dyslipidemia* includes disorders of lipoprotein metabolism that lead to atherosclerosis. These abnormalities arise from genetic and secondary factors and are caused by excessive entry of lipoproteins into the bloodstream or an impairment in their removal, or both. The estrogen component of COCs enhances removal of LDL cholesterol and increases levels of HDL cholesterol. Oral estrogen also increases triglyceride levels; however, in the setting of concomitantly increased HDL and decreased LDL levels, the moderate triglyceride elevations caused by oral estrogen use do not appear to increase the risk of atherogenesis.[249] The progestin component of COCs antagonizes these estrogen-induced lipid changes, which increases LDL levels and decreases HDL and triglyceride levels. Among women taking COCs with an identical dose of estrogen, the choice and dose of the progestin component may affect net lipid changes. COCs formulated with more androgenic progestins raise HDL and triglyceride levels less than formulations with less androgenic progestins.[250] Nevertheless, overall modern COCs have little effect on lipid metabolism in normal-weight women.[251] Similar to COCs, the use of the contraceptive patch and ring does not cause important clinical effects on lipids.[252,253] The USMEC does not recommend routine screening for dyslipidemia prior to initiating hormonal contraceptives.[8,254] Lipids are surrogate measures, and the effect of contraceptives on lipids may not necessarily correlate with effects on cardiovascular disease or mortality risk. It is not known whether the differential lipid effects of distinct hormonal contraceptive formulations or means of administration have any clinical significance in women with normal baseline lipid levels or those with lipid disorders. However, for women with known hyperlipidemias, the type, severity, and presence of other cardiovascular risk factors should be evaluated before using estrogen-containing contraceptives. Because the absolute risk of cardiovascular events is low, most women with controlled dyslipidemia can use COCs formulated with 35 µg estrogen or less. Fasting serum lipid levels should be monitored as frequently as each month after initiating COCs in dyslipidemic women. Less frequent monitoring is appropriate after stabilization of lipid parameters has been observed. In women with uncontrolled LDL cholesterol levels greater than 160 mg/dL or with multiple additional risk factors for cardiovascular disease (including smoking, diabetes, obesity, hypertension, family history of premature coronary artery disease, HDL level <35 mg/dL, or triglyceride level >250 mg/dL), use of non–estrogen-containing contraceptives should be considered.[8]

In contrast to COCs, use of DMPA lowers HDL levels, raises LDL levels, and does not raise triglyceride levels.[255] However, similar to combined hormonal contraception, DMPA is unlikely to cause clinically meaningful changes in normal women. The use of DMPA and other progestin-only contraceptives is appropriate in women with hypertriglyceridemia, who may be at increased risk for pancreatitis if they used COCs. The LNG-IUS and the etonogestrel implant have not been shown to affect circulating lipid or triglyceride levels.[256,257] The USMEC gives all progestin-only contraceptives a category 2 rating for women with known hyperlipidemias, indicating that the benefits outweigh the risks.[8]

Hormonal Contraception in Women with Diabetes

COCs do not appear to impair carbohydrate metabolism or affect vascular disease in diabetic women. A history of gestational diabetes is not a contraindication to hormonal contraceptives.[8] A systematic review concluded that hormonal contraceptives have limited effect on carbohydrate metabolism in women without diabetes. However, studies are limited and do not inform the management of diabetic women who are overweight.[74,258] Although the existing data support the use of combination hormonal contraceptives by women with diabetes, use should be limited to nonsmoking, otherwise healthy women with diabetes who show no evidence of hypertension, nephropathy, retinopathy, or other vascular disease.[8] Similarly, DMPA should be used with caution in diabetics with vascular disease due to its effects on HDL levels. The USMEC states that other progestin-only methods can generally be used in women with diabetes of any severity (category 2) with appropriate follow-up.[8] A clinical trial found that metabolic control was similar in women with uncomplicated diabetes randomized to a copper IUD or the LNG-IUS.[259] The LNG-IUS is an excellent option for women with diabetes.

Hormonal Contraception in Women With Hypercoagulable States

Women with familial thrombophilic syndromes including factor V Leiden mutation; prothrombin G2010 A mutation; and protein C, protein S, or antithrombin deficiencies have an elevated risk for VTE during COC use and pregnancy and can develop VTE earlier during use than lower risk users.[260] Women with factor V Leiden mutation have an increased risk of VTE of about eightfold compared with women without the mutation, and the risk is more than 30 times higher for carriers who used COCs compared with nonusers who are not carriers of the mutation.[261] Approximately 5% of women of European ethnicity are thought to carry the factor V Leiden mutation, but many of them will never experience a thrombotic event. In light of this, screening for factor V Leiden mutations or other thrombophilias is not considered to be cost-effective in the U.S. population considering estrogen-containing contraception in the absence of a clear family or personal history of thrombosis.[9] However, women with known familial thrombophilic conditions should be encouraged to use progestin-only and intrauterine contraception.[8]

Hormonal Contraception in Women Awaiting Surgery

VTE with pulmonary embolism remains a major cause of fatalities associated with surgical (including gynecologic) procedures. There is concern that combined hormonal contraception use around the time of surgery may increase this risk. The procoagulant changes of COCs take 6 weeks or longer to resolve after discontinuation.[262] The benefits associated with stopping combined hormonal contraceptives 1 month or more before major surgery should be balanced against the risks of an unintended pregnancy. The USMEC recommends that COCs be discontinued before major surgery with an anticipated prolonged immobilization postoperatively (category 4).[8] In addition, patients with risk factors for VTE such as prior VTE or undergoing high-risk procedures (such as major abdominal-pelvic surgeries, major orthopedic surgeries, or cancer surgery) may consider discontinuing COCs. Otherwise, for any major surgery for which the patient is expected to be ambulatory immediately after surgery, it is not necessary to discontinue combined hormonal contraceptives. Because of the low perioperative risk of VTE, it is not considered necessary to discontinue combined hormonal contraceptives before

laparoscopic tubal sterilization or other minor surgical procedures not known to be associated with an elevated VTE risk. Progestin-only and intrauterine contraceptives are not expected to be associated with an increased risk of perioperative VTE.

Hormonal Contraception in Women With a History of Thromboembolism

Women with a documented history of unexplained VTE, recurrent VTE, or VTE associated with pregnancy, thrombophilia (including antiphospholipid antibody syndrome), active cancer, or exogenous estrogen use should not use estrogen-containing hormonal contraceptives.[8] Some, but not all, experts allow estrogen use if the woman is taking anticoagulants concomitantly, but there are no published studies on this approach.[263] A COC candidate who experienced a single episode of VTE years earlier associated with a nonrecurring risk factor (e.g., VTE occurring after immobilization after a motor vehicle accident) may not currently be at increased risk for VTE. The decision to initiate estrogen-containing contraceptives in such patients can therefore be individualized. Limited data have assessed the risk of VTE associated with use of progestin-only contraceptives. Most studies have not found an increased VTE risk with use of progestin-only contraception.[231,264,265] The USMEC states that progestin-only contraceptives including the LNG-IUS can generally be used in women with a history of deep vein thrombosis/pulmonary embolism (DVT/PE) or acute DVT/PE (category 2).[8]

Hormonal Contraception in Women Taking Anticoagulation Therapy

The long-term risks of warfarin for reproductive-age women include heavy or prolonged menstrual bleeding and rarely include hemoperitoneum after rupture of ovarian cysts. Warfarin is a teratogen. Because COCs can reduce menstrual blood loss and do not appear to increase the risk of recurrent thrombosis in well-anticoagulated women, some authorities recommend their use in these patients. However, no large studies address the safety of estrogen-containing contraceptives in women taking oral anticoagulation, and many experts recommend the use of progestin-only or intrauterine contraception in this setting.[263] Because use of the copper IUD may increase menstrual flow, use of the LNG-IUS is more appropriate in this situation.[266] Because intramuscular injection of DMPA consistently suppresses ovulation and anecdotal experience has not revealed injection site problems such as hematoma in anticoagulated women,[267] DMPA represents another potential contraceptive choice in this patient population. Finally, another safe option for women on anticoagulation is the etonogestrel implant.[8] There are no data on the risk of hematoma formation at the insertion site of contraceptive implants; however, it is unlikely to be a greater risk than that associated with intramuscular DMPA injections.

Hormonal Contraception for Women With Migraine Headaches

Headaches are common in women of reproductive age. Most of these headaches are tension headaches, not migraines. Some women with migraines experience improvement in their symptoms with the use of hormonal contraceptives, and some women's symptoms worsen. Because the presence of true migraine headaches affects the decision to use estrogen-containing contraception, careful consideration of the diagnosis is important. Neurologists diagnose migraines using the International Classification of Headache Disorders II (ICHD II) criteria, the official criteria of the International Headache Society (IHS).[268]

Most migraines occur without aura. Nausea, vomiting, photophobia, phonophobia, or visual blurring occurring before or during a migraine headache do not constitute aura. Typical auras last 5 to 60 minutes before headache and characteristically are visual. Several reversible visual symptoms indicate the presence of aura: a flickering, uncolored zigzag line progressing laterally to the periphery of one visual field and laterally spreading, scintillating scotoma (i.e., area of lost or depressed vision within a visual field, surrounded by an area of normal or less depressed vision or loss of vision).

The risk of stroke is increased in women who have migraine with aura.[269] Although cerebrovascular events occur rarely among women with migraine with aura who use COCs, the impact of a stroke is so devastating that clinicians should consider the use of progestin-only or intrauterine contraceptives in this setting. According to the USMEC, estrogen-containing contraceptives are contraindicated (category 4) in women migraine sufferers with aura and should be discontinued in patients suffering from migraine without aura if aura symptoms appear.[8] For women older than 35 years with migraines with or without aura, combination estrogen-progestin contraceptives should be avoided in favor of progestin-only and intrauterine methods.

The IHS Task Force on Combined Oral Contraceptives and Hormone Replacement Therapy, however, states that the risks can be individualized to the patient, which is more in line with a category 3 recommendation from the USMEC.[270] Thus, use of combined hormonal contraception in women experiencing migraine with aura is not strictly contraindicated by the IHS. In assessing the risk of combined hormonal contraception in patients who have migraine and migraine with aura, the IHS suggests that other independent risk factors for stroke also be assessed and taken into consideration, including age older than 35 years, tobacco use, dyslipidemia, family history of arterial disease, age younger than 45 years, and other relevant medical comorbid conditions (i.e., obesity [BMI ≥ 30], diabetes, known vascular disease). Of note, some headache specialists are suggesting that today's ultralow-dose COC formulations (e.g., the COC formulated with 10 µg ethinyl estradiol) may be safe and also useful in preventing menstrual-related migraines in migraineurs who are otherwise healthy, normotensive nonsmokers.[271]

Hormonal Contraception in Women With Systemic Lupus Erythematosus

Although effective contraception is important for women with lupus, concerns about increasing disease activity and thrombosis have resulted in clinicians' rarely prescribing combination estrogen-progestin oral contraceptives to women with this disease. Indeed, women with SLE are at higher risk for ischemic heart disease, stroke, and VTE, especially in the presence of antiphospolipid antibodies.[272] Nevertheless, providing effective contraception for women with SLE is extremely important. Pregnancy carries marked maternal and fetal risks, and almost one fourth of women with SLE who conceive choose to terminate their pregnancies.[273] Data indicate that COCs are safe in women with SLE if they have stable, mild disease; are seronegative for antiphospholipid antibodies; and have no history of thrombosis.[274] The USMEC recommends that combined hormonal contraceptives and progestin-only contraceptives may generally be used in women with SLE who have no other cardiovascular risk factors.[8] For women with SLE and antiphospholipid antibodies, combined hormonal contraceptives are contraindicated (category 4), and progestin-only methods should be used with caution (category 3). Prior to initiating contraceptives in women with SLE, the level of disease activity and presence of antiphospholipid antibodies and thrombocytopenia should be established. IUDs remain an option for women with SLE. For women with thrombocytopenia, the levonorgestrel IUD is preferred over the copper IUD.[8] Immunosuppression is no longer considered a contraindication to IUD use.[272]

Hormonal Contraception in Women With Sickle Cell Disease

Similar to pregnancy in SLE patients, pregnancy in women with sickle cell disease increases maternal and fetal morbidity and mortality rates.[8] The safety of hormonal contraceptives in women with homozygous sickle cell (SS) disease has been controversial. Only one small randomized, controlled trial has addressed this issue. Twenty-five patients were given DMPA or intramuscular saline placebo injections once every three months in a crossover design. DMPA users were less likely to experience painful sickle episodes (OR, 0.23; 95% CI, 0.05 to 1.02).[275] No randomized studies have addressed estrogen-containing products.[276] These limited data suggest that DMPA and other progestin-only methods are a safe contraceptive option for women with sickle cell disease.[277]

No well-controlled study has assessed whether VTE risk in oral contraception users with sickle cell disease is higher than in other combination oral contraception users. However, a small U.S. case-control study found that COC use was associated with a nonsignificantly elevated risk of VTE.[278] Cross-sectional studies of women with sickle cell disease have observed no differences in markers for platelet activation, thrombin generation, fibrinolysis, or red blood cell deformability between users of combination oral contraception methods, users of progestin-only methods, and nonusers of hormonal contraception.[279] On the basis of these observations, studies of pregnant women with sickle cell disease, and small observational studies of women with sickle cell disease who use COCs, and on theoretical considerations, the USMEC concludes that pregnancy carries a greater risk than estrogen-containing contraceptive use.[8] This recommendation would change, however, if the woman had concomitant cardiovascular risk factors or pulmonary hypertension, a complication of sickle cell disease.

Although the lack of evidence on IUD use among women with sickle cell disease represents a major gap in the literature, theoretical concerns about IUD use in this population are few. There is no current evidence to support limiting IUD use among women with sickle cell disease.[277] The USMEC rates the levonorgestrel IUD category 1, indicating that there are no restrictions for this method in women with sickle cell disease. The copper IUD is considered category 2, in which benefits outweigh risks, because of the theoretical concern about increased blood loss with menstruation.[8]

Hormonal Contraception in Depression

Depression and mood disorders are extremely common in women of reproductive age.[280] The issues to consider are the impact of hormonal contraceptives on mood and the potential impact of treatments for depression on contraceptive efficacy. Data on the use of hormonal contraceptives in women with depression are limited but usually show no effect.[281] Women with depressive disorders do not

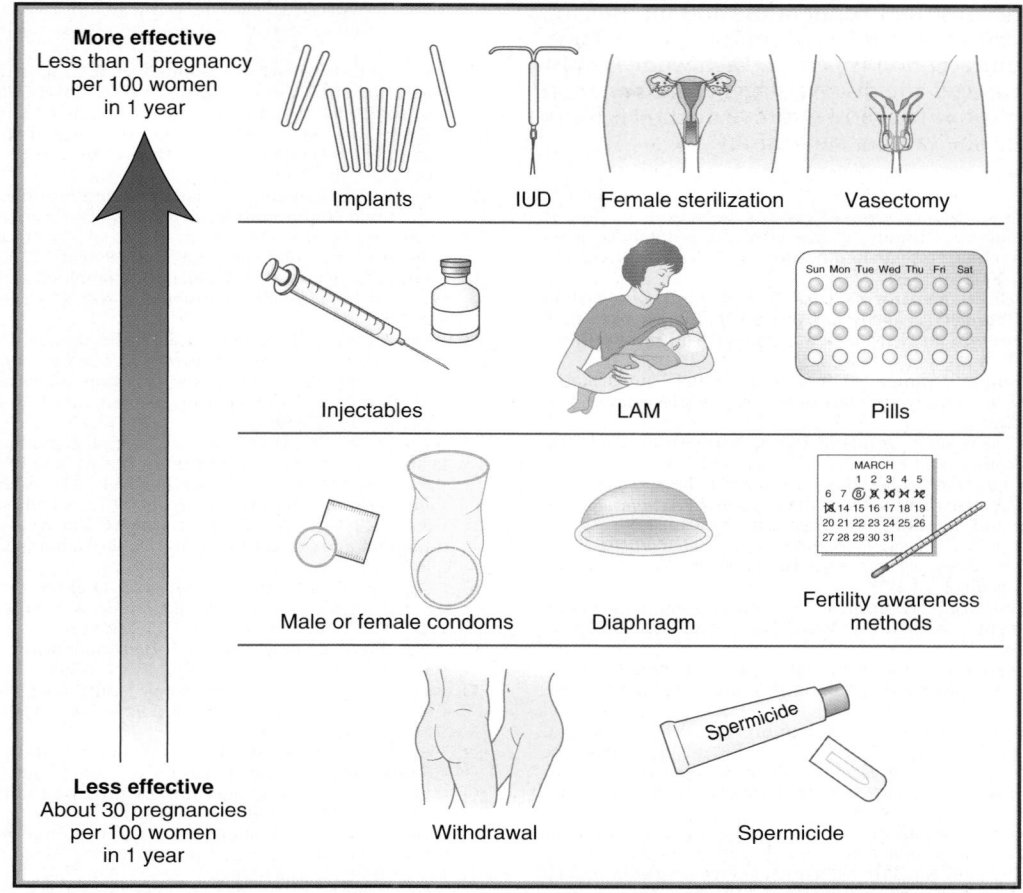

Figure 18-5 Comparing effectiveness of family planning methods. IUD, intrauterine device; LAM, lactational amenorrhea method. (Redrawn from World Health Organization Department of Reproductive Health and Research (WHO/RHR) and Johns Hopkins Bloomberg School of Public Health/Center for Communication Programs (CCP), Knowledge for Health Project. *Family Planning: A Global Handbook for Providers* (2011 update). Baltimore and Geneva: CCP and WHO; 2011.)

appear to suffer worsening of symptoms with use of hormonal methods of contraception including DMPA.[282,283] There are no restrictions on the use of any hormonal contraceptive in women with depressive disorders.[8]

Prescription antidepressants do not affect the efficacy of hormonal contraceptives.[8] Data from randomized, controlled trials of fluoxetine have failed to confirm any effect of COCs on the response to fluoxetine.[284] However, the herbal remedy St. John's wort, a hepatic enzyme inducer, increased progestin and estrogen metabolism, breakthrough bleeding, and the likelihood of ovulation in women using COCs.[285]

CHOOSING A CONTRACEPTIVE METHOD

Given the number of contraceptive options available to women, it is important that providers concentrate their efforts on helping women chose the best contraceptive method and focus on counseling that helps improve continuation. The best birth control method is one that provides the safest and most effective contraceptive for a woman and is the method she chooses to use and has access to. This approach places a strong value on medical considerations but also includes consideration of a woman's lifestyle, preferences, level of prevention desired, and the affordability of the product given her access to health insurance or ability to pay. Long-acting reversible contraceptives (i.e., IUDs and the implant) offer women the

advantages of high contraceptive efficacy and high rates of continuation. When discussing contraception, clinicians should present all suitable options to their patients but outline the options in terms of tiers of effectiveness (Fig. 18-5). Tier 1 includes long-acting reversible contraception and sterilization. Tier 2 includes combined methods (pill, patch, and ring), DMPA, and the POP. Tier 3 includes barrier methods, and tier 4 includes withdrawal and use of spermicides.

When helping women make sound contraceptive decisions, clinicians should consider the patient's age, lifestyle, and other relevant circumstances, including the recognition that contraceptive needs are likely to change during different phases of reproductive life and that the risks and benefits may alter according to age and background health factors. For those considering pregnancy in the future, contraceptive reversibility and time to return of fertility should be discussed. Affordability must be considered, because it may affect continuation rates and therefore affect efficacy.

As with all medications, contraceptives have potential side effects. Candid discussion of these effects and other areas of anticipatory guidance may increase acceptability. The clinician should offer information about adverse events that are individualized and provided in the context of how they compare with the effects of an unplanned pregnancy. Information about contraceptive failure and access to emergency contraception should be given. For those at risk for sexually transmitted diseases, clinicians should encourage consistent condom use and minimizing the number of partners, regardless of contraceptive choice. No method of contraception is perfect. Each woman must consider the advantages and disadvantages of each method in making her decision. The most effective method is likely to be the one that she can use successfully.

REFERENCES

1. Gipson JD, Koenig MA, Hindin MJ. The effects of unintended pregnancy on infant, child, and parental health: a review of the literature. *Stud Fam Plann*. 2008;39:18-38.
2. Gold RB, Sonfield A, Richards C, Frost JJ. *Next Steps for America's Family Planning Program: Leveraging the Potential of Medicaid and Title X in an Evolving Health Care System*. New York, NY: Guttmacher Institute; 2009.
3. Guttmacher Institute. Unintended Pregnancy in the United States, 2013. Available at http://www.guttmacher.org/pubs/FB-unintended-pregnancy-US.html.
4. Singh S, Sedgh G, Hussain R. Unintended pregnancy: worldwide levels, trends, and outcomes. *Stud Fam Plann*. 2010;41:241-250.
5. World Health Organization. *Ensuring Human Rights in the Provision of Contraceptive Information and Services: Guidance and Recommendations*. Geneva, Switzerland: World Health Organization; 2014.
6. Kost K, Henshaw S. *U.S. Teenage Pregnancies, Births and Abortions, 2010: National and State Trends by Age, Race and Ethnicity*. New York, NY: Guttmacher Institute; 2014:1-28.
7. Klein JD, American Academy of Pediatrics Committee on Adolescence. Adolescent pregnancy: current trends and issues. *Pediatrics*. 2005;116:281-286.
8. Centers for Disease Control and Prevention. U.S. Medical Eligibility Criteria for Contraceptive Use, 2010. *MMWR Morb Mortal Wkly Rep*. 2010;59:1-86.
9. Centers for Disease Control and Prevention. U.S. selected practice recommendations for contraceptive use, 2013: adapted from the World Health Organization selected practice recommendations for contraceptive use, 2nd ed. *MMWR Morb Mortal Wkly Rep*. 2013;62:1-60.
10. Cleland K, Peipert JF, Westhoff C, et al. Family planning as a cost-saving preventive health service. *N Engl J Med*. 2011;364:e37.
11. ACOG Practice Bulletin No. 110: Noncontraceptive uses of hormonal contraceptives. *Obstet Gynecol*. 2010;115:206-218.
12. Trussell J. Contraceptive failure in the United States. *Contraception*. 2011;83:397-404.
13. Nelson AL, Cwiak C. Combined oral contraceptives. In: Hatcher RA, Trussell J, Nelson AL, et al., eds. *Contraceptive Technology*. 20th ed. New York, NY: Ardent Media; 2011.
14. Coffee AL, Kuehl TJ, Willis S, Sulak PJ. Oral contraceptives and premenstrual symptoms: comparison of a 21/7 and extended regimen. *Am J Obstet Gynecol*. 2006;195:1311-1319.
15. Allen RH, Cwiak CA, Kaunitz AM. Contraception in women over 40 years of age. *Can Med Assoc J*. 2013;185:565-573.
16. Mosher WD, Jones J. Use of contraception in the United States: 1982-2008. *Vital Health Stat 23*. 2010;(29):1-44.
17. Jensen JT, Burke AE, Barnhart KT, et al. Effects of switching from oral to transdermal or transvaginal contraception on markers of thrombosis. *Contraception*. 2008;78:451-458.
18. Jensen JT. Evaluation of a new estradiol oral contraceptive: estradiol valerate and dienogest. *Expert Opin Pharmacother*. 2010;11:1147-1157.
19. Westhoff C, Kaunitz AM, Korver T, et al. Efficacy, safety, and tolerability of a monophasic oral contraceptive containing nomegestrol acetate and 17beta-estradiol: a randomized controlled trial. *Obstet Gynecol*. 2012;119:989-999.
20. Sulak PJ, Scow RD, Preece C, et al. Hormone withdrawal symptoms in oral contraceptive users. *Obstet Gynecol*. 2000;95:261-266.
21. Edelman A, Gallo MF, Nichols MD, et al. Continuous versus cyclic use of combined oral contraceptives for contraception: systematic Cochrane review of randomized controlled trials. *Hum Reprod*. 2006;21:573-578.
22. Willis SA, Kuehl TJ, Spiekerman AM, Sulak PJ. Greater inhibition of the pituitary-ovarian axis in oral contraceptive regimens with a shortened hormone-free interval. *Contraception*. 2006;74:100-103.
23. Klipping C, Duijkers I, Trummer D, Marr J. Suppression of ovarian activity with a drospirenone-containing oral contraceptive in a 24/4 regimen. *Contraception*. 2008;78:16-25.
24. Vandever MA, Kuehl TJ, Sulak PJ, et al. Evaluation of pituitary-ovarian axis suppression with three oral contraceptive regimens. *Contraception*. 2008;77:162-170.
25. Dinger J, Minh TD, Buttmann N, Bardenheuer K. Effectiveness of oral contraceptive pills in a large U.S. cohort comparing progestogen and regimen. *Obstet Gynecol*. 2011;117:33-40.
26. Van Vliet HA, Grimes DA, Lopez LM, et al. Triphasic versus monophasic oral contraceptives for contraception. *Cochrane Database Syst Rev*. 2011;CD003553.
27. Archer DF. Menstrual-cycle-related symptoms: a review of the rationale for continuous use of oral contraceptives. *Contraception*. 2006;74:359-366.
28. Westhoff C, Heartwell S, Edwards S, et al. Initiation of oral contraceptives using a quick start compared with a conventional start: a randomized controlled trial. *Obstet Gynecol*. 2007;109:1270-1276.
29. Bracken MB. Oral contraception and congenital malformations in offspring: a review and meta-analysis of the prospective studies. *Obstet Gynecol*. 1990;76:552-557.
30. Barnhart KT, Schreiber CA. Return to fertility following discontinuation of oral contraceptives. *Fertil Steril*. 2009;91:659-663.
31. Franks AL, Beral V, Cates W Jr, Hogue CJ. Contraception and ectopic pregnancy risk. *Am J Obstet Gynecol*. 1990;163:1120-1123.
32. Martins SL, Curtis KM, Glasier AF. Combined hormonal contraception and bone health: a systematic review. *Contraception*. 2006;73:445-469.
33. Beral V, Doll R, Hermon C, et al., Collaborative Group on Epidemiological Studies of Ovarian Cancer. Ovarian cancer and oral contraceptives: collaborative reanalysis of data from 45 epidemiological studies including 23,257 women with ovarian cancer and 87,303 controls. *Lancet*. 2008;371:303-314.
34. Antoniou AC, Rookus M, Andrieu N, et al. Reproductive and hormonal factors, and ovarian cancer risk for BRCA1 and BRCA2 mutation carriers: results from the International BRCA1/2 Carrier Cohort Study. *Cancer Epidemiol Biomarkers Prev*. 2009;18:601-610.
35. Grenader T, Peretz T, Lifchitz M, Shavit L. BRCA1 and BRCA2 germ-line mutations and oral contraceptives: to use or not to use. *Breast*. 2005;14:264-268.
36. Cibula D, Zikan M, Dusek L, Majek O. Oral contraceptives and risk of ovarian and breast cancers in BRCA mutation carriers: a meta-analysis. *Expert Rev Anticancer Ther*. 2011;11:1197-1207.
37. ACOG Practice Bulletin No. 103: Hereditary breast and ovarian cancer syndrome. *Obstet Gynecol*. 2009;113:957-966.
38. Faculty of Sexual and Reproductive Health Care. *UK Medical Eligibility Criteria for Contraceptive Use*. London: Faculty of Sexual and Reproductive Healthcare; 2009.
39. The Cancer and Steroid Hormone Study of the Centers for Disease Control and the National Institute of Child Health and Human Development. Combination oral contraceptive use and the risk of endometrial cancer. *JAMA*. 1987;257:796-800.
40. Schlesselman JJ. Risk of endometrial cancer in relation to use of combined oral contraceptives. A practitioner's guide to meta-analysis. *Hum Reprod*. 1997;12:1851-1863.
41. Arowojolu AO, Gallo MF, Lopez LM, Grimes DA. Combined oral contraceptive pills for treatment of acne. *Cochrane Database Syst Rev*. 2012;(7):CD004425.
42. Gallo MF, Lopez LM, Grimes DA, et al. Combination contraceptives: effects on weight. *Cochrane Database Syst Rev*. 2008;CD003987.
43. Grimes DA, Schulz KF. Nonspecific side effects of oral contraceptives: nocebo or noise? *Contraception*. 2011;83:5-9.
44. Halpern V, Lopez LM, Grimes DA, et al. Strategies to improve adherence and acceptability of hormonal methods of contraception. *Cochrane Database Syst Rev*. 2013;(10):CD004317.
45. Gallo MF, Nanda K, Grimes DA, et al. 20 microg versus >20 microg estrogen combined oral contraceptives for contraception. *Cochrane Database Syst Rev*. 2008;(4):CD003989.
46. Sulak PJ, Kuehl TJ, Coffee A, Willis S. Prospective analysis of occurrence and management of breakthrough bleeding during an extended oral contraceptive regimen. *Am J Obstet Gynecol*. 2006;195:935-941.
47. Loder EW, Buse DC, Golub JR. Headache as a side effect of combination estrogen-progestin oral contraceptives: a systematic review. *Am J Obstet Gynecol*. 2005;193:636-649.
48. Hannaford PC, Iversen L, Macfarlane TV, et al. Mortality among contraceptive pill users: cohort evidence from Royal College of General Practitioners' Oral Contraception Study. *BMJ*. 2010;340:c927.
49. Centers for Disease Control and Prevention. Update to CDC's U.S. Medical Eligibility Criteria for Contraceptive Use, 2010: revised recommendations for the use of contraceptive methods during the postpartum period. *MMWR Morb Mortal Wkly Rep*. 2011;60:878-883.
50. Shapiro S, Dinger J. Risk of venous thromboembolism among users of oral contraceptives: a review of two recently published studies. *J Fam Plann Reprod Health Care*. 2010;36(1):33-38.
51. Dinger J. Oral contraceptives and venous thromboembolism: old questions revisited. *J Fam Plann Reprod Health Care*. 2009;35:211-213.
52. Dinger JC, Heinemann LA, Kuhl-Habich D. The safety of a drospirenone-containing oral contraceptive: final results from the European Active Surveillance Study on oral contraceptives based on 142,475 women-years of observation. *Contraception*. 2007;75:344-354.
53. Dinger J, Assmann A, Mohner S, Minh TD. Risk of venous thromboembolism and the use of dienogest- and drospirenone-containing oral contraceptives: results from a German case-control study. *J Fam Plann Reprod Health Care*. 2010;36:123-129.
54. Pomp ER, Rosendaal FR, Doggen CJ. Smoking increases the risk of venous thrombosis and acts synergistically with oral contraceptive use. *Am J Hematol*. 2008;83:97-102.

55. Heinemann LA, Dinger JC. Range of published estimates of venous thromboembolism incidence in young women. *Contraception.* 2007;75:328-336.

56. FDA Drug Safety Communication: Updated information about the risk of blood clots in women taking birth control pills containing drospirenone. 2012. Available at http://www.fda.gov/Drugs/DrugSafety/ucm299305.

57. Heit JA, Kobbervig CE, James AH, et al. Trends in the incidence of venous thromboembolism during pregnancy or postpartum: a 30-year population-based study. *Ann Intern Med.* 2005;143:697-706.

58. Vandenbroucke JP, van der Meer FJ, Helmerhorst FM, et al. Leiden: should we screen oral contraceptive users and pregnant women? *BMJ.* 1996;313:1127-1130.

59. Lidegaard O, Lokkegaard E, Jensen A, et al. Thrombotic stroke and myocardial infarction with hormonal contraception. *N Engl J Med.* 2012;366:2257-2266.

60. Marchbanks PA, McDonald JA, Wilson HG, et al. Oral contraceptives and the risk of breast cancer. *N Engl J Med.* 2002;346:2025-2032.

61. Hannaford PC, Selvaraj S, Elliott AM, et al. Cancer risk among users of oral contraceptives: cohort data from the Royal College of General Practitioner's oral contraception study. *BMJ.* 2007;335:651.

62. Collaborative Group on Hormonal Factors in Breast Cancer. Breast cancer and hormonal contraceptives: further results. *Contraception.* 1996;54:1S-106S.

63. Silvera SA, Miller AB, Rohan TE. Oral contraceptive use and risk of breast cancer among women with a family history of breast cancer: a prospective cohort study. *Cancer Causes Control.* 2005;16:1059-1063.

64. International Collaboration of Epidemiological Studies of Cervical Cancer, Appleby P, Beral V, Berrington de Gonzales A. Cervical cancer and hormonal contraceptives: collaborative reanalysis of individual data for 16,573 women with cervical cancer and 35,509 women without cervical cancer from 24 epidemiological studies. *Lancet.* 2007;370:1609-1621.

65. Petersen JF, Bergholt T, Nielsen AK, et al. Combined hormonal contraception and risk of venous thromboembolism within the first year following pregnancy. Danish nationwide historical cohort 1995-2009. *Thromb Haemost.* 2014;112:1.

66. Truitt ST, Fraser AB, Grimes DA, et al. Hormonal contraception during lactation. Systematic review of randomized controlled trials. *Contraception.* 2003;68:233-238.

67. Panel on Antiretroviral Guidelines for Adults and Adolescents. Guidelines for the use of antiretroviral agents in HIV-1-infected adults and adolescents. 2014. Available at http://aidsinfo.nih.gov/ContentFiles/AdultandAdolescentGL.pdf.

68. Zieman M, Guillebaud J, Weisberg E, et al. Contraceptive efficacy and cycle control with the Ortho Evra/Evra transdermal system: the analysis of pooled data. *Fertil Steril.* 2002;77:S13-S18.

69. Edelman AB, Jensen JT. Obesity and hormonal contraception: safety and efficacy. *Semin Reprod Med.* 2012;30:479-485.

70. van den Heuvel MW, van Bragt AJ, Alnabawy AK, Kaptein MC. Comparison of ethinylestradiol pharmacokinetics in three hormonal contraceptive formulations: the vaginal ring, the transdermal patch and an oral contraceptive. *Contraception.* 2005;72:168-174.

71. Raymond EG, Burke AE, Espey E. Combined hormonal contraceptives and venous thromboembolism: putting the risks into perspective. *Obstet Gynecol.* 2012;119:1039-1044.

72. Jick SS, Hagberg KW, Hernandez RK, Kaye JA. Postmarketing study of ORTHO EVRA and levonorgestrel oral contraceptives containing hormonal contraceptives with 30 mcg of ethinyl estradiol in relation to nonfatal venous thromboembolism. *Contraception.* 2010;81:16-21.

73. O'Connell K, Burkman RT. The transdermal contraceptive patch: an updated review of the literature. *Clin Obstet Gynecol.* 2007;50:918-926.

74. Lopez LM, Grimes DA, Schulz KF. Steroidal contraceptives: effect on carbohydrate metabolism in women without diabetes mellitus. *Cochrane Database Syst Rev.* 2014;(4):CD006133.

75. Creinin MD, Meyn LA, Borgatta L, et al. Multicenter comparison of the contraceptive ring and patch: a randomized controlled trial. *Obstet Gynecol.* 2008;111:267-277.

76. Kaunitz AM, Portman D, Westhoff CL, et al. Low-dose levonorgestrel and ethinyl estradiol patch and pill: a randomized controlled trial. *Obstet Gynecol.* 2014;123:295-303.

77. Shimoni N, Westhoff C. Review of the vaginal contraceptive ring (NuvaRing). *J Fam Plann Reprod Health Care.* 2008;34:247-250.

78. ACOG Committee on Practice Bulletins-Gynecology. ACOG Practice Bulletin No. 73: Use of hormonal contraception in women with coexisting medical conditions. *Obstet Gynecol.* 2006;107:1453-1472.

79. Benagiano G, Primiero FM. Seventy-five microgram desogestrel minipill, a new perspective in estrogen-free contraception. *Ann N Y Acad Sci.* 2003;997:163-173.

80. Korver T, Klipping C, Heger-Mahn D, et al. Maintenance of ovulation inhibition with the 75-microg desogestrel-only contraceptive pill (Cerazette) after scheduled 12-h delays in tablet intake. *Contraception.* 2005;71:8-13.

81. Grimes DA, Lopez LM, O'Brien PA, Raymond EG. Progestin-only pills for contraception. *Cochrane Database Syst Rev.* 2013;(11):CD007541.

82. Eshre Capri Workshop Group. Ovarian and endometrial function during hormonal contraception. *Hum Reprod.* 2001;16:1527-1535.

83. Godsland IF, Crook D, Simpson R, et al. The effects of different formulations of oral contraceptive agents on lipid and carbohydrate metabolism. *N Engl J Med.* 1990;323:1375-1381.

84. Kjos SL, Peters RK, Xiang A, et al. Contraception and the risk of type 2 diabetes mellitus in Latina women with prior gestational diabetes mellitus. *JAMA.* 1998;280:533-538.

85. Committee on Obstetric Practice. ACOG Committee Opinion No. 435: postpartum screening for abnormal glucose tolerance in women who had gestational diabetes mellitus. *Obstet Gynecol.* 2009;113:1419-1421.

86. Raymond EG. Progestin-only pills. In: Hatcher RA, Trussell J, Nelson AL, et al., eds. *Contraceptive Technology.* 20th ed. New York, NY: Ardent Media; 2011.

87. Caird LE, Reid-Thomas V, Hannan WJ, et al. Oral progestogen-only contraception may protect against loss of bone mass in breast-feeding women. *Clin Endocrinol.* 1994;41:739-745.

88. Halderman LD, Nelson AL. Impact of early postpartum administration of progestin-only hormonal contraceptives compared with nonhormonal contraceptives on short-term breast-feeding patterns. *Am J Obstet Gynecol.* 2002;186:1250-1256, discussion 1256-1258.

89. Beasley A, White KO, Cremers S, Westhoff C. Randomized clinical trial of self versus clinical administration of subcutaneous depot medroxyprogesterone acetate. *Contraception.* 2014;89:352-356.

90. Kaunitz AM, Darney PD, Ross D, et al. Subcutaneous DMPA vs. intramuscular DMPA: a 2-year randomized study of contraceptive efficacy and bone mineral density. *Contraception.* 2009;80:7-17.

91. Westhoff C. Depot-medroxyprogesterone acetate injection (Depo-Provera): a highly effective contraceptive option with proven long-term safety. *Contraception.* 2003;68:75-87.

92. Jain J, Jakimiuk AJ, Bode FR, et al. Contraceptive efficacy and safety of DMPA-SC. *Contraception.* 2004;70:269-275.

93. Rickert VI, Tiezzi L, Lipshutz J, et al. Depo now: preventing unintended pregnancies among adolescents and young adults. *J Adolesc Health.* 2007;40:22-28.

94. Borgatta L, Murthy A, Chuang C, et al. Pregnancies diagnosed during Depo-Provera use. *Contraception.* 2002;66:169-172.

95. Rodriguez MI, Kaunitz AM. An evidence-based approach to postpartum use of depot medroxyprogesterone acetate in breastfeeding women. *Contraception.* 2009;80:4-6.

96. Hubacher D, Goco N, Gonzalez B, Taylor D. Factors affecting continuation rates of DMPA. *Contraception.* 1999;60:345-351.

97. Abdel-Aleem H, d'Arcangues C, Vogelsong KM, et al. Treatment of vaginal bleeding irregularities induced by progestin only contraceptives. *Cochrane Database Syst Rev.* 2013;(10):CD003449.

98. Arias RD, Jain JK, Brucker C, et al. Changes in bleeding patterns with depot medroxyprogesterone acetate subcutaneous injection 104 mg. *Contraception.* 2006;74:234-238.

99. Lopez LM, Edelman A, Chen M, et al. Progestin-only contraceptives: effects on weight. *Cochrane Database Syst Rev.* 2013;(7):CD008815.

100. Crosignani PG, Luciano A, Ray A, Bergqvist A. Subcutaneous depot medroxyprogesterone acetate versus leuprolide acetate in the treatment of endometriosis-associated pain. *Hum Reprod.* 2006;21:248-256.

101. Mangan SA, Larsen PG, Hudson S. Overweight teens at increased risk for weight gain while using depot medroxyprogesterone acetate. *J Pediatr Adolesc Gynecol.* 2002;15:79-82.

102. Practice Committee of American Society for Reproductive Medicine. Treatment of pelvic pain associated with endometriosis. *Fertil Steril.* 2008;90:S260-S269.

103. Depot-medroxyprogesterone acetate (DMPA) and risk of epithelial ovarian cancer. The WHO Collaborative Study of Neoplasia and Steroid Contraceptives. *Int J Cancer.* 1991;49:191-195.

104. Depot-medroxyprogesterone acetate (DMPA) and risk of endometrial cancer. The WHO Collaborative Study of Neoplasia and Steroid Contraceptives. *Int J Cancer.* 1991;49:186-190.

105. Depot-medroxyprogesterone acetate (DMPA) and risk of invasive squamous cell cervical cancer. The WHO Collaborative Study of Neoplasia and Steroid Contraceptives. *Contraception.* 1992;45:299-312.

106. Skegg DC, Noonan EA, Paul C, et al. Depot medroxyprogesterone acetate and breast cancer. A pooled analysis of the World Health Organization and New Zealand studies. *JAMA.* 1995;273:799-804.

107. Clark MK, Sowers M, Levy BT, Tenhundfeld P. Magnitude and variability of sequential estradiol and progesterone concentrations in women using depot medroxyprogesterone acetate for contraception. *Fertil Steril.* 2001;75:871-877.

108. Committee Opinion No. 602. Depot medroxyprogesterone acetate and bone effects. *Obstet Gynecol.* 2014;123:1398-1402.

109. Clark MK, Sowers MR, Nichols S, Levy B. Bone mineral density changes over two years in first-time users of depot medroxyprogesterone acetate. *Fertil Steril.* 2004;82:1580-1586.

110. Kaunitz AM, Peipert JF, Grimes DA. Injectable contraception: issues and opportunities. *Contraception.* 2014;89:331-334.

111. Kaunitz AM, Arias R, McClung M. Bone density recovery after depot medroxyprogesterone acetate injectable contraception use. *Contraception.* 2008;77:67-76.

112. Lopez LM, Chen M, Mullins S, et al. Steroidal contraceptives and bone fractures in women: evidence from observational studies. *Cochrane Database Syst Rev.* 2012;(8):CD009849.

113. Clark MK, Sowers M, Levy B, Nichols S. Bone mineral density loss and recovery during 48 months in first-time users of depot medroxyprogesterone acetate. *Fertil Steril.* 2006;86:1466-1474.

114. Scholes D, LaCroix AZ, Ichikawa LE, et al. Change in bone mineral density among adolescent women using and discontinuing depot medroxyprogesterone acetate contraception. *Arch Pediatr Adolesc Med.* 2005;159:139-144.

115. Orr-Walker BJ, Evans MC, Ames RW, et al. The effect of past use of the injectable contraceptive depot medroxyprogesterone acetate on bone mineral density in normal post-menopausal women. *Clin Endocrinol.* 1998;49:615-618.

116. Lanza LL, McQuay LJ, Rothman KJ, et al. Use of depot medroxyprogesterone acetate contraception and incidence of bone fracture. *Obstet Gynecol.* 2013;121:593-600.

117. Vestergaard P, Rejnmark L, Mosekilde L. The effects of depot medroxyprogesterone acetate and intrauterine device use on fracture risk in Danish women. *Contraception.* 2008;78:459-464.

118. Cromer BA, Scholes D, Berenson A, et al. Depot medroxyprogesterone acetate and bone mineral density in adolescents—the Black Box Warning: a Position Paper of the Society for Adolescent Medicine. *J Adolesc Health.* 2006;39:296-301.

119. Kovacs CS. Calcium and bone metabolism disorders during pregnancy and lactation. *Endocrinol Metab Clin North Am.* 2011;40:795-826.

120. Morrison CS, Turner AN, Jones LB. Highly effective contraception and acquisition of HIV and other sexually transmitted infections. *Best Pract Res Clin Obstet Gynaecol.* 2009;23:263-284.

121. Polis CB, Curtis KM. Use of hormonal contraceptives and HIV acquisition in women: a systematic review of the epidemiological evidence. *Lancet Infect Dis.* 2013;13:797-808.

122. Baeten JM, Benki S, Chohan V, et al. Hormonal contraceptive use, herpes simplex virus infection, and risk of HIV-1 acquisition among Kenyan women. *AIDS.* 2007;21:1771-1777.

123. Heffron R, Donnell D, Rees H, et al. Use of hormonal contraceptives and risk of HIV-1 transmission: a prospective cohort study. *Lancet Infect Dis.* 2012;12:19-26.

124. Stringer EM, Kaseba C, Levy J, et al. A randomized trial of the intrauterine contraceptive device vs hormonal contraception in women who are infected with the human immunodeficiency virus. *Am J Obstet Gynecol.* 2007;197:144; e1-144, e8.

125. Polis CB, Phillips SJ, Curtis KM. Hormonal contraceptive use and female-to-male HIV transmission: a systematic review of the epidemiologic evidence. *AIDS.* 2013;27:493-505.

126. Murphy K, Irvin SC, Herold BC. Research gaps in defining the biological link between HIV risk and hormonal contraception. *Am J Reprod Immunol.* 2014;72(2):228-235.

127. Centers for Disease Control and Prevention. Update to CDC's U.S. Medical Eligibility Criteria for Contraceptive Use, 2010: revised recommendations for the use of hormonal contraception among women at high risk for HIV infection or infected with HIV. *MMWR Morb Mortal Wkly Rep.* 2012;61:449-452.

128. Mishell DR Jr. Pharmacokinetics of depot medroxyprogesterone acetate contraception. *J Reprod Med.* 1996;41:381-390.

129. American College of Obstetricians and Gynecologists. ACOG. Practice Bulletin No. 121: Long-acting reversible contraception: implants and intrauterine devices. *Obstet Gynecol.* 2011;118:184-196.

130. Allen RH, Goldberg AB, Grimes DA. Expanding access to intrauterine contraception. *Am J Obstet Gynecol.* 2009;201:456; e1-456, e5.

131. Jensen JT. Contraceptive and therapeutic effects of the levonorgestrel intrauterine system: an overview. *Obstet Gynecol Surv.* 2005;60:604-612.

132. Gemzell-Danielsson K, Schellschmidt I, Apter D. A randomized, phase II study describing the efficacy, bleeding profile, and safety of two low-dose levonorgestrel-releasing intrauterine contraceptive systems and Mirena. *Fertil Steril.* 2012;97:616-622; e1-3.

133. Andersson K, Batar I, Rybo G. Return to fertility after removal of a levonorgestrel-releasing intrauterine device and Nova-T. *Contraception.* 1992;46:575-584.

134. Nelson AL. Contraindications to IUD and IUS use. *Contraception.* 2007;75:S76-S81.

135. Peipert JF, Zhao Q, Allsworth JE, et al. Continuation and satisfaction of reversible contraception. *Obstet Gynecol.* 2011;117:1105-1113.

136. O'Neil-Callahan M, Peipert JF, Zhao Q, et al. Twenty-four-month continuation of reversible contraception. *Obstet Gynecol.* 2013;122:1083-1091.

137. Peipert JF, Madden T, Allsworth JE, Secura GM. Preventing unintended pregnancies by providing no-cost contraception. *Obstet Gynecol.* 2012;120:1291-1297.

138. Mestad R, Secura G, Allsworth JE, et al. Acceptance of long-acting reversible contraceptive methods by adolescent participants in the Contraceptive CHOICE Project. *Contraception.* 2011;84:493-498.

139. ACOG Committee Opinion No. 392. Intrauterine device and adolescents. *Obstet Gynecol.* 2007;110:1493-1495.

140. Stevens-Simon C, Kelly L, Kulick R. A village would be nice but . . . it takes a long-acting contraceptive to prevent repeat adolescent pregnancies. *Am J Prev Med.* 2001;21:60-65.

141. Goodman S, Hendlish SK, Reeves MF, Foster-Rosales A. Impact of immediate postabortal insertion of intrauterine contraception on repeat abortion. *Contraception.* 2008;78:143-148.

142. Baldwin MK, Edelman AB. The effect of long-acting reversible contraception on rapid repeat pregnancy in adolescents: a review. *J Adolesc Health.* 2013;52:S47-S53.

143. Jensen JT, Nelson AL, Costales AC. Subject and clinician experience with the levonorgestrel-releasing intrauterine system. *Contraception.* 2008;77:22-29.

144. Skyla Prescribing Information. Available at http://labeling.bayerhealthcare.com/html/products/pi/Skyla_PI.pdf.

145. Kaunitz AM, Inki P. The levonorgestrel-releasing intrauterine system in heavy menstrual bleeding: a benefit-risk review. *Drugs.* 2012;72:193-215.

146. Heinemann K, Westhoff CL, Grimes DA, Moehner S. Intrauterine devices and the risk of uterine perforations: final results from the EURAS-IUD study. *Obstet Gynecol.* 2014;123(Suppl 1):3S.

147. Hubacher D, Grimes DA, Gemzell-Danielsson K. Pitfalls of research linking the intrauterine device to pelvic inflammatory disease. *Obstet Gynecol.* 2013;121:1091-1098.

148. Farley TM, Rosenberg MJ, Rowe PJ, et al. Intrauterine devices and pelvic inflammatory disease: an international perspective. *Lancet.* 1992;339:785-788.

149. Hubacher D, Lara-Ricalde R, Taylor DJ, et al. Use of copper intrauterine devices and the risk of tubal infertility among nulligravid women. *N Engl J Med.* 2001;345:561-567.

150. Sufrin CB, Postlethwaite D, Armstrong MA, et al. *Neisseria gonorrhea* and *Chlamydia trachomatis* screening at intrauterine device insertion and pelvic inflammatory disease. *Obstet Gynecol.* 2012;120:1314-1321.

151. Lidegaard O, Nielsen LH, Skovlund CW, Lokkegaard E. Venous thrombosis in users of non-oral hormonal contraception: follow-up study, Denmark 2001-10. *BMJ.* 2012;344:e2990.

152. Lethaby AE, Cooke I, Rees M. Progesterone or progestogen-releasing intrauterine systems for heavy menstrual bleeding. *Cochrane Database Syst Rev.* 2005;CD002126.

153. Kaunitz AM, Meredith S, Inki P, et al. Levonorgestrel-releasing intrauterine system and endometrial ablation in heavy menstrual bleeding: a systematic review and meta-analysis. *Obstet Gynecol.* 2009;113:1104-1116.

154. Matteson KA, Rahn DD, Wheeler TL 2nd, et al. Nonsurgical management of heavy menstrual bleeding: a systematic review. *Obstet Gynecol.* 2013;121:632-643.

155. Zapata LB, Whiteman MK, Tepper NK, et al. Intrauterine device use among women with uterine fibroids: a systematic review. *Contraception.* 2010;82:41-55.

156. Sangkomkamhang US, Lumbiganon P, Laopaiboon M, Mol BW. Progestogens or progestogen-releasing intrauterine systems for uterine fibroids. *Cochrane Database Syst Rev.* 2013;(2):CD008994.

157. Kaunitz AM. Progestin-releasing intrauterine systems and leiomyoma. *Contraception.* 2007;75:S130-S133.

158. Sheng J, Zhang WY, Zhang JP, Lu D. The LNG-IUS study on adenomyosis: a 3-year follow-up study on the efficacy and side effects of the use of levonorgestrel intrauterine system for the treatment of dysmenorrhea associated with adenomyosis. *Contraception.* 2009;79:189-193.

159. Bragheto AM, Caserta N, Bahamondes L, Petta CA. Effectiveness of the levonorgestrel-releasing intrauterine system in the treatment of adenomyosis diagnosed and monitored by magnetic resonance imaging. *Contraception.* 2007;76:195-199.

160. Brown J, Farquhar C. Endometriosis: an overview of Cochrane reviews. *Cochrane Database Syst Rev.* 2014;(3):CD009590.

161. Petta CA, Ferriani RA, Abrao MS, et al. Randomized clinical trial of a levonorgestrel-releasing intrauterine system and a depot GnRH analogue for the treatment of chronic pelvic pain in women with endometriosis. *Hum Reprod.* 2005;20:1993-1998.

162. Petta CA, Ferriani RA, Abrao MS, et al. A 3-year follow-up of women with endometriosis and pelvic pain users of the levonorgestrel-releasing intrauterine system. *Eur J Obstet Gynecol Reprod Biol.* 2009;143:128-129.

163. Wildemeersch D, Pylyser K, De Wever N, et al. Endometrial safety after 5 years of continuous combined transdermal estrogen and intrauterine levonorgestrel delivery for postmenopausal hormone substitution. *Maturitas.* 2007;57:205-209.

164. Somboonporn W, Panna S, Temtanakitpaisan T, et al. Effects of the levonorgestrel-releasing intrauterine system plus estrogen therapy in perimenopausal and postmenopausal women: systematic review and meta-analysis. *Menopause.* 2011;18:1060-1066.

165. Chin J, Konje JC, Hickey M. Levonorgestrel intrauterine system for endometrial protection in women with breast cancer on adjuvant tamoxifen. *Cochrane Database Syst Rev.* 2009;CD007245.

166. Committee Opinion No. 601. Tamoxifen and uterine cancer. *Obstet Gynecol.* 2014;123:1394-1397.
167. Luo L, Luo B, Zheng Y, et al. Levonorgestrel-releasing intrauterine system for atypical endometrial hyperplasia. *Cochrane Database Syst Rev.* 2013;(6):CD009458.
168. Orbo A, Vereide A, Arnes M, et al. Levonorgestrel-impregnated intrauterine device as treatment for endometrial hyperplasia: a national multicentre randomised trial. *Br J Obstet Gynaecol.* 2014;121:477-486.
169. Haimovich S, Checa MA, Mancebo G, et al. Treatment of endometrial hyperplasia without atypia in peri- and postmenopausal women with a levonorgestrel intrauterine device. *Menopause.* 2008;15:1002-1004.
170. Gallos ID, Shehmar M, Thangaratinam S, et al. Oral progestogens vs levonorgestrel-releasing intrauterine system for endometrial hyperplasia: a systematic review and metaanalysis. *Am J Obstet Gynecol.* 2010;203:547; e1-547, e10.
171. Montz FJ, Bristow RE, Bovicelli A, et al. Intrauterine progesterone treatment of early endometrial cancer. *Am J Obstet Gynecol.* 2002;186:651-657.
172. Funk S, Miller MM, Mishell DR Jr, et al. Safety and efficacy of Implanon, a single-rod implantable contraceptive containing etonogestrel. *Contraception.* 2005;71:319-326.
173. Hohmann H, Creinin MD. The contraceptive implant. *Clin Obstet Gynecol.* 2007;50:907-917.
174. Darney P, Patel A, Rosen K, et al. Safety and efficacy of a single-rod etonogestrel implant (Implanon): results from 11 international clinical trials. *Fertil Steril.* 2009;91:1646-1653.
175. Harrison-Woolrych M, Hill R. Unintended pregnancies with the etonogestrel implant (Implanon): a case series from postmarketing experience in Australia. *Contraception.* 2005;71:306-308.
176. Xu H, Wade JA, Peipert JF, et al. Contraceptive failure rates of etonogestrel subdermal implants in overweight and obese women. *Obstet Gynecol.* 2012;120:21-26.
177. Mansour D, Korver T, Marintcheva-Petrova M, Fraser IS. The effects of Implanon on menstrual bleeding patterns. *Eur J Contracept Reprod Health Care.* 2008;13(Suppl 1):13-28.
178. Mansour D, Bahamondes L, Critchley H, et al. The management of unacceptable bleeding patterns in etonogestrel-releasing contraceptive implant users. *Contraception.* 2011;83:202-210.
179. Hidalgo MM, Lisondo C, Juliato CT, et al. Ovarian cysts in users of Implanon and Jadelle subdermal contraceptive implants. *Contraception.* 2006;73:532-536.
180. Gurtcheff SE, Turok DK, Stoddard G, et al. Lactogenesis after early postpartum use of the contraceptive implant: a randomized controlled trial. *Obstet Gynecol.* 2011;117:1114-1121.
181. Merki-Feld GS, Imthurn B, Seifert B. Effects of the progestagen-only contraceptive implant Implanon on cardiovascular risk factors. *Clin Endocrinol.* 2008;68:355-360.
182. Leticee N, Viard JP, Yamgnane A, et al. Contraceptive failure of etonogestrel implant in patients treated with antiretrovirals including efavirenz. *Contraception.* 2012;85:425-427.
183. Pymar HC, Creinin MD, Schwartz JL. "Pop-out" method of levonorgestrel implant removal. *Contraception.* 1999;59:383-387.
184. American College of Obstetricians and Gynecologists. ACOG Practice Bulletin No. 112: Emergency contraception. *Obstet Gynecol.* 2010;115:1100-1109.
185. Raymond EG, Trussell J, Polis CB. Population effect of increased access to emergency contraceptive pills: a systematic review. *Obstet Gynecol.* 2007;109:181-188.
186. Trussell J, Schwarz EB, Guthrie K. Research priorities for preventing unintended pregnancy: moving beyond emergency contraceptive pills. *Perspect Sex Reprod Health.* 2010;42:8-9.
187. Grimes DA. Emergency contraception: politics trumps science at the U.S. Food and Drug Administration. *Obstet Gynecol.* 2004;104:220-221.
188. Wood AJ, Drazen JM, Greene MF. A sad day for science at the FDA. *N Engl J Med.* 2005;353:1197-1199.
189. Cleland K, Peipert JF, Westhoff C, et al. Plan B, one step not taken: politics trumps science yet again. *Contraception.* 2012;85:340-341.
190. Levy DP, Jager M, Kapp N, Abitbol JL. Ulipristal acetate for emergency contraception: postmarketing experience after use by more than 1 million women. *Contraception.* 2014;89:431-433.
191. Creinin MD, Schlaff W, Archer DF, et al. Progesterone receptor modulator for emergency contraception: a randomized controlled trial. *Obstet Gynecol.* 2006;108:1089-1097.
192. Schwarz EB, Kavanaugh M, Douglas E, et al. Interest in intrauterine contraception among seekers of emergency contraception and pregnancy testing. *Obstet Gynecol.* 2009;113:833-839.
193. Turok DK, Jacobson JC, Dermish AI, et al. Emergency contraception with a copper IUD or oral levonorgestrel: an observational study of 1-year pregnancy rates. *Contraception.* 2014;89:222-228.
194. Gemzell-Danielsson K, Berger C, Lalitkumar PGL. Emergency contraception—mechanisms of action. *Contraception.* 2013;87:300-308.
195. Davidoff F, Trussell J. Plan B and the politics of doubt. *JAMA.* 2006;296:1775-1778.
196. Cleland K, Zhu H, Goldstuck N, et al. The efficacy of intrauterine devices for emergency contraception: a systematic review of 35 years of experience. *Hum Reprod.* 2012;27:1994-2000.
197. Wilcox AJ, Dunson DB, Weinberg CR, et al. Likelihood of conception with a single act of intercourse: providing benchmark rates for assessment of post-coital contraceptives. *Contraception.* 2001;63:211-215.
198. Raymond E, Taylor D, Trussell J, Steiner MJ. Minimum effectiveness of the levonorgestrel regimen of emergency contraception. *Contraception.* 2004;69:79-81.
199. Cheng L, Gulmezoglu AM, Piaggio G, et al. Interventions for emergency contraception. *Cochrane Database Syst Rev.* 2008;CD001324.
200. Rodrigues I, Grou F, Joly J. Effectiveness of emergency contraceptive pills between 72 and 120 hours after unprotected sexual intercourse. *Am J Obstet Gynecol.* 2001;184:531-537.
201. Glasier AF, Cameron ST, Fine PM, et al. Ulipristal acetate versus levonorgestrel for emergency contraception: a randomised non-inferiority trial and meta-analysis. *Lancet.* 2010;375:555-562.
202. Brache V, Cochon L, Deniaud M, Croxatto HB. Ulipristal acetate prevents ovulation more effectively than levonorgestrel: analysis of pooled data from three randomized trials of emergency contraception regimens. *Contraception.* 2013;88:611-618.
203. Brache V, Cochon L, Jesam C, et al. Immediate pre-ovulatory administration of 30 mg ulipristal acetate significantly delays follicular rupture. *Hum Reprod.* 2010;25:2256-2263.
204. Glasier A, Cameron ST, Blithe D, et al. Can we identify women at risk of pregnancy despite using emergency contraception? Data from randomized trials of ulipristal acetate and levonorgestrel. *Contraception.* 2011;84:363-367.
205. Gemzell-Danielsson K, Trussell J. UPA > LNG, but not good enough. *Contraception.* 2013;88:585-586.
206. Rodriguez MI, Curtis KM, Gaffield ML, et al. Advance supply of emergency contraception: a systematic review. *Contraception.* 2013;87:590-601.
207. Foster DG, Harper CC, Bley JJ, et al. Knowledge of emergency contraception among women aged 18 to 44 in California. *Am J Obstet Gynecol.* 2004;191:150-156.
208. The Emergency Contraception Website. Available at http://ec.princeton.edu/.
209. Skinner SR, Hickey M. Current priorities for adolescent sexual and reproductive health in Australia. *Med J Aust.* 2003;179:158-161.
210. Jumping-Eagle S, Sheeder J, Kelly LS, Stevens-Simon C. Association of conventional goals and perceptions of pregnancy with female teenagers' pregnancy avoidance behavior and attitudes. *Perspect Sex Reprod Health.* 2008;40:74-80.
211. American Academy of Pediatrics Committee on Adolescence, Blythe MJ, Diaz A. Contraception and adolescents. *Pediatrics.* 2007;120:1135-1148.
212. Nelson AL. Combined oral contraceptives. In: Hatcher RA, ed. *Contraceptive Technology.* New York, NY: Ardent Media; 2007.
213. American College of Obstetricians and Gynecologists. ACOG Committee Opinion No. 392: Intrauterine device and adolescents. *Obstet Gynecol.* 2007;110:1493-1495.
214. American College of Obstetricians and Gynecologists Committee on Gynecologic Practice, Long-Acting Reversible Contraception Working Group. ACOG Committee Opinion No. 450: Increasing use of contraceptive implants and intrauterine devices to reduce unintended pregnancy. *Obstet Gynecol.* 2009;114:1434-1438.
215. ACOG Committee Opinion No. 392: Intrauterine device and adolescents. *Obstet Gynecol.* 2007;110:1493-1495.
216. The Guttmacher Institute. State Policies in Brief: Minors' Access to Contraceptive Services. Available at http://www.guttmacher.org/statecenter/spibs/spib_MACS.pdf.
217. Whitaker AK, Gilliam M. Contraceptive care for adolescents. *Clin Obstet Gynecol.* 2008;51:268-280.
218. The National Campaign to Prevent Teen and Unplanned Pregnancy. Bedsider Birth Control Network. Available at www.bedsider.org.
219. American College of Obstetricians and Gynecologists. Committee Opinion No. 460: The initial reproductive health visit. *Obstet Gynecol.* 2010;116:240-243.
220. Workowski KA, Berman S, Centers for Disease Control and Prevention. Sexually transmitted diseases treatment guidelines, 2010. *MMWR Morb Mortal Wkly Rep.* 2010;59:1-110.
221. Rosenstock JR, Peipert JF, Madden T, et al. Continuation of reversible contraception in teenagers and young women. *Obstet Gynecol.* 2012;120:1298-1305.
222. Teal SB. Postpartum contraception: optimizing interpregnancy intervals. *Contraception.* 2014;89:487-488.
223. Phemister DA, Laurent S, Harrison FN Jr. Use of Norplant contraceptive implants in the immediate postpartum period: safety and tolerance. *Am J Obstet Gynecol.* 1995;172:175-179.
224. Gray RH, Campbell OM, Zacur HA, et al. Postpartum return of ovarian activity in nonbreastfeeding women monitored by urinary assays. *J Clin Endocrinol Metab.* 1987;64:645-650.

225. Lopez LM, Hiller JE, Grimes DA. Education for contraceptive use by women after childbirth. *Cochrane Database Syst Rev.* 2010; CD001863.
226. Truitt ST, Fraser AB, Grimes DA, et al. Combined hormonal versus nonhormonal versus progestin-only contraception in lactation. *Cochrane Database Syst Rev.* 2003;CD003988.
227. Schwartz SM, Petitti DB, Siscovick DS, et al. Stroke and use of low-dose oral contraceptives in young women: a pooled analysis of two US studies. *Stroke.* 1998;29:2277-2284.
228. Sidney S, Siscovick DS, Petitti DB, et al. Myocardial infarction and use of low-dose oral contraceptives: a pooled analysis of 2 US studies. *Circulation.* 1998;98:1058-1063.
229. Chakhtoura Z, Canonico M, Gompel A, et al. Progestogen-only contraceptives and the risk of acute myocardial infarction: a meta-analysis. *J Clin Endocrinol Metab.* 2011;96:1169-1174.
230. Chakhtoura Z, Canonico M, Gompel A, et al. Progestogen-only contraceptives and the risk of stroke: a meta-analysis. *Stroke.* 2009;40:1059-1062.
231. Cardiovascular disease and use of oral and injectable progestogen-only contraceptives and combined injectable contraceptives. Results of an international, multicenter, case-control study. World Health Organization Collaborative Study of Cardiovascular Disease and Steroid Hormone Contraception. *Contraception.* 1998;57:315-324.
232. Harlow SD, Gass M, Hall JE, et al. Executive summary of the Stages of Reproductive Aging Workshop + 10: addressing the unfinished agenda of staging reproductive aging. *Fertil Steril.* 2012;97:843-851.
233. Ogden CL, Carroll MD, Kit BK, Flegal KM. Prevalence of obesity among adults: United States, 2011-2012. *NCHS Data Brief.* 2013;1-8.
234. Weiss JL, Malone FD, Emig D, et al. Obesity, obstetric complications and cesarean delivery rate—a population-based screening study. *Am J Obstet Gynecol.* 2004;190:1091-1097.
235. Lopez LM, Grimes DA, Chen M, et al. Hormonal contraceptives for contraception in overweight or obese women. *Cochrane Database Syst Rev.* 2013;(4):CD008452.
236. McNicholas C, Zhao Q, Secura G, et al. Contraceptive failures in overweight and obese combined hormonal contraceptive users. *Obstet Gynecol.* 2013;121:585-592.
237. Trussell J, Schwarz EB, Guthrie K. Obesity and oral contraceptive pill failure. *Contraception.* 2009;79:334-338.
238. Edelman AB, Carlson NE, Cherala G, et al. Impact of obesity on oral contraceptive pharmacokinetics and hypothalamic-pituitary-ovarian activity. *Contraception.* 2009;80:119-127.
239. Abdollahi M, Cushman M, Rosendaal FR. Obesity: risk of venous thrombosis and the interaction with coagulation factor levels and oral contraceptive use. *Thromb Haemost.* 2003;89:493-498.
240. Trussell J, Guthrie KA, Schwarz EB. Much ado about little: obesity, combined hormonal contraceptive use and venous thrombosis. *Contraception.* 2008;77:143-146.
241. Dutton C, Foldvary-Schaefer N. Contraception in women with epilepsy: pharmacokinetic interactions, contraceptive options, and management. *Int Rev Neurobiol.* 2008;83:113-134.
242. Dickinson BD, Altman RD, Nielsen NH, Sterling ML, Council on Scientific Affairs AMA. Drug interactions between oral contraceptives and antibiotics. *Obstet Gynecol.* 2001;98:853-860.
243. UNAIDS report on the global AIDS epidemic 2013. 2013. Available at http://www.unaids.org/en/media/unaids/contentassets/documents/epidemiology/2013/gr2013/UNAIDS_Global_Report_2013_en.pdf.
244. Phillips SJ, Curtis KM, Polis CB. Effect of hormonal contraceptive methods on HIV disease progression: a systematic review. *AIDS.* 2013;27:787-794.
245. Curtis KM, Nanda K, Kapp N. Safety of hormonal and intrauterine methods of contraception for women with HIV/AIDS: a systematic review. *AIDS.* 2009;23(Suppl 1):S55-S67.
246. Cardoso F, Polonia J, Santos A, et al. Low-dose oral contraceptives and 24-hour ambulatory blood pressure. *Int J Gynaecol Obstet.* 1997;59:237-243.
247. Tepper NK, Curtis KM, Steenland MW, Marchbanks PA. Blood pressure measurement prior to initiating hormonal contraception: a systematic review. *Contraception.* 2013;87:631-638.
248. Curtis KM, Mohllajee AP, Martins SL, Peterson HB. Combined oral contraceptive use among women with hypertension: a systematic review. *Contraception.* 2006;73:179-188.
249. Shufelt CL, Bairey Merz CN. Contraceptive hormone use and cardiovascular disease. *J Am Coll Cardiol.* 2009;53:221-231.
250. van Rooijen M, von Schoultz B, Silveira A, et al. Different effects of oral contraceptives containing levonorgestrel or desogestrel on plasma lipoproteins and coagulation factor VII. *Am J Obstet Gynecol.* 2002;186:44-48.
251. Beasley A, Estes C, Guerrero J, Westhoff C. The effect of obesity and low-dose oral contraceptives on carbohydrate and lipid metabolism. *Contraception.* 2012;85:446-452.
252. Sibai BM, Odlind V, Meador ML, et al. A comparative and pooled analysis of the safety and tolerability of the contraceptive patch (Ortho Evra/Evra). *Fertil Steril.* 2002;77:S19-S26.
253. Tuppurainen M, Klimscheffskij R, Venhola M, Dieben TO. The combined contraceptive vaginal ring (NuvaRing) and lipid metabolism: a comparative study. *Contraception.* 2004;69:389-394.
254. Tepper NK, Steenland MW, Marchbanks PA, Curtis KM. Laboratory screening prior to initiating contraception: a systematic review. *Contraception.* 2013;87:645-649.
255. Berenson AB, Rahman M, Wilkinson G. Effect of injectable and oral contraceptives on serum lipids. *Obstet Gynecol.* 2009;114:786-794.
256. Ng YW, Liang S, Singh K. Effects of Mirena (levonorgestrel-releasing intrauterine system) and Ortho Gynae T380 intrauterine copper device on lipid metabolism—a randomized comparative study. *Contraception.* 2009;79:24-28.
257. Dilbaz B, Ozdegirmenci O, Caliskan E, et al. Effect of etonogestrel implant on serum lipids, liver function tests and hemoglobin levels. *Contraception.* 2010;81:510-514.
258. Visser J, Snel M, Van Vliet HA. Hormonal versus non-hormonal contraceptives in women with diabetes mellitus type 1 and 2. *Cochrane Database Syst Rev.* 2013;(3):CD003990.
259. Rogovskaya S, Rivera R, Grimes DA, et al. Effect of a levonorgestrel intrauterine system on women with type 1 diabetes: a randomized trial. *Obstet Gynecol.* 2005;105:811-815.
260. Bloemenkamp KW, Rosendaal FR, Helmerhorst FM, Vandenbroucke JP. Higher risk of venous thrombosis during early use of oral contraceptives in women with inherited clotting defects. *Arch Intern Med.* 2000;160:49-52.
261. Vandenbroucke JP, Rosing J, Bloemenkamp KW, et al. Oral contraceptives and the risk of venous thrombosis. *N Engl J Med.* 2001;344:1527-1535.
262. Robinson GE, Burren T, Mackie IJ, et al. Changes in haemostasis after stopping the combined contraceptive pill: implications for major surgery. *BMJ.* 1991;302:269-271.
263. Culwell KR, Curtis KM. Use of contraceptive methods by women with current venous thrombosis on anticoagulant therapy: a systematic review. *Contraception.* 2009;80:337-345.
264. Heinemann LA, Assmann A, DoMinh T, Garbe E. Oral progestogen-only contraceptives and cardiovascular risk: results from the Transnational Study on Oral Contraceptives and the Health of Young Women. *Eur J Contracept Reprod Health Care.* 1999;4:67-73.
265. Mantha S, Karp R, Raghavan V, et al. Assessing the risk of venous thromboembolic events in women taking progestin-only contraception: a meta-analysis. *BMJ.* 2012;345:e4944.
266. Kadir RA, Chi C. Levonorgestrel intrauterine system: bleeding disorders and anticoagulant therapy. *Contraception.* 2007;75:S123-S129.
267. Sonmezer M, Atabekoglu C, Cengiz B, et al. Depot-medroxyprogesterone acetate in anticoagulated patients with previous hemorrhagic corpus luteum. *Eur J Contracept Reprod Health Care.* 2005;10:9-14.
268. Headache Classification Subcommittee of the International Headache Society. The International Classification of Headache Disorders, 2nd ed. *Cephalalgia.* 2004;24(Suppl 1):9-160.
269. Curtis KM, Mohllajee AP, Peterson HB. Use of combined oral contraceptives among women with migraine and nonmigrainous headaches: a systematic review. *Contraception.* 2006;73:189-194.
270. Bousser MG, Conard J, Kittner S, et al. Recommendations on the risk of ischaemic stroke associated with use of combined oral contraceptives and hormone replacement therapy in women with migraine. The International Headache Society Task Force on Combined Oral Contraceptives & Hormone Replacement Therapy. *Cephalalgia.* 2000;20:155-156.
271. Calhoun A. Combined hormonal contraceptives: is it time to reassess their role in migraine? *Headache.* 2012;52:648-660.
272. Culwell KR, Curtis KM. Contraception for women with systemic lupus erythematosus. *J Fam Plann Reprod Health Care.* 2013;39:9-11.
273. Bermas BL. Oral contraceptives in systemic lupus erythematosus—a tough pill to swallow? *N Engl J Med.* 2005;353:2602-2604.
274. Petri M, Buyon JP. Oral contraceptives in systemic lupus erythematosus: the case for (and against). *Lupus.* 2008;17:708-710.
275. De Ceulaer K, Gruber C, Hayes R, Serjeant GR. Medroxyprogesterone acetate and homozygous sickle-cell disease. *Lancet.* 1982;2:229-231.
276. Manchikanti A, Grimes DA, Lopez LM, Schulz KF. Steroid hormones for contraception in women with sickle cell disease. *Cochrane Database Syst Rev.* 2007;CD006261.
277. Haddad LB, Curtis KM, Legardy-Williams JK, et al. Contraception for individuals with sickle cell disease: a systematic review of the literature. *Contraception.* 2012;85:527-537.
278. Austin H, Lally C, Benson JM, et al. Hormonal contraception, sickle cell trait, and risk for venous thromboembolism among African American women. *Am J Obstet Gynecol.* 2009;200:e1-e3.
279. Yoong WC, Tuck SM, Pasi KJ, et al. Markers of platelet activation, thrombin generation and fibrinolysis in women with sickle cell disease: effects of differing forms of hormonal contraception. *Eur J Haematol.* 2003;70:310-314.
280. Kessler RC. Epidemiology of women and depression. *J Affect Disord.* 2003;74:5-13.

281. Deijen JB, Duyn KJ, Jansen WA, Klitsie JW. Use of a monophasic, low-dose oral contraceptive in relation to mental functioning. *Contraception*. 1992;46:359-367.

282. Poromaa IS, Segebladh B. Adverse mood symptoms with oral contraceptives. *Acta Obstet Gynecol Scand*. 2012;91:420-427.

283. Westhoff C, Wieland D, Tiezzi L. Depression in users of depo-medroxyprogesterone acetate. *Contraception*. 1995;51:351-354.

284. Koke SC, Brown EB, Miner CM. Safety and efficacy of fluoxetine in patients who receive oral contraceptive therapy. *Am J Obstet Gynecol*. 2002;187:551-555.

285. Murphy PA, Kern SE, Stanczyk FZ, Westhoff CL. Interaction of St. John's wort with oral contraceptives: effects on the pharmacokinetics of norethindrone and ethinyl estradiol, ovarian activity and breakthrough bleeding. *Contraception*. 2005;71:402-408.

CHAPTER 19

Testicular Disorders

ALVIN M. MATSUMOTO • WILLIAM J. BREMNER

KEY POINTS

- The testes are critical for normal development of internal and external genitalia in the fetus; for secondary sexual characteristics, sexual function, and initiation of spermatogenesis during puberty; and for maintenance of male body features and function, sexual function, and fertility in the adult.
- Knowledge of the anatomy, physiology, and regulation of the hypothalamic-pituitary-testicular axis forms the basis for understanding the clinical manifestations, diagnosis, and management of the main disorder of testis function, male hypogonadism.
- Male hypogonadism is a clinical syndrome that results from the failure of the testes to produce adequate amounts of testosterone (androgen deficiency) and sperm, or from an isolated impairment of spermatogenesis.
- The consequences of androgen deficiency vary depending on the stage of sexual development. In the fetus, androgen deficiency causes ambiguous genital development; in the child, it causes delayed puberty and eunuchoidism; and in adults, it causes sexual dysfunction, gynecomastia, infertility, and changes in body composition and function that may have profound effects on a man's health.
- Male hypogonadism is common, but the diagnosis should only be made in men with symptoms and signs of androgen deficiency and consistently low testosterone levels, in the absence of conditions that transiently suppress testosterone or alter sex hormone–binding globulin in which free testosterone measurements are needed.
- In men with hypogonadism, gonadotropin levels should be measured to determine whether secondary hypogonadism is present because it may be associated with sella tumor mass effects or anterior pituitary hormone deficiency or excess, functional or potentially reversible causes, and treatable infertility.
- Prior to initiating testosterone replacement in men with hypogonadism, it is important to consider whether management of functional causes would be beneficial, if there are contraindications to therapy, and whether potential benefits outweigh risks.
- Appropriate efficacy and safety monitoring should be performed during testosterone treatment.

The testes have critical physiologic roles during different stages of development. During early fetal life, production of testosterone and antimüllerian hormone (AMH) by the fetal testes is required for the differentiation and development of normal male internal and external genitalia. During puberty, activation of the hypothalamic-pituitary-testicular axis and testosterone production by the testes are necessary for the induction of secondary (adult) male sexual characteristics, stimulation of sexual function, and initiation of sperm production. In adults, testis production of testosterone and sperm is required for the maintenance of adult male characteristics (virilization), sexual function, spermatogenesis, and fertility potential. Therefore, disorders of the testis may result in abnormalities in sexual development and function, body habitus and function, and fertility that have profound effects on health and well-being.

Disorders of the testis are common. Klinefelter syndrome, the most common human sex chromosome abnormality and the primary testicular disorder causing testosterone deficiency and impaired spermatogenesis, affects approximately 1 in 500 to 600 men.[1,2] Isolated disorders of sperm production are the main causes of male infertility, which affects approximately 5% to 6% of otherwise healthy men in the reproductive age group.[3] Testicular disorders resulting in testosterone deficiency may contribute to complaints of reduced libido (sexual interest and desire), erectile dysfunction, gynecomastia (benign breast enlargement), and reduced bone mass (osteoporosis), all of which are common in men, particularly as they age. Finally, disordered hypothalamic-pituitary-testicular function is commonly associated with chronic systemic illnesses, wasting syndromes, morbid obesity, chronic use of certain medications (e.g., glucocorticoids), and aging. These conditions often result in testosterone deficiency that, if severe and prolonged, may contribute to clinical manifestations and morbidity.[4,5]

The treatment of testicular disorders usually results in significant clinical improvements in function and quality of life. In prepubertal boys and adults with severe testosterone deficiency, testosterone therapy results in dramatic transformations in body composition and function.[6] In men with infertility and impaired spermatogenesis due to gonadotropin deficiency, gonadotropin or gonadotropin-releasing hormone (GnRH) therapy may stimulate sperm and testosterone production and effectively restore fertility. Finally, advances in assisted reproductive technology (ART) have permitted previously infertile men with testicular disorders to have children. For example, although men with Klinefelter syndrome and azoospermia (no spermatozoa in their ejaculate) were once thought to have untreatable infertility, testicular sperm extraction using microsurgical techniques combined with intracytoplasmic sperm injection (ICSI) may permit some of these men to father children.[7]

FUNCTIONAL ANATOMY AND HISTOLOGY

The Testis

Adult testes are paired, ovoid organs that hang from the inguinal canal by the *spermatic cord* (which is composed of a neurovascular pedicle, vas deferens, and cremasteric muscle); they are located outside the abdominal cavity within the scrotum. The left testis hangs lower in the scrotum than the right in about 60% of men, and the right testis hangs lower in approximately 30% of men. Each testis has a volume of 15 to 30 mL and measures 3.5 to 5.5 cm in length by 2.0 to 3.0 cm in width.[8,9]

The testis comprises two structurally and functionally distinct compartments: the *seminiferous tubule compartment,* which is composed of Sertoli cells and developing germ cells at various stages of spermatogenesis and accounts for 80% to 90% of the volume of the testis, and the *interstitial compartment,* which is composed of Leydig cells that secrete testosterone, the main male sex steroid hormone, as well as peritubular myoid cells, fibroblasts, neurovascular cells, and macrophages (Fig. 19-1).[10] Because germ cells constitute most of the testis volume, small testes are usually an indication of significantly impaired spermatogenesis.

The testis is surrounded by a fibrous capsule, the *tunica albuginea.* Fibrous septa that emanate from the tunica albuginea separate the parenchyma of the testis into lobules. The arterial blood supply of the testes is derived primarily from the testicular (internal spermatic) arteries that arise from the abdominal aorta and descend through the ingui-

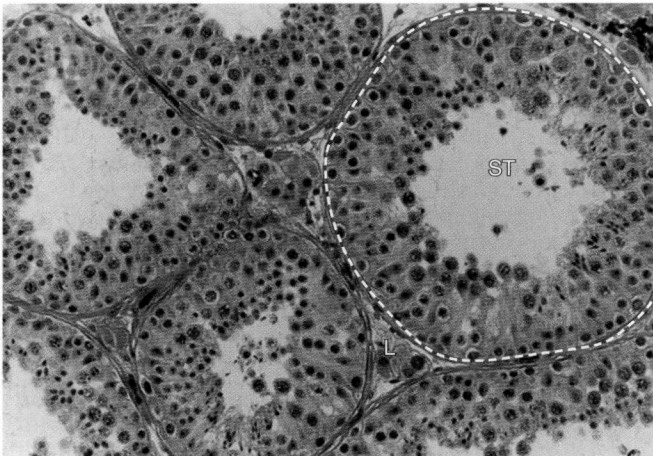

Figure 19-1 Light photomicrograph of the seminiferous tubule and interstitial compartments of the human testes. The seminiferous tubule (ST) compartment makes up the majority of the testis and is composed of developing germ cells enveloped by Sertoli cells. Spermatogonia line the basal lamina of the seminiferous tubules, spermatocytes at various stages of development are present in the middle layers of the tubules, and spermatids at various steps of maturation are present in the luminal aspect of the seminiferous tubules. Within each tubule, there are germ cells at different stages of spermatogenesis. In the interstitial compartment, there are prominent clusters of Leydig cells (L) nestled between seminiferous tubules, peritubular myoid cells within the basal lamina of the tubules, and scattered blood vessels and macrophages. (From Matsumoto AM. Spermatogenesis. In: Adashi EY, Rock JA, Rosenwaks Z, eds. *Reproductive Endocrinology, Surgery, and Technology.* Philadelphia, PA: Lippincott-Raven; 1996:359-384.)

nal canal in the spermatic cord. Collateral blood supply is provided by the cremasteric and deferential arteries. This collateral supply permits survival of the testis after a testicular artery ligation associated with surgical fixation of a high undescended testis into the scrotum (orchiopexy). However, twisting of the spermatic cord, known as *testicular torsion,* results in strangulation of the blood supply to the testis and causes testicular necrosis and infarction after 6 to 8 hours, making this condition a surgical emergency.[11] A testis that has a *bell-clapper deformity* (i.e., is not attached to the scrotal wall) is more susceptible to testicular torsion. Lymphatic drainage from the testes follows the testicular arteries to periaortic lymph nodes; this is a common route for metastasis of testicular cancer.

A network of veins that compose the pampiniform plexus provides venous drainage from the testes. The pampiniform plexus coalesces into the testicular (internal spermatic) vein. The right testicular vein drains into the inferior vena cava, and the left testicular vein empties at a right angle into the left renal vein. One-way valves in testicular veins prevent backflow of blood into the scrotum. Abnormal enlargement of the venous plexus draining a testicle, known as a *varicocele,* occurs if valves are defective or absent or if there is extrinsic venous compression impeding normal venous drainage.[12] Increased pressures associated with the backflow of blood and altered temperature regulation may contribute to testicular dysfunction associated with a varicocele. Ninety-eight percent of varicoceles occur in the left scrotum, possibly because of absent or defective valves in the left testicular vein. The presence of a prominent unilateral right-sided varicocele or new-onset varicocele on either side should prompt evaluation for venous obstruction by an abdominal or pelvic malignancy (e.g., renal cell carcinoma) or lymphadenopathy; a chronic right-sided varicocele may also indicate *situs inversus.* Rarely, an anatomic anomaly of the superior mesenteric artery that compresses the left renal vein causes a left-sided varicocele; this is known as the *nutcracker syndrome.*

Because the testes are located outside the abdominal cavity, they are exposed to temperatures approximately 2° C lower than core body temperature. The position of the testes within the scrotum and the testicular temperature are regulated by the cremasteric muscle. The cremasteric muscle contracts when warming is needed, resulting in shortening of the spermatic cord and drawing of the testis toward the abdomen; when cooling is needed, it relaxes, resulting in lowering of the testis into the scrotum. Also, the pampiniform venous plexus provides a counter-current heat exchange mechanism to cool the testis by surrounding the testicular artery with cooler venous blood. A testis temperature slightly lower than core body temperature is important for normal spermatogenesis. Exposure of the testes to higher temperatures, such as with failure of the testes to descend normally into the scrotum (*cryptorchidism*) or excessive external heat exposure due to frequent hot tub use, impairs spermatogenesis.

Seminiferous Tubule

Seminiferous tubules contain epithelium consisting of Sertoli cells that envelop and support germ cells undergoing progressive differentiation and development into mature spermatozoa. Once released into the lumen, mature spermatozoa are transported within seminiferous tubules, which measure up to 70 cm in length and are tightly coiled within lobules of the testis, to the rete testis, the efferent ducts, the epididymis, and, finally, the vas deferens for ultimate ejaculation. The seminiferous tubules are surrounded by a basal lamina composed of extracellular

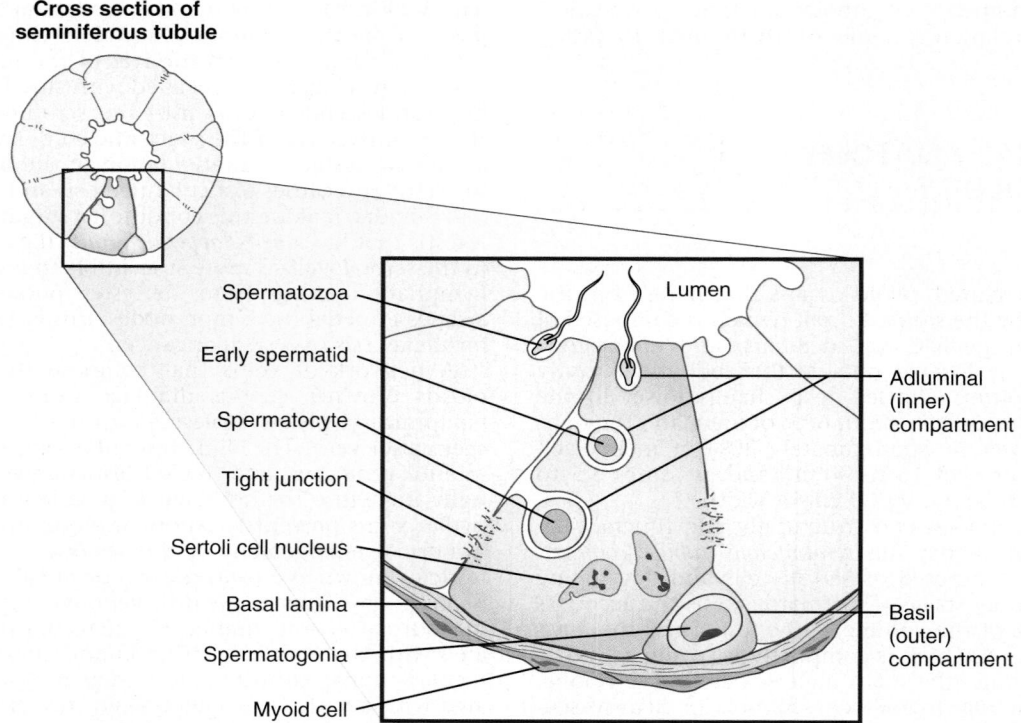

Cross section of seminiferous tubule

Figure 19-2 Schematic diagram of the cells in the seminiferous tubule *(top)*. The seminiferous tubule consists of Sertoli cells that surround developing germ cells *(middle)*. Sertoli cells extend from the basal lamina to the lumen. Tight junctions between adjoining Sertoli cells separate the seminiferous tubule into basal and adluminal compartments and are the anatomic basis for the blood-testis barrier *(bottom)*. The basal compartment, which contains spermatogonia lining the basal lamina and peritubular myoid cells, is exposed to the interstitial compartment, which contains Leydig cells and blood vessels that deliver endocrine regulators of testis function (e.g., gonadotropins). The adluminal compartment contains developing spermatocytes, spermatids, and mature spermatozoa that are released into the lumen of the seminiferous tubule. (From Matsumoto AM. The testis. In: Felig P, Frohman LA, eds. *Endocrinology and Metabolism*, 4th ed. New York, NY: McGraw-Hill; 2001:635-705.)

matrix that serves to separate them from the interstitial compartment, provides structural integrity to the tubules, and regulates the function of cells in contact with it. Histologic examination of a testis biopsy specimen in cross section reveals many different seminiferous tubules surrounded by basal lamina and clusters of Leydig cells in the interstitial compartment between each tubule (see Fig. 19-1).[10]

Sertoli cells extend from the basal lamina to the lumen of tubules, and adjacent Sertoli cells envelop and provide a structural scaffold for germ cells as they differentiate within the tubule (Fig. 19-2).[9] Undifferentiated spermatogenic stem cells, called *spermatogonia*, lie along the basal lamina at the periphery of tubules, interspersed between Sertoli cells. Adjacent Sertoli cells surround spermatogonia and form specialized junctional complexes or tight junctions that divide the seminiferous tubule into the *basal compartment*, in which spermatogonia reside, and the *adluminal compartment*, which is occupied by differentiating germ cells. Sertoli cell tight junctions impede the passage of large molecules, steroids, and ions into the seminiferous tubule and constitute the cytologic basis of the *blood-testis barrier*, analogous to the blood-brain barrier. In the adluminal compartment, *spermatocytes* derived from spermatogonia in the basal compartment undergo meiosis to form *spermatids* that progressively mature *(spermiogenesis)*, with the more mature germ cells occupying positions closer to the lumen, until mature spermatozoa are released into the lumen of the tubule *(spermiation)*.

Because of the blood-testis barrier, only Sertoli cells and spermatogonia are directly accessible to endocrine and paracrine regulation from the circulation and cells of the interstitial compartment, respectively. Sertoli cells need to

synthesize and secrete a number of products, some of which are present in circulation but not accessible to developing germ cells in the adluminal compartment, in order to nurture and regulate spermatogenesis. Sertoli cells contain receptors for follicle-stimulating hormone (FSH) and androgens, and they mediate the regulation of spermatogenesis by circulating FSH and testosterone produced locally by Leydig cells in response to stimulation from circulating luteinizing hormone (LH). Sertoli cells also produce the glycoprotein hormones—antimullerian hormone (AMH), which causes regression of müllerian ducts and prevents the development of female accessory sex organs in the male fetus, and inhibin B, which participates in negative feedback suppression of FSH—and extracellular matrix components.

Spermatogenesis

In male humans, the process of spermatogenesis supports a production rate of approximately 120 million mature spermatozoa per day by the human testis (approximately 1000 per heartbeat!).[13] Spermatogenesis, the process by which stem cells (spermatogonia) differentiate into mature spermatozoa, proceeds in three functionally distinct phases: (1) the *mitotic* or *proliferative phase*, during which the majority of spermatogonia undergo mitosis to renew the stem cell pool and a minority become committed to further differentiation to produce spermatocytes; (2) the *meiotic phase*, during which spermatocytes undergo successive meiotic divisions to produce haploid germ cells (spermatids); and (3) *spermiogenesis*, during which immature, round spermatids differentiate into mature spermatozoa (Fig. 19-3).[10,14]

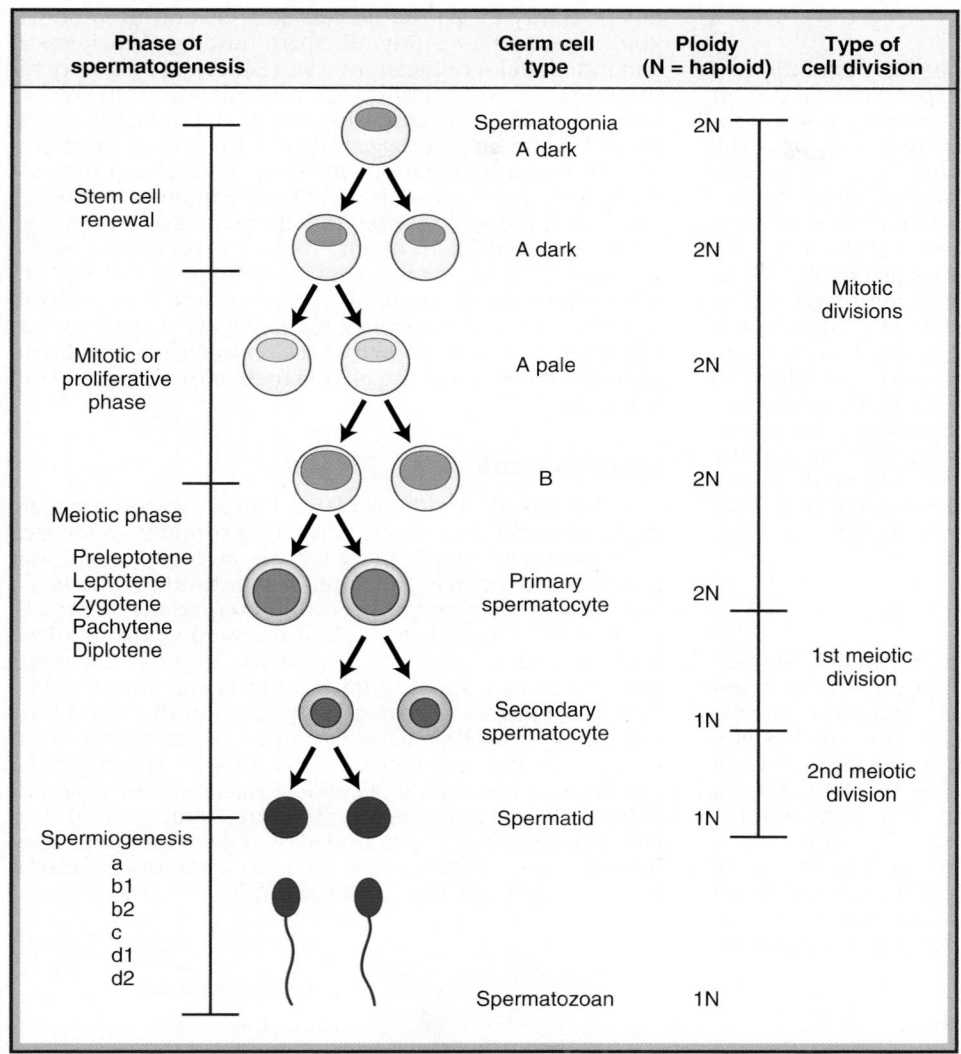

Phase of spermatogenesis		Germ cell type	Ploidy (N = haploid)	Type of cell division
Stem cell renewal		Spermatogonia A dark	2N	
		A dark	2N	
Mitotic or proliferative phase		A pale	2N	Mitotic divisions
Meiotic phase		B	2N	
Preleptotene Leptotene Zygotene Pachytene Diplotene		Primary spermatocyte	2N	
		Secondary spermatocyte	1N	1st meiotic division
Spermiogenesis a b1 b2 c d1 d2		Spermatid	1N	2nd meiotic division
		Spermatozoan	1N	

Figure 19-3 Schematic diagram of human spermatogenesis. Spermatogonial stem cells undergo self-renewal by mitotic division. At the initiation of spermatogenesis, some spermatogonia undergo differentiation into primary spermatocytes, which contain a diploid number of chromosomes (2N = 46 chromosomes). The primary spermatocytes then undergo two successive meiotic divisions to form spermatids, which contain a haploid number of chromosomes (1N = 23 chromosomes). Spermatids undergo spermiogenesis to form mature spermatozoa, which also contain a haploid number of chromosomes. (From Matsumoto AM. Spermatogenesis. In: Adashi EY, Rock JA, Rosenwaks Z, eds. *Reproductive Endocrinology, Surgery, and Technology.* Philadelphia, PA: Lippincott-Raven; 1996:359-384.)

Proliferative Phase

Based on chromatin staining and pattern, spermatogonia may be classified as A dark (A_d), A pale (A_p), or B spermatogonia. Because of their relatively low mitotic rate, A_d spermatogonia are thought to be the spermatogonial stem cells. A_d spermatogonia are relatively resistant to external insults (e.g., ionizing radiation), and in response to such insults, they undergo mitotic proliferation. However, severe or complete depletion of A_d spermatogonia, such as occurs with high-dose x-irradiation or vascular compromise, results in irreversible impairment or loss of sperm production.

A small number of A_d spermatogonia undergo mitotic divisions to form A_p and then B spermatogonia. In humans, the rate of formation of B spermatogonia is low, so that only a small number of B spermatogonia are available to enter meiosis and undergo further differentiation.[15] This limits the efficiency of spermatogenesis in humans. B spermatogonia are the most sensitive germ cells to the effects of ionizing radiation, and their numbers are reduced after irradiation of the testes.[16]

B spermatogonia that become committed to further differentiation undergo mitotic division to form *preleptotene* or *resting* spermatocytes, which enter a prolonged meiotic phase of 24 days. Spermatogonia do not completely separate after mitosis *(incomplete cytokinesis)*. Groups of sper-matogonia remain connected via cytoplasmic bridges, forming a syncytium, and undergo meiosis and spermiogenesis in synchrony.

Meiotic Phase

Preleptotene primary spermatocytes contain a diploid complement of chromosomes (46 chromosomes or 2N, where N is the number of haploid chromosomes), and they are the last germ cells to undergo DNA synthesis. Preleptotene spermatocytes undergo an initial round of meiotic division *(meiosis I)*, lasting longer than 2 weeks, to form secondary spermatocytes that contain a haploid complement of chromosomes (1N). Secondary spermatocytes, which are present for only about 8 hours, undergo a second meiotic division *(meiosis II)* to form haploid spermatids.

Improper segregation of chromosomes *(meiotic nondisjunction)* resulting in an abnormal number of chromosomes *(aneuploidy)* occurs in 0.7% of live births and 50% of first-trimester abortuses.[17,18] Klinefelter syndrome, a common cause of primary hypogonadism, occurs in about 1 in 500 live births and is associated classically with a 47,XXY karyotype caused by paternal meiotic nondisjunction in 50% of cases.[19] Down syndrome (trisomy 21) occurs in approximately 1 in 700 live births and is caused by paternal meiotic nondisjunction in 5% to 20% of cases.[20]

Spermiogenesis

The final phase of spermatogenesis is the maturation of spermatids from round to elongated spermatids and then to mature spermatozoa; this process, known as spermiogenesis, is followed by release of spermatozoa into the lumen of seminiferous tubules (spermiation). The major changes that occur during spermiogenesis include formation of the sperm head with condensation of chromosomes (DNA and nucleoproteins) and formation of the *acrosomal cap*, which contains proteolytic enzymes needed for sperm penetration of the ovum; formation of the sperm tail or *flagellum* (pointing into the lumen), which permits motility; phagocytic removal of excess spermatid cytoplasm (known as the *residual body*) by Sertoli cells; and release of mature spermatozoa into the lumen. Progressive maturation of spermatids is accompanied by progressive movement of more mature spermatids toward the lumen of the seminiferous tubule. Spermiogenesis is directed by the Sertoli cells that sustain and support developing spermatids and by the major endocrine regulators of Sertoli cells, FSH, and testosterone.

Germ Cell Loss

Compared to most other species, the efficiency of spermatogenesis in humans is relatively poor, and the germ cell degeneration and loss that occur predominantly during mitosis and meiosis are major contributors to the low efficiency of sperm production.[21] Significant degrees of germ cell degeneration occurring during meiosis account for a decrease of approximately 40% in the ratio of the number of spermatids to preleptotene spermatocytes. This ratio is reduced further as men age, resulting in a reduction of daily sperm production in elderly men. It is hypothesized that germ cell degeneration prevents abnormal germ cells from further development, thereby serving an important quality control function.

Organization of Spermatogenesis

Histologic examination of a human testis in cross section reveals that germ cells at particular phases of development cluster in six cellular associations, referred to as *stages*, which together constitute a complete *cycle* of spermatogenesis. In most mammals, stages are organized sequentially along the longitudinal axis of the tubules so that all of the germ cells present in a cross section of a tubule are in the same stage of spermatogenesis.[22,23] In contrast, three or more different stages of a cycle may variably be present in a cross section of human testis. Although some have proposed a helical pattern of stages along the tubule to explain this seemingly chaotic arrangement, this has not been confirmed by others.

In humans, the duration of spermatogenesis from A_p spermatogonia to release of mature spermatozoa is 74 ± 4 days.[24] The epididymal transit time of spermatozoa is approximately 12 to 21 days.[25] Therefore, external insults to the testis (e.g., ionizing radiation) or induction of gonadotropin deficiency (e.g., by male contraceptive regimens) that affects early germ cell development and reduces spermatogenesis may not be reflected in reduced sperm counts in the ejaculate until months later.

Sperm Transport and Fertilization

Mature spermatozoa released into the lumen of the seminiferous tubule are transported to the rete testis, to the efferent ducts of the testis, and then to the caput epididymis primarily by peristaltic contractions and intratubular fluid flow. In the epididymis, sperm undergo biochemical and functional modifications that result in the capacity for sustained forward motility. After ejaculation from the vas deferens and penis into the female reproductive tract, human sperm undergo *capacitation* in the uterus; the resulting biochemical alterations in the acrosomal cap increase the fluidity and hyperactivated motility induced by uterine secretory products so that the spermatozoa acquire the capacity to fertilize an ovum.[26,27] After capacitation, as the spermatozoon meets an ovum in the ampulla of the fallopian tube, the sperm binds to the egg and releases hyaluronidase to penetrate the zona pellucida that surrounds the ovum, a process known as the *acrosome reaction*. Fertilization then occurs as the plasma membranes of sperm and ovum fuse.

Spermatozoa

Morphologically, most ejaculated human spermatozoa are composed of an oval-shaped head that contains condensed chromatin and nucleoproteins; an acrosomal cap that covers approximately the anterior two thirds of the head; a short neck that contains centrioles important for attachment of the tail and cleavage of the zygote after fertilization; a middle piece that consists of axial filaments surrounded by a spiral of mitochondria containing oxidative enzymes that provide energy for motility; and a long tail or flagellum that permits normal progressive forward motility of the spermatozoa (Fig. 19-4).[10] The flagellum consists of a microtubule-based cytoskeleton, the *axoneme*, which has a characteristic structure composed of two central microtubules surrounded by nine microtubule doublets ($9 \times 2 + 2$ pattern) that serves as a scaffold for motor protein complexes (i.e., *dynein arms*).[28]

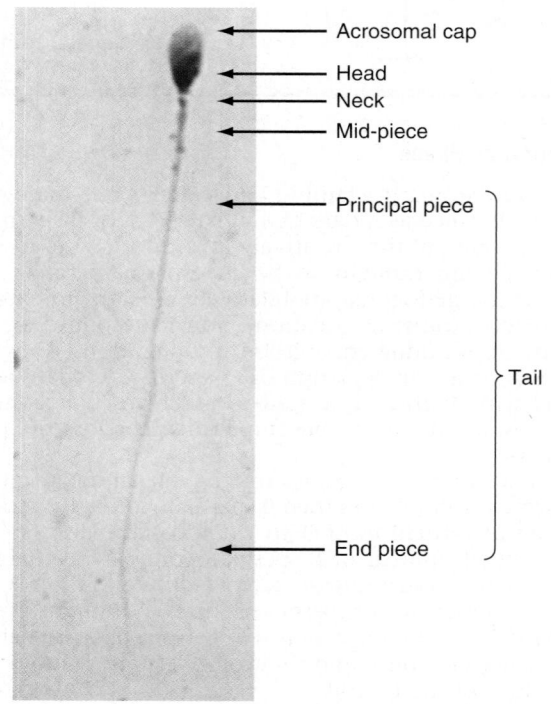

Figure 19-4 Light photomicrograph of an ejaculated mature human spermatozoon, composed of a head, neck, mid-piece, and tail (principal piece and end piece). (From Matsumoto AM. Spermatogenesis. In: Adashi EY, Rock JA, Rosenwaks Z, eds. *Reproductive Endocrinology, Surgery, and Technology.* Philadelphia, PA: Lippincott-Raven; 1996:359-384.)

In humans, the normal sperm concentration in the ejaculate is greater than 15 million/mL, with 4% or more having normal morphologic appearance by strict criteria (≥30% by previous criteria) and 40% or more having total motility, according to the most recent World Health Organization criteria.[29,30] Men with infertility may exhibit morphologic abnormalities of the sperm head (tapered, amorphous, or double-headed forms) or of the tail (coiled forms) and reduced or absent motility. Alterations in the structural or functional components of the axoneme (e.g., absence of dynein arms) result in altered motility, and deficiency of dynein adenosine triphosphatase (ATPase) results in primary ciliary dyskinesia or immotile cilia syndrome.[31]

Interstitium

The interstitial compartment of the testis contains clusters of Leydig cells, the primary sex steroid–producing cells of the testis, which make up only about 5% of testis volume (see Fig. 19-1).[23,32] Leydig cells produce testosterone, which acts as a paracrine regulator within the seminiferous tubules of the testis on Sertoli cells in close proximity to stimulate spermatogenesis. Testosterone is secreted into adjacent testicular capillaries and then into the general circulation to act as an endocrine signal on androgen target organs throughout the body. Leydig cells also produce *insulin-like factor 3 (INSL3)*, a peptide hormone in the relaxin-insulin family, which plays an important role in the first phase of testicular descent from the abdomen into the scrotum during development.[33] INSL3 also may be an important autocrine regulator of Leydig cells and a paracrine regulator of germ cells directly.[34]

Peritubular myoid cells, which surround the seminiferous tubules, are contractile, smooth, muscle-like cells that serve to facilitate forward transport of spermatozoa and testicular fluid within the tubular lumen, provide structural integrity to the tubule, secrete extracellular matrix components and putative regulatory factors such as growth factors, and are involved in retinol metabolism.[23,35] These cells contain androgen receptors (ARs) and are thought to mediate some of the paracrine effects of testosterone on Sertoli cells within the seminiferous tubules, although their precise role in human testicular physiology remains unclear.

The interstitial compartment also contains macrophages that may regulate Leydig cell steroidogenesis by secretion of cytokines and may play a role in phagocytosis of degenerating cells and necrotic debris. The interstitium contains arterioles and a rich network of capillaries that permit secretion of testosterone and other products into the circulation and delivery of the main endocrine regulators of testis function, the gonadotropins LH and FSH.

TESTIS DEVELOPMENT

Fetal Development

During embryogenesis, the Y chromosome directs the development of the testis from an undifferentiated anlage that has the potential to develop into either a testis or an ovary.[36] The *SRY (sex-determining region of the Y chromosome) gene*, located on the pseudoautosomal region of the Y chromosome, encodes a transcription factor that increases the expression of SRY-box 9 (*SOX9*), which in turn drives the formation of Sertoli cells and testis differentiation. *SRY* gene expression is activated by a number of factors, including steroidogenic factor 1 (SF1) and the binding protein

GATA4.[37] *SRY*-independent *SOX9* expression may also be driven by SF1. *SOX9* directs the expression of other genes that are essential in testis differentiation, such as fibroblast growth factor 9 (*FGF9*) and *AMH*, and in repression of ovarian differentiation, such as *WNT4* and *DAX1* (now designated *NROB1*). In the absence of *SRY* or *SRY* action, *SOX9* is repressed by a number of factors, including β-catenin, and development of the follicular cells and ovaries follows.

Primordial germ cells originate in the yolk sac and migrate to the genital ridges. Together with celomic epithelial and mesenchymal cells that eventually differentiate, respectively, into Sertoli cells and interstitial cells (Leydig and peritubular myoid cells), they form the *genital blastema* by 6 weeks of gestation. Primordial germ cells that fail to migrate normally explain the location of extragonadal germ cell cancers in men. Under the influence of gene products activated by *SRY*, primordial germ cells become surrounded by primitive Sertoli cells to form seminiferous or sex cords that eventually develop into seminiferous tubules.

Leydig cells begin to form at 8 weeks of gestation. Then, under the influence of maternal human chorionic gonadotropin (hCG) initially and later LH and FSH from the fetal pituitary gland, immature Leydig cells, Sertoli cells, and germ cells undergo differentiation, proliferation, and organization. Testosterone production from fetal Leydig cells increases progressively and induces development of the epididymis, vas deferens, and seminal vesicles from wolffian or mesonephric ducts. Conversion of testosterone to 5α-dihydrotestosterone (5α-DHT) in the urogenital tract leads to the formation of the prostate from the urogenital sinus, the penis from the genital tubercles and folds, and the scrotum from the urogenital swelling.[38] In the absence of testosterone production or action, female internal and external genitalia develop. AMH secretion from the fetal Sertoli cells causes regression of the müllerian or paramesonephric ducts and prevents the formation of a uterus and fallopian tubes.

Male phenotypic development is complete by about 15 weeks of gestation, after which the proliferation of Sertoli and germ cells arrests and Leydig cells involute until gonadotropin secretion increases at the time of puberty.

Testis Descent

The developing testis is attached to the diaphragm by the craniosuspensory ligament and anchored to the inguinal region by a caudal ligament known as the *gubernaculum*. Descent of the testis occurs in two phases.[33] During the initial *transabdominal phase*, the testis descends within the abdomen to the inguinal region; this occurs between 10 and 23 weeks of gestation. Studies in animals suggest that testis descent during this phase depends on two processes: (1) regression of the craniosuspensory ligament, induced by testosterone, which frees the testes to descend, and (2) thickening of the gubernaculum, which is controlled by INSL3 produced by Leydig cells and its cognate receptor, relaxin family peptide receptor 2 (RXFP2, also known as leucine-rich repeat–containing G protein–coupled receptor 8 [LGR8] or G protein–coupled receptor affecting testis descent [GREAT]). During the *inguinoscrotal phase*, which begins at 26 to 28 weeks of gestation, the testis descends into the scrotum; this process is largely controlled by the effects of testosterone on gubernacular shortening and contractions. The effects of testosterone may be mediated in part by the neurotransmitter, calcitonin gene–related peptide (CGRP), which is released by the genitofemoral nerve. The importance of testosterone, gonadotropins, and INSL3 in testis descent in humans is suggested by the occurrence of undescended testes (cryptorchidism) associated with fetal androgen deficiency or resistance, gonadotropin deficiency, and *INSL3* or *RXFP2* mutations.[34]

Testis descent is usually complete, with the testes entirely within the scrotum, by 7 months of gestation to birth. During testis descent, a herniation of the abdominal cavity, the *processus vaginalis*, develops along the course of the gubernaculum, forming the inguinal ring and canal and descending with the testis into the scrotum. As the abdominal wall and muscles develop, the inguinal rings close, and the processus vaginalis obliterates to form the *tunica vaginalis*, which covers the anterior and lateral portion of the testes. Incomplete closure of the inguinal ring predisposes an individual to *inguinal hernia*, and incomplete obliteration of the processus vaginalis with accumulation of serous fluid results in a *hydrocele*; either of these conditions can manifest as a scrotal mass.

Postnatal Development

During late gestational life, the male fetus is exposed to high concentrations of estrogens from the placenta. With the decline in estrogen levels after birth, the hypothalamic-pituitary-testicular axis is released from negative feedback suppression, resulting in a postnatal surge of gonadotropin that stimulates the testes to produce testosterone and inhibin B.

LH and testosterone levels begin to increase at about 1 week of life and peak 1 to 2 months later, reaching the equivalent of adolescent levels in association with an increase in the number of Leydig cells; they then decline to prepubertal levels by about 6 months of age. Infants with complete androgen insensitivity who lack androgen action due to an AR mutation (see later discussion) do not demonstrate a postnatal gonadotropin surge and have low or undetectable LH and testosterone levels postnatally, suggesting that AR expression is required for the surge.[39] In humans, there is no evidence that the postnatal surge of LH and testosterone has an effect on adult Leydig cell function. However, in infants with hypogonadotropic hypogonadism, lack of a surge in testosterone may play a role in the development of micropenis or cryptorchidism, suggesting a role in postnatal development.[40,41] In infants with micropenis, postnatal hormone testing may permit early identification and possible treatment of isolated hypogonadotropic hypogonadism or hypopituitarism.

FSH and inhibin B levels also begin to rise at 1 week of life, in association with an increase in proliferation of Sertoli cells, and peak at 3 months. FSH then declines to prepubertal levels by 9 months of age. Inhibin B declines more slowly and plateaus at approximately 15 months of age, probably reflecting ongoing Sertoli cell proliferation. Because Sertoli cell number determines spermatogenic potential, the postnatal gonadotropin surge may be important for sperm production in adults. The postnatal testosterone surge also increases the formation of A_d spermatogonia (spermatogonial stem cells) from gonocytes during the first 3 months and increases testis size and seminiferous tubule length during the first year of life, providing further evidence for the importance of the gonadotropin surge on future spermatogenesis and possibly fertility. In men with gonadotropin deficiency, inadequate postnatal gonadotropin stimulation results in inadequate numbers of Sertoli cells and spermatogonia, and this may contribute to the failure of gonadotropin therapy to quantitatively stimulate normal sperm production in men with Kallmann syndrome who are treated as adults.

Pubertal Development

At the onset of puberty, reactivation of hypothalamic GnRH secretion stimulates pituitary LH and testicular Leydig cell testosterone secretion, initially only during the evening (Fig. 19-5) and subsequently throughout the day with FSH secretion.[42,43] Progressive increase in testosterone levels during puberty induces male secondary sexual characteristics and, together with increasing FSH levels, stimulates Sertoli cells to initiate the first wave of spermatogenesis. With increasing germ cell numbers and expansion of seminiferous tubules, testis size increases progressively. Increase in testis size is the first clinical sign of puberty. Also, with the release of mature spermatozoa into the lumen of seminiferous tubules and transport of sperm to the genitourinary tract, sperm begin to appear in the urine *(spermarche)* during early puberty (usually at 12 to 15 years of age).[44]

ADULT PHYSIOLOGY

Hypothalamic-Pituitary-Testicular Axis

The testis is controlled by classic positive feed-forward and negative feedback mechanisms (Fig. 19-6). The major positive regulators of testis function are the gonadotropins LH and FSH, which are synthesized and secreted from the anterior pituitary gland. Secretion of LH and, to a lesser extent, FSH is pulsatile and is driven primarily by episodic release of GnRH from neurons in the hypothalamus.[45] GnRH stimulates gonadotropin-producing cells of the anterior pituitary (gonadotrophs) to secrete both LH and FSH.

LH acts on Leydig cells of the testes to stimulate production of testosterone, the main sex steroid hormone in males. In concert with FSH, testosterone acts locally on Sertoli cells within the seminiferous tubules of the testes to initiate and maintain spermatogenesis. Testosterone secreted into the circulation acts to mediate and promote androgen action on almost every tissue in the body, including negative feedback inhibition of pituitary LH and FSH secretion (primarily via conversion to estradiol) and suppression of GnRH production by the hypothalamus. FSH also stimulates Sertoli cells to produce inhibin B, a peptide hormone that causes negative feedback inhibition of FSH secretion by the anterior pituitary.

Knowledge of the hypothalamic-pituitary-testicular axis is essential in understanding the causes, classification, differential diagnosis, clinical consequences, and treatment of testicular disorders.

Central Nervous System Regulation of Gonadotropin-Releasing Hormone Secretion

The brain plays a vital role in regulation of the testis and of reproductive function through production of the decapeptide, GnRH, by a relatively small number of neurons located primarily in the arcuate nucleus of the medial basal hypothalamus. GnRH is released episodically from axon terminals in the median eminence into capillaries of the hypothalamic hypophyseal portal system, through which it is carried to the anterior pituitary to stimulate synthesis and release of LH and FSH. Because the amount of GnRH in portal blood is low, GnRH concentrations in peripheral blood are very low and cannot be measured reliably for clinical purposes (e.g., to diagnose GnRH deficiency).

The precise mechanism of synchronous episodic release of GnRH from a number of separate GnRH neurons into the hypophyseal portal system to provide pulsatile

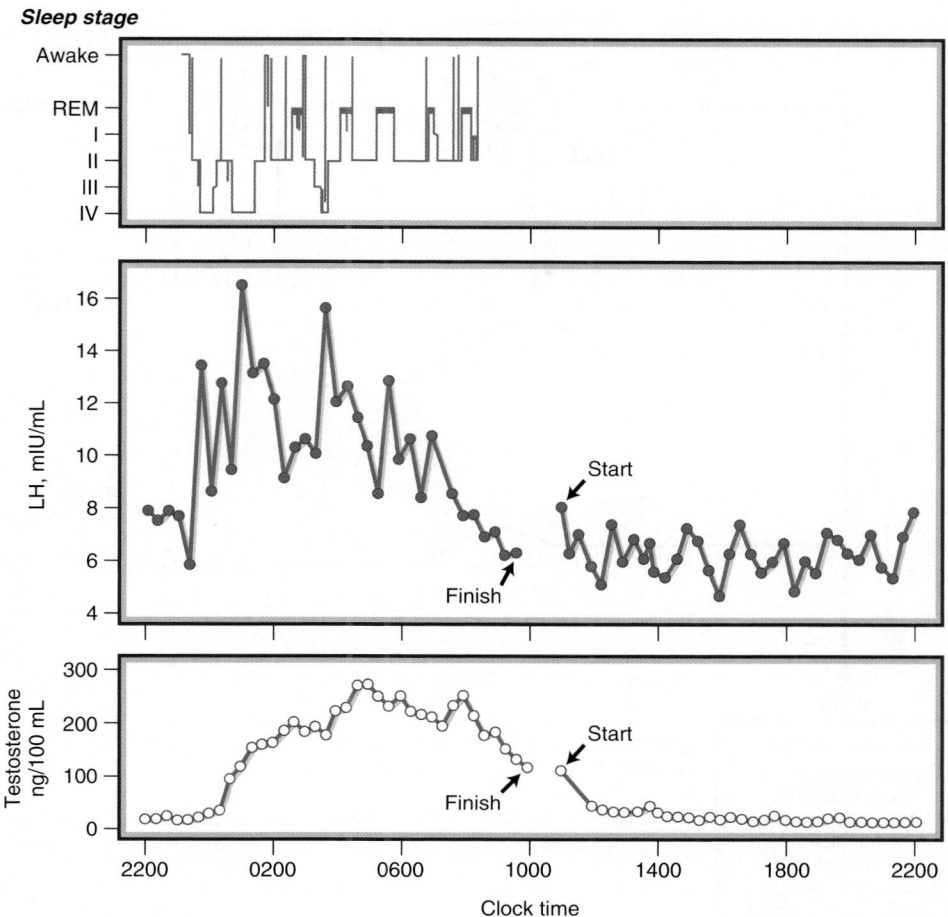

Figure 19-5 Sleep-associated secretion of luteinizing hormone (LH) *(middle)* and testosterone *(bottom)* related to sleep stage *(top)* in a prepubertal boy entering puberty. REM, rapid eye movement sleep. (From Boyar RM, Rosenfeld RS, Kapen S, et al. Human puberty: simultaneous augmented secretion of luteinizing hormone and testosterone during sleep. *J Clin Invest.* 1974;54:609-618.)

stimulation of pituitary gonadotrophs is not clear. There is evidence that pulse generation is a direct consequence of intrinsic periodicity of GnRH or other neurons that synapse on GnRH neurons within the medial basal hypothalamus, such as neurons containing kisspeptin or excitatory or inhibitory neurotransmitters.

The frequency of pulsatile GnRH secretion is temporally coupled with the episodic release of LH, free α-subunit (cosecreted with intact gonadotropins), and FSH.[46] Because the half-lives of LH and free α-subunit in circulation are shorter than that of FSH, levels of LH and α-subunit demonstrate discrete pulses, which are evident with frequent blood sampling (e.g., every 10 minutes for 12 to 24 hours), whereas FSH pulses are not as apparent. The frequency of LH or free α-subunit pulses reflects GnRH pulse frequency and serves as an indicator of synchronous GnRH neuronal activity (pulse generation) in the brain. The amplitude of LH or free α-subunit pulses reflects both the amplitude of GnRH pulses and the responsiveness of the gonadotrophs to GnRH stimulation. Normal men usually demonstrate 12 to 16 LH pulses of varying amplitude over 24 hours (Fig. 19-7). In men with GnRH deficiency (idiopathic hypogonadotropic hypogonadism [IHH] or Kallmann syndrome), there is an absence of LH pulses (most commonly) or abnormalities in LH pulsatility.[47]

Treatment of men who have GnRH deficiency with low-dose pulsatile GnRH normalizes LH and FSH secretion and testicular function. In contrast, continuous low-dose GnRH administration does not stimulate normal gonadotropin secretion in these men.[48] Administration of potent GnRH receptor agonists providing continuous, high-dose GnRH stimulation of the pituitary initially stimulates but then downregulates and profoundly suppresses gonadotropin secretion and testosterone production. This effect has been the basis for the use of potent GnRH agonists to produce medical castration (androgen deprivation therapy) in the men with advanced prostate cancer. These findings underscore the critical importance of pulsatile GnRH control of reproductive function in men.

GnRH neurons receive a number of excitatory and inhibitory inputs from other brain regions (e.g., from kisspeptin neurons) as well as feedback signals from the testes and other circulating endocrine signals. Therefore, the GnRH neuronal system serves an important integrative role in regulation of reproductive and testis function. A large and complex ensemble of neuroregulators mediates GnRH secretion, acting directly on GnRH neurons themselves or indirectly on other neurons that in turn regulate GnRH neurons to stimulate or inhibit GnRH secretion. These central nervous system (CNS) neuromodulatory systems, together with peripheral endocrine regulators, provide the means by which GnRH secretion and testicular function may be altered by environmental factors such as stress (e.g., via corticotropin-releasing hormone, glucocorticoids), nutritional compromise (e.g., via leptin), and medications (e.g., opioid drugs).

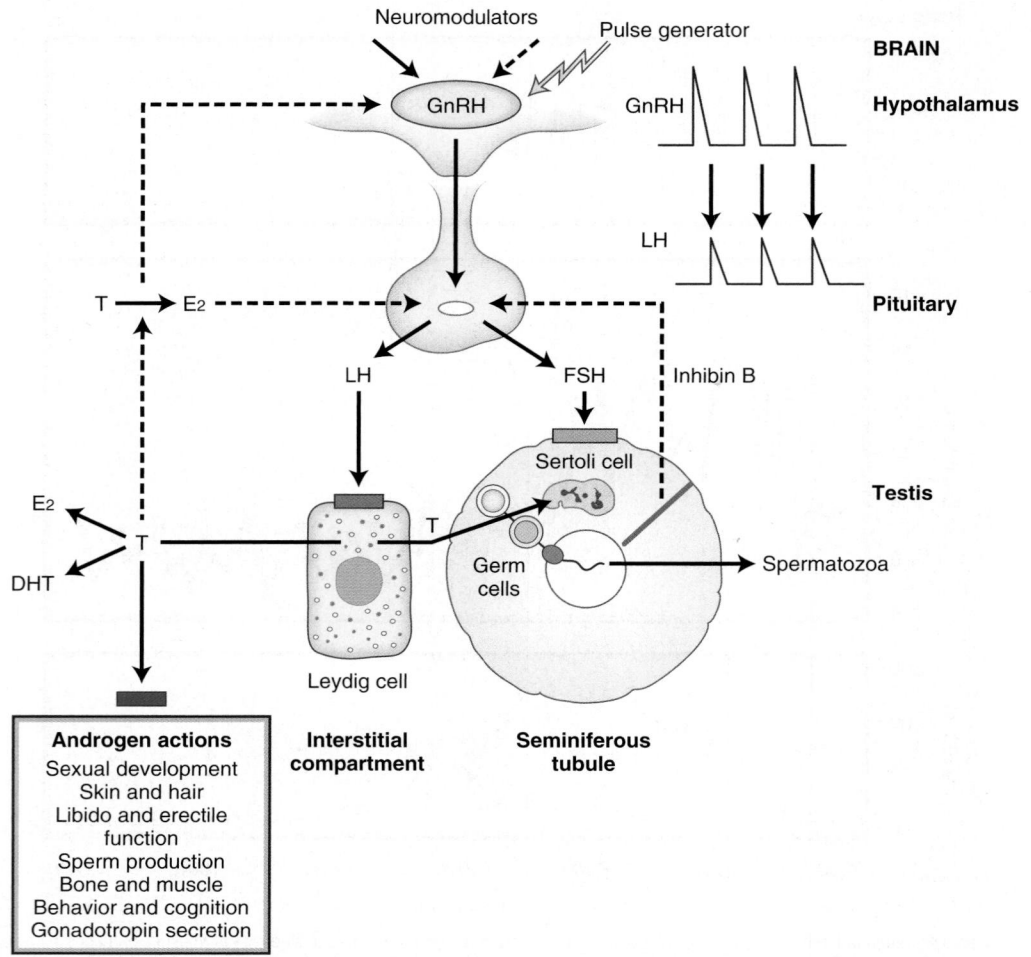

Figure 19-6 Schematic diagram of the hypothalamic-pituitary-testicular axis. Hypothalamic gonadotropin-releasing hormone (GnRH) stimulates the pituitary to produce luteinizing hormone (LH) and follicle-stimulating hormone (FSH). LH stimulates Leydig cells of the testes to produce testosterone (T), which is actively metabolized to estradiol (E_2) and dihydrotestosterone (DHT), resulting in a number of direct and indirect androgen actions. FSH stimulates Sertoli cells of the testes, which together with LH-stimulated testosterone, increases spermatogenesis. LH-stimulated testosterone and E_2 exert negative feedback suppression of GnRH production at the hypothalamus and LH and FSH production at the pituitary, and FSH-stimulated inhibin B exerts negative feedback suppression on FSH secretion by the pituitary. (From Matsumoto AM. The testis. In: Felig P, Frohman LA, eds. *Endocrinology and Metabolism*, 4th ed. New York, NY: McGraw-Hill; 2001:635-705.)

During embryogenesis, GnRH and olfactory neurons originate outside the CNS in the olfactory placode and migrate together along olfactory axons through the cribriform plate of the ethmoid bone to the olfactory bulb, where GnRH neurons diverge and continue to migrate to the medial basal hypothalamus.[49] Abnormalities in the development of the olfactory bulbs and migration of these neurons explain the association between IHH due to GnRH deficiency and the loss or impairment of the sense of smell (anosmia or hyposmia, respectively) that occurs in patients with Kallmann syndrome. Loss-of-function mutations occur in genes that play important roles in the migration and embryologic development of GnRH neurons, such as the genes for Kallmann syndrome 1 *(KAL1), KAL2* (now called *fibroblast growth factor receptor 1 [FGFR1]),* and prokineticin receptor 2 *(PROKR2)* and its ligand, prokineticin 2 *(PROK2).* Similarly, genes that are important in the regulation of GnRH neurons may sustain loss-of-function mutations; examples include the genes for kisspeptin 1 receptor *(KISS1R* [formerly *GPR54])* and its ligand, kisspeptin 1 *(KISS1),* also called metastin; the neurokinin B (tachykinin 3) receptor *(TACR3)* and its ligand *(TAC3);* and the GnRH receptor *(GNRHR)* and its ligand *(GNRH).* All of these result in isolated GnRH deficiency associated with impaired

pubertal development, often in combination with anosmia or hyposmia or other morphologic defects.[50]

Gonadotropin-Releasing Hormone Regulation of Gonadotropin Secretion

GnRH released from the hypothalamus into the hypophyseal portal system binds to G protein–coupled GnRH receptors on anterior pituitary gonadotrophs.[51] In humans, GnRH receptors are coupled primarily to $G_{q/11}$ proteins, which activate phospholipase C-β to produce 1,2-diacylglycerol (DAG) and inositol 1,4,5-triphosphate (IP3). DAG activates protein kinase C (PKC), and IP3 mobilizes intracellular calcium, which binds to the calcium-binding protein, calmodulin. Both PKC and calcium phosphorylate and activate a number of transcription factors, resulting in increased synthesis of the gonadotropin subunits LHβ, FSHβ, and the common α-subunit and release of intact LH and FSH and free α-subunits into the circulation. The GnRH receptor may also be coupled to G_s protein, which activates protein kinase A (PKA), resulting in synthesis and release of gonadotrophs.

LH and FSH, together with another anterior pituitary hormone, thyroid-stimulating hormone (TSH), and a

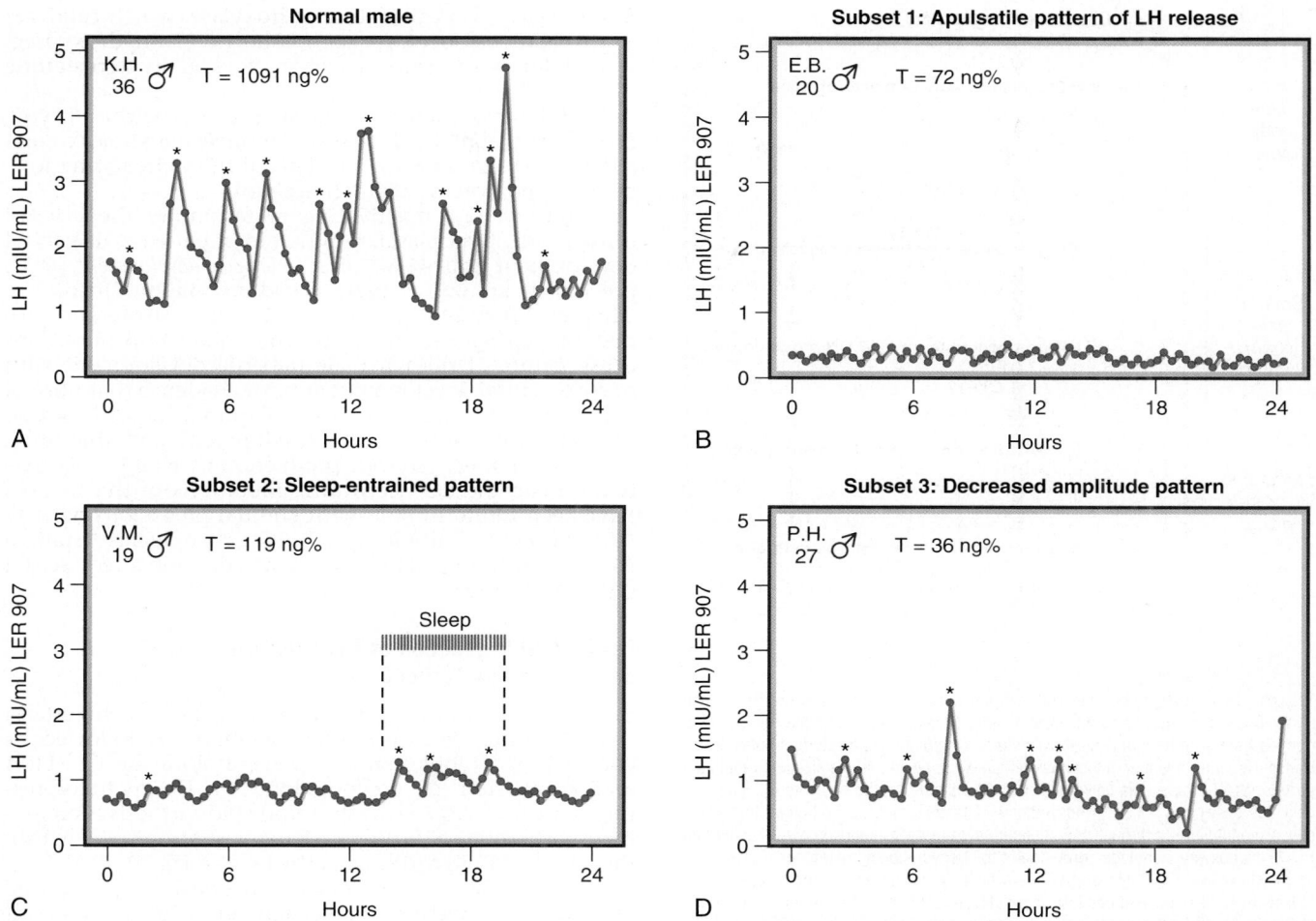

Figure 19-7 Endogenous pulsatile secretion of luteinizing hormone (LH) in a normal man (**A**) and in men with idiopathic hypogonadotropic hypogonadism (**B** through **D**), assessed by blood sampling every 20 minutes for 24 hours. In normal men (**A**), discrete pulses (*) of LH occur approximately every 2 hours, reflecting pulsatile release of gonadotropin-releasing hormone (GnRH) from the hypothalamus, and stimulate normal adult levels of testosterone (T). Most men with idiopathic hypogonadotropic hypogonadism (**B**) demonstrate no detectable LH pulses and have prepubertal testosterone concentrations. Others exhibit primarily sleep-entrained LH pulses of reduced amplitude without significant LH pulsatility during the waking hours (**C**) or LH pulses of reduced amplitude throughout sleep and waking hours (**D**) with pubertal or prepubertal testosterone levels, respectively. (From Santoro N, Filicori M, Crowley WF Jr. Hypogonadotropic disorders in men and women: diagnosis and therapy with pulsatile gonadotropin-releasing hormone. *Endocr Rev.* 1986;7:11-23.)

placental hormone, hCG, are members of the glycoprotein hormone family. Glycoprotein hormones are heterodimers in which two common α-subunits are each linked to a unique β-subunit; this structure confers their ability to bind to their cognate receptors and their biologic specificity. In the pituitary gonadotroph, the common α-subunit and the LHβ- and FSHβ-subunits are products of different genes that are synthesized and regulated differentially.[52] After the subunits are synthesized, an α-subunit combines noncovalently with either an LHβ- or an FSHβ-subunit. After translation, the heterodimer undergoes variable glycosylation wherein oligosaccharide chains (glycans) are attached covalently to specific amino acids, resulting in LH and FSH molecules with a high degree of microheterogeneity (i.e., a large number of LH and FSH isoforms characterized by different glycosylation patterns). The gonadotropin α-subunit is produced in excess relative to the LHβ- and FSHβ-subunits; it too is glycosylated, and free α-subunit is cosecreted into the circulation with LH and FSH. Many nonfunctional and gonadotropin-secreting pituitary adenomas secrete excessive amounts of free α-subunit into the circulation.[53]

The degree of glycosylation of gonadotropins and other glycoprotein hormones alters their clearance rate from circulation and their signal transduction after receptor binding, thereby affecting their biologic activity in vivo. The half-life in circulation of gonadotropins increases with greater degrees of glycosylation: hCG > FSH > LH > free α-subunit. In humans, the initial half-life of disappearance for LH is about 40 minutes, and the secondary half-life of disappearance is about 120 minutes; for FSH, these periods are approximately 4 and 70 hours, respectively.[54,55] Variations in glycosylation of LH and FSH result in substantial microheterogeneity among circulating gonadotropin isoforms, which vary in half-life and biologic activity and may be altered by particular physiologic conditions, such as during puberty, with aging, and with androgen deprivation.

Clinically, serum LH and FSH levels are measured with rapid, nonradioactive, highly sensitive immunoassays that use monoclonal antibodies recognizing two separate epitopes on the gonadotropin molecule. Gonadotropin measurements are essential in the evaluation of men with hypogonadism to distinguish those who have a primary testicular disorder (*primary hypogonadism*, in which gonadotropins are high) from those who have a secondary hypothalamic or a pituitary disorder (*secondary hypogonadism*, in which gonadotropins are low or normal). Specific

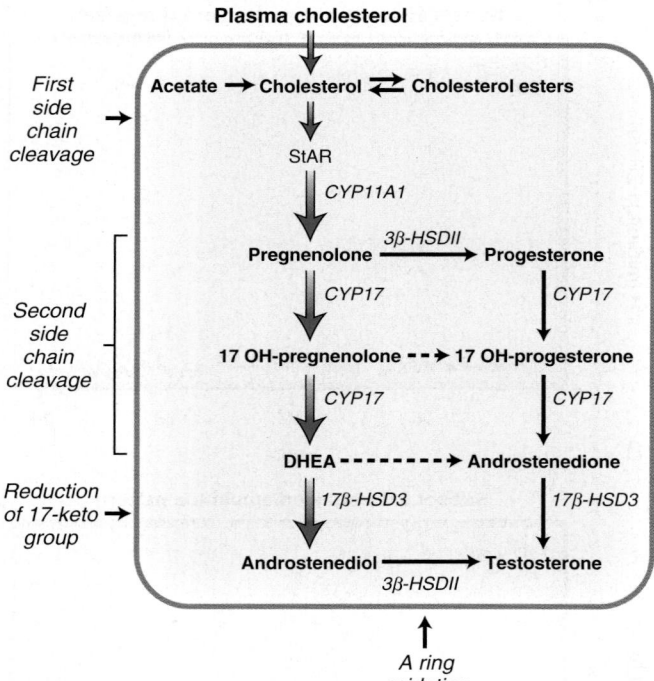

Figure 19-8 Testosterone biosynthetic pathways in the Leydig cell of the human testis. Cholesterol may be synthesized de novo from acetate within the Leydig cell or derived from hydrolysis of cholesterol esters or circulating cholesterol. Cholesterol is transported into the inner mitochondrial membrane by steroidogenic acute regulatory protein (StAR); there it is converted to pregnenolone by the cholesterol side-chain cleavage enzyme (CYP11A1). Biosynthesis of testosterone in the human testis proceeds predominantly through the Δ^5 pathway, in which pregnenolone is converted to 17-hydroxypregnenolone and then to dehydroepiandrosterone (DHEA), by 17α-hydroxylase/17,20 lyase (CYP17), which is converted to androstenediol by 17β-hydroxysteroid dehydrogenase type 3 (17β-HSD3 or HSD17B3) and then to testosterone by 3β-hydroxysteroid dehydrogenase type II (3β-HSDII or HSD3B2). In the Δ^4 pathway, pregnenolone is converted successively to 17-hydroxyprogesterone, androstenedione, and testosterone. (From Bhasin S. Testicular disorders. In: Kronenberg HM, Melmed S, Polonsky KS, et al, eds. *Williams Textbook of Endocrinology*, 11th ed. Philadelphia, PA: Elsevier; 2008:645-698.)

immunoassays for free α-subunit are used to diagnose and monitor patients with nonfunctional and gonadotropin-secreting pituitary adenomas.

Gonadotropin Control of Testicular Function
Luteinizing Hormone Regulation of Leydig Cells

Circulating LH binds to the G protein–coupled receptor for LH and hCG (termed *LHCGR*) on the surface of Leydig cells, resulting in receptor aggregation and a conformational change that activates G_s protein. G_s protein, in turn, results primarily in cyclic adenosine monophosphate (cAMP)-dependent activation of PKA.[56] Activated PKA increases the production of proteins that regulate steroidogenesis and testosterone biosynthesis (Fig. 19-8). The main proteins regulated by LH-stimulated PKA are as follows:

1. *Steroidogenic acute regulatory protein (StAR)*, a transport protein that regulates transfer of cholesterol from the outer to the inner mitochondrial membrane—the rate-limiting step for steroid production
2. *Cytochrome P450 isoenzyme 11a1 (CYP11A1)*, also called cholesterol side-chain cleavage enzyme, within the inner mitochondrial membrane, which catalyzes the conversion of cholesterol delivered by StAR protein to pregnenolone—the first and rate-limiting enzymatic step in steroidogenesis

3. *CYP17A1*, also called 17α-hydroxylase, which catalyzes the conversion of pregnenolone to 17α-hydroxypregnenolone—the second enzymatic step in testosterone biosynthesis[57]

In humans, cholesterol is synthesized within Leydig cells from acetate by *3-hydroxy-3-methylglutaryl-coenzyme A (HMG-CoA) reductase*, or it is derived from circulating low-density lipoprotein (LDL) cholesterol.

Clinically, rare inactivating mutations of the LHCGR cause Leydig hypoplasia, resulting in impaired male genital development and *46,XY disorder of sex development* (DSD, previously known as male pseudohermaphroditism; see Chapter 23) resulting from insufficient testosterone production during fetal development.[58] Rare LHβ mutations cause failure of normal male pubertal development with normal genital development at birth, evidence that normal endogenous LH secretion is not required for male sexual differentiation during fetal development and that hCG stimulation of testosterone production by fetal Leydig cells is the main driver.[59] Activating mutations of the LHCGR have been found in boys with familial precocious puberty *(testotoxicosis)*.[60] Inhibitors of HMG-CoA reductase (statins) used to treat hypercholesterolemia do not affect serum testosterone levels.

Leydig Cell Production of Testosterone and Insulin-like Factor 3

In the human testis, LH-stimulated transport of cholesterol into the inner mitochondrial membrane is followed by conversion of cholesterol to pregnenolone by CYP11A1 and conversion of pregnenolone to 17α-hydroxypregnenolone by CYP17A1. Testosterone biosynthesis then proceeds via a series of further enzymatic steps initially within the Δ^5 steroid biosynthesis pathway (see Fig. 19-8).[57,61]

CYP17A1 also has *17,20-lyase (desmolase)* activity and catalyzes the further conversion of 17α-hydroxypregnenolone to dehydroepiandrosterone (DHEA). DHEA then is converted to Δ^5-androstanediol by *17β-hydroxysteroid dehydrogenase 3* (*17β-HSD3* or *HSD17B3*). DHEA and Δ^5-androstanediol are converted to the Δ^4 steroids, Δ^4-androstenedione and testosterone, respectively, by the enzyme, 3 beta-hydroxysteroid dehydrogenase type II *(3β-HSD)/Δ^{5-4} isomerase (HSD3B2)*.

The early steroid precursors, pregnenolone and 17α-hydroxypregnenolone, also may be converted to progesterone and 17α-progesterone, respectively, by HSD3B1 and then proceed down the Δ^4 pathway to testosterone synthesis. However, in the human testis, the Δ^5 pathway is the predominant early steroid biosynthetic pathway for testosterone production. Testosterone may be converted in the testes to the active metabolites, estradiol (E_2) and DHT, by the enzymes *aromatase (CYP19A1)* and *steroid 5α-reductase type 1 (SRD5A1,* the predominant isoform found in the testes), respectively.

Mutations in testosterone biosynthetic enzymes result in abnormalities of sexual differentiation and varying degrees of 46,XY DSD (male pseudohermaphroditism), depending on the severity of androgen deficiency.[62]

Testosterone is the major androgen produced by the testis. In humans, the average secretion rate of testosterone is approximately 7000 μg/day. The testes also secrete significant but quantitatively smaller amounts of 17α-progesterone, pregnenolone, Δ^4-androstenedione, and progesterone. Very little estradiol (about 10 μg/day) or DHT (about 69 μg/day) is secreted by the testes (Fig. 19-9).[9,63]

In response to pulsatile LH stimulation, testosterone is secreted episodically into the spermatic vein and then into the general circulation. However, testosterone pulses are

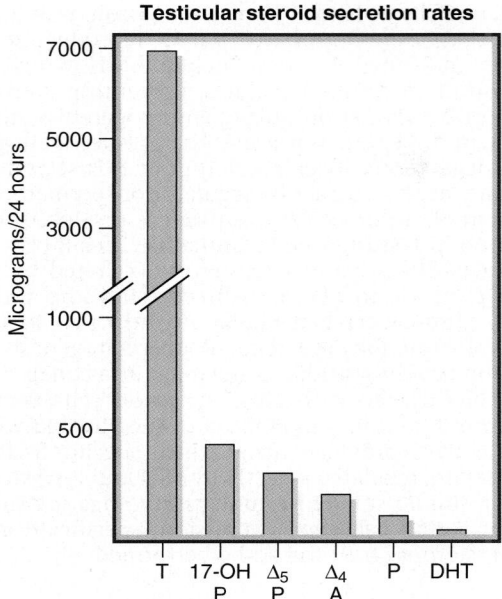

Testicular steroid secretion rates

Figure 19-9 Relative steroid hormone secretion rates from the human testis. Secretion rates were calculated from arteriovenous (AV) differences across the testis of testosterone and other steroids, assuming a testosterone secretion rate of 7000 µg per 24 hours and using the following formula: Secretion rate (SR) = Assumed testosterone SR/testosterone AV difference × AV difference of steroid in question. Testosterone (T) is the main steroid secreted by the testis; much lower amounts of 17-hydroxyprogesterone (17-OHP), pregnenolone (Δ^5P), androstenedione (Δ^4A), progesterone (P), and dihydrotestosterone (DHT) are also secreted. (From Hammond GL, Ruokonen A, Kontturi M, et al. The simultaneous radioimmunoassay of seven steroids in human spermatic and peripheral venous blood. *J Clin Endocrinol Metab.* 1977; 45:16-24.)

less discrete, relatively low in amplitude, and concordant with LH pulses only after a lag time of 80 to 120 minutes, suggesting a relatively sluggish response of Leydig cells to LH stimulation.[45] In addition to this ultradian variation, testosterone levels in young men exhibit a circadian variation characterized by a maximum excursion of 140 ng/dL, with peak testosterone levels occurring at approximately 8 AM and nadir levels at 8 PM.[64] The circadian variation in testosterone levels is blunted but still present in older men, with a maximum excursion of 60 ng/dL. The testosterone response to hCG (LH-like) stimulation is greater in the morning than in the evening, suggesting that diurnal variation in Leydig cell responsiveness may contribute to the circadian variation in testosterone concentrations.[65] Both the ultradian and the circadian variation in testosterone levels contribute to the variability in testosterone measurements within an individual; together with assay variability, this underscores the importance of repeating testosterone measurements during the clinical evaluation of patients with clinical manifestations of male hypogonadism.

INSL3 is a peptide hormone in the relaxin-insulin family that is produced by Leydig cells and secreted into circulation.[66] Serum levels of INSL3 reflect the number and differentiation status of Leydig cells. During puberty, LH induces proliferation and differentiation of Leydig cells and production of INSL3. Serum INSL3 levels increase progressively during puberty, reaching adult levels at about 18 years of age and remaining stable until 35 to 40 years of age, after which they decline steadily with age.

Men with anorchia and bilateral orchidectomy, in whom Leydig cells are absent, and men with chronic gonadotropin suppression induced by GnRH analogues or androgens

have undetectable or very low levels of INSL3. In men with hypogonadotropic hypogonadism, INSL3 levels are undetectable; in these patients, hCG (LH-like) stimulation increases serum testosterone levels within 72 to 96 hours but has no stimulatory effect on INSL3 levels. However, chronic hCG treatment, presumably because of induction of Leydig cell differentiation by longer-term LH-like stimulation, increases both testosterone and INSL3 levels in these men.[67] In men with unilateral orchidectomy, INSL3 levels are intermediate between those in men with bilateral orchidectomy and those in normal men, but testosterone levels are normal, supporting the importance of Leydig cell number for circulating INSL3 concentrations.

Follicle-Stimulating Hormone and Testosterone Regulation of Sertoli Cells

Circulating FSH binds to G protein–coupled FSH receptors on the surface of Sertoli cells, activating G_s protein, which in turn activates cAMP.[68] cAMP then activates PKA and other signal-transduction proteins (e.g., phosphatidylinositol 3-kinase, phospholipase A_2, calcium channel proteins, mitogen-activated protein kinase [MAPK]). Activated PKA activates a number of proteins, including the transcription factor, *cAMP response element–binding protein (CREB)*; these proteins, in turn, regulate gene expression and production of Sertoli cell proteins that play important roles in supporting and regulating spermatogenesis within the seminiferous tubules. In rodents, the expression of FSH receptors in Sertoli cells varies cyclically with the stage of spermatogenesis, being highest in stages XIII through I and lowest in stages VII through VIII.[69] The precise roles of Sertoli cell products in human spermatogenesis are poorly understood and derive from studies using Sertoli cells obtained primarily from immature animals, mostly rodents.

Testosterone produced locally by Leydig cells binds to intracellular ARs in the cytoplasm of Sertoli cells; ligand-bound AR translocates to the nucleus, where it binds to androgen response elements (AREs) and interacts with coregulator proteins to regulate gene expression and production of Sertoli cell proteins that play vital roles in supporting and regulating spermatogenesis. The expression of the AR also varies cyclically with the stage of spermatogenesis, being highest in stage VII, when FSH receptor expression is the lowest.[70]

The major functions of Sertoli cells[71,72] are (1) to maintain seminiferous tubule structure and compartmentalization; (2) to provide nutrients and growth factors to developing germ cells and spermatozoa; (3) to translocate, sculpt, and release developing germ cells; (4) to secrete seminiferous tubule fluid; and (5) to produce reproductive hormones.

Maintenance of Seminiferous Tubule Structure and Compartmentalization. The blood-testis barrier is formed by basal tight junctions between adjacent Sertoli cells; these serve to compartmentalize the seminiferous tubule into basal and adluminal compartments. Compartmentalization provides an environment in which developing germ cells are protected from external insults and the immune system.

Sertoli cells produce a number of junctional complex, structural, and extracellular matrix proteins such as cell adhesion molecules (e.g., claudin 3, which is particularly important for the integrity of Sertoli cell tight junctions), cadherins, laminins, type I and type IV collagen, and proteoglycans including chondroitin and heparin. These proteins are important in maintaining the structural integrity and support for developing germ cells, forming the blood-testis barrier, mediating cell-to-cell interactions, and maintaining polarized secretion of products by Sertoli cells.

Provision of Nutrients and Growth Factors to Developing Germ Cells and Spermatozoa. Although it is protective, the blood-testis barrier also isolates developing germ cells from nutrients, hormones, and growth factors that are present in the systemic circulation. The Sertoli cell has an essential role in producing vital nutrients, cofactors, and proteins that are needed for the normal progression of spermatogenesis and support of spermatozoa being transported within the seminiferous tubule lumen. Sertoli cells produce pyruvate and contain lactate dehydrogenase, which catalyzes the conversion of pyruvate to lactate, the preferred energy substrate of germ cells.

Most of the proteins produced by Sertoli cells are binding or transport proteins for substances (e.g., metals, vitamins, sphingolipids, androgens, hormones, growth factors) that serve as cofactors and regulators of germ cell development within the seminiferous tubule. Binding proteins produced by Sertoli cells include transferrin, an iron-binding protein; ceruloplasmin, a copper-binding protein; glycosphingolipid-binding protein; sulfated glycoprotein 2 (SGP-2), also called clusterin, a lipid-binding protein with other biologic activities; *androgen-binding protein (ABP)*; α_2-macroglobulin, which serves as a binding protein for inhibin and activin; follistatin, a potent binding protein for activin; and insulin-like growth factor–binding proteins (IGFBPs), which bind insulin-like growth factor type 1 (IGF-1).

ABP is a testicular homologue of *sex hormone–binding globulin (SHBG)*, the major circulating ABP, which is synthesized by the liver and encoded by the same gene.[73] Based on studies in rodents, ABP is thought to play a role in regulating local testosterone concentrations in the seminiferous tubule and epididymis. However, one study reported that human SHBG is expressed in germ cells but not in Sertoli cells and that a smaller isoform of SHBG is located between the outer acrosomal membrane and the sperm plasma membrane and is released during capacitation.[74] These findings suggest a potentially different role of SHBG/ABP in humans and rodents and underscore the hazard of extrapolating results from animal studies.

The Sertoli cell also produces a number of growth factors, such as IGF-1, basic fibroblast growth factor, activin A, transforming growth factor-α (TGF-α) and TGF-β, interleukin 1α (IL-1α) and IL-6, stem cell factor (SCF, the KIT ligand), glial cell–derived neurotrophic factor (GDNF), and polyamines (putrescine, spermine, and spermidine), that act both as paracrine regulators of stem cell renewal, germ cell development, and Leydig cell and peritubular myoid cell function and as autocrine regulators.

Translocation, Sculpting, and Release of Developing Germ Cells. Sertoli cells actively move developing germ cells from the basal compartment through the adluminal compartment and release spermatozoa from the seminiferous epithelium into the lumen (spermiation). During translocation, Sertoli cells remove degenerating germ cells, residual cytoplasm from late elongated spermatids (residual body), and seminiferous tubule fluid and contents by phagocytosis and pinocytosis. The Sertoli cell produces proteases and protease inhibitors (e.g., testibumin or SGP-1, tissue plasminogen activators, type IV collagenase, cystatin, α_2-macroglobulin) that are involved in germ cell translocation, removal of degenerating germ cells, and spermiation.

Secretion of Seminiferous Tubule Fluid. Seminiferous tubule fluid serves important roles in the delivery of nutrients to developing germs cells within the seminiferous epithelium, transportation of regulatory factors and nutrients within the seminiferous tubule lumen, and transportation of spermatozoa released into the seminiferous tubule lumen to the rete testis, efferent ducts, and epididymis.

Production of Reproductive Hormones. Sertoli cells produce hormones that are important in male reproductive differentiation and function. These include AMH, which causes regression of the müllerian ducts, preventing uterine and fallopian tube formation during embryogenesis; inhibin B and activin A, peptide hormones that, respectively, participate in negative feedback regulation of FSH secretion and potentially act as a paracrine regulator of spermatogenesis; and estradiol, a potent estrogen that is produced via aromatization of testosterone in immature Sertoli cells.

FSH acts directly and testosterone (secreted by Leydig cells in response to LH) acts directly and also indirectly (e.g., by stimulating peritubular myoid cells) to control Sertoli cell function and regulate spermatogenesis. Gene expression profiling studies using microarray analysis in rat Sertoli cells treated with FSH, in Sertoli cell–specific AR mutant mice, and in GnRH mutant mice treated with testosterone have provided insight into specific Sertoli cell genes that are regulated directly by FSH and testosterone.[75] However, similar studies in humans investigating the regulation of Sertoli cell gene expression, specifically by FSH and testosterone, have yet to be performed.

Paracrine and Autocrine Regulation of Testis Function

As described earlier, gonadotropins, LH, and FSH secreted by the pituitary are the major endocrine regulators, and testosterone produced by Leydig cells in response to LH stimulation is the main paracrine regulator, of testicular function. However, there is evidence, mostly from studies in experimental animals and in vitro studies using isolated testis cell types from animals, that Leydig, Sertoli, and peritubular myoid cells and macrophages in the testis secrete other paracrine and autocrine factors that may be important modulators of testosterone and sperm production.

One of the most important examples of paracrine regulation within the testis is the effect of testosterone, produced locally by Leydig cells, on Sertoli cell function and spermatogenesis. There is evidence that testosterone has both a direct effect on Sertoli cell function and spermatogenesis and an indirect effect (acting through androgen action) on peritubular myoid cells. In GnRH- and gonadotropin-deficient *hpg* mice in which the AR has been knocked out specifically in Sertoli cells, DHT treatment is not able to stimulate spermatogenesis, suggesting that direct androgen action on Sertoli cells is needed to stimulate spermatogenesis.[76] Animals with a peritubular myoid cell–specific AR knockout demonstrate impaired Sertoli function (i.e., reduced seminiferous tubule fluid and Sertoli cell androgen-dependent gene expression), azoospermia, and infertility not explained by alterations in testosterone, LH, and FSH levels.[77] These findings suggest that the paracrine effect of Leydig cell–produced testosterone on Sertoli cell function and regulation of spermatogenesis is mediated in part by androgen-driven interactions between peritubular myoid cells and Sertoli cells. Whether these stromal-epithelial cell interactions occur in humans is not known. At present, the roles of paracrine and autocrine factors other than testosterone in the regulation of human testis function are not clear.

Hormonal Control of Spermatogenesis

FSH and LH are the main hormonal regulators of spermatogenesis in humans. The effect of FSH on spermatogenesis is mediated by a direct endocrine action on Sertoli cells, whereas that of LH is mediated by an action on Leydig cells to produce testosterone, which in turn acts locally within the testes in a paracrine manner, with direct effects on Sertoli cells and possibly indirect effects through peritubular myoid cell regulation of Sertoli cells. The gonadotropin requirements necessary for the initiation of spermatogenesis at the time of puberty differ from those needed for the maintenance of sperm production, once initiated, in adults.[10,78]

Initiation of Spermatogenesis. Usually, both FSH and LH are required to initiate spermatogenesis at the time of puberty. In men with prepubertal gonadotropin deficiency (e.g., IHH), treatment with LH (hCG) is needed to stimulate intratesticular testosterone production sufficient to support spermatogenesis and seminal fluid production by accessory sex glands (seminal vesicles and prostate gland). However, most such patients also require FSH treatment to initiate and complete the first wave of spermatogenesis and to produce sperm in the ejaculate.[79] In some men with incomplete gonadotropin deficiency (usually with evidence of endogenous FSH secretion, such as larger testis volume), LH treatment alone is sufficient to initiate and complete spermatogenesis. FSH treatment without LH (hCG) does not stimulate sperm production in men with prepubertal gonadotropin deficiency.

Natural inactivating mutations of gonadotropin β-subunits and receptors provide some insight into the roles of LH and FSH in initiating spermatogenesis. Men with inactivating mutations of LHβ usually have a lack of pubertal development and arrested spermatogenesis or azoospermia and infertility.[59] Recently, however, a man with an LHβ mutation resulting in a partially active LH molecule (as evidenced by expression of steroidogenic enzymes in a few mature Leydig cells and low intratesticular testosterone concentrations) was reported to have complete and quantitatively normal spermatogenesis.[80] This finding suggests that complete spermatogenesis may be initiated by low concentrations of LH and intratesticular testosterone in the presence of high serum FSH levels, as were present in this case.

Men with inactivating LH receptor mutations present with varying degrees of impaired sexual differentiation or 46,XY DSD (male pseudohermaphroditism), ranging from ambiguous genitalia to perineoscrotal hypospadias, and azoospermia, although defects in sperm production are confounded by the presence of cryptorchidism in many of these men.[58] Recently, a man with a partially inactivating mutation of the LH receptor was reported to have micropenis, delayed puberty, low serum testosterone concentrations, and normal FSH levels but bilaterally normal-sized, descended testes and normal sperm production, albeit with low sperm concentration (oligozoospermia).[81] This finding suggests that spermatogenesis may be initiated by very low LH activity and intratesticular testosterone in the presence of normal FSH levels.

Men with inactivating mutations of FSHβ have been found generally to have azoospermia with low or low-normal testosterone and high LH levels.[82-85] In contrast, men with inactivating FSH receptor mutations have been reported to have moderate to severely reduced sperm counts (but not azoospermia) with normal testosterone and normal to high LH levels.[58,86] The reason for the apparent discrepancy in degree of spermatogenic impairment exhibited by men with FSHβ versus FSH receptor mutations is not clear. It is possible that residual receptor function in men with FSH receptor mutations results in persistent small amounts of FSH activity or that men with FSHβ mutations have greater Leydig cell dysfunction, as evidenced by lower serum concentrations of LH and intratesticular testosterone that result in greater impairment of spermatogenesis.

In summary, findings from the small number of reports of men with inactivating mutations of gonadotropin β-subunits and receptors suggest that initiation of the first wave of spermatogenesis may require only very low levels or activity of either LH (intratesticular testosterone) or FSH in the presence of adequate amounts of the other gonadotropin. Clinically, however, most men with prepubertal gonadotropin deficiency require treatment with both LH and FSH to initiate spermatogenesis during puberty. Because FSH stimulates Sertoli cell proliferation and number during testis development, it plays an important role in determining the capacity for quantitatively normal spermatogenesis.

Maintenance of Spermatogenesis. In men with prepubertal gonadotropin deficiency (e.g., IHH), once spermatogenesis has been initiated with LH (hCG) and FSH treatment, sperm production may be maintained with LH treatment alone without continued FSH administration.[79] However, spermatogenesis is not stimulated by administration of FSH in combination with testosterone (to maintain normal levels of serum testosterone but continued low LH and intratesticular testosterone levels) in men with IHH. Spermatogenesis may be reinitiated with LH (hCG) alone in men with IHH after a period of gonadotropin deficiency associated with exogenous testosterone replacement therapy. Furthermore, in men with gonadotropin deficiency and azoospermia acquired as an adult (e.g., secondary to a pituitary adenoma), spermatogenesis may be reinitiated and maintained with LH (hCG) treatment alone.[79]

In normal men with experimental gonadotropin deficiency induced by high-dose testosterone administration, spermatogenesis may be reinitiated and maintained by either LH or hCG alone, despite markedly suppressed FSH levels, or by FSH alone, despite severely suppressed LH (and presumably low intratesticular testosterone) concentrations. However, sperm production was not stimulated by either LH or FSH alone to the baseline levels that existed before experimental gonadotropin suppression.[87] In this model of gonadotropin deficiency, treatment with both LH (hCG) and FSH restored sperm counts fully to baseline values. Finally, in support of the ability of FSH alone to stimulate sperm production, spermatogenesis was maintained despite undetectable serum gonadotropin levels in a hypophysectomized man who had an activating FSH receptor mutation.[88]

Together, these findings suggest that a normal concentration of either FSH or LH is sufficient for maintenance of qualitatively normal sperm production, but both gonadotropins are necessary for quantitatively normal spermatogenesis in male humans.

The effect of gonadotropins on specific stages of spermatogenesis has been studied in normal men with experimental gonadotropin suppression induced by the administration of high-dose progestin and testosterone. In these gonadotropin-deficient men, selective replacement of either FSH or LH (increasing intratesticular testosterone) supported all stages of spermatogenesis, including spermatogonial maturation, meiosis, spermiogenesis, and spermiation, but each agent had predominant actions on specific stages.[89] FSH exerts a relatively greater effect on maturation of spermatogonia (conversion of spermatogonia A_p to spermatogonia B), early meiosis, and maintenance of pachytene spermatocytes (conversion of spermatogonia to pachytene spermatocytes). LH (stimulating intratesticular testosterone) has predominant effects on the completion of meiosis (conversion of pachytene spermatocytes to round spermatids) and on spermiation (release of mature spermatozoa). FSH and LH (intratesticular testosterone) exert similar effects on spermiogenesis (conversion of round to elongated spermatids).

In normal men, LH stimulates intratestosterone concentrations that are approximately 100- to 200-fold higher than serum testosterone levels and correlate with circulating LH levels. Administration of various combinations of exogenous testosterone, progestin, and GnRH antagonist to induce gonadotropin deficiency in male contraception trials suppressed intratesticular testosterone by 98%, to concentrations comparable to those in serum, and reduced sperm production, producing severe oligozoospermia or azoospermia.[90] Short-term administration of hCG (LH-like activity) in normal men with experimental gonadotropin deficiency resulted in a dose-dependent increase in intratesticular testosterone.[91]

Testosterone replacement therapy in gonadotropin-deficient men does not increase intratesticular testosterone sufficiently to support spermatogenesis. In fact, testosterone treatment suppresses endogenous gonadotropin levels and may suppress sperm production. However, this cannot be assumed to occur in all testosterone-treated gonadotropin-deficient men, especially if testosterone replacement is not adequate. In one study involving a small number of men with acquired hypogonadotropic hypogonadism due to hypothalamic-pituitary disease, half had detectable sperm counts ranging from very low (1 million/mL) to normal (120 million/mL) on testosterone replacement therapy, mostly because of incomplete gonadotropin suppression associated with an inadequate testosterone regimen (200 to 250 mg given by intramuscular [IM] injection every 3 to 4 weeks).[92]

Spermatogenesis is maintained with intratesticular testosterone concentrations that are 10% of normal, but the minimum concentration needed to support sperm production is not known. Intratesticular testosterone is converted within the testes to its active metabolites, estradiol and DHT, by CYP19A1 (aromatase) and 5α-reductase (SRD5A1), respectively. As with testosterone, intratesticular concentrations of estradiol are about 100-fold higher than serum estradiol levels; however, intratesticular concentrations of DHT are only approximately 15-fold higher than levels in circulation.[93] The roles of these relatively high concentrations of estradiol and DHT within the testes in the maintenance of spermatogenesis are not clear.

Negative Feedback Regulation of Gonadotropin Secretion

As described earlier, the feed-forward regulation of testicular function involves hypothalamic GnRH stimulation of pituitary gonadotropin secretion, which in turn stimulates the testes to secrete testosterone and increase sperm production (see Fig. 19-6). An important aspect of hypothalamic-pituitary-testicular axis regulation is the negative feedback suppression of hypothalamic GnRH and pituitary gonadotropin secretion by steroid and peptide hormones produced by the testes. Testosterone, produced by Leydig cells of the testis, and estradiol, its active metabolite, act at both the hypothalamus and the pituitary gland to inhibit GnRH and gonadotropin secretion. Inhibin B, produced by Sertoli cells within seminiferous tubules of the testis, acts primarily on the pituitary to suppress FSH secretion.

Recently, in a series of elegant prospective studies, normal men and GnRH-deficient men with IHH treated with physiologic doses of pulsatile GnRH (i.e., a GnRH clamp) underwent medical castration and aromatase inhibition induced by high-dose ketoconazole plus physiologic doses of testosterone or estradiol. The effects of these interventions on production of FSH and LH were measured. These studies have helped to define the relative roles of testosterone and estradiol in regulating gonadotropin

secretion and the sites of negative feedback by these steroids.[94,95] It appears that both testosterone and estradiol derived from aromatization of testosterone exert negative feedback effects at the hypothalamus to suppress pulsatile GnRH secretion. These studies also demonstrated that negative feedback inhibition of pituitary LH and FSH secretion by testosterone requires aromatization of testosterone to estradiol. The suppression of FSH by estradiol is modest when inhibin B levels are normal and testes are normal, suggesting that inhibin B is the main physiologic negative feedback regulator of FSH secretion.[96] When inhibin B levels are low, as in men with seminiferous tubule failure or anorchia, the negative feedback effect of estradiol derived from testosterone assumes a greater role in suppressing FSH.

Although active metabolism of testosterone to estradiol is important in the negative feedback actions of testosterone, conversion of testosterone to DHT by 5α-reductase types 1 and 2 does not play a major role in steroid feedback. Men with mutations in *SRD5A2* exhibit only modest elevations in gonadotropins and increases in LH pulse amplitude but not frequency.[97] Men with benign prostatic hyperplasia (BPH) and normal men treated with finasteride (an SRD5A2 inhibitor) or dutasteride (an SRD5A1 and SRD5A2 inhibitor) do not demonstrate increases in serum LH and FSH levels.[98] These findings suggest a relatively minor role for DHT in physiologic negative feedback regulation of gonadotropins. However, administration of supraphysiologic amounts of DHT does suppress concentrations of LH (by 30% to 60%) and FSH (by 15% to 30%).[99]

The pituitary gonadotrophs contain estrogen receptor α (ERα), but GnRH neurons appear to lack both ERα and AR. The negative feedback actions of testosterone and estradiol are thought to be mediated indirectly by other neuronal systems that relay steroid feedback signals to GnRH neurons. Studies in animals suggest that neurons that produce *kisspeptin*, a 54–amino acid peptide product of the *KISS1* gene, may be candidate mediators of steroid negative feedback.[100,101] These neurons interact directly with GnRH neurons in the medial basal hypothalamus, the majority of which contains the kisspeptin receptor, *KISS1R*, and release kisspeptin, thereby stimulating GnRH secretion. Kisspeptin neurons may also interact with other neurons (e.g., γ-aminobutyric acid [GABA] neurons) to indirectly regulate GnRH secretion. Kisspeptin neurons contain both AR and ERα. In experimental animals, castration increases kisspeptin expression, coinciding with an increase in GnRH and gonadotropin secretion; sex steroid treatment with testosterone, estradiol, or DHT reverses these changes, and kisspeptin antagonists block the postcastration increase in LH secretion. In humans, mutations in *KISS1* or *KISS1R* cause hypogonadotropic hypogonadism and impaired pubertal development,[102] and there is accumulating evidence in animals that kisspeptin may have an important role in the initiation of puberty.

Inhibins are heterodimeric glycoproteins belonging to the TGF-β superfamily of proteins, which includes activins, inhibins, TGF-β, bone morphogenetic proteins (BMPs), and growth and differentiation factors (GDFs) such as AMH and myostatin.[103] Inhibins are composed of an α-subunit connected by a disulfide bridge to either a β$_A$ or a β$_B$ subunit to form inhibin A or inhibin B, respectively. *Inhibin B* (α-β$_B$ heterodimer) is the physiologically relevant inhibin species in humans. Unlike most proteins in the TGF-β family, which act as local paracrine or autocrine regulators of diverse cellular functions, inhibin B acts as a circulating hormone. Inhibin B is produced by the Sertoli cell in response to FSH stimulation. It binds to a coreceptor composed of the type III TGF-β receptor (TGFBR3 or betaglycan) and the type IIB activin receptor (ACVR2B) and is thought to be the main endocrine negative feedback suppressor of FSH secretion by pituitary gonadotrophs.

In humans, inhibin B levels rise progressively at the time of puberty, correlating with FSH levels and FSH-stimulated Sertoli cell proliferation.[103] Adult levels are reached by mid-puberty. At that time, Sertoli cell function becomes intimately linked to the onset of spermatogenesis, and inhibin B levels assume an inverse relationship with FSH levels as the inhibin B–mediated negative feedback regulation becomes activated. For example, in boys with Sertoli cell–only syndrome, inhibin B levels are normal before puberty as a function of Sertoli cell proliferation but become undetectable at the time of puberty, reflecting the absence of germ cells and Sertoli cell dysfunction. In adults, inhibin B levels are inversely related to the degree of germ cell damage or loss and Sertoli cell dysfunction. This relationship suggests that germ cells regulate Sertoli cell function, although the precise cellular and molecular mechanisms underlying this regulation are not clear. Inhibin B levels have been used as biomarkers of spermatogenesis and Sertoli cell function in research and by some practitioners, but they have not yet been used in routine clinical practice.

Activins include homodimers consisting of two β_A subunits (activin A) or two β_B subunits (activin B) and a heterodimer of one β_A and one β_B subunit (activin AB).[103,104] Activins are produced by gonadotrophs and bind to ACVR2B receptors. They act primarily as autocrine regulators to stimulate FSHβ synthesis and sensitize gonadotrophs to GnRH stimulation, resulting in increased FSH secretion. Inhibin B acts as a selective antagonist of activins in gonadotrophs by binding to ACVR2B receptors. *Follistatins* are glycoproteins produced by gonadotrophs and by folliculostellate cells of the pituitary gland that bind and antagonize the actions of activin. They act as autocrine and paracrine regulators of FSH secretion. Activins and follistatins are also produced in Sertoli cells and germ cells and may act as autocrine and paracrine regulators of testis function.

Negative feedback suppression of gonadotropin production, by pharmacologic doses of androgens or combinations of androgens and progestins or by GnRH antagonists, that is sufficient to result in suppression of sperm production has been the basis for male hormonal contraceptive development strategies.[105]

Testosterone Transport, Metabolism, and Actions

Circulating Testosterone

Like other steroid and thyroid hormones, testosterone secreted into the circulation by Leydig cells is mostly bound to plasma proteins, primarily to SHBG and albumin. In the circulation, *total testosterone* is composed of 0.5% to 3.0% *free testosterone* unbound to plasma proteins, 30% to 44% SHBG-bound testosterone, and 54% to 68% albumin-bound testosterone (Fig. 19-10).[106,107]

Clinically, biologic actions of testosterone, like those of other steroid hormones, are thought to conform to the free hormone hypothesis; that is, the biologic activity of testosterone is mediated only by its free (unbound) concentration or the concentration that is easily dissociable from plasma proteins in circulation.[107,108] Testosterone is tightly bound to SHBG with such high affinity (1.6×10^{-9} mol/L) that it is not easily dissociable and available to target tissues for biologic action. In contrast, testosterone is loosely bound to albumin, with a binding affinity (1.0×10^{-4} mol/L) that is several orders of magnitude less than that of SHBG

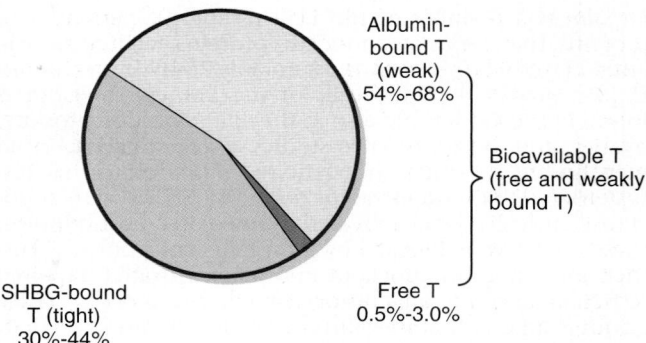

Figure 19-10 Fractions of circulating testosterone in blood. The majority of circulating testosterone (T) is bound to serum proteins: approximately 54% is weakly bound to albumin, and 44% is tightly bound to sex hormone–binding protein (SHBG). Only about 2% of circulating T is free of protein binding. The combination of free and weakly bound (albumin-bound) T is referred to as bioavailable testosterone.

binding. Therefore, albumin-bound testosterone is dissociable and available to target tissues for action. Together, free testosterone and albumin-bound testosterone are referred to as *bioavailable testosterone*, because these fractions are available to diffuse into target tissues, bind AR, and affect gene transcription, resulting in androgen action in those tissues. Recently, the case of a man was reported who had undetectable SHBG and low total testosterone levels due to a missense mutation of the *SHBG* gene that blocked its secretion.[109] Despite symptoms of sexual dysfunction, fatigue, weakness, and depressed mood, his free testosterone and gonadotropin levels and semen analysis were normal and he had normal objective evidence of sexual development. These findings provide support for the free hormone hypothesis.

SHBG, which is synthesized by hepatocytes of the liver, is a homodimeric β-globulin protein composed of a heavy and a light subunit that are identical in peptide sequence and encoded by a single gene but differ in their degree of glycosylation.[73] The *SHBG* gene is also expressed in the testes, and in most mammals, Sertoli cells produce a homologue of SHBG (ABP) under the control of FSH. In the human testis, however, *SHBG* appears to be expressed in germ cells rather than Sertoli cells and to produce a truncated form of SHBG that localizes to the acrosome of spermatozoa.[74] SHBG is a homodimer composed of two identical molecules, and each monomer has two competitive binding sites per molecule; these sites bind DHT and testosterone with high affinity and estradiol less avidly. Previous studies have assumed identical binding affinities of SHBG monomers for testosterone and other ligands. Recent studies suggest that binding of testosterone to one monomer of the SHBG dimer affects the binding affinity of testosterone to the second monomer and that binding can only be characterized by a complex dynamic, multistage, allosteric model.[110] Glycosylation of SHBG is not involved in steroid binding but may prolong the plasma half-life of the protein in circulation. SHBG production by the liver is increased under the influence of estrogens and thyroid and decreased by androgens and insulin.

Counter to the free hormone hypothesis, there is evidence that testosterone bound to SHBG may affect androgen action in some target tissues. In some tissues such as the human prostate, SHBG may bind to a cell surface receptor; testosterone then binds to the SHBG-receptor complex, activating cAMP and affecting target organ function.[111] Glycosylation of SHBG may be important for the interaction of steroid-SHBG complexes with plasma membranes.

Megalin is a member of the LDL receptor superfamily of proteins that serve as endocytic proteins facilitating the entry of steroids into cells (most notably 25-hydroxyvitamin D into proximal tubule cells of the kidney). Megalin is found in the kidney and also in the epididymides, prostate, ovaries, and uterus. In vitro studies in cells that expressed megalin but no other endocytic receptors found that testosterone, DHT, and estradiol bound to SHBG were endocytosed into cells and activated AR-mediated transcription; these effects were blocked by a megalin antagonist.[112] Furthermore, megalin knockout mice demonstrated impaired testicular descent, an androgen-mediated process. These findings suggest that megalin may be important in mediating cellular uptake of androgens into some tissues. However, the importance of testosterone bound to SHBG or endocytic proteins such as megalin in human physiology remains to be determined.

In normal men with an intact hypothalamic-pituitary-testicular axis, alterations in SHBG concentrations and testosterone bound to SHBG do not have an effect on the physiology and action of androgens at steady state. Any acute effects on free testosterone concentration caused by changes in SHBG would alter the negative feedback regulation of gonadotropins, resulting in normalization of free testosterone levels. For example, an acute increase in SHBG levels may transiently decrease free testosterone levels, but the consequent decrease in testosterone negative feedback increases pituitary LH secretion, which increases testosterone production by the testes to restore normal free testosterone levels. In contrast, alterations in SHBG levels may alter free testosterone levels in men with reproductive disorders who have impaired negative feedback regulation or are receiving testosterone replacement therapy.

SHBG concentrations may be decreased or increased in a variety of commonly encountered clinical conditions.[113] Clinically, alterations in SBHG are extremely important to consider in the diagnosis of male hypogonadism (see later discussion). Because serum total testosterone measurements are affected by changes in SHBG levels, accurate measurements of free or bioavailable testosterone are needed to assess the adequacy of Leydig cell function, to determine whether a patient is hypogonadal, and to monitor testosterone replacement in patients with alterations in circulating SHBG concentrations.

Active Metabolism and Catabolism of Testosterone

An important aspect of the effects of testosterone action on target tissues is its active metabolism to *17β-estradiol* (estradiol) by CYP19A1 and to *DHT* by SRD5A1 and SRD5A2; these are the most potent of the endogenous estrogens and androgens (Fig. 19-11).[9] Many of the biologic actions of testosterone are mediated by these active metabolites, acting through mechanisms that are dependent on ERα and ERβ (estradiol) or on AR (DHT). These active metabolites are formed and act locally as paracrine or autocrine regulators, and they also are secreted and act as endocrine regulators of target tissue function.

Aromatization of Testosterone to Estradiol. Aromatase catalyzes the conversion of testosterone to estradiol as well as the conversion of the weaker androgen, Δ⁴-androstenedione, to the weaker estrogen, estrone. These conversions occur predominantly in adipose tissue but also in other tissues, including brain, bone, breast, liver, blood vessels, and testes (Sertoli cells and Leydig cells). Approximately 40 to 50 μg of estradiol is produced daily, primarily by extratesticular aromatization of testosterone to estradiol and of Δ⁴-androstenedione to estrone (which is then converted to estradiol by various isoforms of the enzyme, 17β-HSD).

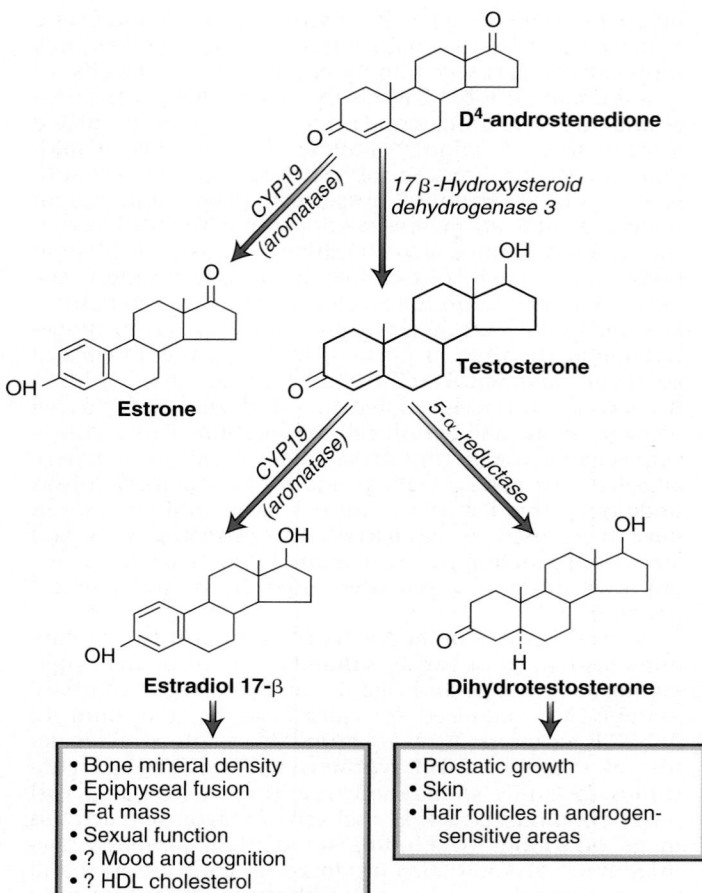

Figure 19-11 Active metabolism of testosterone. Testosterone may be converted to the potent estrogen, 17β-estradiol, by the enzyme aromatase (CYP19) or to the more potent androgen, dihydrotestosterone (DHT), by the enzyme 5α-reductase. The effects of testosterone on prostatic growth, skin, and hair follicles in androgen-sensitive areas require 5α-reduction of testosterone to DHT. The effects of testosterone that require aromatization to estradiol are prevention of bone resorption, increase in bone mineral density, epiphyseal fusion, decrease in fat mass, sexual differentiation of the brain, sexual function, and possibly some aspects of cognitive function, mood, and plasma lipids (high-density lipoprotein [HDL] cholesterol). (Modified from Bhasin S. Testicular disorders. In: Kronenberg HM, Melmed S, Polonsky KS, et al, eds. *Williams Textbook of Endocrinology*, 11th ed. Philadelphia, PA: Elsevier; 2008:645-698.)

Approximately 15% to 25% of circulating estradiol is produced by the testes, primarily by Leydig cells.[114]

Aromatization of testosterone to estradiol mediates the effects of testosterone on epiphyseal closure at the time of puberty, inhibition of bone resorption and maintenance of bone mineral density (BMD), regulation of fat mass accumulation, negative feedback suppression of hypothalamic GnRH secretion and pituitary gonadotropin secretion, sexual function, and possibly regulation of high-density lipoprotein (HDL) cholesterol levels and some aspects of cognitive function and mood.[115,116] Recently, healthy young to middle-aged men with experimental hypogonadism induced by a GnRH agonist were treated with placebo or various dosages of testosterone with or without coadministration of an aromatase inhibitor in order to investigate the relative effects of experimental androgen and estrogen deficiency, respectively.[117] Decreases in lean body mass, muscle size, and strength were induced by androgen deficiency; fat mass accumulation was induced by estrogen deficiency; decline in sexual function was induced by both androgen and estrogen deficiency.

In men, circulating estradiol is regulated primarily by the amount of androgen substrates, testosterone and Δ^4-androstenedione, and by aromatase activity in adipose tissue and other peripheral tissues. Aromatase activity in Leydig cells is controlled primarily by LH. Stimulation of aromatase activity in gonadotropin-deficient men treated with hCG may result in relatively higher concentrations of serum estradiol compared with testosterone and may contribute to benign breast tenderness and enlargement (gynecomastia) during treatment. As in women, men with ER-positive breast cancer may be treated with aromatase inhibitors to reduce estrogen synthesis.

The few men reported with inactivating mutations of the aromatase gene *(CYP19A1)* have demonstrated tall stature, persistent linear growth after puberty, eunuchoidal body proportion, delayed bone age, osteopenia or osteoporosis and progressive *genu valgum*, and variable impairments in glucose and lipid metabolism, including insulin resistance, elevated triglyceride and low HDL-cholesterol levels, abnormal liver enzymes and fatty liver, variable low sperm counts and infertility, and undetectable estradiol levels with normal to elevated serum testosterone and gonadotropin levels.[118] Furthermore, estradiol treatment results in closure of the epiphyses, increased BMD, and increased bone age. Men with a rare inactivating mutation of ERα had a similar phenotype, but in contrast to men with aromatase deficiency, they had high serum estradiol, testosterone, and gonadotropin concentrations, consistent with estrogen resistance.[115] These findings support potentially important roles of estradiol in bone, glucose, and lipid metabolism; liver function; and pituitary and testis function.

5α-Reduction of Testosterone to Dihydrotestosterone. Testosterone is converted to DHT, an androgen that is 2.5 to 3 times more potent than testosterone, by SRD5A1 and SRD5A2. These two isoenzymes of 5α-reductase differ in the optimal pH for their activity and in their expression patterns.[119] SRD5A2 is expressed most highly in prostate, epididymis, seminal vesicles, genital skin, and liver and at lower levels in other tissues such as certain brain regions, nongenital skin, testis, and kidney. SRD5A1 is expressed most highly in nongenital skin (hair follicles), liver, and certain brain regions and at lower levels in prostate, epididymis, seminal vesicles, genital skin, testis, adrenal, and kidney. Approximately 200 to 300 µg of DHT is produced daily, mostly from 5α-reduction of testosterone in peripheral tissues (predominantly skin and liver). The prostate and testis contribute relatively little to concentrations of DHT in blood.

Men with inactivating mutations of *SRD5A2* are born with severe 46,XY DSD (male pseudohermaphroditism) with ambiguous genitalia (clitoris-like phallus, bifid scrotum, pseudovaginal hypospadias, and rudimentary prostate gland) but normal wolffian duct differentiation (normal seminal vesicles, epididymides, and vas deferens) and no müllerian duct structures, supporting the vital role of DHT in external genital differentiation and prostate development.[120] Individuals with SRD5A2 deficiency are usually raised as girls. With the onset of puberty and increase in testosterone to adult male levels, the phallus grows, the scrotum develops, libido and erections are stimulated, and the gender role may change from female to male. Cryptorchidism is common but not invariable and is associated with oligozoospermia or azoospermia. Testes may descend at the time of puberty. Normal sperm counts may occur in individuals with descended testes, and fertility has been reported in men with SRD5A2 deficiency.

However, in adults, the prostate remains underdeveloped and is not palpable, facial and body hair are diminished, sebum is not produced, and male-pattern baldness does not occur, supporting the importance of normal SRD5A2 activity and DHT for hair growth, sebaceous function, and prostate development. Serum DHT concentrations are low, testosterone levels are normal to slightly elevated, and gonadotropin concentrations are normal to modestly elevated.

Within the prostate gland, conversion of testosterone to DHT produces concentrations of DHT that are approximately 10-fold higher than those in serum, serving to amplify androgen activity in the prostate. Intraprostatic androgen concentrations may contribute to prostate disease, such as BPH or prostate cancer.[121]

Inhibitors of SRD5A2 (finasteride) or of both SRD5A1 and SRD5A2 (dutasteride) are used to treat lower urinary tract symptoms, improve urinary flow, and prevent complications related to BPH, as well as to treat male-pattern baldness and androgenic alopecia.[122] Treatment with finasteride or dutasteride reduces, respectively, the prevalence or the incidence of prostate cancer found on biopsy but is possibly associated with a greater number of cancers with high Gleason grade.[123,124] An important aspect of the effect of androgens on the prostate is that intraprostatic androgen concentrations are not reflected in serum levels, underscoring the importance of local paracrine and autocrine actions of androgens in the physiology and pathology of the prostate and probably other androgen target tissues.

Catabolism of Testosterone. The primary site of catabolism of circulating testosterone and 5α-DHT is the liver.[125] Testosterone and 5α-DHT are taken up in the liver, and testosterone is converted to an inactive metabolite, 5β-DHT, by the enzyme 5β-reductase. Both 5α- and 5β-DHT then undergo 3α-reduction by the enzyme 3α-HSD to form 3α,5α-androstanediol (also called 3α-diol) and 3α,5β-androstanediol, respectively; this is followed by 17β-reduction by the enzyme 17β-HSD to form androsterone and etiocholanolone as catabolic products. In peripheral tissues such as skin, 5α-DHT may also be converted to 3α-diol, which is further metabolized in the liver.

In the liver, testosterone, DHT, 3α-androstanediols, androsterone, and etiocholanolone undergo glucuronidation and, to a lesser degree, sulfation to form more hydrophilic conjugates that are released into circulation and excreted in urine and bile. Metabolic inactivation of testosterone primarily involves its conversion to metabolites such as testosterone (about 50%), androsterone (20%), and etiolocholanolone (20%) glucuronides (as well as sulfates) and lesser conversion to 3α-diol glucuronides (3α-diol Gs). Because 3α-diol comes mostly from skin, blood and urine measurements of 3α-diol G have been used as a marker of peripheral androgen action.[125] In men with 5α-reductase deficiency, 3α-diol G concentrations are reduced. The amount of body hair and acne correlates with 3α-diol G levels.

Epitestosterone (17α-hydroxy-4-androsten-3-one) is a biologically inactive 17α-hydroxy epimer of testosterone (17β-hydroxy-4-androsten-3-one) that is produced by the testes in response to LH.[126] The production rate of epitestosterone is about 3% that of testosterone, but its clearance rate is 33% that of testosterone, and there is no interconversion of epitestosterone and testosterone. Similar to testosterone, epitestosterone is conjugated in the liver, primarily to glucuronides and sulfates, and excreted in the urine. Because epitestosterone conjugates are rapidly cleared in the urine, excretion rates of testosterone and epitestosterone are similar, and the ratio of urinary testosterone to epitestosterone (T/E ratio) is approximately 1:1.

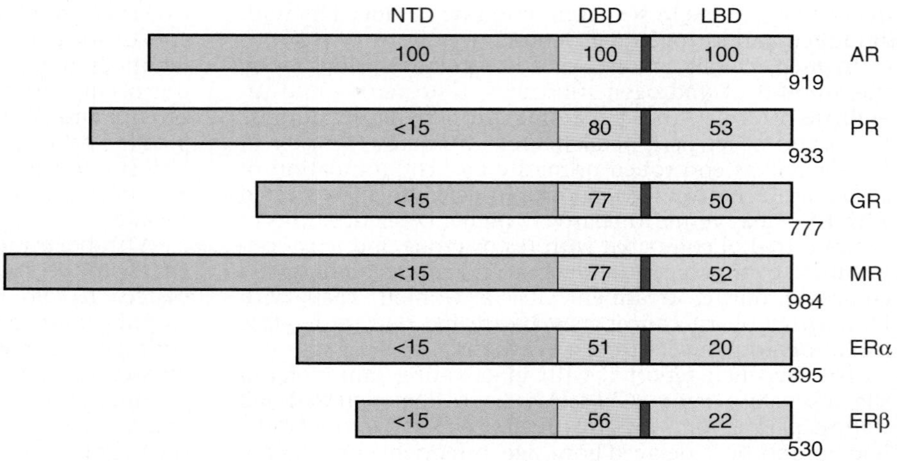

Figure 19-12 Schematic diagram of the structure of the human androgen receptor (AR) gene and homology to other steroid hormone receptors: progesterone receptor (PR), glucocorticoid receptor (GR), mineralocorticoid receptor (MR), estrogen receptor-α (ERα), and estrogen receptor-β (ERβ). The AR is a 919–amino acid protein that is composed of three functional domains: a ligand-binding domain (LBD), a DNA-binding domain (DBD), and an N-terminal transactivation domain (NTD). The DBD shares the greatest degree of homology (>51% versus AR) and the NTD the least degree of homology (<15% versus AR) among steroid hormone receptors. (From Li J, Al-Azzawi F. Mechanism of androgen receptor action. *Maturitas.* 2009;63:142-148.)

Measurements of the T/E ratio and other metabolites in urine by sensitive gas chromatography/mass spectrometry methods are used to detect androgenic anabolic steroid doping, in particular testosterone, by competitive athletes.[126] Administration of androgenic anabolic steroids suppresses the production and clearance of epitestosterone relative to testosterone, resulting in an elevated T/E ratio in urine. The World and United States Anti-Doping Agencies have set a threshold T/E ratio of greater than 4:1 as suspicious for anabolic steroid doping.

Testosterone is glucuronidated primarily by the enzyme uridine diphosphate glucuronyl transferase 2B17 (UGT2B17), whereas epitestosterone is glucuronidated mostly by another UGT isoform, UGT2B7. Although testosterone may be glucuronidated by other UGT isoforms (e.g., UGT2B15), individuals with an inactivating genetic polymorphism of UGT2B17 (common in Asian populations) have reduced testosterone glucuronidation and clearance, resulting in lower T/E ratios that do not reach threshold levels with androgen administration.[125-128] Realization that there were populations with naturally low T/E led to a reduction in the T/E ratio cutoff from the previous threshold for suspicion of doping of (>6:1) to the present one (>4:1). Also, there are individuals with a naturally high T/E ratios, perhaps because of other genetic polymorphisms or environmental factors such as excessive alcohol consumption that may increase T/E ratio transiently, particularly in women.[129] In the absence of environmental perturbations, the T/E ratio in a single individual is remarkably stable over time, and longitudinal measurements of urinary T/E ratio are used to detect illicit androgen use (known as the athlete biologic passport). Coadministration of epitestosterone with testosterone has been used by athletes to avoid detection.

If a urinary T/E ratio is suspicious for doping, exogenous androgen use is confirmed by gas chromatography combustion isotope ratio mass spectrometry (GC/C/IRMS), which can detect small differences in the ratio of carbon-13 to carbon-12 ($^{13}C/^{12}C$) isotopes of testosterone or its metabolites.[126] Because synthetic androgens are synthesized from plant sources (yams or soy), their $^{13}C/^{12}C$ ratio is lower than that of endogenously produced testosterone and other steroids that reflect an animal source or dietary ingestion of both animal and plant products. However, $^{13}C/^{12}C$ IRMS will not detect doping by administration of hCG or LH-like activity to stimulate endogenous testosterone production or administration of androgens derived from animal sources that have a $^{13}C/^{12}C$ ratio similar to that of endogenous testosterone.

Mechanisms of Androgen Action

In androgen target tissues, testosterone and DHT in circulation diffuse through the plasma membrane and bind to intracellular ARs.[130] Binding of androgen to the AR induces a conformational change in the AR that causes dissociation of heat shock proteins bound to AR, permitting translocation into the nucleus, induction of phosphorylation and homodimerization, and interaction with DNA, specifically on AREs located in regulatory sites of target genes. The AR dimer actively recruits tissue-specific coregulators (coactivators and corepressors) to form the transcriptional apparatus necessary to control androgen-regulated gene transcription and subsequent protein synthesis.

The *AR* gene is located on the long arm of the X chromosome (Xq11-12). *AR* is organized into functional domains (Fig. 19-12)[130]: (1) an *N-terminal domain* (NTD) comprising two transactivation domains (AF1 and AF5) that mediate the majority of *AR* transcriptional activity and coregulator interaction and two trinucleotide repeat segments (CAG and GGN, encoding polyglutamine and polyglycine tracts, respectively) of varying number that modify *AR* transactivation; (2) a *DNA-binding domain* (DBD) comprising two finger motifs, the first mediating DNA recognition and binding and the second stabilizing DNA interaction and mediating dimerization of *AR*; (3) a small *hinge region* (H); and (4) a *ligand-binding domain* (LBD) that mediates high-affinity binding of androgen to the AR and also contains another transactivation domain (AF2).

AR is a member of the nuclear receptor superfamily that includes other steroid hormone receptors. It shares approximately 80% sequence homology in the DBD, and 50% in the LBD, with its most closely related steroid receptors, the progesterone receptor (PR), the glucocorticoid receptor (GR), and the mineralocorticoid receptor (MR).[130] This may explain why, for example, some progestins (e.g., medroxyprogesterone acetate) have AR agonist activity, others (e.g., cyproterone acetate) have AR antagonist activity, and a mineralocorticoid antagonist, spironolactone, has AR antagonist activity. Compared with the binding of testosterone, DHT binds to AR with higher affinity, greater stability, and a slower rate of dissociation, conferring greater androgen activity to DHT, the most potent endogenous androgen in humans.

Inactivating mutations of the *AR* may cause qualitative or quantitative abnormalities of receptor function, resulting in variably impaired androgen action.[131] *AR* mutations manifest phenotypic variability, ranging from that of a male who is phenotypically female with normal female external genitalia and breast development *(complete testicular feminization)*, which occurs in individuals with complete androgen insensitivity or resistance, to that of an otherwise normal male with incomplete hypospadias, mild undervirilization, or infertility.

In a normal population, the number of trinucleotide CAG repeats in the first exon of the *AR* gene varies from 11 to 35. In general, the number of CAG repeats appears to correlate inversely with AR function and action, both in vitro and in vivo, in transgenic mice and humans. *Kennedy disease*, or *X-linked spinal and bulbar muscular atrophy (SBMA)*, is a rare adult-onset neurodegenerative disease of motor neurons that results in progressive muscle weakness; it is associated with a markedly expanded number of CAG repeats, varying from 40 to 62, which does not overlap with the normal population.[132] Neurodegeneration in this disorder is thought to be caused by toxicity from intracellular aggregation of the AR and associated cofactors that is worsened by androgen binding to the mutant AR and translocation into the nucleus.

Most men with Kennedy disease also manifest clinical findings of partial androgen resistance, including gynecomastia, reduced libido, erectile dysfunction, decreased facial hair, testicular atrophy, and oligozoospermia or azoospermia in association with high testosterone and high or normal gonadotropin levels.[133] The severity of the latter biochemical indices of androgen insensitivity is directly related to CAG repeat length. Although it is not found consistently, some studies have reported an association between CAG repeat number and manifestations of androgen action in normal men.[134] In these studies, a low number of CAG repeats within the normal range was associated with higher androgenicity (e.g., earlier onset of prostate cancer, male pattern baldness, lower HDL-cholesterol), and a high number of repeats within the normal range was associated with lower androgenicity (e.g., gynecomastia, impaired spermatogenesis, lower bone density, depressive symptoms). CAG repeat number also seems to be associated with the clinical manifestations of men with androgen deficiency due to Klinefelter syndrome and their response to testosterone treatment, the latter suggesting a possible pharmacogenetic influence of this AR polymorphism.

Studies in vitro and in experimental animals suggest that some actions of androgens may occur within seconds to minutes, too rapidly to be caused by classic genomic effects of androgens acting through the AR on gene transcription and subsequent protein synthesis, which usually take hours to produce effects.[135] Rapid, nongenomic effects of androgens may be mediated by cell surface interactions and receptors and by the activation of conventional signal transduction mechanisms, including activation of PKA and PKC, which increase intracellular calcium and MAPK pathways. Binding of androgen to intracellular AR may also activate coregulators that do not require gene transcription to signal, such as the tyrosine kinase, steroid receptor coactivator (SRC). Nongenomic actions of androgens have been described in testis (Sertoli cells), brain, muscle, cardiovascular tissue, prostate, and immune cells. In humans, the rapid vasodilatory effect of testosterone on myocardial ischemia in patients with coronary artery disease is attributed to a direct nongenomic effect of androgens on vascular cells.

Androgen Effects at Various Stages of Sexual Development

Levels of testosterone and its actions differ at various stages of sexual development (Fig. 19-13).[136] During *fetal life*, testosterone is secreted by the fetal testis beginning at 7 weeks of gestation.[36] Testosterone secretion is primarily under the control of maternal hCG, initially, and then LH secreted by the fetal pituitary. During this time, testosterone concentrations increase to almost adult male levels, and testosterone and its conversion to DHT are critical for normal male internal and external genital differentiation (e.g., development of primary sexual characteristics). Testosterone concentrations remain elevated through most of the second trimester, after which they decline.

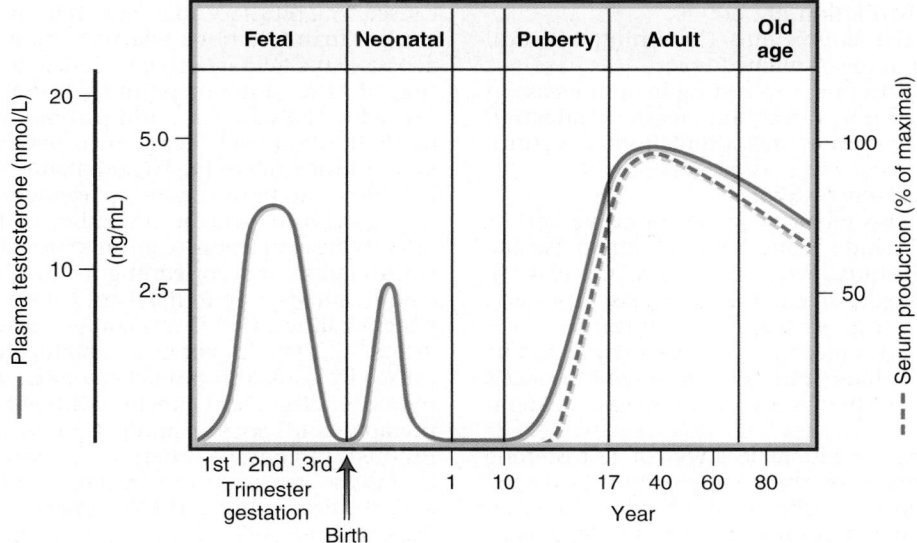

Figure 19-13 Schematic diagram of changes in serum testosterone concentration and sperm production during different phases of life. During fetal life, testosterone levels increase almost to adult male levels, peaking during the first trimester and remaining elevated throughout the second trimester, after which they decline. During neonatal life, testosterone increases almost to adolescent levels at 3 to 6 months of age, then declines to prepubertal levels. During puberty, testosterone concentrations and sperm production increase to adult male levels over several years. With aging, there is a variable, gradual, and progressive decline in serum testosterone levels and sperm production, beginning at age 40 years. (From Griffin JE, Wilson JD. The testis. In: Bondy PK, Rosenberg LE, eds. *Metabolic Control and Disease*, 8th ed. Philadelphia, PA: WB Saunders; 1980:1535-7158.)

Shortly after birth, during *neonatal life*, LH secretion increases and stimulates a second rise in testosterone levels, almost to adolescent concentrations, between 3 and 6 months of age; this is followed by a fall to low prepubertal levels.[137] The neonatal surge in testosterone levels may have a role in the development of normal phallus size and completion of testicular descent. The neonatal increase in testosterone and FSH levels at this time also stimulates Sertoli cell proliferation and spermatogonial development, which may play a role in determining spermatogenic capacity.

During *puberty*, testosterone concentrations increase to adult male levels in response to activation of hypothalamic GnRH secretion and its stimulation of pituitary gonadotropin secretion.[43,138] The progressive increase in testosterone and its active metabolites, estradiol and DHT, is responsible for the development of secondary sexual characteristics (*virilization* or *masculinization*) and other changes. Pubertal changes induced by testosterone may be categorized as those related to body, brain, and sexual function.

Body function changes mediated by testosterone and its active metabolites include the following:

- Growth and development of the penis and scrotum and the appearance of rugal folds and pigmentation in scrotal skin
- Enlargement of the prostate and seminal vesicles and production of accessory sexual gland secretion and seminal fluid
- Androgen-dependent hair growth and development of a male hair distribution—facial (moustache and beard), external auditory canal, chest, axillary, pubic and lower abdomen (male escutcheon), perianal, inner thigh, and leg and arm hair growth and frontal scalp hair recession
- Increase in sebum production
- Stimulation of IGF-1 production together with that of growth hormone (GH)
- Long bone growth and eventually closure of long bone epiphyses resulting in cessation of growth
- Increase in BMD and stimulation of peak bone mass
- Increase in skeletal muscle mass and strength, especially in shoulder and pectoral muscles
- Decrease and redistribution of body fat
- Enlargement of the larynx and thickening of vocal cords, resulting in a lower-pitched voice
- Stimulation of erythropoiesis resulting in an increase in hematocrit, primarily by direct bone marrow induction of erythroid differentiation and stimulation of erythropoietin secretion
- Suppression of HDL-cholesterol

Brain function changes mediated by testosterone and its active metabolites include stimulation of libido (sexual interest, desire, and motivation); increase in motivation, initiative, and social aggressiveness; and increase in aspects of cognitive function (e.g., visuospatial abilities).

Sexual function changes mediated by testosterone and its active metabolites include initiation of spermatogenesis and acquisition of fertility potential and increase in spontaneous erections.

In *adult life*, normal adult male levels of testosterone serve to maintain many of the changes induced during puberty. This includes maintenance of body function changes such as normal amounts of androgen-dependent hair and male hair distribution, sebum production, BMD, muscle mass and strength, hematocrit in the male range (higher than the female range), and HDL-cholesterol in the male range (lower than the female range); brain function changes such as libido, motivation, initiative, social aggressiveness, energy and vitality, mood, and possibly some aspects of cognitive function; and sexual function changes such as sperm production and fertility potential and spontaneous erections. Some of the masculinizing changes induced by testosterone during puberty are permanent. Once they are developed, testosterone is not necessary for maintenance of penis size, scrotal development, linear growth, laryngeal size, vocal cord thickness, or voice pitch.[113]

With *aging*, there is a gradual and progressive decline in serum testosterone concentrations associated with reductions in muscle mass and strength, BMD, libido, energy and vitality, mood, aspects of cognitive function, sperm production and fertility, and erections.[139] However, the contribution of the age-related decline in testosterone levels to these age-associated changes in function is not clear.

MALE HYPOGONADISM

The two major functions of the testis are to produce sufficient amounts of testosterone and of sperm to support the development and maintenance of male sexual function, body function, and fertility. *Male hypogonadism* is a clinical syndrome that results from a failure of the testes to produce adequate amounts of testosterone; this is almost always associated with impaired sperm production (*androgen deficiency and impairment of sperm production*), or an *isolated impairment of sperm production or function* with normal testosterone production. Hypogonadism is the most common disorder of testis function encountered in clinical practice.

Because testis function is controlled by the hypothalamus and the pituitary, male hypogonadism may be caused by a primary disorder of the testis (*primary hypogonadism*); it may be secondary to a disorder of the pituitary or hypothalamus (*secondary hypogonadism*); or in some instances, there may be defects at both levels (*combined primary and secondary hypogonadism*).

Identifying men with secondary hypogonadism has important clinical implications that may affect management.[113] For example, secondary hypogonadism can be caused by a pituitary adenoma that may be associated with clinical manifestations related to tumor mass (e.g., headaches, visual field defects); to deficiency or excessive secretion of other anterior pituitary hormones; or to diabetes insipidus (polyuria) resulting from hypothalamic antidiuretic hormone deficiency. Such patients require management of the underlying hypothalamic or pituitary disorder in addition to testosterone replacement therapy. Secondary hypogonadism may be reversible with treatment of the underlying condition (e.g., nutritional deficiency) or discontinuation of an offending medication (e.g., glucocorticoids, opioids), or it may be associated with a chronic systemic illness that is not curable, such as chronic kidney disease (CKD). Impaired spermatogenesis and infertility caused by gonadotropin deficiency in men with secondary hypogonadism may be treated with gonadotropin or GnRH therapy, and sperm production and fertility may be restored. In contrast, infertility caused by primary testicular disease is usually not treatable with hormone therapy and requires other fertility options, such as the use of donor sperm, ART (e.g., ICSI), or adoption.

Clinical Manifestations
Androgen Deficiency and Impairment in Sperm Production

Because testosterone has different roles during fetal, prepubertal, and adult life, the manifestations of androgen deficiency differ depending on the stage of sexual development.[9,113]

Fetal Androgen Deficiency. During fetal development, testosterone and its conversion to DHT have vital roles in directing male internal and external genital differentiation and development. Fetal androgen deficiency (e.g., from congenital defects in testosterone biosynthesis enzymes) or androgen resistance/insensitivity (e.g., from AR mutations or 5α-reductase deficiency) manifests at birth with varying degrees of ambiguous genitalia and 46,XY DSD (i.e., male pseudohermaphroditism) (Table 19-1).[36,62,140] Depending on the severity of androgen deficiency or resistance/insensitivity, the phenotype of individuals with these disorders may range from that of a normal female to that of an otherwise normal male with microphallus, pseudovaginal perineoscrotal hypospadias, bifid scrotum, and/or cryptorchidism of varying severity. These disorders are described in greater detail in Chapter 23.

Prepubertal Androgen Deficiency. The increase in testosterone levels that occurs at the time of puberty is responsible for development of secondary sexual characteristics; an increase in muscle mass and reduction and redistribution of body fat; long bone growth and eventually closure of epiphyses resulting in cessation of growth; stimulation of sexual interest (libido), spontaneous erections, and sexual activity; and initiation of spermatogenesis and seminal fluid production.[141] Prepubertal androgen deficiency causes *eunuchoidism* (Fig. 19-14; see Table 19-1),[141] which is characterized most notably by infantile genitalia with a small penis and a poorly developed scrotum that lacks rugal folds and pigmentation. The testes are small, usually less than 2 cm in length and from 2 mL to less than 4 mL in volume. Hair is thin and fine, and there is a lack of androgen-dependent hair growth (i.e., absence of a male hair pattern in all body areas) and no temporal hair recession. The pubic hair pattern is more typical of females, with the shape of an inverted triangle in the pubic area (female escutcheon) rather in a diamond shape with hair extending from the pubic area to the umbilicus (male escutcheon), and there is little hair extending to the thighs. Acne does not develop because sebum production is not stimulated by androgens.

Eunuchoidism is typified by a distinctive body habitus, characterized by poor muscle mass development (especially in the shoulders and chest), prepubertal fat distribution (predominantly in the face, chest, and hips), and excessively long arms and legs relative to height. Arm span exceeds height by greater than 5 cm, and the distance from the crown of the head to the symphysis pubis is less than 5 cm than the distance from the symphysis to the floor. The voice is high-pitched in the absence of androgen-dependent laryngeal enlargement and vocal cord thickening. Relatively long arms and legs result from a failure of long bone epiphyses to close; epiphyseal closure is mediated normally by increased estradiol derived from aromatization of the increased testosterone produced at the time of puberty.

Prepubertal androgen deficiency may not be recognized or diagnosed until adulthood. Compromise in peak bone mass accrual due to androgen deficiency may manifest as low BMD for age, and prolonged severe androgen deficiency increases the risk of osteoporosis and fractures as these men become older. Despite the absence of pubertal development, these individuals may develop gynecomastia (benign breast enlargement) that is caused by androgen deficiency rather than by the relatively high ratio of estradiol to testosterone levels associated with pubertal gynecomastia. Motivation and initiative are reduced and, together with poor muscle mass and strength, may contribute to poor physical performance (e.g., in athletics or the

TABLE 19-1

Clinical Manifestations of Androgen Deficiency

Fetal Androgen Deficiency

Symptoms	Signs
Ambiguous genitalia	Ambiguous genitalia (46,XY DSD)
	Normal female genitalia
	Microphallus (resembling clitoromegaly)
	Pseudovaginal perineoscrotal hypospadias
	Bifid scrotum
	Cryptorchidism

Prepubertal Androgen Deficiency

Symptoms	Signs
Delayed puberty	Eunuchoidism
Lack of sexual interest or desire (libido)	Infantile genitalia
Reduced nighttime or morning spontaneous erections	Small testes
Breast enlargement and tenderness	Lack of male hair pattern growth, no acne
Reduced motivation and initiative	Disproportionately long arms and legs relative to height
Diminished strength and physical performance	Pubertal fat distribution
No ejaculate or ejaculation (spermarche)	Poorly developed muscle mass
Inability to father children (infertility)	High-pitched voice
	Reduced peak bone mass, osteopenia or osteoporosis
	Gynecomastia
	Small prostate gland
	Aspermia, severe oligozoospermia or azoospermia

Adult Androgen Deficiency

Symptoms	Signs
Incomplete sexual development	Eunuchoidism
Lack of sexual interest or desire (libido)	Small or shrinking testes
Reduced nighttime or morning spontaneous erections	Loss of male hair (axillary and pubic hair)
Breast enlargement and tenderness	Gynecomastia
Inability to father children (infertility)	Aspermia or azoospermia or severe oligozoospermia
Height loss, history of minimal-trauma fracture	Low bone mineral density (osteopenia or osteoporosis)
Hot flushes, sweats	Height loss, minimal-trauma or vertebral compression fracture
Reduced shaving frequency	Unexplained reduction in prostate size or PSA

Less Specific Symptoms	Less Specific Signs
Decreased energy, vitality	Mild normocytic, normochromic anemia (normal female range)
Decreased motivation, self-confidence	Depressed mood, mild depression or dysthymia
Feeling sad or blue, irritability	Reduced muscle bulk and strength
Weakness, decreased physical or work performance	Increased body fat or body mass index
Poor concentration and memory	Fine facial skin wrinkling (lateral to orbits and mouth)
Increased sleepiness	

DSD, disorders of sex development; PSA, prostate-specific antigen.

military). These men have reduced sexual interest or desire (libido) and lack spontaneous erections at night or on awakening in the morning. Hematocrit remains in the female range due to inadequate androgen stimulation of erythropoiesis. The prostate and seminal vesicles remain small without androgen stimulation, and seminal fluid

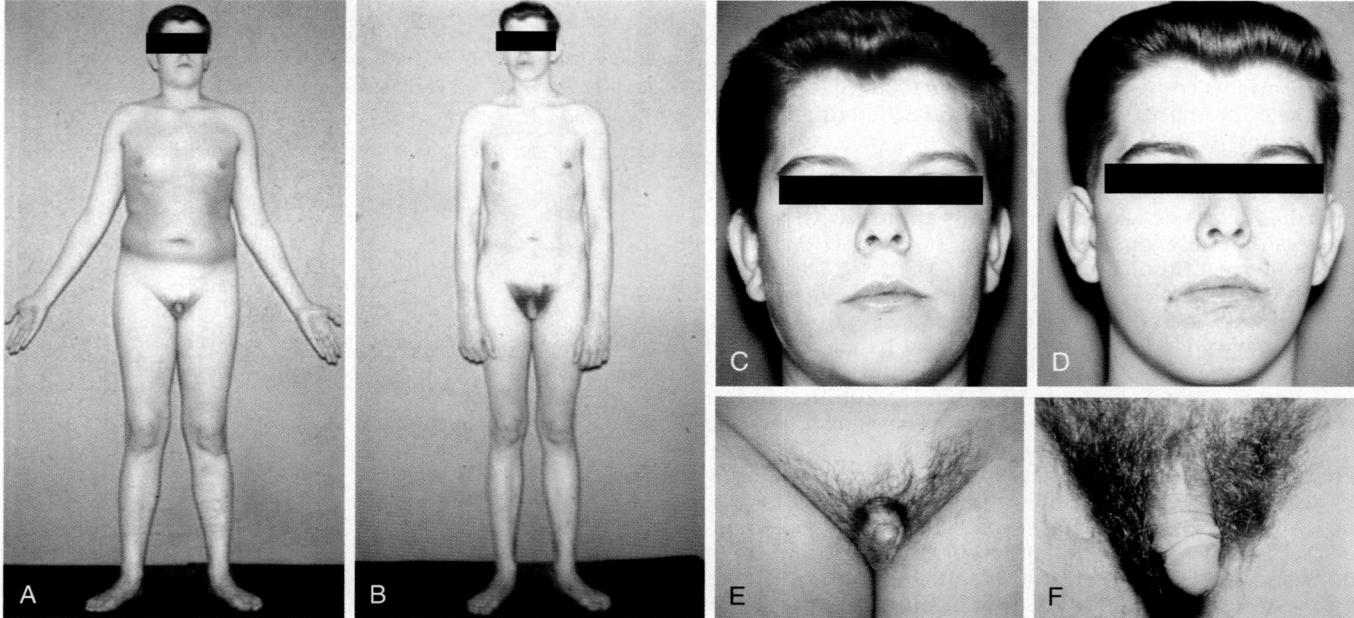

Figure 19-14 A 19-year-old patient with prepubertal androgen deficiency caused by congenital anorchia before (**A**, **C**, and **E**) and after (**B**, **D**, and **F**) 5 years of testosterone treatment. Before testosterone treatment, the patient had features of eunuchoidism, characterized by infantile genitalia (small penis and poorly developed scrotum); lack of chest, pubic, and facial hair; long arms and legs relative to height; and poorly developed muscle mass in the upper body with accumulation of fat in the face, chest, and hips. After testosterone treatment, there was an increase in penis size; an increase in chest, pubic, and facial hair with scalp recession and development of acne; an increase in muscle mass, particularly in the upper body; and loss of fat in the face, chest, and hips. (From Matsumoto AM. The testis. In: Felig P, Frohman LA, eds. *Endocrinology and Metabolism*, 4th ed. New York, NY: McGraw-Hill; 2001:635-705.)

production is absent, resulting in aspermia (lack of ejaculate) and failure to undergo spermarche (first ejaculation). Seminal fluid may be present in men with mild or partial prepubertal androgen deficiency or in those treated with androgens. However, these men usually have severe oligozoospermia or azoospermia, and most are infertile.

Adult Androgen Deficiency. Some individuals with prepubertal androgen deficiency who are not diagnosed or are inadequately treated as boys present as adults with features of eunuchoidism and other manifestations of prepubertal androgen deficiency (see Table 19-1). Their condition is usually clinically obvious because of inadequate sexual development for their chronologic age.

In adults, testosterone is needed to maintain sexual function, some secondary sexual characteristics, muscle and bone mass, and sperm production. Clinical manifestations of androgen deficiency are nonspecific and may be modified by the severity and duration of androgen deficiency, the presence of comorbid illnesses, previous testosterone treatment, or variations in target-organ sensitivity to androgens. Therefore, the clinical diagnosis of androgen deficiency acquired as an adult can be challenging, particularly in older men.[113]

Some clinical symptoms and signs are suggestive of androgen deficiency. Adults most commonly present with *sexual dysfunction* (diminished libido as manifested by reduced sexual interest or desire, reduced spontaneous and sexually evoked erections, and erectile dysfunction); *gynecomastia* (benign breast enlargement that may be accompanied by tenderness); and *infertility* (inability to father children despite unprotected intercourse) associated with oligozoospermia or azoospermia and small or shrinking testes with severe impairment in spermatogenesis. Secondary sexual characteristics do not regress to a prepubertal state; however, with long-standing, severe androgen deficiency, there may be loss of androgen-dependent hair, such as reduced facial hair associated with reduced shaving

frequency and loss of axillary and pubic hair (Fig. 19-15). Men with rapid and profound decreases in testosterone levels (e.g., from GnRH agonist treatment of prostate cancer) may have hot flushes and sweats due to vasomotor instability, similar to those experienced by menopausal women. Because testosterone and its active metabolite, estradiol, have an important role in the maintenance of bone mass, men with chronic androgen deficiency may present with osteopenia or osteoporosis on BMD measurement (e.g., by dual energy x-ray absorptiometry [DXA] scan) or with a minimal-trauma bone or vertebral compression fracture that may be associated with height loss. An unexplained reduction in prostate size or in the level of prostate-specific antigen (PSA) is uncommon but may occur as a result of long-term, severe acquired androgen deficiency.

Other symptoms and signs are much less specific for androgen deficiency but may occur, commonly in conjunction with clinical manifestations described previously that are more suggestive of androgen deficiency. Men with low testosterone concentrations often complain of diminished energy and *joie de vivre* (vitality), poor motivation and social aggressiveness, depressed mood and irritability that may be diagnosed as subsyndromal depression (mild depression or dysthymia), increased sleepiness, or poor concentration and memory. Men with severe androgen deficiency may have a mild hypoproliferative normocytic, normochromic anemia within the female range in the absence of androgen stimulation of erythropoiesis. With long-standing deficiency, reduced muscle bulk and strength associated with weakness and reduced physical and work performance may occur. The latter symptoms may occur in conjunction with an increase in body fat, but androgen deficiency is not a cause of clinically obvious obesity per se. Skin changes and reduced sebum production with severe, long-standing androgen deficiency may be associated with fine facial wrinkling that is particularly noticeable on the lateral corners of the orbits (lateral canthus) and mouth. Testis size may

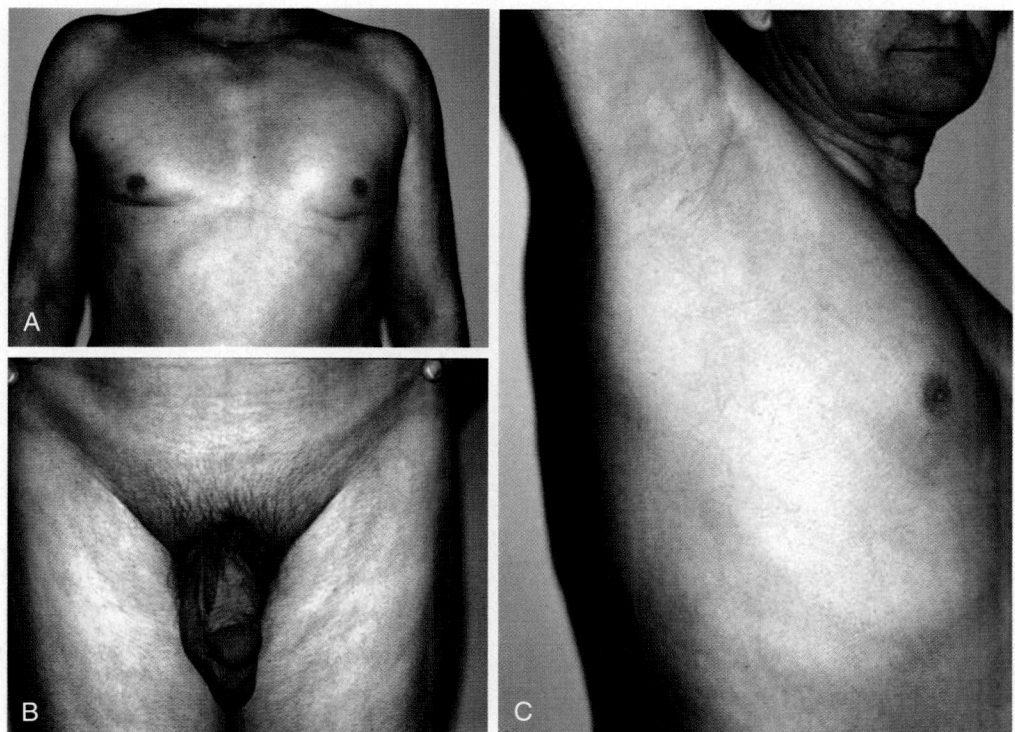

Figure 19-15 A 54-year-old man with adult androgen deficiency caused by hypopituitarism who presented with sexual dysfunction (reduced libido and erectile dysfunction); loss of chest, axillary, and pubic hair (**A**, **B**, and **C**); and gynecomastia (**A**). His penis and testes were normal in size (**B**). He had normal facial hair (**C**), but his shaving frequency was less.

be small, especially with severe impairment of spermatogenesis, but in most men with acquired adult androgen deficiency, testis size is normal to slightly reduced.

Because clinical manifestations are nonspecific, older men may have a number of medical or comorbid conditions and medications that contribute to symptoms and signs that are consistent with androgen deficiency, presenting a particular diagnostic challenge (Fig. 19-16). Symptoms and signs of comorbid illnesses may mask, mimic, or contribute to clinical manifestations of androgen deficiency in older men. Elderly men may present with muscle loss and mobility impairment, fragility fracture or osteoporosis, and reduced vitality and depressed mood. On close examination, however, older men with severe, longstanding androgen deficiency usually manifest objective evidence of androgen deficiency.

Isolated Impairment of Sperm Production or Function

Most men with male infertility have hypogonadism manifested by an isolated impairment of sperm production with normal androgen production. These men present as adults with infertility and demonstrate oligozoospermia or azoospermia, sperm with abnormal morphologic appearance *(teratospermia)* or reduced or absent motility *(asthenospermia)*, or a combination of abnormalities on seminal fluid analysis. They do not have manifestations of androgen deficiency, and serum testosterone concentrations are normal. Testes may be small (if spermatogenesis is severely impaired) or normal sized. Testes may not be palpable if cryptorchidism or anorchia is present.

History and Physical Examination

Clinical evaluation of male hypogonadism involves a careful history and physical examination directed at determining whether there are symptoms and signs of androgen deficiency or isolated impairment of sperm production and at identifying potential common causes of hypogonadism.[9] Because adults with androgen deficiency present commonly with sexual dysfunction, gynecomastia, and infertility, the differential diagnosis of these conditions and causes other than hypogonadism of these presenting complaints should be considered. Laboratory evaluation of serum testosterone, gonadotropins, and seminal fluid (in men who are concerned with infertility) are performed to confirm the diagnosis of hypogonadism and to determine whether there is predominantly primary or secondary hypogonadism.

The *history* should include inquiry regarding symptoms of androgen deficiency. These may be grouped as relating to several areas:

1. *Development:* genital abnormalities and the potential need for surgical correction (e.g., hypospadias, microphallus, cryptorchidism); delayed sexual development or growth and need for hormone therapy; family history of delayed puberty or reproductive disorders; psychological impact of delayed puberty or growth; difficulty in school or learning disability; inability or reduced ability to smell

2. *Sexual function:* poor erections; reduced spontaneous, nighttime, or morning erections; inability to perform sexually; decreased sexual activity; inability to father children despite unprotected sexual intercourse (>1 year); small or shrinking testes

3. *Brain function:* poor general well-being; reduced sexual desire, interest, and motivation (libido); poor energy and vitality and excessive fatigue; poor motivation and initiative, passivity, low self-confidence, and low self-esteem; depressed mood and irritability; difficulty sleeping; hot flushes and sweats; poor concentration and memory

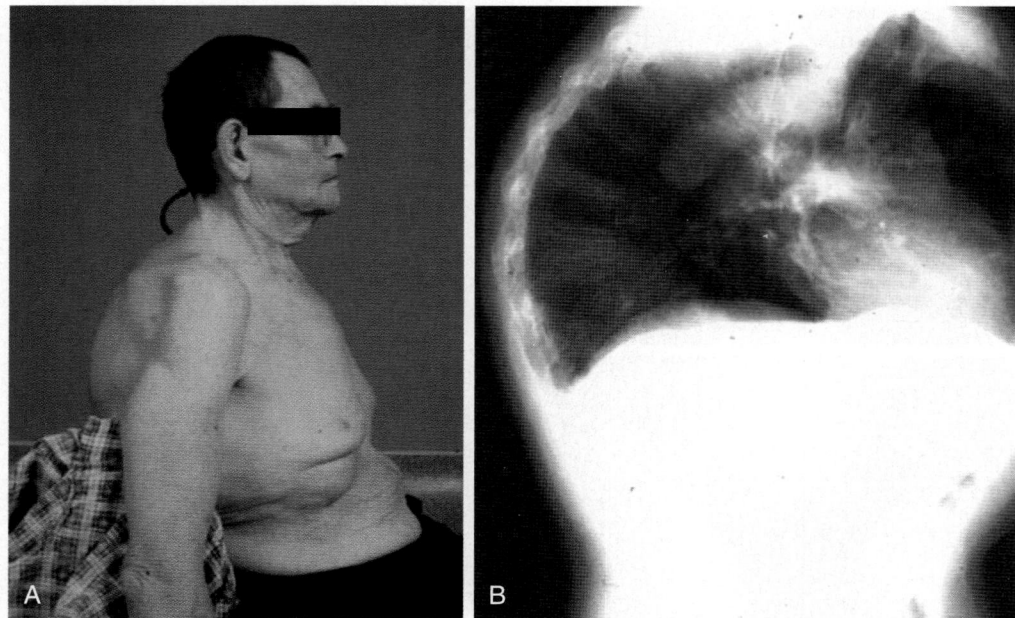

Figure 19-16 A 70-year-old man with severe androgen deficiency caused by Kallmann syndrome (hypogonadotropic hypogonadism and anosmia) who presented to a geriatric evaluation and management unit with functional and mobility disability caused by upper (**A**) and lower extremity muscle wasting and severe back pain from multiple vertebral compression fractures (**B**) due to osteoporosis. He was noted to have gynecomastia and absence of chest, axillary, and pubic hair.

4. *Body function:* decreased muscle bulk and strength; reduced physical activity or performance; breast enlargement or tenderness, especially if recent in onset; height loss, history of low-trauma or vertebral compression fractures, osteopenia, or osteoporosis; body hair loss (chest, axillary, or pubic); reduced beard growth and shaving frequency

The initial history may also include inquiry concerning the potential cause of hypogonadism. With *primary hypogonadism*, there may be a history of mumps involving the testes; testicular trauma, irradiation, or surgery; medication use (spironolactone, ketoconazole, cytotoxic agents); or chronic liver or kidney failure. With *secondary hypogonadism*, headaches, visual complaints or reduced peripheral vision, history of pituitary disease, chronic lung disease or congestive heart failure (CHF), wasting conditions (e.g., acquired immunodeficiency syndrome [AIDS], cancer), nutritional deficiencies, recent acute illness, morbid obesity, or use of certain medications (e.g., opioids, CNS-active drugs, glucocorticoids, anabolic steroids, megestrol acetate, medroxyprogesterone acetate, nutritional supplements) may be noted.

The patient should be questioned regarding conditions that are relative or absolute contraindications to testosterone treatment, including a history of severe BPH and lower urinary tract symptoms as assessed by the American Urological Association (AUA) symptom score or International Prostate Symptom Score (IPSS), history of prostate or breast cancer, history or symptoms of untreated obstructive sleep apnea syndrome (daytime sleepiness, snoring with sleep disruption, witnessed apnea episodes), history of severe CHF, and polycythemia or hyperviscosity.

In patients with suspected prepubertal androgen deficiency, *physical examination* should include measurements of total arm span, height, and the distances from the crown of the head to the symphysis pubis and from the symphysis pubis to the floor to determine whether the patient has excessively long arms and legs (see Fig. 19-14). Eunuchoidal body proportions are characterized by an arm span that

is at least 5 cm greater than height and a crown-to-symphysis distance that is at least 5 cm less than the symphysis-to-floor distance; such proportions are indicative of prepubertal androgen deficiency. Men with Klinefelter syndrome may have disproportionately long legs relative to arms and a greater ratio of lower- to upper-body segment measurements but a relatively normal ratio of arm span to height. Eunuchoidism is also characterized by infantile genitalia (micropenis or small penis, unrugated and nonpigmented scrotum); small testes or, rarely, absence of the testes; cryptorchidism; sparse or absent facial, axillary, chest, extremity, and pubic hair; poorly developed upper body musculature; fat predominance in the face, chest, and hips; and gynecomastia. Patients with Kallmann syndrome may have anosmia or hyposmia that may be tested with an odor identification and threshold test using readily identifiable, common household odorants (e.g., alcohol swab, peppermint, cinnamon, cocoa, coffee, cigarette, orange, soap) or more formally, such as with the University of Pennsylvania scratch and sniff test.

The physical findings of androgen deficiency acquired in adulthood are usually subtler than those of prepubertal androgen deficiency (see Fig. 19-15). In patients with severe, long-standing adult androgen deficiency, there may be loss of androgen-dependent facial, axillary, chest, extremity, and pubic hair; however, there are ethnic variations in body hair in androgen-dependent areas (e.g., less in Asians and Hispanics). The skin may be dry, and there may be fine wrinkling lateral to orbits or mouth in patients with severe, long-standing androgen deficiency. Patients should be carefully examined for the presence of palpable breast tissue or gynecomastia; presence, size, and consistency of the testes; and palpable abnormalities in the scrotum, such as varicocele, epididymal enlargement, or tenderness or absence of the vas deferens. A digital rectal examination (DRE) should be performed primarily to determine whether there are palpable abnormalities, such as a prostate nodule or induration, and also to assess the size of the prostate. Careful examination for kyphosis and measurement of height are useful for detecting significant height loss (>5 cm) associated with osteoporotic vertebral compression fractures that may be asymptomatic.

Proper technique is needed to examine the male breast. The thumb and index finger are used to grasp and gently pinch the periareolar area of the breast and to palpate glandular breast tissue, which is rubbery in consistency and firmer than the surrounding adipose tissue (Fig. 19-17). With this technique, gynecomastia can usually be distinguished from excessive breast adipose tissue, called *pseudogynecomastia*, which is often associated with generalized obesity. Gynecomastia is usually bilateral and relatively symmetric, but occasionally it is asymmetric and more prominent on one side. If present, asymmetric gynecomastia may suggest breast carcinoma, which is usually rockhard and irregular and may be associated with skin dimpling (*peau d'orange*), nipple retraction or discharge, and axillary lymphadenopathy. The diameter of palpable breast tissue is used as an objective measure of gynecomastia. Gynecomastia of recent onset is usually tender on palpation, and men usually complain of nipple irritation associated with rubbing against clothing.

Examination of the testes and scrotum may be performed with the patient either lying on his back or standing, but the latter position is preferred because it relaxes the scrotum, making some abnormalities (e.g., varicocele) more easily detected. In patients with retractile testes positioned high in the scrotum, it may be possible to palpate the testes only after placing the scrotum in warm water, after a warm bath, or by having the patient assume a squatting position. The testes may be very difficult to examine and palpate in morbidly obese men who have excessive folds of fat overlying the scrotum, in the presence of a large hydrocele, if the testis is tender (e.g., with epididymo-orchitis or testicular torsion), or occasionally in some men who are sensitive to palpation for unclear reasons. In these instances, testicular ultrasound may be required to confirm the presence of the testis, estimate its size, and detect abnormalities.

Although ultrasonographic size estimates are more accurate, testis size can be estimated by measuring length and width with a ruler or calipers or by comparing testis volume with that of ellipsoid models of known volume (Prader orchidometer) (Fig. 19-18). Normal testis size varies with age and ethnicity. Normal prepubertal testis size is approximately 1.6 to 2.9 cm in length and 1.0 to 1.8 cm in width, or 1 to 4 mL in volume. Testis size greater than 4 mL suggests the onset of puberty. In adults, normal testes usually measure 3.5 to 5.5 cm in length and 2.0 to 3.0 cm in width or 15 to 30 mL in volume.[8,9] In addition to size, testes should be palpated for consistency or firmness and for presence of a mass representing a benign or malignant testicular tumor. The testicular examination in men with Klinefelter syndrome is notable for very small (usually <3 mL), firm testes.

Differential Diagnosis

Because sexual dysfunction, gynecomastia, and infertility are often presenting complaints in adults with androgen deficiency, it is important to consider the differential diagnosis of these conditions and to be familiar with other common causes of these manifestations when evaluating men who present with these complaints.

Sexual Dysfunction

Normal sexual function requires successive, coordinated physiologic events—libido, erection, ejaculation, orgasm, and detumescence—that occur in a defined sequence and require normal psychological, CNS, peripheral nerve, vascular, and genital function.[142]

Sexual dysfunction may involve specific disorders of libido or sexual desire, erectile dysfunction, ejaculatory

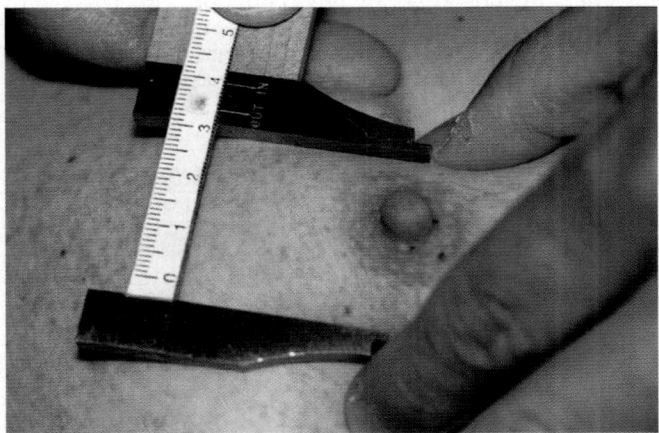

Figure 19-17 The proper method of examining the male breast is to use the thumb and index finger to grasp the periareolar area of the breast and to gently pinch the thumb and index finger together on either side of the breast toward the nipple. Glandular breast tissue feels like a rubbery disc of tissue that extends concentrically from under the nipple and subareolar area and is firmer than the surrounding adipose tissue. The size of gynecomastia is estimated by measurement of the diameter of palpable breast tissue. (From Matsumoto AM. The testis. In: Felig P, Frohman LA, eds. *Endocrinology and Metabolism*, 4th ed. New York, NY: McGraw-Hill; 2001:635-705.)

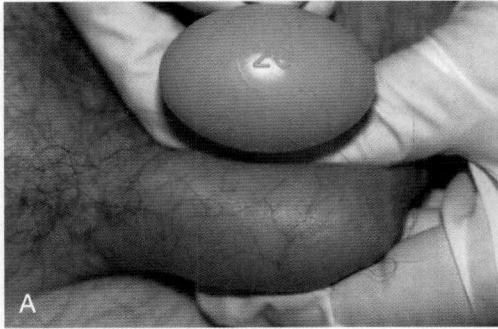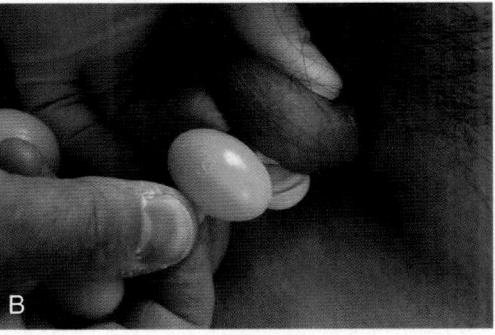

Figure 19-18 The assessment of testis size using a Prader orchidometer in a normal man (**A**), who has a right testis size of 20 mL, and in a man with Kallmann syndrome (**B**), who has a right testis size of 5 mL. Care must be taken not to include the head of the epididymis when estimating testis size. (From Matsumoto AM. The testis. In: Felig P, Frohman LA, eds. *Endocrinology and Metabolism*, 4th ed. New York, NY: McGraw-Hill; 2001:635-705.)

disorders, orgasmic dysfunction, or failure of detumescence. These may occur in isolation, but specific disorders of sexual function commonly occur together because these processes are interrelated and because a specific cause (e.g., androgen deficiency) can affect more than one of the physiologic processes that mediate normal sexual function. Male sexual dysfunction is detailed in Chapter 20. Men with androgen deficiency often present with sexual dysfunction, and it is important to consider the differential diagnosis of this complaint in the evaluation.

Androgen deficiency often results in reduced libido or sexual desire (hypoactive sexual desire disorder), loss or reduction of spontaneous evening and morning or sexually stimulated erections (erectile dysfunction), and, if severe, reduced or absent ejaculation. In many men with androgen deficiency, erectile response to intense erotic stimuli (and, occasionally, spontaneous erections) may be preserved, suggesting that the androgen requirement for sexual function is variable.[143] However, persistent erectile dysfunction may cause performance anxiety, and, together with hypoactive sexual desire and depressed mood associated with androgen deficiency, this may contribute to the eventual loss of erotically stimulated erections and, secondarily, to orgasmic dysfunction. Androgen deficiency may also affect nitric oxide (NO) production and maximal smooth muscle relaxation and vasodilatation within the penis, reducing the ability to produce an erection that is sufficient to satisfactorily complete sexual intercourse and further contributing to the severity of erectile dysfunction.[144,145]

Clinically, men with androgen deficiency most commonly present with hypoactive sexual desire disorder and erectile dysfunction. Severely androgen-deficient men may present with reduced ejaculation, but these individuals usually also complain of hypoactive sexual desire disorder and erectile dysfunction.

Hypoactive Sexual Desire Disorder and Erectile Dysfunction.

Libido, the desire or drive for sexual activity, is generated by external visual, auditory, and tactile stimuli as well as internal psychic stimuli acting on cortical and subcortical brain regions such as the limbic system (amygdala, hippocampus, anterior thalamic nuclei, and prefrontal cortex) and the temporal lobe. Stimuli from these areas are relayed to the medial preoptic area, which serves to integrate central inputs and sends impulses to the paraventricular nuclei; these, in turn, send projections to the thoracolumbar and sacral spinal cord centers that regulate penile erection. This neural pathway explains why brain disorders that cause hypoactive sexual desire disorder are usually accompanied by varying degrees of erectile dysfunction (see later discussion).[142] In particular, there is a loss of the spontaneous evening and morning erections that are associated with brain activation of sexual neural pathways during rapid eye movement (REM) sleep and dreaming. Clinically, libido may be influenced by previous or recent sexual activity and by experiences, psychosocial background, overall state of general health, androgen sufficiency, and brain function.

The neurotransmitter systems that regulate the physiology of normal libido are not known precisely. However, there is evidence that central dopamine neurotransmission may be important in mediating CNS regulation of sexual desire and erections. In humans, treatment with dopamine receptor agonists (e.g., bromocriptine, pergolide) may stimulate spontaneous erections, and in 20% to 30% of men with Parkinson disease, levodopa therapy is associated with stimulation of libido and spontaneous erections. The use of pharmacologic agents with dopamine receptor antagonist activity is frequently associated with reduced libido and erectile dysfunction. However, these agents also affect a number of other neurotransmitter systems. Dopamine antagonism (e.g., by neuroleptic or antipsychotic agents) results in elevated prolactin levels that suppress endogenous gonadotropin and testosterone secretion and may contribute to reduced libido and erectile dysfunction.

Hypoactive sexual desire disorder is defined as persistent or recurrent deficiency or absence of desire for sexual activity resulting in marked personal distress or interpersonal difficulty or both.[142,146,147] It is estimated to affect more than 15% of men. The causes of hypoactive sexual desire disorder are primarily disorders that affect normal brain function and are usually associated with erectile dysfunction, in particular loss of spontaneous evening or morning erections (Table 19-2). *Erectile dysfunction* is defined as the inability to achieve or maintain penile erection that is adequate for completion of satisfactory sexual intercourse or activity.[148] Erectile dysfunction is a common condition that increases with aging. It is estimated to affect fewer than 10% of men younger than 40 years of age but approximately 50% of men between 40 and 70 years of age, with 35% of men in the latter age group having moderate or complete erectile dysfunction.

Hypoactive Sexual Desire Disorder and Erectile Dysfunction Due to Brain Disorders. *Psychogenic disorders* commonly cause hypoactive sexual desire and erectile dysfunction; these disorders include stress or preoccupation associated with life circumstances or situations, illness, marital discord, or underlying maternal transference or gender identity issues; performance anxiety associated with fear of failure or

TABLE 19-2	
Causes of Hypoactive Sexual Desire Disorder and Erectile Dysfunction	
Cause	**Examples**
Brain Disorders	
Psychogenic disorders	Stress or preoccupation, performance anxiety, depression, major psychiatric illness
Chronic systemic illness	Heart, respiratory, kidney, or liver failure; cancer
CNS-active drugs	Alcohol; antihypertensive, narcotic, sedative-hypnotic, anticonvulsant, antidepressant, antipsychotic medications
Structural brain disease	Temporal lobe or limbic system disorders, Parkinson or other neurodegenerative brain disease, vascular brain disorders
Androgen deficiency	Primary and secondary hypogonadism
Other endocrine disorders	Hyperprolactinemia, Cushing syndrome, hyperthyroidism, hypothyroidism
Spinal Cord and Peripheral Disorders	
Spinal cord disorders	Trauma, vascular compromise, spinal stenosis, epidural abscess, tumor, transverse myelitis, multiple sclerosis, other spinal cord lesions
Peripheral nerve disorders	Diabetes mellitus; pelvic, prostate, or retroperitoneal surgery or damage; other causes of peripheral neuropathy
PNS-active drugs	Anticholinergic, antihistamine, antidepressant, sympathomimetic, α-adrenergic agonist, β-adrenergic antagonist medications
Peripheral vascular disease	Aortoiliac atherosclerosis, diabetes mellitus, trauma, surgery, vasculitis, venous incompetence (venous leakage), smoking
Antihypertensive drugs	Diuretics, α- and β-adrenergic antagonists, ACE inhibitors, calcium channel antagonists
Penile abnormalities	Peyronie disease, chordee, micropenis, trauma, priapism, phimosis

ACE, angiotensin-converting enzyme; CNS, central nervous system; PNS, peripheral nervous system.

preoccupation with the adequacy of erections during sexual intercourse; major depression or dysthymia (moderate or complete erectile dysfunction occurs in 60% to 90% of men with moderate to severe depression); and major psychiatric illness such as psychotic or personality disorders.[142,146,147]

Chronic systemic illness (chronic heart disease, respiratory illness, kidney or liver failure, or cancer) and poor general health are usually associated with reduced libido and spontaneous erections.[142,146,147] A number of *CNS-active medications* may cause hypoactive sexual desire disorder and erectile dysfunction, including alcohol, centrally acting antihypertensive medications, narcotics, sedative-hypnotic drugs, anticonvulsants, antidepressants, and antipsychotic medications. In addition to their direct effects on brain neurotransmitter function, both chronic illness and CNS-active medications may also be associated with androgen deficiency. *Structural brain disease*, such as infiltrative or destructive lesions of the temporal lobe or limbic system, Parkinson or other neurodegenerative brain disease, or vascular brain disorders such as stroke or vasculitis, may reduce libido and spontaneous erections.

Androgen deficiency is commonly associated with reduction or loss of libido and spontaneous erections.[149,150] Sexual dysfunction is usually a prominent presenting complaint in young, severely androgen-deficient men and in older men who are treated with medical therapies (e.g., GnRH agonist treatment) or surgical castration for advanced prostate cancer. In contrast, older men with less severe androgen deficiency may have sexual dysfunction that is also related to underlying depression, chronic systemic illness, or use of certain medications.[151] Comorbid conditions contribute to the nonspecificity of presenting complaints of androgen deficiency (e.g., sexual dysfunction) as men age. Testosterone treatment of severe androgen deficiency in young men usually improves sexual desire, interest, and thoughts; attentiveness to erotic stimuli; and the frequency, duration, and rigidity of spontaneous evening and morning erections.[150,152,153]

Other endocrine disorders can cause hypoactive sexual desire disorder and erectile dysfunction; examples include hyperprolactinemia, Cushing syndrome (glucocorticoid excess), hyperthyroidism, and hypothyroidism. In addition to their direct effects on brain function, hyperprolactinemia and glucocorticoid excess also suppress GnRH and gonadotropin secretion and induce androgen deficiency that contributes to sexual dysfunction. Anecdotally, some men with androgen deficiency due to severe hyperprolactinemia who are treated with testosterone alone do not fully recover sexual function and may require additional therapy with dopamine receptor agonists, but this has not been demonstrated conclusively. Dopamine receptor agonists lower elevated prolactin levels and may also have direct affects in the brain to activate neuronal systems involved in stimulating libido and erections.

Erectile Dysfunction Due to Spinal Cord or Peripheral Disorders. External and internal erotic stimuli from the brain are relayed via descending neural pathways in the lateral spinal columns to stimulate the parasympathetic sacral (S2-S4) spinal erection center, resulting in *psychogenic erections.* Efferent parasympathetic nervous system stimulation from the sacral center travels via the nervi erigentes (pelvic splanchnic nerve) and the pelvic plexus and enters the penis via the cavernosal nerve. This stimulation causes relaxation of the smooth muscles that form sponge-like interconnected trabecular spaces within the corpora cavernosa of the penis and vasodilation of the cavernosal arterioles and vascular sinusoids. As a result, blood flow and pressure into the trabecular spaces within the corpora

increase several-fold and cause engorgement of the penis (tumescence). Expansion of the trabecular spaces against the thick fibrous sheath (tunica albuginea) surrounding the corpora compresses subtunical venules and impedes venous outflow, resulting in sustained penile tumescence (i.e., an erection).[142,148]

Afferent somatic (via the pudendal nerve) and parasympathetic impulses in response to sensory stimulation of the penis with sexual intercourse or masturbation also act to stimulate erections via a reflex arc through the sacral spinal erection center, resulting in *reflexogenic erections.* Pudendal nerve stimulation also triggers the reflex contraction of the ischiocavernosus and bulbocavernosus muscles, resulting in vascular compression at the base of the penis, further increasing cavernosal blood pressure and maximal penile rigidity, leading to the plateau phase of erection.

The primary neurotransmitter that mediates penile smooth muscle relaxation and erection is NO. In response to parasympathetic cholinergic (acetylcholine-mediated) stimulation, NO is synthesized from its precursor, L-arginine, by the enzyme nitric oxide synthase (NOS) and is released by corporal sinusoidal endothelial cells and postganglionic noncholinergic, nonadrenergic nerve terminals. NO then enters adjacent smooth muscle cells, where it activates guanylate cyclase and increases intracellular cyclic guanosine monophosphate (cGMP). cGMP activates cGMP-dependent protein kinase, which phosphorylates a number of proteins, including myosin light chains and ion channels that ultimately decrease intracellular calcium concentrations, causing smooth muscle relaxation, increase in penile blood flow, and erection. cGMP is hydrolyzed and inactivated by the enzyme, phosphodiesterase type 5 (PDE5). In addition to cGMP, other neurotransmitters induce cavernosal smooth muscle relaxation, including prostaglandin E_1 (PGE_1), which activates adenylate cyclase and increases cAMP and cAMP-dependent protein kinase.

Knowledge of the neurotransmitter systems that control erections has been used to design pharmacologic treatments for erectile dysfunction (detailed in Chapter 20).[148,154,155] The most commonly used treatments are oral PDE5 inhibitors, such as sildenafil, vardenafil, and tadalafil, which act to inhibit the breakdown of cGMP, resulting in more sustained smooth muscle relaxation and improved penile erection after erotic stimulation. Injection of intracavernosal PGE_1 or insertion of intraurethral PGE_1 pellets acts to increase cavernosal cAMP concentrations and induce smooth muscle relaxation and penile erection even in the absence of sexual stimulation. Intracavernosal injections of papaverine, a nonspecific phosphodiesterase inhibitor (which inhibits the breakdown of both cGMP and cAMP), combined with phentolamine, an α_1- and α_2-adrenergic receptor antagonist vasodilator (bi-mix), or the two combined together with PGE_1 (tri-mix), are also used to induce smooth muscle relaxation and erection.

Studies in experimental animals and in vitro have found that androgen deficiency impairs penile nerve, trabecular smooth muscle, vascular endothelial, and tunica albuginea structure and function; reduces both endothelial and neuronal NOS synthesis and activity; and causes accumulation of adipocytes in the subtunical region of the corpora cavernosa.[145] These changes are reversed with androgen administration, suggesting a direct penile effect of androgens in addition to their central role in maintaining penile erections. In humans, ARs are expressed in the corpora cavernosa tissue. However, there is no conclusive evidence to support the notion that androgen treatment has a direct effect in the penis to enhance the response to PDE5 inhibitor therapy in androgen-deficient men with erectile dysfunction. In practice, symptomatic men with androgen deficiency and sexual dysfunction are usually treated with testosterone replacement, which can variably improve erectile dysfunction, particularly in younger hypogonadal men with severe androgen deficiency and no comorbid illness. If erectile dysfunction does not improve with testosterone treatment alone, they are given additional therapy for erectile dysfunction (e.g., addition of a PDE5 inhibitor). In some hypogonadal men, PDE5 inhibitor treatment alone may be sufficient to improve erectile dysfunction but is not adequate to treat reduced libido or other symptoms of androgen deficiency.[153]

In addition to the brain disorders that cause hypoactive sexual desire disorder and erectile dysfunction, spinal cord and peripheral disorders (e.g., peripheral nervous system disorders, peripheral vascular disease, medications that affect peripheral nerve and vascular function, penile abnormalities) may also cause erectile dysfunction that is usually not associated with hypoactive sexual desire (see Table 19-2). However, long-standing, severe erectile dysfunction may cause performance anxiety or depression, which may secondarily reduce libido. Furthermore, peripheral disorders that cause erectile dysfunction may also affect brain function and alter sexual interest and drive, contributing to erectile dysfunction. Tricyclic antidepressants may affect both peripheral and CNS function.

Spinal cord disorders, such as spinal cord injury due to trauma, vascular compromise, spinal stenosis, epidural abscess, tumor, transverse myelitis, multiple sclerosis, or other spinal cord lesions, usually cause erectile dysfunction. In general, the severity of erectile dysfunction associated with spinal cord injury and the response to treatment vary with the cord level involved, the severity of the lesion (i.e., complete versus incomplete), and the time since the injury. *Peripheral nerve disorders*, particularly those that affect the autonomic nervous system, may disrupt the normal regulation of penile erectile tissue and cause erectile dysfunction. For example, erectile dysfunction may be caused by diabetes mellitus or other diseases that cause peripheral neuropathy (e.g., amyloidosis, vasculitis, heavy metal toxicity, renal failure, multiple system atrophy, acute intermittent porphyria) or by pelvic, prostate, or retroperitoneal surgery or damage (e.g., abdominoperineal resection of the rectum, pelvic lymph node dissection, prostatectomy, aortoiliac bypass, lumbar sympathectomy). Peripheral nervous system medications, including anticholinergic agents, antihistamines, antidepressants, sympathomimetic medications, α-adrenergic agonists, and β-adrenergic antagonists, often impair erectile function by affecting peripheral nervous system regulation of erectile tissue of the penis, and many also cause erectile dysfunction by altering neurotransmitter function in the nervous system and penis.

The blood supply of the penis is derived from the internal iliac (hypogastric) artery, a branch of the common iliac artery that bifurcates from the aorta.[142] The internal iliac artery gives rise to the internal pudendal artery, which branches into the dorsal penile, bulbourethral, and cavernosal arteries. The cavernosal arteries run through the middle of the corpora cavernosa and give off corkscrew-shaped branches, the helicine arteries, that open directly into the lacunar spaces. Smooth muscle relaxation of lacunar spaces increases blood flow into the corpora cavernosa, resulting in penile tumescence. Blood from the lacunar spaces or cavernosal sinusoids collects in the subtunical plexus and is delivered via emissary veins to the deep dorsal vein, which ultimately drains into the internal and common internal iliac veins and then into the inferior vena cava. With filling of the lunar spaces of the corpora

cavernosa and penile tumescence against the fibrous tunica albuginea, venous outflow from the subtunical venous plexus is impeded, and sustained tumescence or erection ensues. Disorders of arterial inflow or venous output may cause erectile dysfunction.

Peripheral vascular disease due to aortoiliac atherosclerosis is probably the most common cause of erectile dysfunction in aging men.[142,148] These men usually have absent or severely diminished femoral artery pulses, and some present clinically with Leriche syndrome (absent femoral pulses, buttock or leg claudication, and erectile dysfunction). Other men with iliac atherosclerosis may be able to achieve an erection, but with penetration and use of the hip muscles for thrusting during sexual intercourse, blood is diverted from the penis to the hips, resulting in premature detumescence and loss of erection; this is known as the *pelvic steal syndrome*. Atherosclerotic large- and small-vessel disease may contribute to erectile dysfunction in men with diabetes mellitus, hypertension, CKD, smoking, and other atherosclerotic risk factors. Erectile dysfunction occurs in about 50% of men with diabetes mellitus. Smoking, specifically nicotine, also causes direct vasoconstriction of the corpora cavernosum and erectile dysfunction. Other conditions that compromise aortoiliac circulation, such as pelvic trauma, irradiation, and vasculitis, are less common causes of erectile dysfunction. Chronic pressure on the pudendal artery from bicycle riding, especially with some bicycle seats, may cause penile ischemia and erectile dysfunction; in addition, pressure on the pudendal nerve may cause penile numbness and contribute to sexual dysfunction. *Penile venous incompetence* (venous leakage) may cause premature loss of erections and inability to maintain erections sufficient to complete intercourse.

Many *antihypertensive medications*, including diuretics, α- and β-adrenergic antagonists, angiotensin-converting enzyme inhibitors, and calcium channel antagonists, have been implicated as causes of erectile dysfunction. *Penile abnormalities*, such as Peyronie disease or chordee (fibrosis or scarring of the tunica albuginea resulting in bending of the penis), micropenis or microphallus, penile trauma, phimosis (inability to retract the foreskin over the penis), and priapism (painful extended erections) may also cause erectile dysfunction.

Evaluation of Erectile Dysfunction. The cause of erectile dysfunction is usually strongly suspected on the basis of a careful medical, psychiatric, and medication history and physical examination.[142,148] Erectile dysfunction of psychogenic origin usually occurs abruptly, is transient, is intermittent or associated with a stressful situation, occurs with only some partners but not with others or does not occur with masturbation. Spontaneous evening and morning erections are usually maintained in psychogenic erectile dysfunction but lost with organic causes. Spontaneous erections may be detected by formal measurements of nocturnal penile tumescence (NPT) in a sleep laboratory or by breakage of wires of different tensile strength in a snap gauge (RigiScan), but these assessments are not routinely performed in practice and usually are not necessary.

Patients with nonpsychogenic brain disorders, spinal cord or peripheral nervous system disorders, vascular disorders, or penile abnormalities that cause organic erectile dysfunction usually exhibit clinical manifestations of the underlying disorder, and offending drugs that impair erectile function are revealed with a careful review of medications. Androgen deficiency is a cause of reduced libido and erectile dysfunction and occurs in 15% to 20% of men who complain of sexual dysfunction in a general medical clinic.[156] Therefore, evaluation of men who present with sexual dysfunction should include inquiry regarding other symptoms of androgen deficiency, examination for signs such as small testis size and gynecomastia, and confirmation of androgen deficiency by measurement of serum testosterone levels (see later discussion).

Peripheral pulses, in particular the presence of femoral pulses, should be tested to assess for peripheral vascular disease. Diagnosis of penile vascular insufficiency may be suspected by Doppler ultrasound measurement of the ratio of penile to brachial systolic blood pressure (penile/brachial index). A penile/brachial index greater than 0.75 is normal, whereas an index of less than 0.60 is suggestive of vascular erectile dysfunction. If there is a clinical suspicion of spinal cord disease, perineal and penile sensation should be assessed. A cremasteric reflex (stroking of the inner thigh associated with contraction of the ipsilateral cremasteric muscle and pulling up of the scrotum and testis) and a bulbocavernosus reflex (squeezing of the glans penis associated with contraction of the anal sphincter) should be elicited to assess spinal cord levels L1-L2 and S2-S4, respectively. Finally, the penis should be examined for abnormalities, such as penile plaques, angulation, or tight, unretractable foreskin.

Ejaculatory Disorders and Orgasmic Dysfunction. After the plateau phase of erection is achieved, sympathetic nervous system stimulation from the thoracolumbar (T10-L2) spinal erection center travels via the hypogastric nerve and pelvic plexus, enters the penis via the cavernosal nerve, and causes α-adrenergic receptor–mediated contraction of the cauda epididymis, vas deferens, accessory sex glands (the bulbourethral or Cowper glands and the urethral glands or glands of Littre), prostate, seminal vesicles, and ejaculatory ducts that moves sperm and semen into the posterior urethra *(emission)*. It also stimulates closure of the internal urethral sphincter to prevent retrograde ejaculation of sperm into the bladder.[142] After emission, continued sensory stimulation of the penis with sexual intercourse or masturbation stimulates reflex rhythmic contractions of the ischiocavernosus and bulbocavernosus muscles, resulting in expulsion of semen from the urethra *(ejaculation)*.[142]

Like erection, ejaculation is under considerable control by higher brain centers, with both voluntary and involuntary regulation.[142] *Premature ejaculation* is ejaculation that occurs before or shortly after vaginal penetration during sexual intercourse and is followed by a rapid loss of erection.[157] The cause of premature ejaculation is usually a psychological disturbance such as performance anxiety; it is rarely the result of an organic cause. There is evidence that serotoninergic neurotransmission inhibits sexual function and ejaculation. Selective serotonin reuptake inhibitors retard ejaculation, an effect that is used therapeutically to treat premature ejaculation.[157,158] Other men with psychological disorders such as excessive anxiety may have *retarded ejaculation* (inability to ejaculate), either in isolation or in combination with impaired libido and erections. The ejaculate is composed of spermatozoa (10%) and seminal fluid (90%), the latter derived mostly from the seminal vesicles (65%) and the prostate gland (30%). Because secretions from these accessory sex glands are androgen dependent, severe androgen deficiency may result in *absent* or *reduced ejaculation*. Absent or reduced ejaculation may also be caused by urethral abnormalities. Autonomic neuropathy, such as that caused by diabetes mellitus, sympatholytic drugs, thoracolumbar sympathectomy, extensive retroperitoneal or pelvic surgery, or bladder neck surgery, may be associated with absent or reduced ejaculation by causing *retrograde ejaculation* into the bladder.

Orgasm, the pleasurable sensation associated with ejaculation, usually occurs simultaneously with ejaculation and is mediated by CNS activation via ascending pathways from the spinal cord erection centers to regions of the temporal lobe and limbic system.[142] Because of impaired libido and erectile dysfunction, men with androgen deficiency may also fail to achieve an orgasm. Isolated absence of orgasm in the presence of normal libido, erections, and ejaculation is relatively rare and is almost always caused by a psychological disorder.

Disorders of Detumescence. After ejaculation, the thoracolumbar sympathetic outflow acts via α-adrenergic receptor stimulation to cause contraction of trabecular smooth muscle, which results in collapse of lacunar spaces, vasoconstriction of arterioles of the corpora cavernosa (reducing blood flow into the penis), and decompression of subtunical venules, leading to an increase in venous outflow and a flaccid penis *(detumescence)*.[142] Premature detumescence may contribute to erectile dysfunction, such as that caused by penile venous incompetence. Intracorporal injection of an α-adrenergic receptor antagonist, phentolamine, together with papaverine and PGE_1, causes sustained lacunar smooth muscle relaxation, arteriole vasodilatation, and penile tumescence and is used to treat erectile dysfunction caused by premature detumescence.

Priapism is failure of detumescence with persistence of erection lasting for longer than 4 hours that is unrelated to sexual stimulation and is usually painful.[142,159] An erection that persists for more than 4 hours is an emergency and may be complicated by ischemia, thrombosis, and vascular damage that contribute further to erectile dysfunction; if ischemia is severe, it can cause gangrene and eventual loss of the penis. Priapism may be idiopathic, or it may be caused by medications (e.g., intracavernosal injection therapy for erectile dysfunction, phenothiazines, trazodone, cocaine), by hematologic disorders such as sickle cell disease or chronic myelogenous leukemia, by neurologic disorders such as spinal cord injury, or by infiltrative diseases such as amyloidosis. The initial treatment is administration of the α-adrenergic receptor agonist, pseudoephedrine; if this is unsuccessful, aspiration of blood from the corpora cavernosa is performed with local anesthesia.

Gynecomastia

Gynecomastia is benign enlargement of the male breast caused by proliferation of glandular breast tissue.[160-162] On inspection, it is difficult to distinguish gynecomastia from increased adipose tissue deposition within the breast in the absence of glandular proliferation (pseudogynecomastia), which is commonly present in obese men and boys. Detection of glandular breast tissue requires a careful and properly performed physical examination (see earlier discussion), feeling for a firm, rubbery, finely lobular, freely mobile disc of tissue that extends concentrically from under the nipple and areola. Initially, gynecomastia of relatively recent and rapid onset may be painful and associated with tenderness. With time, glandular tissue is replaced by fibrous tissue and tenderness resolves, although palpable tissue remains. In contrast, pseudogynecomastia is soft, nondiscrete, and irregularly lobular, similar to subcutaneous fat in the abdomen.

Gynecomastia is usually present bilaterally but may be asymmetric in size and variably symptomatic. If palpable breast tissue is present unilaterally, the major concern is male breast cancer. Breast cancer is usually rock-hard and indurated, eccentrically located from the nipple and areola, and fixed to underlying tissue; it may be associated with skin dimpling with retraction of hair follicles *(peau d'orange)*, nipple retraction, nipple bleeding or discharge, or axillary lymphadenopathy.[163] Other chest wall tumors may cause unilateral breast enlargement, including lipomas, sebaceous or dermoid cysts, hematomas, fat necrosis, lymphangiomas, neurofibromas, and lymphomas.

The primary hormones that regulate breast tissue development are estrogens, which stimulate the growth and differentiation of breast epithelium to form ducts (ductal hyperplasia), and progesterone, which controls acinar development and the formation of glandular buds (glandular formation).[160,162] GH, IGF-1, insulin, thyroid hormone, and cortisol play permissive roles in breast development. Androgens inhibit the growth and differentiation of breast tissue. Prolactin stimulates differentiated breast acinar cells to produce milk, but high progesterone levels inhibit lactogenesis. Therefore, milk production requires a reduction in high progesterone levels in the presence of high prolactin levels, as occurs in the first few days after delivery. Milk production (galactorrhea) is rarely seen in men with hyperprolactinemia and gynecomastia, because progesterone levels are not usually high enough for breast acinar development to occur, and they do not decline in the presence of high prolactin levels to stimulate lactogenesis.

Gynecomastia develops in clinical situations in which the levels or activity of estrogens is relatively high in comparison with androgens (i.e., high estrogen-to-androgen ratio). This hormonal milieu may result from high estrogen or low androgen concentrations or activity. Androgen deficiency, because it decreases the inhibitory influence of androgens on breast development, is a major cause of gynecomastia. However, the differential diagnosis of other causes of gynecomastia should be considered in patients who present with breast enlargement with or without tenderness.

Causes of Gynecomastia. *Physiologic gynecomastia* occurs normally in neonatal and pubertal boys. Transient gynecomastia (neonatal gynecomastia) occurs in 60% to 90% of neonatal boys as a result of exposure in utero to high concentrations of maternal estrogens; it resolves within several weeks after delivery (Table 19-3).[160-162] At the time of puberty, breast enlargement greater than 0.5 cm in diameter, which is often tender, initially occurs in 60% to 70% of boys by 14 years of age and then regresses within 1 to 2 years. This pubertal gynecomastia is thought to be caused by a transient rise in serum concentrations of estrogen relative to testosterone during puberty.

Pathologic gynecomastia may result from excessive estrogen levels or action or from androgen deficiency or resistance/insensitivity in isolation. In some conditions, both estrogen excess and androgen deficiency contribute to proliferation of glandular breast tissue.[160-162] For example, in most conditions that cause gynecomastia as a result of excessive estrogen exposure, high circulating estrogen concentrations inhibit endogenous gonadotropin and testosterone secretion and cause secondary hypogonadism, which also contributes to the growth of breast tissue. Also, some disorders of the testes that cause androgen deficiency (i.e., primary hypogonadism), such as Klinefelter syndrome, result in high circulating LH levels that stimulate aromatase activity in Leydig cells, leading to higher levels of estradiol relative to testosterone and contributing to the pathogenesis of gynecomastia.

Estrogen excess disorders that cause gynecomastia include exposure to exogenous estrogens (e.g., diethylstilbestrol treatment of prostate cancer, contact with an estrogen-containing cream or cosmetic, accidental occupational exposure to estrogens, ingestion of estrogen-containing

TABLE 19-3
Causes of Gynecomastia

Cause	Examples
Physiologic Causes	
Maternal estrogen exposure	Neonatal gynecomastia
Transient increase in estrogen to androgen concentrations	Pubertal gynecomastia
Estrogen Excess	
Estrogens or estrogen receptor agonists	Estrogens, marijuana smoke, digitoxin, testosterone or other aromatizable androgens
Increased peripheral aromatase activity	Obesity, aging, familial
Estrogen-secreting tumors	Adrenal carcinoma, Leydig or Sertoli cell tumor
hCG-secreting tumors hCG treatment	Germ cell, lung, hepatic carcinoma
Androgen Deficiency or Resistance	
Androgen Deficiency Hyperprolactinemia causing androgen deficiency	Primary or secondary hypogonadism
Androgen Resistance Disorders	Congenital and acquired androgen resistance
Drugs that interfere with androgen action	Spironolactone, androgen receptor antagonists, marijuana, 5α-reductase inhibitors, histamine 2 receptor antagonists
Systemic Disorders	
Organ failure	Hepatic cirrhosis, chronic kidney disease
Endocrine disorders	Hyperthyroidism, acromegaly, growth hormone treatment, Cushing syndrome
Nutritional disorders	Refeeding, recovery from chronic illness (hemodialysis, insulin, isoniazid, antituberculous medications, HAART)
Idiopathic Causes	
Drugs	HAART, calcium channel antagonists, amiodarone, antidepressants (SSRIs, tricyclic antidepressants), alcohol, amphetamines, penicillamine, sulindac, phenytoin, omeprazole, theophylline
Adult-onset idiopathic gynecomastia Persistent prepubertal macromastia	

HAART, highly active antiretroviral therapy; hCG, human chorionic gonadotropin; SSRIs, selective serotonin reuptake inhibitors.

nutritional supplements or excessive amounts of phytoestrogens) and exposure to ER agonists such as marijuana smoke (unidentified phenolic components but not active cannabinoids[164]) or digitoxin. Ingestion of normal dietary amounts of phytoestrogens (e.g., soybean isoflavones) does not usually cause gynecomastia.[165] Uncommonly, administration of testosterone or other aromatizable androgens, usually to prepubertal boys or men with long-standing, severe androgen deficiency, induces or worsens gynecomastia by initially causing relatively higher estradiol than testosterone levels.

Increased peripheral aromatase activity with increased conversion of androgens to estrogens in excessive amounts of adipose tissue is thought to cause mild to moderate gynecomastia in men with obesity.[160-162] Also, increased aromatization of androgens to estrogens with increasing amounts of adipose tissue (including that within the breast) probably contributes substantially to the increased prevalence of gynecomastia with aging, which occurs in up to 65% of men 50 to 80 years of age.[160-162] Familial gynecomastia, an autosomal dominant or X-linked genetic disorder caused by constitutive activation of the *CYP19A1* (aromatase) gene that results in increased peripheral conversion of androgen to estrogen, is a very rare cause of gynecomastia that manifests as prepubertal gynecomastia persisting into adulthood.

Estrogen-secreting tumors of the adrenal gland or testis are uncommon causes of gynecomastia. Feminizing adrenal tumors are usually malignant and large, manifesting with a palpable abdominal mass. In contrast, estrogen-secreting Leydig or Sertoli tumors are usually small and benign. Feminizing Sertoli tumors (in particular, the large cell calcifying variety) may occur in isolation or in association with autosomal dominant disorders such as Peutz-Jeghers syndrome (multiple intestinal polyps and mucocutaneous pigmented macules) or the Carney complex (cardiac or cutaneous myxomas, pigmented skin lesions, and endocrinopathy, including functioning endocrine tumors of the adrenal and testis). *hCG-secreting tumors* (e.g., germ cell, lung, gastric, renal cell, or hepatic carcinomas in adults; hepatoblastomas in boys) or *hCG treatment* of gonadotropin deficiency increases aromatase activity in Leydig cells and stimulates excessive secretion of estradiol relative to testosterone, causing relative rapid onset of symptomatic gynecomastia.

Disorders and drugs that cause *androgen deficiency*, such as conditions that cause either primary or secondary hypogonadism (including medications such as cytotoxic agents) or androgen resistance, are major causes of gynecomastia.[160-162] Although prolactin acts on the breast to facilitate milk production in developed glandular tissue, the major mechanism by which hyperprolactinemia causes gynecomastia is inhibition of endogenous gonadotropin and testosterone production (inducing androgen deficiency), which acts indirectly to stimulate breast development by reducing the inhibitory influence of androgens on the breast. Hyperprolactinemia is a main reason that a number of CNS-active medications, such as antipsychotics, antidepressants, and sedatives, are associated with gynecomastia. Drugs that interfere with androgen action, such as spironolactone (in contrast to eplerenone, a selective aldosterone receptor antagonist that does not cause gynecomastia), AR antagonists (e.g., flutamide, bicalutamide, nilutamide), marijuana, and histamine 2 (H_2) receptor antagonists, may cause gynecomastia.

Androgen deficiency contributes to the pathogenesis of gynecomastia in *systemic disorders* such as major organ failure—and, in particular, in hepatic cirrhosis and CKD, which are commonly associated with combined primary and secondary hypogonadism—and in *endocrine disorders* such as acromegaly and Cushing syndrome, which may be associated with secondary hypogonadism.[160-162] In hepatic cirrhosis, there is reduced catabolism of Δ^4-androstenedione, resulting in increased peripheral conversion of Δ^4-androstenedione to estrone and increased circulating estrogen levels. Also, in both hepatic cirrhosis and hyperthyroidism, increased serum concentrations of SHBG, which binds testosterone with greater affinity than estradiol, result in relatively higher free estradiol compared with free testosterone levels and thereby contribute to stimulation of breast tissue and development of gynecomastia. LH levels are often elevated in men with hyperthyroidism, which stimulates relatively more estradiol than testosterone secretion by Leydig cells of the testes. Excessive GH with acromegaly or GH treatment and excessive cortisol with Cushing syndrome directly stimulate breast

tissue growth in addition to causing secondary hypogonadism, both of which contribute to the pathogenesis of gynecomastia.

Gynecomastia often accompanies *nutritional disorders*, in particular during nutritional repletion after a period of starvation and weight loss (refeeding gynecomastia) and analogously during recovery from chronic illness.[160-162] In both starvation and severe chronic illness that is commonly associated with anorexia and weight loss, central GnRH production and concomitant gonadotropin and testosterone secretion are markedly suppressed. With refeeding or restitution of appetite and weight gain, there is activation of the hypothalamic-pituitary-testicular axis and restoration of gonadal function, similar to what occurs during puberty but occurring more rapidly (a "second puberty"), resulting in transiently higher levels of estrogen relative to androgen levels and inducing gynecomastia. Refeeding gynecomastia was described initially in World War II prisoners who developed painful gynecomastia after liberation and nutritional repletion. Analogously, refeeding-like gynecomastia may occur in stage 5 CKD with the initiation of hemodialysis, in type 1 diabetes mellitus (T1DM) with insulin therapy, in tuberculosis with antituberculosis medications, and in human immunodeficiency virus (HIV) infection or AIDS with highly active antiretroviral treatment (HAART). As mentioned, these chronic systemic disorders also cause androgen deficiency that may contribute to the pathogenesis of gynecomastia. HAART also may cause lipohypertrophy and fat accumulation in the breast (pseudogynecomastia), and efavirenz has estrogenic activity.

The mechanisms of gynecomastia associated with a number of *drugs* are not entirely clear, and these cases are usually classified as idiopathic. Such drugs include HAART, calcium channel blockers (e.g., nifedipine, verapamil), amiodarone, antidepressants (selective serotonin reuptake inhibitors, tricyclic antidepressants), alcohol, amphetamines, penicillamine, sulindac, phenytoin, omeprazole (much less commonly than H_2-receptor antagonists), and theophylline.[160-162,166,167]

In a number of cases of adult-onset gynecomastia, the cause remains idiopathic. Most of these cases are probably caused by increased aromatization of androgens to estrogens associated with increased peripheral adiposity, enhanced breast production of estrogens, enhanced sensitivity to estrogens, or some combination of these factors. Rarely, boys may develop severe pubertal gynecomastia (female size breast development, Tanner stage III through V) that persists to adulthood (persistent pubertal macromastia). This disorder is not associated with specific hormonal or receptor abnormalities and remains idiopathic.

Evaluation. Most gynecomastia is asymptomatic and of mild degree but can be appreciated on a properly performed, careful physical examination (as described earlier). Mild, asymptomatic gynecomastia found incidentally on examination and in isolation does not warrant evaluation. However, breast enlargement that is recent and rapid in onset, large (>5 cm in obese men, >2 cm in lean men), symptomatic (i.e., associated with breast pain, tenderness, or galactorrhea), asymmetric, or suspicious for malignancy (eccentrically located, rock-hard, fixed to overlying or underlying tissues, or associated with bloody nipple discharge or lymphadenopathy) should trigger further evaluation.

A careful history, including medication history, and physical examination usually identify potential predisposing conditions or medications causing gynecomastia that in older men may be multifactorial.[160-162] Clinical evaluation should focus on evidence of androgen deficiency;

assessment of prescription and over-the-counter medications, substance abuse, herbal or nutritional supplement intake, cosmetic use, and usual dietary intake; symptoms and signs of systemic illness (e.g., hepatic or renal disease), malignancy, or endocrine disorders (e.g., thyroid, GH, cortisol excess); and history of recent recovery from malnutrition, severe weight loss, or chronic illness. At a minimum, the initial laboratory evaluation comprises serum testosterone, LH, FSH, TSH, and renal and liver function tests. Evaluation also usually includes measurements of estradiol, prolactin, and β-hCG, although elevations of these hormones usually affect testosterone and gonadotropin concentrations. Breast enlargement suspicious for malignancy should be evaluated by mammography and biopsy.

Treatment. Pubertal gynecomastia usually regresses spontaneously without treatment in 1 to 2 years and by age 17 in about 90% of cases. In adults, spontaneous regression of symptoms (breast pain and tenderness, nipple sensitivity) associated with inflammatory glandular proliferation usually occurs within 6 months, after which progressive stromal fibrosis causes more or less permanent palpable breast tissue and only partial regression of gynecomastia by 1 year.

Initial treatment of gynecomastia is directed at correction of the underlying cause of breast enlargement or discontinuation or replacement of a potentially offending medication.[168] Testosterone replacement therapy in androgen-deficient men may result in partial regression of gynecomastia, especially if breast enlargement is of recent onset. Prophylactic low-dose breast irradiation (10 to 15 Gy over 1 to 3 days) may be used before androgen deprivation therapy in men with prostate cancer to prevent the development of gynecomastia; this is more common in surgical orchidectomy and in AR antagonist monotherapy rather than combined therapy with a GnRH agonist or antagonist. ER antagonists (tamoxifen, 10 to 20 mg daily, or raloxifene, 60 mg daily) are effective in treating pubertal and adult gynecomastia and preventing gynecomastia induced by androgen deprivation therapy. For unclear reasons, aromatase inhibitors (e.g., anastrazole) are not effective. Although tamoxifen is not approved for treatment of gynecomastia, it has been shown to be effective in the treatment of idiopathic gynecomastia, resulting in partial regression in approximately 80% and complete regression in about 60% of cases. A gel formulation of DHT, a nonaromatizable androgen, is used to treat gynecomastia in some countries outside the United States.

Gynecomastia of recent onset, during the initial phase of ductal proliferation, periductal inflammation and edema, and subareolar fat accumulation, is usually responsive to medical therapy (e.g., androgen replacement in hypogonadal men, ER antagonist therapy). With long-standing gynecomastia (>1 year), there is progressive stromal fibrosis of the breast that is not responsive to medical treatment. In these cases, surgical reduction mammoplasty (i.e., removal of breast tissue [subcutaneous mastectomy] with or without periareolar adipose tissue [liposuction]) is necessary, especially if breast enlargement is severe, painful, socially embarrassing, or disfiguring.

Infertility

Infertility is defined as the inability of a sexually active couple to achieve conception despite 1 year of unprotected intercourse. The probability of conception in a sexually active couple is approximately 85% by 1 year. Approximately 15% of couples in the reproductive age group are infertile, and a male factor contributes to the cause (either in isolation or in combination with a female factor)

in about half of the cases. Therefore, male infertility is a common condition, affecting approximately 7% of men.[169]

Causes of Male Infertility. In about 80% to 90% of infertile men, infertility is caused by primary or secondary hypogonadism, manifested mostly by an isolated impairment of sperm production or function, much less commonly by androgen deficiency and impaired spermatogenesis, and rarely by androgen resistance (Table 19-4).[170,171] The evaluation and specific causes of hypogonadism are discussed in detail in subsequent sections. Most men with isolated impairment in sperm production have a primary disorder of the testes that is idiopathic in 60% to 70% of cases (if one includes both idiopathic oligozoospermia or azoospermia and varicocele, given that relationship of varicocele to the pathogenesis of infertility is unclear). If isolated impairment of spermatogenesis is severe in men with primary hypogonadism, serum FSH levels may be selectively elevated as a result of reduced negative feedback by inhibin B from Sertoli cells of the testis. In men with less severely impaired spermatogenesis, serum gonadotropin levels are normal, but this is still classified with disorders of primary hypogonadism because gonadotropin treatment has not been demonstrated to improve fertility.

Disorders of spermatogenesis caused by primary hypogonadism may be associated with chromosomal or genetic disorders. There is an 8- to 10-fold increase in the prevalence of chromosomal abnormalities among infertile men

TABLE 19-4	
Causes of Male Infertility	
Cause	**Examples**
Hypogonadism	
Isolated impairment of sperm production or function	
Androgen deficiency and impaired sperm production	
Androgen resistance	
Disorders of Sperm Transport	
Genital tract obstruction	Congenital bilateral absence of the vas deferens, cystic fibrosis, other congenital defects, vasectomy, postinfectious fibrosis, Young syndrome
Accessory gland dysfunction	Androgen deficiency or resistance, infection or inflammation, antisperm antibodies (immunologic)
Sympathetic nervous system dysfunction	Autonomic neuropathy, sympatholytic drugs, sympathectomy, retroperitoneal or abdominopelvic surgery, spinal cord injury or disease, vasovasostomy
Ejaculatory Dysfunction	
Premature or retarded ejaculation	
Retrograde ejaculation	Prostatectomy, bladder neck surgery, autonomic neuropathy, SNS dysfunction
Reduced ejaculation	Androgen deficiency or resistance, SNS dysfunction, ureteral abnormalities
Coital Disorders	
Erectile dysfunction	
Defects in coital technique	Infrequent intercourse, excessive intercourse or masturbation, poor timing in relation to ovulation, premature withdrawal of penis

SNS, sympathetic nervous system.

with impaired spermatogenesis—specifically, sex chromosomal aneuploidy (e.g., Klinefelter syndrome) or Robertsonian translocations of two nonhomologous chromosomes, most commonly involving chromosomes 13 and 14 or chromosomes 14 and 21.[172] The long arm of the Y chromosome (Yq), specifically the azoospermia factor (AZF) region (Yq11), contains a number of genes that encode for proteins that have important roles in spermatogenesis. This region contains highly homologous palindromic DNA repeat sequences that are susceptible to rearrangement and deletions. Small deletions in the AZF region (Y chromosome microdeletions) are the most common genetic cause of impaired sperm production and male infertility; they are found in 5% to 10% of men with azoospermia or severe oligozoospermia (sperm concentration <5 million/mL).[172] Y chromosome microdeletions have been identified in three regions: in the AZFa region, microdeletions are uncommon but are usually associated with azoospermia and Sertoli cell–only histology; in the AZFb region, they are usually associated with severe oligozoospermia and germ cell arrest at the pachytene primary spermatocyte stage; and in the AZFc region, where the majority of Y chromosome microdeletions reside, they are usually associated with germ cell arrest at the spermatid stage or hypospermatogenesis with some mature spermatids present. Occasionally, microdeletions in the AZFb and AZFc regions are associated with azoospermia and Sertoli cell–only histology. Genes encoding a number of candidate proteins for male infertility include DDX3Y (DEAD box Y, an ATP-dependent RNA helicase), RBMY (RNA-binding motif Y-linked, an RNA-binding protein), and DAZ (deleted in azoospermia, another RNA-binding protein) in the AZFa, AZFb, and AZFc regions, respectively.[172,173]

Approximately 15% to 20% of male infertility is caused by disorders of sperm transport from the testes to the urethra, most commonly by genital tract obstruction. Congenital bilateral absence of the vas deferens (CBAVD) is present in 1% to 2% of men with infertility.[172,174,175] Seventy-five percent of men with CBAVD are heterozygous for the cystic fibrosis transmembrane conductance regulator gene (CFTR), which encodes for an epithelial chloride channel, or carry compound heterozygous mutations of CTFR. They do not have obvious clinical manifestations of cystic fibrosis, although some manifest abnormalities on sweat chloride testing and sinopulmonary infections. Conversely, almost all men with cystic fibrosis have CBAVD. CBAVD is also commonly associated with absence of the seminal vesicles, ejaculatory ducts, and epididymides due to fetal atrophy of these wolffian duct derivatives; in 10% of cases, there is also renal agenesis or hypoplasia.

Other causes of genital tract obstruction include other congenital defects of the epididymides and vas deferens (e.g., epididymal cysts associated with prenatal diethylstilbestrol exposure); vasectomy (surgical ligation of the vas deferens); postinfectious fibrosis (e.g., associated with gonorrhea, Chlamydia infection, other sexually transmitted diseases; tuberculosis; leprosy); and Young syndrome, a rare, congenital primary ciliary dyskinesia syndrome characterized by bronchiectasis, recurrent sinopulmonary infections, and obstructive azoospermia caused by thickened, inspissated mucous secretions obstructing the epididymides.

Although a causal link to infertility has not been clearly established, other genital tract abnormalities may contribute to impaired sperm transport and the pathogenesis of infertility in some men. Accessory gland dysfunction, such as reduced seminal vesicle and prostate secretions associated with disorders that cause severe androgen deficiency or resistance, may contribute to reduced fertility, although the main effects of these disorders are to impair spermatogenesis and cause sexual dysfunction. Infection or inflammation of the epididymides, seminal vesicles, or prostate gland may affect fertility directly by impairing sperm maturation or function or secondarily by causing scarring of the genital tract or induction of antisperm antibodies in semen (resulting in sperm agglutination and impaired sperm function).[176,177] Sympathetic nervous system dysfunction (e.g., associated with autonomic neuropathy, sympatholytic drugs, sympathectomy, retroperitoneal or abdominopelvic surgery, spinal cord injury or disease, vasovasostomy) may contribute to impaired sperm transport and male infertility.

Ejaculatory dysfunction may cause or contribute to male infertility by preventing normal or efficient deposition of sperm into the vagina and female genital tract. Premature or retarded ejaculation may contribute to infertility if ejaculation occurs during arousal or foreplay before vaginal penetration or after withdrawal from the vagina. Retrograde ejaculation of semen into the bladder rather than the urethra occurs with neuromuscular failure of normal bladder sphincter contraction during ejaculation. Retrograde ejaculation may be associated with prostatectomy or bladder neck surgery (e.g., transurethral resection of the prostate [TURP]), autonomic neuropathy (e.g., complicating diabetes mellitus), or sympathetic nervous system dysfunction, and in particular with sympatholytic drugs (e.g., α-adrenergic receptor antagonists such as prazosin or terazosin), retroperitoneal or abdominopelvic surgery (e.g., retroperitoneal lymph node dissection), and spinal cord injury or disease. Reduced ejaculation caused by androgen deficiency or resistance, sympathetic nervous system dysfunction, or urethral abnormalities may contribute to reduced sperm delivery to the female genital tract.

Erectile dysfunction may contribute to male infertility by causing unsuccessful completion of intercourse. Coital disorders are uncommon causes of male infertility, but they are potentially correctable with proper education. Infrequent sexual intercourse, excessive intercourse with other partners or masturbation, intercourse during menses rather than just before or around the time of ovulation, and premature withdrawal of the penis during intercourse may contribute to reduced fertility.

Evaluation. Because a coexisting female factor contributes to infertility in 30% of cases, it is important for the female partner to undergo evaluation for ovulation (menstrual periods, androgenization) and for cervical disorders (postcoital testing) and uterine and tubal disorders (hysterosalpingogram, pelvic ultrasound). In men, the history and physical examination are usually able to identify the potential cause of male infertility.[170-172]

In addition to an assessment of general health and medical comorbid conditions, the initial clinical evaluation should focus on the following:
- Symptoms and signs of androgen deficiency or resistance (as detailed elsewhere in this chapter)
- Scrotal examination for presence of a varicocele, presence and size of the testes, and presence or absence of firm, fibrous cords of the vas deferens
- Family history or evidence of cystic fibrosis
- Previous vasectomy or vasovasostomy
- History or manifestations of genitourinary infections
- Medications, particularly ones that cause androgen deficiency or resistance and sympatholytic agents
- Ejaculatory problems, in particular absent or reduced ejaculate
- Autonomic neuropathy (e.g., complicating diabetes mellitus)
- Retroperitoneal or abdominopelvic surgery

- Spinal cord injury or disease
- Erectile dysfunction
- Coital practices and techniques

The initial laboratory evaluation of male infertility should begin with at least two or three seminal fluid analyses performed over a period of a few months (see later discussion) to assess semen volume, sperm count and concentration, and sperm motility and morphologic appearance, with the aim of identifying men who have impaired sperm production or function, the major cause of male infertility. The presence of leukocytes in semen (>10^6/mL, termed *leukospermia* or *pyospermia*) may suggest a genitourinary inflammation or infection, but routine cultures are not usually helpful in guiding treatment. Agglutination of spermatozoa in semen (i.e., sticking of motile sperm to each other) suggests the presence of *antisperm antibodies,* which can be measured in semen and and may indicate an immunologic cause of male infertility.

Seminal fluid fructose is derived mostly from the seminal vesicles (60%) and to a lesser extent from the prostate gland (30%). Absent or low seminal fluid fructose and low semen volume suggest either congenital absence of the vas deferens and seminal vesicles or obstruction of the ejaculatory ducts. Dilated seminal vesicles may be detected on transrectal ultrasonography to confirm the presence of ejaculatory duct obstruction. In men who have little or no ejaculate, a postejaculatory urine specimen should be collected and examined for the presence of sperm, indicating retrograde ejaculation.

If there are clinical manifestations of androgen deficiency, serum testosterone levels should be measured on at least two occasions to confirm androgen deficiency, and measurements of LH and FSH should be performed to determine whether the patient has primary or secondary hypogonadism (see later discussion). Identification of infertile men with secondary hypogonadism potentially has important therapeutic implications. In men with impaired sperm production due to gonadotropin deficiency, spermatogenesis may be stimulated and fertility restored with the use of gonadotropin or GnRH therapy. Secondary hypogonadism is one of few treatable causes of male infertility. Elevated levels of testosterone, LH, and FSH suggest androgen resistance.

Measurements of FSH levels specifically as a marker of Sertoli cell and seminiferous tubule function are useful in identifying men with severe defects in spermatogenesis and impairment of seminiferous tubule and Sertoli cell function; such patients often demonstrate selective elevation in serum FSH concentrations with normal or high-normal LH levels due to loss of negative feedback inhibition of pituitary FSH secretion by inhibin B.[178] However, men with less severe seminiferous tubule dysfunction and impairment of spermatogenesis and those with azoospermia due to genital tract obstruction (obstructive azoospermia) have normal serum FSH levels.

Genetic disorders make up a small but significant proportion of the causes of male infertility. Because ART, and specifically ICSI, which involves direct injection of spermatozoa into the cytoplasm of an ovum (discussed later), is commonly used to treat male infertility, the potential exists for transmission of genetic defects to offspring. Therefore, genetic testing and counseling should be undertaken for men who are considering ICSI, particularly for those with severe oligozoospermia or azoospermia.[170-172]

Men in whom bilateral congenital absence of the vas or genital tract obstruction is suspected (i.e., those with low semen volume, low fructose level, and nonpalpable vas deferens in the scrotum) and those who have unexplained obstructive azoospermia should undergo genetic testing for *CFTR* mutations and genetic counseling before ICSI. In men with severe oligozoospermia (sperm concentration <5 million/mL) or azoospermia, testing for Y chromosome microdeletions in the *AZF* region should be performed routinely. There is a high prevalence of sex chromosome and autosomal chromosome defects, often in the absence of other phenotypic abnormalities, in men with moderately impaired spermatogenesis and infertility. Therefore, karyotyping is recommended before ICSI for infertile men with impaired sperm production, and in particular for those with a sperm concentration of less than 10 million/mL.

In azoospermic men with normal semen volume, a normal fructose level, and a normal FSH level in whom it is unclear whether azoospermia is caused by germ cell failure, genital tract obstruction, or both, surgical exploration of the scrotum and testis biopsy are needed. Biopsy is also used to harvest sperm for ICSI, even in men with known severe impairment in spermatogenesis, such as those with Klinefelter syndrome.[170,171,179,180]

Specialized tests of in vitro sperm function, such as detailed examination of sperm motility using computer-assisted semen analysis (CASA), cervical mucus penetration tests, acrosome reaction, and human zona pellucida binding tests, may be useful in some men who are considering intrauterine insemination or in vitro fertilization. However, these tests should be performed only in highly specialized laboratories that have demonstrated excellent quality control. Even in such laboratories, there is a high rate of clinical false-positive and false-negative results, limiting the clinical utility of these tests.

Treatment. In men with infertility caused by primary hypogonadism (whether due to androgen deficiency and impairment of sperm production or to isolated impairment of sperm production or function), defects in sperm production are not treatable, although spontaneous recovery of spermatogenesis may occur at variable times after discontinuation of cytotoxic drugs or ionizing radiation. Because intratesticular testosterone concentrations are normally approximately 100-fold higher than serum levels, exogenous testosterone treatment of men with androgen deficiency cannot deliver sufficient amounts of testosterone to support sperm production in the testis.

In men with secondary hypogonadism, on the other hand, sperm production can be stimulated with gonadotropin or GnRH treatment, or spermatogenesis may recover sufficiently to restore fertility after discontinuation of drugs that suppress gonadotropins, such as androgenic anabolic steroids, progestins, glucocorticoids, and drugs causing hyperprolactinemia.

Most men with a varicocele and infertility have abnormal seminal fluid. However, varicocele repair has not been demonstrated to be effective in restoring fertility to these men. Therefore, unless a varicocele is very large or symptomatic, surgical repair is not recommended.[12,181] Although the efficacy of treatment is unclear, infertile men with leukospermia or sperm agglutination are usually treated empirically with a 14-day course of antibiotics, such as doxycycline, trimethoprim-sulfamethoxazole, or a fluoroquinolone. Although high-dose prednisone (40 to 60 mg for several months) has been shown to be effective in treating infertile men with antisperm antibodies, the risks of high-dose glucocorticoid treatment are substantial, and this therapy cannot be recommended given the safer alternative of ICSI.

Although ICSI is costly, it is used increasingly to treat male infertility, and it dramatically improves the prognosis for men with impaired sperm production regardless of the cause.[179,180] Spermatozoa that are ejaculated or obtained by testicular biopsy *(testicular sperm extraction [TESE])* or from the epididymis *(microsurgical epididymal sperm aspiration [MESA])* are used for ICSI and other ARTs. With ICSI, fertilization rates of about 60% and pregnancy rates of approximately 20% are achieved, irrespective of the cause of male infertility or source of spermatozoa. ICSI after TESE using microsurgical testis biopsy or fine-needle aspiration to retrieve sperm has been successful in restoring fertility to men with primary hypogonadism who had severe impairments in spermatogenesis and azoospermia that were previously thought to be untreatable (e.g., Klinefelter syndrome, prolonged azoospermia after chemotherapy).[182] Because of the potential for chromosomal abnormalities and transmission of Y chromosome microdeletions and *CFTR* mutations that cause infertility in male offspring, genetic testing and counseling should be conducted if ICSI is being considered (see earlier discussion).[172]

Obstruction of the epididymides or the ejaculatory ducts can be corrected surgically, such as with end-to-end anastomosis of the epididymides or transurethral resection of the ejaculatory ducts. More commonly, MESA is used to obtain spermatozoa that can be incubated with ova in vitro *(in vitro fertilization [IVF])* or directly injected into an ovum (ICSI), and this method is more successful in restoring fertility than surgical options. In contrast, microsurgical reanastomosis of the vas (vasovasostomy) to reverse vasectomy is less costly and more successful in restoring fertility than MESA followed by IVF or ICSI. Return of sperm in the ejaculate occurs in approximately 90% of men who undergo vasectomy reversal, but restoration of fertility occurs in only about 50%, probably because of stenosis or blockage of the previous vasovasostomy, epididymal blockage, or the development of antisperm antibodies in response to the vasectomy.[183]

In men with retrograde ejaculation, collection of spermatozoa in alkalinized postejaculation urine, followed by extensive washing and *intrauterine insemination (IUI)* or ICSI, has been used successfully to treat infertility. With proper education, coital disorders that contribute to infertility may be corrected. Also, the timing of intercourse may be optimized to occur a few days before and after ovulation (the period of highest probability for conception) based on basal body temperature measurements or, more accurately, on commercially available rapid urinary LH kits to estimate the timing of ovulation in the female partner.

If the treatment options described previously are not available or affordable to infertile couples who desire children, artificial insemination with donor sperm or adoption may be considered.

Diagnosis of Male Hypogonadism
Clinical Manifestations of Androgen Deficiency

The diagnosis of male hypogonadism requires clinical manifestations consistent with androgen deficiency and unequivocally low serum testosterone levels. In community-dwelling middle-aged to older men, the crude prevalence of symptomatic androgen deficiency is 2% to 9%, depending on the constellation of symptoms and signs and the biochemical definition of androgen deficiency used (i.e., the threshold used for a single low testosterone level).[184-186] This prevalence increases with age and is much higher in a primary care setting.[187] In community populations, the prevalence of low testosterone levels alone, without consideration of symptoms and signs of androgen deficiency, is much higher than that of clinical androgen deficiency. This underscores the importance of making a diagnosis of hypogonadism only in men who have clinical manifestations and consistently low testosterone levels. Both the

clinical and the biochemical diagnosis of androgen deficiency can be challenging, especially in older adults.

Although the manifestations of fetal androgen deficiency or resistance (ambiguous genitalia and 46,XY DSD) and those of prepubertal androgen deficiency (eunuchoidism) are usually clinically obvious, the clinical diagnosis of androgen deficiency in adults is more difficult. As described previously, the symptoms and signs of androgen deficiency are nonspecific and have a broad differential diagnosis. Moreover, clinical manifestations may be modified by a number of factors, such as the severity and duration of androgen deficiency, age, comorbid illnesses, medications, previous testosterone treatment, and individual variations in androgen sensitivity, all of which contribute to variability in clinical presentation that may confound the diagnosis.[113] Because the manifestations of androgen deficiency in adults are nonspecific, other potential causes (such as depression, comorbid illness, or medications) should be considered in the differential diagnosis to explain clinical features in any individual patient.[188]

The degree and duration of androgen deficiency have impressive effects on clinical manifestations. The severe and relatively rapid suppression of testosterone levels in men with prostate cancer treated with a GnRH agonist or orchidectomy results in prominent clinical manifestations with notable reductions in erectile function, libido, energy, and mood; hot flushes and sleep disturbances; infertility; decreases in muscle mass and strength, BMD (associated with an increase in fracture risk), and body hair; gynecomastia; increases in body fat; anemia; and possibly increases in the risks for diabetes mellitus and for cardiovascular events.[189,190] In contrast, men with mild androgen deficiency may have few or no referable manifestations; such patients have "subclinical" androgen deficiency that may or may not be associated with clinically significant outcomes. The latter situation is analogous to that observed in other endocrine disorders such as subclinical hypothyroidism or asymptomatic primary hyperparathyroidism.

Aging is associated with alterations in body functions, such as declines in sexual function, muscle mass and strength, and BMD, that result in clinical manifestations similar to those of androgen deficiency.[139] These alterations associated with aging may also be caused in part by age-related androgen deficiency. To add to the clinical complexity in older men, age-associated comorbid illnesses and medications used to treat these illnesses may modify the symptoms and signs of androgen deficiency, and in many instances, they may also contribute to the cause of androgen deficiency. Therefore, it is understandable why the diagnosis of clinical androgen deficiency is challenging in older men, and particularly in frail elderly men who have multiple comorbid illnesses and are taking numerous medications.

Previous testosterone treatment that has been discontinued may affect the clinical manifestations of androgen deficiency, depending on the duration of therapy and the time since discontinuation. It is also likely that clinical manifestations of androgen deficiency are affected by individual variations in androgen action on specific target organs. Alterations in androgen sensitivity may result from individual or tissue-specific differences in the activity of the AR or the ER and associated coregulators or from differences in active metabolism to estradiol or DHT, or inactivation of testosterone.

In men with clinical manifestations suggestive of androgen deficiency, the diagnosis of hypogonadism is confirmed biochemically by measurement of consistently low serum testosterone concentrations (Fig. 19-19).[113]

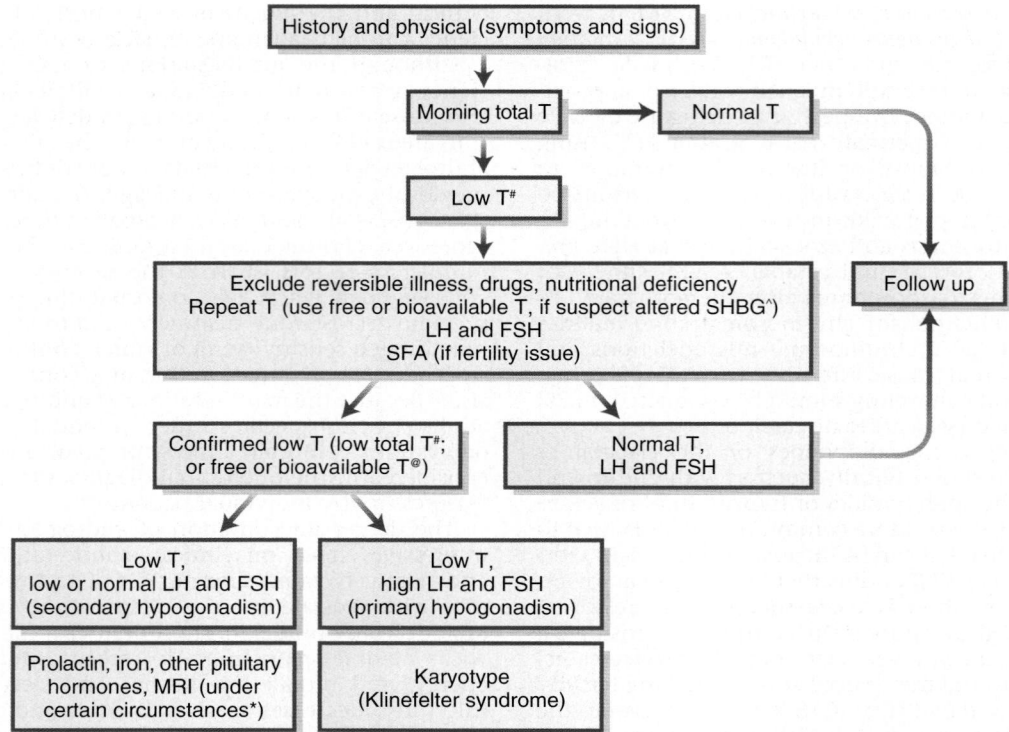

Figure 19-19 Algorithm for the diagnosis and evaluation of suspected androgen deficiency. In men with clinical manifestations (symptoms and signs) consistent with androgen deficiency, a morning serum total testosterone (T) measurement should be obtained. #The normal range for total T in healthy young men varies in different laboratories, but the lower limit of normal for most reliable assays is 280 to 300 ng/dL (9.8 to 10.4 nmol/L). If the initial total T concentration is low, the measurement should be repeated to confirm the presence of biochemical androgen deficiency. Reversible illnesses, drugs, or nutritional deficiencies that can transiently lower T levels should be ruled out before making a diagnosis of male hypogonadism. ^If a condition is present that could cause an alteration in the level of sex hormone–binding globulin (SHBG), an accurate measurement of free or bioavailable T (instead of total T) should be obtained to confirm the presence of biochemical androgen deficiency. @The normal range for accurate measurements of free testosterone (free T by equilibrium dialysis and calculated free T) in healthy young men varies in different laboratories but is usually 5 to 6 ng/dL (0.17 to 0.31 nmol/L). Levels of luteinizing hormone (LH) and follicle-stimulating hormone (FSH) should be obtained with T to determine whether androgen deficiency is caused by secondary hypogonadism (low T with low or normal LH and FSH) or by primary hypogonadism (low T with high LH and FSH). *In men with secondary hypogonadism, assessment of serum prolactin, serum iron, and other pituitary hormones, with or without magnetic resonance imaging (MRI), should be considered for further evaluation. In men with primary hypogonadism and consistent clinical features (e.g., very small testes), a karyotype should be considered to confirm the diagnosis of Klinefelter syndrome. SFA, seminal fluid analysis. (From Bhasin S, Cunningham GR, Hayes FJ, et al. Testosterone therapy in men with androgen deficiency syndromes: an Endocrine Society clinical practice guideline. *J Clin Endocrinol Metab.* 2010;95:2536-2559.)

Testosterone Measurements

As with the clinical manifestations, the biochemical confirmation of androgen deficiency presents its own difficulties. Testosterone levels exhibit both biologic and assay variability. Total testosterone concentrations are affected by alterations in SHBG, and testosterone levels may be suppressed transiently with illness, certain medications, and some nutritional deficiencies.[113] Therefore, the biochemical diagnosis of androgen deficiency requires demonstration of consistently and unequivocally low serum testosterone levels on at least two occasions and preferably measured in the morning. In men who have conditions that alter SHBG, accurate and reliable free or bioavailable testosterone measurements are needed to confirm the diagnosis of hypogonadism. Finally, the diagnosis of hypogonadism should not be made during acute or subacute illness.

The threshold level of circulating total or free testosterone below which symptoms and signs of androgen deficiency occur and for which testosterone treatment will improve clinical manifestations is not known. However, the concept of a single threshold testosterone level is probably not valid, nor is it clinically useful, because thresholds vary with the specific symptom and the androgen target organ or tissue. In general, symptoms and signs of andro-

gen deficiency are more likely to occur with a total testosterone level that is below the lower limit of the normal range for young healthy men (approximately 280 to 300 ng/dL or 2.8 to 3.0 ng/mL [9.7 to 10.4 nmol/L], when using an accurate and reliable assay). The likelihood and severity of clinical manifestations of androgen deficiency increase with a greater decline in testosterone level below normal.

Variability in Testosterone Levels. Because serum testosterone levels exhibit both biologic and assay variability, a single measurement is not a reliable indicator of an individual's average concentration. Serum testosterone levels exhibit both ultradian and circadian variation, providing physiologic sources of biologic variability. Ultradian fluctuations in serum testosterone levels, characterized by peaks of incremental amplitude that average approximately 240 ng/dL (40% fractional amplitude) with a 95-minute duration,[45] have been reported in a small number of young men; more chaotic peaks with lower amplitude have been reported in older men.[191] As described previously, the circadian variation in serum testosterone peaks at about 8 AM and has a maximum excursion averaging 140 ng/dL.[64] The circadian variation in testosterone is blunted but still present in older men, with a maximum excursion averaging 60 ng/dL. In young men, serum testosterone levels are 20% to 25% lower at 4 PM than at 8 AM (i.e., over the course of usual clinic hours).[192] This difference decreases with age: in 70-year-old men, testosterone levels are 10% lower at 4 PM than at 8 AM. Most importantly, many young and old men who have testosterone concentrations that are below normal in the afternoon have consistently normal levels in the morning. Testosterone levels are also suppressed with glucose infusion or food intake,[193,194] and thus measurements should preferably be done in the fasting state. Given these findings and the fact that normal ranges of testosterone concentration are usually based on morning blood samples, testosterone measurements to confirm the diagnosis of hypogonadism should preferably be performed in the morning in the fasting state.

There is also substantial day-to-day variation in serum testosterone concentrations, underscoring the need to repeat the measurement to confirm low levels, particularly if the first result was only moderately below normal. Among men with serum testosterone levels of less than 300 ng/dL on an initial test, 30% to 35% were found to have a normal level on repeat testing.[195] Among community-dwelling middle-aged to older men who had an initial serum testosterone concentration of less than 250 ng/dL, 20% were found to have an average testosterone level higher than 300 ng/dL (i.e., within the normal range) when six samples were drawn over the subsequent 6 months.[196] However, none of the subjects who had an initial average serum testosterone concentration of less than 250 ng/dL on two separate samples obtained 1 to 3 days apart had an average level higher than 300 ng/dL in six samples drawn over the next 6 months. These findings support the need to measure testosterone on at least two occasions to confirm the diagnosis of androgen deficiency.

Total Testosterone Assays. Total testosterone assays are performed in most local laboratories and are readily available to clinicians. Therefore, total testosterone is recommended as the initial measurement for the assessment of androgen deficiency. In local clinical laboratories, total testosterone is usually measured by automated platform-based direct immunoassays on unextracted serum or plasma. However, there is substantial variability in results from different assays, mostly because the accreditation of laboratories has been based on the reproducibility of results in comparison to other laboratories using the same method or kit, rather than on the accuracy of results. For example, when identical quality control samples were assayed by different methods or kits, the reported measured values ranged from 160 to 508 ng/dL. Moreover, the lower limit of the normal range in some assays was as low as 132 to 210 ng/dL (clearly in the hypogonadal range for most conventional assays).[197] In contrast, the lower limit of the normal range based on conventional radioimmunoassays after extraction is approximately 280 to 300 ng/dL.

Most commercial reference laboratories now measure testosterone by liquid chromatography tandem mass spectrometry methods after solid phase extraction that have the potential to be more accurate than immunoassays. To address the problems in the quality control of testosterone assays, the U.S. Centers for Disease Control and Prevention (CDC) has initiated a program to standardize and harmonize testosterone assays using accuracy-based quality control standards to which most commercial reference laboratories participate.[198] Recently, the College of American Pathologists also instituted an accuracy-based quality control program that unfortunately is not mandatory for certification.

The prevalence of low testosterone concentrations is high in a number of clinical conditions, namely, presence of a pituitary or sellar mass; irradiation; disease; use of certain medications, such as opiates or high-dose glucocor-

ticoids; HIV disease with weight loss; late-stage CKD, especially with hemodialysis; moderate to severe chronic lung disease; infertility; BMD levels that reveal osteoporosis or low-trauma fracture; and type 2 diabetes mellitus (T2DM). If clinical manifestations consistent with androgen deficiency are present in men with these conditions, testosterone measurements should be performed.[113]

Total Testosterone Affected by Alterations in Sex Hormone–Binding Globulin. Because a substantial proportion (30% to 40%) of circulating testosterone is bound tightly to SHBG, alterations in SHBG concentration may affect total testosterone levels without altering free or bioavailable testosterone. Conditions that suppress SHBG levels (even within the broad normal range) lower total testosterone (sometimes to below the normal range) without affecting circulating free or bioavailable testosterone levels (Table 19-5).[113] Common conditions that lower SHBG concentrations include moderate obesity, often associated with T2DM; protein-losing states, such as nephrotic syndrome; administration of glucocorticoids, progestins, or androgens; hypothyroidism; acromegaly; and familial SHBG deficiency. SHBG concentrations are increased with increasing age; hepatic cirrhosis and inflammation (hepatitis of any cause); estrogens; hyperthyroidism; anticonvulsants; and HIV disease.

If conditions that affect SHBG concentration are present in a patient or if total testosterone concentrations are close to the lower limit of the normal range, serum free or bioavailable testosterone measurements should be obtained to confirm androgen deficiency. Unfortunately, accurate and reliable assays for free or bioavailable testosterone are not performed routinely in most local clinical laboratories. Although direct free testosterone assays using automated platform-based analogue immunoassay methods are available, these assays are inaccurate and are affected by alterations in SHBG, so they offer no advantage over total testosterone measurements and are not recommended.[199-201]

The gold standard method for measurement of free testosterone levels is equilibrium dialysis or centrifugal ultrafiltration. Free testosterone concentrations may be calculated accurately from measurements of total testosterone, SHBG, and albumin using affinity constants for binding of testosterone to its binding proteins and published formulas. Calculated free testosterone values are comparable to those measured by equilibrium dialysis.[200] However, calculated values depend on the specific testosterone and SHBG assays employed and the formula used to estimate free testosterone.[202] There are a number of formulae used for calculation of free testosterone that all demonstrate some bias relative to the equilibrium dialysis method, largely as a result of assuming a single or

TABLE 19-5

Conditions Associated with Alterations in SHBG Concentrations

Decreased SHBG Concentrations	Increased SHBG Concentrations
Moderate obesity, type 2 diabetes mellitus	Aging
Nephrotic syndrome	Hepatic cirrhosis and hepatitis
Glucocorticoids, progestins, and androgens	Estrogens
Hypothyroidism	Hyperthyroidism
Acromegaly	Anticonvulsants
Familial SHBG deficiency	HIV disease

HIV, human immunodeficiency virus; SHBG, sex hormone–binding globulin.
From Bhasin S, Cunningham GR, Hayes FJ, et al. Testosterone therapy in men with androgen deficiency syndromes; an Endocrine Society clinical practice guideline. *J Clin Endocrinol Metab.* 2010;95:2536-2559.

two identical, noninteracting binding sites on SHBG.[110] However, they all provide reasonable approximations of free testosterone in the normal to low range of values that are less prone to misinterpretation and overdiagnosis of hypogonadism than total testosterone measurements when alterations in SHBG levels are present.

Bioavailable testosterone is measured by ammonium sulfate precipitation of SHBG-bound testosterone and measurement of free and albumin-bound testosterone in the supernatant. Bioavailable testosterone levels may also be calculated from measurements of total testosterone, SHBG, and albumin. These accurate and reliable measurements of free and bioavailable testosterone are available in commercial laboratories and should be used to confirm androgen deficiency in men who have conditions that affect SHBG and in those with total testosterone levels near the lower limit of the normal range. In a recent report, 60% of over 3700 men in a single health care system who had low total testosterone levels were found to have normal calculated free testosterone concentrations using the laboratory reference range that was utilized by practitioners to make clinical decisions. These findings highlight the potential clinical importance of using free testosterone to confirm a biochemical diagnosis of hypogonadism.[203]

Transient Suppression of Testosterone. In evaluating men for a diagnosis of male hypogonadism, it is important to recognize that serum testosterone levels may be suppressed transiently during acute (particularly critical) and subacute illness and recovery; with the short-term use of certain medications, such as opioids, high-dose glucocorticoids, and CNS-active medications or recreational drugs that suppress gonadotropin and testosterone production; and during transient malnutrition, such as that associated with illness, eating disorders, or excessive or prolonged strenuous exercise (resulting in low energy intake relative to energy expenditure). In such situations, measurement of serum testosterone should be delayed until the patient is completely recovered from the illness, the offending drugs are discontinued, the malnutrition is corrected, or the excessive exercise is stopped.[113]

Case-Finding in Androgen Deficiency

In the absence of evidence for long-term clinically meaningful health benefits greater than risks for testosterone treatment of androgen deficiency, screening for androgen deficiency in the general population or in all elderly men is not indicated. Existing case-finding instruments lack sufficient specificity and sensitivity to be clinically useful. In certain clinical conditions, there is a high prevalence of low testosterone concentrations and androgen deficiency, and measurement of serum testosterone should be performed. These conditions include hypothalamic-pituitary mass, disease, surgery, or radiation therapy; medications that suppress testosterone production (e.g., opioids, glucocorticoids); HIV-associated weight loss and other wasting syndromes; and osteoporosis or minimal-trauma fragility fracture, especially in young men. In patients with a chronic disease in which low testosterone and hypogonadism are common (e.g., T2DM, CKD, chronic obstructive pulmonary disease [COPD]), serum testosterone should be measured if symptoms or signs indicative of androgen deficiency (e.g., sexual dysfunction, weakness) are present.[113]

Seminal Fluid Analysis

If infertility is a main complaint, whether or not androgen deficiency is also present, seminal fluid analysis should be performed to determine the presence and degree of impair-

TABLE 19-6

Normal Seminal Fluid Analysis

Parameter	Normal Value
Sperm concentration	≥15 million/mL
Semen volume	≥1.5 mL
Sperm count	≥39 million per ejaculate
Sperm motility	≥40% (progressive sperm motility >32%)
Sperm morphology	≥4% normal forms (by strict criteria excluding sperm with mild abnormalities)

From *WHO Laboratory Manual for the Examination and Processing of Human Semen*, 5th ed. Geneva, Switzerland: World Health Organization; 2010.

ment of sperm production. Seminal fluid analyses are performed on ejaculated semen samples obtained by masturbation after a standardized period (usually 48 hours) of abstinence from ejaculation. Semen collection after withdrawal of the penis from the partner just before ejaculation during sexual intercourse (coitus interruptus) is usually incomplete and is not recommended, but it may be an option if masturbation is not possible or is not permitted for personal or religious reasons. Seminal fluid analyses should be performed in a specialized laboratory that employs standardized procedures, such as those outlined by the World Health Organization (WHO), and is certified and qualified to carry out these procedures.[29]

According to recently revised WHO criteria based on approximately 1800 to 1900 men from 14 countries whose partners became pregnant in 12 months or less (Table 19-6), the lower limit of normal sperm concentration is 15 million/mL; semen volume is 1.5 mL; total sperm count is 39 million per ejaculate; total sperm motility (both progressive and nonprogressive) is 40% and progressive sperm motility is 32%; and the percentage of sperm with normal morphologic forms, using strict criteria to eliminate spermatozoa with even mild abnormalities, is at least 4%.[29] Values below these lower limits may be classified as falling into the subfertile range, and such values are found in independent (unscreened) populations. In another study, the subfertile ranges were defined as follows: sperm concentration, less than 13.5 million/mL; motility, less than 32%; and strict morphologic structure, less than 9%. The respective fertile ranges were greater than 48 million/mL for sperm concentration, 63% for motility, and 12% for strict morphologic structure. Values between these ranges indicated indeterminate fertility.[204]

Sperm counts and concentrations exhibit extreme variability (Fig. 19-20)[9] for a number of reasons, including variations in sexual activity and abstinence, completeness of collection, recent illness (especially febrile illness) that may suppress spermatogenesis, and lifestyle factors such as frequent hot tub use. Therefore, at least two or three seminal fluid analyses, separated by at least 2 weeks, should be performed to assess sperm production adequately. Also, to assess motility, freshly collected semen (within 1 hour of ejaculation) should be used, necessitating collection at or near the laboratory in which the analysis is to be performed.

Gonadotropin Measurements

Androgen Deficiency and Impaired Sperm Production. The diagnosis of hypogonadism is confirmed in men with symptoms and signs consistent with androgen deficiency and in whom low testosterone levels are found on at least two occasions. Testosterone levels should not be measured shortly after an acute illness, medication use, or nutritional deficiency that could transiently lower testosterone. Furthermore, an accurate assay of low free or bioavailable testosterone should be performed for men who have

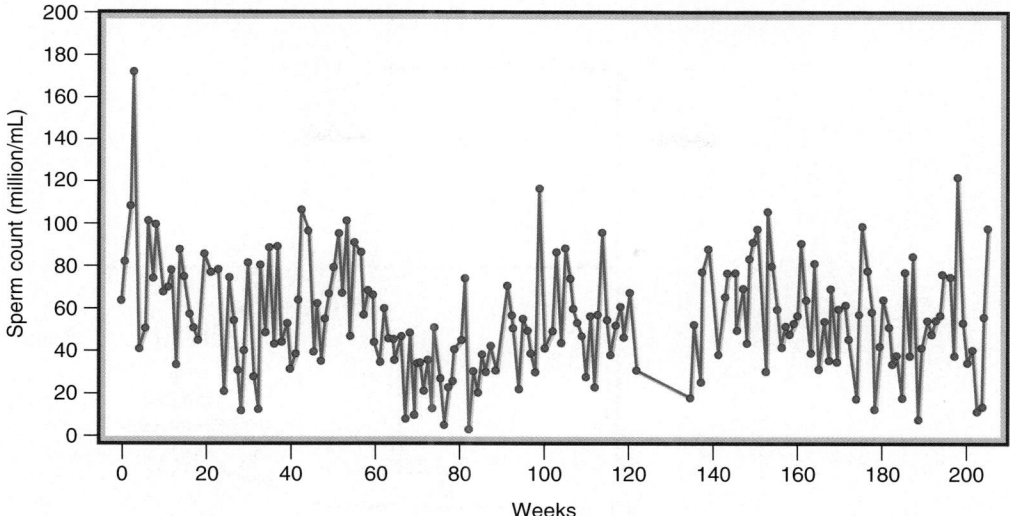

Figure 19-20 Normal variation in sperm concentration (millions of spermatozoa per milliliter of ejaculate) in a healthy young man: results of frequent sampling over a period of 210 weeks. At several times during this period, sperm concentrations dropped below the normal range (15 million/mL). (From Matsumoto AM. The testis. In: Felig P, Frohman LA, eds. *Endocrinology and Metabolism*, 4th ed. New York, NY: McGraw-Hill; 2001:635-705.)

conditions that alter SHBG or a total testosterone level near the lower limit of normal. In men with confirmed hypogonadism, measurements of serum gonadotropins, LH, and FSH should be measured to distinguish primary from secondary hypogonadism (see Fig. 19-19).[113]

Men with primary hypogonadism caused by a disorder of the testis have low serum testosterone in association with elevated LH and FSH levels as a result of reduced negative feedback suppression of gonadotropin secretion by testosterone and inhibin B (Fig. 19-21).[9] In contrast, men with secondary hypogonadism caused by a disorder of the pituitary or the hypothalamus (or both) have low testosterone in association with low gonadotropin levels or inappropriately normal LH and FSH given the presence of low testosterone levels (Fig. 19-22).[9] In most local clinical laboratories, LH and FSH are measured by newer-generation nonradioactive immunoassays that have sufficient sensitivity to distinguish between normal and low concentrations.

Aging, some systemic illnesses (e.g., hemochromatosis), and certain medications (e.g., glucocorticoids) may cause defects in both the testes and the hypothalamus or pituitary, resulting in combined primary and secondary hypogonadism. In most cases, a hormonal pattern consistent with either primary or secondary hypogonadism predominates. For example, men with hemochromatosis have defects in both the pituitary and the testes due to iron overload, but they usually have low testosterone and gonadotropin levels, consistent mostly with secondary hypogonadism. Men with late-stage CKD have both testis and hypothalamic-pituitary dysfunction but usually have low testosterone and elevated LH and FSH concentrations, the latter mostly due to reduced clearance of gonadotropins by the kidney. However, in the presence of comorbid illness, nutritional deficiency, or certain medications, men with CKD may have suppression of gonadotropins and testosterone into the normal range and hormonal pattern consistent with secondary hypogonadism. Some men have more than one disorder influencing the gonadal axis, one affecting the testis and another affecting the hypothalamus or pituitary. This may result in a hormonal pattern that is predominantly consistent with either primary or secondary hypogonadism or in a combined pattern (e.g.,

very low testosterone levels with only slightly elevated or high-normal gonadotropin levels that are lower than expected given the presence of very low testosterone concentrations).

Distinguishing primary from secondary hypogonadism helps to define the specific cause of hypogonadism and has important clinical and therapeutic implications.[9] Secondary hypogonadism may be caused by a destructive process in the pituitary or hypothalamus, such as a pituitary adenoma. A large pituitary adenoma (macroadenoma) may cause space-occupying tumor mass effects such as headaches, visual field defects, hydrocephalus, or cerebrospinal fluid rhinorrhea, or it may result in impaired or excessive secretion of some anterior pituitary hormones, leading to clinical manifestations and therapeutic implications beyond the treatment of androgen deficiency alone. Secondary hypogonadism may be caused by disorders that are transient, such as an acute illness, certain medications (e.g., opioids, glucocorticoids), or malnutrition associated with illness. In such cases, androgen deficiency may resolve with treatment of and recovery from the illness or malnutrition or discontinuation of the offending medication. Finally, in men with secondary hypogonadism who have gonadotropin deficiency but otherwise normal testes, gonadotropin or GnRH treatment may be used to stimulate spermatogenesis and androgen production and to restore fertility in men who wish to father children. In contrast, infertility in men with primary hypogonadism is not treatable with hormone therapy.

Isolated Impairment of Sperm Production or Function. Most men with isolated impairment of sperm production have low sperm counts or abnormalities in sperm motility or morphologic appearance (or both) but no clinical manifestations of androgen deficiency and normal levels of testosterone and gonadotropins. Most men with isolated impairment of sperm production or function are classified as having primary hypogonadism with an isolated defect in the seminiferous tubule compartment of the testes (Table 19-7); in such cases, there is no response to gonadotropin treatment, as there is in secondary hypogonadism. Men with severe seminiferous tubule failure and azoospermia or severe oligozoospermia may demonstrate a selective elevation in FSH levels as a result in reduced negative

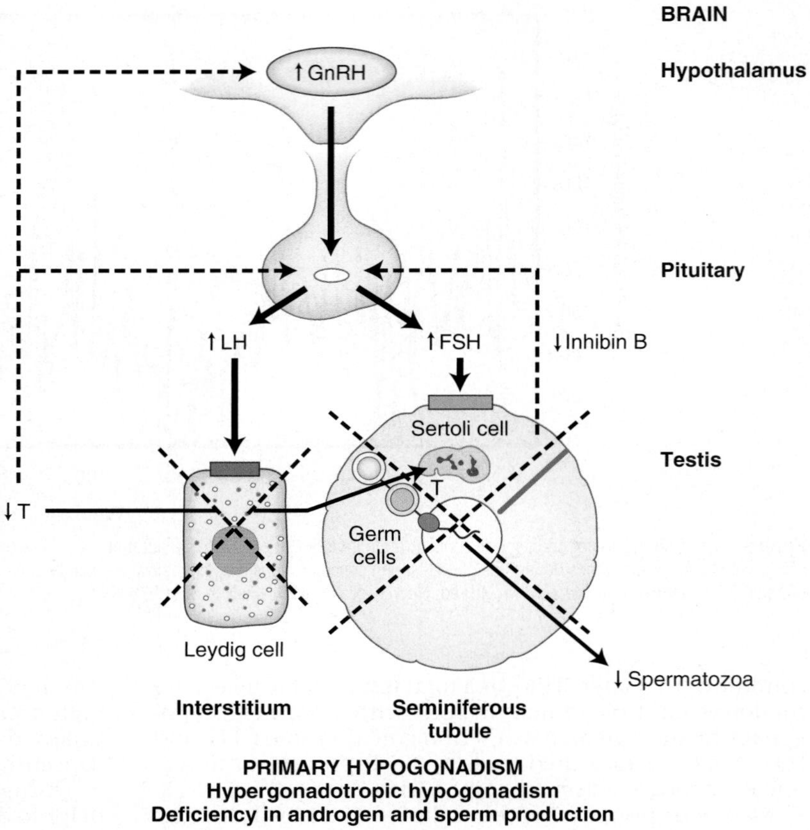

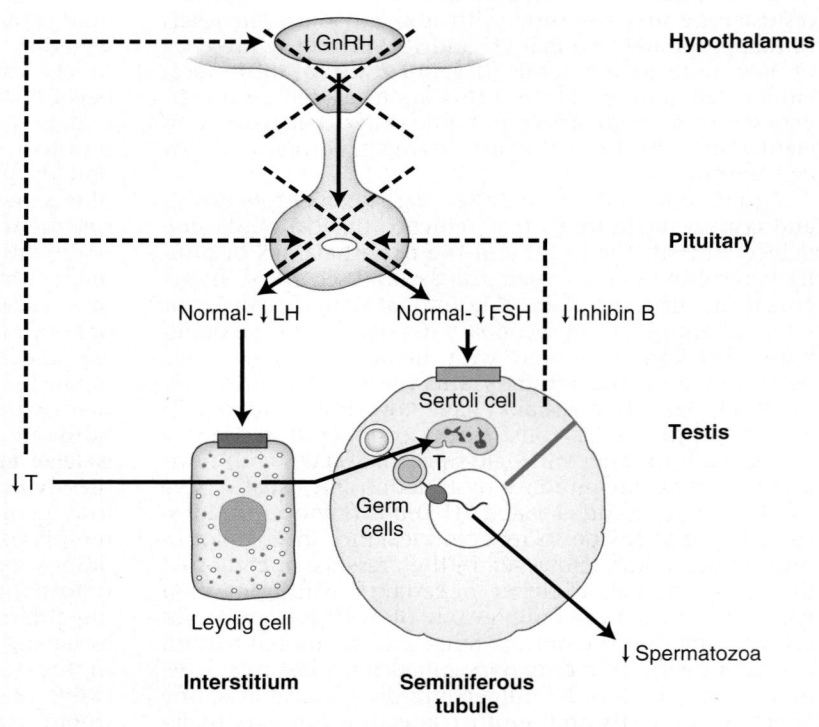

BRAIN

Hypothalamus

Pituitary

↑LH ↑FSH ↓Inhibin B

Sertoli cell

Testis

↓T

Germ cells

T

Leydig cell ↓Spermatozoa

Interstitium **Seminiferous tubule**

PRIMARY HYPOGONADISM
Hypergonadotropic hypogonadism
Deficiency in androgen and sperm production

Figure 19-21 Schematic diagram of alterations in the hypothalamic-pituitary-testicular axis with primary hypogonadism due to testicular disease, which results in both androgen deficiency and impairment of sperm production and elevated luteinizing hormone (LH) and follicle-stimulating hormone (FSH) levels (hypergonadotropic hypogonadism) due to loss of negative feedback regulation of gonadotropins. GnRH, gonadotropin-releasing hormone; T, testosterone. (From Matsumoto AM. The testis. In: Felig P, Frohman LA, eds. *Endocrinology and Metabolism,* 4th ed. New York, NY: McGraw-Hill; 2001:635-705.)

BRAIN

Hypothalamus

Pituitary

Normal-↓LH Normal-↓FSH ↓Inhibin B

Sertoli cell

Testis

↓T

Germ cells

T

Leydig cell ↓Spermatozoa

Interstitium **Seminiferous tubule**

SECONDARY HYPOGONADISM
Hypogonadotropic hypogonadism
Deficiency in androgen and sperm production

Figure 19-22 Schematic diagram of alterations in the hypothalamic-pituitary-testicular axis with secondary hypogonadism due to hypothalamic or pituitary disease, which results in both androgen deficiency and impairment of sperm production and inappropriately normal or low luteinizing hormone (LH) and follicle-stimulating hormone (FSH) levels (hypogonadotropic hypogonadism). GnRH, gonadotropin-releasing hormone; T, testosterone. (From Matsumoto AM. The testis. In: Felig P, Frohman LA, eds. *Endocrinology and Metabolism,* 4th ed. New York, NY: McGraw-Hill; 2001: 635-705.)

TABLE 19-7
Causes of Primary Hypogonadism

Common Causes	Uncommon Causes
Androgen Deficiency and Impairment of Sperm Production	
Congenital or Developmental Disorders	
Klinefelter syndrome (XXY) and variants	Myotonic dystrophy
	Uncorrected cryptorchidism
	Noonan syndrome
	Bilateral congenital anorchia
	Polyglandular autoimmune syndrome
	Testosterone biosynthetic enzyme defects
	CAH (testicular adrenal rest tumors)
	Complex genetic syndromes
	Down syndrome
	LH receptor mutation
Acquired Disorders	
Bilateral surgical castration or trauma	Orchitis
Drugs (spironolactone, ketoconazole, abiraterone, enzalutamide, alcohol, chemotherapy agents)	
Ionizing radiation	
Systemic Disorders	
Chronic liver disease (hepatic cirrhosis)*	Malignancy (lymphoma, testicular cancer)
Chronic kidney disease*	Sickle cell disease*
Aging*	Spinal cord injury
	Vasculitis (polyarteritis)
	Infiltrative disease (amyloidosis, leukemia)
Isolated Impairment of Sperm Prduction or Function	
Congenital or Developmental Disorders	
Cryptorchidism	Myotonic dystrophy
Varicocele	Sertoli cell–only syndrome
Y chromosome microdeletions	Primary ciliary dyskinesia
	Down syndrome
	FSH receptor mutation
Acquired Disorders	
Orchitis	Environmental toxins
Ionizing radiation	
Chemotherapy agents	
Thermal trauma	
Systemic Disorders	
Acute febrile illness	Spinal cord injury
Malignancy (testicular cancer, Hodgkin disease)*	
Idiopathic azoospermia or oligozoospermia	

*Combined primary and secondary hypogonadism.
CAH, congenital adrenal hyperplasia; FSH, follicle-stimulating hormone; LH, luteinizing hormone.

TABLE 19-8
Causes of Secondary Hypogonadism

Common Causes	Uncommon Causes
Androgen Deficiency and Impairment of Sperm Production	
Congenital or Developmental Disorders	
Constitutional delayed puberty	IHH and variants
Hemochromatosis	IHH
	Kallmann syndrome
	Congenital adrenal hypoplasia
	Isolated LH deficiency, LHβ mutations
	Complex genetic syndromes
Acquired Disorders	
Hyperprolactinemia	Hypopituitarism
Opioids	Pituitary or hypothalamic tumor
Androgenic anabolic steroids, progestins, estrogen excess	Surgical hypophysectomy, pituitary or cranial irradiation
GnRH agonist or antagonist	Vascular compromise, traumatic brain injury
	Granulomatous or infiltrative disease
	Infection
	Pituitary stalk disease
	Lymphocytic or autoimmune hypophysitis
Systemic Disorders	
Glucocorticoid excess (Cushing syndrome)*	Chronic systemic illness*
Chronic organ failure*	Spinal cord injury
Chronic liver disease (hepatic cirrhosis), chronic kidney disease, chronic lung disease, chronic heart failure	Transfusion-related iron overload (β-thalassemia)
Chronic systemic illness*	Sickle cell disease
Type 2 diabetes mellitus	Cystic fibrosis
Malignancy	
Rheumatic disease (rheumatoid arthritis)	
HIV disease	
Starvation,* malnutrition,* eating disorders, endurance exercise	
Morbid obesity, obstructive sleep apnea	
Acute and critical illness	
Aging*	
Isolated Impairment of Sperm Production or Function	
Congenital or Developmental Disorders	
	Congenital adrenal hyperplasia (21-hydroxylase deficiency, 11β-hydroxylase deficiency)
	Isolated FSH deficiency, FSHβ mutations
Acquired Disorders	
Testosterone, androgenic anabolic steroids	Androgen- or hCG-secreting tumors
Malignancy (Hodgkin disease, testicular cancer)*	Hyperprolactinemia

*Combined primary and secondary hypogonadism.
FSH, follicle-stimulating hormone; GnRH, gonadotropin-releasing hormone; hCG, human chorionic gonadotropin; HIV, human immunodeficiency virus; IHH, idiopathic hypogonadotropic hypogonadism; LH, luteinizing hormone.

feedback from inhibin B with normal LH levels (Fig. 19-23).[9] Occasionally, isolated impairment in sperm production is caused by gonadotropin deficiency (i.e., secondary hypogonadism) (Table 19-8); this may occur in men who are taking high doses of testosterone and in those who have androgen-secreting tumors, congenital adrenal hyperplasia, or, rarely, isolated FSH deficiency.

Men with nonfunctioning or gonadotropin-secreting pituitary tumors often have secondary hypogonadism with clinical manifestations of androgen deficiency and low testosterone levels.[53] Many of these men secrete excessive amounts of intact FSH and biologically inactive free α-, FSHβ-, and LHβ-subunits but rarely intact LH. Therefore, a gonadotropin-secreting pituitary tumor should be suspected in a man who has clinical manifestations of androgen deficiency, low testosterone, and elevated FSH but normal or low LH (or, rarely, elevated LH but normal or

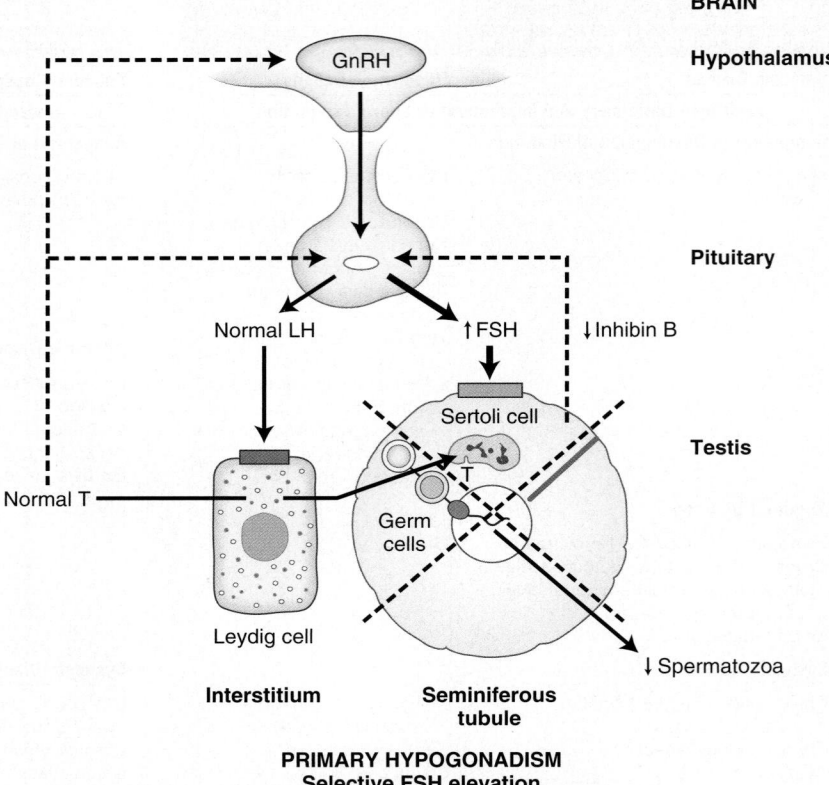

BRAIN

Hypothalamus

Pituitary

Testis

PRIMARY HYPOGONADISM
Selective FSH elevation
Isolated deficiency in sperm production

Figure 19-23 Schematic diagram of alterations in the hypothalamic-pituitary-testicular axis with primary hypogonadism due to an isolated seminiferous tubule defect, which results in isolated impairment of sperm production or function and elevation of follicle-stimulating hormone (FSH) levels with normal luteinizing hormone (LH) levels. With less severe seminiferous tubule defects, both FSH and LH levels are normal. GnRH, gonadotropin-releasing hormone; T, testosterone. (From Matsumoto AM. The testis. In: Felig P, Frohman LA, eds. *Endocrinology and Metabolism*, 4th ed. New York, NY: McGraw-Hill; 2001:635-705.)

TABLE 19-9	
Causes of Androgen Resistance	
Common Causes	**Uncommon Causes**
Congenital or Developmental Disorders	
	Kennedy disease (spinal and bulbar muscular atrophy)
	Partial androgen insensitivity syndrome (AR mutations)
	5α-Reductase type 2 deficiency
	Complete androgen insensitivity syndrome (female phenotype)
Acquired Disorders	
AR antagonists (bicalutamide, nilutamide)	Celiac disease
Drugs (spironolactone, cyproterone acetate, marijuana, histamine 2 receptor antagonists)	

AR, androgen receptor.

low FSH), which is an atypical gonadotropin pattern for men with androgen deficiency.

Rarely, disorders of androgen action or androgen resistance manifest in adults (Table 19-9). These men usually present with clinical manifestations similar to those of men with mild androgen deficiency, usually with an almost normal male phenotype and frequently with varying degrees of hypospadias, cryptorchidism, scrotal abnormalities, or impairment in sperm production. Usually, both serum testosterone and gonadotropin levels are elevated (Fig. 19-24).[9]

Further Evaluation

Testosterone measurements and assessment of sperm production, combined with measurement of gonadotropin levels, allow classification of the causes of male hypogonadism into primary or secondary hypogonadism and subclassification of the latter into disorders causing both androgen deficiency and impairment in sperm production and those causing isolated impairment of sperm production or function (see Tables 19-7 and 19-8).

Once hypogonadism has been classified as primary or secondary hypogonadism, further evaluation includes a history (including medication review), physical examination, and laboratory testing to identify a specific cause or causes of hypogonadism. For example, in men with primary hypogonadism and suggestive clinical manifestations such as very small testes and gynecomastia, low or low-normal testosterone, azoospermia, and markedly elevated gonadotropins, a karyotype may be obtained to confirm the diagnosis of Klinefelter syndrome.

In men with secondary hypogonadism, further evaluation may include measurements of serum prolactin (in almost all cases) to exclude hyperprolactinemia; iron saturation and ferritin to screen for hereditary hemochromatosis, especially in men with other manifestations of iron overload (e.g., liver failure, diabetes, and CHF) and in young men with unexplained selective gonadotropin deficiency; further testing to exclude excessive secretion or deficiency of anterior pituitary hormones; and magnetic resonance imaging (MRI) of the sella turcica to exclude a pituitary or hypothalamic tumor or infiltrative disease. Computed tomography of the sella turcica usually detects a pituitary macroadenoma but is less sensitive than sella MRI in detecting smaller tumors and infiltrative disease.[113]

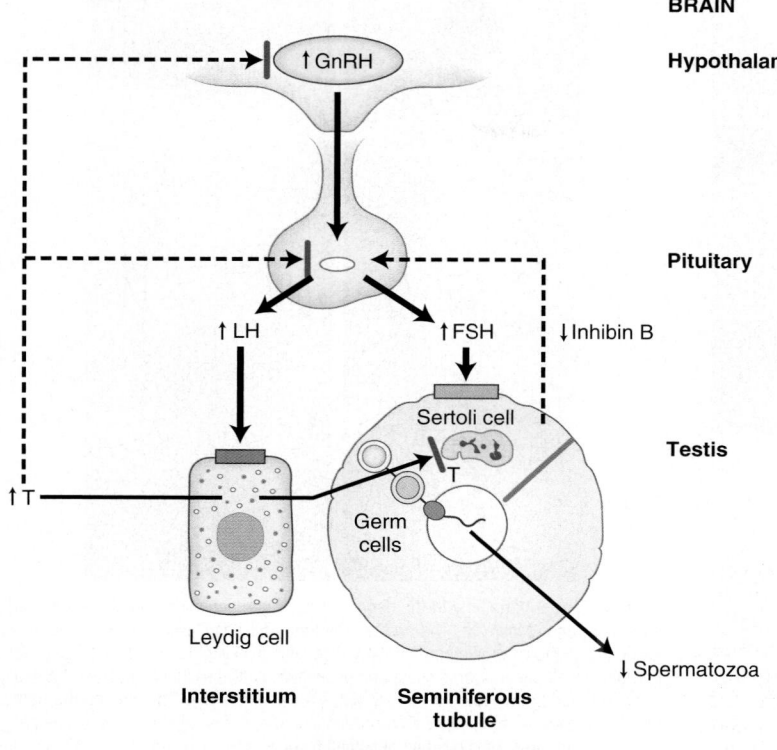

BRAIN

Hypothalamus

Pituitary

Testis

Interstitium   Seminiferous tubule

ANDROGEN RESISTANCE
Hypergonadotropic hypogonadism

Figure 19-24 Schematic diagram of alterations in the hypothalamic-pituitary-testicular axis with androgen resistance due to impaired androgen action (e.g., androgen receptor mutation), which results in high testosterone (T) levels but reduced androgen action. This leads to manifestations of androgen deficiency, impaired sperm production, and elevated luteinizing hormone (LH) and follicle-stimulating hormone (FSH) levels due to impaired androgen-mediated negative feedback regulation of gonadotropins. GnRH, gonadotropin-releasing hormone. (From Matsumoto AM. The testis. In: Felig P, Frohman LA, eds. *Endocrinology and Metabolism*, 4th ed. New York, NY: McGraw-Hill; 2001:635-705.)

It is not cost effective to perform sella MRI in all men with secondary hypogonadism. This modality should be reserved for men with severe androgen deficiency (e.g., serum testosterone <150 ng/dL) due to secondary hypogonadism, particularly with distinctly low gonadotropin levels[205,206]; discordant LH and FSH levels associated with androgen deficiency; hyperprolactinemia (especially with prolactin levels >100 to 200 ng/mL); clinical and biochemical evidence of excessive secretion of other pituitary hormones (e.g., free α-subunit secretion, Cushing syndrome, acromegaly), panhypopituitarism, or diabetes insipidus; tumor mass effects, such as severe headache, visual field defects, or visual impairment; and no obvious functional cause of secondary hypogonadism (e.g., morbid obesity, long-acting opioid, or chronic high-dose glucocorticoid therapy).

In men who have severe androgen deficiency caused by primary or secondary hypogonadism or who have sustained a low-trauma or fragility fracture, DXA scanning to assess BMD should be performed to exclude osteopenia or osteoporosis.[113]

Causes of Primary Hypogonadism

Androgen Deficiency and Impairment in Sperm Production

Congenital or Developmental Disorders

Klinefelter Syndrome. Classically, Klinefelter syndrome is characterized by very small, firm testes; azoospermia and infertility; varying degrees of androgen deficiency and eunuchoidism; and uniformly elevated gonadotropin levels.[207-209] It is the most common sex chromosome abnormality and the most common cause of primary hypogonadism resulting in androgen deficiency and impaired sperm production. It occurs prenatally and neonatally in 1 of every 500 to 700 males, and the prevalence in adults is 1 in 2500.[1,2] Because the syndrome does not cause premature death in boys, the low adult prevalence indicates that Klinefelter syndrome is often overlooked and underdiagnosed in men. This is surprising, given the almost uniform finding of extremely small testes and other phenotypic abnormalities in these men. The risk of having a child with Klinefelter syndrome increases with both maternal and paternal age.

The fundamental chromosomal abnormality in Klinefelter syndrome is the presence of one or more extra X chromosomes due to maternal meiotic nondisjunction (mostly in meiosis I) in approximately 50% of the cases or paternal meiotic nondisjunction in the remaining cases.[207-209] The principal karyotype in 90% of men with Klinefelter syndrome is 47,XXY. Most of the remaining 10% have mosaic Klinefelter syndrome (47,XXY/46,XY), in which there is a 47,XXY karyotype in some tissues and a normal 46,XY karyotype in other tissues. Mosaicism occurs as a result of postfertilization mitotic nondisjunction. Men with mosaic Klinefelter syndrome usually demonstrate a variable and less severe phenotype that depends on the specific tissues in which an extra X chromosome is present. Some men with mosaicism have a normal karyotype in the testis with intact spermatogenesis and fertility. Rarely, men with Klinefelter syndrome have more than one extra X chromosome (e.g., 48,XXXY, 49,XXXXY). Men with these variants manifest a more severe phenotype than is seen in classic Klinefelter syndrome.

Infants with Klinefelter syndrome may manifest micropenis, hypospadias, cryptorchidism, or developmental delay.[210] During childhood, boys with the syndrome commonly have small testes and reduced penile length relative to age-matched normal individuals and may manifest relatively tall stature, clinodactyly, hypertelorism, gynecomastia, elbow dysplasia, high-arched palate, hypotonia, language delay or learning and reading disabilities

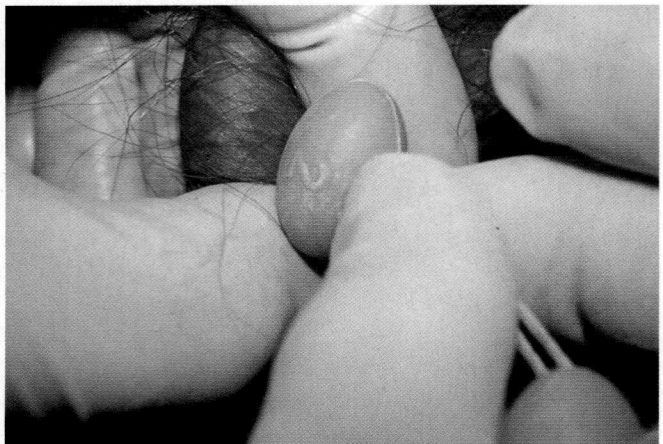

Figure 19-25 Testis size in a man with classic 47,XXY Klinefelter syndrome is characteristically very small (e.g., 2 mL).

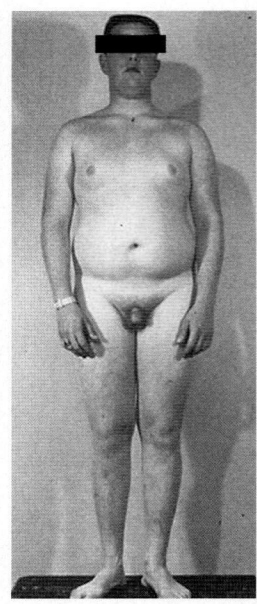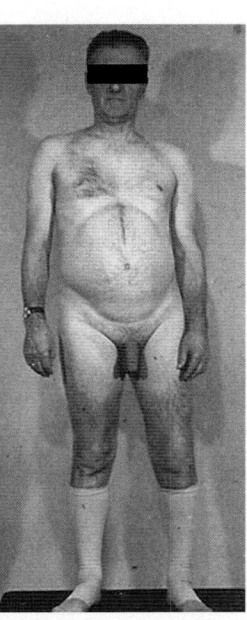

Figure 19-26 Variability in the degree of androgen deficiency manifested in men with Klinefelter syndrome. The man on the left, who has classic 47,XXY Klinefelter syndrome, demonstrates prepubertal androgen deficiency with eunuchoidal body proportions, small penis, sparse chest and pubic hair, poor muscle development, prepubertal fat distribution, and very small testes (2 mL bilaterally). The man on the right, who has mosaic 47,XXY/46,XY Klinefelter syndrome, demonstrates normal body proportions, penis size, and body hair but small testis size (8 mL bilaterally). (From Smyth CM, Bremner WJ. Klinefelter syndrome. *Arch Intern Med.* 1998;158:1309-1314.)

requiring therapy, and behavioral problems.[211] However, these manifestations may be mild and are often missed. Fewer than 10% of boys with Klinefelter syndrome (usually those with the most severe phenotype) are diagnosed before puberty. At puberty, the testes fail to increase in size and become firm due to a progressive loss of germ cells and seminiferous tubule hyalinization and fibrosis; Sertoli cell products, inhibin B, and AMH decline to very low or undetectable levels; testosterone levels increase but to less than normal levels in some boys, resulting in varying degrees of eunuchoidism and gynecomastia; and FSH levels are disproportionately elevated relative to LH levels.

In adults, the most prominent and consistent clinical feature of Klinefelter syndrome is very small testes, less than 4 mL in volume (<2.5 cm in length); this feature is easily detected on examination and should alert the clinician to possibility of Klinefelter syndrome (Fig. 19-25).[8,212] Men with this syndrome may present with a complaint of infertility and subsequently be found to have azoospermia and very small testes.[213] Other manifestations include varying degrees of androgen deficiency, eunuchoidism, and gynecomastia (Fig. 19-26).[209] In contrast to the classic long arms and legs of eunuchoidism seen in patients with prepubertal androgen deficiency, Klinefelter syndrome results in a disproportionate increase in lower- compared with upper-extremity long bone growth. Gynecomastia occurs in 50% to 80% of men with the syndrome and may be quite prominent and embarrassing. Learning and developmental disabilities occur in about 70% of men with Klinefelter syndrome. Character and personality disorders and behavioral problems occur commonly, possibly in part because of the psychosocial consequences of androgen deficiency and learning disabilities. Men with Klinefelter syndrome have intelligence quotient (IQ) scores that are reduced by 10 to 15 points but not into the intellectual disability range. Taurodontism, characterized by enlarged molar teeth resulting from enlargement and extension of the pulp chamber, is present in 40% of men with Klinefelter syndrome.

As described previously, the *AR* gene is located on the X chromosome, and the length of the highly polymorphic CAG repeat in exon 1 of the *AR* gene is inversely related to AR activity. In Klinefelter syndrome, the X chromosome carrying the *AR* gene with a short CAG repeat length (i.e., greater AR activity) undergoes inactivation preferentially.[134] Klinefelter syndrome patients with short CAG repeat lengths were found to have more stable relationships,

higher educational levels, and greater responses to testosterone treatment. In contrast, men with long CAG repeat length (i.e., reduced AR activity) had longer arms and legs, smaller testes, a greater degree of gynecomastia, and lower BMD. Therefore, skewed inactivation of the X chromosome resulting in preferential activity of the long CAG repeat may contribute to phenotypic severity and variability of Klinefelter syndrome.

Most men with mosaic Klinefelter syndrome exhibit less severe clinical manifestations than those with the classic syndrome. Men with more than two extra X chromosomes have more severe manifestations and a higher incidence of intellectual disability and somatic abnormalities such as hypospadias, cryptorchidism, and radioulnar synostosis. Very rarely, some phenotypic males with a 46,XX karyotype exhibit typical clinical manifestations of Klinefelter syndrome except that they have shorter stature and a greater incidence of cryptorchidism, gynecomastia, and androgen deficiency.[214] In most of these cases, there has been a translocation of an SRY-containing segment of the Y chromosome onto an X chromosome.

In addition to infertility, variable androgen deficiency, and gynecomastia, patients with Klinefelter syndrome have an approximately 20-fold increased risk in breast cancer compared with normal men (although the absolute lifetime risk of <1% is low); such patients account for approximately 4% of all cases of male breast cancer.[215] Klinefelter syndrome is also associated with increased risk for mitral valve prolapse; lower-extremity varicose veins, venous stasis ulcers, deep vein thrombosis, and pulmonary embolism; autoimmune diseases such as systemic lupus erythematosus, rheumatoid arthritis, and Sjögren syndrome; other cancers such as extragonadal germ cell cancer and non-Hodgkin lymphoma; T2DM and the metabolic syndrome; and psychiatric illnesses such as depression and schizophrenia. There is a minimal reduction in life

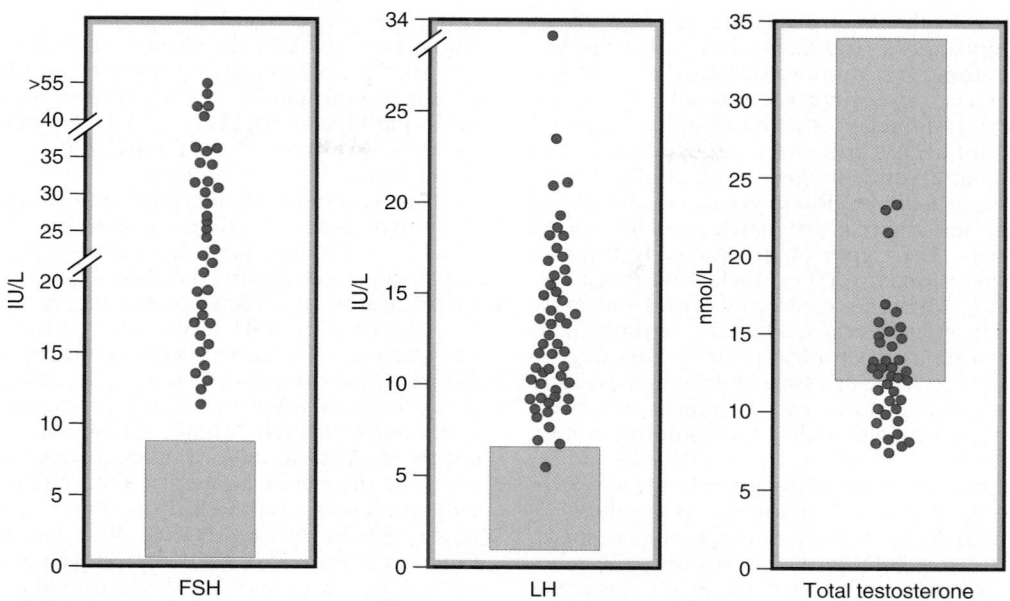

Figure 19-27 Serum levels of follicle-stimulating hormone (FSH, *left*), luteinizing hormone (LH, *middle*), and total testosterone (T, *right*) in men with Klinefelter syndrome *(dots)* compared with normal men (normal range depicted by *shaded boxes*). A substantial proportion of men with Klinefelter syndrome have total testosterone levels within the normal range, but almost all have elevated LH and FSH levels. (From Smyth CM, Bremner WJ. Klinefelter syndrome. *Arch Intern Med.* 1998;158:1309-1314.)

expectancy of approximately 2 years in men with Klinefelter syndrome, associated with a higher rate of deaths due to a variety of common causes.[216,217]

Azoospermia is present in more than 95% of men with classic Klinefelter syndrome and infertility in more than 99%. Serum total testosterone levels are usually low but may fall in the low-normal to mid-normal range in 40% to 50% of cases (Fig. 19-27).[207-209] Relative to normal men, men with Klinefelter syndrome have elevated serum estradiol levels, which probably contributes to the development of gynecomastia, and increased SHBG concentrations. Increased SHBG levels provide a partial explanation for normal total testosterone levels in the presence of low concentrations of free testosterone. Serum FSH levels are almost always elevated; serum LH levels are usually elevated but may fall into the high-normal range in some men (see Fig. 19-27).[207-209] Symptoms of androgen deficiency in the presence of normal total and free testosterone and elevated gonadotropin levels occur in some men with Klinefelter syndrome, suggesting relative androgen deficiency or resistance.

A *Barr body analysis* may be used as a rapid and reliable screening test for Klinefelter syndrome. In a normal female with two X chromosomes, one X chromosome is inactivated and may be detected as sex chromatin (Barr body) on staining of the nucleus in epithelial cells obtained from a scraping of the buccal mucosa (buccal smear). In a normal 46,XY male, the single X chromosome is not inactivated, and no Barr body is present. In contrast, X inactivation occurs in a 47,XXY man with Klinefelter syndrome, resulting in a detectable Barr body. Men with variant syndromes characterized by more than two extra X chromosomes may exhibit more than one Barr body per nucleus; the number of Barr bodies is one less than the number of extra X chromosomes. Although Barr body analysis may be helpful in screening for Klinefelter syndrome, it is subject to false-negative and false-positive results and is no longer commonly performed.

The diagnosis of Klinefelter syndrome is confirmed by *karyotype analysis*, which is usually performed on cultured

peripheral blood lymphocytes. Occasionally, karyotype analysis is performed on cultured skin fibroblasts and testis tissue if mosaicism is suspected. If a fetus is diagnosed on prenatal testing with 47,XY Klinefelter syndrome, genetic counseling should be provided. Despite a reasonably good prognosis, 75% of couples choose termination of a fetus with a prenatal diagnosis of Klinefelter syndrome.

Treatment of Klinefelter syndrome is directed at correction of androgen deficiency. Infants with micropenis may benefit from topical testosterone treatment. For boys with Klinefelter syndrome, early intervention with speech and reading therapy is important if speech delay and dyslexia are present. At puberty, testosterone treatment may be needed for adequate development of secondary sexual characteristics; peak bone mass and BMD; muscle mass and strength; and energy, motivation, mood, and behavior. Adults with Klinefelter syndrome who have clinical manifestations of androgen deficiency and consistently low levels of serum total or free testosterone (or both) should receive testosterone replacement therapy. Also, men who have symptoms and signs of androgen deficiency but normal total and free testosterone levels should be offered a trial of testosterone treatment.

Although azoospermia and infertility are irreversible, TESE permits identification of the relatively few seminiferous tubules that contain active spermatogenesis and harvesting of sperm from the small testes of men with Klinefelter syndrome for use in ICSI; this approach results in live birth rates of approximately 45% in specialized centers.[7] Because there is an increased risk of sex chromosome and autosomal aneuploidy, genetic counseling and prenatal or preimplantation testing should be provided to couples who undergo ICSI.

Prominent gynecomastia does not resolve with testosterone treatment and requires reduction mammoplasty. Psychological counseling for patients and spouses and participation in support groups may be extremely helpful for men with Klinefelter syndrome.

Myotonic Dystrophy. Myotonic dystrophy is an autosomal dominant, multisystem disorder that is characterized by progressive muscle weakness and wasting (particularly in the lower legs, hands, neck, and face) and results in physical disability; myotonia (involuntary sustained contraction of muscles); cataracts; cardiac conduction defects; respiratory insufficiency; dysphagia; testicular atrophy, impaired spermatogenesis, infertility, and androgen deficiency; premature frontal balding; and intellectual disability.[218] Features of the disease usually develop in young adults but can occur at any age, and their severity varies widely among affected individuals. Two types of myotonic dystrophies are caused by expansion of CTG trinucleotide repeats in two different genes. Myotonic dystrophy type 1 has more severe clinical features and is caused by CTG repeat expansion in the dystrophia myotonica protein kinase gene *(DMPK)*; it accounts for 98% of cases. Myotonic dystrophy type 2 is less severe and is caused by CTG repeat expansion in the CCHC-type zinc finger, nucleic acid–binding protein gene *(CNBP)*.

Primary hypogonadism occurs in approximately 80% of young to middle-aged men with myotonic dystrophy.[219,220] Most of these men have isolated impairment of sperm production or function with testicular atrophy, oligozoospermia or azoospermia, moderate to severe testicular damage on testis biopsy, infertility, and disproportionately elevated FSH compared with LH levels. Approximately 20% to 40% of men with myotonic dystrophy have variable degrees of androgen deficiency with low testosterone levels and elevated LH and FSH; testosterone replacement therapy is appropriate for these men. High-dose testosterone therapy has been demonstrated to improve muscle mass but did not affect muscle strength.[221] Infertility is irreversible, and patients who desire children need to pursue ART or other options; genetic counseling and preimplantation or prenatal testing should be provided, given the autosomal dominant nature of the disease.

Cryptorchidism. Cryptorchidism is the failure of one or both testes to descend normally from within the abdomen through the inguinal canal into the scrotum. It is the most common congenital disorder of the male genital tract in children, affecting 2% to 4% of full-term male infants.[222,223] It is more common in premature, low-birth-weight, and small-for-gestational-age infants. Spontaneous descent of the testis occurs during the first year in most infants (probably induced by the neonatal surge of gonadotropins and testosterone), so the prevalence of cryptorchidism in boys and adults is lower, approximately 0.3% to 1.0%. Because a patent processus vaginalis is usually also present, inguinal hernia is found in conjunction with cryptorchidism in 50% to 80% of cases. Both unilateral and bilateral cryptorchidism are associated with impaired sperm production and infertility and an increased risk of testicular cancer.

In contrast to cryptorchidism, *ectopic testes* are located outside the normal path of testicular descent.[224] Ectopic testes may be located anywhere in the perineum or in the femoral or superficial inguinal regions. It is also important to distinguish cryptorchidism from *retractile testes* (pseudocryptorchidism). Retractile testes are located in the scrotum but withdraw into the inguinal canal or abdomen with minimal stimulation due to a hyperactive cremasteric reflex; they are not usually associated with impaired sperm production, infertility, or increased risk of testicular cancer. However, impaired spermatogenesis and fertility have been reported in men with bilateral retractile testes located high in the inguinal canal or, sometimes, in the abdomen.

Bilateral cryptorchidism may be associated with a number of disorders causing primary hypogonadism (including Klinefelter syndrome variants and Noonan syndrome), secondary hypogonadism (including IHH, Kallmann syndrome, and complex genetic disorders associated with multiple congenital anomalies or defects, such as Prader-Labhart-Willi syndrome or Laurence-Moon-Biedl syndrome), and androgen resistance syndromes (e.g., Reifenstein syndrome).[225] Cryptorchidism may also be caused by mutations of the Leydig cell product, INSL3, which controls growth of the gubernaculum, or of its receptor (RXFP2) in up to 5% of cases.

Unilateral or bilateral cryptorchidism that is not related to known causes of hypogonadism or androgen resistance usually results in primary hypogonadism, causing isolated impairment of sperm production associated with low sperm counts, normal testosterone concentrations, a selective elevation in FSH levels, and, occasionally, high LH levels as well.[222,223] Rarely, cryptorchidism causes Leydig cell failure and androgen deficiency (e.g., in adults with uncorrected bilateral cryptorchidism), producing low serum testosterone with high LH and FSH levels.[226,227] Azoospermia occurs in 50% to 60% and oligozoospermia in 75% to 100% of men with bilateral cryptorchidism; among men with unilateral cryptorchidism, these figures are, respectively, 15% to 20% and 20% to 40%. This suggests that the function of both testes is compromised in unilateral cryptorchidism. An underlying developmental or environmental disorder affecting both testes *(testicular dysgenesis)* may contribute to impaired spermatogenesis in these individuals.[222,223] The formation of A_d spermatogonia from neonatal gonocytes is inhibited in undescended testes. Uncommonly, normal testicular descent is impeded by an anatomic abnormality such as a large external inguinal hernia. In this instance, both testes function normally, and correction of the anatomic abnormality with orchiopexy before puberty usually preserves spermatogenesis and fertility.

The risk of testicular cancer in an undescended testis is 2.5- to 8-fold greater than in a scrotal testis, and the risk remains higher even after the testis is surgically relocated into the scrotum, supporting the notion that cryptorchidism is a manifestation of a underlying testicular disorder (i.e., testicular dysgenesis).[222-225] Even though the incidence of testicular cancer is only 1 or 2 per 100,000 males, the lifetime risk of malignancy in a cryptorchid testis is substantial. The prevalence of testicular carcinoma in situ, which is thought to precede testicular cancer, is about 3% in the cryptorchid testis. Testicular cancer usually occurs in men 20 to 40 years of age.

A careful physical examination should be performed to assess the location of testes within the scrotum or inguinal canal; the presence of an inguinal hernia, hydrocele, or other scrotal mass; the cremasteric reflex induced by stroking of the upper medial thigh; and penile size and the position of the urethral meatus. The examination should be performed with the patient standing, squatting, or supine with legs abducted. Scrotal examination may be difficult in a morbidly obese man with a large abdominal panniculus. Techniques that may be helpful in the detection of retractile testes include examination during a Valsalva maneuver, with pressure applied to the lower abdomen, or after scrotal warming or a hot bath to facilitate testicular descent. Also, elicitation of the cremasteric reflex may cause a localized puckering of the scrotal skin if a retractile testis is present in the scrotum. Often, a low undescended testis may be confirmed by pushing with one hand on the lower abdomen, with firm strokes from the anterior superior iliac spine through the groin and to the pubis, toward and into the scrotum, and then grasping the testis with the other hand. After the testis has been held in the scrotum until the cremasteric muscle fatigues, it is released. If the testis then retracts, it is considered a retractile testis; a low cryptorchid testis returns to its undescended position after release. Absence of a palpable testis in the scrotum after repeated examinations may be a result of cryptorchidism, an extremely atrophic testis, or anorchia (absent testis). Up to 50% of men with a unilateral, nonpalpable testis in the scrotum have a severely atrophic or absent testis rather than cryptorchidism; in these instances, the contralateral testis may be relatively large (by about 2 mL). High-resolution ultrasonography or MRI may help to localize testes that are not palpable.

Treatment for persistent cryptorchidism should be started before puberty, when greater germ cell degeneration occurs.[222,223] The exact timing of treatment is controversial, but recent recommendations suggest that treatment should be instituted between 6 and 12 months or up to 24 months of age. Hormonal treatment with hCG or GnRH in prepubertal boys is effective in stimulating descent of a cryptorchid testis in approximately 10% to 20% of cases. A trial of hormonal therapy may be attempted in the hope of avoiding surgery. If hormonal treatment is unsuccessful or not attempted, an orchiopexy (surgical relocation and fixation of the testis into the scrotum with ligation of the hernia sac at the external or internal inguinal ring) should be performed to allow examination of the testes (e.g., as in monitoring for malignancy) and preservation of remaining testis function. Despite orchiopexy, spermatogenesis remains impaired and fertility rates are reduced, particularly with bilateral cryptorchidism (65% paternity rate after orchiopexy). If orchiopexy is performed before puberty, the risk of testicular cancer is reduced but is still increased twofold to threefold. In patients with a history of unilateral cryptorchidism, the risk of malignancy in the contralateral testis is also increased, by about 70%. Because the risk of malignancy is two to six times higher in men who underwent orchiopexy after puberty and the fertility potential is poor, some clinicians recommend orchidectomy for men with cryptorchidism discovered after puberty. The majority of testis cancers found in persistently cryptorchid testes are seminomas, whereas those in cryptorchid testes after orchiopexy are mostly nonseminoma testicular cancers.

Noonan Syndrome. Noonan syndrome is an autosomal dominant or occasional sporadic genetic disorder that is characterized by short stature; unusual facial features (hypertelorism, downward-slanting eyes, ptosis, strabismus, low-set ears with thickened helices, high nasal bridge, micrognathia and triangular-shaped face, high-arched palate, low hairline, dental malocclusion); short, webbed neck; shield-like chest, pectus excavatum or carinatum, scoliosis, cubitus valgus, and joint laxity; intellectual disability; cardiac disease (pulmonary stenosis, hypertrophic cardiomyopathy); hepatosplenomegaly; lymphedema; and cryptorchidism.[228,229]

Because a number of these clinical features resemble those of females with Turner syndrome, Noonan syndrome was previously called male Turner syndrome. However, the karyotype in these men is normal. Noonan syndrome affects approximately 1 in 1000 to 2500 live births and is caused by mutations in genes in the Ras-MAPK signaling pathway.[228,229] Approximately 50% of men with Noonan syndrome have mutations in the *PTPN11* (the protein tyrosine phosphatase nonreceptor type 11) gene, and the remainder have mutations in the *SOS1* (son of sevenless homolog 1), *RAF1*, or *KRAS* genes.

Men with Noonan syndrome may demonstrate primary hypogonadism characterized by androgen deficiency and impaired sperm production with elevated gonadotropin levels; they usually present with delayed puberty.[230] Cryptorchidism is present in more than 50% of men with the syndrome and contributes to the cause of hypogonadism.

Bilateral Congenital Anorchia. Congenital anorchia (also known as functional prepubertal castrate or vanishing testis syndrome) is a rare condition in which one or both testes are absent in a phenotypically and genotypically normal male.[231,232] Normal fetal testis function is needed for normal male internal and external genital differentiation and development during early gestation. The presence of otherwise normal male internal and external genitalia without müllerian duct–derived structures or descent of the spermatic cord structures (e.g., vas deferens, blood vessels) into the scrotum implies that normally functioning testes must have been present during the first 16 weeks of gestation and subsequently lost during fetal or neonatal life. The prevalence of bilateral congenital anorchia is 1 in 20,000, and that of unilateral congenital anorchia is 1 in 5000 males. The cause is not known but is probably heterogeneous. It is hypothesized that congenital anorchia may be caused by spermatic vascular compromise due to torsion or trauma during or after testicular descent.

Infants with bilateral anorchia present with micropenis in almost 50% of cases, supporting a prenatal origin of the disorder.[231,232] Males with congenital anorchia usually present with prepubertal primary hypogonadism with delayed puberty and eunuchoidism (see Fig. 19-14), very low testosterone levels in the castrate range, and elevated gonadotropin levels. On examination, palpable testes are absent but blind-ending spermatic cords and epididymides are usually present. Normal testosterone and gonadotropin concentrations in pubertal or adult patients with absent testes exclude the diagnosis of congenital anorchia and should raise the possibility of bilateral cryptorchidism, which carries an increased risk for testicular malignancy.

An hCG stimulation test may be performed to distinguish congenital anorchia from bilateral cryptorchidism. In patients with congenital anorchia, serum testosterone concentrations do not increase in response to prolonged hCG administration (e.g., 1000 to 2000 IU three times weekly for 2 weeks), whereas most patients with bilateral cryptorchidism respond to hCG. However, lack of testosterone response to hCG administration for 6 weeks has been reported in men with bilateral cryptorchidism.[233] Serum AMH concentrations are usually undetectable in patients with congenital anorchia.[234] Measurements of AMH levels are more sensitive than those of testosterone concentrations but equally specific. If clinical examination and endocrine biochemical tests do not distinguish bilateral anorchia from cryptorchidism, imaging studies (e.g., MRI) and laparoscopy or surgical abdominal exploration may be necessary to confirm the diagnosis.

Treatment of bilateral congenital anorchia consists of testosterone replacement to stimulate penile length in patients with micropenis and to induce and maintain sexual development in boys with delayed puberty and eunuchoidism. Implantation of testicular prostheses in the scrotum may be of psychological and cosmetic value.

Autoimmune Polyglandular Syndrome. Autoimmune polyglandular syndromes are characterized by a clustering of organ-specific autoimmune disorders that involve a number of endocrine and nonendocrine tissues and are associated with circulating autoantibodies to components of these tissues. Autoimmune polyglandular syndrome type 1, also called autoimmune polyendocrinopathy-candidiasis-ectodermal dystrophy (APECED), is a rare autosomal recessive disorder that is caused by a mutation in the autoimmune regulator *(AIRE)* gene.[235,236] Its main features are mucocutaneous candidiasis, hypoparathyroidism, primary adrenal insufficiency, and the presence of autoimmune disorders including primary hypogonadism. The prevalence of primary hypogonadism is much more common in females than in males. In females, hypogonadism is manifested as premature ovarian failure and is present in 35% to 70% of cases, whereas in males, it is present in 8% to 28% of cases and is manifested either by androgen deficiency and impairment in sperm production or isolated impairment in sperm production (azoospermia) with elevated gonadotropin levels.

Autoimmune polyglandular syndrome type 2 is a common polygenic disorder associated with the genes for human leukocyte antigens (HLA) DR3 and DR4.[235,237] It is characterized by autoimmune primary adrenal insufficiency, thyroid disease (Hashimoto or Graves disease), and type 1 diabetes mellitus (T1DM) in addition to other autoimmune disorders including primary hypogonadism (again, more common in females than in males). In autoimmune polyglandular syndrome type 2, primary hypogonadism is associated with circulating steroid-producing cell autoantibodies (SCA) and with specific autoantibodies to CYP11A1 and 17α-hydroxylase.

Defects in Testosterone Biosynthetic Enzymes. Males with uncommon defects in 17,20-lyase/17α-hydroxylase, 17β-HSD/17-ketoreductase type 3, or 3β-HSD type 2, resulting from mutations in the *CYP17*, *HSD17B3*, and *HSD3B2* genes, respectively, usually present at birth as phenotypic females with partial virilization or with ambiguous genitalia. However, patients with incomplete defects in these enzymes may present as phenotypic males with hypospadias, gynecomastia, and primary hypogonadism with androgen deficiency manifested by delayed puberty.

Because 17,20-lyase and 17α-hydroxylase activities reside in the same enzyme, mutations in *CYP17* usually cause deficiencies in both activities, leading to elevated levels of progesterone, corticosterone, and deoxycorticosterone (DOC).[238] Rarely, males exhibiting isolated 17,20-lyase deficiency with elevated 17-hydroxyprogesterone levels have been reported.[239] Patients with 17α-hydroxylase deficiency may have hypertension and hypokalemia due to excessive production of the aldosterone precursor DOC, which has potent mineralocorticoid activity, but this is relatively uncommon in males compared with females. Patients with this deficiency usually do not manifest adrenal insufficiency because of increased production of the cortisol precursor, corticosterone, which has glucocorticoid activity. Males with either 17,20-lyase/17α-hydroxylase deficiency or isolated 17,20-lyase deficiency have primary hypogonadism with low testosterone and elevated LH and FSH levels; they require testosterone treatment at the time of puberty.

Patients with 17β-HSD/17-ketoreductase deficiency may have ambiguous genitalia and be raised as females, but at puberty, their testosterone levels increase sufficiently to induce virilization, resulting in gender reassignment (similar to individuals with androgen resistance due to 5α-reductase deficiency).[240] Serum testosterone levels are low to normal, but androstenedione and gonadotropin levels are increased.

Incomplete deficiency of 3β-HSD is a rare disorder that may manifest in adolescents with mild ambiguous genitalia, delayed virilization, gynecomastia, low testosterone levels, and elevated LH and FSH levels.[241] Levels of pregnenolone, 17-hydroxypregnenolone, and DHEA are elevated. Spontaneous virilization and puberty due to direct effects of high levels of the weak androgen DHEA or conversion of DHEA to testosterone (or both) has been reported. A eugonadal male with partial 3β-HSD deficiency who presented with gynecomastia has also been reported.[242]

Congenital Adrenal Hyperplasia. Adolescent and adult male patients with congenital adrenal hyperplasia due to 21-hydroxylase deficiency may develop *testicular adrenal rest tumors (TARTs)* that resemble Leydig cell tumors but do not contain intracytoplasmic Reinke crystalloids, which

are commonly found (approximately 40%) on histologic analysis in the latter.[243-245] TARTs may be large and easily palpable, or they may be detectable only on testicular ultrasonography. These tumors are thought to originate embryologically from aberrant adrenal tissue, and they are responsive to adrenocorticotropic hormone (ACTH). They regress with adequate glucocorticoid therapy for congenital adrenal hyperplasia and suppression of ACTH, and they grow with inadequate glucocorticoid treatment.

21-Hydroxylase deficiency is an autosomal recessive condition caused by a mutation in the *CYP21* gene. It is the most common enzymatic defect causing congenital adrenal hyperplasia. 21-Hydroxylase deficiency produces an accumulation of steroid substrates (17-hydroxyprogesterone and progesterone) that results in excessive production of adrenal androgens (androstenedione and DHEA), which are subsequently converted to testosterone. In addition, 21-hydroxylase deficiency causes reduced production of cortisol and aldosterone, resulting in deficiency of glucocorticoid and mineralocorticoid, respectively, and increased ACTH secretion (due to reduced cortisol negative feedback). Elevated ACTH secretion stimulates adrenal gland growth, resulting in adrenal hyperplasia. Glucocorticoid treatment suppresses ACTH secretion, reduces excessive adrenal androgen production, treats clinical adrenal insufficiency, and prevents excessive adrenal hyperplasia.

Excessive adrenal androgen production due to untreated or inadequate glucocorticoid therapy for 21-hydroxylase deficiency suppresses gonadotropin secretion by sex steroid negative feedback regulation and causes secondary hypogonadism. Because androgen levels are maintained by excessive adrenal production, men with 21-hydroxylase deficiency may not have clinical androgen deficiency. However, they usually have isolated impairment of sperm production due to gonadotropin deficiency. Adequate glucocorticoid therapy reduces excessive adrenal androgen production and usually restores gonadotropin secretion and normalizes testis function. Adequate and early glucocorticoid treatment also causes regression of adrenal rest tumors, which otherwise may affect testicular function directly or cause mechanical obstruction of seminiferous tubules.[243-245]

If TARTs are present, inadequate glucocorticoid treatment stimulates their growth, often resulting in very large tumors that can cause irreversible testicular damage.[243-245] In this circumstance, although adequate glucocorticoid therapy reduces tumor size, the patient will manifest primary hypogonadism with androgen deficiency due to loss of Leydig cells and impaired sperm production due to loss of seminiferous tubules. On adequate glucocorticoid treatment, tumors may regress completely, but testis size usually remains small, serum testosterone levels and sperm counts low, and gonadotropin levels elevated. Although excessive amounts of glucocorticoid therapy will suppress ACTH production and TART, they will also suppress gonadotropins, and testosterone and sperm production.

Complex Genetic Syndromes. Primary hypogonadism resulting in androgen deficiency and impaired sperm production or in isolated impairment in sperm production or function may occur as a manifestation of complex genetic syndromes, usually in association with a number of congenital anomalies or defects and distinct morphologic developmental manifestations.[246] Examples include the Alström, ataxia telangiectasia, Marinesco-Sjögren, Robinow, Rothmund-Thomson, Sohval-Soffer, Weinstein, Werner, and Wolfram syndromes.[247-256] Prader-Labhart-Willi syndrome (associated with cryptorchidism), Laurence-Moon-Bardet-Biedl syndrome, and Alström syndrome are disorders that are commonly associated with secondary hypogonadism, but primary hypogonadism may also occur in these disorders.[257-260]

Down Syndrome. Down syndrome, or trisomy 21, is a chromosomal disorder in which all or part of an extra chromosome 21 is present.[261] It affects 1 of every 700 to 800 infants and is the most common cause of intellectual disability in children. Down syndrome is characterized by moderate to severe intellectual disability, spontaneous warm and cheerful personality, short stature, characteristic mongoloid facial features (most notably round facies with microgenia, upward-slanting and almond-shaped eyes resulting from bilateral epicanthal folds, macroglossia, and flat nasal bridge), congenital heart defects, hypothyroidism, and defects affecting most other body systems. Males with Down syndrome usually manifest primary hypogonadism, most commonly characterized by isolated impairment in sperm production with normal or selective elevation of FSH levels. Histologically, they may manifest hypospermatogenesis (moderate to severe reduction in all germ cell types), maturation arrest, or Sertoli cell–only syndrome with loss of all germ cells. Less commonly, they demonstrate mild to moderate androgen deficiency with low or low-normal testosterone and elevated LH and FSH levels.

Luteinizing Hormone Receptor Mutations. Inactivating mutations of the LH receptor in males usually cause Leydig cell aplasia or hypoplasia. These patients present with 46,XY DSD characterized by a female phenotype without breast development at puberty (Leydig cell aplasia) or genital ambiguity (hypoplasia) and cryptorchidism.[58] Rarely, partially inactivating LH receptor mutations result in a male phenotype with micropenis, hypospadias, delayed sexual development, undervirilization, low testosterone, impaired sperm production, and high LH levels, consistent with primary hypogonadism. However, they usually have normal FSH levels. An individual with an LH receptor mutation was reported to exhibit normal levels of testosterone and spermatogenesis after hCG stimulation, suggesting that hCG action via the LH receptor may be dissociated from that of LH.[262]

Acquired Disorders

Bilateral Surgical Castration and Trauma. Bilateral surgical castration causes a rapid and profound decline in testosterone levels within hours, resulting in severe clinical manifestations of androgen deficiency, including hot flushes. Severe blunt trauma to the testes and associated vascular compromise may result in testicular atrophy and loss of testis function, including androgen deficiency and impaired spermatogenesis or isolated impairment in sperm production or function.

Drugs and Ionizing Radiation. Certain drugs that affect androgen production may cause androgen deficiency. The antifungal agent ketoconazole and a recently available drug, abiraterone, inhibit 17,20-lyase and 17α-hydroxylase activity at high doses (>400 mg daily and 1000 mg daily, respectively) and have been used, in conjunction with other agents, to lower both adrenal and testicular androgen production in the treatment of prostate cancer.[263-265] Spironolactone, a nonspecific aldosterone antagonist, acts mainly as a competitive AR antagonist and inhibits androgen action.[266] However, it also inhibits 17,20-lyase and 17α-hydroxylase activity and testosterone biosynthesis at high doses. Enzalutamide is a competitive AR antagonist that also inhibits post-receptor AR action (translocation of AR into the nucleus, binding of AR cofactors and DNA binding) that is used to treat castration-resistant prostate cancer.[267] Excessive intake of alcohol inhibits testosterone production, but it may also suppress gonadotropins; it may

be associated with nutritional deficiency or chronic liver disease, which may contribute to androgen deficiency and impairment in sperm production.[268,269]

In general, because spermatogenesis involves active cell replication, the germ cell compartment is much more sensitive to external or environmental influences (e.g., chemotherapy agents, ionizing radiation) than are Leydig cells. Exposure to such agents often results in primary hypogonadism characterized by an isolated impairment in sperm production or function and elevated FSH levels. However, severe testis damage induced by these agents may cause Leydig cell dysfunction or damage, resulting in both androgen deficiency and impairment of sperm production, and elevated LH and FSH levels.

Combination chemotherapy regimens that include alkylating agents (e.g., cyclophosphamide, ifosfamide, procarbazine, busulfan, chlorambucil), such as those used for the treatment of Hodgkin and non-Hodgkin lymphoma and leukemia, or use of alkylating agents, such as cyclophosphamide, in the treatment of systemic rheumatic disorders are particularly toxic to the testes and may result in androgen deficiency in up to 20% of patients.[270,271] High-dose chemotherapy and total-body irradiation before bone marrow transplantation may also cause androgen deficiency in a substantial proportion of men. In contrast, men with testicular cancer who undergo combination chemotherapy that includes platinum drugs (together with unilateral orchidectomy and, often, radiation therapy) have a relatively low prevalence of usually mild androgen deficiency with slightly low to low-normal testosterone levels and elevated LH levels.[271]

Exposure of testes to ionizing irradiation commonly suppresses spermatogenesis in a dose-dependent manner, and doses greater than 600 to 800 cGy may compromise Leydig cell function and reduce testosterone production.[16,272,273]

Orchitis. Viral infection of the testes may result in testicular atrophy, impaired sperm production, and, in severe cases, androgen deficiency. *Mumps orchitis* was common before the introduction of the measles/mumps/rubella (MMR) vaccine in 1968, after which rates of mumps infection decreased profoundly.[274,275] Because of worldwide shortage of the MMR vaccine approximately 15 years ago, there has been a resurgence of mumps infection and orchitis in adolescents and young adults. Prepubertal mumps orchitis is very uncommon and is not associated with subsequent testicular dysfunction. Orchitis is the most common complication of mumps infection in pubertal boys and adults; it usually causes permanent seminiferous tubule damage, impaired spermatogenesis, and, in severe cases, Leydig cell failure and androgen deficiency.

Mumps infection usually manifests with headache, fever, and malaise followed by unilateral or bilateral parotid swelling due to parotiditis.[274,275] Testis pain and swelling due to orchitis occurs in about 10 days or up to 6 weeks after the onset of parotiditis and may be subclinical in up to 50% of cases. Epididymitis accompanies orchitis in 85% of cases. Mumps orchitis is usually unilateral but may be bilateral in 15% of cases in adolescents and in 30% of cases in young adults. Even if orchitis is clinically unilateral, degenerative changes may occur in the apparently unaffected testis. Germ cell sloughing occurs as a result of acute infection, inflammation, and ischemia resulting from pressure induced by swelling of the testes within the tunica albuginea. The acute phase is followed by seminiferous tubule fibrosis and then testicular atrophy (30% to 50% of cases) for the next several months, resulting in impaired spermatogenesis in 25% to 40% of cases. In severe cases, prednisone may be used to reduce inflammation and swelling associated with mumps orchitis, but it does not prevent testis damage.

HIV infection usually causes gonadotropin suppression and secondary hypogonadism, particularly when associated with wasting and systemic illness. However, in 20% to 30% of cases, HIV infection causes primary hypogonadism characterized by low testosterone and elevated gonadotropin levels. The cause of primary hypogonadism is orchitis that is caused by HIV infection of the testis or occurs secondary to opportunistic infection (e.g., by cytomegalovirus [CMV], *Mycobacterium avium intracellulare, Toxoplasma gondii*) associated with the patient's immunocompromised state.[276,277]

Other causes of infectious orchitis usually associated with epididymitis include echovirus, arbovirus, or lymphocytic choriomeningitis infection; gonorrhea or *Chlamydia* infection in young adults and urinary pathogens such as *Escherichia coli* in older men; leprosy and tuberculosis; brucellosis, glanders, and syphilis; and parasitic infections such as filariasis and bilharziasis.[276,278]

Systemic Disorders. Low serum testosterone levels associated with symptoms and signs consistent with androgen deficiency are commonly associated with chronic diseases affecting the liver, kidney, heart, and lungs.[4,5] The underlying cause of both clinical and biochemical hypogonadism in these conditions is complex and multifactorial. The illness itself, associated complications, nutritional compromise, and medications used to treat the illness may contribute to or confound the clinical manifestations of androgen deficiency and also may suppress gonadotropin and testosterone production, thereby playing an etiologic role. Chronic systemic diseases usually have effects both on testis and hypothalamic-pituitary function and cause combined primary and secondary hypogonadism. Clinically, however, measurements of gonadotropin levels usually suggest predominantly primary hypogonadism (i.e., elevated gonadotropins) or secondary hypogonadism (i.e., normal or low gonadotropins). The benefits and risks of testosterone therapy in patients with these systemic disorders have not been evaluated in long-term randomized, controlled outcome studies.

Chronic Liver Disease. In men with chronic liver disease of any cause (and particularly in those with hepatic cirrhosis or liver failure), sexual dysfunction, gynecomastia, and testicular atrophy resulting in impaired androgen and sperm production occur commonly, affecting 50% to 75% of these patients.[4,5,279-281] Total testosterone levels may be low but are often normal or high-normal, because SHBG levels are increased substantially with cirrhosis and chronic active hepatitis. Therefore, measurements of free or bioavailable testosterone using accurate assay methods should be used to assess androgen deficiency. Free and bioavailable testosterone levels are usually low, and LH levels are usually elevated or in the high-normal range in patients with mild to moderate hepatic cirrhosis (Child-Pugh class A or B).

Estrogen (estrone and estradiol) levels are usually high due to increased production (e.g., induced by alcohol excess) and reduced clearance of adrenal androgens (e.g., androstenedione), which provide increased substrates for aromatization of androgens to estrogens. High estrogen levels contribute to the development of gynecomastia (high estrogen-to-androgen ratio), palmar erythema and spider angiomas, and increased prolactin levels. Treatment of ascites and edema with spironolactone may further lower testosterone levels and block androgen action, contributing to gynecomastia and other manifestations of androgen deficiency. High LH levels may be suppressed by high estrogen and prolactin levels and by the malnutrition that occurs commonly in men with hepatic cirrhosis and

liver failure; these factors may contribute a hormonal pattern more consistent with secondary hypogonadism in some men. Oligozoospermia or azoospermia associated with abnormalities in sperm motility and morphologic appearance occurs in approximately 30% to 50% of men with chronic liver disease.

Testosterone treatment of androgen deficiency is usually well tolerated but occasionally may worsen gynecomastia and rarely may increase edema and ascites by causing fluid retention. Because immunosuppressive medications such as prednisone and cyclosporine are used to prevent rejection, liver transplantation only partially reverses hypogonadism associated with chronic liver disease.[279,280]

Chronic Kidney Disease. Late-stage CKD commonly causes combined primary and secondary hypogonadism, resulting in androgen deficiency and impairment in sperm production in 50% to 60% of these patients.[4,5,282] Serum testosterone levels are low, and LH and FSH levels are high, in large part because of markedly reduced renal clearance of gonadotropins as well as increased secretion resulting from reduced negative feedback. SHBG levels are usually not affected by CKD unless nephrotic syndrome is present, in which case levels of SHBG and, consequently, total testosterone may be low. In the latter situation, free or bioavailable testosterone measurements should be performed to assess androgen deficiency. Sperm production is impaired, and sperm motility and the percentage of sperm with normal morphologic appearance are reduced. The Leydig cell response to hCG administration is reduced, consistent with primary testicular dysfunction. The frequency and amplitude of pulsatile LH secretion are altered, suggesting an alteration in hypothalamic-pituitary function as well. Hyperprolactinemia, relative nutritional deficiency, uremia, the proinflammatory state, comorbid conditions that secondarily suppress gonadotropins, and zinc deficiency that affects testicular function may contribute to testicular dysfunction in men with CKD.

Hemodialysis and peritoneal dialysis do not improve testosterone or sperm production.[282,283] Successful renal transplantation usually brings testosterone and sperm production to almost normal levels, although immunosuppression by rapamycin inhibitors (e.g., sirolimus) may impair testis function slightly.[282,284,285]

Aging. After age 40 years, there is a gradual and progressive decline in total testosterone levels (by approximately 1% per year), such that an increasing proportion of older men have low serum testosterone concentrations in the hypogonadal range.[286-288] Because SHBG levels increase with age, free and bioavailable testosterone concentrations decline even more rapidly (2% to 3% per year). Daily sperm production, sperm motility, percentage of sperm with normal morphologic forms, Sertoli cell number, and inhibin B levels also decline with aging.[139] Leydig cell number and testosterone production in response to stimulation by hCG and pulsatile LH are reduced, consistent with primary testicular dysfunction.[139] In older men, circadian variation in testosterone concentration is present but blunted.[64] Furthermore, pulsatile LH secretion is more irregular and disorderly and LH pulse amplitude is reduced in older compared with young men. Pulsatile GnRH administration normalizes pulsatile LH but not testosterone secretion, consistent with an impairment of hypothalamic GnRH secretion occurring in combination with a primary defect in testosterone production by the testis.[289,290]

Serum LH and FSH levels increase (by about 1% to 2% per year) with aging but do not usually rise above the normal range until very old age (>70 years).[286-288,291] Therefore, the most common hormonal profile associated with aging observed in middle-aged to older men is low testosterone with normal LH and FSH levels, consistent with "secondary hypogonadism." As men get older, gonadotropins continue to rise. A hormonal pattern of low testosterone and elevated LH and FSH levels, consistent with "primary hypogonadism," is more prevalent in elderly men, particularly after 70 years of age.

As men age, they may develop chronic organ failure or systemic illnesses, take an increasing number of medications, and develop nutritional deficiency or wasting syndromes that are associated with low testosterone concentrations.[292] It is likely that these comorbid conditions contribute to low testosterone and clinical hypogonadism associated with aging in men. Conversely, the age-related decline in testosterone levels may contribute to the susceptibility to or severity of clinical hypogonadism observed in these conditions.

In community-dwelling middle-aged to older men, the prevalence of low testosterone increased from 12% among men in their 50s to 48% among men older than 80 years of age.[287] The prevalence of clinical androgen deficiency (i.e., symptoms and signs consistent with androgen deficiency and low testosterone levels) was 6% to 9% and increased with age, reaching 18% to 23% among men in their 70s.[184,185] When more stringent criteria for the diagnosis of androgen deficiency associated with aging were used (i.e., three sexual symptoms and a low testosterone level defined as late-onset hypogonadism), the prevalence was 2% and also increased with age, reaching 5% among men in their 70s.[186]

In addition to the decline in testosterone levels, aging is associated with alterations in body function that could be attributable to androgen deficiency.[139] These include a decline in muscle mass and strength associated with reduced physical function and performance; decreased BMD and increased risk of osteoporosis and fractures; increased body fat; reduction in sexual function and activity, including reduced libido and erectile dysfunction; decline in vitality, energy, mood, and cognitive function; and alterations in sleep quality. Similar changes occur in younger hypogonadal men and improve with testosterone treatment, raising the possibility that the decline in testosterone levels that occurs with aging may contribute to these age-associated changes in body function.

Relatively small, short-term (up to 3 years) studies of testosterone treatment in heterogeneous groups of older men with low or low-normal testosterone levels without regard to the presence of symptoms or signs of androgen deficiency have produced conflicting results. Most have found beneficial effects of testosterone treatment on body composition, with increasing lean or muscle mass and decreasing fat mass, but less consistent effects on muscle strength and performance, BMD, sexual function, vitality, and cognitive function. The only adverse effect found in these studies was excessive erythrocytosis in some men. More recent studies of testosterone treatment in frail older men with low testosterone levels found beneficial effects on muscle strength and physical performance,[293,294] but there was an increase in self-reported cardiovascular adverse events in one small study but not in another similar study.[275,276] Meta-analyses of testosterone treatment trials[295-297] and pharmacoepidemiologic studies evaluating cardiovascular events associated with testosterone treatment[298-300] have also been conflicting. Larger, long-term, randomized trials are needed to determine the balance of clinical benefits and risks (particularly as related to prostate cancer and cardiovascular disease) of testosterone treatment in elderly men. Until results from these outcome studies are available, testosterone treatment should be considered only for older men who have

clinically significant manifestations of androgen deficiency and unequivocally low serum testosterone levels, and only after a careful discussion of the uncertainty concerning the long-term benefits and risks of treatment.[113,301]

Other Systemic Disorders. Primary hypogonadism with low testosterone levels or elevated LH levels (or both) occurs in up to 20% of men with *malignancy* such as advanced Hodgkin disease or testicular cancer before gonadotoxic chemotherapy and radiation therapy.[302-304] Impairment of sperm production is found more frequently, in about 30% to 50% of men with Hodgkin disease or testicular cancer before therapy. The mechanism of gonadal dysfunction before treatment is not clear.

Sickle cell disease is an autosomal recessive disorder caused by a point mutation in the β-globulin chain. It results in an abnormal hemoglobin (hemoglobin S) that polymerizes, leading to sickle-shaped, rigid, and fragile red blood cells. The disease is characterized by recurrent episodes of painful, vaso-occlusive events in a variety of organs due to thrombosis, ischemia and infarction, and hemolysis. Sickle cell disease is a common disorder, affecting approximately 1 in 700 African-American infants. Sickle cell disease may cause primary hypogonadism characterized by low to low-normal testosterone concentrations, clinical manifestations consistent with androgen deficiency, testicular atrophy and impaired spermatogenesis, and elevated gonadotropin levels, possibly due to repeated testicular vaso-occlusive events and infarction.[305-307] Hydroxyurea therapy and possibly zinc deficiency may contribute to impaired spermatogenesis. Men with sickle cell disease may experience priapism due to penile vaso-occlusion, and this may be precipitated by restoration of libido with testosterone treatment of hypogonadism.

Within the first few months to 1 year after a *spinal cord injury*, testosterone levels and sperm production are suppressed and gonadotropins are usually normal. However, in some men, LH or FSH levels or both may be elevated in the presence of low to low-normal testosterone, consistent with primary hypogonadism.[308] Chronically after a spinal cord injury, serum testosterone remains low and gonadotropins are usually suppressed or normal, consistent with secondary hypogonadism.[309,310] The latter condition may be caused by hyperprolactinemia associated with medications, nutritional deficiency, obstructive sleep apnea, or debilitation from chronic spinal cord injury. Testis biopsy revealed impaired spermatogenesis in approximately 40% of men with spinal cord injury, but mature sperm that could be used for TESE and ICSI were present in almost 90%.[311]

Vasculitis (e.g., periarteritis nodosa, Wegener granulomatosis, Schönlein-Henoch purpura, Behçet disease) or *infiltrative disease* (e.g., systemic amyloidosis) involving both testes may cause testicular damage and may necessitate orchidectomy, resulting in both androgen deficiency and impaired sperm production.[312-314]

Isolated Impairment of Sperm Production or Function

Congenital or Developmental Disorders. As described previously, cryptorchidism, myotonic dystrophy, and Down syndrome most commonly manifest with primary hypogonadism characterized by isolated impairment in sperm production without androgen deficiency and selectively elevated FSH levels. In men with less severely impaired spermatogenesis, serum gonadotropin levels are normal, but it is most appropriate to classify these men as having primary hypogonadism with isolated impairment in sperm production, because gonadotropin treatment has not been demonstrated to improve fertility.

Varicocele. Varicocele is a dilatation of the pampiniform venous plexus surrounding the spermatic cord in the scrotum. It is caused by retrograde blood flow into the internal spermatic vein, which is usually caused by defective or absent valves in spermatic veins or, rarely, by obstruction of normal venous drainage by extrinsic or intrinsic venous compression (e.g., from a tumor). It usually occurs on the left side, and most cases are asymptomatic. A varicocele is present in 10% to 15% of men in the general population and more frequently in infertile men (up to 30% to 40%).[181,315]

The relationship of varicocele to impaired sperm production and infertility is unclear.[181,315] Approximately 50% of men who have a varicocele demonstrate normal semen analyses, and many are fertile. Men with a large varicocele and infertility usually exhibit low sperm counts with reduced motility and increased numbers of sperm with abnormal morphologic appearance (e.g., tapered or amorphous sperm heads), but these abnormalities are not specific for varicocele. Testis size and serum levels of testosterone, LH, and FSH are usually normal. Varicocele is painful in 2% to 10% of men with infertility. Testis biopsy in men with a varicocele and abnormal semen parameters reveals a spectrum of histopathologic findings, including hypospermatogenesis, maturation arrest, and Sertoli cell–only histology.

It is unclear whether varicocele ligation improves fertility in men who present with infertility. Controlled trials to investigate the efficacy of varicocele ligation have not demonstrated improved fertility. However, these trials were generally small, heterogeneous, and of poor quality. A small number of controlled trials of infertile men with palpable varicocele and at least one abnormal semen parameter have suggested improvement in the spontaneous pregnancy rate with varicocele ligation. Some organizations have recommended surgical ligation for infertile men who have a large, palpable varicocele with an abnormal seminal fluid analysis.[181,315]

Y Chromosome Microdeletion. Yq chromosome (long arm of the Y chromosome) microdeletions are the most common genetic cause of impaired sperm production and male infertility. They are found in 5% to 10% of men with severe oligozoospermia and in 10% to 15% of men with azoospermia.[172] As mentioned earlier, microdeletions have been identified in three regions of the long arm of the Y chromosome (Fig. 19-28).[172,173]

Microdeletions in the *AZFa* region, which contains the *DDX3Y* and *USP9Y* (ubiquitin specific peptidase 9, Y-linked) genes, are usually associated with azoospermia and Sertoli cell–only histology. Microdeletions in the *AZFb* region, which contains multiple copies of the *RBMY* and *PRY* (PTPM13-like, Y-linked) genes, are usually associated with severe oligozoospermia and germ cell arrest at the pachytene primary spermatocyte stage and occasionally with hypospermatogenesis. Microdeletions in the *AZFc* region, which contains the *DAZ* (deleted in azoospermia) gene and is where the majority of Y chromosome microdeletions reside, are usually associated with germ cell arrest at the spermatid stage or with hypospermatogenesis with some mature spermatids present. *AZFc* microdeletions are found in approximately 12% of men with nonobstructive azoospermia and 6% of men with severe oligozoospermia. Microdeletions in both the *AZFb* and the *AZFc* region are usually associated with azoospermia and Sertoli cell–only histology.

Yq microdeletion analysis should be considered for couples who are contemplating ICSI, because these microdeletions have been shown to be transmitted to male offspring with the ICSI procedure.[172] If ICSI is performed in men with Y chromosome microdeletions, genetic counseling and preimplantation or prenatal testing should be considered.

Sertoli Cell–Only Syndrome (Germ Cell Aplasia). Sertoli cell–only syndrome, or germ cell aplasia, is an uncommon histologic diagnosis in which the seminiferous tubules are completely devoid of germ cells and are lined only with Sertoli cells with little to no fibrosis or hyalinization.[316] Men with this disorder present with infertility, normal androgenization, moderately small testes (10 to 20 mL in volume), azoospermia, normal testosterone and LH levels, and selectively elevated FSH levels (indicating severe seminiferous tubule dysfunction).[317] Occasionally, LH levels are slightly high and the testosterone response to hCG stimulation is reduced, suggesting mild Leydig cell dysfunction.

The cause of Sertoli cell–only syndrome is not known, but it is thought to result from congenital absence of germ cells due to a failure of gonocyte migration. In some families, however, germ cells were present before puberty but were subsequently lost during or after puberty. As described previously, a Sertoli cell–only histology may be associated with microdeletions in the long arm of the Y chromosome in the *AZF* regions.[318] Severe germ cell damage and loss occurring with Klinefelter syndrome, mumps orchitis,

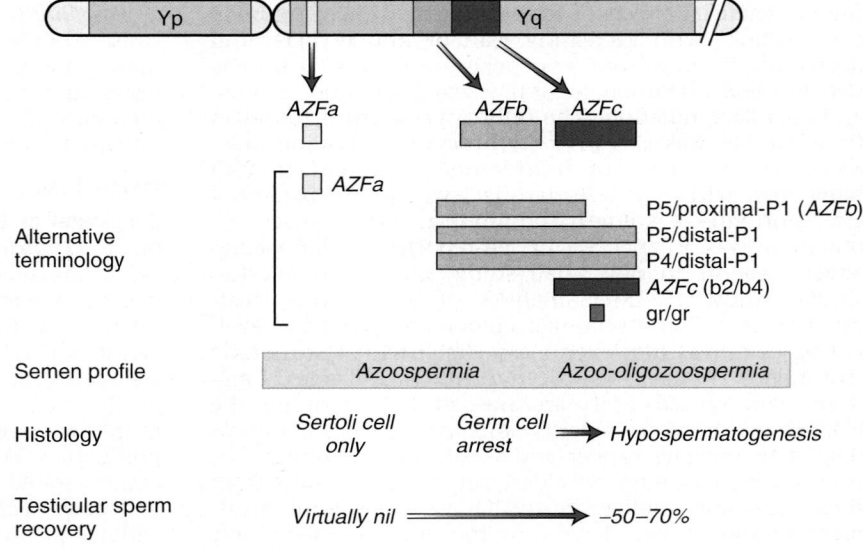

Figure 19-28 Schematic diagram of the short (Yp) and long (Yq) arms of the human Y chromosome. Deletions in regions of Yq, specifically in azoospermia factor (AZF) regions, are associated with severe defects in sperm production. Microdeletions in the AZFa region are usually associated with azoospermia and Sertoli cell–only histology. Microdeletions most commonly affect the AZFc region and may be associated with severe oligozoospermia or azoospermia. However, even if oligozoospermia or azoospermia is present, sperm for use in intracytoplasmic sperm injection (ICSI) are recoverable from half of the patients by testicular sperm extraction (TESE) at biopsy. (From McLachlan RI, O'Bryan MK. Clinical review: state of the art for genetic testing of infertile men. *J Clin Endocrinol Metab.* 2010;95:1013-1024.)

cryptorchidism, ionizing radiation, or alkylating agents may result in seminiferous tubules lined only with Sertoli cells. However, in these cases of acquired Sertoli cell–only syndrome, there is usually extensive seminiferous tubule sclerosis or hyalinization, and the testes are usually smaller. Infertility is irreversible in congenital Sertoli cell–only syndrome, but it may be reversible with time in some cases of acquired Sertoli cell–only syndrome.

Primary Ciliary Dyskinesia (Immotile Cilia Syndrome). Primary ciliary dyskinesia, or immotile cilia syndrome, is a rare, heterogeneous, autosomal recessive genetic disorder of cilia. It is characterized primarily by recurrent respiratory infections (sinusitis and bronchitis) that lead to the development of bronchiectasis, caused by impaired mucociliary clearance due to dyskinesia of respiratory tract cilia, and to infertility caused by asthenozoospermia (nonmotile or poorly motile sperm) due to impaired sperm tail movement.[319,320] In half of the cases, primary ciliary dyskinesia is associated with situs inversus and is known as Kartagener syndrome. Some men exhibit abnormalities of sperm motility in the absence of respiratory tract involvement.

Patients with primary ciliary dyskinesia and impaired sperm motility demonstrate ultrastructural abnormalities of the axoneme, the microtubule cytoskeleton of the sperm flagellum, especially in the dynein arms (motor protein complexes). Almost all men with primary ciliary dyskinesia have mutations of the genes encoding the dynein axonemal heavy chain 5 *(DNAH5)*, dynein intermediate chain 1 *(DNAI1)*, or dynein axonemal heavy chain 11 *(DNAH11)*. These men present with infertility and an isolated impairment in sperm motility with normal sperm counts and morphologic structure and normal testosterone and gonadotropin levels.

Follicle-Stimulating Hormone Receptor Mutations. Rare inactivating FSH receptor mutations have been described in males.[58,86] In contrast to females with FSH receptor mutations, who have primary amenorrhea and infertility, men have a more variable presentation. Some demonstrate severe oligozoospermia, whereas others have moderate oligozoospermia or normal sperm concentrations with abnormal sperm morphologic appearance and some have normal fertility. Serum testosterone levels are normal, FSH levels are elevated, and LH levels are slightly high to normal. It is possible that normal testosterone production within the testes contributes to the persistence of spermatogenesis and fertility in the absence of FSH action.

Acquired Disorders. Because seminiferous tubule function is more susceptible to damage than Leydig cell function, most men with primary hypogonadism due to chemotherapy agents, ionizing radiation, or orchitis caused by mumps or other infections manifest isolated impairment of sperm production without androgen deficiency.

Alkylating agents (e.g., cyclophosphamide, ifosfamide, procarbazine, busulfan, chlorambucil) used in combination chemotherapy regimens to treat lymphoma and leukemia almost uniformly cause azoospermia that recovers after 5 years in up to two thirds of men.[270,321,322] The effect of cyclophosphamide is dose-dependent, and cumulative doses of cyclophosphamide of 10 g/m² for malignancy are likely to result in severe oligozoospermia or azoospermia that may be irreversible.[323] High-dose chemotherapy and total-body irradiation before bone marrow transplantation commonly cause irreversible germ cell damage associated with azoospermia or severe oligozoospermia and elevated FSH levels. Sperm production is suppressed initially in men with testicular cancer who undergo combination chemotherapy that includes platinum drugs, unilateral orchidectomy, and often radiation therapy.[271] However, sperm production recovers in 80% of men by 5 years. Before chemotherapy begins, cryopreservation of sperm for subsequent use in IUI, IVF, or ICSI should be offered to men who desire future fertility. Approaches aimed at suppressing gonadotropins with GnRH agonists or exogenous testosterone administration have not been effective in preventing germ cell damage by chemotherapy.

Methotrexate and sulfasalazine may cause oligozoospermia and low sperm motility and contribute to infertility.[324] The processes of human spermatogenesis, and particularly the spermatogonia, are very sensitive to the effects of exposure to ionizing radiation.[16,272,273] X-radiation doses as low as 15 cGy may suppress sperm production temporarily. The time required to recover spermatogenesis after x-irradiation is dose-dependent. Recovery of sperm counts to baseline takes 9 to18 months after exposure to 100 cGy or less and up to 5 years after 400 to 600 cGy. Although Leydig cell function is more resistant to ionizing radiation, x-irradiation of greater than 800 cGy may cause Leydig cell damage and androgen deficiency. As with chemotherapy, sperm banking before radiation therapy for later use in ART offers hope for subsequent fertility.

Prolonged and repeated *thermal trauma* (e.g., with excessive hot tub use) to the testes may suppress sperm production, usually transiently.[325,326]

A number of chemical agents used in industry and laboratories have been implicated as direct toxins to the testes. Examples of *environmental toxins* include carbon disulfide, a solvent used in rayon production; dibromochloropropane, an insecticide; lead; deuterium oxide; ethyl glycol; cadmium; fluoroacetamide; nitrofurans; dinitropyroles; diamines; and α-chlorohydrin. Furthermore, it is postulated that environmental or xenobiotic agents such as phthalates act as antiandrogens or estrogens to alter reproductive function; these agents have been termed *endocrine disruptors*.[327] Such environmental agents have been implicated in causing the increased incidence of testicular dysgenesis syndrome (i.e., hypospadias, cryptorchidism, declining sperm counts, and testicular cancer).[328]

Systemic Disorders. An acute *febrile illness* may cause a temporary suppression of spermatogenesis.[328] In men with *spinal cord injury* resulting in tetraplegia or paraplegia, impaired sperm production may be caused in part by increased scrotal temperature due to loss of lumbar sympathetic innervations.[308-311] Men with malignancy, in particular Hodgkin lymphoma or testicular cancer, may have impaired spermatogenesis with azoospermia or oligozoospermia in 30% to 80% of cases before treatment (the former possibly related to B symptoms of fever, night sweats, and weight loss).[300,302,304,322]

In the majority of men who present with infertility and an isolated impairment of sperm production, a cause cannot be identified. *Idiopathic oligozoospermia or azoospermia* occurs in 60% to 80% of cases (including men with varicocele).[169-171] If isolated impairment of spermatogenesis is severe in men with primary hypogonadism, serum FSH levels may be selectively elevated. As mentioned earlier, men with less severely impaired spermatogenesis and normal serum gonadotropin levels are still classified as having a disorder of primary hypogonadism, because gonadotropin treatment has not been demonstrated to improve fertility in such cases.

Causes of Secondary Hypogonadism
Androgen Deficiency and Impairment in Sperm Production
Congenital or Developmental Disorders
Constitutional Delay of Growth and Puberty. It is important to consider *constitutional delay of growth and puberty (CDGP)* in the differential diagnosis of secondary hypogonadism

because it is a transient cause of secondary hypogonadism and is the most common cause of pubertal delay usually associated with growth delay and short stature in boys.[141,329,330]

The initial endocrine event that precedes the phenotypic changes of puberty is activation of the CNS mechanisms that regulate GnRH production, which results in pulsatile LH followed by testosterone secretion, initially at night (see Fig. 19-5) and then throughout the day.[42] Under the influence of increasing testosterone concentrations, secondary sexual characteristics appear between 9 and 13 years of age. .

The first physical sign of pubertal development is an increase of testis size to greater than 4 mL in volume (or >2.5 cm in length) and thinning of the scrotum, which is followed by development of rugal folds and increased pigmentation.[141,329,330] Subsequently, penile length increases and pubic hair develops over the next 1 to 2 years, followed by long bone growth (with peak height velocity occurring approximately 3 years later) and development of other secondary sexual characteristics, such as laryngeal enlargement and deepening of the voice. In boys, peak bone mass usually is not reached until the third decade. There is considerable variability in the onset and progression of puberty and the degree of virilization, and this is attributable in large part to an individual's genetic and ethnic background.

Delayed puberty is suspected if there is no evidence of sexual maturation and testis size is less than 4 mL by 14 years of age.[141,329,330] Boys with delayed puberty often experience considerable psychosocial distress due to the lack of sexual and physical development that results in their being considered younger than their peer group and having difficulty competing in athletics. In addition to the lack of sexual development, both boys and their parents are usually also concerned about the boy's failure to undergo a growth spurt and his short stature.

CDGP, or transient secondary hypogonadism, is the cause of delayed puberty in approximately 65% of cases.[141,329,330] Permanent secondary hypogonadism (e.g., due to idiopathic hypogonadotropic hypogonadism (IHH), pituitary or hypothalamic tumors, infiltrative diseases), which initially may be clinically indistinguishable from CDGP, is the cause of delayed puberty in fewer than 10% of cases. Other causes of delayed sexual development and growth, which are usually clinically apparent on presentation, include functional secondary hypogonadism (e.g., due to chronic systemic illness, hypothyroidism, medications) in about 20% and primary hypogonadism (e.g., due to Klinefelter syndrome, mumps, chemotherapy, radiation therapy) or androgen resistance in approximately 5% of cases.

CDGP is a physiologic variant of normal puberty that is characterized by a slowing of the growth rate and of the timing and tempo of pubertal development.[141,329,330] Because there is an increased prevalence of CDGP in families with GnRH deficiency (IHH), CDGP could represent a mild variant of IHH in some cases.[331] No genes or genetic polymorphisms have been identified that determine the variations in the timing of normal puberty. However, a family history of delayed puberty or being a "late bloomer" is found in 80% of boys with CDGP.

Clinically, a boy with this condition typically has a height age (i.e., the age that corresponds to the boy's height at the 50th percentile) and a degree of sexual development (usually prepubertal or early pubertal) that are concordant with his bone age, but all of these measures are similarly delayed with respect to chronologic age; in other words, growth, sexual development, and bone age are all re-

tarded.[141,329,330] Height velocity usually proceeds at a prepubertal rate or slightly more slowly, relative to peers of the same chronologic age whose height velocity has accelerated at 12 to 13 years of age.

In the absence of anosmia, hyposmia, or other morphologic abnormalities, CDGP cannot be distinguished clinically or biochemically from permanent IHH (see later discussion). If spontaneous puberty does not develop by 18 years of age in a normosmic patient, the diagnosis is usually IHH rather than CDGP. However, spontaneous reversal and relapse of hypogonadism has been reported in some men with both anosmic (Kallmann syndrome) and normosmic IHH.[332,333]

Eventually, boys with CDGP undergo normal growth and sexual development but several years after their peers.[141,329,330] Normal height is usually attained, but target midparental height may not be achieved. Also, acquisition of peak bone mass may be compromised in some men. Boys with CDGP may experience severe emotional distress and social exclusion or isolation as a result of immature sexual development and short stature. Therefore, after exclusion of organic causes of delayed puberty, testosterone treatment is usually initiated in boys with CDGP at age 14, or sometimes sooner, to induce sexual maturation and growth that is more consistent with that of their peers. Testosterone is usually started at a low dose and gradually increased over several years; it is stopped intermittently to assess whether spontaneous puberty occurs (see later discussion).

Hereditary Hemochromatosis. Hereditary hemochromatosis is a common autosomal recessive disorder that is characterized by inappropriately high gastrointestinal iron absorption resulting in excessive iron storage in a number of tissues, most prominently liver, pancreas, heart, joints, skin, testes, and pituitary gland.[334,335] In most cases, hereditary hemochromatosis is caused by mutations in the hemochromatosis gene *(HFE)*, most commonly homozygous C282Y/C282Y mutations (70% to 85%) or compound heterozygote C282Y/H63D mutations (5% to 10%), or rarely by other mutations in iron-regulating genes such as transferring receptor 2 *(TFR2)*, hepcidin antimicrobial peptide *(HAMP)*, hemojuvelin *(HJV)*, and solute carrier family 40 A1 *(SLC40A1)*. Homozygous C282Y mutations occur in approximately 1 of every 200 to 400 Caucasians of Northern European descent.

Regardless of the specific mutation causing hereditary hemochromatosis, iron overload results from insufficient hepatic production of hepcidin, a peptide hormone that degrades the iron-exporter protein, ferroportin; this causes unregulated iron absorption in the duodenum and iron overload in tissues.[334,335] Initially, iron overload causes an increase in transferrin iron saturation, followed by an increase in ferritin concentrations in most men with hemochromatosis. Therefore, the biochemical penetrance is high. Evaluation for hemochromatosis should be considered if iron saturation is greater than 45% in men. In the absence of inflammation or cancer, a serum ferritin level higher than 1000 µg/L is associated with greater risk of hepatic cirrhosis in patients with hemochromatosis, and a liver biopsy or MRI for hepatic iron content should be considered.

In contrast to biochemical abnormalities consistent with iron overload, the clinical penetrance of hereditary hemochromatosis is quite low (0.5% to 2.0%), and manifestations of iron overload (hepatic cirrhosis or carcinoma, diabetes mellitus, heart failure or arrhythmias, arthralgias or arthritis, bronzing of skin, hypogonadism) are far less common.[334,335] This may be related to the importance of secondary insults to end organs (e.g., alcoholic liver damage) that contribute to clinical manifestations or to earlier diagnosis with increased awareness and screening. Clinical manifestations, when present, usually appear at between 40 and 60 years of age.

Men with hereditary hemochromatosis almost always manifest secondary hypogonadism resulting in androgen deficiency and impairment in sperm production due to iron overload in the pituitary gland that causes selective gonadotropin deficiency.[336] Serum testosterone levels and sperm counts are low, LH and FSH levels are usually low, and gonadotropin response to GnRH stimulation is absent or markedly attenuated. In the presence of hepatic cirrhosis caused by hemochromatosis, SHBG levels may be elevated; as a result, serum testosterone levels may be normal in the presence of low free testosterone levels. Therefore, accurate and reliable measurements of free testosterone are needed to confirm biochemical androgen deficiency in men with hepatic cirrhosis due to hemochromatosis. Iron deposition in the pituitary may be detected by MRI. Iron overload also occurs in the testes and may occasionally cause a modest reduction in testosterone response to gonadotropin stimulation, resulting in combined primary and secondary hypogonadism. However, in most cases, gonadotropin treatment is able to stimulate normal testicular function, including spermatogenesis and fertility.

After diabetes, secondary hypogonadism is the most common endocrinopathy associated with hereditary hemochromatosis.[334-336] It usually occurs in men with hepatic cirrhosis and ferritin levels higher than 1500 µg/L (i.e., later in the course of iron overload) and diabetes. Because serum SHBG concentrations may be elevated in hepatic cirrhosis, accurate measurements of free rather than total testosterone should be performed to evaluate androgen status in men with hemochromatosis. The prevalence of hypogonadism in iron overload has declined from between 10% and 100% in older reports to approximately 6% more recently, associated with earlier diagnosis and less severe iron overload. Hypogonadism may be reversed with therapeutic phlebotomy, usually early in the course of iron overload.

Idiopathic Hypogonadotropic Hypogonadism. IHH, also referred to as hypogonadotropic eunuchoidism or congenital hypogonadotropic hypogonadism, is an uncommon, clinically heterogeneous group of disorders characterized by isolated gonadotropin deficiency of varying degree with otherwise normal pituitary function.[337] Males with IHH fail to undergo normal puberty, resulting in incomplete sexual maturation or eunuchoidism, androgen deficiency with very low testosterone (usually in the prepubertal range), low to low-normal LH and FSH levels, and impaired sperm production. Gonadotropin deficiency is caused by a defect in normal GnRH production or action, as evidenced by absent or abnormal patterns of pulsatile LH secretion (see Fig. 19-7)[47] and the ability of exogenous pulsatile GnRH treatment to restore normal gonadotropin secretion and testis function. Infants with IHH may have micropenis or cryptorchidism. Rarely, a man with normal virilization develops IHH as an adult.[338]

In approximately 60% of cases, IHH is associated with anosmia or hyposmia and is known as Kallmann syndrome.[337] Developmental failure of olfactory bulbs (detectable on brain MRI) is responsible for the anosmia or hyposmia. The remaining 40% of men have normosmic IHH. In addition, some men with IHH exhibit other developmental defects, including synkinesia (mirror movements), unilateral renal agenesis, cleft lip/palate or high-arched palate, sensorineural hearing loss, digital skeletal abnormalities such as syndactyly or brachydactyly (fourth metacarpal), dental agenesis, eye movement abnor-

malities or color blindness (deuteranopia), and agenesis of the corpus callosum.

The prevalence of Kallmann syndrome is approximately 1 in 8000 to 10,000 men, and there is a marked male predominance (male-to-female ratio, 4:1 to 5:1).[339] X-linked recessive, autosomal dominant, and autosomal recessive modes of inheritance are observed, but many cases are sporadic. Family members of a man with Kallmann syndrome may have variable clinical expressions, such as normosmic IHH, isolated anosmia, or CDGP.[50,340] In approximately 30% to 40% of cases, Kallmann syndrome is caused by a known mutation of genes that play important roles in the migration of GnRH neurons from the olfactory placode to the hypothalamus and in normal development of the olfactory bulbs during fetal development. These include mutations of KAL1 (10% to 20%), FGFR1/KAL2 (10%), PROK2 (5%), and PROKR2 (5%).[50,340]

The KAL1 gene is located on the X chromosome and encodes an extracellular adhesion glycoprotein known as anosmin 1.[50,340] Mutation or deletion of KAL1 results in failure of the normal migration of GnRH neurons from the olfactory placode to the hypothalamus, resulting in severe GnRH deficiency; it is the main cause of X-linked recessive Kallmann syndrome (type 1). The phenotype of Kallmann syndrome caused by KAL1 mutations is more severe and less variable than that of other known genetic defects. Synkinesia is present in 80% and unilateral renal agenesis in 30% of cases. The FGFR1 gene encodes for a fibroblast growth factor receptor that also plays an important role in the migration of GnRH neurons during development.[50,340] Mutations in this gene cause a spectrum of phenotypes, from severe autosomal dominant Kallmann syndrome (type 2) and normosmic IHH to CDGP associated with cleft lip/palate (in 30% of cases), dental agenesis, and skeletal abnormalities such as brachydactyly and syndactyly. PROK2 and PROKR2 encode for a peptide and its G protein–coupled receptor that play important roles in normal GnRH neuronal migration and olfactory bulb development.[50,340] The clinical phenotypes in men with PROK2 or PROKR2 mutations are quite variable, ranging from severe Kallmann syndrome (type 4 or type 3, respectively) to normosmic IHH.

In approximately 30% of cases, normosmic IHH is caused by mutations in genes involved in hypothalamic-pituitary function (particularly during puberty). These include mutations in GNRHR, the GnRH receptor (10% to 20%); KISS1R, which encodes the receptor for kisspeptin 1/metastin, an important GnRH stimulatory neuropeptide particularly at the time of puberty (2% to 5%); TAC3, which encodes neurokinin B, another important GnRH stimulatory neuropeptide, and the gene for its receptor, TAC3R; FGFR1/KAL2 (2% to 5%); PROK2; the genes for leptin (LEP) and its receptor (LEPR), which are associated with massive obesity; and, rarely, the GnRH gene, GNRH1.[50,340]

Hypogonadotropic hypogonadism is a component of complex genetic syndromes associated with specific dysmorphic features or combined hormonal defects. For example, the CHARGE syndrome, characterized by Coloboma of the eye or CNS anomalies, Heart anomalies, nasal choanal Atresia, growth Retardation, Genital defect (hypogonadism), and Ear anomalies (deafness, dysmorphic ears, and hypoplasia of the semicircular canals), may be associated with Kallmann syndrome or normosmic IHH.[341,342] In approximately 60% of cases, CHARGE syndrome is caused by a mutation in the chromodomain helicase DNA binding protein 7 gene (CHD7), which encodes for a chromatin remodeling protein. CDH7 mutations have been found in approximately 3% to 4% of men with Kallmann syndrome or normosmic IHH, and it is hypothesized that IHH may be a mild variant of the CHARGE syndrome.

X-linked congenital adrenal hypoplasia, characterized by adrenal insufficiency due to adrenal hypoplasia and normosmic IHH, is caused by a mutation in the dose-sensitive sex reversal–adrenal hypoplasia (DSS-AHC) critical region on the X chromosome protein 1 gene *(DAX1)*, now known as *NROB1* (nuclear receptor subfamily 0, group B, member 1), which encodes for an orphan nuclear receptor. Mutations of the SF-1 gene *(NR5A1)*, which encodes another orphan nuclear receptor; the prohormone convertase 1 gene *(PC1)*, which encodes an enzyme involved in post-translational processing of pituitary prohormones and neuropeptides; and genes for a number of pituitary transcription factors such as *HESX1* (septo-optic dysplasia or deMorsier syndrome), *LHX3*, *LHX4*, *POUF1*, and *PROP1* cause deficiencies in multiple anterior pituitary and other hormones in addition to gonadotropin deficiency. Mutations in the latter transcription factors may also be associated with specific dysmorphic features. Unlike men with IHH, those with multiple hormone defects usually fail to normalize gonadotropin and testicular function in response to chronic pulsatile GnRH administration.[50,340,343]

In the absence of anosmia, hyposmia, or features of Kallmann syndrome (e.g., synkinesia), it is not possible to confidently distinguish an individual who has normosmic IHH not associated with a complex genetic syndrome from someone who has CDGP.[141,329,330] In both conditions, there may be a family history of delayed puberty, IHH, or Kallmann syndrome; a history of cryptorchidism; clinical manifestations of delayed sexual maturation or eunuchoidism; and low serum testosterone and low to low-normal gonadotropin levels. In contrast to boys with IHH, who have normal height for their chronologic age, those with CDGP usually manifest some growth delay and short stature. Boys with IHH may have a history of micropenis and usually demonstrate pubertal delay after 19 years of age, although some individuals undergo spontaneous puberty after 20 years of age or reversal of IHH in adulthood; a subset of the latter may also relapse with IHH subsequently.[332,333] Currently, there is no diagnostic test that completely and reliably distinguishes isolated normosmic IHH from CDGP.

As discussed previously, after organic causes of delayed puberty (e.g., craniopharyngioma) have been excluded, testosterone therapy is usually initiated in boys with delayed puberty at about 14 years of age to induce sexual maturation and growth.[141,329,330] Testosterone is usually discontinued intermittently to assess whether spontaneous puberty occurs, as determined by an increase in testis size. Boys with IHH usually require continued testosterone treatment to achieve and maintain sexual maturation, whereas those with CDGP do not require further treatment after spontaneous secretion of gonadotropin and testosterone commences. Sustained reversal occurs after discontinuation of therapy in about 10% of men with Kallmann syndrome or normosmic IHH who present initially with absent or partial sexual maturation.[332,333] Therefore, it is reasonable to discontinue treatment briefly to assess the reversibility of hypogonadotropic hypogonadism in all patients.

If fertility is desired, testosterone therapy is stopped and treatment with gonadotropin or, in some specialized centers, pulsatile GnRH is instituted to stimulate sperm production. Previous treatment with testosterone, which might be expected to suppress endogenous gonadotropin further, does not alter the subsequent response of spermatogenesis to gonadotropin therapy.[344,345] Gonadotropin or GnRH therapy is much more likely to stimulate spermatogenesis if there is some evidence of sexual maturation and larger testes at baseline and no history of cryptorchidism or another primary testicular disorder.[338,346] Even in the absence of clinical evidence of hypothalamic-pituitary-testicular disorder, some men with IHH do not have an adequate gonadotropin or testicular response to chronic pulsatile GnRH therapy, suggesting underlying pituitary or testicular defects.[347]

Men with IHH have varying degrees of gonadotropin deficiency, as evidenced by a persistent but abnormal pattern of pulsatile LH secretion (see Fig. 19-7).[47] In some men with IHH, FSH secretion predominates relative to LH secretion, resulting in some germ cell maturation and spermatogenesis and a rare variant form of IHH known as *isolated LH deficiency*, or the "fertile eunuch syndrome."[348-350] This syndrome is characterized by prepubertal androgen deficiency or eunuchoidism caused by LH deficiency but pubertal or almost adult-sized testes in which advanced-stage spermatogenesis is present because of relatively preserved FSH secretion. However, spermatogenesis usually is not completely normal in these men, and they are not fertile, as the name of the syndrome might imply. Because there is only relative gonadotropin deficiency and some spermatogenesis is present, treatment with LH-like activity (hCG) stimulates Leydig cell testosterone production and ameliorates androgen deficiency, stimulating spermatogenesis sufficient for induction of fertility. Men with *isolated FSH deficiency* in the absence of an FSHβ mutation have been reported, but the degree and nature of the defect in pulsatile gonadotropin secretion have not been well documented.[351-353]

Men with inactivating *LHβ mutations* usually demonstrate a lack of pubertal development, impaired spermatogenesis or azoospermia, and infertility.[59,354,355] Recently, however, a man with an LHβ mutation resulting in a partially active LH molecule (as indicated by expression of steroidogenic enzymes in a few mature Leydig cells and low intratesticular testosterone levels) was reported to have complete and quantitatively normal spermatogenesis.[80] Complete spermatogenesis was achieved in the presence of very low LH and intratesticular testosterone concentrations and high serum FSH levels in this man. Men with inactivating *FSHβ mutations* have been found generally to have azoospermia with undetectable FSH, low or low-normal testosterone, and high LH levels.[80,82-85]

Complex Genetic Syndromes. Secondary hypogonadism may be present in a number of complex genetic syndromes, such as Prader-Labhart-Willi, Laurence-Moon-Bardet-Biedl, Alström, Bjornstad, Börjeson-Forssman-Lehmann, Bosma, Chudley, Costello, Gordon-Holmes, Johnson-McMillin, Juberg-Marsidi, LEOPARD (multiple lentigines), Martsof, Moebius-Poland, Roifman, Rud, and Woodhouse-Sakati syndromes.[246,259,356-371] Most of these syndromes are diagnosed by pediatricians and pediatric endocrinologists based on the clustering of specific dysmorphic features and congenital anomalies that are characteristic of the syndrome.[246] Secondary hypogonadism in these disorders usually causes prepubertal androgen deficiency. Many but not all of these syndromes are associated with CNS abnormalities or intellectual disability. Obesity may contribute to the cause of hypogonadism and may alert clinicians to the potential presence of a complex genetic syndrome. Some, such as the Prader-Labhart-Willi, Laurence-Moon-Bardet-Biedl, and Alström syndromes, have been reported to be associated with primary as well as secondary hypogonadism.[249,257,258,260]

Acquired Disorders

Hyperprolactinemia. Hyperprolactinemia is a common cause of secondary hypogonadism. These patients have low testosterone concentrations and low to low-normal gonadotropin levels and present with sexual dysfunction (reduced libido and erectile dysfunction), infertility, and gynecomastia.[372] Because the male breast usually is not exposed to a relatively high estrogen and progestin milieu needed to induce ductal hyperplasia and glandular formation in women, high prolactin levels in men rarely result in galactorrhea. Hyperprolactinemia causes gonadotropin deficiency primarily by suppressing pulsatile hypothalamic GnRH secretion, as evidenced by reduced spontaneous LH pulse frequency and amplitude and restoration of normal LH pulsatility and testosterone levels with dopamine agonist treatment or pulsatile GnRH administration.[373]

Common causes of hyperprolactinemia resulting in clinical secondary hypogonadism are a prolactin-secreting adenoma, pituitary stalk disease (e.g., stalk compression from a non–prolactin-secreting adenoma, traumatic stalk section); hypothalamic disease (e.g., hypothalamic tumors, granulomatous disease); and medications.[372]

In contrast to women who usually present with microadenomas, men with prolactin-secreting adenomas usually present with large macroadenomas because of a lack of symptoms, delay in seeking medical care for symptoms such as sexual dysfunction, or possibly a gender-specific difference in the biologic behavior of the tumor.[374,375] In approximately 10% of cases, there is excessive cosecretion of both prolactin and GH. In men with prolactin-secreting macroadenomas, serum prolactin levels are usually higher than 250 ng/mL, and they can be higher than 1000 ng/mL with tumors larger than 2 cm in diameter. If a patient with a very large pituitary macroadenoma is found to have only modestly elevated prolactin levels, this may be a false-negative result caused by saturation of both the capture and the detection of antibodies used in two-site sandwich immunoassays.[376] This phenomenon is known as the prozone or "hook" effect and necessitates dilution of serum samples.

Diseases affecting the pituitary stalk and hypothalamic diseases may cause hyperprolactinemia because of disruption of the hypothalamic hypophyseal portal tract and transport of dopamine from the hypothalamus to the pituitary in the former condition or loss of hypothalamic dopamine-containing neurons in the latter. Suprasellar extension of a large, non–prolactin-secreting pituitary macroadenoma that compresses the pituitary stalk usually causes hyperprolactinemia with serum prolactin levels in the 20- to 250-ng/mL range, although higher levels are occasionally seen.[372]

Medications that cause hyperprolactinemia (prolactin concentration usually <100 ng/mL) interfere with hypothalamic dopamine production or action or affect the regulation of dopamine secretion by CNS neurotransmitters (e.g., serotonin).[377,378] The medications that most commonly cause hyperprolactinemia are dopamine D_2 receptor antagonists, such as typical antipsychotic drugs (phenothiazines, thioxanthenes, and butyrophenones), some atypical antipsychotic agents (e.g., risperidone, molindone), and gastrointestinal promotility agents (e.g., metoclopramide, domperidone). In contrast, newer atypical antipsychotic medications such as clozapine, olanzapine, quetiapine, ziprasidone, and aripiprazole much less commonly increase prolactin. Other medications that less commonly cause hyperprolactinemia include some tricyclic antidepressants (e.g., clomipramine), monoamine oxidase inhibitors (e.g., pargyline; clorgiline, which is rarely used), and antihypertensive agents (verapamil; α-methyldopa and reserpine, which are rarely used). Selective serotonin and serotonin/norepinephrine reuptake inhibitors in general have minimal to no effect on prolactin levels.

Serum prolactin levels may be elevated in patients with CKD, in proportion to the degree of renal failure, because of both increased secretion and decreased clearance, and this may contribute to the hypogonadism associated with chronic renal failure. The mild hyperprolactinemia associated with primary hypothyroidism does not usually suppress gonadotropin secretion significantly or cause clinical secondary hypogonadism in men. However, if primary hypothyroidism is severe and long-standing, it may cause slight enlargement of the pituitary gland, which may be confused with a pituitary adenoma.

Treatment is aimed initially at the underlying cause of hyperprolactinemia. In men with prolactin-secreting macroadenomas, treatment is initiated with a dopamine agonist medication such as bromocriptine or carbergoline.[372,374,379] Dopamine agonist therapy usually results in a reduction of serum prolactin, decreased tumor size, and improvement in visual field defects. Treatment with these agents may also improve sexual dysfunction, normalize testosterone levels, and improve semen quality. In men who remain persistently hypogonadal despite adequate dopamine agonist treatment, testosterone therapy may be initiated to treat manifestations of androgen deficiency. Testosterone is aromatized to estradiol, which may act directly on lactotrophs in the pituitary and may increase prolactin levels and tumor growth and cause resistance to dopamine agonist therapy.[380] Therefore, careful monitoring of tumor size is required during testosterone replacement therapy.

In some men who do not respond to dopamine agonist treatment alone, gonadotropin or pulsatile GnRH therapy may be necessary to stimulate spermatogenesis sufficient to induce fertility. Surgery or radiation therapy may be needed for tumors that are resistant to dopamine agonists, and urgent surgery may be needed for pituitary apoplexy or rapidly progressive tumor mass effects such as visual loss. Medications that cause hyperprolactinemia may be stopped or switched to ones that do not elevate prolactin. For antipsychotic and antidepressant medications, such changes should be made in consultation with the patient's psychiatrist.[377] If discontinuing or switching drugs is not an option, testosterone treatment may be needed to treat androgen deficiency. Addition of a dopamine agonist while administration of an offending antipsychotic medication is continued should be done with extreme caution, because there is a risk of exacerbating psychosis.

Opioids. Use of opiates or opioid medications, particularly potent, long-acting narcotic analgesics such as methadone (>30 mg daily), controlled-release or intrathecal morphine sulfate or the transdermal fentanyl patch, and drugs of abuse such as heroin (diacetylmorphine) or time-released oxycodone (OxyContin), profoundly suppress gonadotropin secretion, resulting in severe androgen deficiency.[381-384]

Prolonged use of opioids causes symptomatic androgen deficiency, resulting in sexual dysfunction and long-term consequences such as loss of BMD and increased risk of osteoporosis; this is a common cause of secondary hypogonadism associated with androgen deficiency and impairment in sperm production. As such, testosterone treatment should be considered in cases of severe secondary hypogonadism due to chronic use of opioids. However, short-term use of opioids or use of short-acting opioids (e.g., postoperatively) may cause only a transient suppression of gonadotropins and testosterone that does not require treatment.

Administration of opioid antagonists such as naloxone or naltrexone results in an increase in LH pulse frequency in normal men, suggesting that endogenous opioid neuronal systems within the hypothalamus exert a negative regulation on pulsatile GnRH secretion.[385] Therefore, exogenous administration of opioids most likely causes reduced gonadotropin secretion by suppressing hypothalamic GnRH secretion. The action of exogenous opioid on GnRH secretion is probably mediated by μ-opioid receptors. In this regard, the pure μ-opioid receptor agonist, methadone, more severely suppresses gonadotropins and testosterone than does buprenorphine, which is a partial μ-receptor, δ-receptor, and opioid receptor–like 1 (ORL1)/nociceptin receptor agonist and κ-opioid receptor antagonist.[355] Both methadone and buprenorphine are used clinically for detoxification and maintenance treatment of opioid addiction.

In men taking chronic high-dose, long-acting opioids, serum testosterone, LH, and FSH are usually severely suppressed, and sperm production is impaired.[384,386] The most prominent abnormality demonstrated on seminal fluid analysis in men taking methadone is reduced sperm motility (asthenospermia), but abnormalities in sperm morphologic structure (teratospermia) and oligozoospermia are also seen. Functional δ-, κ-, and μ-opioid receptors have been reported to be present on human spermatozoa.[387] Therefore, exogenous opioids may have a direct effect by slowing sperm motility, independent of their effects on the hypothalamic-pituitary-testicular axis.

Sex Steroids. Administration of sex steroids, androgens, progestins, or estrogens suppresses gonadotropin secretion by negative feedback mechanisms at the hypothalamus or the pituitary gland or both; chronic administration may cause secondary hypogonadism, resulting in androgen deficiency and impaired sperm production.

Synthetic androgens (androgenic anabolic steroids) and testosterone are being used increasingly by boys and men to increase muscle bulk and strength and enhance athletic performance or physical appearance. For these purposes, these androgens are used in extremely high doses in a variety of combinations and patterns for prolonged periods. The prevalence of anabolic steroid abuse ranges from approximately 1% to 6% in various populations including high school and college students, young recreational athletes, and competitive athletes.[126,388,389]

During chronic administration of high-dose androgenic anabolic steroids, serum levels of testosterone, LH, and FSH are very low and sperm counts are usually suppressed to severe oligozoospermia or azoospermia.[126,388,389] Unless testosterone is being administered, serum testosterone concentrations are low, because synthetic anabolic steroids do not cross-react in testosterone assays. Although serum testosterone levels are low, abused anabolic steroids are themselves androgens, so individuals taking these agents usually do not complain of androgen deficiency symptoms.

After discontinuation of even prolonged anabolic steroid use, recovery of the hypothalamic-pituitary-testicular axis usually occurs within weeks to months. However, for unclear reasons, some men experience a protracted period of symptomatic hypogonadism that may last for several months to several years, particularly in older men.[126,388,389] It usually is not possible to know whether these men had underlying hypogonadism before taking anabolic steroids; therefore, if secondary hypogonadism is severe, an appropriate workup including sellar imaging is usually needed. Prolonged secondary hypogonadism after androgenic anabolic steroid use often causes sexual dysfunction and depressed mood. Severe symptoms may lead to continued use of these agents and anabolic steroid dependence. Treatment with testosterone to relieve symptoms of androgen deficiency or with gonadotropins (hCG) to stimulate sperm production and induce fertility may be needed. Off-label treatment with clomiphene citrate has also been reported to stimulate gonadotropin and testosterone secretion in these men.[390]

Chronic administration of high doses of progestins such as megestrol acetate or depo-medroxyprogesterone acetate or estrogens such as diethylstilbestrol also suppresses gonadotropins and testicular function, resulting in secondary hypogonadism. Megestrol acetate is used to stimulate appetite in wasting conditions such as cancer and HIV disease. At the doses used for this purpose, it causes severe symptomatic androgen deficiency and suppression of sperm production.[391] Weight gain induced by megestrol acetate is mostly fat rather than lean mass, in part because of the androgen deficiency that it causes.[392] Most importantly, megestrol acetate may cause symptomatic and potentially life-threatening secondary adrenal insufficiency.[391] Both megestrol and depo-medroxyprogesterone acetate have been used to induce medical castration in patients with prostate cancer.[393] Medroxyprogesterone acetate has also been used to reduce libido in psychiatric conditions manifested by deviant sexual behavior (paraphilia), and it is used in combination with testosterone (to prevent androgen deficiency) for suppression of spermatogenesis in male contraceptive development trials.[105,394] Administration of estrogens (e.g., diethylstilbestrol for prostate cancer), exposure to estrogen-containing substances, or excessive estradiol production by estrogen-secreting tumors (e.g., Sertoli cell tumors) suppresses gonadotropin and testosterone production and causes secondary hypogonadism, usually with prominent gynecomastia.[395-397]

Gonadotropin-Releasing Hormone Analogues. GnRH analogues, both agonists and antagonists, severely suppress endogenous gonadotropin and testosterone production (i.e., medical castration); they are used to treat androgen-dependent pathologic states such as locally advanced or metastatic prostate cancer and central precocious puberty.[190,398] Administration of GnRH agonists (e.g., leuprolide, goserelin) produces an initial stimulation of gonadotropin and testosterone secretion (known as a "flare"), which is followed in 1 to 2 weeks by GnRH receptor downregulation and marked suppression of gonadotropins and testosterone to castration levels.[190] The initial surge in testosterone levels has been associated with clinical flares in metastatic prostate cancer, and there have been reports of increased bladder outlet obstruction, bone pain, pathologic fracture, spinal cord compression, and death. However, these complications are very uncommon, and it is not clear that they are directly related to the initial increase in testosterone concentrations. To prevent the potential complications associated with the testosterone flare, AR antagonists (e.g., bicalutamide) are usually coadministered with a GnRH agonist for men with metastatic prostate cancer.[399] In contrast to agonists, GnRH antagonists (e.g., degarelix) cause an immediate suppression of gonadotropin and testosterone secretion without a flare.[398]

Continuous administration of GnRH agonists in men with locally advanced or metastatic prostate cancer induces castration or near-castration testosterone levels and causes symptoms of severe androgen deficiency, including sexual dysfunction with reduced libido and reduced spontaneous erections; diminished energy and motivation; depressed mood and irritability; hot flushes and sleep disturbance; decreased memory and concentration; reduced in muscle mass and strength; increased fat mass and insulin resistance; decreased BMD resulting in osteopenia or osteoporosis; gynecomastia and loss of male hair pattern; and decreased hemoglobin and hematocrit, resulting in significant decline in quality of life.[189,190] As a result, increasingly, GnRH agonist therapy is administered intermittently in the treatment of advanced prostate cancer. However, in a substantial number of men who stop GnRH agonist therapy, testicular function remains suppressed and testosterone levels persist within the castrate or hypogonadal range for prolonged periods (up to 1 to 3 years).[400,401] Risk factors for prolonged testicular suppression are longer duration of GnRH agonist therapy, older age (>70 years), and possibly low testosterone levels and hypogonadism that was present before treatment.

Large population studies have found that prolonged GnRH agonist therapy increases the risk of diabetes mellitus, coronary heart disease, myocardial infarction, sudden cardiac death, stroke, and fractures. Consequently, the U.S. Food and Drug Administration (FDA) has recommended that the risk factors for these diseases should be assessed and the benefits and risks of GnRH agonist therapy weighed before it is used and that monitoring for these conditions should be continued during treatment.[190,398,402,403] A 2011 meta-analysis of randomized trials reported that androgen deprivation therapy of men with unfavorable-prognosis prostate cancer was not associated with an increased risk of cardiovascular mortality but was associated with improved prostate cancer-specific mortality rate.[404]

Hypopituitarism. A destructive or infiltrative lesion of the pituitary gland or hypothalamus commonly causes impaired pituitary hormone production (hypopituitarism) and gonadotropin deficiency resulting in androgen deficiency and impairment in sperm production. The prevalence of hypopituitarism has been estimated to be approximately 1 in 2200.[405,406]

Hypopituitarism is most commonly caused by *pituitary adenomas* and their treatment (hypophysectomy or radiation therapy) or by *hypothalamic* or *parasellar tumors* such as craniopharyngioma, meningioma, optic glioma or astrocytoma, metastatic carcinoma (from breast, lung, colon, or prostate), pinealoma, germinoma, cordoma, and ependymoma; together, these tumors account for approximately 90% of cases.[405,406]

Other conditions of the pituitary or hypothalamus (or both) that cause hypopituitarism include cranial radiation therapy (intracranial tumors, acute lymphoblastic leukemia prophylaxis, nasopharyngeal carcinoma, total-body irradiation); vascular compromise (traumatic brain injury, infarction or pituitary apoplexy, subarachnoid hemorrhage, ischemic stroke, vascular malformation); granulomatous or infiltrative disease (sarcoidosis, histiocytosis X, Wegener granulomatosis, hemochromatosis, transfusion-induced iron overload); infection (tuberculosis, fungal infections such as aspergillosis or coccidioidomycosis, basilar meningitis, encephalitis, syphilis, Whipple disease); pituitary stalk disease (traumatic injury such as basilar skull fracture or surgical pituitary stalk section, granulomatous disease, lymphocytic infundibuloneurohypophysitis, infection, tumor); lymphocytic hypophysitis (in particular, lymphocytic infundibuloneurohypophysitis, which is more common in men, rather than lymphocytic adenohypophysitis, which is more common in women); and autoimmune hypophysitis (with ipilimumab therapy).[405-407] These conditions are discussed in Chapter 9.

Destructive or infiltrative lesions of the pituitary gland (e.g., nonfunctioning pituitary adenoma) usually result in a gradual, progressive loss of anterior pituitary function. In these instances, GH and gonadotropin (FSH and LH) deficiency (i.e., secondary hypogonadism) usually occur initially, followed by deficiencies of TSH (secondary hypothyroidism) and, eventually, ACTH (secondary adrenal insufficiency), resulting in *panhypopituitarism.*[405,406] However, there are many exceptions to this order of loss, depending on the specific location of the pituitary lesion and the nature of the underlying disease process. For example, lymphocytic hypophysitis usually causes ACTH and

TSH deficiency without impairment of gonadotropin production, and ACTH deficiency is more common than TSH deficiency after radiation therapy involving the hypothalamic-pituitary axis. Anterior pituitary hormone loss is even less predictable in disease processes involving the hypothalamus, in part because of the more disperse anatomic arrangement in the hypothalamus of nuclei that produce releasing factors for pituitary hormones. Acute destructive processes such as pituitary apoplexy usually cause panhypopituitarism.

Diseases of the hypothalamus or high in the pituitary stalk may be associated with *diabetes insipidus*, which is caused by destruction or retrograde degeneration of neurons producing arginine vasopressin (AVP) in the supraoptic or the paraventricular nuclei, respectively.[405,406,408] Processes involving only the pituitary gland do not cause diabetes insipidus.

Hypothalamic and pituitary stalk diseases may cause hyperprolactinemia due to loss of dopamine-containing neurons or interruption of the hypothalamic hypophyseal portal tract and transport of dopamine from the hypothalamus to the pituitary. Pituitary microadenomas or macroadenomas may produce prolactin, and suprasellar extension of nonsecretory pituitary macroadenomas or those secreting other hormones (e.g., GH) may cause hyperprolactinemia by interrupting the hypothalamic-hypophyseal portal system.

Prepubertal boys who have hypopituitarism resulting in gonadotropin deficiency present with delayed puberty and eunuchoidism, and men present with adult androgen deficiency and complaints of reduced libido and erectile dysfunction. However, in patients with secondary hypogonadism, clinicians must be alert to the possibility and clinical manifestations of *deficiencies of other pituitary hormones* (ACTH, TSH, GH, and AVP); *excessive pituitary hormone production* by pituitary adenomas and resulting clinical syndromes, such as excessive prolactin production resulting in hyperprolactinemia, ACTH resulting in Cushing syndrome, GH resulting in acromegaly, gonadotropin and free α- and β-subunits (which usually do not result in a hormone excess syndrome but rarely cause precocious puberty), or, rarely, TSH resulting in hyperthyroidism; and *tumor mass effects* such as headache, visual disturbance, and visual field defects (typically bilateral superior quadrantanopia or bitemporal hemianopia, but a unilateral effect and a variety of visual field defects may be present) and, uncommonly, cerebrospinal fluid rhinorrhea, cranial nerve palsies, temporal lobe epilepsy, and personality changes.[405,406] It is important to have a high index of suspicion for the presence of secondary adrenal insufficiency in patients with hypothalamic or pituitary disease, because it is a life-threatening and treatable condition that manifests with nonspecific symptoms and signs. In boys with hypopituitarism who present with a clinical picture of CDGP, GH deficiency may occur in conjunction with gonadotropin deficiency and may contribute to short stature and growth delay.

Usually in men with secondary hypogonadism due to hypopituitarism, the serum testosterone level and sperm count are very low, and LH and FSH levels are distinctly low or, less commonly, in the low-normal to slightly low range. The gonadotropin response to acute or chronic GnRH stimulation is not a clinically useful differential diagnostic test because it does not reliably distinguish between pituitary and hypothalamic disease causing gonadotropin deficiency in hypopituitarism. If hypopituitarism is suspected on the basis of the initial clinical and laboratory evaluation, further evaluation should include hypothalamic-pituitary imaging, preferably an MRI with gadolinium contrast enhancement, which can better define the presence and extent of hypothalamic and pituitary disease compared with a computed tomographic scan (although the latter is able to detect pituitary macroadenoma and microcalcifications found frequently in craniopharyngioma); formal visual field examination; and investigation of anterior pituitary hormone deficiency or excess.[405,406]

Treatment is aimed at the underlying cause of the hypopituitarism and treatment of pituitary hormone deficiency, including treatment of androgen deficiency secondary to gonadotropin deficiency with testosterone replacement therapy.[405,406] With transsphenoidal surgical treatment of pituitary adenomas, pituitary function is improved in approximately 50% of cases. Dopamine agonist treatment of prolactin-secreting pituitary adenomas improves pituitary function in 60% to 75% of cases. If fertility is desired, testosterone treatment is stopped and gonadotropin therapy is initiated, initially with hCG. In men with acquired gonadotropin deficiency without coexisting testicular disease, hCG treatment alone may stimulate spermatogenesis to levels sufficient to restore fertility.[79]

Systemic Disorders

Glucocorticoid Excess (Cushing Syndrome). Excessive levels of either exogenous or endogenous glucocorticoids (the latter due to pituitary Cushing disease or adrenal adenoma) is a common acquired cause of secondary hypogonadism resulting in symptomatic prepubertal or adult androgen deficiency and impaired sperm production.[409-412] In contrast to those patients with adrenal adenoma, some men with glucocorticoid excess due to adrenal carcinoma secrete excessive amounts of androgens (and mineralocorticoids) and do not demonstrate manifestations of androgen deficiency.

Glucocorticoids act primarily to suppress gonadotropins via inhibition of hypothalamic GnRH secretion, but they may also have direct suppressive effects on testis function and therefore produce combined primary and secondary hypogonadism. However, high-dose immunosuppressive glucocorticoid therapy is most commonly associated with a hormone pattern characterized by low testosterone and low-normal gonadotropin levels, consistent with secondary hypogonadism. Occasionally in men receiving glucocorticoid treatment, gonadotropins are high-normal or slightly elevated, suggesting primary hypogonadism.

Although it occurs most commonly with high-dose glucocorticoid treatment, doses as low as 7.5 mg of prednisone may cause hypogonadism, particularly in older men. Because high doses of glucocorticoids may suppress SHBG concentrations, it is important to confirm the biochemical diagnosis of hypogonadism using an accurate measurement of free testosterone (i.e., calculated free testosterone or free testosterone by equilibrium dialysis). In preliminary studies of men receiving chronic glucocorticoid therapy, testosterone treatment was found to improve muscle mass, BMD, and quality of life.[413]

Chronic Organ Failure. Chronic organ failure, such as in hepatic cirrhosis, CKD, chronic lung disease, or CHF, is a common cause of symptomatic secondary hypogonadism.[4,5] As discussed previously, chronic systemic illness commonly affects the hypothalamic-pituitary-testicular axis at multiple levels and usually causes combined primary and secondary hypogonadism, but many disorders are associated with a hormone pattern characterized by low serum testosterone and low to low-normal gonadotropin levels, indicative of secondary hypogonadism.

The cause of clinical and biochemical hypogonadism in these cases is multifactorial and encompasses both the chronic disease itself and its associated conditions of malnutrition, wasting, a proinflammatory state (with elevated cytokines such as IL-1 and tumor necrosis factor-α [TNF-α]), medication use (e.g., alcohol, opiates, glucocorticoids), chronic stress, and other comorbid illnesses. These associated factors play a large role in suppressing gonadotropin levels and contribute to the hormonal pattern of secondary hypogonadism associated with chronic organ failure. The degree to which these factors contribute to the clinical and biochemical manifestations of hypogonadism varies considerably among individuals. Furthermore, biochemical confirmation of low testosterone in patients with chronic organ failure or systemic illness may be confounded by alterations in SHBG. Therefore, accurate and reliable measurements of free testosterone are needed to establish biochemical androgen deficiency in the presence of chronic systemic illness.

Hepatic cirrhosis from any cause (e.g., alcoholic or nonalcoholic liver disease) is commonly associated with a hormone pattern that is consistent with primary hypogonadism (i.e., low free testosterone, high LH, and normal to high-normal FSH levels) in mild to moderate disease (Child-Pugh class A or B) and with secondary hypogonadism (i.e., low free testosterone and low-normal LH and FSH levels) in severe to end-stage liver disease (Child-Pugh class C).[280,281] SHBG concentrations increase progressively with the severity of cirrhosis, resulting in normal or high serum total testosterone levels despite low free testosterone concentrations and clinical manifestations of androgen deficiency. Sperm production is commonly impaired and sperm motility is reduced in men with hepatic cirrhosis.

In alcoholic cirrhosis, serum estrone and estradiol levels are relatively high as a result of increased production of adrenal androgens (e.g., androstenedione) induced by alcohol and its metabolite, acetaldehyde; reduced clearance of these androgens by the liver; and subsequent aromatization of androstenedione to estrone and its conversion to estradiol.[4,5] Relative hyperestrogenism is responsible for a number of the clinical manifestations commonly observed in men with alcoholic compared with nonalcoholic cirrhosis, including gynecomastia, palmar erythema, plethora, spider angiomas, and loss of male body hair (reduced axillary and pubic hair and a female escutcheon). Men with severe alcoholic cirrhosis usually have atrophic testes (usually soft in consistency) due to direct toxic effects of alcohol.

In men with severe hepatic cirrhosis, pulsatile GnRH secretion and the pituitary response to GnRH are diminished, contributing to secondary gonadal failure.[414] Spironolactone, which is used to treat edema and ascites associated with portal hypertension, is an AR antagonist and an androgen biosynthesis inhibitor. Its use may contribute to symptoms of androgen deficiency, gynecomastia, and hypogonadism. Protein-calorie malnutrition, complications of cirrhosis such as infection, and continued alcohol abuse contribute to the clinical manifestations and cause of low testosterone in these chronically ill men. Successful liver transplantation improves but does not normalize gonadal function, probably because of chronic immunosuppressive treatment with glucocorticoids and other agents.[280]

As described in a previous section, *CKD* is commonly associated with a hormone pattern of low serum testosterone and elevated gonadotropin concentrations resulting from reduced renal clearance, consistent with primary hypogonadism.[4,5,282,283,285] However, the amplitude of pulsatile LH secretion is reduced, suggesting impaired hypothalamic-pituitary function in men with CKD.[415]

Gonadotropin secretion may also be suppressed by coexisting uremia, hyperprolactinemia, malnutrition, a proinflammatory state, comorbid conditions (e.g., diabetes), and obesity, and some men demonstrate a hormone pattern that is more consistent with secondary hypogonadism (i.e., with low testosterone and normal to high-normal gonadotropin levels). Successful renal transplantation usually normalizes levels of testosterone and gonadotropins and sperm production.[282,283]

Men with *chronic lung disease*, especially COPD, commonly have low serum testosterone levels.[416-418] The prevalence of biochemical hypogonadism depends on the population studied and varies from 12% in a community-based population to 38% in male veterans, the latter being a population with numerous comorbid conditions. In the population of veterans, approximately 75% of men with COPD with low serum testosterone have low or low-normal gonadotropin levels, consistent with secondary hypogonadism, and the remainder have elevated gonadotropins, indicative of primary hypogonadism.[417] Coexisting factors that contribute to the clinical symptoms and biochemical diagnosis of hypogonadism in men with severe COPD include muscle wasting, inactivity, and deconditioning; malnutrition and cachexia; chronic stress and inflammation; medications (e.g., glucocorticoids); and hypoxia. Hypoxia suppresses gonadotropin and testosterone secretion independent of glucocorticoid therapy in men with COPD or idiopathic pulmonary fibrosis.[416-419] Preliminary studies have demonstrated an increase in lean mass with testosterone treatment in men with COPD and low testosterone levels but inconsistent improvements in muscle strength, including respiratory muscle function, and no effects on endurance or quality of life.

CHF is associated with biochemical androgen deficiency in approximately 25% to 30% of cases.[420-422] Men with CHF who have low serum testosterone usually have normal to low-normal gonadotropin levels, suggesting secondary hypogonadism. However, it is unclear whether men with CHF and low testosterone differ from those with normal testosterone in regard to symptoms and signs or response to testosterone therapy.[421] In limited initial clinical trials in men with CHF, testosterone treatment improved exercise tolerance, muscle strength, and oxygen capacity in men with either low or normal testosterone levels, suggesting a pharmacologic effect of testosterone independent of the presence of androgen deficiency.

Chronic Systemic Illness. A number of chronic systemic illnesses, such as T2DM, malignancy, rheumatic disease, and HIV disease, may also cause secondary hypogonadism characterized by low serum testosterone concentrations and low or low-normal gonadotropin levels.[4,5] As in men with chronic organ failure, the cause of clinical and biochemical hypogonadism is multifactorial due to the chronic illness itself and associated obesity (e.g., with diabetes mellitus) or malnutrition (e.g., with malignancy), wasting, proinflammatory state, medication use (e.g., opiates, glucocorticoids), chronic stress, or other comorbid illnesses. These factors suppress gonadotropin levels and contribute variably to the clinical and biochemical androgen deficiency seen in individuals with systemic illness. Because systemic illnesses and associated comorbid conditions and medications may alter SHBG concentrations, measurements of free testosterone are needed to confirm biochemical androgen deficiency.

Low serum free testosterone and low or low-normal gonadotropin levels, consistent with secondary hypogonadism, occur in 30% to 50% of men with *T2DM*.[423,424] Low testosterone levels are associated with nonspecific clinical manifestations that may be caused by androgen deficiency,

such as sexual dysfunction and reduced vitality. Insulin resistance and moderate obesity are commonly associated with T2DM. In patients with T2DM and moderate obesity, low total testosterone levels may result from reduced SHBG concentrations caused by insulin resistance and action on the liver. Therefore, it is important to confirm biochemical androgen deficiency in these men by using calculated free testosterone values or measurements of free testosterone by equilibrium dialysis.

Secondary hypogonadism and clinical manifestations of androgen deficiency may also be caused by comorbid conditions and complications associated with diabetes, such as obesity, atherosclerotic vascular disease, the proinflammatory state of diabetes, diabetic neuropathy, and CKD. Therefore, testosterone treatment should be considered only in those diabetic men with symptomatic androgen deficiency that has been confirmed by accurate free testosterone measurements. If symptoms do not improve with an adequate trial of testosterone therapy (e.g., 6 months), discontinuation of treatment should be considered, particularly in men who had borderline or slightly low testosterone levels before therapy.

Men with poorly controlled T1DM may have reduced serum testosterone and gonadotropin levels and reduced LH pulse amplitude and frequency, which are not present in those with well-controlled disease and in the absence of obesity.[425,426]

Men with *malignancy* commonly have secondary hypogonadism characterized by low serum testosterone concentrations and low or low-normal gonadotropin levels.[322,427,428] As mentioned previously, some men with malignancy present with low testosterone and elevated gonadotropin concentrations, consistent with primary hypogonadism. Malnutrition, wasting (cancer cachexia), systemic inflammation, medication use (e.g., opioid pain medications, glucocorticoids), chronic stress, and concomitant comorbid illnesses contribute to clinical and biochemical hypogonadism in men with cancer. Because SHBG may be reduced as a result of these associated conditions, free testosterone measurements are needed to confirm androgen deficiency.

Primary or secondary hypogonadism may be present before systemic chemotherapy or radiation therapy as well as after treatment. A low free testosterone concentration with normal or elevated gonadotropin levels was found in 40% to 60% of men with advanced malignancy (i.e., metastatic cancer) presenting with malnutrition and men with various stages of Hodgkin disease before chemotherapy.[303,304,322] Low levels of free testosterone and bioavailable testosterone were present, respectively, in approximately 78% and 66% of men with a variety of cancers, excluding those with androgen-dependent cancer (prostate, breast) or testicular cancer, most of whom received chemotherapy or radiation therapy or both.[322,427] Low testosterone was associated with reduced quality of life and sexual function.[428]

Men with *rheumatic diseases*, in particular the systemic autoimmune disorder rheumatoid arthritis, may manifest symptoms of sexual dysfunction (reduced libido and erectile dysfunction) and low serum free or bioavailable testosterone and gonadotropin levels in approximately 30% of cases.[429] Secondary hypogonadism in rheumatoid arthritis may be due in part to systemic inflammation (with elevated cytokines such as IL-1 and TNF-α), complications such as rheumatoid lung, and treatment with glucocorticoids, but it may also occur early in the course of rheumatoid arthritis in the absence of complications and before glucocorticoid therapy.[429] In men with long-standing rheumatoid arthritis, low free testosterone levels do not normalize after marked suppression of inflammation induced by anti-TNF therapy.[430] Testosterone treatment may improve symptoms of androgen deficiency, but it does not reduce disease activity.[431]

Men with systemic lupus erythematosus also may demonstrate low free testosterone concentrations in conjunction with normal or low-normal gonadotropin levels, indicative of secondary hypogonadism, or elevated gonadotropins, consistent with primary hypogonadism.[432-434] Factors that contribute to gonadotropin suppression and secondary hypogonadism include chronic systemic illness and inflammation, major organ involvement or organ failure (heart, lung, brain, kidney), and glucocorticoid therapy. Factors that contribute to primary testicular dysfunction include systemic and local inflammation or vasculitis, organ failure, and treatment with cytotoxic agents such as cyclophosphamide.

It is also possible that the hypogonadism contributes to the immunologic pathophysiology of rheumatic disorders.[435,436] Autoimmune diseases, and in particular autoimmune rheumatic diseases (e.g., Sjögren syndrome, systemic lupus erythematosus, rheumatoid arthritis), thyroid disease (Hashimoto disease, Graves disease), and autoimmune neurologic diseases (e.g., myasthenia gravis, multiple sclerosis), occur more commonly in women than in men. Sex steroid hormones, primarily estrogens and androgens, modulate immune function by direct actions on immune cell function and may play a role in sex differences in autoimmunity and in the pathophysiology of autoimmune disorders.

Men with *HIV disease* commonly have hypogonadism characterized by symptomatic androgen deficiency and impaired sperm production with low free testosterone levels due to combined primary and secondary hypogonadism.[437,438] Hypogonadism occurred in up to 50% of men with HIV wasting before the advent of HAART. Although androgen deficiency is less common since the advent of HAART, it occurs in approximately 20% of HIV-infected men. In 75% to 90% of cases, low free testosterone is associated with low or low-normal gonadotropin levels, consistent with secondary hypogonadism.[439,440] In the remaining 10% to 25% of cases, gonadotropin concentrations are elevated, indicating primary hypogonadism.

As in other chronic systemic illnesses, the cause of hypogonadism in men with HIV disease is multifactorial.[4,5] In addition to HIV infection itself, gonadotropin suppression and secondary hypogonadism may be caused by malnutrition, wasting, and cachexia; opportunistic infections affecting hypothalamic-pituitary function (e.g., CMV, *T. gondii*); systemic inflammation (with elevated levels of cytokines such as IL-1 and TNF-α); medications (e.g., opiates, glucocorticoids, megestrol acetate); ongoing substance abuse (e.g., alcohol); and acute and chronic illnesses. Conditions that may play a role in causing primary hypogonadism include opportunistic infections affecting the testes (CMV, *M. avium intracellulare, T. gondii*), malignancies involving the testes (Kaposi sarcoma, lymphoma), systemic inflammation, and medications (chemotherapy for secondary neoplasms, ketoconazole).[437-440]

Protein-calorie malnutrition may suppress SHBG concentrations, and advancing HIV infection is associated with increased SHBG levels. Therefore, accurate measurements of free testosterone levels should be used to evaluate men with HIV disease for androgen deficiency.[408,409] Sperm production associated with abnormalities in sperm motility and morphologic structure and testicular atrophy may be present. It is important to recognize that HIV may be present in semen even when it is undetectable in plasma.[438]

In small clinical trials, treatment with testosterone and androgenic anabolic steroid has been demonstrated to improve libido and sexual function; increase muscle mass and strength and BMD; decrease fat mass; improve mood, well-being, and quality of life; and increase hematocrit in HIV-infected men with low serum testosterone levels.[113]

Men with chronic *spinal cord injury* at any level resulting in tetraplegia or paraplegia may have secondary hypogonadism with low serum testosterone and low or normal gonadotropin levels.[309,310] In men with lower spinal cord injury causing paraplegia, there may be a transient suppression of testosterone levels within 4 months after the injury that resolves in most cases.[441] Gonadotropin suppression is caused in part by a number of conditions associated with spinal cord injury, such as acute and chronic trauma and stress associated with the injury and attendant complications; obstructive sleep apnea; obesity or nutritional compromise; hyperprolactinemia (usually associated with medications); and medication use (e.g., glucocorticoids, opioids, CNS-active drugs). The benefits and risks of testosterone treatment in patients with spinal cord injury are not clear.

Thalassemia major, or β-thalassemia, is an autosomal recessive disorder characterized by absent or severely deficient synthesis of β-globulin chains of hemoglobin resulting in severe anemia that requires lifelong blood transfusions. It is common in the Mediterranean region, in India, and in Southeast Asia. Chronic blood transfusions in patients with β-thalassemia cause *transfusion-related iron overload* in tissues and produce clinical manifestations similar to those that occur in patients with hereditary hemochromatosis. Transfusion-related iron overload may also occur in patients with sickle cell anemia, refractory aplastic anemia, or myelodysplastic syndrome.

Iron deposition in the testes and pituitary gland usually causes combined primary and secondary hypogonadism.[442-444] However, males with transfusion-related iron overload usually exhibit a hormonal pattern indicative of secondary hypogonadism, with low serum free testosterone and low to low-normal gonadotropin concentrations in most cases. Hypogonadism due to transfusion-related iron overload may manifest with prepubertal or adult androgen deficiency and impaired sperm production; affected boys usually have short stature and growth delay.[445] Treatment requires iron chelation therapy with agents such as deferoxamine, deferasirox, or deferiprone. In men with long-standing β-thalassemia, chelation therapy does not reverse hypogonadism.[446]

Sickle cell disease may be associated with low serum testosterone and low to low-normal gonadotropin levels, indicative of secondary hypogonadism.[447-449] Gonadotropin suppression may be caused by transfusion-induced iron overload (although much less commonly than in men with β-thalassemia[450]); hypothalamic-pituitary microinfarctions; medications (e.g., opioids for chronic pain); systemic inflammation; nutritional deficiencies; and chronic systemic illness and stress secondary to repeated painful vaso-occlusive events. As discussed earlier, men with sickle cell disease may present with primary hypogonadism due to testicular microinfarctions caused by vaso-occlusive events or iron overload affecting the testes. Priapism, which may occur with vaso-occlusive events, has been reported in patients receiving testosterone therapy.[451]

Uncommonly, boys or men with *cystic fibrosis* have low serum testosterone and low to low-normal gonadotropin concentrations, a hormonal pattern consistent with secondary hypogonadism.[452] Chronic systemic illness and inflammation, malnutrition, and glucocorticoid use may contribute to gonadotropin suppression.

Nutritional Disorders or Endurance Exercise. Starvation, malnutrition, and eating disorders (anorexia nervosa) suppress gonadotropin and testosterone secretion, resulting in symptomatic secondary hypogonadism with androgen deficiency (usually manifested by reduced libido, sexual activity, and performance) and impaired sperm production; these effects are reversed with restoration of food/calorie intake and weight gain. Fasting for periods of 3 to 5 days suppresses gonadotropin and testosterone secretion and decreases LH pulse amplitude and frequency.[453-455] These changes are reversed completely by pulsatile GnRH administration or low-dose recombinant methionyl human leptin replacement, suggesting that short-term starvation suppresses leptin production, which in turn suppresses the hypothalamic GnRH pulse generator.[456,457] Severe protein-calorie malnutrition, often associated with other nutritional deficiencies, may cause severe suppression of testosterone and elevation of gonadotropin levels, indicative of primary hypogonadism.[454,458]

Chronic *endurance exercise* results in low serum testosterone, low to low-normal gonadotropin concentrations, and impaired sperm production and motility, consistent with secondary hypogonadism.[459-461] High-intensity endurance training, such as occurs in the military and with overtraining in athletes, is associated with relative calorie deprivation and intense stress and causes more severe suppression of gonadotropin and testosterone levels than is seen with chronic lower-intensity endurance exercise.[453,459,462] Suppression of the hypothalamic-pituitary-testicular axis resolves with cessation of training and increased calorie intake.[463] Other than reduced spermatogenesis, the clinical consequences of androgen deficiency induced by endurance exercise are not clear.[464] In contrast to chronic endurance exercise, short-term endurance or resistance exercise in some men results in an acute and transient increase in testosterone levels that is modified by the intensity of exercise and prior training and is possibly related to hemoconcentration, reduced metabolic clearance, or increases in serum LH levels.[465]

Mild to moderate obesity results in reduced SHBG and total testosterone levels. Free testosterone is usually normal but may be reduced in association with low or low-normal gonadotropin levels in some men, particularly in those with comorbid conditions such as T2DM or obstructive sleep apnea.[466-468] In men with *morbid obesity,* particularly those with a body mass index (BMI) greater than 40 kg/m^2 or massive obesity (BMI >45 kg/m^2), serum free testosterone is low, gonadotropin levels are low or low-normal, and LH pulse amplitude (but not frequency) is reduced, indicative of secondary hypogonadism.[469] Morbidly and massively obese men often complain of reduced libido and sexual dysfunction, but these symptoms are confounded by obesity and comorbid conditions associated with morbid obesity, such as depression, diabetes, and obstructive sleep apnea. Bariatric surgery and weight loss increase serum testosterone and gonadotropin concentrations.[470-473]

Morbid obesity may be complicated by *obstructive sleep apnea* syndrome. Men with untreated or inadequately treated obstructive sleep apnea have low gonadotropin and testosterone concentrations independent of obesity and age.[467,474] Adequate treatment with continuous positive airway pressure (CPAP) may improve symptoms attributed to androgen deficiency and reverse biochemical secondary hypogonadism in some men, particularly those with massive obesity and comorbid conditions that cause hypogonadism independent of sleep apnea. Whereas obstructive sleep apnea may induce androgen deficiency, treatment of hypogonadism with relatively high doses of testosterone (e.g., doses associated with the use of parenteral testosterone esters) may induce or worsen obstructive sleep apnea

in men with predisposing conditions such as obesity and in older men.[467,475-477]

Acute and Critical Illness. Acute and critical illnesses, including medical and surgical illnesses requiring hospital or intensive care unit admission (e.g., myocardial infarction, respiratory illness, sepsis, burns, surgery, polytrauma, stroke, traumatic brain injury, liver disease), suppress gonadotropin and testosterone secretion as a result of combined primary and secondary testicular dysfunction.[478,479] However, the predominant hormone pattern during acute or critical illness is low serum testosterone with low or low-normal gonadotropin levels, suggesting secondary hypogonadism. Spontaneous LH pulse amplitude is reduced, but pulse frequency is maintained, and pulsatile GnRH administration only partially corrects secondary hypogonadism, underscoring the presence of concomitant pituitary and testicular defects.[480] For unclear reasons, aromatization of testosterone to estradiol and serum levels of estradiol may be increased, sometimes markedly, in patients with acute or critical illness despite low testosterone levels.[481] Estradiol levels are associated with fatality in critically ill and injured patients.[482]

The severity and duration of testosterone suppression are related to the severity of the acute or critical illness, the presence of underlying chronic systemic illnesses, and the medications used (e.g., glucocorticoids, opioids).[478,479] Recovery of testosterone and gonadotropin levels may take several weeks to months, depending on the severity and duration of the acute illness, duration of subacute recovery and rehabilitation, complications including malnutrition, medications, and underlying chronic systemic illnesses or organ failure. In the presence of underlying chronic disease or organ failure, hypogonadism may persist long after recovery from the acute illness. For these reasons, evaluation for underlying hypogonadism should not be performed during acute or subacute illness and recovery. It should be delayed for several months, until recovery to the individual's baseline or near-baseline clinical condition has occurred.

Aging. As discussed earlier, aging is associated with a gradual and progressive decline in total and free testosterone levels; as a result, an increasing proportion of older men have low serum testosterone concentrations in the hypogonadal range.[286-288] The prevalence of clinical androgen deficiency is 6% to 9% and increases with age, reaching 18% to 23% among men in their 70s.[184,185] Serum gonadotropin levels increase with aging but do not usually rise above the normal range until very old age, usually beyond 70 years of age.[288] Therefore, the most common hormonal profile observed clinically in middle-aged to older men is low testosterone with normal LH and FSH levels, indicative of secondary hypogonadism. Pulsatile LH secretion is abnormal and is characterized by disorderly LH pulses of reduced amplitude; it is normalized by exogenous pulsatile GnRH administration, suggesting a defect in hypothalamic GnRH secretion.[290]

The presence of chronic systemic illness or organ failure, medications, or malnutrition or wasting syndromes may contribute to suppression of gonadotropin and testosterone production. Conversely, the age-related decline in testosterone may contribute to the susceptibility and severity of clinical hypogonadism that occur in these conditions.[188,292]

Relatively small, short-term studies of testosterone treatment in heterogeneous populations of older men have produced conflicting results, with most finding beneficial effects of testosterone treatment on body composition (increasing lean mass and decreasing fat mass) but less consistent effects on muscle strength and performance,

BMD, sexual function, vitality, and cognitive function. Larger, long-term, randomized trials are needed to determine the balance of clinical benefits and risks (particularly, prostate cancer and cardiovascular risks) associated with testosterone treatment in elderly men. For now, testosterone treatment should be considered on an individual basis only for older men who have clinically significant symptoms and signs of androgen deficiency and unequivocally low serum testosterone levels and only after a careful discussion of the uncertainty regarding the benefits and risks of treatment.[113]

Isolated Impairment of Sperm Production or Function

Congenital or Developmental Disorders

Congenital Adrenal Hyperplasia. If untreated or inadequately treated with glucocorticoids, congenital adrenal hyperplasia caused by deficiency of 21-hydroxlase or 11β-hydroxylase results in excessive secretion of adrenal androgens (androstenedione and DHEA) that are converted to testosterone. Elevated circulating androgen concentrations suppress gonadotropin secretion by negative feedback regulation, which in turn decreases endogenous testosterone secretion and sperm production, resulting in secondary hypogonadism. Excessive androgen production averts androgen deficiency, so secondary hypogonadism is manifested by isolated impairment of sperm production and function.[483]

Adequate glucocorticoid therapy reduces excessive adrenal androgen production and usually restores gonadotropin secretion and normalizes testis function, including spermatogenesis. However, despite adequate treatment, some men with congenital adrenal hyperplasia continue to manifest impaired sperm production and function, most commonly as a result of long-standing inadequate glucocorticoid treatment and irreversible testicular damage caused by large adrenal rest tumors, or excessive glucocorticoid treatment. As discussed previously, excessive glucocorticoid treatment of congenital adrenal insufficiency also suppresses gonadotropin secretion and results in androgen deficiency and impairment in sperm production.

Isolated Follicle-Stimulating Hormone Deficiency and FSHB Mutations. Rare cases of men with isolated FSH deficiency in the absence of *FSHB* gene mutations have been reported; these patients had isolated impairment in sperm production characterized by azoospermia or severe oligozoospermia, and hypospermatogenesis or maturation arrest was found in the few who underwent testis biopsy.[351-353] These men had normal virilization, normal levels of testosterone and LH, low to undetectable serum FSH levels with poor or no response to GnRH administration, normal LH, and normal inhibin B and activin A levels when tested. In one man, administration of recombinant human FSH (rhFSH) alone resulted in a robust increase in sperm counts and induced fertility on two occasions.

Men with inactivating mutations of *FSHB* have been found generally to have azoospermia with undetectable FSH, low or low-normal testosterone, and high LH levels.[82-85] In one man, rhFSH administration was demonstrated to increase testosterone levels, suggesting that FSH-stimulated Sertoli cells may enhance LH-induced Leydig cell production of testosterone via a paracrine mechanism.[484]

Acquired Disorders

Androgen Administration or Excess. Exogenous testosterone administration (in normal men or in men with partial hypogonadism)[485] or stimulation of endogenous testosterone production by hCG administration[486] or ectopic hCG-secreting tumors (e.g., testis cancer, lung cancer)[487] suppresses pituitary gonadotropin secretion by negative feedback regulation; this in turn suppresses spermatogenesis by the testes in the presence of normal or high serum testosterone levels (i.e., secondary hypogonadism with isolated impairment of sperm production).[488,489] Use of some androgenic anabolic steroids (e.g., nandrolone) may also produce low gonadotropin levels and isolated reduction in spermatogenesis while providing sufficient androgen activity to avoid clinical androgen deficiency; however, endogenous testosterone production is usually also suppressed by androgenic anabolic steroid use, resulting in low serum testosterone levels.

Discontinuation of androgen or hCG administration results in restoration of normal gonadotropin secretion and recovery of normal sperm production and testosterone production by the testis. Long-term anabolic steroid abuse in athletes has been reported to be associated with testicular atrophy and severe oligozoospermia or azoospermia that persists for several months to years after discontinuation of the performance-enhancing agents. Suppressed sperm production induced by anabolic steroids may respond to treatment with hCG or with clomiphene citrate (off-label use).[390,490] Administration of testosterone in combination with progestins in normal men has been the main strategy used to suppress sperm production in recent hormonal male contraceptive development trials.[105]

Malignancy. Malignancies that occur commonly in men of reproductive age (e.g., testicular cancer, Hodgkin disease) manifest with impaired sperm production and function before chemotherapy or radiation therapy in 30% to 80% of cases.[302-304,322] Among men with cancer who provided semen samples for cryopreservation before treatment, approximately 64% had abnormal semen parameters and 12% had no viable sperm.[491]

In population studies, testicular cancer is associated with infertility. This association may reflect abnormal testicular development, termed *testicular dysgenesis syndrome*, caused by exposure to environmental gonadotoxins or endocrine disruptors (e.g., estrogens) or by an underlying genetic predisposition.[302,322,492] Testicular dysgenesis syndrome is also associated with cryptorchidism and hypospadias, and the former is associated with an increased risk of testicular cancer and abnormal spermatogenesis. Ectopic hCG secretion and possibly increased scrotal temperature associated with cancer within the testis may also contribute to impaired spermatogenesis in men with testicular cancer.[492] Hodgkin disease and other lymphomas and leukemias may be associated with fever, weight loss, and systemic inflammation.[492] These cancers may also involve the testis. All of these factors may play a role in impairing sperm production. Men with these cancers who have systemic disease, symptoms, or inflammation may present with low-normal testosterone, suppressed gonadotropin levels, and abnormal semen analysis, consistent with secondary hypogonadism causing isolated impairment of sperm production or function.

Hyperprolactinemia. As discussed previously, men with severe hyperprolactinemia (e.g., prolactin levels >200 ng/mL) develop secondary hypogonadism causing androgen deficiency and impaired sperm production. Mild hyperprolactinemia may be associated with isolated impairment of sperm production.[493] In most of these cases, gonadotropin and testosterone levels are normal and spermatogenesis is not improved with dopamine agonist treatment.[494] Therefore, hyperprolactinemia does not contribute to impairment in sperm production and probably is not clinically significant in most cases. In most instances, abnormal sperm production and function are caused by a primary testicular disorder, such as idiopathic oligozoospermia or azoospermia. Rarely, some men with moderate hyperprolactinemia (e.g., prolactin levels 100 to 200 ng/mL) have low-normal testosterone and gonadotropin levels and isolated impairment of sperm production that respond to dopamine agonist treatment.[493]

Androgen Resistance Syndromes

Congenital Disorders

Congenital androgen resistance and insensitivity syndromes are usually caused by defects in androgen action due to mutations in the *AR* gene or in the steroid 5α-reductase type 2 gene, *SRD5A2*.[120,131,495,496] Males with severe defects in androgen action present at birth either as phenotypic females, as occurs with *complete androgen insensitivity syndrome* (CAIS, previously known as testicular feminization syndrome), or as males with ambiguous genitalia and *46,XY DSD* (previously termed *male pseudohermaphroditism*).[496] Individuals with *partial androgen insensitivity syndrome (PAIS)* present with varying degrees of prepubertal or adult androgen deficiency and mildly to severely disordered male sexual development.

Males with CAIS usually present as females with normal breast development, primary amenorrhea, and absence of body hair.[496] Severe androgen insensitivity results in absence of male facial, axillary, and pubic hair; normal-appearing female external genitalia and distal two thirds of the vagina; and poorly developed or absent male internal genitalia (prostate, epididymides, seminal vesicles, and vasa deferentia) as a result of fetal androgen resistance. In adults with CAIS, female breast development is present due to conversion of normal to high concentrations of testosterone (which are secreted by the testes at puberty) to estradiol, which stimulates breast development. Because testes that are intra-abdominal or inguinal in location secrete AMH during fetal development, female internal genitalia (proximal vagina, uterus, and fallopian tubes) are absent.

There is considerable variation in the presentation of individuals with PAIS.[496] Some of these males present at birth with ambiguous genitalia, whereas others present at puberty or in adulthood with mild genital abnormalities or relatively normal genital development. Clinical manifestations of androgen deficiency and disordered male sexual development range from severe undervirilization to near-normal virilization with infertility. In men with PAIS, manifestations that are indicative of disordered sexual development, such as microphallus, hypospadias, scrotal abnormalities (e.g., bifid scrotum), cryptorchidism, and gynecomastia, are common. Gynecomastia is present in almost all of these individuals.

As a result of the variability in clinical manifestations, PAIS encompasses a number of disorders previously referred to as Reifenstein, Lubs, Rosewater, and Gilbert-Dreyfus syndromes. For example, Reifenstein syndrome is characterized by hypospadias, gynecomastia, undervirilization, a small prostate gland, cryptorchidism, and impaired spermatogenesis. However, even in the same family, different members may have different clinical manifestations. Some family members may not have hypospadias, and others may be normally virilized. Given this degree of variability in manifestations, the older eponyms are not clinically useful.[496]

Some men with PAIS have no evidence of disordered male sexual development and present with isolated impairment of sperm (idiopathic oligozoospermia or azoospermia), occasionally in association with gynecomastia, high to high-normal testosterone levels, and elevated LH levels. This disorder is referred to as *minimal AIS*.[131,495]

In both CAIS and PAIS, serum testosterone levels are high or high-normal and LH concentrations are elevated, but FSH levels are usually normal. Most men with CAIS or PAIS have autosomal recessive mutations of the *AR* gene on the X chromosome that alter its primary sequence and structure (almost always resulting in CAIS) or its function, resulting in impaired androgen binding to AR, AR binding to DNA, or AR transactivation.[131,495] In men with AISs, the correlation of *AR* genotype and clinical phenotype is relatively poor. In some men with PAIS or minimal AIS, no mutations in *AR* are identifiable and are possibly due to high CAG repeat length in the *AR* gene, mutations of *SRD5A2*, or mutations of coactivators or corepressors that regulate AR function.

An increase in the number of trinucleotide CAG repeats in the first exon of the *AR* gene results in expansion of the polyglutamine tract in the NTD of the AR.[134] The CAG repeat length is inversely correlated with AR function and action. Pathologic increase to more than 40 to 62 CAG repeats (normal range, 11 to 35) causes Kennedy disease (SBMA), a rare neurodegenerative disease that is thought to be caused by neurotoxicity from intracellular aggregation of the abnormal AR and associated coregulator proteins (see earlier discussion).[132,133] Men with Kennedy disease have clinical manifestations of partial androgen resistance, including gynecomastia, sexual dysfunction, oligozoospermia or azoospermia, and infertility, associated with high testosterone and high or normal gonadotropin levels. Higher CAG repeat numbers within the normal range have been reported to be associated with decreased virilization, impaired spermatogenesis and infertility, and gynecomastia in some studies but not in others.[134]

5α-Reductase deficiency, caused by an autosomal recessive mutation in *SRD5A2*, is a rare cause of PAIS.[120] Affected individuals typically present with markedly ambiguous genitalia, usually characterized by a clitoris-like phallus, a severely bifid scrotum, an apparent vaginal opening with perineal and scrotal hypospadias (termed *pseudovaginal perineoscrotal hypospadias*), an atrophic prostate, and testes located in the inguinal canal or scrotum or sometimes intra-abdominally (cryptorchidism). In contrast to men with AISs, wolffian duct differentiation is unaffected, and patients with 5α-reductase deficiency have normal epididymides, seminal vesicles, ejaculatory ducts, and vasa deferentia. AMH secretion by the fetal testes causes regression of müllerian duct structures, so no female internal genitalia develop.

Because ambiguous genitalia resemble female more than male external genitalia, individuals with 5α-reductase deficiency are usually raised as females.[120] However, with the marked increase in testosterone production by the testes at puberty, partial virilization occurs (i.e., penile growth, rugation and pigmentation of the scrotum, increased muscle mass and height, deepening of the voice, increase in libido, and spontaneous erections), and some of these individuals take on a male gender role at puberty, depending on complex psychosocial factors and cultural background. Sebum production is normal in these men. Because normal androgen action in the skin and prostate requires conversion of testosterone to DHT by 5α-reductase, men with 5α-reductase deficiency do not develop a male body hair pattern, and the prostate gland remains nonpalpable. Prostate cancer and BPH have not been reported in these men.

Men with 5α-reductase deficiency have high-normal to high serum testosterone and normal to slightly elevated LH and FSH levels. Serum DHT levels are low. Spermatogenesis is impaired (oligozoospermia or azoospermia) as a result of cryptorchidism, but normal sperm production has been reported in some men with descended testes.

Individuals with CAIS are usually raised as females and undergo orchidectomy (particularly if cryptorchidism is present) and treatment with estrogen replacement.[496] In men with PAIS or 5α-reductase deficiency, virilization has been induced with high-dose testosterone treatment, which increases serum testosterone concentrations to above the normal range and normalizes DHT levels.[496]

Acquired Disorders

AR antagonists (flutamide, bicalutamide, and nilutamide) induce androgen resistance and are used to treat androgen-dependent prostate cancer.[497] Drugs such as spironolactone, cyproterone acetate, marijuana, and H_2 receptor antagonists (specifically cimetidine) have AR antagonist activity.[498-502]

Men with *celiac disease* or gluten-sensitive enteropathy may experience manifestations of androgen deficiency, including reduced virilization, sexual dysfunction, impaired sperm production and function, and infertility. They may also demonstrate high to high-normal levels of serum total and free testosterone and high LH levels, indicative of androgen resistance.[503-506] Manifestations of androgen deficiency and biochemical androgen resistance may improve with dietary gluten restriction and improvement in small bowel atrophy in some men.[505] Malnutrition, nutritional deficiencies, chronic systemic illness, and hyperprolactinemia may occur in men with celiac disease and may contribute to their clinical manifestations. Serum DHT concentrations may be low despite high testosterone levels in men with celiac disease, suggesting that partial 5α-reductase deficiency may also be present and may play a role in androgen resistance. The main source of circulating DHT is from conversion of testosterone to DHT by 5α-reductase type 1 in skin and liver.[504] However, 5α-reductase is also present in the gut, so it is possible that loss of enzyme activity in the small bowel with active celiac sprue contributes to low DHT levels.

Treatment of Androgen Deficiency

Functional Versus Organic Causes of Hypogonadism

Once the cause or causes of hypogonadism have been established, prior to initiating testosterone replacement therapy, it is important to consider whether the cause of hypogonadism is functional or organic.[188] *Organic hypogonadism* is caused by congenital/developmental, destructive, or infiltrative disorders of the hypothalamus, pituitary gland, or testes that result in *permanent* hypogonadism. Generally, organic hypogonadism presents with clinically unequivocal severe androgen deficiency (also referred to as *classical hypogonadism*). Most causes of primary hypogonadism and some causes of secondary hypogonadism are organic. *Functional hypogonadism* is caused by nondestructive suppression of hypothalamic, pituitary, or uncommonly, testis function that is *potentially reversible or treatable*. Drug-induced primary hypogonadism is a functional cause. Many causes of secondary and combined primary and secondary hypogonadism are due to functional gonadotropin suppression.

Management or treatment of functional causes of hypogonadism might improve or resolve clinical and biochemical androgen deficiency and should be considered before initiating testosterone replacement therapy. For example, functional hypogonadism caused by hyperprolactinemia may be treated by discontinuation of medications that cause hyperprolactinemia or dopamine agonist therapy; opioids, glucocorticoids, CNS-active medications, or progestins may be reversed by discontinuation of the offending drug; nutritional deficiency may corrected by nutritional supplementation and weight gain; morbid obesity may be improved with diet-induced weight reduction or bariatric surgery; obstructive sleep apnea may be improved by CPAP therapy; type 2 diabetes may be improved by weight loss and reduction in insulin resistance; and alcohol abuse may be improved with treatment of alcohol dependence and abstinence. In many instances, however, functional causes of hypogonadism cannot be treated or managed in a reasonable time frame (e.g., opioid or glucocorticoid therapy for chronic comorbid illnesses), so testosterone treatment should be considered.

Testosterone Replacement Therapy

Therapeutic Goals and Management. The overall goal of testosterone replacement therapy is to correct or improve the clinical manifestations of androgen deficiency in men with primary or secondary hypogonadism. Because specific manifestations vary with the stage of sexual development, the specific goals of testosterone treatment vary depending on whether the patient is a prepubertal boy or an adult.[6,113]

In boys with *prepubertal androgen deficiency* and delayed puberty, the goals of testosterone treatment are the following[141,329,330]:

- To induce and maintain secondary sexual characteristics, including growth of the penis and scrotum, and a male body hair pattern
- To increase muscle mass and strength
- To stimulate BMD, acquisition of peak bone mass, and long bone growth without compromising adult height by inducing premature closure of epiphyses
- To stimulate libido and spontaneous erections
- To improve energy, mood, and motivation
- To induce laryngeal enlargement and deepening of the voice
- To increase red blood cell production into the normal adult male range

Testosterone treatment also stimulates the growth of accessory sex glands (seminal vesicles and prostate), resulting in seminal fluid production and an increase in ejaculate volume, but it does not stimulate sperm production to a degree sufficient for induction of fertility. The most common cause of delayed puberty is not a pathologic condition but rather CDGP. Testosterone therapy in boys who present with delayed puberty utilizes low-dosage testosterone to avoid premature epiphyseal closure and compromise of adult height, and treatment is given intermittently until spontaneous puberty occurs (see later discussion). If spontaneous puberty does not occur, the testosterone dose is increased gradually to adult levels.[141,329,330]

The goals of testosterone therapy in *adult hypogonadism* are the following[6,113]:

- To improve sexual function and activity by restoring libido and improving erectile function
- To increase muscle mass and strength, potentially improving physical function and performance
- To increase BMD, potentially reducing the risk of fractures
- To improve energy, vitality, mood, and motivation
- To increase hematocrit into the normal adult male range
- To restore male hair growth

Recent-onset gynecomastia that is usually symptomatic may respond to testosterone treatment, but severe or long-standing gynecomastia requires surgical excision. Spermatogenesis requires relatively high intratesticular concentrations of testosterone that cannot be achieved by exogenous androgen administration. Therefore, testosterone replacement therapy does not stimulate sperm production or increase testis size, nor does it restore fertility. Treatment of infertility in hypogonadal men is usually possible only in those men with secondary hypogonadism and gonadotropin deficiency; gonadotropin or GnRH therapy is used to induce spermatogenesis and fertility.[507]

The normal adult range of serum testosterone levels is broad and is usually based on results in healthy young men using blood samples drawn in the morning. In young men with androgen deficiency, testosterone replacement therapy produces beneficial clinical effects as serum testosterone concentrations are increased into this normal range. Serum testosterone levels decline gradually and progressively with age, but the physiologic significance of this age-related decline is unclear. Initial studies in older men with low serum testosterone levels demonstrated some clinical beneficial effects with testosterone treatment that increased testosterone levels into the normal young adult range. Therefore, the goal of testosterone treatment of hypogonadism is to restore serum testosterone concentrations to within the normal adult range, irrespective of age.[113]

The dose-response effects of testosterone vary in different target organs and for different clinical outcomes.[508] For example, the action of testosterone on muscle mass demonstrates a continuous dose-response relationship. With testosterone administration, muscle mass increases when testosterone levels are increased from below normal to within the normal range, and it continues to increase as levels are raised from within to above the normal range. In contrast, the actions of testosterone on libido exhibit threshold dose-response characteristics: testosterone administration increases libido when serum testosterone concentrations are increased from low to low-normal levels but does not continue to stimulate libido further as serum testosterone is increased to normal or supraphysiologic levels.

In men with severe, long-standing androgen deficiency, testosterone replacement therapy induces profound alterations in sexuality, behavior, and physical appearance that may be upsetting to patients and their partners and may result in serious adjustment problems. To reduce the likelihood of problems, it is important to inform and counsel hypogonadal men and their partners regarding changes in body characteristics and behavior that are expected during testosterone replacement therapy. In some men with severe, long-standing hypogonadism, initiation of testosterone replacement with a low-dose regimen (e.g., testosterone enanthate or cypionate 100 mg every 2 weeks, testosterone patch 2.5 mg daily, testosterone gel 2.5 g daily) for several months, followed by an increase to full testosterone replacement, may produce a more gradual symptomatic transition from hypogonadism to eugonadism and may result in fewer adjustment difficulties.[509]

Because the metabolic clearance rate of testosterone is reduced in older men with hypogonadism, therapeutic testosterone levels may be achieved with lower doses of testosterone.[510] In some clinical situations, such as severe symptomatic BPH or the presence of a number of comorbid illnesses, full testosterone replacement may be ill advised. In these instances, low-dose testosterone supplementation (e.g., testosterone enanthate or cypionate 50 mg to 100 mg IM injection every 2 weeks, testosterone patch 2.5 mg daily, testosterone gel 2.5 g daily) may be more prudent than full testosterone replacement therapy. Low doses of testosterone may be sufficient to induce some beneficial effects while minimizing potential adverse stimulatory effects on prostate growth.

The potential effectiveness of low-dose testosterone supplementation is suggested by studies of short-acting testosterone formulations (such as oral testosterone undecanoate and sublinqual testosterone cyclodextrin) that produced anabolic effects despite serum testosterone concentrations that were not sustained within the normal range.[511,512] An analogy may be made to the use of hydrocortisone for glucocorticoid replacement therapy, in which the duration of biologic action of hydrocortisone on tissues is not reflected by its serum concentrations. Short-term administration of low-dose testosterone enanthate (50 mg/week IM) was found to increase muscle strength and power in some young men in whom hypogonadism was induced by concomitant GnRH agonist treatment.[513]

Hypogonadism due to gonadotropin deficiency may be caused by hypothalamic-pituitary disease that requires specific management in addition to testosterone replacement. Therefore, careful evaluation to determine the cause of secondary hypogonadism should be performed before testosterone treatment is started. For example, pituitary or hypothalamic tumors may cause mass effects such as visual field defects, or they may be associated with deficiency or excessive secretion of other pituitary hormones. These tumors may require surgery or radiation therapy, additional hormonal replacement, medical therapy, or some combination of these treatments to reduce excessive pituitary hormone secretion. In some cases, treatment of the underlying cause of secondary hypogonadism corrects the androgen deficiency (e.g., stopping a medication that causes hyperprolactinemia or gonadotropin deficiency). In men with gonadotropin deficiency and normal testes who are interested in fathering children, gonadotropin therapy may be used instead of testosterone replacement to stimulate sperm production, restore fertility, and correct androgen deficiency. Similarly, men with secondary hypogonadism due to hypothalamic disease may be treated with pulsatile GnRH to stimulate testosterone and sperm production and restore fertility.

A comprehensive clinical approach is important for optimal management of hypogonadism. It is important to consider causes other than androgen deficiency that might contribute to clinical manifestations and to manage them appropriately. In hypogonadal men who complain primarily of sexual dysfunction, an underlying neurovascular disease or use of certain medications is usually the major cause of erectile dysfunction. In these men, testosterone treatment alone is insufficient to completely restore erections and permit satisfactory sexual intercourse. Additional treatment with a type 5 phosphodiesterase inhibitor (sildenafil, vardenafil, or tadalafil),[153,514] intracavernosal or intraurethral PE₁ (alprostadil [Muse]), or a penile vacuum device may be needed for a satisfactory clinical outcome. In hypogonadal men who present with osteoporosis, it is critical to perform a thorough evaluation for other common causes of bone loss (e.g., vitamin D deficiency, alcohol abuse, smoking, medications, inactivity, primary hyperparathyroidism) and to treat them as well. It is also important to institute measures to prevent falls to reduce the risk of fractures.

Testosterone Formulations. Testosterone formulations that are used to treat male hypogonadism are summarized in Table 19-10.[6,113] In the United States, approved formulations include parenteral testosterone esters that are administered by long- and short-acting IM injection; transdermal testosterone patch and testosterone gels or solutions; a transbuccal testosterone tablet; and an intranasal testosterone gel.

Oral 17α-alkylated testosterone derivatives, such as methyltestosterone and fluoxymesterone, should not be used for testosterone replacement therapy.[6] It is difficult to achieve full androgen replacement with these oral formulations because they are weak androgens that have low bioavailability. They also have the potential for serious hepatotoxicity.[389] 17α-Alkylated androgens most

TABLE 19-10

Treatment of Adult Male Hypogonadism

Formulation	Dosage	Advantages	Disadvantages
		Treatment of Androgen Deficiency	
Formulations Available in the United States			
Parenteral Testosterone Esters			
Testosterone enanthate or cypionate, IM injections	*Adults:* 150-200 mg IM every 2 wk or 75-100 mg IM every wk *Prepubertal boys:* 50-100 mg monthly or 25-50 mg every 2 wk, increasing to 50-100 mg every 2 wk and then to adult replacement dosage over 2-4 yr or until spontaneous pubertal development occurs	Extensive clinical use Inexpensive with self-injection Some dose flexibility	IM injections, discomfort Symptomatic fluctuation of T levels (supraphysiologic after injection to low-normal or low before next injection) Frequent IM injections to reduce fluctuations of T levels More erythrocytosis than with transdermal T
Testosterone undecanoate, IM injections	750 mg at 0 and 4 wk, then every 10 wk	Less frequent IM injections Maintenance of normal T levels for a longer duration No apparent fluctuations in symptoms	REMS: Slow deep IM injection in clinic (no self-injection); 30-min observation for potential pulmonary oil microembolism (POME) and anaphylaxis IM injections, discomfort Large-volume injection (3 mL) Self-injection not possible Rarely, cough immediately after injection Prolonged maintenance of T level after discontinuation if adverse effects develop
Transdermal Testosterone			
Testosterone patch (nonscrotal)	2 mg or 4 mg (one patch) or 6 mg (one 2-mg plus one 4-mg patch) applied daily over nonpressure areas	Low- to mid-normal physiologic T levels Mimics normal circadian variation when applied nightly No injections Less erythrocytosis than with parenteral T Rapid withdrawal of T replacement if adverse effects occur	Frequent skin irritation Low-normal T levels: two patches may be needed Skin adhesion poor with excessive sweating Daily application More expensive than parenteral T
Testosterone gels and solutions	1% T gel: 5-10 g of gel (delivering 5-10 mg of T) applied daily over shoulders or upper arms Available in foil sachets of 2.5 or 5.0 g, tube of 5 g, and metered-dose pump delivering 1.25 g per pump depression 1.62% T gel: 20.25-81 mg (delivering 2.025-8.1 mg of T) applied daily to shoulders or upper arms Available in 20.25-mg and 40.5-mg packets (delivering 2.025 and 4.05 mg of T) or metered-dose pump delivering 20.25 mg (delivering 2.025 mg of T) per pump depression 2% gel: 40-70 mg (delivering 4-7 mg of T) applied daily to inner thighs Available in a metered-dose pump delivering 10 mg (delivering 1 mg of T) per pump depression 2% solution: 30-120 mg applied to underarms Available in a metered-dose pump applicator delivering 30 mg (delivery 3 mg of T) per pump depression	Low- to high-normal steady-state physiologic T levels No injections Little skin irritation Dose flexibility Rapid withdrawal of T replacement if adverse effects occur Same as 1% gel Less gel amount in more concentrated formulations Same as 1% gel Absorption of solution not affected by deodorant or antiperspirant	Potential for contact transfer of T to women or children Daily application More expensive than parenteral T, especially with higher doses Moderately high DHT levels One formulation has a musk odor and another is associated with stickiness or skin dryness Slight skin irritation in some men Solution may drip under arms

TABLE 19-10

Treatment of Adult Male Hypogonadism—cont'd

Formulation	Dosage	Advantages	Disadvantages
Treatment of Androgen Deficiency			
Transbuccal testosterone	30-mg tablet applied between cheek and gum bid	Mid-normal steady-state physiologic T levels No injections, patch or gel application, or their associated disadvantages Rapid withdrawal of T replacement if adverse effects occur	Twice-daily application Gum irritation or inflammation Altered or bitter taste High learning curve for proper application; requires careful instruction or poor acceptability occurs Tablets may be difficult to remove or may fall off prematurely No dose flexibility Moderately high DHT levels More expensive than parenteral T
Testosterone nasal gel	11 mg (delivering 1.1 mg of T) three times daily (every 6-8 hours) for a total daily dose of 33 mg (delivering 3.3 mg of T) daily Available in a metered-dose pump that delivers 5.5 mg (delivering 0.55 mg of T) per pump depression	No injections No interaction with sympathomimetic nasal decongestants	Thrice-daily administration Learning curve for proper administration Fluctuation in T levels from lower to upper normal range after administration No nose blowing or sniffing for 1 hour after administration Discontinue with severe rhinitis Nasal irritation Not recommended with other intranasal drugs or chronic nasal conditions
Testosterone pellets	2-6 pellets (each 3.2 mm diameter × 9 mm in length pellet containing 75 mg of T, for a total of 150-450 mg of T delivered) implanted SC every 3-6 mo (usually 3-4 mo)	Maintenance of normal T levels for a longer duration	Requires surgical incision Extrusion, bleeding, and infection can occur uncommonly Large number of pellets Not easily removed; fibrosis may occur Lack of ability for rapid withdrawal of T replacement if adverse effects occur Infrequent use
Testosterone Formulations Available Outside the United States			
Oral testosterone undecanoate	40-80 mg PO with meals twice a day to three times a day	Oral administration is convenient for many	Twice- or thrice-daily administration Variable T levels and clinical responses Requires administration with meal High DHT levels
Testosterone-in-adhesive matrix patch	Two patches (delivering 4.8 mg of T per day) applied every 2 days	Low- to mid-normal physiologic T levels Duration 2 days No injections	Some skin irritation Two patches needed
Treatment to Initiate and Maintain Sperm Production in Men With Hypogonadotropic Hypogonadism			
Initially to Stimulate Testosterone and Potentially Sperm Production			
Human chorionic gonadotropin (hCG)	500-2000 IU given SC 2-3 times weekly to maintain serum T levels within the normal range for 6-12 mo	Effective in stimulating endogenous T production In men with acquired and some men with partial congenital hypogonadotropic hypogonadism, sperm production may be stimulated with hCG treatment alone SC injections easier than IM injections (smaller needle, injection not as deep) Less fluctuation in T levels compared with IM T ester injections No injection, patch, or buccal tablet	Injections 2-3 times weekly Expensive Higher doses needed in men with concomitant primary testicular disease (e.g., cryptorchidism) Breast tenderness or gynecomastia secondary to high estradiol production by testes May require dilution Occasional burning sensation with injection Ineffective in primary hypogonadism

Continued

TABLE 19-10

Treatment of Adult Male Hypogonadism—cont'd

Formulation	Dosage	Advantages	Disadvantages
Treatment to Initiate and Maintain Sperm Production in Men With Hypogonadotropic Hypogonadism			
Added to hCG to Stimulate Sperm Production			
FSH Human menopausal gonadotropin (hMG), human FSH (hFSH), or recombinant human FSH (rhFSH)	After 6-12 mo of hCG treatment alone resulting in normal T levels, add FSH 75-300 IU given SC three times weekly for an additional 6-12 mo or longer	Effective in stimulating sperm production in men with hypogonadotropic hypogonadism	Injections three times weekly Extremely expensive, prohibitive cost for most Breast tenderness or gynecomastia secondary to high estradiol production by testes May require dilution Occasional burning sensation with injection In men with concomitant primary testicular disease (e.g., cryptorchidism), stimulation of spermatogenesis is not likely
To Stimulate Testosterone and Sperm Production			
Gonadotropin-releasing hormone (GnRH)	5-25 ng/kg SC every 2 hr by programmable infusion pump for 6-12 mo	Effective in stimulating both endogenous T and sperm production	GnRH not readily available Requires pump use and management, usually in a specialized center Expensive Infrequently used except at certain sites Rarely, local irritation, infection

DHT, dihydrotestosterone; FSH, follicle-stimulating hormone; IM, intramuscular; PO, orally; REMS, Risk Evaluation and Mitigation Strategy; SC, subcutaneous; T, testosterone.

commonly cause cholestasis that is reversible with discontinuation. More concerning is the potential for these agents to cause peliosis hepatis (blood-filled cysts in the liver) or benign or malignant hepatic tumors. 17α-Alkylated androgens also lower HDL- and raise LDL-cholesterol, causing a proatherogenic lipid profile, and they are relatively expensive. Therefore, these oral androgens carry greater potential risks with few therapeutic benefits compared with other testosterone formulations, and they should not be used to treat male hypogonadism.

Parenteral Testosterone Esters. Relatively long-acting parenteral 17β-hydroxyl esters of testosterone, *testosterone enanthate* and *testosterone cypionate*, are administered by IM injection. These are effective, safe, and relatively practical and inexpensive preparations that have been used for testosterone replacement in hypogonadal men for decades. Transdermal testosterone gel formulations provide more physiologic testosterone levels and are now used more commonly than testosterone ester injections. However, testosterone esters are preferred over transdermal formulations by some hypogonadal men because they are the least expensive formulation available, require less frequent administration, and usually produce higher average serum testosterone concentrations. Given proper instruction, most hypogonadal men (or a family member) are able to self-administer IM testosterone ester injections. Otherwise, testosterone injections need to be administered in a clinic setting.

Esterification of testosterone at the 17β-hydroxyl group increases its hydrophobicity and solubility within an oil vehicle (sesame oil for testosterone enanthate, cottonseed oil for testosterone cypionate). After IM injection, testosterone esters are released slowly from the oil vehicle within muscle and hydrolyzed rapidly to testosterone, which is released into circulation, resulting in relatively high peak serum testosterone concentrations but an extended duration of release. Testosterone enanthate and testosterone

cypionate have similar pharmacokinetic profiles, duration of action, and therapeutic efficacy, so they are considered clinically equivalent.[515,516]

In adults with hypogonadism, the usual starting dose of testosterone enanthate or cypionate is 150 mg to 200 mg IM injection every 2 weeks. After IM administration of 200 mg of testosterone enanthate, serum testosterone levels usually rise above the normal range for 1 to 3 days and then decline gradually over 2 weeks to the lower end of the normal range, or sometimes to below-normal levels, before the next injection (Fig. 19-29).[517] The extreme rise and fall of serum testosterone concentrations may cause fluctuations in energy, mood, and libido that are disturbing to some men. Shortening the dosing interval to every 10 days and reducing the dose to 150 mg (i.e., 150-mg IM injection every 10 days) may alleviate symptoms associated with nadir testosterone levels occurring before the next injection. Alternatively, some patients prefer changing the dose of testosterone enanthate or cypionate to 75 to 100 mg IM every week to reduce swings in testosterone concentrations and associated symptoms. Administration of testosterone enanthate at doses of 300 mg IM every 3 weeks or 400 mg IM every 4 weeks produces extremely wide fluctuations in serum testosterone concentrations with markedly supraphysiologic levels for several days after an injection and levels below normal 3 weeks after an injection (see Fig. 19-29).[517]

Because CDGP in which puberty eventually occurs spontaneously is clinically indistinguishable from delayed puberty caused by permanent hypogonadotropic hypogonadism (e.g., IHH),[141,329,330] testosterone treatment usually is not initiated in boys with prepubertal androgen deficiency until they are about 14 years of age (with a bone age of at least 10.5 years). Testosterone therapy is administered intermittently to allow determination of spontaneous puberty, if it occurs. Occasionally, testosterone therapy is started at a younger age if delayed genital development

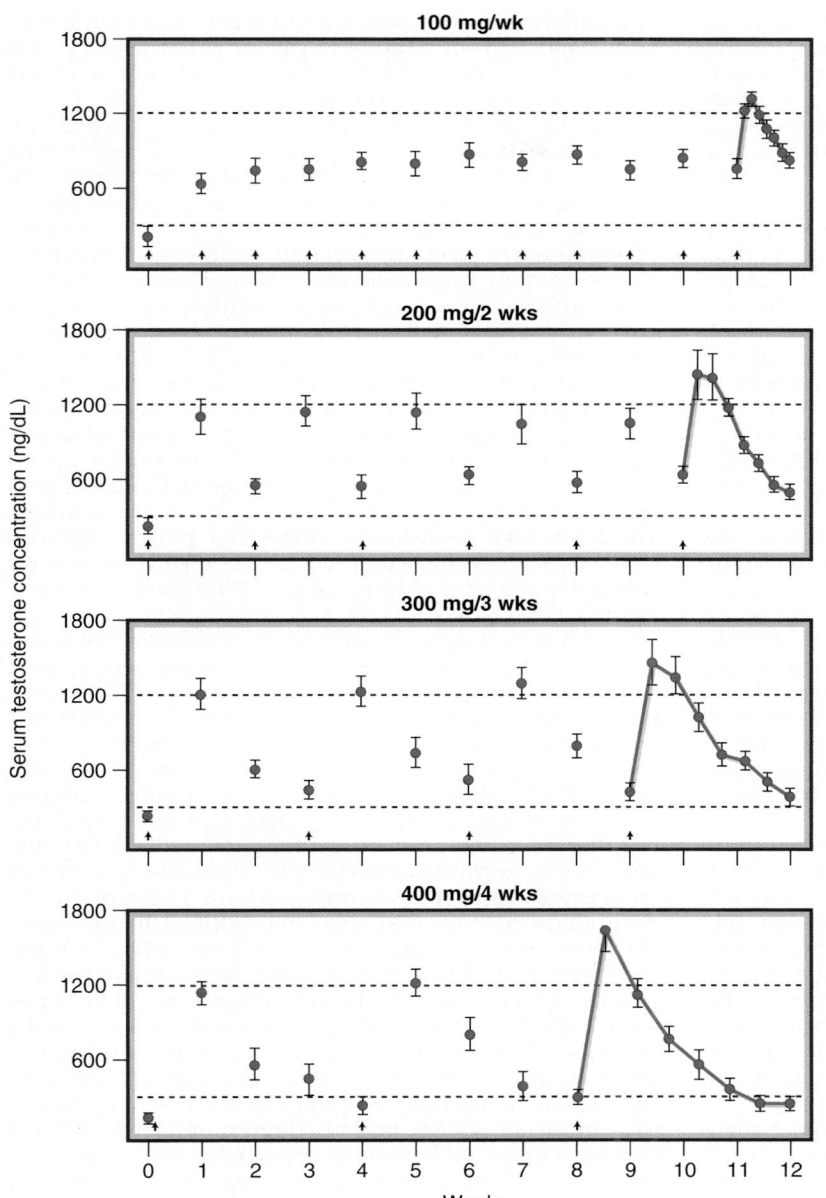

Figure 19-29 Serum total testosterone concentrations in men with primary hypogonadism treated with intramuscular injections of testosterone enanthate for 12 weeks at a dose of 100 mg weekly, 200 mg every 2 weeks, 300 mg every 3 weeks, or 400 mg every 4 weeks. Blood was sampled weekly until the last injection, after which it was sampled more frequently, demonstrating that the optimal dosage to maintain serum testosterone levels within the normal range *(dashed lines)* is 200 mg every 2 weeks or 100 mg every week. (From Snyder PJ, Lawrence DA. Treatment of male hypogonadism with testosterone enanthate. *J Clin Endocrinol Metab.* 1980;51:1335-1339.)

and growth are causing severe psychological distress in affected boys and their families.

In boys with prepubertal androgen deficiency, treatment is initiated with a very low dose of testosterone enanthate or cypionate (e.g., 50 to 100 mg IM injection monthly or 25 to 50 mg every 2 weeks) to prevent premature closure of long bone epiphyses that would compromise adult height.[141,329,330] These low doses of testosterone are sufficient to induce some virilization and long bone growth without interfering with the spontaneous puberty that occurs eventually in boys with CDGP. Testosterone treatment is continued for 3 to 6 months and then stopped for 3 to 6 months to assess whether spontaneous pubertal onset occurs. If there is indication that spontaneous puberty is occurring (e.g., testis size > 8 mL), testosterone therapy is discontinued. If there is no evidence of spontaneous puberty, intermittent testosterone treatment is continued. The dose of testosterone enanthate or cypionate is increased gradually to 50 to 100 mg IM every 2 weeks and then to full adult replacement doses over the next several

years to mimic the gradual increase in testosterone concentrations that occurs during puberty.

At present, transdermal testosterone formulations are not approved for use in boys with delayed puberty. However, because they circumvent the need for IM injections, low-dose transdermal testosterone patches and gels would provide very useful alternatives for the treatment of prepubertal androgen deficiency in boys, and they are currently not approved for this indication.

A formulation of *testosterone undecanoate* in castor oil (*Aveed*, Endo Pharmaceuticals, Malvern, PA) was approved in 2014 for use in the United States for treatment of male hypogonadism. This formulation is administered by slow IM injection into the gluteus muscle at a dose of 750 mg in 3 mL of castor oil initially, followed by another injection of the same dose 4 weeks later and then every 10 weeks to produce and maintain serum testosterone levels within the normal range in most hypogonadal men.[518] Steady state is achieved after the third injection, and mean testosterone levels peak in the high-normal range at 7 days after injection and gradually decline over the next 10 weeks to mean nadir levels just above the normal range. Despite this decline in testosterone levels, fluctuations in or recurrence of symptoms of androgen deficiency have not been reported. Although some men experience discomfort with large-volume injections, they are generally tolerated well and have the advantage of fewer injections than shorter-acting testosterone ester formulations.

A different formulation of testosterone undecanoate in a castor oil vehicle (*Nebido*; Bayer Schering Pharma AG, Berlin, Germany) has been approved and is used in Europe and other countries for testosterone replacement therapy in hypogonadal men.[519] It is administered at a dose of 1000 mg in 4 mL IM, followed by another injection of the same dose 6 weeks later and then every 10 to 14 weeks.

Because of the large volume of drug administered and the need for proper injection technique, self-administration of intramuscular testosterone undecanoate is not possible. Coughing may occur in a small number of men immediately after injection of testosterone undecanoate (this also occurs with shorter-acting testosterone ester injections). Although there is no direct evidence for the cause of coughing, it is conjectured to be related to pulmonary oil micro-embolism (POME) emanating from the large volume of castor oil vehicle that is injected into the muscle with this formulation. For these reasons, the FDA has required a Risk Evaluation and Mitigation Strategy (REMS) for use of testosterone undecanoate that requires training of personnel and certification of the health care facility to ensure proper injection technique (slow IM injection) and adequate monitoring (for 30 minutes) and treatment capability for potential POME or anaphylaxis following injection.

Transdermal Testosterone. Transdermal testosterone formulations available for testosterone replacement therapy for male hypogonadism include an adhesive testosterone patch; two 1% testosterone gels; a 1.62% testosterone gel; a 2% testosterone gel; and a 2% testosterone solution (see Table 19-10). Transdermal delivery of testosterone is used in hypogonadal men who prefer this method or are unable to tolerate or self-administer IM injections of testosterone ester. Currently, testosterone gel is the most frequently used formulation for treatment of male hypogonadism in the United States.

In contrast to testosterone ester injections, which produce transient supraphysiologic testosterone levels, patch, gel, and solution formulations produce a more physiologic range of testosterone concentrations; use of the patch results in a normal circadian variation, and the gel formulations produce steady-state serum testosterone levels.

Testosterone stimulates red blood cell production, and testosterone replacement therapy may result in excessive erythrocytosis. In men with hypogonadism, excessive erythrocytosis occurs less commonly with testosterone patch therapy than with testosterone enanthate injections, suggesting that physiologic testosterone levels produced by transdermal testosterone therapy may be associated with fewer androgenic adverse effects.[520] Compared with testosterone ester injections, transdermal formulations have a short half-life in subcutaneous tissue and in the circulation; consequently, their discontinuation results in a rapid fall in serum testosterone concentrations and a shorter duration of action. Therefore, an advantage of transdermal testosterone is the ability to withdraw androgen replacement relatively rapidly if adverse effects such as excessive erythrocytosis develop or prostate cancer is detected.

Disadvantages of transdermal formulations include the requirement for daily application, greater expense compared with testosterone ester injections, skin irritation or rash with testosterone patches[521] (less common with testosterone gels and solution), and the potential with gel and solution formulations for transfer of testosterone to others through skin contact at the application site.

The first transdermal testosterone delivery system for treatment of male hypogonadism was a scrotal testosterone patch.[522] Treatment required daily application of two relatively large, nonadhesive patches to clean, dry, and preferably shaven scrotal skin and the use of brief-style underwear to hold them in place. These requirements were not acceptable to some hypogonadal men. Also, in some men with long-standing, severe prepubertal androgen deficiency, the scrotum was too small to accommodate even the smaller-sized testosterone patch. Because of poor adherence to scrotal skin, thin adhesive strips were added as an option to this patch. Some men using this testosterone patch experienced skin irritation and itching. The scrotal testosterone patch produced serum DHT levels in the upper-normal range or above the normal range as a result of high 5α-reductase activity within sexual skin of the scrotum. The nonscrotal testosterone patch and testosterone gels have supplanted the scrotal testosterone patch for testosterone replacement therapy, and it is no longer available in the United States.

A nonscrotal testosterone patch, *Androderm* (Watson, Corona, CA), is available for testosterone replacement therapy in male patients with hypogonadism.[523] This patch is composed of a central reservoir containing testosterone and permeation enhancers in an alcohol-based gel surrounded by an adhesive patch that is applied to the skin of the back, abdomen, upper arms, or thighs, avoiding areas over a bony prominence. When applied at night, the testosterone patch produces serum testosterone levels that peak in the morning, mimicking the circadian variation of endogenous testosterone concentrations in normal men. Androderm patches were available initially in two sizes, delivering either 2.5 mg (37 cm^2) or 5 mg (44 cm^2) of testosterone daily. Subsequently, it was reformulated into a smaller, lower dose patches delivering 2 mg (32 cm^2) or 4 mg (39 cm^2) of testosterone daily. Long-term use of the testosterone patch usually maintains serum testosterone levels within the mid- to low-normal range and improves the clinical manifestations of androgen deficiency. Usually, to achieve consistent mid- to high-normal testosterone concentrations, application of two patches was necessary—either one 2.5-mg patch plus one 5-mg patch or two 5-mg patches.[524] Whether the newer formulation would also require two patches is not clear, but likely.

The major limitation of Androderm is skin irritation or rash of varying severity; this side effect occurs in at least 30% to 60% of patients.[521] Mild to moderate erythema and irritation are almost always present, probably because of a skin reaction to the permeation-enhancing agent or adhesive. Uncommonly, severe contact dermatitis or burn-like skin reactions occur. Pretreatment of the skin under the reservoir of the patch with a topical corticosteroid such as triamcinolone acetonide 0.1% cream reduces the incidence and severity of skin irritation produced by testosterone patches.[525]

Two transdermal formulations containing testosterone in a 1% hydroalcoholic gel, *AndroGel* (Abbott, Abbott Park, IL) and *Testim* (Auxilium, Norristown, PA), are available for testosterone replacement therapy in hypogonadal men.[526] AndroGel was the first testosterone gel formulation to be marketed, and it has rapidly become the testosterone formulation most frequently used for treatment of male hypogonadism in the United States.

AndroGel is dispensed into the palm of the hand and applied daily in the morning to clean, dry skin over the shoulders and upper arms preferably or the abdomen and flanks but not on the scrotum.[6] The alcohol-based gel dries rapidly after application, and testosterone is absorbed into the subcutaneous space, where it is released steadily over the remainder of the day, producing relatively steady-state testosterone levels. Residual testosterone remains on the surface of the skin of the hands and at the sites of application. Therefore, the hands should be washed with soap and water after application, the sites of gel application should be covered with clothing, and skin contact with these sites by others (especially women and children) should be avoided to prevent transfer of testosterone.[527] Because of reports of contact transfer of testosterone to children, these instructions and caution to avoid contact transfer are now in an FDA black box warning in the prescribing information for all transdermal testosterone formulations. Residual testosterone on the skin at application sites may be washed off (e.g., by showering or bathing), but this should be avoided for the first 5 to 6 hours after application (or 1 to 2 hours if done infrequently) to maximize testosterone absorption.

Long-term use of AndroGel in hypogonadal men maintains steady-state physiologic serum testosterone concentrations and improves the clinical manifestations of androgen deficiency (Fig. 19-30).[195,528,529] AndroGel was available initially in foil sachets at two different doses: 2.5 g of gel containing 25 mg of testosterone or 5 g of gel containing 50 mg of testosterone. (Because only about 10% of the medication is absorbed, these sachets deliver, respectively, 2.5 mg or 5.0 mg of testosterone.) The starting dose of AndroGel is 5 g daily. Based on testosterone levels or clinical response, approximately 2 weeks after initiation of therapy, the dose may be increased to 7.5 g (i.e., one 2.5-g packet plus one 5.0-g packet) or to 10.0 g (two 5.0-g packets) daily or decreased to 2.5 g daily. A metered-dose pump delivering increments of 1.25 g (delivering 1.25 mg of testosterone) of AndroGel per pump depression is also available to provide greater flexibility in dose adjustment. Also, AndroGel is now available in a more concentrated reformulation of 1.62% that is deliv-

ered by a metered-dose pump that contains 20.25 mg of testosterone (delivering 2.025 mg of testosterone) per acuation, or foil packets of 20.25 mg or 40.5 mg (delivering 2.025 and 4.05 mg of testosterone, respectively). With titration, the dosage of AndroGel 1.62% ranges from 20.25 mg to 80.1 mg (2.025 mg to 8.1 mg of testosterone delivered, respectively).

In contrast to testosterone patches, local skin irritation with testosterone gel and solution formulations is relatively uncommon, occurring in fewer than 5% of men, and is probably related mostly to drying of the skin by the alcohol. Some men complain of stickiness of the skin after the alcohol-based gel dries. AndroGel produces serum DHT levels at the upper end or above the normal range as a result of 5α-reductase activity in the relatively large surface area of skin over which the gel is applied. A major limitation to the use of AndroGel for testosterone replacement therapy is its expense, particularly if more than one packet is needed daily for adequate testosterone replacement. The cost may be prohibitive for patients who do not have adequate third-party medication coverage.

Testim (Auxilium Pharmaceuticals, Chesterbrook, PA) is the other 1% hydroalcoholic testosterone gel that is available for treatment of male hypogonadism.[530] It is applied daily in the morning to intact, clean, dry skin over the shoulders and arms but not over the abdomen or on scrotal skin. Like AndroGel, Testim produces steady-state testosterone levels over 24 hours and has the potential for contact transfer of residual testosterone on the skin surface at application sites. Similar precautions are recommended to prevent contact transfer, and washing off of residual testosterone on the skin surface should be avoided for at least 2 hours to maintain normal testosterone levels.

In short-term, placebo-controlled trials, Testim maintained steady-state physiologic serum testosterone levels in hypogonadal men and improved the clinical manifestations of androgen deficiency.[531] After the initial application of Testim, serum testosterone levels are approximately 30% higher than those achieved after application of AndroGel. However, no direct comparison of steady-state testosterone levels with long-term use of the two testosterone gels is available.

Testim is packaged in a 5-g tube containing 50 mg of testosterone and delivering approximately 5 mg of testosterone (i.e., 10% absorption). The starting dose of Testim is 5 g daily. Based on testosterone levels or clinical response approximately 2 weeks after initiation of therapy, the dose may be increased to 10 g (two tubes) daily. In contrast to AndroGel, Testim is not available in a dose of 2.5 g or in a metered-dose dispenser, limiting dose adjustments with this formulation.

Although AndroGel is odorless, Testim has a musk-like scent. Depending on the individual patient and his partners, this odor may be thought of as pleasant or objectionable. Testim contains a skin emollient and is less drying to the skin than AndroGel. However, both testosterone gels are tolerated well with very little skin irritation compared to the testosterone patch. Like AndroGel, Testim produces high-normal to slightly high serum DHT levels and is expensive.

Recently, two new transdermal formulations for the treatment of male hypogonadism were approved in the United States: *Fortesta* (Endo Pharmaceuticals, Malvern, PA) is a 2% testosterone gel that is applied to the inner thighs at a dosage of 40 to 70 mg (delivering 4-7 mg of testosterone) daily by a metered-dose pump that delivers 10 mg per pump depression (delivering 1 mg of testosterone).[532] *Axiron* (Eli Lilly, Indianapolis, IN) is a 2% testosterone solution that is applied to axillary skin at a dosage of 30 to

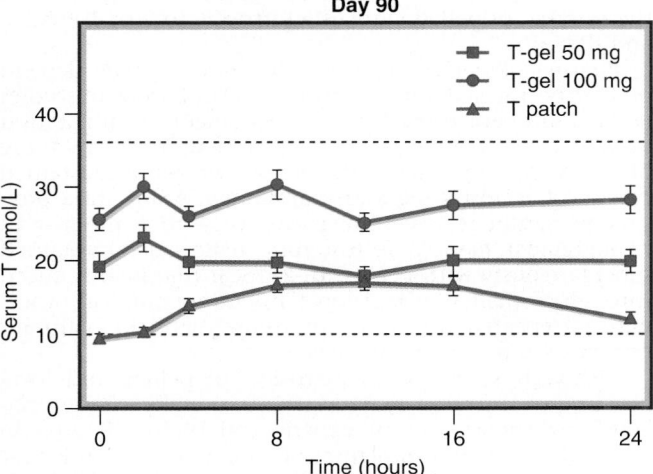

Figure 19-30 Serum total testosterone (T) levels after application of T-gel 50 mg (5 g of gel containing 50 mg of T and delivering approximately 5 mg of T) daily, or T-gel 100 mg (10 g of gel containing 100 mg of T and delivering approximately 10 mg of T) daily, or two T patches (delivering a total 5 mg of T) daily in hypogonadal men treated for 90 days. All three treatments achieved T levels within the low-normal, mid-normal, and upper-normal range *(dashed lines)* over the first 24 hours after application. (From Swerdloff RS, Wang C, Cunningham G, et al. Long-term pharmacokinetics of transdermal testosterone gel in hypogonadal men. *J Clin Endocrinol Metab.* 2000;85:4500-4510.)

120 mg (delivering 3-12 mg of testosterone) daily using a metered-dose pump applicator that delivers 30 mg (delivering 3 mg of testosterone) per pump depression.[533] Both of these transdermal testosterone formulations are able to achieve and maintain relatively steady-state serum testosterone levels within the normal range in hypogonadal men. The advantages and disadvantages of these formulations are similar to 1% and 1.62% testosterone gels. Some men complain of dripping of the 2% testosterone solution from the axilla.

With all transdermal testosterone formulations, serum testosterone levels may vary considerably both within and between individuals and from day to day so that it is difficult to judge the adequacy of a particular dose in maintaining testosterone levels using single measurements of testosterone.

Transbuccal Testosterone. A transbuccal testosterone tablet, *Striant* (Columbia Laboratories, Livingston, NJ), is available for testosterone replacement therapy in hypogonadal men (see Table 19-10).[534,535] This formulation is a small mucoadhesive tablet that contains 30 mg of testosterone in an oil-water emulsion carrier vehicle. The tablet contains polycarbophil, which, after application, remains attached to buccal mucosa until epithelial cells turn over (approximately 12 to 15 hours). The tablet is placed in the mouth between the inner cheek and gum, above the incisors, with the monoconvex side toward the gum and the flat side toward the cheek. After placement, the tablet softens and swells with hydration and becomes gelatinous and sticky, causing it to adhere to the gum. Testosterone is released at a controlled and sustained, constant rate from the tablet through the buccal mucosa into the systemic circulation, circumventing first-pass hepatic metabolism.

Striant tablets are placed on the buccal mucosa twice daily, with one tablet applied in the morning and removed after 12 hours and another applied in the evening on the opposite side.[534,535] Use of Striant requires careful instruction to orient the tablet with the rounded side against the gum and to hold it firmly in place with a finger over the lip for approximately 30 seconds. If the tablet falls off or is dislodged, a new tablet should be applied and left in place until the next regularly scheduled dose. Swallowing of the tablet is not harmful. The buccal tablet is removed by gently sliding it downward toward the incisor to avoid scratching the gum.

Application of a Striant tablet containing 30 mg of testosterone every 12 hours produces average steady-state testosterone levels in the mid-normal range throughout the day.[534,535] Although a formal study has not been conducted, unrestricted intake of food and beverage (including alcohol), tooth-brushing, mouth-washing, and gum-chewing did not appear to affect the absorption of testosterone in pharmacokinetic studies. Contact transfer of testosterone in saliva to others has not been reported to occur. Like the transdermal testosterone gels, Striant produces high-normal to high serum DHT concentrations, probably because of 5α-reductase activity in the buccal mucosa. In general, transbuccal testosterone tablets are tolerated well. Approximately 10% to 15% of men developed gum or mouth irritation or inflammation, and 5% experienced an altered or bitter taste in the mouth.[534]

Like the transdermal testosterone formulations, Striant is relatively expensive compared with testosterone ester injections. Initially, patients are aware and bothered by the tablet between their cheek and gum, resulting in premature discontinuation of the formulation. However, with continued use, the unusual sensation and awareness of the buccal tablet diminish and they become less bothersome. Twice-daily application of Striant is required to sustain physio-

logic testosterone levels, and this makes compliance challenging. Informing patients that awareness of the buccal tablet diminishes over time and linking application of the transbuccal tablet to a routine daily activity such as morning and evening tooth-brushing may help to improve and maintain compliance.

Testosterone Nasal Gel. Recently, a 1% testosterone nasal gel formulation, *Natesto* (Trimel Biopharma, Durants, Barbados), was approved by the FDA to treat men with hypogonadism.[536] This formulation is administered intranasally at a dosage of 11 mg (delivering 1.1 mg of testosterone) three times daily (every 6-8 hours) by a metered-dose pump that delivers 5.5 mg (delivering 0.55 mg of testosterone) per pump depression; the total daily dose is therefore 33 mg (delivering 3.3 mg of testosterone). It is advised that there should be no nose blowing or sniffing for 1 hour after administration, and treatment should be discontinued temporarily during episodes of severe rhinitis. Although there is no interaction with symphathomimetic nasal decongestants, potential interaction with other intranasally administered medications is not known, so use with other nasal drugs is not recommended. It is also not recommended for patients with chronic nasal conditions. When administered to hypogonadal men, mean serum testosterone levels peak in high-normal range approximately 1 hour after administration and decline over 6 to 8 hours to levels at or slightly below normal.

Testosterone Pellets. Subcutaneous testosterone pellets are used infrequently in the United States but more commonly in Australia and some European countries for testosterone replacement therapy in men with hypogonadism.[537,538] In the United States, *Testopel Pellets* (Auxilium Pharmaceuticals, Chesterbrook, PA) are available for testosterone replacement (see Table 19-10). These are cylindrical pellets, 3.2 mm in diameter by 8 to 9 mm in length, that contain 75 mg of testosterone. Testopel Pellets are recommended at doses that range from 150 to 450 mg testosterone (i.e., two to six 75-mg pellets) and are implanted every 3 to 4 months.[537] However, a recent report of implantation of 6 to 12 pellets (450 mg to 900 mg of testosterone) found that decline in serum testosterone levels to below normal occurred by 3 to 4 months after implantation regardless of the number of pellets implanted (from 6 to 9 or 10 to 12) and BMI.[539]

Pharmacokinetic profiles for testosterone pellets depend on the specific pellet formulation.[538,540] In European studies using a different formulation, subcutaneous implantation of three to six 200-mg pellets (for a total of 600 to 1200 mg of testosterone) produced the almost zero-order, sustained release of testosterone and maintained steady-state physiologic serum testosterone levels for 4 to 6 months in hypogonadal men.[540] Testosterone pellets are implanted subcutaneously with the use of a trocar that is introduced through a small skin incision. This minor surgical procedure is repeated three to four times yearly to maintain normal serum testosterone levels.

Although spontaneous extrusion of pellets and local bleeding or infection may occur occasionally, these problems are uncommon in experienced hands. If adverse effects develop after implantation, a major concern is that removal of the testosterone pellets will be difficult, if not impossible. Therefore, the use of testosterone pellets is inappropriate for testosterone replacement in older patients, who are predisposed to erythrocytosis and prostate disease during treatment, and is not an acceptable formulation for many physicians and patients.

Testosterone Formulations Available Outside the United States
Oral Testosterone Undecanoate. In many countries outside the United States, an oral 17β-hydroxyl ester of testosterone,

testosterone undecanoate (Andriol Testocaps; Organon, Oss, Netherlands), is available to provide testosterone replacement therapy in hypogonadal men.[541,542] Testosterone undecanoate, which is formulated in a castor oil vehicle, is absorbed directly from the gastrointestinal tract into the lymphatic system and then into the systemic circulation, thereby avoiding first-pass hepatic accumulation and inactivation. Serum testosterone concentrations peak approximately 5 hours after administration of testosterone undecanoate and fall to pretreatment levels within 8 to 12 hours. For testosterone replacement therapy, it is administered at relatively high doses, 40 to 80 mg two to three times daily (total dose, 80 to 240 mg daily). The frequency of administration makes compliance difficult for many men. Absorption of testosterone undecanoate requires concomitant food ingestion, and serum testosterone levels and clinical responses are highly variable. Because of 5α-reductase activity in the gastrointestinal tract, serum DHT concentrations are often very high.

The use of castor oil and propylene glycol laurate instead of oleic acid, the vehicle used in the original formulation, permits storage at room temperature and extends the shelf-life of Andriol Testocaps for up to 3 years while maintaining pharmacokinetic and pharmacodynamic characteristics similar to those of the original formulation. Testosterone levels fall quickly after discontinuation of testosterone undecanoate. Therefore, it may be particularly useful for testosterone replacement therapy in older men with clinically significant prostate disease and comorbid conditions, in whom rapid withdrawal of androgen action is desirable if adverse effects develop, and in those for whom only low-dose testosterone supplementation is needed.

Transdermal Testosterone Formulations. A *testosterone-in-adhesive matrix patch* (*Testopatch,* Pierre Fabre, Castres, France) is available in a number of countries in Europe for testosterone replacement therapy in patients with male hypogonadism.[543,544] This patch is composed of an adhesive matrix that contains testosterone (0.5 mg/cm^2) and excipients that comes in three sizes—30, 45, and 60 cm^2. Two 60-cm^2 patches (delivering approximately 4.8 mg of testosterone daily) are applied to the skin of the arms, trunk, or thighs every 2 days to maintain serum testosterone levels in the normal range in hypogonadal men. Skin irritation has been reported to occur in about 20% of patients using this patch.

Selective Androgen Receptor Modulators.

There is considerable interest in the development of selective androgen receptor modulators (SARMs), nonsteroidal molecules that interact with AR and have differential effects on various androgen target organs.[545,546] The goal is to develop an orally active, nonsteroidal SARM that will maintain the beneficial anabolic and androgenic actions of testosterone on muscle, bone, sexual function, and mood but have reduced potential for adverse effects (e.g., on the prostate gland). These novel drugs are being developed primarily for use in muscle-wasting conditions such as age-related sarcopenia and cancer cachexia but not at present for treatment of male hypogonadism. The mechanisms by which SARMs act in a tissue-specific manner are unclear. It is possible that SARMs have less stimulatory effect on the prostate because they are not actively metabolized by 5α-reductase, or they may act by unique interactions with tissue-specific AR coactivator and corepressor molecules.

Nonsteroidal SARMs have been developed that have anabolic actions in muscle and bone but reduced stimulatory effects on the prostate gland in animals.[545,546] SARMs do not have intrinsic ER activity, and if they suppress endogenous gonadotropin, testosterone, and estradiol secretion, they will produce a state of relative estrogen deficiency. Therefore, studies evaluating the clinical benefits and risks of an SARM must consider potential adverse effects on target actions that are regulated by estradiol in men, such as effects on BMD, fat mass, sexual function and possibly lipids (HDL-cholesterol), cardiovascular function, and brain function. The importance of estrogens on bone, for example, was underscored by a recent long-term study of the potent, nonaromatizable androgen, DHT gel, administered to older men. Compared with placebo, DHT gel stimulated lean body mass and reduced fat mass but suppressed BMD.[99]

Monitoring Clinical Response and Testosterone Levels.

The clinical responses to testosterone replacement and serum testosterone levels are used to monitor the adequacy of testosterone therapy in androgen-deficient men (Table 19-11).[113] Symptoms and signs of androgen deficiency should be assessed before the initiation of testosterone treatment, 3 to 6 months after starting testosterone, and then yearly. By 3 to 6 months, most hypogonadal men experience improvements in libido, sexual function and activity, energy, vitality, motivation, and mood.[547] Increases in body hair growth, muscle mass and strength, and BMD occur over the subsequent months to years of testosterone therapy.

Serum testosterone concentrations are monitored to determine the adequacy of therapy and to avoid overreplacement or underreplacement. This is particularly important in men treated with transdermal testosterone patch, gels, and solution, because the bioavailability of these formulations is highly variable among individuals; because of this variability, decisions regarding the adequacy of a given dosage of transdermal testosterone should not be made on a single testosterone measurement. The goal of testosterone replacement therapy is to achieve average serum testosterone levels in the mid-normal range.[113]

For testosterone ester injections, testosterone concentrations should be measured at 3 to 6 months of treatment, midway between two injections (e.g., 1 week after an injection if the injections are given every 2 weeks). Serum testosterone levels measured at the nadir of the injection interval (i.e., just before the next injection) may help to document an inadequate dosing interval. For the testosterone patch, testosterone levels should be measured after approximately 3 to 4 weeks of daily use, 8 to 10 hours after application of a patch on the previous evening. For testosterone gels and solution, testosterone levels should be measured after about 2 weeks of daily use, at any time after application of the gel. For buccal testosterone, serum testosterone should be measured 4 to 6 weeks after initiation of therapy, at any time after application of the buccal tablet, preferably in the morning.

Risks and Adverse Effects

Contraindications and Precautions. Testosterone treatment is contraindicated in men with metastatic prostate cancer or breast cancer.[113] The primary concern is that testosterone administration could stimulate the growth of these androgen-dependent malignancies. Testosterone therapy is particularly risky in men with metastatic prostate cancer, in whom rapid growth of metastatic tumors may worsen bone pain or cause spinal cord compression. In fact, the mainstay of treatment for metastatic prostate cancer is androgen-deprivation therapy to reduce endogenous testosterone production and action; this is achieved by GnRH agonist and AR antagonist treatment or by surgical orchidectomy.[548] The effect of testosterone replacement in hypogonadal men with localized prostate cancer is not known. However, in the absence of evidence, testosterone treatment in men with clinical evidence of prostate cancer should be avoided.

TABLE 19-11

Monitoring During Testosterone Treatment

Parameter	Timing	Further Management
Measures of Efficacy		
Symptoms and signs of androgen deficiency	At baseline, after 3-6 mo, and then yearly For men at high risk for fracture, BMD before treatment; for men with osteoporosis or minimal-trauma fracture, BMD after 1-2 yr	Continue testosterone treatment in men with clinical improvement and no adverse effects Consider discontinuing testosterone treatment in men if no clinical improvement Institute appropriate treatment for men with osteoporosis, including calcium and vitamin D
Serum testosterone	Testosterone ester injection: after 3-6 mo, measured midway between injections or at end of dosing interval (if androgen deficiency symptoms are present at that time) Testosterone patch: after 3-4 wk, at 8-10 hr after application Testosterone gel: after 2 wk, at any time after application Buccal testosterone: after 4-6 wk, at any time after application (preferably in the morning) Testosterone pellets: at end of dosing interval Oral testosterone undecanoate: after 1 wk, at 3-5 hr after oral dose Testosterone undecanoate injection: at end of dosing interval	Adjust dose or dosing interval to achieve serum testosterone levels in mid-normal range
Adverse Effects		
Hematocrit	At baseline, after 3-6 mo, and then yearly	If hematocrit >54%, stop or reduce dosage of testosterone until hematocrit declines to normal and reinitiate testosterone at lower dosage Investigate for hypoxic condition such as obstructive sleep apnea, chronic lung disease
PSA level, DRE, and IPSS in men >40 yr	At baseline, after 3-6 mo, and then according to accepted guidelines	Urologic evaluation if any of the following: PSA increase >1.4 ng/mL within any 12-mo period PSA velocity >0.4 ng/mL per year after 6 mo of testosterone treatment (only if 2 yr of PSA values are available) Palpable abnormality (nodule or induration) on DRE IPSS score >19
Obstructive sleep apnea (snoring, witnessed apnea, daytime somnolence, unexplained erythrocytosis, worsening hypertension or edema)	At baseline, after 3-6 mo, and then yearly	Evaluation for obstructive sleep apnea or adjustment of CPAP settings Evaluation of other causes of hypoxia
Formulation-specific adverse effects	At baseline, after 3-6 mo, and then yearly	Discontinue and switch to another formulation
Testosterone ester injections	Discomfort, bleeding, or hematoma with IM injections Fluctuations in energy, mood, libido Allergy to oil vehicle (rare)	Reinstruct on self-injection site technique Consider shortening injection interval if nadir testosterone level low
Testosterone patch	Skin irritation Adhesion to skin	Coadministration of corticosteroid cream may reduce skin irritation
Testosterone gel	Contact transfer to others Skin dryness	Reinstruct on washing hands and covering application area after gel dries or showering 4-6 hr after application, avoiding prolonged skin-to-skin contact of application site with women and children
Buccal testosterone tablets	Gum irritation or inflammation Poor adhesion to gums Altered or bitter taste	Reinstruct on proper application and reassure to complete an adequate trial with correct technique
Subcutaneous testosterone pellets	Pellet extrusion Implantation-site infection, bleeding, fibrosis	Reimplant pellets Treat infection with appropriate drainage and antibiotics

BMD, bone mineral density; CPAP, continuous positive airway pressure; DRE, digital rectal examination; IM, intramuscular; IPSS, International Prostate Symptom Score; PSA, prostate-specific antigen.

The safety of testosterone therapy in hypogonadal men who have been surgically cured of organ-confined, low-grade prostate cancer and have had clinically undetectable disease and an undetectable PSA level for several years also is not clear. Because these men would not have been treated with androgen-deprivation therapy, testosterone replacement to restore eugonadal levels of testosterone seems reasonable. In these patients, a careful discussion of the potential benefits and risks of testosterone replacement should be undertaken, and therapy should be initiated only after informed consent and with careful monitoring by digital rectal examination (DRE) and measurement of PSA levels. It is prudent to avoid testosterone treatment in men with organ-confined high-risk prostate cancer (e.g., Gleason score 8-10, PSA > 20 ng/mL, and clinical stage ≥ T3) despite undetectable PSA levels after surgical or brachytherapy, as these individuals have high likelihood of recurrence and poor outcomes independent of testosterone therapy.

Before testosterone replacement therapy is started in middle-aged and older men (>40 years) with androgen deficiency, a PSA measurement and a careful DRE to look for a suspicious prostate nodule or induration should be performed.[113] Hypogonadal men with an abnormal DRE or a consistently elevated PSA value (e.g., >4 ng/mL in Caucasian men, >3 ng/mL in African-American men and men at high risk for prostate cancer) should have a urologic evaluation that may include a transrectal ultrasound study and biopsy of the prostate before starting testosterone. Older men, African-American men, men with an abnormal DRE, and men with a history of a first-degree relative with prostate cancer have an increased risk of prostate cancer; men with a previous negative prostate biopsy and men who are taking a 5α-reductase inhibitor have a reduced risk. A prostate cancer risk calculator, based on data from placebo-treated men in the Prostate Cancer Prevention Trial, is available to assess the risk of clinical (biopsy-detectable) and high-grade (Gleason score ≥7) prostate cancer according to ethnicity, age, PSA level, family history of prostate cancer, normal or abnormal DRE, results of prior prostate biopsy, and use of a 5α-reductase inhibitor. This calculator is available at http://deb.uthscsa.edu/URORiskCalc/Pages/uroriskcalc.jsp (accessed January 2010).[549,550] Although it has not been validated for men with androgen deficiency, this prostate cancer risk calculator may be helpful in assessing the risk of clinical or high-grade prostate cancer that may be present in a hypogonadal man before testosterone replacement is instituted.

Although breast cancer in men is rare, some disorders that cause androgen deficiency, such as Klinefelter syndrome, are associated with an increased risk of breast cancer.[215] Therefore, a careful breast examination for suspicious masses should be performed in hypogonadal men before starting testosterone treatment. The conversion of testosterone to estradiol may stimulate growth of ER-positive breast cancer.

Relative contraindications to testosterone replacement therapy include the following[113]:

- Untreated obstructive sleep apnea, because higher-dose testosterone treatment may rarely worsen sleep-disordered breathing and its complications
- Baseline hematocrit in the high-normal range (e.g., hematocrit > 50 at or near sea level), because further stimulation of erythropoiesis induced by testosterone therapy may result in erythrocytosis and, potentially, hyperviscosity and vascular complications, particularly in elderly men with underlying vascular disease
- Severe edematous conditions (e.g., uncontrolled or poorly controlled CHF), because the fluid retention associated with testosterone therapy may worsen preexisting edema
- Severe lower urinary tract symptoms (LUTS) due to BPH, such as in men with IPSS greater than 19

Potential Adverse Effects and Monitoring. Monitoring for potential adverse effects of testosterone therapy is summarized in Table 19-11.[113]

Hematocrit. Testosterone replacement stimulates erythropoiesis in hypogonadal men, increasing the hemoglobin concentration and hematocrit from the female range into the normal adult male range.[551] Occasionally, testosterone treatment causes excessive erythrocytosis (e.g., hematocrit > 54%) that may require temporary discontinuation of therapy or lowering of the testosterone dose until the hematocrit declines to normal, reinitiation of testosterone at a lower dose, or sometimes therapeutic phlebotomy.[296]

Excessive erythrocytosis occurs more commonly in older men and in those treated with parenteral testosterone esters rather than transdermal testosterone patches, probably related to the supraphysiologic testosterone levels that are present for a few days after administration and the higher average testosterone concentrations produced by IM testosterone.[520] A greater erythropoietic response to testosterone is associated with greater suppression of hepcidin, a liver-derived peptide that is the main negative regulator of iron bioavailability.[552]

Adverse effects of erythrocytosis induced by testosterone are poorly documented. However, there is concern that an excessive increase in red blood cell volume and blood viscosity could cause vascular complications such as thrombosis, especially older men with underlying atherosclerotic cardiovascular disease, resulting in stroke or myocardial infarction. Therefore, hematocrit should be measured before testosterone therapy is initiated, 3 to 6 months after starting treatment, and then yearly.[113] If erythrocytosis develops during testosterone replacement therapy, testosterone should be stopped and an evaluation should be performed to determine whether an underlying predisposing condition, such as hypoxia due to obstructive sleep apnea syndrome or chronic lung disease, is stimulating or contributing to erythrocytosis. Subsequently, testosterone may be restarted at a lower dosage.

Prostate. Prostate size is reduced in men with androgen deficiency, and testosterone replacement therapy increases prostate volume to that of age-matched eugonadal men.[553] Testosterone therapy does not cause excessive prostate enlargement, and there is no evidence that it worsens LUTS, reduces urinary flow rate, causes urinary retention, or increases the need for invasive intervention for BPH (e.g., TURP). However, long-term, controlled studies have not been performed to evaluate these outcomes in middle-aged to older hypogonadal men, who are most at risk for development of clinically significant, symptomatic BPH. Therefore, in hypogonadal men older than 40 years of age, LUTS should be monitored with the use of the IPSS or the AUA Symptom Index before testosterone treatment, at 3 to 6 months after starting treatment, and then in accordance with accepted guidelines.[113] Concomitant therapy for LUTS (e.g., α-adrenergic receptor antagonists, 5α-reductase inhibitors, surgical bladder outlet procedures) should be considered in hypogonadal men with bothersome severe LUTS that affects quality of life.

There is no evidence that testosterone treatment causes prostate cancer. In middle-aged to older men with androgen deficiency, there is concern that long-term testosterone therapy might stimulate previously unrecognized or clinically undetectable localized or metastatic prostate cancer or accelerate the growth of preexisting subclinical disease into clinically apparent prostate cancer. There is evidence that testosterone treatment stimulates the growth of metastatic prostate cancer, but its effect on progression of subclinical prostate cancer is not known. Small, short-term, controlled studies (up to 3 years in duration) have not found an increased incidence of prostate cancer in older men treated with testosterone.[296] Larger, longer-term, prospective, randomized, controlled trials are needed to determine whether testosterone therapy stimulates the growth and progression of subclinical prostate cancer into clinically evident and significant high-grade disease.

Along with reduced prostate size, serum PSA concentrations in androgen-deficient men are decreased, and testosterone replacement increases PSA to levels observed in age-matched eugonadal men.[553] Because testosterone replacement is a potentially disease-modifying intervention that may alter the natural history of prostate cancer, initial monitoring of PSA is prudent and should be performed to detect marked rises in PSA that might indicate stimulation of previously unrecognized prostate cancer growth.[113] PSA monitoring is distinct from PSA screening for prostate cancer, which is more controversial and has been demonstrated recently to have no effect or only modest effect on mortality rate in the general population of men.[554-556]

Therefore, in men older than 40 years of age, both PSA measurement and DRE should be performed before testosterone therapy is initiated, 3 to 6 months after starting treatment, and then in accordance with accepted guidelines. More intensive PSA monitoring should not be performed, because abnormal levels that would trigger a prostate biopsy are more likely to occur in older hypogonadal men on testosterone therapy, resulting in an increased likelihood of detecting localized prostate cancer, for which the management is unclear.[557] The diagnosis of subclinical or localized low-grade prostate cancer may not affect overall mortality rate, but the potential medical, surgical, psychological, and socioeconomic consequences and morbidity of this diagnosis may be considerable.

Hypogonadal men receiving testosterone therapy who demonstrate a verified increase in PSA greater than 1.4 ng/mL in any 12-month period during therapy; a PSA velocity of greater than 0.4 ng/mL per year using the value at 3 to 6 months as baseline (and only if 2 or more years of PSA values are available); an abnormal finding on DRE (nodule or induration); or an AUA Symptom Index or IPSS greater than 19 should undergo urologic evaluation.[113] Elevated PSA levels should be confirmed with a repeat measurement. If prostatitis or urinary tract infection that can markedly elevate PSA concentrations is suspected, PSA measurements should be repeated after appropriate antibiotic treatment.

Sleep Apnea. Testosterone treatment has been reported to induce or worsen obstructive sleep apnea, but the prevalence of clinically significant obstructive sleep apnea during testosterone replacement therapy is probably very low and may be dose related.[467,476,477] Short-term, high-dose testosterone treatment in older hypogonadal men significantly worsened obstructive sleep apnea, increased the duration of hypoxemia, and shortened total sleep time as assessed by polysomnography. In contrast, older men treated with a scrotal testosterone patch for 3 years did not demonstrate a significant worsening of sleep apnea as assessed by a portable device.[558] As discussed earlier, sleep apnea may conversely cause gonadotropin and testosterone suppression and secondary hypogonadism, probably because of the stress of oxygen desaturation and sleep disturbance.

Sleep apnea is associated with significant morbidity and mortality risks. Therefore, hypogonadal men, and especially those at increased risk (e.g., obese men), should be monitored for symptoms of obstructive sleep apnea syndrome (e.g., loud snoring, apnea witnessed by a bed partner, daytime somnolence, unexplained erythrocytosis, worsening or recent onset of hypertension or edema) before starting testosterone therapy, after 3 to 6 months, and then yearly.[113] If symptoms suggest sleep apnea, a formal sleep study (polysomnography) should be performed. If obstructive sleep apnea is confirmed, appropriate treatment (e.g., CPAP) should be instituted before testosterone treatment is started or continued.

Reduced Sperm Production and Fertility. In men who have androgen deficiency and persistence of some sperm production with either partial primary or secondary hypogonadism, testosterone treatment suppresses gonadotropin production by negative feedback regulation, which in turn suppresses spermatogenesis and may further impair fertility.[485] Suppression of sperm production is most important in men with secondary hypogonadism and normal testes who wish to father children. In these men, testosterone therapy should be discontinued and gonadotropin therapy should be started, initially with hCG alone and then, if necessary, with combined hCG and FSH treatment to stimulate spermatogenesis.[79] In the absence of coexisting testicular disease (e.g., cryptorchidism), prior testosterone therapy does not impair the subsequent induction of sperm production with gonadotropins.[344,345]

Acne and Oily Skin. Boys with prepubertal androgen deficiency who are receiving testosterone therapy to induce puberty and men with severe hypogonadism who are treated with full replacement doses of testosterone may develop acne and increased oiliness of the skin.[141,329,330] These conditions usually respond to local skin measures (e.g., benzoyl peroxide, retinoic acid) and antibiotics, reduction in testosterone dose, or both.

Gynecomastia. Occasionally, breast tenderness or gynecomastia develops or worsens during testosterone replacement therapy, particularly in boys who are receiving testosterone for induction of puberty, men with severe androgen deficiency who are treated with full replacement or high-dose testosterone, and hypogonadal men with predisposing conditions such as hepatic cirrhosis. Gynecomastia is commonly found in boys and men with androgen deficiency before the initiation of testosterone therapy. A careful breast examination should be performed before and again during testosterone replacement therapy to detect the presence or worsening of gynecomastia and the rare occurrence of breast cancer.

Lipids. In hypogonadal men, testosterone replacement results in no change or only a slight decrease in HDL-cholesterol and no change in total cholesterol or LDL-cholesterol levels.[296,559] The reduction in HDL-cholesterol is greater in men with more severe androgen deficiency and in those treated with supraphysiologic testosterone doses or with nonaromatizable, oral 17α-alkylated androgens.[389]

The clinical significance of HDL-cholesterol suppression induced by testosterone in terms of cardiovascular risk is not known. Understanding of the effects of testosterone therapy on major cardiovascular outcomes (e.g., myocardial infarction, stroke, cardiovascular mortality risk) will require larger, longer-term, randomized, controlled studies. Cardiovascular risk and lipid measurements should be evaluated as recommended by available practice guidelines; at present, more intensive monitoring in hypogonadal men receiving therapy is not justified.

Other Potential Adverse Effects. Frontal balding or androgenic alopecia may develop or worsen in genetically predisposed hypogonadal men during testosterone replacement therapy. Mild to moderate *weight gain* usually occurs during testosterone treatment, because of the anabolic actions of testosterone on muscle mass and associated fluid retention. Testosterone therapy usually does not cause clinically significant edema, except occasionally in hypogonadal men with underlying edematous states such as CHF or hepatic cirrhosis.

Stimulation of excessive libido and erections by testosterone is rare and usually occurs in boys or young men with severe, long-standing androgen deficiency who are treated with full replacement or high-dose testosterone therapy. These symptoms usually resolve spontaneously or with a reduction in testosterone dose. Contrary to popular opinion, testosterone treatment does not cause pathologic aggressiveness, anger, or rage.[560,561] Instead, testosterone replacement therapy increases social aggressiveness, motivation, and initiative and reduces irritability and anger.

Profound behavioral and physical changes induced by testosterone treatment in men with severe, long-standing androgen deficiency may be upsetting to both patients and their partners. Therefore, changes that are expected to occur with testosterone replacement should be discussed with patients and their partners before and during treatment. Oral 17α-alkylated androgens may cause cholestasis or potentially serious hepatotoxicity.[389] However, liver toxicity does not occur with testosterone replacement therapy, and routine monitoring of liver enzymes is not necessary in hypogonadal men.

Formulation-Specific Adverse Effects. Testosterone ester injections may cause local discomfort, bleeding, or hematoma at the site of IM injections.[113] Instruction on proper injection technique minimizes the likelihood of these adverse effects. Fluctuations in energy, mood, and libido associated with the peak and nadir swings of testosterone levels after testosterone ester injections may be disturbing to some hypogonadal men and may require reduction of the dose injected and shortening of the injection interval or switching to transdermal testosterone. Rarely, an allergy may occur to the sesame oil (enanthate) or cottonseed oil (cypionate) vehicle used.

Testosterone patches frequently cause local skin erythema, irritation, itching, and contact dermatitis and occasionally lead to more severe reactions.[113] Use of a topical corticosteroid cream under the reservoir of the patch may reduce skin irritation and reactions, but often men prefer to switch to another testosterone formulation. Testosterone patches may adhere poorly to skin, particularly with excessive perspiration.

In contrast to testosterone patches, *testosterone gels* and *solution* cause little to no skin irritation. However, residual testosterone remains on the skin surface at the application sites, and there is a potential for transfer of testosterone to women and children who have prolonged intimate contact with these sites.[113] Precautions to avoid contact transfer of testosterone include washing the hands immediately after application of testosterone gel, covering the application site with clothing, washing off residual testosterone on skin by showering or bathing (4 to 6 hours after application), and avoiding prolonged skin-to-skin contact of the application site with women or children.

Buccal testosterone tablets may cause gum irritation or inflammation or an altered or bitter taste sensation, and they may adhere poorly to gums if not they are not properly applied.[113]

Nasal testosterone gel may cause nasal irritation, nasopharyngitis, rhinorrhea, epistaxis, and nasal scabbing.

Subcutaneous testosterone pellets may uncommonly extrude spontaneously; rarely, there may be bleeding or infection at the site of implantation.[113]

Gonadotropin Therapy

Secondary hypogonadism manifests as prepubertal or adult androgen deficiency and impairment of sperm production due to gonadotropin deficiency. The primary goal of gonadotropin therapy in men with secondary hypogonadism is to initiate and maintain spermatogenesis in order to establish and restore fertility.[509] Because gonadotropin therapy is more complex (requiring multiple injections weekly) and more expensive than testosterone replacement therapy, symptomatic androgen deficiency is usually treated with the latter. In patients with partial gonadotropin deficiency, testosterone treatment may suppress remaining gonadotropin secretion by negative feedback regulation. When fertility is desired and stimulation of sperm production is needed in a man with secondary hypogonadism, testosterone is discontinued and gonadotropin therapy is initiated. Previous testosterone treatment

does not compromise subsequent stimulation of spermatogenesis by gonadotropins.[344,345]

The gonadotropin preparations most commonly used to treat secondary hypogonadism are purified urinary gonadotropins. Human recombinant gonadotropin preparations are now available and have much higher purity than urinary preparations, but they are more expensive. Because urinary gonadotropins are highly effective in treating gonadotropin deficiency, they remain the most commonly used preparations for treatment of secondary hypogonadism.

hCG is used to provide LH-like activity because its half-life is longer than that of LH. In contrast to LH, which would require pulsatile administration approximately every 2 hours, hCG is administered two to three times per week. Purified urinary preparations of hCG (derived from urine of pregnant women) that contain LH-like activity are used almost exclusively in gonadotropin therapy. FSH activity is usually provided by purified urinary *human menopausal gonadotropin* (hMG), which is derived from urine of menopausal women and contains both FSH and LH; by highly purified urinary *human FSH*; or, rarely, by *rhFSH*. FSH preparations are administered three times weekly. hCG and FSH preparations may be administered either intramuscularly or subcutaneously.[562,563] Both are equally effective, but the latter is better tolerated and more easily self-administered.

In patients with prepubertal gonadotropin deficiency, initiation of sperm production requires treatment with both hCG and FSH (Fig. 19-31).[79] Gonadotropin therapy is initiated with administration of hCG alone at a dose of 500 to 2000 IU subcutaneously two to three times weekly to stimulate sufficient endogenous testosterone production to increase and maintain circulating testosterone levels in the normal range and to correct manifestations of androgen deficiency.[6] The dose of hCG is increased until serum testosterone concentrations are within eugonadal range. Despite the more frequent injections, some men with secondary hypogonadism prefer hCG over testosterone treatment because costs are comparable (if purified urinary preparations are used), subcutaneous (SC) injections using smaller needles are better tolerated, and testis size and spermatogenesis may increase slightly, particularly in patients with partial prepubertal gonadotropin deficiency.

Men with gonadotropin deficiency who also have primary testicular disease (e.g., cryptorchidism) or severe prepubertal isolated hypogonadotropic hypogonadism may require larger doses of hCG (e.g., up to 3000 to 5000 IU two to three times weekly or occasionally much more). Men with secondary hypogonadism who have coexisting severe testicular damage may be completely unresponsive to hCG treatment (see Fig. 19-31). Because hCG stimulates Leydig cell aromatase activity within the testes, serum estradiol concentrations may increase disproportionately relative to testosterone levels, resulting in breast tenderness or gynecomastia more frequently than with testosterone replacement therapy. Some men may complain of burning at the site of SC injections of hCG.

hCG stimulates Leydig cell testosterone production, resulting in relatively high intratesticular testosterone concentrations that cause Sertoli cells to mature and sperm production to be initiated to varying degrees. In a small proportion of patients with partial prepubertal deficiency and in almost all men with acquired postpubertal gonadotropin deficiency, treatment with hCG alone may stimulate sperm production (see Fig. 19-31).[79] Evidence for partial gonadotropin deficiency includes testis size larger than 4 mL, physical examination evidence of partial androgenization, low-normal gonadotropin concentrations, and

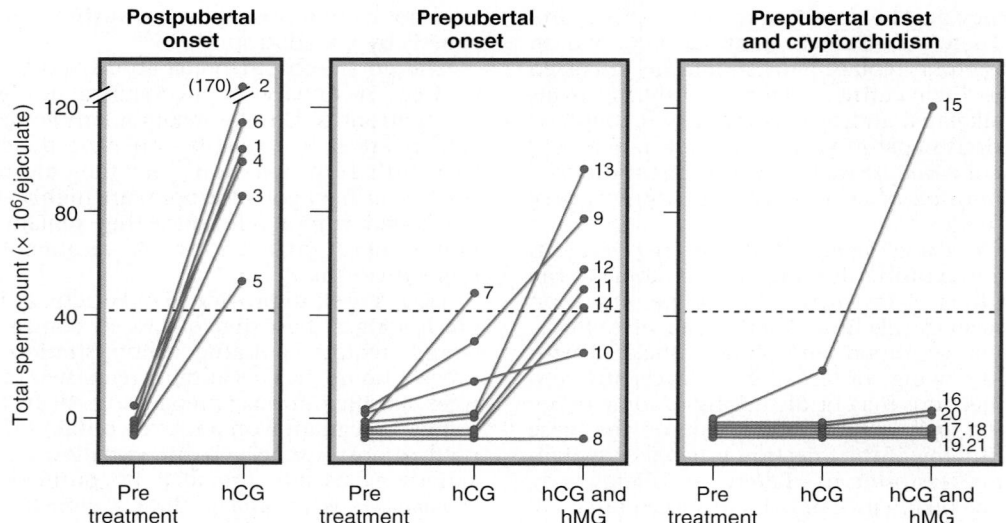

Figure 19-31 Total sperm count response to gonadotropin therapy with human chorionic gonadotropin (hCG) alone or in combination with human menopausal gonadotropin (hMG) in males with hypogonadotropic hypogonadism of postpubertal onset *(left)*, prepubertal onset without cryptorchidism *(middle)*, or prepubertal onset with cryptorchidism *(right)*. Sperm production was induced by hCG alone in all men with postpubertal hypogonadotropic hypogonadism and in some with prepubertal onset who did not have cryptorchidism. Both hCG and hMG treatment was required to increase sperm production above the lower limit of normal *(dashed line)* in patients with prepubertal hypogonadotropic hypogonadism who did not have cryptorchidism. With one exception, men with prepubertal hypogonadotropic hypogonadism who also had cryptorchidism failed to respond to hCG alone or to combined hCG and hMG therapy. (From Finkel DM, Phillips JL, Snyder PJ. Stimulation of spermatogenesis by gonadotropins in men with hypogonadotropic hypogonadism. *N Engl J Med.* 1985;313:651-655.)

low-normal levels of inhibin B.[564-568] Most patients with severe prepubertal gonadotropin deficiency require FSH treatment in addition to hCG to stimulate complete spermatogenesis and induce fertility.[568-571]

If no sperm is present in the ejaculate after 6 to 12 months of treatment with hCG and serum testosterone concentrations in the eugonadal range, hMG or FSH at a dose of 75 IU three times weekly (increasing to 300 IU given subcutaneously three times weekly) is added, in combination with the same dose of hCG, for an additional 6 to 12 months or longer, until spermatogenesis is induced.

The induction of sperm production by gonadotropin therapy may take 12 to 24 months. Factors that limit the duration of gonadotropin treatment are impatience by patients and their partners and the expense of gonadotropins, in particular hMG or FSH preparations, which are very costly. Some couples may opt for alternative means to have children (e.g., adoption). In patients with prepubertal gonadotropin deficiency, sperm output is often low, possibly because of inadequate gonadotropin stimulation of Sertoli cell number and maturation during development.[572] Despite quantitatively low sperm production during gonadotropin therapy, fertility may be possible, sometimes at very low sperm counts (e.g., <1 million/mL).[564] Some patients who have very low sperm counts and remain infertile on gonadotropin treatment may elect to use ejaculated sperm for ICSI.

Once spermatogenesis has been initiated with combined hCG and FSH treatment in patients with prepubertal gonadotropin deficiency, sperm production may be maintained with hCG treatment alone.[507] In men with acquired postpubertal gonadotropin deficiency, reinitiation of spermatogenesis can usually be accomplished with hCG therapy alone.[79]

In men with secondary hypogonadism due to hypothalamic GnRH deficiency (e.g., IHH, Kallmann syndrome), pulsatile GnRH therapy may be used to stimulate production of endogenous gonadotropins (both LH and FSH) and testosterone and to initiate and maintain sperm produc-

tion sufficient for fertility.[47] GnRH is administered subcutaneously with the use of a portable infusion pump that delivers small doses (pulses) of GnRH every few hours (e.g., GnRH 5 to 25 ng/kg subcutaneously every 2 hours, increasing to higher doses if needed); this treatment mimics a near-normal physiologic stimulus to the pituitary gland. In men with IHH, pulsatile GnRH treatment is successful in stimulating gonadotropin, testosterone, and sperm production in approximately 75% of cases; in the other 25% of cases, men fail to respond due to concomitant pituitary or testicular defects.[347] The effectiveness of pulsatile GnRH replacement in stimulating sperm production is comparable to that of gonadotropin therapy. Practically, however, the use of pulsatile GnRH therapy is limited to specialized centers because GnRH is not readily available, the infusion pump requires additional expertise and management, and therapy is expensive.

REFERENCES

1. Bojesen A, Juul S, Gravholt CH. Prenatal and postnatal prevalence of Klinefelter syndrome: a national registry study. *J Clin Endocrinol Metab.* 2003;88(2):622-626.
2. Morris JK, Alberman E, Scott C, Jacobs P. Is the prevalence of Klinefelter syndrome increasing? *Eur J Hum Genet.* 2008;16(2):163-170.
3. Irvine DS. Epidemiology and aetiology of male infertility. *Hum Reprod.* 1998;13(Suppl 1):33-44.
4. Kalyani RR, Gavini S, Dobs AS. Male hypogonadism in systemic disease. *Endocrinol Metab Clin North Am.* 2007;36(2):333-348.
5. Karagiannis A, Harsoulis F. Gonadal dysfunction in systemic diseases. *Eur J Endocrinol.* 2005;152(4):501-513.
6. Matsumoto AM. Androgen treatment of male hypogonadism. In: Kandeel FR, ed. *Male Sexual Function Pathophysiology and Treatment.* New York, NY: Informa Healthcare; 2007:433-452.
7. Ramasamy R, Ricci JA, Palermo GD, et al. Successful fertility treatment for Klinefelter's syndrome. *J Urol.* 2009;182(3):1108-1113.
8. Lubs HA. Testicular size in Klinefelter's syndrome in men over fifty. *N Engl J Med.* 1962;267(7):326-331.
9. Matsumoto AM. The testis. In: Felig P, Frohman LA, eds. *Endocrinology and Metabolism.* 4th ed. New York, NY: McGraw-Hill; 2001:635-705.
10. Matsumoto AM. Spermatogenesis. In: Adashi EY, Rock JA, Rosenwaks Z, eds. *Reproductive Endocrinology, Surgery, and Technology.* Philadelphia, PA: Lippincott-Raven; 1996:359-384.

11. Kapoor S. Testicular torsion: a race against time. *Int J Clin Pract.* 2008;62(5):821-827.
12. Zini A, Boman JM. Varicocele: red flag or red herring? *Semin Reprod Med.* 2009;27(2):171-178.
13. Amann RP, Howards SS. Daily spermatozoal production and epididymal spermatozoal reserves of the human male. *J Urol.* 1980;124(2):211-215.
14. Holstein AF, Schulze W, Davidoff M. Understanding spermatogenesis is a prerequisite for treatment. *Reprod Biol Endocrinol.* 2003;1:107.
15. Russell LD, Ettlin RA, Sinha Hikim AP, Clegg ED. Mammalian spermatogenesis. In: Russell LD, Ettlin RA, Sinha Hikim AP, Clegg ED, eds. *Histological and Histopathological Evaluaton of the Testis.* Clearwater: Cache River Press; 1990:1-40.
16. Rowley MJ, Leach DR, Warner GA, Heller CG. Effect of graded doses of ionizing radiation on the human testis. *Radiat Res.* 1974;59(3):665-678.
17. Hook EB. Maternal age, paternal age, and human chromosome abnormality: nature, magnitude, etiology, and mechanisms of effects. *Basic Life Sci.* 1985;36:117-132.
18. Hook EB, Cross PK, Schreinemachers DM. Chromosomal abnormality rates at amniocentesis and in live-born infants. *JAMA.* 1983;249(15):2034-2038.
19. Wikstrom AM, Dunkel L. Klinefelter syndrome. *Best Pract Res Clin Endocrinol Metab.* 2011;25(2):239-250.
20. Petersen MB, Antonarakis SE, Hassold TJ, et al. Paternal nondisjunction in trisomy 21: excess of male patients. *Hum Mol Genet.* 1993;2(10):1691-1695.
21. Johnson L. Efficiency of spermatogenesis. *Microsc Res Tech.* 1995;32(5):385-422.
22. Clermont Y. The cycle of the seminiferous epithelium in man. *Am J Anat.* 1963;112:35-51.
23. Kerr JB. Functional cytology of the human testis. *Baillieres Clin Endocrinol Metab.* 1992;6(2):235-250.
24. Heller CG, Clermont Y. Spermatogenesis in man: an estimate of its duration. *Science.* 1963;140:184-186.
25. Rowley MJ, Teshima F, Heller CG. Duration of transit of spermatozoa through the human male ductular system. *Fertil Steril.* 1970;21(5):390-396.
26. Geraci E, Giudice G. Sperm activation and sperm-egg interaction. *J Submicrosc Cytol Pathol.* 2006;38(1):11-20.
27. Suarez SS. Control of hyperactivation in sperm. *Hum Reprod Update.* 2008;14(6):647-657.
28. Inaba K. Molecular basis of sperm flagellar axonemes: structural and evolutionary aspects. *Ann N Y Acad Sci.* 2007;1101:506-526.
29. Cooper TG, Noonan E, von Eckardstein S, et al. World Health Organization reference values for human semen characteristics. *Hum Reprod Update.* 2010;16(3):231-245.
30. Menkveld R. Clinical significance of the low normal sperm morphology value as proposed in the fifth edition of the WHO Laboratory Manual for the Examination and Processing of Human Semen. *Asian J Androl.* 2010;12(1):47-58.
31. Leigh MW, Pittman JE, Carson JL, et al. Clinical and genetic aspects of primary ciliary dyskinesia/Kartagener syndrome. *Genet Med.* 2009;11(7):473-487.
32. Haider SG. Cell biology of Leydig cells in the testis. *Int Rev Cytol.* 2004;233:181-241.
33. Hughes IA, Acerini CL. Factors controlling testis descent. *Eur J Endocrinol.* 2008;159(Suppl 1):S75-S82.
34. Foresta C, Zuccarello D, Garolla A, Ferlin A. Role of hormones, genes, and environment in human cryptorchidism. *Endocr Rev.* 2008;29(5):560-580.
35. Maekawa M, Kamimura K, Nagano T. Peritubular myoid cells in the testis: their structure and function. *Arch Histol Cytol.* 1996;59(1):1-13.
36. Biason-Lauber A. Control of sex development. *Best Pract Res Clin Endocrinol Metab.* 2010;24(2):163-186.
37. Sekido R, Lovell-Badge R. Sex determination and sry: down to a wink and a nudge? *Trends Genet.* 2009;25(1):19-29.
38. Tapanainen J, Kellokumpu-Lehtinen P, Pelliniemi L, Huhtaniemi I. Age-related changes in endogenous steroids of human fetal testis during early and midpregnancy. *J Clin Endocrinol Metab.* 1981;52(1):98-102.
39. Quigley CA. Editorial: the postnatal gonadotropin and sex steroid surge-insights from the androgen insensitivity syndrome. *J Clin Endocrinol Metab.* 2002;87(1):24-28.
40. Grumbach MM. A window of opportunity: the diagnosis of gonadotropin deficiency in the male infant. *J Clin Endocrinol Metab.* 2005;90(5):3122-3127.
41. Main KM, Schmidt IM, Skakkebaek NE. A possible role for reproductive hormones in newborn boys: progressive hypogonadism without the postnatal testosterone peak. *J Clin Endocrinol Metab.* 2000;85(12):4905-4907.
42. Boyar RM, Rosenfeld RS, Kapen S, et al. Human puberty. Simultaneous augmented secretion of luteinizing hormone and testosterone during sleep. *J Clin Invest.* 1974;54(3):609-618.
43. Patton GC, Viner R. Pubertal transitions in health. *Lancet.* 2007;369(9567):1130-1139.
44. Nielsen CT, Skakkebaek NE, Richardson DW, et al. Onset of the release of spermatozoa (spermarche) in boys in relation to age, testicular growth, pubic hair, and height. *J Clin Endocrinol Metab.* 1986;62(3):532-535.
45. Veldhuis JD, King JC, Urban RJ, et al. Operating characteristics of the male hypothalamo-pituitary-gonadal axis: pulsatile release of testosterone and follicle-stimulating hormone and their temporal coupling with luteinizing hormone. *J Clin Endocrinol Metab.* 1987;65(5):929-941.
46. Whitcomb RW, O'Dea LS, Finkelstein JS, et al. Utility of free alpha-subunit as an alternative neuroendocrine marker of gonadotropin-releasing hormone (GnRH) stimulation of the gonadotroph in the human: evidence from normal and GnRH-deficient men. *J Clin Endocrinol Metab.* 1990;70(6):1654-1661.
47. Santoro N, Filicori M, Crowley WF Jr. Hypogonadotropic disorders in men and women: diagnosis and therapy with pulsatile gonadotropin-releasing hormone. *Endocr Rev.* 1986;7(1):11-23.
48. Matsumoto AM, Gross KM, Bremner WJ. The physiological significance of pulsatile LHRH secretion in man: gonadotrophin responses to physiological doses of pulsatile versus continuous LHRH administration. *Int J Androl.* 1991;14(1):23-32.
49. Wierman ME, Kiseljak-Vassiliades K, Tobet S. Gonadotropin-releasing hormone (GnRH) neuron migration: initiation, maintenance and cessation as critical steps to ensure normal reproductive function. *Front Neuroendocrinol.* 2010;32:43-52.
50. Brioude F, Bouligand J, Trabado S, et al. Non-syndromic congenital hypogonadotropic hypogonadism: clinical presentation and genotype-phenotype relationships. *Eur J Endocrinol.* 2010;162(5):835-851.
51. Bliss SP, Navratil AM, Xie J, Roberson MS. GnRH signaling, the gonadotrope and endocrine control of fertility. *Front Neuroendocrinol.* 2010;31(3):322-340.
52. Ulloa-Aguirre A, Maldonado A, Damian-Matsumura P, Timossi C. Endocrine regulation of gonadotropin glycosylation. *Arch Med Res.* 2001;32(6):520-532.
53. Greenman Y, Stern N. Non-functioning pituitary adenomas. *Best Pract Res Clin Endocrinol Metab.* 2009;23(5):625-638.
54. Tsatsoulis A, Shalet SM, Robertson WR. Changes in the qualitative and quantitative secretion of luteinizing hormone (LH) following orchidectomy in man. *Clin Endocrinol.* 1988;29(2):189-194.
55. Yen SC, Llerena LA, Pearson OH, Littell AS. Disappearance rates of endogenous follicle-stimulating hormone in serum following surgical hypophysectomy in man. *J Clin Endocrinol Metab.* 1970;30(3):325-329.
56. Ascoli M, Fanelli F, Segaloff DL. The lutropin/choriogonadotropin receptor, a 2002 perspective. *Endocr Rev.* 2002;23(2):141-174.
57. Miller WL. Molecular biology of steroid hormone synthesis. *Endocr Rev.* 1988;9(3):295-318.
58. Latronico AC, Arnhold IJ. Gonadotropin resistance. *Endocr Dev.* 2013;24:25-32.
59. Valdes-Socin H, Salvi R, Daly AF, et al. Hypogonadism in a patient with a mutation in the luteinizing hormone beta-subunit gene. *N Engl J Med.* 2004;351(25):2619-2625.
60. Reiter EO, Norjavaara E. Testotoxicosis: current viewpoint. *Pediatr Endocrinol Rev.* 2005;3(2):77-86.
61. Bhasin S. Testicular disorders. In: Kronenberg HM, Melmed S, Polonsky KS, Larsen PR, eds. *Williams Textbook of Endocrinology.* 11th ed. Philadelphia, PA: Elsevier; 2008:645-698.
62. Mendonca BB, Costa EM, Belgorosky A, et al. 46,XY DSD due to impaired androgen production. *Best Pract Res Clin Endocrinol Metab.* 2010;24(2):243-262.
63. Hammond GL, Ruokonen A, Kontturi M, et al. The simultaneous radioimmunoassay of seven steroids in human spermatic and peripheral venous blood. *J Clin Endocrinol Metab.* 1977;45(1):16-24.
64. Bremner WJ, Vitiello MV, Prinz PN. Loss of circadian rhythmicity in blood testosterone levels with aging in normal men. *J Clin Endocrinol Metab.* 1983;56(6):1278-1281.
65. Nankin HR, Murono E, Lin T, Osterman J. Morning and evening human Leydig cell responses to hCG. *Acta Endocrinol (Copenh).* 1980;95(4):560-565.
66. Ivell R, Anand-Ivell R. Biological role and clinical significance of insulin-like peptide 3. *Curr Opin Endocrinol Diabetes Obes.* 2011;18(3):210-216.
67. Bay K, Hartung S, Ivell R, et al. Insulin-like factor 3 serum levels in 135 normal men and 85 men with testicular disorders: relationship to the luteinizing hormone-testosterone axis. *J Clin Endocrinol Metab.* 2005;90(6):3410-3418.
68. Simoni M, Gromoll J, Nieschlag E. The follicle-stimulating hormone receptor: biochemistry, molecular biology, physiology, and pathophysiology. *Endocr Rev.* 1997;18(6):739-773.
69. Rannikko A, Penttila TL, Zhang FP, et al. Stage-specific expression of the FSH receptor gene in the prepubertal and adult rat seminiferous epithelium. *J Endocrinol.* 1996;151(1):29-35.
70. Bremner WJ, Millar MR, Sharpe RM, Saunders PT. Immunohistochemical localization of androgen receptors in the rat testis: evidence for stage-dependent expression and regulation by androgens. *Endocrinology.* 1994;135(3):1227-1234.

71. Jegou B. The Sertoli cell. *Baillieres Clin Endocrinol Metab*. 1992;6(2): 273-311.

72. Petersen C, Soder O. The Sertoli cell: a hormonal target and "super" nurse for germ cells that determines testicular size. *Horm Res*. 2006; 66(4):153-161.

73. Avvakumov GV, Cherkasov A, Muller YA, Hammond GL. Structural analyses of sex hormone-binding globulin reveal novel ligands and function. *Mol Cell Endocrinol*. 2010;316(1):13-23.

74. Selva DM, Hammond GL. Human sex hormone-binding globulin is expressed in testicular germ cells and not in Sertoli cells. *Horm Metab Res*. 2006;38(4):230-235.

75. McLean DJ, Friel PJ, Pouchnik D, Griswold MD. Oligonucleotide microarray analysis of gene expression in follicle-stimulating hormone-treated rat Sertoli cells. *Mol Endocrinol*. 2002;16(12):2780-2792.

76. O'Shaughnessy PJ, Verhoeven G, De Gendt K, et al. Direct action through the Sertoli cells is essential for androgen stimulation of spermatogenesis. *Endocrinology*. 2010;151(5):2343-2348.

77. Welsh M, Saunders PT, Atanassova N, et al. Androgen action via testicular peritubular myoid cells is essential for male fertility. *FASEB J*. 2009;23(12):4218-4230.

78. Ruwanpura SM, McLachlan RI, Meachem SJ. Hormonal regulation of male germ cell development. *J Endocrinol*. 2010;205(2):117-131.

79. Finkel DM, Phillips JL, Snyder PJ. Stimulation of spermatogenesis by gonadotropins in men with hypogonadotropic hypogonadism. *N Engl J Med*. 1985;313(11):651-655.

80. Achard C, Courtillot C, Lahuna O, et al. Normal spermatogenesis in a man with mutant luteinizing hormone. *N Engl J Med*. 2009;361(19): 1856-1863.

81. Bruysters M, Christin-Maitre S, Verhoef-Post M, et al. A new LH receptor splice mutation responsible for male hypogonadism with subnormal sperm production in the propositus, and infertility with regular cycles in an affected sister. *Hum Reprod*. 2008;23(8):1917-1923.

82. Layman LC. Mutations in the follicle-stimulating hormone-beta (FSH beta) and FSH receptor genes in mice and humans. *Semin Reprod Med*. 2000;18(1):5-10.

83. Layman LC, Porto AL, Xie J, et al. FSH beta gene mutations in a female with partial breast development and a male sibling with normal puberty and azoospermia. *J Clin Endocrinol Metab*. 2002;87(8): 3702-3707.

84. Lindstedt G, Nystrom E, Matthews C, et al. Follitropin (FSH) deficiency in an infertile male due to FSH beta gene mutation. A syndrome of normal puberty and virilization but underdeveloped testicles with azoospermia, low FSH but high lutropin and normal serum testosterone concentrations. *Clin Chem Lab Med*. 1998;36(8):663-665.

85. Phillip M, Arbelle JE, Segev Y, Parvari R. Male hypogonadism due to a mutation in the gene for the beta-subunit of follicle-stimulating hormone. *N Engl J Med*. 1998;338(24):1729-1732.

86. Meduri G, Bachelot A, Cocca MP, et al. Molecular pathology of the FSH receptor: new insights into FSH physiology. *Mol Cell Endocrinol*. 2008;282(1-2):130-142.

87. Matsumoto AM, Bremner WJ. Endocrine control of human spermatogenesis. *J Steroid Biochem*. 1989;33(4B):789-790.

88. Gromoll J, Simoni M, Nieschlag E. An activating mutation of the follicle-stimulating hormone receptor autonomously sustains spermatogenesis in a hypophysectomized man. *J Clin Endocrinol Metab*. 1996;81(4):1367-1370.

89. Matthiesson KL, McLachlan RI, O'Donnell L, et al. The relative roles of follicle-stimulating hormone and luteinizing hormone in maintaining spermatogonial maturation and spermiation in normal men. *J Clin Endocrinol Metab*. 2006;91(10):3962-3969.

90. Page ST, Kalhorn TF, Bremner WJ, et al. Intratesticular androgens and spermatogenesis during severe gonadotropin suppression induced by male hormonal contraceptive treatment. *J Androl*. 2007;28(5):734-741.

91. Roth MY, Page ST, Lin K, et al. Dose-dependent increase in intratesticular testosterone by very low-dose human chorionic gonadotropin in normal men with experimental gonadotropin deficiency. *J Clin Endocrinol Metab*. 2010;95(8):3806-3813.

92. Drincic A, Arseven OK, Sosa E, et al. Men with acquired hypogonadotropic hypogonadism treated with testosterone may be fertile. *Pituitary*. 2003;6(1):5-10.

93. Matthiesson KL, Stanton PG, O'Donnell L, et al. Effects of testosterone and levonorgestrel combined with a 5alpha-reductase inhibitor or gonadotropin-releasing hormone antagonist on spermatogenesis and intratesticular steroid levels in normal men. *J Clin Endocrinol Metab*. 2005;90(10):5647-5655.

94. Pitteloud N, Dwyer AA, DeCruz S, et al. The relative role of gonadal sex steroids and gonadotropin-releasing hormone pulse frequency in the regulation of follicle-stimulating hormone secretion in men. *J Clin Endocrinol Metab*. 2008;93(7):2686-2692.

95. Pitteloud N, Dwyer AA, DeCruz S, et al. Inhibition of luteinizing hormone secretion by testosterone in men requires aromatization for its pituitary but not its hypothalamic effects: evidence from the tandem study of normal and gonadotropin-releasing hormone-deficient men. *J Clin Endocrinol Metab*. 2008;93(3):784-791.

96. Boepple PA, Hayes FJ, Dwyer AA, et al. Relative roles of inhibin B and sex steroids in the negative feedback regulation of follicle-stimulating

97. Canovatchel WJ, Volquez D, Huang S, et al. Luteinizing hormone pulsatility in subjects with 5-alpha-reductase deficiency and decreased dihydrotestosterone production. *J Clin Endocrinol Metab*. 1994;78(4): 916-921.

98. Iranmanesh A, Veldhuis JD. Combined inhibition of types I and II 5 alpha-reductase selectively augments the basal (nonpulsatile) mode of testosterone secretion in young men. *J Clin Endocrinol Metab*. 2005; 90(7):4232-4237.

99. Idan A, Griffiths KA, Harwood DT, et al. Long-term effects of dihydrotestosterone treatment on prostate growth in healthy, middle-aged men without prostate disease: a randomized, placebo-controlled trial. *Ann Intern Med*. 2010;153(10):621-632.

100. Skorupskaite K, George JT, Anderson RA. The kisspeptin-GnRH pathway in human reproductive health and disease. *Hum Reprod Update*. 2014;20(4):485-500.

101. Oakley AE, Clifton DK, Steiner RA. Kisspeptin signaling in the brain. *Endocr Rev*. 2009;30(6):713-743.

102. Silveira LG, Tusset C, Latronico AC. Impact of mutations in kisspeptin and neurokinin B signaling pathways on human reproduction. *Brain Res*. 2010;1364:72-80.

103. de Kretser DM, Buzzard JJ, Okuma Y, et al. The role of activin, follistatin and inhibin in testicular physiology. *Mol Cell Endocrinol*. 2004;225(1-2):57-64.

104. Bilezikjian LM, Blount AL, Donaldson CJ, Vale WW. Pituitary actions of ligands of the TGF-beta family: activins and inhibins. *Reproduction*. 2006;132(2):207-215.

105. Page ST, Amory JK, Bremner WJ. Advances in male contraception. *Endocr Rev*. 2008;29(4):465-493.

106. Dunn JF, Nisula BC, Rodbard D. Transport of steroid hormones: binding of 21 endogenous steroids to both testosterone-binding globulin and corticosteroid-binding globulin in human plasma. *J Clin Endocrinol Metab*. 1981;53(1):58-68.

107. Vermeulen A. Physiology of the testosterone-binding globulin in man. *Ann N Y Acad Sci*. 1988;538:103-111.

108. Mendel CM. The free hormone hypothesis. Distinction from the free hormone transport hypothesis. *J Androl*. 1992;13(2):107-116.

109. Vos MJ, Mijnhout GS, Rondeel JM, et al. Sex hormone binding globulin deficiency due to a homozygous missense mutation. *J Clin Endocrinol Metab*. 2014;99(9):E1798-E1802.

110. Zakharov MN, Bhasin S, Travison TG, et al. A multi-step, dynamic allosteric model of testosterone's binding to sex hormone binding globulin. *Mol Cell Endocrinol*. 2015;399:190-200.

111. Willnow TE, Nykjaer A. Cellular uptake of steroid carrier proteins: mechanisms and implications. *Mol Cell Endocrinol*. 2010;316(1): 93-102.

112. Hammes A, Andreassen TK, Spoelgen R, et al. Role of endocytosis in cellular uptake of sex steroids. *Cell*. 2005;122(5):751-762.

113. Bhasin S, Cunningham GR, Hayes FJ, et al. Testosterone therapy in men with androgen deficiency syndromes: an Endocrine Society clinical practice guideline. *J Clin Endocrinol Metab*. 2010;95(6):2536-2559.

114. Horton R. Sex steroid production and secretion in the male. *Andrologia*. 1978;10(3):183-194.

115. Grumbach MM, Auchus RJ. Estrogen: consequences and implications of human mutations in synthesis and action. *J Clin Endocrinol Metab*. 1999;84(12):4677-4694.

116. Lombardi G, Zarrilli S, Colao A, et al. Estrogens and health in males. *Mol Cell Endocrinol*. 2001;178(1-2):51-55.

117. Finkelstein JS, Lee H, Burnett-Bowie SA, et al. Gonadal steroids and body composition, strength, and sexual function in men. *N Engl J Med*. 2013;369(11):1011-1022.

118. Zirilli L, Rochira V, Diazzi C, et al. Human models of aromatase deficiency. *J Steroid Biochem Mol Biol*. 2008;109(3-5):212-218.

119. Thigpen AE, Silver RI, Guileyardo JM, et al. Tissue distribution and ontogeny of steroid 5 alpha-reductase isozyme expression. *J Clin Invest*. 1993;92(2):903-910.

120. Imperato-McGinley J, Zhu YS. Androgens and male physiology the syndrome of 5-alpha-reductase-2 deficiency. *Mol Cell Endocrinol*. 2002; 198(1-2):51-59.

121. Randall VA. Role of 5 alpha-reductase in health and disease. *Baillieres Clin Endocrinol Metab*. 1994;8(2):405-431.

122. Aggarwal S, Thareja S, Verma A, et al. An overview on 5-alpha-reductase inhibitors. *Steroids*. 2010;75(2):109-153.

123. Andriole GL, Bostwick DG, Brawley OW, et al. Effect of dutasteride on the risk of prostate cancer. *N Engl J Med*. 2010;362(13):1192-1202.

124. Thompson IM, Goodman PJ, Tangen CM, et al. The influence of finasteride on the development of prostate cancer. *N Engl J Med*. 2003; 349(3):215-224.

125. Belanger A, Pelletier G, Labrie F, et al. Inactivation of androgens by UDP-glucuronosyltransferase enzymes in humans. *Trends Endocrinol Metab*. 2003;14(10):473-479.

126. Basaria S. Androgen abuse in athletes: detection and consequences. *J Clin Endocrinol Metab*. 2010;95(4):1533-1543.

127. Schulze JJ, Lorentzon M, Ohlsson C, et al. Genetic aspects of epitestosterone formation and androgen disposition: influence of

polymorphisms in CYP17 and UGT2B enzymes. *Pharmacogenet Genomics.* 2008;18(6):477-485.

128. Swanson C, Mellstrom D, Lorentzon M, et al. The uridine diphosphate glucuronosyltransferase 2B15 D85Y and 2B17 deletion polymorphisms predict the glucuronidation pattern of androgens and fat mass in men. *J Clin Endocrinol Metab.* 2007;92(12):4878-4882.

129. van de Kerkhof DH, de Boer D, Thijssen JH, Maes RA. Evaluation of testosterone/epitestosterone ratio influential factors as determined in doping analysis. *J Anal Toxicol.* 2000;24(2):102-115.

130. Li J, Al-Azzawi F. Mechanism of androgen receptor action. *Maturitas.* 2009;63(2):142-148.

131. Hughes IA, Werner R, Bunch T, Hiort O. Androgen insensitivity syndrome. *Semin Reprod Med.* 2012;30(5):432-442.

132. Finsterer J. Bulbar and spinal muscular atrophy (Kennedy's disease): a review. *Eur J Neurol.* 2009;16(5):556-561.

133. Dejager S, Bry-Gauillard H, Bruckert E, et al. A comprehensive endocrine description of Kennedy's disease revealing androgen insensitivity linked to CAG repeat length. *J Clin Endocrinol Metab.* 2002;87(8): 3893-3901.

134. Zitzmann M. The role of the CAG repeat androgen receptor polymorphism in andrology. *Front Horm Res.* 2009;37:52-61.

135. Rahman F, Christian HC. Non-classical actions of testosterone: an update. *Trends Endocrinol Metab.* 2007;18(10):371-378.

136. Griffin JE, Wilson JD. The testis. In: Bondy PK, Rosenberg LE, eds. *Metabolic Control and Disease.* 8th ed. Philadelphia, PA: WB Saunders; 1980:1535-1578.

137. Chemes HE. Infancy is not a quiescent period of testicular development. *Int J Androl.* 2001;24(1):2-7.

138. Marshall WA, Tanner JM. Variations in the pattern of pubertal changes in boys. *Arch Dis Child.* 1970;45(239):13-23.

139. Kaufman JM, Vermeulen A. The decline of androgen levels in elderly men and its clinical and therapeutic implications. *Endocr Rev.* 2005; 26(6):833-876.

140. Rey RA, Grinspon RP. Normal male sexual differentiation and aetiology of disorders of sex development. *Best Pract Res Clin Endocrinol Metab.* 2011;25(2):221-238.

141. Richmond EJ, Rogol AD. Male pubertal development and the role of androgen therapy. *Nat Clin Pract Endocrinol Metab.* 2007;3(4):338-344.

142. Kandeel FR, Koussa VK, Swerdloff RS. Male sexual function and its disorders: physiology, pathophysiology, clinical investigation, and treatment. *Endocr Rev.* 2001;22(3):342-388.

143. Carani C, Granata AR, Bancroft J, Marrama P. The effects of testosterone replacement on nocturnal penile tumescence and rigidity and erectile response to visual erotic stimuli in hypogonadal men. *Psychoneuroendocrinology.* 1995;20(7):743-753.

144. Corona G, Maggi M. The role of testosterone in erectile dysfunction. *Nat Rev Urol.* 2010;7(1):46-56.

145. Traish AM. Androgens play a pivotal role in maintaining penile tissue architecture and erection: a review. *J Androl.* 2009;30(4):363-369.

146. DeRogatis L, Rosen RC, Goldstein I, et al. Characterization of hypoactive sexual desire disorder (HSDD) in men. *J Sex Med.* 2012;9(3): 812-820.

147. Meuleman EJ, van Lankveld JJ. Hypoactive sexual desire disorder: an underestimated condition in men. *BJU Int.* 2005;95(3):291-296.

148. McVary KT. Clinical practice: erectile dysfunction. *N Engl J Med.* 2007;357(24):2472-2481.

149. Buvat J, Maggi M, Gooren L, et al. Endocrine aspects of male sexual dysfunctions. *J Sex Med.* 2010;7(4 Pt 2):1627-1656.

150. Wylie K, Rees M, Hackett G, et al. Androgens, health and sexuality in women and men. *Maturitas.* 2010;67(3):275-289.

151. Wylie K, Kenney G. Sexual dysfunction and the ageing male. *Maturitas.* 2010;65(1):23-27.

152. Bolona ER, Uraga MV, Haddad RM, et al. Testosterone use in men with sexual dysfunction: a systematic review and meta-analysis of randomized placebo-controlled trials. *Mayo Clin Proc.* 2007;82(1): 20-28.

153. Isidori AM, Buvat J, Corona G, et al. A critical analysis of the role of testosterone in erectile function: from pathophysiology to treatment—a systematic review. *Eur Urol.* 2014;65(1):99-112.

154. Qaseem A, Snow V, Denberg TD, et al. Hormonal testing and pharmacologic treatment of erectile dysfunction: a clinical practice guideline from the American College of Physicians. *Ann Intern Med.* 2009;151(9): 639-649.

155. Tsertsvadze A, Fink HA, Yazdi F, et al. Oral phosphodiesterase-5 inhibitors and hormonal treatments for erectile dysfunction: a systematic review and meta-analysis. *Ann Intern Med.* 2009;151(9):650-661.

156. Buvat J, Bou Jaoude G. Significance of hypogonadism in erectile dysfunction. *World J Urol.* 2006;24(6):657-667.

157. Phillips E, Carpenter C, Oates RD. Ejaculatory dysfunction. *Urol Clin North Am.* 2014;41(1):115-128.

158. Linton KD, Wylie KR. Recent advances in the treatment of premature ejaculation. *Drug Des Devel Ther.* 2010;4:1-6.

159. Tay YK, Spernat D, Rzetelski-West K, et al. Acute management of priapism in men. *BJU Int.* 2012;109(Suppl 3):15-21.

160. Braunstein GD. Clinical practice: gynecomastia. *N Engl J Med.* 2007; 357(12):1229-1237.

161. Johnson RE, Murad MH. Gynecomastia: pathophysiology, evaluation, and management. *Mayo Clin Proc.* 2009;84(11):1010-1015.

162. Narula HS, Carlson HE. Gynaecomastia-pathophysiology, diagnosis and treatment. *Nat Rev Endocrinol.* 2014;10(11):684-698.

163. Gomez-Raposo C, Zambrana Tevar F, Sereno Moyano M, et al. Male breast cancer. *Cancer Treat Rev.* 2010;36(6):451-457.

164. Lee SY, Oh SM, Chung KH. Estrogenic effects of marijuana smoke condensate and cannabinoid compounds. *Toxicol Appl Pharmacol.* 2006;214(3):270-278.

165. Messina M. Soybean isoflavone exposure does not have feminizing effects on men: a critical examination of the clinical evidence. *Fertil Steril.* 2010;93(7):2095-2104.

166. Bowman JD, Kim H, Bustamante JJ. Drug-induced gynecomastia. *Pharmacotherapy.* 2012;32(12):1123-1140.

167. Eckman A, Dobs A. Drug-induced gynecomastia. *Expert Opin Drug Saf.* 2008;7(6):691-702.

168. Gruntmanis U, Braunstein GD. Treatment of gynecomastia. *Curr Opin Investig Drugs.* 2001;2(5):643-649.

169. Gnoth C, Godehardt E, Frank-Herrmann P, et al. Definition and prevalence of subfertility and infertility. *Hum Reprod.* 2005;20(5): 1144-1147.

170. Anawalt BD. Approach to male infertility and induction of spermatogenesis. *J Clin Endocrinol Metab.* 2013;98(9):3532-3542.

171. Krausz C. Male infertility: pathogenesis and clinical diagnosis. *Best Pract Res Clin Endocrinol Metab.* 2011;25(2):271-285.

172. McLachlan RI, O'Bryan MK. Clinical review: state of the art for genetic testing of infertile men. *J Clin Endocrinol Metab.* 2010;95(3):1013-1024.

173. Vogt PH, Falcao CL, Hanstein R, Zimmer J. The AZF proteins. *Int J Androl.* 2008;31(4):383-394.

174. Radpour R, Gourabi H, Dizaj AV, et al. Genetic investigations of CFTR mutations in congenital absence of vas deferens, uterus, and vagina as a cause of infertility. *J Androl.* 2008;29(5):506-513.

175. Walsh TJ, Pera RR, Turek PJ. The genetics of male infertility. *Semin Reprod Med.* 2009;27(2):124-136.

176. Comhaire FH, Mahmoud AM, Depuydt CE, et al. Mechanisms and effects of male genital tract infection on sperm quality and fertilizing potential: the andrologist's viewpoint. *Hum Reprod Update.* 1999;5(5): 393-398.

177. Pellati D, Mylonakis I, Bertoloni G, et al. Genital tract infections and infertility. *Eur J Obstet Gynecol Reprod Biol.* 2008;140(1):3-11.

178. Adamopoulos DA, Koukkou EG. Value of FSH and inhibin-B measurements in the diagnosis of azoospermia: a clinician's overview. *Int J Androl.* 2010;33(1):e109-e113.

179. Hwang K, Walters RC, Lipshultz LI. Contemporary concepts in the evaluation and management of male infertility. *Nat Rev Urol.* 2011;8(2):86-94.

180. Tournaye H. Male factor infertility and art. *Asian J Androl.* 2012;14(1): 103-108.

181. Masson P, Brannigan RE. The varicocele. *Urol Clin North Am.* 2014;41(1): 129-144.

182. Schlegel PN. Nonobstructive azoospermia: a revolutionary surgical approach and results. *Semin Reprod Med.* 2009;27(2):165-170.

183. Nagler HM, Jung H. Factors predicting successful microsurgical vasectomy reversal. *Urol Clin North Am.* 2009;36(3):383-390.

184. Araujo AB, Esche GR, Kupelian V, et al. Prevalence of symptomatic androgen deficiency in men. *J Clin Endocrinol Metab.* 2007;92(11): 4241-4247.

185. Araujo AB, O'Donnell AB, Brambilla DJ, et al. Prevalence and incidence of androgen deficiency in middle-aged and older men: estimates from the Massachusetts Male Aging Study. *J Clin Endocrinol Metab.* 2004;89(12):5920-5926.

186. Wu FC, Tajar A, Beynon JM, et al. Identification of late-onset hypogonadism in middle-aged and elderly men. *N Engl J Med.* 2010;363(2): 123-135.

187. Mulligan T, Frick MF, Zuraw QC, et al. Prevalence of hypogonadism in males aged at least 45 years: the HIM study. *Int J Clin Pract.* 2006; 60(7):762-769.

188. Matsumoto AM. Testosterone administration in older men. *Endocrinol Metab Clin North Am.* 2013;42(2):271-286.

189. Grossmann M, Zajac JD. Androgen deprivation therapy in men with prostate cancer: how should the side effects be monitored and treated? *Clin Endocrinol (Oxf).* 2011;74(3):289-293.

190. Moreau JP, Delavault P, Blumberg J. Luteinizing hormone-releasing hormone agonists in the treatment of prostate cancer: a review of their discovery, development, and place in therapy. *Clin Ther.* 2006;28(10): 1485-1508.

191. Pincus SM, Mulligan T, Iranmanesh A, et al. Older males secrete luteinizing hormone and testosterone more irregularly, and jointly more asynchronously, than younger males. *Proc Natl Acad Sci U S A.* 1996; 93(24):14100-14105.

192. Brambilla DJ, Matsumoto AM, Araujo AB, McKinlay JB. The effect of diurnal variation on clinical measurement of serum testosterone and other sex hormone levels in men. *J Clin Endocrinol Metab.* 2009;94(3): 907-913.

193. Caronia LM, Dwyer AA, Hayden D, et al. Abrupt decrease in serum testosterone levels after an oral glucose load in men: implications

for screening for hypogonadism. *Clin Endocrinol.* 2013;78(2):291-296.

194. Plumelle D, Lombard E, Nicolay A, Portugal H. Influence of diet and sample collection time on 77 laboratory tests on healthy adults. *Clin Biochem.* 2014;47(1-2):31-37.

195. Swerdloff RS, Wang C, Cunningham G, et al. Long-term pharmacokinetics of transdermal testosterone gel in hypogonadal men. *J Clin Endocrinol Metab.* 2000;85(12):4500-4510.

196. Brambilla DJ, O'Donnell AB, Matsumoto AM, McKinlay JB. Intraindividual variation in levels of serum testosterone and other reproductive and adrenal hormones in men. *Clin Endocrinol.* 2007;67(6):853-862.

197. Wang C, Catlin DH, Demers LM, et al. Measurement of total serum testosterone in adult men: comparison of current laboratory methods versus liquid chromatography-tandem mass spectrometry. *J Clin Endocrinol Metab.* 2004;89(2):534-543.

198. Rosner W, Vesper H. Toward excellence in testosterone testing: a consensus statement. *J Clin Endocrinol Metab.* 2010;95(10):4542-4548.

199. Swerdloff RS, Wang C. Free testosterone measurement by the analog displacement direct assay: old concerns and new evidence. *Clin Chem.* 2008;54(3):458-460.

200. Vermeulen A, Verdonck L, Kaufman JM. A critical evaluation of simple methods for the estimation of free testosterone in serum. *J Clin Endocrinol Metab.* 1999;84(10):3666-3672.

201. Winters SJ, Kelley DE, Goodpaster B. The analog free testosterone assay: are the results in men clinically useful? *Clin Chem.* 1998; 44(10):2178-2182.

202. Ly LP, Sartorius G, Hull L, et al. Accuracy of calculated free testosterone formulae in men. *Clin Endocrinol.* 2010;73(3):382-388.

203. Anawalt BD, Hotaling JM, Walsh TJ, Matsumoto AM. Performance of total testosterone measurement to predict free testosterone for the biochemical evaluation of male hypogonadism. *J Urol.* 2012;187(4):1369-1373.

204. Guzick DS, Overstreet JW, Factor-Litvak P, et al. Sperm morphology, motility, and concentration in fertile and infertile men. *N Engl J Med.* 2001;345(19):1388-1393.

205. Citron JT, Ettinger B, Rubinoff H, et al. Prevalence of hypothalamic-pituitary imaging abnormalities in impotent men with secondary hypogonadism. *J Urol.* 1996;155(2):529-533.

206. Dobs AS, El-Deiry S, Wand G, Wiederkehr M. Central hypogonadism: distinguishing idiopathic low testosterone from pituitary tumors. *Endocr Pract.* 1998;4(6):355-359.

207. Groth KA, Skakkebaek A, Host C, et al. Clinical review: Klinefelter syndrome—a clinical update. *J Clin Endocrinol Metab.* 2013;98(1):20-30.

208. Lanfranco F, Kamischke A, Zitzmann M, Nieschlag E. Klinefelter's syndrome. *Lancet.* 2004;364(9430):273-283.

209. Smyth CM, Bremner WJ. Klinefelter syndrome. *Arch Intern Med.* 1998;158(12):1309-1314.

210. Zeger MP, Zinn AR, Lahlou N, et al. Effect of ascertainment and genetic features on the phenotype of Klinefelter syndrome. *J Pediatr.* 2008; 152(5):716-722.

211. Aksglaede L, Skakkebaek NE, Almstrup K, Juul A. Clinical and biological parameters in 166 boys, adolescents and adults with nonmosaic Klinefelter syndrome: a Copenhagen experience. *Acta Paediatr (Oslo, Norway: 1992).* 2011;100(6):793-806.

212. Boisen E. Testicular size and shape of 47,XYY and 47,XXY men in a double-blind, double-matched population survey. *Am J Hum Genet.* 1979;31(6):697-703.

213. Okada H, Fujioka H, Tatsumi N, et al. Klinefelter's syndrome in the male infertility clinic. *Hum Reprod.* 1999;14(4):946-952.

214. Vorona E, Zitzmann M, Gromoll J, et al. Clinical, endocrinological, and epigenetic features of the 46,XX male syndrome, compared with 47,XXY Klinefelter patients. *J Clin Endocrinol Metab.* 2007;92(9):3458-3465.

215. Brinton LA, Carreon JD, Gierach GL, et al. Etiologic factors for male breast cancer in the U.S. Veterans Affairs medical care system database. *Breast Cancer Res Treat.* 2010;119(1):185-192.

216. Bojesen A, Juul S, Birkebaek N, Gravholt CH. Increased mortality in Klinefelter syndrome. *J Clin Endocrinol Metab.* 2004;89(8):3830-3834.

217. Swerdlow AJ, Higgins CD, Schoemaker MJ, et al. Mortality in patients with Klinefelter syndrome in Britain: a cohort study. *J Clin Endocrinol Metab.* 2005;90(12):6516-6522.

218. Turner C, Hilton-Jones D. The myotonic dystrophies: diagnosis and management. *J Neurol Neurosurg Psychiatry.* 2010;81(4):358-367.

219. Al-Harbi TM, Bainbridge LJ, McQueen MJ, Tarnopolsky MA. Hypogonadism is common in men with myopathies. *J Clin Neuromuscul Dis.* 2008;9(4):397-401.

220. Vazquez JA, Pinies JA, Martul P, et al. Hypothalamic-pituitary-testicular function in 70 patients with myotonic dystrophy. *J Endocrinol Invest.* 1990;13(5):375-379.

221. Griggs RC, Pandya S, Florence JM, et al. Randomized controlled trial of testosterone in myotonic dystrophy. *Neurology.* 1989;39(2 Pt 1):219-222.

222. Ashley RA, Barthold JS, Kolon TF. Cryptorchidism: pathogenesis, diagnosis, treatment and prognosis. *Urol Clin North Am.* 2010;37(2):183-193.

223. Lee PA, Houk CP. Cryptorchidism. *Curr Opin Endocrinol Diabetes Obes.* 2013;20(3):210-216.

224. Mathers MJ, Sperling H, Rubben H, Roth S. The undescended testis: diagnosis, treatment and long-term consequences. *Dtsch Arztebl Int.* 2009;106(33):527-532.

225. Virtanen HE, Bjerknes R, Cortes D, et al. Cryptorchidism: classification, prevalence and long-term consequences. *Acta Paediatr (Oslo, Norway: 1992).* 2007;96(5):611-616.

226. Atkinson PM, Epstein MT, Rippon AE. Plasma gonadotropins and androgens in surgically treated cryptorchid patients. *J Pediatr Surg.* 1975;10(1):27-33.

227. Lee PA, Coughlin MT. Leydig cell function after cryptorchidism: evidence of the beneficial result of early surgery. *J Urol.* 2002;167(4):1824-1827.

228. Roberts AE, Allanson JE, Tartaglia M, Gelb BD. Noonan syndrome. *Lancet.* 2013;381(9863):333-342.

229. Romano AA, Allanson JE, Dahlgren J, et al. Noonan syndrome: clinical features, diagnosis, and management guidelines. *Pediatrics.* 2010; 126(4):746-759.

230. Kelnar CJ. Noonan syndrome: the hypothalamo-adrenal and hypothalamo-gonadal axes. *Horm Res.* 2009;72(Suppl 2):24-30.

231. Aynsley-Green A, Zachmann M, Illig R, et al. Congenital bilateral anorchia in childhood: a clinical, endocrine and therapeutic evaluation of twenty-one cases. *Clin Endocrinol.* 1976;5(4):381-391.

232. Zenaty D, Dijoud F, Morel Y, et al. Bilateral anorchia in infancy: occurrence of micropenis and the effect of testosterone treatment. *J Pediatr.* 2006;149(5):687-691.

233. McEachern R, Houle AM, Garel L, Van Vliet G. Lost and found testes: the importance of the hCG stimulation test and other testicular markers to confirm a surgical declaration of anorchia. *Horm Res.* 2004;62(3):124-128.

234. Lee MM, Donahoe PK, Silverman BL, et al. Measurements of serum mullerian inhibiting substance in the evaluation of children with nonpalpable gonads. *N Engl J Med.* 1997;336(21):1480-1486.

235. Cutolo M. Autoimmune polyendocrine syndromes. *Autoimmun Rev.* 2014;13(2):85-89.

236. Husebye ES, Perheentupa J, Rautemaa R, Kampe O. Clinical manifestations and management of patients with autoimmune polyendocrine syndrome type I. *J Intern Med.* 2009;265(5):514-529.

237. Falorni A, Laureti S, Santeusanio F. Autoantibodies in autoimmune polyendocrine syndrome type II. *Endocrinol Metab Clin North Am.* 2002;31(2):369-389, vii.

238. Yanase T. 17 Alpha-hydroxylase/17,20-lyase defects. *J Steroid Biochem Mol Biol.* 1995;53(1-6):153-157.

239. Sherbet DP, Tiosano D, Kwist KM, et al. CYP17 mutation E305G causes isolated 17,20-lyase deficiency by selectively altering substrate binding. *J Biol Chem.* 2003;278(49):48563-48569.

240. Faienza MF, Giordani L, Delvecchio M, Cavallo L. Clinical, endocrine, and molecular findings in 17-beta-hydroxysteroid dehydrogenase type 3 deficiency. *J Endocrinol Invest.* 2008;31(1):85-91.

241. Pang S. Congenital adrenal hyperplasia owing to 3 beta-hydroxysteroid dehydrogenase deficiency. *Endocrinol Metab Clin North Am.* 2001;30(1):81-99, vi-vii.

242. Cavanah SF, Dons RF. Partial 3 beta-hydroxysteroid dehydrogenase deficiency presenting as new-onset gynecomastia in a eugonadal adult male. *Metabolism.* 1993;42(1):65-68.

243. Cabrera MS, Vogiatzi MG, New MI. Long term outcome in adult males with classic congenital adrenal hyperplasia. *J Clin Endocrinol Metab.* 2001;86(7):3070-3078.

244. Claahsen-van der Grinten HL, Otten BJ, Stikkelbroeck MM, et al. Testicular adrenal rest tumours in congenital adrenal hyperplasia. *Best Pract Res Clin Endocrinol Metab.* 2009;23(2):209-220.

245. Stikkelbroeck NM, Otten BJ, Pasic A, et al. High prevalence of testicular adrenal rest tumors, impaired spermatogenesis, and Leydig cell failure in adolescent and adult males with congenital adrenal hyperplasia. *J Clin Endocrinol Metab.* 2001;86(12):5721-5728.

246. Rimoin DL, Conner JM, Pyeritz RE, Korf BR. *Principles and Practice of Medical Genetics.* Philadelphia, PA: Elsevier Health Sciences; 2007.

247. Imura H, Nakao Y, Kuzuya H, et al. Clinical, endocrine and metabolic aspects of the Werner syndrome compared with those of normal aging. *Adv Exp Med Biol.* 1985;190:171-185.

248. Lee PA, Danish RK, Mazur T, Migeon CJ. Micropenis. III. Primary hypogonadism, partial androgen insensitivity syndrome, and idiopathic disorders. *Johns Hopkins Med J.* 1980;147(5):175-181.

249. Marshall JD, Beck S, Maffei P, Naggert JK. Alstrom syndrome. *Eur J Hum Genet.* 2007;15(12):1193-1202.

250. Medlej R, Wasson J, Baz P, et al. Diabetes mellitus and optic atrophy: a study of Wolfram syndrome in the Lebanese population. *J Clin Endocrinol Metab.* 2004;89(4):1656-1661.

251. Molho-Pessach V, Agha Z, Aamar S, et al. The H syndrome: a genodermatosis characterized by indurated, hyperpigmented, and hypertrichotic skin with systemic manifestations. *J Am Acad Dermatol.* 2008; 59(1):79-85.

252. Slavotinek A, Goldman J, Weisiger K, et al. Marinesco-Sjogren syndrome in a male with mild dysmorphism. *Am J Med Genet A.* 2005; 133A(2):197-201.

253. Sohval AR, Soffer LJ. Congenital familial testicular deficiency. *Am J Med*. 1953;14(3):328-348.

254. Weinstein RL, Kliman B, Scully RE. Familial syndrome of primary testicular insufficiency with normal virilization, blindness, deafness and metabolic abnormalities. *N Engl J Med*. 1969;281(18):969-977.

255. Werder EA, Murset G, Illig R, Prader A. Hypogonadism and parathyroid adenoma in congenital poikiloderma (Rothmund-Thomson syndrome). *Clin Endocrinol*. 1975;4(1):75-82.

256. Zadik Z, Levin S, Prager-Lewin R, Laron Z. Gonadal dysfunction in patients with ataxia telangiectasia. *Acta Paediatr Scand*. 1978;67(4):477-479.

257. Hirsch HJ, Eldar-Geva T, Benarroch F, et al. Primary testicular dysfunction is a major contributor to abnormal pubertal development in males with Prader-Willi syndrome. *J Clin Endocrinol Metab*. 2009;94(7):2262-2268.

258. Leroith D, Farkash Y, Bar-Ziev J, Spitz IM. Hypothalamic-pituitary function in the Bardet-Biedl syndrome. *Isr J Med Sci*. 1980;16(7):514-518.

259. Marshall JD, Paisey RB, Carey C, Macdermott S. Alström syndrome. In: Pagan RA, Bird TC, Dolan CR, et al., eds. *GeneReviews [Internet]*. 2003 [updated 2010 Jun 8].

260. Siemensma EP, de Lind van Wijngaarden RF, Otten BJ, et al. Testicular failure in boys with Prader-Willi syndrome: longitudinal studies of reproductive hormones. *J Clin Endocrinol Metab*. 2012;97(3):E452-E459.

261. Hawli Y, Nasrallah M, El-Hajj Fuleihan G. Endocrine and musculoskeletal abnormalities in patients with Down syndrome. *Nat Rev Endocrinol*. 2009;5(6):327-334.

262. Muller T, Gromoll J, Simoni M. Absence of exon 10 of the human luteinizing hormone (LH) receptor impairs LH, but not human chorionic gonadotropin action. *J Clin Endocrinol Metab*. 2003;88(5):2242-2249.

263. Feldman D. Ketoconazole and other imidazole derivatives as inhibitors of steroidogenesis. *Endocr Rev*. 1986;7(4):409-420.

264. Rajfer J, Sikka SC, Rivera F, Handelsman DJ. Mechanism of inhibition of human testicular steroidogenesis by oral ketoconazole. *J Clin Endocrinol Metab*. 1986;63(5):1193-1198.

265. Yin L, Hu Q. Cyp17 inhibitors—abiraterone, C17,20-lyase inhibitors and multi-targeting agents. *Nat Rev Urol*. 2014;11(1):32-42.

266. Loriaux DL, Menard R, Taylor A, et al. Spironolactone and endocrine dysfunction. *Ann Intern Med*. 1976;85(5):630-636.

267. Beer TM, Armstrong AJ, Rathkopf DE, et al. Enzalutamide in metastatic prostate cancer before chemotherapy. *N Engl J Med*. 2014;371(5):424-433.

268. Adler RA. Clinical review 33: clinically important effects of alcohol on endocrine function. *J Clin Endocrinol Metab*. 1992;74(5):957-960.

269. Emanuele MA, Emanuele NV. Alcohol's effects on male reproduction. *Alcohol Health Res World*. 1998;22(3):195-201.

270. Steffens M, Beauloye V, Brichard B, et al. Endocrine and metabolic disorders in young adult survivors of childhood acute lymphoblastic leukaemia (ALL) or non-Hodgkin lymphoma (NHL). *Clin Endocrinol*. 2008;69(5):819-827.

271. Travis LB, Beard C, Allan JM, et al. Testicular cancer survivorship: research strategies and recommendations. *J Natl Cancer Inst*. 2010;102(15):1114-1130.

272. Clifton DK, Bremner WJ. The effect of testicular x-irradiation on spermatogenesis in man. A comparison with the mouse. *J Androl*. 1983;4(6):387-392.

273. Shalet SM, Tsatsoulis A, Whitehead E, Read G. Vulnerability of the human Leydig cell to radiation damage is dependent upon age. *J Endocrinol*. 1989;120(1):161-165.

274. Davis NF, McGuire BB, Mahon JA, et al. The increasing incidence of mumps orchitis: a comprehensive review. *BJU Int*. 2010;105(8):1060-1065.

275. Ternavasio-de la Vega HG, Boronat M, Ojeda A, et al. Mumps orchitis in the post-vaccine era (1967-2009): a single-center series of 67 patients and review of clinical outcome and trends. *Medicine (Baltimore)*. 2010;89(2):96-116.

276. Hagley M. Epididymo-orchitis and epididymitis: a review of causes and management of unusual forms. *Int J STD AIDS*. 2003;14(6):372-377, quiz 8.

277. Pudney J, Anderson D. Orchitis and human immunodeficiency virus type 1 infected cells in reproductive tissues from men with the acquired immune deficiency syndrome. *Am J Pathol*. 1991;139(1):149-160.

278. Trojian TH, Lishnak TS, Heiman D. Epididymitis and orchitis: an overview. *Am Fam Physician*. 2009;79(7):583-587.

279. Floreani A, Mega A, Tizian L, et al. Bone metabolism and gonad function in male patients undergoing liver transplantation: a two-year longitudinal study. *Osteoporos Int*. 2001;12(9):749-754.

280. Foresta C, Schipilliti M, Ciarleglio FA, et al. Male hypogonadism in cirrhosis and after liver transplantation. *J Endocrinol Invest*. 2008;31(5):470-478.

281. Zietz B, Lock G, Plach B, et al. Dysfunction of the hypothalamic-pituitary-glandular axes and relation to Child-Pugh classification in male patients with alcoholic and virus-related cirrhosis. *Eur J Gastroenterol Hepatol*. 2003;15(5):495-501.

282. Handelsman DJ, Liu PY. Androgen therapy in chronic renal failure. *Baillieres Clin Endocrinol Metab*. 1998;12(3):485-500.

283. Prem AR, Punekar SV, Kalpana M, et al. Male reproductive function in uraemia: efficacy of haemodialysis and renal transplantation. *Br J Urol*. 1996;78(4):635-638.

284. Huyghe E, Zairi A, Nohra J, et al. Gonadal impact of target of rapamycin inhibitors (sirolimus and everolimus) in male patients: an overview. *Transpl Int*. 2007;20(4):305-311.

285. Xu LG, Xu HM, Zhu XF, et al. Examination of the semen quality of patients with uraemia and renal transplant recipients in comparison with a control group. *Andrologia*. 2009;41(4):235-240.

286. Feldman HA, Longcope C, Derby CA, et al. Age trends in the level of serum testosterone and other hormones in middle-aged men: longitudinal results from the Massachusetts Male Aging Study. *J Clin Endocrinol Metab*. 2002;87(2):589-598.

287. Harman SM, Metter EJ, Tobin JD, et al. Longitudinal effects of aging on serum total and free testosterone levels in healthy men. Baltimore Longitudinal Study of Aging. *J Clin Endocrinol Metab*. 2001;86(2):724-731.

288. Morley JE, Kaiser FE, Perry HM 3rd, et al. Longitudinal changes in testosterone, luteinizing hormone, and follicle-stimulating hormone in healthy older men. *Metabolism*. 1997;46(4):410-413.

289. Mulligan T, Iranmanesh A, Kerzner R, et al. Two-week pulsatile gonadotropin releasing hormone infusion unmasks dual (hypothalamic and Leydig cell) defects in the healthy aging male gonadotropic axis. *Eur J Endocrinol*. 1999;141(3):257-266.

290. Veldhuis JD, Keenan DM, Liu PY, et al. The aging male hypothalamic-pituitary-gonadal axis: pulsatility and feedback. *Mol Cell Endocrinol*. 2009;299(1):14-22.

291. Tajar A, Forti G, O'Neill TW, et al. Characteristics of secondary, primary, and compensated hypogonadism in aging men: evidence from the European Male Ageing Study. *J Clin Endocrinol Metab*. 2010;95(4):1810-1818.

292. Wu FC, Tajar A, Pye SR, et al. Hypothalamic-pituitary-testicular axis disruptions in older men are differentially linked to age and modifiable risk factors: the European Male Aging Study. *J Clin Endocrinol Metab*. 2008;93(7):2737-2745.

293. Basaria S, Coviello AD, Travison TG, et al. Adverse events associated with testosterone administration. *N Engl J Med*. 2010;363(2):109-122.

294. Srinivas-Shankar U, Roberts SA, Connolly MJ, et al. Effects of testosterone on muscle strength, physical function, body composition, and quality of life in intermediate-frail and frail elderly men: a randomized, double-blind, placebo-controlled study. *J Clin Endocrinol Metab*. 2010;95(2):639-650.

295. Corona G, Rastrelli G, Maggi M. Diagnosis and treatment of late-onset hypogonadism: systematic review and meta-analysis of trt outcomes. *Best Pract Res Clin Endocrinol Metab*. 2013;27(4):557-579.

296. Fernandez-Balsells MM, Murad MH, Lane M, et al. Clinical review 1: adverse effects of testosterone therapy in adult men: a systematic review and meta-analysis. *J Clin Endocrinol Metab*. 2010;95(6):2560-2575.

297. Xu L, Freeman G, Cowling BJ, Schooling CM. Testosterone therapy and cardiovascular events among men: a systematic review and meta-analysis of placebo-controlled randomized trials. *BMC Med*. 2013;11:108.

298. Baillargeon J, Urban RJ, Kuo YF, et al. Risk of myocardial infarction in older men receiving testosterone therapy. *Ann Pharmacother*. 2014;48(9):1138-1144.

299. Finkle WD, Greenland S, Ridgeway GK, et al. Increased risk of non-fatal myocardial infarction following testosterone therapy prescription in men. *PLoS ONE*. 2014;9(1):e85805.

300. Vigen R, O'Donnell CI, Baron AE, et al. Association of testosterone therapy with mortality, myocardial infarction, and stroke in men with low testosterone levels. *JAMA*. 2013;310(17):1829-1836.

301. Wang C, Nieschlag E, Swerdloff R, et al. Investigation, treatment, and monitoring of late-onset hypogonadism in males: ISA, ISSAM, EAU, EAA, and ASA recommendations. *J Androl*. 2009;30(1):1-9.

302. Petersen PM, Giwercman A, Skakkebaek NE, Rorth M. Gonadal function in men with testicular cancer. *Semin Oncol*. 1998;25(2):224-233.

303. Vigersky RA, Chapman RM, Berenberg J, Glass AR. Testicular dysfunction in untreated Hodgkin's disease. *Am J Med*. 1982;73(4):482-486.

304. Viviani S, Ragni G, Santoro A, et al. Testicular dysfunction in Hodgkin's disease before and after treatment. *Eur J Cancer*. 1991;27(11):1389-1392.

305. Abbasi AA, Prasad AS, Ortega J, et al. Gonadal function abnormalities in sickle cell anemia. Studies in adult male patients. *Ann Intern Med*. 1976;85(5):601-605.

306. Brachet C, Heinrichs C, Tenoutasse S, et al. Children with sickle cell disease: growth and gonadal function after hematopoietic stem cell transplantation. *J Pediatr Hematol Oncol*. 2007;29(7):445-450.

307. Parshad O, Stevens MC, Preece MA, et al. The mechanism of low testosterone levels in homozygous sickle-cell disease. *West Indian Med J*. 1994;43(1):12-14.

308. Celik B, Sahin A, Caglar N, et al. Sex hormone levels and functional outcomes: a controlled study of patients with spinal cord injury

compared with healthy subjects. *Am J Phys Med Rehabil.* 2007;86(10): 784-790.

309. Kostovski E, Iversen PO, Birkeland K, et al. Decreased levels of testosterone and gonadotrophins in men with long-standing tetraplegia. *Spinal Cord.* 2008;46(8):559-564.

310. Naderi AR, Safarinejad MR. Endocrine profiles and semen quality in spinal cord injured men. *Clin Endocrinol.* 2003;58(2):177-184.

311. Elliott SP, Orejuela F, Hirsch IH, et al. Testis biopsy findings in the spinal cord injured patient. *J Urol.* 2000;163(3):792-795.

312. Richter JG, Becker A, Specker C, Schneider M. Hypogonadism in Wegener's granulomatosis. *Scand J Rheumatol.* 2008;37(5):365-369.

313. Scalvini T, Martini PR, Obici L, et al. Infertility and hypergonadotropic hypogonadism as first evidence of hereditary apolipoprotein A-I amyloidosis. *J Urol.* 2007;178(1):344-348.

314. Silva CA, Cocuzza M, Carvalho JF, Bonfa E. Diagnosis and classification of autoimmune orchitis. *Autoimmun Rev.* 2014;13(4-5):431-434.

315. Kim HH, Goldstein M. Adult varicocele. *Curr Opin Urol.* 2008;18(6): 608-612.

316. Nistal M, Jimenez F, Paniagua R. Sertoli cell types in the Sertoli-cell-only syndrome: relationships between Sertoli cell morphology and aetiology. *Histopathology.* 1990;16(2):173-180.

317. Micic S, Ilic V, Micic M, et al. Endocrine profile of 45 patients with Sertoli cell only syndrome. *Andrologia.* 1983;15(3):228-232.

318. Kamp C, Huellen K, Fernandes S, et al. High deletion frequency of the complete AZFa sequence in men with Sertoli-cell-only syndrome. *Mol Hum Reprod.* 2001;7(10):987-994.

319. Bush A, Hogg C. Primary ciliary dyskinesia: recent advances in epidemiology, diagnosis, management and relationship with the expanding spectrum of ciliopathy. *Expert Rev Respir Med.* 2012;6(6):663-682.

320. Storm van's Gravesande K, Omran H. Primary ciliary dyskinesia: clinical presentation, diagnosis and genetics. *Ann Med.* 2005;37(6): 439-449.

321. Kiserud CE, Fossa A, Bjoro T, et al. Gonadal function in male patients after treatment for malignant lymphomas, with emphasis on chemotherapy. *Br J Cancer.* 2009;100(3):455-463.

322. Vigano A, Piccioni M, Trutschnigg B, et al. Male hypogonadism associated with advanced cancer: a systematic review. *Lancet Oncol.* 2010; 11(7):679-684.

323. Dohle GR. Male infertility in cancer patients: review of the literature. *Int J Urol.* 2010;17(4):327-331.

324. Grunewald S, Paasch U, Glander HJ. Systemic dermatological treatment with relevance for male fertility. *J Dtsch Dermatol Ges.* 2007;5(1): 15-21.

325. Jung A, Schuppe HC. Influence of genital heat stress on semen quality in humans. *Andrologia.* 2007;39(6):203-215.

326. Wang C, Cui YG, Wang XH, et al. Transient scrotal hyperthermia and levonorgestrel enhance testosterone-induced spermatogenesis suppression in men through increased germ cell apoptosis. *J Clin Endocrinol Metab.* 2007;92(8):3292-3304.

327. Diamanti-Kandarakis E, Bourguignon JP, Giudice LC, et al. Endocrine-disrupting chemicals: an Endocrine Society scientific statement. *Endocr Rev.* 2009;30(4):293-342.

328. Yiee JH, Baskin LS. Environmental factors in genitourinary development. *J Urol.* 2010;184(1):34-41.

329. Dunkel L, Quinton R. Transition in endocrinology: induction of puberty. *Eur J Endocrinol.* 2014;170(6):R229-R239.

330. Harrington J, Palmert MR. Clinical review: distinguishing constitutional delay of growth and puberty from isolated hypogonadotropic hypogonadism: critical appraisal of available diagnostic tests. *J Clin Endocrinol Metab.* 2012;97(9):3056-3067.

331. Waldstreicher J, Seminara SB, Jameson JL, et al. The genetic and clinical heterogeneity of gonadotropin-releasing hormone deficiency in the human. *J Clin Endocrinol Metab.* 1996;81(12):4388-4395.

332. Raivio T, Falardeau J, Dwyer A, et al. Reversal of idiopathic hypogonadotropic hypogonadism. *N Engl J Med.* 2007;357(9):863-873.

333. Sidhoum VF, Chan YM, Lippincott MF, et al. Reversal and relapse of hypogonadotropic hypogonadism: resilience and fragility of the reproductive neuroendocrine system. *J Clin Endocrinol Metab.* 2014;99(3): 861-870.

334. Kanwar P, Kowdley KV. Diagnosis and treatment of hereditary hemochromatosis: an update. *Expert Rev Gastroenterol Hepatol.* 2013;7(6): 517-530.

335. Pietrangelo A. Hereditary hemochromatosis: pathogenesis, diagnosis, and treatment. *Gastroenterology.* 2010;139(2):393-408, e1-e2.

336. McDermott JH, Walsh CH. Hypogonadism in hereditary hemochromatosis. *J Clin Endocrinol Metab.* 2005;90(4):2451-2455.

337. Young J. Approach to the male patient with congenital hypogonadotropic hypogonadism. *J Clin Endocrinol Metab.* 2012;97(3):707-718.

338. Dwyer AA, Hayes FJ, Plummer L, et al. The long-term clinical follow-up and natural history of men with adult-onset idiopathic hypogonadotropic hypogonadism. *J Clin Endocrinol Metab.* 2010;95(9):4235-4243.

339. Pallais JC, Au M, Pitteloud N, et al. Kallmann syndrome. In: Pagan RA, Bird TC, Dolan CR, et al, eds. *GeneReviews [Internet].* 2007 [updated 2011 Jan 4].

340. Layman LC. Clinical genetic testing for Kallmann syndrome. *J Clin Endocrinol Metab.* 2013;98(5):1860-1862.

341. Jongmans MC, van Ravenswaaij-Arts CM, Pitteloud N, et al. CHD7 mutations in patients initially diagnosed with Kallmann syndrome: the clinical overlap with CHARGE syndrome. *Clin Genet.* 2009;75(1): 65-71.

342. Zentner GE, Layman WS, Martin DM, Scacheri PC. Molecular and phenotypic aspects of CHD7 mutation in CHARGE syndrome. *Am J Med Genet A.* 2010;152A(3):674-686.

343. Aminzadeh M, Kim HG, Layman LC, Cheetham TD. Rarer syndromes characterized by hypogonadotropic hypogonadism. *Front Horm Res.* 2010;39:154-167.

344. Burger HG, de Kretser DM, Hudson B, Wilson JD. Effects of preceding androgen therapy on testicular response to human pituitary gonadotropin in hypogonadotropic hypogonadism: a study of three patients. *Fertil Steril.* 1981;35(1):64-68.

345. Ley SB, Leonard JM. Male hypogonadotropic hypogonadism: factors influencing response to human chorionic gonadotropin and human menopausal gonadotropin, including prior exogenous androgens. *J Clin Endocrinol Metab.* 1985;61(4):746-752.

346. Pitteloud N, Hayes FJ, Dwyer A, et al. Predictors of outcome of long-term GnRH therapy in men with idiopathic hypogonadotropic hypogonadism. *J Clin Endocrinol Metab.* 2002;87(9):4128-4136.

347. Sykiotis GP, Hoang XH, Avbelj M, et al. Congenital idiopathic hypogonadotropic hypogonadism: evidence of defects in the hypothalamus, pituitary, and testes. *J Clin Endocrinol Metab.* 2010;95(6):3019-3027.

348. Pitteloud N, Boepple PA, DeCruz S, et al. The fertile eunuch variant of idiopathic hypogonadotropic hypogonadism: spontaneous reversal associated with a homozygous mutation in the gonadotropin-releasing hormone receptor. *J Clin Endocrinol Metab.* 2001;86(6):2470-2475.

349. Shiraishi K, Naito K. Fertile eunuch syndrome with the mutations (Trp8Arg and Ile15Thr) in the beta subunit of luteinizing hormone. *Endocr J.* 2003;50(6):733-737.

350. Smals AG, Kloppenborg PW, van Haelst UJ, et al. Fertile eunuch syndrome versus classic hypogonadotrophic hypogonadism. *Acta Endocrinol (Copenh).* 1978;87(2):389-399.

351. Giltay JC, Deege M, Blankenstein RA, et al. Apparent primary follicle-stimulating hormone deficiency is a rare cause of treatable male infertility. *Fertil Steril.* 2004;81(3):693-696.

352. Mantovani G, Borgato S, Beck-Peccoz P, et al. Isolated follicle-stimulating hormone (FSH) deficiency in a young man with normal virilization who did not have mutations in the FSHbeta gene. *Fertil Steril.* 2003;79(2):434-436.

353. Murao K, Imachi H, Muraoka T, et al. Isolated follicle-stimulating hormone (FSH) deficiency without mutation of the FSHbeta gene and successful treatment with human menopausal gonadotropin. *Fertil Steril.* 2008;90(5):2012, e17-e19.

354. Bhagavath B, Layman LC. The genetics of hypogonadotropic hypogonadism. *Semin Reprod Med.* 2007;25(4):272-286.

355. Lofrano-Porto A, Barra GB, Giacomini LA, et al. Luteinizing hormone beta mutation and hypogonadism in men and women. *N Engl J Med.* 2007;357(9):897-904.

356. Carter MT, Picketts DJ, Hunter AG, Graham GE. Further clinical delineation of the Borjeson-Forssman-Lehmann syndrome in patients with PHF6 mutations. *Am J Med Genet A.* 2009;149A(2):246-250.

357. Chudley AE, Lowry RB, Hoar DI. Mental retardation, distinct facial changes, short stature, obesity, and hypogonadism: a new X-linked mental retardation syndrome. *Am J Med Genet.* 1988;31(4):741-751.

358. Ehara H, Utsunomiya Y, Ieshima A, et al. Martsolf syndrome in Japanese siblings. *Am J Med Genet A.* 2007;143A(9):973-978.

359. Graham JM Jr, Lee J. Bosma arhinia microphthalmia syndrome. *Am J Med Genet A.* 2006;140(2):189-193.

360. Johnson VP, McMillin JM, Aceto T Jr, Bruins G. A newly recognized neuroectodermal syndrome of familial alopecia, anosmia, deafness, and hypogonadism. *Am J Med Genet.* 1983;15(3):497-506.

361. Lopez de Lara D, Cruz-Rojo J, Sanchez del Pozo J, et al. Moebius-Poland syndrome and hypogonadotropic hypogonadism. *Eur J Pediatr.* 2008; 167(3):353-354.

362. Miller JL, Goldstone AP, Couch JA, et al. Pituitary abnormalities in Prader-Willi syndrome and early onset morbid obesity. *Am J Med Genet A.* 2008;146A(5):570-577.

363. Robertson SP, Rodda C, Bankier A. Hypogonadotrophic hypogonadism in Roifman syndrome. *Clin Genet.* 2000;57(6):435-438.

364. Robin G, Jonard S, Vuillaume I, et al. Hypogonadotropic hypogonadism discovered in a patient with cerebellar ataxia. *Ann Endocrinol (Paris).* 2005;66(6):545-551.

365. Saugier-Veber P, Abadie V, Moncla A, et al. The Juberg-Marsidi syndrome maps to the proximal long arm of the X chromosome (Xq12-q21). *Am J Hum Genet.* 1993;52(6):1040-1045.

366. Selvaag E. Pili torti and sensorineural hearing loss: a follow-up of Bjornstad's original patients and a review of the literature. *Eur J Dermatol.* 2000;10(2):91-97.

367. Stoll C, Eyer D. A syndrome of congenital ichthyosis, hypogonadism, small stature, facial dysmorphism, scoliosis and myogenic dystrophy. *Ann Genet.* 1999;42(1):45-50.

368. Swanson SL, Santen RJ, Smith DW. Multiple lentigines syndrome: new findings of hypogonadotrophism, hyposmia, and unilateral renal agenesis. *J Pediatr.* 1971;78(6):1037-1039.

369. Waters AM, Beales PL. Bardet-Biedl syndrome. In: Pagan RA, Bird TC, Dolan CR, et al, eds. *GeneReviews [Internet]*. 2003 [updated 2010 Nov 18].

370. White SM, Graham JM Jr, Kerr B, et al. The adult phenotype in Costello syndrome. *Am J Med Genet A*. 2005;136(2):128-135.

371. Woodhouse NJ, Sakati NA. A syndrome of hypogonadism, alopecia, diabetes mellitus, mental retardation, deafness, and ECG abnormalities. *J Med Genet*. 1983;20(3):216-219.

372. Chahal J, Schlechte J. Hyperprolactinemia. *Pituitary*. 2008;11(2):141-146.

373. Bouchard P, Lagoguey M, Brailly S, Schaison G. Gonadotropin-releasing hormone pulsatile administration restores luteinizing hormone pulsatility and normal testosterone levels in males with hyperprolactinemia. *J Clin Endocrinol Metab*. 1985;60(2):258-262.

374. Casanueva FF, Molitch ME, Schlechte JA, et al. Guidelines of the Pituitary Society for the Diagnosis and Management of Prolactinomas. *Clin Endocrinol*. 2006;65(2):265-273.

375. Klibanski A. Clinical practice: prolactinomas. *N Engl J Med*. 2010;362(13):1219-1226.

376. Frieze TW, Mong DP, Koops MK. "Hook effect" in prolactinomas: case report and review of literature. *Endocr Pract*. 2002;8(4):296-303.

377. Madhusoodanan S, Parida S, Jimenez C. Hyperprolactinemia associated with psychotropics: a review. *Hum Psychopharmacol*. 2010;25(4):281-297.

378. Molitch ME. Medication-induced hyperprolactinemia. *Mayo Clin Proc*. 2005;80(8):1050-1057.

379. Colao A, Di Sarno A, Guerra E, et al. Drug insight: cabergoline and bromocriptine in the treatment of hyperprolactinemia in men and women. *Nat Clin Pract Endocrinol Metab*. 2006;2(4):200-210.

380. Molitch ME. Pharmacologic resistance in prolactinoma patients. *Pituitary*. 2005;8(1):43-52.

381. Abs R, Verhelst J, Maeyaert J, et al. Endocrine consequences of long-term intrathecal administration of opioids. *J Clin Endocrinol Metab*. 2000;85(6):2215-2222.

382. Hallinan R, Byrne A, Agho K, et al. Hypogonadism in men receiving methadone and buprenorphine maintenance treatment. *Int J Androl*. 2009;32(2):131-139.

383. Mendelson JH, Mendelson JE, Patch VD. Plasma testosterone levels in heroin addiction and during methadone maintenance. *J Pharmacol Exp Ther*. 1975;192(1):211-217.

384. Rubinstein AL, Carpenter DM, Minkoff JR. Hypogonadism in men with chronic pain linked to the use of long-acting rather than short-acting opioids. *Clin J Pain*. 2013;29(10):840-845.

385. Veldhuis JD, Rogol AD, Samojlik E, Ertel NH. Role of endogenous opiates in the expression of negative feedback actions of androgen and estrogen on pulsatile properties of luteinizing hormone secretion in man. *J Clin Invest*. 1984;74(1):47-55.

386. Ragni G, De Lauretis L, Bestetti O, et al. Gonadal function in male heroin and methadone addicts. *Int J Androl*. 1988;11(2):93-100.

387. Agirregoitia E, Valdivia A, Carracedo A, et al. Expression and localization of delta-, kappa-, and mu-opioid receptors in human spermatozoa and implications for sperm motility. *J Clin Endocrinol Metab*. 2006;91(12):4969-4975.

388. de Souza GL, Hallak J. Anabolic steroids and male infertility: a comprehensive review. *BJU Int*. 2011;108(11):1860-1865.

389. van Amsterdam J, Opperhuizen A, Hartgens F. Adverse health effects of anabolic-androgenic steroids. *Regul Toxicol Pharmacol*. 2010;57(1):117-123.

390. Rahnema CD, Lipshultz LI, Crosnoe LE, et al. Anabolic steroid-induced hypogonadism: diagnosis and treatment. *Fertil Steril*. 2014;101(5):1271-1279.

391. Dev R, Del Fabbro E, Bruera E. Association between megestrol acetate treatment and symptomatic adrenal insufficiency with hypogonadism in male patients with cancer. *Cancer*. 2007;110(6):1173-1177.

392. Oster MH, Enders SR, Samuels SJ, et al. Megestrol acetate in patients with aids and cachexia. *Ann Intern Med*. 1994;121(6):400-408.

393. Venner P. Megestrol acetate in the treatment of metastatic carcinoma of the prostate. *Oncology*. 1992;49(Suppl 2):22-27.

394. Briken P, Kafka MP. Pharmacological treatments for paraphilic patients and sexual offenders. *Curr Opin Psychiatry*. 2007;20(6):609-613.

395. Aggarwal R, Weinberg V, Small EJ, et al. The mechanism of action of estrogen in castration-resistant prostate cancer: clues from hormone levels. *Clin Genitourin Cancer*. 2009;7(3):E71-E76.

396. Finkelstein JS, McCully WF, MacLaughlin DT, et al. The mortician's mystery: gynecomastia and reversible hypogonadotropic hypogonadism in an embalmer. *N Engl J Med*. 1988;318(15):961-965.

397. Mineur P, De Cooman S, Hustin J, et al. Feminizing testicular Leydig cell tumor: hormonal profile before and after unilateral orchidectomy. *J Clin Endocrinol Metab*. 1987;64(4):686-691.

398. Herbst KL. Gonadotropin-releasing hormone antagonists. *Curr Opin Pharmacol*. 2003;3(6):660-666.

399. Oh WK, Landrum MB, Lamont EB, et al. Does oral antiandrogen use before leutinizing hormone-releasing hormone therapy in patients with metastatic prostate cancer prevent clinical consequences of a testosterone flare? *Urology*. 2010;75(3):642-647.

400. Bong GW, Clarke HS Jr, Hancock WC, Keane TE. Serum testosterone recovery after cessation of long-term luteinizing hormone-releasing hormone agonist in patients with prostate cancer. *Urology*. 2008;71(6):1177-1180.

401. Kaku H, Saika T, Tsushima T, et al. Time course of serum testosterone and luteinizing hormone levels after cessation of long-term luteinizing hormone-releasing hormone agonist treatment in patients with prostate cancer. *Prostate*. 2006;66(4):439-444.

402. Keating NL, O'Malley AJ, Freedland SJ, Smith MR. Diabetes and cardiovascular disease during androgen deprivation therapy: observational study of veterans with prostate cancer. *J Natl Cancer Inst*. 2010;102(1):39-46.

403. Keating NL, O'Malley AJ, Smith MR. Diabetes and cardiovascular disease during androgen deprivation therapy for prostate cancer. *J Clin Oncol*. 2006;24(27):4448-4456.

404. Nguyen PL, Je Y, Schutz FA, et al. Association of androgen deprivation therapy with cardiovascular death in patients with prostate cancer: a meta-analysis of randomized trials. *JAMA*. 2011;306(21):2359-2366.

405. Prabhakar VK, Shalet SM. Aetiology, diagnosis, and management of hypopituitarism in adult life. *Postgrad Med J*. 2006;82(966):259-266.

406. Schneider HJ, Aimaretti G, Kreitschmann-Andermahr I, et al. Hypopituitarism. *Lancet*. 2007;369(9571):1461-1470.

407. Juszczak A, Gupta A, Karavitaki N, et al. Ipilimumab: a novel immunomodulating therapy causing autoimmune hypophysitis: a case report and review. *Eur J Endocrinol*. 2012;167(1):1-5.

408. Rupp D, Molitch M. Pituitary stalk lesions. *Curr Opin Endocrinol Diabetes Obes*. 2008;15(4):339-345.

409. Luton JP, Thieblot P, Valcke JC, et al. Reversible gonadotropin deficiency in male Cushing's disease. *J Clin Endocrinol Metab*. 1977;45(3):488-495.

410. MacAdams MR, White RH, Chipps BE. Reduction of serum testosterone levels during chronic glucocorticoid therapy. *Ann Intern Med*. 1986;104(5):648-651.

411. McKenna TJ, Lorber D, Lacroix A, Rabin D. Testicular activity in Cushing's disease. *Acta Endocrinol (Copenh)*. 1979;91(3):501-510.

412. Reid IR, Ibbertson HK, France JT, Pybus J. Plasma testosterone concentrations in asthmatic men treated with glucocorticoids. *Br Med J (Clin Res Ed)*. 1985;291(6495):574.

413. Crawford BA, Liu PY, Kean MT, et al. Randomized placebo-controlled trial of androgen effects on muscle and bone in men requiring long-term systemic glucocorticoid treatment. *J Clin Endocrinol Metab*. 2003;88(7):3167-3176.

414. Bannister P, Handley T, Chapman C, Losowsky MS. Hypogonadism in chronic liver disease: impaired release of luteinising hormone. *Br Med J (Clin Res Ed)*. 1986;293(6556):1191-1193.

415. Veldhuis JD, Wilkowski MJ, Zwart AD, et al. Evidence for attenuation of hypothalamic gonadotropin-releasing hormone (GnRH) impulse strength with preservation of GnRH pulse frequency in men with chronic renal failure. *J Clin Endocrinol Metab*. 1993;76(3):648-654.

416. Balasubramanian V, Naing S. Hypogonadism in chronic obstructive pulmonary disease: incidence and effects. *Curr Opin Pulm Med*. 2012;18(2):112-117.

417. Laghi F, Antonescu-Turcu A, Collins E, et al. Hypogonadism in men with chronic obstructive pulmonary disease: prevalence and quality of life. *Am J Respir Crit Care Med*. 2005;171(7):728-733.

418. Svartberg J. Androgens and chronic obstructive pulmonary disease. *Curr Opin Endocrinol Diabetes Obes*. 2010;17(3):257-261.

419. Semple PD, Beastall GH, Brown TM, et al. Sex hormone suppression and sexual impotence in hypoxic pulmonary fibrosis. *Thorax*. 1984;39(1):46-51.

420. Iellamo F, Rosano G, Volterrani M. Testosterone deficiency and exercise intolerance in heart failure: treatment implications. *Curr Heart Fail Rep*. 2010;7(2):59-65.

421. Jankowska EA, Biel B, Majda J, et al. Anabolic deficiency in men with chronic heart failure: prevalence and detrimental impact on survival. *Circulation*. 2006;114(17):1829-1837.

422. Malkin CJ, Channer KS, Jones TH. Testosterone and heart failure. *Curr Opin Endocrinol Diabetes Obes*. 2010;17(3):262-268.

423. Dandona P, Dhindsa S. Update: hypogonadotropic hypogonadism in type 2 diabetes and obesity. *J Clin Endocrinol Metab*. 2011;96(9):2643-2651.

424. Grossmann M. Low testosterone in men with type 2 diabetes: significance and treatment. *J Clin Endocrinol Metab*. 2011;96(8):2341-2353.

425. Holt SK, Lopushnyan N, Hotaling J, et al. Prevalence of low testosterone and predisposing risk factors in men with type 1 diabetes mellitus: findings from the DCCT/EDIC. *J Clin Endocrinol Metab*. 2014;99(9):E1655-E1660.

426. Lopez-Alvarenga JC, Zarinan T, Olivares A, et al. Poorly controlled type 1 diabetes mellitus in young men selectively suppresses luteinizing hormone secretory burst mass. *J Clin Endocrinol Metab*. 2002;87(12):5507-5515.

427. Chlebowski RT, Heber D. Hypogonadism in male patients with metastatic cancer prior to chemotherapy. *Cancer Res*. 1982;42(6):2495-2498.

428. Fleishman SB, Khan H, Homel P, et al. Testosterone levels and quality of life in diverse male patients with cancers unrelated to androgens. *J Clin Oncol*. 2010;28:5054-5060.

429. Tengstrand B, Carlstrom K, Hafstrom I. Gonadal hormones in men with rheumatoid arthritis: from onset through 2 years. *J Rheumatol.* 2009;36(5):887-892.

430. Straub RH, Harle P, Atzeni F, et al. Sex hormone concentrations in patients with rheumatoid arthritis are not normalized during 12 weeks of anti-tumor necrosis factor therapy. *J Rheumatol.* 2005;32(7):1253-1258.

431. Hall GM, Larbre JP, Spector TD, et al. A randomized trial of testosterone therapy in males with rheumatoid arthritis. *Br J Rheumatol.* 1996;35(6):568-573.

432. Koller MD, Templ E, Riedl M, et al. Pituitary function in patients with newly diagnosed untreated systemic lupus erythematosus. *Ann Rheum Dis.* 2004;63(12):1677-1680.

433. Mok CC, Lau CS. Profile of sex hormones in male patients with systemic lupus erythematosus. *Lupus.* 2000;9(4):252-257.

434. Vilarinho ST, Costallat LT. Evaluation of the hypothalamic-pituitary-gonadal axis in males with systemic lupus erythematosus. *J Rheumatol.* 1998;25(6):1097-1103.

435. Jimenez-Balderas FJ, Tapia-Serrano R, Fonseca ME, et al. High frequency of association of rheumatic/autoimmune diseases and untreated male hypogonadism with severe testicular dysfunction. *Arthritis Res.* 2001;3(6):362-367.

436. McCombe PA, Greer JM, Mackay IR. Sexual dimorphism in autoimmune disease. *Curr Mol Med.* 2009;9(9):1058-1079.

437. Crum NF, Furtek KJ, Olson PE, et al. A review of hypogonadism and erectile dysfunction among HIV-infected men during the pre- and post-HAART eras: diagnosis, pathogenesis, and management. *AIDS Patient Care STDS.* 2005;19(10):655-671.

438. Lo JC, Schambelan M. Reproductive function in human immunodeficiency virus infection. *J Clin Endocrinol Metab.* 2001;86(6):2338-2343.

439. Moreno-Perez O, Escoin C, Serna-Candel C, et al. The determination of total testosterone and free testosterone (RIA) are not applicable to the evaluation of gonadal function in HIV-infected males. *J Sex Med.* 2010;7(8):2873-2883.

440. Wunder DM, Bersinger NA, Fux CA, et al. Hypogonadism in HIV-1-infected men is common and does not resolve during antiretroviral therapy. *Antivir Ther.* 2007;12(2):261-265.

441. Schopp LH, Clark M, Mazurek MO, et al. Testosterone levels among men with spinal cord injury admitted to inpatient rehabilitation. *Am J Phys Med Rehabil.* 2006;85(8):678-684, quiz 85-87.

442. Ghosh S, Bandyopadhyay SK, Bandyopadhyay R, et al. A study on endocrine dysfunction in thalassaemia. *J Indian Med Assoc.* 2008;106(10):655-656, 658-659.

443. Kim MK, Lee JW, Baek KH, et al. Endocrinopathies in transfusion-associated iron overload. *Clin Endocrinol.* 2013;78(2):271-277.

444. Safarinejad MR. Evaluation of semen quality, endocrine profile and hypothalamus-pituitary-testis axis in male patients with homozygous beta-thalassaemia major. *J Urol.* 2008;179(6):2327-2332.

445. Soliman AT, Nasr I, Thabet A, et al. Human chorionic gonadotropin therapy in adolescent boys with constitutional delayed puberty vs those with beta-thalassemia major. *Metabolism.* 2005;54(1):15-23.

446. Wang C, Tso SC, Todd D. Hypogonadotropic hypogonadism in severe beta-thalassemia: effect of chelation and pulsatile gonadotropin-releasing hormone therapy. *J Clin Endocrinol Metab.* 1989;68(3):511-516.

447. el-Hazmi MA, Bahakim HM, al-Fawaz I. Endocrine functions in sickle cell anaemia patients. *J Trop Pediatr.* 1992;38(6):307-313.

448. Landefeld CS, Schambelan M, Kaplan SL, Embury SH. Clomiphene-responsive hypogonadism in sickle cell anemia. *Ann Intern Med.* 1983;99(4):480-483.

449. Modebe O, Ezeh UO. Effect of age on testicular function in adult males with sickle cell anemia. *Fertil Steril.* 1995;63(4):907-912.

450. Fung EB, Harmatz PR, Lee PD, et al. Increased prevalence of iron-overload associated endocrinopathy in thalassaemia versus sickle-cell disease. *Br J Haematol.* 2006;135(4):574-582.

451. Slayton W, Kedar A, Schatz D. Testosterone induced priapism in two adolescents with sickle cell disease. *J Pediatr Endocrinol Metab.* 1995;8(3):199-203.

452. Leifke E, Friemert M, Heilmann M, et al. Sex steroids and body composition in men with cystic fibrosis. *Eur J Endocrinol.* 2003;148(5):551-557.

453. Friedl KE, Moore RJ, Hoyt RW, et al. Endocrine markers of semistarvation in healthy lean men in a multistressor environment. *J Appl Physiol.* 2000;88(5):1820-1830.

454. Lado-Abeal J, Prieto D, Lorenzo M, et al. Differences between men and women as regards the effects of protein-energy malnutrition on the hypothalamic-pituitary-gonadal axis. *Nutrition.* 1999;15(5):351-358.

455. Wabitsch M, Ballauff A, Holl R, et al. Serum leptin, gonadotropin, and testosterone concentrations in male patients with anorexia nervosa during weight gain. *J Clin Endocrinol Metab.* 2001;86(7):2982-2988.

456. Aloi JA, Bergendahl M, Iranmanesh A, Veldhuis JD. Pulsatile intravenous gonadotropin-releasing hormone administration averts fasting-induced hypogonadotropism and hypoandrogenemia in healthy, normal weight men. *J Clin Endocrinol Metab.* 1997;82(5):1543-1548.

457. Chan JL, Williams CJ, Raciti P, et al. Leptin does not mediate short-term fasting-induced changes in growth hormone pulsatility but

458. increases IGF-I in leptin deficiency states. *J Clin Endocrinol Metab.* 2008;93(7):2819-2827.

458. Smith SR, Chhetri MK, Johanson J, et al. The pituitary-gonadal axis in men with protein-calorie malnutrition. *J Clin Endocrinol Metab.* 1975;41(1):60-69.

459. Di Luigi L, Romanelli F, Sgro P, Lenzi A. Andrological aspects of physical exercise and sport medicine. *Endocrine.* 2012;42(2):278-284.

460. Hackney AC. Endurance exercise training and reproductive endocrine dysfunction in men: alterations in the hypothalamic-pituitary-testicular axis. *Curr Pharm Des.* 2001;7(4):261-273.

461. Hackney AC, Fahrner CL, Gulledge TP. Basal reproductive hormonal profiles are altered in endurance trained men. *J Sports Med Phys Fitness.* 1998;38(2):138-141.

462. Sewani-Rusike CR, Mudambo KS, Tendaupenyu G, et al. Effects of the Zimbabwe Defence Forces training programme on body composition and reproductive hormones in male army recruits. *Cent Afr J Med.* 2000;46(2):27-31.

463. Henning PC, Scofield DE, Spiering BA, et al. Recovery of endocrine and inflammatory mediators following an extended energy deficit. *J Clin Endocrinol Metab.* 2014;99(3):956-964.

464. Arce JC, De Souza MJ. Exercise and male factor infertility. *Sports Med.* 1993;15(3):146-169.

465. Tremblay MS, Copeland JL, Van Helder W. Effect of training status and exercise mode on endogenous steroid hormones in men. *J Appl Physiol.* 2004;96(2):531-539.

466. Allan CA, McLachlan RI. Androgens and obesity. *Curr Opin Endocrinol Diabetes Obes.* 2010;17(3):224-232.

467. Liu PY, Caterson ID, Grunstein RR, Handelsman DJ. Androgens, obesity, and sleep-disordered breathing in men. *Endocrinol Metab Clin North Am.* 2007;36(2):349-363.

468. Mah PM, Wittert GA. Obesity and testicular function. *Mol Cell Endocrinol.* 2010;316(2):180-186.

469. Vermeulen A, Kaufman JM, Deslypere JP, Thomas G. Attenuated luteinizing hormone (LH) pulse amplitude but normal lh pulse frequency, and its relation to plasma androgens in hypogonadism of obese men. *J Clin Endocrinol Metab.* 1993;76(5):1140-1146.

470. Camacho EM, Huhtaniemi IT, O'Neill TW, et al. Age-associated changes in hypothalamic-pituitary-testicular function in middle-aged and older men are modified by weight change and lifestyle factors: longitudinal results from the European Male Ageing Study. *Eur J Endocrinol.* 2013;168(3):445-455.

471. Facchiano E, Scaringi S, Veltri M, et al. Age as a predictive factor of testosterone improvement in male patients after bariatric surgery: preliminary results of a monocentric prospective study. *Obes Surg.* 2013;23(2):167-172.

472. Mora M, Aranda GB, de Hollanda A, et al. Weight loss is a major contributor to improved sexual function after bariatric surgery. *Surg Endosc.* 2013;27(9):3197-3204.

473. Pellitero S, Olaizola I, Alastrue A, et al. Hypogonadotropic hypogonadism in morbidly obese males is reversed after bariatric surgery. *Obes Surg.* 2012;22(12):1835-1842.

474. Yee B, Liu P, Phillips C, Grunstein R. Neuroendocrine changes in sleep apnea. *Curr Opin Pulm Med.* 2004;10(6):475-481.

475. Hoyos CM, Killick R, Yee BJ, et al. Effects of testosterone therapy on sleep and breathing in obese men with severe obstructive sleep apnoea: a randomized placebo-controlled trial. *Clin Endocrinol.* 2012;77(4):599-607.

476. Matsumoto AM, Sandblom RE, Schoene RB, et al. Testosterone replacement in hypogonadal men: effects on obstructive sleep apnoea, respiratory drives, and sleep. *Clin Endocrinol.* 1985;22(6):713-721.

477. Schneider BK, Pickett CK, Zwillich CW, et al. Influence of testosterone on breathing during sleep. *J Appl Physiol.* 1986;61(2):618-623.

478. Spratt DI, Cox P, Orav J, et al. Reproductive axis suppression in acute illness is related to disease severity. *J Clin Endocrinol Metab.* 1993;76(6):1548-1554.

479. Spratt DI, Kramer RS, Morton JR, et al. Characterization of a prospective human model for study of the reproductive hormone responses to major illness. *Am J Physiol Endocrinol Metab.* 2008;295(1):E63-E69.

480. van den Berghe G, Weekers F, Baxter RC, et al. Five-day pulsatile gonadotropin-releasing hormone administration unveils combined hypothalamic-pituitary-gonadal defects underlying profound hypoandrogenism in men with prolonged critical illness. *J Clin Endocrinol Metab.* 2001;86(7):3217-3226.

481. Spratt DI, Morton JR, Kramer RS, et al. Increases in serum estrogen levels during major illness are caused by increased peripheral aromatization. *Am J Physiol Endocrinol Metab.* 2006;291(3):E631-E638.

482. May AK, Dossett LA, Norris PR, et al. Estradiol is associated with mortality in critically ill trauma and surgical patients. *Crit Care Med.* 2008;36(1):62-68.

483. Reisch N, Flade L, Scherr M, et al. High prevalence of reduced fecundity in men with congenital adrenal hyperplasia. *J Clin Endocrinol Metab.* 2009;94(5):1665-1670.

484. Lofrano-Porto A, Casulari LA, Nascimento PP, et al. Effects of follicle-stimulating hormone and human chorionic gonadotropin on gonadal steroidogenesis in two siblings with a follicle-stimulating hormone beta subunit mutation. *Fertil Steril.* 2008;90(4):1169-1174.

485. Matsumoto AM. Effects of chronic testosterone administration in normal men: safety and efficacy of high dosage testosterone and parallel dose-dependent suppression of luteinizing hormone, follicle-stimulating hormone, and sperm production. *J Clin Endocrinol Metab.* 1990;70(1):282-287.

486. Matsumoto AM, Karpas AE, Bremner WJ. Chronic human chorionic gonadotropin administration in normal men: evidence that follicle-stimulating hormone is necessary for the maintenance of quantitatively normal spermatogenesis in man. *J Clin Endocrinol Metab.* 1986; 62(6):1184-1192.

487. de Bruin D, de Jong IJ, Arts EG, et al. Semen quality in men with disseminated testicular cancer: relation with human chorionic gonadotropin beta-subunit and pituitary gonadal hormones. *Fertil Steril.* 2009;91(6):2481-2486.

488. Knuth UA, Behre H, Belkien L, et al. Clinical trial of 19-nortestosterone-hexoxyphenylpropionate (Anadur) for male fertility regulation. *Fertil Steril.* 1985;44(6):814-821.

489. Schurmeyer T, Knuth UA, Belkien L, Nieschlag E. Reversible azoospermia induced by the anabolic steroid 19-nortestosterone. *Lancet.* 1984;1(8374):417-420.

490. Turek PJ, Williams RH, Gilbaugh JH 3rd, Lipshultz LI. The reversibility of anabolic steroid-induced azoospermia. *J Urol.* 1995;153(5): 1628-1630.

491. Hendry WF, Stedronska J, Jones CR, et al. Semen analysis in testicular cancer and Hodgkin's disease: pre- and post-treatment findings and implications for cryopreservation. *Br J Urol.* 1983;55(6):769-773.

492. Magelssen H, Brydoy M, Fossa SD. The effects of cancer and cancer treatments on male reproductive function. *Nat Clin Pract Urol.* 2006;3(6):312-322.

493. Micic S, Dotlic R, Ilic V, Genbacev O. Hormone profile in hyperprolactinemic infertile men. *Arch Androl.* 1985;15(2-3):123-128.

494. Vandekerckhove P, Lilford R, Vail A, Hughes E. Bromocriptine for idiopathic oligo/asthenospermia. *Cochrane Database Syst Rev.* 2000;(2): CD000152.

495. Rajender S, Singh L, Thangaraj K. Phenotypic heterogeneity of mutations in androgen receptor gene. *Asian J Androl.* 2007;9(2):147-179.

496. Werner R, Grotsch H, Hiort O. 46,XY disorders of sex development: the undermasculinised male with disorders of androgen action. *Best Pract Res Clin Endocrinol Metab.* 2010;24(2):263-277.

497. Hirawat S, Budman DR, Kreis W. The androgen receptor: structure, mutations, and antiandrogens. *Cancer Invest.* 2003;21(3):400-417.

498. Barradell LB, Faulds D. Cyproterone: a review of its pharmacology and therapeutic efficacy in prostate cancer. *Drugs Aging.* 1994;5(1):59-80.

499. Doggrell SA, Brown L. The spironolactone renaissance. *Expert Opin Investig Drugs.* 2001;10(5):943-954.

500. Funder JW, Mercer JE. Cimetidine, a histamine H2 receptor antagonist, occupies androgen receptors. *J Clin Endocrinol Metab.* 1979;48(2): 189-191.

501. Peden NR, Boyd EJ, Browning MC, et al. Effects of two histamine H2-receptor blocking drugs on basal levels of gonadotrophins, prolactin, testosterone and oestradiol-17 beta during treatment of duodenal ulcer in male patients. *Acta Endocrinol (Copenh).* 1981;96(4):564-568.

502. Purohit V, Ahluwahlia BS, Vigersky RA. Marihuana inhibits dihydrotestosterone binding to the androgen receptor. *Endocrinology.* 1980; 107(3):848-850.

503. Farthing MJ, Edwards CR, Rees LH, Dawson AM. Male gonadal function in coeliac disease: 1. Sexual dysfunction, infertility, and semen quality. *Gut.* 1982;23(7):608-614.

504. Farthing MJ, Rees LH, Dawson AM. Male gonadal function in coeliac disease: III. Pituitary regulation. *Clin Endocrinol.* 1983;19(6):661-671.

505. Green JR, Goble HL, Edwards CR, Dawson AM. Reversible insensitivity to androgens in men with untreated gluten enteropathy. *Lancet.* 1977;1(8006):280-282.

506. Ozgor B, Selimoglu MA. Coeliac disease and reproductive disorders. *Scand J Gastroenterol.* 2010;45(4):395-402.

507. Matsumoto AM, Bremner WJ. Endocrinology of the hypothalamic-pituitary-testicular axis with particular reference to the hormonal control of spermatogenesis. *Baillieres Clin Endocrinol Metab.* 1987; 1(1):71-87.

508. Bhasin S, Woodhouse L, Casaburi R, et al. Testosterone dose-response relationships in healthy young men. *Am J Physiol Endocrinol Metab.* 2001;281(6):E1172-E1181.

509. Matsumoto AM. Hormonal therapy of male hypogonadism. *Endocrinol Metab Clin North Am.* 1994;23(4):857-875.

510. Coviello AD, Lakshman K, Mazer NA, Bhasin S. Differences in the apparent metabolic clearance rate of testosterone in young and older men with gonadotropin suppression receiving graded doses of testosterone. *J Clin Endocrinol Metab.* 2006;91(11):4669-4675.

511. Gooren LJ, Bunck MC. Androgen replacement therapy: present and future. *Drugs.* 2004;64(17):1861-1891.

512. Wang C, Alexander G, Berman N, et al. Testosterone replacement therapy improves mood in hypogonadal men: a clinical research center study. *J Clin Endocrinol Metab.* 1996;81(10):3578-3583.

513. Bhasin S, Woodhouse L, Casaburi R, et al. Older men are as responsive as young men to the anabolic effects of graded doses of testosterone on the skeletal muscle. *J Clin Endocrinol Metab.* 2005;90(2):678-688.

514. Yassin DJ, Yassin AA, Hammerer PG. Combined testosterone and vardenafil treatment for restoring erectile function in hypogonadal patients who failed to respond to testosterone therapy alone. *J Sex Med.* 2014;11(2):543-552.

515. Schulte-Beerbuhl M, Nieschlag E. Comparison of testosterone, dihydrotestosterone, luteinizing hormone, and follicle-stimulating hormone in serum after injection of testosterone enanthate of testosterone cypionate. *Fertil Steril.* 1980;33(2):201-203.

516. Schurmeyer T, Nieschlag E. Comparative pharmacokinetics of testosterone enanthate and testosterone cyclohexanecarboxylate as assessed by serum and salivary testosterone levels in normal men. *Int J Androl.* 1984;7(3):181-187.

517. Snyder PJ, Lawrence DA. Treatment of male hypogonadism with testosterone enanthate. *J Clin Endocrinol Metab.* 1980;51(6):1335-1339.

518. Wang C, Harnett M, Dobs AS, Swerdloff RS. Pharmacokinetics and safety of long-acting testosterone undecanoate injections in hypogonadal men: an 84-week phase III clinical trial. *J Androl.* 2010;31(5): 457-465.

519. Edelstein D, Basaria S. Testosterone undecanoate in the treatment of male hypogonadism. *Expert Opin Pharmacother.* 2010;11(12):2095-2106.

520. Dobs AS, Meikle AW, Arver S, et al. Pharmacokinetics, efficacy, and safety of a permeation-enhanced testosterone transdermal system in comparison with bi-weekly injections of testosterone enanthate for the treatment of hypogonadal men. *J Clin Endocrinol Metab.* 1999; 84(10):3469-3478.

521. Jordan WP Jr, Atkinson LE, Lai C. Comparison of the skin irritation potential of two testosterone transdermal systems: an investigational system and a marketed product. *Clin Ther.* 1998;20(1):80-87.

522. Amory JK, Matsumoto AM. The therapeutic potential of testosterone patches. *Expert Opin Investig Drugs.* 1998;7(12):1977-1985.

523. Arver S, Dobs AS, Meikle AW, et al. Long-term efficacy and safety of a permeation-enhanced testosterone transdermal system in hypogonadal men. *Clin Endocrinol.* 1997;47(6):727-737.

524. Singh AB, Norris K, Modi N, et al. Pharmacokinetics of a transdermal testosterone system in men with end stage renal disease receiving maintenance hemodialysis and healthy hypogonadal men. *J Clin Endocrinol Metab.* 2001;86(6):2437-2445.

525. Wilson DE, Kaidbey K, Boike SC, Jorkasky DK. Use of topical corticosteroid pretreatment to reduce the incidence and severity of skin reactions associated with testosterone transdermal therapy. *Clin Ther.* 1998;20(2):299-306.

526. Lakshman KM, Basaria S. Safety and efficacy of testosterone gel in the treatment of male hypogonadism. *Clin Interv Aging.* 2009;4: 397-412.

527. de Ronde W. Hyperandrogenism after transfer of topical testosterone gel: case report and review of published and unpublished studies. *Hum Reprod.* 2009;24(2):425-428.

528. Wang C, Swerdloff RS, Iranmanesh A, et al. Transdermal testosterone gel improves sexual function, mood, muscle strength, and body composition parameters in hypogonadal men. *J Clin Endocrinol Metab.* 2000;85(8):2839-2853.

529. Wang C, Swerdloff RS, Iranmanesh A, et al. Effects of transdermal testosterone gel on bone turnover markers and bone mineral density in hypogonadal men. *Clin Endocrinol.* 2001;54(6):739-750.

530. Bouloux P. Testim 1% testosterone gel for the treatment of male hypogonadism. *Clin Ther.* 2005;27(3):286-298.

531. Steidle C, Schwartz S, Jacoby K, et al. AA2500 testosterone gel normalizes androgen levels in aging males with improvements in body composition and sexual function. *J Clin Endocrinol Metab.* 2003;88(6): 2673-2681.

532. Dobs A, Norwood P, Potts S, et al. Testosterone 2% gel can normalize testosterone concentrations in men with low testosterone regardless of body mass index. *J Sex Med.* 2014;11(3):857-864.

533. Wang C, Ilani N, Arver S, et al. Efficacy and safety of the 2% formulation of testosterone topical solution applied to the axillae in androgen-deficient men. *Clin Endocrinol.* 2011;75(6):836-843.

534. Korbonits M, Kipnes M, Grossman AB. Striant SR: a novel, effective and convenient testosterone therapy for male hypogonadism. *Int J Clin Pract.* 2004;58(11):1073-1080.

535. Wang C, Swerdloff R, Kipnes M, et al. New testosterone buccal system (Striant) delivers physiological testosterone levels: pharmacokinetics study in hypogonadal men. *J Clin Endocrinol Metab.* 2004;89(8): 3821-3829.

536. Mattern C, Hoffmann C, Morley JE, Badiu C. Testosterone supplementation for hypogonadal men by the nasal route. *Aging Male.* 2008;11(4):171-178.

537. Cavender RK, Fairall M. Subcutaneous testosterone pellet implant (Testopel) therapy for men with testosterone deficiency syndrome: a single-site retrospective safety analysis. *J Sex Med.* 2009;6(11): 3177-3192.

538. Fennell C, Sartorius G, Ly LP, et al. Randomized cross-over clinical trial of injectable vs. implantable depot testosterone for maintenance of testosterone replacement therapy in androgen deficient men. *Clin Endocrinol.* 2010;73(1):102-109.

539. Pastuszak AW, Mittakanti H, Liu JS, et al. Pharmacokinetic evaluation and dosing of subcutaneous testosterone pellets. *J Androl*. 2012;33(5):927-937.
540. Handelsman DJ, Conway AJ, Boylan LM. Pharmacokinetics and pharmacodynamics of testosterone pellets in man. *J Clin Endocrinol Metab*. 1990;71(1):216-222.
541. Gooren LJ. Advances in testosterone replacement therapy. *Front Horm Res*. 2009;37:32-51.
542. Kohn FM, Schill WB. A new oral testosterone undecanoate formulation. *World J Urol*. 2003;21(5):311-315.
543. Raynaud JP, Aumonier C, Gualano V, et al. Pharmacokinetic study of a new testosterone-in-adhesive matrix patch applied every 2 days to hypogonadal men. *J Steroid Biochem Mol Biol*. 2008;109(1-2):177-184.
544. Raynaud JP, Legros JJ, Rollet J, et al. Efficacy and safety of a new testosterone-in-adhesive matrix patch applied every 2 days for 1 year to hypogonadal men. *J Steroid Biochem Mol Biol*. 2008;109(1-2):168-176.
545. Bhasin S, Jasuja R. Selective androgen receptor modulators as function promoting therapies. *Curr Opin Clin Nutr Metab Care*. 2009;12(3):232-240.
546. Gao W, Dalton JT. Expanding the therapeutic use of androgens via selective androgen receptor modulators (SARMs). *Drug Discov Today*. 2007;12(5-6):241-248.
547. Snyder PJ, Peachey H, Berlin JA, et al. Effects of testosterone replacement in hypogonadal men. *J Clin Endocrinol Metab*. 2000;85(8):2670-2677.
548. Quon H, Loblaw DA. Androgen deprivation therapy for prostate cancer—review of indications in 2010. *Curr Oncol*. 2010;17(Suppl 2):S38-S44.
549. Eyre SJ, Ankerst DP, Wei JT, et al. Validation in a multiple urology practice cohort of the prostate cancer prevention trial calculator for predicting prostate cancer detection. *J Urol*. 2009;182(6):2653-2658.
550. Parekh DJ, Ankerst DP, Higgins BA, et al. External validation of the prostate cancer prevention trial risk calculator in a screened population. *Urology*. 2006;68(6):1152-1155.
551. Coviello AD, Kaplan B, Lakshman KM, et al. Effects of graded doses of testosterone on erythropoiesis in healthy young and older men. *J Clin Endocrinol Metab*. 2008;93(3):914-919.
552. Bachman E, Feng R, Travison T, et al. Testosterone suppresses hepcidin in men: a potential mechanism for testosterone-induced erythrocytosis. *J Clin Endocrinol Metab*. 2010;95(10):4743-4747.
553. Behre HM, Bohmeyer J, Nieschlag E. Prostate volume in testosterone-treated and untreated hypogonadal men in comparison to age-matched normal controls. *Clin Endocrinol*. 1994;40(3):341-349.
554. Andriole GL, Crawford ED, Grubb RL 3rd, et al. Mortality results from a randomized prostate-cancer screening trial. *N Engl J Med*. 2009;360(13):1310-1319.
555. Barry MJ. Screening for prostate cancer: the controversy that refuses to die. *N Engl J Med*. 2009;360(13):1351-1354.
556. Schroder FH, Hugosson J, Roobol MJ, et al. Screening and prostate-cancer mortality in a randomized European study. *N Engl J Med*. 2009;360(13):1320-1328.
557. Calof OM, Singh AB, Lee ML, et al. Adverse events associated with testosterone replacement in middle-aged and older men: a meta-analysis of randomized, placebo-controlled trials. *J Gerontol A Biol Sci Med Sci*. 2005;60(11):1451-1457.
558. Snyder PJ, Peachey H, Hannoush P, et al. Effect of testosterone treatment on bone mineral density in men over 65 years of age. *J Clin Endocrinol Metab*. 1999;84(6):1966-1972.
559. Whitsel EA, Boyko EJ, Matsumoto AM, et al. Intramuscular testosterone esters and plasma lipids in hypogonadal men: a meta-analysis. *Am J Med*. 2001;111(4):261-269.
560. O'Connor DB, Archer J, Wu FC. Effects of testosterone on mood, aggression, and sexual behavior in young men: a double-blind, placebo-controlled, cross-over study. *J Clin Endocrinol Metab*. 2004;89(6):2837-2845.
561. Wang C, Cunningham G, Dobs A, et al. Long-term testosterone gel (androgel) treatment maintains beneficial effects on sexual function and mood, lean and fat mass, and bone mineral density in hypogonadal men. *J Clin Endocrinol Metab*. 2004;89(5):2085-2098.
562. Saal W, Glowania HJ, Hengst W, Happ J. Pharmacodynamics and pharmacokinetics after subcutaneous and intramuscular injection of human chorionic gonadotropin. *Fertil Steril*. 1991;56(2):225-229.
563. Saal W, Happ J, Cordes U, et al. Subcutaneous gonadotropin therapy in male patients with hypogonadotropic hypogonadism. *Fertil Steril*. 1991;56(2):319-324.
564. Burris AS, Clark RV, Vantman DJ, Sherins RJ. A low sperm concentration does not preclude fertility in men with isolated hypogonadotropic hypogonadism after gonadotropin therapy. *Fertil Steril*. 1988;50(2):343-347.
565. Burris AS, Rodbard HW, Winters SJ, Sherins RJ. Gonadotropin therapy in men with isolated hypogonadotropic hypogonadism: the response to human chorionic gonadotropin is predicted by initial testicular size. *J Clin Endocrinol Metab*. 1988;66(6):1144-1151.
566. McLachlan RI, Finkel DM, Bremner WJ, Snyder PJ. Serum inhibin concentrations before and during gonadotropin treatment in men with hypogonadotropic hypogonadism: physiological and clinical implications. *J Clin Endocrinol Metab*. 1990;70(5):1414-1419.
567. Miyagawa Y, Tsujimura A, Matsumiya K, et al. Outcome of gonadotropin therapy for male hypogonadotropic hypogonadism at university affiliated male infertility centers: a 30-year retrospective study. *J Urol*. 2005;173(6):2072-2075.
568. Warne DW, Decosterd G, Okada H, et al. A combined analysis of data to identify predictive factors for spermatogenesis in men with hypogonadotropic hypogonadism treated with recombinant human follicle-stimulating hormone and human chorionic gonadotropin. *Fertil Steril*. 2009;92(2):594-604.
569. Bouloux PM, Nieschlag E, Burger HG, et al. Induction of spermatogenesis by recombinant follicle-stimulating hormone (Puregon) in hypogonadotropic azoospermic men who failed to respond to human chorionic gonadotropin alone. *J Androl*. 2003;24(4):604-611.
570. Farhat R, Al-Zidjali F, Alzahrani AS. Outcome of gonadotropin therapy for male infertility due to hypogonadotrophic hypogonadism. *Pituitary*. 2010;13(2):105-110.
571. Matsumoto AM, Snyder PJ, Bhasin S, et al. Stimulation of spermatogenesis with recombinant human follicle-stimulating hormone (follitropin alfa; GONAL-f): long-term treatment in azoospermic men with hypogonadotropic hypogonadism. *Fertil Steril*. 2009;92(3):979-990.
572. Johnson L, Thompson DL Jr, Varner DD. Role of Sertoli cell number and function on regulation of spermatogenesis. *Anim Reprod Sci*. 2008;105(1-2):23-51.

CHAPTER 20

Sexual Dysfunction in Men and Women

SHALENDER BHASIN • ROSEMARY BASSON

KEY POINTS

- In contrast to the earlier sexual response model, depicting a linear progression of discrete phases, current research conceptualizes sexual response as a motivation/incentive-based cycle comprising phases of physiologic response. These phases of the cycle overlap and their order is variable.
- In middle-aged and older men, sexual dysfunction is often related to comorbid conditions, such as diabetes, coronary artery disease, or a hormonal problem.
- Penile erection results from biochemical and hemodynamic events that are associated with activation of central nervous system sites, cavernosal smooth muscle relaxation, increased blood flow into cavernosal sinuses, and venous occlusion.
- Corporal smooth muscle tone is regulated by transmembrane and intracellular calcium flux, which in turn is regulated by potassium channels, connexin43-derived gap junctions, and cholinergic, adrenergic, and noradrenergic noncholinergic mediators, including nitric oxide.
- Testosterone regulates sexual thoughts and desire, sexual arousal, attentiveness to erotic stimuli, and sleep-entrained erections. Testosterone deficiency is a treatable cause of hypoactive sexual desire in men.
- Selective phosphodiesterase 5 inhibitors are safe and effective and have emerged as first-line therapy for men with erectile disorder (ED).

- Sexual response is understood to be incentive based: multiple reasons for sex motivate receptivity to sexual stimuli that can be appraised as sexually arousing.
- Physical and subjective arousal may diverge. Women complaining of low sexual arousal usually physically respond to sexual stimuli in a laboratory setting. In contrast, men with ED from endothelial or neurologic deficit—the most common cause of men's arousal complaints—typically still experience mental sexual arousal/excitement.
- Women's sexual dysfunctions do not link to androgen deficit.
- Psychological therapies predominate in the treatment of women's sexual dysfunctions with emerging evidence of benefit from mindfulness-based cognitive therapy.
- About 10% to 15% of women have dyspareunia from provoked vestibulodynia—a chronic pain disorder associated with central sensitization of the nervous system and occasionally precipitated by low-dose combined contraceptives.

Endocrine disease and its treatment can frequently disturb sexual function in men and women.[1] In addition, patients may believe, often incorrectly, that their sexual dysfunction must necessarily be due to hormonal imbalance and seek management from endocrinologists.[2] Patients consider their sexual lives to be important; recognizing the importance of sexual function as a determinant of quality of life, the World Health Organization declared sexual health a fundamental right of men and women.

For much of human history, the common beliefs about human sexuality were shaped largely by religious dogma, whose vehemence was rarely justified by the scientific evidence. Alfred C. Kinsey's pioneering epidemiologic investigations provided the first evidence of the considerable variability in sexual practices of American men and women.[3] Excellent epidemiologic surveys, such as the Massachusetts Male Aging Study (MMAS) by Feldman and associates[4] and the National Health and Social Life Survey (NHSLS) by Laumann and colleagues,[5,6] using modern sampling techniques, revealed high prevalence rates of sexual dysfunction among community-dwelling middle-aged and older men. Ongoing and distressing sexual dysfunction affects 10% of people; prevalence rates are even higher in older men.[2,6,7] Temporary or nondistressing dysfunction is frequently reported by up to 40% of the population.

William Masters and Virginia E. Johnson[8] found that both men and women display predictable physiologic responses after sexual stimulation. These landmark descriptions of the human sexual response cycle by Masters and Johnson provided the basis for a rational classification of human sexual disorders[8] (Fig. 20-1A). Sigmund Freud ascribed sexual problems in adult men and women to earlier difficulties in maturation of childhood sexuality and development of parent-child relationships. Recent advances in our understanding of the physiologic and biochemical mechanisms of penile erection and the development of mechanism-specific therapies for ED have largely supplanted Freud's psychoanalytical theories. The 1980s and 1990s witnessed remarkable progress in our understanding of the physicochemical mechanisms that lead to penile tumescence and rigidity. It was recognized that penile erections are the result of cavernosal smooth muscle relaxation

and increased penile blood flow.[9-11] The appreciation of nitric oxide as a key vasodilator in the vascular smooth muscle was a pivotal discovery, recognized later by awarding of the Nobel Prize in Physiology or Medicine to Robert F. Furchgott, Louis J. Ignarro, and Ferid Murad. The recognition that nitric oxide caused cavernosal smooth muscle relaxation by simulating guanylyl cyclase provided the foundation for the discovery of highly effective oral therapies for the treatment of ED.

Historically, the classification and nomenclature for sexual disorders were based on the *Diagnostic and Statistical Manual of Mental Disorders* (DSM), which is primarily a psychiatric nomenclature, reflecting the belief that sexual disorders in men and women are psychogenic in their origin.[12] The DSM and several other expert groups updated the definitions and classification of sexual disorders in the early 1990s.[12,13] In May 2013, the DSM-5 (5th edition)

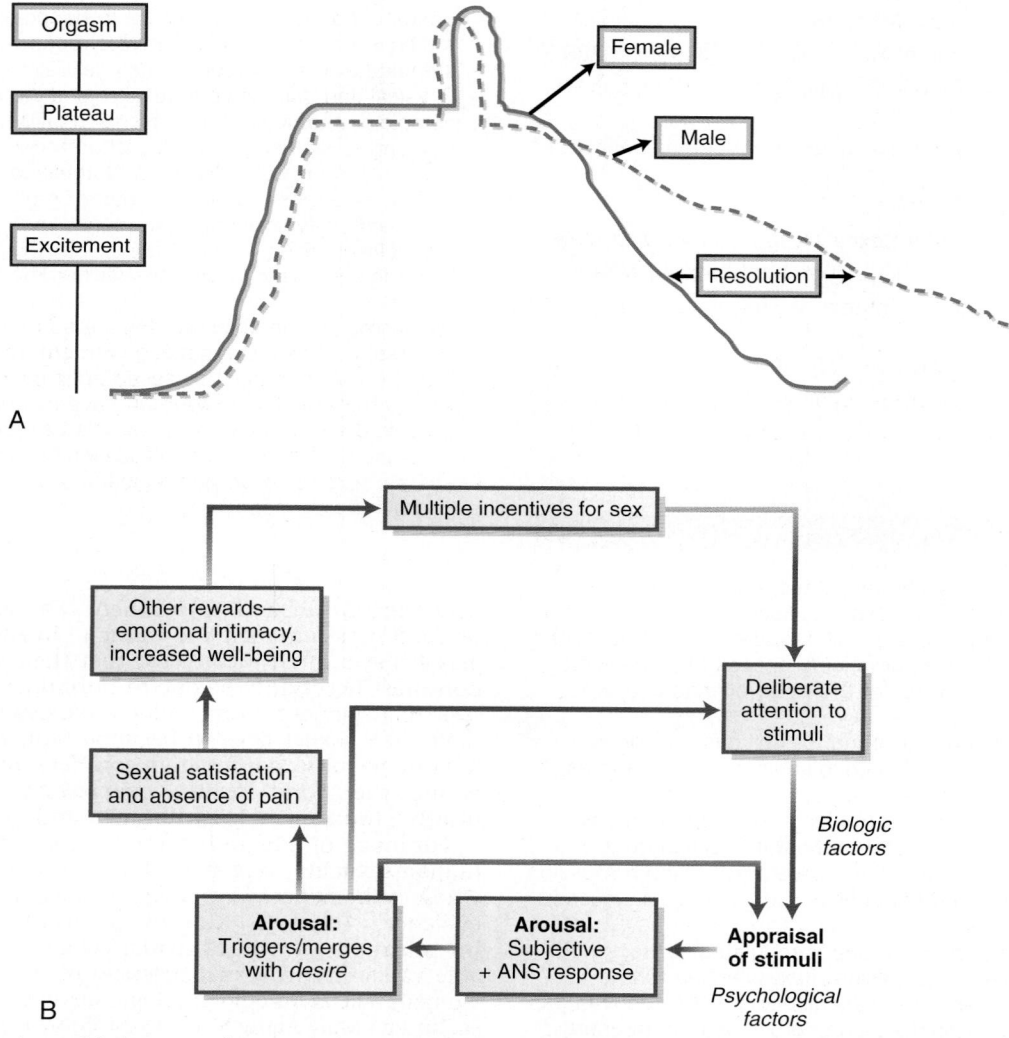

Figure 20-1 A, Four phases of the human sexual response cycle, as postulated by Masters and Johnson. The resolution phase is prolonged considerably in men such that men may experience refractoriness to further stimulation for varying lengths of time before they can achieve another orgasm. As discussed in the text, our views of the female response cycle have evolved substantially since then (see **B**). **B,** Circular human response cycle of overlapping phases. It is being increasingly recognized that there is a lot more complexity, circularity, and flexibility in the human sexual response than is reflected in Masters and Johnson's original model (**A**). Human sexual response is depicted as a motivation/incentive-based cycle of overlapping phases of variable order. A sense of desire may or may not be present initially: it can be triggered alongside the sexual arousal resulting from attending to sexual stimuli. Psychological and biologic factors influence the brain's appraisal of the sexual stimuli. Sexual arousal comprises subjective (pleasure/excitement/wanting more of the same) and physical (genital and nongenital) responses. The merged desire and arousal influence the ongoing attention to and appraisal of further sexual stimulation. The sexual and nonsexual outcomes influence present and future sexual motivation. ANS, autonomic nervous system. (**B,** Adapted from Basson R. The female sexual response: the role of drugs in the management of sexual. dysfunction. *Obstet Gynecol.* 2001;98:350-352.)

further refined the classification and definition of sexual disorders in men and women.[14,15]

The growing recognition that ED is commonly a manifestation of systemic disease and the availability of easy-to-use therapeutic options, including oral and intraurethral drugs, have duly placed sexual disorders in men within the purview of the endocrinologist and the primary care provider. In middle-aged and older men, but less so for women, sexual dysfunction is often related to comorbid medical conditions.[7,9,16-18] Sexual dysfunction can be a manifestation of serious underlying medical disease, such as a pituitary neoplasm, diabetes, or coronary artery disease.[10,19] ED may signal asymptomatic coronary artery disease.[19,20] In women, sexual dysfunction is more strongly linked to mental health.[20-22]

The clinical definitions of sexual dysfunction, especially in women, remain shrouded in debate. In women, there is poor correlation between a clinician's diagnosis of sexual dysfunction and a woman's perception of the problem.[23] For instance, in one study,[23] about 20% of middle-aged women were given a diagnosis of sexual dysfunction even though they reported no problem, whereas a similar number did not receive a diagnosis of sexual dysfunction but reported problematic sex.

This chapter describes the current conceptualization of sexual response in men and women, the underlying pathophysiologic mechanisms, the sexual sequelae of various endocrine disorders, and clinical assessment of sexual dysfunction and its management. Management strategies for sexual dysfunction stemming from hormonal and nonhormonal factors are also outlined.

HUMAN SEXUAL RESPONSE CYCLE

The traditional model of human sexual response stemming from the research of Masters, Johnson, and Kaplan envisioned a linear progression from desire to arousal to a plateau of high arousal followed by orgasm/ejaculation, followed by a phase of resolution (see Fig. 20-1A).[8] In marked contrast to this earlier model depicting a linear invariable progression of discrete phases, recent research conceptualizes sexual response as a motivation/incentive-based cycle comprising phases of physiologic response and subjective experience.[24-28] The phases of the cycle overlap and their order is variable (see Fig. 20-1B). The motivations and incentives for sex are multiple and varied. A wish to both demonstrate and enhance emotional intimacy between the partners is important for both men and women. Depression is a major cause of reduced sexual motivation in otherwise healthy persons and in those with endocrine disease: repeatedly, comorbid depression has been identified as a factor underlying increased sexual dysfunction in women with diabetes.[26,29,30] Even in the absence of clinical depression, low sexual interest is associated with having more depressed and more anxious thoughts and lower sexual self-image than that in control subjects. Endocrine disorders can markedly lessen sexual self-image especially when associated with altered appearances, infertility, or ability to be gainfully employed.[1,26,29,31]

Sexual desire, as in lust or drive, is only one of many reasons people engage in sex and may or may not be sensed initially: desire can be triggered by the sexual excitement (i.e., the subjective sexual arousal in response to sexual stimuli).[24,26,32,33] Some researchers posit that arousal and desire occur exclusively in response to sexually relevant stimuli and that any internal thoughts or fantasies may also stem from something external. In both men and women, the relationship between desire and arousal is vari-able and complex, and both are often unable to separate the two.[34-36] This overlap of phases is in keeping with neuroimaging data of sexual arousal, which have led to the concept that motivation is one facet of sexual arousal and desire is one component of motivation.[37] Many factors, psychological and biologic, influence the brain's appraisal and processing of the sexual stimuli to allow or disallow subsequent arousal.[22,26,30,32-34,36-45] The sexual and nonsexual outcomes influence future sexual motivation. The circle depicted in Figure 20-1B may be partially or completely repeated a number of times during any given sexual encounter (i.e., there is true cyclicity).[24] Variability is marked between individuals and within a person's own sexual life, influenced by multiple factors, including stage of life cycle, age, and relationship duration, and robustly linked to mental health and relationship happiness.[36]

Even with sufficient sexual motivation and the presence of adequate stimuli, the arousal and pleasure may not occur if attention is not focused.[41] Review of the literature on sexual arousal in 2009 confirmed a central role for attentional processes in facilitating the subjective and also the physiologic components of sexual arousal.[41] Sexual information is processed in the mind both automatically and consciously.[42] The sexual nature of the stimuli is processed by the limbic system, allowing genital congestion (observed to be quick and automatic in women and slower but still involuntary in men).[42] Conscious appraisal of the sexual stimuli and the contextual cues can lead to subjective arousal.[42-45] The latter may be further increased by awareness of the genital congestion of arousal, which is more accurately registered and more relevant to men's experience than to women's.[24] The subjective arousal will also be cognitively appraised—for instance, is this pleasurable and safe or is this shameful or likely to have a negative consequence?[42-45] Cognitions such as these continually modify both the physiologic and subjective responses.[42,43]

Focusing on nonerotic thoughts during sexual stimulation, generated possibly by anxiety as first suggested by Barlow, is linked to having sexual problems.[43] A recent study of men and women in long-term relationships found that women tended to report nonerotic thoughts about their body image and the external consequences of sexual activity, whereas men were more likely to report nonerotic thoughts about problematic sexual performance.[44] Both the men and the women in that study had some nonerotic thoughts about the emotional consequences of the sexual activity.[44] Regardless of content, the more frequent the nonerotic thoughts, the more sexual dysfunction. Importantly, the more difficult it was to refocus back on an erotic thought, the more this predicted sexual difficulty. This research is clearly relevant to patients with endocrine disease, which frequently has negative impact upon sexual self-image and sexual functioning.[26,29]

Thus, the current conceptualization of men's and women's sexual responses is in marked contrast to an earlier model depicting a linear invariable progression of discrete phases—from desire, to arousal, to a plateau of high arousal, followed by orgasm/ejaculation, and finally a phase of resolution.[24,25,46] Women's sexual dysfunction typically involves lessened arousal and desire and lessened frequency of orgasm, now reflected in the recently coined *sexual interest/arousal disorder* appearing in the American Psychiatric Association's *Diagnostic and Statistical Manual*, 5th edition (DSM-5) (Table 20-1).[14,15] Although the focus in men has typically been on ED or premature ejaculation, they too may experience a more generalized sexual distress disorder affecting desire, erectile function, and ease of orgasm.[18,45]

TABLE 20-1

Current Definitions of Female Sexual Disorders

Female Sexual Interest/Arousal Disorder

Lack of sexual interest/arousal for a minimum duration of 6 months as manifested by at least three of the following indicators:
1. Absent/reduced frequency or intensity of interest in sexual activity
2. Absent/reduced frequency or intensity of sexual/erotic thoughts or fantasies
3. Absence or reduced frequency of initiation of sexual activity and typically unreceptive to a partner's attempts to initiate
4. Absent/reduced frequency or intensity of sexual excitement/pleasure during sexual activity on all or almost all (approximately 75%) sexual encounters
5. Sexual interest/arousal is absent or infrequently elicited by any internal or external sexual/erotic cues (e.g., written, verbal, visual)
6. Absent/reduced frequency or intensity of genital or nongenital sensations during sexual activity on all or almost all (approximately 75%) sexual encounters

Female Orgasmic Disorder

At least one of the two following symptoms, which must have been present for a minimum duration of approximately 6 months and be experienced on all or almost all (approximately 75%) occasions of sexual activity:
1. Marked delay in, marked infrequency of, or absence of orgasm
2. Markedly reduced intensity of orgasmic sensation

Genitopelvic Pain/Penetration Disorder

Persistent or recurrent difficulties for a minimum duration of approximately 6 months with one or more of the following:
1. Marked difficulty having vaginal intercourse/penetration
2. Marked vulvovaginal or pelvic pain during vaginal intercourse/penetration attempts
3. Marked fear or anxiety either about vulvovaginal or pelvic pain on vaginal penetration
4. Marked tensing or tightening of the pelvic floor muscles during attempted vaginal penetration

Bancroft and colleagues proposed dual control theories for sexual appraisal both in men and women.[47] Their control model envisions a balance between sexual activation and sexual inhibition in an individual's brain, with this balance determining whether sexual stimulation leads to arousal. A questionnaire was used to characterize the specific factors associated with an individual's sexual excitation and sexual inhibition. The latter items were identified as the threat of performance failure and the threat of performance consequences (or both) in men, but in women, relationship importance (reflecting the need for sex to be within a specific type of relationship), concerns about sexual function (worries and distractions about sexual function), and arousal contingency (the potential for arousal to be inhibited by contextual/situational factors) were inhibiting factors.[47]

PHYSIOLOGIC MECHANISMS OF HUMAN SEXUAL RESPONSE

Physiology of Desire and Arousal

Functional Brain Imaging of Sexual Arousal in Men and Women

Although mainly focused on male sexual arousal in response to visual sexual stimuli, functional neuroimaging techniques have clarified some of the neural correlates of sexual response.[48-54] Review of some 73 published studies,

the majority focused on healthy male heterosexual volunteers, has led to a model that includes multiple facets of sexual arousal.[37] Brain imaging during sexual stimulation engages complex circuitry with activation of brain regions related to the different aspects of arousal while other brain regions inhibitory to sexual arousal are deactivated.[48-54]

In keeping with the current circular model of sexual response (depicting sexual incentives/motivations, information processing, overlap of arousal and desire, emphasis on subjective as well as physiologic arousal, plus importance of reward), the model of sexual arousal emanating from the neuroimaging data comprises cognitive, motivational, emotional, and autonomic components[37] (see Fig. 20-1B). The cognitive component includes appraisal of potentially sexual stimuli, focused attention on those stimuli appraised as erotic, and imagery of actual sexual activity. The activations of the right lateral orbitofrontal cortex (OFC), of the right and the left inferior temporal cortices, of the superior parietal lobules, and of areas belonging to the neural network mediating motor imagery (inferior parietal lobules, left ventral premotor area, right and left supplementary motor areas, cerebellum) are considered to be the neural correlates of this cognitive component. The motivational component comprises the processes that direct behavior to a sexual goal, including the perceived urge to express overt sexual behavior. Thus, the motivational component is conceptualized as including the experience of sexual desire. Neural correlates are thought to involve the anterior cingulate cortex (ACC), claustrum, posterior parietal cortex, hypothalamus, substantia nigra, and ventral striatum. The emotional component is the brain activity underlying the pleasure from the mental excitement and the perception of genital and other physical responses. This pleasure comprises *liking* and *wanting*.[55] The left primary and secondary somatosensory cortices, the amygdalae, and the right posterior insula are conceived as neural correlates of this emotional component. The autonomic and neuroendocrine component includes the various responses (e.g., genital, cardiovascular, respiratory, changes in hormonal plasma levels) that allow preparedness for sexual activity: activations in the anterior cingulate cortex, anterior insulae, putamens, and hypothalamus may contribute to this component.

From studying the brain's deactivations with sexual arousal, three components of inhibition are suggested[37]:
1. Inhibition mediated by regions in the temporal lobes and the gyrus rectus of the OFC in the resting state. Patients with lesions in the gyrus rectus are noted to have excessive appetite for sexual and other pleasurable activities.[56] This together with temporal lobe deactivation is exemplified by the marked hypersexuality of Klüver-Bucy syndrome.[57] The deactivated temporal regions are distinct from those activated in response to visual sexual stimuli.
2. Inhibition of arousal once it has begun, to limit its expression because the circumstances are inappropriate, is mediated in the healthy caudate nucleus and putamen. This is consistent with reports of hypersexuality associated with lesions in the head of the caudate nuclei.[58]
3. Activation of the left OFC is thought to undermine sexual stimuli so as to limit their potential to arouse.

It is of interest that these regions thought to mediate inhibition of sexual arousal have been found to be activated during tasks that require moral judgments and those that involve guilt and embarrassment.

Future studies focusing more on women and on nonheterosexual persons are awaited. Of note, men generally show greater responsiveness to visual sexually arousing stimuli than do women.[46] Moreover, the complexity and variability of these systems was reflected in a study of surgically menopausal women who were sexually active but were receiving no hormonal therapy.[49] When these women viewed erotica during functional magnetic resonance imaging (MRI), they failed to display the brain activation observed in premenopausal women or in themselves when they were treated with testosterone and estrogen; yet, they reported sexual arousal from the erotic videos, both without and with hormonal supplementation.[49]

Functional imaging during penile or clitoral stimulation to orgasm indicates that women show more activation in left frontoparietal regions, notably in the posterior parietal cortex and the supplementary motor area—regions associated with making a mental representation of another person's actions.[50] It is suggested that these findings may reflect gender differences in perspective and empathy, and that men and women use different cerebral strategies to reach orgasm—the brain responses during the orgasm(s) themselves being similar in men and women.[50]

Preliminary research has been published into functional and structural neural correlates of persons with low sexual desire. Reduced activation bilaterally in the entorhinal cortices and increased activation in the right medial frontal gyrus and right inferior frontal gyrus and bilaterally in the putamen was observed in women with DSM-IV hypoactive sexual desire disorder (HSDD) as compared to control subjects in response to erotic videos.[51] In keeping with the motivation-based sex response cycle in which processing of sexual information is crucial to subjective and physiologic response, the authors suggest that encoding of erotic stimuli and retrieval of past erotic experiences (entorhinal cortices) differed between the two groups. Additionally, the increased activation in medial and inferior frontal gyri may reflect increased monitoring of sexual responses, which is well documented in women with HSDD. Studying gray matter volume and white matter fractional anisotropy, researchers recently identified changes in women with HSDD as compared to control subjects.[52] Whether this is cause or effect of the sexual dysfunction remains unclear, but the observed changes suggested HSDD to be linked to attribution of reduced importance to sexual stimuli (amygdala and occipitotemporal cortex), reduced awareness of sexual response (insula, anterior temporal cortex), and altered attention to, and inhibition of, sexual responses (anterior cingulate cortex, dorsolateral prefrontal cortex).[52] Evidence of reversal of these changes with effective treatment is awaited. That structural changes associated with chronic pain can reverse with therapy is encouraging and suggests that anatomic as well as functional changes may reflect rather than control experience.[53]

Brain imaging in hypogonadal men before and after treatment suggests that the left OFC might exert a testosterone-dependent inhibitory tonic control on sexual arousal and that this control decreases upon visual sexual stimulation.[54] Also the response of the right anterior insula to visual sexual stimulation was found to depend on the level of plasma testosterone.[54]

Neurotransmitters and Hormones Involved in Sexual Desire and Subjective Arousal

A variety of hormones and peptides are involved in the sexual response. The interplay among androgens and neurotransmitters is complex[59-69]: androgens influence neurotransmitter release, and neurotransmitters may modulate androgen receptor signaling.[46,61,63] The role of testosterone in desire and arousal is better documented in men than in women.[62,63] Serum levels of testosterone do not correlate with women's sexual function according to large epidemiologic studies.[63-66] The radioimmunoassays used to measure testosterone concentrations in many epidemiologic studies were designed to measure the substantially higher levels of testosterone in men and lacked the sensitivity, precision, and accuracy in the low range prevalent in women. When a more sensitive mass spectrometry-based assay was used in a study of women with low desire and low subjective arousal and women in a control group, researchers found no difference in serum testosterone levels between the groups.[66] Additionally, it has been difficult to measure intratissue testosterone levels and activity. Labrie and associates have proposed the measurements of androgen metabolites—most notably androsterone glucuronide (ADT-G)—as markers of ovarian plus intracrine androgen activity. Circulating ADT-G levels decrease with age.[67] Serum ADT-G levels did not differ significantly between 121 women with low desire and 124 women without low desire.[66] Thus, a link between low desire and low androgen activity as reflected by serum testosterone levels or androgen metabolites has not been identified to date.

Animal Models. In animal models, steroid hormones modulate sexual arousal by directing synthesis of the enzymes and the receptors for a number of neurotransmitters, including dopamine, noradrenalin, melanocortin, and oxytocin.[59,60,68-71] Systems that act within the hypothalamus and limbic regions of the brain are involved in the process of arousal, attention, and sexual behavior. It is thought that dopamine transmission in the medial preoptic area (MPOA) and the nucleus accumbens focuses the person's attention on sexual stimuli (the incentives or motivations for sexual activity). It is postulated that the behavioral pattern stimulated by those systems and the subjective feelings that accompany them constitute the phenomenon commonly referred to as *sexual desire* or *arousal* when genital sensations triggered by these systems are subjectively felt. The main part of this neural pathway includes the MPOA and its outputs to the ventral tegmental area. The latter contains dopamine cell bodies that project to various limbic and cortical regions, including the prefrontal cortex, the nucleus accumbens, the anterior cingulate cortex, and the amygdala.

Brain pathways for sexual *inhibition* include opioid, endocannabinoid, and serotonin neural transmissions feeding back to various levels of the excitatory pathways.[60,61] It is thought that the behavioral pattern stimulated by the inhibitory pathways includes both sexual reward and satiety refractoriness.

Exogenous opiates are sexually inhibiting independent of their inhibitory effect on luteinizing hormone (LH), LH-releasing hormone, and testosterone.[70] Endogenous opioids modulate the feedback effects of sex steroids on the hypothalamus and pituitary.[70] β-Endorphin is synthesized in the anterior pituitary, the hypothalamus, and the nucleus of the tractus solitarius in the brainstem. The sexual inhibiting effects of opioids occur mainly through their action in the MPOA and the amygdala.[70] Low doses of opiates can have facilitatory effects, possibly through actions in the ventral tegmental area to activate the mesolimbic dopamine system. Exogenous opiates can induce an intense feeling of pleasure, which has been likened to orgasm, followed by a state of relaxation and calm.[71]

Melanocortins are derived from pro-opiomelanocortin and modulate sexual response through a specific receptor subtype, the melanocortin-4 receptor. Administration of melanocortin receptor agonists has been associated with an increase in spontaneous erections in healthy men and in men with ED, and with increased desire, but not genital responses, in women.[72,73]

Oxytocin levels increase close to orgasm. This hormone is known to be involved in pair bonding in some animal species, but its relevance in humans is unclear.

The physiologic role of prolactin in the human sexual response remains uncertain.[74-76] Because a generalized reduction of dopamine activity in the hypothalamus results in increased prolactin secretion, it has been difficult to distinguish between the effects of raised prolactin itself and the possible effects of the reduced dopamine transmission. High levels of prolactin are associated with impaired sexual function in men and women.[70,76]

The effects of the biologic factors are intertwined with those of the environmental and social factors. For instance, dopamine and progesterone, acting on their cognate receptors in the hypothalamus, can increase sexual behavior in oophorectomized, estrogenized female rats, and the presence of a male animal alongside the cage can cause an identical stimulation of the sexual behavior without the administration of either progesterone or dopamine.[77] In rodents, birds, and fish, complex neural networks enable the animal to assess the context of potential sexual activity and relate it to past experience and to expectation of reward.[78]

Genital Sexual Congestion and Arousal

Men and women differ substantially with respect to the correlation between genital congestion and subjective sexual arousal (excitement). Whereas subjective arousal is typically concordant with genital congestion in men, there is a poor correlation between subjective arousal and measures of genital congestion in women.[79] There are some exceptions in men: sleep-related erections are mostly dissociated from erotic dreams or from subjective sexual arousal.[80] Also psychophysiologic studies have found that men can get erections in response to films of assault or rape while experiencing no subjective arousal.[81] In contrast, a psychophysiologic study identified some 25% of men in a community sample with minimal penile response to an erotic video while their *subjective* arousal was similar to the remaining 75% of men with recorded penile congestion.

Given the consistent finding of low sexual concordance in women, a correlation with reduced interoception (awareness of nonsexual physiologic states, e.g., awareness of heart rate) was suspected but not identified.[82]

In contrast to men's typically accurate assessment of their erections, women's assessment of their degree of genital congestion is less accurate. It is thought that genital congestion in women is a prompt, automatic reflex that occurs within seconds of an erotic stimulus; it may not be deemed at all sexually arousing by the woman, or it may even be deemed emotionally negative.[83] Viewing primates engaging in sexual activity subjectively arouses neither young men nor young women.[79] However, the young women viewing primate sex display marked genital congestion, as measured by vaginal photoplethysmography (VPP), whereas no genital response occurs in the men. Similarly, heterosexual women viewing lesbian women engaged in sexual activity report mostly low subjective arousal but show a prompt vasocongestive response; in contrast, heterosexual men viewing male same-sex activity show minimal genital or subjective response.[79]

Physiologic Mechanisms of Penile Erection
Penile Anatomy and Blood Flow

The erectile tissue of the penis consists of two dorsally positioned corpora cavernosa and a ventrally placed corpus spongiosum.[10,11,84,85] The erectile tissue of both the corpora cavernosa and corpus spongiosum is composed of numerous cavernous spaces separated by trabeculae.[10,11,84,85] These trabeculae are composed mainly of smooth muscle cells that are arranged in a syncytium. Endothelial cells cover the surfaces of the trabeculae.

The penile arterial blood supply is derived from pudendal arteries, which are branches of the internal iliac arteries (Fig. 20-2). The pudendal artery divides into cavernosal, dorsal penile, and bulbourethral arteries. The cavernosal arteries and their branches, the helicine arteries, provide blood flow to corpora cavernosa.[10,11] Dilatation of the helicine arteries increases blood flow and pressure in the cavernosal sinuses.[10,11,84,85]

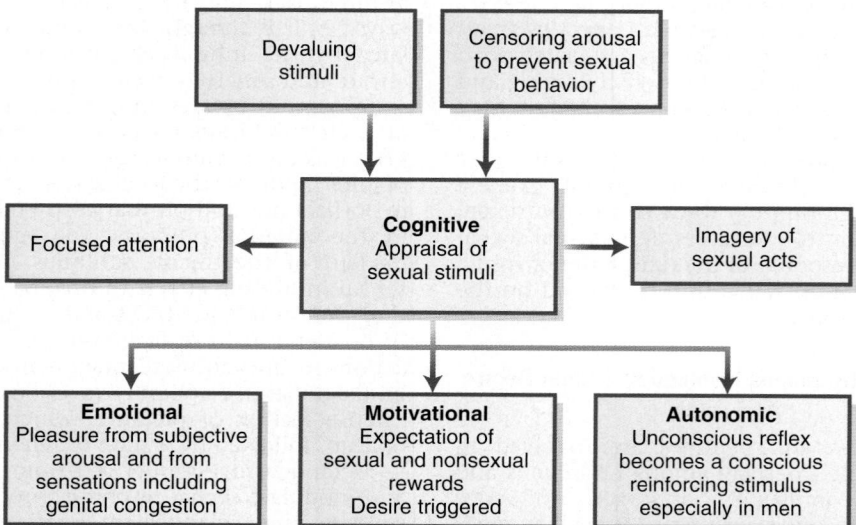

Figure 20-2 Brain areas activated during sexual arousal allow (1) continued focus on sexual stimuli, imaging of sexual behavior, evaluation/censorship, and limitation or prevention of actual behavior despite arousal (all constituting a cognitive component of arousal), (2) sexual feelings (an emotional component), (3) anticipation of reward (a motivational component), and (4) an autonomic/neuroendocrine response of physical sexual arousal. (Adapted from Basson R, Weijmar Schultz W. Sexual sequelae of common medical conditions. *Lancet.* 2007;369:409-424.)

TABLE 20-2

Innervation of the Penis

Types of Fibers	Location of Neurons in the Spinal Cord	Nerves Carrying the Fibers	General Function
Sympathetic	T10-L2	Prevertebral outflow through the hypogastric and cavernous nerves; additionally, paravertebral outflow through the parasympathetic ganglia, and pudendal or pelvic and cavernous nerves	Generally antierectile; sympathetic innervation plays an important role in regulating seminal emission
Parasympathetic	S2-S4	Cavernosal and pelvic nerves	Proerectile
Somatic	S2-S4	Pudendal nerve	Penile sensation, contraction of the striated muscles during ejaculation

Penile Innveration

The neural input to the penis consists of sympathetic (T11-L2), parasympathetic (S2-S4), and somatic nerves (Table 20-2).[85] Sympathetic and parasympathetic fibers converge in the inferior hypogastric plexus where the autonomic input to the penis is integrated and communicated to the penis through cavernosal nerves. In man, the inferior hypogastric ganglionic plexus is located retroperitoneally near the rectum.[11,85]

Several brain regions, including amygdala, MPOA, paraventricular nucleus of the hypothalamus, and periaqueductal gray matter act coordinately to affect penile erections.[85] The MPOA of the hypothalamus serves as the integration site for the central nervous system control of erections; it receives sensory input from the amygdala and sends impulses to the paraventricular nuclei of the hypothalamus and the periaqueductal gray matter. Neurons in paraventricular nuclei project onto the thoracolumbar and sacral nuclei associated with erections.

The parasympathetic input to the penis is proerectile, and sympathetic input is mainly inhibitory.[85] The stimuli from the perineum and lower urinary tract are carried to the penis through the sacral reflex arc.[85]

Hemodynamic Changes During Penile Erection

Penile erection results from a series of biochemical and hemodynamic events that are associated with activation of central nervous system sites involved in regulation of erections, relaxation of cavernosal smooth muscle, increased blood flow into cavernosal sinuses, and venous occlusion resulting in penile engorgement and rigidity.[10,84] Normal penile erection requires coordinated involvement of intact central and peripheral nervous systems, corpora cavernosa and spongiosa, and normal arterial blood supply and venous drainage.[10,84]

As cavernosal smooth muscle relaxes and the blood flow to the penis increases, the increased pooling of blood in the cavernosal spaces results in penile engorgement[10,84] (Fig. 20-3). The expanding corpora cavernosa compress the venules against the rigid tunica albuginea, restricting the venous outflow from the cavernosal spaces.[10,84] This facilitates entrapment of blood in the cavernosal sinuses, imparting rigidity to the erect penis.

Biochemical Regulation of Cavernosal Smooth Muscle Tone

The tone of the corporal smooth muscle cells determines the erectile state of the penis.[10,11,84] When the cavernosal smooth muscle cells are relaxed, the penis is engorged with blood and erect. When the cavernosal smooth muscle cells are contracted, there is predominance of sympathetic neural activity, and the penis is flaccid.[85]

The smooth muscle tone in the corpora cavernosa is maintained by the release of stored intracellular calcium into the cytoplasm and influx of calcium through membrane channels.[86-89] The transmembrane influx of calcium in the cavernosal smooth muscle cells is mediated mostly by L-type voltage-dependent calcium channels, although T-type calcium channels are also expressed in cavernosal smooth muscle cells.[86-89] An increase in intracellular calcium activates myosin light chain kinase resulting in phosphorylation of myosin light chain, actin-myosin interactions, and smooth muscle contraction.[89]

The transmembrane and intracellular calcium flux in the cavernosal smooth muscle cells is regulated by a number of cellular processes that involve K^+ flux through potassium channels, connexin43-derived gap junctions, and a number of cholinergic, adrenergic, and noradrenergic noncholinergic mediators (Figs. 20-4 to 20-6).[86-94] The nonadrenergic noncholinegic mediators include vasoactive intestinal peptide (VIP), calcitonin gene–related peptide (CGRP), and nitric oxide.[94]

Prostaglandin E_1 (PGE$_1$) binding to its cognate receptor results in generation of cyclic adenosine monophosphate (cAMP), which activates protein kinase A. Activated protein kinase A stimulates K^+ channels, resulting in K^+ efflux from the cell (see Fig. 20-4). The protein kinase A–mediated processes also result in a net decrease in intracellular calcium, favoring smooth muscle cell relaxation.

Adrenergic pathways, acting through norepinephrine and α_1-adrenergic receptors, activate phospholipase C, which generates diacyl glycerol and inositol triphosphate (IP$_3$).[89] Diacyl glycerol activates protein kinase C, which inhibits K^+ channels and activates transmembrane calcium influx by activating L-type calcium channels (see Fig. 20-5).[90,91] Inositol triphosphate increases intracellular calcium by promoting the release of calcium from intracellular calcium stores.[90,91] The net increase in intracellular calcium promotes actin-myosin interactions, resulting in smooth muscle contraction and a flaccid penis.

Potassium Channels. At least three types of potassium channels—ATP-sensitive (K_{ATP}), voltage-gated (Kv), and calcium-sensitive K^+ channels (referred to as BK$_{Ca}$ or maxi-K channels)—are expressed in the cavernosal smooth muscle cells.[92,93] Of these, the BK$_{Ca}$ channels are the most important, as they account for 90% of K^+ efflux from the cavernosal smooth muscle cells. BK$_{Ca}$ channel openers have been shown to relax cavernosal smooth muscle cells in vitro.[93] Thus, the strategies that increase BK$_{Ca}$ channel expression in vivo improve erectile capacity in diabetic and older rodents[93-95] and are being explored as therapy for ED. A phase I human gene therapy trial using this approach has shown the feasibility of this approach.[95]

Connexin43 Gap Junctions. The smooth muscle cells in the corpora cavernosa are connected by connexin43 gap junctions that allow the ions and some signaling molecules

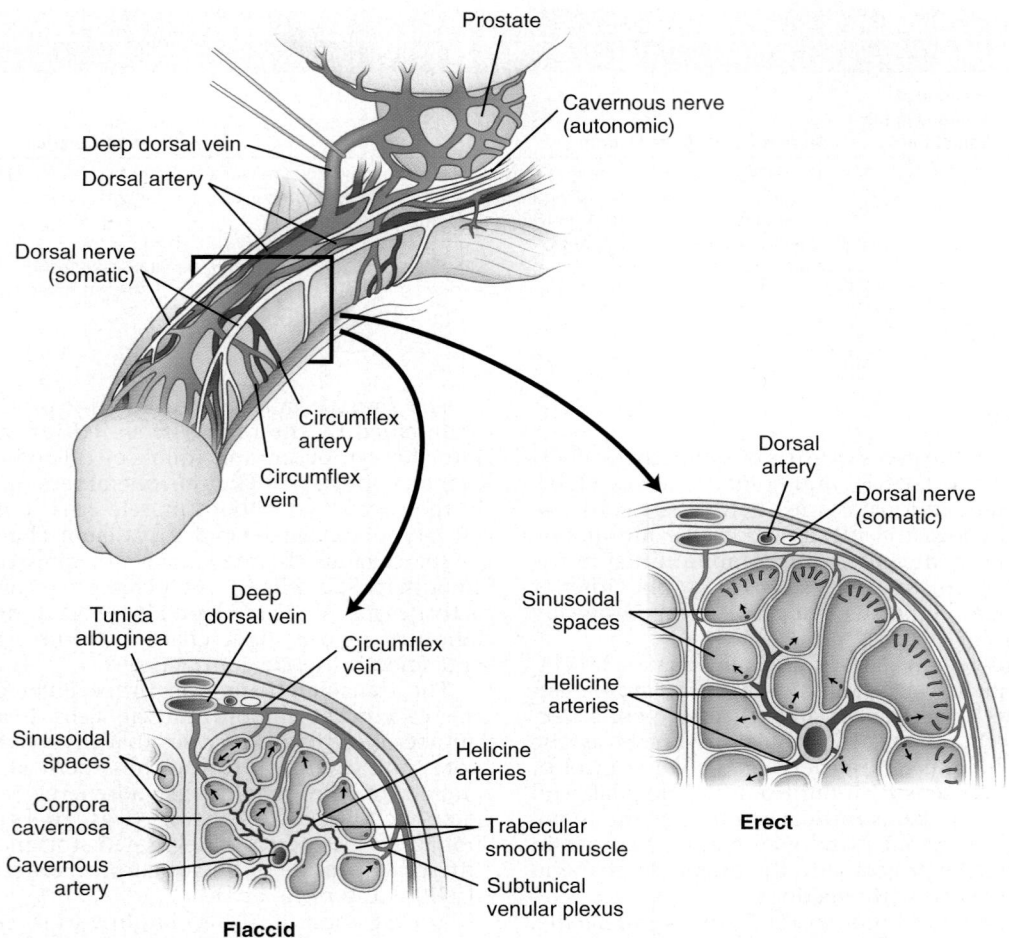

Figure 20-3 Anatomy and mechanism of penile erection. Corpora cavernosa are made up of trabecular spaces that are surrounded by cavernosal smooth muscle. Helicine arteries provide the arterial supply to the cavernosal spaces. The dorsal nerve provides the sensory innervation to the penis. During erection, the relaxation of the trabecular smooth muscle and increased blood flow result in engorgement of the sinusoidal spaces in the corpora cavernosa. The expansion of the sinusoids compresses the venous return against the tunica albuginea, resulting in entrapment of blood, which imparts rigidity to the tumescent penis. (Adapted from Lue TF. Erectile dysfunction. *N Engl J Med.* 2000;342(24):1802-1813.)

such as inositol triphosphate to diffuse freely across smooth muscle cells[96] (Fig. 20-7). The ionic changes induced by a stimulus in one smooth muscle cell are communicated rapidly across other smooth muscle cells, resulting in coordinate regulation of the entire corpora cavernosa.[96] Thus, corpora cavernosa can be viewed functionally as a syncytium of interconnected smooth muscle cells (see Fig. 20-7).[96]

Nitric Oxide. Nitric oxide, derived from the nerve terminals innervating the corpora cavernosa, endothelial lining of penile arteries, and the cavernosal sinuses, is an important biochemical regulator of cavernosal smooth muscle relaxation. Nitric oxide also induces arterial dilatation.[97] The actions of nitric oxide on the cavernosal smooth muscle and the arterial blood flow are mediated through the activation of guanylyl cyclase, the production of cyclic guanosine monophosphate (cGMP), and the activation of cGMP-dependent protein kinase (also called protein kinase G, or PKG) (see Fig. 20-6). cGMP causes smooth muscle relaxation by lowering intracellular calcium. There is some evidence that nitric oxide inhibits Rho kinase–induced cavernosal smooth muscle sensitivity to calcium.[98]

Cyclic Nucleotide Phosphodiesterases. Cyclic nucleotide phosphodiesterases hydrolyze cAMP and cGMP, thus reducing their concentrations within the cavernosal smooth muscle. Of the 13 or more isoforms of cyclic nucleotide phosphodiesterases that have been identified, isoforms 2, 3, 4, and 5 are expressed in the penis.[99-106] Only phosphodiesterase 5 (PDE5) is specific to the nitric oxide/cGMP pathway in the corpora cavernosa.[99-106] Hydrolysis of cGMP by this enzyme results in reversal of the smooth muscle relaxation and reversal of penile erection (see Fig. 20-6). Sildenafil, vardenafil, and tadalafil are potent and selective inhibitors of the activity of PDE5 that prevent breakdown of cGMP and thereby enhance penile erection[9,10] (see Fig. 20-6).

Regulation of Sensitivity to Intracellular Calcium by Rho A/Rho Kinase Signaling. Recently, considerable attention has focused on the role of Rho kinase in modulating the sensitivity of cavernosal smooth muscle to intracellular calcium.[107] A growing body of evidence suggests that sensitization to intracellular calcium is regulated by the balance between phosphorylation of the regulatory light chain of myosin II by a myosin light chain kinase and its dephosphorylation by a myosin light chain phosphatase (Fig. 20-8).[107-112] Phosphorylation of regulatory light chain of myosin II is necessary for activation of myosin II adenosine triphosphatases (ATPases) by actin, and its dephosphorylation prevents activation of myosin II ATPases.[107-112] The ratio of the kinase to phosphatase activities is an

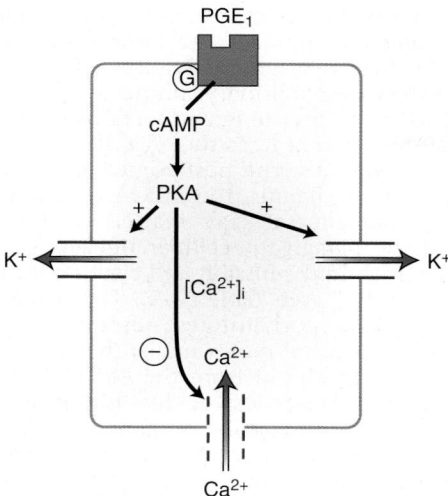

Figure 20-4 Regulation of cavernosal smooth muscle contractility by prostaglandin E_1 (PGE_1). Relaxation of the cavernosal smooth muscle is regulated by intracellular 3',5'-cyclic adenosine monophosphate (cAMP) and cyclic guanosine monophosphate (cGMP). These intracellular second messengers, by activating specific protein kinases, cause sequestration of intracellular calcium (Ca^{2+}) and closure of Ca^{2+} channels and opening of potassium K^+ channels. This results in a net decrease in intracellular Ca^{2+}, leading to smooth muscle relaxation. PGE_1, by binding to PGE_1 receptors, increases the intracellular concentrations of cAMP, which activates protein kinase A (PKA). PKA promotes the sequestration of intracellular Ca^{2+}, inhibits Ca^{2+} influx, and stimulates K^+ channels. The net result is a decrease in intracytoplasmic Ca^{2+} and smooth muscle relaxation. PGE_1 stimulates cAMP generation. (Adapted from Bhasin S, Benson GS. Male sexual function. In: De Kretser D, ed. *Knobil and Neill's Physiology of Reproduction*, 3rd ed. Boston, MA: Academic Press; 2006:1173-1194; and Lue TF. Erectile dysfunction. *N Engl J Med.* 2000;342:1802-1813.)

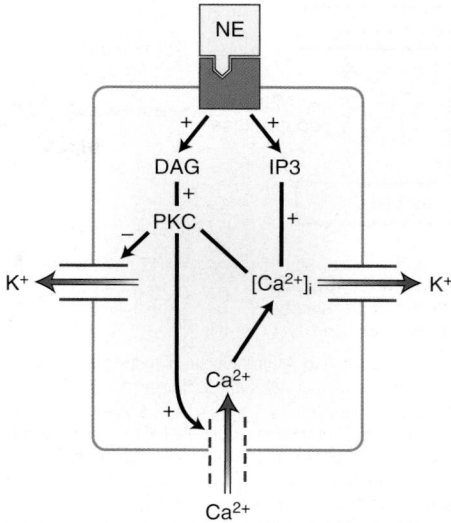

Figure 20-5 Regulation of cavernosal smooth muscle contractility by norepinephrine (NE), which mediates adrenergic signals, binds to adrenergic receptors, and stimulates diacyl glycerol (DAG) and inositol 1,4,5-triphosphate (IP3). DAG stimulates protein kinase C (PKC), which, along with IP3, causes an increase in intracytoplasmic calcium (Ca^{2+}) and inhibition of potassium (K^+) channels. Increased intracellular Ca^{2+} causes cavernosal smooth muscle contraction and loss of penile erection. (Adapted from Bhasin S, Benson GS. Male sexual function. In: De Kretser D, ed. *Knobil and Neill's Physiology of Reproduction*, 3rd ed. Boston, MA: Academic Press; 2006:1173-1194; and Lue TF. Erectile dysfunction. *N Engl J Med.* 2000;342:1802-1813.)

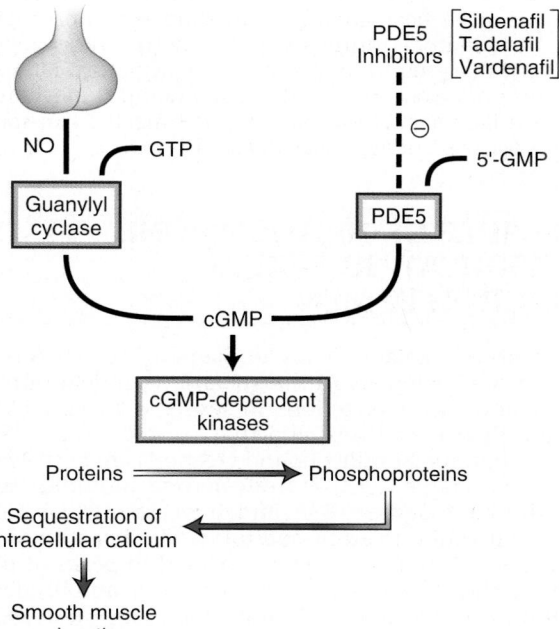

Figure 20-6 Regulation of cavernosal smooth muscle relaxation by nitric oxide (NO). Cyclic guanosine monophosphate (cGMP) regulates cavernosal smooth muscle relaxation by promoting sequestration of cytoplasmic calcium. NO is released from noradrenergic norcholinergic nerve endings and possibly from the endothelium. NO activates guanylyl cyclase, which generates cGMP from guanosine triphosphate (GTP), which in turn activates cGMP-dependent kinases, resulting in sequestration of intracellular calcium and smooth muscle relaxation. cGMP is degraded by cyclic nucleotide phosphodiesterases. Sildenafil, vardenafil, and tadalafil are selective inhibitors of phosphodiesterase isoform 5 (PDE5), which is present in cavernosal smooth muscles. (Adapted from Bhasin S, Benson GS. Male sexual function. In: De Kretser D, ed. *Knobil and Neill's Physiology of Reproduction*, 3rd ed. Boston, MA: Academic Press; 2006:1173-1194; and Lue TF. Erectile dysfunction. *N Engl J Med.* 2000;342:1802-1813.)

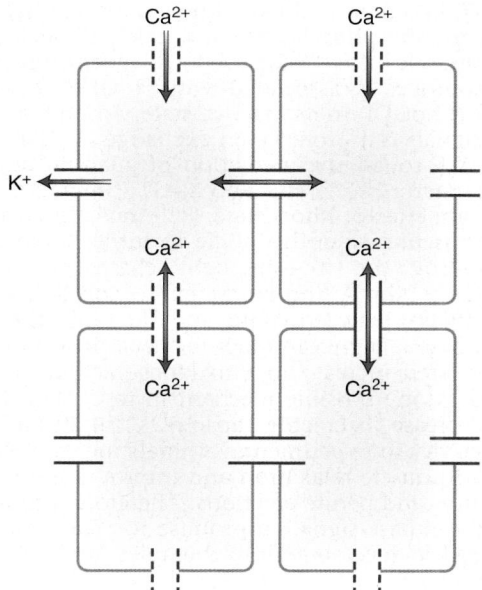

Figure 20-7 The interconnection of cavernosal smooth muscle cells in the penis. Connexin43-derived gap junctions connect adjacent corporal smooth muscle cells and allow flow of ions among interconnected smooth muscle cells. Therefore, alterations in action potential and potassium-channel activity in any myocyte affect the adjacent myocytes. Ca^{2+}, calcium ions; K^+, potassium ions. (Adapted from Melman A, Christ GJ. Integrative erectile biology: the effects of age and disease on gap junctions and ion channels and their potential value to the treatment of erectile dysfunction. *Urol Clin North Am.* 2001;28:217-230.)

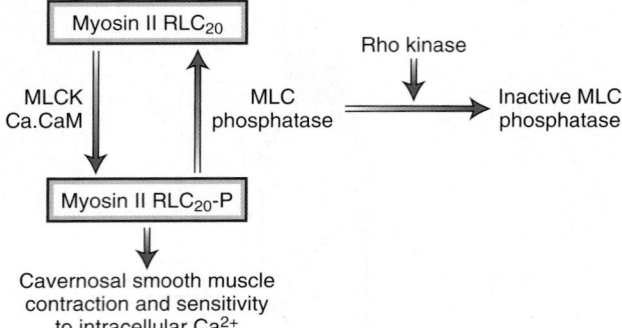

Figure 20-8 The role of Rho A/Rho kinase in regulation of cavernosal smooth muscle sensitivity to intracellular calcium (Ca^{2+}). Sensitivity to calcium and smooth muscle contractility is regulated by the Rho A/Rho kinase system. The balance between phosphorylation (P) of myosin regulatory light-chain (myosin II RLC_{20}) kinase and its dephosphorylation by a myosin light-chain (MLC) phosphatase is a major determinant of the smooth muscle sensitization to Ca^{2+}. By inhibiting the activity of MLC phosphatase, Rho kinase, the downstream effector of Rho A, can regulate smooth muscle responsiveness to calcium. Ca.CaM, calcium calmodulin. (Adapted from Somlyo AP, Somlyo AV. Ca^{2+} sensitivity of smooth muscle and nonmuscle myosin II: modulated by G proteins, kinases, and myosin phosphatase. *Physiol Rev.* 2003;83: 1325-1358.)

important determinant of the contractile sensitivity of the cavernosal smooth muscle cell to intracellular calcium.[109]

Rho A is a guanosine triphosphatase (GTPase) of approximately 20 kDa that modulates Rho kinase activity, myosin light chain phosphorylation, and calcium sensitivity in smooth muscle cells.[107] Rho A–GDP (guanosine diphosphate) complex is associated with a GDP dissociation inhibitor (RhoGDI) in its inactive state. A number of intracellular signals can promote an exchange of GDP for GTP on Rho A through the mediation of guanine nucleotide exchange factors.[107-112] The Rho A–GTP interacts with its downstream effector Rho kinase,[107-112] increasing the sensitivity of vascular smooth muscle to intracellular calcium by inhibiting the myosin light chain phosphatases. Although the Rho A/Rho kinase expression is not significantly different between young and older rats, the activity of Rho kinase is higher in older rats than in young rats[111]; the age-related increase in Rho kinase activity has been proposed as one possible mechanism to explain the age-related decrease in erectile capacity.[111] Inhibition of Rho kinase activity in experimental animals increases cavernosal smooth muscle relaxation and improves intracavernosal pressures and penile erections. Therefore, inhibitors of Rho A/Rho kinase signaling promise to provide attractive targets for the development of therapies for ED.[111,112]

Mechanisms of Ejaculation

The ejaculatory mechanisms consist of three processes: emission, ejection, and orgasm.[113-116] Although orgasm and seminal fluid ejection often occur contemporaneously, these two processes are regulated by separate mechanisms. Emission, the deposition of seminal fluid into the posterior urethra, is dependent upon the integrity of the vasa deferentia, seminal vesicles, prostate gland, and the bladder neck.[115,116] Ejaculation refers to the ejection of seminal fluid containing sperm, and the secretions of seminal vesicles, prostate, and bulbourethral glands from the posterior urethra out through the urethral meatus, and is regulated primarily by the central nervous system activation of the sympathetic nervous system.[115] This emission is ejaculated out of the urethra by the contractions of the *bulbospongiosus* and *levator ani* muscles, the closure of the bladder sphincter due to sympathetic activation, and synchronized opening of the external urinary sphincter.[111] The sensation associated with the rhythmic contractions of these pelvic floor muscles is referred to as the *orgasm*.

The stria terminalis, the posteromedial amygdala, the subparafascicular thalamus, the MPOA of the hypothalamus, the periaqueductal gray matter in the midbrain region, and the paragigantocellular nucleus in the pons integrate seminal fluid emission and ejection during copulatory behavior[117,118] (see Table 20-2). The paragigantocellular nucleus in the pons through serotonergic pathways inhibits the lumbosacral motor nuclei that are involved in ejaculation[118,119]; the input from the MPOA to paragigantocellular nucleus causes loss of this inhibition, resulting in ejaculation.[118,119] An ejaculation generator in the spinal cord integrates the central and peripheral sympathetic and parasympathetic signals to control ejaculation.[113,118] The parasympatheric fibers from the spinal ejaculation generator feed into the sacral parasympathetic nucleus and are carried from there through the pelvic nerve and the major parasympathetic ganglion into the seminal tract.[118] Sympathetic fibers are carried from the spinal ejaculation generator into the dorsal gray commissure and intermediolateral cell column and then through the lumbar sympathetic chain, pelvic nerve, superior hypogastric plexus, and major pelvic ganglion onto the seminal tract.[118]

Neural pathways that utilize serotonin (5-hydroxytryptamine, 5-HT) and dopamine as neurotransmitters play an important role in regulating ejaculation.[115] Thus, administration of selective serotonin reuptake inhibitors (SSRIs) is being explored for the treatment of premature ejaculation.[117-120] At least 14 different serotonin receptor subtypes have been identified in different brain regions; 5-HT1A somatodendritic receptors in the mesencephalic and medullary raphe nuclei reduce ejaculatory latency.[113] A better understanding of the neurochemical mechanisms that regulate ejaculation may provide mechanism-specific targets for treatment of ejaculatory disorders.

THE ROLE OF TESTOSTERONE IN REGULATING SEXUAL FUNCTION IN MEN

Testosterone regulates many domains of sexual function in men and women.[1] Although androgen-deficient men can achieve penile erections in response to visual erotic stimuli, their overall sexual activity is decreased.[121] Spontaneous but not stimulus-bound erections are testosterone-responsive (Table 20-3).[121] Testosterone promotes sexual thoughts and desire[54,121-127] and increases sexual arousal and attentiveness to erotic auditory and other stimuli.[122,123] Nocturnal erections, temporally related to peaks of nighttime testosterone secretion, are of lower amplitude and duration in androgen-deficient men, and testosterone therapy increases the frequency, fullness, and duration of nocturnal penile tumescence.[127,128] Maximum rigidity may require a threshold level of androgen activity.[129-133] Testosterone regulates nitric oxide synthase (NOS) in the cavernosal smooth muscle,[130,131] exerts trophic effects on cavernosal smooth muscle[132] and ischiocavernosus and bulbospongiosus muscles, and is necessary for the veno-occlusive response.[129-132] Androgen-deficient men show delayed orgasm and low ejaculatory volume.[1]

Testosterone therapy in androgen-deficient men improves overall sexual activity, sexual desire, spontaneous

TABLE 20-3
Domains of Sexual Function Regulated by Testosterone*

Domains of Sexual Function That Have Been Shown to Improve in Response to Testosterone Therapy of Androgen-Deficient Men

1. Sexual desire
2. Spontaneous sexual thoughts
3. Attentiveness to erotic auditory stimuli
4. Frequency of nighttime and daytime erections
5. Duration, magnitude, and frequency of nocturnal penile erections
6. Overall sexual activity scores
7. Volume of ejaculate

Domains of Sexual Function That Have Not Been Shown to Improve in Response to Testosterone Therapy or for Which There Is Insufficient or Inconclusive Evidence

1. Erectile response to visual erotic stimulus
2. Erectile function in men who have normal or low-normal testosterone levels
3. Therapeutic response to selective phosphodiesterase inhibitors
4. Ejaculatory dysfunction
5. Orgasms

*Testosterone administration in androgen-deficient men improves overall sexual activity scores through its effects on specific domains of sexuality.
From Bhasin S, Enlzin P, Coviello A, et al. Sexual dysfunction in men and women with endocrine disorders. *Lancet.* 2007;369:597-611, used with permission.

sexual thoughts, and attentiveness to erotic auditory stimuli; frequency of nighttime and daytime erections; duration, magnitude, and frequency of nocturnal penile erections; overall sexual activity scores; and the volume of ejaculate.[1,54,121-124,127-129,133-136] However, testosterone does not improve erectile response to visual erotic stimulus[121] or erectile function in men with ED who have normal testosterone levels.[133-136]

Brain imaging studies suggest that processing of sexual stimuli may be altered in androgen-deficient men with decreased activation in those brain areas that typically are activated in eugonadal men and in androgen-deficient men after testosterone replacement in response to erotic stimuli.[54]

Acting on dopaminergic receptors in the MPOA of the hypothalamus, testosterone elicits reward-seeking behavior in male mammals.[60] This may be the basis for testosterone's motivational effects on mammalian sexual behavior.[60] The roles of cytochrome P450 (CYP19) aromatase and steroid 5α-reductase systems in mediating androgen effects on sexual function remain incompletely understood.[62] Recent studies suggest that 5α-reduction of testosterone to 5α-dihydrotestosterone is not essential for mediating testosterone's effects on desire or erectile function in eugonadal men.[137] Recent investigations, including those in men with mutations of the CYP19A gene suggest that aromatization to estradiol may be important in mediating testosterone's effects on sexual desire.[138-140] Androgen deficiency and ED are two independently distributed disorders that may coexist in middle-aged and older men.[141-143] Selective phosphodiesterase inhibitors (PDE5Is) are highly effective first-line therapies for ED. However, one third of men with ED do not respond to PDE5 inhibitors; some of the men with ED who are PDE5 inhibitor nonresponders have low testosterone levels. Observations that testosterone stimulates penile NOS, increases penile blood flow, and has trophic effects on cavernosal smooth muscle and bulbospongiosus and ischiocavernosus muscles have led to speculation that testosterone therapy might improve erectile response to PDE5 inhibitors.[144-147] Spitzer and associates[148]

evaluated whether the addition of testosterone to sildenafil improves erectile response in men with ED and low testosterone. In this randomized controlled trial, after optimization of sildenafil dose during an initial run-in period, subjects were assigned randomly to 14 weeks of daily testosterone or placebo gel. Sildenafil plus testosterone was not superior to sildenafil plus placebo in improving erectile function in men with ED and low testosterone.[148] In another placebo-controlled trial (TADTEST) of men with ED who were deemed tadalafil (Cialis) failures,[149] the primary analysis of all randomized subjects also did not show a significantly greater improvement in erectile function in the testosterone arm than in the placebo arm. However, in post hoc analysis, erectile function improved with the addition of testosterone in a subset of men with baseline testosterone of 10 nmol/L or less (300 ng/dL).[149] Thus, randomized trials have failed to support the hypothesis that addition of testosterone to PDE5 inhibitor improves erectile function in men with ED. Sildenafil alone raises testosterone levels presumably because of its direct effects on Leydig cell steroidogenesis.[150]

PHYSIOLOGY OF PHYSICAL SEXUAL AROUSAL IN WOMEN: GENITAL CONGESTION

A number of physical changes accompany women's sexual excitement (i.e., their subjective sexual arousal), including genital swelling, increased vaginal lubrication, breast engorgement, and nipple erection; increased skin sensitivity to sexual stimulation; changes in heart rate, blood pressure, muscle tone, breathing, and temperature; and mottling of the skin with a sexual flush of vasodilatation over the chest and face.[151] These changes are reflexive, mediated by the autonomic nervous system. Within seconds there is increased blood flow to the vagina: vasodilatation of the arterioles in the submucosal plexus that increases transudation of interstitial fluid from the capillaries across the epithelium and into the vaginal lumen.[151] Simultaneously, there is relaxation of smooth muscle cells around the clitoral sinusoids, which promotes congestion.

MRI studies have confirmed the presence of extensive clitoral tissue far beyond the visible portion of the clitoris.[152] The clitoris comprises the head, the shaft, the rami that extend along the pubic arch and the periurethral tissue in front of the anterior vaginal wall, as well as the bulbar tissue that surrounds the anterior distal vagina and is contiguous with the periurethral tissue.[152] As the clitoris becomes more swollen, it elevates to lie nearer the symphysis pubis. The vagina lengthens and dilates during arousal, elevating the uterus. The labia become swollen and darker red, and the lower third of the vagina swells.[152]

The autonomic nerves subserving the widespread genital congestion are at risk from gynecologic surgeries that sever the cardinal ligaments and the uterosacral ligaments to potentially injure Frankenhauser's nerve plexus and the uterovaginal nerve plexus.[153,154] Whereas intrafascial abdominal hysterectomy involves an incision and clamping of the pubocervical fascia to sever the dense attachment of cardinal and uterosacral ligaments, thereby interrupting a major support system and nerve plexuses, intrastromal hysterectomy does not involve cutting or clamping the cardinal ligament, uterosacral ligament, or fascia. A 2013 study confirmed ongoing sexual satisfaction after this procedure.[153] Transvaginal tapes for urinary incontinence may also compromise the autonomic nerves between anterior vaginal wall and bladder.[154]

When increases in genital congestion in response to visual erotic stimuli were recorded using vaginal photoplethysmography, the correlation between genital congestion and subjective arousal are found to be highly variable.[50,79] This is true in sexually healthy women and in women reporting a lack of desire or arousal or sexual pain. Women reporting chronic lack of arousal show prompt increases in vaginal congestion, comparable to those in control women, but report no subjective sexual excitement in response to the erotic stimulation. Functional MRI studies show that, unlike in men, activation of the areas organizing genital vasocongestion in women does not correlate with subjective excitement.[50,155]

The neurobiology of the genital vasocongestive response in women is complex and incompletely understood. Involved is release of nitric oxide and VIP from the parasympathetic nerves.[156] Acetylcholine, which blocks noradrenergic vasoconstricting mechanisms and promotes nitric oxide release from the endothelium, is also released. There is communication between the nitric oxide–containing cavernous nerve to the clitoris and the distal portion of the somatic dorsal nerve of the clitoris from the pudendal nerve. Pelvic sympathetic nerves release primarily vasoconstrictive noradrenalin, adrenalin, and adenosine triphosphate (ATP), but some release acetylcholine, nitric oxide, and VIP. The provoked anxiety in the laboratory situation can *increase* the vasocongestive response of the genitalia to erotic stimulation in sexually healthy women.[83] The localization of NOS, cAMP, and cGMP-degrading PDE isoenzymes in human vaginal tissue is established, along with recent identification of cAMP and cGMP-binding proteins. The latter are co-localized with endothelial NOS (eNOS). Close proximity to VIP-positive nerves suggests that cAMP and cGMP work synergistically to control vaginal blood flow.[156] Neuropeptide Y (a vasoconstrictor), CGRP (possibly influencing capillary permeability and sensation), and substance P (a sensory transmitter) also innervate the vaginal microcirculation. The melanocortin-4 receptors and oxytocin also may be involved in clitoral and vaginal efferent pathways.[156]

Intermittency of the vaginal microcirculation due to contraction and relaxation of precapillary sphincters in response to hypoxia and the release of metabolites (PCO_2, lactic acid, ATP), has been termed *vasomotion*. Vasomotion is present in the nonaroused state but decreases within seconds of a sexual stimulus, which increases arterial supply to thereby recruit more capillaries and diminish vasomotion: vaginal vasocongestion follows. Slow oscillations in vaginal blood flow, independent of vaginal vasocongestion, have recently been shown to correlate with subjective arousal in healthy women and to be less marked in women with arousal disorder.[155]

Increased blood flow to the submucosal vaginal capillaries results in increased interstitial fluid production, which diffuses more quickly across the vaginal epithelial cells and onto the lumen: the lubrication fluid in the aroused state thereby contains less potassium and more sodium than in the nonaroused state. How important the contribution of permeability of the epithelial cells is to the process of lubrication is currently unclear. Relaxation of the vaginal wall smooth muscle that enables the vagina to move up into the pelvis is likely mediated by VIP.[155]

The clitoris is the most sexually sensitive area of the body. Immunohistologic studies have identified neurotransmitters thought to be associated with sensation (substance P and CGRP) that are concentrated immediately under the epithelium of the glans clitoris. Nerve terminals in the glans clitoris known as *corpuscular receptors* are thought to be involved. They are mechanoreceptors, and

their density is variable but can be up to 14 times greater than the density of similar receptors on the glans penis.[157] The physiology of nongenital physical changes and their correlation with subjective excitement remain poorly understood.

PHYSIOLOGY OF ORGASM

Orgasm is a brain event, triggered typically by genital stimulation but also by sleep, stimulation of other parts of the body (including breast and nipple), fantasy, certain medications, and in women with spinal cord injury, vibrostimulation of the cervix. Qualitative differences in orgasm, depending on type of stimulation, are reported by some women. Pilot echographic study suggests that vaginal stimulation involves all of the clitoral-urethral complex including the clitoral rami, whereas with clitoral stimulation (i.e., to the shaft and glans), anatomic/circulatory involvement of the clitoral rami is not involved.[151] Men report diminished orgasm intensity subsequent to loss of ejaculation from radical prostatectomy.

Orgasm is a subjective experience in both men and women, and it has been difficult to determine an objective marker. In healthy men, there is the associated ejaculation and, in both genders, involuntary (reflexive) muscular contractions of the striated perineal muscles.[158] One objective and quantitative measure has been established that shows strong correspondence with the subjective experience of orgasm. The researchers performed spectral analysis of rectal pressure data while volunteers imitated orgasm, or tried to achieve orgasm and failed, or experienced orgasm.[158] The most significant and important difference in spectral power between orgasm in both control tasks was found in the alpha band. Outbursts of alpha fluctuations in rectal pressure occurred only during orgasm.[158]

Positron emission tomography (PET) studies during orgasm have shown largely similar brain activations and deactivations in both men and women: activations mainly in the anterior lobe of the cerebellar vermis and deep cerebellar nuclei and deactivations in the left ventromedial and OFC. The only major difference between the genders during orgasm itself was the activation in the periaqueductal gray matter in men.[159,160] The lateral OFC is thought to be involved in urge suppression and behavioral release, whereas the medial parts encode hedonic experiences, becoming activated with increasing satiation and subjective pleasantness and deactivated with feelings of satiety. The medial OFC is part of the neuronal network that includes the amygdala, whose deactivation during orgasm is associated with a more carefree state of mind.[159] More recent PET scanning of the brain during orgasm with comparisons to failed attempts to reach orgasm, and also comparisons to faking an orgasm, has been reported.[160] Insertion of a rectal probe measured involuntary pelvic muscle contractions to identify the occurrence and duration of orgasm. The variations in rectal pressure indicative of orgasm correlated to widespread blood flow changes in the prefrontal cortex.[160,161] The researchers noted specific orgasm-related changes in the mid/anterior OFC and suggest that this fits with the proposed role of the mid-anterior OFC in the experience of pleasure. Failed orgasm significantly enhanced left lateral OFC activity: orgasm was not reached possibly due to excessive behavioral suppression. The researchers suggest that the orgasm-related OFC dynamics may reflect one of the main features of orgasm (i.e., the typical sense of loss of control). Prefrontal but not temporal perfusion was inversely coupled to rectal pressure fluctuations associated with orgasm. These changes in the

OFC (the dorsal and ventral prefrontal divisions) did not show any clear association with arousal but only with these indicators of orgasm. The researchers therefore concluded that the decreased prefrontal cortex activity may be specific to orgasm. Overall the findings of reduced prefrontal metabolism during orgasm are in keeping with the critical role of the prefrontal cortex in behavioral and emotional control. It may be that successful prefrontal regulation is key to reaching orgasm in keeping with experimental data of exaggerated prefrontal activity with associated sexual dysfunction.

Pontine control of female orgasm appears to center on a localized region on the left side of the dorsolateral pontine tegmentum recently termed the *pelvic organ–stimulating center*.[161] Another pontine area, the ventrolateral pontine area, recently termed the *pelvic floor–stimulating center*, is involved in organizing the pelvic floor–contractions during orgasm and has direct projections to pelvic floor motor neurons.

The role of oxytocin and prolactin in orgasm is unclear. Both hormone levels increase at the time of orgasm: PET scanning has confirmed increased pituitary blood flow in women, but not in men, at the moment of orgasm.[162] Both hormones can cause uterine and vaginal smooth muscle contraction, which may contribute to the sensations of orgasm.

THE REVISED DEFINITIONS OF SEXUAL DYSFUNCTION IN MEN

In May 2013, the DSM-5 provided an updated classification and definitions of male sexual disorders.[14] The salient differences of the new DSM-5 classification and definitions from the DSM-IV are the following[15]:
1. DSM-5 includes only four male sexual disorders, as opposed to six in the DSM-IV.[15] The four sexual disorders are the following:
   a. Male hypoactive sexual desire disorder
   b. ED
   c. Premature ejaculation
   d. Delayed ejaculation
2. DSM-5 lists male HSDD as a separate entry.[14,15] Male orgasmic disorder has been renamed *delayed ejaculation*, male ED has been changed to *ED*, and male orgasmic disorder has been changed to *delayed ejaculation*. Premature ejaculation remains unchanged.
3. Male dyspareunia, male sexual pain, sexual aversion disorder, and sexual dysfunction have been removed in the DSM-5.[14,15]
4. Unlike DSM-IV, the DSM-5 includes the requirement of experiencing the disorder 75% to 100% of the time to make a diagnosis of sexual disorder. DSM-5 also requires a minimum duration of approximately 6 months.[14,15]
5. DSM-5 requires that the sexual disorder must have caused significant distress. The DSM-IV requirement of "interpersonal difficulty" has been removed.[14,15]
6. DSM-5 added one new exclusion criterion: the disorder should not be better explained by a "nonsexual mental disorder or a consequence of severe relationship distress or other significant stressors."[14,15]

Male Hypoactive Sexual Desire Disorder

HSDD is the persistent or recurrent deficiency (or absence) of sexual fantasies and desire for sexual activity that causes marked distress and that is not better explained by another disorder, direct physiologic effects of a substance (medication), or general medical condition.[163-166] A diagnosis of HSDD is appropriate *only* if the person reports distress due to low sexual desire.[163-166] Low sexual desire is not necessarily pathologic, as low sexual desire may be an appropriate adaptation to relationship and health-related issues.[163-166]

HSDD is a multifactorial disorder that can result from androgen deficiency, use of medications (SSRIs, antiandrogens, gonadotropin-releasing hormone [GnRH] analogues, antihypertensives, cancer chemotherapeutic agents, anticonvulsants), systemic illness, depression and other psychological problems, other causes of sexual dysfunction, or relationship and differentiation problems. Androgen deficiency is an important, treatable cause of HSDD and should be excluded by measuring serum total testosterone levels.[163-166]

The incidence and prevalence of HSDD in the general population are unknown. In studies of referred patient populations, the prevalence has been estimated at 5% in men and 22% in women.[5-7,165-167] Prevalence increases with age.[165-167] HSDD often coexists with other sexual disorders, such as ED, and may develop as a consequence of other preexisting sexual disorders.[165-167]

Appropriate evaluation and treatment of HSDD are important because evaluation may lead to detection of treatable androgen deficiency. Also, hypoactive sexual desire in one partner can strain the relationship between sexual partners[168] and lead to ED. Low sexual desire may impede or reduce effectiveness of treatments for other sexual dysfunctions.

Erectile Disorder

ED, previously referred to as *impotence* or *male ED*, is the inability to attain or maintain an erection or to achieve penile rigidity sufficient for satisfactory sexual intercourse.[10,11,14,15] DSM-5 requires that the inability to attain or maintain an erection should occur in 75% to 100% of encounters over a period of at least 6 months.[14,15] Sexual dysfunction is a more general term that also includes libidinal, orgasmic, and ejaculatory dysfunction, in addition to the inability to attain or maintain penile erection. The epidemiologic surveys,[4-6,167-175] including the MMAS[4] and the NHSLS,[5,6] revealed a surprisingly high prevalence of ED in men (see later). ED significantly affects quality of life of both the affected individual and his partner. In one study, ED had a negative impact on the sexual life of female partners, specifically on their sexual satisfaction and sexual drive.[168]

Prevalence and Incidence

The best data on the prevalence of ED in men have emerged from two cross-sectional studies that have used population-based sampling techniques, namely the MMAS[4,169,172,173] and the NHSLS.[6,7] The MMAS is a cross-sectional as well as longitudinal, community-based epidemiologic survey in which 1709 men, 40 to 70 years of age, residing in the greater Boston area, were surveyed between 1987 and 1989.[4] This survey revealed that 52% of men between the ages of 40 and 70 were affected by ED of some degree; 17.2% of surveyed men reported minimal ED, 25.2% moderate ED, and 9.6% complete ED.[4,172,173] The NHSLS was a national probability survey of English-speaking Americans, 18 to 59 years of age, living in the United States.[6,7] This survey also revealed a high prevalence of ED in men; the prevalence of ED increased with increasing age.[6,7]

These two landmark studies and data from several other studies are in agreement that ED is a common problem worldwide.[4,6,7,167-174] In the U.S. civilian population, the prevalence of ED in men aged 20 to 39 years has been estimated to be 5.1%, whereas prevalence in men aged 40 to 59 years was almost three times as high (14.8%). In the MMAS, crude incidence of ED was reported at 25.9 cases per 1000 person-years, although that study included only men over the age of 40. ED has been estimated to affect 20 million to 30 million men in the United States alone and 150 million to 200 million men worldwide.[172,173] The prevalence of ED increases with age; it affects fewer than 10% of men younger than 45 years of age but 75% of men over 80 years of age.[4] Men suffering from other medical problems, such as hypertension, diabetes, cardiovascular disease (CVD), and end-stage renal disease, have a significantly higher prevalence of ED than healthy men.[4]

There is a paucity of longitudinal data on the incidence rates of ED in men. In the MMAS, the crude incidence rate of ED in white men in the Boston area was found to be 25.9 cases per 1000 person-years.[169] The incidence rates increased from 12.4 cases per 1000 person-years for men 40 to 49 years of age to 29.8 cases per 1000 person-years for men 50 to 59 years of age and 46.4 per 1000 person-years for men 60 to 69 years of age.[169] In another study, incidence rates were derived from a survey of men seen at a preventive medicine clinic.[7] This study found the incidence rates of ED to be less than 3 cases per 1000 person-years among men less than 45 years of age and 52 cases per 1000 person-years among men 65 years of age or older. These studies suggest that there were 152 million cases of ED in the world in 1995 and that 600,000 to 700,000 men in the United States develop ED each year.[172,173]

Risk Factors for Erectile Disorder

The risk factors for ED include age, diabetes mellitus, hypertension, smoking, medication use, depression, dyslipidemia, and CVD.[4,9-11,175-185] Advancing age is an important risk factor for ED in men[4,6,9-11]: less than 10% of men below the age of 40 and over 50% of men over the age of 70 have ED. In both the MMAS and the NHSLS, the prevalence of ED increased with each decade of life.[4,6]

Among the chronic diseases associated with ED, diabetes mellitus is the most important risk factor. In the MMAS, the age-adjusted risk of complete ED was three times higher in men with history of treated diabetes mellitus than in those without a history of diabetes mellitus.[4,175] Fifty percent of men with diabetes mellitus will experience ED sometime during the course of their illness. In the MMAS, treated heart disease, treated hypertension, and hyperlipidemia were associated with a significantly increased risk of ED. Among men with treated heart disease and hypertension, the probability of ED was more than two times greater for smokers than for nonsmokers.[4-6,9-11] Smoking also increases the risk of ED in men taking medications for CVDs. Cardiovascular disorders, including hypertension, stroke, coronary artery disease, and peripheral vascular disease, are all associated with increased risk of ED. Physical activity is associated with reduced risk of ED.[184]

Several reviews have emphasized the relationship of prescription medications and the occurrence of ED. In the MMAS, the use of antihypertensives, cardiac medication, and oral hypoglycemic drugs was associated with an increased risk of ED.[4] Thiazide diuretics and psychotropic drugs used in the treatment of depression may be the most common drugs associated with ED, simply because of the high prevalence of their use. However, a variety of drugs, including almost all antihypertensives, digoxin, histamine-2

receptor antagonists, anticholinergics, cytotoxic agents, and androgen antagonists, have been implicated in the pathophysiology of ED.[4]

Erectile Disorder as a Marker of Cardiovascular Disease

CVD and ED share common risk factors, such as diabetes mellitus, obesity, hypertension, smoking, and dyslipidemia.[176-184] ED precedes the symptoms of coronary artery disease by 2 to 3 years and cardiovascular events such as myocardial infarction or stroke by 3 to 5 years.[176-184] ED in men is associated with increased risk of death, particularly fatality due to CVD.[178] The presence of ED is a good predictor of subsequent coronary artery disease, especially in younger men, independent of traditional coronary risk factors, although it does not enhance the predictive ability of models that include traditional risk factors, likely reflecting the common pathophysiologic mechanisms of ED and coronary artery disease.[179] Men reporting ED are 1.3 to 1.6 times more likely to experience a cardiovascular event within 10 years than men without ED.[176-184]

Lower Urinary Tract Symptoms and Erectile Disorder

Recent surveys have revealed an association of lower urinary tract symptoms (LUTS) with ED[185-191] even after adjusting for age and other risk factors. The Cologne Male Study and the Multinational Study of Aging Male revealed that the presence and severity of LUTS is an independent predictor of ED independent of age.[186] LUTS and age are stronger predictors of ED than all other risk factors, including diabetes, dyslipidemia, and hypertension. As LUTS and ED are two common conditions in middle-aged and older men, it is possible that this association reflects the coexistence of two highly prevalent conditions. However, there is growing evidence that the two conditions may be mechanistically linked, as the biochemical mechanisms that regulate bladder detrusor and cavernosal smooth muscle function share many similarities.[191,192] K^+ channels, especially calcium-sensitive K^+ channels (BK_{Ca} channels), Rho A/Rho kinase signaling, L-type calcium channels, and gap junctions are important mediators of both detrusor and cavernosal smooth muscle contractility and relaxation.[191,192] Increased myocyte contractility that characterizes both bladder detrusor dysfunction and ED may be mechanistically related to increased Rho kinase activity, impairments of K^+ channel function,[192] α-adrenergic receptor imbalance, and endothelial dysfunction. Additional proposed hypotheses include increased sympathetic activity and autonomic dysfunction, and alterations in nitric oxide generation or protein kinase G activity in the detrusor and cavernosal smooth muscles.[191-193] Some therapies for LUTS such as some types of surgeries and 5α-reductase inhibitors may worsen sexual dysfunction. PDE5 inhibitors are being investigated for the treatment of LUTS.[192-195]

Ejaculatory Disorders

Ejaculatory disorders include premature ejaculation, delayed ejaculation, retrograde ejaculation, anejaculation, and painful ejaculation.[113-116] Recent surveys have highlighted the high prevalence and clinical importance of ejaculatory disorders.[18,113-116,196,197] Although the availability of oral PDE5 inhibitors has increased awareness of ED, ejaculatory disorders are at least as prevalent and may be even more prevalent than ED.[18,197] Premature ejaculation, defined as ejaculation associated with lack of or poor ejaculatory control that causes distress in one or both partners, is the most prevalent sexual disorder in men 18 to 59 years of age.[6,18,197,198] The new DSM-5 definition has now added a time requirement that the ejaculation must occur within approximately 1 minute following vaginal penetration to be deemed premature.[14,15] Delayed ejaculation refers to a man's inability to ejaculate in a reasonable period that interferes with sexual or emotional satisfaction and is associated with distress.

Retrograde ejaculation is the failure of the semen to be ejected out through the urethral meatus; instead the semen is propelled backward into the urinary bladder.[113-116] Retrograde ejaculation can be the result of autonomic neuropathy associated with diabetes mellitus; sympathectomy; therapy with adrenergic antagonists, some types of antihypertensives, antipsychotics, or antidepressants; bladder neck incompetence; or urethral obstruction. Retrograde ejaculation due to diabetes-associated autonomic neuropathy is the second most prevalent ejaculatory disorder.[113-116] Following transurethral resection of the prostate, the bladder neck closure mechanism may be damaged. Patients remain continent because of a second, more distal, continence mechanism that is present in the region of the membranous urethra; however, many patients who have undergone transurethral resection of the prostate experience retrograde ejaculation. Ejaculatory disorders can lead to infertility among men.[113-116]

CURRENT DEFINITIONS OF SEXUAL DISORDERS IN WOMEN

The currently recommended definitions for female sexual disorders in the DSM-5 are shown in Table 20-1.[14,15] A disorder is diagnosed only if there is clinically significant distress or impairment. Disorders are identified as early onset (lifelong) versus late onset (acquired). The sexual dysfunction should not be more attributable to a nonsexual psychiatric disorder, to the effects of a substance (e.g., a drug of abuse, a medication), to a medical condition, or to relationship distress, partner violence, or other significant stressors.[14,15]

Sexual Interest/Arousal Disorder

The definition addressing problematic desire merges sexual interest (motivation) with arousal and focuses away from initial/anticipatory desire.[199,200] Increasing evidence suggests that desire ahead of and at the outset of sexual engagement, although welcomed probably by both partners, is not mandatory for a woman's sexual enjoyment and satisfaction.[25,27,28,201] It is the inability to trigger desire and arousal during sexual engagement (as well as an absence of desire initially) that constitutes disorder. Empirical support for the concept that arousal may precede desire and the two then coexist is now strong and includes data from older and younger women.[26-28] Therefore, merging of sexual and desire difficulties into one disorder appears logical. However, validated questionnaires used to assess sexual function are based on models of sexual response in which desire is assumed necessary at the outset of engagement. This is now acknowledged as a serious limitation to research,[202] and the prevalence of what is currently understood to be *disorder* is quite unclear.[40,201-209] Studies that simply report "low desire and distress" indicate prevalence rates of about 10%, not increasing with age.[40,207] Risk factors include negative feelings for the partner and mood disorders.[204] Depression, either currently or in the past, and, in the absence of any diagnosed depression, more depressive and anxious thoughts and low self-esteem are found significantly more commonly than in control women.[40,207]

Female Orgasmic Disorder

The prevalence of women's orgasmic disorder is also unclear, because many studies include women with low arousal who rarely reach orgasm.[20,40,207] Risk factors include anxiety about the partner's presence, fear of being vulnerable, fear of not being in control, and fear of intimacy.[20] These factors often stem from childhood (nonsexual) experiences.

Genitopelvic Pain/Penetration Disorder

The merging of former terms *vaginismus* and *dyspareunia* has some merit. Some women report typical phobic avoidance of penetration such that a penile introital contact has never been possible, and physical examination has to be deferred until therapy enables a careful inspection and ultimately a complete pelvic examination to be done. When abnormalities other than the reflex muscle tightening are absent, then vaginismus was diagnosed. However, often the condition is complicated. For example, the woman gives a history of phobic avoidance and fear, and subsequent examination confirms vaginistic reaction, but once therapy allows a careful detailed introital examination, allodynia of the vestibule is confirmed. The diagnosis then, prior to DSM-5, was vaginismus by history but provoked vestibulodynia (PVD) on examination.

Reported prevalence of sexual pain varies between 20% and 35%.[210-214] The most common form of pain with penetration, PVD, affects some 16% of mostly premenopausal women, many of whom have had pain consistently from first attempts at penetration.[205] Risk factors for PVD include some personality traits—perfectionism, reward dependency, fear of negative evaluation—as well as harm avoidance, hypervigilance for pain, higher levels of trait anxiety, and shyness.[205] For a small subset, vaginal candidiasis appears to precipitate and maintain the condition.

Vaginismus is now included within genitopelvic pain/penetration disorder.[14] The term had described (phobic) avoidance, involuntary pelvic muscle contraction, and anticipation of, fear of, or the experience of pain—there being no structural or other abnormalities on examination, this having to be deferred until some therapy has begun. Risk factors include depression, anxiety, social phobia, somatization, and hostility. Some studies identify increased catastrophic thinking in women with vaginismus compared with women without pain or women with other forms of pain: moreover, women with vaginismus show greater disgust propensity.[205] Despite the theories, there is no scientific evidence that vaginismus is secondary to religious orthodoxy, negative sexual upbringing, or concerns about sexual orientation. Typically there is extreme fear of vaginal entry, fear that harm will come from something the size of a penis entering the vagina, and fear of damage by vaginal delivery.

Persistent Genital Arousal Disorder

Not included in the DSM-5, but clinically an increasingly common and poorly understood entity, is persistent genital arousal disorder: spontaneous, intrusive, and unwanted genital arousal (e.g., tingling, throbbing, pulsating) in the absence of sexual interest and desire. Any awareness of subjective arousal is typically, but not invariably, unpleasant. The arousal is unrelieved by one or more orgasms, and the feelings of arousal persist for hours or days.[206] Prevalence is unknown and a broad range of symptoms is recognized, from mild (and perhaps pleasant) to intrusive, highly distressing, and markedly interfering with life.

SEXUAL DYSFUNCTION IN THE CONTEXT OF ENDOCRINE DISEASE

We will focus on sexual sequelae of endocrine disease and its treatment, but in any given person nonendocrine factors may be more important. These factors include psychological, relational, contextual, cultural, and nonendocrine medical influences—especially depression, hypertension, neurologic disease, and LUTS.[20] For patients with chronic disease, the disease itself, its treatment, its psychological effects, plus interpersonal, personal, and contextual issues affect sexual response.[20]

In healthy women, factors such as attitudes toward sex, feelings for the partner, past sexual experiences, duration of relationship, and mental and emotional health have been shown to more strongly modulate desire and arousability than do biologic factors.[20] Contrary to gender stereotypes, recent analysis of the 1035 sexually active adults who participated in the NHSLS in 1992 showed that men's physical sexual pleasure was more closely linked to relational factors than was the case for women.[6,40,168] Similarly, in a recent international study of midlife and older couples, men rated the importance of sex for closeness and intimacy to their partner more highly than did their female partners.[40] Qualitative research also suggests that men as well as women note that positive self-esteem and feeling attractive enhance desire and arousal.[40,168] Sexual context is also important for both men and women.[168]

Endocrine Disorders and Sexual Dysfunction in Men

Androgen Deficiency Syndromes

Androgen deficiency in men is a syndrome characterized by a constellation of signs and symptoms associated with consistently low testosterone levels due to disorders of the testes, pituitary, or the hypothalamus.[1,62] Androgen deficiency can occur either because of primary testicular dysfunction or as a result of disorders affecting the hypothalamus or the pituitary.[62] Common causes of primary testicular dysfunction include Klinefelter syndrome, uncorrected cryptorchidism, human immunodeficiency virus (HIV) infection, orchitis, trauma, torsion, and radiation and cancer chemotherapy.[62] Secondary testicular dysfunction can result from systemic illness; excessive exercise; recreational drugs, especially opiates, marijuana, cocaine, and alcohol; pituitary and suprasellar tumors; hemochromatosis; hyperprolactinemia; and infiltrative disorders. Exclusion of these secondary causes of hypogonadism may then justify a diagnosis of idiopathic hypogonadotropic hypogonadism, which is a heterogeneous group of disorders characterized by disordered GnRH secretion.[62] The testosterone levels required to maintain sexual function are close to the lower limit of the normal male range.[64,135,140,215-217] Therefore, some men with pituitary tumors may remain asymptomatic until their tumor has grown substantially and testosterone levels have declined to a level below this threshold.

Androgen deficiency is an important treatable cause of male HSDD. Therefore, the men diagnosed with HSDD should be evaluated for androgen deficiency by measurement of testosterone levels using a reliable assay, preferably in an early morning fasting blood sample.[62] Although ED and androgen deficiency in men are distinct disorders with separate pathophysiologic mechanisms, the two can coexist in the same patient. Testosterone levels should be measured in men presenting with any form of sexual dysfunction because androgen deficiency is treatable, and furthermore, androgen deficiency may be a manifestation of another underlying disease, such as a pituitary tumor, which may require additional evaluation and disease-specific intervention.

Diabetes and Sexual Dysfunction in Men

Men with diabetes mellitus are at increased risk of ED, retrograde ejaculation, and low testosterone levels. Peyronie disease is an important comorbid condition in older diabetic men with ED.[218-225] The men with diabetes have significantly lower scores for sexual desire, activity, arousal, and satisfaction,[219-225] in part due to the medical and psychological factors associated with diabetes, such as the variations in glycemic control, reduced energy, altered self-image, and interpersonal difficulties regarding dietary compliance, glucose monitoring, and medications. Diabetes also is associated with increased risk of low testosterone levels.[62,226-231] In population studies, sex hormone–binding globulin (SHBG) and total testosterone are more strongly associated with diabetes risk than free testosterone levels; these data suggest that the observed association of testosterone with diabetes risk may be related to factors, such as insulin sensitivity and inflammation, that regulate SHBG.[230,231]

The prevalence of ED in men with diabetes increases with age and has been as high as 75% in some studies. ED in men with type 2 diabetes even without other risk factors for coronary artery disease may signal silent cardiac ischemia.[231-235] Among men with diabetes, those with ED are more likely to be older smokers with longer duration of diabetes, poor metabolic control, untreated hypertension, and presence of neuropathy, microalbuminuria and macroalbuminuria, retinopathy, CVD, diuretic treatment, low testosterone levels, and psychological vulnerability.[221-224] Increased physical activity and consumption of small amounts of alcohol have been found to be protective. The risk of ED generally increases with chronic elevation of hemoglobin A_{1c}.[221]

Endothelial and smooth muscle dysfunction, autonomic neuropathy, and psychological and interpersonal issues contribute to sexual dysfunction in men with diabetes.[234,235] Endothelial dysfunction is evident in penile blood vessels as well as in nongenital vascular beds.[189] eNOS is reduced, possibly due to overexpression of arginase or lack of nicotinamide adenine dinucleotide phosphate (NADPH), an essential cofactor for NOS.[235-240] Additionally, accumulation of oxygen free radicals, including those from advanced glycosylation end products (AGEs), quench nitric oxide and attenuate the action of K^+ channels.[239,240] The reduction in NADPH is also associated with increased diacylglycerol and protein kinase C, and consequently, increased smooth muscle contractility.[237] An increased activation of the Rho A/Rho kinase pathway may increase the sensitivity of cavernosal smooth muscle to calcium.[237] Autonomic neuropathy affecting the pelvic nerves may lead to ED as well as ejaculatory dysfunction.[238]

Retrograde ejaculation and partial ejaculatory incompetence affect up to one third of men with diabetes.[241] Autonomic nerve damage in diabetes may be associated with dysfunction of the internal sphincter so that all or a part of the seminal fluid is propelled into the bladder.[238] Partial ejaculatory incompetence refers to the condition in which ejaculatory emission remains intact but the expulsion phase is inhibited; consequently, the semen trickles out of the penis and the experience of orgasm is altered in quality. Both ejaculatory problems may be a cause of infertility.

Sexual Dysfunction Associated With Therapies for Benign Prostatic Hypertrophy

Benign prostatic hypertrophy is frequently associated with LUTS and sexual dysfunction.[185-191] Although treatment with some α_1-adrenergic receptor blockers can improve erectile function, others, such as tamsulosin, are associated with ejaculatory dysfunction.[242,243] Treatment of men with LUTS with 5α-reductase inhibitors has been associated with increased risk of ejaculatory disorder, ED, and decreased libido.[244,245] Several surveys have reported the development of sexual symptoms, including loss of libido, ED, and difficulty with ejaculation in a subset of young men who have taken finasteride for alopecia[246-249]; these symptoms have been reported to persist even after discontinuation of finasteride. Although the causative role of finasteride and the pathophysiology of these symptoms remain to be established, it has been speculated that polymorphisms in androgen receptor or other genes may render these individuals susceptible to off-target actions of finasteride.[250]

Hyperprolactinemia and Sexual Dysfunction

Hyperprolactinemic men often present with decreased libido or ED; 75% of men with macroprolactinomas and 50% of men with microprolactinomas report reduced desire or ED and almost all have subnormal nocturnal penile erections.[251-255] Hyperprolactinemia affects 1% to 5% of men presenting with ED[252]; a fraction of these men have prolactin-secreting pituitary adenomas.

Prolactin lowers testosterone levels through its inhibitory effects on GnRH secretion and on the pituitary response to GnRH. Most, but not all, men with sexual dysfunction and hyperprolactinemia have low testosterone levels.[251,252] Whether and how hyperprolactinemia directly affects erectile function through target organ effects is not well understood. Erectile function generally improves in hyperprolactinemic men following treatment with dopamine agonists.[254,255]

Sexual Dysfunction in Patients With Thyroid Disease

Hypothyroidism has been associated with increased risk of hypoactive sexual desire and ED.[255-260] The exact prevalence of sexual dysfunction in men with hypothyroidism is unknown. Free testosterone levels are lower in hypothyroid men than in control subjects and become normal after thyroxine replacement.[256-260] Serum LH and follicle-stimulating hormone levels are typically not elevated in men with primary hypothyroidism.[259] Hyperprolactinemia is noted in a small fraction of hypothyroid men.[259]

Free testosterone levels are typically normal in men with hyperthyrodism, but SHBG and estradiol levels are elevated, resulting in a high estradiol-to-testosterone ratio and gynecomastia in some hyperthyroid men.[258] Hyperthyroidism has been observed in a small fraction of men with ED.[260]

Sexual Dysfunction in Men With Metabolic Syndrome

The men with metabolic syndrome have a higher prevalence of ED than men without the metabolic syndrome.[261-264] The risk of ED is correlated with the number of identified components of metabolic syndrome.[260-264]

Endocrine Disorders and Sexual Dysfunction in Women

Thyroid Disease in Women

Both hyper- and hypothyroid states have been found to be risk factors for sexual dysfunction, which mostly remits with return to an euthyroid state.[265-267] Studies are few and small, and when mood is also assessed, comorbid depression is found to be associated with sexual dysfunction in the context of thyroid disease.[1,265] There is some evidence that thyroid autoimmunity lessens sexual desire independent of altered thyroid status: euthyroid women with Hashimoto thyroiditis may report persistent loss of desire.[265-267] One research group found women with nodular goiter to have significantly more sexual dysfunction than control subjects. This group also had the highest body mass index.[267]

Hyperprolactinemia in Women

Hyperprolactinemia is associated with increased risk of sexual dysfunction.[76,268] Women with hyperprolactinemia report greater overall dissatisfaction with sexual function and lower scores for sexual desire, arousal, lubrication, and orgasm domains than women with normal prolactin levels. Prolactin inhibits GnRH pulses, attenuates gonadotropin response to GnRH, and is associated with reduced ovarian secretion of estrogen and androgen. Although menstrual disturbance or infertility is more commonly the presenting symptom of hyperprolactinemia, lower scores for sexual function and desire have also been found in women with hyperprolactinemia who have regular menses.[268] However, normal menstruation, younger age, and smaller prolactinoma size are more likely to be associated with normal sexual function than the actual level of prolactin or testosterone.[20] Sexual outcomes of treatment of hyperprolactinemic women with dopamine agonists have not been well studied.

Diabetes in Women

Women's sexual response and satisfaction may be compromised by diabetes-associated changes in their well-being, mood, and self-image, especially if there is unwanted weight gain, recurrent vaginitis from candidiasis, or imposed infertility.[269-282] In addition, there may be a compromised neurovascular genital sexual response from autonomic neuropathy or endothelial dysfunction and microvascular disease. In women with type 1 diabetes, sexual dysfunction is mostly correlated to psychological factors including depression, anxiety, and marital status.[270,271,273,281] The results from a large prospective study of 625 women with type 1 diabetes confirmed depression as the major predictor of dysfunction.[277]

Most studies on women with type 2 diabetes are small, but one larger study of 600 women with type 2 diabetes confirmed only depression and marital status to be independent risk factors for sexual dysfunction.[269] Although sexual dysfunction has been associated with both type 1[20,270,274,277] and type 2[20,271-273,276,278] diabetes, not all studies confirm an association.[273,275,279]

A recent meta-analysis[280] that included 26 studies, 3168 women with diabetes, and 2823 control subjects confirmed sexual dysfunction to be more frequent in women with diabetes. Compared to women without diabetes, the risk of sexual dysfunction was 2.27 and 2.49 times higher in women with type 1 and type 2 diabetes, respectively.[280] The risk for sexual dysfunction was nearly two times higher for women with any form of diabetes. However, postmenopausal women with any form of diabetes did not demonstrate an increased risk of sexual dysfunction. The increased prevalence of sexual dysfunction and lower female sexual function index (FSFI) score in women with diabetes may be related to body weight. This association would be in keeping with other studies showing an increased prevalence of sexual dysfunction in obese women[281-283] and in women with metabolic syndrome.[284,285] Unlike the situation in men with diabetes, sexual dysfunction has not been consistently associated with the presence of diabetic complications in the majority of studies. Type 1 diabetes may be associated with loss of genital sexual sensitivity.[286] Sexual dysfunction in women with diabetes is complex, and the roles of body mass index, fat distribution, diabetic complications, insulin resistance, inflammation, CVD, relationship satisfaction, and depression remain poorly understood.[20,282,283]

Pathogenesis of Sexual Dysfunction in Diabetes. Whereas depression and obesity are the identified major etiologic factors, in the individual woman, neurovascular complications of diabetes may be relevant.[20,287,288] Autonomic and somatic neuropathy may contribute to loss of genital sexual sensitivity. When there is less engorgement of the vascular sinusoidal tissue comprising the shaft, head, rami, and bulbs of the clitoris, massaging the structures during sexual stimulation will fail to elicit typical sexual sensations to compromise arousal and limit the experience of orgasm.[287,288]

In animal studies, diabetes has been shown to impair vaginal smooth muscle relaxation responses to the neurotransmitters, particularly VIP and nitric oxide.[287] These studies also report decreased clitoral and vaginal blood flow to nerve stimulation, diffuse fibrosis of the clitoral and vaginal tissues, as well as reduced muscular layer and epithelial thickness in vaginal tissue. Endothelial dysfunction and reduced clitoral blood flow have been documented in women with diabetes.[288]

Most studies have not found increased prevalence of dyspareunia in women with diabetes. Diabetic women are at higher risk of recurrent candidiasis, which may contribute to dyspareunia.[289]

Metabolic Syndrome in Women

Metabolic syndrome has been shown to have a deleterious effect on women's sexuality, independent of diabetes and obesity.[1,20,289,290] This negative effect seems to be more prevalent in premenopausal than postmenopausal women.[1,20,289,290]

Polycystic Ovary Syndrome

Limited research has shown that women with polycystic ovary syndrome may be less sexually satisfied and may regard themselves as less attractive than control subjects.[291-294] The presumption is that obesity and androgen-related symptoms may contribute to poor body image, which may increase the risk of sexual dysfunction.[1,282] Recent studies show little evidence that polycystic ovary syndrome (as opposed to obesity) is a risk factor for sexual dysfunction.[294,295]

Congenital Adrenal Hyperplasia

Nonclassic forms of congenital adrenal hyperplasia may present with signs of hyperandrogenism in childhood or adulthood, depending on the severity of the 21-hydroxylase enzyme deficiency.[296] The presenting features of 21-hydroxylase enzyme deficiency may include menstrual disorders such as amenorrhea, anovulation, hirsutism, or oligomenorrhea with infertility.[297] Limited research suggests that sexual functioning of women with nonclassic 21-hydroxylase deficiency is not different from that of control subjects. However, women with classic congenital adrenal hyperplasia may show gender-atypical behavior[298]; in one study, male-typical role-playing in childhood correlated with reduced satisfaction with the female gender role and reduced heterosexual interest in adulthood.[299] Disturbed body image, repeated genital examinations, and genital surgery may also affect sexual function in women with congenital adrenal hyperplasia.[298] Caring for these women requires careful individualized treatment with appropriate therapy for signs and symptoms of androgen excess as well as psychosexual counseling.[20]

Pituitary Disease in Women

There is limited research on sexual function in women who have deficiencies of various pituitary hormones. It is known that most women with pituitary disease often report menstrual irregularity or problems with sexual function, including decreased sexual desire and problems with lubrication or orgasm.[76] Although women with hypopituitarism have lower testosterone levels than healthy menstruating women, the short- and long-term effects of testosterone in women with hypopituitarism have not been well studied.[300,301] In one randomized trial of 51 women, testosterone therapy in women who were receiving estrogen therapy was associated with some benefit in sexual function and mood, compared with placebo, but with a higher frequency of androgenic side effects than placebo.[302] The effects of dehydroepiandrosterone (DHEA) on sexual function and mood in women with hypopituitarism are also poorly understood.[301]

Adrenal Insufficiency in Women

In addition to the deficiency of cortisol and aldosterone, women with adrenal insufficiency also have low levels of testosterone and DHEA.[1,303-312] Adrenal insufficiency in women has been associated with low health-related quality of life.[308] However, a 2010 larger study comparing 174 women with Addison disease to 740 age-matched healthy control subjects and to 234 women who had received a risk-reducing bilateral salpingo-oophorectomy (BSO) demonstrated that despite subnormal levels of androgens and androgen metabolites, the women with Addison disease reported higher sexual pleasure and less discomfort with intercourse than the normative control women.[309] Clinical trials of DHEA replacement in women with adrenal insufficiency have been small and mostly negative.[1,303-307,310,312] An earlier small trial in women with primary or secondary adrenal insufficiency reported greater improvements in sexual interest and satisfaction and in mood for women receiving DHEA compared with placebo[303]; however, four subsequent studies did not find significant improvements in sexual function.[304-307] In 2009, a meta-analysis of 10 studies concluded that DHEA therapy in adrenal insufficiency may result in small improvements in health-related quality of life and depression, but it had no effects on anxiety or sexual well-being.[312] Thus, there are insufficient data to support the routine use of DHEA in women with adrenal insufficiency.

Natural Menopause

A majority of women who discontinue postmenopausal estrogen supplementation develop signs of vulvovaginal atrophy, which is a risk factor for sexual dysfunction.[210-214,313,314] However, symptoms from vulvovaginal atrophy may remit spontaneously within 1 year; risk factors for more severe symptoms are diabetes, younger age, and low body mass index.[214,313,314] The traditional notion that maintaining sexual activity will prevent symptomatic vulvovaginal atrophy has been refuted.[314] Subjective symptoms and objective signs of vulvovaginal atrophy correlate poorly.[315] Epidemiologic studies have not shown an increase in the prevalence of dyspareunia with age.[210-212] Clearly not all postmenopausal women develop sexual symptoms of estrogen deficiency: of 1525 women followed from age 47 to 54 years, the vast majority were not affected by the major hormonal shifts.[213] It is likely that multiple factors contribute to sexual symptoms, including variations in the intracrine production of estrogen from adrenal precursors, the number and sensitivity of estrogen receptors, and the degree of sexual arousal or excitement at the time of vulval stimulation and vaginal entry.[316-318] Psychological factors rather than estrogen levels were shown to moderate symptoms when vulvovaginal atrophy is present.[318]

Most studies report a decrease in sexual desire with advancing age[319] that is not easily explained by hormonal deficiency alone. Adaptive changes occur in the brain in response to the reductions in circulating levels of sex hormones associated with age and menopause.[320,321] Sex hormones are produced locally within the brain: in women, steroidogenic enzymes and sex-steroid receptors in the brain are upregulated in response to decreased circulating levels of sex hormones.[320,321] We do not know whether there is biologic adaptation to reduced amounts of sex hormones. In studies of age, menopausal status, and sexual function, the postmenopausal state has generally been negatively associated with desire mainly among women who experienced low emotional intimacy with their partners. Similarly, the negative association between age and sexual desire was particularly pronounced in women experiencing little intimacy.[322]

Surgical Menopause

Surgical menopause is a state of both androgen and estrogen depletion of sudden onset and has often been viewed as a risk factor for sexual dysfunction. However, most women undergoing bilateral BSO for benign clinical indications do not develop sexual dysfunction. Three prospective studies found that women choosing BSO plus hysterectomy for benign indications did not develop sexual dysfunction over the next 1 to 3 years.[323-325]

A national survey of 2207 American women confirmed an increased prevalence of distress about low sexual desire in women with a recent BSO.[319] Thus, in women undergoing nonelective surgery, the thematic context of bilateral oophorectomy may impair sexual desire and function. For example, women who are treated for malignant disease or those who desire to preserve their fertility may experience greater distress about low sexual desire after BSO than those who undergo BSO for benign conditions. In the same survey, both older and younger women with a relatively recent BSO reported low sexual desire per se, as often as age-matched subjects with intact ovaries.[319] Despite their continued hormonal deficit, women older than 45 years who underwent oophorectomy before menopause had fewer complaints of low desire than women of similar age with intact ovaries.[319]

A recent study of 1352 women showed no difference in the report of sexual ideation, sexual function, or sexual problems between women who have had and women who have not had bilateral oophorectomy.[326] Having thoughts about sex is less likely to be affected by contextual details including the sexual relationship than is sexual function or motivation for partnered sex.

The women who carry a BRCA mutation and undergo BSO to lessen the risk of breast, ovarian, or fallopian tube cancer mostly remain satisfied with their decision for surgery.[327] However, studies on sexual response are conflicting. Less sexual pleasure despite the use of local estrogen to alleviate dyspareunia has been noted,[328] whereas another study comparing 234 women who had received a risk-reducing BSO to 740 age-matched control subjects from the general population demonstrated that the women with risk-reducing surgery had greater sexual pleasure and less dyspareunia than the normative control women.[326,329]

Aging-Associated Decline in Sex Hormone Precursors in Women

From the middle 30s to the early 60s, a woman's adrenal production of precursor hormones—DHEA, androstenedione, and DHEA sulfate (DHEAS)—declines by 70%.[65,67] However, the trajectories of decline in these precursor steroids vary among women.[65-67] The relationship of the age-related decline in these circulating precursors to sexual function remains poorly understood. On the population level, variation in circulating levels of sex steroids and their precursors is related to variation in the activities of steroidogenic enzymes such as 3β-hydroxysteroid dehydrogenase (3β-HSD), 17β-HSD, 17,20-lyase, and aromatase and to the variation in the plasma clearance of these hormones and precursors. Labrie and associates have proposed that the androgen metabolites, most notably ADT-G, may serve as useful markers of ovarian as well as tissue production and activity of androgens in women.[67,316,330] A study of 250 women carefully evaluated for sexual dysfunction found that ADT-G levels in the 124 control women were comparable to those in the 121 women with sexual dysfunction.[66]

Selective Estrogen Receptor Modulators

Selective estrogen receptor modulators (SERMs) are a class of ligands that bind estrogen receptor subtypes and induce a unique profile of tissue-specific gene expression. Accordingly, each SERM may also be associated with a unique set of clinical responses. Ospemifene has estrogen antagonist action on breast and endometrium. Ospemifene, but not raloxifene or tamoxifen, can ameliorate the genital sexual symptoms of lack of estrogen.[331] Limited research suggests raloxifene and tamoxifen are not associated with sexual adverse effects.

Hormonal Contraceptives

The estrogen in combined systemic contraceptives increases SHBG and thus decreases available free testosterone. The decrease in sexual desire and subjective arousability in some women receiving oral contraceptives has been attributed to the decrease in free testosterone levels. However, to date low desire has not been associated with testosterone levels, even when mass spectrometry methods are used.[65,66] Hormonal contraceptives exert multiple psychological and biologic actions, some of which may positively affect sexuality, for example, by reducing anxiety about unwanted pregnancy and diminishing dysmenorrhea.[332]

Androgen Insensitivity Syndrome

Research is very limited on sexual function in 46,XY women with androgen insensitivity syndrome due to mutations in the androgen receptor. Women with complete androgen insensitivity syndrome have a female phenotype with full breast development but variable shallow vaginal development, which may require surgical intervention or progressive dilatation. Small cross-sectional studies indicate healthy sexual response with orgasms and experience of self-stimulation and of intercourse.[328,333-336] However, these women are often confronted with complex psychosocial issues related to the mismatch between their genetic sex and their gender role, the timing of diagnosis and timing of disclosure to the woman, and infertility. Reduced sexual confidence, self-esteem, and depression are noted in these studies.

ASSESSMENT OF SEXUAL DYSFUNCTION

Assessment of sexual function is an important part of the general assessment of patients with endocrine diseases. Open-ended, nonjudgmental questions such as, "Many men with diabetes notice changes in their erections or ejaculation—are you having any difficulties?" can facilitate further discussion of sexual problems. When sexual

problems are identified, sensitive and respectful inquiry into their nature and the current and past sexual context is necessary. Evaluating both partners together as well as individually can often uncover problems that may not be apparent in individual interviews (Table 20-4).

Evaluation of Men With Sexual Dysfunction

There are four important considerations in the evaluation of men with HSDDs. First, an important initial step in the evaluation is an interview of the couple to determine whether the patient primarily has ED or a sexual desire problem. Second, ascertain whether the couple has a relationship problem. Establish whether self-stimulation continues despite lack of desire for partnered sex. With the availability of Internet sites, sex alone, possibly on a frequent basis, may allow sexual expression in spite of relationship difficulties. Third, general health evaluation is necessary to exclude systemic illness, depression, and medication use. Last, testosterone levels should be measured to exclude androgen deficiency because androgen deficiency is an important treatable cause of HSDD.

The diagnostic workup of men with ED should start with an evaluation of general health (Tables 20-4 and 20-5).[10,11,337-342] The presence of diabetes mellitus, coronary

TABLE 20-4
Assessment of a Patient With Sexual Dysfunction

Assessment Questions	Comments
Questions Asked of One or Both Partners	
1. Sexual problems and reason for presenting at this time	Ask patients to describe sexual problems in their own words; clarify further with direct questions, giving options rather than leading questions, support and encouragement, acknowledgment of embarrassment, and reassurance that sexual problems are common
2. Duration, consistency, and priority if more than one problem is present	Are problems present in all situations? Which problem is most troubling?
3. Context of sexual problems	Emotional intimacy between partners, activity or behavior just before sexual activity, privacy, sexual communication, time of day and fatigue level, birth control (adequacy, type), risk of STIs, usefulness of sexual stimulation, sexual knowledge
4. Each partner's sexual response in areas other than the given problem area	Both currently and before the onset of the sexual problems
5. Reaction of each partner	How has each reacted emotionally, sexually, and behaviorally?
6. Previous help	Compliance with recommendations and effectiveness
Questions Asked of Each Partner When Seen Alone*	
1. Partner's own assessment of the situation	Sometimes it is easier to disclose symptom severity (e.g., total lack of desire) in the partner's absence
2. Sexual response with self-stimulation	Also inquire about sexual thoughts and fantasies
3. Past sexual experiences	Positive and negative aspects
4. Developmental history	Relationships to others in the home while growing up; losses, traumas, to whom (if anyone) was the patient close; was he or she shown physical affection, love, respect?
5. Past or current sexual, emotional, and physical abuse	Explain that abuse questions are routine and do not necessarily imply causation of the problems; it is helpful to ask whether the patient ever felt hurt or threatened in the relationship and, if so, whether he or she wishes to give more information
6. Physical health, especially conditions leading to debility and fatigue, difficulty with mobility (e.g., in caressing a partner, performing self-stimulation), and difficulties with self-image (e.g., from obesity, Cushing syndrome. hypogonadism)	Specifically, ask about medications with known sexual side effects, including SSRIs, SNRIs, β-blockers, narcotics, antiandrogens, GnRH agonists
7. Evaluation of mood	A significant correlation of sexual function and mood (including anxiety and depression) warrants routine screening for mood disorder using either a questionnaire (e.g., Beck Inventory) or semistructured series of questions

*Items 3 through 5 of the single-patient interview may sometimes be omitted (e.g., for a recent problem after decades of healthy sexual function).
GnRH, gonadotropin-releasing hormone; SSNIs, selective serotonin norepinephrine reuptake inhibitors; SSRIs, selective serotonin reuptake inhibitors; STIs, sexually transmitted infections.
Adapted from Basson R. Sexual dysfunction in women. *N Engl J Med.* 2006;354:1497-1506. Copyright ©2006 Massachusetts Medical Society. All rights reserved.

TABLE 20-5
Directed Diagnostic Evaluation of Erectile Dysfunction

History

Ascertain Psychosexual History
The nature of sexual dysfunction: whether the primary problem is decreased desire, erectile dysfunction, premature or delayed ejaculation, or difficulty in achieving orgasms
The strength of marital relationship and marital discord
Depression
Stress
Sexual performance anxiety
Knowledge and beliefs about sexuality

Ascertain Risk Factors
The presence of diabetes mellitus, hypertension, hyperlipidemia, coronary artery disease, end-stage renal disease, and peripheral vascular disease
History of spinal cord injury, stroke, or Alzheimer disease
Prostate or pelvic surgery
Pelvic injury
Medications such as antihypertensives, antidepressants, antipsychotics, antiandrogens, and inhibitors of androgen production
The use of recreational drugs such as alcohol, cocaine, opiates, and tobacco

Ascertain Factors That Might Affect Choice of Therapy and the Patient's Response to It
Coexisting coronary artery disease and its symptoms and severity
Exercise tolerance
The use of nitrates or nitrate donors
The use of α-adrenergic blockers
The use of vasodilators for hypertension or congestive heart failure
The use of foods (such as cranberry juice) or drugs (such as erythromycin, protease inhibitors, ketoconazole, and itraconazole) that might affect metabolism of PDE5 inhibitors

Physical Examination

Ascertain signs of androgen deficiency, such as loss of secondary sex characteristics, eunuchoidal proportions, small testicular volume, or breast enlargement
Genital and perineal sensation to evaluate neurologic deficit from spinal cord lesion, previous stroke, or peripheral neuropathy
Blood pressure and postural change in blood pressure
Evaluate femoral and pedal pulses and evidence of lower extremity ischemia
Penile examination to exclude Peyronie disease or other penile deformities

Basic Laboratory Evaluation That Should Be Performed in All Men With ED

Fasting blood glucose
Plasma lipids
Serum testosterone level

ED, Erectile dysfunction; PDE5, phosphodiesterase 5.

artery disease, peripheral vascular disease, hypertension, stroke, spinal cord or back injury, multiple sclerosis, depression, or dementia should be verified. Information about use of recreational drugs such as alcohol, marijuana, cocaine, and tobacco; prescription medications, particularly antihypertensives, antiandrogens, antidepressants, and antipsychotic drugs; and nonprescription over-the-counter supplements is important because almost a quarter of all cases of impotence can be attributed to medications. A detailed sexual history including the nature of relationships, partner expectations, situational erectile failure, performance anxiety, and marital discord needs to be elicited. It is important to distinguish between inability to achieve erection, changes in sexual desire, failure to achieve orgasm and ejaculation, and dissatisfaction with the sexual rela-

tionship, as the etiologic factors vary with the type of sexual disorder.

A directed physical examination should focus on secondary sex characteristics, the presence or absence of breast enlargement and testicular volume; evaluation of femoral and pedal pulses; neurologic examination to determine the presence of motor weakness, perineal sensation, anal sphincter tone, and bulbocavernosus reflex; and examination of the penis to evaluate any unusual curvature, palpable plaques, or superficial lesions.[337-342]

The laboratory tests in the evaluation of a man with ED usually include measurements of hemoglobin, blood glucose, blood urea nitrogen and creatinine, plasma lipid, and testosterone levels.

Thus, the initial diagnostic workup in most men presenting with ED consists of general health evaluation; evaluation of cardiovascular risk by the measurements of blood glucose, plasma lipids, and blood chemistries; and measurement of serum testosterone levels. Further evaluation using more invasive diagnostic testing is limited to those men who do not respond to an empiric trial of oral PDE5 inhibitors; these patients should be referred to a specialist for detailed urologic evaluation.

Self-reporting questionnaires are useful because many men with ED do not voluntarily come forward to their physicians and state their sexual complaints for a variety of reasons.[337-340] The International Index of Erectile Function (IIEF), for example, is a multidimensional scale consisting of 15 questions that address relevant domains of male sexual function, including sexual desire, intercourse satisfaction, orgasmic function, and overall satisfaction[337]; a short form is also available.[340]

The diagnosis of androgen deficiency should be made only in men with consistent symptoms and signs and unequivocally low early morning serum testosterone levels that are below the lower limit of the normal range for healthy young men (e.g., testosterone <300 ng/dL in some laboratories) on at least two occasions.[1,11,64] Initial evaluation is directed at excluding systemic illness, eating disorders, excessive exercise, and use of medicines and recreational drugs that can suppress testosterone levels. The measurement of morning total testosterone level by a reliable assay, such as liquid chromatography tandem mass spectrometry (LC-MS/MS), using rigorously derived reference ranges, remains the best initial test.[343-346] The advent of LC-MS/MS, the availability of a testosterone calibrator from the National Institute of Standards and Technologies (NIST), and the institution of Hormone Standardization Program for Testosterone (HoST) has greatly improved the accuracy of testosterone assays and reduced interlaboratory variability among Centers for Disease Control and Prevention (CDC)-certified laboratories.[343-346]

The measurement of free testosterone levels is useful in men with suspected SHBG alteration due to genetic factors, aging, obesity, diabetes, chronic illness, thyroid and liver disease, and HIV or hepatitis B or C infection.[347] Free testosterone levels should be measured using a reliable assay, such as the equilibrium dialysis assay, in a laboratory that has experience in performing this assay.[64] Free testosterone concentrations can also be calculated from total testosterone and SHBG concentrations.[347] However, Zakharov and colleagues[348] have shown that the published linear law of mass action equations based on a linear model of testosterone's binding to SHBG in which one molecule of SHBG binds one molecule of testosterone with a single binding affinity constant are erroneous.[348] These studies have shown that testosterone's binding to SHBG is a dynamic multistep process that includes heterogeneity in circulating isoforms of SHBG dimer, an allosteric interaction between the two binding sites on SHBG such that the binding affinities of the two binding sites on SHBG are not equivalent, and convergence to an energetically favored bound state in which both sites are occupied.[348] The free testosterone levels computed using this dynamic multistep binding with allosteric match closely the values measured directly by equilibrium dialysis.[348]

In men found to be androgen-deficient, measurement of LH levels helps distinguish between testicular (LH elevated) and hypothalamic-pituitary (LH low or inappropriately normal) defects.[64] Men with hypogonadotropic hypogonadism may require measurement of serum prolactin, serum iron, and total iron binding capacity; evaluation of other pituitary hormones; and a pituitary MRI. The diagnostic yield of pituitary imaging to exclude pituitary tumor can be improved by selecting men whose total testosterone level is less than 150 ng/dL or who have panhypopituitarism, persistent hyperprolactinemia, or symptoms of tumor mass.[251,252]

There is considerable debate about the usefulness and cost-effectiveness of hormonal evaluation and the extent to which androgen deficiency should be investigated in men presenting with ED. Between 8% and 10% of men with ED have low testosterone levels; the prevalence of androgen deficiency increases with advancing age.[216,349-351] The prevalence of low testosterone levels is not significantly different among men who present with ED and in an age-matched population.[141] These data are consistent with the proposal that ED and androgen deficiency are two common but independently distributed disorders.[141] However, it is important to exclude androgen deficiency in this patient population. Androgen deficiency is a correctable cause of sexual dysfunction, and some men with ED and low testosterone levels will respond to testosterone replacement. Androgen deficiency may be a manifestation of serious systemic disease and may have additional deleterious effects on the individual's health; for instance, androgen deficiency might contribute to osteoporosis and loss of muscle mass and function. In large studies,[64] only a small fraction of men with ED and low testosterone levels have been found to have space-occupying lesions of the hypothalamic-pituitary region.[251,252] In one large survey, all of the hypothalamic-pituitary lesions were found in men with serum testosterone levels lower than 150 ng/dL.[252] Therefore, the cost-effectiveness of the diagnostic workup to rule out an underlying lesion of the hypothalamic-pituitary region can be increased by limiting the workup to men with serum testosterone levels less than 150 ng/dL.[64]

If the history, physical examination, and laboratory tests do not identify medical problems needing further workup, then a cost-effective approach is to prescribe a trial of oral PDE5 inhibitor provided there are no contraindications (e.g., nitrate use).

Tests that evaluate the integrity of penile vasculature and blood flow[352,353] are not needed in most patients with ED, are reserved for patients in whom the results of these tests would alter the management or prognosis, and should be performed only by those with considerable experience with their use. The penile brachial blood pressure index is a simple and specific, but not a sensitive, index of vascular insufficiency. It is rarely used today in the evaluation of ED.

Intracavernosal injection of a vasoactive agent such as PGE₁ can be useful as a diagnostic as well as a potential therapeutic modality. This procedure can reveal whether the patient will respond to this therapeutic modality and can facilitate patient education about the procedure and its potential side effects. Failure to respond to intracaver-nosal injection can raise the suspicion of vascular insufficiency or a venous leak that might need further evaluation and treatment.

Most men with ED do not need duplex color sonography, cavernosography, or pelvic angiography.[10,11,341,342,352] For instance, angiography could be useful in a young man with arterial insufficiency associated with pelvic trauma. Similarly, suspicion of congenital or traumatic venous leak in a young men presenting with ED would justify a cavernosography. In each instance, confirmation of the vascular lesion might lead to consideration of surgery. Duplex ultrasonography can provide a noninvasive evaluation of vascular function.[352]

Nocturnal penile tumescence testing is not needed for most patients being evaluated for ED and is recommended only for a limited number of patients with a high clinical suspicion of psychogenic ED or situational problems, or to document preoperatively poor penile rigidity, or for medical-legal reasons. Although recording of nocturnal penile tumescence in a sleep laboratory for successive nights can help differentiate organic from psychogenic impotence, this test is expensive and labor intensive. The introduction of portable RigiScan devices in 1985 has provided clinicians with a reliable means of continuously monitoring penile tumescence and rigidity at home.[353] It is a multicomponent device that the patient wears at bedtime for 2 to 3 nights. It has two wire gauge loops that are placed around the base and tip of the penis that record changes in penile circumference and rigidity. Data are stored and downloaded via a software program that allows for interpretation. For most cases, a careful history of nighttime or early morning erections provides a reasonable correlation with nocturnal penile tumescence and RigiScan studies.[353]

Evaluation of Women With Sexual Dysfunction

Sexual dysfunction is diagnosed by clinical interview and, when necessary, physical examination. Sexual function questionnaires can be used to monitor treatment.[354-356] One such instrument is the FSFI.[354,355] Despite the original intention of such questionnaires to monitor treatment progress, they are frequently (mis)used to diagnose sexual dysfunction in women who have not been clinically assessed. Moreover, the FSFI is based on the DSM-IV criteria of sexual disorders, which are grounded in the conceptualization of female sexual response beginning with conscious desire leading to a phase of arousal, then orgasm, and then resolution, these phases being in set order, discrete, and necessary for normal function. The limitations of the FSFI include the lack of recognition of triggered desire and the normality of beginning an experience initially sexually neutral, the possibility of sexual satisfaction without orgasm, and a focus on partnered sex, which interferes with accurate scoring of women who are currently unpartnered.[355] Although the FSFI has been used in most studies of women's sexual function including those of women with endocrine disease, more contemporary instruments such as the National Survey of Sexual Attitudes and Lifestyles (Natsal-3)[356] better reflect the importance of sexual satisfaction in contrast to many previous instruments. This attribute of Natsal-SF instrument is particularly important because patients may report satisfaction despite dysfunction, and dissatisfaction can occur in the context of a functional response[357]: women's satisfaction may or may not include orgasms.[200] A recent study confirms strong links between sexual satisfaction and sexual motivation.[358]

TABLE 20-6
Directed Physical Examination of the Woman With Sexual Dysfunction

General Examination

Signs of systemic disease leading to low energy, low desire, or low arousability, such as anemia, bradycardia, and slow relaxing reflexes of hypothyroidism

Signs of connective tissue disease, such as scleroderma or Sjögren syndrome, that are associated with vaginal dryness

Disabilities that might preclude movements involved in caressing a partner, self-stimulation, or intercourse

Disfigurements or presence of stomas or catheters that may decrease sexual self-confidence leading to low desire, low arousability

External Genitalia

Sparsity of pubic hair suggesting low adrenal androgens

Vulval skin disorders, including lichen sclerosis, that may cause soreness with sexual stimulation and reduce sexual sensitivity

Cracks or fissures in the interlabial folds suggestive of chronic candidiasis

Labial abnormalities that may cause embarrassment or sexual hesitancy

Past genital mutilation: absent labia minora, minimal or no clitoral tissue

Introitus

Vulval disease involving introitus, such as pallor, friability, loss of elasticity and moisture of vulval atrophy; lichen sclerosis; recurrent splitting of the posterior fourchette manifested as just visible white lines perpendicular to the fourchette edge; disfigurement, narrowing from genital mutilation; abnormalities of the hymen, adhesions of the labia minora, swellings in the area of the major vestibular glands, allodynia (pain sensation from touch stimulus) of the crease between the outer hymenal edge and the inner edge of the labia minora—typical of provoked vestibulodynia

Presence of cystocele, rectocele, prolapse interfering with the woman's sexual self-image

Inability to tighten and relax perivaginal muscles often associated with hypertonicity of pelvic muscles and midvaginal dyspareunia; abnormal vaginal discharge associated with burning dyspareunia

Internal Examination

Pelvic muscle tone, presence of tenderness, trigger points on palpation of deep levator ani due to underlying hypertonicity

Full Bimanual Examination

Presence of nodules or tenderness in the cul-de-sac or vaginal fornix and along uterosacral ligaments, retroverted fixed uterus as causes of deep dyspareunia

Tenderness on palpation of posterior bladder wall from anterior vaginal wall suggestive of bladder disease

Adapted from Basson R. Sexual dysfunction in women. *N Engl J Med.* 2006;354:1497-1506, used with permission.

Physical Examination

Physical examination, including pelvic and genital examination, is part of routine care (Table 20-6) and can be reassuring to the patient by confirming normal anatomy and tissue health. Unless dyspareunia is involved, it is not often that physical examination identifies the cause of sexual dysfunction. For some women with a history of coercive or abusive sexual experiences, such examination may cause extreme anxiety. The reason for the examination and an explanation of what will and will not be done should be provided before the examination begins. If the woman would prefer to invite her partner to be present, then the careful examination can be highly educational for both partners. In women with genitopelvic penetration pain disorder with a marked component of vaginismus, the vaginal examination should be delayed until psychological therapy renders it possible and informative for both the patient (and partner if present) and the clinician.

Laboratory Testing

Laboratory testing plays a small role in women's sexual evaluation. Estrogen activity is best evaluated by history and examination. The commercially available estradiol radioimmunoassays lack the sensitivity and precision required to measure the low concentrations present in the older woman; also, these assays do not measure estrone, the major estrogen after menopause. As discussed earlier, serum testosterone levels do not correlate with sexual function, even when LC-MS/MS assays are used.[65,66] The circulating testosterone levels may not reflect intracrine production, metabolism, or activity of androgens. Measurement of testosterone metabolites has been proposed as a marker of intracrine plus gonadal production of testosterone,[67] but the circulating levels of these metabolites have been shown to be similar in women with and without sexual dysfunction.[66] The optimal markers of total androgen activity and the clinical usefulness of these metabolites remain to be demonstrated. Prolactin or thyrotropin should be measured if there are other symptoms that suggest abnormality.

MANAGEMENT OF SEXUAL DYSFUNCTION IN MEN

Treatment of Hypoactive Sexual Desire in Men

There is need to focus on the couple when the patient has a sexual partner. Treating the sexual dysfunction in the male partner improves the female partner's sexual function and satisfaction. Comorbid depression should be treated and relationship difficulties addressed. The efficacy of cognitive and behavioral therapies has not been evaluated systematically in men with HSDD.

Testosterone therapy should be considered in men with HSDD who have androgen deficiency, even though there are no randomized trials of testosterone in men with HSDD. Much of the information about the effects of testosterone on sexual desire has emerged from open-label trials of testosterone in hypogonadal men.[64,124,359-362] These trials recruited men based on the presence of low testosterone levels alone.[124,359-362] Testosterone therapy in these trials has been associated with significant improvements in overall sexual activity, sexual desire, attention to erotic cues, and the duration and frequency of nocturnal penile erections.[64,124,359-362] Meta-analyses of randomized testosterone trials mostly in middle-aged and older men reported greater improvements in nocturnal erections, sexual thoughts and motivation, number of successful intercourses, scores of erectile function, and overall sexual satisfaction in men receiving testosterone than in those receiving placebo.[64,134,136,142,362] A large placebo-controlled randomized trial of testosterone in older men with decreased sexual desire and unequivocally low testosterone levels, funded by the National Institutes of Health, is currently in progress and should provide novel information about the efficacy of testosterone.[363]

Treatment of Erectile Disorder

The current practice employs a stepwise approach that first utilizes minimally invasive therapies that are easy to use

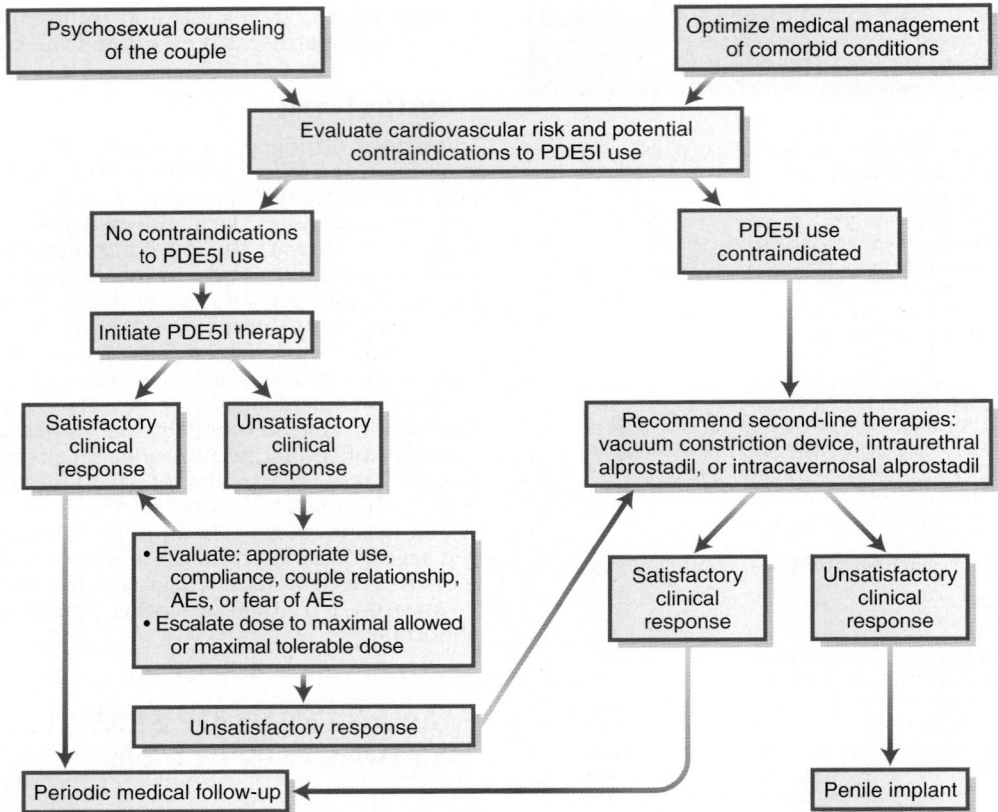

Figure 20-9 An algorithmic approach to the treatment of erectile dysfunction in men. AE, adverse effects; PDE5I, phosphodiesterase 5 inhibitor.

and have fewer adverse effects and progresses to more invasive therapies that may require injections or surgical intervention after the first-line choices have been exhausted (Fig. 20-9). The physician should discuss the risks, benefits, and alternatives of all therapies with the couple. The selection of the therapeutic modality should be based on the underlying cause, patient preference, the nature and strength of the relationship with his sexual partner, and the absence or presence of underlying CVD and other comorbid conditions.[10,11,341,342] All patients with ED can benefit from psychosexual counseling.[10,11,341,342,364-368]

In the execution of good medical practice, treatment of all associated medical disorders should be optimized. In men with diabetes mellitus, efforts to optimize glycemic control should be instituted, although improving glycemic control may not improve sexual function. In men with hypertension, control of blood pressure should be optimized and, if possible, the therapeutic regimen may be modified to remove antihypertensive drugs that impair sexual function. This strategy is not always feasible because almost all antihypertensive agents have been associated with sexual dysfunction; the frequency of this adverse event is less with converting enzyme inhibitors and angiotensin receptor blockers than with other agents.

First-Line Therapies

Psychosexual Counseling. The major goals of psychosexual therapy are to reduce performance anxiety, develop the patient's sexual skills and knowledge, modify negative sexual attitudes, and improve communication between partners.[364] Counseling can be of benefit in both psy-

TABLE 20-7
Goals of Psychosexual Therapy in Men With Sexual Dysfunction

- Reduce performance anxiety; train the couple to avoid "spectatoring" and be "sensate focused"
- Identify relationship problems and improve partner communication and intimacy
- Modify sexual attitudes and beliefs
- Improve couple's sexual skills

Adapted from Rosen RC. Psychogenic erectile dysfunction: classification and management. *Urol Clin North Am.* 2001;28:269-278.

chogenic and organic causes of sexual dysfunction[364-370] (Table 20-7).

An individual's focus on sexual performance rather than erotic stimulation is a major factor in the pathophysiology of psychogenic ED[364,365]; this behavior is referred to as *spectatoring*. Many experts recommend a *sensate focus* treatment approach in which the couple avoids intercourse and engages in nongenital, nondemanding, pleasure-seeking exercises in order to reduce performance anxiety.[364]

Involving the partner in the counseling process helps dispel misperceptions about the problem, decreases stress, enhances intimacy and the ability to talk about sex, and increases the chances of successful outcome.[364] Counseling sessions are also helpful in uncovering conflicts in relationships, psychiatric problems, alcohol and drug abuse, and significant misperceptions about sex. As many men and women may harbor misinformation and unrealistic expectations about sexual performance and age-related changes

TABLE 20-8

Clinical Pharmacology of Selective PDE5 Inhibitors*

Feature	Sildenafil	Vardenafil	Tadalafil	Avanafil
Commercial name	Viagra	Levitra	Cialis	Stendra, Spedra
T_{max}	0.5-2.0 h	0.7-0.9 h	2 h	30-45 min
$T\frac{1}{2}$	3-4 h	4-5 h	16.9 h (young) 21.6 (old)	5 h
Onset of erection (min)	30-60	15-45	20-30 min	15 min
Muscle selectivity (ratio of PDE6 IC_{50}/PDE5 IC_{50})	11 (most selective)	25	187 (least selective)	>100-fold
Retinal selectivity (ratio of PDE11/PDE5 IC_{50}), higher number indicates greater selectivity	780	1160 (most selective)	5 (least selective)	>10,000-fold
Effect of food and alcohol	C_{max} decreased	Minimal change	No change	Absorption delayed
Protein binding	96%	94%	94%	98-99%
Bioavailability	41%	Not available	15%	Not available

Sildenafil Vardenafil Tadalafil Avanafil

*Comparative pharmacokinetic data on the three oral selective PDE5 inhibitors. Selectivity refers to the ratio of the IC_{50} for a PDE isoform other than PDE5 to the IC_{50} for PDE5. A higher number implies greater selectivity. Sildenafil is more selective than tadalafil for PDE5 relative to PDE11, but it is less selective than tadalafil for PDE6 relative to PDE5.
C_{max}, maximum plasma concentration; IC_{50}, 50% inhibitory concentration; PDE, phosphodiesterase; $T\frac{1}{2}$, half-life; T_{max}, time to peak concentration.
Adapted from references 99, 101, 373.

in sexual function, cognitive restructuring techniques are helpful in correcting sexual myths and beliefs.[364] There is a paucity of outcome data on the effectiveness of this psychobehavioral therapy, but meta-analyses have reported benefit from group psychotherapy administered in conjunction with PDE5 inhibitors.[367]

Selective Phosphodiesterase 5 Inhibitors (Tables 20-8 and 20-9). Selective PDE5 inhibitors are safe and effective and have become widely accepted as first-line therapy for patients with ED, except in men for whom these drugs are contraindicated.[9-11,99,101,341,342,370-372] Selective PDE5 inhibitors are contraindicated in men using nitrates on a regular basis, in those with heart disease in whom sexual activity is not recommended, and in those with nonarteritic anterior ischemic optic neuropathy.[10,11,99,101,341,342,371,372]

Mechanisms of Action. Three classes of enzymes—adenylyl cyclase, guanylyl cyclase, and PDEs—play an important role in regulating the intracavernosal concentrations of cAMP and cGMP. PDEs hydrolyze cAMP and cGMP, thus reducing their concentrations within the cavernosal smooth muscle.[100,101,104-106,373-376] Although PDE isoforms 2, 3, 4, and 5 are expressed in the penis, only PDE5 is specific to the nitric oxide/cGMP pathway in the corpora cavernosa.[376] PDE inhibitors sildenafil, vardenafil, tadalafil, avanafil, and udenafil are relatively selective inhibitors of PDE5.[100,101,104-106,373-399] These drugs block the hydrolysis of cGMP induced by nitric oxide, thus promoting cavernosal smooth muscle relaxation. The action of these drugs requires an intact nitric oxide response, as well as constitutive synthesis of cGMP by the smooth muscle cells of the corpora cavernosa. By selectively inhibiting cGMP catabolism in the cavernosal smooth muscle cells, PDE5 inhibitors restore the natural erectile response to sexual stimulation but do not produce an erection in the absence of sexual stimulation.

TABLE 20-9

Common Adverse Effects of Selective Phosphodiesterase Inhibitors

1. Headache
2. Flushing
3. Dyspepsia
4. Nasal and sinus congestion
5. Dizziness
6. Abnormal vision*
7. Back pain*
8. Myalgia*
9. Hearing problems

*These adverse effects are related to nonselective inhibition of phosphodiesterase isoforms in other tissues. Headache, flushing, and nasal congestion are related to the drug's mechanism of vasodilator action.
Adapted from Wespes E, Rammal A, Garbar C. Sildenafil no-responders: hemodynamic and morphometric studies. *Eur Urol.* 2005;48:136-139; Brock GB, McMahon CG, Chen KK, et al. Efficacy and safety of tadalafil for the treatment of erectile dysfunction: results of integrated analyses. *J Urol.* 2002;168:1332-1336; Morales A, Gingell C, Collins M, et al. Clinical safety of oral sildenafil citrate (Viagra) in the treatment of erectile dysfunction. *Int J Impot Res.* 1998;10:69-73; Katz EG, Tan RB, Rittenberg D, Hellstrom WJ. Avanafil for erectile dysfunction in elderly and younger adults: differential pharmacology and clinical utility. *Ther Clin Risk Manag.* 2014;10:701-711.

Clinical Pharmacology (see Table 20-8). Although the three currently available PDE inhibitors have some structural similarities, they differ in their selectivity and pharmacokinetics (see Table 20-8). The common adverse effects of the available PDE5 inhibitors—headache, visual problems, flush, and myalgias—are related to nonselective inhibition of PDE isoforms 6 and 11 in other organ systems[101] (see Table 20-9). The selectivity of PDE5 inhibitor is the ratio of its inhibitory potency for PDE isoforms other than type

5 relative to its inhibitory potency for PDE isoform.[101] For PDE6, tadalafil is the most selective and sildenafil is the least selective; for PDE11, vardenafil is the most selective and tadalafil is the least selective.[101] The retinal side effects of sildenafil are related to inhibition of PDE6 in the retina, whereas muscle aches experienced by a small fraction of men using tadalafil are related to inhibition of PDE11 in the skeletal muscle.[101]

Pharmacokinetics (see Table 20-8). After oral administration of sildenafil, peak plasma concentrations are achieved within 30 to 120 minutes, after which plasma concentrations decline, with a half-life of 4 hours (see Table 20-8).[100,373-382] Vardenafil achieves peak concentrations within 0.7 to 0.9 hour and has a half-life of 4 to 5 hours. The peak concentrations of tadalafil are achieved at 2 hours, and its half-life of 16.9 hours in young men is significantly longer than the half-lives of sildenafil and vardenafil. The half-life of tadalafil is even longer in older men (21.6 hours) than in young men (16.9 hours).[100,373-376] Because of the relatively short half-lives of vardenafil and sildenafil, these drugs should be taken 1 to 4 hours before the planned intercourse; in contrast, tadalafil, because of its longer half-life, does not have to be taken on demand, although it can be.[100,373-376] The second-generation PDE5 inhibitors avanafil and udenafil have a more rapid onset of action than the first-generation PDE5 inhibitors sildenafil, vardenafil, and tadalafil.[377-380]

Food, particularly a high-fat meal and large amounts of alcohol, can delay and decrease the absorption of sildenafil.[381,382] However, early pharmacokinetic studies have not reported changes in maximum serum concentrations or absorption rates of vardenafil or tadalafil due to food or moderate alcohol ingestion.[376]

Efficacy. The orally active, selective PDE5 inhibitors— sildenafil, vardenafil, avanafil, udenafil, and tadalafil— have been shown to be effective and safe in randomized clinical trials of men with ED.[9-11,379-405] In men treated with oral, selective PDE5 inhibitors, the rates of successful intercourse vary from 50% to 65%, and rates of improved erections vary from 70% to 75%.[379-405] The selective PDE5 inhibitors are effective in men of all ethnic groups and ages[379-405] who have ED due to a multitude of causes, although response rates vary in different patient subgroups.[379-405]

Introduced to the U.S. market in March 1998, sildenafil citrate (Viagra, Pfizer, New York, NY) was the first effective oral agent for the treatment of ED.[406] The efficacy of sildenafil has been demonstrated in men with organic, psychogenic, or mixed ED in multiple randomized controlled trials (RCTs)[383-390,406] and confirmed by meta-analyses of randomized trials.[386-388] In these trials, patients receiving sildenafil experienced greater increments in the number of successful attempts per month, penile rigidity, frequency of vaginal penetration, and maintenance of erection than those receiving placebo.[386-388] Increasing doses of sildenafil were associated with higher mean scores for the frequency of penetration and maintenance of erections after sexual penetration. The mean scores for orgasms, intercourse satisfaction, and overall satisfaction were also significantly higher in the sildenafil group than in the placebo group.[386-388] Sildenafil also is an effective treatment for ED in men with diabetes mellitus.[389,390] A meta-analysis of randomized clinical trials of sildenafil confirmed its efficacy in improving erectile function in men with diabetes mellitus.[390]

In the vardenafil efficacy trials, 5-, 10-, and 20-mg doses of vardenafil were all superior to placebo in improving erectile function domain scores; the improvements in erectile function scores were dose-related.[391-397] Vardenafil improved rates of vaginal penetration, penile rigidity, intercourse success, and satisfaction with sexual experience in men with ED from diverse causes.[391-397]

Similarly, in randomized, clinical trials, 2.5-, 5-, 10-, and 20-mg doses of tadalafil were each superior to placebo in improving erectile function scores.[398-402] The beneficial effects of tadalafil were dose-related.[398-402]

Two new PDE5 inhibitors have been introduced recently in clinical practice. Avanafil has a very rapid onset of action because of its rapid absorption, which allows it to reach maximum circulating concentration in about 30 to 45 minutes.[377-379] Therefore, a majority of patients taking avanafil are able to engage in sexual activity within 15 minutes.[377-379] Udenafil also has a relatively rapid onset of action, with a time to maximum serum concentrations of 1.0 to 1.5 hours. It has been approved in Korea, Russia, and the Philippines, but not in the United States.[380]

PDE5 inhibitors are effective in men with ED due to a variety of causes, including spinal cord injury and radical prostatectomy.[389,390] In general, baseline sexual function correlates positively with response to PDE5 inhibitors, and patients with diabetes mellitus or previous prostate surgery respond less well than patients with psychogenic or vasculogenic ED.[389,390] Because there is no baseline characteristic that predicts the likelihood of failure to respond to sildenafil therapy, a therapeutic trial of PDE5 inhibitors should be tried in all patients except in those in whom it is contraindicated.[372]

Adverse Effects (see Table 20-9). In clinical trials, the adverse effects that have been reported with greater frequency in men treated with PDE5 inhibitors than in those treated with placebo include headaches, flushing, rhinitis, dyspepsia, muscle aches, and visual disturbances.[101,372,403-405] The occurrence of headache, flushing, and rhinitis, a direct consequence of nonselective PDE5 inhibition in other organ systems, is related to the administered dose. These drugs do not affect semen characteristics.[407,408] No cases of priapism were noted in the pivotal clinical trials.

Several cases of nonarteritic anterior ischemic optic neuropathy have been reported after ingestion of oral PDE5 inhibitor use.[409,410] This condition is characterized by the sudden onset of monocular visual loss due to acute ischemia of the anterior portion of the optic nerve in the absence of demonstrable arteritis. This may progress to partial or complete infarction of the optic nerve head resulting in permanent visual loss or visual field cuts.[409,410] Although a cause-and-effect relationship with PDE5 inhibitor use has not been established, patients with history of sudden visual loss should not be treated with PDE5 inhibitors without ophthalmologic evaluation.

Recently the U.S. Food and Drug Administration (FDA) noted several reports of sudden hearing loss with and without vestibular symptoms, such as tinnitus, vertigo, or dizziness, in temporal relationship to administration of sildenafil, vardenafil, and tadalafil in postmarketing surveillance. Hearing loss was also reported in a few patients in clinical trials of these drugs.[411,412] Hearing loss has been noted in patients using sildenafil for the treatment of pulmonary arterial hypertension. Although a causal relationship has not been established, the temporal relationship between the use of PDE5 inhibitors and the onset of sudden hearing loss prompted the FDA to recommend change in the product labeling for the drug class. One observational study has reported an association of PDE5 inhibitor use with an increased risk of melanoma.[413]

Cardiovascular and Hemodynamic Effects. In postmarketing surveillance of adverse events associated with sildenafil use, several instances of myocardial infarction and sudden death were reported in men using sildenafil in temporal relation to the ingestion of the drug[414]; many of these deaths occurred in individuals who also were taking nitrates. Because most men presenting with ED also have high prevalence of cardiovascular risk factors, it is unclear whether these events were causally related to the ingestion of sildenafil, underlying heart disease, or both.[414] In controlled studies,[415-418] oral administration of 100 mg of sildenafil to men with severe coronary artery disease produced only a small decrease in systemic blood pressure and no significant changes in cardiac output, heart rate, coronary blood flow, and coronary artery diameter. In a separate pooled analysis of five randomized, placebo-controlled trials of vardenafil,[417] the overall frequency of cardiovascular events was similar in vardenafil-treated men and placebo-treated men. However, vardenafil treatment was associated with a mild reduction in blood pressure (4.6-mm Hg decrease in systolic blood pressure) and a small increase in heart rate (2 beats per minute).[418] This led the American Heart Association and other experts to conclude that preexistent coronary artery disease by itself does not constitute a contraindication for the use of PDE5 inhibitors (Table 20-10).[418-424]

Drug-Drug Interactions. Sildenafil is metabolized mostly by the CYP2C9 and the CYP3A4 pathways. Cimetidine and erythromycin, inhibitors of CYP3A4, increase the plasma concentrations of sildenafil. HIV protease inhibitors may also alter the activity of the CYP3A4 pathway and affect the clearance of sildenafil.[425] Conversely, sildenafil is an inhibitor of the CYP2C9 metabolic pathway, and its administration could potentially affect the metabolism of drugs metabolized by this system, such as warfarin and tolbutamide. Combined administration of sildenafil and ritonavir results in significantly higher plasma levels of sildenafil than sildenafil given alone.[425] There are similar

---

TABLE 20-10

Guidelines for the Use of Selective Phosphodiesterase Inhibitors

1. Do not administer selective PDE5 inhibitors to men taking long-acting or short-acting nitrate drugs on a regular basis.
2. If the patient has stable coronary artery disease, is not taking long-acting nitrates, and uses short-acting nitrates only infrequently, the use of selective PDE5 inhibitor should be guided by careful consideration of risks.
3. Do not administer selective PDE5 inhibitors within 24 hours of the ingestion of any form of nitrate.
4. Advise men about the risks of the potential interaction between selective PDE5 inhibitors and nitrates, nitrate donors, and α-adrenergic blockers. Concurrent use of nitrates, nitrate donors, or α-adrenergic blockers could result in hypotension that could be serious.
5. In men with preexisting coronary artery disease, assess the risk of inducing cardiac ischemia during sexual activity before prescribing PDE5 inhibitors. This assessment may include a stress test.
6. In men who are taking vasodilators and diuretics for the treatment of hypertension or congestive heart failure, consider the potential risk of inducing hypotension because of potential interaction between PDE5 inhibitors and vasodilators, especially in patients with low blood volume.
7. In HIV-infected men, consider potential drug-drug interactions between selective PDE5 inhibitors and antiretroviral drugs and antimicrobial agents.

ACC/AHA, American College of Cardiology/American Heart Association; HIV, human immunodeficiency virus; PDE5, phosphodiesterase isoform 5.
Adapted from Cheitlin MD, Hutter AM Jr, Brindis RG, et al. Use of sildenafil (Viagra) in patients with cardiovascular disease: Technology and Practice Executive Committee [published erratum appears in *Circulation.* 1999;100(23):2389]. *Circulation.* 1999;99(1):168-177; Lue TF, Giuliano F, Montorsi F, et al. Summary of recommendations on sexual dysfunctions in men. *J Sex Med.* 2004;1:6-23.

---

interactions with other drugs, including saquinavir and itraconazole. Therefore, the doses of PDE5 inhibitors should be reduced appropriately in men taking protease inhibitors or erythromycin.

Grapefruit juice can alter oral drug pharmacokinetics by different mechanisms. Grapefruit juice given in normal amounts (e.g., 200-300 mL) or as whole fresh fruit segments can inactivate irreversibly intestinal CYP3A4, thus reducing presystemic metabolism and increasing oral bioavailability of PDE5 inhibitors.[426] Although the magnitude of this problem in clinical practice is unknown, it seems prudent to warn men who are contemplating the use of PDE5 inhibitors not to ingest more than a small amount of grapefruit juice.

The most serious interactions of PDE5 inhibitors are with the nitrates. The vasodilator effects of nitrates are augmented by PDE5 inhibitors; this also applies to inhaled forms of nitrates such as amyl nitrate or nitrites that are sold under the street name "poppers." Concomitant administration of the two vasodilator drugs can cause a potentially fatal decrease in blood pressure.[193-195]

PDE inhibitors should be used carefully in men taking α-adrenergic blockers. In men with congestive heart failure or those receiving vasodilator drugs or those who are using complex regimens of antihypertensive drugs, blood pressure should be monitored after initial administration of PDE5 inhibitors.[193-195] Several trials have demonstrated the safety of administering PDE5 inhibitors in combination with α-adrenergic blockers in men with ED and LUTS.[193-195]

Therapeutic Regimens. Excellent therapeutic guidelines have been published by expert panels from several societies.[99,371,372,419] To minimize the risk of hypotension and adverse cardiovascular events in association with the use of PDE5 inhibitors, the American Heart Association/ American College of Cardiology has published a list of recommendations (see Table 20-10), which should be followed rigorously.[419]

In most men with ED, sildenafil is started at an initial dose of 25 or 50 mg. If this dose does not produce any adverse effects, the dose can be titrated up to 100 mg.[99,371,372,427] Further dose adjustment should be guided by the therapeutic response to therapy and occurrence of adverse effects. Vardenafil should be started at an initial dose of 10 mg; the dose should be increased to 20 mg or decreased to 5 mg depending on the clinical response and the occurrence of adverse effects. Unit doses higher than 20 mg are not recommended. Tadalafil is started at an initial unit dose of 10 mg, with further adjustment of dose based on effectiveness and side effects. Tadalafil need not be taken more frequently than once every 48 hours.

In men taking protease inhibitors (particularly ritonavir and indinavir), erythromycin, ketoconazole, itraconazole, or large amounts of grapefruit, the doses of PDE5 inhibitors should be reduced, and doses greater than 25 mg of sildenafil, 5 mg of vardenafil, or 10 mg of tadalafil are not recommended.

Sildenafil and vardenafil are taken at least 1 hour before sexual intercourse and not more than once in any 24-hour period; because of its longer half-life, tadalafil need not be taken immediately before intercourse.

Based on the results of the randomized clinical trials,[408,428,429] the FDA has approved 2.5 mg or 5 mg tadalafil once daily for the treatment of ED. In the pivotal trials, men using 2.5 mg or 5 mg tadalafil once daily experienced greater improvements in erectile function compared with those taking a placebo.[408,428,429] Subsequent open-label extension studies indicated that once-daily 5 mg tadalafil for up to 2 years was effective in maintaining improvements in erectile function.[408,428,429] Thus, tadalafil may be taken at 2.5 mg or increased to 5 mg, as tolerated. The adverse events associated with once-daily administration of tadalafil included headaches, indigestion, back pain, muscle aches, nasal congestion, and flushing and were similar to those observed with on-demand tadalafil ingestion.[408,428,429] Once-daily regimen of tadalafil had no significant effect on semen or reproductive hormone levels.[408]

The Use of Phosphodiesterase 5 Inhibitors in Men With Coronary Artery Disease (see Table 20-10).[424] Before prescribing PDE5 inhibitors, cardiovascular risk factors should be assessed. If the patient has hypertension or symptomatic coronary artery disease, the treatment of those clinical disorders should be addressed first.[424] The use of nitrates must be ascertained because PDE5 inhibitors are contraindicated in individuals taking any form of nitrates regularly. PDE5 inhibitors should not be used within 24 hours of the use of nitrates or nitrate donors.[10,11,423,424]

Sexual activity can induce coronary ischemia in men with preexisting coronary artery disease[420]; therefore, men contemplating use of ED therapies should undergo assessment of their exercise tolerance. One practical way to assess exercise tolerance is to have the patient climb one or two flights of stairs. If the individual can safely climb one or two flights of stairs without angina or excessive shortness of breath, he can likely engage in sexual intercourse with a stable partner without inducing similar symptoms. Exercise testing before prescribing PDE5 inhibitors may be indicated in some men with significant heart disease to assess the risk of inducing cardiac ischemia during sexual activity.[419-421] Selective PDE inhibitors have been shown not to impair the ability of patients with stable coronary artery disease to engage in exercise at levels equivalent to that attained during sexual intercourse.[419-421] Similarly, each of the three PDE5 inhibitors has been shown not to have significant adverse effects on hemodynamics and cardiac events in carefully selected men with ED who did not have any contraindication for the use of PDE5 inhibitors.[417-424] None of the PDE5 inhibitors adversely affects total exercise time or time to ischemia during exercise testing in men with stable angina.[417-424]

Treatment of Patients Who Do Not Respond to Phosphodiesterase 5 Inhibitors. Although oral PDE5 inhibitor therapy has revolutionized the management of ED, not all men will respond to this treatment. The cumulative probability of intercourse success with sildenafil citrate increases with the number of attempts, reaching a maximum after eight attempts.[430] Based largely on these data,[430] the failure to respond to PDE inhibitor therapy has been defined as the failure to achieve satisfactory response even after eight attempts of either the highest approved dose (e.g., 100 mg sildenafil) or the highest tolerable dose of PDE inhibitor, whichever is lower. Many factors may contribute to apparent treatment failure, including failure to take the medication as recommended, suboptimal dose, dose-limiting adverse effects, psychological issues, partner and relationship issues, incorrect diagnosis, and patient-specific pathophysiologic factors.[430-432] In clinical trials of PDE5 inhibitors, treatment failures were reported predominantly in men who had diabetes mellitus, non-nerve sparing radical prostatectomy, cavernosal nerve damage, venous leak, and high disease severity.[430-432] In an evaluation of cavernosal smooth muscle biopsies in sildenafil nonresponders, Wespes and coworkers[432] found severe vascular lesions and cavernosal smooth muscle atrophy and fibrosis to be the underlying pathologic processes.

Patients may not take the medication appropriately because of inadequate instructions, failure to understand the instructions, adverse effects, or fear of adverse effects.[430-432]

Oral PDE5 inhibitors are taken optimally 1 to 2 hours before planned intercourse. The medication is unlikely to be effective if it is taken immediately before intercourse; a high-fat meal and large amounts of alcohol may further affect the maximal serum concentrations of sildenafil citrate. Similarly, patients may not take the appropriate dose because of side effects or fear of side effects. The men who have been misdiagnosed as having ED and whose primary sexual disorder is unresponsive to PDE5 inhibitors may be incorrectly deemed treatment failures. For instance, men with HSDD, Peyronie disease, or orgasmic or ejaculatory disorder would not be expected to respond to PDE5 inhibitors. The anxiety associated with resumption of sexual activity and unresolved relationship and partner issues can attenuate response to treatment. The sexual partner may not be willing or able to engage in sexual activity because of relationship issues, sexual disorder, or real or perceived health issues.

Patients who report lack of satisfactory response to initial administration of PDE5 inhibitors should be asked about the time of drug administration, the dose taken, and adverse effects experienced. Psychological and partner issues should be evaluated. The dose of PDE5 inhibitor should be increased gradually as tolerated. Should the patient not respond to maximal tolerable doses of PDE5 inhibitors, PDE5 inhibitors can be combined with vacuum devices or intraurethral therapy. Second-line therapies such as intracavernosal injections should be pursued. The men who are unresponsive to oral PDE5 inhibitors and second-line therapies may find penile implant an acceptable alternative.[430]

Cost-Effectiveness of Phosphodiesterase 5 Inhibitor Use for Erectile Disorder. A number of studies have evaluated the economic cost of treating ED in men in managed care health plans.[433-437] One simulation estimated sildenafil citrate cost to be approximately $11,000 per quality-adjusted life year (QALY) that it produces.[435] This amount is less than that for many other accepted treatments for medical disorders that cost less than $50,000 to $100,000 per QALY; thus, the cost-effectiveness of PDE5 inhibitor therapy compares favorably with other accepted medical therapies. Other analyses have concluded that PDE5 inhibitors and vacuum constriction devices are the most cost-effective of all the available therapeutic options.[433-437] Several recent analyses have shown that the financial burden imposed by patients with ED on managed care plans is surprisingly small.[433-437] In one such cost-utility analysis, the monthly cost of providing ED-related treatment services in a health plan with 100,000 members amounted to less than $0.10 per member.[435] Thus, the failure of many insurance companies to cover the cost of PDE5 inhibitor therapy is not informed by cost-utility analyses.

Second-Line Therapies

Vacuum Devices for Inducing Erection. The vacuum devices consist of a plastic cylinder, a vacuum pump, and an elastic constriction band.[438-440] The plastic cylinder fits over the penis and is connected to a vacuum pump. The negative pressure created by the vacuum within the cylinder draws blood into the penis, producing an erection. An elastic band slipped around the base of the penis traps the blood in the penis, maintaining an erection as long as the rubber band is retained. The constriction band should not be left in place for more than 30 minutes. Also, only vacuum devices with a pressure-limiting mechanism should be recommended to prevent injury due to high vacuum.

Limited data on the efficacy of vacuum devices from open-label trials indicate that these devices are safe, relatively inexpensive, and moderately effective.[438-440] They can impair ejaculation, resulting in entrapment of semen. Some couples dislike the lack of spontaneity engendered by the use of these devices. Partner cooperation is important for successful use of these devices.[440]

Intraurethral Therapies. An intraurethral system for delivery of alprostadil called *MUSE* (medicated urethral system for erection; VIVUS, Menlo Park, CA) was released in 1997. Alprostadil is a stable, synthetic form of PGE_1, which results in generation of cAMP and activation of protein kinase A. Activated protein kinase A stimulates K^+ channels, resulting in K^+ efflux from the cell. In addition, protein kinase A–mediated processes also result in a net decrease in intracellular calcium, favoring smooth muscle cell relaxation.

Alprostadil, when applied into the urethra, is absorbed through the urethral mucosa into the corpus cavernosum. In comparison to intracavernosal injection of PGE_1, intraurethral PGE_1 is easier to administer and has a lower frequency of adverse effects, particularly penile fibrosis.

Alprostadil is available in 125-, 250-, 500-, and 1000-μg strengths. Typically, the initial alprostadil dose of 250 μg is applied in the clinician's office to observe changes in blood pressure or urethral bleeding secondary to misapplication of the device into the urethra.

Initial randomized, placebo-controlled studies reported 40% to 60% success rates, defined as having at least one successful sexual intercourse during a 3-month study period.[441-443] In clinical practice, only about a third of men using intraurethral alprostadil will respond.[444]

Common side effects of intraurethral alprostadil are penile pain and urethral burning in up to 30% of patients[441-444]; its use also may cause dizziness, hypotension, and syncope in a small fraction of users. Intraurethral alprostadil can cause mild burning or itching in the vagina of the sexual partner. Intraurethral alprostadil should not be used by men whose partners are pregnant or planning to get pregnant.

Intracavernosal Injection of Vasoactive Agents (Table 20-11). The use of intracavernosal injections of vasoactive agents has been a cornerstone of the medical management of ED since the early 1980s. Patients can be taught to inject a vasoactive agent into their corpora cavernosa using a 27- or 30-gauge needle prior to the planned intercourse. Erections occur typically 15 minutes after intracorporal injection and last 45 to 90 minutes. Although intracavernosal injection therapy is highly effective,[445-452] it is associated with significantly higher complication rates than oral therapy and should be used only by practitioners who are experienced in the use of this therapy and who can provide emergency medical support to their patients in the event of a serious adverse event, such as priapism.

Although several agents—PGE_1, papaverine, and phentolamine—have been used alone or in combination,[445-453] only intracavernosal PGE_1 has been approved for clinical use. The long-term data on the efficacy and safety of intracavernosal therapy are sparse.

Several formulations of alprostadil (PGE_1) are commercially available (Caverject, Pharmacia; Prostin VR, Pharmacia; Edex, Schwarz Pharma). PGE_1 binds to PGE_1 receptors on the cavernosal smooth muscle cells, stimulates adenylyl cyclase, increases the concentrations of cAMP, and is a powerful smooth muscle relaxant. The usual dose is 5 to 20 μg, and response to therapy is dose-related and should be titrated.[445-451]

In one placebo-controlled efficacy trial, the intracavernosal alprostadil injection resulted in satisfactory sexual performance after more than 90% of administrations, and approximately 85% of men and their partners reported satisfactory sexual activity.[445] Intracavernosal alprostadil is more effective than intraurethral alprostadil.[449]

The common adverse effects of intracavernosal therapy include penile pain, occurrence of hematoma, formation of corporal nodules, penile fibrosis, and prolonged erections.[445-452] Despite the effectiveness of this approach in producing rigid erections, many patients do not relish injecting a needle into their penis; therefore, it is not surprising that long-term dropout rates are high.

Intracavernosal injections of papaverine, phentolamine, forskolin, and VIP have also been used, although these agents are not approved by the FDA.[453] Papaverine, derived originally from the poppy seed, is a nonspecific PDE inhibitor, which increases both intracellular cAMP and cGMP. It has a greater propensity to induce priapism and fibrosis with long-term use, and efficacy and long-term safety data from randomized, placebo-controlled trials are lacking. Therefore, there is insufficient information to evaluate its efficacy and safety.

Phentolamine is a competitive α_1- and α_2-adrenergic antagonist that contributes to smooth muscle relaxation. As a single agent it is minimally efficacious, but it has been used to potentiate the effects of papaverine, VIP, and PGE_1.[453] Randomized clinical trial data on its efficacy and safety are lacking. Therefore, there is insufficient information to evaluate its efficacy and safety.

A serious concern with the use of intracavernosal injection therapy is priapism. In patients who develop a prolonged or painful erection with PGE_1, either brethane 5 mg or pseudoephedrine 60 mg, administered orally, may be of benefit. If priapism persists longer than 4 hours, patients should be instructed to seek medical care in which aspiration alone or with the injection of an α-adrenergic agent is used to induce detumescence. If this fails, surgical therapy may be indicated to reverse a prolonged erection; otherwise, anoxic damage to the cavernosal smooth muscle cells and fibrosis can occur.

Third-Line Therapies

Penile Prosthesis. The penile prostheses are invasive and costly, but they can be an effective method for restoring

---

TABLE 20-11

Guidelines for Intracavernosal Therapy

1. Do not prescribe intracavernosal therapy to men who have psychiatric disorders, hypercoagulable states, sickle cell disease; those who are receiving anticoagulant therapy; or those who are unable to comprehend the risks or take appropriate action should complications occur.

2. Designate a physician or a urologist to be available to handle emergencies related to complications of intracavernosal injections such as prolonged erection and priapism.

3. Instruct the patient in the injection technique, the risks of intracavernosal therapy, and the steps to be taken in the event of prolonged erection or priapism.

4. Administer the first injection in the office and observe the blood pressure and heart rate response. This provides an excellent opportunity for educating the patient, observing adverse effects, and determining whether the patient will respond to intracavernosal therapy.

5. Start with a low dose of alprostadil and titrate the dose based on the erectile response and the duration of erection. Adjust the dose of alprostadil to achieve an erection that is sufficient for sexual intercourse but that does not last more than 30 minutes.

6. If the erection does not abate in 30 minutes, the patient should be instructed to take a tablet of pseudoephedrine or brethine or an intracavernosal injection of phenylephrine. If this is not effective, the patient should call the designated physician or the urologist, and come to the emergency room.

erectile function for patients with advanced organic disease who are unresponsive to other medical therapies, have significant structural disorders of the penis (e.g., Peyronie disease), or have suffered corporal loss from cancer or traumatic injury.[454-456]

Penile implants are paired supports that are placed in each of the two erectile bodies. There are two basic types of penile implants: hydraulic (fluid filled), referred to as inflatable prostheses; and malleable, semirigid rods, which are bendable but always remain firm in the penis.[454-456] Penile prostheses come in a variety of lengths and girths. Implantation surgery usually takes less than an hour and in most cases can be done as an outpatient procedure under general or regional anesthesia.

Infection and mechanical malfunction are the most common problems with penile prostheses. With recent improvements in materials and design, the chance of mechanical malfunction has decreased to 5% to 10% in the first 10 years.[454-456] Infection occurs in 1% to 3% of cases, but infection rates can be higher in revision surgery, especially in men with diabetes mellitus.

The total cost of penile prosthesis implantation varies from $3,000 to $20,000, depending on the type of device used and the community in which the procedure is performed. There are no randomized efficacy trials, but retrospective analyses have reported that greater than 80% of patients and 70% of partners are pleased with their prosthesis and the togetherness that it brings to their relationship.[454-457]

Testosterone Replacement in Androgen-Deficient Men Presenting With Erectile Disorder. Testosterone treatment does not improve sexual function in men with ED who have normal testosterone levels.[1,64,134,135,142] It is not known whether testosterone replacement improves sexual function in impotent men with borderline serum testosterone levels. Many, but not all, of the impotent men with low testosterone levels experience improvements in their libido and overall sexual activity with androgen replacement therapy.[1,64,134,135] The response to testosterone therapy even in this group of men is variable, because of the coexistence of other disorders such as diabetes mellitus, hypertension, CVD, and psychogenic factors.[1,134,135,142]

ED in middle-aged and older men is a multifactorial disorder, often associated with other comorbid conditions such as diabetes mellitus, hypertension, medications, peripheral vascular disease, psychogenic factors, and end-stage renal disease. Therefore, it is not surprising that testosterone treatment alone may not improve sexual function in all men with androgen deficiency. Testosterone induces NOS activity,[130,131] has trophic effects on cavernosal smooth muscle and ischiocavernosus and bulbospongiosus muscles,[132] increases penile blood flow,[145] and is essential for achieving venous occlusion in animal models.[129] These observations have led to speculation that testosterone might improve response to PDE5 inhibitors; however, as discussed earlier, data from randomized trials have not shown the superiority of testosterone over placebo in improving erectile function in men with ED who have low testosterone levels and in whom the PDE5 inhibitor dose has been optimized.[148]

Therapies With Either Unproven Efficacy or Limited Efficacy Data. There are insufficient efficacy data to support the use of trazodone[458] or yohimbine[459] in men with ED. The literature on the effectiveness of herbal therapies is difficult to interpret because of lack of consistency in product formulations and potencies, contamination of herbal products with PDE5 inhibitors, poor trial design, and paucity of randomized clinical trial data.[460-464] One randomized trial of Korean red ginseng reported this product to be effective in the treatment of ED[461]; these data need further confirmation. Icariin is a flavonoid, derived from several species of plants, whose extracts have been known in herbal medicine to produce aphrodisiac effects and enhance erectile function.[464] Dipyridamole also inhibits PDE5 and can augment the effects of nitric oxide. 4-Methylpiperazine and pyrazolopyrimidine, components of the lichen *Xanthoparmelia scabrosa*, have also been claimed to inhibit PDE5.[463] The use of these or other herbal therapies is not recommended.[463] Apomorphine also functions as a dopamine agonist and acts centrally to initiate erection; its main adverse effect is nausea.

Gene Therapy and Erectile Disorder. The goal of gene therapy for ED is to introduce novel genetic material into the cavernosal smooth muscle cells to restore normal cellular function and produce a therapeutic effect.[465-467] Gene therapy has been proposed as a treatment option for diseases that have a vascular origin, such as arteriosclerosis, congestive heart failure, and pulmonary hypertension.[465-467] ED may be particularly amenable to gene therapy because of the easily accessible external location of the penis,[465-467] which permits direct injection into the corpora cavernosa. A tourniquet placed around the base of the penis limits entry of the injected material into the systemic circulation. This is a distinct advantage of the gene therapy of penile diseases over gene therapy for other systemic diseases because introduction of the genetic material into the systemic circulation can potentially induce adverse systemic effects due to insertion of the material into an incorrect organ or vascular bed. Additionally, in the penis, only a small number of cells need to be transfected because the interconnection of smooth muscle cells in the corpus cavernosum by gap junctions allows second messenger molecules and ions to be transferred to other interconnected smooth muscle cells.[465-467] The low turnover rate of the vascular smooth muscle cells of the penis allows the desired gene to be expressed for long periods of time.

The current strategies of gene therapy for ED treatment have focused on the molecules that regulate corporal smooth muscle relaxation or neovascularization (Table 20-12).[465-467] A number of candidate genes have been explored, including the penile-inducible NOS, eNOS, VIP, calcitonin-related peptide, maxi-K^+ channel, vascular endothelial growth factor (VEGF), the brain neurotrophic factor, angiopoietin-1, neurturin (a member of the glial cell line–derived neurotrophic factor family), superoxide dismutase, IGF-1, protein kinase G (PKG-1α), and Rho A/Rho kinase[465-475] (see Table 20-12). A number of vectors have been used to transfer exogenous genes, including adenoviruses, adeno-associated viruses, retroviruses, sinbis viruses, replication-deficient retroviruses, liposomes, naked DNA, and gold nanoparticles.[465-481]

Garban and associates[468] first demonstrated that gene therapy can be performed in the penis by utilizing naked cDNA (complementary DNA) encoding the penile-inducible NOS gene leading to physiologic benefit in the aging rat. Christ and colleagues[469] injected hSlo cDNA (which encodes the human smooth muscle maxi-K^+ channel) into the rat corpora cavernosa and demonstrated increased gap junction formation and enhanced erectile responses to nerve stimulation in the aged rat. Adenoviral constructs encoding the eNOS and CGRP genes were shown to reverse age-related ED in rats.[470,471] In these studies, both eNOS and CGRP expression were sustained for at least 1 month in the corpora cavernosa of the rat penis. Five days after transfection with the AdCMVeNOS or AdRSVeNOS viruses, aged rats had significant increases in erectile function as determined by cavernosal nerve stimulation and pharmacologic injection with the endothelium-dependent vasodilator

TABLE 20-12

Physiologic Targets for Gene Therapy

Gene Target	Vector and Mechanism	Reference
Nitric oxide isoforms	Increase eNOS, nNOS, and iNOS activity in the cavernosal smooth muscle	Champion 1999; Bivalacqua 2000, 2003, 2005; Gonzalez-Cadavid 2004; Kendirci 2005; Wessels 2006
Protein inhibitor of NOS (PIN)	Antisense and short hairpin RNA (shRNA) constructs targeting PIN (protein inhibitor of NOS)	Magee et al 2007
Maxi-K$^+$ channel	Transfer of maxi-K$^+$ channels using a plasmid vector that carries the hSlo gene encoding the α-subunit of the maxi K$^+$ channel; first human trial demonstrates the safety and feasibility of gene therapy in humans	Christ et al 2002, 2004, 2004; Melman 2003, 2005, 2006, 2007, 2008; So et al 2007
PKG-1α	Replication-deficient recombinant adenoviruses carrying the PKG-1α	Bivalacqua et al 2007
VEGF	Transfer of VEGF cDNA into rat corpora cavernosa to promote neovascularization	Rogers et al 2003; Buchardt et al 2005; Dall'Era et al 2008
Angiopoietin-1	Adenovirus-mediated transfer of human angiopoietin-1	Ryu et al 2006; Jin et al 2010
BDNF	Transfer of brain-derived neurotrophic factor using adeno-associated virus	Rogers et al 2005; Gholani et al 2003
Neurotrophin 3 gene	Transfer of neurotrophin 3 gene using HSV vector	Bennett et al 2005
Neurturin	Neurturin (NTN), a member of glial cell line–derived neurotrophic factor (GDNF) family	Kato et al 2009
VIP	Transfection of corpora cavernosa of streptozotocin-treated diabetic rats using pcDNA3 carrying VIP cDNA	Shen et al 2005
CGRP	Adenoviral transfer of CGRP in aged rats	Bivalacqua et al 2001; Deng 2004
Superoxide dismutase	Adenoviral-mediated gene transfer of extracellular superoxide dismutase injected into the corpora cavernosa	Bivalacqua 2003; Brown 2006; Lund 2007
Insulin-like growth factor-1	Adenoviral-mediated gene transfer of IGF-1	Pu et al 2007

BDNF, brain-derived neurotrophic factor; cDNA, complementary DNA; CGRP, calcitonin gene–related peptide; HSV, human syncytial virus; IGF-1, insulin-like growth factor 1; NOS, nitric oxide synthase (epithelial [e], inducible [i], or neuronal [n] isoforms); PIN, protein inhibitor of NOS; PKG, protein kinase G; VEGF, vascular endothelial growth factor; VIP, vasoactive intestinal protein.
Adapted from Melman and Davies[481]; Condorelli et al, 2010; Harraz et al[465]; Strong et al[466]; Deng et al.[467]

acetylcholine and the type PDE5 inhibitors.[470,471] In one study, intracavernous injection of adeno-associated virus construct carrying the brain-derived neurotrophic factor gene improved erectile function after cavernosal nerve injury.[475] This neurotrophic factor purportedly restored neuronal NOS in the major pelvic ganglion, thus enhancing the recovery of erectile function after bilateral cavernous nerve injury.[475] In other studies, intracavernosal VEGF injection and adeno-associated virus-mediated VEGF gene therapy were each shown to reverse venogenic ED in rats.[472,473] These preclinical studies and others using additional targets for gene therapy such as CGRP, superoxide dismutase, and Rho A/Rho kinase provide evidence that in vivo gene transfer can be accomplished technically. The translation of these preclinical data into human trials has been slow and unsuccessful so far.

Ion Channel Innovations, Inc. has completed a phase I trial of slow K$^+$ channel in men with ED.[95,477,478] In this trial, hmaxi-K, a "naked" DNA plasmid carrying the human cDNA encoding for the gene for the α-subunit of the human smooth muscle maxi-K channel, was injected directly into the penises of 11 men with ED. Patients who received the highest dose of hmaxi-K experienced significant improvements in their erectile function that was sustained for the 24-week duration of the trial. This trial demonstrated the feasibility and safety of injecting naked DNA into the human penis.[477,478] A trial of hmaxi-K in patients with overactive bladders is ongoing. Phase I gene therapy trials using VEGF and hepatocyte growth factor have been conducted in patients with peripheral vascular disease and chronic limb ischemia and to prevent the development of stent restenosis; these trials have reported low frequency of serious adverse effects. However, phase II studies have not confirmed efficacy. Thus, the early therapeutic promise of gene therapy has yet to be realized. Successful gene therapy may require introduction of multiple gene products using vectors with higher efficiency of transfection of a larger number of target cells and more

prolonged action than can be realized with the current generation of vectors.

The Potential of Stem Cell Therapy for Erectile Disorder. The past decade has seen considerable interest in the transplantation of stem cells derived from bone marrow, adipose tissue, or skeletal muscle into the corpora cavernosa.[482-490] However, it has become apparent that the stem cells, even when injected within the corpora cavernosa, escape rapidly from the penis and hone into the bone marrow.[482-490] The mechanism of the reported improvements in intracavernosal pressure after stem cell injection into the corpora cavernosa remains unclear.[485] The safety and efficacy of stem cell therapy in humans has yet to be demonstrated. We do not know whether transplanted human mesenchymal stem cells (hMSCs) can differentiate into functional cavernosal smooth muscle cells and restore erectile capacity in men with ED. Also, the long-term outcomes including the tumorigenic potential of these transplanted progenitor cells are unknown.

hMSCs may also be attractive gene delivery vehicles because these cells can replicate in vitro as well as in vivo, thus potentially providing a large pool of cells.[486,487] Initial studies have demonstrated that rat mesenchymal stem cells, expanded and transfected ex vivo and implanted into the corpora cavernosa, are capable of expressing the gene product of interest.[482-487] Stem cell therapy using stem cells carrying angiogenic or neurotrophic genes or proteins is also being explored. Although several animal studies have reported improved erectile function with hMSC transplantation, few studies have shown evidence of long-term stem cell survival in the cavernosal smooth muscle or evidence of differentiation of the transplanted stem cells into endothelial cells or cavernosal smooth muscle cells.[482-490]

Management of Retrograde Ejaculation

Case reports have shown benefit from methoxamine, imipramine, midodrine, and ephedrine, although randomized clinical trial data are lacking.[491-493] Induction of fertility in men with retrograde ejaculation may require retrieval of sperm from the urinary bladder after sexual stimulation or electrostimulation of the prostatic nerve plexus per rectum plus assisted reproductive techniques, such as intrauterine insemination or in vitro fertilization with or without intracytoplasmic sperm injection using the retrieved sperm.[494-497]

MANAGEMENT OF SEXUAL DYSFUNCTION IN WOMEN

Psychotherapeutic methods are the mainstay of management of the female sexual dysfunction; Frühauf and coworkers[498] provided a systematic review and meta-analysis of these interventions in 2013.

On an investigational basis a small number of medications have received limited study (see Table 20-13).

Management of Low Desire and Arousal in Women

Management of sexual interest/arousal disorder (SIAD) begins with explaining the circular model of sexual response (see Fig. 20-1B) as a basis for discussing which areas are problematic with one or preferably both partners. When insufficient emotional intimacy is identified, the normality of low interest to be sexual can be clarified; referral for couple counseling may be indicated. When the lack of sexual context and stimuli are contributing factors, simply emphasizing the requirement of appropriate environment and sufficiently erotic stimuli is usually sufficient, but referral to a sex therapist may be appropriate. Nonsexual distractions, fears about sexual outcome, self-monitoring of sexual response, anxiety, low self-image, and depression all interrupt the mental appraisal of stimuli. These issues can be explained and addressed. The main modalities of treatment are cognitive therapy, sex therapy, and psychoeducation.

Psychoeducation

Psychoeducation includes giving information while simultaneously soliciting the woman's input to share thoughts and feelings that emerge in session, which are then addressed and processed. It includes teaching cognitive techniques and can help dispel widespread myths about sexuality in women (e.g., that the absence of desire preceding sexual activity denotes sexual dysfunction). Bibliotherapy with self-help reading material or videos can be helpful.

TABLE 20-13

Investigational Pharmacotherapy for Women's Sexual Dysfunctions

Sexual Dysfunction	Mechanisms of Dysfunction	Drug Type	Off Label/Investigational Drug	Comments
Sexual interest arousal disorder	Loss of brain's sexual arousability to sexual stimuli	Drugs with specific serotonin receptor subtype of agonist/antagonist profile	Flibanserin: 5HT1A agonist and 5HT2A antagonist, weak partial agonist D₄	Recent FDA approval despite marginal benefit and potentially serious side effects[521a]
		Melanocortin agonists	Bremelanotide–synthetic peptide: α-melanocyte-stimulating hormone analogue-agonist at MCR1, MC3R, and MC4R receptors	Small RCT showed benefit for women's arousal disorder with in home use of nasal drug 45 min before sex.[73] Sponsor has discontinued trials
		Dopamine agonists	Bupropion	One small 4-month study, in nondepressed premenopausal women showed increased arousability and sexual response, no increase in initial desire.[110]
Genital arousal disorder: estrogen deplete	Loss of genital vasocongestion in response to sexual stimulation	To provide local substrate for estrogen and testosterone intracrine synthesis	Local vaginal DHEA	Recent phase III RCT showing increased maturation of vaginal epithelium, lower pH and sexual benefit in all domains of response from local vaginal DHEA for 12 weeks[558]
	Loss of genital vasocongestion in response to sexual stimulation	Selective tissue estrogenic activity regulator with androgenic and progestogenic properties	Tibolone	RCT of dysfunctional women showed tibolone marginally superior to 50 μg/140 μg combined transdermal estradiol/norethisterone.[112]
Genital arousal disorder despite estrogen replete	Loss of genital vasocongestion in response to sexual stimulation	To enhance the action of NO-PDEIs	Sildenafil, tadalafil, vardenafil	Major problem is distinguishing the subgroup of women with genital arousal disorder who have reduced genital vasocongestion. Small RCTs in diabetes[146] and MS[116] showed only modest benefit from sildenafil.
Serotonergic antidepressant–associated orgasmic disorder	Former orgasmic response absent or extremely delayed	PDEIs	Sildenafil	Recent 8-week RCT with very strict entry criteria showed benefit from 50-100 mg.[510]

Superscript numbers indicate references at the end of the chapter.
D₄, dopamine 4 receptor; DHEA, dehydroepiandrosterone; 5-HT, serotonin; ISSWSH, International Society for the Study of Women's Sexual Health; MC1R, melanocortin-1 receptor; MS, multiple sclerosis; MSH, melanocyte-stimulating hormone; NO, nitric oxide; PDEIs, phosphodiesterase inhibitors; RCTs, randomized controlled trials.

For some women, information on anatomy and physiology is necessary.

Cognitive Behavioral Therapy

Cognitive behavioral therapy (CBT) can assist the woman to recognize, challenge, and in time, change her negative and often catastrophic self-view imposed by underlying illness, including endocrine conditions or their imposed infertility. Some of the exaggerated or catastrophic thoughts amenable to cognitive therapy include "sex is only for well women," "I am no longer fertile, so I am no longer sexually attractive," and "if intercourse is too painful to include, then no one will want me." Identifying these biased/ maladaptive thoughts is the first step: changing such thoughts to be more evidenced-based is then practiced. Empiric support for benefit from targeting cognitions and emotions during sex in order to increase physical and subjective arousal is emerging.[42,499]

Mindfulness-Based Cognitive Therapy

New to Western medicine is the addition of mindfulness, which is of benefit for medically well women with sexual dysfunction,[500,501] those with pelvic cancer,[502] and those with PVD.[503] Mindfulness is an Eastern practice of meditation: the learned skill is to be fully present and accepting of all that is sensed in that moment. Attention is enhanced by the gradual ability to identify thoughts arising in that moment, be they future- or past-oriented, but not to engage in them but ultimately to view these negative or positive thoughts more distantly as if they are just sensations not dissimilar to physical sensations. The practice of mindfulness focuses the attention on sexual sensations rather than on self-monitoring. Functional brain imaging performed before and after mindfulness training supports the clinical finding that such training lessens self-referencing of sensations and emotions, including pain and anxiety.[504-506] Resources in the community and through the Internet for mindfulness practice can be given.

Recently, an adapted form of CBT blended with mindfulness was defined—the treatment is called *mindfulness-based cognitive therapy* (MBCT). Regular mindfulness practice is an integral component. As with CBT, the skill of detecting maladaptive thoughts including those critical or evaluative is learned but with simple observation of their presence and an acknowledgment that they are just mental events, not necessarily the truth; there is no focus here to change thoughts. MBCT is used to treat or prevent anxiety disorder and depression and has been adapted to treat arousal and desire disorders and chronic pain of PVD.[500,501,503,507]

Current clinical research includes the use of detailed treatment manuals for clinicians with separate versions for patients. The aim is to provide sufficiently detailed manuals for non–mental health professionals and non–sexual medicine specialists to provide CBT and MBCT to small groups of women. This small group format is consistently rated as a major benefit.[508]

Sex Therapy

Sex therapy usually focuses on sensate focus exercises whereby each partner takes turns giving and receiving sensual and, later on, sexual touches, caresses, and kisses. Initially, genital areas and breasts are off-limits. The idea of any goal or expectation is put aside. The couple together with the clinician decides as to when breasts and genital areas are on-limits. Ultimately, the act of intercourse (or vaginal penetration with dildo), may be included—but not as the focus.

Outcome of Psychological Treatments for Women's Sexual Dysfunctions

Data are limited regarding the long-term effects of psychological treatments for women's sexual dysfunction. A systematic review and a meta-analysis of controlled clinical trials for female and male sexual dysfunction published before 2009 was recently conducted.[498] None of these studies targeted patients with endocrine disease. The overall conclusion was that psychosocial interventions for sexual dysfunction were efficacious. For women with sexual dysfunction associated with the hormonal changes arising from breast cancer treatment, a systematic review suggests that the most effective interventions are couple-based psychoeducational interventions that include an element of sex therapy.[509]

Management of Women's Orgasmic Disorder

Although in clinical practice CBT methods and mindfulness training have been used in women with orgasmic disorder, outcome research is sparse. The 2013 meta-analysis found clear evidence of benefit in both symptom severity and sexual satisfaction for women with orgasmic dysfunction, but only three trials were identified.[498] To date there is no pharmacologic treatment for orgasmic disorder. In one trial with highly selective inclusion criteria, sildenafil was reported to improve orgasm dysfunction associated with SSRI use,[510] whereas a recent small trial of transdermal testosterone did not improve sexual function beyond placebo as measured by the Sabbatsberg Sexual Self-Rating Scale as the primary outcome.[511] However, testosterone therapy was associated with statistically significant increase in the number of sexually satisfying events (SSEs) per month. Confirmation of these findings and their clinical relevance is awaited (Table 20-13).

Management of Genitopelvic Pain/Penetration Disorder (Dyspareunia and Vaginismus)

The most common type of dyspareunia is PVD, which affects about 12% to 18% of women.[512] PVD and the other common type of dyspareunia—that stemming from vulvovaginal atrophy—are typically associated with pelvic muscle hypertonicity and reflexive involuntary contractions when penetration is anticipated. DSM-5 therefore merged the previous terms of dyspareunia and vaginismus. The use of pain-free transperineal four-dimensional ultrasound on pelvic floor muscle morphometry in women with PVD confirmed abnormalities both at rest (e.g., small levator hiatus area, small anorectal angle suggesting increased tone) and with maximal contraction. These findings are thought to be consistent with weakness and poor control of pelvic muscle.[513] Pelvic floor physiotherapy is frequently part of sexual pain management.

Management of Provoked Vestibulodynia

There is no definite association between PVD and endocrine status, but recent investigation of the presence of polymorphism in the guanine triphosphate cyclohydrolase gene *(GCH1)* is of interest. Specific single nucleotide polymorphisms (SNPs) in the *GCHI* gene are associated with reduced pain sensitivity. Although no correlation between PVD and the pain-protective *GCH1* SNP combination was found, patients with PVD using oral contraceptives and carrying the specified SNP combination had higher pain sensitivity.[514] This finding is in keeping with the documented clinical experience that some women with PVD benefit from discontinuing oral contraceptives.[515]

Randomized trials of oral and topical medications for PVD including tricyclics, anticonvulsants, lidocaine, fluconazole, cromolyn, and nifedipine gave similar results in analgesic benefit compared to placebo.[516] Investigational botulinum toxin was statistically inferior to placebo in reduction of sexual distress.[516] Because medical treatments for PVD have been unsatisfactory, an interdisciplinary biopsychosexual approach is currently encouraged.[517,518]

Although rarely chosen by women, surgical vestibulectomy can be of benefit; however, exclusion factors are numerous[519] and benefit is obtained mostly in women with acquired as opposed to lifelong histories. Other common negative prognostic factors for successful vestibulectomy include comorbid muscle tightening, widespread allodynia of the introital margin, involvement of the Skene duct openings, unwillingness to have sex therapy if offered, and comorbid depression and anxiety. Negative prognostic factors for all treatment modalities include disgust and contamination sensitivity, erotophobia (the tendency to respond with negative effects to sexual cues), and coexistence of depression and anxiety.[520]

Recent research suggests an expanded stress model of chronic pain,[520,521] focusing on allostasis, which is the physiologic stability maintained by various mechanisms within the body that promote adaptation to stress in the longer term. Allostatic load/overload[522] depicts the wear and tear of body systems, including the brain, from excessive stress. Given the debility and negative consequences of recurrent pain, the stress produced by the pain disorder maintains a vicious cycle. This cycle may be especially applicable to the sexual pain of PVD: a stress-induced and maintenance model for the pain of PVD was recently described,[516] similar to the vicious cycle depicted for migraine.[521] Personality traits of women with PVD, including negative self-evaluation and fear of negative evaluation by others, predisposes to self-labeling as sexually substandard or even sexually inadequate. The stress model of pain posits that sexual stress not only contributes to the chronic pelvic muscle hypertonicity but also maintains a heightened reactivity of the pain circuitry from top-down modulation afforded by neuroplasticity. The cause of the sensitization within the nervous system has not been established with certainty, but internal stress appears to be a likely cause. Women with PVD report higher levels of premorbid depression and anxiety, as well as perfectionism, reward dependency, fear of negative evaluation, increased prevalence of type D personality, self-dislike, harm avoidance, hypervigilance for pain, and shyness compared to women without PVD.[523-527]

Given that mood disorder is so commonly comorbid with PVD, management needs to address both pain and the depression/anxiety. There is evidence of benefit from CBT, which was sustained over the 2 years of follow-up.[528] Catastrophic thinking, amenable to CBT approaches, is particularly common in women with PVD.[529] The lack of self-acceptance apparent in women with PVD, considered to be a pain-maintaining stress, is potentially amenable to MBCT given that a key component of MBCT is acceptance. Significant beneficial effects beyond waitlist control were confirmed from a brief mindfulness-based group intervention on both cotton swab–induced vestibular pain and psychological measures of pain.[503,508]

Management of Phobic Reflex Pelvic Muscle Contractions (Vaginismus)

Heightened pelvic muscle tone, often along with muscle tension elsewhere, may be the only physical findings in women reporting dyspareunia or painful but unsuccessful attempts at penetration. Often guided by pelvic floor physiotherapists, management involves progressive desensitization and progressive vaginal accommodation using a variety of relaxation techniques and vaginal inserts.[530] The term *dilators* is preferably avoided, because women fear that their therapy is going to (painfully) stretch the vagina. Psychotherapies including mindfulness and CBT are often used to reduce anxiety.[531] A 2013 waitlist controlled study of in-clinic physical therapy suggests better outcomes than traditional guidance for insert therapy at home.[532]

Testosterone Therapy for Women With Sexual Dysfunction

As discussed earlier in this chapter, testosterone deficiency has not been demonstrated in women diagnosed with sexual dysfunction, either by measurement of blood levels or by measurement of androgen metabolites. Several randomized trials of testosterone therapy have been conducted, mostly in postmenopausal women. These testosterone trials were conducted largely in women distressed by reduced sexual desire since their menopause. The eligibility criteria for these trials did not meet the diagnostic criteria for DSM-IV, HSDD, or for the newly coined SIAD of DSM-5.

The first series of randomized trials showed a statistically significant improvement in the numbers of SSEs in women receiving testosterone: on average SSEs increased from 2 to 3 per month to 5 per month in women on active drug and to 4 per month in women receiving placebo. Testosterone was given transdermally in the form of a patch with a nominal testosterone delivery of 300 µg/day. Doses of either 150 or 450 µg/day were not effective.[533] Serum testosterone and dihydrotestosterone concentrations exceeded the target high-normal serum concentrations of these hormones in a significant number of women receiving testosterone.[534] Women on active drug reported further improvements in arousal, pleasure, orgasm, self-image, and responsiveness to a statistically significantly greater extent than did women receiving placebo.

These testosterone trials focused mostly on surgically menopausal women, but one testosterone patch study included naturally menopausal women[535] with comparable results. Two testosterone studies recruited naturally and surgically menopausal women who were not receiving estrogen therapy. One of these studies reported a significant increase in SSEs in the naturally menopausal women from the active drug but not in the smaller subgroup of surgically menopausal women.[536] Only 464 of the 814 participants completed treatment, with similar distribution of high discontinuation rates in all three arms. A second study of 272 naturally menopausal women, of whom a total of 73% of the participants were not receiving systemic estrogen therapy, showed a significant increase in SSEs.[537]

On the basis of these studies, all by the same sponsor, the transdermal testosterone patch was approved in Europe, but not in North America or elsewhere, for the treatment of surgically menopausal women with persistently distressing low sexual desire despite adequate systemic estrogen therapy that did not include conjugated equine estrogens. Although approved, the patch is no longer available in Europe because of low sales.

Negative Trials of Testosterone Therapy

In contrast to the previous studies, two large phase III RCTs by a different sponsor of 1172 postmenopausal women, approximately half of whom received systemic estrogen, showed *no* benefit of transdermal testosterone in the form of a gel over placebo.[538] Full study details are not available as these two studies have not been published. The entry criterion of distressingly reduced sexual desire after menopause was similar to the previous randomized trials; end points were numbers of SSEs per month and the level of sexual desire as assessed from a daily diary.

There is very little information available on the effects of testosterone in premenopausal women. One study of 261 women who experienced loss of their former sexual satisfaction reported minimal benefit from testosterone.[539]

Testosterone Plus a Phosphodiesterase Inhibitor

One small study evaluated the efficacy of a pharmacologic dose of testosterone (0.5 mg sublingually) to improve attentiveness for erotic cues in women with low desire.[540] The testosterone was combined with sildenafil, a PDE inhibitor, to facilitate genital congestion. In those women who at baseline already showed high levels of subconscious attention bias for erotic cues (as measured by a masked version of the emotional Stroop task), this drug combination had no effect, and in fact, testosterone alone *reduced* attention to erotic cues. However, the women with lower arousability or sensitivity to erotic cues at baseline showed increased physiologic genital congestion and increased awareness of the genital sensations and of sexual desire when they subsequently viewed an erotic video. The safety of intermittent use of markedly supraphysiologic testosterone therapy is unknown.

Limitations of Trials of Testosterone Therapy in Women

A major limitation of testosterone trials to date is the targeted population. Studies have recruited women with decreased desire since menopause, most of whom retained the ability to be aroused and sexually satisfied on at least some (on average 50%) occasions. Thus, an absence of sexual desire between sexual encounters has been the focus. However, research confirms this to be well within the range of normal female sexual experience. The majority of 3250 multiethnic middle-aged women in the SWAN cohort indicated that although moderately or extremely sexually satisfied, they never or very infrequently felt desire.[541] In an online survey of 3687 younger women, 1865 were assessed to be without evidence of sexual dysfunction, specifically confirming their easy sexual arousal—close to one third of this group rarely or never began a sexual experience with a sense of sexual desire.[542] As noted earlier in this chapter, an incentives/motivations model of human sexual response is now considered to more accurately reflect sexual experience, desire for sex per se being just one of many reasons or incentives for sex. When absent at the beginning of a sexual encounter, desire can be triggered along with arousal after effective stimulation.

Clinical trials have been conducted largely in women who were able to have satisfactory sexual experiences 50% of the time, leading to the criticism that these women probably did not have a biologic cause or consistent sexual dysfunction to merit any hormonal therapy.[543-545] The studies of postmenopausal women showed improvements in desire and response domains using validated sexual questionnaires; however, increasing the degree and frequency of pleasure and arousal currently experienced by study subjects does not necessarily imply that improvements would be observed in women with consistent absence of pleasure and arousal.[543]

There has been criticism of the use of statistical significance alone to evaluate the difference between the powerful placebo effects and active drug treatments in the area of women's sexual dysfunction—especially that of low desire.[546,547] It is suggested that effects might be better reported in terms of percentage of participants no longer meeting criteria for sexual dysfunction.[546] As noted, the women in the testosterone trials were not recruited on the basis of a clinical diagnosis of sexual dysfunction but based on confirmation of low desire after menopause that caused distress.

Risks of Testosterone Therapy

Long-term safety data are lacking; published safety data from trials of up to 12 months' duration are reassuring.[547] There are theoretical reasons to consider exogenous testosterone as either a risk factor or a protective factor for breast cancer; high endogenous testosterone may be associated with an increased risk.[545,548] A high endogenous testosterone-to-estrogen ratio can increase the risk of metabolic syndrome and CVD.[549] However, some data suggest that low SHBG may be related to the risk of diabetes, metabolic syndrome, and CVD.[550] In the Melbourne Women's Midlife Health Project, weight gain and free androgen index, but not total testosterone, were strong predictors of CVD risk.[551] Similar results were observed in 9-year follow-up of the SWAN cohort.[552] In this study, free androgen index was positively and SHBG was negatively associated with the development of obesity. Weight gain preceded changes in the free androgen index and SHBG. The expert panel of the American Endocrine Society noted that the association between the free androgen index, CVD risk factors, and the metabolic syndrome phenotype appears to be more driven by obesity and low SHBG rather than testosterone.[548]

In most randomized trials, testosterone therapy has been administered in the background of concurrent estrogen therapy.[548] However, the present advice, especially in North America, is to limit the duration of estrogen therapy. The Endocrine Society Task Force noted the limited safety data (median follow-up 4 months, range 6 weeks to 2 years). Furthermore, the efficacy data are focused on sexually responsive women without the common comorbid conditions including depression or antidepressant treatment. The task force requested a meta-analysis of transdermal testosterone RCTs; the gel studies, however, were excluded as they are only published in abstract form. Across all trials testosterone, used mostly in sexually responsive women, was associated with a statistically significant improvement in satisfaction, pleasure, orgasm, and libido.[553] The Endocrine Society's recommendations include the following[548]:

1. Most studies of testosterone therapy have targeted women with low desire but with the ability to be aroused and sexually satisfied on at least some (on average 50%) occasions. An incentives/motivations model of human sexual response is now considered to more accurately reflect sexual experience, desire for sex per se being just one of many reasons or incentives for sex. Studies are needed in women with low sexual interest/incentives and low arousal (and typically few orgasms) to reflect the prevalent clinical situation.
2. The expert panel recommended against the generalized use of testosterone by women for infertility or sexual dysfunction (but with the previous caveat in mind, except for a specific diagnosis of DSM-IV HSDD).

3. The expert panel recommended against the routine treatment of women with low androgen levels due to hypopituitarism, adrenal insufficiency, bilateral oophorectomy, or other conditions associated with low androgen levels because of the lack of adequate data supporting efficacy and long-term safety of therapy.

4. The expert panel suggested consideration of a 3- to 6-month trial of a dose of testosterone resulting in a midnormal premenopausal value of plasma testosterone for postmenopausal women who request therapy for properly diagnosed HSDD and in whom therapy is not contraindicated.

Needed Research in the Area of Testosterone Supplementation

Further research is needed in women with low sexual interest/incentives and low arousal (and typically few orgasms) to reflect the prevalent clinical situation and to merit a diagnosis of SIAD. It is of note, however, that in the study of 125 women with and 125 women without HSDD when no group differences in androgen activity were found, 55% of the women with HSDD also met criteria for SIAD.[554]

Women diagnosed with SIAD and in remission from depression but taking antidepressants and women who, despite treatment, still score in the depressive range again reflect the clinical situation. Given that depression typically blunts sexual response, it has been an exclusion factor in clinical trials, as has the use of antidepressant therapy, but the reality is that mood disorder and its treatment commonly accompany complaints of low sexual desire.[554-556] Not only is depression the factor most robustly linked to low desire in otherwise healthy women but also depression frequently determines the presence of sexual dysfunction even when other medical conditions including diabetes are comorbid.[20]

Oral Dehydroepiandrosterone for Sexual Dysfunction in Healthy Women

Small trials of DHEA have been conducted in older healthy women. A recent systematic review and meta-analysis to evaluate the benefits and risks of systemic DHEA therapy for postmenopausal women[557] included 15 randomized trials that were in general considered at high risk of bias and were of short duration. Statistically, DHEA use was marginally significant for desire, and there were no other significant improvements to outcome. The quality of evidence was considered low to moderate for benefit and very low for long-term harm. The recent Endocrine Society Task Force recommended against using DHEA in this setting.[548]

Local DHEA Therapy for Sexual Dysfunction in Healthy Women

A recent phase III randomized trial of local vaginal DHEA therapy in postmenopausal women with vulvovaginal atrophy reported benefit of such therapy in improving vaginal symptoms of dryness and dyspareunia and all domains of sexual function.[558] Moreover, all steroids, measured by mass spectrometry methods, remained in the postmenopausal range. Specifically, ADT-G remained constant. This delivery of precursor hormones to the target tissue may allow strictly local estrogen and androgen actions and may be a preferable choice for women in whom any systemic estrogen therapy is undesirable, such as those receiving aromatase inhibitors for breast cancer who can develop severe vulvovaginal atrophy. Rodent work suggests that local DHEA's beneficial effect on genital sexual sensitivity might stem from its potent stimulatory effect on vaginal nerve fiber density.[559]

Estrogen Therapy for Women With Sexual Dysfunction

Local vaginal therapy is recommended for dyspareunia associated with vulvovaginal atrophy. Low doses of estrogen can be supplied by a Silastic vaginal ring, vaginal cream, or a mucoadhesive vaginal tablet with similar benefit and low systemic absorption. Use of estradiol, 10 µg twice weekly and the estring (a Silastic ring containing estradiol, placed high in the vaginal vault), results in serum levels of 4.6 and 8.0 pg/mL, respectively. Progesterone is usually considered unnecessary for endometrial protection. Smaller doses of these formulations of estrogen are being investigated (e.g., 10 µg rather than 100 µg estradiol cream, 0.03 mg rather than 0.2 mg estriol vaginal pessaries) or have already been approved (e.g., 10-µg rather than 25-µg estradiol vaginal tablets). When local estrogen does not ameliorate postmenopausal vulvovaginal atrophy-associated dyspareunia, comorbid PVD may be present.[560]

Of concern is that women using aromatase inhibitors and vaginal estrogen may show a small increase in serum estradiol levels[561]: a prospective trial of aromatase inhibition plus vaginal estrogen is under way. Investigational vaginal DHEA that appears not to increase serum levels of testosterone or estrogen has not been studied in breast cancer patients but appears promising.[558] Intravaginal testosterone may alleviate symptoms,[562] but any systemic absorption could increase serum estrogen through aromatization. Of particular relevance to women with past breast cancer is a 2013 report of a hyaluronic acid vaginal gel improving dyspareunia in 85% of women, comparable to women receiving vaginal estriol.[563]

When systemic estrogen is needed for other menopausal symptoms, it is sometimes necessary to give additional local estrogen for dyspareunia. In contrast, for some women, ultra-low-dose (0.014 mg/day) systemic transdermal estradiol may be sufficient for all menopausal symptoms including dyspareunia.[564] If systemic supplementation improves insomnia and dyspareunia, sexual motivation would logically be expected to increase, but this has not been vigorously studied. No significant differences were found between estrogen and placebo groups in reported sexual satisfaction in the Women's Health Initiative Trial.[565] However, sexual dysfunction was not a primary focus of that trial; women with marked menopausal symptoms were excluded; and the instruments used to assess sexual function were substandard.

REFERENCES

1. Bhasin S, Enzlin P, Coviello A, Basson R. Sexual dysfunction in men and women with endocrine disorders. *Lancet.* 2007;369(9561):597-611.
2. Mercer CH, Fenton KA, Johnson AM, et al. Sexual function problems and help seeking behaviour in Britain: national probability sample survey. *BMJ.* 2003;327:426-427.
3. Kinsey AC, Pomeroy WB, Martin CE. *Sexual Behavior in the Human Male.* Philadelphia, PA: WB Saunders; 1948.
4. Feldman HA, Goldstein I, Hatzichristou DG, et al. Impotence and its medical and psychosocial correlates: results of the Massachusetts Male Aging Study. *J Urol.* 1994;151:54-61.
5. Laumann EO, Paik A, Rosen RC. The epidemiology of erectile dysfunction: results from the National Health and Social Life Survey. *Int J Impot Res.* 1999;11(Suppl 1):S60-S64.
6. Laumann EO, Paik A, Rosen RC. Sexual dysfunction in the United States: prevalence and predictors. *JAMA.* 1999;281:537-544.
7. Lewis RW, Fugl-Meyer KS, Bosch R, et al. Epidemiology/risk factors of sexual dysfunction. *J Sex Med.* 2004;1(1):35-39.

8. Masters EH, Johnson V. *Human Sexual Response.* Boston, MA: Little, Brown; 1966.
9. Lue TF, Tanagho EA. Hemodynamics of erection. In: Tanagho EA, Lue TF, McClure RD, eds. *Contemporary Management of Impotence and Infertility.* Baltimore, MD: Williams & Wilkins; 1988:28-38.
10. Lue TF. Erectile dysfunction. *N Engl J Med.* 2000;342:1802-1813.
11. Bhasin S, Benson GS. Male sexual function. In: De Kretser D, ed. *Knobil and Neill's Physiology of Reproduction.* 3rd ed. Boston, MA: Academic Press; 2006:1173-1194.
12. American Psychiatric Association. *Diagnostic and Statistical Manual of Mental Disorders.* 4th ed. Washington, DC: American Psychiatric Association; 1994.
13. American Psychiatric Association. *Diagnostic and Statistical Manual of Mental Disorders.* 4th ed, Text Revision. Washington, DC: American Psychiatric Association; 2000.
14. American Psychiatric Association. *Diagnostic and Statistical Manual of Mental Disorders.* 5th ed. Arlington, VA: American Psychiatric Association; 2013.
15. Sungur MZ, Gündüz A. A comparison of DSM-IV-TR and DSM-5 definitions for sexual dysfunctions: critiques and challenges. *J Sex Med.* 2014;11(2):364-373.
16. NIH Consensus Conference. Impotence. NIH Consensus Development Panel on Impotence. *JAMA.* 1993;270:83-90.
17. The Process of Care Consensus Panel. The process of care model for evaluation and treatment of erectile dysfunction. *Int J Impot Res.* 1999;11:59-70, discussion 70-74.
18. Laumann EO, Nicolosi A, Glasser DB, et al. Sexual problems among women and men aged 40-80y: prevalence and correlates identified in the Global Study of Sexual Attitudes and Behaviors. *Int J Impot Res.* 2005;17:39-57.
19. Blumentals WA, Gome-Camninero A, Joo S, Bannappagari V. Should erectile dysfunction be considered as a marker for acute myocardial infarction? Results from a retrospective cohort study. *Int J Impot Res.* 2004;16:350-353.
20. Basson R, Schulz WW. Sexual sequelae of general medical disorders. *Lancet.* 2007;369:409-424.
21. Cyranowski JM, Bromberger J, Youk A, et al. Lifetime depression history and sexual function in women at midlife. *Arch Sex Behav.* 2004;33:539-548.
22. Hartmann U, Philippsohn S, Heiser K, Ruffer-Hesse C. Low sexual desire in midlife and older women: personality factors, psychosocial development, present sexuality. *Menopause.* 2004;11:726-740.
23. King M, Holt V, Nazareth I. Women's view of their sexual difficulties: agreement and disagreement for the clinical diagnoses. *Arch Sex Behav.* 2007;36:281-288.
24. Basson R. Human sex response cycles. *J Sex Marital Ther.* 2001;27(1):33-43.
25. Basson R. The female sexual response: a different model. *J Sex Marital Ther.* 2000;26:51-65.
26. Goldhammer DL, McCabe MP. A qualitative exploration of the meaning and experience of sexual desire among partnered women. *Can J Human Sex.* 2011;20(1-2):19-34.
27. Both S, Everaerd W, Laan E. Desire emerges from excitement: a psychophysiological perspective on sexual motivation. In: Janssen E, ed. *The Psychophysiology of Sex.* Bloomington, IN: Indiana University Press; 2007:327-339.
28. Laan E, Both S. What makes women experience desire? *Feminine Psychol.* 2008;18(4):505-514.
29. Balercia G, Boscaro M, Lombardo F, et al. Sexual symptoms in endocrine diseases: psychosomatic perspectives. *Psychother Psychosom.* 2007;76(3):134-140.
30. Enzlin P, Rosen R, Wiegel M, et al. Sexual dysfunction in women with type-1 diabetes: long-term findings from the DCCT/EDIC study cohort. *Diabetes Care.* 2009;32:780-783.
31. El-Sakka AI. Association of risk factors and medical comorbidities with male sexual dysfunctions. *J Sex Med.* 2007;4:1691-1700.
32. Vannier SA, O'Sullivan LF. Sex without desire: characteristics of occasions of sexual compliance in young adults' committed relationships. *J Sex Res.* 2010;47:429-439.
33. Hayes R. Circular and linear modeling of female sexual desire and arousal. *J Sex Res.* 2011;48:130-141.
34. Janssen E, McBride KR, Yarber W, et al. Factors that influence sexual arousal in men: a focus group study. *Arch Sex Behav.* 2008;37:252-265.
35. Brotto LA, Heiman JR, Tolman D. Narratives of desire in mid-age women with and without arousal difficulties. *J Sex Res.* 2009;16:1-12.
36. Mitchell KR, Wellings KA, Graham C. How do men and women define sexual desire and sexual arousal? *J Sex Marital Ther.* 2014;40(1):17-32.
37. Stoléru S, Fonteille V, Cornélis C, et al. Functional neuroimaging studies of sexual arousal and orgasm in healthy men and women: a review and meta-analysis. *Neurosci Biobehav Rev.* 2012;36:1481-1509.
38. Meston CM, Buss DM. Why humans have sex. *Arch Sex Behav.* 2007;36:477-507.
39. Carpenter LM, Nathanson CA, Kim JY. Physical women, emotional men: gender and sexual satisfaction in midlife. *Arch Sex Behav.* 2009;38:87-107.
40. Heiman JR, Long JS, Smith SN, et al. Sexual behaviour and relationship satisfaction in midlife and older couples in five countries. *J Sex Med.* 2009;6(Suppl 2):72.
41. de Jong DC. The role of attention in sexual arousal: implications for treatment of sexual dysfunction. *J Sex Res.* 2009;46(2-3):237-248.
42. Nobre PJ, Pinto-Gouveia J. Cognitions, emotions, and sexual response: analysis of the relationship among automatic thoughts, emotional responses, and sexual arousal. *Arch Sex Behav.* 2008;37:652-661.
43. Barlow DH. Causes of sexual dysfunction: the role of anxiety and cognitive interference. *J Consult Clin Psychol.* 1986;54:140-148.
44. Nelson AL, Purdon C. Non-erotic thoughts, attentional focus, and sexual problems in a community sample. *Arch Sex Behav.* 2011;40:395-406.
45. Carvalho J, Vieira AL, Nobre P. Latent structures of male sexual functioning. *J Sex Med.* 2011;8:2501-2511.
46. Pfaus JG. Pathways of sexual desire. *J Sex Med.* 2009;6:1506-1533.
47. Bancroft J, Graham C, Janssen E, et al. The dual control model: current status and future directions. *J Sex Res.* 2009;46:121-142.
48. Takahashi H, Yahata N, Koeda M, et al. Brain activation associated with evaluative processes of guilt and embarrassment: an fMRI study. *Neuroimage.* 2004;23(3):967-974.
49. Archer JS, Love-Geffen TE, Herbst-Damm KL, et al. Effect of estradiol versus estradiol and testosterone on brain activation patterns in postmenopausal women. *Menopause.* 2006;13:528-537.
50. Georgiadis JR, Reinders AA, Paans AMJ, et al. Men versus women on sexual brain function: prominent differences during tactile genital stimulation, but not during orgasm. *Hum Brain Mapp.* 2009;30:3089-3101.
51. Arnow BA, Millheiser L, Garrett A, et al. Women with hypoactive sexual desire disorder compared to normal females: a functional magnetic resonance imaging study. *J Neurosci.* 2009;158:484-502.
52. Bloemers J, Scholte S, van Rooij K, et al. Reduced gray matter volume and increased white matter fractional anisotropy in women with hypoactive sexual desire disorder. *J Sex Med.* 2014;11:753-767.
53. Seminowicz DA, Wideman TH, Naso L, et al. Effective treatment of chronic low back pain in humans reverses abnormal brain anatomy and function. *J Neurosci.* 2011;31(20):7540-7550.
54. Redouté J, Stoléru S, Pugeat M, et al. Brain processing of visual sexual stimuli in treated and untreated hypogonadal patients. *Psychoneuroendocrinology.* 2005;30:461-482.
55. Berridge KC. Food reward: brain substrates of wanting and liking. *Neurosci Biobehav Rev.* 1996;20:1-25.
56. Miller B, Cummings J, McIntyre H, et al. Hypersexuality or altered sexual preference following brain injury. *J Neurol Neurosurg Psychiatry.* 1986;49:867-873.
57. Devinsky J, Sacks O, Devinsky O. Kluver-Bucy syndrome, hypersexuality, and the law. *Neurocase.* 2010;16(2):140-145.
58. Richfield E, Twyman R, Berent S. Neurological syndrome following bilateral damage to the head of the caudate nuclei. *Ann Neurol.* 1987;22:768-771.
59. Paredes RG, Agmo A. Has dopamine a physiological role in the control of sexual behavior? A critical review of the evidence. *Prog Neurobiol.* 2004;73:179-226.
60. Hull EM, Muschamp JW, Sato S. Dopamine and serotonin: influences on male sexual behavior. *Physiol Behav.* 2004;83:291-307.
61. Stahl SM. The psychopharmacology of sex: part 2. Effects of drugs and disease on the 3 phases of human sexual response. *J Clin Psychiatry.* 2001;62:147-148.
62. Bhasin S, Cunningham GR, Hayes FJ, et al; Task Force Endocrine Society. Testosterone therapy in men with androgen deficiency syndromes: an Endocrine Society clinical practice guideline. *J Clin Endocrinol Metab.* 2010;95(6):2536-2559.
63. Wierman ME, Basson R, Davis SR, et al. Androgen therapy in women: an Endocrine Society Clinical Practice Guideline. *J Clin Endocrinol Metab.* 2006;1:3697-3710.
64. Santoro N, Torrens J, Crawford S, et al. Correlates of circulating androgens in midlife women: the study of women's health across the nation. *J Clin Endocrinol Metab.* 2005;90(8):4836-4845.
65. Davis SR, Davison SL, Donath S, Bell RJ. Circulating androgen levels in self-reported sexual function in women. *JAMA.* 2005;294:91-96.
66. Basson R, Brotto LA, Petkau J, Labrie F. Role of androgens in women's sexual dysfunction. *Menopause.* 2010;17(5):962-971.
67. Labrie F, Bélanger A, Tusan L, et al. Marked decline in serum concentrations of adrenal C19 sex steroid precursors and conjugated androgen metabolites during aging. *J Clin Endocrinol Metab.* 1997;82:2396-2402.
68. Stahl SM. The psychopharmacology of sex: part 1. Neurotransmitters and the 3 phases of the human sexual response. *J Clin Psychiatry.* 2001;62:80-81.
69. Halaris A. Neurochemical aspects of the sexual response cycle. *CNS Spectr.* 2003;8(3):211-216.
70. van Furth WR, Wolterink G, van Ree JM. Regulation of masculine sexual behavior: involvement of brain opioids and dopamine. *Brain Res Brain Res Rev.* 1995;21(2):162-184.
71. Chessick RD. The "pharmacogenic orgasm" in the drug addict. *Arch Gen Psychiatry.* 1960;3:565-566.

72. Diamond LE, Earle DC, Rosen RC, et al. Double-blind, placebo-controlled evaluation of the safety, pharmacokinetic properties, and pharmacodynamic effects of intranasal PT-141, a melanocortin receptor agonist, in healthy males and patients with mild-to-moderate erectile dysfunction. *Int J Impot Res.* 2004;16:51-59.

73. Diamond LE, Earle DC, Heiman JR, et al. An effect of the subjective sexual response in premenopausal women with sexual arousal disorder by bremelanotide (PT-141), a melanocortin receptor agonist. *J Sex Med.* 2006;3:628-638.

74. Krüger TH, Hartmann U, Schedlowski M. Prolactinergic and dopaminergic mechanisms underlying sexual arousal and orgasm in humans. *World J Urol.* 2005;23:130-138.

75. Corona G, Mannucci E, Fisher AD, et al. Effect of hyperprolactinemia in male patients consulting for sexual dysfunction. *J Sex Med.* 2007;4:1485-1493.

76. Kadioglu P, Yalin AS, Tiryakioglu O, et al. Sexual dysfunction in women with hyperprolactinemia: a pilot study report. *J Urol.* 2005;174:1921-1925.

77. Blaustein JD. Progestin receptors: neuronal integrators of hormonal and environmental stimulation. *Ann N Y Acad Sci.* 2003;1007:238-250.

78. Pfaus JG, Kippin TE, Coria-Avila GA. What can animal models tell us about human sexual response? *Ann Rev Sex Res.* 2003;14:1-63.

79. Chivers ML, Seto MC, Lalumiere ML, et al. Agreement of self-reported and genital measures of sexual arousal in men and women: a meta-analysis. *Arch Sex Behav.* 2010;39(1):5-56.

80. Janssen E, Vorst H, Finn P, et al. The Sexual Inhibition (SIS) and Sexual Excitation (SES) Scales: II. Predicting psychophysiological response patterns. *J Sex Res.* 2002;39:127-132.

81. Janssen E, Goodrich D, Petrocelli J, et al. Psychophysiological response patterns and risky sexual behaviour in heterosexual and homosexual men. *Arch Sex Behav.* 2009;38:538-550.

82. Suschinsky KD, Lalumière ML. The relationship between sexual concordance and interoception in anxious and non-anxious women. *J Sex Med.* 2014;11:942-955.

83. Palace EM, Gorzalka BB. The enhancing effects of anxiety on arousal in sexually dysfunctional and functional women. *J Abnorm Psychol.* 1990;99(4):403-411.

84. Christ GJ. The penis as a vascular organ. The importance of corporal smooth muscle tone in the control of erection. *Urol Clin North Am.* 1995;22:727-745.

85. Benson GS, McConnell J, Lipshultz LI, et al. Neuromorphology and neuropharmacology of the human penis: an in vitro study. *J Clin Invest.* 1980;65:506-513.

86. Christ GJ. Gap junctions and ion channels: relevance to erectile dysfunction. *Int J Impot Res.* 2000;12(Suppl 4):S15-S25.

87. Zeng X, Keyser B, Li M, Sikka SC. T-type (alpha1G) low voltage-activated calcium channel interactions with nitric oxide-cyclic guanosine monophosphate pathway and regulation of calcium homeostasis in human cavernosal cells. *J Sex Med.* 2005;2:620-630, discussion 630-623.

88. Somlyo AP, Somlyo AV. Ca2+ sensitivity of smooth muscle and nonmuscle myosin II: modulated by G proteins, kinases, and myosin phosphatase. *Physiol Rev.* 2003;83:1325-1358.

89. O-Uchi J, Komukai K, Kusakari Y, et al. Alpha1-adrenoceptor stimulation potentiates L-type Ca2+ current through Ca2+/calmodulin-dependent PK II (CaMKII) activation in rat ventricular myocytes. *Proc Natl Acad Sci U S A.* 2005;102:9400-9405.

90. Krall JF, Fittingoff M, Rajfer J. Characterization of cyclic nucleotide and inositol 1,4,5-trisphosphate-sensitive calcium-exchange activity of smooth muscle cells cultured from the human corpora cavernosa. *Biol Reprod.* 1988;39:913-922.

91. Fittingoff M, Krall JF. Changes in inositol polyphosphate-sensitive calcium exchange in aortic smooth muscle cells in vitro. *J Cell Physiol.* 1988;134:297-301.

92. Hewawasam P, Fan W, Ding M, et al. 4-Aryl-3-(hydroxyalkyl)quinolin-2-ones: novel maxi-K channel opening relaxants of corporal smooth muscle targeted for erectile dysfunction. *J Med Chem.* 2003;46:2819-2822.

93. Christ GJ, Day N, Santizo C, et al. Intracorporal injection of hSlo cDNA restores erectile capacity in STZ-diabetic F-344 rats in vivo. *Am J Physiol Heart Circ Physiol.* 2004;287(4):H1544-H1553.

94. Naylor AM. Endogenous neurotransmitters mediating penile erection. *Br J Urol.* 1998;81:424-431.

95. Melman A, Bar-Chama N, McCullough A, et al. The first human trial for gene transfer therapy for the treatment of erectile dysfunction: preliminary results. *Eur Urol.* 2005;48:314-318.

96. Christ GJ, Moreno AP, Melman A, Spray DC. Gap junction-mediated intercellular diffusion of Ca2+ in cultured human corporal smooth muscle cells. *Am J Physiol.* 1992;263:C373-C383.

97. Ignarro LJ, Bush PA, Buga GM, et al. Nitric oxide and cyclic GMP formation upon electrical field stimulation cause relaxation of corpus cavernosum smooth muscle. *Biochem Biophys Res Commun.* 1990;170:843-850.

98. Mills TM, Chitaley K, Lewis RW, Webb RC. Nitric oxide inhibits RhoA/Rho-kinase signaling to cause penile erection. *Eur J Pharmacol.* 2002;439:173-174.

99. Haning H, Niewohner U, Bischoff E. Phosphodiesterase type 5 (PDE5) inhibitors. *Prog Med Chem.* 2003;41:249-306.

100. Wallis RM, Corbin JD, Francis SH, Ellis P. Tissue distribution of phosphodiesterase families and the effects of sildenafil on tissue cyclic nucleotides, platelet function, and the contractile responses of trabeculae carneae and aortic rings in vitro. *Am J Cardiol.* 1999;83:3C-12C.

101. Bischoff E. Potency, selectivity, and consequences of nonselectivity of PDE inhibition. *Int J Impot Res.* 2004;16(Suppl 1):S11-S14.

102. Boolell M, Allen MJ, Ballard SA, et al. Sildenafil: an orally active type 5 cyclic GMP-specific phosphodiesterase inhibitor for the treatment of penile erectile dysfunction. *Int J Impot Res.* 1996;8:47-52.

103. Taher A, Meyer M, Stief CG, et al. Cyclic nucleotide phosphodiesterase in human cavernous smooth muscle. *World J Urol.* 1997;15:32-35.

104. Jeremy JY, Ballard SA, Naylor AM, et al. Effects of sildenafil, a type-5 cGMP phosphodiesterase inhibitor, and papaverine on cyclic GMP and cyclic AMP levels in the rabbit corpus cavernosum in vitro. *Br J Urol.* 1997;79:958-963.

105. Stief CG, Uckert S, Becker AJ, et al. The effect of the specific phosphodiesterase (PDE) inhibitors on human and rabbit cavernous tissue in vitro and in vivo. *J Urol.* 1998;159:1390-1393.

106. Carter AJ, Ballard SA, Naylor AM. Effect of the selective phosphodiesterase type 5 inhibitor sildenafil on erectile dysfunction in the anesthetized dog. *J Urol.* 1998;160:242-246.

107. Gong MC, Iizuka K, Nixon G, et al. Role of guanine nucleotide-binding proteins—ras-family or trimeric proteins or both—in Ca2+ sensitization of smooth muscle. *Proc Natl Acad Sci U S A.* 1996;93:1340-1345.

108. Chikumi H, Fukuhara S, Gutkind JS. Regulation of G protein-linked guanine nucleotide exchange factors for Rho, PDZ-RhoGEF, and LARG by tyrosine phosphorylation: evidence of a role for focal adhesion kinase. *J Biol Chem.* 2002;277:12463-12473.

109. Gong MC, Fujihara H, Somlyo AV, Somlyo AP. Translocation of rhoA associated with Ca2+ sensitization of smooth muscle. *J Biol Chem.* 1997;272:10704-10709.

110. Segraves RT. Bupropion sustained-release for the treatment of hypoactive sexual desire disorder in premenopausal women. *J Clin Psychopharmacol.* 2004;24:339-342.

111. Jin L, Liu T, Lagoda GA, et al. Elevated RhoA/Rho-kinase activity in the aged rat penis: mechanism for age-associated erectile dysfunction. *FASEB J.* 2006;20:536-538.

112. Davis SR, Nijland FA, Weijmar-Schultz W. Tibolone vs transdermal continuous combined estrogen plus progestin in the treatment of female sexual dysfunction in naturally menopausal women: Results from the NETA trial. *Maturitas.* 2006;554S:S1-S112.

113. Lipshultz LI, McConnell J, Benson GS. Current concepts of the mechanisms of ejaculation. Normal and abnormal states. *J Reprod Med.* 1981;26:499-507.

114. McMahon CG, Abdo C, Incrocci L, et al. Disorders of orgasm and ejaculation in men. *J Sex Med.* 2004;1:58-65.

115. Gil-Vernet JM Jr, Alvarez-Vijande R, Gil-Vernet A, Gil-Vernet JM. Ejaculation in men: a dynamic endorectal ultrasonographical study. *Br J Urol.* 1994;73:442-448.

116. Caruso S, Rugolo S, Agmello C, et al. Sildenafil improves sexual functioning in premenopausal women with type 1 diabetes who are affected by sexual arousal disorder: A double-blind, crossover, placebo-controlled pilot study. *Fertil Steril.* 2006;85:1496-1501.

117. Guiliano P, Clement P. Serotonin and premature ejaculation: from physiology to patient management. *Euro Urol.* 2006;50:454-466.

118. Waldinger M. The neurobiological approach to early ejaculation. *J Urol.* 2002;168:2359-2366.

119. Olivier B, Van Oorschot R, Waldinger M. Serotonin, serotonergic receptors, selective serotonin reuptake inhibitors and sexual behavior. *Int Clin Psychopharmacol.* 1998;13(Suppl 6):9.

120. Waldinger MD, Olivier B. Utility of selective serotonin reuptake inhibitors in premature ejaculation. *Curr Opin Investig Drugs.* 2004;5:743-747.

121. Kwan M, Greenleaf WJ, Mann J, et al. The nature of androgen action on male sexuality: a combined laboratory-self-report study on hypogonadal men. *J Clin Endocrinol Metab.* 1983;57:557-562.

122. Alexander GM, Sherwin BB. The association between testosterone, sexual arousal, and selective attention for erotic stimuli in men. *Horm Behav.* 1991;25:367-381.

123. Alexander GM, Swerdloff RS, Wang C, et al. Androgen-behavior correlations in hypogonadal men and eugonadal men. I. Mood and response to auditory sexual stimuli. *Horm Behav.* 1997;31(2):110-119.

124. Arver S, Dobs AS, Meikle AW, et al. Improvement of sexual function in testosterone deficient men treated for 1 year with a permeation enhanced testosterone transdermal system. *J Urol.* 1996;155:1604-1608.

125. King BE, Packard MG, Alexander GM. Affective properties of intramedial preoptic area injections of testosterone in male rats. *Neurosci Lett.* 1999;269:149-152.

126. Bagatell CJ, Heiman JR, Rivier JE, Bremner WJ. Effects of endogenous testosterone and estradiol on sexual behavior in normal young men

[published erratum appears in *J Clin Endocrinol Metab*. 1994;78(6):1520]. *J Clin Endocrinol Metab*. 1994;78(3):711-716.

127. Carani C, Bancroft J, Granata A, et al. Testosterone and erectile function, nocturnal penile tumescence and rigidity, and erectile response to visual erotic stimuli in hypogonadal and eugonadal men. *Psychoneuroendocrinology*. 1992;17:647-654.

128. Cunningham GR, Hirshkowitz M, Korenman SG, Karacan I. Testosterone replacement therapy and sleep-related erections in hypogonadal men. *J Clin Endocrinol Metab*. 1990;70(3):792-797.

129. Mills TM, Lewis RW, Stopper VS. Androgenic maintenance of inflow and veno-occlusion during erection in the rat. *Biol Reprod*. 1998;59(6):1413-1418.

130. Reilly CM, Zamorano P, Stopper VS, Mills TM. Androgenic regulation of NO availability in rat penile erection. *J Androl*. 1997;18(2):110-115.

131. Lugg JA, Rajfer J, Gonzalez-Cadavid NF. Dihydrotestosterone is the active androgen in the maintenance of nitric oxide-mediated penile erection in the rat. *Endocrinology*. 1995;136:1495-1501.

132. Shabsigh R. The effects of testosterone on the cavernous tissue and erectile function. *World J Urol*. 1997;15:21-26.

133. Bhasin S, Cunningham GR, Hayes FJ, et al. Testosterone therapy in adult men with androgen deficiency syndromes: an Endocrine Society clinical practice guideline. *J Clin Endocrinol Metab*. 2006;91:1995-2010.

134. Jain P, Rademaker AW, McVary KT. Testosterone supplementation for erectile dysfunction: results of a meta-analysis. *J Urol*. 2000;164:371-375.

135. Buena F, Swerdloff RS, Steiner BS, et al. Sexual function does not change when serum testosterone levels are pharmacologically varied within the normal male range. *Fertil Steril*. 1993;59:1118-1123.

136. Isidori AM, Giannetta E, Gianfrilli D, et al. Effects of testosterone on sexual function in men: results of a meta-analysis. *Clin Endocrinol (Oxf)*. 2005;63(4):381-394.

137. Bhasin S, Travison TG, Storer TW, et al. Effect of testosterone supplementation with and without a dual 5α-reductase inhibitor on fat-free mass in men with suppressed testosterone production: a randomized controlled trial. *JAMA*. 2012;307(9):931-939.

138. Carani C, Rochira V, Faustini-Fustini M, et al. Role of oestrogen in male sexual behaviour: insights from the natural model of aromatase deficiency. *Clin Endocrinol (Oxf)*. 1999;51(4):517-524.

139. Carani C, Granata AR, Rochira V, et al. Sex steroids and sexual desire in a man with a novel mutation of aromatase gene and hypogonadism. *Psychoneuroendocrinology*. 2005;30(5):413-417.

140. Finkelstein JS, Lee H, Burnett-Bowie SA, et al. Gonadal steroids and body composition, strength, and sexual function in men. *N Engl J Med*. 2013;369(11):1011-1022.

141. Korenman SG, Morley JE, Mooradian AD, et al. Secondary hypogonadism in older men: its relation to impotence. *J Clin Endocrinol Metab*. 1990;71:963-969.

142. Corona G, Isidori AM, Buvat J, et al. Testosterone supplementation and sexual function: a meta-analysis study. *J Sex Med*. 2014;11(6):1577-1592.

143. Kohler TS, Kim J, Feia K, et al. Prevalence of androgen deficiency in men with erectile dysfunction. *Urology*. 2008;71(4):693-697.

144. Shabsigh R, Kaufman JM, Steidle C, Padma-Nathan H. Randomized study of testosterone gel as adjunctive therapy to sildenafil in hypogonadal men with erectile dysfunction who do not respond to sildenafil alone. *J Urol*. 2004;172:658-663.

145. Aversa A, Isidori AM, Spera G, et al. Androgens improve cavernous vasodilation and response to sildenafil in patients with erectile dysfunction. *Clin Endocrinol (Oxf)*. 2003;58(5):632-638.

146. Dasgupta R, Wiseman OJ, Kanabar G, et al. Efficacy of sildenafil in the treatment of female sexual dysfunction due to multiple sclerosis. *J Urol*. 2004;171:1189-1193.

147. Kalinchenko SY, Kozlov GI, Gontcharov NP, Katsiya GV. Oral testosterone undecanoate reverses erectile dysfunction associated with diabetes mellitus in patients failing on sildenafil citrate therapy alone. *Aging Male*. 2003;6:94-99.

148. Spitzer M, Basaria S, Travison TG, et al. Effect of testosterone replacement on response to sildenafil citrate in men with erectile dysfunction: a parallel, randomized trial. *Ann Intern Med*. 2012;157(10):681-691.

149. Buvat J, Montorsi F, Maggi M, et al. Hypogonadal men nonresponders to the PDE5 inhibitor tadalafil benefit from normalization of testosterone levels with a 1% hydroalcoholic testosterone gel in the treatment of erectile dysfunction (TADTEST study). *J Sex Med*. 2011;8(1):284-293.

150. Spitzer M, Bhasin S, Travison TG, et al. Sildenafil increases serum testosterone levels by a direct action on the testes. *Andrology*. 2013;1(6):913-918.

151. Buisson O, Jannini A. Pilot echographic study of the differences in clitoral involvement following clitoral or vaginal sexual stimulation. *J Sex Med*. 2013;10:2734-2740.

152. Oakley SH, Vaccaro CM, Crisp CC, et al. Clitoral size and location in relation to sexual function using pelvic MRI. *J Sex Med*. 2014;11(4):1013-1022.

153. Samimi D, Allam A, Devereaux R, et al. Advantages of nerve-sparing intrastromal total abdominal hysterectomy. *Int J Womens Health*. 2013;5:37-42.

154. Bekker MD, Hogewoning CR, Wallner C, et al. The somatic and autonomic innervation of the clitoris; preliminary evidence of sexual dysfunction after minimally invasive slings. *J Sex Med*. 2012;9:1566-1578.

155. Salonia A, Giraldi A, Chivers ML, et al. Physiology of women's sexual function: basic knowledge and new findings. *J Sex Med*. 2010;7:2637-2660.

156. Uckert S, Albrecht K, Kuczyk MA, et al. Phosphodiesterase type 1, calcitonin gene-related peptide and vasoactive intestinal polypeptide are involved in the control of human vaginal arterial vessels. *Eur J Obstet Gynecol Reprod Biol*. 2013;169(2):283-286.

157. Shih C, Cold CJ, Yang CC. Cutaneous corpuscular receptors of the human glans clitoris: descriptive characteristics and comparison with the glans penis. *J Sex Med*. 2013;10:1783-1789.

158. van Netten JJ, Georgiadis JR, Nieuwenburg A, et al. 8-13 Hz fluctuations in rectal pressure are an objective marker of clitorally-induced orgasm in women. *Arch Sex Behav*. 2008;37:279-285.

159. Hamann S, Herman RA, Nolan CL, et al. Men and women differ in amygdala response to visual sexual stimuli. *Nat Neurosci*. 2004;7(4):411-416.

160. Georgiadis JR, Kringelbach ML. The human sexual response cycle: brain imaging evidence linking sex to other pleasures. *Prog Neurobiol*. 2012;98(1):49-81.

161. Huynh HK, Willemsen ATM, Lovick TA, et al. Pontine control of ejaculation and female orgasm. *J Sex Med*. 2013;10:3038-3048.

162. Huynh HK, Willemsen AT, Holstege G. Female orgasm but not male ejaculation activates the pituitary. A PET-neuro-imaging study. *Neuroimage*. 2013;76:178-182.

163. Beck JG. Hypoactive sexual desire disorder: an overview. *J Consult Clin Psychol*. 1995;63:919-927.

164. Rosen RC, Leiblum SR. Hypoactive sexual desire. *Psychiatr Clin North Am*. 1995;18:107-121.

165. Segraves KB, Segraves RT. Hypoactive sexual desire disorder: prevalence and comorbidity in 906 subjects. *J Sex Marital Ther*. 1991;17:55-58.

166. LoPiccolo J. Diagnosis and treatment of male sexual dysfunction. *J Sex Marital Ther*. 1985;11:215-232.

167. Panser LA, Rhodes T, Girman CJ, et al. Sexual function of men ages 40 to 79 years: the Olmsted County Study of Urinary Symptoms and Health Status Among Men. *J Am Geriatr Soc*. 1995;43(10):1107-1111.

168. Chevret M, Jaudinot E, Sullivan K, et al. Impact of erectile dysfunction (ED) on sexual life of female partners: assessment with the Index of Sexual Life (ISL) questionnaire. *J Sex Marital Ther*. 2004;30:157-172.

169. Johannes CB, Araujo AB, Feldman HA, et al. Incidence of erectile dysfunction in men 40 to 69 years old: longitudinal results from the Massachusetts male aging study. *J Urol*. 2000;163:460-463.

170. Benet AE, Melman A. The epidemiology of erectile dysfunction. *Urol Clin North Am*. 1995;22:699-709.

171. Braun M, Wassmer G, Klotz T, et al. Epidemiology of erectile dysfunction: results of the "Cologne Male Survey." *Int J Impot Res*. 2000;12:305-311.

172. McKinlay JB, Digruttolo L, Glasser D, et al. International differences in the epidemiology of male erectile dysfunction. *Int J Clin Pract Suppl*. 1999;102:35.

173. McKinlay JB. The worldwide prevalence and epidemiology of erectile dysfunction. *Int J Impot Res*. 2000;12(Suppl 4):S6-S11.

174. Ayta IA, McKinlay JB, Krane RJ. The likely worldwide increase in erectile dysfunction between 1995 and 2025 and some possible policy consequences. *BJU Int*. 1999;84:50-56.

175. Selvin E, Burnett AL, Platz EA. Prevalence and risk factors for erectile dysfunction in the US. *Am J Med*. 2007;120(2):151-157.

176. Montorsi P, Ravagnani PM, Galli S, et al. Association between erectile dysfunction and coronary artery disease. Role of coronary clinical presentation and extent of coronary vessels involvement: the COBRA trial. *Eur Heart J*. 2006;27(22):2632-2639.

177. Thompson IM, Tangen CM, Goodman PJ, et al. Erectile dysfunction and subsequent cardiovascular disease. *JAMA*. 2005;294(23):2996-3002.

178. Araujo AB, Travison TG, Ganz P, et al. Erectile dysfunction and mortality. *J Sex Med*. 2009;6(9):2445-2454.

179. Araujo AB, Hall SA, Ganz P, et al. Does erectile dysfunction contribute to cardiovascular disease risk prediction beyond the Framingham risk score? *J Am Coll Cardiol*. 2010;55(4):350-356.

180. Schouten BW, Bohnen AM, Bosch JL, et al. Erectile dysfunction prospectively associated with cardiovascular disease in the Dutch general population: results from the Krimpen Study. *Int J Impot Res*. 2008;20(1):92-99.

181. Jackson G, Boon N, Eardley I, et al. Erectile dysfunction and coronary artery disease prediction: evidence-based guidance and consensus. *Int J Clin Pract*. 2007;61(12):2019-2025.

182. Hodges LD, Kirby M, Solanki J, O'Donnell J. The temporal relationship between erectile dysfunction and cardiovascular disease. *Int J Clin Pract*. 2010;64(7):848-857.

183. Feldman HA, Johannes CB, Derby CA, et al. Erectile dysfunction and coronary risk factors: prospective results from the Massachusetts male aging study. *Prev Med.* 2000;30:328-338.

184. Derby CA, Mohr BA, Goldstein I, et al. Modifiable risk factors and erectile dysfunction: can lifestyle changes modify risk? *Urology.* 2000; 56:302-306.

185. Rosen R, Altwein J, Boyle P, et al. Lower urinary tract symptoms and male sexual dysfunction: the multinational survey of the aging male (MSAM-7). *Eur Urol.* 2003;44:637-649.

186. Braun MH, Sommer F, Haupt G, et al. Lower urinary tract symptoms and erectile dysfunction: co-morbidity or typical "aging male" symptoms? Results of the "Cologne Male Survey." *Eur Urol.* 2003;44: 588-594.

187. Barqawi A, O'Donnell C, Kumar R, et al. Correlation between LUTS (AUA-SS) and erectile dysfunction (SHIM) in an age-matched racially diverse male population: data from the Prostate Cancer Awareness Week (PCAW). *Int J Impot Res.* 2005;17:370-374.

188. Glina S, Santana AW, Azank F, et al. Lower urinary tract symptoms and erectile dysfunction are highly prevalent in ageing men. *BJU Int.* 2006;97:763-765.

189. McVary K. Lower urinary tract symptoms and sexual dysfunction: epidemiology and pathophysiology. *BJU Int.* 2006;97(Suppl 2):23-28, discussion 44-45.

190. Paick SH, Meehan A, Lee M, et al. The relationship among lower urinary tract symptoms, prostate specific antigen and erectile dysfunction in men with benign prostatic hyperplasia: results from the PROSCAR long-term efficacy and safety study. *J Urol.* 2005;173: 903-907.

191. McVary KT. Interrelation of erectile dysfunction and lower urinary tract symptoms. *Drugs Today (Barc).* 2005;41:527-536.

192. Christ GJ, Hodges S. Molecular mechanisms of detrusor and corporal myocyte contraction: identifying targets for pharmacotherapy of bladder and erectile dysfunction. *Br J Pharmacol.* 2006;147(Suppl 2): S41-S55.

193. Carson CC. Combination of phosphodiesterase-5 inhibitors and alpha-blockers in patients with benign prostatic hyperplasia: treatments of lower urinary tract symptoms, erectile dysfunction, or both? *BJU Int.* 2006;97(Suppl 2):39-43, discussion 44-45.

194. Liguori G, Trombetta C, De Giorgi G, et al. Efficacy and safety of combined oral therapy with tadalafil and alfuzosin: an integrated approach to the management of patients with lower urinary tract symptoms and erectile dysfunction. Preliminary report. *J Sex Med.* 2009;6(2):544-545.

195. Kaplan SA, Gonzalez RR, Te AE. Combination of alfuzosin and sildenafil is superior to monotherapy in treating lower urinary tract symptoms and erectile dysfunction. *Eur Urol.* 2007;51(6):1717-1723.

196. Buvat J, Glasser D, Neves RC, et al. Global Study of Sexual Attitudes and Behaviours (GSSAB) Investigators' Group. Sexual problems and associated help-seeking behavior patterns: results of a population-based survey in France. *Int J Urol.* 2009;16(7):632-638.

197. Laumann EO, Glasser DB, Neves RC, Moreira ED Jr. Global Study of Sexual Attitudes and Behaviours Investigators' Group. A population-based survey of sexual activity, sexual problems and associated help-seeking behavior patterns in mature adults in the United States of America. *Int J Impot Res.* 2009;21(3):171-178.

198. Porst H, Montorsi F, Rosen R, et al. The premature ejaculation prevalence and attitudes (PEPA) survey: prevalence, comorbidities, and professional help-seeking. *Eur Urol.* 2007;51:816-824.

199. Brotto L. The DSM diagnostic criteria for hypoactive sexual desire disorder in women. *Arch Sex Behav.* 2010;39:221-239.

200. Graham C. The DSM diagnostic criteria for female sexual arousal disorder. *Arch Sex Behav.* 2010;39:240-255.

201. Carvalho J. Sexual desire in women: an integrative approach regarding psychological, medical, and relationship dimensions. *J Sex Med.* 2010; 7:1807-1815.

202. Althof SE, Dean J, Derogates LR, et al. Current perspectives on the aclinical assessment and diagnosis of female sexual dysfunction and clinical studies of potential therapies: a statement of concern. *J Sex Med.* 2005;2:146-153.

203. Sidi H, Naing L, Midin M, Nik Jaafar NR. The female sexual response cycle: do Malaysian women conform to the circular model? *J Sex Med.* 2008;5:2359-2366.

204. Basson R. Women's sexual desire and arousal disorders. *Prim Psychiatry.* 2008;15:72-81.

205. van Lankveld JJ, Granot M, Weijmar Schultz WC, et al. Women's sexual pain disorders. *J Sex Med.* 2010;7(1 Pt 2):615-631.

206. Basson R, Leiblum S, Brotto L, et al. Definitions of women's sexual dysfunctions reconsidered: advocating expansion and revision. *J Psychosom Obstet Gynaecol.* 2003;24:221-229.

207. Bancroft J, Loftus J, Long JS. Distress about sex: a national survey of women in heterosexual relationships. *Arch Sex Behav.* 2003;32: 193-208.

208. Tiefer L, Hall M, Tavris C. Beyond dysfunction: a new view of women's sexual problems. *J Sex Marital Ther.* 2002;28(Suppl 1):225-232.

209. DeLamater JD, Sill M. Sexual desire in later life. *J Sex Res.* 2005; 42:138-149.

210. Lindau ST, Schumm LP, Laumann EO, et al. The study of sexuality and health among older adults in the United States. *N Engl J Med.* 2007; 357:762-774.

211. Öberg K, Sjögern Fugl-Myer K. On Swedish women's distressing sexual dysfunctions: some concomitant conditions and life satisfaction. *J Sex Med.* 2005;2:169-180.

212. Valadares ALR, Pinto Neto AM, Osis MJD, et al. Dyspareunia: a population based study with Brazilian women between 40 and 65 years old. *Menopause.* 2006;13:P-98-P-1016.

213. Mishra G, Kuh D. Sexual functioning throughout menopause: the perceptions of women in a British cohort. *Menopause.* 2006;13: 880-890.

214. Levine KB, Williams RE, Hartmann KE. Vulvovaginal atrophy is strongly associated with female sexual dysfunction among sexually active postmenopausal women. *Menopause.* 2008;15:661-666.

215. Zitzmann M, Faber S, Nieschlag E. Association of specific symptoms and metabolic risks with serum testosterone in older men. *J Clin Endocrinol Metab.* 2006;91(11):4335-4343.

216. Wu FC, Tajar A, Beynon JM, et al; EMAS Group. Identification of late-onset hypogonadism in middle-aged and elderly men. *N Engl J Med.* 2010;363(2):123-135.

217. Kelleher S, Conway AJ, Handelsman DJ. Blood testosterone threshold for androgen deficiency symptoms. *J Clin Endocrinol Metab.* 2004; 89(8):3813-3817.

218. El-Sakka AI, Tayeb KA. Peyronie's disease in diabetic patients being screened for erectile dysfunction. *J Urol.* 2005;174(3):1026-1030.

219. Corona G, Mannucci E, Mansani R, et al. Organic, relational and psychological factors in erectile dysfunction in men with diabetes mellitus. *Eur Urol.* 2004;46(2):222-228.

220. De Berardis G, Pellegrini F, Franciosi M, et al. QuED (Quality of Care and Outcomes in Type 2 Diabetes) Study Group. Longitudinal assessment of quality of life in patients with type 2 diabetes and self-reported erectile dysfunction. *Diabetes Care.* 2005;28(11):2637-2643.

221. Klein R, Klein BE, Moss SE. Ten-year incidence of self-reported erectile dysfunction in people with long-term type 1 diabetes. *J Diabetes Complications.* 2005;19(1):35-41.

222. Rhoden EL, Ribeiro EP, Riedner CE, et al. Glycosylated haemoglobin levels and the severity of erectile function in diabetic men. *BJU Int.* 2005;95(4):615-617.

223. Kalter-Leibovici O, Wainstein J, Ziv A, et al. Israel Diabetes Research Group (IDRG) Investigators. Clinical, socioeconomic, and lifestyle parameters associated with erectile dysfunction among diabetic men. *Diabetes Care.* 2005;28(7):1739-1744.

224. Xin Z, Yuan SY, Wang ZP, et al. Influencing factors of erectile function in male patients with type 2 diabetes mellitus. *Zhongguo Linchuyang Kangfu.* 2004;8(21):4136-4137.

225. Zheng H, Fan W, Li G, Tam T. Predictors for erectile dysfunction among diabetics. *Diabetes Res Clin Pract.* 2006;71:313-319.

226. Ding EL, Song Y, Malik VS, Liu S. Sex differences of endogenous sex hormones and risks of type 2 diabetes: a systematic review and meta-analysis. *JAMA.* 2006;295:1288-1299.

227. Yeap BB, Chubb SA, Hyde Z, et al. Lower serum testosterone is independently associated with insulin resistance in non-diabetic older men: the Health in Men Study. *Eur J Endocrinol.* 2009;161(4): 591-598.

228. Laaksonen DE, Niskanen L, Punnonen K, et al. Testosterone and sex hormone-binding globulin predict the metabolic syndrome and diabetes in middle-aged men. *Diabetes Care.* 2004;27(5):1036-1041.

229. Dhindsa S, Prabhakar S, Sethi M, et al. Frequent occurrence of hypogonadotropic hypogonadism in type 2 diabetes. *J Clin Endocrinol Metab.* 2004;89(11):5462-5468.

230. Lakshman KM, Bhasin S, Araujo AB. Sex hormone-binding globulin as an independent predictor of incident type 2 diabetes mellitus in men. *J Gerontol A Biol Sci Med Sci.* 2010;65(5):503-509.

231. Bhasin S, Jasjua GK, Pencina M, et al. Sex hormone-binding globulin, but not testosterone, is associated prospectively and independently with incident metabolic syndrome in men: the Framingham Heart Study. *Diabetes Care.* 2011;34(11):2464-2470.

232. Gazzaruso C, Giordanetti S, De Amici E, et al. Relationship between erectile dysfunction and silent myocardial ischemia in apparently uncomplicated type 2 diabetic patients. *Circulation.* 2004;110(1): 22-26.

233. Basu A, Ryder RE. New treatment options for erectile dysfunction in patients with diabetes mellitus [review]. *Drugs.* 2004;64(23):2667-2688.

234. De Vriese AS, Verbeuren TJ, Van de Voorde J, et al. Endothelial dysfunction in diabetes. *Br J Pharmacol.* 2000;130:963-974.

235. Saenz de Tejada I, Angulo J, Cellek S, et al. Pathophysiology of erectile dysfunction. *J Sex Med.* 2005;2:26-39.

236. Seftel AD, Vasin ND, Ni Z, et al. Advanced glycation end products in human penis: elevation in diabetic tissue, site of deposition and possible effect through iNOS or eNOS. *Urology.* 1997;50:1016-1026.

237. Bivalacqua TJ, Champion HC, Usta MF, et al. RhoA/Rho-kinase suppresses endothelial nitric oxide synthase in the penis: a mechanism for diabetes-associated erectile dysfunction. *Proc Natl Acad Sci U S A.* 2004;101(24):9121-9126.

238. Boulton AJM, Vinik AJ, Arezzo JC, et al. Diabetic neuropathies. A statement by the American Diabetes Association. *Diabetes Care*. 2005;28(4):956-962.
239. Bivalacqua TJ, Hellstrom WJ, Kadowitz PJ, Champion HC. Increased expression of arginase II in human diabetic corpus cavernosum: in diabetic-associated erectile dysfunction. *Biochem Biophys Res Commun*. 2001;283(4):923-927.
240. El-Sakka AI, Lin CS, Chui RM, et al. Effects of diabetes on nitric oxide synthase and growth factor genes and protein expression in an animal model. *Int J Impot Res*. 1999;11(3):123-132.
241. Ellenberg M, Weber H. Retrograde ejaculation in diabetic neuropathy. *Ann Intern Med*. 1966;65(6):1237-1246.
242. Seftel AD, Rosen RC, Rosenberg MT, Sadovsky R. Benign prostatic hyperplasia evaluation, treatment and association with sexual dysfunction: practice patterns according to physician specialty. *Int J Clin Pract*. 2008;62(4):614-622.
243. Wilt TJ, Mac Donald R, Rutks I. Tamsulosin for benign prostatic hyperplasia. *Cochrane Database Syst Rev*. 2003;(1):CD002081.
244. Edwards JE, Moore RA. Finasteride in the treatment of clinical benign prostatic hyperplasia: a systematic review of randomised trials. *BMC Urol*. 2002;2:14.
245. Giuliano F. Impact of medical treatments for benign prostatic hyperplasia on sexual function. *BJU Int*. 2006;97(Suppl 2):34-38, discussion 44-45.
246. Ganzer CA, Jacobs AR, Iqbal F. Persistent sexual, emotional, and cognitive impairment post-finasteride: a survey of men reporting symptoms. *Am J Mens Health*. 2015;9(3):222-228.
247. Irwig MS, Kolukula S. Persistent sexual side effects of finasteride for male pattern hair loss. *J Sex Med*. 2011;8(6):1747-1753.
248. Di Loreto C, La Marra F, Mazzon G, et al. Immunohistochemical evaluation of androgen receptor and nerve structure density in human prepuce from patients with persistent sexual side effects after finasteride use for androgenetic alopecia. *PLoS ONE*. 2014;9(6):e100237.
249. Traish AM, Hassani J, Guay AT, et al. Adverse side effects of 5α-reductase inhibitors therapy: persistent diminished libido and erectile dysfunction and depression in a subset of patients. *J Sex Med*. 2011;8(3):872-884.
250. Cecchin E, De Mattia E, Mazzon G, et al. A pharmacogenetic survey of androgen receptor (CAG)n and (GGN)n polymorphisms in patients experiencing long term side effects after finasteride discontinuation. *Int J Biol Markers*. 2014;29(4):e310-e316.
251. Buvat J, Lemaire A. Endocrine screening in 1,022 men with erectile dysfunction: clinical significance and cost-effective strategy [see comments]. *J Urol*. 1997;158:1764-1767.
252. Citron JT, Ettinger B, Rubinoff H, et al. Prevalence of hypothalamic-pituitary imaging abnormalities in impotent men with secondary hypogonadism. *J Urol*. 1996;155:529-533.
253. Carter JN, Tyson JE, Tolis G, et al. Prolactin-screening tumors and hypogonadism in 22 men. *N Engl J Med*. 1978;299(16):847-852.
254. Franks S, Jacobs HS, Martin N, Nabarro JD. Hyperprolactinaemia and impotence. *Clin Endocrinol (Oxf)*. 1978;8(4):277-287.
255. Colao A, Vitale G, Cappabianca P, et al. Outcome of cabergoline treatment in men with prolactinoma: effects of a 24-month treatment on prolactin levels, tumor mass, recovery of pituitary function, and semen analysis. *J Clin Endocrinol Metab*. 2004;89:1704-1711.
256. Krassas GE, Tziomalos K, Papadopoulou F, et al. Erectile dysfunction in patients with hyper- and hypothyroidism: how common and should we treat? *J Clin Endocrinol Metab*. 2008;93(5):1815-1819.
257. Carani C, Isidori AM, Granata A, et al. Multicenter study on the prevalence of sexual symptoms in male hypo- and hyperthyroid patients. *J Clin Endocrinol Metab*. 2005;90:6472-6479.
258. Dumoulin SC, Perret BP, Bennet AP, Caron PJ. Opposite effects of thyroid hormones on binding proteins for steroid hormones (sex hormone-binding globulin and corticosteroid-binding globulin) in humans. *Eur J Endocrinol*. 1995;132(5):594-598.
259. Donnelly P, White C. Testicular dysfunction in men with primary hypothyroidism; reversal of hypogonadotrophic hypogonadism with replacement thyroxine. *Clin Endocrinol (Oxf)*. 2000;52(2):197-201.
260. Veronelli A, Masu A, Ranieri R, et al. Prevalence of erectile dysfunction in thyroid disorders: comparison with control subjects and with obese and diabetic patients. *Int J Impot Res*. 2006;18:111-114.
261. Esposito K, Giugliano D. Obesity, the metabolic syndrome, and sexual dysfunction. *Int J Impot Res*. 2005;17(5):391-398.
262. Koca O, Calışkan S, Oztürk MI, et al. Vasculogenic erectile dysfunction and metabolic syndrome. *J Sex Med*. 2010;7(12):3997-4002.
263. Demir O, Akgul K, Akar Z, et al. Association between severity of lower urinary tract symptoms, erectile dysfunction and metabolic syndrome. *Aging Male*. 2009;12(1):29-34.
264. Demir T, Demir O, Kefi A, et al. Prevalence of erectile dysfunction in patients with metabolic syndrome. *Int J Urol*. 2006;13(4):385-388.
265. Oppo A, Franceschi E, Atzeni F, et al. Effects of hyperthyroidism, hypothyroidism, and thyroid autoimmunity on female sexual function. *J Endocrinol Invest*. 2011;34:449-453.
266. Atis G, Dalkilinc A, Altuntas Y, et al. Hyperthyroidism: a risk factor for female sexual dysfunction. *J Sex Med*. 2011;8(8):2327-2333.
267. Pasquali D, Maiorino MI, Renzullo A, et al. Female sexual dysfunction in women with thyroid disorders. *J Endocrinol Inv*. 2013;36(9):729-733.
268. Wierman M, Nappi R, Avis N, et al. Endocrine aspects of women's sexual function. *J Sex Med*. 2010;7(1 Pt 2):561-585.
269. Esposito K, Maiorino MI, Bellastella G, et al. Determinants of female sexual dysfunction in type 2 diabetes. *Int J Impot Res*. 2010;22:179-184.
270. Maiorino MI, Bellastella G, Esposito K. Diabetes and sexual dysfunction: current perspectives. *Diabetes Metab Syndr Obes*. 2014;7:95-105.
271. Abu Ali RM, Al Hajeri RM, Khader YS, et al. Sexual dysfunction in Jordanian diabetic women. *Diabetes Care*. 2008;31:1580-1581.
272. Olarinoye J, Olarinoye A. Determinants of sexual function among women with type 2 diabetes in a Nigerian population. *J Sex Med*. 2008;5(4):878-886.
273. Wallner LP, Sarma AV, Kim C. Sexual functioning among women with and without diabetes in the Boston Area Community Health Study. *J Sex Med*. 2010;7:881-887.
274. Tagliabue M, Gottero C, Zuffranieri M, et al. Sexual function in women with type 1 diabetes matched with a control group: depressive and psychosocial aspects. *J Sex Med*. 2011;8:1694-1700.
275. Leedom L, Feldman M, Procci W, et al. Symptoms of sexual dysfunction and depression in diabetic women. *J Diabetes Complications*. 1991;5:38-41.
276. Ogbera AO, Chinenye S, Akinlade A, et al. Frequency and correlates of sexual dysfunction in women with diabetes mellitus. *J Sex Med*. 2009;6:3401-3406.
277. Jensen SB. Sexual dysfunction in younger insulin-treated diabetic females. A comparative study. *Diabetes Metab*. 1985;11:278-282.
278. Campbell LV, Redelman MJ, Borkman M, et al. Factors in sexual dysfunction in diabetic female volunteer subjects. *Med J Aust*. 1989;151:550-552.
279. Salonia A, Lanzi R, Scavini M, et al. Sexual function and endocrine profile in fertile women with type 1 diabetes. *Diabetes Care*. 2006;29:312-316.
280. Pontiroli AE, Cortelazzi D, Morabito A. Female sexual dysfunction and diabetes: a systematic review and meta-analysis. *J Sex Med*. 2013;10:1044-1051.
281. Veronelli A, Mauri C, Zecchini B, et al. Sexual dysfunction is frequent in premenopausal women with diabetes, obesity, and hypothyroidism, and correlates with markers of increased cardiovascular risk. A preliminary report. *J Sex Med*. 2009;6:1561-1568.
282. Esposito K, Ciotola M, Giugliano F, et al. Association of body weight with sexual function in women. *Int J Impot Res*. 2007;19(4):353-357.
283. Castellini G, Mannucci E, Mazzei C, et al. Sexual function in obese women with and without binge eating disorder. *J Sex Med*. 2010;7(12):3969-3978.
284. Esposito K, Ciotola M, Marfella R, et al. The metabolic syndrome: a cause of sexual dysfunction in women. *Int J Impot Res*. 2005;17:224-226.
285. Martelli V, Valisella S, Moscatiello S, et al. Prevalence of sexual dysfunction among postmenopausal women with and without metabolic syndrome. *J Sex Med*. 2012;9(2):434-441.
286. Basson RJ, Rucker BM, Laird PG, et al. Sexuality of women with diabetes. *J Sex Reprod Med*. 2001;1(1):11-20.
287. Giraldi A, Persson K, Werkström V, et al. Effects of diabetes on neurotransmission in rat vaginal smooth muscle. *Int J Impot Res*. 2001;13:58-66.
288. Caruso S, Rugolo S, Mirabella D, et al. Changes in clitoral blood flow in premenopausal women affected by type 1 diabetes after single 100-mg administration of sildenafil. *Urology*. 2006;68:161-165.
289. Ponholzer A, Temml C, Rauchenwald M, et al. Is the metabolic syndrome a risk factor for female sexual dysfunction in sexually active women? *Int J Impot Res*. 2008;20:100-104.
290. Kim YH, Kim SM, Kim JJ, et al. Does metabolic syndrome impair sexual function in middle to old-aged women? *J Sex Med*. 2011;8:1112-1130.
291. Elsenbruch S, Hahn S, Kowalsky D, et al. Quality of life, psychosocial well-being, and sexual satisfaction in women with polycystic ovary syndrome. *J Clin Endocrinol Metab*. 2003;88:5801-5807.
292. Hahn S, Janssen OE, Tan S, et al. Clinical and psychological correlates of quality-of-life in polycystic ovary syndrome. *Eur J Endocrinol*. 2005;153:853-860.
293. Janssen OE, Hahn S, Tan S, et al. Mood and sexual function in polycystic ovary syndrome. *Semin Reprod Med*. 2008;26:45-52.
294. Ferraresi SR, Lara LA, Reis RM, et al. Changes in sexual function in women with polycystic ovary syndrome: a pilot study. *J Sex Med*. 2013;10(2):467-473.
295. Ercan CM, Coksuer H, Aydogan U, et al. Sexual dysfunction assessment and hormonal correlations in patients with polycystic ovary syndrome. *Int J Impot Res*. 2013;25(4):127-132.
296. Dewailly D, Vantyghem-Haudiquet MC, Sainsard C, et al. Clinical and biological phenotypes in late-onset 21-hydroxylase deficiency. *J Clin Endocrinol Metab*. 1986;63:418-423.
297. Lobo RA, Goebelsmann U. Adult manifestation of congenital adrenal hyperplasia due to incomplete 21-hydroxylase deficiency mimicking polycystic ovarian disease. *Am J Obstet Gynecol*. 1980;138:720-726.
298. Frisén L, Nordenström A, Falhammar H, et al. Gender role behavior, sexuality, and psychosocial adaptation in women with congenital

adrenal hyperplasia due to CYP21A2 deficiency. *J Clin Endocrinol Metab.* 2009;94:3432-3439.

299. Hines M, Brook C, Conway GS. Androgen and psychosexual development: core gender identity, sexual orientation and recalled childhood gender role behavior in women and men with congenital adrenal hyperplasia (CAH). *J Sex Res.* 2004;41:75-81.

300. Miller KK, Sesmilo G, Schiller A, et al. Androgen deficiency in women with hypopituitarism. *J Clin Endocrinol Metab.* 2001;86(2): 561-567.

301. Wierman M, Arlt W, Basson R, et al. Androgen therapy in women: a reappraisal: an Endocrine Society Clinical Practice Guideline. *J Clin Endocrinol Metab.* 2014;99(10):3489-3510.

302. Miller KK, Biller BM, Beauregard C, et al. Effects of testosterone replacement in androgen-deficient women with hypopituitarism: a randomized, double-blind, placebo-controlled study. *J Clin Endocrinol Metab.* 2006;91:1683-1690.

303. Arlt W, Callies F, van Vlijmen JC, et al. Dehydroepiandrosterone replacement in women with adrenal insufficiency. *N Engl J Med.* 1999;341:1013-1020.

304. Hunt PJ, Gurnell EM, Huppert FA, et al. Improvement in mood and fatigue after dehydroepiandrosterone replacement in Addison's disease in a randomized, double blind trial. *J Clin Endocrinol Metab.* 2000;85: 4650-4656.

305. Gurnell EM, Hunt PJ, Curran SE, et al. Long-term DHEA replacement in primary adrenal insufficiency: a randomized, controlled trial. *J Clin Endocrinol Metab.* 2008;93:400-409.

306. Libè R, Barbetta L, Dall'Asta C, et al. Effects of dehydroepiandrosterone (DHEA) supplementation on hormonal, metabolic and behavioral status in patients with hypoadrenalism. *J Endocrinol Invest.* 2004;27: 736-741.

307. Binder G, Weber S, Ehrismann M, et al. South German Working Group for Pediatric Endocrinology. Effects of dehydroepiandrosterone therapy on pubic hair growth and psychological well-being in adolescent girls and young women with central adrenal insufficiency: a double-blind, randomized, placebo-controlled phase III trial. *J Clin Endocrinol Metab.* 2009;94:1182-1190.

308. Erichsen MM, Løvås K, Skinningsrud B, et al. Clinical, immunological, and genetic features of autoimmune primary adrenal insufficiency: observations from a Norwegian registry. *J Clin Endocrinol Metab.* 2009;94:4882-4890.

309. Erichsen MM, Huseby ES, Michelsen TM, et al. Sexuality and fertility in women with Addison's disease. *J Clin Endocrinol Metab.* 2010;95: 4354-4360.

310. Løvås K, Husebye ES. Replacement therapy in Addison's disease. *Expert Opin Pharmacother.* 2003;4:2145-2149.

311. Van Thiel SW, Romijn JA, Pereira AM, et al. Effects of dehydroepiandrostenedione, superimposed on growth hormone substitution, on quality of life and insulin-like growth factor I in patients with secondary adrenal insufficiency: a randomized, placebo-controlled, cross-over trial. *J Clin Endocrinol Metab.* 2005;91:1683-1690.

312. Alkatib AA, Cosma M, Elamin MB, et al. A systematic review and meta-analysis of randomized placebo-controlled trials of DHEA treatment effects on quality of life in women with adrenal insufficiency. *J Clin Endocrinol Metab.* 2009;94:3676-3681.

313. Huang AJ, Moore EE, Boyko EJ, et al. Vaginal symptoms in post menopausal women: self-reported severity, natural history, and risk factors. *Menopause.* 2010;17:121-126.

314. Santoro N, Komi J. Prevalence and impact of vaginal symptoms among postmenopausal women. *J Sex Med.* 2009;6:2133-2142.

315. Indhavivadhana S, Leerasiri P, Rattanachaiyanont M, et al. Vaginal atrophy and sexual dysfunction in current users of systemic postmenopausal hormone therapy. *J Med Assoc Thai.* 2010;93(6):667-675.

316. Labrie F, Bélanger A, Bélanger P, et al. Androgen glucuronides, instead of testosterone, as the new markers of androgenic activity in women. *J Steroid Biochem.* 2006;99:182-188.

317. Woods NF, Mitchell ES, Tao Y, et al. Polymorphisms in the estrogen synthesis and metabolism pathways and symptoms during the menopausal transition: observations from the Seattle Midlife Women's Health Study. *Menopause.* 2006;13:902-910.

318. Kao A, Binik Y, Amsel R, et al. Biopsychosocial predictors of postmenopausal dyspareunia: the role of steroid hormones, vulvovaginal atrophy, cognitive-emotional factors and dyadic adjustment. *J Sex Med.* 2012;9:2057-2076.

319. West SL, D'Aloisio AA, Agans RP, et al. Prevalence of low sexual desire and hypoactive sexual desire disorder in a nationally representative sample of US women. *Arch Intern Med.* 2008;168:1441-1449.

320. Melcangi RC, Panzica GC. Neuroactive steroids: old players in a new game. *Neuroscience.* 2006;138:733-739.

321. Ishunina TA, Swaab DF. Alterations in the human brain in menopause. *Maturitas.* 2007;57:20-22.

322. Birnbaum GE, Cohen O, Wertheimer V. It is all about intimacy? Age, menopausal status, and women's sexuality. *Pers Relation.* 2007;14: 167-185.

323. Aziz A, Brannstrom M, Bergquist C, et al. Perimenopausal androgen decline after oophorectomy does not influence sexuality or psychological well-being. *Fertil Steril.* 2005;83:1021-1028.

324. Farquar CM, Harvey SA, Yu Y, et al. A prospective study of three years of outcomes after hysterectomy with and without oophorectomy. *Obstet Gynecol.* 2006;194:714-717.

325. Teplin V, Vittinghoff E, Lin F, et al. Oophorectomy in premenopausal women: health-related quality of life and sexual functioning. *Obstet Gynecol.* 2007;109:347-354.

326. Erekson EA, Martin DK, Zhu K, et al. Sexual function in older women after oophorectomy. *Obstet Gynecol.* 2012;120(4):833-842.

327. Finch A, Narod SA. Quality of life and health status after prophylactic salpingo-oophorectomy in women who carry a BRCA mutation: a review. *Maturitas.* 2011;70:261-265.

328. Fliegner M, Krupp K, Brunner F, et al. Sexual life and sexual wellness in individuals with complete androgen insensitivity syndrome (CAIS) and Mayer-Rokitansky-Küster-Hauser Syndrome (MRKHS). *J Sex Med.* 2014;11:729-742.

329. Erekson EA, Martin DK, Ratner ES. Oophorectomy: the debate between ovarian conservation and elective oophorectomy. *Menopause.* 2013;20: 110-114.

330. Labrie F. Intracrinology. *Mol Cell Endocrinol.* 1991;78:C113-C118.

331. Cui Y, Zong H, Yan H, et al. The efficacy and safety of ospemifene in treating dyspareunia associated with postmenopausal vulvar and vaginal atrophy: a systematic review and meta-analysis. *J Sex Med.* 2014;11:487-497.

332. Pastor Z, Holla K, Chmel R. The influence of combined oral contraceptives on female sexual desire: a systematic review. *Eur J Contracept Reprod Health Care.* 2013;18:27-43.

333. Wisniewski AB, Migeon CJ, Meyer-Bahlburg HFL, et al. Complete androgen insensitivity syndrome: long-term medical, surgical, and psychosexual outcome. *J Clin Endocrinol Metab.* 2000;85:2664-2669.

334. Minto CL, Liao KL, Conway GS, et al. Sexual function in women with complete androgen insensitivity syndrome. *Fertil Steril.* 2003;80: 157-164.

335. Hines M, Ahmed SF, Hughes IA. Psychological outcomes and gender-related development in complete androgen insensitivity syndrome. *Arch Sex Behav.* 2003;32:93-101.

336. Köhler B, Kleinemeier E, Lux A, et al. Satisfaction with genital surgery and sexual life of adults with XY disorders of sex development: results from the German Clinical Evaluation Study. *J Clin Endocrinol Metab.* 2012;97:577-588.

337. Cappelleri JC, Rosen RC, Smith MD, et al. Diagnostic evaluation of the erectile function domain of the International Index of Erectile Function. *Urology.* 1999;54:346-351.

338. Lue TF, Giuliano F, Montorsi F, et al. Summary of recommendations on sexual dysfunctions in men. *J Sex Med.* 2004;1:6-23.

339. O'Leary MP, Fowler FJ, Lenderking WR, et al. A brief male sexual function inventory. *Urology.* 1995;46:697-706.

340. Rosen RC, Cappelleri JC, Smith MD, et al. Development and evaluation of an abridged, 5-item version of the International Index of Erectile Function (IIEF-5) as a diagnostic tool for erectile dysfunction. *Int J Impot Res.* 1999;11:319-326.

341. Montague DK, Jarow JP, Broderick GA, et al. Erectile Dysfunction Guideline Update Panel. *J Urol.* 2005;174(1):230-239.

342. Lobo JR, Nehra A. Clinical evaluation of erectile dysfunction in the era of PDE-5 inhibitors. *Urol Clin North Am.* 2005;32(4):447-455.

343. Bhasin S, Pencina M, Jasuja GK, et al. Reference ranges for testosterone in men generated using liquid chromatography tandem mass spectrometry in a community-based sample of healthy nonobese young men in the Framingham Heart Study and applied to three geographically distinct cohorts. *J Clin Endocrinol Metab.* 2011;96(8): 2430-2439.

344. Rosner W, Vesper H. Endocrine Society; American Association for Clinical Chemistry; American Association of Clinical Endocrinologists; Androgen Excess/PCOS Society; American Society for Bone and Mineral Research; American Society for Reproductive Medicine; American Urological Association; Association of Public Health Laboratories; Endocrine Society; Laboratory Corporation of America; North American Menopause Society; Pediatric Endocrine Society. Toward excellence in testosterone testing: a consensus statement. *J Clin Endocrinol Metab.* 2010;95(10):4542-4548.

345. Vesper HW, Botelho JC. Standardization of testosterone measurements in humans. *J Steroid Biochem Mol Biol.* 2010;121(3–5):513-519.

346. Bhasin S, Zhang A, Coviello A, et al. The impact of assay quality and reference ranges on clinical decision making in the diagnosis of androgen disorders. *Steroids.* 2008;73(13):1311-1317.

347. Rosner W, Auchus RJ, Azziz R, et al. Position statement: utility, limitations, and pitfalls in measuring testosterone: an Endocrine Society position statement. *J Clin Endocrinol Metab.* 2007;92(2):405-413.

348. Zakharov MN, Bhasin S, Travison TG, et al. A multi-step, dynamic allosteric model of testosterone's binding to sex hormone binding globulin. *Mol Cell Endocrinol.* 2015;399:190-200.

349. Wu FC, Tajar A, Pye SR, et al; European Male Aging Study Group. Hypothalamic-pituitary-testicular axis disruptions in older men are differentially linked to age and modifiable risk factors: the European Male Aging Study. *J Clin Endocrinol Metab.* 2008;93(7):2737-2745.

350. Harman SM, Metter EJ, Tobin JD, et al; Baltimore Longitudinal Study of Aging. Longitudinal effects of aging on serum total and free

testosterone levels in healthy men. *Baltimore Longitudinal Study of Aging. Clin Endocrinol Metab.* 2001;86(2):724-731.

351. Orwoll E, Lambert LC, Marshall LM, et al. Testosterone and estradiol among older men. *J Clin Endocrinol Metab.* 2006;91(4):1336-1344.

352. Mueller SC, Wallenberg-Pachaly H, Voges GE, Schild HH. Comparison of selective internal iliac pharmaco-angiography, penile brachial index and duplex sonography with pulsed Doppler analysis for the evaluation of vasculogenic (arteriogenic) impotence. *J Urol.* 1990;143:928-932.

353. Brock G. Tumescence monitoring devices: past and present. In: Hellstrom WJ, ed. *Handbook of Sexual Dysfunction.* San Francisco, CA: The American Society of Andrology; 1999:65-69.

354. Rosen RC. Assessment of female sexual dysfunction: review of validated methods. *Fertil Steril.* 2002;77(S4):s89-s93.

355. Brotto LA. The Female Sexual Function Index. *J Sex Marital Ther.* 2009;35:161-163.

356. Mitchell KR, Ploubidis GB, Datta J, et al. The Natsal-SF: a validated measure of sexual function for use in community surveys. *Eur J Epidemiol.* 2012;27:409-418.

357. Dundon CM, Rellini AH. More than sexual function: predictors of sexual satisfaction in a sample of women aged 40-70. *J Sex Med.* 2010;7:896-904.

358. Stephenson KR, Ahrold TK, Meston CM. The association between sexual motives and sexual satisfaction: gender differences and categorical comparisons. *Arch Sex Behav.* 2011;40:607-618.

359. Steidle C, Schwartz S, Jacoby K, et al; North American AA2500 T Gel Study Group. AA2500 testosterone gel normalizes androgen levels in aging males with improvements in body composition and sexual function. *J Clin Endocrinol Metab.* 2003;88(6):2673-2681.

360. Wang C, Swerdloff RS, Iranmanesh A, et al; Testosterone Gel Study Group. Transdermal testosterone gel improves sexual function, mood, muscle strength, and body composition parameters in hypogonadal men. *J Clin Endocrinol Metab.* 2000;85(8):2839-2853.

361. Wang C, Cunningham G, Dobs A, et al. Long-term testosterone gel (AndroGel) treatment maintains beneficial effects on sexual function and mood, lean and fat mass, and bone mineral density in hypogonadal men. *J Clin Endocrinol Metab.* 2004;89(5):2085-2098.

362. Boloña ER, Uraga MV, Haddad RM, et al. Testosterone use in men with sexual dysfunction: a systematic review and meta-analysis of randomized placebo-controlled trials. *Mayo Clin Proc.* 2007;82(1):20-28.

363. Snyder PJ, Ellenberg SS, Cunningham GR, et al. The Testosterone Trials: seven coordinated trials of testosterone treatment in elderly men. *Clin Trials.* 2014;11(3):362-375.

364. Rosen RC. Psychogenic erectile dysfunction. Classification and management. *Urol Clin North Am.* 2001;28:269-278.

365. Abrahamson DJ, Barlow DH, Beck JG. The effects of attentional focus and partner responsiveness on sexual responding: replication and extension. *Arch Sex Behav.* 1985;14:361-371.

366. Kilmann PR, Boland JP, Norton SP, et al. Perspectives of sex therapy outcome: a survey of AASECT providers. *J Sex Marital Ther.* 1986;12:116-138.

367. Melnik T, Soares BG, Nasselo AG. Psychosocial interventions for erectile dysfunction. *Cochrane Database Syst Rev.* 2007;(3):CD004825.

368. Melnik T, Soares BG, Nasello AG. The effectiveness of psychological interventions for the treatment of erectile dysfunction: systematic review and meta-analysis, including comparisons to sildenafil treatment, intracavernosal injection, and vacuum devices. *J Sex Med.* 2008;5(11):2562-2574.

369. Schmidt HM, Munder T, Gerger H, et al. Combination of psychological intervention and phosphodiesterase-5 inhibitors for erectile dysfunction: a narrative review and meta-analysis. *J Sex Med.* 2014;11(6):1376-1391.

370. Hatzimouratidis K, Amar E, Eardley I, et al. Guidelines on male sexual dysfunction: erectile dysfunction and premature ejaculation. *Eur Urol.* 2010;57(5):804-814.

371. Qaseem A, Snow V, Denberg TD, et al; Clinical Efficacy Assessment Subcommittee of the American College of Physicians. Hormonal testing and pharmacologic treatment of erectile dysfunction: a clinical practice guideline from the American College of Physicians. *Ann Intern Med.* 2009;151(9):639-649.

372. Nehra A, Jackson G, Miner M, et al. The Princeton III Consensus recommendations for the management of erectile dysfunction and cardiovascular disease. *Mayo Clin Proc.* 2012;87(8):766-778.

373. Saenz de Tejada I, Angulo J, Cuevas P, et al. The phosphodiesterase inhibitory selectivity and the in vitro and in vivo potency of the new PDE5 inhibitor vardenafil. *Int J Impot Res.* 2001;13:282-290.

374. Yu G, Mason H, Wu X, et al. Substituted pyrazolopyridopyridazines as orally bioavailable potent and selective PDE5 inhibitors: potential agents for treatment of erectile dysfunction. *J Med Chem.* 2003;46:457-460.

375. Seftel AD. Phosphodiesterase type 5 inhibitor differentiation based on selectivity, pharmacokinetic, and efficacy profiles. *Clin Cardiol.* 2004;27:I14-I19.

376. Sussman DO. Pharmacokinetics, pharmacodynamics, and efficacy of phosphodiesterase type 5 inhibitors. *J Am Osteopath Assoc.* 2004;104:S11-S15.

377. Kedia GT, Uckert S, Assadi-Pour F, et al. Avanafil for the treatment of erectile dysfunction: initial data and clinical key properties. *Ther Adv Urol.* 2013;5(1):35-41.

378. Limin M, Johnsen N, Hellstrom WJ. Avanafil, a new rapid-onset phosphodiesterase 5 inhibitor for the treatment of erectile dysfunction. *Expert Opin Investig Drugs.* 2010;19(11):1427-1437.

379. Katz EG, Tan RB, Rittenberg D, Hellstrom WJ. Avanafil for erectile dysfunction in elderly and younger adults: differential pharmacology and clinical utility. *Ther Clin Risk Manag.* 2014;10:701-711.

380. Cho MC, Paick JS. Udenafil for the treatment of erectile dysfunction. *Ther Clin Risk Manag.* 2014;10:341-354.

381. Rajagopalan P, Mazzu A, Xia C, et al. Effect of high-fat breakfast and moderate-fat evening meal on the pharmacokinetics of vardenafil, an oral phosphodiesterase-5 inhibitor for the treatment of erectile dysfunction. *J Clin Pharmacol.* 2003;43:260-267.

382. Nichols DJ, Muirhead GJ, Harness JA. Pharmacokinetics of sildenafil after single oral doses in healthy male subjects: absolute bioavailability, food effects and dose proportionality. *Br J Clin Pharmacol.* 2002;53(Suppl 1):5S-12S.

383. Rendell MS, Rajfer J, Wicker PA, Smith MD. Sildenafil for treatment of erectile dysfunction in men with diabetes: a randomized controlled trial. Sildenafil Diabetes Study Group [see comments]. *JAMA.* 1999;281:421-426.

384. Blanker MH, Thomas S, Bohnen AM. Systematic review of Viagra RCTs. *Br J Gen Pract.* 2002;52:329.

385. Burls A, Gold L, Clark W. Systematic review of randomised controlled trials of sildenafil (Viagra) in the treatment of male erectile dysfunction. *Br J Gen Pract.* 2001;51:1004-1012.

386. Fink HA, Mac Donald R, Rutks IR, et al. Sildenafil for male erectile dysfunction: a systematic review and meta-analysis. *Arch Intern Med.* 2002;162:1349-1360.

387. Montorsi F, McCullough A. Efficacy of sildenafil citrate in men with erectile dysfunction following radical prostatectomy: a systematic review of clinical data. *J Sex Med.* 2005;2:658-667.

388. Moore RA, Derry S, McQuay HJ. Indirect comparison of interventions using published randomised trials: systematic review of PDE-5 inhibitors for erectile dysfunction. *BMC Urol.* 2005;5:18.

389. Jarow JP, Burnett AL, Geringer AM. Clinical efficacy of sildenafil citrate based on etiology and response to prior treatment [see comments]. *J Urol.* 1999;162:722-725.

390. Vardi M, Nini A. Phosphodiesterase inhibitors for erectile dysfunction in patients with diabetes mellitus. *Cochrane Database Syst Rev.* 2007;(1):CD002187.

391. Markou S, Perimenis P, Gyftopoulos K, et al. Vardenafil (Levitra) for erectile dysfunction: a systematic review and meta-analysis of clinical trial reports. *Int J Impot Res.* 2004;16:470-478.

392. Brock G, Nehra A, Lipshultz LI, et al. Safety and efficacy of vardenafil for the treatment of men with erectile dysfunction after radical retropubic prostatectomy. *J Urol.* 2003;170:1278-1283.

393. Donatucci C, Eardley I, Buvat J, et al. Vardenafil improves erectile function in men with erectile dysfunction irrespective of disease severity and disease classification. *J Sex Med.* 2004;1:301-309.

394. Hatzichristou D, Montorsi F, Buvat J, et al. The efficacy and safety of flexible-dose vardenafil (Levitra) in a broad population of European men. *Eur Urol.* 2004;45:634-641, discussion 641.

395. Hellstrom WJ, Gittelman M, Karlin G, et al. Vardenafil for treatment of men with erectile dysfunction: efficacy and safety in a randomized, double-blind, placebo-controlled trial. *J Androl.* 2002;23:763-771.

396. Nehra A, Grantmyre J, Nadel A, et al. Vardenafil improved patient satisfaction with erectile hardness, orgasmic function and sexual experience in men with erectile dysfunction following nerve sparing radical prostatectomy. *J Urol.* 2005;173:2067-2071.

397. Rosen R, Shabsigh R, Berber M, et al. Efficacy and tolerability of vardenafil in men with mild depression and erectile dysfunction: the depression-related improvement with vardenafil for erectile response study. *Am J Psychiatry.* 2006;163:79-87.

398. Brock GB, McMahon CG, Chen KK, et al. Efficacy and safety of tadalafil for the treatment of erectile dysfunction: results of integrated analyses. *J Urol.* 2002;168:1332-1336.

399. Carson C, Shabsigh R, Segal S, et al. Efficacy, safety, and treatment satisfaction of tadalafil versus placebo in patients with erectile dysfunction evaluated at tertiary-care academic centers. *Urology.* 2005;65:353-359.

400. Padma-Nathan H, McMurray JG, Pullman WE, et al. On-demand IC351 (Cialis) enhances erectile function in patients with erectile dysfunction. *Int J Impot Res.* 2001;13:2-9.

401. Porst H, Padma-Nathan H, Giuliano F, et al. Efficacy of tadalafil for the treatment of erectile dysfunction at 24 and 36 hours after dosing: a randomized controlled trial. *Urology.* 2003;62:121-125, discussion 125-126.

402. Saenz de Tejada I, Anglin G, Knight JR, Emmick JT. Effects of tadalafil on erectile dysfunction in men with diabetes. *Diabetes Care.* 2002;25:2159-2164.

403. Morales A, Gingell C, Collins M, et al. Clinical safety of oral sildenafil citrate (Viagra) in the treatment of erectile dysfunction. *Int J Impot Res.* 1998;10:69-73.

404. Coelho OR. Tolerability and safety profile of sildenafil citrate (Viagra) in Latin American patient populations. *Int J Impot Res.* 2002;14(Suppl 2):S54-S59.

405. Giuliano F, Jackson G, Montorsi F, et al. Safety of sildenafil citrate: review of 67 double-blind placebo-controlled trials and the postmarketing safety database. *Int J Clin Pract.* 2010;64(2):240-255.

406. Goldstein I, Lue TF, Padma-Nathan H, et al. Oral sildenafil in the treatment of erectile dysfunction. Sildenafil Study Group [see comments] [published erratum appears in N Engl J Med. 1998;339(1):59]. *N Engl J Med.* 1998;338(20):1397-1404.

407. Aversa A, Mazzilli F, Rossi T, et al. Effects of sildenafil (Viagra) administration on seminal parameters and post-ejaculatory refractory time in normal males. *Hum Reprod.* 2000;15:131-134.

408. Hellstrom WJG, Gittelman M, Jarow J, et al. An evaluation of semen characteristics in men 45 years of age after daily dosing with tadalafil 20 mg: results of a multicenter, randomized, double-blind, placebo-controlled, 9-month study. *Eur Urol.* 2008;53:1058-1065.

409. Hatzichristou DG. Phosphodiesterase 5 inhibitors and nonarteritic anterior ischemic optic neuropathy (NAION): coincidence or causality. *J Sex Med.* 2004;2:751-758.

410. Buono L, Foroozan R, Sergott RC, Savino PJ. Nonarteritic anterior ischemic optic neuropathy. *Curr Opin Ophthalmol.* 2002;13:357-361.

411. Snodgrass AJ, Campbell HM, Mace DL, et al. Sudden sensorineural hearing loss associated with vardenafil. *Pharmacotherapy.* 2010;30(1):112.

412. McGwin G Jr. Phosphodiesterase type 5 inhibitor use and hearing impairment. *Arch Otolaryngol Head Neck Surg.* 2010;136(5):488-492.

413. Li WQ, Qureshi AA, Robinson KC, Han J. Sildenafil use and increased risk of incident melanoma in US men: a prospective cohort study. *JAMA Intern Med.* 2014;174:964-970.

414. Feenstra J, Drie-Pierik RJ, Lacle CF, Stricker BH. Acute myocardial infarction associated with sildenafil [letter] [see comments]. *Lancet.* 1998;352:957-958.

415. Zusman RM, Morales A, Glasser DB, Osterloh IH. Overall cardiovascular profile of sildenafil citrate. *Am J Cardiol.* 1999;83:35C-44C.

416. Herrmann HC, Chang G, Klugherz BD, Mahoney PD. Hemodynamic effects of sildenafil in men with severe coronary artery disease. *N Engl J Med.* 2000;342:1622-1626.

417. Thadani U, Smith W, Nash S, et al. The effect of vardenafil, a potent and highly selective phosphodiesterase-5 inhibitor for the treatment of erectile dysfunction, on the cardiovascular response to exercise in patients with coronary artery disease. *J Am Coll Cardiol.* 2002;40:2006-2012.

418. Jackson G. Hemodynamic and exercise effects of phosphodiesterase 5 inhibitors. *Am J Cardiol.* 2005;96:32M-36M.

419. Cheitlin MD, Hutter AM Jr, Brindis RG, et al. Use of sildenafil (Viagra) in patients with cardiovascular disease. Technology and Practice Executive Committee [published erratum appears in Circulation. 1999;100(23):2389] [see comments]. *Circulation.* 1999;99(1):168-177.

420. Muller JE, Mittleman A, Maclure M, et al. Triggering myocardial infarction by sexual activity. Low absolute risk and prevention by regular physical exertion. Determinants of Myocardial Infarction Onset Study Investigators [see comments]. *JAMA.* 1996;275:1405-1409.

421. Conti CR, Pepine CJ, Sweeney M. Efficacy and safety of sildenafil citrate in the treatment of erectile dysfunction in patients with ischemic heart disease. *Am J Cardiol.* 1999;83:29C-34C.

422. Carson CC 3rd. Cardiac safety in clinical trials of phosphodiesterase 5 inhibitors. *Am J Cardiol.* 2005;96:37M-41M.

423. Kloner RA. Novel phosphodiesterase type 5 inhibitors: assessing hemodynamic effects and safety parameters. *Clin Cardiol.* 2004;27:I20-I25.

424. Vlachopoulos C, Jackson G, Stefanadis C, Montorsi P. Erectile dysfunction in the cardiovascular patient. *Eur Heart J.* 2013;34(27):2034-2046.

425. Highleyman L. Protease inhibitors and sildenafil (Viagra) should not be combined. *BETA.* 1999;12(2):3.

426. Bailey DG, Dresser GK. Interactions between grapefruit juice and cardiovascular drugs. *Am J Cardiovasc Drugs.* 2004;4:281-297.

427. McCullough AR, Barada JH, Fawzy A, et al. Achieving treatment optimization with sildenafil citrate (Viagra) in patients with erectile dysfunction. *Urology.* 2002;60:28-38.

428. McMahon C. Comparison of efficacy, safety, and tolerability of on-demand tadalafil and daily dosed tadalafil for the treatment of erectile dysfunction. *J Sex Med.* 2005;2(3):415-425, discussion 425-427.

429. Porst H, Rajfer J, Casabé A, et al. Long-term safety and efficacy of tadalafil 5 mg dosed once daily in men with erectile dysfunction. *J Sex Med.* 2008;5:2160-2169.

430. Lau DHW, Kommu S, Mumtaz FH, et al. The management of phosphodiesterase inhibitor failure. *Curr Vasc Pharmacol.* 2006;4:89-93.

431. Martinez JM. Prognostic factors for response to sildenafil in patients with erectile dysfunction. *Eur Urol.* 2001;40:641-646.

432. Wespes E, Rammal A, Garbar C. Sildenafil no-responders: hemodynamic and morphometric studies. *Eur Urol.* 2005;48:136-139.

433. McGarvey MR. Tough choices: the cost-effectiveness of sildenafil [editorial; comment]. *Ann Intern Med.* 2000;132:994-995.

434. Smith KJ, Roberts MS. The cost-effectiveness of sildenafil [see comments]. *Ann Intern Med.* 2000;132:933-937.

435. Tan HL. Economic cost of male erectile dysfunction using a decision analytic model: for a hypothetical managed-care plan of 100,000 members. *Pharmacoeconomics.* 2000;17:77-107.

436. Sun P, Seftel A, Swindle R, et al. The costs of caring for erectile dysfunction in a managed care setting: evidence from a large national claims database. *J Urol.* 2005;174:1948-1952.

437. Plumb JM, Guest JF. Annual cost of erectile dysfunction to UK Society. *Pharmacoeconomics.* 1999;16:699-709.

438. Vrijhof HJ, Delaere KP. Vacuum constriction devices in erectile dysfunction: acceptance and effectiveness in patients with impotence of organic or mixed aetiology. *Br J Urol.* 1994;74:102-105.

439. Cookson MS, Nadig PW. Long-term results with vacuum constriction device. *J Urol.* 1993;149:290-294.

440. Lewis JH, Sidi AA, Reddy PK. A way to help your patients who use vacuum devices. *Contemp Urol.* 1991;3:15-21.

441. Engelhardt PF, Plas E, Hubner WA, Pfluger H. Comparison of intraurethral liposomal and intracavernosal prostaglandin-E1 in the management of erectile dysfunction. *Br J Urol.* 1998;81:441-444.

442. Kim ED, McVary KT. Topical prostaglandin-E1 for the treatment of erectile dysfunction [see comments]. *J Urol.* 1995;153:1828-1830.

443. Peterson CA, Bennett AH, Hellstrom WJ, et al. Erectile response to transurethral alprostadil, prazosin and alprostadil-prazosin combinations. *J Urol.* 1998;159:1523-1527.

444. Fulgham PF, Cochran JS, Denman JL, et al. Disappointing initial results with transurethral alprostadil for erectile dysfunction in a urology practice setting. *J Urol.* 1998;160:2041-2046.

445. Linet OI, Ogrinc FG. Efficacy and safety of intracavernosal alprostadil in men with erectile dysfunction. The Alprostadil Study Group. *N Engl J Med.* 1996;334:873-877.

446. El-Sakka AI. Intracavernosal prostaglandin E1 self vs office injection therapy in patients with erectile dysfunction. *Int J Impot Res.* 2006;18:180-185.

447. Heaton JP, Lording D, Liu SN, et al. Intracavernosal alprostadil is effective for the treatment of erectile dysfunction in diabetic men. *Int J Impot Res.* 2001;13:317-321.

448. Tsai YS, Lin JS, Lin YM. Safety and efficacy of alprostadil sterile powder (S. Po., CAVERJECT) in diabetic patients with erectile dysfunction. *Eur Urol.* 2000;38:177-183.

449. Shabsigh R, Padma-Nathan H, Gittleman M, et al. Intracavernous alprostadil alfadex is more efficacious, better tolerated, and preferred over intraurethral alprostadil plus optional actis: a comparative, randomized, crossover, multicenter study. *Urology.* 2000;55:109-113.

450. Chew KK. Intracavernosal injection therapy. Does it still have a role in erectile dysfunction? *Aust Fam Physician.* 2001;30:43-46.

451. The European Alprostadil Study Group. The long-term safety of alprostadil (prostaglandin-E1) in patients with erectile dysfunction. *Br J Urol.* 1998;82:538-543.

452. Dinsmore WW, Gingell C, Hackett G, et al. Treating men with predominantly nonpsychogenic erectile dysfunction with intracavernosal vasoactive intestinal polypeptide and phentolamine mesylate in a novel auto-injector system: a multicentre double-blind placebo-controlled study. *BJU Int.* 1999;83:274-279.

453. Mulhall JP, Daller M, Traish AM, et al. Intracavernosal forskolin: role in management of vasculogenic impotence resistant to standard 3-agent pharmacotherapy. *J Urol.* 1997;158:1752-1758, discussion 1758-1759.

454. Hellstrom WJ, Usta MF. Surgical approaches for advanced Peyronie's disease patients. *Int J Impot Res.* 2003;15(Suppl 5):S121-S124.

455. Carson CC, Mulcahy JJ, Govier FE. Efficacy, safety and patient satisfaction outcomes of the AMS 700CX inflatable penile prosthesis: results of a long-term multicenter study. AMS 700CX Study Group. *J Urol.* 2000;164:376-380.

456. Wilson SK, Cleves MA, Delk JR 2nd. Comparison of mechanical reliability of original and enhanced Mentor Alpha I penile prosthesis. *J Urol.* 1999;162:715-718.

457. Usta MF, Bivalacqua TJ, Sanabria J, et al. Patient and partner satisfaction and long-term results after surgical treatment for Peyronie's disease. *Urology.* 2003;62:105-109.

458. Fink HA, MacDonald R, Rutks IR, Wilt TJ. Trazodone for erectile dysfunction: a systematic review and meta-analysis. *BJU Int.* 2003;92:441-446.

459. Lebret T, Herve JM, Gorny P, et al. Efficacy and safety of a novel combination of L-arginine glutamate and yohimbine hydrochloride: a new oral therapy for erectile dysfunction. *Eur Urol.* 2002;41:608-613, discussion 613.

460. Fleshner N, Harvey M, Adomat H, et al. Evidence for pharmacological contamination of herbal erectile function products with type 5 phosphodiesterase inhibitors (abstract). *J Urol.* 2004;171:314.

461. Hong B, Ji YH, Hong JH, et al. A double-blind crossover study evaluating the efficacy of Korean red ginseng in patients with erectile dysfunction: a preliminary report. *J Urol.* 2002;168:2070-2073.

462. Jang DJ, Lee MS, Shin BC, et al. Red ginseng for treating erectile dysfunction: a systematic review. *Br J Clin Pharmacol.* 2008;66(4):444-450.

463. Ho CC, Tan HM. Rise of herbal and traditional medicine in erectile dysfunction management. *Curr Urol Rep.* 2011;12(6):470-478.

464. Shindel AW, Xin ZC, Lin G, et al. Erectogenic and neurotrophic effects of icariin, a purified extract of horny goat weed (*Epimedium* spp.) in vitro and in vivo. *J Sex Med.* 2010;7(4 Pt 1):1518-1528.

465. Harraz A, Shindel AW, Lue TF. Emerging gene and stem cell therapies for the treatment of erectile dysfunction. *Nat Rev Urol.* 2010;7(3): 143-152.

466. Strong TD, Gebska MA, Burnett AL, et al. Endothelium-specific gene and stem cell-based therapy for erectile dysfunction. *Asian J Androl.* 2008;10(1):14-22.

467. Deng W, Bivalacqua TJ, Hellstrom WJ, Kadowitz PJ. Gene and stem cell therapy for erectile dysfunction. *Int J Impot Res.* 2005;17(Suppl 1):S57-S63.

468. Garban H, Marquez D, Magee T, et al. Cloning of rat and human inducible penile nitric oxide synthase. Application for gene therapy of erectile dysfunction. *Biol Reprod.* 1997;56:954-963.

469. Christ GJ, Rehman J, Day N, et al. Intracorporal injection of hSlo cDNA in rats produces physiologically relevant alterations in penile function. *Am J Physiol.* 1998;275:H600-H608.

470. Bivalacqua TJ, Champion HC, Mehta YS, et al. Adenoviral gene transfer of endothelial nitric oxide synthase (eNOS) to the penis improves age-related erectile dysfunction in the rat. *Int J Impot Res.* 2000;12(Suppl 3):S8-S17.

471. Champion HC, Bivalacqua TJ, Hyman AL, et al. Gene transfer of endothelial nitric oxide synthase to the penis augments erectile responses in the aged rat. *Proc Natl Acad Sci U S A.* 1999;96:11648-11652.

472. Burchardt M, Burchardt T, Anastasiadis AG, et al. Application of angiogenic factors for therapy of erectile dysfunction: protein and DNA transfer of VEGF 165 into the rat penis. *Urology.* 2005;66:665-670.

473. Rogers RS, Graziottin TM, Lin CS, et al. Intracavernosal vascular endothelial growth factor (VEGF) injection and adeno-associated virus-mediated VEGF gene therapy prevent and reverse venogenic erectile dysfunction in rats. *Int J Impot Res.* 2003;15:26-37.

474. Deng W, Bivalacqua TJ, Chattergoon NN, et al. Adenoviral gene transfer of eNOS: high-level expression in ex vivo expanded marrow stromal cells. *Am J Physiol Cell Physiol.* 2003;285:C1322-C1329.

475. Gholami SS, Rogers R, Chang J, et al. The effect of vascular endothelial growth factor and adeno-associated virus mediated brain derived neurotrophic factor on neurogenic and vasculogenic erectile dysfunction induced by hyperlipidemia. *J Urol.* 2003;169(4):1577-1581.

476. Deng W, Bivalacqua TJ, Chattergoon NN, et al. Engineering ex vivo-expanded marrow stromal cells to secrete calcitonin gene-related peptide using adenoviral vector. *Stem Cells.* 2004;22:1279-1291.

477. Melman A, Bar-Chama N, McCullough A, et al. Plasmid-based gene transfer for treatment of erectile dysfunction and overactive bladder: results of a phase I trial. *Isr Med Assoc J.* 2007;9(3):143-146.

478. Melman A, Bar-Chama N, McCullough A, et al. hMaxi-K gene transfer in males with erectile dysfunction: results of the first human trial. *Hum Gene Ther.* 2006;17(12):1165-1176.

479. Magee TR, Kovanecz I, Davila HH, et al. Antisense and short hairpin RNA (shRNA) constructs targeting PIN (Protein Inhibitor of NOS) ameliorate aging-related erectile dysfunction in the rat. *J Sex Med.* 2007;4(3):633-643.

480. Condorelli RA, Calogero AE, Vicari E, et al. Vascular regenerative therapies for the treatment of erectile dysfunction: current approaches. *Andrology.* 2013;1(4):533-540.

481. Melman A, Davies K. Gene therapy for erectile dysfunction: what is the future? *Curr Urol Rep.* 2010;11(6):421-426.

482. Garcia MM, Fandel TM, Lin G, et al. Treatment of erectile dysfunction in the obese type 2 diabetic ZDF rat with adipose tissue-derived stem cells. *J Sex Med.* 2010;7(1 Pt 1):89-98.

483. Bivalacqua TJ, Deng W, Kendirci M, et al. Mesenchymal stem cells alone or ex vivo gene modified with endothelial nitric oxide synthase reverse age-associated erectile dysfunction. *Am J Physiol Heart Circ Physiol.* 2007;292(3):H1278-H1290.

484. Abdel Aziz MT, El-Haggar S, Mostafa T, et al. Effect of mesenchymal stem cell penile transplantation on erectile signaling of aged rats. *Andrologia.* 2010;42(3):187-192.

485. Lin CS, Xin Z, Dai J, et al. Stem-cell therapy for erectile dysfunction. *Expert Opin Biol Ther.* 2013;13(11):1585-1597.

486. Lin CS, Xin ZC, Wang Z, et al. Stem cell therapy for erectile dysfunction: a critical review. *Stem Cells Dev.* 2012;21(3):343-351.

487. Albersen M, Kendirci M, Van der Aa F, et al. Multipotent stromal cell therapy for cavernous nerve injury-induced erectile dysfunction. *J Sex Med.* 2012;9(2):385-403.

488. Kim Y, de Miguel F, Usiene I, et al. Injection of skeletal muscle-derived cells into the penis improves erectile function. *Int J Impot Res.* 2006; 18(4):329-334.

489. Song YS, Lee HJ, Park IH, et al. Potential differentiation of human mesenchymal stem cell transplanted in rat corpus cavernosum toward endothelial or smooth muscle cells. *Int J Impot Res.* 2007;19:378-385.

490. Nolazco G, Kovanecz I, Vernet D, et al. Effect of muscle-derived stem cells on the restoration of corpora cavernosa smooth muscle and erectile function in the aged rat. *BJU Int.* 2008;101:1156-1164.

491. Tomasi PA, Fanciulli G, Delitala G. Successful treatment of retrograde ejaculation with the alpha1-adrenergic agonist methoxamine: case study. *Int J Impot Res.* 2005;17(3):297-299.

492. Ochsenkühn R, Kamischke A, Nieschlag E. Imipramine for successful treatment of retrograde ejaculation caused by retroperitoneal surgery. *Int J Androl.* 1999;22(3):173-177.

493. Safarinejad MR. Midodrine for the treatment of organic anejaculation but not spinal cord injury: a prospective randomized placebo-controlled double-blind clinical study. *Int J Impot Res.* 2009;21(4): 213-220.

494. Kamischke A, Nieschlag E. Treatment of retrograde ejaculation and anejaculation. *Hum Reprod Update.* 1999;5:448-474.

495. Webster L. Management of sexual problems in diabetic patients. *Br J Hosp Med.* 1994;51(9):465-468.

496. Gerig NE, Meacham RB, Ohl DA. Use of electroejaculation in the treatment of ejaculatory failure secondary to diabetes mellitus. *Urology.* 1997;49(2):239-242.

497. Zhao Y, Garcia J, Jarow JP, Wallach EE. Successful management of infertility due to retrograde ejaculation using assisted reproductive technologies: a report of two cases. *Arch Androl.* 2004;50(6):391-394.

498. Frühauf S, Gerger H, Maren Schmidt H, et al. Efficacy of psychological interventions for sexual dysfunction: a systematic review and meta-analysis. *Arch Sex Behav.* 2013;42:915-933.

499. Middleton LS, Kuffel SW. Effects of experimentally adopted sexual schemas on vaginal response and subjective sexual arousal: a comparison between women with arousal disorder and sexually healthy women. *Arch Sex Behav.* 2008;37:950-961.

500. Brotto LA, Basson R, Luria M. A mindfulness research group psychoeducational intervention targeting sexual arousal disorder in women. *J Sex Med.* 2008;5:1646-1659.

501. Brotto LA, Basson R. Group mindfulness-based therapy significantly improves sexual desire in women. *Behav Res Ther.* 2014;57:43-54.

502. Brotto L, Heiman J, Goff B, et al. A psychoeducational intervention for sexual dysfunction in women with gynecologic cancer. *Arch Sex Behav.* 2008;37(2):317-329.

503. Brotto LA, Basson R, Driscoll M, et al. Mindfulness-based group therapy for women with provoked vestibulodynia. *Mindfulness.* 2014;6:417-432.

504. Zeidan F, Gordon NS, Merchant J, et al. The effects of brief mindfulness meditation training on experimentally induced pain. *J Pain.* 2010; 11(3):199-209.

505. Zeidan F, Martucci KT, Kraft RA, et al. Brain mechanisms supporting the modulation of pain by mindfulness meditation. *J Neurosci.* 2011; 31(14):5540-5548.

506. Ives-Deliperi VL, Solms M, Meintjes EM. The neural substrates of mindfulness: an fMRI investigation. *Soc Neurosci.* 2011;6(3):231-242.

507. Basson R, Smith KB. Incorporating mindfulness meditation into the treatment of provoked vestibulodynia. *Curr Sex Health Rep.* 2013; DOI 10. 1007/s1 1930-013-008-0.

508. Brotto LA, Basson R, Carlson M, et al. Impact of an integrated mindfulness and cognitive behavioural treatment for provoked vestibulodynia (IMPROVED): a qualitative study. *Sex Rel Ther.* 2013;28:3-19.

509. Harley TS. Interventions for sexual problems following treatment for breast cancer: a systematic review. *Breast Cancer Res Treat.* 2011;130: 711-724.

510. Nurnberg HG, Hensley PL, Heiman JR, et al. Sildenafil treatment of women with antidepressant-associated sexual dysfunction: a randomized controlled trial. *JAMA.* 2008;300:395-404.

511. Fooladi E, Bell RJ, Jane F, et al. Testosterone improves antidepressant-emergent loss of libido in women: findings from a randomized, double-blind, placebo-controlled trial. *J Sex Med.* 2014;11:831-839.

512. Danielsson I, Sjoberg I, Stelund H, et al. Prevalence and incidence of prolonged and severe dyspareunia in women: results from a population study. *Scand J Public Health.* 2003;31:113-118.

513. Morin M, Bergeron S, Khalifé S. Morphometry of the pelvic floor muscles in women with and without provoked vestibulodynia using 4D ultrasound. *J Sex Med.* 2014;11:776-785.

514. Heddini U, Bohm-Starle N, Gronbladh A, et al. GCH1-polymorphism and pain sensitivity among women with provoked vestibulodynia. *Mol Pain.* 2012;8:68.

515. Bouchard C, Brisson J, Fortier M, et al. Use of oral contraceptive pills and vulvar vestibulitis: a case-control study. *Am J Epidemiol.* 2002;156: 254-261.

516. Basson R. The recurrent pain and sexual sequelae of provoked vestibulodynia: a perpetuating cycle. *J Sex Med.* 2012;9:2077-2092.

517. Desrochers G, Bergeron S, Khalife S, et al. Provoked vestibulodynia: psychological predictors of topical and cognitive-behavioral treatment outcome. *Behav Res Ther.* 2010;48:106-115.

518. Spoelstra SK, Dijkstra JR, van Driel MF, et al. Long-term results of an individualized, multifaceted, and multidisciplinary therapeutic approach to provoked vestibulodynia. *J Sex Med.* 2011;8:489-496.

519. Tommola P, Unkila-Kallio L, Paavonen J. Surgical treatment of vulvar vestibulitis: a review. *Acta Obstet Gynecol Scand.* 2010;89:1385-1395.

520. Vachon-Presseau E, Roy M, Martel MO, et al. The stress model of chronic pain: evidence from basal cortisol and hippocampal structure and function in humans. *Brain.* 2013;136:815-827.

521. Borsook D, Maleki N, Becerra L, et al. Understanding migraine through the lens of maladaptive stress responses: a model disease of allostatic load. *Neuron.* 2012;73(2):219-234.

521a. Basson R, Driscoll M, Correia S. Flibanserin for low sexual desire in women: a molecule from bench to bed? *E BioMed.* 2015;2:772-773.

522. McEwen BS, Stellar E. Stress and the individual. Mechanisms leading to disease. *Arch Intern Med.* 1993;153:2903-3101.

523. Khandker M, Brady SS, Vitonis AF, et al. The influence of depression and anxiety on risk of adult onset vulvodynia. *J Women's Health.* 2011; 20:1445-1451.

524. Brotto LA, Basson R, Gehring D. Psychological profiles among women with vulvar vestibulitis syndrome: a chart review. *J Psychosom Obstet Gynecol.* 2003;24:195-203.

525. Danielsson I, Sjoberg I, Wikman M. Vulvar vestibulitis: medical, psychosexual and psychosocial aspects, a case control study. *Acta Obstet Gynecol Scand.* 2000;79:872-878.

526. Jantos M, White G. The vestibulitis syndrome: medical and psychosexual assessment of a cohort of patients. *J Reprod Med.* 1997;42: 145-152.

527. Ehrström S, Kornfeld D, Rylander E, et al. Chronic stress in women with localized provoked vulvodynia. *J Psychosom Obstet Gynecol.* 2009;30:73-79.

528. Bergeron S, Khalifé S, Glazer HI, et al. Surgical and behavioral treatments for vestibulodynia: two-and-one-half year follow-up and predictors of outcome. *Obstet Gynecol.* 2008;111:159-166.

529. Schweinhardt P, Kuchinad A, Pukall CF, et al. Increased gray matter density in young women with chronic vulvar pain. *Pain.* 2008;140: 411-419.

530. van Lankveld JJ, ter Kuile MM, de Groot HE, et al. Cognitive-behavioral therapy for women with lifelong vaginismus: a randomized waiting-list controlled trial of efficacy. *J Consult Clin Psychol.* 2006;74:168-178.

531. Rosenbaum TY. An integrated mindfulness-based approach to the treatment of women with sexual pain and anxiety: promoting autonomy and mind/body connection. *Sex Rel Ther.* 2013;28:20-28.

532. Ter Kuile MM, Melles R, de Groot HE, et al. Therapist-aided exposure for women with lifelong vaginismus: a randomized waiting-list control of efficacy. *J Consult Clin Psychol.* 2013;81(6):1127-1136.

533. Braunstein GD, Sundwall DA, Katz M, et al. Safety and efficacy of a testosterone patch for the treatment of hypoactive sexual desire disorder in surgically menopausal women: a randomized, placebo-controlled trial. *Arch Intern Med.* 2005;165:1582-1589.

534. Arlt W. Androgen therapy in women. *Eur J Endocrinol.* 2006;154: 1-11.

535. Shifren JL, Davis SR, Moreau M, et al. Testosterone patch for the treatment of hypoactive sexual desire disorder in naturally menopausal women: results from the INTIMATE NM1 Study. *Menopause.* 2006;13: 770-779.

536. Davis SR, Moreau M, Kroll R, et al. Testosterone for low libido in postmenopausal women not taking estrogen. *N Engl J Med.* 2008;359: 2005-2017.

537. Panay N, Al-Azzawi F, Bouchard C, et al. Testosterone treatment of HSDD in naturally menopausal women: the ADORE study. *Climacteric.* 2010;13(2):121-131.

538. Snabes MC, Zborowski J, Simes S. Libigel (testosterone gel) does not differentiate from placebo therapy in the treatment of hypoactive sexual desire in postmenopausal women. *J Sex Med.* 2012;S3:S171.

539. Davis S, Papalia MA, Norman RJ, et al. Safety and efficacy of a testosterone metered-dose transdermal spray for treatment of decreased sexual satisfaction in premenopausal women: a placebo-controlled randomized, dose ranging study. *Ann Intern Med.* 2008;148:569-577.

540. Van der Nadem F, Bloemers J, Yassem WE, et al. The influence of testosterone combined with a PDE5-inhibitor on cognitive, effective, and physiological sexual functioning in women suffering from sexual dysfunction. *J Sex Med.* 2009;6:777-790.

541. Cain VS, Johannes CB, Avis NE, et al. Sexual functioning and practices in a multi-ethnic study of midlife women: baseline results from SWAN. *J Sex Res.* 2003;40:266-276.

542. Carvalheira AA, Brotto LA, Leal I. Women's motivations for sex: exploring the diagnostic and statistical manual, fourth edition, text revision criteria for hypoactive sexual desire and female sexual arousal disorders. *J Sex Med.* 2010;7:1454-1463.

543. Basson R. Testosterone supplementation to improve women's sexual satisfaction: complexities and unknowns [editorial]. *Ann Intern Med.* 2008;148:620-621.

544. Padero MC, Bhasin S, Friedman TC. Androgen supplementation in older women: too much hype, not enough data. *J Am Geriatr Soc.* 2002;50:1131-1140.

545. Schover LR. Androgen therapy for loss of desire in women: is the benefit worth the breast cancer risk? *Fertil Steril.* 2008;90:129-140.

546. Bradford A, Meston CM. Placebo response in the treatment of women's sexual dysfunctions: a review and commentary. *J Sex Marital Ther.* 2009;35:164-181.

547. Braunstein GD. Management of female sexual dysfunction in postmenopausal women by testosterone administration: safety issues and controversies. *J Sex Med.* 2007;4(4 Pt 1):859-866.

548. Wierman M, Arlt W, Basson R, et al. Androgen therapy in women: a reappraisal: an Endocrine Society clinical practice guideline. *J Clin Endocrinol Metab.* 2014;99(10):3489-3510.

549. Wild RA. Endogenous androgens and cardiovascular risk. *Menopause.* 2007;14:609-610.

550. Bell RJ, Davison SL, Papalia MA, et al. Endogenous androgen levels and cardiovascular risk profile in women across the adult life span. *Menopause.* 2007;14:630-638.

551. Guthrie JR, Dennerstein L, Taffe JR, et al. The menopausal transition: a 9-year prospective population-based study. The Melbourne Women's Midlife Health Project. *Climacteric.* 2004;7:375-389.

552. Sutton-Tyrrell K, Zhao X, Santoro N, et al. Reproductive hormones and obesity: 9 years of observation from the Study of Women's Health Across the Nation. *Am J Epidemiol.* 2010;171:1203-1213.

553. Elraiyah T, Sonbol MB, Wang Z, et al. The benefits and harms of systemic testosterone therapy in postmenopausal women with normal adrenal function. A systematic review and meta-analysis. *J Clin Endocrinol Metab.* 2014;99:3543-3550.

554. Brotto LA, Petkau AJ, Labrie F, Basson R. Predictors of sexual desire disorders in women. *J Sex Med.* 2011;8:742-753.

555. Dennerstein L, Dudley E, Burger H. Are changes in sexual functioning during midlife due to aging or menopause? *Fertil Steril.* 2011;76: 456-460.

556. Woods NF, Mitchell ES, Smith-Di Julio K. Sexual desire during menopause transition and early postmenopause: observations from the Seattle Midlife Women's Health Study. *J Women's Health.* 2010;19: 209-218.

557. Elraiyah T, Sonbol MB, Wang Z, et al. Clinical review: The benefits and harms of systemic dehydroepiandrosterone (DHEA) in postmenopausal women with normal adrenal function. A systematic review and meta-analysis. *J Clin Endocrinol Metab.* 2014;99:3536-3542.

558. Labrie F, Archer D, Bouchard C, et al. Effect of intravaginal prasterone (DHEA) on libido and sexual dysfunction in postmenopausal women. *Menopause.* 2009;16:923-931.

559. Pelletier G, Ouillet J, Martel C, et al. Effects of ovariectomy and dehydroepiandrosterone (DHEA) on vaginal wall thickness and innervation. *J Sex Med.* 2012;9:2525-2533.

560. Kao A, Binik YM, Amsel R, et al. Challenging atrophied perspectives on postmenopausal dyspareunia: a systematic description and synthesis of clinical pain characteristics. *J Sex Marital Ther.* 2012;38: 128-150.

561. Kendal A, Dowsett M, Folkerd E, et al. Caution: vaginal estradiol appears to be contraindicated in postmenopausal women on adjunct aromatase inhibitors. *Ann Oncol.* 2006;17:584-587.

562. Krychman ML, Katz A. Breast cancer and sexuality: multi-modal treatment options. *J Sex Med.* 2012;9:5-213.

563. Chen J, Geng L, Song X, et al. Evaluation of the efficacy and safety of hyaluronic acid vaginal gel to ease vaginal dryness: a multicenter, randomized, controlled, open-label, parallel-group, clinical trial. *J Sex Med.* 2013;10:1575-1584.

564. Bachman GA, Schaefers M, Uddin A, et al. Microdose transdermal estrogen therapy for relief of vulvovaginal symptoms in postmenopausal women. *Menopause.* 2009;16:877-882.

565. Hays J, Ockene JK, Brunner RL, et al. Effects of estrogen plus progestin on health-related quality of life. *N Engl J Med.* 2003;348:1839-1854.

Section VI

Endocrinology and the Life Span

CHAPTER 21

Endocrine Changes in Pregnancy

SARAH L. BERGA • JOSHUA F. NITSCHE • GLENN D. BRAUNSTEIN

KEY POINTS

- The impact of pregnancy on the endocrine system is profound and begins very early with the production of human chorionic gonadotropin (hCG) from the trophoblast at implantation.
- It is important to remember that only a small portion of the recommended weight gain is due to an increase in maternal adipose stores.
- It is important to consider the increase in glomerular filtration rate (GFR) and blood volume when treating women with medications that are cleared in the kidney.
- Although these increases in cardiac demand are easily met by most pregnant women, for some, particularly those with preexisting coronary artery or structural heart disease, the added strain can threaten the health of both mother and baby.
- Numerous changes in maternal metabolism occur in pregnancy to ensure the fetus has a consistent supply of metabolic fuel during in utero development. These changes include hyperinsulinemia, insulin resistance, increased plasma lipids, and more efficient plasma amino acid transport.

PLACENTAL DEVELOPMENT

Normal placentation requires a coordinated series of events, beginning with fertilization. The fertilization rate following unprotected regular intercourse during a single menstrual cycle is 25% to 30%. However, in approximately one third of conceptions there is either failure of implantation or clinical or subclinical spontaneous abortion.[1]

For the first 5 days, preimplantation development takes place within the fallopian tube. During this period, the zygote undergoes cleavage division, and, at least through the 8-cell stage, the blastomeres remain totipotential. In the 16-cell stage, differentiation of the innermost cells into the *inner cell mass* and the surrounding cells into the *trophectoderm* occurs. The inner cell mass develops into the fetus, and the trophectoderm gives rise to the placenta and

membranes. On approximately day 5 or 6 after fertilization, the blastocyst enters the uterus, but implantation does not occur for another 1 to 2 days. Implantation occurs after the zona pellucida disappears from around the embryo.[2]

Implantation is a complex process that involves apposition of the microvilli present on the trophectoderm cells with pinocytes (fused microvilli) on the endometrial cells, followed by removal of fluid between the cells through pinocytosis by the endometrial cells, a process stimulated by progesterone.[3] Progesterone synthesis by the corpus luteum is stimulated and sustained during this time and for the first 6 to 7 weeks of pregnancy by secretion of hCG by the trophoblast cells. The hCG is first detected in the maternal serum 6 to 9 days after conception.[4] Attachment of the embryo is enhanced through the expression of a variety of adhesion molecules, including mucins, integrins, and trophinin, a trophoblast-specific cell membrane adhesion protein, as well as cytokines, growth factors, and a variety of transcription factors encoded by homeobox genes.[3,5]

After the trophoblast attaches to the endometrium during the window of implantation 6 to 10 days after ovulation, the embryo invades the endometrium through a complex process involving matrix metalloproteinases and differentiation of the trophectoderm into *cytotrophoblasts* or *syncytiotrophoblasts*. The syncytiotrophoblasts are multinucleated cells formed by the fusion of cytotrophoblasts. The cytotrophoblasts form a column of cells that invade the endometrium, form anchoring villi, and enter the maternal vasculature, eventually replacing the endothelial layer of the endometrial and myometrial spiral arterioles with a layer of cytotrophoblasts (vascular trophoblasts).[6] This process converts the high-resistance, low-capacity uterine vessels into low-resistance, high-volume vessels, which are essential for growth of the placenta and fetus.[7] At the site of implantation, the endometrial cells undergo decidualization, enlarging and increasing their metabolic activity with enhanced production of tissue inhibitors or metalloproteinase, extracellular matrix proteins, cytokines, and growth factors that modulate the extent of trophoblast invasion and influence trophoblast function.[3,4,8]

The trophoblast cells secrete several angiogenic proteins, including vascular endothelial growth factor (VEGF), platelet-derived growth factor (PDGF), and basic fibroblast growth factor (bFGF), which stimulate blood vessel development within the villi.[9] The syncytiotrophoblasts form an outer layer of cells in the chorionic villi, between the cytotrophoblast cells and the maternal blood space on the exterior surface. Only three tissues separate the fetal blood from maternal blood: (1) the endothelium of the fetal vessels in the villi, (2) connective tissue, and (3) the trophoblasts; this form of placentation is referred to as *hemochorial*. Thus, in addition to hCG secretion, which is responsible for maintaining early pregnancy; progesterone secretion, which is required for continuation of pregnancy after the luteal-placental shift; and the synthesis and secretion of other hormones and growth factors (Table 21-1), the syncytiotrophoblasts provide the major site for transportation of oxygen and nutrients to and removal of waste from the fetus.

Substances are transferred across the placenta through transcellular pathways that include carrier-mediated transport (e.g., immunoglobulin G through the Fcγ receptor) and simple extracellular diffusion. The degree of transpla-

TABLE 21-1
Hormones, Peptides, and Growth Factors Produced by the Placenta

Hypothalamic Analogues

Gonadotropin-releasing hormone
Corticotropin-releasing hormone
Urocortin
Somatostatin
Growth hormone–releasing hormone
Ghrelin
Thyrotropin-releasing hormone
Dopamine
Neuropeptide Y
Enkephalin

Pituitary Analogues

Chorionic gonadotropin
Placental lactogen
Chorionic corticotropin
β-Endorphin
α-Melanocyte-stimulating hormone
Placental variant growth hormone
Oxytocin

Steroid Hormones

Estrogens
Progesterone

Growth Factors and Other Hormones

Activins
Inhibins
Follistatin
Relaxin
Calcitonin
Leptin
Parathyroid hormone–related protein
Erythropoietin
Renin
Interleukins
Nitric oxide
Transforming growth factor-β
Tumor necrosis factor-α
Epidermal growth factor
Insulin-like growth factor type 1
Insulin-like growth factor type 2
Insulin-like growth factor binding protein 1
Colony-stimulating factor 1
Basic fibroblast growth factor
Corticotropin-releasing hormone–binding protein
Platelet-derived growth factor
Vascular endothelial growth factor
Endothelin 1
Anadamide (endocannabinoid)
Hepatocyte growth factor
Oncomodulin

cental passage of a hormone from the mother to the fetus through diffusion depends on (1) the rate of placental blood flow, (2) the maternal concentration of the free or readily disassociatable hormone, and (3) the molecular mass, lipid solubility, charge, and degree of placental metabolic degradation of the hormone. Maternal-to-fetal transfer occurs for hormones smaller than 700 Da, but the placenta is not permeable to hormones larger than 1200 Da.[10]

The trophoblast also anchors the placenta and fetus to the uterus and helps to protect the fetus, which contains paternal antigens, from rejection by the maternal immune system. This immunologic protection may be mediated by high concentrations of progesterone at the trophoblast fetal-maternal interface and the expression by the trophoblasts of a histocompatibility complex antigen, human leukocyte antigen G (HLA-G), which exhibits reduced polymorphism in comparison with other major HLA antigens.[11] The mass of the trophoblast increases logarithmically during the first trimester, followed by a more gradual increase throughout the remainder of pregnancy. Trophoblastic mass closely correlates with maternal serum concentrations of human placental lactogen (hPL) and pregnancy-specific β_1-glycoprotein throughout pregnancy and with hCG during the first trimester but not during the subsequent trimesters.[12]

MATERNAL ADAPTATIONS TO PREGNANCY

To some extent every maternal organ system is altered in pregnancy. The impact of pregnancy on the endocrine system is profound and begins very early with the production of hCG from the trophoblast at implantation. The effects on many other organ systems are more gradual and may not appear until later in pregnancy. Although the vast majority of these changes are hormonally mediated, some organ systems are also affected by the anatomic alterations caused by the enlarging uterus or the physiologic increase in maternal blood volume. It is critically important for the clinician to understand these changes when caring for pregnant women because many physical examination findings, laboratory values, and imaging findings that would be viewed as abnormal and of great concern outside pregnancy can be normal and reassuring in pregnant women.

Physiologic Adaptations

During pregnancy some amount of weight gain is expected, with overweight and obese women expected to gain less than normal or underweight women. Excessive gestational weight gain has been associated with a number of adverse neonatal[13,14] and maternal outcomes.[15-19] Given this association and the increasing prevalence of obesity among women of childbearing age the Institute of Medicine (IOM) has recommended an updated set of guidelines regarding weight gain in pregnancy based on the woman's prepregnancy body mass index (BMI) (Table 21-2).[20]

Recently, experts and medical professional organizations with a stake in the obesity epidemic have proposed further subdividing obesity (BMI > 30) into class I (BMI 30-34), class II (BMI 35-39), and class III (BMI 40+).[21] The IOM guidelines did not further refine their recommendations for weight gain based on level of obesity, citing a lack of evidence regarding proper weight gain in women with very high BMI. Although this more specific classification system is helpful for consistency in categorizing patients

TABLE 21-2				
Recommended Weight Gain in Pregnancy				
	Total Weight Gain		**Rates of Weight Gain During Second and Third Trimesters**	
Prepregnancy Body Mass Index	**Range in kg**	**Range in lb**	**Mean (Range) in kg/Week**	**Mean (Range) in lb/Week**
Underweight (<18.5 kg/m²)	12.5-18	28-40	0.51 (0.44-0.58)	1 (1-1.3)
Normal weight (18.5-24.9 kg/m²)	11.5-16	25-35	0.42 (0.35-0.50)	1 (0.8-1)
Overweight (25.0-29.9 kg/m²)	7-11.5	15-25	0.28 (0.23-0.33)	0.6 (0.5-0.7)
Obese (≥30.0 kg/m²)	5-9	11-20	0.22 (0.17-0.27)	0.5 (0.4-0.6)

From the Institute of Medicine Guidelines.

for epidemiologic or clinical studies, it is not clinically meaningful because the impact of obesity on maternal health has a much more linear relationship than the abrupt classification system would suggest. As with the BMI classification schema proposed by the IOM, the subclassification of obesity also groups large numbers of patients into the high end of the scale, such as class III (BMI 40+). Such patients are often encountered in current clinical practice as the prevalence of women of childbearing age with BMI over 40 is approximately 7.5% overall and as high as 15% among certain ethnic groups.[22]

It is important to remember that only a small portion of the recommended weight gain is due to an increase in maternal adipose stores. For example, in a normal weight woman with a weight gain of 12.5 kg, 9.25 kg are due to factors other than maternal adipose stores (fetus accounts for about 3.4 kg, placenta for 0.65 kg, amniotic fluid for 0.8 kg, uterus for 1 kg, breasts for 0.4 kg, blood for 1.5 kg, extravascular fluid for 1.5 kg).[13] Thus, only 3.25 kg is due to the increase in maternal adipose stores. If one considers the weight gain goal for overweight and obese women (5-9 kg) and assumes that most will be expected to gain 9.25 kg of nonadipose weight during pregnancy, there should be a negligible increase and potentially a decrease in adipose stores in these women if IOM guidelines are followed.

The volume of the uterine cavity increases from 10 mL in the nonpregnant state to an average of 5 L at term, and blood flow through the uteroplacental circulation reaches 450 to 650 mL/minute, approximately a 10-fold increase.[23] To maintain appropriate perfusion of the mother and the fetal-placental unit, systemic blood volume increases throughout pregnancy and is 40% to 45% higher at term than in the nonpregnant state. The plasma volume increases by about 45% to 50% as a result of aldosterone-stimulated sodium and water retention. The red blood cell mass increases approximately 20% because of increased production resulting from a twofold to threefold increase in erythropoietin secretion. The net effect is a physiologic decrease in the hematocrit by about 15% at term.[23]

The increase in uterine blood flow, although essential to maintain the fetus and placenta during pregnancy, carries a risk of severe hemorrhage surrounding delivery. Laceration of a vessel during a vaginal delivery can lead to heavy bleeding due to the high rate of blood flow to the uterus, cervix, and vagina. Bleeding can be life threatening if it tracks into the retroperitoneum, where a large amount of blood can accumulate before symptoms prompt an evaluation and confirmation of the diagnosis. Damage to a branch of the uterine artery during a cesarean section can lead to bleeding rapid enough to require intraoperative blood transfusion to replace ongoing blood loss. For these reasons elective operations are typically avoided in the third trimester. Fortunately, there are also maternal adaptations that lessen the potential impact of blood loss. The physiologic drop in hematocit during pregnancy leads to less red blood cell mass lost per a given volume of blood. This allows women to maintain oxygen-carrying capacity after volumes of blood loss that would lead to advanced stages of shock in nonpregnant individuals.[24]

The renal blood flow and GFR increase rapidly and peak during the second trimester, and a 50% increase in creatinine clearance results in a reduction in the serum creatinine level. Atrial natriuretic peptide (ANP) levels increase during pregnancy and may in part be responsible for increased renal blood flow, GFR, 24-hour urine volume, and natriuresis.[25] An alteration in the osmotic thresholds for the release of vasopressin and activation of the hypothalamic thirst centers, possibly caused by an extragonadal effect of hCG, lead to an approximately 4% reduction in serum osmolality (approximately 10 mOsm/kg).[26]

It is important to consider the increase in GFR and blood volume when treating women with medications that are cleared in the kidney. Many medications, both prescription and over the counter, are cleared in this way, including amnioglycosides, β-lactams, antiviral agents, antifungal agents, H₁ blockers, and H₂ blockers, among others. Some of these medications require dose adjustments because of the increased GFR of pregnancy. Adjustments in dose are particularly relevant for antiepileptic drugs, the plasma levels of which can become subtherapeutic if not monitored and steadily increased over the course of pregnancy. Although not all the reasons for the increased drug requirement in pregnancy are clear, it is likely that the increase in the volume of distribution is a contributing factor.[27] This is also true of low-molecular-weight heparins, a preferred anticoagulant in pregnancy. Although only a small portion of the drug is cleared in the kidney, the increased GFR of pregnancy is thought to contribute to the much larger doses required in pregnant women to maintain effectiveness.[28]

Several hemodynamic changes are induced by the low-resistance, high-capacity uteroplacental vasculature, which in many respects act like an arteriovenous shunt in pregnancy. The large quantities of estrogens, progesterone, prostaglandins, and angiotensin present during pregnancy are thought to mediate these changes. Other changes include an increase in the heart rate by 10 to 15 beats per minute, a 30% to 50% increase in cardiac output resulting from increased stroke volume in early pregnancy and heart rate during the third trimester, a reduction in diastolic blood pressure of 10 to 15 mm Hg with little or no change in systolic pressure, and an approximately 20% reduction in peripheral vascular resistance.[23]

Although these increases in cardiac demand are easily met by most pregnant women, for some, particularly those with preexisting coronary artery or structural heart disease, the added strain can threaten the health of both mother and baby. Although women with a history of myocardial infarction (MI) with normal left ventricular function tolerate pregnancy well, women with poor hemodynamics with significant left ventricular injury are discouraged from attempting pregnancy as maternal morbidity and mortality rates are markedly increased.[29] In women with structural heart disease, particularly Eisenmenger syndrome, the increase in cardiac output and blood volume can overwhelm an already impaired heart, leading to arrhythmia, congestive heart failure, pregnancy loss, and maternal death.[30]

In pregnancy the pulmonary vascular resistance is reduced by about one third and pulmonary tidal volume increases by about 30%. The latter results in a respiratory alkalosis that is compensated by increased bicarbonate excretion by the kidneys and causes increases in minute ventilatory volume by 30% to 40%. There are no changes in respiratory rate, maximum breathing capacity, or forced or timed vital capacity. However, there is an approximately 40% reduction in the expiratory reserve because of the elevation of the diaphragm by the enlarged uterus.[23]

Although these changes do not increase the risk of pregnant women contracting respiratory infections such as influenza and bacterial pneumonia, their morbidity and mortality risks are notably increased during pregnancy. This was most recently noted in the 2009 H1N1 pandemic, in which pregnant women accounted for 5% of the deaths but made up only 1% of the affected population.[31] Pregnant women were also more likely to be hospitalized with pneumonia[32] but did not appear to be at an increased risk of infection compared to the general population.[33]

Gastrointestinal tract function is altered during pregnancy. Gastric emptying time is unchanged until labor, when it becomes prolonged. Reduced lower esophageal sphincter tone and displacement of the abdominal contents by the pregnant uterus result in a marked increase in gastroesophageal reflux. Motility of the intestine is also reduced, contributing to nausea and vomiting early in pregnancy and constipation that is common later in pregnancy. Decreased motility of the gallbladder leads to an increased gallbladder volume and reduced emptying of bile after meals, producing a more lithogenic bile and increasing cholelithiasis risk during pregnancy.[23]

Metabolic Adaptations

Numerous changes in maternal metabolism occur in pregnancy to ensure the fetus has a consistent supply of metabolic fuel during in utero development. These changes include hyperinsulinemia, insulin resistance, increased plasma lipids, and more efficient plasma amino acid transport.[34] As a result of these alterations maternal energy requirements are met predominantly by lipolysis, allowing glucose and other carbohydrates to supply the energy needs of the fetus. This shift in maternal fuel utilization can be conceptualized as an accelerated starvation. Although carbohydrates are readily available in the maternal circulation, the insulin resistance reduces entry of glucose into maternal cells, thereby limiting her use of carbohydrates for energy. To compensate, maternal cells turn toward lipid metabolism for energy-producing levels of ketones similar to those seen after prolonged fasting.[35] The increased levels of maternal low-density lipoprotein (LDL) and very low-density lipoprotein (VLDL) that occur in pregnancy[36,37] are also thought to be the main cholesterol supply for steroid hormone production in the placenta, as the placenta has very low hydroxymethylglutaryl–coenzyme A reductase activity and thus limited ability to produce cholesterol from acetate in situ.[38]

The underlying causes of the shift in metabolic fuels during pregnancy are largely understood, but significant gaps in knowledge persist. It is clear that the increasing levels of hPL and human placental growth hormone (hPGH) reduce insulin receptors and glucose transport.[39] However, to what extent glucagon and cortisol, which demonstrate strong diabetogenic effects outside pregnancy, play a role in this process has not been thoroughly investigated.

Maternal Endocrine Alterations
Pituitary Gland

The anterior pituitary gland enlarges by an average of 36% during pregnancy, primarily because of a 10-fold increase in lactotroph size and number. This enlargement increases the height and convexity of the pituitary gland, which can be observed on magnetic resonance imaging. Numbers of somatotrophs and gonadotrophs are reduced, and there are no changes in corticotrophs or thyrotrophs.[40] The size of the posterior pituitary gland diminishes during pregnancy.[41]

The marked increase in estrogen levels during pregnancy enhances prolactin synthesis and secretion, and maternal serum prolactin levels increase in parallel with the enlargement of the lactotrophs. At term, the mean serum prolactin concentration is 207 ng/mL (range, 35-600 ng/mL), in contrast to a mean of 10 ng/mL in nonpregnant, premenopausal women.[42] Prolactin also is present in the amniotic fluid and appears to be primarily of decidual origin because the decidua actively synthesizes prolactin. Amniotic fluid prolactin levels are 10 to 100 times higher than in the maternal circulation in early pregnancy. Serum prolactin levels return to the baseline of nonpregnancy approximately 7 days after delivery in the absence of breastfeeding. With breastfeeding, the basal prolactin levels remain elevated for several months but gradually decrease; however, with suckling, there is a brisk rise in prolactin levels within 30 minutes.[40]

Although rare, pituitary tumors do occur in women of childbearing age. Although most are diagnosed prior to pregnancy, some are diagnosed for the first time in pregnancy. The most common type of tumor is a prolactinoma, which as the name implies, is due to an overgrowth of lactotrophs. Prolactinomas, and other pituitary tumors, are typically classified based on size, with those less 10 mm in diameter designated as microadenomas and those greater than 10 mm in diameter designated macroadenomas. The increase in pituitary size during pregnancy can lead to complications in women with prolactinomas. In a study of 352 women with untreated microadenomas, 2.3% experienced visual disturbances, 4.8% experienced headaches, and 0.6% experienced diabetes insipidus. The rates of complications were much higher in 144 women with macroadenomas, with 15.3% experiencing visual disturbances, 15.3% experiencing headache, and 2.14% experiencing diabetes insipidus.[43] In cases of symptomatic tumor expansion in pregnancy, the dopamine agonist bromocriptine can be safely used and is successful in reducing tumor size and symptoms in the majority of cases.[44] Cabergoline, a more selective dopamine 2 receptor agonist and the preferred treatment outside pregnancy, also appears safe, but there is less experience with this drug in pregnancy. Transsphenoidal resection of the pituitary is occasionally needed if rapid tumor growth occurs or symptoms persist despite bromocriptine treatment.

Growth hormone (GH) levels in maternal serum remain unchanged throughout pregnancy, although the source of immunoreactive GH during gestation does change as a result of placental production of the hormone. Relaxin, secreted by the corpus luteum of pregnancy, and estrogens stimulate GH secretion during early pregnancy.[45]

Pituitary GH is known as *GH1* or *hGH-N*; GH1 messenger ribonucleic acid (mRNA) and secretion decrease after the 25th week of pregnancy, and beginning in the fourth month of gestation, the placental syncytiotrophoblast secretes a variant of GH (*GH2* or *hGH-V*) in a nonpulsatile pattern. In concert with the different sources of GH during the first and second halves of pregnancy, the GH response to provocative stimuli differs in each half. Insulin hypoglycemia or arginine infusion results in an enhanced GH response during the first half of gestation, and during the second half, the response is decreased compared with the response in nonpregnant women.[40]

Maternal serum concentrations of insulin-like growth factor type 1 (IGF-1) are elevated during the second half of pregnancy, probably through the combined effect of the placental GH variant and hPL, which is evolutionarily related to GH and prolactin. hPL has somatotropic biologic activity, and its serum concentration increases throughout pregnancy, paralleling that of IGF-1.[46] It is likely that the suppression of GH1 synthesis and secretion is caused by the high IGF-1 concentrations, which in late pregnancy are five times higher than those in nonpregnant women.[47]

Although the placenta synthesizes and secretes biologically active gonadotropin-releasing hormone (GnRH), pituitary gonadotropin production decreases throughout pregnancy, as indicated by a marked reduction in gonadotropin immunoreactivity in the gonadotrophs beginning at 10 weeks' gestation and by a reduction in serum levels of luteinizing hormone (LH) and follicle-stimulating hormone (FSH).[40] Suppression is probably mediated through the elevated blood levels of ovarian and placental sex steroid hormones and by placental production of inhibin. Suppression is incomplete because administration of exogenous GnRH leads to release of gonadotropins, although the response is blunted compared with that of nonpregnant women and does not return to normal until a month after birth.[47]

The mean concentrations of human thyroid-stimulating hormone (thyrotropin, or hTSH) during the first trimester are significantly lower than in the second and third trimesters or in the nonpregnant state.[48] Much of this early decrease may be accounted for by the intrinsic thyrotropic activity of hCG. The maximal biologic thyrotropic activity in maternal serum corresponds to the peak concentration of hCG at 10 to 12 weeks after the last menstrual period, when there is a reciprocal relationship between the rising hCG levels and falling hTSH concentrations[48,49] (Fig. 21-1). The only time during pregnancy when the free thyroxine (T_4) concentration in the maternal serum is elevated corresponds to the time of peak hCG and lowest hTSH, suggesting that the depressed hTSH is the result of feedback suppression by T_4. Despite the lower mean hTSH during early pregnancy, the hTSH response to exogenous thyrotropin-releasing hormone (TRH) is normal.[40]

Maternal adrenocorticotropic hormone (ACTH, or corticotropin) levels rise during pregnancy, increasing fourfold over concentrations in the nonpregnant state between 7 and 10 weeks' gestation. There is a further gradual rise to weeks 33 to 37, when a mean fivefold increase over prepregnancy values is found, followed by a 50% drop just before parturition and a marked 15-fold increase during the stress of delivery.[50] The ACTH concentration returns to the prepregnancy level within 24 hours of delivery. The pituitary gland and placenta are sources of circulating ACTH during pregnancy, and exogenous corticotropin-releasing hormone (CRH) stimulates the release of ACTH from both tissues in a dose-dependent manner.[23] Biologically active CRH is synthesized and secreted by the placenta and, to a lesser extent, by the decidual and fetal membranes, but

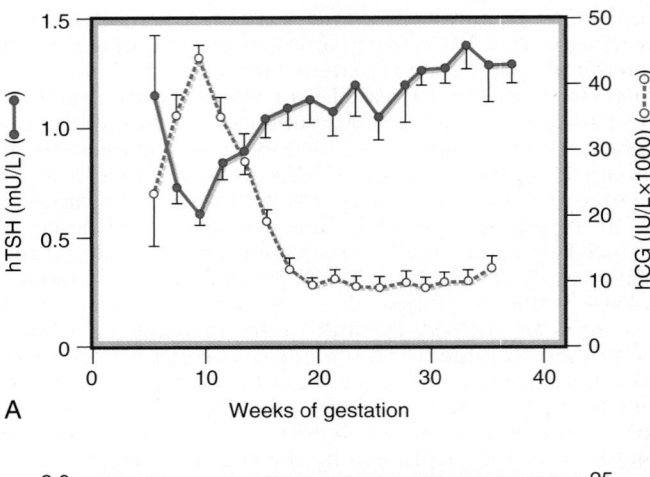

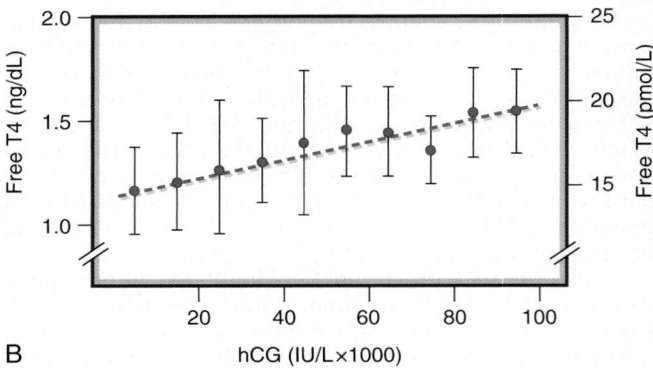

Figure 21-1 A, Concentrations of serum thyrotropin (hTSH, *filled circles*) and human chorionic gonadotropin (hCG, *open circles*) throughout pregnancy. Between 8 and 14 weeks of gestation, there is a significant negative correlation between the individual hTSH and hCG levels ($p < 0.001$). Each point represents the mean (± standard error). **B,** Linear regression of maternal serum free thyroxine (T_4) and hCG concentrations during the first half of gestation ($p < 0.001$). (From Glinoer D, de Nayer P, Bourdoux P, et al. Regulation of maternal thyroid during pregnancy. *J Clin Endocrinol Metab.* 1990;71:276.)

unlike the inhibitory effect on pituitary CRH, glucocorticoids stimulate the expression of placental CRH.[51]

There appears to be a disconnect between CRH and ACTH during pregnancy. Although biologically active CRH would be expected to stimulate ACTH production, the qualitative patterns of CRH production, which show an exponential rise during the sixth month of gestation, and ACTH secretion, which demonstrates a more gradual rise during pregnancy, are quite different. The lack of a significant correlation between maternal plasma CRH and ACTH during pregnancy suggests that factors such as the elevated levels of free cortisol in the maternal serum may modulate the response to CRH. The circadian rhythm and the ability to respond to stress are maintained throughout pregnancy; however, the ACTH response to exogenous CRH during the third trimester is blunted, whereas the responsiveness to vasopressin is maintained, suggesting that the elevation of CRH in the maternal serum downregulates the responsiveness to CRH.[50]

Arginine vasopressin (AVP) concentrations in the maternal serum are similar to those in nonpregnant women. During pregnancy, however, there is increased synthesis of AVP, which is offset by the increased metabolic clearance of the hormone through destruction by a trophoblast-derived cysteine aminopeptidase (i.e., vasopressinase), which rises throughout pregnancy in parallel with the increase in trophoblastic mass.[52,53] The osmolar set-point for thirst is reduced, and the release of AVP is related to the 10-mOsm/kg average decrease in plasma osmolality during pregnancy, possibly reflecting an extragonadotropic effect of hCG.[26] Taking into account the reduced set-point, the AVP response to dehydration and water loading is normal.

Oxytocin levels progressively increase in the maternal blood and parallel the increase in maternal serum levels of estradiol and progesterone. The levels increase further with cervical dilation and vaginal distention during labor and delivery, stimulating contraction of the uterine smooth muscles and enhancing fetal expulsion.[54] Uterine oxytocin receptors also increase throughout pregnancy, resulting in a 100-fold increase in oxytocin binding at term in the myometrium.[55]

Thyroid Gland

The thyroid gland enlarges by an average of 18% during pregnancy.[48] Enlargement is associated with an increase in the size of the follicles with increased amounts of colloid and enhanced blood volume. This enlargement may be a response to the thyrotropic effect of hCG and asialo-hCG, which may account for some of the increase in serum thyroglobulin concentrations observed during pregnancy. Although clinically contraindicated, experimental evidence suggests that enhanced ^{131}iodine uptake by the maternal thyroid gland reflects the combined effects of hCG stimulation and reduction of the blood levels of iodide by increased renal iodide clearance.[48]

Rising estrogen concentrations during pregnancy induce increased hepatic synthesis of thyroxine-binding globulin (TBG) and enhanced sialylation of TBG, which decreases its metabolic clearance rate.[49] The results are a twofold increase in TBG and increased total T_4 and triiodothyronine (T_3) levels in maternal serum throughout pregnancy,[49] whereas for most of the gestation, the free T_4 and free T_3 concentrations remain normal. There are no significant changes in the levels of thyroxine-binding prealbumin, but albumin levels are decreased because of the increase in vascular volume.

Although hyperthyroidism is rather rare, hypothyroidism is relatively common in women of childbearing age. In managing a pregnancy complicated by hypothyroidism it is important to note that the pregnant woman is the source of T_4 and T_3 for the fetus throughout the first trimester. As a result, the maternal thyroid hormone replacement requirements increase as early as the fifth week of gestation. Although requirements often plateau in the second trimester, they continue to increase well into the third trimester in many patients. Increased doses of thyroid hormone are needed in 50% to 85% of women, and the total dose may increase as much as 50%.[56,57] Thus, in women with preexisting hypothyroidism, it is necessary to check thyroid function at the first prenatal visit to determine if additional thyroid hormone replacement is necessary. Alternatively the dose can be empirically increased when pregnancy is confirmed prior to any laboratory assessment of thyroid function.[58] Intermittent monitoring throughout pregnancy is warranted every 4 to 8 weeks to make certain replacement remains adequate as gestation progresses. Routine screening for undiagnosed hypothyroidism in pregnancy is controversial and is not currently endorsed by the American Thyroid Association, American College of Obstetricians and Gynecologists (ACOG), or Endocrine Society.[59-61] Instead, a targeted screening approach has been adopted based on risk factors such as family or personal history of thyroid disease, prior head or neck radiation, morbid obesity, and age greater than 30 years.

Parathyroid Glands

During pregnancy, approximately 30 g of calcium is transferred from the maternal compartment to the fetus, with most of the transfer occurring during the last trimester. Maternal total serum calcium levels decrease during pregnancy, with a nadir at 28 to 32 weeks related to the decrease in albumin levels that accompanies the increase in vascular volume. However, the albumin-adjusted total calcium and the ionized calcium concentrations actually rise slightly above the level in the nonpregnant state.[62] The urinary calcium excretion rate increases in parallel with the increased GFR, and intestinal calcium absorption undergoes a twofold increase.[62]

Although some studies have suggested that parathyroid hormone (PTH) levels increase during pregnancy, measurements of intact PTH levels by two-site immunometric assays indicate that they are within the normal, nonpregnancy range throughout pregnancy. In contrast, the circulating concentrations of PTH-related protein (PTHrp) increase throughout pregnancy.[63] Many normal tissues produce this protein and the source of the elevated levels during pregnancy is unclear, although the two most likely sites are the mammary tissue and the placenta.[63] This protein is probably involved in placental and mammary gland calcium transport.

The serum levels of 25-hydroxyvitamin D are unchanged during pregnancy, but the estrogen-induced rise in vitamin D–binding globulin results in a twofold increase in 1,25-dihydroxyvitamin D concentrations in maternal serum.[62] There is also a rise in the biologically active free fraction of 1,25-dihydroxyvitamin D, which may reflect both increased maternal renal 1α-hydroxylase activity and the synthesis and secretion of 1,25-dihydroxyvitamin D by the placenta.[62] This increase in the active metabolite of vitamin D may be responsible in part for the enhanced intestinal calcium absorption.

Although hyper- and hypoparathyroidism are uncommon, they both can lead to serious complications in pregnancy. Pregnancy is somewhat protective in women with hyperparathyroidism as calcium uptake by the fetus helps lower maternal calcium levels. Although women with hypercalcemia in pregnancy often have mild to moderate symptoms of nausea, vomiting, pain, and renal colic,[64] some experience more serious complications such as nephrolithiasis, pancreatitis, hypertension, bone disease, and hypercalcemic crisis.[65] A crisis can be difficult to treat as many of the agents used in nonpregnant patients, such as bisphosphonates and plicamycin, are avoided because of concern for fetal harm. Calcitonin can potentially be used because it does not cross the placenta; however, its benefits and safety in pregnancy have not been sufficiently investigated.[66]

Hypoparathyroidism in general poses a much less serious risk but can lead to both maternal and fetal fractures if sufficiently severe.[67,68] These complications can generally be prevented with sufficient oral calcium and vitamin D supplementation. As mentioned earlier, a significant amount of maternal calcium is consumed by the fetus during gestation. This often requires a steady increase in calcium (1.0 to 1.5 mg of elemental calcium per day) and vitamin D (up to 50,000 to 100,000 units/day or more) intake throughout pregnancy to maintain normal maternal serum calcium homeostasis.[69]

Pancreas

Hyperplasia and hypertrophy of the beta cells in the islets of Langerhans are probably the result of stimulation by estrogen and progesterone.[70] During early pregnancy, the glucose requirements of the fetus lead to enhanced transport of glucose across the placenta by facilitated diffusion, and maternal fasting hypoglycemia may be present. Although basal insulin levels may be normal, there is hypersecretion of insulin in response to a meal. Because the half-life ($t_{1/2}$) of insulin is not altered during pregnancy,[71] this increase represents an increase in synthesis and secretion. The results are enhanced glycogen storage and decreased hepatic glucose production.

As pregnancy progresses, the levels of hPL rise, as do the levels of glucocorticoids, leading to the insulin resistance found during the last half of pregnancy.[72] Thus, in late pregnancy, glucose ingestion results in higher and more sustained levels of glucose and insulin and a greater degree of glucagon suppression than in the nonpregnant state.

Adrenal Glands

As a result of the hyperestrogenemia of pregnancy, hepatic production of cortisol-binding globulin is increased. The increased production results in a doubling of the maternal serum levels of cortisol-binding globulin, which in turn result in decreased metabolic clearance of cortisol and a threefold rise in total plasma cortisol by week 26, when the levels reach a plateau until they rise at the onset of labor.[50,73] The rate of cortisol production is increased, and the plasma free cortisol concentrations are also increased.[74] The enhanced cortisol production is due to an increase in the maternal plasma ACTH concentrations and hyperresponsiveness of the adrenal cortex to ACTH stimulation during pregnancy.[50] Cortisol secretion follows that of ACTH, and the diurnal rhythm is maintained during pregnancy.[73] Despite the elevated free cortisol levels, pregnant women do not develop the stigma of glucocorticoid excess, possibly because of the antiglucocorticoid activities of the elevated concentrations of progesterone.

Levels of androstenedione and testosterone, whether they are of adrenal or ovarian origin, are elevated because of the estrogen-induced increase in hepatic synthesis of sex hormone–binding globulin. However, the free androgen levels remain normal or low. The adrenal production rates of dehydroepiandrosterone (DHEA) and dehydroepiandrosterone sulfate (DHEAS) are increased twofold, but the maternal serum concentration of DHEAS is reduced to one third to one half the nonpregnancy levels because of the enhanced 16-hydroxylation and placental utilization of 16-hydroxydehydroepiandrosterone sulfate in estrogen formation. Adrenal medullary function remains normal throughout pregnancy. Thus, 24-hour urine catecholamine and plasma epinephrine and norepinephrine levels are similar to concentrations in the nonpregnant state.[75]

Fortunately, hypercortisolism is rare in pregnancy as the disorder often leads to menstrual disturbance and infertility. Although outside pregnancy hypercortisolism is most commonly caused by an ACTH-producing pituitary[76] adenoma (so-called Cushing disease), when encountered in pregnancy it is more likely due to primary adrenal hyperplasia (so-called Cushing syndrome). This discrepancy may be due to the lower degree of menstrual disturbance in patients with primary adrenal hyperplasia.[77] The high levels of cortisol in both conditions can lead to hypertension, diabetes, preeclampsia, and even maternal death. Cushing syndrome in pregnancy is also associated with a 43% risk of preterm delivery and a 6% risk of stillbirth.[50]

Renin-Angiotensin System

Plasma renin substrate levels are increased as a consequence of the effects of estrogen on the liver. Renin levels are also increased, and increased renin activity results in increased levels of angiotensin II, which lead to an 8-fold to 10-fold increase in aldosterone production and serum aldosterone levels.[50] The aldosterone levels peak in mid-pregnancy and are maintained until delivery.

Despite their baseline elevations, the various components of the renin-angiotensin-aldosterone system demonstrate normal responses to positional changes, sodium restriction, and sodium loading. The elevated aldosterone levels do not lead to an increase in serum sodium, a decrease in serum potassium, or an increase in blood pressure, which again may reflect the high progesterone concentrations, which are capable of displacing aldosterone from its renal receptors. Another mineralocorticoid, 11-deoxycorticosterone, shows a 6-fold to 10-fold increase in concentration at term.[21] Elevated levels of this hormone are due to estrogen-induced extraglandular 21-hydroxylation of progesterone produced by the placenta.[78]

The prevalence of hypertension in women of childbearing age has steadily increased over time and is now a common problem encountered by obstetric providers. Outside pregnancy angiotensin-converting enzyme inhibitors (ACEIs) and angiotensin receptor blockers (ARBs) are widely used in the treatment of hypertension, particularly in people with diabetes, because they have been shown to slow the progression of diabetic nephropathy.[79] ACEIs have been linked to oligohydramnios, fetal renal dysplasia, and fetal calvarial hypoplasia.[80] As a result, this group of medications is avoided in pregnancy. Although ARBs have not been shown to have the same adverse fetal effects, they are also typically avoided in pregnancy.[81] Patients on these medications should be switched to alternative agents prior to or in the first trimester of pregnancy. Methyldopa is the best studied antihypertensive medication in pregnancy and is safe for use at any point in gestation.[82] Although less well studied, the calcium channel blocker nifedipine appears to be safe for the fetus and is often used in pregnancy.[83] Beta blockers are often used, but these medications have been associated with an increased risk of fetal growth restriction.[84]

PLACENTAL HORMONE PRODUCTION

Sex-Steroid Production From the Maternal-Fetal-Placental Unit

Sex steroid production in the adult ovary has been classically described as a two-cell process in which the theca cells convert cholesterol to progesterone, testosterone, and other androgens but are then unable to produce estrogen because the theca cells lack the crucial enzyme aromatase. This enzymatic obstacle is overcome by the nearby granulosa cells, which have an abundance of aromatase and take up androgens and rapidly convert them to estrogens.[85] A similar strategy using multiple locations and cell types is also used in the massively increased sex steroid machinery of pregnancy. In this system both the maternal and fetal adrenal glands interact with the placenta to produce very large amounts of progesterone and estrogens. This dependence has led to the concept of the *maternal-fetal-placental unit*.[86] These interactions are outlined in Figure 21-2.[87,88]

The placenta, like the theca cell of the ovary, has the enzymes necessary to produce progesterone. However, the placenta has very low levels of hydroxymethylglutaryl-coenzyme A activity so it utilizes cholesterol from the maternal circulation as a substrate for progesterone production.[89] Cholesterol is delivered to the placenta by VLDL, LDL, and high-density lipoproteins (HDL) as receptors for

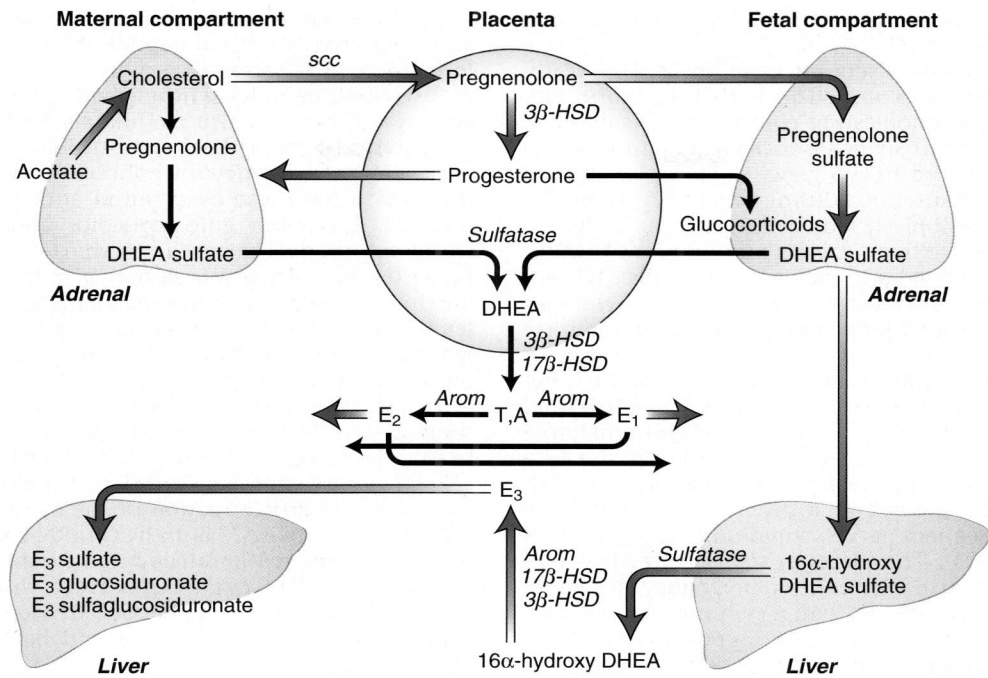

Figure 21-2 Steroidogenesis in the maternal-fetal-placental unit. A, androstenedione; Arom, aromatase-enzyme complex; DHEA, dehydroepiandrosterone; E_1, estrone; E_2, estradiol; E_3, estriol; HSD, hydroxysteroid dehydrogenase; SCC, cholesterol side-chain cleavage enzyme; T, testosterone.

all these lipoproteins are present in the syncytiotrophoblast. Cholesterol is converted to pregnenolone by the enzyme CYP11A1,[86,90] which is in turn converted to progesterone by 3β-hydroxysteroid dehydrogenase (3β-HSD). The placenta also lacks the enzyme 17α-hydroxylase and cannot convert progesterone to androgens even though it has sufficient aromatase activity to convert androgens into estrogens.[91] Thus, progesterone is not further modified in the placenta, and approximately 90% is released into the maternal circulation. However, placental progesterone is also an important substrate for production of glucocorticoids and mineralocorticoids in the fetal adrenal glands.[86,90]

The trophoblast lacks 17α-hydroxylase and 17,20-lyase (CYP17) activities and therefore cannot directly convert progesterone to estrogen. Pregnenolone produced in the placenta enters the fetal compartment, where it is taken up by the fetal zone of the adrenal cortex, which also synthesizes pregnenolone from fetal LDL cholesterol. Pregnenolone is conjugated with sulfate by fetal steroid sulfotransferase in the fetal liver and adrenals to form pregnenolone sulfate and is converted in the fetal adrenals to 17α-hydroxypregnenolone sulfate and then DHEAS by 17α-hydroxylase and 17,20-lyase (CYP17) activities.[74]

The DHEAS enters the fetal circulation and undergoes hydroxylation in the fetal liver to form 16α-hydroxy-DHEAS, which is converted to 16α-DHEA in the placenta through the action of placental sulfatase. Further metabolism in the trophoblast by 3β-HSD1, 17β-HSD, and aromatase (CYP19) leads to the generation of estriol, which is quantitatively the major estrogen in the maternal circulation during pregnancy. The maternal liver actively conjugates estriol with glucosiduronate and sulfate, which are excreted into the urine. Approximately 90% of the estriol present in the maternal serum and urine is derived from fetal precursors, and therefore measurement of estriol levels in serum or urine serves as an index of fetal well-being.[74]

DHEAS from both the fetus and mother is also taken up by the placenta and converted to estradiol by the actions of sulfatase, 3β-HSD1, 17β-HSD, and aromatase or to estrone by sulfatase, 3β-HSD1, and aromatase. An estrogen unique to pregnancy, estetrol, is generated by 15α-hydroxylation of 16α-DHEAS in the fetal adrenal followed by enzymatic conversion by placental sulfatase, 3β-HSD1, 17β-HSD, and aromatase.[74]

Protein Hormones

Human Chorionic Gonadotropin

Chemistry. hCG is a glycoprotein composed of two dissimilar subunits, α and β, which are noncovalently linked through hydrophobic bonding. This molecule shares structural homology with the other glycoprotein hormones, human LH (hLH), hFSH, and hTSH. These hormones have α-subunits that contain the same sequence of 92 amino acids and differ only in their carbohydrate composition; the β-subunits differ in both amino acid and carbohydrate structure and are responsible for the biologic and immunologic specificity of the heterodimeric (intact) hormones. The 22,200-Da β-subunit of hCG is composed of 145 amino acids. Approximately 80% of the first 115 amino acids are homologous to those in the β-subunit of hLH. hCG has an additional 24 amino acids on its carboxy-terminal end that enhance its biologic activity.

Both subunits of hCG contain two oligosaccharide chains attached to asparagine residues through N-glycosidic linkages, and the β-subunit contains in addition four O-serine-linked oligosaccharide units in the carboxy-terminal peptide. The carbohydrate composition of hCG contains microheterogeneity and affects hormone clearance and biologic activity. The tertiary structure of hCG is determined by the carbohydrate composition and multiple disulfide bonds within each subunit. The α-subunit contains five disulfide bonds; the β-subunit has six. In each of the subunits, three of the disulfide bonds form a cystine knot, similar to that found in PDGF-β and transforming growth factor-β (TGF-β).[92]

Biosynthesis. The single α-subunit gene, located on chromosome 6, is actively expressed in both the cytotrophoblast and syncytiotrophoblast. In contrast, the β-subunit is encoded by a cluster of six genes located on chromosome 19 in proximity to the hLH-β gene. Three of the hCG-β genes are actively transcribed during pregnancy, primarily in the syncytiotrophoblast, which thus has the ability to synthesize and secrete free subunits and intact hCG. After synthesis of the protein core, each subunit is glycosylated, undergoes further post-translational modification through trimming of the carbohydrate, and then combines to form intact hCG.[92]

Secretion of hCG differs from that of many of the other placental proteins, whose secretory pattern parallels that of the trophoblastic mass. hCG is first detected in maternal serum 6 to 9 days after conception.[4] The levels rise in a logarithmic fashion, peaking 8 to 10 weeks after the last menstrual period, followed by a decline to a nadir at 18 weeks, with subsequent levels remaining constant until delivery[93] (Fig. 21-3). The placenta also secretes free subunits. During the first 13 weeks of pregnancy, relatively more β-subunit is synthesized than α-subunit, and throughout the remainder of pregnancy the opposite occurs.[94] In addition, a hyperglycosylated form of α-subunit (*big α*) that is unable to combine with free β-subunit is secreted into the maternal serum.

The physiologic factors that regulate hCG secretion in vivo are unknown. Much of the data concerning factors that stimulate or inhibit hCG synthesis and secretion have been derived from in vitro studies and are difficult to extrapolate to the in vivo situation. There is strong circumstantial evidence that GnRH, synthesized in both the cytotrophoblast and syncytiotrophoblast, may be an important factor in hCG secretion. This peptide is identical to hypothalamic GnRH and stimulates placental hCG production both in vitro and in vivo, whereas GnRH antagonists decrease basal hCG secretion.[92,95,96]

Immunohistochemical staining for GnRH in placental tissue is highest at 8 weeks of gestation and lower afterward,[97] roughly paralleling the pattern of hCG production, as do the circulating levels of GnRH measured in maternal serum.[96] In addition, the placenta contains GnRH receptors.[98] Placental GnRH release is stimulated by cyclic adenosine monophosphate (cAMP), prostaglandin E₂, prostaglandin F₂, epinephrine, epidermal growth factor, insulin, and vasoactive intestinal peptide (VIP), factors also noted to increase hCG secretion in vitro.[92,95,99]

Two other peptides synthesized by the cytotrophoblast, activin and inhibin, also modulate GnRH and hCG secretion; activin increases both, and inhibin inhibits the action of GnRH on the syncytiotrophoblast.[95] Increases in hCG production have also been found after trophoblast exposure to FGF, calcium, glucocorticoids, and phorbol esters.[95] Decreased production occurs with TGF-β, follistatin, and progesterone.[95] The decidua may also influence hCG production through paracrine mechanisms.[8] Decidual interleukin 1 stimulates hCG secretion in cultured trophoblasts,[100] whereas decidual prolactin and an 8- to 10-kDa decidual protein inhibit hCG production.[101]

Finally, hCG may autoregulate its own production to some extent. hCG receptors are present on the surface of trophoblastic cells, and the addition of hCG to placental cells in culture stimulates cAMP production as well as proliferation and differentiation of the cytotrophoblasts into syncytiotrophoblasts.[92] Both hCG mRNA and hCG production are stimulated by analogues of cAMP or agents that activate adenylate cyclase, probably through a protein kinase.[92,95] Thus, the net effect of an increase in syncytiotrophoblast mass and cAMP would be enhancement of hCG secretion.

The placenta is not the only site of hCG synthesis. Immunoreactive hCG has been found by immunocytochemistry or by immunoassay of extracts of a wide variety of normal tissues, including spermatozoa, testes, endometrium, kidney, liver, colon, gastric tissue, lung, spleen, heart, fibroblast, brain, and pituitary gland,[102] and the hormone has been shown to be synthesized in some fetal tissues.[92] The pituitary gland appears to be the major source of hCG or an hCG-like material present in nonpregnant individuals. Immunoactive and bioactive hCG has been partially purified from pituitary glands; the material is secreted in vitro by fetal pituitary cells and is shown by immunocytochemistry to be present in gonadotroph-type cells that do not contain hLH or human FSH.[102,103]

Immunoreactive hCG has been measured in sera from normal, nonpregnant individuals, with the highest concentrations found in postmenopausal women.[103,104] In postmenopausal women, this material is secreted in a pulsatile fashion in parallel with hLH pulses, and during the normal menstrual cycle the immunoreactive hCG shows a midcycle peak concomitant with the hLH peak.[105] In both men and postmenopausal women, GnRH stimulates secretion of the hormone, whereas its secretion is inhibited by oral contraceptives in women and by a GnRH agonist in agonadal men.[104,106]

Both gestational and nongestational trophoblastic tumors secrete hCG and its free subunits. The sources of hCG secretion in nongestational trophoblastic neoplasms are the syncytiotrophoblastic cells and in seminomas are the trophoblastic giant cells.[106] In many instances, the tumors produce incomplete forms of hCG or its subunits, and differences in carbohydrate content from the hCG in pregnancy have been especially apparent. A wide variety of nontrophoblastic tumors also secrete hCG, although the predominant moiety appears to be the free β-subunit of hCG.[106,107]

Metabolism. After it is secreted, hCG exhibits a biexponential clearance from the circulation with a fast $t_{1/2}$ of 6 hours and a slow $t_{1/2}$ of close to 36 hours. In contrast, the free β-subunit has a 41-minute fast $t_{1/2}$ and a slow $t_{1/2}$ of 4 hours, and the free α-subunit has a 13-minute fast $t_{1/2}$ and a 76-minute slow $t_{1/2}$.[108] Approximately 22% of the intact hormone appears in the urine unchanged; the rest

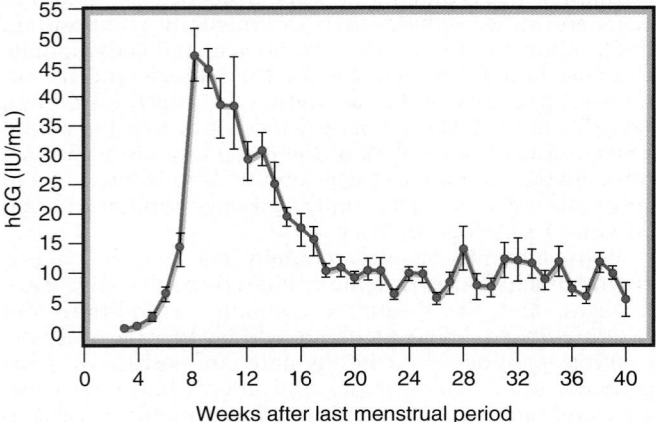

Figure 21-3 Mean (± standard error) levels of maternal serum human chorionic gonadotropin (hCG) throughout normal pregnancy. (From Braunstein GD, Rasor J, Danzer H, et al. Serum human chorionic gonadotropin levels throughout normal pregnancy. *Am J Obstet Gynecol.* 1976;126:678.)

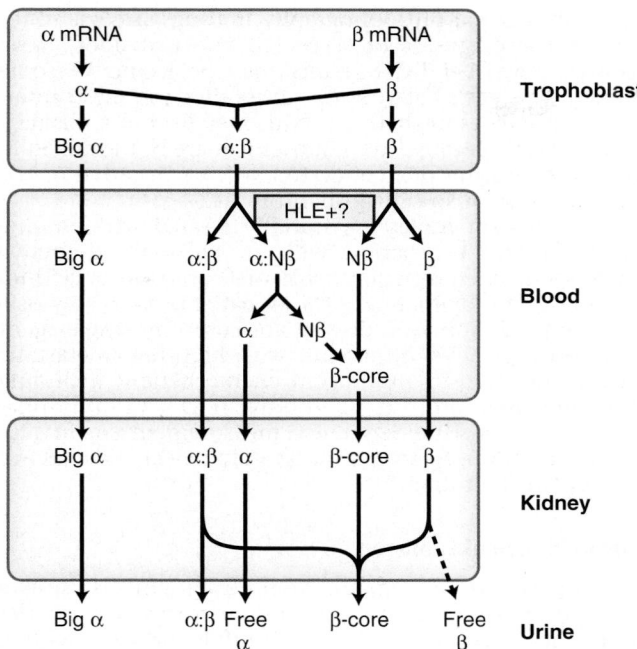

Also contains α:Nβ, Nβ, CTP fragment, α fragments

Figure 21-4 Proposed pathways for metabolism of human chorionic gonadotropin (hCG). α:β, intact hCG; α:Nβ, hCG with nicked β-subunit; Big α: hyperglycosylated form of the α-subunit; HLE, human leukocyte elastase; Nβ, free nicked β-subunit; CTP fragment, carboxy-terminal fragment; mRNA, messenger RNA. (From Braunstein GD. Physiologic functions of human chorionic gonadotropin during pregnancy. In: Mochizuki M, Hussa R, eds. *Placental Protein Hormones.* Amsterdam: Elsevier Science; 1988:33.)

undergoes metabolic degradation (Fig. 21-4). One of the early steps is proteolytic cleavage (nicking) of the β-subunit at Val44-Leu45 and Gly47-Val48. Human leukocyte elastase, present in macrophages and leukocytes, appears to be responsible for some of the nicking of the β-subunit.[108]

Nicked hCG is unstable and dissociates into free α-subunit and nicked free β-subunit. The latter is further metabolized, primarily in the kidney, to produce the β-core fragment, which is composed of the β-subunit amino acids 6 to 40 disulfide-bridged to amino acids 55 to 92, trimmed of a portion of carbohydrate, and with a molecular mass of 10,479 Da.[109] This fragment is the major form of immunoreactive hCG present in the urine in pregnancy. In normal pregnancy, the urine also contains variable quantities of the hyperglycosylated form of α-subunit, free α-subunit, free β-subunit, nicked hCG, nicked free β-subunit, carboxy-terminal fragments of the β-subunit, and fragments of the α-subunit.[108]

Physiologic Functions. Most, if not all, of the physiologic functions of hCG occur after interaction of the hormone with the hLH-hCG receptor. The receptor gene is located on chromosome 2 and encodes for a G protein–coupled receptor with seven hydrophobic transmembrane domains and a large extracellular amino terminus that binds to hCG (and hLH). The receptor is part of a superfamily of receptors, including those for hFSH, hTSH, AVP, VIP, PTH, and receptors for a variety of biogenic amines and neurotransmitters.[92] The hCG-receptor interaction results in increased cAMP production and, in some tissues, increased phosphoinositide turnover.[108]

Because of the close structural homology of the hLH-hCG receptor with the other glycoprotein hormone receptors, hCG may interact with the hTSH and hFSH receptors and

thus has weak intrinsic hTSH and hFSH biologic activity. As previously noted, the hTSH-like activity of hCG is clinically manifested during normal pregnancy by the reciprocal decrease in maternal hTSH at the time of the hCG peak between 8 and 12 weeks after the last menstrual period. It is especially important in patients with hydatidiform moles and other forms of trophoblastic disease in which hCG levels may exceed 100,000 IU/L and result in clinical thyrotoxicosis[48,49] (see Fig. 21-1).

One of the major functions of hCG during pregnancy is the "rescue" of the corpus luteum during the conception cycle.[110] During a menstrual cycle without conception, progesterone concentrations in the serum increase for the first 6 to 7 days of the luteal phase, followed by a 3- to 4-day plateau and then a decrease, resulting in shedding of the endometrial lining. After conception and implantation, the corpus luteum continues to secrete progesterone and 17-hydroxyprogesterone for another 4 to 6 weeks. The maternal serum progesterone and 17-hydroxyprogesterone concentrations then decrease, indicating a marked diminution in corpus luteum function.[111] The fall in 17-hydroxyprogesterone concentrations continues, but the drop in progesterone levels is only transient. This marks the transition from dependence on ovarian progesterone production to placental progesterone secretion (the luteal-placental shift). As previously noted, luteectomy during the first 50 days after the last menstrual period is associated with a decline in progesterone levels and expulsion of the products of conception. After a therapeutic abortion, progesterone levels also drop rapidly.

Thus, the fetal-placental unit is responsible for the signal to maintain the corpus luteum. The data supporting the idea that hCG is that physiologic signal include the following:

- The presence of hLH-hCG receptors on the corpus luteum
- The early production of hCG by the implanting trophoblast
- The dose-dependent increase in cAMP, progesterone, and estradiol from luteal cells cultured in vitro after exposure to hCG
- The parallel rise of progesterone and hCG in early pregnancy
- The enhanced progesterone secretion and prolongation of the menstrual cycle in nonpregnant women given exogenous hCG during their luteal phase

The inability of hCG to prolong the life of the corpus luteum of pregnancy beyond the sixth to eighth weeks of pregnancy appears to be due to homologous desensitization of the adenylate cyclase system and the inhibitory effects of the high estrogen levels on progesterone synthesis through inhibition of 3β-HSD and Δ^{5-4}-isomerase in the corpus luteum.

Another physiologic role for hCG is in the differentiation of fetal male genitalia through stimulation of the hLH-hCG receptors on the fetal testicular Leydig cells during the period when differentiation of wolffian duct structures and development of the external genitalia occur. The maximum testosterone production per unit weight of the testes coincides with the maximum binding of ^{125}I-labeled hCG to the fetal testicular receptors at 10 to 12 weeks of development, and fetal Leydig cells produce cAMP and testosterone in vitro after exposure to hCG. The hCG concentrations in fetal serum parallel the fetal testicular testosterone levels at a time when the amount of fetal pituitary hLH is not sufficient to stimulate the testosterone production.[112]

There are several other possible actions of hCG during normal pregnancy. In vitro, hCG stimulates the differentiation of cytotrophoblast to syncytiotrophoblast and hence may play an important paracrine role in regulating syncytiotrophoblast mass and production of trophoblast hormones.[101,113] Additional data supporting this autoregulatory effect of hCG include the in vitro stimulation of placental synthesis of cAMP, activation of glycogen phosphorylase, and incorporation of radiolabeled galactose and leucine into placental proteins upon exposure to hCG.[112] hCG stimulates the secretion of VEGF from the cytotrophoblast, which may be important for placental angiogenesis.[92] Vasodilatation of myometrial blood vessels mediated by hCG binding to vascular hCG receptors may enhance uterine blood flow in early pregnancy.[92] The fetal zone of the adrenal releases DHEAS in response to hCG exposure in vitro, and therefore, hCG may have adrenocorticotropic activities in concert with fetal pituitary ACTH and placental ACTH.[112]

It has also been suggested that hCG plays a role in the immunosuppression that occurs during pregnancy. Many early studies on this topic were hampered by the use of impure preparations of hCG or the presence of preservatives such as phenol that may alter the end points of the test systems used to define immunosuppression. In addition, the immunosuppressive effects may be due to gonadal steroid secretion in response to the hCG in the in vivo models used in some of the studies.[114] Relaxin secretion from the corpus luteum is stimulated by hCG both in vivo and in vitro.[92]

Finally, the decrease in osmotic threshold for thirst and AVP release during pregnancy is clearly related to hCG.[53] Whether this decrease is due to a direct effect of hCG or an indirect effect through stimulation of gonadal steroids or interaction with hLH-hCG receptors present in vascular smooth muscle is unclear.

Gestational Trophoblastic Disease. Gestational trophoblastic disease (GTD) includes complete and partial hydatidiform moles, choriocarcinoma, and placental-site trophoblastic tumor.[115] Complete molar pregnancy is the most common variety, occurring in 1 to 2 in 1000 pregnancies. Patients usually present with vaginal bleeding, a uterus that is larger than expected for the duration of the pregnancy, anemia, and excessive vomiting. Pathologically, trophoblast hyperplasia, marked edema of the chorionic villi, and absence of fetal tissues are observed. In contrast, partial moles demonstrate focal trophoblast hyperplasia and villous swelling and often have fetal tissues with congenital malformations. Approximately 20% of patients with complete moles develop persistent trophoblastic disease, whereas only 2% to 4% of patients develop persistent disease after partial molar pregnancy. Persistent trophoblastic disease also can occur after a normal term pregnancy as well as pregnancies that end in spontaneous or induced abortion.

Choriocarcinoma is the most aggressive malignant form of persistent trophoblastic disease and may involve complications from local uterine disease, such as bleeding and rupture of the uterus, or from the effects of metastases, especially those involving the liver, lungs, and brain. The least common form of GTD is placental-site trophoblastic tumor, which is derived from the intermediate trophoblast and is often associated with vaginal bleeding and amenorrhea.[115]

All of these neoplasms secrete hCG, free β-subunit, and often additional forms of these molecules. With the exception of placental-site trophoblastic tumor, which secretes relatively low amounts of hCG, the serum and urine concentrations of hCG roughly parallel the tumor burden and also provide prognostic information. Thus, hCG measurements in concert with clinical and radiologic findings,

especially vaginal ultrasonography findings, are useful for making the diagnosis of GTD. On rare occasions, false-positive, low-level hCG results may be found in some women who have heterophilic antibodies and other interfering substances in their sera. This may lead to a misdiagnosis of GTD. Because these substances are not excreted in the urine, a urine pregnancy test will be negative in the presence of such so-called phantom hCG.[115]

Hydatidiform moles are initially treated with uterine dilatation and evacuation with or without adjunctive single-agent chemotherapy with methotrexate or actinomycin D. Approximately 90% of patients with low-risk, persistent trophoblastic disease are cured by single-agent chemotherapy; 75% of patients with high-risk, metastatic disease are cured by multiagent chemotherapy, including etoposide, methotrexate, actinomycin D, cyclophosphamide, and vincristine. Serial hCG measurements are invaluable for monitoring as they accurately reflect the effect of therapy on the tumor.[115]

Human Placental Lactogen

Also called chorionic somatomammotropin, hPL is a single-chain, nonglycosylated polypeptide composed of 191 amino acid residues and two disulfide bridges, with a molecular mass of 21,600 Da.[46] It is closely related chemically and biologically to both GH (85% amino acid homology) and prolactin (13% amino acid homology). The hGH-hPL gene cluster is located on the long arm of chromosome 17 and consists of five genes—one coding for hGH-N, one for hGH-V, and three for placental hPL (hPL-L, hPL-A, and hPL-B, of which only hPL-A and hPL-B are transcribed).[116]

hPL is synthesized and secreted by the syncytiotrophoblast and is detected in maternal serum between 20 and 40 days of gestation. The maternal serum levels rise rapidly and peak at 34 weeks, followed by a plateau[46] (Fig. 21-5). Both the serum concentrations and placental hPL mRNA concentrations are closely correlated with placental weight and syncytiotrophoblastic mass.[117] The maternal serum concentrations at term average between 6 and 7 μg/mL; at that time, on the basis of the 9- to 15-minute $t_{1/2}$ of disappearance from the circulation, the placental production rate of hPL is in excess of 1 g/day. The fetal serum levels are $\frac{1}{50}$ to $\frac{1}{100}$ of the maternal levels.[116]

The physiologic in vivo regulation of hPL synthesis and secretion, other than the constitutive production related to placental mass, is unknown. Several studies have examined the possible role of nutrients in hPL secretion in pregnant women. Neither acute hyperglycemia nor hypoglycemia appeared to alter the hPL concentrations, although prolonged glucose infusions decreased and prolonged fasting increased the concentrations.[46,95] Arginine infusions, dexamethasone administration, and changes in plasma free fatty acid levels did not affect the maternal hPL concentrations.[118,119] Glucose, estrogens, glucocorticoids, prostaglandins, epinephrine, oxytocin, TRH, GnRH, and L-dopa have been examined in in vitro systems and found to be without consistent effects.[120-123]

Angiotensin II, IGF-1, phospholipase A$_2$, arachidonic acid, and epidermal growth factor stimulated hPL release in vitro.[95,124] Epidermal growth factor probably enhances production through promotion of cytotrophoblast-to-syncytiotrophoblast differentiation.[124] Apolipoprotein AI also stimulated hPL synthesis and release through cAMP-dependent and arachidonic acid–dependent pathways.[46,125,126] Because changes in the maternal plasma apolipoprotein AI concentrations parallel those of hPL during pregnancy, it is likely that this apoprotein, alone and as

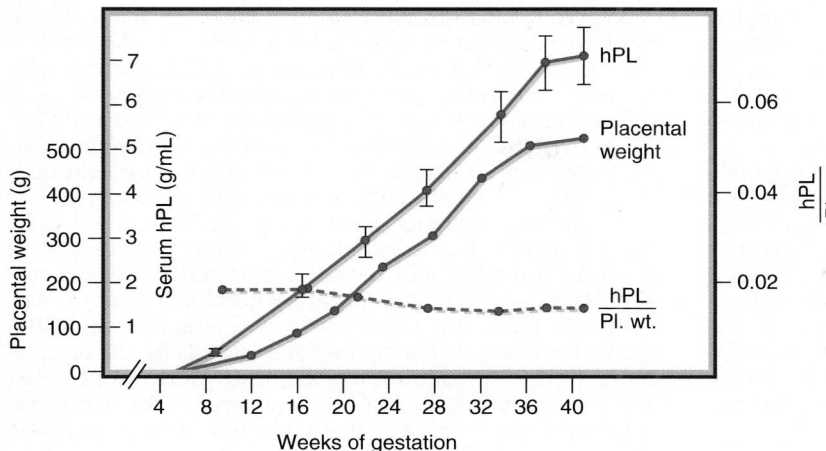

Figure 21-5 Placental weight (Pl. wt.), maternal serum concentrations of human placental lactogen (hPL), and the ratio of hPL to Pl. wt. during pregnancy. (From Selenkow HA, Saxena BN, Dana CL. Measurement and pathophysiologic significance of human placental lactogen. In: Pecile A, Finzi C, eds. *The Feto-Placental Unit.* Amsterdam: Excerpta Medica; 1969:340.)

part of circulating HDL, is important in the secretion of hPL.[126]

hPL has a number of biologic activities that are qualitatively similar to those of hGH and prolactin and can bind to both the hGH and prolactin receptors.[127] In various bioassay systems, hPL had weak somatotropic and lactogenic effects.[127,128] It appears to be a major regulator of IGF-1 production, and during pregnancy, hPL concentrations are correlated with those of IGF-1.[46,128] HPL also affects the metabolism of maternal nutrients. It stimulates pancreatic islet insulin secretion, both directly and after carbohydrate administration,[127] and is a diabetogenic factor during pregnancy through its promotion of insulin resistance. It enhances lipolysis, leading to a rise in free fatty acids, which may in part be responsible for the insulin resistance.[127]

The various biologic activities of hPL have led to the hypothesis that the role of hPL during pregnancy is to provide the fetus with a constant supply of glucose and amino acids.[127] The hPL-stimulated lipolysis allows the mother to utilize free fatty acids for energy during fasting, allowing glucose, amino acids, and ketone bodies to cross the placenta for use by the fetus. In addition, hPL has actions in the fetus, promoting amino acid uptake by muscle and stimulating protein production, IGF-1 production, and glycogen synthesis.[128]

Despite the proposed importance of hPL in maternal and fetal metabolic homeostasis during pregnancy, its absence does not appear to impair pregnancy. Deficient or absent hPL production related to gene defects has been described in several women who experienced normal pregnancies and delivered normal infants.[129]

Placental Growth Hormone

hGH-V is synthesized and secreted by the syncytiotrophoblast.[46] Alternate splicing of the hGH-V gene results in two nonglycosylated isoforms with molecular masses of 22 and 26 kDa.[46,116] The 22-kDa variant may also be glycosylated and circulate as a 26-kDa protein.[116] HGH-V is detected in the maternal plasma from 10 weeks of gestation and peaks during the third trimester[46,130,131] (Fig. 21-6).

hGH-V has somatotropic activity and stimulates IGF-1 production, and the increase in IGF-1 concentrations may in turn be responsible for the suppression of maternal pituitary hGH secretion[128] (see Fig. 21-6). Unlike pituitary hGH, hGH-V is not secreted in a pulsatile fashion, nor is it released from the trophoblast by growth hormone–releasing hormone (GHRH), but it is inhibited by glucose.

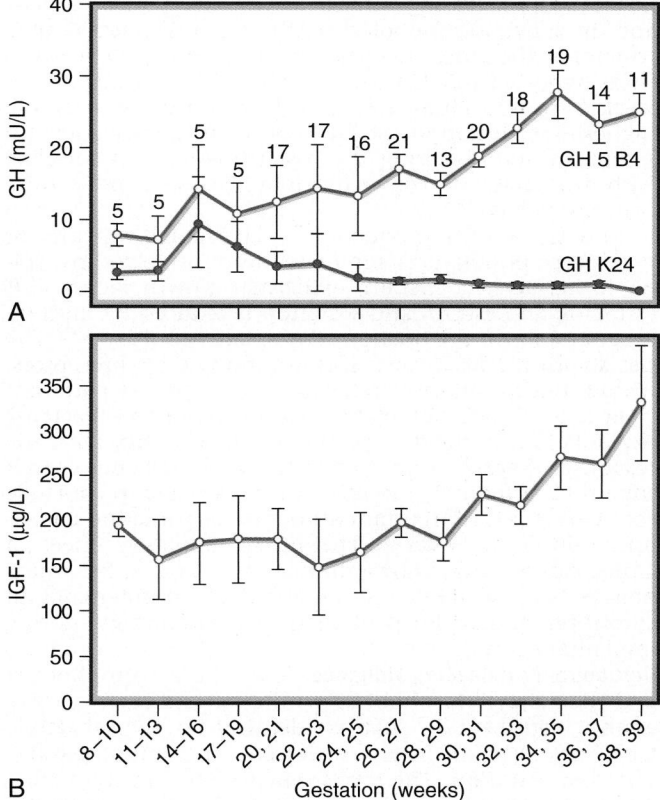

Figure 21-6 Mean (± standard error) of plasma human growth hormone (GH) (**A**) and insulin-like growth factor type 1 (IGF-1) (**B**) levels throughout pregnancy. The number of individual assays of GH and IGF-1 at each gestational stage is indicated in A at the top of vertical bars. GH 5 B4, placental GH (GH2); GH K24, pituitary GH (GH1). (From Mirlesse V, Frankenne F, Alsat E, et al. Placental growth hormone levels in normal pregnancy and in pregnancies with intrauterine growth retardation. *Pediatr Res.* 1993;34:39.)

It has been estimated that at term, 85% of the GH biologic activity in maternal serum is due to hGH-V, 12% to hPL, and only 3% to pituitary hGH.[132] Within 48 hours of delivery, pituitary hGH secretion returns to normal.

Human Chorionic Corticotropin

The syncytiotrophoblast synthesizes an ACTH-like peptide, human chorionic corticotropin (hCC), as well as several pro-opiomelanocortin-derived peptides, including β-lipotropin, β-endorphin, and α-melanocyte-stimulating hormone.[50] The maternal serum concentrations of ACTH increase as pregnancy progresses, and the elevation of free cortisol levels during pregnancy may be related in part to both placental hCC and pituitary ACTH production.[50]

HCC secretion is stimulated by CRH, which is probably the most important factor regulating the local production of the peptide through paracrine or autocrine mechanisms, or both, because it is also produced by both the cytotrophoblast and the syncytiotrophoblast. Unlike the situation with the pituitary, glucocorticoids and oxytocin also stimulate hCC release from placental cultures.[51] Indeed, the resistance of maternal plasma ACTH concentrations to suppression after glucocorticoid administration may reflect the placental hCC contribution to the total pool of circulating immunoreactive ACTH.[50]

Hypothalamic Peptides

Gonadotropin-Releasing Hormone. Both the cytotrophoblast and the syncytiotrophoblast synthesize and secrete GnRH, which has the same chemical structure and biologic activity as hypothalamic GnRH.[95,97] Although the GnRH mRNA levels in the placenta are similar throughout gestation, the highest concentrations of the peptide in the placenta and serum are found during the first trimester and correlate with the mass of the cytotrophoblast and peak hCG concentrations.[97,133]

In vitro, GnRH production by placental explants or purified trophoblasts is stimulated by prostaglandins, epinephrine, activin, insulin, epidermal growth factor, VIP, estradiol, and estriol, and secretion is reduced by inhibin, progesterone, and κ-opiate and μ-opiate agonists.[132,134] The syncytiotrophoblast contains low-affinity GnRH receptors, whose concentrations parallel the hCG secretory pattern.[98]

Because GnRH stimulates hCG secretion by placental explants and purified trophoblast cells in vitro, with the response of early to midtrimester placentas being greater than that of term trophoblast, it is reasonable to conclude that GnRH is an important autocrine or paracrine regulator of hCG secretion.[132] The hCG-stimulatory effect of GnRH can be blocked by administration of a GnRH antagonist.[135] Because GnRH stimulates metalloproteinases in cytotrophoblasts, the peptide may be important during implantation.[136]

Corticotropin-Releasing Hormone. Both the cytotrophoblast and the syncytiotrophoblast synthesize and secrete a 41–amino acid peptide that is identical to hypothalamic CRH.[95,137] CRH mRNA is first detected in trophoblast at 7 weeks of gestation. The levels remain low during the first 30 weeks of pregnancy but rise 20-fold during the final 5 weeks, a pattern that is parallel to the rise of CRH content in the placenta and concentrations in maternal plasma.[101] In maternal plasma, CRH circulates bound to a 37-kDa protein that is synthesized by the placenta, liver, and brain and that reduces the biologic activity of the CRH.[51,137]

In vitro, placental CRF production is stimulated by prostaglandins (E_2 and F_{2a}), norepinephrine, acetylcholine, oxytocin, neuropeptide Y, AVP, angiotensin II, and interleukin 1. Glucocorticoids have been shown to increase both CRH mRNA and peptide, whereas in the hypothalamus suppression is found. CRH secretion is reduced by progesterone and nitric oxide donors. The placenta contains CRH binding sites, and the addition of CRH to cultured placental cells results in a dose-dependent increase in hCC, β-endorphin, and α-melanocyte-stimulating hormone secretion.[50,95,137] Thus, it is likely that CRH has an autocrine or paracrine effect in the placenta.

Whether CRH has a physiologic effect on the maternal pituitary secretion of ACTH is unclear; the circulating CRH may be biologically inactive because of the binding protein. However, just before parturition, the binding protein concentration decreases by approximately 50% and the CRH levels rise.[50,137] At this time, CRH stimulates the synthesis and release of prostaglandins from the decidua, amnion, and chorion, which enhances cervical ripening.[138] The myometrium contains CRH receptors, and CRH may increase myometrial contractility.[101] Thus, CRH may have a role in initiating and promoting parturition. CRH may also stimulate the fetal pituitary production of ACTH, which, in turn, may lead to increased fetal adrenal DHEA production and ultimately estriol synthesis by the fetoplacental unit.[137] In addition to CRH, the syncytiotrophoblast and fetal membranes secrete urocortin 1, which in vitro stimulates placental ACTH, PGE_2, and activin secretion through the CRH receptor.[139]

THE ENDOCRINOLOGY OF PREGNANCY AND PARTURITION

The Role of Estrogen and Progesterone

Although it is an oversimplification, it is helpful to view the maintenance of pregnancy versus the initiation of labor as a balance between the effects of progesterone and estrogen in order to conceptualize this very complicated process. Progesterone has long been known to be essential for pregnancy; in fact, its name is a contraction of the term *proges*tational *ster*oid horm*one*. It is essential from the very beginning of pregnancy as interruption of its production prior to 7 weeks of pregnancy leads to pregnancy loss.[140] Later in pregnancy is it thought to maintain uterine quiescence by limiting the production of prostaglandins and the expression of genes such as ion channels, oxytocin receptors, prostaglandin receptors, and ion channels involved in the contraction machinery of the uterus.[141,142] Progesterone's role in maintaining uterine quiescence is also illustrated in the benefits of progesterone supplementation to prevent preterm birth, which is now the standard of care in women at high risk for preterm birth.[143]

Estrogen clearly has a role in the endocrinology of pregnancy, but it appears less important than progesterone during both pregnancy and labor. During pregnancy estrogen enhances the uptake of LDL in the syncytiotrophoblast to aid in steroid production, increases uterine blood flow to allow for adequate gas exchange and nutrient transport across the placenta, and causes hypertrophy of mammary tissue to prepare the breasts for lactation.[85]

In many animal models it has been clearly demonstrated that a decline in progesterone concentration, either spontaneous or induced, is sufficient to initiate labor.[144] However, in women there is no clear spontaneous drop in progesterone levels in the weeks leading up to labor. Although this may seem contradictory at first, there is mounting evidence that functional progesterone withdrawal does occur in humans despite a constant level of the hormone throughout late gestation. The progesterone receptor (PR) has two distinct isoforms: PR-A and PR-B. PR-B is thought to mediate most of progesterone's effects of uterine quiescence by activating progesterone-responsive genes and suppressing estrogen receptor (ER) production. PR-A, on the other hand, predominantly acts as a repressor of PR-B. The onset of labor is associated with an increase in the relative levels of PR-A compared to PR-B in the myometrium, suggesting that a functional decrease in progesterone activity occurs in humans as it does in other mammals.[145-149]

This functional decrease occurs in concert with an increase in ER expression, which in turn produces a contractile uterine phenotype in preparation for labor, including an increase in myometrial gap junctions and prostaglandin production. Although important, estrogen has a nonessential role in pregnancy and in labor, which is demonstrated in pregnancies complicated by placental sulfatase deficiency. These pregnancies generally continue to term, despite the very low estrogen production throughout pregnancy. Although there is a delay in the onset of labor and the uterus is relatively refractory to prostaglandins and oxytocin, labor does ultimately occur spontaneously and induction of labor, although difficult, can be successfully carried out.[150]

The Role of Prostaglandins

There is overwhelming evidence for the role of prostaglandins as mediators of labor.[141,142] Their production is carefully compartmentalized within the uterus, with PGE_2 confined to the fetal membranes, $PGF_{2\alpha}$ in the decidua, and PGI_2 in the myometrium. Although structurally very similar, the different prostaglandin species can have opposing effects, adding to the complexity of how prostaglandins regulate uterine activity. Although the PGE_2 produced by the fetal membranes and the PGI_2 produced by the myometrium inhibit uterine activity, the $PGF_{2\alpha}$ produced by the decidua is a potent uterotonic,[151] an action that is exploited in the treatment of postpartum hemorrhage. $PGF_{2\alpha}$ production is suppressed in pregnancy, with prostaglandin levels in the gravid uterus being lower than those found in the nongravid uterus at any time during the menstrual cycle.[152,153] Later in pregnancy, and particularly at term with the onset of labor, $PGF_{2\alpha}$ levels of prostaglandins increase in maternal serum and amniotic fluid.[151]

The physiology of prostaglandins in the labor process is exploited extensively in modern obstetrics. Procontractile prostaglandins, such as PGE_1, are commonly used for cervical ripening and induction of labor.[109] Postpartum hemorrhage due to uterine atony is very effectively treated by administration of PGE_1 or $PGF_{2\alpha}$.[154] Furthermore, inhibitors of prostaglandin synthesis, such as indomethacin, are among the most potent tocolytic agents used in the treatment of preterm labor.[155]

The Role of Oxytocin

Oxytocin is a polypeptide hormone produced in the hypothalamus and stored in the posterior pituitary gland. It is one of the first endogenous compounds discovered to play a role in human labor and is one of the few medications to receive Food and Drug Administration (FDA) approval for specific use in pregnancy. It has long been known to produce uterine contractions and is frequently used for induction of labor and to treat postpartum hemorrhage due to uterine atony.[154] Oxytocin mediates its effects by binding to G protein–coupled receptors that are present throughout the uterus. The receptors are preferentially distributed in the uterine fundus, with lower levels found in the lower uterine segment and cervix, corresponding to the increased contractility of the fundus compared to the lower uterine segment.[156] Although the levels of oxytocin do not increase perceptively throughout pregnancy until late in the second stage of labor,[156] receptor concentrations increase up to 100-fold in the first trimester and up to 300-fold in the third trimester of pregnancy.[156] The increase in receptors, mediated predominantly by estrogen, leads to

the increased sensitivity of the myometrium to oxytocin in the second trimester.[156]

THE USE OF PLACENTAL HORMONES IN GENETIC SCREENING

Modern biochemical screening tests for Down syndrome, other aneuploidies, and less common genetic disorders rely heavily on assessing hormones and other proteins produced by the placenta. For example, maternal levels of hCG and pregnancy-associated plasma protein A (PAPP-A) are combined with a measurement of fetal nuchal translucency in first trimester screening. In general, hCG levels are higher in pregnancies affected by Down syndrome and lower in pregnancies affected by trisomy 18 than euploid pregnancies. PAPP-A levels are lower in pregnancies affected by the common aneuploidies (i.e., Down syndrome, trisomy 13, trisomy 18) than in euploid pregnancies.[157,158] For screening in the second trimester hCG is combined with estriol and inhibin A—all of which are produced by the placenta—and α-fetoprotein, which is predominantly produced by the fetus. Estriol is lower in pregnancies affected by Down syndrome and other trisomies; whereas levels of inhibin A are higher in pregnancies affected by Down syndrome compared to euploid pregnancies.[159] Although not designed to do so, the hormone levels assayed in these genetic screening tests can provide some clues to other genetic conditions and even help predict future pregnancy complications. For example, very low levels of estriol are seen in pregnancies complicated by placental sulfatase[160] deficiency and Smith-Lemli-Opitz syndrome,[161] a disorder in which an enzymatic defect in the cholesterol synthesis pathway leads to a disturbance of all steroid hormones, including estriol. These analyte patterns are summarized in Table 21-3.

Abnormalities in maternal serum analytes used in genetic screening are associated with pregnancy complications later in pregnancy in euploid nonanomalous fetuses. The association is strongest for elevated maternal serum alpha-fetoprotein (MSAFP) and inhibin A, which are both associated with an increased risk of fetal growth disturbance and intrauterine fetal death. Elevated inhibin A is also associated with increased risk of preterm birth.[160,162,163] Once discovered, these pregnancies are often monitored by serial fetal ultrasound tests to assess for growth disturbance and ongoing documentation of fetal well-being if abnormal growth is found. Although the association is less well established, an abnormally low PAPP-A in a euploid pregnancy is associated with growth restriction and stillbirth, preterm birth, and preeclampsia.[164] Both a low first trimester PAPP-A and an increased second trimester inhibin A have been associated with an increased risk of preeclampsia. The correlations between abnormal serum analytes and pregnancy complications are outlined in Table 21-4.

TABLE 21-3
Serum Analyte Patterns for Genetic Disorders

	PAPP-A	hCG	AFP	uE3	Inh A
Genetic Disorder					
Down syndrome	↓	↑	↓	↓	↑
Trisomy 18	↓	↓	↓	↓	—
Trisomy 13	↓	↓	—	—	—
Smith-Lemli-Opitz syndrome	—	↓	—	—	—
Placental sulfatase deficiency	—	↓	—	—	—

AFP, alpha-fetoprotein; hCG, human chorionic gonadotropin; Inh A, inhibin A; PAPP-A, pregnancy-associated plasma protein A; uE3, unconjugated estriol; ↓, decreased; ↑, increased.

TABLE 21-4
Serum Analytes and Pregnancy Outcomes

Analyte	Preeclampsia	Growth Restriction	Fetal Demise	Preterm Birth
PAPP-A (<0.42 MoM)	↑	↑	↑	↑
Free hCG (<0.021 MoM)	—	↑	↑	—
AFP (>2.0 MoM) first trimester	—	↑	↑	—
hCG (>2.0 MoM) second trimester	—	—	↑	—
uE3 (<0.5 MoM)	—	↑	↑	—
Inh A (>2.0 MoM)	↑	↑	↑	↑

AFP, alpha-fetoprotein; hCG, human chorionic gonadotropin; Inh A, inhibin A; MoM, multiples of the median; PAPP-A, pregnancy-associated plasma protein A; uE3, unconjugated estriol; ↓, decreased; ↑, increased.

REFERENCES

1. Wilcox AJ, Weinberg CR, O'Connor JF, et al. Incidence of early loss of pregnancy. *N Engl J Med.* 1988;319:189-194.
2. Norwitz ER, Schust DJ, Fisher SJ. Implantation and the survival of early pregnancy. *N Engl J Med.* 2001;345:1400-1408.
3. Kodaman PH, Taylor HS. Hormonal regulation of implantation. *Obstet Gynecol Clin North Am.* 2004;31:745-766, ix.
4. Braunstein GD, Grodin JM, Vaitukaitis J, Ross GT. Secretory rates of human chorionic gonadotropin by normal trophoblast. *Am J Obstet Gynecol.* 1973;115:447-450.
5. Dey SK, Lim H, Das SK, et al. Molecular cues to implantation. *Endocr Rev.* 2004;25:341-373.
6. Cross JC, Werb Z, Fisher SJ. Implantation and the placenta: key pieces of the development puzzle. *Science.* 1994;266:1508-1518.
7. Greiss FC Jr, Anderson SG, Still JG. Uterine pressure-flow relationships during early gestation. *Am J Obstet Gynecol.* 1976;126:799-808.
8. Tabibzadeh S. Human endometrium: an active site of cytokine production and action. *Endocr Rev.* 1991;12:272-290.
9. Gordon JD, Shifren JL, Foulk RA, et al. Angiogenesis in the human female reproductive tract. *Obstet Gynecol Surv.* 1995;50:688-697.
10. Fisher DA. Endocrinology of fetal development. In: Kronenberg PR, Melmed S, Polansky KS, eds. *Williams Textbook of Endocrinology.* 10th ed. Philadelphia, PA: WB Saunders; 2003:811.
11. Szekerese-Bartho J. Immunological relationship between the mother and the fetus. *Int Rev Immunol.* 2002;24:471.
12. Braunstein GD, Rasor JL, Engvall E, Wade ME. Interrelationships of human chorionic gonadotropin, human placental lactogen, and pregnancy-specific beta 1-glycoprotein throughout normal human gestation. *Am J Obstet Gynecol.* 1980;138:1205-1213.
13. Hedderson MM, Weiss NS, Sacks DA, et al. Pregnancy weight gain and risk of neonatal complications: macrosomia, hypoglycemia, and hyperbilirubinemia. *Obstet Gynecol.* 2006;108:1153-1161.
14. Kim SY, Sharma AJ, Sappenfield W, et al. Association of maternal body mass index, excessive weight gain, and gestational diabetes mellitus with large-for-gestational-age births. *Obstet Gynecol.* 2014;123:737-744.
15. de la Torre L, Flick AA, Istwan N, et al. The effect of new antepartum weight gain guidelines and prepregnancy body mass index on the development of pregnancy-related hypertension. *Am J Perinatol.* 2011;28:285-292.
16. Hedderson MM, Gunderson EP, Ferrara A. Gestational weight gain and risk of gestational diabetes mellitus. *Obstet Gynecol.* 2010;115:597-604.
17. Johnson J, Clifton RG, Roberts JM, et al. Pregnancy outcomes with weight gain above or below the 2009 Institute of Medicine guidelines. *Obstet Gynecol.* 2013;121:969-975.
18. Macdonald-Wallis C, Tilling K, Fraser A, et al. Gestational weight gain as a risk factor for hypertensive disorders of pregnancy. *Am J Obstet Gynecol.* 2013;209:327, e1-17.
19. Nehring I, Lehmann S, von Kries R. Gestational weight gain in accordance to the IOM/NRC criteria and the risk for childhood overweight: a meta-analysis. *Pediatr Obes.* 2013;8:218-224.
20. Rasmussen KM, Yaktine AL, eds. *Weight Gain During Pregnancy: Reexamining the Guidelines.* Washington, DC: National Academies Press; 2009.
21. Obesity: preventing and managing the global epidemic. Report of a WHO consultation. *World Health Organ Tech Rep Ser.* 2000;894:i-xii, 1-253.
22. Flegal KM, Carroll MD, Kit BK, Ogden CL. Prevalence of obesity and trends in the distribution of body mass index among US adults, 1999-2010. *JAMA.* 2012;307:491-497.
23. Cunningham FG, Leveno KJ, Bloom S, et al. Maternal physiology. In: Cunningham FG, Leveno KJ, Bloom S, eds. *Williams Obstetrics.* 22nd ed. New York, NY: McGraw-Hill; 2005:121.
24. Ueland K. Cardiorespiratory physiology of pregnancy. In: Sciarra J, ed. *Gynecology and Obstetrics.* Baltimore, MD: Harper & Row; 1979.
25. Castro LC, Hobel CJ, Gornbein J. Plasma levels of atrial natriuretic peptide in normal and hypertensive pregnancies: a meta-analysis. *Am J Obstet Gynecol.* 1994;171:1642-1651.
26. Lindheimer MD, Davison JM. Osmoregulation, the secretion of arginine vasopressin and its metabolism during pregnancy. *Eur J Endocrinol.* 1995;132:133-143.
27. Aminoff MJ. Neurological disorders of pregnancy. In: Creasy RK, Resnick R, Iams JD, et al, eds. *Creasy and Resnick's Maternal-Fetal Medicine: Principles and Practice.* 6th ed. Philadelphia, PA: Elsevier; 2009.
28. Barbour LA, Oja JL, Schultz LK. A prospective trial that demonstrates that dalteparin requirements increase in pregnancy to maintain therapeutic levels of anticoagulation. *Am J Obstet Gynecol.* 2004;191:1024-1029.
29. Janion-Sadowska A, Sadowski M, Kurzawski J, et al. Pregnancy after acute coronary syndrome: a proposal for patients' management and a literature review. *Biomed Res Int.* 2013;2013:957027.
30. Drenthen W, Pieper PG, Roos-Hesselink JW, et al. Outcome of pregnancy in women with congenital heart disease: a literature review. *J Am Coll Cardiol.* 2007;49:2303-2311.
31. Siston AM, Rasmussen SA, Honein MA, et al. Pandemic 2009 influenza A(H1N1) virus illness among pregnant women in the United States. *JAMA.* 2010;303:1517-1525.
32. Mosby LG, Rasmussen SA, Jamieson DJ. 2009 pandemic influenza A (H1N1) in pregnancy: a systematic review of the literature. *Am J Obstet Gynecol.* 2011;205:10-18.
33. Jamieson DJ, Honein MA, Rasmussen SA, et al. H1N1 2009 influenza virus infection during pregnancy in the USA. *Lancet.* 2009;374:451-458.
34. Butte NF. Carbohydrate and lipid metabolism in pregnancy: normal compared with gestational diabetes mellitus. *Am J Clin Nutr.* 2000;71:1256S-1261S.
35. Homko CJ, Sivan E, Reece EA, Boden G. Fuel metabolism during pregnancy. *Semin Reprod Endocrinol.* 1999;17:119-125.
36. Brizzi P, Tonolo G, Esposito F, et al. Lipoprotein metabolism during normal pregnancy. *Am J Obstet Gynecol.* 1999;181:430-434.
37. Piechota W, Staszewski A. Reference ranges of lipids and apolipoproteins in pregnancy. *Eur J Obstet Gynecol Reprod Biol.* 1992;45:27-35.
38. Simpson ER, Burkhart MF. Regulation of cholesterol metabolism by human choriocarcinoma cells in culture: effect of lipoproteins and progesterone on cholesteryl ester synthesis. *Arch Biochem Biophys.* 1980;200:86-92.
39. Ciaraldi TP, Kettel M, el-Roeiy A, et al. Mechanisms of cellular insulin resistance in human pregnancy. *Am J Obstet Gynecol.* 1994;170:635-641.
40. Foyouzi N, Frisbaek Y, Norwitz ER. Pituitary gland and pregnancy. *Obstet Gynecol Clin North Am.* 2004;31:873-892, xi.
41. Elster AD, Sanders TG, Vines FS, Chen MY. Size and shape of the pituitary gland during pregnancy and post partum: measurement with MR imaging. *Radiology.* 1991;181:531-535.
42. Lehtovirta P, Ranta T. Effect of short-term bromocriptine treatment on amniotic fluid prolactin concentration in the first half of pregnancy. *Acta Endocrinol (Copenh).* 1981;97:559-561.
43. Albrecht BH. Prolactin-secreting pituitary tumors and pregnancy. In: Olesfsy JM, Robbins JM, eds. *Contemporary Issues in Endocrinology and Metabolism: Prolactinomas.* New York, NY: Churchill Livingstone; 1986:195.
44. Molitch ME. Pituitary disorders during pregnancy. *Endocrinol Metab Clin North Am.* 2006;35:99-116, vi.
45. Emmi AM, Skurnick J, Goldsmith LT, et al. Ovarian control of pituitary hormone secretion in early human pregnancy. *J Clin Endocrinol Metab.* 1991;72:1359-1363.
46. Handwerger S, Brar A. Placental lactogen, placental growth hormone, and decidual prolactin. *Semin Reprod Endocrinol.* 1992;10:106.
47. Alsat E, Guibourdenche J, Luton D, et al. Human placental growth hormone. *Am J Obstet Gynecol.* 1997;177:1526-1534.
48. Glinoer D. The regulation of thyroid function in pregnancy: pathways of endocrine adaptation from physiology to pathology. *Endocr Rev.* 1997;18:404-433.
49. Glinoer D, de Nayer P, Bourdoux P, et al. Regulation of maternal thyroid during pregnancy. *J Clin Endocrinol Metab.* 1990;71:276-287.
50. Lindsay JR, Nieman LK. The hypothalamic-pituitary-adrenal axis in pregnancy: challenges in disease detection and treatment. *Endocr Rev.* 2005;26:775-799.
51. Jones SA, Brooks AN, Challis JR. Steroids modulate corticotropin-releasing hormone production in human fetal membranes and placenta. *J Clin Endocrinol Metab.* 1989;68:825-830.
52. Davison JM, Sheills EA, Barron WM, et al. Changes in the metabolic clearance of vasopressin and in plasma vasopressinase throughout human pregnancy. *J Clin Invest.* 1989;83:1313-1318.

53. Davison JM, Shiells EA, Philips PR, Lindheimer MD. Serial evaluation of vasopressin release and thirst in human pregnancy. Role of human chorionic gonadotrophin in the osmoregulatory changes of gestation. *J Clin Invest.* 1988;81:798-806.

54. Leake RD, Weitzman RE, Glatz TH, Fisher DA. Plasma oxytocin concentrations in men, nonpregnant women, and pregnant women before and during spontaneous labor. *J Clin Endocrinol Metab.* 1981; 53:730-733.

55. Zeeman GG, Khan-Dawood FS, Dawood MY. Oxytocin and its receptor in pregnancy and parturition: current concepts and clinical implications. *Obstet Gynecol.* 1997;89:873-883.

56. Alexander EK, Marqusee E, Lawrence J, et al. Timing and magnitude of increases in levothyroxine requirements during pregnancy in women with hypothyroidism. *N Engl J Med.* 2004;351:241-249.

57. Vadiveloo T, Mires GJ, Donnan PT, Leese GP. Thyroid testing in pregnant women with thyroid dysfunction in Tayside, Scotland: the thyroid epidemiology, audit and research study (TEARS). *Clin Endocrinol (Oxf).* 2013;78:466-471.

58. Yassa L, Marqusee E, Fawcett R, Alexander EK. Thyroid hormone early adjustment in pregnancy (the THERAPY) trial. *J Clin Endocrinol Metab.* 2010;95:3234-3241.

59. Stagnaro-Green A, Abalovich M, Alexander E, et al. Guidelines of the American Thyroid Association for the diagnosis and management of thyroid disease during pregnancy and postpartum. *Thyroid.* 2011; 21:1081-1125.

60. Surks MI, Ortiz E, Daniels GH, et al. Subclinical thyroid disease: scientific review and guidelines for diagnosis and management. *JAMA.* 2004;291:228-238.

61. Committee on Patient Safety and Quality Improvement; Committee on Professional Liability. ACOG Committee Opinion No. 381: subclinical hypothyroidism in pregnancy. *Obstet Gynecol.* 2007;110(4): 959-960.

62. Kovacs CS. Calcium and bone metabolism in pregnancy and lactation. *J Clin Endocrinol Metab.* 2001;86:2344-2348.

63. Strewler GJ. The physiology of parathyroid hormone-related protein. *N Engl J Med.* 2000;342:177-185.

64. Kristoffersson A, Dahlgren S, Lithner F, Jarhult J. Primary hyperparathyroidism in pregnancy. *Surgery.* 1985;97:326-330.

65. Mestman JH. Parathyroid disorders of pregnancy. *Semin Perinatol.* 1998;22:485-496.

66. Murray JA, Newman WA 3rd, Dacus JV. Hyperparathyroidism in pregnancy: diagnostic dilemma? *Obstet Gynecol Surv.* 1997;52: 202-205.

67. Fleischman AR. Fetal parathyroid gland and calcium homeostasis. *Clin Obstet Gynecol.* 1980;23:791-802.

68. Loughead JL, Mughal Z, Mimouni F, et al. Spectrum and natural history of congenital hyperparathyroidism secondary to maternal hypocalcemia. *Am J Perinatol.* 1990;7:350-355.

69. Nader S. Other endocrine disorders of pregnancy. In: Creasy RK, Resnick R, Iams JD, et al, eds. *Creasy and Resnick's Maternal-Fetal Medicine: Principles and Practice.* 6th ed. Philadelphia, PA: Elsevier; 2009:1015-1040.

70. Costrini NV, Kalkhoff RK. Relative effects of pregnancy, estradiol, and progesterone on plasma insulin and pancreatic islet insulin secretion. *J Clin Invest.* 1971;50:992-999.

71. Lind T, Bell S, Gilmore E, et al. Insulin disappearance rate in pregnant and non-pregnant women, and in non-pregnant women given GHRIH. *Eur J Clin Invest.* 1977;7:47-52.

72. Galerneau F, Inzucchi SE. Diabetes mellitus in pregnancy. *Obstet Gynecol Clin North Am.* 2004;31:907-933, xi-xii.

73. Carr BR, Parker CR Jr, Madden JD, et al. Maternal plasma adrenocorticotropin and cortisol relationships throughout human pregnancy. *Am J Obstet Gynecol.* 1981;139:416-422.

74. Ryan KJ. Placental synthesis of steroid hormones. In: Tulchinsky D, Ryan KJ, eds. *Maternal-Fetal Endocrinology.* Philadelphia PA: WB Saunders; 1980:3.

75. Tunbridge RD, Donnai P. Plasma noradrenaline in normal pregnancy and in hypertension of late pregnancy. *Br J Obstet Gynaecol.* 1981; 88:105-108.

76. Lydakis C, Lip GY, Beevers M, Beevers DG. Atenolol and fetal growth in pregnancies complicated by hypertension. *Am J Hypertens.* 1999; 12:541-547.

77. Buescher MA, McClamrock HD, Adashi EY. A case report of prostaglandin E2 termination of pregnancy complicated by Cushing's syndrome. *Am J Obstet Gynecol.* 1991;165:1412-1413.

78. Rainey WE, Rehman KS, Carr BR. Fetal and maternal adrenals in human pregnancy. *Obstet Gynecol Clin North Am.* 2004;31:817-835, x.

79. Chobanian AV, Bakris GL, Black HR, et al. The Seventh Report of the Joint National Committee on Prevention, Detection, Evaluation, and Treatment of High Blood Pressure: the JNC 7 report. *JAMA.* 2003; 289(19):2560-2572.

80. Barr M Jr. Teratogen update: angiotensin-converting enzyme inhibitors. *Teratology.* 1994;50:399-409.

81. Alwan S, Polifka JE, Friedman JM. Angiotensin II receptor antagonist treatment during pregnancy. *Birth Defects Res A Clin Mol Teratol.* 2005; 73(2):123-130.

82. Cockburn J, Moar VA, Ounsted M, Redman CW. Final report of study on hypertension during pregnancy: the effects of specific treatment on the growth and development of the children. *Lancet.* 1982;1: 647-649.

83. Smith P, Anthony J, Johanson R. Nifedipine in pregnancy. *BJOG.* 2000;107(3):299-307.

84. Xie RH, Guo Y, Krewski D, et al. Beta-blockers increase the risk of being born small for gestational age or of being institutionalised during infancy. *BJOG.* 2014;121(9):1090-1096.

85. Armstrong DT, Goff AK, Dorrington JH. Regulation of follicular estrogen biosynthesis. In: Midgley AR, Sadler WA, eds. *Ovarian Follicular Development and Function.* New York, NY: Raven Press; 1979: 169-182.

86. Pepe GJ, Albrecht ED. Actions of placental and fetal adrenal steroid hormones in primate pregnancy. *Endocr Rev.* 1995;16:608-648.

87. Tulchinsky D, Hobel CJ, Yeager E, Marshall JR. Plasma estrone, estradiol, estriol, progesterone, and 17-hydroxyprogesterone in human pregnancy. I. Normal pregnancy. *Am J Obstet Gynecol.* 1972;112: 1095-1100.

88. Levitz M, Young BK. Estrogens in pregnancy. *Vitam Horm.* 1977; 35:109-147.

89. Simpson ER, MacDonald PC. Endocrine physiology of the placenta. *Annu Rev Physiol.* 1981;43:163-188.

90. Kallen CB. Steroid hormone synthesis in pregnancy. *Obstet Gynecol Clin North Am.* 2004;31:795-816, x.

91. Voutilainen R, Tapanainen J, Chung BC, et al. Hormonal regulation of P450scc (20,22-desmolase) and P450c17 (17 alpha-hydroxylase/17,20-lyase) in cultured human granulosa cells. *J Clin Endocrinol Metab.* 1986;63:202-207.

92. Keay SD, Vatish M, Karteris E, et al. The role of hCG in reproductive medicine. *BJOG.* 2004;111:1218-1228.

93. Braunstein GD, Rasor J, Danzer H, et al. Serum human chorionic gonadotropin levels throughout normal pregnancy. *Am J Obstet Gynecol.* 1976;126:678-681.

94. Ozturk M, Bellet D, Manil L, et al. Physiological studies of human chorionic gonadotropin (hCG), alpha hCG, and beta hCG as measured by specific monoclonal immunoradiometric assays. *Endocrinology.* 1987;120:549-558.

95. Sullivan MH. Endocrine cell lines from the placenta. *Mol Cell Endocrinol.* 2004;228:103-119.

96. Siler-Khodr TM, Khodr GS, Vickery BH, Nestor JJ Jr. Inhibition of hCG, alpha hCG and progesterone release from human placental tissue in vitro by a GnRH antagonist. *Life Sci.* 1983;32:2741-2745.

97. Miyake A, Sakumoto T, Aono T, et al. Changes in luteinizing hormone-releasing hormone in human placenta throughout pregnancy. *Obstet Gynecol.* 1982;60:444-449.

98. Currie AJ, Fraser HM, Sharpe RM. Human placental receptors for luteinizing hormone releasing hormone. *Biochem Biophys Res Commun.* 1981;99:332-338.

99. Petraglia F, Santuz M, Florio P, et al. Paracrine regulation of human placenta: control of hormonogenesis. *J Reprod Immunol.* 1998;39: 221-233.

100. Masuhiro K, Matsuzaki N, Nishino E, et al. Trophoblast-derived interleukin-1 (IL-1) stimulates the release of human chorionic gonadotropin by activating IL-6 and IL-6-receptor system in first trimester human trophoblasts. *J Clin Endocrinol Metab.* 1991;72:594-601.

101. Ren SG, Braunstein GD. Decidua produces a protein that inhibits choriogonadotropin release from human trophoblasts. *J Clin Invest.* 1991;87:326-330.

102. Braunstein GD, Kamdar V, Rasor J, et al. Widespread distribution of a chorionic gonadotropin-like substance in normal human tissues. *J Clin Endocrinol Metab.* 1979;49:917-925.

103. Odell WD, Griffin J, Bashey HM, Snyder PJ. Secretion of chorionic gonadotropin by cultured human pituitary cells. *J Clin Endocrinol Metab.* 1990;71:1318-1321.

104. Stenman UH, Alfthan H, Ranta T, et al. Serum levels of human chorionic gonadotropin in nonpregnant women and men are modulated by gonadotropin-releasing hormone and sex steroids. *J Clin Endocrinol Metab.* 1987;64:730-736.

105. Odell WD, Griffin J. Pulsatile secretion of human chorionic gonadotropin in normal adults. *N Engl J Med.* 1987;317:1688-1691.

106. Braunstein GD. Placental proteins as tumor markers. In: Herberman RB, Mercer DW, eds. *Immunodiagnosis of Cancer.* New York, NY: Marcel Dekker; 1991:673.

107. Stenman UH, Alfthan H, Hotakainen K. Human chorionic gonadotropin in cancer. *Clin Biochem.* 2004;37:549-561.

108. Braunstein GD. Beta core fragment: structure, production, metabolism, and clinical utility. In: Lustbader JW, Puett D, Ruddon RW, eds. *Glycoprotein Hormones.* New York, NY: Springer-Verlag; 1994:293.

109. Alfirevic Z, Aflaifel N, Weeks A. Oral misoprostol for induction of labour. *Cochrane Database Syst Rev.* 2014;6:CD001338.

110. Braunstein GD. Evidence favoring human chorionic gonadotropin as the physiological "rescuer" of the corpus luteum during early pregnancy. *Early Pregnancy.* 1996;2(3):183-190.

111. Yoshimi T, Strott CA, Marshall JR, Lipsett MB. Corpus luteum function in early pregnancy. *J Clin Endocrinol Metab.* 1969;29:225-230.

112. Braunstein GD. Physiologic functions of human chorionic gonadotropin during pregnancy. In: Mochizuki M, Hussa R, eds. *Placental Protein Hormones*. Amsterdam: Elsevier Science; 1988:33.

113. North RA, Whitehead R, Larkins RG. Stimulation by human chorionic gonadotropin of prostaglandin synthesis by early human placental tissue. *J Clin Endocrinol Metab*. 1991;73:60-70.

114. Nisula BC, Bartocci A. Choriogonadotropin and immunity: a reevaluation. *Ann Endocrinol (Paris)*. 1984;45:315.

115. Soper JT, Mutch DG, Schink JC, American College of Obstetricians and Gynecologists. Diagnosis and treatment of gestational trophoblastic disease: ACOG Practice Bulletin No. 53. *Gynecol Oncol*. 2004;93(3): 575-585.

116. Barrera-Saldana HA. Growth hormone and placental lactogen: biology, medicine and biotechnology. *Gene*. 1998;211:11-18.

117. Hoshina M, Boothby M, Boime I. Cytological localization of chorionic gonadotropin alpha and placental lactogen mRNAs during development of the human placenta. *J Cell Biol*. 1982;93:190-198.

118. Morris HH, Vinik AI, Mulvihal M. Effects of acute alterations in maternal free fatty acid concentration on human chorionic somatomammotropin secretion. *Am J Obstet Gynecol*. 1974;119:224-229.

119. Ylikorkala O, Kauppila A. Effect of dexamethasone on serum levels of human placental lactogen during the last trimester of pregnancy. *J Obstet Gynaecol Br Commonw*. 1974;81(5):368-370.

120. Niven PA, Buhi WC, Spellacy WN. The effect of intravenous oestrogen injections on plasma human placental lactogen levels. *J Obstet Gynaecol Br Commonw*. 1974;81:466-468.

121. Belleville F, Lasbennes A, Nabet P. Study of compounds capable of intervening in the in vitro regulation of secretion of chorionic samatomammotropin by placenta in culture. *C R Seances Soc Biol Fil*. 1974; 168:1057.

122. Handwerger S, Barrett J, Tyrey L, Schomberg D. Differential effect of cyclic adenosine monophosphate on the secretion of human placental lactogen and human chorionic gonadotropin. *J Clin Endocrinol Metab*. 1973;36:1268-1270.

123. Hershman JM, Kojima A, Friesen HG. Effect of thyrotropin-releasing hormone on human pituitary thyrotropin, prolactin, placental lactogen, and chorionic thyrotropin. *J Clin Endocrinol Metab*. 1973; 36:497-501.

124. Wilson EA, Jawad MJ, Vernon MW. Effect of epidermal growth factor on hormone secretion by term placenta in organ culture. *Am J Obstet Gynecol*. 1984;149:579-580.

125. Handwerger S, Quarfordt S, Barrett J, Harman I. Apolipoproteins AI, AII, and CI stimulate placental lactogen release from human placental tissue. A novel action of high density lipoprotein apolipoproteins. *J Clin Invest*. 1987;79:625-628.

126. Desoye G, Schweditsch MO, Pfeiffer KP, et al. Correlation of hormones with lipid and lipoprotein levels during normal pregnancy and postpartum. *J Clin Endocrinol Metab*. 1987;64:704-712.

127. Eberhardt NL, Jiang SW, Shepard AR, et al. Hormonal and cell-specific regulation of the human growth hormone and chorionic somatomammotropin genes. *Prog Nucleic Acid Res Mol Biol*. 1996;54:127-163.

128. Handwerger S, Freemark M. The roles of placental growth hormone and placental lactogen in the regulation of human fetal growth and development. *J Pediatr Endocrinol Metab*. 2000;13:343-356.

129. Sideri M, De Virgiliis G, Guidobono F, et al. Immunologically undetectable human placental lactogen in a normal pregnancy. Case report. *Br J Obstet Gynaecol*. 1983;90:771-773.

130. Mirlesse V, Frankenne F, Alsat E, et al. Placental growth hormone levels in normal pregnancy and in pregnancies with intrauterine growth retardation. *Pediatr Res*. 1993;34:439-442.

131. Lonberg U, Damm P, Andersson AM, et al. Increase in maternal placental growth hormone during pregnancy and disappearance during parturition in normal and growth hormone-deficient pregnancies. *Am J Obstet Gynecol*. 2003;188:247-251.

132. Petraglia F, Lim AT, Vale W. Adenosine 3′,5′-monophosphate, prostaglandins, and epinephrine stimulate the secretion of immunoreactive gonadotropin-releasing hormone from cultured human placental cells. *J Clin Endocrinol Metab*. 1987;65:1020-1025.

133. Kelly AC, Rodgers A, Dong KW, et al. Gonadotropin-releasing hormone and chorionic gonadotropin gene expression in human placental development. *DNA Cell Biol*. 1991;10:411-421.

134. Petraglia F, Vaughan J, Vale W. Steroid hormones modulate the release of immunoreactive gonadotropin-releasing hormone from cultured human placental cells. *J Clin Endocrinol Metab*. 1990;70:1173-1178.

135. Siler-Khodr TM, Khodr GS, Valenzuela G. Immunoreactive gonadotropin-releasing hormone level in maternal circulation throughout pregnancy. *Am J Obstet Gynecol*. 1984;150:376-379.

136. Chou CS, Zhu H, MacCalman CD, Leung PC. Regulatory effects of gonadotropin-releasing hormone (GnRH) I and GnRH II on the levels of matrix metalloproteinase (MMP)-2, MMP-9, and tissue inhibitor of metalloproteinases-1 in primary cultures of human extravillous cytotrophoblasts. *J Clin Endocrinol Metab*. 2003;88:4781-4790.

137. Fadalti M, Pezzani I, Cobellis L, Springolo F. Placental corticotrophin-releasing factor. *Ann N Y Acad Sci*. 2000;900:89.

138. Jones SA, Challis JR. Local stimulation of prostaglandin production by corticotropin-releasing hormone in human fetal membranes and placenta. *Biochem Biophys Res Commun*. 1989;159:192-199.

139. Florio P, Vale W, Petraglia F. Urocortins in human reproduction. *Peptides*. 2004;25:1751-1757.

140. Csapo AI, Pulkkinen M. Indispensability of the human corpus luteum in the maintenance of early pregnancy. Luteectomy evidence. *Obstet Gynecol Surv*. 1978;33:69-81.

141. Norwitz ER, Robinson JN, Challis JR. The control of labor. *N Engl J Med*. 1999;341:660-666.

142. Challis JR, Matthews SG, Gibb W, Lye SJ. Endocrine and paracrine regulation of birth at term and preterm. *Endocr Rev*. 2000;21: 514-550.

143. Dodd JM, Jones L, Flenady V, et al. Prenatal administration of progesterone for preventing preterm birth in women considered to be at risk of preterm birth. *Cochrane Database Syst Rev*. 2013;7:CD004947.

144. Nathanielsz PW. Comparative studies on the initiation of labor. *Eur J Obstet Gynecol Reprod Biol*. 1998;78:127-132.

145. Haluska GJ, Wells TR, Hirst JJ, et al. Progesterone receptor localization and isoforms in myometrium, decidua, and fetal membranes from rhesus macaques: evidence for functional progesterone withdrawal at parturition. *J Soc Gynecol Investig*. 2002;9:125-136.

146. Madsen G, Zakar T, Ku CY, et al. Prostaglandins differentially modulate progesterone receptor-A and -B expression in human myometrial cells: evidence for prostaglandin-induced functional progesterone withdrawal. *J Clin Endocrinol Metab*. 2004;89:1010-1013.

147. Mesiano S. Myometrial progesterone responsiveness and the control of human parturition. *J Soc Gynecol Investig*. 2004;11:193-202.

148. Mesiano S, Chan EC, Fitter JT, et al. Progesterone withdrawal and estrogen activation in human parturition are coordinated by progesterone receptor A expression in the myometrium. *J Clin Endocrinol Metab*. 2002;87:2924-2930.

149. Ni X, Hou Y, Yang R, et al. Progesterone receptors A and B differentially modulate corticotropin-releasing hormone gene expression through a cAMP regulatory element. *Cell Mol Life Sci*. 2004;61:1114-1122.

150. Shozu M, Akasofu K, Harada T, Kubota Y. A new cause of female pseudohermaphroditism: placental aromatase deficiency. *J Clin Endocrinol Metab*. 1991;72:560-566.

151. Fuchs AR. Plasma, membrane receptors regulating myometrial contractility and their hormonal modulation. *Semin Perinatol*. 1995;19: 15-30.

152. Phaneuf S, Europe-Finner GN, Varney M, et al. Oxytocin-stimulated phosphoinositide hydrolysis in human myometrial cells: involvement of pertussis toxin-sensitive and -insensitive G-proteins. *J Endocrinol*. 1993;136:497-509.

153. Molnar M, Hertelendy F. Regulation of intracellular free calcium in human myometrial cells by prostaglandin F2 alpha: comparison with oxytocin. *J Clin Endocrinol Metab*. 1990;71:1243-1250.

154. Mousa HA, Blum J, Abou El Senoun G, et al. Treatment for primary postpartum haemorrhage. *Cochrane Database Syst Rev*. 2014;2:CD003249.

155. Garrioch DB. The effect of indomethacin on spontaneous activity in the isolated human myometrium and on the response to oxytocin and prostaglandin. *Br J Obstet Gynaecol*. 1978;85:47-52.

156. Fuchs AR, Fuchs F. Endocrinology of human parturition: a review. *Br J Obstet Gynaecol*. 1984;91:948-967.

157. Wald NJ, Rodeck C, Hackshaw AK, et al. First and second trimester antenatal screening for Down's syndrome: the results of the Serum, Urine and Ultrasound Screening Study (SURUSS). *J Med Screen*. 2003;10(2):56-104.

158. Malone FD, Canick JA, Ball RH, et al. First-trimester or second-trimester screening, or both, for Down's syndrome. *N Engl J Med*. 2005;353: 2001-2011.

159. Wald NJ, Huttly WJ, Hackshaw AK. Antenatal screening for Down's syndrome with the quadruple test. *Lancet*. 2003;361:835-836.

160. Yaron Y, Cherry M, Kramer RL, et al. Second-trimester maternal serum marker screening: maternal serum alpha-fetoprotein, beta-human chorionic gonadotropin, estriol, and their various combinations as predictors of pregnancy outcome. *Am J Obstet Gynecol*. 1999;181:968-974.

161. Rabe T, Hosch R, Runnebaum B. Sulfatase deficiency in the human placenta: clinical findings. *Biol Res Pregnancy Perinatol*. 1983;4: 95-102.

162. Florio P, Ciarmela P, Luisi S, et al. Pre-eclampsia with fetal growth restriction: placental and serum activin A and inhibin A levels. *Gynecol Endocrinol*. 2002;16:365-372.

163. D'Anna R, Baviera G, Corrado F, et al. Is mid-trimester maternal serum inhibin-A a marker of preeclampsia or intrauterine growth restriction? *Acta Obstet Gynecol Scand*. 2002;81:540-543.

164. Dugoff L, Hobbins JC, Malone FD, et al. First-trimester maternal serum PAPP-A and free-beta subunit human chorionic gonadotropin concentrations and nuchal translucency are associated with obstetric complications: a population-based screening study (the FASTER Trial). *Am J Obstet Gynecol*. 2004;191:1446-1451.

CHAPTER 22

Endocrinology of Fetal Development

MEHUL T. DATTANI • EVELIEN F. GEVERS

KEY POINTS

- The placental-fetal endocrine environment is created by a spectrum of placental hormones and growth factors and a variety of fetal endocrine adaptations to the intrauterine environment.
- Disorders of development of a number of structures such as the thyroid, parathyroid, pituitary, pancreas, and gonads can be associated with clinical endocrine phenotypes.
- The fetal adrenal cortex, the para-aortic chromaffin system, and the intermediate lobe of the pituitary are prominent fetal endocrine glands.
- Fetal adrenocorticotropic hormone (ACTH) is required for adrenal cortex steroidogenesis. Paradoxically, adrenal steroidogenesis leads to production of mostly inactive steroids such as pregnenolone and dehydroepiandrosterone (DHEA).
- Some of the adrenal steroids are converted by the fetal adrenal gland and fetal liver to provide substrates for placental estrone and estradiol production.
- The anterior and posterior pituitary lobes develop from oral ectoderm and ventral diencephalon. Pituitary hormone secretion starts at 8 to 10 weeks of gestation.
- Thyroid hormone synthesis starts at 11 weeks of gestation. Circulating thyroxine (T_4) increases to maximal levels at 35 to 40 weeks, but maturation of hypothalamic pituitary control and response of thyroid gland to thyroid-stimulating hormone (TSH, thyrotropin) develops in the third trimester.
- In the presence of SRY (the sex-determining region of the Y chromosome), male gonadal differentiation starts at 7 weeks of gestation. Development of Leydig cells leads to an increase in fetal testosterone production from week 10 and stimulates differentiation of the primitive mesonephric ducts into bilateral ductus deferens, epididymides, seminal vesicles, and ejaculatory ducts. Dihydrotestosterone stimulates male differentiation of the urogenital sinus and external genitalia.
- Active calcium transport across the placenta takes place in the third trimester to maintain fetal calcium concentrations and is dependent on parathyroid hormone–related protein (PTHrP).

- Calcium-sensing receptor (CaSR) and fibroblast growth factor 23 (FGF23) are required for normal calcium and phosphate metabolism in the neonate.

The unfolding of our understanding of mammalian pregnancy and fetal development represents one of the dramatic chapters of scientific progress during the past half-century. Successful pregnancy involves complex genetic, cellular, and hormonal interactions facilitating implantation, placentation, embryonic and fetal development, parturition, and fetal adaptation to extrauterine life. An array of signaling molecules, transcription factors, and epigenetic events programs embryogenesis and fetal development in concert with autocrine, paracrine, and endocrine networks of hormones and growth factors that provide the cellular communication coordinating maternal-placental-fetal interactions and fetal maturation. Unique features of the placental-fetal endocrine environment include a growing spectrum of placental hormones and growth factors and a variety of fetal endocrine adaptations to the intrauterine environment (Table 22-1).[1] The fetal adrenal cortex, the para-aortic chromaffin system including the paired organs of Zuckerkandl, and the intermediate lobe of the pituitary are prominent among these elements. Vasotocin (VT), the parent neurohypophyseal hormone in submammalian species, is expressed transiently during fetal life, and calcitonin, a largely vestigial hormone in adult mammals, plays a significant role in fetal calcium and bone metabolism.

In addition, the active adrenal glucocorticoid, cortisol, and the thyroid hormones are largely inactive during much of fetal life because of the production of inactive analogues. Hormones and growth factors that play prominent roles in the fetus include catecholamines, PTHrP, antimüllerian hormone (AMH), insulin-like growth factor 1 (IGF-1), IGF-2, transforming growth factor beta (TGF-β), and the neuroregulins (growth factors that stimulate ErbB receptors). In the perinatal period, cortisol serves to modulate the functional adaptations that are required for extrauterine survival. In addition, hormonal programming during the fetal-perinatal period conditions the adult functional characteristics of selected endocrine systems. This chapter reviews the current status of our understanding of the maternal-placental-fetal endocrine and growth factor milieu, maturation of the fetal endocrine systems, and adaptations of the fetal endocrine systems to extrauterine life.

PLACENTAL HORMONE TRANSFER

The fetal endocrine milieu is largely independent of maternal hormones because the placenta is impermeable to most peptide hormones. Hormones larger than 0.7 to 1.2 kDa

TABLE 22-1

Features of the Fetal Endocrine Environment

Placental Hormone Production

Estrogens
Progesterone
Neuropeptides
Growth factors

Neutralization of Hormone Actions

Growth hormone
Cortisol
Thyroxine
Catecholamines

Unique Fetal Endocrine Systems

Fetal adrenal cortex
Para-aortic chromaffin system
Intermediate lobe of the pituitary

Prominent Fetal Hormones or Metabolites

Vasotocin
Calcitonin
Cortisone
Reverse triiodothyronine (rT$_3$)
Sulfated iodothyronines
Ectopic neuropeptides

Fetal Endocrine System Adaptations

Adrenal-placental interactions
Testicular control of male phenotypic differentiation
Developmentally regulated growth factor control of fetal growth
Neuropeptides and fetal water metabolism
Parathyroid glands and placental calcium transport
Catecholamine and vasopressin responses to hypoxia
Cortisol programming for extrauterine exposure
Catecholamine and cortisol control of extrauterine adaptation
Perinatal hormonal programming

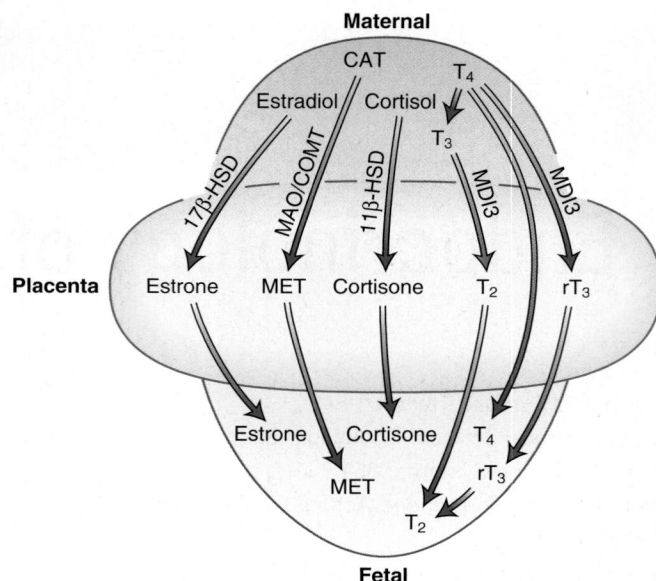

Figure 22-1 Placental neutralization of biologic activity of hormones during maternal-fetal transfer. The neutralizing enzymes, 17β-hydroxysteroid dehydrogenase (17β-HSD) and 11β-HSD, are shown. See text for details. CAT, catecholamines; COMT, catechol O-methyltransferase; MAO, monoamine oxidase; MDI3, type 3 iodothyronine monodeiodinase; MET, metanephrines; rT$_3$, 3,3'5' (reverse)-triiodothyronine; T$_2$, diiodothyronine; T$_3$, 3,5,3'-triiodothyronine; T$_4$, thyroxine.

have little or no access to the fetal compartment.[2] The exception is immunoglobulin G, which is actively transported from mother to fetus during the latter half of gestation.[3] Steroid and thyroid hormones and catecholamines do cross the placenta, but several of them are metabolized en route, including cortisol, estradiol, T$_4$, triiodothyronine (T$_3$), and catecholamines.[4-8]

In particular, the placental cells contain an active 11β-hydroxysteroid dehydrogenase type 2 (11β-HSD2) that catalyzes the conversion of most of the maternal cortisol to inactive cortisone.[5,6] This is important considering the steep gradient between the maternal cortisol concentration and that of the fetus—almost a 10-fold difference. This enzymatic inactivation can be bypassed with dexamethasone, leading to fetal exposure to glucocorticoid, which, in rodent models, has adverse effects on blood pressure, blood glucose, and memory.[9,10] This altered metabolism is used to promote glucocorticoid maturation of the fetal lung in cases of preterm delivery in humans and in the management of fetuses affected by a virilizing form of congenital adrenal hyperplasia. Single doses appear to be safe for mother and child,[11] but more chronic exposure may be less safe. Use in pregnancy to reduce virilization of an unborn child with congenital adrenal hyperplasia should therefore take place in a research setting only and requires auditing.[12,13]

Placental 17β-HSD is considered to prevent passage of excessive estrogens to the fetus by catalyzing inactivation of estradiol to estrone.[7] Placental tissue also contains an iodothyronine inner ring monodeiodinase, which deiodinates most of the T$_4$ to inactive reverse triiodothyronine (rT$_3$) and converts active 3,5,3-T$_3$ to inactive diiodothyro-

nine (T$_2$).[8,14] Nonetheless, there is some transplacental passage of T$_4$ to the fetus in early pregnancy, and this may be of importance, because observational studies have suggested altered intellectual function and behavior, albeit mild, in infants born to mothers with mild untreated or subclinical hypothyroidism.[15-17] although this may also be due to placental passage of thyroid peroxidase (TPO) antibodies.[18]

Catecholamine-degrading enzymes in placental tissue include monoamine oxidase and catechol O-methyltransferase, and both metanephrine and dihydroxymandelic acid metabolites of catecholamines are present in placental homogenates (Fig. 22-1).[19]

ECTOPIC FETAL HORMONE PRODUCTION

Kidney, liver, and testes from 16- to 20-week-old human fetuses produce immunoreactive and bioactive human chorionic gonadotropin (hCG) in vitro.[20,21] Kidney tissue produces almost half as much hCG per milligram of protein as placenta; liver activity is lower. ACTH-like immunoreactivity is present in relatively high concentrations in neonatal rat pancreas and kidney.[22] This material is presumably derived from a pro-opiomelanocortin (POMC) parent molecule. Hypothalamic neuropeptides are present in a variety of adult tissues, particularly in the pancreas and gut.[23-27] In the fetus, hypothalamic neuropeptides are also present in the gut and tissues derived from it. High concentrations of thyrotropin-releasing hormone (TRH) and somatostatin immunoreactivity have been reported in neonatal rat pancreas and gastrointestinal tract tissues, whereas hypothalamic concentrations of these immunoreactive substances are low.[28,29] These neuropeptides have immunoreactive and chromatographic properties similar to those of the synthetic hypothalamic peptides. Ghrelin, expressed mostly in

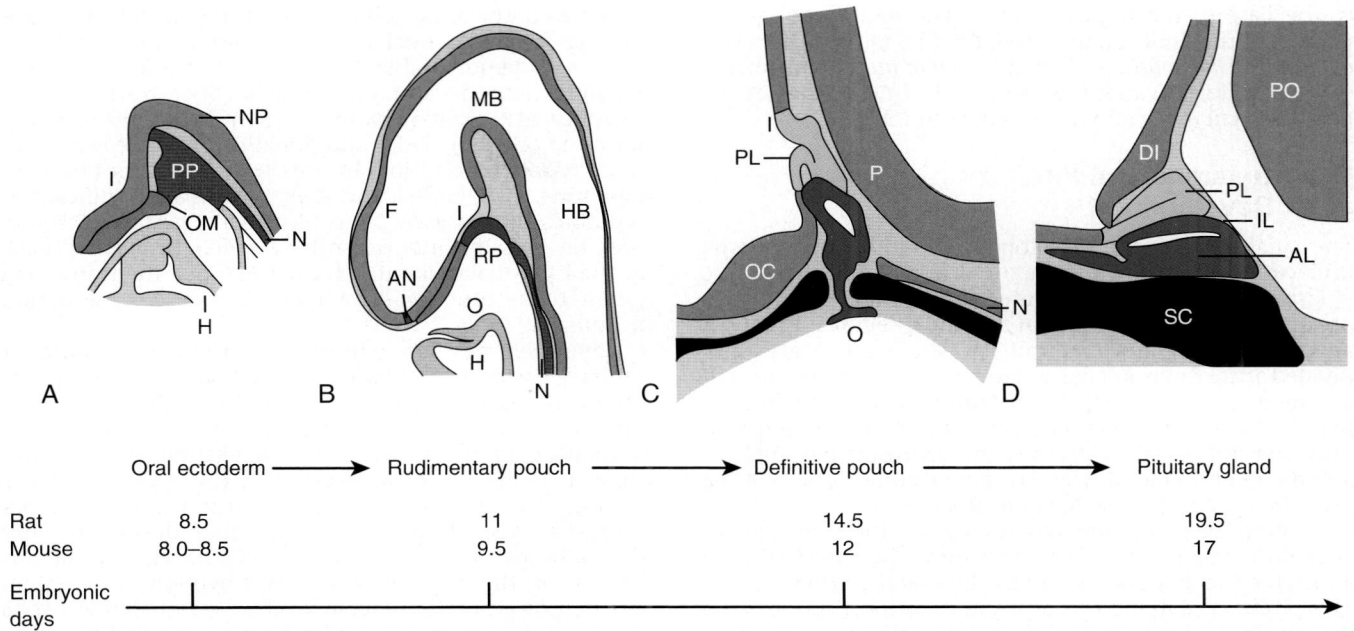

Figure 22-2 Schematic representation of the developmental processes implicated in pituitary development. **A,** Development of the hypophyseal placode, a thickening of the ectoderm in the midline of the anterior neural ridge. **B,** The placode invaginates dorsally to form a rudimentary Rathke's pouch, the primordium of the anterior and intermediate lobe. **C,** The overlying neural ectoderm evaginates to form the infundibulum, from which the posterior pituitary and pituitary stalk will derive, which comes into direct contact with Rathke's pouch. **D,** At 12.5 dpc it is completely separated from the underlying oral ectoderm. The lumen of the pouch persists as the pituitary cleft, separating the anterior and intermediate lobes in the mature gland. See text for details. AL, anterior lobe; AN, anterior neural pore; DI, diencephalon; F, forebrain; H, heart; HB, hindbrain; I, infundibulum; IL, intermediate lobe; MB, midbrain; N, notochord; NP, neural plate; O, oral cavity; OC, optic chiasma; OM, oral membrane; P, pontine flexure; PL, posterior lobe; PO, pons; PP, prechordal plate; RP, Rathke's pouch; SC, sphenoid cartilage. (Based on Sheng HZ, Westphal H. Early steps in pituitary organogenesis. *Trends Genet.* 1999;15:236-240. As adapted in Gevers EF, Fisher DA, Dattani MT. Fetal and neonatal endocrinology. In: Jameson JL, De Groot LJ, eds. *Endocrinology: Adult and Pediatric,* 7th ed. Philadelphia, PA: Elsevier; 2016.)

stomach and hypothalamus postnatally, is more abundant in the fetal pancreas than the fetal stomach and is also present in fetal lung.[30]

Encephalectomy does not alter the circulating TRH levels in the neonatal rat, whereas significant reductions are produced by pancreatectomy. In the sheep fetus, thyroid hormones modulate pancreatic and gut TRH concentrations, pointing to thyroid hormone control of extrahypothalamic *TRH* gene transcription or translation in the fetus.[31] TRH and somatostatin also are present in the human neonatal pancreas and in blood of the human newborn, with both hormones derived mostly from extrahypothalamic sources.[32-35] The presence of TRH at high concentrations in fetal ovine blood and the modulation of fetal pancreatic, placental, and blood TRH levels by thyroid hormones suggest a role for extrahypothalamic TRH in the control of fetal pituitary TSH secretion before the near-term maturation of hypothalamic TRH.[31] The role of extraneural somatostatin in the fetus remains undefined.

FETAL ENDOCRINE SYSTEMS

Anterior Pituitary and Target Organs

The three lobes of the mature pituitary gland have a dual embryonic origin; the anterior and intermediate lobes are derived from oral ectoderm, and the posterior pituitary originates from the infundibulum, a specific region of the developing central nervous system (CNS) that forms in the midline of the ventral diencephalon. Much information has been derived from the mouse as a model organism for pituitary development in mammals, given the increasing number of mouse mutants that have been analyzed in

which morphogenesis of the pituitary has been affected. However, fate map studies have shown that these processes are similar in all vertebrate species studied, including zebrafish, amphibians, chicks, and rodents.[36-39] In the mouse, the first sign of pituitary development occurs at 7.5 days post coitum (dpc) with the development of the hypophyseal placode, a thickening of the ectoderm in the midline of the anterior neural ridge (Fig. 22-2). During the next 24 hours, as the anterior neural tube bends and rapidly expands, the hypophyseal placode is displaced ventrally to become situated under, and in contact with, the prospective forebrain within the ectoderm at the roof of the future oral cavity. At approximately 9 dpc, the placode invaginates dorsally to form a rudimentary Rathke's pouch, the primordium of the anterior and intermediate lobe. By 10.5 dpc, the overlying neural ectoderm then evaginates to form the infundibulum, from which the posterior pituitary and pituitary stalk will derive, which comes into direct contact with Rathke's pouch. The juxtaposition of Rathke's pouch and the diencephalon is maintained throughout the early stages of pituitary organogenesis. This close relationship is required for tissue interactions between neural and oral ectoderm, which are critical for the initial stages of pituitary specification. By 10.5 dpc the pouch is fully invaginated to form a definitive structure, and at 12.5 dpc it is completely separated from the underlying oral ectoderm. The lumen of the pouch persists as the pituitary cleft, separating the anterior and intermediate lobes in the mature gland. The iterative nature of the inductive interactions required for pituitary morphogenesis makes it very sensitive to both loss-of-function and gain-of-function mutations.[40]

The posterior lobe comprises axonal projections of neurons that traverse the pituitary stalk and median eminence at the base of the hypothalamus. The neurons originate from hypothalamic magnocellular bodies termed the *supra-optic, suprachiasmatic,* and *paraventricular nuclei.* The former two nuclei release arginine vasopressin (AVP), whereas the paraventricular nuclei release oxytocin (OT).[41]

Hypothalamus and Pituitary Stalk Development

The anatomy of the developed hypothalamus is well understood. It extends from the anteriorly located optic chiasm to the posteriorly located mammillary body and is organized into distinct rostral-to-caudal regions: preoptic, anterior, tuberal, and mammillary. The organ is also sub-divided into three medial-to-lateral regions: periventricular, medial, and lateral.[42] Contained within the medial region is the medial preoptic nucleus, anterior hypothalamus, the dorsomedial nucleus, the ventromedial nucleus, and the mammillary nuclei. The lateral zone consists of the preoptic area and hypothalamic area.[42]

As Rathke's pouch invaginates, part of the ventral diencephalon evaginates ventrally to form the infundibulum and later the posterior pituitary lobe and pituitary stalk. The pituitary stalk acts as a physical connection between the pituitary gland and brain and contains the hypophyseal (hypothalamic-pituitary) portal system, as well as the neuronal connections traversing across the hypothalamic median eminence. These neurons originate from the supra-optic, suprachiasmatic, and paraventricular nuclei, which are large hypothalamic magnocellular bodies located within the periventricular region of the hypothalamus.[42] Within the median eminence itself at the base of the hypothalamus is the capillary bed, into which the widely dispersed hypothalamic parvocellular neurons secrete hypophysiotrophic hormones. These neurons stimulate the release of the seven anterior/intermediate pituitary lobe hormones via the hypophyseal portal system. Interestingly, the parvocellular neurons also secrete OT and AVP, although at much lower concentrations than the magnocellular neurons, with the parvocellular-derived AVP acting synergistically with corticotropin-releasing hormone (CRH) in regulating ACTH release. It is therefore evident that the hypothalamus is the central mediator of growth, reproduction, and homeostasis, acting through the pituitary gland.[43]

Interestingly, however, deciphering hypothalamic development during embryogenesis has proved problematic, perhaps due to its anatomic complexity and highly diverse collection of cell groups and neuronal subtypes, for which there is a dearth of literature defining the genetics and signaling and marker molecules involved in their delineation and identification.[44,45] Furthermore, genetic expression studies within the hypothalamus have knock-on effects on multiple neuronal subtypes and downstream physiologic processes. However, studies are slowly elucidating hypothalamic development.

Human Hypothalamic-Pituitary Development

The human fetal forebrain is identifiable by 3 weeks of gestation, the diencephalon and telencephalon by 5 weeks. Rathke's pouch, the buccal precursor of the anterior pituitary gland, separates from the primitive pharyngeal stomodeum by 5 weeks of gestation.[43,46,47] The neural components of the transducer system (hypothalamus, pituitary stalk, and posterior pituitary) are largely developed by 7 weeks of gestation, and the bony floor of the sella turcica is also present by that time, separating the adenohypophysis from the primitive gut.

The hypothalamic cell condensations, which represent the hypothalamic nuclei, and the interconnecting fiber tracts are demonstrable by 15 to 18 weeks.[43,46] Hypothalamic neurons and diencephalic fiber tracts for the neuropeptides somatostatin, growth hormone–releasing hormone (GHRH), TRH, and gonadotropin-releasing hormone (GnRH) are visible by this time. Concentrations of dopamine, TRH, GnRH, and somatostatin are significant in hypothalamic tissue by 10 to 14 weeks of gestation. Therefore, the anatomy and biosynthetic mechanisms that make up the hypothalamic-pituitary neuroendocrine transducer appear to be functional by 12 to 17 weeks of gestation in humans.

Capillaries develop within the proliferating anterior pituitary tissue around Rathke's pouch and the diencephalon by 8 weeks of gestation, and intact hypothalamic-pituitary portal vessels are present by 12 to 17 weeks. Maturation of the pituitary portal vascular system continues through 30 to 35 weeks, and the system becomes functional with portal vascular extension into the hypothalamus. Recent work suggests that local OT and fibroblast growth factors FGF8 and FGF10 regulate the formation of the hypothalamic-neurohypophyseal system and neurovascular contact between hypothalamic axons and neurohypophyseal capillaries by stimulating endothelial morphogenesis and by attracting hypothalamic-neurohypophyseal neurons.[48,49]

The definitive Rathke's pouch comprises proliferative progenitors that will gradually relocate ventrally, away from the lumen as they differentiate. A proliferative zone containing SRY-box 2 (*SOX2*)-expressing progenitors is maintained in the mouse embryo in a periluminal area and persists in the adult.[50-52] These progenitors are capable of giving rise to all of the cell types within the anterior pituitary.

Specialized anterior pituitary cell types, including lacto-trophs, somatotrophs, corticotrophs, thyrotrophs, and gonadotrophs, can be recognized in the human anterior pituitary between 7 and 16 weeks.[46] Secretory granules are present within anterior pituitary cells by 10 to 12 weeks, and pituitary hormones, including growth hormone (GH), prolactin (PRL), TSH, luteinizing hormone (LH), follicle-stimulating hormone (FSH), ACTH, OT, VT, and AVP, can be identified by immunoassay between 10 and 17 weeks.[46,53] Thus, the anatomy and biosynthetic mechanisms that make up the hypothalamic-pituitary neuroendocrine transducer appear functional by 12 to 17 weeks of gestation.

Hormone-producing terminally differentiated cells in the adult anterior pituitary are organized in three-dimensional homotypic cell networks. In the embryo, the first differentiated cells appear as isolated cells, which rapidly aggregate with other cells, producing the same hormone into strands of cells and then into three-dimensional networks. The first hormone-producing network to appear is the POMC lineage at E13 in the mouse, followed by the somatotroph/lactotroph and gonadotroph network. A network of thyrotroph cells has not been visualized thus far.[54]

Genes Involved in Pituitary Development and Disease

Complex genetic interactions dictate normal pituitary development. A cascade of signaling molecules and transcription factors plays a crucial role in organ commitment, cell proliferation, cell patterning, and terminal differentiation, and the final product is a culmination of this coordinated process (Fig. 22-3). Initially, cells within the primordium of the pituitary gland are competent to differentiate into all cell types. After expression of the

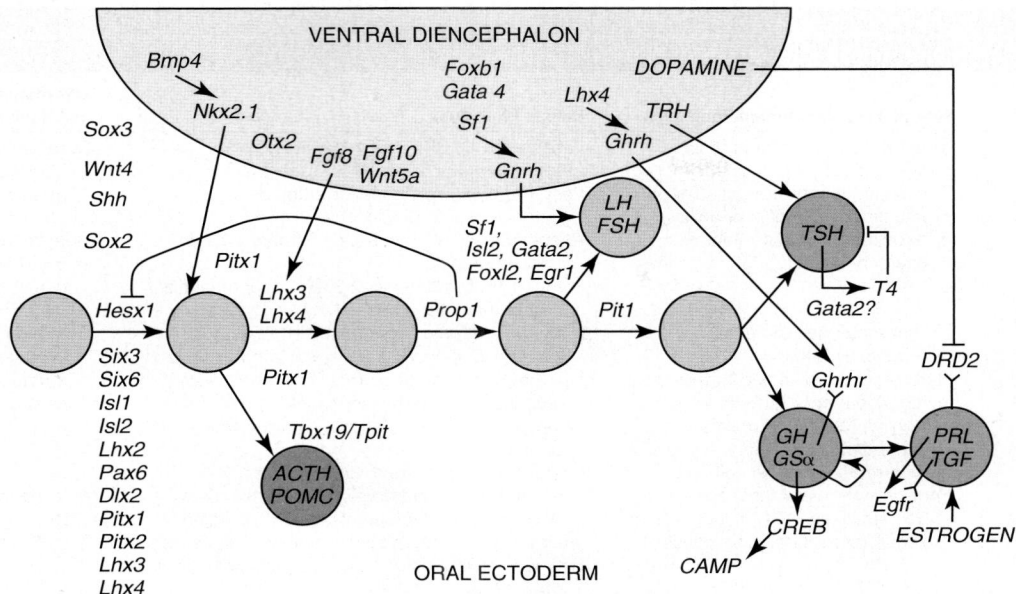

Figure 22-3 Schematic representation of the developmental cascade of genes implicated in human pituitary development with particular reference to pituitary cell differentiation.

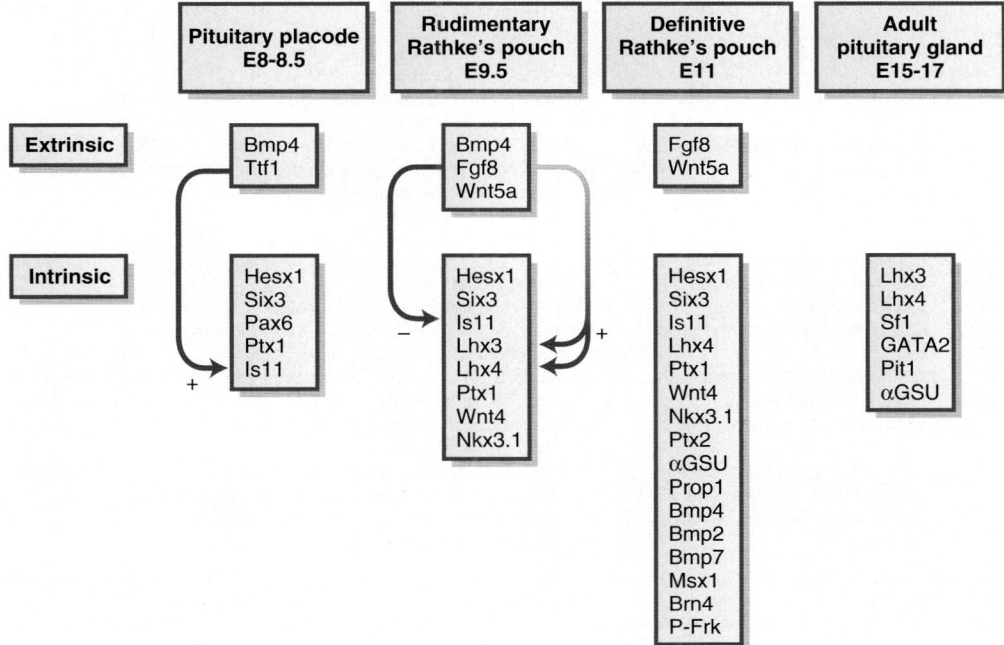

Figure 22-4 Transcription factors and signaling molecules involved in anterior pituitary development.

earliest markers of pituitary gland development, such as homeobox gene expressed in embryonic stem (ES) cells *(Hesx1)*, further signaling pathways are established from within the gland and ventral diencephalon that direct these cells toward terminal differentiation into mature hormone-secreting cell types. Signaling molecules and transcription factors are expressed sequentially at critical periods of pituitary development, and expression of many of these factors is attenuated subsequently (Fig. 22-4). Genes that are expressed early are implicated in organ commitment but are also implicated in repression and activation of downstream target genes that have specific roles in directing the cells toward a particular fate.

Spontaneous or artificially induced mutations in the mouse have led to significant insights into human pituitary disease, and identification of mutations associated with human pituitary disease have, in turn, been invaluable in defining the genetic cascade responsible for the development of this embryologic tissue. Mutations involved specifically in human hypothalamic-pituitary disease are listed in Table 22-2 and are briefly discussed here.

Extrinsic molecules within the ventral diencephalon and surrounding structures, such as bone morphogenetic proteins 2 and 4 (BMP2, BMP4), FGF8, sonic hedgehog (Shh), wingless (Wnt4), thyroid transcription factor 1 (TTF-1; also called Nkx2-1), and molecules involved in

TABLE 22-2

Comparison of Murine and Human Phenotypes in Pituitary Development

Gene	Protein	Murine Loss-of-Function Phenotype	Human Phenotype	Inheritance (Murine and Human)
HESX1	HESX1	Anophthalmia or microphthalmia, agenesis of corpus callosum, absence of septum pellucidum, pituitary dysgenesis or aplasia	Variable: SOD, CPHD, IGHD with EPP Anterior pituitary hypoplastic or absent Posterior pituitary ectopic or eutopic Frequency of mutations: <1%	Dominant or recessive in humans, recessive in mouse
OTX2	OTX2	Lack of forebrain and midbrain, olfactory placode, optic placodes	Anophthalmia, APH, ectopic posterior pituitary, absent infundibulum Frequency of mutations: 2-3% of anophthalmia/microphthalmia cases	Heterozygous: haploinsufficiency/dominant negative
SOX2	SOX2	Homozygous null mutants: embryonic lethal Heterozygous mice and further dose reduction: poor growth, reduced fertility, CNS abnormalities, anophthalmia; pituitary hypoplasia with reduction in all cell types	Hypogonadotropic hypogonadism; APH, abnormal hippocampi, bilateral anophthalmia/microphthalmia, abnormal corpus callosum, learning difficulties, esophageal atresia, sensorineural hearing loss, hypothalamic hamartoma Frequency of mutations: 8/235	De novo haploinsufficiency in humans, heterozygous mutation associated with haploinsufficiency in mouse
SOX3	SOX3	Poor growth, weakness, craniofacial abnormalities, ACC, hypothalamic and infundibular abnormalities	IGHD and mental retardation, hypopituitarism; APH, infundibular hypoplasia, EPP, midline abnormalities, persistent craniopharyngeal canal Frequency of mutations: 6% (duplications), 1.5% (mutations)	X-linked recessive in both mice and humans
GLI2	GLI2	N/A	Holoprosencephaly, hypopituitarism, craniofacial abnormalities, polydactyly, single nares, single central incisor, partial ACC Frequency of mutations: 1.5%	Haploinsufficiency in humans
LHX3	LHX3	Hypoplasia of Rathke's pouch	GH, TSH, gonadotropin deficiency with pituitary hypoplasia ACTH insufficiency variable Short, rigid cervical spine Variable sensorineural hearing loss Frequency of mutations: 1.3%	Recessive in both
LHX4	LHX4	Mild hypoplasia of anterior pituitary	GH, TSH, cortisol deficiency, persistent craniopharyngeal canal and abnormal cerebellar tonsils; APH, ectopic/eutopic posterior pituitary, absent infundibulum Frequency of mutations: 1.2%	Recessive in mouse, dominant in humans
PROP1	PROP1	Hypoplasia of anterior pituitary with reduced somatotrophs, lactotrophs, thyrotrophs, corticotrophs, and gonadotrophs	GH, TSH, PRL, and gonadotropin deficiency Evolving ACTH deficiency Enlarged pituitary with later involution Frequency of mutations: 1.1% sporadic cases, 29.5% familial cases	Recessive in both
POU1F1	POU1F1 (PIT1)	Anterior pituitary hypoplasia with reduced somatotrophs, lactotrophs, and thyrotrophs	Variable anterior pituitary hypoplasia with GH, TSH, and PRL deficiencies Frequency of mutations: 3.8% sporadic cases, 18% familial cases	Recessive in mouse, dominant/recessive in humans
ARNT2	ARNT	Anterior pituitary hypoplasia, TRH, somatostatin, oxytocin and CRH deficiencies, reduced vasopressin neurons	TSH, GH, ACTH deficiencies, DI, small anterior pituitary, vesicoureteric reflux, renal impairment, visual impairment, neonatal seizures with progressive microcephaly	Recessive in humans

ACC, agenesis of corpus callosum; ACTH, adrenocorticotropic hormone; APH, anterior pituitary hypoplasia; CNS, central nervous system; CPHD, combined pituitary hormone deficiencies; CRH, corticotropin-releasing hormone; DI, diabetes insipidus; EPP, ectopic posterior pituitary; GH, growth hormone; IGHD, isolated growth hormone deficiency; N/A, not applicable; PRL, prolactin; SOD, septo-optic dysplasia; TRH, thyrotropin-releasing hormone; TSH, thyroid-stimulating hormone.

Notch signaling play critical roles in early organogenesis.[43,47,55] Recent studies in the mouse have shown that a close interaction between oral ectoderm and neural ectoderm is critical for initial development of the pituitary gland. Rathke's pouch develops in a two-step process that requires at least two sequential inductive signals from the diencephalon. First, induction and formation of the rudimentary pouch are dependent upon BMP4, and second, FGF8 activates two key regulatory genes, LIM homeobox 3 (LHX3) and LIM homeobox 4 (LHX4), that are essential for subsequent development of the rudimentary pouch into a definitive pouch.

BMP4 and FGF8 are present only in the diencephalon and not in Rathke's pouch. Murine mutations within the TTF-1/Nkx2-1 (also called thyroid-specific enhancer binding protein), which is expressed only in the presumptive ventral diencephalon, can cause severe defects in the development of the diencephalon and the anterior pituitary gland. Conditional deletion of RBPJ, which encodes the major mediator of the Notch pathway, leads to conversion of the late (pituitary-specific transcription factor 1 [Pit-1]) lineage into the early (corticotroph) lineage. Notch signaling is required for maintaining expression of PROP1 (prophet of Pit-1), which is required for generation of the Pit-1 lineage. Attenuation of Notch signaling is necessary for terminal differentiation in Pit-1 cells and for maturation and proliferation of the GH-producing somatotrophs.[55]

Mutations of the sonic hedgehog *(SHH)* signaling pathway (SHH, TGIF, ZIC2, PTCH1, GLI2) and the transcription factors SIX3, TDGF1 (teratocarcinoma-derived growth factor 1), and *FOXH1/FAST1* have been identified in patients with holoprosencephaly, with and without hypothalamic-pituitary defects.[56-61] Mutations in *FGF8* have also been identified in association with both holoprosencephaly associated with diabetes insipidus and with Kallmann syndrome.[62,63] Mutations in *HESX1* have been identified in patients with septo-optic dysplasia (SOD; a combination of pituitary, eye, and midline forebrain defects), combined pituitary hormone deficiencies (CPHD), and isolated growth hormone deficiency (IGHD).[43,64] Mutations in *SOX2* and *OTX2* have been described in association with severe eye defects, hypogonadotropic hypogonadism, and variable hypopituitarism.[65-69] Mutations and genomic duplications in *SOX3* have been identified in patients with hypopituitarism with and without learning defects.[70]

Mutations in the gene encoding the LIM homeodomain transcription factor LHX3 have been identified in patients with hypopituitarism, neck abnormalities, and sensorineural deafness, whereas mutations in *LHX4* have been identified in patients with hypopituitarism and cerebellar abnormalities.[71-73] Mutations in genes expressed later in pituitary development, such as *PROP1* and *POU1F1* (previously known as *PIT1*), are associated with more specific pituitary phenotypes (variable GH, TSH, ACTH, PRL, and gonadotropin deficiencies and often a large anterior pituitary that later involutes with *PROP1* mutations; GH, TSH, and PRL deficiencies with *POU1F1* mutations), in keeping with a role for these genes in cellular proliferation and differentiation and hormone secretion.[43,74-76] Mutations in the T-box transcription factor *TBX19/TPIT* have been described in patients with early-onset isolated ACTH deficiency.[77] Mutations in TSHβ have been associated with central hypothyroidism.[78] More recently, mutations and deletions of *IGSF1* have been associated with TSH and variable GH and PRL deficiencies associated with macro-orchidism. IGSF1 (immunoglobulin superfamily, member 1) is a glycoprotein that is expressed in the pituitary and in testis. The function of the gene remains unclear but it may be involved in TRH signaling.[79,80]

The hypothalamic-pituitary-gonadal axis is the key regulator of sex development and reproduction, processes that are initiated through the decapeptide GnRH. GnRH is produced and released after the successful migration during embryogenesis of the GnRH neurons from the olfactory placode, across the cribriform plate, to the hypothalamic arcuate nucleus, where they are detectable from about 9 weeks of gestation. These neurons are then projected into the hypothalamic median eminence. A functional connection with respect to GnRH is detected by 16 to 20 weeks of human gestation. This hormone is released in a pulsatile fashion and binds to its receptors on pituitary gonadotrophs, which in turn respond by synthesizing and releasing the gonadotropins LH and FSH. These bind to their cognate receptors in the gonads, where they stimulate the production of sex steroids, such as androgens or estrogens, and stimulate gametogenesis. The sex steroids then regulate gonadotropin secretion via negative feedback at the level of the hypothalamus or pituitary. Congenital disorders of gonadotropin secretion include hypogonadotropic hypogonadism and Kallmann syndrome, a disorder characterized by hypogonadotropic hypogonadism, anosmia/hyposmia, cleft lip/plate, sensorineural hearing loss, dental anomalies, synkinesia, and renal abnormalities.

A number of genes have been reported to date in Kallmann syndrome, namely, by chronologic order of discovery: *KAL1, FGFR1, PROKR2* and *PROK2, FGF8, CHD7,* *WDR11, HS6ST1, SEMA3A, NELF,* and *SOX10.*[63,81] More recently, mutations have also been identified in *FGF17, IL17RD, DUSP6, SPRY4,* and *FLRT3,* all of which have been implicated in FGF signaling.[82] Variants in *PROKR2* and *PROK2,* encoding prokineticin receptor-2 and prokineticin-2, respectively, have been identified in approximately 9% of patients with Kallmann syndrome.[83] Prokineticins are secreted cysteine-rich proteins that possess diverse biologic activities including effects on neuronal survival, gastrointestinal smooth muscle contraction, circadian locomotor rhythm, and appetite regulation.[83] Prokineticins PROK1 and PROK2 act through their G protein–coupled receptors PROKR1 and PROKR2, which are expressed in the olfactory bulbs. PROK2 functions as a chemoattractant for neuronal progenitors, which follow a rostral migratory stream. *Prokr2−/−* mice have reduced LH in the pituitary, small gonads, and abnormal olfactory bulb formation, but *Prokr2* seems to be dispensable for normal pituitary formation.[84,85] Variations in *PROKR2* have also been associated with hypopituitarism, pituitary stalk interruption syndrome, and septo-optic dysplasia but are unlikely to be causative in isolation and likely only contribute to the phenotype, including Kallmann syndrome, in combination with other genetic mutations or environmental factors.

Mutations in a number of genes have also been identified in association with normosmic hypogonadotropic hypogonadism, and these mutations include genes encoding for GnRH1 and its receptor GnRHR, kisspeptin *(KISS1)* and its receptor KISS1R, and neurokinin B (encoded by tachykinin 3, TAC3) and its receptor TAC.[86-90]

More recently, mutations in genes such as *RNF216, OTUD4, STUB1,* and *PNPLA6* have been found in syndromic forms of GnRH deficiency that have associated features such as ataxia and dementia, as part of Gordon Holmes syndrome *(RNF216, OTUD4, STUB1)* and Boucher-Neuhäuser syndrome *(PNPLA6).*[91-93] *RNF216, OTUD4,* and *STUB1* are involved in protein ubiquitination; *PNPLA6* encodes an enzyme involved in the production of the neurotransmitter acetylcholine.

Other genes implicated in syndromic forms of hypothalamic-pituitary disease include *GLI3,* part of the sonic hedgehog signaling pathway, haploinsufficiency of which results in Pallister-Hall syndrome associated with polydactyly, hypothalamic disorganization, hypothalamic hamartoma, and hypopituitarism.[94,95] *PITX2* mutation has been identified as one cause of Axenfeld-Rieger syndrome involving ocular, dental, and hypothalamic abnormalities.[96] *Pitx2* knockout mice have pituitary hypoplasia and decreased GHRH receptor, GH, FSH, LH, and TSH gene expression.[96]

Rare isolated pituitary hormone deficiencies have been associated with mutations in the respective hypothalamic releasing hormones or the releasing hormone receptors, for example, familial GH deficiency due to *GHRHR* mutations, TSH deficiency due to *TRHR* mutations, and gonadotropin deficiency due to *GNRHR* mutations.[87,97,98]

No genetic cause has been identified in most cases of congenital hypopituitarism to date, suggesting a role for other, unidentified genes or environmental factors. However, it is also likely that further genes implicated in hypothalamic-pituitary disease will be identified that play a role in hypothalamic development. Indeed, we have recently identified mutations in *ARNT2* that are associated with severe pituitary insufficiency, including GH, TSH, and ACTH deficiencies as well as diabetes insipidus, together with progressive microcephaly, seizures, severe visual impairment, and severe learning difficulties and abnormalities of the renal and urinary tracts.[99] ARNT2 (aryl hydrocarbon receptor nuclear translocator 2) is a basic helix-loop-helix transcription factor that is critical for normal development of the paraventricular and supraoptic nuclei. The discovery of genetic factors implicated in the formation of the hypothalamus and pituitary has recently been used by Suga and associates, who performed experiments that led to the efficient self-formation of three-dimensional anterior pituitary tissue in an aggregate culture of mouse ES cells.[100] ES cells were stimulated to differentiate into non-neural head ectoderm and hypothalamic neuroectoderm in adjacent layers within the aggregate and treated with agonists of hedgehog signaling. Self-organization of Rathke's pouch–like three-dimensional structures occurred at the interface of these two epithelia. Various endocrine cells were subsequently produced, and these cells were able to respond to trophic hormones. This seminal study showed that functional anterior pituitary tissue self-forms in culture after manipulation of ES cells, recapitulating local tissue interactions, and hence opens up the possibility of novel future treatments for hypopituitarism.[100]

Growth Hormone and Prolactin

The human fetal pituitary gland can synthesize and secrete GH by 8 to 10 weeks of gestation. Pituitary GH content increases from about 1 nmol (20 ng) at 10 weeks to 45 nmol (1000 ng) at 16 weeks of gestation. Fetal plasma GH concentrations in cord blood samples are in the range of 1 to 4 nmol/L during the first trimester and increase to a mean peak of approximately 6 nmol/L at midgestation. Plasma GH concentrations fall progressively during the second half of gestation, to a mean value of 1.5 nmol/L at term.[46] Pituitary GH messenger ribonucleic acid (mRNA) and GH content generally parallel the increase in plasma GH concentration between 16 and 24 weeks of gestation.[101] This pattern of ontogenesis of plasma GH reflects a progressive maturation of hypothalamic-pituitary and forebrain function. The responses of plasma GH to somatostatin and GHRH and to insulin and arginine are mature at term in human infants.[46,102]

The high plasma GH concentrations at midgestation after development of the pituitary portal vascular system may reflect unrestrained secretion.[46] Studies of 9- to 16-week-old human fetal pituitary cells in culture showed a predominant response to GHRH and a limited effect of somatostatin, suggesting that the inhibitory action of somatostatin develops later in gestation.[103] This interpretation was substantiated by in vivo studies in the sheep fetus, which showed a failure of somatostatin to inhibit GHRH-stimulated GH release early in the third trimester and maturation of the inhibitory effect of somatostatin near term.[46] The predominant GHRH enhancement and limited somatostatin inhibition of GH secretion at midgestation presumably relate to a limited capacity for inhibition of GH release by somatomedin feedback. In addition, there may be unrestrained GH secretion at the pituitary cell level, or immaturity of limbic and forebrain inhibitory circuitry that modulates hypothalamic function, or both.[46] Whatever the mechanisms, control of GH secretion matures progressively during the last half of gestation and the early weeks of postnatal life, so that mature responses to sleep, glucose, and L-dopa are present by 3 months of age. GH secretion is already pulsatile soon after birth in humans,[104] but trough concentrations are still higher than in later life, so random GH sampling can be used to detect GH deficiency in the neonatal period, something that is not possible at a later age.

The ontogenesis of fetal plasma PRL differs significantly from that of GH; concentrations are low until 25 to 30 weeks of gestation and increase to a mean peak value of approximately 11 nmol/L at term (Fig. 22-5).[46] Pituitary PRL content increases progressively from 12 to 15 weeks, and in vitro fetal pituitary cells from midgestation fetuses show limited autonomous PRL secretion, although PRL release increases in response to TRH and decreases in response to dopamine. Brain and hypothalamic control of PRL matures late in gestation and during the first months of extrauterine life.[46,102] Estrogen stimulates PRL synthesis and release by pituitary cells, and the marked increase in fetal plasma PRL concentration in the last trimester parallels the increase in fetal plasma estrogen concentrations, although lagging by several weeks.[46,102] Anencephalic fetuses have plasma PRL concentrations in the normal or low-normal range. These data support a role for estrogen in stimulating fetal PRL release. The fetal sheep exhibits a similar pattern of fetal plasma PRL concentrations, indicating that maturation and integration of brain and hypothalamic mechanisms modulating PRL release develop late in gestation and in the postnatal period, accounting for the delayed postnatal fall in plasma PRL concentration in the neonate of this species.[46]

There is a general tendency toward hypersecretion of fetal pituitary hormones during the last half of gestation,

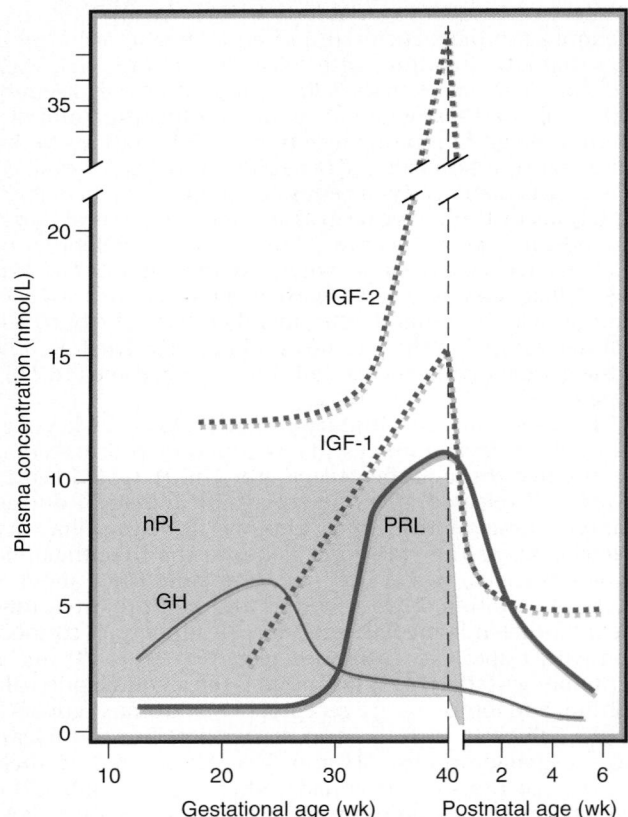

Figure 22-5 Patterns of change of fetal plasma human placental lactogen (hPL), growth hormone (GH), prolactin (PRL), insulin-like growth factor 1 (IGF-1), and insulin-like growth factor 2 (IGF-2) during gestation and in the neonatal period. The shaded area indicates the range of fetal plasma hPL concentrations. (Data from Bennett A, Wilson DM, Liu R, et al. Levels of insulin-like growth factors I and II in human cord blood. *J Clin Endocrinol Metab.* 1983;57:609-612; Kaplan SL, Grumbach MM, Aubert ML. The ontogenesis of pituitary hormones and hypothalamic factors in the human fetus: maturation of central nervous system regulation of anterior pituitary function. *Recent Prog Horm Res.* 1976;32:161-243; Bala RM, Lopatka J, Leung A, et al. Serum immunoreactive somatomedin levels in normal adults, pregnant women at term, children at various ages, and children with constitutionally delayed growth. *J Clin Endocrinol Metab.* 1981;52:508-512.)

and pituitary hormones found at high concentrations in cord blood from aborted human fetuses and premature human infants include GH, TSH, ACTH, β-endorphin, β-lipotropin, LH, and FSH.[46,102] Development of hypothalamic-pituitary control is complex, involving maturational events in the cortex and midbrain, hypothalamus and hypothalamic-pituitary portal vascular system, peripheral endocrine systems, and the placenta itself, including hormone, growth factor, and neuropeptide production. The fetal pituitary hyperfunction appears to be related more to relatively delayed maturation of the CNS and hypothalamic control with unrestrained secretion of stimulating hypothalamic hormones than to the action of placental neuropeptides.[46]

Postnatally, GH acts through receptors in liver and other tissues to stimulate production of IGF-1 and, to a lesser degree, IGF-2. Prenatally, GH receptor mRNA levels and receptor binding are low in fetal liver, although receptor mRNA is present in other fetal tissues.[46] The growth of anencephalic fetuses is almost normal, suggesting that factors other than GH stimulate fetal IGF production. Nutrition plays an important role.[105,106]

PRL receptors are present in most fetal tissues during the first trimester of gestation, and it is likely that lactogenic hormones have a significant role in organ and tissue development early in gestation.[53,105] The coordinated increase in fetal adipose tissue and the adipose tissue PRL receptors PRLR1 and PRLR2 suggests that PRL may play a role in growth and maturation of fetal adipose tissue later in gestation.[107] PRL may also play a role in fetal skeletal maturation.[107] Ovine placental lactogen stimulates glycogen synthesis in fetal ovine liver, and human placental lactogen (hPL) stimulates amino acid transport, DNA synthesis, and IGF-1 production in human fetal fibroblasts and muscle cells. GH and PRL have little activity in these tissues (see "Fetal Growth").[53]

Human chromosome 17q22-24 contains a growth hormone/placental lactogen (GH/PL) gene cluster containing five related genes: *GH-N* encodes pituitary GH, *GH-V* encodes placental GH, and *hPL-A*, *hPL-B*, and *hPL-L* encode placental lactogens (also called *human chorionic somato-mammotropins*, HCS). The major circulating placental lactogens derive from the *hPL-A* and *hPL-B* genes. GH-V differs in 13 of the 191 amino acids of GH-N and is produced in the syncytiotrophoblast.[108] It rises sharply after midgestation to a peak at 34 to 37 weeks, and within 1 hour after delivery of the placenta, it disappears from the circulation.[109] GH-V is not secreted into the fetal circulation and exclusively plays a role in maternal and possibly uteroplacental physiology. Placental GH-V is secreted into the maternal circulation and reduces insulin sensitivity in the mother and so spares glucose and other nutrients for transplacental delivery and fetal growth. As a counterbalance, insulin production and beta-cell mass increase during pregnancy.[110]

hPL is structurally homologous to GH but functionally closer to PRL and is secreted directly into both fetal and maternal circulations. hPL is first detected in the mother at 6 weeks of gestation to reach a peak of 5000 to 7000 ng/mL at 32 to 35 weeks; fetal hPL concentrations, however, approximate 20 to 50 ng/mL at term. hPL concentrations increase with placental mass and are higher in twin than singleton pregnancies. In the mother, lactogens affect insulin production, hypothalamic gene expression, and leptin action and so maintain metabolic homeostasis while providing the substrates for nutrition for the fetus and newborn infant. Maternal fat deposition derives from increases in food intake and insulin-dependent lipogenesis, and studies in rodents suggest that the hyperphagia is mediated by progesterone and PRL.[108] At least in rodents, evidence suggests that PRL and placental lactogen signaling through the PRL receptor is essential for the increase in beta-cell mass. A surge in PRL concentration in the perinatal period parallels an increase in beta-cell replication, and a whole-body knockout of the PRL receptor reduces beta-cell mass and insulin secretion in the perinatal period.[111]

Adrenal System

Embryology

The primordia of the adrenal glands can be recognized just cephalad of the bilaterally developing mesonephros by 3 to 4 weeks of gestation.[112,113] The adrenal cortex is derived from a thickening of the intermediate mesoderm at 4 to 5 weeks of gestation in humans, in contrast to the adrenal medulla, which derives from the ectoderm. This region, known as the *gonadal ridge*, contains adrenogonadal progenitor cells that give rise to the steroidogenic cells of the adrenal gland and the gonad. The gonadal cells migrate caudally. Cells destined to become adrenal tissue migrate retroperitoneally to the upper pole of the mesonephros. They are then infiltrated at 7 to 8 weeks of gestation by sympathetic cells derived from the neural crest that will form the adrenal medulla. Encapsulation of the adrenal gland occurs after 8 weeks of gestation and results in the formation of a distinct organ just above the developing kidney.

Following the neural crest invasion, the adrenal primordium becomes encapsulated within a population of mesenchymal cells.[114] The presumptive cortical and medullary populations proliferate rapidly and sort into a central medulla and surrounding cortex, all encased in a stromal capsule that is several cell layers thick. The cells of the definitive adrenal gland segregate into three concentric steroid-producing zones. The zona glomerulosa (ZG), which produces the mineralocorticoid aldosterone under the control of the renin-angiotensin system (RAS), is the outer zone. The zona fasciculata (ZF) produces glucocorticoids in response to signals from the hypothalamus and pituitary, develops before the ZG, and comprises the inner zone. The fetal adrenal glands also contain a much larger inner fetal zone, the zona reticularis, capable of producing significant amounts of C19 androgens such as DHEA and dehydroepiandrosterone sulfate (DHEAS), which are then converted to estrogens by the placenta. The large eosinophilic cells of the fetal zone are well differentiated by 9 to 12 weeks of gestation and are capable of active steroidogenesis. The fetal adrenal glands grow rapidly and progressively in mass and form 0.4% of body weight at term; the combined glandular weight is approximately 8 g at term, when the fetal zone makes up about 80% of the mass of the gland with a relative size 10- to 20-fold that of the adult adrenal gland.[20,112,113] The fetal zone is identified only in higher primates. The adrenal gland undergoes rapid involution postnatally, largely due to regression of the fetal zone, which is absent by 6 months of age in most cases.

Genetic Regulation of Adrenal Development

Fetal adrenal cortical development is under the control of several genes and growth factors. Much of our understanding of adrenal development derives from studies of transgenic mice and of patients with various forms of adrenal hypoplasia. The earliest stages of adrenal development may be regulated by a number of transcription factors (e.g., SALL1, FOXD2, PBX1, WT1, SF1 [NR5A1], DAX1 [NROB1]), coregulators (e.g., CITED2), signaling molecules

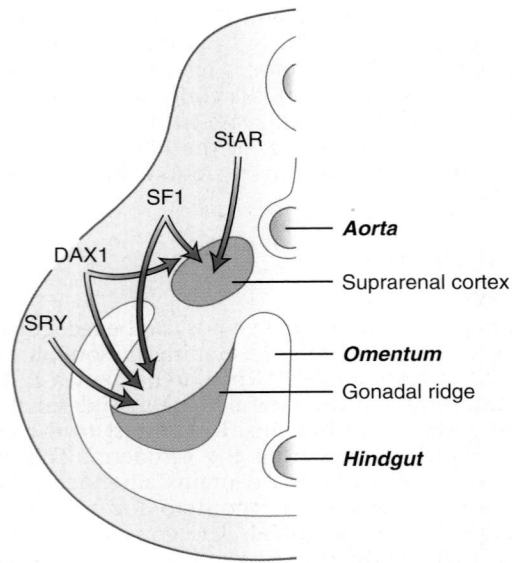

Figure 22-6 Partial cross section of a 5-week human embryo showing the locations of the adrenal primordia (suprarenal cortices) and gonadal ridges. The developmental genes programming adrenal and gonadal embryogenesis are indicated. Steroidogenic factor 1 (SF1) is involved in testicular and ovarian development. SRY is the single critical regulator of testicular embryogenesis. Inactivation of the *DAX1* gene leads to adrenal hypoplasia. The steroidogenic acute regulatory protein (StAR) is the rate-limiting factor for adrenal steroidogenesis. See text for details.

(e.g., Hedgehog/GLI3, WNT3/WNT4/WNT11, midkine), matrix proteins (e.g., SPARC), and regulators of telomerase activity (e.g., ACD). Of these molecules, the genes encoding the orphan nuclear receptors SF1 (steroidogenic factor 1) and DAX1 (dosage-sensitive sex reversal, adrenal hypoplasia congenita [AHC], X-chromosome factor)[115-117] appear to be critical for early development (Fig. 22-6). These genes show coordinated expression in adrenal cortex, testis, ovary, hypothalamus, and pituitary tissues.

Wt1 knockout mice have renal and gonadal abnormalities and lack adrenal glands.[116] *SF1* gene knockout mice manifest adrenal and gonadal agenesis, gonadotropin deficiency, and absence of the hypothalamic ventromedial nucleus.[116] Inactivating *Dax1/DAX1* gene mutations are associated with adrenal hypoplasia and gonadotropin deficiency in mice and humans.[116] Sonic hedgehog signaling is also required for normal adrenal development at a later stage than SF1 and DAX1. Shh expression marks cortical progenitors, and Shh expressing cells give rise to all steroidogenic (glucocorticoid and mineralocorticoid) cells in cortical zones but not in the capsule or medulla; Shh mutant mice have a thin capsule and a small cortex.[118]

Several other transcription factors including *Pbx1*, *Lim1*, and *Wnt4* are involved earlier in the complex genetic cascade programming adrenal gland organogenesis from the celomic epithelium and urogenital ridge.[116,117] *Pbx1* knockout mice die in utero with multiple organ defects that include adrenal agenesis and impaired testis development, whereas *Wnt4* gene disruption leads to abnormal adrenal development, masculinization of XX females, and müllerian duct agenesis. Several growth factors also play an important role in later adrenal development. FGF signaling interacts with SF1 and Shh signaling. *Fgfr2* and *Fgfr4* are expressed in the developing adrenal cortex, and deletion of *Fgfr2-IIIb* leads to reduced adrenal growth and impaired expression of SF1 and steroidogenic enzymes.[118] Epidermal growth factor (EGF) stimulates proliferation of both the fetal and definitive zones. The fetal adrenal

expresses high levels of IGF-2 mRNA and protein, which are responsive to ACTH.[20,119] IGF-2 augments ACTH-stimulated expression of steroidogenic enzymes and stimulates steroid hormone production in fetal adrenal cortical cells. The pattern of enzyme maturation in the fetal adrenal suggests that cortisol production by the definitive zone does not occur de novo from cholesterol until 30 weeks of gestation, but some production using progesterone as precursor probably occurs earlier.[20,119]

CDKN1C (cyclin-dependent kinase inhibitor 1 C, *P57KIP2*) is a paternally imprinted gene, located on chromosome 11p.15, and encoding for the CDKN1C protein, an inhibitor of cell cycle progression. Variations in *CDKN1C* or its genomic imprinting can lead to adrenal pathology. Loss-of-function of *CDKN1C* results in Beckwith-Wiedemann syndrome, an overgrowth syndrome with increased susceptibility to adrenal carcinoma. IMAGe syndrome is a rare multisystem disorder that mirrors the features of Beckwith-Wiedemann syndrome and is caused by gain-of-function mutations in *CDKN1C*. It is characterized by intrauterine growth restriction, metaphyseal dysplasia, congenital adrenal hypoplasia, and genital anomalies.[120]

The steroidogenic acute regulatory protein (StAR) is a rate-limiting factor in adrenal steroidogenesis. StAR knockout mice manifest glucocorticoid and mineralocorticoid deficiency and female genitalia in XY animals.[121] In humans, inactivating *StAR* mutations cause adrenal hypoplasia and adrenal hormone insufficiency; however, in humans, 46,XY males with normal male genitalia have been described in association with *StAR* mutations.[121,122]

Adrenal Steroidogenesis

The fetal adrenal gland expresses the same five steroidogenic apoenzymes as the adult gland. One microsomal enzyme has 17-hydroxylase/17-20-lyase (CYP17A1 or P450c17) activities, and another has 21-hydroxylase (CYP21A2 or P450c21) activity. Two mitochondrial cytochrome P450 enzymes provide cholesterol side-chain cleavage (CYP11A1 or P450scc) and C11/C18 hydroxylation of the parent steroid structure (CYP11B1/CYP11B2 or P450c11/aldosterone synthase). A fifth enzyme, expressed by the smooth endoplasmic reticulum, exhibits both 3β-HSD and Δ^4, Δ^5-isomerase activities.[112,113] Quantitative differences in the relative activities of these enzymes are found between cells derived from the fetal versus the definitive zones, and these differences are largely due to regulated steroidogenic gene transcription.[112]

The fetal zone has relatively high steroid sulfotransferase activity, and because of the low 3β-HSD and high sulfotransferase activity, the major steroid products of the fetal adrenal gland are DHEA, DHEAS, pregnenolone sulfate, several $\Delta^5$3β-hydroxysteroids, and limited amounts of $\Delta^5$3-ketosteroids, including cortisol and aldosterone.[112,113] The definitive zone contributes only a small fraction of total fetal adrenal steroid output. Glucocorticoids are synthesized in the first trimester due to transient expression of type 2 3β-hydroxysteroid dehydrogenase (HSD3B2), which is maximal between 8 and 9 months of gestation.[123] The hypothalamic-pituitary-adrenal axis is sensitive to glucocorticoid-mediated feedback at this time; 46,XX fetuses with steroidogenic defects (e.g., in CYP21 or CYP11) lack cortisol and have an elevated ACTH drive that results in excess production of fetal androgens at a time when the genital and scrotal folds are sensitive to androgen exposure, resulting in virilization of female genitalia.[123]

Cholesterol, the major substrate for fetal adrenal steroidogenesis, is derived from circulating low-density lipoprotein (LDL) and from de novo adrenal synthesis. LDL cholesterol, largely of fetal liver and testicular origin, contributes 70% of the total. The fetal zone contains more LDL binding sites and manifests a greater rate of de novo cholesterol synthesis than does the definitive zone, in keeping with its greater steroidogenic activity. Both ACTH and angiotensin II receptors (AT_1 and AT_2) are present on fetal adrenal cells early in gestation. ACTH stimulates steroid production by activating StAR and increasing delivery of substrate cholesterol to P450scc; angiotensin II inhibits 3β-HSD activity and promotes DHEA production in the fetal zone.[112] Both fetal adrenal cortisol and placental estradiol regulate hepatic synthesis of cholesterol in the fetus.

The major stimulus to fetal adrenal function is fetal pituitary ACTH.[20,112,124] Although placental hCG may support early adrenal growth, the involution of the adrenal gland that occurs after 15 weeks in the anencephalic fetus suggests a crucial role for pituitary-derived factors. CRH protein has been demonstrated in fetal baboon pituitary, adrenal gland, liver, kidney, and lung tissues during the last third of gestation. The levels are highest in the pituitary (300 to 500 pg/mg protein); levels in adrenal and lung average 20 to 30 pg/mg protein, and those in liver and kidney tissues average 5 to 10 pg/mg protein.[125] CRH gene knockout in mice leads to neonatal death due to pulmonary hypoplasia, suggesting that CRH-stimulated glucocorticoid production is essential for adrenergic chromaffin and normal lung development.[126] Circulating CRH levels are elevated in the fetus, largely from extrahypothalamic and placental sources.[20,125,127] Maternal levels of CRH are elevated during the last trimester of gestation and reach values of 0.5 to 1 nmol/L at term; normal values in nonpregnant women are lower than 0.01 nmol/L.[128] This placental CRH is bioactive, and levels correlate with maternal cortisol concentrations, suggesting that this circulating placental CRH plays a role in stimulating maternal corticotropin release. Fetal plasma CRH levels at term are approximately 0.03 nmol/L; relative to the presumably high level in pituitary portal blood, plasma CRH probably has little role in modulating fetal corticotropin release. Midgestation fetal plasma corticotropin concentrations average about 55 pmol/L (250 pg/mL), levels that maximally stimulate fetal adrenal steroidogenesis, and concentrations are higher throughout gestation than in postnatal life, although they fall near term (Fig. 22-7).[20,112] AVP and catecholamines also are significant stimuli for fetal ACTH secretion.[129]

The paradox of human fetal adrenal function is that steroidogenesis is programmed largely to production of inactive products.[112] The gland is maximally stimulated to maintain fetal cortisol levels and ACTH feedback homeostasis but is programmed by the steroidogenic enzyme expression pattern (e.g., relative 3-HSD deficiency) to produce inactive DHEA and pregnenolone and their sulfate conjugates. Much of the DHEA is converted to 16-hydroxy-DHEAS by the fetal adrenal and fetal liver. As already discussed, this programming is designed to provide DHEA substrate for placental estrone and estradiol production: 16-hydroxy-DHEA undergoes metabolism to estriol in the placenta. Fetal DHEAS production and maternal estriol concentrations increase progressively to term; DHEAS production approximates to 200 mg/day near term.[20] In the anencephalic fetus, placental estrogen production is reduced to about 10% of normal.[20,112] In pregnant baboons with placental estrogen production suppressed by administration of an aromatase inhibitor, the volume of the fetal zone of the fetal adrenal increased markedly.[130] This effect was reversed by administration of inhibitor plus estrogen, suggesting that estrogen selectively suppresses fetal zone growth and development during the second half of primate

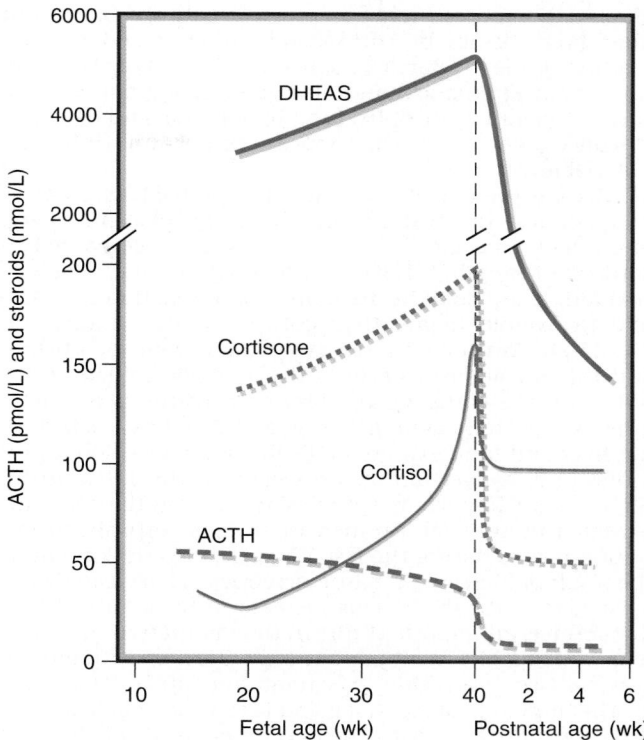

Figure 22-7 Patterns of change of fetal plasma adrenocorticotropic hormone (ACTH), cortisol, cortisone, and dehydroepiandrosterone sulfate (DHEAS) during gestation and in the neonatal period. The trend of average values is shown for each hormone in nanomoles per liter. Notice the broken scale for DHEAS. (Data from Geller and Miller[113] and Winters AJ, Oliver C, Colston C, et al. Plasma ATH levels in the human fetus and neonate as related to age and parturition. *J Clin Endocrinol Metab.* 1974;39:269-273; Murphy BEP. Human fetal serum cortisol levels related to gestational age: evidence of a midgestational fall and a steep late gestational rise, independent of sex or mode of delivery. *Am J Obstet Gynecol.* 1982;144:276-282; Beitins IZ, Bayard F, Ances FIG, et al. The metabolic clearance rate, blood production, interconversion and transplacental passage of cortisol and cortisone in pregnancy near term. *Pediatr Res.* 1973;7:509-513.)

pregnancy. It is proposed that this represents a feedback system to regulate secretion of fetal adrenal DHEA, thereby maintaining normal fetal-placental function and development.[130] Near term, the fetal cortisol production rate in blood, per unit body weight, is similar to that in the adult.[112] About two thirds of fetal cortisol is derived from the fetal adrenal glands, and one third is derived from placental transfer.[112] The metabolic clearance of cortisol in the fetus is rapid; 80% is oxidized in fetal tissues or placenta to cortisone or further metabolites.[112]

The corticotropin feedback control system matures progressively during the second half of gestation and the early neonatal period. Dexamethasone can suppress the human fetal pituitary-adrenal axis at term but not at 18 to 20 weeks of gestation.[112] In fetal sheep, hypothalamic and pituitary glucocorticoid receptors (GRs) are present at midgestation, and corticotropin suppressibility can be demonstrated by the midpoint of the third trimester of gestation.[131] The number of GRs in the sheep fetal hypothalamus increases at term, at the time of increasing glucocorticoid levels, suggesting that some process in the fetus allows the normal autoregulation of GRs to be overridden at term.[132]

Adrenal hormone receptors, including GRs and mineralocorticoid receptors (MRs), are members of the nuclear receptor superfamily of steroid hormone, thyroid hormone, vitamin D, and retinoid receptors.[133] GRs are present in most body tissues by the second trimester and play an important role in fetal development. Mice lacking GR function manifest enlarged and disorganized adrenal cortices, adrenal medullary atrophy, lung hypoplasia, and defective gluconeogenesis.[128,133] They appear normal at birth but are not viable.

GRs are present at birth and are probably present at midgestation in most tissues, including placenta, lung, brain, liver, and gut.[112,132,134] Fetal cortisol is converted to cortisone through 11HSDB2 in fetal tissues, and levels of circulating cortisone in the fetus at midgestation are fourfold to fivefold higher than cortisol concentrations (see Fig. 22-7). Cortisone is a relatively inactive glucocorticoid, and this metabolism protects the anabolic milieu of the fetus, because cortisol can retard both placental and fetal growth.[135] As term approaches, selected fetal tissues including liver and lung express 11HSDB1, a reductase that promotes local conversion of cortisone to cortisol.[112] Cortisol serves as an important stimulus to prepare the fetus for extrauterine survival. An increase in fetal cortisol concentration occurs during the last 10 weeks of gestation and is the result of increased cortisol secretion and decreased conversion to cortisone.[112] This increase in fetal cortisol production has an important role in the maturation of several fetal systems or functions that are critical to extrauterine survival (see "Transition to Extrauterine Life").[112,136]

The human fetal adrenal gland is capable of aldosterone secretion near term with the development of the ZG, and fetal plasma aldosterone concentrations in infants who are born by cesarean section are threefold to fourfold higher than maternal levels.[112,137] Vaginal delivery and maternal salt restriction increase concentrations in both mother and infant. The increased aldosterone concentrations in the fetus are a result of increased fetal adrenal secretion and persist during the first year of extrauterine life.[137] However, there is a poor correlation between plasma renin activity (PRA) and aldosterone concentrations in cord blood.[138] Aldosterone secretion is low in the midgestation human fetal adrenal gland and is unresponsive to the secretagogues that are known to modulate aldosterone production in the adult. In sheep, fetal aldosterone becomes responsive to PRA and angiotensin II in the neonatal period.[139] In this species, in which late fetal aldosterone levels are also high compared with adult levels, furosemide stimulates PRA but not aldosterone during the third trimester; the aldosterone response to furosemide (and PRA) is delayed until the neonatal period.[139,140] This situation also appears to be the case in the human fetus and neonate.

MRs are present in fetal tissues from 12 to 16 weeks of gestation.[141] MR immunoreactivity is detectable in fetal kidney, skin, hair follicles, trachea and bronchioles, esophagus, stomach, small intestine, colon, and pancreatic exocrine ducts. The role of MRs in these fetal tissues remains unclear. MR knockout mice appear normal at birth but demonstrate defects in mineralocorticoid and RAS functions in the postnatal period.[142]

Angiotensin II concentrations in the sheep fetus are similar to maternal values, and blockade of fetal production with angiotensin-converting enzyme inhibitors decreases the fetal glomerular filtration rate.[140] Both subtypes of angiotensin receptors, AT_1 and AT_2, are detectable in various tissues early in fetal development.[143] AT_1 receptor mRNA expression in the fetal sheep kidney is low early in gestation, increases in the latter third of pregnancy, and decreases postnatally. AT_2 mRNA levels are high at midgestation and decrease during the third trimester.[143] These changes are believed to reflect growth factor–mediated changes in cells that contain AT in various tissues. Hormonal factors modulate fetal renal AT gene expression in sheep: angiotensin II suppresses both AT_1 and AT_2, and cortisol increases AT_1 gene expression in kidney and lungs.[143,144]

The role of the fetal RAS is not clear; rather than modulating renal sodium excretion through aldosterone, it may maintain renal excretion of salt and water into amniotic fluid to prevent oligohydramnios.[140] This renal effect is presumably mediated by modulation of arterial pressure. The mechanism for the high aldosterone concentrations in the fetal and neonatal periods remains unclear. Atrial natriuretic peptide (ANP), a cardiac hormone, is known to inhibit aldosterone secretion. Because plasma atrial natriuretic factor concentrations (ANP, brain natriuretic peptide [BNP], and C-type natriuretic peptide [CNP]) are high in the fetus, the increased PRA and aldosterone concentrations are not caused by relative atrial natriuretic factor deficiency.[145]

Aldosterone affects renal sodium excretion in the fetal sheep and in premature infants.[112,139] Manifestations of mineralocorticoid deficiency in the newborn term infant can occur as a result of aldosterone deficiency or competition for binding to renal MRs by other steroids such as 17-hydroxyprogesterone.[112] Relatively reduced glomerular filtration in the newborn limits sodium loss initially, but by 1 week of age, aldosterone deficiency produces the characteristic manifestations of hyponatremia, hyperkalemia, and volume depletion.

Defects of Adrenal Steroidogenesis

Adrenal insufficiency may occur secondary to ACTH deficiency, or it may be primary, resulting from adrenal failure. The mature ACTH peptide is cleaved from the larger precursor molecule, POMC, together with other small peptides such as β-endorphin and α- and β-melanocyte-stimulating hormone (MSH). Defects in ACTH synthesis, processing, or release can lead to secondary adrenal hypoplasia resulting in neonatal hypoglycemia, prolonged jaundice, or collapse. Given that mineralocorticoid secretion is largely independent of ACTH secretion, it is preserved, and salt loss is therefore unusual. Nevertheless, mineralocorticoid deficiency can be an issue in some patients with ACTH insensitivity. Low serum concentrations of ACTH, absence of hyperpigmentation, and the presence of associated features such as pale skin, red hair, diarrhea, and obesity (POMC/PC1 mutations) are important diagnostic clues.

The presence of multiple pituitary hormone deficiencies (e.g., GH, ACTH, TSH, gonadotropins, vasopressin, and PRL) may point to a diagnosis of multiple pituitary hormone deficiency, often in association with structural abnormalities of the pituitary gland, eye abnormalities, and forebrain abnormalities (septo-optic dysplasia). Signs such as those of congenital hypothyroidism, hypoglycemia, congenital hypogonadotropic hypogonadism (micropenis, undescended testes), and severe postnatal growth failure may be suggestive of the diagnosis. A number of single-gene defects have now been associated with congenital hypopituitarism (e.g., mutations in HESX1, SOX3, OTX2, GLI2, ARNT2, LHX3, LHX4, PROP1).[43,99,146] Occasionally, ACTH insufficiency may not be present at the time of diagnosis but may develop progressively with time.

Recessive mutations in the T-box factor TPIT (TBX19) have been identified in patients with severe, early-onset isolated ACTH deficiency with profound hypoglycemia, prolonged jaundice, and sudden neonatal death.[77] TPIT is required for the specification, maturation, and maintenance of both precorticotroph and premelanotroph populations and for the suppression of gonadotroph fate. It is also required to activate the expression of POMC in conjunction with the transcription factor PTX1. Murine transgenesis resulted in ACTH and glucocorticoid deficiencies, adrenal hypoplasia, and pigmentation defects in mice deleted for *TPit*.[77] Sixty-five percent of patients with severe congenital isolated ACTH deficiency are found to have *TBX19* mutations, but mutations are not found in partial or later-onset ACTH deficiency.[147]

ACTH resistance can occur in a number of well-defined entities, such as defects in the ACTH receptor (melanocortin 2 receptor [MC2R], familial glucocorticoid deficiency [FGD] type 1), in MC2R accessory protein (MRAP, FGD type 2), or as part of the triple-A syndrome (alacrimia, achalasia, addisonism; also known as Allgrove syndrome, caused by defects in ALADIN/*AAAS*). These disorders are characterized by isolated glucocorticoid deficiency, hyperpigmentation, and markedly elevated concentrations of ACTH.[148,149] Nevertheless, approximately 15% of individuals with triple-A syndrome have evidence of mineralocorticoid insufficiency, those with the most severe loss of function manifesting hyponatremia on presentation. Recently, mutations in *NNT* (nicotinamide nucleotide transhydrogenase), *GPX1* (glutathione peroxidase 1), and *MCM4* (mini-chromosome maintenance-deficient-4 homologue) have been found as a cause of FGD.[150-152] Mutations in *MCM4* were found in an Irish traveler community and result in late-onset, less severe glucocorticoid deficiency, short stature, and natural killer cell deficiency due to increased chromosomal breakage. Mutations in *GPX1* and *NNT*, involved in detoxification of reactive oxygen species, can also result in FGD.[153]

Primary adrenal failure may be caused by congenital adrenal hypoplasia (or AHC).[154] This results in severe salt-losing primary adrenal failure in early infancy or childhood, although milder, delayed-onset forms of the condition exist. The most common form of the condition is X-linked. Patients have mutations in the nuclear receptor DAX1 *(NROB1)*, and in addition to adrenal failure, the males suffer from hypogonadotropic hypogonadism. Rarely, patients present with isolated mineralocorticoid deficiency with normal cortisol concentrations; however, glucocorticoid deficiency usually develops later. *DAX1* is expressed in ES cells, steroidogenic tissues (gonads and adrenals), the ventromedial hypothalamus (VMH), and pituitary gonadotrophs. It acts as a transcriptional repressor of other nuclear receptor pathways but is also involved in maintenance of pluripotency of stem cells.[155]

Heterozygous and homozygous mutations in SF1 have been associated with adrenal failure in 46,XY phenotypic females, as well as in at least one 46,XX girl, although the latter phenotype is rare.[154] Mutations in SF1 have also been associated with gonadal dysgenesis in 46,XY individuals in the absence of adrenal insufficiency.[156] Additionally, SF1 mutations have been associated with primary ovarian failure, but this is rare.[157,158]

Various forms of congenital adrenal hyperplasia may be associated with variable adrenal failure (e.g., mutations in *CYP11A1*, *StAR*, *HSD3B2*, *CYP17*, *CYP21A2*, *CYP11B1*) with varying degrees of genital ambiguity. The enzyme P450c11 (aldosterone synthase), which is found in the ZG, has 11β-hydroxylase, 18-hydroxylase, and 18-methyloxidase activities and catalyzes all the reactions needed to convert 11-deoxycorticosterone (DOC) to aldosterone. Mutations in the gene encoding the enzyme are associated with isolated mineralocorticoid deficiency. Functional mineralocorticoid deficiency with severe salt loss resulting in hyponatremia and hyperkalemia may also arise as a result of mutations in the MR or in the gene encoding the epithelial sodium channel (ENaC).

Thyroid System
Embryology

The thyroid gland is a derivative of the primitive buccopharyngeal cavity and develops from contributions of two anlagen: a midline thickening of the pharyngeal floor (median anlage) that acts as the precursor of the T_4-producing follicular cells and paired caudal extensions of the fourth pharyngobranchial pouches (lateral anlagen) that give rise to the parafollicular calcitonin-secreting cells (C cells).[159,160] These structures are discernible by 16 to 17 days of gestation, and by 24 days the median anlage develops a thin, flask-like diverticulum extending from the floor of the buccal cavity, at a point that is later known as the *foramen cecum* on the developing tongue, to the fourth branchial arch. At 24 to 32 days, this median anlage has already become a bilobed structure, and by 50 days of gestation, the median and lateral anlagen have fused and the buccal stalk has ruptured.

During this period, the thyroid gland, which initially consists of a round cluster of cells, migrates caudally from the pharyngeal floor, through the anterior midline of the neck, to its definitive location in the anterior neck; during this time, the cells multiply. Data suggest that localization of growing thyroid tissue along the anteroposterior axis is linked to the development of the ventral aorta in the zebrafish; in other words, vessels provide guidance cues in zebrafish thyroid morphogenesis.[161] In mouse thyroid development, the midline primordium bifurcates and two lobes relocalize cranially along the bilateral pair of carotid arteries. In *Shh*-deficient mice, thyroid tissue always develops along the ectopically and asymmetrically positioned carotid arteries, suggesting that in mice, as in zebrafish, codeveloping arteries define the presence of the thyroid.[161]

Additionally, Fagman and colleagues[162] implicated *Tbx1* in the development of the thyroid gland, although it cannot be detected in the thyroid primordium at any embryonic stage. In *Tbx1*[-/-] mice, the downward translocation of *Titf1/Nkx2.1*-expressing thyroid progenitor cells is much delayed. In late mutant embryos, the thyroid fails to form symmetric lobes but persists as a single mass that is approximately one quarter of the normal size. The hypoplastic gland mostly attains a unilateral position resembling thyroid hemiagenesis. The data suggest that failure of the thyroid primordium to reestablish contact with the aortic sac is a major factor in the prevention of normal growth of the midline anlage along the third pharyngeal arch arteries. This interaction may be facilitated by *Tbx1*-expressing mesenchyme filling the gap between the pharyngeal endoderm and the detached thyroid primordium.[162] Conditional ablation of *Fgf8* in *Tbx1*-expressing cells caused an early thyroid phenotype similar to that of *Tbx1*[-/-] mice. In addition, expression of an *Fgf8* complementary DNA in the *Tbx1* domain rescued the early size defect of the thyroid primordium in *Tbx1* mutants. These data suggest that a *Tbx1-Fgf8* pathway in the pharyngeal mesoderm is a key regulator of mammalian thyroid development.[162]

At 51 days, the gland exhibits its definitive external form, with an isthmus connecting the two lateral lobes, and it reaches its final position below the thyroid cartilage by the 7th week of embryonic life in humans. At the same time, connection of the median anlage with the ultimobranchial body, developed from the endoderm of the fourth pharyngeal pouch, occurs, resulting in incorporation of the C cells into the thyroid. During its descent, the developing thyroid gland retains an attachment to the pharynx by a narrow epithelial stalk known as the thyroglossal duct.[163] By 37 days, this structure that connects the median thyroid anlage with the point of origin of its migration on the floor of the pharynx has usually disappeared,[164] and normally the only remnant of the thyroglossal duct is the foramen cecum itself. An ectopic thyroid and persistent thyroglossal duct or cyst may occur as a consequence of abnormalities of thyroid descent.

Usually, the terminal differentiation of thyroid follicular cells—as evidenced by expression of the genes encoding the TSH receptor *(TSHR)*, the sodium-iodide symporter *(NIS)*, thyroglobulin *(TG)*, and thyroid peroxidase *(TPO)* and the formation of follicles—occurs in the normal embryo only after migration is complete.[165] Gene expression studies performed on thyroid tissues derived from human embryos and fetuses showed that *TITF1, FOXE1, PAX8, TSHR,* and *DUOX2* were stably expressed from the 7th to the 33rd gestational weeks.[166-169] Genes encoding thyroglobulin (Tg), TPO, and pendrin were expressed as early as 7 weeks' gestational age. NIS expression appeared last. Immunohistochemical studies detected TITF1, TSHR, and Tg in unpolarized thyrocytes before follicle formation. T_4 and NIS labeling were found in developing follicles from the 11th gestational week onward. These studies suggest a key role for NIS in the onset of human thyroid function.[166]

By 70 days of gestation, colloid is visible histologically, and Tg synthesis and iodide accumulation can be demonstrated within the gland. During the final follicular phase of development, colloid spaces increase in size, and there is progressive cell growth and accumulation of thyroid hormones. Terminal differentiation of the human thyroid is characterized by the onset of follicle formation and thyroid hormone synthesis at 11 weeks' gestation. At 12 weeks of gestation, the fetal thyroid gland weighs about 80 mg, and at term it weighs 1 to 1.5 g. The parathyroid glands develop between 5 and 12 weeks of gestation from the third and fourth pharyngeal pouches.

At least five developmental genes are involved in thyroid and parathyroid gland embryogenesis. These include the genes for thyroid transcription factors HEX, TTF1 (*Titf1/Nkx2.1*), FOXE1 (*Titf2/Foxe1*), NKX2-5, and PAX8 (Fig. 22-8).[160,167-170] *Hex$^{-/-}$* mice have thyroid agenesis or severe hypoplasia. *Ttf2* knockout results in thyroid dysgenesis and cleft palate. *Ttf1* knockout leads to pulmonary hypoplasia and thyroid agenesis. Inactivating *Pax8* mutations lead to thyroid hypoplasia and renal anomalies. *Ttf1* knockout is also associated with parafollicular C-cell aplasia. The *HOX* genes appear to be important in the expression of *Ttf1* and *Pax8*. *HOX15* gene disruption in mice results in parathyroid gland aplasia.[171] *TTF1/NKX2-1* and *PAX8* also play a role in the survival of thyroid cell precursors and regulation of thyroid-specific gene expression, whereas *FOXE1/TTF2* is critical for cellular migration. Overexpression of the transcription factors Nkx2-1 and PAX8 is sufficient to direct mouse embryonic stem cell (mESC) differentiation into thyroid follicular cells that organized into three-dimensional follicular structures when treated with TSH.[172]

TTF1, TTF2, PAX8, NKX2-5, SHH, TBX1, and *TSHR* gene mutations account for fewer than 10% of patients with familial thyroid dysgenesis and congenital hypothyroidism; no mutations have been identified in *HEX* as yet.[169] Most cases of congenital hypothyroidism occur sporadically, and the pathogenesis in these cases remains unclear. It is known that signaling molecules such as those in the FGF pathway and the SHH pathway are also implicated in murine thyroid development.[171] In late organogenesis, the *SHH* gene appears to have an important role in the symmetric bilobation of the thyroid; it also suppresses the ectopic expression of thyroid follicular cells.[161] Congenital hypothyroidism appears to be increasing in incidence

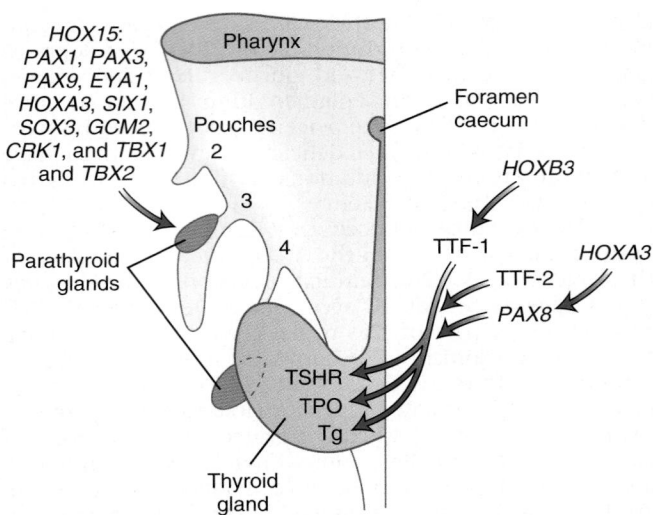

Figure 22-8 Homeobox genes that program development of the thyroid and parathyroid glands. *HEX* is involved early in the integrated cascade that programs thyroid gland embryogenesis. *HOXB3* and *HOXA3* may be responsible for activation of thyroid transcription factors TTF-1 and TTF-2, respectively, during early embryogenesis. *PAX8* is essential in the cascade. These factors are also involved in thyroid follicular cell function, promoting thyroglobulin (Tg), thyroid peroxidase (TPO), and thyroid-stimulating hormone receptor (TSHR) gene transcription. *HOX15* gene knockout in mice causes parathyroid gland aplasia. See text for details.

(from 1:2900 to 1:2450 in Canada), but this is due to increased stringency of screening strategies, and the greatest increase has been in mildly affected children with normal location of the thyroid.[173]

In the rat, at fetal day 15, despite early evidence of *Tg, TPO,* and *TSHR* gene expression, the thyroid gland is difficult to distinguish from the surrounding structures, and iodine organification, thyroid hormonogenesis, and evidence of a follicular structure are absent. Expression of the *TSHR* gene is significantly upregulated on fetal day 17, and this is accompanied by significant growth and rapid development in terms of structure and function. The expression of *Tg* and *TPO* is increased, and thyroid follicles are seen with thyroid hormonogenesis, suggesting that the TSHR has an important role to play in these events. Murine mutation of the *TSHR* gene is associated with the *hyt/hyt* phenotype in mice, which exhibits severe hypothyroidism and a hypoplastic but normally located thyroid gland with a poorly developed follicular structure. In humans, a similar phenotype is observed in babies of mothers with potent TSHR-blocking antibodies and in babies with severe loss-of-function mutations in *TSHR*.

Embryogenesis is largely complete by 10 to 12 weeks' gestation, equivalent to fetal day 15 to 17 in the rat, and thyroid follicle precursors are first seen at this stage. Tg is also detected in follicular spaces, and evidence of iodine uptake and organification is obtained at this stage. Pituitary and plasma TSH concentrations begin to increase during the second trimester in the human fetus, at about the time that pituitary portal vascular continuity develops (Fig. 22-9).[166,174] Plasma TSH concentrations increase progressively during the last half of gestation. Plasma concentrations of T_4-binding globulin and total T_4 increase progressively, from low levels at 16 to 18 weeks of gestation to maximal levels at 35 to 40 weeks. Free T_4 concentrations also increase as a consequence of the increase in T_4 production. The increases in plasma TSH and T_4 concentrations during the third trimester reflect a progressive maturation of hypothalamic pituitary control and of thyroid gland

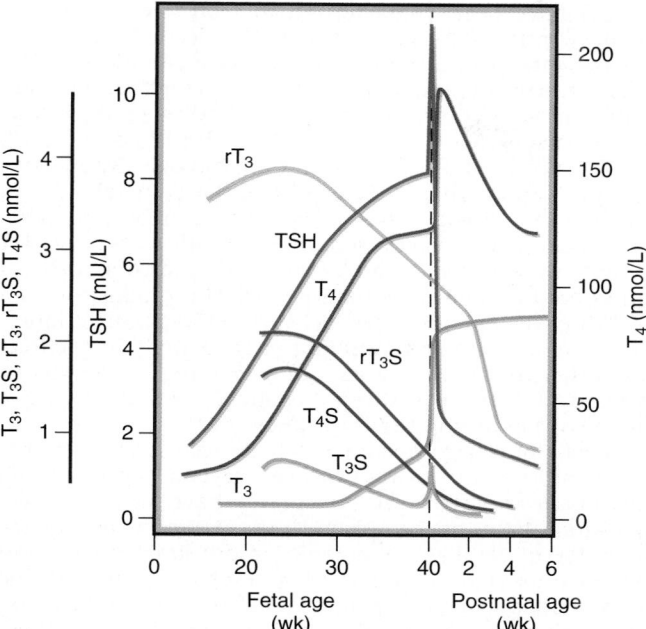

Figure 22-9 Patterns of change of fetal plasma thyroid-stimulating hormone (TSH), thyroxine (T$_4$), triiodothyronine (T$_3$), reverse T$_3$ (rT$_3$), and iodothyronine sulfates (T$_4$S, rT$_3$S, and T$_3$S) during gestation and in the neonatal period. The patterns for T$_4$S and rT$_3$S are based on limited 30-week data. (Data from Roti[175] and Fisher DA, Klein AH. Thyroid development and disorders of thyroid function in the newborn. *N Engl J Med.* 1981;304:702-712; Santini F, Chiovato L, Ghirri P, et al. Serum iodothyronines in the human fetus and the newborn: evidence for an important role of placenta in fetal thyroid hormone homeostasis. *J Clin Endocrinol Metab.* 1999;84:493-498.)

responsiveness to TSH. Pituitary TSH secretion is responsive to hypothyroxinemia and to TRH early in the third trimester.[169] Hypothyroxinemia results in an elevated fetal serum TSH concentration, whereas hyperthyroidism due to maternal Graves disease is associated with a suppressed fetal TSH concentration. Premature infants born at 26 to 28 weeks of gestation respond to exogenous TRH with an increase in plasma TSH concentration comparable to that in adults.[175] However, their TSH response to extrauterine exposure is reduced, indicating hypothalamic immaturity. Neonatal free T$_4$ increments are reduced (compared with term infants) in premature infants born at 31 to 34 weeks, attenuated at 28 to 30 weeks, and absent in 23- to 27-week-old infants, reflecting a relative hypothalamic-pituitary-thyroid system immaturity, inversely correlated in severity with gestational age.[176] Age-specific changes in thyroid function in children who are small for gestational age and who are normal birth weight from birth to adulthood are available.[177] Several patterns of thyroid dysfunction can occur in preterm neonates. Transient hypothyroxinemia of prematurity is identified by a low free T$_4$ and normal TSH and is seen in 50% of preterms born before 28 weeks and does not require treatment. Indeed, treatment has been associated with a lower IQ (intelligence quotient) in more mature infants. Very low birth weight (VLBW) infants have a higher risk of primary hypothyroidism and can exhibit a pattern of delayed TSH rise, although in a considerable number of these infants the hypothyroidism is transient. When primary hypothyroidism is suspected, thyroid hormone treatment should be instituted. Once treatment has been instituted, it should continue at least until thyroid hormone–dependent brain maturation has completed at approximately 3 years of age, when thyroid function can be reassessed. In addition, preterm infants are at risk of

hypothyroidism due to iodine excess, for example, from iodine-containing antiseptic and contrast agents. Preterm infants are also at risk of iodine deficiency because they have small iodine stores; fetal iodine stores are laid down in the third trimester, and enteral and parenteral forms of nutrition contain little iodine. Nonthyroidal illness also leads to thyroid function alterations, often with low T$_4$, T$_3$, and TSH, and again, treatment is not indicated but repeat testing every 1 to 2 weeks until normal thyroid function is achieved is recommended.[173,178]

Thyroid Hormonogenesis

Hypothalamic-pituitary-thyroid control matures during an interval corresponding to the late third trimester and early neonatal period of human development.[174,179] The period of parallel increases in fetal TSH and free T$_4$ concentrations during the latter half of gestation is followed by the sequential TSH and free T$_4$ surges in the early neonatal period and a final slow equilibration of the TSH/free T$_4$ ratio to adult values during infancy and childhood.[176,177,179,180] This maturation includes coordinated maturation of hypothalamic TRH secretion, pituitary TRH sensitivity, TSH negative-feedback control, and thyroid follicular cell responsiveness to TSH. Fetal serum TRH levels are higher than in maternal blood as a consequence of extrahypothalamic (placenta and pancreas) TRH production and decreased TRH degradation in fetal serum. Functionally, the fetus progresses from a state of both primary (thyroidal) and tertiary (hypothalamic) hypothyroidism at midgestation, through a state of mild tertiary hypothyroidism during the final weeks in utero, to a fully mature hypothalamic-pituitary-thyroid axis by 2 months after birth.

The adult thyroid follicular cell can modify iodine transport or uptake with changes in dietary iodine intake, independent of variations in serum TSH concentrations.[181,182] Before 36 to 40 weeks of gestation, the thyroid gland lacks this autoregulatory mechanism and is susceptible to iodine-induced inhibition of thyroid hormone synthesis.[175,182] The fetal thyroid follicular cell, when exposed to high circulating levels of iodide, is unable to reduce iodide trapping and prevent the high intracellular iodide concentrations that produce the blockade of hormone synthesis referred to as the *Wolff-Chaikoff effect*. Failure of the immature thyroid to exhibit autoregulation is probably due to failure of downregulation of thyroid cell membrane NIS units, which may be related to the absence or reduced iodination of an 8- to 10-kDa protein in the thyroid follicular cell.[181,182] In addition to maturation of autoregulation, thyroidal responsiveness to TSH increases during the last trimester.[160]

The metabolism of thyroid hormones occurs through a progressive series of monodeiodinations.[174,183] Three deiodinase enzymes act to remove an iodine atom from the outer (phenolic) ring or the inner (tyrosyl) ring of the tetraiodothyronine (T$_4$) molecule, thus, respectively, activating or inactivating the hormone. The deiodinases are encoded by separate genes and share sequence homology. Most of the circulating biologically active T$_3$ in adults is derived by outer-ring monodeiodination of T$_4$ in liver and other nonthyroidal tissues; biologically inactive rT$_3$ derives from inner-ring deiodination of T$_4$ in peripheral tissues. The type I enzyme (D1), an outer-ring monodeiodinase, is a high–Michaelis constant (K$_m$) enzyme inhibited by propylthiouracil and stimulated by thyroid hormone. It deiodinates T$_4$ to T$_3$ and rT$_3$ to T$_2$. D1 also has inner-ring deiodinase activity, converting T$_3$ to T$_2$. Activity of D1 is low throughout gestation. The type 2 outer-ring monodeiodinase (D2) is a low-K$_m$ enzyme that is insensitive to propylthiouracil and inhibited by thyroid hormone. It deiodinates T_4 to T_3 and rT_3 to T_2, and it is highly expressed in brain and pituitary. Type 3 monodeiodinase (D3) inactivates T_4 and T_3 via inner-ring deiodination of T_4 to rT_3 and of T_3 to T_2; it is highly expressed in fetal tissues and placenta. D1 is largely responsible for the production of T_3 that escapes from the cells, especially liver and kidney, into the circulation, whereas D2 is responsible for the production of local tissue T_3. Inactive rT_3 also diffuses out of most tissues to appear in plasma.

Iodothyronine deiodinases belong to a family of selenoproteins. Selenium is an essential trace element required for the biosynthesis of selenoproteins. Selenocysteine insertion sequence (SECIS) binding protein 2 (SBP2) represents a key factor for the insertion of selenocysteine into selenoproteins. Recently, mutations in the *SBP2* gene have been described that lead to a multisystem disorder with deficiencies of multiple selenoproteins, resulting in growth retardation, myopathy and skin photosensitivity, nonketotic hypoglycemia, colitis, and infertility.[184,185] Due to abnormal D2 activity, T_3 is low, T_4 and rT_3 are increased, and TSH is slightly elevated. As selenoproteins also serve as antioxidants, tissue damage may be related to increased concentrations of reactive oxygen species (ROS).[185,186]

The distribution of the deiodinases has been characterized in rodent and human tissues (Table 22-3).[183] D2 is detectable by midgestation and plays an important role in supplying T_3 to developing brain tissue, regulating thermogenesis in brown adipose tissue in the neonatal period, and regulating pituitary TSH secretion. D3 activity is present in placenta, liver, and perhaps fetal skin, accounting for the higher concentrations of rT_3 in the fetus and limiting the metabolic effects of thyroid hormones during much of fetal life. There is little conversion of T_4 to circulating T_3 via D1 deiodination until midgestation in the human fetus; plasma T_3 concentrations are low (<0.2 nmol/L or <15 ng/dL) until 30 weeks of gestation, after which the mean value increases to 0.7 nmol/L (50 ng/dL) at term (see Fig. 22-7).[187] On the other hand, fetal brain T_3 concentrations are 60% to 80% of those in the adult by fetal age 20 to 26 weeks owing to D2 activity. In the presence of fetal hypothyroidism, D2 increases while D3 decreases in an effort to maintain near-normal brain T_3 concentrations.

Sulfation is active in fetal tissues, and the predominant thyroid hormone metabolites in the fetus are iodothyronine sulfates.[174,188,189] High levels of phenolsulfotransferases (SULT) have been characterized in fetal liver, lung, and brain by midgestation. SULT activities decrease rapidly in the neonatal period.[189] In the last third of gestation in fetal sheep, the mean plasma production rates for T_4 and metabolites (in micrograms per kilogram of body weight per day) are as follows: T_4, 40; T_4 sulfate (T_4S), 10; rT_3, 5; rT_3S, 12; T_3, 2; and T_3S, 2. All metabolites are biologically inactive except T_3 and perhaps T_3S, so 90% of the T_4 metabolites in the fetus are biologically inactive.[188] The sulfated metabolites accumulate in fetal serum as a result of the low D1 activity in fetal tissues and because the sulfated iodothyronines are not substrates for D3.[181,188] The production rate of T_3 increases progressively between 30 weeks of gestation and term because of maturation of D1 activity in the liver and other tissues and because of decreasing D3 activity in placenta.[160,190] In fetal sheep, hepatic D1 activity increases progressively during the last trimester.[191]

It has long been assumed that thyroid hormones passively diffuse into cells. However, several classes of cell membrane iodothyronine transporters have been described, questioning this hypothesis.[192-194] These transporters belong to different families of organic anion, amino acid, and monocarboxylate solute carriers, including the organic anion transporting polypeptide (OATP) family and the solute carrier family 21 (SLC21).[192-194] The significance of these transporters is not yet clear, but mutation of the human monocarboxylate transporter 8 (MCT8), a member of the SLC21 family shown to be a specific thyroid hormone transporter present in developing brain, leads to a syndrome of combined thyroid dysfunction and psychomotor retardation (X-linked Allan-Herndon-Dudley syndrome).[193,194] *Mct8* expression in neonatal mice has been localized to neurons in the olfactory bulb, cerebral cortex, hippocampus, and amygdala. Presumably, all thyroid hormone–sensitive cell populations express iodothyronine membrane transporters. A cell surface T_4 receptor has been characterized as an $\alpha_V\beta_3$ integrin that serves as the initiation site for T_4-induced activation of the mitogen-activated protein kinase (MAPK) pathway for angiogenesis and perhaps actin polymerization and neuronal migration.[195] The ontogenesis and significance of these cell surface receptors and membrane transporters in fetal development remain to be further defined. Recent studies have suggested that MCT8 is also required for normal thyroid hormone secretion, in addition to its role as a thyroid hormone transporter.[196]

Thyroid Hormone Action

Classic thyroid hormone actions are mediated via functional thyroid hormone nuclear receptors (TRs), members of the steroid/retinoid/vitamin D family of nuclear transcription factors. Two genes code for the receptors: *THRA* on chromosome 17 encodes TRα, and *THRB* on chromosome 3 encodes TRβ.[197] These genes code for four classic receptor isoforms (TRα1, TRα2, TRβ1, and TRβ2), three of which bind thyroid hormones (T_3/T_4 affinity 10:1) and bind to DNA to effect gene transcription. The TRα2 isoform does not bind thyroid hormone but binds to DNA and can inhibit binding of other TRs. The TRs exist as monomers, homodimers, and heterodimers with other nuclear receptor family members such as retinoid X (RXR). Other TR transcripts, including TRΔα1 and TRΔα2, have been characterized; they do not bind DNA or T_3 but can inhibit TR and retinoid receptor activities.[198]

The TRs are expressed developmentally and differentially in various fetal and adult tissues. TRα proteins are present in most tissues. TRβ1 is expressed in liver, kidney, and lung and in developing brain, cochlea, and pituitary. TRβ2 expression is restricted largely to the pituitary gland,

TABLE 22-3

Deiodinase Expression in Human and Rodent Tissues

Tissue	D1	D2	D3
Brain	X	X	X
Pituitary	X	X	
Thyroid	X	X*	
Liver	X		X†
Kidney	X		
Ovary	X		X
Ear		X*	
Heart		X*	
Muscle		X†	
Skin		X	X
Testes		X	X
Uterus		X	X
Brown fat		X	

*Expressed in human only.
†Expressed only in fetus.
Modified from St. Germain DL, Hernandez A, Schneider MJ, et al. Insights into the role of deiodinases from studies of genetically modified animals. *Thyroid.* 2005;15:905-916.

TABLE 22-4
Predominant Thyroid Hormone Receptor Subtype Functions in Developing Mice

Brain	Thermogenesis
TRα1, TRβ1	TRα1, TRβ1, TRβ2
Pituitary TSH secretion	Inner ear
	TRα1, TRβ2
	TRβ2, TRα1
Pituitary GH secretion	Retina
	TRβ2
	TRα1
Bone maturation	Intestine
TRα1	TRα1
Liver	Heart
TRβ1	TRα1

GH, growth hormone; TR, thyroid hormone receptor; TSH, thyroid-stimulating hormone.

Modified from Yen P. Genomic and nongenomic actions of thyroid hormones. In: Braverman LE, Utiger RD, eds. *The Thyroid*, 9th ed. Philadelphia, PA: Lippincott Williams & Wilkins; 2005:135-150; and Flamant F, Samarut J. Thyroid hormone receptors: lessons from knockout and knockin mutant mice. *Trends Endocrinol Metab.* 2005;14:85-90; Ortiga-Carvalho TM, Sidhaye AR, Wondisford FE. Thyroid hormone receptors and resistance to thyroid hormone disorders. *Nat Rev Endocrinol.* 2014;10:582-591.

retina, and cochlea.[160,197] The receptors function redundantly, as indicated by knockout studies in mice, but predominant effects of one or another TR have been characterized (Table 22-4). Knockout of both the TRα and TRβ genes in mice is not lethal but results in elevated TSH concentrations, deafness, bradycardia, and decreased postnatal growth with delayed bone maturation.[160,197,198] Lethality occurs because of improper intestinal development associated with persistent TRΔα isoforms in TRα or combined TRα and TRβ knockout mice.[198] In the fetal rat brain, TRα1 mRNA and receptor binding are detectable by 12 to 14 days of gestation (term is 21 days), increasing to maximal levels at birth. The TRβ1 isoform is detected at birth and increases approximately 40-fold in the early postnatal period.[160,199] In human fetal brain, TRα1 and TRβ1 isoforms and receptor binding are present by 8 to 10 weeks of gestation; TRα1 transcripts and receptor occupancy increase 8- to 10-fold by 16 to 18 weeks.[160,200,201] Liver, heart, and lung receptor binding can be identified by 13 to 18 weeks.[160,201,202]

Heterozygous missense mutations in *THRA*, coding for the TRα1, have recently been described in association with short stature, developmental delay, and chronic constipation. The mutations act in a dominant negative fashion. The clinical phenotype is in line with the TRα1 being the predominant subtype receptor in bone, the gastrointestinal tract, cardiac and skeletal muscle, and the CNS.[203,204]

Ontogeny of Thyroid Hormone Secretion

The role of maternal thyroid hormone during fetal development remains controversial. The high placental concentration of D3 inactivates most of the thyroid hormone presented from the maternal circulation. The iodide released in this manner is used for fetal thyroid hormone synthesis. Despite the limited maternal-fetal placental transfer of T_4 and the predominant production of inactive thyroid hormone metabolites in the human fetus, significant levels of free T_4 are present in fetal fluids, from placental transfer early in gestation and from fetal thyroid production during later gestation.[160,199] Early in gestation, placental transfer is the only source of T_4 in fetal fluids and is essential for normal fetal neurodevelopment. T_4 is detectable in human celomic fluid at levels of 0.5 to 2 nmol/L between 6 and 11 weeks of gestation, before the onset of fetal thyroid function.[205] Low concentrations of T_4 are detectable in the fetal brain at about 10 weeks of gestation. Significant placental transfer continues to term, when serum T_4 levels in the athyroid fetus range from 30 to 70 nmol/L (2.3 to 5.4 µg/dL).[206] Isotopic equilibrium studies with pregnant rats at term suggest that 15% to 20% of the T_4 in fetal tissues is of maternal origin.[207] As indicated, thyroid hormones cross the placenta early in gestation, supplying the low levels of free T_4 that are essential for brain development between 12 and 20 weeks, before the onset of fetal thyroid hormone production.[199] Most thyroid hormone in the fetal compartment is inactivated to sulfated and deiodinated analogues until the perinatal period.[174,188,189] This neutralization of active circulating thyroid hormone maintains the low T_3 metabolic state, facilitating fetal growth and programmed tissue maturation.

Thyroid hormone–programmed development of selective fetal tissues requires the interaction of local tissue D1, D2, thyroid receptors, receptor coactivators, and thyroid-responsive genes. In most responsive tissues, the timing of maturation events is controlled by the state of the thyroid receptors acting as a molecular switch.[198,208] In the absence of T_3, the unliganded receptor (aporeceptor) recruits corepressors, repressing gene transcription. Non–T_3-binding receptors also can repress transcription by inhibiting receptor DNA binding. Local tissue maturation events are initiated by the coincident availability of T_3, liganded T_3 receptor, T_3-mediated receptor exchange of corepressor with coactivators for creation of an active holoreceptor, and activation of responsive gene transcription.

These programming events have been investigated in studies of transgenic mice, including brain, liver, heart, intestine, and bone tissues, thermogenesis, and spleen erythropoiesis.[208-214] The timing of these events in the mouse range from early midbrain neuronal development at gestational day 15; through perinatal activation of hepatic enzymes, cardiac ion channels, and spleen erythropoiesis; to postnatal brain, intestinal, and bone maturation and thermogenesis. Parturition occurs at a gestational age equivalent to human midgestation. In hypothyroid mice, repressive effects of aporeceptors have been shown to delay tissue maturation in brain, bone, intestine, spleen, and heart.[211] The increase in circulating T_3 levels associated with parturition in mice and humans normally triggers development of tissue functions essential to postnatal metabolism and homeostasis (e.g., hepatic, intestinal, and cardiac functions and brown fat thermogenesis). Thyroid hormone–stimulated maturation of vision and hearing appear to be triggered by the local expression of D2, mediating local T_3 production, postnatally in the mouse and probably toward the end of the second midtrimester in the human fetus.[183]

In humans, T_3-mediated maturation of fetal tissues, including liver, heart, brown adipose tissue, and bone, allows them to become thyroid hormone–responsive during late gestation and in the perinatal period. Paracrine actions of thyroid hormone are critical for normal fetal development—for example, in the cochlea, where D2 is expressed in connective tissue immediately adjacent to the sensory epithelium and spiral ganglion, where thyroid hormone receptors are located. This implies that D2-containing cells in the connective tissue take up T_4 from the circulation, convert it to T_3, and then release D3 to adjacent responsive cells. Similarly, in the brain, D2 is expressed predominantly in glial cells, whereas TRs are expressed in adjacent neurons and oligodendrocytes. In other areas of the brain, such as the pituitary gland, hippocampus, and caudate nucleus, there is coexpression of

D2 and TRs. On the other hand, D3 is coexpressed with TRs in neurons, thereby protecting sensitive tissues from the effects of excess thyroid hormone.

The actions of thyroid hormones and their developmental regulation in the brain are complex. Functionally, thyroid hormones are critical for the establishment of neural circuits during a critical window of brain development. They provide inductive cues for the differentiation and maturation of a number of processes such as neurogenesis and neural cell migration (occurring between 5 and 24 weeks of gestation), neuronal differentiation, dendritic and axonal growth, synaptogenesis (late fetal period to 6 months postpartum), myelination (second trimester to 24 months postpartum), and neurotransmitter enzyme synthesis. TRs are found in highest concentration in developing neurons and in multiple areas of the fetal brain, including the cerebrum, the cerebellum, and the auditory and visual cortices. The hormones bind to receptors and stimulate a number of genes such as myelin, neurotropins and their receptors, cytoskeletal components, transcription factors, extracellular matrix proteins and adhesion molecules, intracellular signaling molecules, and mitochondrial and cerebellar genes.

Thyroid hormone is also important for normal bone growth. T_3 regulates endochondral ossification and controls chondrocyte differentiation in the growth plate both in vivo and in vitro. TRs are expressed on osteoblasts and growth plate chondrocytes, and T_3 target genes have been identified in bone. T_3 stimulates skull suture closure in vivo.[215]

In the perinatal period, thyroid hormone stimulates the transcription of thermogenin (also known as uncoupling protein 1 [UCP1]), a protein that uncouples nucleotide phosphorylation and the storage of energy as adenosine triphosphate (ATP), actions that are important for nonshivering thermogenesis by brown adipose tissue.

Congenital Hypothyroidism

Classic signs of congenital hypothyroidism (jaundice, lethargy, feeding difficulties, macroglossia, myxedema, hypothermia, growth retardation, and progressive developmental delay and IQ deterioration) accrue during the early weeks and months of extrauterine life as maternal T_4 becomes unavailable and the non-CNS tissues become responsive to thyroid hormone.[160,174] Rarely, hypothyroidism is associated with respiratory distress in the neonatal period. Maternal hypothyroxinemia has been associated with attention deficit/hyperactivity disorder and with 5 to 10 points of IQ deficit in the offspring of such pregnancies.[15,160,199] The period of brain dependency for thyroid hormone extends postnatally to 2 to 3 years of age, but the early weeks and months of life are most critical. Untreated thyroid agenesis is associated with a loss of 5 to 7 IQ points monthly during the first months of postnatal life, and over 6 to 8 months this can amount to a 30- to 40-point IQ deficit.[199] Most countries, therefore, have a rigorous screening program to ensure early diagnosis and treatment.

In congenital hypothyroidism, there is an increased net flux of maternal thyroid hormone to the fetus, resulting in cord T_4 concentrations that are 25% to 50% of normal. There is increasing evidence of maternal-fetal T_4 transfer in the first half of pregnancy, when fetal thyroid hormone levels are low.[216] The transplacental passage of thyroid hormone, in conjunction with adjustments in brain deiodinase activity, has a critical role in minimizing the adverse effects of fetal hypothyroidism and helps explain the normal or near-normal outcome of hypothyroid fetuses (provided that prompt and adequate treatment of hypo-

thyroidism ensues postnatally) as well as the relatively normal clinical appearance of the majority of babies with congenital hypothyroidism at birth. On the other hand, in the presence of both maternal and fetal hypothyroidism—such as that observed in the presence of potent TSHR–blocking antibodies, maternal and fetal POU1F1 deficiency, and severe iodine deficiency—there is severe neurocognitive impairment despite early and adequate commencement of thyroid replacement. Importantly, the presence of maternal hypothyroxinemia or inadequately controlled hypothyroidism is also associated with significant neurocognitive deficit in the offspring that is not reversible by early postnatal therapy.[15,217] Table 22-5 shows mechanisms resulting in congenital hypothyroidism due to abnormal thyroid development, dyshormonogenesis, abnormal thyroid hormone transport or action, and genes involved in these mechanisms.[173,218] International guidelines for treatment of congenital hypothyroidism are available.[219]

Pituitary-Gonadal Axis

The mammalian gonad originates from the intermediate mesoderm from which the bipotential genital ridge differentiates. The gonad is derived from two tissue anlagen:

TABLE 22-5
Mechanisms Involved in Congenital Hypothyroidism

Thyroid dysgenesis (1 in 4500)
Isolated thyroid aplasia, hemiagenesis, hypoplasia, or ectopy
  Transcription factor defect (PAX8)
  Unknown*
Associated with other developmental abnormalities
  Transcription factor defect (TTF-1, FOXE1 [TTF-2], NKX2-5, SHH, Tbx1)
Inborn errors of thyroid hormonogenesis (1 in 35,000)
Abnormal iodide uptake via Na-I transporter (NIS, SLC5A5)
Abnormal concentration of iodine
Abnormal organification of iodine
Abnormal iodination of thyroglobulin catalyzed by thyroid peroxidase (TPO)
Abnormal H_2O_2 generation (THOX, DUOX2, DUOXA2)
Efflux of iodide into colloid via apical anion channel (Pendred syndrome, SLC26A4)
Defective thyroglobulin synthesis or transport
Abnormal iodotyrosine deiodinase (DEHAL1)
Abnormal thyroid hormone transport in the brain (MCT8)
Abnomal selenium incorporation (SECISBP2)
Secondary and tertiary hypothyroidism (1 in 50,000 to 100,000)
Hypothalamic abnormality
  Isolated TRH deficiency
  Multiple hypothalamic hormone deficiencies
  Isolated hypothalamic defect
  Associated with other midline facial/brain dysmorphic features (e.g., SOD, cleft lip/palate)
Pituitary abnormality
  Isolated TSH deficiency (IGSF1)
  TRH resistance
  Abnormal TSHβ molecule
  Multiple pituitary hormone deficiencies
  Posterior pituitary eutopic (transcription factor defect, e.g., POU1F-1, PROP1, LHX3)
  Posterior pituitary ectopic (idiopathic, transcription factor defect, e.g., HESX1, SOX3, LHX4, OTX2)
TSH resistance
TSH receptor gene mutation (TSHR)
Postreceptor defect?
$G_s\alpha$ gene mutation (GNAS)
Thyroid hormone resistance (1 in 100,000)

*Most common.

the primordial germ cells of the yolk sac wall and the somatic, stromal cells that migrate from the primitive mesonephros.[220,221] By 4 to 5 weeks of gestation, the germ cells have begun their migration from the yolk sac, and the gonadal ridge has appeared as a derivative of the mesonephros. The germ cells are incorporated into the developing gonadal ridge during the 6th week, when the primitive gonad is composed of a surface epithelium, primitive gonadal cords continuous with the epithelium, and a dense cellular mass referred to as the *gonadal blastema*, which includes the steroidogenic cell precursors.[220]

Until the appearance of testicular cords made up of Sertoli cells at 6 weeks, the fetal testis and ovary are indistinguishable. Embryogenesis of the gonads is programmed by genes encoding the male sexual determinant SRY as well as SF1, SOX9, and DAX1.[222,223] SRY is a critical regulator of male gonadal differentiation. Three other genes—*WT1*, *SOX9*, and *SF1*—are expressed in the bipotential gonadal ridge during its differentiation from the intermediate mesoderm and are critical for normal male sexual differentiation. *WT1*, the Wilms tumor suppressor gene located at 11p13, is expressed in both the primitive kidney and the genital ridge. Its expression is related to the transition from mesenchyme to epithelium. WT1 is a transcription factor that contains four zinc fingers and binds to an EGR1 consensus binding sequence. It is a zinc finger DNA-binding protein that acts as a transcriptional activator or repressor, depending on the cellular or chromosomal context. Alternative splicing results in several WT1 isoforms that contain or lack a KTS sequence and have separate functions. WT1 isoforms associate and synergize with SF1 to promote expression of AMH. WT1 missense mutations associated with 46,XY DSD in Denys-Drash syndrome fail to synergize with SF1.[224] In addition, WT1 binds to and activates the SRY promoter.

SF1 is required for testicular and ovarian development and mediates müllerian-inhibiting hormone (AMH) gene expression and gonadotropin production. SF1 and DAX1 are orphan receptors of the steroid/thyroid hormone family of nuclear receptors and appear to interact as heterodimers coordinately involved in the regulation of target genes in the adrenal glands and in hypothalamic gonadotroph cells and the ventromedial hypothalamic nucleus.[222,223] Both SF1 and DAX1 are required for normal gonadal development. SF1 also regulates the expression of the cytochrome P450 enzymes. Recent data suggest that SRY binds to multiple elements within a SOX9 gonad-specific enhancer in mice and that it does so along with SF1. SF1 and SRY cooperatively upregulate SOX9; then, together with SF1, SOX9 also binds to the enhancer to help maintain its own expression after that of SRY has declined.[225]

The expression of SRY is transcriptionally regulated by WT1, SF1, GATA-4 and its cofactor zinc finger protein FOG-2 (also called ZFPM2), and chromobox protein homolog 2 (CBX2).[226] SRY is thought to have evolved from SOX3. Loss-of-function mutations of *SOX3* do not affect sex determination, but *SOX3* overexpression in murine XX gonads leads to testis differentiation, and in humans, *SOX3* duplication or rearrangements of the *SOX3* regulatory region have been found in 46,XX individuals with dysgenetic testes.[227]

INSL3 and its G protein–coupled receptor relaxin family peptide receptor 2 (RXFP2) play a role in testicular descent. Insl3 is produced in Leydig cells, is secreted in the circulation, and may prove to be a biomarker of Leydig cell function. Rare mutations have been described in cryptorchidism.[228,229]

In the presence of SRY, male gonadal differentiation begins at 7 weeks of gestation with organization of the gonadal blastema into interstitium and germ cell–containing testicular cords. The primitive cords lose their connections with the epithelium, primitive Sertoli cells and spermatogonia become visible within the cords, and the epithelium differentiates to form the tunica albuginea.[230] Leydig cells derived from the undifferentiated interstitium are visible by the end of the 8th week of gestation and are capable of androgen synthesis at that time. By 14 weeks of gestation, these cells make up as much as 50% of the cell mass, but as the tubules develop, they account for a smaller percentage of the tissue. The fetal testes grow from approximately 20 mg at 14 weeks of gestation to 800 mg at birth; at 5 to 6 months they descend into the inguinal canal in association with the epididymis and the ductus deferens.[230] The gonad, adrenal gland, and kidney all initially develop in close proximity, and as the testes descend, they may carry rests of adrenocortical cells with them. These adrenal rests may become hyperplastic with resulting testicular enlargement if subjected to prolonged ACTH stimulation (e.g., in patients with poorly controlled congenital adrenal hyperplasia). In the mouse, testicular descent is regulated by Insl3, which is a member of the insulin-like family and is secreted by Leydig cells.[231] Targeted disruption of the *Insl3* gene is associated with maldevelopment of the gubernaculum and bilateral cryptorchidism.[231] *Insl3* is also secreted by theca cells of the postnatal ovary, and females homozygous for *Insl3* mutations are subfertile with deregulation of the estrous cycle.

In human females, differentiation of ovaries begins during the 7th week of gestation, in the absence of *SRY*. The gonadal blastema differentiates into interstitium and medullary cords containing the primitive germ cells, referred to as *oogonia*. The cords degenerate, and cortical layers of surface epithelium, containing individual small oogonia, appear. By 11 to 12 weeks of gestation, clusters of dividing oogonia are surrounded by cord cells within the cortex; the medulla at this time consists largely of connective tissue.[232] At 12 weeks of gestation, primitive granulosa cells begin to replicate, and many of the large oogonia in the deepest layers of the cortex enter their first meiotic division. Primordial follicles are first observed at about 18 weeks of gestation, and the number increases rapidly thereafter.[233] However, the number of oocytes progressively declines, from a peak of 3 million to 6 million at 5 months' gestation to approximately 2 million at term.[20,233] Germ cell proliferation and apoptosis are ongoing simultaneously. Proliferating oocytes cluster, but the clusters break down with the development of follicles because only those oocytes enfolded by developing granulosa cells (as primordial follicles) survive.[20,233] From 5 months of gestation, stroma-derived thecal cells develop around the primordial follicles as they mature to primary follicles. This process continues after birth, again progressing toward the superficial layers. Each fetal ovary weighs about 15 mg at 14 weeks of gestation and 300 to 350 mg at birth.[232] The number of surviving primary follicles at birth correlates with the duration of subsequent postpubertal ovulation. Interstitial cells with characteristics of steroid-producing cells are present after 12 weeks, and during the third trimester theca cells with steroidogenic capacity surround the developing follicles.[20] Significant aromatase activity also is present, but few if any steroids are produced by the ovary during development.[20,232]

The specific genetic mechanisms dictating ovarian development are being unraveled, and some of the most powerful regulators include the WNT/FZD/β-catenin, FOXO/FOXL2, and TGFβ/SMAD pathways.[226,234] *FOXL2*, encoding a forkhead transcription factor, is required for ovarian development.[235] DMRT1, expressed in testis, prevents expression of FOXL2, and hence female programming, in the postnatal testis.[236] In the XX gonad, *RSPO1*, *WNT4*, *CTNNB1*, *FOXL2*, and *FST* are also expressed in a female-specific manner so as to promote ovarian development and repress testicular development. In humans and mice, R-spondin-1 (encoded by *RSPO1*) augments β-catenin signaling, possibly via WNT4.[237] Homozygous mutations in *RSPO1* result in a syndrome with palmoplantar hyperkeratosis and 46,XX DSD with sex reversal and dysgenetic testes or ovotestes.[238,239] Aberrations of the *WNT4* gene cause Mayer-Rokitansky syndrome or SERKAL syndrome (*sex reversal, dysgenetic kidneys, adrenals and lung*).[233,240]

In the male, the development of Leydig cells leads to an increase in fetal testosterone production between gestational weeks 10 and 20 (Fig. 22-10).[230] In vitro studies in the rat have shown that hCG binding to fetal testis cells does not downregulate LH receptors. If this is true in vivo in the human, continuous exposure of the Leydig cell to hCG would not desensitize the fetal testis and would allow the maintenance of augmented testosterone production during development. Fetal LH may contribute to fetal Leydig cell function, but quantitatively hCG is the predominant gonadotropin. Testosterone itself, acting through the androgen receptor, stimulates differentiation of the primitive mesonephric ducts into bilateral ductus deferens, epididymides, seminal vesicles, and ejaculatory ducts. Androgen receptors appear in the mesenchyme of urogenital structures at 8 weeks of gestation, followed by appearance of the receptors in the epithelium during development

at 9 to 12 weeks.[240] There was no difference in receptor expression in male and female fetuses. Dihydrotestosterone stimulates male differentiation of the urogenital sinus and external genitalia, including differentiation of the prostate, growth of the genital tubercle to form a phallus, and fusion of the urogenital folds to form the penile urethra. Dihydrotestosterone is formed from testosterone by the 5α-reductase enzyme within the urogenital sinus and urogenital tubercle, and it acts through the same androgen receptor that mediates the action of testosterone in the wolffian ducts. Mutations in the gene encoding the enzyme 5α-reductase are associated with variable disorders of sex development with 46,XY phenotypes.

The fetal testis also produces AMH, which causes dedifferentiation of the müllerian duct system in the male fetus.[241,242] AMH is a glycoprotein with a monomer molecular size of approximately 72 kDa and multimer sizes ranging from 145 to 235 kDa. It is a member of the TGF-β family. It is produced by testicular Sertoli cells and reaches the müllerian ducts largely by diffusion; duct regression in vitro requires a 24- to 36-hour exposure to AMH. AMH is synthesized early in gestation, with production peaking at the time of müllerian duct regression; biosynthesis continues throughout gestation and decreases after birth. *AMH* gene expression is activated by the *SRY* and *SF1* genes.[241] AMH also has autocrine and paracrine effects on testicular steroidogenic function during fetal life.[242] Male phenotypic differentiation is mediated by testicular testosterone and AMH and occurs between 8 and 14 weeks of gestation. In the female fetus, the müllerian duct system differentiates in the absence of AMH, the mesonephric ducts fail to develop in the absence of testosterone, and the undifferentiated urogenital sinus and external genitalia mature into female structures. Mutation of the AMH gene results in a persistent müllerian duct syndrome in the XY fetus.[241]

Estrogen effects are mediated by cognate receptors, members of the large family of steroid and thyroid hormone, vitamin D, and retinoid receptors.[243,244] Two estrogen receptors, ERα and ERβ, have been identified, with 96% and 58% homology in the DNA-binding and ligand-binding domains, respectively. ERα is encoded by *ESR1* on chromosome 6 and ERβ by *ESR2* on chromosome 14. Expression profiles of mRNAs of both receptors have been characterized in the 16- to 23-week human fetus. One or both receptor mRNAs are present in most tissues. The ERβ message is predominant, particularly in testis, ovary, spleen, thymus, adrenal gland, brain, kidney, and skin. The ERα message is prominent in the uterus, with relatively low levels in most other tissues.[243,244] The significance of ERs in fetal development is unclear. Knockout of the *ERα* gene in mice does not impair fetal development of any tissue, but adult females are infertile, with hypoplastic uteri and polycystic ovaries, and adult males manifest decreased fertility.[244] ERβ knockout mice develop normally, and female adults are fertile with normal sexual behavior; adult males reproduce normally but have prostate and bladder hyperplasia.[243] It is known that estrogens regulate DHEA production in the baboon and human fetal adrenal gland.[243] Knockout of both *ERα* and *ERβ* genes also has little impact on fetal development, but after birth the uterus, fallopian tubes, vagina, and cervix in females are hypoplastic and unresponsive to estrogen.[244] In humans ERα mutations in males are associated with tall stature, osteoporosis, and insulin insensitivity.[245]

Both androgens and estrogens are involved in the structural development of the rat brain.[246] Gonadal hormones also control gonadotropin production in the brain that results in cyclic ovarian function and normal function of the testes.[247,248] Testosterone administration to neonatal

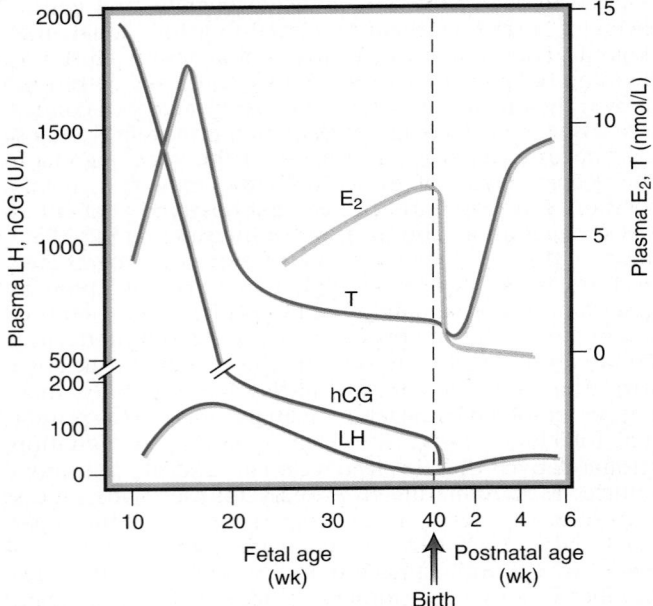

Figure 22-10 Patterns of change of plasma concentrations of human chorionic gonadotropin (hCG), luteinizing hormone (LH), testosterone (T), and estradiol (E₂) in a male fetus during gestation and in the neonatal period. (Data from Mann and associates[424] and Reyes FI, Boroditsky RS, Winter JS, et al. Studies on human sexual development: II. Fetal and maternal serum gonadotropin and sex steroid concentrations. *J Clin Endocrinol Metab.* 1974;38:612-617; Kaplan SL, Grumbach MM, Aubert ML. The ontogenesis of pituitary hormones and hypothalamic factors in the human fetus: maturation of central nervous system regulation of anterior pituitary function. *Recent Prog Horm Res.* 1976;32:161-243; Winter JS, Faiman C, Hobson WC, et al. Pituitary-gonadal relations in infancy: I. Patterns of serum gonadotropin concentrations from birth to four years of age in man and chimpanzee. *J Clin Endocrinol Metab.* 1975;40:545-551; Forest MG, Cathiard AM. Pattern of plasma testosterone and delta4-androstenedione in normal newborns; evidence for testicular activity at birth. *J Clin Endocrinol Metab.* 1975;41:977-980.)

female rats produces permanent inhibition of cyclic hypothalamic control through local aromatization to estradiol and ER binding. In primates and humans, estrogens seem to be more effective in this regard. However, there is no evidence for permanent programming in the primate, and there appear to be no major tissue biochemical differences between the sexes in utero to account for sexual dimorphic behavioral or gonadotropic programming.[248] Therefore, the mechanisms for these effects are not yet clear in the primate and human fetus.

A current view of the pathways for genes programming gonadal differentiation is shown in Figure 22-11. The full menu of downstream gene targets remains to be defined, but the net result is the highly organized pattern of gonadal development and phenotypic sexual differentiation. Fetal pituitary gonadotropins are not required for gonadal development or sexual differentiation; LH or FSH receptor knockout mice are born phenotypically normal.[249]

Human mutations in several of the genes programming gonadal differentiation have been described.[221] Loss-of-function mutations of SRY or SOX9 produce XY sex reversal, whereas gain-of-function mutations or duplications produce XX sex reversal. Mutations in SOX9 are associated with campomelic dysplasia and 46,XY sex reversal. SF1 mutations have been associated with 46,XY sex reversal with gonadal dysgenesis, with or without adrenal failure. More recently, the phenotypic spectrum of SF1 mutations

has widened to encompass gonadal dysgenesis, premature ovarian failure, male infertility, and the vanishing testis syndrome.[156,157,250] Mutations may be heterozygous or recessive, the former likely to be associated with a more severe loss of function. WT1 mutations produce several syndromes associated with abnormal testicular embryogenesis (WAGR syndrome [Wilms tumor, aniridia, genitourinary anomalies, and mental retardation], Denys-Drash syndrome, and Frasier syndrome) and renal abnormalities such as Wilms tumor or glomerulosclerosis. WNT4 gain-of-function mutations result in XX sex reversal, whereas DAX1 duplication is associated with XY sex reversal.[221] Mutations in CBX2 are also associated with 46,XY DSD with gonadal dysgenesis and ovarian development.[251]

Intermediate Lobe of the Pituitary

The intermediate lobe of the pituitary gland is prominent in both the human and the sheep fetus. Intermediate lobe cells begin to disappear near term and are virtually absent in the adult human pituitary, although the intermediate lobe in the adult of some lower species is anatomically and functionally distinct.[252] The major secretory products of the intermediate lobe are α-MSH and β-endorphin, both derived from cleavage of the POMC molecule.[253] Cleavage of POMC in the anterior lobe results predominantly in corticotropin and β-lipotropin formation. In rhesus monkeys and humans, the fetal pituitary contains high concentrations of compounds resembling α-MSH and corticotropin-like intermediate lobe peptide (CLIP).[254] In the human fetus, α-MSH levels decrease with increasing fetal age.[255] The circulating levels of β-endorphin and β-lipotropin are high in the fetal lamb, and the ratio of β-endorphin to β-lipotropin increases during hypoxic stimulation of the anterior pituitary.[255] Because hypoxia provokes corticotropin release and β-lipotropin production from the anterior pituitary, these data have been interpreted to suggest that basal β-endorphin levels in the fetus originate in the intermediate lobe. α-MSH and CLIP may play a role in fetal adrenal activation, and α-MSH may play a role in fetal growth.[256,257] However, these effects are probably minor. The processing of pituitary POMC in the human fetus by the end of the second trimester is similar to that in the adult, but the role of these intermediate lobe peptides in the fetus remains obscure.[258]

Posterior Pituitary

The fetal neurohypophysis is well developed by 10 to 12 weeks of gestation and contains both AVP (also called *antidiuretic hormone*) and oxytocin (OT).[259,260] In addition, arginine vasotocin (AVT), the parent neurohypophyseal hormone in submammalian vertebrates, is present in the fetal pituitary and pineal glands and in adult pineal glands from several mammalian species, including humans.[261] AVT is present in the pituitary during fetal life from 11 to 19 weeks, is secreted by cultured human fetal pineal cells during the second trimester, and disappears in the neonatal period.[260,261] In adult mammals, instillation of AVT into cerebrospinal fluid inhibits gonadotropin and corticotropin release, stimulates PRL release by the anterior pituitary, and induces sleep; however, the physiologic importance of these effects remains unclear. The role of AVT in the fetal pineal gland is unknown. Recent work shows a role for OT in the development of the neurovascular interface in the posterior pituitary.[48] The genetic programming of transcription factors underlying the development of the neurohypophysis is shown in Figure 22-2. By 40 weeks, the concentrations of AVP and OT approximate 20% of those

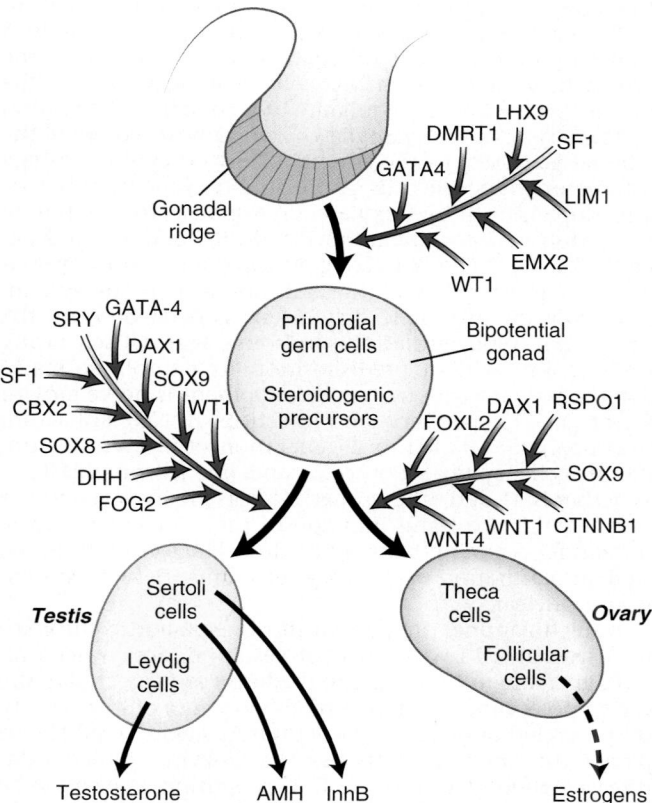

Figure 22-11 Summary of the molecular and cellular events of gonadal differentiation. AMH, antimüllerian hormone (or müllerian inhibiting substance); DHH, desert hedgehog; InhB, inhibin B. See text for details. (Molecular cascades developed from Harley VR, Clarkson MJ, Argentaro A. The molecular action and regulation of the testis-determining factors, SRY (sex determining region of the Y chromosome) and SOX9 (SRY-related high-mobility group [HMG] Box 9). *Endocr Rev.* 2003;24:466-487; and Park SY, Jameson JL. Minireview: transcriptional regulation of gonadal development and differentiation. *Endocrinology.* 2005;146:1035-1042.)

in adults. Fetal pituitary OT concentration, detectable by 11 to 15 weeks, exceeds AVP concentration by 19 weeks. The AVP-OT ratio falls progressively thereafter.

In fetal sheep, the baseline fetal plasma AVP concentrations are similar to maternal levels after midgestation. During the last trimester of gestation, fetal hypothalamic and pituitary responsiveness to both volume and osmolar stimuli for AVP secretion are well developed, and AVP exerts antidiuretic effects on the fetal kidney.[259,260] Baseline plasma levels of AVT in fetal sheep during the last trimester approximate values for AVP and OT.[261] Presumably this AVT is derived from the posterior pituitary, but the stimuli for AVT secretion in the fetus are not defined. The neurohypophyseal peptides are synthesized as large precursor molecules (neurophysins) and processed to bioactive amidated peptides.[262] Enzymatic processing involves progressive cleavage of carboxy terminal–extended peptides, sequentially producing (for OT) OT-glycine-lysine-arginine (OTGKR), OTGK, OTG, and OT. Similar progressive processing yields AVPG and AVP from the AVP neurophysin. Enzymatic processing of neurophysins matures progressively in the fetus so that early in gestation fetal plasma contains relatively large concentrations of the extended peptides. For OT, the ratio of OT-extended peptides to OT in fetal sheep serum is approximately 35:1 early in gestation and 3:1 late in gestation.[262]

In the fetus, AVP appears to function as a stress-responsive hormone. Perhaps the major potential stress for the fetus is hypoxia, and the response of AVP to hypoxia is increased compared with the maternal response and with fetal AVP responses to osmolar stimuli.[260,263-265] Plasma AVP concentrations in human cord blood are elevated in association with intrauterine bradycardia and meconium passage.[264] The vasopressor action of AVP may be important in the maintenance of fetal circulatory homeostasis during hemorrhage and hypoxia; AVP has a limited effect on fetoplacental blood flow.[259,265] Fetal hypoxia is also a major stimulus for catecholamine release. There is little information on interactions between AVP and catecholamines during fetal hypoxia, but both fetal hypoxia and AVP stimulate anterior pituitary function.[265] A role for AVP as a CRH is established in the adult, and the ovine fetal pituitary responds separately and synergistically to AVP and CRH early in the third trimester.[266] The role of AVP in controlling fetal corticotropin release seems to decrease with gestational age. It is not known whether AVT functions as a CRH in the fetus.

OT receptors have been demonstrated in human fetal membranes at term, and AVP receptors have been found in the renal medullary membranes of newborn sheep.[267-269] Both AVP and AVT evoke antidiuretic actions in the sheep fetus during the last third of gestation, and both hormones act to conserve water for the fetus by inhibiting fluid loss into amniotic fluid through the lungs and kidneys.[259,260] Aquaporin-1, -2, and -3 water channel receptors are present in the human fetal and newborn kidney, and the ability of the newborn infant to regulate free water clearance in response to volume and osmolar stimuli has been demonstrated.[270,271] Whether AVT exerts its effects through AVP receptors or separate fetal AVT receptors is not clear. Maximal concentrating capacity by the fetal kidney is limited to about 600 mmol/L. This limitation is not related to inadequate AVP stimulation but rather to inherent immaturity of the renal tubules.

Lack of AVP is associated with diabetes insipidus and with a failure to retain water in the body, leading to polyuria and polydipsia. Although most cases of diabetes insipidus are from acquired causes such as pituitary germinoma, craniopharyngioma, or Langerhans cell histiocytosis, the condition may rarely be due to mutations in the AVP-neurophysin gene or to other congenital causes such as septo-optic dysplasia or holoprosencephaly. Mutations in *WFS1* are associated with autosomal recessive Wolfram syndrome that includes diabetes insipidus, diabetes mellitus, optic atrophy, and sensorineural hearing loss.[272]

Fetal Autonomic Nervous System

The primordia of the sympathetic trunk ganglia are visible in the human fetus by 6 to 7 weeks of gestation. The preaortic sympathetic primordia at that time are composed of primitive sympathetic neurons and chromaffin cells, which condense into chains of cell masses along the abdominal aorta. By 10 to 12 weeks of gestation, the paired adrenal masses are well developed. In addition, numerous extramedullary paraganglia (derived from preaortic condensations of sympathetic neurons and chromaffin cells) are scattered throughout the abdominal and pelvic sympathetic plexuses.[273] Each of these extramedullary paraganglia may reach a maximal diameter of 2 to 3 mm by 28 to 30 weeks of gestation. The largest of the paraganglia, the organs of Zuckerkandl near the origin of the inferior mesenteric arteries, enlarge to 10 to 15 mm in length at term. After birth, the paraganglia gradually atrophy and disappear by 2 to 3 years of age. With increasing gestational age, there is progressive growth of the adrenal medullae, increasing catecholamine content of the adrenal medullae, and progressive maturation of medullary functional capacity. Histologically, the adrenal medullae are somewhat immature at birth, but by 1 year they resemble the adult glands.

Both chromaffin and sympathetic nerve cells are derived from common neuroectodermal stem cells. In mice, the sympathoadrenal progenitor cells first aggregate at the dorsal aorta, where they migrate in a dorsolateral direction to form sympathetic ganglia or ventrally to colonize the adrenal glands.[274] In the adrenal glands, they differentiate into neuroendocrine cells, expressing tyrosine hydroxylase and dopamine β-hydroxylase in response to a series of transcription factors including PHOX2B, MASH1, PHOX2A, and dHAND.[274] The *PHOX2B* gene is pivotal in the development of most relays of the autonomic nervous system; mutation of this gene has been associated with the congenital hypoventilation syndrome, with Hirschsprung disease, and with a predisposition to neuroblastoma.[275] Sympathetic nervous system development is nerve growth factor (NGF) dependent, and injections of NGF antiserum into neonatal rats led to degeneration of immature chromaffin cells, sympathetic cells, and pheochromoblasts.[276] Whether NGF and other growth factors are involved in the transient life span and function of the paraganglia in the human fetus and neonate is not clear. The role of placental NGF in maturation of the fetal autonomic nervous system is also unclear.

Catecholamines are present in the para-aortic chromaffin tissue by 10 to 15 weeks of gestation, and concentrations increase until term. The predominant catecholamine is norepinephrine (NE), presumably because of low activity of phenylethanolamine *N*-methyltransferase (PNMT) in para-aortic chromaffin tissue. This enzyme, which catalyzes the methylation of NE to epinephrine, appears to be activated by the high levels of cortisol that diffuse into the adrenal medulla from the adrenal cortex; in contrast, cortisol levels in extramedullary chromaffin tissue are low.[273,277,278] In fetal mammals, the chromaffin cells of the adrenal medulla can respond directly to asphyxia, long before splanchnic innervation develops, by secreting NE; the noninnervated para-aortic tissue responds similarly. In the fetal sheep, a similar developmental transition occurs between days 120 and 135 of the 150-day gestation.[273,277,278] The CNS responds to stimuli that evoke sympathetic nervous system responses before the adrenomedullary splanchnic innervation, but the adrenal medulla is relatively unresponsive to such stimuli. The transition is heralded by an adrenomedullary response to hypoglycemia mediated by the CNS.[277] This response is present in developing sheep, monkeys, and human fetuses during the third trimester of gestation.[279-281] Central and adrenal enkephalins are also involved in fetal autonomic nervous system function, and pretreatment with naloxone potentiates and methadone inhibits the catecholamine response to hypoxia.[273,278]

Basal plasma epinephrine, NE, and dopamine levels during the last third of gestation in sheep decrease as term approaches.[281,282] The metabolic clearance rate of epinephrine increases with gestational age, whereas the production rate remains unchanged, indicating that the decrease in basal catecholamine levels that occurs with fetal age is due to maturation of clearance mechanisms.[282] The fetal sheep responds to maternal exercise or hypoxia with increased catecholamine levels.[283] The human neonate responds to parturition with an increase in plasma epinephrine and NE concentrations, and these responses are augmented by hypoxia and acidosis.[283-285] In the newborn infant, catecholamine secretion also increases after cold exposure and hypoglycemia.[277,280]

Catecholamines are critical for fetal cardiovascular function and fetal survival. Gene knockout studies in mice, targeting either tyrosine hydroxylase or dopamine β-hydroxylase, produced fetal catecholamine deficiency and midgestation fetal death in 90% of the mutant embryos.[284,285] In addition, fetal catecholamines are the major stress hormones in the fetus.[277-280] The fetal adrenal and the para-aortic chromaffin masses discharge large amounts of catecholamines directly into the circulation in response to fetal hypoxia.[277] Moreover, the defense against fetal hypoxia involves catecholamine actions mediated through cardiac α-receptors that are unique to immature animals. α-Adrenergic receptors predominate in immature cardiac tissue and gradually decline in number as β-adrenergic receptors increase with maturation. Chromaffin tissue in the fetus is also innervated by opiate receptors and contains relatively large amounts of opiate peptides that appear to be cosecreted with the catecholamines.[277] The extent to which these peptides or pituitary endorphins are involved in modulating fetal catecholamine secretion remains unclear.

Parathyroid Hormone/Calcitonin System

Parathyroid gland development from the third and fourth pharyngeal pouches proceeds in synchrony with thyroid embryogenesis.[159,160] The third pouches encounter the migrating thyroid anlage, and the parathyroid anlagen are carried caudally with the thyroid gland, finally coming to rest at the lower poles of the thyroid lobes as the inferior parathyroid glands. The fourth pouches encounter the thyroid anlage later and come to rest at the upper poles of the thyroid lobes as the superior parathyroid glands. The individual parathyroid glands increase in diameter from less than 0.1 mm at 14 weeks of gestation to 1 to 2 mm at birth. The fifth pouches contribute paired ultimobranchial bodies that are incorporated into the developing thyroid gland as the parafollicular or C cells that secrete calcitonin. Both endocrine systems are functional during the second and third trimesters (see Fig. 22-8). Near term, fetal parathyroid cells are largely composed of inactive chief cells, with only a few intermediate chief cells containing occa-

sional secretory granules. C cells are particularly prominent in the neonatal thyroid gland, and the calcitonin content is as high as 540 to 2100 mU/g of tissue, values as much as 10 times those observed in the normal adult gland.[286]

Figure 22-8 shows the genetic cascade programming normal thyroid-parathyroid development.[287,288] Disruption of the HOX15 gene in mice results in parathyroid gland aplasia, indicating that this gene functions as part of the genetic cascade programming normal thyroid-parathyroid gland development. Targeted disruption of the murine homeobox gene Hoxa3 results in parathyroid agenesis. Additional transcription factors involved in parathyroid gland embryogenesis in the mouse include Pax1, Pax3, Pax9, Eya1, Six1, Sox3, Gcm2, Crk1, and Tbx1 and Tbx2.[288] CRK1 and TBX1 mutations have been associated with 22q11 deletion syndrome.[289] GCM2 mutation leads to isolated hypoparathyroidism.[287]

Complex human disorders with congenital hypoparathyroidism have been found in association with mutations and deletions of TBX1, GATA3 (hypoparathyroidism, sensorineural deafness, and renal disease [HDR]), AIRE1 (APECED), TBCE (Kenny-Caffey syndrome), PTH/PTHrP (Blomstrand chondrodysplasia), and GNAS1 (pseudohypoparathyroidism). Isolated hypoparathyroidism can be found in association with mutations in PTH, GCMB, and SOX3.[288] SOX3 mutations are generally associated with variable hypopituitarism, but recent studies have implicated the gene in parathyroid development.[290]

At birth, the body contains approximately 30 g calcium. Studies in fetal sheep and monkeys and measurements in human preterm and term infants indicate that high concentrations of fetal calcium (averaging 2.75 to 3 mmol/L in the last trimester) are maintained by active placental transport, against a concentration gradient, from maternal blood.[291,292] The transport of calcium occurs across the syncytiotrophoblast. A three-step model (Fig. 22-12) has been proposed involving voltage-dependent Ca channels (primarily TRPV6 [transient receptor potential vanilloid]) at the apical brush-border membrane of the trophoblast cells (at the maternal-placental interface); intracellular calcium-binding proteins (primarily calbindin D9K), which ferry calcium to the basal membrane; and a basolateral membrane ATP-dependent Ca pump (PMCA3, at the placental-fetal interface), which transports calcium into the fetal circulation.[292,293] The set-point for fetal serum calcium is higher than the maternal set-point, and the middle part of PTHrP, secreted by the fetal parathyroids and the placenta, is critical for maintaining this level.[292,294] Fetal serum phosphate is also higher than maternal levels, but little is known about its placental transport. NaPi-2b, a member of the family of sodium-dependent inorganic phosphate transporters, is expressed in embryonic visceral and parietal endoderm as well as in labyrinthine cells of the placenta and likely has a role in fetal phosphate homeostasis (see Fig. 22-12).[293]

The placenta is impermeable to parathyroid hormone (PTH), PTHrP, and calcitonin, but 25-hydroxyvitamin D and 1,25-dihydroxyvitamin D (calcitriol) are transported across the placenta, and free vitamin D concentrations in fetal blood are similar to or higher than maternal values.[291,292] The principal PTH receptor is PTHR1, which has equal affinity for PTH and PTHrP. A second receptor, PTHR2, is present in CNS and binds PTH but not PTHrP, whereas PTHrP action in the placenta occurs most likely through a distinct receptor that binds PTHrP but not PTH.[293,295]

Thyroparathyroidectomy in fetal sheep causes a rapid decrease in fetal plasma calcium concentration and a loss of the placental calcium gradient.[291] In mice, knockout of PTHrP abolishes the maternal-fetal calcium gradient and

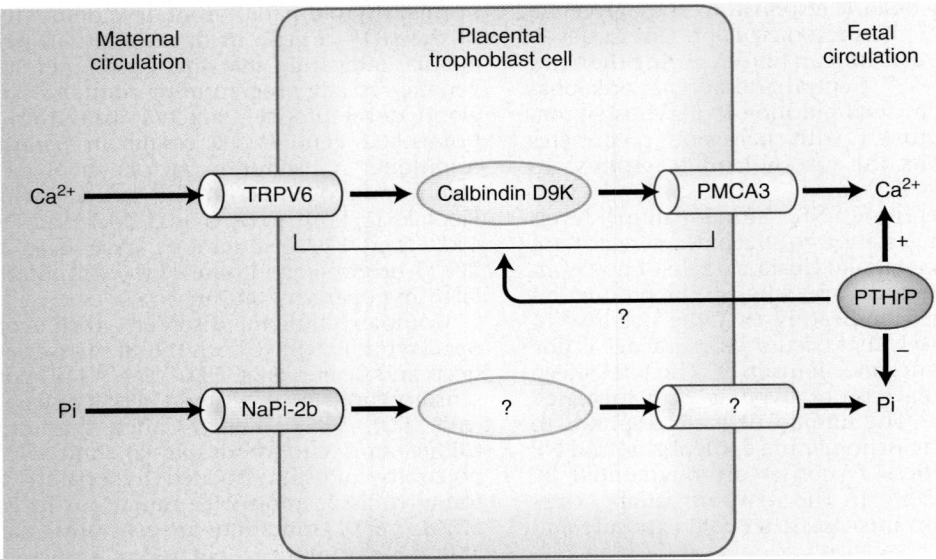

Figure 22-12 Calcium enters the placental trophoblast at the brush-border membrane primarily via the TRPV6 channel. Transport is facilitated by calbindin D9K, and calcium is released to the fetal circulation through the calcium pump PMCA3. Inorganic phosphate (Pi) enters the trophoblast likely via the sodium-phosphate cotransporter NaPi-2b. See discussion in text. PTHrP, parathyroid hormone–related protein. (From Mitchell DM, Juppner H. Regulation of calcium homeostasis and bone metabolism in the fetus and neonate. *Curr Opin Endocrinol Diabetes Obes.* 2010;17:25-30.)

reduces placental transport of calcium.[292,296] Placental calcium transport in these models is restored by the mid-molecule fragment of PTHrP (amino acids 67 to 86) but not by PTH or the PTHrP(1-34) fragment, both of which activate the PTH/PTHrP receptor.[294,296] Therefore, a second, as yet unidentified PTHrP receptor recognizing the PTHrP(38-94) ligand appears to be involved in placental calcium pump activation.[292]

Other factors are also involved in maintenance of fetal serum calcium levels, because knockout of the mouse gene for PTH-PTHrP also results in hypocalcemia in the presence of normal or increased placental calcium transport.[291,297] PTH and PTHrP, through the PTH/PTHrP receptor, presumably modulate fetal skeletal calcium flux, calcium excretion through the fetal kidney, and perhaps reabsorption of calcium from amniotic fluid. PTHrP has a major role in fetal bone development and metabolism as well as fetal calcium homeostasis. PTHrP knockout mice display increased ossification of the basal portion of the skull, long bones, vertebral bodies, and pelvic bones and mineralization of the normally cartilaginous portions of the ribs and sternum; as a result of the cartilaginous mineralization, the animals die of asphyxiation in the early neonatal period.[292,294,296,298] The skeletal chondrodysplasia is more severe in combined PTH plus PTHrP or PTH/PTHrP receptor gene–ablated animals.[299,300] In the mouse model, knockout of the calcitonin gene or the vitamin D receptor gene leads to postnatal osteosclerosis or osteomalacia, respectively; the pups appear normal at birth.[301]

Fetal sheep have low circulating concentrations of PTH but can increase serum PTH concentrations in response to a fall in serum calcium concentration induced by ethylenediaminetetraacetic acid (EDTA) and can respond promptly to infused calcium with increased serum calcito-

nin concentrations. In this model, as noted, fetal parathyroidectomy decreases placental calcium transport and lowers fetal serum calcium. Although PTH has no effect on placental calcium transport, PTHrP is present in fetal tissues and placenta and stimulates calcium transport. Nephrectomy in the fetal sheep reduces fetal serum calcium concentrations, and this hypocalcemia can be prevented by prior administration of 1,25-dihydroxyvitamin D. Moreover, infusion into the sheep fetus of antibody to $1,25(OH)_2D$ reduced the placental calcium gradient.[291] The fetal kidney can produce 1,25-dihydroxyvitamin D, and the placenta contains 1,25-dihydroxyvitamin D receptors, as well as a vitamin D–dependent calcium-binding protein.[298] Dihydroxyvitamin D production in the fetal sheep is sixfold greater than in the maternal ewe. The metabolic clearance of $1,25(OH)_2D$ was also higher in the fetus than in the mother.

The fetal parathyroid-placental axis promotes maternal-fetal transfer of bone mineral and accretion of fetal bone mineral. It seems likely that fetal PTH and presumably PTHrP act on the fetal kidney to stimulate 1α-hydroxylation of 25-hydroxyvitamin D and that 1,25-dihydroxyvitamin D participates in modulating placental calcium transport. $1,25(OH)_2D$ or $24,25(OH)_2D$ also plays a role in fetal cartilage growth and bone mineral accretion.[302] Thus, PTHrP and to a lesser extent PTH in the ovine fetus appear to augment maternal-to-fetal calcium transport across the placenta and thus provide for the high rate of bone mineral accretion in the latter half of pregnancy (Fig. 22-13). The high blood concentrations of calcitonin in the fetus, probably resulting from the chronic stimulation by fetal hypercalcemia, are thought to contribute to the fetal bone mineral accretion.[291,299] A prominent effect of calcitonin is to inhibit bone resorption, and the high fetal serum

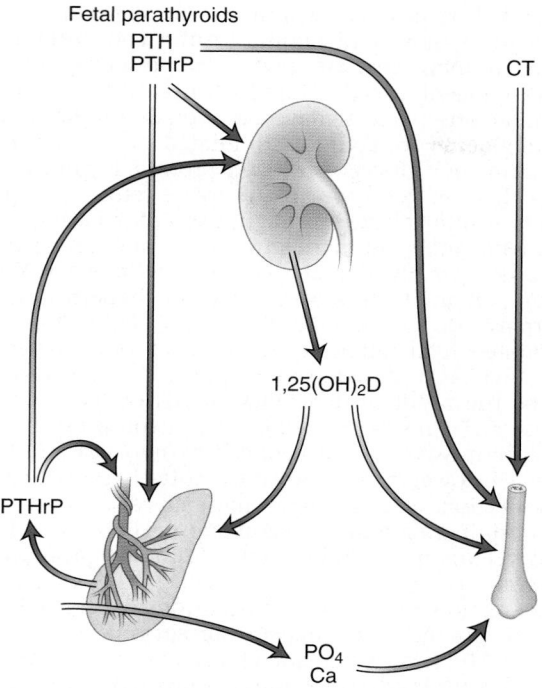

Figure 22-13 Proposed actions of parathyroid hormone (PTH), PTH-related protein (PTHrP), and calcitonin (CT) in the fetus. PTHrP and perhaps PTH from the parathyroid glands and PTHrP from the placenta act on the placenta to promote calcium (Ca) and phosphate (PO₄) transport from the maternal to the fetal circulation to maintain the relative fetal hypercalcemia and the high rate of fetal bone formation during the last half of gestation. PTHrP also acts on the kidney to promote 1-hydroxylation of 25-hydroxycholecalciferol to 1,25(OH)₂D (1,25-dihydroxyvitamin D, calcitriol), which augments placental calcium transport and promotes fetal bone growth. High fetal CT levels tend to promote bone accretion. See text for details. (From Kovacs CS. Bone metabolism in the fetus and neonate. *Pediatr Nephrol.* 2014;29:793-803.)

calcium concentrations coupled with high circulating calcitonin promote bone mineral anabolism.[299] Placental calcitonin production may contribute to the calcitonin in fetal plasma, but the persistence of high plasma concentrations in neonatal plasma argues for predominant fetal production (see Fig. 22-13).

Calcium-Sensing Receptor and Fibroblast Growth Factor 23

The CaSR, a G protein–coupled receptor, serves to maintain a constant level of blood calcium concentration by modulating the production and secretion of calcium-regulating hormones such as PTH, calcitonin, FGF23, and vitamin D.[303,304] The CaSR is present in parathyroid glands, renal tubules, bone and cartilage, and multiple other tissues. Magnesium also binds to the CaSR and influences PTH secretion. Mutations within the *CASR* gene result in either inactivation or overactivaton of the receptor, resulting in hypercalcemia or hypocalcemia, respectively.[305] Inactivating mutations lead to a switching off of PTH secretion at a lower calcium concentration than usual, and hypercalcemia ensues. Renal calcium secretion is reduced. This condition is known as FBH (familial benign hypercalcemia) or FHH (familial hypocalciuric hypercalcemia). In contrast, activating *CASR* mutations cause autosomal dominant hypercalciuric hypocalcemia (ADH). An online database to keep track of described mutations is available.[306]

A few conditions are of particular importance in the neonatal period. When a neonate presents with abnormal calcium concentrations, assessment of calcium, albumin, phosphate, creatinine, alkaline phosphatase, vitamin D, and urine calcium-creatinine ratio and phosphate reabsorption, in both the child and parents, will help to formulate the underlying diagnosis. Hypocalcemia resulting from fetal and maternal vitamin D deficiency is relatively common. Occasionally, severe neonatal vitamin D deficiency can be associated with a dilated cardiomyopathy, which is reversible.[307,308] Asphyxia can result in subcutaneous fat necrosis, which is due to release of 1,25-dihydroxyvitamin D from macrophages, and leads to hypercalcemia. Hyperhydration, steroid therapy, low-calcium milk, and occasionally bisphosphonate treatment may be needed to reduce calcium concentrations. FBH and FHH can present in neonates with mild to moderately elevated calcium concentrations, high-normal (nonsuppressed) PTH, and a low urine calcium/creatinine ratio.[309] FHH may also present as neonatal hyperparathyroidism leading to bone disease and variable symptoms of hypercalcemia. This scenario occurs especially if an affected infant has inherited the inactivating *CASR* mutation from the father, but the mother is normal. The fetus will consider the mother as hypocalcemic and therefore will overproduce PTH. Cinacalcet therapy may help to bind calcium and settle the hyperparathyroidism, but parathyroidectomy is occasionally necessary. Hypo- and hypercalcemic disorders may also be due to mutations in G protein subunit alpha11, *AP2S1* (involved in G protein internalization), and calcium channels *TRPV5* and *TRPV6*.[310,311]

FGF23 is the principal hormone that regulates phosphate transport. It is primarily produced and secreted into the circulation by osteocytes and, after its activation through glycosylation by GALNT3, acts through receptors FGFR1c and FGFR4 on renal tubules to increase phosphate excretion through the sodium-phosphate exchanger (NaPi-2C, SLC34A3).[312] Alpha-Klotho acts as a cofactor for FGF23 to bind to FGFR1c, increasing specificity of FGFR1c for FGF23. FGF23 is inactivated by cleavage by subtilisin/furin-like enzyme. PHEX (phosphate-regulating gene with homologies to endopeptidases on the X chromosome) regulates cleavage of FGF23, and *PHEX* mutations therefore render FGF23 constitutively active. Besides increasing renal tubular phosphate excretion, FGF23 inhibits 1α-hydroxylase, thus reducing 1,25-hydroxyvitamin D activity. Gain-of-function and loss-of-function mutations in various components of this FGF23 network result in hypophosphatemic rickets (*FGF23, PHEX, SLC34A3,* subtilisins [*PCSKs*], phosphate transporters *NPT2A* and *NPT2C*) or hyperphosphatemic syndromes (*GALNT3, FGF23, alpha-Klotho*).[313]

Endocrine Pancreas: Insulin and Glucagon

Embryogenesis of the pancreas is mediated in the mouse by a series of homeobox genes and transcription factors that program pancreatic budding from the gut tube, development of branching ducts and undifferentiated epithelium, differentiation of exocrine and endocrine cell lineages that originate from endodermal tissue, and organization of the endocrine cells into islets of Langerhans. The process begins at day 8 of the 21-day gestation and extends 2 to 3 weeks after birth.[314-316] Studies in mice have shown that knockout of the *Pdx1, Mnx1 (HlxB9), Isl1,* or *Hes1* genes results in pancreatic agenesis or dysgenesis. *Nkx2.2, Nkx6.1, Pax4,* or *Pax6* loss of function results in endocrine cell agenesis or hypogenesis.[315-317] *Ngn3* or *Hnf1b* gene knockout in the mouse leads to marked beta-cell dysplasia and hypoplasia, whereas knockout of the lower pathway genes will impair specific islet cell differentiation.[314] *Gata4* and *Gata6* have recently been shown to play a role in pancreatic progenitor cell development.[318] More recent studies have compiled gene regulatory networks for pancreas development, integrating data from multiple studies including mutation analysis, gene expression, cell lineage tracing, and biochemical gene regulation. These networks include all previous mentioned genes but also include other genes such as *Tle2*, *Dll*, *Onecut1*, *BMP7*, *SOX9*, and *FOXO1*.[316]

In humans, mutations in *GLIS3*, *NeuroD1*, *PDX1*, *PTF1A*, and *GATA6* are associated with neonatal diabetes mellitus due to pancreatic agenesis, and mutations in *EIF2AK3*, *HNF1B*, *MNX1*, *NKX2-2*, and *RFX6* lead to neonatal diabetes due to pancreatic hypoplasia.[319-322] Recently, recessive mutations in a distal enhancer of *PTF1A* were also found to cause pancreas agenesis.[323] In mice, *Ngn3* or *Beta2* knockout leads to complete absence of endocrine cells, whereas knockout of the lower pathway genes impairs specific islet cell differentiation.[314] Members of the EGF family of growth factors, laminin, and perhaps other growth factors including the IGFs also contribute to pancreatic growth and differentiation.[324,325]

The human fetal pancreas is identifiable by 4 weeks of gestation, and alpha and beta cells can be recognized by 8 to 9 weeks. Insulin, glucagon, somatostatin, and pancreatic polypeptide are measurable by 8 to 10 weeks of gestation.[326] Alpha cells are more numerous than beta cells in the early fetal pancreas and reach a relative peak at midgestation; beta cells continue to increase throughout the second half of gestation so that, by term, the ratio of alpha to beta cells is approximately 1:1. The insulin content of the pancreas increases from less than 3.6 pmol/g (0.5 U/g) at 7 to 10 weeks to 30 pmol/g (4 U/g) at 16 to 25 weeks of gestation and 93 pmol/g (13 U/g) near term; the concentration in the adult pancreas is approximately 14 pmol/g (2 U/g).[327] Endocrine cells are dispersed throughout the exocrine tissues by 20 weeks, and the islets of Langerhans are clearly differentiated by 31 weeks.

The beta cell is functional by 14 weeks of human gestation, and fetal pancreatic insulin content exceeds that of the adult throughout most of gestation. However, fetal glucose metabolism is largely independent of the glucoregulatory hormones insulin and glucagon.[317,328] In physiologic doses, glucagon does not increase hepatic glucose production, probably because of a paucity of hepatic glucagon receptors in the fetus.[329] Insulin receptors are present in a variety of fetal tissues at levels generally exceeding those of the adult. However, downregulation of insulin receptor binding does not occur during fetal hyperinsulinemia, in contrast with observations in adult animals. Acute hypoglycemia or hyperglycemia is not associated with significant alterations in either insulin or glucagon concentrations.

Although the fetal beta cell is functional by 14 to 24 weeks of gestation, secretion of insulin into the bloodstream by the fetal pancreas is low. Insulin release from the fetal rat pancreas in vitro in response to glucose or pyruvate is minimal but can be stimulated by leucine, arginine, tolbutamide, or potassium chloride, indicating that parts of the secretory mechanism are functional in the fetus.[327,330,331] Insulin secretion in adult islets is mediated by two or more mechanisms, including stimulation of the adenylate cyclase system with production of cyclic adenosine monophosphate (cAMP) and inhibition of potassium efflux, which leads to depolarization of the cell membrane and opening of voltage-dependent calcium channels. The former mechanism, although suppressed in the fetal islets, can be augmented by theophylline, but calcium channel activation does not occur in fetal islets in response to initiators of insulin release that cause depolarization of adult islet cells.[331] Infusion of glucose or arginine to pregnant women fails to provoke fetal insulin secretion at midgestation or near term, and plasma insulin concentrations in the late human fetus are relatively unresponsive to high glucose concentrations before the onset of labor.[327]

Similar observations have been made in the monkey: neither glucose nor arginine stimulated fetal insulin release near term, but glucagon evoked prompt insulin production.[327] Late in gestation in the ovine fetus, epinephrine inhibits insulin release through a receptor pathway.[327] In the anencephalic human fetus, the endocrine pancreas develops normally if maternal carbohydrate metabolism is not impaired; however, beta-cell hypertrophy and hyperplasia do not occur in the anencephalic fetus nor in decapitated fetal rabbits exposed to chronic hyperglycemia. This lack of beta-cell response to hyperglycemia may be the result of deficiency of GH or IGF-1 or both, because GH stimulates insulin gene expression and may play a permissive role in beta-cell hyperplasia and hypertrophy.[325] However, in contrast to acute changes in glucose concentration, chronic fetal hyperglycemia does evoke hyperinsulinemia and glucagon suppression, and chronic hypoglycemia may inhibit fetal insulin and promote fetal glucagon release.[316]

Pancreatic glucagon concentrations are relatively high in fetal plasma and increase progressively with fetal age.[327,330] The fetal pancreatic glucagon content at midgestation is approximately 6 µg/g, compared with an adult level of 2 µg/g. As is true for insulin, the capacity for glucagon secretion is blunted in the fetus. Hyperglycemia does not suppress fetal plasma glucagon concentrations in rats, monkeys, or sheep, and acute hypoglycemia does not evoke glucagon secretion in the rat fetus. Amino acids, which are important secretagogues for insulin and glucagon in the adult, probably have little role in modulating insulin and glucagon secretion in the preterm fetus. However, infusion of alanine into women at term increases both maternal and cord blood glucagon concentrations, indicating a fetal glucagon response to amino acids in the term fetus. Catecholamines also evoke glucagon release in the near-term ovine fetus.[327]

Therefore, the fetal pancreatic islet cells, although histologically mature and capable of hormone synthesis and hyperplasia, are relatively immature functionally at birth with regard to their capacity to secrete insulin and glucagon. The rapid maturation of responsiveness to glucose in the neonatal period in both premature and mature infants suggests that this blunted state may be a secondary result of the relatively stable fetal serum glucose concentrations maintained by placental transfer of maternal glucose rather than a primary, temporally fixed maturation process. Alternatively, the lack of any enteric signal to the pancreas from feeding via release of incretins may also account for this stability. The blunted capacity for insulin and glucagon secretion has been related to a deficient capacity of the fetal pancreatic islet cells to generate cAMP or to rapid destruction of cAMP by phosphodiesterase, or both.[327]

In rodents, a period of a rapid increase in beta-cell mass at the time of birth and shortly thereafter has been observed, and this rapid change is attenuated by a period of apoptosis before adult mass is achieved. Beta-cell mass is more difficult to determine from a developmental standpoint in humans. At birth in the human, there are some 200 to 300 × 10^6 beta cells, which is approximately one third of the population present in adulthood. However, most of the actual mass change takes place in the newborn period and is associated with changes in beta-cell size rather than number.[332] Thereafter, there is rapid further expansion in terms of cell numbers, but the waxing and waning of the beta-cell mass, particularly with pregnancy, is poorly understood. How much beta-cell mass is a determinant of predisposition to type 2 diabetes mellitus is unclear.

Insulin and glucagon are normally not necessary for substrate metabolism in the fetus.[330] Glucose is obtained by placental transfer through facilitated diffusion. The fetal respiratory quotient is approximately 1, which suggests that glucose is the primary energy substrate for the fetus. Other substrates, such as amino acids and lactate, may also be utilized in the human as in the sheep fetus. However, at least early in gestation, hepatic metabolism and substrate utilization appear to be independent of insulin and to be modulated in an autoregulatory fashion by glucose.[327] In addition, the constant supply of glucose normally precludes the necessity for endogenous gluconeogenesis, and gluconeogenic enzyme activities are low in the fetal liver.

Glycogen storage in the fetus is modulated by fetal glucocorticoids and probably by placental lactogen (hPL). Fetal insulin plays a role near term, when insulin also has the capacity to increase fetal glucose uptake and lipogenesis.[327,330] Insulin receptors are present on most fetal cells in higher numbers than on adult cells; moreover, hyperinsulinemia fails to downregulate fetal insulin receptors.[327] Fetal hepatic glucagon receptors, in contrast, are reduced in number, and fetal liver is relatively resistant to the glycemic effect of glucagon. These conditions tend to potentiate the fetal anabolic milieu during the period of rapid growth in the last trimester of gestation.

During the newborn period, the placental source of glucose is abolished, and plasma glucagon concentrations rise in association with a rapid increase in functionally coupled glucagon receptors. The increase in plasma catecholamines coincident with parturition may be responsible for some of these changes; catecholamines both stimulate glucagon release and inhibit insulin release.[317,329,333] Phosphoenolpyruvate carboxykinase (PEPCK) activity also increases during this period. Thus, gluconeogenesis is readily demonstrable in the newborn, in which nearly 10% of glucose utilization is accounted for by gluconeogenesis from alanine. Plasma free fatty acid concentrations rise postnatally as a result of the effects of catecholamines and chemical thermogenesis. Oxidation of fatty acids probably provides cofactors (acetyl coenzyme A and the reduced form of nicotinamide adenine dinucleotide) required for gluconeogenesis, as well as sparing glucose for utilization by crucially dependent tissues such as the brain.[317]

Poorly controlled maternal diabetes mellitus is associated with fetal macrosomia, an increased risk of spontaneous abortion, and fetal malformation. Maternal hyperglycemia also leads to hyperinsulinism and beta-cell hyperplasia in the infant. Infants of diabetic mothers are prone to polycythemia, renal vein thrombosis, hypocalcemia, respiratory distress syndrome, jaundice, persistent fetal circulation, cardiomyopathy, congenital heart disease, and malformations of other organs.

Neonatal Diabetes

Neonatal diabetes is defined as diabetes that develops in the first 6 months of life. Two types exist, one that shows spontaneous remission before 18 months of age (60% of cases) and one that is permanent, both with an incidence of approximately 1:200,000 to 1:250,000.[334] Transient neonatal diabetes mellitus (TNDM) may be due to overexpression of an imprinted gene on chromosome 6q24 in the majority of cases, whereas activating mutations of KCNJ11 and ABCC8, encoding for the two subunits (Kir6.2 and sulfonylurea receptor 1, SUR1) of the pancreatic beta cell ATP-sensitive inward rectifier potassium (K-ATP) channel

account for 25% of cases. Mutations in the INS gene, encoding pre-proinsulin, are rarer, as are mutations in ZPF57, which regulates gene methylation. A genetic cause can be identified in approximately half of patients with NDM. Intrauterine growth retardation (IUGR) is another feature of TNDM, although not in TNDM due to K-ATP channelopathies. After remission, diabetes mellitus recurs in approximately 50% of cases.

Permanent neonatal diabetes mellitus (PNDM) is most often due to activating mutations in KCNJ11 or ABCC8, resulting in overactivation of potassium channels and thus impaired insulin secretion. These patients are responsive to sulfonylurea therapy and do not require insulin treatment. Other causes of PNDM include INS and GCK mutations. Mutations in EIF2AK3 (eukaryotic translation initiation factor 2 alpha kinase 3) lead to Wolcott-Rallison syndrome of which other features include skeletal abnormalities, liver dysfunction, cardiac and renal abnormalities, developmental delay, epilepsy, and neutropenia. FOXP3 mutations result in IPEX (immune dysregulation, polyendocrinopathy, on X chromosome), which can lead to PNDM. Other monogenic causes of PNDM include mutations in genes encoding for zinc finger protein GLIS3, PAX6, the thiamine transporter SLC19A2, glucose transporter GLUT2 (encoded by SLC2A2),[335] NeuroG3, and NeuroD1, and genes important for pancreas development: PTF1A (hypoplasia of pancreas and cerebellum), PDX1 (pancreas agenesis, endocrine and exocrine hormone deficiency),[336] RFX6, acting downstream of NeuroG3 (hypoplasia of pancreas, gallbladder, intestinal atresia, intractable diarrhea),[337,338] GATA4,[339] and GATA6.[336] Recently, mutations in MNX1 (previously called HLXB9) and NKX2-2, coding for key transcription factors for pancreas development, were identified as monogenic causes for PNDM in humans.[322] Neonatal diabetes that does not respond to sulfonylurea therapy is best treated with continuous subcutaneous insulin infusion via a pump using rapid-acting insulin analogues. Dilution of insulin to fill the pump is often required for neonates and infants. Demand of insulin is so small, and feeding so frequent that treatment with multiple daily injections is difficult.[340,341]

Hyperinsulinemic Hypoglycemia of Infancy

Hyperinsulinemic hypoglycemia is the most frequent cause of persistent and recurrent hypoglycemia in neonates and infants. It is due to unregulated secretion of insulin and can be transient or permanent. Transient forms lasting for days are associated with maternal diabetes mellitus, maternal sulfonylurea treatment, and glucose infusions during labor. Transient hyperinsulinism due to IUGR, perinatal asphyxia, and Beckwith-Wiedemann syndrome can last for days to months and may require diazoxide treatment. Permanent hyperinsulinism can histologically be divided into focal and diffuse forms that are inherited in, respectively, a sporadic or autosomal manner. Mutations have been described in eight genes: ABCC8, KCNJ11, GLUD1, GCK, HADH, SLC16A1, HNF4A, and UCP2. ABCC8 and KCNJ11 encode for the subunits (Kir6.2 and SUR1) of the pancreatic beta cell ATP-sensitive K+ channel.[342] Owing to their sensitivity to ATP, K+ channels convert intracellular metabolic signals to membrane excitability in the following cascade. Glucose is transported into the cell by glucose transporters; intracellular glucokinase catalyzes an essential irreversible step for glycolysis. Intracellular glucose metabolism raises the cytosol ATP/ADP ratio, which inhibits the SUR1 component of the K+ channel, resulting in K+ channel closure, which subsequently results in membrane depolarization, opening of voltage-gated calcium channels and calcium influx, which then triggers the release of insulin from stored granules. Mutations in *ABCC8* and *KCNJ11* can thus result in oversecretion of insulin. The hyperinsulinism/hyperammonemia syndrome (HI/HA) is due to gain-of-function mutations in glutamate dehydrogenase (GDH) and is characterized by both fasting hypoglycemia and hyperinsulinemic hypoglycemia due to protein ingestion.[343] Certain syndromes have been associated with hyperinsulinism: overgrowth syndromes (Beckwith-Wiedemann, Sotos, Simpson-Golabi-Behmel), chromosomal abnormalities (trisomy 13, mosaic Turner syndrome), growth failure syndromes (Kabuki syndrome, Costello syndrome), syndromes with abnormal calcium homeostasis (Timothy syndrome), congenital disorders of glycosylation, congenital hypoventilation syndrome, and a contiguous gene deletion including *ABCC8* (Usher syndrome).[344]

At the time of hypoglycemia, a hypoglycemia screen including glucose, insulin, C-peptide, acetoacetate and β-hydroxybutyrate will easily identify congenital hyperinsulinism.

Diagnostic criteria are a glucose infusion rate more than 8 mg/kg/minute, a laboratory blood glucose less than 3 mmol/L with detectable serum insulin or C-peptide, low serum ketone bodies, and low serum fatty acids.

First-line treatment is diazoxide and chlorothiazide, and second-line treatment is octreotide and glucagon. Patients who are diazoxide insensitive need further investigation with a combined computed tomography (CT)/^{18}F-DOPA PET scan to assess for focal or diffuse lesions. Focal lesions can be cured with surgery, whereas diffuse lesions require near-total pancreatectomy, which usually does not result in a cure and may lead to diabetes mellitus.[342] More recently, the use of sirolimus, a mammalian target of rapamycin (mTOR) inhibitor, has been advocated.[345]

NEUTRALIZATION OF HORMONE ACTIONS IN THE FETUS

After the period of embryogenesis, the fetal milieu is programmed to optimize body growth and organ development through an array of generalized and specialized growth factors (see "Fetal Growth"). These factors function in a stable metabolic environment with substrate supply maintained by the placenta. The endocrine and metabolic systems characterizing the extrauterine environment are programmed to maintain metabolic stability in a changing external environment with intermittent substrate provision. Hormonal systems in the fetus are programmed to maintain anabolism with minimal hormonal perturbation. Therefore, production of catabolic and thermogenic hormones is limited, and the effects of the hormones altering metabolic substrate supply and distribution pathways are muted (Table 22-6).

Limitation of Hormone Secretion

The human fetal pancreas is functional during the second trimester, but secretion of insulin in response to glucose or pyruvate is minimal until the neonatal period.[327,330] Glucagon secretion is also blunted, although fetal blood glucagon concentrations are relatively high. Fetal islet hyperplasia and increased insulin secretion occur in response to chronic hyperglycemia (e.g., in the infant of a diabetic mother), and insulin release can be stimulated by acute fetal infusions of leucine, arginine, or tolbutamide.[327,331] Moreover, responsiveness of both insulin and glucagon secretion to glucose develops rapidly in the neonatal period.[327] It is not

TABLE 22-6

Neutralization of Hormone Actions in the Fetus*

Production of Inactive Metabolites	
Active Hormone	**Inactive Metabolites**
Cortisol	Cortisone
Thyroxine (T_4)	rT_3, T_4S, rT_3S
Triiodothyronine (T_3)	T_3S, T_2
Delayed Expression or Neutralization of Receptors	
Active Hormone	**Receptor**
Growth hormone (GH)	GHR
Thyroid hormone	$TR\alpha$, $TR\beta$
Catecholamines	α-AR
Estrogens	$ER\alpha$, $ER\beta$
Glucagon	GR
Limited Hormone Secretion	
Active Hormone	**Secretory Cell**
Insulin	Islet cell beta
Glucagon	Islet cell alpha

*See text for details.
AR, adrenergic receptor; T_2, diiodothyronine; rT_3, reverse T_3; T_4S, T_4 sulfate.

clear whether the limited fetal islet cell responsiveness results from the relatively stable fetal serum glucose levels or from a temporally fixed maturation process (see earlier discussion).

Production of Inactive Hormone Metabolites

Throughout the second half of gestation, cortisol is metabolized in fetal tissues to inactive cortisone through the activity of HSD11B2. The placenta is permeable to steroid hormones, including cortisol. During midgestation, placental HSD11B2 activity is low, and some cortisol is transferred to the fetus. Placental HSD11B2 activity increases during the second half of pregnancy under the control of placental estrogens, and enzyme activity near term is high.[20,346] Maternal-fetal cortisol transfer decreases progressively. In addition, although many adult tissues can convert cortisone to cortisol, conversion is limited during most of fetal life. Consequently, most of the cortisol that crosses the placenta or is produced by the fetus is inactivated to cortisone by the placenta or by fetal tissues.

Concentrations of cortisone in fetal plasma exceed those of cortisol by threefold to fourfold until after 30 weeks of gestation (see Fig. 22-7). Teleologically, this would help preserve the anabolic and growth-promoting milieu of the fetus and minimize premature maturational and parturitional effects of cortisol. After 30 weeks, the ratio of cortisol to cortisone in fetal tissues and plasma increases as a result of increased fetal secretion and decreased conversion of cortisol to cortisone within the placenta and fetal tissues.[346] Cortisol has an important maturational action on several fetal tissues near term (see later discussion).

Fetal thyroid hormone metabolism is characterized by conversion of active thyroid hormones to inactive rT_3 and inactive sulfated iodothyronines and by limited receptor and postreceptor responsiveness to thyroid hormone in selected tissues.[174,188] The placenta contains an iodothyronine inner-ring monodeiodinase that catalyzes conversion of maternal T_4 to rT_3. The fetal sheep liver and kidney, in contrast to the adult liver and kidney, manifest low levels of D1 outer-ring monodeiodinase activity, so conversion of T_4 to active T_3 is limited, and large amounts of inactive iodothyronine sulfoconjugates accumulate.[174,190] As a consequence, plasma T_3 levels in the fetus remain low until the last few weeks of gestation (see Fig. 22-9). Selected fetal tissues (brain, brown adipose tissue) have active D2 outer-ring monodeiodinase activities that contribute to local tissue T_3 concentrations; local T_3 is important in development, particularly in the hypothyroid fetus.[174,347] Near term and in the neonatal period in the human fetus, the dramatic increase in plasma T_3 levels, and presumably in T_3 production, heralds the onset of thyroid hormone actions on growth and development and on metabolism (see Fig. 22-9).

Neutralization of Receptor Response

Selected ovine fetal tissues seem relatively unresponsive to thyroid hormones. Fetal ovine liver and kidney thermogenesis—as evidenced by oxygen consumption, sodium-potassium pump (Na^+/K^+-ATPase) activity, and mitochondrial α-glycerophosphate activity—is unresponsive to exogenous T_3 during the third trimester, and thyroid hormone responsiveness in a number of tissues (cardiac, hepatic, renal, and skin) develops only during the perinatal period.[348] β-Adrenergic receptor binding in heart and lung of the ovine fetus is unresponsive to T_3 late in the third trimester but increases in response to T_3 in the neonatal period.[160,348] In rodent species, in which development at birth is comparable to human fetal development at midgestation, pituitary GH concentrations become responsive to thyroid hormone only during the first weeks of extrauterine life.[349] Mouse submandibular gland EGF and NGF levels become responsive to thyroid hormone during the second week of life, as do urine and kidney EGF concentrations and hepatic EGF receptor levels.[350,351] Mouse skin EGF levels and EGF receptors are responsive during the first neonatal week.[352,353] Therefore, despite the presence of nuclear T_3 receptors in significant concentrations in developing rat and sheep fetuses, many thyroid hormone actions in these species are delayed.[354] The mechanism of this delayed thyroid hormone responsiveness is not clear; developmental programming of iodothyronine monodeiodinase expression and gene expression programming via unliganded TRs or TR-interacting corepressors probably all play a role.

The effect of the high circulating concentrations of GH in the fetus is also limited. Fetal somatic growth is only partially GH dependent; indeed, the GH-deficient fetus has little or no growth retardation.[53,355] The paucity of fetal GH effects is due to delayed maturation of GH receptors or postreceptor mechanisms. In animals such as sheep, hepatic GH receptor binding appears only during the neonatal period.[53] Receptor deficiency may also be a factor in the limited PRL bioactivity in the fetus near term.[53]

There is less information on fetal hormone responsiveness in other systems. β-Adrenergic receptor binding in the heart and lung of the sheep fetus is relatively low near term and increases in the neonatal period in response to thyroid hormones.[348] Premature lambs have an augmented plasma catecholamine surge at birth but have a relatively mild increase in plasma free fatty acid levels, which suggests reduced catecholamine responsiveness.[356] The high concentrations of progesterone and estrogens in fetal blood also seem to have limited effects in the fetus. Progesterone receptors are present in low concentration in fetal guinea pig kidney, lung, and uterus at midgestation and increase progressively until term.[357] ERs appear in neonatal rat uterus, oviduct, cervix, and vagina during the first 10 days of extrauterine life, and both ERα and ERβ mRNAs are present in human fetal tissues during the second trimester.[243,358] The human neonate often manifests mild breast enlargement at birth, and vaginal estrogenization may be evident in female infants at birth. Estrogen effects otherwise appear to be limited (see Table 22-6).

FETAL GROWTH

The hormones most important for postnatal growth, including T_4, GH, and gonadal steroids, have a limited role in fetal growth even though TR and GHR are expressed in many embryonic tissues including the growth plates.[1] Placental hormones including the human GH variant and hPLs play a limited role; hPL may promote early embryonic growth and may stimulate IGF and insulin production.[1] IGF-1 and IGF-2 are produced by the placenta and may exert autocrine-paracrine actions on placental growth. IGF-1, IGF-2, and the IGF-1 and IGF-2 receptors (IGF1R, IGF2R) are widely expressed in fetal tissues of mesenchymal, ectodermal, and endodermal origin and play a critical role in modulating normal fetal growth, including the nervous system.[359,360]

Insulin-like Growth Factors

The IGFs are involved in regulation of uterine and placental growth during pregnancy. In early embryonic and fetal development, IGF-1, EGF, and estrogens are mitogens for endometrial stromal cells, and the endometrial contents of IGF-1 and IGF-1 mRNA are high at implantation and during early embryogenesis in the sow.[361] Uterine IGF-1 and IGF-1 mRNA levels decrease progressively with advancing gestation.[361] Placental tissue also contains IGF-1 and IGF-2 mRNAs, significant concentrations of the respective proteins, and IGF1Rs.[20] Autocrine and paracrine roles for the IGFs in uterine and placental tissues are postulated. IGF-1 and insulin are produced by embryonic tissues during the prepancreatic stage of mouse development, and both factors stimulate growth of embryonic mouse cells.[362]

IGF-2 is genomically imprinted and paternally expressed in the fetus and placenta. The mature IGF-2 protein is generated from the biologically inactive pro-IGF-2 peptide by the action of proprotein convertase 4. Recent studies have shown a role of IGF-2 in determining placental nutrient supply and, hence, fetal growth.[363] In mutant mice lacking the imprinted placental-specific IGF-2 transcript, growth of the placenta is altered from early gestation, but fetal growth is normal until late gestation, suggesting functional adaptation of the placenta to meet the fetal demands. It is believed that this adaptation may be mediated by the altered expression of placental transporters GLUT3 and Slc38a4.[364]

Studies of transgenic mice with null mutations of the genes encoding IGF-1, IGF-2, or IGF1R have defined the role of these somatomedins; the birth weight of the embryos lacking IGF-1 or IGF-2 is only 60% that of control mice. When both genes are inactive, birth weight is reduced by another 30%, and mice lacking the IGF1R have birth weights averaging 45% of control values.[105] IGF-2–deficient mice also manifest IUGR in association with a small placenta. They have near-normal postnatal growth but delayed bone development.[105] IGF2R knockout fetal mice are 30% overweight, suggesting a negative growth-modulating effect of this receptor.

The normal growth in fetuses with both IGF1R and IGF2R knockout is caused by IGF-1 signaling via the insulin receptor; combined IGF-1, IGF-2, and insulin receptor knockout results in severe IUGR and fetal death. Knockout of individual IGF binding proteins (IGFBPs) has little effect on fetal or placental growth.[105] In humans, mutations in *IGF1* or *IGF1R* are associated with IUGR,[365,366] suggesting that IGF-1 signaling contributes significantly to fetal growth. Apart from growth retardation, these children also suffer from developmental delay, microcephaly, hypoglycemia, and sensorineural hearing loss.[364,365] Indeed, there is a relation between umbilical IGF-1 concentration and birth weight in humans; maternal smoking reduces both umbilical IGF-1 and birth weight.[367,368] Recent work in mice suggests that IGF-1 and IGF1R are required for late gestational lung maturation.[369] Hypomethylation of the 11p15-imprinted region has been associated with the phenotype of Silver-Russell syndrome.[370] This results in the relaxation of imprinting and biallelic expression of *H19* and downregulation of *IGF2*. Additionally, abnormal processing of IGF-2 by proprotein convertase 4 in the placenta has been implicated in the cause of fetal growth restriction.[371] Pregnant women carrying fetuses with IUGR (low birth weight for gestational age) had higher levels of pro-IGF-2 compared with control subjects. More recently, Murphy and colleagues reported severe IUGR and atypical diabetes mellitus secondary to insulin resistance in association with disruption of regulation of the *IGF2* gene.[372] On the other hand, overexpression of IGF-2 as a result of loss of imprinting associated with uniparental paternal disomy, *CDKN1C* gene loss of function, alteration in the KvLQT1 differentially methylated region (DMR), or microdeletions in the human H19 DMR is associated with overgrowth in the form of Beckwith-Wiedemann syndrome.[373]

IGFBPs are present as early as 5 weeks of gestation; prenatally and postnatally, the IGFs circulate in association with binding proteins.[105] High concentrations of circulating IGFBP1 are associated with fetal growth restriction in the mouse, as is overexpression of fetal IGFBP1 in the human.[374,375] IGFBP4 is expressed in the maternal decidua, is cleaved by its protease PAPP-A (pregnancy-associated plasma protein A), and inhibits IGF action. High maternal concentrations of IGFBP4 were recently shown to be related to fetal growth restriction.[376] During fetal and postnatal life, plasma concentrations of IGFs are relatively high compared with tissue concentrations. In the fetus, IGF-2 concentrations are five to six times higher than those of IGF-1, in contrast to these concentrations in children and adults, and concentrations of both increase progressively throughout gestation.[377] Fetal concentrations of both peptides at term are 30% to 50% of the adult concentrations.

In most studies, cord blood IGF-1 concentrations correlate with birth size.[105] Despite the fetal growth–enhancing effects of IGF-2, blood concentrations are only weakly related to size at birth, largely because of the inhibiting effect of soluble IGF2R[360] but also because IGF-2 appears to exert most of its growth effects in the earlier part of gestation. Soluble IGF2R is derived through proteolytic cleavage of the transmembrane region of the receptor in many tissues. IGF receptors have been identified as early as 5 weeks of gestation and are widespread in fetal tissues.[105] IGF-1 stimulates glycogenesis in cultured fetal rat hepatocytes and induces formation of myotubes in cultured myoblasts. IGF-2 is active in cultured muscle and neonatal rat astroglial cells. Insulin receptors are increased in fetal cells and are resistant to downregulation.

As discussed earlier, the control of IGF production differs in fetal and postnatal life. GH receptors are present, but receptors for hPL predominate in fetal tissues,[53,107] and GH, which stimulates IGF-1 production after birth, has a limited role in fetal IGF production.[359] GH does play a minor role in fetal growth, as reflected in the low IGF concentrations and slight reduction in birth weight and length in infants with GH resistance (Laron dwarfism) and GH deficiency.[355] hPL stimulates IGF-1 production and augments amino acid transport and DNA synthesis in human fetal fibroblasts

and muscle cells.[53] IGF-1 and IGF-2 concentrations are reduced in fetuses of protein-starved pregnant rats, and the low IGF-2 concentrations are reversed by hPL.[378] Thyroidectomy of the third-trimester sheep fetus impairs skeletal muscle growth in association with a decrease in muscle GH receptor mRNA and IGF-1 mRNA without an effect on IGF-2 levels.[379] Glucocorticoids can inhibit fetal growth, presumably by inhibiting IGF gene transcription, but may also affect growth plate chondrocytes directly.[379] The in utero environment (e.g., insulin exposure) plays a role in modulating IGF synthesis in the fetus.[380] Indeed, nutrition is the major factor modulating IGF production in the fetus. IGF concentrations fall in suckling rats deprived of milk, and IGF-1 and IGF-2 concentrations are reduced in fetuses of protein-starved pregnant rats and placentally restricted sheep.[105,106] Recent work suggests that light stimuli alter circulating and brain IGF-1 concentration and control neuronal migration through increased IGF-1 signaling.[381] Weekly intra-amniotic injections increase fetal growth of intrauterine growth-restricted sheep.[382] These data support the view that the IGFs are important in embryonic and fetal growth and that in the fetus they are regulated, at least in part, by hPL and by nutritional substrate derived transplacentally. The high concentrations of IGF-2 in fetal rat serum, the high levels of IGF-2 mRNA in fetal tissues, and the presence of a truncated form of IGF-1 in human fetal brain tissue suggest unique developmental actions of these peptides.

Insulin

Insulin has been proposed to act as a fetal growth factor. Infants born to women with diabetes mellitus may have hyperinsulinemia associated with increased birth weight.[383] Most of this increased weight is accounted for by body fat; there is little increase in body length, but some organomegaly may occur. Infants with hyperinsulinemia caused by congenital hyperinsulinism or the Beckwith-Wiedemann syndrome may also have increased somatic growth in utero. Conversely, the human fetus with pancreatic agenesis is small and has decreased muscle bulk and little or no adipose tissue.[383]

Mice with insulin or insulin receptor gene mutations have a 10% decrease in birth weight and early neonatal death with hyperglycemia and ketonemia.[105] Insulin receptor mutations in humans lead to severe IUGR and limited postnatal weight gain.[105] In contrast to mice, the human fetus during the latter half of gestation has a significant increase in adipose mass, and adipose tissue is highly sensitive to insulin. Treatment with IGF-1 improves the clinical condition to some extent.[384]

In clinical conditions associated with fetal hyperinsulinemia, the human neonate is born large for gestational age, primarily due to increased lipogenesis mediated by insulin or IGF-1 receptors.

Epidermal Growth Factor/Transforming Growth Factor System

The EGF/TGF-α system has been characterized in considerable detail.[385,386] EGF is a 6-kDa peptide product of a large, 1207–amino acid precursor molecule and acts through a 170-kDa membrane receptor glycoprotein. This receptor, like the IGF receptor, has intrinsic tyrosine kinase activity, and tyrosine kinase–mediated autophosphorylation is a critical event in EGF signal transduction. TGF-α, which has 35% amino acid homology with murine EGF and 44% homology with human EGF, also acts through the EGF receptor system.[385,386] Several additional family members have been characterized, including amphiregulin, heparin-binding EGF, betacellulin, and neuregulins.[386] Three additional receptors are referred to as ErbB2, ErbB3, and ErbB4 in animals; the human receptors are called human EGF receptor 2 (HER2), HER3, and HER4.[386]

EGF, pre-pro-EGF mRNA, and EGF receptors are present in most tissues in the postnatal rodent, but mRNA levels are highest in salivary glands and kidneys. EGF and pre-pro-EGF mRNA levels are absent or low in the fetal mouse and remain low in mouse tissues during the early neonatal period.[387] Nonetheless, the EGF receptor knockout mouse exhibits epithelial immaturity and multiorgan failure with early death.[387] Tissue concentrations of both EGF and EGF mRNA increase in the mouse during the first 2 months of postnatal life; indeed, concentrations of EGF in the salivary glands increased by several thousand-fold between 3 weeks and 3 months of age. Mouse urinary levels increase 200-fold and kidney concentrations increase 10-fold between 1 week and 2 months of age. EGF concentrations in mouse ocular tissues increase 100-fold during the first week of life.[385] Liver EGF concentrations increase more slowly, as do serum levels, and there is a high degree of correlation between serum and liver EGF levels in the developing mouse.[385] Therefore, the production of EGF in the rodent is accelerated during the early neonatal period, and it is during this time that most hormone-stimulated growth and development occur.

Fetal mouse and human tissues have high concentrations of TGF-α.[386,388,389] Immunoreactive TGF-α concentrations in mice are measurable at relatively high levels in lung, brain, liver, and kidney tissues in the fetal/neonatal rat, and the ontogenic pattern of TGF-α is tissue specific; most late fetal tissues studied contained TGF-α, and levels persisted or increased in most tissues through the period of growth and development.[388] In rodents and sheep, EGF provokes precocious eyelid opening and tooth eruption in neonatal animals; stimulates lung maturation; promotes palatal development in organ culture; stimulates gastrointestinal maturation; evokes secretion of pituitary hormones including GH, PRL, and corticotropin; and stimulates secretion of chorionic gonadotropin and placental lactogen by the placenta.[385,387] Both EGF and TGF-α compete for binding to the EGF receptor, and both factors accelerate eye opening and tooth eruption in the neonatal rodent, presumably through interaction with the same EGF receptor.[385]

Considerable evidence suggests a role for the EGF family of growth factors in mammalian CNS development.[390] EGF, TGF-α, neuregulins, and the EGF receptors are widely distributed in the nervous system.[385,391-394] EGF promotes proliferation of astroglial cells, acts as an astroglial differentiation factor, and enhances survival and outgrowth of selected neuronal cells.[391,392] Transgenic mice with a deficiency of neuregulin, ErbB2, ErbB3, or ErbB4 die in utero with cardiac anomalies and developmental anomalies of the hindbrain, midbrain, and ventral forebrain (see Table 22-6).[393,394]

EGF also plays an important role in rodent pregnancy. Maternal salivary gland and plasma EGF concentrations in the mouse increase fourfold to fivefold during pregnancy.[395] Removal of the salivary glands prevents the increase in plasma EGF; moreover, salivary gland removal reduces the number of mice completing term pregnancy (by 50%), decreases the percentage of live pups, and decreases the crown-rump length of fetuses delivered.[395] Administration of EGF antiserum to pregnant mice without salivary glands further increases the abortion rate, whereas administration of EGF improves pregnancy outcome.[395] Because maternal EGF is too large a molecule to traverse the placental barrier, an effect on maternal metabolism or on the placenta is likely.[395] The placenta is richly endowed with EGF receptors, and placental tissue binds and degrades EGF to constituent amino acids.[385] TGF-α is also produced by the maternal deciduus in rodents and stimulates proliferation of decidual tissue and decidual PRL production.

Nerve Growth Factor

NGF is a 13-kDa protein that is present at high concentrations in mouse salivary gland and at low concentrations in many adult tissues.[386] It is also produced by human placental tissue. It is the original member of an expanding family of neurotropic growth factors that now includes brain-derived neurotropic factor, neurotropin 3, and two less well-characterized factors; these ligands act via two receptors, NGF and NGF2 (or Trk).[386,396] NGF binds to high-affinity plasma membrane receptors and is internalized and transported to subcellular organelles, including the nucleus, in neurons of the peripheral nervous system. It promotes neurite outgrowth and enhances tyrosine hydroxylase and dopamine β-hydroxylase activities in developing sympathetic neurons. NGF acts on undifferentiated sympathetic cell precursors to evoke both hyperplastic and hypertrophic effects and plays a permissive role in stimulating the development of immature autonomic neurons along either a sympathetic or a cholinergic pathway.[386,397]

The injection of NGF in neonatal mice causes a marked increase in the volume of the superior cervical ganglia and increases the nerve supply of body organs. Likewise, injection of NGF antiserum during early neonatal life results in a decrease in the size of the superior cervical ganglia, reduction in tyrosine hydroxylase activity, and permanent sympathectomy.[397] Maternal NGF autoantibodies in rats and rabbits impair autonomic nervous system development in utero.[398] This impairment affects sympathetic and dorsal root ganglia and autonomic innervation of peripheral organs. NGF is produced by neonatal mouse astroglial cells in tissue culture, is present in developing mouse brain tissue, and together with brain-derived neurotropic factor and neurotropin 3, plays an important role in brain development.[395,396,399] Thyroid hormones and testosterone modulate postnatal NGF levels in the submandibular gland of the mouse. Thyroid hormones increase NGF, neurotropin 3, and brain-derived neurotropic factor mRNA levels in adult rat brain.[385,390]

Other Factors

Additional growth factors are involved in fetal growth and development, including hematopoietic growth factors, platelet-derived growth factors (PDGFs), FGFs, vascular endothelial growth factor (VEGF), and members of the TGF-β family.[105,386] The TGF-β superfamily of extracellular growth factors comprises more than 35 members, including TGF-β, the BMPs, growth and differentiation factors, activins, inhibins, müllerian inhibiting substance, nodal proteins, and lefty proteins.[400] These ligands activate some 12 transmembrane serine/threonine kinase receptors expressed in a variety of tissues. The family is critical for early embryonic development, left-right asymmetry, heart and vascular system development, craniofacial development, nervous system development, and skeletal morphogenesis and plays an important role in body composition and growth.

Hematopoietic growth factors are also active in the fetus during development; erythropoietin in fetal sheep is produced by the liver rather than the kidney, and erythropoietin gene expression in fetal sheep is regulated by glucocorticoids.[401] A switch to kidney production occurs after parturition.[402] Postnatally, thyroid hormones, testosterone, and hypoxia modulate erythropoietin production. PDGF represents a family of homodimers and heterodimers of PDGFA and PDGFB chains derived from two gene loci.[403] Two PDGF receptors have been characterized, PDGFα and PDGFβ. The genes for PDGF and its receptors are expressed in many tissues. *PDGFA* gene inactivation in mice leads to defects in lung, skin, intestine, testes, and brain that result in early postnatal death.[403] *PDGFB* gene inactivation leads to microvessel disruption and leakage with hemorrhage, edema, and intrauterine death.

The FGF family of heparin-binding growth factors now includes 17 members with diverse effects on development, angiogenesis, wound healing, and other biologic systems.[404,405] These effects are mediated by ligand-activated tyrosine protein kinase receptors (FGFRs) transcribed from four related genes. Several receptor isoforms are products of alternative RNA splicing.[106,386] Targeted disruptions of *FGF* and *FGFR* genes in mice have defined critical roles in development.[386,404] FGF3-deficient mice show tail and inner ear defects. Knockout of the *FGF4* gene is lethal, leading to early death. Knockout of the *FGFR1* gene also leads to early fetal death. *FGF10* knockout mice die at birth because of pulmonary agenesis. Deficiency of FGF4, FGF8, FGF9, FGF10, or FGF17 is associated with limb deformities. FGF8 deficiency leads to abnormal left-right axis patterning. In mice, *FGFR3* knockout results in chondrocyte hypertrophy and increased bone length.[386] In humans, a variety of gain-of-function *FGFR* mutations are associated with chondrodysplasias and craniosynostosis syndromes.[386] On the other hand, loss-of-function mutations in both *FGFR1* and *FGF8* are associated with Kallmann syndrome or hypogonadotropic hypogonadism; *FGF8* mutations are also associated with holoprosencephaly.[62,406,407] FGF, like EGF, stimulates the production of hCG from a choriocarcinoma cell line.[405] These observations and the fact that the placenta contains FGF, NGF, TGF-α, TGF-β, IGF-1, and IGF-2 suggest that the placenta plays an important role in modulating fetal growth.

Last, Wnt signaling, Notch signaling, BMP signaling, and hedgehog signaling play major roles in embryogenesis and fetal organ growth and development. These signaling pathways are also involved in bone development and growth and thus have a major effect on fetal size.[408]

TRANSITION TO EXTRAUTERINE LIFE

The transition to extrauterine life involves abrupt delivery from the protected intrauterine environment and succor by the placenta into the relatively hostile extrauterine environment. The neonate must initiate air breathing and defend against hypothermia, hypoglycemia, and hypocalcemia as the placental supply of energy and nutritional substrate is removed. Both the adrenal cortex and the autonomic nervous system, including the para-aortic chromaffin system, are essential for extrauterine adaptation. Longer-term transition requires adaptation to an environment of intermittent nutrient supply and transient substrate deficiency and requires maturation of the secretory control mechanisms for the PTH-calcitonin system and the endocrine pancreas.

Cortisol Surge

In most mammals, a cortisol surge occurs near term and is mediated by increased cortisol production by the fetal adrenal and a decreased rate of conversion of cortisol to cortisone. Pepe and Albrecht have proposed that the preterm fetal cortisol surge is due to the progressive stimulation by estrogens of placental HSD11B2 activity and the subsequent increase in placental conversion of cortisol to cortisone.[346] The resulting decrease in maternal-to-fetal cortisol transfer results in stimulation of fetal CRH and corticotropin secretion through the negative-feedback control loop. The concomitant estrogen-stimulated increase in HSD11B2 activity in fetal tissues potentiates the relative fetal cortisol deficiency and the CRH-corticotropin response.[346] Placental CRH may also potentiate fetal adrenal activation. Recent data suggest an increase in HSD11B1 expression and activity in placenta and intrauterine fetal membranes during late gestation, with a consequent increase in local cortisol production in preparation for parturition.[409]

The cortisol surge augments surfactant synthesis in lung tissue; increases lung liquid reabsorption; increases adrenomedullary PNMT activity, which in turn increases methylation of NE to epinephrine; increases hepatic iodothyronine outer-ring monodeiodinase activity and hence conversion of T_4 to T_3; decreases sensitivity of the ductus arteriosus to prostaglandins, facilitating ductus closure; induces maturation of several enzymes and transport processes of the small intestine; and stimulates maturation of hepatic enzymes (Fig. 22-14).[136,410] In some cases, these events involve increased synthesis of specific proteins or enzymes. In other instances, such as the action on the ductus arteriosus, the mechanism remains obscure.

Secondary effects of cortisol also promote extrauterine adaptations. The increased T_3 levels stimulate β-adrenergic receptor binding, potentiate surfactant synthesis in lung tissue, and increase the sensitivity of brown adipose tissue to NE. The significance of prenatal cortisol is demonstrated by the effects of gene-targeted CRH or GR deficiency in mice; the progeny of homozygous CRH-deficient or GR-deficient animals die in the first 12 hours with lung dysplasia and surfactant deficiency.[126,411]

The adaptational effects of the prenatal cortisol surge have led to the current recommendation for prenatal corticosteroid therapy in pregnancies threatened by the risk of preterm delivery. Generally, preterm infants prenatally exposed to augmented glucocorticoid concentrations have lower overall morbidity and mortality rates than untreated infants.

Catecholamine Surge

Parturition also evokes a dramatic catecholamine surge in the newborn, resulting in extraordinarily high levels of NE, epinephrine, and dopamine in cord blood.[273] As discussed earlier, plasma NE concentrations exceed epinephrine concentrations because of peripheral and adrenomedullary and para-aortic catecholamine release. Cord blood NE concentrations of 15 nmol/L (2500 pg/mL) and epinephrine concentrations of 2 nmol/L (370 pg/mL) are common after spontaneous delivery of term infants.[273] Concentrations of 25 nmol/L (4200 pg/mL) of NE and 35 nmol/L (640 pg/mL) of epinephrine are common in cord blood of premature infants. These changes evoke critical cardiovascular adaptations, including increased blood pressure and increased cardiac inotropic effects; increased glucagon secretion; decreased insulin secretion; increased thermogenesis in brown adipose tissue and increased plasma free fatty acid levels; and pulmonary adaptation, including mobilization of pulmonary fluid and increased surfactant release.[273,277,409]

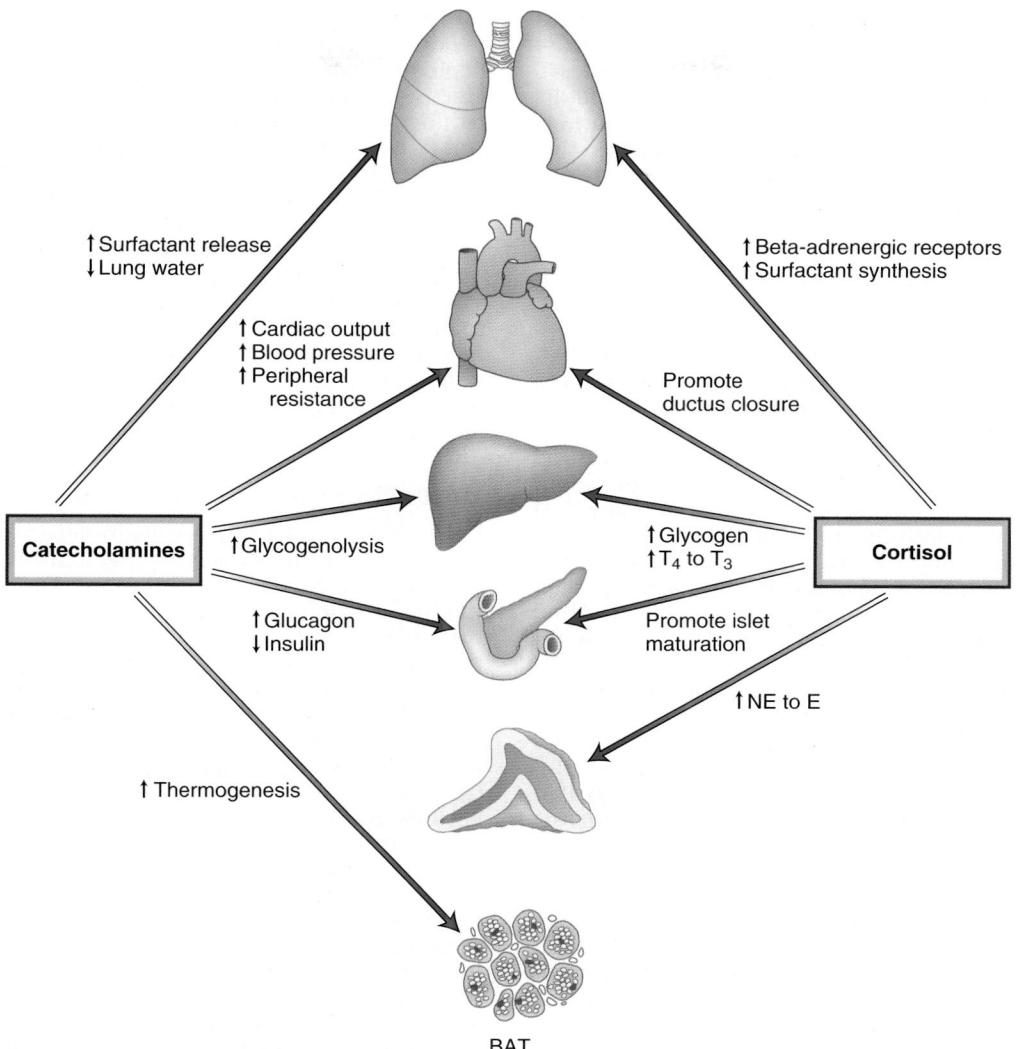

Figure 22-14 Actions of cortisol and catecholamines during fetal adaptation to the extrauterine environment. The prenatal cortisol surge acts to promote functional maturation of several organ systems. The neonatal catecholamine surge triggers or potentiates a number of the extrauterine cardiopulmonary and metabolic functional adaptations that are critical to extrauterine survival. See text for details. BAT, brown adipose tissue; E, epinephrine; NE, norepinephrine; T_3, triiodothyronine; T_4, thyroxine.

Thermogenesis in Neonatal Brown Adipose Tissue

Brown adipose tissue is the major site of thermogenesis in the newborn and is especially prominent in the mammalian fetus. The largest accumulations of brown adipose tissue envelop the kidneys and adrenal glands, and smaller amounts surround the blood vessels of the mediastinum and neck.[412] The mass of brown adipose tissue peaks at the time of birth and gradually decreases during the early weeks of life. Surgical removal of this tissue leads to neonatal hypothermia. NE, through β-adrenergic receptors, stimulates thermogenesis by brown adipose tissue, and optimal responsiveness of this tissue to NE is dependent on thyroid hormone.[412,413] Brown adipose tissue is rich in mitochondria, containing a unique 32-kDa protein (thermogenin) that uncouples oxidation and phosphorylation of adenosine diphosphate, reduces ATP production, and consequently enhances thermogenesis.[412,414] Thermogenin is T_3 dependent, and brown adipose tissue contains a 5′-monoiodothyronine deiodinase that deiodinates

T_4 locally to T_3.[412,414] Full maturation of catecholamine-stimulated cellular respiration in brown adipose tissue occurs before delivery in the ovine fetus and requires thyroid hormone.[412,415] Fetal thyroidectomy in this species leads to marked hypothermia, with low plasma free fatty acid levels and increased plasma epinephrine concentrations.[415] In vitro, basal brown adipose tissue thermogenesis and NE-stimulated and dibutyryl cAMP-stimulated thermogenesis are decreased by fetal thyroidectomy.

The rapid onset of thermogenesis in brown adipose tissue is essential for survival in newborn infants. Catecholamine release is the stimulus for brown adipose tissue thermogenesis in the early neonatal period, and responsiveness to catecholamines is markedly increased by cutting of the umbilical cord.[413] Fetal hypoxia and placental inhibitors, including prostaglandin E_2 and adenosine, appear to inhibit brown adipose tissue thermogenesis in utero.[413] Cord cutting, neonatal cooling, catecholamine stimulation, and augmented conversion of T_4 to T_3 in brown adipose tissue in the neonatal period are the essential features that mediate and condition newborn thermogenesis. It was previously thought that brown adipose tissue involuted soon after birth, but combined [^{18}F]fluorodeoxyglucose positron emission tomography ([^{18}F]FDG-PET) and CT scans have identified active brown adipose tissue in adults and shown a strong positive correlation between brown adipose tissue activity and the basal metabolic rate.[416-418]

Calcium Homeostasis

In utero, active calcium transport from the mother to the fetus takes place through the placenta, responsible for approximately 20% to 30% of calcium stores in the fetus. The neonate must adjust rapidly from a high-calcium environment regulated by PTHrP and calcitonin to a low-calcium environment that requires regulation by PTH and vitamin D. With removal of the placenta in term infants, plasma total calcium concentration falls, reaching a nadir of approximately 2.3 mmol/L (9 mg/dL),[292] and the ionized calcium concentration reaches a low level of about 1.2 mmol/L (4.8 mg/dL) by 24 hours of life.[419] Plasma PTH concentrations are relatively low in the neonatal period and are minimally responsive to hypocalcemia during the first 2 to 3 days of life. Calcitonin concentrations are high in cord blood (approximately 2000 ng/L), increase further during the early neonatal period, and remain high for several days after birth.[292,420] The relatively obtunded PTH response and the high calcitonin concentrations lead to a 2- to 3-day period of transient neonatal hypocalcemia.[420,421] Inhibition of calcitonin secretion and stimulation of PTH secretion gradually result in increased serum calcium concentrations in the neonate. The disappearance of PTHrP in the neonatal lamb is approximately coincident with the time of restoration of calcium levels to the adult range.[292] The mechanism of transition from PTHrP to PTH secretion by the neonatal parathyroid glands is not clear.

Calcium homeostasis is also affected in the human newborn by the low level of glomerular filtration that persists for several days.[420,421] In addition, renal responsiveness to PTH is reduced in the first few days of life. These factors limit phosphate excretion and predispose the neonate to hyperphosphatemia, particularly if the diet includes high-phosphate milk such as unmodified cow milk. Premature infants, compared with term infants, tend to have lower PTH and higher calcitonin concentrations and more immature kidney function; in these infants, neonatal hypocalcemia may be more marked and prolonged, and the incidence of symptomatic hypocalcemia is higher. Birth asphyxia also predisposes the neonate to hypocalcemia.[421] Infants born to mothers with hypercalcemia related to hyperparathyroidism have a high incidence of symptomatic hypocalcemia. These infants have a more marked suppression of parathyroid function and a longer period of transient hypoparathyroidism in the neonatal period. PTH secretion and calcium homeostasis usually return to normal in 1 to 2 weeks in full-term infants and within 2 to 3 weeks in the small premature infant.

Glucose Homeostasis

The abrupt withdrawal of the placental glucose supply leads to a prompt fall in plasma glucose in the term neonate.[327,330] The low glucose and high catecholamine levels stimulate glucagon secretion, and the plasma glucagon concentration peaks within 2 hours after birth.[327,330] Plasma insulin concentrations are low at birth and tend to fall further with hypoglycemia. The early glucagon response is short-lived; however, concentrations remain at about 100 ng/L for the first 12 to 24 hours, and the glucagon/insulin ratio is high enough to stabilize glucose levels in the range of 2.8 to 4 mmol/L (50 to 70 mg/dL) during this period. The early glucagon and catecholamine surges deplete hepatic glycogen stores, so the return of plasma glucose concentrations to normal after 12 to 18 hours requires maturation of hepatic gluconeogenesis under the stimulus of a high plasma glucagon/insulin ratio.[330] Glucagon secretion gradually increases during the early hours after birth, especially with protein feeding, which stimulates gut glucagon release and pancreatic glucagon secretion.[327,330] Premature infants have more severe and more prolonged hypoglycemia because of reduced glycogen stores and impaired hepatic gluconeogenesis. Infants born to diabetic mothers have more severe neonatal hypoglycemia because of relative hyperinsulinism. In the healthy term infant, glucose homeostasis is achieved within 5 to 7 days of life; in premature infants, 1 to 2 weeks may be required.

Other Hormonal Adaptations

Delivery of the placenta results in decreases in fetal blood concentrations of estrogens, progesterone, hCG, and hPL. The fall in estrogen concentrations presumably removes the major stimulus to fetal pituitary PRL release, and PRL concentrations decrease within several weeks. The relatively delayed fall may be due to lactotroph hyperplasia in the fetal pituitary or to delayed maturation of hypothalamic dopamine secretion. The gradual fall of GH concentrations during the early weeks of life is due to delayed maturation of hypothalamic-pituitary feedback control of GH release.[46] In the neonatal primate, there are concomitant decreases in plasma GH concentrations and GH responsiveness to exogenous GHRH.[422] The mechanisms remain unclear; changes in secretion or in pituitary sensitivity to GHRH or somatostatin, or both, may be involved. IGF-1 and IGF-2 concentrations fall to infantile values within a few days, presumably because of the removal of placental hPL and placental IGF production (see Fig. 22-5).

In male infants (see Fig. 22-10), after a transient fall in testosterone concentrations as the hCG stimulus abates, pituitary LH secretion rebounds modestly, and there is a secondary surge of plasma testosterone that persists at significant levels for several weeks.[46,423] This surge is mediated by hypothalamic GnRH; blockade of neonatal activation of the pituitary-testicular axis with a GnRH agonist in neonatal monkeys ablates the neonatal increments in LH and testosterone.[424] Such a blockade also results in subnormal increments in plasma LH and testosterone concentrations and subnormal testicular enlargement at puberty in these animals, suggesting that neonatal GnRH release with pituitary-testicular activation may be critical for normal sexual maturation of male primates.[424] In females, a transient, secondary surge in FSH may transiently elevate estrogen concentrations.

Delivery results in a reversal of the high fetal cortisone/cortisol ratio, and plasma cortisol concentrations are higher in the neonate despite relatively lower plasma corticotropin concentrations (see Fig. 22-7). Presumably, this increase is due to decreased inhibition of adrenal 3β-HSD by estrogen and perhaps to removal of a placental CRH action on fetal pituitary corticotropin release. Plasma DHEAS and DHEA concentrations fall as the fetal adrenal atrophies.

The increase in serum TSH concentrations during the early minutes after birth is due to cooling of the neonate in the extrauterine environment.[160,174] In term infants, the TSH surge peaks at 30 minutes at a concentration of about 70 mU/L (see Fig. 22-9). This peak evokes increased secretion of T$_4$ and T$_3$ by the thyroid gland. In addition, increased conversion of T$_4$ to T$_3$ by the liver and other tissues maintains the T_3 concentration in the extrauterine range of 1.6 to 3.4 nmol/L (105 to 220 ng/dL). The re-equilibration of TSH concentrations to the normal extrauterine range is probably a result of the readjustment of prevailing serum T_3 concentrations and maturation of feedback control of TSH by thyroid hormones during the early weeks of life.[160,179] Production of rT_3 by fetal and neonatal tissues abates by 3 to 4 weeks of age, at which time serum rT_3 reaches adult concentrations.

PROGRAMMING OF DEVELOPING ENDOCRINE SYSTEMS

During the past several decades, the concept of the plasticity of fetal endocrine systems has evolved from experiments in several mammalian species, indicating that hormonal programming occurs during a critical fetal or perinatal period of development. There is a growing list of examples. In the female rodent, transient neonatal androgen administration masculinizes the pattern of hypothalamic control of GnRH secretion and pituitary gonadotropin secretion, masculinizes adult behavior and adult sexual activity, permanently alters the pattern of GH secretion, increases longitudinal bone growth and body weight, and masculinizes the pattern of hepatic steroid metabolism.[425,426] Prenatal androgens program the timing of neuroendocrine puberty in sheep: the higher the dose of prenatal testosterone, the earlier the initiation of the pubertal LH rise.[427] Estrogen administration to pregnant rats during the last third of gestation produces cryptorchid male offspring and may permanently suppress spermatogenesis in adult males.[428] Transient levothyroxine administration to neonatal rodents leads to growth retardation, delayed puberty, decreased adult pituitary weight, decreased pituitary TRH concentrations, low serum TSH levels, and decreased TSH responsiveness to propylthiouracil challenge.[429,430] Administration of insulin or alloxan to neonatal rats produces permanent alteration of glucose tolerance.[431] A single dose of vasopressin to the neonatal rat permanently enhances the adult response to vasopressin.[432] Fetal exposure to high maternal glucocorticoid levels in the rat inhibits fetal growth and leads to subsequent hypertension in the offspring.[9] Moreover, it has been observed that the permanent programming can be transmitted to later generations, leading to the concept of epigenetic effects.[431,433]

The concept of fetal programming was extended with the observation of ecologic associations between fetal and early life health indicators (e.g., birth size, infant mortality) and adult diseases. The concept, advanced in the 1980s, that adult diseases have fetal and perinatal genesis has been referred to as the *Barker hypothesis*.[434] There is now extensive documentation of the association of IUGR with an increased risk of later hypertension, insulin resistance, diabetes, and cardiovascular and coronary heart disease.[435-442] The programming involves epigenetic, neuroendocrine, hormonal receptor, and metabolic alterations involving the placenta and fetus.[443-451]

Epigenetic effects include genetic imprinting. Imprinted genes are a class of genes in placental mammals and marsupials whose expression depends on the parental origin.[443-449] Imprinting is controlled epigenetically (by such factors as nutrition) via DNA methylation and chromatin modifications. In mice, imprinted genes in the placenta regulate the supply of nutrients; in the fetus, they control nutrient metabolism.[443] In mice, approximately 60 imprinted genes have been identified, and for most the imprinting status is conserved in humans; many of these genes are involved in the control of fetal growth.[449] Paternally expressed imprinted genes tend to enhance and maternally expressed genes tend to suppress fetal growth. Knockout of paternally expressed genes for IGF-2, PEG1, PEG2, and insulin result in IUGR, whereas knockout of the maternal genes *H19*, *IGF2R*, or overexpression of *IGF2* results in fetal overgrowth.[443] Other genetic alterations including modification of tandem repeats in the insulin gene have been described.[444]

Hormones in the fetus are derived from the placenta, from the mother, from fetal endocrine glands, and from circulating precursors in fetal or placental tissues. These extensive networks linking maternal-placental-fetal endocrine interactions, and the apparent plasticity of developing endocrine and metabolic systems, facilitate endocrine system programming. As discussed earlier, the programming may be relatively system limited.[9,425-432] Other examples include the observation many years ago that diethylstilbestrol administration to pregnant women increased the prevalence of vaginal adenocarcinoma in female offspring during the second and third decades of life.[440] More recently, it was shown that prenatal or neonatal diethylstilbestrol exposure in hamsters and mice perturbs normal uterine development by affecting the genetic pathways programming uterine differentiation and results in hyperplastic and neoplastic uterine lesions with increased levels of cJun, cFos, Myc, Bax, and Bcl-x.[452,453] Excessive androgen exposure during fetal life has been associated with later polycystic ovary syndrome.[440] Hormonal programming also is demonstrable in cell lines and in unicellular organisms, in which a single exposure to a hormone can produce persistent alteration of the hormonal response characteristics or of prohormone processing.[454,455] Undernutrition during pregnancy in the rat results in the development of obesity, hyperinsulinemia, and hyperleptinemia during adult life; this phenotype is potentiated when the offspring are fed a high-fat diet.[456] Neonatal leptin treatment normalized the programmed phenotype, indicating that metabolic programming may be reversible during the period of developmental plasticity.[456]

The effects of maternal undernutrition and fetal IUGR extend to several systems, and it is hypothesized that excessive maternal-fetal glucocorticoids play a significant programming role. Glucocorticoids have wide-ranging effects in the fetus, altering receptors, enzymes, ion channels, and transporters in a variety of cells and tissues in the late-gestation fetus, and can induce programming of other endocrine systems. Throughout gestation, they modify *GLUT* gene expression in placenta and fetus, influence IGF and GR gene expression in various tissues, affect expression of several transcription factors, and affect a wide variety of enzymes in placenta, liver, kidney, intestine, and lung.[446] Maternal undernutrition, stress, and placental dysfunction are associated with increased maternal and fetal glucocorticoid levels, which contribute importantly to IUGR and programmed alterations in adult endocrine systems and metabolism.[438,446,447]

MATERNAL AND FETAL MEDICINE

We describe our current understanding of the intrauterine endocrine milieu and highlights progress in this challenging frontier of medicine. This progress has set the stage for fetal endocrine disease diagnosis, therapy for fetal endocrine and metabolic disorders, management of disorders of fetal growth, and diagnosis and management of perinatal or neonatal endocrine dysfunction. In addition, understanding of developmental endocrinology is increasingly relevant to management strategies for premature infants and infants and children with fetal growth retardation and for understanding of the pathogenesis of adult endocrine and metabolic diseases.

We are now entering an era of direct access to and management of the intrauterine environment with provision of medical and surgical fetal therapy, entailing both potential advantages and risks.[457] With expansion of the application and scope of amniotic fluid fetal cell sampling, maternal plasma DNA analysis, and the advent of fetal visualization and intrauterine fetal blood sampling, direct access for fetal diagnosis is now possible.[458-461] Intrauterine diagnosis and treatment of fetal adrenal and thyroid disorders have become the standard of care.[462,463] Intravenous nutritional supplementation of fetal sheep can prevent some forms of growth retardation, and chronic fetal therapy through indwelling pumps is feasible in animal fetuses.[464] These approaches, coupled with increasing availability of synthetic hormones and growth factor agonists and antagonists, facilitate direct fetal endocrine therapy. In addition, intrauterine stem cell transplantation has been successful in the correction of congenital hematologic disease. The fetus in early gestation is a favorable recipient of cellular therapy, and fetal cell transplantation may be applicable to therapy for selected endocrine and metabolic disease.[465,466] Finally, there is a growing experience with fetal and neonatal gene therapy in animals.[467]

REFERENCES

1. Murphy VE, Smith R, Giles WB, et al. Endocrine regulation of human fetal growth: the role of the mother, placenta, and fetus. *Endocrine Rev.* 2006;27:141-169.
2. Fisher DA. Fetal and neonatal endocrinology. In: DeGroot LJ, Jameson JL, eds. *Endocrinology.* 5th ed. Philadelphia, PA: Elsevier Saunders; 2006:3369-3386.
3. Palfi M, Selbing A. Placental transport of maternal immunoglobulin G. *Am J Reprod Immunol.* 1998;39:24-26.
4. Sodha RJ, Proegler M, Schneider H. Transfer and metabolism of norepinephrine studied from maternal to fetal and fetal to maternal sides in the in vitro perfused human placental life. *Am J Obstet Gynecol.* 1984;148:474-481.
5. Benediktsson R, Calder A, Edwards CRW, et al. Placental 11β-hydroxysteroid dehydrogenase: a key regulator of fetal glucocorticoid exposure. *Clin Endocrinol (Oxf).* 1997;46:161-166.
6. Murphy BEP. Cortisol and cortisone in human fetal development. *J Steroid Biochem.* 1979;11:509-513.
7. Takeyama J, Sasano H, Suzuki T, et al. 17β-Hydroxysteroid dehydrogenase types 1 and 2 in human placenta: an immunohistochemical study with correlation to placental development. *J Clin Endocrinol Metab.* 1998;83:3710-3715.
8. Krysina E, Brzezinska-Slebodzinska E, Slebodzinski AB. Divergent deiodination of thyroid hormones in the separated parts of the fetal and maternal placenta in pigs. *J Endocrinol.* 1997;155:295-303.
9. Benediktsson R, Lindsay RD, Noble J, et al. Glucocorticoid exposure in utero: new model for adult hypertension. [Erratum in *Lancet.* 1993;341:572]. *Lancet.* 1993;341(8841):339-341.
10. Yau JL, Olsson T, Morris RG, et al. Glucocorticoids, hippocampal corticosteroid receptor gene expression and antidepressant treatment: relationship with spatial learning in young and aged rats. *Neuroscience.* 1995;66:571-581.
11. Roberts D, Dalziel SR. Antenatal corticosteroids for accelerating fetal lung maturation for women at risk of preterm birth. *Cochrane Database Syst Rev.* 2006;(3):CD004454.
12. Speiser PW, Azziz R, Baskin LS, et al; Endocrine Society. Congenital adrenal hyperplasia due to steroid 21-hydroxylase deficiency: an Endocrine Society clinical practice guideline. *J Clin Endocrinol Metab.* 2010;95:4133-4160.
13. Hindmarsh PC. Endocrine Society congenital adrenal hyperplasia guidelines: great content but how to deliver? *Clin Endocrinol.* 2012;76: 465-466.
14. Roti E, Gnudi A, Braverman LE. The placental transport, synthesis and metabolism of hormones and drugs which affect thyroid function. *Endocr Rev.* 1983;4:131-149.
15. Haddow JE, Palomaki GE, Allan WC, et al. Maternal thyroid deficiency during pregnancy and subsequent neuropsychological development of the child. *N Engl J Med.* 1999;341:549-555.
16. Li Y, Shan Z, Teng W, et al. Abnormalities of maternal thyroid function during pregnancy affect neuropsychological development of their children at 25-30 months. *Clin Endocrinol.* 2010;72:825-829.
17. Ghassabian A, Bongers-Schokking JJ, Henrichs J, et al. Maternal thyroid function during pregnancy and behavioral problems in the offspring: the Generation R study. *Pediatr Res.* 2011;69:454-459.
18. Ghassabian A, Bongers-Schokking JJ, de Rijke YB, et al. Maternal thyroid autoimmunity during pregnancy and the risk of attention deficit/hyperactivity problems in children: the Generation R Study. *Thyroid.* 2012;22:178-186.
19. Iisalo E, Castren O. The enzymatic inactivation of noradrenaline in human placental tissue. *Ann Med Exp Biol Fenn.* 1967;45:253-257.
20. Mesiano S, Jaffe RB. Neuroendocrine-metabolic regulation of pregnancy. In: Strauss JF III, Barbieri RL, eds. *Reproductive Endocrinology.* 5th ed. Philadelphia, PA: WB Saunders; 2004:327-366.
21. Goldsmith PC, McGregor WG, Raymoure WJ, et al. Cellular localization of chorionic gonadotropin in human fetal liver and kidney. *J Clin Endocrinol Metab.* 1983;57:654-661.
22. Kapcala LP. Immunoassayable adrenocorticotropin in peripheral organs: concentrations during early development. *Life Sci.* 1985;37: 2283-2290.
23. Martino E, Lernmark A, Seo H, et al. High concentration of thyrotropin releasing hormone in pancreatic islets. *Proc Natl Acad Sci U S A.* 1978;75:4265-4267.
24. Pekary AE, Meyer NV, Vaillant C, et al. Thyrotropin releasing hormone and a homologous peptide in the male rat reproductive system. *Biochem Biophys Res Commun.* 1980;95:993-1000.
25. Suda T, Tomori N, Tozawa F, et al. Distribution and characterization of immunoreactive corticotropin-releasing factor in human tissues. *J Clin Endocrinol Metab.* 1984;59:861-866.
26. Thompson RC, Seasholtz AF, Herbert E. Rat corticotropin releasing hormone gene: sequence and tissue specific expression. *Mol Endocrinol.* 1987;1:363-370.
27. Shibaski T, Kiyosawa Y, Masuda A, et al. Distribution of growth hormone releasing hormone-like immunoreactivity in human tissue extracts. *J Clin Endocrinol Metab.* 1984;59:263-268.
28. Wu P, Jackson IMD. Identification, characterization and localization of thyrotropin releasing hormone precursor peptides in perinatal rat pancreas. *Regul Pept.* 1988;22:347-360.
29. Koshimizu T. The development of pancreatic and gastrointestinal somatostatin-like immunoreactivity and its relationship to feeding in neonatal rats. *Endocrinology.* 1983;112:911-916.
30. Steculorum SM, Bouret SG. Developmental effects of ghrelin. *Peptides.* 2011;32:2362-2366.
31. Polk DH, Reviczky AL, Lam RW, et al. Thyrotropin releasing hormone in the ovine fetus: ontogeny and effect of thyroid hormone. *Am J Physiol.* 1991;23:E53-E58.
32. Rahier J, Wallon J, Henquin JC. Abundance of somatostatin cells in the human neonatal pancreas. *Diabetologia.* 1980;18:251-254.
33. Leduque P, Aratan-Spire S, Czernichow P, et al. Ontogenesis of thyrotropin-releasing hormone in the human fetal pancreas. *J Clin Invest.* 1986;78:1028-1034.
34. Saito H, Saito S, Sano T, et al. Fetal and maternal plasma levels of immunoreactive somatostatin at delivery: evidence for its increase in the umbilical artery and its arteriovenous gradient in the fetoplacental circulation. *J Clin Endocrinol Metab.* 1983;56:567-571.
35. Koshimizu T, Ohyama Y, Yokota Y, et al. Peripheral plasma concentrations of somatostatin-like immunoreactivity in newborns and infants. *J Clin Endocrinol Metab.* 1985;61:78-82.
36. Kawamura K, Kouki T, Kawahara G, Kikuyama S. Hypophyseal development in vertebrates from amphibians to mammals. *Gen Comp Endocrinol.* 2002;126:130-135.
37. Rubenstein JL, Shimamura K, Martinez S, Puelles L. Regionalization of the prosencephalic neural plate. *Annu Rev Neurosci.* 1998;21:445-477.
38. Osumi-Yamashita N, Ninomiya Y, Doi H, Eto K. The contribution of both forebrain and midbrain crest cells to the mesenchyme in the frontonasal mass of mouse embryos. *Dev Biol.* 1994;164:409-419.
39. Pogoda HM, Hammerschmidt M. Molecular genetics of pituitary development in zebrafish. *Semin Cell Dev Biol.* 2007;18:543-558.
40. Davis SW, Ellsworth BS, Perez Millan MI, et al. Pituitary gland development and disease: from stem cell to hormone production. *Curr Top Dev Biol.* 2013;106:1-47.
41. Pearson CA, Placzek M. Development of the medial hypothalamus: forming a functional hypothalamic-neurohypophyseal interface. *Curr Top Dev Biol.* 2013;106:49-88.
42. Szarek E, Cheah PS, Schwartz J, Thomas P. Molecular genetics of the developing neuroendocrine hypothalamus. *Mol Cell Endocrinol.* 2010; 323:115-123.
43. Kelberman D, Rizzoti K, Lovell-Badge R, et al. Genetic regulation of pituitary gland development in human and mouse. *Endocr Rev.* 2009; 30:790-829.
44. Blackshaw S, Scholpp S, Placzek M, et al. Molecular pathways controlling development of thalamus and hypothalamus: from neural specification to circuit formation. *J Neurosci.* 2010;30:14925-14930.
45. Tosches MA, Arendt D. The bilaterian forebrain: an evolutionary chimaera. *Curr Opin Neurobiol.* 2013;23:1080-1089.

46. Grumbach MM, Gluckman PD. The human fetal hypothalamus and pituitary gland: the maturation of neuroendocrine mechanisms controlling secretion of fetal pituitary growth hormone, prolactin, gonadotropins, adrenocorticotropin-related peptides, and thyrotropin. In: Tulchinsky D, Little AB, eds. *Maternal Fetal Endocrinology*. 2nd ed. Philadelphia, PA: WB Saunders; 1994:193-261.

47. Cohen LE, Radovik S. Molecular basis of combined pituitary hormone deficiencies. *Endocr Rev*. 2002;23:431-442.

48. Gutnick A, Blechman J, Kaslin J, et al. The hypothalamic neuropeptide oxytocin is required for formation of the neurovascular interface of the pituitary. *Dev Cell*. 2011;21:642-654.

49. Liu F, Pogoda HM, Pearson CA, et al. Direct and indirect roles of Fgf3 and Fgf10 in innervation and vascularisation of the vertebrate hypothalamic neurohypophysis. *Development*. 2013;140:1111-1122.

50. Rizzoti K, Lovell-Badge R. Early development of the pituitary gland: induction and shaping of Rathke's pouch. *Rev Endocr Metab Disord*. 2005;6:161-172.

51. Fauquier T, Rizzoti K, Dattani M, et al. SOX2-expressing progenitor cells generate all of the major cell types in the adult mouse pituitary gland. *Proc Natl Acad Sci U S A*. 2008;105:2907-2912.

52. Castinetti F, Davis SW, Brue T, Camper SA. Pituitary stem cell update and potential implications for treating hypopituitarism. *Endocr Rev*. 2011;32:453-471.

53. Gluckman PD, Pinal CS. Growth hormone and prolactin. In: Polin RA, Fox WW, Abman SH, eds. *Fetal and Neonatal Physiology*. 3rd ed. Philadelphia, PA: WB Saunders; 2004:1891-1895.

54. Mollard P, Hodson DJ, Lafont C, et al. A tridimensional view of pituitary development and function. *Trends Endocrinol Metab*. 2012;23: 261-269.

55. Zhu X, Zhang J, Tollkuhn J, et al. Sustained Notch signaling in progenitors is required for sequential emergence of distinct cell lineages during organogenesis. *Genes Dev*. 2006;20:2739-2753.

56. Roessler E, Belloni E, Gaudenz K, et al. Mutations in the human sonic hedgehog gene cause holoprosencephaly. *Nat Genet*. 1996;14:357-360.

57. Brown SA, Warburton D, Brown LY, et al. Holoprosencephaly due to mutation in ZIC1, a homologue of *Drosophila* odd-paired. *Nat Genet*. 1998;20:180-183.

58. Roessler E, Muenke M. The molecular genetics of holoprosencephaly. *Am J Med Genet C Semin Med Genet*. 2010;154C(1):52-61.

59. Cohen MM Jr. Holoprosencephaly: clinical, anatomic, and molecular dimensions. Birth defects research Part A. *Clin Mol Teratol*. 2006;76: 658-673.

60. Mercier S, Dubourg C, Garcelon N, et al. New findings for phenotype-genotype correlations in a large European series of holoprosencephaly cases. *J Med Genet*. 2011;48:752-760.

61. Roessler E, Ouspenskaia MV, Karkera JD, et al. Reduced NODAL signaling strength via mutation of several pathway members including FOXH1 is linked to human heart defects and holoprosencephaly. *Am J Hum Genet*. 2008;83:18-29.

62. McCabe MJ, Gaston-Massuet C, Tziaferi V, et al. Novel FGF8 mutations associated with recessive holoprosencephaly, craniofacial defects, and hypothalamo-pituitary dysfunction. *J Clin Endocrinol Metab*. 2011;96: E1709-E1718.

63. Valdes-Socin H, Rubio Almanza M, Tome Fernandez-Ladreda M, et al. Reproduction, smell, and neurodevelopmental disorders: genetic defects in different hypogonadotropic hypogonadal syndromes. *Front Endocrinol (Lausanne)*. 2014;5:109.

64. Dattani MT, Martinez-Barbera JP, Thomas PQ, et al. Mutations in the homeobox gene HESX1/Hesx1 associated with septo-optic dysplasia in human and mouse. *Nat Genet*. 1998;19:125-133.

65. Kelberman D, Rizzoti K, Avilion A, et al. Mutations within Sox2/SOX2 are associated with abnormalities in the hypothalamo-pituitary-gonadal axis in mice and humans. *J Clin Invest*. 2006;116:2442-2455.

66. Kelberman D, de Castro SC, Huang S, et al. SOX2 plays a critical role in the pituitary, forebrain and eye during human embryonic development. *J Clin Endocrinol Metab*. 2008;93:1865-1873.

67. Tajima T, Ohtake A, Hoshino M, et al. OTX2 loss of function mutation causes anophthalmia and combined pituitary hormone deficiency with a small anterior and ectopic posterior pituitary. *J Clin Endocrinol Metab*. 2008;94:314-319.

68. Dateki S, Fukami M, Sato N, et al. OTX2 mutation in a patient with anophthalmia, short stature, and partial growth hormone deficiency: functional studies using the IRBP, HESX1, and POU1F1 promoters. *J Clin Endocrinol Metab*. 2008;93:3697-3702.

69. Diaczok D, Romero C, Zunich J, et al. A novel dominant negative mutation of OTX2 associated with combined pituitary hormone deficiency. *J Clin Endocrinol Metab*. 2008;93:4351-4359.

70. Woods KS, Cundall M, Turton J, et al. Over- and underdosage of SOX3 is associated with infundibular hypoplasia and hypopituitarism. *Am J Hum Genet*. 2005;76:833-849.

71. Netchine I, Sobrier ML, Krude H, et al. Mutations in LHX3 result in a new syndrome revealed by combined pituitary hormone deficiency. *Nat Genet*. 2000;25:182-186.

72. Rajab A, Kelberman D, de Castro SC, et al. Novel mutations in LHX3 are associated with hypopituitarism and sensorineural hearing loss. *Hum Mol Genet*. 2008;17:2150-2159.

73. Machinis K, Pantel J, Netchine I, et al. Syndromic short stature in patients with a germline mutation in the LIM homeobox LHX4. *Am J Hum Genet*. 2001;69:961-968.

74. Wu W, Cogan JD, Pfaffle RW, et al. Mutations in PROP1 cause familial combined pituitary hormone deficiency. *Nat Genet*. 1998;18:147-149.

75. Radovick S, Nations M, Du Y, et al. A mutation in the POU-homeodomain of Pit-1 responsible for combined pituitary hormone deficiency. *Science*. 1992;257:1115-1118.

76. Ohta K, Nobukuni Y, Mitsubuchi H, et al. Mutations in the Pit-1 gene in children with combined pituitary hormone deficiency. *Biochem Biophys Res Commun*. 1992;189:851-855.

77. Pulichino AM, Vallette-Kasic S, Couture C, et al. Human and mouse TPIT gene mutations cause early onset pituitary ACTH deficiency. *Genes Dev*. 2003;17:711-716.

78. Ramos HE, Labedan I, Carre A, et al. New cases of isolated congenital central hypothyroidism due to homozygous thyrotropin beta gene mutations: a pitfall to neonatal screening. *Thyroid*. 2010;20:639-645.

79. Sun Y, Bak B, Schoenmakers N, et al. Loss-of-function mutations in IGSF1 cause an X-linked syndrome of central hypothyroidism and testicular enlargement. *Nat Genet*. 2012;44:1375-1381.

80. Joustra SD, Schoenmakers N, Persani L, et al. The IGSF1 deficiency syndrome: characteristics of male and female patients. *J Clin Endocrinol Metab*. 2013;98:4942-4952.

81. Pingault V, Bodereau V, Baral V, et al. Loss-of-function mutations in SOX10 cause Kallmann syndrome with deafness. *Am J Hum Genet*. 2013;92:707-724.

82. Miraoui H, Dwyer AA, Sykiotis GP, et al. Mutations in FGF17, IL17RD, DUSP6, SPRY4, and FLRT3 are identified in individuals with congenital hypogonadotropic hypogonadism. *Am J Hum Genet*. 2013;92: 725-743.

83. Dode C, Rondard P. PROK2/PROKR2 Signaling and Kallmann syndrome. *Front Endocrinol (Lausanne)*. 2013;4:19.

84. Matsumoto S, Yamazaki C, Masumoto KH, et al. Abnormal development of the olfactory bulb and reproductive system in mice lacking prokineticin receptor PKR2. *Proc Natl Acad Sci U S A*. 2006;103: 4140-4145.

85. McCabe MJ, Gaston-Massuet C, Gregory LC, et al. Variations in PROKR2, but not PROK2, are associated with hypopituitarism and septo-optic dysplasia. *J Clin Endocrinol Metab*. 2013;98:E547-E557.

86. Bouligand J, Ghervan C, Tello JA, et al. Isolated familial hypogonadotropic hypogonadism and a GNRH1 mutation. *N Engl J Med*. 2009; 360:2742-2748.

87. de Roux N, Young J, Misrahi M, et al. A family with hypogonadotropic hypogonadism and mutations in the gonadotropin-releasing hormone receptor. *N Engl J Med*. 1997;337:1597-1602.

88. Seminara SB, Messager S, Chatzidaki EE, et al. The GPR54 gene as a regulator of puberty. *N Engl J Med*. 2003;349:1614-1627.

89. Topaloglu AK, Tello JA, Kotan LD, et al. Inactivating KISS1 mutation and hypogonadotropic hypogonadism. *N Engl J Med*. 2012;366:629-635.

90. Topaloglu AK, Reimann F, Guclu M, et al. TAC3 and TACR3 mutations in familial hypogonadotropic hypogonadism reveal a key role for neurokinin B in the central control of reproduction. *Nat Genet*. 2009;41:354-358.

91. Margolin DH, Kousi M, Chan YM, et al. Ataxia, dementia, and hypogonadotropism caused by disordered ubiquitination. *N Engl J Med*. 2013;368:1992-2003.

92. Shi CH, Schisler JC, Rubel CE, et al. Ataxia and hypogonadism caused by the loss of ubiquitin ligase activity of the U box protein CHIP. *Hum Mol Genet*. 2013;23(4):1013-1024.

93. Synofzik M, Gonzalez MA, Lourenco CM, et al. PNPLA6 mutations cause Boucher-Neuhauser and Gordon Holmes syndromes as part of a broad neurodegenerative spectrum. *Brain*. 2014;137:69-77.

94. Johnston JJ, Olivos-Glander I, Killoran C, et al. Molecular and clinical analyses of Greig cephalopolysyndactyly and Pallister-Hall syndromes: robust phenotype prediction from the type and position of GLI3 mutations. *Am J Hum Genet*. 2005;76:609-622.

95. Demurger F, Ichkou A, Mougou-Zerelli S, et al. New insights into genotype-phenotype correlation for GLI3 mutations. *Eur J Hum Genet*. 2014;23(1):92-102.

96. Semina EV, Reiter R, Leysens NJ, et al. Cloning and characterization of a novel bicoid-related homeobox transcription factor gene, RIEG, involved in Rieger syndrome. *Nat Genet*. 1996;14:392-399.

97. Alatzoglou KS, Turton JP, Kelberman D, et al. Expanding the spectrum of mutations in GH1 and GHRHR: genetic screening in a large cohort of patients with congenital isolated growth hormone deficiency. *J Clin Endocrinol Metab*. 2009;94:3191-3199.

98. Collu R, Tang J, Castagne J, et al. A novel mechanism for isolated central hypothyroidism: inactivating mutations in the thyrotropin-releasing hormone receptor gene. *J Clin Endocrinol Metab*. 1997;82: 1561-1565.

99. Webb EA, AlMutair A, Kelberman D, et al. ARNT2 mutation causes hypopituitarism, post-natal microcephaly, visual and renal anomalies. *Brain*. 2013;136:3096-3105.

100. Suga H, Kadoshima T, Minaguchi M, et al. Self-formation of functional adenohypophysis in three-dimensional culture. *Nature*. 2011;480: 57-62.

101. Mulchahey JJ, DiBlasio AM, Martin MC, et al. Hormone production and peptide regulation of the human fetal pituitary gland. *Endocr Rev.* 1987;8:406-425.

102. Suganuma N, Seo H, Yamamoto N, et al. The ontogeny of growth hormone in the human fetal pituitary. *Am J Obstet Gynecol.* 1989; 160:729-733.

103. Goodyear CG, Sellen JM, Fuks M, et al. Regulation of growth hormone secretion from human fetal pituitaries, interactions between growth hormone releasing factor and somatostatin. *Reprod Nutr Dev.* 1987; 27:461-470.

104. Adcock CJ, Ogilvy-Stuart AL, Robinson IC, et al. The use of an automated microsampling system for the characterization of growth hormone pulsatility in newborn babies. *Pediatr Res.* 1997;42:66-71.

105. DeLeon DD, Cohen P, Katz LEL. Growth factor regulation of fetal growth. In: Polin RA, Fox WW, Abman SH, eds. *Fetal and Neonatal Physiology.* 3rd ed. Philadelphia, PA: WB Saunders; 2004:1880-1890.

106. Kind KL, Owens JA, Robinson JS, et al. Effect of restriction of placental growth on expression of IGFs in fetal sheep: relationship to fetal growth, circulating IGFs and binding proteins. *J Endocrinol.* 1995; 146:23-34.

107. Clement-Lacroix P, Ormandy C, Lepescheux L, et al. Osteoblasts are a new target for prolactin analysis of bone formation in prolactin receptor knockout mice. *Endocrinology.* 1999;140:3404-3410.

108. Newbern D, Freemark M. Placental hormones and the control of maternal metabolism and fetal growth. *Curr Opin Endocrinol Diabetes Obes.* 2011;18:409-416.

109. Ho Y, Liebhaber SA, Cooke NE. Activation of the human GH gene cluster: roles for targeted chromatin modification. *Trends Endocrinol Metab.* 2004;15:40-45.

110. Lacroix MC, Guibourdenche J, Frendo JL, et al. Human placental growth hormone—a review. *Placenta.* 2002;23(Suppl A):S87-S94.

111. Auffret J, Freemark M, Carre N, et al. Defective prolactin signaling impairs pancreatic beta-cell development during the perinatal period. *Am J Physiol Endocrinol Metab.* 2013;305:E1309-E1318.

112. Winter JSD. Fetal and neonatal adrenocortical physiology. In: Polin RA, Fox WW, Abman SH, eds. *Fetal and Neonatal Physiology.* Philadelphia, PA: WB Saunders; 2004:1915-1925.

113. Geller DH, Miller WL. Molecular development of the adrenal gland. In: Pescovitz OH, Eugster EA, eds. *Pediatric Endocrinology.* Philadelphia, PA: Lippincott Williams & Wilkins; 2004:548-567.

114. Keegan CE, Hammer GD. Recent insights into organogenesis of the adrenal cortex. *Trends Endocrinol Metab.* 2002;13:200-208.

115. Ikeda Y, Swain A, Weber TH, et al. Steroidogenic factor 1 and DAX-1 localize in multiple cell lineages: potential links in endocrine development. *Mol Endocrinol.* 1996;10:1261-1272.

116. Hammer GD, Parker KL, Schimmer BP. Minireview: transcriptional regulation of adrenocortical development. *Endocrinology.* 2005;146: 1018-1024.

117. Fujieda K, Tajima T. Molecular basis of adrenal insufficiency. *Pediatric Res.* 2005;57:62R-69R.

118. Laufer E, Kesper D, Vortkamp A, King P. Sonic hedgehog signaling during adrenal development. *Mol Cell Endocrinol.* 2012;351:19-27.

119. Fisher DA. Endocrinology of fetal development. In: Kronenberg HM, Melmed S, Polonsky KS, eds. *Williams Textbook of Endocrinology.* Philadelphia, PA: WB Saunders; 2008:755-782.

120. Arboleda VA, Lee H, Parnaik R, et al. Mutations in the PCNA-binding domain of CDKN1C cause IMAGe syndrome. *Nat Genet.* 2012;44: 788-792.

121. Miller WL. Steroid hormone biosynthesis and actions in the materno-feto-placental unit. *Clin Perinatol.* 1998;25:799-817.

122. Baker BY, Lin L, Kim CJ, et al. Nonclassic congenital lipoid adrenal hyperplasia: a new disorder of the steroidogenic acute regulatory protein with very late presentation and normal male genitalia. *J Clin Endocrinol Metab.* 2006;91:4781-4785.

123. Goto M, Piper Hanley K, Marcos J, et al. In humans, early cortisol biosynthesis provides a mechanism to safeguard female sexual development. *J Clin Invest.* 2006;116:953-960.

124. Leavitt MG, Albrecht EO, Pepe GJ. Development of the baboon fetal adrenal gland: regulation of the ontogenesis of the definitive and transitional zones by adrenocorticotropin. *J Clin Endocrinol Metab.* 1999;84:3831-3835.

125. Dotzler DA, Digeronimo JJ, Yoder BA, et al. Distribution of corticotrophin releasing hormone in the fetus, newborn, juvenile and adult baboon. *Pediatr Res.* 2004;55:120-125.

126. Cole TJ, Blendy JA, Monaghan AD, et al. Targeted disruption of the glucocorticoid receptor gene blocks adrenergic chromaffin development and severely retards lung maturation. *Genes Dev.* 1995;9: 1608-1625.

127. Thompson M, Smith R. The action of hypothalamic and placental corticotrophin releasing factor on the corticotrope. *Mol Cell Endocrinol.* 1989;62:1-12.

128. Goland RS, Wardlow SL, Blum M, et al. Biologically active corticotropin-releasing hormone in maternal and fetal plasma during pregnancy. *Am J Obstet Gynecol.* 1988;159:884-890.

129. Rivier C, Vale W. Neuroendocrine interactions between corticotrophin releasing factor and vasopressin on adrenocorticotropic hormone secretion in the rat. In: Schrier WW, ed. *Vasopressin.* New York, NY: Raven; 1985:181-188.

130. Albrecht ED, Aberdeen GW, Pepe GJ. Estrogen elicits cortical zone specific effects on development of the primate fetal adrenal gland. *Endocrinology.* 2005;146:1737-1744.

131. Rose JC, Turner CS, Ray De W, et al. Evidence that cortisol inhibits basal adrenocorticotropin secretion in the sheep fetus by 0.70 gestation. *Endocrinology.* 1988;123:1307-1313.

132. Yang K, Jones SA, Challis JRG. Changes in glucocorticoid receptor number in the hypothalamus of the sheep fetus with gestational age and after adrenocorticotropin treatment. *Endocrinology.* 1990;126: 11-17.

133. McKenna NT, Moore DD. Nuclear receptors: structure, function and cofactors. In: DeGroot LJ, Jameson JL, eds. *Endocrinology.* 5th ed. Philadelphia, PA: Elsevier Saunders; 2006:277-287.

134. Pavlik A, Buresova M. The neonatal cerebellum: the highest level of glucocorticoid receptors in the brain. *Dev Brain Res.* 1984;12:13-20.

135. Johnson JW, Mitzner W, Beck JC, et al. Long term effects of beta-methasone in fetal development. *Am J Obstet Gynecol.* 1981;141: 1053-1064.

136. Liggins GC. The role of cortisol in preparing the fetus for birth. *Reprod Fertil Dev.* 1994;6:141-150.

137. Beitins IZ, Graham GG, Kowarski A, et al. Adrenal function in normal infants and in marasmus and kwashiorkor: plasma aldosterone concentration and aldosterone secretion rate. *J Pediatr.* 1974;84:444-451.

138. Katz FH, Beck P, Makowski EL. The renin-aldosterone system in mother and fetus at term. *Am J Obstet Gynecol.* 1974;118:51-55.

139. Siegel SR, Fisher DA. Ontogeny of the renin-angiotensin-aldosterone system in the fetal and newborn lamb. *Pediatr Res.* 1980;14:99-102.

140. Lumbers ER. Functions of the renin-angiotensin system during development. *Clin Exp Pharmacol Physiol.* 1995;22:499-505.

141. Berger S, Bleich M, Schmid N, et al. Mineralocorticoid receptor knockout mice: pathophysiology of Na+ metabolism. *Proc Natl Acad Sci U S A.* 1998;95:9424-9429.

142. Hirasawa G, Sasano H, Suzuki T, et al. 11β-Hydroxysteroid dehydrogenase type 2 and mineralocorticoid receptor in human fetal development. *J Clin Endocrinol Metab.* 1999;84:1453-1458.

143. Robillard JE, Page WV, Matthews MS, et al. Differential gene expression and regulation of renal angiotensin II receptor subtypes (AT1 and AT2) during fetal life in sheep. *Pediatr Res.* 1995;38:896-904.

144. Chen K, Carey LC, Liu J, et al. The effect of hypothalamo-pituitary disconnection on the renin-angiotensin system in the late gestation sheep. *Am J Physiol Regul Integr Comp Physiol.* 2005;288:R1279-R1287.

145. Walther T, Schultheiss HP, Tschope C, et al. Natriuretic peptide system in fetal heart and circulation. *J Hypertens.* 2002;20:785-791.

146. Bancalari RE, Gregory LC, McCabe MJ, Dattani MT. Pituitary gland development: an update. *Endocr Dev.* 2012;23:1-15.

147. Couture C, Saveanu A, Barlier A, et al. Phenotypic homogeneity and genotypic variability in a large series of congenital isolated ACTH-deficiency patients with TPIT gene mutations. *J Clin Endocrinol Metab.* 2012;97:E486-E495.

148. Clark AJ, Chan LF, Chung TT, et al. The genetics of familial glucocorticoid deficiency. *Best Pract Res Clin Endocrinol Metab.* 2009;23: 159-165.

149. Cooray SN, Chan L, Metherell L, et al. Adrenocorticotropin resistance syndromes. *Endocr Devel.* 2008;13:99-116.

150. Hughes CR, Guasti L, Meimaridou E, et al. MCM4 mutation causes adrenal failure, short stature, and natural killer cell deficiency in humans. *J Clin Invest.* 2012;122:814-820.

151. Gineau L, Cognet C, Kara N, et al. Partial MCM4 deficiency in patients with growth retardation, adrenal insufficiency, and natural killer cell deficiency. *J Clin Invest.* 2012;122:821-832.

152. Meimaridou E, Kowalczyk J, Guasti L, et al. Mutations in NNT encoding nicotinamide nucleotide transhydrogenase cause familial glucocorticoid deficiency. *Nat Genet.* 2012;44:740-742.

153. Kowalczyk JC, Meimaridou E, Novoselova T, et al. Digenic inheritance of mutations in antioxidant pathway genes causing familial glucocorticoid deficiency? *Endocr Rev.* 2013;34:SAT-49.

154. Ferraz-de-Souza B, Achermann JC. Disorders of adrenal development. *Endocr Dev.* 2008;13:19-32.

155. Jadhav U, Harris RM, Jameson JL. Hypogonadotropic hypogonadism in subjects with DAX1 mutations. *Mol Cell Endocrinol.* 2011;346: 65-73.

156. Kohler B, Lin L, Ferraz-de-Souza B, et al. Five novel mutations in steroidogenic factor 1 (SF1/Ad4BP, NR5A1) are associated with 46XY disorders of sex development with normal adrenal function. *Hum Mutat.* 2008;29:59-64.

157. Lourenco D, Brauner R, Lin L, et al. Mutations in NR5A1 associated with ovarian insufficiency. *N Engl J Med.* 2009;360:1200-1210.

158. Kohler B, Achermann JC. Update—steroidogenic factor 1 (SF-1, NR5A1). *Minerva Endocrinol.* 2010;35(2):73-86.

159. Santisteban P. Development and anatomy of the hypothalamic-pituitary axis. In: Braverman LE, Utiger RD, eds. *The Thyroid.* 9th ed. Philadelphia, PA: JB Lippincott; 2005:8-25.

160. Brown RS, Huang SA, Fisher DA. The maturation of thyroid function in the perinatal period and during childhood. In: Braverman LE, Utiger

RD, eds. *The Thyroid.* 9th ed. Philadelphia, PA: JB Lippincott; 2005: 1013-1028.

161. Alt B, Elsalini OA, Schrumpf P, et al. Arteries define the position of the thyroid gland during its developmental relocalization. *Development.* 2006;133:3797-3804.

162. Fagman H, Liao J, Westerlund J, et al. The 22q11 deletion syndrome candidate gene Tbx1 determines thyroid size and positioning. *Hum Mol Genet.* 2007;16:276-285.

163. O'Rahilly R. The timing and sequence of events in the development of the human endocrine system during the embryonic period proper. *Anat Embryol (Berlin).* 1983;166:439-451.

164. Sprinzl GM, Koebke J, Wimmers-Klick J, et al. Morphology of the human thyroglossal tract: a histologic and macroscopic study in infants and children. *Ann Otol Rhinol Laryngol.* 2000;109(12 Pt 1): 1135-1139.

165. Macchia P. Recent advances in understanding the molecular basis of primary congenital hypothyroidism. *Mol Med Today.* 2000;6:36-42.

166. Szinnai G, Lacroix L, Carre A, et al. Sodium/iodide symporter (NIS) gene expression is the limiting step for the onset of thyroid function in the human fetus. *J Clin Endocrinol Metab.* 2007;92:70-76.

167. Parlato R, Rosica A, Rodriguez-Mallon A, et al. An integrated regulatory network controlling survival and migration in thyroid organogenesis. *Dev Biol.* 2004;276:464-475.

168. Trueba SS, Auge J, Mattei G, et al. PAX8, TITF1 and FOXE1 gene expression patterns during human development: new insights into human thyroid development and thyroid dysgenesis-associated malformations. *J Clin Endocrinol Metab.* 2005;90:455-462.

169. De Felice M, Di Lauro R. Thyroid development and its disorders: genetics and molecular mechanisms. *Endocr Rev.* 2004;25:722-746.

170. Dentice M, Cordeddu V, Rosica A, et al. Missense mutation in the transcription factor NKX2-5: a novel molecular event in the pathogenesis of thyroid dysgenesis. *J Clin Endocrinol Metab.* 2006;91:1428-1433.

171. Chisaka O, Capecchi MR. Regionally restricted developmental defects resulting from targeted disruption of the mouse homeobox gene hox-1.5. *Nature.* 1991;350:473-479.

172. Antonica F, Kasprzyk DF, Opitz R, et al. Generation of functional thyroid from embryonic stem cells. *Nature.* 2012;491:66-71.

173. Wassner AJ, Brown RS. Hypothyroidism in the newborn period. *Curr Opin Endocrinol Diabetes Obes.* 2013;20(5):449-454.

174. Burrow GN, Fisher DA, Larsen PR. Maternal and fetal thyroid function. *N Engl J Med.* 1994;331:1072-1078.

175. Roti E. Regulation of thyroid stimulating hormone (TSH) secretion in the fetus and neonate. *J Endocrinol Invest.* 1988;11:145-158.

176. Williams FLR, Simpson J, Delahunty C, et al. Developmental trends in cord and postpartum serum thyroid hormones in preterm infants. *J Clin Endocr Metab.* 2004;89:5314-5320.

177. Lem AJ, de Rijke YB, van Toor H, et al. Serum thyroid hormone levels in healthy children from birth to adulthood and in short children born small for gestational age. *J Clin Endocrinol Metab.* 2012;97:3170-3178.

178. Korzeniewski SJ, Kleyn M, Young WI, et al. Screening for congenital hypothyroidism in newborns transferred to neonatal intensive care. *Arch Dis Child Fetal Neonatal Ed.* 2013;98(4):F310-F315.

179. Fisher DA, Nelson JC, Carlton EI, et al. Maturation of human hypothalamic-pituitary-thyroid function and control. *Thyroid.* 2000; 10:229-234.

180. Murphy N, Home R, vanToor H, et al. The hypothalamic-pituitary-thyroid axis in preterm infants: changes in the first 24 hours of postnatal life. *J Clin Endocrinol Metab.* 2004;89:2824-2831.

181. Eng PHK, Cardona GR, Fang SL, et al. Escape from the acute Wolff-Chaikoff effect is associated with a decrease in thyroid sodium/iodide symporter messenger ribonucleic acid and protein. *Endocrinology.* 1999;140:3404-3410.

182. Sherwin JR. Development of regulatory mechanisms in the thyroid: failure of iodide to suppress iodide transport activity. *Proc Soc Exp Biol Med.* 1982;169:458-462.

183. St. Germain DL, Hernandez A, Schneider MJ, et al. Insights into the role of deiodinases from studies of genetically modified animals. *Thyroid.* 2005;15:905-916.

184. Schoenmakers E, Agostini M, Mitchell C, et al. Mutations in the selenocysteine insertion sequence-binding protein 2 gene lead to a multisystem selenoprotein deficiency disorder in humans. *J Clin Invest.* 2010;120:4220-4235.

185. Dumitrescu AM, Refetoff S. Inherited defects of thyroid hormone metabolism. *Ann Endocrinol (Paris).* 2011;72:95-98.

186. Dumitrescu AM, Di Cosmo C, Liao XH, et al. The syndrome of inherited partial SBP2 deficiency in humans. *Antioxid Redox Signal.* 2010; 12(7):905-920.

187. Hume R, Simpson J, Delahunty C, et al. Human fetal and cord serum thyroid hormones: developmental trends and interrelationships. *J Clin Endocrinol Metab.* 2004;89:4097-4103.

188. Polk DH, Reviczky A, Wu SY, et al. Metabolism of sulfoconjugated thyroid hormone derivatives in developing sheep. *Am J Physiol.* 1994; 266:E892-E896.

189. Kerry R, Hume R, Kaptein E, et al. Sulfation of thyroid hormone and dopamine during human development: ontogeny of phenol sulfo-

transferases and arylsulfatase in liver, lung, and brain. *J Clin Endocrinol Metab.* 2001;86:2734-2742.

190. Richard K, Hume R, Kaptein E, et al. Ontogeny of iodothyronine deiodinases in human liver. *J Clin Endocrinol Metab.* 1998;83: 2868-2874.

191. Polk DH, Wu WY, Wright C, et al. Ontogeny of thyroid hormone effect on tissue 5'-monodeiodinase activity in fetal sheep. *Am J Physiol.* 1988;254:E337-E341.

192. Jansen J, Friesema ECH, Milici C, et al. Thyroid hormone transporters in health and disease. *Thyroid.* 2005;15:757-768.

193. Heuer H, Maier ML, Iden S, et al. The monocarboxylate transporter 8 linked to human psychomotor retardation is highly expressed in thyroid hormone-sensitive neuron populations. *Endocrinology.* 2005; 146:1701-1706.

194. Dumitrescu AM, Liao XH, Best TB, et al. A novel syndrome combining thyroid and neurological abnormalities is associated with mutations in a monocarboxylate transporter gene. *Am J Hum Genet.* 2004;74: 168-175.

195. Bergh JJ, Lin HY, Lansing L, et al. Integrin αVβ3 contains a cell surface receptor site for thyroid hormone that is linked to activation of mitogen-activated protein kinase and induction of angiogenesis. *Endocrinology.* 2005;146:2864-2871.

196. Di Cosmo C, Liao XH, Dumitrescu AM, et al. Mice deficient in MCT8 reveal a mechanism regulating thyroid hormone secretion. *J Clin Invest.* 2010;120:3377-3388.

197. Yen P. Genomic and nongenomic actions of thyroid hormones. In: Braverman LE, Utiger RD, eds. *The Thyroid.* 9th ed. Philadelphia, PA: Lippincott Williams & Wilkins; 2005:135-150.

198. Flamant F, Samarut J. Thyroid hormone receptors: lessons from knockout and knockin mutant mice. *Trends Endocrinol Metab.* 2005;14: 85-90.

199. Morreale de Escobar G, Obregon MJ, Escobar del Rey F. Role of thyroid hormone during early brain development. *Eur J Endocrinol.* 2004;151: U25-U37.

200. Kilby MD, Giltoes N, McCabe C, et al. Expression of thyroid receptor isoforms in the human fetal central nervous system and the effects of intrauterine growth retardation. *Clin Endocrinol (Oxf).* 2000;53:469-477.

201. Iskaros J, Pickard M, Evans I, et al. Thyroid hormone receptor gene expression in first trimester human fetal brain. *J Clin Endocrinol Metab.* 2000;85:2620-2623.

202. Rajatapiti P, Kester MHA, de Krijger RR, et al. Expression of glucocorticoid, retinoid, and thyroid hormone receptors during human lung development. *J Clin Endocrinol Metab.* 2005;90:4309-4314.

203. Bochukova E, Schoenmakers N, Agostini M, et al. A mutation in the thyroid hormone receptor alpha gene. *N Engl J Med.* 2012;366:243-249.

204. van Mullem A, van Heerebeek R, Chrysis D, et al. Clinical phenotype and mutant TRalpha1. *N Engl J Med.* 2012;366:1451-1453.

205. Contempre B, Jauniaux E, Calvo R, et al. Detection of thyroid hormones in human embryonic cavities during the first trimester of pregnancy. *J Clin Endocrinol Metab.* 1993;77:1719-1722.

206. Vulsma T, Gons MH, de Vijlder JJ. Maternal-fetal transfer of thyroxine in congenital hypothyroidism due to a total organification defect or thyroid agenesis. *N Engl J Med.* 1989;321:13-16.

207. Morreale De Escobar G, Calvo R, Obregon MJ, et al. Contribution of maternal thyroxine to fetal thyroxine pools in normal rats near term. *Endocrinology.* 1990;126:2765-2767.

208. Sadow PM, Chassande O, Koo EK, et al. Regulation of expression of thyroid hormone receptor isoforms and coactivators in liver and heart by thyroid hormone. *Mol Cell Endocrinol.* 2003;203:65-75.

209. Quignodon L, Legrand C, Allioli N, et al. Thyroid hormone signaling is highly heterogeneous during pre- and postnatal brain development. *J Mol Endocrinol.* 2004;33:467-476.

210. Plateroti M, Gauthier K, Domon-Dell C, et al. Functional interference between thyroid hormone receptor α (TRα) and natural truncated TRα isoforms in the control of intestinal development. *Mol Cell Biol.* 2001;21:4761-4772.

211. Mai W, Janier MF, Allioli N, et al. Thyroid hormone receptor α is a molecular switch of cardiac function between fetal and postnatal life. *Proc Natl Acad Sci U S A.* 2004;101:10332-10337.

212. Harvey CB, O'Shea PJ, Scott AJ, et al. Molecular mechanisms of thyroid hormone effects on bone growth and function. *Mol Gen Metab.* 2002; 75:17-30.

213. Marrit H, Schifman A, Stepanyan Z, et al. Temperature homeostasis in transgenic mice lacking thyroid receptor α gene products. *Endocrinology.* 2004;146:2872-2884.

214. Angelin-Duclos C, Domenget C, Kolbus A, et al. Thyroid hormone T3 acting through the thyroid hormone α receptor is necessary for implementation of erythropoiesis in the neonatal spleen environment in the mouse. *Development.* 2005;132:925-934.

215. Williams GR. Thyroid hormone actions in cartilage and bone. *Eur Thyroid J.* 2013;2(1):3-13.

216. Morreale de Escobar G, Obregon MJ, Escobar del Rey F. Is neuropsychological development related to maternal hypothyroidism or to maternal hypothyroxinemia? *J Clin Endocrinol Metab.* 2000;85: 3975-3987.

217. Pop VJ, Brouwers EP, Vader HL, et al. Maternal hypothyroxinaemia during early pregnancy and subsequent child development: a 3-year follow-up study. *Clin Endocrinol (Oxf).* 2003;59:282-288.

218. Grasberger H, Refetoff S. Genetic causes of congenital hypothyroidism due to dyshormonogenesis. *Curr Opin Pediatr.* 2011;23:421-428.

219. Leger J, Olivieri A, Donaldson M, et al. European Society for Paediatric Endocrinology consensus guidelines on screening, diagnosis, and management of congenital hypothyroidism. *J Clin Endocrinol Metab.* 2014;99:363-384.

220. Erickson RP, Blecher SR. Genetics of sex determination and differentiation. In: Polin RA, Fox WW, Abman SH, eds. *Fetal and Neonatal Physiology.* 3rd ed. Philadelphia, PA: WB Saunders; 2004:1935-1941.

221. Lee MM. Molecular genetic control of sex differentiation. In: Pescovitz OH, Eugster EA, eds. *Pediatric Endocrinology.* Philadelphia, PA: Lippincott Williams & Wilkins; 2004:231-242.

222. Harley VR, Clarkson MJ, Argentaro A. The molecular action and regulation of the testis-determining factors, SRY (sex determining region of the Y chromosome) and SOX9 (SRY-related high-mobility group [HMG] Box 9.). *Endocr Rev.* 2003;24:466-487.

223. Park SY, Jameson JL. Minireview: transcriptional regulation of gonadal development and differentiation. *Endocrinology.* 2005;146:1035-1042.

224. Larson A, Nokoff NJ, Travers S. Disorders of sex development: clinically relevant genes involved in gonadal differentiation. *Discov Med.* 2012; 14(78):301-309.

225. Sekido R, Lovell-Badge R. Sex determination involves synergistic action of SRY and SF1 on a specific Sox9 enhancer. *Nature.* 2008; 453:930-934.

226. Ono M, Harley VR. Disorders of sex development: new genes, new concepts. *Nat Rev Endocrinol.* 2013;9:79-91.

227. Sutton E, Hughes J, White S, et al. Identification of SOX3 as an XX male sex reversal gene in mice and humans. *J Clin Invest.* 2011;121:328-341.

228. Bay K, Main KM, Toppari J, Skakkebaek NE. Testicular descent: INSL3, testosterone, genes and the intrauterine milieu. *Nat Rev Urol.* 2011;8: 187-196.

229. Ivell R, Anand-Ivell R. Biological role and clinical significance of insulin-like peptide 3. *Curr Opin Endocrinol Diabetes Obes.* 2011;18: 210-216.

230. Aslan AR, Kogan BA, Gondos B. Testicular development. In: Polin RA, Fox WW, Abmans SH, eds. *Fetal and Neonatal Physiology.* 3rd ed. Philadelphia, PA: WB Saunders; 2004:1950-1955.

231. Nef S, Parada LF. Cryptorchidism in mice mutant for Insl3. *Nat Genet.* 1999;22:295-299.

232. Byskov AG, Westergaard LG. Differentiation of the ovary. In: Polin RA, Fox WW, Abman SH, eds. *Fetal and Neonatal Physiology.* 3rd ed. Philadelphia, PA: WB Saunders; 2004:1941-1949.

233. Fulton N, da Silva SJM, Bayne RAL, et al. Germ cell proliferation and apoptosis in the developing human ovary. *J Clin Endocrinol Metab.* 2005;90:4664-4670.

234. Richards JS, Pangas SA. The ovary: basic biology and clinical implications. *J Clin Invest.* 2010;120:963-972.

235. Uhlenhaut NH, Jakob S, Anlag K, et al. Somatic sex reprogramming of adult ovaries to testes by FOXL2 ablation. *Cell.* 2009;139:1130-1142.

236. Matson CK, Zarkower D. Sex and the singular DM domain: insights into sexual regulation, evolution and plasticity. *Nat Rev Genet.* 2012; 13:163-174.

237. Biason-Lauber A. WNT4, RSPO1, and FOXL2 in sex development. *Semin Reprod Med.* 2012;30:387-395.

238. Tomaselli S, Megiorni F, De Bernardo C, et al. Syndromic true hermaphroditism due to an R-spondin 1 (RSPO1) homozygous mutation. *Hum Mutat.* 2008;29(2):220-226.

239. Parma P, Radi O, Vidal V, et al. R-spondin 1 is essential in sex determination, skin differentiation and malignancy. *Nat Genet.* 2006;38: 1304-1309.

240. Sajjad Y, Quenby S, Nickson P, et al. Immunohistochemical localization of androgen receptors in the urogenital tracts of human embryos. *Reproduction.* 2004;128:331-339.

241. Josso N, Belville C, Dicard JY. Mutations in AMH and its receptors. *Endocrinology.* 2003;13:247-251.

242. Roviller Fabre V, Carmona S, Abou Merhi A, et al. Effect of anti-müllerian hormone on Sertoli and Leydig cell functions in fetal and immature rats. *Endocrinology.* 1998;139:1213-1220.

243. Brandenberger AW, Tee MK, Lee JY, et al. Tissue distribution of estrogen receptors alpha (ERα) and beta (ERβ) mRNA in the midgestation human fetus. *J Clin Endocrinol Metab.* 1997;82:3509-3512.

244. Couse JF, Korach KS. Estrogen receptor null mice: what have we learned and where will they lead us? *Endocrine Rev.* 1999;20:358-417.

245. Smith EP, Boyd J, Frank GR, et al. Estrogen resistance caused by a mutation in the estrogen-receptor gene in a man. *N Engl J Med.* 1994; 331:1056-1061.

246. Falgueras AG, Pinos H, Collado P, et al. The role of the androgen receptor in CNS masculinization. *Brain Res.* 2005;1035:13-23.

247. Naftolin F, Brawer JB. The effect of estrogens on hypothalamic structure and function. *Am J Obstet Gynecol.* 1978;132:758-765.

248. Sholl SA, Goy RW, Kim KL. 5α-Reductase, aromatase, and androgen receptor levels in the monkey brain during fetal development. *Endocrinology.* 1989;124:627-634.

249. Zang FP, Poutanen M, Wilbertz J, et al. Normal prenatal but arrested postnatal sexual development of luteinizing hormone receptor knockout (LURKO) mice. *Mol Endocrinol.* 2001;15:172-183.

250. Philibert P, Zenaty D, Lin L, et al. Mutational analysis of steroidogenic factor 1 (*NR5a1*) in 24 boys with bilateral anorchia: a French collaborative study. *Hum Reprod.* 2007;22:3255-3261.

251. Biason-Lauber A, Konrad D, Meyer M, et al. Ovaries and female phenotype in a girl with 46,XY karyotype and mutations in the CBX2 gene. *Am J Hum Genet.* 2009;84:658-663.

252. Visser M, Swaab DF. Life span changes in the presence of alpha-melanocyte-stimulating-hormone-containing cells in the human pituitary. *J Dev Physiol.* 1979;1:161-178.

253. Perry RA, Mulvogue HM, McMillen IC, et al. Immunohistochemical localization of ACTH in the adult and fetal sheep pituitary. *J Dev Physiol.* 1985;7:397-404.

254. Silman RE, Holland T, Chard T, et al. The ACTH family tree of the rhesus monkey changes with development. *Nature.* 1978;276:526-528.

255. Charles MA, Suh H, Hjalt TA, et al. PITX genes are required for cell survival and Lhx3 activation. *Mol Endocrinol.* 2005;19:1893-1903.

256. Glickman JA, Carson GD, Challis JRG. Differential effects of synthetic adrenocorticotropin and melanocyte stimulating hormone on adrenal formation in human and sheep fetus. *Endocrinology.* 1979;104:34-39.

257. Swaab DF, Martin JT. Functions of alpha melanotropin and other opiomelanocortin peptides in labour, intrauterine growth and brain development. *Ciba Found Symp.* 1981;81:196-217.

258. Facchinetti F, Storchi AR, Petraglia F, et al. Ontogeny of pituitary β-endorphin and related peptides in the human embryo and fetus. *Am J Obstet Gynecol.* 1987;156:735-739.

259. Leake RD, Fisher DA. Ontogeny of vasopressin in man. In: Czernichow P, Robinson AG, eds. *Diabetes Insipidus in Man: Frontiers in Hormone Research,* Vol. 13. Basel: S Karger; 1985:42-51.

260. Leake RD. The fetal-maternal neurohypophysial system. In: Polin RA, Fox WW, eds. *Fetal and Neonatal Physiology.* 2nd ed. Philadelphia, PA: WB Saunders; 1998:2442-2446.

261. Ervin MG, Leake RD, Ross MG, et al. Arginine vasotocin in ovine maternal and fetal blood, fetal urine, and amniotic fluid. *J Clin Invest.* 1985;75:1696-1701.

262. Morris M, Castro M, Rose JC. Alterations in prohormone processing during early development in the fetal sheep. *Am J Physiol.* 1992; 263:R738-R740.

263. Zhao X, Nijland MJM, Ervin G, et al. Regulation of hypothalamic arginine vasopressin content in fetal sheep: effect of acute tonicity alterations and fetal maturation. *Am J Obstet Gynecol.* 1998;179:899-905.

264. DeVane GW, Porter JC. An apparent stress-induced release of arginine vasopressin by human neonates. *J Clin Endocrinol Metab.* 1980;51: 1412-1416.

265. Matthews SG, Challis JRG. Regulation of CRH and AVP mRNA in the developing ovine hypothalamus: effects of stress and glucocorticoids. *Am J Physiol.* 1995;268:E1096-E1107.

266. Brooks AN, White A. Activation of pituitary adrenal function in fetal sheep by corticotrophin-releasing factor and arginine vasopressin. *J Endocrinol.* 1990;124:27-35.

267. Benedetto MT, DeCicco F, Rossiello F, et al. Oxytocin receptor in human fetal membranes at term and during labor. *J Steroid Biochem.* 1990;35:205-208.

268. Tribollet E, Charpak S, Schmidt A, et al. Appearance and transient expression of oxytocin receptors in fetal, infant and peripubertal rat brain studied by autoradiography and electrophysiology. *J Neurosci.* 1989;9:1764-1773.

269. Ervin MG, Miller SJ, Ramseyer LJ, et al. Renal arginine vasopressin receptors in newborn and adult sheep. *Clin Res.* 1990;38:170A.

270. Devuyst O, Burrow CR, Smithe BL, et al. Expression of aquaporins 1 and 2 during nephrogenesis and in autosomal dominant polycystic kidney disease. *Am J Physiol.* 1996;271:F169-F183.

271. Baum MA, Ruddy MK, Hosselet CA, et al. The perinatal expression of aquaporin-2 and aquaporin-3 in developing kidney. *Pediatr Res.* 1998;43:783-790.

272. Cryns K, Sivakumaran TA, Van den Ouweland JM, et al. Mutational spectrum of the WFS1 gene in Wolfram syndrome, nonsyndromic hearing impairment, diabetes mellitus and psychiatric disease. *Hum Mutat.* 2003;22(4):275-287.

273. Padbury JF. Functional maturation of the adrenal medulla and peripheral sympathetic nervous system. *Baillieres Clin Endocrinol Metab.* 1989; 33:689-705.

274. Huber K, Karch N, Ernsberger U, et al. The role of PHOX2B in chromaffin cell development. *Dev Biol.* 2005;279:501-508.

275. Gaultier C, Trang H, Dauger S, et al. Pediatric disorders with autoimmune dysfunction: What role for PHOX2B? *Pediatr Res.* 2005;58: 1-6.

276. Aloe L, Levi-Montalcini R. Nerve growth factor-induced transformation of immature chromaffin cells in vivo into sympathetic neurons: effect of antiserum to nerve growth factor. *Proc Natl Acad Sci U S A.* 1979;76:1246-1250.

277. Slotkin TA, Seidler FJ. Adrenomedullary catecholamine release in the fetus and newborn: secretory mechanisms and their role in stress and survival. *J Dev Physiol.* 1988;10:1-16.

278. Stonestreet BS, Piasecki GJ, Susa JB, et al. Effects of insulin infusion on catecholamine concentration in fetal sheep. *Am J Obstet Gynecol.* 1989;160:740-745.
279. Cohen WR, Piasecki GJ, Cohn HE, et al. Plasma catecholamines in the hypoxaemic fetal rhesus monkey. *J Dev Physiol.* 1987;9:507-515.
280. Pryds O, Christensen NJ, Friis-Hansen B. Increased cerebral blood flow and plasma epinephrine in hypoglycemic, preterm neonates. *Pediatrics.* 1990;85:172-176.
281. Palmer SM, Oakes GK, Lam RW, et al. Catecholamine physiology in the ovine fetus. I: gestational age variation in basal plasma concentrations. *Am J Obstet Gynecol.* 1984;149:420-425.
282. Palmer SM, Oakes GK, Lam RW, et al. Catecholamine physiology in the ovine fetus. II: Metabolic clearance rate of epinephrine. *Am J Physiol.* 1984;246:E350-E355.
283. Palmer SM, Oakes GK, Champion JA, et al. Catecholamine physiology in the ovine fetus. III: Maternal and fetal response to acute maternal exercise. *Am J Obstet Gynecol.* 1984;149:426-434.
284. Zhou QY, Ouaife CJ, Palmiter RD. Targeted disruption of the tyrosine hydroxylase gene reveals that catecholamines are required for mouse fetal development. *Nature.* 1995;374:640-643.
285. Thomas SA, Matsumoto AM, Palmiter RD. Noradrenaline is essential for mouse fetal development. *Nature.* 1995;374:643-646.
286. Wolfe HJ, DeLellis RA, Voelkel EF, Tashjian AH Jr. Distribution of calcitonin-containing cells in the normal neonatal human thyroid gland: a correlation of morphology with peptide content. *J Clin Endocrinol Metab.* 1975;41:1076-1081.
287. Kameda Y, Arai Y, Nishimaki T, Chisaka O. The role of Hoxa3 gene in parathyroid gland organogenesis of the mouse. *J Histochem Cytochem.* 2004;52(5):641-651.
288. Grigorieva IV, Thakker RV. Transcription factors in parathyroid development: lessons from hypoparathyroid disorders. *Ann N Y Acad Sci.* 2011;1237:24-38.
289. Papangeli I, Scambler P. The 22q11 deletion: DiGeorge and velocardio-facial syndromes and the role of TBX1. *Wiley Interdiscip Rev Dev Biol.* 2013;2(3):393-403.
290. Bowl MR, Nesbit MA, Harding B, et al. An interstitial deletion/insertion involving chromosomes 2p25.3 and Xq27.1 near SOX3 causes X-linked recessive hypoparathyroidism. *J Clin Invest.* 2005;115:2822-2831.
291. Prada JA. Calcium-regulating hormones. In: Polin RA, Fox WW, eds. *Fetal and Neonatal Physiology.* 2nd ed. Philadelphia, PA: WB Saunders; 1998:2287-2296.
292. Kovacs CS, Kronenberg HM. Maternal-fetal calcium and bone metabolism during pregnancy, puerperium and lactation. *Endocr Rev.* 1997;18(6):832-872.
293. Mitchell DM, Juppner H. Regulation of calcium homeostasis and bone metabolism in the fetus and neonate. *Curr Opin Endocrinol Diabetes Obes.* 2010;17:25-30.
294. Kovacs CS, Lanske B, Hunzelman JL, et al. Parathyroid hormone-related peptide (PTHrP) regulates fetal-placental calcium transport through a receptor distinct from the PTH/PTHrP receptor. *Proc Natl Acad Sci U S A.* 1996;93:15233-15238.
295. Vilardaga JP, Romero G, Friedman PA, Gardella TJ. Molecular basis of parathyroid hormone receptor signaling and trafficking: a family B GPCR paradigm. *Cell Mol Life Sci.* 2011;68:1-13.
296. Karaplis AC, Luz A, Glowacki J, et al. Lethal skeletal dysplasia from targeted disruption of the parathyroid hormone-related protein gene. *Genes Dev.* 1994;8:277-289.
297. Care AD, Abbas SK, Pickard DW, et al. Stimulation of ovine placental transport of calcium and magnesium by mid-molecule fragments of human parathyroid hormone-related protein. *J Exp Physiol.* 1990;75:605-608.
298. Kovacs CS. Bone metabolism in the fetus and neonate. *Pediatr Nephrol (Berlin, Germany).* 2014;29(5):793-803.
299. Miao D, He B, Karaplis C, et al. Parathyroid hormone is essential for normal fetal bone formation. *J Clin Invest.* 2002;109:1173-1182.
300. Lanske B, Amling M, Neff L, et al. Ablation of the PTHrP gene or the PTH/PTHrP receptor gene leads to distinct abnormalities in bone development. *J Clin Invest.* 1999;104:399-407.
301. Hoff AO, Catala-Lehnen P, Thomas PM, et al. Increased bone mass is an unexpected phenotype associated with deletion of the calcitonin gene. *J Clin Invest.* 2002;110:1849-1857.
302. Ross R, Halbert K, Tsang RC. Determination of the production and metabolic clearance rates of 1,25-dihydroxyvitamin D_3 in the pregnant sheep and its chronically catheterized fetus by primed infusion technique. *Pediatr Res.* 1989;26:633-638.
303. Brown EM. Role of the calcium-sensing receptor in extracellular calcium homeostasis. *Best Pract Res Clin Endocrinol Metab.* 2013;27:333-343.
304. Riccardi D, Brennan SC, Chang W. The extracellular calcium-sensing receptor, CaSR, in fetal development. *Best Pract Res Clin Endocrinol Metab.* 2013;27:443-453.
305. Hannan FM, Thakker RV. Calcium-sensing receptor (CaSR) mutations and disorders of calcium, electrolyte and water metabolism. *Best Pract Res Clin Endocrinol Metab.* 2013;27:359-371.
306. Calcium-Sensing Receptor Database. Montreal, Quebec, Canada.: McGill University. Available at: <http://www.casrdb.mcgill.ca>.
307. Bansal B, Bansal M, Bajpai P, Garewal HK. Hypocalcemic cardiomyopathy-different mechanisms in adult and pediatric cases. *J Clin Endocrinol Metab.* 2014;99:2627-2632.
308. Maiya S, Sullivan I, Allgrove J, et al. Hypocalcaemia and vitamin D deficiency: an important, but preventable, cause of life-threatening infant heart failure. *Heart.* 2008;94(5):581-584.
309. Hannan FM, Nesbit MA, Zhang C, et al. Identification of 70 calcium-sensing receptor mutations in hyper- and hypo-calcaemic patients: evidence for clustering of extracellular domain mutations at calcium-binding sites. *Hum Mol Genet.* 2012;21:2768-2778.
310. Nesbit MA, Hannan FM, Howles SA, et al. Mutations affecting G-protein subunit alpha11 in hypercalcemia and hypocalcemia. *N Engl J Med.* 2013;368:2476-2486.
311. Nesbit MA, Hannan FM, Howles SA, et al. Mutations in AP2S1 cause familial hypocalciuric hypercalcemia type 3. *Nat Genet.* 2013;45:93-97.
312. Hu MC, Shiizaki K, Kuro-o M, Moe OW. Fibroblast growth factor 23 and Klotho: physiology and pathophysiology of an endocrine network of mineral metabolism. *Annu Rev Physiol.* 2013;75:503-533.
313. Christov M, Juppner H. Insights from genetic disorders of phosphate homeostasis. *Semin Nephrol.* 2013;33:143-157.
314. Habener JF, Kemp DM, Thomas MJ. Mini review: transcriptional regulation in pancreatic development. *Endocrinology.* 2005;146:1025-1034.
315. Cano DA, Soria B, Martin F, Rojas A. Transcriptional control of mammalian pancreas organogenesis. *Cell Mol Life Sci.* 2014;71:2383-2402.
316. Arda HE, Benitez CM, Kim SK. Gene regulatory networks governing pancreas development. *Dev Cell.* 2013;25:5-13.
317. Girard J, Ferre P, Pegorier JP, Duee PH. Adaptations of glucose and fatty acid metabolism during perinatal period and suckling-weaning transition. *Physiol Rev.* 1992;72:507-562.
318. Carrasco M, Delgado I, Soria B, et al. GATA4 and GATA6 control mouse pancreas organogenesis. *J Clin Invest.* 2012;122:3504-3515.
319. Haldorsen IS, Raeder H, Vesterhus M, et al. The role of pancreatic imaging in monogenic diabetes mellitus. *Nat Rev Endocrinol.* 2012;8:148-159.
320. Franco B, Guioli S, Pragliola A, et al. A gene deleted in Kallmann's syndrome shares homology with neural cell adhesion and axonal path-finding molecules. *Nature.* 1991;353:529-536.
321. Lango Allen H, Flanagan SE, Shaw-Smith C, et al. GATA6 haploinsufficiency causes pancreatic agenesis in humans. *Nat Genet.* 2012;44:20-22.
322. Flanagan SE, De Franco E, Lango Allen H, et al. Analysis of transcription factors key for mouse pancreatic development establishes NKX2-2 and MNX1 mutations as causes of neonatal diabetes in man. *Cell Metab.* 2014;19:146-154.
323. Weedon MN, Cebola I, Patch AM, et al. Recessive mutations in a distal PTF1A enhancer cause isolated pancreatic agenesis. *Nat Genet.* 2014;46:61-64.
324. Jiang FX, Harrison LC. Laminin-1 and epidermal growth factor family members co-stimulate fetal pancreas cell proliferation and colony formation. *Differentiation.* 2005;73:45-49.
325. Formby B, Ullrich A, Coussens L, et al. Growth hormone stimulates insulin gene expression in cultured human fetal pancreatic islets. *J Clin Endocrinol Metab.* 1988;66:1075-1079.
326. Edlund H. Pancreatic organogenesis: developmental mechanisms and implications for therapy. *Nat Rev Genet.* 2002;3:524-532.
327. Sperling MA. Carbohydrate metabolism: insulin and glucagons. In: Tulchinsky D, Little AB, eds. *Maternal-Fetal Endocrinology.* 2nd ed. Philadelphia, PA: WB Saunders; 1994:380-400.
328. Rao PN, Shashidhar A, Ashok C. In utero fuel homeostasis: lessons for a clinician. *Indian J Endocrinol Metab.* 2013;17(1):60-68.
329. Aldoretta PW, Hay WW Jr. Metabolic substrates for fetal energy metabolism and growth. *Clin Perinatol.* 1995;22(1):15-36.
330. Girard J. Control of fetal and neonatal glucose metabolism by pancreatic hormones. *Baillieres Clin Endocrinol Metab.* 1989;3:817-836.
331. Ammon HP, Glocker C, Waldner RG, et al. Insulin release from pancreatic islets of fetal rats mediated by leucine, b-BCH, tolbutamide, glibenclamide, arginine, potassium chloride, and theophylline does not require stimulation of Ca^{2+} net uptake. *Cell Calcium.* 1989;10:441-450.
332. Meier JJ, Butler AE, Saisho Y, et al. Beta-cell replication is the primary mechanism subserving the postnatal expansion of beta-cell mass in humans. *Diabetes.* 2008;57:1584-1594.
333. Guenther MA, Bruder ED, Raff H. Effects of body temperature maintenance on glucose, insulin, and corticosterone responses to acute hypoxia in the neonatal rat. *Am J Physiol Regul Integr Comp Physiol.* 2012;302(5):R627-R633.
334. Kanakatti Shankar R, Pihoker C, Dolan LM, et al. Permanent neonatal diabetes mellitus: prevalence and genetic diagnosis in the SEARCH for Diabetes Youth Study. *Pediatr Diabetes.* 2013;14:174-180.
335. Sansbury FH, Flanagan SE, Houghton JA, et al. SLC2A2 mutations can cause neonatal diabetes, suggesting GLUT2 may have a role in human insulin secretion. *Diabetologia.* 2012;55:2381-2385.
336. De Franco E, Shaw-Smith C, Flanagan SE, et al. Biallelic PDX1 (insulin promoter factor 1) mutations causing neonatal diabetes without exocrine pancreatic insufficiency. *Diabet Med.* 2013;30:e197-e200.

337. Smith SB, Qu HQ, Taleb N, et al. Rfx6 directs islet formation and insulin production in mice and humans. *Nature*. 2010;463:775-780.

338. Spiegel R, Dobbie A, Hartman C, et al. Clinical characterization of a newly described neonatal diabetes syndrome caused by RFX6 mutations. *Am J Med Genet A*. 2011;155A(11):2821-2825.

339. Shaw-Smith C, De Franco E, Lango Allen H, et al. GATA4 mutations are a cause of neonatal and childhood-onset diabetes. *Diabetes*. 2014;63:2888-2894.

340. Karges B, Meissner T, Icks A, et al. Management of diabetes mellitus in infants. *Nat Rev Endocrinol*. 2012;8:201-211.

341. Vaxillaire M, Bonnefond A, Froguel P. The lessons of early-onset monogenic diabetes for the understanding of diabetes pathogenesis. *Best Pract Res Clin Endocrinol Metab*. 2012;26:171-187.

342. Senniappan S, Shanti B, James C, Hussain K. Hyperinsulinaemic hypoglycaemia: genetic mechanisms, diagnosis and management. *J Inherit Metab Dis*. 2012;35:589-601.

343. Palladino AA, Stanley CA. The hyperinsulinism/hyperammonemia syndrome. *Rev Endocr Metab Disord*. 2010;11:171-178.

344. Kapoor RR, James C, Hussain K. Hyperinsulinism in developmental syndromes. *Endocr Dev*. 2009;14:95-113.

345. Senniappan S, Alexandrescu S, Tatevian N, et al. Sirolimus therapy in infants with severe hyperinsulinemic hypoglycemia. *N Engl J Med*. 2014;370:1131-1137.

346. Pepe GJ, Albrecht ED. Actions of placental and fetal adrenal steroid hormones in primate pregnancy. *Endocr Rev*. 1995;16:608-648.

347. Ruiz de Ona C, Obregon MJ, Escobar del Rey F, et al. Developmental changes in rat brain 5′-deiodinase and thyroid hormones during the fetal period: the effects of fetal hypothyroidism and maternal thyroid hormones. *Pediatr Res*. 1988;24:588-594.

348. Polk DH, Cheromcha D, Reviczky A, et al. Nuclear thyroid hormone receptors: ontogeny and thyroid hormone effects in sheep. *Am J Physiol*. 1989;256:E543-E549.

349. Coulombe P, Ruel J, Dussault JH. Effects of neonatal hypo- and hyperthyroidism on pituitary growth hormone content in the rat. *Endocrinology*. 1980;107:2027-2033.

350. Lakshmanan J, Perheentupa J, Macaso T, et al. Acquisition of urine, kidney and submandibular gland epidermal growth factor responsiveness to thyroxine administration in neonatal mice. *Acta Endocrinol*. 1985;109:511-516.

351. Alm J, Scott SM, Fisher DA. Epidermal growth factor receptor ontogeny in mice with congenital hypothyroidism. *J Dev Physiol*. 1986;8:377-385.

352. Hoath SB, Lakshmanan J, Fisher DA. Thyroid hormone effects on skin and hepatic epidermal growth factor concentrations in neonatal and adult mice. *Biol Neonate*. 1984;45:49-52.

353. Hoath SB, Lakshmanan J, Fisher DA. Epidermal growth factor binding to neonatal mouse skin explants and membrane preparations: effect of triiodothyronine. *Pediatr Res*. 1985;19:277-280.

354. Perez Castillo A, Bernal J, Ferriero B, et al. The early ontogenesis of thyroid hormone receptor in the rat fetus. *Endocrinology*. 1985;117:2457-2461.

355. Mehta A, Hindmarsh PC, Stanhope RG, et al. The role of growth hormone in determining birth size and early postnatal growth, using congenital growth hormone deficiency (GHD) as a model. *Clin Endocrinol (Oxf)*. 2005;63:223-231.

356. Padbury JF, Lam RW, Newnham JP, et al. Neonatal adaptation: greater neurosympathetic system activity in preterm than full term sheep at birth. *Am J Physiol*. 1985;248:E443-E449.

357. Pasqualini JR, Sumida C, Gelly C, et al. Progesterone receptors in the fetal uterus and ovary of the guinea pig: evolution during fetal development and induction and stimulation in estradiol-primed animals. *J Steroid Biochem*. 1976;7:1031-1038.

358. Yamashita S, Newbold RR, McLachlan JA, et al. Developmental pattern of estrogen receptor expression in female mouse genital tracts. *Endocrinology*. 1989;125:2888-2896.

359. Russo VC, Gluckman PD, Feldman EL, Werther GA. The insulin-like growth factor system and its pleiotropic functions in brain. *Endocr Rev*. 2005;26:916-943.

360. Ong K, Kratzsch J, Kiess W, et al. Size at birth and cord blood levels of insulin, insulin-like growth factor I (IGF-I), IGF-II, IGF-binding protein-1 (IGFBP-1), IGFBP-3, and the soluble IGF-II/mannose-6-phosphate receptor in term human infants. The ALSPAC Study Team. Avon Longitudinal Study of Pregnancy and Childhood. *J Clin Endocrinol Metab*. 2000;85(11):4266-4269.

361. Simmen FA, Simmon RCM, Letcher LR, et al. IGFs in pregnancy: developmental expression in uterus and mammary gland and paracrine actions during embryonic and neonatal growth. In: LeRoith D, Raizada MK, eds. *Molecular and Cellular Biology of Insulin-Like Growth Factors and Their Receptors*. New York, NY: Plenum; 1989:195-208.

362. Spaventi R, Antica M, Pavelic K. Insulin and insulin-like growth factor I (IGF I) in early mouse embryogenesis. *Development*. 1990;108:491-495.

363. Sibley CP, Coan PM, Ferguson-Smith AC, et al. Placental-specific insulin-like growth factor 2 (IGF2) regulates the diffusional exchange characteristics of the mouse placenta. *Proc Natl Acad Sci U S A*. 2004;101:8204-8208.

364. Constancia M, Angiolini E, Sandovici I, et al. Adaptation of nutrient supply to fetal demand in the mouse involves interaction between the Igf2 gene and placental transporter systems. *Proc Natl Acad Sci U S A*. 2005;102:19219-19224.

365. Woods KA, Camacho-Huebner C, Savage MO, et al. Intrauterine growth retardation and postnatal growth failure associated with deletion of the insulin-like growth factor 1 gene. *N Engl J Med*. 1996;335:1383-1387.

366. Abuzzahab MJ, Schneider A, Goddard A, et al. IGF-1 receptor mutations resulting in intrauterine and postnatal growth retardation. *N Engl J Med*. 2003;349:2211-2222.

367. Geary MP, Pringle PJ, Rodeck CH, et al. Sexual dimorphism in the growth hormone and insulin-like growth factor axis at birth. *J Clin Endocrinol Metab*. 2003;88:3708-3714.

368. Pringle PJ, Geary MP, Rodeck CH, et al. The influence of cigarette smoking on antenatal growth, birth size, and the insulin-like growth factor axis. *J Clin Endocrinol Metab*. 2005;90:2556-2562.

369. Epaud R, Aubey F, Xu J, et al. Knockout of insulin-like growth factor-1 receptor impairs distal lung morphogenesis. *PLoS ONE*. 2012;7:e48071.

370. Gicquel C, Rossignol S, Cabrol S, et al. Epimutation of the telomeric imprinting center region on chromosome 11p15 in Silver-Russell syndrome. *Nat Genet*. 2005;37:1003-1007.

371. Qiu Q, Basak A, Mbikay M, et al. Role of pro-IGF-11 processing by proprotein convertase 4 in human placental development. *Proc Natl Acad Sci U S A*. 2005;102:11047-11052.

372. Murphy R, Baptista J, Holly J, et al. Severe intrauterine growth retardation and atypical diabetes associated with a translocation breakpoint disrupting regulation of the insulin-like growth factor 2 gene. *J Clin Endocrinol Metab*. 2008;93:4373-4380.

373. Sparago A, Cerrato F, Vernucci M, et al. Microdeletions in the human H19 DMR result in loss of IGF2 imprinting and Beckwith-Wiedemann syndrome. *Nat Genet*. 2004;36:958-960.

374. Watson CS, Bialek P, Arizo M, et al. Elevated circulating insulin-like growth factor-binding protein-1 is sufficient to cause fetal growth restriction. *Endocrinology*. 2006;147:1175-1186.

375. Ben Lagha N, Seurin D, Le Bouc Y, et al. Insulin-like growth factor-binding protein (IGFBP-1) involvement in intrauterine growth retardation: study on IGFBP-1 overexpressing transgenic mice. *Endocrinology*. 2006;147:4730-4737.

376. Qiu Q, Bell M, Lu X, et al. Significance of IGFBP-4 in the development of fetal growth restriction. *J Clin Endocrinol Metab*. 2012;97:E1429-E1439.

377. Forhead AJ, Li J, Gilmour RS, et al. Thyroid hormone and the mRNA of the GH receptor and IGFs in skeletal muscle of fetal sheep. *Am J Physiol Endocrinol Metab*. 2002;282:E80-E86.

378. Pilistine SJ, Moses AC, Munro HN. Placental lactogen administration reverses the effect of low protein diet on maternal and fetal somatomedin levels in the pregnant rat. *Proc Natl Acad Sci U S A*. 1984;81:5853-5857.

379. Gohlke BC, Fahnenstich H, Dame C, et al. Longitudinal data for intrauterine levels of fetal IGF-I and IGF-II. *Horm Res*. 2004;61:200-204.

380. Randhawa R, Cohen P. The role of the insulin-like growth factor system in prenatal growth. *Mol Genet Metab*. 2005;86:84-90.

381. Li Y, Komuro Y, Fahrion JK, et al. Light stimuli control neuronal migration by altering insulin-like growth factor 1 (IGF-1) signaling. *Proc Natl Acad Sci U S A*. 2012;109:2630-2635.

382. Wali JA, de Boo HA, Derraik JG, et al. Weekly intra-amniotic IGF-1 treatment increases growth of growth-restricted ovine fetuses and up-regulates placental amino acid transporters. *PLoS ONE*. 2012;7:e37899.

383. Accili D, Drago J, Lee EJ, et al. Early neonatal death in mice homozygous for a null allele of the insulin receptor gene. *Nat Genet*. 1996;12:106-109.

384. Semple RK, Savage DB, Cochran EK, et al. Genetic syndromes of severe insulin resistance. *Endocr Rev*. 2011;32:498-514.

385. Fisher DA, Lakshmanan J. Metabolism and effects of EGF and related growth factors in mammals. *Endocr Rev*. 1990;11:418-442.

386. Rotwein P. Peptide growth factors other than insulin-like growth factors or cytokines. In: DeGroot LJ, Jameson JL, eds. *Endocrinology*. 5th ed. Philadelphia, PA: Elsevier Saunders; 2006:675-695.

387. Meittinen PJ, Berger JE, Menesses J, et al. Epithelial immaturity and multiorgan failure in mice lacking epidermal growth factor receptor. *Nature*. 1995;376:337-341.

388. Brown PI, Lam R, Lakshmanan J, et al. Transforming growth factor alpha in developing rats. *Am J Physiol*. 1990;259:E256-E260.

389. Hemmings R, Langlais J, Falcone T, et al. Human embryos produce transforming growth factor α activity and insulin-like growth factor II. *Fertil Steril*. 1992;58:101-104.

390. Giordano T, Pan JB, Casuto D, et al. Thyroid hormone regulation of NGF, NT3 and BDNF RNA in the adult rat brain. *Mol Brain Res*. 1992;16:239-245.

391. Mazzoni IE, Kenigsberg RL. Effects of epidermal growth factor in the mammalian central nervous system. *Drug Dev Res*. 1992;26:111-128.

392. Kitchens DL, Snyder EY, Gottlieb DI. FGF and EGF are mitogens for immortalized neural progenitors. *J Neurobiol*. 1990;21:356-375.

393. Santa-Olalla J, Covarrubias L. Epidermal growth factor, transforming growth factor-α, and fibroblast growth factor differentially influence neural precursor cells of mouse embryonic mesencephalon. *J Neurosci Res.* 1995;42:172-183.

394. Lee KF, Simon H, Chen C, et al. Requirement for neuregulin receptor erbB2 in neural and cardiac development. *Nature.* 1995;378:394-398.

395. Kamei Y, Tsutsumi O, Kuwabara Y, et al. Intrauterine growth retardation and fetal losses are caused by epidermal growth factor deficiency in mice. *Am J Physiol.* 1993;264:R597-R600.

396. Yan Q, Elliott J, Snider WD. Brain derived neurotrophic factor rescues spinal motor neurons from axotomy-induced cell death. *Nature.* 1992;360:753-755.

397. Gospodarowicz D. Epidermal and nerve growth factors in mammalian development. *Annu Rev Physiol.* 1981;43:251-263.

398. Padbury JF, Lam RW, Polk DH, et al. Autoimmune sympathectomy in fetal rabbits. *J Dev Physiol.* 1986;8:369-376.

399. Tarris RH, Weichsel ME Jr, Fisher DA. Synthesis and secretion of a nerve growth stimulating factor by neonatal mouse astrocyte cells in vitro. *Pediatr Res.* 1986;20:367-372.

400. Weiss A, Attisano L. The TGFbeta superfamily signaling pathway. *Wiley Interdisc Rev Dev Biol.* 2013;2:47-63.

401. Lim GB, Dodic M, Earnest L, et al. Regulation of erythropoietin gene expression in fetal sheep by glucocorticoids. *Endocrinology.* 1996;137:1658-1663.

402. Moritz KM, Lim GB, Wintour EM. Developmental regulation of erythropoietin and erythropoiesis. *Am J Physiol.* 1997;273:R1829-R1844.

403. Betsholtz C. Functions of platelet-derived growth factor and its receptors deduced from gene inactivation in mice. *J Clin Ligand Assay.* 2000;23:206-213.

404. Lewandoski M, Sun X, Martin GR. Fgf8 signalling from the AER is essential for normal limb development. *Nat Genet.* 2000;26:460-463.

405. Oberbauer AM, Linkhart TA, Mohan S, et al. Fibroblast growth factor enhances human chorionic gonadotropin synthesis independent of mitogenic stimulation in Jar choriocarcinoma cells. *Endocrinology.* 1988;123:2696-2700.

406. Dode C, Levilliers J, Dupont JM, et al. Loss-of-function mutations in FGFR1 cause autosomal dominant Kallmann syndrome. *Nat Genet.* 2003;33:463-465.

407. Falardeau J, Chung WC, Beenken A, et al. Decreased FGF8 signaling causes deficiency of gonadotropin-releasing hormone in humans and mice. *J Clin Invest.* 2008;118:2822-2831.

408. Dwivedi PP, Lam N, Powell BC. Boning up on glypicans—opportunities for new insights into bone biology. *Cell Biochem Funct.* 2013;31:91-114.

409. Alfaidy N, Li W, Macintosh T, et al. Late gestation increase in 11beta-hydroxysteroid dehydrogenase 1 expression in human fetal membranes: a novel intrauterine source of cortisol. *J Clin Endocrinol Metab.* 2003;88:5033-5038.

410. Wallace MJ, Hooper SB, Harding R. Effects of elevated fetal cortisol concentrations on the volume, secretion, and reabsorption of lung liquid. *Am J Physiol.* 1995;269:R881-R887.

411. Muglia L, Jacobson L, Dikkes P, et al. Corticotropin-releasing hormone deficiency reveals major fetal but not adult glucocorticoid need. *Nature.* 1995;373:427-432.

412. Polk DH. Thyroid hormone effects on neonatal thermogenesis. *Semin Perinatol.* 1988;12:151-156.

413. Gunn TR, Gluckman PD. Perinatal thermogenesis. *Early Hum Dev.* 1995;42:169-183.

414. Obregon MJ, Pitamber R, Jacobsson A, et al. Euthyroid status is essential for the perinatal increase in thermogenin mRNA in brown adipose tissue of rat pups. *Biochem Biophys Res Commun.* 1987;148:9-14.

415. Polk DH, Padbury JF, Callegari CC, et al. Effect of fetal thyroidectomy on newborn thermogenesis in lambs. *Pediatr Res.* 1987;21:453-457.

416. Cypess AM, Kahn CR. The role and importance of brown adipose tissue in energy homeostasis. *Curr Opin Pediatr.* 2010;22:478-484.

417. van Marken Lichtenbelt WD, Vanhommerig JW, Smulders NM, et al. Cold-activated brown adipose tissue in healthy men. *N Engl J Med.* 2009;360:1500-1508.

418. Lidell ME, Betz MJ, Dahlqvist Leinhard O, et al. Evidence for two types of brown adipose tissue in humans. *Nat Med.* 2013;19:631-634.

419. Longhead JL, Minouni F, Tsang RC. Serum ionized calcium concentrations in normal neonates. *Am J Dis Child.* 1988;142:516-518.

420. Venkataraman PS, Tsang RC, Chen IW, et al. Pathogenesis of early neonatal hypocalcemia: studies of serum calcitonin, gastrin and plasma glucagon. *J Pediatr.* 1987;110:599-603.

421. Mimoumi F, Tsang RC. Perinatal mineral metabolism. In: Tulchinsky D, Little AB, eds. *Maternal-Fetal Endocrinology.* 2nd ed. Philadelphia, PA: WB Saunders; 1994:402-417.

422. Wheeler MD, Styne DM. Longitudinal changes in growth hormone response to growth hormone-releasing hormone in neonatal rhesus monkeys. *Pediatr Res.* 1990;28:15-18.

423. Penny R, Parlow AF, Frasier SD. Testosterone and estradiol concentrations in paired maternal and cord sera and their correlation with the concentration of chorionic gonadotropin. *Pediatrics.* 1979;64:604-608.

424. Mann DR, Gould KG, Collins DC, et al. Blockade of neonatal activation of the pituitary-testicular axis: effect on peripubertal luteinizing hormone and testosterone secretion and on testicular development in male monkeys. *J Clin Endocrinol Metab.* 1989;68:600-607.

425. Dohler KD. The special case of hormonal imprinting: the neonatal influence on sex. *Experientia.* 1986;42:759-769.

426. Resko JA, Roselli CE. Prenatal hormones organize sex differences in the neuroendocrine reproductive system: observations on guinea pigs and nonhuman primates. *Cell Mol Neurobiol.* 1997;17:627-648.

427. Kosut SS, Wood RI, Herbosa-Encaracion C, et al. Prenatal androgens time neuroendocrine puberty in the sheep: effect of testosterone dose. *Endocrinology.* 1997;138:1072-1077.

428. Grocock CA, Charlton HM, Pike MC. Role of fetal pituitary in cryptorchidism induced by exogenous maternal oestrogen during pregnancy in mice. *J Reprod Fertil.* 1988;83:295-300.

429. Martin SM, Moberg GP. Effects of early neonatal thyroxine treatment on development of the thyroid and adrenal axes in rats. *Life Sci.* 1981;29:1683-1688.

430. Walker P, Courtin F. Transient neonatal hyperthyroidism results in hypothyroidism in the adult rat. *Endocrinology.* 1985;116:2246-2250.

431. Csaba G, Inczefi-Gonda A, Dobozy O. Hereditary transmission in the F_1 generation of hormonal imprinting (receptor memory) induced in rats by neonatal exposure to insulin. *Acta Physiol Hung.* 1984;63:93-99.

432. Csaba G, Ronai A, Laszlo V, et al. Amplification of hormone receptors by neonatal oxytocin and vasopressin treatment. *Horm Metab Res.* 1980;12:28-31.

433. Drake AJ, Walker BR, Seckl JR. Intergenerational consequences of fetal programming by in utero exposure to glucocorticoids in rats. *Am J Physiol Regul Integr Comp Physiol.* 2005;288:R34-R38.

434. Lackland DR. Fetal and early life determinants of hypertension in adults: implications for study. *Hypertension.* 2004;44:811-812.

435. Barker DJP. Fetal programming of coronary heart disease. *Trends Endocrinol Metab.* 2002;13:364-368.

436. Barker DJP. The developmental origins of chronic adult disease. *Acta Paediatr Suppl.* 2004;336:26-33.

437. Ozanne SE, Hales CN. Early programming of glucose-insulin metabolism. *Trends Endocrinol Metab.* 2002;13:368-373.

438. Matthews SG. Early programming of the hypothalamo-pituitary-adrenal axis. *Trends Endocrinol Metab.* 2002;13:373-380.

439. Young BS. Programming of sympatho-adrenal function. *Trends Endocrinol Metab.* 2002;13:381-385.

440. Davies MJ, Norman RJ. Programming and reproductive function. *Trends Endocrinol Metab.* 2002;13:386-392.

441. Holt RIG. Fetal programming of the growth hormone–insulin-like growth factor axis. *Trends Endocrinol Metab.* 2002;13:392-402.

442. Dodic M, Moritz K, Koukoulas I, et al. Programmed hypertension: kidney, brain or both. *Trends Endocrinol Metab.* 2002;13:403-408.

443. Reik W, Constancia M, Fowdey A, et al. Regulation of supply and demand for maternal nutrients in mammals by imprinted genes. *J Physiol.* 2003;547:35-44.

444. Ibanez L, Ong K, Potau N, et al. Insulin gene variable number of tandem repeat genotype and the low birth weight, precocious pubarche, and hyperinsulinism sequence. *J Clin Endocrinol Metab.* 2001;86:5788-5793.

445. Ijzerman RG, Stehouwer CDA, de Geus EJ, et al. Low birth weight is associated with increased sympathetic activity: dependence on genetic factors. *Circulation.* 2003;108:566-571.

446. Fowden AL, Forhead AJ. Endocrine mechanisms of intrauterine programming. *Reproduction.* 2004;127:515-526.

447. Slone-Wilcoxon J, Redei EE. Maternal-fetal glucocorticoid milieu programs hypothalamic-pituitary-thyroid function of adult offspring. *Endocrinology.* 2004;145:4068-4072.

448. Lavcola L, Perrini S, Belsanti G, et al. Intrauterine growth restriction in humans is associated with abnormalities in placental insulin-like growth factor signaling. *Endocrinology.* 2005;146:1498-1505.

449. Waterland RA, Jirtle RL. Early nutrition, epigenetic changes at transposons and imprinted genes, and enhanced susceptibility to adult chronic diseases. *Nutrition.* 2004;20:63-68.

450. McMullen S, Langley-Evans SC. Maternal low-protein diet in rat pregnancy programs blood pressure through sex-specific mechanisms. *Am J Physiol Regul Integr Physiol.* 2005;288:R85-R90.

451. Bunt JC, Tataranni PA, Salbe AD. Intrauterine exposure to diabetes is a determinant of hemoglobin A(1)c and systolic blood pressure in Pima Indian children. *J Clin Endocrinol Metab.* 2005;90:3225-3229.

452. Zheng X, Hendry WJ III. Neonatal stilbestrol treatment alters the estrogen-related expression of both cell proliferation and apoptosis-related proto-oncogene (c-jun, dfos, cmyc, bax, bcl-2 and bcl-x) in the hamster uterus. *Cell Growth Diff.* 1997;8:425-434.

453. Huang WW, Yin Y, Bi Q, et al. Developmental diethylstilbestrol exposure alters genetic pathways of uterine cytodifferentiation. *Mol Endocrinol.* 2005;19:669-682.

454. Csaba G. Receptor ontogeny and hormonal imprinting. *Experientia.* 1986;42:750-759.

455. Sato SM, Mains MI, Adzick MS, et al. Plasticity in the adrenocorticotropin-related peptides produced by primary cultures of neonatal rat pituitary. *Endocrinology.* 1988;122:68-77.
456. Vickers MH, Gluckman PD, Coveny HH, et al. Neonatal leptin treatment reverses developmental programming. *Endocrinology.* 2005;146:4211-4216.
457. Flake AW. Fetal therapy: medical and surgical approaches. In: Creasy RK, Resnik R, eds. *Maternal-Fetal Medicine.* 4th ed. Philadelphia, PA: WB Saunders; 1999:365-377.
458. Harman CR. Assessment of fetal health. In: Creasy RK, Resnik R, eds. *Maternal-Fetal Medicine.* 5th ed. Philadelphia, PA: WB Saunders; 2004:357-401.
459. Resnick R, Creasy RK. Intrauterine growth restriction. In: Creasy RK, Resnick R, eds. *Maternal Fetal Medicine.* 5th ed. Philadelphia, PA: WB Saunders; 2004:495-512.
460. Bianchi DW. Prenatal exclusion of recessively inherited disorders: should maternal plasma analysis precede invasive techniques. *Clin Chem.* 2002;48:689-690.
461. Manning FA. General principles and applications of ultrasonography. In: Creasy RK, Resnik R, eds. *Maternal-Fetal Medicine.* 5th ed. Philadelphia, PA: WB Saunders; 2004:315-355.
462. Fisher DA. Fetal thyroid function: diagnosis and management of fetal thyroid disorders. *Clin Obstet Gynecol.* 1997;40:16-31.
463. New MI, Carlton A, Obeid J, et al. Update: prenatal diagnosis for congenital adrenal hyperplasia in 595 pregnancies. *Endocrinologist.* 2003;13:233-239.
464. Charlton V, Johengen M. Fetal intravenous nutritional supplementation ameliorates the development of embolization-induced growth retardation in sheep. *Pediatr Res.* 1987;22:55-61.
465. Flake AW, Zanjani ED. In utero hematopoietic stem cell transplantation. *JAMA.* 1997;278:932-937.
466. Lin RY, Kubo A, Keller GM, et al. Committing embryonic stem cells to differentiate into thyrocyte-like cells in vitro. *Endocrinology.* 2003;144:2644-2649.
467. Waddington SN, Kennea NL, Buckley SMK, et al. Fetal and neonatal gene therapy: benefits and pitfalls. *Gene Ther.* 2004;11:592-597.

CHAPTER 23

Pediatric Disorders of Sex Development

JOHN C. ACHERMANN • IEUAN A. HUGHES

KEY POINTS

- Disorders of sex development (DSDs) can present to different health professionals at different ages, but pediatric and adult endocrinologists play a central role in diagnosis, support, and management.
- DSDs represent a broad range of conditions with many underlying causes; understanding the basic biology of sex development and steroidogenesis can help in elucidating the causes of these conditions.
- Achieving a diagnosis is important for predicting the natural history of specific conditions, identifying associated features, monitoring endocrine function and tumor risk, and counseling families about inheritance patterns. In some situations a diagnosis might influence sex assignment or gender.
- A range of special biochemical tests and genetic analyses can help reach a specific diagnosis in most steroidogenesis disorders. Currently, a genetic diagnosis is reached in fewer than half of children with gonadal dysgenesis.
- A multidisciplinary team approach is key in providing coordinated management from diagnosis through later life. An experienced psychologist or allied professional can help support families and young people in the early years, as well as following transition to adult services. Support groups also play an important role.
- A subset of DSDs presents in teenage years or even in adulthood. Adult endocrinologists have a crucial role to play in managing young people who present in adulthood, as well as for long-term follow up of individuals with DSDs from childhood. A supportive and sensitive approach is essential.

Disorders of (or differences in) sex development represent a broad range of conditions that can present to many different health professionals at different stages of life.

In the newborn period, approximately 1 in every 4500 babies has atypical (ambiguous) genitalia and cannot be immediately assigned to male or female without further expert evaluation or investigations. However, DSDs can present in many other ways, such as karyotype-phenotype discordance prenatally; bilateral hernia or associated syndromic features (e.g., renal) in childhood; virilization, absent puberty, or primary amenorrhea in teenage years; or even later in life with infertility. Therefore, many different health professionals could be involved in DSDs, and all should be aware of the range of conditions, how they might present, and the principles of their management.[1,2]

The investigation and management of DSDs require a multidisciplinary team with experience in these conditions.[2,3] The pediatric endocrinologist plays a key role within this team in the childhood and teenage years, whereas adult endocrinologists need to be involved in transitioning care and in the management of long-term issues such as hormone replacement and bone health. In addition to input from urologists, gynecologists, biochemists, and geneticists, it is becoming increasingly clear that experienced psychological support is essential for families and individuals with DSDs at key points in their lives. DSD still has significant stigma. The past decade has seen changing terminology and attitudes (Table 23-1), but this is an ever-evolving area, and engagement with support groups and the DSD community is increasingly important to define the best pathways of care at local and national levels.

In keeping with previous editions of this textbook, this chapter will first describe the development of the reproductive systems, then present an overview of the range of conditions that can be classified as DSDs, and will finally consider approaches to investigation and management of DSDs at different ages.[4]

DEVELOPMENT OF REPRODUCTIVE SYSTEMS

Reproductive system development begins at 4 to 5 weeks' gestation in humans and is complete with the achievement of secondary sexual characteristics and fertility (i.e., production of viable gametes) after puberty. Sex development is a dynamic process that requires the interaction of many genes, proteins, signaling molecules, paracrine factors, and

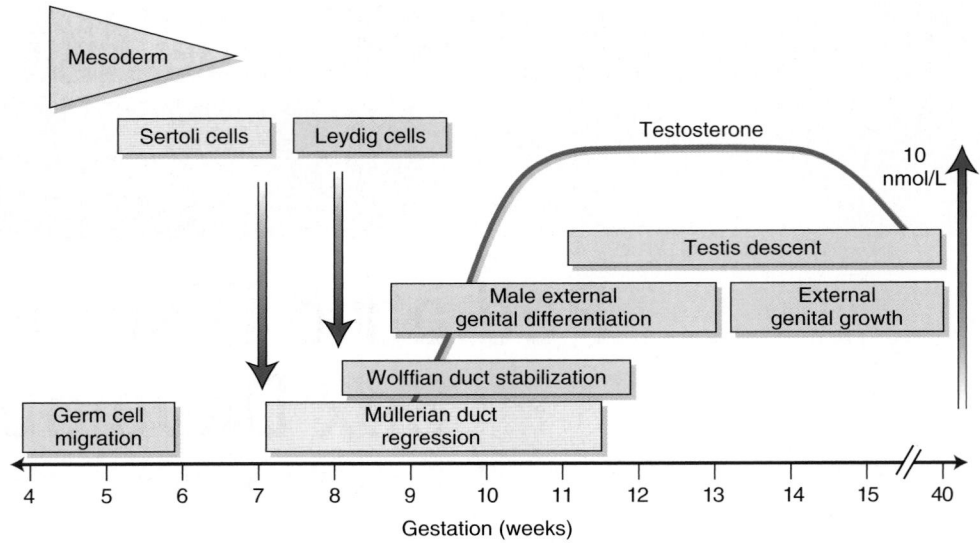

Figure 23-1 Events temporally related to sex differentiation in the male fetus. Mesoderm refers to the tissue source for Sertoli and Leydig cell formation. The continuous line depicts the rise in fetal serum testosterone, with a peak concentration of about 10 nmol/L (300 ng/dL).

TABLE 23-1
Proposed Revised Nomenclature

Previous Terms	Proposed Terms
Intersex	Disorders of sex development (DSDs)
Male pseudohermaphrodite Undervirilization of an XY male Undermasculinization of an XY male	46,XY DSD
Female pseudohermaphrodite Overvirilization of an XX female Masculinization of an XX female	46,XX DSD
True hermaphrodite	Ovotesticular DSD
XX male or XX sex reversal	46,XX testicular DSD
XY sex reversal	46,XY complete gonadal dysgenesis

Reproduced with permission from Hughes IA, Houk C, Ahmed SF, et al. Consensus statement on management of intersex disorders. *Arch Dis Child.* 2006;91:554-562.

endocrine stimuli.[5-9] Marked differences in the basic mechanisms of sex determination, differentiation, and reproductive strategy have evolved in different species, with variability in sex chromosome complement, gonad development, and gametogenesis throughout the animal kingdom.[10,11] In this chapter, we focus on the basic mechanisms of reproductive development in humans. We also include some important insights obtained from studies of normal and transgenic mice, although these are reviewed extensively elsewhere. More detailed explanation of pituitary gonadotrope development is provided in Chapter 22 and of normal and disordered puberty in Chapter 25.

Sex Determination and Sex Differentiation

Sex determination is the process whereby the bipotential gonad develops into a testis or an ovary. *Sex differentiation* requires the developing gonad to function appropriately to produce peptide hormones and steroids with a consequent effect on the developing genitalia.

In the typical male, the process of sex differentiation involves regression of müllerian structures (uterus, fallo-

pian tubes, and the upper one third of the vagina), stabilization of wolffian structures (seminal vesicles, vasa deferentia, and epididymides), androgenization of the external genitalia (penis and scrotum), and descent of the testes from their origin in the urogenital ridge to their final position in the scrotum (Fig. 23-1).

In the typical female, the ovary usually is steroidogenically quiescent until the time of puberty, when estrogen synthesis stimulates breast and uterine development and follicular development results in regular menstrual cycles. Defects in ovarian development therefore usually manifest in adolescence with absent puberty. Consequently, ovarian development and differentiation have been viewed in the past as a default or passive process. Although male sex differentiation is undoubtedly a more active developmental process—as defined in the classic experiments of Alfred Jost[12]—studies of gene expression show that a specific complement of genes is implicated in ovarian development and integrity, some of which (e.g., *RSPO1*) may actively antagonize testis differentiation.[6,13,14] Even the concept of a fixed and quiescent population of ovarian germ cells at birth, or absent ovarian steroidogenesis, has been challenged.[15,16] Therefore, ovarian development probably involves many active processes.

Classically, sex determination and sex differentiation can be divided into three major components: chromosomal sex (i.e., presence of a Y or X chromosome), gonadal sex (i.e., presence of a testis or ovary), and phenotypic or anatomic sex (i.e., presence of male or female external and internal genitalia) (Fig. 23-2). None of these processes absolutely defines a person's sex, and psychosexual or gender development ("brain sex") is an outcome of several biologic factors, as well as environmental and social influences. The presence or absence of a Y chromosome or well-formed testes should not be the focus of how a physician views an individual with a DSD after a diagnosis or management plan has been established. However, consideration of sex development in terms of chromosomal sex, gonadal sex, and phenotypic (or anatomic) sex can be a useful way of understanding the processes involved in reproductive development, and it can be a helpful construct for the investigation and diagnosis of individuals with these conditions, especially because the (somatic)

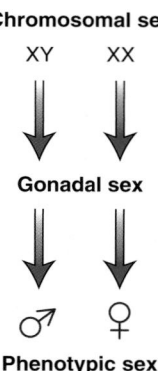

Chromosomal sex

XY   XX

Gonadal sex

♂   ♀

Phenotypic sex

Figure 23-2 Division of sex development into three major components provides a useful framework for diagnosis and classification. Chromosomal sex refers to the karyotype (46,XX, 46,XY, or variants). Gonadal sex refers to the presence of a testis or ovary after the process of sex determination. Phenotypic (anatomic) sex refers to the appearance of the external genitalia and internal structures after the process of sex differentiation.

karyotype is usually readily available. The chromosomal-gonadal-phenotypic model is described in this chapter.

Chromosomal Sex

Chromosomal sex describes the complement of sex chromosomes present in an individual (e.g., 46,XY; 46,XX). In humans, the usual complement of 46 chromosomes consists of 22 pairs of autosomes (identified numerically from 1 to 22 based on decreasing size) and a pair of sex chromosomes (XX or XY) (Fig. 23-3). Other species have different numbers of chromosomes, or they may have sexually dimorphic autosomes.[10,11]

In humans, chromosomal sex usually is determined at the time of fertilization, when two haploid gametes (ova and sperm, with 23 chromosomes each) fuse to generate a diploid zygote (46 chromosomes). Gametes are ultimately derived from germ cells, which initially replicate their chromosome complement and then undergo a series of two meiotic divisions, meiosis I (reduction division) and

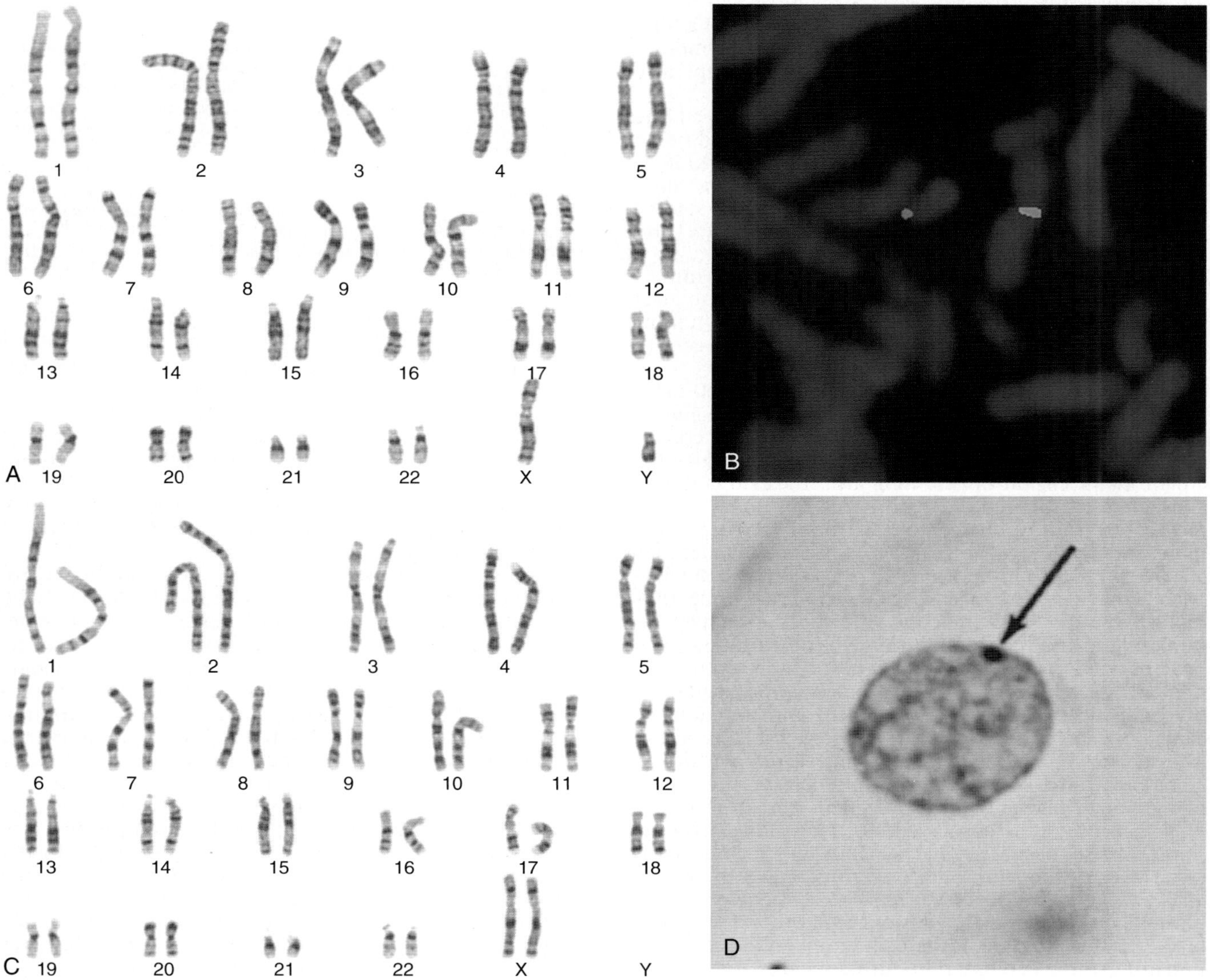

Figure 23-3 Cytogenetic and fluorescence in situ hybridization (FISH) studies. **A,** Male (46,XY) G-banded karyotype. **B,** FISH analysis of a male (46,XY) using fluorescent probes directed against SRY (sex-determining region on the Y chromosome, spectrum red) and against the X centromere (spectrum green). **C,** Female (46,XX) G-banded karyotype. **D,** Photomicrograph shows the X chromatin body (Barr body, *arrow*) in the nucleus of buccal mucosa cells from a 46,XX female (thionine stain; original magnification, ×2000). (A through C courtesy of Lee Grimsley and Jonathan Waters, MD, North East London Regional Cytogenetics Laboratory, Great Ormond Street Hospital NHS Trust, London, UK.)

meiosis II, to produce haploid ova or sperm. Normal ova have a single X chromosome. Normal sperm contain a single Y chromosome or a single X chromosome, resulting, respectively, in a 46,XY or 46,XX zygote after fertilization.

Nondisjunction is the failure of either of a pair of sister chromatids to separate during anaphase.[17,18] *Meiotic nondisjunction* during gametogenesis can result in ova or sperm with gain or loss of sex chromosomal material. Fertilization by such gametes can give rise to a zygote with an imbalance in sex chromosome number, called *sex chromosome aneuploidy*. For example, a zygote with a single X chromosome (i.e., 45,X) has Turner syndrome, and the presence of an extra X causes Klinefelter syndrome (47,XXY) or triple X syndrome (47,XXX).[18] Zygotes with no X chromosomal material (45,Y) are nonviable.

Mitotic nondisjunction can occur in the zygote (i.e., after fertilization), resulting in an imbalance in sex chromosome number in a *subset* of cells, and this is called *sex chromosome mosaicism* (e.g., 45,X/46,XY). In such cases, the two (or more) cell lines originate from a single zygote. This situation differs from *chimerism*, which is the existence of two or more cell lines with different genetic origins in one individual. Chimerism can occur through several mechanisms, including double fertilization (dispermy) of a binucleate ovum, fusion of two complete zygotes or morulae before implantation, or fertilization by separate sperm of an ovum and its polar body.

Chimerism is difficult to detect if the separate cell lines have the same sex chromosomes. However, if the different cell lines have different sex chromosomes, a 46,XX/46,XY karyotype occurs. This form of true *sex chromosome chimerism* is very rare in humans. The consequences of some of these events in humans are discussed later (see "Sex Chromosome Disorders of Sex Development").

The Y Chromosome. Although the Y chromosome was initially thought to be inert, detection of a 46,XY karyotype in males and a 47,XXY karyotype in men with Klinefelter syndrome provided evidence that the Y chromosome carries a gene (or genes) responsible for male sex determination.

The human Y chromosome is approximately 60 megabases (Mb) long and represents only 2% of the human genome DNA (Fig. 23-4).[19,20] The Y chromosome consists of the highly variable and largely genetically inactive heterochromatic region on the long arm, the remnants of a conserved male-specific region, and autosomal-derived regions that are estimated to have been added approximately 80 to 130 million years ago. It is thought that there are around 200 Y-chromosomal genes, at least 72 of which encode proteins. The male-specific regions are undergoing rapid evolution, with marked differences even between humans and chimpanzees.[21] Although some of these genes have putative roles in growth, cognition, and tooth development, several genes in the male-specific region are involved in reproductive development and function. For example, a cluster of genes at Yq11.22 (e.g., the *AZF*c region) is essential for spermatogenesis, and genes within the gonadoblastoma locus (e.g., *TSPY*) increase the risk of malignancy when present in dysgenetic gonads.[22,23]

The euchromatic (conserved) portion of the Y chromosome consists of a Y-specific segment and regions at the distal ends of the short and long arms, called the *pseudoautosomal regions* (PARs) (see Fig. 23-4).[19,24] These PARs are homologous to the distal ends of the short and long arms of the X chromosome and are the only regions involved in pairing and recombination during meiosis. This process is essential for proper distribution of recombined sex chromosomal material to daughter cells and for maintaining dosage sensitivity of X-Y pairs. PAR1 (distal short arm, Yp and Xp) contains at least 10 genes, including the homeo-

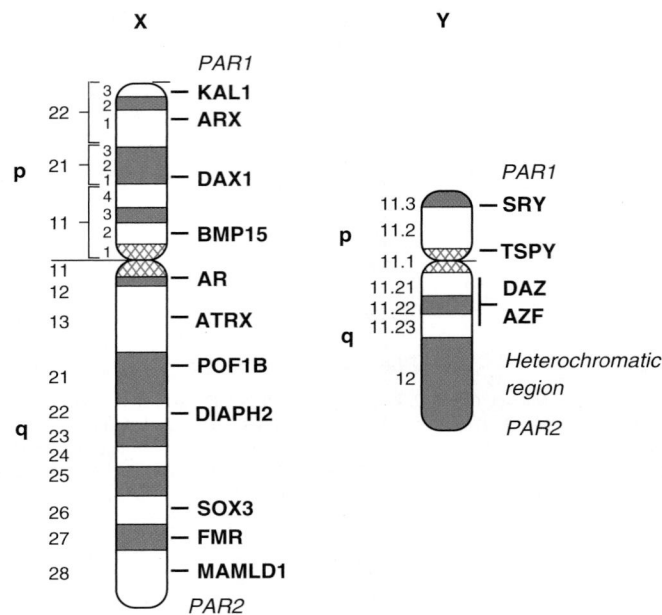

Figure 23-4 Schematic diagrams of the X chromosome *(left)* and Y chromosome *(right)* show key regions and genes involved in sex development and reproduction. AR, androgen receptor; ARX, aristaless-related homeobox, X-linked; ATRX, α-thalassemia, X-linked mental retardation; AZF, azoospermia factor; BMP15, bone morphogenetic protein 15; DAX1, dosage-sensitive sex reversal congenital adrenal hypoplasia critical region on the X chromosome type 1; DAZ, deleted in azoospermia; DIAP2, human homolog of the *Drosophila* diaphanous gene; FMR, fragile X, mental retardation; KAL1, Kallmann syndrome type 1; MAMLD1, mastermind-like domain containing 1 (CXorf6); p, short arm; PAR, pseudoautosomal region; POF1B, actin-binding protein, 34 kDa; q, long arm; SOX3, SRY-related HMG box 3; SRY, sex-determining region Y; TSPY, testes-specific protein Y.

box gene *SHOX* (formerly called *PHOG*). SHOX haploinsufficiency contributes to the short stature associated with Turner syndrome, Xp– or Yp– deletions, and Léri-Weill syndrome (i.e., dyschondrosteosis). These regions are not subject to dosage compensation (i.e., gene inactivation). PAR2 (distal long arm) contains genes that mostly encode growth factors and signaling molecules. These regions may potentially play a role in maintaining male viability and in sex-specific health and disease traits.

The search for a testis-determining factor on the Y chromosome began more than 50 years ago. The discovery by Eichwald and Silmser in 1955 of a male cell membrane-specific antigen that causes rejection of skin grafts by female mice led to pursuit of the H-Y antigen as a candidate testis-determining factor.[25] In 1987, Mardon and Page proposed that the sex-determining function of the Y chromosome is located within a 140-kb segment of the short arm, within the Y-specific euchromatic portion.[26] A zinc finger transcription factor, ZFY, was the initial candidate in this region. However, in 1989, Palmer and colleagues described several 46,XX *males* who had Y-to-X translocations of Y chromosomal material that was distal (telomeric) to the ZFY locus; this focused attention on a 35-kb region of the Y chromosome close to the pseudoautosomal boundary.[27] This region contained a putative transcription factor subsequently called *sex-determining region Y (SRY)* that was expressed in appropriate tissues (see Fig. 23-4).

A series of elegant studies in mice and humans established *SRY* as the primary Y-chromosomal testis-determining gene.[28-30] The first definitive proof came with the generation of transgenic XX mice specifically expressing the *SRY*

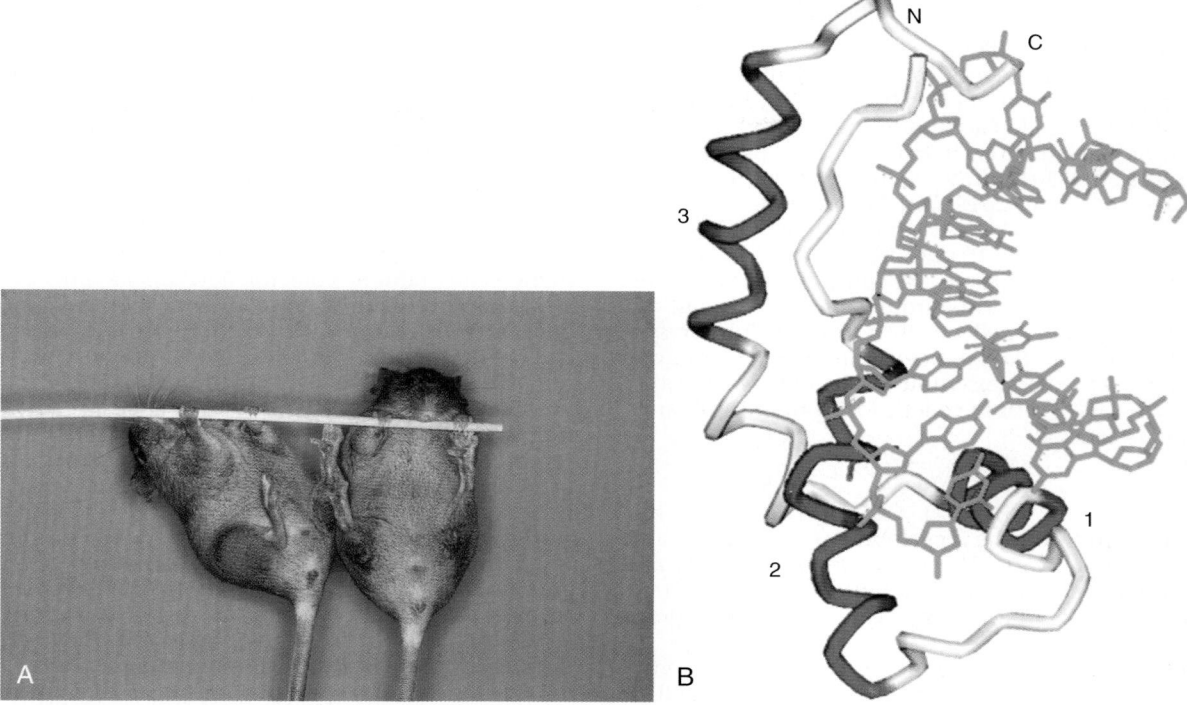

Figure 23-5 A, The XXSRY⁺ mouse *(right)* has testis development and a male phenotype, providing convincing evidence that SRY (sex-determining region on the Y chromosome) is a testis-determining gene. A normal XY male littermate is shown for comparison *(left)*. **B,** Model of the structure of the SRY high-mobility group (HMG) box bound to DNA. The HMG domain contains three α-helices *(red)*, which adopt an L-shaped conformation. Binding of this region of SRY to the minor groove of DNA *(green)* causes it to bend and unwind. (A courtesy of Professor Robin Lovell-Badge, National Institute of Medical Research, London, UK; B from Harley VR, Clarkson MJ, Argentaro A. The molecular action and regulation of the testis-determining factors, SRY [sex-determining region on the Y chromosome] and SOX9 [SRY-related high-mobility group (HMG) box 9]. *Endocr Rev.* 2003;24:466-487, used with permission of The Endocrine Society, copyright 2003.)

locus (14 kb); some of these mice had a male phenotype, developed testes (without spermatogenesis), and showed male sexual mating behavior (Fig. 23-5).[31] This work was supported by reports of deletions and loss-of-function mutations in *SRY* in humans with 46,XY complete gonadal dysgenesis (Swyer syndrome) (see later discussion).[29,32,33]

The X Chromosome. The X chromosome is a relatively large and gene-rich chromosome compared with the Y chromosome, and it consists of about 160 Mb of genomic DNA (see Fig. 23-4).[19,34,35] This DNA contains 5% of the haploid genome and more than 1200 expressed genes, of which at least 800 encode proteins. Genes on the X chromosome play an important role in sex development in males and females at the level of the gonad and gametogenesis and also in hypothalamic-pituitary (gonadotrope) function (e.g., androgen receptor *[AR]*, *KAL1*, DAX1 *[NR0B1]*, *MAMLD1*, *SOX3*). More than 100 X-chromosome genes are expressed in the testis and germ cells.[34] However, most X-linked genes are unrelated to sex development and have a diverse range of cellular functions.

The X chromosome contains PARs at the distal end of each arm, similar to the Y chromosome (see Fig. 23-4).[19] These regions and several genes in their boundaries do not undergo X inactivation; they function in an autosomal fashion with their homologs on the Y-chromosome PARs. A large number of genes on the X chromosome are located outside the PARs and do not have homologs on the Y chromosome. Because many of these genes are involved in a wide range of cellular processes unrelated to sex development or sex-specific function, a process must exist to maintain the balance in expressed copy number (i.e., gene dosage) of these genes in both males with a single X chromosome and females with two X chromosomes.

The first insight into *X inactivation* came after the identification in 1949 of the X chromatin body (i.e., Barr body) in a proportion of cells in females (see Fig. 23-3). This X chromatin is derived from only one of the two X chromosomes in interphase nuclei of these somatic cells. Grumbach and colleagues showed that the X chromosome giving rise to X chromatin completes DNA synthesis later than any other chromosome.[36] These findings led to the concept that only one X chromosome is genetically active during interphase, whereas the other X chromosome is heterochromatinized and relatively inactive. This change in activation state occurs in early gestation in humans (12 to 18 days, late blastocyte stage) and is a multistep process leading to stable epigenetic silencing of genes on all X chromosomes in excess of one (Lyon hypothesis).[37] However, female germ cells beyond the stage of oogonia are exempt from X inactivation, in keeping with the need for a second X chromosome for germ cell and ovarian development.

X inactivation occurs randomly in different cells.[38] After inactivation has occurred, the inactive state of that particular X chromosome is transmitted to all descendants of that cell so that females effectively function as genetic mosaics insofar as X-linked traits are concerned. If the initial population of cells is small, skewed X inactivation can occur as a chance event despite random inactivation. In these situations, heterozygous female carriers of an X-linked disorder may manifest symptoms of the condition. A subset of genes on the X chromosome may also be imprinted.

It was originally suggested that genes involved in ovary development and function would be located on the X chromosome and that studying families with ovarian failure or women with Turner syndrome who have chromosomal variations such as partial loss of X-chromosome material would lead to identification of the loci for key genes.[39,40] Several X-chromosomal loci and genes for premature ovarian failure (POF) or primary ovarian insufficiency (POI) have been identified, including those for POF1 (*FMR1* premutations on Xq26-q28), POF2A (*DIAPH2* on Xq22), POF2B (*POF1B* [an actin-binding protein] on Xq21), and POF4 (*BMP15* on Xp11.2). However, many other genes are autosomal: POF3 (*FOXL2*) on 3q23; POF5 (*NOBOX*) on 7q35; POF6 (*FIGLA*) on 2p12; POF7 (steroidogenic factor 1 [SF1], *NR5A1*) on 9q33; POF8 (*STAG3*) on 7q22; POF9 (*HFM1*) on 1p22; and POF10 (*MCM8*) on 20p12.[41-50] Certain variants of Turner syndrome are more likely to involve ovarian dysfunction (e.g., isochromosome for Xq), but it is likely that the accelerated oocyte atresia in Turner syndrome also reflects impaired meiosis and subsequent germ cell apoptosis caused by sex chromosome imbalance, rather than only the loss of certain genetic loci containing ovarian development genes.[39]

Gonadal Sex

Gonadal sex refers to the development of the gonadal tissue as testis or ovary. The principal embryologic and morphologic changes involved in gonad development are shown in Figure 23-6 and have been described in detail elsewhere.[6-8]

The Bipotential Gonad. The primitive gonad arises from a condensation of the medioventral region of the urogenital ridge at approximately 4 to 5 weeks after conception in humans (see Fig. 23-6). The primitive gonad separates from the adrenal primordium at about 5 weeks but remains bipotential (indifferent) until about 42 days after conception. Testes and ovaries are morphologically indistinguishable from each other until approximately the 6th week of postconception (13-mm stage).

Several important genes are expressed in the developing urogenital ridge in mice that facilitate formation of the bipotential gonad; they include *Emx2, Lim1, Lhx9, M33/CBX2, Pod1, Six1/4, Map3k4, Wt1 (+KTS),* and *Nr5a1/Sf1.*[51-57] Deletion of these genes causes gonadal dysgenesis in mice and can be associated with other abnormalities (e.g., kidney, brain). Only some of them have been associated with human DSDs to date (e.g., *WT1, CBX2, NR5A1/SF1*), possibly through their effects on multiple components of gonad development and function.[58]

Several other transcription factors and signaling pathways present in the primordial gonad may play a role ultimately in regulating *Sry* expression and testis development. *Gata4* (and its cofactor, *Fog2/Zfpm2*) encodes a transcriptional regulator involved in early gonadal and cardiac development. Mice with deletions of these genes have cardiac defects and variable gonadal phenotypes.[59,60] Haploinsufficiency and point mutations in *GATA4* have been identified in patients with cardiac defects, and human mutations associated with gonadal dysgenesis have been reported.[61] Disruption of FOG2/ZFPM2 has also recently been described associated with testicular dysgenesis in humans.[62]

Deletions of multiple components of the insulin signaling pathway (i.e., insulin receptor, insulin-related receptor, and insulin-like growth factor 1 receptor) disrupt the early stages of testis development and downstream *Sry* expression in mice, whereas alterations in *Map3k1* and *Map3k4* (formerly called *Mekk4*) affect mitogen-activated protein kinase kinase kinase signaling, resulting in impaired gonadal growth, altered mesonephric cell migration, and reduced *Sry* and *Sox9* expression.[57,63,64]

The role of key transcription factors such as the product of the Wilms tumor 1 gene (*WT1*) and SF1 (*NR5A1*) in early gonad development has become better understood as murine models are characterized, and alterations in these genes have been found in patients with impaired gonad development (see "46,XY Disorders of Sex Development" and Fig. 23-7).

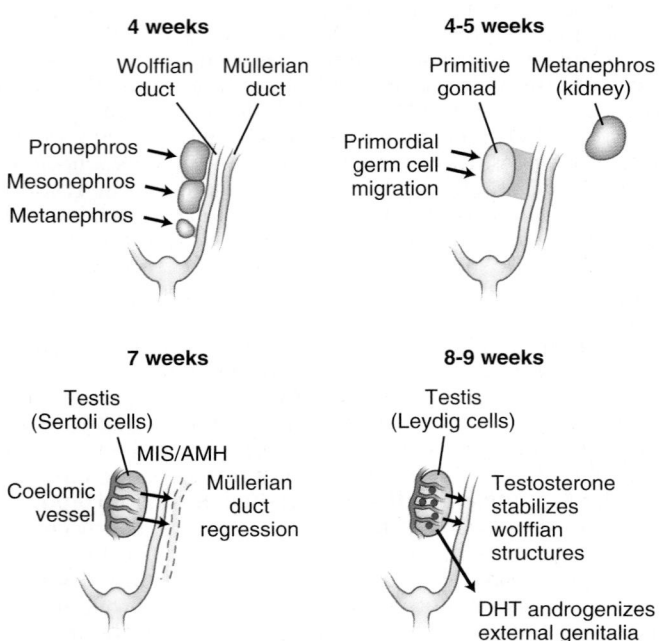

Figure 23-6 Schematic representation of the principal morphologic and functional events during early gonad or testis development in humans. DHT, dihydrotestosterone; MIS/AMH, müllerian inhibiting substance/antimüllerian hormone. (Modified from Achermann JC, Jameson JL. Testis determination. *Top Endocrinol.* 2003;22:10-14, used with permission of Chapterhouse Codex.)

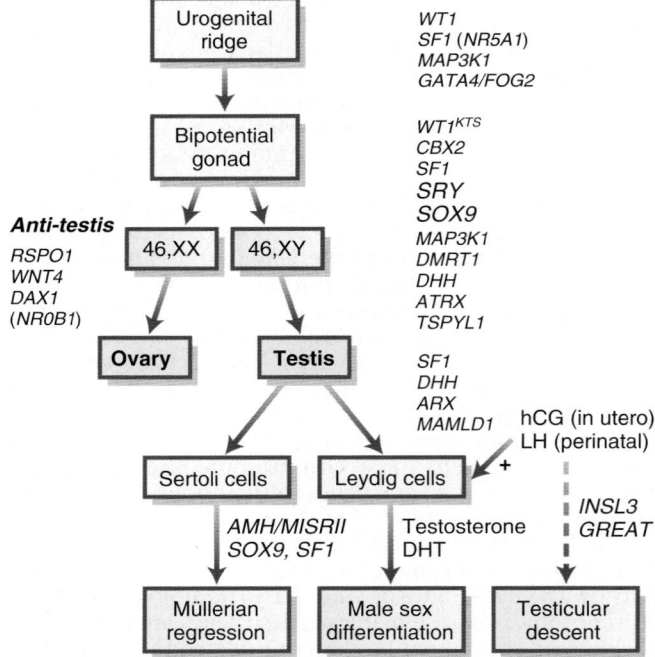

Figure 23-7 The flow chart provides an overview of the major events involved in sex determination and sex differentiation. Mutations or deletions in the genes reported to cause disorders of sex development in humans are shown. hCG, human chorionic gonadotropin; LH, luteinizing hormone.

The *WT1* gene (11p13) encodes a four–zinc finger transcription factor expressed in the developing genital ridge, kidney, gonads, and mesothelium.[65] Homozygous deletion of the gene encoding Wt1 in mice prevents gonad and kidney development.[66] The WT1 protein is subject to complex post-translational modification and splicing processes, and it is thought that at least 24 WT1 isoforms exist.[67] The two most common variants are an isoform with alternative splicing of exon 5 and insertion of an additional 17 amino acids in the middle of the protein and an isoform that uses an alternative splice donor site for exon 9, resulting in the addition of three amino acids (lysine, threonine, and serine; called +KTS) between zinc fingers 3 and 4. It is thought that +KTS and –KTS isoforms have different cellular functions and differential effects on gonad and renal development.[68] The ratio of +KTS to –KTS isoforms may be important in testis development, with the +KTS isoform having a cell-autonomous role in regulating SRY expression and influencing cellular proliferation and Sertoli cell differentiation.[69] WT1 also regulates expression of *Sf1* and *Sox9* in mice and may oppose β-catenin pathways. Although significant insight into the roles of different WT1 isoforms is being obtained from transgenic mice, the overall role of WT1 in cellular biology is complex and incompletely understood.

In humans, WT1 transcripts can be detected in the indifferent gonadal ridge when it first forms at 32 days after ovulation.[70] Deletions or mutations of WT1 cause well-defined syndromes in humans. Haploinsufficiency of WT1 due to deletion of the chromosomal locus containing *WT1* and *PAX6* (11p13) causes WAGR syndrome (Wilms tumor, aniridia, genitourinary abnormalities, and mental retardation).[71] Dominant negative point mutations in *WT1* cause Denys-Drash syndrome (gonadal dysgenesis, genital ambiguity, nephropathy, and predisposition to Wilms tumor),[72] whereas mutations in the exon 9 splice site of *WT1*, causing an altered ratio of +KTS to –KTS isoforms of WT1, result in Frasier syndrome (gonadal dysgenesis, late-onset nephropathy, and predisposition to gonadoblastoma) (see "46,XY Disorders of Sex Development" and see Fig. 23-19).[73,74] Although these isoforms may play different roles in regulating various stages of renal and gonad development, it is likely some phenotypic overlap in the latter two conditions exists.

Another key transcription factor expressed in the urogenital ridge is steroidogenic factor 1 (SF1, *NR5A1*).[75] SF1 is a member of the nuclear receptor superfamily that regulates the transcription of at least 30 genes known to be involved in gonadal development, adrenal development, steroidogenesis, and reproduction. In mice, complete deletion of the gene encoding Sf1 results in apoptosis of the developing gonad and adrenal gland during early embryonic development.[76] Other features of these homozygous-deleted animals include persistent müllerian structures and impaired androgenization in XY animals, hypogonadotropic hypogonadism, abnormalities of the ventromedial hypothalamus, altered stress responses, and late-onset obesity in adult animals rescued by adrenal transplantation.[77] Heterozygous animals have reduced gonadal size and impaired adrenal stress responses.[78]

SF1 is expressed during the early stages of urogenital ridge formation in humans (32 days after ovulation), where it is involved in maintaining gonadal integrity and permitting testicular differentiation.[70] Consistent with the mouse phenotype, heterozygous or homozygous loss-of-function mutations have been described in three patients with primary adrenal failure, severe 46,XY gonadal dysgenesis, and persistent müllerian structures (see later discussion).[79,80] Haploinsufficiency of SF1 is emerging as a relatively frequent cause of 46,XY DSD.[7,81] Data for mice suggest that Sf1 plays a critical role in testis development and facilitates SRY regulation of *SOX9* expression.[82] Although SF1 was originally thought to play a less significant role in the ovary compared with the testis, studies in mice and humans show that SF1 is also an important regulator of ovarian integrity and function.[47,83,84]

In addition to the single-gene defects outlined previously, several chromosomal duplications or deletions have been associated with impaired gonad development in patients. Dosage-sensitive overexpression or underexpression of key factors in these regions may interfere with sex development. For example, duplication of a region of the X chromosome (Xp21, dosage-sensitive sex reversal) containing the gene encoding DAX1 *(NR0B1)* has been reported in several 46,XY patients with impaired testicular development or ovotestes.[85] These reports suggest that the orphan nuclear receptor DAX1 may act to antagonize testis development as an anti-testis gene. This concept was supported by studies in mice *(Mus poshiavinus)* in which overexpression of *Dax1* caused impaired testis development in the presence of a weakened *Sry* locus.[86] However, targeted deletion of *Dax1* in a similar mouse strain also caused impaired testis development or ovotestis. Patients with X-linked adrenal hypoplasia congenita due to mutations in DAX1 have abnormal testis architecture and infertility, suggesting that critical doses of these factors have important roles; underactivity or overactivity could have deleterious effects at different stages of gonadal development.[87]

Impaired gonadal development has been described in a 46,XY individual with duplication of 1p35 that resulted in overexpression of the signaling molecules WNT4 and RSPO1, further supporting the concept that genes in certain loci have a role in opposing testis development, mostly likely through opposing SOX9 and testis determination pathways (see later).[88]

In addition to these regions of genomic duplication, many chromosomal rearrangements and deletions have been described in individuals with reproductive disorders. The most frequent ones associated with abnormalities of testis development (i.e., 9p24, 10q25-qter, Xq13) are considered in later sections of this chapter.

Primordial Germ Cell Migration. Primordial germ cells (PGCs) are the embryonic precursors of gametes (spermatocytes or ova). Surprisingly, in all species, PGCs arise some distance from the developing gonad and undergo a process of migration during the early stages of embryogenesis.[89,90] In humans, PGCs arise from pluripotent epiblast cells and are initially located in the 24-day embryo in a region of the dorsal endoderm of the yolk sac, close to the allantoic evagination (see Fig. 23-6). After mitotic division, PGCs migrate into the primitive gonad (between 4 and 5 weeks' gestation) under the influence of signaling molecules, receptors, and extracellular matrix proteins such as KIT, the KIT ligand KITLG (formerly called Steel), β$_1$-integrin, E-cadherin, Wnt5a/Ror2, KIF13B, interferon-induced transmembrane protein 1 (IFITM1), and IFITM3.[91,92] Hindgut expansion may also regulate or facilitate this process. Gonadal colonization is mediated by CXCL12 (previously called SDF1) and its receptor CXCR4 and influenced by CXCR7.

In the first few months of gestation, PGCs undergo multiple cycles of mitotic division. In the testis, a self-renewing population of germ cells exists. These undifferentiated PGCs are maintained by factors such as POU5F1 (also called OCT4), but they commit to differentiation in response to the expression of specific signaling molecules and transcription factors. After several cycles of mitotic division, these cells enter mitotic arrest.[93] Subsequent testicular

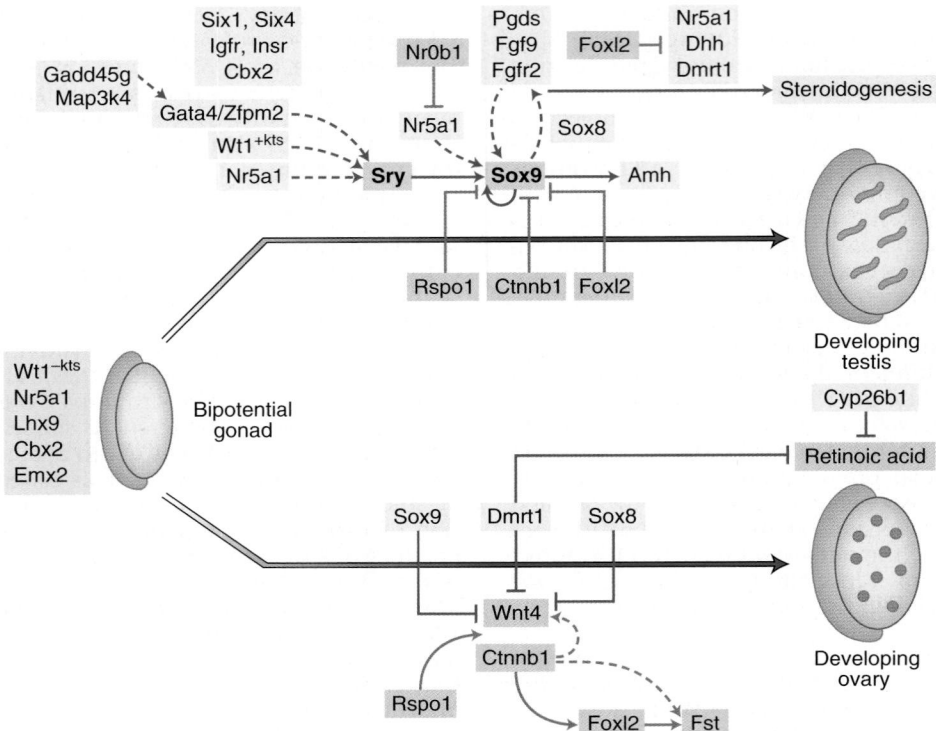

Figure 23-8 Overview of some of the molecular events thought to be involved in the development of the bipotential gonad, as well as in testis determination and ovary development. These data are based mostly on studies in mice. Sry is the principal testis-determining factor, but many other factors interact downstream to support testis development and repress ovary development, or vice versa.

development can occur in the absence of this germ cell population.[94] Meiosis occurs only during the progress of spermatogenesis during puberty (see Chapter 19).

In the developing ovary, primordial ova (oogonia) undergo mitotic expansion in the first few months of gestation (5 to 24 weeks), followed by meiotic division (8 to 36 weeks) and a process of meiotic arrest (oocytes). Although it was originally thought that entry into meiosis occurred autonomously, data suggest that retinoic acid signaling from the mesonephros stimulates this process.[95,96] Male germ cells may be protected from this signal by their location within the testis cord and by Sertoli cell expression of the cytochrome P450 isoenzyme 26B1 (CYP26B1), which breaks down retinoic acid. Meiotic arrest occurs in the first prophase, when the chromatids of homologous pairs have begun to separate but are fixed by chiasmata (diplotene stage). The presence of these PGCs and subsequent meiotic oocytes is critical for differentiation of prefollicular cells into follicular cells and for the maintenance of ovarian development (see Chapter 17).

More than 6 million oogonia and prophase oocytes exist in the developing ovary at about 16 weeks' gestation, and formation of oogonia from PGCs ceases by the 7th month. At that stage, some oocytes remain in undifferentiated nests, whereas others associate with somatic pregranulosa cells to form primitive or primordial follicles. However, approximately 80% of oogonia fail to form follicles and undergo apoptosis, so that only 1 million germ cells are present in the ovary at the time of birth. These resting primordial follicles can remain in that stage of development throughout the woman's reproductive life, and meiosis progresses only in response to ovulation of the graafian follicle (approximately 400 times in a woman's reproductive lifetime).

Testis Determination. Testis determination is an active process that begins at about 6 weeks after conception in humans and consists of several distinct genetic and morphologic events.[5-8] One of the first and most significant events in testis determination is a transient wave of SRY expression through the undifferentiated gonad (Fig. 23-8). SRY expression must reach a certain threshold within a definite time window for testis development to occur.[97,98] Initially, this occurs centrally, followed by expression in cells located at the cranial and caudal poles.

In humans, *SRY* is a single-exon gene (Yp11.3) that encodes a 204–amino acid, high-mobility group (HMG)–box transcription factor.[97] Mutations and deletions in *SRY* tend to cluster within the region encoding the HMG box and have been reported in approximately 10% to 15% of patients with sporadic or familial 46,XY gonadal dysgenesis (see "46,XY Disorders of Sex Development" and Fig. 23-20). As described earlier, translocation or transgenic expression of *SRY* is sufficient to induce testis development in XX patients and mice (see "The Y Chromosome" and see Fig. 23-5).

In humans, *SRY* is first detected in the XY gonad at approximately 42 days after conception, just before differentiation of the bipotential gonad into a testis.[99] Expression levels peak from approximately day 44, when testicular cords are first visible. Low-level *SRY* expression in humans is confined to Sertoli cells (day 52), where it persists into adulthood.

The HMG box of human SRY is a 79–amino acid structure that has moderate homology with SRY in other species (approximately 70%) and with the HMG box of related SOX (SRY-like HMG box) proteins (60%) (see "46,XY Disorders of Sex Development" and see Fig. 23-20).[97] The HMG box consists of three α-helices, which are able to adopt an L-shaped or boomerang-shaped configuration (see Fig. 23-5). The HMG box binds to variations on specific response elements (AACAAT/A) in the minor groove of DNA and induces a 40- to 85-degree structural bend in its target, depending on the sequence. The precise function of protein-directed DNA bending is not known, although this interaction results in minor groove expansion, DNA unwinding, and altered base stacking. These effects likely alter DNA architecture in chromatin and may permit the interaction of other protein complexes with the DNA, resulting in activation or repression. Other important domains in SRY are two nuclear localization signals that can interact with calmodulin and importin-β to regulate cellular localization; several serine residues in the amino (N)-terminal of SRY that can undergo phosphorylation and influence DNA binding; and a carboxy (C)-terminal, 7–amino acid motif that interacts with PDZ domains of SRY-interacting protein 1 (SIP1).[100-104] SRY expression is thought to switch the fate of the progenitor cells to that of pre-Sertoli cells; elegant studies of chimeric XX-XY gonads have shown that most Sertoli cells are XY derived.[105,106] These SRY-positive cells can signal to other cell lineages to induce male-specific differentiation, possibly via platelet-derived growth factor receptor α (PDGFRα).[7] The onset of SRY expression is followed by marked cellular proliferation and the migration of mesonephric cells into the developing testis (Fig. 23-9).[5,105-106] These mesonephric cells are thought to form endothelial cells of the vasculature, whereas the exact origins of Leydig and peritubular myoid cells remains unknown.[7] Furthermore, although SRY was shown convincingly to be the primary testis-determining gene more than 20 years ago, relatively little is known about the regulation of SRY expression. Some studies have shown that SF1, WT1, and GATA4 can all regulate SRY

promoter activity in vitro, and MAP3K4 and insulin-related signaling pathways may be important, but the exact mechanisms that activate SRY in vivo remain poorly understood.[107] The downstream targets of SRY are also unknown, although SOX9 is an obvious candidate. SRY and SF1 can synergistically regulate SOX9 expression through a testis-specific enhancer region (TESCO).[82,108] It is unclear whether other direct SRY target genes exist or whether SRY also acts as a negative regulator of factors involved in testis repression, such as R-spondin 1 or β-catenin.

SOX9 is an SRY-related HMG box factor comprising 3 exons (509 amino acids) that shows upregulation and nuclear localization in the developing testis shortly after the initial wave of SRY expression.[109-112] In humans, SOX9 becomes strongly localized to the developing sex cords at 44 to 52 days after ovulation and is expressed in Sertoli cells thereafter.[99] SOX9 is also expressed in the developing cartilage under the regulation of parathyroid hormone–related protein (PTHRP)/Indian hedgehog signaling pathways. Heterozygous mutations or deletions in SOX9 cause camptomelic dysplasia, a form of severe skeletal dysplasia associated with variable gonadal dysgenesis in approximately 75% of patients.[109,110] Mutations have been found in the HMG box of SOX9, in the C-terminal transactivation domain, and in a region that interacts with heat shock proteins (e.g., HSP70) (see "46,XY Disorders of Sex Development" and see Fig. 23-20).[111,112]

Although SOX9 is a key target of SRY, SOX9 can be a testis-determining factor in its own right, as overexpression of SOX9 due to duplication of 17q24.3-q25.1 has been reported in a 46,XX individual with ambiguous genitalia or ovotesticular DSD.[113,114] Furthermore, transgenic expression of Sox9 in mice results in testis development in XX animals, and the XX odsex (Ods) mouse develops as a male

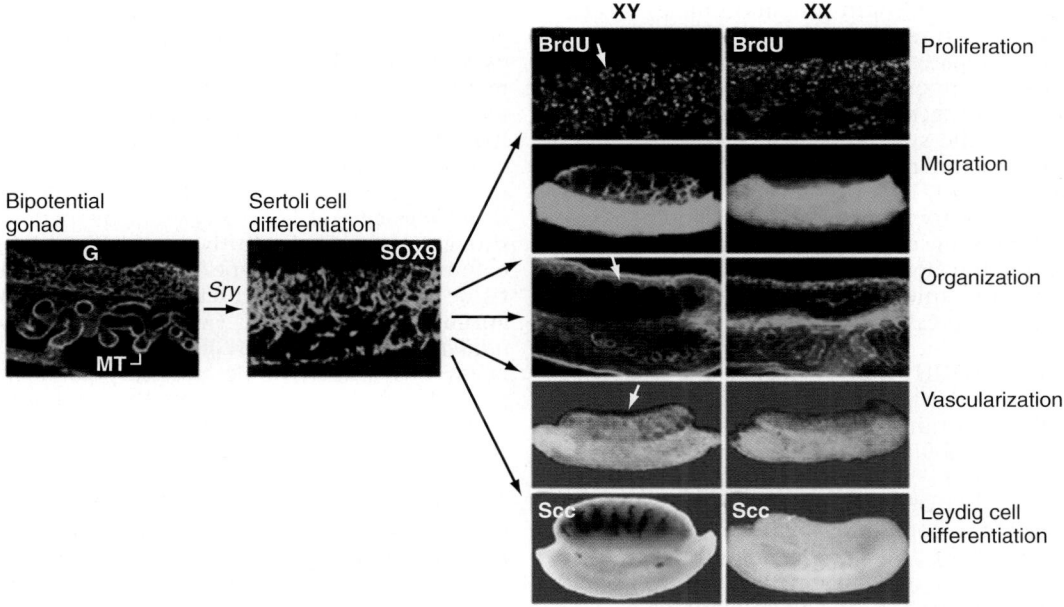

Figure 23-9 Key morphologic changes in the developing testis in mice. No morphologic differences between the XY and XX gonad are seen during the bipotential gonad stage at 10.5 to 11.5 days postcoitum (dpc) *(far left)*. In XY gonads, *SRY* expression is followed by expression and nuclear localization of SOX9 *(blue)* in pre-Sertoli cells *(middle)*, resulting in Sertoli cell differentiation by 11.5 dpc (vasculature and germ cells are labeled with platelet endothelial cell adhesion molecule [PECAM] and appear *green*). Between 11.5 and 12.5 dpc, distinct changes occur in the XY gonad *(near right column)*, which are not seen in the XX gonad *(far right)*. These changes include proliferation of coelomic epithelial cells (measured by BrdU incorporation; *red, arrow*); migration of cells from the mesonephros (shown by recombinant culture of a wild-type gonad and a mesonephros in which the cells express green fluorescent protein); structural organization of testis cords (detected by laminin deposition, *green*); male-specific vascularization (by light microscopy with blood cells indicated by an *arrow*); and Leydig cell differentiation (detected by mRNA in situ hybridization for the steroidogenic enzyme P450scc). BrdU, bromodeoxyuridine; MT, basal lamina of mesonephric tubules; G, gonad. (From Brennan J, Capel B. One tissue, two fates: molecular genetic events that underlie testis versus ovary development. *Nat Rev Genet.* 2004;5:509-521, used with permission of Macmillan Publishers, Ltd.)

owing to disruption of a regulatory element 1 Mb upstream of *Sox9* that causes testis-specific overexpression of Sox9 during development.[115,116] Similar disruption of an upstream *cis*-regulatory region resulting in SOX9 overexpression causes 46,XX testicular DSD.[117] The regulatory region of the *SOX9* promoter is very large. Breakpoints have been reported up to 350 kb from the start of the *SOX9* gene in patients with camptomelic dysplasia and gonadal dysgenesis. In mice, *Sox9* may mediate its effects through direct interactions with other target genes (e.g., *Fgf9, Ptgds, Amh*) and through the mutual degradation of β-catenin, thereby promoting testis development pathways rather than those opposing testis development (see Fig. 23-8). Autoregulatory loops may also be important in maintaining SOX9 expression.

Around the time of SRY and SOX9 expression (and nuclear localization), the developing testis undergoes a series of distinct cellular and morphologic changes (see Fig. 23-9). Understanding of these processes has resulted largely from studies in mice.[5] As outlined earlier, the first stage of testis development in mice involves a proliferation of Sf1-positive somatic cells that results in an increase in Sertoli cell precursors and Sertoli cell differentiation. This process is influenced by growth factors such as fibroblast growth factor (Fgf9) and the receptor Fgfr2. These primitive Sertoli cells coalesce with peritubular myoid cells to form primary sex cords, which then condense to form primitive seminiferous cords (at about 7 weeks after conception in humans). Sex cord development is supported by a striking reorganization of the gonadal vasculature in the developing testis but not in the ovary (see Fig. 23-9).[5,118] These changes include the development of a discrete coelomic vessel, restriction of endothelial cells to the interstitial space between the sex cords, and increased branching of blood vessels. The development of these vascular systems is influenced by growth factor signaling systems, such as PDGFRα/PTGDS (prostaglandin D2 synthase), and can be repressed by the Wnt4/β-catenin/follistatin systems in mice.[118] These changes in vascular architecture play an important role in determining cellular patterning and organization in the developing testis, in supporting paracrine interactions, and in the export of androgens from the developing Leydig cells to the perineal and systemic circulation.

Although the expression of SRY plays a crucial role as a testis-determining factor, it is becoming clear that many other factors are necessary for early testis development (see Figs. 23-7 and 23-8). Some of these factors may be expressed exclusively within the developing testis, whereas others may play a facilitative role in supporting gonad development and are also expressed in other developing tissues (e.g., brain).

Desert hedgehog (DHH) is a member of the hedgehog signaling pathway that is expressed in mouse embryonic Sertoli cells and interstitium, and it plays a key role in the differentiation of peritubular myoid cells through its action on the Patched receptor.[119] The peritubular myoid cells are flat, smooth muscle–like cells that ensheath the testis cords and are necessary for cord development and structural integrity. Deletion of the *Dhh* gene in the mouse leads to impaired differentiation of peritubular myoid cells and Leydig cells and to impaired androgenization in males.[119,120] In humans, *DHH* mutations have been reported in patients with impaired testicular development, with or without minifascicular neuropathy.[121,122]

DMRT1 (double sex, Mab3–related transcription factor 1; 9p24.3) encodes a 373–amino acid protein that is homologous to the sex-development *double sex* gene of *Drosophila* and the *Mab3* gene of *Caenorhabditis elegans*. *DMRT1* shows a male-specific pattern expression in the developing genital ridge and is expressed in the developing Sertoli cells by 7 weeks after conception.[123] Deletion of *Dmrt1* in the mouse results in normal androgenization but regression of testes later in embryonic development.[124] A dominant negative point mutation in *DMRT1* has recently been described in humans, and impaired gonadal development and 46,XY DSDs are well-established features of the 9p deletion syndrome.[125-127]

ARX (aristaless-related homeobox, X-linked gene) encodes a transcription factor that regulates neuronal migration, brain development, and Leydig cell development. Deletion of *Arx* in the mouse causes abnormal neuronal development and a block in Leydig cell differentiation.[128] Mutations in *ARX* in humans cause a condition known as *X-linked lissencephaly and ambiguous genitalia* (XLAG).[128] *MAMLD1* (mastermind-like domain–containing 1; previously called *CXORF6*) is a regulator of fetal Leydig cell function. Defects in *MAMLD1* have been reported in infants with severe hypospadias.[129] Signaling through Pdgf and the Pdgfrα also has been shown to be important in fetal and adult Leydig cell differentiation after deletion of these genes in mice.[130]

Other genes proposed to play a role in early testis development have been identified from chromosome deletions or differential expression studies. For example, ATRX (Xq13.3; also known as *XH2* or *XNP*) is a transcription factor deleted in the α-thalassemia mental retardation syndrome.[131] The syndrome includes a range of genital phenotypes from partial gonadal dysgenesis to micropenis. The locus containing *SOX8* is deleted in the ATR-16 (α-thalassemia mental retardation) syndrome affecting the tip of chromosome 16p,[132] and terminal deletions of chromosome 10 (10q25-qter) are frequently associated with urogenital abnormalities and sometimes with complete gonadal dysgenesis.[133] More than 50 syndromic conditions or human chromosomal rearrangements have been associated with a range of urogenital phenotypes.[134,135] Furthermore, gene expression profiling in the embryonic mouse gonad is revealing a host of expressed and differentially expressed genes involved in testicular and ovarian development. Higher resolution analysis of chromosomal changes using techniques such as array comparative genome hybridization is allowing the identification of much smaller chromosomal deletions, duplications, and rearrangements that may affect genes related to sex development.[136,137]

Ovary Development. For many years, ovary development was thought to be a constitutive (default) process, because an external female phenotype occurs in the absence of gonadal tissue and müllerian structures persist in the absence of antimüllerian hormone (AMH; also known as *müllerian inhibiting substance* [MIS]). Although the presence of PGCs was known to be necessary to maintain ovarian integrity, evidence now shows that ovarian development is an active process that requires expression of a set of specific genes and factors necessary to actively prevent testis development.

Several genes, including *Dazl, Bmp8b, Smad5, Gja4* (previously known as *Cx37*), *Foxl2*, and the POF family of genes listed previously, have been implicated in ovarian and follicular development in mice.[8,41-50] Studies comparing gene expression profiles in the testes and ovaries of mice at critical stages of fetal development (e10.5 to e13.5) have shown that a specific subset of ovarian genes (e.g., follistatin, cyclin kinase inhibitors) are turned on soon after the onset of testis determination.[13] It is unclear whether any ovary-determining genes exist or whether these factors play a role in maintaining ovarian development in the absence of testis-determining gene expression. However, it seems likely that certain active processes are involved, because many of the genes and proteins (e.g., Wnt4, Rspo1/β-catenin, Foxl2, estrogen receptors), as well as meiotic germ cells, may antagonize testis development or prevent development of a male-type cell lineage (see Fig. 23-8).[138-142] Data in mice suggest that these processes may be ongoing, even in the postnatal ovary.[143]

Phenotypic or Anatomic Sex

The developing gonad produces several steroid and peptide hormones that mediate sexual differentiation and result in the phenotypic sex seen at birth. Alfred Jost first showed the importance of fetal testicular androgens in this process in 1947.[12] In his classic experiments, Jost demonstrated that surgical removal of the gonads during embryonic development of the rabbit resulted in development of female reproductive characteristics, regardless of the chromosomal sex of the embryo.

Male Sexual Differentiation

Sertoli Cells and Müllerian Regression. Sertoli cells play a key role in supporting germ cell survival, and they produce two important peptide hormones: AMH and inhibin B. AMH, a glycoprotein homodimer, is a member of the transforming growth factor-β (TGF-β) superfamily and is first secreted in humans from about 7 to 8 weeks after conception under the regulation of key transcription factors such as SOX9, SF1, WT1, and GATA4 (see Figs. 23-1 and 23-6).[144,145] AMH causes regression of müllerian structures (e.g., fallopian tubes, uterus, upper two thirds of the vagina) by its paracrine action on the AMH type 2 receptor (AMHR2).

Müllerian structures appear to be maximally sensitive to AMH between 9 and 12 weeks' gestation, a time when the developing testis is producing peak concentrations of AMH but before the onset of significant AMH production by the developing ovary. Consequently, boys with mutations in the *AMH* or *AMHR2* genes can present with persistent müllerian duct syndrome (PMDS) and undescended testes but otherwise normal external genitalia. In contrast, severe forms of 46,XY gonadal dysgenesis can result in persistent müllerian structures due to impaired Sertoli cell development and AMH release. In some cases, a hemiuterus is present if testicular development is more severely affected on that same side, but it is likely that androgenization of the external genitalia also is impaired so that these children present with atypical genitalia. Defects confined to Leydig cell steroidogenesis in 46,XY DSD are not associated with persistent müllerian structures, because Sertoli cell production of AMH is unaffected. In boys, a small müllerian remnant sometimes persists as a testicular appendage, and a utriculus or utricular remnant is a frequent finding in many children with 46,XY DSD. Inhibin B suppresses pituitary follicle-stimulating hormone (FSH) activity, but its local role during testis development is less clear. AMH and inhibin B may have important functions throughout life at multiple levels of the hypothalamic-pituitary-gonadal (HPG) axis.[146]

Fetal Leydig Cells and Steroidogenesis. Fetal Leydig cells develop within the interstitium of the developing testis and secrete androgens by 8 to 9 weeks after conception (see Fig. 23-1).[147] An expansion in fetal Leydig cells occurs between 14 and 18 weeks' gestation, resulting in marked increase in testosterone secretion at about 16 weeks.[147,148] Fetal Leydig cell steroidogenesis is stimulated by placental human chorionic gonadotropin (hCG) during the first two trimesters of pregnancy, but the developing hypothalamic-gonadotroph system produces significant amounts of luteinizing hormone (LH) from about 20 weeks' gestation.[149,150]

The pathways of testicular steroidogenesis are shown in Figure 23-10. The role of individual enzymes is discussed in relation to individual steroidogenic defects later in this chapter and in several excellent reviews.[151] In brief, cholesterol is taken up into Leydig cells by low-density lipoprotein or high-density lipoprotein receptors or is generated de novo by cholesterol synthesis pathways or from cholesterol ester. Stimulation of the LH/hCG receptor by the appropriate glycoprotein hormone increases the ability of steroidogenic acute regulatory protein (StAR) to facilitate movement of cholesterol from the outer to the inner mitochondrial membrane.[152] The first and rate-limiting step in steroid hormone synthesis involves three distinct reactions: 20α-hydroxylation, 22-hydroxylation, and cleavage of the cholesterol side chain to generate pregnenolone and isocaproic acid. These steps are catalyzed by a single enzyme, P450scc (CYP11A1).

Pregnenolone is converted to progesterone by the microsomal enzyme 3β-hydroxysteroid dehydrogenase type 2 (HSD3B2), or it can undergo 17α-hydroxylation by P450c17 (CYP17) to yield 17-hydroxypregnenolone. CYP17 also has 17,20-lyase activity, which can cleave the C17,20 carbon bond of 17-hydroxypregnenolone to generate dehydroepiandrosterone (DHEA). This 17,20-lyase activity is favored by the presence of Δ^5-substrates, redox partners such as P450 oxidoreductase (POR) and cytochrome b_5, and serine phosphorylation. These reactions are facilitated by the relative abundance of these factors in Leydig cells in humans, and the main pathway to androgen production is through conversion of 17-hydroxypregnenolone to DHEA rather than through conversion of 17-hydroxyprogesterone (17-OHP) to androstenedione.[153] Subsequent testosterone production can occur through conversion of DHEA to androstenedione (by HSD3B2), followed by the actions of HSD17B3 to generate testosterone, or by the intermediate metabolite androstenediol (see Fig. 23-10). During male sex development, testosterone undergoes local conversion to dihydrotestosterone (DHT) by 5α-reductase type 2. DHT's high-affinity action on the androgen receptor results in androgenization of the external genitalia. Studies based on the phenotype of patients with POR deficiency and the fetal tammar wallaby have proposed that an alternative pathway to DHT production may exist in the human fetal testis (see "P450 Oxidoreductase Deficiency"): the so-called backdoor pathway (Fig. 23-11).[154,155]

Local production of testosterone stabilizes wolffian structures such as the epididymides, vasa deferentia, and seminal vesicles, whereas the potent metabolite DHT induces androgenization of the external genitalia and urogenital sinus (Fig. 23-12). In the male, the urogenital sinus develops into the prostate and prostatic urethra, the genital tubercle develops into the glans penis, the urogenital (urethral) folds fuse to form the shaft of the penis, and the urogenital (labioscrotal) swellings form the scrotum (Figs. 23-13 and 23-14).[156] The distinction between a clitoris and a penis at this stage is based primarily on size and whether the labia minora fuse to form a corpus spongiosum.

Testosterone and DHT mediate their effects through the androgen receptor (AR; Xq11-q12), which is a transcription factor. A more detailed description of the androgen receptor and its actions is provided later (see "46,XY Disorders of Sex Development"). Surprisingly little is known about AR targets in the developing wolffian structures (testosterone responsive) and in the key target tissues (DHT responsive). Studies in mice have revealed a number of factors that are necessary for development of the wolffian ducts (e.g., Gdf7, Bmps4, Bmps7, Bmps8a, Bmps8b, Hoxa10, Hoxa11) and for growth of the genital tubercle (e.g., Fgfs, Shh, Wnts, Hoxa13, Hoxd13, Bmp/noggin, ephrin

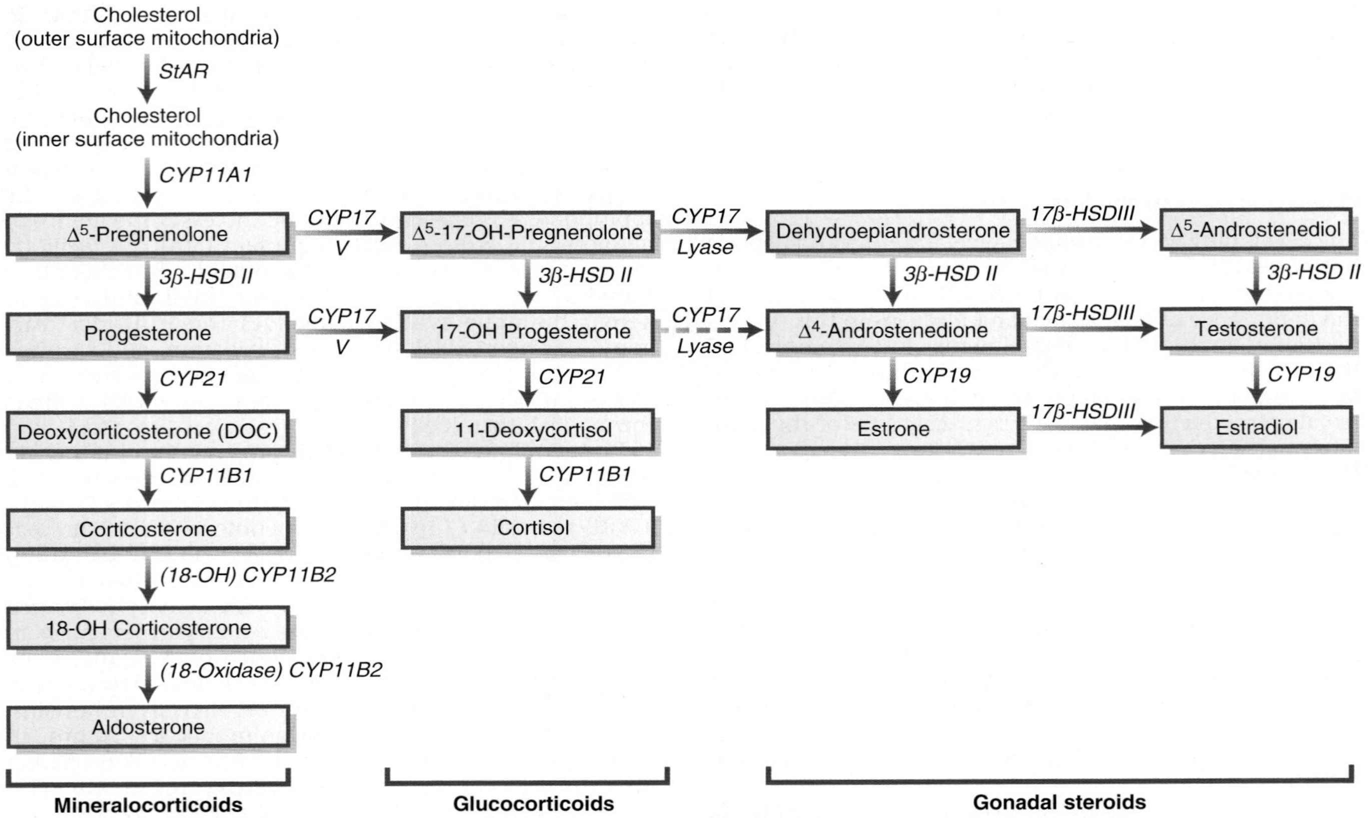

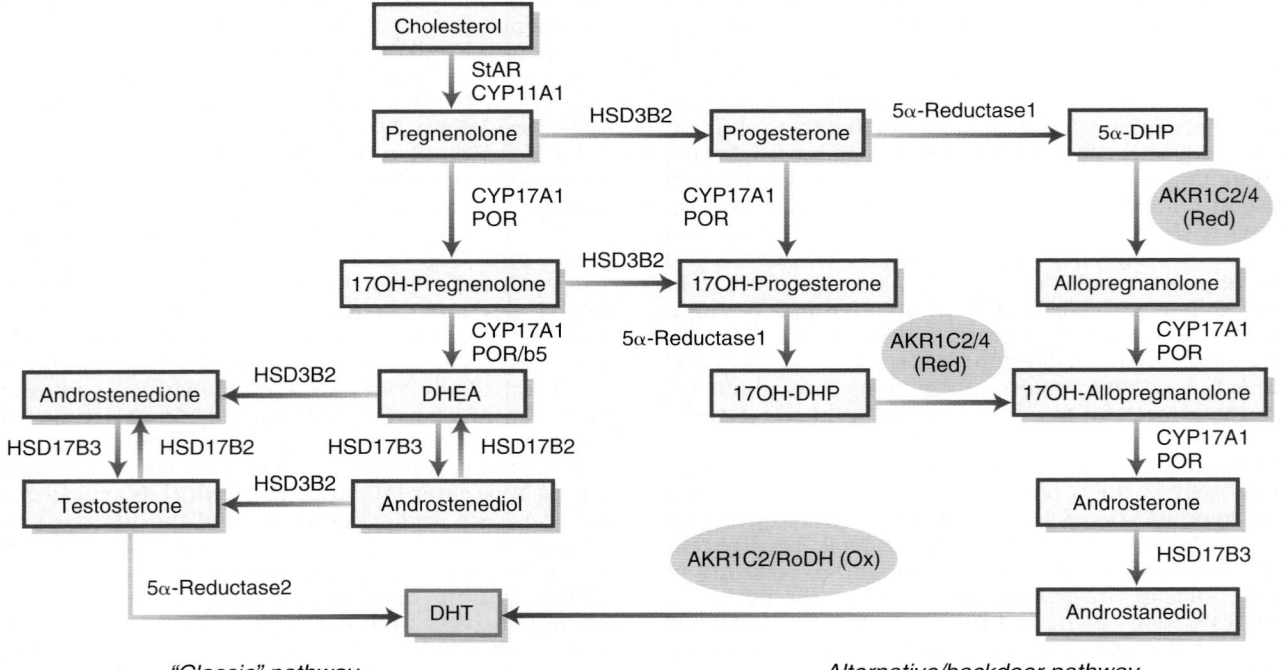

Cholesterol
(outer surface mitochondria)

StAR

Cholesterol
(inner surface mitochondria)

CYP11A1

| Δ^5-Pregnenolone | $\xrightarrow{CYP17 \atop V}$ | Δ^5-17-OH-Pregnenolone | $\xrightarrow{CYP17 \atop Lyase}$ | Dehydroepiandrosterone | $\xrightarrow{17\beta\text{-}HSDIII}$ | Δ^5-Androstenediol |

3β-HSD II | *3β-HSD II* | *3β-HSD II* | *3β-HSD II*

| Progesterone | $\xrightarrow{CYP17 \atop V}$ | 17-OH Progesterone | $\dashrightarrow{CYP17 \atop Lyase}$ | Δ^4-Androstenedione | $\xrightarrow{17\beta\text{-}HSDIII}$ | Testosterone |

CYP21 | *CYP21* | *CYP19* | *CYP19*

Deoxycorticosterone (DOC) 11-Deoxycortisol Estrone $\xrightarrow{17\beta\text{-}HSDIII}$ Estradiol

CYP11B1 | *CYP11B1*

Corticosterone Cortisol

(18-OH) CYP11B2

18-OH Corticosterone

(18-Oxidase) CYP11B2

Aldosterone

Mineralocorticoids **Glucocorticoids** **Gonadal steroids**

Figure 23-10 Schematic diagram shows the steroid biosynthetic pathways leading to androgen production in the testis. In humans, the main pathway to androgen production is through conversion of 17-hydroxypregnenolone to dehydroepiandrosterone (DHEA) rather than through conversion of 17-hydroxyprogesterone to androstenedione. Subsequent testosterone biosynthesis can occur through conversion of DHEA to androstenedione (by 3β-hydroxysteroid dehydrogenase type 2 [3β-HSD II]), followed by the actions of 17α-hydroxysteroid dehydrogenase type 3 (17β-HSD III) to generate testosterone, or through the intermediate metabolite androstenediol. During male sex development, testosterone undergoes local conversion to dihydrotestosterone by 5α-reductase type 2 (not shown). The high-affinity action of dihydrotestosterone on the androgen receptor results in androgenization of the external genitalia. The pathways responsible for mineralocorticoid and glucocorticoid synthesis are present in the adrenal gland. Additional or alternative pathways to dihydrotestosterone production may exist in the fetal testis.

"Classic" pathway *Alternative/backdoor pathway*

Figure 23-11 The classic and alternative (backdoor) pathways of dihydrotestosterone (DHT) synthesis. The classic pathway leading to synthesis of DHT is shown on the left. The alternative pathway potentially involved in DHT synthesis is shown on the right. The alternative pathway involves the actions of additional enzymes: 5α-reductase, type 1 (5α-reductase 1, encoded by *SRD5A1*), AKR1C2 (3α-reductase, type 3) and possibly AKR1C4 (3α-reductase, type 1), and RoDH (3-hydroxyepimerase, encoded by *HSD17B6*). DHEA, dehydroepiandrosterone; DHP, dihydroprogesterone; HSD, hydroxysteroid dehydrogenase; POR, P450 oxidoreductase; StAR, steroidogenic acute regulatory protein. (From Flück CE, Meyer-Böni M, Pandey AV, et al. Why boys will be boys: two pathways of fetal testicular androgen biosynthesis are needed for male sexual differentiation. *Am J Hum Genet*. 2011;89:201-218, used with permission of Elsevier, Inc.)

Indifferent stage

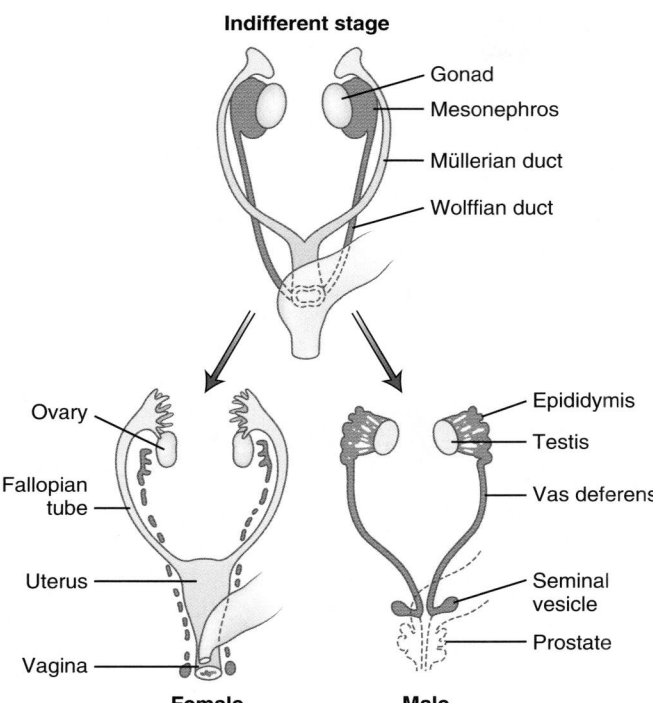

Figure 23-12 Embryonic differentiation of female and male genital ducts from wolffian and müllerian primordial tissue before descent of the testes into the scrotum. In females, müllerian structures persist to form the fallopian tubes, uterus, and upper portion of the vagina. The lower portion of the vagina and urethra are derived from the urogenital sinus. In males, wolffian structures develop into the epididymides, vasa deferentia, and seminal vesicles, whereas the prostate and prostatic urethra are derived from the urogenital sinus. In some cases, a small müllerian remnant can persist in males as a testicular appendage.

TABLE 23-2	
Terminology for Gender-Related Behavior	
Term	**Explanation**
Gender identity	Identification of sex as male or female
Gender role	Expression of sexually dimorphic behavior
	Aggression
	Parenting rehearsal
	Peer and group interactions
	Labeling (e.g., "tomboy")
	Grooming behavior
Sexual orientation	Choice of sexual partner

signaling). Impaired androgen action occurs in several syndromic conditions and may reflect defects in genes that mediate target-tissue responsiveness and genital tubercle growth (e.g., *HOXA10*, *HOXA13*).

Testis Descent. Testicular descent is a two-stage process that starts at about 8 weeks' gestation and is usually complete by the middle of the third trimester.[157] The initial *transabdominal* stage of testicular descent (8 to 15 weeks) involves contraction and thickening of the gubernacular ligament and degeneration of the craniosuspensory ligament. This stage is mediated by the testis itself after secretion of factors such as insulin-like 3 (INSL3, a relaxin-like factor) and its G protein–coupled receptor, GREAT (also called LGR8 or RXFP2).[158] Other testicular factors are likely to be involved in testicular descent, because most dysgenetic testes are intra-abdominal. The subsequent transinguinal (or inguinoscrotal) phase of testicular descent (25 to 35 weeks) is primarily driven by androgens. The genito-femoral nerve and its neurotransmitter, calcitonin gene–related peptide (CGRP), have also been implicated in this process.

Subsequent Testicular Development. During the second and third trimesters, the testes show several distinct morphologic changes, including a reduction in fetal Leydig cell mass and elongation and coiling of seminiferous cords. There is no further significant development of germ cells during this time, and seminiferous cords do not canalize until later in childhood. Nevertheless, certain developmental insults can affect the testis at this stage. For example, vanishing (absent) testis syndrome is most likely a late fetal event, because boys with this condition have adequate androgenization and no müllerian structures.

Female Sexual Differentiation. The processes of female sexual differentiation are less obvious than in the male and do not involve significant changes in the external genitalia. Müllerian structures persist to form the fallopian tubes, uterus, and upper portion of the vagina (see Fig. 23-12). Normal uterine development in mice occurs in the absence of the ovary, but it is not a passive process, because a host of factors are required for uterine development (e.g., Pax2, Lim1, Emx2, Wnt4/Lp, Hoxa13) and differentiation (e.g.,Wnt7a, Hoxa10, Hoxa11, Hoxa13, progesterone and estrogen receptors).[159] The lack of local testosterone production leads to degeneration of wolffian structures. The urogenital sinus develops into the urethra and lower portion of the vagina, the genital tubercle develops into the clitoris, the urogenital (urethral) folds form the labia minora, and the urogenital (labioscrotal) swellings form the labia majora (see Figs. 23-12 and 23-13).

In contrast to the testis, the developing ovary does not express FSH and LH/hCG receptors until after 16 weeks' gestation. At about 20 weeks' gestation, plasma concentrations of FSH reach a peak and the first primary follicles are formed.[150] By 25 weeks' gestation, the ovary has developed definitive morphologic characteristics. Folliculogenesis can proceed, and a few graafian follicles have developed by the third trimester.[8] Although some studies have suggested that the early fetal ovary can produce steroids, the amount of estrogen secreted by the developing ovary is likely to be insignificant compared with placental estrogen synthesis, and the ovary is thought to remain generally quiescent until activation at the time of puberty.[16]

Several conditions can affect female sexual development in utero. Exposure of the fetus to androgens results in androgenization of the external genitalia. A uterus is present, but the local testosterone concentration typically is not sufficient to stabilize wolffian structures because the androgens are usually adrenal in origin. Most frequently, androgenization of the 46,XX fetus results from disorders of adrenal steroidogenesis (e.g., 21-hydroxylase [CYP21] deficiency, 11β-hydroxylase deficiency, POR deficiency) or from mild androgenic effects after conversion of excess DHEA in HSD3B2 deficiency (discussed later). Rare causes of androgenization include aromatase deficiency, glucocorticoid resistance, ovotesticular DSD, and maternal virilizing tumors (e.g., luteoma of pregnancy). Exposure to certain chemical agents in pregnancy has been proposed as a cause of fetal androgenization, but data are limited. For other developmental abnormalities of the female genital tract (e.g., Mayer-Rokitansky-Küster-Hauser syndrome) see "46,XX Disorders of Sex Development."

Psychosexual Development

Psychosexual development is traditionally viewed as having several distinct components (Table 23-2). *Gender*

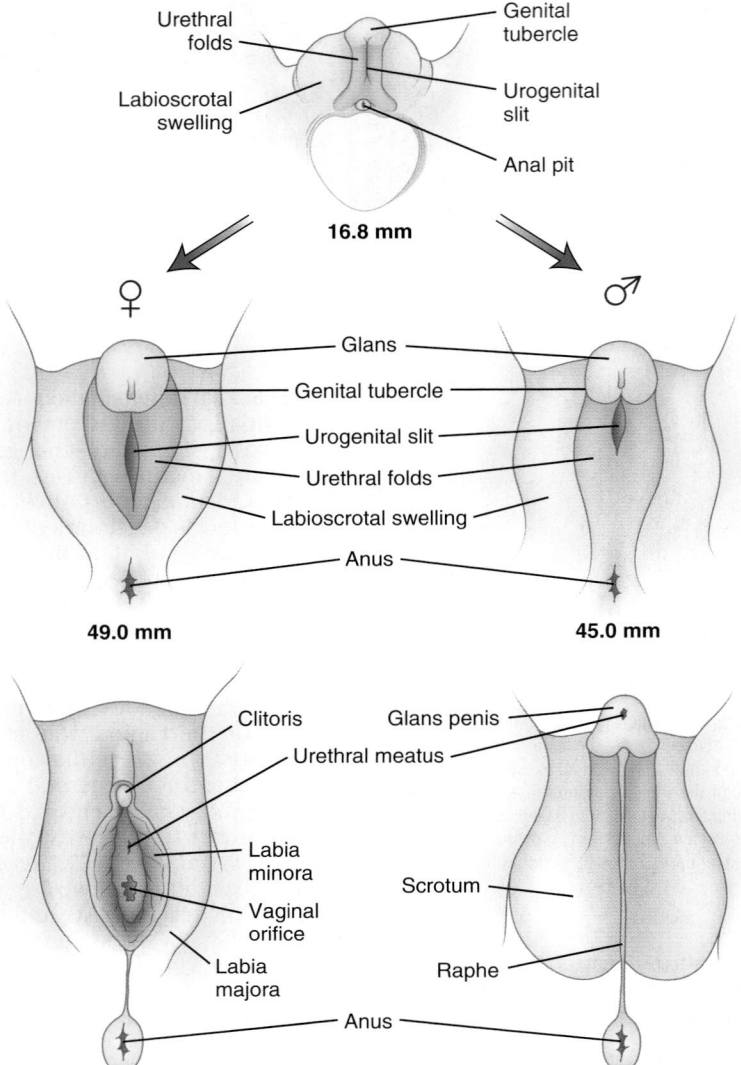

Figure 23-13 Differentiation of male and female external genitalia. (Adapted from Spaulding MH. The development of the external genitalia in the human embryo. *Contrib Embryol Carnegie Inst.* 1921;13:69-88.)

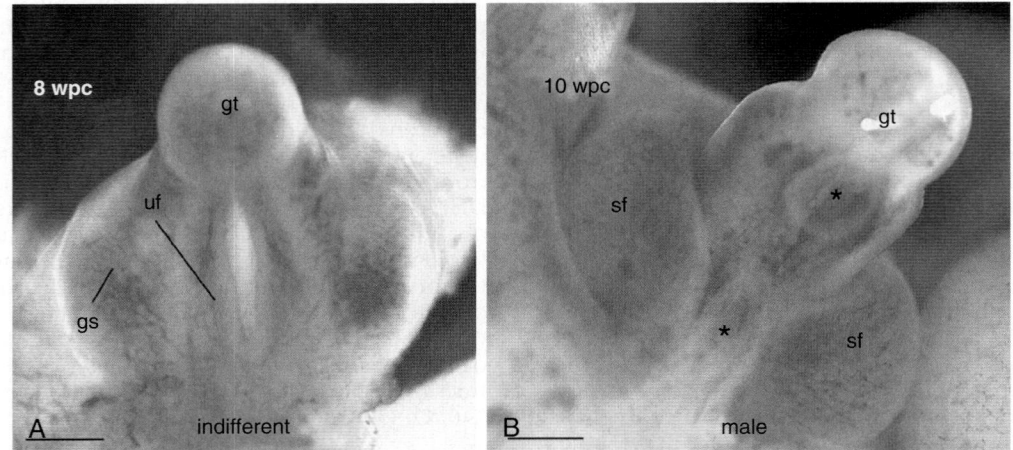

Figure 23-14 Differentiation of male external genitalia in humans between 8 and 10 weeks postconception (wpc). **A,** Undifferentiated human external genitalia at 8 wpc. **B,** Differentiation of scrotal folds and fusion of the urethral folds (asterisks indicate patent regions on either side) at 10 wpc. gs, genital swelling; gt, genital tubercle; sf, scrotal folds; uf, urethral folds. Scale bars: 500 μm. (From Goto M, Piper Hanley K, Marcos J, et al. In humans, early cortisol biosynthesis provides a mechanism to safeguard female sexual development. *J Clin Invest.* 2006;116:872-874, used with permission of the American Society for Clinical Investigation, copyright 2006.)

identity refers to a person's self-representation or identification as male or female (with the caveat that some individuals may not identify exclusively with a binary model). *Gender role* (sex-typical behaviors) describes the expression or portrayal of psychological characteristics that are sexually dimorphic within the general population, such as toy preferences and physical aggression. *Sexual orientation* refers to choice of sexual partner and erotic interest (e.g., heterosexual, bisexual, homosexual) and includes behavior, fantasies, and attractions.

The past 50 years have seen a number of opposing theories about the origins of psychosexual development and debate about the relative contributions of chromosomes, hormones, brain structure, and societal and family influences on the various components. Much of this work has focused on the study of rodents and nonhuman primate species. For example, Young and colleagues first showed in 1959 that exposure of guinea pigs to testosterone during pregnancy resulted in altered mating behavior of female offspring.[160] These effects may be most pronounced during a critical window of exposure and, in rodents and some primates, may depend in part on aromatization of the androgens to estrogens, receptor availability, and social environment.[161] More recently, interest has focused on the role of genes and chromosomes in sex behavior. For example, studies of differential gene expression patterns in the developing mouse brain have shown upregulation of different X and Y chromosomal genes in early embryonic life, even before the onset of significant androgen secretion by the developing testis in males.[162] Studies of mice in which *Sry* was deleted (XYSRY⁻) or transgenically expressed (XXSRY) showed certain neuroanatomic differences between XY and XX mice independent of gonad development and endocrine status.[163] These findings suggest that factors related to chromosome complement have at least the potential to affect psychosexual development independent of sex hormone action, and a model integrating classic organizational and activational effects with sex chromosome effects may be more appropriate.[164]

Understanding the complex issues related to human psychosexual development is much more challenging, especially because gender identity is a component of psychosexual development that cannot readily be assessed in nonhuman species. For many years, it was thought that gender identity would be concordant with assigned sex, provided that the child was raised unambiguously and appropriate surgical procedures and hormone therapies were instituted concordant with the gender chosen. This theory assumed psychosexual neutrality at birth, but it has been challenged by a refocusing on the potential importance of prenatal (e.g., endocrine) and innate (e.g., chromosomal) influences on psychosexual development.[165,166] Direct data to assess such effects in humans are limited, but studies in women with complete androgen insensitivity syndrome (CAIS) argue against a strong behavioral role for Y chromosome genes alone in human psychosexual development, because the karyotype is 46,XY but psychosexual development is almost always female.[167] However, the gender characteristics of individuals with a Y chromosome and a degree of androgen exposure or responsiveness (e.g., partial androgen insensitivity syndrome [PAIS], 17β-hydroxysteroid dehydrogenase deficiency, 5α-reductase deficiency) can vary, and long-term gender identity can be difficult to predict.[168,169]

Prenatal exposure to androgens can also influence certain aspects of psychosexual development in 46,XX individuals.[166,170] Girls with congenital adrenal hyperplasia (CAH) who harbor more severe mutations and have more marked genital androgenization are more likely to play more with boys' toys, with long-term effects evident into adulthood.[171] Prenatal androgen exposure can also be associated with other psychological characteristics, such as sexual orientation.[172] However, the association between high prenatal androgen exposure and gender *identity* is generally less marked, except perhaps in some cases of testicular DSD.[173] Although gender dissatisfaction (i.e., unhappiness with assigned sex) is more common in individuals with DSD, more than 90% of 46,XX individuals with CAH who are assigned female gender in infancy later identify as female.[166,174] The small number of 46,XX men with CAH usually have been raised male and diagnosed late, although more cross-gender identification may occur than originally thought.[175,176] The causes of gender dissatisfaction are poorly understood and are sometimes hard to predict from karyotype, prenatal androgen exposure, degree of genital virilization, or assigned gender. Because gender identity, sex-typical behavior, and sexual orientation are separate components of psychosexual development, it is important to appreciate that an interest in same-sex relationships (relative to sex of rearing) or strong cross-sex interest in an individual with DSD is not necessarily an indication of incorrect gender assignment.[3]

Challenges in assessing gender identity in young children make it difficult to know when this is established, although it is thought to be between 18 and 36 months and possibly younger.[177] Many of the sexually dimorphic differences in brain structures reported at late childhood, puberty, or adulthood are not seen in early childhood and are therefore not useful for guiding gender assignment.[178,179] Potential plasticity in psychosexual development may exist, as is evident from studies of some patients with conditions such as 5α-reductase deficiency who may change their gender role in adolescence. A better understanding of the processes of human psychosexual development and of the influences of different forms of DSD is needed to help make early gender assignment decisions and to guide psychological support in the future. Some individuals with DSD do not fit into a binary model of gender. In several countries, important legal changes have taken place to acknowledge this, such as the option not to define gender as male or female on passports. Nevertheless, many societies still have a very binary view of gender, and freedom of expression is difficult for people who do not feel they fit a binary model.

Development of the Hypothalamic-Pituitary-Gonadal Axis in the Fetus

Fetal hypothalamic-gonadotrope development occurs from 6 weeks after conception in humans, in parallel with the processes of sex determination and differentiation. This involves migration of gonadotropin-releasing hormone (GnRH)-producing neurons from the cribriform plate to the fetal hypothalamus; development of the hypothalamic nuclei; formation of the anterior pituitary from Rathke's pouch; and specification and maturation of pituitary gonadotropes that are capable of releasing LH and FSH as part of a functional HPG axis. These mechanisms are described in Chapter 22. Defects in these systems can result in a range of clinical conditions such as Kallmann syndrome, congenital isolated hypogonadotropic hypogonadism (HH), or gonadotropin insufficiency as part of a multiple pituitary hormone deficiency, which are reviewed elsewhere (Chapters 8, 22, and 25).

Although development of the HPG axis occurs in parallel with human sex development, it is generally thought that pulsatile release of LH and FSH does not occur and therefore influence the gonad until about 20 weeks after conception.[150] The main effects of gonadotropins are to support the latter stages of testicular steroidogenesis involved in elongation of the penis as well as supporting the transinguinal aspects of testicular descent. Consequently, boys with congenital gonadotropin insufficiency tend to have a small penis (micropenis) and bilaterally undescended testis. These children might need monitoring for important associated features such as renal agenesis in Kallmann syndrome or growth hormone or adrenocorticotropic hormone (ACTH) insufficiency (causing hypoglycemia) in panhypopituitarism. Classically, boys with hypothalamic or pituitary gonadotropin insufficiency do not have hypospadias as fusion of urethral folds has occurred before 20 weeks. Very rarely, hypospadias does occur with HPG disorders, potentially reflecting loss of a common and as yet unknown regulatory factor or factors.

The Hypothalamic-Pituitary-Gonadal Axis in Infancy and Childhood

At birth, the infant is removed from the influence of maternal and placental hormones and undergoes a series of distinct endocrine changes.

Postnatal Endocrine Changes in Boys

In boys, low concentrations of testosterone can be detected by standard assays at birth, but these levels fall during the first few days of life. Thereafter, a reactivation of the HPG axis occurs, beginning at about 6 weeks of age, which results in peaks of testosterone nearing midpubertal levels between 2 and 3 months after birth (Fig. 23-15).[180,181] This peak of testosterone is associated with an acceleration in penile growth and may be linked in part to early postnatal maturation of gonocytes in the testis.[181] The HPG axis then becomes relatively quiescent by 6 months of age until the onset of puberty in late childhood.

Inhibin B concentrations are high at birth and fall during the first 2 years of life before rising with the onset of puberty between 11 and 15 years of age (see Fig. 23-15).[182,183] In contrast, AMH concentrations remain high from birth through childhood and decline to low concentrations with the onset of puberty (see Fig. 23-15).[144,145] AMH and inhibin B can be useful markers of active testicular tissue in boys with cryptorchidism, anorchia, and 46,XY DSD. INSL3 assays may provide a useful additional marker of testicular integrity in the future.[184,185]

Postnatal Endocrine Changes in Girls

The early postnatal endocrine events in girls are less well understood. Placental estrogen exposure can result in breast development before birth, and a small episode of menstrual bleeding can occur several days after birth from withdrawal of estrogen and progesterone. It is likely that girls also have a discrete activation of the HPG axis in infancy. However, detectable concentrations of estradiol (5 to 20 pg/mL [20 to 80 pmol/L]) and inhibin B (50 to 200 pg/mL) can be measured in the first few months of life, and surprisingly high concentrations of FSH with marked interindividual variability can be found during infancy and early childhood (median, 3.8 IU/L; range, 1.2 to 18.8 IU/L [2.5% to 97.5%] at 3 months of age in healthy term girls).[186] Inhibin A has been proposed as a test of ovarian tissue in the newborn period in children with possible ovotesticular DSD, but this hormone is below the limits of detection in many normal term newborn girls, and FSH stimulation may be needed to detect it.[187]

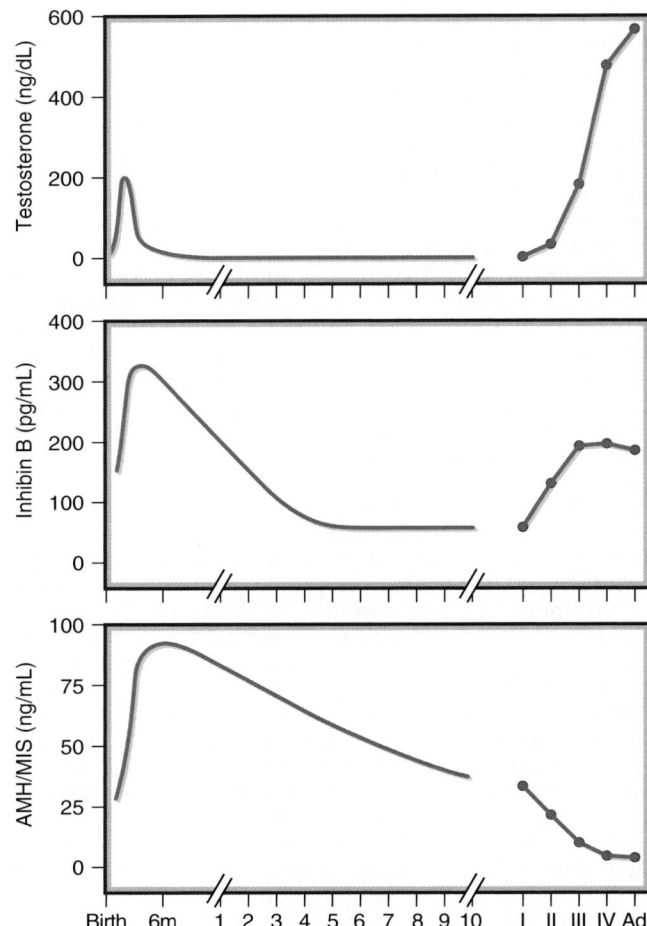

Figure 23-15 Typical postnatal changes are shown for testosterone, antimüllerian hormone (AMH/MIS), and inhibin B in normal males from birth to adulthood. Pubertal stages (I through IV) are indicated. Conversions: testosterone, ng/dL × 0.0347 for nmol/L; AMH/MIS, ng/mL × 7.14 for pmol/L; ranges may vary with the assay, so only indicative values are provided to show trends over time.

DISORDERS (DIFFERENCES) OF SEX DEVELOPMENT

DSDs can have a wide range of presenting phenotypes depending on the underlying condition and its severity. Individuals with these conditions can present to many different health care professions, including neonatologists, geneticists, urologists, gynecologists, and internists. When an infant is born with ambiguous genitalia, the need for further investigation is usually clear. However, 46,XY individuals with complete 17α-hydroxylase/17,20-lyase deficiency may first present in early adolescence with hypertension and delayed puberty, or a young woman with CAIS (46,XY) may first present to a gynecologist with amenorrhea.

Significant progress in understanding of the molecular basis of gonad development has occurred during the past 20 years. Although several single-gene disorders causing gonadal dysgenesis in humans have been described and many more candidate genes are emerging from studies in mice, the percentage of patients with disorders of gonad development who can be diagnosed at the molecular level remains disappointingly low (around 25%). In contrast, molecular diagnosis of classic disorders of steroidogenesis can be reached in most situations. Defining the exact bases of different DSDs can have important implications for gender assignment, predicting response to treatment (e.g., androgen supplementation), assessing associated features (e.g., adrenal dysfunction) or the risk of tumorigenesis, and determining likely fertility options and long-term counseling for the individual and family. However, long-term outcome studies are often inadequate, and an evidence-based approach to management is not possible in many cases.

Nomenclature and Classification of Disorders of Sex Development

DSD has been defined as "congenital conditions in which development of chromosomal, gonadal, or anatomic sex is atypical."[1] This definition is wide ranging enough to cover conditions such as cloacal extrophy but sufficiently specific not to embrace, for example, disorders of puberty. Table 23-3 shows how such a classification system can be applied to DSDs. The list is not exhaustive but provides a framework for the following discussion of the more common causes of DSD, which classifies them as sex chromosome variations (sex chromosome DSD), disorders of testis development and androgenization (46,XY DSD), and disorders of ovary development and androgen excess (46,XX DSD) (see Fig. 23-2). As stated earlier, the karyotype does define someone's gender. However, rapid assessment of karyotype can be a very useful stepping stone for focusing investigations and to help counsel the family about likely causes and outcomes. The aim is to reach a specific diagnosis for each child, even if it remains a broad one such as testicular dysgenesis.

Sex Chromosome Disorders of Sex Development

Differences in the number of sex chromosomes (i.e., sex chromosome aneuploidy) can be considered *sex chromosome DSDs*. These conditions include Klinefelter syndrome (47,XXY and its variants), Turner syndrome (45,X and its variants), 45,X/46,XY mosaicism and its variants (sometimes referred to as mixed gonadal dysgenesis), and true sex chromosome chimerism (46,XY/46,XX) (Table 23-4). A 45,Y cell line is nonviable.

Sex chromosome chimerism and 45,X/46,XY mosaicism can manifest with ambiguous genitalia at birth, but such a presentation is unlikely in Klinefelter syndrome unless multiple X chromosomes are present or in Turner syndrome unless there is a Y fragment. In many cases of classic sex chromosome aneuploidy, the diagnosis is made in adolescence or adult life as a result of associated features, impaired pubertal development, or infertility. More detailed descriptions of the long-term management of some of these conditions are provided in the relevant chapters (e.g., Turner syndrome and Klinefelter syndrome in Chapter 25).

Klinefelter Syndrome and Its Variants

Klinefelter syndrome and its variants are the most common forms of sex chromosome aneuploidy, with a reported incidence of 1 in 500 to 1 in 1000 live births.[188] This incidence

TABLE 23-3
Example of a DSD Classification System

Sex Chromosome DSD	46,XY DSD	46,XX DSD

A: 47,XXY (Klinefelter syndrome and variants)
B: 45,X (Turner syndrome and variants)
C: 45,X/46,XY (mixed gonadal dysgenesis)
D: 46,XX/46,XY (chimerism)
	A: Disorders of gonadal (testis) development
	  1. Complete or partial gonadal dysgenesis (e.g., *SF1/NR5A1, WT1, GATA4, FOG2/ZFPM2, CBX2, SRY, SOX9, MAP3K1, DMRT1, TSPYL1, DHH, ARX, MAMLD1/CXorf6*)
	  2. Ovotesticular DSD
	  3. Testis regression
	B: Disorders in androgen synthesis or action
	  1. Disorders of androgen synthesis
	    Luteinizing hormone (LH) receptor mutations
	    Smith-Lemli-Opitz syndrome
	    StAR protein mutations
	    Cholesterol side-chain cleavage *(CYP11A1)*
	    3β-Hydroxysteroid dehydrogenase 2 *(HSD3B2)*
	    17α-Hydroxylase/17,20-lyase *(CYP17)*
	    P450 oxidoreductase *(POR)*
	    Cytochrome b_5 *(CYB5A)*
	    Aldo-keto reductase 1C2 *(AKR1C2)*
	    17β-Hydroxysteroid dehydrogenase *(HSD17B3)*
	    5α-Reductase 2 *(SRD5A2)*
	  2. Disorders of androgen action
	    Androgen insensitivity syndrome
	    Drugs and environmental modulators
	C: Other
	  1. Syndromic associations of male genital development (e.g., cloacal anomalies, Robinow, Aarskog, hand-foot-genital, popliteal pterygium)
	  2. Persistent müllerian duct syndrome
	  3. Vanishing testis syndrome
	  4. Isolated hypospadias
	  5. Congenital hypogonadotropic hypogonadism
	  6. Cryptorchidism *(INSL3, GREAT)*
	  7. Environmental influences
		A: Disorders of gonadal (ovary) development
		  1. Gonadal dysgenesis
		  2. Ovotesticular DSD
		  3. Testicular DSD (e.g., *SRY⁺*, dup *SOX9*, dup *SOX3, RSPO1, WNT4*)
		B: Androgen excess
		  1. Fetal
		    3β-Hydroxysteroid dehydrogenase 2 *(HSD3B2)*
		    21-Hydroxylase *(CYP21A2)*
		    P450 oxidoreductase *(POR)*
		    11β-Hydroxylase *(CYP11B1)*
		    Glucocorticoid receptor mutations
		  2. Fetoplacental
		    Aromatase *(CYP19)* deficiency
		    Oxidoreductase *(POR)* deficiency
		  3. Maternal
		    Maternal virilizing tumors (e.g., luteomas)
		    Androgenic drugs
		C: Other
		  1. Syndromic associations (e.g., cloacal anomalies)
		  2. Müllerian agenesis/hypoplasia (e.g., MKRH)
		  3. Uterine abnormalities (e.g., MODY5)
		  4. Vaginal atresias (e.g., McKusick-Kaufman)
		  5. Labial adhesions

CYP, cytochrome P450 isoenzyme; DSD, disorders of sex development; MODY5, maturity-onset diabetes of the young type 5; MURCS, müllerian, renal, and cervical spine syndrome; StAR, steroidogenic acute regulatory (protein).

TABLE 23-4
Clinical Features of Sex Chromosome DSDs

Condition	Karyotype	Gonad	Internal Genitalia	Features
Klinefelter syndrome	47,XXY and variants	Hyalinized testes	No uterus	Small testis, azoospermia, hypoandrogenemia; tall stature and increased leg length; increased incidence of learning difficulties, obesity, breast tumors, varicose veins, impaired glucose tolerance
Turner syndrome	45,X and variants	Streak gonad or immature ovary	Uterus	*Childhood:* Lymphedema, shield chest, web neck, low hairline; cardiac defects and coarctation of the aorta; renal and urinary abnormalities; short stature, cubitus valgus, hypoplastic nails, scoliosis; otitis media and hearing loss; ptosis and amblyopia; nevi; autoimmune thyroid disease; visuospatial learning difficulties *Adulthood:* Pubertal failure, primary amenorrhea; hypertension; aortic root dilatation and dissection; sensorineural hearing loss; increased risk of CVD, IBD, colon cancer, thyroid disease, glucose intolerance and diabetes mellitus, osteoporosis (note that some of these may be related to estrogen deficiency)
Mixed gonadal dysgenesis	45,X/46,XY and variants	Testis or dysgenetic gonad	Variable	Increased risk of gonadal tumors; short stature; features of Turner syndrome may be present
Ovotesticular DSD	46,XX/46,XY chimerism	Testis, ovary, or ovotestis	Variable	Possible increased risk of gonadal tumors

CVD, cardiovascular disease; DSDs, disorders of sex development; IBD, inflammatory bowel disease.

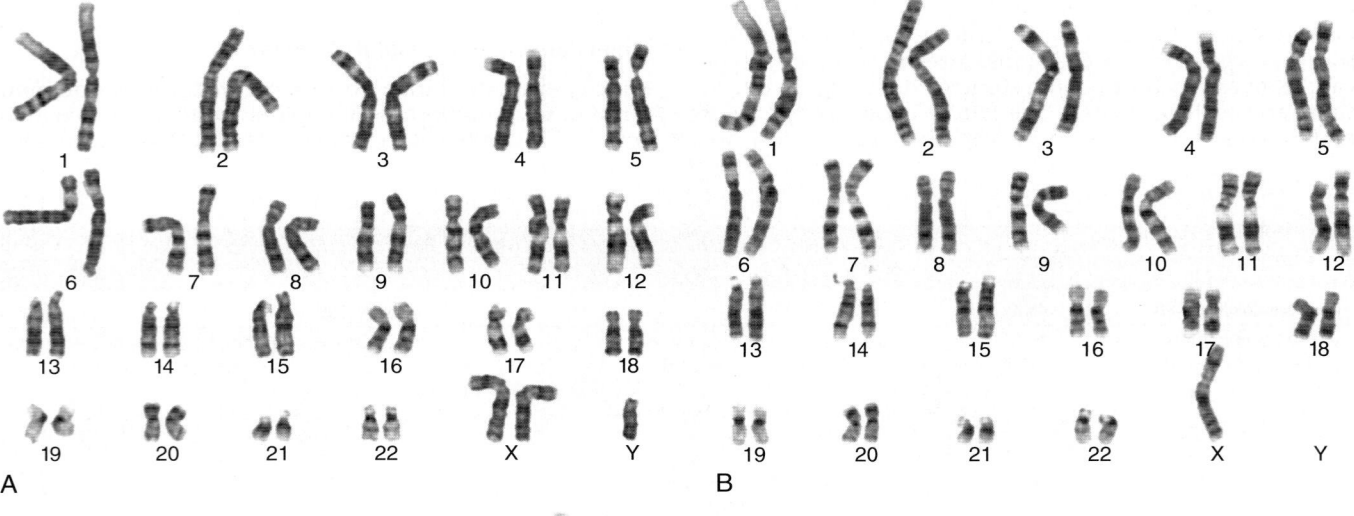

Figure 23-16 G-banded karyotypes of Klinefelter syndrome (47,XXY) (**A**) and Turner syndrome (45,X) (**B**). **C,** Structural changes of the X chromosome seen in variants of Turner syndrome (*from left to right:* normal X; ring chromosome [r(X)(p22.3q22)]; short-arm deletion [del(X)(p21)]; long-arm deletion [del(X)(q21.31)]; isochromosome [I(X)(q10)]). (Images courtesy of Lee Grimsley and Jonathan Waters, MD, North East London Regional Cytogenetics Laboratory, Great Ormond Street Hospital NHS Trust, London, UK.)

may be increasing.[189] The classic form of Klinefelter syndrome is associated with a 47,XXY karyotype and is caused by meiotic nondisjunction of the sex chromosomes during gametogenesis (Fig. 23-16).[18] This abnormality occurs during spermatogenesis in approximately 40% of patients and during oogenesis in approximately 60%. Mosaic forms of Klinefelter syndrome (46,XY/47,XXY) represent mitotic nondisjunction within the developing zygote and are thought to occur in approximately 10% of individuals. Other chromosomal variants associated with Klinefelter syndrome (e.g., 48,XXXY) have been reported.

The clinical features of Klinefelter syndrome and its variants are summarized in Table 23-4.[188] In the most severe situations, a young man may be diagnosed because of small testes, gynecomastia, poor androgenization at puberty, eunuchoid proportions, or infertility. Diagnosis before puberty is the exception. Other features, such as learning difficulties, speech and language delay, behavioral issues, and altered motor development, may occur, and early educational support focusing on any specific areas of difficulty is important.[190,191] However, it is likely that the clinical detection of Klinefelter syndrome based on postnatal karyotyping is biased toward detection of those individuals with a more severe phenotype. As few as 25% of men with Klinefelter syndrome may be diagnosed throughout their life span.

The development of testes and a male phenotype in individuals with Klinefelter syndrome provides important evidence for the key role of the Y chromosome in testis determination and subsequent prenatal androgen production. However, micropenis and hypospadias may be presenting features in some cases, and some studies report mildly elevated FSH concentrations during the postnatal "minipuberty" together with testoterone levels in the lower half of the normal range.[192]

A more predictable elevation in gonadotropin concentrations (e.g., FSH, LH) occurs in the periadolescent period in patients with Klinefelter syndrome, after activation of the HPG axis.[193,194] By midadolescence, plasma concentrations of FSH are increased in 90% of patients with Klinefelter syndrome, and plasma concentrations of LH are increased in 80%. Other serum markers of testicular function (e.g., peripubertal inhibin B, midpubertal INSL3) are often below the normal ranges.[185,194] Although some androgenization usually occurs at the start of puberty in classic Klinefelter syndrome, plasma testosterone is decreased in 50% to 75% of young men, often around the middle of puberty. Testes usually remain small and firm; the median length and volume are 2.5 cm and 4 mL, but most are smaller than 3.5 cm (12 mL).[193] Testes typically appear inappropriately small for the degree of androgenization. The serum estradiol concentration is often elevated, which contributes to the gynecomastia observed during the adolescent period.

Testicular biopsy is not warranted clinically, because the diagnosis can usually be made on karyotyping from peripheral blood cells. However, studies in which testicular histologic examination has been obtained report germ cell depletion, progressive hyalinization of seminiferous tubules, and Leydig cell hyperplasia after chronic LH stimulation.[193] Testosterone levels need careful surveillance during puberty.[194] A significant proportion of men with Klinefelter syndrome receive testosterone supplementation to fully induce puberty and to support sexual characteristics, libido, and bone mineralization into adult life. Psychological support and educational support may be needed, as well as attention to potential long-term issues such as diabetes. Management of Klinefelter syndrome in adolescence and adulthood is discussed in Chapters 19 and 25.

Although some cases of spontaneous fertility have been reported for mosaic forms of Klinefelter syndrome (46,XY/47,XXY), the prospects for fertility in classic Klinefelter syndrome have been thought to be poor. Occasionally, sperm can obtained from ejaculate and this should always be assessed. However, in the past decade testicular sperm extraction (TESE or micro-TESE) combined with intracytoplasmic sperm injection (ISCI) has led to successful pregnancy for approximately 50% of men with classic Klinefelter syndrome (47,XXY) in specialist centers.[193,195] The potential risk of transmission of the sex chromosome aneuploidy must be considered, and preimplantation genetic diagnosis is often offered; the risk seems to be low, although an increase in some other chromosomal changes

is seen. At present there appear to be very few predictors of success other than age. Even testicular volume, testosterone levels, or inhibin B do not consistently correlate with outcome. The lower success with age supports the concept that progressive deterioration in testicular function is a feature of Klinefelter syndrome.

Turner Syndrome and Its Variants

Turner syndrome is the second most frequent form of sex chromosome aneuploidy, with an incidence of approximately 1 woman in 2500.[39] The classic form of Turner syndrome is associated with a 45,X karyotype, which occurs in approximately one half of individuals with this condition (see Fig. 23-16). Mosaic forms of Turner syndrome (45,X/46,XX) account for approximately one fourth of the patients, and the remainder have structural abnormalities of the X chromosome, such as long-arm or short-arm deletions, isochromosomes, or ring chromosomes (see Fig. 23-16).[39,196]

A 45,X chromosome constitution may be the consequence of nondisjunction or chromosome loss during gametogenesis in either parent that results in a sperm or ovum that lacks a sex chromosome. Although errors in mitosis in normal zygotes often lead to mosaicism, a purely 45,X constitution may arise at the first cleavage division from anaphase lag with loss of a sex chromosome or, less often, from mitotic nondisjunction with failure of the complementary 47,XXX or 47,XYY cell line to survive.[17] An estimated 2% of all zygotes have a 45,X karyotype, and approximately 7% of spontaneous abortuses have a 45,X karyotype, making this the most frequent chromosomal anomaly in humans.

The clinical features of Turner syndrome are highly variable and depend on the age of the child and time of diagnosis. For example, a prenatal diagnosis of Turner syndrome may be made incidentally after amniocentesis or chorionic villous sampling for another reason, such as advanced maternal age, or after the detection of increased nuchal translucency on fetal ultrasound scanning.[196] In early infancy, the diagnosis should be considered in females with lymphedema, nuchal folds, low hair line, or left-sided cardiac defects. Unexplained growth failure or somatic features (e.g., abnormal nails, shield chest, abnormal carrying angle, recurrent ear infections) may point to the diagnosis during childhood, and Turner syndrome should be considered in all girls with pubertal delay or pubertal failure. The clinical features of Turner syndrome are summarized in Table 23-4, and diagnosis and management are discussed in Chapter 25. Timely and appropriate introduction of estrogens is necessary in adolescence to ensure adequate breast and uterine development, thereby optimizing the opportunity to potentially carry a pregnancy by ovum donation in the future.[196-198] However, careful assessment of cardiovascular risk in pregnancy in needed.[199] Women with Turner syndrome benefit from dedicated transition in adolescence and long-term follow-up with a focus on issues such as cardiovascular, bone, and reproductive health and hearing.[39,196,200,201]

Girls with classic Turner syndrome show ovarian dysgenesis. Studies of Turner syndrome embryos have shown normal germ cell migration and normal ovarian development until the third month of gestation.[202] Then, accelerated germ cell apoptosis and subsequent oocyte atresia occur, resulting in progressive degeneration of the ovary in the prenatal or postnatal period. With these gonadal changes, LH and FSH tend to rise in late childhood, after activation of the hypothalamic pulse generator. Nevertheless, sufficient estrogen synthesis for puberty to commence in adolescence occurs in approximately 25% of girls with Turner syndrome (10% of those with 45,X; 30% to 40% of those with 45,X/46,XX mosaicism), and menstruation occurs in about 2% of cases.[39,203] AMH may be a useful marker of ovarian reserve and predictor of ovarian insufficiency.[204] Gonadectomy is not usually required except when a Y fragment containing the *TSPY* locus is present; in such patients, the risk of gonadoblastoma is increased.[205] It is unclear whether follicular tissue can be usefully cryopreserved for girls in whom spontaneous puberty has occurred, although oocyte cryopreservation has been used successfully in several women with Turner mosaicism.[206,207] More detailed studies of ovarian cryopreservation or oocyte maturation in Turner syndrome are needed.[208]

45,X/46,XY Mosaicism and Variants

A mosaic 45,X/46,XY karyotype, sometimes referred to as *mixed gonadal dysgenesis*, probably arises through anaphase lag during mitosis in the zygote, although Y chromosomal abnormalities are sometimes seen, and interchromosomal rearrangements with loss of structural abnormal Y material may be a common mechanism for variants of this condition. Although the classic form of this condition is associated with 45,X/46,XY mosaicism, 45,X/47,XYY or 45,X/46,XY/47,XYY mosaic karyotypes have also been reported.

The clinical phenotype associated with a 45,X/46,XY mosaicism is highly variable, and the true prevalence of this condition is unknown (see Table 23-4). Historically, individuals with the most severe forms of 45,X/46,XY mosaicism have been referred for further assessment, and most series of patients reported in the literature have probably reflected this bias, as studies based on nonselected prenatal karyotyping have shown that most children with 45,X/46,XY mosaicism appear male.[209-211]

Reported genital phenotypes associated with 45,X/46,XY mosaicism range from female external genitalia or mild clitoromegaly through all stages of ambiguous genitalia to hypospadias or a normal penis.[209,212-215] Gonadal phenotypes range from streak gonads through dysgenetic testes to testes with normal histologic architecture. In rare cases, ovarian-like stroma and sparse primordial follicles may be present. The gonads may be positioned anywhere along the pathway of testicular descent, with streak gonads more likely to be intra-abdominal and well-formed testes more likely to be in the inguinoscrotal region. Müllerian structures may be present in the most severe cases because of impaired AMH production by Sertoli cells. Marked differences in gonadal development and histologic appearance can be seen between the right and the left sides or even within a single gonad (hence, the term *mixed gonadal dysgenesis*), often resulting in an asymmetry of the external genitalia.[215] The presence of a hemiuterus and fallopian tube on the side of the most severely affected gonad in some cases provides important evidence for the paracrine actions of AMH on developing müllerian structures.

Somatic features associated with a 45,X/46,XY karyotype are highly variable and do not always correlate well with the gonadal phenotype.[209,213-215] Approximately 40% of children have additional, clinical features reminiscent of Turner syndrome, such as short stature, nuchal folds, low-set hairline, and cardiac and renal abnormalities.[215] Detailed evaluation and long-term follow-up of these patients may be warranted, as for Turner syndrome (see Chapter 10). In other cases, a reduction in predicted height may be the only somatic manifestation. Ongoing monitoring for features associated with Turner syndrome (e.g., thyroid function, hearing, cardiac anomalies) may be required for this group of individuals, and many families benefit from the psychological support and education that can be linked to specialist services.

Gender assignment can be difficult in individuals with 45,X/46,XY, and several factors should be considered, including genital appearance and urogenital anatomy, risk of gonadal malignancy, fertility and reproductive options, potential need for hormone replacement, and probable gender identity, sex role behavior, and psychosexual functioning.

Most infants with female or minimally androgenized genitalia are raised as female, and the presence of a uterus or hemiuterus allows the potential for pregnancy by ovum donation in the future, though predicting future function can be difficult. Intra-abdominal streak and dysgenetic gonads are thought to pose a significant risk of malignancy and should be removed because of a higher germ-cell tumor risk in dysgenetic structures.[212,214,216] Estrogen replacement is required to induce breast and uterine development in adolescence, and the addition of progestins allows menstruation when a uterus is present. Growth-promoting agents have been used on an individual basis when short stature or Turner syndrome–like features are present. No large trials have been performed to assess this group of patients, although there can be a significant loss of growth during puberty and some studies have suggested use of GH from earlier in childhood may optimize growth potential if this is a concern.[213,214,217] Similarly, no long-term outcome data on gender identity or psychosexual functioning are available.

Infants with hypospadias and reasonable phallic development are usually raised as male. Testosterone can sometimes be given to promote phallic growth in infancy, and hypospadias repair is usually offered as a two-stage procedure. Attempts should be made to perform orchidopexy as a one- or two-stage procedure, because there may be a significant risk of malignancy in these gonads, and careful monitoring of testes is necessary. Gonads that cannot be placed within the scrotum are usually removed.[212,214] Gonads that can be secured within the scrotum need careful monitoring by palpation and biopsy in adolescence to assess for carcinoma in situ. Some studies have suggested that regular testicular ultrasound in adolescence can be used to detect changes such as microlithiasis.[212,214] Puberty should be carefully monitored to ensure adequate endogenous testosterone production, and in some cases, testosterone supplementation is needed. Most boys enter puberty spontaneously but some then develop androgen insufficiency and are typically likely to undergo urogenital surgery.[214] Reduced final height is invariable but there is beneficial response to growth hormone in some boys.[213,214,217]

Assignment of gender and management of a 45,X/46,XY child with *highly ambiguous genitalia* can be a difficult situation for parents and physicians, and long-term outcome data for this group are not available. Limited data suggest that approximately 60% of infants with this phenotype are raised female, but they are infertile, have no uterus, require gonadectomy, and are likely to undergo urogenital surgery. In contrast, those raised as male often undergo multiple hypospadias operations, may have poor corporal tissue, are infertile if dysgenetic gonads are present that need to be removed, and may have a significantly reduced height potential. Detailed assessment of each child is important and an individualized approach by an experienced multidisciplinary team is important for management and for long-term monitoring and support. Long-term outcome data from larger studies may provide better guidance on the management of this group of individuals in the future.

In addition to the most severe cases described earlier, a 45,X/46,XY mosaic karyotype can be associated with a male phenotype and apparently normal testis development. Initial cases of normal males with a 45,X/46,XY karyotype were described after screening of family members as potential bone marrow transplant donors, but later studies of amniocentesis showed that 90% of fetuses diagnosed as 45,X/46,XY by amniocentesis and confirmed as having this karyotype have normal male genitalia and apparently normal testes postnatally.[210,211] Moreover, there seems to be limited correlation between the degree of mosaicism on peripheral blood sampling and gonadal or somatic phenotype. Follow-up data on this cohort are limited, HPG function has not been reported in detail, and fertility outcome and tumor risk are not known. Although a 45,X/46,XY karyotype is an uncommon finding in men presenting with testicular tumors or in the infertility clinic, more detailed long-term studies of the 45,X/46,XY male cohort are required to know whether extensive follow-up is necessary. It may seem prudent to monitor gonadal function in this cohort and to assess for evidence of testicular carcinoma in situ in adolescence, but evidence for the best approach is lacking.

Ovotesticular Disorders of Sex Development: 46,XX/46,XY Chimerism and Variants

The diagnosis of ovotesticular DSD (true hermaphroditism) requires the presence of ovarian tissue (containing follicles) and testicular tissue in the same or the opposite gonad (Fig. 23-17; see Table 23-4). Gonadal stroma arranged in whorls, similar to those found in the ovary but lacking oocytes, is a common finding in dysgenetic or streak testis and is not considered sufficient evidence to designate the rudimentary gonad as an ovary.

Ovotesticular DSD is an uncommon condition that has been reported in approximately 500 individuals worldwide and in our experience occurs in around 1% of babies referred because of atypical genitalia. Although 46,XX/46,XY chimerism (sometimes caused by double fertilization or ovum fusion; see "Chromosomal Sex") does occur in a proportion of these patients, especially in North America

and Europe, most individuals with this condition do not have 46,XX/46,XY chimerism (Table 23-5).[218] Rather, most patients with ovotesticular DSD, especially those in South and Western Africa, have a 46,XX karyotype.[218,219] The molecular basis of this disorder is not known. Rare genetic causes include SRY translocation (although usually this causes 46,XX testicular DSD), RSPO1 mutations (in association with palmar-plantar hyperkeratoderma and skin tumors), and chromosomal alterations that cause upregulation of expression of SOX9 (chromosome 17q24).[220,221] Ovotesticular DSD associated with a 46,XY karyotype is much less prevalent and may represent cryptic gonadal mosaicism for a Y chromosome deletion or early sex-determining gene mutation. Patients with ovotesticular DSD may be subclassified according to the type and location of the gonads.[4] Lateral cases (20%) have a testis on one side and an ovary on the other. Bilateral cases (30%) have testicular and ovarian tissue present bilaterally, usually as ovotestes. Unilateral cases (50%) have an ovotestis present on one side and an ovary or testis on the other. The ovary (or ovotestis) is more frequently found on the left side of the body, whereas the testis (or ovotestis) is found more often on the right. An ovary is likely to be in its normal anatomic position, whereas a testis or ovotestis can be anywhere along the pathway of testicular descent and is often found in the right inguinal region.

Differentiation of the genital tract and development of secondary sex characteristics vary in ovotesticular DSD.[222-223] Most patients who present early have ambiguous genitalia or significant hypospadias. Cryptorchidism is common, but at least one gonad is palpable, usually in the labioscrotal fold or inguinal region, and often associated with an inguinal hernia. The differentiation of the genital ducts usually follows that of the gonad, and a hemiuterus or rudimentary uterus is often present on the side of the ovary or ovotestis.

Breast development at the time of puberty is common in ovotesticular DSD.[223] Menses occurs in a significant proportion of cases, and ovulation and pregnancy have been reported in a number of patients with a 46,XX karyotype, especially when an ovary is present. However, progressive androgenization can occur in girls with testicular tissue, which can result in voice changes and clitoral enlargement during adolescence if left untreated. Individuals reared as male often present with hypospadias and undescended testes, although bilateral scrotal ovotestes have been reported. These individuals can experience significant estrogenization at the time of puberty and may have cyclic hematuria if a uterus is present. Spermatogenesis is rare, and interstitial fibrosis of the testis is common. Fertility requires Y chromosomal genes other than SRY, so boys with 46,XX ovotesticular DSD will be infertile.

Although ovotesticular DSD is rare, the diagnosis should be considered in all patients with ambiguous genitalia. A

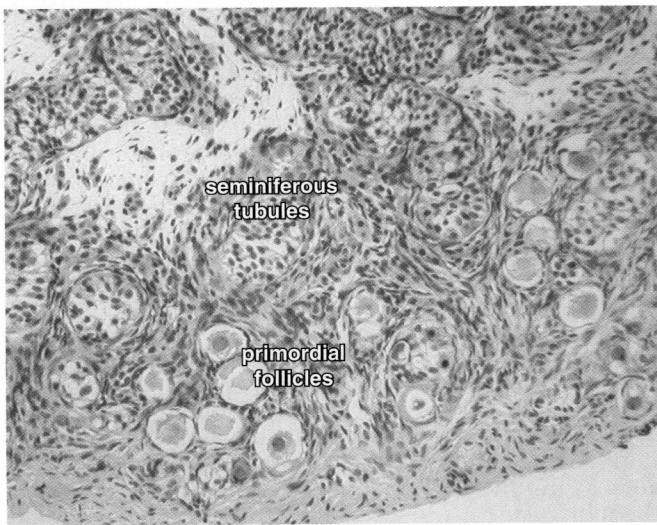

Figure 23-17 Ovotestis, showing immature seminiferous tubules lined with Sertoli cells and germ cells *(upper left)* and ovarian tissue with primordial follicles *(lower right)* (hematoxylin-eosin stain; original magnification, ×400). (Courtesy of Neil Sebire, MD, Great Ormond Street Hospital NHS Trust, London, UK.)

TABLE 23-5			
Relative Frequency (%) of Different Karyotypes in Ovotesticular DSD (True Hermaphroditism)			
Location	**46,XX/46,XY**	**46,XX**	**46,XY**
North America	21	72	7
Europe	41	52	7
Africa	—	97	—

DSD, disorders of sex development.
Adapted from Krob G, Braun A, Kuhnle U. True hermaphroditism: geographical distribution, clinical findings, chromosomes and gonadal histology. *Eur J Pediatr.* 1994;153:2-10.

46,XX/46,XY karyotype strongly supports the diagnosis, but the detection of a 46,XX or 46,XY karyotype does not exclude the diagnosis, especially if a 46,XX baby has genital asymmetry. Pelvic imaging with ultrasound or magnetic resonance imaging (MRI) is useful for visualizing internal genitalia. The presence of testicular tissue may be detected by measurement of basal testosterone, AMH, and inhibin B in the first months of life and by measuring basal AMH thereafter. Ovarian tissue is more difficult to detect in early childhood, although estradiol, inhibin A, and follicular response to repeated injection of recombinant human FSH can provide useful information.[187] Examination under anesthesia and laparoscopy may provide the most detailed information about internal structures and allow a biopsy to confirm the diagnosis of ovotesticular DSD when other forms of DSD have been excluded.[224,225] However, the biopsy sometimes does not sample all the tissues present in a gonad.[225]

The management of ovotesticular DSD depends on the age at diagnosis, genital development, internal structures, and reproductive capacity. Male or female assignment may be appropriate for the young infant in whom a strong gender identity has not been established. Individuals with a 46,XX karyotype and a uterus are likely to have functional ovarian tissue, and female assignment is likely to be appropriate. Potentially functional testicular tissue should be removed before puberty and monitored postoperatively by measuring serum AMH levels or by demonstrating a lack of testosterone response to hCG stimulation. The risk of malignant transformation in ovarian tissue of 46,XX patients is not known.

A male gender assignment may be more appropriate if there is reasonable phallic development and testicular tissue, and müllerian structures are absent or very poorly formed. Ovarian tissue is usually removed to prevent estrogenization at puberty, and remnant müllerian structures can be removed by an experienced surgeon if appropriate. The prevalence of gonadoblastoma or germinoma arising in the testicular tissue of patients with 46,XX ovotesticular DSD has been estimated at 3% to 4%. Because the ovotesticular tissue is usually dysgenetic, removal of this testicular tissue has been advocated.[22] However, management of a histologically normal, scrotally positioned testis is more difficult, and careful monitoring and biopsy for carcinoma in situ in adolescence may be an appropriate strategy, especially if endogenous testosterone is being produced.

Gender identity is an important consideration in patients with ovotesticular DSD who first present in late childhood or adolescence due to androgenization in girls or estrogenization in boys. In most cases, gender identity is consistent with sex of rearing. After appropriate counseling, the discordant gonad and dysgenetic tissue should be removed to prevent further androgenization in girls and estrogenization in boys. Sex hormone supplementation may be required for complete pubertal development.

46,XY Disorders of Sex Development

The 46,XY DSDs can be categorized as disorders of testis development, disorders of androgen synthesis, disorders of androgen action, and other conditions affecting sex development (Table 23-6; see also Fig. 23-7).

Disorders of Testis Development

Disorders of testis development can have a spectrum of phenotypes and presentations. *Complete testicular dysgenesis* is associated with a complete lack of androgenization of the external genitalia and persistent müllerian structures

due to insufficient AMH production—a condition sometimes called *Swyer syndrome*. In contrast, *partial gonadal dysgenesis* may be associated with clitoromegaly or ambiguous or atypical genitalia. A uterus or uterine remnant and vagina or common urogenital sinus may be present. Subtle forms of testicular dysgenesis can present with isolated hypospadias, testicular regression, a small penis, or potentially even male infertility.

Several single-gene disorders have been described in patients with various degrees of testicular dysgenesis. Table 23-6 summarizes these factors, and the role of many of these factors in development has already been discussed (see "Testis Determination"). Although associated features can sometimes help to direct genetic analysis, often there are no other findings and a genetic diagnosis is currently reached in only 20% to 30% of individuals with 46,XY testicular dysgenesis.

Single-Gene Disorders

Steroidogenic Factor 1: NR5A1. SF1 (encoded by *NR5A1*) is a member of the nuclear receptor superfamily that regulates the transcription of at least 30 genes involved in gonadal development, adrenal development, steroidogenesis, and reproduction.[75] Complete deletion of the gene encoding Sf1 in mice results in apoptosis of the developing gonad and adrenal gland during early embryonic development.[76] XY animals are phenotypically female and have persistent müllerian structures. Abnormalities of the ventromedial hypothalamus and variable HH are also described.

SF1 mutations were first reported in two 46,XY individuals with female external genitalia, persistent müllerian structures, and primary adrenal failure.[79,80] These changes resulted in impaired DNA binding. The first variant was a de novo heterozygous p.Gly35Glu change in the P-box primary DNA-binding region of SF1, and the second was a recessively inherited homozygous p.Arg92Gln mutation in the A-box secondary DNA-binding region (Fig. 23-18). This combined gonadal and adrenal phenotype is not common and it initially seemed that disruption of SF1 would be a rare cause of DSD in humans.

However, the past decade has seen a different picture emerging as an ever-increasing number of heterozygous nonsense, frameshift, and missense mutations in *NR5A1* have been associated with a spectrum of 46,XY DSD conditions in individuals with normal adrenal function (see Fig. 23-18).[75,81,226] These changes usually result in haploinsufficiency of SF1. A range of phenotypes is seen, most commonly mild gonadal dysgenesis and significantly impaired androgenization, where alterations in SF1 are found in approximately 15% of cases.[75] These variations usually arise de novo but may be inherited from the mother in a sex-limited dominant fashion (i.e., the mother carries the mutation but is unaffected) and occasionally may be autosomal recessive.[80] In some situations, there is a family history of ovarian insufficiency, or females in the family may be identified who are at risk of developing ovarian insufficiency in the future.[47] Loss of SF1 function also is reported in some boys with severe hypospadias and undescended testes (approximately 5%), bilateral anorchia, and a small penis and in men with infertility (approximately 2%).[227-229] Therefore, variable loss of SF1 activity is associated primarily with testicular dysfunction or different degrees of ovarian dysfunction in humans. Adrenal function may need to be monitored over time, but at present adrenal insufficiency does not seem prevalent. Defining the molecular basis in different families can be important for counseling, especially the potential risk of ovarian insufficiency, and for identifying those males who might need surveillance for potential androgen insufficiency or a decline in fertility with age.

TABLE 23-6

Overview of Important Genes Involved in DSDs

A. Causes of 46,XY DSD

Disorders of Gonadal (Testicular) Development: Single-Gene Disorders

Gene	Protein	OMIM	Locus	Inheritance	Gonad	Müllerian Structures	External Genitalia	Associated Features/Variants
WT1	TF	607102	11p13	AD	Dysgenetic testis	±	Female, ambiguous or hypospadias	Wilms tumor, renal abnormalities, gonadal tumors (WAGR, Denys-Drash, and Frasier syndromes)
NR5A1 (SF1)	Nuclear receptor TF	184757	9q33.3	AD/AR (SLD)	Dysgenetic testis (variable)	±	Female, ambiguous, or hypospadias	More severe phenotypes include primary adrenal failure; milder phenotypes have isolated partial gonadal dysgenesis or impaired androgenization or both
GATA4	TF	600576	8p23.1	AD (SLD)	Dysgenetic testis (variable)	–	Female, ambiguous, or hypospadias/micropenis	Cardiac defects (e.g., septal defects, tetralogy of Fallot)
ZFPM2 (FOG2)	Co-regulator	603693	8q23.1	AD	Dysgenetic testis (variable)	–	Female	
CBX2	Polycomb protein	602770	17q25.3	AR	Ovary (one case)	+	Female	
SRY	TF	480000	Yp11.3	Y	Dysgenetic testis or ovotestis	±	Female or ambiguous	
SOX9	TF	608160	17q24-q25	AD	Dysgenetic testis or ovotestis	±	Female or ambiguous	Camptomelic dysplasia (17q24 rearrangements have a milder phenotype than point mutations)
MAP3K1	Signaling molecule	600982	5q11.2	AD	Dysgenetic testis (variable)	±	Female, ambiguous, or hypospadias/micropenis	
DMRT1	TF	602424	9q24.3	AD	Dysgenetic testis	+	Female	
TSPYL1	? Chromatin remodeling	604714	6q22.1	AR	Dysgenetic testis	–	Female or ambiguous	Sudden infant death
DHH	Signaling molecule	605423	12q13.1	AR	Dysgenetic testis, testis	–	Female	Minifascicular neuropathy in several patients
ARX	TF	300382	Xp22.13	X	Dysgenetic testis	–	Ambiguous	X-linked lissencephaly, epilepsy, temperature instability
MAMLD1 (CXORF6)	Unknown	300120	Xq28	X	Normal (Leydig cell dysfunction)	–	Hypospadias	

Disorders of Gonadal (Testicular) Development: Chromosomal Changes Involving Key Candidate Genes*

Gene	Protein	OMIM	Locus	Inheritance	Gonad	Müllerian Structures	External Genitalia	Associated Features/Variants
DMRT1	TF	602424	9p24.3	Monosomic deletion	Dysgenetic testis	±	Female or ambiguous	Mental retardation
ATRX	Helicase (? chromatin remodeling)	300032	Xq13.3	X	Dysgenetic testis	–	Female, ambiguous, or male	α-Thalassemia, mental retardation
NR0B1 (DAX1)	Nuclear receptor TF	300018	Xp21.3	dupXp21	Dysgenetic testis or ovary	±	Female or ambiguous	
WNT4	Signaling molecule	603490	1p36.12	dup1p35	Dysgenetic testis	+	Ambiguous	Mental retardation

Continued

TABLE 23-6

Overview of Important Genes Involved in DSDs—cont'd

Gene	Protein	OMIM	Locus	Inheritance	Gonad	Müllerian Structures	External Genitalia	Associated Features/Variants
Disorders in Hormone Synthesis or Action								
DHCR7	Enzyme	602858	11q13.4	AR	Testis	−	Variable	Smith-Lemli-Opitz syndrome: coarse facies, second-third toe syndactyly, failure to thrive, developmental delay, cardiac and visceral abnormalities
LHCGR	G protein receptor	152790	2p16.3	AR	Testis	−	Female, ambiguous, or micropenis	Leydig cell hypoplasia
STAR	Mitochondrial associated protein	600617	8p11.2	AR	Testis	−	Female, ambiguous, or micropenis	Lipoid CAH (primary adrenal failure), pubertal failure
CYP11A1	Enzyme	118485	15q24.1	AR	Testis	−	Female or ambiguous	CAH (primary adrenal failure), pubertal failure
HSD3B2	Enzyme	201810	1p13.1	AR	Testis	−	Ambiguous	CAH, primary adrenal failure, ↑ Δ⁵:Δ⁴ ratio
CYP17A1	Enzyme	202110	10q24.3	AR	Testis	−	Female, ambiguous, or micropenis	CAH, hypertension due to DOC (except in isolated 17,20-lyase deficiency)
POR (P450 oxidoreductase)	CYP enzyme electron donor	124015	7q11.2	AR	Testis	−	Male or ambiguous	Mixed features of 21-hydroxylase deficiency, 17α-hydroxylase/17,20-lyase deficiency, and aromatase deficiency; sometimes associated with Antley-Bixler craniosynostosis
CYB5A	Cofactor	613218	18q22.3	AR	Testis	−	Ambiguous or hypospadiac	Methemoglobinemia
AKR1C2 (AKR1C4)	Enzyme	600450	10p15.1	AR (? digenic)	Testis	−	Variable	
HSD17B3	Enzyme	605573	9q22.23	AR	Testis	−	Female or ambiguous	Partial androgenization at puberty, ↑ ratio of androstenedione to testosterone
SRD5A2	Enzyme	607306	2p23.1	AR	Testis	−	Ambiguous or micropenis	Partial androgenization at puberty, ↑ ratio of testosterone to DHT
Androgen receptor (*NR3C4*)	Nuclear receptor TF	313700	Xq12	X	Testis	−	Female, ambiguous, micropenis, or normal male	Phenotypic spectrum from complete AIS (female external genitalia) to partial AIS (ambiguous) to normal male genitalia/infertility
AMH	Signaling molecule	600957	19p13.3	AR	Testis	+	Normal male	Persistent müllerian duct syndrome (PMDS)
AMH receptor	Serine/threonine kinase transmembrane receptor	600956	12q13.13	AR	Testis	+	Normal male	Male external genitalia, bilateral cryptorchidism

B. Causes of 46,XX DSD

Disorders of Gonadal (Ovarian) Development

Gene	Protein/function	OMIM	Locus	Inheritance	Gonads	+/–	Phenotype	Additional features
SRY	TF	480000	Yp11.3	Translocation	Testis or ovotestis	–	Male or ambiguous	
SOX9	TF	608160	17q24	dup17q24 or deletion of regulatory region	Not determined	–	Male or ambiguous	Additional features if large duplication
SOX3	TF	313430	Xq27.1	dup Xq27 or del of regulatory region	Testis (variable)	–	Male	
RSPO1	Thrombospondin (Wnt signaling)	609595	1p34.3	AR	Testis or ovotestis	–	Male	Palmar-plantar hyperkeratosis, squamous cell carcinoma
WNT4	Wnt signaling	611812	1p36.12	AR	Testis or ovotestis	–	Male or ambiguous	SERKAL syndrome

Androgen Excess

Gene	Protein/function	OMIM	Locus	Inheritance	Gonads	+/–	Phenotype	Additional features
HSD3B2	Enzyme	201810	1p13.1	AR	Ovary	+	Clitoromegaly (mild)	CAH, primary adrenal failure, partial androgenization due to ↑ conversion of DHEA
CYP21A2	Enzyme	201910	6p21.33	AR	Ovary	+	Ambiguous; rarely Prader V	CAH, phenotypic spectrum from severe salt-losing forms associated with adrenal failure to simple virilizing forms with compensated adrenal function, ↑ 17-OHP
CYP11B1	Enzyme	202010	8q24.3	AR	Ovary	+	Ambiguous; rarely Prader V	CAH, hypertension due to ↑ 11-deoxycorticosterone
POR (P450 oxidoreductase)	CYP enzyme electron donor	124015	7q11.23	AR	Ovary	+	Normal or ambiguous	Mixed features of 21-hydroxylase deficiency, 17α-hydroxylase/17,20-lyase deficiency and aromatase deficiency; associated with Antley-Bixler craniosynostosis
CYP19	Enzyme	107910	15q21.2	AR	Ovary	+	Ambiguous	Maternal androgenization during pregnancy, absent breast development at puberty except in partial cases
Glucocorticoid receptor† (NR3C1)	Nuclear receptor TF	138040	5q31.3	AR	Ovary	+	Normal or ambiguous	↑ ACTH, 17-OHP, cortisol, mineralocorticoids, and androgens; failure of dexamethasone suppression

*Chromosomal rearrangements likely to include key genes are included.

†Note: Patient heterozygous for a mutation in CYP21.

–, absent; +, present; ACTH, adrenocorticotropic hormone; AD, autosomal dominant (often de novo mutation); SLD, sex-limited dominant; AIS, androgen insensitivity syndrome; AR, autosomal recessive; CAH, congenital adrenal hyperplasia; CYP, cytochrome P450 enzyme; DHEA, dehydroepiandrosterone; DOC, 11-deoxycorticosterone; DSDs, disorders of sex development; 17-OHP, 17-hydroxyprogesterone; LHCGR, the luteinizing hormone (LH) or human chorionic gonadotropin (hCG) receptor; OMIM, *Online Mendelian Inheritance in Man*; SERKAL, sex-reversal with kidney, adrenal, and lung dysgenesis; TF, transcription factor; WAGR, Wilms tumor, aniridia, genitourinary anomalies, and mental retardation.

Adapted from Achermann JC, Ozisik G, Meeks JJ, et al. Genetic causes of human reproductive disease. *J Clin Endocrinol Metab.* 2002;87:2447-2454, used with permission. © 2002 The Endocrine Society.

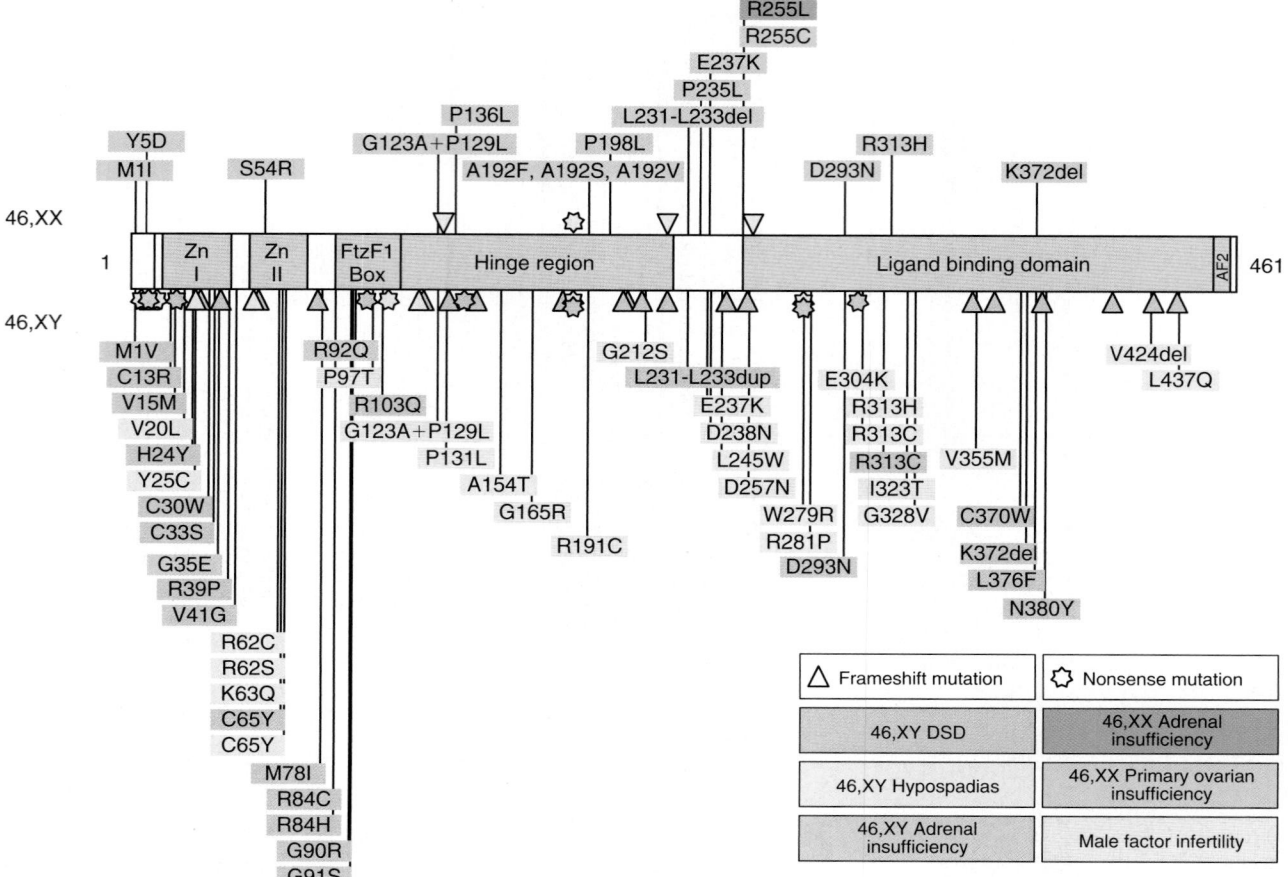

Figure 23-18 Schematic diagram of steroidogenic factor 1 (SF1) shows key domains and mutations associated with a gonadal phenotype. The Gly35Glu (heterozygous) and Arg92Gln (homozygous) changes affect DNA-binding regions of the protein and are associated with marked underandrogenization, dysgenetic gonads, müllerian structures, and primary adrenal failure. Heterozygous frameshift *(triangles)* and nonsense mutations *(stars)*, as well as missense mutations, have been described in 46,XY individuals with a spectrum of disorders of sex development (DSD) phenotypes *(below the structure drawing)* and in women with primary ovarian insufficiency *(above he structure drawing)*. (Modified from Lin L, Philibert P, Ferraz-de-Souza B, et al. Heterozygous missense mutations in steroidogenic factor-1 [SF1/Ad4BP, NR5A1] are associated with 46,XY disorders of sex development with normal adrenal function. *J Clin Endocrinol Metab.* 2007;92:991-999, used with permission of The Endocrine Society, copyright 2007.)

Wilms Tumor 1 Gene: WT1. WT1 (11p13) is a four–zinc finger transcription factor expressed in the developing genital ridge, kidney, gonads, and mesothelium.[65] Homozygous deletion of *Wt1* in mice prevents development of the gonads and kidneys.[66] The WT1 protein has several different isoforms that have complex roles in sex development, as outlined previously and shown in Figure 23-19. The important role of WT1 in human testis development has been confirmed through the description of various WT1 mutations in patients with WAGR syndrome, Denys-Drash syndrome, and Frasier syndrome.

WAGR syndrome is caused by deletion of a region of chromosome 11p13.[230] The resultant phenotype is likely to be the consequence of haploinsufficiency of *WT1*, together with loss of developmental genes such as *PAX6*, which is involved in eye development.[71] Renal abnormalities typically include childhood Wilms tumor in about half of children, although renal agenesis has been reported and renal dysfunction often occurs after adolescence. Genitourinary abnormalities are usually relatively mild and include bilateral cryptorchidism, micropenis, and occasionally hypospadias. Careful ophthalmic support is needed for the aniridia or iridic hypoplasia and cataracts or corneal clouding can occur. Developmental delay can occur with larger chromosomal deletions, and obesity is postulated if

the deletion is large and includes the *BDNF* gene (WAGRO syndrome).

Denys-Drash syndrome is characterized by gonadal dysgenesis, severe congenital or early-onset nephropathy (i.e., diffuse mesangial sclerosis), and predisposition to Wilms tumor.[72] Most 46,XY patients with Denys-Drash syndrome present with genital ambiguity or severe penoscrotal hypospadias in the newborn period, although normal male or female phenotypes have been described. The presence or absence of müllerian structures depends on the degree of Sertoli cell dysfunction. Denys-Drash syndrome usually results from heterozygous de novo point mutations in *WT1* that have a dominant negative effect on the function of the wild-type protein. These point mutations usually affect the DNA-binding region (zinc fingers) of WT1. The risk of early-onset renal failure is high, and Wilms tumor usually develops in the first few years of life. Gonadoblastoma occurs in fewer than 10% of cases. The prevalence of *WT1* mutations in boys with penoscrotal hypospadias and undescended testes has been reported to be as high as 7%.[231]

Frasier syndrome usually results from heterozygous mutations in the donor splice site of exon 9 of *WT1*.[73,74] These changes are predicted to result in an imbalance in the ratio of +KTS to −KTS isoforms of WT1. Frasier syndrome is typically characterized by streak gonads, a 46,XY

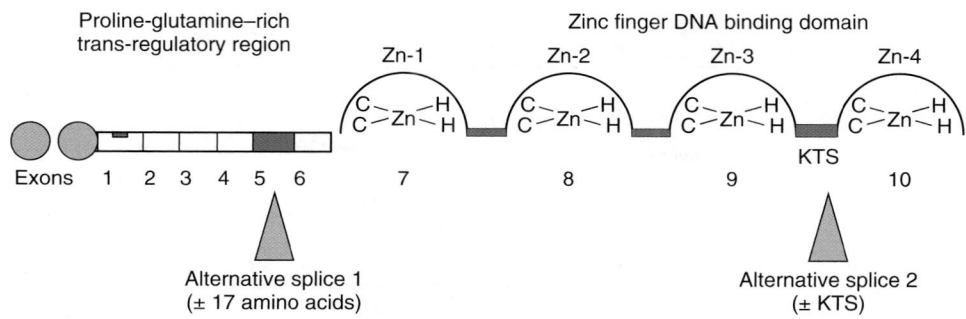

Figure 23-19 Schematic diagram shows the structure of WT1 and the changes associated with exon 5 and exon 9 (addition of lysine, threonine, and serine) in +KTS isoforms. Many point mutations associated with Denys-Drash syndrome are located within zinc fingers 2 and 3 (especially Arg394). Mutations affecting the exon 9 splice site are associated with Frasier syndrome. (Modified from Koziell A, Grundy R. Frasier and Denys-Drash syndromes: different disorders or part of a spectrum? *Arch Dis Child.* 1999;81:365-369, used with permission of the BMJ Publishing Group, copyright 1999.)

female phenotype with müllerian structures, and later-onset nephropathy (i.e., focal segmental glomerulosclerosis) that usually causes renal failure in the second decade of life. There is a high risk of gonadal tumors such as gonadoblastoma in patients with Frasier syndrome.[22] In practice, Denys-Drash syndrome and Frasier syndrome may represent a continuum of phenotypes rather than distinct conditions.[232] Severe forms of these conditions can present with congenital nephrotic syndrome, whereas milder variants have been reported, for example, in a man with hypospadias and late-onset nephropathy.[233] Taken together, these cases highlight the importance of considering this diagnosis in 46,XY DSD and of performing urinalysis for proteinuria in children with 46,XY DSD.

Management of patients with *WT1* mutations includes monitoring and treatment of renal function and assessment for Wilms tumor, as well as gonadectomy in individuals with Frasier syndrome and in patients with Denys-Drash syndrome who have a Y chromosome if the gonads cannot be monitored.[22] Meacham syndrome (i.e., DSD, cardiac defects, and diaphragmatic hernia) also may result from changes in *WT1*.[234]

Gata-Binding Protein 4: GATA4. GATA4 is a four–zinc finger transcription factor involved in early testis development and heart development. Haploinsufficiency of *GATA4* or heterozygous loss-of-function changes are well established in a range of cardiac defects such as atrial and ventricular septal defects, and more recently, heterozygous *GATA* mutations have been shown to cause testicular dysgenesis with or without cardiac anomalies.[61] These mutations can be transmitted by a mother in a sex-limited dominant manner. Reported changes may disrupt interactions between GATA4 and its cofactor, friend of GATA 2 (FOG2, also known as ZFPM2).

Friend of GATA2 (FOG2): ZFPM2. FOG2 is a key coregulator, and recently missense mutations in the genes encoding FOG2 *(ZFPM2)* have been described two individuals with 46,XY gonadal dysgenesis.[62] The point mutations affect interactions with GATA4 and, in one case, have been described previously in patients with cardiac defects, highlighting the very variable penetrance of gonadal and cardiac phenotypes following disruption of the GATA4/FOG2 complex.

Chromobox Homolog 2: CBX2. Chromobox homolog 2 *(CBX2)* is a human homolog of the polycomb protein M33. Deletion of its gene causes XY sex reversal in mice. Loss-of-function mutations in *CBX2* were described in a 46,XY girl with a uterus and ovaries who was diagnosed by prenatal karyotyping, but at present *CBX2* variants in humans are rare.[58]

Sex-Determining Region of the Y Chromosome: SRY. The sequence of events leading to the identification of *SRY* as the primary testis-determining gene and the actions of SRY in testis development were described earlier. SRY is a 204–amino acid HMG box transcription factor that is encoded by a single exon on the Y chromosome (Yp11.3) (see Fig. 23-5).[97] The discovery of inactivating mutations in SRY in patients with 46,XY gonadal dysgenesis confirmed the key role played by this factor in testis determination in humans.[32]

Approximately 10% of individuals with the complete form of 46,XY gonadal dysgenesis have inactivating mutations in *SRY*.[97] Most of the mutations occur in the HMG box DNA-binding domain of the SRY protein (Fig. 23-20), a region that is involved in binding and bending of DNA.[97] Rare mutations in the 5' and 3' flanking regions lead, respectively, to complete and partial gonadal dysgenesis.[235] The HMG box contains at least two nuclear localization signals that bind calmodulin/exportin 4 and importin B. Mutations in these nuclear localization signal domains in the HMG box of SRY result in failure to transport the SRY protein into the nucleus and subtle alterations in nuclear import and export can lead to XY gonadal dysgenesis.[101] Most individuals with *SRY* mutations are girls who have no pubertal development (Swyer syndrome). Gonadoblastoma risk in this group is high.

SRY Box 9: SOX9. Heterozygous mutations of the autosomal *SOX9* gene (17q24-q25) cause camptomelic dysplasia.[101,109,110] Features of this condition include bowed long bones, hypoplastic scapula, a deformed pelvis, 11 pairs of ribs, a small thoracic cage, cleft palate, macrocephaly, micrognathia, hypertelorism, and a variety of cardiac and renal defects. Death from respiratory distress often occurs in the neonatal period, but long-term survival has been reported.

SOX9 is emerging as an important testis-determining gene in its own right, and it may be one of the key regulators of testis determination downstream of *SRY* (see "Testis Determination"). Consistent with this hypothesis, three fourths of affected 46,XY patients have dysgenetic gonads, but a complete spectrum of genital phenotypes can be seen, from completely male to completely female appearance.[97] Histologic examination of the gonads from 46,XY patients with ambiguous or female external genitalia shows various degrees of testicular dysgenesis extending to streak gonads with primordial follicles or even ovaries.[236] Müllerian structures may or may not be present, depending on the degree of gonadal dysgenesis. Affected 46,XX females have normal external genitalia and apparently normal ovaries.

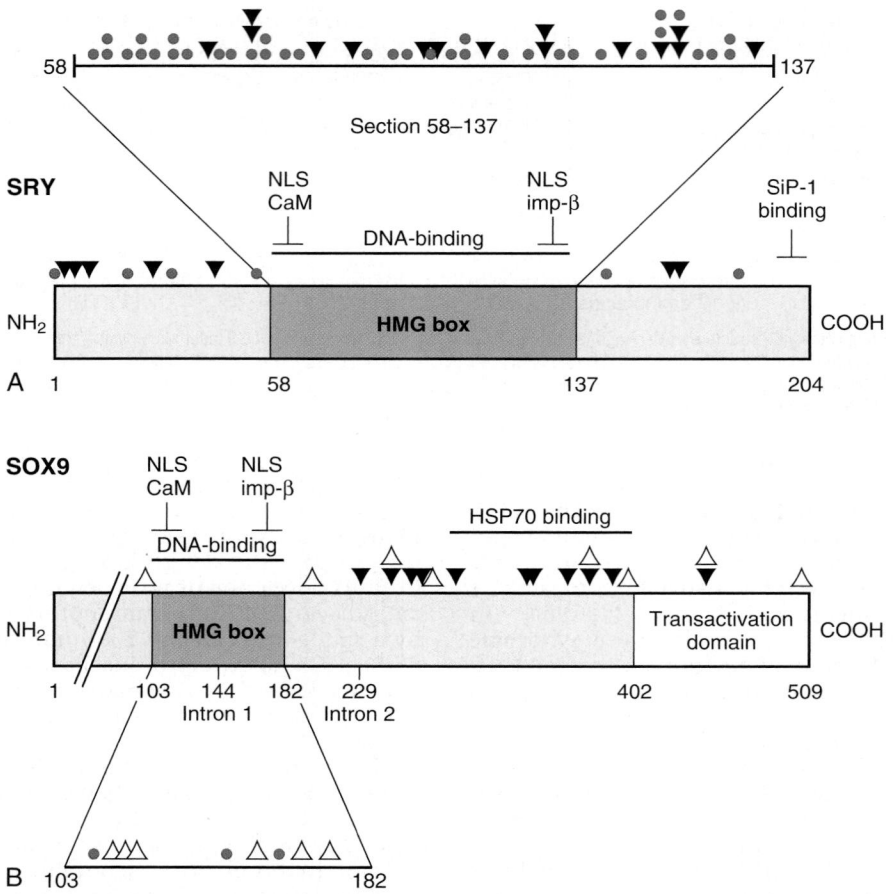

Figure 23-20 Structure of human SRY and SOX9 proteins and a selection of reported mutations. **A,** Diagram of SRY. The high-mobility group (HMG) box is an 80–amino acid, DNA-binding domain with nuclear localization signals (NLSs) at either end, one of which binds calmodulin (CaM) or exportin-4 and the other importin-β (imp-β). The last seven amino acids of SRY can bind to either of the PDZ domains found in SRY-interacting protein 1 (SiP-1). The *solid circles* indicate missense mutations reported in the SRY protein that affect testicular development and cluster within the HMG box. Nonsense and frameshift mutations in SRY are indicated by *solid triangles.* **B,** Diagram of SOX9. SOX9 has an HMG box with two NLSs, similar to SRY. However, SOX9 is encoded by three exons, binds to heat shock protein 70 (HSP70), and has a transactivation domain at the carboxy-terminal end, unlike SRY. Selected mutations causing 46,XY DSD and camptomelic dysplasia are indicated by the *solid circles* (missense) and solid triangles (nonsense and frameshift). Mutations that cause only camptomelia or a bony phenotype in 46,XY males or affect 46,XX females are indicated by *open triangles.*

The locus for camptomelic dysplasia with 46,XY DSD was mapped to 17q24.3-q25.1 after studies of three patients with balanced, de novo reciprocal translocations and the proposal of *SOX9* as a candidate gene based on expression studies in the mouse. Subsequently, missense, nonsense, frameshift, and splice junction mutations have been detected in *SOX9* in patients with camptomelic dysplasia with or without gonadal dysgenesis.[97] These mutations are usually heterozygous de novo changes. In one kindred, multiple siblings were affected due to germline mosaicism for a *SOX9* mutation in a parent.[236] The gonadal phenotype in this kindred varied in the two affected 46,XY siblings: one of them had dysgenetic gonads, and the other was reported to have normal ovaries.

The *SOX9* gene has three exons and two introns; it encodes a 509-residue protein that contains an HMG box with 71% homology to that of the SRY protein and a C-terminal, *trans*-activation domain (see Fig. 23-20). Unlike SRY, in which most mutations are located within the HMG box, SOX9 mutations are located throughout the protein, with little relation between functional domains and phenotype. Chromosomal translocations that disrupt regulatory elements upstream of the *SOX9* promoter can be associated with a less severe phenotype or camptomelic dysplasia without gonadal abnormalities. Heterozygous

changes that allow residual DNA binding and transactivation may also be associated with the acamptomelic variant and variable or absent DSD.

Mitogen-Activated Protein Kinase Kinase Kinase-1: MAP3K1. MAP3K1 is one of several kinase signaling pathways involved in organogenesis, and heterozygous splice site or point mutations in MAP3K1 have been described in several families and individuals with impaired testis development.[64] MAP3K1 is expressed in early testis cords and Sertoli cells in mice, and disruption of *MAP3K1* has been described in diverse phenotypes ranging from 46,XY complete testicular dysgenesis to hypospadias and micropenis with cryptorchidism. Familial cases have a clear autosomal dominant inheritance. In two individuals with nonfamilial gonadal dysgenesis, changes in codon 189 (p.Leu189Pro, p.Leu189Arg) were found that altered the phosphorylation of the downstream targets, p38 and ERK1/2, and enhanced binding of RHOA to the MAP3K1 complex.

Desert Hedgehog: DHH. The hedgehog signaling pathways play an important role in many aspects of neuronal, skeletal, and endocrine development. A homozygous mutation in the desert hedgehog gene *(DHH)* was reported in a patient with partial gonadal dysgenesis and minifascicular neuropathy.[121] Subsequently, a number of *DHH* changes were reported in patients with complete 46,XY gonadal dysgenesis or Leydig cell defects, with or without apparent neurologic features.[122]

Aristaless-Related Homeobox, X-Linked Gene: ARX. ARX is a transcription factor that plays a central role in neuronal migration, and the *Arx* knockout mouse has a profound myelination defect. *ARX* was considered a candidate gene for the X-linked lissencephaly ambiguous genitalia (XLAG) syndrome, and mutations in *ARX* have been described in several patients with this condition.[128] This unusual form of lissencephaly is associated with severe epilepsy and thermal instability. The genital abnormality most likely represents a defect in Leydig cell function. Additional *ARX* mutations have been described in patients with neurologic defects (e.g., infantile spasms) without significant DSDs.

Testis-Specific Protein, Y-Linked–like 1 Gene: TSPYL1. An association between 46,XY gonadal dysgenesis and sudden infant death syndrome was characterized in a large Amish kindred and named *sudden infant death, dysgenetic testes* (SIDDT).[237] An autosomal recessive gene responsible for this condition, *TSPYL1*, encodes a protein of unknown function that may be involved in chromatin remodeling. Additional variants of *TSPYL1* and 46,XY DSD have been described.[238]

Mastermind-like Domain-Containing 1: MAMLD1. *MAMLD1* (formerly called *CXORF6*) is a gene on the X chromosome that encodes a protein expressed in the developing testes. Hemizygous mutations in *MAMLD1* were originally described in boys with isolated severe hypospadias, although a range of severities has been described.[129,239] *MAMLD1* disruption results in a defect in fetal Leydig cell development and function.

Chromosomal Rearrangements Associated with Gonadal Dysgenesis. Abnormalities of genital development are associated with a number of chromosomal deletions, duplications, and rearrangements. The most frequently seen changes are deletions of 9p24-pter, 10q25-qter, and Xq13 and duplications of Xp21.

Deletions of 9p24-pter likely disrupt *DMRT1*, a gene with sex-specific homologs in *Drosophila* (*double sex* gene) and *Caenorhabditis elegans* (*Mab3*) that is expressed in early gonad development (see "Normal Sex Development").[123,124] Impaired gonadal development and 46,XY DSD are well-established features of the 9p-deletion syndrome, suggesting that haploinsufficiency of the *DMRT* locus may be a cause of testicular dysgenesis in humans.[127] Very recently, a partial deletion of *DMRT1* and dominant negative point mutation in *DMRT1* causing DSD have been seen.[125,126]

Terminal deletions of chromosome 10 (10q25-qter) are frequently associated with urogenital abnormalities and sometimes with complete gonadal dysgenesis.[133] The gene in this locus has not been identified.

Deletions of Xq13.3 and of the tip of chromosome 16p cause α-thalassemia mental retardation (ATR) syndromes that may have gonadal dysgenesis as part of the phenotype.[131] The Xq13.3 locus contains the transcription factor gene *ATRX* (also known as *XH2* or *XNP*), and the *SOX8* gene is located on 16p.[132]

Duplications of the Xp21.3 region that contains the *DAX1 (NROB1)* gene can cause abnormal testis development in some cases.[86] The role of *DAX1* and the *WNT4* pathway (duplication 1p35) in opposing testis development was discussed previously (see "Development of Reproductive Systems").[86,88]

Several other studies using array comparative genomic hybridization or single-nucleotide polymorphism (SNP) analysis have been reported and have proposed other candidate regions for testicular dysgenesis.[136,137]

Syndromic Causes of 46,XY Disorders of Sex Development. In addition to the specific syndromes outlined earlier, various degrees of testicular dysgenesis and impaired genital development (e.g., hypospadias, cryptorchidism, scrotal transposition) are seen in many discrete syndromes.[134,135] In some situations, a genetic basis has been identified, but in many cases the cause is unknown. Syndromic associations of 46,XY DSD may be more prevalent than originally thought and have been reviewed in detail elsewhere.[134,135]

46,XY DSD is often associated with intrauterine growth restriction (IUGR). Monozygotic twins can show disparate genital development, with the growth-restricted twin having ambiguous genitalia and the larger twin appearing as a normal male. The mechanism of this association is unclear and may represent a shared genetic cause, or a common epigenetic or developmental event affecting fetal growth, placental function, and reproductive development. More common genetic causes of 46,XY DSD (e.g., mutations of SRY, SF1, androgen receptor, and steroidogenic enzymes) are rarely found in this group of IUGR patients (personal observation).

Disorders of Androgen Synthesis

Defects anywhere along the pathway of androgen synthesis and target organ action can result in impaired androgenization and 46,XY DSD (formerly referred to as male pseudohermaphroditism) (see Table 23-6 and Fig. 23-10).

Cholesterol Synthesis Defects: Smith-Lemli-Opitz Syndrome. Smith-Lemli-Opitz syndrome has a broad phenotypic spectrum but typically includes microcephaly, developmental delay, cardiac defects, ptosis, upturned nose, micrognathia, cleft palate, polydactyly, syndactyly of toes (especially the second and third toes), severe hypospadias, micropenis, and growth failure.[240] The abnormalities of the external genitalia in approximately 65% of 46,XY patients vary from micropenis and hypospadias to complete failure of androgenization, resulting in a female phenotype.

Smith-Lemli-Opitz syndrome is caused by a deficiency of 7-dehydrocholesterol reductase (3β-hydroxysterol Δ7-reductase [DHCR7]), the phylogenetically conserved sterol-sensing domain–containing enzyme required for the last step in the biosynthetic pathway from acetate to cholesterol. Cholesterol is necessary as a substrate for steroid synthesis, and intermediates of cholesterol synthesis may have important interactions with hedgehog signaling pathways.

The syndrome is diagnosed by finding elevated plasma levels of 7-dehydrocholesterol (7-DHC) and low levels of cholesterol. The *DHCR7* gene maps to 11q12-q13, and more than 150 mutations have been described.[241] Measurement of serum 7-DHC should be considered in all underandrogenized males with relevant phenotypic features, however mild. Testis development is apparently normal, and normal, elevated, or low concentrations of plasma testosterone have been described in affected male infants with intact HPG function. Compromised adrenal function can sometimes occur.

Luteinizing Hormone Receptor Mutations. Mutations in the LH/hCG receptor cause impaired responsiveness to hCG and LH, resulting in Leydig cell agenesis or hypoplasia.[242] Phenotypically, the external genitalia vary from a female appearance to a male with a micropenis (Table 23-7). Müllerian derivatives are absent in patients, and rudimentary wolffian derivatives may be present, even in some patients with severely underandrogenized external genitalia. This finding may reflect some early hCG-independent mechanisms of testosterone synthesis between 8 and 10 weeks' gestation.[4] Small, undescended testes are usually found in the inguinal region in the most severe forms of this Leydig cell hypoplasia. Patients with milder phenotypes may have appropriately descended testes of relatively normal size because the Leydig cell population contributes only about 10% to testicular volume. On histologic examination, the testes lack distinct Leydig cells in prepubertal patients. Postpubertal patients have absent or decreased numbers of Leydig cells without Reinke crystalloids, normal-appearing

Sertoli cells, and discrete seminiferous tubules with spermatogenic arrest. This observation highlights the important role of intratesticular androgen in the final stages of sperm maturation.

The typical biochemical profile of patients with Leydig cell hypoplasia includes elevated basal and luteinizing hormone–releasing hormone (LHRH)–stimulated LH (and FSH) levels in early infancy or at puberty. In childhood, when the GnRH pulse generator is quiescent, basal LH levels may sometimes be detected above the normal range. Plasma levels of 17-OHP, androstenedione, and testosterone are low, with little or no response to prolonged hCG stimulation. Plasma LH falls after testosterone administration. Less marked biochemical changes can occur with milder forms of this condition.

More than 30 different homozygous or compound heterozygous mutations have been reported in the LH/hCG receptor gene (LHCGR) in individuals with various forms of this condition (Fig. 23-21).[243,244] The original reports of Kremer and colleagues[243] and Latronico and associates[244] described homozygous Ala593Pro and Arg554Stop mutations, respectively, in 46,XY phenotypic females with Leydig cell hypoplasia, hypergonadotropic hypogonadism, and no testosterone response to hCG stimulation. An affected 46,XX sister showed normal sexual maturation at puberty but an elevated LH level and amenorrhea, demonstrating that the LH receptor is not necessary for estrogen

TABLE 23-7
Clinical Features of Leydig Cell Hypoplasia in 46,XY Individuals

Karyotype	46,XY
Inheritance	Autosomal recessive; mutations in *LHCGR* gene
Genitalia	Female, hypospadias, or micropenis
Wolffian duct derivatives	Hypoplastic
Müllerian duct derivatives	Absent
Gonads	Testes
Biochemical features	Underandrogenization with variable insufficiency of sex hormone production at puberty
Hormone profile	Low T and DHT; elevated LH (and FSH); exaggerated LH response to LHRH stimulation; poor T and DHT response to hCG stimulation

DHT, dihydrotestosterone; FSH, follicle-stimulating hormone; hCG, human chorionic gonadotropin; LH, luteinizing hormone; LHCGR, the LH or hCG receptor; LHRH, luteinizing hormone–releasing hormone; T, testosterone.

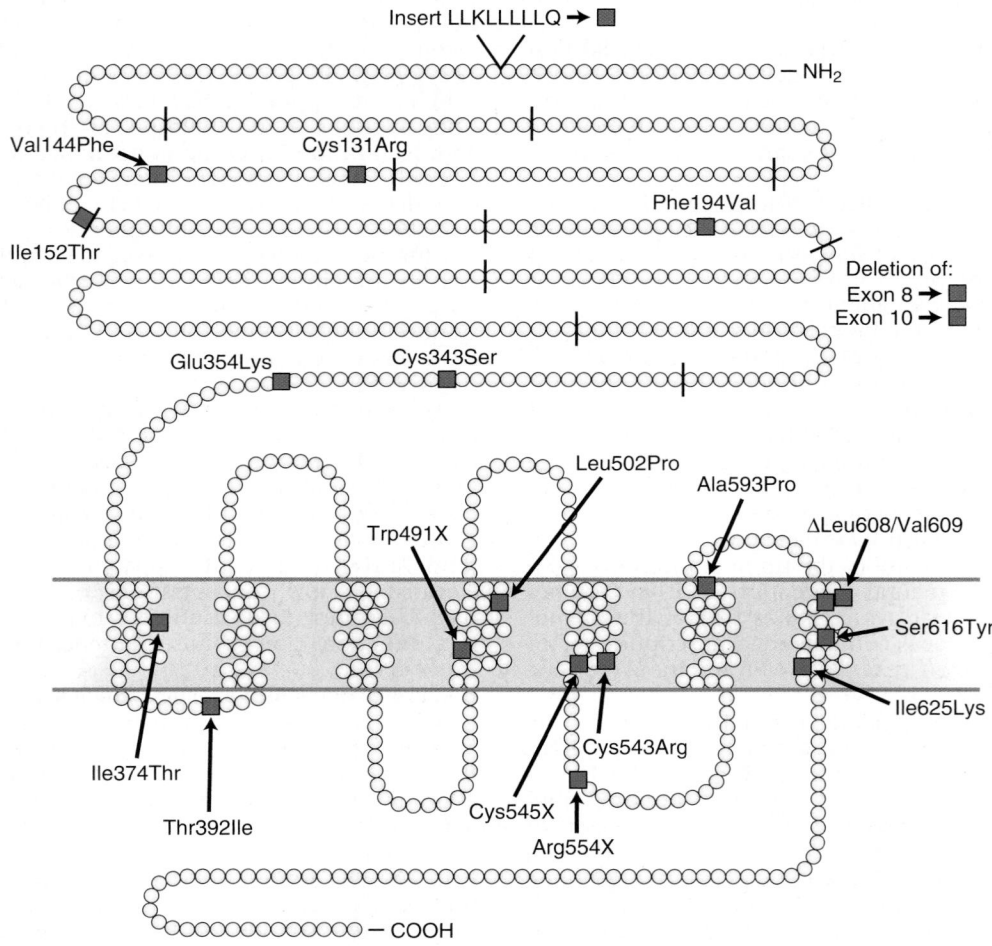

Figure 23-21 Diagram of the seven transmembrane domain of the luteinizing hormone/human chorionic gonadotropin (LH/hCG) receptor with selected inactivating missense mutations shown by squares. Most of these changes are associated with marked underandrogenization. However, the changes at residues 616 and 625 in the seventh transmembrane domain are associated with a milder phenotype of micropenis.

synthesis but is necessary for normal ovulation in females. These mutations impair hCG stimulation of intracellular cyclic adenosine monophosphate (cAMP) in in vitro studies through disturbances in hCG binding, intracellular signaling, or receptor stability and trafficking, depending on the nature of the change. Defects in a novel cryptic exon of the LH receptor (exon 6A) have also been described as a cause of 46,XY DSD.[245] Partial loss-of-function mutations in the LH/hCG receptor causing milder phenotypes such as micropenis have tended to localize within the seventh transmembrane domain (Ser616Tyr, Ile625Lys) (see Fig. 23-21).[244,246] Individuals with complete Leydig cell hypoplasia are usually reared as females and require estrogens at puberty. Gonadectomy is usually performed. If a male gender assignment is chosen, testosterone supplements may be given in early infancy and to support puberty. The risk of gonadal malignancy is unknown.

Steroidogenic Acute Regulatory Protein Defects. Steroidogenic acute regulatory protein (StAR) is a 30-kDa mitochondrial protein that is present in the adrenal gland and gonads. It plays a key role in facilitating the rapid movement of cholesterol from the outer to the inner mitochondrial membrane.[152,247] This process is necessary to allow de novo steroid biosynthesis in response to an increase in ACTH or angiotensin II in the adrenal gland or an LH pulse in the gonad. The exact mechanism by which StAR facilitates this movement is unclear, but it is likely that the protein remains on the mitochondrial surface in a molten globule structure. Although a limited amount of cholesterol transfer is StAR independent (14%), this protein certainly plays a central role in the acute regulation of adrenal and gonadal steroidogenesis.

Consistent with these actions, patients with recessively inherited defects in StAR develop a severe form of primary adrenal failure called *lipoid congenital adrenal hyperplasia* (lipoid CAH).[248,249] Patients with this condition tend to present with severe glucocorticoid deficiency (e.g., hypoglycemia, hyperpigmentation) early in life and progressive mineralocorticoid insufficiency resulting in hyponatremia, hyperkalemia, dehydration, acidosis, and collapse (Table 23-8). Little or no C18, C19, and C21 steroids are detectable in plasma or urine, even after corticotropin or hCG

stimulation. Females (46,XX) with lipoid CAH have normal genitalia and a uterus. In 46,XY individuals, mutations in *STAR* typically cause a marked deficiency in testosterone synthesis by fetal Leydig cells so that female-typical genitalia are seen. Testes may be abdominal, inguinal, or labial. A blind vaginal pouch is present, and müllerian structures have regressed. A karyotype should be performed in all apparent girls presenting with early-onset adrenal failure.

The typical finding in lipoid CAH is lipid accumulation within steroidogenic cells. In the steroid-deficient state, the tropic drive by ACTH, angiotensin II, and LH causes increased cholesterol uptake and synthesis by steroidogenic cells. Coupled with the inability of StAR to facilitate cholesterol movement into mitochondria, this leads to marked accumulation of cholesterol in cells and results in the appearance of enlarged, lipid-laden adrenal glands sometimes seen on MRI or computed tomography (CT). Eventually, cholesterol accumulation causes engorgement and results in disruption of the structural and functional integrity of the cell—the two-hit hypothesis (Fig. 23-22).[249] StAR is not necessary for placental progesterone production, unlike P450scc (CYP11A1).

The two-hit hypothesis also explains why 46,XX girls with lipoid CAH show evidence of estrogenization and breast development at puberty but have progressive hypergonadotropic hypogonadism.[249,250] Follicular cells are relatively quiescent in utero and before puberty and are therefore undamaged. At the beginning of each cycle, they are recruited, and a small amount of estradiol can be produced as a result of StAR-independent mechanisms. This can occur until the follicular cells are engorged and rendered nonfunctional. Puberty can occur, but any cycles are anovulatory because progesterone synthesis in the latter half of the cycle is disturbed. Without treatment, polycystic ovaries and progressive ovarian failure usually ensue.

Although more than 40 different StAR mutations have been described in patients from around the world, lipoid CAH is especially prevalent in Japan and Korea, where it is the second most common steroidogenic disorder after CYP21 deficiency (Fig. 23-23). Most Japanese patients and virtually all Korean patients harbor the Gln258Stop mutation, which is estimated to be carried by 1 in 300 Japanese people.[251] Other geographic clusters include the Leu260Pro mutation in patients of Swiss ancestry, Arg182His in Eastern Saudi Arabia, and Arg182Leu in Palestinians. Most of these mutations show complete loss of function. However, a nonclassic form of lipoid CAH has been described that is caused by point mutations in StAR and retains approximately 20% function.[252] These patients present with progressive glucocorticoid deficiency between 2 and 4 years of age; affected males have normal androgenization of the external genitalia but may be at risk of hypoandrogenism or reduced fertility later in life. StAR mutations with intermediate function may also be associated with hypospadias and milder adrenal failure.[253] These partial loss-of-function changes tend to affect amino acids (codons 187, 188, 192, 221) around the cholesterol binding pocket.[254]

Management of classic lipoid CAH includes glucocorticoid and mineralocorticoid replacement and salt supplementation in early life. Gonadectomy is usually performed in individuals with a 46,XY karyotype. Males with nonclassic CLAH need careful follow-up to ensure adequate testosterone production in puberty and adulthood. Estrogen treatment is given to induce puberty and is administered to 46,XX females when gonadal failure occurs.

P450 Side-Chain Cleavage Enzyme Deficiency. P450scc (CYP11A1) is the mitochondrial enzyme that converts cholesterol to pregnenolone by three distinct enzymatic reactions: 20α-hydroxylation, 22-hydroxylation, and cleavage

TABLE 23-8	
Clinical Features of Lipoid CAH in 46,XY Individuals	
Karyotype	46,XY
Inheritance	Autosomal recessive; mutations in *STAR* gene
Genitalia	Female; sometimes ambiguous, hypospadias, or male
Wolffian duct derivatives	Hypoplastic or normal
Müllerian duct derivatives	Absent
Gonads	Testes
Biochemical and physiologic features	Severe adrenal insufficiency in infancy with salt loss; lack of pubertal development; rare nonclassic cases associated with isolated glucocorticoid deficiency
Hormone profile	Usually deficiency of glucocorticoids, mineralocorticoids, and sex steroids except in nonclassic cases in which a predominant defect in glucocorticoid production is seen (similar to familial glucocorticoid deficiency)

CAH, congenital adrenal hyperplasia; StAR, steroidogenic acute regulatory (protein).

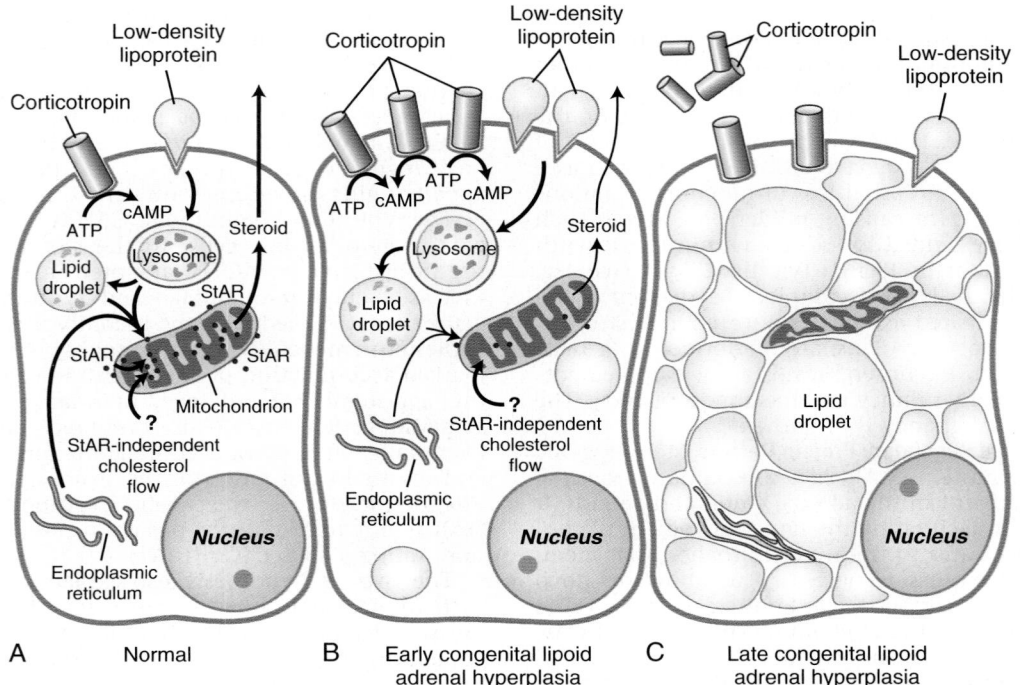

Figure 23-22 Model of the steroid-synthesizing cell (adrenal/gonadal) showing conversion of cholesterol to steroids. **A,** Cholesterol from low-density lipoprotein, from cholesterol esters stored in lipid droplets, and from endogenous synthesis in the endoplasmic reticulum is transported from the outer mitochondrial membrane to the inner membrane. This transport is facilitated by the steroidogenic acute regulatory protein (StAR) and by other, StAR-independent, mechanisms. In the mitochondria, steroid synthesis begins with the conversion of cholesterol to Δ^5-pregnenolone by the enzyme CYP11A1 (P450scc). **B,** In patients with lipoid congenital adrenal hyperplasia, a mutation in the gene encoding StAR results in little or no activity of the mutant StAR, greatly reducing cholesterol transport into the mitochondria. Low levels of steroidogenesis by mechanisms independent of StAR can occur; however, increased secretion of corticotropin (or luteinizing hormone or follicle-stimulating hormone) results in cholesterol accumulation in the cells as lipid droplets. **C,** Continued stimulation and resultant accumulation of cholesterol causes engorgement of these cells, with mechanical and chemical perturbation of cell function. This results in primary adrenal insufficiency and impaired androgen biosynthesis by fetal Leydig cells. Females with lipoid congenital adrenal hyperplasia feminize at puberty and menstruate but have progressive hypergonadotropic hypogonadism. This may occur because the follicular cells are relatively quiescent in utero and before puberty and therefore are undamaged. At the beginning of each cycle, follicles are recruited, and a small amount of estradiol can be produced as a result of StAR-independent mechanisms. This can occur until the follicular cells are engorged and rendered nonfunctional. ATP, adenosine triphosphate; cAMP, cyclic adenosine monophosphate. (From Bose HS, Sujiwara T, Strauss JF III, et al. The pathophysiology and genetics of congenital lipoid adrenal hyperplasia. *N Engl J Med.* 1996;335:1870-1878, used with permission of the Massachusetts Medical Society, copyright 1996.)

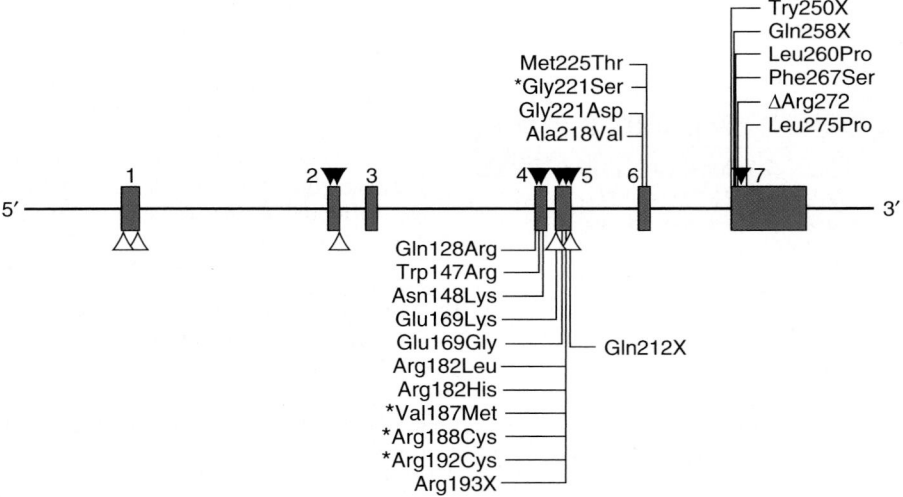

Figure 23-23 Diagram of selected mutations identified in the *STAR* gene associated with lipoid congenital adrenal hyperplasia. Numbered *solid boxes* depict the exons. The three-letter abbreviations for amino acids are used to indicate the position of missense mutations; X indicates a nonsense (stop) mutation; insertions and deletions resulting in frameshift mutations *(solid triangles)* and splice site mutations *(open triangles)* are shown. Although *STAR* mutations are common in Japan, Korea, and regions of the Middle East, an increasing number of sporadic changes in the steroidogenic acute regulatory (StAR) protein are being detected in other countries. Missense mutations at residues 187,188, 192, and 221 *(asterisks)* have been associated with a nonclassic late-onset phenotype of glucocorticoid insufficiency.

TABLE 23-9
Clinical Features of CYP11A1 Deficiency in 46,XY Individuals

Karyotype	46,XY
Inheritance	Autosomal recessive; mutations in CYP11A1 gene
Genitalia	Female; rarely ambiguous or hypospadias
Wolffian duct derivatives	Hypoplastic or normal
Müllerian duct derivatives	Absent
Gonads	Testes (or absent)
Biochemical and physiologic features	Severe adrenal insufficiency in infancy with salt loss ranging to milder adrenal insufficiency with onset in childhood; prematurity associated in one case
Hormone profile	Usually deficiency of glucocorticoids, mineralocorticoids, and sex steroids

CYP11A1, cytochrome P450 side-chain cleavage enzyme.

TABLE 23-10
Clinical Features of HSD3B2 Deficiency in 46,XY Individuals

Karyotype	46,XY
Inheritance	Autosomal recessive; mutations in HSD3B2 gene
Genitalia	Ambiguous; hypospadias
Wolffian duct derivatives	Normal
Müllerian duct derivatives	Absent
Gonads	Testes
Biochemical and physiologic features	Severe adrenal insufficiency in infancy; poor virilization at puberty with gynecomastia *Mild form:* no mineralocorticoid deficiency, premature adrenarche → mild virilization
Hormone profile	Increased concentrations of Δ^5 C21- and C19-steroids (e.g., 17-hydroxypregnenolone/cortisol ratio response to corticotropin, 17-hydroxypregnenolone, DHEA suppressible by dexamethasone)

DHEA, dehydroepiandrosterone; HSD3B2, 3β-hydroxysteroid dehydrogenase type 2.

of the cholesterol side chain. P450scc is therefore responsible for the first and rate-limiting step in steroid synthesis, which is necessary for pregnenolone production by the placenta and for mineralocorticoid, glucocorticoid, and androgen production by the adrenal glands and gonads.

Although a natural model of lipoid CAH due to P450scc deficiency exists in the rabbit, it was thought that severe loss of P450scc activity in humans would be incompatible with survival. Placental progesterone production is necessary to support pregnancy (i.e., luteoplacental shift) after the second trimester in higher primates but not in rodents. However, complete disruption of P450 activity due to a homozygous frameshift mutation in *CYP11A1* has been reported in a 46,XY infant with a female phenotype and severe early-onset, salt-losing adrenal failure.[255] An increasing number of other mutations in P450scc have also been described, initially in 46,XY phenotypic females with severe salt-losing adrenal failure (Table 23-9).[256,257] More recently, partial loss-of-function defects in P450scc have been described in boys with hypospadias who developed adrenal failure in late childhood, and milder changes in *CYP11A1* have been reported in children with primary adrenal insufficiency without DSD.[258-260] This condition is now well established as a cause of combined adrenal and gonadal failure, as well as isolated adrenal insufficiency. Long-term follow-up of these adrenal insufficient patients may be needed to monitor testicular function and fertility with time. Molecular analysis is needed to differentiate this P450scc deficiency from StAR deficiency, though it seems that patients with P450scc deficiency rarely have significant lipoid enlargement of the adrenal glands.[257]

3β-Hydroxysteroid Dehydrogenase/Δ⁴,⁵-Isomerase Type 2 Deficiency.
3β-HSD deficiency is a rare cause of CAH and is one of the steroidogenic deficiencies that affects both adrenal and gonadal steroid production. The autosomal recessive disorder is a consequence of mutations in *HSD3B2*, the gene encoding the 3β-HSD/Δ⁴,⁵-isomerase type 2 isozyme, which is expressed mainly in the adrenals and gonads. This enzyme catalyzes a crucial step in the biosynthesis of all steroid hormones, the conversion of Δ^5- to Δ^4-steroids (see Fig. 23-10).[261] The other 3β-HSD isoenzyme in humans, HSD3B1, is expressed in the placenta and in peripheral tissues such as the skin (mainly sebaceous glands), breast, and prostate; it is not associated with CAH.

Classic HSD3B2 deficiency is subdivided into salt-losing and non–salt-losing forms (Table 23-10). Severely disruptive changes in HSD3B2 cause salt-losing adrenal insufficiency soon after birth. The external genitalia are usually atypical, with a small penis, severe hypospadias, partial labioscrotal fusion, a urogenital sinus, and a blind vaginal

pouch. Examples of mutations that severely disrupt enzymatic activity usually present with salt loss (Fig. 23-24).[262-264] Sometimes these mutations are found in a compound heterozygous state. In contrast, mutations such as Ala245Pro retain considerable enzyme activity (2-10%) and have been found in males with penoscrotal hypospadias and no salt loss. A late-onset form of HSD3B2 deficiency usually manifests as premature pubarche and idiopathic hirsutism in females. The biochemical profile of classic HSD3B2 deficiency is based on an elevated ratio of Δ^5- to Δ^4-steroids, determined in plasma or urine. The most specific plasma analyte to confirm the diagnosis is 17-hydroxypregnenolone, which is present at levels greater than 100 nmol/L basally or after ACTH stimulation.[265] However, this steroid is measured only in specialist laboratories. The concentrations of Δ^4-steroids such as 17-OHP and androstenedione may also be elevated in HSD3B2 deficiency because of peripheral HSD3B1 activity. In a neonatal screening program, an elevated 17-OHP level in a salt-losing person with HSD3B2 deficiency may be potentially misdiagnosed as CYP21 deficiency.[266,267]

Children with HSD3B2 deficiency need glucocorticoid and sometimes mineralocorticoid replacement. A recent study of the Amish population, where the c.35G>A founder effect is seen, has suggested that some children need standard doses to supress ACTH, whereas others need higher doses.[267] Undertreatment can be associated with advanced skeletal maturation and early puberty due to sex steroid excess in childhood, whereas overtreatment is associated with iatrogenic complications.[267] Gynecomastia can occur at puberty in affected males and females. This is presumably the result of HSD3B1-mediated peripheral conversion of Δ^5-C19-steroids to Δ^4-C19-steroids and aromatization to estrogens.[268] Normal puberty has been reported in males with a null mutation in the *HSD3B2* gene, but puberty needs close monitoring to ensure adequate androgens are produced, and data on fertility are still limited.[268]

17α-Hydroxylase/17,20-Lyase Deficiency.
P450c17 (CYP17) is a microsomal enzyme with 17α-hydroxylase and 17,20-lyase activity that is expressed in the adrenals and gonads but not in the placenta or in ovarian granulosa cells.[269,270] The 17α-hydroxylase action of P450c17 catalyzes the conversion of pregnenolone (Δ^5) to 17-hydroxypregnenolone and the conversion of progesterone (Δ^4) to 17-OHP (see

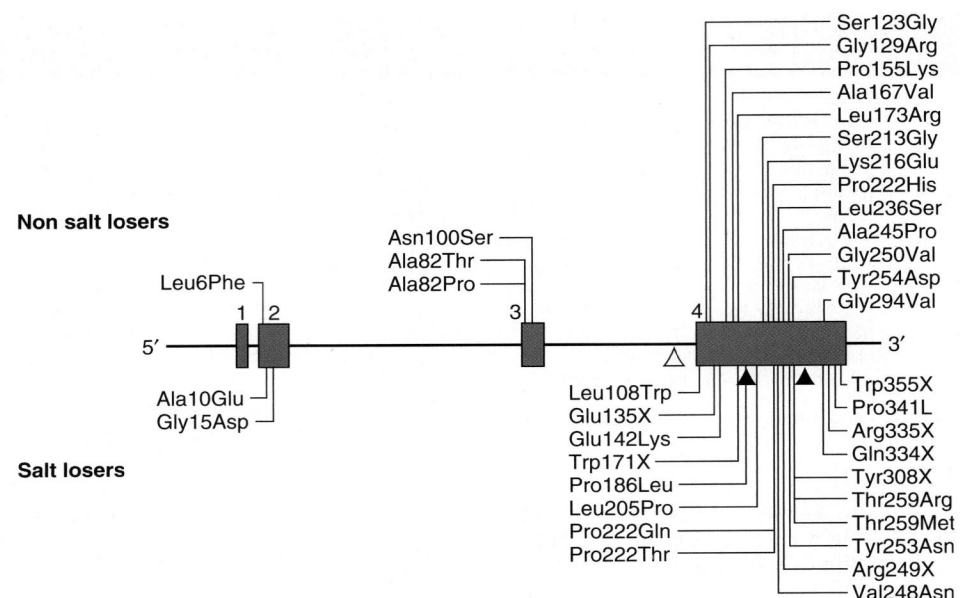

Figure 23-24 Diagram of the 3β-hydroxysteroid dehydrogenase type 2 gene *(HSD3B2)* shows the mutations that result in deficiency of the enzyme. Changes associated with salt loss are shown below and non–salt loss above. The numbered *solid boxes* depict the exons. Mutations are subdivided according to their association with salt-losing and non–salt-losing states. The three-letter abbreviations for amino acids are used to indicate the position of missense mutations; X indicates a nonsense (stop) mutation; insertions and deletions resulting in frameshift mutations *(solid triangles)* and splice site mutations *(open triangles)* are shown.

Fig. 23-10). The 17,20-lyase action of P450c17 can convert 17-hydroxypregnenolone (Δ^5) to DHEA and 17-OHP (Δ^4) to androstenedione (see Fig. 23-10). P450c17 is bound to the smooth endoplasmic reticulum, where it accepts electrons from a specific flavoprotein, reduced nicotinamide adenine dinucleotide phosphate (NADPH)-POR. The 17,20-lyase activity of P450c17 is favored by the presence of Δ^5 substrates, redox partners such as POR and cytochrome b_5, and serine phosphorylation. Unlike in rodents, the Δ^5-17,20-lyase activity of human P450c17 is 50 times more efficient than its Δ^4-17,20-lyase activity; therefore, very little androstenedione is formed directly from 17-OHP, and the principal pathway to androgen production is through DHEA.[153] P450c17 also has 16α-hydroxylase activity.

Defects in P450c17 action can result in two different forms of CAH. Most often, combined 17α-hydroxylase/17,20-lyase deficiency is seen, but rare cases of isolated 17,20-lyase deficiency have been reported (Tables 23-11 and 23-12).[271]

Combined 17α-hydroxylase/17,20-lyase deficiency is an uncommon form of CAH, although an increasing number of cases are being reported from many different countries.[272] A prevalence of approximately 1 case per 50,000 individuals is reported in some areas, but in general the prevalence is lower than this. The classic phenotype of complete combined 17α-hydroxylase/17,20-lyase deficiency is that of a phenotypic female (46,XX, or underandrogenized 46,XY) who presents with an absence of secondary sexual characteristics (i.e., hypergonadotropic hypogonadism) at puberty and is found to have low-renin hypertension and hypokalemic alkalosis (see Table 23-11).

The classic phenotype and underlying biochemistry can be explained by the enzyme deficiency (see Fig. 23-10).[271] A defect in 17α-hydroxylation in the adrenal cortex and gonads results in impaired synthesis of 17-OHP and 17-hydroxypregnenolone and therefore of cortisol, androgens, and estrogens. Decreased cortisol synthesis causes increased corticotropin secretion, which results in excessive secretion of 17-deoxysteroids by the adrenal cortex,

TABLE 23-11	
Clinical Features of Combined CYP17 Deficiency in 46,XY Individuals	
Karyotype	46,XY
Inheritance	Autosomal recessive; mutations in *CYP17* gene
Genitalia	Female, ambiguous, or hypospadias
Wolffian duct derivatives	Absent or hypoplastic
Müllerian duct derivatives	Absent
Gonads	Testes
Physiologic features	Absent or poor virilization at puberty, gynecomastia, hypertension
Hormone profile	Decreased T; increased LH and FSH; increased plasma deoxycorticosterone, corticosterone, and progesterone; decreased plasma renin activity
	Low renin hypertension with hypokalemic alkalosis

CYP17, 17α-hydroxylase/17,20-lyase; FSH, follicle-stimulating hormone; LH, luteinizing hormone; T, testosterone.

including the mineralocorticoids 11-deoxycorticosterone (DOC), corticosterone, and 18-hydroxycorticosterone. Excess DOC secretion leads to hypertension, hypokalemic alkalosis, and suppression of the renin-angiotensin system. Diminished aldosterone synthesis and secretion are sometimes reported. Corticosterone is a weak glucocorticoid; the high plasma concentrations in this disorder prevent the signs and symptoms of cortisol deficiency (e.g., hypoglycemia) and modulate the secretion of corticotropin.

Affected 46,XX females have normal female internal and external genital tracts, but the ovaries cannot secrete estrogens at puberty, resulting in absent breast development and hypogonadism with elevated plasma FSH and LH levels. The lack of adrenal and ovarian androgens can result in little or no growth of pubic and axillary hair. In affected 46,XX individuals, the ovaries have a high proportion of atretic follicles, and some ovaries contain an increased number of enlarged follicular cysts.

Affected 46,XY individuals with complete combined 17α-hydroxylase/17,20-lyase deficiency who are diagnosed in adolescence usually have female external genitalia and a blind vaginal pouch (see Table 23-11). Testes may be intra-abdominal, in the inguinal canal, or in the labioscro-

tal folds. Inguinal hernias are common, müllerian structures are absent, and wolffian derivatives are hypoplastic. Bone age is frequently delayed, and prolonged linear growth can lead to tall stature. Pubic and axillary hair is absent or sparse, and hypergonadotropic hypogonadism is associated with a failure to develop secondary sexual characteristics at puberty. Excessive secretion of DOC and corticosterone usually leads to low-renin hypertension and hypokalemic alkalosis, as in 46,XX girls with this condition.

Complete 17α-hydroxylase/17,20-lyase deficiency is associated with a variety of mutations in the *CYP17* gene that cause complete loss of function in assays of enzyme activity. These changes include a range of missense, frameshift, and nonsense mutations (Fig. 23-25). A common mutation is the 4-bp duplication in exon 8, which is shared by Mennonites and individuals in the Friesland region of the Netherlands and is attributed to a founder effect originating in Friesland. Other geographic clusters include an in-frame deletion of residues 487 to 489 in Southeast Asia and the Arg362Cys and Trp406Arg missense mutations found among Brazilians of Portuguese and Spanish ancestry, respectively.[272] However, many different changes occur in other populations and are located throughout the enzyme.[273]

Partial forms of combined 17α-hydroxylase/17,20-lyase deficiency have been described. This condition most frequently manifests in a 46,XY infant with ambiguous genitalia or severe hypospadias for whom the steroid profile is consistent with the diagnosis of P450c17 deficiency. Hypertension may or may not be present in partial forms of combined 17α-hydroxylase/17,20-lyase deficiency, and aldosterone secretion may be normal or even elevated. Corticosterone levels, which are usually 50- to 100-fold

TABLE 23-12

Clinical Features of Isolated 17,20-Lyase Deficiency in 46,XY Individuals

Karyotype	46,XY
Inheritance	Autosomal recessive; mutations in *CYP17* gene, usually affecting key redox domains
Genitalia	Female, ambiguous, or hypospadias
Wolffian duct derivatives	Absent or hypoplastic
Müllerian duct derivatives	Absent
Gonads	Testes
Physiologic features	Absent or poor virilization at puberty; gynecomastia
Hormone profile	Decreased plasma T, DHEA, androstenedione, and estradiol; abnormal increase in plasma 17-hydroxyprogesterone and 17-hydroxypregnenolone; increased LH and FSH; increased ratio of C21-deoxysteroids to C19-steroids (DHEA, androstenedione) after hCG stimulation

CYP17, 17α-hydroxylase/17,20-lyase; DHEA, dehydroepiandrosterone; FSH, follicle-stimulating hormone; hCG, human chorionic gonadotropin; LH, luteinizing hormone; T, testosterone.

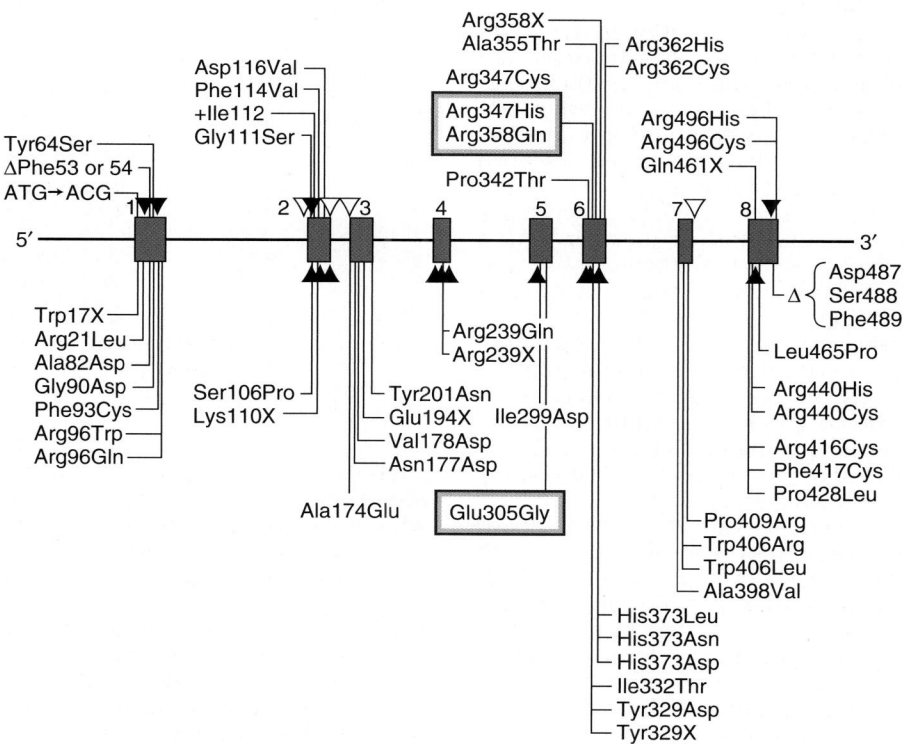

Figure 23-25 Diagram of selected mutations in the *CYP17* gene causing 17α-hydroxylase/17,20-lyase deficiency. The numbered *solid boxes* depict the exons. The three-letter abbreviations for amino acids are used to indicate the position of missense mutations; X indicates a nonsense (stop) mutation; insertions and deletions resulting in frameshift and splice site mutations are shown by *solid triangles* and *open triangles*, respectively. All of these mutations cause 17α-hydroxylase deficiency. Several missense mutations, such as those at codons 305, 347, and 358 *(boxes)*, have been associated with isolated 17,20-lyase deficiency.

higher than normal, provide adequate glucocorticoid effects and prevent symptoms of cortisol deficiency. The development of male secondary sexual characteristics at puberty may be incomplete, and gynecomastia is often seen. This rare condition has been associated with a phenylalanine deletion at codon 53 or 54 and several missense changes.[271,274]

Isolated 17,20-lyase activity has been reported in a small number of patients.[271,275,276] These 46,XY individuals usually have genital ambiguity, normal secretion of glucocorticoids and mineralocorticoids, and marked reduction in sex steroid synthesis (see Table 23-12). The first two patients shown to have a molecular defect in P450c17 harbored homozygous point mutations in the enzyme (Arg347His, Arg358Gln) that specifically interfered with 17,20-lyase activity by changing the distribution of surface charges in the redox-partner binding site.[277] Other patients have been reported with similar mutations or with a point mutation (Glu305Gly) that specifically alters the conformation of the substrate binding site.[278]

The diagnosis of 17α-hydroxylase deficiency should be suspected in all cases of 46,XY DSD, and it is strongly supported by the discovery of hyporeninemic hypertension and hypokalemic alkalosis and by a lack of secondary sex characteristics at puberty. Plasma concentrations of corticotropin, DOC, corticosterone, and progesterone are high, and those of 17α-OHP, cortisol, and gonadal steroids are low. Replacement therapy with physiologic doses of glucocorticoids suppresses DOC and corticosterone secretion and normalizes serum potassium levels, blood pressure, and plasma renin and aldosterone levels. The hypokalemia can be associated with life-threatening cardiac arrhythmia, so careful monitoring and treatment in the acute phase are needed. Gonadectomy is usually performed in 46,XY patients who have a female gender assignment once this is established. Appropriate gonadal steroid replacement therapy is indicated at puberty.

Cytochrome b_5 Deficiency. A splice site mutation in the 17,20-lyase redox partner cytochrome b_5 was first reported in a 46,XY child with ambiguous genitalia and methemoglobinemia, although extensive hormone data were not reported.[279] However, homozygous nonsense and missense mutations in this gene (CYB5A) have now been described in 46,XY children with severe hypospadias and a biochemical profile consistent with isolated 17,20-lyase deficiency and in a family with multiple affected members and a range of genital phenotypes.[280,281] Methemoglobin was elevated above the normal range in all these cases, but it did not result in clinical signs.

P450 Oxidoreductase Deficiency. POR is a membrane-bound flavoprotein that plays a central role in electron transfer from NADPH to P450 enzymes (Fig. 23-26).[282] POR is crucial in the 17,20-lyase reaction of P450c17, and it interacts with all 57 microsomal P450 enzymes, including P450c21 (21-hydroxylase) and P450c19 (aromatase), and with many others involved in hepatic drug metabolism.

A potential role for POR in human steroidogenesis emerged after the description of several patients with apparent combined deficiencies of CYP17 and CYP21.[283] Ambiguous genitalia and unusual patterns of combined steroidogenic defects have been described in a subset of patients with Antley-Bixler syndrome, a form of skeletal dysplasia that is characterized by craniosynostosis, brachycephaly, midface hypoplasia, proptosis, choanal stenosis, radioulnar or radiohumeral synostosis, bowed femora, and arachnodactyly.

The first recessively inherited human mutations in POR were described in 2004, and a significant number of changes have been described in patients with marked

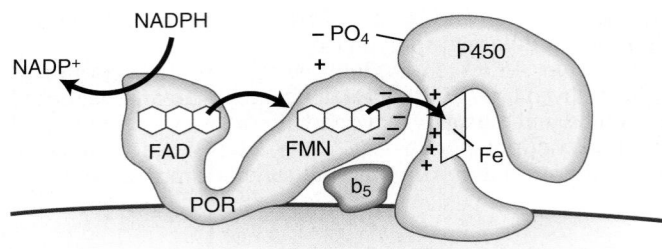

Figure 23-26 Role of P450 oxidoreductase (POR) in electron transfer to microsomal (type II) P450 enzymes. Reduced nicotinamide adenine dinucleotide phosphate (NADPH) interacts with POR, which is bound to the endoplasmic reticulum, and transfers a pair of electrons to the FAD moiety. This change in charge results in altered conformation, which allows the electrons to pass from the FAD to the FMN moiety. After further realignment, the FMN domain can interact with the redox partner binding site of the P450 enzyme (e.g., P450c17, P450c21, P450c19), permitting electron transfer to the active heme group of the enzyme, which results in substrate catalysis. The interaction of POR and the P450 enzymes is coordinated by negatively charged acidic residues on the surface of the FMN domain of POR and positively charged basic residues in the redox partner binding site of the P450 enzyme. In the case of human P450c17, this interaction is facilitated by the allosteric action of cytochrome b_5 and by serine phosphorylation of P450c17. FAD, flavin adenine dinucleotide; FMN, flavin mononucleotide. (From Miller WL. Minireview: regulation of steroidogenesis by electron transfer. *Endocrinology.* 2005;146:2544-2550, used with permission of The Endocrine Society, copyright 2005.)

TABLE 23-13

Clinical Features of P450 Oxidoreductase Deficiency in 46,XY Individuals

Karyotype	46,XY
Inheritance	Autosomal recessive; mutations in *POR* gene
Genitalia	Ambiguous; hypospadias or male
Wolffian duct derivatives	Absent or hypoplastic
Müllerian duct derivatives	Absent
Gonads	Testes
Biochemical and physiologic features	Variable androgenization at birth; variable virilization at puberty, especially in girls; glucocorticoid deficiency; no severe mineralocorticoid deficiency; features of Antley-Bixler syndrome (craniosynostosis, skeletal dysplasia) in some cases
Hormone profile	Evidence of combined CYPC17 and CYPC21 insufficiency; normal or low cortisol with poor response to ACTH stimulation; elevated 17-OHP; T low

ACTH, adrenocorticotropic hormone; CYP, cytochrome P450 enzyme; 17-OHP, 17-hydroxyprogesterone; POR, P450 oxidoreductase; T, testosterone.

phenotypic variations (Table 23-13).[154,284,285] At the most severe end of the spectrum are Antley-Bixler syndrome with ambiguous genitalia and apparent combined CYP17 and CYP21 deficiency with no skeletal phenotype. Milder defects in POR have also been seen in women with a form of polycystic ovary syndrome and in men with mild gonadal insufficiency. A range of POR activity is associated with this spectrum of phenotypes, and skeletal features can be subtle. Two common mutations are emerging: Arg-287Pro is the most prevalent mutation in patients of European ancestry, whereas the Arg457His mutation is common in Japan.[285,286] Activating mutations in fibroblast growth factor receptor 2 (FGFR2) have also been reported in association with Antley-Bixler syndrome; these patients do not have ambiguous genitalia or steroidogenic defects.

Most patients with POR deficiency have normal electrolytes and mineralocorticoid function (see Table 23-13). Cortisol insufficiency may be present, or if basal levels are adequate, the response to ACTH stimulation is reduced.[286] The serum 17-OHP concentration is usually elevated, with a variable response to ACTH stimulation, and levels of sex steroids tend to be low, especially outside the early neonatal period. POR deficiency can be associated with ambiguous genitalia in both sexes (46,XY and 46,XX). Underandrogenization of 46,XY males can occur and may result from disturbed 17,20-lyase activity during fetal Leydig cell steroidogenesis. The partial androgenization of 46,XX infants is more prevalent and may be the result of a disturbance in aromatase activity, because POR is an electron donor for this enzyme and aromatase deficiency causes prenatal androgenization of the developing 46,XX fetus (see "Aromatase Deficiency"). Alternatively, a backdoor pathway of androgen biosynthesis has been described in certain species, such as the fetal tammar wallaby.[154,155] In this model system, 17-OHP can be converted to DHT without the use of androstenedione or testosterone as an intermediate. Emerging data indicate that this pathway may also be functional during human development. Puberty can be variable in children with POR deficiency, with delayed or disordered puberty especially common in girls. This diagnosis should be considered in any child with skeletal features or hypospadias (46,XY)/clitoromegaly (46,XX) who does not progress through puberty.[287]

3α-Reductase Type 3 and 3α-Reductase Type 1: AKR1C2 and AKR1C4.
Variations in AKR1C2 (aldo-keto reductase family 1 member C2), sometimes in combination with changes in AKR1C4, have been described in several members of a family with various degrees of 46,XY underandrogenization, who were originally thought to have 17,20-lyase deficiency.[288] Compound heterozygous variants or rearrangements in AKR1C2 were found in another unrelated child with 46,XY DSD. These variants were inherited in a sex-imited recessive manner and affect enzymes that have been implicated in the backdoor pathway for DHT synthesis (see Fig. 23-11).[155,288] These findings were taken as evidence that this alternative pathway plays a role in human fetal androgen synthesis, too. These studies also highlight that biochemical 17,20-lyase deficiency can have several molecular causes: CYP17A1, CYB5A, POR, and AKR1C2.[276]

17β-Hydroxysteroid Dehydrogenase Type 3 Deficiency.
The 17β-hydroxysteroid dehydrogenase type 3 (HSD17B3) reaction is mediated by isozymes that catalyze the reduction of androstenedione, DHEA, and estrone to testosterone, Δ^5-androstenediol, and estradiol, respectively, as well as the reverse reaction (see Fig. 23-10). The HSD17B3 enzyme uses NADPH as a cofactor. The *HSD17B3* gene contains 11 exons and is located on chromosome 9q22. The type 3 isoenzyme is expressed primarily in the testes, where it favors the conversion of the weak androgen substrate, androstenedione, to the more biologically active testosterone (see Fig. 23-10). HSD17B3 does not play a role in estrogen synthesis in the ovary. Rather, the family of 17β-HSDs comprises at least 14 isoenzymes that have physiologic relevance to a range of human tissues and disorders such as breast cancer, prostate cancer, and endometriosis.

A deficiency of HSD17B3, which is also called 17-ketosteroid reductase, was first reported as a cause of 46,XY DSD by Saez and colleagues (Fig. 23-27).[289] Many cases have been reported, and the phenotype is well characterized (Table 23-14).[290,291] Most affected children (46,XY) have female-typical external genitalia at birth, although a few infants present with clitoromegaly or ambiguous genitalia. The testes are usually located in the inguinal canal and there is a blind vaginal pouch. The wolffian ducts are often stabilized to form epididymides, vas deferens, seminal vesicles, and ejaculatory ducts, which likely reflects the paracrine androgenic effects of high concentrations of androstenedione.[292,293] Affected infants are usually assigned a female sex and may mistakenly be assumed to have CAIS.

TABLE 23-14
Clinical Features of HSD17B3 Deficiency in 46,XY Individuals

Karyotype	46,XY
Inheritance	Autosomal recessive; mutations in *HSD17B3* gene
Genitalia	Female → ambiguous; blind vaginal pouch
Wolffian duct derivatives	Present
Müllerian duct derivatives	Absent
Gonads	Testes (usually undescended)
Physiologic features	Virilization at puberty (phallus enlargement, deepening of voice, and development of facial and body hair); gynecomastia variable
Hormone profile	Increased plasma estrone and androstenedione; decreased ratio of plasma testosterone/androstenedione after hCG stimulation test; increased plasma FSH and LH levels

FSH, follicle-stimulating hormone; hCG, human chorionic gonadotropin; HSD17B3, 17β-hydroxysteroid dehydrogenase 3; LH, luteinizing hormone.

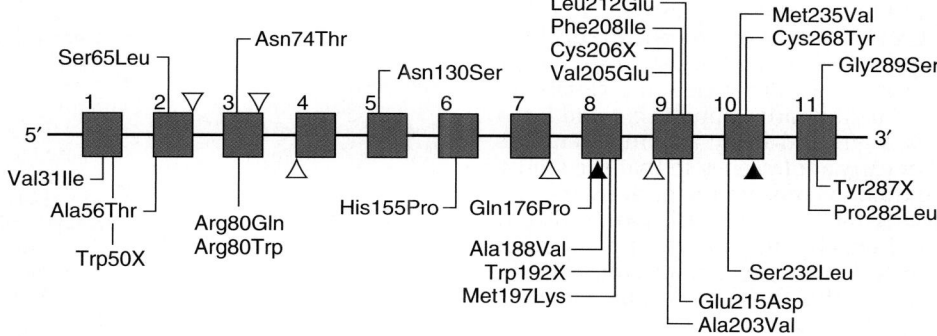

Figure 23-27 Diagram of the 17β-hydroxysteroid dehydrogenase type 3 gene *(HSD17B3)* shows the mutations that result in deficiency of the enzyme. The numbered *solid boxes* depict the exons. The three-letter abbreviations for amino acids are used to indicate the position of missense mutations; X indicates a nonsense (stop) mutation; insertions and deletions resulting in frameshift mutations *(solid triangles)* and splice site mutations *(open triangles)* are shown.

Significant virilization usually occurs at puberty in HSD17B3 deficiency in the form of clitoral enlargement, hirsutism, deepening of the voice, and muscle development. These symptoms and signs may be the presenting features of this condition if it has not been diagnosed earlier in life.[294] The pubertal increase in testosterone is mostly from extraglandular conversion from androstenedione. It has been speculated that this is mediated by genetic or environmental induction of enzyme activities of AKR1C, such as the 17β-HSD17B5 type 5 isoenzyme, also known as AKR1C3.[295] The androstenedione substrate is increased at puberty, and the testes have partial HSD17B3 activity in some cases. In a large cohort of patients from a consanguineous population in the Gaza Strip, the phallus was described as reaching lengths of 4 to 8 cm.[296] The HSD17B3 mutation reported in this population (Arg80Gln) is associated with 15% to 20% retention of normal HSD17B3 activity (see Fig. 23-27). The development of gynecomastia at puberty occurs because of estrogens derived from the conversion of androstenedione by aromatase in extraglandular tissue and the action of the HSD17B1 or HSD17B2 isoenzymes.

The typical biochemical profile in HSD17B3 deficiency is an elevated androstenedione level relative to testosterone (see Table 23-14). Expressed as a ratio of testosterone to androstenedione (after an hCG stimulation test before puberty), values less than 0.8 are typically found in these patients, but findings can be variable.[291,297,298] Testicular vein sampling at the time of gonadectomy shows a markedly increased androstenedione gradient relative to testosterone, though this test is not routinely performed. Early genetic analysis can be useful and can avoid the need for hCG stimulation in some children.[299,300]

The range of mutations reported in patients with HSD17B3 deficiency is shown in Figure 23-27. Most are missense mutations, and some patients are compound heterozygotes. Expression studies of the mutant enzymes in heterologous cells usually show complete absence of activity in the conversion of androstenedione to testosterone compared with the normal enzyme. Women homozygous or compound heterozygous for HSD17B3 mutations are asymptomatic and are fertile. When the mother is homozygous/compound heterozygous and when the father is a heterozygous carrier there is a 50% chance of a 46,XY child being affected. If both parents are heterozygous, then there is a 25% chance of having an affected 46,XY child.

Sex assignment can be difficult in children with HSD17B3 deficiency and needs careful consideration of many factors, such as the degree of androgenization, likely activity of the enzyme and effects at puberty, social and cultural aspects, and the family and child's role in decision making. When the diagnosis is made soon after birth in a child with female-typical genitalia, some babies have had early gonadectomy and been brought up as girls. In other settings, such as in Gaza, it has been proposed that these patients be given male sex assignment at diagnosis and be treated with early testosterone, although some variability in outcome is seen.[301] An alternative approach could be to bring the child up as a girl and delay any interventions until late childhood or early adolescence so that the family and child have more time to consider the options and the child's gender is more established. Careful monitoring is needed for the onset of puberty and androgen production if the child is to remain as female, and gonadectomy would typically be undertaken at this time if a female gender is appropriate.

Those children who first present with virilization at puberty may undergo gender reassignment from female to male in some cases. Gender changes at puberty have been reported in 39% to 64% of patients reared as girls in one study, but the numbers of subjects on which these figures were based were fewer than for 5α-reductase deficiency, and in our experience the rates are lower.[168,169,302] Patients presenting as androgenized females at puberty who feel they have a female gender usually undergo gonadectomy. Sometimes androgenization has been blocked in the short term with antiandrogens and puberty suppression to allow appropriate counseling and to ensure the young person is involved in the decision making. Other young people may feel they want to reassign as males or may occasionally feel nonbinary. Careful assessment and support from a multidisciplinary team and experienced psychologist are important.

Long-term follow-up is also important for hormone replacement and support. One recent study from a single center specializing in adult DSD found that approximately one fourth of the cohort of women with partially virilized 46,XY DSD were found to have mutations in HSD17B3.[302] The degree of androgenization was less than that typically seen in 5α-reductase deficiency, and many had been labeled as having PAIS. The diagnosis could only be made by genetic analysis after gonadectomy.

Steroid 5α-Reductase Type 2 Deficiency. Steroid 5α-reductase type 2 deficiency is also characterized by a 46,XY karyotype, normally differentiated testes, and male internal ducts but external genitalia that may be more ambiguous at birth than in 17β-HSD deficiency. There is a striking degree of virilization at puberty in patients reared as female with gonads retained. Classic features of this enzyme deficiency are summarized in Table 23-15.

The description of a genetic variant in SRD5A2 in the Dominican Republic and Mexico and analysis of the biochemical and molecular features underline the importance of DHT in the development of the male phenotype.[303-305] At birth, there is typically a bifid scrotum, a urogenital sinus, a blind vaginal pouch, and a clitoris-like, hypospadiac phallus. Testes differentiate normally and are located in the inguinal canal or in the labioscrotal folds. No müllerian structures are present. The wolffian ducts are stabilized so that the epididymides, vasa deferentia, and seminal vesicles are well differentiated; the ejaculatory ducts usually terminate in the blind vaginal pouch. The prostate is hypoplastic. Up to a third of cases may present with isolated hypospadias.[306]

TABLE 23-15

Clinical Features of 5α-Reductase Type 2 Deficiency in 46,XY Individuals

Karyotype	46,XY
Inheritance	Autosomal recessive; mutations in SRD5A2 gene
Genitalia	Usually ambiguous with small, hypospadiac phallus; blind vaginal pouch
Wolffian duct derivatives	Normal
Müllerian duct derivatives	Absent
Gonads	Normal testes
Physiologic features	Decreased facial and body hair, no temporal hair recession, prostate not palpable
Hormone profile	Decreased ratio of 5α/5β C21 and C19 steroids in urine; increased T/DHT ratio before and after hCG stimulation; modest increase in plasma LH; decreased conversion of T to DHT in vitro

DHT, dihydrotestosterone; hCG, human chorionic gonadotropin; LH, luteinizing hormone; SRD5A2, steroid-5α-reductase type 2; T, testosterone.

Individuals assigned male gender virilize to various degrees at puberty. The voice deepens, muscle mass increases, the phallus lengthens to 4 to 8 cm, the bifid scrotum becomes rugated and pigmented, and the testes enlarge and descend into the labioscrotal folds. Postpubertal affected males do not have acne, temporal hair recession, or enlargement of the prostate, and they do not develop gynecomastia. There is normal libido with penile erections. Histologic examination of the testes shows Leydig cell hyperplasia and decreased spermatogenesis. Infertility is caused by a composite of failure to transform spermatogonia into spermatocytes, the adverse effect of a cryptorchid testis, and the specific role of DHT in regulating semen volume and viscosity.[307] Nevertheless, some members of the Dominican cohort had a normal sperm count. One man fathered a child after intrauterine insemination, and two affected brothers in a Swedish family were spontaneously fertile after hypospadias repair performed in childhood.[308,309] Gender role changes occur frequently in 5α-reductase deficiency, particularly where clusters of cases occur in geographic regions. Overall, gender role is changed in 56% to 63% of cases.[168,169] Male sex assignment is now increasingly chosen when the diagnosis is made in infancy.[310] An alternative approach similar to that sometimes used for 17β-hydroxysteroid dehydrogenase deficiency could be to rear the child as female with the gonads kept intact pending further informed discussions before puberty. Females (46,XX) homozygous for 5α-reductase deficiency undergo normal puberty but delayed menarche, and fertility is normal.[311]

The biochemical profile in 5α-reductase deficiency typically shows an elevated testosterone-to-DHT ratio basally or after hCG stimulation when investigations are undertaken before puberty (see Table 23-15). Various ratios have been suggested as diagnostic but none is unequivocal. A ratio exceeding 10:1 had a sensitivity and specificity of 78% and 72%, respectively, in a cohort of 90 patients investigated for this enzyme deficiency.[312] Serum LH and FSH levels may be normal or elevated after puberty. The most reliable biochemical test (undertaken after 3 months of age) is analysis of a urinary steroid profile by gas chromatography and mass spectrometry to demonstrate a diminished ratio of urinary 5α- to 5β-reduced C19 and C21 steroids.[313,314] The diagnosis can still be confirmed biochemically after gonadectomy because of persistent effects on 5α/5β-reduced C21 steroids.[315]

Early diagnosis of 5α-reductase type 2 deficiency is important because of its bearing on sex assignment. The natural history of this condition, with a tendency for change to a male gender role with virilization at puberty, indicates that male gender assignment is now a frequent option even when the external genitalia are relatively severely undermasculinized at birth.[316] The enzyme deficiency can masquerade as PAIS in newborns.[317] DHT, which may be applied topically as a cream, increases penile length and facilitates repair of the hypospadias.[318]

5α-Reductase type 2 deficiency is transmitted as an autosomal recessive trait. Two microsomal 5α-reductase enzymes catalyze the NADPH-dependent conversion of testosterone to DHT. 5α-Reductase type 2 is a 254–amino acid protein encoded by the SRD5A2 gene on chromosome 2p23. The type 2 isozyme is expressed predominantly in the primordia of the prostate and external genitalia but not in the wolffian ducts until after their differentiation into the male internal genital ducts.[319] The type 1 isoenzyme is expressed in skin, including human genital skin fibroblasts. The action of this isoenzyme may contribute to the virilization that occurs in 5α-reductase–deficient patients at puberty.[320]

The 5α-reductase type 2 deficiency is genetically heterogeneous, and the more than 60 mutations detected in the SRD5A2 gene are distributed among all five exons (Fig. 23-28). Most are missense mutations, and a complete gene deletion is found in the New Guinea population. There is

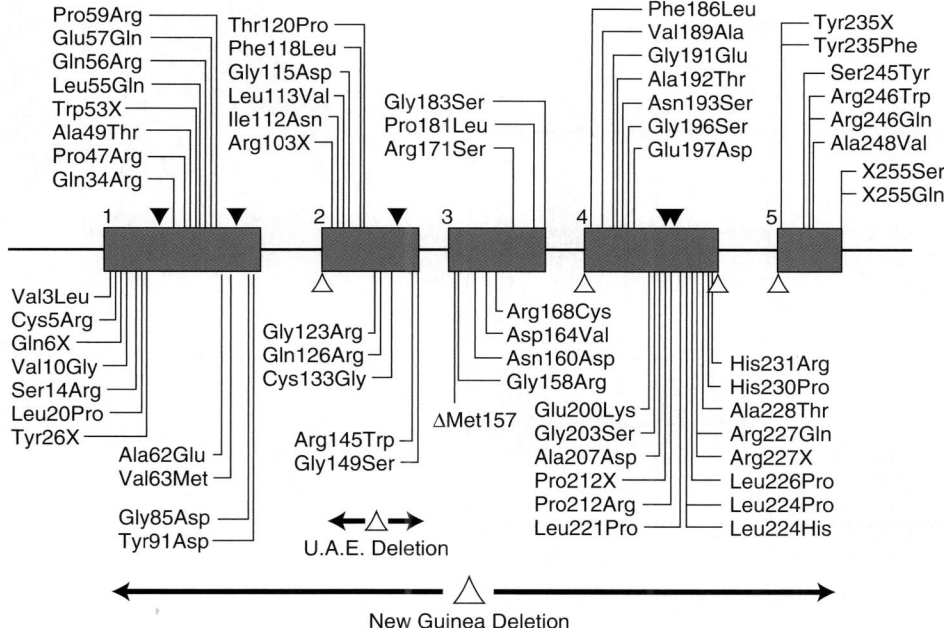

Figure 23-28 Diagram of the 5α-reductase type 2 gene (SRD5A2) shows the mutations that result in 5α-reductase deficiency. The numbered *solid boxes* depict the exons. The three-letter abbreviations for amino acids are used to indicate the position of missense mutations; X indicates a nonsense (stop) mutation; insertions and deletions resulting in frameshift and splice site mutations are shown by *solid triangles* and *open triangles*, respectively. Large deletions found in affected United Arab Emirates (U.A.E.) and New Guinea populations are shown. (Adapted from Grumbach MM, Hughes IA, Conte FA. Disorders of sex differentiation. In: Larsen PR, Kronenberg HM, Melmed S, et al, eds. *Williams Textbook of Endocrinology*, 10th ed. Philadelphia, PA: Saunders; 2003, with additional data provided courtesy of Dr. Julianne Imperato-McGinley, Department of Medicine, Weill Medical College of Cornell University, Ithaca, NY.)

a predominance of mutations in exon 4, mostly localized between codons 197 and 230, where the effect is complete inactivation of the mutant enzyme. A significant number of cases are compound heterozygotes, and consanguinity is common. Male heterozygotes are not affected. The use of plasma testosterone or urinary profile screening in elite female athletes has shown a number of individuals with this enzyme deficiency who hitherto had been undiagnosed.[321] The result of subsequent clinical assessment showed primary amenorrhea, a tall, muscular habitus, and evidence of clitoromegaly with labial fusion. The plasma testosterone level was well within the adult male range. Clearly, this contributes to a significant advantage when competing against nonaffected female athletes. This has resulted in the International Association of Athletics Federations (IAAF) establishing an expert medical panel to review female athletes with evidence of hyperandrogenism. Such athletes would be allowed to continue competing as normal once the cause of their hyperandrogenism

(such as 5α-reductase deficiency) has been treated to result in a plasma testosterone level less than 10 nmol/L, the lower end of the normal adult male range.

Disorders of Androgen Action

Androgen insensitivity syndrome (AIS) is the paradigm of a clinical disorder resulting from hormone resistance.[322] Male fetal sex differentiation, the development of secondary sex characteristics at puberty, and the subsequent onset of spermatogenesis are all the result of androgens binding to a single intracellular androgen receptor (AR) ubiquitously expressed in target tissue. The AR is a member of the ligand-dependent transcription factor superfamily of nuclear receptors encoded by a gene (AR, also known as *NR3C4*) on the X chromosome.[322] It shares structural similarities with other nuclear receptors, including a highly conserved central DNA-binding domain (DBD) and a C-terminal ligand-binding domain (LBD) (Fig. 23-29). In

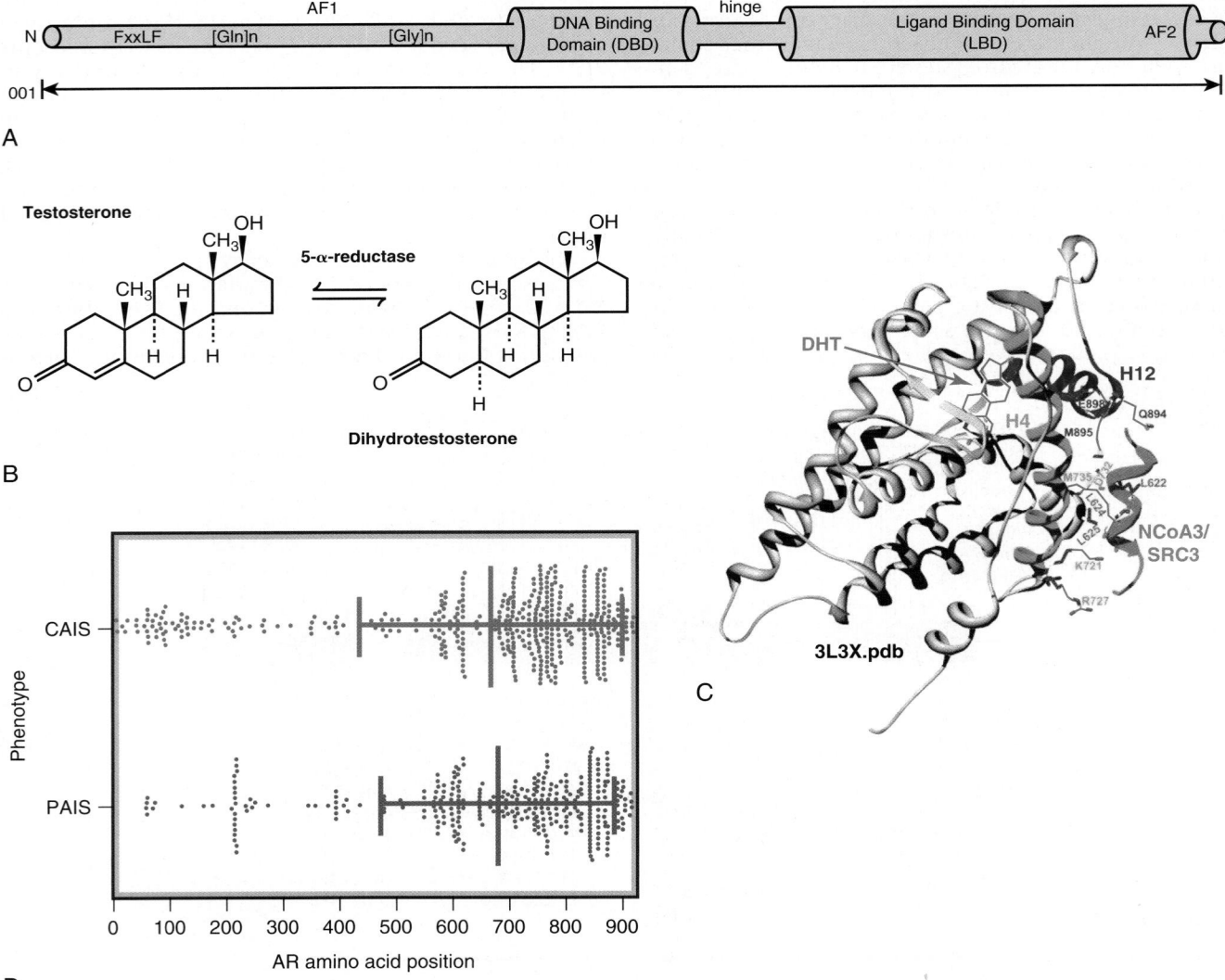

Figure 23-29 A and **B,** Structure of the androgen receptor (AR) in keeping with nuclear receptors in general. The AR uniquely has an extended amino-terminal domain, which contains the FxxLF, polyglutamine, and polyglycine motifs, which influence transactivation in response to testosterone and its 5α-reduced metabolite, dihydrotestosterone. **C,** The crystal structure of the LBD (ligand-binding domain) is shown bound to the ligand, DHT, which initiates a conformational change involving helix 12 and enables recruitment of coactivators such as NCoA3/SRC3. **D,** The gene distribution of mutations associated with CAIS and PAIS are shown (see also Fig. 23-30). CAIS, complete androgen insensitivity syndrome; PAIS, partial androgen insensitivity syndrome. (From Mongan NP, Tadokoro-Cuccaro R, Bunch T, Hughes IA. Androgen insensitivity syndrome. *Best Pract Res Clin Endocrinol Metab.* 2015;29(4):569-580, used with permission of Elsevier, Inc.)

addition, the AR uniquely contains an extended N-terminal domain (NTD) that includes polymorphic polyglutamine (CAG) and polyglycine (GGN) repeats. These residues modulate AR activity. The DBD contains cysteine residues that coordinate zinc atoms to form two zinc fingers, the first of which contains a P box that enters the major groove of DNA to form specific base-pair contacts that are identical for all classic steroid receptors. The second zinc finger containing the D box is involved in protein-protein interactions and stabilizes the unit for receptor dimerization. This binding requires preferential recognition of androgen response elements (AREs) composed of an inverted repeat of DNA sequences related to 5'-AGAACA-3'.[323]

Activation of transcription involves motif activation function 1 (AF1) in the NTD and motif activation function 2 (AF2) in the LBD. AF1 is ligand independent, whereas AF2 is ligand dependent and interacts with p160 steroid receptor coactivators such as NCOA1, NCOA2, and NCOA3.[324] N-terminal and C-terminal (N-C) interaction is a relatively unique feature of the AR. In the presence of its primary physiologic ligands, testosterone and DHT, the AR recruits multiple enzymatically diverse epigenetic coregulators that cooperate in the activation of transcription of androgen-regulated genes (see Fig. 23-29). N-terminal sequences comprising amino acid residues 23 to 27 (FQNLF) and residues 435 to 439 (WHTLF) participate in the AR N-C terminal interactions to stabilize the AR and slow down dissociation of ligand. Further modulation of AR function occurs post-translationally by processes such as phosphorylation and sumoylation.

The AR in the unliganded state is located in the cytoplasm complexed to heat shock proteins such as HSP70 and HSP90 and complexed to co-chaperone proteins such as FKBP4 (also called FKBP52). Binding of ligand to its receptor initiates dissociation from these complexes to allow translocation of the AR into the nucleus, where it binds to DNA as a homodimer. The action of the AR is further modulated by interaction with coregulatory proteins that function as coactivators or corepressors.[324] The crucial role of agonist-induced changes in LBD organization enables coactivator recruitment through their LXXLL motifs.[325] The AR exhibits a selective preference for the ARA70, ARA55, and ARA54 coregulators, which contain FXXLF motifs related to the aforementioned amino acid residues in the N-terminal.

The crystal structure of the AR LBD bound to natural and synthetic androgens is shown in Figure 23-29C. Helix 12, in the presence of ligand, undergoes a conformational change to fold back on top of the ligand hydrophobic pocket to capture the ligand, thus slowing the rate of ligand-receptor dissociation. This trapping effect by helix 12 enables recruitment of coactivators.

Complete Androgen Insensitivity Syndrome. CAIS is an X-linked condition that typically presents in an adolescent female who has breast development with a pubertal growth spurt but who has not had her menarche (Table 23-16). Pubic and axillary hair is absent or scanty and the uterus is absent as a result of normal AMH action, although there may be müllerian remnants. The wolffian ducts are stabilized in many patients, with well-developed vas deferens and epididymis observed when gonadectomy is performed.[293] Estimates of the prevalence of CAIS range from 1 case in 20,400 to 1 in 99,000 individuals with a 46,XY karyotype.[326] The main differential diagnosis at this age is XY complete gonadal dysgenesis (Swyer syndrome), which is distinguished by poor breast development, taller stature, decreased ratio of upper to lower body segments, and a different hormone profile.[327] CAIS may present in early infancy with bilateral inguinal or labial swellings. 17β-HSD

deficiency may also manifest in this manner. Bilateral inguinal hernias are rare in girls, of whom 1% to 2% are estimated to have CAIS.[328] The diagnosis should be considered in girls with this type of hernia and the presence of a Y chromosome checked by fluorescence in situ hybridization (FISH) or a full karyotype. If the hernial sac contains gonads, a biopsy should be performed together with the cytogenetic studies.[329] A history of an older female sibling who had an inguinal hernia repair in infancy and, when tested, was found to have an XY karyotype is not unusual. Presently, with fetal sex determination so commonplace, a mismatch between the predicted infant sex and the birth phenotype can be the presenting feature of CAIS.

Partial Androgen Insensitivity Syndrome. This form of AIS is characterized by incomplete masculinization resulting from a partial biologic response to androgens (Table 23-17). The prototypic phenotype for PAIS comprises penoscrotal hypospadias, micropenis, and a bifid scrotum. The testes may be undescended. The most severe form of PAIS manifests as isolated clitoromegaly. The milder end of the spectrum includes isolated hypospadias; PAIS does not present as isolated micropenis.

TABLE 23-16

Clinical Features of Complete Androgen Insensitivity Syndrome

Karyotype	46,XY
Inheritance	X-linked recessive; mutations in *AR* gene
Genitalia	Female with blind vaginal pouch
Wolffian duct derivatives	Often present, depending on mutation type
Müllerian duct derivatives	Absent or vestigial
Gonads	Testes
Physiologic findings	Scant or absent pubic and axillary hair; breast development at puberty; primary amenorrhea
Hormone and metabolic profile	Increased LH and testosterone levels; increased estradiol (for male reference range); FSH levels often normal or slightly increased; resistance to androgenic and metabolic effects of testosterone

AR, androgen receptor; FSH, follicle-stimulating hormone; LH, luteinizing hormone.

TABLE 23-17

Clinical Features of Partial Androgen Insensitivity Syndrome

Karyotype	46,XY
Inheritance	X-linked recessive; mutations in *AR* gene
External genitalia	Ambiguous with blind vaginal pouch → isolated hypospadias → male with infertility (mild AIS)
Wolffian duct derivatives	Often normal
Müllerian duct derivatives	Absent
Gonads	Testes (usually undescended)
Physiologic features	Decreased to normal axillary and pubic hair, beard growth, and body hair; gynecomastia common at puberty
Hormone and metabolic profile	Increased LH and testosterone concentrations; increased estradiol (for men); FSH levels may be normal or slightly increased
	Partial resistance to androgenic and metabolic effects of testosterone

AIS, androgen insensitivity syndrome; AR, androgen receptor; FSH, follicle-stimulating hormone; LH, luteinizing hormone.

The list of causes for a PAIS-like phenotype is lengthy. Alternative diagnoses include partial gonadal dysgenesis, a defect in androgen biosynthesis (e.g., LH receptor, SF1, 17β-HSD, and 5α-reductase deficiencies), 45,X/46,XY mosaicism, and ovotesticular DSD.

Minimal or Mild Androgen Insensitivity Syndrome. This category of AIS is generally associated with normal male development but gynecomastia at puberty and infertility in adulthood.[330] Cancer of the breast is rare in males, but the risk is increased in MAIS and in those with PAIS raised male. In contrast, breast cancer has not been reported in women with CAIS. A mild form of androgen insensitivity is also found in spinal and bulbar muscular atrophy (Kennedy syndrome), a condition caused by hyperexpansion of the N-terminal polyglutamine repeat region.[331]

Hormone Profiles in Androgen Insensitivity Syndromes. Serum testosterone is within or above the adult male range with an inappropriately increased concentration of LH consistent with hormone resistance. Serum estradiol is increased from abundant aromatization of androgens.[332] Concentrations of sex hormone–binding globulin (SHBG) are sexually dimorphic, with levels in patients with CAIS similar to those found in normal females. Serum AMH concentration is typically increased in CAIS, whereas the levels are low in gonadal dysgenesis.[333]

Male infants have an LH-induced surge in serum testosterone concentrations during the first few months of life, whereas the surge is absent in CAIS.[334] Testosterone levels do increase after hCG stimulation. In contrast, infants with PAIS have a spontaneous neonatal testosterone surge.

Molecular Pathogenesis of Androgen Insensitivity Syndromes. Information about mutations that affect the AR is recorded on an International Mutation Database at McGill University[335] (Fig. 23-30). More than 400 germline mutations are recorded for AIS; the database also records somatic mutations associated with prostate cancer. There is no specific hot spot of mutations, but certain locations, such as exons 5 and 7 within the LBD, are affected more frequently. Approximately 20% of mutations are located in the DBD. The most common functional AR defect results from disruption of the hydrophobic ligand-binding pocket, which is necessary for repositioning of helix 12 to form the AF2 coregulator interaction surface.

The phenotype of individuals with AIS can vary according to different substitutions at the same codon. For example, phenylalanine at codon 754 in helix 5 has a side chain that points away from the ligand-binding pocket. When substituted for a valine, the mutant AR is transcriptionally inactive and causes CAIS.[336] In contrast, serine and leucine substitutions result in a PAIS phenotype, explained

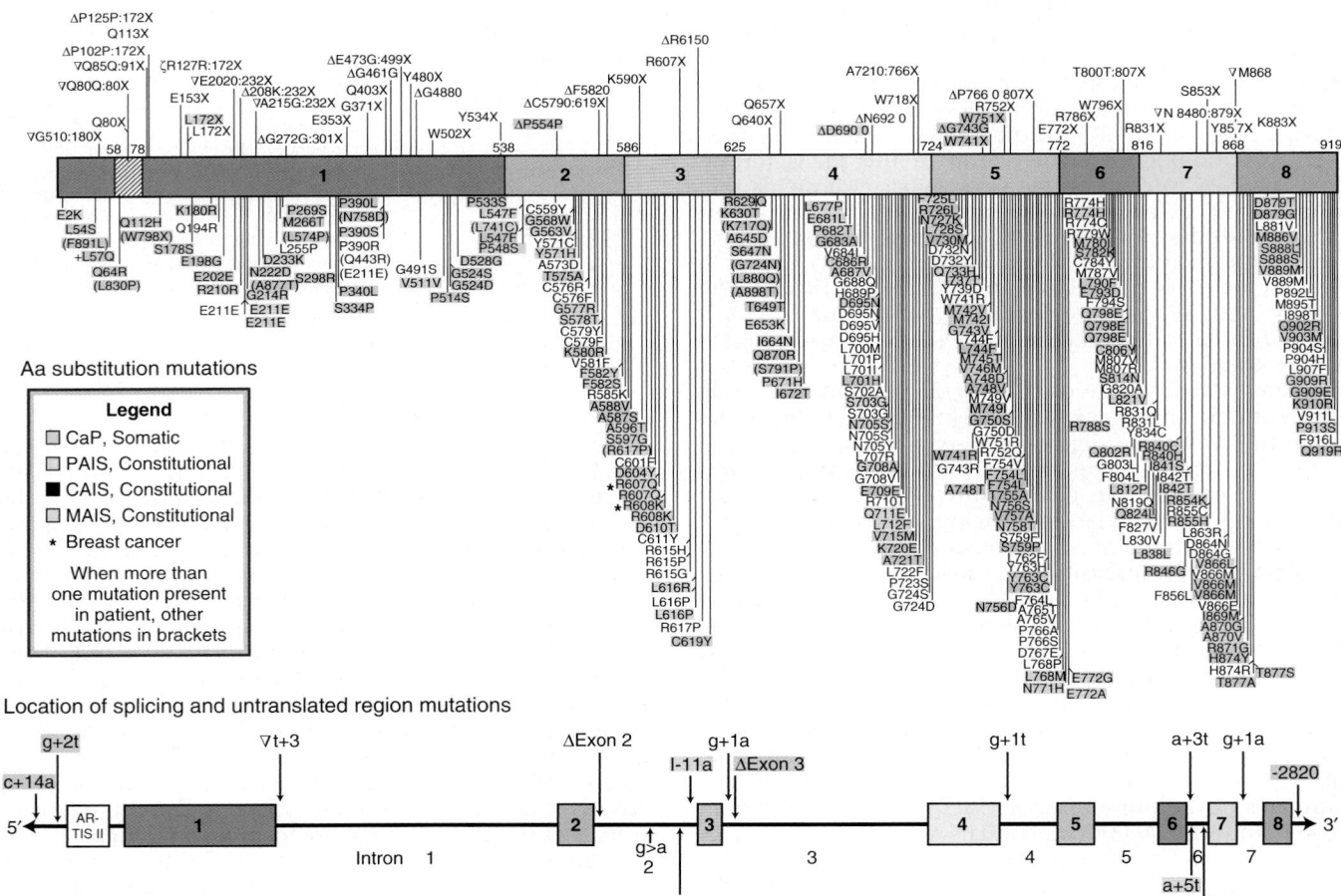

Figure 23-30 Overview of androgen receptor (AR) mutations that cause different forms of androgen insensitivity syndrome (AIS). CAIS, complete androgen insensitivity syndrome; MAIS, minimal or mild androgen insensitivity syndrome; PAIS, partial androgen insensitivity syndrome. (From the McGill Androgen Receptor Gene Mutation Database. Available at http://www.androgendb.mcgill.ca.)

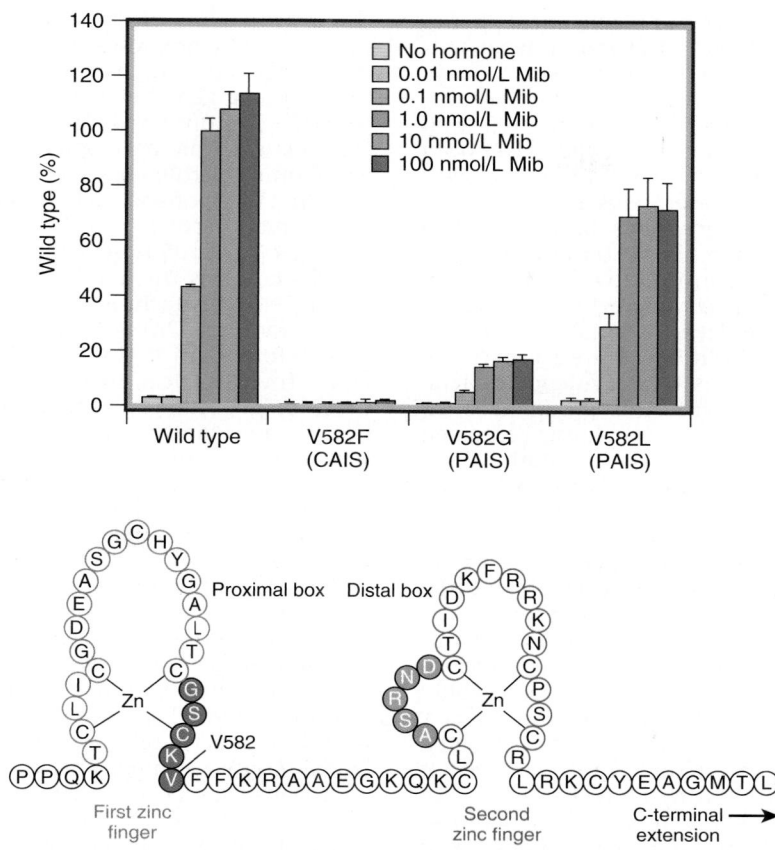

Figure 23-31 Phenotypes differing according to mutation at codon 582 in first zinc finger of the DNA-binding domain (DBD). The effects of substitution of a valine (V) with phenylalanine (F), glycine (G), and leucine (L) are shown in a transactivation assay *(upper panel)* with the synthetic androgen, mibolerone. The linear stretch of amino acids composing the DBD is shown in the lower panel. CAIS, complete androgen insensitivity syndrome; PAIS, partial androgen insensitivity syndrome. (From Hughes IA, Davies JD, Bunch TI, et al. Androgen insensitivity syndrome. *Lancet.* 2012;380:1419-1428, used with permission of Elsevier, Inc.)

by some residual transcriptional activity as measured in vitro. Linking the DBD to the LBD is a flexible hinge region defined by residues 628 to 669. This region stabilizes receptor interaction with selective androgen response elements and signals nuclear localization. Deletion of the hinge region by site-directed mutagenesis results in enhanced gene transcription, suggesting that it has a role in repression.[337]

There can be considerable heterogeneity in the phenotypic expression of a particular mutation, sometimes even within families. A mutation at codon 703 in exon 4 of the LBD, which changes a serine to a glycine, is reported in four individuals listed in the McGill database. One patient had a normal female phenotype consistent with CAIS. The other three all had ambiguous genitalia consistent with PAIS, but the degree of androgenization of the external genitalia was sufficiently variable that two were raised male and the other was raised female.[338] About 30% of mutations in AIS are de novo. Such mutations arise as a single mutational event in a parental germ cell (the mother in the case of AIS) or as germ cell mosaicism in the maternal gonad. When the mutation arises at the postzygotic stage, the index case is a somatic mosaic. This gives rise to expression of mutant and wild-type ARs in different target tissues, including the external genitalia. Perhaps one third of de novo mutations arise at the postzygotic stage, giving rise to expression of mutant and wild-type AR in different target tissues. This may explain some of the variable phenotype in PAIS.[339]

Identifying an AR mutation generally requires proof of pathogenicity when it is novel and particularly with a

PAIS phenotype. A promoter-luciferase system applied after transient transfection into a receptor-negative cell line such as Cos-1, Hela, CV-1, or the PC3 prostate cancer cell line is commonly used as a transactivation assay. Figure 23-31 illustrates the application of such an assay for analysis of three different amino acid substitutions at codon 582 in the DBD.[340] A range of phenotypes from CAIS to severe and mild PAIS is found, depending on the nature of the substitution. Furthermore, the data provide an indication of potential mutant AR recovery over a range of androgen concentrations. This has particular relevance for subjects with PAIS who are raised male and may require large doses of androgens to induce puberty or to stimulate spermatogenesis. Allied to functional studies in vitro, structure-guided modeling of the nuclear receptor can be used to predict the likely consequences of a mutant AR (see Fig. 23-31). The NTD has a disordered flexible structure that has yet to be analyzed by crystallography. Nonsense mutations have long been identified in the NTD, but improved sequencing techniques have now identified a number of missense mutations generally associated with the milder forms of AIS. It is possible that the structural flexibility of the NTD enables the AR to tolerate amino acid substitutions with little functional consequence. Analysis of such mutations provides a means to better define the structure-function relationship of the N-terminal domain.[340] The discovery of novel mutations is more common now that full sequencing of the *AR* gene is more straightforward.[341]

Androgen Insensitivity Syndromes Without an Androgen Receptor Mutation. An *AR* gene mutation is identified in about

95% of subjects when the clinical and biochemical phenotype is consistent with CAIS.[342] Multiple ligation-dependent probe amplification (MLPA) is a useful ancillary test to detect exon deletions sometimes found in AIS.

The yield of mutations is less than 25% in PAIS, even when other causes of a similar phenotype have been excluded.[338] There is evidence that the AR can interact with more than 200 unique coregulator proteins, but in contrast to prostate cancer, no mutations have been identified when screening these proteins in AIS.[343] So the vast majority of cases with a phenotype consistent with PAIS do not have a mutation in the *AR* gene coding region. The genital phenotype, as based on a validated external masculinization score, is identical to PAIS infants with a proven AR mutation.[344,345] However, there is clear evidence of fetal growth restriction associated with this group as birth weight for gestational age is significantly lower compared with PAIS infants who have an *AR* gene mutation.[346] It has been suggested that this form of XY DSD with fetal growth restriction is a defined category that as yet remains unexplained.

Management of Androgen Insensitivity Syndromes. Gender assignment and sex of rearing is uniformly female in CAIS. Inguinal hernias need repair when presenting in infancy. There is an option then to perform gonadectomy at this early stage, although there is no uniform practice concerning early versus late gonadectomy, and many people would opt to keep their gonads to enable spontaneous puberty to occur. If gonadectomy is performed before puberty, hormone induction of puberty is similar to that used for girls with Turner syndrome, starting at 10 to 11 years of age. In the absence of a uterus, hormone replacement can be continuous, unopposed estrogen. Some adults with CAIS report improved well-being when androgen replacement is also given. The mechanism of this androgenic effect is not understood. A straightforward explanation would be an estrogenic effect from aromatization of testosterone. However, androgens are reported to have nongenomic effects through activation of protein kinase A and protein kinase C and the MAP kinase pathway.[347] One small double-blind trial of testosterone undecanoate treatment in gonadectomized women with CAIS showed no clear effects on psychosexual function and mood scores.[348] Bone mineral density is lower in women with CAIS, indicative of the direct effect of androgens on bone mineralization.[349] The effect is similar whether gonadectomy occurs before or after puberty.

There is an increased risk of gonadal germ cell tumors in XY DSD, including AIS. The majority of tumors are categorized as type II germ cell tumors and include seminoma, dysgerminoma, and various types of nonseminoma/nongerminoma.[350] These tumors arise from embryonic stem cells that fail to mature within an abnormal microenvironment characterized by androgen resistance in the case of AIS. There is a precursor in situ neoplastic change called carcinoma in situ (CIS), also referred to as *intratubular germ cell neoplasia unclassified* (ITGNU). CIS cells originate from primordial germ cells (i.e., gonocytes) and express immunohistochemical markers such as placenta-like alkaline phosphatase (PLAP), KIT (the receptor for the stem cell factor KITLG), POU5F1 (a protein encoded by the OCT3/4 transcription factor), and NANOG. Immunohistochemical detection of POU5F1 is the most sensitive and specific marker for CIS. The risk of developing a germ cell tumor before puberty in CAIS is low, of the order of 0.8% to 2.0%.[351] Hence, there is a general preference to delay gonadectomy until young adulthood to enable spontaneous puberty to occur. The risk of malignancy increases with age, although precise estimates are not available. Some

adults with CAIS elect to retain the gonads. Nearly all CIS eventually progresses to germ cell cancer. Monitoring tumor markers, which requires gonadal biopsy, is sometimes undertaken after resiting the gonads in the inguinal region.[352] Noninvasive monitoring may potentially become available with the development of techniques to measure embryonic microRNAs in serum.[353] Other common findings in CAIS gonads include Sertoli cell adenomas and epididymal cysts.[354]

Surgery in CAIS is generally confined to gonadectomy. Self-dilatation is the first-line approach for vaginal hypoplasia.[355,356] This technique is effective in lengthening the vagina for most CAIS women but should be started some time before a girl is thinking about sexual relations, and when there is clear focus and motivation. A specialist nurse or gynecologist with experience of vaginal dilatation is important to provide support and guidance, and several useful written materials are becoming available. In situations in which self-dilatation is not appropriate or possible, alternative forms to vaginoplasty may be offered. This is best undertaken by a laparoscopic Vecchietti procedure.[355]

The early management of PAIS centers on gender assignment and the subsequent plan and timing for surgery. There has been an increasing trend in recent decades to choose male sex of rearing.[357] Several surgical procedures may be required to correct hypospadias and relocate the testes in a scrotal sac. Androgen supplementation, either to induce puberty or to enhance virilization after puberty, is commonly required. Oral or parenterally administered androgens may be required in high doses, reflecting the degree of androgen resistance. Topical DHT gel is also used. Gynecomastia is an invariable feature of PAIS in adolescent boys. This may respond to aromatase inhibitors or to an antiestrogen, but surgical reduction mammoplasty is often needed. The risk of germ cell tumor of the testis is 15% or greater in patients with PAIS if the gonad is nonscrotal in position.[358] When scrotal in position, testes should be monitored by regular self-examination and periodic imaging by ultrasound. It is suggested that bilateral testicular biopsies are undertaken after puberty to determine the presence of CIS.[359] In view of its malignant progression in the majority of cases, gonadectomy is advised, although an alternative may be irradiation of in situ lesions.

When an infant with PAIS is assigned female gender, gonadectomy will be required before puberty to avoid virilization and subsequently a genitoplasty. Estrogen replacement is needed to induce puberty and for hormone replacement thereafter. Sex assignment in MAIS is male. Clinical presentation occurs in adolescence either because of gynecomastia or for investigation of male factor infertility in adulthood. Reduction mammoplasty is required for the gynecomastia.

Other Conditions Affecting 46,XY Sex Development

Persistent Müllerian Duct Syndrome. AMH is a glycoprotein homodimer that is secreted by the Sertoli cells of the developing testes from approximately 7 weeks after conception. It acts through the AMH type 2 receptor (AMHR2) between 8 and 12 weeks after conception to cause regression of the müllerian duct (see "Development of Reproductive Systems").[144]

AMH is encoded by a 2.75-kb gene containing 5 exons in the region of chromosome 19p13.3. The AMHR2 is a serine/threonine kinase with a single transmembrane domain that is encoded by an 11-exon gene on 12q13. Exons 1 to 3 code for the signal sequence and the extracellular domain of the AMHR2, exon 4 codes for the transmembrane domain, and exons 5 through 11 code for the intracellular serine/threonine domain.

Persistent müllerian duct syndrome (PMDS), also known as *hernia uteri inguinale,* is a condition in which 46,XY males have well-developed testes and normal male ducts and external genitalia but also have müllerian duct derivatives. The diagnosis is often not made until a fallopian tube and uterus are encountered in patients undergoing inguinal hernia repair, orchiopexy, or abdominal surgery. There are two anatomic forms. In the more prevalent form, a hernia contains a partially descended or scrotal testis, and the ipsilateral tube and uterus are in the hernia. In some instances, the contralateral testis and tube also are present in the hernial sac; the presence of transverse testicular ectopia should suggest PMDS. In the second form, the uterus, tubes, and testes are in the pelvis.

Approximately one half of all genetically proven cases of PMDS result from defects in AMH, and half are caused by mutations in its receptor (Fig. 23-32).[360,361] *AMH* gene mutations are most commonly found in Mediterranean, Northern African, and Middle Eastern countries,[362] and most familial mutations are homozygous. In contrast, mutations in the gene encoding AMHR2 are more commonly found in France and Northern Europe and are often compound heterozygous mutations, sometimes involving a 27-bp deletion in exon 10.[363,364] Measurement of serum AMH levels can provide a useful means for guiding genetic analysis; patients with PMDS caused by mutations of the *AMH* gene typically have low or undetectable levels of serum AMH, whereas AMH concentrations are often high-normal or elevated in patients with mutations of *AMHR2*.

The main aim of management of PMDS is to preserve fertility in males, which can be difficult because of the anatomic findings. An increased prevalence of testicular degeneration has been described, which probably results from torsion of the testes. Anatomic abnormalities of the epididymis and the vas deferens are common. Infertility may result from late orchiopexy or from mechanical problems associated with entrapment of the vas deferens in the müllerian derivatives. Early orchiopexy, proximal salpingectomy (leaving the epididymis attached to the fimbriae of the fallopian tube), dissection of the vas deferens from the lateral walls of the uterus, and a complete hysterectomy have been attempted, but these structures can be left in place if there is risk of damage to the genital ducts or blood supply. Men with high pelvic testes rarely have successful orchiopexy, and many of these individuals are androgen deficient.

Hypospadias. Hypospadias is incomplete fusion of the penile urethra defined by an arrest in development of the urethral spongiosum and ventral prepuce.[365] The normal embryologic correction of penile curvature is also interrupted. It is a common congenital anomaly, with an estimated birth prevalence of 3 to 4 cases per 1000 live births. Although it has been suggested that the rates of hypospadias have been increasing, this is not borne out in contemporaneous studies.[366] The cause is unknown in most cases, but it is assumed that there is an interplay of genetic and

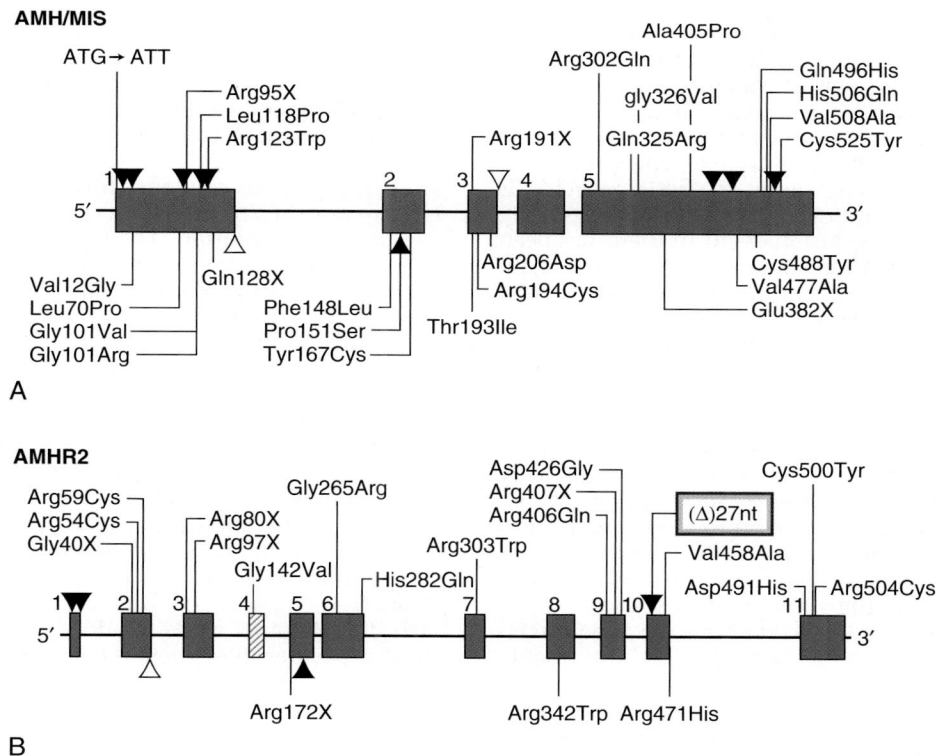

Figure 23-32 A, Diagram of the mutations in the antimüllerian hormone (AMH/MIS) gene that cause persistent müllerian duct syndrome. The numbered solid boxes depict the exons. The three-letter abbreviations for amino acids are used to indicate the positions of missense mutations; X indicates a nonsense (stop) mutation; insertions and deletions resulting in frameshift and splice site mutations are shown by *solid triangles* and *open triangles,* respectively. **B,** Diagram of selected mutations in the gene for the AMH receptor type 2 *(AMHR2).* The numbered solid boxes depict the exons. Exons 1 to 3 encode the extracellular domain of the receptor. Exon 4 *(diagonal lines)* encodes the transmembrane domain, and exons 5 through 11 encode the intracytoplasmic domain. Different forms of mutation are depicted, as in part A. The Δ27nt *(open box)* is a 27-nucleotide deletion, the most common *AMHR2* mutation causing the persistent müllerian duct syndrome. (A redrawn from Imbeaud S, Carré Eusebe D, Rey R, et al. Molecular genetics of the persistent müllerian duct syndrome: a study of 19 families. *Hum Mol Genet.* 1994;3:125-131, used with permission of Oxford University Press. B redrawn from Imbeaud S, Belville C, Messike-Zeitoun L, et al. A 27 base-pair deletion of the antimüllerian type II receptor gene is the most common cause of the persistent müllerian duct syndrome. *Hum Mol Genet.* 1996;5:1269-1277, used with permission of Oxford University Press.)

environmental factors.[367-369] Mutations in candidate genes such as *MAMLD1* and the *AR* are found in a minority of cases.[370] There is a familial clustering of cases in hypospadias, with a 7% incidence of one or more additional affected family members.[371] Four chromosomal regions have been identified in familial hypospadias by fine mapping analysis that involve genes in steroid metabolism.[372]

Hypospadias is associated with increased maternal age, multiple births, maternal exposure to diethylstilbestrol in utero, paternal subfertility, maternal vegetarian diet, maternal smoking, assisted reproductive techniques, paternal exposure to pesticides, and fetal growth restriction.[373] The association with low birth weight is remarkably consistent across all studies of idiopathic hypospadias.[374]

Management is generally surgical. The urethral meatus is relocated to the glans, and the penis is straightened by correcting any chordee to give a normal, forward-directed urinary stream and the ability to have satisfactory sexual intercourse. Numerous techniques are described; repairs may require more than one stage, usually starting at 6 to 12 months of age. The severity of the hypospadias may not be apparent until release of the chordee. Complications include fistula formation, meatal stenosis, urethral stricture, and residual chordee. Follow-up studies in adulthood indicate a less satisfactory cosmetic appearance compared to control subjects, shorter penile length, more dysfunction with voiding, and a lower urinary flow rate.[375] These problems were more evident in the severe form of hypospadias.

Anorchia and Cryptorchidism. The term *vanishing testis syndrome* was coined for the phenotype of bilateral anorchia in an otherwise normally developed male infant. The phenotype is consistent with the presence of testes in early gestation functioning appropriately to induce müllerian duct regression, stabilize wolffian duct development, and differentiate male external genitalia. Bilateral anorchia with a normally differentiated but small phallus (micropenis) is a variant of the syndrome and may represent a form of testicular dysgenesis. The cause of classic anorchia is unknown, but an interruption of the testis blood supply by a torsion or vascular occlusion event in utero has been proposed. Surgical exploration and histologic findings typically show nubbins of fibrous tissue devoid of any testicular tissue attached to a blind-ending vas deferens.

Diagnosis is based on a combination of biochemical tests, imaging studies, and surgical exploration. An undetectable serum AMH level is a reliable marker when evaluating infants with nonpalpable gonads. This, coupled with elevated serum levels of gonadotropins (particularly FSH) and no testosterone response to hCG stimulation, is highly predictive of the absence of testes.[376] Such findings would question the need for surgical exploration in bilateral anorchia. Androgen replacement is required to induce puberty at around 11 to 12 years of age. Testicular prostheses can be inserted if and when the young person desires.

Testes that have not descended at birth (i.e., cryptorchidism) present the most common congenital abnormality in boys, affecting 2% to 9% of term infants.[157,377] There is epidemiologic evidence of an increasing prevalence to 6% in populations studied in the United Kingdom.[378] Longitudinal studies demonstrate the expected spontaneous descent of the testis in early infancy but an unexpected re-ascent of the testis to a cryptorchid position in later childhood. It is now recognized that there are just as many boys with acquired cryptorchidism as there are with congenital cryptorchidism.[379] There is a strong association with low birth weight, disorders of the pituitary-gonadal axis, and a number of syndromes, but in the majority of situations the cause of maldescent is unknown. Mutations in

INSL3 and the gene for its receptor, *RXFP2*, factors involved in the transabdominal phase of testis descent, are found in a few boys with cryptorchidism.[380] Cord blood levels of INSL3 but not testosterone are decreased in idiopathic cryptorchidism, particularly in infants whose testes descended by 3 months of age.[381]

Congenital and acquired forms of cryptorchidism differ in their management. Orchidopexy is the recommended treatment in the former after 6 months but no later than 12 to 18 months of age according to the American Urological Association guidelines.[382] Hormonal treatment with gonadotropins or GnRH analogues is no longer recommended. The guidelines also recommend orchidopexy for acquired cryptorchidism within a year of its presentation. An alternative approach is to wait until puberty because in 50% of cases the testes descend spontaneously at this time.[383] There is substantial evidence to indicate that the relative risk of germ cell tumor development in adulthood associated with cryptorchidism is more than halved if orchidopexy is undertaken before puberty.[384] Early orchidopexy is also beneficial for testis development and spermatogenesis, although the evidence that this is translated into improved fertility is lacking.[385]

Endocrine Disruptors. The proposed increase in male reproductive tract disorders (testis cancer, abnormal spermatogenesis, cryptorchidism, and hypospadias) led to the concept that testicular dysgenesis syndrome (TDS) of fetal origin might be triggered by lifestyle factors and exposure to endocrine-disrupting chemicals (EDCs) operating during the fetal and perinatal periods.[386,387] The U.S. Environmental Protection Agency has defined an EDC as an exogenous agent that interferes with synthesis, secretion, transport, metabolism, binding action, or elimination of natural blood-borne hormones that are present in the body and are responsible for homeostasis, reproduction, and developmental processes.[388] Such a broad definition and the ubiquity of thousands of compounds in the environment which may have endocrine-disrupting effects poses an enormous challenge for scientific studies to prove that adverse health effects occur in humans and, if so, measures for prevention. The types of compounds generically include detergents, pesticides, and cosmetics with postulated modes of action comprising estrogenic and antiandrogenic effects.

Use of classic toxicologic methods in animals is not apposite for human studies, but application of a phenotypic marker long used by toxicologists testing EDCs in animals has now been validated in humans for epidemiologic studies.[389] Anogenital distance (AGD) is significantly reduced in isolated hypospadias and cryptorchidism in comparison with normative data (Fig. 23-33).[390] As an exemplar of the application of this marker in epidemiologic studies in reproductive development, prenatal exposure to phthalates widely used as plasticizers in many products was associated with reduced AGD in males at birth.[391,392] Another angle to adopt is the study of occupational exposure where there is evidence of increased risk of hypospadias and cryptorchidism in offspring of parents working with pesticides, industrial chemicals, cosmetics, and several other potentially toxic substances.[393,394]

The relevance of these epidemiologic findings to the assessment of an individual child with DSD remains uncertain. There is no consensus yet about low-dose effects on health from the combination of a myriad of chemicals to which humans are exposed over the lifespan and what is the optimal toxicologic approach to measure exposure.[395,396] An expert panel has identified compelling evidence for male infertility attributable to phthalate exposure and estimated the financial burden that accrues to the European

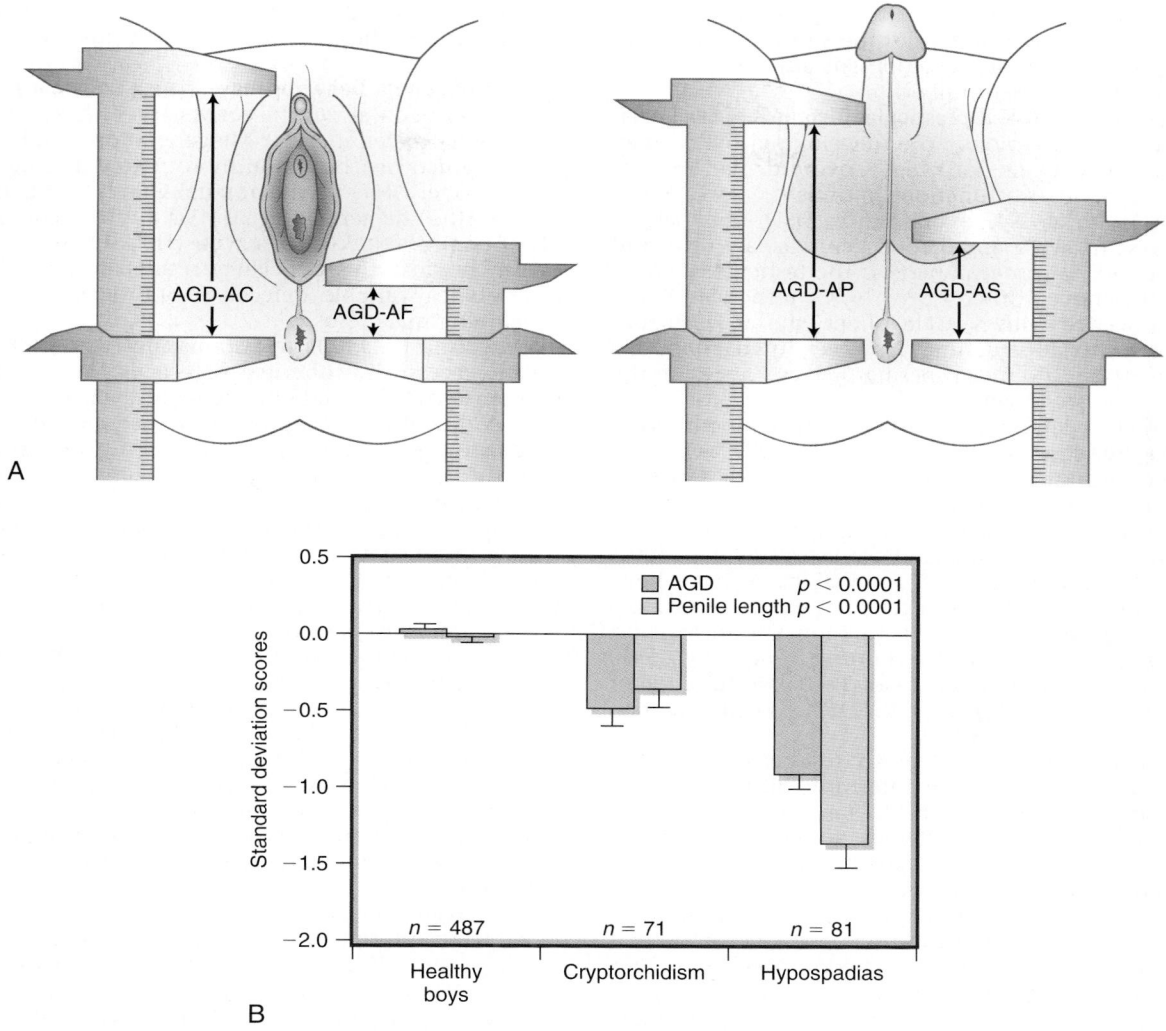

Figure 23-33 Measurement of anogenital distance (AGD). **A,** Different landmarks used for measurement in female and male infants. The distance from the posterior fourchette (AF) and the clitoris (AC) to the midpoint of the anus in females and from the junction of the scrotal (AS) and perineal (AP) skin to the midpoint of the anus in males are commonly used methods to determine AGD in epidemiologic studies. **B,** Measurements of penile length and AGD in boys with cryptorchidism and hypospadias compared with normal male infants. (Redrawn from Thankamony A, Lek N, Carroll D, et al. Anogenital distance and penile length in infants with hypospadias or cryptorchidism; comparison with normative data. *Environ Health Perspect.* 2014;122:207-211, used with permission of Environmental Health Perspectives.)

Union from the consequences of needing additional assisted reproductive technology procedures.[397] A similar analysis can be undertaken to estimate the additional cases of cryptorchidism requiring orchidopexies. Adopting the precautionary principle to reduce exposure to chemicals to as low as is reasonably practicable is a sensible approach in the face of so much uncertainty about the adverse effects of EDCs on human health.

46,XX Disorders of Sex Development

46,XX DSDs can be divided into disorders of ovary development, disorders of androgen synthesis, and other conditions affecting sex development (see Table 23-3).

Disorders of Ovary Development

Disorders of ovary development (i.e., ovarian dysgenesis or resistance) usually manifest as absent puberty due to absent estrogenization production. Other disorders of gonadal development can result in a 46,XX individual with an ovary containing testicular tissue (i.e., 46,XX ovotesticular DSD) or a testis capable of producing enough androgen for a male phenotype and sufficient AMH to regress the uterus (i.e., 46,XX testicular DSD).

Ovarian Dysgenesis. Ovarian dysgenesis most often occurs as a result of sex chromosome aneuploidy (e.g., Turner syndrome; 45,X and variants) with progressive ovarian apoptosis. Ovarian resistance results from mutations in the FSH receptor. Ovarian dysfunction can also occur with a wide range of multisystem syndromes, often involving DNA repair mechanisms (e.g., Perrault, Maximilian, Quayle and Copeland, Pober, Malouf, Nijmegen, Cockayne, Rothmund-Thompson, Werner syndromes; ataxia-telangiectasia). Several nonmetabolic causes of POI or POF have been described,[43-50] including POF1, Xq26-q28, *FMR* premutations; POF2A, Xq22, *DIAPH2*; POF2B, Xq21, POF1B (actin-binding protein); POF3, 3q22, *FOXL2*; POF4, Xp11.2, *BMP15*; POF5, 7q35, *NOBOX*; POF6, 2p12, *FIGLA*; POF7, 9q33, *NR5A1*; POF8, 7q22, *STAG3*; POF9, 1p22, *HFM1*; and POF10, 20p12, *MCM8*, as well as mitochondrial disorders such as mutations in POLG.[398] Although these conditions usually manifest with POI and early menopause, more severe forms of some of these disorders can interfere with earlier aspects of ovarian development and function and can present due to absent puberty.

46,XX Ovotesticular and 46,XX Testicular Disorders of Sex Development. In rare situations, the developing ovary may contain testicular tissue (i.e., 46,XX ovotesticular DSD) or may even develop as a functioning testis (i.e., 46,XX testicular DSD). In 46,XX ovotesticular DSD, the patient usually presents with ambiguous genitalia at birth and progressive virilization at puberty if the testicular component is not removed. In contrast, 46,XX testicular DSD is usually associated with a male phenotype at birth and absence of müllerian structures. However, infertility occurs in both situations as crucial spermatogenesis genes on the Y chromosome are absent.

A detailed review of the presentation, endocrinology, and management of 46,XX ovotesticular DSD was given earlier (see "Sex Chromosome Disorders of Sex Development") as many of the issues faced are similar to those with 46,XX/46,XY chimerism. A 46,XX karyotype is the most frequent finding in ovotesticular DSD, especially in patients from sub-Saharan Africa.[218,219] Familial cases have been described, and it is likely that a genetic basis exists in some cases, although the exact cause is unknown. Translocation and upregulation of testis-determining genes (e.g., *SRY*, *SOX9*) have been found in rare cases. Partial dysfunction of the ovarian-testis repressor gene *RSPO1* has been described in 46,XX ovotesticular DSD.[221]

In contrast, patients with 46,XX testicular DSD often present first with male factor infertility, although sometimes hypospadias is present. In some cases, a family history is found. Because different family members can have different phenotypes, it is possible that 46,XX testicular DSD represents the most severe end of the spectrum of ovarian transdifferentiation phenotypes. Up to 80% of 46,XX males harbor translocations of Y-chromosomal material containing SRY, the testis-determining factor. This finding helped considerably in mapping the *SRY* gene in the first instance (see "Development of Reproductive Systems"), and in some situations, residual ovarian tissue (ovotestis) develops. Individuals with *SRY* translocations can be diagnosed by FISH analysis using a probe directed to that gene (see Fig. 23-3). A number of *SRY*-negative cases have been reported. Often these arise from duplication of the genetic locus containing *SOX9* or deletions or rearrangements in distant regulatory regions that result in *SOX9* overexpression.[113,114,117] Alterations in the X chromosome resulting in overexpression of *SOX3* have also been described.[399] Loss-of-function mutations in *RSPO1* (an ovarian gene encoding R-spondin 1) have been reported in individuals with 46,XX testicular DSD with palmar-plantar hyperkeratosis and squamous cell carcinoma.[14] This factor, which mediates the WNT4 signaling pathway, was the first ovarian-specific repressor of testis development to be described. Loss of function of R-spondin 1 in the developing gonad of 46,XX individuals results in testis development and an infertile male phenotype. It is likely that additional factors may act as repressors of SRY and testis determination. Severe disruption of WNT4 can result in 46,XX sex reversal as part of the SERKAL syndrome, which consists of female-to-male sex reversal and renal, adrenal, and lung dysgenesis.[400]

Disorders of Androgen Excess

The steroid biosynthetic disorders causing androgen excess and 46,XX DSD are summarized in Table 23-6. Although CYP21 deficiency is by far the most common form of this condition, alternative diagnoses should be considered because approaches to counseling and management may vary.

3β-Hydroxysteroid Dehydrogenase Type 2 Deficiency. 3β-HSD/$\Delta^{4,5}$-isomerase catalyzes the conversion of Δ^5-steroids to Δ^4-steroids and is required for the generation of mineralocorticoids, glucocorticoids, and more potent androgens (e.g., testosterone, DHT) by the adrenal glands and gonads (see Fig. 23-10). The actions of 3β-HSD and the consequences of deficiency of the type 2 enzyme (HSD3B2) were described earlier, because this deficiency results in adrenal insufficiency with variable defects in androgenization of the developing male fetus.

Defects in HSD3B2 can also manifest in 46,XX females. Severe, recessively inherited defects in enzyme function can cause mild clitoral enlargement at birth in girls with glucocorticoid deficiency (with or without salt loss). This mild androgenization occurs not as a direct androgenic effect of the excess DHEA but as a result of its conversion and that of other Δ^5-3β-hydroxy-C19-steroids to testosterone by HSD3B1 in the placenta and in the peripheral tissues of the fetus. This conversion, coupled with the limited capacity of the placenta to aromatize androgens to estrogens early in gestation, can increase circulating levels of androgens in the female fetus and cause modest clitoromegaly in a minority of patients. Other girls have normal genitalia but show adrenal features. Milder, nonclassic forms of HSD3B2 deficiency can cause premature pubarche in girls. Breast development can occur at puberty in affected females, presumably by peripheral conversions of Δ^5-C19-steroids to Δ^4-C19-steroids by HSD3B1 expressed principally in peripheral tissues and by the subsequent aromatization of androgens to estrogens. The presence of menses has been reported in treated females with this condition.

The diagnosis of HSD3B2 deficiency can be challenging in nonclassic forms of this condition.[266] The levels of Δ^5-steroids (e.g., 17-hydroxypregnenolone, DHEA, and its sulfate, DHEAS) usually are increased, and the ratio of Δ^5-steroids to Δ^4-steroids (e.g., the ratio of 17-OHP to cortisol) is markedly increased, especially after stimulation with intravenous ACTH. The urinary steroid profile can also be informative, because 17-ketosteroids and especially DHEAS and 16-hydroxy-DHEAS are elevated. Basal plasma concentrations of 17-OHP can be increased as a result of peripheral conversion of Δ^5-17-hydroxypregnenolone to 17-OHP by the type 1 enzyme. This finding may lead to confusion with alternative forms of CAH, such as CYP21 deficiency or POR deficiency. Mild forms of HSD3B2 deficiency may manifest in a fashion similar to that of virilizing adrenal tumors. Suppression of the increased plasma and urinary levels of C19 and C21 3β-hydroxysteroids by glucocorticoids distinguishes 3β-HSD deficiency in such cases. Treatment for 3β-HSD deficiency is glucocorticoid, mineralocorticoid, and salt supplementation, as appropriate, and estrogen replacement to induce puberty if needed.[269]

21-Hydroxylase Deficiency. In the context of DSD, CYP21 deficiency (see Fig. 23-10) is one of the most common causes of ambiguous genitalia of the newborn. It is primarily a disorder of adrenal steroidogenesis that affects around 1 in 18,000 children in the first year of life, with most 46,XX girls presenting at birth due to virilization of the genitalia (see Chapter 15).[401,402]

A female fetus with CYP21 deficiency can become androgenized to various degrees, as illustrated by the Prader classification (Fig. 23-34). Serum concentrations of testosterone are invariably within the adult male range and sometimes higher in CAH caused by CYP21 deficiency. High fetal concentrations of 17-OHP, androstenedione, and testosterone are the hallmark of androgenization in CAH due to CYP21 deficiency. More than 75% of patients are also salt losers because of their inability to synthesize sufficient mineralocorticoids. The two forms are readily explained by the nature of the mutation, which affects the *CYP21* gene on chromosome 6p21.3. The concordance between genotype and phenotype for the single-gene disorder is remarkably precise (Fig. 23-35). In patients who are compound heterozygotes, the phenotype usually is concordant with the milder allele. More than 90% of cases result from *CYP21* deletion or one of nine mutations derived from the nonfunctional pseudogene *CYP21P* (see Fig. 23-35). About 5% of *CYP21* mutations arise spontaneously.[403] Worldwide, around 100 non–pseudogene-derived mutations are reported for the *CYP21A2* allele.

The diagnosis of CYP21 deficiency in a newborn with ambiguous genitalia is readily confirmed by markedly elevated serum 17-OHP concentrations (>300 nmol/L) after the first 48 hours. Sick, preterm infants can have moderately increased steroid levels, so ACTH stimulation may be needed to resolve any diagnostic confusion. The affected male usually has no alerting clinical signs at birth and, if a salt loser, does not decompensate with hypokalemia, hyperkalemia, and weight loss until 1 to 2 weeks after birth.[402] Newborn screening programs to measure blood spot 17-OHP concentrations soon after birth have been introduced in some countries.[404] Elevated 17-OHP can also be seen in conditions such as 3β-HSD deficiency, 11β-hydroxylase deficiency, and P450 oxidoreductase deficiency, although the levels are usually not as high as in 21-hydroxylase deficiency.

Of major relevance to DSD is the potential to prevent ambiguous genitalia of the newborn through prenatal treatment with dexamethasone.[405,406] Androgenization can be prevented if dexamethasone is administered to the mother early enough in gestation, indicating an intact fetal pituitary-adrenal axis that is responsive to negative-feedback regulation. This model is based on studies of human fetal adrenal explants that synthesize cortisol, androstenedione, and testosterone under ACTH regulation, which is subject to negative feedback by glucocorticoids.[156] Treatment is effective if dexamethasone is started by 6 to 7 weeks' gestation. However, in current practice, karyotype analysis and *CYP21* genotype analysis is not available until approximately 5 weeks later. Seven unaffected or male fetuses would need to be treated with dexamethasone during this initial period for every one affected female fetus who might benefit.

Several concerns have been raised about the potential effects of dexamethasone on the developing fetus. Although cognitive and motor development based on questionnaires appeared not to be adversely affected by exposure to dexamethasone, direct examination of children who had been exposed to dexamethasone from gestational age 6 to 7 weeks did show adverse effects on verbal working memory compared with control subjects.[407-410] All of these studies were observational, and a meta-analysis emphasized the paucity of good-quality, long-term follow-up data to inform a risk/benefit analysis.[411] This aspect should be considered when counseling families about prenatal treatment. Clinical practice guidelines have suggested that prenatal therapy should only be undertaken using protocols approved by institutional review boards and at centers capable of collecting long-term outcome data as part of multicenter studies.[412,413]

Recent advances in the detection of circulating free fetal DNA in the maternal serum have increased the sensitivity and specificity of determining fetal sex much earlier in

Scoring external genitalia

Prader stage

Normal ♀   I   II   III   IV   V   Normal ♂

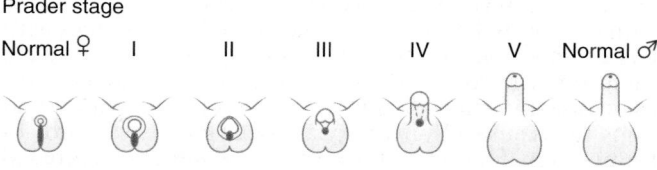

Figure 23-34 Prader classification of the degree of androgenization in a female with congenital adrenal hyperplasia.

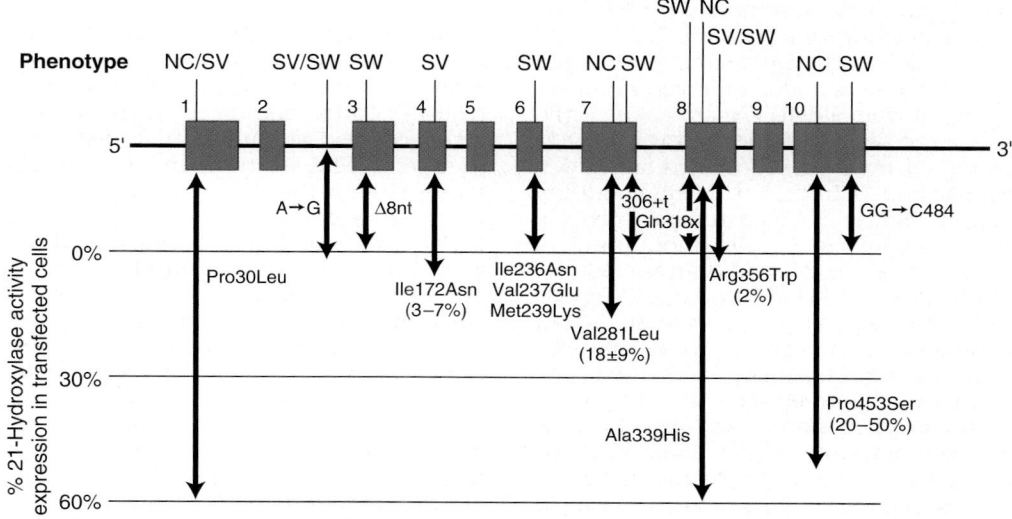

Figure 23-35 Diagram of the *CYP21* gene and locations of the mutations that cause more than 90% of cases of 21-hydroxylase deficiency. The numbered boxes depict the exons. The three-letter abbreviations for amino acids are used; X indicates a nonsense (stop) mutation. An adenine (A) to guanine (G) transition in intron 2 causes a common splice site mutation. Other mutations include an 8-nucleotide deletion (Δ8nt) in exon 3, a thymidine insertion at codon 306 (306+t), and a guanine (G) to cytosine (C) transition at codon 484. The activities of the mutant enzymes, expressed as a percentage of the wild type, are indicated on the vertical axis and in parentheses for some missense mutations. NC, nonclassic form; SV, simple virilizing; SW, salt wasting.

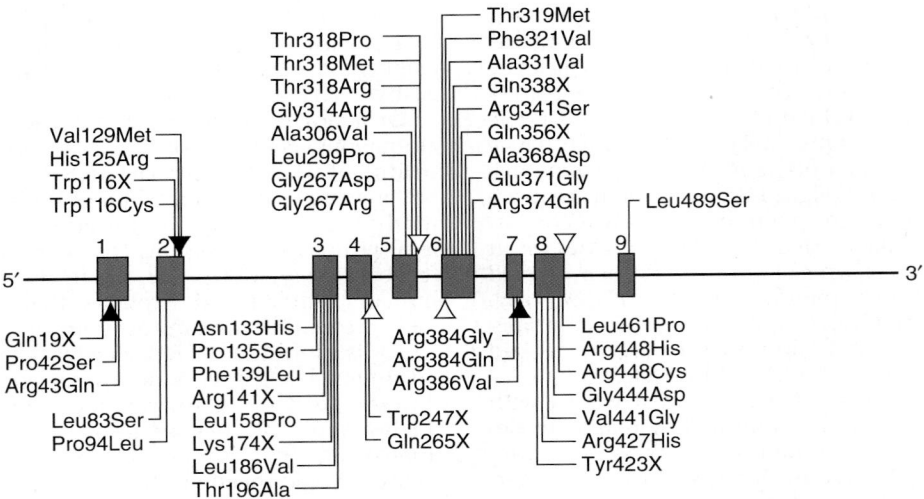

Figure 23-36 Diagram of the *CYP11B1* gene and locations of the mutations causing 11β-hydroxylase deficiency. The numbered solid boxes depict the exons. The three-letter abbreviations for amino acids are used; X indicates a nonsense (stop) mutation. A deletion of cytosine (C) at codon 32 and the addition of two nucleotides at codon 394 cause frameshift mutations; insertions and deletions resulting in a frameshift and splice site are shown by *solid triangles* and *open triangles*, respectively.

pregnancy.[414] This would mean that only female fetuses would be treated and would allow some reduction in unnecessary exposure to dexamethasone in male fetuses. Furthermore, using parental haplotype analysis by targeted massively parallel sequencing of the *CYP21* locus, it has been possible to determine the genotype of the fetus earlier in pregnancy so that fewer unaffected females would be treated.[415] These are all potentially promising advances to prevent exposure of unaffected babies to dexamethasone, or to limit the exposure in affected girls, if parents do decide to have dexamethasone treatment in pregnancy in a center that offers it.

P450 Oxidoreductase Deficiency. POR is a membrane-bound flavoprotein that plays a central role in electron transfer from NADPH to all microsomal P450 enzymes, including CYP17, CYP21, and CYP19 (aromatase) (see Fig. 23-26). Defects in POR can cause apparent combined CYP17 and CYP21 deficiency, with or without Antley-Bixler syndrome, a form of craniosynostosis. These conditions were described earlier (see "Disorders of Androgen Synthesis").[285,287] POR deficiency can be associated with ambiguous genitalia in both 46,XX and 46,XY infants. The androgenization of 46,XX fetuses may result from a defect in aromatase activity or occur through a proposed backdoor pathway of DHT production that does not involve androstenedione or testosterone as intermediates.[155] Children with this condition usually have cortisol deficiency, but mineralocorticoid function is relatively preserved. Careful monitoring of puberty is needed as this can be delayed or disrupted.[288]

11β-Hydroxylase Deficiency. 11β-Hydroxylase (CYP11B1) deficiency is a disorder of adrenal steroidogenesis. It can cause profound androgenization in an affected female fetus and accounts for 5% to 8% of patients with CAH.[416,417] 11β-Hydroxylase deficiency typically presents with ambiguous genitalia in the 46,XX newborn, although in some situations the androgenization may be so severe that the baby is thought to be a boy with a small penis and undescended testes.[418] Subsequently in childhood there can be hyperandrogenism and precocious puberty, with accelerated growth and skeletal maturation. Hypertension occurs in two thirds of cases as prolonged accumulation of 11-deoxycorticosterone leads to salt and fluid retention, and plasma renin is suppressed. Milder changes in

11β-hydroxylase cause a nonclassic form of the condition, similar to nonclassic 21-hydroxylase deficiency, which presents mostly with hyperandrogenism.[419] The biochemical diagnosis can be made by urine steroid profile and through a pattern of reduced cortisol and elevated intermediates such as 11-deoxycorticosterone.

11β-Hydroxylase is encoded by the *CYP11B1* gene, which is located on chromosome 8q21-22 in tandem with *CYP11B2*, which encodes aldosterone synthase, the enzyme catalyzing the conversion of deoxycorticosterone to corticosterone and then to aldosterone. Some *CYP11B1* mutations that cause 11β-hydroxylase deficiency are shown in Figure 23-36. Most changes are missense mutations. Arg448 appears to be a relative hot spot for mutations, with Arg448His possibly a founder mutation in the Moroccan Jewish population. Treatment of 11β-hydroxylase deficiency includes glucocorticoid replacement to reduce ACTH drive and in some situations antihypertensive treatment.

Familial Glucocorticoid Resistance. Glucocorticoid resistance is a rare disorder that is usually caused by sporadic heterozygous mutations in the glucocorticoid receptor α-isoform (GRα).[420] Partial end-organ insensitivity to glucocorticoid action coupled with impaired feedback mechanisms results in excess ACTH secretion and elevated circulating cortisol levels without the clinical features of Cushing syndrome. In many cases, elevated levels of mineralocorticoids cause hypertension and hypokalemia, and elevated levels of adrenal androgens cause hirsutism and acne. One homozygous *NR3C1* mutation (Val571Ala) was reported in a Brazilian girl who had a large clitoris, posterior labioscrotal fusion, and a urogenital sinus at birth.[421] This mutation caused marked reduction in GRα function without complete loss of receptor activity. She also harbored a heterozygous mutation in *CYP21*. More severe GRα mutations may manifest as mild 46,XX DSD, although the phenotype might have been modified in this case by the coexistence of a heterozygous CYP21 change.

Aromatase Deficiency. Aromatase (CYP19A1) is the only cytochrome P450 enzyme known to catalyze the conversion of androgens (C19 steroids) to estrogens (C18 steroids) in vertebrate species.[422] Aromatase is expressed in many tissues, including the placenta, ovary, brain, bone, vascular

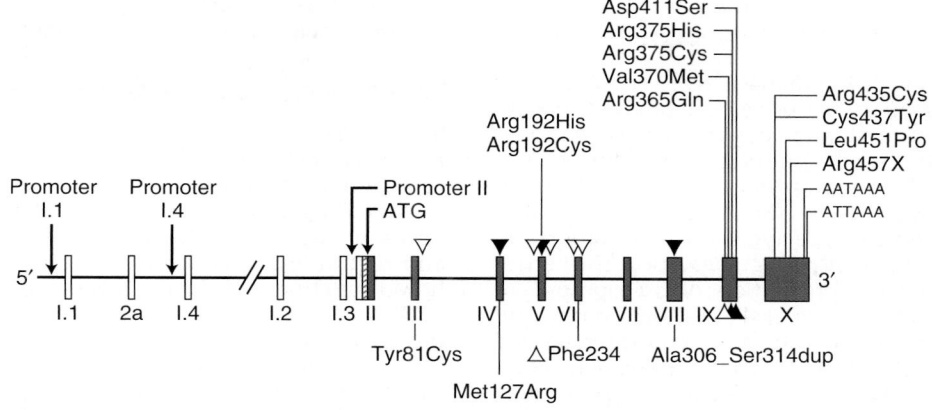

Figure 23-37 Diagram of the *CYP19* gene and selected mutations causing aromatase deficiency. The numbered solid boxes represent translated exons. The septum in the open box in exon II represents the 3′ acceptor splice junction for the untranslated exons. Multiple alternative promoters and the untranslated exons *(open boxes)* are indicated. The three-letter abbreviations for amino acids are used to indicate the positions of missense mutations; X indicates a nonsense (stop) mutation; insertions and deletions resulting in frameshift and splice site mutations are shown by *solid triangles* and *open triangles*, respectively. In addition to the mutations causing classic aromatase deficiency, a homozygous Arg435Cys mutation and deletion of a phenylalanine residue at position 234 are both associated with a partial aromatase insufficiency phenotype. (Modified from Morishima A, Grumbach MM, Simpson ER, et al. Aromatase deficiency in male and female siblings caused by a novel mutation and the physiological role of estrogens. *J Clin Endocrinol Metab.* 1995;80:3689-3698, used with permission of The Endocrine Society, copyright 1995.)

endothelium, breast, and adipose tissue, where it is regulated by a number of tissue-specific promoters to convert testosterone to estradiol and androstenedione to estrone (Fig. 23-37). Aromatase plays a crucial role in the local production of estrogens and in the synthesis of circulating estrogens from the ovary at the time of puberty.

Aromatase deficiency due to recessively inherited mutations in *CYP19* has been described in approximately 25 girls with 46,XX DSD (see Fig. 23-37). The clinical and biochemical features of this condition underscore the key role aromatase plays in the fetoplacental unit, and this condition is sometimes referred to as *placental aromatase deficiency*. Aromatase plays a critical role in protecting the fetus from excessive androgen exposure in utero (Fig. 23-38). In the absence of aromatase, estrogen cannot be synthesized by the placenta, and large quantities of placental testosterone and androstenedione are transferred to the fetal and maternal circulation, resulting in androgenization of the female fetus and virilization of the mother during pregnancy.[423]

Females (46,XX) with aromatase insufficiency are born with clitoromegaly, various degrees of posterior fusion, scrotalization of the labioscrotal folds, and, in some infants with a urogenital sinus, a single perineal orifice.[424-426] There is often a striking history of maternal virilization after the second trimester of pregnancy (e.g., acne, hair growth, voice changes) coupled with elevated maternal androgen levels, which usually resolve after the infant is born, but it is also emerging that maternal virilization does not always occur.[427-428] As expected for a steroidogenic defect, affected girls (46,XX) have normal müllerian structures. The histologic picture of the ovaries in infancy is normal, but under increased FSH stimulation in the absence of ovarian aromatase, multiple, enlarged follicular cysts develop. At puberty, affected females have hypergonadotropic hypogonadism, typically fail to develop female secondary sexual characteristics, and exhibit progressive virilization. Plasma androstenedione and testosterone levels are elevated, and estrone and estradiol levels are low or not measurable. The ovaries enlarge and develop multiple cysts at puberty; in one affected female, polycystic ovaries were detected in infancy. The hypergonadotropism and the multiple ovarian

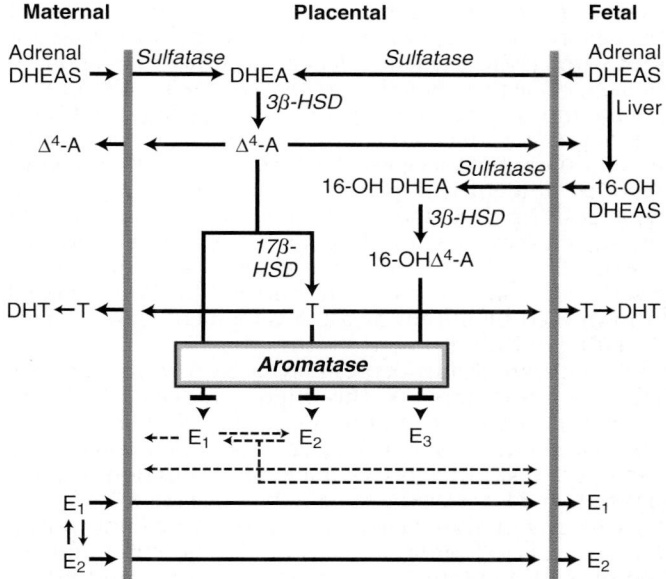

Figure 23-38 Aromatase plays a crucial role in protecting the fetus from excessive androgen exposure in utero. The placenta lacks CYP17 enzymatic activity and cannot convert C21 steroids such as progesterone to C19 steroids and thereafter to estrogens. During gestation, large quantities of dehydroepiandrosterone sulfate (DHEAS) are produced in the fetal and maternal adrenal glands. DHEAS is 16α-hydroxylated in the fetal adrenal and liver. The 16α-hydroxy-DHEAS from the fetus and DHEAS from the fetus and mother are transferred to the placental unit, where the sulfate moiety is cleaved by placental sulfatase. These steroids can then be converted to androstenedione (A) and 16α-hydroxyandrostenedione by 3β-hydroxysteroid dehydrogenase (HSD) type 1/Δ4,5-isomerase; to testosterone and 16α-hydroxytestosterone by 17β-HSD; and to estrogens (mainly estriol from 16α-hydroxy-DHEA) by placental aromatase. Androstenedione and 16α-hydroxyandrostenedione may be aromatized directly to estrogens. DHT, dihydrotestosterone; E1, estrone; E2, estradiol; E3, estriol; T, testosterone. (Modified and redrawn from Conte FA, Grumbach MM, Ito Y, et al. A syndrome of female pseudohermaphrodism, hypergonadotropic hypogonadism, and multicystic ovaries associated with missense mutations in the gene encoding aromatase (P450arom). *J Clin Endocrinol Metab.* 1994;78:1287-1292, used with permission of The Endocrine Society, copyright 1994.)

cysts respond to estrogen replacement therapy, but in some cases, temporary treatment with an antiandrogen is necessary.

In addition to a role in the reproductive axis, aromatase deficiency has implications for bone development, metabolism, and immune function, as determined by the long-term follow-up of the small numbers of women (46,XX) and men (46,XY) with aromatase deficiency and by studies of aromatase-knockout mice. Males present only after puberty and have tall stature, delayed bone maturation and epiphyseal fusion, and osteopenia, suggesting that estrogens are essential for the prevention of osteoporosis in males and females and for normal skeletal maturation and proportions.[429] Hyperinsulinemia and abnormal plasma lipids have also been reported in aromatase deficiency, which may in part reflect estrogen insufficiency but may also reflect specific actions of aromatase itself. The finding of apparently normal psychosexual development in the three aromatase-deficient adolescent or adult patients and in the man with an estrogen receptor defect suggests that estrogen does not play a critical role in sex differentiation of the human brain, as has been reported in nonprimate mammals.

CYP19A1 mutations have been described in males and females with aromatase deficiency, are inherited in a recessive fashion, and are present in a homozygous or compound heterozygous state (see Fig. 23-37). Functional assays of aromatase activity have shown severe loss of enzyme function (approximately 0.3%) in all cases associated with classic aromatase deficiency, other than approximately 1% activity for the Arg435Cys change found in a compound heterozygote together with the null Cys437Tyr mutation.[426] Partial aromatase deficiency has also been described; a homozygous Arg435Cys change has been reported in a girl who presented with androgenized genitalia at birth but showed limited breast development during puberty, and deletion of a single phenylalanine residue (Phe234del) causing partial loss of aromatase activity was described in an androgenized 46,XX individual who showed significant breast development (Tanner stage 4) during puberty.[430]

A spectrum of phenotypes may be seen with aromatase insufficiency in humans. This important diagnosis should be considered in all androgenized 46,XX infants when more common forms of CAH (e.g., CYP21 deficiency) have been excluded. A history of maternal virilization in pregnancy should always be sought but may not always be present, and increased levels of Δ^4-androstenedione, testosterone, and DHT and low levels of plasma estriol, urinary estriol, and amniotic fluid estrone, estradiol, and estriol may be detected. The diagnosis can be difficult to make during childhood years, when the HPG axis is quiescent, and genetic analysis may be needed.

Maternal Androgen Excess. Maternal sources of androgens that may virilize a female fetus may be endogenous from adrenal and ovarian tumors or exogenous from maternal ingestion of androgenic compounds. Danazol, a synthetic derivative of ethisterone with androgenic, antiestrogenic, and antiprogestogenic activities, is used in diverse conditions such as endometriosis, benign fibrocystic breast disease, and hereditary angioedema and in women with unexplained subfertility. It crosses the placenta and is contraindicated in pregnancy in view of reports that a female fetus may become androgenized.[431] Ovarian causes of virilization include primary malignancy, benign lesions such as luteoma and hyperreactio luteinalis, and polycystic ovary syndrome. Recurrence in subsequent pregnancies and maternal virilization can occur with luteomas.[432] As in fetal aromatase deficiency, a similar pattern of recurrent

hyperandrogenization without evidence of placental aromatase deficiency has been reported.[433]

Other Conditions Affecting 46,XX Sex Development

Several syndromic associations can cause developmental genital abnormalities in 46,XX females, although these are less common than the syndromic associations resulting in underandrogenization in 46,XY males. Complex urogenital anomalies such as cloacal extrophy can affect both sexes and require major reconstructive surgery for bladder and bowel function and for the lower genital system.

Abnormalities in uterine development can result in bicornate uterus (i.e., Fryns syndrome), uterine hemiagenesis or hypoplasia, or uterine agenesis. These conditions can be associated with renal, cardiac, and cervical spinal abnormalities as part of Mayer-Rokitansky-Küster-Hauser (MRKH) syndrome or MURCS (müllerian, renal, and cervical spine syndrome).[434,435] The cause of these conditions is unknown for most women, although some familial cases have been described, and a mutation in *WNT4* was reported in a patient with absent müllerian structures (uterus and upper vagina), unilateral renal agenesis, and mild hyperandrogenemia.[436] Uterine abnormalities have also been associated with maturity-onset diabetes of the young type 5 (MODY5, *HNF1B*) and with vaginal abnormalities in patients with hand-foot-genital syndrome (*HOXA13*) and McKusick-Kaufman syndrome (*MKKS*, formerly called *BBS6*). Because a prominent clitoris can be associated with conditions such as Fraser syndrome or neurofibromatosis, careful evaluation is necessary before a hyperandrogenic cause is diagnosed.

Other common conditions that may be mistaken for a more serious underlying disorder include apparent clitoromegaly seen in premature or former premature babies or when little labial adipose tissue is present. Assessment by a surgeon or physician with experience of normal variability in clitoral size is important. Sometimes this form of isolated clitoromegaly can persist into childhood.[437] Labial adhesions are a common finding in female newborns. They often resolve spontaneously, although estrogen cream can be used to accelerate the process. Transient menstrual bleeding during the first week of life can be seen frequently in female infants with the withdrawal of large amounts of estrogens and progesterones after birth. This finding can be alarming for parents, but it rapidly resolves, and no treatment is needed.

INVESTIGATION AND MANAGEMENT OF DISORDERS OF SEX DEVELOPMENT

DSDs can present at many ages and to a wide range of different health professionals. Some of the most common presentations are shown in Table 23-18, and the range of conditions discussed in our center over a 2-year period is shown in Table 23-19. The potential diagnosis of DSD has major implications for the child and the family. Most people will never have heard of DSD or will not have thought they may be faced with a situation, for example, in which they cannot be told immediately whether their newborn is a boy or a girl. Talking about such issues can be difficult. Sensitive and positive support and education from all health professionals is essential to provide parents with knowledge and confidence.[438]

Specialist multidisciplinary team (MDT) involvement with families, young people, and adults with DSD is important.[1-3,313,439] These specialists are usually based only at large centers, so effective communication between the team and those health professionals dealing with the initial presentation is crucial. Although there is often uncertainty at the start, a general diagnosis can usually be reached following a series of careful assessments and basic investigations. Reaching a more specific diagnosis can be important

in some situations and may take longer and involve more detailed investigations or genetic tests (discussed later). Every person is different, and many DSD-related conditions can have a spectrum of presentations, so it is also important to take an individualized approach to the child and the family.

The following is a discussion of the investigation and management of DSDs at different ages. Several overarching themes are subsequently highlighted. More extensive detail of specific conditions is discussed previously in this chapter.

Prenatal Diagnosis

Prenatal diagnosis of DSD is increasingly common as fetal ultrasonography improves and as more people have karyotype analysis or cell-free fetal DNA (cffDNA) for various reasons in pregnancy.[440] Although some prospective parents choose not to know the sex of their baby, many couples ask whether they are having a boy or a girl, and issues can arise when the genital appearances are unclear on the scan or when the appearance of the genitals is discordant with the known karyotype. These situations can generate great anxiety, and early contact with the DSD MDT is helpful to support the couple. Genital appearance at birth can differ from that seen on prenatal scans, so support to deal with this uncertainty and a time frame of what will happen if their baby does have atypical genitalia are important. A potential prenatal diagnosis of DSD can have benefits as it gives parents time to learn about possible conditions and to think how they will deal with the situation as long as support is provided in a sensitive manner.

The Newborn with Atypical Genitalia

The most established presentation of DSD occurs when a newborn baby has atypical (or ambiguous) genitalia, and

TABLE 23-18
Common Presentations of DSDs at Different Ages

Presentation	Feature	Examples
Prenatal	Karyotype-phenotype discordance	Many
Neonatal	Atypical genitalia	Many
	Salt-losing crisis	21-Hydroxylase deficiency, 3β-HSD deficiency (46,XX) StAR, CYP11A1, 3β-HSD deficiency, SF1/NR5A1 (46,XY)
Childhood	Hernia	Complete AIS
	Androgenization	21-Hydroxylase deficiency, 11β-hydroxylase deficiency
	Associated features	Wilms tumor
Puberty	Androgenization	17β-HSD deficiency, 5α-reductase deficiency (rarely SF1/NR5A1, partial AIS, ovotestes)
	Absent puberty	Swyer syndrome (complete gonadal dysgenesis), 17α-hydroxylase deficiency
Postpuberty	Amenorrhea	Complete AIS
Adult	Infertility ?Tumors	Minimal AIS, SF1/NR5A1, etc.

AIS, androgen insensitivity syndrome; CYP, cytochrome P450 enzyme; DSDs, disorders of sex development; HSD, hydroxysteroid dehydrogenase; SF1, steroidogenic factor 1; StAR, steroidogenic acute regulatory (protein).

TABLE 23-19
The Range of Diagnoses of DSD Seen in a Single Center Over 2 Years

Sex Chromosome DSD (n = 13)	46,XY DSD (n = 65)	46,XX DSD (n = 23)
A: 47,XXY (Klinefelter syndrome and variants) (2) B: 45,X (Turner syndrome and variants) (2) (both Y fragment) C: 45,X/46,XY mosaicism (mixed gonadal dysgenesis and variants) (8) D: 46,XX/46,XY (chimerism/mosaicism) (1)	A: Disorders of gonadal (testis) development 1. Complete gonadal dysgenesis (7) 2. Partial gonadal dysgenesis (8) 3. Steroidogenic factor 1 (2) B: Disorders in androgen synthesis or action 1. Disorders of androgen biosynthesis StAR (1) 17β-HSD III (2) 5α-Reductase II (6) 2. Disorders of androgen action CAIS (6) PAIS (5) C: Other 1. Syndromic associations of male genital development (11) (e.g., chromosomal variants, skeletal, lung, skin, gastrointestinal, Cornelia de Lange, CHARGE) 2. Cloacal anomalies (1) 3. IUGR/preterm/hypospadias (4) 4. Persistent müllerian duct syndrome (3) 5. Vanishing testis syndrome (2) 6. Isolated severe hypospadias (4) 7. Micropenis (1) 8. Bilateral undescended testes (2)	A: Disorders of gonadal (ovary) development 1. Ovotesticular DSD (1) 2. Testicular DSD (1) B: Androgen excess 1. Fetal 21-Hydroxylase (10) 11β-Hydroxylase (2) 2. Fetoplacental 3. Maternal C: Other 1. Syndromic associations (e.g., cloacal anomalies) (1) 2. Müllerian agenesis (1) 3. Clitoromegaly, possible clitoromegaly or clitoral variants (6) 4. Ovarian cysts (1)

CAIS, complete androgen insensitivity syndrome; CHARGE, coloboma, heart defect, atresia chonanae, retarded growth and development, genital hypoplasia, ear anomalies (deafness); DSDs, disorders of sex development; IUGR, intrauterine growth restriction; PAIS, partial androgen insensitivity syndrome; StAR, steroidogenic acute regulatory (protein).
From Brain CE, Creighton SM, Mushtaq I, et al. Holistic management of DSD. *Best Pract Res Clin Endocrinol Metab.* 2010;24:335-354, used with permission of Elsevier, Inc.

TABLE 23-20

Problems in Newborns That Merit Investigation for DSDs

Ambiguous (atypical) genitalia
Apparent female genitalia
   Enlarged clitoris
   Posterior labial fusion
   Inguinal/labial mass
Apparent male genitalia
   Nonpalpable testes
   Isolated penoscrotal hypospadias
   Severe hypospadias, undescended testes, micropenis
Family history of DSD, such as complete AIS
Discordance between genital appearance and prenatal karyotype

AIS, androgen insensitivity syndrome; DSDs, disorders of sex development.

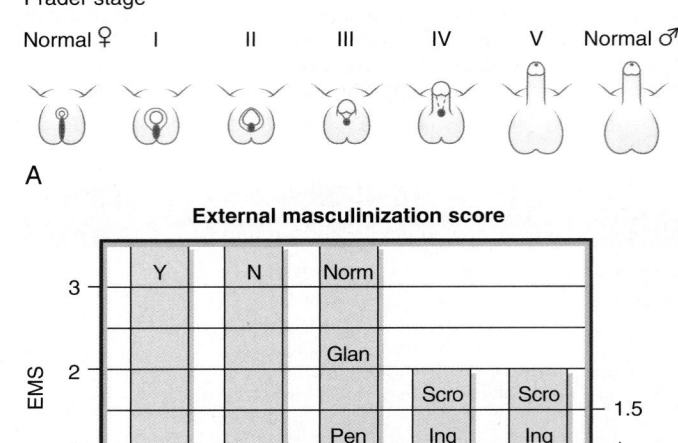

Figure 23-39 A, Prader staging for scoring the degree of androgenization of the external genitalia in a female infant with congenital adrenal hyperplasia. **B,** The external masculinization score (EMS) is used to assess degree of underandrogenization in an individual with 46,XY disorder of sex development. The score is based on the presence or absence of a micropenis and bifid scrotum, the location of the urethral meatus (normal, glandular, penile, perineal), and the position of the testes (scrotal, inguinal, abdominal, absent). (B from Ahmed SF, Khwaja O, Hughes JA. The role of a clinical score in the assessment of ambiguous genitalia. *BJU Int.* 2000;85;120-124.)

it is not possible to say immediately and with certainty whether the baby is a boy or a girl. Further investigations such as a karyotype are usually needed, and specialist review may be required. It is estimated that around 1 in 4500 babies cannot be immediately assigned a sex at birth, although the exact incidence is not known. In some situations there may be confusion due to labial swelling after a breech delivery, or undescended testes, or a mild hypospadias, which can affect up to 1 in 300 male infants. However, in many situations it is not so obvious. Some of the genital features that need further consideration are outlined in Table 23-20. Any child with hypospadias and nonpalpable testes needs careful review because this child could—rarely, but importantly—be a 46,XX baby with severe CAH. Sometimes atypical genital features are first picked up on a newborn examination rather than at birth.

Examination and History

A careful examination is needed but should be done sensitively and only after the parents have had some time to be with their baby. Genital appearances can be misleading because of chordee (bending and tethering of the phallus) or if there is a large suprapubic fat pad, so palpation as well as observation is important. Key features to note are the length of the phallus; the consistency of the corpora and glans; extent of chordee and scrotal transposition; features of the foreskin (hooded, excess skin); position of the urethral opening; rugosity (scrotalization) and midline fusion of the labioscrotal folds; and size and position of any palpable gonads (likely to be testes). The external masculinization score (EMS) is one way of recording findings and is useful for research purposes, but individual features are important, too (Fig. 23-39).[344] For example, asymmetry of the genitalia can suggest 45,X/46,XY mosaicism or partial gonadal dysgenesis (previously referred to as mixed gonadal dysgenesis). Other features such as evidence of IUGR, position of the anus, skeletal or cardiac anomalies, or dysmorphic features are important. Hyperpigmentation is a rare but important sign of primary adrenal insufficiency due to elevated ACTH, but increased local pigmentation can often be seen in babies of Asian or African ancestry.

A careful history is important but must be done sensitively and rarely points to an immediate diagnosis. Key points to consider include family history of adrenal conditions, such as CAH or known DSD; aspects of the pregnancy, such as growth restriction and preeclampsia (IUGR and hypospadias); maternal acne or hair growth in pregnancy (aromatase deficiency); and any prenatal tests or scans performed. Medications and drugs can have a theoretical effect on the fetus (e.g., 5α-reductase inhibitors), and assisted reproduction or the need for fertility treat-

ment might indicate an underlying and variably penetrant genetic cause. A history of hypospadias, DSD, or infertility in the extended family may be relevant but may not be known or widely discussed. It is important to understand the parents' thoughts and beliefs and not to generate additional anxiety by insensitive questions.

The Initial Approach to the Baby With Atypical Genitalia

A useful mnemonic for the initial approach is BASIC: Bonding, Adrenal insufficiency, Sex assignment, Imaging, and Cytogenetics.

Bonding between the parents and baby can be disrupted by the shock of the situation or if the newborn is taken away to an intensive care nursery without good reason. Focusing on their baby is important, and putting the genital issue aside at times is key. Staff members who do not have experience with DSD may feel uncomfortable. Nursing staff can play a crucial role in helping families initially by engaging with them and acknowledging the stress that uncertainty can bring. Allowing privacy is important but avoiding contact is unprofessional. These parents need support and guidance in many aspects of caring for their baby, such as establishing feeding, changing diapers, and sleeping, as would any new parents. Parents may find this situation particularly challenging if this baby is their first child.

Adrenal insufficiency is an important and potentially life-threatening association of DSD. This most commonly occurs in a 46,XX baby with 21-hydroxylase deficiency, which affects about 15% to 20% of babies with atypical genitalia. Adrenal insufficiency can also occur in 46,XY babies (e.g., StAR, CYP11A, HSD3B2, CYP17A1, NR5A1) but is rare. Monitoring for hypoglycemia, hyponatremia, and hyperkalemia is necessary, but the electrolyte changes usually take several days to manifest. The baby is losing whole-body sodium during this time, but regular, rather than excessive, monitoring is appropriate, for which the infant can be kept with its mother if otherwise well.

Sex assignment should be undertaken as soon as possible but without rushed decisions being made. Babies whose sex is not clear need input from specialists and a rapid assessment of sex chromosomes. In the interim, it is advisable to use neutral terms rather than penis or clitoris, and to speak in terms of their "baby" or "little one" rather than "he" or "she." Parents sometimes have strong preconceptions about their baby, especially if they have been told they are expecting a boy or girl prenatally, or may want a child of a specific sex to fit their desired family structure. If wrong decisions are made, it can be very traumatic to reverse them, so keeping an open mind from the start is helpful.[441]

Imaging is useful but can be confusing in nonspecialist hands. Pelvic ultrasound or MRI can show internal structures, but a utricular remnant, which is commonly found in boys with hypospadias, can be confused with a uterus, and lymph nodes can be confused with testes.[224,442] Parents need to know the limitations of these tests.

Cytogenetics or a rapid assessment of sex chromosome complement is essential. This testing has been done traditionally by FISH for X-chromosome and Y-chromosome markers (such as SRY) (see Fig. 23-3), but in some centers is now being performed by quantitative fluorescent polymerase chain reaction (qfPCR) on DNA. The relevant laboratories should be informed of the urgency of the test and samples should be transported quickly. An attempt to look for mosaicism should be made, although sometimes this test needs a full mosaic screen on cultured cells. Rapid karyotyping can help with the next stages of management and investigation, and a result is usually available within 2 working days.

Support for the Parents

Providing parents with adequate support in the first days while results are awaited is essential.[438] It can be useful to stress that many other parents are in a similar position each year, that specialists who have knowledge and experience are available, and that the situation will become clearer in the next days. Parents need to be provided with information about the tests performed and a realistic expectation of when results will be available. They should be encouraged to ask questions and to rediscuss information that is not clear or difficult to understand. Sometimes recording conversations can be helpful so that families have an opportunity to listen to information again. Being asked by family and friends if they have a boy or a girl is highly stressful. There is no single strategy that suits all parents, but many seek the safe haven of the hospital and will try to delay announcing the birth until the situation is clearer. It is reasonable to ask friends for some private time and to say that they will be in touch soon with more information. It often helps parents to confide in one or two close friends or family members; sometimes fathers can be under pressure with work, and siblings may have questions or need care. Several resources have been developed to help support parents during this time.[443] It is important that parents look after themselves, too.

The Multidisciplinary Team

The MDT (or interdisciplinary team) includes specialists with experience in DSDs. The pediatric (or adult) endocri-nologist plays a central role in the team with support from psychologists, urologists, and other health professionals (Fig. 23-40).[3,439,444] The structure and available expertise vary depending on the center. Sometimes regional or national networks are needed to provide support where the population is scattered geographically or to link experts in different centers together (e.g., the Scottish Genital Anomalies Network), with meetings held by teleconference rather than in person.[445] It is important to keep the primary care physician informed. It is also useful for families to have a clearly defined point of contact if they need to ask further questions or if information about further steps in management is unclear.

Assigning Sex

Most people feel that a child should be brought up as either a boy or a girl in Western societies, although in some situations the child may choose another path later in life. Sufficient information should be gathered so that parents can be informed and educated to make the best decisions for their child. This should be done as quickly as practical but without rushing decisions. The karyotype per se does not make anyone male or female, but it is a useful starting point for focusing investigations and reaching a diagnosis (see the classification of DSD, Table 23-3). A broad diagnosis is often sufficient for assigning sex, but a more specific diagnosis can be reached later. Within the context of the karyotype and diagnosis, useful points to consider are the child's future gender identity; functional anatomic aspects such as likely urologic and sexual function; whether endocrine function (consistent with assigned sex) is possible; whether there may be fertility options; and whether the tumor risk of retaining gonads is acceptable. Many of these questions are difficult to answer, and in some situations more investigations may be undertaken to inform the parents, but usually the choice is relatively straightforward once the baby is reviewed in light of the karyotype. Particularly challenging situations arise in babies with limited phallic development and a 46,XY karyotype who have potential testosterone responsiveness (such as 17β-hydroxysteroid dehydrogenase deficiency, 5α-reductase deficiency, partial testicular dysgenesis, and SF1-associated DSD) or when mixed internal and external phenotypes can occur (e.g., 45,X/46,XY or various forms of ovotesticular DSD). In the past there was a greater focus on the genitalia and a tendency to bring some children with a very small phallus up as female. More recently, there has been a trend to raise more 46,XY children as male and to look at other aspects of the child such as likely gender identity, possible fertility, and endocrine function.[357] Sometimes, cultural influences can be important for the parents.[446] In most countries there is a time limit to register the birth of a baby (e.g., 42 days in England and Wales), but this is rarely a problem and can usually be deferred or the registration done without defining sex (e.g., Germany).

Investigations for DSDs

Once the initial analysis of sex chromosomes is available, several investigations can be undertaken to reach a more specific diagnosis or to obtain a more detailed assessment of urogenital anatomy and future function.[2,439] It is difficult to develop rigid guidelines for investigations because local availability and affordability of tests around the world vary greatly.[447] Details of some of the commonly used tests for DSD are shown in Table 23-21, and potential investigations based on karyotype are shown in Figure 23-41. It is important to consider what the likelihood of a specific diagnosis

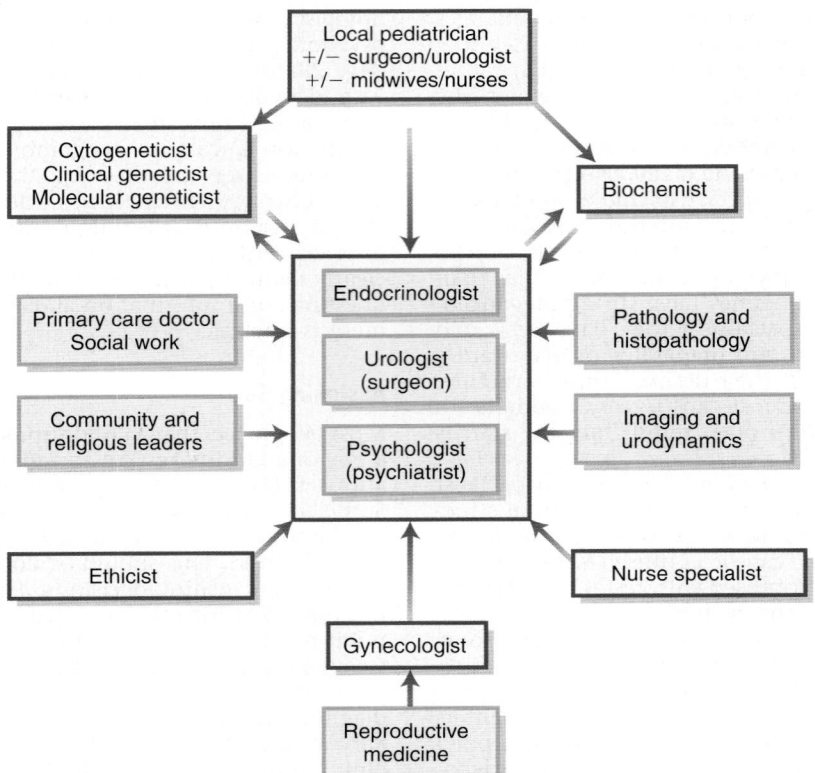

Figure 23-40 Overview of the multidisciplinary team (MDT). (From Brain CE, Creighton SM, Mushtaq I, et al. Holistic management of DSD. *Best Pract Res Clin Endocrinol Metab.* 2010;24:335-354, used with permission of Elsevier, Inc.)

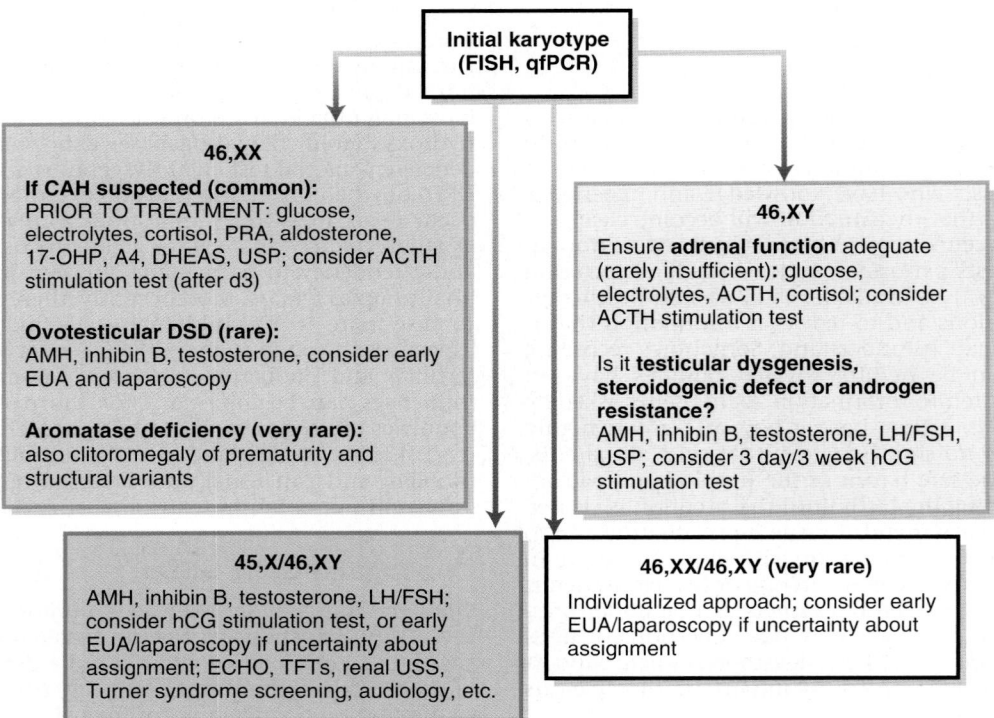

Figure 23-41 Overview of potential investigations for a newborn with atypical genitalia or disorders of sex development (DSD) once the initial karyotype or assessment of sex chromosome complement has been made. A4, androstenedione; ACTH, adrenocorticotropic hormone; AMH, antimüllerian hormone; CAH, congenital adrenal hyperplasia; DHEAS, dehydroepiandrosterone sulfate; ECHO, echocardiogram; EUA, examination under anesthetic; FISH, fluorescent in situ hybridization; FSH, follicle-stimulating hormone; hCG, human chorionic gonadotropin; LH, luteinizing hormone; 17-OHP, 17-hydroxyprogesterone; PRA, plasma renin activity; qfPCR, quantitative fluorescent polymerase chain reaction; TFT, thyroid function test; USP, urine steroid profiling; USS, ultrasound screening.

TABLE 23-21

Potential Investigations for DSDs

Approach	Test	Uses
Genetics	FISH* (X- and Y-specific probes)	Rapid analysis of sex chromosome complement on cells
	qfPCR*	Rapid analysis of sex chromosome signal in DNA
	Karyotype*	Analysis of sex chromosomes and autosomes in cells with ability to look for mosaicism by screening multiple cells, as well as detection of major deletions, duplications, and balanced translocations
	Array CGH or SNP microarray*	Analysis of chromosome signal across the genome, with ability to detect smaller copy number variants but not balanced translocations, using DNA
	Multiple ligation probe-dependent amplification	Analysis of the loss of gain of specific exons or whole genes on a predefined panel of probes, such as for DSD genes, using DNA
	Single-gene analysis	Sanger sequencing and analysis of individual genes that are highly likely to be the cause of DSD based on incidence and clinical and biochemical features (e.g., *CYP21A2*)
	Targeted panel sequencing	Analysis of large numbers of known DSD-causing genes using high throughput sequencing of DNA
	Whole exome sequencing	Analysis of all the coding exons in the DNA, which may show changes in known, putative, or novel DSD-associated genes, using high-throughput sequencing
Endocrine	Routine serum biochemistry*; urinalysis*	May reveal a salt-losing crisis or associated renal disorder (e.g., WT1)
	17-Hydroxyprogesterone,* 11-deoxycortisol, 17-hydroxypregnenolone	May help to diagnose CAH or reveal a specific block in an adrenal pathway relevant to DSD
	Renin, ACTH	May show a salt-losing state or primary adrenal insufficiency
	Testosterone,* androstenedione, DHT	Indicates the degree of androgen production and ratios of androgens in the basal state or following hCG stimulation and may help to diagnose a block in androgen production consistent with a specific diagnosis (e.g., 17β-HSD or 5α-reductase deficiencies); can also reveal androgen production in ovotesticular DSD
	Gonadotropins	May indicate an underlying block in steroidogenesis or androgen insensitivity (LH), or impaired Sertoli cell function (FSH)
	AMH, inhibin B	Can be useful markers of testicular integrity: AMH is detectable throughout childhood and in reduced in testicular dysgenesis or absent if streak gonads or anorchia occurs; AMH may be high in AIS or reduced androgen production due to steroidogenic defects; AMH may help to reveal the presence of testicular tissue in 46,XX ovotesticular DSD
	Urinary steroids by GC/MS	Can be used to diagnose specific steroidogenic defects in the newborn period (e.g., 21-hydroxylase deficiency, 11β-hydroxylase deficiency, 3β-hydroxysteroid dehydrogenase deficiency, P450 oxidoreductase deficiency, 17α-hydroxylase deficiency); can reveal 5α-reductase deficiency only after 3-6 months of life
	Dynamic tests: ACTH stimulation	Used to assess the adrenal gland stress response (quantitative) and can be coupled with measurement of steroid metabolites or poststimulation urine steroid analysis to study ratios of metabolites (diagnostic)
	hCG stimulation	Used in short (3-day) or prolonged (3-week) formats to assess androgen production (quantitative) and androgen biosynthesis pathways (diagnostic); can also be used to assess for the presence of testicular tissue (e.g., anorchia, ovotestis), although AMH is now more often used initially
	FSH stimulation test	Rarely used to investigate the presence of ovarian tissue by measuring inhibin A and estradiol response
Imaging	Abdominopelvic and renal ultrasound*	Can reveal the size, position, and structure of gonads (especially testes), the presence of müllerian structures, and associated changes (such as renal size or anomalies)
	MRI	Sometimes used to assess internal structures, especially in adolescence
	Cystourethroscopy, sinogram	Can reveal the structure of the bladder, vagina, and common channel
Surgical	Laparoscopy	Can reveal internal structures by direct visualization, such as gonads and müllerian structures
	Gonadal biopsies	Can be used to determine the nature of gonads, especially if dysgenetic testes or ovotestes are suspected

ACTH, adrenocorticotropic hormone; AIS, androgen insensitivity syndrome; AMH, antimüllerian hormone; CAH, congenital adrenal hyperplasia; CGH, comparative genomic hybridization; DHT, dihydrotestosterone; DSDs, disorders of sex development; FISH, fluorescent in situ hybridization; FSH, follicle-stimulating hormone; GC-MS, gas chromatography–mass spectrometry; hCG, human chorionic gonadotropin; LH, luteinizing hormone; MRI, magnetic resonance imaging; qfPCR, quantitative fluorescent polymerase chain reaction; SNP, single-nucleotide polymorphism.
*Indicates first-line investigations for which results are available within days. For images of G-banded karyotypes and FISH analysis, see Figure 23-3.

might be. An overview of diagnoses discussed in our setting is shown in Table 23-19, but in areas of the world with greater consanguinity the relative prevalence of recessive conditions such as CAH is greater. There may also be "hotspots" of specific diagnoses due to founder effects (e.g., 5α-reductase in the Dominican Republic), so knowledge of the local prevalence of certain conditions is important. Genetic testing is more widely available and might sometimes avoid the need for invasive tests or prolonged endocrine stimulation, but it has certain drawbacks, which are discussed later.[300]

In our experience, approximately 10% to 15% of newborn referrals have a chromosomal DSD (usually 45,X/ 46,XY) and an individualized approach is needed.[3,215] This includes assessment of anatomy and gonadal functional, as well as screening for potential Turner syndrome–associated features (e.g., renal and cardiac conditions) (see Fig. 23-41). Sometimes an early examination under anesthesia and laparoscopy is performed to assess anatomy and to determine gonadal characteristics and histologic features.

Approximately 20% to 25% have a 46,XX karyotype. The majority of these babies have 21-hydroxylase deficiency, although other rarer forms of CAH, ovotesticular DSD, and clitoromegaly associated with prematurity are seen. Children have variable genital appearances; sometimes the baby may have a clitoris that is naturally large (Table 23-22) or appears slightly more prominent or with excess clitoral skin. However, any 46,XX baby must be assumed to be at risk of adrenal insufficiency until proved otherwise. Serial electrolytes should be monitored and tests to confirm or refute the diagnosis should be undertaken according to local protocol or availability (such as 17-OHP, basal and stimulated cortisol, ACTH, plasma renin activity, and urine steroid profiling). Results can be inaccurate before 3 days of age using conventional assays, although liquid chromatography/tandem mass spectrometry (LC/MS-MS) assays may be more useful if available.[448,449] Steroid replacement treatment can be started once the diagnosis is clear and any additional samples obtained. Of note, 17-OHP can be mildly elevated in other forms of CAH (e.g., 11β-hydroxylase deficiency, 3β-HSD, POR), and investigation of steroid intermediates (e.g., 11-deoxycortisol, 11-deoxycorticosterone) and urine steroid profiling can be useful in these situations.[314] If all adrenal investigations are negative, rare diagnoses such as 46,XX ovotesticular DSD and aromatase deficiency should be considered, and AMH/MIS measured to investigate for testicular tissue.[439] The presence of ovarian tissue can be difficult to assess in early infancy without laparoscopy or even biopsy. Occasionally follicles can be seen on imaging or there can be a rise in estradiol and inhibin A following recombinant FSH stimulation, but such tests are rarely performed.[187]

The most common newborn karyotype in our experience is 46,XY, which occurs in approximately 60% of babies. These children can have a range of conditions, including variable forms of partial testicular dysgenesis, disorders of androgen synthesis and action, or other diagnoses such as severe penoscrotal hypospadias of unknown cause or a DSD-associated syndrome. In some situations the diagnosis might influence decision making. For example, some clinicians would advocate bringing a baby with 5α-reductase deficiency up as a boy and giving dihydrotestosterone cream, whereas a child with androgen resistance causing a more severe form of PAIS might be reared as a girl. Basic investigations in the 46,XY baby can include karyotype or array analysis looking for established chromosomal alterations (e.g., 9q deletion, 10p deletion, Xp21 duplication) and basal assessment of testis integrity (e.g., AMH/MIS, androgens).[2,145] Adrenal disorders do occur but are rare. Most children with complete blocks in steroid production (e.g., StAR, CYP11A1) do not present with atypical genitalia but rather present as a phenotypic girl with a salt-losing crisis, and the 46,XY karyotype is only found afterward. Atypical genitalia at birth can be a sign of partial defects in high steroidogenic enzymes (e.g., partial StAR, CYP11A1) or partial 17α-hydroxylase insufficiency (CYP17A1), as well as classic presentations of 3β-hydroxysteroid dehydrogenase deficiency (HSD3B2) or P450 oxidoreductase deficiency (POR). It is currently unclear whether detailed investigations of adrenal function are justified in all boys with 46,XY DSD, but an adrenal diagnosis should at least be considered. Additional diagnostic tests include basal androgens (DHEA, androstenedione, testosterone, DHT), and short- and long-term hCG-stimulated androgens.[450] The ratios of intermediates can be useful in diagnosing specific blocks, especially 17β-hydroxysteroid dehydrogenase deficiency (testosterone:androstenedione ratio often less than 0.8) and 5α-reductase deficiency (testosterone:dihydrotestosterone ratio often greater than 10 to 20).[313] However, these assays may not be accurate in the first few days of life unless performed by LC/MS-MS, and diagnosing 5α-reductase deficiency by

TABLE 23-22

Anthropometric Measurements of the External Genitalia (Mean ± SD)

Population	Age	Stretched Penile Length (cm) or Clitoral Length	Penile Width (cm) or Clitoral Width	Testicular Volume (mL) or Perineum Length
Males				
United States	30 wk GA	2.5 ± 0.4		
United States	Full term	3.5 ± 0.4	1.1 ± 0.1	0.52 (median)
Japan	Term to 14 yr.	2.9 ± 0.4 to 8.3 ± 0.8		
Australia	24 to 36 wk GA	2.27 + (0.16 GA)		
China	Term	3.1 ± 0.3	1.07 ± 0.09	
India	Term	3.6 ± 0.4	1.14 ± 0.07	
North America	Term	3.4 ± 0.3	1.13 ± 0.08	
Europe	10 yr	6.4 ± 0.4		0.95 to 1.20
Europe	Adult	13.3 ± 1.6		16.5 to 18.2
Females				
United States	Full term	4.0 ± 1.24 mm	3.32 ± 0.78 mm	
United States	Adult, nulliparous	15.4 ± 4.3 mm		
United States	Adult	19.1 ± 8.7 mm	5.5 ± 1.7 mm	31.3 ± 8.5 mm

GA, gestational age; SD, standard deviation.

From Hughes IA, Houk C, Ahmed SF, Lee PA. Consensus statement on management of intersex disorders. *Arch Dis Child*. 2006;91:554-562, used with permission.

Data from Cheng PK, Chanoine JP. Should the definition of micropenis vary according to ethnicity? *Horm Res*. 2001;55:278-281; Feldman KW, Smith DW. Fetal phallic growth and penile standards for newborn male infants. *J Pediatr*. 1975;86:395-398; Fujieda K, Matsuura N. Growth and maturation in the male genitalia from birth to adolescence. II. Change of penile length. *Acta Paediatr Jpn*. 1987;29:220-223; Lloyd J, Crouch NS, Minto CL, et al. Female genital appearance: "normality" unfolds. *BJOG*. 2005;112:643-646; Oberfield SE, Mondok A, Shahrivar F, et al. Clitoral size in full-term infants. *Am J Perinatol*. 1989;64:53-54; Schonfield WA, Beebe GW. Normal growth and variation in the male genitalia from birth to maturity. *J Urol*. 1942;48:759-777; Tuladhar R, Davis PG, Batch J, et al. Establishment of a normal range of penile length in preterm infants. *J Paediatr Child Health*. 1998;34:471-473; Verkauf BS, Von Thron J, O'Brien WF. Clitoral size in normal women. *Obstet Gynecol*. 1992;80:41-44; Zachmann M, Prader A, Kind HP, et al. Testicular volume during adolescence: cross-sectional and longitudinal studies. *Helv Paediatr Acta*. 1974;29:61-72.

androgen ratios or urine steroid profiling can be difficult in the first few months of life, possibly because of other pathways or isoenzymes influencing the results.[314]

Presentation During Childhood

DSD can occasionally present during childhood years. Sometimes a parent may notice genital differences for the first time in childhood or feel inguinal masses that turn out to be testes in a child with 46,XY chromosomes. A small proportion of inguinal hernias in girls are found to contain testes, most often due to CAIS. Sometimes associated features first present in childhood; for example, a small proportion of boys with penoscrotal hypospadias develop an abdominal mass due to a Wilms tumor and are found to have Denys-Drash syndrome *(WT1)*.

Presentation During Adolescence

Another common time for DSD to present is during the adolescence period. Young people with 46,XY chromosomes present in three well-recognized ways: (1) a girl who virlizes at puberty, (2) a girl with absent puberty development, and (3) a girl who has primary amenorrhea.[2] Although the situation is not as urgent as in the newborn, it is equally if not more important to handle the situation with sensitivity, as the young person is aware of the issues as well as the parents and must be involved in decision making and consent.

The conditions that are typically associated with virlization at puberty are 5α-reductase deficiency type 2 and 17β-hydroxysteroid dehydroxygenase deficiency type 3. Alternative diagnoses include mutations in SF1 *(NR5A1)*[451] or in cases in which previous clitoromegaly may have been overlooked in partial gonadal dysgenesis, partial androgen insensitivity syndrome, or ovotesticular DSD. Usually the diagnosis is relatively straightforward based on ratios of androgens, urine steroid profiling (if available, for 5α-reductase deficiency), and in some situations genetic testing.[2] It is best to avoid further stimulation with hCG tests, and some have proposed that puberty can be blocked for several months with antiandrogens and a GnRH analogue in order to obtain a genetic diagnosis and to have time to counsel the young person and the family. An MDT approach is invaluable, and the input of an experienced psychologist or expert in gender medicine is key. A proportion of young people with 5α-reductase deficiency will choose to transition from female to male, and it has been reported that some girls with 17β-hydroxysteroid dehydroxygenase deficiency may wish to change gender, too.[168,169] Many girls with these conditions want to stay as females and would want to have gonads removed. Puberty would then need to be induced with estrogens. Gathering and sharing the information and obtaining psychological support over a period of time can help ensure that the young person makes the best choices for the future.

Another presentation in adolescence is a girl who does not have any pubertal development. Although this situation may represent many diagnoses in the 46,XX girl (e.g., extreme delayed puberty, hypogonadotropic hypogonadism, or primary ovarian insufficiency) or with Turner syndrome (45,X), it may rarely be the presenting feature of a girl (46,XY) with complete gonadal (testicular) dysgenesis or 17α-hydroxylase/17,20-lyase deficiency. In complete testicular dysgenesis (sometimes known as Swyer syndrome) there is usually an immature uterus that may be difficult to see, even on MRI scan, but it may be demonstrated following estrogen treatment (the clandestine uterus).[452] Streak or dysgenetic gonads are usually present and gener-

ally have a high tumor risk. The underlying cause may be a range of genetic conditions (see Table 23-6), but at present a cause is not often found. Puberty is usually induced with estrogens, which are required in the long term, and gonads are removed on account of the tumor risk. In contrast, 46,XY girls with 17α-hydroxylase/17,20-lyase deficiency do not have a uterus. The block in adrenal steroidogenesis can be associated with hypertension and hypokalemia, which can cause arrhythmias, so this is a rare but important diagnosis to make. Estrogen treatment is needed, and gonads are usually removed.

The third common presentation is with primary amenorrhea in a girl who has developed in puberty. A karyotype and pelvic ultrasound are useful initial investigations.[2] The diagnosis is most likely a form of uterine agenesis such as Mayer-Rokitansky-Küster-Hauser (MRKH) syndrome if the karyotype is 46,XX, and complete androgen insensitivity syndrome (CAIS) if the karyotype is 46,XY. Girls with CAIS often have reduced pubic and axillary hair. Detailed discussion about the management of these conditions is provided earlier in this chapter.

Presentation During Adulthood

Occasionally, DSD may first present in adulthood. Examples include mild variants in DSD genes associated with male factor infertility or ovarian insufficiency (e.g., NR5A1), conditions such as persistent müllerian duct syndrome (PMDS) when a uterine-like structure is found incidentally in a man, or when a person with a more typical form of DSD only presents to health professionals later in life, sometimes after migration from rural areas to a city or from one country to another.

Information Sharing, Transitioning, and Adult Services

Information sharing (disclosure) is an important part of educating people about their condition and giving them understanding and insight into the future. In the past there was more secrecy around DSD, but most research supports sharing information in an age-appropriate manner over time.[453] Sometimes parents need considerable help in how to deal with questions and concerns, and psychological support is important to allow them to feel confident in discussing these issues with their child over time.[438,454,455] Education is an ongoing process, and understanding changes with the child's cognitive development.[453] Different families may prefer different strategies but usually being prepared for an open dialogue in stages when the opportunity arises works well. Sometimes a psychologist or pediatric endocrinologist can provide information at key stages and support the family in reinforcing information or answering questions as they come up.

Transitioning the care of young people from pediatric to adult services is important.[456,457] Often the pediatric endocrinologist will induce puberty before transfer to an adult endocrinologist, but it may be useful to involve the gynecologist at an earlier stage so that the young person can build trust with the doctor. In childhood and later, any genital examinations should be performed only when necessary and ideally by someone with experience who will be involved in long-term care. Photography should be avoided unless absolutely necessary and then only with consent.

As more young people transition into adult services, the need for specialist adult centers for DSDs is becoming apparent. The team still largely includes an endocrinologist, psychologist, urologist, and gynecologist, but radiologists can be important team members, especially when discussing young people with retained gonads or complex anatomy. Multidisciplinary clinics in which all team members are available are useful and reduce the number of hospital visits and time away from work. The key issues in long-term management of DSDs include hormone replacement, bone health, sexual activity, relationship issues, urinary issues, psychological well-being, and other factors that contribute to overall quality of life.[458-460] Some data are now emerging on outcome in adulthood for general medical issues and quality of life (see later).

Support Groups and Information

Support groups can also have a very important role in providing additional information for adults with DSD and for bringing members of the community together.[461] There are well-established support groups in several countries for general aspects of DSD as well as for specific conditions such as CAH and AIS. Examples include Accord Alliance (USA), the CARES foundation (USA), livingwithCAH (UK), the Androgen Insensitivity Support Group (AISSG) (UK), and GrApSIA (Spain). Increasingly accessible information about DSD is becoming available through the Internet, such as the biology of DSDs,[462] support for families (e.g., dsdfamilies),[443,463] and information for young people about DSDs (e.g., dsdteens).[464] It is useful to guide young people and families in how to search for information, as general search terms such as "sex" can result in many inappropriate hits.

Genetic Testing and DSDs

Genetic testing can play an important role for reaching a specific diagnosis, counseling individuals and families about recurrence in other family members, defining the need to look for associated features, and in some situations, providing guidance on issues such as potential gender identity, endocrine function, and tumor risk.[299] Reaching a specific genetic diagnosis can provide a sense of resolution and reduce uncertainty but may generate anxiety if no cause is found or if incidental genetic information is uncovered. Individuals and families should have a clear understanding about what genetic tests are being performed and what the potential benefits and risks might be. Genetic testing can be expensive and may not be available or affordable locally, especially as a clinical service.[299]

Approaches to genetic testing are changing rapidly with new technologies, for the analysis of chromosomes as well as individual genes. In some centers sex chromosome FISH is being replaced by qfPCR, and microarray or array-based CGH (comparative genomic hybridization) approaches are being used to replace or supplement traditional karyotype analysis. These technologies can detect much smaller copy number variations than traditional G-banded karyotypes but do not detect balanced translocations and may miss low levels of mosaicism. Multiplex ligation-dependent probe amplification (MLPA) is a method of looking for specific copy number changes in known DSD genes (e.g., duplication of *NR0B1*, or loss of exons of other genes) that are too small to be picked up on arrays.

Analysis of single genes is also changing with the development of next generation sequencing (NGS) approaches. Traditionally, individual candidate genes for a condition were amplified by PCR and analyzed by Sanger sequencing. This approach is relatively time-consuming and expensive, but it is sometimes available as a clinically approved service. Direct sequencing is still the method of choice when there is a clear candidate gene from biochemical analysis (e.g., *HSD17B3*, *SRD5A2*), especially when the presence of a pseudogene can make sequencing difficult (e.g., *CYP21A2*).[299] Newer approaches involve sequencing panels of genes relevant to DSD at the same time using NGS or sequencing all the exomes or even whole genomes.[465,466] These methods can provide high throughput analysis but are still expensive, generate large amounts of data (including "bystander" data for other genes that may or may not be desired), and are still mostly only available as research tools. However, positive findings can be backed up by focused clinical testing, which can then provide useful information for the family and clinician.

Given the advances in genetics, and increasing recognition that DSD can be a feature of many well-defined syndromes, a clinical geneticist can be a very valuable member of the MDT, especially when a child needs to be reviewed for additional features or when the family needs to be counseled about genetic testing and the significance of any results.

Tumor Risk and DSDs

The gonads of individuals with DSD are at risk of malignant change, but the prevalence can vary widely depending on the underlying diagnosis (Table 23-23). In general, dysgenetic gonads (containing germ cells) are at greater risk of premalignant and malignant changes than streak gonads, especially if they are intra-abdominal. These changes are initially intratubular germ cell neoplasia (ITGN)/carcinoma in situ but can progress to gonadoblastoma or other malignant tumors. Onset is greatest at or after the time of puberty, but life-course data for the development of these changes are not available.[22,359] The risk in conditions affecting steroidogenesis is much lower, but not negligible, and other tumors such as Sertoli cell adenomas are common in CAIS. Standard circulating tumor markers (e.g., α-fetoprotein, β-hCG, lactate dehydrogenase) and imaging are not very sensitive at detecting early tumors, although microcalcification may be one early sign. Novel serum biomarkers such as microRNAs (e.g., miR371-3/367) are being investigated.[359]

Surgery and DSDs

Surgical approaches to DSD were once regarded as standard management, but there is much greater consideration now about the need for surgery and its timing.[467] Some procedures are functionally important (e.g., to prevent hematocolpos, if there is urinary pooling or high tumor risk), whereas others such as clitoral reduction surgery might be viewed as cosmetic. Some people believe that early surgery can be beneficial because the tissues are easier to operate on and heal better, whereas others feel that surgery should be deferred until a time when a young person can be part of the decision-making process and consent.[468,469] The psychological implications of these decisions can be great. Some parents experience great stress because of the appearance of their child's genitals.[470] Performing early surgery to normalize the appearance of the genitalia may make some parents feel more comfortable, but the child may later regret these decisions, especially if there is reduced sensation or further surgeries are required. On the other hand, bringing up a child with very atypical genitalia protects the child's rights to bodily integrity but needs strong positive parenting and support, and it is not yet known how well young people cope in these situations as they grow up.

In a child born with atypical genitalia and raised female the parents need to have a balanced discussion about all options. In a baby with CAH there is often considerable

TABLE 23-23

Risk of Germ Cell Malignancy According to Diagnosis

Risk Group	Disorder	Malignancy Risk (%)	Recommended Action	No. Studies	No. Patients
High	GD* (+Y)[†] intra-abdominal	15-35	Gonadectomy[‡]	12	350
	Partial AIS nonscrotal	50	Gonadectomy[‡]	2	24
	Frasier syndrome	60	Gonadectomy[‡]	1	15
	Denys-Drash syndrome (+Y)	40	Gonadectomy[‡]	1	5
Intermediate	Turner syndrome (+Y)	12	Gonadectomy[‡]	11	43
	17β-HSD	28	Watchful waiting	2	7
	GD (+Y)[†] scrotal	Unknown	Biopsy[§] and irradiation?	0	0
	Partial AIS scrotal gonad	Unknown	Biopsy[§] and irradiation?	0	0
Low	Complete AIS	2	Biopsy[§] and ?	2	55
	Ovotesticular DSD	3	Testis tissue removal?	3	426
	Turner syndrome (−Y)	1	None	11	557
No (?)	5α-Reductase	0	Unresolved	1	3
	Leydig cell hypoplasia	0	Unresolved	1	2

*GD including disorders not further specified, 46XY, 45X/46XY, mixed, partial, and complete.
[†]GBY region positive, including the *TSPY* gene.
[‡]At time of diagnosis.
[§]At puberty, allowing investigation of at least 30 seminiferous tubules, preferentially diagnosis based on OCT3/4 immunohistochemistry.
AIS, androgen insensitivity syndrome; DSDs, disorders of sex development; GD, gonadal dysgenesis; 17β-HSD, 17β-hydroxysteroid dehydrogenase.
Reproduced with permission from Hughes IA, Houk C, Ahmed SF, et al. Consensus statement on management of intersex disorders. *Arch Dis Child.* 2006;91:554-562.

reduction in the size of the enlarged clitoris once androgen exposure is reduced by adrenal suppression, or the clitoris may become less prominent as the child grows, so a period of time is needed and parents should not rush into surgery in an attempt to "fix" the appearance.[468] Psychological support in dealing with worries such as diaper changing should be provided, and in many situations surgery may not be considered necessary. Outcome studies involving assessment of genital sensitivity and sexual function in women with CAH show impairment related to previous feminizing genital surgery.[469,471] Although surgical procedures have changed, with greater emphasis on nerve sparing, these data have had a bearing on decisions taken during infancy and childhood for the surgical management of conditions such as CAH, and long-term outcome data are awaited for newer approaches. It is generally accepted that clitoroplasty should be reserved only for the most severe degree of clitoromegaly, and in many situations vaginal surgery is deferred until after puberty. The long-term outcome of vaginal reconstruction procedures performed before puberty for a variety of conditions (e.g., CAH, AIS, mixed gonadal dysgenesis, persistent cloaca) suggests that complications may be reduced by undertaking the surgery later.[468,469,471] In adulthood, vaginal length in conditions such as CAIS and the MRKH syndrome can often be normalized by dilator treatment alone.[355] Alternative approaches to vaginoplasty such as the Vecchietti procedure are often preferred.

Subjects with DSD raised male usually undergo surgery to correct hypospadias and orchidopexy for testis maldescent. Hypospadias repair usually is scheduled for between 6 and 18 months of age. More than one procedure is often required. It is the surgeon's responsibility to map out these procedures for the parents and to ensure that their expectations are realistic.[472] Many boys with severe hypospadias undergo surgery in early life, as performing these approaches in adolescence may be more difficult, but there is a lack of data for optimal timing.[473] Open discussions with the parents and later with the child are needed and boys may need more support in adolescence than is usually currently offered.

The topic of gonadectomy planned before puberty in 46,XY individuals raised female to prevent virilization and in others with DSD to avoid gonadal tumors was covered earlier. The irreversible nature of such a procedure has created uncertainty among professionals, particularly when the procedure is performed before the affected child can be engaged in discussions. This is another issue that requires the collective discussion of the multidisciplinary team and often includes input from an ethicist. The practice of cryopreserving excised gonads with unrealistic expectations for preservation of reproductive potential should be viewed cautiously, especially because current knowledge is based primarily on the gonadal effects of cancer therapies. However, reproductive technologies are changing rapidly, and there are highly publicized stem cell approaches such as germ cell reprogramming reported in animals.[474] Whether these technologies will eventually provide useful clinical alternatives remains to be seen.

DSD in Resource-Limited Countries

Many of our approaches to DSD are being developed within the context of large medical centers and experienced multidisciplinary teams with ready access to biochemical assays such as AMH/MIS, imaging, and state of the art genetic tests. In reality, many children and adults with DSDs grow up in countries with less access to resources or with different social and cultural pressures.[447] Each clinician needs to work with the tests that are available and affordable to optimize their ability to assess and diagnose DSDs. Knowledge of the local prevalence of certain forms of DSDs can be very important, as well as relevant social, cultural, and religious factors that might influence the way a child and the family view DSD.

Outcome Studies

There is such a range of conditions included under the umbrella of DSDs that it is difficult to obtain an overarching impression on the health and quality of life in adulthood for individuals who have lived with DSD from childhood. There is a plethora of data regarding sexual function and quality of life in women with CAH who had various genitoplasty procedures during their childhood.[475,476] The debate continues regarding the timing of any surgery for girls with CAH and whether one-stage or two-stage surgery is the preferred option.[477]

Adult endocrinologists are now undertaking detailed studies of the comorbid conditions associated with CAH and its medical treatment (see also Chapter 15, The Adrenal Cortex). The CaHASE (United Kingdom Congenital Adrenal Hyperplasia Adult Study Executive) studies on cohorts of more than 200 adults show poorer health status relating to increased obesity, hypertension, insulin resistance, osteoporosis, impaired fertility, and reduced quality of life.[478-480] Despite improvements in growth achievement in recent years, shorter adult height was associated with the adverse outcomes, particularly in relation to hypertension. Similar findings were found in outcome studies of a Swedish population of adults with CAH.[481] The Swedish population also had lower educational achievement and reduced income, increased disability allowance and sick leave, were less often married and with fewer children, compared to control subjects.[482] The medical comorbid conditions may result from long-standing inadequate control of CAH by replacement glucocorticoids, estimated to be the case in more than a third of adults. Studies of modified-release hydrocortisone preparations that mimic more closely the cortisol circadian rhythm are showing promising results, with a reduction in the total hydrocortisone daily dose required for adequate adrenal androgen suppression.[483]

There are fewer outcome studies available for adults with conditions within the category of 46,XY DSD, but data are beginning to emerge. Quality of life studies have recently been reported in populations of German, Italian, and Brazilian mixed individuals with 46,XX DSD and 46,XY DSD and of either male or female social sex, so study cohorts are quite heterogeneous.[484-486] In general, quality of life was satisfactory, there was no evidence of gender dysphoria, and psychosocial adjustment was better in younger people when compared with an older generation of DSD individuals. Among the 46,XY DSD group in the Brazilian population, those with a male social sex had a better quality of life than those with a female social sex (e.g., the group with CAIS). There were more difficulties overall in partnerships and sexual relationships. Another study from Germany, which included both XX and XY DSD individuals, showed evidence of dissatisfaction with health care services available, especially in the group with 46,XY DSD.[487] In a study that focused on comparing women with either CAIS or MRKHS, there was greater lack of sexual confidence and sexual satisfaction in CAIS women, whereas those with MRKHS, while apprehensive in sexual situations, reported being satisfied with their sex life.[488]

As discussed previously, a recent study of more than 400 46,XY subjects subdivided according to clinical diagnoses of PAIS, disorders of gonadal development (partial gonadal dysgenesis), and disorders of androgen synthesis (such as 5α-reductase deficiency) has shown an increasing trend for babies with atypical genitalia to be brought up as boys.[357] Therefore, outcome studies are needed for these groups of individuals. A recent generic review of 46,XY DSD provided mainly anecdotal data on issues such as gender identity and sex reassignment, whether males were satisfied with the appearance of their genitalia, and the prevalence of sexual dysfunction.[489] Overall, males were satisfied with their gender and rarely did male-to-female gender reassignment occur in adulthood. Most males had some concern about the appearance of the genitalia, and many were dissatisfied with sexual function. Another small Dutch study reported poor outcome in terms of penile size and sexual function, although their overall body image and psychosexual functioning was no different from control subjects.[490]

There is a paucity of information about outcome in specific causes of 46,XY DSD, such as PAIS. Often, this label is applied without confirmation that the phenotype is due to a mutation in the *AR* gene. A French multicenter study reported on 15 adults with PAIS who had been monitored since birth.[491] The EMS (see Fig. 23-39) was very low and penile length was markedly reduced in adulthood irrespective of additional androgen treatment. All boys developed gynecomastia in adolescence, and sexual function was severely impaired. A more recent study from Denmark of 14 males with PAIS also confirmed universal development of gynecomastia and reduced penile size that, in some, did respond to androgens.[492] The EMS at birth in this cohort was higher, suggesting that the EMS at birth in PAIS (and perhaps in other causes of 46,XY DSD) may predict development of male sexual characteristics at puberty and young adulthood. No data were available on sexual function as this cohort was younger, but as expected, the typical endocrine profile for androgen resistance was markedly prominent at puberty.

Evidence shows that there has been considerable progress in many aspects of DSD since the previous edition of this chapter. What is clearly needed now are outcome studies in larger cohorts of individuals with DSD, particularly within the 46,XY DSD category. A major step toward that goal is the establishment of international registries for DSD studies (I-DSD) and allied activities such as sustainable improvement in clinical care of DSD patients (DSD-Life), an information network for DSD (DSDnet), and DSD Translational Research Network (DSD-TRN).[493] Such networking should provide the means to gather more data on the individual rare causes of DSDs across the lifespan and thereby be translated into improved management and outcome.

ACKNOWLEDGMENTS

We recognize the major contributions made to this chapter by previous editors Melvin Grumbach, MD, and Felix Conte, MD. John C. Achermann holds a Wellcome Trust Senior Research Fellowship in Clinical Science (098513). Ieuan A. Hughes is supported by the NIHR Cambridge Biomedical Research Centre for his work on disorders of sex development.

REFERENCES

1. Hughes IA, Houk C, Ahmed SF, et al. Consensus statement on management of intersex disorders. *Arch Dis Child.* 2006;91:554-563.
2. Ahmed SF, Achermann JC, Arlt W, et al. UK guidance on the initial evaluation of an infant or an adolescent with a suspected disorder of sex development. *Clin Endocrinol (Oxf).* 2011;75:12-26.
3. Brain CE, Creighton SM, Mushtaq I, et al. Holistic management of DSD. *Best Pract Res Clin Endocrinol Metab.* 2010;24:335-354.
4. Grumbach MM, Hughes IA, Conte FA. Disorders of sex differentiation. In: Larsen PR, Kronenberg HM, Melmed S, et al., eds. *Williams Textbook of Endocrinology.* 10th ed. Philadelphia, PA: WB Saunders; 2003: 842-1002.
5. Brennan J, Capel B. One tissue, two fates: molecular genetic events that underlie testis versus ovary development. *Nat Rev Genet.* 2004;5: 509-521.
6. Eggers S, Ohnesorg T, Sinclair A. Genetic regulation of mammalian gonad development. *Nat Rev Endocrinol.* 2014;10:673-683.
7. Svingen T, Koopman P. Building the mammalian testis: origins, differentiation, and assembly of the component cell populations. *Genes Dev.* 2013;27:2409-2426.
8. Smith P, Wilhelm D, Rodgers RJ. Development of mammalian ovary. *J Endocrinol.* 2014;221:R145-R161.
9. Arboleda VA, Sandberg DE, Vilain E. DSDs: genetics, underlying pathologies and psychosexual differentiation. *Nat Rev Endocrinol.* 2014;10:603-615.
10. Marshall Graves JA. Weird animal genomes and the evolution of vertebrate sex and sex chromosomes. *Annu Rev Genet.* 2008;42:565-586.
11. Livernois AM, Waters SA, Deakin JE, et al. Independent evolution of transcriptional inactivation on sex chromosomes in birds and mammals. *PLoS Genet.* 2013;9:e1003635.

12. Jost A. Recherches sur la differentiation sexuelle de l'embryo de lapin. *Arch Anat Microsc Morphol Exp.* 1947;36:271-315.
13. Nef S, Schaad O, Stallings NR, et al. Gene expression during sex determination reveals a robust female genetic program at the onset of ovarian development. *Dev Biol.* 2005;287:361-367.
14. Parma P, Radi O, Vidal V, et al. R-spondin1 is essential in sex determination, skin differentiation and malignancy. *Nat Genet.* 2006;38:1304-1309.
15. Tilly JL, Sinclair DA. Germline energetics, aging, and female infertility. *Cell Metab.* 2013;17:838-850.
16. Fowler PA, Anderson RA, Saunders PT, et al. Development of steroid signaling pathways during primordial follicle formation in the human fetal ovary. *J Clin Endocrinol Metab.* 2011;96:1754-1762.
17. Hall H, Hunt P, Hassold T. The origin of human aneuploidy: where we have been, where we are going. *Hum Mol Genet.* 2007;16:R203-R208.
18. Thomas NS, Hassold TJ. Aberrant recombination and the origin of Klinefelter syndrome. *Hum Reprod Update.* 2003;9:309-317.
19. Ross MT, Bentley DR, Tyler-Smith C. The sequences of the human sex chromosomes. *Curr Opin Genet Dev.* 2006;16:213-218.
20. Tilford CA, Kuroda-Kawaguchi T, Skaletsky H, et al. A physical map of the human Y chromosome. *Nature.* 2001;409:943-945.
21. Hughes JF, Skaletsky H, Pyntikova T, et al. Chimpanzee and human Y chromosomes are remarkably divergent in structure and gene content. *Nature.* 2010;463:536-539.
22. Cools M, Wolffenbuttel KP, Drop SL, et al. Gonadal development and tumor formation at the crossroads of male and female sex determination. *Sex Dev.* 2011;5:167-180.
23. Kratz CP, Mai PL, Greene MH. Familial testicular germ cell tumours. *Best Pract Res Clin Endocrinol Metab.* 2010;24:503-513.
24. Bellott DW, Hughes JF, Skaletsky H, et al. Mammalian Y chromosomes retain widely expressed dosage-sensitive regulators. *Nature.* 2014;508:494-499.
25. Goldberg E. HY antigen and sex determination. *Philos Trans R Soc Lond B Biol Sci.* 1988;322:72-81.
26. Mardon G, Page DC. The sex determining region of the mouse Y chromosome encodes a protein with a highly acidic domain and 13 zinc fingers. *Cell.* 1989;56:765-770.
27. Palmer MS, Sinclair AH, Berta P, et al. Genetic evidence that ZFY is not the testis-determining factor. *Nature.* 1989;342:937-939.
28. Sinclair AH, Berta P, Palmer MS, et al. A gene from the human sex determining region encodes a protein with homology to a conserved DNA-binding motif. *Nature.* 1990;346:240-244.
29. Berta P, Hawkins RJ, Sinclair AH, et al. Genetic evidence equating SRY and the testis determining factor. *Nature.* 1990;348:448-450.
30. Koopman P, Munsterberg A, Capel B, et al. Expression of a candidate sex determining gene during mouse testis differentiation. *Nature.* 1990;348:450-452.
31. Koopman P, Gubbay J, Vivian N, et al. Male development of chromosomally female mice transgenic for SRY. *Nature.* 1991;351:117-121.
32. Jager RJ, Anvret M, Hall K, et al. A human XY female with a frame shift mutation in the candidate testis-determining gene SRY. *Nature.* 1990;348:452-454.
33. Goodfellow PN, Lovell-Badge R. SRY and sex determination in mammals. *Annu Rev Genet.* 1993;27:271-292.
34. Ross MT, Grafham DV, Coffey AJ, et al. The DNA sequence of the human X chromosome. *Nature.* 2005;434:325-337.
35. Harsha HC, Suresh S, Amanchy R, et al. A manually curated functional annotation of the human X chromosome. *Nat Genet.* 2005;37:331-332.
36. Grumbach MM, Morishima A, Taylor JH. Human sex chromosome abnormalities in relation to DNA replication and heterochromatinization. *Proc Natl Acad Sci U S A.* 1963;49:581-589.
37. Lyon MF. The X inactivation centre and X chromosome imprinting. *Eur J Hum Genet.* 1994;2:255-261.
38. Deng X, Berletch JB, Nguyen DK, et al. X chromosome regulation: diverse patterns in development, tissues and disease. *Nat Rev Genet.* 2014;15:367-378.
39. Elsheikh M, Dunger DB, Conway GS, et al. Turner's syndrome in adulthood. *Endocr Rev.* 2002;23:120-140.
40. Schlessinger D, Herrera L, Crisponi L, et al. Genes and translocations involved in POF. *Am J Med Genet.* 2002;222:328-333.
41. Murray A, Webb J, Grimley S, et al. Studies of FRAXA and FRAXE in women with premature ovarian failure. *J Med Genet.* 1998;35:637-640.
42. Sala C, Arrigo G, Torri G, et al. Eleven X chromosome breakpoints associated with premature ovarian failure (POF) map to a 15-Mb YAC contig spanning Xq21. *Genomics.* 1997;40:123-131.
43. Lacombe A, Lee H, Zahed L, et al. Disruption of POF1B binding to nonmuscle actin filaments is associated with premature ovarian failure. *Am J Hum Genet.* 2006;79:113-119.
44. Di Pasquale E, Beck-Peccoz P, Persani L. Hypergonadotropic ovarian failure associated with an inherited mutation of human bone morphogenetic protein-15 (BMP15) gene. *Am J Hum Genet.* 2004;75:106-111.
45. Moumné L, Batista F, Benayou BA, et al. The mutations and potential targets of the forkhead transcription factor FOXL2. *Mol Cell Endocrinol.* 2008;282:2-11.
46. Qin Y, Choi Y, Zhao H, et al. NOBOX homeobox mutation causes premature ovarian failure. *Am J Hum Genet.* 2007;81:576-581.
47. Lourenço D, Brauner R, Lin L, et al. Mutations in NR5A1 associated with ovarian insufficiency. *N Engl J Med.* 2009;360:1200-1210.
48. Caburet S, Arboleda VA, Llano E, et al. Mutant cohesin in premature ovarian failure. *N Engl J Med.* 2014;370:943-949.
49. Wang J, Zhang W, Jiang H, et al. Mutations in HFM1 in recessive primary ovarian insufficiency. *New Engl J Med.* 2014;370:972-974.
50. AlAsiri S, Basit S, Wood-Trageser MA, et al. Exome sequencing reveals MCM8 mutation underlies ovarian failure and chromosomal instability. *J Clin Invest.* 2015;125:258-262.
51. Miyamoto N, Yoshida M, Kuratani S, et al. Defects of urogenital development in mice lacking Emx2. *Development.* 1997;124:1653-1664.
52. Shawlot W, Behringer RR. Requirement for Lim1 in head-organizer function. *Nature.* 1995;374:425-430.
53. Birk OS, Casiano DE, Wassif CA, et al. The LIM homeobox gene *Lhx9* is essential for mouse gonad formation. *Nature.* 2000;403:909-913.
54. Katoh-Fukui Y, Tsuchiya R, Shiroishi T, et al. Male-to-female sex reversal in M33 mutant mice. *Nature.* 1998;393:688-692.
55. Cui S, Ross A, Stallings N, et al. Disrupted gonadogenesis and male-to-female sex reversal in Pod1 knockout mice. *Development.* 2004;131:4095-4105.
56. Fujimoto Y, Tanaka SS, Yamaguchi YL, et al. Homeoproteins six1 and six4 regulate male sex determination and mouse gonadal development. *Dev Cell.* 2013;26:416-430.
57. Bogani D, Siggers P, Brixey R, et al. Loss of mitogen-activated protein kinase kinase kinase 4 (MAP3K4) reveals a requirement for MAPK signalling in mouse sex determination. *PLoS Biol.* 2009;7:e1000196.
58. Biason-Lauber A, Konrad D, Meyer M, et al. Ovaries and female phenotype in a girl with 46,XY karyotype and mutations in the CBX2 gene. *Am J Hum Genet.* 2009;84:658-663.
59. Tevosian SG, Albrecht KH, Crispino JD, et al. Gonadal differentiation, sex determination and normal *SRY* expression in mice require direct interaction between transcription partners GATA4 and FOG2. *Development.* 2002;129:4627-4634.
60. Bouma GJ, Washburn LL, Albrecht KH, et al. Correct dosage of Fog2 and Gata4 transcription factors is critical for fetal testis development in mice. *Proc Natl Acad Sci U S A.* 2007;104:14994-14999.
61. Lourenço D, Brauner R, Rybczynska N, et al. Loss-of-function mutation in *GATA4* causes anomalies of human testicular development. *Proc Natl Acad Sci U S A.* 2011;102:1597-1602.
62. Bashamboo A, Brauner R, Bignon-Topalovic J, et al. Mutations in the FOG2/ZFPM2 gene are associated with anomalies of human testis determination. *Hum Mol Genet.* 2014;23:3657-3665.
63. Pitetti JL, Calvel P, Romero Y, et al. Insulin and IGF1 receptors are essential for XX and XY gonadal differentiation and adrenal development in mice. *PLoS Genet.* 2013;9:e1003160.
64. Pearlman A, Loke J, Le Caignec C, et al. Mutations in *MAP3K1* cause 46,XY disorders of sex development and implicate a common signal transduction pathway in human testis development. *Am J Hum Genet.* 2010;87:898-906.
65. Pritchard-Jones K, Fleming S, Davidson D, et al. The candidate Wilms' tumor gene is involved in genitourinary development. *Nature.* 1990;346:194-197.
66. Kreidberg JA, Sariola H, Loring JM, et al. WT1 is required for early kidney development. *Cell.* 1993;74:679-691.
67. Toska E, Roberts SG. Mechanisms of transcriptional regulation by WT1 (Wilms' tumour 1). *Biochem J.* 2014;461:15-32.
68. Nachtigal MW, Hirokawa Y, Enyeart-VanHouten DL, et al. Wilms' tumor 1 and Dax-1 modulate the orphan nuclear receptor SF-1 in sex-specific gene expression. *Cell.* 1998;93:445-454.
69. Bradford ST, Wilhelm D, Bandiera R, et al. A cell-autonomous role for WT1 in regulating SRY in vivo. *Hum Mol Genet.* 2009;18:3429-3438.
70. Hanley NA, Ball SG, Clement-Jones M, et al. Expression of steroidogenic factor 1 and Wilms' tumour 1 during early human gonadal development and sex determination. *Mech Dev.* 1999;87:175-180.
71. Francke U, Holmes LB, Atkins L, et al. Aniridia–Wilms' tumor association: evidence for specific deletion of 11p13. *Cytogenet Cell Genet.* 1979;24(3):185-192.
72. Pelletier J, Bruening W, Kashtan CE, et al. Germline mutations in the Wilms tumor suppressor gene are associated with abnormal urogenital development in Denys-Drash syndrome. *Cell.* 1991;67:437-447.
73. Barbaux X, Niandet P, Gubler MC, et al. Donor splice-site mutations in WT1 are responsible for Frasier syndrome. *Nat Genet.* 1997;17:467-470.
74. Klamt B, Koziell A, Poulat F, et al. Frasier syndrome is caused by defective alternative splicing of WT1 leading to an altered ratio of WT1 +/−KTS splice isoforms. *Hum Mol Genet.* 1998;7:709-714.
75. Ferraz-de-Souza B, Lin L, Achermann JC. Steroidogenic factor-1 (SF-1, NR5A1) and human disease. *Mol Cell Endocrinol.* 2011;336:198-205.
76. Luo X, Ikeda Y, Parker KL. A cell-specific nuclear receptor is essential for adrenal and gonadal development and sexual differentiation. *Cell.* 1994;77:481-490.
77. Majdic G, Young M, Gomez-Sanches E, et al. Knockout mice lacking steroidogenic factor 1 are a novel genetic model of hypothalamic obesity. *Endocrinology.* 2002;143:607-614.

78. Park SY, Meeks JJ, Raverot G, et al. Nuclear receptors Sf1 and Dax1 function cooperatively to mediate somatic cell differentiation during testis development. *Development.* 2005;132:2415-2423.

79. Achermann JC, Ito M, Ito M, et al. A mutation in the gene encoding steroidogenic factor-1 causes XY sex reversal and adrenal failure in humans. *Nat Genet.* 1999;22(2):125-126.

80. Achermann JC, Ozisik G, Ito M, et al. Gonadal determination and adrenal development are regulated by the orphan nuclear receptor, steroidogenic factor-1 in a dose dependent manner. *J Clin Endocrinol Metab.* 2002;87:1829-1833.

81. Lin L, Pascal P, Ferraz-de-Souza B, et al. Heterozygous missense mutations in steroidogenic factor 1 (SF1/Ad4BP, NR5A1) are associated with 46,XY disorders of sex development with normal adrenal function. *J Clin Endocrinol Metab.* 2007;92:991-999.

82. Sekido R, Lovell-Badge R. Sex determination involves synergistic action of SRY and SF1 on a specific SOX9 enhancer. *Nature.* 2008; 453:930-934.

83. Biason-Lauber A, Schoenle EJ. Apparently normal ovarian differentiation in a prepubertal girl with transcriptionally inactive steroidogenic factor 1 (NR5A1/SF-1) and adrenocortical insufficiency. *Am J Hum Genet.* 2000;67:1563-1568.

84. Pelusi C, Ikeda Y, Zubair M, et al. Impaired follicle development and infertility in female mice lacking steroidogenic factor 1 in ovarian granulosa cells. *Biol Reprod.* 2008;79:1074-1083.

85. Bardoni B, Zanaria E, Guioli S, et al. A dosage sensitive locus at chromosome Xp21 is involved in male to female sex reversal. *Nat Genet.* 1994;7:497-501.

86. Swain A, Narvaez V, Burgoyne P, et al. Dax1 antagonizes SRY action in mammalian sex determination. *Nature.* 1998;391:761-767.

87. Meeks JJ, Weiss J, Jameson JL. Dax1 is required for testis determination. *Nat Genet.* 2003;34:32-33.

88. Jordan BK, Mohammed M, Ching ST, et al. Up-regulation of WNT-4 signaling and dosage-sensitive sex reversal in humans. *Am J Hum Genet.* 2001;68:1102-1109.

89. Molyneaux KA, Stallock J, Schaible K, et al. Time-lapse analysis of living mouse germ cell migration. *Dev Biol.* 2001;240:488-498.

90. Richardson BE, Lehmann R. Mechanisms guiding primordial germ cell migration: strategies from different organisms. *Nat Rev Mol Cell Biol.* 2010;11:37-49.

91. Laird DJ, Altshuler-Keylin S, Kissner MD, et al. Ror2 enhances polarity and directional migration of primordial germ cells. *PLoS Genet.* 2011;7:e1002428.

92. Chawengsaksophak K, Svingen T, Ng ET, et al. Loss of Wnt5a disrupts primordial germ cell migration and male sexual development in mice. *Biol Reprod.* 2012;86:1-12.

93. McLaren A. Germ and somatic cell lineages in the developing gonad. *Mol Cell Endocrinol.* 2000;163:3-9.

94. Kurohmaru M, Kanai Y, Hayashi Y. A cytological and cytoskeletal comparison of Sertoli cells without germ cell and those with germ cells using the W/WV mutant mouse. *Tissue Cell.* 1992;24:895-903.

95. Bowles J, Knight D, Smith C, et al. Retinoid signaling determines germ cell fate in mice. *Science.* 2006;312:596-600.

96. Feng CW, Bowles J, Koopman P. Control of mammalian germ cell entry into meiosis. *Mol Cell Endocrinol.* 2014;382:488-497.

97. Harley VR, Clarkson MJ, Argentaro A. The molecular action and regulation of the testis-determining factors, SRY (sex-determining region on the Y chromosome) and SOX9 (SRY-related high-mobility group [HMG] box 9). *Endocr Rev.* 2003;24:466-487.

98. Hiramatsu R, Matoa S, Kanai-Azuma M, et al. A critical time window of SRY action in gonadal sex determination in mice. *Development.* 2009;136:129-138.

99. Hanley NA, Hagan DM, Clement-Jones M, et al. SRY, SOX9, and DAX1 expression patterns during human sex determination and gonadal development. *Mech Dev.* 2000;91:403-407.

100. Sim H, Argentaro A, Harley VR. Boys, girls and shuttling of SRY and SOX9. *Trends Endocrinol Metab.* 2008;19:213-222.

101. Chen YS, Racca JD, Phillips NB, et al. Inherited human sex reversal due to impaired nucleocytoplasmic trafficking of SRY defines a male transcriptional threshold. *Proc Natl Acad Sci U S A.* 2013;110:E3567-E3576.

102. Sim H, Argentaro A, Czech DP, et al. Inhibition of SRY-calmodulin complex formation induces ectopic expression of ovarian cell markers in developing XY gonads. *Endocrinology.* 2011;152:2883-2893.

103. Desclozeaux M, Poulat F, de Santa Barbara P, et al. Phosphorylation of an N-terminal motif enhances DNA-binding activity of the human SRY protein. *J Biol Chem.* 1998;273:7988-7995.

104. Poulat F, Barbara PS, Desclozeaux M, et al. The human testis determining factor SRY binds a nuclear factor containing PDZ protein interaction domains. *J Biol Chem.* 1997;272:7167-7172.

105. Burgoyne PS, Buehr M, Koopman P. Cell-autonomous action of the testis-determining gene: Sertoli cells are exclusively XY in XX-XY chimaeric mouse testes. *Development.* 1988;102:443-450.

106. Albrecht KH, Eicher EM. Evidence that SRY is expressed in pre-Sertoli cells and Sertoli and granulosa cells have a common precursor. *Dev Biol.* 2001;240:92-107.

107. Larney C, Bailey TL, Koopman P. Switching on sex: transcriptional regulation of the testis-determining gene Sry. *Development.* 2014;141: 2195-2205.

108. Li Y, Zheng M, Lau YF. The sex-determining factors SRY and SOX9 regulate similar target genes and promote testis cord formation during testicular differentiation. *Cell Rep.* 2014;8:723-733.

109. Foster JW, Dominguez-Steglich MA, Guioli S, et al. Camptomelic dysplasia and autosomal sex reversal caused by mutations in an SRY-related gene. *Nature.* 1994;372:525-530.

110. Wagner T, Wirth J, Meyer J, et al. Autosomal sex reversal and camptomelic dysplasia are caused by mutations in and around the *SRY*-related gene *SOX9. Cell.* 1994;79:1111-1120.

111. Morais da Silva S, Hacker A, Harley V, et al. SOX 9 expression during gonadal development implies a conserved role for the gene in testis differentiation in mammals and birds. *Nat Genet.* 1996;14:62-68.

112. Südbeck P, Schmitz ML, Baeuerle PA, et al. Sex reversal by loss of the C-terminal transactivation domain of human SOX9. *Nat Genet.* 1996; 13:230-232.

113. Huang B, Wang S, Ning Y, et al. Autosomal XX sex reversal caused by duplication of SOX9. *Am J Med Genet.* 1999;87:349-353.

114. Cox JJ, Willatt L, Homfray T, et al. A SOX9 duplication and familial 46,XX developmental testicular disorder. *N Engl J Med.* 2011;364:91-93.

115. Vidal VP, Chaboissier MC, de Rooij DG, et al. SOX9 induces testis development in XX transgenic mice. *Nat Genet.* 2001;28:216-217.

116. Bishop CE, Whitworth DJ, Qin Y, et al. A transgenic insertion upstream of SOX9 is associated with dominant XX sex reversal in the mouse. *Nat Genet.* 2000;26:490-494.

117. Hyon C, Chantot-Bastaraud S, Harbuz R, et al. Refining the regulatory region upstream of SOX9 associated with 46,XX testicular disorders of sex development (DSD). *Am J Med Genet A.* 2015;167(8):1851-1858.

118. Coveney D, Cool J, Oliver T, et al. Four-dimensional analysis of vascularization during primary development of an organ, the gonad. *Proc Natl Acad Sci U S A.* 2008;105:7212-7217.

119. Yao HH, Whoriskey W, Capel B. Desert Hedgehog/Patched 1 signaling specifies fetal Leydig cell fate in testis organogenesis. *Genes Dev.* 2002;16(11):1433-1440.

120. Park SY, Tong M, Jameson JL. Distinct roles for steroidogenic factor 1 and desert hedgehog pathways in fetal and adult Leydig cell development. *Endocrinology.* 2007;148:3704-3710.

121. Umehara F, Tate G, Itoh K, et al. A novel mutation of desert hedgehog in a patient with 46,XY partial gonadal dysgenesis accompanied by minifascicular neuropathy. *Am J Hum Genet.* 2000;67:1302-1305.

122. Werner R, Merz H, Birnbaum W, et al. 46,XY Gonadal dysgenesis due to a homozygous mutation in desert hedgehog (DHH) identified by exome sequencing. *J Clin Endocrinol Metab.* 2015;100:E1022-E1029.

123. Moniot B, Berta P, Scherer G, et al. Male specific expression suggests role of DMRT1 in human sex determination. *Mech Dev.* 2000;91: 323-325.

124. Raymond CS, Murphy MW, O'Sullivan MG, et al. Dmrt1, a gene related to worm and fly sexual regulators, is required for mammalian testis differentiation. *Genes Dev.* 2000;14:2587-2595.

125. Murphy MW, Lee JK, Rojo S, et al. An ancient protein-DNA interaction underlying metazoan sex determination. *Nat Struct Mol Biol.* 2015;22: 442-451.

126. Ledig S, Hiort O, Wünsch L, et al. Partial deletion of DMRT1 causes 46,XY ovotesticular disorder of sexual development. *Eur J Endocrinol.* 2012;167:119-124.

127. Barbaro M, Balsamo A, Anderlid BM, et al. Characterization of deletions at 9p affecting the candidate regions for sex reversal and deletion 9p syndrome by MLPA. *Eur J Hum Genet.* 2009;17:1439-1447.

128. Kitamura K, Yanazawa M, Sugiyama N, et al. Mutation of ARX causes abnormal development of forebrain and testes in mice and X-linked lissencephaly with abnormal genitalia in humans. *Nat Genet.* 2002;32: 359-369.

129. Fukami M, Wada Y, Miyabayashi K, et al. CXorf6 is a causative gene for hypospadias. *Nat Genet.* 2006;38:1369-1371.

130. Brennan J, Tilmann C, Capel B. Pdgfr-α mediates testis cord organization and fetal Leydig cell development in the XY gonad. *Genes Dev.* 2003;17:800-810.

131. Bagheri-Fam S, Argentaro A, Svingen T, et al. Defective survival of proliferating Sertoli cells and androgen receptor function in a mouse model of the ATR-X syndrome. *Hum Mol Genet.* 2011;20:2213-2224.

132. Pfeifer D, Poulat F, Holinski-Feder E, et al. The SOX8 gene is located within 700 kb of the tip of chromosome 16p and is deleted in a patient with ATR-16 syndrome. *Genomics.* 2000;63:108-116.

133. Waggoner DJ, Chow CK, Dowton SB, et al. Partial monosomy of distal 10q: three new cases and a review. *Am J Med Genet.* 1999;86:1-5.

134. Cox K, Bryce J, Jiang J, et al. Novel associations in disorders of sex development: findings from the I-DSD Registry. *J Clin Endocrinol Metab.* 2014;99:E348-E355.

135. Hutson JM, Grover SR, O'Connell M, et al. Malformation syndromes associated with disorders of sex development. *Nat Rev Endocrinol.* 2014; 10:476-487.

136. White S, Ohnesorg T, Notini A, et al. Copy number variation in patients with disorders of sex development due to 46,XY gonadal dysgenesis. *PLoS ONE.* 2011;6:e17793.

137. Ledig S, Hiort O, Scherer G, et al. Array-CGH analysis in patients with syndromic and non-syndromic XY gonadal dysgenesis: evaluation of array CGH as diagnostic tool and search for new candidate loci. *Hum Reprod.* 2010;25:2637-2646.

138. Yao HH, DiNapoli L, Capel B. Meiotic germ cells antagonize mesonephric cell migration and testis cord formation in mouse gonads. *Development.* 2003;130:5895-5902.

139. Vainio S, Heikkila M, Kispert A, et al. Female development in mammals is regulated by Wnt-4 signalling. *Nature.* 1999;397:405-409.

140. Chassot AA, Gregoire EP, Magliano M, et al. Genetics of ovarian differentiation: Rspo1, a major player. *Sex Dev.* 2008;2:219-227.

141. Liu CF, Bingham N, Parker K, et al. Sex specific roles of beta-catenin in mouse gonadal development. *Hum Mol Genet.* 2009;18:405-417.

142. Couse JF, Hewitt SC, Bunch DO, et al. Postnatal sex reversal of the ovaries in mice lacking estrogen receptors alpha and beta. *Science.* 1999;286:2328-2331.

143. Uhlenhaut NH, Jakob S, Anlag K, et al. Somatic sex reprogramming of adult ovaries to testes by FOXL2 ablation. *Cell.* 2009;139:1130-1142.

144. Teixeira J, Maheswaran S, Donahoe PK. Müllerian inhibiting substance: an instructive developmental hormone with diagnostic and possible therapeutic applications. *Endocr Rev.* 2001;22:657-674.

145. Josso N, Rey RA, Picard JY. Anti-müllerian hormone: a valuable addition to the toolbox of the pediatric endocrinologist. *Int J Endocrinol.* 2013;2013:674105.

146. Bedecarrats GY, O'Neill FH, Norwitz ER, et al. Regulation of gonadotropin gene expression by müllerian inhibiting substance. *Proc Natl Acad Sci U S A.* 2003;100:9348-9353.

147. Siiteri PK, Wilson JD. Testosterone formation and metabolism during male sexual differentiation in the human embryo. *J Clin Endocrinol Metab.* 1974;38:113-125.

148. Murray TJ, Fowler PA, Abramovich DR, et al. Human fetal testis: second trimester proliferative and steroidogenic capacities. *J Clin Endocrinol Metab.* 2000;85:4812-4817.

149. Tapanainen JS, Kellokumpu-Lehtinen P, Pelliniemi L, et al. Age-related changes in endogenous steroids of human fetal testis during early and midpregnancy. *J Clin Endocrinol Metab.* 1981;52:98-102.

150. Kaplan SL, Grumbach MM. Pituitary and placental gonadotrophins and sex steroids in the human and sub-human primate fetus. *Clin Endocrinol Metab.* 1978;7:487-511.

151. Miller WL, Auchus RJ. The molecular biology, biochemistry, and physiology of human steroidogenesis and its disorders. *Endocr Rev.* 2011;32:81-151.

152. Papadopoulos V, Miller WL. Role of mitochondria in steroidogenesis. *Best Pract Res Clin Endocrinol Metab.* 2012;26:771-790.

153. Flück CE, Miller WL, Auchus RJ. The 17,20-lyase activity of cytochrome p450c17 from human fetal testis favors the delta5 steroidogenic pathway. *J Clin Endocrinol Metab.* 2003;88:3762-3766.

154. Arlt W, Walker EA, Draper N, et al. Congenital adrenal hyperplasia caused by mutant P450 oxidoreductase and human androgen synthesis: analytical study. *Lancet.* 2004;363:2128-2135.

155. Biason-Lauber A, Miller WL, Pandey AV, et al. Of marsupials and men: "Backdoor" dihydrotestosterone synthesis in male sexual differentiation. *Mol Cell Endocrinol.* 2013;371:124-132.

156. Goto M, Piper Hanley K, Marcos J, et al. In humans, early cortisol biosynthesis provides a mechanism to safeguard female sexual development. *J Clin Invest.* 2006;116:953-960.

157. Hutson JM, Southwell BR, Li R, et al. The regulation of testicular descent and the effects of cryptorchidism. *Endocr Rev.* 2013;34:725-752.

158. Zimmermann S, Steig G, Emmen JM, et al. Targeted disruption of the Insl3 gene causes bilateral cryptorchidism. *Mol Endocrinol.* 1999;13:681-691.

159. Mullen RD, Behringer RR. Molecular genetics of Müllerian duct formation, regression and differentiation. *Sex Dev.* 2014;8:281-296.

160. Phoenix CH, Goy RW, Gerall AA, Young WC. Organizing action of prenatally administered testosterone proprionate on the tissues mediating mating behaviour in the female guinea pig. *Endocrinology.* 1959;65:369-382.

161. Wallen K, Hassett JM. Sexual differentiation of behaviour in monkeys: role of prenatal hormones. *J Neuroendocrinol.* 2009;21:421-426.

162. Dewing P, Shi T, Horvath S, et al. Sexually dimorphic gene expression in mouse brain precedes gonadal differentiation. *Brain Res Mol Brain Res.* 2003;118:82-90.

163. Arnold AP, Chen X. What does the "four core genotypes" mouse model tell us about sex differences in the brain and other tissues? *Front Neuroendocrinol.* 2009;30:1-9.

164. Arnold AP. The organizational-activational hypothesis as the foundation for a unified theory of sexual differentiation in all mammalian tissues. *Horm Behav.* 2009;55:570-578.

165. McCarthy MM, Arnold AP. Sex differences in the brain: the not so inconvenient truth. *J Neurosci.* 2012;32:2241-2247.

166. Berenbaum SA, Meyer-Bahlburg HF. Gender development and sexuality in disorders of sex development. *Horm Metab Res.* 2015;47:361-366.

167. Hines M, Ahmed F, Hughes IA. Psychological outcomes and gender-related development in complete androgen insensitivity syndrome. *Arch Sex Behav.* 2003;32:93-101.

168. Wisniewski AB, Mazur T. 46,XY DSD with female or ambiguous external genitalia at birth due to androgen insensitivity syndrome, 5alpha-reductase-2 deficiency, or 17beta-hydroxysteroid dehydrogenase deficiency: a review of quality of life outcomes. *Int J Pediatr Endocrinol.* 2009;2009:567430.

169. Chuang J, Vallerie A, Breech L, et al. Complexities of gender assignment in 17β-hydroxysteroid dehydrogenase type 3 deficiency: is there a role for early orchiectomy? *Int J Pediatr Endocrinol.* 2013;2013(1):15.

170. Cohen-Bendahan CCC, van de Beek C, Berenbaum SA. Prenatal sex hormone effects on child and adult sex-typed behavior: methods and findings. *Neurosci Biobehav Rev.* 2005;29:353-384.

171. Frisén L, Nordenström A, Falhammar H, et al. Gender role behavior, sexuality, and psychosocial adaptation in women with congenital adrenal hyperplasia due to CYP21A2 deficiency. *J Clin Endocrinol Metab.* 2009;94:3432-3439.

172. Meyer-Bahlburg HF, Dolezal C, Baker SW, et al. Sexual orientation in women with classical or non-classical congenital adrenal hyperplasia as a function of degree of prenatal androgen excess. *Arch Sex Behav.* 2008;37:85-99.

173. Meyer-Bahlburg HF, Dolezal C, Baker SW, et al. Prenatal androgenization affects gender-related behavior but not gender identity in 5-12-year-old girls with congenital adrenal hyperplasia. *Arch Sex Behav.* 2004;33:97-104.

174. Dessens AB, Slijper FM, Drop SL. Gender dysphoria and gender change in chromosomal females with congenital adrenal hyperplasia. *Arch Sex Behav.* 2005;32:389-397.

175. Lee PA, Houk CP. Review of outcome information in 46,XX patients with congenital adrenal hyperplasia assigned/reared male: what does it say about gender assignment? *Int J Pediatr Endocrinol.* 2010;2010:982025.

176. Pasterski V, Zucker KJ, Hindmarsh PC, et al. Increased cross-gender identification independent of gender role behavior in girls with congenital adrenal hyperplasia: results from a standardized assessment of 4- to 11-year-old children. *Arch Sex Behav.* 2015;44:1363-1375.

177. Martin CL, Ruble DN, Szkrybalo J. Cognitive theories of early gender development. *Psychol Bull.* 2002;128:903-933.

178. Raznahan A, Shaw PW, Lerch JP, et al. Longitudinal four-dimensional mapping of subcortical anatomy in human development. *Proc Natl Acad Sci U S A.* 2014;111:1592-1597.

179. Lombardo MV, Ashwin E, Auyeung B, et al. Fetal testosterone influences sexually dimorphic gray matter in the human brain. *J Neurosci.* 2012;32:674-680.

180. Forest MG, Sizonenko PC, Cathiard AM, et al. Hypophyso-gonadal function in humans during the first year of life: 1. Evidence for testicular activity in early infancy. *J Clin Invest.* 1974;53:819-828.

181. Boas M, Boisen KA, Virtanen HE, et al. Postnatal penile length and growth rate correlate to serum testosterone levels: a longitudinal study of 1962 normal boys. *Eur J Endocrinol.* 2006;154:125-129.

182. Crofton PM, Illingworth PJ, Groome NP, et al. Changes in dimeric inhibin A and B during normal early puberty in boys and girls. *Clin Endocrinol.* 1997;46:109-114.

183. Kubini K, Zachmann M, Albers N, et al. Basal inhibin B and the testosterone response to human chorionic gonadotropin correlate in prepubertal boys. *J Clin Endocrinol Metab.* 2000;85:134-138.

184. Bay K, Virtanen HE, Hartung S, et al. Insulin-like factor 3 levels in cord blood and serum from children: effects of age, postnatal hypothalamic-pituitary-gonadal axis activation, and cryptorchidism. *J Clin Endocrinol Metab.* 2007;92:4020-4027.

185. Wikstrom AM, Bay K, Hero M, et al. Serum insulin-like factor 3 levels during puberty in healthy boys and boys with Klinefelter syndrome. *J Clin Endocrinol Metab.* 2006;91:4705-4708.

186. Chellakooty M, Schmidt IM, Haavisto AM, et al. Inhibin A, inhibin B, follicle-stimulating hormone, luteinizing hormone, estradiol, and sex hormone-binding globulin levels in 473 healthy infant girls. *J Clin Endocrinol Metab.* 2003;88:3515-3520.

187. Steinmetz L, Rocha MN, Longui CA, et al. Inhibin A production after gonadotropin stimulus: a new method to detect ovarian tissue in ovotesticular disorder of sex development. *Horm Res.* 2009;71:94-99.

188. Groth KA, Skakkebæk A, Høst C, et al. Clinical review: Klinefelter syndrome—a clinical update. *J Clin Endocrinol Metab.* 2013;98:20-30.

189. Morris JK, Alberman E, Scott C, et al. Is the prevalence of Klinefelter syndrome increasing? *Eur J Hum Genet.* 2008;16:163-170.

190. Ross JL, Roeltgen DP, Stefanatos G, et al. Cognitive and motor development during childhood in boys with Klinefelter syndrome. *Am J Med Genet A.* 2008;146(A):708-719.

191. Ross JL, Roeltgen DP, Kushner H, et al. Behavioral and social phenotypes in boys with 47,XYY syndrome or 47,XXY Klinefelter syndrome. *Pediatrics.* 2012;129:769-778.

192. Cabrol S, Ross JL, Fennoy I, et al. Assessment of Leydig and Sertoli cell functions in infants with nonmosaic Klinefelter syndrome: insulin-like peptide 3 levels are normal and positively correlated with LH levels. *J Clin Endocrinol Metab.* 2011;96:E746-E753.

193. Aksglaede L, Juul A. Testicular function and fertility in men with Klinefelter syndrome: a review. *Eur J Endocrinol.* 2013;168:R67-R76.

194. Gies I, Unuane D, Velkeniers B, et al. Management of Klinefelter syndrome during transition. *Eur J Endocrinol.* 2014;171:R67-R77.

195. Schiff JD, Palermo GD, Veeck LL, et al. Success of testicular sperm extraction and intracytoplasmic sperm injection in men with Klinefelter syndrome. *J Clin Endocrinol Metab.* 2005;90:6263-6267.

196. Bondy CA, Turner Syndrome Study Group. Care of girls and women with Turner syndrome: a guideline of the Turner Syndrome Study Group. *J Clin Endocrinol Metab.* 2007;92:10-25.

197. Davenport ML. Approach to the patient with Turner syndrome. *J Clin Endocrinol Metab.* 2010;95:1487-1495.

198. Lee MC, Conway GS. Turner's syndrome: challenges of late diagnosis. *Lancet Diabetes Endocrinol.* 2014;2:333-338.

199. Hagman A, Loft A, Wennerholm UB, et al. Obstetric and neonatal outcome after oocyte donation in 106 women with Turner syndrome: a Nordic cohort study. *Hum Reprod.* 2013;28:1598-1609.

200. Devernay M, Ecosse E, Coste J, et al. Determinants of medical care for young women with Turner syndrome. *J Clin Endocrinol Metab.* 2009; 94:3408-3413.

201. Backeljauw PF, Bondy C, Chernausek SD, et al. Proceedings from the Turner Resource Network symposium: The crossroads of health care research and health care delivery. *Am J Med Genet A.* 2015;167(9): 1962-1971.

202. Singh RF, Carr DH. The anatomy and histology of XO human embryos and fetuses. *Anat Rec.* 1966;155:369-384.

203. Pasquino AM, Passeri F, Pucarelli I, et al. Spontaneous pubertal development in Turner's syndrome. Italian Study Group for Turner's syndrome. *J Clin Endocrinol Metab.* 1997;82:1810-1813.

204. Lunding SA, Aksglaede L, Anderson RA, et al. AMH as predictor of premature ovarian insufficiency: a longitudinal study of 120 Turner syndrome patients. *J Clin Endocrinol Metab.* 2015;100:E1030-E1038.

205. Gravholt CH, Fedder J, Naeraa RW, et al. Occurrence of gonadoblastoma in females with Turner syndrome and Y chromosome material: a population study. *J Clin Endocrinol Metab.* 2000;85:3199-3202.

206. El-Shawarby SA, Sharif F, Conway G, et al. Oocyte cryopreservation after controlled ovarian hyperstimulation in mosaic Turner syndrome: another fertility preservation option in a dedicated UK clinic. *BJOG.* 2010;117:234-237.

207. Oktay K, Rodriguez-Wallberg KA, Sahin G. Fertility preservation by ovarian stimulation and oocyte cryopreservation in a 14-year-old adolescent with Turner syndrome mosaicism and impending ovarian failure. *Fertil Steril.* 2010;94:753.e15-753.e19.

208. Hewitt JK, Jayasinghe Y, Amor DJ, et al. Fertility in Turner syndrome. *Clin Endocrinol.* 2013;79:606-614.

209. Telvi L, Lebbar A, Del Pino O, et al. 45,X/46,XY mosaicism: report of 27 cases. *Pediatrics.* 1999;104:304-308.

210. Hsu LY. Prenatal diagnosis of 45,X/46,XY mosaicism: a review and update. *Prenat Diagn.* 1989;9:31-48.

211. Chang HJ, Clark RD, Bachman H. The phenotype of 45,X/46,XY mosaicism: an analysis of 92 prenatally diagnosed cases. *Am J Hum Genet.* 1990;46:156-167.

212. Cools M, Pleskacova J, Stoop H, et al. Gonadal pathology and tumor risk in relation to clinical characteristics in patients with 45,X/46,XY mosaicism. *J Clin Endocrinol Metab.* 2011;96:E1171-E1180.

213. Lindhardt JM, Hagen CP, Rajpert-De Meyts E, et al. 45,X/46,XY mosaicism: phenotypic characteristics, growth, and reproductive function— a retrospective longitudinal study. *J Clin Endocrinol Metab.* 2012;97: E1540-E1549.

214. Martinerie L, Morel Y, Gay CL, et al. Impaired puberty, fertility, and final stature in 45,X/46,XY mixed gonadal dysgenetic patients raised as boys. *Eur J Endocrinol.* 2012;166:687-694.

215. Farrugia MK, Sebire NJ, Achermann JC, et al. Clinical and gonadal features and early surgical management of 45,X/46,XY and 45,X/47,XYY chromosomal mosaicism presenting with genital anomalies. *J Pediatr Urol.* 2013;9:139-144.

216. Müller J, Skakkebaek NE, Ritzen M, et al. Carcinoma in situ of the testis in children with 45,X/46,XY gonadal dysgenesis. *J Pediatr.* 1985;106: 431-436.

217. Tosson H, Rose SR, Gartner LA. Children with 45,X/46,XY karyotype from birth to adult height. *Horm Res Paediatr.* 2010;74:190-200.

218. Krob G, Braun A, Kuhnle U. True hermaphroditism: geographical distribution, clinical findings, chromosomes and gonadal histology. *Eur J Pediatr.* 1994;153:2-10.

219. Wiersma R, Ramdial PK. The gonads of 111 South African patients with ovotesticular disorder of sex differentiation. *J Pediatr Surg.* 2009;44: 556-560.

220. McElreavey K, Rappaport R, Vilain E, et al. A minority of 46,XX true hermaphrodites are positive for the Y DNA sequence including SRY. *Hum Genet.* 1992;90:121-125.

221. Tomaselli S, Megiorni F, De Bernardo C, et al. Syndromic true hermaphroditism due to an R-spondin (RSPO1) homozygous mutation. *Hum Mutat.* 2008;29:220-226.

222. Damiani D, Fellous M, McElreavey K, et al. True hermaphroditism: clinical aspects and molecular studies in 16 cases. *Eur J Endocrinol.* 1997;136:201-204.

223. Sircili MH, Denes FT, Costa EM, et al. Long-term followup of a large cohort of patients with ovotesticular disorder of sex development. *J Urol.* 2014;191:1532-1536.

224. Steven M, O'Toole S, Lam JP, et al. Laparoscopy versus ultrasonography for the evaluation of Mullerian structures in children with complex disorders of sex development. *Pediatr Surg Int.* 2012;28:1161-1164.

225. Moriya K, Morita K, Mitsui T, et al. Impact of laparoscopy for diagnosis and treatment in patients with disorders of sex development. *J Pediatr Urol.* 2014;10:955-961.

226. Correa RV, Domenice S, Bingham NC, et al. A microdeletion in the ligand binding domain of human steroidogenic factor 1 causes XY sex reversal without adrenal insufficiency. *J Clin Endocrinol Metab.* 2004;89: 1767-1772.

227. Köhler B, Lin L, Mazen I, et al. The spectrum of phenotypes associated with mutations in steroidogenic factor 1 (SF-1, NR5A1, Ad4BP) includes severe penoscrotal hypospadias in 46,XY males without adrenal insufficiency. *Eur J Endocrinol.* 2009;161:237-242.

228. Philibert P, Zenaty D, Lin L, et al. Mutational analysis of steroidogenic factor 1 (NR5a1) in 24 boys with bilateral anorchia: a French collaborative study. *Hum Reprod.* 2007;22:3255-3261.

229. Bashamboo A, Ferraz-de-Souza B, Lourenço D, et al. Human male infertility associated with mutations in NR5A1 encoding steroidogenic factor 1. *Am J Hum Genet.* 2010;87:505-512.

230. Fischbach BV, Trout KL, Lewis J, et al. WAGR syndrome: a clinical review of 54 cases. *Pediatrics.* 2005;116:984-988.

231. Köhler B, Biebermann H, Friedsam V, et al. Analysis of the Wilms' tumor suppressor gene (WT1) in patients 46,XY disorders of sex development. *J Clin Endocrinol Metab.* 2011;96:E1131-E1136.

232. Lipska BS, Ranchin B, Iatropoulos P, et al. Genotype-phenotype associations in WT1 glomerulopathy. *Kidney Int.* 2014;85:1169-1178.

233. Köhler B, Schumacher V, l'Allemand D, et al. Germline Wilms tumor suppressor gene (WT1) mutation leading to isolated genital malformation without Wilms tumor or nephropathy. *J Pediatr.* 2001;138: 421-424.

234. Suri M, Kelehan P, O'Neill D, et al. WT1 mutations in Meacham syndrome suggest a coelomic mesothelial origin of the cardiac and diaphragmatic malformations. *Am J Med Genet A.* 2007;143A:2312-2320.

235. Hawkins JR, Taylor A, Goodfellow PN, et al. Evidence for increased prevalence of SRY mutations in XY females with complete rather than partial gonadal dysgenesis. *Am J Hum Genet.* 1992;51:979-984.

236. Cameron FJ, Hageman RM, Cooke-Yarborough C, et al. A novel germ line mutation in SOX9 causes familial camptomelic dysplasia and sex reversal. *Hum Mol Genet.* 1996;5:1625-1630.

237. Puffenberger EG, Hu-Lince D, Parod JM, et al. Mapping of sudden infant death with dysgenesis of the testes syndrome (SIDDT) by a SNP genome scan and identification of TSPYL loss of function. *Proc Natl Acad Sci U S A.* 2004;101:11689-11694.

238. Vinci G, Brauner R, Tar A, et al. Mutations in the TSPYL1 gene associated with 46,XY disorder of sex development and male infertility. *Fertil Steril.* 2009;92:1347-1350.

239. Kalfa N, Fukami M, Philibert P, et al. Screening of MAMLD1 mutations in 70 children with 46,XY DSD: identification and functional analysis of two new mutations. *PLoS ONE.* 2012;7:e32505.

240. Porter FD. Smith-Lemli-Opitz syndrome: pathogenesis, diagnosis and management. *Eur J Hum Genet.* 2008;16:535-541.

241. Waterham HR, Hennekam RC. Mutational spectrum of Smith-Lemli-Opitz syndrome. *Am J Med Genet C Semin Med Genet.* 2012;160C: 263-284.

242. Berthezene F, Forest MG, Grimaud JA, et al. Leydig cell agenesis: a cause of male pseudohermaphroditism. *N Engl J Med.* 1976;295: 969-972.

243. Kremer H, Kraaij R, Toledo S, et al. Male pseudohermaphroditism due to a homozygous missense mutation of the luteinizing hormone receptor gene. *Nat Genet.* 1995;9:160-164.

244. Latronico AC, Anasti J, Arnhold IJP, et al. Brief report: testicular and ovarian resistance to luteinizing hormone caused by homozygous inactivating mutations of the luteinizing hormone receptor gene. *N Engl J Med.* 1996;334:507-512.

245. Kossack N, Simoni M, Richter-Unruh A, et al. Mutations in a novel, cryptic exon of the luteinizing hormone/chorionic gonadotropin receptor gene cause male pseudohermaphroditism. *PLoS Med.* 2008;5: e88.

246. Martens JWM, Verhoef-Post M, Abelin N, et al. A homozygous mutation in the luteinizing hormone receptor causes partial Leydig cell hypoplasia: correlation between receptor activity and phenotype. *Mol Endocrinol.* 1998;12:775-784.

247. Lin D, Sugawara T, Strauss JF III, et al. Role of steroidogenic acute regulatory protein in adrenal and gonadal steroidogenesis. *Science.* 1995; 267:1828-1831.

248. Prader A, Gurtner HP. Das Syndrom des Pseudohermaphroditismus masculinus bei kongenitaler NebennierenrindenHyperplasie ohne Androgenuberproduktion (adrenaler Pseudohermaphrotidismus masculinus). *Helv Paediatr Acta.* 1955;10(4):397-412.

249. Bose HS, Sugawara T, Strauss JF III, et al. The pathophysiology and genetics of congenital lipoid adrenal hyperplasia. *N Engl J Med.* 1996; 335:1870-1878.

250. Bose HS, Pescouitz OH, Miller WL. Spontaneous feminization in a 46,XX female patient with adrenal hyperplasia due to a homozygous

frame shift mutation in the steroidogenic reactive protein. *J Clin Endocrinol Metab.* 1997;82:1511-1515.

251. Nakae J, Tajima T, Sugawara T, et al. Analysis of the steroidogenic acute regulatory protein (StAR) gene in Japanese patients with congenital lipoid adrenal hyperplasia. *Hum Mol Genet.* 1997;6:571-576.

252. Baker BY, Lin L, Kim CJ, et al. Nonclassic congenital lipoid adrenal hyperplasia: a new disorder of the steroidogenic acute regulatory protein with very late presentation and normal male genitalia. *J Clin Endocrinol Metab.* 2006;91:4781-4785.

253. Sahakitrungruang T, Soccio RE, Lang-Muritano M, et al. Clinical, genetic, and functional characterization of four patients carrying partial loss-of-function mutations in the steroidogenic acute regulatory protein (StAR). *J Clin Endocrinol Metab.* 2010;95:3352-3359.

254. Flück CE, Pandey AV, Dick B, et al. Characterization of novel StAR (steroidogenic acute regulatory protein) mutations causing non-classic lipoid adrenal hyperplasia. *PLoS ONE.* 2011;6:e20178.

255. Hiort O, Holterhus PM, Werner R, et al. Homozygous disruption of P450 side-chain cleavage (CYP11A1) is associated with prematurity, complete 46,XY sex reversal, and severe adrenal failure. *J Clin Endocrinol Metab.* 2005;90:538-541.

256. Kim CJ, Lin L, Huang N, et al. Severe combined adrenal and gonadal deficiency caused by novel mutations in the cholesterol side chain cleavage enzyme, P450scc. *J Clin Endocrinol Metab.* 2008;93:696-702.

257. Tee MK, Abramsohn M, Loewenthal N, et al. Varied clinical presentations of seven patients with mutations in CYP11A1 encoding the cholesterol side-chain cleavage enzyme, P450scc. *J Clin Endocrinol Metab.* 2013;98:713-720.

258. Rubtsov P, Karmanov M, Sverdlova P, et al. A novel homozygous mutation in CYP11A1 gene is associated with late-onset adrenal insufficiency and hypospadias in a 46,XY patient. *J Clin Endocrinol Metab.* 2009;94:936-939.

259. Sahakitrungruang T, Tee MK, Blackett PR, et al. Partial defect in the cholesterol side-chain cleavage enzyme P450scc (CYP11A1) resembling nonclassic congenital lipoid adrenal hyperplasia. *J Clin Endocrinol Metab.* 2011;96:792-798.

260. Parajes S, Kamrath C, Rose IT, et al. A novel entity of clinically isolated adrenal insufficiency caused by a partially inactivating mutation of the gene encoding for P450 side chain cleavage enzyme (CYP11A1). *J Clin Endocrinol Metab.* 2011;96:E1798-E1806.

261. Simard J, Ricketts ML, Gingras S, et al. Molecular biology of the 3beta-hydroxysteroid dehydrogenase/delta^5-delta^4 isomerase gene family. *Endocr Rev.* 2005;26(4):525-582.

262. Rheaume E, Simard J, Morel Y, et al. Congenital adrenal hyperplasia due to point mutations in the type II 3 beta-hydroxysteroid dehydrogenase gene. *Nat Genet.* 1992;1:239-245.

263. Moisan AM, Ricketts ML, Tardy V, et al. New insight into the molecular basis of 3β-hydroxysteroid dehydrogenase deficiency: identification of eight mutations in the HSD3B2 gene eleven patients from seven new families and comparison of the functional properties of twenty-five mutant enzymes. *J Clin Endocrinol Metab.* 1999;84:4410-4425.

264. Codner E, Okuma C, Iniguez G, et al. Molecular study of the 3 beta-hydroxysteroid dehydrogenase gene type II in patients with hypospadias. *J Clin Endocrinol Metab.* 2004;89:957-964.

265. Mermejo LM, Elias LL, Marui S, et al. Refining hormonal diagnosis of type II 3 beta-hydroxysteroid dehydrogenase deficiency in patients with premature pubarche and hirsutism based on HSD3B2 genotyping. *J Clin Endocrinol Metab.* 2005;90:1287-1293.

266. Johannsen TH, Mallet D, Dige-Petersen H, et al. Delayed diagnosis of congenital adrenal hyperplasia with salt wasting due to type II 3β-hydroxysteroid dehydrogenase deficiency. *J Clin Endocrinol Metab.* 2005;90:2076-2080.

267. Benkert AR, Young M, Robinson D, et al. Severe salt-losing 3β-hydroxysteroid dehydrogenase deficiency: treatment and outcomes of HSD3B2 c.35G>A homozygotes. *J Clin Endocrinol Metab.* 2015;100(8):E1105-E1115.

268. Alos N, Moisan AM, Ward L, et al. A novel A10E homozygous mutation in the HSD3B2 gene causing severe salt-wasting 3β-hydroxysteroid dehydrogenase deficiency in 46,XX and 46,XY French-Canadians: evaluation of gonadal function after puberty. *J Clin Endocrinol Metab.* 2000;85:1968-1974.

269. New MI. Male pseudohermaphrodism due to a 17-alpha-hydroxylase deficiency. *J Clin Invest.* 1970;49:1930-1941.

270. Winter JSD, Couch RM, Muller J, et al. Combined 17-hydroxylase and 17/20 desmolase deficiencies: evidence for synthesis of a defective cytochrome P450c17. *J Clin Endocrinol Metab.* 1989;68:309-316.

271. Marsh CA, Auchus RJ. Fertility in patients with genetic deficiencies of cytochrome P450c17 (CYP17A1): combined 17-hydroxylase/17, 20-lyase deficiency and isolated 17,20-lyase deficiency. *Fertil Steril.* 2014;101:317-322.

272. Costa-Santos M, Kater CE, Auchus RJ, Brazilian Congenital Adrenal Hyperplasia Multicenter Study Group. Two prevalent CYP17 mutations and genotype-phenotype correlations in 24 Brazilian patients with 17-hydroxylase deficiency. *J Clin Endocrinol Metab.* 2004;89:49-60.

273. Dhir V, Reisch N, Bleicken CM, et al. Steroid 17alpha-hydroxylase deficiency: functional characterization of four mutations (A174E,

274. V178D, R440C, L465P) in the CYP17A1 gene. *J Clin Endocrinol Metab.* 2009;94:3058-3064.

274. Yanase T, Kagimoto M, Suzuki B, et al. Deletion of a phenylalanine in the N-terminal region of human cytochrome P-450(17α) results in combined 17α-hydroxylase/17,20-lyase deficiency. *J Biol Chem.* 1989; 264:18076-18082.

275. Geller DH, Auchus RJ, Mendonca BB, et al. The genetic and functional basis of isolated 17,20 lyase deficiency. *Nat Genet.* 1997;17:201-205.

276. Miller WL. The syndrome of 17,20 lyase deficiency. *J Clin Endocrinol Metab.* 2012;97:59-67.

277. Geller DH, Auchus RJ, Miller WL. P450c17 mutations R347H and R358Q selectively disrupt 17,20-lyase activity by disrupting interactions with P450 oxidoreductase and cytochrome b5. *Mol Endocrinol.* 1999;13:167-175.

278. Sherbert DP, Tosiano D, Kwist KM, et al. CYP17 mutation E305G causes isolated 17,20-lyase deficiency by selectively altering substrate binding. *J Biol Chem.* 2003;278:48563-48569.

279. Giordano SJ, Kaftory A, Steggles AW. A splicing mutation in the cytochrome b_5 gene from a patient with congenital methemoglobinemia and pseudohermaphrodism. *Hum Genet.* 1994;93:568-570.

280. Kok RC, Timmerman MA, Wolffenbuttel KP, et al. Isolated 17,20-lyase deficiency due to the cytochrome b5 mutation W27X. *J Clin Endocrinol Metab.* 2010;95:994-999.

281. Idkowiak J, Randell T, Dhir V, et al. A missense mutation in the human cytochrome b5 gene causes 46,XY disorder of sex development due to true isolated 17,20 lyase deficiency. *J Clin Endocrinol Metab.* 2012;97: E465-E475.

282. Miller WL. Minireview: regulation of steroidogenesis by electron transfer. *Endocrinology.* 2005;146:2544-2550.

283. Peterson RE, Imperato-McGinley J, Gautier T, et al. Male pseudohermaphroditism due to multiple defects in steroid-biosynthetic microsomal mixed-function oxidases: a new variant of congenital adrenal hyperplasia. *N Engl J Med.* 1985;313:1182-1191.

284. Flück CE, Tajima T, Pandey AV, et al. Mutant P450 oxidoreductase causes disordered steroidogenesis with and without Antley-Bixler syndrome. *Nat Genet.* 2004;36:228-230.

285. Fukami M, Nishimura G, Homma K, et al. Cytochrome P450 oxidoreductase deficiency: identification and characterization of biallelic mutations and genotype-phenotype correlations in 35 Japanese patients. *J Clin Endocrinol Metab.* 2009;94:1723-1731.

286. Krone N, Reisch N, Idkowiak J, et al. Genotype-phenotype analysis in congenital adrenal hyperplasia due to P450 oxidoreductase deficiency. *J Clin Endocrinol Metab.* 2012;97:E257-E267.

287. Idkowiak J, O'Riordan S, Reisch N, et al. Pubertal presentation in seven patients with congenital adrenal hyperplasia due to P450 oxidoreductase deficiency. *J Clin Endocrinol Metab.* 2011;96:E453-E462.

288. Flück CE, Meyer-Böni M, Pandey AV, et al. Why boys will be boys: two pathways of fetal testicular androgen biosynthesis are needed for male sexual differentiation. *Am J Hum Genet.* 2011;89:201-218.

289. Saez JM, de Perett E, Morera AM, et al. Familial male pseudohermaphroditism with gynaecomastia due to a testicular 17-ketosteroid reductase defect: I. In vivo studies. *J Clin Endocrinol Metab.* 1971;32:604-610.

290. Andersson S, Geissler WM, Wu L, et al. Molecular genetics and pathophysiology of 17 beta-hydroxysteroid dehydrogenase 3 deficiency. *J Clin Endocrinol Metab.* 1996;81:130-136.

291. Boehmer AL, Brinkmann AO, Sandkuijl LA, et al. 17 Beta-hydroxysteroid dehydrogenase-3 deficiency: diagnosis, phenotypic variability, population genetics, and worldwide distribution of ancient and de novo mutations. *J Clin Endocrinol Metab.* 1999;84:4713-4721.

292. Moghrabi N, Hughes IA, Dunaif A, et al. Deleterious missense mutations and silent polymorphism in the human 17beta-hydroxysteroid dehydrogenase 3 gene (HSD17B3). *J Clin Endocrinol Metab.* 1998;83: 2855-2860.

293. Hannema SE, Scott IS, Hodapp J, et al. Residual activity of mutant androgen receptors explains wolffian duct development in the complete androgen insensitivity syndrome. *J Clin Endocrinol Metab.* 2004; 89:5815-5822.

294. Lee YS, Kirk JM, Stanhope RG, et al. Phenotypic variability in 17β-hydroxysteroid dehydrogenase-3 deficiency and diagnostic pitfalls. *Clin Endocrinol (Oxf).* 2007;67:20-28.

295. Qiu W, Zhou M, Labrie F, et al. Crystal structures of the multispecific 17beta-hydroxysteroid dehydrogenase type 5: critical androgen regulation in human peripheral tissues. *Mol Endocrinol.* 2004;18:1798-1807.

296. Rösler A. Steroid 17 beta-hydroxysteroid dehydrogenase deficiency in man: an inherited form of male pseudohermaphrodism. *J Steroid Biochem Mol Biol.* 1992;43:989-1002.

297. Faisal SF, Iqbal A, Hughes IA. The testosterone: androstenedione ratio in male undermasculinization. *Clin Endocrinol.* 2000;53:697-702.

298. Khattab A, Yuen T, Yau M, et al. Pitfalls in hormonal diagnosis of 17-beta hydroxysteroid dehydrogenase III deficiency. *J Pediatr Endocrinol Metab.* 2015;28:623-628.

299. Achermann JC, Domenice S, Bachega TA, et al. Disorders of sex development: effect of molecular diagnostics. *Nat Rev Endocrinol.* 2015;11: 478-488.

300. Baetens D, Mladenov W, Delle Chiaie B, et al. Extensive clinical, hormonal and genetic screening in a large consecutive series of 46,XY

neonates and infants with atypical sexual development. *Orphanet J Rare Dis*. 2014;9:209.

301. Gross DJ, Landau H, Kohn G, et al. Male pseudohermaphroditism due to 17 beta-hydroxysteroid dehydrogenase deficiency: gender assignment in early infancy. *Acta Endocrinol*. 1986;112:238-246.

302. Phelan N, Williams EL, Cardamone S, et al. Screening for mutations in 17β-hydroxysteroid dehydrogenase and androgen receptor in women presenting with partially virilised 46,XY disorders of sex development. *Eur J Endocrinol*. 2015;172:745-751.

303. Imperato-McGinley J, Guerrero L, Gautier T, et al. Steroid 5α-reductase deficiency in man: an inherited form of male pseudohermaphroditism. *Science*. 1974;186:1213-1215.

304. Andersson S, Berman DM, Jenkins EP, et al. Deletion of steroid 5-alpha-reductase 2 gene in male pseudohermaphroditism. *Nature*. 1991;354:159-161.

305. Vilchis F, Ramos L, Mendez JP, et al. Molecular analysis of the SRD5A2 in 46,XY subjects with incomplete virilization: the P212R substitution of the steroid 5α-reductase-2 may constitute an ancestral founder mutation in Mexican patients. *J Androl*. 2009;31:358-364.

306. Cheng J, Lin R, Zhang W, et al. Phenotype and molecular characteristics in 45 Chinese children with 5α-reductase type 2 deficiency from South China. *Clin Endocrinol (Oxf)*. 2015;83(4):518-526.

307. Kang HJ, Imperato-McGinley J, Zhu YS, Rosenwaks Z. The effect of 5α-reductase-2 deficiency's effect on human fertility. *Fertil Steril*. 2014;101(2):310-316.

308. Katz MD, Kligman I, Cai LQ, et al. Paternity by intrauterine insemination with sperm from a man with 5α-reductase-2 deficiency. *N Engl J Med*. 1997;336:994-997.

309. Nordenskjold A, Ivarsson SA. Molecular characterization of 5 alpha-reductase type 2 deficiency and fertility in a Swedish family. *J Clin Endocrinol Metab*. 1998;83:3236-3238.

310. Herdt GH, Davidson J. The Sambia "turnim-man": sociocultural and clinical aspects of gender formation in male pseudohermaphrodites with 5-alpha-reductase deficiency in Papua, New Guinea. *Arch Sex Behav*. 1988;17:33-56.

311. Katz MD, Cai LQ, Zhu YS, et al. The biochemical and phenotypic characterization of females homozygous for 5 alpha-reductase 2 deficiency. *J Clin Endocrinol Metab*. 1995;80:3160-3167.

312. Hughes IA. Consequences of the Chicago DSD Consensus: a personal perspective. *Horm Metab Res*. 2015;47:394-400.

313. Krone N, Hughes BA, Lavery GG, et al. Gas chromatography/mass spectrometry (GC/MS) remains a pre-eminent discovery tool in clinical steroid investigations even in the era of fast liquid chromatography tandem mass spectrometry (LC/MS/MS). *J Steroid Biochem Mol Biol*. 2010;121:496-504.

314. Chan AOK, But BWM, Lee CY, et al. Diagnosis of 5α-reductase 2 deficiency: is measurement of dihydrotestosterone essential? *Clin Chem*. 2013;59:798-806.

315. Berra M, Williams EL, Muroni B, et al. Recognition of 5α-reductase-2 deficiency in an adult female 46XY DSD clinic. *Eur J Endocrinol*. 2011;164:1019-1025.

316. Costa EM, Domenice S, Sircili MH, et al. DSD due to 5α-reductase 2 deficiency: from diagnosis to long term outcome. *Semin Reprod Med*. 2012;30(5):427-431.

317. Maimoun L, Philibert P, Cammas B, et al. Undervirilization in XY newborns may hide a 5alpha-reductase deficiency: report of three new SRD5A2 gene mutations. *Int J Androl*. 2010;33:841-847.

318. Charmandari E, Dattani MT, Perry LA, et al. Kinetics and effect of percutaneous administration of dihydrotestosterone in children. *Horm Res*. 2001;56:177-181.

319. Levine AC, Wang JP, Ren M, et al. Immunohistochemical localization of steroid 5 alpha-reductase 2 in the human male fetal reproductive tract and adult prostate. *J Clin Endocrinol Metab*. 1996;81:384-389.

320. Thiele S, Hoppe U, Holterhus P-M, et al. Isoenzyme type 1 of 5alpha-reductase is abundantly transcribed in normal human genital skin fibroblasts and may play an important role in masculinisation of 5alpha-reductase type 2 deficient males. *Eur J Endocrinol*. 2005;152:875-880.

321. Fenichel P, Paris F, Philibert P, et al. Molecular diagnosis of 5a-reductase deficiency in 4 elite young athletes through hormonal screening for hyperandrogenism. *J Clin Endocrinol Metab*. 2013;98:E1055-E1059.

322. Hughes IA, Davies JD, Bunch TI, et al. Androgen insensitivity syndrome. *Lancet*. 2012;380:1419-1428.

323. De Bruyn R, Bollen R, Claessens F. Identification and characterization of androgen response elements. *Methods Mol Biol*. 2011;776:81-93.

324. Stashi E, York B, O'Malley B. Steroid receptor coactivators: servants and masters for control of systems metabolism. *Trends Endocrinol Metab*. 2014;25:337-347.

325. Bevan CL, Hoare S, Claessens F, et al. The AF1 and AF2 domains of the androgen receptor interact with distinct regions of SRC1. *Mol Cell Biol*. 1999;19:8383-8392.

326. Boehmer AL, Brinkmann AO, Bruggenwirth H, et al. Genotype versus phenotype in families with androgen insensitivity syndrome. *J Clin Endocrinol Metab*. 2001;86:4151-4160.

327. Han TS, Goswami D, Trikudanathan S, et al. Comparison of bone mineral density and body proportions between women with complete androgen insensitivity syndrome and women with gonadal dysgenesis. *Eur J Endocrinol*. 2008;159:179-185.

328. Hurme T, Lahdes-Vasama T, Makela E, et al. Clinical findings in prepubertal girls with inguinal hernia with special reference to the diagnosis of androgen insensitivity syndrome. *Scand J Urol Nephrol*. 2009;43:42-46.

329. Deeb A, Hughes IA. Inguinal hernia in female infants: a cue to check the sex chromosomes? *BJU Int*. 2005;96:401-403.

330. Yong EL, Loy CJ, Sim KS. Androgen receptor gene and male infertility. *Hum Reprod Update*. 2003;9:1-7.

331. Grunseich C, Rinaldi C, Fishbeck KH. Spinal and bulbar muscular atrophy: pathogenesis and clinical management. *Oral Dis*. 2014;20:6-9.

332. Ahmed SF, Cheng A, Hughes IA. Assessment of the gonadotropin-gonadal axis in androgen insensitivity syndrome. *Arch Dis Child*. 1999;80:324-329.

333. Boukari K, Meduri G, Brailly-Tabard S, et al. Lack of androgen receptor expression in Sertoli cells accounts for the absence of anti-müllerian hormone repression during early human testis development. *J Clin Endocrinol Metab*. 2009;94:1818-1825.

334. Bouvattier C, Carel JC, Lecointre C, et al. Postnatal changes of T, LH, and FSH in 46,XY infants with mutations in the AR gene. *J Clin Endocrinol Metab*. 2002;87:29-32.

335. Androgen Receptor Gene Mutations Database. Jewish General Hospital, McGill University, Montreal, Quebec, Canada. Available at: <http://www.androgendb.mcgill.ca>.

336. Tadokoro R, Bunch T, Schwabe JW, et al. Comparison on the molecular consequences of different mutations at residue 754 and 690 of the androgen receptor (AR) and androgen insensitivity syndrome (AIS) phenotype. *Clin Endocrinol*. 2009;71:253-260.

337. Deeb A, Jääskeläinen J, Dattani M, et al. A novel mutation in the human androgen receptor suggests a regulatory role for the hinge region in amino-terminal and carboxy-terminal interactions. *J Clin Endocrinol Metab*. 2008;93:3691-3696.

338. Deeb A, Mason C, Lee YS, et al. Correlation between genotype, phenotype and sex of rearing in 111 patients with partial androgen insensitivity syndrome. *Clin Endocrinol*. 2005;63:56-62.

339. Köhler B, Lumbroso S, Leger J, et al. Androgen insensitivity syndrome: somatic mosaicism of the androgen receptor in seven families and consequences for sex assignment and genetic counselling. *J Clin Endocrinol Metab*. 2005;90:106-111.

340. Tadokoro-Cuccaro R, Davies J, Mongan NP, et al. Promoter-dependent activity on androgen receptor N-terminal domain mutations in androgen insensitivity syndrome. *Sex Dev*. 2014;8:339-349.

341. Audi L, Fernandez-Caneio M, Carrascosa A, et al. Novel (60%) and recurrent (40%) androgen receptor gene mutations in a series of 59 patients with a 46,XY disorder of sex development. *J Clin Endocrinol Metab*. 2010;95:1876-1888.

342. Tadokoro-Cuccaro R, Hughes IA. Androgen insensitivity syndrome. *Curr Opin Endocrinol Diabetes Obes*. 2014;21:499-503.

343. Mongan NP, Tadokoro-Cuccaro R, Bunch T, et al. Androgen insensitivity syndrome. *Best Pract Res Clin Endocrinol Metab*. 2015;29(4):569-580. doi:10.1016/j.beem.2015.04.005.

344. Ahmed SF, Khwaja O, Hughes IA. The role of a clinical score in the assessment of ambiguous genitalia. *BJU Int*. 2000;85:120-124.

345. Ahmed SF, Cheng A, Dovey L, et al. Phenotypic features, androgen receptor binding, and mutational analysis in 278 clinical cases reported as androgen insensitivity syndrome. *J Clin Endocrinol Metab*. 2000;85:658-665.

346. Lek N, Miles H, Bunch T, et al. Low frequency of androgen receptor gene mutations in 46 XY DSD and fetal growth restriction. *Arch Dis Child*. 2014;99:358-361.

347. Chang C, Lee SO, Wang RS, et al. Androgen receptor (AR) physiological roles in male and female reproductive systems: lessons learned from AR-knockout mice lacking AR in selective cells. *Biol Reprod*. 2013;89:21.

348. Slob AK, van der Werff ten Bosch IJ, van Hall EV, et al. Psychosexual functioning in women with complete androgen insensitivity syndrome: is androgen replacement therapy preferable to estrogen? *J Sex Marital Ther*. 1993;19:201-209.

349. Danilovic DL, Correa PH, Costa EM, et al. Height and bone mineral density in androgen insensitivity syndrome with mutations in the androgen receptor gene. *Osteoporos Int*. 2007;18:369-374.

350. van der Zwan YG, Biermann K, Wolffenbuttel KP, et al. Gonadal maldevelopment as risk factor for germ cell cancer: towards a clinical decision model. *Eur Urol*. 2015;67:692-701.

351. Hannema SE, Scott IS, Rajpert-De Meyts E, et al. Testicular development in the complete androgen insensitivity syndrome. *J Pathol*. 2006;208:518-527.

352. Wunsch L, Holterhus PM, Wessel L, et al. Patients with disorders of sex development (DSD) at risk of gonadal tumour development: management based on laparoscopic biopsy and molecular diagnosis. *BJU Int*. 2012;110:E958-E965.

353. Rigilaarsdam MA, van Agthoven T, Gillis AJ, et al. Embryonic micro-RNAs in serum that discriminate germ cell cancer from controls for seminoma and non-seminoma germ cell tumours. *Andrology*. 2015;3:85-91.

354. Nakhal RS, Hall-Craggs M, Freeman A, et al. Evaluation of retained testes in adolescent girls and women with complete androgen insensitivity syndrome. *Radiology*. 2013;268:153-160.

355. Callens N, De Cuypere G, De Sutter P, et al. An update on surgical and non-surgical treatment for vaginal hypoplasia. *Hum Reprod Update*. 2014;20:775-801.

356. Ismail-Pratt IS, Bikoo M, Liao LM, et al. Normalization of the vagina by dilator treatment alone in complete androgen insensitivity syndrome and Mayer-Rokitansky-Kuster-Hauser syndrome. *Hum Reprod*. 2007;22(7):2020-2024.

357. Kolesinska Z, Ahmed SF, Niedziela M, et al. Changes over time in sex assignment for disorders of sex development. *Pediatrics*. 2014;134: e710-e715.

358. Pleskacova J, Hersmus R, Oosterhuis JW, et al. Tumor risk in disorders of sex development. *Sex Dev*. 2010;4:259-269.

359. Cools M, Looijenga LHJ, Wolffenbuttal KP, et al. Managing the risk of germ cell tumourigenesis in disorders of sex development patients. *Endocr Dev*. 2014;27:185-196.

360. Josso N, Belville C, de Clemente N, et al. AMH and AMH receptor defects in persistent müllerian duct syndrome. *Hum Reprod Update*. 2005;11:351-356.

361. Josso N, Rey R, Picard JY. Testicular anti-Mullerian hormone: clinical applications in DSD. *Semin Reprod Med*. 2012;30:364-373.

362. Imbeaud S, Carre-Eusebe D, Rey R, et al. Molecular genetics of the persistent müllerian duct syndrome: a study of 19 families. *Hum Mol Genet*. 1994;13:125-131.

363. Imbeaud S, Faure E, Lamarre I, et al. Insensitivity to anti müllerian hormone due to a mutation in the human antimüllerian hormone receptor. *Nat Genet*. 1995;11:382-388.

364. Imbeaud S, Belville C, Messika-Zeitoun L, et al. A 27 base pair deletion of the antimüllerian type II receptor gene is the most common cause of the persistent müllerian duct syndrome. *Hum Mol Genet*. 1996;5: 1269-1277.

365. Baskin LS, Ebbers MB. Hypospadias: anatomy, etiology, and technique. *J Pediatr Surg*. 2006;41:463-472.

366. Bergman JE, Loanne M, Vrijheid M, et al. Epidemiology of hypospadias in Europe; a registry-based study. *World J Urol*. [Epub 2015 Feb 25].

367. George M, Schneuer FJ, Jamieson SE, Holland AJA. Genetic and environmental factors in the aetiology of hypospadias. *Pediatr Surg Int*. 2015;31:519-527.

368. van der Zanden LF, van Rooij IA, Feitz WF, et al. Common variants in DGKK are strongly associated with risk of hypospadias. *Nat Genet*. 2011;43:48-50.

369. Geller F, Feenstra B, Carstensen L, et al. Genome-wide association analyses identify variants in developmental genes associated with hypospadias. *Nat Genet*. 2014;46:957-963.

370. Ogata T, Sano S, Nagata E, et al. MAMLD1 and 46,XY disorders of sex development. *Semin Reprod Med*. 2012;30:410-416.

371. Fredell L, Kockum I, Hansson E, et al. Heredity of hypospadias and the significance of low birth weight. *J Urol*. 2002;167:1423-1427.

372. Soderhall C, Korberg IB, Thei HT, et al. Fine mapping analysis confirms and strengthens linkage of four chromosomal regions in familial hypospadias. *Eur J Hum Genet*. 2015;23:516-522.

373. Brouwers MM, van der Zanden LF, de Gier RP, et al. Hypospadias: risk factor patterns and different phenotypes. *BJU Int*. 2010;105:254-262.

374. Chen MJ, Macias CG, Gunn SK, et al. Intrauterine growth restriction and hypospadias; is there a connection? *Int J Pediatr Endocrinol*. 2014; 2014(1):20.

375. Ortqvist L, Fossum M, Andersson M, et al. Long-term follow up of men born with hypospadias: urological and cosmetic results. *J Urol*. 2015; 193:975-981.

376. Teo AQA, Khan AR, Williams MP, et al. Is surgical exploration necessary in bilateral anorchia? *J Pediatr Urol*. 2013;9:e78-e81.

377. Bay K, Main KM, Toppari J, et al. Testicular descent: INSL3, testosterone, genes and the intrauterine milieu. *Nat Rev Urol*. 2011;8:187-196.

378. Acerini CL, Miles HL, Dunger DB, et al. The descriptive epidemiology of congenital and acquired cryptorchidism in a UK infant cohort. *Arch Dis Child*. 2009;94:868-872.

379. Wohlfahrt-Veje C, Boisen KA, Boas M, et al. Acquired cryptorchidism is frequent in infancy and childhood. *Int J Androl*. 2009;32:423-428.

380. Ferlin A, Zuccarello D, Garolla A, et al. Mutations in INSL3 and RXFP2 genes in cryptorchid boys. *Ann N Y Acad Sci*. 2009;1160:213-214.

381. Fenichel P, Lahlou N, Coquillards P, et al. Cord blood insulin–like peptide 3 (INSL3) but not testosterone is reduced in idiopathic cryptorchidism. *Clin Endocrinol*. 2015;82:242-247.

382. Toppari J. New cryptorchidism guidelines reach a consensus. *Nat Rev Urol*. 2014;11:432-433.

383. van der Plas EM, van Brakel J, Meij-de Vries A, et al. Acquired undescended testes and fertility potential: is orchidopexy at diagnosis better than awaiting spontaneous descent? *Andrology*. 2015;3(4):677-684.

384. Pettersson A, Richiardi L, Nordenskjold A, et al. Age at surgery for undescended testes and risk of testicular cancer. *N Engl J Med*. 2007; 356:1835-1841.

385. Kollin C, Ritzen EM. Cryptorchidism: a clinical perspective. *Pediatr Endocrinol Rev*. 2014;11(Suppl 2):240-250.

386. Main KM, Skakkebaek NE, Virtanen HE, et al. Genital anomalies in boys and the environment. *Best Pract Res Clin Endocrinol Metab*. 2010;24:279-289.

387. Juul A, Almstruo K, Andersson AM, et al. Possible fetal determinants of male infertility. *Nat Rev Endocrinol*. 2014;10:553-562.

388. Diamanti-Kandarakis E, Bourguinon JP, Guidice LC, et al. Endocrine-disrupting chemicals: an Endocrine Society Statement. *Endocr Rev*. 2009;30:293-342.

389. Thankamony A, Ong KK, Dunger DB, et al. Anogenital distance from birth to 2 years: a population study. *Environ Health Perspect*. 2009; 117:1786-1790.

390. Thankamony A, Lek N, Carroll D, et al. Anogenital distance and penile length in infants with hypospadias or cryptorchidism; comparison with normative data. *Environ Health Perspect*. 2014;122:207-211.

391. Bornehag CG, Carlstedt F, Jonsson BA, et al. Prenatal phthalate exposures and anogenital distance in Swedish boys. *Environ Health Perspect*. 2015;123:101-107.

392. Swan SH, Sathyanarayana S, Barrett ES, et al. First trimester phthalate exposure and anogenital distance in newborns. *Hum Reprod*. 2015; 30:963-972.

393. Jorgensen KT, Jensen MS, Toft GV, et al. Risk of cryptorchidism among sons of horticultural workers and farmers in Denmark. *Scand J Work Environ Health*. 2014;40:323-330.

394. Kalfa N, Paris F, Philibert P, et al. Is hypospadias associated with prenatal exposure to endocrine disruptors? A French collaborative controlled study of a cohort of 300 consecutive children without genetic defect. *Eur Urol*. [Epub 2015 May 23].

395. Zoeller RT, Bergman A, Becher G, et al. A path forward in the debate over health impacts of endocrine disrupting chemicals. *Environ Health*. 2014;14:118.

396. Kortenkamp A. Low dose mixture effects of endocrine disruptors and their implications for regulatory thresholds in chemical risk assessment. *Curr Opin Pharmacol*. 2014;19:105-111.

397. Hauser R, Skakkabaek NE, Hass U, et al. Male reproductive disorders, diseases, and costs of exposure to endocrine-disrupting chemicals in the European Union. *J Clin Endocrinol Metab*. 2015;100:1267-1277.

398. Pagnamenta AT, Taanman JW, Wilson CJ, et al. Dominant inheritance of premature ovarian failure associated with mutant mitochondrial DNA polymerase gamma. *Hum Reprod*. 2006;21:2467-2473.

399. Sutton E, Hughes J, White S, et al. Identification of SOX3 in XX male sex reversal gene in mice and humans. *J Clin Invest*. 2011;121:318-341.

400. Mandel H, Shemer R, Borochowitz ZU, et al. SERKAL syndrome: an autosomal-recessive disorder caused by a loss-of-function mutation in WNT4. *Am J Hum Genet*. 2008;82:39-47.

401. White PC, Bachega TA. Congenital adrenal hyperplasia due to 21 hydroxylase deficiency: from birth to adulthood. *Semin Reprod Med*. 2012;30:400-409.

402. Khalid JM, Oerton JM, Dezateux C, et al. Incidence and clinical features of congenital adrenal hyperplasia in Great Britain. *Arch Dis Child*. 2012;97:101-106.

403. Robins T, Bellanne-Chantelot C, Barbaro M, et al. Characterization of novel missense mutations in CYP21 causing congenital adrenal hyperplasia. *J Mol Med*. 2007;85:243-251.

404. White PC. Medscape. Neonatal screening for congenital adrenal hyperplasia. *Nat Rev Endocrinol*. 2009;5:490-498.

405. Nimkarn S, New MI. Congenital adrenal hyperplasia due to 21-hydroxylase deficiency: a paradigm for prenatal diagnosis and treatment. *Ann N Y Acad Sci*. 2010;1192:5-11.

406. New MI, Carlson A, Obeid J, et al. Prenatal diagnosis for congenital adrenal hyperplasia in 532 pregnancies. *J Clin Endocrinol Metab*. 2001; 86:5651-5657.

407. Hirvikoski T, Nordenström A, Lindholm T, et al. Cognitive functions in children at risk for congenital adrenal hyperplasia treated prenatally with dexamethasone. *J Clin Endocrinol Metab*. 2007;92:542-548.

408. Lajic S, Nordenström A, Hirvikoski T. Long-term outcome of prenatal dexamethasone treatment of 21-hydroxylase deficiency. *Endocr Dev*. 2011;20:96-105.

409. Meyer-Bahlburg HF, Dolezal C, Baker SW, et al. Cognitive and motor development of children with and without congenital adrenal hyperplasia after early-prenatal dexamethasone. *J Clin Endocrinol Metab*. 2004;89:610-614.

410. Meyer-Bahlburg HF, Dolezal C, Haggerty R, et al. Cognitive outcome of offspring from dexamethasone-treated pregnancies at risk for congenital adrenal hyperplasia due to 21-hydroxylase deficiency. *Eur J Endocrinol*. 2012;167:103-110.

411. Fernández-Balsells M, Muthusamy K, Smushkin G, et al. Prenatal dexamethasone use for the prevention of virilization in pregnancies at risk for classical congenital adrenal hyperplasia due to 21 hydroxylase (CYP21A2) deficiency: a systematic review and meta-analyses. *Clin Endocrinol*. 2010;73:436-444.

412. Speiser PW, Azziz R, Baskin LS. Congenital adrenal hyperplasia due to 21-hydroxylase deficiency: an Endocrine Society clinical practice guideline. *J Clin Endocrinol Metab*. 2010;95:4133-4160.

413. Miller WL, Witchel SF. Prenatal treatment of congenital adrenal hyperplasia: risks outweigh benefits. *Am J Obstet Gynecol*. 2013;208: 354-359.

414. Tardy-Guidollet V, Menassa R, Costa JM, et al. New management strategy of pregnancies at risk of congenital adrenal hyperplasia using fetal sex determination in maternal serum: French cohort of 258 cases (2002-2011). *J Clin Endocrinol Metab*. 2014;99:1180-1188.

415. New MI, Tong YK, Yuen T, et al. Noninvasive prenatal diagnosis of congenital adrenal hyperplasia using cell-free fetal DNA in maternal plasma. *J Clin Endocrinol Metab*. 2014;99:E1022-E1030.

416. Nimkarn S, New MI. Steroid 11beta-hydroxylase deficiency congenital adrenal hyperplasia. *Trends Endocrinol Metab*. 2008;19:96-99.

417. Parajes S, Loidi L, Reisch N, et al. Functional consequences of seven novel mutations in the CYP11B1 gene: four mutations associated with nonclassic and three mutations causing classic 11beta-hydroxylase deficiency. *J Clin Endocrinol Metab*. 2010;95:779-788.

418. Soardi FC, Penachioni JY, Justo GZ, et al. Novel mutations in CYP11B1 gene leading to 11 beta-hydroxylase deficiency in Brazilian patients. *J Clin Endocrinol Metab*. 2009;94:3481-3485.

419. Reisch N, Högler W, Parajes S, et al. A diagnosis not to be missed: nonclassic steroid 11β-hydroxylase deficiency presenting with premature adrenarche and hirsutism. *J Clin Endocrinol Metab*. 2013;98: E1620-E1625.

420. Charmandari E, Kino T, Ichijo T, et al. Generalized glucocorticoid resistance: clinical aspects, molecular mechanisms, and implications of a rare genetic disorder. *J Clin Endocrinol Metab*. 2008;93:1563-1572.

421. Mendonca BB, Leite MV, de Castro M, et al. Female pseudohermaphroditism caused by a novel homozygous missense mutation of the GR gene. *J Clin Endocrinol Metab*. 2002;87:1805-1809.

422. Santen RJ, Brodie H, Simpson ER, et al. History of aromatase: saga of an important biological mediator and therapeutic target. *Endocr Rev*. 2009;30:343-375.

423. Shozu M, Akasofu K, Harada T, et al. A new cause of female pseudohermaphroditism: placental aromatase deficiency. *J Clin Endocrinol Metab*. 1991;72:560-566.

424. Belgorosky A, Guercio G, Pepe C, et al. Genetic and clinical spectrum of aromatase deficiency in infancy, childhood and adolescence. *Horm Res*. 2009;72:321-330.

425. Ito Y, Fisher CR, Conte FA, et al. Molecular basis of aromatase deficiency in an adult female with sexual infantilism and polycystic ovaries. *Proc Natl Acad Sci U S A*. 1993;90:11673-11677.

426. Conte FA, Grumbach MM, Ito Y, et al. A syndrome of female pseudohermaphrodism, hypergonadotropic hypogonadism, and multicystic ovaries associated with missense mutations in the gene encoding aromatase (P450arom). *J Clin Endocrinol Metab*. 1994;78:1287-1292.

427. Mullis PE, Yoshimura N, Kuhlmann B, et al. Aromatase deficiency in a female who is compound heterozygote for two new point mutations in the P450arom gene: impact of estrogens on hypergonadotropic hypogonadism, multicystic ovaries, and bone densitometry in childhood. *J Clin Endocrinol Metab*. 1997;82:1739-1745.

428. Bouchoucha N, Samara-Boustani D, Pandey AV, et al. Characterization of a novel CYP19A1 (aromatase) R192H mutation causing virilization of a 46,XX newborn, undervirilization of the 46,XY brother, but no virilization of the mother during pregnancies. *Mol Cell Endocrinol*. 2014;390:8-17.

429. Carani C, Qin K, Simoni M, et al. Effect of testosterone and estradiol in a man with aromatase deficiency. *N Engl J Med*. 1997;337:91-95.

430. Lin L, Ercan O, Raza J, et al. Variable phenotypes associated with aromatase (CYP19) insufficiency in humans. *J Clin Endocrinol Metab*. 2007;92:982-990.

431. Brunskill J. The effects of fetal exposure to danazol. *Br J Obstet Gynaecol*. 1992;99:212-214.

432. VanSlooten AJ, Rechner SF, Dodds WG. Recurrent maternal virilization during pregnancy caused by benign androgen-producing ovarian lesions. *Am J Obstet Gynecol*. 1992;167:1342-1343.

433. Holt HB, Medbak S, Kirk D, et al. Recurrent severe hyperandrogenism during pregnancy: a case report. *J Clin Pathol*. 2005;58:439-442.

434. Oppelt P, Renner SP, Kellermann A, et al. Clinical aspects of Mayer-Rokitansky-Kuester-Hauser syndrome: recommendations for clinical diagnosis and staging. *Hum Reprod*. 2006;21:792-797.

435. Rall K, Eisenbeis S, Henninger V, et al. Typical and atypical associated findings in a group of 346 patients with Mayer-Rokitansky-Kuester-Hauser syndrome. *J Pediatr Adolesc Gynecol*. 2014;28(5):362-368.

436. Biason-Lauber A, Konrad D, Navratil F, et al. A WNT4 mutation associated with müllerian-duct regression and virilization in a 46,XX woman. *N Engl J Med*. 2004;351:792-798.

437. Williams CE, Nakhal RS, Achermann JC, et al. Persistent unexplained congenital clitoromegaly in females born extremely prematurely. *J Pediatr Urol*. 2013;9:962-965.

438. Magritte E. Working together in placing the long term interests of the child at the heart of the DSD evaluation. *J Pediatr Urol*. 2012;8:571-575.

439. Hiort O, Birnbaum W, Marshall L, et al. Management of disorders of sex development. *Nat Rev Endocrinol*. 2014;10:520-529.

440. Chitty LS, Chatelain P, Wolffenbuttel KP, et al. Prenatal management of disorders of sex development. *J Pediatr Urol*. 2012;8:576-584.

441. Pasterski V, Mastroyannopoulou K, Wright D, et al. Predictors of posttraumatic stress in parents of children diagnosed with a disorder of sex development. *Arch Sex Behav*. 2014;43:369-375.

442. Wünsch L, Buchholz M. Imaging, endoscopy and diagnostic surgery. *Endocr Dev*. 2014;27:76-86.

443. Magritte E, Achermann JC. When your baby is born with genitals that look different . . . the early days. Available at: <www.dsdfamilies.org>.

444. Auchus RJ, Witchel SF, Leight KR, et al. Guidelines for the development of comprehensive care centers for congenital adrenal hyperplasia: guidance from the CARES Foundation Initiative. *Int J Pediatr Endocrinol*. 2010;2010:275213.

445. Ahmed SF, Bryce J, Hiort O. International networks for supporting research and clinical care in the field of disorders of sex development. *Endocr Dev*. 2014;27:284-292.

446. Warne GL, Raza J. Disorders of sex development (DSDs), their presentation and management in different cultures. *Rev Endocr Metab Disord*. 2008;9:227-236.

447. Raza J, Mazen I. Achieving diagnostic certainty in resource-limited settings. *Endocr Dev*. 2014;27:257-267.

448. Kulle AE, Welzel M, Holterhus PM, et al. Implementation of a liquid chromatography tandem mass spectrometry assay for eight adrenal C-21 steroids and pediatric reference data. *Horm Res Paediatr*. 2013; 79:22-31.

449. Kamrath C, Wudy SA, Krone N. Steroid biochemistry. *Endocr Dev*. 2014;27:41-52.

450. Ahmed SF, Keir L, McNeilly J, et al. The concordance between serum anti-müllerian hormone and testosterone concentrations depends on duration of hCG stimulation in boys undergoing investigation of gonadal function. *Clin Endocrinol*. 2010;72:814-819.

451. Tantawy S, Lin L, Akkurt I, et al. Testosterone production during puberty in two 46,XY patients with disorders of sex development and novel NR5A1 (SF-1) mutations. *Eur J Endocrinol*. 2012;167:125-130.

452. Michala L, Aslam N, Conway GS, et al. The clandestine uterus: or how the uterus escapes detection prior to puberty. *BJOG*. 2010;117:212-215.

453. Nordenström A, Thyen U. Improving the communication of healthcare professionals with affected children and adolescents. *Endocr Dev*. 2014;27:113-127.

454. Rolston AM, Gardner M, Vilain E, et al. Parental reports of stigma associated with child's disorder of sex development. *Int J Endocrinol*. 2015;2015:980121.

455. Wisniewski AB, Sandberg DE. Parenting children with disorders of sex development (DSD): a developmental perspective beyond gender. *Horm Metab Res*. 2015;47:375-379.

456. Auchus RJ, Quint EH. Adolescents with disorders of sex development (DSD): lost in transition? *Horm Metab Res*. 2015;47:367-374.

457. Crouch NS, Creighton SM. Transition of care for adolescents with disorders of sex development. *Nat Rev Endocrinol*. 2014;10:436-442.

458. Berra M, Liao LM, Creighton SM, et al. Long-term health issues of women with XY karyotype. *Maturitas*. 2010;65:172-178.

459. Hewitt J, Zacharin M. Hormone replacement in disorders of sex development: current thinking. *Best Pract Res Clin Endocrinol Metab*. 2015; 29:437-447.

460. Birnbaum W, Bertelloni S. Sex hormone replacement in disorders of sex development. *Endocr Dev*. 2014;27:149-159.

461. Baratz AB, Sharp MK, Sandberg DE. Disorders of sex development peer support. *Endocr Dev*. 2014;27:99-112.

462. Sex Development: Genetics and Biology. National Health and Medical Research Council, Australia. Available at: <www.dsdgenetics.org>.

463. Accord Alliance. Clinical Guidelines for Management of Disorders of Sex Development in Childhood. Available at: <www.accordalliance.org>.

464. dsdteens. Available at: <www.dsdteens.org>.

465. Tobias ES, McElreavey K. Next generation sequencing for disorders of sex development. *Endocr Dev*. 2014;27:53-62.

466. Baxter RM, Arboleda VA, Lee H, et al. Exome sequencing for the diagnosis of 46,XY disorders of sex development. *J Clin Endocrinol Metab*. 2015;100(2):E333-E344.

467. Creighton S, Chernausek SD, Romao R, et al. Timing and nature of reconstructive surgery for disorders of sex development—introduction. *J Pediatr Urol*. 2012;8:602-610.

468. Wolffenbuttel KP, Crouch NS. Timing of feminising surgery in disorders of sex development. *Endocr Dev*. 2014;27:210-221.

469. Köhler B, Kleinemeier E, Lux A, et al. Satisfaction with genital surgery and sexual life of adults with XY disorders of sex development: results from the German clinical evaluation study. *J Clin Endocrinol Metab*. 2012;97:577-588.

470. Suorsa KI, Mullins AJ, Tackett AP, et al. Characterizing early psychosocial functioning of parents of children with moderate to severe genital ambiguity due to a disorder of sex development (DSD). *J Urol*. [Epub 2015 Jul 18].

471. Crouch NS, Liao LM, Woodhouse CR, et al. Sexual function and genital sensitivity following feminizing genitoplasty for congenital adrenal hyperplasia. *J Urol*. 2008;179:634-638.

472. Callens N, Hoebeke P. Phalloplasty: a panacea for 46,XY disorder of sex development conditions with penile deficiency? *Endocr Dev*. 2014; 27:222-233.

473. Springer A, Baskin LS. Timing of hypospadias repair in patients with disorders of sex development. *Endocr Dev*. 2014;27:197-202.

474. Moreno I, Míguez-Forjan JM, Simón C. Artificial gametes from stem cells. *Clin Exp Reprod Med*. 2015;42:33-44.

475. Nordenstrom A. Adult women with 21-hydroxylase deficient congenital adrenal hyperplasia, surgical and psychological aspects. *Curr Opin Pediatr.* 2011;23:436-442.

476. Michala L, Liao LM, Wood D, et al. Practice changes in childhood surgery for ambiguous genitalia? *J Pediatr Urol.* 2014;10:934-939.

477. Eckoldt-Wolke F. Timing of surgery for feminizing genitoplasty in patients suffering from congenital adrenal hyperplasia. *Endocr Dev.* 2014;27:203-209.

478. Arlt W, Willis DS, Wild SH, et al. Health status of adults with congenital adrenal hyperplasia: a cohort study of 203 patients. *J Clin Endocrinol Metab.* 2010;95:5110-5121.

479. Han TS, Walker BR, Arlt W, et al. Treatment and health outcomes in adults with congenital adrenal hyperplasia. *Nat Rev Endocrinol.* 2014; 10:115-124.

480. Han TS, Conway GS, Willis DS, et al. Relationship between final height and health outcomes in adults with congenital adrenal hyperplasia. *J Clin Endocrinol Metab.* 2014;99:E1547-E1555.

481. Falhammar H, Frisen L, Hirschberg A, et al. Increased cardiovascular and metabolic morbidity in patients with 21-hydroxylase deficiency: a Swedish population-based national cohort study. *J Clin Endocrinol Metab.* 2015;100(9):3520-3528. doi:10.1210/JC.2015-2093.

482. Strandqvist A, Falhammar H, Lichtenstein P, et al. Suboptimal psychosocial outcomes in patients with congenital adrenal hyperplasia; epidemiological studies in a nonbiased national cohort in Sweden. *J Clin Endocrinol Metab.* 2014;99:1425-1432.

483. Nallappa A, Sinaii N, Kumar P, et al. A phase 2 study of Chronocort, a modified-release formulation of hydrocortisone, in the treatment of adults with congenital adrenal hyperplasia. *J Clin Endocrinol Metab.* 2015;100:1137-1145.

484. Jurgensen M, Kleinemeiser E, Lux A, et al. Psychosexual development in adolescents and adults with disorders of sex development-results from the German clinical evaluation study. *J Sex Med.* 2013;10: 2703-2714.

485. Cassia Amaral RC, Inacio M, Brito VN, et al. Quality of life in a large cohort of adult Brazilian patients with 46,XX and 46,XY disorders of sex development from a single tertiary centre. *Clin Endocrinol.* 2015; 82:274-279.

486. D'Alberton F, Assante MT, Foresti M, et al. Quality of life and psychological adjustment of women living with 46,XY differences of sex development. *J Sex Med.* 2015;12:1440-1449.

487. Thyen U, Lux A, Jurgensen M, et al. Utilization of health care services and satisfaction with care in adults affected by disorders of sex development (DSD). *J Gen Intern Med.* 2014;29(Suppl 3):S752-S759.

488. Fliegner M, Krupp K, Brunner F, et al. Sexual life and sexual wellness in individuals with complete androgen insensitivity syndrome (CAIS) and Mayer-Rokitansky-Kuster-Hauser syndrome (MRKHS). *J Sex Med.* 2014;11:729-742.

489. Massanyi EZ, DiCarlo HN, Migeon CJ, et al. Review and management of 46,XY disorders of sex development. *J Pediatr Urol.* 2013;9:368-379.

490. van der Zwan YG, Callens N, van Kuppenfeld J, et al. Long-term outcomes in males with disorders of sex development. *J Urol.* 2013;190: 1038-1042.

491. Bouvattier C, Mignot B, Lefevre H, et al. Impaired sexual activity in male adults with partial androgen insensitivity. *J Clin Endocrinol Metab.* 2006;91:3310-3315.

492. Hellmann P, Christiansen P, Johannsen TH, et al. Male patients with partial androgen insensitivity syndrome: a longitudinal follow-up of growth, reproductive hormones and the development of gynaecomastia. *Arch Dis Child.* 2012;97:403-409.

493. Sandberg DE, Callens N, Wisniewski AB. Disorders of sex development (DSD): networking and standardization considerations. *Horm Metab Res.* 2015;47:387-393.

CHAPTER 24

Normal and Aberrant Growth in Children

DAVID W. COOKE • SARA A. DiVALL • SALLY RADOVICK

KEY POINTS

- Height is an important "vital sign" to obtain in childhood because deviations from the normal linear growth pattern may indicate an underlying disorder.
- An intact hypothalamic (GHRH; growth hormone-releasing hormone)/pituitary (GH; growth hormone)/IGF-1 (insulin-like growth factor 1) axis, adequate nutrition, and absence of significant systemic disease are requirements for normal linear growth.
- A comprehensive past medical, family, and social history with assessment of an accurate growth velocity is required for the initial investigation of abnormal growth. Laboratory and radiologic investigations include an evaluation for occult systemic disease and exclusion of hormonal abnormalities.
- Successful treatment of the underlying disorder or correction of hormone deficiency(ies) improves linear growth.
- Treatment of short stature with growth-promoting agents may improve linear growth in select patients with intact GHRH/GH/IGF-1 axis function.

NORMAL GROWTH

Overview

Growth is a fundamental, intrinsic aspect of childhood health. It is also a complex yet tightly regulated process. An individual's final height and the path taken to reach that end point are significantly determined by that person's genetic composition. But growth and final height can also be affected by external factors, including the quality and quantity of nutrition, and by psychosocial factors. This process is regulated by multiple hormones and growth factors interacting with an array of membrane receptors that activate seemingly redundant intracellular signaling cascades. And yet, as complex as this process is, 1 standard

deviation (SD) of adult height represents about only 4% of the mean adult height.

Whether linear growth occurs as a continuous process or with periodic bursts of growth and arrest[1-4] has been hard to characterize definitively. There do appear to be seasonal variations of growth, with slower growth in autumn and winter and greater growth in spring and early summer.[5,6] Some normal children have a broad growth channel, with many showing diverse but characteristic growth tracks.[7] Nonetheless, even though the process of growth is multifactorial and complex, children usually grow in a remarkably predictable manner. Deviation from such a normal pattern of growth can be the first manifestation of a wide variety of disease processes, including endocrine and nonendocrine disorders and involving virtually any organ system of the body. Therefore, frequent and accurate assessment of growth is of primary importance in the care of children.

Measurement

Assessment of growth requires accurate and reproducible determinations of height. Supine length is routinely measured in children younger than 2 years of age, and erect height is assessed in older children. It can be useful to measure both length and height in children between 2 and 3 years of age to allow comparisons with prior length measurements and to begin to record height measurement for ongoing comparisons. The inherent inaccuracies involved in measuring length in infants are often obscured by the rapid skeletal growth during this period. For measurement of supine length (Fig. 24-1), it is best to use a firm box with an inflexible board, against which the head lies, and a movable footboard, on which the feet are placed perpendicular to the plane of the supine length of the infant. Optimally, the child should be relaxed, the legs should be fully extended, and the head should be positioned in the Frankfurt plane, with the line connecting the outer canthus of the eyes and the external auditory meatus perpendicular to the long axis of the trunk.

When children are old enough (and physically capable) to stand erect, it is best to employ a wall-mounted Harpenden stadiometer similar to that designed by Tanner and Whitehouse for the British Harpenden Growth Study. The traditional measuring device of a flexible arm mounted to a weight balance is notoriously unreliable and does not provide accurate serial measurements.

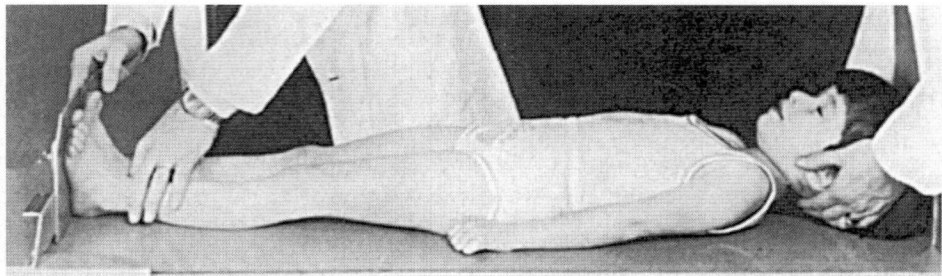

Figure 24-1 Technique for measuring recumbent length. (A device suitable for measurement of length of infants can be purchased from Raven Equipment Limited, Essex, UK.) (Photograph courtesy of Noel Cameron.)

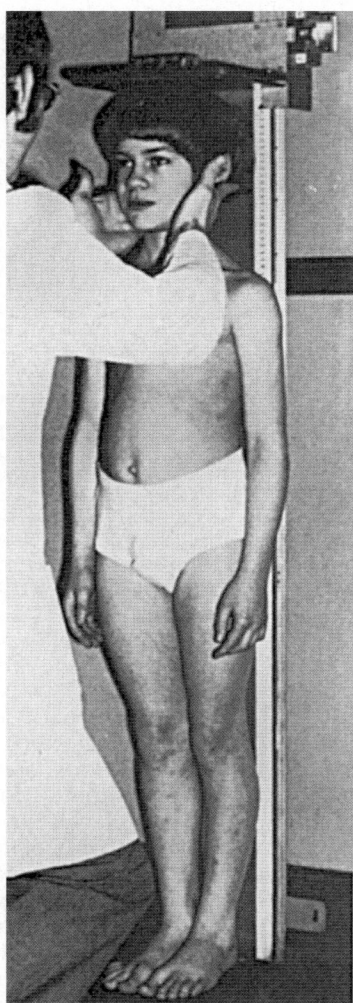

Figure 24-2 Technique for measuring erect height using the Harpenden stadiometer with direct digital display of height. (Devices of this type are available from Holtain Ltd, Wales, UK, and Seritex Inc., Carlstadt, NJ.)

As with length measurements in infants, positioning of the child in the stadiometer is critical (Fig. 24-2). The child should be fully erect, with the head in the Frankfurt plane; the back of the head, thoracic spine, buttocks, and heels should touch the vertical axis of the stadiometer; and the heels should be together. Every effort should be made to correct discrepancies related to lordosis or scoliosis. Ideally, serial measurements should be made at the same

time of day, because standing height may undergo diurnal variation.

Height determinations should be performed by a trained individual rather than an inexperienced member of the staff. We recommend that lengths and heights be measured in triplicate, that variation should be no more than 0.3 cm, and that the mean height should be recorded. For determination of height velocity when several measurements are being made within a short period, the same individual should perform the determinations to eliminate interobserver variability. Even when every effort is made to obtain accurate height measurements, a minimum interval of 6 months is necessary for meaningful height velocity computation. Nine to 12 months of data are preferable so that errors of measurement are minimized and the seasonal variation in height velocity is assimilated into the data.

Growth Charts

Evaluation of a child's height must be done in the context of normal standards. Most American pediatric endocrine clinics use the cross-sectional data provided by the National Center for Health Statistics (NCHS), which were originally introduced in 1977. Revised and updated growth charts have been available on the Centers for Disease Control (CDC) website since 2000 (www.cdc.gov/growthcharts; Figs. 24-3 through 24-8).[8] The data for these charts encompass measurements obtained in the United States between 1963 and 1995, and they include a broader representation of the U.S. population for all measures than was available in earlier charts. Growth charts based on the WHO data that were gathered from 1997 throughout 2003 should be used to monitor the growth of children under 2 years of age. While the data on length are very similar between the CDC and WHO curves, the CDC curves describe higher weight gain that, among other things, reflects the lower prevalence of breastfed infants in the CDC data and is not felt to represent optimal growth.[9]

These charts allow comparison of individual children with the 3rd, 10th, 25th, 50th, 75th, 90th, and 97th percentiles of normal American children. There are, however, two limitations of these charts when applied to the individual child. First, they do not satisfactorily define children below the 3rd or above the 97th percentiles—the very children in whom it is most critical to define the degree to which they deviate from the normal growth centiles. However, the NCHS data tables (also available on the CDC website) can be used to compute standard deviation scores (SDS). For example, a short child below the 3rd percentile can be described more precisely as being approximately 4.2 SDS below the mean for age. A height SDS for age is calculated as follows: the SDS equals the child's height, minus the mean height for normal children

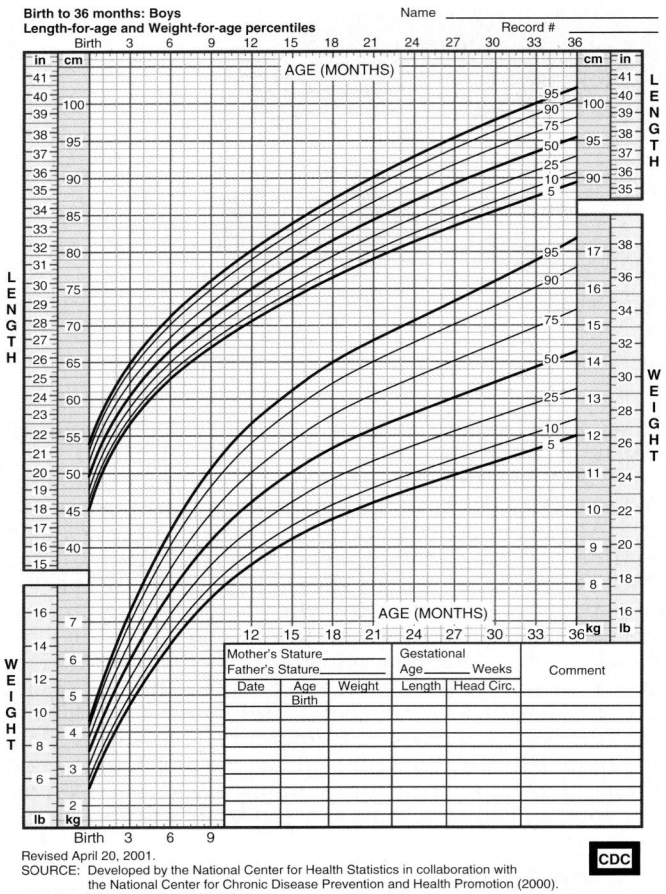

Figure 24-3 Length-for-age and weight-for-age percentiles for boys (birth to 36 months). (Developed by the National Center for Health Statistics in collaboration with the National Center for Chronic Disease Prevention and Health Promotion, 2000. Available at http://www.cdc.gov/growthcharts; accessed October 2010.)

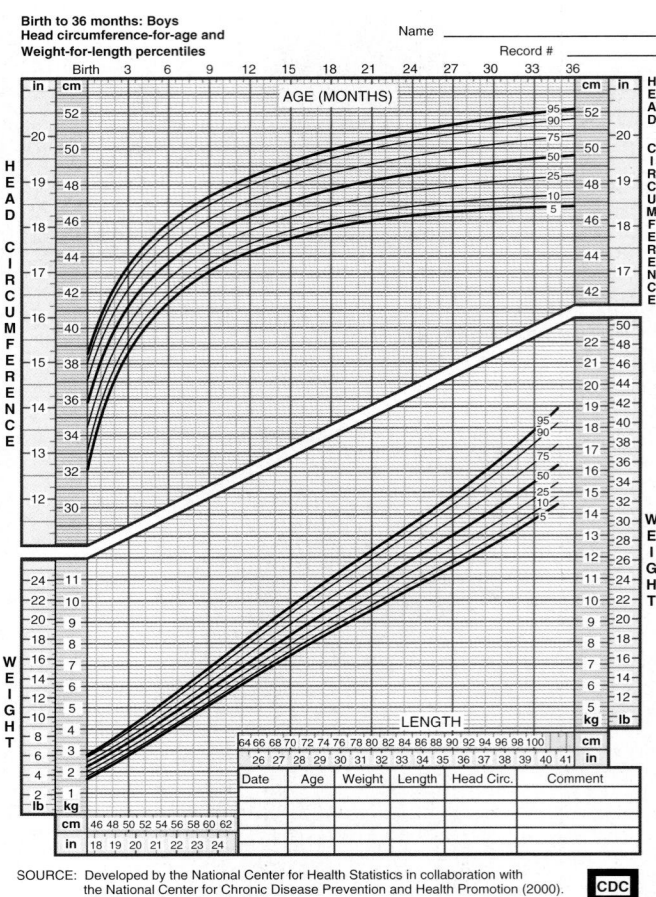

Figure 24-4 Head circumference-for-age and weight-for-length percentiles for boys (birth to 36 months). (Developed by the National Center for Health Statistics in collaboration with the National Center for Chronic Disease Prevention and Health Promotion, 2000. Available at http://www.cdc.gov/growthcharts; accessed October 2010.)

of the child's age and gender, divided by the SD of the height for normal children of this age and gender. Second, cross-sectional data are of greater value during infancy and childhood than in adolescence, because differences in the timing of pubertal onset can considerably influence normal growth rates. To address this issue, Tanner and Davies[10] developed longitudinal growth charts in an effort to construct the curve shapes with centile widths obtained from a large cross-sectional survey, thus accounting for variability in the timing of puberty. Such charts are of particular value in assessing growth during adolescence and puberty and for plotting sequential growth data for any individual child.

The data from cross-sectional and longitudinal growth studies have been employed to develop *height velocity* standards (Figs. 24-9 and 24-10). It is important to emphasize that carefully documented height velocity data are invaluable in assessing a child with abnormalities of growth. There is considerable variability in normal height velocity of children at different ages; however, between the age of 2 years and the onset of puberty, children grow with remarkable fidelity relative to the normal growth curves. Any crossing of percentile curves on the height chart during this age period should be considered abnormal and warrants further evaluation.

Syndrome-specific growth curves have been developed for a number of clinical conditions associated with growth failure, such as Turner syndrome (TS),[11] achondroplasia,[12] and Down syndrome.[13] Such growth profiles are invaluable for tracking the growth of children with these clinical conditions. Deviation of growth from the appropriate disease-related growth curve suggests the possibility of a second underlying cause, such as acquired autoimmune hypothyroidism in children with Down syndrome or TS.

Body Proportions

Many abnormal growth states, including both short stature and excessive stature, are characterized by *disproportionate* growth. The following determinations should be made as part of the evaluation of short stature:
1. Occipitofrontal head circumference
2. Lower body segment: distance from top of pubic symphysis to the floor
3. Upper body segment: the difference between total height and lower body segment (it can also be measured as the sitting height, subtracting the height of the chair or stool)
4. Arm span

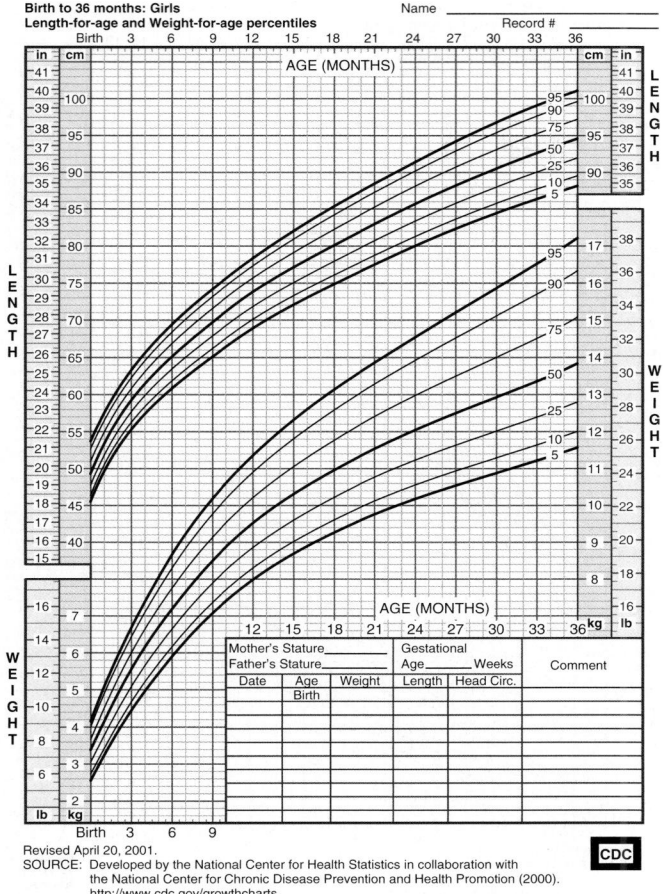

Figure 24-5 Length-for-age and weight-for-age percentiles for girls (birth to 36 months). (Developed by the National Center for Health Statistics in collaboration with the National Center for Chronic Disease Prevention and Health Promotion, 2000. Available at http://www.cdc.gov/growthcharts; accessed October 2010.)

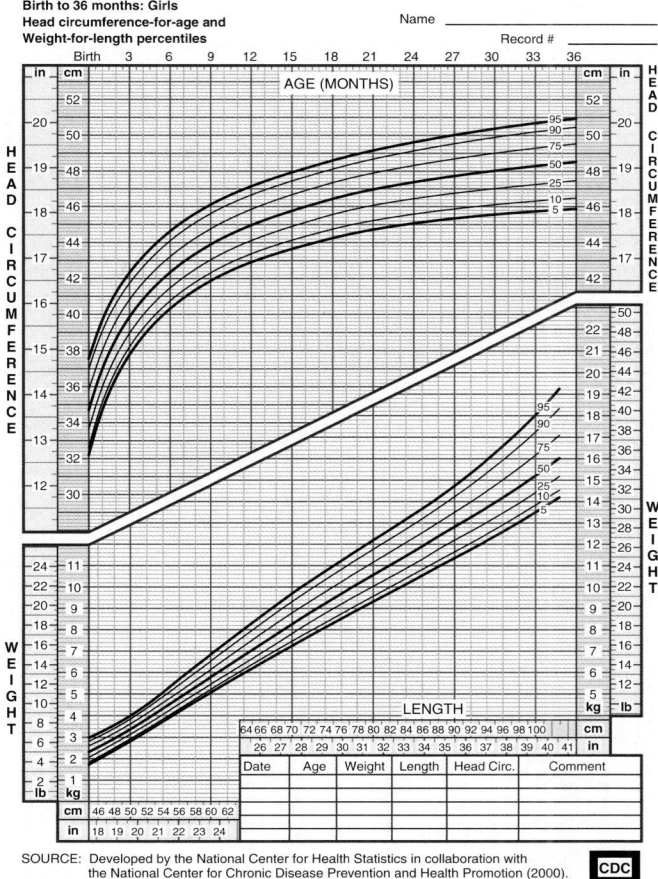

Figure 24-6 Head circumference-for-age and weight-for-length percentiles for girls (birth to 36 months). (Developed by the National Center for Health Statistics in collaboration with the National Center for Chronic Disease Prevention and Health Promotion, 2000. Available at http://www.cdc.gov/growthcharts; accessed October 2010.)

Published standards exist for these body proportion measurements, which must be evaluated relative to the patient's age.[14] The ratio of upper segment to lower segment ranges from 1.7 in the neonate to slightly less than 1.0 in the adult (Fig. 24-11).

Parental Target Height

Genetic factors are important determinants of growth and height potential. Therefore, it is useful to assess a patient's stature relative to that of siblings and parents. Tanner and associates developed a growth chart that factored parents' heights into the evaluation of the heights of children ages 2 to 9 years.[15] One can also calculate a child's expected final height based on the parents' heights by calculating the midparental height. This is the average of the parents' heights, after accounting for the average difference in height between adult men and women (13 cm). In other words, a boy's midparental height equals the average of his parents' heights plus 6.5 cm, and a girl's midparental height equals the average of her parents' heights minus 6.5 cm.

Because of regression to the mean,[16,17] children of short parents are likely to be less short than their parents, and children of tall parents are likely to be less tall than their parents. Therefore, a child's genetic *target height range* centers on the point that represents 80% of the difference between the child's midparental height and the mean adult height for the child's gender.[16] For example, if a boy's father is 168 cm tall and his mother is 153 cm tall, his midparental height is 167 cm, which is 10 cm below the mean height of adult men (177 cm). Therefore, the boy's target height range centers on 169 cm, which is 8 cm below the mean adult height for men. In more than 95% of children, the adult height falls within 10 cm of the point thus calculated.[15,16] In children with extremely short stature (≥3 SD), the father's height may more strongly correlate with the patient's height, and the mother's height may more greatly influence birth length.[18]

Skeletal Maturation

The growth potential in the tubular bones can be assessed by evaluation of the progression of ossification within the epiphyses. The ossification centers of the skeleton appear and progress in a predictable sequence in normal children, and this skeletal maturation can be compared with normal age-related standards. This forms the basis of the *bone age* or *skeletal age*, a quantitative determination of net somatic maturation that serves as a mirror of the tempo of growth and maturation. The bone age also reflects the degree of growth plate senescence and therefore is a useful adjunct

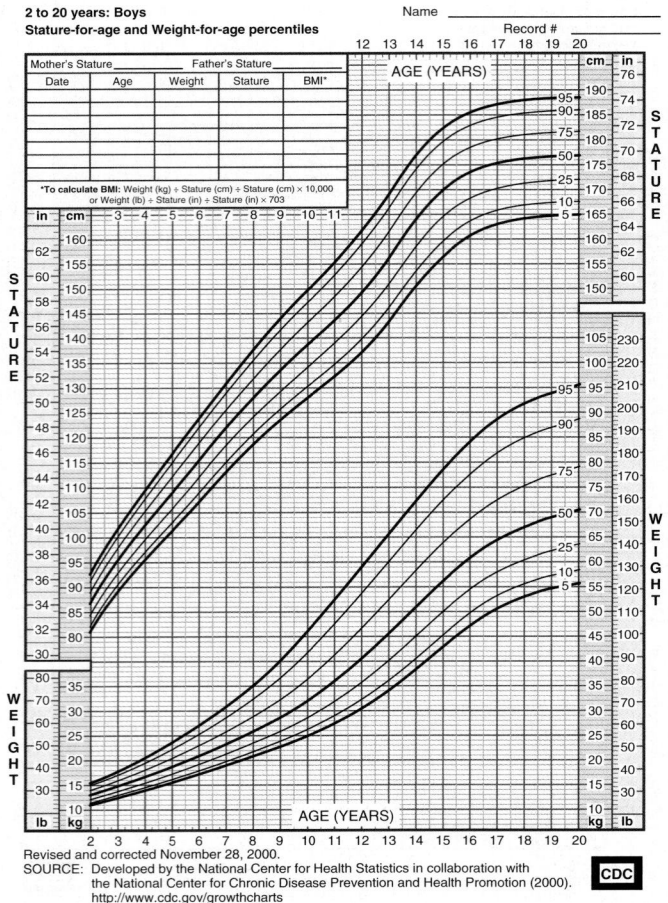

Figure 24-7 Stature-for-age and weight-for-age percentiles for boys (2 to 20 years). (Developed by the National Center for Health Statistics in collaboration with the National Center for Chronic Disease Prevention and Health Promotion, 2000. Available at http://www.cdc.gov/growthcharts; accessed October 2010.)

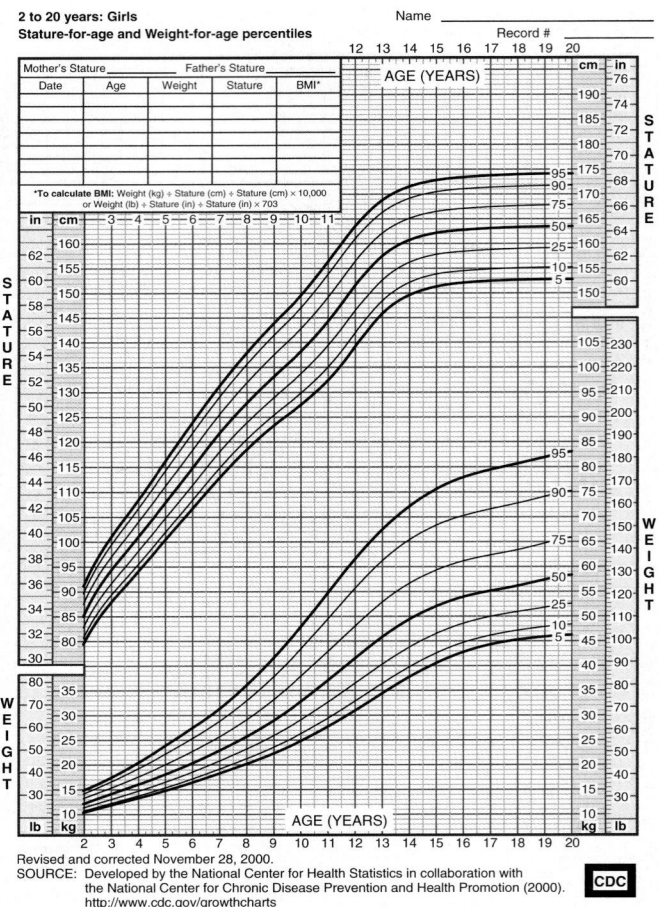

Figure 24-8 Stature-for-age and weight-for-age percentiles for girls (2 to 20 years). (Developed by the National Center for Health Statistics in collaboration with the National Center for Chronic Disease Prevention and Health Promotion, 2000. Available at http://www.cdc.gov/growthcharts; accessed October 2010.)

in estimating growth opportunity (i.e., the ultimate adult height), as discussed later in this chapter.

Not all of the factors that determine the normal pattern of skeletal maturation have been identified, but genetic factors and multiple hormones, including thyroxine, growth hormone (GH), and gonadal steroids, are involved.[19] Ultimately, growth cessation occurs after exhaustion of the proliferative capacity of the growth plate chondrocyte.[20] Estrogen plays an important role in this process: animal studies have indicated that estrogen accelerates growth plate senescence,[21] and studies in patients with mutations of the gene for the estrogen receptor[22] or for the aromatase enzyme[23,24] demonstrated that estrogen is primarily responsible for epiphyseal fusion.[25]

Phases of Normal Growth

Growth occurs at differing rates during intrauterine life, early and middle childhood, and adolescence and then ceases after fusion of long bone and vertebral epiphyseal growth plates. Karlberg and associates resolved the normal linear growth curve into three additive, partially superimposable phases[26,27]: an "infancy" phase, starting in midgestation and then rapidly decelerating until about 3 to 4 years of age; a "childhood" phase, of slowly decelerating growth through early adolescence; and a sigmoid-shaped

"puberty" phase that comprises the adolescent growth spurt. Prenatal growth averages 1.2 to 1.5 cm per week but varies dramatically (Fig. 24-12); the midgestational length growth velocity of 2.5 cm per week falls to almost 0.5 cm per week immediately before birth. Growth velocity (see Figs. 24-9 and 24-10) averages about 15 cm per year during the first 2 years of life; it then slows to approximately 6 cm per year during middle childhood. During this time, a normal child's height, plotted on a growth curve, typically remains within a given growth channel; that is, it does not cross percentile lines on the growth curve.

Prepubertal growth is similar between boys and girls. The height difference between men and women, an average of 13 cm, is accounted for by two factors. First, boys grow for an average of 2 years longer than girls do, because girls have an earlier onset of puberty and, consequently, earlier cessation of growth. Therefore, prepubertal growth is greater for boys; they are 8 to 10 cm taller when their puberty starts, compared with girls' heights when their puberty starts.[16] Second, boys achieve a greater maximal pubertal growth velocity than girls do, giving them 3 to 5 cm greater pubertal growth. The time of onset of puberty varies in normal children, resulting in a normal variation in the timing of the pubertal growth spurt. However, in most normal children, the final height is not influenced by the chronologic age at onset of the pubertal growth spurt,

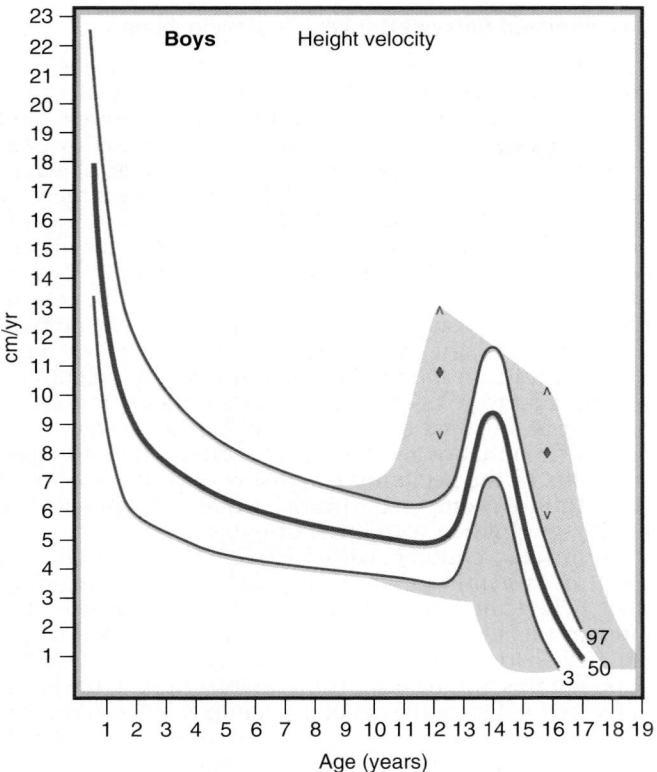

Figure 24-9 Height velocity chart for boys constructed from longitudinal observations of British children. The 97th, 50th, and 3rd percentile curves define the general pattern of growth during puberty. Shaded areas indicate velocities in those children with peak velocities occurring up to 2 standard deviations before or after the average age depicted by the percentile lines. (*Up arrows, diamonds,* and *down arrows* mark, respectively, the 97th, 50th, and 3rd percentiles of peak velocity when the peak occurs at these early or late limits.) (Modified from charts prepared by J.M. Tanner and R.H. Whitehouse from data published in references 10 and 30. Reproduced with permission of J.M. Tanner and Castlemead Publications, Ward's Publishing Services, Herts, UK.)

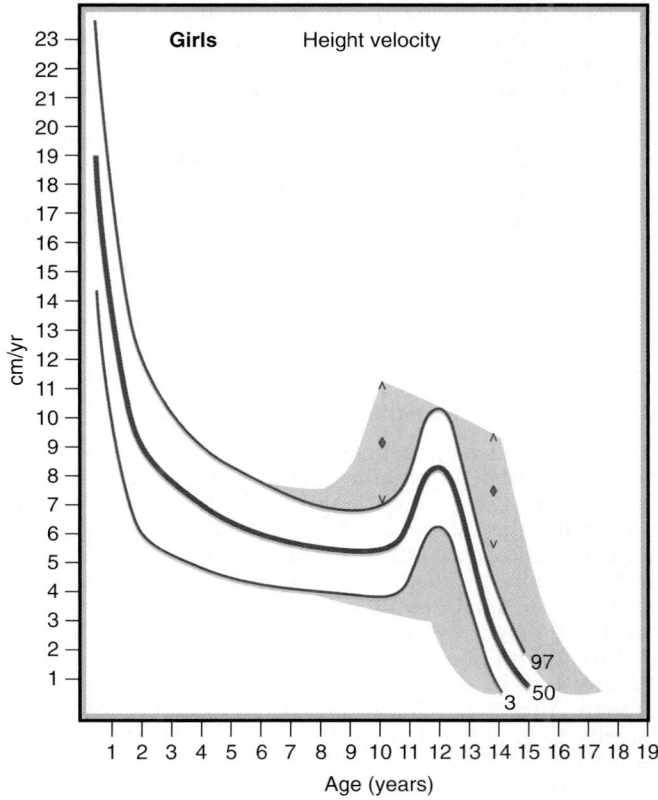

Figure 24-10 Height velocity chart for girls constructed from longitudinal observations of British children. The 97th, 50th, and 3rd percentile curves define the general pattern of growth during puberty. Shaded areas indicate velocities in those children with peak velocities occurring up to 2 standard deviations before or after the average age depicted by the percentile lines. (*Up arrows, diamonds,* and *down arrows* mark, respectively, the 97th, 50th, and 3rd percentiles of peak velocity when the peak occurs at these early or late limits.) (Modified and reproduced with permission of J.M. Tanner and Castlemead Publications, Ward's Publishing Services, Herts, UK.)

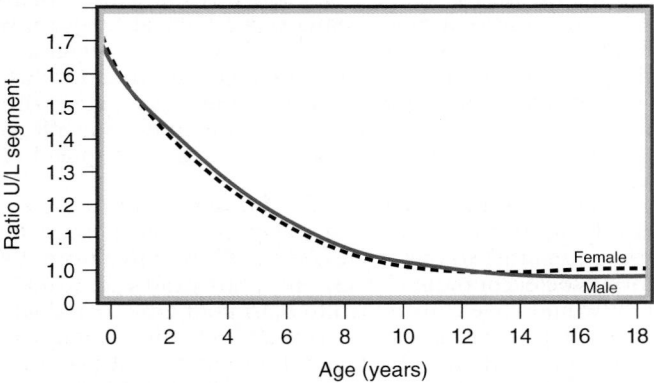

Figure 24-11 Upper/lower segment ratio from birth to 18 years of age. (Data from Wilkins L. *The diagnosis and treatment of endocrine disorders in childhood and adolescence.* Springfield, IL: Charles C. Thomas, 1957.)

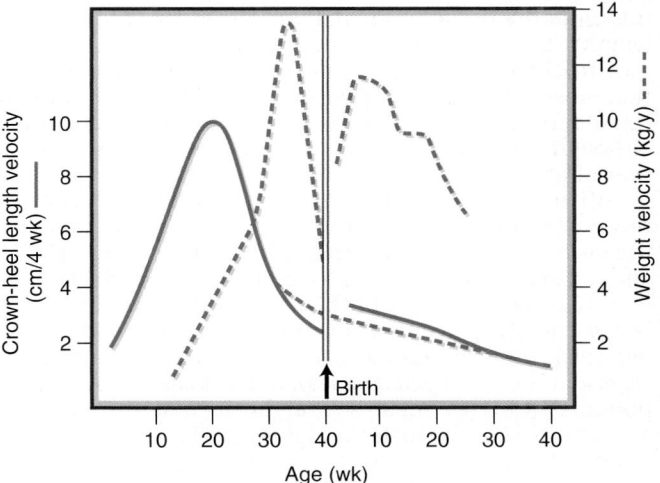

Figure 24-12 Rate of linear growth and weight gain in utero and during first 40 weeks after birth. Length velocity is expressed in centimeters per week. The solid line depicts the actual linear growth rate; the dashed line connecting the prenatal and postnatal length velocity lines depicts the theoretical curve for no uterine restriction late in gestation. The lighter dashed line depicts weight velocity. (From data in Tanner JM. *Fetus into Man.* Cambridge, MA: Harvard University Press; 1978.)

because the additional time for prepubertal growth that occurs when puberty is late is balanced by the fact that pubertal growth is smaller the later it occurs (see Figs. 24-9 and 24-10). After puberty, chondrocyte proliferation in the growth plate slows and senescence occurs due to depletion of stem-like cells in the resting zone of the growth plate.[28,29]

There are two variants of normal growth whose characteristic patterns are such that children exhibiting these growth variants are often evaluated for a growth disorder. These two variants are crossing linear percentiles of infancy and constitutional delay of growth and development (CDGD). In many cases, it is difficult to differentiate children with these normal growth variants from children with a growth disorder.

Crossing Linear Percentiles of Infancy

As in postnatal growth, genetic and environmental factors are important determinants of fetal growth and of the size of an infant (weight and length) at birth. However, there are significant differences between the factors affecting birth size and those affecting childhood growth and adult stature. There is much less correlation between length at birth and ultimate adult height than between length at birth and height in the later years of childhood.[30]

Parental stature affects birth length, as it does adult stature; this is an indicator of the genetic influence on growth. Although maternal and paternal stature contribute equally to childhood growth and adult stature, the effect of maternal stature may predominate over that of paternal stature on length at birth.[31,32] However, some studies have found equal effects of maternal and paternal stature on birth size.[33] Maternal nutrition and health have significant effects on fetal growth. Maternal weight has a positive effect, and smoking during pregnancy has a negative effect. Maternal diabetes has a strong positive effect on fetal growth. It is possible for the prenatal determinants of growth to result, for example, in a child who will ultimately grow to below-average stature but is above average size at birth. For this reason, it is common for infants' lengths to cross percentiles on the growth curve. Indeed, it is more common for the growth of an infant to cross percentiles than to follow a single percentile from birth into childhood: approximately one third of infants have lengths that cross percentiles moving upward on the growth curves, and approximately one third have lengths that cross percentiles moving downward.[32,34] Most normal infants crossing percentiles do so in the first 6 to 12 months, although some normal infants cross percentiles after 1 year of age.

Infants who are small at birth can be divided into (1) those who are small only because of prematurity and are therefore of a size appropriate for gestational age (AGA) and (2) those who are small for gestational age (SGA). SGA is usually defined as a birth weight or length (or both) below the 3rd percentile (or, sometimes, below the 10th percentile) for gestational age.[35] Some infants born SGA represent the small percentage of individuals whose genetic potential leads to small size at birth, and they can be expected to remain small throughout childhood and adulthood. However, many infants are SGA due to intrauterine growth retardation (IUGR) and have a genetic potential that would not be expected to result in small adult stature. Most infants who are born small, either AGA or SGA, have catch-up growth and achieve lengths greater than the 3rd percentile within the first 2 years of life. However, up to 10% of SGA infants do not show such catch-up growth.[36,37] The pathologic aspects of IUGR and of SGA in infants who do not have catch-up growth are discussed later.

Constitutional Delay of Growth and Development

CDGD is a normal variant of growth.[38] It describes the growth pattern of children who will experience a later than average timing of puberty. Their birth size is normal, and their final height is within their genetic potential. However, during most of their childhood, they grow at a height percentile below that expected based on their genetic potential. Typically, these children have a low growth velocity during the first years of life, crossing downward on the length percentile growth curves, so that by 2 years of age their heights are at or slightly below the 5th percentile. After age 3 years, their growth rate is typically normal, so that their height growth usually remains parallel to the 5th percentile until adolescence, although the height SDS may gradually drift slightly lower during the middle childhood years in some cases.[38,39] Their height diverges even further from that of average children during the early teen years due to the declining prepubertal growth velocity of these children compared with the accelerating growth rate of average children with onset of puberty.

Ultimately, children with CDGD have a late growth spurt, consistent with their late puberty, and this brings their height into the normal adult range. Final height is often in the lower part of the parental target height range, and few patients exceed the parental target height,[40-42] although this finding is probably, at least in part, the result of a selection bias of the children examined for such studies. However, there is evidence that a delayed growth spurt may adversely affect growth of the spine, resulting in a decrease in the final ratio of the upper to the lower segment and perhaps contributing to a limited final height.[43] Studies have also reported that prepubertal boys with CDGD have decreased bone mineral density (BMD),[44] although by young adulthood the majority of the BMD deficit is lost.[45,46]

Secular Changes in Height

There are surprisingly few data concerning the stature of modern humans before the measurement of military recruits became customary in the 18th century. Skeletal remains from the last ice age appear to indicate that adult stature 10,000 to 20,000 years ago was not substantially different from that of contemporary adults, although this record is obviously fragmentary.[47] It has been suggested that a reduction in stature was observed with the introduction of agriculture approximately 5000 years ago, with growth attenuation resulting from the combined effects of nutrient deficiency, population growth, and spread of infectious diseases.

Military recruits in the 18th and 19th centuries were clearly shorter than those of today, although it must be recognized that soldiers were commonly recruited from the lower socioeconomic classes, and poor health and nutrition would have contributed to both poor growth and late maturity.[48] Whereas men in the 20th century averaged 5 to 10 cm greater in height than those in the 18th century for whom we have records, much of this height gain has occurred over the past 100 years and probably reflects the dramatic improvement in overall nutrition and health seen in the Western world. This upward trend in height appears to have stopped in many developed countries in the early 21st century.[49]

Therefore, secular changes in height appear to reflect fundamental alterations in the standard of living rather than major genomic differences among populations; future economic advances in developing countries can be predicted to lead to improvement in adult stature and a reduction in international differences in growth.

ENDOCRINE REGULATION OF GROWTH

The Hypothalamic-Pituitary Axis: Embryogenesis and Anatomy

The pituitary gland is central to the regulation of mammalian growth. The pituitary gland develops from oral ectoderm in response to inductive signals from the neuroepithelium of the ventral diencephalon and intrinsic signaling gradients determining expression patterns of pituitary-specific transcription factors in the developing anterior pituitary gland.[50] The primordium of the anterior pituitary, Rathke's pouch, forms as an upward invagination of a single-cell-thick layer of ectoderm that contacts the neuroectoderm of the primordium of the ventral hypothalamus at embryonic day 8.5 (E8.5) in the mouse embryo[51] and can be identified by the third week of pregnancy in humans. The neurohypophysis (posterior pituitary) originates in the neural ectoderm of the floor of the forebrain, which also develops into the third ventricle. During anterior pituitary development, overlapping but regionally specific and temporally distinct patterns of homeobox transcription factor expression lead to the sequential appearance of the terminally differentiated cell types from E12.5 to birth.[51]

The initiation of anterior pituitary gland development depends on the competency of the oral ectoderm to respond to inducing factors from the neural epithelium of the ventral diencephalon.[52] The bone morphogenetic protein 4 (BMP4) signal from the ventral diencephalon is the critical dorsal neuroepithelial signal required for organ commitment of the anterior pituitary gland. Wnt5a and fibroblast growth factor 8 (FGF8) are also expressed in the diencephalon in distinct overlapping patterns with BMP4. Subsequently, a BMP2 signal arises from the boundary of a region of oral ectoderm in which Sonic hedgehog (SHH) expression, initially expressed uniformly in the oral ectoderm, is selectively excluded from the developing Rathke's pouch. The ventral-dorsal BMP2 signal and the dorsal-ventral FGF8 signal appear to create opposing activity gradients that are suggested to dictate overlapping patterns of specific transcription factors underlying cell lineage specification. The various extensions of these transcription factors in their fields are theorized to combinatorially determine the specific cell types. The FGF8 gradient determines the dorsal cell phenotypes,[52,53] and dorsally expressed transcription factors include Nkx-3.1, Six3, Pax6,[54] and prophet of PIT1 (PROP1).[55] Temporally specific attenuation of the BMP2 signal is required for terminal differentiation of the ventral cell types, and ventrally expressed transcription factors include islet-1 (Isl1), Brn4, P-Frk, and GATA2.[52,55,56] PIT1 (encoded by the gene POU1F1) is required for somatotroph, lactotroph, and thyrotroph development,[57,58] whereas the orphan nuclear receptor steroidogenic factor 1 (SF1) is selectively expressed in the gonadotrophs.[59,60]

The ventral-dorsal gradient induces GATA2 in a corresponding gradient in presumptive gonadotrophs and thyrotrophs, and high levels of GATA2 in the most ventral aspect of the developing anterior pituitary directly or indirectly restrict expression of POU1F1 out of the presumptive gonadotrophs. In the absence of PIT1, GATA2 expression appears sufficient to induce the entire set of transcription factors that are typical of the gonadotroph cell type, including SF-1, P-Frk, and Isl-1. Conversely, the absence of GATA2 dorsally is critical for differentiation of PIT1-positive cells to somatotroph/lactotroph fates. It is hypothesized that the level of GATA2 expression in the

thyrotrophs is below the threshold required to inhibit activation of the POU1F1 gene early enhancer, permitting the emergence of a PIT1+, GATA2+ cell that results in the thyrotroph fate.[56] Pax6 has a role in the sharp boundary of attenuation of the ventral signals that dictate thyrotroph and gonadotroph cell lineages. In the absence of Pax6, the ventral lineages, particularly thyrotrophs, become dorsally extended at the expense of somatotroph and lactotroph cell types,[54] and Pax6 mutant mice are GH and PRL deficient.[61]

The earliest marker of the anterior pituitary is expression of the glycoprotein α-subunit (αGSU), which appears at E11.5 in the mouse. These αGSU-positive cells also express the transcription factor Isl1 and mark a population of differentiating thyrotrophs that disappears after birth.[53,57,62,63] αGSU is expressed in mature thyrotrophs and gonadotrophs. At E12.5, corticotrophs start to differentiate and produce pro-opiomelanocortin (POMC).[53,63] Intensified cell proliferation within Rathke's pouch results in formation of a visible nascent anterior pituitary lobe on E12.5.[51] Definitive thyrotrophs are observed at 14.5 dpc (days post coitum), characterized by the expression of Tshb at E14.5 and followed by the expression of GH and prolactin (PRL) in somatotrophs and lactotrophs, respectively, at E15.5. The gonadotrophs are the last cell type to develop, at E16.5, marked by expression of luteinizing hormone (LH) and later by follicle-stimulating hormone (FSH). Eventually, the mature gland is populated by at least five highly differentiated cell types; ventrally to dorsally, they are the gonadotrophs, thyrotrophs, somatotrophs, lactotrophs, and corticotrophs.[52] Ultimately, some of these same transcription factors are also involved in the cell-specific expression and regulation of the gene products of these pituitary cell types, with corticotrophs producing adrenocorticotropin (ACTH), thyrotrophs producing thyrotropin (thyroid-stimulating hormone, TSH), gonadotrophs producing gonadotropins (LH and FSH), somatotrophs producing GH, and lactotrophs producing PRL. The developmental factors that play an in vivo role in pituitary gland development and differentiation are shown in Figure 24-13.

In humans, GH-producing cells can be found in the anterior pituitary gland by 9 weeks of gestation,[64] and vascular connections between the anterior lobe of the pituitary and the hypothalamus develop at about the same time,[65] although hormone production can occur in the pituitary in the absence of connections with the hypothalamus. Somatotrophs can be demonstrated in the pituitary in anencephalic newborns.[66]

In the newborn, the pituitary weighs about 100 mg. In the adult, the mean weight is about 600 mg, with a range of 400 to 900 mg; the pituitary is slightly heavier in women than in men and increases during pregnancy.[67] The mean adult pituitary size is 13 × 9 × 6 mm.[68] The anterior pituitary normally constitutes 80% of the weight of the pituitary. The pituitary resides in the sella turcica, immediately above and partially surrounded by the sphenoid bone. The volume of the sella turcica is a good index of pituitary size and may be reduced in the child with pituitary hypoplasia. The optic chiasm is located superior to the pituitary gland, so suprasellar growth of a pituitary tumor may initially manifest with visual complaints or evidence of decreases in peripheral vision. Furthermore, development of the neurohypophysis and the pituitary are intimately related, leading to potential anatomic associations of central nervous system (CNS) abnormalities with pituitary hypoplasia. For example, septo-optic dysplasia is associated with several CNS anatomic abnormalities and pituitary hormone deficiencies. For this reason, children with

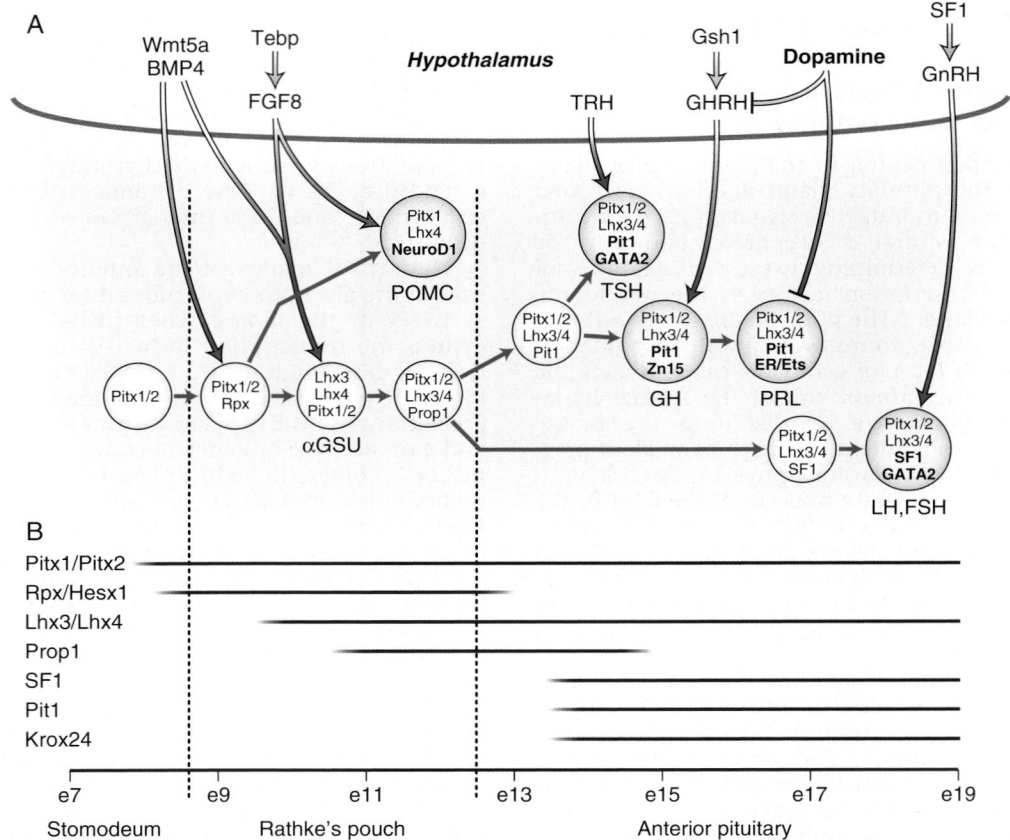

Figure 24-13 Development of pituitary cell lineages. **A,** Schematic representation of pituitary cell precursors shows the expression of prevalent transcription factors at each stage of development. Terminally differentiated cells are shown as larger and shaded circles together with the hormones produced (lineage-specific transcription factors are highlighted in bold in these cells). The interaction with transcription factors and signaling molecules in the hypothalamus is also depicted. Transcription factors are represented in lowercase (except for SF1 and GATA2), whereas signaling molecules appear in uppercase. **B,** The timing of appearance and disappearance of pituitary transcription factors during mouse embryogenesis. BMP4, bone morphogenic protein 4; e, embryonic day; ER, estrogen receptor; FGF8, fibroblast growth factor 8; FSH, follicle-stimulating hormone; GHRH, growth hormone–releasing hormone; GnRH, gonadotropin-releasing hormone; αGSU, glycoprotein α-subunit; LH, luteinizing hormone; POMC, pro-opiomelanocortin; PRL, prolactin; SF1, steroidogenic factor 1; TRH, thyrotropin-releasing hormone; TSH, thyroid-stimulating hormone (thyrotropin); Wmt5a, wingless type MMTV integration site family, member 5A; Hesx1, homeobox expressed in ES1 cells (Rathke's pouch homeobox, Rpx). (Reprinted with permission from Lopez-Bermejo A, Buckway CK, Rosenfeld RG. Genetic defects of the growth hormone-insulin-like growth factor axis. *Trends Endocrinol.* 2000;11:43.)

congenital blindness or nystagmus should be monitored for hypopituitarism.

The anterior pituitary receives controlling signals from the hypothalamus through the portal circulatory system (Fig. 24-14).[65] The hypothalamus integrates signals from other brain regions and the environment, resulting in the release of factors that control pituitary hormone synthesis and secretion. Hypothalamic neurons that synthesize peptides terminate in the infundibulum, enter the primary plexus of the hypophyseal portal circulation, and are transported via the hypophyseal portal veins to the capillaries of the anterior pituitary. This portal system in the pituitary stalk provides a means of communication between the neurons of the hypothalamus and the anterior pituitary. Magnetic resonance imaging (MRI) of the pituitary stalk conveys important anatomic information in patients with hypopituitarism.

Growth Hormone

Human GH is produced as a single-chain, 191–amino acid, 22-kDa protein containing two intramolecular disulfide bonds (Fig. 24-15). GH shares sequence homology with PRL, chorionic somatomammotropin (CS, placental lactogen), and a 22-kDa GH variant (GH-V) that is secreted only

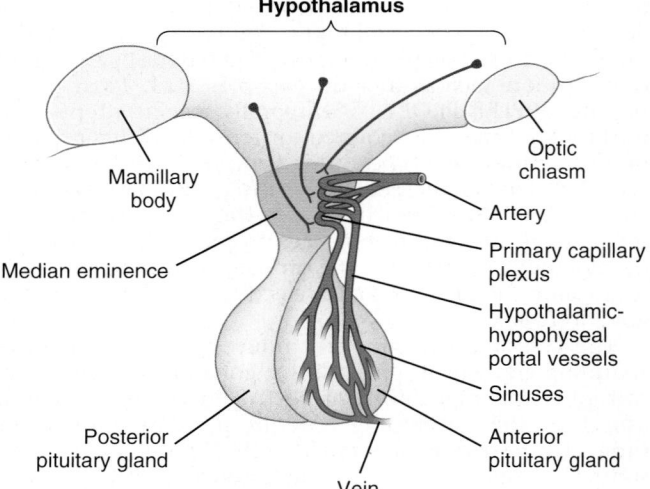

Figure 24-14 The main components of the hypothalamic-pituitary portal system. (From Guyton AC, Hall JC. *Human Physiology and Mechanisms of Disease*, 6th ed. Philadelphia, PA: WB Saunders; 1997:600, used with permission.)

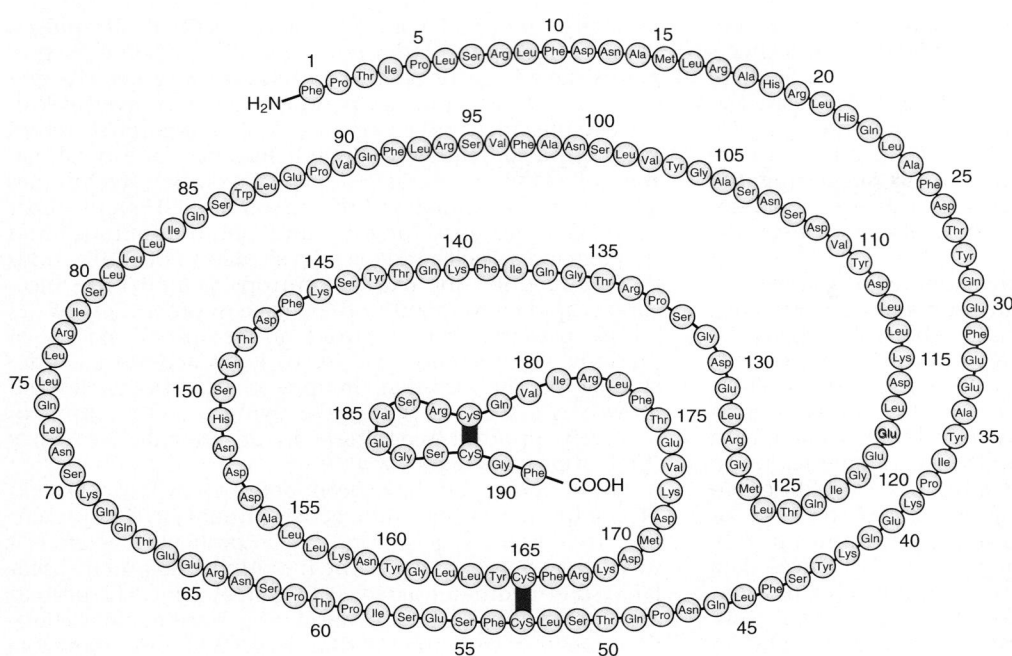

Figure 24-15 Covalent structure of human growth hormone. (From Chawla RK, Parks JS, Rudman D. Structural variants of human growth hormone: biochemical, genetic and clinical aspects. *Annu Rev Med.* 1983;34:519-547.)

by the placenta and differs from pituitary GH by 13 amino acids. The genes encoding these proteins most likely evolved from a common ancestral gene, despite being located on different chromosomes (chromosome 6 for PRL and chromosome 17 for GH).[69] The genes for GH, PRL, and placental lactogen share a common structural organization, with four introns separating five exons. The GH subfamily contains five members, with genes located on a 78-kilobase (kb) section of chromosome 17; the 5′ to 3′ order of the genes is GH, a CS pseudogene, CS-A, GH-V, and CS-B. Normally, about 75% of GH produced by the pituitary is of the mature, 22-kDa form. Alternative splicing of the second codon results in deletion of amino acids 32 through 46, yielding a 20-kDa form that normally accounts for 5% to 10% of pituitary GH.[69] The remainder of pituitary GH includes desamidated and *N*-acetylated forms and various GH oligomers.

The pulsatile pattern characteristic of GH secretion reflects the interplay of two hypothalamic regulatory peptides, growth hormone–releasing hormone (GHRH) and somatostatin (also called somatotropin release–inhibiting factor, or SRIF), with modulation by other putative GH-releasing factors.[70,71] GHRH is secreted from nerve cells within the hypothalamus and binds to receptors in the anterior pituitary to stimulate somatotroph cell proliferation, differentiation, and growth[72,73] and to stimulate the secretion and synthesis of GH.[74,75] Regulation of GH production by GHRH is mediated largely at the level of transcription and is enhanced by increases in intracellular cyclic adenosine monophosphate (cAMP) levels. The GHRH receptor is a member of the G protein–coupled receptor family B-III.[76] In a dwarf transgenic mouse model with diminished GHRH production, pituitary somatotroph proliferation is markedly decreased.[77,78] Transgenic mice that overexpress GHRH grow at a faster rate than control mice.[79]

Somatostatin appears to have its major effect on the timing and amplitude of pulsatile GH secretion and lesser effects on the regulation of GH synthesis. The pulsatile secretion of GH in vivo is believed to result from a simultaneous reduction in hypothalamic somatostatin release and increased GHRH release.[80] Conversely, a trough of GH secretion occurs when somatostatin is released in the face of diminished GHRH activity. The coordinated secretion of GH pulses in response to GH secretagogues results from a continuum of GH cells geographically connected by adherens junctions as revealed by three-dimensional reconstructive microscopy.[81]

Regulation of the reciprocal secretion of GHRH and somatostatin is imperfectly understood. The hypothalamus integrates signals for stress, sleep, hemorrhage, fasting, hypoglycemia, and exercise through the secretion of multiple neurotransmitters and neuropeptides to regulate the release of these hypothalamic factors and ultimately to influence GH secretion. This physiologic phenomenon forms the basis for a number of GH-stimulatory tests employed in the evaluation of GH secretory capacity or reserve. GH secretion is also influenced by a variety of nonpeptide hormones, including androgens,[82] estrogens,[83] thyroxine,[84] and glucocorticoids.[85,86] The mechanisms by which these hormones regulate GH secretion may involve actions at the hypothalamus and the pituitary. For example, hypothyroidism and glucocorticoid excess may each blunt spontaneous and provocative GH secretion. Gonadal steroids appear to be responsible for the rise in GH secretion that characterizes puberty.

Synthetic hexapeptides capable of stimulating GH secretion are termed GH secretagogues.[76] These peptides stimulate GH release and enhance the GH response to GHRH, although they work at receptors distinct from those for GHRH, at hypothalamic and pituitary sites. Kojima and colleagues[87] identified a natural ligand called *ghrelin*, a 28–amino acid protein with the serine 3 residue *n*-octanoylated. It is produced mainly by the oxyntic cells of the stomach (and throughout the gastrointestinal tract[88]) and in the hypothalamus, heart, lung, and adipose tissue. Ghrelin has a potent, dose-related, GH-releasing effect[89] and potentiates the GHRH-dependent secretion of GH. GH release results from the binding of ghrelin to the growth hormone secretagogue 1a receptor (GHSR-1a) on somatotrophs in the pituitary[89] and on GHRH-containing neurons in the hypothalamus.[90] Many studies have demonstrated that ghrelin has a wide range of effects, including immune function, cognition, gonadal axis regulation, bone metabolism, gastrointestinal motility, cell proliferation, and effects on the cardiovascular system.[91] However, it is difficult to separate the direct effects of ghrelin from those related to GH secretion. Although ghrelin has documented physiologic effects in vivo, GHSR-1a knockout mice have a phenotype similar to that of wild-type animals, suggesting that ghrelin does not have a role in growth. However, compensatory mechanisms may provide an explanation for these findings.[92,93]

More recently, studies have documented a positive correlation between ghrelin and anthropometric parameters in the first months of life, a finding that strengthens the hypothesis that ghrelin exerts an influence on growth.[94] Two reports of mutations in GHSR-1a in familial short stature provide evidence to the contrary.[95,96] Further studies indicate that the aging process may be associated with decreased expression of GHSRs in the hypothalamus [97] and with systemic concentration of ghrelin.[98] In addition to direct effects on linear growth, ghrelin has been shown to increase energy stores by stimulating appetite and affecting peripheral glucose and lipid metabolism.[99-101] These data suggest that ghrelin is an important stimulus for nutrient allocation for growth and metabolism and a central component of the GH regulatory system. Orally active ghrelin analogues have been considered as therapeutic agents in the treatment of GH deficiency (GHD), because they may provide a more physiologic approach to increasing the pulsatile release of endogenous GH compared with a single daily dose of recombinant human GH. However, there has been no definite evidence of the therapeutic efficacy of ghrelin analogues in the treatment of GHD states.

Pituitary adenylate cyclase–activating polypeptide (PACAP) is a hypothalamic peptide that has been shown to be effective in releasing GH from cultured pituitary cells. It belongs to a superfamily of hormones that includes glucagon, secretin, glucagon-like peptide 1 (GLP1), GLP2, GHRH, vasoactive intestinal polypeptide (VIP), peptide histidine methionine (PHM), and glucose-dependent insulinotropic polypeptide (GIP). Gene knockout of the specific PACAP receptor (PAC1R) resulted in a 60% mortality rate in the PAC1R null mice in the first 4 weeks after birth, providing insight into the importance of PACAP even though other superfamily members may compensate some of its functions.[102] The surviving knockout mice showed reduced glucose-stimulated insulin release and glucose intolerance. This observation suggests that PACAP is important in carbohydrate metabolism, potentially through GH.

The synthesis and secretion of GH are also regulated by the insulin-like growth factor (IGF) peptides. Receptors specific for IGF-1 and IGF-2 have been identified in the hypothalamus and pituitary.[103] Inhibition of GH secretion by IGF-1 or IGF-2 or both has been demonstrated,[104,105] and spontaneous GH secretion is diminished in humans treated with synthetic IGF-1.[106]

Growth Hormone Secretion in Humans

The episodic release of GH from the pituitary somatotrophs results in intermittent increases in serum levels of GH separated by periods of low or undetectable levels, during which time GH secretion is minimal.[80,107] The pulsatile nature of GH secretion has been demonstrated by frequent serum sampling coupled with the use of sensitive immunofluorometric or chemoluminescent assays of GH.[107] Under normal circumstances, serum GH levels are less than 0.04 mg/L between secretory bursts. It is impractical to assess GH secretion by random serum sampling. Extensive sampling studies at different ages in normal persons and

in many abnormal conditions have defined GH pulses, basal secretion, and diurnal variability. Computer programs have been developed to indicate whether changes in GH levels in various life periods and under diverse clinical circumstances occur because of a change of secretory mass or pulse frequency, altered clearance, or a combination of these processes.[107,108] Deconvolution techniques allow accurate estimates of the quantity of GH secreted per burst, GH clearance kinetics, and pulse amplitudes and frequencies, as well as an overall calculation of endogenous GH production. Approximate entropy, a model-free measure, is applied to quantify the degree of orderliness of GH release patterns.[109] The impact of the specific nature of pulsatile GH secretion on its biologic actions is under study.[107,108] For example, it appears that better statural growth is associated with large swings of GH output of relatively uniform magnitude in an irregular sequence (high approximate entropy).[110,111]

GH-secreting cells have been identified by 9 to 12 weeks of gestation, and immunoreactive pituitary GH is present by 7 to 9 weeks of gestation.[112] Fetal pituicytes secrete GH in vitro by 5 weeks, before the hypothalamic-portal vascular system is differentiated. PIT1 mRNA and PIT1 protein are expressed by at least 6 weeks of gestation; their abundant presence early in gestation suggests an important role in cytodifferentiation and cell proliferation.[113] GH can be identified in fetal serum by the end of the first trimester, with peak levels of approximately 150 mg/L in midgestation.[112] Serum levels fall throughout the latter part of pregnancy and are lower in full-term than in premature infants, perhaps reflecting feedback by the higher serum levels of IGF peptides that characterize the later stages of gestation.[114]

Mean levels of GH decrease from values of 25 to 35 mg/L in the neonatal period to approximately 5 to 7 mg/L through childhood and early puberty.[115] Twenty-four-hour GH secretion peaks during adolescence, undoubtedly contributing to the high serum levels of IGF-1 that are characteristic of puberty. The increase in GH production during middle to late puberty is caused by enhanced pulse amplitude and increased mass of GH per secretory burst, rather than by a change in pulse frequency (Figs. 24-16 and

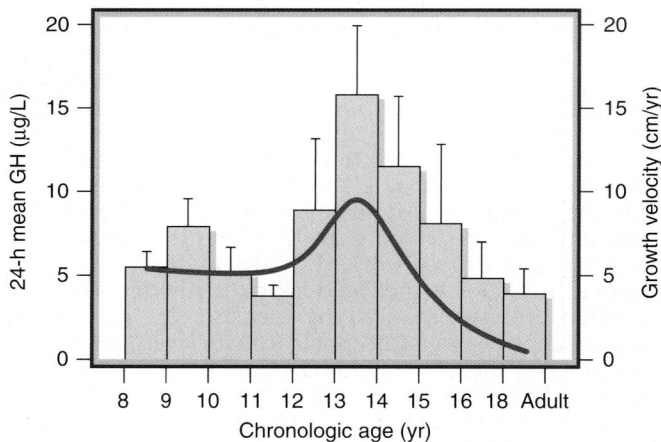

Figure 24-16 Relation between 24-hour mean growth hormone (GH) levels and age in boys and men. The bars represent the 24-hour mean and standard error (+SE) values of GH *(left axis)* obtained from 60 24-hour GH profiles of healthy boys and men subdivided according to chronologic age. An idealized growth velocity curve reproduced from the 50th percentile values for whole-year height velocity of North American boys[15] is superimposed. (From Martha PM Jr, Rogol AD, Veldhuis JD, et al. Alterations in the pulsatile properties of circulating growth hormone concentrations during puberty in boys. *J Clin Endocrinol Metab.* 1989;69:563-570.)

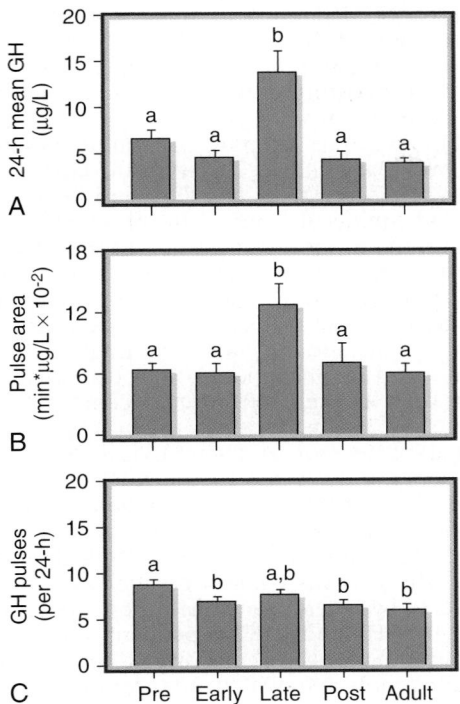

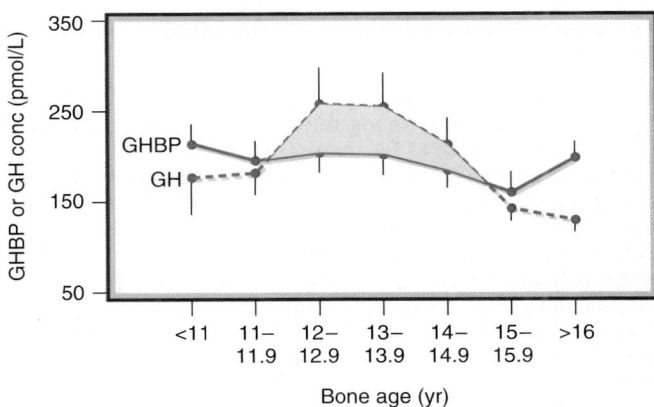

Figure 24-18 Levels of growth hormone (GH) and growth hormone–binding protein (GHBP) measured in normal pubertal boys throughout adolescence. The GHBP levels do not significantly change during puberty, but there is a significant increment of GH production and, therefore, of GH levels during this same time. These data suggest that there may be greater amounts of "free GH" during this period, leading to greater production of insulin-like growth factor 1. (Based on data from Martha and associates, in references 147 and 1021.)

Figure 24-17 A, The 24-hour and standard error (+SE) levels of growth hormone (GH) for groups of normal boys at varied stages of pubertal maturation. **B,** The mean (+SE) area under the GH concentration-versus-time curve for individual GH pulses, as identified by the cluster pulse detection algorithm. **C,** The number of GH pulses (+SE), as detected by the cluster algorithm, in the 24-hour GH concentration profiles for boys in each of the pubertal study groups. Notice that the mean 24-hour GH concentration changes are largely mediated by changes in the amount of GH secreted per pulse, rather than the frequency of pulses. In each panel, bars bearing the same letter are statistically indistinguishable. (From Martha PM Jr, Rogol AD, Veldhuis JD, et al. Alterations in the pulsatile properties of circulating growth hormone concentrations during puberty in boys. *J Clin Endocrinol Metab.* 1989;69:563-570.)

24-17).[108,109,115] Greater irregularity in GH secretion corresponds to greater linear growth.[116] In the face of stable levels of the growth hormone–binding protein (GHBP),[117] the enhanced pubertal GH production appears to be associated with higher levels of "free" GH (Fig. 24-18), potentially facilitating the delivery of IGF-1 to target tissues. This enhanced activity of the GH-IGF axis contributes to the insulin resistance that occurs during puberty.[118] Production of GH and IGF begins to decline by late adolescence and continues to fall throughout adult life. Normal young adult men experience 6 to 10 GH secretory bursts per 24 hours, a value similar to that observed in younger children and adolescents.[107,115] On the other hand, 24-hour GH production rates for normal men range from 0.25 to 0.52 mg/m^2 surface area,[86] about 20% to 30% of pubertal levels; this is largely due to decreased GH pulse amplitude with age.[115] Indeed, puberty may be considered, with some justification, a period of "physiologic acromegaly," whereas aging, with its decrease in GH secretion, has been termed *the somatopause*.[83,119]

Physiologic states that affect GH secretion, in addition to maturation and aging, include sleep,[120] nutritional status,[70,121] fasting, exercise,[122] stress,[122] and gonadal steroids. Maximal GH secretion occurs during the night, especially at the onset of the first slow-wave sleep period (stages III and IV). Rapid eye movement (REM) sleep, on the other hand, is associated with low GH secretion.[120] A circadian rhythm of somatostatin secretion, upon

which is superimposed episodic bursts of GHRH release, may help explain the nocturnal augmentation of GH production.[123]

When testosterone was administered to boys with delayed puberty, spontaneous GH release was enhanced, but such a change was not duplicated by administration of nonaromatizable androgens, emphasizing the possible unique importance of estrogen in GH secretion.[124] The effects of testosterone on serum IGF-1 levels may in part be independent of GH, because individuals with mutations of the GH receptor (GHR) still experience a modest rise in serum IGF-1 during puberty.[125] With a combination of deconvolution analysis, approximate entropy, and cosine regression analysis, Veldhuis and associates[109,124] carefully evaluated intensive GH sampling data derived from measurements in sensitive GH assays in prepubertal and pubertal children of both genders. In addition to the amplified secretory burst mass caused by jointly increased GH pulse amplitude and duration, they found that sex steroids selectively affect facets of GH neurosecretory control: estrogen increases the basal GH secretion rate and the irregularity of GH release patterns, whereas testosterone stimulates greater GH secretory burst mass and greater IGF-1 concentrations.

Obesity is characterized by lowered GH production, reflected by a diminished number of GH secretory bursts and shorter half-life duration.[126,127] Obesity in childhood and adolescence is characterized by decreased GH production with normal IGF and increased GHBP levels and often by increased linear growth.[127] The hyperinsulinism associated with obesity causes lowered levels of IGF-binding protein 1 (IGFBP-1) and, perhaps, higher levels of "free" IGF-1.[128] Endogenous GH secretion and levels achieved during provocative tests in obese subjects[129] approximated the diagnostic range of GHD. Fasting increased both the number and the amplitude of GH secretory bursts, presumably reflecting decreased somatostatin secretion and enhanced GHRH release, while lowering GHBP concentrations. Rapid changes in levels of IGFBPs in response to altered nutrition and changes in insulin levels may modify the effect of IGF-1 on its negative feedback and effector sites.[121,127] Body mass also influences GH production in normal prepubertal and pubertal children and adults.[130-132]

The Growth Hormone Receptor and Growth Hormone Binding Protein

The gene for the human GHR is located on chromosome 5p13.1-p12, where it spans more than 87 kb.[133] The GHR gene *(GHR)* contains 10 exons: exon 1 contains the 5′ untranslated region, whereas exons 2 through 10 encode the three domains of the GHR—the extracellular ligand-binding domain, a single transmembrane domain, and a cytoplasmic domain for signal transduction.[134] The highest level of *GHR* expression is in the liver, followed by muscle, fat, kidney, and heart. Although ubiquitously expressed transcription factors have been found to bind the *GHR* promoter, little is known about how these transcription factors coordinate regulation of *GHR* expression. The receptor is 620 amino acids long, with a predicted molecular weight of 70 kDa before glycosylation.

Two isoforms of the *GHR* have been found in humans—a full-length form and a form that has a deletion of exon 3 *(GHRd3)* with a loss of a 22–amino acid segment of the extracellular domain of the receptor.[135] The *GHRd3* allele is present in approximately 33% of the general population.[135] Several studies have investigated the clinical significance of the *GHRd3* allele on growth and GH responsiveness in specific disease states.

GH must bind to a homodimer complex of GHR to activate its intracellular signaling pathways (Fig. 24-19). Whether dimerization of the GHR subunits occurs before or after GH binding is a matter of debate. It was initially thought that dimerization would occur only after GH binding; GH would bind to the first subunit, after which the GH-GHR complex would diffuse within the membrane until contacted by a second subunit, leading to receptor activation.[136] However, it was shown in live cells that the subunits of the GHR are constitutively dimerized in an inactive (i.e., unbound) state.[137] The two subunits are joined by their transmembrane domains through leucine zipper interactions, with steric hindrance from extracellular domains preventing interactions between identical receptor partners. The GH binding sites on the extracellular domains of the two subunits are placed asymmetrically.

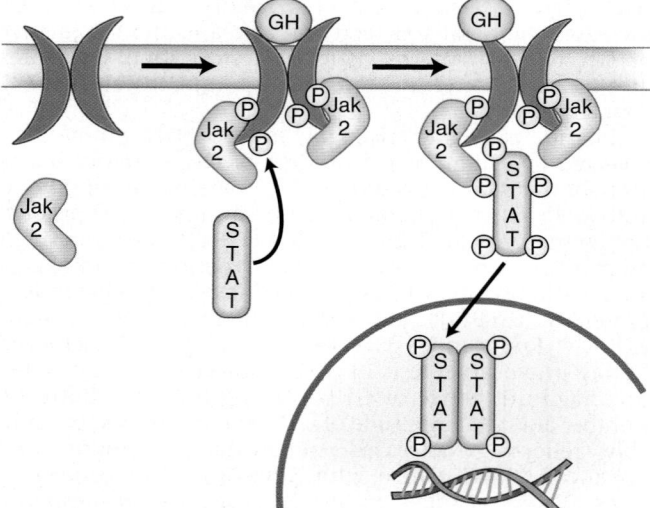

Figure 24-19 A model depicting intracellular signaling intermediates induced by binding of growth hormone (GH) with the GH receptor (GHR). Jak, Janus kinase; P, phosphorylation; STAT, signal transducer and activator of transcription. (From Le Roith DC, Bondy S, Yakar J-L, et al. The somatomedin hypothesis: 2001. *Endocrine Rev.* 2001;22:53-74.)

Therefore, once GH binds to the constitutive dimer, it induces rotation of the two subunits of the dimer that is transmitted via the transmembrane domain to the intracellular domain, allowing downstream kinase activation by transphosphorylation.

After binding to its receptor, GH stimulates phosphorylation of JAK2 (Janus kinase 2), a tyrosine kinase associated with the GHR (see Fig. 24-19). On recruitment or activation, the JAK2 molecule causes phosphorylation of critical tyrosines on the intracellular portion of the GHR, a sort of transphosphorylation. The phosphorylated tyrosines on the GHR provide docking sites for critical intermediary STAT proteins (signal transducers and activators of transcription).[136] STAT proteins dock, via their SRC homology 2 (SH2) domain to phosphotyrosines on ligand-activated receptors, such as the GHR. After docking, phosphorylation occurs on single tyrosines at the carboxy-terminus (C-terminal) of the protein. Then STATs dissociate from the GHR, dimerize, translocate to the nucleus, and bind to DNA through their DNA-binding domain to regulate gene transcription. There are seven known mammalian STATs; of these, STAT5B appears to be most critically involved in mediating the growth-promoting actions of the GHR, as was indicated by several gene disruption studies in rodent models.[138,139] GH- and JAK2-dependent phosphorylation and activation have been demonstrated for many cytoplasmic signaling molecules which, after forming homodimers or heterodimers, translocate into the nucleus, bind DNA, and activate transcription.[140]

It has been shown that GHR signaling can also lead to activation of extracellular-regulated kinase 1 (ERK1) and ERK2 to increase transcription.[141] How GHR activation leads to ERK1/2 activation is a matter of debate. A JAK2-independent but SRC-dependent phosphorylation has been modeled,[130] as has a JAK2-dependent but SRC-independent mechanism.[142] Experiments were conducted in different cell lines, so it is possible that the mechanisms of ERK1/2 activation by GHR are different in different cell lines. It is unclear what role these pathways play in the GH stimulation of growth.

Inhibition of GH signaling by several members of the GH-inducible suppressor of the cytokine signaling (SOCS) family has been reported.[143] The importance of SOCS proteins in controlling growth is demonstrated by the finding of gigantism in *Socs2* knockout mice,[144] an effect that appears to require the presence of GH and activation of STAT5B.[145]

GHBP prolongs the half-life of GH, presumably by impairing glomerular filtration, and modulates its binding to the GHR. It binds GH with high specificity and affinity but with low capacity; only about 45% of circulating GH is bound.[117] GHBP is derived from proteolytic cleavage of the extracellular domain of the receptor.[146] GHBP levels reflect GHR levels and activity; that is, low levels are associated with states of GH insensitivity.[117] Levels of GHBP are low early in life, rise through childhood, and plateau during the pubertal years and adulthood.[147,148] Levels are constant for an individual once puberty is reached and correlate inversely with 24-hour GH production.[147] Impaired nutrition, diabetes mellitus, hypothyroidism, chronic liver disease, and inherited abnormalities of the GHR are associated with low levels of GHBP, whereas obesity, refeeding, early pregnancy, and estrogen treatment are associated with elevated levels of GHBP.[117] In general, GHBP levels reflect GHR levels and activity. Patients with GH insensitivity due to defects of the extracellular domain of the GHR have low GHBP levels, and GHBP levels therefore can be useful in identifying these individuals. Patients with GH insensitivity due to nonreceptor abnormalities, defects of the intracellular domain of the GHR, or inability of the receptor to dimerize may have normal levels of GHBP.[125]

GHR signaling affects the transcription of many genes immediately (<3 hours after stimulation) and other genes over a longer period of stimulation. After acute GH stimulation in GH-deficient rats, hepatic genes immediately induced by GH included signal transducers (STAT3, gp130, p38), DNA repair proteins, receptor proteases, and metabolic regulators such as Igf1, Igfbp3, and Mct1.[149] Studies indicate that GHR signaling is involved in regulation of expression of genes involved in carbohydrate, fat, and steroid metabolism.[126,150,151]

The development of mice that lack *Ghr* or downstream components of GHR signaling has shed light on the role of GH in normal physiology. *Ghr*[−/−] mice exhibit normal size at birth but have attenuated postnatal growth, with body weight about half of normal and length about two thirds of normal.[152] *Ghr*[−/−] mice also exhibit delayed pubertal maturation, longer life span, and increased insulin sensitivity compared with a control group.

To determine which cytoplasmic regions of the GHR are involved in growth-promoting actions, mice with truncated *Ghr* were engineered via homologous recombination (so-called knock-in mice). One knock-in mouse had a mutation that resulted in removal of the C-terminal region of the receptor (mutant 569), including some recognized Stat5 and Socs2 recruitment sites; a second knock-in mouse had a mutation that resulted in truncation of the receptor downstream from the Jak2, mitogen-activated protein (MAP) kinase, and phosphatidylinositol 3 (PI3) kinase interaction sites, a region that included the majority of Stat5 recruitment sites (mutant 391).[150] Homozygous mutant 569 mice exhibited a body size 44% of that of wild-type mice on loss of 70% of Stat5 signaling and with IGF-1 levels 80% lower than in the wild-type mouse. As expected, homozygous mutant 391 mice had more severe growth attenuation, with a body size 11% of that of wild-type mice on complete loss of Stat5 signaling. The fact that these mice had some growth implicates other signaling pathways, such as MAP kinase, in growth-promoting roles.

Mice with *Ghr* deleted only in the liver were produced and were found to have low IGF-1 levels and high GH levels. These mice exhibited normal growth but had significantly lower bone density than controls. They also exhibited liver steatosis with insulin resistance and elevated serum free fatty acid levels.[153] This mouse model sheds light on the metabolic function of excessive GHR signaling independent of serum IGF-1 signaling.

Deletion of *Jak2* in mice is embryonically lethal,[154] as is deletion of *Stat3*. Deletion of *Stat1* or *Stat5a* does not affect body size. However, deletion of *Stat5b* leads to decreased size in male but not female mice. The *Stat5a/b*[−/−] mouse is smaller than the *Stat5b*[−/−] mouse.[155] Deletion of *Socs2*,[144] but not of other *Socs* genes,[145] produced gigantism in mice, indicating the specific role of *Socs2* in the negative regulation of GHR action. The combined *Igf1* and *Ghr*[−/−] mouse had a more severe attenuation of postnatal growth than mice with knockout of either gene alone, indicating that GH and IGF-1 promote growth by both common and independent functions.[156] The liver-specific IGF-1 knockout mouse with extremely low serum IGF-1 levels has normal linear growth, suggesting IGF-independent actions of GH or paracrine production and effects of IGF-1, or both.[157]

Historically, the anabolic actions of GH were thought to be mediated entirely by the IGF peptides (the so-called somatomedin hypothesis).[127] Although a majority of GH actions are mediated by IGFs, the opposite effects of GH and IGFs on metabolism and in knockout mouse models

suggest that there are IGF-independent actions of GH. Indeed, the "diabetogenic" actions of GH are contradictory to the glucose-lowering effects of IGFs. In vitro studies suggest potential IGF-independent action of GH in the following tissues:
1. Epiphysis—stimulation of epiphyseal growth
2. Bone—stimulation of osteoclast differentiation and activity, stimulation of osteoblast activity, and increase in bone mass through endochondral bone formation
3. Adipose tissue—acute insulin-like effects, followed by increased lipolysis, inhibition of lipoprotein lipase, stimulation of hormone-sensitive lipase, decreased glucose transport, and decreased lipogenesis[128]
4. Muscle—increased amino acid transport, increased nitrogen retention, increased lean tissue, and increased energy expenditure[129]

The concept of IGF-independent actions of GH is supported by results of in vivo studies in which IGF-1 could not duplicate all of the effects of GH, such as nitrogen retention and insulin resistance.[131]

Insulin-like Growth Factors
Historical Background

The IGFs (somatomedins) are a family of peptides that are, in part, GH dependent and mediate many of the anabolic and mitogenic actions of GH. They were originally identified in 1957 by their ability to stimulate [^{35}S]-sulfate incorporation into rat cartilage and were called *sulfation factors*.[127] In 1972, that term was replaced with *somatomedin*,[132] and purification of somatomedin from human serum yielded a basic peptide (somatomedin C) and a neutral peptide (somatomedin A).[158] In 1978, Rinderknecht and Humbel[159,160] isolated two active somatomedins from human plasma and, after demonstrating a striking structural resemblance to proinsulin, renamed them *insulin-like growth factors* (IGFs).

IGF Genes and Protein Structure

There are two IGFs circulating in humans, IGF-1 and IGF-2. IGF-1 is a basic peptide of 70 amino acids, and IGF-2 is a peptide of 67 amino acids. The two peptides share 45 of 73 possible amino acid positions and have 50% amino acid homology to insulin.[127,159,160] Like insulin, both IGFs have A and B chains connected by disulfide bonds. The connecting C-peptide region is 12 amino acids for IGF-1 and 8 amino acids for IGF-2, bearing no homology for the C-peptide region of proinsulin. The D-peptide region contains C-terminal extensions of 8 amino acids for IGF-1 and 6 amino acids for IGF-2. The E-peptide is a trailer peptide that is cleaved in post-translational processing. The structural similarity explains the ability of both IGFs to bind to the insulin receptor and the ability of insulin to bind to the type I IGF receptor (encoded by *IGF1R*). On the other hand, structural differences probably explain the failure of insulin to bind with high affinity to the IGFBPs.

Insulin-like Growth Factor 1

Gene Regulation. The human IGF-1 gene (*IGF1*) is located on the long arm of chromosome 12 and contains at least six exons (Fig. 24-20). Exons 1 and 2 encode alternative signal peptides, each containing several transcription start sites; that is, the multiple existing *IGF1* transcripts consist of either exon 1 or exon 2. Two different promoters regulated in a tissue-specific manner[161] control the use of exon 1 or 2. Exons 3 and 4 encode the remaining signal peptide, the remainder of the mature IGF-1 molecule, and part of the trailer peptide (E peptide). Exons 5 and 6 encode

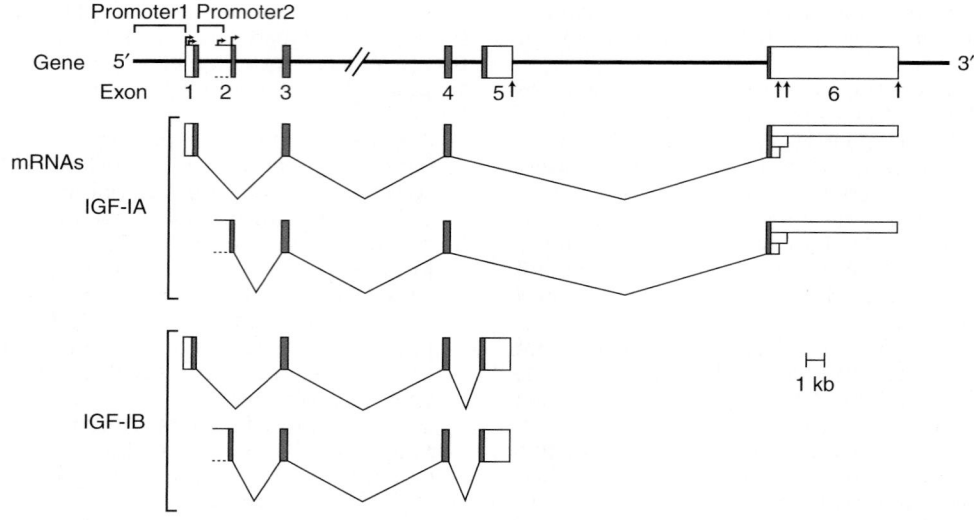

Figure 24-20 Structure and expression of the human insulin-like growth factor 1 (IGF-1) gene. The structure of the different human IGF-1 messenger RNAs (mRNAs) is displayed below the map of the gene. Sites of pre-mRNA processing are indicated by the thin lines. Sites of differential polyadenylation are marked at the 3′ end of the gene by vertical arrows and in the mRNAs by horizontal boxes of varying length. (From Rotwein P. Structure, evolution, expression and regulation of insulin-like growth factors I and II. *Growth Factors.* 1991;5:3-18.)

alternatively used segments of the trailer peptide and 3′ untranslated sequences with multiple different polyadenylation sites. As a result, multiple mRNA species exist, allowing for tissue-specific, developmental, and hormonal regulation of *IGF1* gene expression.

GH appears to be the primary regulator of *Igf1* transcription, which begins as early as 30 minutes after intraperitoneal injection of GH into hypophysectomized rats.[151] Transcriptional activation by GH results in a 20-fold rise in *Igf1* mRNA, but there may be tissue-to-tissue variability in extent of GH-induced expression of *Igf1* mRNA.[162,163] Another influential factor is estrogen, as its administration to a *Ghr*−/− mouse can stimulate hepatic *Igf1* synthesis and growth.[152] The sex-steroid effects on *IGF1* transcription play a role in the pubertal rise of IGF-1 levels in humans[164] (see later discussion).

The mechanisms involved in regulation of IGF gene expression include the existence of multiple promoters, heterogeneous transcription initiation within each of the promoters, alternative splicing of various exons, differential RNA polyadenylation, and variable mRNA stability. Translation of *IGF1* may also be under complex control. The transcription factor STAT5B is the most critical mediator of GH-induced activation of *IGF1* transcription, as detailed earlier. Two adjacent STAT5B binding sites have been identified in the second intron of the rat *Igf1* gene, within a region previously identified as undergoing acute changes in chromatin structure after GH treatment.[139]

Once translated, IGF-1 pre-propeptides require processing to form the mature IGF-1 peptide (Fig. 24-21). After processing, all transcript isoforms result in an identical 70–amino acid protein containing the A, B, C, and D domains. Pro-IGF-1 also contains the E peptide. Proteases from the subtilisin-related proprotein convertase family (SPC) cleave pro-IGF-1 at Arg71, located in the D portion of the peptide.[165] Pro-IGF-1 is secreted from fibroblasts and other cells,[166] although the biologic significance of the pro-IGF-1 peptide is unclear.

Serum Levels. In human fetal serum, IGF-1 levels are relatively low and are positively correlated with gestational age.[167] There is a reported correlation between fetal cord serum IGF-1 levels and birth weight,[168] but this relationship is controversial.[169] IGF-1 levels in newborn serum are

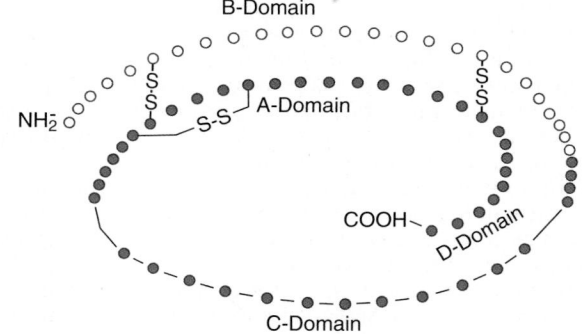

Figure 24-21 Structure of the insulin-like growth factor 1 (IGF-1) peptide. See discussion in text. (From Yakar S, Wu Y, Setser J, et al. The role of circulating IGF-1. *Endocrine.* 2002;19:239-248.)

typically 30% to 50% of adult levels. Serum levels rise during childhood. During puberty, IGF-1 levels rise to two to three times the adult range. Levels during adolescence correlate better with Tanner stage or bone age than with chronologic age.[170-172] The pubertal rise in gonadal steroids may stimulate IGF-1 production indirectly by contributing to a rise in GH secretion and directly by augmenting liver synthesis and secretion of IGF-1. Girls with gonadal dysgenesis show no adolescent increase in serum IGF-1, providing evidence of the association of the pubertal rise in IGF-1 with the production of gonadal steroids.[173] As further evidence, patients with GH insensitivity due to GHR mutations exhibit a modest rise in IGF-1 during puberty despite a decline in GH levels. After 20 to 30 years of age, serum IGF-1 levels gradually and progressively fall.[174] The age-associated decline in IGF-1 levels has been implicated in the negative nitrogen balance, decrease in muscle mass, and osteoporosis of aging.[174]

Insulin-like Growth Factor 2

Gene Regulation. The gene for IGF-2 (*IGF2*) is located on the short arm of chromosome 11, adjacent to the insulin gene, and contains 9 exons (Fig. 24-22). Exons 1 through 6 encode 5′ untranslated RNA, exon 7 encodes the signal

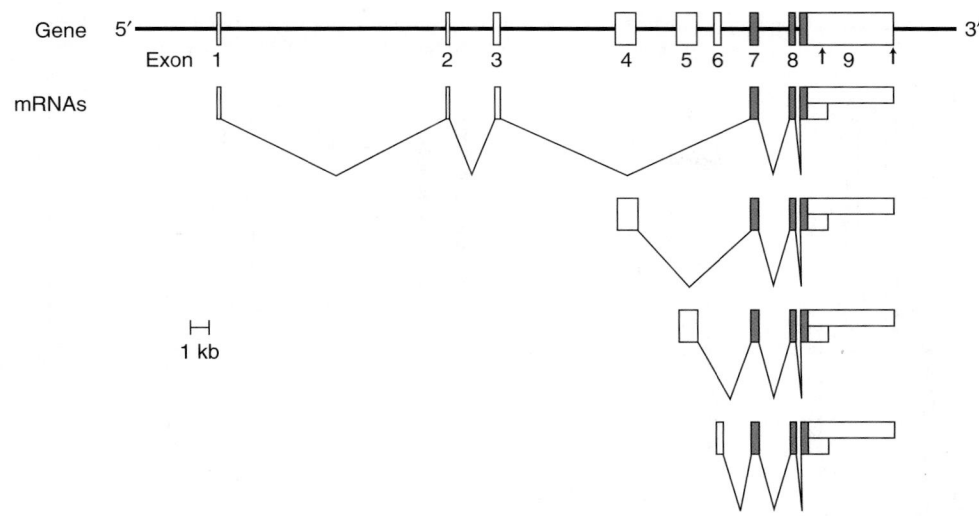

Figure 24-22 Structure and expression of the human insulin-like growth factor 2 (IGF-2) gene. The structure of different human IGF-2 messenger RNAs (mRNAs) is displayed below the map of the gene. The patterns of mRNA processing are indicated by the thin lines. Sites of differential polyadenylation are marked at the 3′ end of the gene by vertical arrows and in the mRNAs by horizontal boxes of varying length. (From Rotwein P. Structure, evolution, expression and regulation of insulin-like growth factors 1 and 2. *Growth Factors.* 1991;5:3-18.)

peptide and most of the mature protein, and exon 8 encodes the C-terminal portion of the protein. As with *IGF1*, multiple mRNA species exist to allow for developmental and hormonal regulation of expression. *IGF2* mRNA expression is high in fetal life and has been detected as early as the blastocyst stage in mice.[175] Fetal tissues generally have high *IGF2* mRNA levels that decline postnatally.

IGF2 is imprinted—that is, only one allele is active, depending on parental origin. In the case of *IGF2*, only the paternally expressed allele is active. Most imprinted genes occur in clusters with reciprocally imprinted genes, and *IGF2* is no exception. The noncoding gene *H19* is downstream from *IGF2* and is oppositely imprinted, meaning that only the maternal allele is expressed and the paternal allele is inactive. The promoters of *IGF2* and *H19* share a set of enhancers that act on either gene. On the paternal allele, the *H19* promoter region is methylated and thus inactivated (so-called epigenetic regulation of expression).[176] The *IGF2* promoter does not contain regions that can be methylated. Instead, upstream from the *H19* and *IGF2* promoter region is a so-called differentially methylated region (DMR). When it is methylated, binding of CCCTC binding factor (CTCF) is prevented, allowing enhancers to act on the *IGF2* promoter to activate transcription.[177] On the maternal chromosome, the DMR is not methylated, allowing CTCF to bind and preventing transcription (Fig. 24-23).[178]

The fact that *IGF2* is monoallelically expressed emphasizes the importance of gene dosage to normal physiology and development. Loss of imprinting of *IGF2* can lead to constitutively expressed *IGF2* mRNA and excessive IGF-2. *IGF2* mRNA is expressed constitutively in a number of mesenchymal and embryonic tumors, including Wilms tumor,[179] rhabdomyosarcoma, neuroblastoma, pheochromocytoma, hepatoblastoma, leiomyoma, leiomyosarcoma, liposarcoma, and colon carcinoma.[180] Loss of imprinting has been demonstrated as the cause for dysregulated expression in some of these tumors. Production of *IGF2* variants by these tumors can cause non–islet cell tumor hypoglycemia (NICTH).[181] Loss of imprinting of *IGF2* resulting in biallelic gene expression has also been found in Beckwith-Weidemann syndrome (BWS), which is characterized by fetal and neonatal overgrowth and an increased

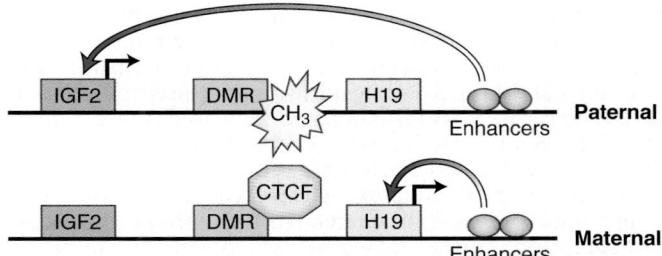

Figure 24-23 Schematic of the imprinted region of the insulin-like growth factor 2 *(IGF2)-H19* locus. CTCF, CCCTC binding factor; CH3, methylation; DMR, differentially methylated region. (Adapted from Chao W, D'Amore P. IGF2: epigenetic regulation and role in development and disease. *Cytokine Growth Factor Rev.* 2008;19: 111-120.)

risk of childhood cancers. Loss of imprinting in BWS can result from mutations that effect imprinting in the region of chromosome 11 that contains *IGF2*,[182] methylation defects that cause hypermethylation of the region or duplication of the expressed paternal allele resulting in increased *IGF2* expression, or paternal uniparental disomy (i.e., inheritance of only the expressing paternal allele).

Variant peptides of IGF-2 have been identified in normal human serum, the significance of which is uncertain. A variant peptide with the Ser29 replaced by Arg-Leu-Pro-Gly has also been identified in human plasma, presumably from the liver.[183] Other IGF-2 variants have been identified that are longer than the predominant IGF-2 species.[184] The significance of these larger forms of IGF-2 is uncertain. In general, these variants appear capable of binding to IGF and insulin receptors and to IGFBPs, and they can participate in formation of the 150-kDa IGF–IGFBP3–acid-labile subunit (ALS) ternary complex (discussed later). Large IGF-2 variants have been shown to be produced by mesenchymal tumors and cause NICTH. In a patient with leiomyosarcoma and recurrent hypoglycemia, 70% of serum IGF-2 consisted of the higher-molecular-weight forms.[181] Removal of the tumor decreased the fraction of the large IGF-2 forms and serum and corrected the hypoglycemia. It has been documented that the total serum IGF-2 in NICTH

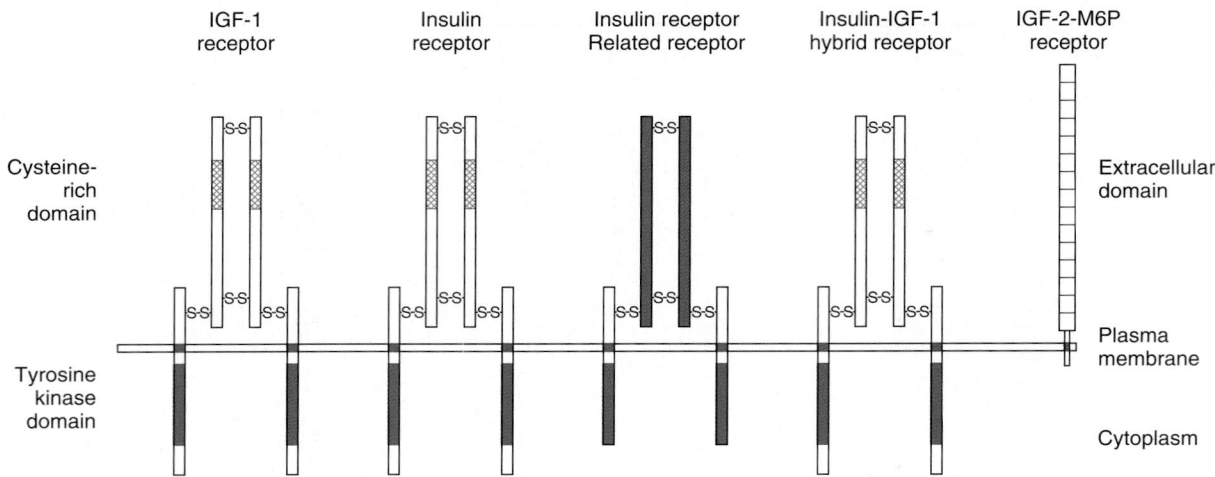

Figure 24-24 Structure of the insulin-like growth factor (IGF) receptors. The insulin receptor and the IGF type 2 receptor are both heterotetrameric complexes composed of extracellular α-subunits that bind the ligands and β-subunits that anchor the receptor in the membrane and contain tyrosine kinase activity in their cytoplasmic domains. The tyrosine kinase domain of the insulin receptor–related receptor (IRR) is homologous to the tyrosine kinase domains of the insulin and IGF-1 receptors. The carboxyl-terminal domain is deleted in the IRR. Hybrids consist of a hemireceptor from both insulin and IGF-1 receptors. The IGF type 2/mannose-6-phosphate (M6P) receptor is not structurally related to the IGF-1 and insulin receptors or to the IRR, having a short cytoplasmic tail and no tyrosine kinase activity. (From LeRoith D, Werner H, Geitner-Johnson D, et al. Molecular and cellular aspects of the insulin-like growth factor I receptor. *Endocr Rev.* 1995;16:143-163.)

is normal, yet the fraction of the larger forms is larger. Zapf[185] proposed that NICTH occurs when secretion of large IGF-2 forms results in suppression of GH, insulin, and the normal 7-kDa IGF-2, leading to decreased production of IGF-1, IGFBP3, and the ALS and increased production of IGFBP2. This produces a shift in the distribution of IGF-2 from the IGF-2–IGFBP ternary complex to the lower-molecular-weight complex. The result is increased bioavailability of IGF-2 to target tissues, enhanced glucose consumption, and decreased hepatic glucose production. **Serum Levels.** Human newborn levels of IGF-2 are typically 50% of adult levels. By 1 year of age, adult levels are attained, and there is little, if any, subsequent decline, even up to the seventh or eighth decade.[186]

Insulin-like Growth Factor Receptors

There are two types of IGF receptors, type I and type II (Fig. 24-24). Structural characterization of these receptors has provided documentation of the differences between these two forms.[187] The type I IGF receptor is closely related to the insulin receptor; both are heterotetramers comprising two membrane-spanning α-subunits and two intracellular β-subunits. The α-subunits contain the binding sites for IGF-1 and are linked by disulfide bonds. The β-subunits contain a transmembrane domain, an adenosine triphosphate (ATP)-binding site, and a tyrosine kinase domain, which constitute the presumed signal transduction mechanism for the receptor. One mole of the full heterotetrameric receptor appears to bind 1 mole of ligand.

Although the type I IGF receptor has been commonly termed the *IGF-1 receptor*, this receptor binds both IGF-1 and IGF-2 with high affinity, and both IGF peptides can activate tyrosine kinase by binding to the type I receptor. In studies involving transfection and overexpression of the type I IGF receptor complementary DNA (cDNA), the dissociation constant for IGF-1 is typically 0.2 to 1.0 nmol/L, whereas the affinity for IGF-2 is usually slightly less, although it varies from study to study.[188] The affinity of the type I IGF receptor for insulin is usually 100-fold less, explaining the relatively weak mitogenic effect of insulin.

The mature IGF receptor peptide has 1337 amino acids with a predicted molecular mass of 151,869 kDa (Fig.

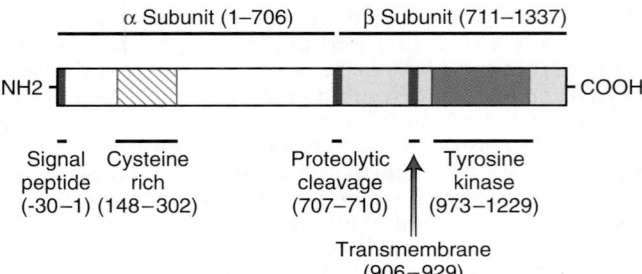

Figure 24-25 Structure of the human insulin-like growth factor type I receptor precursor. Molecular cloning of human IGF-1 receptor complementary DNAs isolated from a placental library revealed the presence of an open reading frame of 4101 nucleotides. The 1367–amino acid polypeptide contains, at its NH2-terminus, a 30–amino acid hydrophobic signal peptide that is responsible for the transfer of the nascent protein chain into the endoplasmic reticulum. After digestion by endopeptidases at a proteolytic cleavage site (Arg-Lys-Arg-Arg) located at residues 707 through 710, α- and β-subunits are released and linked by disulfide bonds to yield the configuration of the mature heterotetrameric receptor. Also shown are the cysteine-rich domain of the α-subunit and the transmembrane and tyrosine kinase domains of the β-subunit. (From LeRoith D, Werner H, Beitner-Johnson D, et al. Molecular and cellular aspects of the insulin-like growth factor I receptor. *Endocr Rev.* 1995;16:143-163.)

24-25). The translated αβ heterodimer is cleaved at an Arg-Lys-Arg-Arg sequence at positions 707 through 710. The released α- and β-subunits, linked by disulfide bonds, then form the mature $(\alpha\beta)_2$ receptor, in which two α chains are joined by secondary disulfide bonds. The α-subunits are extracellular and contain a cysteine-rich domain that is critical for IGF binding. The β-subunit has a short extracellular domain, a hydrophobic transmembrane domain, and the intracellular tyrosine kinase domain with the ATP-binding site.

The gene for the type I IGF receptor *(IGF1R)* spans more than 100 kb of genomic DNA, with 21 exons; the genomic organization resembles that of the insulin receptor gene.[189] Exons 1 through 3 encode for the 5′ untranslated region and the cysteine-rich domain of the α-subunit that is involved in ligand binding. The remainder of the α-subunit is encoded by exons 4 through 10. The peptide cleavage site involved in generation of the α- and β-subunits is

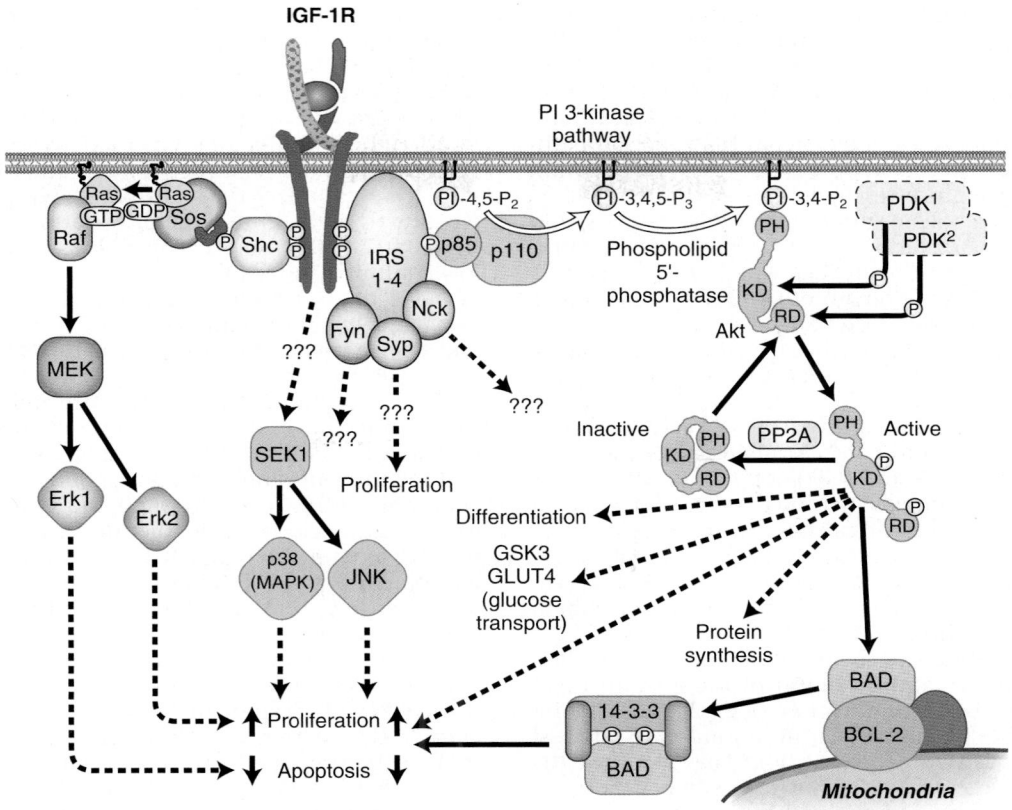

Figure 24-26 Schematic representation of intracellular signaling pathways of the insulin-like growth factor type 1 (IGF-1) receptor. On binding of IGF-1, the IGF receptor undergoes autophosphorylation at multiple tyrosine residues. The intrinsic kinase activity of the receptor also phosphorylates insulin receptor substrate 1 (IRS1) at multiple tyrosine residues. Various SH domain–containing proteins, including phosphatidylinositol 3 (PI 3) kinase, Syp, Fyn, and Nck associate with specific phosphotyrosine-containing motifs within IRS1. These docking proteins recruit diverse other intracellular substrates, which then activate a cascade of protein kinases including Raf-1 and one or more related kinases including mitogen-activated protein kinase (MAPK), mitogen and extracellular signal-related kinase (MEK), and others. These protein kinases, in turn, activate various other elements, including nuclear transcription factors. Alterations in expression of various IGF-1–responsive genes result in longer-term effects of IGF-1, including growth and differentiation. This model of signal transduction cascades also shows a potential mechanism for inhibition of apoptosis. BAD, BCL2-associated agonist of cell death; Erk, extracellular signal-regulated kinase; GDP, guanosine diphosphate; GLUT4, glucose transporter 4; GTP, guanosine triphosphate; JNK, c-Jun N-terminal kinase; KD, catalytic kinase domain of Akt; MEK, mitogen-activated protein kinase; P, phosphorylation; PH, pleckstrin homology domain of Akt; PP2A, protein phosphatase 2A; RD, regulatory C-terminal tail of Akt; SEK1, serum- and glucocorticoid-inducible protein kinase 1. (From Le Roith D, Bondy C, Yakar S, et al. The somatomedin hypothesis: 2001. *Endocr Rev.* 2001;22:53-74.)

encoded by exon 11, and the tyrosine kinase domain of the β-subunit is encoded by exons 16 through 20. It is in the latter region that *IGF1R* and the insulin receptor gene share the greatest sequence homology, ranging from 80% to 95%. Exon 21 encodes the 3′ untranslated sequences.

IGF1R mRNA has been identified in virtually every tissue except liver.[190] The mRNA is most abundant in embryonic tissues and appears to decrease with age. *IGF1R* expression is present at the embryonic 8-cell stage, whereas expression of the type II IGF receptor gene is first demonstrable at the 2-cell stage. *IGF1R* becomes widely expressed after implantation, consistent with the observation that this receptor is essential for normal fetal growth.

As with other growth factor receptor tyrosine kinases, binding of ligand (IGF-1 or IGF-2) induces receptor autophosphorylation of critical tyrosine residues in the type I IGF receptor.[149] Specifically, ligand binding to the α-subunits leads to activation of the tyrosine kinase domain of the β-subunits. Mutations of the ATP-binding site or of critical tyrosine residues (Tyr1131, Tyr1135, and Tyr1136)[149] in the tyrosine kinase domain of the β-subunit result in loss of IGF-stimulated thymidine incorporation and glucose uptake. Autophosphorylation appears to occur by trans-phosphorylation of sites on the opposite β-subunit.[191] A

tyrosine proximal to the tyrosine kinase domain, Tyr 950, is part of a motif that, when deleted, reduces receptor autophosphorylation, affects receptor internalization, and inhibits postreceptor signaling. The adapter proteins Shc and insulin receptor substrate 1 (IRS1) bind to this domain.

Autophosphorylation and activation of the cytoplasmic region of the IGF type I receptor promotes recruitment or activation of several docking proteins, each of which activate distinct signaling pathways, with some overlap (Fig. 24-26). Proteins that can dock onto the activated IGF type I receptor include members of the IRS family, Shc, 14-3-3e, p85 subunit of PI3 kinase, tyrosine phosphatase PTP1D, and mGRB10. Of these docking proteins, the pathways involving IRS and Shc are best characterized. IRS1 is a 185-kDa protein that, when phosphorylated, contains specific phosphotyrosine motifs that can associate with proteins containing SRC homology 2 (SH2) domains such as the p85 subunit of PI3 kinase, growth factor receptor–bound protein 2 (Grb2), Syp (a phosphotyrosine phosphatase), and Nck (an oncogenic protein). Activation of Shc and Grb2 results in activation of the Ras, Raf, MAP kinase kinase, and S6 kinase pathways.[192]

Phosphorylation of IRS1 by either the type I IGF receptor or the insulin receptor activates multiple signaling cascades that ultimately influence nuclear transcription and gene expression. Mice with a null deletion for the *IRS1* gene have poor growth in addition to insulin resistance.[193] Binding of the p85 subunit of PI3 kinase leads to activation of the p110 subunit of PI3 kinase. This process then activates downstream phospholipid signal transduction pathways that include Akt. Activation of Akt leads to regulation of diverse cellular processes including apoptosis, glucose transport and metabolism, protein synthesis, mitosis, and differentiation.[194] Activation of the type I IGF receptor leads to phosphorylation of Shc, which then acts as a docking site for the Sh2 domain of Grb2. Grb2 then binds SOS, a guanine nucleotide exchange factor that converts inactive Ras guanosine diphosphate (GDP) into guanosine triphosphate (GTP). GTP-bound Ras then recruits Raf, and Raf subsequently activates MAP kinase and mitogen and extracellular signal-related kinases (MEK) 1 and 2. Activation of these proteins ultimately regulates gene transcription. Given that insulin and IGF peptides activate similar signaling pathways through their own specific receptors, it is unclear how the cell distinguishes among these overlapping ligands. Whether the consequences merely reflect the relative levels of receptors or whether divergent downstream pathways exist for insulin and IGF action remain questions for future investigation.[195]

The α- and β-subunit of the IGF receptor can form heterodimer with the α- and β-subunit of the insulin receptor, forming hybrid receptors (see Fig. 24-24). Hybrid receptors have been found in significant amounts in most tissues. There is a high degree of homology between the insulin and IGF receptor, which facilitates hybrid receptor formation. The hybrid receptor can bind either insulin of IGF-1, but IGF-1 may bind with higher affinity. No matter the ligand bound, autophosphorylation of the β-subunit of the insulin or IGF-1 receptor occurs.[196] The physiologic significance of these hybrid receptors is unknown. Studies thus far have been performed in vitro, and thus, the in vitro significance of the binding characteristics is not known.

The type II IGF receptor bears no structural homology with either the insulin receptor or type I IGF receptors (see Fig. 24-24). The receptor does not contain an intrinsic tyrosine kinase domain or any other recognized signal transduction mechanism. The type II IGF receptor is identical to the cation-independent mannose-6-phosphate (M6P) receptor, a protein involved in the intracellular lysosomal targeting of acid hydrolases and other mannosylated proteins.[197] This common receptor is often referred to as the IGF-2/M6P receptor. The gene for the IGF-2/M6P receptor (*IGF2R*) is located on the long arm of chromosome 6. Exons 1 through 46 encode the extracellular region of the receptor, which contains 15 repeat sequences of 147 residues each. Exons 47 and 48 encode the 23-residue transmembrane domain and a small cytoplasmic domain consisting of only 164 residues.[198] In mice, gene expression is maternally imprinted, but for humans the expression is biallelic.[199] Like *IGF2*, the *IGF2R* gene is expressed at highest levels early in fetal development and declines to lower levels postnatally.[198]

The IGF-2/M6P receptor has an apparent molecular weight of 220,000 under nonreducing conditions and 250,000 after reduction, indicating that it is a monomeric protein.[200] The 15 repeat sequences contain cysteines to form intramolecular disulfide bonds necessary for receptor folding.[198] Repeat 11 binds IGF-2, whereas repeats 3, 5, and 9 bind M6P.[198] Because of receptor folding, it appears that the IGF-2 binding site is on the opposite face to the M6P binding site.[201] A truncated form of the receptor, missing the cytoplasmic domain, has been observed to be soluble

in serum.[202] The soluble form is able to bind IGF-2[203] and is able to inhibit cell responses to IGF-2 in vitro.[204]

The IGF-2/M6P receptor binds a variety of M6P-containing proteins, including lysosomal enzymes, transforming growth factor-β (TGF-β),[205] and leukemia inhibitory factor (LIF).[206] Unlike the type I IGF receptor, which binds both IGF peptides with high affinity and insulin with 100-fold lower affinity, the IGF-2/M6P receptor binds only IGF-2 with high affinity, the dissociation constant ranging from 0.017 to 0.7 nmol/L; IGF-1 binds to this receptor with lower affinity, and insulin does not bind at all.[207] One mole of IGF-2 binds 1 mole of receptor. It participates in lysosomal enzyme trafficking between the trans-Golgi network and the extracellular space, regulates extracellular IGF-2 and LIF levels, and plays a role in TGF-β activation (reviewed by El-Shewy and colleagues[208]). Mice null for the type II IGF receptor have macrosomia and fetal death, consistent with a potential role in IGF-2 degradation.[209]

The mitogenic and metabolic actions of IGF-1 and IGF-2 appear to be mediated through the type I IGF receptor, because monoclonal antibodies directed against the IGF-1 binding site on the type I IGF receptor inhibit the ability of both IGF-1 and IGF-2 to stimulate thymidine incorporation and cell replication.[210] Polyclonal antibodies that block IGF-2 binding to the IGF-2/M6P receptor do not block IGF-2 actions.[211-213] IGF-2 analogues with decreased affinity for the type I IGF receptor but reserved affinity for the IGF-2/M6P receptor are less potent than IGF-2 in stimulating DNA synthesis.[159] However, there is evidence that some of the mitogenic actions of IGF-2 may be mediated by the IGF-2/M6P receptor.[208] IGF-2 may stimulate the growth of a human erythroleukemia cell line, an action not duplicated by either IGF-1 or insulin. IGF-2 may be able to act as an autocrine growth factor and cell motility factor for human rhabdomyosarcoma cells, actions apparently mediated through the type II receptor. Additionally, it has been reported that IGF-2 activates a calcium-permeable cation channel via the IGF-2/M6P receptor, perhaps through coupling to a pertussis toxin–sensitive guanine nucleotide binding protein (G$_i$ protein).[208]

Function-Targeted Disruption of IGF and IGF Receptor Genes

The role of the IGF axis in prenatal and postnatal growth was firmly established by a series of studies involving IGF and IGF receptor gene null mutations.[214] Unlike *Gh* or *Ghr* null mice that are near-normal at size at birth, mice with deletions of *Igf1* or *Igf2* have birth weights approximately 60% of normal.[215] Fetal size is proportionately reduced, but mice with deletion of *Igf1* have a higher neonatal death rate. *Igf2* null mice also exhibit smaller placentas. Growth delay begins on day E11 for mice with deletion of *Igf2* and on day E13.5 for mice with deletion of *Igf1*. Postnatally, mice with deletion of *Igf1* who survive the neonatal period continue to have growth failure, with weights 30% of normal by 2 months of age. A similar prenatal and postnatal growth phenotype was observed in the reported case of an *Igf1* deletion[216] and in the case of a bioinactive IGF-1 molecule resulting from a missense mutation.[217] When both *Igf1* and *Igf2* were disrupted, weight at birth was only 30% of normal and all animals died shortly after birth, apparently from respiratory insufficiency secondary to muscular hypoplasia (Fig. 24-27).

Mice lacking *Igf1* and the *Ghr* are only 17% of normal size.[156] Therefore, both IGF-1 and IGF-2 are important in fetal growth, but GHR signaling may have IGF-independent actions on growth as well. The postnatal growth of *Igf1*$^{-/-}$ mice was poorer than that observed in mice with *Ghr* or

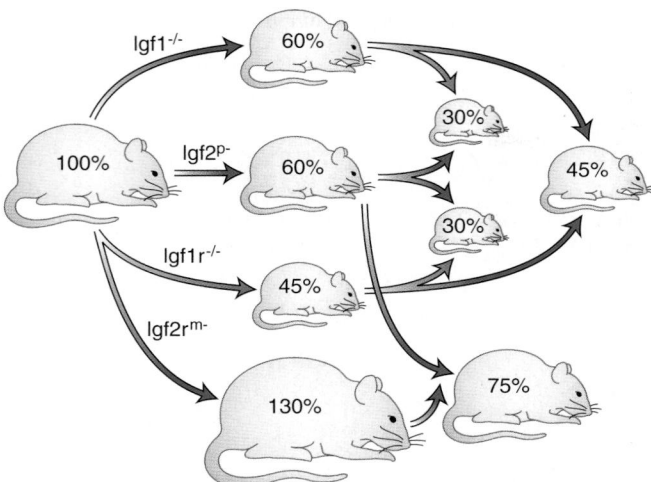

Figure 24-27 Effects of the disruption of one or more genes of the insulin-like growth factor *(Igf)* system on fetal growth in mice, expressed as percentage of normal body weight. Igf1[-/-], Igf1 gene null mice; Igf2[p-], Igf2 paternal allele null mice; Igf1r[-/-], Igf1r gene null mice; Igf2r[m-], Igf2r maternal allele null mice. Mice with two source arrows are the combined genotype of the source arrow mice. (From Gicquel C, LeBouc Y. Hormonal regulation of fetal growth. *Horm Res.* 2006;65:28-33.)

Ghrh receptor mutations, indicating that both GH-dependent and GH-independent effects of IGF-1 are necessary for normal growth.

Specific ablation of hepatic IGF-1 production through the Cre/LoxP recombination system confirmed that the liver is the principal source of circulating IGF-1, but the resulting 80% reduction in serum IGF-1 levels had no effect on postnatal growth,[157,218,219] suggesting that postnatal growth is relatively independent of hepatic IGF-1 production. Presumably, production of IGF-1 from local chondrocytes or other tissues maintains adequate endocrine sources of IGF-1 to account for growth preservation. Supportive data for the predominant role in growth of locally produced IGF-1 include the fact that only modest decrement of postnatal growth is seen in mice null for *Igfals* (the gene encoding ALS).[220] The hormonal profile of the murine models is complex, with reduced IGFBP3 levels despite increased GH. Free IGF-1 levels have been reported to be normal in these animals, even though GH levels are elevated.[219]

By crossing the liver-derived IGF-1 gene–deleted mice with ALS gene–deleted mice, 85% to 90% reduction in serum IGF-1 was achieved, and early postnatal growth retardation was observed.[221] These findings suggest that postnatal growth is dependent on both hepatic and tissue IGF-1, although definite conclusions are problematic in the face of elevated GH production and perturbations of the IGFBP system observed in these studies.

Deletion of *Igf1r* resulted in birth weights 45% of normal with 100% neonatal lethality.[222] In humans, two cases of mutations in the *IGF1R* gene have been reported; these patients had IUGR and postnatal growth failure with elevated IGF-1 levels. One patient had a compound for point mutations in exon 2 of the *IGFR1* gene, leading to decreased receptor affinity for IGF-1, whereas the other patient had a nonsense mutation of one allele, resulting in reduced numbers of IGF type I receptors.[223] Concurrent deletion of *Igf1* and the *Igf1r* resulted in no further reduction in birth size compared with deletion of *Igf1r* alone; this is consistent with the hypothesis that all IGF-1 actions are mediated via the IGF type I receptor.[214]

Deletion of *Igf2r* in mice causes an increase in birth weight but death in late gestation or at birth.[209] Because this receptor normally degrades IGF-2, increased growth reflects excess IGF-2 acting through the IGF type I receptor, with variable accumulation of IGF-2 in tissues. Deletion of *Igf2r* plus *Igf2* results in a birth weight 60% of normal, similar to the size of mice with knockout of *Igf2* alone, with no effect on neonatal survival.[224] Simultaneous knockout of the genes for *Igf2* and *Igf1r* causes further reduction of birth size to 30% of normal, suggesting that some of the fetal anabolic actions of IGF-2 are mediated by another mechanism such as via placental growth or interactions with the insulin receptor. Indeed, specific deletion of *Igf2* in the placenta causes small placenta and growth retardation.[225]

These studies allow the following conclusions: (1) IGF-1 is important for both fetal and postnatal growth; (2) IGF-2 is a major fetal growth factor but has little, if any, role in postnatal growth; (3) the IGF type I receptor mediates anabolic actions of both IGF-1 and IGF-2; (4) the IGF type II receptor is bifunctional, serving to target lysosomal enzymes and to enhance IGF-2 turnover; (5) IGF-2 deletion results in impaired placental growth; and (6) IGF-1 is the major mediator of GH effects on postnatal growth, although GH and GHR may have small IGF-1-independent effects. Whether these effects apply to humans is not yet known.

Insulin-like Growth Factor–Binding Proteins

In contrast to insulin, the IGFs circulate in plasma complexed to a family of binding proteins that extend the serum half-life of the IGF peptides, transport the IGFs to target cells, and modulate the interactions of the IGFs with surface membrane receptors.[226] In addition to these effects, the IGFBPs have been found to have effects on cells independent of IGFs. The presence and various actions of the IGFBPs provide layers of regulation to the GH-IGF axis, greatly increasing its complexity (Fig. 24-28). In the following paragraphs, the structure of the IGFBP family is described first, followed by the role of IGFBPs in IGF physiology and the characteristics of individual IGFBPs.

Structure of IGFBPs. Six distinct human IGFBPs have been cloned, and their highly conserved amino acid sequences have been determined. The six IGFBPs share structural homology in the N-terminal and C-terminal domains but have highly variable midsections, which probably accounts for the more specialized properties of the individual IGFBPs, such as cell dissociation, IGF-binding enhancement, and IGF-independent actions. In each of the conserved N- and C-terminal domains, there are a high number of cysteine-rich residues with a conserved spatial order, implying that the disulfide bond–dependent secondary structure of the IGFBPs is also conserved.[227] Reduction of the disulfide proteins results in loss of IGF binding, further demonstrating the importance of the cysteine-rich region.

The N-terminal domain contains residues that have been shown to be essential for IGF binding to IGFBPs 1, 3, and 4.[228] Whether this binding is important for IGF-independent effects of the IGFBPs is unknown. The exact sequences in the C-terminal domain that are responsible for binding may differ among the IGFBPs; for example, the arginine-glycine-aspartic acid sequence in the C-terminal of IGFBPs 1 and 2, which is putatively necessary for binding to cellular surfaces,[229] is not present on IGFBP3, which can also bind cell membranes.[230] The highly variable midregion segment of the IGFBPs is the site of post-translational modifications such as glycosylation and phosphorylation and of proteolysis. Both the primary structure of IGFBPs and their post-translational modifications are responsible for

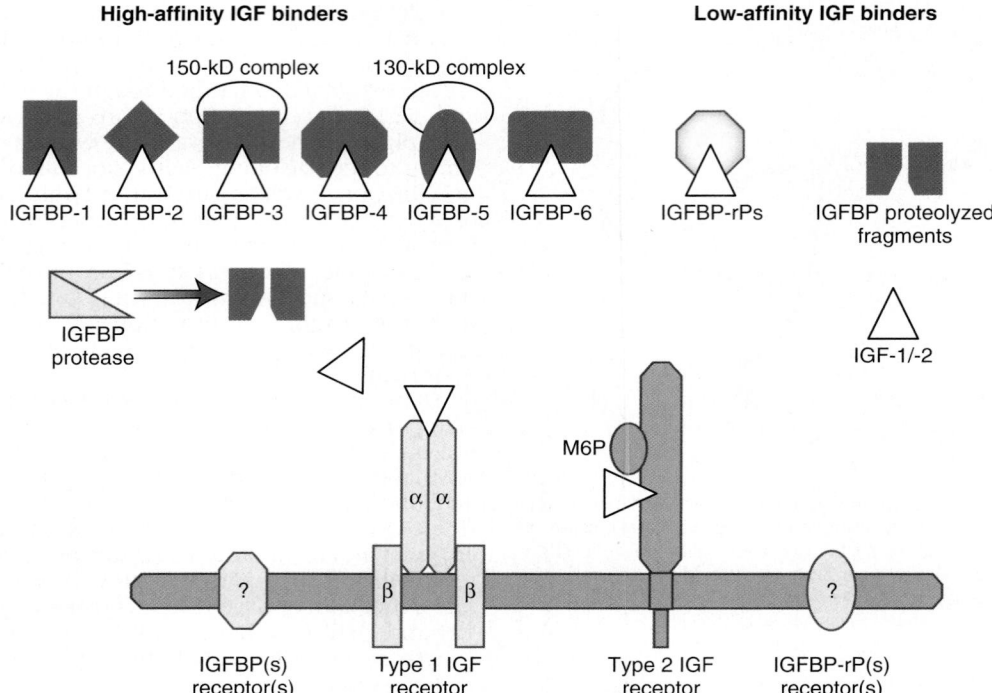

High-affinity IGF binders

Low-affinity IGF binders

Figure 24-28 Schematic representation of the insulin-like growth factor (IGF) system, including IGF ligands (IGF receptors 1 and 2), binding proteins (both high- and low-affinity binders), IGF-binding protein (IGFBP) proteases, type 1 and type 2 IGF receptors, and potential receptors for other IGFBPs and IGFBP-related proteins (IGFBP-rPs). M6P, mannose-6-phosphate. (From Hwa V, Oh Y, Rosenfeld RG. The insulin-like growth factor–binding protein [IGFBP] superfamily. *Endocr Rev.* 1999;20:761-787, copyright © Endocrine Society.)

the differential targeting to tissues: glycosylation can affect cell interactions, phosphorylation can affect IGF-1 binding affinity and susceptibility to proteases, and proteolysis can affect IGF/IGF receptor–dependent and –independent actions.[231]

The three-dimensional structure of IGFBPs 1, 2, 4, and 5 have been determined, confirming the presence of IGF-binding sites in the N- and C-terminal domains. Crystallography has shown that the structure of the N-terminal domain is critical for IGF binding, whereas the C-terminal domain is important for inhibiting interactions between IGF-1 and its receptor.[232,233]

Several groups of cysteine-rich proteins that contain domains similar to the IGFBPs have been discovered, leading to the proposal of an IGFBP superfamily.[234] This superfamily includes the six high-affinity IGFBPs and a number of IGFBP-related proteins (IGFBP-rPs). Three of these proteins—Mac25 (IGFBP-rP1), connective tissue growth factor (CTGF/IGFBP-rP2), and NovH (IGFBP-rP3)—have been shown to bind IGFs, although with considerably lower affinity than the IGFBPs. The role, if any, of IGFBP-rPs in normal IGF physiology is unclear.

Analysis of IGFBPs is complicated by the presence of IGFBP proteases that degrade IGFBP (Fig. 24-29).[235,236] Proteolysis of IGFBPs complicates their assay and must be taken into consideration when measuring the various IGFBPs in biologic fluids. Proteases for IGFBPs 2, 3, 4, and 5 are present in serum and urine.[236] It is likely that multiple IGFBP proteases exist, including calcium-dependent serine proteases, kallikreins, cathepsin, and matrix metalloproteases.[237,238] It is postulated that proteolysis of IGFBPs releases IGFs to interact with cell surface receptors, thereby enhancing the mitogenic and anabolic effects of IGF peptides. There is some evidence that the proteolytic fragments of IGFBP3 and IGFBP5 have IGF-1-independent effects.[239,240]

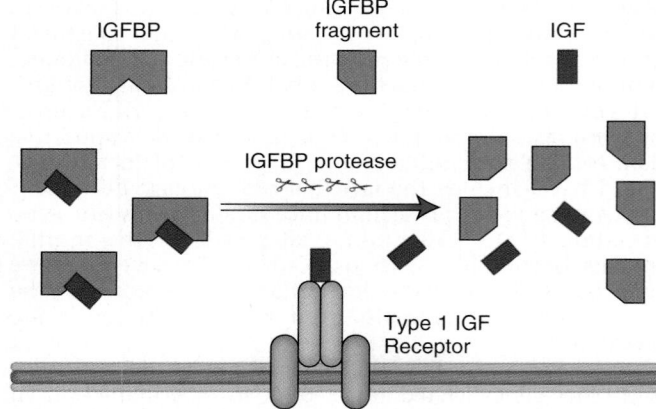

Figure 24-29 Schematic representation of the effect of insulin-like growth factor (IGF)-binding protein (IGFBP) proteases on IGF action. In this model, proteolysis of IGFBPs results in a reduction in their affinity for IGF ligands, leading to enhanced binding of IGF peptides by IGF receptors. (From Cohen P, Rosenfeld RG. The IGF axis. In Rosenbloom AL, ed. *Human Growth Hormone: Basic and Scientific Aspects.* Boca Raton, FL: CRC Press; 1995:43-58.)

Role of IGFBPs in IGF Physiology

IGFBPs as Carrier Proteins. The IGFBPs complex almost all of the circulating IGF-1 and IGF-2 secondary to their high affinity for the IGFs (10^{-10} to 10^{-11} mol/L).[241] In adults, 75% to 80% of IGFs are carried in a ternary complex consisting of 1 molecule of IGF plus 1 molecule of IGFBP3 plus 1 molecule of the protein ALS.[242] This 150-kDa ternary complex is too large to leave the vascular compartment and extends the half-life of IGF peptides from approximately 10 minutes for IGF alone to 12 to 15 hours for IGF

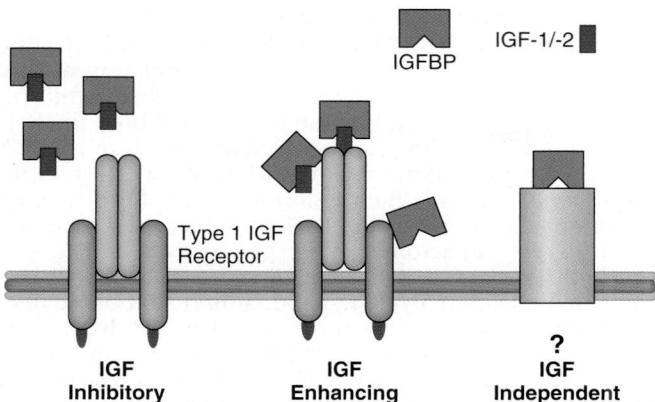

Figure 24-30 Theoretical mechanisms of cellular actions of insulin-like growth factor (IGF)-binding proteins (IGFBPs). See text for details.

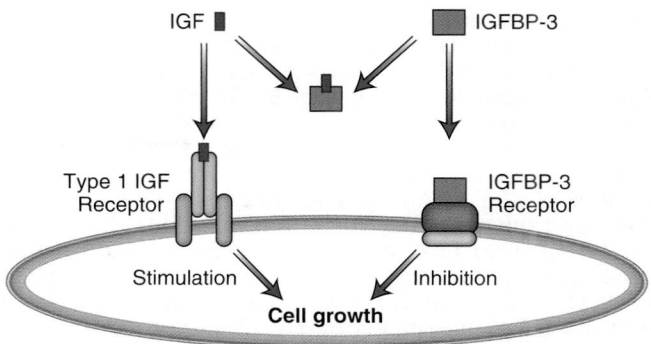

Figure 24-31 Schematic diagram of insulin-like growth factor (IGF)-dependent and IGF-independent actions of IGF-binding protein 3 (IGFBP3), the latter being mediated through a putative membrane-associated IGFBP3 receptor.

in the ternary complex.[243] Binding of IGF to IGFBP3 in a binary complex extends the half-life of IGF to 1 to 2 hours. When IGFs bind as a binary complex to the IGFBPs, diffusion out of the vascular compartment may occur; this has been observed for IGF-binding proteins 1, 2, and 4.[244]

Both IGFBP3 and ALS are GH dependent, providing an additional mechanism for GH regulation of the IGF axis. Whereas GH administration to GH-deficient patients shifts IGF from a 40- to 50-kDa form to the ternary complex,[245] this shift does not occur after IGF-1 treatment. No sustained increase in levels of IGFBP3 occurs after administration of IGF-1,[107] but ALS levels may decrease after IGF-1 administration, possibly reflecting IGF feedback inhibition of pituitary GH secretion.[246] In serum of patients with GHD or GH insensitivity, little IGF is present in the 150-kDa ternary complex; the IGF present is in the IGF-IGFBP3 binary complex or is bound by other IGFBPs such as IGFBPs 1, 2, 4, or 5.[186,235]

IGFBPs as Modulators of IGF Action. IGFBPs also regulate biologic actions by modulating the availability of IGFs (Fig. 24-30). The binding affinity of IGFs for IGFBPs is higher than for IGF receptors, and dissociation of IGFs from IGFBPs is required for IGFs to interact with IGF receptors.[241] Additionally, the concentration of IGFBPs is in excess, compared with IGFs, in many bodily fluids.[247] Dissociation of IGFs from IGFBPs is achieved by mass action, proteolysis, or other unknown mechanisms. Alterations in the interaction between IGF-1 and its receptor can result in inhibition or potentiation of IGF effects on cell proliferation.[248] Inhibition of IGF-1 action by the presence of IGFBP4 has been demonstrated in vitro and in vivo,[249] because IGF analogues with decreased affinity for IGFBP4 have increased biologic potency. IGFBPs 1, 3, and 5 have been shown to have potentiating effects on IGF action, perhaps by facilitating the delivery of IGF to target receptors, as has been shown for IGFBP3.[250]

The enhancing effects of IGFBP5 were shown to involve binding of IGFBP5 to extracellular matrix proteins, which reduces the affinity of IGFBP5 for IGF. Possibly, IGFBP5 binding to the extracellular matrix brings IGF close to the cell surface in a low-affinity complex, from which it can be released slowly to bind neighboring IGF receptors.[251] To complicate matters, it appears that the same IGFBP can potentiate or inhibit IGF action in vitro, depending on cell culture conditions, cell type, IGFBP dose, and post-translational modifications such as phosphorylation state.[248] It has been proposed that IGFBP3 and IGFBP5 may have their own receptors that, when activated, interact with IGF receptor signaling pathways.

It has also been proposed that IGFBP-IGF complexes can be stored in tissues to act in a paracrine manner. This has been demonstrated for IGFBP5 and bone matrix. IGFBP5 is produced by osteoblasts, and the IGFBP5-IGF complex can bind hydroxyapatite. It has been proposed that the complex participates in bone turnover.[252]

IGFBP proteases, which degrade IGFBPs, are postulated to play a role in altering IGF availability by lowering affinities of IGFBPs for their ligand, thereby increasing the availability of IGFs to cell membrane receptors.

IGF-Independent Actions of IGFBPs. IGFBPs also have IGF-independent actions, such as growth inhibition of certain cell types, growth stimulation of tissues, direct induction of apoptosis, and modulation of the effects of other, non-IGF growth factors. The mechanisms of IGF-independent actions are slowly being unraveled and include binding to IGFBP-specific cell surface receptors, binding to other cell surface receptors, and interaction with nuclear receptors (Fig. 24-31).

IGF-independent actions have been characterized for IGFBPs 1, 2, 3, and 5. IGFBP1 has been implicated in cell motility and adhesion while IGFBP2 has mitogenic actions independent of IGF-1 binding. IGFBP3 also appears to have intrinsic inhibitory effects on cells. In in vitro studies, IGFBP3 administration or overexpression inhibits DNA synthesis and cell proliferation in conditions in which IGF-1 or the IGF type I receptor is neutralized, suggesting IGF-independent inhibition by IGFBP3.[253] IGFBP3 is more effective than immunoneutralization of IGF-1 in inhibiting serum-stimulated DNA synthesis in cultured ovarian granulosa cells, with or without added IGF.[254] IGFBP3 has been demonstrated to induce apoptosis in fibroblasts lacking functional IGF receptors, an IGFBP3 that does not bind IGF stimulates apoptosis in these fibroblasts and in wild-type fibroblasts.[231] IGFBP5 also has IGF-independent effects on osteoblasts. In osteoblasts cultured from mice null for the IGF-1 gene, the presence of IGFBP5 increased cell growth, alkaline phosphatase activity, and osteocalcin expression to levels similar to those of wild-type osteoblasts.[231] In addition, IGFBP5 administered to bone of *IGF1* null mice was associated with an increase in markers of bone formation.

The IGFBPs have IGF-independent effects via binding to IGFBP-specific membrane receptors for IGFBP3, IGFBP5, or other receptors such as the TGF-β receptor type V.[231] The downstream signaling pathways activated by the IGFBP-specific receptors are unknown, as are the possible interactions with IGF receptor signaling. IGFBP3 and IGFBP5 also contain nuclear localization signals, and these proteins have been localized to the nucleus in vitro.[255,256] IGFBP proteases can also generate IGFBP3 fragments with enhanced affinity for cell surface IGFBP3 receptors.[257]

Characteristics of IGFBPs 1 through 6. IGFBP1 was the first of the IGFBPs to be purified and to have its cDNA cloned. Its gene is 5.2 kb long, is located on the short arm of chromosome 7, and comprises four exons.[258] The mature protein is 30 kDa and is not glycosylated. Messenger RNA is strongly expressed in decidua, liver, and kidney. It is the major IGFBP in fetal serum in early gestation, reaching levels as high as 3000 µg/L by the second trimester. Levels of IGFBP1 in newborn serum are inversely correlated with birth weight, suggesting an inhibitory role on fetal IGF action.

IGFBP1 may be involved in reproductive function, including endometrial cycling, oocyte maturation, and fetal growth.[259] It also appears to have an important metabolic role, in that its gene expression is enhanced in catabolic states[186] while insulin suppresses IGFBP1 mRNA levels. It is thought that the high IGFBP1 levels in fasting bind IGF-1 to reduce the insulin-like activity of IGF-1 on metabolism. Serum IGFBP1 levels correlate with insulin sensitivity. Low levels are associated with lower insulin sensitivity. Fasting levels predict risk of diabetes development in longitudinal cohorts.[260] IGFBP1 null mice have normal glucose homeostasis, but IGFBP1 transgenic mice are protected against insulin resistance when challenged with a high-fat diet. The cellular target(s) of IGFBP1 that mediate these effects are not known, as IGFBP1 can have IGF-1-independent effects.

Although most in vitro studies consistently show an inhibitory effect of IGFBP1 on IGF action, presumably reflecting interference with IGF ligand-receptor interactions,[226] IGFBP1 potentiates IGF effects in certain cell systems, possibly as a result of the binding of IGFBP1 to cell membranes through its Arg-Gly-Asp sequence.[229] The ability of IGFBP1 to inhibit or potentiate IGF action may depend on post-translational modifications of IGFBP1, such as phosphorylation, which appears to enhance the affinity of IGFBP1 for IGF-1, thereby inhibiting IGF action.[226]

The *IGFBP2* gene is located on the long arm of chromosome 2 and encodes for a mature protein of 34 kDa.[261] Like IGFBP1, IGFBP2 is highly expressed in fetal tissues, particularly in the CNS.[262] It is also expressed in the liver, adipocytes, and reproductive system. It is the second most abundant IGFBP in the serum, behind IGFBP3. Unlike IGFBP1, its expression does not change with feeding. IGFBP2 transgenic mice have diminished postnatal weight gain and slightly reduced fasting insulin levels with protection against age-related insulin resistance.[260]

The *IGFBP3* gene is located on chromosome 7. It contains four exons homologous to *IGFBP1* and *IGFBP2* and a fifth exon consisting of 3′ untranslated sequences. Messenger RNA levels are high in the liver, most notably in the hepatic endothelia and Kupffer cells, compared with ALS, which is high in hepatocytes.[263] The mature, unglycosylated IGFBP3 protein has a molecular weight of approximately 29 kDa and comprises 264 amino acids. IGFBP3 is composed of the conserved N-terminal and C-terminal domains and the variable midsection. The midsection is the site of N-linked glycosylation, which is not present in IGFBP1 or IGFBP2, and this is why it normally migrates as a doublet-triplet of 40 to 46 kDa. Glycosylation does not appear to alter its affinity for IGF-1 or IGF-2.[231] The midsection is also the site of phosphorylation. Studies have shown that this midsection is the site responsible for interaction with cell surfaces.[264]

IGFBP3 is the predominant IGFBP in adult serum, where it carries approximately 75% of the total IGF, primarily as part of the 150-kDa ternary complex consisting of IGF-1, IGFBP3, and ALS. IGFBP3 and IGFBP5 are the only IGFBPs to form this complex. It is believed that formation of this ternary complex limits IGF access to target cells, while at the same time prolonging serum half-lives of both the IGF peptide and its binding protein.[265] Serum levels of IGFBP3 and ALS are reduced in patients with GHD or GH insensitivity, conditions in which assays for serum IGFBP3 have important diagnostic value. IGFBP3 is increased in states of GH excess and acromegaly.

IGFBP3 action is GH dependent, either directly or through regulation by IGF. IGF-1 administration to hypophysectomized rats increases serum levels of IGFBP3.[266] IGF-1 treatment of patients with GH insensitivity, however, does not greatly alter serum IGFBP3 levels,[106] and GH treatment of GH-deficient patients does not increase serum levels. Whether these observations mean that GH has a direct effect on IGFBP3 or reflects GH regulation of ALS and ternary complex formation is unclear, although it appears likely that both factors are contributory.

IGFBP3 associates with cell membrane proteins in a specific, cation-dependent manner and with high affinity.[231] Whether the cell membrane proteins constitute genuine IGFBP3 receptors remains to be determined, although they may mediate IGF-independent actions of IGFBP3. Alternatively, IGFBP3 may associate with heparin-containing proteoglycans in the extracellular matrix and in the cell membrane, because it contains heparin-binding consensus sequences in the C-terminus.[267] It has been suggested that IGFBP3 is a ligand of the serine/theonine kinase type V TGF-β receptor, with the resultant interaction leading to cell growth inhibition.[231]

IGFBP3 can also translocate to the cell nucleus from the extracellular compartment. It has a consensus nuclear translocation sequence, and translocation is facilitated by importin-B.[268] IGFBP3 can bind the nuclear RXRα. This feature is important to the IGFBP3 effect on apoptosis.[269]

IGFBP3 expression can be induced by cell cycle regulators and growth-inhibitory factors such as TNF-α, TNF-β, retinoic acid, vitamin D, antiestrogens, and antiandrogens.[270] In many cases, modulation of *IGFBP3* expression has been shown to be crucial to the antiproliferative effects of factors in vitro.[270] *IGFBP3* expression is also activated by the tumor suppression gene p53[271] in tumor cell lines treated with chemotherapeutic agents.[272] Like many genes, *IGFBP3* expression is affected by methylation and histone modification. Numerous studies have shown that abnormal methylation or histone modification of the *IGFBP3* gene is present in many different types of human cancers (reviewed by Jogie-Brahim and colleagues[270]).

The *IGFBP4* gene is located on chromosome 17 and contains four exons. It is present mostly as a nonglycosylated form of 24 kDa, with the glycosylated form being 29 kDa. Similar to IGFBP3, its glycosylation site is in the highly variable midregion of the protein. It is widely expressed in embryonic tissues, fibroblasts, osteoblastic cells, prostatic cells, ovarian cells, and liver. The circulating form is derived mostly from the liver. Evidence suggests that IGFBP4 is the only IGFBP that does not have IGF-independent effects. In vitro, IGFBP4 inhibits IGF action, and in vivo studies have demonstrated that the inhibitory action of IGFBP4 on cellular processes is IGF-1-dependent.[273,274] The inhibitory effects of IGFBP4 are reduced by proteolysis, similar to IGFBP3. IGFBP4 proteases are present in a wide variety of cells, including neuroblastoma, smooth muscle, fibroblasts, osteoblasts, and prostatic epithelium.[274,275] Activation of IGFBP4 proteolysis occurs in the presence of IGF-1 or IGF-2, presumably reflecting a conformational change in IGFBP4 resulting from IGF occupancy.[276] The protease pregnancy-associated plasma protein-A (PPAP-A) has been shown to degrade IGFBPs 2, 4, and 5, but not IGFBP3,[277] and it has been associated with the decline of IGFBP4 during ovarian follicular growth.[278] Proteolysis of IGFBP4 by PPAP-A in developing ovarian follicles has been postulated to play a role in the development of dominant follicles.[278]

The *IGFBP5* gene is located on chromosome 5 and contains four exons. It is 28 kDa and contains a glycosylation site in the highly variable midregion of the protein. In contrast to the other glycosylated IGFBPs, IGFBP5 is O-glycosylated rather than N-glycosylated. IGFBP5 has been shown to bind extracellular matrix proteins such as types III and IV collagen, laminin, and fibronectin, and it does so in response to binding of IGF-1.[279] The affinity of IGFBP5 is reduced about sevenfold when the binding protein is associated with extracellular matrix, providing a potential mechanism for release of IGFs to cell surface receptors. Association of IGFBP5 with extracellular matrix also appears to protect it from proteolysis.[280] Unlike proteolysis of IGFBP4, which is enhanced by the addition of IGFs, degradation of IGFBP5 is inhibited by the binding of IGF peptides.[281] Proteolytic fragments of IGFBP5 have been shown to have IGF-independent effects on mitogenesis, possibly by binding an IGFBP5-specific cell surface receptor.[282]

The *IGFBP6* gene is located on chromosome 12 and contains four exons. The mature peptide contains 216 amino acids and is 23 kDa, although it may undergo O-glycosylation, similar to IGFBP5.[283] Although IGFBP6 binds both IGF-1 and IGF-2, it has a significantly greater affinity for IGF-2.[284] IGFBP6 is found in high levels in cerebrospinal fluid, as is IGFBP2, which also binds IGF-2 with high affinity. IGFBP6 may have a role in regulating ovarian activity, perhaps by functioning as an antigonadotropin.[285]

Mice null for the individual IGFBPs have been generated. Only modest, if any, effects on growth have been found. Modest decreases in organ size have been noted in IGFBP2 null mice,[286] whereas growth in IGFBP4 null mice is 85% to 90% of normal. Increases in other IGFBP levels were noted in these mice. Triple knockout mice null for IGFBPs 3, 4, and 5 have been generated,[287] and they exhibit lengths 80% of normal with IGF-1 levels 45% that of the wild type. Transgenic mice overexpressing the IGFBPs 1, 2, 3, and 4 have also been generated,[288] and they exhibit growth retardation to varying degrees, demonstrating the role of the IGFBPs in sequestering IGF-1 or inhibiting its actions. In addition, mice overexpressing IGFBP1 and IGFBP3 also exhibit impaired glucose tolerance and decreased fertility, further implicating a role for IGF-1 or a separate role for these IGFBPs in glucose metabolism and reproduction.

Gonadal Steroids

Androgens and estrogens affect growth predominantly through two mechanisms: regulation of the GH/IGF-1 axis and maturation of the epiphyseal growth plates. The adolescent rise in serum gonadal steroid levels is an important part of the pubertal growth spurt. In addition, it is the stimulation of epiphyseal fusion by the pubertal rise of gonadal steroid production that results in the ultimate cessation of linear growth. The details of the roles of androgens and estrogens in enhancing GH secretion and directly stimulating IGF-1 production were discussed earlier.

Both androgens and estrogens increase skeletal maturation and accelerate growth plate senescence. However, most of these effects are due to the action of estrogen, with androgens acting indirectly after their conversion to estro-gens by aromatase in extraglandular tissues, including locally within the growth plate. The primacy of the role of estrogen comes from animal studies[21] as well as reports of human subjects with mutations. A mutation of the estrogen receptor in a man was associated with tall stature and open epiphyses,[22] and similar findings were reported in patients with mutations of the gene encoding the aromatase enzyme.[289] In addition, variants of the estrogen receptor have been associated with height in males[290] and in females,[291] and increased aromatase expression results in short adult stature in males.[292,293]

Whereas most of the effects of androgen on growth are mediated through actions that occur after their aromatization to estrogen, there is evidence of androgen-specific effects. Notably, dihydrotestosterone, a nonaromatizable androgen, can accelerate linear growth in boys. This effect of androgen does not appear to be mediated by either GH or circulating IGF-1, but it may be mediated by an increase in local IGF-1 production.[294]

Gonadal steroids, along with GH and IGF-1, contribute to the attainment of peak bone mass in adults. Again, this sex hormone effect is largely mediated by estrogen action.[295-297]

Thyroid Hormone

Thyroid hormone is of relatively little importance in the growth of the fetus, but it has significant effects on postnatal growth and bone maturation. Patients with hypothyroidism have decreased spontaneous GH secretion and blunted responses to GH provocative tests. Thyroid hormone also has a direct effect on chondrocytes and osteoblasts, which both express thyroid hormone receptors. Thyroid hormone regulates chondrocyte proliferation and stimulates terminal differentiation, mineralization, and angiogenesis.[298,299] In particular, thyroid hormone is essential for hypertrophic chondrocyte differentiation.[300] Postnatally, hypothyroidism can cause growth failure and delayed skeletal maturation, whereas hyperthyroidism can accelerate linear growth and skeletal maturation.

Glucocorticoids

Glucocorticoids have both stimulatory and inhibitory effects on GH secretion, with the absolute effect depending on the timing and the glucocorticoid concentration. Glucocorticoid deficiency, as in Addison disease, leads to a decrease in GH secretion due to decreased expression of GHRH and GH secretagogue receptors.[301] Acute exposure to supraphysiologic levels of glucocorticoids decreases GH secretion within 1 hour followed by a subsequent transient increase in GH secretion.[301,302] Ongoing glucocorticoid excess then causes ongoing suppression of GH secretion. This decrease in GH secretion is due to an increase in somatostatin tone.[301] Glucocorticoids can also impair growth through direct actions at the growth plate, by inhibiting local IGF-1 production through suppression of chondrocyte GHR expression, impairment of chondrocyte IGF-1 receptor expression,[301,303] alterations in IGFBP levels, and impairment of intracellular signaling.[304] Finally, glucocorticoids may stimulate apoptosis of growth plate chondrocytes.[294]

Additional indirect effects of excess glucocorticoids on growth can result from glucocorticoid inhibition of calcium absorption and reabsorption, with the development of secondary hyperparathyroidism.[299] In pubertal children, glucocorticoid excess can induce sex hormone deficiency, causing a loss of the normal growth stimulatory effect of these hormones.[299]

TABLE 24-1

Causes of Growth Retardation

I. Disorders of the GH/IGF-1 axis
   A. GH deficiency
      1. Hypothalamus
         a. Congenital disorders
         b. Acquired disorders
      2. Pituitary
         a. Congenital disorders
            (1) Combined pituitary hormone deficiencies
            (2) Isolated GH deficiency (IGHD)
         b. Acquired disorders
            (1) Craniopharyngiomas and other tumors
            (2) Histiocytosis X
   B. GH insensitivity
      1. Mutations in GHR signaling proteins and acid-labile subunit (ALS)
   C. Abnormalities of IGF-1 and IGF-1 receptor signaling
II. Growth disorders outside the GH/IGF-1 axis
   A. Malnutrition
   B. Chronic disease
   C. Endocrine disorders
   D. Osteochondrodysplasias
   E. Chromosomal abnormalities
   F. Small for gestational age (SGA)
   G. Maternal and placental factors
III. Idiopathic short stature (ISS)

GH, growth hormone; IGF-1, insulin-like growth factor 1.

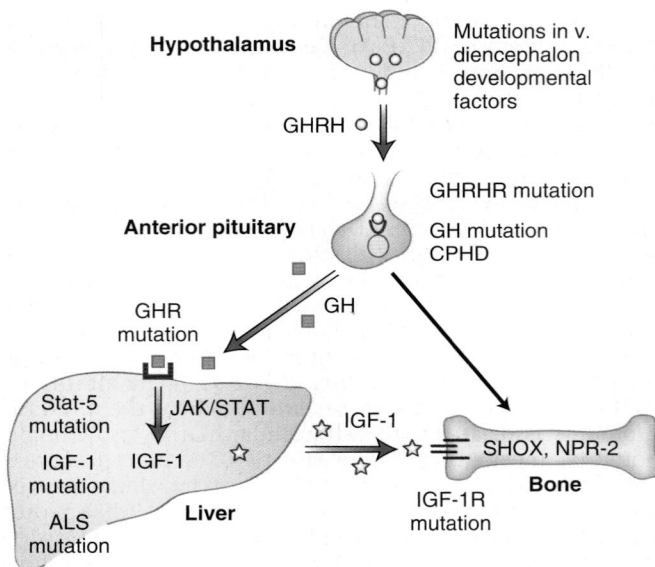

Figure 24-32 The hypothalamic-pituitary-IGF axis: sites of established mutations. ALS, acid-labile subunit; CPHD, combined pituitary hormone deficiency; GH, growth hormone; GHRH, GH-releasing hormone; GHRHR, GHRH receptor; IGF-1, insulin-like growth factor 1; IGF-1R, IGF-1 receptor; JAK, Janus kinase; NPR-2, natriuretic peptide receptor 2; SHOX, short homeobox; STAT, signal transducer and activator of transcription; v, ventral. (Reprinted with permission from Lopez-Bermejo A, Buckway CK, Rosenfeld RG. Genetic defects of the growth hormone-insulin-like growth factor axis. *Trends Endocrinol Metab.* 2000;11:43.)

PATHOLOGIC BASIS OF GROWTH RETARDATION

A classification of growth retardation is presented in Table 24-1. Growth disorders can also be subdivided into (1) disorders of the hypothalamic-pituitary axis resulting in deficiency of GH, (2) disorders resulting in deficiency or resistance to the action of IGF-1, (3) growth disorders that primarily affect the growth plate or are caused by chronic disease, and (4) idiopathic short stature (ISS), which is considered separately but may have a pathogenic basis in the GH/IGF-1 axis or at the growth plate. A schematic diagram of known defects in the GH/IGF-1 axis is shown in Figure 24-32, and the known involved genes are listed in Table 24-2.

Disorders of the GH/IGF-1 Axis

Growth Hormone Deficiency

Although it is not always possible to establish definitively whether hypothalamic or pituitary dysfunction is responsible for the hormone deficiency, these compartments are differentiated to facilitate discussion of the pathology. Table 24-3 indicates possible causes for deficiency in the GH-IGF axis. The term *idiopathic* is often used to designate lack of understanding of the basis for the GHD. Developmental or functional abnormalities of the hypothalamus account for most "idiopathic" cases of hypopituitarism, and recent molecular studies have begun to elucidate the molecular bases of these disorders. It is anticipated that most cases of idiopathic hypopituitarism will be defined at the genetic level in the future.

The Hypothalamus

Congenital Disorders. The primary hypothalamic neuropeptide responsible for synthesis and release of GH is GHRH. Somatostatin plays an antagonistic role in GH release. Synthesis of these two hypothalamic proteins is controlled by a series of neurochemicals, and the balance between them

is responsible for the tight neuroendocrine control of GH biosynthesis. Mutations of some of the genes encoding hypothalamic peptides explain some cases of GHD due to hypothalamic dysfunction.

As noted earlier, patients with early-diagnosed congenital GHD frequently have an abnormal pituitary stalk, ectopia of the posterior pituitary, and hypoplasia of the anterior pituitary (Fig. 24-33). Anencephaly results in a pituitary gland that is small or abnormally formed and is frequently ectopic. Despite the loss of hypothalamic regulation, somatotrophs differentiate and proliferate, although in diminished overall mass.[66] During intrauterine life, serum GH and IGF-1 levels are 30% to 50% of the normal range,[114] and pituitary GH content at birth is about 15% to 20% of normal,[112,114] with similarly low neonatal plasma GH levels.[305]

In most patients, so-called idiopathic hypopituitarism or GHD is presumed to be due to abnormalities of synthesis or secretion of hypothalamic hypophysiotropic factors.[306,307] In a number of reports, idiopathic GHD is associated with MRI findings of an ectopic neurohypophysis, pituitary stalk dysgenesis, and hypoplasia or aplasia of the anterior pituitary. Overall, those patients with the most striking abnormalities of the hypothalamic-pituitary region, largely those with CPHD, had the smallest anterior pituitary glands.[308] Patients with more severe deficiencies of GH have greater frequency of significant morphologic abnormalities.[309]

Although the increased incidence of breech presentation and birth trauma with neonatal asphyxia in congenital idiopathic hypopituitarism has led some to suggest an etiologic role for these occurrences,[310] the syndrome of pituitary stalk dysgenesis with congenital hypopituitarism is probably the result of abnormal development, and the perinatal difficulties are likely the consequence rather than the cause of the abnormalities. Findings of a similar MRI appearance in patients with septo-optic dysplasia,[112,311] in

TABLE 24-2

Genetic Defects of the GH-IGF Axis Resulting in Somatotroph Dysfunction and GH Deficiency

Factor	Gene Function	Affected Cell Types	Clinical Phenotype	Mode of Inheritance
	Mutations in Factors Resulting in Growth Hormone and Associated Hormone Deficiencies			
Hesx1	• Paired-like homeobox gene • Early marker for pituitary primordium and Rathke's pouch • Requires Lhx3 for maintenance and PROP1 for repression	Somatotrophs, thyrotrophs, gonadotrophs (posterior pituitary may also be affected)	• Isolated GH deficiency or multiple hormone deficiency (including diabetes insipidus) • Puberty may be delayed • Associated with septo-optic dysplasia • Abnormal MRI findings: pituitary hypoplasia, ectopic posterior pituitary, midline forebrain abnormalities	AD, AR
Lhx3 (Lim3, P-LIM)	• Member of LIM-homeodomain family of gene regulatory proteins • Required for survival and proliferation of Rathke's pouch • Activates αGSU promoter • Acts with PIT1 to activate TSHβ gene promoter	Somatotrophs, lactotrophs, thyrotrophs, gonadotrophs, possibly corticotrophs	• Patients may present with rigid cervical spine causing limited neck rotation • Hypoplastic anterior/intermediate pituitary lobe	AR
Lhx4	• An LIM protein with close resemblance to Lhx3 • Important for proliferation and differentiation of cell lineages • May have overlapping function with PROP1 and POU1F1	Somatotrophs, lactotrophs, thyrotrophs, gonadotrophs, corticotrophs	• Combined pituitary hormone deficiencies with predominant GH deficiency • Severe anterior pituitary hypoplasia, ectopic neurohypophysis	AD
SIX6	• Member of the *SIX/sine oculis* family of homeobox genes • Expressed early in hypothalamus, later in Rathke's pouch, neural retina, and optic chiasma	Somatotrophs, gonadotrophs	• Bilateral anophthalmia • Pituitary hypoplasia • Associated with deletion at chromosome 14q22-23	Unknown
PITX2 (RIEG1)	• Bicoid-related homeobox gene expressed early in Rathke's pouch • Important in maintaining expression of *Hesx1* and *PROP1*	Somatotrophs, lactotrophs, thyrotrophs, reduced expression of gonadotrophs	• Associated with Rieger syndrome: • Anterior-chamber eye anomalies • Dental hypoplasia • A protuberant umbilicus • Mental retardation • Pituitary dysfunction	AD
PROP1 (Prophet of PIT1)	• Paired-like homeodomain transcription factor required for *PIT1* expression • Coexpressed with *Hesx1*	Somatotrophs, lactotrophs, thyrotrophs, gonadotrophs, corticotrophs (delayed)	• Combined pituitary deficiencies (GH, TSH, PRL, and late-onset ACTH reported) • Gonadotropin insufficiency or normal puberty with later onset of deficiency • Several mutations noted in nonconsanguineous families	AR
POU1F1 (PIT1)	• Member of the POU transcription factor family • Important for activation of *GH1*, *PRL*, and *TSHβ* genes	Somatotrophs, lactotrophs, thyrotrophs	• Combined pituitary deficiencies (GH, TSH, PRL, and late-onset ACTH reported); TSH secretion may initially be normal • Pituitary hypoplasia	AD, AR
Otx2	• Bicoid-type homeodomain gene required for forebrain and eye development • Antagonizes *FGF8* and *SHH* expression • May have importance in activation of *Hesx1*	Somatotrophs, thyrotrophs, corticotrophs, and probably gonadotrophs	• Severe ocular malformation including anophthalmia • Combined pituitary hormone deficiencies with LH/FSH deficiency • Anterior pituitary hypoplasia with ectopic posterior pituitary	Unknown
SOX2	• Member of SOXB1 subfamily as *SOX1* and *SOX3* expressed early in development	Somatotrophs, gonadotrophs (and, in animal models, thyrotrophs)	• Hypogonadotropic hypogonadism • Anterior pituitary hypoplasia • Bilateral anophthalmia/microphthalmia • Midbrain defects including corpus callosum and hippocampus • Sensorineural defects • Esophageal atresia and learning difficulty	De novo
SOX3	• Member of SOX (SRY-related HMG box) • Developmental factor expressed in developing infundibulum and hypothalamus	Somatotrophs, additional anterior pituitary cell types	• Duplications of Xq26-27 in affected males (female carriers unaffected) • Variable mental retardation • Hypopituitarism with abnormal MRI • Anterior pituitary hypoplasia • Infundibular hypoplasia • Ectopic/undescended posterior pituitary • Abnormal corpus callosum • Murine studies suggest SOX3 dosage critical for normal pituitary development	X-linked

Continued

TABLE 24-2

Genetic Defects of the GH-IGF Axis Resulting in Somatotroph Dysfunction and GH Deficiency—cont'd

Factor	Gene Function	Affected Cell Types	Clinical Phenotype	Mode of Inheritance
		Isolated Growth Hormone Deficiency		
GLI2	• Member of the *GLI* gene family; transcription factors that mediate SHH signaling	Somatotrophs	• Heterozygous loss-of-function mutations in patients with holoprosencephaly • Penetrance variable • Pituitary dysfunction accompanied by variable craniofacial abnormalities	Unknown
GHRHr	• Encodes GHRH receptor	Somatotrophs	• Short stature • Anterior pituitary hypoplasia	AR
GH1	• Encodes GH peptide • Several mutations shown to affect GH secretion or function	Somatotrophs	• Short stature • Abnormal facies • Presentation includes bioinactive GH	AR, AD, or X-linked

ACTH, adrenocorticotropic hormone; AD, autosomal dominant; AR, autosomal recessive; FSH, follicle-stimulating hormone; GH, growth hormone; GHRH, growth hormone–releasing hormone; αGSU, glycoprotein α-subunit; HMG, high mobility group; IGF, insulin-like growth factor; LH, luteinizing hormone; MRI, magnetic resonance imaging; PRL, prolactin; SHH, Sonic hedgehog; TSH, thyroid-stimulating hormone (thyrotropin).

TABLE 24-3

GH/IGF-1 Deficiency Syndromes

Congenital Growth Hormone Deficiency

GH deficiency resulting from hypothalamic dysfunction
Holoprosencephaly and septo-optic dysplasia
GH deficiency resulting from pituitary dysfunction
GH deficiency resulting from mutations of the GHRH receptor and GH
GH deficiency resulting from CPHD
Bioactive GH

Acquired Growth Hormone Deficiency

GH deficiency resulting from CNS tumors, trauma, or inflammation
Circulating antibodies to GH that inhibit GH action

Congenital IGF-1 Deficiency

Abnormalities of the GHR
STAT5 mutations
ALS mutations
IGF1 gene mutations
IGF-1 receptor mutations

Acquired IGF-1 Deficiency

Circulating antibodies to the GHR
Chronic disease states

ALS, acid-labile subunit; CHPD, combined pituitary hormone deficiencies; CNS, central nervous system; GH, growth hormone; GHR, growth hormone receptor; GHRH, growth hormone–releasing hormone; IGF-1, insulin-like growth factor 1.

association with type I Arnold-Chiari syndrome and syringomyelia,[112,308] and possibly in holoprosencephaly[112] and the occurrence of micropenis with congenital hypopituitarism[112,312,313] all support the concept that congenital hypopituitarism is a genetic or developmental malformation, not a birth injury. Further indirect evidence in studies[314] of isolated, complete anterior pituitary aplasia indicates that hypothalamic hypopituitarism and breech delivery are consequences of congenital midline brain defects, although perinatal residua of breech delivery may exacerbate ischemic damage to the hypothalamic-pituitary unit.

The MRI findings described for early-diagnosed patients with hypopituitarism are also found in children diagnosed at a later age. Most of these children have hypothalamic dysfunction as the cause of diminished pituitary hormone secretion. In the older group, as in the infants, structural, acquired hypothalamic, stalk, or pituitary abnormalities must be considered.

Holoprosencephaly. Holoprosencephaly, which is caused by abnormal midline development of the embryonic forebrain, usually results in hypothalamic insufficiency and has been associated with mutations in developmental proteins.[315-319] These mutations are associated with diminished signaling by SHH, a critical factor in forebrain development.[318] Hedgehog ligands bind to and activate the transmembrane receptor Patched (PTCH), which results in release of the coreceptor, Smoothened (SMO), activating GLI transcription factors. SHH and FGF8 play a role in the induction of BMP2 and LHX, which are important for proliferation in the developing pituitary gland and are influenced by loss-of-function mutations of the *GL12* gene.[317,318]

Facial dysmorphism of holoprosencephaly ranges from cyclopia to hypertelorism and is accompanied by absence of the nasal septum, midline clefts of the palate or lip, and sometimes a single central incisor. GHD may be accompanied by other pituitary hormone insufficiencies.[320] The incidence of GHD is increased in cases of simple clefts of the lip or palate (or both),[321] and children with cleft palates who grow abnormally require further evaluation.

Septo-optic Dysplasia. In its complete form, the rare syndrome of *septo-optic dysplasia* (SOD) combines hypoplasia or absence of the optic chiasm or optic nerves (or both), agenesis or hypoplasia of the septum pellucidum or corpus callosum (or both), and hypothalamic insufficiency.[311,322,323] The extent of the anatomic and functional abnormalities can vary but usually are in parallel to each other.[322,323] GHD can occur by itself or in combination with deficiencies of TSH, ACTH, or gonadotropins. About 50% to 70% of children with severe anatomic defects have hypopituitarism or, at least, identifiable abnormalities of the GH-IGF axis,[324] and the diagnosis should be considered in any child who has growth failure associated with pendular or rotatory nystagmus or impaired vision and a small optic nerve disc. In some patients, a hypoplastic or interrupted pituitary stalk and ectopic posterior pituitary placement have been identified by MRI.[112,311,322] An increasing number of mutations in developmental transcription factors including HESX1, SOX2, SOX3, and OTX2 are implicated in the pathogeneses of septo-optic dysplasia. The varying conditions of environment and genetics likely contribute to the variable phenotype.[325,326] There is an increased incidence in offspring of young mothers, in first-born children, in areas of high unemployment, and in babies exposed to intrauterine medications, smoking, alcohol, or diabetes.[327]

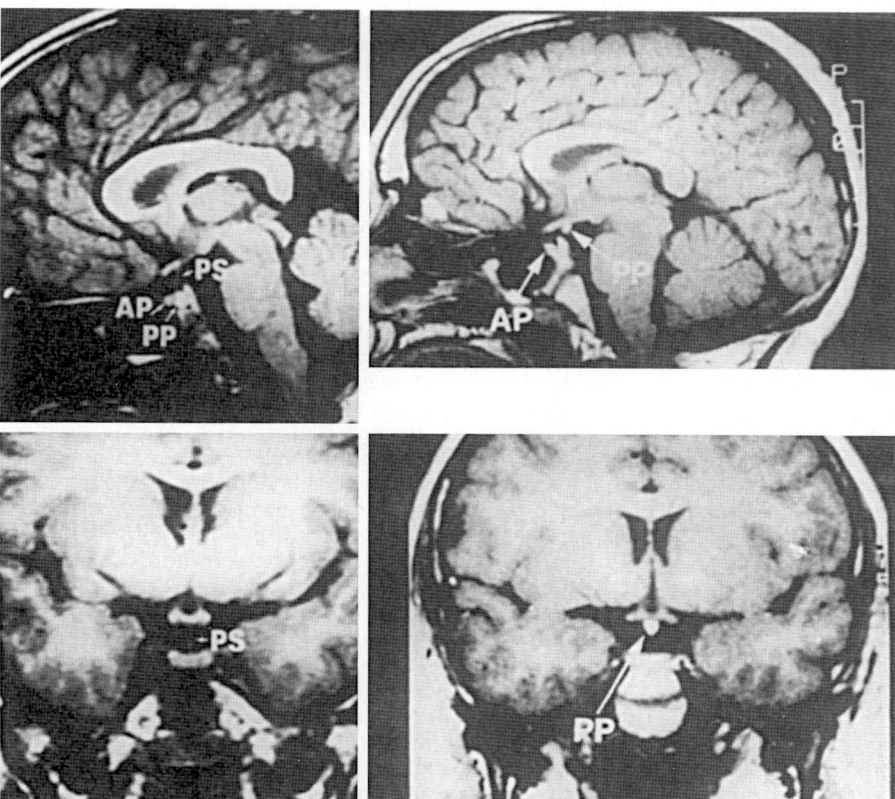

Figure 24-33 Magnetic resonance imaging of infundibular dysgenesis. **A,** T1-weighted sagittal and coronal images of the hypothalamic-pituitary area in a normal 8-year-old girl. The anterior (AP) and posterior pituitary (PP) lobes and the pituitary stalk (PS) are marked. **B,** T1-weighted sagittal and coronal images of the hypothalamic-pituitary area of a 17-year-old boy with isolated growth hormone deficiency. The anterior pituitary lobe (AP) is hypoplastic, the posterior pituitary (PP) is ectopic, and the pituitary stalk is absent. (From Root AW, Martinez CR. Magnetic resonance imaging in patients with hypopituitarism. *Trends Endocrinol Metab.* 1992;3:283-287.)

HESX1. Mutations of *HESX1*, a paired-like homeodomain gene that is expressed early in pituitary and forebrain development, are associated with familial forms of septo-optic dysplasia.[325,328-330] *HESX1*, also referred to as *RPX* (Rathke's pouch homeobox), is a member of the paired-like class of homeobox genes and is essential for normal forebrain and pituitary formation.[331] It is one of the earliest known specific markers for the pituitary primordium and encodes for a developmental repressor with localization to the Rathke's pouch.[332] TLE1 (the mammalian ortholog of the *Drosophila* protein Groucho) and the nuclear corepressor NCOR1 bind to HESX1 to exert repression.[333-334] *HESX1* downregulation is required for cell determination mediated by PROP1 to occur.[335] The LIM homeodomain proteins LHX1 and LHX3 are required for activation of the HESX1 promoter.[336]

Hesx1 null mutant mice display abnormalities in the forebrain, eyes, and other anterior structures such as the pituitary.[328] Mouse embryos heterozygous for both *Hesx1* and *Six3* null mutations have a mild phenotype, suggesting that these developmental factors control a switch in progenitor proliferation between repression by HESX1 and activation of PROP1.[337] These defects have similarity with human phenotypes such as septo-optic dysplasia and CPHD. Patients with septo-optic dysplasia may present with a wide spectrum of phenotypes associated with congenital hypopituitarism. Several homozygous and heterozygous mutations have been identified in *HESX1* (Online Mendelian Inheritance in Man [OMIM] no. 601802) in patients with hypopituitarism with variable phenotypes.[328,330,332,338-343]

Two siblings (born to consanguineous parents) with a severe septo-optic dysplasia phenotype including anterior pituitary hypoplasia, an ectopic posterior lobe, agenesis of the corpus callosum, absent septum pellucidum, and optic nerve hypoplasia were found to have a homozygous mutation at a highly conserved arginine residue of the homeodomain (p.R160C) that resulted in loss of DNA binding of the mutant protein. Another homozygous mutation, a threonine/isoleucine substitution at residue 26 (p.I26T), was identified in a child with GH and gonadotropin deficiency that later evolved to deficiencies of ACTH and TSH. She had no forebrain abnormalities and normal optic nerves, but on MRI had hypoplasia of the anterior pituitary and an undescended posterior pituitary. This mutation lies in a highly conserved engrailed homology domain (eh-1) that is required for transcriptional repression. Loss of repressor function was found to be caused by impaired interaction with the TLE1 corepressor. To determine the mechanisms by which these mutations cause the disorder, mice homozygous for these mutations were generated.[344] Mice homozygous for the p.R160C mutation displayed pituitary and forebrain defects similar to those in the *Hesx1* null embryos, indicating the critical role of HESX1 interactions with DNA in transcriptional repression during development. Mice homozygous for the p.I26T allele displayed pituitary defects and ocular abnormalities suggestive of a hypomorph allele, indicating the important role of TLE interaction in pituitary and ocular development.

Heterozygous mutations of *HESX1* have been identified in patients with hypopituitarism and septo-optic dysplasia and are usually associated with less affected phenotypes. Approximately 850 patients were studied for mutations in *HESX1*, including more than 300 patients with septo-optic dysplasia; 410 with isolated pituitary dysfunction, optic nerve hypoplasia, or midline neurologic abnormalities; and 126 with familial inheritance. The incidence of coding region mutations in *HESX1* within this population was about 1%, suggesting that mutations in *HESX1* are a rare cause of hypopituitarism and septo-optic dysplasia.[338]

OTX2. Mutations in other genes have been associated with CNS anatomic abnormalities and hypopituitarism. *OTX2* is a homeobox gene that is expressed earliest in the neuroectoderm[345] cells of the forebrain and midbrain and encodes a transcription factor belonging to the orthodenticle family. This factor also plays a role in ocular development. Murine models harboring mutant *Otx2* genes demonstrate abnormal primitive streak organization and a headless phenotype.[345] OTX2 has a role in regulating early expression of HESX1 and is expressed in the pituitary to regulate POU1F1 (PIT1). Dateki and colleagues[346] identified a frameshift *OTX2* mutation in a patient with bilateral anophthalmia and partial isolated GHD (IGHD) with minimal transactivation activity. A heterozygous *OTX2* mutation was described in two unrelated patients with hypopituitarism; although initial studies demonstrated normal binding to HESX1 binding sites, the mutant *OTX2* gene was demonstrated to have decreased activation of the *HESX1* promoter, suggesting a dominant negative effect leading to CPHD.[347] This relationship between the transcription factors OTX2 and HESX1 emphasizes the complexities of pituitary development and suggests that genetic causes may be multifactorial. Further studies have revealed two frameshift mutations, a nonsense mutation in two unrelated patients and a heterozygous microdeletion in a fifth patient.[346]

SOX3. A syndrome of X-linked hypopituitarism and mental retardation involving duplications of Xq26-27 encompassing *SOX3* (OMIM 313430) has been described in several pedigrees. The affected males have anterior pituitary and infundibular hypoplasia with an undescended posterior pituitary and abnormalities of the corpus callosum. The GHD may also be associated with deficiencies of ACTH, TSH, or gonadotropins. Because *Sox3* is not expressed in Rathke's pouch in the mouse, the anterior pituitary developmental defects are probably secondary to disruption of infundibular development.[325,348-351] Female carriers appear to be clinically unaffected, and no mutations have been found in patients with sex reversal, gonadal dysgenesis, or infertility.[352,353]

SOX2. Heterozygous mutations within *SOX2* in males have been associated with anophthalmia or microphthalmia and anterior pituitary hypoplasia. The resulting hormonal abnormalities include GH and gonadotropin deficiency. Some patients also present with genital abnormalities.[354] A wide variety of additional abnormalities may be present, including hypoplasia of the corpus callosum, hypothalamic hamartoma, hippocampal malformation, esophageal atresia, sensorineural hearing loss, and learning difficulties.[355-358] In addition to de novo heterozygous mutations, nonsynonymous changes have been identified in individuals who inherited the variant from a clinically unaffected parent.[354,358] A perplexing case of a patient with isolated hypogonadotropic hypogonadism but without anterior pituitary hypoplasia suggests that *SOX2* may be independently involved in hypothalamic neuronal development. The expression of *SOX2* has been found to overlap with that of *LHX3* and *HESX1* within Rathke's pouch.[344,354,359]

Acquired Disorders

Inflammation of the Brain or Hypothalamus. Bacterial, viral, or fungal infections may result in hypothalamic/pituitary insufficiency, and the hypothalamus or pituitary or both may also be involved in sarcoidosis.[360]

Tumors of the Brain or Hypothalamus. Brain tumors are a major cause of hypothalamic insufficiency,[361] especially midline brain tumors such as germinomas, meningiomas, gliomas, ependymomas, and gliomas of the optic nerve.[362] Although short stature and GHD are most often associated with suprasellar lesions in neurofibromatosis, they may also exist without such lesions. Whether growth impairment antedates the pathologic findings is not yet clear.[361] Metastases from extracranial carcinomas are rare in children, but hypothalamic insufficiency can result from local extension of craniopharyngeal carcinoma or Hodgkin disease of the nasopharynx. The laboratory diagnosis of GHD in children with brain tumors can be difficult because levels of IGF-1 type I and IGFBP3 are poor predictors, especially in pubertal patients.[363] Craniopharyngiomas and histiocytosis can cause hypothalamic dysfunction (see later discussion).

Trauma of the Brain or Hypothalamus. Head trauma, resulting from boxing and various injuries, can cause IGHD or multiple anterior pituitary deficiencies. Some series of patients with GHD have indicated an increased incidence of birth trauma, such as breech deliveries, extensive use of forceps, prolonged labor, or abrupt delivery. Although GHD can be a consequence of a difficult delivery or hypoxemic perinatal period, it is more commonly associated with developmental deficiencies (discussed previously) or head trauma later in life. In a series of 22 head-injured adolescents and adults, almost 40% had some degree of hypopituitarism.[364-366]

Psychosocial Dwarfism. An extreme form of failure to thrive is termed *psychosocial dwarfism* or *emotional deprivation dwarfism.*[367-370] Most cases of failure to thrive can be traced back to a poor home environment and indadequate parenting, with improved weight gain and growth upon removal of the infant from the dysfunctional home. Some children have been reported, however, to show dramatic behavioral manifestations beyond those in the typical failure-to-thrive infant, namely, bizarre eating and drinking habits, such as drinking from toilets, social withdrawal, and primitive speech.[367] Hyperphagia and abnormalities of GH production may be associated.[368] GH secretion is low in response to pharmacologic stimuli but returns to normal upon removal from the home. Concomitantly, eating and behavioral habits returned to normal, and a period of catch-up growth ensued. Careful assessment of endogenous GH secretion showed reversal of the GH insufficiency within 3 weeks, including enhancement of GH pulse amplitude and a variable increase of pulse frequency.[368] The reversibility of GH secretory defects and the later growth increment in the context of the clinical findings described previously confirm the diagnosis of psychosocial dwarfism.[368]

The neuroendocrinologic mechanisms involved in psychosocial swarfism remain to be elucidated. GH secretion is abnormal and ACTH and TSH levels may also be low, although some patients have high plasma cortisol levels. Even when GH secretion is reduced, treatment with GH is not usually of benefit until the psychosocial situation is improved. Management of the environmental causes of the growth failure is imperative and often associated with substantial growth. In our experience, although psychosocial dysfunction is a common cause of failure to thrive in infancy, the constellation of bizarre behaviors described in psychosocial dwarfism is rare.

The fact that GH production is impaired in adults with varied psychiatric disorders and the growth aberrations of functional GHD with psychosocial dwarfism together suggest that children with emotional problems may have impaired GH secretion and growth.[369] Indeed, depression in children, as adults, can lower GH production,[370] and in girls, anxiety disorders predict a modest height loss in adults.[369]

The Anterior Pituitary

As discussed earlier, many of the disease processes that impair hypothalamic regulation of GH secretion also impair pituitary function. Another group of abnormalities specifically affect pituitary somatotroph development and function.

Congenital Disorders. As many as 3% to 30% of patients with GHD have an affected parent, sibling, or child.[371] Inborn errors of the genes for nuclear transcription factors affecting hypothalamic-pituitary development, the GHRH receptor, or the GH gene can cause GHD and IGF deficiency.

Combined Pituitary Hormone Deficiency. During pituitary development, a series of transcription factors are expressed in a specific timeframe and in a spatial context. The result of cell differentiation and proliferation is a mature anterior pituitary gland with five distinct cell types.[326]

PITX2. PITX2 (also known as *RIEG*) is a member of the bicoid-like homeobox transcription factor family that is closely related to the mammalian OTX genes expressed in the rostral brain during development; it is required at many stages of pituitary development.[326] Studies have shown that activation of the WNT signaling pathway or constitutive activation of β-catenin can induce *PITX2* expression. Further, protein inhibitors of activated STAT (PIAS) modulate PITX2 expression.[372] *PITX2* is expressed in thyrotrophs, gonadotrophs, somatotrophs, and lactotrophs but not in corticotrophs.[373]

PITX2 acts to activate the promoters of pituitary hormone target genes.[374,375] Homozygous loss of *PITX2* results in early embryonic lethality with pituitary development severely affected.[376-379] This is thought to be related to the control of cell cycle regulatory genes by PITX2.[380,381] Furthermore, the lack of *PITX2* also results in excessive cell death during early pituitary development, suggesting a role in cell survival.[382] A mouse line expressing a hypomorphic allele of *Pitx2* provided evidence that the extent of pituitary hypoplasia and cellular differentiation is proportional to the reduced dosage of *Pitx*.[379,383] In this model, the gonadotroph lineage was primarily affected and the numbers of differentiated somatotrophs and thyrotrophs were reduced, but the corticotroph population was unaffected.[383]

In a *Pitx2* overexpression model, the gonadotroph population was expanded, probably because of the role of *Pitx2* in the expression of gonadotroph-specific transcription factors GATA2, EGR1, and NR5A1 (SF1).[382] Mutations of *PITX2* have been described in patients diagnosed with Rieger syndrome, an autosomal dominant condition with variable manifestations including anomalies of the anterior chamber of the eye, dental hypoplasia, a protuberant umbilicus, mental retardation, and pituitary abnormalities. PHX2 has been further associated with a role in left-right signaling, odontogenesis, cardiac development, and atrial fibrillation.[384-386] Mutations of *PITX2*, located within the homeodomain responsible for DNA binding, have been described, and several of these mutations show loss of DNA binding capacity.[387] A heterozygous mutation that changes the lysine at position 50 to glutamic acid in the homeodomain has been found to impart a dominant negative effect leading to a pronounced phenotype.[388]

SOX2. Heterozygous mutations in SOX2 (sex-determining region Y box 2) have been associated with eye abnormalities (i.e., anophthalmia, microphthalmia, and coloboma) and hypopituitarism characterized by anterior pituitary hypoplasia associated with GH and gonadotropin deficiency. Numerous nonsense, frameshift, and missense mutations, as well as chromosome deletions of SOX2, resulting in expression of SOX2 proteins with impaired function, have been identified.[326]

LHX3. LHX3 is a member of the LIM-type homeodomain protein family of transcription factors that feature two LIM domains in their amino terminus (N-terminal) and a centrally located homeodomain used to interact with specific DNA elements on target genes. During development, expression of *LHX3*, which persists in the adult pituitary, is seen in the anterior and intermediate lobes of the pituitary, spinal cord, and medulla.[389] Murine models with targeted disruption of *Lhx3*, reporter transgenic mice, and mutants of LHX3[390] show depletion of thyrotrophs, gonadotrophs, and somatotrophs, suggesting that *Lhx3* is important for cell specification and proliferation.[391] Three LHX3 isoforms have been identified in humans: LHX3a, LHX3b, and M2-LHX3.[392] Of these, LHX3a displays the greatest ability to activate the promoters of pituitary genes. LHX3 interacts with components of the inhibitor of histone acetyltransferase (INHAT) to modulate chromatin structure.[393] Patients with reported mutations in *LHX3* have deficits of GH, PRL, TSH, and gonadotropins, as well as abnormal pituitary morphology along with a rigid cervical spine that limits head rotation.[394-396] *LHX3* mutations are a rare cause of reported hypopituitarism, and one study reported that the incidence of a homozygous *LHX3* mutation in patients studied with CPHD was 2.2%.[397] Several other novel *LHX3* mutations in patients with CPHD demonstrating autosomal recessive inheritance have been reported and characterized.[398-400]

LHX4. LHX4 is another LIM homeodomain protein with homology to LHX3, and it is also expressed in the developing brain, including the cortex, pituitary, and spinal cord.[401] Despite similarities in protein structure, the role of LHX4 in development is distinct from that of LHX3, as demonstrated by single and combined gene-deletion targeting in mice. Murine models with targeted deletion of *Lhx4* form a definitive Rathke's pouch that arrests and results in a hypoplastic pituitary. In contrast to *Lhx3* gene knockout mice, *Lhx4*[−/−] mice contain all five differentiated cell types.[402,403] *Lhx3* expression is impaired in the *Lhx4* mutants, suggesting that *Lhx4* is required for cell survival, expansion of the pouch, and differentiation of pituitary-specific cell lineages.

Several reports have described CPHD patients with evidence of a hypoplastic pituitary who harbored *LHX4* mutations.[389,404,405] These heterozygous mutations have been shown to result in proteins that are unable to bind DNA and activate pituitary gene expression.[406] Further studies have demonstrated a functional relationship between POU1F1 and LHX4 in the regulation of POU1F1 expression in specific pituitary cell types.[407] Also, several studies have suggested that LHX4 and PROP1 have overlapping functions in pituitary development.[402] Finally, in addition to pituitary hormone deficiencies, *LHX4* mutations have been implicated in structural abnormalities; patients with an *LHX4* mutation have been reported with abnormal MRI findings including a hypoplastic anterior pituitary, ectopic posterior lobe, poorly developed sella turcica, and Chiari malformation.[408]

SIX6. SIX6 is a member of the SIX/sine oculis family of homeobox genes that is expressed in retina, optic nerve, hypothalamus, and pituitary.[409] Murine expression studies of the TCF/LEF family of transcription factors during pituitary development demonstrated that *Six6* plays a role in proliferation of cells during early formation of Rathke's pouch.[410] *SIX6* has also been shown to interact with the Groucho family of transcriptional repressors.[411,412] Mice lacking *SIX6* demonstrate infertility.[413] *SIX6* has been mapped to chromosome 14q22-23, and patients with deletions of this chromosomal region display bilateral anophthalmia and pituitary anomalies.[414,415] Patients with anophthalmia/microphthalmia were shown to have several frequent polymorphisms of *Six6* and one potential causative missense mutation.[409] One case report implicated *SIX6* haploinsufficiency as being responsible for ocular and pituitary maldevelopment. Despite its importance in early development, further studies are required to determine whether *SIX6* mutations are present in patients with pituitary hormone deficiency.

ISL1. ISL1 is a member of the LIM homeodomain family of transcription factors, which are characterized by two tandemly repeated cysteine/histidine-rich LIM domains that are involved in protein-protein interactions. ISL1 has been shown to be a transcriptional regulator of LHX3.[416] Its expression is restricted to cells that will express the pituitary of glycoprotein hormone α-subunit (αGSU) gene.[417,418] Homozygous loss of *Isl1* in mice results in developmental arrest with no pouch formation.[419] To date, no human mutations in *ISL1* have been identified.

PROP1. Mutations in *PROP1*, a paired-like homeodomain transcription factor with expression restricted to the anterior pituitary during development, have also been found to result in CPHD.[420] Mutation of this gene is responsible for a form of murine pituitary-dependent dwarfism known as the Ames mouse.[421] The pituitary gland appears to be enlarged in mice bearing mutations in *Prop1*, although the mechanism is unclear.[421-424] In the end, a decrease in proliferation and apoptosis results in pituitary hypoplasia, similar to that seen in humans.[402,422-426] The switch from repression of target gene expression by HESX1 to activation by PROP1 is important for development of the POU1F1 (GH, PRL, and TSH) and gonadotroph lineages.[334,424,427] PROP1 and β-catenin have been shown to form a complex that represses *Hesx1* while activating *Pou1f1* expression.[428] PROP1 bends to a palindrome TAAT sequence as a dimer to actuate target gene expression.[429,430] The gonadotropin deficiency in the Ames dwarf remains unexplained, although treatment with thyroxine (T₄) or GH (or both) restored fertility in some male mice and restored sexual maturation, but not fertility, in female mice.[431,432]

Mutations of *PROP1* in humans result in GH, PRL, and TSH deficiencies, although failure in all cell lineages, including gonadotrophs and corticotrophs, has been reported.[433-435] The characterization of *PROP1* mutations is complex, because the phenotypes are variable and dynamic and hormone deficiencies may develop over time even in patients with similar genetic backgrounds.[433,436,437] Gonadotropin abnormalities are particularly diverse in that approximately 30% of patients have spontaneous pubertal development, including menarche, before ultimately developing hypogonadotropic hypogonadism.[433,438] Apparently normal growth without GH has also been found in a child with PROP1 deficiency.[439,440] The ACTH deficiency may develop in the fourth or fifth decade of life.[441] Striking variability has been described in pituitary size, with very large glands, possibly arising from the intermediate lobe,[442] producing a hyperintense T1-weighted signal occasionally demonstrated by MRI.[434,443,444] These glands may undergo involution, leaving a large empty sella in patients with complete anterior hypopituitarism including ACTH deficiency.[445-447]

Many *PROP1* (chromosome 5q35, OMIM 601538) abnormalities have been identified, including missense, frameshift, and splicing mutations. A GA repeat in exon 2 (295-CGA-GAG-AGT-303) has been reported to be a "hot spot" in *PROP1;* any combination of a GA or AG deletion in this repeat region results in a frameshift in the coding sequence and premature termination at codon 109.[438,448] Similar abnormalities result from homozygous lesions at other sites on exon 2 and affect codons 73, 88, and 149.[438,448]

Compound heterozygosity for two mutations was detected in 36% of children from four families; two different common deletions both led to a stop codon at position 109.[449] These mutations are predicted to result in loss of the DNA-binding and C-terminal transactivating domains of *PROP1*. Some missense mutations have been shown to retain partial activity.[434,435,450] Two mutations in the transactivating domain, not the DNA binding domain (W194 X Prop1, S156 insTProp1), were shown to differentially affect DNA binding and transactivation.[451]

There does not appear to be strong correlation between phenotype and genotype.[438] A screen of 73 subjects (36 families) diagnosed with CPHD by Deladoey and associates identified 35 patients with *PROP1* gene defects, including three different missense mutations, two frameshift mutations, and one splice site mutation. In 12 of 36 unrelated families, defects were located in the region nt296 through nt302, suggesting a possible hot spot for *PROP1* mutations in CPHD.[438] Although *PROP1* mutations appear to be rare in sporadic cases, their prevalence is 29.5% in familial cases of CHPD, as reported by Turton and colleagues.[353,452] Nyström and associates reported compound heterozygous mutations in the *PROP1* gene in twins with hypopituitarism and late ACTH deficiency.[453]

POU1F1. The *POU1F1* gene (chromosome 3p11, OMIM 173110) encodes PIT1, a member of a large family of transcription factors referred to as POU-domain proteins that is responsible for pituitary-specific transcription of genes for GH, PRL, TSH, and the GHRH receptor.[58,454-456] PIT1, a 290–amino acid protein, contains two domains, the POU-specific and the POU-homeo domains; both are necessary for DNA binding and activation of GH and PRL genes and for regulation of the PRL, TSH-β, and POU1F1 genes.[457] Its expression is restricted to the anterior pituitary to control differentiation, proliferation, and survival of somatotrophs, lactotrophs, and thyrotrophs.[371,456-458] PIT1 regulates target genes by binding to response elements and recruiting coactivator proteins, such as cAMP response element–binding protein (CREB)-binding protein (CBP).[459] Gene expression microarray assays combined with chromatin immunoprecipitation (CHIP) were used to detect targets of POUIFI.[273]

Two mouse models were first reported to have GH, PRL, and TSH deficiencies associated with mutations or rearrangements of the *Pit1* gene; these were the Snell (dw/dwS) and the Jackson (dw/dwJ) dwarf mice.[460,461] Many different mutations of the *POU1F1* gene have been found internationally in families with GHD and PRL deficiency and variable defects in TSH expression.[462-465] These mutations are transmitted as autosomal recessive or dominant traits and cause variable peptide hormone deficiencies with or without anterior pituitary hypoplasia.[462-468]

The most common mutation is an R271W substitution that affects the POU homeodomain, encoding a mutant protein that binds normally to DNA and acts as a dominant inhibitor of transcription.[468-471] Vertical transmission of the R271W mutation was shown, emphasizing the importance of diagnostic and theraputic management during pregnancy.[472] Evidence from a patient with the R271W mutation suggests that PIT1 may have a role in cell survival.[471] Indeed, the mutation was used to target cell proliferation tumoral model systems. A patient diagnosed with GHD, along with dysregulation of PRL and TSH, was reported to have a lysine-to–glutamic acid mutation at codon 216 (K216E).[457] This mutant PIT1 binds to DNA and appears not to inhibit basal activation of GH and PRL genes; however, the mutant is unable to support retinoic acid induction of *POU1F1* gene expression. Another report suggested that CBP (p300) recruitment and PIT1 dimerization are necessary for target gene activation and that disruption of this process may account for the pathogenesis of CPHD.[473] All of the reported mutations involve sites affecting *POU1F1* DNA-binding, dimerization, or target gene transactivation.

Phenotypic variability occurs among patients with apparently similar genotypes. It does not appear that ACTH or gonadotropin deficiencies occur, as is frequently the case with *PROP1* defects,[452] but adrenarche has been reported to be absent or delayed in patients with a POU1F1 mutation.[474] Circulating antibodies against Pit1 have been identified to be responsible for hypopituitarism similar to that caused by mutations.[475]

Isolated Growth Hormone Deficiency. The incidence of IGHD is estimated to be 1 in every 3480 to 10,000 live births.[78,476-478] In most children with IGHD, no cause can be identified, and this group is often referred to as having idiopathic GHD. However, there is increasing recognition that genetic defects underlie some cases of GHD. Patients with GHD may develop deficiencies of additional anterior pituitary hormones.[479] Four forms of IGHD have been reported (see Table 24-2).[480] The classification system is based on clinical characteristics, inheritance patterns, and GH secretion but not necessarily on disease causation. IGHD was most recently reviewed by Alatzoglou and associates.[481]

The gene encoding GH *(GH1)* is located on chromosome 17q23 in a cluster that includes two genes for placental lactogen (hPL), a pseudogene for hPL, and the *GH2* gene that encodes placental GH. *GH1* and *GH2* differ in mRNA splicing pattern: *GH1* generates 20- and 22-kDa proteins (of approximately equal bioactivity), whereas *GH2* yields a protein that differs from *GH1* by 13 amino acid residues.

IGHD Type I. IGHD type IA results primarily from large deletions, with rare microdeletions and single base-pair substitutions of the *GH1* gene that prevent synthesis or secretion of the hormone.[481,482] IGHD IA is inherited as an autosomal recessive trait, and affected individuals have profound congenital GHD. Because GH is not produced even in fetal life, patients are immunologically intolerant of GH and typically develop anti-GH antibodies when treated with either pituitary-derived or recombinant DNA–derived GH. When antibodies prevent patients from responding to GH, IGHD IA can be viewed as a form of GH insensitivity, and such patients are candidates for IGF-1 therapy.

The less severe form of autosomal recessive GHD, termed IGHD type IB, also may result from mutations or rearrangements of the *GH1* gene that cause production of an aberrant GH molecule that retains some function or at least generates immune tolerance. The phenotypic variability is greater than in IGHD IA.[480,481] These patients usually respond to exogenous GH therapy without antibody production. The very low frequency (1.7%) of *GH1* gene mutations in familial type IB IGHD suggests the importance of studying the *GH1* gene promoter region in patients with unexplained GHD.[483] In a group of 65 children with IGHD IB, the GHRH receptor gene *(GHRHR)* was normal in domains coding for the extracellular region,[484] but mutations in transmembrane and intracellular gene domains were found in 10% of families with IGHD IB.[485]

IGHD Type II. IGHD type II is inherited as an autosomal dominant trait. The most common cause appears to be mutations that inactivate the 5′ splice donor site of intron 3 of the *GH1* gene, resulting in skipping of exon 3 and producing a molecule that cannot fold normally. It is likely that the 17.5-kDa GH isoform mutant functions in a dominant-negative manner to suppress intracellular accumulation and secretion of wild-type GH.[486-488] In patients

with missense mutations in exon 4 or 5, clinical presentation is quite variable, with some evidence for reversibility of the impairment of intracellular GH storage and secretion by GH treatment.[489] Mullis and coworkers[490] studied 57 subjects from 19 families and found that patients with IGHD type II not only have a variable phenotype in terms of onset, severity, and progression of GHD but also may demonstrate later onset of ACTH or TSH deficiencies and pituitary hypoplasia. An extensive assessment of *GH1* gene mutations in short children with and without GHD revealed a substantial number of heterozygous mutations.[490] Recent studies characterizing the mechanism of the GH secretory defects and the increased expression of the 17.5-kDa isoform may lead to novel molecular therapies.[491]

Mutations in *GHRHR* are also classified as IGHD type IB. The GHRH receptor is G protein coupled with seven transmembrane domains and is found predominantly in the pituitary gland. Mutation of the gene for *Ghrhr* in its ligand-binding domain has been identified in the *little mouse (lit/lit)*[486] and results in dwarfism and decreased numbers of somatotrophs.[456,492,493] In this model, the fetal somatotroph mass is normal, and hypoplasia (but not absence) of the somatotrophs is evident only postnatally.[456,458,492,493] Such data suggest that GHRH is not an essential factor for fetal differentiation of the somatotrophs and that GHRH-independent cells persist or that mutation does not cause total loss of GHRH function. The human *GHRHR* gene is 15 kb with 13 exons. The GHRHR protein is encoded by a 1.3-kb cDNA.[72,494-496]

Wajnrajch and colleagues reported the first human cases of a mutation in the *GHRHR* gene in two cousins in a consanguineous Indian Muslim family with IGF deficiency and profound growth failure.[497] The gene defect, a nonsense mutation that introduced a stop codon at position 72 (E72X), resulted in a markedly truncated GHRHR protein that lacked the membrane-spanning regions and the G protein–binding site. The affected children had undetectable GH release during standard provocative tests and after exogenous GHRH administration but responded to GH treatment. The same mutation was also identified in a reportedly unrelated Tamoulean kindred in Sri Lanka,[498] in a consanguineous kindred in Pakistan ("dwarfism of Sindh"),[499,500] and in 17 patients from one Muslim and four Hindu families in Western India.[501] The largest kindred in which a mutation of *GHRHR* was identified was a Brazilian family with a homozygous donor splice mutation (G to A at position +1) of exon 1.[78] This mutation disrupts the highly conserved consensus GT of the 50-donor splice site, generating a truncated GHRHR.[502,503]

A *GHRHR* missense mutation in exon 11 (R357C) was described in two consanguineous Israeli Arab families.[504] Patients in all of the groups had early growth failure with short stature (−4.5 to −8.6 SD), a high-pitched voice, and increased abdominal fat accumulation.[499,503] As expected, all of the patients demonstrated severely reduced or undetectable serum concentrations of GH in response to provocative GH stimulation, as well as very low serum concentrations of IGF-1, IGFBP3, and ALS.[503] The adults manifest an unfavorable cardiovascular risk profile, which includes increased levels of low-density lipoprotein cholesterol and total cholesterol, elevated C-reactive protein, elevated blood pressure, and abdominal obesity. However, a perplexing study found no evidence of premature atherosclerosis or premature myocardial ischemia in these patients with *GHRHR* mutations.[505] The patients respond well to exogenous GH without antibody formation. Heterozygotes may have minimal height deficits and may show moderate biochemical deficiencies of the GH-IGF axis.[499] Despite extensive study, the geographic separation and ethnic differences among these patient groups do not suggest recent (>200 years) contact among the families from the Indian subcontinent. At present, the likely explanation for all four families is that of a "founder effect" or one-time mutation in each group followed by propagation within a geographically isolated gene pool.[78] In an analysis of 30 families with IGHD type IB, Salvatori and colleagues[485] found new missense mutations in transmembrane and intracellular domains of the *GHRHR* in three families (10%), with two affected members in each. Transfection experiments indicated normal cellular expression of these mutant receptors. Mutations in GHRH were recently reviewed by Corazzini and Salvatori.[506]

IGHD Type III. IGHD type III, transmitted as an X-linked trait with associated hypogammaglobulinemia,[507] has not yet been related to a mutation of the *GH1* gene. A large Australian kindred demonstrated GHD with a variable spectrum of pituitary hormonal deficiencies that may have been caused by duplication of the Xq25-Xq28 region.[508]

Bioactive GH. Serum GH exists in multiple molecular forms, reflecting the consequences of alternative post-transcriptional or post-translational processing of the mRNA or protein, respectively. Some of these forms are presumed to have defects in the amino acid sequences required for binding of GH to its receptor, and different molecular forms of GH may have varying potencies for stimulating skeletal growth, although this remains to be rigorously proved. Short stature with normal GH immunoreactivity but reduced biopotency has been suggested,[509,510] but the molecular abnormalities have been characterized in relatively few patients, and many cases of suspected bioinactive GH have not been rigorously proved.[511,512]

In one child with extreme short stature (−6.1 SDS), a mutant GH caused by a single missense heterozygous mutation (cysteine to arginine, codon 77 of *GH1*) bound with greater affinity than normal to GHBP and the GHR and inhibited the action of normal GH. The child grew more (6 versus 3.9 cm/year) during a period of exogenous GH in moderate dosage. The father was found to have the same genetic abnormality but did not express the mutant hormone. In a second patient[512] with marked short stature (−3.6 SDS), a heterozygous alanine-to-glycine substitution in exon 4 of GH led to a substitution of glycine for arginine. This mutation was located in site 2 of GH molecular binding with its receptor and apparently led to failure of appropriate molecular rotation of the dimerized receptor and subsequent diminished tyrosine phosphorylation and the GH-mediated intracellular cascade of events. Bioactivity determined in a mouse B-cell lymphoma line was about 33% of immunoreactivity.[513] Exogenous GH substantially increased growth velocity (from 4.5 to 11.0 cm/year).

An Ile179Met substitution found in a short child was characterized by normal STAT5 activation but a 50% decrement in ERK activation.[141] This novel finding demonstrated the complexity of the functional interaction of GH with its receptor, but because STAT5B is clearly the major (if not the sole) GH-dependent mediator of *IGF1* gene transcription, the role of this mutation is not clear. Six GH heterozygous variants with evidence of impairment of JAK/STAT activation were found by screening of short children, suggesting that further studies are needed to determine the mechanism of interaction of GH with its receptor.[514] Because these variants occur in heterozygotes, the genotype-phenotype correlations are unclear. In one of the more convincing cases of bioinactive GH reported to date, Besson and associates[515] found a homozygous missense mutation (G705C) in a short child (−3.6 SDS) that resulted in absence

of two disulfide bridges. Both GHR binding and JAK2/STAT5 signaling activity were markedly reduced.

Some patients demonstrate a decrease in bioactivity (when measured by sensitive in vitro assays) but not in immunoreactivity. The absence of mutations suggests that abnormal post-translational modifications of GH or other peripheral mechanisms may be responsible.[516,517]

Acquired Disorders

Craniopharyngiomas and Other Tumors. Many tumors that impair hypothalamic function also affect pituitary secretion of GH. In addition, *craniopharyngiomas* are a major cause of pituitary insufficiency. These tumors arise from remnants of Rathke's pouch, the diverticulum of the roof of the embryonic oral cavity that normally gives rise to the anterior pituitary. The diagnosis and treatment of craniopharyngioma has been recently reviewed. This tumor is a congenital malformation present at birth and gradually grows over the ensuing years. The tumor arises from rests of squamous cells at the junction of the adenohypophysis and neurohypophysis and forms a cyst as it enlarges; the cyst contains degenerated cells and may calcify but does not undergo malignant degeneration. The cyst fluid ranges from the consistency of machine oil to a shimmering, cholesterol-laden liquid, and the calcifications may be microscopic or gross. About 75% of craniopharyngiomas arise in the suprasellar region; the remainder resemble pituitary adenomas. Mutations in β-catenin have been found in patients with adamantinomatous craniopharyngiomas.[518]

Craniopharyngiomas can cause manifestations at any age from infancy to adulthood but usually manifest in middle childhood. The most common presentation results from increased intracranial pressure and includes headaches, vomiting, and oculomotor abnormalities. Visual field defects result from compression of the optic chiasm, and papilledema or optic atrophy may be present. Visual and olfactory hallucinations have been reported, as have seizures and dementia. Most children with craniopharyngiomas have evidence of growth failure at the time of presentation, and they are often found retrospectively to have had reduced growth since infancy.[519] GH and the gonadotropins are the most commonly affected pituitary hormones in children and adults, but deficiency of TSH and ACTH may also occur, and diabetes insipidus is present in 25% to 50% of patients.[519] Between 50% and 80% of patients have abnormalities of at least one anterior pituitary hormone at diagnosis.

Cystic and solid components can be identified by MRI, and anatomic relationships can be delineated to help plan a rational operative approach. Operative intervention via craniotomy or transsphenoidal resection may result in partial or almost complete removal of the lesion. Postoperative irradiation is commonly used, especially if tumor resection was incomplete. In some patients, particularly those who become obese, a syndrome of normal linear growth without GH may occur. The metabolic syndrome, with evidence of insulin insensitivity and increased body mass index (BMI), is common and is a predictor of potential major long-term morbidity.[519-521] The long-term childhood and adolescent consequences of craniopharyngioma are substantial, with many quality-of-life issues exacerbating the hypopituitarism. Patients with a history of hypothalamic obesity associated with craniopharyngiomas undergoing brain surgery were favored to have sustained weight loss.

Pituitary adenomas (see Chapter 9) are infrequent during childhood and adolescence, accounting for fewer than 5% of patients undergoing surgery at large centers. Almost two thirds of tumors immunochemically stain for

PRL, and a small number stain for GH. GH-secreting pituitary adenomas are exceedingly unusual in youth. There is a variable experience as to the invasive nature of pituitary adenomas, but the prevailing opinion is that they are less aggressive in children than in adults. In 56 patients at the Mayo Clinic with non–ACTH-secreting adenomas removed transsphenoidally, macroadenomas were about one third more frequent than microadenomas, with cases in girls outnumbering those in boys 3.3 to 1. The patients with macroadenoma had an approximately 50% incidence of hypopituitarism, compared with zero incidence in those patients with microadenomas; long-term cure rates were between 55% and 65% for both tumor sizes. Familial isolated pituitary adenoma (FIPA) accounts for about 2% of pituitary adenomas and is associated with aryl hydrocarbon receptor interacting protein (AIP) gene mutations. Gigantism is a feature of some patients with somatotropinomas.[522]

Histiocytosis X. The localized or generalized proliferation of mononuclear macrophages (histiocytes) characterizes Langerhans cell histiocytosis, a diverse disorder that occurs in patients of all ages, with a peak incidence at ages 1 to 4 years. Endocrinologists are more familiar with the term *histiocytosis X,* which includes three related disorders: solitary bony disease (eosinophilic granuloma), Hand-Schüller-Christian disease (chronic disease with diabetes insipidus, exophthalmos, and multiple calvarial lesions), and disseminated histiocytosis X (Letterer-Siwe disease, with widespread visceral involvement). These syndromes are characterized by an infiltration and accumulation of Langerhans cells in the involved areas, such as skull, hypothalamic-pituitary stalk, CNS, and viscera. Although these disorders, especially Hand-Schüller-Christian disease, are classically associated with diabetes insipidus, approximately 50% to 75% of patients in selected series have growth failure and GHD at the time of presentation. The degree of pituitary stalk thickness has been shown to correlate with long-term risk outcomes.[523] In contrast, a French national registry (*n* = 589) found GHD in 61 subjects, with overall endocrine dysfunction in 148. In the latter group, an evolving neurodegenerative syndrome (identified in 10% of patients with 15-year follow-up) seemed to be associated with pituitary involvement.[524] Only 1% of unselected children with Langerhans cell histiocytosis living in Canada during a 15-year period had GHD.[525]

Growth Hormone Insensitivity

Mutations in GHR Signaling Proteins and ALS. Conditions of GH insensitivity, also referred to as *primary IGF-1 deficiency,* encompass a variety of genetic conditions characterized by growth failure, high serum GH levels, and very low serum IGF-1 levels.[526] These findings, first described in siblings in 1966 by Laron and colleagues,[527] are also known collectively as *Laron syndrome.* Fewer than 500 cases of true GH insensitivity have been identified worldwide, with most individuals from pedigrees of Mediterranean or Middle Eastern descent. Members of a well-described pedigree from Ecuador were from an inbred population with Mediterranean origins.[528]

The phenotypic characteristics of GH insensitivity include growth failure evident at birth[527] with postnatal subnormal growth velocities and stature −4 to −10 SD below the mean (Fig. 24-34).[526] Patients also have a subnormal head circumference, protruding forehead, abnormal upper- to lower-body ratio, short extremities, and sparse hair (Table 24-4). There is delayed motor development, indicating the importance of IGF-1 in cerebral development. The genitalia are small, and puberty is delayed, but fertility is normal. Metabolically, the most striking feature

of IGF-1 deficiency is hypoglycemia with later development of obesity, relative hyperinsulinemia, and insulin resistance.[529] Individuals do not respond to exogenous GH, as determined by growth velocity, hypoglycemia incidence, or serum IGF-1 or IGFBP1 levels.[530] In addition, GHBP activity is usually undetectable in sera of these patients,[531,532] but measurable levels correspond to higher final heights.

Almost 20 years after the original description of GH insensitivity, liver biopsy performed on two affected patients demonstrated that microsomal cells did not bind recombinant GH, suggesting a defect in the GHR.[533] Subsequently, both deletions and homozygous point mutations (missense, nonsense, and abnormal splicing) in the GHR were described in persons with GH insensitivity.[534-536] The initially described gene deletion involved exons 3, 5, and 6.[537] Deletion of exons 5 and 6 results in a frameshift and a premature translational stop signal with consequent encoding of a receptor lacking most of the extracellular GH-binding domain.

More than 60 distinct mutations of the *GHR* gene resulting in GH insensitivity have been reported to date.[538] Most of the mutations are in the extracellular (GH-binding) domain of the receptor and result in impaired ability of GH to bind to the receptor; this leads to a deficiency of circulating GHBP, which is derived from the extracellular domain of the receptor. One reported mutation of the extracellular domain does not affect GH binding to the receptor but prevents dimerization of the receptor.[539] Homozygous mutations have also been reported in the transmembrane domain.[540,541] These mutations result in GH insensitivity with normal GH binding but lack of receptor transduction. Because the extracellular domain is intact and the mutant receptor protein apparently becomes detached from the cell receptor surface, GHBP levels are normal to elevated.

Mutations affecting the intracellular domain of the GHR have also been found. Two defects directly involving the intracellular domain have been reported to result in dominantly inherited GH insensitivity.[542-547] In the two heterozygous mutations reported, truncation of the GHR results in absence of the intracellular domain. In vitro, the GHR molecule behaves in a dominant negative manner, presumably by retaining an ability to dimerize with the normal GHR and thereby inhibiting GH-induced tyrosine phosphorylation of STAT5.[544,546,547] Mutations resulting in C-terminal deletions of the intracellular domain of the GHR have been shown to exhibit normal GH binding and JAK2 phosphorylation but impaired phosphorylation of STAT5B.[548,549]

That a dominant negative effect has been described for some mutations raises the question of whether heterozygosity for defects of the extracellular domain can also result in short stature. Heterozygosity for defects of *GHR* has been reported to cause some degree of relative GH insensitivity, with modest growth improvement occurring only with high doses of GH.[550-553] In addition, a truncated *GHR* splice variant has been described that functions as a dominant negative inhibitor of the full-length receptor and results in large amounts of GHBP, further downregulating GHR function.[554]

The most extensively studied polymorphism in the *GHR* gene is the deletion of exon 3 (*GHRd3*), which is present in up to 50% of Caucasians. It has been proposed that GHRs without exon 3 bind GH with comparable affinity[555,556] but may transduce the signal with a different intensity in vitro.[555,556] In an observational study, GH treatment of short children with GHD found that those with one or two copies of the *GHRd3* variant grew faster than other children after correction for GH dosing.[555,556] Similar

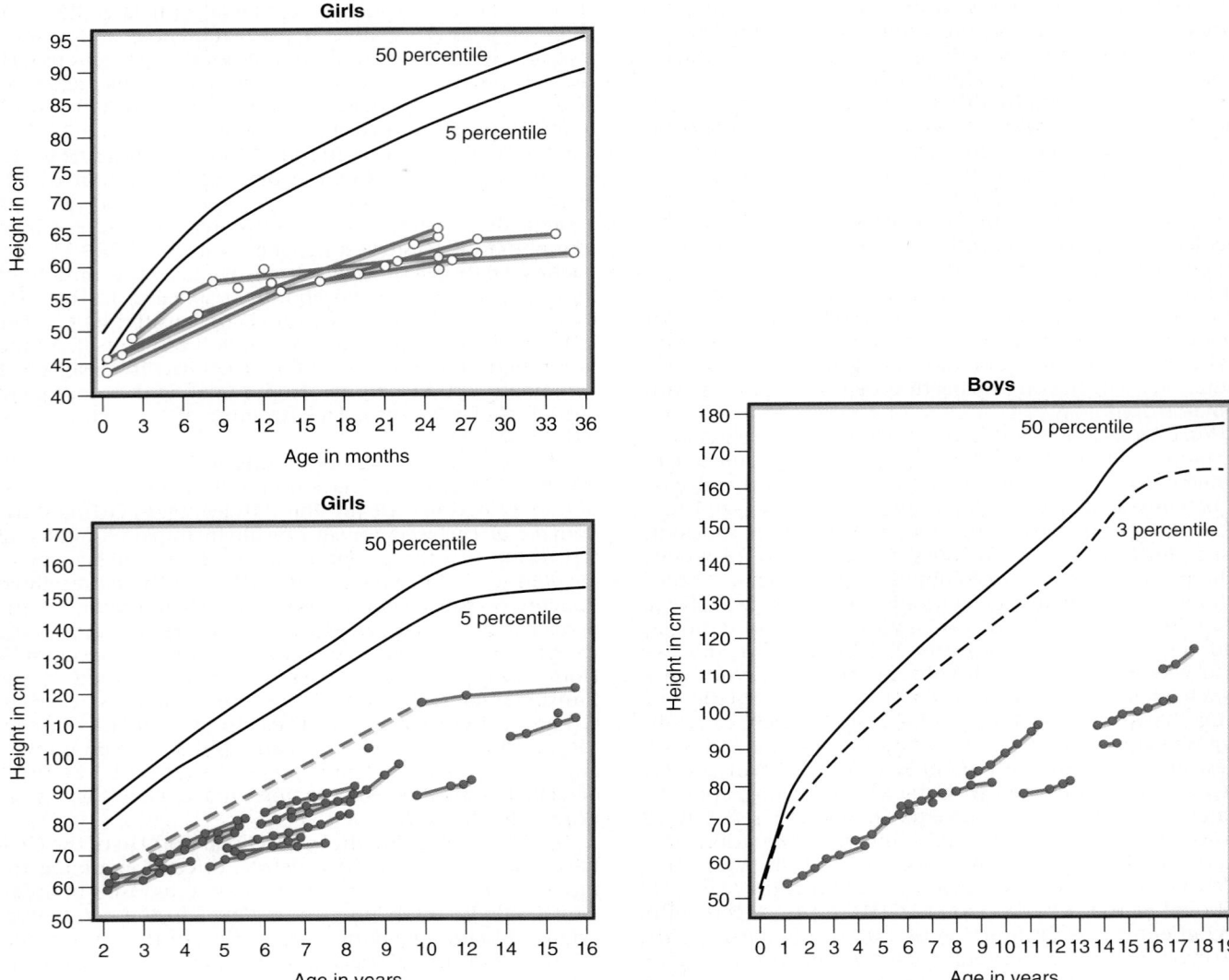

Figure 24-34 Height measurements for Ecuadorian children with insulin-like growth factor (IGF) deficiency resulting from growth hormone (GH) insensitivity. (From Rosenfeld RG, Rosenbloom AL, Guevara-Aguirre J. Growth hormone [GH] resistance due to primary GH receptor deficiency. *Endocr Rev.* 1994;15:369-390.)

observations were reported in studies of patients with TS and children with SGA.[555,556] Different studies reported different findings on whether GH-deficient children with the *GHRd3* variant experience faster growth.[557-559] Different GH dosing among studies and differences among the populations studied could account for the varying results.

Some patients with the phenotype of GH insensitivity but without mutations of the *GHR* gene have been found to have mutations in downstream GHR signaling molecules. Homozygous mutations in the *Stat5B* gene have been found to cause GH insensitivity either by decreasing the phosphorylation of tyrosine[560] with resultant inability to dock with phosphotyrosines on GH-activated receptors or to stably bind DNA[561] or by causing an insertion in exon 10 leading to early protein termination.[562] A mutation in the SH2 domain of *Stat5b* has also been described, leading to inability to induce gene transcription.[563] Patients with mutations in *Stat5b* have evidence of immune dysfunction and recurrent pulmonary infections, presumably because Stat5B is involved in downstream signaling for multiple cytokines. To date, no mutations of the genes for JAK2 or MAP kinase have been implicated in GH insensitivity.

Deletion of Jak2 in mice is embryonically lethal, as detailed earlier.

Markedly reduced serum concentrations of IGF-1 and IGFBP3 have been observed in two cases involving mutations of the ALS gene.[564,565] Even though IGF-1 and IGFBP3 were as low as in patients with classic GH insensitivity, the index case attained an adult height within the normal range. Whether the relatively normal growth of these patients reflects the greater importance of locally produced IGF-1 or altered kinetics of serum IGF-1 in the face of reduced concentrations of binding proteins remains uncertain.

Abnormalities of IGF-1 and IGF-1 Receptor Signaling. Woods and colleagues[566] described a 15-year-old boy with deletion of exons 4 and 5 of the *IGF1* gene that resulted in a truncated IGF-1 molecule. The boy exhibited severe prenatal and postnatal (approximately −7 SDS) growth retardation unresponsive to GH in addition to sensorineural deafness, mental retardation, and microcephaly. He had normal IGFBP3 and GHBP levels, undetectable IGF-1 levels, and hyperinsulinism. On treatment with IGF-1, the child experienced growth and improved metabolic parameters.[567]

TABLE 24-4

Clinical Features of Growth Hormone Insensitivity

Parameter	Clinical Finding
Growth and Development	
Birth weight	Near-normal
Birth length	May be slightly decreased
Postnatal growth	Severe growth failure
Bone age	Delayed, but may be advanced relative to height age
Genitalia	Micropenis in childhood; normal for body size in adults
Puberty	Delayed 3 to 7 years
Sexual function and fertility	Normal
Craniofacies	
Hair	Sparse before age 7 years
Forehead	Prominent; frontal bossing
Skull	Normal head circumference; craniofacial disproportion due to small facies
Facies	Small
Nasal bridge	Hypoplastic
Orbits	Shallow
Dentition	Delayed eruption
Sclerae	Blue
Voice	High-pitched
Musculoskeletal/Metabolic/Miscellaneous	
Blood glucose	Hypoglycemia in infants and children; fasting symptoms in some adults
Walking and motor milestones	Delayed
Hips	Dysplasia; avascular necrosis of femoral head
Elbow	Limited extensibility
Skin	Thin, prematurely aged
Bone mineral density	Osteopenia

Disruption of one allele of the *IGF1* gene has been associated with short stature. In one report of a kindred of members with height SDS -4.0 and low but detectable IGF-1, heterozygous mutation in the *IGF1* gene caused splicing of exon 4 and resultant protein truncation.[568] A second report of a child with height of –2.7 SDS and an IGF-1 level in the low normal range was found to have a 260-kb heterozygous deletion of chromosome 12, which includes the *IGF1* gene.[569]

Inactivating Mutation of the IGF1 Gene. An adult was identified who had the same phenotype as the boy with the *IGF1* deletion but with markedly elevated serum IGF-1 levels.[217] A homozygous point mutation in the *IGF1* gene was found. This mutation resulted in an IGF-1 molecule with markedly reduced affinity for the IGF-1 receptor that poorly stimulated autophosphorylation of the IGF-1 receptor and activation of AKT or ERK.[570] Family members heterozygous for this mutation were found to have significantly lower birth weight, final height, and head circumference, suggesting an effect of heterozygosity for this mutation on IGF-1 function.

Primary Defects of IGF Transport and Clearance. An extremely short boy (–6 SDS) with increased GH, normal IGF-1, and 20- to 30-fold elevated IGFBP1 levels had improvement in growth and suppression of IGFBP1 levels with GH administration. The growth failure was hypothesized to result from inhibition of IGF-1 action by IGFBP1. Tollefson and colleagues identified a child with growth failure whose fibroblasts were resistant to IGF-1.[571] The fibroblasts were able to be stimulated with an IGF variant that exhibited a 600-fold lower binding affinity for IGFBPs and secreted more IGFBPs than normal, suggesting an IGFBP inhibition of IGF-1 action.

Primary Defects of IGF-1 Receptor Production or Responsiveness. Patients with IUGR and postnatal growth failure, microcephaly, and mental retardation with normal to elevated serum IGF-1 levels have been reported to have reduced binding of IGF-1 to its receptor.[223,572] Studies in the African Efe pygmies demonstrated extreme insensitivity to the in vitro growth-enhancing effects of IGF-1.[573] Explanations for these findings include reduced IGF-1 receptor transcripts and sites with resultant diminished tyrosine phosphorylation and postreceptor signaling. Fang and associates published a report of a patient with height –5.9 SDS with elevated IGF-1 levels and resultant decreased activation of downstream signaling pathways.[574]

In leprechaunism, a syndrome of growth failure and insulin receptor dysfunction, there is variable IGF-1 insensitivity.[575,576] The profound abnormality of the insulin receptor suggests that heterodimeric insulin and IGF-1 receptor combinations might lead to failed activation of the IGF-1 signaling cascade. The IGF-1 receptor gene resides on 15q, so persons with deletions of the distal long arm of chromosome 15 or ring chromosome 15 have heterozygosity of the IGF-1 receptor.[576,577] These patients may have IUGR and postnatal growth failure, but lack of a biologic response to IGF-1 has not been conclusively demonstrated.[577] Therefore, whether the growth failure is caused by altered levels of IGF-1 receptor or is a result of the loss of other genes located on 15q remains to be determined.

Disorders Outside the Growth Hormone/IGF Axis

Many systemic disorders, if severe enough, can cause growth failure in children. Those that primarily alter hormones that directly regulate growth (e.g., thyroid hormone, glucocorticoids) can be understood based on the known actions of those hormones. Even in those disorders in which the pathology is not primarily within the endocrine system, there is often an underlying hormonal abnormality contributing to the growth failure. In some cases, the underlying disorder produces a secondary hormone deficiency. Those disorders in which a hormone deficiency cannot be identified may be thought of as demonstrating hormone resistance, because these children have growth failure in the presence of normal GH production.

Malnutrition

Given the worldwide presence of undernutrition, inadequate intake of energy (calories), protein, or both is the most common cause of growth failure. *Marasmus* refers to an overall deficiency of calories including protein malnutrition. Subcutaneous fat is minimal, and protein wasting is marked. *Kwashiorkor* refers specifically to inadequate protein intake, although it may also be characterized by some caloric undernutrition. Frequently, the two conditions overlap. Decreased weight growth usually precedes the failure of linear growth by a very short time in the neonatal period and by several years at older ages. Stunting of growth due to caloric or protein malnutrition in early life often has lifelong consequences, including diminished skeletal growth.[578]

Both acute and chronic malnutrition affect the GH/IGF-1 system. The impaired growth seen in malnutrition is usually associated with elevated basal or stimulated serum GH levels,[579,580] although in some cases of generalized malnutrition (marasmus) the GH levels are normal or low.[581] In both conditions, serum IGF-1 levels are reduced.[580,582]

The increase in GH levels is caused by a decrease in negative feedback by IGF-1 and a decrease in somatostatin tone.[583] Malnutrition also results in increased ghrelin levels,[584,585] which could also contribute to an increase in GH secretion, although the role of ghrelin in regulating GH secretion remains unclear.[586] With serum IGF-1 levels reduced despite normal or elevated GH levels, malnutrition is a form of GH insensitivity.[580] One cause of this insensitivity is a decrease in GHR expression, which is reflected in decreased serum GHBP levels.[579,587] This GH insensitivity may be an adaptive response, diverting scarce energy resources from growth toward use for acute metabolic needs. The low IGF-1 minimizes stimulation of anabolism, whereas the direct actions of the elevated GH levels (e.g., lipolysis, insulin antagonism) may increase the availability of energy substrates.[580,588,589] These adaptive mechanisms are accompanied by changes in serum IGFBPs that further limit IGF action during periods of malnutrition.[579,590]

Inadequate calorie or protein intake complicates many chronic diseases that are characterized by growth failure. Anorexia is a common feature of renal failure and inflammatory bowel disease, and it also occurs with cyanotic heart disease, congestive heart failure, CNS disease, and other illnesses. Some of these conditions may be further characterized by deficiencies of specific dietary components, such as zinc, iron, and vitamins necessary for normal growth and development.

Undernutrition may also be voluntary, as occurs with dieting and food fads (Fig. 24-35).[591] Caloric restriction is especially common in girls during adolescence, in whom it may be associated with anxiety concerning obesity, and in gymnasts and ballet dancers. Anorexia nervosa and bulimia are extremes of "voluntary" caloric deprivation that are commonly associated with impaired growth before epiphyseal fusion, which may result in diminished final adult height.[592,593] Adolescent bone mineral accretion is impaired, and significant osteopenia may persist into adulthood.[594] Later in adolescence, malnutrition may cause delayed puberty or menarche or both, as well as a variety of metabolic alterations. In anorexia nervosa, hormonal profiles are similar to those in protein-energy malnutrition,[592,593,595] with high basal levels of GH. However, in contrast to chronic critical illness, in which there is an increase in nonpulsatile secretion but a decrease in pulsatile GH secretion, in anorexia both nonpulsatile and pulsatile secretion of GH are increased.[583] The GH secretion stimulated by insulin-induced hypoglycemia, dopaminergic agents, or acute administration of dexamethasone is impaired in patients with anorexia nervosa, whereas clonidine and arginine elicit normal GH responses. Finally, a paradoxical increase in GH release to intravenous glucose infusion has been described.[583] As in malnutrition in general, low levels of IGF-1 and IGFBP3 are found in anorexia nervosa, indicating GH resistance. Similarly, GHBP levels are decreased,[583] indicating a decrease in GHR expression as a contributing factor to the GH resistance. The hormones of the GH/IGF-1 axis return to normal levels with refeeding.[579,592,596]

A rare cause of failure to thrive in infants and young children is the diencephalic syndrome.[597] This syndrome is characterized by a marked impairment of weight gain, or even weight loss, but with normal linear growth (at least initially). It is caused by hypothalamic tumors. Similar to the findings in other causes of low weight for length or height, increased GH levels have been found in patients with diencephalic syndrome. As in patients with anorexia nervosa, GH levels paradoxically increase in response to a glucose load. However, in contrast to the increased GH secretion seen in malnutrition or anorexia nervosa, IGF-1

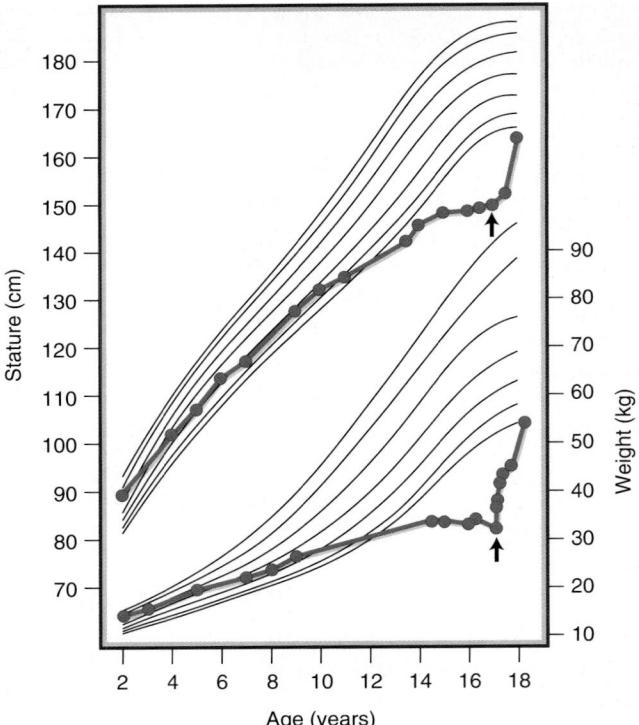

Figure 24-35 Curves of weight and height for a child who had growth failure resulting from prolonged self-imposed caloric restriction due to a fear of becoming obese. Notice that crossing of percentiles on the weight curve preceded that on the height curve, and that, after caloric intake was normalized *(arrow)*, gain in weight occurred before improvement in linear growth. At the end of the prolonged period of caloric restriction, weight age (10.2 years) was less than height age (12 years). (From Pugliese MT, Lifshitz F, Grad G, et al. Fear of obesity: a cause of short stature and delayed puberty. *N Engl J Med.* 1983;309:513-518. Reprinted by permission of the *New England Journal of Medicine.*)

levels are normal rather than decreased.[597] Therefore, diencephalic syndrome does not demonstrate GH resistance in the way that these other disorders do.

Chronic or Systemic Diseases

Malabsorption and Gastrointestinal Diseases. Intestinal disorders that impair absorption of calories or protein cause growth failure, for many of the same reasons as malnutrition per se.[588,598,599] Growth retardation may predate other manifestations of malabsorption or chronic inflammatory bowel disease. Celiac disease (gluten-induced enteropathy) and regional enteritis (Crohn disease) should be considered in the differential diagnosis of unexplained growth failure. Serum levels of IGF-1 may be reduced,[588,600] reflecting the malnutrition, and it is critical to discriminate between these conditions and disorders related to GHD. Documentation of malabsorption requires demonstration of fecal wasting of calories, especially fecal fat, along with other measures of gut dysfunction such as the D-xylose or breath hydrogen studies.

In celiac disease, an immune-mediated disorder in which the intestinal mucosa is damaged by dietary gluten (Fig. 24-36), impaired linear growth may be the first manifestation of disease.[588] The degree of growth impairment may be similar in patients with or without gastrointestinal symptoms.[588] Celiac disease has an increased incidence in individuals with TS, insulin-dependent (type 1) diabetes mellitus (IDDM), Down syndrome, or Williams syndrome. The prevalence of celiac disease in children being evaluated for short stature is approximately 5%.[601] The onset and

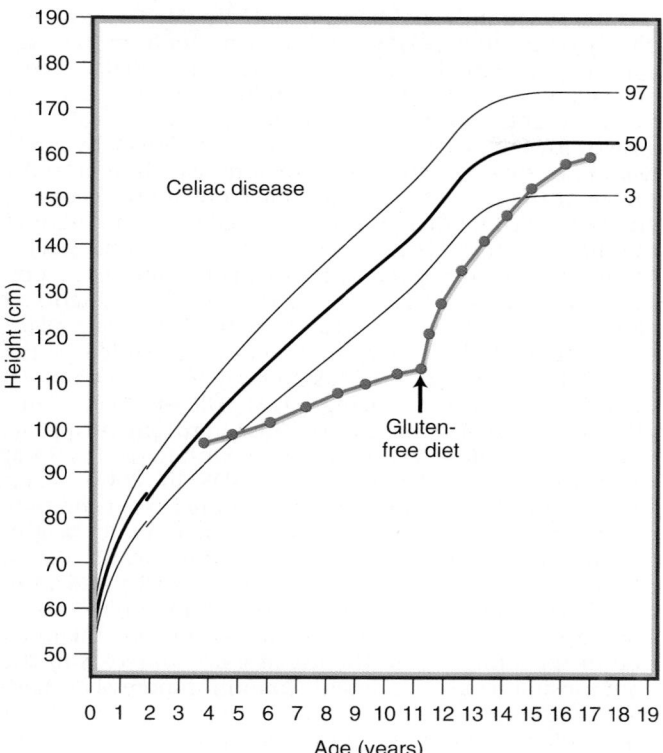

Figure 24-36 Catch-up growth in a girl with gluten-induced enteropathy (celiac disease). After 8 years of growth impairment, the patient was placed on a gluten-free diet and demonstrated substantial catch-up growth, returning to the previous growth percentiles. (Courtesy of J.M. Tanner.)

progression of puberty may be delayed, and menarche may be late.[602] Measurement of an immunoglobulin A (IgA) tissue transglutaminase antibody (tTG-IgA)[603] is the currently recommended screening test. This test has a sensitivity of up to 99%, with much higher specificity than IgA gliadin antibodies (AGA-IgA). However, tTG-IgA has significantly lower sensitivity in children younger than 18 months of age,[604] in whom it may be preferable to also measure AGA-IgA. When measuring IgA antibodies, it is necessary to measure total IgA levels to exclude IgA deficiency, particularly because IgA deficiency has an increased incidence in patients with celiac disease.[605] (In subjects with IgA deficiency, tTG-IgG may be used.[605]) Nonetheless, the diagnosis of celiac disease ultimately requires demonstration of the characteristic mucosal flattening in small bowel biopsy. The incidence of childhood celiac disease in the United States is about 0.9%.[606] Gluten withdrawal is a highly effective treatment for celiac disease and results in rapid catch-up growth and decreased clinical symptoms during the first 6 to 12 months of treatment.[588,602] Low IGF-1 and IGFBP3 levels return to normal during this period.[600,607] Most children who receive appropriate dietary management ultimately achieve a normal final height.[608,609]

Growth failure in Crohn disease, which correlates with disease severity,[610] is probably due to a combination of malnutrition from malabsorption, anorexia, nutrient loss, chronic inflammation,[599,610] inadequacy of trace minerals in the diet, and use of glucocorticoids. IGF-1 levels are low, especially with impaired growth.[588,599] In an animal model, approximately one half of the decrease in IGF-1 levels was accounted for by undernutrition, with the other half attributable to the effects of inflammation.[611] One third to two thirds or more of children with Crohn disease have impaired growth at diagnosis. In some patients, the growth failure precedes clinical symptoms of bowel disease by a few years, with a significant number showing linear growth failure before any weight loss.[588,599,610,612,613] Adequate nutritional supplementation and surgical resection of the diseased intestine can lead to improved growth, but surgery is not always an option.[614-616] Osteopenia is common.[617,618] An elevated erythrocyte sedimentation rate, anemia, and low serum albumin are useful clues, but diagnosis of Crohn disease ultimately requires colonoscopy and biopsy, along with gastrointestinal imaging studies. Permanent impairment of linear growth and deficits of final height may occur in 30% of patients.[619] Approximately 20% of patients at adult height are more than 8 cm below the midparental target height.[620] Small, mostly uncontrolled trials of GH treatment in children with Crohn disease have had conflicting results: some have shown improved growth velocity,[621,622] but others have not.[623] Some have shown improved body composition and BMD.[622] None of the reports, however, has extended beyond 2 years of treatment to determine whether there is a long-term benefit.

Chronic Liver Disease. Chronic liver disease in childhood can cause impaired linear growth. Decreased food intake, fat and fat-soluble vitamin malabsorption, and trace element deficiencies contribute to growth failure.[624-627] In addition, these children show evidence of GH resistance, having decreased levels of IGF-1 and IGFBP3 and increased GH secretion.[628-631] IGF-2 levels are also decreased, and IGFBP1 levels are increased.[628-630] Although the low IGF-1 levels might be due to the impaired synthetic capacity of the liver, there is decreased expression of the GHR in cirrhotic liver, just as in malnutrition.[632] However, despite provision of adequate calories, insensitivity to the action of GH persists,[627,629] suggesting that the GH resistance of liver failure is not due solely to malnutrition. Liver transplantation prolongs life expectancy, and linear growth is variably improved in the early post-transplantation years.[626,630,633,634] Exogenous glucocorticoid administration presumably plays a major role in the continued growth retardation[626,634]; GH and IGF-1 production are normal, but the amount of "free IGF" may be decreased, because IGFBP3 levels are relatively high.[630,633] Post-transplantation growth is inversely correlated with age and directly correlated with the degree of growth impairment at transplantation.[625,626,633] Exogenous GH treatment enhances growth rates and increases median height SDS by 0.3 to 0.6 unit after 1 year of treatment,[420,635,636] with continued increases in height SDS for up to 5 years during treatment.[420]

Cardiovascular Disease. Congenital heart disease with cyanosis or chronic congestive heart failure can cause growth failure.[637-639] Although some children with congenital heart disease will have growth failure related to an underlying genetic disorder, the disease itself can cause growth failure. The growth failure in children with CHD is often due to malnutrition, which can have a number of causes in children with CHD. Frequently this is due to inadequate calorie intake due to feeding difficulties associated with the heart disease.[637,638,640] In addition, chronic congestive heart failure is associated with malabsorption that includes protein-losing enteropathy, intestinal lymphangiectasia, and steatorrhea. Greater cardiac and respiratory work requirement and the relatively higher ratio of metabolically active, energy-utilizing brain and heart tissue to the growth-retarded body mass (cardiac cachexia) cause an increased basal metabolic rate in these children.[642,643] Thus, food intake that appears adequate for the child's weight is often inadequate for normal growth. Finally, in children with cyanotic CHD, the hypoxemia impairs cellular metabolism and growth. Decreased levels of IGF-1 and IGFBP3[643-645] and normal levels of GH and hepatic GHRs in chronically hypoxemic newborn sheep[645] suggest GH insensitivity distal to the GHR.

In the past, up to 30% of children with congenital heart disease had heights and weights that fell below the 3rd percentile for age.[646] In the developing world, up to 90% of children with CHD continue to suffer growth failure.[647] In contrast, in the developed world the impact of CHD on the growth of children has been nearly eliminated owing to the ability to make an early diagnosis, as well on improvements in supportive care and the early surgical correction of these lesions. The nutrional management of these infants before surgical correction includes the use of calorie-dense feedings because of the need to restrict fluids, calcium supplementation because of the use of diuretics that can cause calcium loss in the urine, and iron to maintain an enhanced rate of erythropoiesis. Early surgical correction restores normal growth, frequently after a phase of catch-up growth with normalization of energy expenditure.[637,639,642,648]

Renal Disease. All conditions that impair renal function can impair growth.[649-652] Uremia and renal tubular acidosis can cause growth failure before other clinical manifestations become evident. The growth impairment results from multiple mechanisms, including inadequate formation of 1,25-dihydroxycholecalciferol (1,25-dihydroxyvitamin D_3, calcitriol) with resultant osteopenia, decreased caloric intake, loss of electrolytes necessary for normal growth, metabolic acidosis, protein wasting, insulin resistance, chronic anemia, compromised cardiac function, and impairment of GH and IGF production and action. In nephropathic cystinosis, acquired hypothyroidism contributes to the inadequate growth.[653] Between 60% and 75% of patients with chronic renal failure treated before the GH therapeutic era had final adult heights more than 2 SD below the mean.[654]

The effects of renal failure on the GH/IGF-1 axis are complex, and there is evidence for both GH and IGF-1 resistance. Children and adolescents have normal or elevated circulating levels of GH, depending on the degree of renal failure.[649,650,655-657] The increased GH levels result from both an increase in GH secretory bursts and a decrease in renal GH clearance.[658] Serum IGF-1 and IGF-2 levels are usually normal in patients with renal failure.[649,657,659,660] Early reports of decreased serum IGF levels in uremia were an artifact caused by inadequate separation of IGF from IGFBPs before assay.[661] However, the normal IGF-1 levels in the face of elevated GH levels denotes GH resistance, which is also indicated by the finding of decreased hepatic IGF-1 production.[662] The mechanism for GH resistance includes decreased GHR gene expression in the liver and in the growth plate.[659,663] There is also evidence that the uremic state causes a postreceptor defect in GH signal transduction by diminishing phosphorylation and nuclear translocation of GH-activated STAT proteins.[658,664] Although a defect in IGF-1 receptor signaling has been demonstrated in renal failure,[663] the more important mechanism for decreased IGF-1 action in renal failure is alterations in the serum level of IGFBPs that decrease the bioavailability of IGF-1. IGFBPs 1, 2, 4, and 6 are increased.[649,650,663,665-668] In addition, low-molecular-weight IGFBP3 fragments, which have decreased affinity for IGF-1, accumulate as a result of reduced renal clearance.[663] In nephrotic syndrome, an additional contribution to growth failure may come from reduced serum levels of IGF-1 and IGFBP3 resulting from urinary loss of IGF-IGFBP complexes.[651] Finally, glucocorticoid therapy that may be used for treatment of the renal disease can exacerbate growth retardation by diminishing GH release and blunting IGF-1 action at growth plates.[667,669,670]

After successful renal transplantation, growth may completely return to normal.[671,672] Based on data from the large cohort of patients in the North American Pediatric Renal Transplant Cooperative Study, children who underwent transplantation before 6 years of age showed catch-up growth for the subsequent 1 to 2 years, followed by a plateauing of their growth rate.[673] In contrast, children older than 6 at the time of transplant have not shown catch-up growth; their final height is determined by their height at the time of transplantation.[673] In spite of this, final height in children requiring renal transplant has improved dramatically in the past 25 years so that the final heights of children in the North American Pediatric Renal Transplant Cooperative Study registry that were transplanted in the years 2002-2010 had a final height of −0.94 SDS, compared with final heights averaging −1.93 SDS in those transplanted between 1987 and 1991. This improvement appears to be driven almost completely by the improved height at the time of transplantation: −1.5 SDS in 2009 versus −2.5 SDS in 1987.[673] The importance of height at the time of transplantation in determining final adult height, despite the complex post-transplantation health issues, confirms the value of improving growth velocity and absolute height before transplantation. Additional factors that impact growth after transplantation include the function of the allograft and the use of glucocorticoids in the immunosuppressive regimen. Immunosuppressive regimens with alternate-day glucocorticoid treatment, rather than daily treatment,[672,673] utilizing a glucocorticoid withdrawal approach,[673,674] and regimens that avoid glucocorticoids have all been associated with improved post-transplant growth rates.[673] There are conflicting data on whether sirolimus impairs growth in comparison to tacrolimus.[673] Growth-retarded post-transplantation children receiving daily or alternate-day glucocorticoid treatment have decreased GH secretion, normal levels of IGF-1 and IGFBP1, and elevated levels of IGFBP3. They differ from patients with end-stage renal disease in that IGFBP1 levels are not strikingly elevated, perhaps because of altered glucose tolerance and hyperinsulinism due to chronic glucocorticoid therapy.[667]

Hematologic Disorders. Chronic anemias, such as sickle cell disease, are characterized by growth failure.[675] In general, the decrease in height and weight is greater in adolescent years than earlier because the onset of the adolescent growth spurt is delayed and menarche is late.[675-677] However, the adolescent growth and final adult height in patients with sickle cell disease may be normal.[677] The causes of growth retardation probably include suboptimal nutrition and hypogonadism.[678] Impaired oxygen delivery to tissues, increased work of the cardiovascular system, and energy demands of increased hematopoiesis are likely contributors to the impaired nutrition. Long-term chronic transfusion therapy as part of stroke prevention treatment is associated with enhanced growth.[679] The GH/IGF-1 system probably does not have a primary role in the growth impairment of sickle cell anemia, although abnormalities in the GH/IGF-1 system have been described.[680]

In thalassemia, in addition to the consequences of chronic anemia, endocrine deficiencies can result from chronic transfusions and accompanying hemosiderosis.[681] Despite vigorous efforts to maintain hemoglobin levels near normal and to avoid iron overload, growth failure is still a common feature of thalassemia, especially in male adolescents.[682] The patients tend to show body disproportion, with truncal shortening but normal leg length. It is likely that anemia, impaired IGF-1 synthesis, hypothyroidism, gonadal failure, and hypogonadotropic hypogonadism all contribute to growth failure in this disorder. GH insensitivity in some cases is suggested by generally adequate GH production with low IGF-1 levels.[683,684] Several groups have reported data on treatment of thalassemia patients in whom GH production seemed diminished. In most patients, GH treatment increased growth, at least initially.[683,685] In a longer-term study (average duration, 59 months) starting with young patients (7.2 years of age), an increased growth velocity was maintained throughout the treatment period[686]; when treatment was initiated at an older age (13.6 years), final height was not improved.[687] A small number of adults with thalassemia are found to have continued GHD, so GH treatment for cardiac and bone health reasons may be important in this disease.[688]

About half of the patients in the International Fanconi Anemia Registry have short stature. GHD was demonstrated by provocative testing (22 of 48 patients) or with assessment of endogenous secretion (13 of 13) in a group with a mean height of −2.23 SDS.[689] In pure red blood cell aplasia,[690] approximately 30% of patients demonstrated growth retardation. The frequency increased with age (42% in individuals >16 years) and with treatment programs such as chronic transfusions or glucocorticoids.

Inborn Errors of Metabolism. Inborn errors of metabolism are often accompanied by growth failure that may be pronounced. Glycogen storage disease, the mucopolysaccharidoses, glycoproteinoses, and mucolipidoses are characterized by poor growth. Many inborn metabolic disorders are also associated with significant skeletal dysplasia. In a small number of patients with organic acidoses, such as methylmalonic and propionic acidurias, IGF-1 levels are low and GH levels are normal, suggesting a possible state of GH insensitivity related to nutritional status.[691] Preliminary data suggest that exogenous GH treatment may improve the metabolic status of such children.[691,692]

Pulmonary Disease. Growth can be retarded in children with asthma, including those who have not received glucocorticoid therapy. The lowered growth in asthmatic children does not appear to be associated with abnormalities of the GH/IGF-1 axis.[693] Impaired nutrition and increased energy requirements, along with chronic stress, especially with nocturnal asthma and enhanced endogenous glucocorticoid production, cause poor linear growth. However, despite this growth impairment, there is at most only a small difference in final height achieved by those with asthma, with the majority of the growth failure due to a delay in puberty.[694] Systemic glucocorticoid therapy, which is rarely required, can be expected to impair growth. Intermittent glucocorticoid therapy is usually not associated with impaired final height. Alternate-day or aerosolized glucocorticoid therapy often ameliorates growth retardation and can be associated with an accelerated catch-up phase.[695,696] The large Childhood Asthma Management Program investigated the effect of inhaled corticosteroids (ICS) on the growth of children with asthma. Although growth rate declined with the initiation of ICS, it subsequently normalized, and the final height in children treated with ICS for 4 to 6 years was only 1.2 cm below that in control subjects.[697] ICS can, however, suppress the hypothalamic-pituitary axis, and investigation for this is appropriate in children who have a more marked suppression of growth with ICS treatment.[694]

Bronchopulmonary dysplasia (BPD), a sequela of neonatal respiratory distress syndrome and prematurity, has an incidence as high as 35% in infants with very low birth weight (<1500 g).[698] The use of dexamethasone in the treatment of BPD in neonates causes a transient cessation of growth[699] and has engendered long-term concern for neurodevelopment and somatic growth.[700] Growth in surviving infants is poor through early childhood,[701-703] but the defect usually disappears by 8 years of age.[704-706] Long-term hypoxemia, poor nutrition, chronic pulmonary infections, and reactive airway disease are responsible for the poor early growth.

In patients with cystic fibrosis (CF), chronic pulmonary infection with bronchiectasis, pancreatic insufficiency with exocrine and endocrine inadequacy, malabsorption, and malnutrition all contribute to decreased growth and late sexual maturation. Over 20% of individuals with CF under 25 years of age will have heights or weights below the 10th percentile.[707] With newborn screening for CF the failure to thrive that was a common presenting feature is now less likely to be seen, although these infants still demonstrate some growth failure.[708] Infants who are not identified by newborn screening often show marked growth failure before diagnosis followed by catch-up growth after diagnosis. The linear growth rate during childhood is generally normal before puberty,[709] followed by delayed puberty, including a delayed and attenuated pubertal growth spurt. Adult height in individuals with CF is slightly decreased compared with population norms by approximately −0.2 to −0.7 SD.[709-711] The GH/IGF-1 axis in CF patients shows evidence for some degree of acquired GH insensitivity with lowered mean IGF-1 and elevated GH levels.[712] The degree of growth retardation is related most closely to the severity and variability of the pulmonary disease rather than to pancreatic dysfunction.[713,714] While the degree of steatorrhea does not correlate well with growth impairment, improved nutrition programs do enhance the overall clinical picture.[715,716] Endocrine abnormalities, such as failure of both alpha and beta islet cells with decreased glucagon and insulin production, do not seem to influence prepubertal growth patterns in children with CF. Alterations of vitamin D metabolism, while potentially affecting skeletal mineralization, do not diminish growth.[717]

There is the potential for the anabolic effects of GH treatment to improve the health in patients with CF. A number of short-term trials of up to 12 months with GH treatment have been reported.[707,718,719] These studies have demonstrated that GH treatment of CF patients increases height, weight, and lean body mass. In addition, some measures of lung function are slightly improved, notably forced vital capacity, although this improvement did not always exceed that expected based on the improved growth.[718] Although some studies have demonstrated a decreased rate of hospitalization in GH-treated patients, there has not been clear evidence of a decrease in pulmonary exacerbations.[718,719] These studies, as well as reports of uncontrolled treatments of up to 4 years, have not raised serious safety concerns of GH treatment in CF patients. Specifically, there has not been an increase in glucose intolerance or diabetes mellitus, although in some studies fasting glucose levels were increased.[718-720] Although the current data demonstrate the possibility that GH treatment will benefit patients with CF, there are not yet sufficient data to indicate that GH treatment improves long-term health outcomes in these patients.

Chronic Inflammation and Infection. Poor growth is a characteristic feature of chronic inflammatory disease and recurrent serious infection. The impaired growth associated with such disorders as Crohn disease, CF, and asthma, in which inflammatory processes may be significant, has already been discussed. Inflammatory states are associated with increased levels of numerous cytokines. Interleukin 6 (IL-6), specifically, has been implicated in this growth impairment. De Benedetti and colleagues,[721] studying juvenile rheumatoid arthritis in humans and in a transgenic murine model expressing excessive IL-6, demonstrated an

IL-6–mediated decrease in IGF-1 production. IL-6 has been demonstrated to activate SOCS3; this provides a pathway for inflammation to inhibit IGF-1 production because SOCS3 is a negative regulator of the JAK2/STAT5 GH signal transduction pathway.[611,722,723] IL-6 may also cause a decrease in serum IGF-1 levels by increasing its clearance through a decrease in IGFBP3 levels.[611] In addition, cytokines can affect the endocrine system at many other levels,[724,725] impairing mineral and nutrient metabolism and the growth and remodeling of bone.[726]

Exposure to human immunodeficiency virus (HIV) in children and adolescents occurs through perinatal transmission, blood transfusions, drug usage, and sexual contact. Growth failure is a cardinal feature of childhood acquired immunodeficiency syndrome (AIDS).[727-731] However, HIV-infected infants and children show growth failure even before demonstrating severe immune dysfunction.[732,733] Weight, length, and head circumference are all affected, although weight-for-height may be normal.[729,731,734] Before the era of highly active antiretroviral therapy (HAART), height growth velocity was associated with survival, independent of either CD4+ T-cell lymphocyte count or viral load, with HAART therapy normalizing growth in most studies.[734] Studies of the GH/IGF-1 axis in HIV-infected children have shown evidence of decreased GH secretion, GH resistance, and IGF-1 resistance; both normal and low levels of GH and IGF-1 are seen.[732] Lipodystrophy associated with HAART therapy occurs in children, although less commonly than in adults, and decreased GH secretion has been demonstrated in HIV-associated lipodystrophy,[732] potentially contributing to impaired growth. HIV-infected children frequently have delayed puberty, which could contribute to their linear growth failure. In a short-term treatment trial with standard doses of GH, height and weight growth increased and protein catabolism diminished, without any adverse effect on viral burden.[735]

Endocrine Disorders

Hypothyroidism. Untreated severe congenital hypothyroidism results in profound growth failure. With proper treatment, however, children with congenital hypothyroidism reach a height appropriate for their genetic potential.[736]

Acquired hypothyroidism during childhood may also result in growth failure that can range from subtle to profound, depending on the severity and duration of the hypothyroidism. Growth failure may be the most prominent manifestation of hypothyroidism in children.[737] The poor growth is more apparent in height than in weight gain, so these children tend to be overweight for height. Rivkees and coworkers[737] reported a mean 4.2-year delay between slowing of growth and the diagnosis of hypothyroidism; at diagnosis, girls were 4.04 SD below and boys 3.15 SD below the mean height for their age. Skeletal maturation is delayed in those children in whom the hypothyroidism was sufficient to retard growth, with the bone age at diagnosis corresponding to the age at onset of the hypothyroidism.[737] Body proportion is immature, with an increased upper- to lower-body segment ratio. Although chronic hypothyroidism is usually associated with delayed puberty, precocious puberty and premature menarche can occur in hypothyroid children (see Chapter 13).

In those children with severe growth failure, treatment with thyroid hormone results in rapid catch-up growth. This growth is typically accompanied by marked skeletal maturation. In cases of prolonged severe hypothyroidism, the advancement of skeletal maturation with treatment can exceed the growth acceleration, resulting in a compromised adult height.[737] The deficit in adult stature correlates with the duration of hypothyroidism before initiation of treatment. Catch-up growth may be particularly compromised if therapy is initiated near puberty.[738]

As expected, hyperthyroidism has effects on growth opposite to those of hypothyroidism: it results in accelerated growth and epiphyseal maturation. Children with hyperthyroidism present with an increased height and advanced bone age. In neonates, hyperthyroidism can result in craniosynostosis. However, despite the advanced bone age at diagnosis, the final height of children treated for hyperthyroidism remains normal in relation to genetic potential.[739]

Diabetes Mellitus. Although weight loss may occur immediately before the onset of clinically apparent IDDM, children with new-onset diabetes are frequently taller than their peer group, possibly because GH and insulin levels are increased during the preclinical evolution of the disease.[740-742] Most children with IDDM, even those with marginal control,[743] grow quite normally, especially in prepubertal years, although growth velocity may decrease during puberty.[744] However, growth failure can occur in diabetic children with long-standing poor glycemic control.[745,746] The Mauriac syndrome[747] describes children with poorly regulated IDDM, severe growth failure, and hepatosplenomegaly due to excess hepatic glycogen deposition. This type of growth retardation has become increasingly rare with modern diabetes care.

Many pathophysiologic processes, including malnutrition, chronic intermittent acidosis, increased glucocorticoid production, hypothyroidism, impaired calcium balance, and end-organ unresponsiveness to either GH or IGF, may contribute to growth failure in IDDM.[740,748-750] IGF-1 and IGFBP3 levels are diminished in the face of enhanced GH production,[751-755] reflecting acquired GH insensitivity. GHBP levels are decreased,[748,754] supporting the concept of impaired GHR number or function. Furthermore, IGFBP1 is normally suppressed by insulin, and hypoinsulinemia results in elevated serum IGFBP1 levels that may inhibit IGF action.[524,754,756-758] In contrast to the situation in adolescents and adults, IGFBP1 levels are not elevated in well-growing prepubertal children.[758] On the contrary, increased IGFBP3 proteolysis may enhance the bioactivity of the available IGF-1.[525,755] Most children with IDDM attain normal cellular nutrition and growth factor action despite intermittent hypoinsulinemia and derangements of peripheral indices of the GH/IGF-1 system.

Even though glycemic control is inversely correlated with IGF-1 level,[749,751,754,759] the correlation between glycemic control and growth is weak. After conflicting reports as to the influence of glycemic regulation on growth,[740,741,760,761] a longitudinal study[761] of 46 children whose diabetes began before age 10 indicated that initial heights at diagnosis were normal and that the final height SDS was minimally reduced from that at onset. In boys, despite a delay of about 2.5 years in onset of puberty, total pubertal height gain was normal. In girls with diabetes, however, total pubertal height gain was diminished and the age at menarche was delayed; the effects of altered insulin and IGF-1 levels on ovarian function have not been assessed in such patients. Chronic metabolic control did not correlate with the pubertal height gain or with the normal final height. Nevertheless, good glycemic control may improve growth at certain maturational periods such as puberty.[740,753,762]

Cushing Syndrome: Glucocorticoid Excess. Glucocorticoid excess impairs skeletal growth, interferes with normal bone metabolism by inhibiting osteoblastic activity, and enhances bone resorption.[763-765] These effects are related to the duration of steroid excess,[766] regardless of whether the

Cushing syndrome is due to ACTH hypersecretion, adrenal tumor, or glucocorticoid administration.

Even modest doses of oral glucocorticoids can inhibit growth; these doses may be as low as 3 to 5 mg/m² per day of prednisone or 12 to 15 mg/m² per day of hydrocortisone (i.e., only slightly above what is considered physiologic replacement).[767] The "toxic" effects of glucocorticoids on the epiphysis may persist to some degree after correction of chronic glucocorticoid excess, and patients frequently do not attain their target height.[768,769] The longer the duration and the greater the intensity of glucocorticoid excess, the less likely is catch-up growth to be completed. Alternate-day glucocorticoid treatment decreases but does not eliminate the risk of growth suppression.[696,770,771] Inhaled glucocorticoids given for the treatment of asthma have an even lower risk of growth suppression, but even at modest doses (e.g., 400 µg/day of beclomethasone,[772] 200 µg/day of fluticasone,[772] or 400 µg/day of budesonide[697]) they can cause at least temporary slowing of growth. However, inhaled corticosteroids do not appear to significantly impair final height.[697]

GH therapy can overcome some of the growth-inhibiting effects of excess glucocorticoids. The GH-induced increase in growth rate is inversely related to the glucocorticoid dose,[773] with one small study finding no benefit of GH treatment for prednisone doses greater than 0.35 mg/kg per day.[774] GH or IGF-1 administration can diminish many of the catabolic effects of excess glucocorticoids.[764,775,776]

Adrenal tumors secreting large amounts of glucocorticoids can produce excess androgens, which may mask the growth-inhibitory effects of glucocorticoids. In addition, Cushing syndrome in children may not cause all the clinical signs and symptoms associated with the disorder in adults and may manifest with growth arrest. However, Cushing syndrome is an unlikely diagnosis in children with obesity, because exogenous obesity is associated with normal or even accelerated skeletal growth and growth deceleration is usually evident by the time other signs of Cushing syndrome appear (Fig. 24-37). In a series of 10 children and adolescents treated for Cushing disease with surgery and cranial irradiation, post-therapy GHD was common and mean final height was −1.36 SDS.[777]

Pseudohypoparathyroidism: Albright Hereditary Osteodystrophy. Albright hereditary osteodystrophy (AHO) is caused by mutations in the stimulatory GTP-binding protein, $G_s\alpha$. It exists both with and without multihormone resistance—termed *pseudohypoparathyroidism type 1A* (PHP-1A) and *pseudo-pseudohypoparathyroidism* (pseudo-PHP). This condition is discussed in detail in Chapter 28 but is included here because short adult height is a common feature.[778] AHO is characterized by obesity (more marked in PHP-1A than in pseudo-PHP[779]), short metacarpals, subcutaneous ossifications, round facies, and cognitive impairments. Patients with AHO, whether they have PHP-1A or pseudo-PHP, typically have short adult stature. Many patients with PHP-1A demonstrate GHD due to resistance to GHRH.[780,781] Interestingly, patients with PHP-1B, which is caused by a methylation defect in the *GNAS* gene that encodes $G_s\alpha$, have PTH and TSH resistance like PHP-1A patients, but they do not have the AHO phenotype and do not demonstrate GHRH resistance.[782] However, although AHO patients have evidence of GHD, their growth pattern suggests that there is another contributor to growth failure because they often have only modest growth failure in early and middle childhood, with early epiphyseal fusion contributing to their short final height.[780,783] Consistent with this likely multifactorial cause for short stature, preliminary data in patients with PHP-1A found an increase in growth rate with GH treatment, but without an increase in final height, as the

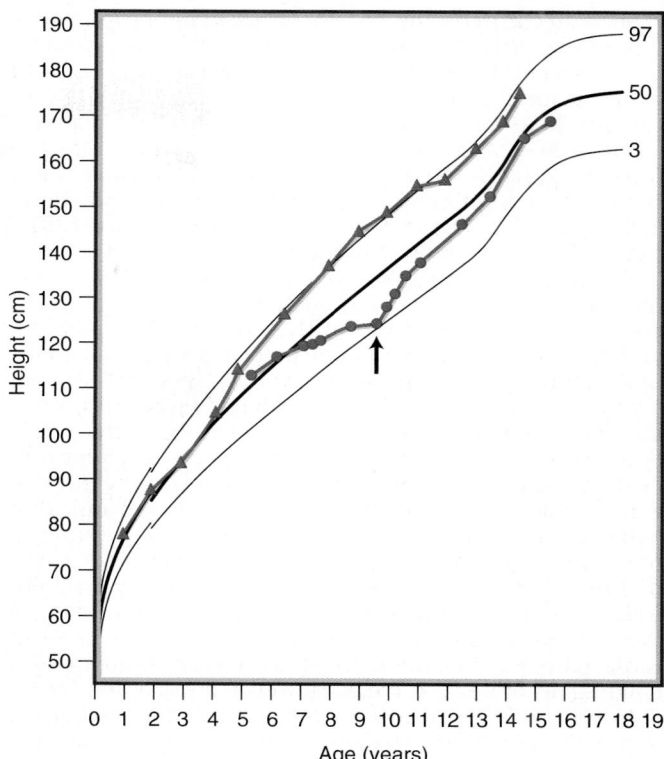

Figure 24-37 Growth curves of two boys with obesity. The boy depicted by the circles had cortisol excess related to Cushing disease. He had onset of rapid weight gain associated with a decrease in linear growth velocity at age 7. The diagnosis was made, and an adrenalectomy *(arrow)* was performed at age 9½ years, with an almost immediate increase in growth rate and striking catch-up growth. The boy whose growth is depicted by triangles had exogenous obesity. At age 9½, his weight was approximately the same as that of the patient with Cushing disease, but his height was at the 97th percentile, reflecting the enhancement of linear growth in individuals with exogenous obesity.

few children reaching final height appeared to have an absence of a pubertal growth spurt.[784]

Rickets. In the past, hypovitaminosis D was a major cause of short stature and was often associated with other causes of growth failure, such as malnutrition, prematurity, malabsorption, hepatic disease, or chronic renal failure (see Chapter 28). In isolated vitamin D deficiency, breastfed infants typically have poor exposure to sunlight and are not nutritionally supplemented with vitamin D. Characteristic skeletal manifestations of rickets include frontal bossing, craniotabes, rachitic rosary, and bowing of the legs. Such children usually begin to synthesize 1,25-dihydroxyvitamin D_3 as they become older, broaden their diet, and have increased exposure to sunlight, with amelioration of the transient early decrease of linear growth velocity. The association of vitamin D receptor gene polymorphism with birth length, growth rate, adult stature, and BMD[785-789] further emphasizes the importance of vitamin D in normal growth. Additionally, vitamin D and estrogen receptor genotypes appear to interactively affect infant growth, especially in males.[787,790] The presence of high-affinity binding sites for the vitamin D receptor DNA-binding domain in the GH promoter suggests that the vitamin D receptor may actually modulate GH expression.[791]

Hypophosphatemic Rickets. Hypophosphatemic rickets is an X-linked dominant disorder caused by decreased renal tubular reabsorption of phosphate related to mutations in the phosphate-regulating endopeptidase gene, *PHEX,* located on chromosome Xp22.1. Other hypophosphatemic syndromes include autosomal-dominant hypophosphatemic rickets, hereditary hypophosphatemic rickets with hypercalciuria, and tumor-induced osteomalacia (see Chapter 28).[792] In all of these conditions, there are increased levels of FGF23, a major phosphaturic agent.[793] The features are usually more severe in boys and include short stature,[690,794] prominent bowing of the legs, and sometimes rachitic signs.[795] The metabolic and skeletal abnormalities cannot be overcome by vitamin D therapy alone.

Treatment of hypophosphatemic rickets requires oral phosphate replacement, but such therapy may result in poor calcium absorption from the intestine. The addition of calcitriol to oral phosphate increases intestinal phosphate absorption and prevents hypocalcemia and secondary hyperparathyroidism. Such combined therapy improves the rickets but does not necessarily correct growth.[792,796,797] Potential growth-related benefits of this regimen appear to be dependent on the initiation of therapy in early infancy, which leads to achievement of greater childhood and adult height.[794] There is no clear association between endogenous GH secretion, IGF-1, or phosphate levels and height in this disorder.[798-800] Nevertheless, GH therapy in eight trials including 83 patients resulted in an enhancement of skeletal growth and improvement in BMD.[801-803] In 14 of those patients, treatment for 4 to 5 years resulted in a height gain of up to 1.2 SDS. However, a Cochrane review did not find conclusive evidence that GH treatment improved growth in patients with hypophosphatemic rickets.[804] One report cautioned that GH treatment appeared to exaggerate disproportionate truncal growth.[805]

Osteochondrodysplasias

The osteochondrodysplasias encompass a heterogeneous group of disorders characterized by intrinsic abnormalities of cartilage and bone.[806] These disorders include abnormalities in the size or shape of bones in the limbs, spine, or skull, often with abnormalities seen on radiographic evaluation. More than 100 osteochondrodysplasias have been identified based on physical characteristics and radiographic characteristics (Table 24-5).

Diagnosis of osteochondrodysplasias can be difficult, with clinical and radiologic evaluation central to the diagnosis. The family history is critical, although many cases are caused by de novo mutations, and this is generally the case in autosomal-dominant achondrodysplasia and hypochondrodysplasia. Measurement of body proportions should include arm span, sitting height, upper and lower body segments, and head circumference. Radiologic evaluation should be used to determine whether involvement is of the long bones, skull, or vertebrae and whether abnormalities are primarily at the epiphyses, metaphyses, or diaphyses. The osteochondrodysplasias most commonly encountered in endocrine practice are discussed in the following paragraphs.

Achondrodysplasia is the most common of the osteochondrodysplasias, with a frequency of 1 in 26,000 individuals. Characteristic abnormalities of the skeleton include megalocephaly, low nasal bridge, lumbar lordosis, short trident hand, and rhizomelia (shortness of the proximal legs and arms) with skin redundancy. Radiologic findings include small, cuboid-shaped vertebral bodies with short pedicles and progressive narrowing of the lumbar interpedicular distance. The small foramen magnum may lead to hydrocephalus, and spinal cord and root compression may result from kyphosis, stenosis of the spinal canal, or disk lesions.[807] Diminished growth velocity is present from infancy, although short stature may not be evident until

TABLE 24-5

Classification of Osteochondrodysplasias

I. Defects of the tubular (and flat) bones and axial skeleton
  A. Achondroplasia group
  B. Achondrogenesis
  C. Spondylodysplastic group (perinatally lethal)
  D. Metatropic dysplasia group
  E. Short rib dysplasia group (with or without polydactyly)
  F. Atelosteogenesis/diastrophic dysplasia group
  G. Kniest-Stickler dysplasia group
  H. Spondyloepiphyseal dysplasia congenita group
  I. Other spondyloepiphyseal/metaphyseal dysplasias
  J. Dysostosis multiplex group
  K. Spondylometaphyseal dysplasias
  L. Epiphyseal dysplasias
  M. Chondrodysplasia punctata (stippled epiphyses) group
  N. Metaphyseal dysplasias
  O. Brachyrachia (short spine dysplasia)
  P. Mesomelic dysplasias
  Q. Acro/acromesomelic dysplasias
  R. Dysplasias with significant (but not exclusive) membranous bone involvement
  S. Bent bone dysplasia group
  T. Multiple dislocations with dysplasias
  U. Osteodysplastic primordial dwarfism group
  V. Dysplasias with increased bone density
  W. Dysplasias with defective mineralization
  X. Dysplasias with increased bone density
II. Disorganized development of cartilaginous and fibrous components of the skeleton
III. Idiopathic osteolysis

after 2 years of age. Mean adult heights in males and females are 130 and 120 cm, respectively. GH secretion is comparable to that in normal subjects.

Achondrodysplasia is caused by mutations in the transmembrane domain of the FGF receptor 3 gene (FGFR3).[810] It is transmitted in an autosomal dominant manner, but 80% to 90% of cases are caused by de novo mutations. Most of the cases are the result of activating mutations at nucleotide 1138 of the FGFR3 gene, which creates new recognition sites for restriction enzymes, thus easing the molecular diagnosis. The mutation rate reported at this site is very high, and FGFR3 has been labeled the most mutable gene in the genome. As a result of the upregulation of receptor activity, there is abnormal chondrogenesis and osteogenesis during endochondral ossification, leading to the typical phenotypic findings. The homogeneity of the mutation in achondroplasia probably explains the minimal heterogeneity in the phenotype. Infants homozygous for the mutation have severe disease, typically dying in infancy from respiratory insufficiency due to a small thorax. In mice with the equivalent Fgfr3 mutation, there is ligand-independent dimerization and phosphorylation of Fgfr3 with activation of Stat proteins and upregulation of cell cycle inhibition.

Hypochondroplasia is also autosomal dominant, and 70% of affected individuals are heterozygous for mutations in the FGFR3 gene, frequently at amino acid position 1620.[812] The facial features of achondroplasia are absent, and both short stature and rhizomelia are less pronounced. Adult heights are typically in the 120- to 150-cm range. Poor growth may not by evident until after 2 years of age, but stature then deviates progressively from normal. Occasionally, the disproportionate short stature is not apparent until adulthood. Outward bowing of the legs may be accompanied by genu varum. On radiologic evaluation, lumbar interpedicular distances are diminished between L1 and L5, and there may be flaring of the pelvis and narrow sciatic notches. The diagnosis can be difficult to make, with mild variants of the syndrome difficult to distinguish from normal.

The short stature homeobox-containing (SHOX) gene is located in the pseudoautosomal region of distal Xp and Yp. Mutations or deletion of *SHOX* is associated with syndromes of poor growth and skeletal dysplasia, including Léri-Weill dyschondrosteosis (LWD), TS, and Langer mesomelic dysplasia (LMD).[813] Findings include short stature, Madelung deformity, increased carrying angle, tibial bowing, scoliosis, and high arched palate. The auxologic finding of relatively short limbs suggests a defect in *SHOX*, because the SHOX protein may affect cellular proliferation and apoptosis of chondrocytes at the growth plate.[814] Indeed, the skeletal manifestations have been associated with areas in which there is intrauterine expression of *SHOX*.[814] LWD is caused by homozygous gene defects, whereas TS and LMD are caused by haploinsufficiency. The profound findings in LWD, compared with TS, may reflect the impact of pubertal estrogen exposure in LWD.[813]

Endochondral growth is regulated by multiple endocrine, paracrine, and autocrine factors, and many inborn errors have been identified. In the syndrome of acromesomelic dysplasia, growth is remarkably impaired, leading to adult heights that may be more than 5 SD below the mean. A homozygous mutation in the homodimeric transmembrane natriuretic peptide receptor B (NPR-B) that impairs binding of the ligand C-type natriuretic peptide has been found in some affected individuals.[815] Obligatory heterozygotes are significantly shorter than normal but have normal skeletal anatomy.[816] Therefore, heterozygous mutations of NPR-B demonstrate that a subset of children with unexplained short stature may, in fact, have mild forms of osteochondrodysplasias.

Chromosomal Abnormalities

Abnormalities of autosomes or sex chromosomes can cause growth retardation without evidence of skeletal dysplasia, frequently with somatic abnormalities and developmental delay. In many cases, the precise cause of growth failure is not clear because the genetic defects do not affect known components of the GH/IGF-1 system. Chromosomal lesions may directly influence normal tissue growth and development or indirectly modulate local responsiveness to IGF or other growth factors at the growth plate.

Down Syndrome. Trisomy 21, or Down syndrome, is probably the most common chromosomal disorder associated with growth retardation, affecting approximately 1 in 600 neonates. On average, newborns with Down syndrome have birth weights 500 g below normal and are 2 to 3 cm shorter than normal. Growth failure continues postnatally and is typically associated with delayed skeletal maturation and a delayed and incomplete pubertal growth spurt. Adult heights range from 135 to 170 cm in men and 127 to 158 cm in women.[13] The cause of growth failure in Down syndrome is unknown, and attempts to find underlying hormonal explanations for growth retardation have been unsuccessful. Marginal levels of GH secretion and low-normal serum levels of IGF-1 has been reported in patients with Down syndrome. Exogenous GH has been tried in some of these patients and has produced increases in growth velocity, but the long-term effects on final adult height have not been studied. In addition, no improvement in gross motor or mental development was noted.[817,818] Hashimoto thyroiditis is common in individuals with Down syndrome and should be sought and treated promptly. Because of the concern for development of leukemia, which is more common in individuals with Down syndrome, GH use is generally not recommended.

Turner Syndrome. In girls with TS, short stature is the single most common feature, occurring more frequently than delayed puberty, cubitus valgus, or webbing of the neck.[819-821] Short stature occurs in 95% to 100% of girls with a 45,X karyotype.[822-825] Mean adult heights in the United States and Europe range from 142.0 to 146.8 cm, with important genetic and ethnic influences on growth of girls in different regions. Parental height correlates well with final adult height,[825,826] and a cross-cultural study in 15 countries demonstrated a very strong correlation between final height in TS and in the normal population, with an approximate 20-cm deficit.[822] Several distinct phases of growth have been identified in girls with TS[827,828]:

1. Mild IUGR with a mean birth weight of 2800 g and a mean birth length of 48.3 cm
2. Slow growth recognized during early infancy and reaching −3 SDS by 3 years of age[829]
3. Delayed onset of the "childhood" phase of growth[26,27,830] and progressive decline in height velocity from age 3 years until approximately 14 years, resulting in further deviation from normal height percentiles
4. A prolonged adolescent growth phase, characterized by a partial return toward normal height, followed by delayed epiphyseal fusion

These girls have many features of skeletal dysplasia such as Madelung deformity and are haploinsufficient for the *SHOX* gene, which is located in the pseudoautosomal region of the short arm of the X chromosome.[831] When heights of girls with TS are compared with those of girls with LWD, which involves a *SHOX* deletion, it appears that the *SHOX* defect may account for about two thirds of the height deficit in TS.[832] Girls with TS have normal GH and IGF levels during childhood; reports of low levels of GH or IGF, or both, in adolescents are likely due to low serum levels of gonadal steroids.[833] Multiple studies have shown that GH therapy is capable of accelerating short-term growth and increasing final adult height.[824,834,835] GH treatment in TS is discussed in detail later in the chapter.

Noonan Syndrome. Individuals with Noonan syndrome have postnatal growth failure, right-sided cardiac abnormalities (most often pulmonary valve abnormalities), webbing of the neck, low posterior hairline, ptosis, cubitus valgus, and malformed ears. Microphallus and cryptorchidism are common, and puberty may be delayed or incomplete. Cognitive delay of variable degrees is present in about 25% to 50% of patients. Although this disorder shares phenotypic features with TS, the two are clearly distinct.[836,837] Therefore, oft-used terms such as "Turner-like syndrome" or "male Turner syndrome" are misleading. In Noonan syndrome, the sex chromosomes are normal and transmission is autosomal dominant, although about 50% of cases are sporadic. Noonan syndrome is caused by heterozygous activating mutations in the genes of proteins in the RAS-MAPK pathway, including *PTPN11*, *SOS1*, *RAF1*, *KRAS*, and *NRAS*, with approximately half of patients having mutations in *PTPN11*.[838,839] Through much of childhood, mean growth in length and weight is below the third percentile.[840-842] GH secretory abnormalities do not account for the short stature, although endogenous GH production may be slightly reduced.[842,843] The protein product of the *PTPN11* gene is the nonreceptor type 2 tyrosine phosphatase (SHP2). SHP2 dephosphorylates JAK2, suggesting that the growth failure of Noonan syndrome might be due to growth hormone resistance from the enhanced action of SHP2.[844-846] However, SHP2 is a positive regulator of the RAS-MAPK pathway, and the development of Noonan syndrome from activating mutations in other proteins in this pathway suggests that alterations in RAS-MAPK signaling are responsible for the phenotype. GH therapy has been used in the treatment of patients with Noonan syndrome who have short stature, as discussed in detail later.

Prader-Willi Syndrome. In Prader-Willi syndrome (PWS), growth failure may be evident at birth but is more pronounced postnatally.[847] This syndrome is discussed at length in a later section of this chapter.

Other Syndromes. Other syndromes associated with moderate to profound growth failure include Bloom syndrome, de Lange syndrome, leprechaunism, Ellis–van Creveld syndrome, Aarskog syndrome, Rubinstein-Taybi syndrome, mulibrey nanism, Dubowitz syndrome, progeria, Cockayne syndrome, and Johanson-Blizzard syndrome.[848]

Small for Gestational Age

Historically, infants born SGA have composed a heterogeneous group with birth weight or length below the 3rd, 5th, or 10th percentile for gestational age, depending on the study.[35] As the growth and metabolic consequences of being born SGA have been observed and characterized, studies have more consistently used the definition of SGA as birth weight or length (or both) at least 2 SD below the mean for gestational age (usually at or below the 2.3 percentile for a population). The term *IUGR* has been used interchangeably with SGA to describe these infants. However, it has been proposed that, because IUGR implies a known underlying pathologic process, that term should be reserved for infants whose abnormal prenatal growth has been confirmed by intrauterine growth assessments and whose growth restriction can be attributed to a specific cause.[849] The reason for abnormal fetal growth is unclear in up to 40% of cases[850]; known underlying reasons are listed in Table 24-6. Accurate assessment of an infant as SGA depends on accurate gestational dating and weight and length measurements, which can be difficult in both developed and developing countries.

Most SGA infants exhibit catch-up growth (as defined by a growth velocity greater than the median for chrono-

TABLE 24-6

Factors Associated with Small for Gestational Age (SGA) Births

I. Intrinsic Fetal Factors

A. Chromosomal disorders
B. Syndromes
  1. Russell-Silver syndrome
  2. Seckel syndrome
  3. Progeria
  4. Cockayne syndrome
  5. Bloom syndrome
  6. Rubinstein-Taybi syndrome

II. Placental Abnormalities

A. Abnormal implantation of the placenta
B. Placental vascular insufficiency; infarction
C. Vascular malformations

III. Maternal Disorders

A. Malnutrition
B. Constraints on uterine growth
C. Vascular disorders
  1. Hypertension
  2. Toxemia
  3. Severe diabetes mellitus
D. Uterine malformations
E. Drug ingestion
  1. Tobacco
  2. Alcohol
  3. Narcotics

logic age and gender) by 2 years of age. Catch-up growth occurs during the first 6 months of life in approximately 80% of infants born SGA.[36] Approximately 10% to 15% of infants born SGA exhibit slow, attenuated growth with persistent height deficits in childhood and adolescence. The remaining 5% to 10% exhibit a slower catch-up growth pattern, reaching heights 2 SD below the mean between 3 and 5 years of age. These estimations vary by study; in a population of severely affected infants with SGA who required care in a neonatal intensive care unit, 27% had not achieved catch-up growth by 6 years of age.[851]

Low-birth-weight premature babies who are appropriate for gestational age (AGA) invariably experience catch-up growth in the first 2 years of life. Final adult height of all children born SGA is –0.8 to –0.9 SDS, a mean deficit of 3.6 to 4 cm when adjusted for family stature.[852] It has been estimated that the 10% to 15% of SGA children with short stature account for as much as 20% of all short children. In the United States, 2.3% of the population fitting the definition of SGA represents roughly an incidence of 1 in 43 neonates. Therefore, SGA children have a fivefold to sevenfold greater possibility of short stature than AGA children.[35]

Normal fetal growth depends on a complex interplay of maternal and fetal genetic and external environmental influences. Abnormal intrauterine growth can result from pathologic processes in the fetus, the placenta, or the mother. Growth in length occurs early in fetal life, whereas weight gain occurs later in fetal life[853]; first-trimester growth failure has been closely associated with low birth weight and low-birth-weight percentile.[854] Because there is a differential effect on weight and length depending on the fetal period when the pathologic processes occur, IUGR has been subclassified into symmetric and asymmetric types. The symmetric type of IUGR results from an insult early in the pregnancy, often due to fetal genetic factors or syndromes, congenital infections, or toxic effects; asymmetric IUGR results from an insult occurring late in gestation, often due to fetoplacental insufficiency. Historically, it was thought that infants with symmetric IUGR do not experience catch-up growth, whereas those with asymmetric IUGR who have normal head circumference and length yet low birth weight usually experience catch-up growth postnatally.[853] However, studies have suggested that infants with asymmetric IUGR have worse perinatal outcomes than those with symmetric IUGR[855,856] and that both types of growth restrictions can arise in the second trimester of pregnancy.[857,858] Therefore, the subclassification of IUGR, like the term *IUGR* itself, is controversial.

Endocrine-related causes account for a small fraction of the many contributors to fetal growth abnormalities, but hormonal disorders associated with fetal and neonatal growth restriction shed light on the endocrine mechanisms of growth in the fetus. Although GH plays a major role in postnatal growth, it has less of a role in fetal growth; infants with neonatal GHD are typically –0.5 to –1.5 SD below the mean in length and are heavy for this length.[859,860] An adequate nutrient supply is the main determinant of fetal growth, but growth factors such as insulin, IGF-1, and IGF-2 also play a role. Defects of insulin secretion or action are associated with impaired fetal growth.[853] Congenital defects of insulin secretion such as glucokinase deficiency[861] or pancreatic agenesis[862] are associated with severe IUGR. Leprechaunism is caused by defects in the insulin receptor and is associated with severe insulin resistance and IUGR.[26] The initial case of a deletion of the IGF-1 gene had profound intrauterine growth failure.[216,566] Polymorphisms of the *IGF1* gene have also been reported to be associated with IUGR.[216,863,864]

Neonates who are SGA exhibit hormonal patterns consistent with insensitivity to GH and IGF-1 and insulin action. In neonates with IUGR, GH levels are elevated[865] and IGF-1 and IGFBP3 levels are low.[114,865-868] IGFBP1 and IGFBP2 levels have been reported to be higher than in AGA infants,[235] a pattern seen in individuals with insulin resistance. Similar patterns are found in the first week of life after severe fetal malnutrition.[869] Exogenous GH treatment has little or no effect on growth, body composition, or energy expenditure[870,871] in the neonatal period. In most infants with SGA, normalization of GH, IGF-1, and IGFBP3 levels occurs by 3 months of age, with normal response to GH stimulation testing in childhood.[872] In measurement of spontaneous GH secretion, high pulse frequency with attenuated pulse amplitude and elevated trough values of GH have been noted in SGA children.[873-875] Serum IGF-1 levels in children with short stature born SGA are slightly but significantly lower than in children with catch-up growth.[872,873,875]

SGA children who have striking weight gain during the first several years of life can develop endocrine disorders later in childhood, including premature adrenarche, insulin resistance, polycystic ovary syndrome, and an attenuated growth spurt.[876] This subset of SGA children have increased risks of hypertension, maturity-onset diabetes, and cardiovascular disease later in life.[877,878] This is consistent with the Barker hypothesis, which states that fetal metabolic responses to a nutritionally hostile intrauterine environment may lead to inappropriate extrauterine consequences.[877,879] These problems do not appear to occur in SGA babies without catch-up growth, although insulin resistance has been described.[880] Whether being SGA is causally related to these disorders or is a symptom of an underlying inborn metabolic disorder is not yet known.

Russell-Silver syndrome (RSS) was independently described by Russell[881] and by Silver.[882] Findings include IUGR with postnatal growth failure, congenital hemihypertrophy, and small, triangular facies.[883] Other nonspecific findings include clinodactyly, delayed closure of the fontanel, delayed bone age, and precocious puberty.[884-886] Adults are short, with final heights approximately −4 SD below the mean.[883] The incidence is between 1 in 50,000 and 1 in 100,000 live births. Endogenous GH secretion in prepubertal RSS children is similar to that in other short IUGR children and less than in AGA short children.[873,887] Maternal uniparental disomy of chromosome 7 is present in 7% to 10% of cases.[883,888] Although there are a number of imprinted genes or factors involved in growth and development on chromosome 7, numerous studies have not detected any pathologic mutations in the candidate genes. A gene on chromosome 7p, *GRB10*, is involved in regulation of insulin and IGF-1 receptor signaling and is mainly expressed from the maternal allele; loss of the maternal allele results in fetal and placental overgrowth.[888,889] Mutations that could cause overexpression of *GRB10* have not been found in patients with RSS.

A small number of patients with RSS have duplication of the maternal allele of the 11p15 region[890]; duplication of the paternal allele in this region is associated with BWS and overexpression of IGF-2. The 11p15 region contains two imprinting control regions (ICR), ICR1 and ICR2 (Fig. 24-38). ICR1 comprises the *IGF2* and *H19* genes. The noncoding gene *H19* is downstream from *IGF2* and is oppositely imprinted, meaning that only the maternal allele is expressed and the paternal allele is inactive. The promoters of the *IGF2* and *H19* genes share a set of enhancers that act on either gene. On the paternal allele, the *H19* promoter region is methylated and therefore inactivated.[176]

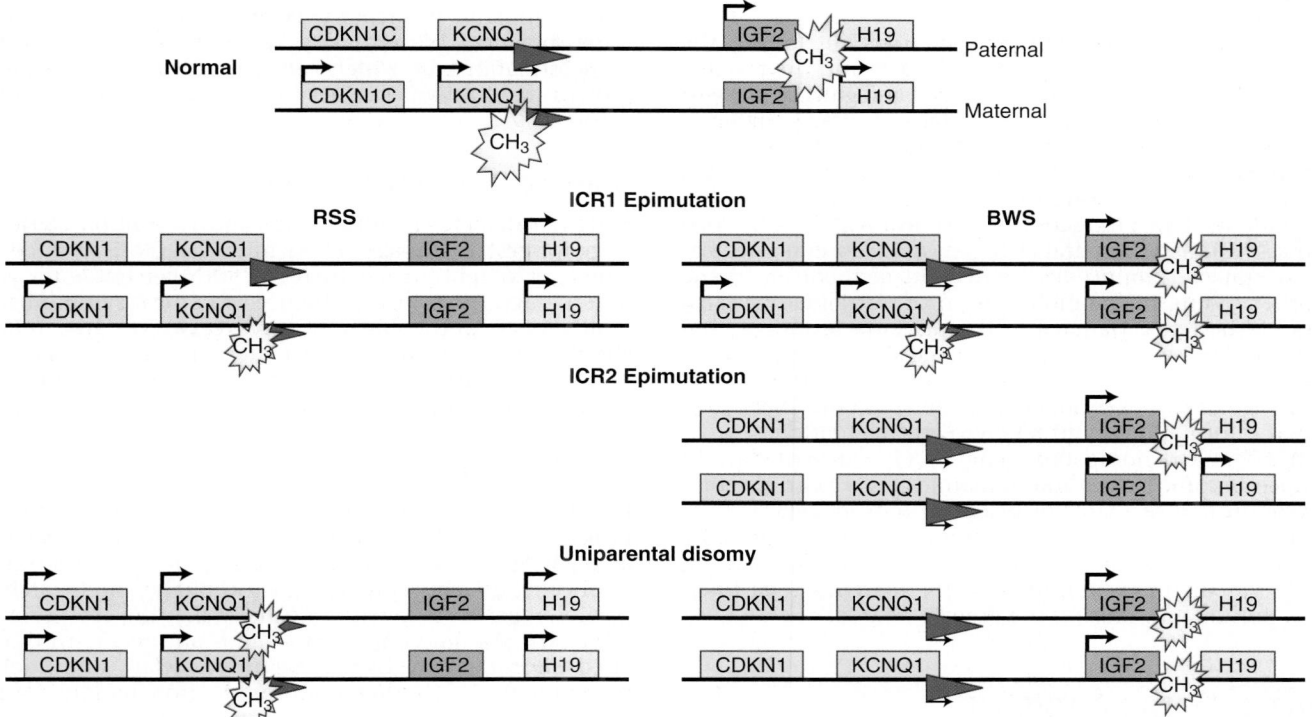

Figure 24-38 Schematic representation of the 11p15 region and the epigenetic mutations associated with Russell-Silver syndrome and Beckwith-Weidemann syndrome. Red and pink boxes represent genes of imprinting control region 1 (1CR1), and green boxes represent genes of 1CR2. The arrow represents the presence of gene transcription. Dark triangeles represent anti-sense transcripts that can repress transcription of *ICR2* genes. When methylated (represented by CH₃), the transcripts cannot be formed, allowing transcription of *ICR2* genes and reciprocal suppression of transcription of downstream genes (i.e., *IGF2*). (Adapted from Eggerman T. Silver-Russell and Beckwith-Weidemann syndromes: opposite (epi)mutations in 11p15 result in opposite clinical pictures. *Horm Res.* 2009;71(Suppl 2):30-35.)

Upstream from the *H19* and *IGF2* promoter region is a paternally methylated region that prevents binding of CTCF, allowing enhancers to act on the *IGF2* promoter to activate transcription.[177] On the maternal chromosome, this region is not methylated, allowing CTCF to bind and preventing transcription.[178] In this ICR1 region, mutations causing hypomethylation of the *H19* promoter region have been described in approximately 40% of patients with RSS.[891] Oppositely, hypermethylation of the ICR1 region has been associated with BWS. Disruption of ICR2 has been described in BWS (described later) but not in RSS. Reduced *IGF2* expression has been demonstrated in fibroblasts of patients with RSS in vitro,[891] but serum levels of IGF-2 in patients with RSS are normal.[892] Mice with a null mutation of IGF-2 have prenatal growth retardation but normal postnatal growth; how reduced expression of IGF-2 contributes to postnatal growth failure in RSS has yet to be elucidated.

Maternal and Placental Factors

Maternal factors and placental insufficiency can impair fetal growth and likely account for most cases of asymmetric IUGR. Maternal nutrition is an important contributor to fetal growth and to growth during the first year of life.[893] Fetal growth retardation may result from use of alcohol,[894] cocaine,[895] marijuana,[895] or tobacco[896] during pregnancy. The mechanisms for drug-induced fetal growth retardation are unclear but may include uterine vasoconstriction and vascular insufficiency, placental abruption, or premature rupture of membranes. The maternal hormonal milieu is affected by placental steroids and peptides. Maternal IGF-1 affects placental function and may facilitate transport of nutrients to the fetus. Maternal IGF-1 levels have been found to correlate with fetal growth.[897,898] Increased levels of free IGF-1 are found during normal human pregnancy.[899]

The placenta has multiple functions, including the transport of nutrients, oxygen, and waste and the production of hormones. It consumes oxygen and glucose brought by the uterine circulation. Placental GH affects maternal IGF production, which in turn affects placental function. A woman with GHD due to *PIT1* mutation exhibited normal levels of placental GH and IGF-1, demonstrating the independent production of GH and IGF-1 by the placenta.[900] Human placental lactogen (hPL) is a major regulator of glucose, amino acid, and lipid metabolism in the mother, aiding in the mobilization of nutrients for transport to the fetus. Damage to the placenta resulting from vascular disease, infection, or intrinsic abnormalities of the syncytiotrophoblasts can impair these important functions. At times, examination of the placenta may yield causal information about fetal growth retardation.

An X-linked homeobox gene, *ESX1*, detected only in extraembryonic tissues and human testes, is a chromosomally imprinted regulator of placental morphogenesis.[901-903] Heterozygous and homozygous mutant mice are born 20% smaller than normal and have large edematous placentas.[901] Vasculature is abnormal at the maternal-fetal interface, presumably causing the growth retardation.

PATHOLOGIC BASIS OF EXCESS GROWTH

Although by definition there are as many children with heights greater than 2 SD above the mean as those with heights less than 2 SD below the mean, tall stature as a

TABLE 24-7
Differential Diagnosis of Statural Overgrowth
Fetal Overgrowth
Maternal diabetes mellitus
Cerebral gigantism (Sotos syndrome)
Weaver syndrome
Beckwith-Wiedemann syndrome
Other insulin-like growth factor 2 (IGF-2) excess syndromes
Postnatal Overgrowth Leading to Childhood Tall Stature
Familial (constitutional) tall stature
Cerebral gigantism
Beckwith-Wiedemann syndrome
Exogenous obesity
Excess growth hormone (GH) secretion (pituitary adenoma with gigantism)
McCune-Albright syndrome or multiple endocrine neoplasia (MEN) associated with excess GH secretion
Precocious puberty
Marfan syndrome
Klinefelter syndrome (XXY karyotype)
Weaver syndrome
Fragile X syndrome
Homocystinuria
XYY karyotype
Hyperthyroidism
Postnatal Overgrowth Leading to Adult Tall Stature
Familial (constitutional) tall stature
Androgen or estrogen deficiency/estrogen resistance (in males)
Testicular feminization
Excess GH secretion
Marfan syndrome
Klinefelter syndrome (XXY karyotype)
XYY karyotype

chief complaint is encountered much less often in endocrine practice. Nevertheless, it is critical to identify those situations in which tall stature or an accelerated growth rate provides clues of an underlying disorder (Table 24-7).

Statural Overgrowth in the Fetus

Maternal diabetes mellitus is the most common cause of large-for-gestational-age (LGA) infants. LGA is defined as length or weight greater than the 90th percentile for gestational age. Even in the absence of clinical symptoms or family history, the birth of an excessively large infant should lead to evaluation for maternal or gestational diabetes. Two relatively rare syndromes, Sotos syndrome and BWS, can also cause LGA infants.

Sotos Syndrome

Children with cerebral gigantism (Sotos syndrome) are typically above the 90th percentile for length and weight at birth.[904-906] Clinical features also include a prominent forehead; dolichocephaly; macrocephaly; high arched palate; hypertelorism with unusually slanting eyes; prominent ears, jaw, and chin; large hands and feet with thickened subcutaneous tissue; cognitive delay; and motor incoordination. Children continue to grow rapidly during early childhood, but puberty is usually early, with premature epiphyseal fusion. Therefore, most children with Sotos syndrome have a final height within the normal range.[906] GH secretion and serum IGF levels are normal, and no specific cause of the overgrowth has been identified. About 80% of patients have a loss-of-function mutation in the

NSD1 gene whose product is a nucleus-localized basic transcription factor.[907]

Beckwith-Weidemann Syndrome

BWS is the most common (1 of every 13,700 live births) of the overgrowth disorders, the group of disorders associated with excessive somatic and specific organ growth. It is characterized by fetal macrosomia with omphalocele[908] and other clinical features secondary to organomegaly, such as macroglossia, renal medullary hyperplasia, and neonatal hypoglycemia due to islet cell hyperplasia.[909] Excessive childhood growth ultimately leads to earlier puberty and early epiphyseal fusion with resultant normal adult height.[910]

Various lines of evidence have shown that BWS is associated with loss of imprinting of the genes on chromosome 11p15.5, home of the *IGF2* gene (see Fig. 24-38). Under normal conditions, the paternally derived *IGF2* gene is expressed and the maternally transmitted gene is not active, as described in detail earlier in this chapter. BWS has been associated with uniparental disomy or duplication of the paternal 11p15 region and resultant overexpression of the *IGF2* gene.[911] The ICR1 region of 11p15 contains the *IGF2* and *H19* genes; the noncoding gene *H19* is located downstream from *IGF2* and is oppositely imprinted. The promoters of the *IGF2* and *H19* genes share a set of enhancers that act on either gene. On the paternal allele, the *H19* promoter region is methylated and therefore inactivated.[176] Upstream from the *H19* and *IGF2* promoter region is a paternally methylated region that prevents binding of CTCF, allowing enhancers to act on the *IGF2* promoter to activate transcription.[177] On the maternal chromosome, this region is not methylated, allowing CTCF to bind and preventing transcription.[178] Hypermethylation of the *H19* promoter region with resultant loss of imprinting and biallelic expression of IGF-2 has been associated with fewer than 10% of the cases of BWS.[182,912] Point mutations in the ICR1 region have been identified in patients with BWS. These mutations alter binding of OCT (octamer) transcription factors to the region leading to hypermethylation of the promoter.[913] Hypomethylation of this region is associated with RSS, a syndrome associated with prenatal and postnatal growth failure (see earlier discussion).

ICR2, located 5′ of ICR1, contains the genes for cyclin-dependent kinase inhibitor 1C *(CDKN1C)* and potassium channel KQT family member 1 *(KCNQ1)*, among others that are methylated on the maternal allele. Associated with these two genes is an antisense transcript with paternal expression that may suppress transcription; it has been postulated that this cluster of genes is in "expression competition" with the *IGF2/H19* cluster.[914] Up to 25% of familial cases of BWS are associated with mutations in the *CDKN1C* or *KCNQ1* gene,[915] but there is debate about whether loss of imprinting of the *IGF2* gene convincingly occurs with most of the mutations. Four children with somatic overgrowth but not the diagnostic features of BWS had *IGF2* gene overexpression.[916] Additionally, mutations in *GPC3*, a glypican gene that codes for an IGF-2 neutralizing membrane receptor, cause the related Simpson-Golabi-Behmel overgrowth syndrome.[917,918]

Postnatal Statural Overgrowth

As in the case of the child with growth failure, crossing of height percentiles between infancy and the onset of puberty is an indication for further evaluation because it can indicate serious underlying pathology. As with short stature, children with tall stature must be evaluated in the context of familial growth and pubertal patterns.

Tall Stature

GH secretion and levels of IFG-1 and IGFBP3 in familial tall stature are often in the upper-normal range.[919] Tauber and colleagues[920] divided 65 children with familial tall stature into a subset with high GH secretion rates and frequent secretory bursts and another subset with lower GH secretion and fewer episodic spikes. IGF-1 levels were higher among those producing more GH and normal in the low-GH group. The authors postulated that both enhanced secretion of GH and greater efficiency of GH-mediated IGF-1 production might be potential causes of familial tall stature.

Tall stature is also a characteristic of certain syndromes. Marfan syndrome, an autosomal dominant disorder of collagen metabolism, is characterized by hyperextensible joints, dislocation of the lens, kyphoscoliosis, dissecting aortic aneurysm, and long, thin bones that result in arachnodactyly and moderately tall stature. It is caused by mutations in the fibrillin-1 gene *(FBN1)*. The abnormal FBN1 monomers from the mutated gene disrupt the normal aggregation of FBN1, impairing microfibril formation. Homocystinuria is an autosomal recessive disorder that phenotypically resembles Marfan syndrome, but patients also have cognitive disabilities. Tall stature has also been found in patients with familial ACTH resistance due to a defective ACTH receptor.[921]

Dosage effects of the *SHOX* gene may result in tall stature.[922] In females with three copies of the *SHOX* gene and gonadal dysgenesis, adult stature was +2 to +2.9 SDS.[923] In women with the 47,XXX karyotype, mean final heights are 5 to 10 cm taller than population means, and men with the 47,XXY karyotype (Klinefelter syndrome) are about 3.5 cm taller than population means.[30,924] Males with an XYY karyotype may also have moderately tall stature. In addition to SHOX effects, the variable degree of estrogen production in these syndromes may also influence skeletal maturation and final height.[25]

Failure to enter puberty and complete sexual maturation may result in sustained growth during adult life with ultimate tall stature and a characteristic eunuchoid habitus. The description of tall stature with open epiphyses resulting from mutation of the estrogen receptor or from aromatase deficiency[22,23,925] underscores the fundamental role of estrogen in promoting epiphyseal fusion and termination of normal skeletal growth.

Obesity

Obesity is frequently associated with rapid skeletal growth and early onset of puberty.[926] Rapid early postnatal weight gain has been associated with taller stature at 8 years of age than that predicted from the midparental target height.[927] Others have shown that early postnatal growth is associated with altered tempo of development, but sudden weight gain in middle childhood has little effect on height trajectory.[928] Patients with obesity tend to have diminished overall GH production but normal to high GHBP, and IGF-1 levels appear to be capable of maintaining adequate or enhanced linear growth velocity. Bone age is usually modestly accelerated, so that both puberty and epiphyseal fusion occur early and adult height is normal. This association between obesity and rapid growth is so characteristic that a child with obesity and short stature should always be evaluated for underlying pathology, such as hypothyroidism, GHD, Cushing syndrome, or PWS.

Tumors

Pituitary gigantism is a rare condition, analogous to acromegaly in the adult (see Chapter 9).[929-931] GH-secreting tumors of the pituitary are typically eosinophilic or chromophobic adenomas. Their cause is uncertain, although many result from somatic mutations that generate constitutively activated G proteins with reduced GTPase activity (see Chapter 9).[932] The resulting increase in intracellular cAMP in the pituitary leads to increased GH secretion. Somatotropic tumors with excess GH secretion may occur in McCune-Albright syndrome, which is caused by mutations resulting in constitutive activation of G proteins.[933,934] GH-secreting tumors have also been reported in multiple endocrine neoplasia (MEN) and in association with neurofibromatosis and tuberous sclerosis.[935]

GH excess that occurs before epiphyseal fusion results in rapid growth and attainment of adult heights above expected adult potential. When GH hypersecretion is accompanied by gonadotropin deficiency, accelerated linear growth may persist for decades, as was the case for the Alton giant, who reached a height of 280 cm by the time of his death in his 20s.[936] Manifestations typical of acromegaly may also appear, such as soft tissue swelling; enlargement of the nose, ears, and jaw with coarsening of facial features; pronounced increases in hand and foot size; diaphoresis; galactorrhea; and menstrual irregularity.

EVALUATION AND TREATMENT OF GROWTH ABNORMALITIES

Clinical Evaluation of Growth Retardation

The most important parameter in assessing children with growth failure is careful clinical evaluation, including accurate serial assessment of height and height velocity. Consideration of a growth disorder is raised when a child's length or height falls below the normal range (<3rd percentile), the growth velocity is subnormal (indicated by length or height measurements that cross percentiles on the growth curve or by an annual growth velocity less than the 3rd percentile for age), or the child's height is below the range expected based on the parents' heights. To grow along the 3rd percentile for height, a child must maintain a height velocity at the 25th percentile for age.[937] Therefore, a height velocity consistently below the 25th percentile in a short child suggests abnormal growth. However, because of the greater error intrinsic to assessment of growth velocity compared with height velocity,[938] a single height velocity measurement above the 25th percentile for age, even based on annual height data, cannot fully exclude a growth abnormality in a short child.[938]

GH is relatively less important as a growth factor prenatally compared with its role postnatally. However, GH is not without impact on prenatal growth, so that although many of these children have lengths and weights within the normal range, the average size of infants with congenital GH deficiency is decreased, with a mean birth length of −1.3 SDS and a mean birth weight of −1.0 SDS.[939] Growth velocity over the first year averages near −2 SD, so that over half of these infants have a length more than 2 SD below the mean at 1 year of age.[939]

Table 24-8 provides an algorithm for evaluation of the child with growth failure. Although one third of healthy infants will cross downward on the length percentile growth curve (discussed previously), this is normal only in relatively large infants born to small parents or in those

---

TABLE 24-8

Clinical and Biochemical Evaluation of Growth Failure: Evaluating the GH/IGF-1 Axis

Step 1: Defining the Risk of IGF Deficiency Syndrome

Auxologic abnormalities
  Severe short stature (height SDS < −3 SD)
  Severe growth deceleration
    Height < −2 SD and height velocity < −1.0 SD over 2 years
    Height < −1.5 SD and height velocity < −1.5 SD over 2 years
Risk factors
  History of a brain tumor, cranial irradiation, or other documented organic or congenital hypothalamic-pituitary abnormality
  Incidental finding of hypothalamic-pituitary abnormality on MRI
  If any of the above exists, proceed with Step 2; if not, follow clinically and return to Step 1 in 6 months

Step 2: Screening for IGF Deficiency and Other Diseases

A. Order a laboratory panel including a bone age, free T_4, TSH, chromosomes (in females), and nonendocrine tests; if indicated, refer back to primary care physician or treat diagnosed conditions as appropriate.
B. Order an IGF-1 and IGFBP3 level.
  If IGF-1/IGFBP3 are both above the −1 SD, follow clinically and return to Step 1 in 6 months.
  If IGF-1/IGFBP3 are both below −2 SD, proceed to Step 4. If MRI is abnormal, GH provocative testing is optional (see Table 23-11).
  Otherwise, proceed to Step 3. If this is a patient with delayed adolescence, consider sex steroid treatment prior to Step 3.

Step 3: Testing GH Secretion

This step can be bypassed if a clear GHD risk factor and a severe IGF deficiency are identified.
Perform two of the following GH stimulation tests (if appropriate, estrogen prime) (see Table 23-9):
  Clonidine
  Arginine
  Insulin
  Glucagon
  L-Dopa
  Propranolol
If all GH levels are below 10 ng/mL, go to Step 4.
If peak GH > 15 ng/mL, obtain GHBP; if GHBP < −2 SD, consider an IGF-generation test and, if abnormal, IGF treatment.
If peak GH > 15 ng/mL and GHBP is normal, follow clinically and return to Step 1 in 6 months. If peak GH is between 10 and 15 ng/mL, go back to Step 1 in 6 months.
If peak GH is between 10 and 15 ng/mL, go back to Step 2 in 6 months.

Step 4: Evaluating the Pituitary

Perform MRI, with particular emphasis on hypothalamic-pituitary anatomy.
Test HPA, if not already done (CRH stimulation of ITT), and teach cortisol supplementation as needed (must do this if MRI is abnormal).
Consider molecular evaluation of GH, GHR, or GHRHR and other potential genetic defects (see Fig. 24-2).

Step 5: Treating for Growth Promotion

Initiate GH treatment at appropriate dose levels.
If GHIS is suspected, consider IGF therapy, if available.
Regularly evaluate growth parameters, IGF-1, and IGFBP3, as well as compliance and safety (see Table 24-14).
GH secretion should be retested, according to adult GH assessment protocols, at the end of growth.

CRH, corticotropin-releasing hormone; GH, growth hormone; GHD, growth hormone deficiency; GHIS, growth hormone insensitivity; GHR, growth hormone receptor; GHRHR, growth hormone–releasing hormone receptor; HPA, hypothalamic-pituitary axis; IGF-1, insulin-like growth factor 1; IGFBP3, IGF-binding protein 3; ITT, insulin tolerance test; MRI, magnetic resonance imaging; SD, standard deviation; SDS, standard deviation score; T_4, thyroxine; TSH, thyroid-stimulating hormone (thyrotropin).

infants who are following a growth pattern of CDGD (see later discussion). In other situations, the infant who is crossing downward on the length percentile curve should be investigated in the same way as other children with subnormal growth velocities.

History and Physical Examination

The many illness-related causes of diminished growth were discussed in earlier sections of this chapter. A growth pattern in which weight gain is impaired before linear growth or in which there is greater impairment of weight gain than of length/height gain suggests an impairment of nutrition, such as inadequate intake, malabsorption, or increased energy requirements. Nonhormonal causes of growth failure should be investigated based on data obtained from a careful history and physical examination. In addition, careful evaluation of the growth curve in the context of the family history may suggest a normal variant growth pattern, such as crossing linear percentiles of infancy, familial short stature, or CDGD. In such cases, careful observation may be all that is required. One third of all infants have growth parameters that cross percentiles downward on the growth curve, and 3% of the all children have a length or height below the 3rd percentile. Most of these children have no disease or growth disorder and will demonstrate this by having a normal growth velocity on continued observation.

The physical examination should look for evidence of an underlying organ-specific or systemic disease. It should also evaluate for clues specific to growth disorders, such as findings suggestive of genetic disorders such as Noonan syndrome, RSS, or TS. In addition, body proportions should be measured, because skeletal disproportion suggests a skeletal dysplasia.

Findings on the history and examination may point to an increased likelihood of the presence of GHD (Table 24-9). Micropenis in a male newborn should always lead to an evaluation of the GH/IGF-1 axis. Nystagmus, indicating neonatal blindness, suggests hypopituitarism due to its association with optic nerve hypoplasia in the syndrome of septo-optic dysplasia. A history of other midline defects, such as cleft lip and cleft palate,[940] or a single central incisor increases concern for hypopituitarism. Unexplained neonatal hypoglycemia, hepatitis, or prolonged jaundice should prompt an evaluation of pituitary function. Older children with GHD have less impaired weight gain than height gain, resulting in an increased weight for height; they are often described as having a "cherubic" appearance. Increased weight for height with growth failure is also characteristic of hypothyroidism. If the weight gain is dramatic, Cushing syndrome should be considered. (However, linear growth acceleration with excess weight gain is not consistent with Cushing syndrome.) Finally, GHD should be suspected in children with known or suspected CNS pathology (e.g., tumors, prior radiation therapy to the CNS, malformations, infection, trauma) or with documented deficiency of TSH, ACTH, antidiuretic hormone, or gonadotropin.

Laboratory Testing

If the history and physical examination do not suggest a specific disorder causing growth failure and the growth pattern and family history do not provide sufficient reassurance that the growth is following a normal variant growth pattern, it is necessary to perform laboratory testing. In many cases, the testing does not identify an abnormality, and the child either is ultimately found to

TABLE 24-9

Key History and Physical Examination Findings That Suggest the Diagnosis of Growth Hormone Deficiency*

Findings That Suggest the Diagnosis of GHD

In the Neonate
Hypoglycemia
Prolonged jaundice
Hepatitis
Microphallus
Traumatic delivery

In a Child with Short Stature or Growth Failure
Cranial irradiation
Head trauma or central nervous system infection
Consanguinity or an affected family member
Craniofacial midline abnormalities

Findings That Support Immediate Investigation for GHD

In a Child with Short Stature
Signs indicative of an intracranial lesion
Neonatal symptoms and signs of GHD
Auxologic findings
  Severe short stature (<−3 SD)
  Height < −2 SD and height velocity over 1 year of < −1 SD
  A decrease in height SD of >0.5 over 1 year in children >2 years of age
  A height velocity below −2 SD over 1 year
  A height velocity >1.5 SD below the mean sustained velocity over 2 years
Signs of multiple pituitary hormone deficiency (MPHD)

GHD, growth hormone deficiency; SD, standard deviation.
*The Growth Hormone Research Society 2000 Criteria.
From Growth Hormone Research Society. Consensus guidelines for the diagnosis and treatment of growth hormone (GH) deficiency in childhood and adolescence: summary statement of the GH research society. *J Clin Endocrinol Metab*. 2000;85:3990-3993.

have a normal variant growth pattern or falls into the classification of ISS. The laboratory tests can be divided into those screening for disorders outside the GH/IGF-1 axis and those evaluating that axis.

Screening Tests

Because a number of illnesses can cause growth failure either before or in the absence of other signs or symptoms, it is necessary to screen for these disorders in children with abnormal growth. A complete blood count looks for evidence of anemia, chronic infection, and inflammation. A complete blood chemistry panel provides evidence for silent renal disease (including renal tubular acidosis), liver disease, and disorders of calcium and phosphorus. The erythrocyte sedimentation rate is measured to look for evidence of disorders involving chronic inflammation, such as presymptomatic juvenile idiopathic arthritis and inflammatory bowel disease. A urinalysis is obtained to look for renal disease and chronic urinary tract infection. Tissue transglutaminase IgA (and total serum IgA) is measured to screen for celiac disease. In girls in whom no other explanation for short stature is found, a karyotype should be obtained to exclude TS. This is done even in the absence of other physical features of TS, because growth failure may be the only evident feature, particularly in cases of significant mosaicism.

Hypothyroidism should be screened for in children with growth failure. Because of the importance of thyroid hormone on brain development in infants, this possibility should be considered early in the evaluation of an infant with growth failure in order to correct identified hypothyroidism quickly. In addition, hypothyroidism results in lower serum IGF-1 levels and decreases GH levels during provocative testing.[941-943] Therefore, it is necessary to ensure that thyroid function is normal before evaluating for GHD. TSH is measured because it is the most sensitive indicator of primary hypothyroidism. However, because central hypothyroidism must also be considered as a cause for growth failure in children, the thyroxine level should also be measured.

Bone Age. After the neonatal period, a bone age determination can be useful in the evaluation of children with growth disorders. A radiograph of the left hand and wrist is commonly used for comparison with the published standards of Greulich and Pyle.[944] An alternative method for assessing bone age from radiographs of the left hand involves a scoring system for developmentally identified stages of each of 20 individual bones,[945] a technique that has been adapted for computerized assessment.[946,947] The left hand is used because radiographs of the entire skeleton would be tedious and expensive and would involve additional radiation exposure. However, the hand does not contribute to height, and accurate evaluation of growth potential may require radiographs of the legs and spine.

Although the bone age result does not identify a specific diagnosis in a child with a growth disorder, it can be used to classify the child's growth in relation to groups of diagnoses. Growth disorders caused by an underlying illness or hormone disorder (e.g., renal disease, malnutrition, glucocorticoid excess) are associated with a delayed bone age—that is, a bone age that is younger than the patient's chronologic age. Similarly, hypothyroidism and GHD are associated with a delayed bone age. If short stature is intrinsic to the condition, however, bone age is not delayed and is within the range of normal for the chronologic age. This is true for genetic disorders such as TS, Noonan syndrome, and RSS and also for familial short stature. In CDGD, the bone age is delayed, consistent with the future delay in puberty and late epiphyseal fusion. Given the lack of precise diagnostic laboratory tests for GHD, a lack of bone age delay argues against this diagnosis. On the other hand, the fact that patients with CDGD have a delayed bone age does not help in the sometimes difficult discrimination between this condition and GHD.

A number of important caveats concerning bone age must be considered. Experience in determination of bone age is essential to minimize intraobserver variance, and clinical studies involving bone age benefit from having a single reader perform all interpretations. The normal rate of skeletal maturation differs between boys and girls and among different ethnic groups. The standards of Greulich and Pyle are separable by sex but were developed in American white children between 1931 and 1942. Both those and the Tanner and Whitehouse standards are based on normal children[948] and may not be applicable to children with skeletal dysplasias, endocrine abnormalities, or other forms of growth retardation or acceleration.

Prediction of Adult Height. The extent of skeletal maturation observed in an individual can be used to predict the ultimate height potential. Such predictions are based on the observation that the more delayed the bone age (relative to the chronologic age), the longer the time before epiphyseal fusion prevents further growth. The most commonly used method for height prediction, based on Greulich and Pyle's *Radiographic Atlas of Skeletal Development*,[944] was developed by Bayley and Pinneau[949] and relies on bone age, height, and a semiquantitative allowance for chronologic age (Table 24-10). The system of Tanner and colleagues[945] uses measurements of height, bone age, chronologic age, and, during puberty, height and bone age increments during the previous year, as well as menarchal status.

Roche, Wainer, and Thissen[950] used the combination of height, bone age, chronologic age, midparental height, and weight (RWT method). Attempts have been made to calculate final height predictions without requiring the determination of skeletal age[951] by using multiple regression analyses with available data such as height, weight, birth measurements, and midparental stature. All of these systems are, by nature, empiric and are not absolute predictors. Indeed, the 90% confidence intervals for the predictions are approximately ±6 cm at younger ages. The more advanced the bone age, the greater the accuracy of the adult height prediction, because a more advanced bone age places a patient closer to his or her final height.

All methods of predicting adult height are based on data from normal children, and none has been documented to be accurate in children with growth abnormalities. For this kind of precision, it would be necessary to develop disease-specific atlases of skeletal maturation (e.g., for achondroplasia or TS). In addition, height predictions will clearly be inaccurate in predicting the final height in the case of a growth-impairing process that is not adequately treated. In addition, height predictions must be used with care in assessing height outcomes during treatment. For example, in patients with precocious puberty treated with GnRH agonists, height prediction is known to overpredict the actual final height.[952] Thus, height predictions should only be considered a reasonable estimate.

Tests of the GH/IGF-1 Axis

In children with growth retardation in whom other causes have been excluded, the possibility of GHD should be considered. However, these tests can have poor specificity, so clinical assessment must always play an important part in the evaluation of abnormalities in the GH/IGF-1 axis. For example, a child growing consistently just below the 3rd percentile for height, with a growth rate that is accordingly above the 25th percentile for age, is very unlikely to be GH deficient. Abnormal test results in this situation would most likely represent false-positive results.

Testing of the GH/IGF-1 axis begins with "static" testing of GH function, measuring IGF-1. It may also be helpful to measure IGFBP3. In some cases—if the clinical presentation is highly suggestive of GHD (see Table 24-9)[953] and the IGF-1 level (and the IGFBP3 level, if obtained) also indicates a high likelihood of GHD—it is appropriate to proceed directly to the dynamic tests of GH secretion. In most cases, however, unless there is an abnormality identified on the screening tests, it is appropriate to monitor the child's growth for a period of 6 to 12 months to accurately assess the child's growth rate. Then, based on the complete clinical picture, including the growth rate and the IGF-1 level, the decision is made to proceed with dynamic testing of GH secretion or to continue monitoring the child's growth.

There is no test that definitively diagnoses GHD. Because there is no "gold standard," it is impossible to precisely define the sensitivity or specificity of any test for GHD. Some information on specificity can be obtained by comparing the results with those obtained in normal children, although, for the more complicated tests, these data can be difficult to obtain in children. Sensitivity relies on comparing positive results from one test with those of another—for example, comparing low IGF-1 concentrations to failed results on provocative GH tests. Poor sensitivity of IGF-1 as an indicator of GHD has been based on results from children with normal IGF-1 concentrations who have abnormal results on provocative GH tests.[954] However, because of the known limited specificity of these

TABLE 24-10

Prediction of Adult Stature

	Fraction of Adult Height Attained at Each Bone Age*					
	Girls			Boys		
Bone Age (yr-mo)	Retarded	Average	Advanced	Retarded	Average	Advanced
6-0	0.733	0.720		0.680		
6-3	0.742	0.729		0.690		
6-6	0.751	0.738		0.700		
6-9	0.763	0.751		0.709		
7-0	0.770	0.757	0.712	0.718	0.695	0.670
7-3	0.779	0.765	0.722	0.728	0.702	0.676
7-6	0.788	0.772	0.732	0.738	0.709	0.683
7-9	0.797	0.782	0.742	0.747	0.716	0.689
8-0	0.804	0.790	0.750	0.756	0.723	0.696
8-3	0.813	0.801	0.760	0.765	0.731	0.703
8-6	0.823	0.810	0.771	0.773	0.739	0.709
8-9	0.836	0.821	0.784	0.779	0.746	0.715
9-0	0.841	0.827	0.790	0.786	0.752	0.720
9-3	0.851	0.836	0.800	0.794	0.761	0.728
9-6	0.858	0.844	0.809	0.800	0.769	0.734
9-9	0.866	0.853	0.819	0.807	0.777	0.741
10-0	0.874	0.862	0.828	0.812	0.784	0.747
10-3	0.884	0.874	0.841	0.816	0.791	0.753
10-6	0.896	0.884	0.856	0.819	0.795	0.758
10-9	0.907	0.896	0.870	0.821	0.800	0.763
11-0	0.918	0.906	0.883	0.823	0.804	0.767
11-3	0.922	0.910	0.887	0.827	0.812	0.776
11-6	0.926	0.914	0.891	0.832	0.818	0.786
11-9	0.929	0.918	0.897	0.839	0.827	0.800
12-0	0.932	0.922	0.901	0.845	0.834	0.809
12-3	0.942	0.932	0.913	0.852	0.843	0.818
12-6	0.949	0.941	0.924	0.860	0.853	0.828
12-9	0.957	0.950	0.935	0.869	0.863	0.839
13-0	0.964	0.958	0.945	0.880	0.876	0.850
13-3	0.971	0.967	0.955		0.890	0.863
13-6	0.977	0.974	0.963		0.902	0.875
13-9	0.981	0.978	0.968		0.914	0.890
14-0	0.983	0.980	0.972		0.927	0.905
14-3	0.986	0.983	0.977		0.938	0.918
14-6	0.989	0.986	0.980		0.948	0.930
14-9	0.992	0.988	0.983		0.958	0.943
15-0	0.994	0.990	0.986		0.968	0.958
15-3	0.995	0.991	0.988		0.973	0.967
15-6	0.996	0.993	0.990		0.976	0.971
15-9	0.997	0.994	0.992		0.980	0.976
16-0	0.998	0.996	0.993		0.982	0.980
16-3	0.999	0.996	0.994		0.985	0.983
16-6	0.999	0.997	0.995		0.987	0.985
16-9	0.9995	0.998	0.997		0.989	0.988
17-0	1.00	0.999	0.998		0.991	0.990
17-3					0.993	
17-6		0.9995	0.9995		0.994	
17-9					0.995	
18-0		1.00			0.996	
18-3					0.998	
18-6					1.00	

*The column headed "Retarded" is used when bone age is >1 year below chronologic age; the column headed "Advanced" is used when bone age is >1 year greater than chronologic age.

Table derived from Richman RA, Kirsch LR. Testosterone treatment in adolescent boys with constitutional delay in growth and development. *N Engl J Med.* 1988;319:1563-1567. Based on the data of Bayley and Pinneau.[949] Predicted final height is calculated by dividing the current height by the fraction of adult height achieved determined from the table.

provocative tests (discussed later), one cannot determine whether the discrepant results are due to the poor sensitivity of the IGF-1 test or the poor specificity of the provocative GH test. Again, it is critical to interpret all results together and in the context of the clinical data.

Insulin-like Growth Factor 1. GHD is associated with low serum concentrations of IGF-1 (Fig. 24-39). Unlike GH levels, which rise and fall with its pulsatile secretion, the IGF-1 level in blood has minimal diurnal variation. The GH dependency of the IGFs was established in the initial report from Salmon and Daughaday[127] and was further clarified with the development of sensitive and specific immunoassays that distinguish between IGF-1 and IGF-2.[955] IGF-1 levels are more GH-dependent than IGF-2 levels and are more likely to reflect subtle differences in GH secretory patterns. However, serum IGF-1 levels are also influenced by age,[170-172] degree of sexual maturation, and nutritional status. Therefore, IGF-1 levels must be compared with age-specific ranges (Fig. 24-40), and with ranges defined by stage of sexual maturation. Some clinicians evaluate IGF-1

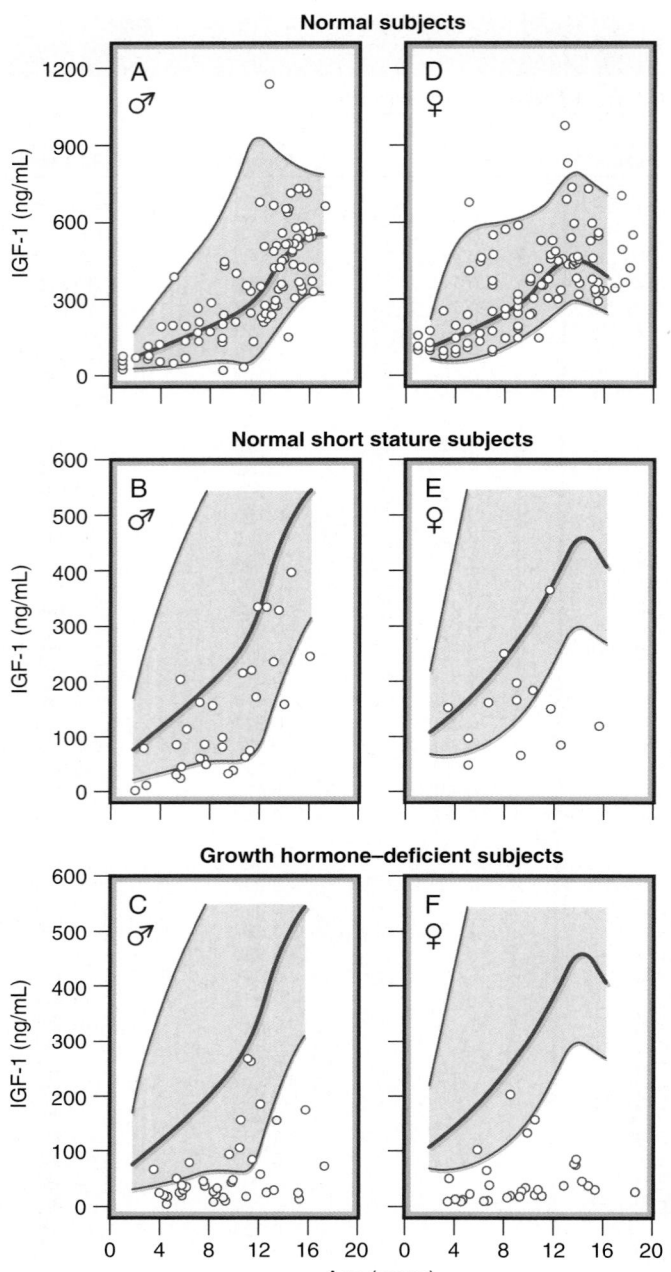

Figure 24-39 Serum levels of insulin-like growth factor 1 (IGF-1) in normal patients and in patients with growth disorders. Circles represent IGF-1 levels in normal subjects *(A, D)*, normal short stature subjects *(B, E)*, and growth hormone–deficient subjects *(C, F)*. The lines represent the 5th, 50th, 95th percentiles for log-normalized IGF-1 levels in normal subjects. (From Rosenfeld RG, Wilson DM, Lee PD, et al. Insulin-like growth factors I and II in the evaluation of growth retardation. *J Pediatr.* 1986;109:428-433.)

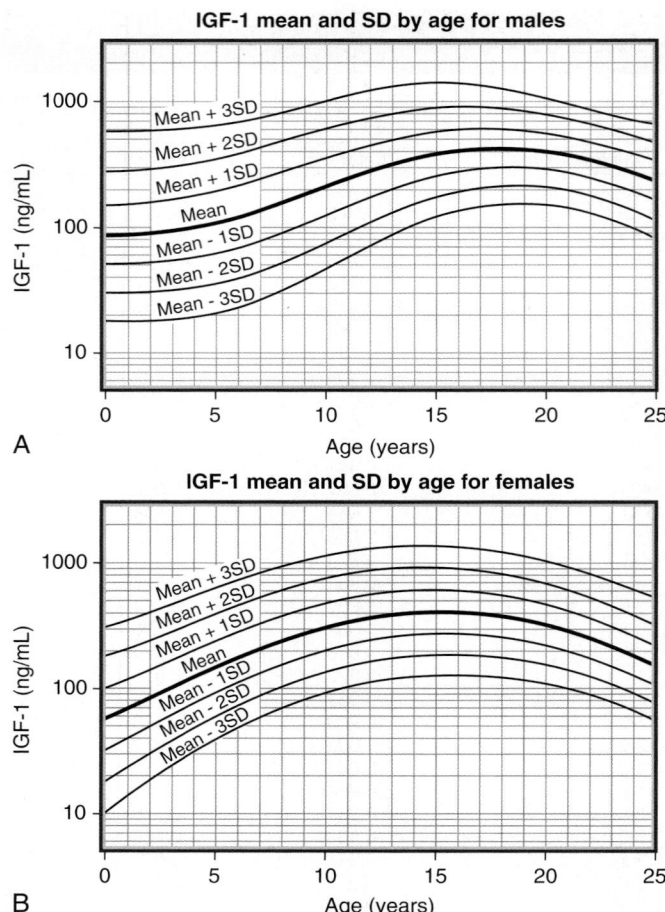

Figure 24-40 Normal serum levels of insulin-like growth factor 1 (IGF-1) for males (**A**) and females (**B**). SD, standard deviation. (Data courtesy of Diagnostic Systems Laboratories, Inc., Webster, TX.)

results against the reference range based on bone age (rather than the chronologic age). This may improve the specificity of this test for GHD, although there are no data to address the validity of this approach.

IGF-1 levels in normal children younger than 5 or 6 years of age are low. This leads to poor sensitivity of IGF-1 levels for identifying GHD in young children. As few as 40% to 50% of young, short children with evidence of GHD on provocative tests have IGF-1 levels below the lower level of the reference range.[956,957] IGF-1 levels increase with age, resulting in better separation of IGF-1 levels in GH-deficient children from those in normal children and a higher sensitivity of IGF-1 levels for GHD. However, although sensitivities of 85% to 100% have been reported in some studies,[957,958] in others it has averaged approximately 70%.[941,958-961] Again, the lack of a gold standard means that some of the false-negative findings obtained by measurement of IGF-1 levels might rather represent false-positives on provocative GH testing.

IGF-1 levels also suffer from a lack of specificity in diagnosing GHD. In general, IGF-1 levels have higher specificity in younger children, with declining specificity in older children. Juul and Skakkebaek[961] found that IGF-1 levels had a specificity for GHD of 98% in children younger than 10 years of age but a specificity of only 67% in those older than 10 years. Similarly, Cianfarani and colleagues[956] found a specificity of 100% in children younger than 9 years of age that dropped to 76% in older children. Thus, the overall specificity of a low IGF-1 measurement may only be approximately 70%.[941,958,959]

In addition to the specific challenges of accurately quantitating IGF-1 levels in serum (see later discussion), the nutritional dependence of IGF-1 levels significantly affects the accuracy of this test in evaluating for GHD. Even a few days of decreased caloric intake can lower IGF-1 levels.[941,962] This probably contributes to the finding that IGF-1 levels can vary by as much as 38% from day to day in a given patient.[962,963]

Early quantitation of IGFs used bioassays based on [^{35}S]-sulfate incorporation (hence, "sulfation factor" as an early synonym for IGF/somatomedin C); on stimulation of the synthesis of DNA, RNA, or protein; or on glucose uptake.[964,965] Development of specific antibodies permitted the development of accurate and specific measurement of IGF-1 and IGF-2.[955,959,966,967] However, the presence of IGFBPs results in a significant technical challenge for the accurate quantitation of IGF-1 (and IGF-2) in serum.[941,964,968] Interference is a particular problem in conditions with a relatively high IGFBP/IGF peptide ratio and at the extremes of the assay (i.e., GHD, acromegaly). In uremia, IGFBPs artifactually lower IGF-1 levels and increase IGF-2 levels in assays that do not eliminate this interference.[661]

The most effective way to deal with IGFBPs is to separate them from IGF peptides by chromatography under acidic conditions.[969] This labor-intensive procedure has occasionally been replaced by an acid ethanol extraction procedure.[970] Although the latter method may be reasonably effective for most serum samples, it is problematic in conditions of high IGFBP/IGF peptide ratios, such as conditioned media from cell lines and sera from newborns or from subjects with GHD or uremia. A number of alternative approaches to addressing the interference from the IGFBs have been developed, including the use of tracers that do not bind to IGFBPs[971] and "sandwich" assay methods.[972] Automated IGF-1 immunometric (IRMA) or immunochemiluminometric (ICMA) assays typically add an excess of IGF-2 to the assay to displace the IGFBPs and use highly specific IGF-1 antibodies.[941,964,973] Although current IGF-1 assays significantly minimize the interference from IGBPs, it is important that each assay develop reference ranges that match the clinical samples to be tested, because ethnic variations and nutritional and environmental factors can affect "normal" serum IGF-1 concentrations.

A number of assays have been developed that purport to measure "free" or "free dissociable" IGF-1 as a means of assessing concentrations of IGF-1 peptides that circulate unbound to IGFBPs.[974] Both the accuracy and the physiologic relevance of these determinations remain open to debate.[172,941,974]

Insulin-like Growth Factor–Binding Protein 3. Measurement of the serum level of IGBP3, the major serum carrier of IGF peptides, is a potential additional tool for evaluating GH function.[666,975,976] The advantages of assaying IGFBP3 concentration include the following:

1. IGFBP3 levels are GH dependent.
2. IGFBP3 levels are constant throughout the day.
3. The immunoassay of IGFBP3 is technically simple and does not require separation of the binding protein from IGF peptides.
4. Normal serum levels of IGFBP3 are high, typically in the 1- to 5-mg/L range, so that assay sensitivity is not an issue. (The molar concentration of IGFBP3 approximates the sum of the molar concentration of IGF-1 and IGF-2.)
5. Serum IGFBP3 levels vary with age to a lesser degree than is the case for IGF-1 (Fig. 24-41). Even in infants, serum IGFBP3 levels are sufficiently high to allow discrimination of low values from the normal range.
6. Serum IGFBP3 levels are less dependent on nutrition than serum IGF-1, reflecting the "stabilizing" effect of IGF-2 levels.

Like IGF-1 levels, determination of the sensitivity and specificity of IGBP3 levels for identifying GHD suffers from the lack of a gold standard. With that limitation in mind, Blum and colleagues[666] initially found that low IGFBP3 levels had both high sensitivity (97%) and high specificity (95%) for GHD. Most subsequent studies confirmed the

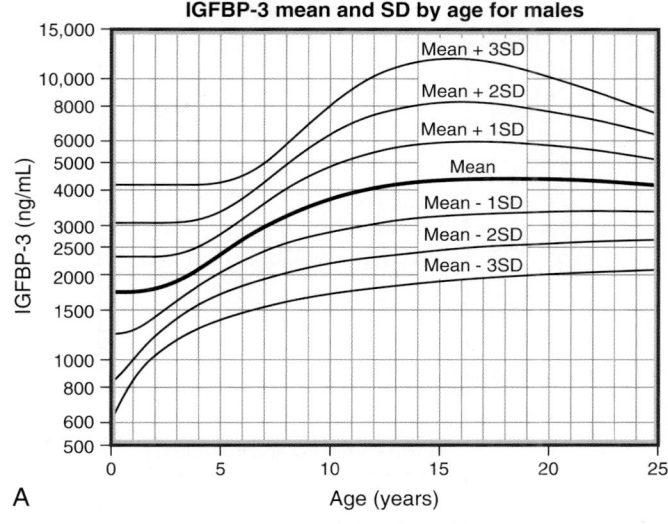

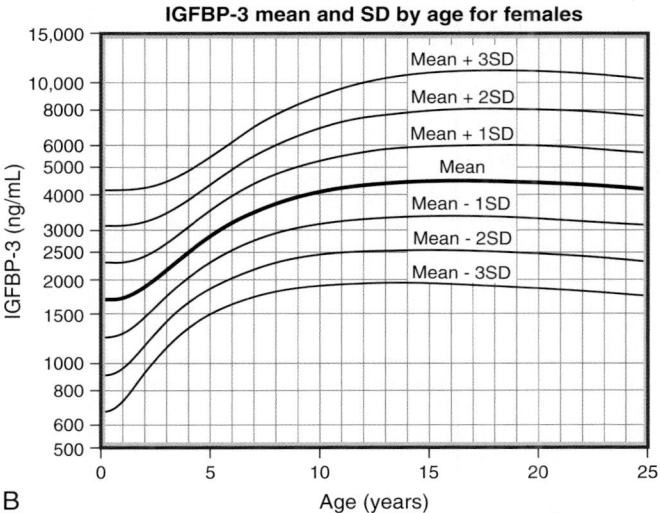

Figure 24-41 Normal serum levels of insulin-like growth factor–binding protein 3 (IGFBP3) for males (**A**) and females (**B**). (Data courtesy of Diagnostic Systems Laboratories, Inc., Webster, TX.)

high specificity, with values generally greater than 80% to 90%.[941,956,958,960,961] However, most studies have found that many children diagnosed with GHD on the basis of provocative GH testing actually have normal IGFBP levels, and the sensitivity of this test is less than 60%. In a study by Cianfarani and colleagues,[956] only 7% (2/28) of children younger than 14 years of age with GHD had an IGFBP3 level more than 1 SD below the mean. Low IGFBP3 levels may be an indicator of more severe GHD. For example, in one study the sensitivity of the IGFBP3 assay was 93% if the peak GH was less than 5 µg/L on provocative testing, but when the peak GH was 5 to 10 µg/L, the sensitivity was only 43%.[977]

Insulin-like Growth Factor 2. IGF-2 levels are higher than those of IGF-1. Levels increase rapidly after birth, but thereafter IGF-2 levels are less age dependent than those of IGF-1. However, although GHD is associated with low IGF-2 levels, IGF-2 is much less GH dependent than IGF-1 (Fig. 24-42). In two studies, IGF-2 levels were more than 2 SD below the mean in only 21% and 31% of children defined as GH deficient based on provocative GH testing.[956,978]

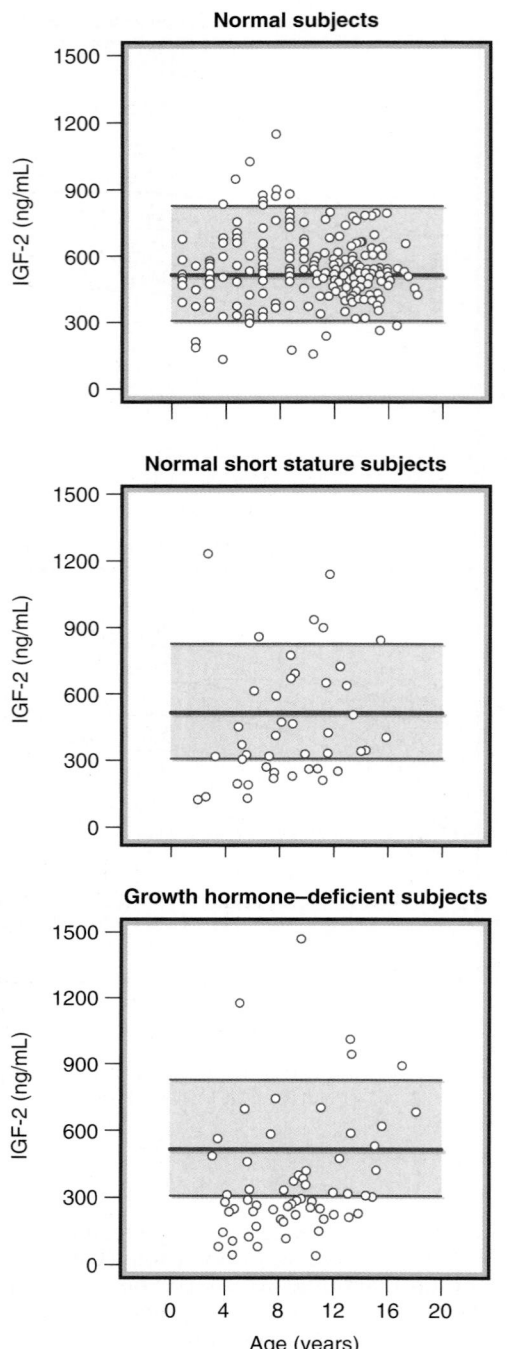

Figure 24-42 Serum insulin-like growth factor 2 (IGF-2) levels in normal patients and in patients with growth disorders. (From Rosenfeld RG, Wilson DM, Lee PD, et al. Insulin-like growth factors I and II in the evaluation of growth retardation. *J Pediatr.* 1986;109:428-433.)

Rosenfeld and colleagues[959] found low IGF-2 levels in 52% of GH-deficient children and in 35% of normal short children. However, only 4% of GH-deficient children and 11% of normal short children had normal plasma levels of both IGF-1 and IGF-2, showing a similar sensitivity and specificity to combined IGF-1/IGFBP3 testing.

Growth Hormone. Assessment of pituitary GH production is difficult because GH secretion is pulsatile, with the most consistent surges occurring at times of slow-wave electroencephalographic rhythms during stage 3 and stage 4 of sleep. Spontaneous GH secretion varies with gender, age,

pubertal stage, and nutritional status, all of which must be factored into the evaluation of GH production.

Between normal pulses of GH secretion, serum GH levels are low (often <0.1 µg/L), below the limits of sensitivity of most conventional assays (typically <0.2 µg/L). Accordingly, measurement of random serum GH concentrations is almost useless in diagnosing GHD but may be useful in the diagnosis of GH insensitivity and GH excess. Measurement of GH "secretory reserve" relies on the use of physiologic or pharmacologic stimuli, and such provocative tests have formed the basis for diagnosis of GHD for more than 30 years.[979,980]

Assay Limitations. One of the biggest confounders in the evaluation of GH secretion is the variability of measured GH levels across different assays. Many studies have demonstrated as much as threefold variability in the measurement of serum GH levels among established laboratories.[981,982] A recent study found an inter-assay coefficient of variation of 24.3% among 9 current assays for values within the range of 5 to 10 ng/mL and a maximal difference for a given sample as high as 11.4 ng/mL.[983] This variability is explained, in part, by the presence of several molecular forms of GH in serum. Circulating GH consists of monomers of the two secreted GH isoforms (with approximately 43% existing as the monomeric 22-kDa isoform and 8% as the monomeric 20-kDa isoform), along with dimers and higher-order oligomers of the two isoforms, acetylated forms of GH, desamidated GH, and peptide fragments of GH.[941] Therefore, much of the variability in results is due to the use of different monoclonal or polyclonal antibodies, including variability in recognition of the different circulating forms of GH by these antibodies. Additionally, variations in the choice of standards, labeling techniques, and assay buffers (matrix) are also contributory.[941] Consequently, a child who is determined to have GHD by one assay may be considered normal by another.[983]

Provocative Tests. Because random GH levels cannot be used to diagnose GHD, evaluation of GH secretion requires that samples be obtained after an expected stimulation of GH secretion. Physiologic stimuli include fasting, sleep, and exercise, and pharmacologic stimuli include levodopa, clonidine, glucagon, propranolol, arginine, and insulin. Standard provocative GH tests are summarized in Table 24-11. GH levels are measured on multiple specimens obtained after the stimulus. Failure to increase serum GH above a defined cutoff level is believed to indicate GHD.

Although provocative GH testing has been the foundation for the diagnosis of GHD since GH assays first became available, they have a number of weaknesses when they are used to identify GHD.[979,984,985] Most important, there is no clear cutoff level that discriminates a normal response from a deficient response, and second, these provocative tests have poor specificity.

Determination of the "Subnormal" Response to Provocative Tests. GH secretion has a continuous distribution; there is not a bimodal distribution of either spontaneous GH secretion or peak GH levels after provocative tests that would clearly separate normal from deficient secretion. The initial levels of GH during provocative testing that were used to define GHD were based on the study of patients with profound classic findings or organic destruction of the adenohypophysis.[986] In addition, partly because of the limited supply of GH, one goal was to identify the most severely affected children.

Initially, a cutoff level of 2.5 µg/L was used; this was later increased to 5 µg/L and subsequently to 7 µg/L. After the development of recombinant DNA-derived GH eliminated the limits on GH supply, many pediatric endocrinologists considered a peak GH level lower than 10 µg/L

TABLE 24-11
Tests to Provoke Growth Hormone Secretion

Stimulus	Dosage	Times Samples Are Taken (min)	Comments
Sleep	Obtain sample from indwelling catheter	60-90 min after onset of sleep	
Exercise	Step climbing; exercise cycle for 10 minutes	0, 10, 20	Observe child closely when on the steps
Levodopa	<15 kg: 125 mg 10-30 kg: 250 mg >30 kg: 500 mg	0, 60, 90	Nausea, rarely emesis
Clonidine	0.15 mg/m²	0, 30, 60, 90	Tiredness, postural hypotension
Arginine HCl (IV)	0.5 g/kg (max 30 g) 10% arginine HCl in 0.9% NaCl over 30 min	0, 15, 30, 45, 60	
Insulin (IV)*	0.05 to 0.1 unit/kg	0, 15, 30, 60, 75, 90, 120	Hypoglycemia, requires close supervision
Glucagon (IM)	0.03 mg/kg (max 1 mg)	0, 30, 60, 90, 120, 150, 180	Nausea, occasional emesis
GHRH (IV)†	1 μg/kg	0, 15, 30, 45, 60, 90, 120	Flushing, metallic taste

Patients must be euthyroid at the time of testing. Tests should be performed after an overnight fast. For prepubertal children, pretreating with sex hormones increases the specificity of the tests (see text).

*Insulin-induced hypoglycemia is a potential risk of this procedure, which is designed to lower the blood glucose by at least 50%. Documentation of appropriate lowering of blood glucose is recommended. If GHD is suspected, the lower dosage of insulin is usually administered, especially in infants. A solution of 10% dextrose in water (D₁₀W) and glucagon should be available.

†The cutoff used for tests involving GHRH is higher than that for other tests. (Maghnie M, Cavigioli F, Tinelli C, et al. GHRH plus arginine in the diagnosis of acquired GH deficiency of childhood-onset. *J Clin Endocrinol Metab.* 2002;87:2740-2744; and Pandian R, Nakamoto JM. Rational use of the laboratory for childhood and adult growth hormone deficiency. *Clin Lab Med.* 2004;24:141-174.)

Table derived from Post EM, Richman RA. A condensed table for predicting adult stature. *J Pediatr.* 1981;989:440-442, based on the data of Bayley and Pinneau.[949] Predicted final height is calculated by dividing the current height by the fraction of adult height achieved, determined from the table.

to be indicative of GHD. The higher cutoff level can be partially justified by the desire to identify children with GHD that is less complete (i.e., partial GHD). Nonetheless, there have been few data validating the higher cutoff values.[985,987]

Further confounding the determination of an evidence-based cutoff level is the variability in GH levels measured across different assays (discussed earlier). Many new GH assays give results that are 33% to 50% lower than earlier assays, but there has not been a systematic reassessment of the "new normal" GH cutoff levels, nor has there been a critical evaluation by many endocrinologists of which assay their center might be using.[988,989] The same cutoff level has been applied without regard to the stimulus used. However, the peak GH levels obtained are only modestly different for many of these agents, with the exception of GHRH, which leads to substantially higher levels of GH,[990-992] indicating a need for a higher cutoff value for such tests.

Specificity of Provocative Tests for Growth Hormone Deficiency. The data that are available suggest a low specificity for the provocative tests, with a substantial number of normal children having peak GH levels lower than 7 to 10 μg/L.[984] Ghigo and colleagues[991] studied 472 healthy, normal chil-

dren, including 296 with normal stature and 177 with normal short stature. Excluding tests that used GHRH (which has generally not been used in the evaluation of GH function in children), they found that between 10% and 25% of their subjects had peak GH levels lower than 7 μg/L and 23% to 49% had peak levels lower than 10 μg/L. Similar results were found in other studies.[993-996] Because of this poor specificity, failure on two provocative tests should be obtained before GHD is diagnosed on the basis of provocative testing. This approach significantly improves the specificity of provocative testing, although it remains imperfect. In the study of Ghigo and colleagues,[991] two tests were performed on 78 children, and 10% had peak GH levels lower than 10 μg/L on both tests (2.6% had peak GH levels <7 μg/L on both tests).

The specificity of provocative GH tests can be increased by using a lower cutoff point to define a normal response. However, this is undesirable if it excludes individuals with less severe degrees of GHD. Because of the continuous nature of GH secretion across individuals and the lack of a gold standard test for GHD, the conflict between specificity and sensitivity cannot be completely resolved. However, two reports have examined multiple clinical and laboratory characteristics of short children who were divided into three groups based on their results on GH stimulation testing: a group whose results were low (<5 or <7 μg/L), fulfilling criteria for GHD; a group whose results were greater than 10 μg and therefore were believed not to have GHD; and a group whose results were intermediate between these high and low cutoff points. In both of these studies, the group with the lowest peak GH levels differed significantly from both the intermediate-level and the high-level GH groups on numerous measures.[997,998] However, the intermediate group was indistinguishable from the group without GHD, rather than having characteristics intermediate between the other two groups, as might be expected if they had a less severe degree of GHD.

Sex Hormone Priming. Serum GH levels rise during puberty, with GH secretion stimulated by the rise in estrogen produced from the ovary or from aromatization of testosterone.[115,999] This same process results in higher peak GH levels during provocative testing in pubertal children (compared with prepubertal children)[994,1000] and in children who have received treatment with estrogen or testosterone.[954,994,1000-1002] In a study by Marin and colleagues,[994] 61% of normal prepubertal children and 44% of normal children in early puberty (Tanner stage I) had GH levels lower than 7 μg/L on provocative testing; based on these results (but not on their heights), they would have met criteria for a diagnosis of GHD. However, after 2 days of treatment with estrogen, 95% of these children had a peak GH level higher than 7 μg/L. Therefore, the specificity of GH provocative tests can be improved by pretreating ("priming") the pediatric patients with exogenous gonadal steroids.[1003,1004] In a placebo-controlled comparison, the specificity of GH provocative tests (using 9 μg/L as a cutoff point on a polyclonal GH assay) increased from 80% to 98% after estrogen priming.[954] In a study of 50 growth-retarded boys who had subnormal results on provocative GH tests without testosterone priming but normal results after priming, final height (without intervention) was greater than the midparental height, consistent with normal GH function in these children.[1005]

Another factor to consider when evaluating provocative GH testing is the impact of body weight on GH secretion. In both adults[107,1006-1008] and children,[1009,1010] obese individuals have decreased spontaneous and stimulated GH levels, compared with nonobese individuals. Even within the normal range, the BMI SDS is inversely associated with peak GH level on provocative tests in children.[1011] Therefore, particular care must be taken when interpreting GH stimulation test results in obese individuals.

Although there are limitations to the information gained from provocative GH tests, they continue to be helpful in evaluating a child for GHD. The tests should be performed after an overnight fast, and the patient needs to be euthyroid at the time of testing. Testing should not be performed if the patient is taking supraphysiologic doses of glucocorticoid (i.e., >15 mg/m^2 per day of hydrocortisone or the equivalent of a synthetic glucocorticoid), because these drugs can suppress the GH response. The tests are generally safe, although appropriate precautions must be taken. Specifically, tests involving insulin administration carry the risk of hypoglycemia and seizures and should be performed only by experienced medical personnel and under appropriate patient supervision. Deaths have been reported from insulin-induced hypoglycemia and from its overly vigorous correction with parenteral glucose.[1012] The specificity of the tests can be increased by pretreating the child with estrogen or testosterone (e.g., 1-2 mg of micronized estradiol[954] or 50-100 µg/day of ethinyl estradiol for 3 consecutive days before testing, or 100 mg of depot testosterone 3 days before testing) and by carefully selecting the lower limit for a normal response.

Tests of Spontaneous Growth Hormone Secretion. Another diagnostic approach to evaluate GH secretion involves measurement of spontaneous GH secretion. This can be done either by multiple sampling (every 5 to 30 minutes) over a 12- to 24-hour period or by continuous blood withdrawal over 12 to 24 hours.[86,1013-1015] The former method allows one to evaluate and characterize GH pulsatility, whereas the latter only permits determination of the mean GH concentration. Both methods are subject to many of the same limitations as provocative GH testing. The problems of expense and discomfort are obvious, and, although it was thought that this approach might be more reproducible than provocative GH tests, variability remains a problem.[1016-1018] The ability of such tests to discriminate between children with GHD and those with normal short stature is very limited because of significant overlap of each of the parameters measured between normal children and children with GHD. Rose and coworkers[1019] reported that measurement of spontaneous GH secretion identified only 57% of children with GHD as defined by provocative testing. Similarly, Lanes[1020] reported that one fourth of normally growing children have low overnight GH levels, and a longitudinal study of normal boys through puberty demonstrated a wide intersubject variance, including many "low" 24-hour GH production rates in children with fully normal growth.[115,1021] Therefore, measurement of spontaneous GH secretion does not appear to offer advantages over alternative means of evaluating GH function.

Summary. Despite the many problems associated with GH measurement methods, there continues to be value in determining GH secretory capacity in the diagnostic evaluation of a child with growth failure. Documentation of GH levels as being decreased, normal, or increased helps in discriminating among GHD, non–GH/IGF-1–related growth failure (including ISS), and GH insensitivity. Results supporting the presence of GHD alert the clinician to the possibility of other pituitary deficiencies. The presence of pituitary dysfunction mandates clinical and radiologic evaluation for evidence of congenital or acquired structural defects of the hypothalamus or pituitary, including the possibility of intracranial tumors. Finally, documentation of GHD, either alone or combined with other pituitary deficiencies, may warrant evaluation for molecular defects of GH production.

Growth Hormone–Binding Protein. Mutation of the GHR can impair GH signaling, resulting in GH insensitivity. The most severe mutations cause profound growth failure (Laron dwarfism). The extracellular portion of the GHR is cleaved from the remaining portion and circulates in the blood as GHBP. GHBP levels can be measured in serum. Low levels, particularly undetectable levels, may be diagnostic of GH insensitivity due to GHR mutations.

GHBP levels are not low in all forms of GH insensitivity. The levels may be normal, or even increased, with mutations in the GHR that do not alter the GHBP portion of the protein (i.e., mutations in the transmembrane or intracellular domains) or with defects that are downstream of the GHR.

IGF-1 and IGFBP Generation Tests. IGF-1 and IGFBP3 generation tests are designed to evaluate for the presence of GH insensitivity.[1022] When patients with GH insensitivity are treated with GH for several days, the levels of IGF-1 and IGFBP do not increase as they would in normal individuals.[1023,1024] Criteria for a response indicating GH insensitivity have included a rise in IGF-1 of less than two times the intra-assay variation (approximately 10%)[529] or a failure to increase IGF-1 by at least 15 µg/L.[662] However, Laron dwarfism is extremely rare outside specific communities, so the role of these tests in clinical practice is limited.

The utility of these tests in identifying subtler forms of GH insensitivity in children with ISS has been explored,[1025] but at this time additional data are needed to determine the usefulness of this test in such cases. It will also be important to know the limitations of the test in such instances, including understanding of potential confounders. For example, studies have indicated that the IGF-1 response to GH is related to BMI and adiposity[1000] and to pubertal stage.[950]

Interpretation of Tests

Neonate. GH levels in the neonate are much higher than levels seen after this period. Levels are highest in cord blood and within the first days of life.[1026] Cornblath and colleagues reported in 1965 an average GH concentration in cord blood of 66 µg/L; this fell over the first week to an average of 16 to 20 µg/L in infants 7 to 55 days of age.[1026] However, even under the assay conditions used, the range of levels reported included measurements as low as 1 µg/L. Subsequent studies confirmed the high GH levels in neonates, with many documenting cord blood levels in the range of 20 to 40 µg/L, although other studies using similar assays found levels of 13 to 18 µg/L.[1027] Other studies also confirmed that GH levels fall during the first week of life so that low basal values are seen by 1 to 2 months of age.[1027,1028] GH levels in preterm infants have generally been found to be even higher than those in full-term infants.[1026]

The neonatal period is one period during which random measurement of GH levels may be useful. However, low values can be found in healthy neonates.[1028] Therefore, although a high value can exclude GHD, a single low value is not diagnostic of GHD—except, perhaps, for the first few days of life. There have been no studies reporting GH levels in GH-deficient infants compared with normal infants. However, after the first few days of age, if the clinical findings in a neonate raise concern for GHD (see Table 24-9), multiple random GH levels that are all below the cutoff value used to define normal GH secretion during provocative testing would be supportive of the diagnosis of GHD. GH levels that are obtained during an episode of spontaneous hypoglycemia or during a glucagon stimulation test should also increase at least above the same cutoff value. An IGFBP3 measurement is of value for the diagnosis of neonatal GHD and should be measured in infants with suspected GHD; IGF-1 levels are rarely helpful.[1029]

Growth Hormone Deficiency. Both clinical and laboratory evaluation must be utilized when considering the diagnosis of GHD in a child being evaluated because of short stature or growth failure.[953] As discussed earlier, there is no definitive test for the diagnosis for GHD. In addition, the laboratory tests for GHD have poor specificity and should be performed only in children who have a clinical presentation consistent with GHD. Short children who have well-documented normal height velocities usually do not require evaluation of GH function. Therefore, the evaluation starts with identifying those children who may have GHD based on risk factors or growth parameters (see Tables 24-8 and 24-9).

In a child with a history and growth pattern that indicate a risk for GHD and in whom other causes for growth failure (including hypothyroidism) have been excluded, testing for GHD begins with measurement of the IGF-1 level and proceeds to GH provocation tests in selected patients (see Table 24-8). In some cases, particularly in younger children, it may also be helpful to measure the IGFBP3 level. If IGHD is suspected, two GH provocation tests (given sequentially or on separate days) are required. A patient is diagnosed with classic GHD when the IGF-1 (or IGFBP3) level is below the normal range (i.e., >2 SD below the mean for age and pubertal status) and peak GH levels on two provocative tests are below the cutoff value that supports a diagnosis of GHD. The diagnosis is more firmly established if the child is pretreated with estrogen or testosterone before the provocative GH tests. In a patient with defined CNS pathology, a history of irradiation, CPHD, or a genetic defect, one provocative GH test suffices. In patients who have had cranial irradiation or malformations of the hypothalamic-pituitary unit, GHD may evolve over years, and its diagnosis may require serial testing.

Some patients with auxology suggestive of GHD may have IGF-1 or IGFBP3 levels below the normal range on repeated tests but GH responses in provocation tests above the cutoff level. Such children do not have classic GHD but may have an abnormality of the GH/IGF-1 axis. The child with a history of cranial irradiation, decreased height velocity, and reduced serum levels of IGF-1 and IGFBP3 may have GHD (or GH insensitivity) even in the face of normal provocative tests.[1030] Other children may have GHD that is not supported by the results of nonphysiologic provocative tests (perhaps a milder degree of GHD than in those who fail the provocative tests), or they may have GH insensitivity (discussed later). Systemic disorders affecting the synthesis or action of IGF-1 must again be considered and excluded.

A difficult clinical situation to resolve is that of the short child with a persistently subnormal growth velocity whose IGF-1 and IGFBP3 levels are normal. One can reasonably exclude consideration of GHD if the IGF-1 level is higher than 1 SD below the normal mean. However, because up to 30% of children with GHD identified by GH stimulation testing have had IGF-1 levels that were not low,[941,958-961] it is appropriate to consider provocative GH testing in those children with persistent growth failure who have an IGF-1 level between –1 SD and –2 SD for age and puberty status, with abnormal results on two tests indicating a diagnosis of GHD. In this situation in particular, it would be appropriate to pretreat the child with testosterone or estrogen in order to maximize the specificity of the provocative tests.

A cranial MRI scan with particular attention to the hypothalamic-pituitary region should be carried out in any child who is diagnosed as having GHD. In addition, documentation of abnormal pituitary GH secretion should

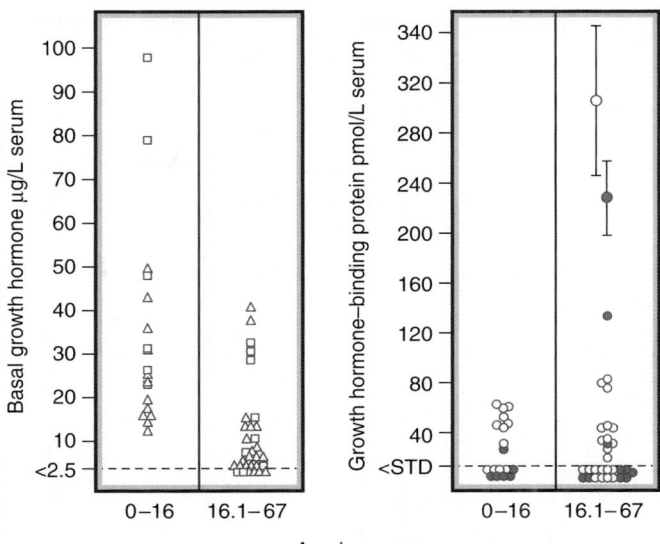

Figure 24-43 GH assays were performed by radioimmunoassay *(squares)* and by immunoradiometric assay *(triangles)*. For GHBP levels, open circles represent females, and closed circles represent males. Standard error of the mean (±SD) for GHBP levels in adult Ecuadorian control subjects are shown. STD, assay standard. (From Rosenfeld RG, Rosenbloom AL, Guevara-Acquirre J. Growth hormone [GH] resistance due to primary GH receptor deficiency. *Endocr Rev.* 1994;15:369-390.)

prompt evaluation for other pituitary hormone deficiencies. Based on the clinical scenario, one may also consider molecular evaluation of GH, GHR, GHRHR, and other potential genetic defects.

Growth Hormone Insensitivity. GH insensitivity is characterized by low serum IGF-1 concentrations in the presence of normal (or increased) production of GH (Figs. 24-43 and 24-44). As discussed earlier, GH insensitivity can be caused by defects of the GHR (Laron syndrome), the GH signaling cascade, IGFBPs, IGF-1, or the IGF-1 receptor.[538] If GH insensitivity is defined more broadly as growth failure in the absence of GHD, then defects in IGFBPs, IGF-1, and the type I IGF receptor can also be considered forms of GH insensitivity; IGF-1 levels may or may not be low in these disorders.[538] GH insensitivity should be considered in a patient with growth failure who has a low IGF-1 level but evidence of increased GH secretion based on increased basal or stimulated GH levels (e.g., basal GH levels >5 µg/L or stimulated levels >15 µg/L). This pattern is also seen with malnutrition, a form of physiologic GH insensitivity. If GH insensitivity is suspected, GHBP and ALS can be measured: low values support the diagnosis of GH insensitivity due to mutations in the genes for the GHR or ALS. IGF-1/IGFBP3 generation studies may demonstrate GH insensitivity, but they cannot completely discriminate among its various causes. In addition, there is limited normative data or standardization of such tests, so their ability to identify defects other than the severe insensitivity of Laron syndrome is not yet known.

Savage and colleagues[529] devised a scoring system for use in evaluating short children for the diagnosis of GHR deficiency based on five parameters: (1) basal serum GH level greater than 10 mU/L (approximately 5 µg/L); (2) serum IGF-1 level less than 50 µg/L; (3) height SDS less than –3; (4) serum GHBP less than 10% (based on binding of [^{125}I] GH); and (5) a rise in serum IGF-1 levels after GH administration of less than two times the intra-assay variation (approximately 10%). Blum and associates[662] proposed that these criteria could be strengthened by (1) evaluating GH

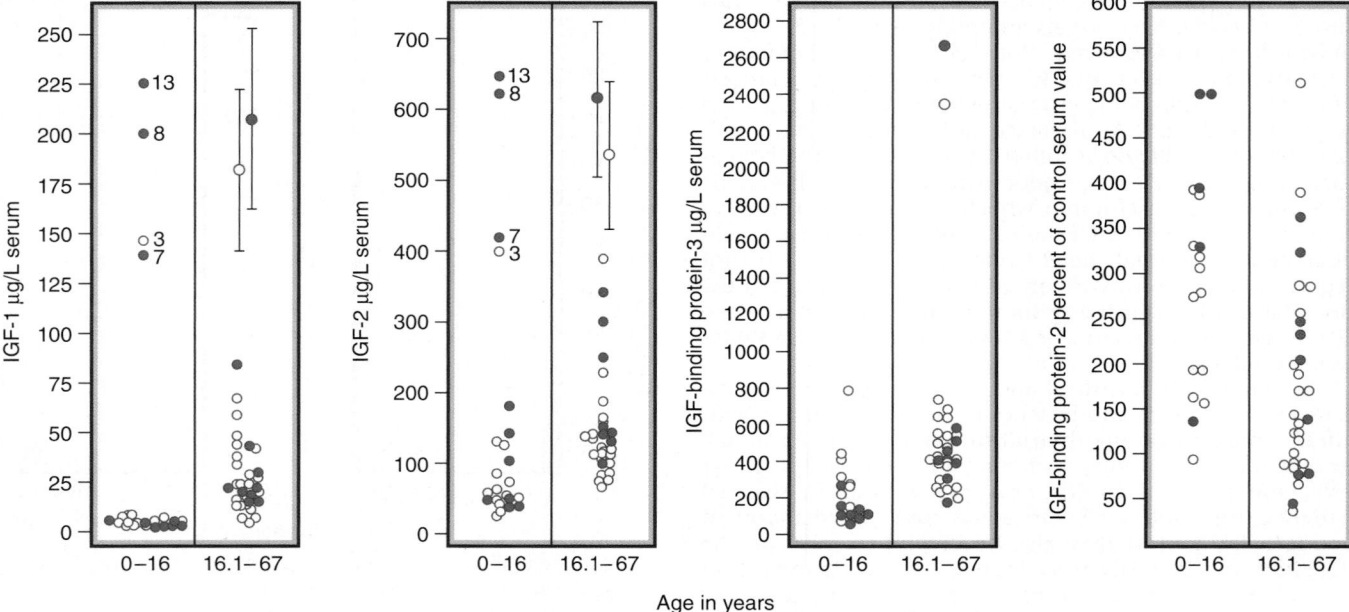

Figure 24-44 Serum levels of insulin-like growth factors (IGF) and IGF-binding proteins in patients from Ecuador with growth hormone receptor deficiency. Open circles represent females, closed circles represent males. Control values for Ecuadorian adults are shown as mean ±SD for males and females, except for IGFBP-3, for which large circles represent pooled male *(closed circle)* and female *(open circle)* control sera. Numbers adjacent to circles represent normal Ecuadorian children 3, 7, 8, and 13 years of age. (From Rosenfeld RG, Rosenbloom AL, Guevara-Acquirre J. Growth hormone [GH] resistance due to primary GH receptor deficiency. *Endocr Rev.* 1994;15:369-390.)

secretory profiles rather than isolated basal levels; (2) employing an age-dependent range and the 0.1 percentile as the cutoff level for evaluation of serum IGF-1 concentrations; (3) employing highly sensitive IGF-1 immunoassays and defining a failed GH response as the inability to increase serum IGF-1 levels by at least 15 μg/L; and (4) measuring both basal and GH-stimulated IGFBP3 levels. These criteria fit well with findings in the population of GHR-deficient patients in Ecuador, but that is a homogeneous population with severe GH insensitivity.[125] The applicability of these criteria elsewhere remains to be evaluated. An important biochemical marker is the response of IGF-1 (and, possibly, IGFBP3) to GH stimulation.[1023]

Additional considerations related to GH insensitivity include the following:

1. The presence of IUGR (in addition to postnatal growth failure) suggests *IGF1* gene deletions, bioactive IGF-1, or IGF type I receptor abnormalities.
2. Low GHBP suggests a defect in the extracellular domain of the GHR, but normal (or increased) GHBP may be seen in some patients with defects of the GHR or the GH signaling cascade.
3. An elevated IGF-1 level (in a child with growth failure) may suggest a defect in the IGF type I receptor; markedly elevated levels suggest bioactive IGF-1.[217]
4. IGFBP3 and ALS concentrations may be increased in patients with molecular defects of IGF-1.
5. STAT5B defects should be suspected in a child with evidence of GH insensitivity who has evidence of immune deficiency; an elevated PRL level has also been reported in the presence of STAT5B mutation.[1031]

Constitutional Delay of Growth and Development. The term *constitutional delay of growth and development* describes children who have a normal variant of maturational tempo characterized by short stature with relatively normal growth rates during childhood, delayed puberty with a late and attenuated pubertal growth spurt, and attainment of a normal adult height that is also within the target height range

TABLE 24-12
Criteria for Presumptive Diagnosis of Constitutional Delay of Growth and Development

1. No history of systemic illness
2. Normal nutrition
3. Normal physical examination, including body proportions
4. Normal thyroid and growth hormone levels
5. Normal complete blood count, sedimentation rate, electrolytes, blood urea nitrogen
6. Height ≤3rd percentile but with annual growth rate >5th percentile for age
7. Delayed puberty: in males, failure to achieve Tanner G2 stage by age 13.8 years or P2 by 15.6 years; in females, failure to achieve Tanner B2 stage by age 13.3 years
8. Delayed bone age
9. Normal predicted adult height: in males, >163 cm (64″); in females, >150 cm (59″)

based on parental heights (Table 24-12).[38,1032] In childhood, such patients have heights that are lower than expected based on parental heights. CDGD aggregates in families.[1033] The diagnosis of CDGD may be suspected in a child with short stature if one or both parents have a history of a late timing of puberty. Bone age is usually delayed, so the predicted final height is in the normal range and is within the child's target height range, although the correlation between predicted and final height is imperfect and must be viewed with caution.[43,1034,1035] The predicted final height, especially when the skeletal age is extremely delayed, is greater than that usually achieved but is difficult to reliably anticipate.[43,1035,1036] Although the findings described can lead to a presumptive diagnosis of CDGD, the diagnosis can only be made retrospectively, once the child demonstrates a late timing for puberty and completes his or her growth in the normal range and at a height consistent with the parents' heights.

Because of the estrogen stimulation associated with GH secretion that occurs during puberty, children with CDGD can be expected to have decreased GH secretion and lower IGF-1 levels compared with their pubertal, age-matched peers. However, IGF-1 levels should be normal for pubertal stage, and GH levels on provocative tests should be normal after pretreatment with gonadal steroids.[1003,1036-1038] Overnight GH secretion is usually normal in these children when control groups are carefully matched.[1039]

It is often difficult to differentiate CDGD from GHD. Both groups of patients have height SDS below their target height SDS range, and both have delayed bone ages. As the child with CDGD enters the usual age for puberty, his or her growth rate can be too low to exclude GHD on that basis. (The growth rate normally declines throughout childhood until it increases at the time of the pubertal growth spurt; a child with CDGD and delayed pubertal growth spurt may have an additional 2 or more years of declining growth velocity, which can result in growth velocities <4 cm/year.) If there is a clear family history of CDGD, the likelihood is high that the child also has CDGD, and careful continued observation may be all that is needed. An increase in growth velocity after treatment with a short course of sex hormone can be taken as evidence against the presence of GHD.[1040] In some cases, however, a laboratory investigation to exclude GHD is necessary. In such children, levels of IGF-1 and IGFBP3 that are low for pubertal stage or skeletal age and a poor GH response to provocative testing after priming with gonadal steroids would raise concern for GHD and would mandate the appropriate investigation for underlying disease (e.g., intracranial tumor).

Genetic (Familial) Short Stature. The control of growth in childhood and the final height attained are polygenic in nature. Familial height affects the growth of an individual, and evaluation of a specific growth pattern must be placed in the context of familial growth and stature. As discussed at the beginning of this chapter, calculations can be made to determine whether a child's growth pattern is appropriate based on his or her parents' heights. As a general rule, a child who is growing at a rate that is inconsistent with that of siblings or parents warrants further evaluation.

Genetic short stature (GSS), also called familial short stature, is a normal growth pattern that describes the growth of healthy individuals who fall at the lower extreme of the distribution of height (i.e., below the 3rd percentile). Their height is appropriate for their genetic potential based on the parents' heights; that is, their height SDS is within the target height SDS range. Particularly when the midparental height is significantly above or below the mean, it is important to include adjustment for regression toward the mean when calculating this target height range.

Although the differentiation may not be complete, children with GSS are generally distinguished from children with CDGD: those with GSS will have a final height that is below the 3rd percentile, whereas children with CDGD will achieve a final height in the normal range. The midparental height of children with GSS is lower than that of children with CDGD; often, height in both parents is below the 10th percentile. Growth in children with GSS is at or below the 3rd percentile, but the velocity is usually normal. The onset and progression of puberty are normal, so the skeletal age is concordant with chronologic age. Final heights in these individuals are in the target height range for the family.[42] By definition, the GH/IGF-1 system is normal (as are all other systems).

Many diseases characterized by growth retardation are genetically transmitted, including GH insensitivity due to mutations of the *GHR* gene; *GH* gene deletions; mutations of the *PROP1*, *POUF1*, or *SHOX* genes; pseudohypoparathyroidism; and some forms of hypothyroidism. Inherited nonendocrine diseases characterized by short stature include osteochondrodysplasias and dysmorphic syndromes associated with IUGR (both described earlier), inborn errors of metabolism, renal disease, and thalassemia. Identifying a patient's short stature as inherited does not, by itself, relieve the clinician of responsibility for determining the underlying cause of growth failure. Moreover, a parent's short stature may be the result of an uncharacterized genetic difference that has been transmitted to the child and is causing the child's short stature. Because height is normally distributed in the population, it can be arbitrary whether one characterizes such genetic differences as mutations or as allelic variants. However, the further the parents' and the child's heights are from the mean, the more reasonable it is to consider such genetic alterations as abnormal.

Idiopathic Short Stature. ISS is defined as "a condition in which the height of the individual is more than 2 SD below the corresponding mean height for a given age, sex and population group, and in whom no identifiable disorder is present."[1031] This definition includes children with CDGD, those with GSS, and short children who will not have delayed puberty and whose height is not consistent with parental heights. Therefore, this definition includes both normal, healthy children (those with GSS and CDGD) and children who are presumed to have an unidentified disorder impairing their growth. It is not always a simple matter to distinguish among these possibilities: CDGD can be definitively diagnosed only at the completion of growth, and GSS does not exclude inherited disorders of growth.

Children with ISS may have undiagnosed disorders outside the GH/IGF-1 axis (e.g., an uncharacterized chondrodystrophy), or they may have subtler disorders of the hypothalamic-pituitary-IGF axis than those that are identified by the currently available diagnostics tests.[538,551] Because of the lack of a gold standard for the diagnosis of GHD, the distinction between isolated partial GHD and ISS is somewhat arbitrary, relying heavily on the results of the nonphysiologic provocative stimulation tests. The activity of different GH promoter haplotypes can differ as much as sixfold.[514,1041] Some children with ISS may have GH neurosecretory dysfunction that cannot be detected with current diagnostic tests.[1013,1014] Similarly, although the severe GH insensitivity of Laron syndrome can be identified by laboratory testing, partial GH insensitivity may be an unrecognized cause of ISS.[1042]

Heterozygous mutations in the GHR have been found in significant numbers of children with ISS.[550,553,1033] In heterozygotes, protein from the mutant allele may disrupt the normal dimerization and rotation that is needed for normal GHR activation, leading to diminished GH action and growth impairment.[137] In addition, GHBP expression may be decreased in patients with ISS, 20% of whom have serum levels of GHBP below the normal range.[1042-1044] Other potential causes for partial GH insensitivity in ISS include heterozygous mutations in other components of the growth system, a relatively greater preponderance of blockers of the GH-signaling cascade (e.g., enhanced intracellular phosphatase activity, production of such signaling factors as SOC2 and CIS), gene-mediated alterations in patterns of GH or IGF production, or other possibilities yet to be discovered.[1045]

Treatment of Growth Failure

When growth failure is the result of a chronic underlying disease, such as renal failure, CF, or malabsorption, therapy must first be directed at treatment of the underlying condition. Although growth acceleration may occur in such children with GH or IGF-1 therapy, complete catch-up requires correction of the primary medical problem. If treatment of the underlying condition involves glucocorticoids, growth failure may be profound and is unlikely to be correctable until steroids are reduced or discontinued.

Correction of growth failure associated with chronic hypothyroidism requires appropriate thyroid replacement. As discussed earlier, thyroid therapy causes dramatic catch-up growth but also markedly accelerates skeletal maturation, potentially limiting adult height.

Treatment of Constitutional Delay

CDGD is a normal growth variant with delayed pubertal maturation and a normal adult height. Most subjects can be managed by careful evaluation to rule out other causes of abnormal growth or delayed puberty combined with appropriate explanation and counseling. A family history of CDGD is frequently a source of reassurance. The skeletal age and Bayley-Pinneau table are often helpful in explaining the potential for normal growth to the patient and parents. The predicted final height is usually greater than that achieved, especially when the skeletal age is extremely delayed, but this is difficult to reliably anticipate.[43,1034,1046]

On occasion, the stigmata of short stature and delayed maturation are psychologically disabling for a preadolescent or teenage patient. Some adolescents with delayed puberty have poor self-image and limited social involvement.[1047] In such patients and in some in whom pubertal delay is predicted based on the overall clinical picture, there may be a role for judicious short-term treatment with androgen.

Androgen (Oxandrolone and Testosterone). Two aspects of CDGD in boys are addressed by androgen treatment: short stature, especially in boys 10 to 14 years of age, and delayed puberty after age 14. In the younger group, in whom CDGD is the presumed cause of short stature, the orally administered synthetic androgen oxandrolone has been used extensively to accelerate growth so that height increases into (or closer to) the normal range sooner than it would without treatment.[1048] In several controlled studies,[1032,1049-1053] oxandrolone therapy for 3 months to 4 years increased linear growth velocity by 3 to 5 cm/year without adverse effects and without decreasing either actual[1053-1055] or predicted[1050,1054,1056] final height. (This treatment does not increase the final height of these boys.) The growth-promoting effects of oxandrolone appear to be related to its androgenic and anabolic effects rather than to augmentation of the GH/IGF-1 axis.[1057,1058] The lack of a measurable effect on the GH/IGF-1 axis probably reflects the fact that oxandrolone cannot be aromatized to estrogen. Currently recommended treatment is 0.05 to 0.1 mg/kg orally per day.

Oxandrolone is a relatively weak androgen, and its use stimulates only minimal pubertal masculinization. In older boys in whom the delayed pubertal maturation is highly stressful and anxiety-provoking, testosterone enanthate has been administered intramuscularly with success.[1048,1049,1059] Criteria for treatment in such adolescents should include (1) a minimum age of 14 years; (2) height below the 3rd percentile; (3) prepubertal or early Tanner G2 stage with an early-morning serum testosterone level of less than 3.5 nmol/L (<1 ng/mL); and (4) a poor self-image that does not respond to reassurance alone. Therapy consists of intramuscular testosterone enanthate, 50 to 100 mg every 3 to 4 weeks, for a total of four to six injections.[1047,1057,1059,1060] Patients typically show early secondary

sex characteristics by the fourth injection and grow an average of 10 cm in the ensuing year. Testosterone enhances growth velocity by direct actions, increases GH production, and may have a direct effect on IGF-1 secretion.[999,1037,1057,1061-1063] Brief testosterone regimens do not cause overly rapid skeletal maturation, compromise adult height, or suppress pubertal maturation.[1064] It is important to emphasize to the patient that he is normal, that therapy is short-term and is designed to provide some pubertal development earlier than he would on his own, and that treatment will not increase his final adult height. In such situations, the combination of short-term androgen therapy, reassurance, and counseling can help boys with CDGD to cope with a difficult adolescence.

The availability of several new forms of testosterone, which are approved for adults with hypogonadism, provides adolescents with an opportunity for a choice among different androgen replacement therapies. Testosterone gel is painless and easy to apply and has proved popular since its release.[1065] However, there are concerns about environmental contamination, including reports of precocious puberty in children caused by topical testosterone use by an adult in the household.[1066-1068] If topical testosterone is prescribed, careful instruction must be given to avoid such inadvertent exposure of others. Testosterone patches also avoid the need for injections, but they are often poorly tolerated because of local skin reactions. The most recent testosterone products include a solution applied in the axilla and a nasal gel. Another disadvantage of these topical testosterone preparations and the transdermal patches is the need for daily application. The dosing of these alternative forms of therapy in children and adolescents has not been established, and care must be taken to avoid treating with too high a dose, which risks compromising final height.

Patients must be reevaluated to ensure that they enter "true" puberty. One year after testosterone treatment, boys should have testicular enlargement and a serum testosterone level in the pubertal range. If this is not the case, a diagnosis of hypothalamic-pituitary insufficiency or hypogonadotropic hypogonadism should be considered. Although the diagnosis of constitutional growth delay remains most likely in such patients, some eventually prove to be gonadotropin deficient, especially if they are still prepubertal late in adolescence.

Referrals for CDGD are more common in boys than girls. When CDGD is a problem in girls, short-term estrogen therapy may be employed, but the acceleration of skeletal maturation is a greater hazard at doses that enhance growth velocity and sexual maturation.

Growth Hormone. The final height of a child with CDGD will be in the normal range and appropriate for the child's genetic potential. No treatment is needed for these children to achieve a normal height. However, as discussed earlier, the diagnosis of CDGD cannot be confirmed until a late puberty and normal height are achieved. Therefore, it can be difficult in some cases to distinguish these children from children with ISS or GHD. In such cases, there may be uncertainty about whether the final height will be in the normal range, and treatment to try to increase final height may be considered. If laboratory studies support a diagnosis of GHD, then GH treatment would be appropriate. If there is no evidence of GHD, the consideration regarding treatment with GH would be the same as that regarding the use of GH to treat ISS (discussed later).

The Food and Drug Administration (FDA) indication for GH treatment includes in its definition of ISS the criterion that the child has "growth rate[s] unlikely to permit attainment of normal adult height." A child with CDGD, who is expected to achieve a normal adult height, would not fit within this definition. Nonetheless, partly because of the uncertainty of the diagnosis and the inability to perfectly predict final height, the database on outcomes of children treated with GH for ISS includes within it data on the treatment of children with CDGD. ISS GH treatment trials may include children with significant bone age delay,[1069,1070] at least some of whom have CDGD. For this reason, the outcome data for GH treatment of ISS (see later) can be taken as an indication of the expected outcome of GH treatment of CDGD. Moreover, because estimated final height gain with GH treatment of ISS is proportional to the bone age delay at the time of initiation of treatment,[1071] height gain with GH treatment of CDGD may be greater than that for treatment of ISS. However, a retrospective study specifically reporting the outcome of GH treatment in CDGD found no difference in adult height between those treated with GH and those receiving either no treatment or testosterone treatment.[1072]

Aromatase Inhibitor. In view of the important role of estrogen in the process of skeletal maturation, aromatase inhibitors could be used in conjunction with androgen therapy to prevent an acceleration of bone age and further enhance final adult height.[808,1073] The one report of combined use of an aromatase inhibitor (letrozole) and testosterone did not provide a clear answer as to whether the addition of aromatase inhibitor increased final height in boys with CDGD. Whereas the near-final height in the boys treated with letrazole plus testosterone was higher than that of boys treated with testosterone alone, the letrazole-treated boys were a year older at the time of these height measurements and had higher pretreatment and midparental heights.[1073] In addition, the boys treated with testosterone alone achieved a near-final height within the normal range (consistent with the diagnosis of CDGD). Given the lack of long-term safety data on the use of aromatase inhibitors in pubertal boys, there are insufficient data to suggest a role for aromatase inhibitors in CDGD.

Treatment of Growth Hormone Deficiency

Nomenclature and Potency Estimation. The nomenclature for the various biosynthetic GH preparations reflects the source and the chemical composition of the product. *Somatropin* refers to GH of the same amino acid sequence as that in naturally occurring human GH. Somatropin from human pituitary glands is abbreviated *GH* or *pit-GH;* somatropin of recombinant origin is termed *recombinant GH* or *rGH.* *Somatrem* refers to the methionine derivative of recombinant GH and is abbreviated *met-rGH.* Although the latter is a more antigenic preparation, that propensity is not clinically relevant; despite the presence of anti-GH antibodies, growth responses to met-rGH were similar to those in patients treated with rGH.[1074,1075] This derivative of GH is no longer available for use. In this discussion, we refer to the biosynthetic preparations as GH.

The biopotency of commercially available biosynthetic GH preparations, expressed as international units per milligram of the second World Health Organization (WHO) recombinant GH reference reagent for somatropin 98/574, is 3 IU/mg.[1076] It was necessary to standardize the early GH preparations by bioassay because of variable production techniques (e.g., extraction, column purification). The most common bioassays have been the hypophysectomized rat weight-gain assay, the tibial width assay, and the more sensitive Nb2 rat lymphoma proliferation assay.[1077-1079] With the availability of purified and essentially equivalent recombinant GH products, the requirement for bioassays has become an FDA requisite to substantiate biologic activity rather than to assess potential

differences among preparations. The bioassays are likely to be replaced by in vitro binding assays using GHRs or GHBP derived from molecular techniques.

Historical Perspective. Because untreated patients with GHD have profound short stature (averaging almost 5 SDS[1080,1081]), the clinical urgency to use GH therapy as soon as it became available is understandable.[987] The action of GH is highly species-specific, and humans do not respond to animal-derived GH (except that from other primates).[1082] Human cadaver pituitary glands were for many years the only practical source of primate GH for treatment of GHD, and more than 27,000 children with GHD worldwide were treated with pit-GH.[1083] The limited supplies of pit-GH, the low doses used, and interrupted treatment regimens resulted in incomplete growth increments; usually, therapy was discontinued in boys who reached a height of 5 feet 5 inches and in girls who reached 5 feet. Nonetheless, this treatment did increase linear growth and in many patients enhanced final adult height. The dose-response relationship and the relation of age to GH response were recognized during this period.[1084]

Distribution of pit-GH was halted in the United States and most of Europe in 1985 because of concern about a causal relationship with Creutzfeldt-Jakob disease (CJD), a rare and fatal spongiform encephalopathy that had been previously reported to be capable of iatrogenic transmission through human tissue. In North America and Europe, this disorder has an incidence of approximately 1 case per 1 million in the general population, and it is exceedingly rare before the age of 50 years. To date, more than 200 young adults who had received human cadaver pituitary products have been diagnosed with CJD, with the sad likelihood that all affected patients will die of the disease.[1085-1087] The onset of CJD has occurred 5 to 42 years after treatment, with a mean incubation of 17 years.[1087] No cases of CJD have been identified in Americans who began treatment after new methods of purifying the hormone came into use in the United States in 1977.

By the time the risks of pituitary-derived GH were discovered, biosynthetic GH was being tested for safety and efficacy.[1074,1088,1089] The original recombinant GH mimicked pit-GH in regard to both anabolic and metabolic actions and was scrupulously scrutinized for monoisomerism, antigenic bacterial products, and toxins of any sort. GH has universally replaced pit-GH as the accepted treatment for children with GHD.

Treatment Regimens. The recommended therapeutic starting dose of GH in children with GHD is 0.18 to 0.35 mg/kg body weight per week, administered in seven daily doses.[1090] Alternative regimens include a 6-day/week and a 3-day/week schedule, with the same weekly dosage, but they are not as successful. In general, the growth response to GH is a function of the log-dose given, so increasing dosages further enhance growth velocities,[1083,1084,1091] but daily dosing may be the most important treatment parameter.[1092] Subcutaneous and intramuscular administration has equivalent growth-promoting activity[1093]; the former is now used exclusively. At this time, all of the commercially available GH preparations yield comparable growth outcomes.

Growth responses to exogenous GH vary, depending on the frequency of administration, dosage, age (greater absolute gain in a younger child, although not necessarily greater growth velocity SDS), weight, GHR type and amount (as assessed by serum GHBP levels), and, perhaps, seasonality.[557,1094-1097] Nevertheless, the general regimen of daily GH at the recommended doses typically accelerates growth in a GH-deficient child from a pretreatment rate of 3 to 4 cm/year to 10 to 12 cm/year in year 1 of therapy to 7 to 9 cm/

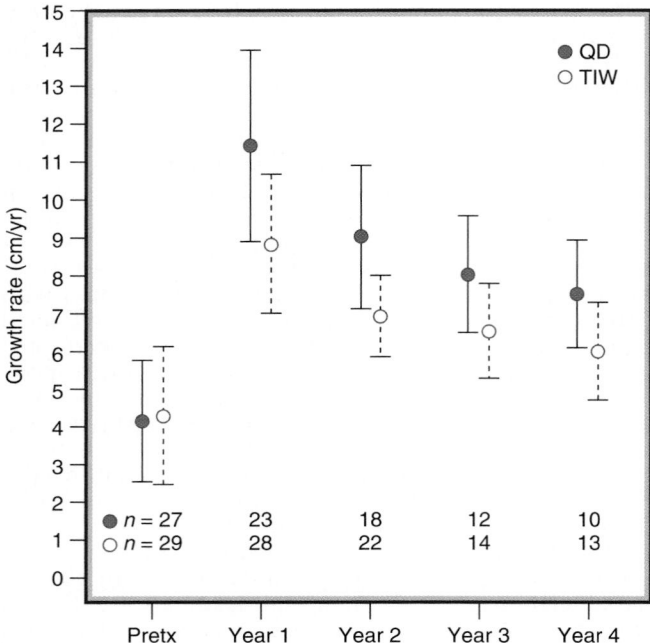

Figure 24-45 Annual growth velocity (mean ± standard deviation) for prepubertal patients with growth hormone (GH) deficiency before and during 4 years of GH treatment, contrasting results from daily (QD) versus thrice-weekly (TIW) injections. The mean annual growth velocity in the QD group was significantly greater than that in the TIW group during each year, although significance diminished from year 1 to year 4. (From MacGillivray MH, Baptista J, Johanson A. Outcome of a four-year randomized study of daily versus three times weekly somatropin treatment in prepubertal naive growth hormone deficient children. *J Clin Endocrinol Metab.* 1996;81:1806-1809. Reproduced by permission of M.H. MacGillivray.)

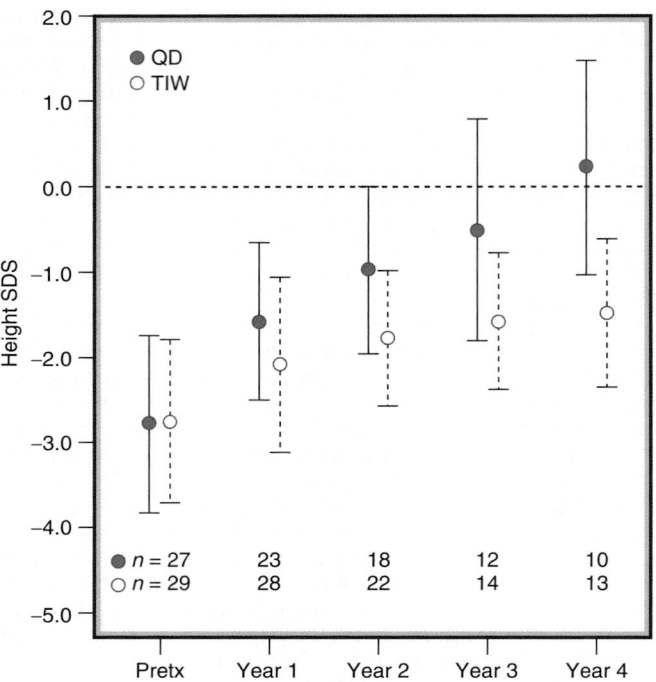

Figure 24-46 Height standard deviation score (SDS) for prepubertal patients with growth hormone (GH) deficiency before and during 4 years of GH treatment, contrasting results (mean ± standard deviation) with daily (QD) versus thrice-weekly (TIW) injections. The mean SDS in the QD group was significantly greater throughout the treatment period. Younger patients had the greatest increase in height SDS, and the effect of age was more marked in the QD group. (From MacGillivray MH, Baptista J, Johanson A. Outcome of a four-year randomized study of daily versus three times weekly somatropin treatment in prepubertal naive growth hormone deficient children. *J Clin Endocrinol Metab.* 1996;81:1806-1809. Reproduced by permission of M.H. MacGillivray.)

year in years 2 and 3. Progressive waning of GH efficacy occurs and is poorly understood. The importance of dosage frequency is illustrated (Figs. 24-45 and 24-46) by data from a carefully done assessment of growth responses in prepubertal naïve GH-deficient children randomly assigned to receive thrice-weekly or daily GH at the same total weekly dose (0.30 mg/kg per week).[1092] The mean total height gain during this period was 9.7 cm greater in the patients treated daily (38.4 versus 28.7 cm, *p* < 0.0002), with similar increments in skeletal maturation and no acceleration of the onset of puberty. Mean height SDS at the end of 4 years was +0.2, or at the midpoint of normal for age. Studies using varying dosing of GH based on gender, growth responsivity, and growth factor concentrations have suggested the need for greater sophistication and individualization of the current treatment regimens.[1098,1099]

Sophisticated mathematical models[1091,1100] have examined many laboratory and auxologic parameters that influence response to GH therapy. Because age at onset of treatment is inversely correlated with growth responses, and because the smaller, lighter child requires less GH (with marked economic benefit), it is important to assess growth data in children treated early. In short-term studies of 134 patients[1101-1103] treated before age 3 years, marked early catch-up growth occurred, with a mean height gain of about 3 SDS by 4 years of therapy, allowing most children to reach their normal height range by middle childhood. Mean height in one study[1101] reached −0.4 SDS after 8 years of treatment. Near-adult height in 13 patients treated before 5 years of age[1104] did not differ significantly from the midparental target height (−0.9 versus −0.7 SDS). In a group of 25 children treated before 12 months of age,[1105] adult height also matched the target height despite

low dosage and less frequent administration. In an analysis of postmarketing data for development of a growth prediction model, a greater height gain per GH amount occurred in the very young children, but a seemingly lowered sensitivity to endogenous GH in early infancy adds complexity to interpretation of these data.[1106]

Adult Height Outcomes. Treatment of growth-deficient children with pit-GH significantly increased their final heights, although the majority had final heights below −2 SD.[1107] This was likely due to the lower doses used, as well to treatment interruptions and the shorter duration compared to current treatment.

Patients treated with biosynthetic GH[987,1104,1107-1116] have improved final adult height SDS, with average final height in more than 1400 patients approximating −1.3 SD. Data from the two largest databases,[1108,1110,1115-1117] representing the North American and European experiences as reported by pediatric endocrinologists, are shown in Table 24-13.

Despite the use of GH therapy, long-term studies still show that most patients fail to reach their genetic target heights. Evaluation of adult heights in 121 patients with childhood GHD treated in the Genentech GH research trials indicated a mean adult height in both male and female patients of −0.7 SDS, with 106 patients being within 2 SDS for normal adult Americans.[1113] Even in these closely monitored patients, however, a difference of −0.4 to −0.6 SDS from midparental target height still occurred. The achievement of the genetic target is possible, however: a Swedish subgroup (in the Kabi International Growth Study [KIGS] database) of consistently treated patients reached a median final height SDS of −0.32, which was equivalent to

TABLE 24-13

Adult Height in Children with Growth Hormone Deficiency Treated with Biosynthetic Growth Hormone

Study	Gender	N	GH Dose (mg/kg/wk)	Duration (yr)	Age (yr)	Height SDS	Change in Height SDS	Height vs. MPH
KIGS*								
	M	351	0.22	7.5	18.2	−0.8	+1.6	−0.2
	F	200	0.20	6.9	16.6	−1.0	+1.6	−0.5
KIGS (Sweden)†								
	M	294	0.23	8.4	18.5	−0.9	+1.8	+0.2
	F	107	0.23	8.5	17.4	−0.7	+2.1	+0.2
NCGS‡								
	M	2095	0.28	5.2	18.2	−1.1	+1.4	−0.7
	F	1116	0.29	5.0	16.7	−1.3	+1.6	−0.9

F, female; GH, growth hormone; KIGS, Pharmacia Kabi International Growth Study; M, male; MPH, midparental target height; NCGS, Genentech National Cooperative Growth Study; SDS, standard deviation score.

*Data from Reiter EO, Price DA, Wilton P, et al. Effect of growth hormone (GH) treatment on the near-final height of 1258 patients with idiopathic GH deficiency: analysis of a large international database. *J Clin Endocrinol Metab.* 2006;91:2047-2054.

†Data from Westphal O, Lindberg A, Swedish KIGS National Board. Final height in Swedish children with idiopathic growth hormone deficiency enrolled in KIGS treated optimally with growth hormone. *Acta Paediatr.* 2008;97:1698-1706.

‡Data from August GP, Julius JR, Blethen SL. Adult height in children with growth hormone deficiency who are treated with biosynthetic growth hormone: the National Cooperative Growth Study experience. *Pediatrics.* 1998;102(2 Pt 3):512-516; updated NCGS data from Dana K, Baptista J, Blethen SL (personal communication, 2001).

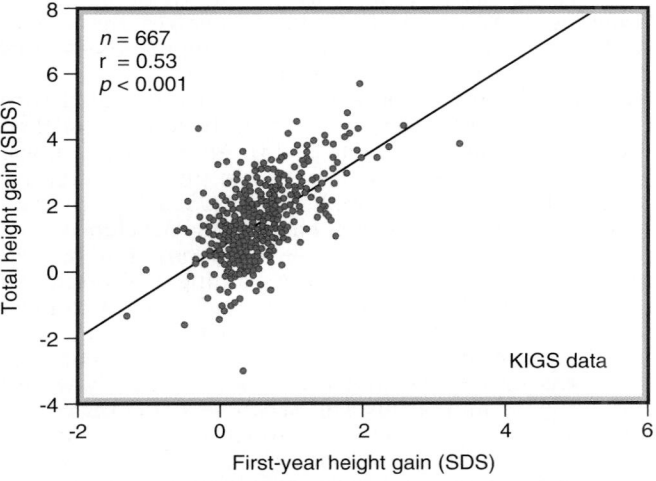

Figure 24-47 Relationship between first-year change in height standard deviation score (SDS) and total change in height SDS between start of growth hormone (GH) treatment and near-final height in children with idiopathic isolated GH deficiency. KIGS, Kabi International Growth Study database. (Modified with permission from Reiter EO, Price DA, Wilton P, et al. Effect of growth hormone [GH] treatment on the final height of 1258 patients with idiopathic GH deficiency: analysis of a large international database. *J Clin Endocrinol Metab.* 2006;91:2047-2054.)

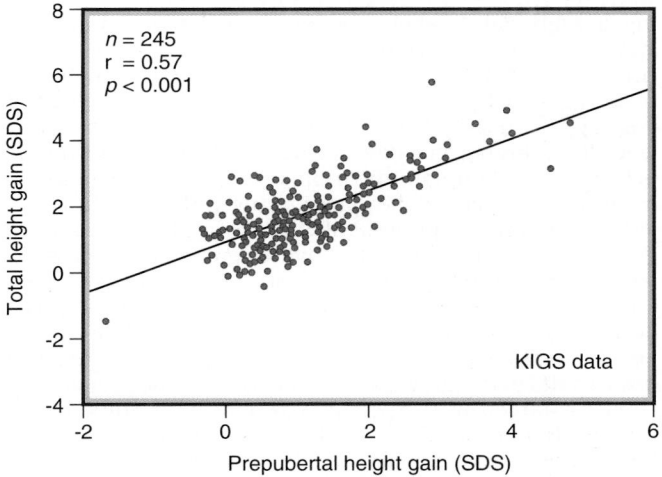

Figure 24-48 Relationship between prepubertal change in height standard deviation score (SDS) and total change in height SDS between start of growth hormone (GH) treatment and near-final height in children with idiopathic isolated GH deficiency. KIGS, Kabi International Growth Study database. (Modified with permission from Reiter EO, Price DA, Wilton P, et al. Effect of growth hormone [GH] treatment on the final height of 1258 patients with idiopathic GH deficiency: analysis of a large international database. *J Clin Endocrinol Metab.* 2006;91:2047-2054.)

the midparental target height.[1117] A more recent study of the Swedish subgroup actually found a final height SDS greater than midparental target height by +0.2 (see Table 24-13).[1108]

Factors that have been found to correlate with enhanced adult height in GH-treated, GH-deficient children include baseline height, younger age at onset of treatment, longer treatment duration (especially during prepubertal years), and a greater growth velocity during the first year of treatment (Figs. 24-47 and 24-48).[1116] Increased height velocity and subsequent superior adult height outcome, although with considerable overlap, were demonstrated in children with GHD who carried one or both *GHRd3* alleles (i.e., with an exon 3 deletion).[557,1118,1119] Data from National Cooperative Growth Study (NCGS) and KIGS showed that the height gained during puberty in patients with GHD was generally comparable to that in healthy children with delayed bone age.[1115,1120] As might be expected based on that observation, final height correlates with height at the

onset of puberty in GHD patients.[1096,1112,1121-1123] Therefore, every effort should be made to enhance growth before puberty, and delays in diagnosis and initiation of therapy probably contribute to the compromised adult heights still reported in many studies.

GH treatment of children who develop GHD as a result of cranial irradiation represents a special case when evaluating final height outcomes. In these children, who have received cranial irradiation for the treatment of malignancy, GH treatment is not initiated until there is no evidence of active tumor; this results in a delay between the diagnosis of GHD and the initiation of treatment. Final height is negatively correlated with the length of that lag time.[1124] In addition, those who have received spinal irradiation in addition to the cranial irradiation have a lower final height due to impairment of spinal growth after irradiation.[1124,1125]

In an effort to increase final height in GHD patients, the use of high-dose GH during puberty has been studied, based on the rationale that GH secretion normally rises twofold to fourfold during the pubertal growth spurt, with dramatic concomitant increases in serum IGF-1 levels, and the pubertal growth spurt normally accounts for approximately 17% of adult male height and 12% of adult female height. Earlier studies by Stanhope and associates[1126,1127] indicated that little difference in height gain could be observed when adolescent patients were treated with 30 versus 15 IU/m² per week of GH (approximately 0.04 versus 0.02 mg/kg per day). Mauras and colleagues[1128] evaluated higher pubertal GH doses (0.1 versus 0.043 mg/kg per day) and found that the higher dosage resulted in a 4.6-cm increase in near-final height. Mean height SDS achieved in the group receiving 0.043 mg/kg per day of GH (as in the earlier report[1113]) was −0.7 ± 0.9, but in the group receiving 0.1 mg/kg per day it was 0.0 ± 1.2. The higher GH dosage did not result in more rapid acceleration of skeletal maturation.

Another approach that has been taken to attempt to increase final height in GH-treated patients has been to adjust the dose of GH to reach a target IGF-1 level rather than treating with a fixed, weight-based dose.[1129,1130] A study reported by Cohen and colleagues found that targeting a high IGF-1 level (reaching a mean IGF-1 SDS of approximately +1.5) resulted in an increase in growth rate compared with the two comparator groups, which had mean IGF-1 SDS of approximately +1.[1129] It required a GH dose approximately three times higher to reach this IGF-1 level (0.11 mg/kg per day versus 0.041 and 0.033 mg/kg per day for the comparator groups).[1129] In the study reported by Marchisotti and colleagues,[1130] the difference in IGF-1 levels between groups (+0.8 SDS versus −0.3 SDS) was even greater than that in the report by Cohen and colleagues,[1129] but the Marchisotti study did not find a difference in growth rate between the two groups. The difference in GH dose was much smaller, however (0.038 versus 0.30 mg/kg per day). Therefore, as would be expected, a higher GH dose results in a higher growth rate, but it is not yet known whether targeting a specific IGF-1 level results in an increased final height; nor is it known whether these higher doses have adverse effects not seen with the more usual doses currently used. An interesting finding was the wide range of doses required to reach a given IGF-1 level: the high-IGF-1 targeted group required GH doses ranging from less than 0.025 mg/kg per day to greater than 0.25 mg/kg per day, whereas the low-IGF-1 targeted group required doses ranging from less than 0.025 to 0.15 mg/kg per day.[1129]

The impact of treatments to alter sex hormone levels (e.g., GnRH agonists, aromatase inhibitors) with the aim of improving final height in GHD and other conditions is discussed later.

Combined Pituitary Hormone Deficiencies. If GHD is part of a combined pituitary deficiency syndrome, it is necessary to address each endocrine deficiency, both for general medical reasons and to ensure maximal effect of GH therapy. TSH deficiency is often "unmasked" during the initial phase of therapy, and thyroid function should be assessed before the onset of therapy, during the first 3 months of GH treatment,[1131] and at least on an annual basis thereafter. The pituitary-adrenal axis can be evaluated during the insulin stimulation test in the workup for GHD or separately if GHD is identified with the use of a different provocative test. If ACTH secretion is impaired, patients may be placed on the lowest safe maintenance dose of glucocorticoids, certainly no more than 10 mg/m² per day of hydrocortisone, and less if possible. Higher doses impair the growth response to GH therapy but should be given during times of stress. It is critical to monitor the long-term evolution

of glucocorticoid deficiency, especially in those with *PROP1* mutations (discussed earlier). However, Lange and colleagues studied 24 adults with a prior history of idiopathic isolated childhood GHD and identified adrenal insufficiency in 10 of them, half of whom did not have evidence of ongoing GHD[1132]; this suggests a need to consider monitoring for impaired ACTH secretion even in those patients with presumed IGHD.

Gonadotropin deficiency may be evident in the infant with microphallus. This can be treated with three or four monthly injections of 25 mg of testosterone enanthate in the first months of life.[1133] Management at puberty can be more complicated, in that the physical and psychological benefits of promoting sexual maturation must be balanced against the effects of epiphyseal fusion. When GH therapy is initiated in childhood and growth is normal before adolescence, it is appropriate to begin gonadal steroid replacement at a normal age (11 to 12 years of age in girls, 12 to 13 years of age in boys). In boys, this can be done by beginning with monthly injections of 50 to 100 mg of testosterone enanthate, gradually increasing to 200 mg per month, and eventually moving to the appropriate adult replacement regimen as determined by monitoring of plasma testosterone levels. In girls, therapy involves the use of conjugated estrogens or ethinyl estradiol and eventual cycling with estrogen and progesterone.

Monitoring Growth Hormone Therapy. Patients treated with GH should be seen every 3 to 6 months to monitor their response to treatment (Table 24-14). An increase in linear growth velocity should be seen within the first 6 months. Height SDS should increase at least 0.25 SDS in the first year.[1090] Treatment models have been developed that predict the expected growth rate in response to GH treatment.[1091,1100,1134-1136] A model[1091] explaining 61% of growth response variability in the first year of therapy includes inverse relationships with maximum GH response during provocative testing, age, and height SDS minus midparental height SDS and positive correlation with body weight SDS, GH dose, and birthweight SDS.[1137,1138] The single most important predictive factor for growth in years 2 through 4 is the first-year height velocity. These models can be used to quantify whether the individual patient is responding appropriately to GH treatment. If a patient's initial growth response is lower than predicted, the clinician should consider whether the diagnosis of GHD was correct, whether additional growth disorders (e.g., hypothyroidism) are present, and whether there is lack of compliance with the treatment.[1135]

It is appropriate to monitor the IGF-1 levels after initiation of GH treatment and perhaps yearly thereafter.[1090,1139] A failure of IGF-1 levels to increase into the normal range with treatment, together with an inadequate growth response, suggests compliance failure or the presence of

TABLE 24-14
Monitoring Growth Hormone Therapy

Close follow-up with a pediatric endocrinologist every 3-6 months
Determination of growth response (change in height SDS)
Evaluation of compliance
Screening for potential adverse effects
Interval measurements of serum IGF-1 and IGFBP3
Annual assessment of thyroid function
Consideration of dose adjustment based on IGF values, growth response, and comparison with growth prediction models
Periodic reevaluation of adrenal and thyroid function

IGF, insulin-like growth factor; IGBP, insulin-like growth factor–binding protein; SDS, standard deviation score.

GH insensitivity. Because of the association of elevated IGF-1 levels with certain cancers (see later discussion), a reduction in GH dose should be considered for patients with serum IGF-1 levels substantially above the normal range after the first 2 years of therapy.[1090] Whether the IGF-1 level should be used to guide GH dosing awaits additional studies (see earlier discussion).

CPHD may evolve over several years, so children who are initially diagnosed with IGHD may develop CPHD. Thyroxine levels should be assessed after GH treatment has been initiated, and annually thereafter, to identify the development of central hypothyroidism during treatment. Periodic reevaluation for ACTH deficiency should be performed. It is not necessary to routinely monitor fasting insulin and glucose levels, but if impaired glucose control is suspected, a fasting glucose level and glycosylated hemoglobin (HbA_{1c}) should be measured.

The growth response to GH typically attenuates after several years but should continue to be equal to or greater than the normal height velocity for age throughout treatment. Use of statistical growth treatment models can prove valuable in judging therapeutic efficacy.[1140-1142] A suboptimal response to GH can result from several causes: (1) poor compliance, (2) improper preparation of GH for administration or incorrect injection techniques, (3) subclinical hypothyroidism, (4) coexisting systemic disease, (5) excessive glucocorticoid therapy, (6) prior irradiation of the spine, (7) epiphyseal fusion, (8) anti-GH antibodies, or (9) incorrect diagnosis of GHD as the explanation for growth retardation (particularly in a patient with idiopathic IGHD and normal findings on MRI). Although 10% to 20% of recipients of recombinant GH develop anti-GH antibodies, growth failure is rarely caused by such antibodies, except in the case of individuals who have GHD as a result of GH gene deletion.[1143-1145]

Treatment During the Transition to Adulthood and in Adulthood. A growing challenge in the management of patients with GHD has been the issues surrounding their care after the growth process has ceased.[1146] This period, from the middle to late teenage years until the mid-20s, is a normal physiologic phase during which peak bone and muscle mass is achieved and the independence and self-sufficiency characteristics of adulthood are attained. It is also a time during which care of pediatric patients is transferred to endocrinologists who treat adults.

Clinical consequences of GHD in adults and the potential benefits of GH therapy in such patients have already been described.[1147,1148] Signs and symptoms of adult GHD include reduced lean body mass and musculature, increased body fat, reduced BMD, reduced exercise performance, and increased plasma cholesterol. Adults with GHD have a significantly increased risk of death from cardiovascular causes, a finding potentially linked to increased visceral adiposity and other cardiovascular risk factors.[1149] Adults with GHD have been found to have "impaired psychological well-being and quality of life."[1150] Several placebo-controlled studies have demonstrated that GH therapy for adult GHD results in marked alterations in body composition, fat distribution, bone density, and sense of well-being.[1148]

Given the metabolic derangements associated with untreated GHD, continuation of GH treatment in late adolescence in the patient who shows persistent GHD is an important issue. Documentation of persistent GHD is important. Among almost 500 patients with IGHD, 207 (44%) had normal GH levels on provocative retesting.[1151,1152] In contrast, approximately 96% of patients with CPHD, with or without structural abnormalities of the hypothalamic-pituitary area, had sustained GHD.[1151,1152]

The presence of multiple anterior pituitary hormone deficiencies or structural disease would seem to obviate the need for retesting. The data are not absolute, so clinical judgment is of paramount importance. The strict pharmacologic definition of GHD in this age group is difficult, as was shown by Maghnie and colleagues,[1153] who suggested that the much lower GH responses to testing that characterize older adults should not be used in this population. The issue of testing validity may have influenced the dichotomy observed between the IGD and CPHD patient populations in testing "positive" on the provocative tests. As in the childhood population, it seems reasonable not to rely solely on artificial cutoffs in pharmacologic provocative tests but to include broader clinical and laboratory data.[1146]

Many patients do not wish to continue the daily GH regimen, but the data support consideration for sustained treatment. After 1 to 2 years off GH therapy, IGF-1 and IGFBP3 levels decrease substantially below baseline levels.[1147,1154,1155] Resumption of GH normalizes these levels, although there is a strong suggestion of a gender-based difference in GH requirements, with females needing higher GH doses.[1147,1154,1155] Loss of energy and strength may occur, and some quality-of-life data suggest age-specific psychological issues in patients with untreated severe GHD during the transition to adulthood.[1156] Quality-of-life data with rigorous study designs are lacking in GH-treated childhood GHD.[1157] In untreated patients, total body fat and abdominal fat increase significantly and lean body mass is lost, compared with control subjects, comparable GH-treated patients, and patients who have reinstituted therapy.[1158,1159]

Because bone mass accrual is not completed until the third decade, late adolescence is an important time for GH sufficiency, to prevent later osteopenia.[617,1146] There have been numerous GH treatment studies carried out in the transition age group to assess the impact on bone mineralization.[1155,1158,1160,1161] Differences in age at onset of re-treatment, duration of therapy, GH dosage, and gender distribution have led to variations in results. In general, however, the data affirm the concept that reinstitution of treatment for 2 years in the transition period prevents deterioration in bone mineral density as experienced by untreated young adults with persistent GHD.

The cardiovascular risk of stopping GH treatment has also been examined. Colao and associates showed modest left ventricular ejection fraction decrements that paralleled IGF levels when stopping and restarting GH therapy in a group of adolescents with GHD.[1162] The overall IGF levels were rather low, so cardiac changes were relatively modest. It should be recalled that GH treatment during childhood alters cardiac size but does not seem to change cardiac function.[1163] Mauras and associates used a wide array of functional studies in a similar transition-age group and were unable to demonstrate cardiac changes,[1155] but their patients had relatively high IGF-1 levels (mean, 427 ng/mL) at GH discontinuation, suggesting a degree of "protectiveness" in the subsequent period off GH treatment. Nonetheless, abnormal cardiovascular risk factors, such as elevated concentrations of lipids, fibrinogen, inflammatory markers, and homocysteine, and platelet hyperactivation may occur in adolescents with untreated GHD.[1164] In prepubertal children with GHD, normalization of homocysteine levels and of markers of oxidative stress is achieved with GH treatment,[1165,1166] buttressing the notion of important effects of GH on cardiovascular health. Therefore, cardiac function and those factors affecting vascular biology are targets in the spectrum of GH-mediated body compositional changes.

These studies support the continuation of GH treatment in late adolescence, albeit at lower doses than in childhood, to prevent the development of adverse cardiovascular risk, diminished bone mineralization, and a deterioration in quality of life. Whether the diversity of treatment and response data relates to the efficacy of the childhood GH therapeutic process is not clear, but the period of time off GH and the degree of persistent GHD would seem likely predictors of clinical status at the time of reinitiation of GH treatment.

After the adolescent with GHD has completed skeletal growth, the persistence of GHD is evaluated.[1167,1168] If the patient has a high probability of persistent GHD (i.e., CPHD, IGHD with structural abnormalities, or confirmed genetic mutations), a presumption of persistent GHD is made. Otherwise, GH therapy should be halted for 2 to 3 months, followed by a thorough reevaluation. A recommended algorithm for this evaluation is shown in Figure 24-49.[1169]

As in childhood GHD, laboratory testing is imperfectly precise for diagnosis of ongoing GHD. Some patients have results that neither indicate nor eliminate ongoing GHD but are intermediate, suggesting either probable or partial GHD. If ongoing GHD is considered to be present or

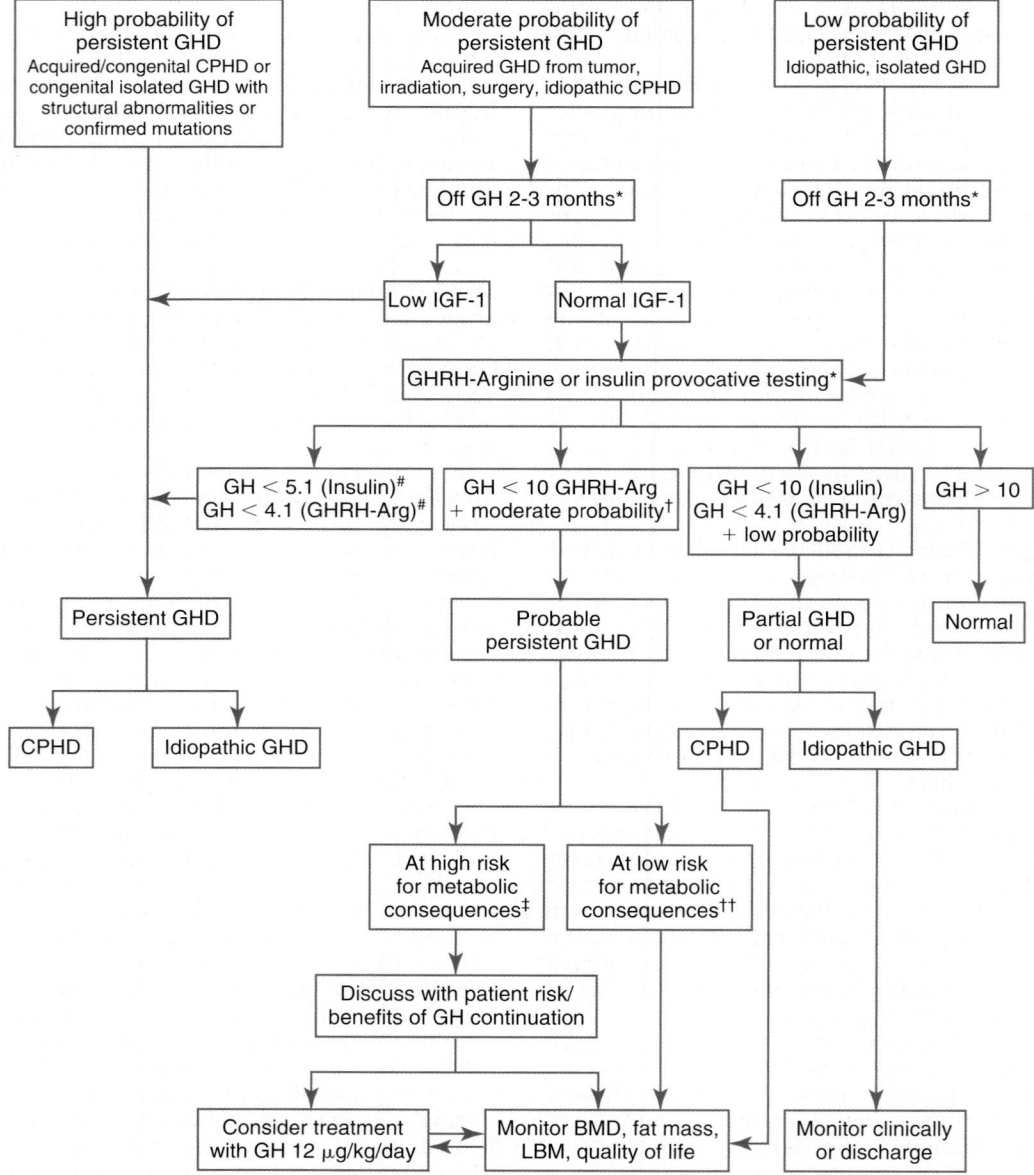

Figure 24-49 Algorithm for evaluating patients diagnosed with GHD during childhood at the completion of growth. *, Based on consensus and clinical practice guidelines. GH, growth hormone; GHD, growth hormone deficiency; CPHD, combined pituitary hormone deficiencies; BMD, bone mineral density; LBM, lean body mass. (From Molitch ME, Clemmons DR, Malozowski S, et al. Evaluation and treatment of adult growth hormone deficiency: an Endocrine Society Clinical Practice Guideline. *J Clin Endocrinol Metab.* 2006;91:1621-1634 and Growth Hormone Research Society. Consensus guidelines for the diagnosis and treatment of growth hormone (GH) deficiency in childhood and adolescence: summary statement of the GH Research Society. *J Clin Endocrinol Metab.* 2000;85:3990-3993. #Threshold values that achieve a sensitivity of 95% and specificity 91-92% for diagnosing GHD in adults; from Biller BMK, Samuels MH, Zagar A, et al. Sensitivity and specificity of six tests for the diagnosis of adult GH deficiency. *J Clin Endocrinol Metab.* 2002;87:2067-2079. †Based upon data indicating that patients with irradiation-induced CPHD can have hypothalamic dysfunction causing GHD; from Darzy KH, Aimaretti G, Wieringa G, et al. The usefulness of the combined growth hormone (GH)-releasing hormone and arginine stimulation test in the diagnosis of radiation-induced GH deficiency is dependent on the post-irradiation time interval. *J Clin Endocrinol Metab.* 2003;88:95-102. ‡Those at high risk for metabolic complications include patients with abnormal BMD, high fat mass, low LBM. ††Those at low risk for metabolic complications include patients with normal BMD, fat mass, and LBM.)

probable, assessment of body composition, BMD, and fasting lipid levels should be determined. The decision to reinitiate GH treatment is then based on a discussion with the patient and family regarding the risks and benefits in light of the laboratory test results and the risk for metabolic consequences (see Fig. 24-49).[1169] In addition, caution should be exercised in considering whether to continue GH therapy when there is a known risk of diabetes or malignancy. This is also an opportunity for a thorough clinical reassessment and a determination of the need for replacement of other hormones. The transition to adult GH replacement should be arranged as a close collaboration between endocrinologists who treat pediatric patients and those who treat adult patients and should include discussion with the patient and family. A discussion of many transition issues was reported by Clayton and associates from a European consensus meeting.[1146]

Growth Hormone Treatment of Other Forms of Short Stature

Prader-Willi Syndrome. Guidelines for the clinical management of PWS were published after an international multidisciplinary expert meeting in 2013.[1170] Short stature due to GH insufficiency is almost always present in children with PWS. In a large cohort of 1135 children with PWS starting GH treatment, median height SDS was −2.2 (range, −4.1 to −0.3) at a median age of 6.4 years (range, 1.3 to 12.9 years).[1171] Growth standards for infants with PWS have been pubished.[1172]

Serum levels of IGF-1 are reduced in most children with PWS.[1173-1176] Studies have shown that spontaneous GH secretion is reduced, and 70% of children with PWS have GH peaks of less than 10 µg/L during pharmacologic stimulation tests.[1177] Most experts agree that prior GH testing is not required before GH treatment is initiated. GH treatment of growth failure in PWS is an FDA-approved indication. GH treatment in children with PWS aims to improve childhood growth, final adult height, and body composition (see review by Burman and associates[1177]).[1178] Numerous clinical trials have documented the efficacy of GH therapy. In randomized, controlled studies there were significant increases in height and growth velocity and a significant decrease in percent body fat, as well as increased percentage of fat-free mass, improved muscle strength and agility, and increased fat oxidation during the first year of GH treatment.[1174,1179] Stabilization of these parameters occurs after the second year of therapy. Lean body mass increased significantly during the first 2 years in children with PWS who received GH treatment, compared with no treatment.[1180,1181] GH therapy for 2 additional years resulted in continued beneficial effects on body composition. When the dose of GH was reduced to 0.3 mg/m^2 per day, these improvements were not maintained.[1180] Beneficial effects continued after 8 years of GH treatment.[1182]

BMD improves in children with PWS treated with GH. In two German cohorts, the mean spontaneous adult heights were reported in one study as 162 cm in boys and 150 cm in girls[1183] and the other as 159 cm in boys and 149 cm in girls.[1184] In the KIGS database, 33 patients (21 boys and 12 girls) reached adult height, and two thirds of them were above −2 SDS; the median adult height was −1 SDS after a mean duration of 8.4 years.[1185] Another study with 21 adults (13 boys, 8 girls) revealed a mean adult height of 0.3 SDS after a mean duration of 7.9 years of GH treatment.[1185] In this cohort, the strength and agility that were evident during the initial 2 years continued into adulthood. The patients also reported a higher quality of life and reduced depression.[1186] In 55 children monitored during 4 years of continuous GH treatment (1 mg/m^2 per day), body composition was significantly improved, mean height normalized, head circumference increased, and BMI significantly decreased. GH treatment had no adverse effects on bone maturation, blood pressure, glucose homeostasis, and serum lipids.[1187] Improved body composition and metabolic status was demonstrated in adults treated with GH in childhood and adolescence.[1188]

Before GH therapy is begun, screening for hypothyroidism is indicated because of the association with primary and central hypothyroidism.[1189,1190] Continued screening is also recommended. Treatment with GH beginning as early as 2 years of age is recommended, but there may be additional benefits to starting therapy between 6 and 12 months of age. Several studies have found improvements in motor development, muscle tone, head circumference, and, possibly, cognition and behavior.[1191,1192] A recent review documents the benefits of GH therapy including an increase in female height, improved body composition, and increased exercise tolerance.[1193] Cognitive function was improved in children with treated GH.[1194]

Since October 2002, several reports of unexpected deaths in infants and children with PWS have been published.[1195-1197] Between 1985 and 2006, the NCGS monitored the safety and efficacy of recombinant human GH in 54,996 children. Two deaths were reported in patients with PWS.[1198] Although death from presumed obesity-induced hypoventilation or apneic events in PWS without GH treatment is well described, the occurrence of such deaths during GH administration raises the question of whether GH exacerbates this condition.[1199,1200] Tonsillar hypertrophy and fluid retention associated with GH therapy are potential risk factors. Most of the deaths, with or without GH treatment, were related to obesity or to a complicated course of a relatively mild respiratory tract infection, sleep apnea, adenoid or tonsillar hypertrophy (or both), hypoventilation, and aspiration. The obesity-hypoventilation syndrome is the more likely etiologic factor, suggesting that ventilatory and pulmonary function should be assessed with polysomnographic studies before and during GH treatment.[1199,1201]

In a review that included 64 children (42 boys and 22 girls, 28 receiving GH treatment), the highest death risk occurred during the first 9 months of GH treatment.[1197] Therefore, it is recommended that GH treatment be started at a low dose (e.g., 0.25 to 0.30 mg/m^2 per day or 0.009 to 0.012 mg/kg per day) and increased during the first weeks and months to reach the standard replacement dosage of approximately 1 mg/m^2 per day or 0.24 mg/kg per week. Patients should be monitored for sleep apnea and IGF-1 levels. The GH dose should be decreased if there is evidence of high IGF-1 levels, especially if associated with edema, worsening or new onset of snoring, headache, or acromegalic clinical features. A longitudinal observational study evaluated 75 children with PWS and showed an increase in the apnea-hypoxia index (AHI) after GH treatment.[1202]

Five prospective studies have evaluated the effects of GH treatment on breathing disorders in PWS.[1203-1206] Carbon dioxide responsiveness, resting ventilation, and airway occlusion pressure improved during 6 to 9 months of GH treatment,[1206] and the inspiratory and expiratory muscle strength improved during 12 months of GH treatment, compared with control subjects.[1204] In a double-blind, placebo-controlled, crossover study, AHI was found to decrease in 12 children with PWS, compared with control subjects, after 6 months of GH therapy although the difference was not statistically significant.[1203] Another study found a decrease in AHI in most of the adults and children studied after 6 weeks of GH therapy.[1207] A subset of patients had an increased AHI with more obstructive events, but most of these latter patients had upper respiratory tract infections and adenoid/tonsil hypertrophy, and two of them had high IGF-1 levels. In another study in 35 prepubertal children with PWS, the AHI did not significantly change during 6 months of GH therapy.[1208] However, four of these children had an increase in the number of episodes of obstructive apnea during an upper respiratory illness; these episodes were not present after recovery. Therefore, it is recommended that obesity-related sleep and breathing problems be evaluated before and vigilantly monitored after GH treatment begins. Polysomnography and ear, nose, and throat evaluations should be performed as necessary. A longitudinal review of polysomnography data suggests that children younger than 2 years of age are most vulnerable to sleep-related disordered breathing (SRDB) after initiation of GH therapy.[1209]

A recent study[1210] showed that 60% of PWS patients had central adrenal insufficiency. This may explain the high rate of sudden death especially during infection-related stress. The authors concluded that patients with PWS should be treated with hydrocortisone during stress until adrenal insufficiency can be ruled out.[1210,1211]

Between 30% and 70% of children with PWS have scoliosis.[1212-1217] Weight control is a vital part of its prevention and management. Therefore, before GH treatment is initiated, spinal radiographs and, if appropriate, orthopedic assessment are recommended. Reports of scoliosis worsening during GH treatment reflect the natural history of this condition rather than a side effect of treatment in most cases, and discontinuation of GH is not indicated.

In view of the childhood findings of low lean body mass and high fat content, osteopenia, and some degree of glucose intolerance ameliorated by GH, the issue of long-term therapy through adulthood must be considered and studied.[1218-1220] After growth is complete, attainment of a normal peak bone mass, continued improvement of muscle mass and strength, reduction of body fat, prevention of cardiovascular morbidity, and improvement in well-being and quality of life are potential benefits of continued GH therapy.[1221] Adult GHD and low IGF-1 levels have been reported in patients with PWS.[1176,1222] Short-term GH treatment in GH-naïve adults with PWS has been reported to modestly improve body composition, cognition, motor performance, and social status.[1222] Further long-term studies are needed on adolescents with PWS transitioning to adult therapies.

Chronic Renal Disease. Chronic renal disease (CRD) is regarded as indication for the commencement of GH administration. Short stature is more severe in children with congenital renal disorders than in children with acquired renal diseases.[650,1223,1224] Even after renal transplantation, final height is below the lower limit of normal in about 50% of children.[1225] GH treatment is able to increase height velocity and height SDS[660,1226,1227] and significantly improves final height[1228-1230] in patients with CRD (Figs. 24-50 and 24-51). The therapy should be implemented if short stature persists for longer than 6 months and in subjects with marked deceleration of growth velocity, and it should be continued until transplantation is performed.[1231] Typical growth patterns for the year after GH initiation have been devised. A growth velocity less than -1 SDS for age (in a child without dialysis or transplant) is inadequate and indicates presence of confounding factors that require investigation.[1232]

GH accelerates growth in children with CRD, at least over 5 years of therapy.[1233-1236] Using a GH dosage of 0.05 mg/kg per day, Fine and colleagues[1226] reported a mean first-year growth rate of 10.7 cm in GH recipients and 6.5 cm in the placebo group; in the second year, GH-treated patients had a mean growth rate of 7.8 cm/year compared with 5.5 cm/year in placebo recipients, resulting

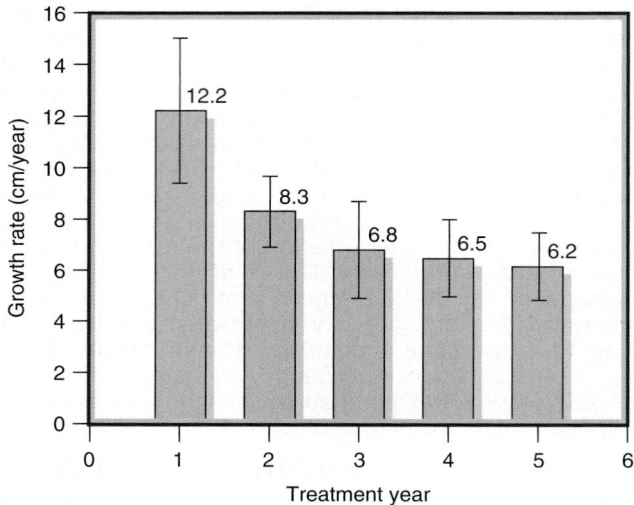

Figure 24-50 Annual growth velocity (mean ± standard deviation) in 20 growth-retarded prepubertal patients with chronic renal insufficiency who were treated with growth hormone. (From Fine RN, Kohaut E, Brown D, et al. Long-term treatment of growth retarded children with chronic renal insufficiency with recombinant human growth hormone. *Kidney Int.* 1996;49:781-785. Reproduced with permission of R.N. Fine.)

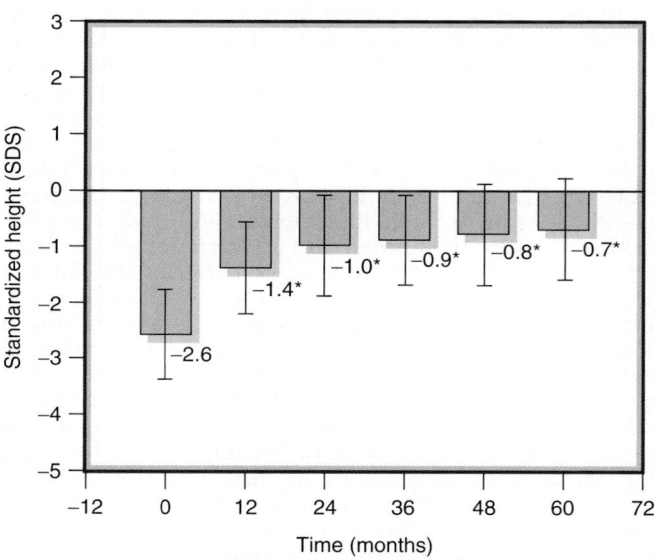

Figure 24-51 Height standard deviation score (SDS) in 20 growth-retarded prepubertal patients with chronic renal insufficiency (mean ± standard deviation). Note that the basal height is outside the normal range (at −2.6 SDS), enters the normal range within 1 year of treatment initiation, and is not different from the mean by the fifth year of growth hormone therapy. (From Fine RN, Kohaut E, Brown D, et al. Long-term treatment of growth retarded children with chronic renal insufficiency with recombinant human growth hormone. *Kidney Int.* 1996;49:781-785. Reproduced with permission of R.N. Fine.)

in an improvement of height SDS from −2.9 to −1.5. Twenty patients who were treated for 5 years reached a normal height SDS of −0.7, with a mean height increase of 40 cm.[1236] The youngest patients (<2.5 years of age) had the most impressive growth response to GH therapy (14.1 cm/year). Doses recommended in children with CRD are higher than in GHD patients (i.e., about 0.35 mg/kg per week) because growth patterns in these patients are dose dependent. Deleterious effects on renal function and progression of osteodystrophy were not observed.[1237] This treatment regimen does not adversely affect renal graft function after transplantation, nor is there significant "catch-down" growth after the transplantation.[1238] The final height in 38 German children treated with GH for an average of 5.3 years was −1.6 ± 1.2 SDS, an increment of 1.4 SDS over the pretreatment baseline. The final height of an untreated control group was −2.1 ± 1.2, or 0.6 SDS below baseline.[1229]

More recently, adult heights of 178 French patients treated with GH were reported. Mean adult height was 162.2 cm in men and 152.9 cm in women, and 46% were more than −2 SDS for height. Adult height SDS was correlated with height SDS and spontaneous height velocity before treatment and with the effect of treatment. These adult heights were significantly better when compared with historical cohorts of patients not treated with GH.[1239]

In 2009, a review of longitudinal data from 7189 patients enrolled in the chronic renal insufficiency registry of the North American Pediatric Renal Trials and Collaborative Studies (NAPRTCS) revealed that 827 patients (11.5%) had received GH. A total of 787 children with CRD who were previously naïve to GH treatment and received recombinant human GH for 1 to 4 years (median, 1.5 years) were paired with 787 control patients and monitored for 4 years. The GH-treated group had a significantly greater height velocity SDS than the control group at 2.5 years. Among 220 pairs evaluated at 2 years, the height SDS of the GH-treated group was 0.56 SDS higher than that of the control group ($p < 0.05$). Treatment with GH had no significant impact on BMI or estimated glomerular filtration rate (GFR).[1240]

The magnitude of response to GH treatment depends on the GH dosage. A dose of 0.35 mg/kg per week appears to be optimal for short patients with CRD; half of this dose was less effective, and doubling did not significantly improve the response in double-blind studies.[1234] Long-term GH treatment has also been shown to be safe and effective for extremely short (−4.0 SDS) children with nephropathic cystinosis and should be considered if nutrition and cysteamine treatment do not prevent growth failure.[1224] Because children are often short at the time of renal transplantation, have hormone findings of relative GH insensitivity, and receive chronic prednisone therapy, GH is sometimes administered in the post-transplantation period. Data after 1 and 2 years of treatment of such children and adolescents[1241] indicated a large increment of growth velocity at year 1 and a smaller benefit at year 2. As with GH treatment of CRD, the pharmacologic regimen overcomes the relative GH insensitivity. Individual patients show a wide variation in response, and predictors include age, GFR, need for dialysis treatment, target height, and pretreatment growth rate.[1242]

A mathematical model for prediction of the individual response to GH in prepubertal children with CRD was developed from the KIGS.[11] Thirty-seven percent of the variation in the first-year growth response was explained by this model, with the greatest first-year response in younger children who had no weight reduction, no hereditary renal disorder, and high residual renal function. There was a small GH dose effect during the first treatment year.[11] Such models, using clinical variables, may allow individualized GH treatment decisions in children with CRD.

Considerable assessment must yet be undertaken to demonstrate whether there is increased growth over a longer term, that renal function does not deteriorate during therapy, and that the risk of rejection is not enhanced. GH treatment does not appear to cause an accelerated decline of allograft function[1243-1245] or changes in histopathologic findings.[1246] Use of nonsteroid-based immunosuppressive regimens may obviate the need for post-transplantation GH treatment.

A short-term study in chronic well-nourished dialysis patients showed that combined administration of moderate doses of GH with recombinant human IGF-1 (rhIGF-1) had a complementary effect on protein metabolism.[1247] This approach is theoretically reasonable; however, the safety profile of this intervention is unknown.

Juvenile Idiopathic Arthritis. Juvenile idiopathic arthritis (JIA) is often complicated by growth deficiency. The decrease in linear growth usually correlates with the severity of the disease, although catch-up growth may not occur during remissions. The final height is less than −2 SDS in 11% of patients with polyarticular JIA and in 40% of those with systemic JIA.[1248] Serum GH levels are normal or low, usually with low plasma IGF-1 levels.[1249] The pathogenesis of short stature is thought to be GH insensitivity associated with both the inflammatory process and glucocorticoid treatment.[1250] Several trials have been conducted to determine whether GH replacement therapy is effective in patients with JIA.[1167,1251,1252] Trial of GH replacement using GH dosages ranging from 0.1 to 0.46 mg/kg per week increased serum levels of IGF-1 and linear growth velocity. However, the trials all had significant interindividual variability.[1253] GH therapy for up to 3 years was notable for a decrease in the loss of growth velocity associated with the active phase of JIA.[1167]

In a randomized, controlled trial of GH therapy (0.33 mg/kg per week for 4 years) in 31 children with JIA, a height increase of 1 SDS was found, compared with a decrease of 0.7 SDS in the untreated control group.[1252] The GH-treated patients had a significantly greater final height compared with untreated control patients (−1.6 ± 0.25 SDS versus −3.4 ± 2.0 SDS; $p < 0.001$).[1254] As expected, the severity of inflammation negatively affected the efficacy of GH therapy.[1252,1254] In a randomized trial of normal-height children with JIA treated with high-dose GH therapy (0.46 mg/kg per week) starting within 12 to 15 months after initiation of glucocorticoid therapy, the 3-year follow-up showed that the heights of GH-treated children remained normal (−1.1 SDS at baseline and −0.3 SDS after 3 years) while linear growth of the control patients declined from −1.0 SDS to −2.1 SDS.[1255] In the randomized, controlled trials published to date, patients were followed for up to 7 years, and no substantial differences were found in disease activity variables, including worsening of preexisting bone deformities, between GH-treated and control patients.[1167,1250-1252]

In a longitudinal study of patients treated for a mean of greater than 5 years, GH increased and normalized final height and improved bone and muscle mass.[1256] Because chronic inflammation, glucocorticoid treatment, and GH therapy are all associated with decreased sensitivity to insulin, children with JIA are at risk for impaired glucose homeostasis.[303,1253,1257] Therefore, monitoring of glucose tolerance using blood glucose, fasting insulin, and HbA$_{1c}$ assays at 6- to 12-month intervals is recommended. More intensive monitoring with oral glucose tolerance tests at baseline and then once yearly during treatment may be indicated.

Turner Syndrome. Patients with TS have a final height averaging 143 cm in the United States,[11,824] about 20 cm lower than the mean final height of normal women.[822] The goals of growth-promoting therapies are to attain a normal height for age as early as possible, to progress through puberty at a normal age, and to attain a normal adult height.

Before the availability of recombinant GH, there were conflicting data concerning its efficacy in this disorder, but

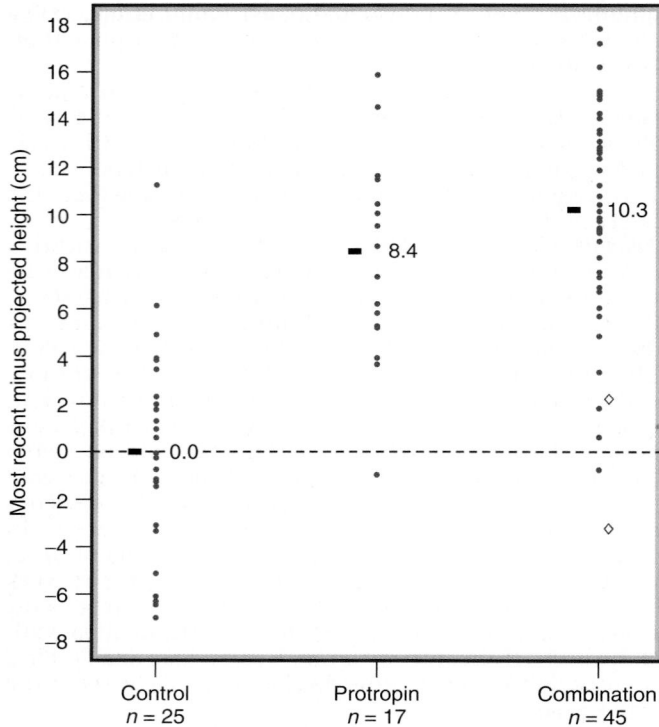

Figure 24-52 Adult heights of patients with Turner syndrome treated with growth hormone (GH) or with a combination of GH plus oxandrolone and of historical control subjects, relative to each subject's projected adult height (indicated by the *dotted zero line*). The mean increments in relative adult height are indicated. The diamond symbols in the combination group indicate two subjects with poor compliance who terminated treatment early. (From Rosenfeld RG, Attie KM, Frane J, et al. Growth hormone therapy of Turner syndrome: beneficial effect on adult height. *J Pediatr.* 1998;132:319-324.)

the ability of GH to accelerate growth has now been demonstrated in multiple reports. Growth responses are not affected by the karyotype. In 1983, a randomized, controlled North American study of treatment with GH (at a dose of 0.375 mg/kg per week) with or without added oxandrolone was initiated, with a mean age at onset of treatment of approximately 9 years.[1258] Analysis of all 62 girls enrolled in the study at near-final height showed a mean stature of 152.1 cm in the group treated with GH plus oxandrolone (a gain of 10.3 cm compared with the height predictions derived from Lyon and colleagues),[11] whereas girls receiving GH alone averaged 150.4 cm (a gain of 8.4 cm) (Fig. 24-52).[824] In another arm of this study, addition of estrogen to the GH regimen before age 15 years lowered the final height gain from 8.4 cm to 5.1 cm.[1259] In a reassessment of North American data in the NCGS, early initiation of GH treatment was shown to allow estrogen administration at a physiologic age without loss of adult height.[1260,1261]

Several other studies[834,1262] using higher doses of GH showed even greater gains in adult height outcomes. In a multicenter trial, Sas and coworkers used a maximum GH dose of approximately 0.63 mg/kg per week for 4.8 estrogen-free GH treatment years beginning at a mean age of 8.1 years, resulting in a gain of 16 cm over the modified Lyon and colleagues' projection.[11,834] In the same study, the group receiving a GH dose similar to that in the American studies achieved a height gain of 12.5 cm by age 16 with 4.8 estrogen-free GH treatment years starting at 7.9 years. In these girls, induction of puberty at a normal (not delayed) age was associated with these excellent height

outcomes.[1263] Carel and colleagues,[1262] using 0.7 mg/kg per week in a group that received 5.1 estrogen-free GH treatment years beginning at 10.2 years, gained 10.6 cm over the projections of Lyon and colleagues.[11] The group receiving a conventional dose (0.3 mg/kg per week) gained only 5.2 cm with 3.0 estrogen-free GH treatment years starting at 11 years. Because girls with TS usually have a normal GH secretory pattern, provocative GH testing should be performed only in those whose growth is clearly abnormal relative to that expected for patients with TS, as determined by plotting lengths and heights on TS-specific growth curves.[11,827,831,1264]

Although it was well established that GH therapy was effective in increasing final adult height, the magnitude of the gain in height varied in the earlier studies, depending on study design and treatment parameters. In 2005, in the first randomized, controlled trial to follow GH-treated subjects with TS to final height, the Canadian Growth Hormone Advisory Committee corroborated the increases in adult stature reported by studies with historical control subjects.[824,1263,1265,1266] In the Canadian study, girls with TS (age 7 to 13 years) who were randomized to receive GH (0.3 mg/kg per week; maximum weekly dose, 15 mg) achieved a final adult stature 7.2 cm taller than that seen in the control group after an average of 5.7 years. Factors predictive of taller adult stature include a relatively tall height at initiation of therapy, tall parental heights, young age at initiation of therapy, a long duration of therapy, and a high GH dose.[834,1261,1267,1268]

Although the optimal age for initiation of GH treatment has not been established, preliminary data from the Toddler Turner Study, in which 88 girls between the ages of 9 months and 4 years were randomized to receive GH or no GH therapy, showed that GH therapy is effective beginning as early as 9 months, with a safety profile similar to that in older children with TS.[1269] Treatment with GH should be considered as soon as growth failure is evident. GH therapy in the United States is typically initiated at the FDA-approved dose of 0.375 mg/kg per week. The dose can be changed in response to the patient's growth response and IGF-1 levels. Growth prediction models may be helpful in determining the potential effects of changes in dosing.[1267]

Studies have shown that higher doses produce a relatively small gain in final height, although there is no apparent increase in short-term adverse events.[1270] In a study by the Dutch Working Group, the mean gain in final height with 4 IU/m² per day (0.045 mg/kg per day), 6 IU/m² per day, and 8 IU/m² per day averaged 11.9 ± 3.6, 15.7 ± 3.5, and 16.9 ± 5.2 cm, respectively.[1263] However, when GH was given at the higher doses, IGF-1 levels were often above the normal range, which theoretically could lead to long-term adverse effects.[1271]

In girls naïve to GH who are older than 9 years of age and in those with extreme short stature, consideration can be given to using higher doses of GH and adding a nonaromatizable anabolic steroid, such as oxandrolone.[824] The maximum suggested dose of oxandrolone is 0.05 mg/kg per day, because higher doses have been associated with virilization and accelerated skeletal maturation. Liver enzymes should be monitored. Therapy may be continued until a satisfactory height has been attained (bone age >14 years) or until the yearly growth velocity falls to less than 2 cm/year. The children should be monitored at 3- to 6-month intervals.[1272]

The substantial variations in GH-induced growth increments in these studies were presumably related to GH dose, duration of estrogen-free GH treatment years, and age at initiation of GH and estrogen administration, as well as the population and parental adult heights. Additionally, the

GHRd3 polymorphism has been reported to be associated with increased responsivity to GH in girls with TS.[1273] Transdermal or depot estrogen administration, as opposed to oral estrogen, may also contribute positively to growth outcomes.[1274,1275] In these higher-dose treatment studies, hyperinsulinism with presumed insulin resistance was evident but reversible.[1262,1276] Other data suggest that impaired insulin secretion may ultimately be the significant issue in patients with TS,[1277,1278] although long-term GH therapy has been well tolerated.

None of these studies was placebo-controlled to adult height, and some studies have yielded much poorer height outcomes,[835] so some uncertainty existed until the randomized, controlled, multicentered Canadian study, in which the mean height gain ascribed to GH treatment was 7.3 cm at 1 year after cessation of the treatment protocol. Estrogen was initiated at 13 years of age.[1265] Another temporally matched control study from Italy showed a gain of 8.1 cm.[1266] These studies corroborated and supported the information that had accumulated from historical data on natural growth in TS juxtaposed to the available GH treatment results. Such data, in aggregate, provides convincing support that GH can both accelerate growth velocity and increase adult height.

Recommendations include seeking the diagnosis vigorously at any age in every girl with otherwise unexplained short stature and initiating therapy at that young age (i.e., at diagnosis or in early childhood). One must bear in mind that growth velocity in girls with untreated TS can be slowed as early as the 1- to 3-year-old period.[828,830] Treatment with the FDA-approved GH dosage of 0.375 mg/kg per week should be initiated and compliance should be monitored with auxologic and IGF-1 measurements; continued normal thyroid status should be assured. Oxandrolone may be added to the regimen in the late-diagnosed girl. Estrogen therapy should be initiated at an appropriate physiologic age in girls who started GH therapy at a young age, but it should be delayed as long as clinically reasonable in those whose GH therapy was initiated at a late age. Often, growth-promoting and pubertal needs must be balanced, and the therapeutic approach should be individualized. The diminished areal bone density in TS is enhanced by GH, but estrogen therapy is needed to normalize volumetric density (i.e., not simply size).[1279] Absence of an adverse impact of GH on aortic diameters is reassuring, given the predisposition of such patients for dissecting aneurysms.[474] Use of statistical prediction models for long-term growth in TS may permit a more quantitative assessment of individual therapeutic efficacy.[1267]

Despite evidence for aggressive GH treatment of girls with TS to achieve adequate adult heights and relatively high quality-of-life assessments in adulthood,[1280,1281] health-related issues continue to imperil outcomes. Carel and colleagues[1282] reviewed health outcomes of 568 adult French women (in their mid-20s) with GH-treated TS who had a mean height of 150.9 cm (having gained about 9 cm over prediction) and found that neither height nor height gain was associated with quality-of-life scores. Rather, issues regarding cardiologic and otologic health concerns and delay of pubertal initiation beyond 15 years were of greater concern. In contrast, a long-term follow-up assessment of 49 women from the Netherlands who had reached a mean adult height of 160.7 cm (a gain of >15 cm), suggested that the high quality-of-life scores were related to height gain and adequate estrogenization.

The NCGS recently published data on the efficacy and safety of GH therapy in 5220 children with TS treated during the past 20 years. A total of 442 adverse events were reported for these patients, including 117 that were considered to be serious. Seven deaths occurred, including five from aortic dissection or rupture. The incidences of intracranial hypertension, slipped capital femoral epiphysis, scoliosis, and pancreatitis were increased compared with other patients in the registry who did not have TS. Ten new-onset malignancies occurred, including six in patients without known risk factors. The number of patients who developed IDDM also appeared to be increased. It is believed that these adverse events are likely to be unrelated to treatment with GH. The incidence of aortic dissection or rupture reflects the higher baseline risk in TS.[1283]

Two echocardiography studies reported normal left ventricular morphology and function in girls with GH-treated TS[1284,1285] and two MRI studies found no deleterious effect of GH treatment on aortic diameter.[474,1272,1286,1287] Because GH treatment can alter craniofacial proportions, all girls with TS treated with GH should receive periodic orthodontic follow-up.[1288] These studies were not controlled, but their findings emphasize the broad range of health concerns in women with TS and affirm the need for multidisciplinary follow-up care.

Small for Gestational Age. Studies employing GH in short children born SGA have been hampered by the heterogeneity of this group of patients, whose poor growth may reflect maternal factors, chromosomal disorders, dysmorphic syndromes (e.g., RSS, Dubowitz syndrome), toxins, and idiopathic factors.[1289] A 2001 consensus statement recommended that SGA be defined as a birth weight or length at least 2 SD below the mean.[1290] Almost 90% of infants born SGA undergo catch-up growth within the first 2 years of life, and those who do not would then be eligible for GH treatment.[36,37,852,887,1289,1291,1292] Based on these proportions, and because the prevalence of "short SGA" is 2 to 3 per 1000 children, between 1 in 300 and 1 in 500 children are eligible for GH treatment, as approved in the United States in 2001 and in Europe in 2003. It appears that GH mediates the postnatal catch-up growth.[1293] Children born SGA appear to grow at a low-normal growth velocity during childhood,[1294] but puberty tends to occur at a somewhat earlier age and to progress rapidly, resulting in decreased pubertal height gain and an adult height about 1 SD (approximately 7 cm) below the mean[37,885,887,1295-1298] and about 4 cm below the midparental target height.[852]

The impaired postnatal growth observed in children born SGA is probably due to many factors, including generalized cellular hypoplasia,[1299] altered diurnal GH secretion patterns,[167,873,875,1294,1300] and, potentially, abnormalities in the GH-IGF axis resulting from GH sensitivity as determined by the presence or absence of exon 3 of the GHR.[1301-1303] Deletions and mutations of the *IGF1* gene have been reported in patients with profound IUGR, microcephaly, deafness, and postnatal growth failure.[216,217,1304] SGA patients have also been reported to have *IGF1* gene polymorphisms or missense mutations resulting in low serum IGF-1 concentrations.[863,864,887,1303,1305,1306] Reduced levels of IGF-2 expression, associated with hypomethylation of the telomeric domain of chromosome 11p15 were found in a cohort of SGA patients who had RSS.[891] Mutations in the type I IGF receptor gene (one compound heterozygous, one nonsense) were found in two patients with IUGR and poor postnatal growth (one with elevated IGF-1).[223]

The low levels of IGF-1 and IGFBP3 in many infants with IUGR, apparently related to fetal malnutrition, do not seem to predict the degree of subsequent growth impairment,[872] although continuing low levels are associated with poor catch-up growth.[1307] Short children born SGA make up a substantial portion of growth-retarded patients seen in pediatric endocrine practices.[852,887,1308] Because these children may have heights in the range seen in IGF deficiency syndrome, therapeutic attempts are appropriate, assuming that the insulin resistance noted in these thin, small children[880] does not become a clinical issue. Encouraging growth responses have been obtained with GH treatment.

The FDA approval of GH for the long-term treatment of growth failure in children born SGA who fail to manifest catch-up growth by age 2 was based on data obtained from four randomized, controlled, open-label, clinical trials that enrolled 209 patients between the ages of 2 and 8 years. Height velocity was determined after 1 year without treatment, and then patients were randomized to receive either GH treatment (34 or 69 mg/kg per day [0.24 or 0.48 mg/kg per week]) or no treatment for 2 years, after which a crossover design occurred. Children who received the higher GH dose had an increase of about 0.5 SDS in height after 2 years, compared with the children who received the lower dose, although both treated groups had significant increases in height velocity compared with untreated children (prescribing information for Genotropin somatropin of recombinant DNA origin for injection, Pfizer, Inc., New York, 2006). In Europe, the criteria for treatment differ from those in the United States: height SDS below −2.5, height velocity SDS below 0 during the previous year, and age greater than 4 years.

The data documenting efficacy in regard to adult height continues to be limited despite European regulatory authorities' requiring this evidence before approval. A meta-analysis of final height data for 56 children born SGA was performed at the request of European authorities and demonstrated a mean height increase of 1.9 SDS for subjects treated with GH at 34 mg/kg per day versus 2.2 SDS for 69 mg/kg per day. A meta-analysis of three randomized studies of 28 patients reported that GH treatment for 7 to 10 years, initiated at doses of 34 to 69 mg/kg per day, can be expected to increase adult height by about 1.0 to 1.4 SDS.[1309] A larger, randomized, controlled study of 91 GH-treated and 33 untreated French adolescents (mean age, 12 years) reported a lower intergroup difference of 0.6 SDS in adult height after 2.7 years of treatment.[1310]

The many studies documenting efficacy of GH therapy in thousands of children with SGA are far too numerous to report in detail here and have been reviewed elsewhere.[1309,1311,1312] Although results vary, it appears that GH treatment can be expected to result in a 1-cm increment in height gain each year. The factors that can increase the gain in height include a greater height deficit relative to the midparental height, a higher GH dose, initiation of therapy at an earlier age, longer treatment duration, and the proposed presence of the *GHRd3* allele.[1273,1290,1311,1313] In a prediction model derived from KIGS SGA data, Ranke and coworkers[1313] found that age and GH dose were strong predictors of initial growth but that growth achieved during the first year was a powerful predictor of later growth.

Children born SGA, especially those who have rapid postnatal weight gain, have reduced insulin-mediated glucose uptake and are more likely to have insulin resistance.[880,1314-1319] However, there have been no solid data documenting an increased risk of non-IDDM.[1318] There have been reports of several children in GH registration studies who had mild, transient hyperglycemia (prescribing information for Genotropin somatropin of recombinant DNA origin for injection, Pfizer, Inc., New York, 2006). Insulin resistance during GH treatment in children born SGA has been reported[1270,1320,1321] and typically resolves after discontinuation of GH.[1322] In a large database of children treated with GH, no differences in glucose regulation were found in 1900 children born SGA compared with

children with ISS.[1323] With 6000 patient-years of exposure, no cases of diabetes mellitus have been reported during GH treatment.[1323-1326]

The European product labeling for GH treatment of children born SGA reads, "The management of these patients should follow accepted clinical practice and include safety monitoring of fasting insulin and blood glucose before treatment and annually during treatment."[1312] In addition to insulin resistance alone, children born SGA have an increased risk of metabolic syndrome.[1325,1327-1329] The current literature provides no information on whether GH treatment in childhood increases risks for adult metabolic disease. Long-term follow-up studies are needed to determine the metabolic risk associated with GH treatment.

Osteochondrodysplasias. GH therapy has been studied in several skeletal dysplasias. The largest published study in achondroplasia involved 40 children; during the first year of treatment, the height velocity increased from 3.8 to 6.6 cm/year, and in the second year it decreased to approximately 5 cm/year.[1330] A modest improvement was seen in the ratio of lower limb length to height. Although GH was well tolerated, atlantoaxial dislocation during GH therapy was reported in one patient. In another study, normal growth velocity was achieved for up to 6 years in 35 subjects, with a significant increment in height SDS for at least 4 years[1330,1331]; in that study, vertebral growth was disproportionately greater than limb growth.

Bridges and Brook[1332] reported on the effects of GH therapy in 27 patients with hypochondroplasia; response was maximal during the first year of treatment, but substantial benefit was seen through 4 years of treatment in pubertal subjects.

Experience with GH treatment is limited in other skeletal disorders, such as dyschondrosteosis, hereditary multiple exostoses, osteogenesis imperfecta, and Ellis–van Creveld syndrome.

SHOX Haploinsufficiency and Léri-Weill Syndrome. Patients with mutations or deletions of the *SHOX* gene have variable degrees of short stature with or without mesomelic skeletal dysplasia. If untreated, short patients with SHOX deficiency remain short in adulthood. The *SHOX* gene is located in the pseudoautosomal region 1 (PAR1) on the distal end of the X and Y chromosomes at Xp22.3 and Yp11.3.[1333] Because genes in PAR1 do not undergo X inactivation, normal individuals express two copies of the *SHOX* gene. This gene encodes a homeodomain transcription factor that is expressed during early fetal life in the growth plate and functions in the regulation of chondrocyte differentiation and proliferation.[814,1334] SHOX haploinsufficiency (or deficiency) is the primary cause of short stature in patients with LWD (see earlier discussion).[848,1335] *SHOX* mutations and deletions are also found in patients with short stature without clinical evidence of dyschondrosteosis.[1336]

Clinical manifestations of SHOX deficiency include bowing of the forearms and lower legs, cubitus valgus, Madelung deformity or partial dislocation of the ulna at the wrist and elbow, short fourth and fifth metacarpals, and a high-arched palate along with characteristic radiologic signs.[813,848,1335] In a randomized 2-year study of 52 prepubertal subjects with a *SHOX* gene defect, the first-year height velocity in the GH-treated group was significantly greater than in the untreated control group (mean ± standard error of the mean [SE], 8.7 ± 0.3 versus 5.2 ± 0.2 cm/year; $p < 0.001$) and was similar to the first-year height velocity to GH-treated subjects with TS (8.9 ± 0.4 cm/year; $p < 0.592$). GH-treated subjects with SHOX deficiency also had significantly greater second-year height velocity (7.3 ±

0.2 versus 5.4 ± 0.2 cm/year; $p < 0.001$), second-year height SDS (−2.1 ± 0.2 versus −3.0 ± 0.2; $p < 0.001$), and second-year height gain (16.4 ± 0.4 versus 10.5 ± 0.4 cm; $p < 0.001$) compared with untreated subjects.[1337] Data on 28 persons with SHOX deficiency who received GH for a mean of 4.5 years through to adult height indicate that adjusted final height was −2.1 SDS, similar to girls with TS enrolled in the study. Calculated height SDS gain was 1.3, again similar to girls with TS.[1338]

Turner Syndrome and Langer Mesomelic Dysplasia. Homozygous mutation of the *SHOX* gene results in the Langer type of mesomelic dwarfism (i.e., LMD). A child with LMD and TS was found to have a *SHOX* gene abnormality resulting from a downstream allele deletion in her normal X chromosome. Although there have been numerous studies documenting growth improvement with GH therapy in patients with TS[824,1262,1283] and in those with heterozygous *SHOX* gene deletions,[1335] only one case of growth response to GH therapy in the rare condition of LMD with TS has been found. Growth rates of 3.46, 3.87, 2.3, and 0.7 cm/year were observed in the first, second, third, and fourth years of GH therapy, respectively, and there was no clinical deterioration of the skeletal deformities in this patient. Because there was a failure to achieve growth improvement with GH therapy, the authors concluded that GH therapy was not beneficial in patients with the severe short stature caused by combined TS and LMD resulting from homozygous *SHOX* deficiency.[1339]

Noonan Syndrome. Since 1994, when a gene for Noonan syndrome was mapped to chromosome 12 (12q24.1) and a mutation in the protein tyrosine phosphatase nonreceptor type 11 *(PTPN11)* was identified and characterized in familial cases, at least three other gene mutations have been identified.[839,840,1340-1343] While contributing to the broad heterogeneity of NS, these mutations have not completely localized the cause of the short stature. However, several genotype-phenotype correlations are relevant to patient management. Patients with *PTPN11* mutations often have normal or elevated GH levels and low serum IGF-1 concentrations.[845] The *PTPN11* genetically modified mouse model had a GH-stimulated increase in ERK activation, and growth was stimulated by inhibition of ERK1/2.[1344] Several studies have reported effects of GH on near-adult height in patients with Noonan syndrome,[1345-1349] but all involved small numbers of patients with varied enrollment ages, treatment durations, GH doses, and responses. The largest study of the response to GH in children with Noonan syndrome came from the NCGS, a postmarketing observational study of recombinant human GH treatment in children with various disorders. A total of 370 patients with Noonan syndrome (mean enrollment age, 11.6 years) received GH (mean dosage, 0.33 mg/kg per week) for a mean of 5.6 years. In the 65 patients with data to derive near-adult height, the mean gain above the projected height was 10.9 ± 4.9 cm in boys and 9.2 ± 4.0 cm in girls. Duration of prepubertal recombinant human GH therapy and height SDS at puberty were important contributors to the near-adult height. No new adverse events were observed. The authors suggested that greater growth optimization would be possible with earlier initiation of therapy.[1350] This height increase was similar to the change observed in patients with TS but significantly less in those with idiopathic GHD in the same study.

Most experience with GH treatment of short stature in Noonan syndrome has been limited to small, uncontrolled studies in which few patients reached final height.[837,1351,1352] The clinical diagnosis of a dysmorphic syndrome potentially makes the treatment groups heterogeneous, although identification of a mutant *PTNN11* gene[1353] helps with characterization. Overall, treatment results for 3 to 4 years are similar to those attained in patients with TS; mean growth velocities improve by 2 to 4 cm/year (over baseline rates of approximately 4 cm/year) during the first 4 years of therapy, with patients gaining from about −3.5 to −1.7 SDS of stature without inordinate advancement of bone age.[836,837,846,1352] Those children with identifiable *PTPN11* mutations are reported to have a poorer response to GH treatment in terms of growth and IGF production, suggesting impaired efficiency of phosphorylation-dependent GH signaling pathways.[844-846] Although the initial anecdotal experience suggested progression of ventricular hypertrophic cardiomyopathy, this was not confirmed in larger, carefully monitored studies.[837,1354,1355] However, it has been suggested that children with Noonan syndrome receiving GH be monitored for hypertrophic cardiomyopathy and hematologic abnormalities.[838]

Idiopathic Short Stature (Subtle Errors Throughout the Growth Axis). Although children with ISS, by definition, are without an identifiable cause of growth retardation, the term clearly encompasses a heterogeneous group that may include children with constitutional growth delay, genetic short stature, or subtle defects of the GH-IGF axis. Even though they are often grouped in one category, children with ISS have been shown to have a broad range of provocative GH responses, ranging from normal to elevated, and a wide range of serum IGF concentrations, from normal to IGF deficient. This group may also include children with unidentified syndromes or unidentified chronic illnesses or endocrine disorders. Children with ISS may experience stressful behavioral circumstances, but studies suggest that the relationship of psychosocial problems to the short stature is variable.[1356-1358] Nonetheless, hormonal intervention to enhance growth, with the aim of diminishing such difficulties, has been used.

Although the specific etiologies are often unknown, GH treatment has been used widely. Important questions have been raised about the financial, ethical, and psychosocial impact of GH therapy in "normal" short children.[1354,1359,1360] Given the cost of GH, the financial implications of treating such children are considerable. The point is well taken that 5% of the population will always be below the 5th percentile, whether we treat with GH or not, and that focusing on short stature could potentially handicap an otherwise normal child psychologically and socially. No convincing data have been presented to show that GH treatment of short children definitively improves psychological, social, or educational function.[1360-1362] A possible exception is the improved intellectual function in SGA children treated with GH.[1363] Furthermore, final adult height in the subset of children with CDGD (probably a common inclusion, although not ISS as defined in the FDA approval) may be adequate without any treatment.[40-42]

Finally, the known and unknown treatment risks of GH therapy in otherwise apparently normal children, even if exceedingly small, are a legitimate concern.[1364] The failure to report levels of IGF-1, IGFBP3, and GHBP in many studies and differing interpretations of endogenous GH secretion studies (e.g., assay variance, control group size), as well as the heterogeneity of the patient groups, confounds assessment of response data. Nevertheless, it is clear that many children who do not meet conventional criteria for the diagnosis of GHD and who fall under the heading of ISS have as great a degree of growth retardation as children with bona fide GHD and might be considered suitable candidates for growth-promoting therapy.

Members of the Growth Hormone Research Society, the Lawson Wilkins Pediatric Endocrine Society, and the European Society for Pediatric Endocrinology meeting in 2007 published a manuscript detailing their agreement on the evidence-based evaluation and management of ISS in children. They agreed that the primary goal of therapy should be the attainment of normal adult height. They also agreed that the expectation from patients and their families that taller stature is associated with positive changes in quality of life should be discouraged.[1359] Physicians should inform families about the available therapeutic options and provide a realistic expectation for height gain with therapy, including the fact that there may be variability in the outcome, and the psychological counseling options should be discussed. In addition, the patient and family should be aware that therapy may be discontinued if the growth response is poor or if the child no longer provides assent. The physician is responsible for continued monitoring of efficacy and safety and should provide flexibility in treatment options.

The studies that ultimately led to approval of GH treatment in the United States included the long-term, randomized, double-blind, placebo-controlled trial at the National Institutes of Health by Leschek and associates[1070] and the randomized dosing trial of the European Idiopathic Short Stature Study Group.[1365] In the former trial, which used a less optimal regimen of 0.22 mg/kg per week given thrice weekly in subjects with a mean starting height of almost −3 SDS, the treated children had mean final height gain of 3.7 cm over the control group.[1070] In the latter randomized study, GH doses of 0.24 and 0.37 mg/kg per week, given as a regimen of six doses per week in children with a mean starting height of −3.0 to −3.4 SDS, the improvement in the higher-dose group exceeded that in the lower-dose group by 3.6 cm, with subjects achieving a final height of −1.12 SDS.[1365] When the data from the two trials were combined, there was a cumulative gain of 7.3 cm in the group treated with 0.37 mg/kg per week, compared with placebo.

In a meta-analysis looking at an aggregate group of 1089 children, there were four controlled trials that presented adult height data showing treatment benefits ranging from 0.54 to 0.84 SDS, corresponding to a mean effect on growth of 5 to 6 cm.[1366]

Concerns had been raised that GH treatment might accelerate pubertal onset and progression in children with ISS, resulting in failure to improve height SDS for bone age and offsetting the positive responses observed during the early years of GH treatment. In the European ISS study,[1367] there was no evidence of accelerated pubertal or skeletal maturation in the group receiving the higher dose, in contrast to data reported by Kamp and colleagues[1368] with a 30% greater GH dose. This hypothetical effect of advancing maturation has not been substantiated by additional studies.[1369-1372] Taken together, these data show that GH treatment of prepubertal children with ISS increases growth velocity and final height.

The auxologic criteria for GH therapy in the United States are based on FDA approval of GH treatment for children shorter than −2.25 SDS (1.2 percentile). Some believe that children should be treated if their height is below −2.0 SDS and more than 2.0 SDS below their midparental target height or if their predicted height is below −2.0 SDS (or both). Although there is no consensus on the age for initiating treatment, most studies of GH therapy in children with ISS have involved children from 5 years to early puberty. There are no accepted biochemical criteria for initiating GH treatment in ISS. The bone age is used to predict adult height, although in a longitudinal study of ISS subjects, bone age delay had an effect on the precision of the prediction. In children with a bone age delay of about 2 years, the average adult height was almost equal to the predicted height; in children with no bone age delay, the adult height was greater than the initial predicted height; and if the bone age was delayed by more than 2 years, the adult height was significantly below the predicted adult height.[1373] The psychological benefits of GH therapy in children with ISS are unproved,[1374] but medical and psychological interventions should be considered for the child who seems to suffer from his or her short stature.

The clinical trials of the treatment of ISS with GH in the literature often did not contain long-term control groups; hence, the results show variable growth responses.[1364,1375] Most short children treated with GH experience growth acceleration that is usually sustained over the first several years of therapy, with attenuation of the treatment response over time. In general, a slower pretreatment growth velocity and a higher weight-to-height ratio—factors suggestive of GHD and, to a lesser degree, bone age retardation—are associated with better early growth responses. Three thousand children were classified as having ISS in the KIGS database, with 153 having reached final height.[1370] GH treatment (0.2 to 0.25 mg/kg per week) resulted in achievement of target height in patients with familial short stature, although they continued to have short stature as adults (−1.7 SDS in males and −2.2 SDS in females), with a mean gain during therapy of 0.6 to 0.9 SDS. In children who did not have familial short stature, the mean final height was greater for males (−1.4 SDS), although not for females (−2.3 SDS), with average gains of 1.3 and 0.9 SDS, respectively. These attained heights were quite different from the midparental target heights, which were near 0 SDS. Hintz and colleagues[1069] assessed adult height in 80 North American children with ISS who were treated for up to 10 years at a GH dose of 0.3 mg/kg per week. At the conclusion of the study, the mean height SDS was −1.4 SDS with a gain of 1.3 SDS, results quite similar to those from the KIGS database. Although the Hintz study was not placebo controlled, the data were compared with predicted and actual final heights in two groups of untreated short children followed for similar periods. Compared to untreated children, treated boys achieved a mean of 9.2 cm and girls 5.7 cm stature above predicted heights.

Several additional studies have documented the increase in final height with GH therapy in children with ISS, although the responses have been highly variable and dose dependent. The mean increase in adult height in children with ISS is 3.5 to 7.5 cm (with an average duration of therapy of 4 to 7 years) when compared with historical control subjects,[1069,1376] with patients' pretreatment predicted adult heights, or with nontreatment or placebo control groups.[1070,1366] Multiple factors affect the growth response to GH, and the best response is seen in children who are younger or heavier, those receiving higher GH doses, and those who are shortest relative to their target height. Adult height outcome is influenced negatively by age at initiation of therapy and positively by midparental height, initial height, delayed bone age, and the magnitude of the first-year response to GH.[809,1373] A 2-year study suggested that an increase in IGF-1 correlates with height gain.[1070] Recently, a review of the literature on ISS was published, concluding that GH therapy increases height in some children; however, the cost-benefit ratio and long-term safety are concerning.[1377]

Studies using monotherapy with GnRH agonists have shown only a small and variable effect on final adult height, so GnRH agonist therapy is not recommended. Furthermore, GnRH agonists have been shown to have short-term adverse effects on BMD.[1378] However, combination therapy with a GnRH agonist and GH has potential value in increasing final height, but only with treatment lasting at least 3 years.[1379,1380] However, in a randomized study, children treated with a combination of GnRH agonist and GH and control subjects had no difference in adult height.[1380]

Monitoring of GH treatment should include height, weight, pubertal development, and adverse effects (scoliosis, tonsillar hypertrophy, papilledema, and slipped capital femoral epiphysis) two to three times per year. After 1 year of therapy, the height velocity SDS and the change in height SDS should be calculated. The bone age may be obtained to reassess height prediction and if one is considering intervention to delay puberty. IGF-1 levels may be helpful in guiding GH dose adjustment. Because elevated blood glucose levels in patients with GH-treated ISS have not been reported, routine monitoring of glucose metabolism is not advised.

The FDA-approved dose for GH in ISS is 0.3 to 0.37 mg/kg per week.[1381] The dose may be increased if the growth response is inadequate and compliance was assured. However, there are no data regarding the long-term safety of GH doses higher than 0.5 mg/kg per week in children with ISS. IGF-1 levels may be helpful in assessing compliance and GH sensitivity. IGF-1 levels that are elevated (>2.5 SDS) should prompt consideration of GH dose reduction. IGF-based dose adjustments in children with ISS increased short-term growth when higher IGF targets were selected, but long-term studies with respect to efficacy, safety, and cost effectiveness have not been done.[1368] If the growth rate continues to be inadequate, GH treatment should be stopped and alternative therapies considered. The duration of treatment is controversial, with consideration given for stopping treatment when near-adult height is achieved (height velocity <2 cm/year or bone age >16 years in boys or >14 years in girls) if height is in the normal adult range (above −2 SDS). Stopping therapy may be influenced by satisfaction of the patient and family with the resulting height, an ongoing cost/benefit analysis, or desire of the child to stop for other reasons (e.g., dissatisfaction with daily injections).

The possible side effects in GH-treated children with ISS are similar to those previously reported in children receiving GH therapy for other indications, with no long-term adverse effects documented.[1382,1383] Post-treatment surveillance with a focus on cancer prevalence and metabolic side effects is advisable.

The average cost of GH treatment of children with ISS is $10,000 to $20,000 per centimeter of growth improvement.[1376] The benefits are less clear,[1376] because it is unknown whether a gain in height improves quality of life. Therefore, recommendations for treatment that increases adult height should be balanced against the high cost of these therapies.

Miscellaneous Causes of Growth Failure. In addition to the clinical conditions described earlier, GH has been employed in the treatment of short stature associated with a variety of other conditions involving postnatal growth failure. In general, such trials have been uncontrolled and have not included sufficient numbers of subjects for efficacy to be evaluated. Examination of such treatments should be continued in the large international databases.

Down Syndrome. The encouraging results of GH trials in TS led to studies of GH therapy in children with Down syndrome. In several preliminary studies, GH accelerated growth in such patients, although ethical issues were raised concerning the appropriateness of such therapy.[1384-1387] In the uncontrolled NCGS experience, 23 children experienced a 1.3-SDS height gain over the first 4 years of GH therapy.[1351] No convincing data exist that GH improves neurologic or intellectual function in such patients. The

increased risks of diabetes mellitus and leukemia in children with Down syndrome could be augmented by GH therapy.[1388] A review of GH therapy given to 15 children with Down syndrome reported an increase in mean height but no effect on mental development. They do not recommend GH therapy and call for further controlled studies.[817]

Normal Aging and Other Catabolic States. Detailed consideration of the potential use of GH in normal aging is beyond the scope of this chapter. The rationale for such therapy is based on the concept of the *somatopause,* a term that highlights the progressive decline in GH secretion after 30 years of age, as reflected in decreasing IGF-1 levels. Aging can be viewed as a catabolic state, with the potential that GH therapy might reverse or retard the loss of muscle mass and strength and the decrease in bone density that occur with aging. There is no evidence that GH supplementation during aging improves muscle strength or quality of life.[1389]

Growth failure, often with impaired final adult height, is a characteristic clinical finding in endogenous or exogenous Cushing syndrome. Excess glucocorticoids cause a catabolic state characterized by increased proteolysis, decreased protein synthesis, lowered osteoblastic and increased osteolytic activity, and insulin resistance.[1143] GH treatment blunts some of these catabolic actions but increases the insulin resistance.[1144] Mauras and Beaufrere[776] showed that IGF-1 therapy similarly induces an anabolic response, despite excess glucocorticoids, but does not cause insulin resistance. GH treatment after transplantation[1243-1245] and in other glucocorticoid-treated children[765] causes some height increments but does not produce as good a response as in individuals not taking glucocorticoids. GH does enhance bone formation and increases osteoblastic activity in such children.[1390] The marked increase in IGF-1 levels during GH treatment may be sufficient to overcome the local insensitivity to IGF action.[259,668,669,1391]

GH therapy is also being investigated in catabolic states such as burns, tumor cachexia, major abdominal surgery, AIDS, sepsis, metabolic acidosis, and situations requiring total parenteral alimentation. GH should not be used in critically ill patients, because a randomized, controlled trial demonstrated increased morbidity and mortality rates with GH treatment of such patients.[1392] The FDA-approved indications for the use of GH for purposes other than stimulation of growth are (1) GHD in adults, (2) AIDS-associated wasting or cachexia, and (3) short-bowel syndrome requiring total parenteral nutrition.

Adverse Effects of Growth Hormone

Pituitary-derived human GH had an enviable safety record for a quarter of a century but proved to be an agent for transmission of the fatal spongiform encephalopathy, CJD.[1085-1087] Although pit-GH was removed from use in the United States in 1985, and later throughout the world, more than 200 patients with GH-derived CJD have been identified.[1085-1087] Although recombinant DNA–derived GH does not carry this risk, the experience with pit-GH serves as a grim reminder of the potential toxicity that can reside in products used for physiologic replacement.

Extensive experience with recombinant GH over nearly 30 years has been encouraging.[987,1198,1393-1395] Concerns have been raised about a number of potential complications, which clearly require continued follow-up and assessment. This evaluation has been facilitated by the extensive databases that have been established by GH manufacturers, for example, Genentech (NCGS)[1198] and Pharmacia (KIGS).[1324,1396] An important limitation of these registries, however, is that although they have provided valuable information about the risks of disease during GH use, they were not designed to provide data on adverse effects after discontinuation of GH use.

Development of Leukemia and Other Malignancies. A report in 1998 of five cases of leukemia that developed in GH-treated Japanese children raised concern that GH therapy could increase the risk of leukemia.[1397] One difficulty in assessing the role of GH treatment in this disorder is that many GH-deficient children have conditions that predispose to the development of leukemia, such as prior malignancy, a history of irradiation, or concurrent syndromes that themselves are associated with the development of leukemia (e.g., Bloom syndrome, Down syndrome, Fanconi anemia). After the intial concerns about the role of GH treatment in the development of leukemia, long-term data have shown that GH treatment does not increase the incidence of leukemia in children who are not already at an increased risk of leukemia,[1198,1398-1400] does not increase the risk of leukemia as a subsequent neoplasm in cancer survivors,[1401] and does not increase the rate of leukemia relapse.[1324,1398,1402] Although it is not possible to determine if GH treatment increases the incidence of leukemia in children at increased risk for reasons other than prior malignancy, the incidence of leukemia in these at-risk children does not appear to be out of line with the expected rate.[1399] Nonetheless, care should be used in prescribing GH therapy for children with a past history of leukemia or lymphoma or other disorders conveying an increased risk of leukemia.

With respect to malignancies other than leukemia, data from more than 88,000 GH-treated patients with more than 275,000 patient-years at risk did not reveal an increased risk for nonleukemic extracranial neoplasms.[1198,1332,1394] However, an increased risk of posttransplant lymphoproliferative disease (odds ratio 1.88; 95% confidence interval [CI] 1.00-3.55, $p = 0.05$) was found in children treated with GH before transplant for growth failure related to their end-stage renal disease.[1403] And a statistically nonsignificant increase in malignancies was found in GH-treated girls with TS (standardized incidence ratio compared with the age-matched general population of 2.1; 95% CI, 0.76-4.49.)[1283]

Recurrence of Central Nervous System Tumors. Because many recipients of GH have acquired GHD due to CNS tumors or their treatment, the possibility of tumor recurrence with therapy is of obvious importance. Estimates of CNS tumor recurrence rates in non–GH-treated children and adolescents are difficult to obtain, bearing in mind the vast array of treatment programs used in the past 4 decades. In a total of 1083 patients compiled from 11 reports who were not treated with GH, 209 (19.3%) had recurrences.[1140,1402,1404-1412] Such data in a heterogeneous group, including patients with craniopharyngiomas, gliomas, ependymomas, medulloblastomas, and germ cell tumors, provide a background for assessing recurrence rates in GH-treated youth. Reports from nine centers, encompassing 390 patients, indicated recurrence in 64 patients (16.4%) at the time of publication,[821,1402,1404-1412-1417] which is not much different from the recurrence rate observed in a much larger number of untreated patients. In a particularly well-done comparative study at three pediatric neuro-oncology centers comprising 1071 brain tumor patients, 180 patients were treated with GH for a mean of 6.4 years, and 31 of them were monitored for more than 10 years; the relative risk of recurrence or death was similar with and without GH treatment.[1416] In a study of 361 cancer survivors (including 172 brain tumor patients), disease recurrence of all cancers in GH-treated children did not differ from recurrence in those children not treated with GH.[1401] A single center study of 110 previously irradiated brain tumor patients found no difference

in recurrence in GH-treated patients compared to matched control subjects after approximately 15 years of follow-up.[1418] Finally, extensive analysis of 4410 patients with a history of brain tumor or craniopharyngioma before GH therapy in the NCGS and KIGS databases[1324,1394,1419] showed a similar lack of increased tumor recurrence. In the NCGS series, recurrence rates of the most common CNS neoplasms, craniopharyngioma (6.4%), primary neuroectodermal tumors (medulloblastoma and ependymoma, 7.2%), and lowgrade glioma (18.1%) were lower than or similar to those reported in non–GH-treated children.[1141,1402,1420]

Development of Subsequent Neoplasms. Children who have survived cancer are at an increased risk of developing a second neoplasm because of either an underlying genetic predisposition or the consequences of the treatment for the primary malignancy, including radiation therapy and treatment with alkylating agents. Because of the mitogenic and antiapoptotic effects of GH and IGF-1, there is concern that GH treatment could increase the rate of subsequent neoplasms. This has been monitored through both the large NCGS and KIGS GH treatment databases, as well as through the Childhood Cancer Survivor Study (CCSS) group. The CCSS studies followed 361 GH-treated cancer survivors, and the initial report found an overall increased risk of 3.21 (95% CI, 1.88-5.46) for second neoplasms.[1401] Although the majority of these second neoplasms were meningiomas, there were 3 children who developed osteogenic sarcoma out of 122 leukemia/lymphoma survivors who had not been treated with GH. A similar increased risk for second neoplasms, also largely meningiomas, was found in a study of 60 GH-treated adult patients.[1421] And in 2500 GH-treated cancer survivors in the NCGS database, there was also an increased incidence in secondary malignances, predominantly CNS tumors (glioblastoma/glioma, astrocytoma, meningioma) and osteogenic sarcoma.[1198] However, the most recent follow-up of the CCSS found that the rate of meningioma in those children not treated with GH had risen over time to equal that of survivors treated with GH. Therefore, the CCSS data found that the rate of subsequent CNS neoplasms was not increased by GH treatment,[1422] with an adjusted rate of 1.0 for any CNS secondary neoplasm, 0.8 for meningiomas, and 1.9 (95% CI, 0.7-4.8; $p = 0.21$) for gliomas. The equalization of the rate ratio for meningiomas with longer follow-up raised the possibility that GH treatment may accelerate the manifestation of these tumors, rather than increase the absolute rate. Another possible explanation, however, is that the GH-treated patients had more intense surveillance because of their GH treatment and were therefore identified at an earlier stage.

Pseudotumor Cerebri. Pseudotumor cerebri (idiopathic intracranial hypertension) has been reported in GH-treated patients.[1198,1324,1394,1423] The disorder may develop within months after treatment starts or as long as 5 years into the course; it appears to be more frequent in patients with renal failure than in those with GHD.[1198,1394] The mechanism for the effect is unclear but may reflect changes in fluid dynamics within the CNS. Pseudotumor has also been described after thyroid hormone replacement in patients with hypothyroidism. In any case, clinicians should be alert to complaints of headache, nausea, dizziness, ataxia, or visual changes. Significant fluid retention with edema or hypertension is rare.[1424] Because of the possible association of pseudopapilledema with GHD, perhaps representing a variant of optic nerve hypoplasia,[1425] careful ophthalmologic evaluation should be undertaken in patients with suspected GH therapy–associated pseudotumor cerebri to avoid overdiagnosis and invasive treatments.

Slipped Capital Femoral Epiphysis. Slipped capital femoral epiphysis is associated with both hypothyroidism and GHD. Whether GH therapy plays a role in this disorder has been difficult to determine, in part because the incidence of slipped capital femoral epiphysis varies with age, gender, race, and geographic locale. The reported incidence is between 2 and 142 cases per 100,000 population; the data in the KIGS and NCGS studies are in this range.[1198,1324,1394] Accordingly, although slipped capital femoral epiphysis cannot be attributed to GH therapy per se, complaints of hip and knee pain or limp should be evaluated carefully. The occurrence of such pain in a GH-treated child with an exceedingly rapid growth rate should lead to consideration of this diagnosis.

Scoliosis. Both progression of preexisting scoliosis and new-onset scoliosis have been described in children treated with GH.[1198] The numbers are extremely small, with only 238 reported cases among 54,996 patients in the NCGS database. There is specific concern for GH effects on scoliosis in TS and PWS patients, in whom the underlying rate of scoliosis is increased. Although the rate of scoliosis in GH-treated TS patients was higher than in other GH-treated patients, it remained rare, being reported in only 0.69% of patients.[1283] PWS by itself has a rate of scoliosis of 30% to 80%, and GH treatment does not appear to increase the rate or severity of scoliosis in PWS patients.[1217,1426]

Diabetes Mellitus. The association of GH treatment with insulin resistance is well documented.[1427] In addition, candidates for GH therapy include some who are known to have increased risk of type 2 diabetes mellitus (T2DM) including patients with TS, PWS, or those born IUGR. Data from the NCGS database estimated the incidence of T2DM in GH-treated patients as approximately 14 cases per 100,000 patient-years,[1198,1324] and data from KIGS and from GeNeSIS (Genetic and Neuroendocrinology of Short Stature International Study; another large pharmaceutical company sponsored postmarketing surveillance database) found the incidence of T2DM in GH-treated children to be approximately 30 cases per 100,000 patient-years.[1428,1429] The incidence found in the KIGS and GeNeSIS studies was 6 to 6.5 times higher than the expected incidence.[1428,1429] Many of these children did have risk factors for T2DM, although not all of them were obese.[43,44,1394] In some, but not all, of the subjects who developed T2DM, there was resolution of the diabetes on discontinuation of GH treatment,[1398,1428,1429] likely highlighting both the underlying risk of diabetes in these individuals, as well as supporting a causative role of GH treatment in the development of diabetes. Therefore, the reduction of insulin sensitivity induced by GH is a concern that demands close assessment, particularly in high-risk patients such as those with PWS or TS or a history of IUGR.

Miscellaneous Side Effects.[1198,1324,1394] Other potential side effects of GH therapy include prepubertal gynecomastia,[1430] pancreatitis,[1431] growth of nevi[1432,1433] (although typically without evidence of malignant degeneration[1398]), behavioral changes, worsening of neurofibromatosis, hypertrophy of tonsils and adenoids, and sleep apnea. A report[1434] of reduced testicular volume and elevated gonadotropin levels in four young adult men previously treated with GH for ISS was not confirmed by a double-blind, placebo-controlled study,[1435] nor by the international databases.[1436] This list of side effects is only partial. It is best for the clinician to remember that GH and the peptide growth factors it regulates are potent mitogens with diverse metabolic and anabolic actions. All patients receiving GH treatment, even as replacement therapy, must be carefully monitored for side effects.

For the most part, the side effects of GH are minimal and rare. When they do occur, a careful history and physical examination are adequate to identify their presence. Management of these side effects may include transient reduction of dosage or temporary discontinuation of GH.[953] In the absence of other risk factors, there is no evidence that the risk of leukemia, brain tumor recurrence, or slipped capital femoral epiphysis is increased in recipients of long-term GH treatment. Any patient receiving GH who has a second major medical condition (e.g., being a tumor survivor) should be followed up in conjunction with an appropriate specialist such as an oncologist or neurosurgeon. Whereas GH has been shown to increase the mortality rate of critically ill patients in intensive care units,[1392] there is no evidence that GH replacement therapy needs to be discontinued during intercurrent illness in children with GHD.

The Question of Long-Term Cancer Risk. Several epidemiologic studies have suggested an association between high serum IGF-1 levels and an increased incidence of malignancies.[1437-1439] Such studies have found an association of higher IGF-1 levels with breast, prostate, and colon cancer.[1439-1441] In contrast, higher IGFBP3 levels have been associated with a decreased risk of prostate and breast cancer, although other studies found no association of IGFB3 levels and cancer[1439] or found a positive association.[1439,1441] Because GH increases production of both IGF-1 and IGFBP3, the studies that found the highest association with cancer with high IGF-1 and low IGFBP3 levels do not suggest a simple relationship between GH and cancer risk.

Epidemiologic studies assessing the risk of malignancy in patients with acromegaly found differing results, with some,[1441-1444] but not others,[1445,1446] identifying significant associations between acromegaly and colon cancer risk. The small size and uncontrolled retrospective nature of these studies and the multiple possible sources of bias make these reports difficult to interpret. The largest study to date, reviewing more than 1000 patients, indicated no overall increased cancer incidence in acromegaly.[1447] Although colon cancer risk was also not increased in that study, the mortality rate was higher, suggesting an effect of GH or IGF on established tumors.[1448] A prospective analysis of colon cancer and colonic polyps in acromegalics did not observe an association between these two diseases when using either autopsy series or prospective colonoscopy screening series for the control population.[1449] Acromegaly is associated with a marked increase in the incidence of benign hyperplasia in several organs, including colonic polyps.[1450] Such findings suggest that the GH/IGF-1 axis may lead to symptomatic benign proliferative disease, which could be associated with symptoms, such as rectal bleeding, that would lead to a potential detection (or ascertainment) bias.

Children receiving GH do not appear to have a greater risk of de novo or recurrent tumors.[987,1198,1324,1394] A cohort of 1848 patients treated with GH in the United Kingdom was assessed after as long as 40 years and found to have increased rates of colorectal cancer and Hodgkin disease, but the tumor-associated deaths were so few that a single patient death would markedly alter the risk ratios.[1451,1452] No increased incidence of cancer was found in GH recipients among adults who were treated for GHD.[1453,1454] Other long-term follow up studies of adults treated with GH during childhood also did not find an increase in cancer-related deaths,[1455,1456] although there was an increased mortality rate from bone tumors in the French study.[1455] These reports represent imperfect, uncontrolled studies, but the overall data do not indicate a clear association of GH therapy with the future development of neoplasms in the absence of other risk factors.

The use of IGF-1 and IGFBP3 in the monitoring of GH recipients, both adult and pediatric, has been recommended and endorsed by international bodies such as the Growth Hormone Research Society[952] and the Drug and Therapeutics Committees of the Lawson Wilkins Pediatric Endocrine Society and the European Society of Pediatric Endocrinology.[1451,1452] Until the issue of cancer risk in GH therapy is fully resolved, the prudent approach appears to be regular monitoring of both IGF-1 and IGFBP3 and alteration of the GH dose to ensure that the theoretical risk profile induced by GH therapy is favorable. This can be done by avoiding the unlikely situation of a GH-treated patient with an IGF-1 level at the upper end of the normal range and an IGFBP3 level at the lower end of the normal range.

Long-Term Mortality with GH Treatment. The effect of GH deficiency and GH treatment on overall mortality is complex. Subjects with untreated congenital GH deficiency from mutations in *PROP1* appear to have increased lifespan.[1439] In contrast, individuals with GH deficiency from *GH1* gene deletion have a decreased lifespan, with increased cardiovascular and infectious disease mortality rates,[1439] yet subjects with GH deficiency from *GHRH* mutations have no change in mortality rate compared with the local population.[1439] The background mortality rates of the gene deletion and *GHRH* mutation ethnic populations were quite different, which may account for some of the mortality discrepancy. Untreated Laron patients have been found to have a marked decrease in cancer mortality rate.[1439] Mortality data on GH-treated Laron patients are not available. Mortality risk is increased in adults with untreated GH deficiency (due to increased mortality rate from cardiovascular disease) but also in adults with GH excess (due to an increase in cardiovascular, cerebrovascular, and respiratory deaths).[1439] In 2012, investigators reported on the all-cause mortality rate of French children treated with GH for isolated GH deficiency. GH treatment in this cohort was begun between 1985 and 1996, with a mean age at follow-up of 28 years. They found an increase in all-cause mortality rate when compared to the French general population, with a standardized mortality ratio of 1.33 (95% CI 1.08-1.64).[1455] The diseases contributing to this increase in mortality rate were diseases of the circulatory system and subarachnoid or intracerebral hemorrhage. In response to this report investigators looked at all-cause mortality rate in GH-treated children in Sweden, Belgium, and the Netherlands.[1456] These patients started treatment between 1985 and 1997 and had a mean age of 27 to 29 years at follow-up. In this cohort, no subjects died from cancer or cardiovascular disease. Thus, the data do not give a clear answer to the long-term effects of GH treatment on longevity, including whether the impact would differ based on the indication for GH treatment.

IGF-1 Treatment

In 2005, the FDA approved the use of rhIGF-1 for "long term treatment of growth failure in children with severe primary IGF-1 deficiency and in children with GH gene deletions who have developed neutralizing antibodies to GH. Severe primary IGF-1 deficiency is defined by height SD score less than –3.0 and a basal IGF-1 SD score less than –3.0 and normal or elevated GH. Severe primary IGF-1 deficiency includes patients with mutations in the GHR, post-GHR receptor signaling pathway, and IGF-1 gene defects" (Increlex [rhIGF-1] prescribing information, 2009, Tercica, Inc.). Clinical trials to study the safety and efficacy of rhIGF-1 therapy have been conducted mostly in individuals with proven mutations in the *GHR*; fewer than 10%

of enrollees have had GH insensitivity due to GH antibodies. Because of the rarity of *GHR* mutations, the clinical trials have been small. When all clinical trials are combined, the total number of children treated to date is less than 200.

A number of short-term growth-related studies with subcutaneous IGF-1 treatment at varied doses have been reported. Despite slight differences in IGF-1 dosage and inclusion criteria, the short-term effects of IGF-1 on growth in GH insensitivity were consistent: growth increased from pretreatment rates of 3 to 5 cm/year to 8 to 11 cm/year on average. In five children with GHR deficiency, single daily doses of 150 μg/kg for 3 to 10 months resulted in growth acceleration to rates of 8.8 to 13.6 cm/year.[1457] Wilton[1142] reported collaborative data on the treatment of 30 patients, ages 3 to 23 years, with GH insensitivity due to GHR deficiency or IGHD type IA with anti-GH antibodies; the dose of IGF-1 varied from 40 to 120 μg/kg twice daily. With the exception of the two oldest individuals, growth rates increased in Wilton's subjects by at least 2 cm/year. A mean increment of more than 4 cm/year in growth velocity was found in 11 prepubertal children treated with 80 μg/kg twice daily.[1458] This study also demonstrated a significant inverse relationship between growth response to exogenous IGF-1 and the severity of the GH insensitivity phenotype.

Longer-term studies of IGF-1 treatment of GH insensitivity demonstrated a progressive waning effect of IGF-1 on growth velocity.[1459] Data from 17 patients in a European collaborative trial who were treated for at least 4 years showed an increase in mean height SDS from –6.5 to –4.9, with two adolescents reaching the 3rd percentile. Children who received rhIGF-1 for 2 years or less had a higher growth velocity than those children who received rhIGF-1 for longer periods. In the longest treatment study of 58 children with GH receptor mutations, GH antibodies, or biochemical evidence of GH insensitivity without documented mutation,[1460] outcomes were similar to those in the European study, with an initial burst of growth (from 3.1 to 8.0 cm/year) followed by slowing to just above baseline (4.8 cm/year) by the fourth year of therapy. Height SDS improved from –6.5 to –5.2 after 5 to 6 years of therapy. Data on 21 of these patients at or near adult height with average treatment duration of 10 years ranged from –8.0 to –6.2 SDS, lower for those persons with GH antibodies as the underlying cause for their GH resistance.[1461]

These limited data indicate that rhIGF-1 is effective in increasing statural growth, but the growth response is neither as robust nor as sustained as the growth response to GH among children with GHD. The suboptimal growth response to rhIGF-1 compared with recombinant human GH has been attributed to (1) inability of rhIGF-1 to increase IGFBP3 and ALS levels, leading to decreased delivery of IGF-1 to target tissues; (2) lack of GH-induced proliferation of prechondrocytes in the growth plate; (3) absence of GH-induced local IGF-1 at the growth plate; and (4) difficulty in using higher doses of IGF-1 because of the risk of hypoglycemia.

IGF-1 treatment has also been administered to individuals with *IGF1* gene deletion[566] and post-GHR signaling defects with growth patterns similar to those of children with GH insensitivity due to GHR deficiency. First-year results from an open-label trial of 124 children with low serum IGF-1 and height SDS < –2 without biochemical evidence of GH insensitivity indicate that growth velocity increased for the year of therapy (from 5 cm/year to 7 cm/year).[1145]

The most common adverse effect of rhIGF-1 is hypoglycemia. In some studies, it occurred in almost half of the patients with GH insensitivity treated with rhIGF-1,[1460] usually within the first month of therapy. Importantly, individuals with GHR defects, the highest proportion of enrollees in these treatment studies, have baseline hypoglycemia. In a 6-month, placebo-controlled trial, 67% of children receiving placebo experienced hypoglycemia, compared with 85% of children receiving rhIGF-1—a difference that was not statistically significant.[1168] In a study of 23 patients with GH insensitivity, hypoglycemia was noted before the start of treatment; after 3 months, 2.6% of glucose values in those receiving placebo were less than 50 mg/dL, compared with 5.5% of glucose values in those receiving rhIGF-1.[1460] The hypoglycemia was not to be avoidable with adequate food intake. In children with low IGF-1 but without GH insensitivity, 20% of subjects who received the higher IGF-1 dose experienced symptoms attributed to hypoglycemia; documentation of hypoglycemia was only noted in one subject.[1145]

Patients with GH insensitivity treated with rhIGF-1 have also experienced lymphoid tissue hypertrophy, encompassing tonsillar/adenoidal growth and associated snoring and sleep apnea, and thymic and splenic enlargement.[1460] The hypertrophy occurred in 22% of patients, with 10% of patients requiring tonsillectomy/adenoidectomy. Coarsening of the face was observed in patients of pubertal age.[1460] Studies have reported an increase in BMI with treatment and a twofold to threefold increase in body fat as assessed by dual-energy x-ray absorptiometry (DEXA).[1462] The study to adult height did not note this significant increase in body fat.[1461] Intracranial hypertension with associated papilledema has also been observed in as many as 5% of treated patients. In the study by Midyett and coworkers, two out of 100 patients receiving IGF-1 had documented intracranial hypertension.[1145] Anti–IGF-1 antibodies develop in about half of treated patients during the first year, but they have no effect on the response.[1460] As with recombinant human GH treatment, an increased cancer risk with rhIGF-1 treatment is an unknown but legitimate concern, considering the role of IGF-1 in neoplasias and the increased cancer risk associated with hypersomatotropism.[1463]

Approval by the FDA and the European Agency for the Evaluation of Medical Products of rhIGF-1 has ignited debate about expansion of the diagnosis of severe IGF-1 deficiency and consequent expanded use of rhIGF-1 beyond those patients with neutralizing GH antibodies or documented mutations in the *GHR*, GHR signaling pathways, or the IGF-1 gene. Some advocate that individuals with ISS, low serum IGF-1, or poor response to a GH trial may have unidentified subtle alterations in GHR signaling and could benefit from treatment with rhIGF-1.[1464] Others express reservations about expanding the diagnosis of IGF-1 deficiency and rhIGF-1 use, postulating that the response of children with ISS to rhIGF-1 may be minimal considering the lower long-term growth response of children with GHR defects treated with IGF-1 compared with GH-deficient children treated with GH. Another theoretical concern regards negative feedback of rhIGF-1 on GH secretion, which leads to diminished IGF-1–independent effects of GH on growth.[1465]

Other Treatments to Promote Growth

GnRH Agonists

Increasing Adult Height of Children with Idiopathic Short Stature. The effect of GnRH agonist therapy on adult height has been studied in girls with ISS and normal puberty (8 to 10 years of age); there was a mean gain of 0 to 4.2 cm, compared with predicted height.[1364,1466-1477] In boys with rapidly progressing puberty, GnRH agonist therapy increased adult height compared with predicted height,[1478,1479] with mean

gains of 4.4 to 10 cm in those receiving the combination therapy, compared with 0.5 to 6.1 cm in untreated control subjects.[1366,1480]

In these studies, the effects of GH cannot be separated definitively from those of the GnRH agonist. In two randomized studies of adopted girls with normal puberty, treatment with a GnRH agonist plus GH was compared with GnRH agonist alone, and a 3-cm height gain was demonstrated with the combination therapy.[1481,1482]

Disadvantages of the use of GnRH agonists in children with ISS include absence of pubertal growth acceleration, delayed puberty with potential psychosocial disadvantage, and decreased BMD. Long-term follow-up studies are lacking. A panel of experts concluded that GnRH agonist therapy alone in children with ISS and normally timed puberty is minimally effective in increasing adult height, may compromise BMD, and cannot be suggested for routine use.[1483] Combined GnRH agonist and GH therapy leads to a significant height gain but may have adverse effects. Routine use of GnRH agonists in children with ISS being treated with GH cannot be suggested (level of evidence, C-III).

Increasing Adult Height of Children Born Small for Gestational Age. Short children born SGA usually have a normal pubertal timing, although some of them have rapidly progressing puberty and may be treated with GH.[1484] Data on the additional effect of treatment with GnRH agonists are limited. Routine use of the combination of a GnRH agonist and GH in children born SGA cannot be suggested.

Increasing Adult Height of Children with Growth Hormone Deficiency. Some children with GHD are short at the start of puberty and at risk for short adult stature. Retrospective studies evaluating the addition of GnRH agonists to GH therapy involved a limited number of subjects and provided controversial results.[1485,1486] Three prospective studies that reported near-adult or adult heights showed a height gain of −1 SDS.[1487-1489] Routine use of combined therapy with a GnRH agonist and GH in GH-deficient children with low predicted adult height at onset of puberty cannot be suggested (level of evidence, C-III).

Aromatase Inhibitors. Men with estrogen deficiency due to aromatase gene defects or estrogen resistance due to inactive estrogen receptors experience growth into the third decade, demonstrating the role of estrogen in growth plate fusion.[22,289] The aromatase enzyme catalyzes aromatization of testosterone and androstenedione to estradiol and estrone, respectively. Various studies have been conducted to explore the efficacy of the aromatase inhibitor class of drugs delaying growth plate fusion and increasing height in disorders associated with short stature in boys. Studies to date have been small, and many have used adjuvant treatments, including GH, GnRH agonist, or testosterone, so the singular effect of the aromatase inhibitor has been unclear. Additionally, most studies to date have been short term and have measured changes in predicted adult height, with only one study investigating the effect on final adult height.

Aromatase inhibitors were first tried in disorders of sex steroid excess and precocious puberty, with only modest, if any, effects on predicted adult height. Treatment of boys with familial male-limited precocious puberty with testolactone, a first-generation aromatase inhibitor, resulted in an improvement in predicted adult height only after 5 to 6 years of treatment.[1490] The improvement in predicted adult height after 6 years was robust, however, at 12.9 cm compared with untreated control subjects. In contrast, first- and second-generation aromatase inhibitors have not significantly affected predicted adult height in patients with McCune-Albright syndrome.[1491-1493] Final height data are not available.

Aromatase inhibitors have also been used in boys with CDGD. Available studies had a small number of subjects enrolled, and boys with CDGD who received the second-generation aromatase inhibitor letrozole, in combination with testosterone, for 12 months experienced an increase in predicted adult height of 5.1 cm compared with control subjects treated with testosterone alone.[808] When followed to adult height, those boys who received letrozole in addition to testosterone achieved a final adult height 5.7 cm higher than that of boys receiving testosterone alone.[1073] In GH-deficient boys treated with GH, the addition of anastrozole for 3 years increased predicted adult height by 6.7 cm, compared with an increase of 1.0 cm in boys treated with GH alone.[809] The results of these preliminary, small trials indicate that aromatase inhibitors may be able to increase adult height, but larger, longer trials are needed to determine the optimal conditions and duration of treatment to significantly increase adult height. In addition, longer follow-up will be needed to demonstrate the safety of such treatments in peripubertal and pubertal boys.

Given the observation of decreased BMD in males with defects in estrogen synthesis or action, the effects of short-term aromatase inhibitor therapy on BMD were investigated in these treatment studies. None of the studies found a difference in BMD as assessed by DEXA scans in patients who received aromatase inhibitor or placebo for up to 3 years.[809,811] However, mild vertebral abnormalities were noted in boys who received the aromatase inhibitor compared with placebo[1494]; it is unknown whether the deformities are due to treatment effects and whether they resolve upon longer duration letrozole therapy. In light of these effects, aromatase inhibitors must be used with caution. Clearly, longitudinal follow-up is needed to better characterize the safety and efficacy of aromatase inhibitors to promote growth.

Oxandrolone. Oxandrolone, an anabolic steroid, has been used to increase growth velocity in a number of disorders. Because it cannot be aromatized to estrogen, it should not accelerate skeletal maturation. In general, studies evaluating the effect of oxandrolone on growth have found that it increases growth velocity but is not associated with an increase in final height.

Clinical Trials of Efficacy. Numerous studies have investigated oxandrolone therapy in boys with CDGD. The studies have found that oxandrolone increases growth velocity in these boys.[1032,1050] The typical response is an increase in growth velocity from approximately 4 to 4.5 cm/year up to 8 to 9 cm/year. Although treatment does not decrease final height, as might occur with accelerated skeletal maturation from excessive sex hormone exposure, neither does it increase final height.[1050] Therefore, oxandrolone can be used to accelerate the growth of boys with CDGD to allow them to increase their height sooner than they would naturally, but it does not increase their final adult height. There have been no trials comparing efficacy of oxandrolone versus testosterone treatment in boys with CDGD.

Oxandrolone has been studied in girls with TS, both as a single agent and as combined therapy with GH. As in boys with CDGD, oxandrolone increases the growth rate in girls with TS.[1495,1496] Although some studies found no effect on final height with oxandrolone treatment alone,[1497] others found a mean increase in final height of up to 5.2 cm with oxandrolone treatment.[1496] Results of three controlled trials testing the effects of combination therapy with GH versus GH alone on adult height were reviewed.[1498] The studies had different average age at treatment start and used different GH and oxandrolone doses.[1499-1501] In general, the studies reported a positive effect of oxandro-

lone when added to standard GH therapy, with the effect on adult height varying between 2.3 and 4.6 cm.

Side Effects. No significant side effects have been reported in boys treated with oxandrolone for CDGD. Although oxandrolone has significantly fewer androgenic effects than testosterone, mild virilization has been reported in girls taking oxandrolone, including clitoromegaly. This is less of a concern at lower doses.[1498] There are also reports of a delay in breast development that improves upon higher estrogen dosing. Hepatic dysfunction has been reported with oxandrolone treatment, manifested by alterations in HDL cholesterol, and thus monitoring of lipids is suggested.[1498]

Diagnosis and Treatment of Excess Growth and Tall Stature

Diagnosis

The normal distribution of height predicts that 2.5% of the population will be taller than 2 SD above the mean. The most common cause of tall stature is familial, and the diagnostic evaluation centers on distinguishing tall or constitutional stature from rare pathologic causes of tall stature. As with short stature, children with tall stature must be evaluated relative to familial growth patterns and parental target heights. When a family history of tall stature is available and the growth rate and physical examination findings are normal, support and reassurance are frequently all that is needed without further testing. A careful assessment of pubertal status and bone age facilitates prediction of adult height and discussions with the patient and family. If the history suggests an underlying disorder or growth rate is accelerated, additional testing should be done to investigate the GH-IGF-1 axis, chromosomal disorders, puberty, or other rare causes.

In GH excess, serum IGF-1 levels are elevated, although high IGF-1 levels may be a normal manifestation of puberty. Basal serum GH levels may be normal to increased, but serum GH is not suppressed by administration of glucose (1.75 g/kg body weight up to a maximum of 100 g). Although abnormalities of the sella turcica can be evident on lateral skull films, the demonstration of increased GH-IGF secretion should lead to radiologic evaluation of the hypothalamus and pituitary by MRI or computed tomography.

Treatment

Definitive treatment of GH-secreting tumors requires surgical ablation, either transsphenoidally or with a more aggressive surgical approach if large. As described in Chapter 9, somatostatin analogues, dopamine agonists, and GH-receptor antagonists are important components of treatment programs for GH excess.

In the past, most patients treated for familial tall stature were females. The numbers of patients treated in the United States has fallen markedly over the past 4 decades as tall stature in girls has become increasingly acceptable socially and psychologically. Treatment regimens were generally with estrogen prior to pubertal onset to induce early epiphyseal maturation[1502] and considered girls with predicted heights greater than 183 cm (6 feet 0 inches). Treatment regimens varied considerably, and there are no randomized trials testing treatment effectiveness. Controversy surrounds the treatment of girls with tall stature, especially in light of long-term studies that raised the possibility of effects on fertility.[1503] One fifth of pediatric endocrinologists reported use of estrogens for treatment of tall stature in 1999,[1504] a percentage that is likely diminishing.

In males, androgens have been used to accelerate skeletal maturation via aromatization to estrogen, but virilization is rapid.

REFERENCES

1. Heinrichs C, Munson PJ, Counts DR, et al. Patterns of human growth. *Science.* 1995;268(5209):442-447.
2. Lampl M, Veldhuis JD, Johnson ML. Saltation and stasis: a model of human growth. *Science.* 1992;258(5083):801-803.
3. Lampl M, Cameron N, Veldhuis JD, et al. Patterns of human growth: response. *Science.* 1995;268:445-447.
4. Tillmann V, Thalange NK, Foster PJ, et al. The relationship between stature, growth, and short-term changes in height and weight in normal prepubertal children. *Pediatr Res.* 1998;44(6):882-886.
5. Thalange NK, Foster PJ, Gill MS, et al. Model of normal prepubertal growth. *Arch Dis Child.* 1996;75(5):427-431.
6. Gelander L, Karlberg J, Albertsson-Wikland K. Seasonality in lower leg length velocity in prepubertal children. *Acta Paediatr.* 1994;83(12):1249-1254.
7. Hermanussen M, Lange S, Grasedyck L. Growth tracks in early childhood. *Acta Paediatr.* 2001;90(4):381-386.
8. Ogden CL, Kuczmarski RJ, Flegal KM, et al. Centers for Disease Control and Prevention 2000 growth charts for the United States: improvements to the 1977 National Center for Health statistics version. *Pediatrics.* 2002;109(1):45-60.
9. Grummer-Strawn LM, Reinold C, Krebs NF, Centers for Disease Control and Prevention (CDC). Use of World Health Organization and CDC growth charts for children aged 0-59 months in the United States. *MMWR Recomm Rep.* 2010;59(RR-9):1-15.
10. Tanner JM, Davies PS. Clinical longitudinal standards for height and height velocity for North American children. *J Pediatr.* 1985;107(3):317-329.
11. Lyon AJ, Preece MA, Grant DB. Growth curve for girls with Turner syndrome. *Arch Dis Child.* 1985;60(10):932-935.
12. Horton WA, Rotter JI, Rimoin DL, et al. Standard growth curves for achondroplasia. *J Pediatr.* 1978;93(3):435-438.
13. Cronk C, Crocker AC, Pueschel SM, et al. Growth charts for children with Down syndrome: 1 month to 18 years of age. *Pediatrics.* 1988;81(1):102-110.
14. Bayer LM, Bayley L. *Growth Diagnosis.* Chicago, IL: University of Chicago Press; 1959.
15. Tanner JM, Goldstein H, Whitehouse RH. Standards for children's height at ages 2-9 years allowing for heights of parents. *Arch Dis Child.* 1970;45(244):755-762.
16. Tanner JM. Auxology. In: Kappy MS, Blizzard RM, Migeon CJ, eds. *The Diagnosis and Treatment of Endocrine Disorders.* Springfield, IL: Charles C Thomas; 1994.
17. Wright CM, Cheetham TD. The strengths and limitations of parental heights as a predictor of attained height. *Arch Dis Child.* 1999;81(3):257-260.
18. Giacobbi V, Trivin C, Lawson-Body E, et al. Extremely short stature: influence of each parent's height on clinical-biological features. *Horm Res.* 2003;60(6):272-276.
19. Reiter EO, Rosenfeld RG. Normal and aberrant growth. In: Kronenberg HM, Melmed S, Polonsky KS, Larsen PR, eds. *Williams Textbook of Endocrinology.* 11th ed. Philadelphia, PA: Saunders Elsevier; 2008.
20. Emons JA, Boersma B, Baron J, Wit JM. Catch-up growth: testing the hypothesis of delayed growth plate senescence in humans. *J Pediatr.* 2005;147(6):843-846.
21. Weise M, De-Levi S, Barnes KM, et al. Effects of estrogen on growth plate senescence and epiphyseal fusion. *Proc Natl Acad Sci U S A.* 2001;98(12):6871-6876.
22. Smith EP, Boyd J, Frank GR, et al. Estrogen resistance caused by a mutation in the estrogen-receptor gene in a man. *N Engl J Med.* 1994;331(16):1056-1061.
23. Conte FA, Grumbach MM, Ito Y, et al. A syndrome of female pseudohermaphrodism, hypergonadotropic hypogonadism, and multicystic ovaries associated with missense mutations in the gene encoding aromatase (P450arom). *J Clin Endocrinol Metab.* 1994;78(6):1287-1292.
24. Bilezikian JP, Morishima A, Bell J, Grumbach MM. Increased bone mass as a result of estrogen therapy in a man with aromatase deficiency. *N Engl J Med.* 1998;339(9):599-603.
25. Grumbach MM, Auchus RJ. Estrogen: consequences and implications of human mutations in synthesis and action. *J Clin Endocrinol Metab.* 1999;84(12):4677-4694.
26. Karlberg J, Engstrom I, Karlberg P, Fryer JG. Analysis of linear growth using a mathematical model. I. From birth to three years. *Acta Paediatr Scand.* 1987;76(3):478-488.
27. Karlberg J, Fryer JG, Engstrom I, Karlberg P. Analysis of linear growth using a mathematical model. II. From 3 to 21 years of age. *Acta Paediatr Scand Suppl.* 1987;337:12-29.
28. Schrier L, Ferns SP, Barnes KM, et al. Depletion of resting zone chondrocytes during growth plate senescence. *J Endocrinol.* 2006;189(1):27-36.
29. Parfitt AM. Misconceptions (1): epiphyseal fusion causes cessation of growth. *Bone.* 2002;30(2):337-339.
30. Tanner JM, Whitehouse RH, Takaishi M. Standards from birth to maturity for height, weight, height velocity, and weight velocity: British children, 1965. I. *Arch Dis Child.* 1966;41(219):454-471.
31. Wingerd J, Schoen EJ. Factors influencing length at birth and height at five years. *Pediatrics.* 1974;53(5):737-741.
32. Smith DW, Truog W, Rogers JE, et al. Shifting linear growth during infancy: illustration of genetic factors in growth from fetal life through infancy. *J Pediatr.* 1976;89(2):225-230.
33. Knight B, Shields BM, Turner M, et al. Evidence of genetic regulation of fetal longitudinal growth. *Early Hum Dev.* 2005;81(10):823-831.
34. Mei Z, Grummer-Strawn LM, Thompson D, Dietz WH. Shifts in percentiles of growth during early childhood: analysis of longitudinal data from the California Child Health and Development study. *Pediatrics.* 2004;113(6):e617-e627.
35. Lee PA, Kendig JW, Kerrigan JR. Persistent short stature, other potential outcomes, and the effect of growth hormone treatment in children who are born small for gestational age. *Pediatrics.* 2003;112(1 Pt 1):150-162.
36. Hokken-Koelega AC, De Ridder MA, Lemmen RJ, et al. Children born small for gestational age: do they catch up? *Pediatr Res.* 1995;38(2):267-271.
37. Karlberg J, Albertsson-Wikland K. Growth in full-term small-for-gestational-age infants: from birth to final height. *Pediatr Res.* 1995;38(5):733-739.
38. Horner JM, Thorsson AV, Hintz RL. Growth deceleration patterns in children with constitutional short stature: an aid to diagnosis. *Pediatrics.* 1978;62(4):529-534.
39. Du Caju MV, Op De Beeck L, Sys SU, et al. Progressive deceleration in growth as an early sign of delayed puberty in boys. *Horm Res.* 2000;54(3):126-130.
40. Crowne EC, Shalet SM, Wallace WH, et al. Final height in boys with untreated constitutional delay in growth and puberty. *Arch Dis Child.* 1990;65(10):1109-1112.
41. LaFranchi S, Hanna CE, Mandel SH. Constitutional delay of growth: expected versus final adult height. *Pediatrics.* 1991;87(1):82-87.
42. Ranke MB, Grauer ML, Kistner K, et al. Spontaneous adult height in idiopathic short stature. *Horm Res.* 1995;44(4):152-157.
43. Albanese A, Stanhope R. Predictive factors in the determination of final height in boys with constitutional delay of growth and puberty. *J Pediatr.* 1995;126(4):545-550.
44. Moreira-Andres MN, Canizo FJ, de la Cruz FJ, et al. Bone mineral status in prepubertal children with constitutional delay of growth and puberty. *Eur J Endocrinol.* 1998;139(3):271-275.
45. Bertelloni S, Baroncelli GI, Ferdeghini M, et al. Normal volumetric bone mineral density and bone turnover in young men with histories of constitutional delay of puberty. *J Clin Endocrinol Metab.* 1998;83(12):4280-4283.
46. Darelid A, Ohlsson C, Nilsson M, et al. Catch up in bone acquisition in young adult men with late normal puberty. *J Bone Miner Res.* 2012;27(10):2198-2207.
47. Ruff C. Variation in human size and shape. *Annu Rev Anthropol.* 2002;31:211-232.
48. Tanner JM. *A history of the study of human growth.* Cambridge, MA: Cambridge University Press; 1981.
49. Schonbeck Y, Talma H, van Dommelen P, et al. The world's tallest nation has stopped growing taller: the height of Dutch children from 1955 to 2009. *Pediatr Res.* 2013;73(3):371-377.
50. Kioussi C, Carriere C, Rosenfeld MG. A model for the development of the hypothalamic-pituitary axis: transcribing the hypophysis. *Mech Dev.* 1999;81(1-2):23-35.
51. Gage PJ, Camper SA. Pituitary homeobox 2, a novel member of the bicoid-related family of homeobox genes, is a potential regulator of anterior structure formation. *Hum Mol Genet.* 1997;6(3):457-464.
52. Treier M, Gleiberman AS, O'Connell SM, et al. Multistep signaling requirements for pituitary organogenesis in vivo. *Genes Dev.* 1998;12(11):1691-1704.
53. Ericson J, Norlin S, Jessell TM, Edlund T. Integrated FGF and BMP signaling controls the progression of progenitor cell differentiation and the emergence of pattern in the embryonic anterior pituitary. *Development.* 1998;125(6):1005-1015.
54. Kioussi C, O'Connell S, St-Onge L, et al. Pax6 is essential for establishing ventral-dorsal cell boundaries in pituitary gland development. *Proc Natl Acad Sci U S A.* 1999;96(25):14378-14382.
55. Sornson MW, Wu W, Dasen JS, et al. Pituitary lineage determination by the prophet of pit-1 homeodomain factor defective in Ames dwarfism. *Nature.* 1996;384(6607):327-333.
56. Dasen JS, O'Connell SM, Flynn SE, et al. Reciprocal interactions of Pit1 and GATA2 mediate signaling gradient-induced determination of pituitary cell types. *Cell.* 1999;97(5):587-598.
57. Simmons DM, Voss JW, Ingraham HA, et al. Pituitary cell phenotypes involve cell-specific pit-1 mRNA translation and synergistic

interactions with other classes of transcription factors. *Genes Dev.* 1990;4(5):695-711.

58. Li S, Crenshaw EB 3rd, Rawson EJ, et al. Dwarf locus mutants lacking three pituitary cell types result from mutations in the POU-domain gene pit-1. *Nature.* 1990;347(6293):528-533.

59. Ingraham HA, Lala DS, Ikeda Y, et al. The nuclear receptor steroidogenic factor 1 acts at multiple levels of the reproductive axis. *Genes Dev.* 1994;8(19):2302-2312.

60. Luo X, Ikeda Y, Lala DS, et al. A cell-specific nuclear receptor plays essential roles in adrenal and gonadal development. *Endocr Res.* 1995; 21(1-2):517-524.

61. Bentley CA, Zidehsarai MP, Grindley JC, et al. Pax6 is implicated in murine pituitary endocrine function. *Endocrine.* 1999;10(2): 171-177.

62. Japon MA, Rubinstein M, Low MJ. In situ hybridization analysis of anterior pituitary hormone gene expression during fetal mouse development. *J Histochem Cytochem.* 1994;42(8):1117-1125.

63. Lamolet B, Pulichino AM, Lamonerie T, et al. A pituitary cell-restricted T box factor, tpit, activates POMC transcription in cooperation with pitx homeoproteins. *Cell.* 2001;104(6):849-859.

64. Goodyer CG. Ontogeny of pituitary hormone secretion. In: Collu R, Ducharme JR, Guyda HJ, eds. *Pediatric Endocrinology.* New York, NY: Raven; 1989.

65. Gorczyca W, Hardy J. Arterial supply of the human anterior pituitary gland. *Neurosurgery.* 1987;20(3):369-378.

66. Pilavdzic D, Kovacs K, Asa SL. Pituitary morphology in anencephalic human fetuses. *Neuroendocrinology.* 1997;65(3):164-172.

67. Scheithauer BW, Sano T, Kovacs KT, et al. The pituitary gland in pregnancy: a clinicopathologic and immunohistochemical study of 69 cases. *Mayo Clin Proc.* 1990;65(4):461-474.

68. Thorner MO, Vance ML, Horvath E. The anterior pituitary. In: Wilson JD, Foster DW, eds. *Williams Textbook of Endocrinology.* Philadelphia, PA: WB Saunders; 1991.

69. Cooke NE, Ray J, Watson MA, et al. Human growth hormone gene and the highly homologous growth hormone variant gene display different splicing patterns. *J Clin Invest.* 1988;82(1):270-275.

70. Cordoba-Chacon J, Gahete MD, Castano JP, et al. Somatostatin and its receptors contribute in a tissue-specific manner to the sex-dependent metabolic (fed/fasting) control of growth hormone axis in mice. *Am J Physiol Endocrinol Metab.* 2011;300(1):E46-E54.

71. Frohman LA, Kineman RD, Kamegai J, et al. Secretagogues and the somatotrope: signaling and proliferation. *Recent Prog Horm Res.* 2000; 55:269-290, discussion 290-291.

72. Lin C, Lin SC, Chang CP, Rosenfeld MG. Pit-1-dependent expression of the receptor for growth hormone releasing factor mediates pituitary cell growth. *Nature.* 1992;360(6406):765-768.

73. Mayo KE, Hammer RE, Swanson LW, et al. Dramatic pituitary hyperplasia in transgenic mice expressing a human growth hormone-releasing factor gene. *Mol Endocrinol.* 1988;2(7):606-612.

74. Barinaga M, Yamonoto G, Rivier C, et al. Transcriptional regulation of growth hormone gene expression by growth hormone-releasing factor. *Nature.* 1983;306(5938):84-85.

75. Frohman LA, Jansson JO. Growth hormone-releasing hormone. *Endocr Rev.* 1986;7(3):223-253.

76. Smith RG, Palyha OC, Feighner SD, et al. Growth hormone releasing substances: types and their receptors. *Horm Res.* 1999;51(Suppl 3): 1-8.

77. Kineman RD, Aleppo G, Frohman LA. The tyrosine hydroxylase-human growth hormone (GH) transgenic mouse as a model of hypothalamic GH deficiency: growth retardation is the result of a selective reduction in somatotrope numbers despite normal somatotrope function. *Endocrinology.* 1996;137(11):4630-4636.

78. Salvatori R, Hayashida CY, Aguiar-Oliveira MH, et al. Familial dwarfism due to a novel mutation of the growth hormone-releasing hormone receptor gene. *J Clin Endocrinol Metab.* 1999;84(3):917-923.

79. Hammer RE, Brinster RL, Rosenfeld MG, et al. Expression of human growth hormone-releasing factor in transgenic mice results in increased somatic growth. *Nature.* 1985;315(6018):413-416.

80. Hartman ML, Faria AC, Vance ML, et al. Temporal structure of in vivo growth hormone secretory events in humans. *Am J Physiol.* 1991;260(1 Pt 1):E101-E110.

81. Bonnefont X, Lacampagne A, Sanchez-Hormigo A, et al. Revealing the large-scale network organization of growth hormone-secreting cells. *Proc Natl Acad Sci U S A.* 2005;102(46):16880-16885.

82. Zeitler P, Argente J, Chowen-Breed JA, et al. Growth hormone-releasing hormone messenger ribonucleic acid in the hypothalamus of the adult male rat is increased by testosterone. *Endocrinology.* 1990;127(3):1362-1368.

83. Ho KY, Evans WS, Blizzard RM, et al. Effects of sex and age on the 24-hour profile of growth hormone secretion in man: importance of endogenous estradiol concentrations. *J Clin Endocrinol Metab.* 1987; 64(1):51-58.

84. Katz HP, Youlton R, Kaplan SL, Grumbach MM. Growth and growth hormone. 3. Growth hormone release in children with primary hypothyroidism and thyrotoxicosis. *J Clin Endocrinol Metab.* 1969;29(3): 346-351.

85. Frantz AG, Rabkin MT. Human growth hormone. Clinical measurement, response to hypoglycemia and suppression by corticosteroids. *N Engl J Med.* 1964;271:1375-1381.

86. Thompson RG, Rodriguez A, Kowarski A, Blizzard RM. Growth hormone: metabolic clearance rates, integrated concentrations, and production rates in normal adults and the effect of prednisone. *J Clin Invest.* 1972;51(12):3193-3199.

87. Kojima M, Hosoda H, Date Y, et al. Ghrelin is a growth-hormone-releasing acylated peptide from stomach. *Nature.* 1999;402(6762): 656-660.

88. Date Y, Kojima M, Hosoda H, et al. Ghrelin, a novel growth hormone-releasing acylated peptide, is synthesized in a distinct endocrine cell type in the gastrointestinal tracts of rats and humans. *Endocrinology.* 2000;141(11):4255-4261.

89. Malagon MM, Luque RM, Ruiz-Guerrero E, et al. Intracellular signaling mechanisms mediating ghrelin-stimulated growth hormone release in somatotropes. *Endocrinology.* 2003;144(12):5372-5380.

90. Popovic V, Miljic D, Micic D, et al. Ghrelin main action on the regulation of growth hormone release is exerted at hypothalamic level. *J Clin Endocrinol Metab.* 2003;88(7):3450-3453.

91. Higgins SC, Gueorguiev M, Korbonits M. Ghrelin, the peripheral hunger hormone. *Ann Med.* 2007;39(2):116-136.

92. Sun Y, Ahmed S, Smith RG. Deletion of ghrelin impairs neither growth nor appetite. *Mol Cell Biol.* 2003;23(22):7973-7981.

93. Sun Y, Wang P, Zheng H, Smith RG. Ghrelin stimulation of growth hormone release and appetite is mediated through the growth hormone secretagogue receptor. *Proc Natl Acad Sci U S A.* 2004;101(13): 4679-4684.

94. Savino F, Grassino EC, Fissore MF, et al. Ghrelin, motilin, insulin concentration in healthy infants in the first months of life: relation to fasting time and anthropometry. *Clin Endocrinol (Oxf).* 2006;65(2): 158-162.

95. Pantel J, Legendre M, Cabrol S, et al. Loss of constitutive activity of the growth hormone secretagogue receptor in familial short stature. *J Clin Invest.* 2006;116(3):760-768.

96. Wang HJ, Geller F, Dempfle A, et al. Ghrelin receptor gene: identification of several sequence variants in extremely obese children and adolescents, healthy normal-weight and underweight students, and children with short normal stature. *J Clin Endocrinol Metab.* 2004; 89(1):157-162.

97. Muccioli G, Ghe C, Ghigo MC, et al. Specific receptors for synthetic GH secretagogues in the human brain and pituitary gland. *J Endocrinol.* 1998;157(1):99-106.

98. Akamizu T, Murayama T, Teramukai S, et al. Plasma ghrelin levels in healthy elderly volunteers: the levels of acylated ghrelin in elderly females correlate positively with serum IGF-I levels and bowel movement frequency and negatively with systolic blood pressure. *J Endocrinol.* 2006;188(2):333-344.

99. Cummings DE, Purnell JQ, Frayo RS, et al. A preprandial rise in plasma ghrelin levels suggests a role in meal initiation in humans. *Diabetes.* 2001;50(8):1714-1719.

100. Shiiya T, Nakazato M, Mizuta M, et al. Plasma ghrelin levels in lean and obese humans and the effect of glucose on ghrelin secretion. *J Clin Endocrinol Metab.* 2002;87(1):240-244.

101. Tschop M, Smiley DL, Heiman ML. Ghrelin induces adiposity in rodents. *Nature.* 2000;407(6806):908-913.

102. Jamen F, Persson K, Bertrand G, et al. PAC1 receptor-deficient mice display impaired insulinotropic response to glucose and reduced glucose tolerance. *J Clin Invest.* 2000;105(9):1307-1315.

103. Rosenfeld RG, Ceda G, Wilson DM, et al. Characterization of high affinity receptors for insulin-like growth factors I and II on rat anterior pituitary cells. *Endocrinology.* 1984;114(5):1571-1575.

104. Ceda GP, Davis RG, Rosenfeld RG, Hoffman AR. The growth hormone (GH)-releasing hormone (GHRH)-GH-somatomedin axis: evidence for rapid inhibition of GHRH-elicited GH release by insulin-like growth factors I and II. *Endocrinology.* 1987;120(4):1658-1662.

105. Romero CJ, Pine-Twaddell E, Sima DI, et al. Insulin-like growth factor 1 mediates negative feedback to somatotroph GH expression via POU1F1/CREB binding protein interactions. *Mol Cell Biol.* 2012; 32(21):4258-4269.

106. Vaccarello MA, Diamond FB Jr, Guevara-Aguirre J, et al. Hormonal and metabolic effects and pharmacokinetics of recombinant insulin-like growth factor-I in growth hormone receptor deficiency/Laron syndrome. *J Clin Endocrinol Metab.* 1993;77(1):273-280.

107. Veldhuis JD, Liem AY, South S, et al. Differential impact of age, sex steroid hormones, and obesity on basal versus pulsatile growth hormone secretion in men as assessed in an ultrasensitive chemiluminescence assay. *J Clin Endocrinol Metab.* 1995;80(11): 3209-3222.

108. Hartman ML, Veldhuis JD, Thorner MO. Normal control of growth hormone secretion. *Horm Res.* 1993;40(1-3):37-47.

109. Veldhuis JD, Roemmich JN, Rogol AD. Gender and sexual maturation-dependent contrasts in the neuroregulation of growth hormone secretion in prepubertal and late adolescent males and females—a general clinical research center-based study. *J Clin Endocrinol Metab.* 2000;85(7):2385-2394.

110. Gill MS, Thalange NK, Foster PJ, et al. Regular fluctuations in growth hormone (GH) release determine normal human growth. *Growth Horm IGF Res.* 1999;9(2):114-122.

111. Tillmann V, Gill MS, Thalange NK, et al. Short-term changes in growth and urinary growth hormone, insulin-like growth factor-I and markers of bone turnover excretion in healthy prepubertal children. *Growth Horm IGF Res.* 2000;10(1):28-36.

112. Grumbach MM, Gluckman PD. The human fetal hypothalamic and pituitary gland: the maturation of neuroendocrine mechanisms controlling secretion of fetal pituitary growth hormone, prolactin, gonadotropin, adrenocorticotropin-related peptides and thyrotropin. In: Tulchinsky D, Little AB, eds. *Maternal and Fetal Endocrinology.* Philadelphia, PA: WB Saunders; 1994.

113. Puy LA, Asa SL. The ontogeny of pit-1 expression in the human fetal pituitary gland. *Neuroendocrinology.* 1996;63(4):349-355.

114. Arosio M, Cortelazzi D, Persani L, et al. Circulating levels of growth hormone, insulin-like growth factor-I and prolactin in normal, growth retarded and anencephalic human fetuses. *J Endocrinol Invest.* 1995;18(5):346-353.

115. Martha PM Jr, Gorman KM, Blizzard RM, et al. Endogenous growth hormone secretion and clearance rates in normal boys, as determined by deconvolution analysis: relationship to age, pubertal status, and body mass. *J Clin Endocrinol Metab.* 1992;74(2):336-344.

116. Pincus SM, Veldhuis JD, Rogol AD. Longitudinal changes in growth hormone secretory process irregularity assessed transpubertally in healthy boys. *Am J Physiol Endocrinol Metab.* 2000;279(2):E417-E424.

117. Baumann G, Shaw MA, Amburn K. Circulating growth hormone binding proteins. *J Endocrinol Invest.* 1994;17(1):67-81.

118. Moran A, Jacobs DR Jr, Steinberger J, et al. Association between the insulin resistance of puberty and the insulin-like growth factor-I/growth hormone axis. *J Clin Endocrinol Metab.* 2002;87(10):4817-4820.

119. Rudman D, Kutner MH, Rogers CM, et al. Impaired growth hormone secretion in the adult population: relation to age and adiposity. *J Clin Invest.* 1981;67(5):1361-1369.

120. Van Cauter E, Caufriez A, Kerkhofs M, et al. Sleep, awakenings, and insulin-like growth factor-I modulate the growth hormone (GH) secretory response to GH-releasing hormone. *J Clin Endocrinol Metab.* 1992;74(6):1451-1459.

121. Veldhuis JD, Iranmanesh A, Ho KK, et al. Dual defects in pulsatile growth hormone secretion and clearance subserve the hyposomatotropism of obesity in man. *J Clin Endocrinol Metab.* 1991;72(1):51-59.

122. Schalch DS. The influence of physical stress and exercise on growth hormone and insulin secretion in man. *J Lab Clin Med.* 1967;69(2):256-269.

123. Jaffe CA, Turgeon DK, Friberg RD, et al. Nocturnal augmentation of growth hormone (GH) secretion is preserved during repetitive bolus administration of GH-releasing hormone: potential involvement of endogenous somatostatin—a clinical research center study. *J Clin Endocrinol Metab.* 1995;80(11):3321-3326.

124. Veldhuis JD, Metzger DL, Martha PM Jr, et al. Estrogen and testosterone, but not a nonaromatizable androgen, direct network integration of the hypothalamo-somatotrope (growth hormone)-insulin-like growth factor I axis in the human: evidence from pubertal pathophysiology and sex-steroid hormone replacement. *J Clin Endocrinol Metab.* 1997;82(10):3414-3420.

125. Rosenfeld RG, Rosenbloom AL, Guevara-Aguirre J. Growth hormone (GH) insensitivity due to primary GH receptor deficiency. *Endocr Rev.* 1994;15(3):369-390.

126. Tollet-Egnell P, Flores-Morales A, Stahlberg N, et al. Gene expression profile of the aging process in rat liver: normalizing effects of growth hormone replacement. *Mol Endocrinol.* 2001;15(2):308-318.

127. Salmon WD Jr, Daughaday WH. A hormonally controlled serum factor which stimulates sulfate incorporation by cartilage in vitro. *J Lab Clin Med.* 1990;116(3):408-419.

128. Gerich JE, Lorenzi M, Bier DM, et al. Effects of physiologic levels of glucagon and growth hormone on human carbohydrate and lipid metabolism. Studies involving administration of exogenous hormone during suppression of endogenous hormone secretion with somatostatin. *J Clin Invest.* 1976;57(4):875-884.

129. Hjalmarson A, Isaksson O, Ahren K. Effects of growth hormone and insulin on amino acid transport in perfused rat heart. *Am J Physiol.* 1969;217(6):1795-1802.

130. Ling L, Zhu T, Lobie PE. Src-CrkII-C3G-dependent activation of Rap1 switches growth hormone-stimulated p44/42 MAP kinase and JNK/SAPK activities. *J Biol Chem.* 2003;278(29):27301-27311.

131. Griffin EE, Miller LL. Effects of hypophysectomy of liver donor on net synthesis of specific plasma proteins by the isolated perfused rat liver. Modulation of synthesis of albumin, fibrinogen, alpha 1-acid glycoprotein, alpha 2-(acute phase)-globulin, and haptoglobin by insulin, cortisol, triiodothyronine, and growth hormone. *J Biol Chem.* 1974;249(16):5062-5069.

132. Daughaday WH, Hall K, Raben MS, et al. Somatomedin: proposed designation for sulphation factor. *Nature.* 1972;235:107.

133. Barton DE, Foellmer BE, Wood WI, Francke U. Chromosome mapping of the growth hormone receptor gene in man and mouse. *Cytogenet Cell Genet.* 1989;50(2-3):137-141.

134. Kelly PA, Djiane J, Postel-Vinay MC, Edery M. The prolactin/growth hormone receptor family. *Endocr Rev.* 1991;12(3):235-251.

135. Pantel J, Machinis K, Sobrier ML, et al. Species-specific alternative splice mimicry at the growth hormone receptor locus revealed by the lineage of retroelements during primate evolution. *J Biol Chem.* 2000; 275(25):18664-18669.

136. Waters MJ, Hoang HN, Fairlie DP, et al. New insights into growth hormone action. *J Mol Endocrinol.* 2006;36(1):1-7.

137. Brown RJ, Adams JJ, Pelekanos RA, et al. Model for growth hormone receptor activation based on subunit rotation within a receptor dimer. *Nat Struct Mol Biol.* 2005;12(9):814-821.

138. Udy GB, Towers RP, Snell RG, et al. Requirement of STAT5b for sexual dimorphism of body growth rates and liver gene expression. *Proc Natl Acad Sci U S A.* 1997;94(14):7239-7244.

139. Woelfle J, Chia DJ, Rotwein P. Mechanisms of growth hormone (GH) action. identification of conserved Stat5 binding sites that mediate GH-induced insulin-like growth factor-I gene activation. *J Biol Chem.* 2003;278(51):51261-51266.

140. Schindler C, Darnell JE Jr. Transcriptional responses to polypeptide ligands: the JAK-STAT pathway. *Annu Rev Biochem.* 1995;64:621-651.

141. Lewis MD, Horan M, Millar DS, et al. A novel dysfunctional growth hormone variant (Ile179Met) exhibits a decreased ability to activate the extracellular signal-regulated kinase pathway. *J Clin Endocrinol Metab.* 2004;89(3):1068-1075.

142. Jin H, Lanning NJ, Carter-Su C. JAK2, but not src family kinases, is required for STAT, ERK, and akt signaling in response to growth hormone in preadipocytes and hepatoma cells. *Mol Endocrinol.* 2008;22(8):1825-1841.

143. Hansen JA, Lindberg K, Hilton DJ, et al. Mechanism of inhibition of growth hormone receptor signaling by suppressor of cytokine signaling proteins. *Mol Endocrinol.* 1999;13(11):1832-1843.

144. Metcalf D, Greenhalgh CJ, Viney E, et al. Gigantism in mice lacking suppressor of cytokine signalling-2. *Nature.* 2000;405(6790):1069-1073.

145. Greenhalgh CJ, Bertolino P, Asa SL, et al. Growth enhancement in suppressor of cytokine signaling 2 (SOCS-2)-deficient mice is dependent on signal transducer and activator of transcription 5b (STAT5b). *Mol Endocrinol.* 2002;16(6):1394-1406.

146. Trivedi B, Daughaday WH. Release of growth hormone binding protein from IM-9 lymphocytes by endopeptidase is dependent on sulfhydryl group inactivation. *Endocrinology.* 1988;123(5):2201-2206.

147. Martha PM Jr, Rogol AD, Blizzard RM, et al. Growth hormone-binding protein activity is inversely related to 24-hour growth hormone release in normal boys. *J Clin Endocrinol Metab.* 1991; 73(1):175-181.

148. Massa G, de Zegher F, Vanderschueren-Lodeweyckx M. Serum growth hormone-binding proteins in the human fetus and infant. *Pediatr Res.* 1992;32(1):69-72.

149. Gronborg M, Wulff BS, Rasmussen JS, et al. Structure-function relationship of the insulin-like growth factor-I receptor tyrosine kinase. *J Biol Chem.* 1993;268(31):23435-23440.

150. Rowland JE, Lichanska AM, Kerr LM, et al. In vivo analysis of growth hormone receptor signaling domains and their associated transcripts. *Mol Cell Biol.* 2005;25(1):66-77.

151. Flores-Morales A, Stahlberg N, Tollet-Egnell P, et al. Microarray analysis of the in vivo effects of hypophysectomy and growth hormone treatment on gene expression in the rat. *Endocrinology.* 2001;142(7):3163-3176.

152. Zhou Y, Xu BC, Maheshwari HG, et al. A mammalian model for Laron syndrome produced by targeted disruption of the mouse growth hormone receptor/binding protein gene (the Laron mouse). *Proc Natl Acad Sci U S A.* 1997;94(24):13215-13220.

153. Fan Y, Menon RK, Cohen P, et al. Liver-specific deletion of the growth hormone receptor reveals essential role of growth hormone signaling in hepatic lipid metabolism. *J Biol Chem.* 2009;284(30):19937-19944.

154. Neubauer H, Cumano A, Muller M, et al. Jak2 deficiency defines an essential developmental checkpoint in definitive hematopoiesis. *Cell.* 1998;93(3):397-409.

155. Levy DE. Physiological significance of STAT proteins: investigations through gene disruption in vivo. *Cell Mol Life Sci.* 1999;55(12):1559-1567.

156. Lupu F, Terwilliger JD, Lee K, et al. Roles of growth hormone and insulin-like growth factor 1 in mouse postnatal growth. *Dev Biol.* 2001;229(1):141-162.

157. Yakar S, Liu JL, Stannard B, et al. Normal growth and development in the absence of hepatic insulin-like growth factor I. *Proc Natl Acad Sci U S A.* 1999;96(13):7324-7329.

158. Hall K, Takano K, Fryklund L. Sievertsson H. Somatomedins. *Adv Metab Disord.* 1975;8:19-46.

159. Rinderknecht E, Humbel RE. The amino acid sequence of human insulin-like growth factor I and its structural homology with proinsulin. *J Biol Chem.* 1978;253(8):2769-2776.

160. Rinderknecht E, Humbel RE. Primary structure of human insulin-like growth factor II. *FEBS Lett.* 1978;89(2):283-286.

161. Adamo ML, Neuenschwander S, LeRoith D, Roberts CT Jr. Structure, expression, and regulation of the IGF-I gene. *Adv Exp Med Biol.* 1993;343:1-11.

162. Yoon JB, Berry SA, Seelig S, Towle HC. An inducible nuclear factor binds to a growth hormone-regulated gene. *J Biol Chem.* 1990;265(32):19947-19954.

163. Lowe WL Jr, Roberts CT Jr, Lasky SR, LeRoith D. Differential expression of alternative 5' untranslated regions in mRNAs encoding rat insulin-like growth factor I. *Proc Natl Acad Sci U S A.* 1987;84(24):8946-8950.

164. Bonioli E, Taro M, Rosa CL, et al. Heterozygous mutations of growth hormone receptor gene in children with idiopathic short stature. *Growth Horm IGF Res.* 2005;15(6):405-410.

165. Duguay SJ, Lai-Zhang J, Steiner DF. Mutational analysis of the insulin-like growth factor I prohormone processing site. *J Biol Chem.* 1995;270(29):17566-17574.

166. Conover CA, Baker BK, Bale LK, et al. Human hepatoma cells synthesize and secrete insulin-like growth factor-1a prohormone under growth hormone control. *Regul Pept.* 1993;48(1-2):1-8.

167. Bennett A, Wilson DM, Liu F, et al. Levels of insulin-like growth factors I and II in human cord blood. *J Clin Endocrinol Metab.* 1983;57(3):609-612.

168. Lassarre C, Hardouin S, Daffos F, et al. Serum insulin-like growth factors and insulin-like growth factor binding proteins in the human fetus. Relationships with growth in normal subjects and in subjects with intrauterine growth retardation. *Pediatr Res.* 1991;29(3):219-225.

169. Hall K, Hansson U, Lundin G, et al. Serum levels of somatomedins and somatomedin-binding protein in pregnant women with type I or gestational diabetes and their infants. *J Clin Endocrinol Metab.* 1986;63(6):1300-1306.

170. Luna AM, Wilson DM, Wibbelsman CJ, et al. Somatomedins in adolescence: a cross-sectional study of the effect of puberty on plasma insulin-like growth factor I and II levels. *J Clin Endocrinol Metab.* 1983;57(2):268-271.

171. Cara JF, Rosenfield RL, Furlanetto RW. A longitudinal study of the relationship of plasma somatomedin-C concentration to the pubertal growth spurt. *Am J Dis Child.* 1987;141(5):562-564.

172. Bidlingmaier M, Friedrich N, Emeny RT, et al. Reference intervals for insulin-like growth factor-1 (IGF-I) from birth to senescence: results from a multicenter study using a new automated chemiluminescence IGF-I immunoassay conforming to recent international recommendations. *J Clin Endocrinol Metab.* 2014;99(5):1712-1721.

173. Cuttler L, Van Vliet G, Conte FA, et al. Somatomedin-C levels in children and adolescents with gonadal dysgenesis: differences from age-matched normal females and effect of chronic estrogen replacement therapy. *J Clin Endocrinol Metab.* 1985;60(6):1087-1092.

174. Rudman D, Feller AG, Nagraj HS, et al. Effects of human growth hormone in men over 60 years old. *N Engl J Med.* 1990;323(1):1-6.

175. Rappolee DA, Sturm KS, Behrendtsen O, et al. Insulin-like growth factor II acts through an endogenous growth pathway regulated by imprinting in early mouse embryos. *Genes Dev.* 1992;6(6):939-952.

176. Thorvaldsen JL, Duran KL, Bartolomei MS. Deletion of the H19 differentially methylated domain results in loss of imprinted expression of H19 and IGF2. *Genes Dev.* 1998;12(23):3693-3702.

177. Bell AC, Felsenfeld G. Methylation of a CTCF-dependent boundary controls imprinted expression of the IGF2 gene. *Nature.* 2000;405(6785):482-485.

178. Ohlsson R, Renkawitz R, Lobanenkov V. CTCF is a uniquely versatile transcription regulator linked to epigenetics and disease. *Trends Genet.* 2001;17(9):520-527.

179. Reeve AE, Eccles MR, Wilkins RJ, et al. Expression of insulin-like growth factor-II transcripts in Wilms' tumour. *Nature.* 1985;317(6034):258-260.

180. Rainier S, Johnson LA, Dobry CJ, et al. Relaxation of imprinted genes in human cancer. *Nature.* 1993;362(6422):747-749.

181. Daughaday WH, Emanuele MA, Brooks MH, et al. Synthesis and secretion of insulin-like growth factor II by a leiomyosarcoma with associated hypoglycemia. *N Engl J Med.* 1988;319(22):1434-1440.

182. Sparago A, Cerrato F, Vernucci M, et al. Microdeletions in the human H19 DMR result in loss of IGF2 imprinting and Beckwith-Wiedemann syndrome. *Nat Genet.* 2004;36(9):958-960.

183. Jansen M, van Schaik FM, van Tol H, et al. Nucleotide sequences of cDNAs encoding precursors of human insulin-like growth factor II (IGF-II) and an IGF-II variant. *FEBS Lett.* 1985;179(2):243-246.

184. Gowan LK, Hampton B, Hill DJ, et al. Purification and characterization of a unique high molecular weight form of insulin-like growth factor II. *Endocrinology.* 1987;121(2):449-458.

185. Zapf J. Insulinlike growth factor binding proteins and tumor hypoglycemia. *Trends Endocrinol Metab.* 1995;6(2):37-42.

186. Donovan SM, Oh Y, Pham H, Rosenfeld RG. Ontogeny of serum insulin-like growth factor binding proteins in the rat. *Endocrinology.* 1989;125(5):2621-2627.

187. Oh Y, Muller HL, Neely EK, et al. New concepts in insulin-like growth factor receptor physiology. *Growth Regul.* 1993;3(2):113-123.

188. LeRoith D, Werner H, Beitner-Johnson D, Roberts CT Jr. Molecular and cellular aspects of the insulin-like growth factor I receptor. *Endocr Rev.* 1995;16(2):143-163.

189. Abbott AM, Bueno R, Pedrini MT, et al. Insulin-like growth factor I receptor gene structure. *J Biol Chem.* 1992;267(15):10759-10763.

190. Werner H, Woloschak M, Adamo M, et al. Developmental regulation of the rat insulin-like growth factor I receptor gene. *Proc Natl Acad Sci U S A.* 1989;86(19):7451-7455.

191. Treadway JL, Morrison BD, Soos MA, et al. Transdominant inhibition of tyrosine kinase activity in mutant insulin/insulin-like growth factor I hybrid receptors. *Proc Natl Acad Sci U S A.* 1991;88(1):214-218.

192. Werner H, Le Roith D. The insulin-like growth factor-I receptor signaling pathways are important for tumorigenesis and inhibition of apoptosis. *Crit Rev Oncog.* 1997;8(1):71-92.

193. Kadowaki T, Tamemoto H, Tobe K, et al. Insulin resistance and growth retardation in mice lacking insulin receptor substrate-1 and identification of insulin receptor substrate-2. *Diabet Med.* 1996;13(9 Suppl 6):S103-S108.

194. Marte BM, Downward J. PKB/Akt: connecting phosphoinositide 3-kinase to cell survival and beyond. *Trends Biochem Sci.* 1997;22(9):355-358.

195. Chao MV. Growth factor signaling: where is the specificity? *Cell.* 1992;68(6):995-997.

196. Belfiore A, Frasca F, Pandini G, et al. Insulin receptor isoforms and insulin receptor/insulin-like growth factor receptor hybrids in physiology and disease. *Endocr Rev.* 2009;30(6):586-623.

197. MacDonald RG, Pfeffer SR, Coussens L, et al. A single receptor binds both insulin-like growth factor II and mannose-6-phosphate. *Science.* 1988;239(4844):1134-1137.

198. Braulke T. Type-2 IGF receptor: a multi-ligand binding protein. *Horm Metab Res.* 1999;31(2-3):242-246.

199. Kalscheuer VM, Mariman EC, Schepens MT, et al. The insulin-like growth factor type-2 receptor gene is imprinted in the mouse but not in humans. *Nat Genet.* 1993;5(1):74-78.

200. Ludwig T, Tenscher K, Remmler J, et al. Cloning and sequencing of cDNAs encoding the full-length mouse mannose 6-phosphate/insulin-like growth factor II receptor. *Gene.* 1994;142(2):311-312.

201. Olson LJ, Hancock MK, Dix D, et al. Mutational analysis of the binding site residues of the bovine cation-dependent mannose 6-phosphate receptor. *J Biol Chem.* 1999;274(52):36905-36911.

202. Causin C, Waheed A, Braulke T, et al. Mannose 6-phosphate/insulin-like growth factor II-binding proteins in human serum and urine. Their relation to the mannose 6-phosphate/insulin-like growth factor II receptor. *Biochem J.* 1988;252(3):795-799.

203. Scott CD, Weiss J. Soluble insulin-like growth factor II/mannose 6-phosphate receptor inhibits DNA synthesis in insulin-like growth factor II sensitive cells. *J Cell Physiol.* 2000;182(1):62-68.

204. Scott CD, Ballesteros M, Madrid J, Baxter RC. Soluble insulin-like growth factor-II/mannose 6-P receptor inhibits deoxyribonucleic acid synthesis in cultured rat hepatocytes. *Endocrinology.* 1996;137(3):873-878.

205. Dennis PA, Rifkin DB. Cellular activation of latent transforming growth factor beta requires binding to the cation-independent mannose 6-phosphate/insulin-like growth factor type II receptor. *Proc Natl Acad Sci U S A.* 1991;88(2):580-584.

206. Blanchard F, Duplomb L, Raher S, et al. Mannose 6-phosphate/insulin-like growth factor II receptor mediates internalization and degradation of leukemia inhibitory factor but not signal transduction. *J Biol Chem.* 1999;274(35):24685-24693.

207. Rosenfeld RG, Conover CA, Hodges D, et al. Heterogeneity of insulin-like growth factor-I affinity for the insulin-like growth factor-II receptor: comparison of natural, synthetic and recombinant DNA-derived insulin-like growth factor-I. *Biochem Biophys Res Commun.* 1987;143(1):199-205.

208. El-Shewy HM, Luttrell LM. Insulin-like growth factor-2/mannose-6 phosphate receptors. *Vitam Horm.* 2009;80:667-697.

209. Lau MM, Stewart CE, Liu Z, et al. Loss of the imprinted IGF2/cation-independent mannose 6-phosphate receptor results in fetal overgrowth and perinatal lethality. *Genes Dev.* 1994;8(24):2953-2963.

210. Beukers MW, Oh Y, Zhang H, et al. Leu[27] insulin-like growth factor II is highly selective for the type-II IGF receptor in binding, cross-linking and thymidine incorporation experiments. *Endocrinology.* 1991;128(2):1201-1203.

211. Mottola C, Czech MP. The type II insulin-like growth factor receptor does not mediate increased DNA synthesis in H-35 hepatoma cells. *J Biol Chem.* 1984;259(20):12705-12713.

212. Kiess W, Haskell JF, Lee L, et al. An antibody that blocks insulin-like growth factor (IGF) binding to the type II IGF receptor is neither an agonist nor an inhibitor of IGF-stimulated biologic responses in L6 myoblasts. *J Biol Chem.* 1987;262(26):12745-12751.

213. Adashi EY, Resnick CE, Rosenfeld RG. Insulin-like growth factor-I (IGF-I) hormonal action in cultured rat granulosa cells: mediation via type I but not type II IGF receptors. *Endocrinology.* 1989;126:216-222.

214. Efstratiadis A. Genetics of mouse growth. *Int J Dev Biol.* 1998;42(7):955-976.

215. Baker J, Liu JP, Robertson EJ, Efstratiadis A. Role of insulin-like growth factors in embryonic and postnatal growth. *Cell.* 1993;75(1):73-82.

216. Woods KA, Camacho-Hubner C, Savage MO, Clark AJ. Intrauterine growth retardation and postnatal growth failure associated with deletion of the insulin-like growth factor I gene. *N Engl J Med.* 1996;335(18):1363-1367.

217. Walenkamp MJ, Karperien M, Pereira AM, et al. Homozygous and heterozygous expression of a novel insulin-like growth factor-I mutation. *J Clin Endocrinol Metab.* 2005;90(5):2855-2864.

218. Sjogren K, Liu JL, Blad K, et al. Liver-derived insulin-like growth factor I (IGF-I) is the principal source of IGF-I in blood but is not required for postnatal body growth in mice. *Proc Natl Acad Sci U S A.* 1999;96(12):7088-7092.

219. Le Roith D, Bondy C, Yakar S, et al. The somatomedin hypothesis: 2001. *Endocr Rev.* 2001;22(1):53-74.

220. Ueki I, Ooi GT, Tremblay ML, et al. Inactivation of the acid labile subunit gene in mice results in mild retardation of postnatal growth despite profound disruptions in the circulating insulin-like growth factor system. *Proc Natl Acad Sci U S A.* 2000;97(12):6868-68673.

221. Yakar S, Rosen CJ, Beamer WG, et al. Circulating levels of IGF-1 directly regulate bone growth and density. *J Clin Invest.* 2002;110(6):771-781.

222. Liu JP, Baker J, Perkins AS, et al. Mice carrying null mutations of the genes encoding insulin-like growth factor I (IGF-1) and type 1 IGF receptor (IGF1r). *Cell.* 1993;75(1):59-72.

223. Abuzzahab MJ, Schneider A, Goddard A, et al. IGF-I receptor mutations resulting in intrauterine and postnatal growth retardation. *N Engl J Med.* 2003;349(23):2211-2222.

224. Filson AJ, Louvi A, Efstratiadis A, Robertson EJ. Rescue of the T-associated maternal effect in mice carrying null mutations in igf-2 and igf2r, two reciprocally imprinted genes. *Development.* 1993;118(3):731-736.

225. Constancia M, Hemberger M, Hughes J, et al. Placental-specific IGF-II is a major modulator of placental and fetal growth. *Nature.* 2002;417(6892):945-948.

226. Jones JI, Clemmons DR. Insulin-like growth factors and their binding proteins: biological actions. *Endocr Rev.* 1995;16:3-34.

227. Bach LA, Headey SJ, Norton RS. IGF-binding proteins—the pieces are falling into place. *Trends Endocrinol Metab.* 2005;16(5):228-234.

228. Buckway CK, Wilson EM, Ahlsen M, et al. Mutation of three critical amino acids of the N-terminal domain of IGF-binding protein-3 essential for high affinity IGF binding. *J Clin Endocrinol Metab.* 2001;86(10):4943-4950.

229. Jones JI, Gockerman A, Busby WH Jr, et al. Insulin-like growth factor binding protein 1 stimulates cell migration and binds to the alpha 5 beta 1 integrin by means of its arg-gly-asp sequence. *Proc Natl Acad Sci U S A.* 1993;90(22):10553-10557.

230. Oh Y, Muller HL, Lamson G, Rosenfeld RG. Insulin-like growth factor (IGF)-independent action of IGF-binding protein-3 in Hs578T human breast cancer cells. Cell surface binding and growth inhibition. *J Biol Chem.* 1993;268(20):14964-14971.

231. Firth SM, Baxter RC. Cellular actions of the insulin-like growth factor binding proteins. *Endocr Rev.* 2002;23(6):824-854.

232. Sitar T, Popowicz GM, Siwanowicz I, et al. Structural basis for the inhibition of insulin-like growth factors by insulin-like growth factor-binding proteins. *Proc Natl Acad Sci U S A.* 2006;103(35):13028-13033.

233. Kuang Z, Yao S, McNeil KA, et al. Cooperativity of the N- and C-terminal domains of insulin-like growth factor (IGF) binding protein 2 in IGF binding. *Biochemistry.* 2007;46(48):13720-13732.

234. Hwa V, Oh Y, Rosenfeld RG. The insulin-like growth factor-binding protein (IGFBP) superfamily. *Endocr Rev.* 1999;20(6):761-787.

235. Giudice LC, de Zegher F, Gargosky SE, et al. Insulin-like growth factors and their binding proteins in the term and preterm human fetus and neonate with normal and extremes of intrauterine growth. *J Clin Endocrinol Metab.* 1995;80(5):1548-1555.

236. Lee DY, Park SK, Yorgin PD, et al. Alteration in insulin-like growth factor-binding proteins (IGFBPs) and IGFBP-3 protease activity in serum and urine from acute and chronic renal failure. *J Clin Endocrinol Metab.* 1994;79(5):1376-1382.

237. Conover CA, De Leon DD. Acid-activated insulin-like growth factor-binding protein-3 proteolysis in normal and transformed cells. Role of cathepsin D. *J Biol Chem.* 1994;269(10):7076-7080.

238. Fowlkes JL, Enghild JJ, Suzuki K, Nagase H. Matrix metalloproteinases degrade insulin-like growth factor-binding protein-3 in dermal fibroblast cultures. *J Biol Chem.* 1994;269(41):25742-25746.

239. Zadeh SM, Binoux M. The 16-kDa proteolytic fragment of insulin-like growth factor (IGF) binding protein-3 inhibits the mitogenic action of fibroblast growth factor on mouse fibroblasts with a targeted disruption of the type 1 IGF receptor gene. *Endocrinology.* 1997;138(7):3069-3072.

240. Andress DL, Loop SM, Zapf J, Kiefer MC. Carboxy-truncated insulin-like growth factor binding protein-5 stimulates mitogenesis in osteoblast-like cells. *Biochem Biophys Res Commun.* 1993;195(1):25-30.

241. Oh Y, Muller HL, Lee DY, et al. Characterization of the affinities of insulin-like growth factor (IGF)-binding proteins 1-4 for IGF-I, IGF-II, IGF-I/insulin hybrid, and IGF-I analogs. *Endocrinology.* 1993;132(3):1337-1344.

242. Leong SR, Baxter RC, Camerato T, et al. Structure and functional expression of the acid-labile subunit of the insulin-like growth factor-binding protein complex. *Mol Endocrinol.* 1992;6(6):870-876.

243. Guler HP, Zapf J, Schmid C, Froesch ER. Insulin-like growth factors I and II in healthy man. Estimations of half-lives and production rates. *Acta Endocrinol (Copenh).* 1989;121(6):753-758.

244. Bar RS, Boes M, Clemmons DR, et al. Insulin differentially alters transcapillary movement of intravascular IGFBP-1, IGFBP-2 and endothelial cell IGF-binding proteins in the rat heart. *Endocrinology.* 1990;127(1):497-499.

245. Gargosky SE, Tapanainen P, Rosenfeld RG. Administration of growth hormone (GH), but not insulin-like growth factor-I (IGF-I), by continuous infusion can induce the formation of the 150-kilodalton IGF-binding protein-3 complex in GH-deficient rats. *Endocrinology.* 1994;134(5):2267-2276.

246. Walker JL, Baxter RC, Young S, et al. Effects of recombinant insulin-like growth factor I on IGF binding proteins and the acid-labile subunit in growth hormone insensitivity syndrome. *Growth Regul.* 1993;3(1):109-112.

247. Rajaram S, Baylink DJ, Mohan S. Insulin-like growth factor-binding proteins in serum and other biological fluids: regulation and functions. *Endocr Rev.* 1997;18(6):801-831.

248. Mohan S, Baylink DJ. IGF-binding proteins are multifunctional and act via IGF-dependent and -independent mechanisms. *J Endocrinol.* 2002;175(1):19-31.

249. Miyakoshi N, Richman C, Qin X, et al. Effects of recombinant insulin-like growth factor-binding protein-4 on bone formation parameters in mice. *Endocrinology.* 1999;140(12):5719-5728.

250. Cohen P, Lamson G, Okajima T, Rosenfeld RG. Transfection of the human IGFBP-3 gene into Balb/c fibroblasts: a model for the cellular functions of IGFBPs. *Growth Regul.* 1993;3(1):23-26.

251. Clemmons DR, Busby W, Clarke JB, et al. Modifications of insulin-like growth factor binding proteins and their role in controlling IGF actions. *Endocr J.* 1998;45(Suppl):S1-S8.

252. Nicolas V, Mohan S, Honda Y, et al. An age-related decrease in the concentration of insulin-like growth factor binding protein-5 in human cortical bone. *Calcif Tissue Int.* 1995;57(3):206-212.

253. Oh Y, Muller HL, Pham H, Rosenfeld RG. Demonstration of receptors for insulin-like growth factor binding protein-3 on Hs578T human breast cancer cells. *J Biol Chem.* 1993;268(35):26045-26048.

254. Bicsak TA, Shimonaka M, Malkowski M, Ling N. Insulin-like growth factor-binding protein (IGF-BP) inhibition of granulosa cell function: effect on cyclic adenosine 3′,5′-monophosphate, deoxyribonucleic acid synthesis, and comparison with the effect of an IGF-I antibody. *Endocrinology.* 1990;126(4):2184-2189.

255. Radulescu RT. Nuclear localization signal in insulin-like growth factor-binding protein type 3. *Trends Biochem Sci.* 1994;19(7):278.

256. Amaar YG, Thompson GR, Linkhart TA, et al. Insulin-like growth factor-binding protein 5 (IGFBP-5) interacts with a four and a half LIM protein 2 (FHL2). *J Biol Chem.* 2002;277(14):12053-12060.

257. Lalou C, Lassarre C, Binoux M. A proteolytic fragment of insulin-like growth factor (IGF) binding protein-3 that fails to bind IGFs inhibits the mitogenic effects of IGF-I and insulin. *Endocrinology.* 1996;137(8):3206-3212.

258. Brinkman A, Groffen CA, Kortleve DJ, Drop SL. Organization of the gene encoding the insulin-like growth factor binding protein IBP-1. *Biochem Biophys Res Commun.* 1988;157(3):898-907.

259. Unterman TG, Simmons RA, Glick RP, Ogata ES. Circulating levels of insulin, insulin-like growth factor-I (IGF-I), IGF-II, and IGF-binding proteins in the small for gestational age fetal rat. *Endocrinology.* 1993;132(1):327-336.

260. Wheatcroft SB, Kearney MT. IGF-dependent and IGF-independent actions of IGF-binding protein-1 and -2: implications for metabolic homeostasis. *Trends Endocrinol Metab.* 2009;20(4):153-162.

261. Wood TL, Rogler L, Streck RD, et al. Targeted disruption of IGFBP-2 gene. *Growth Regul.* 1993;3(1):5-8.

262. Lamson G, Pham H, Oh Y, et al. Expression of the BRL-3A insulin-like growth factor binding protein (rBP-30) in the rat central nervous system. *Endocrinology.* 1989;125(2):1100-1102.

263. Chin E, Zhou J, Dai J, et al. Cellular localization and regulation of gene expression for components of the insulin-like growth factor ternary binding protein complex. *Endocrinology.* 1994;134(6):2498-2504.

264. Yamanaka Y, Fowlkes JL, Wilson EM, et al. Characterization of insulin-like growth factor binding protein-3 (IGFBP-3) binding to human breast cancer cells: kinetics of IGFBP-3 binding and identification of receptor binding domain on the IGFBP-3 molecule. *Endocrinology.* 1999;140(3):1319-1328.

265. Janosi JB, Ramsland PA, Mott MR, et al. The acid-labile subunit of the serum insulin-like growth factor-binding protein complexes. Structural determination by molecular modeling and electron microscopy. *J Biol Chem.* 1999;274(33):23328-23332.

266. Zapf J, Hauri C, Waldvogel M, et al. Recombinant human insulin-like growth factor I induces its own specific carrier protein in

hypophysectomized and diabetic rats. *Proc Natl Acad Sci U S A.* 1989; 86(10):3813-3817.

267. Booth BA, Boes M, Andress DL, et al. IGFBP-3 and IGFBP-5 association with endothelial cells: role of C-terminal heparin binding domain. *Growth Regul.* 1995;5(1):1-17.

268. Schedlich LJ, Le Page SL, Firth SM, et al. Nuclear import of insulin-like growth factor-binding protein-3 and -5 is mediated by the importin beta subunit. *J Biol Chem.* 2000;275(31):23462-23470.

269. Liu B, Lee KW, Li H, et al. Combination therapy of insulin-like growth factor binding protein-3 and retinoid X receptor ligands synergize on prostate cancer cell apoptosis in vitro and in vivo. *Clin Cancer Res.* 2005;11(13):4851-4856.

270. Jogie-Brahim S, Feldman D, Oh Y. Unraveling insulin-like growth factor binding protein-3 actions in human disease. *Endocr Rev.* 2009; 30(5):417-437.

271. Buckbinder L, Talbott R, Velasco-Miguel S, et al. Induction of the growth inhibitor IGF-binding protein 3 by p53. *Nature.* 1995; 377(6550):646-649.

272. Grimberg A, Coleman CM, Burns TF, et al. p53-dependent and p53-independent induction of insulin-like growth factor binding protein-3 by deoxyribonucleic acid damage and hypoxia. *J Clin Endocrinol Metab.* 2005;90(6):3568-3574.

273. Herman JP, Jullien N, Guillen S, et al. Research resource: a genome-wide study identifies potential new target genes for POU1F1. *Mol Endocrinol.* 2012;26(8):1455-1463.

274. Conover CA, Kiefer MC, Zapf J. Posttranslational regulation of insulin-like growth factor binding protein-4 in normal and transformed human fibroblasts. Insulin-like growth factor dependence and biological studies. *J Clin Invest.* 1993;91(3):1129-1137.

275. Durham SK, Kiefer MC, Riggs BL, Conover CA. Regulation of insulin-like growth factor binding protein 4 by a specific insulin-like growth factor binding protein 4 proteinase in normal human osteoblast-like cells: implications in bone cell physiology. *J Bone Miner Res.* 1994; 9(1):111-117.

276. Neely EK, Rosenfeld RG. Insulin-like growth factors (IGFs) reduce IGF-binding protein-4 (IGFBP-4) concentration and stimulate IGFBP-3 independently of IGF receptors in human fibroblasts and epidermal cells. *Endocrinology.* 1992;130(2):985-993.

277. Rivera GM, Fortune JE. Selection of the dominant follicle and insulin-like growth factor (IGF)-binding proteins: evidence that pregnancy-associated plasma protein A contributes to proteolysis of IGF-binding protein 5 in bovine follicular fluid. *Endocrinology.* 2003;144(2): 437-446.

278. Hourvitz A, Kuwahara A, Hennebold JD, et al. The regulated expression of the pregnancy-associated plasma protein-A in the rodent ovary: a proposed role in the development of dominant follicles and of corpora lutea. *Endocrinology.* 2002;143(5):1833-1844.

279. Jones JI, Gockerman A, Busby WH Jr, et al. Extracellular matrix contains insulin-like growth factor binding protein-5: potentiation of the effects of IGF-I. *J Cell Biol.* 1993;121(3):679-687.

280. Clemmons DR, Nam TJ, Busby WH, et al. Modification of IGF action by insulin-like growth factor binding protein-5. In: Baxter RC, Gluckman PD, Rosenfeld RG, eds. *The Insulin-like Growth Factors and Their Regulatory Proteins.* Amsterdam: Elsevier; 1994.

281. Conover CA, Kiefer MC. Regulation and biological effect of endogenous insulin-like growth factor binding protein-5 in human osteoblastic cells. *J Clin Endocrinol Metab.* 1993;76(5):1153-1159.

282. Andress DL, Birnbaum RS. Human osteoblast-derived insulin-like growth factor (IGF) binding protein-5 stimulates osteoblast mitogenesis and potentiates IGF action. *J Biol Chem.* 1992;267(31):22467-22472.

283. Bach LA, Thotakura NR, Rechler MM. Human insulin-like growth factor binding protein-6 is O-glycosylated. *Growth Regul.* 1993; 3(1):59-62.

284. Roghani M, Lassarre C, Zapf J, et al. Two insulin-like growth factor (IGF)-binding proteins are responsible for the selective affinity for IGF-II of cerebrospinal fluid binding proteins. *J Clin Endocrinol Metab.* 1991;73(3):658-666.

285. Rohan RM, Ricciarelli E, Kiefer MC, et al. Rat ovarian insulin-like growth factor-binding protein-6: a hormonally regulated theca-interstitial-selective species with limited antigonadotropic activity. *Endocrinology.* 1993;132(6):2507-2512.

286. Wood TL, Rogler LE, Czick ME, et al. Selective alterations in organ sizes in mice with a targeted disruption of the insulin-like growth factor binding protein-2 gene. *Mol Endocrinol.* 2000;14(9): 1472-1482.

287. Ning Y, Schuller AG, Bradshaw S, et al. Diminished growth and enhanced glucose metabolism in triple knockout mice containing mutations of insulin-like growth factor binding protein-3, -4, and -5. *Mol Endocrinol.* 2006;20(9):2173-2186.

288. Silha JV, Murphy LJ. Insights from insulin-like growth factor binding protein transgenic mice. *Endocrinology.* 2002;143(10):3711-3714.

289. Morishima A, Grumbach MM, Simpson ER, et al. Aromatase deficiency in male and female siblings caused by a novel mutation and the physiological role of estrogens. *J Clin Endocrinol Metab.* 1995; 80(12):3689-3698.

290. Lorentzon M, Lorentzon R, Backstrom T, et al. Estrogen receptor gene polymorphism, but not estradiol levels, is related to bone density in healthy adolescent boys: a cross-sectional and longitudinal study. *J Clin Endocrinol Metab.* 1990;84:4597-4601.

291. Lehrer S, Rabin J, Stone J, Berkowitz GS. Association of an estrogen receptor variant with increased height in women. *Horm Metab Res.* 1994;26(10):486-488.

292. Demura M, Martin RM, Shozu M, et al. Regional rearrangements in chromosome 15q21 cause formation of cryptic promoters for the CYP19 (aromatase) gene. *Hum Mol Genet.* 2007;16(21):2529-2541.

293. Martin RM, Lin CJ, Nishi MY, et al. Familial hyperestrogenism in both sexes: clinical, hormonal, and molecular studies of two siblings. *J Clin Endocrinol Metab.* 2003;88(7):3027-3034.

294. Nilsson O, Marino R, De Luca F, et al. Endocrine regulation of the growth plate. *Horm Res.* 2005;64(4):157-165.

295. Matkovic V. Skeletal development and bone turnover revisited. *J Clin Endocrinol Metab.* 1996;81(6):2013-2016.

296. Abrams SA, O'Brien KO, Stuff JE. Changes in calcium kinetics associated with menarche. *J Clin Endocrinol Metab.* 1996;81(6):2017-2020.

297. Slemenda CW, Reister TK, Hui SL, et al. Influences on skeletal mineralization in children and adolescents: evidence for varying effects of sexual maturation and physical activity. *J Pediatr.* 1996;125: 201-207.

298. Wexler JA, Sharretts J. Thyroid and bone. *Endocrinol Metab Clin North Am.* 2007;36(3):673-705, vi.

299. Robson H, Siebler T, Shalet SM, Williams GR. Interactions between GH, IGF-I, glucocorticoids, and thyroid hormones during skeletal growth. *Pediatr Res.* 2002;52(2):137-147.

300. Siebler T, Robson H, Shalet SM, Williams GR. Glucocorticoids, thyroid hormone and growth hormone interactions: implications for the growth plate. *Horm Res.* 2001;56(Suppl 1):7-12.

301. Mazziotti G, Giustina A. Glucocorticoids and the regulation of growth hormone secretion. *Nat Rev Endocrinol.* 2013;9(5):265-276.

302. Veldhuis JD, Lizarralde G, Iranmanesh A. Divergent effects of short term glucocorticoid excess on the gonadotropic and somatotropic axes in normal men. *J Clin Endocrinol Metab.* 1992;74(1):96-102.

303. Jux C, Leiber K, Hugel U, et al. Dexamethasone impairs growth hormone (GH)-stimulated growth by suppression of local insulin-like growth factor (IGF)-I production and expression of GH- and IGF-I-receptor in cultured rat chondrocytes. *Endocrinology.* 1998;139(7): 3296-3305.

304. Hochberg Z. Mechanisms of steroid impairment of growth. *Horm Res.* 2002;58(Suppl 1):33-38.

305. Grumbach MM, Kaplan SL. Fetal pituitary hormones and the maturation of central nervous system regulation of anterior pituitary function. In: Gluck L, ed. *Modern Perinatal Medicine.* Chicago, IL: Year Book Medical Publishers; 1974.

306. Pombo M, Barreiro J, Penalva A, et al. Absence of growth hormone (GH) secretion after the administration of either GH-releasing hormone (GHRH), GH-releasing peptide (GHRP-6), or GHRH plus GHRP-6 in children with neonatal pituitary stalk transection. *J Clin Endocrinol Metab.* 1995;80(11):3180-3184.

307. Nagel BH, Palmbach M, Petersen D, Ranke MB. Magnetic resonance images of 91 children with different causes of short stature: pituitary size reflects growth hormone secretion. *Eur J Pediatr.* 1997;156(10): 758-763.

308. Argyropoulou M, Perignon F, Brauner R, Brunelle F. Magnetic resonance imaging in the diagnosis of growth hormone deficiency. *J Pediatr.* 1992;120(6):886-891.

309. Kornreich L, Horev G, Lazar L, et al. MR findings in growth hormone deficiency: correlation with severity of hypopituitarism. *AJNR Am J Neuroradiol.* 1998;19(8):1495-1499.

310. Maghnie M, Larizza D, Triulzi F, et al. Hypopituitarism and stalk agenesis: a congenital syndrome worsened by breech delivery? *Horm Res.* 1991;35(3-4):104-108.

311. Hellstrom A, Wiklund LM, Svensson E, et al. Midline brain lesions in children with hormone insufficiency indicate early prenatal damage. *Acta Paediatr.* 1998;87(5):528-536.

312. Wit JM, van Unen H. Growth of infants with neonatal growth hormone deficiency. *Arch Dis Child.* 1992;67(7):920-924.

313. De Luca F, Bernasconi S, Blandino A, et al. Auxological, clinical and neuroradiological findings in infants with early onset growth hormone deficiency. *Acta Paediatr.* 1995;84(5):561-565.

314. de Zegher F, Kaplan SL, Grumbach MM, et al. The foetal pituitary, postmaturity and breech presentation. *Acta Paediatr.* 1995;84(10): 1100-1102.

315. Roessler E, Muenke M. Holoprosencephaly: a paradigm for the complex genetics of brain development. *J Inherit Metab Dis.* 1998; 21(5):481-497.

316. Brown SA, Warburton D, Brown LY, et al. Holoprosencephaly due to mutations in ZIC2, a homologue of *Drosophila* odd-paired. *Nat Genet.* 1998;20(2):180-183.

317. Roessler E, Du YZ, Mullor JL, et al. Loss-of-function mutations in the human GLI2 gene are associated with pituitary anomalies and holoprosencephaly-like features. *Proc Natl Acad Sci U S A.* 2003; 100(23):13424-13429.

318. Treier M, O'Connell S, Gleiberman A, et al. Hedgehog signaling is required for pituitary gland development. *Development*. 2001;128(3): 377-386.

319. Roessler E, Muenke M. The molecular genetics of holoprosencephaly. *Am J Med Genet C Semin Med Genet*. 2010;154C(1):52-61.

320. Solomon BD, Pineda-Alvarez DE, Raam MS, et al. Analysis of component findings in 79 patients diagnosed with VACTERL association. *Am J Med Genet A*. 2010;152A(9):2236-2244.

321. Pineda-Alvarez DE, Dubourg C, David V, et al. Current recommendations for the molecular evaluation of newly diagnosed holoprosencephaly patients. *Am J Med Genet C Semin Med Genet*. 2010;154C(1): 93-101.

322. Hahn JS, Barnes PD. Neuroimaging advances in holoprosencephaly: refining the spectrum of the midline malformation. *Am J Med Genet C Semin Med Genet*. 2010;154C(1):120-132.

323. Mehta A, Dattani MT. Developmental disorders of the hypothalamus and pituitary gland associated with congenital hypopituitarism. *Best Pract Res Clin Endocrinol Metab*. 2008;22(1):191-206.

324. Ahmad T, Garcia-Filion P, Borchert M. Endocrinological and auxological abnormalities in young children with optic nerve hypoplasia: a prospective study. *J Pediatr*. 2006;148:78-84.

325. McCabe MJ, Alatzoglou KS, Dattani MT. Septo-optic dysplasia and other midline defects: the role of transcription factors: HESX1 and beyond. *Best Pract Res Clin Endocrinol Metab*. 2011;25(1):115-124.

326. Kelberman D, Rizzoti K, Lovell-Badge R, et al. Genetic regulation of pituitary gland development in human and mouse. *Endocr Rev*. 2009;30(7):790-829.

327. Patel L, McNally RJ, Harrison E, et al. Geographical distribution of optic nerve hypoplasia and septo-optic dysplasia in northwest England. *J Pediatr*. 2006;148(1):85-88.

328. Dattani MT, Martinez-Barbera JP, Thomas PQ, et al. Mutations in the homeobox gene HESX1/Hesx1 associated with septo-optic dysplasia in human and mouse. *Nat Genet*. 1998;19(2):125-133.

329. Hermesz E, Mackem S, Mahon KA. Rpx: a novel anterior-restricted homeobox gene progressively activated in the prechordal plate, anterior neural plate and Rathke's pouch of the mouse embryo. *Development*. 1996;122(1):41-52.

330. Sobrier ML, Netchine I, Heinrichs C, et al. Alu-element insertion in the homeodomain of HESX1 and aplasia of the anterior pituitary. *Hum Mutat*. 2005;25(5):503.

331. Dattani MT, Robinson IC. HESX1 and septo-optic dysplasia. *Rev Endocr Metab Disord*. 2002;3(4):289-300.

332. Carvalho LR, Woods KS, Mendonca BB, et al. A homozygous mutation in HESX1 is associated with evolving hypopituitarism due to impaired repressor-corepressor interaction. *J Clin Invest*. 2003;112(8): 1192-1201.

333. Thomas PQ, Johnson BV, Rathjen J, Rathjen PD. Sequence, genomic organization, and expression of the novel homeobox gene Hesx1. *J Biol Chem*. 1995;270(8):3869-3875.

334. Dasen JS, Martinez Barbera JP, Herman TS, et al. Temporal regulation of a paired-like homeodomain repressor/TLE corepressor complex and a related activator is required for pituitary organogenesis. *Genes Dev*. 2001;15(23):3193-3207.

335. Cohen RN, Cohen LE, Botero D, et al. Enhanced repression by HESX1 as a cause of hypopituitarism and septooptic dysplasia. *J Clin Endocrinol Metab*. 2003;88(10):4832-4839.

336. Chou SJ, Hermesz E, Hatta T, et al. Conserved regulatory elements establish the dynamic expression of Rpx/HesxI in early vertebrate development. *Dev Biol*. 2006;292(2):533-545.

337. Gaston-Massuet C, Andoniadou CL, Signore M, et al. Genetic interaction between the homeobox transcription factors HESX1 and SIX3 is required for normal pituitary development. *Dev Biol*. 2008;324(2): 322-333.

338. McNay DE, Turton JP, Kelberman D, et al. HESX1 mutations are an uncommon cause of septooptic dysplasia and hypopituitarism. *J Clin Endocrinol Metab*. 2007;92(2):691-697.

339. Brickman JM, Clements M, Tyrell R, et al. Molecular effects of novel mutations in Hesx1/HESX1 associated with human pituitary disorders. *Development*. 2001;128(24):5189-5199.

340. Sobrier ML, Maghnie M, Vie-Luton MP, et al. Novel HESX1 mutations associated with a life-threatening neonatal phenotype, pituitary aplasia, but normally located posterior pituitary and no optic nerve abnormalities. *J Clin Endocrinol Metab*. 2006;91(11):4528-4536.

341. Coya R, Vela A, Perez de Nanclares G, et al. Panhypopituitarism: genetic versus acquired etiological factors. *J Pediatr Endocrinol Metab*. 2007;20(1):27-36.

342. Tajima T, Hattorri T, Nakajima T, et al. Sporadic heterozygous frameshift mutation of HESX1 causing pituitary and optic nerve hypoplasia and combined pituitary hormone deficiency in a Japanese patient. *J Clin Endocrinol Metab*. 2003;88(1):45-50.

343. Radovick S, Cohen LE, Wondisford FE. The molecular basis of hypopituitarism. *Horm Res*. 1998;49(Suppl 1):30-36.

344. Sajedi E, Gaston-Massuet C, Signore M, et al. Analysis of mouse models carrying the I26T and R160C substitutions in the transcriptional repressor HESX1 as models for septo-optic dysplasia and hypopituitarism. *Dis Model Mech*. 2008;1(4-5):241-254.

345. Kurokawa D, Takasaki N, Kiyonari H, et al. Regulation of Otx2 expression and its functions in mouse epiblast and anterior neuroectoderm. *Development*. 2004;131(14):3307-3317.

346. Dateki S, Kosaka K, Hasegawa K, et al. Heterozygous orthodenticle homeobox 2 mutations are associated with variable pituitary phenotype. *J Clin Endocrinol Metab*. 2010;95(2):756-764.

347. Diaczok D, Romero C, Zunich J, et al. A novel dominant negative mutation of OTX2 associated with combined pituitary hormone deficiency. *J Clin Endocrinol Metab*. 2008;93(11):4351-4359.

348. Lagerstrom-Fermer M, Sundvall M, Johnsen E, et al. X-linked recessive panhypopituitarism associated with a regional duplication in Xq25-q26. *Am J Hum Genet*. 1997;60(4):910-916.

349. Hol FA, Schepens MT, van Beersum SE, et al. Identification and characterization of an Xq26-q27 duplication in a family with spina bifida and panhypopituitarism suggests the involvement of two distinct genes. *Genomics*. 2000;69(2):174-181.

350. Woods KS, Cundall M, Turton J, et al. Over- and underdosage of SOX3 is associated with infundibular hypoplasia and hypopituitarism. *Am J Hum Genet*. 2005;76(5):833-849.

351. Laumonnier F, Ronce N, Hamel BC, et al. Transcription factor SOX3 is involved in X-linked mental retardation with growth hormone deficiency. *Am J Hum Genet*. 2002;71(6):1450-1455.

352. Lim HN, Berkovitz GD, Hughes IA, Hawkins JR. Mutation analysis of subjects with 46, XX sex reversal and 46, XY gonadal dysgenesis does not support the involvement of SOX3 in testis determination. *Hum Genet*. 2000;107(6):650-652.

353. Raverot G, Lejeune H, Kotlar T, et al. X-linked sex-determining region Y box 3 (SOX3) gene mutations are uncommon in men with idiopathic oligoazoospermic infertility. *J Clin Endocrinol Metab*. 2004; 89(8):4146-4148.

354. Kelberman D, Rizzoti K, Avilion A, et al. Mutations within Sox2/SOX2 are associated with abnormalities in the hypothalamo-pituitary-gonadal axis in mice and humans. *J Clin Invest*. 2006;116(9): 2442-2455.

355. Fantes J, Ragge NK, Lynch SA, et al. Mutations in SOX2 cause anophthalmia. *Nat Genet*. 2003;33(4):461-463.

356. Williamson KA, Hever AM, Rainger J, et al. Mutations in SOX2 cause anophthalmia-esophageal-genital (AEG) syndrome. *Hum Mol Genet*. 2006;15(9):1413-1422.

357. Chassaing N, Gilbert-Dussardier B, Nicot F, et al. Germinal mosaicism and familial recurrence of a SOX2 mutation with highly variable phenotypic expression extending from AEG syndrome to absence of ocular involvement. *Am J Med Genet A*. 2007;143(3):289-291.

358. Faivre L, Williamson KA, Faber V, et al. Recurrence of SOX2 anophthalmia syndrome with gonosomal mosaicism in a phenotypically normal mother. *Am J Med Genet A*. 2006;140(6):636-639.

359. Kelberman D, Dattani MT. Role of transcription factors in midline central nervous system and pituitary defects. *Endocr Dev*. 2009;14: 67-82.

360. Falorni A, Minarelli V, Bartoloni E, et al. Diagnosis and classification of autoimmune hypophysitis. *Autoimmun Rev*. 2014;13(4-5):412-416.

361. Carpinteri R, Patelli I, Casanueva FF, Giustina A. Pituitary tumours: inflammatory and granulomatous expansive lesions of the pituitary. *Best Pract Res Clin Endocrinol Metab*. 2009;23(5):639-650.

362. Sklar CA. Childhood brain tumors. *J Pediatr Endocrinol Metab*. 2002; 15(suppl 2):669-673.

363. Weinzimer SA, Homan SA, Ferry RJ, Moshang T. Serum IGF-I and IGFBP-3 concentrations do not accurately predict growth hormone deficiency in children with brain tumours. *Clin Endocrinol (Oxf)*. 1999;51(3):339-345.

364. Rose SR, Auble BA. Endocrine changes after pediatric traumatic brain injury. *Pituitary*. 2012;15(3):267-275.

365. Hannon MJ, Sherlock M, Thompson CJ. Pituitary dysfunction following traumatic brain injury or subarachnoid haemorrhage in "endocrine management in the intensive care unit." *Best Pract Res Clin Endocrinol Metab*. 2011;25(5):783-798.

366. Gasco V, Prodam F, Pagano L, et al. Hypopituitarism following brain injury: when does it occur and how best to test? *Pituitary*. 2012; 15(1):20-24.

367. Powell GF, Brasel JA, Raiti S, Blizzard RM. Emotional deprivation and growth retardation simulating idiopathic hypopituitarism. II. Endocrinologic evaluation of the syndrome. *N Engl J Med*. 1967;276(23): 1279-1283.

368. Skuse D, Albanese A, Stanhope R, et al. A new stress-related syndrome of growth failure and hyperphagia in children, associated with reversibility of growth-hormone insufficiency. *Lancet*. 1996;348(9024): 353-358.

369. Pine DS, Cohen P, Brook J. Emotional problems during youth as predictors of stature during early adulthood: results from a prospective epidemiologic study. *Pediatrics*. 1996;97(6 Pt 1):856-863.

370. Jensen JB, Garfinkel BD. Growth hormone dysregulation in children with major depressive disorder. *J Am Acad Child Adolesc Psychiatry*. 1990;29(2):295-301.

371. Bancalari RE, Gregory LC, McCabe MJ, Dattani MT. Pituitary gland development: an update. *Endocr Dev*. 2012;23:1-15.

372. Wang J, Sun Z, Zhang Z, et al. Protein inhibitors of activated STAT (Pias1 and piasy) differentially regulate pituitary homeobox 2 (PITX2) transcriptional activity. *J Biol Chem*. 2013;288(18):12580-12595.

373. Drouin J, Lamolet B, Lamonerie T, et al. The PTX family of homeodomain transcription factors during pituitary developments. *Mol Cell Endocrinol*. 1998;140(1-2):31-36.

374. Tremblay JJ, Lanctot C, Drouin J. The pan-pituitary activator of transcription, Ptx1 (pituitary homeobox 1), acts in synergy with SF-1 and Pit1 and is an upstream regulator of the lim-homeodomain gene Lim3/Lhx3. *Mol Endocrinol*. 1998;12(3):428-441.

375. Tremblay JJ, Goodyer CG, Drouin J. Transcriptional properties of Ptx1 and Ptx2 isoforms. *Neuroendocrinology*. 2000;71(5):277-286.

376. Lin CR, Kioussi C, O'Connell S, et al. Pitx2 regulates lung asymmetry, cardiac positioning and pituitary and tooth morphogenesis. *Nature*. 1999;401(6750):279-282.

377. Lu MF, Pressman C, Dyer R, et al. Function of Rieger syndrome gene in left-right asymmetry and craniofacial development. *Nature*. 1999; 401(6750):276-278.

378. Kitamura K, Miura H, Miyagawa-Tomita S, et al. Mouse Pitx2 deficiency leads to anomalies of the ventral body wall, heart, extra- and periocular mesoderm and right pulmonary isomerism. *Development*. 1999;126(24):5749-5758.

379. Gage PJ, Suh H, Camper SA. Dosage requirement of Pitx2 for development of multiple organs. *Development*. 1999;126(20):4643-4651.

380. Kioussi C, Briata P, Baek SH, et al. Identification of a Wnt/Dvl/beta-catenin → Pitx2 pathway mediating cell-type-specific proliferation during development. *Cell*. 2002;111(5):673-685.

381. Briata P, Ilengo C, Corte G, et al. The Wnt/beta-catenin → Pitx2 pathway controls the turnover of Pitx2 and other unstable mRNAs. *Mol Cell*. 2003;12(5):1201-1211.

382. Charles MA, Suh H, Hjalt TA, et al. PITX genes are required for cell survival and Lhx3 activation. *Mol Endocrinol*. 2005;19(7):1893-1903.

383. Suh H, Gage PJ, Drouin J, Camper SA. Pitx2 is required at multiple stages of pituitary organogenesis: pituitary primordium formation and cell specification. *Development*. 2002;129(2):329-337.

384. Zhang Z, Gutierrez D, Li X, et al. The LIM homeodomain transcription factor LHX6: a transcriptional repressor that interacts with pituitary homeobox 2 (PITX2) to regulate odontogenesis. *J Biol Chem*. 2013;288(4):2485-2500.

385. Franco D, Kelly RG. Contemporary cardiogenesis: new insights into heart development. *Cardiovasc Res*. 2011;91(2):183-184.

386. John LB, Trengove MC, Fraser FW, et al. Pegasus, the "atypical" ikaros family member, influences left-right asymmetry and regulates pitx2 expression. *Dev Biol*. 2013;377(1):46-54.

387. Amendt BA, Semina EV, Alward WL. Rieger syndrome: a clinical, molecular, and biochemical analysis. *Cell Mol Life Sci*. 2000;57(11): 1652-1666.

388. Saadi I, Semina EV, Amendt BA, et al. Identification of a dominant negative homeodomain mutation in Rieger syndrome. *J Biol Chem*. 2001;276(25):23034-23041.

389. Colvin SC, Malik RE, Showalter AD, et al. Model of pediatric pituitary hormone deficiency separates the endocrine and neural functions of the LHX3 transcription factor in vivo. *Proc Natl Acad Sci U S A*. 2011;108(1):173-178.

390. Prince KL, Colvin SC, Park S, et al. Developmental analysis and influence of genetic background on the Lhx3 W227ter mouse model of combined pituitary hormone deficiency disease. *Endocrinology*. 2013; 154(2):738-748.

391. Park S, Mullen RD, Rhodes SJ. Cell-specific actions of a human LHX3 gene enhancer during pituitary and spinal cord development. *Mol Endocrinol*. 2013;27(12):2013-2027.

392. Sloop KW, Dwyer CJ, Rhodes SJ. An isoform-specific inhibitory domain regulates the LHX3 LIM homeodomain factor holoprotein and the production of a functional alternate translation form. *J Biol Chem*. 2001;276(39):36311-36319.

393. Hunter CS, Malik RE, Witzmann FA, Rhodes SJ. LHX3 interacts with inhibitor of histone acetyltransferase complex subunits LANP and TAF-1beta to modulate pituitary gene regulation. *PLoS ONE*. 2013; 8(7):e68898.

394. Bechtold-Dalla Pozza S, Hiedl S, Roeb J, et al. A recessive mutation resulting in a disabling amino acid substitution (T194R) in the LHX3 homeodomain causes combined pituitary hormone deficiency. *Horm Res Paediatr*. 2012;77(1):41-51.

395. Sobrier ML, Brachet C, Vie-Luton MP, et al. Symptomatic heterozygotes and prenatal diagnoses in a nonconsanguineous family with syndromic combined pituitary hormone deficiency resulting from two novel LHX3 mutations. *J Clin Endocrinol Metab*. 2012;97(3): E503-E509.

396. Bonfig W, Krude H, Schmidt H. A novel mutation of LHX3 is associated with combined pituitary hormone deficiency including ACTH deficiency, sensorineural hearing loss, and short neck—a case report and review of the literature. *Eur J Pediatr*. 2011;170(8):1017-1021.

397. Pfaeffle RW, Savage JJ, Hunter CS, et al. Four novel mutations of the LHX3 gene cause combined pituitary hormone deficiencies with or without limited neck rotation. *J Clin Endocrinol Metab*. 2007;92(5): 1909-1919.

398. Bhangoo AP, Hunter CS, Savage JJ, et al. Clinical case seminar: a novel LHX3 mutation presenting as combined pituitary hormonal deficiency. *J Clin Endocrinol Metab*. 2006;91(3):747-753.

399. Kristrom B, Zdunek AM, Rydh A, et al. A novel mutation in the LIM homeobox 3 gene is responsible for combined pituitary hormone deficiency, hearing impairment, and vertebral malformations. *J Clin Endocrinol Metab*. 2009;94(4):1154-1161.

400. Rajab A, Kelberman D, de Castro SC, et al. Novel mutations in LHX3 are associated with hypopituitarism and sensorineural hearing loss. *Hum Mol Genet*. 2008;17(14):2150-2159.

401. Mullen RD, Colvin SC, Hunter CS, et al. Roles of the LHX3 and LHX4 LIM-homeodomain factors in pituitary development. *Mol Cell Endocrinol*. 2007;265-266:190-195.

402. Raetzman LT, Ward R, Camper SA. Lhx4 and Prop1 are required for cell survival and expansion of the pituitary primordia. *Development*. 2002;129(18):4229-4239.

403. Sheng HZ, Moriyama K, Yamashita T, et al. Multistep control of pituitary organogenesis. *Science*. 1997;278(5344):1809-1812.

404. Takagi M, Ishii T, Inokuchi M, et al. Gradual loss of ACTH due to a novel mutation in LHX4: comprehensive mutation screening in Japanese patients with congenital hypopituitarism. *PLoS ONE*. 2012;7(9): e46008.

405. Dateki S, Fukami M, Uematsu A, et al. Mutation and gene copy number analyses of six pituitary transcription factor genes in 71 patients with combined pituitary hormone deficiency: identification of a single patient with LHX4 deletion. *J Clin Endocrinol Metab*. 2010;95(8):4043-4047.

406. Pfaeffle RW, Hunter CS, Savage JJ, et al. Three novel missense mutations within the LHX4 gene are associated with variable pituitary hormone deficiencies. *J Clin Endocrinol Metab*. 2008;93(3):1062-1071.

407. Machinis K, Amselem S. Functional relationship between LHX4 and POU1F1 in light of the LHX4 mutation identified in patients with pituitary defects. *J Clin Endocrinol Metab*. 2005;90(9):5456-5462.

408. Tajima T, Hattori T, Nakajima T, et al. A novel missense mutation (P366T) of the LHX4 gene causes severe combined pituitary hormone deficiency with pituitary hypoplasia, ectopic posterior lobe and a poorly developed sella turcica. *Endocr J*. 2007;54(4):637-641.

409. Gallardo ME, Rodriguez De Cordoba S, et al. Analysis of the developmental SIX6 homeobox gene in patients with anophthalmia/microphthalmia. *Am J Med Genet A*. 2004;129A(1):92-94.

410. Brinkmeier ML, Potok MA, Davis SW, Camper SA. TCF4 deficiency expands ventral diencephalon signaling and increases induction of pituitary progenitors. *Dev Biol*. 2007;311(2):396-407.

411. Zhu CC, Dyer MA, Uchikawa M, et al. Six3-mediated auto repression and eye development requires its interaction with members of the groucho-related family of co-repressors. *Development*. 2002;129(12): 2835-2849.

412. Lopez-Rios J, Tessmar K, Loosli F, et al. Six3 and Six6 activity is modulated by members of the groucho family. *Development*. 2003;130(1): 185-195.

413. Larder R, Clark DD, Miller NL, Mellon PL. Hypothalamic dysregulation and infertility in mice lacking the homeodomain protein Six6. *J Neurosci*. 2011;31(2):426-438.

414. Nolen LD, Amor D, Haywood A, et al. Deletion at 14q22-23 indicates a contiguous gene syndrome comprising anophthalmia, pituitary hypoplasia, and ear anomalies. *Am J Med Genet A*. 2006;140(16): 1711-1718.

415. Martinez-Frias ML, Ocejo-Vinyals JG, Arteaga R, et al. Interstitial deletion 14q22.3-q23.2: genotype-phenotype correlation. *Am J Med Genet A*. 2014;164A(3):639-647.

416. Mullen RD, Park S, Rhodes SJ. A distal modular enhancer complex acts to control pituitary- and nervous system-specific expression of the LHX3 regulatory gene. *Mol Endocrinol*. 2012;26(2):308-319.

417. Susa T, Ishikawa A, Cai LY, et al. The highly related LIM factors, LMO1, LMO3 and LMO4, play different roles in the regulation of the pituitary glycoprotein hormone alpha-subunit (alpha GSU) gene. *Biosci Rep*. 2009;30(1):51-58.

418. Cai Y, Xu Z, Nagarajan L, Brandt SJ. Single-stranded DNA-binding proteins regulate the abundance and function of the LIM-homeodomain transcription factor LHX2 in pituitary cells. *Biochem Biophys Res Commun*. 2008;373(2):303-308.

419. Takuma N, Sheng HZ, Furuta Y, et al. Formation of Rathke's pouch requires dual induction from the diencephalon. *Development*. 1998; 125(23):4835-4840.

420. Puustinen L, Jalanko H, Holmberg C, Merenmies J. Recombinant human growth hormone treatment after liver transplantation in childhood: the 5-year outcome. *Transplantation*. 2005;79(9):1241-1246.

421. Pfaffle R, Klammt J. Pituitary transcription factors in the aetiology of combined pituitary hormone deficiency. *Best Pract Res Clin Endocrinol Metab*. 2011;25(1):43-60.

422. Chen J, Crabbe A, Van Duppen V, Vankelecom H. The notch signaling system is present in the postnatal pituitary: marked expression and regulatory activity in the newly discovered side population. *Mol Endocrinol*. 2006;20(12):3293-3307.

423. Kita A, Imayoshi I, Hojo M, et al. Hes1 and Hes5 control the progenitor pool, intermediate lobe specification, and posterior lobe formation in the pituitary development. *Mol Endocrinol*. 2007;21(6):1458-1466.

424. Gage PJ, Brinkmeier ML, Scarlett LM, et al. The Ames dwarf gene, df, is required early in pituitary ontogeny for the extinction of rpx transcription and initiation of lineage-specific cell proliferation. *Mol Endocrinol*. 1996;10(12):1570-1581.

425. Ward RD, Raetzman LT, Suh H, et al. Role of PROP1 in pituitary gland growth. *Mol Endocrinol*. 2005;19(3):698-710.

426. Ward RD, Stone BM, Raetzman LT, Camper SA. Cell proliferation and vascularization in mouse models of pituitary hormone deficiency. *Mol Endocrinol*. 2006;20(6):1378-1390.

427. Andersen B, Pearse RV 2nd, Jenne K, et al. The Ames dwarf gene is required for pit-1 gene activation. *Dev Biol*. 1995;172(2):495-503.

428. Olson LE, Tollkuhn J, Scafoglio C, et al. Homeodomain-mediated beta-catenin-dependent switching events dictate cell-lineage determination. *Cell*. 2006;125(3):593-605.

429. Nakayama M, Kato T, Susa T, et al. Dimeric PROP1 binding to diverse palindromic TAAT sequences promotes its transcriptional activity. *Mol Cell Endocrinol*. 2009;307(1-2):36-42.

430. Ikeshita N, Kawagishi M, Shibahara H, et al. Identification and analysis of prophet of pit-1-binding sites in human pit-1 gene. *Endocrinology*. 2008;149(11):5491-5499.

431. Bartke A. Histology of the anterior hypophysis, thyroid and gonads of two types of dwarf mice. *Anat Rec*. 1964;149:225-235.

432. Bartke A. The response of two types of dwarf mice to growth hormone, thyrotropin, and thyroxine. *Gen Comp Endocrinol*. 1965;5(4):418-426.

433. Fluck C, Deladoey J, Rutishauser K, et al. Phenotypic variability in familial combined pituitary hormone deficiency caused by a PROP1 gene mutation resulting in the substitution of arg → Cys at codon 120 (R120C). *J Clin Endocrinol Metab*. 1998;83(10):3727-3734.

434. Osorio MG, Kopp P, Marui S, et al. Combined pituitary hormone deficiency caused by a novel mutation of a highly conserved residue (F88S) in the homeodomain of PROP-1. *J Clin Endocrinol Metab*. 2000;85(8):2779-2785.

435. Kelberman D, Turton JP, Woods KS, et al. Molecular analysis of novel PROP1 mutations associated with combined pituitary hormone deficiency (CPHD). *Clin Endocrinol (Oxf)*. 2009;70(1):96-103.

436. Lebl J, Vosahlo J, Pfaeffle RW, et al. Auxological and endocrine phenotype in a population-based cohort of patients with PROP1 gene defects. *Eur J Endocrinol*. 2005;153(3):389-396.

437. Vieira TC, da Silva MR, Abucham J. The natural history of the R120C PROP1 mutation reveals a wide phenotypic variability in two untreated adult brothers with combined pituitary hormone deficiency. *Endocrine*. 2006;30(3):365-369.

438. Deladoey J, Fluck C, Buyukgebiz A, et al. "Hot spot" in the PROP1 gene responsible for combined pituitary hormone deficiency. *J Clin Endocrinol Metab*. 1999;84(5):1645-1650.

439. Dattani MT. GH deficiency might be associated with normal height in PROP1 deficiency. *Clin Endocrinol (Oxf)*. 2002;57(2):157-158.

440. Arroyo A, Pernasetti F, Vasilyev VV, et al. A unique case of combined pituitary hormone deficiency caused by a PROP1 gene mutation (R120C) associated with normal height and absent puberty. *Clin Endocrinol (Oxf)*. 2002;57(2):283-291.

441. Pavel ME, Hensen J, Pfaffle R, et al. Long-term follow-up of childhood-onset hypopituitarism in patients with the PROP-1 gene mutation. *Horm Res*. 2003;60(4):168-173.

442. Voutetakis A, Argyropoulou M, Sertedaki A, et al. Pituitary magnetic resonance imaging in 15 patients with Prop1 gene mutations: pituitary enlargement may originate from the intermediate lobe. *J Clin Endocrinol Metab*. 2004;89(5):2200-2206.

443. Rosenbloom AL, Almonte AS, Brown MR, et al. Clinical and biochemical phenotype of familial anterior hypopituitarism from mutation of the PROP1 gene. *J Clin Endocrinol Metab*. 1999;84(1):50-57.

444. Mendonca BB, Osorio MG, Latronico AC, et al. Longitudinal hormonal and pituitary imaging changes in two females with combined pituitary hormone deficiency due to deletion of A301,G302 in the PROP1 gene. *J Clin Endocrinol Metab*. 1999;84(3):942-945.

445. Agarwal G, Bhatia V, Cook S, Thomas PQ. Adrenocorticotropin deficiency in combined pituitary hormone deficiency patients homozygous for a novel PROP1 deletion. *J Clin Endocrinol Metab*. 2000;85(12):4556-4561.

446. Asteria C, Oliveira JH, Abucham J, Beck-Peccoz P. Central hypocortisolism as part of combined pituitary hormone deficiency due to mutations of PROP-1 gene. *Eur J Endocrinol*. 2000;143(3):347-352.

447. Bottner A, Keller E, Kratzsch J, et al. PROP1 mutations cause progressive deterioration of anterior pituitary function including adrenal insufficiency: a longitudinal analysis. *J Clin Endocrinol Metab*. 2004;89(10):5256-5265.

448. Vallette-Kasic S, Barlier A, Teinturier C, et al. PROP1 gene screening in patients with multiple pituitary hormone deficiency reveals two sites of hypermutability and a high incidence of corticotroph deficiency. *J Clin Endocrinol Metab*. 2001;86(9):4529-4535.

449. Fofanova O, Takamura N, Kinoshita E, et al. Compound heterozygous deletion of the PROP-1 gene in children with combined pituitary hormone deficiency. *J Clin Endocrinol Metab*. 1998;83(7):2601-2604.

450. Wu W, Cogan JD, Pfaffle RW, et al. Mutations in PROP1 cause familial combined pituitary hormone deficiency. *Nat Genet*. 1998;18(2):147-149.

451. Shibahara H, Ikeshita N, Sugiyama Y, et al. W194XProp1 and S156insTProp1, both of which have intact DNA-binding domain, show a different DNA-binding activity to the Prop1-binding element in human pit-1 gene. *Mol Cell Endocrinol*. 2010;323(2):167-171.

452. Turton JP, Reynaud R, Mehta A, et al. Novel mutations within the POU1F1 gene associated with variable combined pituitary hormone deficiency. *J Clin Endocrinol Metab*. 2005;90(8):4762-4770.

453. Nyström HF, Saveanu A, Barbosa EJ, et al. Detection of genetic hypopituitarism in an adult population of idiopathic pituitary insufficiency patients with growth hormone deficiency. *Pituitary*. 2011;14(3):208-216.

454. Nelson C, Albert VR, Elsholtz HP, et al. Activation of cell-specific expression of rat growth hormone and prolactin genes by a common transcription factor. *Science*. 1988;239(4846):1400-1405.

455. Mangalam HJ, Albert VR, Ingraham HA, et al. A pituitary POU domain protein, pit-1, activates both growth hormone and prolactin promoters transcriptionally. *Genes Dev*. 1989;3(7):946-958.

456. Lin SC, Lin CR, Gukovsky I, et al. Molecular basis of the little mouse phenotype and implications for cell type-specific growth. *Nature*. 1993;364(6434):208-213.

457. Cohen LE, Zanger K, Brue T, et al. Defective retinoic acid regulation of the pit-1 gene enhancer: a novel mechanism of combined pituitary hormone deficiency. *Mol Endocrinol*. 1999;13(3):476-484.

458. Montminy M. Cell differentiation. The road not taken. *Nature*. 1993;364(6434):190-191.

459. Xu L, Lavinsky RM, Dasen JS, et al. Signal-specific co-activator domain requirements for pit-1 activation. *Nature*. 1998;395(6699):301-306.

460. Pfaffle RW, DiMattia GE, Parks JS, et al. Mutation of the POU-specific domain of pit-1 and hypopituitarism without pituitary hypoplasia. *Science*. 1992;257(5073):1118-1121.

461. Buckwalter MS, Katz RW, Camper SA. Localization of the panhypopituitary dwarf mutation (df) on mouse chromosome 11 in an intersubspecific backcross. *Genomics*. 1991;10(3):515-526.

462. Cogan JD, Phillips JA 3rd, Schenkman SS, et al. Familial growth hormone deficiency: a model of dominant and recessive mutations affecting a monomeric protein. *J Clin Endocrinol Metab*. 1994;79(5):1261-1265.

463. Cohen LE, Wondisford FE, Salvatoni A, et al. A "hot spot" in the pit-1 gene responsible for combined pituitary hormone deficiency: clinical and molecular correlates. *J Clin Endocrinol Metab*. 1995;80(2):679-684.

464. Tatsumi K, Miyai K, Notomi T, et al. Cretinism with combined hormone deficiency caused by a mutation in the PIT1 gene. *Nat Genet*. 1992;1(1):56-58.

465. Pellegrini-Bouiller I, Belicar P, Barlier A, et al. A new mutation of the gene encoding the transcription factor pit-1 is responsible for combined pituitary hormone deficiency. *J Clin Endocrinol Metab*. 1996;81(8):2790-2796.

466. Snabboon T, Plengpanich W, Buranasupkajorn P, et al. A novel germline mutation, IVS4+1G>A, of the POU1F1 gene underlying combined pituitary hormone deficiency. *Horm Res*. 2008;69(1):60-64.

467. Miyata I, Vallette-Kasic S, Saveanu A, et al. Identification and functional analysis of the novel S179R POU1F1 mutation associated with combined pituitary hormone deficiency. *J Clin Endocrinol Metab*. 2006;91(12):4981-4987.

468. Radovick S, Nations M, Du Y, et al. A mutation in the POU-homeodomain of pit-1 responsible for combined pituitary hormone deficiency. *Science*. 1992;257(5073):1115-1118.

469. Arnhold IJ, Nery M, Brown MR, et al. Clinical and molecular characterization of a Brazilian patient with pit-1 deficiency. *J Pediatr Endocrinol Metab*. 1998;11(5):623-630.

470. Kelberman D, Dattani MT. Hypopituitarism oddities: congenital causes. *Horm Res*. 2007;68(Suppl 5):138-144.

471. Pellegrini I, Roche C, Quentien MH, et al. Involvement of the pituitary-specific transcription factor pit-1 in somatolactotrope cell growth and death: an approach using dominant-negative pit-1 mutants. *Mol Endocrinol*. 2006;20(12):3212-3227.

472. Pine-Twaddell E, Romero CJ, Radovick S. Vertical transmission of hypopituitarism: critical importance of appropriate interpretation of thyroid function tests and levothyroxine therapy during pregnancy. *Thyroid*. 2013;23(7):892-897.

473. Cohen RN, Brue T, Naik K, et al. The role of CBP/p300 interactions and pit-1 dimerization in the pathophysiological mechanism of combined pituitary hormone deficiency. *J Clin Endocrinol Metab*. 2006;91(1):239-247.

474. Bondy CA, Van PL, Bakalov VK, Ho VB. Growth hormone treatment and aortic dimensions in Turner syndrome. *J Clin Endocrinol Metab*. 2006;91(5):1785-1788.

475. Yamamoto M, Iguchi G, Takeno R, et al. Adult combined GH, prolactin, and TSH deficiency associated with circulating PIT-1 antibody in humans. *J Clin Invest.* 2011;121(1):113-119.

476. Rona RJ, Tanner JM. Aetiology of idiopathic growth hormone deficiency in England and Wales. *Arch Dis Child.* 1977;52(3):197-208.

477. Vimpani GV, Vimpani AF, Lidgard GP, et al. Prevalence of severe growth hormone deficiency. *Br Med J.* 1977;2(6084):427-430.

478. Lindsay R, Feldkamp M, Harris D, et al. Utah growth study: growth standards and the prevalence of growth hormone deficiency. *J Pediatr.* 1994;125(1):29-35.

479. Blum WF, Deal C, Zimmermann AG, et al. Development of additional pituitary hormone deficiencies in pediatric patients originally diagnosed with idiopathic isolated GH deficiency. *Eur J Endocrinol.* 2013;170(1):13-21.

480. Mullis PE. Genetic control of growth. *Eur J Endocrinol.* 2005;152(1):11-31.

481. Alatzoglou KS, Webb EA, Le Tissier P, Dattani MT. Isolated growth hormone deficiency (GHD) in childhood and adolescence: recent advances. *Endocr Rev.* 2014;35(3):376-432.

482. Illig R, Prader A, Ferrandez A, et al. Hereditary prenatal growth hormone deficiency with increased tendency to growth hormone antibody formation ("A-type" of isolated growth hormone deficiency). *Acta Paediatr Scand.* 1971;60:607.

483. Wagner JK, Eble A, Hindmarsh PC, Mullis PE. Prevalence of human GH-1 gene alterations in patients with isolated growth hormone deficiency. *Pediatr Res.* 1998;43(1):105-110.

484. Cao Y, Wagner JK, Hindmarsh PC, et al. Isolated growth hormone deficiency: testing the little mouse hypothesis in man and exclusion of mutations within the extracellular domain of the growth hormone-releasing hormone receptor. *Pediatr Res.* 1995;38(6):962-966.

485. Salvatori R, Fan X, Phillips JA 3rd, et al. Three new mutations in the gene for the growth hormone (GH)-releasing hormone receptor in familial isolated GH deficiency type IB. *J Clin Endocrinol Metab.* 2001;86(1):273-279.

486. Gaylinn BD, Dealmeida VI, Lyons CE Jr, et al. The mutant growth hormone-releasing hormone (GHRH) receptor of the little mouse does not bind GHRH. *Endocrinology.* 1999;140(11):5066-5074.

487. Lee MS, Wajnrajch MP, Kim SS, et al. Autosomal dominant growth hormone (GH) deficiency type II: the Del32-71-GH deletion mutant suppresses secretion of wild-type GH. *Endocrinology.* 2000;141(3):883-890.

488. Binder G, Keller E, Mix M, et al. Isolated GH deficiency with dominant inheritance: new mutations, new insights. *J Clin Endocrinol Metab.* 2001;86(8):3877-3881.

489. Deladoey J, Stocker P, Mullis PE. Autosomal dominant GH deficiency due to an Arg183His GH-1 gene mutation: clinical and molecular evidence of impaired regulated GH secretion. *J Clin Endocrinol Metab.* 2001;86(8):3941-3947.

490. Mullis PE, Robinson IC, Salemi S, et al. Isolated autosomal dominant growth hormone deficiency: an evolving pituitary deficit? A multicenter follow-up study. *J Clin Endocrinol Metab.* 2005;90(4):2089-2096.

491. Miletta MC, Lochmatter D, Pektovic V, Mullis PE. Isolated growth hormone deficiency type 2: from gene to therapy. *Endocr Dev.* 2012;23:109-120.

492. Godfrey P, Rahal JO, Beamer WG, et al. GHRH receptor of little mice contains a missense mutation in the extracellular domain that disrupts receptor function. *Nat Genet.* 1993;4(3):227-232.

493. Mayo KE, Godfrey PA, Suhr ST, et al. Growth hormone-releasing hormone: synthesis and signaling. *Recent Prog Horm Res.* 1995;50:35-73.

494. Gaylinn BD. Molecular and cell biology of the growth hormone-releasing hormone receptor. *Growth Horm IGF Res.* 1999;9(Suppl A):37-44.

495. Mayo KE. Molecular cloning and expression of a pituitary-specific receptor for growth hormone-releasing hormone. *Mol Endocrinol.* 1992;6(10):1734-1744.

496. Gaylinn BD, Harrison JK, Zysk JR, et al. Molecular cloning and expression of a human anterior pituitary receptor for growth hormone-releasing hormone. *Mol Endocrinol.* 1993;7(1):77-84.

497. Wajnrajch MP, Gertner JM, Harbison MD, et al. Nonsense mutation in the human growth hormone-releasing hormone receptor causes growth failure analogous to the little (lit) mouse. *Nat Genet.* 1996;12(1):88-90.

498. Netchine I, Talon P, Dastot F, et al. Extensive phenotypic analysis of a family with growth hormone (GH) deficiency caused by a mutation in the GH-releasing hormone receptor gene. *J Clin Endocrinol Metab.* 1998;83(2):432-436.

499. Maheshwari HG, Silverman BL, Dupuis J, Baumann G. Phenotype and genetic analysis of a syndrome caused by an inactivating mutation in the growth hormone-releasing hormone receptor: dwarfism of Sindh. *J Clin Endocrinol Metab.* 1998;83(11):4065-4074.

500. Baumann G, Maheshwari H. The dwarfs of Sindh: severe growth hormone (GH) deficiency caused by a mutation in the GH-releasing hormone receptor gene. *Acta Paediatr Suppl.* 1997;423:33-38.

501. Kamijo T, Hayashi Y, Seo H, et al. A nonsense mutation (E72X) in growth hormone releasing hormone receptor (GHRHR) gene is the major cause of familial isolated growth hormone deficiency in western region of India: founder effect suggested by analysis of dinucleotide repeat polymorphism close to GHRHR gene. *Growth Horm IGF Res.* 2004;14(5):394-401.

502. Yokoyama Y, Narahara K, Tsuji K, et al. Growth hormone deficiency and empty sella syndrome in a boy with dup(X) (q13.3-q21.2). *Am J Med Genet.* 1992;42(5):660-664.

503. Aguiar-Oliveira MH, Gill MS, de A Barretto ES, et al. Effect of severe growth hormone (GH) deficiency due to a mutation in the GH-releasing hormone receptor on insulin-like growth factors (IGFs), IGF-binding proteins, and ternary complex formation throughout life. *J Clin Endocrinol Metab.* 1999;84(11):4118-4126.

504. Haskin O, Lazar L, Jaber L, et al. A new mutation in the growth hormone-releasing hormone receptor gene in two Israeli Arab families. *J Endocrinol Invest.* 2006;29(2):122-130.

505. Menezes Oliveira JL, Marques-Santos C, Barreto-Filho JA, et al. Lack of evidence of premature atherosclerosis in untreated severe isolated growth hormone (GH) deficiency due to a GH-releasing hormone receptor mutation. *J Clin Endocrinol Metab.* 2006;91(6):2093-2099.

506. Corazzini V, Salvatori R. Molecular and clinical aspects of GHRH receptor mutations. *Endocr Dev.* 2013;24:106-117.

507. Fleisher TA, White RM, Broder S, et al. X-linked hypogammaglobulinemia and isolated growth hormone deficiency. *N Engl J Med.* 1980;302(26):1429-1434.

508. Solomon NM, Nouri S, Warne GL, et al. Increased gene dosage at Xq26-q27 is associated with X-linked hypopituitarism. *Genomics.* 2002;79(4):553-559.

509. Valenta LJ, Sigel MB, Lesniak MA, et al. Pituitary dwarfism in a patient with circulating abnormal growth hormone polymers. *N Engl J Med.* 1985;312(4):214-217.

510. Kowarski AA, Schneider J, Ben-Galim E, et al. Growth failure with normal serum RIA-GH and low somatomedin activity: somatomedin restoration and growth acceleration after exogenous GH. *J Clin Endocrinol Metab.* 1978;47(2):461-464.

511. Takahashi Y, Kaji H, Okimura Y, et al. Brief report: short stature caused by a mutant growth hormone. *N Engl J Med.* 1996;334(7):432-436.

512. Takahashi Y, Shirono H, Arisaka O, et al. Biologically inactive growth hormone caused by an amino acid substitution. *J Clin Invest.* 1997;100(5):1159-1165.

513. Ishikawa M, Nimura A, Horikawa R, et al. A novel specific bioassay for serum human growth hormone. *J Clin Endocrinol Metab.* 2000;85(11):4274-4279.

514. Millar DS, Lewis MD, Horan M, et al. Novel mutations of the growth hormone 1 (GH1) gene disclosed by modulation of the clinical selection criteria for individuals with short stature. *Hum Mutat.* 2003;21(4):424-440.

515. Besson A, Salemi S, Deladoey J, et al. Short stature caused by a biologically inactive mutant growth hormone (GH-C53S). *J Clin Endocrinol Metab.* 2005;90(5):2493-2499.

516. Ross M, Francis GL, Szabo L, et al. Insulin-like growth factor (IGF)-binding proteins inhibit the biological activities of IGF-1 and IGF-2 but not des-(1-3)-IGF-1. *Biochem J.* 1989;258(1):267-272.

517. Radetti G, Bozzola M, Pagani S, et al. Growth hormone immunoreactivity does not reflect bioactivity. *Pediatr Res.* 2000;48(5):619-622.

518. Brastianos PK, Taylor-Weiner A, Manley PE, et al. Exome sequencing identifies BRAF mutations in papillary craniopharyngiomas. *Nat Genet.* 2014;46(2):161-165.

519. Muller HL, Emser A, Faldum A, et al. Longitudinal study on growth and body mass index before and after diagnosis of childhood craniopharyngioma. *J Clin Endocrinol Metab.* 2004;89(7):3298-3305.

520. Geffner M, Lundberg M, Koltowska-Haggstrom M, et al. Changes in height, weight, and body mass index in children with craniopharyngioma after three years of growth hormone therapy: analysis of KIGS (Pfizer international growth database). *J Clin Endocrinol Metab.* 2004;89(11):5435-5440.

521. Srinivasan S, Ogle GD, Garnett SP, et al. Features of the metabolic syndrome after childhood craniopharyngioma. *J Clin Endocrinol Metab.* 2004;89(1):81-86.

522. Beckers A, Aaltonen LA, Daly AF, Karhu A. Familial isolated pituitary adenomas (FIPA) and the pituitary adenoma predisposition due to mutations in the aryl hydrocarbon receptor interacting protein (AIP) gene. *Endocr Rev.* 2013;34(2):239-277.

523. Di Iorgi N, Allegri AE, Napoli F, et al. Central diabetes insipidus in children and young adults: etiological diagnosis and long-term outcome of idiopathic cases. *J Clin Endocrinol Metab.* 2014;99(4):1264-1272.

524. Taylor AM, Dunger DB, Preece MA, et al. The growth hormone independent insulin-like growth factor-I binding protein BP-28 is associated with serum insulin-like growth factor-I inhibitory bioactivity in adolescent insulin-dependent diabetics. *Clin Endocrinol (Oxf).* 1990;32(2):229-239.

525. Bereket A, Lang CH, Blethen SL, et al. Insulin-like growth factor binding protein-3 proteolysis in children with insulin-dependent

diabetes mellitus: a possible role for insulin in the regulation of IGFBP-3 protease activity. *J Clin Endocrinol Metab.* 1995;80(8): 2282-2288.

526. Laron Z. The essential role of IGF-I: lessons from the long-term study and treatment of children and adults with Laron syndrome. *J Clin Endocrinol Metab.* 1999;84(12):4397-4404.

527. Laron Z, Pertzelan A, Mannheimer S. Genetic pituitary dwarfism with high serum concentration of growth hormone—a new inborn error of metabolism. *Isr J Med Sci.* 1966;2(2):152-155.

528. Rosenbloom AL, Guevara Aguirre J, Rosenfeld RG, Fielder PJ. The little women of Loja—growth hormone-receptor deficiency in an inbred population of southern Ecuador. *N Engl J Med.* 1990;323(20): 1367-1374.

529. Savage MO, Blum WF, Ranke MB, et al. Clinical features and endocrine status in patients with growth hormone insensitivity (Laron syndrome). *J Clin Endocrinol Metab.* 1993;77(6):1465-1471.

530. Golde DW, Bersch N, Kaplan SA, et al. Peripheral unresponsiveness to human growth hormone in Laron dwarfism. *N Engl J Med.* 1980; 303(20):1156-1159.

531. Daughaday WH, Trivedi B. Absence of serum growth hormone binding protein in patients with growth hormone receptor deficiency (Laron dwarfism). *Proc Natl Acad Sci U S A.* 1987;84(13):4636-4640.

532. Baumann G, Shaw MA, Winter RJ. Absence of the plasma growth hormone-binding protein in Laron-type dwarfism. *J Clin Endocrinol Metab.* 1987;65(4):814-816.

533. Eshet R, Laron Z, Pertzelan A, et al. Defect of human growth hormone receptors in the liver of two patients with Laron-type dwarfism. *Isr J Med Sci.* 1984;20(1):8-11.

534. Woods KA, Dastot F, Preece MA, et al. Phenotype: genotype relationships in growth hormone insensitivity syndrome. *J Clin Endocrinol Metab.* 1997;82(11):3529-3535.

535. Amselem S, Duquesnoy P, Attree O, et al. Laron dwarfism and mutations of the growth hormone-receptor gene. *N Engl J Med.* 1989; 321(15):989-995.

536. Berg MA, Guevara-Aguirre J, Rosenbloom AL, et al. Mutation creating a new splice site in the growth hormone receptor genes of 37 Ecuadorean patients with Laron syndrome. *Hum Mutat.* 1992;1(1): 24-32.

537. Godowski PJ, Leung DW, Meacham LR, et al. Characterization of the human growth hormone receptor gene and demonstration of a partial gene deletion in two patients with Laron-type dwarfism. *Proc Natl Acad Sci U S A.* 1989;86(20):8083-8087.

538. Rosenfeld RG. Molecular mechanisms of IGF-I deficiency. *Horm Res.* 2006;65(Suppl 1):15-20.

539. Duquesnoy P, Sobrier ML, Duriez B, et al. A single amino acid substitution in the exoplasmic domain of the human growth hormone (GH) receptor confers familial GH resistance (Laron syndrome) with positive GH-binding activity by abolishing receptor homodimerization. *EMBO J.* 1994;13(6):1386-1395.

540. Woods KA, Fraser NC, Postel-Vinay MC, et al. A homozygous splice site mutation affecting the intracellular domain of the growth hormone (GH) receptor resulting in Laron syndrome with elevated GH-binding protein. *J Clin Endocrinol Metab.* 1996;81(5):1686-1690.

541. Silbergeld A, Dastot F, Klinger B, et al. Intronic mutation in the growth hormone (GH) receptor gene from a girl with Laron syndrome and extremely high serum GH binding protein: extended phenotypic study in a very large pedigree. *J Pediatr Endocrinol Metab.* 1997;10(3):265-274.

542. Kaji H, Nose O, Tajiri H, et al. Novel compound heterozygous mutations of growth hormone (GH) receptor gene in a patient with GH insensitivity syndrome. *J Clin Endocrinol Metab.* 1997;82(11):3705-3709.

543. Ayling RM, Ross R, Towner P, et al. A dominant-negative mutation of the growth hormone receptor causes familial short stature. *Nat Genet.* 1997;16(1):13-14.

544. Iida K, Takahashi Y, Kaji H, et al. Functional characterization of truncated growth hormone (GH) receptor-(1-277) causing partial GH insensitivity syndrome with high GH-binding protein. *J Clin Endocrinol Metab.* 1999;84(3):1011-1016.

545. Gastier JM, Berg MA, Vesterhus P, et al. Diverse deletions in the growth hormone receptor gene cause growth hormone insensitivity syndrome. *Hum Mutat.* 2000;16(4):323-333.

546. Milward A, Metherell L, Maamra M, et al. Growth hormone (GH) insensitivity syndrome due to a GH receptor truncated after Box1, resulting in isolated failure of STAT 5 signal transduction. *J Clin Endocrinol Metab.* 2004;89(3):1259-1266.

547. Tiulpakov A, Rubtsov P, Dedov I, et al. A novel C-terminal growth hormone receptor (GHR) mutation results in impaired GHR-STAT5 but normal STAT-3 signaling. *J Clin Endocrinol Metab.* 2005;90(1): 542-547.

548. Horikawa R, Hellmann P, Cella SG, et al. Growth hormone-releasing factor (GRF) regulates expression of its own receptor. *Endocrinology.* 1996;137(6):2642-2645.

549. Szabo M, Butz MR, Banerjee SA, et al. Autofeedback suppression of growth hormone (GH) secretion in transgenic mice expressing a human GH reporter targeted by tyrosine hydroxylase 5′-flanking sequences to the hypothalamus. *Endocrinology.* 1995;136(9):4044-4048.

550. Goddard AD, Covello R, Luoh SM, et al. Mutations of the growth hormone receptor in children with idiopathic short stature. The growth hormone insensitivity study group. *N Engl J Med.* 1995; 333(17):1093-1098.

551. Rosenfeld RG. Broadening the growth hormone insensitivity syndrome. *N Engl J Med.* 1995;333(17):1145-1146.

552. Attie KM. Mutations of the growth hormone receptor—widening the search. *J Clin Endocrinol Metab.* 1996;81(5):1683-1685.

553. Sanchez JE, Perera E, Baumbach L, Cleveland WW. Growth hormone receptor mutations in children with idiopathic short stature. *J Clin Endocrinol Metab.* 1998;83(11):4079-4083.

554. Ross RJ, Esposito N, Shen XY, et al. A short isoform of the human growth hormone receptor functions as a dominant negative inhibitor of the full-length receptor and generates large amounts of binding protein. *Mol Endocrinol.* 1997;11(3):265-273.

555. Urbanek M, Russell JE, Cooke NE, Liebhaber SA. Functional characterization of the alternatively spliced, placental human growth hormone receptor. *J Biol Chem.* 1993;268(25):19025-19032.

556. Sobrier ML, Duquesnoy P, Duriez B, et al. Expression and binding properties of two isoforms of the human growth hormone receptor. *FEBS Lett.* 1993;319(1-2):16-20.

557. Jorge AA, Marchisotti FG, Montenegro LR, et al. Growth hormone (GH) pharmacogenetics: influence of GH receptor exon 3 retention or deletion on first-year growth response and final height in patients with severe GH deficiency. *J Clin Endocrinol Metab.* 2006;91(3): 1076-1080.

558. Pilotta A, Mella P, Filisetti M, et al. Common polymorphisms of the growth hormone (GH) receptor do not correlate with the growth response to exogenous recombinant human GH in GH-deficient children. *J Clin Endocrinol Metab.* 2006;91(3):1178-1180.

559. Blum WF, Machinis K, Shavrikova EP, et al. The growth response to growth hormone (GH) treatment in children with isolated GH deficiency is independent of the presence of the exon 3-minus isoform of the GH receptor. *J Clin Endocrinol Metab.* 2006; 91(10):4171-4174.

560. Kofoed EM, Hwa V, Little B, et al. Growth hormone insensitivity associated with a STAT5b mutation. *N Engl J Med.* 2003;349(12): 1139-1147.

561. Fang P, Kofoed EM, Little BM, et al. A mutant signal transducer and activator of transcription 5b, associated with growth hormone insensitivity and insulin-like growth factor-I deficiency, cannot function as a signal transducer or transcription factor. *J Clin Endocrinol Metab.* 2006;91(4):1526-1534.

562. Hwa V, Little B, Adiyaman P, et al. Severe growth hormone insensitivity resulting from total absence of signal transducer and activator of transcription 5b. *J Clin Endocrinol Metab.* 2005;90(7):4260-4266.

563. Scaglia PA, Martinez AS, Feigerlova E, et al. A novel missense mutation in the SH2 domain of the STAT5B gene results in a transcriptionally inactive STAT5b associated with severe IGF-I deficiency, immune dysfunction, and lack of pulmonary disease. *J Clin Endocrinol Metab.* 2012;97(5):E830-E839.

564. Domene HM, Bengolea SV, Martinez AS, et al. Deficiency of the circulating insulin-like growth factor system associated with inactivation of the acid-labile subunit gene. *N Engl J Med.* 2004;350(6): 570-577.

565. Hwa V, Haeusler G, Pratt KL, et al. Total absence of functional acid labile subunit, resulting in severe insulin-like growth factor deficiency and moderate growth failure. *J Clin Endocrinol Metab.* 2006; 91(5):1826-1831.

566. Woods KA, Camacho-Hubner C, Barter D, et al. Insulin-like growth factor I gene deletion causing intrauterine growth retardation and severe short stature. *Acta Paediatr Suppl.* 1997;423:39-45.

567. Camacho-Hubner C, Woods KA, Miraki-Moud F, et al. Effects of recombinant human insulin-like growth factor I (IGF-I) therapy on the growth hormone-IGF system of a patient with a partial IGF-I gene deletion. *J Clin Endocrinol Metab.* 1999;84(5):1611-1616.

568. Fuqua JS, Derr M, Rosenfeld RG, Hwa V. Identification of a novel heterozygous IGF1 splicing mutation in a large kindred with familial short stature. *Horm Res Paediatr.* 2012;78(1):59-66.

569. Batey L, Moon JE, Yu Y, et al. A novel deletion of IGF1 in a patient with idiopathic short stature provides insight into IGF1 haploinsufficiency. *J Clin Endocrinol Metab.* 2014;99(1):E153-E159.

570. Denley A, Wang CC, McNeil KA, et al. Structural and functional characteristics of the Val44Met insulin-like growth factor I missense mutation: correlation with effects on growth and development. *Mol Endocrinol.* 2005;19(3):711-721.

571. Tollefsen SE, Heath-Monnig E, Cascieri MA, et al. Endogenous insulin-like growth factor (IGF) binding proteins cause IGF-1 resistance in cultured fibroblasts from a patient with short stature. *J Clin Invest.* 1991;87(4):1241-1250.

572. Raile K, Klammt J, Schneider A, et al. Clinical and functional characteristics of the human Arg59Ter insulin-like growth factor I receptor (IGF1R) mutation: implications for a gene dosage effect of the human IGF1R. *J Clin Endocrinol Metab.* 2006;91(6):2264-2271.

573. Hattori Y, Vera JC, Rivas CI, et al. Decreased insulin-like growth factor I receptor expression and function in immortalized African pygmy T cells. *J Clin Endocrinol Metab.* 1996;81(6):2257-2263.

574. Fang P, Cho YH, Derr MA, et al. Severe short stature caused by novel compound heterozygous mutations of the insulin-like growth factor 1 receptor (IGF1R). *J Clin Endocrinol Metab.* 2012;97(2):E243-E247.

575. Jain S, Golde DW, Bailey R, Geffner ME. Insulin-like growth factor-I resistance. *Endocr Rev.* 1998;19(5):625-646.

576. Wertheimer E, Lu SP, Backeljauw PF, et al. Homozygous deletion of the human insulin receptor gene results in leprechaunism. *Nat Genet.* 1993;5(1):71-73.

577. Siebler T, Lopaczynski W, Terry CL, et al. Insulin-like growth factor I receptor expression and function in fibroblasts from two patients with deletion of the distal long arm of chromosome 15. *J Clin Endocrinol Metab.* 1995;80(12):3447-3457.

578. Liu Y, Albertsson-Wikland K, Karlberg J. Long-term consequences of early linear growth retardation (stunting) in Swedish children. *Pediatr Res.* 2000;47(4 Pt 1):475-480.

579. Zamboni G, Dufillot D, Antoniazzi F, et al. Growth hormone-binding proteins and insulin-like growth factor-binding proteins in protein-energy malnutrition, before and after nutritional rehabilitation. *Pediatr Res.* 1996;39(3):410-414.

580. Fazeli PK, Klibanski A. Determinants of GH resistance in malnutrition. *J Endocrinol.* 2014;220(3):R57-R65.

581. Beas F, Contreras I, Maccioni A, Arenas S. Growth hormone in infant malnutrition: the arginine test in marasmus and kwashiorkor. *Br J Nutr.* 1971;26(2):169-175.

582. Soliman AT, Hassan AE, Aref MK, et al. Serum insulin-like growth factors I and II concentrations and growth hormone and insulin responses to arginine infusion in children with protein-energy malnutrition before and after nutritional rehabilitation. *Pediatr Res.* 1986;20(11):1122-1130.

583. Scacchi M, Ida Pincelli A, Cavagnini F. Nutritional status in the neuroendocrine control of growth hormone secretion: the model of anorexia nervosa. *Front Neuroendocrinol.* 2003;24(3):200-224.

584. Altinkaynak S, Selimoglu MA, Ertekin V, Kilicarslan B. Serum ghrelin levels in children with primary protein-energy malnutrition. *Pediatr Int.* 2008;50(4):429-431.

585. El-Hodhod MA, Emam EK, Zeitoun YA, El-Araby AM. Serum ghrelin in infants with protein-energy malnutrition. *Clin Nutr.* 2009;28(2):173-177.

586. Dimaraki EV, Jaffe CA. Role of endogenous ghrelin in growth hormone secretion, appetite regulation and metabolism. *Rev Endocr Metab Disord.* 2006;7(4):237-249.

587. Thissen JP, Ketelslegers JM, Underwood LE. Nutritional regulation of the insulin-like growth factors. *Endocr Rev.* 1994;15(1):80-101.

588. Mayer E, Stern M. Growth failure in gastrointestinal diseases. *Baillieres Clin Endocrinol Metab.* 1992;6(3):645-663.

589. Phillips LS. Nutrition, somatomedins, and the brain. *Metabolism.* 1986;35(1):78-87.

590. Donovan SM, Atilano LC, Hintz RL, et al. Differential regulation of the insulin-like growth factors (IGF-I and -II) and IGF binding proteins during malnutrition in the neonatal rat. *Endocrinology.* 1991;129(1):149-157.

591. Pugliese MT, Lifshitz F, Grad G, et al. Fear of obesity. A cause of short stature and delayed puberty. *N Engl J Med.* 1983;309(9):513-518.

592. Golden NH, Kreitzer P, Jacobson MS, et al. Disturbances in growth hormone secretion and action in adolescents with anorexia nervosa. *J Pediatr.* 1994;125(4):655-660.

593. Russell GF. Premenarchal anorexia nervosa and its sequelae. *J Psychiatr Res.* 1985;19(2-3):363-369.

594. Miller KK, Klibanski A. Clinical review 106: amenorrheic bone loss. *J Clin Endocrinol Metab.* 1999;84(6):1775-1783.

595. Postel-Vinay MC, Saab C, Gourmelen M. Nutritional status and growth hormone-binding protein. *Horm Res.* 1995;44(4):177-181.

596. Counts DR, Gwirtsman H, Carlsson LM, et al. The effects of anorexia nervosa and refeeding on growth hormone-binding protein, the insulin-like growth factors (IGFs), and the IGF-binding proteins. *J Clin Endocrinol Metab.* 1992;75:762-766.

597. Fleischman A, Brue C, Poussaint TY, et al. Diencephalic syndrome: a cause of failure to thrive and a model of partial growth hormone resistance. *Pediatrics.* 2005;115(6):e742-e748.

598. Preece MA, Law CM, Davies PS. The growth of children with chronic paediatric disease. *Clin Endocrinol Metab.* 1986;15(3):453-477.

599. Savage MO, Beattie RM, Camacho-Hubner C, et al. Growth in Crohn's disease. *Acta Paediatr Suppl.* 1999;88(428):89-92.

600. Locuratolo N, Pugliese G, Pricci F, et al. The circulating insulin-like growth factor system in children with coeliac disease: an additional marker for disease activity. *Diabetes Metab Res Rev.* 1999;15(4):254-260.

601. Catassi C, Fasano A. Celiac disease as a cause of growth retardation in childhood. *Curr Opin Pediatr.* 2004;16(4):445-449.

602. Auricchio S, Greco L, Troncone R. Gluten-sensitive enteropathy in childhood. *Pediatr Clin North Am.* 1988;35(1):157-187.

603. Hill ID, Dirks MH, Liptak GS, et al. Guideline for the diagnosis and treatment of celiac disease in children: recommendations of the North American Society for Pediatric Gastroenterology, Hepatology and Nutrition. *J Pediatr Gastroenterol Nutr.* 2005;40(1):1-19.

604. Lagerqvist C, Dahlbom I, Hansson T, et al. Antigliadin immunoglobulin A best in finding celiac disease in children younger than 18 months of age. *J Pediatr Gastroenterol Nutr.* 2008;47(4):428-435.

605. Zawahir S, Safta A, Fasano A. Pediatric celiac disease. *Curr Opin Pediatr.* 2009;21(5):655-660.

606. Hoffenberg EJ, MacKenzie T, Barriga KJ, et al. A prospective study of the incidence of childhood celiac disease. *J Pediatr.* 2003;143(3):308-314.

607. Hernandez M, Argente J, Navarro A, et al. Growth in malnutrition related to gastrointestinal diseases: coeliac disease. *Horm Res.* 1992;38(Suppl 1):79-84.

608. Bode SH, Bachmann EH, Gudmand-Hoyer E, Jensen GB. Stature of adult coeliac patients: no evidence for decreased attained height. *Eur J Clin Nutr.* 1991;45(3):145-149.

609. Cacciari E, Corazza GR, Salardi S, et al. What will be the adult height of coeliac patients? *Eur J Pediatr.* 1991;150(6):407-409.

610. Shamir R, Phillip M, Levine A. Growth retardation in pediatric Crohn's disease: pathogenesis and interventions. *Inflamm Bowel Dis.* 2007;13(5):620-628.

611. Walters TD, Griffiths AM. Mechanisms of growth impairment in pediatric Crohn's disease. *Nat Rev Gastroenterol Hepatol.* 2009;6(9):513-523.

612. Cezard JP, Touati G, Alberti C, et al. Growth in paediatric Crohn's disease. *Horm Res.* 2002;58(Suppl 1):11-15.

613. Kanof ME, Lake AM, Bayless TM. Decreased height velocity in children and adolescents before the diagnosis of Crohn's disease. *Gastroenterology.* 1988;95(6):1523-1527.

614. Rosenthal SR, Snyder JD, Hendricks KM, Walker WA. Growth failure and inflammatory bowel disease: approach to treatment of a complicated adolescent problem. *Pediatrics.* 1983;72(4):481-490.

615. Homer DR, Grand RJ, Colodny AH. Growth, course, and prognosis after surgery for Crohn's disease in children and adolescents. *Pediatrics.* 1977;59(5):717-725.

616. Griffiths AM, Nguyen P, Smith C, et al. Growth and clinical course of children with Crohn's disease. *Gut.* 1993;34(7):939-943.

617. Soyka LA, Fairfield WP, Klibanski A. Clinical review 117: hormonal determinants and disorders of peak bone mass in children. *J Clin Endocrinol Metab.* 2000;85(11):3951-3963.

618. Cowan FJ, Warner JT, Dunstan FD, et al. Inflammatory bowel disease and predisposition to osteopenia. *Arch Dis Child.* 1997;76(4):325-329.

619. Kirschner BS. Growth and development in chronic inflammatory bowel disease. *Acta Paediatr Scand Suppl.* 1990;366:98-104, discussion 105.

620. Sawczenko A, Ballinger AB, Savage MO, Sanderson IR. Clinical features affecting final adult height in patients with pediatric-onset Crohn's disease. *Pediatrics.* 2006;118(1):124-129.

621. Wong SC, Kumar P, Galloway PJ, et al. A preliminary trial of the effect of recombinant human growth hormone on short-term linear growth and glucose homeostasis in children with Crohn's disease. *Clin Endocrinol (Oxf).* 2011;74(5):599-607.

622. Mauras N, George D, Evans J, et al. Growth hormone has anabolic effects in glucocorticosteroid-dependent children with inflammatory bowel disease: a pilot study. *Metabolism.* 2002;51(1):127-135.

623. Calenda KA, Schornagel IL, Sadeghi-Nejad A, Grand RJ. Effect of recombinant growth hormone treatment on children with Crohn's disease and short stature: a pilot study. *Inflamm Bowel Dis.* 2005;11(5):435-441.

624. Wasserman D, Zemel BS, Mulberg AE, et al. Growth, nutritional status, body composition, and energy expenditure in prepubert children with Alagille syndrome. *J Pediatr.* 1999;134(2):172-177.

625. Viner RM, Forton JT, Cole TJ, et al. Growth of long-term survivors of liver transplantation. *Arch Dis Child.* 1999;80(3):235-240.

626. Bartosh SM, Thomas SE, Sutton MM, et al. Linear growth after pediatric liver transplantation. *J Pediatr.* 1999;135(5):624-631.

627. Bucuvalas JC, Cutfield W, Horn J, et al. Resistance to the growth-promoting and metabolic effects of growth hormone in children with chronic liver disease. *J Pediatr.* 1990;117(3):397-402.

628. Donaghy A, Ross R, Gimson A, et al. Growth hormone, insulinlike growth factor-1, and insulinlike growth factor binding proteins 1 and 3 in chronic liver disease. *Hepatology.* 1995;21(3):680-688.

629. Quirk P, Owens P, Moyse K, et al. Insulin-like growth factors I and II are reduced in plasma from growth retarded children with chronic liver disease. *Growth Regul.* 1994;4(1):35-38.

630. Holt RI, Jones JS, Stone NM, et al. Sequential changes in insulin-like growth factor I (IGF-I) and IGF-binding proteins in children with end-stage liver disease before and after successful orthotopic liver transplantation. *J Clin Endocrinol Metab.* 1996;81(1):160-168.

631. Maghnie M, Barreca A, Ventura M, et al. Failure to increase insulin-like growth factor-I synthesis is involved in the mechanisms of growth retardation of children with inherited liver disorders. *Clin Endocrinol (Oxf).* 1998;48(6):747-755.

632. Shen XY, Holt RI, Miell JP, et al. Cirrhotic liver expresses low levels of the full-length and truncated growth hormone receptors. *J Clin Endocrinol Metab.* 1998;83(7):2532-2538.

633. Sarna S, Sipila I, Vihervuori E, et al. Growth delay after liver transplantation in childhood: studies of underlying mechanisms. *Pediatr Res*. 1995;38(3):366-372.

634. Codoner-Franch P, Bernard O, Alvarez F. Long-term follow-up of growth in height after successful liver transplantation. *J Pediatr*. 1994;124(3):368-373.

635. Sarna S, Sipila I, Ronnholm K, et al. Recombinant human growth hormone improves growth in children receiving glucocorticoid treatment after liver transplantation. *J Clin Endocrinol Metab*. 1996;81(4):1476-1482.

636. Rodeck B, Kardorff R, Melter M, Ehrich JH. Improvement of growth after growth hormone treatment in children who undergo liver transplantation. *J Pediatr Gastroenterol Nutr*. 2000;31(3):286-290.

637. Schuurmans FM, Pulles-Heintzberger CF, Gerver WJ, et al. Long-term growth of children with congenital heart disease: a retrospective study. *Acta Paediatr*. 1998;87(12):1250-1255.

638. Okoromah CA, Ekure EN, Lesi FE, et al. Prevalence, profile and predictors of malnutrition in children with congenital heart defects: a case-control observational study. *Arch Dis Child*. 2011;96(4):354-360.

639. Cheung MM, Davis AM, Wilkinson JL, Weintraub RG. Long term somatic growth after repair of tetralogy of Fallot: evidence for restoration of genetic growth potential. *Heart*. 2003;89(11):1340-1343.

640. McLean WC. Protein energy malnutrition. In: Grand RJ, Sutphen JL, Dietz WH, eds. *Pediatric Nutrition: Theory and Practice*. Stoneham, MA: Butterworths; 1987.

641. Schuurmans FM, Pulles-Heintzberger CF, Gerver WJ, et al. Long-term growth of children with congenital heart disease: a retrospective study. *Acta Paediatr*. 1998;87(12):1250-1255.

642. Leitch CA, Karn CA, Ensing GJ, Denne SC. Energy expenditure after surgical repair in children with cyanotic congenital heart disease. *J Pediatr*. 2000;137(3):381-385.

643. Leitch CA, Karn CA, Peppard RJ, et al. Increased energy expenditure in infants with cyanotic congenital heart disease. *J Pediatr*. 1998;133(6):755-760.

644. Barton JS, Hindmarsh PC, Preece MA. Serum insulin-like growth factor 1 in congenital heart disease. *Arch Dis Child*. 1996;75(2):162-163.

645. Bernstein D, Jasper JR, Rosenfeld RG, Hintz RL. Decreased serum insulin-like growth factor-I associated with growth failure in newborn lambs with experimental cyanotic heart disease. *J Clin Invest*. 1992;89(4):1128-1132.

646. Cheung MM, Davis AM, Wilkinson JL, Weintraub RG. Long term somatic growth after repair of tetralogy of Fallot: evidence for restoration of genetic growth potential. *Heart*. 2003;89(11):1340-1343.

647. Okoromah CA, Ekure EN, Lesi FE, et al. Prevalence, profile and predictors of malnutrition in children with congenital heart defects: a case-control observational study. *Arch Dis Child*. 2011;96(4):354-360.

648. Carmona F, Hatanaka LS, Barbieri MA, et al. Catch-up growth in children after repair of tetralogy of Fallot. *Cardiol Young*. 2012;22(5):507-513.

649. Kohaut EC. Chronic renal disease and growth in childhood. *Curr Opin Pediatr*. 1995;7(2):171-175.

650. Mehls O, Blum WF, Schaefer F, et al. Growth failure in renal disease. *Baillieres Clin Endocrinol Metab*. 1992;6(3):665-685.

651. Lee DY, Park SK, Kim JS. Insulin-like growth factor-I (IGF-I) and IGF-binding proteins in children with nephrotic syndrome. *J Clin Endocrinol Metab*. 1996;81(5):1856-1860.

652. Kuizon BD, Salusky IB. Growth retardation in children with chronic renal failure. *J Bone Miner Res*. 1999;14(10):1680-1690.

653. Kimonis VE, Troendle J, Rose SR, et al. Effects of early cysteamine therapy on thyroid function and growth in nephropathic cystinosis. *J Clin Endocrinol Metab*. 1995;80(11):3257-3261.

654. Warady BA, Jabs K. New hormones in the therapeutic arsenal of chronic renal failure. growth hormone and erythropoietin. *Pediatr Clin North Am*. 1995;42(6):1551-1577.

655. Hokken-Koelega AC, Hackeng WH, Stijnen T, et al. Twenty-four-hour plasma growth hormone (GH) profiles, urinary GH excretion, and plasma insulin-like growth factor-I and -II levels in prepubertal children with chronic renal insufficiency and severe growth retardation. *J Clin Endocrinol Metab*. 1990;71(3):688-695.

656. Schaefer F, Hamill G, Stanhope R, et al. Pulsatile growth hormone secretion in peripubertal patients with chronic renal failure. Cooperative study group on pubertal development in chronic renal failure. *J Pediatr*. 1991;119(4):568-577.

657. Tonshoff B, Veldhuis JD, Heinrich U, Mehls O. Deconvolution analysis of spontaneous nocturnal growth hormone secretion in prepubertal children with preterminal chronic renal failure and with end-stage renal disease. *Pediatr Res*. 1995;37(1):86-93.

658. Mahan JD, Warady BA. Consensus Committee. Assessment and treatment of short stature in pediatric patients with chronic kidney disease: a consensus statement. *Pediatr Nephrol*. 2006;21(7):917-930.

659. Tonshoff B, Eden S, Weiser E, et al. Reduced hepatic growth hormone (GH) receptor gene expression and increased plasma GH binding protein in experimental uremia. *Kidney Int*. 1994;45(4):1085-1092.

660. Hokken-Koelega AC, Stijnen T, de Muinck Keizer-Schrama SM, et al. Placebo-controlled, double-blind, cross-over trial of growth hormone treatment in prepubertal children with chronic renal failure. *Lancet*. 1991;338(8767):585-590.

661. Powell DR, Rosenfeld RG, Baker BK, et al. Serum somatomedin levels in adults with chronic renal failure: the importance of measuring insulin-like growth factor I (IGF-I) and IGF-II in acid-chromatographed uremic serum. *J Clin Endocrinol Metab*. 1986;63(5):1186-1192.

662. Blum WF, Ranke MB, Savage MO, Hall K. Insulin-like growth factors and their binding proteins in patients with growth hormone receptor deficiency: suggestions for new diagnostic criteria. The Kabi Pharmacia Study Group on insulin-like growth factor I treatment in growth hormone insensitivity syndromes. *Acta Paediatr Suppl*. 1992;383:125-126.

663. Roelfsema V, Clark RG. The growth hormone and insulin-like growth factor axis: its manipulation for the benefit of growth disorders in renal failure. *J Am Soc Nephrol*. 2001;12(6):1297-1306.

664. Rabkin R, Sun DF, Chen Y, et al. Growth hormone resistance in uremia, a role for impaired JAK/STAT signaling. *Pediatr Nephrol*. 2005;20(3):313-318.

665. Rees L, Maxwell H. The hypothalamo-pituitary-growth hormone insulin-like growth factor 1 axis in children with chronic renal failure. *Kidney Int Suppl*. 1996;53:S109-S114.

666. Blum WF, Ranke MB, Kietzmann K, et al. Growth hormone resistance and inhibition of somatomedin activity by excess of insulin-like growth factor binding protein in uraemia. *Pediatr Nephrol*. 1991;5(4):539-544.

667. Hokken-Koelega AC, Stijnen T, de Muinck Keizer-Schrama SM, et al. Levels of growth hormone, insulin-like growth factor-I (IGF-I) and -II, IGF-binding protein-1 and -3, and cortisol in prednisone-treated children with growth retardation after renal transplantation. *J Clin Endocrinol Metab*. 1993;77(4):932-938.

668. Hanna JD, Santos F, Foreman JW, et al. Insulin-like growth factor-I gene expression in the tibial epiphyseal growth plate of growth hormone-treated uremic rats. *Kidney Int*. 1995;47(5):1374-1382.

669. Unterman TG, Phillips LS. Glucocorticoid effects on somatomedins and somatomedin inhibitors. *J Clin Endocrinol Metab*. 1985;61(4):618-626.

670. Allen DB. Growth suppression by glucocorticoid therapy. *Pediatr Rounds*. 1995;(4):1-5.

671. Laster ML, Fine RN. Growth following solid organ transplantation in childhood. *Pediatr Transplant*. 2014;18(2):134-141.

672. Hokken-Koelega AC, Van Zaal MA, de Ridder MA, et al. Growth after renal transplantation in prepubertal children: impact of various treatment modalities. *Pediatr Res*. 1994;35(3):367-371.

673. Laster ML, Fine RN. Growth following solid organ transplantation in childhood. *Pediatr Transplant*. 2014;18(2):134-141.

674. Ellis D. Growth and renal function after steroid-free tacrolimus-based immunosuppression in children with renal transplants. *Pediatr Nephrol*. 2000;14(7):689-694.

675. Bennett EL. Understanding growth failure in children with homozygous sickle-cell disease. *J Pediatr Oncol Nurs*. 2011;28(2):67-74.

676. Collett-Solberg PF, Fleenor D, Schultz WH, Ware RE. Short stature in children with sickle cell anemia correlates with alterations in the IGF-I axis. *J Pediatr Endocrinol Metab*. 2007;20(2):211-218.

677. Singhal A, Thomas P, Cook R, et al. Delayed adolescent growth in homozygous sickle cell disease. *Arch Dis Child*. 1994;71(5):404-408.

678. Smiley D, Dagogo-Jack S, Umpierrez G. Therapy insight: metabolic and endocrine disorders in sickle cell disease. *Nat Clin Pract Endocrinol Metab*. 2008;4(2):102-109.

679. Wang WC, Morales KH, Scher CD, et al. Effect of long-term transfusion on growth in children with sickle cell anemia: results of the STOP trial. *J Pediatr*. 2005;147(2):244-247.

680. Collett-Solberg PF, Fleenor D, Schultz WH, Ware RE. Short stature in children with sickle cell anemia correlates with alterations in the IGF-I axis. *J Pediatr Endocrinol Metab*. 2007;20(2):211-218.

681. Saka N, Sukur M, Bundak R, et al. Growth and puberty in thalassemia major. *J Pediatr Endocrinol Metab*. 1995;8(3):181-186.

682. Filosa A, Di Maio S, Baron I, et al. Final height and body disproportion in thalassaemic boys and girls with spontaneous or induced puberty. *Acta Paediatr*. 2000;89(11):1295-1301.

683. Low LC, Kwan EY, Lim YJ, et al. Growth hormone treatment of short Chinese children with beta-thalassaemia major without GH deficiency. *Clin Endocrinol (Oxf)*. 1995;42(4):359-363.

684. DeLuca G, Maggiolini M, Bria M, et al. GH secretion in thalassemia patients with short stature. *Horm Res*. 1995;44(4):158-163.

685. Scacchi M, Danesi L, De Martin M, et al. Treatment with biosynthetic growth hormone of short thalassaemic patients with impaired growth hormone secretion. *Clin Endocrinol (Oxf)*. 1991;35(4):335-339.

686. Masala A, Atzeni MM, Alagna S, et al. Growth hormone secretion in polytransfused prepubertal patients with homozygous beta-thalassemia. effect of long-term recombinant GH (recGH) therapy. *J Endocrinol Invest*. 2003;26(7):623-628.

687. Cavallo L, De Sanctis V, Cisternino M, et al. Final height in short polytransfused thalassemia major patients treated with recombinant growth hormone. *J Endocrinol Invest*. 2005;28(4):363-366.

688. La Rosa C, De Sanctis V, Mangiagli A, et al. Growth hormone secretion in adult patients with thalassaemia. *Clin Endocrinol (Oxf)*. 2005; 62(6):667-671.

689. Wajnrajch MP, Gertner JM, Huma Z, et al. Evaluation of growth and hormonal status in patients referred to the International Fanconi Anemia Registry. *Pediatrics*. 2001;107(4):744-754.

690. McNair SL, Stickler GB. Growth in familial hypophosphatemic vitamin-D-resistant rickets. *N Engl J Med*. 1969;281(10):512-516.

691. Marsden D, Barshop BA, Capistrano-Estrada S, et al. Anabolic effect of human growth hormone: management of inherited disorders of catabolic pathways. *Biochem Med Metab Biol*. 1994;52(2):145-154.

692. Bain MD, Nussey SS, Jones M, Chalmers RA. Use of human somatotrophin in the treatment of a patient with methylmalonic aciduria. *Eur J Pediatr*. 1995;154(10):850-852.

693. Crowley S, Hindmarsh PC, Matthews DR, Brook CG. Growth and the growth hormone axis in prepubertal children with asthma. *J Pediatr*. 1995;126(2):297-303.

694. Doull IJ. The effect of asthma and its treatment on growth. *Arch Dis Child*. 2004;89(1):60-63.

695. Russell G. Asthma and growth. *Arch Dis Child*. 1993;69(6):695-698.

696. Nassif E, Weinberger M, Sherman B, Brown K. Extrapulmonary effects of maintenance corticosteroid therapy with alternate-day prednisone and inhaled beclomethasone in children with chronic asthma. *J Allergy Clin Immunol*. 1987;80(4):518-529.

697. Kelly HW, Sternberg AL, Lescher R, et al. Effect of inhaled glucocorticoids in childhood on adult height. *N Engl J Med*. 2012;367(10): 904-912.

698. Avery ME, Tooley WH, Keller JB, et al. Is chronic lung disease in low birth weight infants preventable? A survey of eight centers. *Pediatrics*. 1987;79(1):26-30.

699. Gibson AT, Pearse RG, Wales JK. Growth retardation after dexamethasone administration: assessment by knemometry. *Arch Dis Child*. 1993;69(5 Spec No):505-509.

700. Finer NN, Craft A, Vaucher YE, et al. Postnatal steroids: short-term gain, long-term pain? *J Pediatr*. 2000;137(1):9-13.

701. Kurzner SI, Garg M, Bautista DB, et al. Growth failure in infants with bronchopulmonary dysplasia: nutrition and elevated resting metabolic expenditure. *Pediatrics*. 1988;81(3):379-384.

702. Yu VY, Orgill AA, Lim SB, et al. Growth and development of very low birthweight infants recovering from bronchopulmonary dysplasia. *Arch Dis Child*. 1983;58(10):791-794.

703. Meisels SJ, Plunkett JW, Roloff DW, et al. Growth and development of preterm infants with respiratory distress syndrome and bronchopulmonary dysplasia. *Pediatrics*. 1986;77(3):345-352.

704. Vrlenich LA, Bozynski ME, Shyr Y, et al. The effect of bronchopulmonary dysplasia on growth at school age. *Pediatrics*. 1995;95(6): 855-859.

705. Ross G, Lipper EG, Auld PA. Growth achievement of very low birth weight premature children at school age. *J Pediatr*. 1990;117(2 Pt 1):307-309.

706. Robertson CM, Etches PC, Goldson E, Kyle JM. Eight-year school performance, neurodevelopmental, and growth outcome of neonates with bronchopulmonary dysplasia: a comparative study. *Pediatrics*. 1992;89(3):365-372.

707. Thaker V, Haagensen AL, Carter B, et al. Recombinant growth hormone therapy for cystic fibrosis in children and young adults. *Cochrane Database Syst Rev*. 2013;(6):CD008901.

708. Scaparrotta A, Di Pillo S, Attanasi M, et al. Growth failure in children with cystic fibrosis. *J Pediatr Endocrinol Metab*. 2012;25(5-6):393-405.

709. Assael BM, Casazza G, Iansa P, et al. Growth and long-term lung function in cystic fibrosis: a longitudinal study of patients diagnosed by neonatal screening. *Pediatr Pulmonol*. 2009;44(3):209-215.

710. Patel L, Dixon M, David TJ. Growth and growth charts in cystic fibrosis. *J R Soc Med*. 2003;96(Suppl 43):35-41.

711. Hardin DS. GH improves growth and clinical status in children with cystic fibrosis—a review of published studies. *Eur J Endocrinol*. 2004; 151(Suppl 1):S81-S85.

712. Laursen EM, Juul A, Lanng S, et al. Diminished concentrations of insulin-like growth factor I in cystic fibrosis. *Arch Dis Child*. 1995;72(6):494-497.

713. Lapey A, Kattwinkel J, Di Sant'Agnese PA, Laster L. Steatorrhea and azotorrhea and their relation to growth and nutrition in adolescents and young adults with cystic fibrosis. *J Pediatr*. 1974;84(3): 328-334.

714. Mearns M. Growth and development. In: Hodson E, Norman A, Batten J, eds. *Cystic Fibrosis*. London: Bailliere Tindall; 1983.

715. Shepherd RW, Holt TL, Thomas BJ, et al. Nutritional rehabilitation in cystic fibrosis: controlled studies of effects on nutritional growth retardation, body protein turnover, and course of pulmonary disease. *J Pediatr*. 1986;109(5):788-794.

716. Reiter EO, Brugman SM, Pike JW, et al. Vitamin D metabolites in adolescents and young adults with cystic fibrosis: effects of sun and season. *J Pediatr*. 1985;106(1):21-26.

717. Reiter EO, Gerstle RS. Cystic fibrosis in puberty and adolescence. In: Lerner RM, Petersen AC, Brooks-Gunn J, eds. *Encyclopedia of Adolescence*. New York: Garland Publishing; 1991.

718. Stalvey MS, Anbar RD, Konstan MW, et al. A multi-center controlled trial of growth hormone treatment in children with cystic fibrosis. *Pediatr Pulmonol*. 2012;47(3):252-263.

719. Phung OJ, Coleman CI, Baker EL, et al. Recombinant human growth hormone in the treatment of patients with cystic fibrosis. *Pediatrics*. 2010;126(5):e1211-e1226.

720. Zemel BS, Jawad AF, FitzSimmons S, Stallings VA. Longitudinal relationship among growth, nutritional status, and pulmonary function in children with cystic fibrosis: analysis of the Cystic Fibrosis Foundation national CF patient registry. *J Pediatr*. 2000;137(3):374-380.

721. De Benedetti F, Alonzi T, Moretta A, et al. Interleukin 6 causes growth impairment in transgenic mice through a decrease in insulin-like growth factor-I. A model for stunted growth in children with chronic inflammation. *J Clin Invest*. 1997;99(4):643-650.

722. Bazan JF. Haemopoietic receptors and helical cytokines. *Immunol Today*. 1990;11(10):350-354.

723. Lang CH, Hong-Brown L, Frost RA. Cytokine inhibition of JAK-STAT signaling: a new mechanism of growth hormone resistance. *Pediatr Nephrol*. 2005;20(3):306-312.

724. McCann SM, Lyson K, Karanth S, et al. Role of cytokines in the endocrine system. *Ann N Y Acad Sci*. 1994;741:50-63.

725. Vassilopoulou-Sellin R. Endocrine effects of cytokines. *Oncology (Williston Park)*. 1994;8(10):43-49, discussion 49-50.

726. Skerry TM. The effects of the inflammatory response on bone growth. *Eur J Clin Nutr*. 1994;48(Suppl 1):S190-S197, discussion S198.

727. McKinney RE Jr, Robertson JW. Effect of human immunodeficiency virus infection on the growth of young children. Duke pediatric AIDS clinical trials unit. *J Pediatr*. 1993;123(4):579-582.

728. Saavedra JM, Henderson RA, Perman JA, et al. Longitudinal assessment of growth in children born to mothers with human immunodeficiency virus infection. *Arch Pediatr Adolesc Med*. 1995;149(5): 497-502.

729. McKinney RE Jr, Wilfert C. Growth as a prognostic indicator in children with human immunodeficiency virus infection treated with zidovudine. AIDS clinical trials group protocol 043 study group. *J Pediatr*. 1994;125(5 Pt 1):728-733.

730. Gertner JM, Kaufman FR, Donfield SM, et al. Delayed somatic growth and pubertal development in human immunodeficiency virus-infected hemophiliac boys: hemophilia growth and development study. *J Pediatr*. 1994;124(6):896-902.

731. Moye J Jr, Rich KC, Kalish LA, et al. Natural history of somatic growth in infants born to women infected by human immunodeficiency virus. Women and infants transmission study group. *J Pediatr*. 1996; 128(1):58-69.

732. Majaliwa ES, Mohn A, Chiarelli F. Growth and puberty in children with HIV infection. *J Endocrinol Invest*. 2009;32(1):85-90.

733. Isanaka S, Duggan C, Fawzi WW. Patterns of postnatal growth in HIV-infected and HIV-exposed children. *Nutr Rev*. 2009;67(6):343-359.

734. Chantry CJ, Frederick MM, Meyer WA 3rd, et al. Endocrine abnormalities and impaired growth in human immunodeficiency virus-infected children. *Pediatr Infect Dis J*. 2007;26(1):53-60.

735. Hardin DS, Rice J, Doyle ME, Pavia A. Growth hormone improves protein catabolism and growth in prepubertal children with HIV infection. *Clin Endocrinol (Oxf)*. 2005;63(3):259-262.

736. Chiesa A, Gruneiro de Papendieck L, Keselman A, et al. Growth follow-up in 100 children with congenital hypothyroidism before and during treatment. *J Pediatr Endocrinol*. 1994;7(3):211-217.

737. Rivkees SA, Bode HH, Crawford JD. Long-term growth in juvenile acquired hypothyroidism: the failure to achieve normal adult stature. *N Engl J Med*. 1988;318(10):599-602.

738. Boersma B, Otten BJ, Stoelinga GB, Wit JM. Catch-up growth after prolonged hypothyroidism. *Eur J Pediatr*. 1996;155(5):362-367.

739. Cassio A, Corrias A, Gualandi S, et al. Influence of gender and pubertal stage at diagnosis on growth outcome in childhood thyrotoxicosis: results of a collaborative study. *Clin Endocrinol (Oxf)*. 2006; 64(1):53-57.

740. Malone JI. Growth and sexual maturation in children with insulin-dependent diabetes mellitus. *Curr Opin Pediatr*. 1993;5(4):494-498.

741. Thon A, Heinze E, Feilen KD, et al. Development of height and weight in children with diabetes mellitus: report on two prospective multicentre studies, one cross-sectional, one longitudinal. *Eur J Pediatr*. 1992;151(4):258-262.

742. Bognetti E, Riva MC, Bonfanti R, et al. Growth changes in children and adolescents with short-term diabetes. *Diabetes Care*. 1998;21(8): 1226-1229.

743. Hjelt K, Braendholt V, Kamper J, Vestermark S. Growth in children with diabetes mellitus. the significance of metabolic control, insulin requirements and genetic factors. *Dan Med Bull*. 1983;30(1):28-33.

744. Jackson RL, Holland E, Chatman ID, et al. Growth and maturation of children with insulin-dependent diabetes mellitus. *Diabetes Care*. 1978;1(2):96-107.

745. Vanelli M, de Fanti A, Adinolfi B, Ghizzoni L. Clinical data regarding the growth of diabetic children. *Horm Res*. 1992;37(Suppl 3):65-69.

746. Rogers DG, Sherman LD, Gabbay KH. Effect of puberty on insulinlike growth factor I and HbA1 in type I diabetes. *Diabetes Care*. 1991; 14(11):1031-1035.

747. Mandell F, Berenberg W. The Mauriac syndrome. *Am J Dis Child.* 1974;127(6):900-902.

748. Menon RK, Arslanian S, May B, et al. Diminished growth hormone-binding protein in children with insulin-dependent diabetes mellitus. *J Clin Endocrinol Metab.* 1992;74(4):934-938.

749. Froesch ER, Hussain M. Metabolic effects of insulin-like growth factor I with special reference to diabetes. *Acta Paediatr Suppl.* 1994;399:165-170.

750. Malone JI, Lowitt S, Duncan JA, et al. Hypercalciuria, hyperphosphaturia, and growth retardation in children with diabetes mellitus. *Pediatrics.* 1986;78(2):298-304.

751. Clayton KL, Holly JM, Carlsson LM, et al. Loss of the normal relationships between growth hormone, growth hormone-binding protein and insulin-like growth factor-I in adolescents with insulin-dependent diabetes mellitus. *Clin Endocrinol (Oxf).* 1994;41(4):517-524.

752. Bereket A, Lang CH, Blethen SL, et al. Effect of insulin on the insulin-like growth factor system in children with new-onset insulin-dependent diabetes mellitus. *J Clin Endocrinol Metab.* 1995;80(4):1312-1317.

753. Rudolf MC, Sherwin RS, Markowitz R, et al. Effect of intensive insulin treatment on linear growth in the young diabetic patient. *J Pediatr.* 1982;101(3):333-339.

754. Munoz MT, Barrios V, Pozo J, Argente J. Insulin-like growth factor I, its binding proteins 1 and 3, and growth hormone-binding protein in children and adolescents with insulin-dependent diabetes mellitus: clinical implications. *Pediatr Res.* 1996;39(6):992-998.

755. Bereket A, Lang CH, Wilson TA. Alterations in the growth hormone-insulin-like growth factor axis in insulin dependent diabetes mellitus. *Horm Metab Res.* 1999;31(2-3):172-181.

756. Dunger DB. Insulin and insulin-like growth factors in diabetes mellitus. *Arch Dis Child.* 1995;72(6):469-471.

757. Suikkari AM, Koivisto VA, Rutanen EM, et al. Insulin regulates the serum levels of low molecular weight insulin-like growth factor-binding protein. *J Clin Endocrinol Metab.* 1988;66(2):266-272.

758. Batch JA, Baxter RC, Werther G. Abnormal regulation of insulin-like growth factor binding proteins in adolescents with insulin-dependent diabetes. *J Clin Endocrinol Metab.* 1991;73(5):964-968.

759. Winter RJ, Phillips LS, Klein MN, et al. Somatomedin activity and diabetic control in children with insulin-dependent diabetes. *Diabetes.* 1979;28(10):952-954.

760. Clarson D, Daneman D, Ehrlich RM. The relation of metabolic control to growth and pubertal development in children with insulin-dependent diabetes. *Diabetes Res.* 1985;2:237-241.

761. Du Caju MV, Rooman RP, op de Beeck L. Longitudinal data on growth and final height in diabetic children. *Pediatr Res.* 1995;38(4):607-611.

762. Tamborlane WV, Hintz RL, Bergman M, et al. Insulin-infusion-pump treatment of diabetes: influence of improved metabolic control on plasma somatomedin levels. *N Engl J Med.* 1981;305(6):303-307.

763. Reid IR. Pathogenesis and treatment of steroid osteoporosis. *Clin Endocrinol (Oxf).* 1989;30(1):83-103.

764. Giustina A, Bussi AR, Jacobello C, Wehrenberg WB. Effects of recombinant human growth hormone (GH) on bone and intermediary metabolism in patients receiving chronic glucocorticoid treatment with suppressed endogenous GH response to GH-releasing hormone. *J Clin Endocrinol Metab.* 1995;80(1):122-129.

765. Allen DB, Goldberg BD. Stimulation of collagen synthesis and linear growth by growth hormone in glucocorticoid-treated children. *Pediatrics.* 1992;89(3):416-421.

766. Schatz M, Dudl J, Zeiger RS, et al. Osteoporosis in corticosteroid-treated asthmatic patients: clinical correlates. *Allergy Proc.* 1993;14(5):341-345.

767. Kerrebijn KF, de Kroon JP. Effect of height of corticosteroid therapy in asthmatic children. *Arch Dis Child.* 1968;43(231):556-561.

768. Mosier HD Jr, Smith FG Jr, Schultz MA. Failure of catch-up growth after Cushing's syndrome in childhood. *Am J Dis Child.* 1972;124(2):251-253.

769. Leong GM, Mercado-Asis LB, Reynolds JC, et al. The effect of Cushing's disease on bone mineral density, body composition, growth, and puberty: a report of an identical adolescent twin pair. *J Clin Endocrinol Metab.* 1996;81(5):1905-1911.

770. Reimer LG, Morris HG, Ellis EF. Growth of asthmatic children during treatment with alternate-day steroids. *J Allergy Clin Immunol.* 1975;55(4):224-231.

771. Lai HC, FitzSimmons SC, Allen DB, et al. Risk of persistent growth impairment after alternate-day prednisone treatment in children with cystic fibrosis. *N Engl J Med.* 2000;342(12):851-859.

772. Sharek PJ, Bergman DA. The effect of inhaled steroids on the linear growth of children with asthma: a meta-analysis. *Pediatrics.* 2000;106(1):E8.

773. Allen DB, Julius JR, Breen TJ, Attie KM. Treatment of glucocorticoid-induced growth suppression with growth hormone. national cooperative growth study. *J Clin Endocrinol Metab.* 1998;83(8):2824-2829.

774. Rivkees SA, Danon M, Herrin J. Prednisone dose limitation of growth hormone treatment of steroid-induced growth failure. *J Pediatr.* 1994;125(2):322-325.

775. Horber FF, Haymond MW. Human growth hormone prevents the protein catabolic side effects of prednisone in humans. *J Clin Invest.* 1990;86(1):265-272.

776. Mauras N, Beaufrere B. Recombinant human insulin-like growth factor-I enhances whole body protein anabolism and significantly diminishes the protein catabolic effects of prednisone in humans without a diabetogenic effect. *J Clin Endocrinol Metab.* 1995;80(3):869-874.

777. Lebrethon MC, Grossman AB, Afshar F, et al. Linear growth and final height after treatment for Cushing's disease in childhood. *J Clin Endocrinol Metab.* 2000;85(9):3262-3265.

778. Schwindinger WF, Levine MA. Albright hereditary osteodystrophy. *Endocrinologist.* 1994;4:17-27.

779. Long DN, McGuire S, Levine MA, et al. Body mass index differences in pseudohypoparathyroidism type 1a versus pseudopseudohypoparathyroidism may implicate paternal imprinting of galpha(s) in the development of human obesity. *J Clin Endocrinol Metab.* 2007;92(3):1073-1079.

780. Germain-Lee EL. Short stature, obesity, and growth hormone deficiency in pseudohypoparathyroidism type 1a. *Pediatr Endocrinol Rev.* 2006;3(Suppl 2):318-327.

781. Mantovani G, Maghnie M, Weber G, et al. Growth hormone-releasing hormone resistance in pseudohypoparathyroidism type Ia: new evidence for imprinting of the gs alpha gene. *J Clin Endocrinol Metab.* 2003;88(9):4070-4074.

782. Mantovani G, Bondioni S, Linglart A, et al. Genetic analysis and evaluation of resistance to thyrotropin and growth hormone-releasing hormone in pseudohypoparathyroidism type Ib. *J Clin Endocrinol Metab.* 2007;92(9):3738-3742.

783. Plagge A, Kelsey G, Germain-Lee EL. Physiological functions of the imprinted gnas locus and its protein variants galpha(s) and XLalpha(s) in human and mouse. *J Endocrinol.* 2008;196(2):193-214.

784. Mantovani G, Ferrante E, Giavoli C, et al. Recombinant human GH replacement therapy in children with pseudohypoparathyroidism type Ia: first study on the effect on growth. *J Clin Endocrinol Metab.* 2010;95(11):5011-5017.

785. Minamitani K, Takahashi Y, Minagawa M, et al. Difference in height associated with a translation start site polymorphism in the vitamin D receptor gene. *Pediatr Res.* 1998;44(5):628-632.

786. Lorentzon M, Lorentzon R, Nordstrom P. Vitamin D receptor gene polymorphism is associated with birth height, growth to adolescence, and adult stature in healthy Caucasian men: a cross-sectional and longitudinal study. *J Clin Endocrinol Metab.* 2000;85(4):1666-1670.

787. Suarez F, Zeghoud F, Rossignol C, et al. Association between vitamin D receptor gene polymorphism and sex-dependent growth during the first two years of life. *J Clin Endocrinol Metab.* 1997;82(9):2966-2970.

788. Kanan RM, Varanasi SS, Francis RM, et al. Vitamin D receptor gene start codon polymorphism (FokI) and bone mineral density in healthy male subjects. *Clin Endocrinol (Oxf).* 2000;53(1):93-98.

789. Arai H, Miyamoto K, Taketani Y, et al. A vitamin D receptor gene polymorphism in the translation initiation codon: effect on protein activity and relation to bone mineral density in Japanese women. *J Bone Miner Res.* 1997;12(6):915-921.

790. Suarez F, Rossignol C, Garabedian M. Interactive effect of estradiol and vitamin D receptor gene polymorphisms as a possible determinant of growth in male and female infants. *J Clin Endocrinol Metab.* 1998;83(10):3563-3568.

791. Alonso M, Segura C, Dieguez C, et al. High affinity binding sites to the vitamin D receptor DNA binding domain in the human growth hormone promoter. *Biochem Biophys Res Commun.* 2000;247:882-887.

792. Cho HY, Lee BH, Kang JH, et al. A clinical and molecular genetic study of hypophosphatemic rickets in children. *Pediatr Res.* 2005;58(2):329-333.

793. Liao E. FGF23 associated bone diseases. *Front Med.* 2013;7(1):65-80.

794. Makitie O, Doria A, Kooh SW, et al. Early treatment improves growth and biochemical and radiographic outcome in X-linked hypophosphatemic rickets. *J Clin Endocrinol Metab.* 2003;88(8):3591-3597.

795. Chan JC. Renal hypophosphatemic rickets—a review. *Int J Pediatr Nephrol.* 1982;3(4):305-310.

796. Petersen DJ, Boniface AM, Schranck FW, et al. X-linked hypophosphatemic rickets: a study (with literature review) of linear growth response to calcitriol and phosphate therapy. *J Bone Miner Res.* 1992;7(6):583-597.

797. Balsan S, Tieder M. Linear growth in patients with hypophosphatemic vitamin D-resistant rickets: influence of treatment regimen and parental height. *J Pediatr.* 1990;116(3):365-371.

798. Jasper H, Cassinelli H. Growth hormone and insulin-like growth factor I plasma levels in patients with hypophosphatemic rickets. *J Pediatr Endocrinol.* 1993;6(2):179-184.

799. Saggese G, Baroncelli GI, Bertelloni S, Perri G. Growth hormone secretion in poorly growing children with renal hypophosphataemic rickets. *Eur J Pediatr.* 1994;153(8):548-555.

800. Bistritzer T, Chalew SA, Hanukoglu A, et al. Does growth hormone influence the severity of phosphopenic rickets? *Eur J Pediatr.* 1990;150(1):26-29.

801. Wilson DM. Growth hormone and hypophosphatemic rickets. *J Pediatr Endocrinol Metab.* 2000;13(Suppl 2):993-998.

802. Wilson DM, Lee PD, Morris AH, et al. Growth hormone therapy in hypophosphatemic rickets. *Am J Dis Child.* 1991;145(10):1165-1170.

803. Baroncelli GI, Bertelloni S, Ceccarelli C, Saggese G. Effect of growth hormone treatment on final height, phosphate metabolism, and bone mineral density in children with X-linked hypophosphatemic rickets. *J Pediatr.* 2001;138(2):236-243.

804. Huiming Y, Chaomin W. Recombinant growth hormone therapy for X-linked hypophosphatemia in children. *Cochrane Database Syst Rev.* 2005;(1):CD004447.

805. Haffner D, Nissel R, Wuhl E, Mehls O. Effects of growth hormone treatment on body proportions and final height among small children with X-linked hypophosphatemic rickets. *Pediatrics.* 2004;113(6):e593-e596.

806. Hall CM. International Nosology and Classification of Constitutional Disorders of Bone (2001). *Am J Med Genet.* 2002;113(1):65-77.

807. Hecht JT, Bodensteiner JB, Butler IJ. Neurologic manifestations of achondroplasia. *Handb Clin Neurol.* 2014;119:551-563.

808. Wickman S, Sipila I, Ankarberg-Lindgren C, et al. A specific aromatase inhibitor and potential increase in adult height in boys with delayed puberty: a randomised controlled trial. *Lancet.* 2001;357(9270):1743-1748.

809. Mauras N, Gonzalez de Pijem L, Hsiang HY, et al. Anastrozole increases predicted adult height of short adolescent males treated with growth hormone: a randomized, placebo-controlled, multicenter trial for one to three years. *J Clin Endocrinol Metab.* 2008;93(3):823-831.

810. Vajo Z, Francomano CA, Wilkin DJ. The molecular and genetic basis of fibroblast growth factor receptor 3 disorders: the achondroplasia family of skeletal dysplasias, Muenke craniosynostosis, and Crouzon syndrome with acanthosis nigricans. *Endocr Rev.* 2000;21:23-39.

811. Hero M, Makitie O, Kroger H, et al. Impact of aromatase inhibitor therapy on bone turnover, cortical bone growth and vertebral morphology in pre- and peripubertal boys with idiopathic short stature. *Horm Res.* 2009;71(5):290-297.

812. Ramaswami U, Rumsby G, Hindmarsh PC, Brook CG. Genotype and phenotype in hypochondroplasia. *J Pediatr.* 1998;133(1):99-102.

813. Ross JL, Kowal K, Quigley CA, et al. The phenotype of short stature homeobox gene (SHOX) deficiency in childhood: contrasting children with Leri-Weill dyschondrosteosis and Turner syndrome. *J Pediatr.* 2005;147(4):499-507.

814. Marchini A, Marttila T, Winter A, et al. The short stature homeodomain protein SHOX induces cellular growth arrest and apoptosis and is expressed in human growth plate chondrocytes. *J Biol Chem.* 2004;279(35):37103-37114.

815. Bartels CF, Bukulmez H, Padayatti P, et al. Mutations in the transmembrane natriuretic peptide receptor NPR-B impair skeletal growth and cause acromesomelic dysplasia, type maroteaux. *Am J Hum Genet.* 2004;75(1):27-34.

816. Olney RC, Bukulmez H, Bartels CF, et al. Heterozygous mutations in natriuretic peptide receptor-B (NPR2) are associated with short stature. *J Clin Endocrinol Metab.* 2006;91(4):1229-1232.

817. Anneren G, Tuvemo T, Gustafsson J. Growth hormone therapy in young children with Down syndrome and a clinical comparison of Down and Prader-Willi syndromes. *Growth Horm IGF Res.* 2000;10(suppl B):S87-S91.

818. Annerén G1, Tuvemo T, Carlsson-Skwirut C, et al. Growth hormone treatment in young children with Down's syndrome: effects on growth and psychomotor development. *Arch Dis Child.* 1999;80(4):334-338.

819. Rosenfeld RG, Grumbach MM. *Turner Syndrome.* New York: Marcel Dekker; 1990.

820. Turner syndrome: growth promoting therapies. *Proceedings of a Workshop on Turner Syndrome.* Amsterdam: Excerpta Medica; 1991.

821. Basic and clinical approach to Turner syndrome. *Proceedings of the 3rd International Symposium on Turner Syndrome.* Amsterdam: Excerpta Medica; 1993.

822. Rochiccioli P, David M, Malpuech G, et al. Study of final height in Turner's syndrome: ethnic and genetic influences. *Acta Paediatr.* 1994;83(3):305-308.

823. Nilsson KO, Albertsson-Wikland K, Alm J, et al. Improved final height in girls with Turner's syndrome treated with growth hormone and oxandrolone. *J Clin Endocrinol Metab.* 1996;81(2):635-640.

824. Rosenfeld RG, Attie KM, Frane J, et al. Growth hormone therapy of Turner's syndrome: beneficial effect on adult height. *J Pediatr.* 1998;132(2):319-324.

825. Brook CG, Gasser T, Werder EA, et al. Height correlations between parents and mature offspring in normal subjects and in subjects with Turner's and Klinefelter's and other syndromes. *Ann Hum Biol.* 1977;4(1):17-22.

826. Massa G, Vanderschueren-Lodeweyckx M, Malvaux P. Linear growth in patients with Turner syndrome: influence of spontaneous puberty and parental height. *Eur J Pediatr.* 1990;149(4):246-250.

827. Ranke MB, Pfluger H, Rosendahl W, et al. Turner syndrome: spontaneous growth in 150 cases and review of the literature. *Eur J Pediatr.* 1983;141(2):81-88.

828. Davenport ML, Punyasavatsut N, Gunther D, et al. Turner syndrome: a pattern of early growth failure. *Acta Paediatr Suppl.* 1999;88(433):118-121.

829. Davenport ML, Punyasavatsut N, Stewart PW, et al. Growth failure in early life: an important manifestation of Turner syndrome. *Horm Res.* 2002;57(5-6):157-164.

830. Even L, Cohen A, Marbach N, et al. Longitudinal analysis of growth over the first 3 years of life in Turner's syndrome. *J Pediatr.* 2000;137(4):460-464.

831. Blaschke RJ, Rappold GA. SHOX: Growth, Leri-Weill and Turner syndromes. *Trends Endocrinol Metab.* 2000;11(6):227-230.

832. Ross JL, Scott C Jr, Marttila P, et al. Phenotypes associated with SHOX deficiency. *J Clin Endocrinol Metab.* 2001;86(12):5674-5680.

833. Ross JL, Long LM, Loriaux DL, Cutler GB Jr. Growth hormone secretory dynamics in Turner syndrome. *J Pediatr.* 1985;106(2):202-206.

834. Sas TC, de Muinck Keizer-Schrama SM, Stijnen T, et al. Normalization of height in girls with Turner syndrome after long-term growth hormone treatment: results of a randomized dose-response trial. *J Clin Endocrinol Metab.* 1999;84(12):4607-4612.

835. Saenger P. Growth-promoting strategies in Turner's syndrome. *J Clin Endocrinol Metab.* 1999;84(12):4345-4348.

836. Collins E, Turner G. The Noonan syndrome—a review of the clinical and genetic features of 27 cases. *J Pediatr.* 1973;83(6):941-950.

837. Kelnar CJ. Growth hormone therapy in Noonan syndrome. *Horm Res.* 2000;53(Suppl 1):77-81.

838. Roberts AE, Allanson JE, Tartaglia M, Gelb BD. Noonan syndrome. *Lancet.* 2013;381(9863):333-342.

839. Zenker M. Genetic and pathogenetic aspects of Noonan syndrome and related disorders. *Horm Res.* 2009;72(Suppl 2):57-63.

840. Patton MA. Noonan syndrome: a review. *Growth Genet Horm.* 1994;10:1-3.

841. Ranke MB, Heidemann P, Knupfer C, et al. Noonan syndrome: growth and clinical manifestations in 144 cases. *Eur J Pediatr.* 1988;148(3):220-227.

842. Witt DR, Keena BA, Hall JG, Allanson JE. Growth curves for height in Noonan syndrome. *Clin Genet.* 1986;30(3):150-153.

843. Bernardini S, Spadoni GL, Cianfarani S, et al. Growth hormone secretion in Noonan's syndrome. *J Pediatr Endocrinol.* 1991;4:217-221.

844. Ferreira LV, Souza SA, Arnhold IJ, et al. PTPN11 (protein tyrosine phosphatase, nonreceptor type 11) mutations and response to growth hormone therapy in children with Noonan syndrome. *J Clin Endocrinol Metab.* 2005;90(9):5156-5160.

845. Binder G, Neuer K, Ranke MB, Wittekindt NE. PTPN11 mutations are associated with mild growth hormone resistance in individuals with Noonan syndrome. *J Clin Endocrinol Metab.* 2005;90(9):5377-5381.

846. Limal JM, Parfait B, Cabrol S, et al. Noonan syndrome: relationships between genotype, growth, and growth factors. *J Clin Endocrinol Metab.* 2006;91(1):300-306.

847. Bray GA, Dahms WT, Swerdloff RS, et al. The Prader-Willi syndrome: a study of 40 patients and a review of the literature. *Medicine (Baltimore).* 1983;62(2):59-80.

848. Jones KL. *Smith's Recognizable Patterns of Human Malformation.* Philadelphia, PA: WB Saunders; 1988.

849. Saenger P, Czernichow P, Hughes I, Reiter EO. Small for gestational age: short stature and beyond. *Endocr Rev.* 2007;28(2):219-251.

850. Lepercq J, Mahieu-Caputo D. Diagnosis and management of intrauterine growth retardation. *Horm Res.* 1998;49(Suppl 2):14-19.

851. Seminara S, Rapisardi G, La Cauza F, et al. Catch-up growth in short-at-birth NICU graduates. *Horm Res.* 2000;53(3):139-143.

852. Leger J, Limoni C, Collin D, Czernichow P. Prediction factors in the determination of final height in subjects born small for gestational age. *Pediatr Res.* 1998;43(6):808-812.

853. Rappaport R. Fetal growth. In: Bertrand J, Rappaport R, Sizonenko PC, eds. *Pediatric Endocrinology: Physiology, Pathophysiology, and Clinical Aspects.* 2nd ed. Baltimore, MD: Williams & Wilkins; 1993.

854. Smith GC, Smith MF, McNay MB, et al. First-trimester growth and the risk of low birth weight. *N Engl J Med.* 1999;339:1817-1822.

855. Patterson RM, Pouliot MR. Neonatal morphometrics and perinatal outcome: who is growth retarded? *Am J Obstet Gynecol.* 1987;157(3):691-693.

856. Campbell S, Thoms A. Ultrasound measurement of the fetal head to abdomen circumference ratio in the assessment of growth retardation. *Br J Obstet Gynaecol.* 1977;84(3):165-174.

857. Hindmarsh PC, Geary MP, Rodeck CH, et al. Intrauterine growth and its relationship to size and shape at birth. *Pediatr Res.* 2002;52(2):263-268.

858. Vik T, Markestad T, Ahlsten G, et al. Body proportions and early neonatal morbidity in small-for-gestational-age infants of successive births. *Acta Obstet Gynecol Scand Suppl.* 1997;165:76-81.

859. Gluckman PD, Gunn AJ, Wray A, et al. Congenital idiopathic growth hormone deficiency associated with prenatal and early postnatal growth failure. The international board of the Kabi Pharmacia International Growth Study. *J Pediatr.* 1992;121(6):920-923.

860. DeLuca F, Bernasconi S, Blandino A, et al. Auxological, clinical, and neuroradiological findings in infants with early onset growth hormone deficiency. *Acta Paediatr Scand.* 1995;84:561-565.

861. Hattersley AT, Beards F, Ballantyne E, et al. Mutations in the glucokinase gene of the fetus result in reduced birth weight. *Nat Genet.* 1998;19(3):268-270.

862. Warshaw JB. Intrauterine growth restriction revisited. *Growth Genet Horm.* 1992;8:5-8.

863. Vaessen N, Janssen JA, Heutink P, et al. Association between genetic variation in the gene for insulin-like growth factor-I and low birthweight. *Lancet.* 2002;359(9311):1036-1037.

864. Arends N, Johnston L, Hokken-Koelega A, et al. Polymorphism in the IGF-I gene: clinical relevance for short children born small for gestational age (SGA). *J Clin Endocrinol Metab.* 2002;87(6):2720.

865. de Zegher F, Kimpen J, Raus J, Vanderschueren-Lodeweyckx M. Hypersomatotropism in the dysmature infant at term and preterm birth. *Biol Neonate.* 1990;58(4):188-191.

866. Spencer JA, Chang TC, Jones J, et al. Third trimester fetal growth and umbilical venous blood concentrations of IGF-1, IGFBP-1, and growth hormone at term. *Arch Dis Child Fetal Neonatal Ed.* 1995;73(2):F87-F90.

867. Leger J, Oury JF, Noel M, et al. Growth factors and intrauterine growth retardation. I. Serum growth hormone, insulin-like growth factor (IGF)-I, IGF-II, and IGF binding protein 3 levels in normally grown and growth-retarded human fetuses during the second half of gestation. *Pediatr Res.* 1996;40(1):94-100.

868. Cianfarani S, Germani D, Rossi L, et al. IGF-I and IGF-binding protein-1 are related to cortisol in human cord blood. *Eur J Endocrinol.* 1998;138(5):524-529.

869. Cance-Rouzaud A, Laborie S, Bieth E, et al. Growth hormone, insulin-like growth factor-I and insulin-like growth factor binding protein-3 are regulated differently in small-for-gestational-age and appropriate-for-gestational-age neonates. *Biol Neonate.* 1998;73(6):347-355.

870. Wollmann HA, Ranke MB. GH treatment in neonates. *Acta Paediatr.* 1996;85(4):398-400.

871. van Toledo-Eppinga L, Houdijk EC, Cranendonk A, et al. Effects of recombinant human growth hormone treatment in intrauterine growth-retarded preterm newborn infant on growth, body composition and energy expenditure. *Acta Paediatr.* 1996;85(4):476-481.

872. Leger J, Noel M, Limal JM, Czernichow P. Growth factors and intrauterine growth retardation. II. Serum growth hormone, insulin-like growth factor (IGF) I, and IGF-binding protein 3 levels in children with intrauterine growth retardation compared with normal control subjects: prospective study from birth to two years of age. Study group of IUGR. *Pediatr Res.* 1996;40(1):101-107.

873. Boguszewski M, Rosberg S, Albertsson-Wikland K. Spontaneous 24-hour growth hormone profiles in prepubertal small for gestational age children. *J Clin Endocrinol Metab.* 1995;80(9):2599-2606.

874. Ackland FM, Stanhope R, Eyre C, et al. Physiological growth hormone secretion in children with short stature and intra-uterine growth retardation. *Horm Res.* 1988;30(6):241-245.

875. de Waal WJ, Hokken-Koelega AC, Stijnen T, et al. Endogenous and stimulated GH secretion, urinary GH excretion, and plasma IGF-I and IGF-II levels in prepubertal children with short stature after intrauterine growth retardation. The Dutch working group on growth hormone. *Clin Endocrinol (Oxf).* 1994;41(5):621-630.

876. Ibanez L, Dimartino-Nardi J, Potau N, Saenger P. Premature adrenarche—normal variant or forerunner of adult disease? *Endocr Rev.* 2000;21(6):671-696.

877. Varvarigou AA. Intrauterine growth restriction as a potential risk factor for disease onset in adulthood. *J Pediatr Endocrinol Metab.* 2010;23(3):215-224.

878. Osmond C, Barker DJ. Fetal, infant, and childhood growth are predictors of coronary heart disease, diabetes, and hypertension in adult men and women. *Environ Health Perspect.* 2000;108(Suppl 3):545-553.

879. Langley-Evans SC, McMullen S. Developmental origins of adult disease. *Med Princ Pract.* 2010;19(2):87-98.

880. Hofman PL, Cutfield WS, Robinson EM, et al. Insulin resistance in short children with intrauterine growth retardation. *J Clin Endocrinol Metab.* 1997;82(2):402-406.

881. Russell A. A syndrome of intra-uterine dwarfism recognizable at birth with cranio-facial dysostosis, disproportionately short arms, and other anomalies (5 examples). *Proc R Soc Med.* 1954;47(12):1040-1044.

882. Silver HK. Asymmetry, short stature, and variations in sexual development. A syndrome of congenital malformations. *Am J Dis Child.* 1964;107:495-515.

883. Wakeling EL. Silver-Russell syndrome. *Arch Dis Child.* 2011;96(12):1156-1161.

884. Angehrn V, Zachmann M, Prader A. Silver-Russell syndrome. Observations in 20 patients. *Helv Paediatr Acta.* 1979;34(4):297-308.

885. Davies PS, Valley R, Preece MA. Adolescent growth and pubertal progression in the Silver-Russell syndrome. *Arch Dis Child.* 1988;63(2):130-135.

886. Saal HM, Pagon RA, Pepin MG. Reevaluation of Russell-Silver syndrome. *J Pediatr.* 1985;107(5):733-737.

887. Albertsson-Wikland K, Boguszewski M, Karlberg J. Children born small-for-gestational age: postnatal growth and hormonal status. *Horm Res.* 1998;49(Suppl 2):7-13.

888. Monk D, Wakeling EL, Proud V, et al. Duplication of 7p11.2-p13, including GRB10, in Silver-Russell syndrome. *Am J Hum Genet.* 2000;66(1):36-46.

889. Miyoshi N, Kuroiwa Y, Kohda T, et al. Identification of the Meg1/Grb10 imprinted gene on mouse proximal chromosome 11, a candidate for the Silver-Russell syndrome gene. *Proc Natl Acad Sci U S A.* 1998;95(3):1102-1107.

890. Eggermann T, Meyer E, Obermann C, et al. Is maternal duplication of 11p15 associated with Silver-Russell syndrome? *J Med Genet.* 2005;42(5):e26.

891. Gicquel C, Rossignol S, Cabrol S, et al. Epimutation of the telomeric imprinting center region on chromosome 11p15 in Silver-Russell syndrome. *Nat Genet.* 2005;37(9):1003-1007.

892. Binder G, Seidel AK, Weber K, et al. IGF-II serum levels are normal in children with Silver-Russell syndrome who frequently carry epimutations at the IGF2 locus. *J Clin Endocrinol Metab.* 2006;91(11):4709-4712.

893. Edwards LE, Alton IR, Barrada MI, Hakanson EY. Pregnancy in the underweight woman. Course, outcome, and growth patterns of the infant. *Am J Obstet Gynecol.* 1979;135(3):297-302.

894. Patra J, Bakker R, Irving H, et al. Dose-response relationship between alcohol consumption before and during pregnancy and the risks of low birthweight, preterm birth and small for gestational age (SGA)—a systematic review and meta-analyses. *BJOG.* 2011;118(12):1411-1421.

895. Zuckerman B, Frank DA, Hingson R, et al. Effects of maternal marijuana and cocaine use on fetal growth. *N Engl J Med.* 1989;320(12):762-768.

896. Abel EL. Smoking during pregnancy: a review of effects on growth and development of offspring. *Hum Biol.* 1980;52(4):593-625.

897. Hall K, Enberg G, Hellem E, et al. Somatomedin levels in pregnancy: longitudinal study in healthy subjects and patients with growth hormone deficiency. *J Clin Endocrinol Metab.* 1984;59(4):587-594.

898. Mirlesse V, Frankenne F, Alsat E, et al. Placental growth hormone levels in normal pregnancy and in pregnancies with intrauterine growth retardation. *Pediatr Res.* 1993;34(4):439-442.

899. Hasegawa T, Hasegawa Y, Takada M, Tsuchiya Y. The free form of insulin-like growth factor I increases in circulation during normal human pregnancy. *J Clin Endocrinol Metab.* 1995;80(11):3284-3286.

900. Verhaeghe J, Bougoussa M, Van Herck E, et al. Placental growth hormone and IGF-I in a pregnant woman with pit-1 deficiency. *Clin Endocrinol (Oxf).* 2000;53(5):645-647.

901. Li Y, Behringer RR. Esx1 is an X-chromosome-imprinted regulator of placental development and fetal growth. *Nat Genet.* 1998;20(3):309-311.

902. Li Y, Lemaire P, Behringer RR. Esx1, a novel X chromosome-linked homeobox gene expressed in mouse extraembryonic tissues and male germ cells. *Dev Biol.* 1997;188(1):85-95.

903. Fohn LE, Behringer RR. ESX1L, a novel X chromosome-linked human homeobox gene expressed in the placenta and testis. *Genomics.* 2001;74(1):105-108.

904. Sotos JF, Cutler EA, Dodre P. Cerebral gigantism. *Am J Dis Child.* 1977;131(6):625-627.

905. Wit JM, Beemer FA, Barth PG, et al. Cerebral gigantism (Sotos syndrome). Compiled data of 22 cases. Analysis of clinical features, growth and plasma somatomedin. *Eur J Pediatr.* 1985;144(2):131-140.

906. Agwu JC, Shaw NJ, Kirk J, et al. Growth in Sotos syndrome. *Arch Dis Child.* 1999;80(4):339-342.

907. Waggoner DJ, Raca G, Welch K, et al. NSD1 analysis for Sotos syndrome: insights and perspectives from the clinical laboratory. *Genet Med.* 2005;7(8):524-533.

908. Sotelo-Avila C, Gonzalez-Crussi F, Starling KA. Wilms' tumor in a patient with an incomplete form of Beckwith-Wiedemann syndrome. *Pediatrics.* 1980;66(1):121-123.

909. Elliott M, Bayly R, Cole T, et al. Clinical features and natural history of Beckwith-Wiedemann syndrome: presentation of 74 new cases. *Clin Genet.* 1994;46(2):168-174.

910. Weng EY, Moeschler JB, Graham JM Jr. Longitudinal observations on 15 children with Wiedemann-Beckwith syndrome. *Am J Med Genet.* 1995;56(4):366-373.

911. Kubota T, Saitoh S, Matsumoto T, et al. Excess functional copy of allele at chromosomal region 11p15 may cause Wiedemann-Beckwith (EMG) syndrome. *Am J Med Genet.* 1994;49(4):378-383.

912. Prawitt D, Enklaar T, Gartner-Rupprecht B, et al. Microdeletion and IGF2 loss of imprinting in a cascade causing Beckwith-Wiedemann syndrome with Wilms' tumor. *Nat Genet.* 2005;37(8):785-786, author reply 786-787.

913. Poole RL, Leith DJ, Docherty LE, et al. Beckwith-Wiedemann syndrome caused by maternally inherited mutation of an OCT-binding motif in the IGF2/H19-imprinting control region, ICR1. *Eur J Hum Genet.* 2012;20(2):240-243.

914. Brannan CI, Bartolomei MS. Mechanisms of genomic imprinting. *Curr Opin Genet Dev.* 1999;9(2):164-170.

915. Reik W, Constancia M, Dean W, et al. IGF2 imprinting in development and disease. *Int J Dev Biol.* 2000;44(1):145-150.
916. Morison IM, Becroft DM, Taniguchi T, et al. Somatic overgrowth associated with overexpression of insulin-like growth factor II. *Nat Med.* 1996;2(3):311-316.
917. Cano-Gauci DF, Song HH, Yang H, et al. Glypican-3-deficient mice exhibit developmental overgrowth and some of the abnormalities typical of Simpson-Golabi-Behmel syndrome. *J Cell Biol.* 1999;146(1): 255-264.
918. Veugelers M, Cat BD, Muyldermans SY, et al. Mutational analysis of the GPC3/GPC4 glypican gene cluster on Xq26 in patients with Simpson-Golabi-Behmel syndrome: identification of loss-of-function mutations in the GPC3 gene. *Hum Mol Genet.* 2000;9(9):1321-1328.
919. Joss EE, Temperli R, Mullis PE. Adult height in constitutionally tall stature: accuracy of five different height prediction methods. *Arch Dis Child.* 1992;67(11):1357-1362.
920. Tauber M, Pienkowski C, Rochiccioli P. Growth hormone secretion in children and adolescents with familial tall stature. *Eur J Pediatr.* 1994;153(5):311-316.
921. Elias LL, Huebner A, Metherell LA, et al. Tall stature in familial glucocorticoid deficiency. *Clin Endocrinol (Oxf).* 2000;53(4):423-430.
922. Ogata T, Kosho T, Wakui K, et al. Short stature homeobox-containing gene duplication on the der(X) chromosome in a female with 45,X/46,X, der(X), gonadal dysgenesis, and tall stature. *J Clin Endocrinol Metab.* 2000;85(8):2927-2930.
923. Nakamura Y, Suehiro Y, Sugino N, et al. A case of 46,X,der(X) (pter → q21::P21 → pter) with gonadal dysgenesis, tall stature, and endometriosis. *Fertil Steril.* 2001;75(6):1224-1225.
924. Ogata T, Matsuo N. Sex chromosome aberrations and stature: deduction of the principal factors involved in the determination of adult height. *Hum Genet.* 1993;91(6):551-562.
925. Morishima A, Grumbach MM, Ito Y, et al. A syndrome of female pseudohermaphrodism. Hypergonadotropic hypogonadism and multicystic ovaries associated with missense mutations in the gene encoding aromatase (P450arom). *J Clin Endocrinol Metab.* 1994;78:1287.
926. Forbes GB. Nutrition and growth. *J Pediatr.* 1977;91(1):40-42.
927. Ong KK, Ahmed ML, Emmett PM, et al. Association between postnatal catch-up growth and obesity in childhood: prospective cohort study. *BMJ.* 2000;320(7240):967-971.
928. Cole TJ. The secular trend in human physical growth: a biological view. *Econ Hum Biol.* 2003;1(2):161-168.
929. Spence HJ, Trias EP, Raiti S. Acromegaly in a 9-and-one-half-year-old boy. Pituitary function studies before and after surgery. *Am J Dis Child.* 1972;123(5):504-506.
930. AvRuskin TW, Sau K, Tang S, Juan C. Childhood acromegaly: successful therapy with conventional radiation and effects of chlorpromazine on growth hormone and prolactin secretion. *J Clin Endocrinol Metab.* 1973;37(3):380-388.
931. DeMajo SF, Onativia A. Acromegaly and gigantism in a boy: comparison with three overgrown non-acromegalic children. *Pediatrics.* 1960;57:382-390.
932. Lefkowitz RJ. G proteins in medicine. *N Engl J Med.* 1995;332(3): 186-187.
933. Lightner ES, Winter JS. Treatment of juvenile acromegaly with bromocriptine. *J Pediatr.* 1981;98(3):494-496.
934. Geffner ME, Nagel RA, Dietrich RB, Kaplan SA. Treatment of acromegaly with a somatostatin analog in a patient with McCune-Albright syndrome. *J Pediatr.* 1987;111(5):740-743.
935. Hoffman WH, Perrin JC, Halac E, et al. Acromegalic gigantism and tuberous sclerosis. *J Pediatr.* 1978;93(3):478-480.
936. Daughaday WH. Extreme gigantism. Analysis of growth velocity and occurrence of severe peripheral neuropathy and neuropathic arthropathy (Charcot joints). *N Engl J Med.* 1977;297(23):1267-1269.
937. Hindmarsh PC, Brook CG. Auxological and biochemical assessment of short stature. *Acta Paediatr Scand Suppl.* 1988;343:73-76.
938. Voss LD, Wilkin TJ, Bailey BJ, Betts PR. The reliability of height and height velocity in the assessment of growth (the Wessex growth study). *Arch Dis Child.* 1991;66(7):833-837.
939. Mayer M, Schmitt K, Kapelari K, et al. Spontaneous growth in growth hormone deficiency from birth until 7 years of age: development of disease-specific growth curves. *Horm Res Paediatr.* 2010;74(2): 136-144.
940. Rudman D, Davis T, Priest JH, et al. Prevalence of growth hormone deficiency in children with cleft lip or palate. *J Pediatr.* 1978; 93(3):378-382.
941. Pandian R, Nakamoto JM. Rational use of the laboratory for childhood and adult growth hormone deficiency. *Clin Lab Med.* 2004; 24(1):141-174.
942. Akin F, Yaylali GF, Turgut S, Kaptanoglu B. Growth hormone/insulin-like growth factor axis in patients with subclinical thyroid dysfunction. *Growth Horm IGF Res.* 2009;19(3):252-255.
943. Purandare A, Co Ng L, Godil M, et al. Effect of hypothyroidism and its treatment on the IGF system in infants and children. *J Pediatr Endocrinol Metab.* 2003;16(1):35-42.
944. Greulich WW, Pyle SI. *Radiographic Atlas of Skeletal Development of the Hand and Wrist.* Stanford, CA: Stanford University Press; 1959.
945. Tanner JM, Whitehouse RH, Cameron N, et al. *Assessment of Skeletal Maturity and Prediction of Adult Height (TW2 Method).* New York: Academic Press; 1983.
946. Tanner JM, Oshman D, Lindgren G, et al. Reliability and validity of computer-assisted estimates of Tanner-Whitehouse skeletal maturity (CASAS): comparison with the manual method. *Horm Res.* 1994; 42(6):288-294.
947. Van Teunenbroek A, De Waal W, Roks A, et al. Computer-aided skeletal age scores in healthy children, girls with Turner syndrome, and in children with constitutionally tall stature. *Pediatr Res.* 1996; 39(2):360-367.
948. Roche AF, Davila GH, Eyman SL. A comparison between Greulich-Pyle and Tanner-Whitehouse assessments of skeletal maturity. *Radiology.* 1971;98(2):273-280.
949. Bayley N, Pinneau SR. Tables for predicting adult height from skeletal age: revised for use with the Greulich-Pyle hand standards. *J Pediatr.* 1952;40(4):423-441.
950. Roche AF, Wainer H, Thissen D. The RWT method for the prediction of adult stature. *Pediatrics.* 1975;56(6):1027-1033.
951. Khamis HJ, Roche AF. Predicting adult stature without using skeletal age: the Khamis-Roche method. *Pediatrics.* 1994;94(4 Pt 1): 504-507.
952. Oerter KE, Manasco P, Barnes KM, et al. Adult height in precocious puberty after long-term treatment with deslorelin. *J Clin Endocrinol Metab.* 1991;73(6):1235-1240.
953. Growth Hormone Research Society. Consensus guidelines for the diagnosis and treatment of growth hormone (GH) deficiency in childhood and adolescence: summary statement of the GH Research Society. *J Clin Endocrinol Metab.* 2000;85(11):3990-3993.
954. Martinez AS, Domene HM, Ropelato MG, et al. Estrogen priming effect on growth hormone (GH) provocative test: a useful tool for the diagnosis of GH deficiency. *J Clin Endocrinol Metab.* 2000;85(11): 4168-4172.
955. Baxter RC, Axiak S, Raison RL. Monoclonal antibody against human somatomedin-C/insulin-like growth factor-I. *J Clin Endocrinol Metab.* 1982;54(2):474-476.
956. Cianfarani S, Liguori A, Boemi S, et al. Inaccuracy of insulin-like growth factor (IGF) binding protein (IGFBP)-3 assessment in the diagnosis of growth hormone (GH) deficiency from childhood to young adulthood: association to low GH dependency of IGF-II and presence of circulating IGFBP-3 18-kilodalton fragment. *J Clin Endocrinol Metab.* 2005;90(11):6028-6034.
957. Cianfarani S, Boemi S, Spagnoli A, et al. Is IGF binding protein-3 assessment helpful for the diagnosis of GH deficiency? *Clin Endocrinol (Oxf).* 1995;43(1):43-47.
958. Cianfarani S, Liguori A, Germani D. IGF-I and IGFBP-3 assessment in the management of childhood onset growth hormone deficiency. *Endocr Dev.* 2005;9:66-75.
959. Rosenfeld RG, Wilson DM, Lee PD, Hintz RL. Insulin-like growth factors I and II in evaluation of growth retardation. *J Pediatr.* 1986; 109(3):428-433.
960. Cianfarani S, Tondinelli T, Spadoni GL, et al. Height velocity and IGF-I assessment in the diagnosis of childhood onset GH insufficiency: do we still need a second GH stimulation test? *Clin Endocrinol (Oxf).* 2002;57(2):161-167.
961. Juul A, Skakkebaek NE. Prediction of the outcome of growth hormone provocative testing in short children by measurement of serum levels of insulin-like growth factor I and insulin-like growth factor binding protein 3. *J Pediatr.* 1997;130(2):197-204.
962. Clemmons DR. Commercial assays available for insulin-like growth factor I and their use in diagnosing growth hormone deficiency. *Horm Res.* 2001;55(Suppl 2):73-79.
963. Milani D, Carmichael JD, Welkowitz J, et al. Variability and reliability of single serum IGF-I measurements: impact on determining predictability of risk ratios in disease development. *J Clin Endocrinol Metab.* 2004;89(5):2271-2274.
964. Rosenfeld RG, Gargosky SE. Assays for insulin-like growth factors and their binding proteins: practicalities and pitfalls. *J Pediatr.* 1996;128(5 Pt 2):S52-S57.
965. Daughaday WH, Rotwein P. Insulin-like growth factors I and II. peptide, messenger ribonucleic acid and gene structures, serum, and tissue concentrations. *Endocr Rev.* 1989;10(1):68-91.
966. Furlanetto RW, Underwood LE, Van Wyk JJ, D'Ercole AJ. Estimation of somatomedin-C levels in normals and patients with pituitary disease by radioimmunoassay. *J Clin Invest.* 1977;60(3):648-657.
967. Zapf J, Walter H, Froesch ER. Radioimmunological determination of insulinlike growth factors I and II in normal subjects and in patients with growth disorders and extrapancreatic tumor hypoglycemia. *J Clin Invest.* 1981;68(5):1321-1330.
968. Daughaday WH, Kapadia M, Mariz I. Serum somatomedin binding proteins: physiologic significance and interference in radioligand assay. *J Lab Clin Med.* 1986;109:355-363.
969. Horner JM, Liu F, Hintz RL. Comparison of [125I]somatomedin A and [125I]somatomedin C radioreceptor assays for somatomedin peptide content in whole and acid-chromatographed plasma. *J Clin Endocrinol Metab.* 1978;47(6):1287-1295.

970. Daughaday WH, Mariz IK, Blethen SL. Inhibition of access of bound somatomedin to membrane receptor and immunobinding sites: a comparison of radioreceptor and radioimmunoassay of somatomedin in native and acid-ethanol-extracted serum. *J Clin Endocrinol Metab.* 1980;51(4):781-788.

971. Bang P, Eriksson U, Sara V, et al. Comparison of acid ethanol extraction and acid gel filtration prior to IGF-I and IGF-II radioimmunoassays: improvement of determinations in acid ethanol extracts by the use of truncated IGF-I as radioligand. *Acta Endocrinol (Copenh).* 1991;124(6):620-629.

972. Khosravi MJ, Diamandi A, Mistry J, Lee PD. Noncompetitive ELISA for human serum insulin-like growth factor-I. *Clin Chem.* 1996;42(8 Pt 1):1147-1154.

973. Gluckman PD, Johnson-Barrett JJ, Butler JH, et al. Studies of insulin-like growth factor -I and -II by specific radioligand assays in umbilical cord blood. *Clin Endocrinol (Oxf).* 1983;19(3):405-413.

974. Bang P, Ahlsen M, Berg U, Carlsson-Skwirut C. Free insulin-like growth factor I: are we hunting a ghost? *Horm Res.* 2001;55(Suppl 2):84-93.

975. Gargosky SE, Pham HM, Wilson KF, et al. Measurement and characterization of insulin-like growth factor binding protein-3 in human biological fluids: discrepancies between radioimmunoassay and ligand blotting. *Endocrinology.* 1992;131(6):3051-3060.

976. Baxter RC, Martin JL. Radioimmunoassay of growth hormone-dependent insulinlike growth factor binding protein in human plasma. *J Clin Invest.* 1986;78(6):1504-1512.

977. Hasegawa Y, Hasegawa T, Aso T, et al. Usefulness and limitation of measurement of insulin-like growth factor binding protein-3 (IGFBP-3) for diagnosis of growth hormone deficiency. *Endocrinol Jpn.* 1992;39(6):585-591.

978. Rikken B, van Doorn J, Ringeling A, et al. Plasma levels of insulin-like growth factor (IGF)-I, IGF-II and IGF-binding protein-3 in the evaluation of childhood growth hormone deficiency. *Horm Res.* 1998;50(3):166-176.

979. Rosenfeld RG, Albertsson-Wikland K, Cassorla F, et al. Diagnostic controversy: the diagnosis of childhood growth hormone deficiency revisited. *J Clin Endocrinol Metab.* 1995;80(5):1532-1540.

980. Frasier SD. A review of growth hormone stimulation tests in children. *Pediatrics.* 1974;53:929-937.

981. Celniker AC, Chen AB, Wert RM Jr, Sherman BM. Variability in the quantitation of circulating growth hormone using commercial immunoassays. *J Clin Endocrinol Metab.* 1989;68(2):469-476.

982. Amed S, Delvin E, Hamilton J. Variation in growth hormone immunoassays in clinical practice in Canada. *Horm Res.* 2008;69(5):290-294.

983. Muller A, Scholz M, Blankenstein O, et al. Harmonization of growth hormone measurements with different immunoassays by data adjustment. *Clin Chem Lab Med.* 2011;49(7):1135-1142.

984. Gandrud LM, Wilson DM. Is growth hormone stimulation testing in children still appropriate? *Growth Horm IGF Res.* 2004;14(3):185-194.

985. Reiter EO, Martha PM Jr. Pharmacological testing of growth hormone secretion. *Horm Res.* 1990;33(2-4):121-126, discussion 126-127.

986. Kaplan SL, Abrams CA, Bell JJ, et al. Growth and growth hormone. I. Changes in serum level of growth hormone following hypoglycemia in 134 children with growth retardation. *Pediatr Res.* 1968;2(1):43-63.

987. Grumbach MM, Bin-Abbas BS, Kaplan SL. The growth hormone cascade: progress and long-term results of growth hormone treatment in growth hormone deficiency. *Horm Res.* 1998;49(Suppl 2):41-57.

988. Guyda HJ. Growth hormone testing and the short child. *Pediatr Res.* 2000;48(5):579-580.

989. Guyda HJ. Four decades of growth hormone therapy for short children: what have we achieved? *J Clin Endocrinol Metab.* 1999;84(12):4307-4316.

990. Corneli G, Di Somma C, Prodam F, et al. Cut-off limits of the GH response to GHRH plus arginine test and IGF-I levels for the diagnosis of GH deficiency in late adolescents and young adults. *Eur J Endocrinol.* 2007;157(6):701-708.

991. Ghigo E, Bellone J, Aimaretti G, et al. Reliability of provocative tests to assess growth hormone secretory status. Study in 472 normally growing children. *J Clin Endocrinol Metab.* 1996;81(9):3323-3327.

992. Maghnie M, Cavigioli F, Tinelli C, et al. GHRH plus arginine in the diagnosis of acquired GH deficiency of childhood-onset. *J Clin Endocrinol Metab.* 2002;87(6):2740-2744.

993. Tillmann V, Buckler JM, Kibirige MS, et al. Biochemical tests in the diagnosis of childhood growth hormone deficiency. *J Clin Endocrinol Metab.* 1997;82(2):531-535.

994. Marin G, Domene HM, Barnes KM, et al. The effects of estrogen priming and puberty on the growth hormone response to standardized treadmill exercise and arginine-insulin in normal girls and boys. *J Clin Endocrinol Metab.* 1994;79(2):537-541.

995. Slover RH, Klingensmith GJ, Gotlin RW, Radcliffe J. A comparison of clonidine and standard provocative agents of growth hormone. *Am J Dis Child.* 1984;138(3):314-317.

996. Loche S, Cappa M, Ghigo E, et al. Growth hormone response to oral clonidine test in normal and short children. *J Endocrinol Invest.* 1993;16(11):899-902.

997. Nwosu BU, Coco M, Jones J, et al. Short stature with normal growth hormone stimulation testing: lack of evidence for partial growth hormone deficiency or insensitivity. *Horm Res.* 2004;62(2):97-102.

998. Smyczynska J, Lewinski A, Hilczer M, et al. Partial growth hormone deficiency (GHD) in children has more similarities to idiopathic short stature than to severe GHD. *Endokrynol Pol.* 2007;58(3):182-187.

999. Mauras N, Blizzard RM, Link K, et al. Augmentation of growth hormone secretion during puberty: evidence for a pulse amplitude-modulated phenomenon. *J Clin Endocrinol Metab.* 1987;64(3):596-601.

1000. Coutant R, de Casson FB, Rouleau S, et al. Divergent effect of endogenous and exogenous sex steroids on the insulin-like growth factor I response to growth hormone in short normal adolescents. *J Clin Endocrinol Metab.* 2004;89(12):6185-6192.

1001. Chalew SA, Udoff LC, Hanukoglu A, et al. The effect of testosterone therapy on spontaneous growth hormone secretion in boys with constitutional delay. *Am J Dis Child.* 1988;142(12):1345-1348.

1002. Moll GW Jr, Rosenfield RL, Fang VS. Administration of low-dose estrogen rapidly and directly stimulates growth hormone production. *Am J Dis Child.* 1986;140(2):124-127.

1003. Gourmelen M, Pham-Huu-Trung MT, Girard F. Transient partial hGH deficiency in prepubertal children with delay of growth. *Pediatr Res.* 1979;13(4 Pt 1):221-224.

1004. Lippe B, Wong SL, Kaplan SA. Simultaneous assessment of growth hormone and ACTH reserve in children pretreated with diethylstilbestrol. *J Clin Endocrinol Metab.* 1971;33(6):949-956.

1005. Gonc EN, Kandemir N, Ozon A, Alikasifoglu A. Final heights of boys with normal growth hormone responses to provocative tests following priming. *J Pediatr Endocrinol Metab.* 2008;21(10):963-971.

1006. Iranmanesh A, Lizarralde G, Veldhuis JD. Age and relative adiposity are specific negative determinants of the frequency and amplitude of growth hormone (GH) secretory bursts and the half-life of endogenous GH in healthy men. *J Clin Endocrinol Metab.* 1991;73(5):1081-1088.

1007. Bonert VS, Elashoff JD, Barnett P, Melmed S. Body mass index determines evoked growth hormone (GH) responsiveness in normal healthy male subjects: diagnostic caveat for adult GH deficiency. *J Clin Endocrinol Metab.* 2004;89(7):3397-3401.

1008. Williams T, Berelowitz M, Joffe SN, et al. Impaired growth hormone responses to growth hormone-releasing factor in obesity. A pituitary defect reversed with weight reduction. *N Engl J Med.* 1984;311(22):1403-1407.

1009. Misra M, Bredella MA, Tsai P, et al. Lower growth hormone and higher cortisol are associated with greater visceral adiposity, intramyocellular lipids, and insulin resistance in overweight girls. *Am J Physiol Endocrinol Metab.* 2008;295(2):E385-E392.

1010. Argente J, Caballo N, Barrios V, et al. Multiple endocrine abnormalities of the growth hormone and insulin-like growth factor axis in prepubertal children with exogenous obesity: effect of short- and long-term weight reduction. *J Clin Endocrinol Metab.* 1997;82:2076-2083.

1011. Stanley TL, Levitsky LL, Grinspoon SK, Misra M. Effect of body mass index on peak growth hormone response to provocative testing in children with short stature. *J Clin Endocrinol Metab.* 2009;94(12):4875-4881.

1012. Shah A, Stanhope R, Matthew D. Hazards of pharmacological tests of growth hormone secretion in childhood. *BMJ.* 1992;304(6820):173-174.

1013. Bercu BB, Shulman D, Root AW, Spiliotis BE. Growth hormone (GH) provocative testing frequently does not reflect endogenous GH secretion. *J Clin Endocrinol Metab.* 1986;63(3):709-716.

1014. Spiliotis BE, August GP, Hung W, et al. Growth hormone neurosecretory dysfunction. A treatable cause of short stature. *JAMA.* 1984;251(17):2223-2230.

1015. Zadik Z, Chalew SA, Raiti S, Kowarski AA. Do short children secrete insufficient growth hormone? *Pediatrics.* 1985;76(3):355-360.

1016. Zadik Z, Chalew SA, Gilula Z, Kowarski AA. Reproducibility of growth hormone testing procedures: a comparison between 24-hour integrated concentration and pharmacological stimulation. *J Clin Endocrinol Metab.* 1990;71(5):1127-1130.

1017. Tassoni P, Cacciari E, Cau M, et al. Variability of growth hormone response to pharmacological and sleep tests performed twice in short children. *J Clin Endocrinol Metab.* 1990;71(1):230-234.

1018. Donaldson DL, Hollowell JG, Pan FP, et al. Growth hormone secretory profiles: variation on consecutive nights. *J Pediatr.* 1989;115(1):51-56.

1019. Rose SR, Ross JL, Uriarte M, et al. The advantage of measuring stimulated as compared with spontaneous growth hormone levels in the diagnosis of growth hormone deficiency. *N Engl J Med.* 1988;319(4):201-207.

1020. Lanes R. Diagnostic limitations of spontaneous growth hormone measurements in normally growing prepubertal children. *Am J Dis Child.* 1989;143(11):1284-1286.

1021. Martha PM Jr, Rogol AD, Veldhuis JD, et al. Alterations in the pulsatile properties of circulating growth hormone concentrations during puberty in boys. *J Clin Endocrinol Metab.* 1989;69(3): 563-570.

1022. Blum WF, Cotterill AM, Postel-Vinay MC, et al. Improvement of diagnostic criteria in growth hormone insensitivity syndrome: solutions and pitfalls. pharmacia study group on insulin-like growth factor I treatment in growth hormone insensitivity syndromes. *Acta Paediatr Suppl.* 1994;399:117-124.

1023. Buckway CK, Guevara-Aguirre J, Pratt KL, et al. The IGF-I generation test revisited: a marker of GH sensitivity. *J Clin Endocrinol Metab.* 2001;86(11):5176-5183.

1024. Rosenfeld RG, Buckway C, Selva K, et al. Insulin-like growth factor (IGF) parameters and tools for efficacy: the IGF-I generation test in children. *Horm Res.* 2004;62(Suppl 1):37-43.

1025. Buckway CK, Selva KA, Burren CP, et al. IGF generation in short stature. *J Pediatr Endocrinol Metab.* 2002;15(Suppl 5):1453-1454.

1026. Cornblath M, Parker ML, Reisner SH, et al. Secretion and metabolism of growth hormone in premature and full-term infants. *J Clin Endocrinol Metab.* 1965;25:209-218.

1027. Hawkes CP, Grimberg A. Measuring growth hormone and insulin-like growth factor-I in infants: what is normal? *Pediatr Endocrinol Rev.* 2013;11(2):126-146.

1028. Shimano S, Suzuki S, Nagashima K, et al. Growth hormone responses to growth hormone releasing factor in neonates. *Biol Neonate.* 1985;47(6):367-370.

1029. Bhala A, Harris M, Cohen P. Insulin-like growth factors and their binding proteins in critically ill infants. *J Pediatr Endocrinol.* 1998; 11:451-459.

1030. Stubberfield TG, Byrne GC, Jones TW. Growth and growth hormone secretion after treatment for acute lymphoblastic leukemia in childhood. 18-gy versus 24-gy cranial irradiation. *J Pediatr Hematol Oncol.* 1995;17(2):167-171.

1031. Wit JM, Clayton PE, Rogol AD, et al. Idiopathic short stature: definition, epidemiology, and diagnostic evaluation. *Growth Horm IGF Res.* 2008;18(2):89-110.

1032. Clayton PE, Shalet SM, Price DA, Addison GM. Growth and growth hormone responses to oxandrolone in boys with constitutional delay of growth and puberty (CDGP). *Clin Endocrinol (Oxf).* 1988;29(2): 123-130.

1033. Sedlmeyer IL, Hirschhorn JN, Palmert MR. Pedigree analysis of constitutional delay of growth and maturation: determination of familial aggregation and inheritance patterns. *J Clin Endocrinol Metab.* 2002; 87(12):5581-5586.

1034. Blethen SL, Gaines S, Weldon V. Comparison of predicted and adult heights in short boys: effect of androgen therapy. *Pediatr Res.* 1984;18(5):467-469.

1035. Volta C, Ghizzoni L, Buono T, et al. Final height in a group of untreated children with constitutional growth delay. *Helv Paediatr Acta.* 1988;43(3):171-176.

1036. Eastman CJ, Lazarus L, Stuart MC, Casey JH. The effect of puberty on growth hormone secretion in boys with short stature and delayed adolescence. *Aust N Z J Med.* 1971;1(2):154-159.

1037. Martha PM Jr, Reiter EO. Pubertal growth and growth hormone secretion. *Endocrinol Metab Clin North Am.* 1991;20(1):165-182.

1038. Deller JJ Jr, Boulis MW, Harriss WE, et al. Growth hormone response patterns to sex hormone administration in growth retardation. *Am J Med Sci.* 1970;259(4):292-297.

1039. Rose SR, Municchi G, Barnes KM, Cutler GB Jr. Overnight growth hormone concentrations are usually normal in pubertal children with idiopathic short stature—a clinical research center study. *J Clin Endocrinol Metab.* 1996;81(3):1063-1068.

1040. Kaplowitz PB. Diagnostic value of testosterone therapy in boys with delayed puberty. *Am J Dis Child.* 1989;143(1):116-120.

1041. Horan M, Millar DS, Hedderich J, et al. Human growth hormone 1 (GH1) gene expression: complex haplotype-dependent influence of polymorphic variation in the proximal promoter and locus control region. *Hum Mutat.* 2003;21(4):408-423.

1042. Attie KM, Carlsson LM, Rundle AC, Sherman BM. Evidence for partial growth hormone insensitivity among patients with idiopathic short stature. The National Cooperative Growth Study. *J Pediatr.* 1995; 127(2):244-250.

1043. Carlsson LM, Attie KM, Compton PG, et al. Reduced concentration of serum growth hormone-binding protein in children with idiopathic short stature. National Cooperative Growth Study. *J Clin Endocrinol Metab.* 1994;78(6):1325-1330.

1044. Davila N, Moreira-Andres M, Alcaniz J, Barcelo B. Serum growth hormone-binding protein is decreased in prepubertal children with idiopathic short stature. *J Endocrinol Invest.* 1996;19(6):348-352.

1045. Rosenfeld RG. The molecular basis of idiopathic short stature. *Growth Horm IGF Res.* 2005;15(Suppl A):S3-S5.

1046. Krajewska-Siuda E, Malecka-Tendera E, Krajewski-Siuda K. Are short boys with constitutional delay of growth and puberty candidates for rGH therapy according to FDA recommendations? *Horm Res.* 2006; 65(4):192-196.

1047. Rosenfeld RG, Northcraft GB, Hintz RL. A prospective, randomized study of testosterone treatment of constitutional delay of growth and development in male adolescents. *Pediatrics.* 1982;69(6):681-687.

1048. Blizzard RM, Hindmarsh PC, Stanhope R. Oxandrolone therapy: 25 years experience. *Growth Genet Horm.* 1991;7:1-6.

1049. Buyukgebiz A, Hindmarsh PC, Brook CG. Treatment of constitutional delay of growth and puberty with oxandrolone compared with growth hormone. *Arch Dis Child.* 1990;65(4):448-449.

1050. Joss EE, Schmidt HA, Zuppinger KA. Oxandrolone in constitutionally delayed growth, a longitudinal study up to final height. *J Clin Endocrinol Metab.* 1989;69(6):1109-1115.

1051. Marti-Henneberg C, Niirianen AK, Rappaport R. Oxandrolone treatment of constitutional short stature in boys during adolescence: effect on linear growth, bone age, pubic hair, and testicular development. *J Pediatr.* 1975;86(5):783-788.

1052. Stanhope R, Buchanan CR, Fenn GC, Preece MA. Double blind placebo controlled trial of low dose oxandrolone in the treatment of boys with constitutional delay of growth and puberty. *Arch Dis Child.* 1988;63(5):501-505.

1053. Wilson DM, McCauley E, Brown DR, Dudley R. Oxandrolone therapy in constitutionally delayed growth and puberty. Bio-technology general corporation cooperative study group. *Pediatrics.* 1995;96(6): 1095-1100.

1054. Tse WY, Buyukgebiz A, Hindmarsh PC, et al. Long-term outcome of oxandrolone treatment in boys with constitutional delay of growth and puberty. *J Pediatr.* 1990;117(4):588-591.

1055. Papadimitriou A, Wacharasindhu S, Pearl K, et al. Treatment of constitutional growth delay in prepubertal boys with a prolonged course of low dose oxandrolone. *Arch Dis Child.* 1991;66(7):841-843.

1056. Hochberg Z, Korman S. Oxandrolone therapy for short stature. *Pediatr Endocrinol (Isr).* 1987;(2):115-120.

1057. Link K, Blizzard RM, Evans WS, et al. The effect of androgens on the pulsatile release and the twenty-four-hour mean concentration of growth hormone in peripubertal males. *J Clin Endocrinol Metab.* 1986;62(1):159-164.

1058. Malhotra A, Poon E, Tse WY, et al. The effects of oxandrolone on the growth hormone and gonadal axes in boys with constitutional delay of growth and puberty. *Clin Endocrinol (Oxf).* 1993;38(4):393-398.

1059. Kulin HE, Reiter EO. Managing the patient with delay in puberty development. *Endocrinologist.* 1992;2:231-239.

1060. Richman RA, Kirsch LR. Testosterone treatment in adolescent boys with constitutional delay in growth and development. *N Engl J Med.* 1988;319(24):1563-1567.

1061. Keenan BS, Richards GE, Ponder SW, et al. Androgen-stimulated pubertal growth: the effects of testosterone and dihydrotestosterone on growth hormone and insulin-like growth factor-I in the treatment of short stature and delayed puberty. *J Clin Endocrinol Metab.* 1993;76(4):996-1001.

1062. Metzger DL, Kerrigan JR. Estrogen receptor blockade with tamoxifen diminishes growth hormone secretion in boys: evidence for a stimulatory role of endogenous estrogens during male adolescence. *J Clin Endocrinol Metab.* 1994;79(2):513-518.

1063. Metzger DL, Kerrigan JR. Androgen receptor blockade with flutamide enhances growth hormone secretion in late pubertal males: evidence for independent actions of estrogen and androgen. *J Clin Endocrinol Metab.* 1993;76(5):1147-1152.

1064. Wilson DM, Kei J, Hintz RL, Rosenfeld RG. Effects of testosterone therapy for pubertal delay. *Am J Dis Child.* 1988;142(1):96-99.

1065. Wang C, Swerdloff RS, Iranmanesh A, et al. Transdermal testosterone gel improves sexual function, mood, muscle strength, and body composition parameters in hypogonadal men. *J Clin Endocrinol Metab.* 2000;85(8):2839-2853.

1066. Stephen MD, Jehaimi CT, Brosnan PG, Yafi M. Sexual precocity in a 2-year-old boy caused by indirect exposure to testosterone cream. *Endocr Pract.* 2008;14(8):1027-1030.

1067. Franklin SL, Geffner ME. Precocious puberty secondary to topical testosterone exposure. *J Pediatr Endocrinol Metab.* 2003;16(1):107-110.

1068. Yu YM, Punyasavatsu N, Elder D, D'Ercole AJ. Sexual development in a two-year-old boy induced by topical exposure to testosterone. *Pediatrics.* 1999;104(2):e23.

1069. Hintz RL, Attie KM, Baptista J, Roche A. Effect of growth hormone treatment on adult height of children with idiopathic short stature. Genentech Collaborative Group. *N Engl J Med.* 1999;340(7): 502-507.

1070. Leschek EW, Rose SR, Yanovski JA, et al. Effect of growth hormone treatment on adult height in peripubertal children with idiopathic short stature: a randomized, double-blind, placebo-controlled trial. *J Clin Endocrinol Metab.* 2004;89(7):3140-3148.

1071. Wit JM, Reiter EO, Ross JL, et al. Idiopathic short stature: management and growth hormone treatment. *Growth Horm IGF Res.* 2008; 18(2):111-135.

1072. Zucchini S, Wasniewska M, Cisternino M, et al. Adult height in children with short stature and idiopathic delayed puberty after different management. *Eur J Pediatr.* 2008;167(6):677-681.

1073. Hero M, Wickman S, Dunkel L. Treatment with the aromatase inhibitor letrozole during adolescence increases near-final height in boys with constitutional delay of puberty. *Clin Endocrinol (Oxf)*. 2006; 64(5):510-513.

1074. Kaplan SL, Underwood LE, August GP, et al. Clinical studies with recombinant-DNA-derived methionyl human growth hormone in growth hormone deficient children. *Lancet*. 1986;1(8483):697-700.

1075. Underwood LE, Moore WV. Antibodies to growth hormone: measurement and meaning. *Growth Genet Horm*. 1987;3:1-3.

1076. Bristow AF, Jespersen AM. The second international standard for somatropin (recombinant DNA-derived human growth hormone): preparation and calibration in an international collaborative study. *Biologicals*. 2001;29(2):97-106.

1077. Marx W, Simpson ME, Evans HM. Bioassay of growth hormone at anterior pituitary. *Endocrinology*. 1942;30:1-10.

1078. Wilhelmi AE. Measurement: bioassay. In: Berson SA, Yalow RS, eds. *Peptide Hormones: Methods in Investigative and Diagnostic Endocrinology*. New York: North-Holland Publishing; 1973.

1079. Binder G, Benz MR, Elmlinger M, et al. Reduced human growth hormone (hGH) bioactivity without a defect of the GH-1 gene in three patients with rhGH responsive growth failure. *Clin Endocrinol (Oxf)*. 1999;51(1):89-95.

1080. Wit JM, Kamp GA, Rikken B. Spontaneous growth and response to growth hormone treatment in children with growth hormone deficiency and idiopathic short stature. *Pediatr Res*. 1996;39(2):295-302.

1081. Ranke MB. A note on adults with growth hormone deficiency. *Acta Paediatr Scand Suppl*. 1987;331:80-82.

1082. Blizzard RM. Growth hormone as a therapeutic agent. *Growth Genet Horm*. 2005;21:49-54.

1083. Frasier SD. Human pituitary growth hormone (hGH) therapy in growth hormone deficiency. *Endocr Rev*. 1983;4(2):155-170.

1084. Frasier SD, Costin G, Lippe BM, et al. A dose-response curve for human growth hormone. *J Clin Endocrinol Metab*. 1981;53(6): 1213-1217.

1085. Tintner R, Brown P, Hedley-Whyte ET, et al. Neuropathologic verification of Creutzfeldt-Jakob disease in the exhumed American recipient of human pituitary growth hormone: epidemiologic and pathogenetic implications. *Neurology*. 1986;36(7):932-936.

1086. Hintz RL. The prismatic case of Creutzfeldt-Jakob disease associated with pituitary growth hormone treatment. *J Clin Endocrinol Metab*. 1995;80(8):2298-2301.

1087. Brown P, Brandel JP, Sato T, et al. Iatrogenic Creutzfeldt-Jakob disease, final assessment. *Emerg Infect Dis*. 2012;18(6):901-907.

1088. Rosenfeld RG, Aggarwal BB, Hintz RL, Dollar LA. Recombinant DNA-derived methionyl human growth hormone is similar in membrane binding properties to human pituitary growth hormone. *Biochem Biophys Res Commun*. 1982;106(1):202-209.

1089. Hintz RL, Rosenfeld RG, Wilson DM, et al. Biosynthetic methionyl human growth hormones is biologically active in adult man. *Lancet*. 1982;1(8284):1276-1279.

1090. Wilson TA, Rose SR, Cohen P, et al. Update of guidelines for the use of growth hormone in children: the Lawson Wilkins Pediatric Endocrinology Society Drug and Therapeutics Committee. *J Pediatr*. 2003; 143(4):415-421.

1091. Ranke MB, Lindberg A, Chatelain P, et al. Derivation and validation of a mathematical model for predicting the response to exogenous recombinant human growth hormone (GH) in prepubertal children with idiopathic GH deficiency. KIGS international board. Kabi Pharmacia International Growth Study. *J Clin Endocrinol Metab*. 1999; 84(4):1174-1183.

1092. MacGillivray MH, Baptista J, Johanson A. Outcome of a four-year randomized study of daily versus three times weekly somatropin treatment in prepubertal naive growth hormone-deficient children. Genentech study group. *J Clin Endocrinol Metab*. 1996;81(5): 1806-1809.

1093. Wilson DM, Baker B, Hintz RL, Rosenfeld RG. Subcutaneous versus intramuscular growth hormone therapy: growth and acute somatomedin response. *Pediatrics*. 1985;76(3):361-364.

1094. Martha PM Jr, Reiter EO, Davila N, et al. The role of body mass in the response to growth hormone therapy. *J Clin Endocrinol Metab*. 1992;75(6):1470-1473.

1095. Martha PM Jr, Reiter EO, Davila N, et al. Serum growth hormone (GH)-binding protein/receptor: an important determinant of GH responsiveness. *J Clin Endocrinol Metab*. 1992;75(6):1464-1469.

1096. Price DA, Ranke MB. Final height following growth hormone treatment. In: Ranke MB, Gunnarsson R, eds. *Progress in Growth Hormone Therapy: 5 Years of KIGS*. Mannheim, Germany: J&J Verlag; 1994.

1097. Land C, Blum WF, Stabrey A, Schoenau E. Seasonality of growth response to GH therapy in prepubertal children with idiopathic growth hormone deficiency. *Eur J Endocrinol*. 2005;152(5):727-733.

1098. Cohen P, Bright GM, Rogol AD, et al. Effects of dose and gender on the growth and growth factor response to GH in GH-deficient children: implications for efficacy and safety. *J Clin Endocrinol Metab*. 2002;87(1):90-98.

1099. Cohen P, Rogol AD, Howard C, et al. IGF-based dosing of growth hormone accelerates the growth velocity of children with growth hormone deficiency (GHD) and idiopathic short stature. *Horm Res*. 2005;64(Suppl 1):48.

1100. Wikland KA, Kristrom B, Rosberg S, et al. Validated multivariate models predicting the growth response to GH treatment in individual short children with a broad range in GH secretion capacities. *Pediatr Res*. 2000;48(4):475-484.

1101. Huet F, Carel JC, Nivelon JL, Chaussain JL. Long-term results of GH therapy in GH-deficient children treated before 1 year of age. *Eur J Endocrinol*. 1999;140(1):29-34.

1102. Boersma B, Rikken B, Wit JM. Catch-up growth in early treated patients with growth hormone deficiency. Dutch growth hormone working group. *Arch Dis Child*. 1995;72(5):427-431.

1103. Rappaport R, Mugnier E, Limoni C, et al. A 5-year prospective study of growth hormone (GH)-deficient children treated with GH before the age of 3 years. French Serono Study Group. *J Clin Endocrinol Metab*. 1997;82(2):452-456.

1104. De Luca F, Maghnie M, Arrigo T, et al. Final height outcome of growth hormone-deficient patients treated since less than five years of age. *Acta Paediatr*. 1996;85(10):1167-1171.

1105. Carel JC, Huet F, Chaussain JL. Treatment of growth hormone deficiency in very young children. *Horm Res*. 2003;60(Suppl 1):10-17.

1106. Ranke MB, Lindberg A, Albertsson-Wikland K, et al. Increased response, but lower responsiveness, to growth hormone (GH) in very young children (aged 0-3 years) with idiopathic GH deficiency: analysis of data from KIGS. *J Clin Endocrinol Metab*. 2005;90(4): 1966-1971.

1107. MacGillivray MH, Blethen SL, Buchlis JG, et al. Current dosing of growth hormone in children with growth hormone deficiency: how physiologic? *Pediatrics*. 1998;102(2 Pt 3):527-530.

1108. Westphal O, Lindberg A, Swedish KIGS National Board. Final height in Swedish children with idiopathic growth hormone deficiency enrolled in KIGS treated optimally with growth hormone. *Acta Paediatr*. 2008;97(12):1698-1706.

1109. Birnbacher R, Riedl S, Frisch H. Long-term treatment in children with hypopituitarism: pubertal development and final height. *Horm Res*. 1998;49(2):80-85.

1110. Cutfield W, Lindberg A, Albertsson Wikland K, et al. Final height in idiopathic growth hormone deficiency: the KIGS experience. KIGS International Board. *Acta Paediatr Suppl*. 1999;88(428):72-75.

1111. Bramswig JH, Schlosser H, Kiese K. Final height in children with growth hormone deficiency. *Horm Res*. 1995;43(4):126-128.

1112. Severi F. Final height in children with growth hormone deficiency. *Horm Res*. 1995;43(4):138-140.

1113. Blethen SL, Baptista J, Kuntze J, et al. Adult height in growth hormone (GH)-deficient children treated with biosynthetic GH. the Genentech growth study group. *J Clin Endocrinol Metab*. 1997;82(2):418-420.

1114. Bernasconi S, Arrigo T, Wasniewsk M, et al. Long-term results with growth hormone therapy in idiopathic hypopituitarism. *Horm Res*. 2000;53(Suppl 1):55-59.

1115. August GP, Julius JR, Blethen SL. Adult height in children with growth hormone deficiency who are treated with biosynthetic growth hormone: the National Cooperative Growth Study experience. *Pediatrics*. 1998;102(2 Pt 3):512-516.

1116. Reiter EO, Price DA, Wilton P, et al. Effect of growth hormone (GH) treatment on the near-final height of 1258 patients with idiopathic GH deficiency: analysis of a large international database. *J Clin Endocrinol Metab*. 2006;91(6):2047-2054.

1117. Cutfield WS, Lindberg A, Chatelain P, et al. Final height following growth hormone treatment of idiopathic growth hormone deficiency in KIGS. In: Ranke MB, Wilton P, eds. *Growth Hormone Therapy in KIGS—10 Years' Experience*. Heidelberg-Leipzig: Johann Ambrosius Barth Verlag; 1999.

1118. Wassenaar MJ, Dekkers OM, Pereira AM, et al. Impact of the exon 3-deleted growth hormone (GH) receptor polymorphism on baseline height and the growth response to recombinant human GH therapy in GH-deficient (GHD) and non-GHD children with short stature: a systematic review and meta-analysis. *J Clin Endocrinol Metab*. 2009; 94(10):3721-3730.

1119. Rosenfeld RG. Editorial: The pharmacogenomics of human growth. *J Clin Endocrinol Metab*. 2006;91(3):795-796.

1120. Ranke MB, Price DA, Albertsson-Wikland K, et al. Factors determining pubertal growth and final height in growth hormone treatment of idiopathic growth hormone deficiency. Analysis of 195 patients of the Kabi Pharmacia International Growth Study. *Horm Res*. 1997;48(2): 62-71.

1121. Frisch H, Birnbacher R. Final height and pubertal development in children with growth hormone deficiency after long-term treatment. *Horm Res*. 1995;43(4):132-134.

1122. Burns EC, Tanner JM, Preece MA, Cameron N. Final height and pubertal development in 55 children with idiopathic growth hormone deficiency, treated for between 2 and 15 years with human growth hormone. *Eur J Pediatr*. 1981;137(2):155-164.

1123. Bourguignon JP, Vandeweghe M, Vanderschueren-Lodeweyckx M, et al. Pubertal growth and final height in hypopituitary boys: a minor role of bone age at onset of puberty. *J Clin Endocrinol Metab*. 1986; 63(2):376-382.

1124. Beckers D, Thomas M, Jamart J, et al. Adult final height after growth hormone therapy for irradiation-induced growth hormone deficiency in childhood survivors of brain tumours: the Belgian experience. *Eur J Endocrinol.* 2010;162:483-490.

1125. Xu W, Janss A, Moshang T. Adult height and adult sitting height in childhood medulloblastoma survivors. *J Clin Endocrinol Metab.* 2003; 88(10):4677-4681.

1126. Stanhope R, Uruena M, Hindmarsh P, et al. Management of growth hormone deficiency through puberty. *Acta Paediatr Scand Suppl.* 1991;372:47-52, discussion 53.

1127. Stanhope R, Albanese A, Hindmarsh P, Brook CG. The effects of growth hormone therapy on spontaneous sexual development. *Horm Res.* 1992;38(Suppl 1):9-13.

1128. Mauras N, Attie KM, Reiter EO, et al. High dose recombinant human growth hormone (GH) treatment of GH-deficient patients in puberty increases near-final height: a randomized, multicenter trial. Genentech, Inc., cooperative study group. *J Clin Endocrinol Metab.* 2000; 85(10):3653-3660.

1129. Cohen P, Rogol AD, Howard CP, et al. Insulin growth factor-based dosing of growth hormone therapy in children: a randomized, controlled study. *J Clin Endocrinol Metab.* 2007;92(7):2480-2486.

1130. Marchisotti FG, Jorge AA, Montenegro LR, et al. Comparison between weight-based and IGF-I-based growth hormone (GH) dosing in the treatment of children with GH deficiency and influence of exon 3 deleted GH receptor variant. *Growth Horm IGF Res.* 2009;19(2): 179-186.

1131. Lippe BM, Van Herle AJ, LaFranchi SH, et al. Reversible hypothyroidism in growth hormone-deficient children treated with human growth hormone. *J Clin Endocrinol Metab.* 1975;40(4):612-618.

1132. Lange M, Feldt-Rasmussen U, Svendsen OL, et al. High risk of adrenal insufficiency in adults previously treated for idiopathic childhood onset growth hormone deficiency. *J Clin Endocrinol Metab.* 2003; 88(12):5784-5789.

1133. Guthrie RD, Smith DW, Graham CB. Testosterone treatment for micropenis during early childhood. *J Pediatr.* 1973;83(2):247-252.

1134. Lechuga-Sancho A, Lechuga-Campoy JL, del Valle-Nunez J, Rivas-Crespo F. Predicting the growth response of children with idiopathic growth hormone deficiency to one year of recombinant growth hormone treatment: derivation and validation of a useful method. *J Pediatr Endocrinol Metab.* 2009;22(6):501-509.

1135. Ranke MB, Lindberg A. Predicting growth in response to growth hormone treatment. *Growth Horm IGF Res.* 2009;19(1):1-11.

1136. de Ridder MA, Stijnen T, Drop SL, et al. Validation of a calibrated prediction model for response to growth hormone treatment in an independent cohort. *Horm Res.* 2006;66(1):13-16.

1137. Achermann JC, Hamdani K, Hindmarsh PC, Brook CG. Birth weight influences the initial response to growth hormone treatment in growth hormone-insufficient children. *Pediatrics.* 1998;102(2 Pt 1): 342-345.

1138. Cacciari E, Zucchini S, Cicognani A, et al. Birth weight affects final height in patients treated for growth hormone deficiency. *Clin Endocrinol (Oxf).* 1999;51(6):733-739.

1139. Tillmann V, Patel L, Gill MS, et al. Monitoring serum insulin-like growth factor-I (IGF-I), IGF binding protein-3 (IGFBP-3), IGF-I/IGFBP-3 molar ratio and leptin during growth hormone treatment for disordered growth. *Clin Endocrinol (Oxf).* 2000;53(3):329-336.

1140. Torres CF, Rebsamen S, Silber JH, et al. Surveillance scanning of children with medulloblastoma. *N Engl J Med.* 1994;330(13):892-895.

1141. Weiss M, Sutton L, Marcial V, et al. The role of radiation therapy in the management of childhood craniopharyngioma. *Int J Radiat Oncol Biol Phys.* 1989;17(6):1313-1321.

1142. Wilton P. Treatment with recombinant human insulin-like growth factor I of children with growth hormone receptor deficiency (Laron syndrome). Kabi Pharmacia Study Group on insulin-like growth factor I treatment in growth hormone insensitivity syndromes. *Acta Paediatr Suppl.* 1992;383:137-142.

1143. Robinson IC, Gabrielsson B, Klaus G, et al. Glucocorticoids and growth problems. *Acta Paediatr Suppl.* 1995;411:81-86.

1144. Reusz GS, Hoyer PF, Lucas M, et al. X linked hypophosphataemia: treatment, height gain, and nephrocalcinosis. *Arch Dis Child.* 1990; 65(10):1125-1128.

1145. Midyett LK, Rogol AD, Van Meter QL, et al. Recombinant insulin-like growth factor (IGF)-I treatment in short children with low IGF-I levels: first-year results from a randomized clinical trial. *J Clin Endocrinol Metab.* 2010;95(2):611-619.

1146. Clayton PE, Cuneo RC, Juul A, et al. Consensus statement on the management of the GH-treated adolescent in the transition to adult care. *Eur J Endocrinol.* 2005;152(2):165-170.

1147. Attanasio AF, Bates PC, Ho KK, et al. Human growth hormone replacement in adult hypopituitary patients: long-term effects on body composition and lipid status—3-year results from the HypoCCS database. *J Clin Endocrinol Metab.* 2002;87(4):1600-1606.

1148. Molitch ME, Clemmons DR, Malozowski S, et al. Evaluation and treatment of adult growth hormone deficiency: an Endocrine Society clinical practice guideline. *J Clin Endocrinol Metab.* 2011;96(6): 1587-1609.

1149. Maison P, Griffin S, Nicoue-Beglah M, et al. Impact of growth hormone (GH) treatment on cardiovascular risk factors in GH-deficient adults: a metaanalysis of blinded, randomized, placebo-controlled trials. *J Clin Endocrinol Metab.* 2004;89(5):2192-2199.

1150. Hull KL, Harvey S. Growth hormone therapy and quality of life: possibilities, pitfalls and mechanisms. *J Endocrinol.* 2003;179(3):311-333.

1151. Maghnie M, Strigazzi C, Tinelli C, et al. Growth hormone (GH) deficiency (GHD) of childhood onset: reassessment of GH status and evaluation of the predictive criteria for permanent GHD in young adults. *J Clin Endocrinol Metab.* 1999;84(4):1324-1328.

1152. Tauber M, Moulin P, Pienkowski C, et al. Growth hormone (GH) retesting and auxological data in 131 GH-deficient patients after completion of treatment. *J Clin Endocrinol Metab.* 1997;82(2):352-356.

1153. Maghnie M, Aimaretti G, Bellone S, et al. Diagnosis of GH deficiency in the transition period: accuracy of insulin tolerance test and insulin-like growth factor-I measurement. *Eur J Endocrinol.* 2005; 152(4):589-596.

1154. Shalet SM, Shavrikova E, Cromer M, et al. Effect of growth hormone (GH) treatment on bone in postpubertal GH-deficient patients: a 2-year randomized, controlled, dose-ranging study. *J Clin Endocrinol Metab.* 2003;88(9):4124-4129.

1155. Mauras N, Pescovitz OH, Allada V, et al. Limited efficacy of growth hormone (GH) during transition of GH-deficient patients from adolescence to adulthood: a phase III multicenter, double-blind, randomized two-year trial. *J Clin Endocrinol Metab.* 2005;90(7):3946-3955.

1156. Attanasio AF, Shavrikova EP, Blum WF, Shalet SM. Quality of life in childhood onset growth hormone-deficient patients in the transition phase from childhood to adulthood. *J Clin Endocrinol Metab.* 2005; 90(8):4525-4529.

1157. Sandberg DE. Health-related quality of life as a primary endpoint for growth hormone therapy. *Horm Res.* 2006;65(5):250-252, discussion 252.

1158. Attanasio AF, Shavrikova E, Blum WF, et al. Continued growth hormone (GH) treatment after final height is necessary to complete somatic development in childhood-onset GH-deficient patients. *J Clin Endocrinol Metab.* 2004;89(10):4857-4862.

1159. Cowan FJ, Evans WD, Gregory JW. Metabolic effects of discontinuing growth hormone treatment. *Arch Dis Child.* 1999;80(6):517-523.

1160. Drake WM, Carroll PV, Maher KT, et al. The effect of cessation of growth hormone (GH) therapy on bone mineral accretion in GH-deficient adolescents at the completion of linear growth. *J Clin Endocrinol Metab.* 2003;88(4):1658-1663.

1161. Underwood LE, Attie KM, Baptista J. Genentech Collaborative Study Group. Growth hormone (GH) dose-response in young adults with childhood-onset GH deficiency: a two-year, multicenter, multiple-dose, placebo-controlled study. *J Clin Endocrinol Metab.* 2003;88(11): 5273-5280.

1162. Colao A, Di Somma C, Salerno M, et al. The cardiovascular risk of GH-deficient adolescents. *J Clin Endocrinol Metab.* 2002;87(8): 3650-3655.

1163. Salerno M, Esposito V, Spinelli L, et al. Left ventricular mass and function in children with GH deficiency before and during 12 months GH replacement therapy. *Clin Endocrinol (Oxf).* 2004;60(5): 630-636.

1164. Lanes R, Paoli M, Carrillo E, et al. Cardiovascular risk of young growth-hormone-deficient adolescents. Differences in growth-hormone-treated and untreated patients. *Horm Res.* 2003;60(6):291-296.

1165. Mohn A, Marzio D, Giannini C, et al. Alterations in the oxidant-antioxidant status in prepubertal children with growth hormone deficiency: effect of growth hormone replacement therapy. *Clin Endocrinol (Oxf).* 2005;63(5):537-542.

1166. Esposito V, Di Biase S, Lettiero T, et al. Serum homocysteine concentrations in children with growth hormone (GH) deficiency before and after 12 months GH replacement. *Clin Endocrinol (Oxf).* 2004;61(5): 607-611.

1167. Simon D, Lucidarme N, Prieur AM, et al. Effects on growth and body composition of growth hormone treatment in children with juvenile idiopathic arthritis requiring steroid therapy. *J Rheumatol.* 2003;30(11): 2492-2499.

1168. Guevara-Aguirre J, Vasconez O, Martinez V, et al. A randomized, double blind, placebo-controlled trial on safety and efficacy of recombinant human insulin-like growth factor-I in children with growth hormone receptor deficiency. *J Clin Endocrinol Metab.* 1995;80(4): 1393-1398.

1169. Radovick S, DiVall S. Approach to the growth hormone-deficient child during transition to adulthood. *J Clin Endocrinol Metab.* 2007; 92(4):1195-1200.

1170. Deal CL, Tony M, Hoybye C, et al. Growth Hormone Research Society workshop summary: consensus guidelines for recombinant human growth hormone therapy in Prader-Willi syndrome. *J Clin Endocrinol Metab.* 2013;98(6):E1072-E1087.

1171. Fridman C, Kok F, Koiffmann CP. Hypotonic infants and the Prader-Willi syndrome. *J Pediatr (Rio J).* 2000;76(3):246-250.

1172. Butler MG, Sturich J, Lee J, et al. Growth standards of infants with Prader-Willi syndrome. *Pediatrics.* 2011;127(4):687-695.

1173. Eiholzer U, Stutz K, Weinmann C, et al. Low insulin, IGF-I and IGFBP-3 levels in children with Prader-Labhart-Willi syndrome. *Eur J Pediatr*. 1998;157(11):890-893.

1174. Lindgren AC, Hagenas L, Muller J, et al. Growth hormone treatment of children with Prader-Willi syndrome affects linear growth and body composition favourably. *Acta Paediatr*. 1998;87(1):28-31.

1175. Corrias A, Bellone J, Beccaria L, et al. GH/IGF-I axis in Prader-Willi syndrome: evaluation of IGF-I levels and of the somatotroph responsiveness to various provocative stimuli. Genetic obesity study group of Italian Society of Pediatric Endocrinology and Diabetology. *J Endocrinol Invest*. 2000;23(2):84-89.

1176. Tauber M, Barbeau C, Jouret B, et al. Auxological and endocrine evolution of 28 children with Prader-Willi syndrome: effect of GH therapy in 14 children. *Horm Res*. 2000;53(6):279-287.

1177. Burman P, Ritzen EM, Lindgren AC. Endocrine dysfunction in Prader-Willi syndrome: a review with special reference to GH. *Endocr Rev*. 2001;22(6):787-799.

1178. Wolfgram PM, Sarrault J, Clark S, Lee JM. State-to-state variability in Title V coverage for children with diabetes. *J Pediatr*. 2013;162(4):873-875.

1179. Lindgren AC, Lindberg A. Growth hormone treatment completely normalizes adult height and improves body composition in Prader-Willi syndrome: experience from KIGS (Pfizer international growth database). *Horm Res*. 2008;70(3):182-187.

1180. Carrel AL, Myers SE, Whitman BY, Allen DB. Benefits of long-term GH therapy in Prader-Willi syndrome: a 4-year study. *J Clin Endocrinol Metab*. 2002;87(4):1581-1585.

1181. Allen DB, Carrel AL. Growth hormone therapy for Prader-Willi syndrome: a critical appraisal. *J Pediatr Endocrinol Metab*. 2004;17 (Suppl 4):1297-1306.

1182. Bakker NE, Kuppens RJ, Siemensma EP, et al. Eight years of Growth hormone treatment in children with Prader-Willi syndrome: maintaining the positive effects. *J Clin Endocrinol Metab*. 2013;98(10):4013-4022.

1183. Wollmann HA, Schultz U, Grauer ML, Ranke MB. Reference values for height and weight in Prader-Willi syndrome based on 315 patients. *Eur J Pediatr*. 1998;157(8):634-642.

1184. Hauffa BP, Schlippe G, Roos M, et al. Spontaneous growth in German children and adolescents with genetically confirmed Prader-Willi syndrome. *Acta Paediatr*. 2000;89(11):1302-1311.

1185. Tauber M. Effects of growth hormone treatment in children presenting with Prader-Willi syndrome: the KIGS experience. In: Ranke MB, Price DA, Reiter EO, eds. *Growth Hormone Therapy in Pediatrics—20 Years of KIGS*. Basel: Karger; 2007.

1186. Whitman BY, Myers MG, Carrel AL, et al. The behavioral impact of growth hormone treatment for children and adolescents with Prader-Willi syndrome: a 2-year controlled study. *Pediatrics*. 2005;109(e35):308-309.

1187. de Lind van Wijngaarden RF, Siemensma EP, Festen DA, et al. Efficacy and safety of long-term continuous growth hormone treatment in children with Prader-Willi syndrome. *J Clin Endocrinol Metab*. 2009;94(11):4205-4215.

1188. Coupaye M, Lorenzini F, Lloret-Linares C, et al. Growth hormone therapy for children and adolescents with Prader-Willi syndrome is associated with improved body composition and metabolic status in adulthood. *J Clin Endocrinol Metab*. 2013;98(2):E328-E335.

1189. Miller JL, Goldstone AP, Couch JA, et al. Pituitary abnormalities in Prader-Willi syndrome and early onset morbid obesity. *Am J Med Genet A*. 2008;146A(5):570-577.

1190. Butler MG, Theodoro M, Skouse JD. Thyroid function studies in Prader-Willi syndrome. *Am J Med Genet A*. 2007;143(5):488-492.

1191. Carrel AL, Moerchen V, Myers SE, et al. Growth hormone improves mobility and body composition in infants and toddlers with Prader-Willi syndrome. *J Pediatr*. 2004;145(6):744-749.

1192. Festen DA, Wevers M, Lindgren AC, et al. Mental and motor development before and during growth hormone treatment in infants and toddlers with Prader-Willi syndrome. *Clin Endocrinol (Oxf)*. 2008;68(6):919-925.

1193. Bridges N. What is the value of growth hormone therapy in Prader Willi syndrome? *Arch Dis Child*. 2014;99(2):166-170.

1194. Siemensma EP, de Lind van Wijngaarden RF, et al. Testicular failure in boys with Prader-Willi syndrome: longitudinal studies of reproductive hormones. *J Clin Endocrinol Metab*. 2012;97(3):E452-E459.

1195. Bakker B, Maneatis T, Lippe B. Sudden death in Prader-Willi syndrome: brief review of five additional cases. Concerning the article by Eiholzer U. Deaths in children with Prader-Willi syndrome. A contribution to the debate about the safety of growth hormone treatment in children with PWS (*Horm Res* 2005;63:33-39). *Horm Res*. 2007;67(4):203-204.

1196. Whittington JE, Holland AJ, Webb T, et al. Population prevalence and estimated birth incidence and mortality rate for people with Prader-Willi syndrome in one UK health region. *J Med Genet*. 2001;38(11):792-798.

1197. Tauber M, Diene G, Molinas C, Hebert M. Review of 64 cases of death in children with Prader-Willi syndrome (PWS). *Am J Med Genet A*. 2008;146(7):881-887.

1198. Bell J, Parker KL, Swinford RD, et al. Long-term safety of recombinant human growth hormone in children. *J Clin Endocrinol Metab*. 2010;95(1):167-177.

1199. Eiholzer U. Deaths in children with Prader-Willi syndrome. A contribution to the debate about the safety of growth hormone treatment in children with PWS. *Horm Res*. 2005;63(1):33-39.

1200. Van Vliet G, Deal CL, Crock PA, et al. Sudden death in growth hormone-treated children with Prader-Willi syndrome. *J Pediatr*. 2004;144(1):129-131.

1201. Nagai T, Obata K, Tonoki H, et al. Cause of sudden, unexpected death of Prader-Willi syndrome patients with or without growth hormone treatment. *Am J Med Genet A*. 2005;136(1):45-48.

1202. Berini J, Spica Russotto V, Castelnuovo P, et al. Growth hormone therapy and respiratory disorders: long-term follow-up in PWS children. *J Clin Endocrinol Metab*. 2013;98(9):E1516-E1523.

1203. Haqq AM, Stadler DD, Jackson RH, et al. Effects of growth hormone on pulmonary function, sleep quality, behavior, cognition, growth velocity, body composition, and resting energy expenditure in Prader-Willi syndrome. *J Clin Endocrinol Metab*. 2003;88(5):2206-2212.

1204. Myers SE, Carrel AL, Whitman BY, Allen DB. Sustained benefit after 2 years of growth hormone on body composition, fat utilization, physical strength and agility, and growth in Prader-Willi syndrome. *J Pediatr*. 2000;137(1):42-49.

1205. Festen D, Hokken-Koelega A. Breathing disorders in Prader-Willi syndrome: the role of obesity, growth hormone treatment and upper respiratory tract infections. *Exp Rev Endocrinol Metab*. 2007;2:529-537.

1206. Lindgren AC, Hellstrom LG, Ritzen EM, Milerad J. Growth hormone treatment increases CO_2 response, ventilation and central inspiratory drive in children with Prader-Willi syndrome. *Eur J Pediatr*. 1999;158(11):936-940.

1207. Miller J, Silverstein J, Shuster J, et al. Short-term effects of growth hormone on sleep abnormalities in Prader-Willi syndrome. *J Clin Endocrinol Metab*. 2006;91(2):413-417.

1208. Festen DA, de Weerd AW, van den Bossche RA, et al. Sleep-related breathing disorders in prepubertal children with Prader-Willi syndrome and effects of growth hormone treatment. *J Clin Endocrinol Metab*. 2006;91(12):4911-4915.

1209. Al-Saleh S, Al-Naimi A, Hamilton J, et al. Longitudinal evaluation of sleep-disordered breathing in children with Prader-Willi syndrome during 2 years of growth hormone therapy. *J Pediatr*. 2013;162(2):263-268, e1.

1210. de Lind van Wijngaarden RF, Otten BJ, Festen DA, et al. High prevalence of central adrenal insufficiency in patients with Prader-Willi syndrome. *J Clin Endocrinol Metab*. 2008;93(5):1649-1654.

1211. de Lind van Wijngaarden RF, Joosten KF, van den Berg S, et al. The relationship between central adrenal insufficiency and sleep-related breathing disorders in children with Prader-Willi syndrome. *J Clin Endocrinol Metab*. 2009;94(7):2387-2393.

1212. Angulo MA, Castro-Magana M, Lamerson M, et al. Final adult height in children with Prader-Willi syndrome with and without human growth hormone treatment. *Am J Med Genet A*. 2007;143A(13):1456-1461.

1213. Butler JV, Whittington JE, Holland AJ, et al. Prevalence of, and risk factors for, physical ill-health in people with Prader-Willi syndrome: a population-based study. *Dev Med Child Neurol*. 2002;44(4):248-255.

1214. Nagai T, Obata K, Ogata T, et al. Growth hormone therapy and scoliosis in patients with Prader-Willi syndrome. *Am J Med Genet A*. 2006;140(15):1623-1627.

1215. de Lind van Wijngaarden RF, de Klerk LW, Festen DA, Hokken-Koelega AC. Scoliosis in Prader-Willi syndrome: prevalence, effects of age, gender, body mass index, lean body mass and genotype. *Arch Dis Child*. 2008;93(12):1012-1016.

1216. Odent T, Accadbled F, Koureas G, et al. Scoliosis in patients with Prader-Willi syndrome. *Pediatrics*. 2008;122(2):e499-e503.

1217. de Lind van Wijngaarden RF, de Klerk LW, Festen DA, et al. Randomized controlled trial to investigate the effects of growth hormone treatment on scoliosis in children with Prader-Willi syndrome. *J Clin Endocrinol Metab*. 2009;94(4):1274-1280.

1218. Hoybye C, Thoren M. Somatropin therapy in adults with Prader-Willi syndrome. *Treat Endocrinol*. 2004;3(3):153-160.

1219. Hoybye C, Frystyk J, Thoren M. The growth hormone-insulin-like growth factor axis in adult patients with Prader Willi syndrome. *Growth Horm IGF Res*. 2003;13(5):269-274.

1220. Festen DA, de Lind van Wijngaarden R, van Eekelen M, et al. Randomized controlled GH trial: effects on anthropometry, body composition and body proportions in a large group of children with Prader-Willi syndrome. *Clin Endocrinol (Oxf)*. 2008;69(3):443-451.

1221. Hoybye C, Thoren M, Bohm B. Cognitive, emotional, physical and social effects of growth hormone treatment in adults with Prader-Willi syndrome. *J Intellect Disabil Res*. 2005;49(Pt 4):245-252.

1222. Partsch CJ, Lammer C, Gillessen-Kaesbach G, Pankau R. Adult patients with Prader-Willi syndrome: clinical characteristics, life circumstances and growth hormone secretion. *Growth Horm IGF Res*. 2000;10(Suppl B):S81-S85.

1223. Schaefer F, Wingen AM, Hennicke M, et al. Growth charts for prepubertal children with chronic renal failure due to congenital renal disorders. European study group for nutritional treatment of chronic renal failure in childhood. *Pediatr Nephrol.* 1996;10(3):288-293.

1224. Wuhl E, Haffner D, Offner G, et al. Long-term treatment with growth hormone in short children with nephropathic cystinosis. *J Pediatr.* 2001;138(6):880-887.

1225. Hokken-Koelega AC, van Zaal MA, van Bergen W, et al. Final height and its predictive factors after renal transplantation in childhood. *Pediatr Res.* 1994;36(3):323-328.

1226. Fine RN, Kohaut EC, Brown D, Perlman AJ. Growth after recombinant human growth hormone treatment in children with chronic renal failure: report of a multicenter randomized double-blind placebo-controlled study. Genentech cooperative study group. *J Pediatr.* 1994;124(3):374-382.

1227. Tonshoff B, Mehls O, Heinrich U, et al. Predicting GH response in short uremic children. *J Clin Endocrinol Metab.* 2010;95:686-692.

1228. Fine RN, Stablein D. Long-term use of recombinant human growth hormone in pediatric allograft recipients: a report of the NAPRTCS transplant registry. *Pediatr Nephrol.* 2005;20(3):404-408.

1229. Haffner D, Schaefer F, Nissel R, et al. Effect of growth hormone treatment on the adult height of children with chronic renal failure. German study group for growth hormone treatment in chronic renal failure. *N Engl J Med.* 2000;343(13):923-930.

1230. Hokken-Koelega A, Mulder P, De Jong R, et al. Long-term effects of growth hormone treatment on growth and puberty in patients with chronic renal insufficiency. *Pediatr Nephrol.* 2000;14(7):701-706.

1231. Wuhl E, Schaefer F. Effects of growth hormone in patients with chronic renal failure: experience in children and adults. *Horm Res.* 2002;58(Suppl 3):35-38.

1232. Mehls O. Treatment with growth hormone for growth impairment in renal disorders. In: Ranke MB, Gunnarsson R, eds. *Progress in Growth Hormone Therapy: 5 Years of KIGS.* Mannheim, Germany: J&J Verlag; 1996.

1233. Mardh G, Lundin K, Borg B, et al. Growth hormone replacement therapy in adult hypopituitary patients with growth hormone deficiency: combined data from 12 European placebo-controlled clinical trials. *Endocrinol Metab.* 1994;1(Suppl A):43-49.

1234. Hokken-Koelega AC, Stijnen T, De Jong MC, et al. Double blind trial comparing the effects of two doses of growth hormone in prepubertal patients with chronic renal insufficiency. *J Clin Endocrinol Metab.* 1994;79(4):1185-1190.

1235. Mehls O, Broyer M. Growth response to recombinant human growth hormone in short prepubertal children with chronic renal failure with or without dialysis. The European/Australian study group. *Acta Paediatr Suppl.* 1994;399:81-87.

1236. Fine RN, Kohaut E, Brown D, et al. Long-term treatment of growth retarded children with chronic renal insufficiency, with recombinant human growth hormone. *Kidney Int.* 1996;49(3):781-785.

1237. Watkins SL. Bone disease in patients receiving growth hormone. *Kidney Int Suppl.* 1996;53:S126-S127.

1238. Fine RN, Sullivan EK, Kuntze J, et al. The impact of recombinant human growth hormone treatment during chronic renal insufficiency on renal transplant recipients. *J Pediatr.* 2000;136(3):376-382.

1239. Berard E, Andre JL, Guest G, et al. Long-term results of rhGH treatment in children with renal failure: experience of the French Society of Pediatric Nephrology. *Pediatr Nephrol.* 2008;23(11):2031-2038.

1240. Seikaly MG, Waber P, Warady BA, Stablein D. The effect of rhGH on height velocity and BMI in children with CKD: a report of the NAPRTCS registry. *Pediatr Nephrol.* 2009;24(9):1711-1717.

1241. Ingulli E, Tejani A. An analytical review of growth hormone studies in children after renal transplantation. *Pediatr Nephrol.* 1995;9(Suppl):S61-S65.

1242. Nissel R, Lindberg A, Mehls O, et al. Factors predicting the near-final height in growth hormone-treated children and adolescents with chronic kidney disease. *J Clin Endocrinol Metab.* 2008;93(4):1359-1365.

1243. Fine RN. Allograft rejection in growth hormone and non-growth hormone treated children. *J Pediatr Endocrinol.* 1994;7(2):127-133.

1244. Chavers BM, Doherty L, Nevins TE, et al. Effects of growth hormone on kidney function in pediatric transplant recipients. *Pediatr Nephrol.* 1995;9(2):176-181.

1245. Benfield MR, Parker KL, Waldo FB, et al. Growth hormone in the treatment of growth failure in children after renal transplantation. *Kidney Int Suppl.* 1993;43:S62-S64.

1246. Laine J, Krogerus L, Sarna S, et al. Recombinant human growth hormone treatment. Its effect on renal allograft function and histology. *Transplantation.* 1996;61(6):898-903.

1247. Guebre-Egziabher F, Juillard L, Boirie Y, et al. Short-term administration of a combination of recombinant growth hormone and insulin-like growth factor-I induces anabolism in maintenance hemodialysis. *J Clin Endocrinol Metab.* 2009;94(7):2299-2305.

1248. Simon D, Fernando C, Czernichow P, Prieur AM. Linear growth and final height in patients with systemic juvenile idiopathic arthritis treated with longterm glucocorticoids. *J Rheumatol.* 2002;29(6):1296-1300.

1249. Allen RC, Jimenez M, Cowell CT. Insulin-like growth factor and growth hormone secretion in juvenile chronic arthritis. *Ann Rheum Dis.* 1991;50(9):602-606.

1250. Bergad PL, Schwarzenberg SJ, Humbert JT, et al. Inhibition of growth hormone action in models of inflammation. *Am J Physiol Cell Physiol.* 2000;279(6):C1906-C1917.

1251. Touati G, Prieur AM, Ruiz JC, et al. Beneficial effects of one-year growth hormone administration to children with juvenile chronic arthritis on chronic steroid therapy. I. Effects on growth velocity and body composition. *J Clin Endocrinol Metab.* 1998;83(2):403-409.

1252. Bechtold S, Ripperger P, Hafner R, et al. Growth hormone improves height in patients with juvenile idiopathic arthritis: 4-year data of a controlled study. *J Pediatr.* 2003;143(4):512-519.

1253. Simon D. rhGH treatment in corticosteroid-treated patients. *Horm Res.* 2007;68(1):38-45.

1254. Bechtold S, Ripperger P, Dalla Pozza R, et al. Growth hormone increases final height in patients with juvenile idiopathic arthritis: data from a randomized controlled study. *J Clin Endocrinol Metab.* 2007;92(8):3013-3018.

1255. Simon D, Prieur AM, Quartier P, et al. Early recombinant human growth hormone treatment in glucocorticoid-treated children with juvenile idiopathic arthritis: a 3-year randomized study. *J Clin Endocrinol Metab.* 2007;92(7):2567-2573.

1256. Bechtold S, Ripperger P, Dalla Pozza R, et al. Dynamics of body composition and bone in patients with juvenile idiopathic arthritis treated with growth hormone. *J Clin Endocrinol Metab.* 2010;95(1):178-185.

1257. Mushtaq T, Farquharson C, Seawright E, Ahmed SF. Glucocorticoid effects on chondrogenesis, differentiation and apoptosis in the murine ATDC5 chondrocyte cell line. *J Endocrinol.* 2002;175(3):705-713.

1258. Rosenfeld RG, Hintz RL, Johanson AJ, et al. Three-year results of a randomized prospective trial of methionyl human growth hormone and oxandrolone in Turner syndrome. *J Pediatr.* 1988;113(2):393-400.

1259. Chernausek SD, Attie KM, Cara JF, et al. Growth hormone therapy of Turner syndrome: the impact of age of estrogen replacement on final height. Genentech, Inc., collaborative study group. *J Clin Endocrinol Metab.* 2000;85(7):2439-2445.

1260. Reiter EO, Baptista J, Price L, et al. Effect of the age at initiation of GH treatment on estrogen use and near adult height in Turner syndrome. In: Saenger PH, Pasquino AM, eds. *5th International Turner Symposium: Optimizing Health Care for Turner Patients in the 21st Century.* Amsterdam, The Netherlands: 2000.

1261. Reiter EO, Blethen SL, Baptista J, Price L. Early initiation of growth hormone treatment allows age-appropriate estrogen use in turner's syndrome. *J Clin Endocrinol Metab.* 2001;86(5):1936-1941.

1262. Carel JC, Mathivon L, Gendrel C, et al. Near normalization of final height with adapted doses of growth hormone in Turner's syndrome. *J Clin Endocrinol Metab.* 1998;83(5):1462-1466.

1263. van Pareren YK, de Muinck Keizer-Schrama SM, Stijnen T, et al. Final height in girls with Turner syndrome after long-term growth hormone treatment in three dosages and low dose estrogens. *J Clin Endocrinol Metab.* 2003;88(3):1119-1125.

1264. Stahnke N, Keller E, Landy H, Serono Study Group. Favorable final height outcome in girls with Ullrich-Turner syndrome treated with low-dose growth hormone together with oxandrolone despite starting treatment after 10 years of age. *J Pediatr Endocrinol Metab.* 2002;15(2):129-138.

1265. Stephure DK, Canadian Growth Hormone Advisory Committee. Impact of growth hormone supplementation on adult height in Turner syndrome: results of the Canadian randomized controlled trial. *J Clin Endocrinol Metab.* 2005;90(6):3360-3366.

1266. Pasquino AM, Pucarelli I, Segni M, et al. Adult height in sixty girls with Turner syndrome treated with growth hormone matched with an untreated group. *J Endocrinol Invest.* 2005;28(4):350-356.

1267. Ranke MB, Lindberg A, Chatelain P, et al. Prediction of long-term response to recombinant human growth hormone in Turner syndrome: development and validation of mathematical models. KIGS International Board. Kabi International Growth Study. *J Clin Endocrinol Metab.* 2000;85(11):4212-4218.

1268. Quigley CA, Crowe BJ, Anglin DG, Chipman JJ. Growth hormone and low dose estrogen in Turner syndrome: results of a United States multi-center trial to near-final height. *J Clin Endocrinol Metab.* 2002;87(5):2033-2041.

1269. Davenport ML, Quigley CA, Bryant CG, et al. Effect of early growth hormone (GH) treatment in very young girls with Turner syndrome (TS). Seventh Joint European Society for Paediatric Endocrinology/Lawson Wilkins Pediatric Endocrine Society Meeting, Lyon, France, 2005.

1270. Sas TC, de Muinck Keizer-Schrama SM, Stijnen T, et al. Carbohydrate metabolism during long-term growth hormone (GH) treatment and after discontinuation of GH treatment in girls with Turner syndrome participating in a randomized dose-response study. Dutch advisory group on growth hormone. *J Clin Endocrinol Metab.* 2000;85(2):769-775.

1271. Park P, Cohen P. The role of insulin-like growth factor I monitoring in growth hormone-treated children. *Horm Res*. 2004;62(Suppl 1):59-65.

1272. Bondy CA, Turner Syndrome Study Group. Care of girls and women with Turner syndrome: a guideline of the Turner syndrome study group. *J Clin Endocrinol Metab*. 2007;92(1):10-25.

1273. Binder G, Baur F, Schweizer R, Ranke MB. The d3-growth hormone (GH) receptor polymorphism is associated with increased responsiveness to GH in Turner syndrome and short small-for-gestational-age children. *J Clin Endocrinol Metab*. 2006;91(2):659-664.

1274. Soriano-Guillen L, Coste J, Ecosse E, et al. Adult height and pubertal growth in Turner syndrome after treatment with recombinant growth hormone. *J Clin Endocrinol Metab*. 2005;90(9):5197-5204.

1275. Rosenfield RL, Devine N, Hunold JJ, et al. Salutary effects of combining early very low-dose systemic estradiol with growth hormone therapy in girls with Turner syndrome. *J Clin Endocrinol Metab*. 2005;90(12):6424-6430.

1276. Van Pareren YK, De Muinck Keizer-Schrama SM, Stijnen T, et al. Effect of discontinuation of long-term growth hormone treatment on carbohydrate metabolism and risk factors for cardiovascular disease in girls with Turner syndrome. *J Clin Endocrinol Metab*. 2002;87(12):5442-5448.

1277. Radetti G, Pasquino B, Gottardi E, et al. Insulin sensitivity in Turner's syndrome: influence of GH treatment. *Eur J Endocrinol*. 2004;151(3):351-354.

1278. Bakalov VK, Cooley MM, Quon MJ, et al. Impaired insulin secretion in the Turner metabolic syndrome. *J Clin Endocrinol Metab*. 2004;89(7):3516-3520.

1279. Bertelloni S, Cinquanta L, Baroncelli GI, et al. Volumetric bone mineral density in young women with Turner's syndrome treated with estrogens or estrogens plus growth hormone. *Horm Res*. 2000;53(2):72-76.

1280. Carel JC. Growth hormone in Turner syndrome: twenty years after, what can we tell our patients? *J Clin Endocrinol Metab*. 2005;90(6):3793-3794.

1281. Bannink EM, Raat H, Mulder PG, de Muinck Keizer-Schrama SM. Quality of life after growth hormone therapy and induced puberty in women with Turner syndrome. *J Pediatr*. 2006;148(1):95-101.

1282. Carel JC, Ecosse E, Bastie-Sigeac I, et al. Quality of life determinants in young women with Turner's syndrome after growth hormone treatment: results of the StaTur population-based cohort study. *J Clin Endocrinol Metab*. 2005;90(4):1992-1997.

1283. Bolar K, Hoffman AR, Maneatis T, Lippe B. Long-term safety of recombinant human growth hormone in Turner syndrome. *J Clin Endocrinol Metab*. 2008;93(2):344-351.

1284. Radetti G, Crepaz R, Milanesi O, et al. Cardiac performance in Turner's syndrome patients on growth hormone therapy. *Horm Res*. 2001;55(5):240-244.

1285. Sas TC, Cromme-Dijkhuis AH, de Muinck Keizer-Schrama SM, et al. The effects of long-term growth hormone treatment on cardiac left ventricular dimensions and blood pressure in girls with Turner's syndrome. Dutch working group on growth hormone. *J Pediatr*. 1999;135(4):470-476.

1286. van den Berg J, Bannink EM, Wielopolski PA, et al. Aortic distensibility and dimensions and the effects of growth hormone treatment in the Turner syndrome. *Am J Cardiol*. 2006;97(11):1644-1649.

1287. Donaldson MD, Gault EJ, Tan KW, Dunger DB. Optimising management in Turner syndrome: from infancy to adult transfer. *Arch Dis Child*. 2006;91(6):513-520.

1288. Russell KA. Orthodontic treatment for patients with Turner syndrome. *Am J Orthod Dentofacial Orthop*. 2001;120(3):314-322.

1289. Albertsson-Wikland K, Karlberg J. Postnatal growth of children born small for gestational age. *Acta Paediatr Suppl*. 1997;423:193-195.

1290. Lee PA, Chernausek SD, Hokken-Koelega AC, et al. International Small for Gestational Age Advisory Board consensus development conference statement: management of short children born small for gestational age, April 24-October 1, 2001. *Pediatrics*. 2003;111:1253-1261.

1291. Karlberg JP, Albertsson-Wikland K, Kwan EY, et al. The timing of early postnatal catch-up growth in normal, full-term infants born short for gestational age. *Horm Res*. 1997;48(Suppl 1):17-24.

1292. Karlberg J, Albertsson-Wikland K, Kwan CW, Chan FY. Early spontaneous catch-up growth. *J Pediatr Endocrinol Metab*. 2002;15(Suppl 5):1243-1255.

1293. Chatelain P, Job JC, Blanchard J, et al. Dose-dependent catch-up growth after 2 years of growth hormone treatment in intrauterine growth-retarded children. Belgian and French pediatric clinics and Sanofi-Choay (France). *J Clin Endocrinol Metab*. 1994;78(6):1454-1460.

1294. de Zegher F, Francois I, van Helvoirt M, Van den Berghe G. Clinical review 89: small as fetus and short as child: from endogenous to exogenous growth hormone. *J Clin Endocrinol Metab*. 1997;82(7):2021-2026.

1295. Vicens-Calvet E, Espadero RM, Carrascosa A, Spanish SGA Collaborative Group. Small for gestational age: longitudinal study of the pubertal growth spurt in children born small for gestational age without

1296. Job JC, Rolland A. Natural history of intrauterine growth retardation: pubertal growth and adult height. *Arch Fr Pediatr*. 1986;43(5):301-306.

1297. Lazar L, Pollak U, Kalter-Leibovici O, et al. Pubertal course of persistently short children born small for gestational age (SGA) compared with idiopathic short children born appropriate for gestational age (AGA). *Eur J Endocrinol*. 2003;149(5):425-432.

1298. Rogol A. Growth, puberty and therapeutic interventions [abstract S1–15]. Presented at the 45th European Society for Pediatric Endocrinology Annual Meeting, Helsinki, Finland, 2006.

1299. Wollmann HA. Intrauterine growth restriction: definition and etiology. *Horm Res*. 1998;49(Suppl 2):1-6.

1300. Ogilvy-Stuart AL, Hands SJ, Adcock CJ, et al. Insulin, insulin-like growth factor I (IGF-I), IGF-binding protein-1, growth hormone, and feeding in the newborn. *J Clin Endocrinol Metab*. 1998;83(10):3550-3557.

1301. Audi L, Esteban C, Espadero R, et al. D-3 growth hormone receptor polymorphism (d3-GHR) genotype frequencies differ between short small for gestational age children (SGA) (n 1/4 247) and a control population with normal adult height (n 1/4 289) (CPNAH) [abstract S1–15]. Presented at the 45th European Society for Pediatric Endocrinology Annual Meeting, Helsinki, Finland, 2006.

1302. Jensen RB, Viewerth S, Larsen T, et al. High prevalence of d3-growth hormone gene polymorphism in adolescents born SGA/IUGR: association with intrauterine growth velocity, birth weight, postnatal catch-up growth and near-final height [abstract FC1–42]. Presented at the 45th European Society for Pediatric Endocrinology Annual Meeting, Helsinki, Finland, 2006.

1303. Tenhola S, Halonen P, Jaaskelainen J, Voutilainen R. Serum markers of GH and insulin action in 12-year-old children born small for gestational age. *Eur J Endocrinol*. 2005;152(3):335-340.

1304. Bonapace G, Concolino D, Formicola S, Strisciuglio P. A novel mutation in a patient with insulin-like growth factor 1 (IGF1) deficiency. *J Med Genet*. 2003;40(12):913-917.

1305. Cianfarani S, Maiorana A, Geremia C, et al. Blood glucose concentrations are reduced in children born small for gestational age (SGA), and thyroid-stimulating hormone levels are increased in SGA with blunted postnatal catch-up growth. *J Clin Endocrinol Metab*. 2003;88(6):2699-2705.

1306. Johnston LB, Dahlgren J, Leger J, et al. Association between insulin-like growth factor I (IGF-I) polymorphisms, circulating IGF-I, and pre- and postnatal growth in two European small for gestational age populations. *J Clin Endocrinol Metab*. 2003;88(10):4805-4810.

1307. Ali O, Cohen P. Insulin-like growth factors and their binding proteins in children born small for gestational age: implication for growth hormone therapy. *Horm Res*. 2003;60(Suppl 3):115-123.

1308. Strauss RS, Dietz WH. Growth and development of term children born with low birth weight: effects of genetic and environmental factors. *J Pediatr*. 1998;133(1):67-72.

1309. de Zegher F, Hokken-Koelega A. Growth hormone therapy for children born small for gestational age: height gain is less dose dependent over the long term than over the short term. *Pediatrics*. 2005;115(4):e458-e462.

1310. Carel JC, Chatelain P, Rochiccioli P, Chaussain JL. Improvement in adult height after growth hormone treatment in adolescents with short stature born small for gestational age: results of a randomized controlled study. *J Clin Endocrinol Metab*. 2003;88(4):1587-1593.

1311. de Zegher F, Ong KK, Ibanez L, Dunger DB. Growth hormone therapy in short children born small for gestational age. *Horm Res*. 2006;65(Suppl 3):145-152.

1312. Ong K, Beardsall K, de Zegher F. Growth hormone therapy in short children born small for gestational age. *Early Hum Dev*. 2005;81(12):973-980.

1313. Ranke MB, Lindberg A, Cowell CT, et al. Prediction of response to growth hormone treatment in short children born small for gestational age: analysis of data from KIGS Pharmacia International growth database. *J Clin Endocrinol Metab*. 2003;88(1):125-131.

1314. Leger J, Levy-Marchal C, Bloch J, et al. Reduced final height and indications for insulin resistance in 20 year olds born small for gestational age: regional cohort study. *BMJ*. 1997;315(7104):341-347.

1315. Barker DJ, Hales CN, Fall CH, et al. Type 2 (non-insulin-dependent) diabetes mellitus, hypertension and hyperlipidaemia (syndrome X): relation to reduced fetal growth. *Diabetologia*. 1993;36(1):62-67.

1316. Crowther NJ, Cameron N, Trusler J, Gray IP. Association between poor glucose tolerance and rapid postnatal weight gain in seven-year-old children. *Diabetologia*. 1998;41(10):1163-1167.

1317. Jaquet D, Gaboriau A, Czernichow P, Levy-Marchal C. Insulin resistance early in adulthood in subjects born with intrauterine growth retardation. *J Clin Endocrinol Metab*. 2000;85(4):1401-1406.

1318. Veening MA, Van Weissenbruch MM, Delemarre-Van De Waal HA. Glucose tolerance, insulin sensitivity, and insulin secretion in children born small for gestational age. *J Clin Endocrinol Metab*. 2002;87(10):4657-4661.

1319. Soto N, Bazaes RA, Pena V, et al. Insulin sensitivity and secretion are related to catch-up growth in small-for-gestational-age infants at age 1 year: results from a prospective cohort. *J Clin Endocrinol Metab.* 2003;88(8):3645-3650.

1320. de Zegher F, Maes M, Gargosky SE, et al. High-dose growth hormone treatment of short children born small for gestational age. *J Clin Endocrinol Metab.* 1996;81(5):1887-1892.

1321. de Zegher F, Ong K, van Helvoirt M, et al. High-dose growth hormone (GH) treatment in non-GH-deficient children born small for gestational age induces growth responses related to pretreatment GH secretion and associated with a reversible decrease in insulin sensitivity. *J Clin Endocrinol Metab.* 2002;87(1):148-151.

1322. van Pareren Y, Mulder P, Houdijk M, et al. Effect of discontinuation of growth hormone treatment on risk factors for cardiovascular disease in adolescents born small for gestational age. *J Clin Endocrinol Metab.* 2003;88(1):347-353.

1323. Cutfield WS, Lindberg A, Rapaport R, et al. Safety of growth hormone treatment in children born small for gestational age: the US trial and KIGS analysis. *Horm Res.* 2006;65(Suppl 3):153-159.

1324. Wilton P. Adverse events during GH treatment: 10 years' experience with KIGS, a pharmacoepidemiological survey. In: Ranke MB, Wilton P, eds. *Growth Hormone Therapy in KIGS: 10 Years' Experience.* Heidelberg-Leipzig: Johann Ambrosius Barth Verlag; 1999.

1325. Sas T, Mulder P, Hokken-Koelega A. Body composition, blood pressure, and lipid metabolism before and during long-term growth hormone (GH) treatment in children with short stature born small for gestational age either with or without GH deficiency. *J Clin Endocrinol Metab.* 2000;85(10):3786-3792.

1326. Czernichow P. Treatment with growth hormone in short children born with intrauterine growth retardation. *Endocrine.* 2001;15(1):39-42.

1327. Simeoni U, Zetterstrom R. Long-term circulatory and renal consequences of intrauterine growth restriction. *Acta Paediatr.* 2005;94(7):819-824.

1328. Chatelain P. Children born with intra-uterine growth retardation (IUGR) or small for gestational age (SGA): long term growth and metabolic consequences. *Endocr Regul.* 2000;34(1):33-36.

1329. Levy-Marchal C, Czernichow P. Small for gestational age and the metabolic syndrome: which mechanism is suggested by epidemiological and clinical studies? *Horm Res.* 2006;65(Suppl 3):123-130.

1330. Seino Y, Yamate T, Kanzaki S, et al. Achondroplasia: effect of growth hormone in 40 patients. *Clin Pediatr Endocrinol.* 1994;3(Suppl 4):41-45.

1331. Ramaswami U, Rumsby G, Spoudeas HA, et al. Treatment of achondroplasia with growth hormone: six years of experience. *Pediatr Res.* 1999;46(4):435-439.

1332. Bridges NA, Brook CG. Progress report: growth hormone in skeletal dysplasia. *Horm Res.* 1994;42(4-5):231-234.

1333. Rao E, Weiss B, Fukami M, et al. Pseudoautosomal deletions encompassing a novel homeobox gene cause growth failure in idiopathic short stature and Turner syndrome. *Nat Genet.* 1997;16(1):54-63.

1334. Clement-Jones M, Schiller S, Rao E, et al. The short stature homeobox gene SHOX is involved in skeletal abnormalities in Turner syndrome. *Hum Mol Genet.* 2000;9(5):695-702.

1335. Binder G, Renz A, Martinez A, et al. SHOX haploinsufficiency and Leri-Weill dyschondrosteosis: prevalence and growth failure in relation to mutation, sex, and degree of wrist deformity. *J Clin Endocrinol Metab.* 2004;89(9):4403-4408.

1336. Rappold GA, Fukami M, Niesler B, et al. Deletions of the homeobox gene SHOX (short stature homeobox) are an important cause of growth failure in children with short stature. *J Clin Endocrinol Metab.* 2002;87(3):1402-1406.

1337. Rappold G, Blum WF, Shavrikova EP, et al. Genotypes and phenotypes in children with short stature: clinical indicators of SHOX haploinsufficiency. *J Med Genet.* 2007;44(5):306-313.

1338. Blum WF, Ross JL, Zimmermann AG, et al. GH treatment to final height produces similar height gains in patients with SHOX deficiency and Turner syndrome: results of a multicenter trial. *J Clin Endocrinol Metab.* 2013;98(8):E1383-E1392.

1339. Shah BC, Moran ES, Zinn AR, Pappas JG. Effect of growth hormone therapy on severe short stature and skeletal deformities in a patient with combined Turner syndrome and Langer mesomelic dysplasia. *J Clin Endocrinol Metab.* 2009;94(12):5028-5033.

1340. Jamieson CR, van der Burgt I, Brady AF, et al. Mapping a gene for Noonan syndrome to the long arm of chromosome 12. *Nat Genet.* 1994;8(4):357-360.

1341. Schubbert S, Zenker M, Rowe SL, et al. Germline KRAS mutations cause Noonan syndrome. *Nat Genet.* 2006;38(3):331-336.

1342. Roberts AE, Araki T, Swanson KD, et al. Germline gain-of-function mutations in SOS1 cause Noonan syndrome. *Nat Genet.* 2007;39(1):70-74.

1343. Pandit B, Sarkozy A, Pennacchio LA, et al. Gain-of-function RAF1 mutations cause Noonan and LEOPARD syndromes with hypertrophic cardiomyopathy. *Nat Genet.* 2007;39(8):1007-1012.

1344. De Rocca Serra-Nedelec A, Edouard T, Treguer K, et al. Noonan syndrome-causing SHP2 mutants inhibit insulin-like growth factor 1 release via growth hormone-induced ERK hyperactivation, which contributes to short stature. *Proc Natl Acad Sci U S A.* 2012;109(11):4257-4262.

1345. Raaijmakers R, Noordam C, Karagiannis G, et al. Response to growth hormone treatment and final height in Noonan syndrome in a large cohort of patients in the KIGS database. *J Pediatr Endocrinol Metab.* 2008;21(3):267-273.

1346. Kirk JM, Betts PR, Butler GE, et al. Short stature in Noonan syndrome: response to growth hormone therapy. *Arch Dis Child.* 2001;84(5):440-443.

1347. Osio D, Dahlgren J, Wikland KA, Westphal O. Improved final height with long-term growth hormone treatment in Noonan syndrome. *Acta Paediatr.* 2005;94(9):1232-1237.

1348. Municchi G, Pasquino AM, Pucarelli I, et al. Growth hormone treatment in Noonan syndrome: report of four cases who reached final height. *Horm Res.* 1995;44(4):164-167.

1349. Noordam C, Peer PG, Francois I, et al. Long-term GH treatment improves adult height in children with Noonan syndrome with and without mutations in protein tyrosine phosphatase, non-receptor-type 11. *Eur J Endocrinol.* 2008;159(3):203-208.

1350. Romano AA, Dana K, Bakker B, et al. Growth response, near-adult height, and patterns of growth and puberty in patients with Noonan syndrome treated with growth hormone. *J Clin Endocrinol Metab.* 2009;94(7):2338-2344.

1351. Rosenfeld RG, Buckway CK. Should we treat genetic syndromes? *J Pediatr Endocrinol Metab.* 2000;13:971-981.

1352. Romano AA, Blethen SL, Dana K, Noto RA. Growth hormone treatment in Noonan syndrome: the National Cooperative Growth Study experience. *J Pediatr.* 1996;128(5 Pt 2):S18-S21.

1353. Tartaglia M, Mehler EL, Goldberg R, et al. Mutations in PTPN11, encoding the protein tyrosine phosphatase SHP-2, cause Noonan syndrome. *Nat Genet.* 2001;29(4):465-468.

1354. Cotterill AM, McKenna WJ, Brady AF, et al. The short-term effects of growth hormone therapy on height velocity and cardiac ventricular wall thickness in children with Noonan's syndrome. *J Clin Endocrinol Metab.* 1996;81(6):2291-2297.

1355. Rauen KA, Schoyer L, McCormick F, et al. Proceedings from the 2009 genetic syndromes of the Ras/MAPK pathway: from bedside to bench and back. *Am J Med Genet A.* 2010;152A(1):4-24.

1356. Voss LD. Growth hormone therapy for the short normal child: who needs it and who wants it? The case against growth hormone therapy. *J Pediatr.* 2000;136(1):103-106.

1357. Voss LD, Mulligan J. Bullying in school: are short pupils at risk? Questionnaire study in a cohort. *BMJ.* 2000;320(7235):612-613.

1358. Saenger P. The case in support of GH therapy. *J Pediatr.* 2000;136(1):106-109, discussion 109-110.

1359. Allen DB, Fost N. hGH for short stature: ethical issues raised by expanded access. *J Pediatr.* 2004;144(5):648-652.

1360. Sandberg DE, Colsman M. Growth hormone treatment of short stature: status of the quality of life rationale. *Horm Res.* 2005;63(6):275-283.

1361. Ross JL, Sandberg DE, Rose SR, et al. Psychological adaptation in children with idiopathic short stature treated with growth hormone or placebo. *J Clin Endocrinol Metab.* 2004;89(10):4873-4878.

1362. Voss LD, Sandberg DE. The psychological burden of short stature: evidence against. *Eur J Endocrinol.* 2004;151(Suppl 1):S29-S33.

1363. van Pareren YK, Duivenvoorden HJ, Slijper FS, et al. Intelligence and psychosocial functioning during long-term growth hormone therapy in children born small for gestational age. *J Clin Endocrinol Metab.* 2004;89(11):5295-5302.

1364. Cuttler L. Safety and efficacy of growth hormone treatment for idiopathic short stature. *J Clin Endocrinol Metab.* 2005;90(9):5502-5504.

1365. Wit JM, Rekers-Mombarg LT, Cutler GB, et al. Growth hormone (GH) treatment to final height in children with idiopathic short stature: evidence for a dose effect. *J Pediatr.* 2005;146(1):45-53.

1366. Finkelstein BS, Imperiale TF, Speroff T, et al. Effect of growth hormone therapy on height in children with idiopathic short stature: a meta-analysis. *Arch Pediatr Adolesc Med.* 2002;156(3):230-240.

1367. Crowe BJ, Rekers-Mombarg LT, Robling K, et al. Effect of growth hormone dose on bone maturation and puberty in children with idiopathic short stature. *J Clin Endocrinol Metab.* 2006;91(1):169-175.

1368. Kamp GA, Waelkens JJ, de Muinck Keizer-Schrama SM, et al. High dose growth hormone treatment induces acceleration of skeletal maturation and an earlier onset of puberty in children with idiopathic short stature. *Arch Dis Child.* 2002;87(3):215-220.

1369. Buchlis JG, Irizarry L, Crotzer BC, et al. Comparison of final heights of growth hormone-treated vs. untreated children with idiopathic growth failure. *J Clin Endocrinol Metab.* 1998;83(4):1075-1079.

1370. Wit J. Growth hormone treatment of idiopathic short stature. In: Ranke MB, Wilton P, eds. *Growth Hormone Therapy in KIGS: 10 Years' Experience.* Heidelberg-Leipzig: Johann Ambrosius Verlag; 1999.

1371. Saenger P, Attie KM, DiMartino-Nardi J, et al. Metabolic consequences of 5-year growth hormone (GH) therapy in children treated with GH for idiopathic short stature. Genentech collaborative study group. *J Clin Endocrinol Metab.* 1998;83(9):3115-3120.

1372. Kelnar CJ, Albertsson-Wikland K, Hintz RL, et al. Should we treat children with idiopathic short stature? *Horm Res.* 1999;52(3):150-157.

1373. Wit JM, Rekers-Mombarg LT, Dutch Growth Hormone Advisory Group. Final height gain by GH therapy in children with idiopathic short stature is dose dependent. *J Clin Endocrinol Metab.* 2002;87(2):604-611.

1374. Visser-van Balen H, Geenen R, Kamp GA, et al. Long-term psychosocial consequences of hormone treatment for short stature. *Acta Paediatr.* 2007;96(5):715-719.

1375. Weise KL, Nahata MC. Growth hormone use in children with idiopathic short stature. *Ann Pharmacother.* 2004;38(9):1460-1468.

1376. Bryant J, Baxter L, Cave CB, Milne R. Recombinant growth hormone for idiopathic short stature in children and adolescents. *Cochrane Database Syst Rev.* 2007;(3):CD004440.

1377. Cohen LE. Idiopathic short stature: a clinical review. *JAMA.* 2014;311(17):1787-1796.

1378. Yanovski JA, Rose SR, Municchi G, et al. Treatment with a luteinizing hormone-releasing hormone agonist in adolescents with short stature. *N Engl J Med.* 2003;348(10):908-917.

1379. Tanaka T. Sufficiently long-term treatment with combined growth hormone and gonadotropin-releasing hormone analog can improve adult height in short children with isolated growth hormone deficiency (GHD) and in non-GHD short children. *Pediatr Endocrinol Rev.* 2007;5(1):471-481.

1380. van Gool SA, Kamp GA, Visser-van Balen H, et al. Final height outcome after three years of growth hormone and gonadotropin-releasing hormone agonist treatment in short adolescents with relatively early puberty. *J Clin Endocrinol Metab.* 2007;92(4):1402-1408.

1381. Food and Drug Administration, 2008. Available from <www.accessdata.fda.gov/drugsatfda_docs/label/2008/0202805060Ibl.pdf>.

1382. Tanaka T, Cohen P, Clayton PE, et al. Diagnosis and management of growth hormone deficiency in childhood and adolescence—part 2: growth hormone treatment in growth hormone deficient children. *Growth Horm IGF Res.* 2002;12(5):323-341.

1383. Quigley CA, Gill AM, Crowe BJ, et al. Safety of growth hormone treatment in pediatric patients with idiopathic short stature. *J Clin Endocrinol Metab.* 2005;90(9):5188-5196.

1384. Anneren G, Tuvemo T, Carlsson-Skwirut C, et al. Growth hormone treatment in young children with Down's syndrome: effects on growth and psychomotor development. *Arch Dis Child.* 1999;80(4):334-338.

1385. Anneren G, Gustafsson J, Sara VR, Tuvemo T. Normalized growth velocity in children with Down's syndrome during growth hormone therapy. *J Intellect Disabil Res.* 1993;37(Pt 4):381-387.

1386. Neyzi O, Darendeliler F. Growth hormone treatment in syndromes with short stature including Down syndrome, Prader Labhardt-Willi syndrome, von Recklinghausen syndrome, Williams syndrome and others. In: Ranke MB, Gunnarsson R, eds. *Progress in Growth Hormone Therapy: 5 Years of KIGS.* Mannheim: J&J Verlag; 1994.

1387. Torrado C, Bastian W, Wisniewski KE, Castells S. Treatment of children with Down syndrome and growth retardation with recombinant human growth hormone. *J Pediatr.* 1991;119(3):478-483.

1388. Allen DB, Frasier SD, Foley TP Jr, Pescovitz OH. Growth hormone for children with Down syndrome. *J Pediatr.* 1993;123(5):742-743.

1389. Sattler FR. Growth hormone in the aging male. *Best Pract Res Clin Endocrinol Metab.* 2013;27(4):541-555.

1390. Sanchez CP, Goodman WG, Brandli D, et al. Skeletal response to recombinant human growth hormone (rhGH) in children treated with long-term corticosteroids. *J Bone Miner Res.* 1995;10(1):2-6.

1391. Luo JM, Murphy LJ. Dexamethasone inhibits growth hormone induction of insulin-like growth factor-I (IGF-I) messenger ribonucleic acid (mRNA) in hypophysectomized rats and reduces IGF-I mRNA abundance in the intact rat. *Endocrinology.* 1989;125(1):165-171.

1392. Takala J, Ruokonen E, Webster NR, et al. Increased mortality associated with growth hormone treatment in critically ill adults. *N Engl J Med.* 1999;341(11):785-792.

1393. Wilton P. Adverse events during growth hormone treatment: 5 years' experience. In: Ranke MB, Gunnarsson R, eds. *Progress in Growth Hormone Therapy: 5 Years of KIGS.* Mannheim: J&J Verlag; 1994.

1394. Maneatis T, Baptista J, Connelly K, Blethen S. Growth hormone safety update from the National Cooperative Growth Study. *J Pediatr Endocrinol Metab.* 2000;13(Suppl 2):1035-1044.

1395. Cowell CT, Dietsch S. Adverse events during growth hormone therapy. *J Pediatr Endocrinol Metab.* 1995;8(4):243-252.

1396. Ranke MB, Wilton PM. *Growth Hormone Therapy in KIGS: 10 Years' Experience.* Heidelberg-Leipzig: Johann Ambrosius Barth Verlag; 1999.

1397. Watanabe S, Yamaguchi N, Tsunematsu Y, Komiyama A. Risk factors for leukemia occurrence among growth hormone users. *Jpn J Cancer Res.* 1989;80(9):822-825.

1398. Blethen SL, Allen DB, Graves D, et al. Safety of recombinant deoxyribonucleic acid-derived growth hormone: the National Cooperative Growth Study experience. *J Clin Endocrinol Metab.* 1996;81(5):1704-1710.

1399. Blethen SL. Leukemia in children treated with growth hormone. *Trends Endocrinol Metab.* 1999;9:367-370.

1400. Nishi Y, Tanaka T, Takano K, et al. Recent status in the occurrence of leukemia in growth hormone-treated patients in Japan. GH treatment study committee of the Foundation For Growth Science, Japan. *J Clin Endocrinol Metab.* 1999;84(6):1961-1965.

1401. Sklar CA, Mertens AC, Mitby P, et al. Risk of disease recurrence and second neoplasms in survivors of childhood cancer treated with growth hormone: a report from the childhood cancer survivor study. *J Clin Endocrinol Metab.* 2002;87(7):3136-3141.

1402. Ogilvy-Stuart AL, Ryder WD, Gattamaneni HR, et al. Growth hormone and tumour recurrence. *BMJ.* 1992;304(6842):1601-1605.

1403. Dharnidharka VR, Talley LI, Martz KL, et al. Recombinant growth hormone use pretransplant and risk for post-transplant lymphoproliferative disease—a report of the NAPRTCS. *Pediatr Transplant.* 2008;12(6):689-695.

1404. Arslanian SA, Becker DJ, Lee PA, et al. Growth hormone therapy and tumor recurrence. findings in children with brain neoplasms and hypopituitarism. *Am J Dis Child.* 1985;139(4):347-350.

1405. Bloom HJ, Glees J, Bell J, et al. The treatment and long-term prognosis of children with intracranial tumors: a study of 610 cases, 1950-1981. *Int J Radiat Oncol Biol Phys.* 1990;18(4):723-745.

1406. Davis CH, Joglekar VM. Cerebellar astrocytomas in children and young adults. *J Neurol Neurosurg Psychiatry.* 1981;44(9):820-828.

1407. Halperin EC. Pediatric brain stem tumors: patterns of treatment failure and their implications for radiotherapy. *Int J Radiat Oncol Biol Phys.* 1985;11(7):1293-1298.

1408. Hoffman HJ, De Silva M, Humphreys RP, et al. Aggressive surgical management of craniopharyngiomas in children. *J Neurosurg.* 1992;76(1):47-52.

1409. Lapras C, Patet JD, Mottolese C, et al. Craniopharyngiomas in childhood: analysis of 42 cases. *Prog Exp Tumor Res.* 1987;30:350-358.

1410. Nishio S, Fukui M, Takeshita I, et al. Recurrent medulloblastoma in children. *Neurol Med Chir (Tokyo).* 1986;26(1):19-25.

1411. Schuler D, Somlo P, Borsi J, et al. New drug combination for the treatment of relapsed brain tumors in children. *Pediatr Hematol Oncol.* 1988;5(2):153-156.

1412. Uematsu Y, Tsuura Y, Miyamoto K, et al. The recurrence of primary intracranial germinomas. Special reference to germinoma with STGC (syncytiotrophoblastic giant cell). *J Neurooncol.* 1992;13(3):247-256.

1413. Clayton PE, Shalet SM, Gattamaneni HR, Price DA. Does growth hormone cause relapse of brain tumours? *Lancet.* 1987;1(8535):711-713.

1414. Rodens KP, Kaplan SL, Grumbach MM, et al. Does growth hormone therapy increase the frequency of tumor recurrence in children with brain tumors? *Acta Endocrinol.* 1987;28(Suppl):188-189.

1415. Moshang T Jr. Is brain tumor recurrence increased following growth hormone treatment? *Trends Endocrinol Metab.* 1995;6(6):205-209.

1416. Swerdlow AJ, Reddingius RE, Higgins CD, et al. Growth hormone treatment of children with brain tumors and risk of tumor recurrence. *J Clin Endocrinol Metab.* 2000;85(12):4444-4449.

1417. Karavitaki N, Warner JT, Marland A, et al. GH replacement does not increase the risk of recurrence in patients with craniopharyngioma. *Clin Endocrinol (Oxf).* 2006;64(5):556-560.

1418. Mackenzie S, Craven T, Gattamaneni HR, et al. Long-term safety of growth hormone replacement after CNS irradiation. *J Clin Endocrinol Metab.* 2011;96(9):2756-2761.

1419. Darendeliler F, Karagiannis G, Wilton P, et al. Recurrence of brain tumours in patients treated with growth hormone: analysis of KIGS (Pfizer international growth database). *Acta Paediatr.* 2006;95(10):1284-1290.

1420. Packer RJ, Sutton LN, Elterman R, et al. Outcome for children with medulloblastoma treated with radiation and cisplatin, CCNU, and vincristine chemotherapy. *J Neurosurg.* 1994;81(5):690-698.

1421. Jostel A, Mukherjee A, Hulse PA, Shalet SM. Adult growth hormone replacement therapy and neuroimaging surveillance in brain tumour survivors. *Clin Endocrinol (Oxf).* 2005;62(6):698-705.

1422. Patterson BC, Chen Y, Sklar CA, et al. Growth hormone exposure as a risk factor for the development of subsequent neoplasms of the central nervous system: a report from the childhood cancer survivor study. *J Clin Endocrinol Metab.* 2014;99(6):2030-2037.

1423. Malozowski S, Tanner LA, Wysowski D, Fleming GA. Growth hormone, insulin-like growth factor I, and benign intracranial hypertension. *N Engl J Med.* 1993;329(9):665-666.

1424. Ranke MB. Effects of growth hormone on the metabolism of lipids and water and their potential in causing adverse events during growth hormone treatment. *Horm Res.* 1993;39(3-4):104-106.

1425. Collett-Solberg PF, Liu GT, Satin-Smith M, et al. Pseudopapilledema and congenital disc anomalies in growth hormone deficiency. *J Pediatr Endocrinol Metab.* 1998;11(2):261-265.

1426. Fillion M, Deal C, Van Vliet G. Retrospective study of the potential benefits and adverse events during growth hormone treatment in children with Prader-Willi syndrome. *J Pediatr.* 2009;154(2):230-233.

1427. Alford FP, Hew FL, Christopher MC, Rantzau C. Insulin sensitivity in growth hormone (GH)-deficient adults and effect of GH replacement therapy. *J Endocrinol Invest.* 1999;22(5 Suppl):28-32.

1428. Child CJ, Zimmermann AG, Scott RS, et al. Prevalence and incidence of diabetes mellitus in GH-treated children and adolescents: analysis from the GeNeSIS observational research program. *J Clin Endocrinol Metab.* 2011;96(6):E1025-E1034.

1429. Cutfield WS, Wilton P, Bennmarker H, et al. Incidence of diabetes mellitus and impaired glucose tolerance in children and adolescents receiving growth-hormone treatment. *Lancet.* 2000;355(9204):610-613.

1430. Malozowski S, Stadel BV. Prepubertal gynecomastia during growth hormone therapy. *J Pediatr.* 1995;126(4):659-661.

1431. Malozowski S, Hung W, Scott DC, Stadel BV. Acute pancreatitis associated with growth hormone therapy for short stature. *N Engl J Med.* 1995;332(6):401-402.

1432. Bourguignon JP, Pierard GE, Ernould C, et al. Effects of human growth hormone therapy on melanocytic naevi. *Lancet.* 1993;341(8859):1505-1506.

1433. Pierard GE, Pierard-Franchimont C. Morphometric evaluation of the growth of nevi. *Ann Dermatol Venereol.* 1993;120(9):605-609.

1434. Bertelloni S, Baroncelli GI, Viacava P, et al. Can growth hormone treatment in boys without growth hormone deficiency impair testicular function? *J Pediatr.* 1999;135(3):367-370.

1435. Leschek EW, Troendle JF, Yanovski JA, et al. Effect of growth hormone treatment on testicular function, puberty, and adrenarche in boys with non-growth hormone-deficient short stature: a randomized, double-blind, placebo-controlled trial. *J Pediatr.* 2001;138(3):406-410.

1436. Frasier SD. A red flag unfurled? Growth hormone treatment and testicular function. *J Pediatr.* 1999;135(3):278-279.

1437. Chan JM, Stampfer MJ, Giovannucci E, et al. Plasma insulin-like growth factor-I and prostate cancer risk: a prospective study. *Science.* 1998;279(5350):563-566.

1438. Hankinson SE, Willett WC, Colditz GA, et al. Circulating concentrations of insulin-like growth factor-I and risk of breast cancer. *Lancet.* 1998;351(9113):1393-1396.

1439. Pekic S, Popovic V. GH therapy and cancer risk in hypopituitarism: what we know from human studies. *Eur J Endocrinol.* 2013;169(5):R89-R97.

1440. Ma J, Pollak MN, Giovannucci E, et al. Prospective study of colorectal cancer risk in men and plasma levels of insulin-like growth factor (IGF)-I and IGF-binding protein-3. *J Natl Cancer Inst.* 1999;91(7):620-625.

1441. Renehan AG, Zwahlen M, Minder C, et al. Insulin-like growth factor (IGF)-I, IGF binding protein-3, and cancer risk: systematic review and meta-regression analysis. *Lancet.* 2004;363(9418):1346-1353.

1442. Ron E, Gridley G, Hrubec Z, et al. Acromegaly and gastrointestinal cancer. *Cancer.* 1991;68(8):1673-1677.

1443. Popovic V, Damjanovic S, Micic D, et al. Increased incidence of neoplasia in patients with pituitary adenomas. The pituitary study group. *Clin Endocrinol (Oxf).* 1998;49(4):441-445.

1444. Bengtsson BA, Eden S, Ernest I, et al. Epidemiology and long-term survival in acromegaly. *Acta Med Scand.* 1998;223:327-335.

1445. Delhougne B, Deneux C, Abs R, et al. The prevalence of colonic polyps in acromegaly: a colonoscopic and pathological study in 103 patients. *J Clin Endocrinol Metab.* 1995;80(11):3223-3226.

1446. Ladas SD, Thalassinos NC, Ioannides G, Raptis SA. Does acromegaly really predispose to an increased prevalence of gastrointestinal tumours? *Clin Endocrinol (Oxf).* 1994;41(5):597-601.

1447. Orme SM, McNally RJ, Cartwright RA, Belchetz PE. Mortality and cancer incidence in acromegaly: a retrospective cohort study. United Kingdom acromegaly study group. *J Clin Endocrinol Metab.* 1998;83(8):2730-2734.

1448. Sonksen P, Jacobs H, Orme S, Belchetz P. Acromegaly and colonic cancer. *Clin Endocrinol (Oxf).* 1997;47(6):647-648.

1449. Renehan AG, O'Dwyer ST, Shalet SM. Colorectal neoplasia in acromegaly: the reported increased prevalence is overestimated. *Gut.* 2000;46(3):440-441.

1450. Colao A, Balzano A, Ferone D, et al. Increased prevalence of colonic polyps and altered lymphocyte subset pattern in the colonic lamina propria in acromegaly. *Clin Endocrinol (Oxf).* 1997;47(1):23-28.

1451. Sperling MA, Saenger PH, Ray H, et al. LWPES Executive Committee and the LWPES Drug and Therapeutics Committee. Growth hormone treatment and neoplasia-coincidence or consequence? *J Clin Endocrinol Metab.* 2002;87(12):5351-5352.

1452. Swerdlow AJ, Higgins CD, Adlard P, Preece MA. Risk of cancer in patients treated with human pituitary growth hormone in the UK, 1959-85: A cohort study. *Lancet.* 2002;360(9329):273-277.

1453. Abs R, Bengtsson BA, Hernberg-Stahl E, et al. GH replacement in 1034 growth hormone deficient hypopituitary adults: demographic and clinical characteristics, dosing and safety. *Clin Endocrinol (Oxf).* 1999;50(6):703-713.

1454. Tuffli GA, Johanson A, Rundle AC, Allen DB. Lack of increased risk for extracranial, nonleukemic neoplasms in recipients of recombinant deoxyribonucleic acid growth hormone. *J Clin Endocrinol Metab.* 1995;80(4):1416-1422.

1455. Carel JC, Ecosse E, Landier F, et al. Long-term mortality after recombinant growth hormone treatment for isolated growth hormone deficiency or childhood short stature: preliminary report of the French SAGHE study. *J Clin Endocrinol Metab.* 2012;97(2):416-425.

1456. Savendahl L, Maes M, Albertsson-Wikland K, et al. Long-term mortality and causes of death in isolated GHD, ISS, and SGA patients treated with recombinant growth hormone during childhood in Belgium, the Netherlands, and Sweden: preliminary report of 3 countries participating in the EU SAGhE study. *J Clin Endocrinol Metab.* 2012;97(2):E213-E217.

1457. Laron Z, Anin S, Klipper-Aurbach Y, Klinger B. Effects of insulin-like growth factor on linear growth, head circumference, and body fat in patients with Laron-type dwarfism. *Lancet.* 1992;339(8804):1258-1261.

1458. Azcona C, Preece MA, Rose SJ, et al. Growth response to rhIGF-I 80 microg/kg twice daily in children with growth hormone insensitivity syndrome: relationship to severity of clinical phenotype. *Clin Endocrinol (Oxf).* 1999;51(6):787-792.

1459. Ranke MB, Savage MO, Chatelain PG, et al. Long-term treatment of growth hormone insensitivity syndrome with IGF-I. Results of the European multicentre study. the working group on growth hormone insensitivity syndromes. *Horm Res.* 1999;51:128-134.

1460. Chernausek SD, Backeljauw PF, Frane J, et al. Long-term treatment with recombinant insulin-like growth factor (IGF)-I in children with severe IGF-I deficiency due to growth hormone insensitivity. *J Clin Endocrinol Metab.* 2007;92(3):902-910.

1461. Backeljauw PF, Kuntze J, Frane J, et al. Adult and near-adult height in patients with severe insulin-like growth factor-I deficiency after long-term therapy with recombinant human insulin-like growth factor-I. *Horm Res Paediatr.* 2013;80(1):47-56.

1462. Laron Z, Ginsberg S, Lilos P, et al. Long-term IGF-I treatment of children with Laron syndrome increases adiposity. *Growth Horm IGF Res.* 2006;16(1):61-64.

1463. Perry JK, Emerald BS, Mertani HC, Lobie PE. The oncogenic potential of growth hormone. *Growth Horm IGF Res.* 2006;16(5-6):277-289.

1464. Bright GM, Mendoza JR, Rosenfeld RG. Recombinant human insulin-like growth factor-1 treatment: ready for primetime. *Endocrinol Metab Clin North Am.* 2009;38(3):625-638.

1465. Rosenbloom AL. The role of recombinant insulin-like growth factor I in the treatment of the short child. *Curr Opin Pediatr.* 2007;19(4):458-464.

1466. Lazar L, Padoa A, Phillip M. Growth pattern and final height after cessation of gonadotropin-suppressive therapy in girls with central sexual precocity. *J Clin Endocrinol Metab.* 2007;92:3483-3489.

1467. Arrigo T, Cisternino M, Galluzzi F, et al. Analysis of the factors affecting auxological response to GnRH agonist treatment and final height outcome in girls with idiopathic central precocious puberty. *Eur J Endocrinol.* 1999;141:140-144.

1468. Klein KO, Barnes KM, Jones JV, et al. Increased final height in precocious puberty after long-term treatment with LHRH agonists: the National Institutes of Health experience. *J Clin Endocrinol Metab.* 2001;86:4711-4716.

1469. Carel JC, Lahlou N, Roger M, et al. Precocious puberty and statural growth. *Hum Reprod Update.* 2004;10:135-147.

1470. Pasquino AM, Pucarelli I, Accardo F, et al. Long-term observation of 87 girls with idiopathic central precocious puberty treated with gonadotropin-releasing hormone analogs: impact on adult height, body mass index, bone mineral content, and reproductive function. *J Clin Endocrinol Metab.* 2008;93:190-195.

1471. Mul D, Oostdijk W, Otten BJ, et al. Final height after gonadotrophin releasing hormone agonist treatment for central precocious puberty: the Dutch experience. *J Pediatr Endocrinol Metab.* 2000;13(Suppl 1):765-772.

1472. Cassio A, Cacciari E, Balsamo A, et al. Randomised trial of LHRH analogue treatment on final height in girls with onset of puberty aged 7.5-8.5 years. *Arch Dis Child.* 1999;81:329-332.

1473. Antoniazzi F, Cisternino M, Nizzoli G, et al. Final height in girls with central precocious puberty: comparison of two different luteinizing hormone-releasing hormone agonist treatments. *Acta Paediatr.* 1994;83:1052-1056.

1474. Carel JC, Hay F, Coutant R, et al. Gonadotropin-releasing hormone agonist treatment of girls with constitutional short stature and normal pubertal development. *J Clin Endocrinol Metab.* 1996;81:3318-3322.

1475. Bouvattier C, Coste J, Rodrigue D, et al. Lack of effect of GnRH agonists on final height in girls with advanced puberty: a randomized long-term pilot study. *J Clin Endocrinol Metab.* 1999;84:3575-3578.

1476. Lanes R, Soros A, Jakubowicz S. Accelerated versus slowly progressive forms of puberty in girls with precocious and early puberty: gonadotropin suppressive effect and final height obtained with two different analogs. *J Pediatr Endocrinol Metab.* 2004;17:759-766.

1477. Tuvemo T. Treatment of central precocious puberty. *Expert Opin Investig Drugs.* 2006;15:495-505.

1478. Lazar L, Pertzelan A, Weintrob N, et al. Sexual precocity in boys: accelerated versus slowly progressive puberty gonadotropin-suppressive therapy and final height. *J Clin Endocrinol Metab.* 2001;86:4127-4132.

1479. Carel JC. Management of short stature with GnRH agonist and co-treatment with growth hormone: a controversial issue. *Mol Cell Endocrinol.* 2006;254-255:226-233.

1480. Pasquino AM, Pucarelli I, Roggini M, et al. Adult height in short normal girls treated with gonadotropin-releasing hormone analogs and growth hormone. *J Clin Endocrinol Metab.* 2000;85:619-622.

1481. Tuvemo T, Jonsson B, Gustafsson J, et al. Final height after combined growth hormone and GnRH analogue treatment in adopted girls with early puberty. *Acta Paediatr.* 2004;93:1456-1462.

1482. Mul D, Oostdijk W, Waelkens JJ, et al. Final height after treatment of early puberty in short adopted girls with gonadotrophin releasing hormone agonist with or without growth hormone. *Clin Endocrinol (Oxf).* 2005;63:185-190.

1483. Carel JC, Eugster EA, Rogol A, et al. ESPE-LWPES GnRH Analogs Consensus Conference Group, consensus statement on the use of gonadotropin-releasing hormone analogs in children. *Pediatrics.* 2009;123:e752-e762.

1484. Clayton PE, Cianfarani S, Czernichow P, et al. Management of the child born small for gestational age through to adulthood: a consensus statement of the International Societies of Pediatric Endocrinology and the Growth Hormone Research Society. *J Clin Endocrinol Metab.* 2007;92(3):804-810.

1485. Carel JC, Ecosse E, Nicolino M, et al. Adult height after long term treatment with recombinant growth hormone for idiopathic isolated growth hormone deficiency: observational follow up study of the French population based registry. *BMJ.* 2002;325(7355):70.

1486. Reiter EO, Lindberg A, Ranke MB, et al. The KIGS experience with the addition of gonadotropin-releasing hormone agonists to growth hormone (GH) treatment of children with idiopathic GH deficiency. *Horm Res.* 2003;60(Suppl 1):68-73.

1487. Mericq MV, Eggers M, Avila A, et al. Near final height in pubertal growth hormone (GH)-deficient patients treated with GH alone or in combination with luteinizing hormone-releasing hormone analog: results of a prospective, randomized trial. *J Clin Endocrinol Metab.* 2000;85(2):569-573.

1488. Saggese G, Federico G, Barsanti S, Fiore L. The effect of administering gonadotropin-releasing hormone agonist with recombinant-human growth hormone (GH) on the final height of girls with isolated GH deficiency: results from a controlled study. *J Clin Endocrinol Metab.* 2001;86(5):1900-1904.

1489. Tanaka T, Satoh M, Yasunaga T, et al. When and how to combine growth hormone with a luteinizing hormone-releasing hormone analogue. *Acta Paediatr Suppl.* 1999;88(428):85-88.

1490. Leschek EW, Jones J, Barnes KM, et al. Six-year results of spironolactone and testolactone treatment of familial male-limited precocious puberty with addition of deslorelin after central puberty onset. *J Clin Endocrinol Metab.* 1999;84(1):175-178.

1491. Feuillan PP, Jones J, Cutler GB Jr. Long-term testolactone therapy for precocious puberty in girls with the McCune-Albright syndrome. *J Clin Endocrinol Metab.* 1993;77(3):647-651.

1492. Nunez SB, Calis K, Cutler GB Jr, et al. Lack of efficacy of fadrozole in treating precocious puberty in girls with the McCune-Albright syndrome. *J Clin Endocrinol Metab.* 2003;88(12):5730-5733.

1493. Feuillan P, Calis K, Hill S, et al. Letrozole treatment of precocious puberty in girls with the McCune-Albright syndrome: a pilot study. *J Clin Endocrinol Metab.* 2007;92(6):2100-2106.

1494. Hero M, Toiviainen-Salo S, Wickman S, et al. Vertebral morphology in aromatase inhibitor-treated males with idiopathic short stature or constitutional delay of puberty. *J Bone Miner Res.* 2010;25(7):1536-1543.

1495. Rudman D, Goldsmith M, Kutner M, Blackston D. Effect of growth hormone and oxandrolone singly and together on growth rate in girls with X chromosome abnormalities. *J Pediatr.* 1980;96(1):132-135.

1496. Joss E, Zuppinger K. Oxandrolone in girls with Turner's syndrome. A pair-matched controlled study up to final height. *Acta Paediatr Scand.* 1984;73(5):674-679.

1497. Sybert VP. Adult height in Turner syndrome with and without androgen therapy. *J Pediatr.* 1984;104(3):365-369.

1498. Sas TC, Gault EJ, Zeger Bardsley M, et al. Safety and efficacy of oxandrolone in growth hormone-treated girls with Turner syndrome: evidence from recent studies and recommendations for use. *Horm Res Paediatr.* 2014;81(5):289-297.

1499. Menke LA, Sas TC, de Muinck Keizer-Schrama SM, et al. Efficacy and safety of oxandrolone in growth hormone-treated girls with Turner syndrome. *J Clin Endocrinol Metab.* 2010;95(3):1151-1160.

1500. Zeger MP, Shah K, Kowal K, et al. Prospective study confirms oxandrolone-associated improvement in height in growth hormone-treated adolescent girls with Turner syndrome. *Horm Res Paediatr.* 2011;75(1):38-46.

1501. Gault EJ, Perry RJ, Cole TJ, et al. Effect of oxandrolone and timing of pubertal induction on final height in Turner's syndrome: randomised, double blind, placebo controlled trial. *BMJ.* 2011;342:d1980.

1502. de Waal WJ, Greyn-Fokker MH, Stijnen T, et al. Accuracy of final height prediction and effect of growth-reductive therapy in 362 constitutionally tall children. *J Clin Endocrinol Metab.* 1996;81(3):1206-1216.

1503. Venn A, Bruinsma F, Werther G, et al. Oestrogen treatment to reduce the adult height of tall girls: long-term effects on fertility. *Lancet.* 2004;364(9444):1513-1518.

1504. Barnard ND, Scialli AR, Bobela S. The current use of estrogens for growth-suppressant therapy in adolescent girls. *J Pediatr Adolesc Gynecol.* 2002;15(1):23-26.

CHAPTER 25

Physiology and Disorders of Puberty

DENNIS M. STYNE • MELVIN M. GRUMBACH

KEY POINTS

- Puberty is not a de novo event but rather a phase in the continuum of development of gonadal function and the ontogeny of the hypothalamic-pituitary-gonadal system from the fetus to full sexual maturation and fertility.
- During puberty, secondary sexual characteristics appear, and the adolescent growth spurt occurs, resulting in the striking sex dimorphism of mature individuals; fertility is achieved, and profound psychological effects ensue.
- Gonadarche, or the awakening of gonadal sex steroid secretion, and adrenarche, or the awakening of adrenal androgen secretion, are separate processes that must be evaluated individually, as the customary chronologic relationship between the events may vary considerably among individuals.
- The age of onset of female puberty has decreased over the past several decades according to international data, and the obesity epidemic may be one of the factors responsible for this secular trend toward earlier female puberty.
- The discovery of new genes involved in the regulation of the hypothalamic control of pubertal development greatly expands our understanding of the cause of delayed and precocious puberty, but the complex mechanisms that initiate normal pubertal development at a given age remain largely unknown.
- Evaluation of puberty in children and adolescents must involve the use of highly specific and sensitive assays with pediatric standards; sex steroids must be measured in high-performance liquid chromatography tandem mass spectroscopy (HPLC-MS/MS) methods unless painstaking extraction and manual immunoassays are invoked.
- The remarkable success in the treatment of childhood neoplasia has led to secondary effects on pubertal development, either advancing or delaying the age of onset of puberty and often impairing fertility.

Puberty is not a de novo event but rather a phase in the continuum of development of gonadal function and the ontogeny of the hypothalamic-pituitary-gonadal system from the fetus to full sexual maturation and fertility. During puberty, secondary sexual characteristics appear, and the adolescent growth spurt occurs, resulting in the striking sex dimorphism of mature individuals; fertility is achieved, and profound psychological effects ensue.[1] These changes result from stimulation of the gonads by pituitary gonadotropins and a subsequent increase in gonadal steroid output.

Humans have evolved into the most reproductively successful of mammals, and many anthropologists have attributed this success to the prolonged pattern of human growth and development and to the delay in attaining full sexual maturity.[2] The human scheme of growth involves a childhood stage and an adolescent stage that includes an adolescent or pubertal growth spurt (Fig. 25-1). Not even our closest biologic relative, the chimpanzee, which matures twice as rapidly as the human, unequivocally exhibits these two stages, including the unique human adolescent growth spurt. Learning and practice of adult behaviors related to sex and childrearing, particularly provisioning children (not just infants) with food, which is unique to humans, is considered a critical part of human success: "the building of a better, healthier body and the developing of greater biological, behavioral, and cultural resilience prior to sexual maturity that leads to greater adult health, fitness, and longevity."[2] Tool making preceded the evolutionary development of adolescence, suggesting that the evolution and value of human childhood and adolescence and this unique pattern of growth and development have had significant roles in the reproductive success of humans.

In the developed world, reproductive maturity occurs years earlier than psychosocial maturation, causing a mismatch between biologic stages and psychosocial expectations and roles (Fig. 25-2).[3] In past eras, such as the Neolithic, Greek, or Roman periods, there was not such a mismatch, because menarche occurred at an age close to that of reproductive maturity. With increased population, the advent of agriculture, and the growth of cities and later urban centers, menarche occurred later, and the complexity of life led to a delay in the attainment of an adult role in society. In modern times, the age of menarche has decreased, but the age of social adulthood still occurs later, causing a discrepancy that probably has not occurred previously in human history. The study of human evolution adds to the understanding of many modern medical conditions as well as puberty, and the discipline of evolutionary biology is now recommended as a required premedical course by the American Association of Medical Colleges.[4]

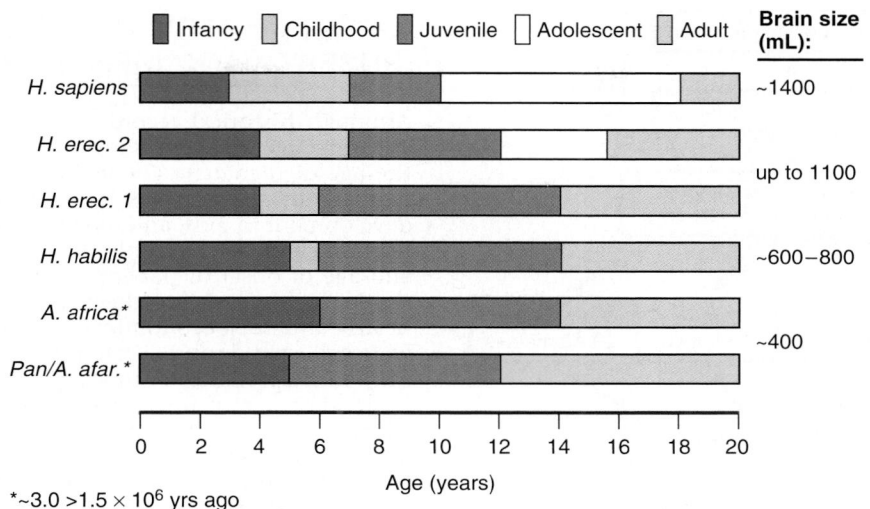

Figure 25-1 Evolution of the human pattern of postnatal growth and development during the first 20 years of life. Specimens include A. afar. *Australopithecus afarensis*, a "bipedal chimpanzee"; A. africa, *Australopithecus africanus*; H. habilis, *Homo habilis*, the toolmaker; H. erec. 1, early *Homo erectus*; H. erec. 2, late *Homo erectus*; H. sapiens, *Homo sapiens*. The early hominid australopithecine specimens from South Africa date to about 3.0 to 1.5 million years ago. *H. afarensis*, although a hominid (family of all human species), retained many anatomic features of nonhominid species, such as an adult brain size of about 400 mL compared with *H. habilis* (650 to 800 mL), early *H. erectus* (850 to 900 mL), late *H. erectus* (up to 1100 mL), and modern *H. sapiens* (about 1400 mL). Infancy is the period when the mother's breast milk is the sole or most important source of nutrition, and in preindustrialized societies, it ends at about 36 months. Childhood is the period after weaning, when the child depends on others for food and protection; this period ends when the growth of the brain in weight is almost complete, at about age 7 years. The juvenile stage is defined as prepubertal individuals who are no longer dependent on their parents for survival. The adolescent stage, which begins with the onset of puberty, ends when adult height is attained (Moggi-Cecchi; Conroy and Kuykendall). The pattern in *A. afarensis* is no different from that of the chimpanzee *(Pan troglodytes)*. Notice the first appearance of the childhood stage in *H. habilis* (arising about 2 million years ago) and the first appearance of the adolescent stage in *H. erectus* 2 (about 500,000 years ago); *H. sapiens* arose about 120,000 to 150,000 years ago. (Modified from Bogin B. Growth and development: recent evolutionary and biocultural research. In: Boaz NT, Wolfe LD, eds. *Biological Anthropology: The State of the Science.* Bend, OR: International Institute for Human Evolutionary Research; 1995:49-70; addional data from Moggi-Cecchi J. Questions of growth. *Nature.* 2001;414:595-597; and Conroy GC, Kuykendall K. Paleopediatrics: or when did human infants really become human? *Am J Phys Anthropol.* 1995;98:121-131.)

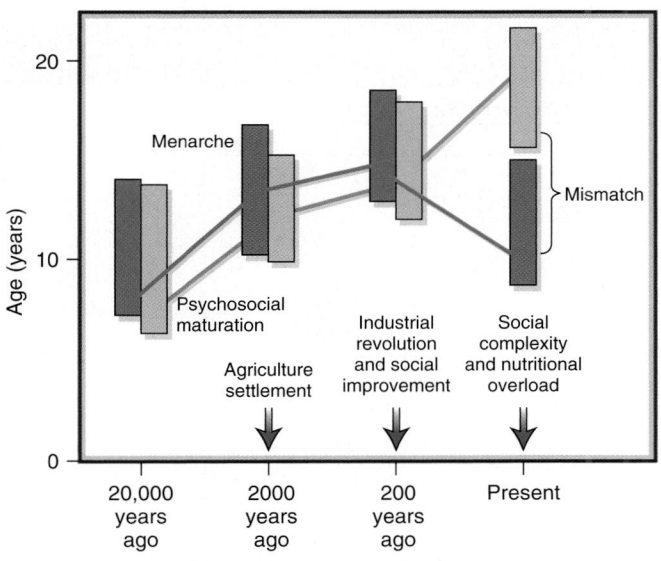

Figure 25-2 The relationship between the likely range of ages of menarche *(purple)* and achievement of psychosocial maturity *(pink)* from 20,000 years ago to the current day. The mismatch in timing between these two processes is a novel phenomenon. (From Gluckman PD, Hanson MA. Evolution, development, and timing of puberty. *Trends Endocrinol Metab.* 2006;17:7-12.)

FETAL ORIGINS OF ADULT DISEASE

There are long-lasting effects of abnormalities in fetal and neonatal growth. As seen in longitudinal studies, low birth weight followed by rapid weight gain in infancy (i.e., catch-up growth) leads to tall childhood stature and early pubertal development. Poor prenatal nutrition and small-for-gestational-age (SGA) status tends to advance the age of menarche and the age of adrenarche,[5] and a secondary effect of increased postnatal nutrition, often leading to overweight or obesity, also lowers the age of puberty. Figure 25-3 describes the relationship between excessive adipose tissue and early puberty. A prospective study demonstrated that a lower expected birth weight ratio (i.e., ratio of observed infant's birth weight to median birth weight appropriate for maternal age, weight, height, parity, infant sex, and gestational age) and a higher body mass index (BMI) at 8 years led to an earlier age of menarche.[6] Girls who are longer and lighter at birth and subsequently have greater BMI values at 8 years tend to have earlier menarche.[7] Rapid weight gain in the second to ninth months but not thereafter correlated with a greater BMI at 10 years and with earlier menarche in a longitudinal study.[8]

Many international studies find a relationship between low birth weight or catch-up growth and chronic diseases in adulthood. Birth weight and rate of postnatal growth—not prematurity alone—are inversely related to cardiovascular mortality risk and prevalence of insulin resistance syndrome (i.e., metabolic syndrome or syndrome X), which consists of hypertension, impaired glucose tolerance, and elevated triglyceride levels, among a growing list of other features. This outcome is attributed to fetal and neonatal metabolic programming, in which early adjustments to enhance survival in difficult intrauterine circumstances set the stage for later disorders. Insulin resistance, which may be the basis for most of these complications or may be just one feature of the syndrome, may spare nutrients from use in muscle, leaving them available for the brain. This mechanism can minimize central nervous system (CNS) damage in the fetus during periods of malnutrition.

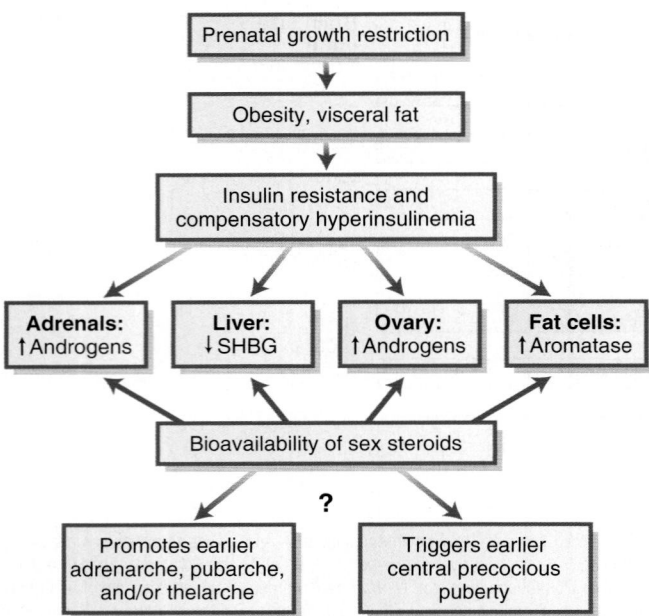

Figure 25-3 Proposed endocrine pathways linking childhood obesity and insulin resistance to early pubertal onset and maturation. Childhood obesity and the predisposition to visceral adiposity after intrauterine growth restraint lead to insulin resistance and peripheral hyperinsulinemia. Insulin acts on various organs, including the adrenals, liver, ovary, and fat cells, to increase sex steroid bioavailability. Elevated circulating and tissue sex steroid levels in obese prepubertal children can have only mild local effects or activate early hypothalamic-pituitary puberty and early reproductive maturation. SHBG, sex hormone–binding globulin. (From Ahmed ML, Ong KK, Dunger DB. Childhood obesity and the timing of puberty. *Trends Endocrinol Metab.* 2009;20:237-242.)

DETERMINANTS OF THE AGE OF PUBERTY AND MENARCHE

Although historical records show that puberty occurs at an earlier age today, most evidence derives from reports of the age of menarche (Table 25-1).[9,10] Age of menarche is removed by several years from the first sign of secondary development in girls, and modern studies demonstrate correlation coefficients of only 0.37 between age of menarche and age of onset of puberty, suggesting both unique and similar factors exerting effects on these ages.[11] Changes in health and socioeconomic status in regions where data were collected during different decades lead to complexity in the interpretation of modern national data.

Recalled age of menarche is considered to be accurate within 1 year (in 90% of cases) up to 30 years after the event.[12] Contemporaneous recordings are performed with the probit method of asking for a response of "Yes" or "No" to the question, "Are you menstruating?" However, the results are subject to social pressures of the culture and socioeconomic group considered.[13]

Physical examination with palpation of gonads or breasts by trained observers is the most accurate method of assessment of pubertal development. Detection of the onset of stage 2 breast development in an overweight girl on physical examination may be difficult even for a trained observer (although stage 3 usually is obvious). Visual observation of the stage of development in person (not by photographs) is one step removed from physical examination and palpation; errors in the evaluation of breast tissue in obese girls or the stage of testicular enlargement in boys may occur. Visual observation by multiple observers was

TABLE 25-1
Comparison of Menarcheal Ages Reported by Various Studies

Study	Year	Plan	Evaluation	n	Overall	W	B	M	Comments
Britain	1969	Long	Probit	192 (W)		13.5			
NHES III	1963-1970	Cross	Recalled	3272		Born 1940-1960: 12.8	12.52		
						Born 1890-1910: 13.5			
NHANES III	1988-1994	Cross	Yes/No Probit	330 (W) 419 (B) 419 (M)		12.7	12.3	12.5	Men. age black < white
NHANES III	1988-1994	Cross	Yes/No Probit	2510 710 (W) 917 (B) 883 (M)	12.43	12.6	12.06	12.3	Men. age black < white
PROS	1992-1993	Cross	Status Quo Probit	17077 (W) 1638 (B)		12.9	12.16		Men. age black < white
NHLB Growth	1987-1997	Long	Recalled	1092 (W) 1164 (B)		12.7	12.1		Men. age black < white BMI inversely proportional to men. age
Bogalusa	1973-1974	Cross		5552		12.7	12.9		
	1992-1994	Cross				12.5	12.1		
	1973-1994	Long		2508		12.6	12.3		Men. age black < white BMI inversely proportional to men. age
NHES	1963-1970	Status Quo	Yes/No Status Quo	3272	12.75	12.8	12.48		
	1988-1994	Status Quo	Median Yes/N	1414	12.54	12.6	12.14		Men. age NHANES III < NHES Growing difference in men. age white-black BMI inversely proportional to men. age

B, black; BMI, body mass index; Cross, cross sectional; Long, longitudinal; M, Mexican American; men., menarcheal; NHANES, National Health and Nutrition Examination Surveys; NHES, National Health Examination Survey; NHLB Growth, National Heart, Lung, and Blood Institute Growth and Health Study; PROS, Pediatric Research in Office Settings; W, white.
From Styne DM. Puberty, obesity and ethnicity. *Trends Endocrinol Metab.* 2004;15:472-478.

used in the Third National Health and Nutrition Examination Survey (NHANES III) (and in the National Health Examination Survey [NHES] that occurred more than 20 years earlier), and visual observation is subject to interobserver variation. In a study by Pediatric Research in the Office Setting (PROS), a network fostered by the American Academy of Pediatrics, specially trained pediatricians, nurse practitioners, or physician assistants (225 offices) used palpation for 30% of the study population and visual inspection for all members of a convenience sample of 17,070 girls across the United States.[14]

The availability of only limited numbers of trained personnel for examination or subjects' refusal of embarrassing examinations sometimes leads to the use of proxy measures. Photographs or drawings of pubertal development allow self-reporting or parental reporting of pubertal progress, but correlations range widely from 0.48 to 0.91 compared with physicians' examinations or visual observation of subjects.[15] The answers to self-assessment may be influenced by the subjects' wishes to conform with their understanding of normal development and may be less accurate in some ethnic groups than others, similar to reported menarcheal age. Obese girls may overestimate breast developmental stage, and boys may overestimate pubic hair development. Individuals with learning disabilities, chronic diseases (e.g., cystic fibrosis, Crohn disease), or psychological conditions (e.g., anorexia nervosa) may have less accurate pubertal staging.[16] Self-report is related to testosterone values for boys and girls and is said to be accurate enough if precision is not needed.[17] With all of its difficulties, physical examination remains the best method to accurately evaluate large populations.

The Secular Trend in Puberty and Menarche
The Developed World

The average age of menarche in industrialized European countries has decreased by 2 to 3 months per decade over the past 150 years, and in the United States, the decrease has been approximately 2 to 3 months per decade during the past century[9,18] (Fig. 25-4). However, this secular trend slowed in developed countries such as the United States, Australia, and Western Europe between approximately 1940 and 1970, presumably due to improved socioeconomic status, better health, and the benefits of urbanization. There is a relatively small range of ages of menarche in the well-off developed world, where lower socioeconomic classes do not have an increased burden of disease or malnutrition. Chronic diseases previously increased the age of menarche, and delay in menarche is still associated with serious conditions (e.g., celiac disease, asthma) that are not adequately treated. The standard deviation of the mean age of menarche also decreased, suggesting a diminished number of those maturing very late, as might be found among disadvantaged people.[19] Teasing out the various factors involved in any remaining and subtler secular trends will require further long-term study and newer methodologic approaches in areas where nutrition and health are optimal or close to it.[20] Remarkably, a reverse secular trend is reported in certain areas of Europe, leading to a later age of menarche. This has been attributed to a resurgence of physical and psychological stress, as was seen in previous eras (e.g., World War II).[20]

There are cross-sectional and longitudinal data from the late 20th century demonstrating a resurgence of a secular trend in the United States, including ethnic influences.[21,22] The age of menarche in the United States was 12.8 years according to the 1973 U.S. National Center for Health Statistics National Health Education Study, and data from

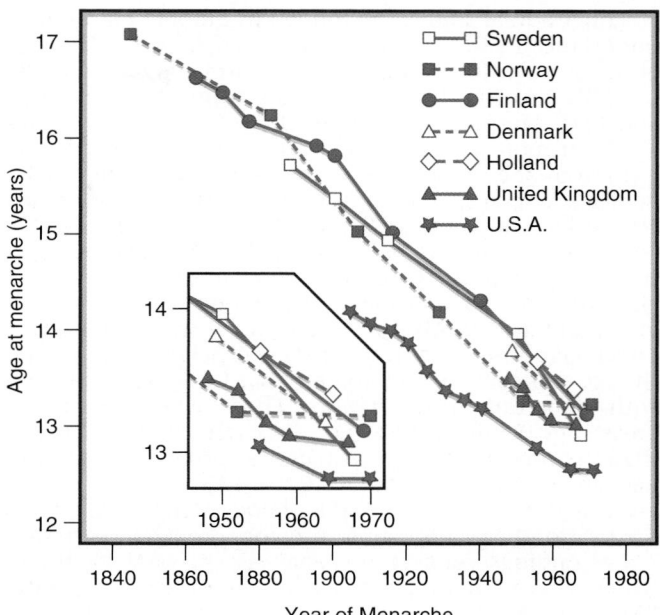

Figure 25-4 The changes in age at menarche between 1840 and 1978 illustrate the advance in the age at menarche in Western Europe and the United States since 1840 and slowing of this trend since about 1965. (Modified from Tanner M, Eveleth PB. Variability between populations in growth and development at puberty. In: Berenberg SR, ed. *Puberty, Biologic and Psychosocial Components.* Leiden, The Netherlands: H.E. Stenfert Kroese; 1975:256-273.)

NHANES III, 1988-1994 indicate that the median age at that time was 12.43 years, 0.37 year earlier than in 1973.[23] During a 20-year period in the Bogalusa Heart Study, the median menarcheal age decreased by approximately 9.5 months among African-American girls compared with 2 months among white girls,[24] leading to a 4-month difference. Between the ages of 5 and 9 years, African-American girls in the Bogalusa study had taller stature and greater weight, factors that were predictive of menarche before age 11 years. African-American girls have advanced secondary sexual development compared with white American girls of the same age during the first three stages of puberty, and they have an advanced bone age; this may be related to the higher prevalence of obesity among African-American girls and to an ethnic-specific genetic influence.[25-27]

Obesity is defined as a BMI (calculated as weight in kilograms divided by height in meters squared) above the 95th percentile for age, and overweight is defined by the Centers for Disease Control and Prevention (CDC) as a BMI greater than the 85th percentile for age. Many studies have reported on the effect of the epidemic of childhood obesity and overweight on age of menarche.[28,29] Most cross-sectional and longitudinal studies found an inverse relationship between menarcheal age or other stages of puberty and BMI or other reflections of adiposity.[30,31] If the population in the 1970s had had the same range of BMI values as was found in the 1990s, the projected age of menarche would have been the same in the 1970s as it was in the 1990s.[32] Girls had a greater prevalence of overweight or obesity between the ages of 8 and 10 years if they were in puberty or had advanced breast development.[33] A study of the age at onset of puberty in U.S. boys of various ethnic groups indicated an earlier age of onset between 6 months and 2 years depending upon indicator and ethnic group.[34] Except for a delay in pubertal development with BMI less than 15% there was no effect of overweight or obesity in these boys as was found in girls in other studies.

Longitudinal studies are limited in number but of great importance in the evaluation of a secular trend. The longitudinal National Heart, Lung, and Blood Institute (NHLBI) Growth and Health Study followed 1266 white and 1313 African-American girls from 9 or 10 years of age for 10 or more years. A recent report of a sample of 1239 girls from the study noted that 10.4% of white, 23.4% of black non-Hispanic, and 14.9% of Hispanic girls had attained breast stage 2 at 7 years; 18.3%, 42.9%, and 30.9%, respectively, attained breast stage 2 at 8 years, younger than data from 10 to 30 years ago. In a sample of 1155 girls, the mean age of menarche among whites was 12.7 years, and among African Americans, it was 12.1 years; a direct relationship was found between weight and BMI and the age of menarche.[26] Of these girls, 51.6% started puberty with only one manifestation. Those who experienced breast development first (i.e., thelarche pattern), rather than the appearance of pubic hair (i.e., adrenarche pattern), had an earlier menarche (12.6 vs. 13.1 years); this was associated with a greater BMI and body weight, which was not true for those girls manifesting the adrenarche pattern.[35] These findings support the analysis of NHANES III, in which girls with earlier breast development had greater BMI values at the time of menarche than those with adrenarche occurring first.[36]

African-American girls in the National Longitudinal Study of Adolescent Health (Add Health) were 1.55 times more likely than white girls to have menarche before 11 years[37] of age, and Mexican Americans were 1.76 times more likely to do so than whites. Asians were 1.65 more likely than whites to mature later than 14 years. Those undergoing early menarche were twice as likely to be overweight, and African-American girls had a 2.57-fold greater risk for overweight if they had menarche before they were 11 years old. Among early menarcheal African Americans, 57.5% had a BMI greater than the 85th percentile, and 32.5% had a BMI greater than the 95th percentile. A longitudinal study of 180 girls between the ages of 5 and 9 years demonstrated that those with a higher percentage of body fat at 5 years; those with a higher percentage of body fat, higher BMI percentile, or larger waist circumference at 7 years; those with larger increases in the percentage of body fat from 5 to 9 years; and those with larger increases in waist circumference from 7 to 9 years old were more likely to exhibit earlier pubertal development at 9 years.[38]

During the past 40 years, menarcheal age in the white subjects in the Fels Longitudinal Study has remained stable even as BMI has increased, with no relationship shown between the two. Subjects with early menarche had a tendency to increase BMI after menarche,[39] demonstrating that increased weight appears to be a consequence rather than determinant of the age at menarche and that secular changes in BMI and in mean age at menarche may be independent phenomena. There was a rise in BMI, waist circumference, hip circumference, and serum levels of luteinizing hormone (LH), androstenedione, testosterone, and dehydroepiandrosterone sulfate (DHEAS) during the years immediately after menarche in a shorter longitudinal study.[40]

International data support the effects of BMI on puberty, but earlier onset of pubertal growth and a tall stature in childhood does not lead to a taller adult height.[41] Children studied longitudinally in Denmark showed earlier breast development (estimated mean age: 9.86 years compared to 10.88 years and menarche (13.42 compared to 13.13 years) in 2006 compared to 1991, which could not be explained by BMI or even by a difference in gonadotropin values suggesting other factors were at work.[42]

The Developing World

The interaction of socioeconomic conditions, nutrition, energy expenditure, states of health, and puberty is of particular importance in areas of the world where nutrition is suboptimal; where the most rapid improvement is found, such as in Oaxaca, Greenland, or South Korea, the age of menarche decreases more rapidly. Where standards of living do not change, neither does the age of menarche. In South America and Africa, some rural children fare better and have earlier puberty and taller stature than urban children, demonstrating a trend of adverse health and nutritional conditions in crowded urban centers. Malnourished individuals have later age of menarche across the world.[43]

As a whole, these reports indicate that populations existing in the most difficult conditions who experience improvement in socioeconomic status demonstrate a greater decrease in the age of menarche. Once a minimum nutritional status or state of health is reached, the effects of socioeconomic status on the age of menarche are minimized or eliminated, but increased BMI can lower the age of menarche further.

Factors Affecting the Age of Puberty and Menarche

The composition of diet and the number of calories in the diet may relate to menarche. The prospective, longitudinal Harvard Longitudinal Studies of Childhood Health and Development found that girls had earlier menarche if they were taller and consumed more animal protein and less vegetable protein as early as 3 to 5 years old and that they had earlier peak growth velocity if they had higher dietary fat intake at 1 to 2 years old and higher animal protein intake at 6 to 8 years. Peak height velocity (PHV) increased, controlling for body size, if more calories and animal protein were consumed 2 years before peak growth. The correlation between higher animal protein intake and lower age of menarche is confirmed in Germany and Britain.[44,45] A positive relationship between high fiber intake and age of menarche held true in a comparison of 46 countries,[46] and a longitudinal study demonstrated a later onset of puberty and PHV in girls with higher isoflavone intakes, suggesting a lower risk for breast cancer with a high fiber prepubertal diet.[47] On the other hand, lifelong vegetarian dietary intake does not affect the age of menarche,[48] and a low-fat diet in otherwise healthy, prepubertal, 8- to 10-year-old children with elevated low-density lipoprotein (LDL) cholesterol produced no difference in age of menarche or pubertal progression.[49] Phytoestrogen (flavinol but not lignan) intake delays breast development, particularly in girls with lower BMI values.[50,51]

Another influence of the age of menarche is the maternal environment. Macrosomia due to maternal diabetes or obesity is associated with increased BMI in childhood, which itself is related to earlier puberty and menarche. Increased or decreased weight gain in pregnancy likewise decreases the age of menarche according to data from the Nurses Health Study II.[52] Heavy maternal smoking of cigarettes but not of marijuana leads to earlier male puberty but not female puberty in offspring.[53] Maternal tea drinking but not coffee drinking had a later age of menarche and puberty in girls as did daughters of mothers who were more physically active during pregnancy.[54]

Stress and Puberty. Life history theories aiming to explain influences on the age of puberty address energetics, stress suppression, psychosocial acceleration, paternal investment, and child development, each of which may have various effects on the timing and progression of pubertal development.[55] Evolution optimizes allocation of limited resources to maximize fitness and allow reproductive success.[56]

Stress is variably reported to increase or decrease the age of menarche, depending on the study. The absence of a father or lower parental education increases the likelihood of early menarche; however, there is evidence that the exposure to paternal psychopathology that precedes the absence of the father might be causative in such situations.[57] War increases the age of voice breaking in boys (e.g., in Bach's choir during the War of Austrian Succession in 1727-1749), and the age of menarche increased during World War II and during more recent hostilities in the former Yugoslavia.[58] Sexual abuse is associated with earlier onset of puberty and earlier menarche compared with a control population in a large U.S. national study, although it is difficult to eliminate the effect of family dysfunction in this situation as well.[59] Child abuse of various types is associated with delayed puberty and menarche in a large British study, and sexual abuse in this cohort led to both early and late menarche.[60]

Genetic Effects on Puberty and Menarche. There remains a difference in age at attainment of stages of puberty in different countries even with stability in socioeconomic factors; for example, Japanese boys undergo changes in testicular size about 1 year earlier than Swiss boys do.[61] When socioeconomic and environmental factors lead to good nutrition, general health, and infant care, 60% to 80% of the determination of the age at onset of puberty in normal children appears to be due to genetic causes.

The important role played by genetic factors in the onset of puberty is illustrated by the similar age of menarche in members of an ethnic population and in mother-daughter and sibling or twin pairs.[62] The correlation between mother and daughter patterns should theoretically be equal to sister-sister age at menarche if only genetic factors are operative, but because sister-sister correlations are higher than mother-daughter correlations, environmental influences must provide an additional influence beyond genetic factors; the secular trend and nutritional factors may be invoked.

Concordance of ages of pubertal developmental stages and menarche is closer between monozygotic than dizygotic twins, supporting the influence of genetic factors. Monozygotic twins reared together have more similar ages of menarche than those reared apart, and dizygotic twins reared together are less similar than either of the monozygotic groups, pointing to environmental influences on genetic factors. Some twin research suggests that additive genetic factors account for 96% of the variance in the age of puberty in girls and 88% of the variance in boys (although other sources from the United States, Australia, Great Britain, Finland, and Norway have found genetic effects accounting for between 50% and 80% of the variance), with the remainder resulting from shared and nonshared environmental influences.[63,64]

Investigations of genes now involve genome-wide association study (GWAS) techniques to approach the greatly complex question of the genetic control of puberty and growth. Alleles near 6q21 (T) at rs7759938 *(LIN28B)* correlated with earlier puberty and shorter prepubertal childhood height, as well as age of menarche.[65,66] A meta-analysis of GWAS data for 17,510 women demonstrated the strongest signal related to age of menarche × 10⁻⁹, where the nearest genes include *TMEM38B, FKTN, FSD1L, TAL2,* and *ZNF462*, and the next strongest signal near the *LIN28B* gene (rs7759938; $p = 7.0 \times 10^{-9}$), which also influences adult height and cancer risk.[67] Studies of thousands of European individuals linked locus upstream of myocardin-like 2 *(MKL2)* ($p = 8.9 \times 10^{-9}$) with earlier puberty with reduced

pubertal growth ($p = 4.6 \times 10^{-5}$) and short adult stature ($p = 7.5 \times 10^{-6}$) in both males and females.[68] Variants near *MAPK3, PXMP3,* and *VGLL3* linked taller prepubertal stature with earlier menarche, and a variant near *ADCY3-POMC* was associated with increased BMI, reduced pubertal growth, and earlier puberty.[68]

Gonadotropin-releasing hormone type I (GnRH-I) and its receptor (GnRHR) are only modestly related to the age of menarche.[69] The *LEP1875* and XbaI and PvuII polymorphisms of the estrogen receptor α (ERα) gene *(ESR1)* and maternal age at birth (i.e., >30 or <30 years) were associated with age of menarche.[70,71] High-activity *CYP17* alleles involved in estrogen formation and high-activity *CYP1A2* and *CYP1B1* alleles, whose gene products metabolize estradiol, are not associated with pubertal stage,[72] whereas the high activity *CYP3A4** 1B/1B girls had an earlier age of onset of normal puberty alleles. The variant rs10235235 of *CYP3* is associated with a reduction in breast cancer risk for women who had their menarche age at 15 years or older but not for those with menarche younger than 11 years.[73] Girls with longer (>8) TAAAA repeats in their sex hormone–binding globulin gene *(SHBG)* have a later age of menarche than those with fewer repeats.[74] Further study is required to clarify the most important relationships.

Other Factors. Seasonality of menarche has been observed. In a U.S. cohort of 3000 college students, those born after 1970 had an earlier age of menarche and a more pronounced frequency peak in July. Factors hypothesized to contribute to seasonality of menarche include stress and the photoperiod.[75] In Peru, puberty begins at a later age, and pubertal development lasts longer at high altitudes than at low altitudes even when nutritional status is similar. There is a north-to-south decrease in the age of menarche in Europe[17] that results from environmental factors or genetic influences.[19]

The Comorbid Conditions of Early Puberty

Many international studies show that earlier age at menarche is associated with a greater risk of development of breast cancer by a factor of 1.050 (95% confidence interval [CI] 1.044-1.057; $p < 0.0001$) for every year younger at menarche.[76] The risk of premenopausal breast cancer decreases 9% per year of delay in menarche, and the risk for postmenopausal breast cancer decreases 4%.[77] In disease-discordant monozygotic twins, the one with cancer recalled puberty to be earlier, and in disease-concordant twins, the one with earlier menarche had the earlier diagnosis of breast cancer.[78] Women with breast cancer were taller and leaner in childhood and had increased height velocity at age 4 to 7 years and age 11 to 15 years; higher BMI increased this risk. These variables were particularly significant in women with early menarche (at age <12.5 years).[79] Remarkably, another study of 117,415 women found that increased birth weight, height at 8 years of age, peak growth at an early age, taller stature at 14 years of age, and low BMI at 14 years of age were independent risk factors for breast cancer but there was no effect of age of menarche[80]; increased body weight at 8 years also appears to decrease the risk of breast cancer.[81]

There is indirect evidence relating earlier menarche to increasing likelihood of hepatocellular carcinoma. On the other hand, later age of menarche (>14 years) is associated with an increased risk of glioma or non-Hodgkin lymphoma.[82,83]

Evidence from the Fels Longitudinal Study of white females revealed that girls with self-reported menarcheal age of less than 11.9 years (classified as early menarche; 23% of the sample) had adverse cardiovascular risk factors such as elevated blood pressure and glucose intolerance unrelated to body composition.[84]

National Trends in Pubertal Development
Limits of Normal Pubertal Development

The U.S. Health Examination Survey (HES) enrolled subjects who were 12 years old; although it is useful for defining the upper limits of normal pubertal development, the survey is uninformative about the lower limits of the age at onset of puberty.[25,85] A longitudinal study (Tables 25-2 and 25-3) that enrolled 9.5-year-old white boys and girls added much to the determination of the mean age at

attainment of stages of puberty[86]; however, it started too late to include normal children entering puberty at an earlier age. Two studies used data from NHANES III. One found onset of stage 2 breast development for African Americans, Mexican Americans, and whites to occur at 9.5, 9.8, and 10.3 years, respectively, and pubic hair stage 2 to occur at 9.5, 10.3, and 10.5 years, respectively, using a sample of 1623 girls.[87] The other study reported that the ages for onset of stage 2 breast development were 9.5 years for African Americans, 9.8 years for Mexican Americans, and 10.4 years for white Americans, whereas the onset of stage 2 pubic hair occurred at 10.4 years for white Americans, 9.4 years for African Americans, and 10.6 years for Mexican Americans in a sample of 2145 girls.[88]

Because the PROS started at 3 years of age but ended at 12 years of age, it excluded a proportion of normal children who enter puberty at a later age, although the probit statistical method can estimate events even when only a portion of the population has achieved the event.[14] This study was criticized because the subjects from the convenience sample were not matched for the many factors considered in a national study such as NHANES. The standard deviation of the longitudinal study described earlier was low, 1.0 years or less in most cases, whereas the cross-sectional study PROS had a larger standard deviation of approximately 2 years. Any study of puberty will demonstrate a limit in the spread of the upper end of the age at onset of puberty curve, because rarely do individuals with the most severe constitutional delay of puberty (CDP) spontaneously enter puberty after 18 years of age. There may be a skewing of the normal age at onset of puberty to an earlier spread of ages.

A study of the age of pubertal stages in children in NHANES revealed that in those with normal BMI values, pubertal signs occurred before 8.0 years of age in fewer than 5% of the non-Hispanic white, female population, although thelarche occurred before age 8.0 in 12% to 19% of normal-BMI, non-Hispanic black and Mexican American girls; the 5th percentile for menarche was 0.8 years earlier for non-Hispanic black than non-Hispanic white subjects.[31] Although the appearance of pubic hair occurred in up to 3% of 8.0-year-old girls with normal BMI values in all ethnicities, it did occur significantly earlier in the minority groups. Girls with the higher BMI values had a significantly higher prevalence of thelarche between the ages of 8.0 and 9.6 years and pubarche from the ages of 8.0 to 10.2 years,

TABLE 25-2
Descriptive Statistics for the Timing of Sexual Maturity Stages in Females

	Breast Stages			
	Onset of Stage		Mean Age for Stage	
Stage	Mean	SD	Mean	SD
Stage 2				
Roche et al (Ohio)	11.2	0.7	11.3	1.1
Herman-Giddens et al (USA)				
African-American	8.9	1.9		
White	10.0	1.8		
Stage 3				
Roche et al (Ohio)	12.0	1.0	12.5	1.5
Herman-Giddens et al (USA)				
African-American	10.2	1.4		
White	11.3	1.4		
Stage 4				
Roche et al (Ohio)	12.4	0.9		
	Tanner Pubic Hair			
Tanner Stage 2				
Roche et al (Ohio)	11.0	0.5		
Herman-Giddens et al (USA)				
African-American	8.8	2.0		
White	10.5	1.7		
Tanner Stage 3				
Roche et al (Ohio)	11.8	1.0		
Herman-Giddens et al (USA)				
African-American	10.4	1.6		
White	11.5	1.2		
Tanner Stage 4				
Roche et al (Ohio)	12.4	0.8		
	Menarche			
Herman-Giddes et al (USA)				
African-American	12.2	1.2		
White	12.9	1.2		
Percent Menstruating	**At Age 11**		**At Age 12**	
African-American	27.9%*		62.1%	
White	13.4%*		35.2%	
Onset of Axillary Hair (Stage 2)				
African-American	10.1 ± 2.0			
White	11.8 ± 1.9			

*African-American girls enter puberty approximately 1 to 1½ years earlier than white girls and begin menses 8½ months earlier. Data from Roche AF, Weilens R, Attie KM, et al. The timing of sexual maturation in a group of U.S. white youths. *J Pediatr Endocrinol*. 1995;8:11-18; Herman-Giddens ME, Slora EJ, Wasserman RC, et al. Secondary sexual characteristics and menses in young girls seen in office practice: a study from the Pediatric Research in Office Settings network. *Pediatrics*. 1997;99:505-512.

TABLE 25-3
Descriptive Statistics for the Timing of Sexual Maturity Stages in White Males (Ohio)

	Age at Onset of Stage (Yr)		Age for Stage (Yr)	
Stage	Mean	SD	Mean	SD
Genital Stage				
2	11.2	0.7	11.3	1.0
3	12.1	0.8	12.6	1.0
4	13.5	0.7	14.5	1.1
5	14.3	1.1	—	—
Pubic Hair Stages				
2	11.2	0.8	11.3	0.9
3	12.1	1.0	12.4	1.0
4	13.4	0.9	13.7	0.9
5	14.3	0.8	14.8	1.0
6	15.3	0.8	—	—

From Roche AF, Wellens R, Attie KM, et al. The timing of sexual maturation in a group of U.S. white youths. *J Pediatr Endocrinol*. 1995;8:11-18.

compared with girls with normal BMI values. Menarche was significantly more likely to occur in younger girls with elevated BMI values. In boys with normal BMI values, pubic hair appeared in fewer than 2% before 10.0 years. The study authors concluded that pubertal development in girls with normal BMI values before 8.0 years of age is premature. These data support other analyses of NHANES III, in which the heaviest girls tended to have thelarche before pubarche and the heaviest boys had pubarche before gonadarche.[36]

The latest and largest multiracial and ethnic study of the age at onset of puberty in a convenience sample of 4131 American boys between the ages of 6 and 16 years found the mean ages for onset of Tanner 2 genital development for non-Hispanic white boys was 10.14, African-American boys was 9.14, and Hispanic boys was 10.04 years; and for stage 2 pubic hair, the ages were 11.47, 10.25, and 11.43 years, respectively. Mean ages for achieving testicular volumes of greater than 3 mL were 9.95 for white, 9.71 for African-American, and 9.63 for Hispanic boys; and for greater than 4 mL ages were 11.46, 11.75, and 11.29, respectively.[34]

Taking these data as a whole, it seems reasonable to set the lower range of normal puberty at 8 years in girls and 9 years in boys. The influence of BMI must be taken into account. Obese boys characteristically enter puberty early, especially when there is an *MCR4* mutation, but obesity is also associated with delayed puberty.

Spanish investigators demonstrated that the earlier normal girls entered puberty, the longer the duration of puberty before menarche. In one of these studies, girls who started puberty at 9, 10, 11, 12, and 13 years of age experienced menarche 2.77, 2.27, 1.78, 1.44, and 0.65 years later, respectively, demonstrating a normalizing trend that keeps the age of menarche relatively stable in the group as a whole.[89] These data may suggest that earlier onset of the first stages of puberty may not exert major effects on the age of menarche. This contrasts with a suggestion of a decrease in the time required to transit puberty from start to end in Dutch and Swedish boys and girls.[19]

In sum, the data show that African-American girls develop before white girls, regardless of socioeconomic issues. There is evidence that rising BMI values in childhood are associated with earlier pubertal maturation, which may explain some of the increasing age differences between these ethnic groups. This suggests that an irrefutable decrease in the age at puberty in the overall population of girls may be realized in the future due to the increased BMI percentiles. Environmental disruptors may also play a role. Although there is evidence for earlier menarche, a secular trend toward earlier puberty in girls in the absence of increased BMI cannot be supported from these data because of the different ages studied and lack of comparable studies over past decades.[22,90]

The United States is lacking a comprehensive, large, longitudinal study that would start early enough to include the youngest normal pubertal subjects and last long enough to include the oldest and that would be based on direct physical examination rather than observation. Such a study must be balanced in terms of ethnic groups, and the planners must use the predicted increase of certain ethnic populations in the United States to avoid the unfortunate position we now have as we look back and try to draw conclusions about secular trends without sufficient data from various ethnic groups.[22]

From all of the longitudinal and some of the cross-sectional data, we may consider the mean age at onset of puberty in boys to be 11 years, with the normal limits being 9 to 14 years.[86] It is possible that some normal boys,

especially African-American boys, will enter puberty or adrenarche between 8 and 9 years of age.

Guidelines for the normal variation in pubertal development for girls in the United States are controversial. In the cross-sectional, convenience sample study, 3.0% of white girls had stage 2 breast development in their sixth year and 5.0% by the seventh year, whereas 6.4% of African Americans had stage 2 breast development by the sixth year and 15.4% by the seventh year. African-American girls have an earlier onset of pubertal development by about 1 year, even though their average age at menarche in the cross-sectional study was only 8.5 months different (12.2 years for African Americans and 12.9 for whites). We may combine these findings and set the normal range for age at puberty in white girls at 7 to 13 years and in African-American girls at 6 to 13 years. However, some girls in this early range may have a loss-of-function *MKRN3* mutation, possibly in a familial pattern; testing is available only in research laboratories at present but may be available for clinical diagnosis in the future.

These guidelines help the decision of which children with early onset of puberty are candidates for expensive diagnostic tests and for consideration of long-term therapy, because many of those children who appeared to have mild sexual precocity in years past may now be considered to represent a normal variation. We emphasize that family history, the rapidity of development of secondary sex characteristics, the rate of growth, and the presence or absence of CNS or other types of diseases must enter into the decision to evaluate a child. We recommended these ideas in previous editions of this textbook, and the Drug and Therapeutics and Executive Committees of the Lawson Wilkins Pediatric Endocrine Society support such a revision of the lower limit of the normal age at onset of puberty to age 7 for white girls and age 6 for African-American girls, with no changes in the current guidelines for evaluating boys, which target those with signs of puberty developing before 9 years of age.[91]

Several studies indicate the likelihood of missing serious endocrine disorders if the new guidelines are followed.[92-94] With all of these studies, it may be inferred that if the examining physician looks for signs and symptoms of disease rather than just relying on the age criteria, somewhat less than 10% of true precious puberty will be missed; of those cases, some (probably many) will be so mild as to not need intervention and may represent variations of normal. A multinational study from Europe suggested that valid indications for magnetic resonance imaging (MRI) of the CNS in the diagnosis of precocious puberty are puberty onset in girls before 6 years of age, in agreement with our recommendations, and an estradiol value higher than the 45th percentile (in the laboratory performing the diagnostic tests) for girls with central precocious puberty (CPP), a new criterion.[95]

SECONDARY SEXUAL CHARACTERISTICS AND PHYSICAL CHANGES OF PUBERTY

Female Development

Two distinct phenomena occur in the female. The development of the breast and its modified apocrine glands is primarily under the control of estrogens secreted by the ovaries (Fig. 25-5); the growth of pubic and axillary hair (Fig. 25-6) is mainly under the influence of androgens secreted by the adrenal cortex and the ovary. Breast cancer

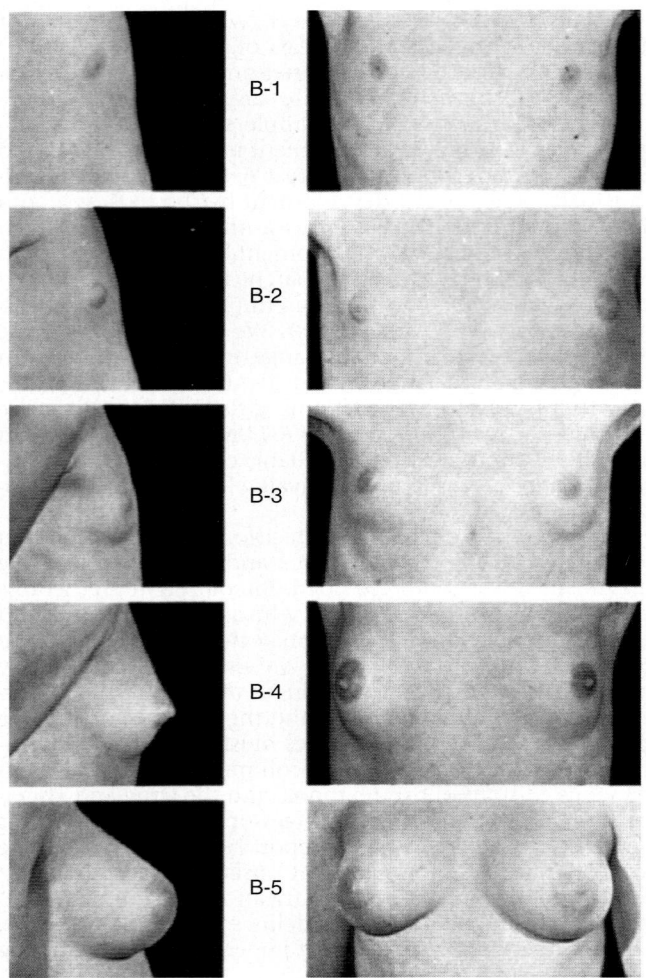

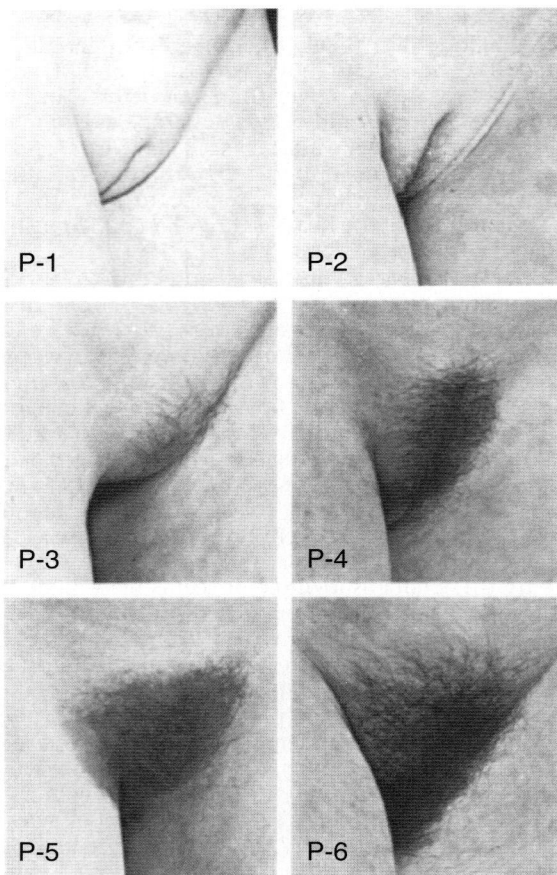

Figure 25-5 Stages of breast development according to Marshall and Tanner (1969). Stage 1: preadolescent; elevation of papilla only. Stage 2: breast bud stage; elevation of breast and papilla as a small mound, with enlargement of the areolar diameter. Stage 3: further enlargement of the breast and areola, with no separation of their contours. Stage 4: projection of the areola and papilla to form a secondary mound above the level of the breast. Stage 5: mature stage; projection of the papilla only, resulting from recession of the areola to the general contour of the breast. (Photographs from Van Wieringen JD, Wafelbakker F, Verbrugge HP, et al. *Growth Diagrams 1965 Netherlands: Second National Survey on 0-24 Year Olds.* Netherlands Institute for Preventative Medicine TNO. Groningen, The Netherlands: Wolters-Noordhoff; 1971. Additional data from Marshall WA, Tanner JM. Variations in pattern of pubertal changes in girls. *Arch Dis Child.* 1969;44:291-303.)

Figure 25-6 Stages of female pubic hair development according to Marshall and Tanner (1969). Stage 1: preadolescent; the vellus over the pubes is not further developed than that over the anterior abdominal wall; there is no pubic hair. Stage 2: sparse growth of long, slightly pigmented, downy hair that is straight or only slightly curled, appearing chiefly along the labia. This stage is difficult to see on photographs. Stage 3: hair is considerably darker, coarser, and curlier. The hair spreads sparsely over the junction of the pubic region. Stage 4: hair is adult in type, but the area covered by it is still considerably smaller than in most adults. There is no spread to the medial surface of the thighs. Stage 5: hair is adult in quantity and type, distributed as an inverse triangle of the classic feminine pattern. The spread is to the medial surface of the thighs but not up the linea alba or elsewhere above the base of the inverse triangle. (Photographs from Van Wieringen JD, Wafelbakker F, Verbrugge HP, et al. *Growth Diagrams 1965 Netherlands: Second National Survey on 0-24 Year Olds.* Netherlands Institute for Preventative Medicine TNO. Groningen, The Netherlands: Wolters-Noordhoff; 1971. Additional data from Marshall WA, Tanner JM. Variations in pattern of pubertal changes in girls. *Arch Dis Child.* 1969;44:291-303.)

develops in rodents exposed to environmental toxins (e.g., endocrine disruptors) that alter normal mammary development, and this same relationship is postulated to occur in girls exposed to endocrine-disrupting chemicals, especially if development occurs early.[96] Aromatase is present in adipose tissue, and estrogen produced in excess adipose tissue may stimulate breast development at an earlier age in obese girls. Peripubertal girls also demonstrated elevated values of androgens, especially just before the onset of puberty and in the early stages, but there is also decreased LH secretion, suggesting that central pubertal development may not be the cause of the physical signs of pubertal development.[97,98]

The five stages of breast development described by Tanner are the most widely used staging mechanism (see Fig. 25-5). Initial breast development may be unilateral for several months, causing unfounded concern by girls or parents. Needless surgical biopsies are carried out for this

normal variation, and an ultrasound examination may preempt unfounded concerns about breast cancer. If concern arises about breast cancer during puberty (a rare event), ultrasound evaluation is suggested because of the dense nature of the tissue at this stage. Inherited or sporadic agenesis of the breast allows no glandular or fat enlargement, regardless of the level of estrogen stimulation. Virginal breast hypertrophy, an extreme and rapid increase in breast size at the onset of puberty, is rare but is attributed in part to increased sensitivity to estrogen action or to increased local estrogen synthesis and growth factors.

Changes in the diameter of the papilla of the nipple are sequential and are linked to stages of pubertal development. Nipple papilla diameter (3 to 4 mm) does not increase much during pubic hair stage 1 to 3 or breast stage 1 to 3 but does increase after breast stage 3, providing an objective method of differentiating stage 4 from[99] stage 5 (final diameter, approximately 9 mm). The stage of breast

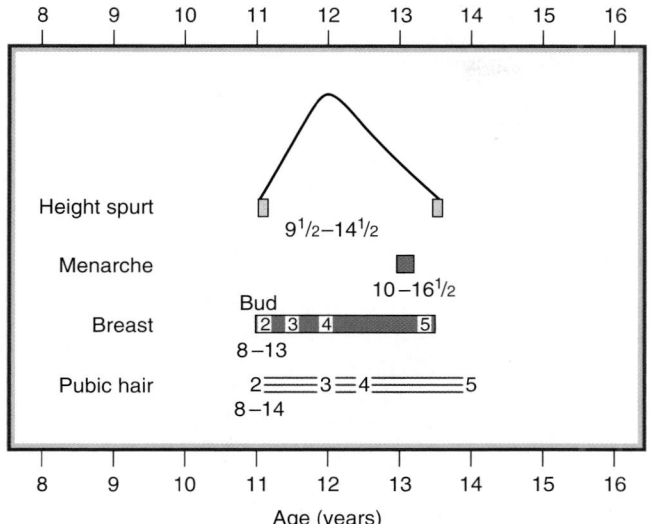

Figure 25-7 The sequence of events at puberty in females. Diagram of the sequence of events at puberty in males. An average is represented in relation to the scale of ages; the range of ages within which some of the changes occur is indicated by the numbers below. The ages are from British girls 40 years in the past, so the sequence of changes, rather than the ages, is the important factor. (From Marshall WA, Tanner JM. Variations in pattern of pubertal changes in girls. *Arch Dis Child.* 1969;44:291-303.)

development usually progresses along with the stage of pubic hair development in normal girls, but because different endocrine organs control these two processes, discordance can occur. Therefore, breast and pubic hair developmental stages should be classified separately for greatest accuracy (Table 25-2 and Fig. 25-7).

Dulling and thickening of the vaginal mucosa from the prepubertal reddish, glistening appearance occurs as the lining cells cornify and the secretion of clear or whitish discharge increases in the months before menarche as a result of estrogen action. Girls may notice light-colored discharge on their underwear at this stage. The vaginal pH decreases as menarche approaches due to the increase in lactic acid produced by lactobacilli in the vaginal flora. The length of the vagina increases from about 8 cm at onset of puberty to 11 cm at menarche. Thickening, protrusion, and rugation of the labia majora and minora occur. Fat is deposited in the area of the mons pubis, and the appearance of the labia majora becomes wrinkled. Occasionally, the labia minora may enlarge on one or both sides enough to suggest a tumor; childhood asymmetric labium majus enlargement is a disorder of prepuberty or early puberty.[100] The clitoris enlarges slightly, and the urethral opening becomes more prominent. Photographic atlases of normal female prepubertal genitalia are available and include standards for the variation in appearance of the hymenal opening; this information is invaluable in the evaluation of a victim of suspected child abuse.

Ovarian Development

The peak cohort of germ cells in the fetal ovary is attained at 16 to 20 weeks of gestation. Primordial follicles start to appear at 20 weeks of fetal life, and primary follicles soon follow; they constitute the lifelong store of follicles for the individual, which decreases with development and aging.[101] Follicle-stimulating hormone (FSH) receptors have not been detected in midtrimester human fetal ovaries; fetal pituitary FSH is not required for proliferation of oogonia, oocyte differentiation, or formation of primordial folli-

cles.[102] During fetal life and childhood, follicular growth to the large antral stage occurs, but before menarche, all developing follicles are destined to undergo atresia (Fig. 25-8). Large preovulatory follicles are rarely present before puberty.

The ultrasound appearance of the prepubertal ovary changes with pulsatile gonadotropin secretion, and a multicystic appearance occurs with more than six follicles of at least 4 mm in diameter; this appearance differs from that found in the polycystic ovary syndrome (PCOS). During prepuberty, the ovarian volume is 0.2 to 1.6 mL on ultrasound scans, and after the onset of puberty, the volume increases to 2.8 to 15 mL. Tall girls have greater ovarian volume than average-size girls.

The uterus grows until the age of 16 years under the influence of estradiol, progesterone, growth hormone (GH),[103] and insulin-like growth factor 1 (IGF-1). Ultrasound studies (Fig. 25-9) show that the corpus of the uterus increases during pubertal progression, from an initial tubular shape to a bulbous structure; the length of the uterus increases from 2 to 3 cm to 5 to 8 cm; and the volume increases from 0.4 to 1.6 mL to 3 to 15 mL.[104] Decreased uterine size is found in patients with Turner syndrome, childhood exposure to radiotherapy, and abnormalities in *HOX* and *WNT* gene expression, and maternal cigarette smoking can decrease uterine size at adolescence. Smaller uterine size is associated with an increased risk of miscarriage and failed implantation.

Uterine ultrasonography measurements are proposed to aid the clinician in differentiating premature thelarche from precocious puberty. The addition of color Doppler studies may improve accuracy of the diagnosis of precocious puberty and can differentiate the condition from premature thelarche. A Doppler study showed the lowest impedance of the uterine artery to be in girls with established CPP.[105]

Endometriosis is considered to be an estrogen-dependent process, although it has been reported in premenarcheal girls. It was suggested that this cause for chronic abdominal pain is more common than previously considered. One proposed explanation for early-onset endometriosis is that the condition results from müllerian rests.[106]

Menarche and Teenage Pregnancy

Menarche usually occurs in the 6-month period preceding or following the fusion of the second and first distal phalanges and the appearance of the sesamoid bone; this corresponds to Tanner stage 4 in most cases. The 95th percentile for menarche is 14.5 years, although many textbooks define primary amenorrhea as absence of menses at 16 years. Reconsideration of the age at onset of female puberty may lead to a reconsideration of the definition of primary amenorrhea. Anovulatory cycles are common in the first years after menarche. There is a reported prevalence of 55% anovulation in the first 2 years after menarche that decreases to 20% anovulatory cycles by the fifth year; others have observed a lower number of ovulatory events shortly after menarche and 5 years after the event. With the high prevalence of PCOS, it is unclear how often delayed regularity is an early sign of PCOS or normal variation. The number of pregnancies for U.S. teenagers 15 to 19 years old decreased almost 50% since 1991 and 22% since 2009; it was 31.3 per 1000 women in 2011.[107] However, there is an ethnic specific difference as the rate for Hispanic was 49.6 per 1000, non-Hispanic black was 47.3, American Indian/Alaska Native (AIAN) was 36.1, non-Hispanic white was 21.7, and American Pacific Islanders (API) was 10.2. The decline is attributed to pregnancy prevention messages, and there is evidence of increased use of contraception.

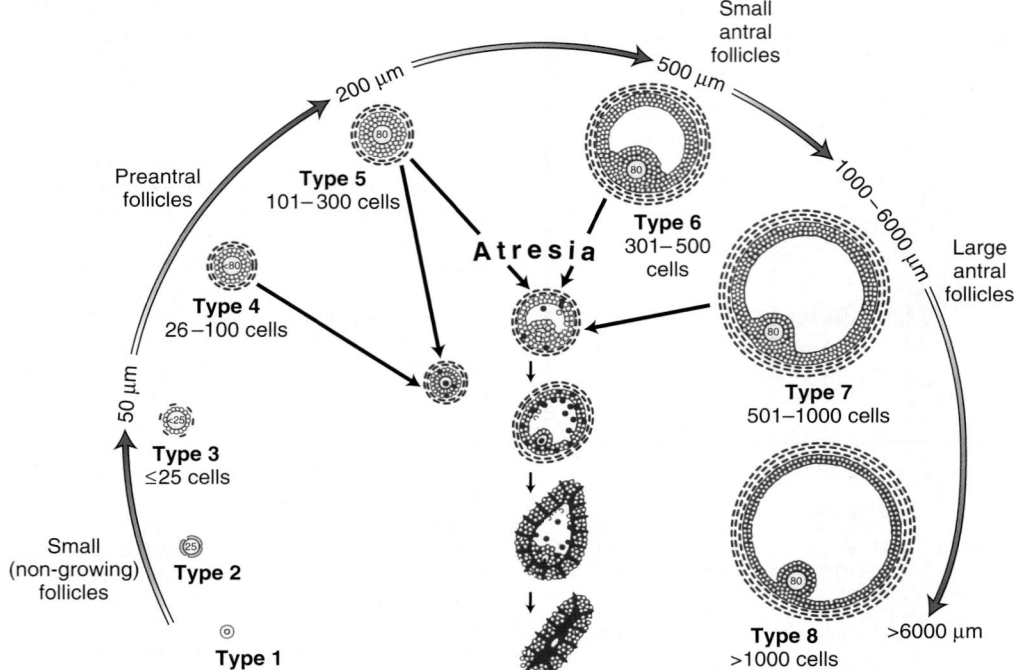

Figure 25-8 Schematic representation of the growth of ovarian follicles during infancy and childhood. Type 1 (primordial follicle) and type 2 (primary follicle) are composed of a small oocyte and a few to a ring of flat granulosa cells. In the diplotene (nesting) stage of prophase, primary follicles are the predominant form of oocyte and constitute the reservoir of cells from which follicular growth occurs. Types 3 to 5 (preantral follicles) are follicles that have entered the growth phase; the oocyte is enlarging and is surrounded by a zona pellucida, and granulosa cells increase in number and differentiate. The growth of the oocyte is complete by the end of the preantral stage, and the increased follicular size is caused by follicular growth and fluid accumulation. Types 6 to 8 represent antral follicles (graafian follicles) and contain a fully grown oocyte, a large number of granulosa cells, a fluid-filled cavity, and a well-developed theca external to the basement membrane. Large preovulatory follicles are absent (10,000 to 15,000 μm). Follicular growth and atresia take place throughout childhood. All follicles that enter the growth phase become atretic, and this can occur at any stage in their development but mainly involves large antral follicles. (From Peters H, Byskov AG, Grinsted J. Follicular growth in fetal and prepubertal ovaries of humans and other primates. *Clin Endocrinol Metab.* 1978;7:469-485.)

Male Development

The growth and maturation of the penis usually correlate closely with pubic hair development, because both features are under androgen control. However, the stages of pubic hair development and genital development should be determined independently, because discordant stages provide clues to potential disease states of the adrenal gland or testes (Figs. 25-10 and 25-11 and Table 25-3).

Growth of the testes is usually the first sign of puberty in the male, and it begins approximately 6 months after the average chronologic age of initiation of breast development in girls (see Fig. 25-4). Pubertal testicular enlargement is indicated when the longitudinal measurement of a testis is greater than 2.5 cm (excluding the epididymis) or the volume is greater than 3 mL. The testicular volume index ([(length × width of right testis) + (length × width of left testis)]/2) and testicular volume, measured by comparing the testes with ellipsoids of known volume, correlate with the stages of puberty.[108,109] A longitudinal study supported the utility of adding a stage 2a when testicular volume is 3 mL; further pubertal progression occurred within 6 months in 82% of boys who had reached this 3-mL phase[110] (Table 25-4). The most significant changes in serum testosterone and calculated free testosterone occur at the transitions of testicular volume between 1 and 2 mL, 2 and 3 mL, 6 and 8 mL, and 10 and 15 mL, suggesting the denotation of stages pre-1 (testis, 1 mL), pre-2 (testis, 2 mL), early (testis, 3 to 6 mL), middle (testis, 8 to 12 mL), late-1 (testis, 15 to 25 mL, the boy has not reached final height), and late-2 (testis, 15 to 25 mL, the boy has reached final height).[111] The right testis is normally larger

TABLE 25-4

Correlation of Testicular Volume (TV) With Stage of Pubertal Development

Parameter	Pubertal Stage				
	1	2	3	4	5
TV Index*					
Burr et al and August et al	1.8	4.5	8.2	10.5	—
Volume (cm³)					
Zachmann et al†	2.5	3.4	9.1	11.8	14
Waaler et al‡	1.8	4.2	10.0	11.0	15
Waaler et al§	1.8	5.0	9.5	12.5	17

*TV index calculated as follows: [(length × width of right testis) + (length × width of left testis)] ÷ 2.
†Volume estimated by comparison with ellipsoid of known volume (orchidometer) that is equal to or smaller than the testes.
‡Volume by comparison with orchidometer.
§Measurement with calipers and average volume of both testes calculated as follows: 0.52 × longitudinal axis × transverse axis.
Data from August GP, Grumbach, MM, Kaplan SL. Hormonal changes in puberty: correlation of plasma testosterone, LH, FSH, testicular size, and bone age with male pubertal development. J Clin Endocrinol. 1972 Feb;34(2):319-326. No abstract available; Burr IM, Sizonenko PC, Kaplan SL, Grumbach MM. Hormonal changes in puberty: correlation of serum luteinizing hormone and follicle stimulating hormone with stages of puberty, testicular size, and bone age in normal boys. Pediatr Res.1970 Jan;4(1):25-35. No abstract available; Waaler PE, Thorsen T, Stoa KF, Aarskog D. Studies in normal male puberty. *Acta Paediatr Scand Suppl.* 1974;249:1-36; Zachmann M, Prader A, Kind HP, Hafliger H, Budliger H, et al. Testicular volume during adolescence. Cross-sectional and longitudinal studies. *Helv Paediatr Acta.* 1974;29(1):61-72.

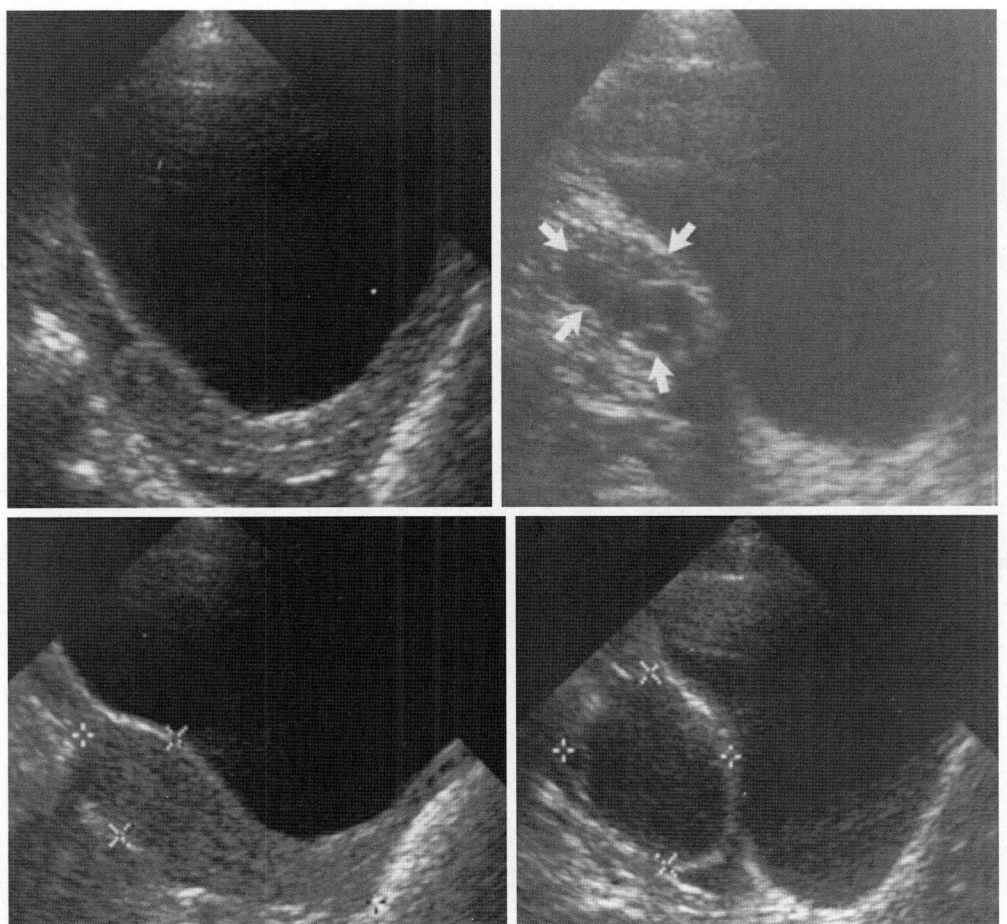

Figure 25-9 High-resolution pelvic ultrasonography. *Top left*, Prepubertal uterus. *Top right*, Prepubertal ovary demonstrating four small follicular cysts *(arrows)*. *Bottom left*, Pubertal postmenarchal uterus. *Bottom right*, Ovarian cyst in a girl with true precocious puberty.

than the left testis, and the left testis is located lower in the scrotum than the right testis.

The phallus should be measured while stretched and in the flaccid state, because there is much variation among individuals in the length of the unstretched penis. The length of the erectile tissue (excluding the foreskin) increases from an average of 6.2 cm in the prepubertal state to 12.4 ± 2.7 cm in the white adult. Ethnic differences have been identified; the mean value in African-American men is 14.6 cm, and in Asians it is 10.6 cm.[112]

As in girls, the areolar diameter increases in boys during puberty, with a distinct separation between the sexes occurring in stage 4, when female areolar diameter increases much more than in the male. In gynecomastia, the areolar diameter increases to above-normal values.

Male Testicular Development in Puberty

The testes are active during the prepubertal period albeit at a lower level than during pubertal development.[113] During pubertal development, the testes increase in size, principally because of the growth of the seminiferous tubules associated with the onset of spermatogenetic activity and mitosis of Sertoli cells, and testosterone production increases (Fig. 25-12 and Table 25-5). The Sertoli cells are the major cell type in the seminiferous cords in prepuberty and early puberty, but in the adult, germ cells predominate. During progression through puberty, the Sertoli cells cease

to undergo mitosis, differentiate into adult-type Sertoli cells, and form occlusive junctions with the development of the blood-testes barrier. Although Leydig cells are found in early gestation and during the neonatal period of testosterone secretion, the interstitial tissue is composed principally of undifferentiated mesenchyme-type cells during childhood. With pubertal development and rising serum LH levels, adult-type Leydig cells appear (Table 25-6). It is suggested that three phases of Leydig cell maturation correspond with ages of increased testosterone production: 14 to 18 weeks of fetal life, 2 to 3 months after birth, and puberty through adulthood.[114] The seminal vesicle enlarges through childhood to puberty to hold 3.4 to 4.5 mL, or 70% of the seminal fluid. The mean blood flow in the testes increases to adult values (measured by Doppler sonography) in boys, with a testicular volume greater than 4 mL.

Spermatogenesis

The first histologic evidence of spermatogenesis appears between ages 11 and 15 years (see Figs. 25-6, 25-9, and 25-13). Spermaturia may be the first sign of pubertal development, but the presence of sperm in urine is intermittent and therefore not a reliable indicator in all boys. Spermaturia is more prevalent in early puberty than in late puberty, suggesting that there may be a continuous flow of sperm through the urethra in early puberty but that ejaculation is necessary for sperm to appear in the urine in late puberty.

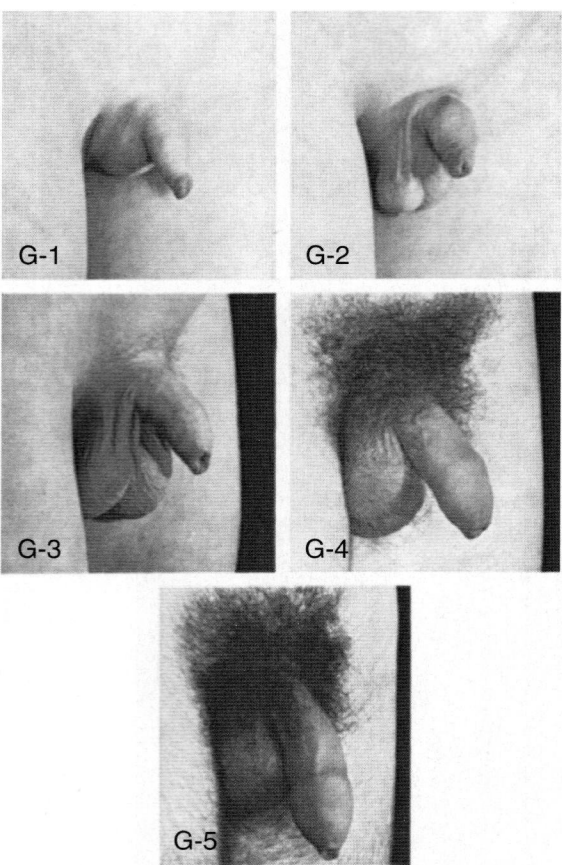

Figure 25-10 Stages of male genital development and pubic hair development according to Marshall and Tanner (1969). Genital development: stage 1: preadolescent. Testes, scrotum, and penis are about the same size and proportion as in early childhood. Stage 2: the scrotum and testes have enlarged; the scrotal skin shows a change in texture and some reddening. Stage 3: growth of the penis has occurred, at first mainly in length but with some increase in breadth; there is further growth of the testes and scrotum. Stage 4: the penis is further enlarged in length and breadth, along with development of the glans. The testes and scrotum are further enlarged. The scrotal skin has further darkened. Stage 5: genitalia are adult in size and shape. No further enlargement takes place after stage 5 is reached. Pubic hair development: stage 1: preadolescent; the vellus over the pubic region is not further developed than that over the abdominal wall; there is no pubic hair. Stage 2: sparse growth of long, slightly pigmented, downy hair that is straight or slightly curled, appearing chiefly at the base of the penis. Stage 3: hair is considerably darker, coarser, and curlier and spreads sparsely over the junction of the pubes. Stage 4: hair is adult in type, but the area it covers is still considerably smaller than in most adults. There is no spread to the medial surface of the thighs. Stage 5: hair is adult in quantity and type, distributed as an inverse triangle. The spread is to the medial surface of the thighs but not up the linea alba or elsewhere above the base of the inverse triangle. Most men will have further spread of the pubic hair. (Photographs from Van Wieringen JD, Wafelbakker F, Verbrugge HP, et al. *Growth Diagrams 1965 Netherlands: Second National Survey on 0-24 Year Olds.* Netherlands Institute for Preventative Medicine TNO. Groningen, The Netherlands: Wolters-Noordhoff; 1971. Additional data from Marshall WA, Tanner JM. Variations in pattern of pubertal changes in girls. *Arch Dis Child.* 1969;44:291-303.)

Spermaturia in the first morning urine specimen occurs at a mean chronologic age of 13.3 years, and at a mean pubic hair stage 2 to 3 in one study (or 16 years in another study), but may be found in normal boys with bilateral testicular volumes of only 3 mL and no signs of puberty.[115] Normospermia (i.e., normal sperm concentration, morphologic appearance, and motility) is not present until a bone age of 17 years. The first conscious ejaculation occurs at a mean chronologic age of 13.5 years in normal boys and at a mean bone age of 13.5 years in boys with delayed puberty.[116] The

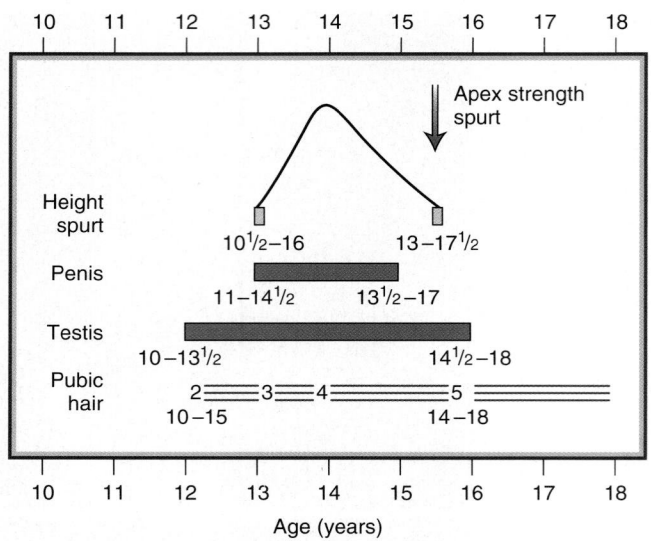

Figure 25-11 Diagram of the sequence of events at puberty in males. An average is represented in relation to the scale of ages, and the range of ages within which some of the changes occur is indicated by the numbers below. The ages are from British boys 40 years in the past, so the sequence of changes, rather than the ages, is the important factor. (From Marshall WA, Tanner JM. Variations in the pattern of pubertal changes in boys. *Arch Dis Child.* 1970;45:13-23.)

potential for fertility is reached before an adult phenotype is attained, before adult plasma testosterone concentrations are reached, and before PHV occurs.

Other Physical and Biochemical Changes of Puberty

The gender difference in voice develops during puberty. In the peripubertal period, the length of the vocal cords in boys and girls is about 12 to 15 mm, of which the membranous portion is 7 to 8 mm.[117] In adult men, the vocal cords attain a length of 18 to 23 mm (membranous portion, 12 to 16 mm), whereas in women, the cords enlarge only slightly (13 to 18 mm). During puberty, the male larynx, cricothyroid cartilage, and laryngeal muscles enlarge, leading to the appearance of an Adam's apple. The largest changes in singing and speaking frequencies occur between Tanner genital stages 3 and 4; breaking of the voice occurs at approximately 13 years, and the adult voice is achieved by about 15 years.

Facial hair in boys is first apparent on the corners of the upper lip and the upper cheeks; it then spreads to the midline of the lower lip and finally to the sides and the lower border of the chin. The first stage of facial hair development usually occurs during pubic hair stage 3 (average age of 14.9 years in the United States), and the last stage occurs after pubic hair stage 5 and genital stage 5.

Axillary hair appears at approximately 14 years in boys. Ninety-three percent of African-American girls have axillary hair by age 12, in contrast to 68% of white girls.[14] Axillary sweat glands begin to function as the hair appears. The appearance of circumanal hair slightly precedes that of axillary hair in boys.

Comedones, acne, and seborrhea of the scalp appear as a result of the increased secretion of gonadal and adrenal sex steroids.[118] Early-onset acne correlates with the development of severe acne later in puberty. Acne vulgaris, the most prevalent skin disorder in adolescence, appears at a mean age of 12.2 ± a standard deviation (SD) of 1.4 years (range, 9 to 15 years) in boys and progresses with

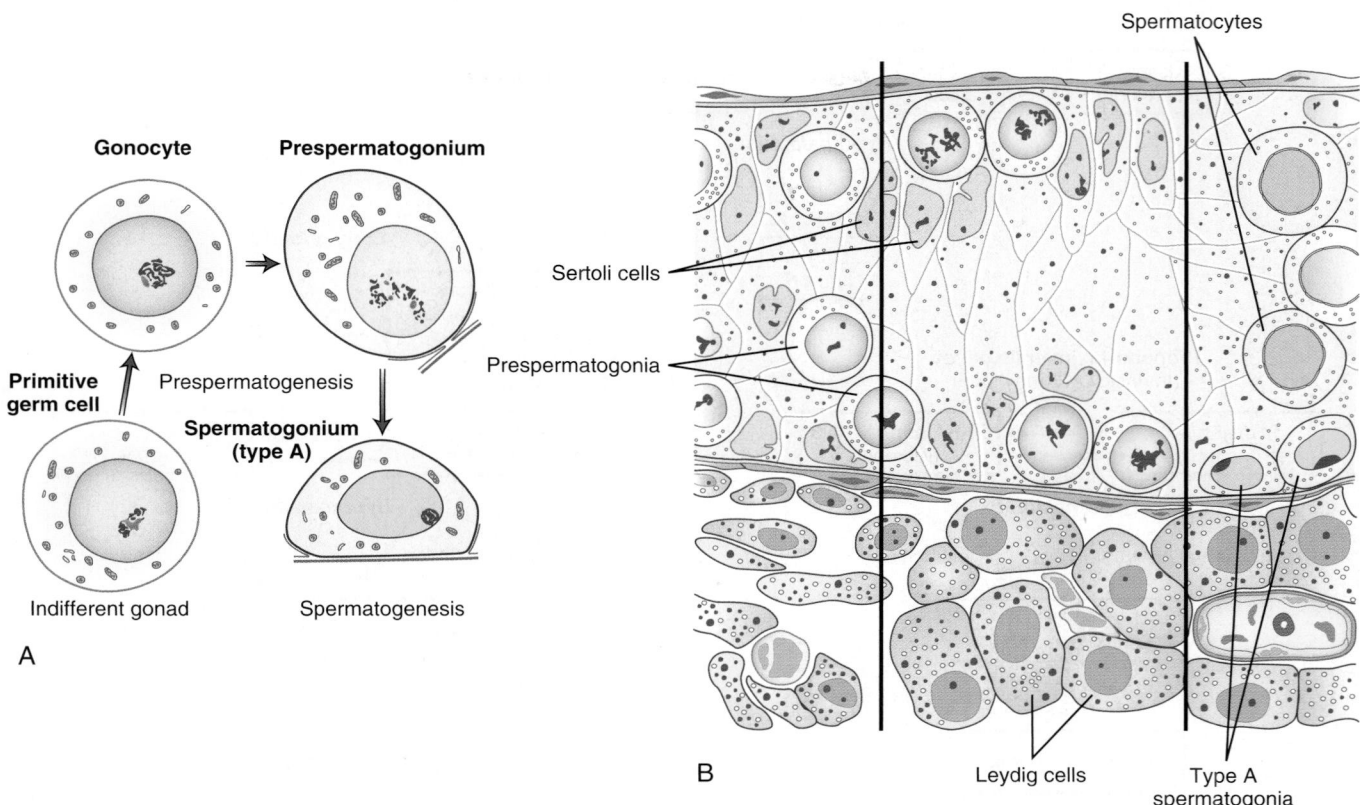

Figure 25-12 A, The diagram shows the developmental stages of testicular germ cells based on electron microscopic findings in the rabbit. Notice the differences between prespermatogonium and spermatogonium. **B,** The diagram shows maturation of testicular cell types in the rabbit from prepubertal appearance *(left)* to onset of spermatogenesis *(right)*. Interstitial cells undergo changes in shape, size, and arrangement in the process of Leydig cell differentiation. (From Gondos B. Testicular development. In: Johnson AD, Gomes WR, eds. *The Testis*, vol 4. New York, NY: Academic Press; 1977:1-37.)

TABLE 25-5

Mean Values of Various Body Measurements and Serum Hormone Levels by Pubertal Stage in Boys (Ohio)*

Variable	PS1	PS2a	PS2b	PS3	PS4	PS5
Age (yr)	11.44 (NS)	12.18	12.79	13.74	14.63	15.19
Height (cm)	144.2	149.8	154.6	162.3	169.9	173.3
Weight (kg)	38.18	41.65	47.27	54.67	61.11	66.88
Body mass index (kg/m²)	18.1	18.4	19.5	20.6	21.0	22.2
Testosterone (nmol/L [ng/dL])						
Blacks	0.8 (23)	3.0 (86)	4.9 (141)	11.5 (331)	13.4 (338)	15.5 (449)
Whites	0.6 (16)	2.9 (83)	4.6 (132)	9.7 (281)	13.3 (383)	14.6 (422)
Free testosterone (pmol/L [ng/dL])	11 (0.33)	60 (1.74)	114 (3.28)	294 (8.49)	413 (11.9)	504 (14.5)
DHEAS (µmol/L [µg/dL])	2.71 (99.7)	3.31 (121.8)	4.04 (148.7)	4.75 (175.0)	5.08 (187.0)	5.89 (217.0)
TeBG (nmol/L)	34.6 (NS)	33.3 (NS)	28.4	21.5	14.4	10.7

*Subjects were 515 boys from Ohio, including 237 blacks and 278 whites, aged 10-15 years at intake, who were monitored every 6 months for 3 years. All values were significant by Duncan post-hoc analysis at $p < 0.01$ except those marked NS. Pubertal stages were defined as follows: PS1, absence of pubic hair, testicular volume < 3 mL; PS2a, absence of pubic hair, testicular volume ≥ 3 mL; PS2b, Tanner stage 2 pubic hair; PS3 to PS5, Tanner pubic hair stages 3 to 5.
DHEAS, dehydroepiandrosterone sulfate; NS, not significant; TeBG, testosterone-binding globulin.
Modified from Biro FM, Lucky AW, Hoster GA, et al. Pubertal staging in boys. *J Pediatr.* 1995;127:40-46.

TABLE 25-6

Cellular Activity in Human Testis at Various Stages of Development

Stage	Germ Cells	Sertoli Cells	Leydig Cells
Prepubertal	Prespermatogenic cells are present	Predominant cells in seminiferous cords	Scattered, partially differentiated cells are present
Pubertal	Initiation of spermatogenesis	Increased complexity, formation of occlusive junctions	Fully differentiated cells appear
Adult	Active spermatogenesis, predominant cells	Individual cells associated with groups of germ cells	Groups of fully differentiated cells are present

From Gondos B, Kogan S. Testicular development during puberty. In: Grumbach MM, Sizonenko PC, Aubert ML, eds. *Control of the Onset of Puberty.* Baltimore, MD: Williams & Wilkins; 1990:387-398. © 1990, the Williams & Wilkins Co., Baltimore.)

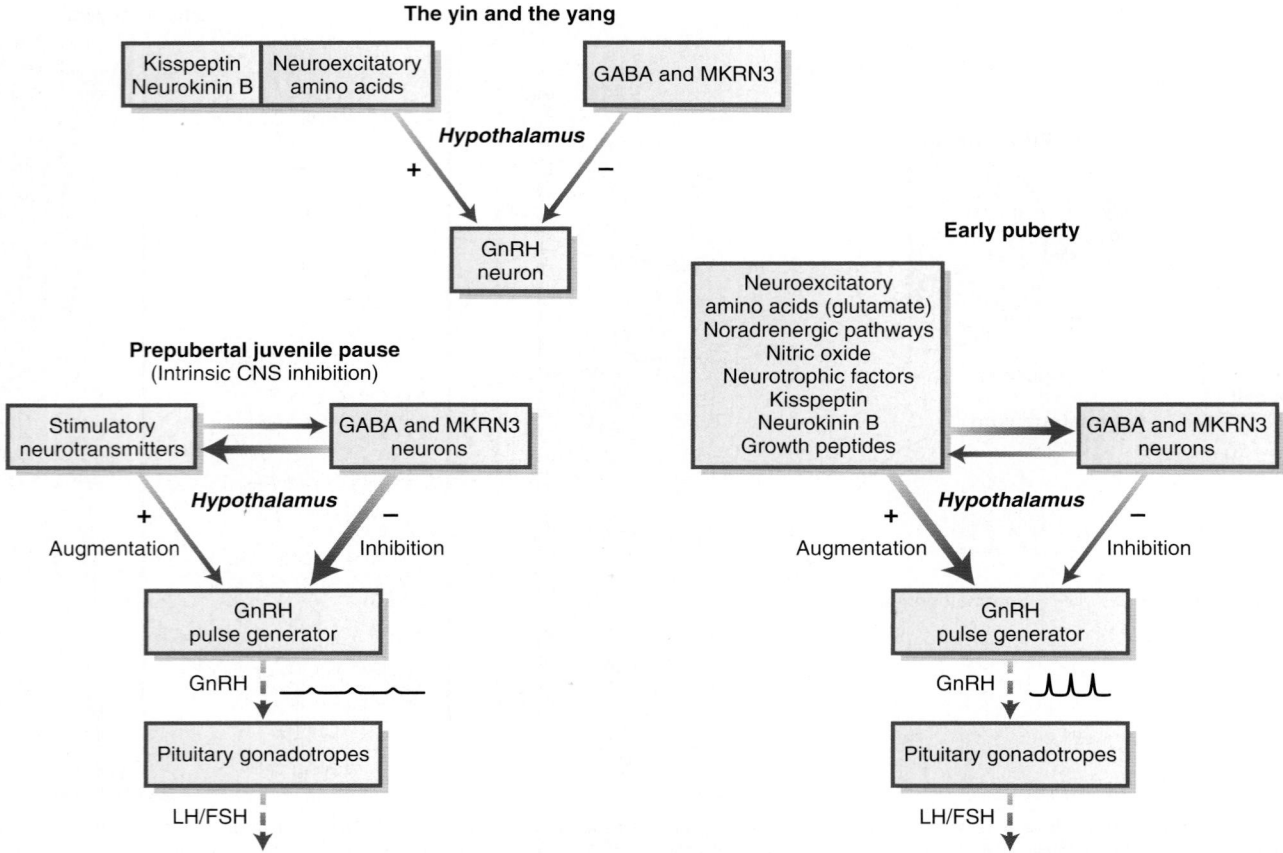

The yin and the yang

Figure 25-13 The yin and yang of the neuroendocrinology of the prepubertal juvenile pause and its intrinsic central inhibition of the gonadotropin-releasing hormone (GnRH) pulse generator and the reversal of this inhibition and termination of the juvenile pause, which leads to the onset of puberty. The GABAergic neuronal network and its neurotransmitter γ-aminobutyric acid (GABA) constitute the most ubiquitous inhibitory transmitter in the hypothalamus and the brain. During the prepubertal juvenile pause, this neurotransmitter system appears to play the major neural role in inhibiting the GnRH pulse generator. Suppression of GABA inhibition during this period promptly results in reactivation of the suppressed GnRH pulse generator in the rhesus monkey. With the approach of puberty, GABA inhibition of the GnRH pulse generator wanes, and its reactivation gradually occurs. This reactivation likely is augmented by stimulatory neurotransmitters (e.g., kisspeptin, excitatory amino acids), some of which depend on increased gonadal steroids for their activation, and by neurotrophic factors and growth peptides. A critical component of the reawakening of the GnRH neuronal network is the increase, independent of sex steroids, in KISS1 messenger ribonucleic acid (mRNA) expression in kisspeptinergic neurons in the medial basal hypothalamus and the secretion of kisspeptins, the cognate ligands for the kisspeptin receptor (KISS1R, formerly GPR54) on the surface of the GnRH neuron (Shahab et al). As a consequence, the amplitude and, to a lesser extent, the frequency of GnRH pulses increase, which leads to increased pulsatile secretion of follicle-stimulating hormone (FSH) and luteinizing hormone (LH) and the activation of the ovary and testis. As shown experimentally in monkeys, the GnRH pulse generator can function in the absence of hypothalamic stimulatory factors. The nature of and factor or factors responsible for this transition from central inhibition and the postulated dominance of GABA in the release of inhibition and reactivation of the GnRH pulse generator are unknown. (Additional data from Shahab M, Mastronardi C, Seminara SB, et al. Increased hypothalamic GPR54 signaling: a potential mechanism for initiation of puberty in primates. *Proc Natl Acad Sci U S A.* 2005;102:2129-2134.)

advancement through puberty. However, acne vulgaris can be the first notable sign of puberty in a girl, preceding pubic hair and breast development.[118] Analysis of the Nurses Study indicates that intake of milk and skim milk is related to the development of acne, an association suggested to reflect the hormone content of milk.[119] At late prepuberty, comedones are present in many boys, and 100% of boys have comedones by genital stage 5.

Facial morphologic appearance changes with pubertal development, leading to the mature appearance. The mandible and nose enlarge more in boys, but they and the maxilla, brow, frontal sinuses, and middle and posterior fossae enlarge in both sexes, mainly during the pubertal growth spurt. Children with isosexual precocity (ISP) have the facial appearance of older children, and individuals with delayed puberty have faces of younger children. There is a greater change in various measurements of the face compared with measurements of the skull, with the jaw showing the most increase.[120]

The size of the thyroid gland evaluated by ultrasonography normally increases roughly 40% to 50% with growth in height, weight, surface area, and fat-free mass during puberty but not with BMI.[121] This may lead an examiner to wrongly conclude there is a thyroid disorder due to the physiologic change. Lymphoid tissue growth reaches a maximum at about age 12 and thereafter decreases with pubertal progression.

A host of other physiologic and biochemical measurements change with the onset of puberty and must be interpreted in terms of the stage of pubertal development. Age-related standards should be used in all laboratories but often are not, and the interpreting clinician must turn to a textbook of pediatrics or the *Harriet Lane Handbook*. For example, hemoglobin levels increase at puberty in boys; the effect appears to be mediated by androgen, because treatment of boys with CDP with testosterone and letrozole (to block aromatization to estrogen) resulted in increased hemoglobin levels, even in the absence of a rise in IGF-1.[122]

The use of biomarkers of pubertal onset and progression will be studied in the U.S. National Child Health Study that longitudinally follows children from conception to adulthood to determine normal changes and the effects of environmental exposures, among other factors.[123]

Adolescent Growth

Pubertal Growth Spurt

The pubertal growth spurt may be divided for purposes of comparison into three stages: the time of prespurt minimal growth velocity in peripuberty just before the spurt (takeoff velocity); the time of most rapid growth, or PHV; and the stage of decreased velocity and cessation of growth at epiphyseal fusion. The greatest postnatal growth occurs in infancy; growth decreases to the nadir known as the minimal prespurt velocity, the slowest period of growth in childhood, immediately before the pubertal growth spurt.

During puberty, boys and girls experience a growth velocity greater than at any postnatal age since infancy (but paling in comparison to fetal growth, when one fertilized cell grows to 7 pounds in 9 months). Boys reach PHV approximately 2 years later than girls and are taller at takeoff (Fig. 25-14); PHV occurs during stage 3 to 4 of puberty in most boys (see Fig. 25-11) and is completed by stage 5 in more than 95% of boys. Boys achieve a PHV of 9.5 cm/year at a mean of about 13.5 years, with a greater PHV in those who mature earlier than in those who mature later.[124] The pubertal growth spurt in girls (PHV in girls is approximately 8.3 cm/year at a mean chronologic age of 11.5 years) occurs between stages 2 and 3 (see Fig. 25-7). Boys grew a mean of 28 cm, and girls grew 25 cm between takeoff and cessation of growth in a study in the United Kingdom.[125] Although the 8 to 11 cm of increased height gained during the pubertal growth spurt in boys has been held mainly responsible for the difference in adult height between the sexes,[124] twin studies of bone morphologic appearance indicate that the difference in adult height results more from the later onset of pubertal growth in boys rather than a difference in growth rate between the genders. The difference in bone widths between boys and girls is in large part established before puberty.[126]

A mathematical model that attempts to define the various stages of the pubertal growth curve based on longitudinal data separates the infancy, childhood, and pubertal phases of growth and allows evaluation of growth despite variation in the age at onset of puberty. A slowly decelerating childhood component is the base, with a sigmoidal pubertal component added during secondary sexual development (see Fig. 25-14C). The infancy-childhood-puberty (ICP) model detected the onset of the pubertal growth spurt, predicted the actual magnitude of the pubertal growth spurt, and predicted adult height using only the age at onset of puberty and a measurement of height.[127] Tanner and Davies constructed growth curves for American children using data from the National Center for Health Statistics, and data calculated from theoretical growth curves can be adjusted for time of PHV.[128]

Daily, meticulous observations of girls during puberty over 120 to 150 days show stasis periods in each girl (three to seven events lasting between 7 and 22 consecutive days); steep changes in each girl (one to four episodes, with the sum of these steep changes calculated as a percentage of total growth during the study period ranging from 15.3% to 42.9%); and continuous growth the remainder of time, with no rhythms or cycles found.[129] Clinicians observe an integrated growth rate during puberty, rather than these various complex patterns occurring during shorter periods of observation.

In a large Swedish registry, faster linear growth during infancy and childhood was associated with earlier PHV during adolescence but less height gain between 8 and 18 years, although greater height and BMI at birth were associated with later PHV in adolescence and more height gain between the ages of 8 and 18 years.[130]

Because girls reach PHV about 1.3 years before menarche, there is limited growth potential after menarche; most girls grow only about 2.5 cm taller after menarche, although there is a variation from 1 to 7 cm. The ages at menarche, takeoff, and PHV are not good predictors of adult height because the duration of pubertal growth is the more important determinant. Later onset of puberty and consequent increase in height at takeoff of the pubertal growth spurt can be balanced by a decrease in actual height achieved during PHV and result in no net change in adult height. However, early onset of puberty can diminish ultimate adult stature, prolonged delay of puberty can increase stature, and an older age at menarche leads to taller adult height in women. The age at PHV and the age at initiation of puberty correlate well with the rate of passage through the stages of pubertal development in normal children. Physical examination of a boy can reveal that he is likely to have significant growth left (if he is in early puberty), whereas limited growth is likely in boys who are in late puberty.

Stature and the upper-to-lower (U/L) segment ratio, defined as the length from the top of the pubic ramus to the top of the head divided by the distance from the top of the pubic ramus to the sole of the foot, change markedly during the peripubertal and early pubertal periods because of the elongation of the extremities.[131] At birth, the U/L ratio is about 1.7; at 1 year, it is 1.4; and at 10 years, it is 1.0 in a normal healthy individual. The legs begin to grow before the trunk, although late in puberty, during the growth spurt, growth of the legs is similar to growth of the upper torso.[132]

The mean U/L segment ratio of white adults is 0.92, and that of African-American adults is 0.85. There are no differences in U/L segment ratio between the sexes. In general, hypogonadal patients have delayed epiphyseal fusion and lack a pubertal growth spurt; therefore, their extremities grow for a prolonged period, leading to a decreased U/L segment ratio and an increased span for height, a condition known as *eunuchoid proportions*. Eunuchoid proportions are found in subjects with defects in estrogen synthesis and estrogen receptor deficiency, but normal proportions occur in patients with complete androgen insensitivity syndrome, demonstrating the primary role of estrogen in mitigating or establishing these proportions.[133-135] The distal parts of the extremities, the hands and feet, grow before the proximal parts; a rapid increase in shoe size is a harbinger of the pubertal growth spurt. Boys with Klinefelter syndrome have long legs but not long arms, a physical feature that can assist diagnosis before the onset of puberty. The shoulders become wider in boys, and the hips enlarge more in girls. The female pelvic inlet widens, mainly because of growth of the os acetabuli. The size of the head approaches the adult size by age 10 years, and the brain reaches 95% of adult size by the onset of puberty.

Bone Age

Skeletal maturation is assessed by comparing radiographs of the hand, the knee, or the elbow with standards of maturation in a normal population.[136,137] Ossification centers appear in early life, the bones mature in shape and size and develop articulation of surfaces; ultimately, the epiphyses or growth plates fuse with their shafts. Bone age,

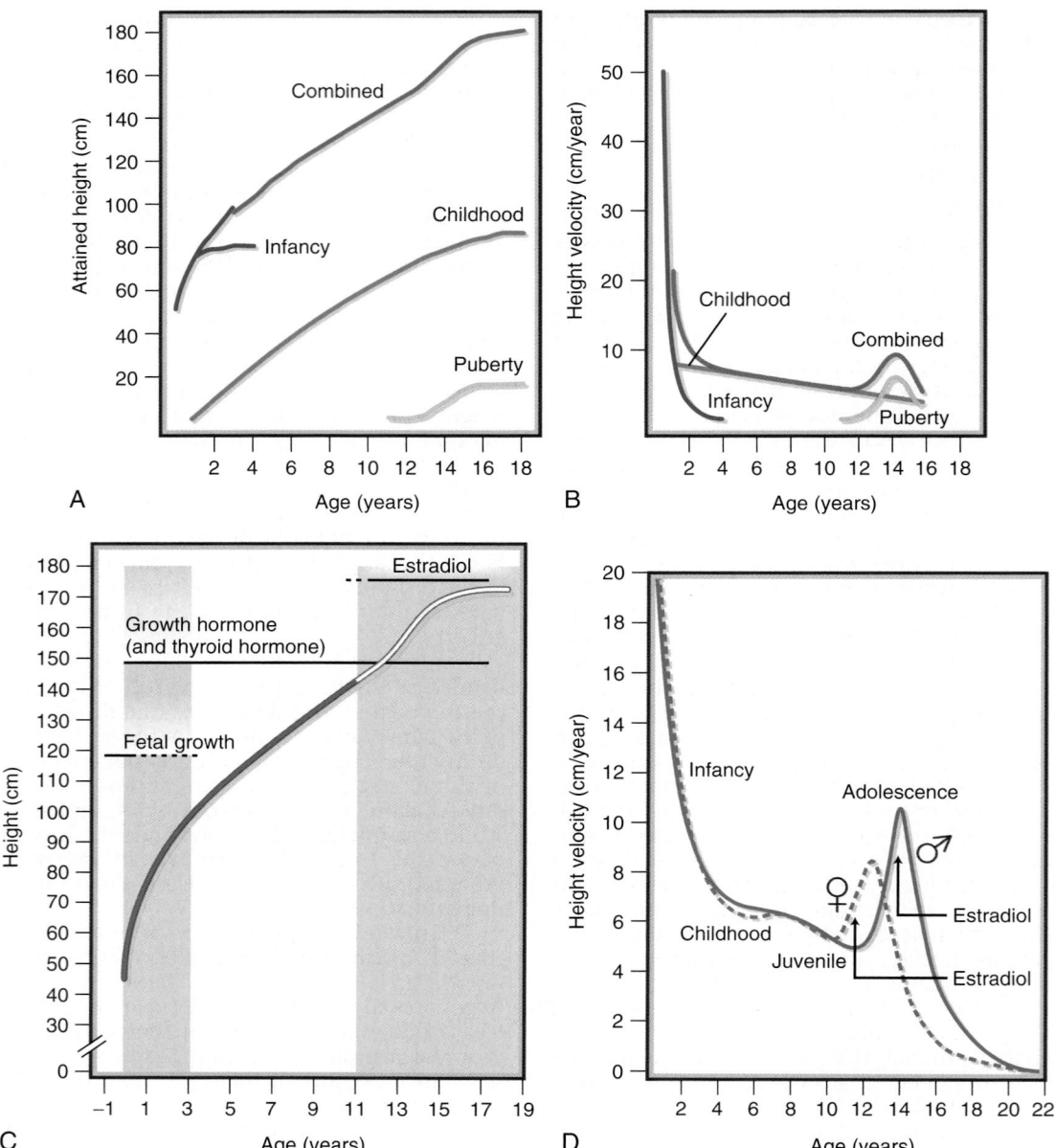

Figure 25-14 The infancy-childhood-puberty (ICP) model of Karlberg for mean attained height (**A**) and height velocity (**B**) for boys. The mean value for each component (infancy, childhood, and puberty) and their sums (combined growth [**A**] and combined velocity [**B**]) are plotted. The growth curve for an individual represents the additive effect of the three biologic phases of the growth process (ICP). Karlberg has provided mathematical functions for each component of his model. *Infancy:* This component starts before birth and falls off by age 3 to 4 years. It can be described by the exponential function $y = a + b[1 - \exp(-ct)]$. Average total gain in height for Swedish boys is 79.0 cm (44.0% of final height) and for girls is 76.8 cm (46.2%). *Childhood:* This phase begins at the end of the first year of life and continues to mature height. A second-degree polynomial function describes this component: $y = a + bt + ct^2$. Average total gain in height for boys is 85.2 cm (47.4%) and for girls is 78.4 cm (47.3%). *Puberty:* The model for the pubertal growth spurt is a logistic function: $y = a/[1 + \exp(-b(t - t_v))]$. Average total gain in height for boys is 15.4 cm (8.6%) and for girls is 10.9 cm (6.5%); y designates attained height at time t in years from birth; a, b, and c are constants; t_v is the age at peak height velocity. **C,** A schematic male growth chart shows the features of the ICP pattern overlaid and illustrates the predominant endocrine mechanisms controlling each phase of growth. The first *shaded area* emphasizes the decreasing velocity of infantile growth as the individual leaves the rapid growth phase of fetal life. The *open area* is the childhood phase, which continues and magnifies the decreased velocity of growth into a plateau of rather constant growth during childhood. These two phases depend largely on the effects of growth hormone (GH) and thyroid hormone, with no or little effect derived from gonadal steroids. In the next period of the pubertal growth spurt, gonadal steroids exert their direct and indirect effects. Gonadal steroids exert direct effects on the bone by stimulating the generation of insulin-like growth factor 1 (IGF-1) and other growth factors locally, and they exert indirect effects by stimulating increased GH secretion, which exerts its own effects on bone and stimulates the production of IGF-1. In the female, the major gonadal steroid involved in the pubertal growth spurt is estradiol, whereas in the male, testosterone and estradiol (arising mainly from the aromatization of testosterone) are the major gonadal steroids. **D,** The adolescent growth spurt in girls and boys (growth velocity curves). Notice the later onset of the pubertal growth spurt in boys and the approximately 2-year difference in peak height velocity and the greater magnitude of peak height velocity compared with girls. The timing of the effects of estradiol is indicated. Progressive epiphyseal fusion terminates the growth spurt and leads to final or adult height. (A and B modified from Karlberg J. On the construction of the infancy-childhood-puberty growth standard. *Acta Paediatr Scand Suppl.* 1989;356:26-37; C and D from Grumbach MM. Estrogen, bone, growth, and sex: a sea change in conventional wisdom. *J Pediatr Endocrinol Metab.* 2000;13[Suppl 6]:1439-1455.)

an index of physiologic maturation, does not have a well-defined relationship in normal children to the onset of puberty because it appears to be more variable than chronologic age.[138] In addition, the bone age evaluator must have experience with the method or an erroneous reading may occur; smaller hospitals/radiology offices will not likely have such experience. However, bone age is still used for predicting the age of menarche, and in boys, the onset of normal, premature, and delayed puberty correlates better with the onset of secondary sexual development than does chronologic age.

A difference between bone age and chronologic age must exceed 2 SDs to be of biologic significance. Standard deviations may range from a few months in infancy to 1 year in later adolescence; a 2-year variation of bone age from chronologic age is within normal limits in middle teenage years. As commonly estimated, bone age is imprecise and is a qualitative rather than a quantitative measure.[139] The development of techniques for scanning radiographs coupled with computer analysis is now approved in Europe and may improve accuracy of assessment.[140] African-American children have reportedly had slightly more advanced bone ages than do white children of the same chronologic age,[141] but recent evidence suggests that Asian and Hispanic children have more advanced bone ages than African Americans or Caucasians at the same chronologic age.[142]

Bone age, height, and chronologic age can be used for prediction of adult height from the Bayley-Pinneau tables[143] or by the use of the Roche-Wainer-Thissen,[144] Khamis-Roche[145] (for healthy whites only), or Tanner-Whitehouse techniques, TW2[132] and TW3.[146] Skeletal maturation is more advanced in girls than in boys of the same chronologic age because the early pubertal bone ages of 11 years in girls and 13 years in boys are equivalent stages of bone maturation by the hand-wrist method. There are reportedly considerable variations in height prediction between the methods, so the subjective manner of prediction must be borne in mind.[147]

Skeletal Density

Prevailing views locate the determinants of adult bone density in large part in genetic tendencies and the appropriate acquisition of bone mineral in childhood during growth. Osteoporosis and osteopenia are important conditions of the adult that are held to have antecedents in youth, and increasing interest focuses on bone health in children and adolescents, including the effects of age of menarche, nutrition, exercise, and genetics on normal skeletal development.[148,149] A relationship of bone density exists between generations if the effects of age and puberty are eliminated: 60% to 80% of variance in peak bone mass is attributed to genetic factors.[150] Clinical studies and animal models lead to the conclusion that distant-past patterns of bone growth are less important than recent conditions and that childhood bone growth does not exert a strong effect on adult bone density.[151] Thus, even with poor diet in childhood and adolescence, improvement in bone density may be possible later in life.

Areal bone mineral density (BMD) represents a two-dimensional image and is a function of the size of bone; this is the measurement most often available clinically with commercial dual-energy x-ray absorptiometry (DXA) devices. Smaller bones attenuate the radiation beam less than larger bones, and this factor must be considered in the interpretation when measuring bone density using commercial DXA devices. BMD of the total body, lumbar spine, and femoral neck measured by DXA increases at a mean annualized rate of 0.047 g/cm^2 for boys and 0.039 g/cm^2 for girls (Fig. 25-15A). Longitudinal studies of total-body DXA assessments indicate that boys accumulate 407 g/year and girls 322 g/year of mineral (i.e., 359 mg/day for boys and 284 mg/day for girls); 26% of adult calcium is laid down during the adolescent years of peak calcium accretion—14 years (mean) for boys and 12.5 years for girls.[152] BMD approaches a maximum accretion in girls by the age of 16 years, and in boys by about 17 years, with the difference in timing related to the disparity in PHV; the

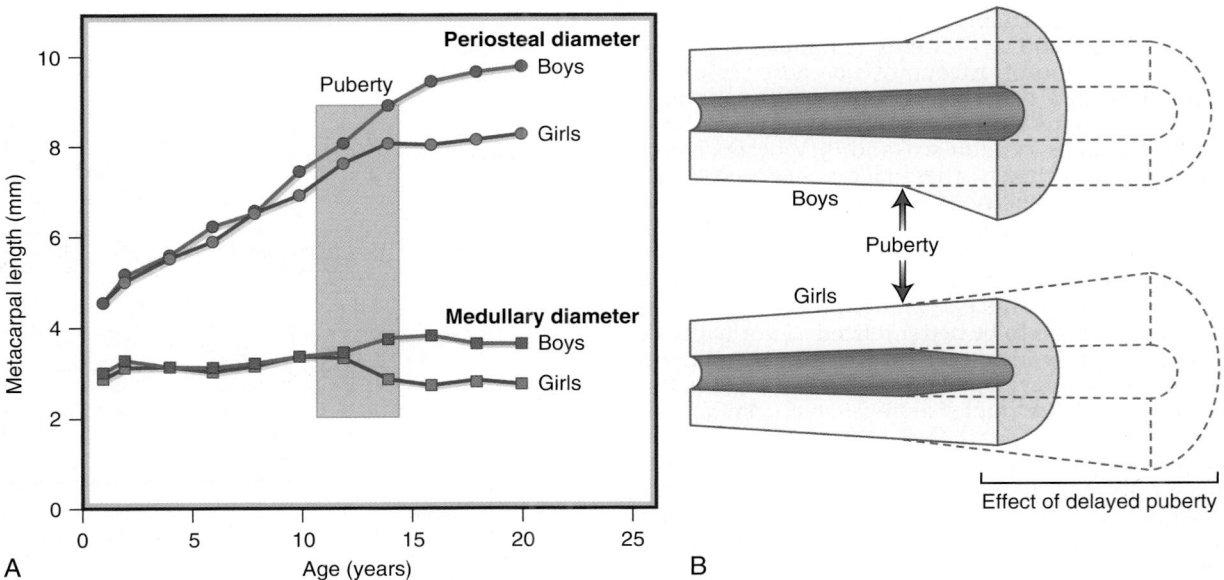

Figure 25-15 A, Periosteal diameter of the metacarpal bones does not differ before puberty in boys and girls. During puberty, the periosteal diameter expands in boys and ceases to expand in girls, whereas medullary diameter remains fairly constant in boys throughout growth but contracts in girls. **B,** In boys, delayed puberty may reduce periosteal apposition, leaving a smaller bone with a thinner cortex but normal medullary diameter *(top)*. In girls, delayed puberty may result in reduced endocortical apposition, leaving a normal or larger bone (if periosteal apposition continues in the absence of the inhibitory effect of estrogen) with a thinner cortex and larger medullary diameter *(bottom)*. (From Seeman E. Pathogenesis of bone fragility in women and men. *Lancet.* 2002;359:1841-1850.)

rate then decreases, reaching a plateau in the third decade of life.[153]

Quantitative computed tomography (CT) is at present a research technique but provides important information about the material aspects of bone.[154] Although quantitative CT demonstrates an increase in the cortical bone density of the lumbar spine with age, less increase in cancellous bone density with age occurs until the later stages of puberty.

Increased BMD correlates well with height, weight (a main determinant of bone density in adolescent and postpubertal females), age, pubertal development, and BMI but has less relationship with serum IGF-1 levels. Some consider that the concept of age at peak bone density attainment is too simplistic and prefer to consider the strength of the bone and its geometry.[155]

Volumetric bone density (bone mineral apparent density [BMAD]) represents the amount of bone within the periosteal envelope and is of more physiologic importance, because it does not rely on the size of the bone that is changing during growth, particularly pubertal growth (see Fig. 25-15A). Volumetric bone density grows in a region-specific pattern, and conditions in childhood and adolescence that affect the accrual of bone mineral have different effects based on the length of time the affected bone has left to achieve its maximum bone mineral content (BMC); deficits may occur in limb dimensions (prepuberty), spine dimensions (early puberty), or volumetric bone density by interference with mineral accrual (late puberty).[156]

Calculations for BMAD are made as follows:

$$\text{Spine BMAD} = \text{spine BMC} \div (\text{spine area})^{1.5}$$

$$= \text{spine BMC} \div \text{the square root of } (\text{spine area})^3$$

$$\text{Femoral neck BMAD} = \text{femoral neck BMC} \div (\text{femoral neck area})^2$$

$$\text{Whole-body BMAD} = \text{BMC} \div \text{height (cm) as a means of correcting for bone size}$$

The patterns of areal or volumetric bone density differ during development.[157]

DXA device manufacturers do not always provide standards for children and adolescents. Children are often referred for evaluation of osteoporosis because their DXA results are compared with young adult values although they have not come close to reaching maximal bone density. Bone reaches its adult size and PHV occurs before maximal BMC is reached[158]; these factors may result in a period of increased fragility and susceptibility to trauma characteristic of adolescence. Lean body mass (LBM) is related to skeletal density (stronger in boys than girls) and fat mass and skeletal density (stronger in girls than in boys).[159] Standards are available to interpret BMC in terms of LBM, which appears to be better related to normal bone growth than to chronologic age; muscle stress is an important factor in the development of bone.[160] Normative data for pediatric DXA studies are available from various centers.[153,160,161]

An applet available on the Stanford University website generates a Z-score for BMD or BMAD measurements at the lumbar spine (L2-4), hip, or whole body using the Hologic 1000W with respect to the age, gender, and ethnicity of the subject.[162]

Quantitative ultrasound standards are available for children and adolescents.[163] Because they do not require radiation exposure, they may achieve wider use in childhood.

Seeman presented what he considers to be two fallacies in the interpretation of densitometry.[157] The first is the concept that volumetric BMD increases during growth. It does not. Growth builds a bigger, not denser, skeleton. Second is the idea that peak volumetric BMD is higher in men than in women. It is not. Bone size is greater and is underestimated in patients with larger bones than controls. The misconceptions occur because the result of areal bone density is the BMC per unit projected bone area of bone in the coronal plane, or an areal BMC (g/cm²). Too often, the "areal" element is deleted, and "content" is replaced by density, so that BMC per unit projected area is called BMD, even though volumetric bone density is the desired measurement. Although BMC may normally be higher in boys than in girls and rises with development, volumetric bone density of the long bones is identical in boys and girls. In contrast to the long bones, volumetric bone density increases at the spine in both sexes.[153,156,157]

The increase in BMD during the prepubertal and pubertal years reflects the increase in the size of the long bones. Legs grow more rapidly than the trunk in prepubertal girls, but during puberty, there is more truncal growth. Boys develop greater bone size due to increased periosteal apposition (increasing bone strength) and endosteal resorption compared with girls; girls add bone on the endocortical surface, which may serve as a reservoir for calcium for later lactation and pregnancy.[164]

Birth weight, weight gain during infancy, and weight gain during the years 9 through 12 influence bone mass achieved at 21 years.[165] The BMD at the beginning of puberty predicted the peak bone mass at sexual maturity and appeared to predict the likelihood of osteoporosis as an adult in longitudinal studies, suggesting a method of identification of those most in need of intervention[166] (Fig. 25-16). The mechanostat concept posits that developmental changes in bone strength result from the increasing loads imposed by larger muscle forces, which stimulate bone mineral acquisition. In a longitudinal study, a rise in LBM occurred before peak BMC, and fat mass later exerted more influence.[167] Increased physical activity is generally beneficial for bone health, but excessive running, gymnastics, and cheerleading are progressively more likely to lead to stress fractures,[168] and excessive exercise can lead to the

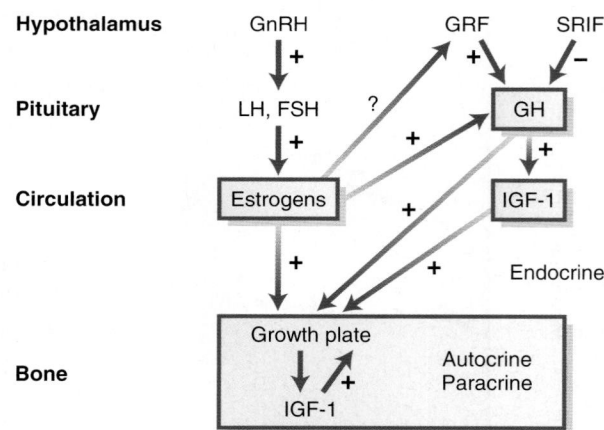

Figure 25-16 Interactions of the major growth-promoting hormones during puberty. Plus (+) indicates stimulatory action; minus (−) indicates inhibitory action. Circulating insulin-like growth factor 1 (IGF-1) arises mainly from liver, but other tissues also contribute (i.e., endocrine action). Growth hormone (GH) and gonadal steroids have a direct stimulatory effect on the generation of IGF-1 (i.e., paracrine action) locally in bone and cartilage cells. For simplification, the feedback loops for IGF-1 and gonadal steroids on the hypothalamic pituitary unit are omitted. FSH, follicle-stimulating hormone; GnRH, gonadotropin-releasing hormone; GRF, growth hormone–releasing factor; LH, luteinizing hormone; SRIF, somatotropin release–inhibiting factor.

female athletic triad (discussed later). Femoral head strength increases markedly during puberty, and the femoral neck increases in density more with impact load sports such as running (compared with active load sports such as swimming); only 3 to 12 minutes of daily exercise increases femoral bone density in early pubertal children,[169] with greater increases occurring during puberty.

Prepubertal girls engaged in gymnastics have increased bone density in the limbs that are more often used, and this occurs in a dose-response manner.[170] A longitudinal study of gymnasts and their mothers found that these effects do not mainly result from genetic influences. Female adolescent athletes have increased bone density, although the effects last only as long as the activity continues.

Calcium intake during puberty has been documented to strongly affect bone density later in life in most studies[150]; the effect of increased ingestion of calcium may last only as long as the calcium is administered. Pubertal girls are estimated to get well below the recommended intake levels, and even recommended levels may be too low for optimal mineralization. Children who avoid dairy products and are without calcium supplementation have an increased prevalence of fractures in the prepubertal period, even with minor trauma.[171] Early pubertal girls cannot increase gastrointestinal calcium absorption enough to compensate for a poor diet, as older individuals may. African-American children retain more calcium than white children do, and the bone structure is thicker in African-American children; the difference in vertebral bone density between ethnic groups appears to develop by late puberty. Randomized, placebo-controlled clinical trials between 1985 and 2005 that enrolled normal children for at least 3 months revealed a small effect of calcium supplementation in the upper limb, but the increase in BMD was not thought to influence the likelihood of a fracture later in life.[172] However, the lack of effects applies only to normal children, and studies of subjects with disorders of puberty that affect bone development may reveal other findings. Remarkably, calcium intake is directly related to the rate of bone age advancement to a degree.[173] Increased sodium intake at the expense of calcium intake adversely affects bone accretion. Adequate zinc intake is another factor related to BMD in puberty.

Vitamin D status is a concern, because 32% of girls with low calcium intake were also vitamin D deficient and had elevated serum concentrations of parathyroid hormone (PTH) and thyroid hormone receptor–associated protein 5b (TRAP-5b), as well as significantly lower cortical volumetric BMD of the distal radius and tibia shaft, and another 46% had low-normal concentrations of vitamin D.[174] Deficient calcium and vitamin D can lead to secondary hyperparathyroidism in adolescence.

Girls with heterozygote ERα genotype (Pp) and high levels of physical activity had significantly higher bone mass, higher BMD, and thicker cortex at loaded bone sites (compared with the distal radius, which is not a weight-bearing bone) than their counterparts[175] with low physical activity. These results suggest that high physical activity benefits those with heterozygous ER genotypes, and the less favorable Pp genotype may be compensated by increasing the amount of leisure-time physical activity at early puberty.

Studies of male athletes are less common than those of girls, but 16- to 19-year-old athletic boys can still gain more bone mass in the spine and femora than nonathletic control subjects.[176] Abnormalities of puberty impair bone accretion in both sexes and are mainly consequences of estrogen deficiency due to decreased secretion or peripheral aromatization of androgens (see Fig. 25-15B). A 1.9-year increase in mean age at menarche in young women was associated with lower radial areal BMD T-scores; lower trabecular number, thickness, and spacing; and cortical thickness without a reduction in cross-sectional area, a finding compatible with less endocortical accrual and a possible explanation of how late menarche is a risk factor for forearm osteoporosis.[177] Urinary adrenal hormone metabolites are related to the achievement of increased proximal radial diaphyseal bone strength; the level of urinary androstenediol at about 8 years of age is an early predictor of diaphyseal bone strength in late puberty (about 16 years of age).[178] Peripheral conversion of adrenarchal dehydroepiandrosterone (DHEA) by 17β-hydroxysteroid dehydrogenase (17β-HSD) to androstenediol may be associated with radial bone accretion during growth.

Testosterone administration to normal prepubertal boys increases calcium retention and bone growth and also increases bone density in adolescents with CDP, testosterone-deficient Klinefelter syndrome, or male hypogonadotropic hypogonadism. Bone density is increased in females with excess androgens, whereas girls with anorexia nervosa, hypothalamic amenorrhea, or ovarian failure have decreased bone density.

Serum levels of inorganic phosphate, alkaline phosphatase, serum osteocalcin (Gla-protein level), collagen type I cross-linked N-terminal telopeptides (NTX),[179] and procollagen type I C-terminal propeptide (PICP); the cross-linked C-terminal telopeptide of type I collagen (ICTP), procollagen type III N-terminal propeptide (P3NP), and tartrate-resistant acid phosphatase isoform 5b; and urinary pyridinoline, deoxypyridinoline, and galactosyl-hydroxylysine excretion reflect the increased osteoblastic activity and growth rate during childhood and pubertal growth in both sexes, with values reaching a peak at midpuberty and decreasing thereafter.[180]

Body Composition

Just as endocrine changes bring about remarkable changes in secondary sexual development and growth, body composition is dramatically affected. GH and gonadal steroids play major roles in this process.[181] LBM, skeletal mass, and body fat are equal in prepubertal boys and girls, but by maturity, men have 1.5 times the LBM and almost 1.5 times the skeletal mass of women, whereas women have twice as much body fat (25%) as men (13%), producing a gynecoid (woman-like) or android (man-like) appearance.[182] LBM increases by the age of 6 years in girls and 9.5 years in boys. Boys acquire fat-free mass more quickly and for a longer period than girls during puberty; stability is attained by 15 to 16 years in girls and 2 to 3 years later in boys.[124] Fat mass increases in girls at an average rate of 1.14 kg/year, but the fat mass does not change in boys during the pubertal years, leading to the greater fat value in girls than boys with age.[124]

The generalized distribution of fat in males (central fat, apple-shaped, android), which is different from that in females (lower body fat predominance, pear-shaped, gynecoid), develops largely during puberty as males become more android than they were in prepuberty, although girls start and remain gynecoid. There are ethnic differences in the pattern of change, and Asians have the most significant changes.[183]

A strength spurt occurs during puberty after the pubertal growth spurt. Muscle mass is 54% of body weight in adolescent boys and 42% of body weight in adolescent girls, with the difference partly due to the presence of more muscle cells and larger muscle cells in men. There is little gender difference before 8 years of age, but by 14 years, boys usually have developed greater lean leg mass and greater power than girls.[184]

Obesity, Puberty, and the Metabolic Syndrome

Between NHANES II and NHANES III, a period of roughly 20 years, there was more than a tripling of the prevalence of children and adolescents above the 95th percentile in weight (denoted by the CDC as overweight), to a prevalence of 17.1%, and a 50% increase in those above the 85th percentile (denoted as at risk for overweight).[185]

Weight is not an adequate reflection of body fat. The BMI is now invoked in describing the shape of the body in age-adjusted terms and is used as a better, if imperfect, reflection of body fat in childhood and adolescence.[28] BMI changes with age, and there is no specific number indicating normal or abnormal BMI at all stages of development, as there is for adults. Reference charts of BMI compared with age and gender between the 3rd and 97th percentiles are available online for interpretation of BMI values.[186]

Increased visceral fat (i.e., intra-abdominal adipose tissue, or IAAT) in obese teenagers is associated with hypertriglyceridemia, decreased high-density lipoprotein (HDL) cholesterol, and small, dense, cholesterol-laden very low-density lipoprotein (VLDL) particles. Subcutaneous fat is associated with large, lipid-laden VLDL particles, which are removed directly from the circulation and pose less risk. The subcutaneous adipose tissue that leads to visibly different body forms is only an imperfect reflection of this internal distribution of fat cells, because increased IAAT may cause metabolic derangements without increasing total-body fat. Studies support the role of increased intra-abdominal fat in children as a cause of insulin resistance and dyslipidemia, with small adipocytes demonstrating limited storage ability, leading to increased ectopic fat deposition in myocytes and hepatocytes.[187,188] Waist-to-hip ratios may not reflect IAAT in children and adolescents, because subcutaneous abdominal fat may be low despite increased visceral fat.[187] Although there is interest in waist circumference in children as a reflection of IAAT and standards are available there is question if the waist circumference adds to the determination of IAAT more than BMI alone.[189]

DXA is used to determine the percentage of body fat, water, and bone mineral with great accuracy but cannot differentiate visceral from subcutaneous adipose tissue. CT was used until the validation of MRI to determine intra-abdominal and subcutaneous fat distribution without the use of radiation. Excessive body fat during childhood and adolescence has significant medical effects early and later in life. Obesity, glucose intolerance, and hypertension in childhood are strongly associated with increased rates of premature death among Native Americans, but childhood hypercholesterolemia is not.[190]

Serum Lipids in Normal Puberty and in Obesity and the Metabolic Syndrome. In normal puberty, testosterone increases serum levels of LDL-cholesterol and decreases HDL-cholesterol concentrations, accounting for the adverse LDL/HDL ratio in men compared with women.[191] Postheparin hepatic lipase activity is increased by exogenous androgens (and decreased by estrogens), accounting for the decrease in HDL after androgen treatment or after a rise in endogenous androgen secretion. Standards for lipid levels in childhood differ from adult values.[192]

The epidemic of obesity has led to the advent of the metabolic syndrome in youth. Diagnosis of metabolic syndrome varies among studies, and a generally accepted definition is needed.[193] Elevated cholesterol levels in children and adolescents track to adult values in longitudinal studies. Although familial hypercholesterolemia leads to carotid intimal plaques by puberty, random autopsies demonstrate macroscopic or microscopic evidence of arteriosclerosis in normal youth without familial hypercholesterolemia, and the tendency is increased by obesity. By 15 to 19 years, 2% of autopsied males had advanced (American Heart Association grade 4 or 5) atherosclerotic coronary artery lesions associated with increased serum cholesterol, obesity, and hypertension.[194]

Insulin and Insulin Resistance. Insulin resistance is a hallmark of obesity and is thought to be the cause of or an associated factor in the metabolic syndrome associated with cardiac disease.[195] Euglycemic clamp techniques are the gold standard for measurement of insulin resistance. Fasting insulin concentrations offer little insight into insulin resistance in an individual, and equations such as the homeostatic model assessment (HOMA) that are based on fasting insulin levels offer little more; however, fasting insulin values are used in epidemiologic studies and offer more useful information.[196] The fasting insulin concentration increases twofold to threefold with PHV, insulin secretion after a glucose load increases over prepubertal levels, and insulin-mediated glucose disposal in peripheral tissues decreases in the hyperinsulinemic euglycemic clamp or the minimal model frequently sampled intravenous glucose tolerance test (IVGTT), showing increased insulin resistance during normal puberty. Insulin sensitivity is inversely related to pubertal stage and BMI.

The response of insulin to an oral glucose tolerance test is greater in African-American subjects than in white subjects at all stages of pubertal development; this ethnic difference in insulin resistance is suggested as a cause for the increased incidence of type 2 diabetes among African-American adults compared with white adults and appears to offer a similar explanation of the ethnic disparity in youth, with white teenagers having greater insulin sensitivity than African-American or Hispanic youth.[197,198] Insulin resistance occurs early in the course of Turner syndrome and thalassemia major, but even in Turner syndrome, in which there is an underlying increase in insulin resistance, there seems to be low or no risk of these conditions developing with GH treatment.

With the increased prevalence of type 2 diabetes (non–insulin-dependent diabetes mellitus, or NIDDM), proposed screening criteria are being evaluated. Currently, children with a BMI higher than the 85th percentile should be screened if they (1) have a family history of type 1 diabetes, (2) have signs of insulin resistance (e.g., acanthosis nigricans, functional ovarian hyperandrogenism, hypertension, dyslipidemia), or (3) belong to one of several specific ethnic groups (e.g., African American, Native American, Hispanic American, Asian American). If a fasting plasma glucose level is higher than 126 mg/dL or a 2-hour postprandial value is higher than 200 mg/dL, or if there are symptoms such as weight loss, polyuria, or polydipsia and a casual plasma glucose level is higher than 200 mg/dL, the diagnosis of diabetes is likely, and determination of the type of diabetes (type 1 or 2) is appropriate.

Patients with type 1 diabetes (insulin-dependent diabetes mellitus, or IDDM) usually require an increase in the dose of insulin for euglycemic control at puberty. The cause of insulin resistance has been attributed in part to increased fat oxidation at puberty, which correlates with rising serum IGF-1 levels and may be linked to increased GH secretion. However, there is no evidence that GH treatment alone increases the likelihood of development of type 2 diabetes or impaired glucose tolerance. Weight gain increases in children with type 1 diabetes during puberty, leading to a higher incidence of obesity in children with IDDM than would be expected from family patterns. Some adolescents with IDDM, predominantly girls, reduce their insulin use in order to lose weight, with dire consequences. Retinopathy due to IDDM characteristically appears in the teenage years or later, but duration and control of diabetes in the prepubertal years are contributing factors. The American Diabetes Association recommends screening for microalbuminuria, an indicator of the development of diabetic nephropathy during puberty.

A normal individual adapts to the changes in the physiologic rise in pubertal insulin resistance, but an individual at genetic risk for type 2 diabetes, with the accompanying defect in pancreatic beta cell function,[199] may not adapt to the insulin resistance and, with the additional insulin resistance characteristic of obesity, may develop clinical type 2 diabetes during the pubertal years or earlier. Type 2 diabetes in children or adolescents should not be confused with the various forms of monogenetic diabetes (previously called maturity-onset diabetes of the young, MODY), which are inherited as autosomal dominant traits.[200]

Although PCOS is common, several rare syndromes of severe insulin resistance combine hyperglycemia and virilization.[201] The Kahn type A syndrome features include a lean, muscular adolescent female phenotype with acanthosis nigricans, hirsutism, oligomenorrhea or amenorrhea, and ovarian hyperthecosis and stromal hyperplasia associated with abnormalities of the insulin receptor gene. Hyperandrogenism, insulin resistance, acanthosis nigricans (HAIR-AN) syndrome, and PCOS are less severe than Kahn type A and usually manifest in adolescent females. Persons with Rabson-Mendenhall syndrome have severe insulin resistance (possibly leading to diabetic ketoacidosis), dysmorphic facies, acanthosis nigricans, thickened nails, hirsutism, dental dysplasia, abdominal distention, and phallic or clitoral enlargement. The Rabson-Mendenhall syndrome, similar to the Donahue (leprechaunism) syndrome, which shares some of these features, is caused by homozygous or compound heterozygote defects in the insulin receptor gene. Kahn type B syndrome is caused by inhibitory or stimulatory antibodies to the insulin receptor gene and sometimes occurs with acanthosis nigricans and ovarian hyperandrogenism. This syndrome can occur with ataxia-telangiectasia syndrome or in otherwise normal adolescents. Individuals with the Berardinelli-Seip syndrome combine lipodystrophy and severe insulin resistance and complete or partial absence of subcutaneous fat with increased growth and skeletal maturation, muscle hypertrophy, acanthosis nigricans, hypertrichosis, organomegaly, and mild hypertrophy of the external genitalia.

Most of these NIDDM syndromes can be treated with oral hypoglycemic agents initially; progression of the disorder may require the use of insulin. Several girls with these syndromes of insulin resistance have been described to have low serum gonadotropin values during puberty without response to GnRH but with enlarged ovaries, suggesting a direct role for insulin in stimulating the growth of the ovary. The hypoleptinemic state found in various degrees of lipodystrophy does not appear to affect pubertal progression, but administration of leptin has led to resumption of menstrual periods in some females and adjustment of testosterone production toward normal levels in males.[202]

Blood Pressure. Blood pressure is related to the age, gender, and height of the child using appropriate standards.[203] Blood pressure increases with pubertal maturation, related to increased stature and synchronized with the pubertal growth spurt, suggesting some relationship in the control of the two processes.[204] Hypertension is becoming common in puberty as a comorbid condition of obesity. Increased blood pressure at puberty depends on BMI and height,

factors that are interrelated. Blood pressure in childhood and adolescence is predictive of adult blood pressure (tracking). Blood pressure rises in African-American children at lower BMIs than in white children, making the problem worse in the African-American population. In sexual precocity, blood pressure rises above prepubertal levels to values commensurate with body size and BMI.

CENTRAL NERVOUS SYSTEM ANATOMY, FUNCTION, PSYCHOLOGY, AND ELECTROENCEPHALOGRAPHIC RHYTHM IN PUBERTY

Brain anatomy and function change substantially during late childhood and adolescence (Fig. 25-17). Behavior or psychopathology that becomes evident at this time has its basis in these changes and exposures dating from early life and the prenatal period, all interacting against a genetic background. Puberty is the time of appearance of the ability to solve complex problems in a mature manner. An increase in cortical metabolic rate in infancy is followed by a late childhood decline to adult levels; this decline ceases by the end of the second decade. The prefrontal association cortex, an area of the brain that is concerned with forward planning and regulatory control of emotional behavior, continues to develop until the age of 20 to 25 years.[205] Stress at various stages of development, even in early childhood, may cause psychological manifestations during puberty.

The anatomic changes revealed by functional MRI studies of the prefrontal cortex, an area that is involved with emotional regulation and planning, occur during a time of physical maturation and are likely to relate to many of the characteristic behavior changes of puberty. The volume of white matter increases linearly between 4 and 22 years of age owing to an increase in myelination during development.[206] A reduction in cortical synaptic density and neuronal density, analogous to programmed cell death, occurs between 2 and 16 years of age, and this pruning of synapses appears to be linked to improved memory. This change in gray matter follows an inverted U-shaped curve of increase from the age of 6 years. Longitudinal studies using dynamic mapping of human cortical development demonstrate that higher order association cortices (e.g., those involved in executive function, attention, and motor coordination) mature after lower-order somatosensory, motor, and visual cortices mature, and those areas that are phylogenetically older mature before newer ones.[207,208] Intrauterine excess of androgens leads to enlargement of the amygdala, and girls reach greater mass of gray matter 2 years before boys during puberty, demonstrating aspects of the effects of sex steroids on brain growth and remodeling in human beings. Increased LH levels are related to areas of increased white matter density, including the cingulum, middle temporal gyrus, and splenium of the corpus callosum; there is a genetic overlay to this relationship. Gray matter volume, at least in girls, appears to be related to a pubertal increase in estradiol[209] levels.

Brain plasticity decreases during puberty. Examples include the inability to learn to speak a foreign language without an accent after puberty and recovery of a child from the effects of a CNS injury that in an adult might have led to aphasia. Loss of plasticity may be maladaptive to our rapidly changing world and extended life span compared with prehistoric times.[210] Plasticity allowed developmental learning before puberty, but lack of plasticity and a standard response to conditions in the adult allowed success in that static environment of the past.

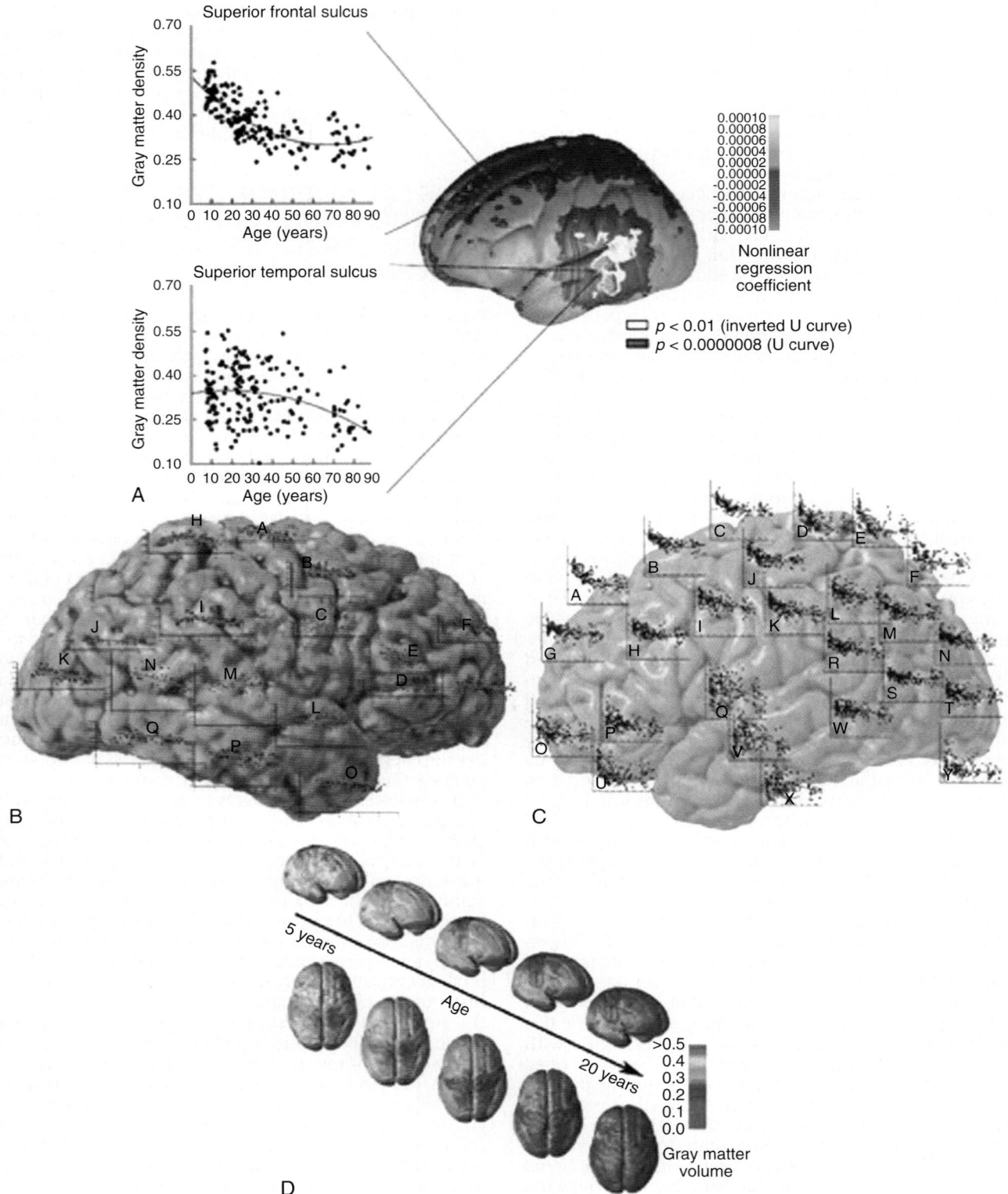

Figure 25-17 Mapping brain change over time. Brain changes in development can be identified by fitting time-dependent statistical models to data collected from subjects cross-sectionally (i.e., across a group of subjects at a particular time) or longitudinally (i.e., following individual subjects as they aged), or both. Measurements such as cortical thickness are then plotted onto the cortex using a color code. Trajectory of gray matter loss over the human life span is based on a cohort of 176 subjects between 7 and 78 years of age.[8] **A** represents a region in which the gray matter density decreases rapidly during adolescence (i.e., superior frontal sulcus in which the decrease in gray matter is described by a quadratic equation represented by an inverted U-shaped curve), or follows a more steadily declining time course during the life span (i.e., superior temporal sulcus in which the decrease in gray matter is described by a quadratic equation represented by a U-shaped curve). In **B** and **C**, plots superimposed on the brain show how gray matter density decreases for particular regions with age, with the regions denoted by different letters. Brain maturation and change in gray matter density is mapped by year of age in **D** with fractional change in gray matter shown by color coding (**C** and **D**). (From Sowell ER, Peterson BS, Thompson PM, et al. Mapping cortical change across the human life span. *Nat Neurosci.* 2003;6:309-315; Toga AW, Thompson PM, Sowell ER. Mapping brain maturation. *Trends Neurosci.* 2006;29:146-159.)

Mania, depression, obsessive-compulsive disorders, and schizophrenia are more common after puberty. They are postulated to be related to alterations of the normal changes in brain architecture and function that occur during puberty.

Sleep Patterns in Puberty

Increased sleep is characteristic of the period of growth and development across species. Because sleep is a time of vulnerability, threats leading to stress are antithetical to normal sleep, and a feeling of safety is thought to be necessary to allow sleep to proceed normally as the adolescent is preparing for independence and increased self-care in a possibly hostile world. Rising complexity of brain function during puberty is reflected in increases in the amplitude and frequency of delta waves (0- to 3-Hz electroencephalographic waves) found during deep sleep, which appears more related to age than to pubertal development or growth.[211] The function of deep sleep (i.e., slow-wave or non–rapid eye movement sleep) is thought to be restorative to learning and other activities of the waking state, and the most restorative portion is high-amplitude delta-wave sleep. During adolescence, the time spent in deep (stage 4) sleep declines by 40% to 50%, and increased (19.7%) stage 2 sleep occurs with pubertal development. The decline of slow-wave sleep during adolescence may reflect developmental changes of the brain.

When an individual is allowed to "run free," the period is entrained (synchronized) close to the earth's 24-hour light-dark cycle. Because human beings had little to do after dark, evolution favored an early bedtime, but within this schedule, developmental changes occur. One-year-old infants sleep an average of 11 hours per day, and by age 18, if circumstances permit, the mean is 8 hours. Older people have earlier waking times and rate themselves as more morning-like than adolescents or young adults; because children are also morning-like, there is an inverted U-shaped curve of preferred times of awakening across the span of development.[212] This change to evening from morning alertness during puberty appears to be related to biologic factors, in contrast to social factors; in the past, social factors were thought to be more important.

Without the pressure of work or school, adolescents would stay up longer and awaken hours later than a normal weekday schedule would dictate, a schedule far different from the one they followed at a younger age. Adolescents with early school starts awaken earlier than those with later school starts, but they do not change the time they go to sleep, leading to great variation in the amount of sleep attained. Data from the Add Health study showed decreased self-reported sleep duration during self-reported pubertal development, with girls reporting more problems with sleep (e.g., insomnia, insufficient sleep, awakening tired) as puberty progressed but with no such relationship seen in boys.[213] There is an increase in daytime sleepiness during adolescence, particularly during midpuberty up to stage 3 to 4, even if total sleep time is held constant during longitudinal multiple-year studies.[214] With voluntary sleep deprivation (e.g., with late-night homework habits), sleepiness can reach levels seen in narcolepsy and sleep apnea. Adolescents adapt more poorly to changes in sleep patterns than other age groups; this is manifested in the difference in hours awake between the school week and the weekend. Adolescents are able to shift to a later schedule more easily than to an earlier schedule. When self-selected bedtimes are late during summer but have to be changed to allow school attendance, the adjustment is particularly lengthy and difficult.

After study of 27,000 individuals, it was proposed that the point of inflection from evening alertness during adolescence (after a morning-like pattern in childhood) to morning alertness in adulthood might be used as a marker of the end of adolescence, a sign that developmental remodeling of brain pathways is completed.[215] The age of this inflection point is about 20.9 years in males and 19.5 years in females, who have an earlier change in this and other aspects of puberty than males (Fig. 25-18).

Characteristics of Adolescence

Most of this chapter deals with the biochemical and physical changes of the period we denote as puberty, but there are also profound psychosocial changes during this period, usually denoted as adolescence. Although the attainment of an adult role in society occurs within a few years after achievement of reproductive maturity in non-Western societies, the more technologically advanced the society, the more protracted the time allowed for adolescent psychosocial development. The prolonged period of adolescence in current society, ranging from 11 to 20 years in the United States, arose recently in human history, beginning no more than 100 years ago in Western society.

As expressed by Remschmidt, the most important psychological and psychosocial changes in adolescence are the emergence of abstract thinking, the growing ability to absorb the perspectives or viewpoints of others, an increased capacity for introspection, the development of personal and sexual identity, the establishment of a system of values, increasing autonomy from family and personal independence, greater importance of peer relationships of sometimes subcultural quality, and the emergence of skills and coping strategies to overcome problems and crises.[216]

Adolescence may be divided into three periods (early, middle, and late) by chronologic age. However, these periods may be reached at different maturational ages, because rates of physiologic maturation differ among individuals in these age groups.[217]

Early adolescence (age 11 to 15 years) encompasses most of the physical changes of puberty and in American society includes a profound social change from the sheltered, single-classroom environment of elementary school to the multiple-classroom and multiple-teacher experience of middle school or junior high school. The individual develops a maturing, but not mature, capacity for abstract thought and decision-making processes in contrast to the concrete reasoning of childhood.

Middle adolescence (ages 15 to 17 years) is the period of the high school years, a calmer period than early adolescence. The school experience is not a striking change, and many of the most prominent biologic and physical changes of puberty have been accomplished. There is acceptance of some increased autonomy (e.g., drivers' permits and licenses are allowed), but the individual still lives at home. The individual emotionally moves away from the family and is less influenced by his or her peer group than are early adolescents; friendships assume an increasingly important role.

Late adolescence starts at the senior year of high school and is the age of acceptance of adult roles in work, family, and community. If the individual attends college, this stage is prolonged.

Behavior and Normal Puberty

Almost 100 years ago, G. Stanley Hall, without using what would be considered contemporary research techniques, characterized the maturing child as experiencing Sturm

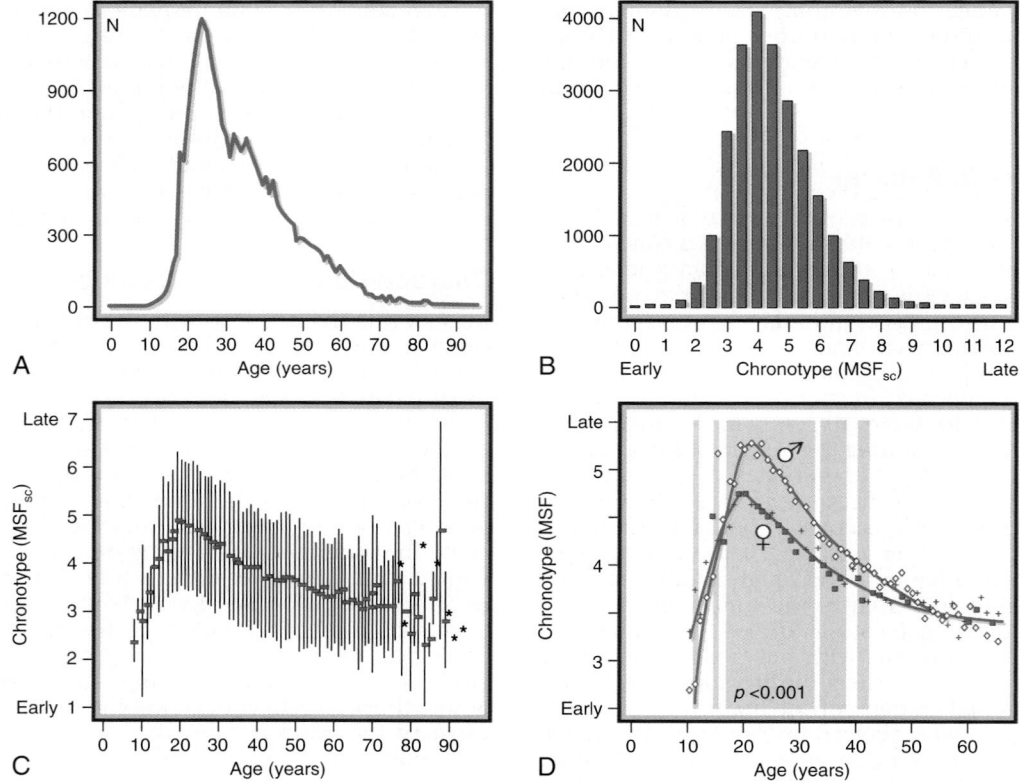

Figure 25-18 Assessment of chronotype (time of awakening in the absence of external cues) using the MCTQ database ($N \approx 25,000$). Age distribution within the database (**A**). Distribution of chronotypes (**B**). Age-dependent changes (**C**) in average chronotype (± SD [standard deviation]) are highly systematic (except for the age groups of 19, 21, 22, and 23, all other age-dependent averages ± SD are significantly different from that of age group 20; t-test, $p < 0.001$). Age-dependent changes of the chronotype (**D**) are different for males and females (*filled circles and black line*: females; *open circles* and *gray line*: males). Gray areas indicate significant male-female differences (t-test, $p < 0.001$). (From Roenneberg T, Kuehnle T, Pramstaller PP, et al. A marker for the end of adolescence. *Curr Biol.* 2004;14:R1038-R1039.)

und Drang (i.e., storm and stress), which is normally restrained by cultural influences.[218] Contrary to this view, most recent empiric studies describe adolescent development as a continuous, adaptive phase of emotional growth characterized more by stability rather than disorder and more by harmonious relationships between generations rather than conflict. Although mood changes are normally more rapid (occurring over hours or days) and marked in teenagers than in adults, these shifts must be differentiated from long-standing mood and behavior changes associated with serious psychopathology.

Turmoil, or truly tumultuous behavior, in adolescence is not a normal phase but may reflect psychopathology that requires diagnosis and treatment. It is often misdiagnosed as a temporary problem of adjustment reactions of adolescence. When the conditions extend from adolescence to the adult stage, they are more severe. A 4-year longitudinal study of normal first-year U.S. high school students showed that 25% experienced continuous growth, characterized by smooth, well-adjusted functioning despite stressful situations; 34% experienced surgent growth, demonstrating good adaptation in general and short periods of difficulty and distress after some stressful situations. Twenty-one percent were judged to be in turmoil, characterized by mood swings, anxiety, and depression; these teenagers mainly came from homes characterized by conflict, familial mental illness, and socioeconomic distress.[219] Many with adolescent turmoil had not "grown out of it" when studied 5 years later and eventually were diagnosed with unipolar and bipolar depressive disorders. It may be concluded that 80% to 90% of adolescents do well

psychologically during puberty and are happy individuals, but 10% to 20% have significant difficulties.

Mood and Self-Image in Puberty

Young girls at the beginning of puberty frequently exhibit a negative self-image but a positive body image; positive peer relationships and superior adjustment improvement are observed with continued breast development. Mood in adolescence is not closely related to stage of puberty, but a significant curvilinear trend is seen for depressive affect (i.e., an increase followed by a decrease), for impulse control (a decrease followed by an increase), and according to the level of serum estradiol. These data suggest that hormonal changes may be more important than physical changes as determinants of certain mood and behavior patterns during adolescence.

Behavior in Variations of the Normal Age at Onset of Puberty

Within the normal limits of pubertal development, early-maturing girls and late-maturing boys have the greatest prevalence of adjustment reactions in puberty and thereafter. Boys and girls who mature earlier are at increased risk for abuse.[220]

Early-developing boys are perceived to be more mature, attractive, and smart and are given more leadership roles; late-developing boys are more insecure, more susceptible to lower levels of self-esteem and body image, and more vulnerable to peer pressure, especially in working-class and minority groups. Most of these difficulties of late maturation focus on the decreased height of the individual rather than the lack of sexual development. Social maturation lags even after androgen treatment in patients with severe CDP. Delayed social maturation may put boys at risk for missing educational opportunities.

In contrast, early-maturing girls tend to experience more difficulty, especially in the junior high school setting, where they may attract the attention of older, more mature boys and have a higher prevalence of internalizing symptoms and disorders. Early puberty may lead to negative body image in girls, compared with boys, in whom the effect is positive. Early maturation may increase a propensity to violent behavior, which is fostered by living in a disadvantaged neighborhood. Early pubertal maturation in girls may be related to a small intelligence quotient (IQ) advantage over late-maturing girls. Late-maturing girls are often more comfortable, remaining with the support of their families longer, and they are less often brought to medical attention than late-maturing boys. Early- and late-maturing girls have a tendency to engage in health-risking behaviors involving strategies to lose weight, strategies to increase muscle, disordered eating, use of food supplements and steroids, and exercise dependence—tendencies not found in boys at the same developmental stages.

Risk-Taking Behavior

Adolescents who function at lower levels of cognitive complexity or concrete thinking and have an early onset of puberty demonstrate an increase in risk-taking behavior. The age at onset of cigarette smoking and alcohol use is proportional to the age at onset of puberty in girls: early-maturing girls partake earlier, and boys may follow the same pattern.

Sexuality During Puberty

The percentage of adolescents who have had sex rises from less than 2% by 12 years of age, 16% by age 15, 33% by 16, 48% by 17, 61% by 18, and 71% by 19-year-olds for either sex. Teenagers are waiting longer to have sex than they did in the recent past. Factors such as the onset of puberty, weak self-concept, having tried smoking or drinking, and not being overweight were significantly associated with early sexual activity in girls. For boys, older age, a poor relationship with parents, low household income, and having tried smoking were factors significantly associated with sexual activity. Add Health revealed that adolescents at the upper and lower ends of the intelligence distribution were less likely to have sex.

Fertility is reached well before adult phenotype is acquired in boys and girls. The number of pregnancies for U.S. girls aged 15 to 19 years is 41.5 per 1000.[221] Sexuality appears to be correlated with testosterone production in boys in some studies, but in others, it appears to be modified by the social effects of pubertal maturation. Religious activity may decrease the likelihood of sexual activity.

The social pressures are more mixed in their messages to girls, both encouraging sexuality and restricting it in a way more disparate than that encountered by boys. The earlier onset of puberty today compared with previous centuries has had a profound effect on societal norms of sexual behavior.[3]

A randomized, double-blind, placebo-controlled, cross-over clinical trial of boys and girls with delayed puberty addressing the effects of administration of oral conjugated estrogen to girls and testosterone enanthate to boys at three dose levels that were intended to simulate early,

middle, and late pubertal levels demonstrated modest or no effects. Boys had increased nocturnal emission and touching behaviors at the middle and high doses but no other effects. Girls demonstrated a significant increase in necking related to the administration of estrogen only at the late pubertal dose and no other effects.

HORMONAL AND METABOLIC CHANGES IN PUBERTY

Increased amplitude and alterations of the patterns of GnRH secretion at puberty initiate and regulate the sequential increases in secretion of pituitary gonadotropins and gonadal steroids that culminate in fertility.

Gonadotropins

Because of the pulsatile secretion of GnRH, gonadotropin secretion is also episodic. The newer immunometric supersensitive assays allow accurate measurement in small pediatric samples. The results are lower than previously reported by the older assays.

During the first 2 years after birth, plasma levels of LH and FSH rise intermittently to adult values and occasionally higher but then remain low until puberty. Ultrasensitive assays and third-generation assays for LH and FSH confirm earlier evidence of pulsatile secretion of the gonadotropins in prepuberty and indicate that the basal immunoreactive levels of LH are much lower than previously reported.[222,223] The serum FSH level is higher than the LH level in prepubertal boys and girls.[224] There is a more striking rise in serum LH amplitude by at least 1 year before the onset of puberty (i.e., the peripubertal period immediately preceding the appearance of signs of sexual maturation) that reaches an early plateau, whereas FSH rises more consistently through male puberty rather than before, with increased pulse amplitude. An increased amplitude of LH and FSH secretion occurs at night in prepubertal boys and girls by 5 years of age; the amplitude and frequency of such peaks increase, and daytime secretion increases with the progression of pubertal development.

In girls, FSH levels rise during the early stages of puberty, and LH levels tend to rise in the later stages; from beginning to late puberty, the LH concentration rises more than 100-fold (Figs. 25-19 and 25-20).

Disorderly patterns of secretion of LH, but not FSH, were noted just before the onset of puberty; this was followed by, first, increased orderliness in early puberty and, then, increased disorderliness again in later puberty. This suggests that a more integrated feedback system operates in early puberty and is then followed by less stability.[225]

Doses of exogenous GnRH that are relatively ineffective in stimulating gonadotropin or gonadal steroid secretion before puberty become effective with the onset of puberty; an amplification occurs in the hypothalamic-pituitary-gonadal axis with progression of puberty.[226] Although the GnRH or GnRH agonist test usually requires multiple sampling after the administration of GnRH, a single determination at 60 or 24 minutes now suffices with the new, sensitive assays.[227-230] The basal values of serum LH and FSH measured in modern supersensitive assays are reported to predict the onset of pubertal development as well as GnRH testing does; a value of serum LH greater than 4 mIU/mL measured by immunochemiluminometric (ICMA) assay is consistent with the onset of puberty. Moreover, the use of these ultrasensitive assays to determine concentrations of LH and FSH in urine reveals a pattern of a fivefold rise in

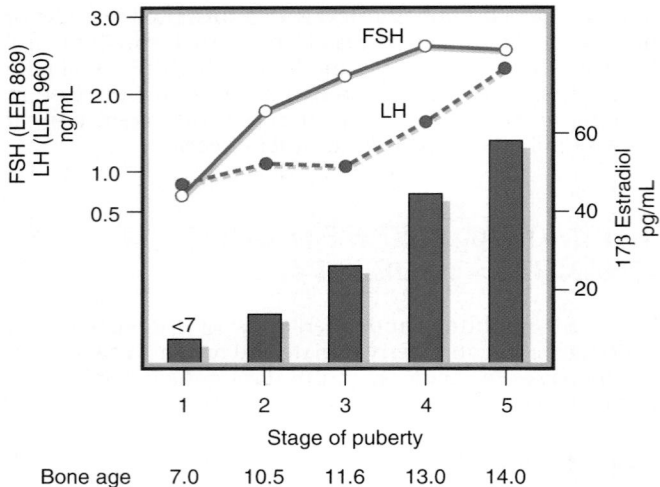

Figure 25-19 Mean plasma estradiol, follicle-stimulating hormone (FSH), and luteinizing hormone (LH) concentrations in prepubertal and pubertal females by pubertal stage of maturation (1, prepubertal; 5, menstruating adolescents) and the mean bone age for each stage. Single daytime values of gonadotropins have limited usefulness because of pulsatility of gonadotropin release and the increased amplitude of LH pulses during sleep throughout puberty. The gonadal steroid values, however, are useful in determining the stage of pubertal development. To convert FSH values (LER-869) to international units per liter, multiply by 8.4. To convert LH values (LER-960) to international units per liter, multiply by 3.8. To convert estradiol values to picomoles per liter, multiply by 3.671. (From Grumbach MM. Onset of puberty. In: Berenberg SR, ed. *Puberty, Biologic and Social Components.* Leiden, The Netherlands: H.E. Stenfert Kroese; 1975:1-21. Reprinted by permission of Kluwer Academic Publishers.)

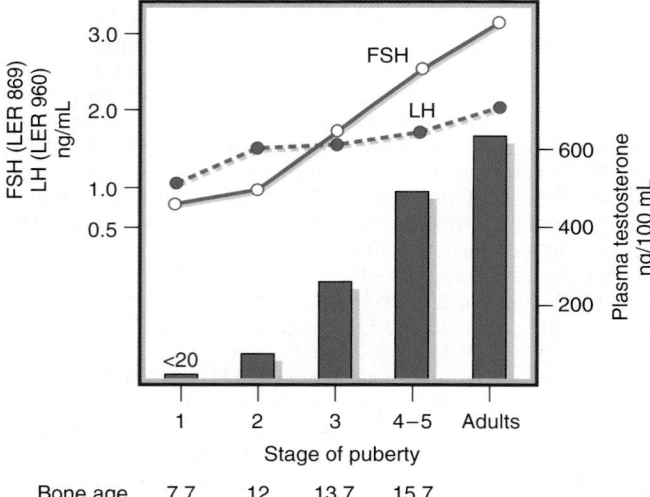

Figure 25-20 Mean plasma testosterone (after solvent extraction and chromatography) and gonadotropin levels in normal boys by stage of maturation (1, prepubertal) and mean bone age for each stage (see Fig. 25-19). To convert testosterone values to nanomoles per liter, multiply by 0.03467. (From Grumbach MM. Onset of puberty. In: Berenberg SR, ed. *Puberty, Biologic and Social Components.* Leiden, The Netherlands: H.E. Stenfert Kroese; 1975:1-21. Reprinted by permission of Kluwer Academic Publishers.)

urinary FSH in boys and girls, with a 50-fold rise in urinary LH in boys and a 100-fold rise in girls during puberty.[231]

In addition to the well-defined quantitative changes that occur in the pattern of FSH and LH in the pituitary gland, serum, and urine during development, qualitative changes occur. The pattern of glycosylation of the α- and the β-subunits of the gonadotropins is influenced by

maturation, GnRH secretion, and the effects of gonadal steroids on the pituitary gonadotrophs. Variation in glycosylation that affects the size and charge of the hormone is the principal cause of the heterogeneity of FSH and LH and the large number of isoforms that vary according to the more acidic or more basic charge.[232] This pleomorphism has an important effect on biologic half-life and biologic activity and provides an additional mechanism of regulating the biologic activity of the gonadotropins. Discrepancies between serum bioactivity and immunoactivity of LH during pubertal development have been reported by some but not all researchers. However, a change in the isoforms of FSH released during puberty may favor the secretion of increased bioactive FSH, which may favor reproductive development.[232]

Gonadal Steroids

Only recently has it been appreciated that many actions on linear skeletal growth, skeletal maturation, and accretion of bone mass thought to be due to testosterone in the male are mainly attributable to its peripheral aromatization to estrogen (Table 25-7).

Testosterone

The Leydig cells of the testes produce testosterone and, in lesser amounts, androstenedione, α5-androstenediol, dihydrotestosterone, and estradiol, although a small amount of testosterone is derived from extraglandular conversion of androstenedione secreted by the testes and the adrenal. In the female, extraglandular conversion of ovarian and adrenal androstenedione accounts for almost all of the circulating testosterone.

Previous methods of determination of low levels of sex steroids have been demonstrated to be inaccurate.[233,234]

This insensitivity is mainly due to the presence of interfering substances and relative insensitivity of antibodies used in assays. Now, larger national laboratories are beginning to use HPLC-MS/MS, which allows the accurate measurement of extremely low values present in pediatric samples.[235] These newer techniques may lead to revision of some of the results (described here) obtained by older methods. Measurement of testosterone and estradiol by HPLC-MS/MS in laboratories with pediatric standards is the preferred method to measure gonadal steroids to investigate disorders of puberty.

Prepubertal boys and girls have plasma testosterone concentrations of less than 0.3 nmol/L except during the first 3 to 5 months of infancy in the male, when pubertal levels are found. Nighttime elevations of serum testosterone levels are detectable in the male by 5 years of age, before the onset of physical signs of puberty, and increase during early puberty after the appearance of sleep-entrained secretion of LH and increased pituitary sensitivity to GnRH. The 60-minute lag between the peak of LH and the increase in testosterone is presumably due to synthesis and secretion of the steroid. In the daytime, increases in testosterone levels are detectable after the testis volume is greater than 4 mL, with a consistent increase throughout puberty. The steepest increment in testosterone concentration occurs between pubertal stages 2 and 3 in males (see Fig. 25-20 and Table 25-5). The ratio of testosterone to epitestosterone in the urine, which is used to evaluate doping of athletes, may be elevated normally during puberty.

Free testosterone measurements may be determined by dialysis or by calculation using testosterone values and available protein binding sites; the accuracy of the testosterone assay can be problematic.[235] Nonetheless, if the total testosterone concentration on which the free testosterone level is based is measured by a highly specific assay, free or bioavailable testosterone determinations are helpful in evaluation of PCOS or nonclassic congenital adrenal hyperplasia (CAH) in girls.

A sensitive mammalian cell recombinant bioassay for androgen bioactivity strongly correlates with serum immunoreactive testosterone concentration and demonstrates a rise with pubertal development in concert with progression of pubic hair and penile development in patients with CDP.[236] In contrast to this specific bioassay, a novel, highly sensitive transcriptional androgen receptor (AR)-mediated bioassay system demonstrated higher circulating values of bioactive androgen in menopausal women and may be directed toward children in he future.[237]

The values of sex steroids measured in saliva are much lower than in the serum, but trauma (even tooth brushing) that leads to blood in the specimen can influence the results, and the accuracy of the basic assay is critical (see earlier discussion).[235] The steroid level in saliva is not a direct representation of free steroid in the serum, as is often claimed. Testosterone in saliva is said in some reports to correlate well with serum levels of testosterone in normal subjects and in patients with chronic disease (e.g., cystic fibrosis). Salivary progesterone is said to rise with the progression of puberty. Salivary DHEA is higher after the onset of puberty than before. Salivary steroid measurements, if accurate, can increase the ability of investigators to address the relationship between development and behavior in a noninvasive manner, but it may take the use of LC/MS-MS in salivary assays to achieve such accuracy.

Estrogens

In the female, estradiol is secreted principally (90%) by the ovary; a small fraction of circulating estradiol arises from the extraglandular conversion of testosterone and androstenedione. In the male, approximately 75% of estradiol is derived from extraglandular aromatization of testosterone and (indirectly) androstenedione, and 25% is from testicular secretion.

In the fetus and at term, estrogen is high due to conversion of fetal and maternal adrenal C19-steroids to estrogen by the placenta, but they drop precipitously during the first few days of life. Plasma estradiol levels are so low in prepuberty that detection by standard immunoassays is difficult, but a rise through puberty and a diurnal rhythm is seen with a sensitive radioimmunoassay (Table 25-8; see Fig. 25-19). Estrone levels rise early and reach a plateau by midpuberty. A highly sensitive bioassay demonstrated higher estradiol concentrations in girls than in boys before puberty, with a rise through puberty until the pubertal growth spurt and a decrease thereafter. There is a significant correlation between peak growth velocity and the rise in estradiol concentration; the rise is earlier in girls than in boys, but bioactive estradiol levels are equivalent at peak growth velocity.[134,238] The higher estrogen levels in girls may be an important factor in the more advanced levels of skeletal maturation in girls compared with boys and may play a part in their earlier onset of sexual maturation. A human cell bioassay measuring total estrogenic bioactivity (rather than estradiol alone) in children has an extremely sensitive detection limit of less than 1 pg/mL.[239]

The daily peak of estradiol in early pubertal girls occurs about 6 to 9 hours after the peak of serum LH detected during the night, apparently related to time required for synthesis. In all stages of puberty, boys have higher concentrations of estrone than estradiol, and levels of both estrogens are lower than those measured in girls at comparable stages.

Protein Products of the Gonads
Inhibin, Activin, and Follistatin

Inhibin, a heterodimeric glycoprotein product of the Sertoli cell of the testes and the ovarian granulosa cell (as well as the placenta and other tissues), exerts negative feedback action on the secretion of FSH from the pituitary. Inhibin is composed of an α-subunit and one of two β-subunits, β_A or β_B, which, respectively, form inhibin A or inhibin B, dimers with apparently identical function. Inhibin is a member of the transforming growth factor-β (TGF-β) superfamily that includes antimüllerian hormone (AMH) and the dimers of two inhibin subunits, activin A and activin B, which stimulate the release of FSH from pituitary cells.[240] Synthesis and secretion of gonadal inhibin are induced by FSH. Inhibin plays a role in the feedback regulation of FSH secretion during puberty in males and females.

Like inhibin, follistatin inhibits, whereas activin stimulates, FSH β-subunit expression and therefore affects FSH biosynthesis and secretion. Inhibin may also be an inhibitor of LH release in the follicular phase.[241] These hormones are synthesized in a variety of tissues in addition to the gonads and have diverse activities apart from those on the reproductive apparatus.

Two distinct binding proteins for inhibin and activin are present in the circulation, the gonads, and other tissues: α_2-macroglobulin, a high-capacity, low-affinity binding protein; and follistatin, a glycosylated, single-peptide chain that functions as a high-affinity binding protein and as a regulator of activin bioactivity (e.g., in the pituitary gland, a site of synthesis of activin and follistatin).

During pregnancy, the placenta secretes inhibin A, and the fetal membranes secrete inhibin A and inhibin B, but for at least the first 20 weeks of gestation, only inhibin A

TABLE 25-8

Plasma Gonadal Steroid Values in Children

Steroid and Assay	Age	Normal Values		Sample Volume (Pediatric Minimums)
		Males	Females	
Testosterone, by LC-MS/MS (ng/dL)	Term infant	75-400	20-64	0.18 mL serum (Quest) 0.5 mL serum (Esoterix) 0.15 mL serum (ARUP)
	1-7 mo	Levels decrease rapidly in first week to 20-50, then increase to 60-400 between 20 and 60 days; levels then decline to prepubertal range by 7 mo	Levels decrease during the first month to <10 and remain at that level until puberty	
	7-12 mo	<16	<11	
	Tanner stage I	<16	<16	
	Tanner stage II	<167	<40	
	Tanner stage III	7-762*	<60	
	Tanner stage IV	25-912	<62	
	Tanner stage V	110-975	<68*	
Androstenedione, by RIA after extraction (ng/dL)	Term infant	20-290; levels decrease to 10-80 after 1 week	20-290 ng/dL; levels decrease to 10-80 after 1 week	0.25 mL serum (Esoterix) 0.5 mL serum (Quest)
	1-11 mo	6-68	6-68	
	Prepubertal	8-50	8-50	
	Tanner I	8-50	8-50	
	Tanner II	31-65	42-100	
	Tanner III	50-100	80-190	
	Tanner IV	48-140	77-225	
	Tanner V	65-210	80-240	
DHT, by extraction chromatography, RIA (ng/dL)	1-6 mo	12-85	<5	0.5 mL serum (Esoterix) 1.1 mL serum (Quest)
	Prepubertal	<5	<5	
	Tanner II-III	3-33	5-19	
	Tanner IV-V	22-75	3-30	
Estradiol, by LC-MS/MS (ng/dL)	Newborn	Levels are markedly elevated and fall during first week to <1.5	Levels are markedly elevated and fall during first week to <1.5	1.2 mL serum (Esoterix)
	1-11 mo	Levels increase to 1-3.2 between 1 and 2 mo, then decrease to <1.5 by 6 mo	Levels increase to 0.5-5 between 1 and 2 mo, then decrease to <1.5 during the first year	
	Prepubertal	<1.5	<1.5	
	Tanner I	0.5-1.1	0.5-2	
	Tanner II	0.5-1.6	1-2.4	
	Tanner III	0.5-2.5	0.7-6	
	Tanner IV	1-3.6	2.1-8.5	
	Tanner V	1-3.6	3.4-17	
Estradiol, by extraction chromatography, RIA (ng/dL)	Tanner stage I	0.3-1.5	0.5-1	0.6 mL (Quest)
	Tanner stage II	0.3-1	0.5-11.5	
	Tanner stage III	0.5-1.5	0.5-18	
	Tanner stage IV	0.3-4	2.5-34.5	
	Tanner stage V	1.5-4.5	2.5-41	
Estradiol, chemiluminescent immunoassay (ng/dL)	0-8	0.7-0.8	0.7-1.4	0.2 mL serum (ARUP)
	9-10	0.7-1.1	0.7-3.2	
	11-12	0.7-2.2	0.7-3.8	
	13-14	0.7-2.4	1-9.1	
	15-16	1.1-3.3	1.7-18.1	
	17-40	1.8-6.7	2.3-17.0	
Extrone, by LC-MS/MS (ng/dL)		Levels are markedly elevated at birth, then decrease during first week to <1.5	Levels are markedly elevated at birth, then decrease during first week to <1.5	1.2 mL serum (Esoterix)
	Prepubertal	<1.5	<1.5	
	Tanner I	0.5-1.7	0.4-2.9	
	Tanner II	1.0-2.5	1-3.3	
	Tanner III	1.5-2.5	1.5-4.3	
	Tanner IV	1.5-4.5	1.6-7.7	
	Tanner V	2-4.5	2.9-10.5	

*Because this chart combines values from different laboratories, the ranges are larger in the aggregate than would be found in the specific laboratories' standards. Please consult the laboratory being used to interpret results for clinical decisions.

DHT, dihydrotestosterone; LC-MS/MS, liquid chromatography tandem mass spectrometry; RIA, radioimmunoassay.

From Albrecht L, Styne D. Laboratory testing of gonadal steroids in children. *Pediatr Endocrinol Rev.* 2007;5(Suppl 1):599-607.

is detected in maternal serum. In umbilical cord serum from term female newborn infants, no inhibin dimer was detected, whereas cord serum from male newborns contained inhibin B, the only inhibin detected in adult males.[242] In the human fetal testis, α and β$_B$ (but not β$_A$) subunits were present in Sertoli and Leydig cells at 16 weeks' gestation; by 24 weeks' gestation, immunoexpression of both subunits was greater in the Sertoli cells. Postnatally, the expression of both subunits was decreased by 4 months of age. Inhibin subunits were not detected in the fetal ovary, nor was immunoreactive follistatin present in fetal or neonatal gonads.[243]

In large cross-sectional studies using highly specific inhibin B and inhibin A immunoassays that correlate with the bioactivity of inhibin and distinguish inhibin B from inhibin A, the mean concentration of serum inhibin B in males increased between prepuberty (a stage when it is higher than the undetectable levels in castrated men)[244] and the first stage of puberty; when the strong correlation with chronologic age was taken into account, a correlation with LH and testosterone values remained. From genital stage 2 of puberty on, inhibin B levels were relatively constant, despite a rise in the mean concentration of serum FSH between stages 2 and 3, after which the FSH value was relatively unchanged. The rise in inhibin B is mirrored by a drop in AMH in early puberty, apparently reflecting Sertoli cell maturation.[245] By genital stage 3, a negative partial correlation between inhibin B and FSH was found that persisted as puberty advanced, and by genital stage 4, there was a clear negative correlation of inhibin with serum FSH. Dimeric inhibin B rises twice during development, reflecting the two periods of Sertoli cell proliferation in infancy and in early puberty, whereas an inverse relationship between inhibin and FSH is seen at midpuberty and thereafter, indicating the development of negative feedback inhibition. In the early stages of puberty, inhibin B values are closely related to LH and testosterone levels, but in stage 3, when inhibin B values peak, this relationship is lost, and inhibin B values become more closely related to FSH levels.[246]

Serum levels of inhibin A and B increase early in puberty in girls, although there are individual increases in the prepubertal period directly related to FSH levels, demonstrating sporadic follicular development in the infant and child due to FSH stimulation. Inhibin B is predominant in the follicular phase, as is inhibin A during the luteal phase. Inhibin A and inhibin B peak in midpuberty, and inhibin B is thereafter decreased. During the early stages of puberty, inhibin B values are related to estradiol and FSH values, but these relationships diminish with the progression of puberty.[247] Although there is no significant change in activin during female puberty, follistatin decreases from a midpuberty peak to later values that fall below prepubertal values.

Serum values of FSH regulating proteins follow circadian patterns, with higher values of LH and FSH overnight, just after a nadir of inhibin B. Follistatin concentrations were found to reach their greatest value in early morning, and activin A concentrations declined coincident with the nighttime increase in FSH levels in pubertal girls.[248] Diurnal variation of inhibin B in boys in the peripubertal or early pubertal period demonstrates a fall in inhibin during the night as LH and, subsequently, testosterone rise, showing the negative feedback effect of testosterone on inhibin B secretion.[249] Recombinant FSH treatment, which raises testosterone secretion, suppresses inhibin B, demonstrating the ability of testosterone to negatively influence inhibin B secretion.[250] Administration of a GnRH agonist led to an increase in the FSH level by 30 minutes as well as an increase in the inhibin B level in girls older than 5 years of age by 8 hours and in boys by 20 hours.[251] The baseline inhibin B concentration was greater in boys than in girls, baseline activin A concentrations were greater in girls, and activin did not change with GnRH administration. Testosterone administration to boys in Tanner stage 2 led to decreased FSH and LH, increased activin, and decreased inhibin B levels but caused no change in follistatin. Estradiol administered to girls in Tanner stage 1 or 2 led to decreased LH and FSH and increased activin A levels

but no change in inhibin B or follistatin concentrations, whereas administration of estradiol to girls with Tuner syndrome led to decreased serum levels of FSH, although the effectively nondetectable levels of activin and inhibin did not change.[252]

A low concentration of inhibin B in men and pubertal boys is an indicator of impaired seminiferous tubule function.[253] Early pubertal boys with testicular defects have higher FSH concentrations and low inhibin levels. Inhibin B is the form most closely related to testicular function, and it is absent in orchidectomized men. Inhibin B is related to Sertoli cell function in prepuberty, but a developmental change occurs during puberty so that later in life, inhibin B concentration is related to spermatogenesis. Prepubertal boys with the Sertoli cell–only syndrome had normal inhibin B levels, whereas postpubertal affected boys and men with Sertoli cell–only syndrome and early-stage spermatogenic arrest had undetectable or low levels of inhibin B, whereas those with late-stage spermatogenic arrest or obstructive azoospermia had normal or near-normal levels of serum inhibin B.[244] In prepuberty, the α and the β_B inhibin subunits are expressed in Sertoli cells, but during puberty and in men, fully differentiated Sertoli cells express only the α-subunit; the β-subunit is expressed in germ cells. Inhibin B in the adult appears to be a product of germ and Sertoli cells. In prepubertal boys, basal plasma inhibin B concentrations have a high correlation with the incremental testosterone response to administration of human chorionic gonadotropin (hCG), and they provide a useful assessment of the presence of testes and their function.[254]

Antimüllerian Hormone

AMH (also called müllerian inhibiting substance [MIS] or factor [MIF]), a 14-kDa homodimeric glycoprotein that is structurally related to the subunit of inhibin and TGF-β, is produced by the Sertoli cells of the fetal testis after 7 weeks, the prepubertal testis and causes the regression of the müllerian ducts in boys during early fetal development and later in gestation by granulosa cells of the fetal ovary. Immunoassayable concentrations of AMH values rise from birth to relatively high levels during the first year of life in males, decrease by age 10 years, and decrease further during puberty.[255] Newborn females have low or nondetectable serum levels of AMH, which rise only slightly thereafter; serum AMH concentrations are virtually nondetectable in most girls just before puberty. Serum levels of AMH and of estradiol after GnRH analogue stimulation are increased in low-birth-weight and high-birth-weight female infants, suggesting altered follicular development.[256] Increased poststimulation FSH levels and low adiponectin concentrations are observed only in high-birth-weight infants, indicating that altered ovarian function occurs by a different mechanism than that found in low-birth-weight infants.

Serum levels of AMH and inhibin B are inversely related to androgen concentrations in pubertal boys,[245] and values in boys with CPP are appropriate for pubertal stage rather than chronologic age.[255] Elevated serum AMH concentrations occur in the newborn period, at puberty, and thereafter in androgen resistance. Treatment with recombinant FSH and hCG in hypogonadotropic hypogonadism increases testosterone and decreases the elevated levels of serum AMH (due to immature Sertoli cells) and inhibin B, further demonstrating this relationship.[250] AMH is slightly higher in boys with delayed puberty than in pubertal age-matched control subjects and lower in those with testicular dysgenesis associated with impaired virilization than in normal boys. Boys with isolated cryptorchidism have normal values of AMH, and AMH and inhibin B are absent in anorchia, allowing a differential diagnosis during the first month after birth.[257] Dysgenetic testes secrete only low serum AMH levels; the testosterone response to hCG indicates the presence of testicular tissue.[258]

AMH is elevated in girls with PCOS and in girls with oligomenorrhea without classic AMH. This finding suggests that oligomenorrheic adolescents may have increased antral follicle number, similar to that observed in girls with PCOS.[259] AMH is a useful gonadal tumor marker because values are elevated in males with primitive Sertoli-like tumors and in girls and women with granulosa cell tumors.

Adrenal Androgens

A progressive increase in plasma levels of Δ^5-steroids, DHEA, and DHEAS in boys and girls begins before age 8 (skeletal age of 6 to 8 years) and continues through early adulthood (Table 25-9). The increase in the secretion of adrenal androgen and its precursors is known as *adrenarche,* and the appearance of pubic hair caused by adrenarche is known as *pubarche.* Plasma DHEA levels have a diurnal rhythm similar to that of cortisol, but plasma levels of DHEAS show less variation and are a useful biochemical marker of adrenarche.

DHEA is the predominant precursor to more potent androgens in females, and DHEAS cannot be converted. DHEAS is produced from DHEA by the action of the sulfotransferase enzyme SULT2A1, mainly in the adrenal glands and the liver. The sulfate donor phosphoadenosine phosphosulfate (PAPS) is required by SULT2A1, and in human beings, PAPS is synthesized by the two isoforms of PAPS synthase, PAPSS1 and PAPSS2.[260]

Testosterone-Binding Globulin

Between 97% and 99% of circulating testosterone and estradiol is reversibly bound to testosterone-binding globulin (TeBG) (i.e., sex steroid–binding globulin); prepubertal levels of TeBG are approximately equal in boys and girls, but a decrease in TeBG level occurs with advancing prepubertal age and the concomitant increase in the plasma gonadal steroid levels.[261] At puberty, there is a small decrease in TeBG levels in girls; as a consequence of testosterone, there is a greater decrease in boys, although the drop observed in normal boys is attenuated by treatment with tamoxifen, even with advancing pubertal development. The rise in adrenal androgen levels at adrenarche may explain the early drop in TeBG levels, which allows more circulating free hormone at a given concentration of testosterone. Although the plasma concentration of testosterone is 20 times greater in men than in women, the concentration of free testosterone is 40 times greater. Boys with hypogonadotropic hypogonadism and patients with the androgen resistance syndrome show the same characteristic fall in TeBG levels at puberty, but values are intermediate between those of normal adult males and females.

Prolactin

Prolactin levels rise in girls during puberty. Prepubertal mean (± standard error) plasma prolactin concentrations are 4.0 ± 0.5 µg/L in boys and 4.5 ± 0.6 µg/L in girls. Late pubertal girls and adult women have higher concentrations of prolactin (7.5 ± 0.7 and 8.3 ± 0.7 µg/L, respectively), whereas the mean concentration in adult men is 5.2 ± 0.4 µg/L.[262] This sex difference is probably a consequence of the higher estradiol levels during puberty in girls and in women.

Insulin-like 3 Protein

During puberty, serum levels of insulin-like 3 (INSL3), a protein produced by the Leydig cells, rise in normal boys under LH stimulation and in those in whom increased secretion is induced by letrozole treatment.[263,264] Values do not increase in Klinefelter syndrome, in which the initial rise levels off during midpuberty.[264] INSL3 is as sensitive as testosterone as an indication of Leydig cell function.[265]

Prostate-Specific Antigen

Prostate-specific antigen (PSA) is detectable in male and female cord blood and in the serum of infants, but PSA concentrations decrease to undetectable levels during childhood. PSA concentrations rise to the measurable range with the onset of puberty in the male and correlate with the progression of pubertal stage, the size of the testes, serum LH and testosterone concentrations, and, presumably, the size of the prostate.[266,267] PSA values are increased to the pubertal range in boys with idiopathic CPP, and they decrease with GnRH agonist treatment.

Hormonal Control of the Pubertal Growth Spurt

Postnatal growth follows a specific pattern: an extremely high growth rate just after birth is followed by a declaration that continues until 3 years of age; next, there is a slower phase of deceleration until puberty. The subsequent pubertal growth spurt, the second greatest period of postnatal growth, is followed by maturation of the spine and long bones until adult height is reached.[125] Many factors influence the growth plate.[268] The adolescent growth spurt in

TABLE 25-9

Mean Serum Concentrations (mmol/L [ng/mL]) of DHEAS During Childhood

	6-8 yr	8-10 yr	10-12 yr	12-14 yr	14-16 yr	16-20 yr
By Chronologic Age						
Boys	0.5 (188)	1.6 (586)	3.4 (1260)	3.6 (1330)	7.2 (2640)	7.2 (2640)
Girls	0.8 (306)	3.2 (1170)	3.1 (1130)	4.6 (1690)	6.9 (2540)	6.3 (2320)
By Bone Age						
Boys	0.98 (360)	1.6 (574)	3.4 (1250)	5.8 (2150)	10.9 (4030)	
Girls	0.73 (276)	3.1 (1130)	4.33 (1560)	7.1 (2610)	3.9 (1450)	

DHEAS, dehydroepiandrosterone sulfate.
Modified from Reiter EO, Fuldauer VG, Root AW. Secretion of the adrenal androgen, dehydroepiandrosterone sulfate, during normal infancy, childhood, and adolescence, in sick infants, and in children with endocrinologic abnormalities. *J Pediatr.* 1977;90:766-770.

normal girls and boys depends on estradiol and GH levels, among other factors.

Hormonal control of the pubertal growth spurt is complex (see Figs. 25-15 and 25-16). GH is involved in increasing growth at puberty through stimulation of IGF-1 production. Gonadal steroids have two effects on pubertal growth: (1) induction of an increase in GH secretion, with a consequent increase in IGF-1 production, thereby indirectly stimulating pubertal growth, and (2) a direct effect on cartilage and bone through stimulation of local production of IGF-1 and other local factors.[134,269]

Gonadal Steroids[133,134]

In the developing human skeleton, gonadal steroids have growth-promoting and maturational effects on chondrocytes, osteoblasts, and other bone constituents.[133,134] This action, which eventually leads to epiphyseal fusion and the cessation of longitudinal growth in boys and girls, is mediated mainly by estrogen that is directly secreted (in girls) or arises from the conversion of testosterone and androstenedione to estrogen in peripheral tissues by aromatase (see Table 25-8). Detection of estrogen resistance resulting from a null mutation in the gene encoding the estrogen receptor and from derangements in the *CYP19A1* gene, leading to severe cytochrome P450 aromatase deficiency, has highlighted the cardinal role of estradiol (but not testosterone) in both boys and girls in the pubertal growth spurt, completion of epiphyseal maturation, and normal skeletal proportions and mineralization. Individuals with a mutation in the ERα gene *(ESR1)* or the *CYP19A1* gene encoding aromatase continue to grow, lack a pubertal growth spurt, and have open epiphyses and osteopenia.[270-272] Estrogen treatment of men with aromatase deficiency leads to epiphyseal closure, cessation of growth, and a striking increase in bone mass.[273-275] Patients with aromatase excess, who produce excess estrogen, have advanced skeletal maturation and rapid growth and ultimately reach short adult stature.[276]

Although estradiol secreted by the ovary has long been recognized as the major sex steroid responsible for the pubertal growth spurt, skeletal maturation, and bone mineral accrual in females, until the detection of the rare human genetic defects in estrogen synthesis or action, conventional wisdom dictated that testosterone mediated these maturational changes during puberty in males. Now it is known that estrogen (not androgen) is the critical sex hormone in males and females in the pubertal growth spurt, skeletal maturation, accrual of peak bone mass, and maintenance of bone mass in the adult. Estrogen stimulates chondrogenesis in the epiphyseal growth plate, increasing pubertal linear growth.[240] At puberty, estrogen promotes skeletal maturation and the gradual progressive closure of the epiphyseal growth plate.[133] The use of a supersensitive assay for plasma estradiol in prepubertal and pubertal boys revealed a high positive correlation between estradiol concentrations and peak growth velocity (but not serum GH level), which was greatest about 3 years after the onset of puberty,[238] further implicating estrogen in the pubertal growth spurt and skeletal maturation of boys and girls.

There are estrogen receptors, both ERα and ERβ, in the growth plate chondrocytes.[268] Histologic studies of the bone and cartilage of rodents treated with corticosteroids or estrogen and clinical evaluations of children with precocious puberty support the theory that senescence of the growth plate occurs because of estrogen exposure in precocious puberty, causing decreased growth during treatment with GnRH agonists.[277]

The high rate of bone turnover in early puberty followed by a decrease in periosteal apposition and endosteal resorption within cortical bone and decreased bone remodeling within cortical and cancellous bone mediated by apoptosis of chondrocytes in the growth plate and osteoclasts within cortical and cancellous bone is mediated in part by estrogen. This leads to a reduction in bone turnover markers at menarche, reflecting the closure of the epiphyseal growth plates.[278]

Girls with Turner syndrome without estrogen exposure retain elevated markers of bone turnover. Prepubertal girls with Turner syndrome tend to lose bone, but that ceases when estrogen therapy begins; administration of estrogen may best be started earlier in these patients.[279] During puberty and into the third decade, estrogen has an anabolic effect on the osteoblast and an apoptotic effect on the osteoclast, increasing bone mineral acquisition in the axial and appendicular skeletons. Evolutionary theory suggests that positive effects of estrogen on bone density, added to mechanical loading, allow women to carry increased weight for pregnancy and lactation; this process is unnecessary after reproduction, and osteoporosis becomes more common at menopause.[280]

Testosterone may also have a direct action on bone in the human male, because ARs are found in human tibial growth plates in osteoblasts and chondrocytes, osteocytes, mononuclear cells, and endothelial cells of blood vessels in the bone marrow.[281] Androgens that cannot be aromatized to estrogen still cause an increase in growth rate, presumably due to interaction with these receptors. The greater increase in periosteal bone deposition, the resultant thickening of cortical bone and greater bone strength, and the greater bone dimensions in boys probably result from direct effects of testosterone. Androgens may protect men against osteoporosis by maintenance of cancellous bone mass and expansion of cortical bone.

A pubertal growth spurt leading to adult height close to that of genotypic men occurs in individuals with the complete form of androgen resistance, demonstrating the critical role of estrogen rather than androgen in the adolescent growth spurt in boys. A modest decrease in BMD Z-scores occurs in the spine but not in the hip based on age-specific female standard values, but the reductions are greater when male standards are used. Affected women have an increased prevalence of fractures, even with estrogen replacement. This suggests that lack of a direct effect of testosterone on the skeleton, especially the spine, has a part in the defects in bone mineralization observed in women with complete androgen insensitivity[282] (see Table 25-8).

Growth Hormone and Growth Factors

GH secretion approximately doubles during puberty in boys and girls in the basal state or after stimulation but decreases after pubertal development. Remarkably, peak values after hexarelin, a 6–amino acid GH-releasing peptide (or GH secretagogue) stimulates as much GH secretion in prepuberty as in puberty. The greater elevation in girls starts at an earlier age and pubertal stage than in boys due to the earlier onset of puberty in girls. GH secretion increases coincident with the onset of breast development (Tanner stage 2) and is maximal at Tanner stage 3 to 4 breast development; in boys, GH rises later and peaks at stage 4 genital development. GH secretion and IGF-1 levels decrease after late puberty in both sexes. Adolescents of normal height have an inverse relationship between weight and GH levels. Increased GH pulse amplitude and content of GH secreted per pulse (not but frequency, metabolic clearance rate, or intersecretory burst interval and half-life of GH) in the basal state are mainly responsible for the augmented GH levels.[283]

The increase in estradiol at puberty, which in boys results from testicular secretion and extraglandular synthesis from testosterone and androstenedione and in girls from secretion by the ovaries, is the principal mediator of the increase in pulse amplitude and amount of GH secreted per pulse. Administration of exogenous androgens in delayed puberty raises GH secretion. Transdermal application of testosterone increases spontaneous GH secretion overnight independent of growth hormone–releasing hormone (GHRH), because infusion of GnRH antagonist does not affect this phenomenon.[284] The effect of testosterone is mediated mainly through its conversion to estradiol, because treatment of late pubertal boys with tamoxifen, an estrogen receptor blocker, causes smaller GH secretory peaks and fewer GH secretory episodes. Exogenous estrogen increases the peak GH reached after insulin-induced hypoglycemia, exercise, and arginine, a priming effect that is used in clinical practice, because estrogen administered before a provocative test in prepubertal subjects increases the GH response. Androgens that cannot be aromatized to estrogen (e.g., oxandrolone, dihydrotestosterone) have less effect on GH secretion; however, androgen blockade with flutamide increases GH secretion. Dihydrotestosterone, which is not aromatized to estrogen, does not increase GH secretion or the plasma concentration of IGF-1 and may decrease the integrated GH secretion, but it still stimulates increased growth rate, suggesting a possible direct effect of androgen on pubertal growth independent of GH or estradiol.[269] Increased GH secretion also occurs in sexual precocity. GH secretion decreases with the fall in gonadal steroid levels after treatment of CPP with potent GnRH agonists.[285]

GH deficiency or GH resistance causes an attenuated pubertal growth spurt, indicating the importance of GH and IGF-1 in this process. Severe primary or secondary hypogonadism leads to a minimal or absent growth spurt, demonstrating the primary role of gonadal steroids in pubertal growth. Hypopituitary patients deficient in GH and gonadotropins do not have an adolescent growth spurt when GH alone is replaced; gonadal steroids must also be given, substantiating the interaction of GH and gonadal steroids in the pubertal growth spurt. In normal puberty, neither the magnitude of the increase in GH secretion nor the concentration of plasma IGF-1 correlates with the PHV of the pubertal growth spurt. Although a threshold level of GH secretion is necessary, the extent of the growth spurt correlates with gonadal sex steroid secretion. Individuals with both CPP and GH deficiency (usually as a consequence of cranial irradiation for a brain tumor) have a growth spurt clinically indistinguishable from that of CPP and normal GH secretion.[269] After treatment with a GnRH agonist for sexual precocity, growth velocity in patients with GH deficiency and CPP is decreased and pubertal progression is suppressed, illustrating the direct effect of gonadal steroids, principally estradiol, on the pubertal growth spurt.

Urinary GH excretion reflects serum levels and changes occurring with pubertal development. A peak is reached at pubertal stage 3 to 4. The level is higher in boys than in girls.

Growth Hormone–Binding Protein

Growth hormone–binding protein (GHBP) has the same amino acid sequence as the extracellular component of the GH receptor (GHR), and serum concentrations are directly related to the number of GHRs. In normal children, the plasma GHBP level is inversely related to 24-hour GH secretion. The serum GHBP level rises early in childhood and also through puberty in some cross-sectional studies, but not in others. Because plasma GHBP does not change appreciably with the onset of puberty, at the time of the pubertal growth spurt there is a relative increase in unbound (free) GH in relation to GH bound to GHBP. GHBP is related to adiposity, and it may be this factor that accounts for the increased levels of GHBP in girls compared with boys, the rise in GHBP in girls with precocious puberty, and the negative influence of testosterone on GHBP levels.[286]

Insulin-like Growth Factor Type 1

Concentrations of IGF-1 rise during puberty to levels higher than those of prepuberty or adulthood; they remain elevated past the time of PHV, with a peak attained 1 or 2 years after the pubertal growth spurt (later in boys than in girls) and then fall to normal adult levels.[285,287] The pattern of the GH-dependent serum levels of IGF-binding protein 3 (IGFBP3) in pubertal development is similar to that of serum[288] IGF-1. However, serum IGFBP3 concentrations correlate with BMI even though IGF-1 does not. Measurement of free IGF-1 shows the same pattern of change with development as does that of total IGF-1, a slow rise in serum free IGF-1 in prepuberty followed by a steeper rise during puberty. A decrease of free IGF-1 is associated with age in the later stages of puberty.[288,289] The increase in the serum ratio of IGF-1 to IGFBP3 at the time of the pubertal growth spurt appears to result from production, because proteolysis of IGFBP3 does not change in puberty in normal children. The testosterone level in boys and the estradiol level in girls correlate with the rise in IGF-1 concentration, but gonadal steroids are not the direct cause of the increase in circulating IGF-1 levels; rather, GH secretion approximately doubles during puberty owing to the effect of estrogen causing augmented release of GH.

Plasma IGF-1 concentrations are high for chronologic age in sexual precocity and low in delayed puberty. Estrogen mediates the pubertal increase in IGF-1 concentration through increased secretion of GH, with an additional effect through the gonadal steroid–induced local generation of IGF-1 in cartilage and bone. Treatment with GnRH agonist in a 16-year-old boy with a homozygous mutation in the WSXWS-like motif of the human GHR causing Laron syndrome led to a further decrease in the already low serum levels of IGF-1 and IGFBP3, which did not reverse with dihydrotestosterone treatment, suggesting a direct effect of estradiol on IGF-1 production.[268,290] Children with CPP treated with a GnRH agonist showed suppression of the untreated elevated serum GH concentrations and a decrease in plasma IGF-1 concentrations, although not to prepubertal values, supporting the concept that GH is the major (but not the only) factor that raises circulating IGF-1 levels in puberty.[285]

A confounding factor is the relative roles of hepatic-generated circulating IGF-1 (i.e., endocrine role) and of locally produced IGF-1 (i.e., paracrine/autocrine role) in linear growth. For example, mice with a totally deleted hepatic IGF-1 gene have strikingly reduced circulating levels of IGF-1 but normal postnatal body and bone growth.[291]

GH stimulates local IGF-1 production in resting zone chondrocytes, located at the epiphyseal end of the growth plate in the area known as the reserve zone or stem cell zone, through GHRs in the chondrocytes. This IGF-1 production stimulates, through autocrine and paracrine effects, the clonal expansion of proliferating chondrocytes derived from the resting chondrocyte or germ cells. GH and IGF-1 can reduce the stem cell cycle time, proliferating cell cycle time and duration of the hypertrophic phase, a phase that leads to apoptosis, leaving the cells serving as a scaffold for the mineralization and production of new bone.

Other Hormones

There are glucocorticoid receptors in human growth plates, mostly in hypertrophic chondrocytes. However, children with chronic adrenal insufficiency who receive appropriate replacement therapy have a normal pubertal growth spurt despite deficient adrenal androgen secretion, indicating a minimal impact of these adrenal androgens on normal growth at puberty.[259]

Hypothyroid subjects lack a pubertal growth spurt even when the disorder is accompanied by sexual precocity.[292] Thyroid hormone has a permissive role in the pubertal growth spurt but is a requisite for normal growth. Hypothyroidism decreases GH secretion and affects growth indirectly. However, thyroid hormone also interacts with the thyroid hormone receptors α1 and β, whose proteins are found in early proliferating chondrocytes of the human growth plate, and the messenger ribonucleic acid (mRNA) found in other developing stages of chondrocytes and osteoblasts. Thyroid hormones also interact with the local effects of IGF-1 and GH at the growth plate.[268]

CENTRAL NERVOUS SYSTEM AND PUBERTY

Two independent but associated processes (controlled by different mechanisms but closely linked temporally) are involved in the increased secretion of sex steroids in the peripubertal and pubertal periods. In the first process, adrenarche, the increase in adrenal androgen secretion[270,293] precedes by approximately 2 years the second process, gonadarche, which is a consequence of the pubertal reactivation of the hypothalamic-pituitary gonadotropin-gonadal apparatus.[259,293,294]

The onset of puberty is a consequence of maturational changes, including the development of secondary sexual characteristics, the adolescent growth spurt, the attainment of fertility, and psychosocial changes, all emanating from the disinhibition or reaugmentation of the hypothalamic GnRH pulse generator and gonadotropin secretion, causing an increase in gonadal steroid secretion[226,295] (Table 25-10). The events characterizing the development of gonadal function can be viewed as a continuum extending from sexual differentiation and the ontogenesis of the hypothalamic-pituitary gonadotropin-gonadal system during fetal life and early infancy,[102,224,294,295] through a juvenile pause (in which the system is suppressed to a low level of activity,[294] discussed later), to the attainment of full sexual maturation and fertility during puberty, leading to the ability to procreate (Fig. 25-21). In this light, puberty does not represent the initiation or first occurrence of pulsatile secretion of GnRH or pituitary gonadotropins but the reactivation or disinhibition of GnRH neurosecretory neurons in the medial basal hypothalamus and the endogenous, apparently self-sustaining oscillatory secretion of GnRH after the period of quiescent activity during childhood. An increase in the pulsatile release of GnRH heralds the onset of puberty in primates and other mammals.[102,295-297] The CNS, and not the hypothalamic GnRH pulse generator, pituitary gland, gonads, or gonadal steroid target tissues,

TABLE 25-10

Hypothesis of the Control of the Onset of Human Puberty

1. *Central Dogma:* The CNS exercises the only major restraint on the onset of puberty. The neuroendocrine control of puberty is mediated by the hypothalamic GnRH-secreting neurosecretory neurons in the medial basal hypothalamus, which act as an endogenous pulse generator (oscillator).
2. The development of reproductive function is a continuum extending from sexual differentiation and the ontogeny of the hypothalamic-pituitary-gonadal system in the fetus to the attainment of full sexual maturation and fertility.
3. In the prepubertal child the GnRH pulse generator, operative in the fetus and infant, functions at a low level of activity (the juvenile pause) because of steroid-independent and steroid-dependent inhibitory mechanisms.
4. Puberty represents the *reactivation* (disinhibition) of the CNS suppressed GnRH pulse generator characteristic of late infancy and childhood, leading to increased amplitude and frequency of GnRH pulsatile discharges, to increased stimulation of the pituitary gonadotropes, and finally to gonadal maturation. Hormonally, puberty is initiated by the recrudescence of augmented pulsatile GnRH and gonadotropin secretion, mainly at night.

CNS, central nervous system; GnRH, gonadotropin-releasing hormone.
From Grumbach MM, Kaplan SL. The neuroendocrinology of human puberty: an ontogenetic perspective. In: Grumbach MM, Sizonenko PC, Aubert ML, eds. *Control of the Onset of Puberty.* Baltimore, MD: Williams & Wilkins, 1990:1-68. © 1990, the Williams & Wilkins Co., Baltimore.

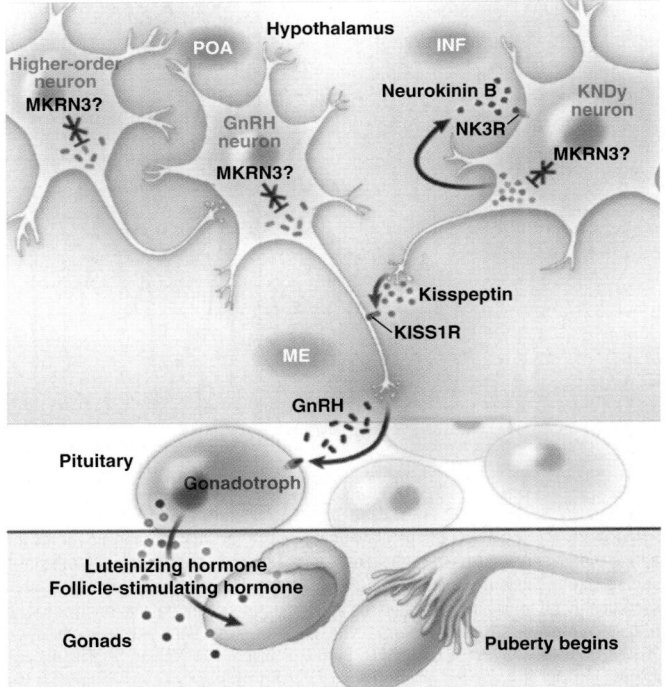

A

Figure 25-21 Timing of puberty. A pivotal event in the onset of puberty in mammals is the resumption of pulsatile release of gonadotropin-releasing hormone (GnRH) from neurons of the hypothalamus. Known influences on the timing of the onset of puberty in mammals include the photoperiod, leptin levels, and the increased expression of neurokinin. **A,** Kisspeptin, and their receptors (NK3R and KISS1R, respectively). Abreu and associates[387] implicate MKRN3, a protein that is believed to mediate ubiquitination, in puberty onset. In contrast with kisspeptin and neurokinin B, which stimulate the commencement of puberty, MKRN3 seems to inhibit puberty: Abreu and associates[387] show that mutations in MKRN3 predicted to cause loss of function of the protein cause central precocious puberty. INF, infundibular nucleus; KNDy, kisspeptin–neurokinin B–dynorphin; MBH, medial basal hypothalamus; ME, median eminence; POA, preoptic area.

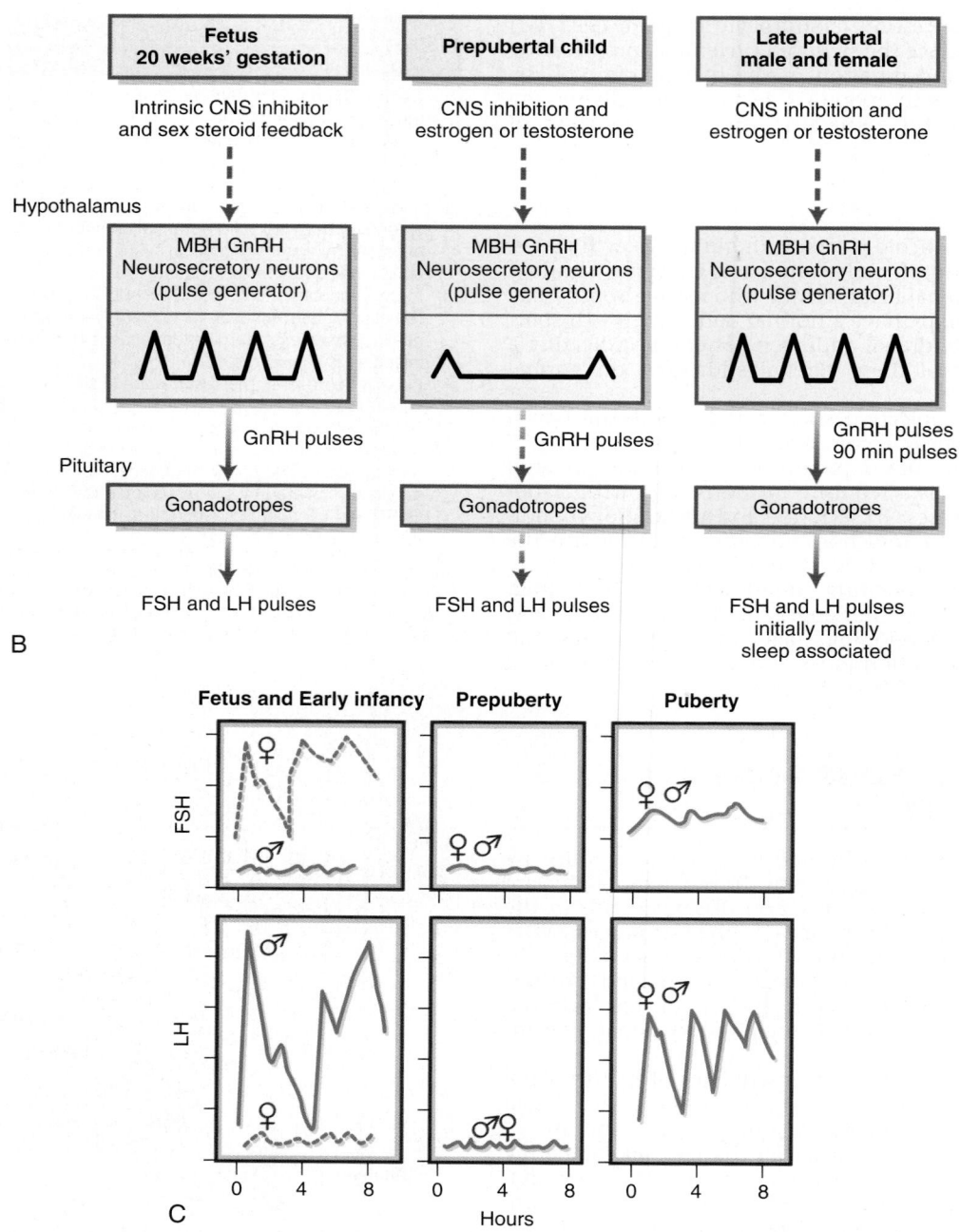

Figure 25-21, cont'd B, Postulated ontogeny of the dual mechanism for the inhibition of puberty. *Dashed arrows* indicate inhibition. Notice the action of both components during the juvenile pause (i.e., prepuberty) (see Fig. 25-39 for the relative roles of these two mechanisms during development). **C,** Change in the pattern of pulsatile follicle-stimulating hormone (FSH) and luteinizing hormone (LH) secretion in the fetus and early infancy, prepuberty, and puberty (data from Waldhauser et al). Notice the pulsatile secretion in the fetus and infant and the striking difference in the amplitude of FSH and LH pulses between male and female infants. After infancy, the amplitude and frequency of gonadotropin pulses decrease greatly for almost a decade (i.e., juvenile pause) until the onset of puberty. (A from Hughes IA. Releasing the brake on puberty. *N Engl J Med.* 2013;368:2513-2515; B and C modified from Grumbach MM, Kaplan SL. The neuroendocrinology of human puberty: an ontogenetic perspective. In: Grumbach MM, Sizonenko PC, Aubert ML, eds. *Control of the Onset of Puberty.* Baltimore, MD: Williams & Wilkins; 1990:1-68; additional data from Waldhauser F, Weissenbacher G, Frisch H, Pollak A. Pulsatile secretion of gonadotropins in early infancy. *Eur J Pediatr.* 1981;137:71-74.)

restrains activation of the hypothalamic-pituitary-gonadal system during the prepubertal years.

Certain CNS lesions involving the hypothalamus and nearby structures can advance or delay the onset of human puberty.[226,294] CPP, including cyclic ovulation in girls and spermatogenesis in boys, can result from a variety of CNS disorders. Several regulatory systems control puberty (Fig. 25-22):

1. In primates, the neural component controlling gonadotropin secretion resides in the medial basal hypothalamus, including the arcuate region. There are about 1500 to 2000 transducer GnRH neurosecretory neurons, which are not segregated into a specific nucleus but are functionally interconnected. These GnRH neurons comprise the GnRH pulse generator, which drives and controls the pituitary gonadal components, stimulates the

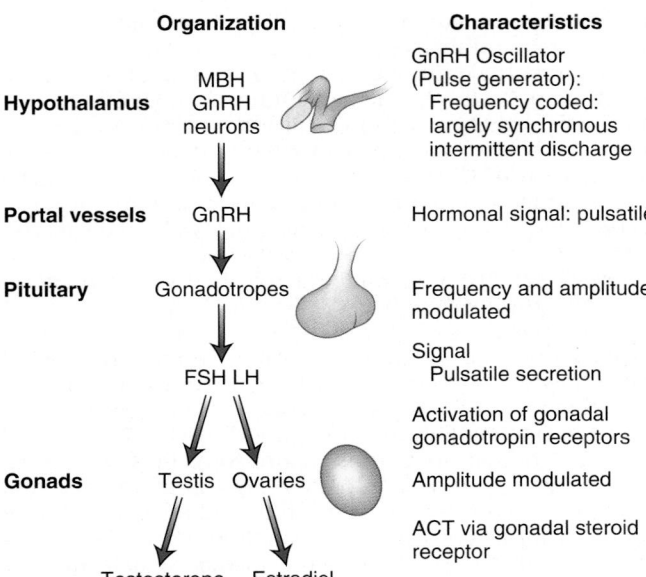

Organization		Characteristics
Hypothalamus	MBH GnRH neurons	GnRH Oscillator (Pulse generator): Frequency coded: largely synchronous intermittent discharge
Portal vessels	GnRH	Hormonal signal: pulsatile
Pituitary	Gonadotropes	Frequency and amplitude modulated
	FSH LH	Signal Pulsatile secretion
		Activation of gonadal gonadotropin receptors
Gonads	Testis Ovaries	Amplitude modulated
		ACT via gonadal steroid receptor
	Testosterone Estradiol	

Figure 25-22 Organization and characteristics of the hypothalamic-pituitary gonadotroph-gonadal system. The medial basal hypothalamus (MBH) contains the transducer gonadotropin-releasing hormone (GnRH) neurosecretory neurons. These neurons translate neural signals into a periodic, oscillatory chemical signal, GnRH. This MBH complex functions as a GnRH pulse generator (oscillator), which is frequency coded and releases GnRH from its axon terminals at the median eminence as a largely synchronous, intermittent discharge into the primary capillary plexus of the hypothalamic-hypophyseal portal circulation. The GnRH pulse generator is influenced by biogenic amine neurotransmitters, peptidergic neuromodulators, neuroexcitatory amino acids, and neural pathways. During the follicular phase in women and men, a GnRH pulse (estimated indirectly by monitoring luteinizing hormone [LH] pulses in peripheral blood) occurs approximately every 90 to 120 minutes throughout the day. Changes in the frequency and probably in the amplitude of the GnRH secretory episodes modulate the pattern of LH and follicle-stimulating hormone (FSH). The major site of action of testosterone and progesterone is on the GnRH pulse generator, because these two classes of steroids decrease LH pulse frequency, but a pituitary site of action has also been described. Estrogens have major direct inhibitory and stimulatory effects on the GnRH-primed pituitary gonadotroph; the inhibitory or negative feedback action is associated with a decrease in the frequency and the amplitude of pituitary LH secretion. Evidence supports the negative and positive feedback action of estrogen on the GnRH pulse generator. Inhibin has a direct inhibitory effect on the pituitary gland and the secretion of FSH. The secretion of gonadal steroids by the gonads is controlled mainly by the amplitude of the gonadotropin signal. (Modified from Grumbach MM, Kaplan SL. The neuroendocrinology of human puberty: an ontogenetic perspective. In: Grumbach MM, Sizonenko PC, Aubert ML, eds. *Control of the Onset of Puberty.* Baltimore, MD: Williams & Wilkins; 1990:1-68.)

release of LH and FSH, and translates neural signals into a periodic, oscillatory chemical signal, GnRH, in a coordinated manner. These pulses appear to be generated by a propagated depolarization, the firing of action potentials in individual cells, and the resulting influx of calcium through L-type calcium channels.[298]

2. In response to the GnRH rhythmic signal, the pituitary gonadotrophs, which contain the seven-transmembrane domain G_s-coupled LH/hCG receptors (LHCGRs),[299] release LH and FSH in a pulsatile manner. Each LH and FSH pulse is induced by a pulse of GnRH.
3. The gonads, which are modulated primarily by the amplitude of the gonadotropin pulse, transmit the episodic gonadotropin signal into pulsatile secretion of gonadal steroids.[300]

This control mechanism is common to all mammalian species. At the last two levels—the pituitary gland and the gonad—the target cells contain receptors for the peptide hormones that mediate the cellular response to the signal.[299,300] Diverse adaptive mechanisms and strategies

have evolved among species and between the sexes that influence the biology and timing of puberty. Photoperiodicity and seasonal breeding, biologic clocks, and pheromones are integral parts of the pubertal process in some species but not humans. The most enlightening studies on the neuroendocrinology of human puberty have emerged from studies of humans and nonhuman primates.[296,297]

Pattern of Gonadotropin Secretion
Tonic Secretion
Tonic, or basal, secretion is regulated by a negative, or inhibitory, feedback mechanism in which changes in the concentration of circulating gonadal steroids and inhibin result in reciprocal changes in the secretion of pituitary gonadotropins. This is the pattern of secretion in the male and one of the control mechanisms in the female. Clinical studies reveal that testosterone and estradiol in the male have independent effects on LH secretion. Inhibition of LH by testosterone requires aromatization for its pituitary but not its hypothalamic effects, and estradiol-induced negative feedback on LH occurs at the level of the hypothalamus.[301]

In the female, cyclic secretion involves a positive, or stimulatory, feedback mechanism in which an increase in circulating estrogens, to a critical level and of sufficient duration, initiates the synchronous release of LH and FSH (i.e., preovulatory LH surge) that is characteristic of the normal adult woman before menopause.

Pulsatile Secretion
The GnRH Pulse Generator
GnRH. Generation of the GnRH pulse is an intrinsic property of the GnRH neurosecretory neuronal network, and other factors modulate the fundamental autorhythmicity of the GnRH neuron, including the downstream effects of cyclic adenosine monophosphate (cAMP)-gated cation channels on the regulation of pulsatility by cAMP.[302] The immortalized GnRH neurosecretory neuronal cell line and cultured monkey GnRH-I neurons exhibit spontaneous pulsatile release of GnRH at a frequency similar to that observed in vivo. Patch-clamped primary GnRH neurons show disordered patterns of release that are sensitive to increased extracellular potassium; firing activity can be stimulated by exposure to estrogen in a manner that appears to function through the estrogen receptor.[303]

The secretion of FSH and LH is always pulsatile or episodic, regardless of developmental stage, due to the pulsatility of the GnRH pulse generator. The pulsatile secretion of immunoreactive FSH in normal adults is less prominent than that of LH; this is attributed in part to the longer half-life of FSH compared with LH, to differences in the factors that modulate the action of GnRH on FSH and LH release by the gonadotrophs (especially gonadal steroids, inhibin, and possibly activin and follistatin), and to intrinsic differences in the secretory pattern of the two gonadotropins. For example, a change in the frequency of GnRH pulses can modify the ratio of FSH to LH released; midfollicular-phase concentrations of estradiol and adult male concentrations of plasma testosterone have a greater inhibitory effect on the response of FSH to pulsatile injections of GnRH, compared with that of LH.

Intermittent or pulsatile administration (e.g., GnRH, 1 μg/minute for 6 minutes every hour) induces pulsatile release of LH and FSH in adult monkeys in which hypothalamic lesions have obliterated the arcuate nucleus region and eliminated endogenous GnRH secretion.[304] Continuous infusion of GnRH inhibits gonadotropin

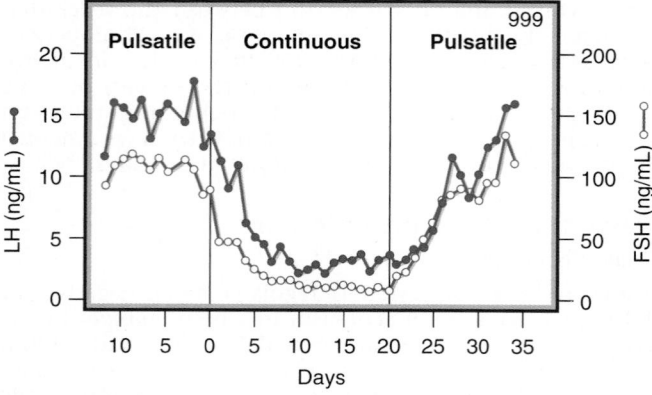

Figure 25-23 The Knobil paradigm. Effect of pulsatile administration of gonadotropin-releasing hormone (GnRH) in contrast to continuous infusion of GnRH in adult oophorectomized rhesus monkeys in which gonadotropin secretion has been abolished by lesions that ablated the medial basal hypothalamic GnRH pulse generator. Notice the high concentrations of plasma luteinizing hormone (LH) and follicle-stimulating hormone (FSH) in monkeys given one GnRH pulse per hour, the suppression of gonadotropin secretion by continuous infusion of GnRH even though the total dose of GnRH was the same, and the restoration of FSH and LH secretion when the pulsatile mode of GnRH administration was reinitiated. (From Belchetz PE, Plant TM, Nakai Y, et al. Hypophysial responses to continuous and intermittent delivery of hypothalamic gonadotropin releasing hormone. *Science.* 1978;202:631-633.)

secretion because of desensitization of GnRH receptors on the gonadotroph. Pulsatile GnRH administration reestablished gonadotropin secretion in animals in which gonadotropin secretion was suppressed by the continuous infusion of GnRH (Fig. 25-23). The GnRH signal to the pituitary gonadotrophs of the adult is frequency coded.

The GnRH neurosecretory neurons of the hypothalamic GnRH pulse generator that arise in the olfactory placode exhibit spontaneous autorhythmicity and function intrinsically as a neuronal oscillator for entrainment of the repetitive release of GnRH. The autorhythmicity in the GnRH neurosecretory neurons involves cAMP and cyclic nucleotide-gated cation channels associated with oscillatory increases in intracellular calcium ions (Ca^{2+}), a hallmark of neurosecretion and gap junctional communication.[305] Moreover, the immortalized GnRH neuronal cell line contains neuronal nitric oxide (NO) synthase, and NO generated by GnRH neurons may act as an intercellular or intracellular messenger.[306] GnRH acting as an autocrine factor may play a role in the synchronization mechanism. GnRH is synthesized in these neurons and released episodically from axon terminals at the median eminence into the primary plexus of the hypothalamic-hypophyseal portal circulation; it is then transported by the portal vessels to the anterior pituitary gland to produce the pulsatile LH and FSH secretion. Remarkably, GnRH neurons exhibit characteristics of both axons and dendrites and are known as *dendrons.*[307] Ionotropic γ-aminobutyric acid (GABA) and glutamate receptors on the dendrons can be stimulated to depolarize the cells to produce action potentials.

Gonadotropin-Inhibitory Hormone. Gonadotropin-inhibitory hormone (GnIH), a peptide first described in quail but now homologues of GnIH are known in most animals, is a member of the RFamide family that has an RFamide (Arg-Phe-NH2) motif at the C-terminus.[308] The family is called *RFamide–related peptides* (RFRPs); kisspeptin is one of the neurotransmitters belonging to this family. The human homologue is known as *RFRP-3* and is coded for by the *NPVF* gene. The mammalian receptor for RFP-3 is GPR147,

a seven-transmembrane domain G protein–coupled receptor.[309] RFP-3 and its receptor is found in the human dorsomedial hypothalamus with axons terminating both on the GnRH neuron and the median eminence, suggesting a role on the hypothalamus and the pituitary in human beings. Surprisingly, the first survey of isolated hypogonadotropic hypogonadism (IHH) and CPP in a well-characterized cohort of patients noted a 3-nucleotide in-frame deletion in the *NPVF* gene (p.I71K72), associated with a reduced risk for the occurrence of CPP.[310] Further study is needed to determine if RFP-3 may play a role in the treatment of disorders of puberty.

Kisspeptins and KISS1R. Description of the role of kisspeptins and their receptors (KISS1R or GRP54) in the CNS hypothalamic-pituitary-gonadal axis led to a flurry of investigation into this factor, which also is released in a pulsatile manner (Figs. 25-24 and 25-25; see Fig. 25-21).[311,312] *KISS1* is a human metastasis suppressor gene at gene map locus 19p13.3, and *KISS1* mRNA is found in placenta, testes, pancreas, liver, small intestine, and the brain, mainly in the hypothalamus and basal ganglion.[313,314] *KISS1* mRNA is present in the primate in the medial arcuate nucleus only, but in the mouse, it occurs in the arcuate, periventricular, and anteroventral periventricular (AVPV) nuclei, regions important in reproductive function.[315,316] The product of the *KISS1* gene is a 145–amino acid peptide, but the cleaved and secreted product is a 54–amino acid protein known as *metastin* or *kisspeptin,* which binds to an endogenous receptor.

The KISS1 receptor, KISS1R (formerly called GPR54), is a G protein–coupled receptor found in the brain, mainly in the hypothalamus and basal ganglia, and in the placenta, from which it was first isolated and sequenced. KISS1R is coexpressed within GnRH neurons in the rat, in the medial and lateral sections of the arcuate nucleus and the ventral aspect of the ventromedial hypothalamus in mice, and in primates.[315,317] Although the expression of KISS1R mRNA does not increase with development in the mouse, kisspeptin mRNA increases dramatically in the AVPV nucleus, and the number of receptors responsive to kisspeptin increase with development.[318] Activation of GnRH neurons by kisspeptin at puberty in the mouse reflects a dual process involving an increase in kisspeptin input from the AVPV and a post-transcriptional change in KISS1R signaling within the GnRH neuron. Increases in kisspeptin lead to increased GnRH release by means of an interneuron, rather than acting directly on the GnRH-secreting neurons.[319]

Mice transfected with mutant KISS1R genes exhibited hypogonadotropic hypogonadism, although they had normal content of GnRH in their hypothalamus and were responsive to GnRH or gonadotropin administration, suggesting normal function of the gonadotroph GnRH receptors and the gonadal LH and FSH receptors despite the mutation.[320] The intact mouse also releases significant LH boluses after kisspeptin administration, an effect that is abolished in the $KISS1R^{-/-}$ mouse, which lacks the receptor.[317]

Underfed prepubertal mice have decreased hypothalamic KISS1, but kisspeptin administration leads to increases in KISS1R mRNA, which in turn leads to increased in vivo LH secretion and in vitro GnRH secretion.[321] Chronic kisspeptin administration to these underfed mice restores vaginal opening and enhances gonadotropin and estrogen responses.

Administration of kisspeptin into the rostral preoptic area (RPOA), medial preoptic area (MPOA), paraventricular nuclei (PVN), and arcuate nuclei of the hypothalamus of male adult rats increased plasma LH and testosterone

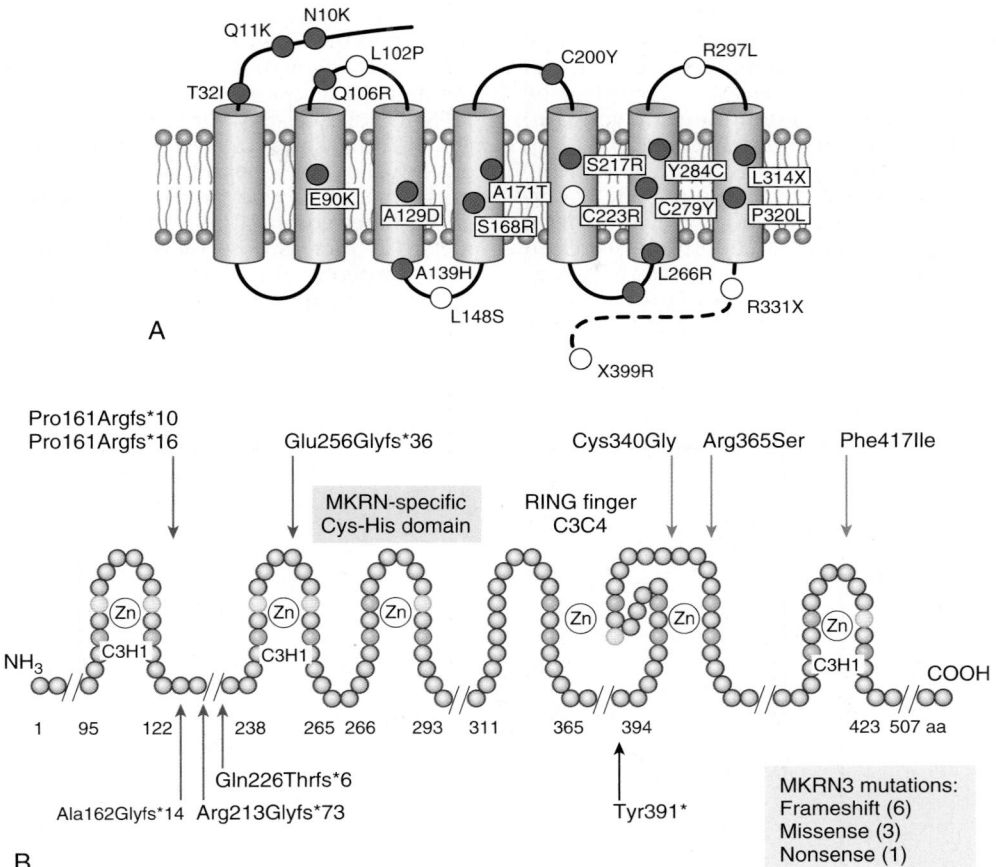

Figure 25-24 A, Inactivating mutations of the gonadotropin-releasing hormone receptor GnRHR *(closed circles)* and the kisspeptin receptor (KISS1R, formerly GPR54) *(open circles)* were identified in patients with isolated hypogonadotropic hypogonadism. The *dashed line* indicates the intracellular domain of KISS1R. The seven-transmembrane G protein–coupled receptor model is used for illustration of both receptors. **B,** Schematic illustration of mutations found in the *MKRN3* gene causing precocious puberty. The amino acid positions in the protein are noted by the numbers and frameshift mutations are indicated by red arrows, a nonsense mutation is indicated by a black arrow, and the 3 missense mutations are indicated by green arrows. (A from de Roux N. GnRH receptor and GPR54 inactivation in isolated gonadotropic deficiency. *Best Pract Res Clin Endocrinol Metab.* 2006;20:515-528. B from Macedo DB, Brito VN, Latronico AC. New causes of central precocious puberty: the role of the genetic factors. *Neuroendocrinology.* 2014;100(1):1-8.)

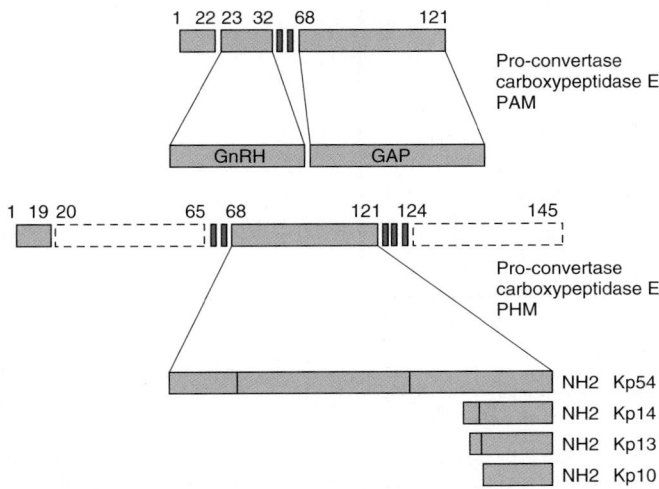

Figure 25-25 Post-translational maturation of gonadotropin-releasing hormone (GnRH) *(top)* and kisspeptins (Kp). Doublets of basic residues and glycine are indicated by *shaded vertical bars.* Enzymes involved in the normal maturation are indicated. GAP, GnRH-associated peptide; PAM, peptidyl glycine α-amidating monooxygenase; PHM, peptidyl α-hydroxylating monooxygenase. (From de Roux N. GnRH receptor and GPR54 inactivation in isolated gonadotropic deficiency. *Best Pract Res Clin Endocrinol Metab.* 2006;20:515-528.)

substantially,[322] and intracerebral kisspeptin administration stimulated the release of FSH, albeit at a far higher dose than needed to stimulate LH release.[323,324] Because the release of FSH is abolished with blockade of GnRH, GnRH modulates the central actions of kisspeptin in the rodent. In the rat, the mRNA for kisspeptin and its receptor increase at puberty, and administration of intracerebral injection of kisspeptin in prepubertal female rats caused large peaks of LH and advanced vaginal opening as a sign of pubertal development and premature ovulation.[325,326] The ovulation elicited by peripheral kisspeptin in the prepubertal female rat is abolished by blockade of GnRH.[327]

KISS1 and KISS1R mRNA expression is found in the posterior two thirds of the arcuate nucleus of the monkey.[328] Kisspeptin-beaded axons make only infrequent contacts with GnRH neurons in the medial basal hypothalamus, whereas in the median eminence, kisspeptin and GnRH axons were found in extensive and intimate association with GnRH contacts on kisspeptin perikarya and dendrites were observed. Nonsynaptic pathways of communication in the median eminence may offer a possible mechanism of kisspeptin regulation of GnRH release and provide an anatomic basis for reciprocal control of kisspeptin neuronal activity by GnRH.[329] Although KISS1 increases with puberty in intact male and female monkeys, KISS1R mRNA levels increase in intact females but not in agonadal male monkeys. Administration of KISS1 through intracerebral catheters to GnRH-primed juvenile female rhesus monkeys stimulates GnRH release, but this release is abolished by infusion of GnRH antagonist. These findings have led to the postulation that KISS1 signaling through KISS1R of primate hypothalamus may be activated at the end of the juvenile pause and may contribute to the pubertal resurgence of pulsatile GnRH release at puberty.[315] Short-term administration of kisspeptin raises gonadotropin secretion in men and nonhuman primates (Fig. 25-26A). Just as continuous infusion of GnRH suppresses GnRH release, continuous infusion of kisspeptin decreased the response

of gonadotrophs in the agonadal male monkey to boluses of kisspeptin. However, the release of FSH and LH after a bolus of N-methyl-D-aspartate (NMDA) or GnRH was maintained demonstrated that the desensitization of the KISS1Rs was selective for kisspeptin administration[330] (see Fig. 25-26B). This is in contrast to the finding that continuous infusion of kisspeptin in men and a woman with *TAC3* mutations and hypogonadotropic hypogonadism experienced renewed pulsatile release of gonadotropins and the men had increased secretion of inhibin B.[331] Treatment with kisspeptin for a variety of disorders of puberty and reproduction appears promising, but the pattern of optimal administration is not yet clear.

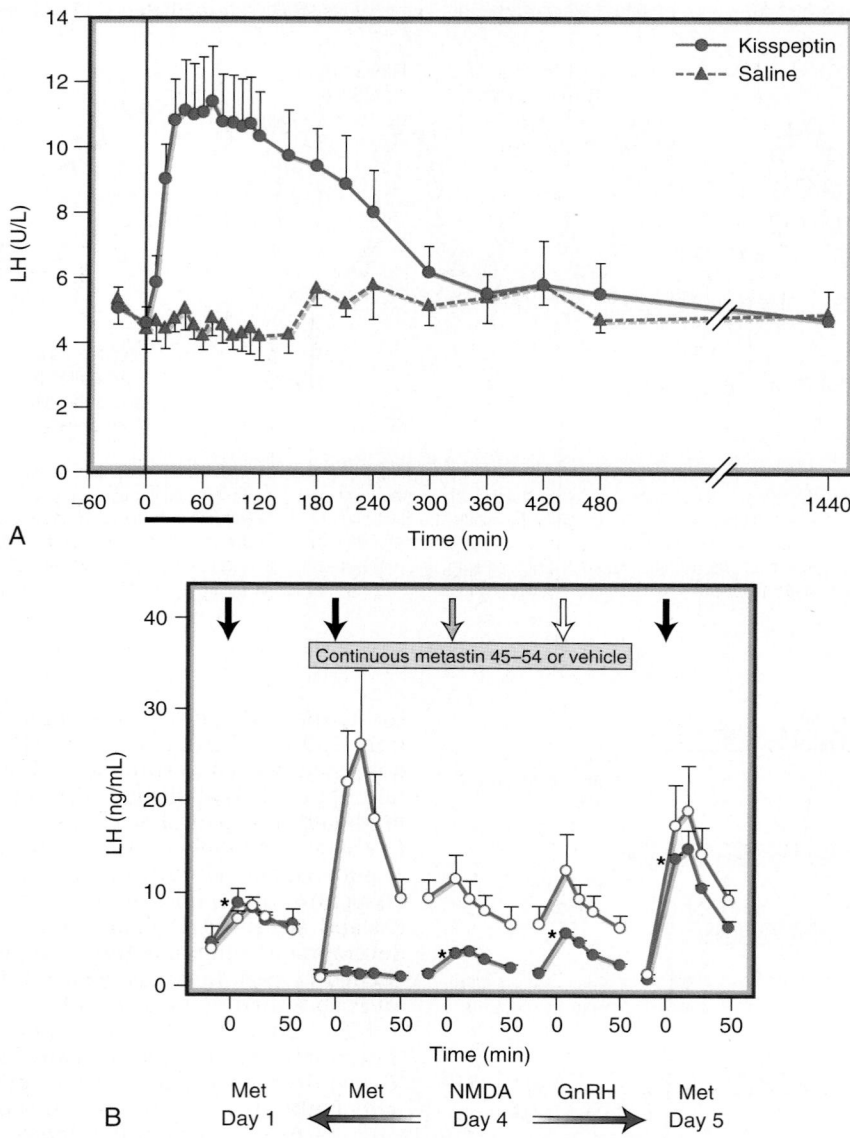

Figure 25-26 **A,** Effects of kisspeptin-54 (4 pmol/kg/minute) or saline infusion in male volunteers ($n = 6$) on mean plasma. Each volunteer received both kisspeptin-54 and saline infusions and acted as their own controls. **B,** Effect of single sequential boluses of human metastin 45-54 (Met-Kisspeptin 10) *(black arrow)*, N-methyl-D-aspartate (NMDA) *(gray arrow)*, and gonadotropin-releasing hormone (GnRH) *(white arrow)* on plasma luteinizing hormone (LH) concentrations (mean ± SEM [standard error of the mean]) during the last 3 hours of the 98-hour intravenous infusion *(shaded box)* of human metastin 45-54 at a dose of 100 μg/hour *(closed circles)* or vehicle compared with the LH response to the same bolus of human metastin 45-54 1 hour before (day 1) and 21 hours after (day 5) the termination of continuous human metastin 45-54 or vehicle infusion. Infusion of human metastin 45-54 *(asterisk)* was significantly different ($p < 0.05$) from the preinjection mean; $n = 3$. (A from Dhillo WS, Chaudhri OB, Patterson M, et al. Kisspeptin-54 stimulates the hypothalamic-pituitary gonadal axis in human males. *J Clin Endocrinol Metab.* 2005;90:6609-6615; B from Seminara SB, Dipietro MJ, Ramaswamy S, et al. Continuous human metastin 45-54 infusion desensitizes G protein-coupled receptor 54-induced gonadotropin-releasing hormone release monitored indirectly in the juvenile male rhesus monkey *(Macaca mulatta):* a finding with therapeutic implications. *Endocrinology.* 2006;147[5]:2122-2126.)

Administration of testosterone to castrated young male monkeys led to decreased kisspeptin mRNA in the medio-basal hypothalamus but not in the preoptic area. There was no change in KISS1R expression. This suggests that feedback inhibition of gonadotropin secretion by testosterone is mediated by kisspeptin upstream of the GnRH network.[332]

KISS1R mRNA is expressed in the pituitary gland, and there is evidence that kisspeptin can act directly on the gonadotroph to prompt LH secretion.[323] In sheep, kisspeptin colocalizes to a high proportion of GnRH receptor cells in the preoptic area as well as various neuronal fibers within the external neurosecretory zone of the median eminence. This raises the possibility that both kisspeptin and GnRH are secreted into the pituitary portal system to affect the pituitary gland.[333] There are also single-labeling KISSP1R cells in the preoptic area, and the number rises with ovariectomy.

In addition to neurons that specifically secrete kisspepetin, other infundibular nucleus neurons in the human being that coexpress kisspeptin and neurokinin B as well as B-dynorphin (an opioid inhibitor) are known as *kisspeptin-neurokinin* (KNDy) neurons.[334] KNDy cells have receptors for neurokinin B, and B-dynorphin axons connect with their own KNDy cell and other KNDy cells as well as GnRH neurons. It appears that the stimulatory role of neurokinin B and the inhibitory action of dynorphin auto-synaptically coordinate the pulsatile release of kisspeptin, which in turn stimulates the pulsatile release of GnRH.[334] There are no steroid receptors on GnRH neurons but there are on kisspeptin and KNDy neurons, which appear to modulate both the feedback inhibition and positive feedback effects of estrogen on gonadotropin secretion.

Spontaneous mutations in the KISS1/KISS1R axis in human beings are rare but instructive in elucidating the role of KISS1 in pubertal development; hypogonadotropic hypogonadism and CPP occur with different mutations of KISS1R (see later). Plasma concentrations of kisspeptin are higher in children than adults, and preliminary studies indicate that a rise occurs at puberty in boys and girls.[335] These cases, augmented with studies of various animal species, suggest that kisspeptin acting through the KISS1R stimulates GnRH secretion.

With the demonstrated importance of KISS/KISSR in human reproduction, it is interesting to note that in mice alterative pathways operate. Thus, elimination of KISS signaling by knockout of *KISS* (5% remained) and of *KISSR* genes (90% remained) did not eliminate puberty or fertility in developing female mice, although acute ablation of the axis in adult mice did eliminate fertility.[336] Alternative studies demonstrated that retention of 5% of the KISS/KISSR axis in male mice allowed fertility but conversely demonstrated decreased fertility in female mice.[336] The discrepancy in the female mouse results may be due to variatons in techniques used in the studies but is not yet resolved. However, it does appear clear that there are far more KISS or KISSR neurons than are needed for fertility and that redundancy is invoked to ensure the vital role of reproduction can occur.

Ontogeny

In all vertebrates examined, GnRH neurons arise in the embryo from the epithelium of the olfactory placode and migrate in a rostrocaudal direction by an ordered spatiotemporal course along the pathway of the nervus terminalis-vermonasal complex to the forebrain.[337] The terminalis-vermonasal complex also originates in the olfactory placode and forms a connection between the nasal septum and the forebrain. This contrasts to the pattern of growth hormone–releasing factor (GRF), thyrotropin-releasing factor (TRF), or corticotropin-releasing factor (CRF) neurosecretory neurons, which originate from ventricular zones within the embryonic forebrain.[338]

The GnRH green fluorescent protein model demonstrates an increase in dendritic and somal spines in adult mice compared with juveniles, suggesting an increase in direct excitatory inputs to GnRH neurons and increased glutamatergic stimulation of GnRH neurons across the time of puberty.[339] Embryonic GnRH neurons of the olfactory placode and the hypothalamus coexpress mRNAs for GnRH and the type 1 GnRH receptor. These neurons demonstrate spontaneous electrical pulsatile activity, which can be stimulated by GnRH agonist and abolished by GnRH antagonist in the same pattern as GnRH pulses, all in a calcium-dependent manner (i.e., the intracellular calcium responses are stimulated by the agonist and inhibited by the antagonist).[321]

Human Fetus

GnRH immunoreactivity was observed in the epithelium of the medial aspect of the olfactory placode of the normal human fetus by 42 days of gestation but not at 28 to 32 days[337] (Table 25-11). No GnRH neurosecretory neurons were found in the brain, including the hypothalamus, of a 19-week gestational male human fetus with Kallmann syndrome,[340] and the olfactory bulbs were absent. However, dense clusters of GnRH cells and fibers were present in the nose, including the nasal septum and cribriform plate, and within the dural layers of the meninges under the forebrain. The GnRH neurosecretory neurons migrate from the olfactory placode to the hypothalamus in normal humans and other mammals.

Aberrant migration of the GnRH neurons leads to delayed or absent pubertal development due to hypogonadotropic hypogonadism, and anosmia or hyposmia is a cardinal feature of some forms of the Kallmann syndrome and the CHARGE syndrome (*c*olobomas, *h*eart anomalies, choanal *a*tresia, *r*etardation, *g*enital and *e*ar anomalies) (see later discussion).

The number of the GnRH neurons and the GnRH mRNA levels in nonhuman primates and mice do not appear to change during pubertal development. The ability of the GnRH neuron to respond to electrical or neurochemical (e.g., glutamatergic, kisspeptinergic) stimuli does not change with pubertal development.[341]

GnRH has been detected in human embryonic brain extracts by 4.5 weeks and in the fetal hypothalamus by 6 weeks (see Table 25-11); the fetal pituitary gonadotrophs are responsive to GnRH. The hypothalamic-hypophyseal portal system is functional by 11.5 weeks' gestation, and by 16 weeks, axon fibers that contain GnRH are present in the median eminence and terminate in contact with capillaries of the portal system.[102,224,294,295] The available data are consistent with the development of a human fetal hypothalamic GnRH pulse generator by at least the end of the first trimester.[103,295]

The human fetal gonad is affected by placental gonadotropins and by fetal pituitary FSH and LH.[295] The placental gonadotropin hCG may play an important role in the secretion of testosterone by the Leydig cells of the fetal testes during masculinization of the wolffian ducts and the external genitalia at 8 to 13 weeks' gestation. However, it is uncertain whether functional hCG/LH and FSH receptors are present in the fetal testis by 12 weeks of gestation and whether the early fetal testis responds to hCG. Fetal Leydig cells are a unique population of Leydig cells limited to the

TABLE 25-11

Early Development of the Human Fetal Pituitary and Hypothalamus

Gestational Age (wk)	Hypothalamus	Pituitary	Portal Circulation
3	Forebrain appears		
4		Rathke's pouch in contact with stomodeum	
5	Diencephalon differentiated	Rathke's pouch separated from stomodeum and in contact with infundibulum; pituitary in culture can secrete corticotropin, prolactin, GH, FSH	
6	Premammillary preoptic nucleus; GnRH detected	Intermediate-lobe primordia; cell cords penetrate mesenchyme around Rathke's pouch	
7	Arcuate, supraoptic nucleus	Sphenoidal plate forms	
8	Median eminence differentiated: TRH detected	Basophils appear	Capillaries in mesenchyme
9	Paraventricular nucleus; dorsal medial nucleus	Pars tuberalis formed: β-endorphin detected*	
10	Serotonin and norepinephrine detected*	Acidophils appear	
11	Mammillary nucleus; primary (hypothalamic) portal plexus present; β-endorphin and opioidergic neurons detected*	Secondary (pituitary) portal plexus present; catecholamines detected by IF	Functional hypothalamic hypophyseal portal system
12	Dopamine present		
13	Corticotropin-releasing hormone detected*	α-Melanocyte-stimulating hormone detected	
14	Fully differentiated hypothalamus	Adult form of hypophysis developed	

*Hormone is detected at this gestational age but may be present earlier.
FSH, follicle-stimulating hormone; GH, growth hormone; GnRH, gonadotropin-releasing hormone; IF, immunofluorescence; TRH, thyrotropin-releasing hormone.
Modified from Gluckman P, Grumbach MM, Kaplan SL. The human fetal hypothalamus and pituitary gland. In: Tulchinsky D, Ryan KJ, eds. *Maternal-Fetal Endocrinology*. Philadelphia, PA: WB Saunders, 1980:196-232.

fetus and infant, which regress to be followed by the differentiation of adult-type Leydig cells in the peripubertal period.[342] Fetal testosterone and hCG levels, but not LH levels, were decreased in fetuses studied after elective second-trimester abortions between 11 and 19 weeks' gestation, with no significant change in testicular responsiveness. The proportion of nonfunctional LHCGR transcripts in fetal testes was 2.3-fold lower than in adults, so available ligand may exert a greater effect. Fetal hCG was reduced, and the ratio of inactive to active LHCGR isoforms was lowered by maternal smoking. Second-trimester fetal testosterone levels appear to decrease due to decreasing maternal hCG, because Leydig cell LH/hCG responsiveness remains constant. Even with the decrease of fetal hCG caused by maternal cigarette smoking, because the ratio of inactive to active LHCGR isoforms is reduced, testosterone remains normal due to fetal gonadotropin stimulation.

Compared with the adult type, fetal Leydig cells form tightly opposed clusters joined by gap junctions and lack Reinke crystals; they are resistant to hCG/LH-induced desensitization (hCG/LH produce upregulation of LHCGRs); and they contain little aromatase activity and few estradiol receptors. In contrast to the fetal testis, FSH receptors in the fetal ovary appear only late in the second trimester, well after completion of male phenotypic differentiation, demonstrating a sex difference in the stage of gestation at which fetal pituitary gonadotropins have an important effect on the development of the fetal gonad. In the anencephalic fetus (which is deficient in hypothalamic GHRH, resulting in deficiency of pituitary gonadotropins), the testes appear hypoplastic by early in the third trimester; however, the ovaries in this disorder are normal until at least 32 weeks' gestation.[102,295] AR mRNA expression is lower, and AMH mRNA expression is higher in fetal testicular Sertoli cells than in adult testes. This may explain the failure of testicular testosterone to support spermatogenesis and to suppress AMH at that stage; patients with androgen insensitivity syndrome also have an increase in circulating testosterone and AMH and have combined gonadotropin stimulation that is consistent with a failure of testosterone to repress AMH in the absence of AR signaling.[343] AR was expressed in peritubular and Leydig cells.

The human fetal pituitary gland contains FSH and LH by 10 weeks, secretion begins by 11 to 12 weeks, and the gonadotropin content increases until approximately 25 to 29 weeks of gestation.[102,224,295] Fetal serum LH and FSH concentrations rise to peak levels by midgestation and then decrease to low values in umbilical venous blood at term. The serum concentrations of FSH and LH and of bioactive FSH at 17 to 24 weeks' gestation are strikingly higher in female than in male fetuses, and in both sexes, they decrease remarkably between 25 and 40 weeks of gestation. Mean FSH and LH concentrations are elevated at the beginning of the third trimester and decrease with advancing gestational age to undetectable values in term fetuses. Mean FSH values are higher in female fetuses between 26 and 36 weeks, whereas the mean LH level is higher in males. In the ovine fetus, LH and FSH are secreted in a pulsatile manner in response to the episodic secretion of fetal hypothalamic GnRH; human fetal pituitary gonadotropins are probably released in the same mode. The mean FSH and LH content of fetal pituitary glands is greater in female than in male fetuses at midgestation. This difference has been ascribed to the higher concentration of plasma testosterone between 11 and 24 weeks in the male fetus (the only major difference in gonadal steroids between the male and female fetus) and to fetal testicular inhibin.[102,295] The decrease in serum FSH and LH concentrations during late gestation and near term is attributed to maturation of the negative feedback mechanism, the development of gonadal steroid receptors in the hypothalamic-pituitary unit,[224] and the effect of inhibin.[102,295]

In vitro studies indicate that the human fetal pituitary gland is responsive to GnRH as early as 10 weeks' gestation; the GnRH-stimulated release of LH is greater in second trimester fetal pituitary cells cultured from females than in those cultured from males and is augmented by estradiol in both sexes.[322] In vivo studies during middle and late gestation demonstrate the stimulating action of exogenous GnRH on fetal FSH and LH release by 16 weeks, with a striking sex difference in the FSH response and a fall in responsiveness to GnRH in late gestation. Anencephalic infants and some infants with neonatal hypothalamic hypopituitarism have an absent or diminished gonadotropin response to GnRH,[102,224,295] in contrast to the brisk increase demonstrated in the normal infant.

A pattern of increasing synthesis and secretion of FSH and LH leading to peak serum concentrations at castrate levels, probably the result of relatively autonomous, unrestrained activity of the fetal hypothalamic GnRH pulse generator and subsequent stimulation of the fetal gonadotrophs by GnRH, is followed by a decline after midgestation that persists to term, probably due to maturation of the negative feedback mechanism and increasing sensitivity of the GnRH pulse generator to the inhibitory effects of the high concentration of sex steroids (estrogens and progesterone from the placenta and, in the male, testosterone from the fetal testes) the fetal circulation; in the male fetus, there is also a contributory effect on the decrease in FSH by testicular inhibin in late gestation. The increasing CNS control of gonadotropin secretion seems to require the maturation of gonadal steroid receptors (intracellular or on the cell surface, or both) in the fetal hypothalamus and in the pituitary gonadotrophs.[224]

Sheep Fetus

In fetal sheep, the hypothalamus secretes GnRH in a pulsatile manner.[294] By 0.6 gestation, the secretion of fetal LH and FSH is pulsatile, mediated by the hypothalamic GnRH pulse generator.[294] A sex difference in gonadotropin secretion occurs in ovine and human fetuses, and orchiectomy (but not oophorectomy) in the ovine fetus leads to increased pulsatile secretion of LH and, to a lesser degree, of FSH.[344] Opioidergic neurons have a tonic suppressive effect on the pulsatile release of GnRH in the ovine fetus,[345] and the excitatory amino acid analogue NMDA evokes an LH pulse mediated by GnRH.[346] The excitatory amino acids, glutamate and aspartate, can stimulate the GnRH pulse generator directly or indirectly. Glutamate is present in abundance in the hypothalamus and is released from glutamatergic neurons by exocytosis in an adenosine triphosphate- and calcium-dependent process. FSH stimulates inhibin synthesis by the ovine fetal testis and ovary, and administration of an inhibin-rich extract inhibits fetal FSH but not LH secretion, evidence of the functional capacity of the FSH-fetal gonadal inhibin feedback system.[347] These observations provide support for the central role of this process in the regulation of the CNS in the hypothalamic GnRH-pituitary gonadotropin unit.

Human Neonate and Infant[294]

In both sexes, the concentration of plasma FSH and LH is low in cord blood as a consequence of the inhibitory effect of the high levels of placental-derived estrogens, but within a few minutes after birth, the concentration of LH increases abruptly in peripheral blood (about 10-fold) in the male neonate, but not in the female; this is followed by an increase in serum testosterone concentration during the first 3 hours that persists for 12 hours or longer.[294,348] After the fall in circulating levels of steroids of placental origin (especially estrogens) during the first few days after birth, the serum concentrations of FSH and LH increase and exhibit a pulsatile pattern with wide perturbations during the first few months of life. FSH pulse amplitude is much greater in the female infant and is associated with a larger FSH response to GnRH throughout childhood; LH pulses are of greater magnitude in the male. This striking sex difference also is present in agonadal male and female infants and in infant rhesus monkeys.[294,349,350] This sex difference may in part be related to the effect of testosterone in

the male fetus on the development and function of the hypothalamic-pituitary apparatus.[102,295]

The high gonadotropin concentrations are associated with a proliferation of Sertoli cells and gonocytes (and their transformation into spermatogonia) and with a transient second wave of differentiation of fetal-type Leydig cells and increased serum testosterone levels in male infants during the first few postnatal months and increased estradiol levels intermittently during the first year of life and part of the second year in females.[342] The mean FSH concentration is higher in females than in males during the first few years of life. By approximately 6 months of age for boys and 2 to 3 years for girls, the concentration of plasma gonadotropins decreases to the low levels that are present until the onset of puberty (earlier in boys than girls) in the juvenile pause.

The neonatal-to-midinfancy surge in pulsatile gonadotropin secretion, sex hormones, and inhibin—the postnatal surge or mini-puberty of infancy—is attributable to an increase in GnRH pulse amplitude and is associated in the male infant with the following[295]:
1. Increase in testicular volume (by direct measurement) due to increased seminiferous tubule length (about a sixfold increase in year 1)
2. Rapid expansion of the Sertoli cell population (which makes up 85% to 95% of seminiferous tubular cell mass)
3. High concentration of circulating inhibin B (low in hypogonadotropic hypogonadism)
4. Sertoli cell number, including postnatal proliferation, as a determinant of spermatogenic function

The increase in circulating testosterone in the normal male infant may lead to facial comedones and even to acneiform lesions, and the increase in gonadotropins may lead to a transient increase in testicular size, but there may be subtler changes. An LH and testosterone surge is absent in those with the complete androgen insensitivity syndrome.

The postnatal surge apparently is not essential for masculine-typical psychosexual development. The brain in patients with congenital hypogonadotropic hypogonadism, including Kallmann syndrome, is masculinized by testosterone therapy at puberty despite the lack of an infantile surge in gonadotropins and testosterone.

The transient postnatal to midinfancy function of the GnRH pulse generator in the male infant may be related to future spermatogenic function and fertility.[351,352] Sertoli cells and germ cells proliferate for about 100 days after birth (indicating mitotic activity and the transformation of gonocytes into adult dark (Ad) spermatogonia, the stem cells for spermatogenesis), with a subsequent decrease, mainly by apoptosis, after about 6 months of age, coincident with the waning of gonadotropins and testosterone.

Neural Control

Maturation of the CNS is the outcome or consequence of the totality of environmental and genetic factors that retard or accelerate the onset of puberty. It is a provocative but unproven hypothesis that a metabolic signal related to body composition is an important factor in the maturation or activation of the hypothalamic GnRH pulse generator and not a result of the early hormonal and body composition changes in human puberty. In either event, clinical and experimental data support the contention that the factors influencing the timing of puberty are expressed finally through CNS regulation of the onset of puberty.[226,294] In humans, the pineal gland and melatonin do not appear to have a major effect on this control system.[294,353]

Timing and Onset of Puberty
Genetic Neural Control

Because many levels control the onset of pubertal development, a systems biology approach holds promise in characterizing the complex components of this neural and neuroendocrine network. It appears that normal and some types of abnormal puberty are under polygenic control. Although the increased pulsatile release of GnRH is most frequently considered, this change is caused by a balance in the inhibitory and excitatory factors through coordinated changes in transsynaptic and glial-neuronal communication, increased stimulatory factors (most prominently glutamate and kisspeptin), and decreased inhibitory tone, mostly through GABAergic neurons (i.e., those secreting γ-aminobutyric acid [GABA]), opioidergic neurons, and MKRN3 expression all controlled by gene expression. Glial cells affect GnRH secretion through growth factor–dependent cell-cell signaling coordinated by numerous unrelated genes. A second level of genes is postulated to control cell-cell interaction. The third highest level of control occurs through transcriptional regulation of the subordinate genes by other higher level genes that maintain the function and integration of the network.

The activation of GnRH release at puberty involves many different cellular phenotypes and intracellular and cell-to-cell signaling molecules, which is controlled by a highly coordinated and interactive regulatory system involving more than hundreds of gene products; a systems biology approach is proposed to explain how these networks are organized in a hierarchical fashion.[354] This theory states that there are transcriptional regulators that direct expression of downstream subordinate genes in order to allow stability and to coordinate the cellular networks involved in controlling the onset of puberty. Epigenetic mechanisms sesnative to external inputs such as nutrition or endocrine disruptors are posited to integrate the response of these gene networks.[355]

Although the action of multiple genes (i.e., quantitative or polygenic inheritance) on the time of onset of puberty (e.g., on stature) has long been recognized, little is known about the gene loci involved in this complex quantitative trait or the effect of gene interactions on this paradigm of complex traits.[356] Genetic factors are estimated to account for 50% to 80% of the variation in the onset of normal puberty. These complex traits have been analyzed by linkage analyses (in which quantitative trait loci have been shown to relate to the age of menarche) and by large-scale haplotype-based association studies. Pedigree analyses have revealed relative risks for delay of puberty in kindreds with histories of CDP compared with those without such a history; for example, for first-degree relatives, the risk for a 2-SD delay in the onset of puberty is 4.8. There are clear genetic influences on the time of onset of puberty in monogenetic disorders, such as *KAL1, KISS, KISS1R (GRP54), MKRN3* and mutations and other influences, that can prevent or advance pubertal development (see later discussion).

Nutrition and Metabolic Control

The genetic effects on the time of onset of puberty and its course are influenced by environmental factors (e.g., socioeconomic factors, nutrition, general health, geography) operating through the CNS. It has long been postulated that some alteration of body metabolism linked to energy metabolism may affect the CNS restraints on pubertal onset and progression, because of the earlier age of menarche in moderately obese girls, delayed menarche in states of malnutrition and chronic disease and with early rigorous athletic or ballet training, and changes in gonadotropin secretion and amenorrhea in girls with anorexia nervosa, voluntary weight loss, and strenuous physical conditioning.

An invariant mean weight (48 kg) for initiation of the pubertal spurt in weight, the maximal rate of weight gain, and menarche in healthy girls regardless of chronologic age was proposed in the 1970s, but the concept generated controversy and criticism, in part because the empiric estimations and the equations used to determine fat mass were challenged and because no direct measurements supported the theory.[357] A more recent, 5-year longitudinal study of 469 girls revealed that there was a similar percentage of body fat associated with the onset of puberty, although there was a spread of chronologic ages at onset.[358] Body composition in the 2 years before puberty had a modest impact on the age of pubertal growth, but higher fat mass led to more rapid progress through pubertal stages.[359]

The relationships of adipose tissue mass, fat metabolism, and energy balance to reproduction were illuminated by the discovery of the genes encoding leptin, an adipocyte satiety factor,[360,361] and its receptor.[362] Considerable interest has focused on the potential role of leptin in the control of the onset of puberty—from a proposal that it was an essential, if not a key, factor in triggering the onset of puberty to one in which it had a more subsidiary role. Leptin is a well-established afferent satiety factor in humans; it acts on the hypothalamus, including nuclei controlling appetite, to suppress appetite. Leptin reflects body fat and therefore energy stores and has an important role in the control of body weight and the regulation of metabolism.

Ob/ob mice (which lack leptin) and db/db mice (which lack leptin receptors) are obese and exhibit hypogonadotropic hypogonadism, providing evidence for an important role of leptin in reproduction. Administration of recombinant leptin to hypogonadal ob/ob mice and to rats experiencing pubertal delay associated with food restriction in the rat partially reverses the hypogonadism. However, leptin administration to normal prepubertal rats did not advance the time of onset of puberty. A critical threshold level of leptin was necessary for puberty to begin and advance, but leptin alone (as in administration to normal rodents) was insufficient to promote puberty; it was but one among several permissive factors.[363]

The site of action of leptin in its effect on the hypothalamic GnRH-pituitary gonadotropin apparatus was clarified by experiments in the mouse.[364] Even though leptin receptors (LepR) were reported to be expressed in immortalized mouse GnRH (GT1) cells, leptin receptors are not expressed on GnRH neurons in vivo.[365] Mice with selective deletion of the long form (signaling) of the leptin receptor underwent normal puberty and fertility. Kiss1 neurons express the leptin receptor (Ob-Rb isoform), and the suggestion was advanced that the effect of leptin on puberty onset and fertility was mediated through the Kiss1/Kiss1n complex. Mice with selective deletion of the leptin receptor from Kiss1 neurons underwent normal puberty and fertility, strongly suggesting that the action of leptin on the hypothalamic GnRH-pituitary gonadotropin system is not mediated through Kiss1 neurons.[366,367] The leptin receptor is expressed at a high level in ventral premammillary neurons, which express the excitatory neurotransmitter glutamate, which stimulates either GnRH neurons or GnRH terminals in the median eminence or both sites. These observations dissociate the action of leptin on reproductive function and on nutrition (Fig. 25-27).

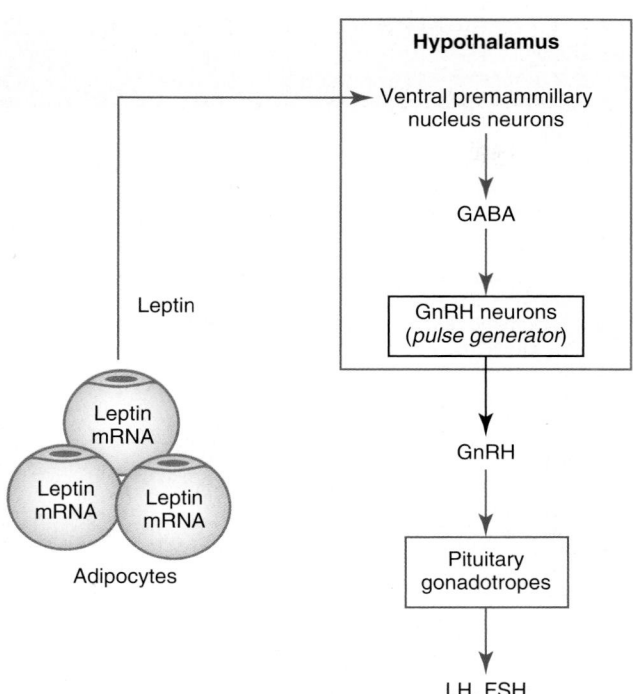

Figure 25-27 The leptin receptor is expressed in ventral premammillary neurons (PMV). Leptin secreted by adipocytes evokes release of the excitatory neurotransmitter glutamate from the PMV leading to activation of gonadotropin-releasing hormone (GnRH) neurons. Leptin functions as a permissive factor, not a trigger, in the onset of human puberty. In rodents, leptin advances the onset of puberty and plays a key role in initiating puberty and infertility. The hypothalamic pathway that regulates energy expenditure and food intake by leptin is independent of the effect of leptin on reproduction. FSH, follicle-stimulating hormone; LH, leutinizing hormone; mRNA, messenger ribonucleic acid.

Leptin levels in the male rhesus monkey were similar during the advancement of prepuberty to puberty. In peripubertal 3- to 5-year-old rhesus monkeys fasted for 2 days, the administration of leptin prevented the decrease in plasma gonadotropins detected in the untreated animals. Continuous infusion of leptin into the lateral ventricle of agonadal male monkeys failed to evoke an increase in GnRH on gonadotropin secretion.[296]

Is leptin the peripheral, somatic trigger for the onset of puberty to the CNS, or does it have a permissive role, signaling the hypothalamus and the GnRH pulse generator that a critical energy store has been attained? A longitudinal study of serum leptin levels in prepubertal and pubertal boys and girls showed leptin to increase gradually during the prepubertal years, with similar levels in the two sexes.[368] During puberty, leptin continued to rise in girls, whereas in boys, the leptin mean levels peaked at Tanner stage 2 and decreased to prepubertal concentrations by genital stage 5.[369] This decrease is attributed to the effect of testosterone on leptin secretion.[370] Adipose tissue mass, percentage of body fat, and age correlated with leptin levels, among other variables,[368,371] but there was no correlation between 24-hour serum estradiol and leptin concentrations in nonobese and obese prepubertal and early pubertal girls. Serum leptin levels rose after administration of pulsatile GnRH administration for 36 hours to children with delayed puberty but not after a single dose of buserelin, a GnRH agonist, suggesting that, rather than puberty's being triggered by leptin, pubertal increase in GnRH pulsatility increases leptin.[372]

Leptin circulates in both a free form and a high-molecular-weight, bound form. Leptin-binding activity in serum is highest in childhood and decreases to relatively low levels during puberty. Free leptin is postulated to have more relevance to reproductive development than total leptin measured in the circulation; the soluble leptin receptor appears to be higher in males than in females and is inversely related to leptin levels later in development in females.[373] A study of a 132 monozygotic female twin pairs and 48 dizygotic female twin pairs demonstrated a rise in leptin throughout puberty and a decrease in the soluble leptin receptor between stages 1 and 2, leading to a rise in the free leptin index between stages 1 and 2; there was greater heritability for the soluble leptin receptor than leptin,[374] and there was also high heritability of free IGF-1 values. There is no known relationship between leptin and leptin receptor gene polymorphism and CDP; however, the presence of a short allele of leptin was associated with heavier weight, whereas those who were thin, had significant bone age delay, and had increased frequency of parental pubertal delay were less likely to have this leptin short allele.[375]

As in the ob/ob mouse, human beings with a homozygous mutation in the leptin gene[376] or the leptin receptor[377] have morbid obesity and a striking delay in puberty because of hypogonadotropic hypogonadism. In a pedigree affected by a stop codon mutation in the gene encoding leptin, a 23-year-old man failed to attain puberty because of hypogonadotropic hypogonadism, and two affected women were prepubertal and amenorrheic, one until 29 years of age, after which she began to have irregular, scanty periods, and the other until age 36 years, at which time she began to menstruate monthly. A 9-year-old girl with a bone age of 13 years who was affected with congenital leptin deficiency lost weight and had an early pubertal pattern of LH release in response to the administration of GnRH after treatment with recombinant leptin.[378] A 4-year-old affected relative of this 9-year-old girl benefited from the metabolic improvement that occurred with leptin administration but did not undergo early pubertal development, indicating the permissive nature of leptin on puberty.

Boys with CDP have lower mean levels of leptin than expected and can enter puberty without an increase in circulating leptin. Two women with congenital lipoatrophic diabetes (Berardinelli-Seip syndrome), which is associated with absence of subcutaneous and visceral adipose tissue, did not have a delay in menarche despite severe hypoleptinemia, and one of the women had three unaffected children.[379] Severe leptin deficiency causes hypogonadotropic hypogonadism, suggesting that a critical level of leptin and a leptin signal are required to achieve puberty, but a rise in leptin is not required to trigger puberty. In summary, leptin is a permissive factor (tonic mediator) and not a trigger (phasic mediator) in the onset of human puberty (Table 25-12).

In a longitudinal study of boys leading up to an increase in morning salivary testosterone concentrations, they had a relatively constant ratio of basal metabolic rate (BMR) to LBM but an increase in the ratio of BMR to total daily energy expenditure. A subtle energy-dependent process is in play, possibly related to an increase in brain BMR as a secondary phenomenon at the initiation of puberty or indicating that a central rise in BMR is a signal for the onset of puberty.

Ghrelin is the natural ligand for the GH secretagogue receptor but also serves as an orexigenic signal that is increased after food deprivation; ghrelin is usually negatively correlated with BMI. Ghrelin administration delays pubertal development in rats because of gonadal and

TABLE 25-12

Leptin and Puberty: A Permissive Factor, Not a Trigger for the Onset of Puberty

Pro-Trigger Evidence

Congenital leptin deficiency or congenital leptin resistance related to mutations is associated with delayed puberty and gonadotropin deficiency, evidence that the virtual absence of leptin or the leptin signal leads to severe hypogonadotropic hypogonadism.

In congenital leptin deficiency, administration of leptin led to a reduction in weight and an early pubertal pattern of luteinizing hormone release in an affected prepubertal girl.

Pro-Permissive Evidence

A sharp rise in circulating leptin does not occur at the onset of puberty.

In prepubertal and early pubertal girls, the rise in serum leptin did not correlate with the increase in serum estradiol.

In constitutional delay in growth and adolescence, an increase in prepubertal leptin levels is not essential for the onset of puberty.

In congenital lipoatrophic diabetes, despite the absence of subcutaneous and visceral adipose tissue and, as a consequence, severe hypoleptinemia, puberty can occur at the usual age and fertility is reported.

Supportive experimental data exist in rodents, sheep, and nonhuman primates.

From Grumbach MM. The neuroendocrinology of human puberty revisited. *Horm Res.* 2002;57(Suppl 2):2-14.

central effects, suggesting a link between malnutrition and the decrease in reproductive development or function.[380]

Adiponectin is an adipocytokine produced in fat cells that has antidiabetic, antiatherogenic, and anti-inflammatory effects. Adiponectin decreases in the face of excess fat mass in obesity and is suppressed by rising testosterone and DHEAS levels. The concentration of adiponectin falls during pubertal development in males but remains rather stable in females with advancing Tanner stage.[381]

Resistin is an adipocytokine belonging to the resistin-like molecular family of cysteine-rich molecules (RELMs). Values increase with pubertal development in boys, and this appears to be true in girls as well, although the evidence is weaker. Because resistin serum levels were elevated in mouse models of obesity, it was considered to be a potential link between insulin resistance and obesity, but serum resistin levels appear to relate more to pubertal development than to insulin resistance.[382]

Mechanisms of Control

Diverse strategies and adaptive mechanisms have evolved to control puberty in different species.[296,350] In rodents, exteroceptive factors and cues, including light, olfaction, and pheromones, have an important influence by way of the CNS on gonadotropin secretion. In seasonal-breeding species such as sheep, the length of the light-dark cycle is critical, and the pattern of gonadotropin secretion is different. In contrast, male and female primates exhibit an estrogen-provoked LH surge.

In humans and nonhuman primates, after the initial development and function in the fetus, the infantile surge of increased LH and FSH secretion occurs; this is followed by a decade of suppression (but not absence) of activity of the hypothalamic GnRH pulse generator and the resulting quiescence of the pituitary gonadotropin-gonadal axis, known as the prepubertal period or juvenile pause (Table 25-13).[102,294,296,350] Then there is gradual disinhibition and reactivation, mainly at night during late child-

TABLE 25-13

Potential Components of the Intrinsic Central Nervous System Inhibitory Mechanism ("Juvenile Pause")

I. Inhibitory

A. Inhibitory central neurotransmitter-neuromodulatory pathways
  1. γ-Aminobutyric acid (the main inhibitory factor)
  2. Endogenous opioid peptides

II. Stimulatory

A. Stimulatory central neurotransmitter-neuromodulatory pathways
  1. Excitatory amino acids
  2. Calcium-mobilizing agonists
  3. Noradrenergic
  4. Dopaminergic
  5. Neuropeptide Y
  6. Nitric oxide
  7. Prostaglandins (PGE$_2$)
B. Other brain peptides
  1. Neurotrophic and growth peptides
  2. Activin A
  3. Endothelin-1, -2, -3

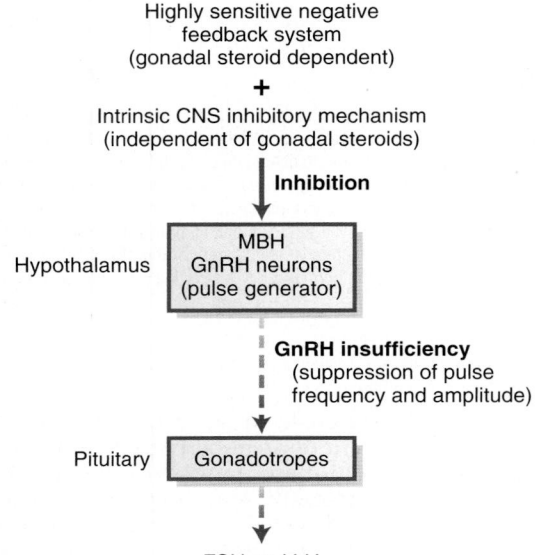

Figure 25-28 Postulated dual mechanism of restraint of puberty involves gonadal steroid-dependent and gonadal steroid-independent processes (i.e., intrinsic central nervous system [CNS] inhibitory mechanism). FSH, follicle-stimulating hormone; GnRH, gonadotropin-releasing hormone; LH, luteinizing hormone; MBH, medial basal hypothalamus. (Modified from Grumbach MM, Kaplan SL. The neuroendocrinology of human puberty: an ontogenetic perspective. In: Grumbach MM, Sizonenko PC, Aubert ML, eds. *Control of the Onset of Puberty.* Baltimore, MD: Williams & Wilkins; 1990: 1-68.)

hood,[294,296,350,383] and, finally, the increased amplitude of the GnRH pulses, reflected in the progressively increased and changing pattern of circulating LH pulses that occurs with the approach of and during puberty. Two interacting mechanisms have been proposed to explain the juvenile pause [294,383] (Fig. 25-28).

Gonadal Steroid–Dependent Negative Feedback Mechanism. There are three lines of evidence for an operative negative feedback mechanism in prepubertal[226,294] children[228,295]:

1. The pituitary of the prepubertal child secretes small amounts of FSH and LH, showing a low level of activity of the hypothalamic-pituitary-gonadal complex.
2. In agonadal infants and prepubertal children (e.g., in Turner syndrome), secretion of FSH and, to a lesser

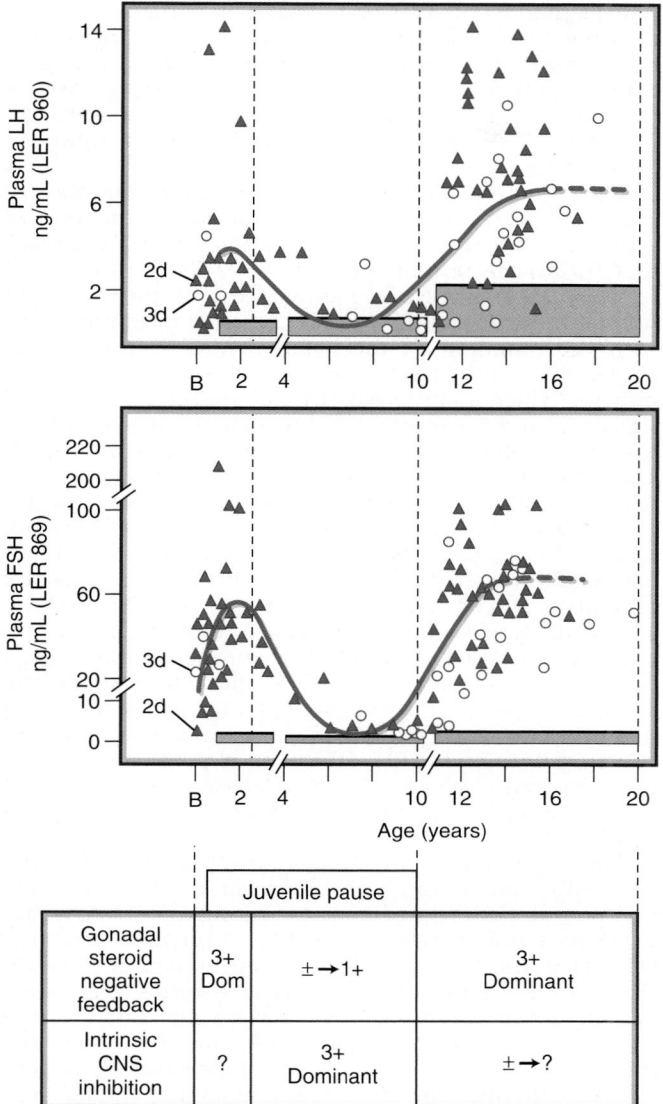

		Juvenile pause	
Gonadal steroid negative feedback	3+ Dom	± → 1+	3+ Dominant
Intrinsic CNS inhibition	?	3+ Dominant	± → ?

Figure 25-29 Interaction of the negative feedback mechanism and the putative intrinsic central nervous system (CNS) inhibitory mechanism in restraining puberty as extrapolated from the pattern of change in the concentrations of follicle-stimulating hormone (FSH) and luteinizing hormone (LH) in agonadal infants, children, and adolescents. *Triangles* designate patients with the 45,X karyotype. *Circles* indicate Turner syndrome patients with X chromosome mosaicism or structural abnormalities of the X chromosome, or both. Notice the values for the 2- and 3-day-old infants. The *solid line* represents a regression line of best fit. The *hatched area* indicates the mean plasma values for normal females. To convert FSH values to international units per liter, multiply by 8.4. For about the first 3 years of life, the sensitive gonadal steroid negative feedback mechanism has a dominant role in restraining gonadotropin secretion, as exemplified by the high gonadotropin concentrations in this age group in the absence of gonads (and gonadal steroid feedback). A major role of the intrinsic CNS inhibitory mechanism in this age group is unlikely in light of the rise in gonadotropins to castrate levels in the absence of functional gonads. From 4 to 6 years of age, the postulated intrinsic CNS inhibitory mechanism is dominant, as indicated by the fall in FSH and LH concentrations in the absence of gonads. Even in this age group, the augmented gonadotropin response evoked by gonadotropin-releasing hormone (GnRH) and the slightly higher mean basal gonadotropin concentrations in agonadal individuals support a role, although a subsidiary one, for gonadal steroid negative feedback in the suppression of gonadotropin secretion during this period of the juvenile pause. The investigators suggested that the intrinsic CNS inhibitory mechanism suppresses the functional GnRH pulse generator. After about 10 years of age, the CNS inhibition gradually wanes, resulting in disinhibition of the GnRH pulse generator. The gonadal steroid negative feedback mechanism with an adult-type set-point and inhibin plays a dominant role in regulating the GnRH pulse generator and pituitary gonadotropin system. For conversion to SI units, see Figure 25-19. (Modified from Grumbach MM, Kaplan SL. The neuroendocrinology of human puberty: an ontogenetic perspective. In: Grumbach MM, Sizonenko PC, Aubert ML, eds. *Control of the Onset of Puberty.* Baltimore, MD: Williams & Wilkins; 1990:1-68; and Conte FA, Grumbach MM, Kaplan SL. A diphasic pattern of gonadotropin secretion in patients with the syndrome of gonadal dysgenesis. *J Clin Endocrinol Metab.* 1975;40:670-674. Copyright by The Endocrine Society.)

degree, LH is increased, suggesting that even low levels of hormones secreted by the normal prepubertal gonad inhibit gonadotropin secretion by a sensitive, functional, tonic, negative feedback mechanism[226,294,383] (Fig. 25-29).

3. The low level of gonadotropin secretion in childhood is shut off by administration of small amounts of gonadal steroids, showing that the hypothalamic-pituitary gonadotropin unit is highly sensitive (approximately 6 to 15 times more sensitive than in the adult) to the feedback effect of gonadal steroids.[228,295]

Gonadal Steroid–Independent (Intrinsic) Central Nervous System Inhibitory Mechanism. The diphasic pattern of basal and GnRH-induced FSH and LH secretion from infancy to adulthood is similar in normal individuals and in agonadal patients, but in the latter, gonadotropin concentrations are higher, except during the middle childhood nadir.[355,356,383] The high plasma concentrations of FSH and LH in agonadal children between infancy and about 4 years of age and the increased gonadotropin reserve reflect the absence of gonadal steroid inhibition (see Fig. 25-29) of the hypothalamic-pituitary unit by the low plasma levels of

gonadal steroids.[294,295] However, the striking fall in gonadotropin secretion between the ages of 4 and 11 years suggests the presence of a CNS inhibitory mechanism that restrains the hypothalamic GnRH pulse generator, independent of gonadal steroid secretion. The resulting fall in gonadotropin secretion in agonadal children does not result from gonadal steroid feedback (because functional gonads are lacking) nor from increased secretion of adrenal steroids (because concentrations are low and glucocorticoid suppression of the adrenal does not augment the concentration of circulating gonadotropins.[294,295] A CNS steroid-independent inhibitory mechanism for suppression of the hypothalamic GnRH pulse generator seems to be the dominant factor in restraint of puberty between[294,384] the ages of 4 and 11 years,[295,357] and a gradual loss of this intrinsic CNS inhibitory mechanism leads to disinhibition or reactivation of the GnRH pulse generator at puberty.

Interaction of the Negative Feedback Mechanism and the Intrinsic Central Nervous System Inhibitory Mechanism. The negative feedback mechanism and the intrinsic CNS inhibitory mechanism appear to interact in restraining puberty (see Fig. 25-29). During the first 2 to 3 years of life, the gonadal-steroid negative feedback mechanism seems to be dominant, but beginning at about 3 years of age, the intrinsic CNS inhibitory mechanism becomes dominant and remains so during the rest of the juvenile pause, as evidenced by the fall in FSH and LH levels between the ages of 3 and 10 years despite the lack of functional gonads. The negative feedback mechanism remains operative during the juvenile pause; agonadal patients in this age group have higher mean plasma FSH levels than normal prepubertal children and a greater FSH and LH response to the acute administration of GnRH.[355,356,383] As puberty approaches, the CNS inhibitory mechanism gradually wanes, initially during nighttime sleep, and the hypothalamic GnRH pulse generator becomes less sensitive to gonadal steroid negative feedback (see Fig. 25-29).[294,295] After the onset of puberty, gonadal-steroid negative feedback becomes the dominant mechanism in restraining gonadotropin secretion (along with inhibin), as reflected in the increased gonadotropin concentrations that are characteristic of the adolescent with severe primary hypogonadism.[296] The postulated ontogeny of this dual mechanism of restraint of puberty is illustrated in Figure 25-29.

Potential Components of the Intrinsic Central Nervous System Inhibitory Mechanism. The intrinsic CNS inhibitory mechanism long remained elusive.[350] In the rhesus monkey, despite the damping of the GnRH pulse generator during the juvenile pause, the content of hypothalamic GnRH and GnRH mRNA during this phase is similar to that in the infant or the adult monkey. Low-amplitude LH and FSH pulses are detectable by sensitive and specific immunoradiometric assays in the juvenile pause, demonstrating a low level of activity of the GnRH pulse generator.[298,350] The end of the juvenile pause is marked by an increase in LH pulse amplitude that is most evident during the early hours of sleep.

Children with CPP associated with posterior hypothalamic neoplasms (usually a pilocytic astrocytoma), irradiation of the CNS, midline CNS developmental abnormalities such as septo-optic dysplasia with deficiency of one or more pituitary hormones, or other CNS lesions provide indirect evidence for an inhibitory neural component located in or projecting through the posterior hypothalamus. These lesions compromise the neural pathway, which inhibits the hypothalamic GnRH pulse generator and results in its disinhibition and activation leading to CPP.[294] For example, a suprasellar arachnoid cyst can cause CPP by compressing and distorting the hypothalamus,[294] but the puberty is reversed with regression of the hormonal and physical features of puberty after decompression of the cyst due to reversal of the disinhibition of the CNS inhibitory mechanism of the posterior pituitary (Fig. 25-30). Precocious sexual maturation can be induced in the juvenile female rhesus monkey by posterior hypothalamic lesions; such lesions advance the age at onset of a pubertal increase in LH secretion and the time of the first positive feedback effects of estrogen.[350]

The GnRH-secreting hypothalamic hamartoma, a heterotypic mass of nervous tissue that contains GnRH neurosecretory neurons attached to the tuber cinereum or the floor of the third ventricle, can cause CPP.[385,386] The GnRH neurons within the hamartoma with their axon fibers projecting to the median eminence secrete GnRH in pulsatile fashion. We consider the hypothalamic hamartoma to be an ectopic GnRH pulse generator that functions independently of the CNS inhibitory mechanism, which normally restrains the hypothalamic GnRH pulse generator (Fig. 25-31).[294,386] An analogy can be drawn between the GnRH-secreting hypothalamic hamartoma and the rescue of fertility in GnRH-deficient hypogonadal (hyp/hyg) mice by

transplantation of fetal or neonatal hypothalamic tissue into the third ventricle. Some rare, large hypothalamic hamartomas that cause CPP contain TGF-α, an astroglia-derived growth factor, with few or no GnRH neurosecretory neurons, raising the possibility that the secretion of TGF-α may interact directly or indirectly to stimulate GnRH release.

The recent discovery of families with precocious puberty associated with loss of function mutations in the *MKRN3* gene has led to important insights into the CNS "brake" that intrinsically restrains puberty.[387,388] *MKRN3* is imprinted as the maternal allele is methylated and suppressed in normal individuals and only the paternal gene functions; with the mutation in the paternal *MKRN3* there is no longer function. *MKRN3* encodes makorin RING-finger protein, which is involved with ubiquitination and cell signaling, and is expressed in the arcuate nucleus, a location where other genes involved with puberty are found. *MKRN3* decreases in mice at the same time that KISS and neurokinin B rise to promote puberty. At present, 10 different loss-of-function mutations of *MKRN3* have been described in 22 patients with CPP from 13 multiplex families, including eight frameshift defects, three missense mutations, and one nonsense mutation[389] (see Fig. 25-24B).

Noradrenergic, dopaminergic, serotoninergic, and opioidergic pathways; inhibitory neurotransmitters (e.g., GABA); excitatory amino acids (e.g., glutamic acid, aspartic acid); nitrergic transmitters; other brain peptides, including neurotrophic and growth factors; and corticotropin-releasing hormone (CRH) affect the hypothalamic GnRH pulse generator (see Table 25-13). Melatonin is not a critical restraining factor in primates, nor are endogenous opioid peptides.[294,296,346]

The GnRH pulse generator is inhibited by GABA (the most important inhibitory neurotransmitter in the primate brain) and GABAergic neurons during prepuberty, but exogenous administration of GABA in prepuberty is ineffective because of the high local endogenous GABA levels[297] (Fig. 25-32).[298] Both GAD65 and GAD67 forms of glutamic acid decarboxylase (GAD), the enzyme that catalyzes the conversion of glutamate to GABA, are present in the mediobasal hypothalamus, the site of the GnRH pulse generator. Antisense oligodeoxynucleotides for GAD67 and GAD65 mRNAs infused into the stalk median eminence of prepubertal monkeys induced a striking increase in GnRH release, whereas nonsense D-oligos did not. These studies provided additional support for GABA arising from interneurons as the intrinsic CNS inhibitor during the juvenile pause of prepuberty.

GABA acting through GABA$_A$ and GABA$_B$ receptors affects GnRH secretion in the perifused mouse GT1 GnRH-releasing neuronal cell line. Stimulation of GABA$_B$ receptors also inhibits kisspeptin secretion in the adult mouse.[390] Conversely, chronic, repetitive administration of bicuculline, a GABA inhibitor, into the base of the third ventricle of a prepubertal monkey caused premature menarche and the onset of the first ovulation.[297] Although GABA is inhibitory in the juvenile and adult brain it is excitatory early in brain development through the postnatal period.[391] The switch from dominance of the gonadal steroid-dependent negative feedback mechanism in infancy and early childhood to dominance of the intrinsic CNS inhibitory mechanism may be associated with the developmental switch of GABAergic synaptic transmission from excitatory to inhibitory.

The onset of puberty in the rhesus monkey is characterized by a decrease in GABAergic (and possibly neuropeptide Y [NPY]) inhibition of the hypothalamic GnRH pulse generator and increased release of glutamate,[298] the major

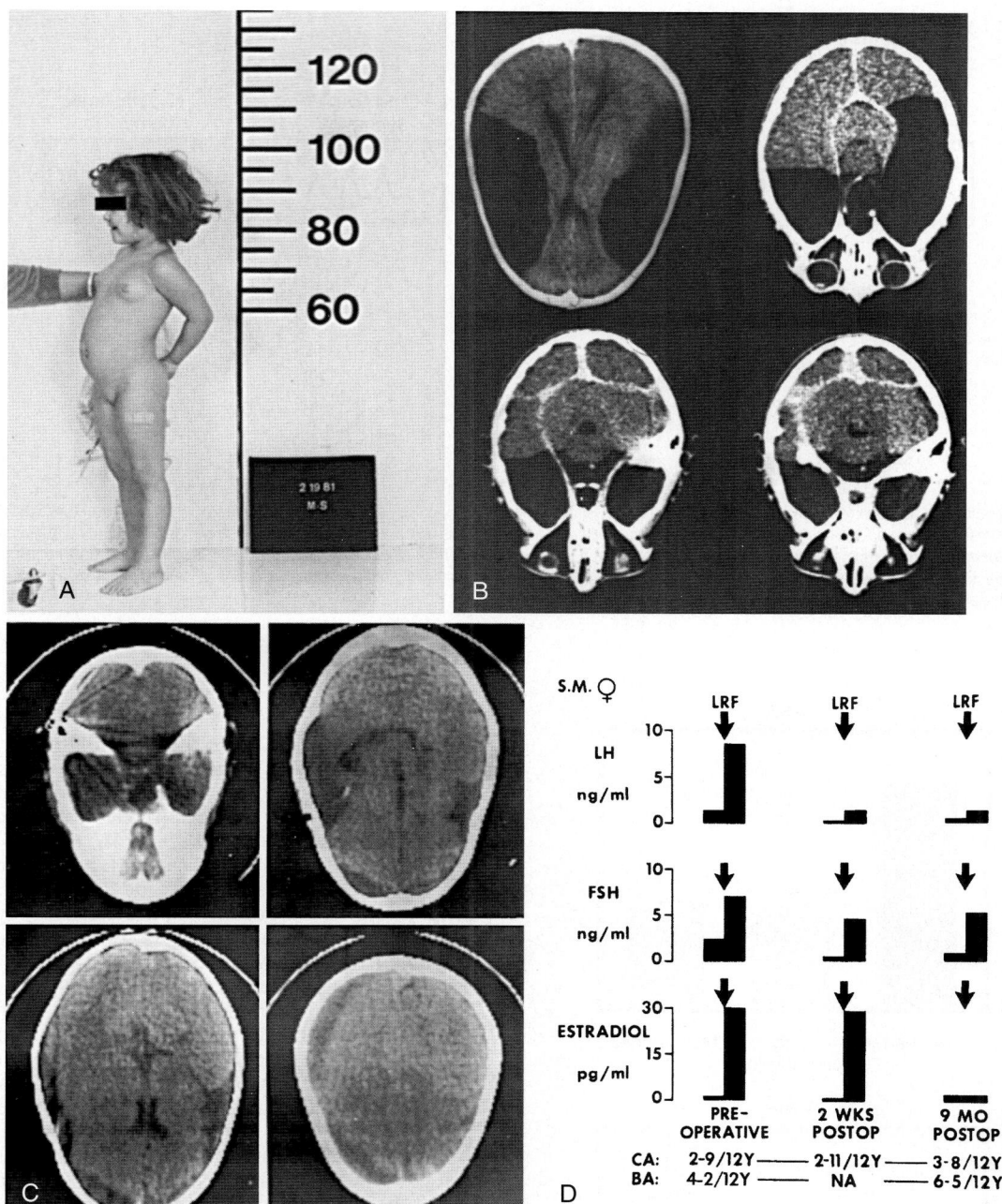

Figure 25-30 A, True precocious puberty in a 2.75-year-old girl is caused by a large, bilateral, congenital suprasellar arachnoid cyst. Signs of sexual precocity were observed during the preceding year. The head circumference was +5 SD above the mean value for age, and frontal bossing was present. Breasts were Tanner stage 3. The serum estradiol level was 26 pg/mL, the estrone level was 38 pg/mL, and the dehydroepiandrosterone sulfate (DHEAS) level was less than 3 μg/dL. The serum luteinizing hormone (LH) concentration rose from 1.4 to 8.7 ng/mL (LER-960) after intravenous administration of gonadotropin-releasing hormone (GnRH), which constitutes a pubertal response. Bone age was 3.5 years. Pelvic ultrasonography showed pubertal-size uterus and ovaries. To convert estrone values to picomoles per liter, multiply by 3.699. To convert DHEAS values to micromoles per liter, multiply by 0.02714. For other conversions, see Figure 25-19. **B,** Cranial computed tomography (CT) scans show a low-density fluid collection in the middle cranial fossa, thinning of the cortex, and striking compression of the lateral and third ventricles. **C,** Cranial CT scans 8 months later, after decompression of the arachnoid cyst and creation of a communication between the cyst and the basal cerebrospinal fluid cisterns and a cystoperitoneal shunt. Notice the striking decrease in size of the fluid collections and expansion of the cerebral cortex. **D,** Basal and peak LH and follicle-stimulating hormone (FSH) concentrations after GnRH administration in SM and serum estradiol values before surgical decompression and 2 weeks and 9 months after surgical decompression of the arachnoid cyst. Notice the prepubertal LH response to GnRH and fall in serum estradiol level by 9 months after surgery. The bone age had increased by 3 years over an 11-month period, but the velocity returned to normal. The patient remained prepubertal during follow-up. LRF, luteinizing hormone-releasing factor; SD, standard deviation. (From Grumbach MM, Kaplan SL. The neuroendocrinology of human puberty: an ontogenetic perspective. In: Grumbach MM, Sizonenko PC, Aubert ML, eds. *Control of the Onset of Puberty.* Baltimore, MD: Williams & Wilkins; 1990:1-68.)

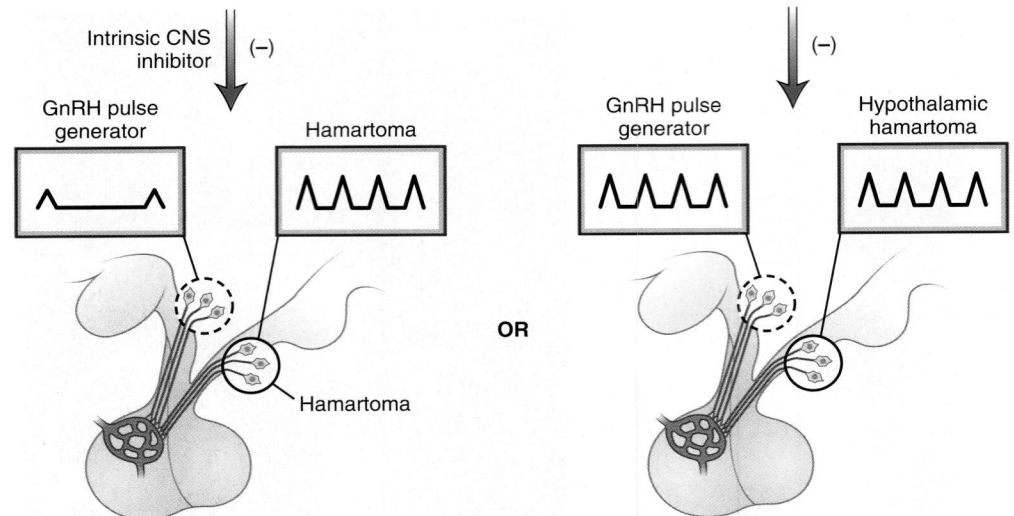

Figure 25-31 Hypothalamic hamartoma as an ectopic gonadotropin-releasing hormone (GnRH) pulse generator that escapes the intrinsic central nervous system (CNS) inhibitory mechanism and results in true precocious puberty. Two possible mechanisms are proposed. *Left,* The GnRH neurosecretory neurons in the hamartoma are functioning as a GnRH pulse generator without activation of the suppressed, normally located GnRH pulse generator. *Right,* The hamartoma acts as an ectopic GnRH pulse generator but communicates with and activates (possibly through axonic connections or by GnRH itself) the normally located hypothalamic GnRH pulse generator, which then functions synchronously with the hamartoma.

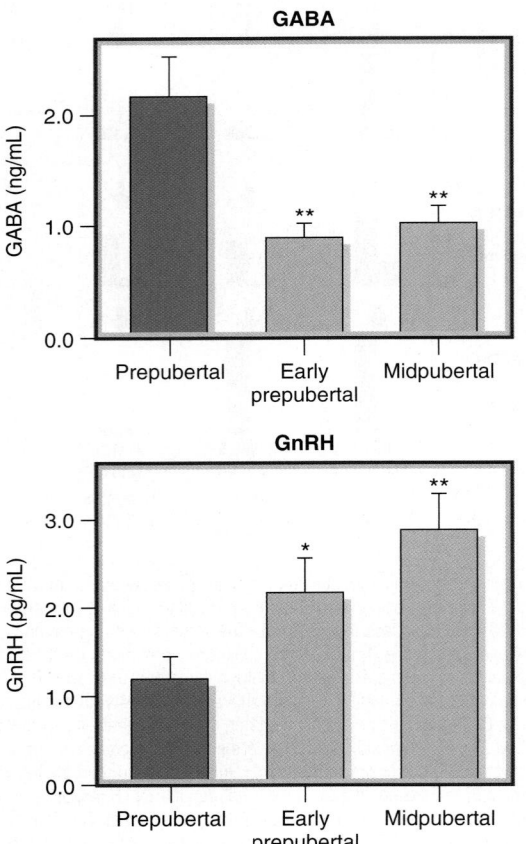

Figure 25-32 The striking developmental changes in γ-aminobutyric acid (GABA) and gonadotropin-releasing hormone (GnRH) release between the prepubertal and the pubertal rhesus monkey as measured in 10-minute perfusate samples from the stalk of the median eminence. Multiple samples were obtained from each animal. Mean ± SEM (standard error of the mean); **$p < 0.01$; *$p < 0.05$ versus prepubertal monkeys. (From Mitsushima D, Hei DL, Terasawa E. γ-Aminobutyric acid is an inhibitory neurotransmitter restricting the release of luteinizing hormone-releasing hormone before the onset of puberty. *Proc Natl Acad Sci U S A.* 1994;91:395-399.)

excitatory amino acid neurotransmitter in the hypothalamus.[297] The sensitivity to the stimulatory glutamatergic input into the GnRH pulse generator increases strikingly after the onset of puberty, but it is the reduction in GABA-ergic inhibition that is the critical factor in disinhibition of the GnRH pulse generator.[298]

A persistent question has been how a single central signal can activate GnRH neurons to cause LH release and bring about ovulation by simultaneous suppression of GABA and stimulation of glutamate release, both of which converge in the AVPV nucleus. Most neurons in the AVPV of female rats express both vesicular glutamate transporter 2 (VGLUT2), a marker of hypothalamic glutamatergic neurons, and GAD and vesicular GABA transporter (VGAT), markers of GABAergic neurons. These dual-phenotype neurons are twice as prevalent in females than in males and are the main targets of the E2 binding site in the region.[392] Moreover, dual-phenotype synaptic terminals contact GnRH neurons, and at the time of the surge, VGAT-containing vesicles decrease and VGLUT2-containing vesicles increase in these terminals. Dual-phenotype GABA/glutamate neurons may act as central transducers of hormonal and neural signals to GnRH neurons to simultaneously decrease GABA and increase glutamate release.

NELL2, a protein containing epidermal growth factor (EGF)-like repeats, is selectively expressed in the glutamatergic neurons containing VGLUT1 and in those expressing VGLUT2 in the postnatal rodent brain. NELL2 mRNA abundance increases selectively in the medial basal hypothalamus of the female rat, reaching a peak at the end of the juvenile period, and declines at the time of puberty with less change observed in the preoptic area. Intraventricular administration of antisense oligodeoxynucleotides to NELL2 reduced GnRH release from the medial basal hypothalamus and delayed the initiation of female puberty. Therefore, NELL2 plays an important role in glutamate-dependent processes of neuroendocrine regulation in puberty.[393]

Excitatory NMDA stimulates LH release in neonatal and adult rats, fetal sheep, and prepubertal and adult rhesus monkeys, and its receptors are widely distributed throughout the CNS, including the hypothalamus. NMDA evoked GnRH secretion from rat hypothalamic explants from a GnRH neuronal cell line and acutely stimulated the GnRH pulse generator in the ovine fetus but did not have a direct effect on pituitary gonadotrophs.[296,346,350,394]

Immortalized GnRH neurons contain inotropic NMDA receptors that mediate the release of GnRH by NMDA.[367] The prepubertal male rhesus monkey may be forced to enter puberty by repetitive intravenous administration of NMDA; in the prepubertal and pubertal female rhesus monkey, NMDA administered centrally and peripherally induced the release of GnRH.[395]

NPY has been suggested as a component of the central restraint mechanism in the male rhesus monkey. A small study of girls demonstrated higher NPY concentrations in those with CDP than in those with normal onset of puberty, supporting this relationship.[296,396]

These observations provide additional evidence that the hypothalamic GnRH neurosecretory neuron is not a limiting factor in puberty, as is the GnRH pulse generator; the anterior pituitary gland, gonads, and gonadal steroid end organs are functionally intact in the fetus and prepubertally and can be fully activated by the appropriate stimulus. CNS restraint of puberty lies therefore above the level of the autorhythmic GnRH neurosecretory neurons in the hypothalamus. Figure 25-13 contrasts the direct and indirect effects of the GABA inhibitory and excitatory amino acid stimulatory neurotransmitters (as represented by NMDA and other glutamate receptors) on GnRH release. In the primate, the GABA hypothalamic neural network seems to be the major component of the intrinsic CNS inhibitory mechanism during the juvenile pause.

Sleep-Associated Luteinizing Hormone Release and Onset of Puberty

In sensitive radioimmunoassays, a diurnal rhythm of serum LH, FSH, and testosterone is already demonstrable in 5- to 6-year-olds, short but otherwise normal girls, demonstrating that preparation for the changes of puberty starts long before the physical features and classic endocrine markers of puberty appear.[222,294] Although adult men and women during most phases of the menstrual cycle have little difference in the amplitude or frequency of LH pulses over a 24-hour period, sleep-associated pulsatile release of LH is prominent in early and midpuberty; only in late puberty are prominent LH-secretory episodes detected during the day, but they are still less than during sleep until the adult pattern is achieved. Augmented LH release during sleep leads to a rise in the plasma concentration of testosterone at night in boys, in children with CPP, in glucocorticoid-treated children with CAH who have an advanced bone age and early onset of true puberty, and in agonadal patients during the pubertal age period, suggesting that it does not depend on gonadal function. There is significantly increased excretion of urinary LH in prepubertal children at night compared with the day.

Sleep-enhanced LH secretion can be viewed as a maturational phenomenon related to changes in the CNS and in the hypothalamic restraint of GnRH release. Episodic release of gonadotropins is suppressed by anti-GnRH antibodies and by the administration of gonadal steroids or certain catecholaminergic agonists and antagonists and is augmented by the opioid antagonist naloxone. Naloxone does not alter the testosterone-mediated suppression of LH, nor does it alter the testosterone effect on LH pulsatility in boys in early to middle puberty. We have suggested that an increase in endogenous GnRH secretion at puberty has a priming effect on the gonadotroph and leads to increased sensitivity of the pituitary to endogenous or exogenous GnRH.[226] In monkeys, a striking increase in pulse amplitude and a lesser increase in pulse frequency occurs between prepuberty and puberty.[296,297] Sleep-associated LH release in the peripubertal period correlates with increased sensitivity of the pituitary gonadotrophs to administration of GnRH in the peripubertal period and in puberty and is an indication that the hypothalamic GnRH pulse generator initially is less inhibited during sleep, even in prepubertal children.

Pituitary and Gonadal Sensitivity to Tropic Stimuli

Endogenous GnRH secretion is estimated indirectly and qualitatively by determining the pulsatile pattern of LH and by the gonadotropin response to exogenous GnRH at different stages[388] and in disorders of the hypothalamic-pituitary-gonadal system. The release of LH after administration of GnRH is minimal in prepubertal children beyond infancy, increases during the peripubertal period and puberty (Fig. 25-33), and is still greater in adults (depending on the phase of the menstrual cycle in women).[226] These results support the concept that the prepubertal state is characterized by functional GnRH deficiency. FSH release after the administration of GnRH is comparable in prepubertal, pubertal, and adult males, indicating similar pituitary sensitivity to GnRH, but females release more FSH than males at all stages of sexual maturation. There is a striking reversal of the FSH/LH ratio after administration of GnRH to males or females between prepuberty and puberty (see Fig. 25-33).

These observations suggest a striking change in pituitary sensitivity to GnRH in prepubertal and pubertal individuals and indicate a sex difference in the dynamic reserve of pituitary FSH because the pituitary gonadotrophs of prepubertal females are more sensitive to GnRH than those of prepubertal males, even though the concentration of circulating gonadal steroids is very low in both sexes at that stage of maturation.[226] Prepubertal girls have a larger readily releasable pool of pituitary FSH than prepubertal or pubertal males, possibly related in part to the higher concentration of inhibin B in prepubertal boys (see Fig. 25-33). These may be factors in the higher frequency of idiopathic CPP in girls and in the occurrence of premature thelarche.[397] The available data are consistent with the hypothesis that less GnRH is required for FSH than for LH release.

This change in responsiveness of the gonadotrophs is apparently mediated by increased pulsatile secretion of GnRH[226,294]; the increased LH response to synthetic GnRH is one of the earliest hormonal markers of puberty onset. Studies of the effects of acute and chronic administration of synthetic GnRH in hypergonadotropic hypogonadism, hypogonadotropic hypogonadism, constitutionally delayed growth and adolescence, and idiopathic precocious puberty indicate that the degree of previous exposure of gonadotrophs to endogenous GnRH appears to affect both the magnitude and the quality of LH responses—a self-priming phenomenon.[226] With the approach of puberty, the derepression of the hypothalamic GnRH pulse generator, and the increased pulsatile secretion of GnRH augment pituitary sensitivity to GnRH and enlarge the reserve of LH. Reduction in the frequency of exogenous GnRH pulses (from one per hour to one every 3 hours) in adult rhesus monkeys with ablative hypothalamic lesions that eliminated endogenous GnRH secretion increased the FSH/LH ratio, suggesting that GnRH pulse frequency is one factor affecting relative secretion of FSH and LH. Inhibin and endogenous gonadal steroids may also affect this ratio

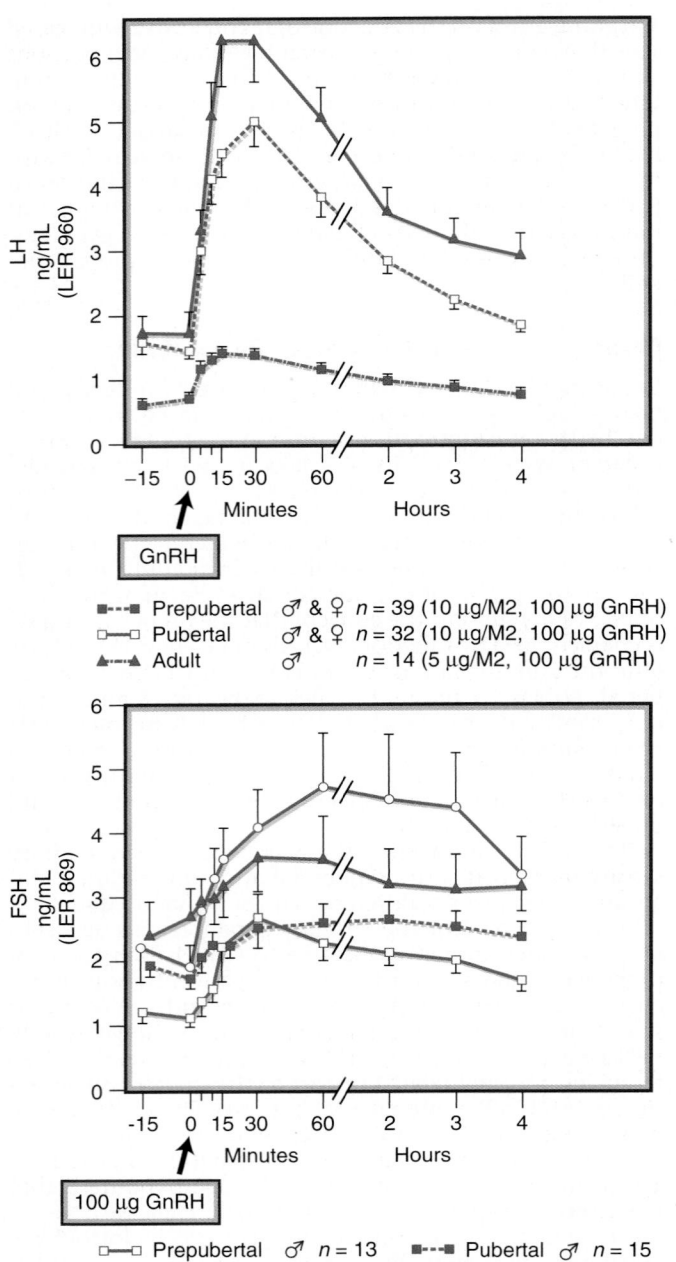

Figure 25-33 Changes in plasma luteinizing hormone (LH) *(top)* and follicle-stimulating hormone (FSH) *(bottom)* levels in prepubertal, pubertal, and adult individuals. Notice the limited LH response in prepubertal children compared with that of pubertal and adult subjects. The FSH response to gonadotropin-releasing hormone (GnRH) is similar in prepubertal, pubertal, and adult males. In females, the FSH response is significantly greater than that of prepubertal, pubertal, or adult males. For conversion to SI units, see Figure 25-19. (Modified from Grumbach MM, Roth JC, Kaplan SL, et al. Hypothalamic pituitary regulation of puberty in man: evidence and concepts derived from clinical research. In: Grumbach MM, Grave GD, Mayer FE, eds. *Control of the Onset of Puberty.* New York, NY: John Wiley & Sons; 1974:115-166.)

through action on the hypothalamus or the pituitary or both.

Pulsatile administration of GnRH to prepubertal monkeys promptly initiates puberty (and ovulatory menstrual cycles in females) and restores complete gonadal function in adult monkeys with hypothalamic lesions.[296,398] Similar studies in humans yielded comparable results for prepuber-

tal children, patients with anorexia nervosa, and adults with hypothalamic-hypogonadotropic hypogonadism.[399] These results provide further support for reactivation of the hypothalamic GnRH pulse generator as the first hormonal change in the onset of puberty.

Responsiveness of the gonads to gonadotropins increases during puberty. For example, the augmented testosterone secretion in response to administration of hCG at puberty in boys is probably a consequence of the priming effect of the increase in endogenous secretion of LH (in the presence of FSH) on the Leydig cells.

Maturation of Positive Feedback Mechanism

Estrogen exerts suppressive effects from late fetal life to peripuberty, when the positive action of endogenous (or exogenous) estradiol on gonadotropin release is not demonstrated.[226,294] A positive feedback effect, which is required for ovulation, is a late maturational event in puberty and probably does not occur before midpuberty in normal girls. The positive feedback effect requires an increased concentration of plasma estradiol for a sufficient length of time during the latter part of the follicular phase in later pubertal and adult women.[304]

Among the requirements for the positive feedback action of estradiol on gonadotropin release at puberty are ovarian follicles that are primed by FSH to secrete sufficient estradiol to reach and maintain a critical level in the circulation, a pituitary gland that is sensitized to GnRH and contains a large enough pool of releasable LH to support an LH surge, and sufficient GnRH stores for the GnRH neurosecretory neurons to respond with an acute increase in GnRH release in addition to the usual adult pattern of pulsatile GnRH secretion (this last requirement is controversial in humans but not in lower animals).[226]

Estrogen exerts effects at the anterior pituitary and the hypothalamus.[400] In the rhesus monkey, positive and negative feedback can occur in adult ovariectomized females in whom the medial basal hypothalamus is surgically disconnected from the remainder of the CNS.[296] In monkeys with hypothalamic lesions, unvarying, intermittent GnRH administration leads to sufficient estradiol release from the ovary to induce an ovulatory LH surge in the absence of an increase in the dose of the[304,398] GnRH pulses. Estradiol has a positive feedback effect directly on the pituitary gland in normal women, and prolonged administration of estradiol is accompanied by an augmented LH response to GnRH administration. The fact that the major positive feedback action on the pituitary gland is demonstrable in the absence of an increase in pulsatile GnRH secretion suggests that the failure to elicit positive feedback action with administration of estradiol to prepubertal girls may be related to the inadequate GnRH pulses or insufficient LH reserve or both.

Gonadotropin cyclicity and estradiol-induced positive feedback can be demonstrated by midpuberty and before menarche but may be insufficient to induce an ovulatory LH surge even when there is an adequate pituitary store of readily releasable LH and FSH.[1,226] The ovary does not secrete estradiol at a high level or long enough to induce an ovulatory LH surge. We visualize the process leading to ovulation as a gradual one in which the ovary (i.e., the zeitgeber for ovulation[304]) and the hypothalamic-pituitary-gonadal complex become progressively more integrated and synchronous until an ovary primed for ovulation secretes sufficient estradiol to induce an ovulatory LH surge.

As many as 55% to 90% of cycles are anovulatory during the first 2 years after menarche, but the proportion decreases to less than 20% of cycles by 5 years after menarche.[401] The mechanism of ovulation seems unstable and immature, and it does not appear to have attained the fine tuning and synchronization that are requisite for maintenance of regular ovulatory cycles. However, the prevalence of PCOS adds to the irregularity of menses and anovulation in puberty.

Overview of Current Concept

Puberty is not an immutable process; it can be arrested or reversed. Environmental factors and certain disorders that affect the onset or progression of puberty mediate their effects by direct or indirect suppression of the hypothalamic GnRH pulse generator and its periodic oscillatory signal, GnRH. Table 25-14 lists some of these factors.

ADRENAL ANDROGENS AND ADRENARCHE

Speculation has focused on the mechanism of adrenarche (the adrenal component of pubertal maturation), the fact that adrenarche occurs earlier than gonadarche (the maturation of the hypothalamic-pituitary-gonadal system), and the interaction between adrenal and gonadal hormones at puberty.[259,293,402]

Nature and Regulation of Adrenal Androgens

The major adrenal androgen precursors secreted by the adrenal cortex are DHEA, DHEAS, and androstenedione, which can undergo extraglandular metabolism to produce physiologically active testosterone and estradiol[133]; however, adrenal androgens do not directly activate the AR. DHEA and especially DHEAS (which binds avidly to serum proteins, particularly albumin) are useful biochemical markers of adrenal androgen secretion and the onset of adrenarche. Androstenedione is the major androgen secreted by the ovary during and after puberty, and it is more readily converted to potent androgens than DHEA or DHEAS.

Cross-sectional and longitudinal studies have demonstrated a progressive increase in the plasma concentration of DHEA and DHEAS in boys and girls starting by 3 years of age and becomes more noticeable approximately 2 years before the increase in gonadotropin and gonadal steroid secretion that continues through puberty (13 to 15 years),[259,293,403,404] reaches a peak at age 20 to 30 years, and then gradually decreases (Fig. 25-34).[402] The increase is not associated with increased sensitivity of the pituitary gonadotrophs to GnRH[390] or with sleep-associated LH secretion and occurs at an age when the hypothalamic-pituitary-gonadal complex is functioning at a low level.[259,397] The importance of adrenarche is a matter of long-term debate. DHEA is a neurosteroid with parallel patterns of increase along with cortical maturation from approximately age 6 years to the middle 20s, suggesting that adrenarche affects brain development. DHEAS may increase activity of the amygdala and hippocampus and promote synaptogenesis within the cortex, with effects on fearfulness, anxiety, and memory that increase social interaction with unfamiliar individuals and shape cognitive development.[405]

Associated with the increase in adrenal secretion of DHEA and DHEAS (and independent of a change in the secretion of cortisol or aldosterone) is the appearance and growth of the zona reticularis (i.e., the principal source of DHEA and DHEAS) that occurs coincidently with adrenarche (Fig. 25-35).

TABLE 25-14

Postulated Ontogeny of the Hypothalamic-Pituitary-Gonadal Circuit

Fetus

Medial basal hypothalamic GnRH neurosecretory neurons (pulse generator) operative by 80 days of gestation
Pulsatile secretion of FSH and LH by 80 days of gestation
Initially unrestrained secretion of GnRH (100 to 150 days of gestation)
Maturation of negative gonadal steroid feedback mechanism by 150 days of gestation—sex difference
Low level of GnRH secretion at term

Early Infancy

Hypothalamic GnRH pulse generator highly functional after 12 days of age
Prominent FSH and LH episodic discharges until approximately age 6 mo in males and 18 mo in females, with transient increases in plasma levels of testosterone in males and estradiol in females

Late Infancy and Childhood

Intrinsic CNS inhibition of hypothalamic GnRH pulse generator operative; predominant mechanism in childhood; maximal sensitivity by approximately 4 yr of age
Negative feedback control of FSH and LH secretion highly sensitive to gonadal steroids (low set-point)
GnRH pulse generator inhibited; low amplitude and frequency of GnRH discharges
Low secretion of FSH, LH, and gonadal steroids

Late Prepubertal Period

Decreasing effectiveness of intrinsic CNS inhibitory influences and decreasing sensitivity of hypothalamic-pituitary unit to gonadal steroids (increased set-point)
Increased amplitude and frequency of GnRH pulses, initially most prominent with sleep (nocturnal)
Increased sensitivity of gonadotrophs to GnRH
Increased secretion of FSH and LH
Increased responsiveness of gonad to FSH and LH
Increased secretion of gonadal hormones

Puberty

Further decrease in CNS restraint of hypothalamic GnRH pulse generator and in the sensitivity of negative feedback mechanism to gonadal steroids
Prominent sleep-associated increase in episodic secretion of GnRH gradually changes to adult pattern of pulses about every 90 min
Pulsatile secretion of LH follows pattern of GnRH pulses
Progressive development of secondary sexual characteristics
Spermatogenesis in males
Middle to late puberty—operative positive feedback mechanism and capacity to exhibit an estrogen-induced LH surge
Ovulation in females

CNS, central nervous system; FSH, follicle-stimulating hormone; LH, luteinizing hormone; GnRH, gonadotropin-releasing hormone.
Modified from Grumbach MM, Roth JC, Kaplan SL, et al. Hypothalamic-pituitary regulation of puberty in man: evidence and concepts derived from clinical research. In: Grumbach MM, Grave GD, Mayer FE, eds. *Control of the Onset of Puberty.* New York, NY: John Wiley & Sons; 1974:115-166.

In contrast to the zona glomerulosa and fasciculata, four main features distinguish the zona reticularis:
1. There is a low level of expression of 3β-HSD/Δ^{4,5}-isomerase type 2 and CYP21 mRNAs and enzyme activities.
2. Abundant DHEA (hydroxysteroid) sulfotransferase activity is found.
3. There is a relative increase in 17,20-lyase versus 17α-hydroxylase activity of CYP17, the enzyme that catalyzes both activities. These characteristics are shared by the fetal zone of the fetal adrenal cortex.

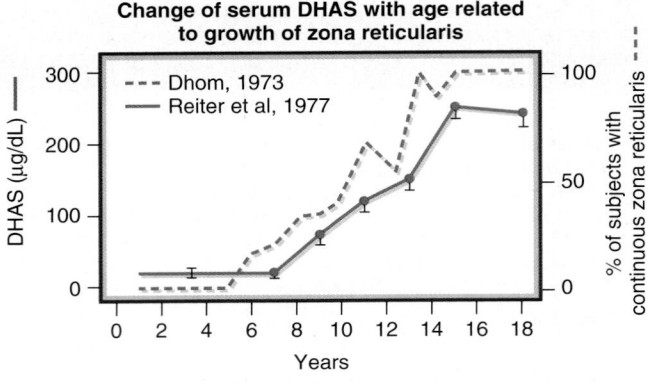

Change of serum DHAS with age related to growth of zona reticularis

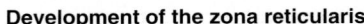

Development of the zona reticularis

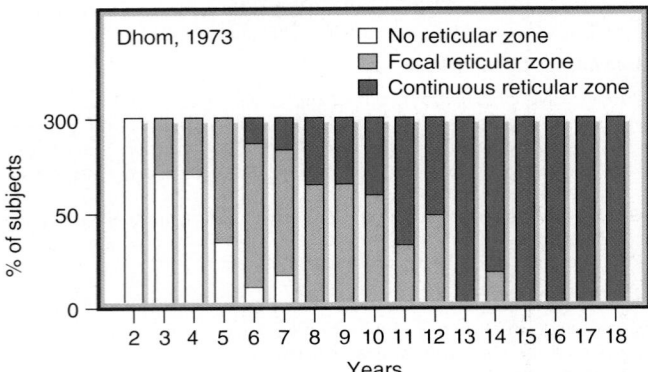

Growth of the adrenal

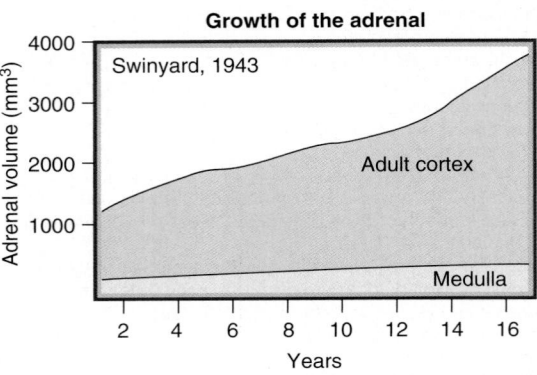

Figure 25-34 Relation of plasma dehydroepiandrosterone sulfate (DHEAS [DHAS]) levels to growth of the zona reticularis and increase in adrenal volume with age. *Top,* The close correlation between the development of the zona reticularis and the increase in the plasma DHEAS level. *Middle,* The age at which focal islands of reticular tissue or a continuous reticular zone was found in a series of patients with sudden death who had not had an antecedent illness. *Bottom,* The increase in adrenal volume at the time of puberty. For conversion to SI units, see Figure 25-19. (From Grumbach MM, Richards HE, Conte FA, et al. Clinical disorders of adrenal function and puberty: assessment of the role of the adrenal cortex and abnormal puberty in man and evidence for an ACTH-like pituitary adrenal androgen stimulating hormone. In: James VHT, Serio M, Giusti G, et al, eds. *The Endocrine Function of the Human Adrenal Cortex.* New York, NY: Academic Press; 1978:583-612.)

4. There is expression of major histocompatibility complex (MHC) class II (HLA-DR) antigens, which are not expressed in the fetal zone of the fetal adrenal cortex.

In contrast to the zona fasciculata, the zona reticularis has an increased ratio of 17,20-lyase to 17α-hydroxylase. An Arg347Ala mutation in human CYP17 resulted in strikingly decreased 17,20-lyase activity but retention of 17α-hydroxylase activity. Two XY phenotypic females with hypergonadotropic hypogonadism and normal mineralo-

corticoid and glucocorticoid function had isolated 17,20-lyase deficiency due to homozygous mutations at the Arg347 or the Arg358 residue in CYP17.

In contrast to these observations of loss of 17,20-lyase activity with retention of 17α-hydroxylase activity, the ratio of human 17,20-lyase to 17α-hydroxylase activities was increased by increased phosphorylation of serine and threonine residues on the CYP17 enzyme and by the increased abundance of redox partners such as cytochrome P450 oxidoreductase and by cytochrome b_5, which preferentially promotes 17,20-lyase activity by allosterically affecting the interaction between CYP17 and P450 oxidoreductase.[406] These studies provided a provisional hypothesis of the mechanisms that appear to be involved in the relatively increased 17,20-lyase activity of the zona reticularis, although not its regulation (see Fig. 25-35).

Regulation of adrenal androgen secretion in the zona reticularis is postulated to be based on a dual-control mechanism. First, corticotropin (ACTH, adrenocorticotropic hormone) is obligatory, as evidenced by the findings in cases of ACTH deficiency or resistance. Second, the mechanism requires the action of an unidentified adrenal androgen-stimulating factor, possibly pituitary in origin or from a nonadrenal source, or an intra-adrenal event.[270] This concept is illustrated in Figure 25-36.[403]

CRH has been advanced as an adrenal androgen secretagogue that has stimulatory action on the zona reticularis. The intravenous infusion of human CRH into dexamethasone-suppressed young men increased DHEA, DHEAS, and androstenedione secretion within 3 hours. Similar results were obtained in adolescent girls with hyperandrogenism and a history of premature adrenarche. CRH directly stimulates DHEAS secretion and the expression of CYP17 by the fetal adrenal cortical cells.[407] Leptin in vitro vigorously stimulates 17,20-lyase activity and transiently stimulates 17α-hydroxylase activity of the microsomal enzyme CYP17, implying a role in adrenarche,[408] but no clinical evidence suggests a pivotal role of leptin in adrenarche. Therefore, a distinct hormone or factor that in addition to ACTH stimulates the zona reticularis and adrenal androgen secretion has not been isolated, and the mechanism regulating adrenarche remains unknown.[293]

A distinct adrenal androgen-stimulating factor, whether of pituitary, intra-adrenal, or other origin, may explain the following observations[270]:

1. The spurt in adrenal growth and the differentiation and growth of the zona reticularis at adrenarche occur independently of an increase in ACTH or cortisol secretion but correlate with the increase in plasma levels of DHEAS (see Fig. 25-35).
2. Cortisol and adrenal androgen secretions vary independently with age, during normal and premature adrenarche, and in Cushing disease, starvation, malnutrition, anorexia nervosa, and chronic disease.
3. Unlike cortisol secretion, the secretion of DHEA and DHEAS in response to ACTH administration varies with age.
4. Dissociation of adrenarche and gonadarche occurs in a variety of disorders of sexual maturation (see Fig. 25-36), including premature adrenarche (i.e., onset of pubic or axillary hair before 8 years of age), chronic adrenal insufficiency, CPP (when the onset is before age 6 years), primary hypogonadism, isolated gonadotropin deficiency, and anorexia nervosa.[402]

A longitudinal study of 42 children demonstrated that an increase in BMI (but not the value itself at any age) was related to the rise in urinary excretion of DHEAS, suggesting that a change in nutritional status is one physiologic regulator of adrenarche.[404,409]

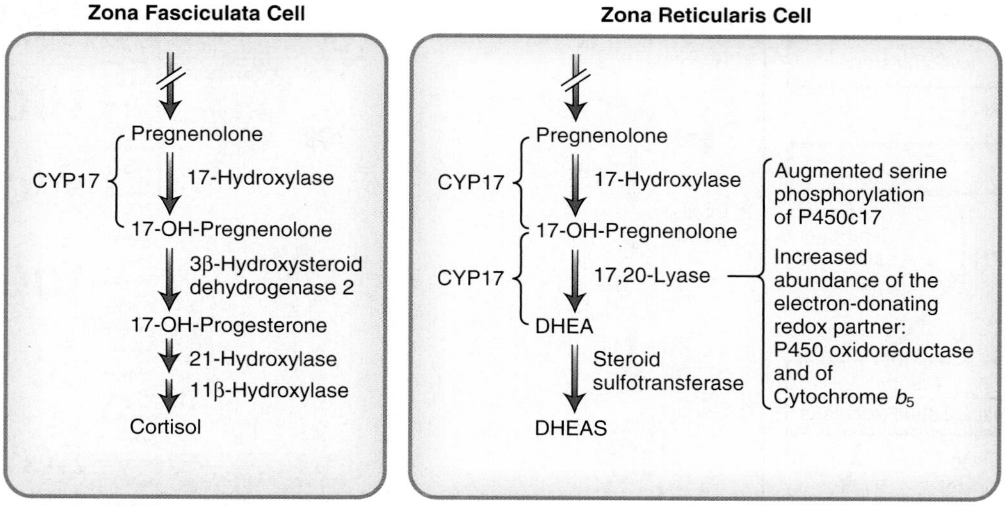

Zona Fasciculata Cell

Zona Reticularis Cell

Figure 25-35 Adrenarche and the zona reticularis. The rise in circulating dehydroepiandrosterone sulfate (DHEAS) levels is the biochemical hallmark of adrenarche. The diagram compares and contrasts the major steroidogenic pathway in the zona fasciculata with that in the zona reticularis. In contrast to the zona fasciculata, the expression of 3β-hydroxysteroid, $\Delta^{4,5}$ isomerase type 2 messenger ribonucleic acid (mRNA), and its activity (the enzyme that irreversibly traps Δ^5 precursors into Δ^4 steroids) is very low in the zona reticularis, whereas the expression of and activity of steroid sulfotransferase is high. A single gene, *CYP17* (now designated *CYP17A1*), encodes a single enzyme that has 17α-hydroxylase and 17,20-lyase activity, but the ratio of 17,20-lyase to 17α-hydroxylase activity is relatively high in the zona reticularis compared with that in the zona fasciculata. Some of the factors that seem to amplify the increased 17,20-lyase activity of *CYP17* are the augmented serine phosphorylation of the enzyme and the apparent increased abundance of the electron-donating redox partner, including P450 reductase and of cytochrome b_5.

The increase in DHEA before and at adrenarche might suggest a similarity to the actions of the fetal adrenal zone; indeed the histologic finding and biochemistry are similar in both the fetal adrenal zone and the zona reticularis. However, the fetal adrenal zone undergoes involution at birth; in addition biomarkers such as enzyme AKR1C3 (17β-hydroxysteroid dehydrogenase type 5, 17β-HSD5) are higher in the zona reticularis than the fetal adrenal zone.[293]

Adrenal Androgens and Puberty

The earlier onset of adrenarche than gonadarche and the contribution of adrenal androgens to the growth of pubic and axillary hair have led some to suggest that adrenal androgens in normal children are an important factor in the onset of puberty and the maturation of the hypothalamic-pituitary-gonadal complex.

Although CPP may occur when the prepubertal child has previously been exposed to excessive levels of androgens from an endogenous or exogenous source (e.g., after the initiation of glucocorticoid therapy in congenital virilizing adrenal hyperplasia or after removal of a sex steroid–secreting adrenal or gonadal neoplasm[259,410]), there is little evidence that adrenal androgens play an important qualitative or rate-limiting role in the onset of puberty in normal children.[259] Most patients with premature adrenarche, who secrete excessive amounts of adrenal androgens for their age, enter puberty and experience menarche within the normal age range.[259] Moreover, prepubertal children who have congenital or acquired chronic adrenal insufficiency (i.e., Addison disease) and consequently have deficient or absent adrenal androgen secretion usually have a normal onset and normal progression through puberty when given appropriate glucocorticoid and mineralocorticoid replacement therapy.[259] Studies of children with chronic adrenal insufficiency, isolated gonadotropin deficiency, hypergonadotropic hypogonadism, or androgen resistance suggest that adrenal androgens in girls and boys are not essential for the adolescent growth spurt, whereas gonadal steroids secreted by the testis and ovary are essential and act in concert with GH.[259] The transient increase in height velocity (about 1.5 cm/year in both sexes) that occurs in middle childhood (6 to 7 years) and lasts about 2 years terminates while the serum DHEAS level continues to increase. This increase in height velocity is related to the cyclic pattern of prepubertal growth and to genetic regulation of growth rather than to an increase in adrenal androgen or GH secretion.[411]

DISORDERS OF PUBERTY

Delayed Puberty and Sexual Infantilism

The upper limits of the normal age of onset of puberty are 14 years for boys and 13 years for girls (Table 25-15). Functionally, delayed puberty can be divided into disorders that affect the operation of the GnRH pulse generator, the pituitary gland, or the gonad.

Idiopathic or Constitutional Delay in Growth and Puberty

Otherwise healthy girls who spontaneously enter puberty after the age of 13 years and boys who begin after 14 years have constitutional delay in growth and adolescence, the most common diagnosis for delayed puberty. Affected individuals usually are short (2 SD below the mean value of height for age) at evaluation and have been shorter than their classmates for years, although growth velocity and height are usually appropriate for bone age (Fig. 25-37 and Table 25-16). Family history in as many as 77% of cases reveals a mother who had delayed menarche or a father (or sibling) who entered puberty late (i.e., age 14 to 18 years), and the pattern in some cases suggests dominant inheritance with incomplete penetrance.[412,413] Constitutional delay in development is physiologic immaturity with a slow tempo of maturation; full sexual maturity will be reached, but the process takes longer than usual. Because of delay in reactivation of the GnRH pulse generator, there is functional deficiency of GnRH for chronologic age but

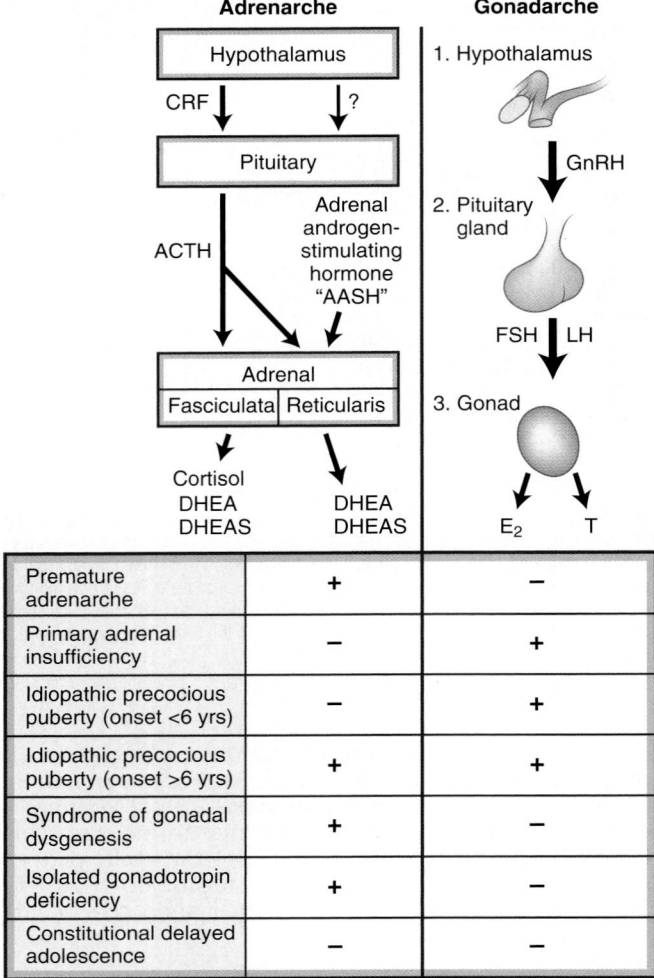

Figure 25-36 Hypothesis of the control of pituitary adrenal androgen secretion by a putative separate adrenal androgen-stimulating hormone acting on a corticotropin (ACTH)-primed adrenal cortex. Although this diagram suggests that adrenal androgen-stimulating hormone (AASH) arises from the pituitary gland, a distinct pituitary factor with AASH activity has not been isolated; an extrapituitary factor is not excluded. The lower part of the diagram shows the relationship of adrenarche to gonadarche, including dissociation in various clinical disorders of sexual development (+, present; −, absent). CRF, corticotropin-releasing factor; DHEA, dehydroepiandrosterone; DHEAS, DHEA sulfate; E2, estradiol; FSH, follicle-stimulating hormone; GnRH, gonadotropin-releasing hormone; T, testosterone. (Modified from Sklar CA, Kaplan SL, Grumbach MM. Evidence for dissociation between adrenarche and gonadarche: studies in patients with idiopathic precocious puberty, gonadal dysgenesis, isolated gonadotropin deficiency, and constitutionally delayed puberty. *J Clin Endocrinol Metab.* 1980;51:548-556. Copyright by The Endocrine Society.)

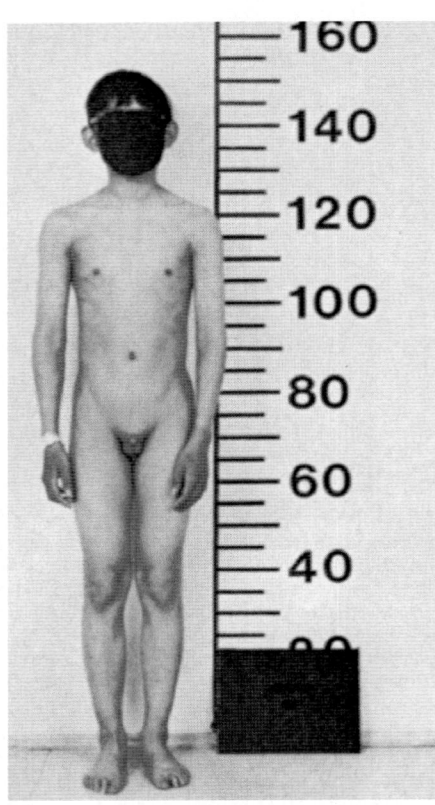

Figure 25-37 A boy age 16 years and 2 months has constitutional delay in growth and puberty. His height is 149.5 cm (4 SD [standard deviation] below the mean value for age); upper-to-lower body ratio is 1.1 (retarded for age); phallus is 6.0 × 1.6 cm; testes are 2.5 × 1.4 cm; and the scrotum showed early thinning. At a chronologic age of 15 years and 4 months, the bone age was 11 years and the sella turcica was normal. The plasma concentration of luteinizing hormone (LH) was 0.7 ng/mL (LER-960); the concentration of follicle-stimulating hormone (FSH) was 0.5 ng/mL (LER-869). On gonadotropin-releasing hormone (GnRH) testing, the plasma concentration of LH increased to 2.2 ng/mL (an increment of 1.5 ng/mL), and the testosterone level rose from 52 to 77 ng/dL. The testes subsequently spontaneously enlarged, and the patient progressed through puberty. For conversion to SI units, see Figures 25-19 and 25-20. (From Styne DM, Grumbach MM. Puberty in the male and female: its physiology and disorders. In: Yen SCC, Jaffe RB, eds. *Reproductive Endocrinology*, 2nd ed. Philadelphia, PA: WB Saunders; 1986:313-384.)

not for the stage of physiologic development. Adrenarche and gonadarche occur later in individuals with constitutional (idiopathic) delay in growth and adolescence,[412] whereas adrenarche usually occurs at a normal age in patients with isolated gonadotropin deficiency.[402] Bone age is delayed at presentation, but after a bone age of approximately 12 to 14 years for boys or 11 to 13 years for girls is achieved, sexual maturation begins (although bone age is not a fully reliable indicator).

Most of these patients with CDP are thin, but 25% are above the 85th percentile in BMI for age, and their bone age is less delayed than in classic thin patients (i.e., they tend to achieve taller adult stature[412]). Prepubertal boys who meet the criteria for diagnosis with delayed bone age

have greater total energy expenditure (TEE) and increased nutritional needs possibly due to an alteration in mitochondrial metabolism or increased nonexercise activity thermogenesis (NEAT); increased nutrition increased energy intake but TEE rose as well, continuing the need for high energy intake.[414] There is no impairment of olfaction, as in Kallmann syndrome, and undescended testes occur in the rate found in the general population. Plasma gonadal steroid levels are low in pediatric assays at the time of presentation, but as bone age advances, the serum gonadotropin concentration and the amplitude of LH pulses increase (initially at night); the basal serum gonadotropin concentrations measured by third-generation assays and the LH response to GnRH or GnRH agonists reflect maturation of the hypothalamic-pituitary system.

The first signs of secondary sexual development occur within 1 year after LH rises to pubertal levels in response to administration of 100 μg of intravenous synthetic GnRH or subcutaneous GnRH agonist or within 1 year after gonadotropin and testosterone or estradiol concentrations begin to increase spontaneously above prepubertal values.[226,294] An 8 AM serum testosterone value of 0.7 nmol/L

TABLE 25-15
Classification of Delayed Puberty and Sexual Infantilism

Idiopathic (Constitutional) Delay in Growth and Puberty (Delayed Activation of Hypothalamic LRF Pulse Generator)	Malnutrition
	Anorexia nervosa
Hypogonadotropic Hypogonadism: Sexual Infantilism Related to Gonadotropin Deficiency	Bulimia
	Psychogenic amenorrhea
CNS Disorders	Impaired puberty and delayed menarche in female athletes and ballet dancers (exercise amenorrhea)
Tumors	Hypothyroidism
Craniopharyngiomas	Diabetes mellitus
Germinomas	Cushing disease
Other germ cell tumors	Hyperprolactinemia
Hypothalamic and optic gliomas	Marijuana use
Astrocytomas	Gaucher disease
Pituitary tumors (including MEN-1, prolactinoma)	**Hypergonadotropic Hypogonadism**
	Males
Other Causes	The syndrome of seminiferous tubular dysgenesis and its variants (Klinefelter syndrome)
Langerhans histiocytosis	Other forms of primary testicular failure
Postinfectious lesions of the CNS	Chemotherapy
Vascular abnormalities of the CNS	Radiation therapy
Radiation therapy	Testicular steroid biosynthetic defects
Congenital malformations especially associated with craniofacial anomalies	Sertoli-only syndrome
Head trauma	LH receptor mutation
Lymphocytic hypophysitis	Anorchia and cryptorchidism
Isolated Gonadotropin Deficiency	Trauma/surgery
Kallmann syndrome	**Females**
With hyposmia or anosmia	The syndrome of gonadal dysgenesis (Turner syndrome) and its variants
Without anosmia	XX and XY gonadal dysgenesis
LHRH receptor mutation	Familial and sporadic XX gonadal dysgenesis and its variants
Congenital adrenal hypoplasia (*DAX1* mutation)	Familial and sporadic XY gonadal dysgenesis and its variants
Isolated LH deficiency	Aromatase deficiency
Isolated FSH deficiency	Other forms of primary ovarian failure
Prohormone convertase 1 deficiency (PCI)	Premature menopause
Idiopathic and Genetic Forms of Multiple Pituitary Hormone Deficiencies Including PROP1 Mutation	Radiation therapy
	Chemotherapy
Miscellaneous Disorders	Autoimmune oophoritis
Prader-Willi syndrome	Galactosemia
Laurence-Moon and Bardet-Biedl syndromes	Glycoprotein syndrome type 1
Functional gonadotropin deficiency	Resistant ovary
Chronic systemic disease and malnutrition	FSH receptor mutation
Sickle cell disease	LH/hCG resistance
Cystic fibrosis	Polycystic ovarian disease
Acquired immunodeficiency syndrome (AIDS)	Trauma/surgery
Chronic gastroenteric disease	Noonan or pseudo-Turner syndrome
Chronic renal disease	Ovarian steroid biosynthetic defects

CNS, central nervous system; hCG, human chorionic gonadotropin; LHRH, luteinizing hormone-releasing hormone; LRF, luteinizing hormone-releasing factor; MEN, multiple endocrine neoplasia.

TABLE 25-16
Constitutional Delay in Growth and Adolescence

A variation of normal
Males more often seek assistance
Family history of delayed menarche or delayed secondary sexual characteristics
Height is often below the 5th percentile, but growth rate is normal for skeletal age
Onset of adrenarche is delayed
The combination of genetic short stature and constitutional delay leads to more profound short stature
Final height is less than predicted

(20 ng/dL) heralds the development of phenotypic puberty in boys within 12 to 15 months.[415] INSL3 is produced by the testes in the fetal, neonatal, and pubertal periods and holds promise for diagnosis of CDP as it appears to be as sensitive as testosterone measurements in determining testicular function.[265]

CDP is more common in boys and may be a counterpart of idiopathic CPP, a condition that is many times more common in girls. Familial short stature is a physiologic variant of growth in which the velocity of development and bone age are normal but stature is decreased, in contrast to CDP, which is a disorder of tempo that secondarily impairs growth. The combination of CDP and familial short stature leads to conspicuous shortness during adolescence, especially when other children increase their growth velocity, and referrals occur more often with this combination than with either condition alone. Because no single test reliably distinguishes between CDP and isolated hypogonadotropic hypogonadism (IHH), watchful waiting is usually in order.

The growth rate before the actual onset of puberty in constitutional delay is often suboptimal for chronologic age, but growth velocity usually increases to normal levels after puberty begins.[416] Affected boys seem to be more distressed by short stature than by delay in sexual development.

GH release in the basal state and in response to GH secretagogues, including the administration of GHRH, is low for age and may be decreased further in children with CDP, but the amplitude of GH secretion and the GH response to GHRH is greater after administration of exogenous (aromatizable) androgens or estrogens. Therefore, CDP may constitute a temporary state of functional GH insufficiency for chronologic age but not for bone age. IGF-1 interacts with gonadotropins in the ovary and testis, and the relatively low secretion of GH (and presumably intragonadal IGF-1) in CDP may impair the gonadal response to gonadotropins.

Patients with constitutional delay in adolescence and growth often do not reach their predicted height. When the genetic tendency for growth is greater, subjects with CDP reach taller adult stature, but the patients most likely to be referred are those that combine genetic short stature with CDP. Girls with CDP have a mean deficit in adult height of 2.4 cm below the mean predicted height, although the range of adult height varies about 10 cm above or below predictions. The magnitude of the catch-up in linear growth during puberty in boys is a major determinant of adult height. Heavier individuals with CDP reach greater height than those who are thinner.[412] Adult height is lower if affected individuals show decreased height SDS in earlier life.[417,418] The role of bone density in CDP was discussed earlier.

Because 15% to 20% of adult height is gained during puberty, many approaches have been tried to increase stature in otherwise normal, short children. Delaying the onset or progression with puberty by the use of GnRH agonists was suggested by some, but a decrease in bone density 1 year after cessation led to warnings that routine administration of this treatment carries substantial risk.[419] The additional psychological risk of delaying puberty in otherwise normal children should also be considered, and this treatment is neither established nor recommended.[420]

The U.S. Food and Drug Administration (FDA) approved GH treatment for children who are predicted to reach an adult height less than the 1st percentile (160 cm), which includes some children with CDP, and some studies reported an increase in adult height with this treatment. Because endogenous GH level rises during pubertal development, the FDA approved GH therapy in larger doses for subjects with GH deficiency during puberty. However, there are only moderate effects of increased GH doses during puberty on adult height, and both overshadow, although male gender has a positive effect and age at onset of puberty has a negative effect, the effects of the change in dose on adult[421] height. GH therapy is approved for idiopathic short stature but is not specifically approved by the FDA for CDP alone.

The combination of GnRH agonist therapy with GH treatment in attempts to increase adult height in children who were normal except for genetic short stature and in SGA children led to inconclusive results or to increased predicted or near-final height, which does not necessarily translate into increased adult height. This approach to treatment remains experimental. Review of a large database from a postmarketing survey did not support the efficacy of this approach,[422] and there was no good follow-up evaluation of adult height. This combination therapy cannot be supported by substantial evidence.[423]

The cost of GH for treatment of non–GH-deficient short stature is exceptionally high: $14,000 per cm or $35,000 per inch gained.[424] Payers are reluctant in many cases to cover the cost of the GH therapy for those without confirmed GH deficiency. There are few controlled studies of adult height, but available results demonstrate either increase in adult height or gain of several centimeters; more studies are strongly recommended to better determine the efficacy of this treatment in short, normal children.[425]

Because the critical role of estradiol in skeletal maturation was appreciated, treatment with a potent aromatase inhibitor to increase adult height by inhibiting skeletal maturation[133,134,272] aroused interest. A double-blind, randomized, placebo-controlled study enrolled boys with CDP who were treated with 6 months of monthly testosterone or testosterone plus an added 12-month trial of daily oral letrozole (a potent fourth-generation aromatase inhibitor). The results revealed a mean increase in predicted adult height of 5.1 cm in the letrozole plus testosterone group[414]; a subsequent study supported these promising effects on increasing the time of pubertal growth height without affecting the development of male secondary sex characteristics, but there are few data on actual adult height. The boys in the group treated with testosterone and letrozole developed increased bioactive testosterone, analyzed by a cellular assay, compared with control boys.[236] Serum testosterone measured by HPLC-MS/MS can reach levels of more than 1000 ng/dL. However, markers of bone turnover decrease, and vertebral abnormalities may develop with the use of these agents in idiopathic short stature.[426] A 1-year study of the aromatase inhibitor anastrozole plus GH, compared with GH treatment alone, in boys demonstrated no ill effects on body composition, plasma lipids, bone metabolism, or the tempo of puberty (although estrogen decreased, as expected, with the use of anastrozole), and the predicted height was increased.[427] This treatment has not been supported by long-term studies observing patients up to adult height, and concerns about possible effects on bone density must be addressed, probably until the patients are at least 20 to 25 years old, and as well as a decrease in serum HDL-cholesterol levels and increase of erythrocytosis before this off-label therapy can be recommended.[428,429]

Hypogonadotropic Hypogonadism: Sexual Infantilism Related to Gonadotropin Deficiency

Insufficient pulsatile secretion of GnRH and the resulting FSH and LH deficiency lead to delayed sexual maturation, which is usually permanent. The phenotype in hypogonadotropic hypogonadism can vary from severe sexual infantilism to apparent CDP. Both conditions may be found in the same family or hypogonadotropic hypogonadism may first appear to be CDP as a homozygous R262Q mutation in GNRHR presented with constitutional delay but later was associated with oligospermia[430]). There may be an absolute or relative quantitative deficiency of pulsatile GnRH, or the deficiency may be qualitative, especially in females; it may involve abnormalities in amplitude or frequency of GnRH pulses or in both components (Fig. 25-38).

Patients with IHH usually are of normal height in early or middle adolescent years, whereas patients with CDP usually have a normal growth rate for bone age but are short for chronologic age. In contrast to CDP patients, those with hypogonadotropic hypogonadism usually do not respond to GnRH stimulation, nor do they have a pulsatile LH profile commensurate with bone age. Although serum concentrations of plasma FSH and LH and urinary gonadotropins are low, the differences are relative rather than absolute and are not diagnostic for an individual.

Hypogonadotropic hypogonadism can involve puberty and reproduction alone or can be a manifestation of a life-threatening condition. Hypogonadotropic hypogonadism

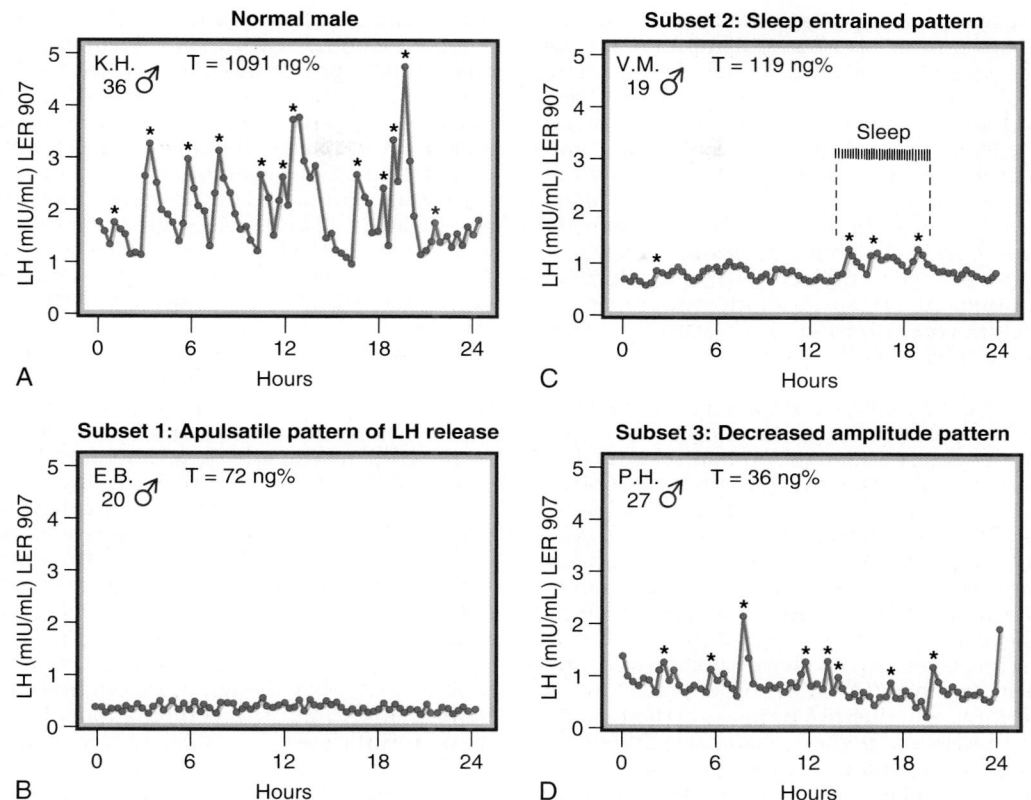

Figure 25-38 Various patterns of pulsatile luteinizing hormone (LH) secretion that can occur in isolated hypogonadotropic hypogonadism (**B** to **D**) are compared with LH secretion in a normal man (**A**). **A,** Discrete LH pulses occur about every 2 hours in a normal 36-year-old man. **B,** Typical apulsatile LH pattern is associated with a low testosterone (T) concentration usually found in isolated hypogonadotropic hypogonadism. **C,** Pattern of developmental arrest with low-amplitude nocturnal LH pulses is apparent only during sleep. **D,** Low-amplitude LH pulse pattern occurs during sleep and wake periods. To convert LH values to international units per liter, multiply by 1.0. (From Spratt DI, Crowley WF. Hypogonadotropic hypogonadism: GnRH therapy. In: Krieger DT, Bardin CW, eds. *Current Therapy in Endocrinology and Metabolism, 1985-1986.* Toronto, Canada: BC Decker; 1985:155-159.)

may result from a genetic or developmental defect present at birth but remain undetected until the age of expected puberty, or it may be caused by a tumor, inflammatory process, vascular lesion, irradiation, or trauma to the hypothalamus. Similarly, hypogonadotropic hypogonadism may arise from lesions or defects that involve the pituitary gland directly. When GH is affected as well as gonadotropins, impaired growth is manifested by decreased growth velocity, especially during the expected pubertal growth spurt, and short stature.

Central Nervous System Tumors

Extrasellar masses may interfere with GnRH synthesis, secretion, or stimulation of pituitary gonadotrophs. Most patients with hypothalamic-pituitary tumors causing gonadotropin deficiency have one or more additional pituitary hormone deficiencies (or an increased serum prolactin level with prolactinomas). Those with GH deficiency due to a neoplasm have late onset of growth failure compared with those who have idiopathic and familial hypopituitarism, in which growth failure starts early in life. The presence of anterior and posterior pituitary deficiencies in infancy suggests a midline developmental defect, but the development of this combination after infancy ominously suggests an expanding CNS lesion.

Craniopharyngioma. Craniopharyngioma is a rare embryonic malformation of nonglial origin in childhood (0.5-2.0 new cases per 1 million population annually, or 1.2-4% of pediatric intracranial tumors), a common CNS neoplasm.[431] It is, however, the most common brain tumor associated with hypothalamic-pituitary dysfunction and sexual infantilism and accounts for 80% to 90% of neoplasms found in the pituitary and up to 15% of all intracranial tumors in childhood.[432] Symptoms usually arise before the age of 20 years with a peak incidence between the ages of 6 and 14 years with about 30% to 50% occurring in the pediatric age range. Harvey Cushing introduced the term *craniopharyngioma* and said that they were "the most formidable of intracranial tumors."[433]

Various theories of the embryologic origin of this nonglial intracranial tumor are current: one theory favors development from ectodermal remnants of Rathke's pouch and another development from residual embryonic epithelium of the anterior pituitary gland and of the anterior infundibulum. Craniopharyngiomas may reside within or above the sella turcica, or more rarely, they may be found in the nasopharynx or the third ventricle.

Craniopharyngioma appears to be a monoclonal tumor, and about 50% have cytogenetic abnormalities such as gains in 1q, 12q, and 17q. About 70% of cases of craniopharygioma in childhood are the adamantinomatous type with cyst formation. These types have dysregulation of the Wnt signaling pathway and a mutation in the β-catenin gene *(CTNNB1)* in contrast to the papillary type of craniopharyngioma that has *BRAF* mutations and is more often found in adult patients.[433,434]

CNS signs of craniopharyngiomas develop as the tumor encroaches on surrounding structures. Symptoms of craniopharyngioma include headache, visual disturbances, short stature, diabetes insipidus, vomiting, and weakness of one or more limbs. Visual defects (including bilateral temporal field deficits), optic atrophy or papilledema, and signs of GH deficiency, delayed puberty, and hypothyroidism are features of craniopharyngiomas. Although most patients are below the mean in height and height velocity at diagnosis, a long, indolent course is possible. Deficiencies of gonadotropins, GH, thyrotropin (TSH, thyroid-stimulating hormone), ACTH, and arginine vasopressin are common. The serum concentration of prolactin is normal or increased. Delayed bone age is common and may point to the onset of tumor growth.

About 70% of patients with a craniopharyngioma have suprasellar or intrasellar calcification (found in fewer than 1% of normal individuals) and an abnormal sella turcica, which are sometimes found on radiographs taken for other indications, including orthodontia. CT (but not MRI) reveals fine calcifications that are not apparent on lateral skull radiographs. MRI scans before and after gadolinium are the diagnostic procedures of choice for suspected craniopharygioma and can determine whether the tumor is cystic or solid and indicate the presence of hydrocephalus; if necessary a CT scan can be used to search for calcifications, and CT or MRI with contrast (the diagnostic procedure of choice) can determine whether the tumor is cystic or solid and indicate the presence of hydrocephalus (Fig. 25-39).

Smaller craniopharyngiomas, usually intrasellar, can be treated by transsphenoidal microsurgery, but larger or suprasellar masses usually require craniotomy, and the approach must be individualized. The reported postsurgical 5-year overall survival rate is 88% to 94%, and the reported 10-year overall survival rate is 70% to 92% with a 20-year survival rate of 76%. The combination of limited tumor removal and radiation therapy leads to a satisfactory neurologic prognosis, better cognitive outcome, and better endocrine outcome compared with attempts at complete surgical extirpation. Frequent and early tumor relapse after apparently complete resection and tumor progression after incomplete resection suggest the wisdom of radiation therapy after surgery. Alternative approaches include proton beam therapy and in mainly cystic craniopharyngioma cases, instillation of radioisotopes or sclerosing substances such as bleomycin or interferon-α are being investigated.[431] Nonetheless, the preferred manner of treatment to retain the best quality of life is not yet established, but longitudinal studies such as the randomized multinational trial KRANIOPHARYNGEOM 2007 may answer this question.

Postoperative hyperphagia and obesity (BMI >5 SD above normal) can be striking and correlate with the magnitude of hypothalamic damage on cranial MRI. Injury to the hypothalamic ventromedial nuclei (associated with increased parasympathetic activity and hyperinsulinemia) or to the PVN may cause these findings, and insulin suppression may be helpful. Short-term follow-up studies demonstrate the efficacy of bariatric surgery in the management of obesity in affected patients.[435] Hypothalamic sparing surgery decreases the risk of postoperative hyperphagia and obesity.[436] Aberrant sleep patterns and even narcolepsy and daytime somnolence may follow surgical treatment of craniopharyngiomas, with melatonin improving sleep patterns in some.[437] Although the endocrine complications are more manageable, the combination of antidiuretic hormone insufficiency (i.e., diabetes insipidus) and impaired sense of thirst remains a complex management problem.

A Rathke cleft cyst is often discovered as an incidental finding on MRI, but it can produce symptoms and signs indistinguishable from those of a craniopharyngioma, such as precocious or delayed puberty.[438] Surgical drainage and excision of the cyst wall are customary approaches.

Other Extrasellar Tumors

Germinomas. Germinomas (i.e., pinealomas, ectopic pinealomas, atypical teratomas, or dysgerminomas) and other

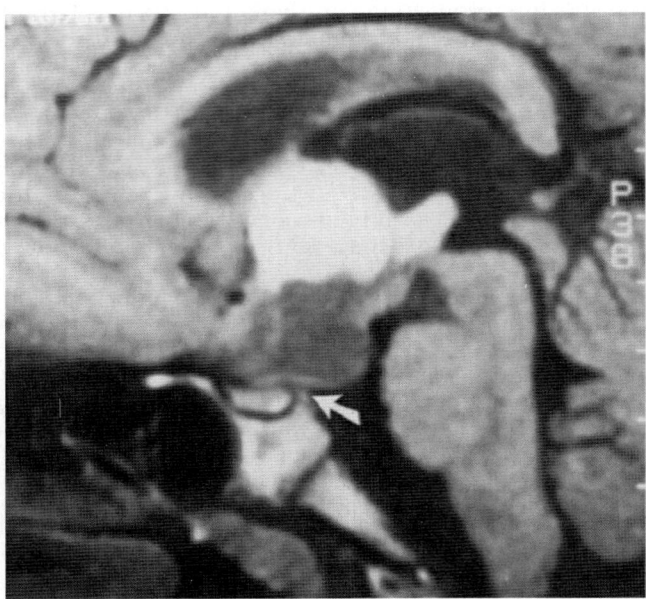
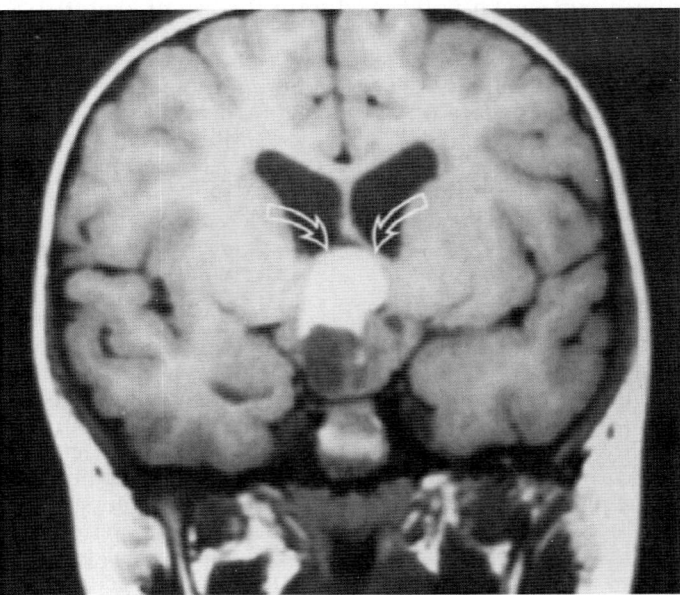

Figure 25-39 Craniopharyngioma in a short 5-year-old girl with a history of frontal headaches, impaired vision, and poor growth. *Left,* Midline, sagittal, T1-weighted image shows a hyperintense region superiorly and an inferior hypointense region. The combination of hyperintense and hypointense areas in a non–contrast-enhanced examination is the most characteristic finding for craniopharyngioma. Notice the erosion of dorsum sellae *(solid arrow)* and posterior pituitary bright spot. *Right,* Coronal, T1-weighted image shows tumor extending upward to the inferior frontal horns, narrowing the foramen of Monro, and causing mild hydrocephalus. The *open arrows* indicate the upper border of the hyperintense area of the tumor.

germ cell tumors of the CNS are the most common extra-sellar tumors that arise in the suprasellar hypothalamic region and in the pineal region that commonly cause sexual infantilism. Germinomas constitute 66% of all intracranial germ cell tumors (GCTs), which make up 3% to 11% of pediatric brain tumors. About 84% are found in the pineal and the neurohypophyseal regions. Peak incidences occur in the second decade and during infancy. They are found more often in males.[439] Polydipsia and polyuria are the most common symptoms, followed by visual difficulties and abnormalities of growth and puberty or movement disorders. Diagnosis is often delayed for months to years because the findings are attributed to psychiatric disorders. Deficiencies of vasopressin and GH are most common, but other anterior pituitary hormone deficiencies (including gonadotropin deficiency) and elevated serum prolactin levels are also frequent. Determination of the concentration of hCG in spinal fluid and in serum and assessment of α-fetoprotein levels provide useful tumor markers in children and adolescents with germ cell tumors. Germ cell tumors in boys cause isosexual GnRH-independent sexual precocity (GISP) by secretion of hCG (see "Sexual Precocity"). Tumors secreting hCG cause precocious puberty in boys, and there has been one case report of an affected girl.

Subependymal spread of germ cell tumors along the lining of the third ventricle is common, and seeding may involve the lower spinal cord and corda equina. MRI with contrast enhancement is useful in the detection of isolated enlargement of the pituitary stalk, an early finding that requires periodic MRI monitoring, especially in patients with diabetes insipidus.[440] The size of the pituitary gland increases by 100% between year 1 and year 15, but the pineal gland does not normally change in size after the first year of life; any later enlargement indicates a mass lesion. Pineal cysts are a rare cause of CPP.

Irradiation is the preferred treatment for pure germ cell tumors such as germinomas; surgery is rarely indicated, except for biopsy to establish a tissue diagnosis.[440] However, attempts to decrease the long-term morbidity of radiation therapy leads to consideration of chemotherapy. Chemotherapy alone is inadequate, but the combination of chemotherapy and radiation therapy can be successful,[441,442] and both treatment methods are recommended for a mixed germ cell tumor. Because testicular germ cell tumors are occasionally found years after successful therapy for CNS germ cell tumors, long-term surveillance is indicated.[443,444]

Hypothalamic and optic gliomas or astrocytomas, occurring as part of neurofibromatosis (von Recklinghausen disease) or arising independently, can also cause sexual infantilism. Gliomas and meningiomas are the most common CNS tumors to develop in childhood cancer survivors treated with CNS radiation, often the young adult or even late teenage years.[445]

Pituitary Adenomas. Only 2% to 6% of all surgically treated pituitary tumors occur in childhood and adolescence, with about 1 in 1 million children affected.[432] Most functional pituitary adenomas are ACTH secreting, with prolactinomas or GH secreting or nonfunctioning adenomas occurring less commonly. Most pituitary tumors are monoclonal lesions caused by mutations of *GNAS*. Adolescent onset of pituitary team tumors may be the first manifestation of multiple endocrine neoplasia type I or familial isolated pituitary adenoma (FIPA).[446] With higher sensitive imaging techniques the presence of a pituitary incidentaloma, a previously unsuspected pituitary lesion that is discovered on an imaging study performed for an unrelated reason, may be discovered.[447] Evaluation of secretory activity of such a lesion, consideration of mass effects and follow-up

to monitor a change in size are important, but some lesions detected will not be related to the pubertal abnormality.

Incidence of prolactinoma is low in childhood but 1 in 5 present in the 15- to 24-year-old age group.[448] A survey of 44 cases reported that 61% of prolactinomas were macroadenomas (more often in boys; hypopituitarism and growth failure were common) and 39% were microadenomas (more often in girls; delayed puberty was common).[449] Only 2 of these 29 patients had delayed onset of puberty, although primary amenorrhea was the presenting symptom in 13 of 20 pubertal females. Presenting symptoms included oligomenorrhea and galactorrhea in the girls and headache in the boys. Galactorrhea may be demonstrable only by manual manipulation of the nipples (blood samples for prolactin should be obtained before examination or many hours later, because manipulation of the nipples raises prolactin levels).

Dopaminergic therapy is often successful in decreasing prolactin values. The dopamine agonist bromocriptine may decrease serum prolactin concentrations and decrease tumor size, which is a useful approach before surgery of large macroprolactinomas is undertaken and when resection of the adenoma is incomplete. Transsphenoidal resection of microprolactinomas in children and adolescents is an effective treatment. Pubertal progression and normal menstrual function in girls usually follows reduction of serum prolactin levels. Pituitary apoplexy followed cabergoline treatment of a macroprolactinoma in a 16-year-old girl[450]; this complication has been seen in adults treated with bromocriptine, and tricuspid regurgitation may be a cumulative effect.[451] High serum levels of macroprolactin, a complex of immunoglobulin G and monomeric prolactin with little biologic activity in vivo, cross-react in commercial prolactin assays, leading to a finding of pseudohyperprolactinemia; high prolactin values should be rechecked with subfractionation after polyethylene glycol precipitation.[452]

Other Central Nervous System Disorders Leading to Delayed Puberty

Langerhans Cell Histiocytosis. Langerhans cell histiocytosis (i.e., Hand-Schüller-Christian disease or histiocytosis X) is a clonal proliferative disorder of Langerhans histiocytes or their precursors. It is characterized by the infiltration of lipid-laden histiocytic cells or foam cells in skin, viscera, and bone.[453] The cause is not clear, because there are features of a neoplasm and features of a reactive immunologic disorder. Diabetes insipidus, caused by infiltration of the hypothalamus or the pituitary stalk, is the most common endocrine manifestation, with GH deficiency and delayed puberty possible. The lung, liver, and spleen, cystlike areas in flat and long bones, and the dorsolumbar spine may be involved. "Floating teeth" within rarefied bone of the mandible, absent or loose teeth, and exophthalmos due to infiltration of the orbit are seen. Mastoid or temporal bone involvement may lead to chronic otitis media. Treatment with glucocorticoids, antineoplastic agents, and radiation therapy is promising in terms of survival, but more than 50% of patients have late sequelae or disease progression. The natural waxing and waning course of this rare disease makes evaluation of therapy difficult and highlights the importance of national treatment protocols.[453]

Postinfectious Inflammatory Lesions of the Central Nervous System, Vascular Abnormalities, and Head Trauma. Tuberculous or sarcoid granulomas of the CNS are associated with delayed puberty. The original case of adiposogenital dystrophy, or Fröhlich syndrome, is thought to have been caused by tuberculosis infection rather than a neoplasm.

Hydrocephalus may cause delayed puberty that can be reversed with decompression, as may pressure from a subarachnoid cyst.

Irradiation of the Central Nervous System. Irradiation of the CNS for treatment of tumors, leukemia, or neoplasms of the head and face may result in the gradual onset of hypothalamic-pituitary failure.[454] Although GH deficiency is the most common hormone disorder resulting from irradiation, gonadotropin deficiency, hypothyroidism, and decreased bone density also occur.[455] Self-reported fertility was reported to be lower in women who received CNS radiotherapy for acute lymphoblastic leukemia at about the time of menarche,[456] although the average age of women in this long-term study was in the early 20s, and longer follow-up of fertility may change the results. Irradiation of the CNS in early life predisposes the patient to later onset of secondary CNS tumors sometimes in just a few years after treatment of the first tumor.[445]

Fröhlich Syndrome. Fröhlich syndrome or adiposodysgenesis is a constellation of endocrine abnormalities, combining findings of obesity and hypogonadism due to a hypothalamic-pituitary disorder. Remarkably, the original description involved a patient with tuberculosis involving the hypothalamic-pituitary axis.

Isolated Hypogonadal Hypogonadism

A defect involving the GnRH pulse generator or gonadotrophs without an anatomic lesion causes selective deficiency of gonadotropins, producing IHH (Tables 25-17 and 25-18).[457] Puberty fails to begin by 14 years in boys and 13 years in girls, or pubertal maturation is incomplete or transient. In boys, micropenis (the penis is normally formed but stretched length is less than 2 cm in length, which is 2.5 SD below the mean length in average newborn males) or undescended testes or both signs are evidence of a fetal testosterone deficiency caused by gonadotropin deficiency. Prepubertal concentration of gonadal sex steroid values (testosterone in boys; estradiol in girls) and low serum gonadotropin levels or values within the normal range (i.e., normal in the basal state but not in the secretory state) are characteristic. Concentrations of gonadal sex steroids and gonadotropins are low, pulsatile LH secretion is often virtually absent, and the LH response to GnRH or GnRH agonist administration is deficient in the severe form. The testes are small and may be hard to find, and serum inhibin B, an estimate of seminiferous tubule function, is lower than in CDP in initial studies.[458]

IHH may occur in families (about 20% to 30% of patients), or it may occur sporadically. In contrast to CNS tumors (in which patients usually have GH deficiency and growth failure) and to CDP (in which patients are short for chronologic age), height is appropriate for age in patients with IHH (Fig. 25-40). Because the levels of gonadal steroids, particularly estradiol, are too low to cause epiphyseal fusion at the normal age, increased arm span for height and a decreased ratio of upper to lower body segments (i.e., eunuchoid body proportions) are present. If the condition is left untreated, growth continues, and adult height is tall.[440,441,459]

Remarkably, about 20% of affected males with IHH and severe delay of puberty spontaneously increase their testicular size and enter full puberty.[460] Thus, long-term follow-up is essential. However, this does not mean indefinite waiting is in order when puberty does not start by the upper limit of normal, hoping for such a reversal to occur, as many years may pass if indeed reversal does occur.

Kallmann Syndrome

Anosmia or hyposmia resulting from agenesis or hypoplasia of the olfactory lobes or sulci is associated with GnRH deficiency in Kallmann syndrome, the most common form of IHH[461] (see Table 25-18). The condition was first observed in 1856, in the autopsy of a 40-year-old man with micropenis, small cryptorchid testes, and absence of the olfactory bulbs, but Kallmann described a familial pattern in

---

TABLE 25-17

Isolated Gonadotropin Deficiency

Males more commonly affected

Familial (more common in females) or sporadic (more common in males)

Height normal for age; tall adult height if untreated

Eunuchoid skeletal proportions

Delayed bone age

Small, often cryptorchid testes: diameter <2.5 cm prepubertal size; phallus may be small

Normal adrenarche

Examine for anosmia or hyposmia (Kallmann syndrome)

Look for associated malformations (facial, central nervous system, skeletal, renal)

TABLE 25-18

Features of Kallmann Syndrome

Clinical

GnRH deficiency: absent or arrested puberty

Anosmia or hyposmia

In infancy: microphallus; cryptorchidism

Normal stature and growth in childhood

Normal adrenarche

Eunuchoid proportions

Associated midline defects (e.g., cleft lip, cleft palate, midline cranial anomalies)

MRI: aplasia or hypoplasia of olfactory bulbs and/or sulci

Prevalence

Approximately 1 in 7500 males, 1 in 50,000 females; 10% prevalence of Klinefelter syndrome

Inheritance

Sporadic and familial cases; genetic heterogeneity

X linked

X-linked recessive (Kallmann et al)

X chromosome deletion: Xp22.3 (Meitinger et al)

Autosomal

Dominant (sex limitation) (Santen and Paulsen; Merriam et al)

Recessive (White et al)

Anatomy

Developmental field defect

Aplasia or hypoplasia of olfactory bulb and sulcus

Arrested migration of GnRH neurosecretory neurons from olfactory placode to medial basal hypothalamus

GnRH, gonadotropin-releasing hormone; MRI, magnetic resonance imaging.
Data from Kallmann F, Schonfeld WA, Barrera SW. Genetic aspects of primary eunuchoidism. *Am J Ment Defic.* 1944;48:203-236; Meitinger T, Heye B, Petit C, et al. Definitive localization of X-linked Kallmann's syndrome (hypogonadotropic hypogonadism and anosmia) to Xp22.3: close linkage to the hypervariable repeat sequence CRI-S232. *Am J Hum Genet.* 1990;47:664-669; Merriam GR, Beitins IZ, Bode HH. Father-to-son transmission of hypogonadism with anosmia: Kallmann's syndrome. *Am J Dis Child.* 1977;131:1216-1219; Santen RJ, Paulsen CA. Hypogonadotropic eunuchoidism. I. Clinical study of the mode of inheritance. *J Clin Endocrinol Metab.* 1973;36:47-54; White BJ, Rogal AD, Brown KS, et al. The syndrome of anosmia with hypogonadotropic hypogonadism: a genetic study of 18 new families and a review. *Am J Med Genet.* 1983;15:417-435.

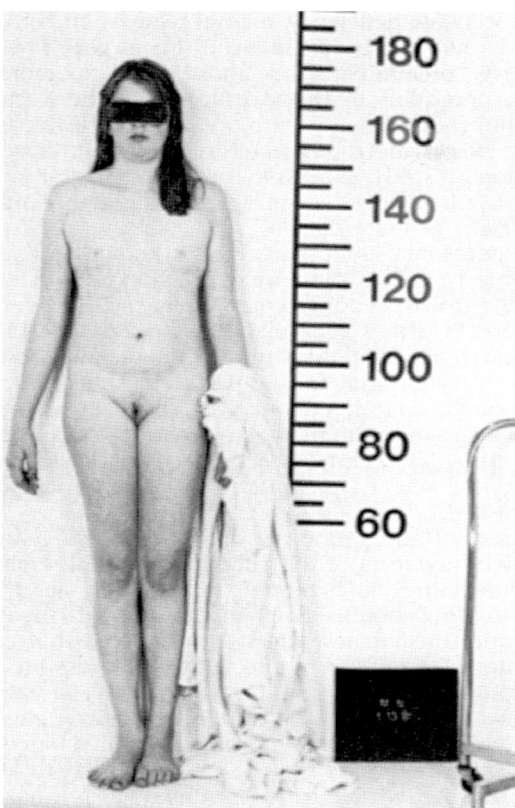

Figure 25-40 A girl aged 18 years and 8 months has isolated gonadotropin deficiency (i.e., sexual infantilism and primary amenorrhea). Her height is 173 cm (+1 SD [standard deviation]), weight was 66.5 kg (+1 SD), and the skeletal age was 13 years. Adrenarche with pubic hair development occurred at age 13.5 years. At the time of the photograph, pubic hair was in stage 3, and there was slight breast and nipple development resulting from a previous short course of estrogen therapy. Immature labia minora and majora were observed, and no estrogen effect was seen on the vaginal mucosa. Olfactory testing results were normal. The plasma luteinizing hormone (LH) (LER-960) level after gonadotropin-releasing hormone (GnRH) administration rose from 0.5 to 1.8 ng/mL (a prepubertal response). Serum estradiol was undetectable. The dehydroepiandrosterone sulfate (DHEAS) level was 92 μg/dL (appropriate for pubic hair stage 2). Notice the discrepancy between adrenarche and gonadarche. For conversion to SI units, see Figures 25-19 and 25-30. (From Styne DM, Grumbach MM. Puberty in the male and female: its physiology and disorders. In: Yen SCC, Jaffe RB, eds. *Reproductive Endocrinology*, 2nd ed. Philadelphia, PA: WB Saunders; 1986:313-384.)

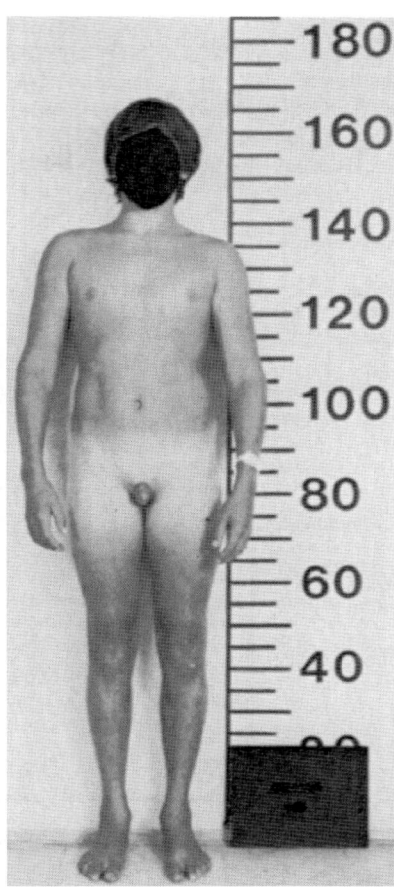

Figure 25-41 A boy aged 15 years and 10 months had isolated gonadotropin deficiency and anosmia (Kallmann syndrome). He had undescended testes, but after administration of 10,000 U of human chorionic gonadotropin (hCG), the testes descended and were palpable in the scrotum. His height was 163.9 cm (+1.5 SD [standard deviation]); the upper-to-lower body ratio was 0.86, which is eunuchoid. The phallus measured 6.3 × 1.8 cm, and the testes were 1.2 × 0.8 cm. The concentration of plasma luteinizing hormone (LH) was less than 0.3 ng/mL; the follicle-stimulating hormone (FSH) level was 1.2 ng/mL; and the testosterone level was 16 ng/dL. After 100 μg of gonadotropin-releasing hormone (GnRH), the plasma LH level (LER-960) was 0.7 ng/mL, and the FSH level (LER-869) was 2.4 ng/mL. For conversion to SI units, see Figures 25-19 and 25-20. (From Styne DM, Grumbach MM. Puberty in the male and female: its physiology and disorders. In: Yen SCC, Jaffe RB, eds. *Reproductive Endocrinology*, 2nd ed. Philadelphia, PA: WB Saunders; 1986: 313-384.)

1944 (Fig. 25-41). The prevalence is 1 of every 10,000 males and 1 of every 40,000 females. Although the loss of olfaction usually correlates with the degree of GnRH deficiency, even in complete anosmia, the GnRH deficiency may be partial (see "Isolated Luteinizing Hormone Deficiency").[462] Because affected individuals often do not notice impaired olfaction, testing with graded dilutions of pure scents is necessary to determine partial anosmia. Patients with Kallmann syndrome have no or diminished nocturnal pulses of gonadotropins found in normal prepubertal boys, although daytime values are equal. Undescended testes are common in this and all types of hypogonadotropic hypogonadism in boys.[459] The magnitude of the GnRH deficiency correlates with the size of the testes. Micropenis occurs in about one half of males with Kallmann syndrome as a result of absence of the elevated pituirary gonadotropins characteristic of normal fetal life (Fig. 25-42).

Associated defects that are inconstantly present include cleft lip, cleft palate, imperfect facial fusion, seizure disor-

ders, short metacarpals, pes cavus, neurosensory hearing loss (rarely found in the X-linked form, cerebellar ataxia and nystagmus, ocular motor abnormalities, unilateral or rarely bilateral renal aplasia or dysplasia, and mirror movements of the upper extremities (i.e., bimanual synkinesia), limited to the X-linked form (see Table 25-18).

In classic, X-linked KAL1, fetal GnRH neurosecretory neurons do not migrate from the olfactory placode to the medial basal hypothalamus, where they should constitute the GnRH pulse generator, but instead end in a tangle around the cribriform plate and in the dural layers adjacent to the meninges beneath the forebrain.[340] Abnormal or absent olfactory bulbs or folds are seen on MRI scans with other changes in brain morphometry resulting.[463] Coronal and axial cranial MRI scans of the olfactory bulbs and sulci, unilaterally or bilaterally, reflect this defect in about 90% of cases and can point to the diagnosis, especially in affected infants and prepubertal-age children (Fig. 25-43).

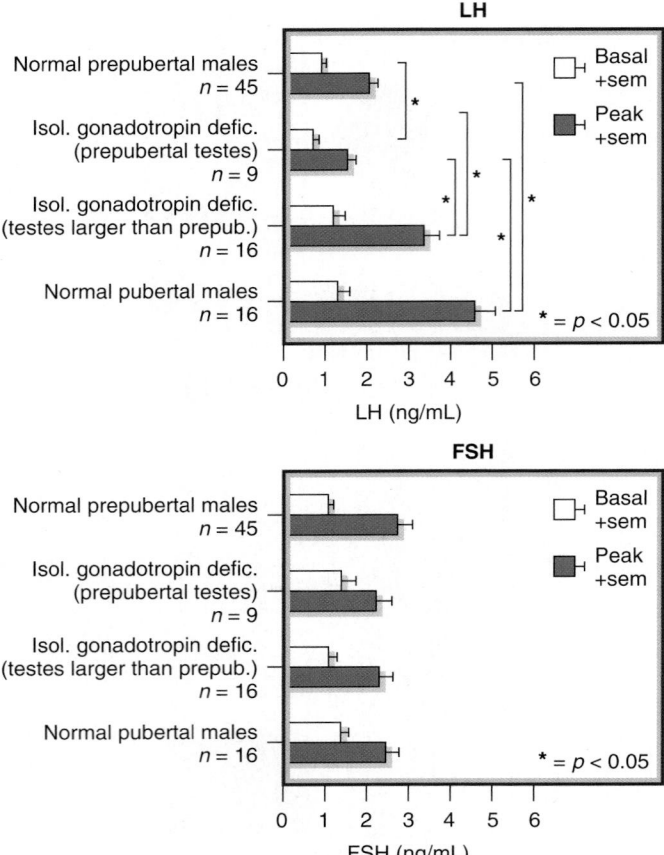

Figure 25-42 Serum luteinizing hormone (LH) and follicle-stimulating hormone (FSH) responses to the administration of gonadotropin-releasing hormone (GnRH) in 25 males with an isolated gonadotropin deficiency with or without anosmia were segregated according to whether the volume of the testes was prepubertal or greater than 2.5 cm³. Testicular volume in those with testes larger than 2.5 cm³ was as large as 4 cm³. Basal and GnRH-stimulated gonadotropin levels after the intravenous injection of 100 μg GnRH (peak value) are shown ($p < 0.05$). For conversion to SI units, see Figure 25-16. sem, standard error of the mean. (From Van Dop C, Burstein S, Conte FA, et al. Isolated gonadotropin deficiency in boys: clinical characteristics and growth. *J Pediatr.* 1987;111:684-692.)

An increasing number of genes are implicated in Kallmann syndrome, starting from the classic *KAL1* gene in the X-linked form first described, but only 30% of patients can be shown to have an identifiable gene defect. Further digenetic and oligogenetic inheritance is now recognized and may explain the genetic heterogeneity of the syndrome and the variation in phenotype encountered within a family. Recently mutations in genes "synexpressed" with fibroblast growth factor 8 (FGF8) were found in IHH and Kallmann syndrome (*FGF17, IL17RD, DUSP6, SPRY4,* and *FLRT3*), supporting thie oligogenetic nature of the condition.[464]

A variety of deletions and mutations of the *KAL1* gene have been described, including large and small (exon) deletions, point mutations, and a variety of nonsense mutations leading to frameshift and premature stop codons. The *KAL1* mutations are more prevalent in Japanese than in white patients, and they can be associated with normal olfactory function.[465] The defect in some rare patients with no *KAL1* mutation but X-linked inheritance may be located in the promoter region of the *KAL1* gene. Kallmann syndrome associated with X-linked ichthyosis caused by

steroid sulfatase deficiency, mental retardation, and chondroplasia punctata occurs in a contiguous gene syndrome. Only 14% of familial cases and 11% of sporadic cases involve mutations in the *KAL1* gene on the X chromosome, but these patients are more likely to have complete absence of gonadotropin secretory pulses and absence of migration of GnRH neurons to the hypothalamus.[466] Hypogonadotropic hypogonadism is rarely caused by a mutation in the *KAL1* gene in females.

The autosomal dominant form is known as Kallmann syndrome type 2 (KAL2), and the associated gene is the fibroblast growth factor receptor 1 gene, *FGFR1* (previously called *KAL2*) with a gene map locus of 8p11.2-p11.1 and its ligand FGF8. Mutations result in autosomal dominant Kallmann syndrome, autosomal dominant normosmic hypogonadotropic hypogonadism, or delayed puberty. KAL2 is associated with mental retardation, choanal atresia, short stature, congenital heart defects, and sensorineural hearing loss, and its presentations are more varied than those of KAL1.

The loss-of-function mutation of the *FGFR1* gene interferes with migration of the olfactory cells to the olfactory bulb. Anosmin 1, a neuronal protein, may act through *FGFR1* to bring about FGF signaling. KAL1 partially escapes inactivation in females, and it is postulated that enough KAL1 may be produced in affected females, despite *FGFR1* haploinsufficiency, to maintain adequate FGF signaling and allow olfactory function and GnRH neuron migration. One kindred of Kallmann syndrome contained four women with *FGFR1* mutations that were transmitted to affected male offspring, although the mothers had normal reproduction and olfaction.[467]

Although gain-of-function mutations of the *FGFR1* gene are associated with craniosynostosis, a loss-of-function mutation is not associated with lack of fusion of the cranial sutures. One kindred with an *FGFR1* mutation (Arg622X) in the tyrosine kinase domain, in which some of the manifestations were temporary, has been reported; the mother of the proband had delayed puberty, and the maternal grandmother had anosmia, whereas the proband with KAL2 exhibited normal LH levels, testosterone production, and spermatogenesis after prior testosterone therapy.[468]

Studies of mice revealed that the early emergence of GnRH neurons from the embryonic olfactory placode requires FGF8 signaling as a ligand mediated through *FGFR1*.[469] About 30% of FGF8/FGFR1 loss-of-function mutations are associated with cleft palate, whereas *FGFR1* mutations may rarely lead to cartilage abnormalities in the ears, nose, or digits.[470] An unusual kindred with a proband demonstrating severe ear anomalies, mandibular hypoplasia, thoracic dystrophia, and other usual findings was associated with an Arg622 mutation in the *FGFR1* gene, and investigation for hypogonadism is indicated when such facial abnormalities occur.[471] Prevalence of *FGFR1* mutations in the Japanese population is equal to the prevalence among whites. Although renal aplasia is characteristic of KAL1 mutations and cleft palate and dental agenesis are characteristic of *FGFR1* mutations in KAL2, these findings can occur in Kallmann patients without KAL1 or *FGFR1* mutations.[465]

Apparent autosomal recessive inheritance characterizes other kindreds with Kallmann syndrome type 3 (KAL3), for which the affected gene is *PROKR2*. Unilateral renal agenesis, hypotelorism, cleft lip and palate, and a midline cranial fusion defect occur. Fibrous dysplasia, sleep disorder, severe obesity, synkinesia, and epilepsy have been described in patients with *PROK2* or *PROKR2* mutations, and 3% of IHH patients were affected in one study. Knockout mice lacking the *PROK2* gene (formerly called KAL4),

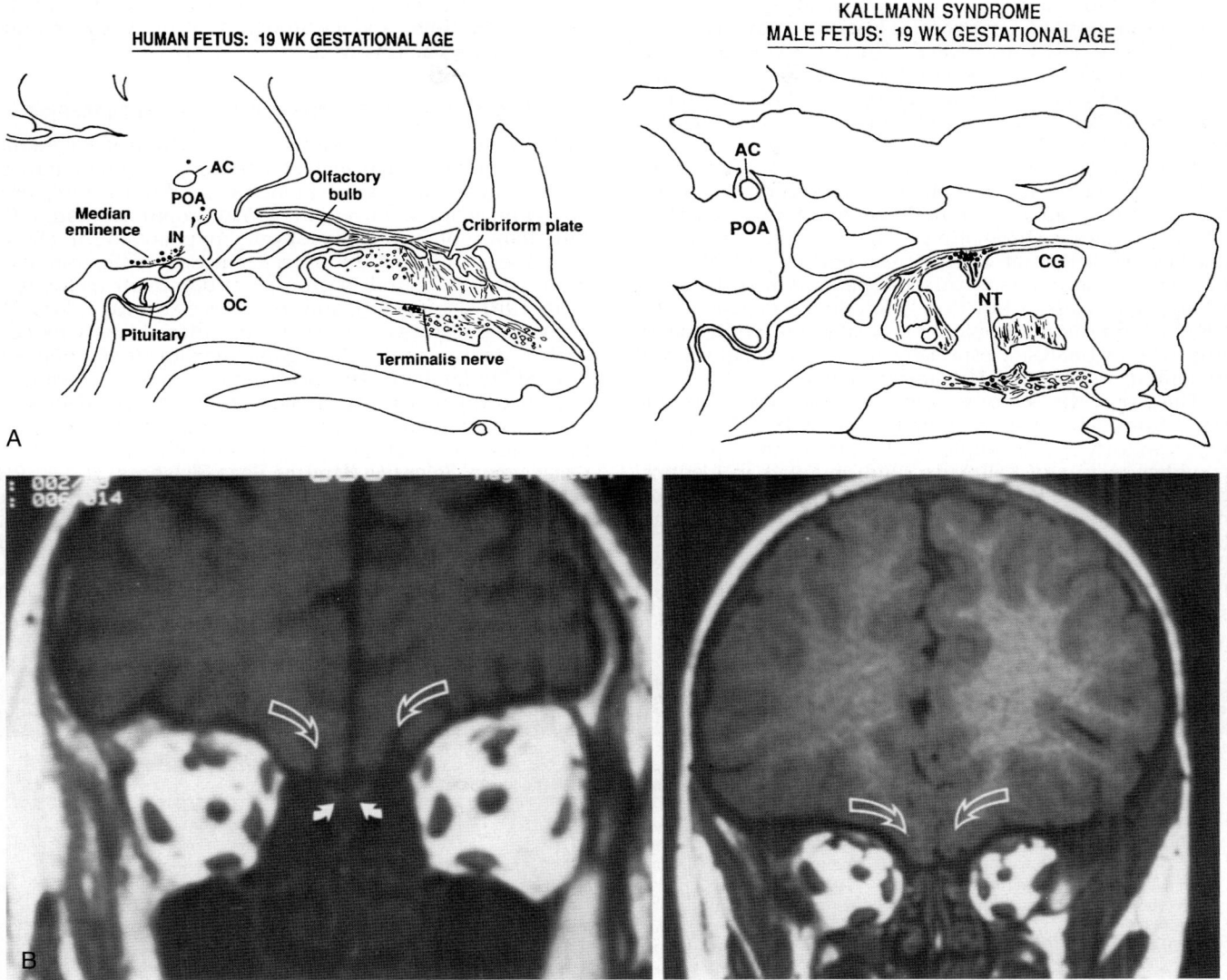

HUMAN FETUS: 19 WK GESTATIONAL AGE

KALLMANN SYNDROME
MALE FETUS: 19 WK GESTATIONAL AGE

A

B

Figure 25-43 Comparison of the brain and nasal cavities of a normal 19-week-old male fetus *(upper left)* and those of a male fetus of similar age with Kallmann syndrome caused by an X chromosome deletion at Xp22.3 *(upper right)*. In the normal fetal brain, the gonadotropin-releasing hormone (GnRH) neurosecretory neurons *(black dots)* are located in the hypothalamic area, including the medial basal hypothalamus, the anterior hypothalamic area, and of interest regarding hypothalamic hamartoma as an ectopic GnRH pulse generator, the premammillary and retromammillary areas. A small cluster of GnRH neurons exists among the fibers of the terminalis nerve on the floor of the nasal septum. In the male fetus with Kallmann syndrome, no GnRH neurons were detected in the hypothalamic region, including the basal hypothalamus, median eminence, and preoptic area. The GnRH cells fail to migrate to and enter the brain from their origin in the nose; these cells end in a tangle beneath the forebrain on the dorsal surface of the cribriform plate and in the nasal cavity. AC, anterior commissure; CG, crista galli; IN, infundibular nucleus; NT, terminalis nerve; OC, optic chiasm; POA, preoptic area. Lower panels show magnetic resonance imaging scans of brain (coronal section, TI-weighted image). *Lower left,* normal olfactory sulci *(open arrows)* and bulbs *(solid arrows)* in a 15-year-old boy. *Lower right,* absent olfactory sulci *(open arrows)* and bulbs in a 17-year-old, anosmic, sexually infantile boy with Kallmann syndrome.

which encodes prokineticin 2, an 81–amino acid peptide that signals through the G protein–coupled product of the *PROKR2* gene (formerly called KAL3), had defective development of the olfactory bulbs and failed migration of GnRH neurons.[472] This model led to demonstration of loss-of-function mutations in *PROKR2* or *PROK2* in 9% of patients with Kallmann syndrome,[473] who were mostly heterozygous, although homozygous and compound heterozygous mutations were also described. Some families appear to have autosomal dominant inheritance.

The human equivalent of the mouse nasal embryonic GnRH factor gene *(Nelf)* is *NELF*; a mutation of this gene is found in patients with IHH and in Kallmann syndrome.[474]

Mutations in the binding domain of the membrane coreceptor neuropilin-1 *(SEMA3A)* gene is found in Kallmann syndrome in an autosomal dominant pattern.[475] This mutation was found in some patients who already had mutations in other Kallmann syndrome genes, further suggesting the oligogenic nature of the disorder.

About 30% of Kallmann syndrome patients have hearing impairment, and of those about 38% were shown to have heterogeneous mutations of the *SOX10* gene.[476] Deafness may also be found in the CHARGE syndrome (discussed later), but in the absence of other CHARGE findings a search for a mutation in *SOX10* is indicated.

Mutations in heparin sulfate 6-O-sulfotransferase 1 *(HS6ST1)* are found in patients and families with IHH and Kallmann syndrome.[477] This abnormality is found in complex inheritance patterns as patients may also have mutations in *FGF1* and *NELF*. Thus, *HS6ST1* mutations may not be sufficient to cause disease but may add to it.

Recently Kallmann syndrome has been linked to mutations in *HESX1* (found in septo-optic dysplasia, discussed later)[478] and *FEZF1*.[479]

The CHARGE syndrome includes IHH and hyposmia, including absent olfactory bulbs. In autosomal dominant familial cases, causative mutations were found in *CHD7*, which encodes a chromatin-remodeling factor, which in a small percentage of cases were found in patients with Kallmann syndrome and in some patients with IHH due to apparent loss-of-function mutations. Patients with CHARGE syndrome should be evaluated for hypogonadotropic hypogonadism, especially if there is deafness and hypoplasia of the semicircular canals.[480]

Therefore, the various forms of Kallmann syndrome result from heterogeneous mutations in which the phenotype can vary. For example, a 20-year-old man with the complete picture of Kallmann syndrome had an identical twin brother (proved by genetic fingerprinting) with anosmia but a normal adult phenotype and normal plasma testosterone and gonadotropin concentrations.

Other postulated defects that may interfere with GnRH neuron migration are mutations in the genes for neural cell adhesion molecules (NCAM) and related proteins, such as tenascin, laminin, and phosphacan. Various glycoconjugates may also be involved.

Other Forms of Isolated Hypogonadotropic Hypogonadism

Only about 15% of normosmic hypogonadotropic patients have a definable genetic defect. The combination of human genetic studies and mouse models has led to the discovery of many genes involved in gonadotropin regulation.[481] Inheritance of hypogonadotropic hypogonadism (Table 25-19) with none of the other features of Kallmann syndrome may be found in autosomal dominant (gene map locus 19p13.3, 9q34.3), autosomal recessive (8p21-p11.2), or X-linked recessive (Xp21)[482,483] disorders. Males with cerebellar ataxia and deficient gonadotropin production are reported in kindreds with X-linked inheritance (possibly a variant form of Kallmann syndrome), and hypogonadotropic hypogonadism may be associated with the multiple lentigines and basal cell nevus syndromes.

Gonadotropin-Releasing Hormone Gene Mutations. The GnRH gene *(GNRH1)* would seem a likely candidate for the cause of hypogonadotropic hypogonadism, but although mutations of the GnRH receptor gene *(GNRHR)* were identified years ago, mutations in the *GNRH1* gene were not demonstrated until 2009. An autosomal recessive form had been

TABLE 25-19

Molecular Basis for Developmental Disorders Associated With Hypogonadotropic Hypogonadism

Gene	Phenotype	Complex Phenotype
	Isolated Hypogonadotropic Hypogonadism	
Kallmann Syndrome or Normosmic IHH (With the Same Mutant Gene)		
KAL1 (Xp22.3)	X-linked Kallmann syndrome	Anosmia/hyposmia, renal agenesis, dyskinesia
FGFR1 (KAL2) (8p11.2)	Autosomal dominant Kallmann syndrome (± recessive)	Anosmia/hyposmia, cleft lip/palate
FGF8 (ligand for FGFR1) (10q25)		
NELF (9q34.3)	Autosomal dominant (?) Kallmann syndrome	
PROK2 (3p21.1)	Autosomal recessive Kallmann syndrome	
*PROKR2** (20p12.3)		
CHD7 (8p12.1)	Autosomal dominant (some)	CHARGE syndrome includes hyposmia
Normosmic Isolated Hypogonadotropic Hypogonadism		
GNRH1 (8p21-11.2)	Autosomal recessive	
*GNRHR** (4q13.2-3)	Autosomal recessive (± dominant)	
*GPR54** (19p13.3)	Autosomal recessive	
SNRPN		Prader-Willi syndrome
Lack of function of paternal 15q11-q13 region or maternal uniparental disomy		Obesity
LEP (7q31.3)	Autosomal recessive	Obesity
LEPR (1p31)	Autosomal recessive	Obesity
NR0B1 (DAX1) (X21.3-21.2)	X-linked recessive	Adrenal hypoplasia
TAC3 (12q13-12)	Autosomal recessive	
TACR3 (4q25)	Autosomal recessive	
Multiple Pituitary Hormone Deficiencies		
PROP1 (POU1F1)	Autosomal recessive GH, PRL, TSH, and LH/FSH (less commonly, later-onset ACTH deficiency)	
HESX1 (RPX)	Autosomal recessive; and heterozygous mutations Multiple pituitary deficiencies including diabetes insipidus, but LH/FSH uncommon	Septo-optic dysplasia
LHX3	Autosomal recessive GH, PRL, TSH, FSH/LH	Rigid cervical spine
PHF6	X-linked; GH, TSH, ACTH, LH/FSH	Borjeson-Lehmann syndrome: mental retardation; facies

*A G-protein–coupled receptor.

ACTH, corticotropin; CHD7, chromatin-remodeling factor; DAX1, dosage-sensitive sex reversal-adrenal hyperplasia congenita critical region on the X chromosome, gene 1; FGF, fibroblast growth factor; FSH, follicle-stimulating hormone; GH, growth hormone; GNRH, gonadotropin-releasing hormone; GPR54, kisspeptin G protein–coupled receptor 54; *HESX1*, homeobox gene expressed in ES cells; IHH, idiopathic hypogonadotropic hypogonadism; LEP, leptin; LH, luteinizing hormone; *LHX3*, lim homeobox gene 3; NELF, nasal embryonic luteinizing hormone–releasing factor; NR0B1, nuclear receptor family 0, group B, member 1; *PHF6*, plant homeodomain–like finger gene; PRL, prolactin; PROK2, prokineticin 2; PROP1, prophet of Pit-1; R, receptor; SNRPN, small nuclear ribonucleoprotein polypeptide SmN; TAC3, neurokinin 3; TSH, thyroid-stimulating hormone.

described in the mouse (hyg/hyg), in which there is a deletion of part of the *Gnrh* gene. There appears to be normal migration of GnRH neurons to the medial basal hypothalamus based on information from the mouse model.[486]

GNRH1 mutation is a very rare condition with a prevalence of under 1% in isolated populations and probably far lower in the general population. A homozygous *GNRH1* frameshift mutation in human beings, characterized by the insertion of an adenine at nucleotide position 18 (c.18-19insA) in the sequence encoding the N-terminal region of the signal peptide–containing protein precursor of GnRH (prepro-GnRH), was found in a teenage brother and sister who had normosmic IHH.[485] When expressed in vitro, the mutant peptide did not demonstrate immunoreactive GnRH. One patient of 310 with severe, congenital, normosmic IHH (with micropenis, bilateral cryptorchidism, and absent puberty) had a homozygous frameshift mutation that is predicted to disrupt the three C-terminal amino acids of the GnRH decapeptide and to produce a premature stop codon.[486] Of four patients with normosmic IHH, one had a nonsynonymous missense mutation in the eighth amino acid of the GnRH decapeptide; one had a nonsense mutation that causes premature termination within the GnRH-associated peptide (GAP), which lies C-terminal to the GnRH decapeptide within the GnRH precursor; and two had sequence variants that cause nonsynonymous amino acid substitutions in the signal peptide and GnRH-associated peptide.

Gonadotropin-Releasing Hormone Receptor Mutations. Mutations of the gene encoding the type 1 GnRH receptor (*GNRHR*, gene map locus 4q21.2) that affect the G protein–coupled, seven-transmembrane segments lead to various degrees of familial and sporadic hypogonadotropic hypogonadism with normosmia. A *GNRHR* mutation is found in about 40% to 50% of cases of familial, autosomal recessive, normosmic IHH and in about 17% of sporadic cases of normosmic IHH.

Mutations in hypergonadal hypogonadism with amino acid substitutions in the extracellular N-terminal domain (Thr32Ile), the second extracellular loop (Cys200Tyr), the third intracellular loop (Leu266Arg), and the sixth transmembrane helix (Cys279Tyr) were found to affect specific GnRH binding.[487,488] Except for Thr32Ile, there was no significant inositol phosphate accumulation after GnRH stimulation, demonstrating loss of function even if binding was accomplished. However, an increased dose of GnRH allowed stimulation of the gonadotropin subunit and GnRHR promoters and the ability to partially activate extracellular signal-regulated kinase 1 and stimulate cAMP response element (CRE)–luciferase activity. A higher dose of GnRH caused the Cys200Tyr mutant to stimulate gonadotropin subunit and GnRHR promoter activity because this mutant reduces cell surface receptor expression.

Another human GnRH receptor *(GNRHR)* gene mutation of a highly conserved sequence located in the second-transmembrane helix impairs *GNRHR* effector coupling due to loss of surface expression of the receptor and leads to a severe manifestation of IHH.[489]

Certain GnRH receptor defects may be rescued by membrane-permeant pharmacologic agents that can act as a folding template, chaperones, that rescue the structural defects caused by the mutations and allowing function to occur (i.e., ligand binding and restoration of receptor coupling to effector).[490] This approach may allow a therapeutic approach to conditions caused by this and other mutations in receptors that result in protein misfolding.

The clinical presentation of patients with mutations in the GnRH receptor is heterogeneous, and impairment of signal transmission is highly variable (e.g., severe features of IHH, sexual infantilism, long-delayed puberty with reversal in adulthood, relatively mild hypogonadism and infertility), even within the same pedigree and especially in patients with compound heterozygous mutations. When the mutation is homozygous the phenotype is related to the number of mutations. However, when it is monoallelic there is no relationship, which indicates that other genes interact with the single allic mutation in *GNRH1*.[491]

In all types of congenital gonadotropin deficiencies, male patients are likely to manifest micropenis (penile length <2.0 cm at birth and in infancy) due to lack of fetal gonadotropin stimulation of fetal testes during the last half of gestation. Boys with congenital GH deficiency have micropenis even if gonadotropin function is normal. Because testosterone therapy is effective in increasing penile size (see later discussion), sex reversal is not indicated in these cases of microphallus.[492]

KISS1/KISS1R Axis Mutations. The KISS1/KISS1R axis plays a role in the increased amplitude of GnRH signaling in puberty. KISS1/KISS1R axis mutations are rare but instructive. Of 30 normosmic subjects with hypogonadotropic hypogonadism who were evaluated, one person had two missense mutations in KISS1R (Cys223Arg in the fifth transmembrane helix and Arg297Leu in the third extracellular loop); the former had no activity, and the latter manifested as mildly decreased signaling ability.[493] Homozygous deletions of 155 nucleotides in the *KISS1R* gene encompassing the splicing acceptor site of the intron 4–exon 5 junction and part of exon 5 were found in all affected family members with IHH,[494] but unaffected family members had no deletion or only one mutant allele. Another kindred had a Leu48Ser mutation in the second intracellular loop (IL2) of KISS1R, and another had two separate mutations in the gene,[320] Arg331Xaa and Xaa399Arg. The latter patient had decreased secretion of GnRH and decreased response to GnRH administration. A line of mice transfected with the affected gene exhibited hypogonadotropic hypogonadism with decreased GnRH in the hypothalamus but were responsive to GnRH or gonadotropin administration. Agonist stimulation may stabilize the switch II region of Gα to promote the opening of Gα switch II to facilitate exchange of guanosine diphosphate (GDP) and guanosine triphosphate (GTP).[495] The Leu148Ser mutation does not affect the expression, ligand-binding properties, or protein interaction network of KISS1R, but diverse KISS1R functional responses are markedly inhibited.

X-Linked Congenital Adrenal Hypoplasia and Hypogonadotropic Hypogonadism. A rare deletion or mutation in the dosage-sensitive sex reversal-A (DSS) adrenal hypoplasia congenita gene on the X chromosome gene 1 (*NROB1*, formerly called *DAX1*; gene map locus Xp21.3-p21.2) leads to an X-linked recessive disorder of adrenocortical organogenesis.[496] The gene encodes an orphan receptor, a member of the nuclear receptor superfamily, that is a putative transcriptional repressor mapping to the Xp21 locus. A double dose of *NROB1* is associated with a female phenotype or ambiguous genitalia in 46,XY males. The NROB1 protein has a novel domain in the N-terminus that contains two putative unique zinc finger motifs, and the C-terminus contains a conserved ligand-binding domain that binds DNA, localizes in the nucleus, and contains a transcriptional silencing domain that antagonizes the steroidogenic factor 1 (SF1, also called NR5A1) transactivation function. NROB1 has an SF1 response element in the 5′-promoter region that is another orphan member of the nuclear hormone receptor superfamily. Both NROB1 and SF1 are expressed in the adrenals, gonads, pituitary, and hypothalamus, raising the possibility of an important interaction between these two genes and their products.

Rare abnormalities of NR0B1 are characterized by severe glucocorticoid, mineralocorticoid, and at puberty, androgen deficiency. The abnormal structure of the adrenal cortex resembles that of the fetal zone because it consists of disorganized, vacuolated, cytomegalic cells with a normal mature cortex. The severe primary adrenal insufficiency with hyponatremia, hyperkalemia, acidosis, and hypoglycemia is characterized by failure to thrive, vomiting, poor feeding, dehydration, circulatory collapse, and increased pigmentation and is lethal if not treated early in life in affected boys.

Adrenoleukodystrophy may manifest with adrenal failure long before neurologic symptoms develop, and some cases of X-linked Addison disease may represent this diagnosis. This condition is in the differential diagnosis of adrenal hypoplasia. Plasma renin activity is high; plasma cortisol and aldosterone levels are low. Symptomatic adrenal insufficiency may first manifest in later childhood. In male infants, signs of salt wasting are usually the most prominent feature, but cortisol deficiency is detectable, and adrenal insufficiency includes deficient secretion of the zona reticularis steroids, DHEA and DHEAS. An early sign of elevated ACTH is increased skin pigmentation. The testes are undescended in fewer than one half of patients; micropenis is rare, but urogenital abnormalities and hearing loss occasionally are present. Boys who do not present with clinical evidence of adrenal insufficiency in infancy often have a more insidious onset during childhood or adulthood.

In a pedigree in which two affected boys had a hemizygous NR0B1 nonsense mutation and neonatal onset of adrenal insufficiency, a maternal aunt who was homozygous for the mutation had sexual infantilism and primary amenorrhea, but even after decades of follow-up, she maintained normal adrenal function. A maternal grandfather who carried the same mutation was asymptomatic.[497] This pedigree highlights the limitations and complexities of genotype and phenotype correlations. Most commonly, due to hypogonadotropic hypogonadism, signs of sexual maturation at the age of puberty (e.g., pubic and axillary hair, testicular enlargement) are lacking, and the concentrations of serum FSH, LH, and testosterone are low. Delayed puberty is a manifestation in some female carriers of a NR0B1 mutation.

Intragenic mutations in NR0B1 (i.e., frameshift mutations, nonsense mutations, and missense mutations) indicate that the hypogonadotropic hypogonadism is an intrinsic characteristic of the disorder, a manifestation of the single-gene mutation and not a result of involvement of a contiguous gene. The NR0B1 gene is expressed in the adrenal cortex, in testes (and weakly in the ovary), and in the hypothalamus and pituitary. There is evidence of GnRH deficiency and an abnormality in the gonadotrophs, yielding a mixed picture of hypothalamic and intrinsic gonadotroph defects with absent or erratic pulsatile secretion of LH. Even if basal immunoreactive LH and FSH levels are normal, gonadotropins seem to lack bioactivity. In some affected boys, the GnRH pulse generator and pituitary gonadotropin apparatus is intact and functional in infancy and early childhood, and the GnRH-gonadotroph defects do not manifest until later in childhood or during the peripubertal period. Azoospermia unresponsive to gonadotropin treatment was detected in a few affected men.[480,482,498,499]

A deletion of the adrenal hypoplasia congenita locus (at Xp21) can include the glycerol kinase (GK) and Duchenne muscular dystrophy (DMD) genes if it extends centromerically or produce mental retardation if there is extension toward the telomere, leading to contiguous gene syndromes.

Other mutations of the X chromosome may be associated with IHH. Two brothers were reported who had hypogonadotropic hypogonadism, obesity, and short stature associated with a maternally inherited pericentric inversion (X) (p11.4q11.2). Because the breakpoint is not related to other genes associated with pubertal disorders, it is not clear whether this is a functional relationship or a coincidence.[500]

Other Presentations of Hypogonadotropic Hypogonadism

Neurokinin B (encoded by TAC3) is a member of the tachykinin superfamily of 127 neuropeptides that includes substance P and neurokinin A. Its cognate G protein–coupled receptor 126 is NK3R, which is encoded by TACR3. Studies demonstrate loss-of-function mutations in this system in familial, congenital hypogonadotropic hypogonadism; administration of pulsatile GnRH caused resumption of gonadotropin secretion[501,502] (Fig. 25-44). A survey of 345 patients with normosmic hypogonadotropic hypogonadism found 13 rare, distinct nucleotide sequence coding variants (three 108 nonsense, six nonsynonymous, and four synonymous mutations [one predicted to affect splicing]) in TACR3 and one 109 homozygous single-base-pair deletion, resulting in complete loss of neurokinin B. Of the 16 males for whom phenotype information was available, 15 had microphallus, and none of the females had spontaneous thelarche. When subjects were assessed after discontinuation of therapy, six of seven males and four of five females demonstrated evidence for reversibility of their hypogonadotropism.[503] Continuous infusion of kisspeptin to two patients with loss-of-function mutations in neurokinin B (TAC3) or its receptor (TAC3R) led to pulsatile gonadotropin secretion, indicating that pulsatile administration of kisspeptin is not necessary to institute pulsatile GnRH secretion.[331]

Mutations in the prohormone convertase 1 gene (PCSK1, also called PC1) lead to extreme childhood obesity, hypocortisolemia, defects in conversion of proinsulin to insulin leading to hypoglycemia, diabetes insipidus, and isolated partial hypogonadotropic hypogonadism, allowing spontaneous pubertal development but primary amenorrhea. The hypogonadal hypogonadism probably resulted from impaired processing of GnRH or neuropeptides involved in its secretion. Findings in another subject extended to gastrointestinal disturbance, small intestinal malabsorption related to monosaccharide and fats, and elevation in progastrin and proglucagon levels, showing that prohormone processing in enteroendocrine cells was abnormal.[504]

Isolated Luteinizing Hormone Deficiency. Isolated LH deficiency (fertile eunuch syndrome) is associated with deficient testosterone production (which responds to hCG administration) and decreased virilization in the presence of mature testicular size and variable spermatogenesis; the disorder may be idiopathic or may result from a hypothalamic pituitary neoplasm. A homozygous Gln106Arg mutation in the first extracellular loop of the GnRH receptor at gene map locus 4q21.2 was associated with normal testicular volume (17 mL) but with apulsatile, low gonadotropin values and low testosterone[505] values in one subject. After hCG stimulation, he developed adequate spermatogenesis to father a child, and after cessation of hCG treatment, he demonstrated adult testosterone values and pulsatile gonadotropin secretion, an example of reversibility of the syndrome.

Isolated Follicle-Stimulating Hormone Deficiency. Homozygous or compound heterozygous mutations in the FSH β-subunit have been reported in three females and two

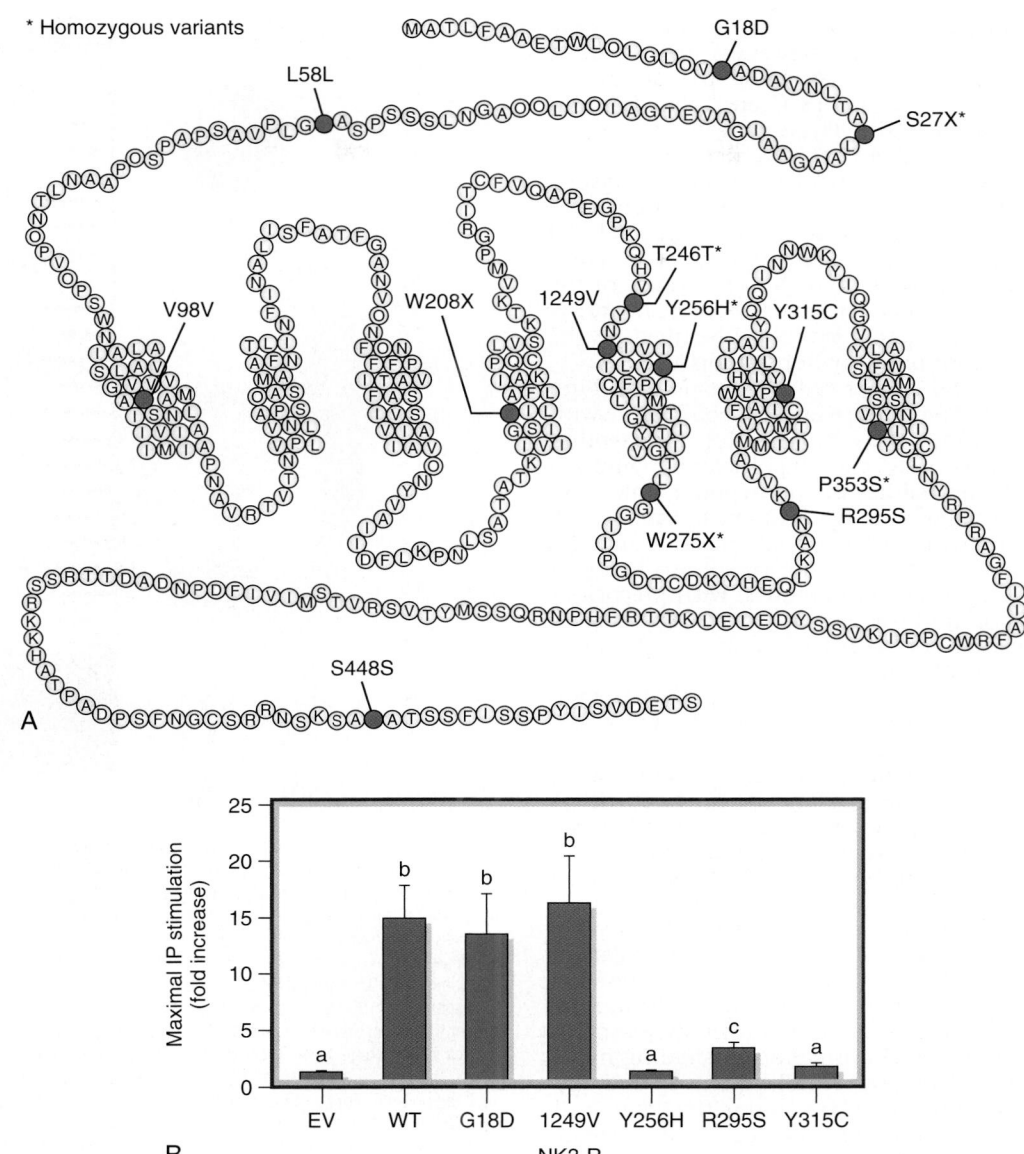

Figure 25-44 A, Schematic of mutations in the NK3-R, which is encoded by *TAC3*. **B,** Effects of mutations in *TACR3* on neurokinin B (NKB)-mediated activation of signal transduction. COS-7 cells transfected with wild-type (WT) G18D, I249V, Y256H, R295S, and Y315C NK3-R or empty vector (EV) were treated with NKB (10-7 M) for 1 hour. A significant increase in inositol phosphate (IP) accumulation occurred in cells transfected with WT, G18D, or I249V NK3-R. In contrast, there was a marked reduction in NKB-stimulated IP production in cells transfected with Y256H, R295S, or Y315C NK3-R, or with EV. *a, b,* and *c* denote significantly different fold increases in IP accumulation. (From Gianetti E, Tusset C, Noel SD, et al. *TAC3/TACR3* mutations reveal preferential activation of gonadotropin-releasing hormone release by neurokinin B in neonatal life followed by reversal in adulthood. *J Clin Endocrinol Metab.* 2010;95:2857-2867.)

males with delayed puberty or poorly developed secondary sex characteristics and with primary amenorrhea but normal adrenarche in the women.[506] The LH concentration was elevated, the serum level of estradiol was low, and immunoactive FSH was absent. Two of the three women had a homozygous nonsense mutation (Val61X) in the FSH β-subunit gene at gene map locus 11p13, and the other was a compound heterozygote (Cys51Gly/Val61X). The women had antral follicles but no progression, demonstrating that FSH action may not be necessary for development to the antral stage. The two men had azoospermia; small, soft testes; and absence of serum FSH. One had normal puberty and normal LH and testosterone values, with a missense mutation (Cys82Arg), and the other had slightly delayed puberty, low testosterone and inhibin B levels, high LH levels, and a nonsense mutation (Val61X). The low testos-

terone may indicate a necessity for FSH to promote testosterone production.

Follicle-Stimulating Hormone Receptor Mutations. Hypergonadotropic hypogonadism is noted with rare mutations in FSH receptors.[506] Women may have several mutations but only five men are described as homozygous for the Finnish p.Ala189Val *FSHR* gene mutation. Although the affected women had amenorrhea, some of the men were fertile and all progressed through puberty with normal or slightly small testes. The defect in the FSH receptor appears to be less severe than the absence of the ligand.

Developmental Defect of the Midline

Septo-optic or optic dysplasia is caused by abnormal development of the prosencephalon, leading to small, dysplastic, pale optic discs with a double outline and pendular (evenly moving side to side) nystagmus; blindness may occur. A midline hypothalamic defect may cause GH deficiency, diabetes insipidus, and ACTH, TSH, and gonadotropin deficiency. Short stature and delayed puberty may result, although CPP is an alternative.[507] The septum pellucidum is often absent in association with optic hypoplasia or dysplasia, which is readily demonstrable by imaging techniques.[508] In the University of California at San Francisco (UCSF) series, the syndrome was associated with decreased maternal age. The pituitary may be hypoplastic because of the lack of hypothalamic stimulatory factors, and the neurohypophysis may have an ectopic location identified by the location of the posterior pituitary hot spot on MRI.

Abnormalities of the corpus callosum and cerebellum are common on MRI. Four groups are described: those with normal MRI results, those with abnormalities of the septum pellucidum and with a normal hypothalamic pituitary area, those with abnormalities of the hypothalamic pituitary area and a normal septum pellucidum, and those with abnormalities in both areas.[509] No endocrine abnormalities were described in the first group, but the others had progressively more endocrine abnormalities, with precocious puberty most common in the second group. Early diagnosis is important because of the risk of sudden death associated with adrenal insufficiency.

The condition is usually sporadic, but inherited cases invoving transcription factors HESX1, SOX2, SOX3, and OTX2 are reported.[510]

The solitary median maxillary incisor syndrome is associated with the eponymous midline defect and with a prominent midpalatal ridge (torus palatinus) and hypopituitarism. The defect in this autosomal dominant condition is in the sonic hedgehog gene *(SHH)* at gene map locus 7q3.[511]

Other congenital midline defects ranging from complete dysraphism and holoprosencephaly to cleft palate or lip are associated with hypothalamic-pituitary dysfunction. Delayed puberty is rarely described in duplication of the hypophysis. Myelomeningocele (myelodysplasia) is associated with endocrine abnormalities, including hypothalamic hypothyroidism, hyperprolactinemia, and elevated gonadotropin concentrations, and with CPP.

Long-term follow-up of hypogonadotropic hypogonadism or partial pubertal development revealed that even with defined genetic defects, restoration of normal gonadal function, including pulsatile LH secretion and spermatogenesis in adulthood, may occur in up to 20% of cases.[443,512] Of the 15 patients described, 4 had anosmia, 6 had absent puberty, 9 had partial puberty at first, and all had abnormal GnRH-induced LH secretion. Three of 13 evaluated with genetic analysis who reversed their hypogonadotropic hypogonadism had mutations in *FGFR1* or *GNRHR*. Long-term follow-up is necessary, even for patients with established genetic defects.

Idiopathic Hypopituitary Dwarfism

In addition to *HESX1* mutations, autosomal recessive mutations in homeobox genes encoding transcription factors involved in the early aspects of pituitary development lead to hypogonadotropic hypogonadism and other pituitary hormone deficiencies.[513,514] *PROP1* mutations at gene map locus 5q cause GH and TSH deficiency and produce delayed puberty or late onset of secondary hypogonadism in adulthood and rarely cause ACTH deficiency (Fig. 25-45).[515] In one study of 73 patients with idiopathic multiple pituitary hormone deficiencies, 35 had a mutation in *PROP1*. Homozygous Arg73Cys mutation of PROP1

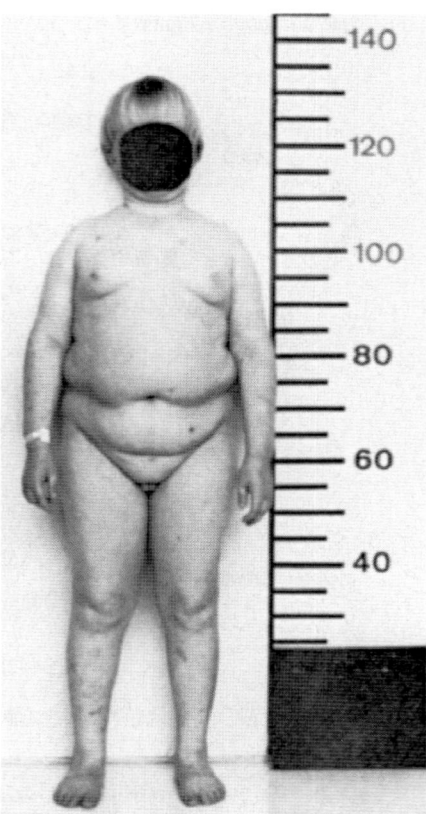

Figure 25-45 A 20-year-old man with idiopathic hypopituitary dwarfism and deficiencies of gonadotropins, thyrotropin, corticotropin, and growth hormone had a history of arrested hydrocephalus. His height was 129 cm (−8 SD [standard deviation]), the phallus was 2 cm long, and the testes measured 1.5 × 1 cm. He had received thyroid hormone and glucocorticoid replacement. The basal luteinizing hormone (LH) level was less than 0.2 ng/mL (LER-960), follicle-stimulating hormone (FSH) level was 0.5 ng/mL (LER-869), and testosterone level was less than 0.1 ng/mL. In response to 100 μg of gonadotropin-releasing hormone (GnRH), the plasma LH concentration increased slightly to 0.6 ng/mL, and there was no increase in the plasma testosterone level. The excretion of urinary 17-ketosteroids was 1.1 mg/24 hours. The bone age was 10 years, and the volume of the sella turcica was small on skull radiographs. For conversion to SI units, see Figures 25-19 and 25-20. (From Styne DM, Grumbach MM. Puberty in the male and female: its physiology and disorders. In: Yen SCC, Jaffe RB, eds. *Reproductive Endocrinology*, 2nd ed. Philadelphia, PA: WB Saunders; 1986:313-384.)

allowed spontaneous puberty in 2 of 10 affected family members. ACTH deficiency is more rarely a feature of PROP1 deficiency.

Homozygous mutations occur in the *LHX3* gene at gene map locus 9q34.3. It encodes a member of the LIM class of homeodomain proteins, which are associated with multiple pituitary hormone deficiencies, including LH and FSH, and often with severe restriction of head rotation.[516] *LH4* and *GLI2* mutations may cause isolated GH deficiency or combined pituitary hormone deficiencies including gonadotropin deficiency.[517,518]

The familial forms of multiple pituitary hormone deficiencies with autosomal recessive or X-linked inheritance are less common. The degree of hormone deficit and the age at onset of pituitary hormone deficiencies may vary within a single kindred having the same genetic defect.

The X-linked form of hypopituitarism can be associated with duplication of the *SOX3* gene.[519] Deficiency of SOX2, a transcription factor involved in early hypothalamic-pituitary embryonic development, leads to anterior pituitary hypoplasia. Patients with *SOX2* mutations have major eye abnormalities, including anophthalmia, microphthalmia, and coloboma. They also have hypogonadotropic hypogonadism as the most common pituitary defect, in contrast to most other types of pituitary hypoplasias, demonstrating GH deficiency most frequently.[520]

There is an association between breech delivery (especially for male infants), perinatal distress, and idiopathic hypopituitarism.[102] Malformations of the pituitary stalk demonstrable by MRI are common in these patients. Other types of birth traumas or complications may lead to hypopituitarism as well.

Common to many patients with congenital hypopituitary dwarfism is early onset of growth failure; late onset of diminished growth is an ominous finding, suggesting the presence of a CNS tumor.

Isolated GH deficiency allows spontaneous pubertal development when the bone age reaches the pubertal stage of 11 to 13 years, usually after the corresponding chronologic age is reached. Associated gonadotropin deficiency does not allow spontaneous puberty, even when the bone age advances to the pubertal stage during GH therapy.

Miscellaneous Conditions
Prader-Willi Syndrome

Prader-Willi syndrome is an autosomal dominant disorder that combines a tendency for intrauterine growth retardation, delayed onset and poor fetal activity, infantile central hypotonia, and lethargy, followed by early-onset childhood hyperphagia, pathologic obesity, and carbohydrate intolerance (leading to type 2 diabetes in 25% of patients at a mean age of 20 years). Features include short stature, small hands and feet, mild to moderate mental retardation, and emotional instability, including perseveration, obsessions, and compulsions. Almond-shaped eyes, a triangular mouth, and narrow bifrontal diameter combined with delayed puberty and hypogonadotropic hypogonadism caused by combined hypothalamic and gonadal dysfunction are characteristic.[521] Despite the late or absent puberty, there is a tendency to early adrenarche (14%) or even precocious puberty rarely (3.6%).

Affected boys usually have a micropenis and cryptorchidism (100% in a large series[522]), and an underdeveloped scrotum (69%) is common. In a study of 37 adults with Prader-Willi syndrome, none achieved full genital development, and primary testicular defects were suggested.[523] Serum AMH levels were near the lower limits of normal, inhibin B levels were consistently low or undetectable, and in the adults, FSH levels were high, although LH levels were normal. Two adults had undetectable levels of LH and FSH, but in contrast to the others, they had high AMH levels. Female subjects exhibit underdevelopment of the labia majora, labia minora, or clitoris (76%). Amenorrhea occurs in about one half of cases (53%), and irregular menses or spotting are common in others. Weight reduction may lead to menarche in some females, because severe obesity may play a role in the impaired puberty in some patients. Dietary therapy during years 2 through 10 can provide effective treatment of obesity but may decrease growth, although contemporaneous GH therapy may overcome slow growth.[524]

The role of relative GH deficiency in this disorder is uncertain and controversial. The FDA approved Prader-Willi syndrome as an indication for recombinant human GH treatment without a requirement for assessing GH secretion. Genetic testing is used to confirm the clinical diagnosis of the syndrome. GH treatment (in a dose of 0.24 mg/kg per week subcutaneously given six to seven times per week) was shown in long-term, randomized, controlled trials to decrease body fat; increase fat utilization, LBM, linear growth, and energy expenditure; and possibly to improve physical strength and motor development.[525] Children with Prader-Willi syndrome are at risk for sudden death due to gastrointestinal, respiratory, or cardiac complications.[526] However, the report of sudden deaths due to respiratory complications during GH treatment led to a recommendation for evaluation for sleep apnea or respiratory difficulties before instituting GH therapy. More recent data cast doubt on the beneficial effects of GH on body composition and BMI, but higher parental educational status was correlated with better clinical outcome.[527]

This distinct genetic disorder, with a frequency of about 1 case in 15,000 to 30,000 individuals, is rarely familial (i.e., the recurrence risk depends on the type of the genetic defect). It is caused by abnormalities involving the long arm of chromosome 15 in the q11-q13 region. Approximately 70% of Prader-Willi cases are caused by a paternal deletion of 15q11-q13 (commonly 3 to 5 mega-base pairs long); 20% to 25% of cases involve maternal uniparental disomy (isodisomy or heterodisomy) in which both chromosomes 15 are derived from the mother, possibly by nondisjunction during maternal meiosis, representing a striking example of genomic imprinting.[521] In 2% to 5% of cases, an imprinting center defect has been detected. Lack of a functional paternal 15q11-q13 region, caused by any of a variety of genetic mechanisms, can result in the syndrome. One imprinted gene, that for small nuclear ribonucleoprotein-associated polypeptide SmN (*SNRPN*), which is implicated in splicing pre-mRNA, is expressed in the brain, including the hypothalamus, and has been advanced as one explanation of the syndrome.

Elevated serum concentrations of the GH secretagogue and orexigenic gastrointestinal hormone ghrelin are found in the basal state in Prader-Willi syndrome.[528] Increased levels are identified after meals, when values should be suppressed, and are a possible cause of the insatiable appetite. Administration of the somatostatin analogue octreotide leads to a decrease in basal ghrelin values and some decrease in values after meals, but no change in appetite was demonstrated as yet.

Laurence-Moon and Bardet-Biedl Syndromes

The Laurence-Moon syndrome and the Bardet-Biedl syndrome were previously separated as rare autosomal recessive traits, with retinitis pigmentosum and hypogonadism of various types. Currently the conditions are considered as one and the present term is *Bardet-Biedl syndrome*. The estimated incidence is 1:160,000 in northern European populations and 1:13,500 in some Arab populations.[529] The findings are developmental delay, spastic paraplegia, postaxial polydactyly, onset of obesity (usually in early infancy), and renal dysplasia. Hypogonadism is characteristic and males are infertile as are most females. The genetically and phenotypically heterogenous Bardet-Biedl syndrome is linked to 16 genes, which account for 80% of cases. The basic defect is a ciliopathy. The Biemond syndrome II has similar features, with iris coloboma, hypogenitalism, obesity, polydactyly, and developmental delay, but it is a distinct entity.

Functional Gonadotropin Deficiencies

The effects of malnutrition, which can lead to functional hypogonadotropic hypogonadism, should be separated from the primary effects of chronic systemic disease, some of which have direct effects on the function of the hypothalamic-pituitary unit or the gonads. Even if nutrition is adequate, puberty may be affected. Weight loss of any cause to less than 80% of ideal weight for height can lead to gonadotropin deficiency and low serum leptin levels; weight regain usually restores hypothalamic-pituitary gonadal function over a variable period, although the weight needed to restart menstrual periods varies among individuals and is related to the weight at which menstruation first ceased.[530]

If adequate nutrition and body weight are maintained in patients with regional enteritis or chronic pulmonary disease, gonadotropin secretion is usually adequate. Cystic fibrosis is also associated with delay in puberty and the age of PHV, in large part through malnutrition; improved management has increased PHV and advanced the age of PHV but neither has reached normal values.[531] The age of menarche in girls with cystic fibrosis is related to maternal age, as expected, but it is delayed by approximately 1 year compared with menarche in the mother, an effect that is mainly related to nutritional status.[532] However, even with normal pubertal progression, boys with cystic fibrosis almost universally have oligospermia caused by obstruction of the spermatic ducts, which is unrelated to nutritional status. The greater prevalence of reproductive difficulties in male patients with cystic fibrosis compared with female patients may reflect the greater prevalence of the cystic fibrosis transmembrane regulator (CFTR) in male reproductive tissues (e.g., epididymis, vas deferens), and more viscid luminal contents, which ultimately damage the testes and can lead to absence of the epididymides and the vasa deferentia. Normal ovaries do not express CFTR, and endometrial tissue expresses it only after puberty, with variable levels found in cervical epithelium and the fallopian tubes. Even though the *CFTR* gene and its protein are expressed in the human hypothalamus, mutations in the corresponding gene did not appear to affect LH and FSH secretion in an immortalized mouse hypothalamic GnRH-secreting cell line.

Boys and girls with sickle cell disease have delayed pubertal development by about 2 years and delayed menarche of about 6 months even with modern treatment techniques.[533] This may be due to nutritional status. Boys with sickle cell anemia often exhibit impaired Leydig cell function caused by ischemia of the testes or gonadotropin deficiency or both.

Thalassemia carries the risk of hemochromatosis due to transfusional iron deposition in the pituitary and hypothalamus; as a consequence, 60% to 80% patients may have hypogonadotropic hypogonadism and impairment of growth.[534] The gonads can be stimulated by exogenous gonadotropins, and satisfactory sexual development, including fertility, can be promoted by the use of hCG and human FSH in many patients without gonadal damage, although pituitary and gonadal damage may be severe in children with poorly controlled disease. Primary hypothyroidism is prevalent in this condition, but it is only part of the problem of sexual maturation. Desferrioxamine therapy may cause skeletal dysplasia and compromise pubertal growth, and growth failure due to GH deficiency may also affect pubertal growth.[535] Decreased BMD in thalassemia makes early recognition and treatment of the problem all the more important.

Cytotoxic effects of the alkylating agents used to prepare patients for bone marrow transplantation in this condition add to the problem. Treatment after the onset of puberty is safer for gonadal function in boys but not necessarily in girls. Girls with early bone marrow transplantation and apparently normal pubertal development have elevated serum FSH levels and menstrual abnormalities ranging up to amenorrhea,[536] suggesting that gonadal impairment is universal in girls with thalassemia major after bone marrow transplantation.

Puberty is significantly delayed in children with prenatally acquired human immunodeficiency virus (HIV) infection compared to those exposed but not affected.[537] Modern treatment regimens are predicted to decrease this delay.

Chronic gastrointestinal disease (e.g., Crohn disease) is often accompanied by delayed puberty, and therapy to restore nutrition, if successful, enables puberty to progress. The pubertal growth spurt is compromised by active inflammatory bowel disease, especially if glucocorticoid therapy is necessary. Celiac disease decreases the growth rate in childhood and adolescence, but with appropriate dietary restrictions, adult height appears to be normal.

Chronic renal disease is associated with delayed pubertal development and decreased pulsatile gonadotropin secretion due to a decrease in the mass of bioactive and immunoactive LH secreted rather than an alteration of the frequency. Successful renal transplantation usually restores gonadotropin secretion and improves growth. Immunoreactive gonadotropin concentrations may be elevated, presumably because of impaired renal clearance, but the response to GnRH is blunted in severe renal impairment. TeBG is elevated in chronic renal failure, and the level of free testosterone is low. Survivors of renal transplantation who are undergoing immune suppression and alternate-day steroid treatment often have delayed onset of puberty and decreased pulsatility of GH and gonadotropins at night.

Patients with nephrotic syndrome have poor pubertal growth, poor secondary sexual development, and deficient gonadotropin secretion in a pattern resembling CDP. Glomerulonephritis treated with alternate-day glucocorticoid therapy leads to a late, diminished, but prolonged pubertal growth spurt that can result in a normal final height.

Children with early onset of leukemia and long-term remission experience puberty at an appropriate age or with only a slight delay, whereas patients with initial symptoms of leukemia in late childhood may have considerable delay of pubertal development. Radiation treatment to the CNS may cause hypogonadotropic hypogonadism or GH deficiency or both, and irradiation of the abdomen or pelvis and certain types of chemotherapies, especially if administered during puberty, may impair gonadal function and cause primary hypogonadism, although ovarian function may return even in the face of elevated serum gonadotropin levels.[538] Total-body irradiation for bone marrow transplantation exerts the most significant effects, such as severe GH deficiency in 50%, hypothyroidism in 56%, and hypogonadism in 83% of males, and 100% of women had ovarian failure; insulin resistance was found in 83% and dyslipidemia in 61%.[539] Children with leukemia treated with CNS irradiation had a diminished pubertal growth spurt and diminished final height. Long-term follow-up studies demonstrate the rising incidence of the metabolic syndrome survivors and high lifetime risk for cardiovascular disease in childhood cancer.[540]

Hypothyroidism may delay the onset of puberty or menarche (except in extreme cases in which puberty starts early); treatment with levothyroxine reverses this pattern, but there is likely to be a permanent loss of height if the diagnosis is delayed. Poorly controlled diabetes mellitus can lead to poor growth, fatty infiltration of the liver, and sexual infantilism (i.e., Mauriac syndrome), which is probably related to poor nutritional status. Prepubertal children are most vulnerable to poor glycemic control, and pubertal subjects exhibit normal growth unless severe hyperglycemia occurs. The degree of control necessary to avoid these complications cannot be exactly quantified, but adolescents with even moderately poor control frequently manifest some degree of growth impairment and delayed puberty or irregular menses. Cushing disease can be associated with delayed onset or arrest of gonadarche, although excessive virilization is an alternative finding.

Anorexia Nervosa and Variants[541,542]

Anorexia Nervosa. Anorexia nervosa,[543] a common cause of gonadotropin deficiency in adolescence, is a functional disorder. Prevalence is increased among girls (it is the third most common chronic disease of adolescent girls), and it starts at ever-younger ages, but it is rare in boys. This condition has the highest mortality rate of all psychiatric disorders[544]; weighted mortality rates (i.e., deaths per 1000 person-years) were 5.1 for anorexia nervosa, and 1.7 standardized mortality ratios were 5.86 for anorexia nervosa. It is characterized by a distorted body image, obsessive fear of obesity, and food avoidance that can cause severe self-induced weight loss (to less than 85% of normal weight for age and height or a BMI <17.5 kg/m^2 after cessation of growth), primary or secondary amenorrhea in affected females, widespread endocrine disorders, and even death. Specific diagnostic details are provided in the *Diagnostic and Statistical Manual of Mental Disorders*, fourth edition (DSM-IV) criteria of the American Psychiatric Association[542]:

A. Restriction of energy intake relative to requirements, leading to a significantly low body weight in the context of age, sex, developmental trajectory, and physical health. Significantly low weight is defined as a weight that is less than minimally normal or, for children and adolescents, less than that minimally expected.

B. Intense fear of gaining weight or of becoming fat, or persistent behavior that interferes with weight gain, even though at a significantly low weight.

C. Disturbance in the way in which one's body weight or shape is experienced, undue influence of body weight or shape on self-evaluation, or persistent lack of recognition of the seriousness of the current low body weight.

Subtype:

Restricting type

Binge-eating/purging type

The onset of amenorrhea precedes the onset of severe weight loss. Other common features include onset in middle adolescence, hyperactivity, defective thermoregulation with hypothermia and sensitivity to cold, constipation, bradycardia and hypotension, decreased BMR, dry skin, fine or downy hypertrichosis, peripheral edema, and parotid enlargement. The pathogenesis is multifactorial and includes a genetic factor and a well-characterized psychological component. Before the diagnosis of anorexia nervosa is made, organic disease must be excluded; for example a girl with macroprolactinoma may present with signs consistent with anorexia nervosa. The prevalence of anorexia nervosa is increased among individuals with Turner syndrome.

Anorexia nervosa has considerable endocrine ramifications.[545] The concentrations of plasma FSH, LH, leptin, and estradiol and the excretion of urinary gonadotropins are characteristically low. There may be a reversion to a circadian rhythm of LH secretion and to the sleep-associated increase in episodic LH secretion or LH response to GnRH characteristic of early puberty, or the amplitude of the pulsatile episodes may be diminished, as in the pattern of prepubertal children, if onset occurs during puberty. Pulsatile administration of intravenous GnRH at 90- to 120-minute intervals can produce LH pulses that are indistinguishable from the normal pubertal pattern, demonstrating functional GnRH deficiency. Serum leptin levels are low, consistent with the strikingly decreased mass of adipose tissue, and increase with regain of weight. Other hormonal changes include increased mean concentrations of plasma GH and plasma cortisol; low levels of plasma IGF-1, DHEAS, and triiodothyronine (T$_3$) with normal levels of thyroxine (T$_4$) (unless the low thyroxine syndrome is present) and TSH; a decreased rise in serum prolactin after administration of thyrotropin-releasing hormone (TRH) or insulin-induced hypoglycemia; and a diminished capacity to concentrate urine. This condition must be considered in the differential diagnosis of growth failure in younger subjects.

Lower heart rates are characteristic and a dangerous sign of severe disease and not to be confused with an athletic bradycardia in view of the excessive exercise the patient engages in. A lower systolic blood pressure, lower body temperature, anemia, and leukopenia are found in persons with anorexia nervosa. The ratio of bone age to chronologic age is significantly lower in girls with anorexia nervosa and correlates positively with duration of illness and markers of nutritional status. All measures of BMD are lower, and the most significant predictors of bone density are LBM, BMI, and age at menarche. Treatment of decreased bone density in these individuals is accomplished with improved nutrition, and a degree of catch-up in bone density occurs, although reversion to normal may not occur.

Normal endocrine and metabolic function may follow weight gain, but amenorrhea may persist for months, suggesting persistent hypothalamic dysfunction. In view of the associated mortality rate, parenteral alimentation may be indicated in resistant patients with severe weight loss, especially in those with infection or an electrolyte imbalance. However, refeeding syndrome with attendant hypophosphatemia may result if not handled appropriately. Treatment of this disorder requires skillful management, understanding, patience, and psychiatric consultation in a team approach. Unfortunately, evidence-based approach to optimal treatment is not plentiful, and the difficulty in obtaining therapy in uninsured individuals remains.[546]

Functional hypothalamic amenorrhea is defined as the absence of menses, low or normal gonadotropin levels, and normal gonadotropin response to GnRH stimulation but lack of or an inadequate midcycle LH surge and a decrease in normal pulsatile secretion (amplitude or frequency, or both) of gonadotropins and hypoestrogenemia without organic abnormality.[547] This condition can occur in women with normal weight but decreased percentage of body fat. These patients have higher than average cortisol values; decreased levels of free T$_4$, free T$_3$, and total T$_4$ with normal TSH levels; and decreased leptin concentrations that are probably caused by subtle dysfunction of eating patterns and altered energy expenditure. The consequences range from severe estrogen deficiency to anovulation to a short luteal phase. Reduced bone density is a concern. Genes involved in the cause of hypogonadotropic hypogonadism such as *GNRHR*, *KAL1*, and *PROKR2* are found in heterozygous patterns in women with functional hypothalamic amenorrhea, suggesting a genetic susceptibility to the condition that is brought out by various types of stresses[547]; thus, functional amenorrhea may not be simply functional.[548,549]

Bulimia Nervosa. Bulimia nervosa is now separated from the diagnosis of anorexia nervosa[543]; DSM-IV diagnostic criteria are as follows:

A. Recurrent episodes of binge eating. An episode of binge eating is characterized by both of the following:

1. Eating, in a discrete period of time (e.g., within any 2-hour period), an amount of food that is definitely

larger than what most individuals would eat in a similar period of time under similar circumstances.

2. A sense of lack of control over eating during the episode (e.g., a feeling that one cannot stop eating or control what or how much one is eating).

B. Recurrent inappropriate compensatory behaviors in order to prevent weight gain, such as self-induced vomiting; misuse of laxatives, diuretics, or other medications; fasting; or excessive exercise.

C. The binge eating and inappropriate compensatory behaviors both occur, on average, at least once a week for 3 months.

D. Self-evaluation is unduly influenced by body shape and weight.

E. The disturbance does not occur exclusively during episodes of anorexia nervosa.

Bulimia occurs in about 1.5% of young women. A hand lesion from the induced vomiting (i.e., Russell sign) and an abnormal level of serum electrolytes are useful clinical markers. Abuse of laxatives, diet pills, and diuretics is frequent. Although weight loss is not frequent, amenorrhea is common. Bulimia is especially prevalent in female high school and college students. A history of childhood sexual abuse is more common than in unaffected adolescents. Cessation of growth can occur in infants and young children with psychosocial dwarfism. Stressful social situations can also inhibit growth and physical pubertal development at adolescence.

Exercise, Hypo-ovarianism, and Amenorrhea: The Female Athlete Triad. In 1992, the American College of Sports Medicine defined the female athletic triad as primary or secondary amenorrhea, disordered eating, and osteoporosis.[543] Although there are substantial endocrine effects of excessive athletic training in girls, elite prepubertal and pubertal female athletes suffer relatively few physical injuries. Because there is no demonstrable effect on pubertal development from moderate exercise in subelite female runners, moderate exercise should not be discouraged during adolescence. However, extensive training (10 to 12 hours/week) may be excessive for prepubertal girls.

Bulimia, anorexia nervosa, or anorexia athletica is most often found in girls engaged in sports that emphasize weight.[550] Teenage ballet dancers are lighter, have less body fat, and have a high incidence of delayed puberty and of primary and secondary amenorrhea than less physically active girls. Factors other than decreased body weight can impair pubertal progression and delay menarche through inhibition of the hypothalamic GnRH pulse generator in healthy ballet dancers and female athletes such as swimmers who are not underweight.

Athletes who began strenuous training before menarche have a delay in menarcheal age.[551] However, genetic influences overlie changes due to weight or activity because there is a positive correlation between the delayed menarche found in athletic girls and the age of menarche of their mothers. Although some studies of artistic and rhythmic gymnasts found delayed menarche when compared with their mothers and sisters, with a more significant delay in artistic gymnasts,[552-554] a recent survey of the literature by a committee of the Scientific Commission of the International Gymnastics Federation found that "(1) Adult height or near adult height of female and male artistic gymnasts is not compromised by intensive gymnastics training. (2) Gymnastics training does not appear to attenuate growth of upper (sitting height) or lower (legs) body segment lengths. (3) Gymnastics training does not appear to attenuate pubertal growth and maturation, neither rate of growth nor the timing and tempo of the growth spurt. (4) Available data are inadequate to address the issue of intensive gymnastics training and alterations within the endocrine system."[555] These athletes may be shorter and delayed in puberty due to self-selection.

Higher bone density is reported in the femurs of gymnasts compared with those of ballet dancers and control subjects, but lower radial bone density in the gymnasts and ballet dancers reflects the effect of the application of force on bone remodeling; a positive relationship between serum leptin and tibial bone density is found.[556] The bone density of female long distance runners is greater in those with regular menses than in those with menstrual irregularities. Osteopenia in later life may result from amenorrhea in ballet dancers, even with estrogen replacement, and nutrition therapy is considered important to improve outcome.[557]

Thinness and strenuous physical activity appear to act synergistically, but strenuous exercise training by itself may inhibit the GnRH pulse generator, mediated in part by endogenous opioidergic pathways involving β-endorphin. When the strenuous physical activity is interrupted (e.g., by injury), puberty advances, and menarche often occurs within a few months in those with amenorrhea, in some cases before a significant change in body composition or weight. Even though gonadarche is retarded, adrenarche is not delayed.

Female athletes of normal weight who have less fat and more muscle than nonathletic girls (e.g., ice skaters, swimmers) are also at risk for delayed puberty and for primary and secondary amenorrhea. However, the mechanism apparently is different from the hypothalamic amenorrhea in runners and ballet dancers. In swimmers, menstrual cycles frequently are irregular and anovulatory rather than absent, and the plasma concentrations of DHEAS and LH were higher than normal, but plasma estrogen levels were normal.

Prospective study of gymnasts contrasted with swimmers demonstrated decreased growth velocity, stunting in leg length growth, and in some studies, decreased height prediction in the gymnasts.[558]

Prolactin levels may be elevated in women athletes and may contribute to the delayed menarche found in this group. Osteopenia can result from the associated chronic hypoestrogenism.[551]

Scoliosis in girls usually develops during the pubertal growth spurt and more often occurs in girls with a more rapid pubertal growth spurt. Ballet dancers have a higher incidence of scoliosis than the general population and often have delayed puberty and delayed menarche. These girls have decreased leptin levels, but soluble leptin receptor and adiponectin levels were increased throughout puberty; these changes were related to changes in LBM rather than BMI. Idiopathic scoliosis in the general population is associated with a statistically earlier age of menarche and an early adolescent growth spurt. The strongest association with scoliosis is taller stature at the time of the pubertal growth spurt. Adult height in familial constellations of scoliosis does not vary from the family norm.

Although men are less affected than women, men may also be affected by rigorous physical training. They may have decreased LH response to GnRH and decreased spontaneous LH pulse frequency and amplitude; the serum testosterone level is normal or low with extreme activity levels.

Other Causes of Delayed Puberty

Marijuana use has been associated with gynecomastia and is a putative cause of pubertal delay. Untreated Gaucher disease causes delay in pubertal development, but early treatment with enzyme replacement allows puberty to begin on time.[559] Girls with familial dysautonomia have delayed menarche and often have a severe premenstrual syndrome. The condition is ultimately compatible with pregnancy. Chronic infections may delay the onset of puberty.

Diabetes mellitus type 1 is associated with delayed menarche.[560] Remarkably, this may occur no matter the degree of glycemic control. Mauriac syndrome is characterized by poorly controlled diabetes, hepatomegaly, and delayed puberty.[561]

Hypergonadotropic Hypogonadism: Sexual Infantilism Caused by Primary Gonadal Disorders

The most common forms of primary gonadal failure are associated with sex chromosome abnormalities and characteristic physical findings.[553,562] Testicular or ovarian dysfunction as an isolated finding is less commonly a cause of pubertal hypergonadotropic hypogonadism.

Boys

Klinefelter Syndrome and Its Variants (see Chapter 23). Klinefelter syndrome (i.e., syndrome of seminiferous tubular dysgen-esis) and its variants occur in approximately 1 in 1000 males, and they are the most common forms of male hypogonadism.[562-564] The invariable clinical features include small, firm testes as an adult (<3.5 cm long); impaired spermatogenesis; and a male phenotype, usually with gynecomastia and long legs but not long arms[562] (Fig. 25-46). Prepubertally, patients can be detected by the disproportionate length of the extremities, decreased U/L body ratio without an increase in arm span rather than eunuchoid proportions, in which arm span and leg length are increased; however, less than 10% are diagnosed prepubertally. With increasing use of karyotype determination in children with behavior problems and in pregnancy for various reasons, diagnosis earlier in life may increase. Tall stature for family size is common in this disorder due to the disproportionate growth of the legs and appears to be related to multiple copies of the *SHOX* gene[565]; however, normal or short stature does not eliminate the diagnosis.

Infants with Klinefelter syndrome have normal INSL3 levels transiently increased at 2 to 3 months of age during the minipuberty of infancy, testosterone levels were below the median of control subjects but within the normal

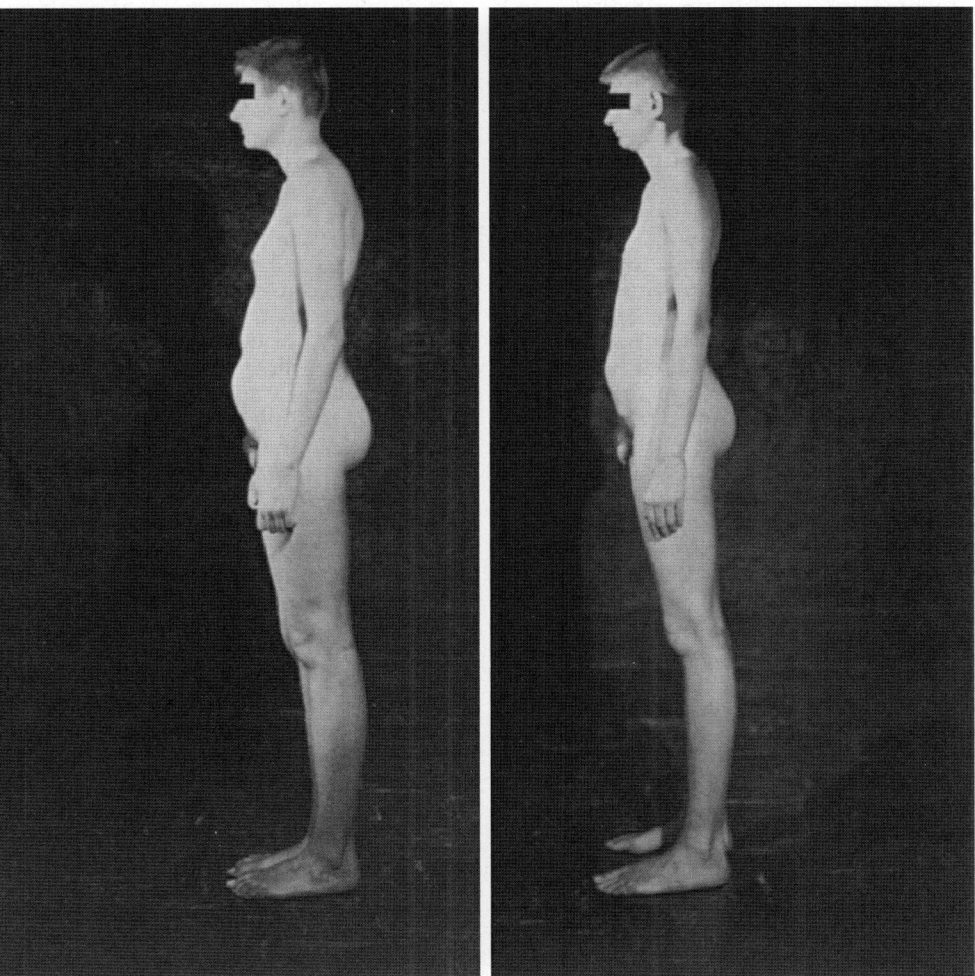

Figure 25-46 47,XXY Klinefelter syndrome in 17-year-old identical twins. At age 15, gynecomastia was observed. The twins had a eunuchoid habitus and poorly developed male secondary sexual characteristics. Both were 187 cm tall; arm spans were 187 cm and 189.5 cm; the voices were high pitched; the testes measured 1.8 × 1.5 cm; and penis length was 7.5 cm. Gynecomastia and signs of androgen deficiency were more evident in the twin on the left. Urinary gonadotropin levels were greater than 50 mU/24 hours. The testes exhibited extensive tubular fibrosis, small dysgenetic tubules, and clumping or pseudoadenomatous formation of Leydig cells; germ cells were rare. The microscopic appearance was typical of seminiferous tubule dysgenesis. (Patient data from Grumbach MM, Barr ML. Cytologic tests of chromosome sex in relation to sexual anomalies in man. *Recent Prog Horm Res.* 1958;14:255-324.)

range, and inhibin B and AMH levels were also within normal range.[565] However, FSH levels were above normal in 25% of patients, indicating early evidence of testicular deficiency. Muscle tone is also lower in some.[566]

There is a normal increase in the concentrations of testosterone, INSL3, and inhibin B before puberty. By midpuberty testosterone and INSL3 concentrations remain in the low-normal range, AMH levels were undetectable in XXY adolescents but decreased at an age later than in normal boys, and inhibin B levels decreased from normal to the low levels characteristic of adult Klinefelter syndrome during late puberty after an unequivocal increase in serum testosterone (>2.5 nmol/L) levels and degeneration of Sertoli cells.[567] Serum LH and FSH usually rise by midpuberty. Rarely, low gonadotropin concentrations occur when hypogonadotropic hypogonadism is associated with 47,XXY Klinefelter syndrome or coexisting constitutional delay.

Prepubertal testes show only subtle histologic changes, although the testes are small, and the germ cell content is reduced, whereas Sertoli cells are normal in abundance and appearance before 2 years of age. Older prepubertal subjects have normal seminiferous tubules. Hyalinization and fibrosis of the seminiferous tubules and pseudoadenomatous changes of the Leydig cells develop after puberty; adult-type spermatogonia are found in peripubertal boys, but older boys had no germ cells; and the testes degenerate in an accelerated manner at the onset of puberty.[568] However, there is a 44% success rate for sperm retrieval from testicular tissues and a 55% success rate for use of microdissection testicular sperm aspiration. Intracytoplasmic sperm injection led to the birth of 101 children, in whom there was no apparent increase in congenital or genetic defects.[569] Cryopreservation of testicular tissue is recommended before degeneration progresses[570] although coverage for such procedure may be difficult to obtain.

There is variation in Leydig cell function among childhood and pubertal subjects, but the plasma concentration of testosterone fails to rise to normal adult levels. The onset of puberty usually is not delayed, but impaired Leydig cell reserve and low testosterone levels may lead to slow progression or arrest of pubertal changes. Testosterone replacement should be considered when the LH level rises above the normal range of values but is not necessary in all subjects in early puberty.[571] Serum estradiol-to-testosterone ratios and TeBG levels are higher than those in normal males, which indicates an increased estrogen effect and decreased testosterone effect that may account in part for the gynecomastia characteristic of Klinefelter syndrome. Testosterone administration does not appear to reduce the gynecomastia, but dihydrotestosterone may help. Aromatase inhibitors or estrogen receptor antagonists do not seem to be effective treatment for the gynecomastia of Klinefelter syndrome. If the gynecomastia does not regress within 2 years, reduction mammoplasty is required. Monitoring for breast cancer is important in these susceptible individuals.

The AR gene is located on the X chromosome and encodes a ligand-dependent transcription factor with highly polymorphic CAGn trinucleotide repeats in the coding sequence of the first exon. The length of the translated polyglutamate tract in the N-terminal transactivation domain of the resulting protein and the length of this polyglutamate tract is inversely proportional to receptor transactivation activity. The shorter the repeat sequence within the range of normal variation, the more active the AR, and small changes in this activity may result in more significant effects in Klinefelter syndrome, in which testosterone secretion may already be impaired. A negative

correlation between CAGn repeat length and penile length, but not testicular size, in children has been reported.[560,572] Another study found a positive association between CAGn repeat length and body height, an inverse relationship to bone density and arm span to body height, and the presence of longer CAGn repeats for gynecomastia and smaller testes[573] in adults. A paternal origin of the extra X chromosome is associated with later onset of puberty and longer CAG repeats.[568]

Behavior and Development in Klinefelter Syndrome. Neurobehavioral abnormalities, primarily in language, speech, learning, and frontal executive functions, are common, even universal, in Klinefelter syndrome, but severe retardation is uncommon.[218] These problems may lead to evaluation in childhood and the prepubertal recognition of the syndrome. The prevalence of adjustment problems in adolescence is increased. Adults with Klinefelter syndrome have shorter education, lower income, earlier retirement, and increased unemployment, and more rarely marry than the national average. Fatality among Klinefelter syndrome men was significantly increased (hazard ratio, 1.9).[574] The crime rates for sexual abuse and arson are significantly increased, whereas traffic offenses and drug-related crime are significantly decreased.

The global IQ in unselected populations of Klinefelter syndrome subjects is normal or near normal, but verbal IQ, in contrast to that of patients with Turner syndrome, is usually lower (e.g., 10 to 20 points) than performance IQ.

Prepubertal Klinefelter syndrome patients have reduced left hemisphere specialization for verbal tasks and enhanced right hemisphere specialization for nonverbal tasks. However, these abnormalities tended to normalize after puberty began, suggesting hemispheric reorganization during puberty. Hypotheses are advanced supporting the effect of prenatal testosterone on cerebral dominance and on language and reading pathology.

There is controversy about the indication for testosterone treatment of infants or adolescents with Klinefelter syndrome. Although there is a growing feeling among parents that testosterone treatment in the infancy or early pubertal period improves language, reading, behavior, and self-image in boys with Klinefelter syndrome, no well-controlled studies supporting this contention are available, and long-term studies are needed.[575]

Other Aspects of Klinefelter Syndrome. Conditions associated with Klinefelter syndrome include aortic valvular disease and ruptured berry aneurysms (six times the normal rate); breast carcinoma (20 times the rate in normal men and one fifth that of women); other malignancies such as acute leukemia, lymphoma, and germ cell tumors at any midline site; systemic lupus erythematosus; and osteoporosis in about 25% of affected adults. There is an increased risk of diabetes mellitus, thyroid disease, fatigue, varicose veins, and essential tremor.

About 20% of mediastinal germ cell tumors are associated with Klinefelter syndrome, and they occur at a younger age than the mediastinal germ cell tumors that are not associated with the syndrome. With rare exceptions, these germ cell tumors, which may be located in the midline anywhere from the CNS to the pelvis, secrete hCG and induce sexual precocity. Klinefelter syndrome needs to be considered in boys with hCG-secreting germ cell tumors, especially if the tumor is located in the mediastinum or CNS.

Other Forms of Primary Testicular Failure
Cancer Survivors
Chemotherapy. Chemotherapy and direct radiotherapy affect testicular function, and as more children survive with effective therapy for cancer, delayed puberty and adult infertility will result. Cancer therapy, especially

irradiation of the gonads or the use of alkylating chemotherapeutic agents, affects testicular function and can lead to adult infertility.[576] Some courses of therapy can cause severe damage to germinal cells without apparent effect on Leydig cells. Chemotherapy for childhood Hodgkin disease, including chlorambucil, vinblastine, Mustargen (mechlorethamine), Oncovin (vincristine), procarbazine, and prednisone (COPP/MOPP), may allow spontaneous progression through puberty, but FSH and LH concentrations may be elevated, and the inhibin B concentrations decrease during puberty. The basal serum FSH level and rise in LH and FSH levels after GnRH correlate with the dose of cyclophosphamide. COPP/MOPP chemotherapy for Hodgkin disease can cause severe damage to Sertoli and germinal cells, but it has less effect on Leydig cells, even if therapy occurred in the prepubertal period. Lower dosing or limiting therapy to less than three courses is suggested to decrease these complications.[577] Normal basal LH values may raise hope that Leydig cell function is normal, but if there is an exaggerated rise of the LH level after GnRH, compensated Leydig cell damage is present. The combination of Adriamycin (doxorubicin), bleomycin, vinblastine, and dacarbazine (ABVD regimen) can cause germ cell depletion. Although initially it was thought that some degree of prepubertal gonadal maturation was necessary before these drugs could cause gonadal damage, gonadal damage can occur earlier as a result of therapy in the prepubertal period but may not be demonstrable until the age of puberty. Chemotherapeutic agents used in the treatment of nephrotic syndrome or leukemia, such as cyclophosphamide or chlorambucil, have led to Sertoli cell, Leydig cell, and germ cell damage in prepubertal patients; these effects are sometimes reversible. indicative of gonadal damage.

Radiation Therapy. Radiation to the gonads can cause primary testicular failure, usually resulting in azoospermia, although normal testosterone secretion may be associated with elevated LH and FSH values (compensated Leydig cell failure); the gonads must be shielded from the treatment, if possible. Preservation of sperm by freezing is being investigated for pediatric cancer patients (in Klinefelter syndrome patients), but the ethical and logistics problems of collecting sperm from adolescents remain substantial, all the more in prepubertal children. Not all sperm may be affected by treatment, and functional sperm may be recovered by microdissection of seminiferous tubules even in individuals who appear to have testicular failure. This may allow fertilization by successful intracytoplasmic sperm injection even if the quantity of sperm is low. The genes responsible for apoptosis are activated when DNA damage from radiation or chemotherapy occurs; manipulation of such genes may allow reestablishment of fertility in the future. Oncofertility is a new field of investigation that aims to preserve fertility in children and teenagers subject to cancer therapy, and new methods will undoubtedly appear. Survey of adults who were not offered fertility preservation or with whom such an issue was not even discussed at time of diagnosis shows that they feel considerable distress. However, sperm banking in puberty or prepuberty presents ethical concerns as to the procedure, the cost of banking, and the uncertainty of outcome and is not presently standard therapy.[578]

Concern for decreased bone density and risk for fractures is also raised in cancer survivors who have undergone radiation treatment of the hypothalamic-pituitary axis.

Testicular Biosynthetic Defects. The 46,XY disorder of sex development is caused by 17α-hydroxylase/17,20-lyase deficiency resulting from mutations in CYP17A1 at gene map locus 10q24.3; it is associated with sexual infantilism and a female phenotype.[579] The testosterone biosynthetic defect blocks the synthesis of testosterone and adrenal androgens, impairing masculinization at all stages of development. Associated cortisol deficiency and increased mineralocorticoid secretion in this condition lead to hypertension, decreased serum potassium levels, and metabolic alkalosis. Elevated serum progesterone levels and decreased plasma renin activity are helpful diagnostic features.[580] Glucocorticoid replacement suppresses ACTH and mineralocorticoid excess and corrects the electrolyte abnormalities, but no sexual development occurs unless exogenous gonadal steroids are administered. Less severe deficiencies are associated with ambiguous genitalia. CYP17A1 mutations leading to isolated 17,20-lyase deficiency are rare.

A rare autosomal recessive condition is steroidogenic acute regulatory protein (StAR) deficiency, in which the ability to produce C21-, C19-, and C18-steroids is lost and a severe impairment of the conversion of cholesterol to pregnenolone results; severely affected patients have lipid-laden adrenal glands.[581] The large adrenal glands may be visualized on ultrasound, CT, or MRI. Death often occurs in infancy if untreated because of unrecognized glucocorticoid and mineralocorticoid deficiencies. Affected individuals physically appear to be sexually infantile females, whether their karyotype is 46,XY or 46,XX; because of the absence of gonadal or adrenal androgen production, the affected XY phenotypic females do not develop secondary sexual characteristics, including pubic hair.[562] However, XX females with a null mutation develop female sex characteristics at puberty, including pubic hair and multicystic ovaries, but they also have primary or secondary amenorrhea. In contrast to the fetal testis, the fetal ovary, which is insensitive to FSH and steroidogenically inactive, is undamaged in fetal life and remains so until the onset of puberty. Under FSH stimulation during puberty and with recruitment of ovarian follicles, the ovaries undergo progressive damage and cyst formation. Ovarian damage and impairment of ovarian StAR-independent steroidogenesis appear to be related to lipid deposition in the ovary.[582]

Luteinizing Hormone Resistance. Presumptive evidence of LH resistance caused by an LH receptor abnormality on the Leydig cell was reported in an 18-year-old boy with a male phenotype, no male secondary sexual development, gynecomastia, elevated plasma LH levels, and early pubertal plasma testosterone concentrations that did not increase after hCG administration; there was no elevation of testosterone precursor levels.[583] The testes were prepubertal in size and had the microscopic appearance of normal prepubertal testes. Plasma membrane receptor preparations from the testes bound only one half as much radiolabeled hCG as control testes.

In affected males, this autosomal recessive disorder is caused by a mutation in LHCGR, the gene encoding the G protein–coupled, seven-transmembrane LH/hCG cell receptor at gene map locus 2p21. Mutations that cause a more severe compromise in LHCGR function are associated with XY disorders of sex development. Homozygous deletion of exon 10 or the homozygous missense mutations Ser616Tyr and Ile625Lys of the LH receptor are associated with micropenis (but not hypospadias) due to partial impairment of LH receptor function, leading to a discordance with a poor response to LH but not to hCG. Nephropathic cystinosis in boys leads to hypergonadotropic hypogonadism.

Anorchia and Cryptorchidism. Cryptorchidism is the condition in which one or both testes have not reached the bottom of the scrotum before birth. Animal and human data demonstrate that testicular descent is influenced by testosterone and INSL3; for example, androgen resistance leads to lack of descent, as also occurs in transgenetic mice without

INSL3. When testes are not descended they may be located in high scrotal, suprascrotal, or inguinal positions or can be nonpalpable, which includes ectopic testes as well.[584] Data collection is variable but analysis of the literature shows the undescended testis rate in term appropriate weight for gestational age (AGA) babies is 1.0% to 4.6%, whereas in premature or SGA infants it is 1.1% to 45.3%.[585] By 1 year the undescended testis rate in term AGA boys was 1.0% to 1.5%, at 6 years 0.0% to 2.6, at 11 years 0.0% to 6.6%, and at 15 years 1.6% to 2.2% of boys. Testes may ascend after birth, ascensus testis, which leads to a higher prevalence of undescended testes in prepuberty than at birth in several international reports, and these patients are not always included in cryptorchidism surveys. Study of more than 1 million Danish boys showed the concordance rate of cryptorchidism was 3.4% for paternal half-brothers, 6.0% for maternal half-brothers, 8.8% for full brothers, 24.1% for dizygotic twin brothers, and 27.3% for monozygotic twin brothers demonstrating effects of genetics and intrauterine environment.[586]

A 46,XY male without palpable testes may have intra-abdominal testes, which carry an increased risk of malignant degeneration; anorchia (i.e., vanishing testes syndrome, caused by perinatal torsion), in which no testes are found at laparotomy; or retractile testes, a variation of normal. About 50% of bilateral, nonpalpable testes are undescended, and the other 50% are testicular remnants from vanishing testes that usually do not contain germ cells, are found in the scrotum, are not at risk for carcinoma, and need not be removed if the history is certain.[587] If there is a male phenotype and male internal ducts, functioning fetal testes capable of secreting testosterone and AMH were present early during fetal life but degenerated thereafter. Serum gonadotropins follow the normal U-shaped curve of high values in infancy and puberty with lower values in midchildhood in anorchia, although the values are above normal.[588] Serum AMH and inhibin B are nondetectable in anorchia.[589] Ultrasound is often used to located undescended testes, but the accuracy is poor: a meta-analysis demonstrated that a positive ultrasound result increases and negative ultrasound result decreases the probability that a nonpalpable testis is located within the abdomen from 55% to 64% and 49%, respectively.[590] Laparoscopy, however, is recommended in diagnosis of nonpalpable testes.[591]

Discovery of unilateral cryptorchidism may represent the presence of a descended testis on one side and none on the other side, and this presents a diagnostic dilemma. Compensatory hypertrophy occurs if there is no contralateral testis, and this aids the diagnosis. A Japanese study demonstrated that the mean contralateral testicular length and volume in the boys with an absent testis were 22.4 mm and 2.20 mL compared with 16.6 mm and 1.10 mL in boys with a testis present and 16.6 mm and 1.18 mL in control subjects; the optimal cutoff value of 21 mm in length and 1.6 mL in volume led to a predictive accuracy for an absent testis of 87.3%, sensitivity of 81.8%, and specificity of 95.5%, with 85.5%, 84.8%, and 86.4% for the volume, respectively.[592] Because the finding does not universally predict monorchia, laparoscopy can be used for diagnosis of this condition if ultrasound is unsuccessful. If there is an unilateral undescended testis, the increased relative risk of carcinoma in the contralateral descended testis is 1.74 (95% CI, 1.01 to 2.98), which is lower than in the unilateral undescended testes (6.33; 95% CI, 4.30 to 9.31).[593]

Hormonal treatment of undescended testes may be successful in causing descent, but evidence is scarce and meta-anaysis is difficult owing to variation in dosage and length of treatment. There is no compelling evidence that hormonal therapy in the short term is harmful, but unsuccessful medical therapy should not be allowed to significantly delay surgical therapy. In one schema, a single dose of 1500 IU hCG is administered intramuscularly, and serum levels of LH, FSH, testosterone, inhibin B, and AMH are measured at baseline and at 72 hours afterward. The test was positive in Prader-Willi syndrome when the maximum testosterone level after 72 hours was 2 to 20 times higher than baseline levels in infants aged 3 to 12 months and 5 to 10 times higher, between 2.5 and 9.0 nmol/L, in infants aged 1 to 4 years.[594] Administration of an hCG dose, 250 IU for infants aged 3 to 12 months of age and 500 IU intramuscularly for infants aged 1 to 4 years, twice a week for 6 weeks led to a descent of testes in 62% who had a positive stimulation test, and 23% of the testes reached a stable scrotal position. There are studies of longer-term administration of hCG or GnRH to either foster a rise in testosterone for diagnosis or for descent of testes for treatment of boys without Prader-Willi syndrome with variable results. The lack of a rise in testosterone concentration, in conjunction with an increased plasma concentration of FSH and LH or an augmented gonadotropin response to GnRH, and descreased AMH and inhibin B are evidence for the diagnosis of bilateral anorchia. Because testicular descent normally occurs by 1 year of age, orchidopexy is recommended between 6 and 12 months in those whose have testes that do not descend with medical treatment or upon discovering cryptorchidism after 12 months of age.[600] One study linked testicular descent to an adequate neonatal surge of LH and testosterone by 4 months in AGA infants and by 6 months in premature infants; these study authors recommended treatment be considered earlier than at 1 year.

Cryptorchidism is associated with an increased risk of infertility. Cryptorchid testes may demonstrate congenital abnormalities and may not function normally even if brought into the scrotum early in life. Two critical steps in the maturation of germ cells are described in the normal prepubertal testis that do not occur in the unilaterally undescended testes. First, at 2 to 3 months of age, the gonocytes (primitive spermatogonia) in the fetal stem cell pool transform into the adult dark spermatogonia, which become the adult stem pool (possibly related to the early infancy surge in LH, FSH, and testosterone). Second, at 4 to 5 years of age, meiosis begins, and primary spermatocytes appear. The contralateral descended testis is affected but less so than the undescended testis. Identification of the gonocyte transformation has influenced recommendations on the timing of orchidopexy. Postpubertal orchidopexy is associated with a greater than 85% prevalence of azoospermia or oligospermia. It has been surmised that cryptorchid testes, even if replaced in the scrotum, may never have normal spermatogenic function as a consequence of an early abnormality in germ cell maturation, vascular damage to the testicular circulation during orchidopexy, or an intrinsic testicular defect. Fertility potential varies depending upon preoperative history and laboratory results. Testicular dysgenesis may be indicated by increased gonadotropin levels and early surgery may be indicated; normal gonadotropin levels and a decreased germ cell number, may indicate transient hypothalamus-pituitary-gonadal hypofunction with a poor fertility prognosis; and if there are normal gonadotropins, inhibin B, and germ cell number, there is a good fertility prognosis.[595] A study of men with cryptorchidism reported a paternity rate of 65% for men who had had bilateral cryptorchidism, compared with 90% for the formerly unilateral cryptorchid men and 93% for control men; the reduction in fertility was supported by semen and hormone analyses.[596] Successful fertilization was reported by the use of intracytoplasmic injection of sperm extracted from the testes of cryptorchid men who had orchiopexy after puberty.[597] Patients undergoing orchiopexy may sustain subtle damage to the vas deferens, leading to the later production of antibodies to sperm that may result in infertility.

Cryptorchidism is associated with an increased risk of cancer of the testes, which is rising. The incidence of testicular carcinoma in England at all ages increased from 2 per 100,000 in 1909 to 4.4 per 100,000 in 1999, with a rise noticed during puberty.[598] Such data are nation specific, and there is an approximately 10-fold range between countries.[587] A recent Swedish study reported the overall relative risk of testicular carcinoma in cryptorchidism is 2.5 to 8, with the highest risk associated with intra-abdominal rather than inguinal testes and higher risks observed for those with abnormal chromosomes, syndromes, or late or no orchiopexy. Undescended testes remain at a higher temperature than descended testes, and undescended testes have a maturation arrest at the conversion of the gonocytes to spermatogonia, which appears to direct the testes toward malignant degeneration. There is a very small risk of carcinoma of the testes in prepuberty, but the absence of carcinoma in situ in prepuberty is not an assurance that carcinoma will not develop in adult life. Periodic sonography of the testis of affected patients is recommended after the onset of puberty.

Adverse environmental factors may be important in the apparent increase in testis cancer, cryptorchidism, hypospadias, and low semen quality, which are all qualities described in the the testicular dysgenesis syndrome (TDS).[599] The complexities of clustering such findings without a pathophysiologic explanation has led to criticism of the concept.[600] This remains an important area of research.

Retractile testes can descend into the scrotum but then reascend. They are considered a normal variation, but a requirement for orchiopexy was reported for 22.7% in a series of 150. The finding of one case of testicular carcinoma in a boy with spontaneous descent in this series led to a suggestion of following such cases in the long term.[601] The risk of breast cancer associated with gynecomastia is increased in men with a history of undescended testes, orchiopexy, orchitis, testicular injury, infertility, or any cause of delayed puberty.

Small for Gestational Age. SGA predisposes males to reproductive problems and is also associated with the TDS. Males born SGA tend to have smaller testes and lower testosterone and higher LH[602] levels, suggesting an impairment of fertility, as is found in SGA females. Adult males born SGA have increased aromatase and 5α-reductase activities, leading to elevated levels of estradiol and dihydrotestosterone.[603] Of most concern is the fact that elevated estradiol levels in males increase the risk of testicular cancer and do not provide the protective effect on cardiovascular health as found in females. The level of inhibin B is elevated in significantly SGA boys (i.e., mean birth weights more than 2 SD below the mean for gestational age), although other studies with higher-birth-weight SGA boys demonstrated no such chages.[588,604]

Girls

Syndrome of Gonadal Dysgenesis and Its Variants.[562] The most common form of hypergonadotropic hypogonadism in the female is the syndrome of gonadal dysgenesis (Turner syndrome and its variants), a sporadic disorder with an incidence of 1 per 2500 liveborn girls in which all (i.e., X chromosome monosomy with haploinsufficiency) or part of the second sex chromosome (i.e., partial sex chromosome monosomy) is absent.[553,589] About 99% of 45,X conceptuses abort spontaneously, and 1 in 15 spontaneous abortions has a 45,X karyotype. The 45,X karyotype is associated with female phenotype, short stature, sexual infantilism, and various somatic abnormalities.

Sex chromosome mosaicism or structural abnormalities of an X or Y chromosome (affects about 40% of individuals with Turner syndrome) may modify the features of this syndrome. The syndrome of gonadal dysgenesis and its variants are found in a continuum ranging from the typical 45,X phenotype to a normal male or female phenotype.[553,562] Comprehensive recommendations for the diagnosis and management of Turner syndrome were presented by an international committee.[590]

45,X Turner Syndrome. Short stature and sexual infantilism are typical features of sex chromatin–negative 45,X gonadal dysgenesis (Turner syndrome), which is the karyotype found in approximately 60% of cases[562] (Fig. 25-47). The short stature is caused by loss of a homeobox-containing gene that is located on the pseudoautosomal region (PAR1) of the short arms of the X (p22) and Y (p11.3) chromosomes and encodes an osteogenic factor. This short stature homeobox-containing gene[605] (SHOX) was previously called the *pseudoautosomal homeobox osteogenic gene (PHOG)*. Because it is located on the PAR1 of the short arm of the X and Y chromosomes, it escapes X-chromosome inactivation. SHOX haploinsufficiency is responsible for, in addition to abnormal growth, mesomelic growth retardation, and Madelung deformity of the wrist (i.e., bilateral bowing of the radius with a dorsal subluxation of the distal ulna in Leri-Weill dyschondrosteosis (i.e., SHOX haploinsufficiency). Langer mesomelic dysplasia, which includes severe dwarfism with striking hypoplasia or aplasia of the ulnar and fibula, is caused by SHOX nullizygosity. SHOX haploinsufficiency appears to be responsible for 2.0 SD of the approximately 3.0 SD deficit in stature and the skeletal abnormalities in Turner syndrome. On the other hand, patients with complete gonadal dysgenesis and tall stature had a 45,X/46,X der(X) and three doses of the SHOX gene due to the SHOX duplication on the der(X) chromosome.

Turner syndrome may be recognized in the newborn period or before. More than 90% of Turner fetuses spontaneously abort. The 45,X abortuses have edema and large hygromas of the neck that may be seen on prenatal ultrasound studies. This lymphatic defect is the basis for the loose skinfolds that ultimately form the webbed neck (i.e., pterygium colli). Affected newborn infants may also have lymphedema of the extremities; the term *Bonnevie-Ullrich syndrome* has been applied to newborn infants with these features of Turner syndrome.

Frequent features are distinct facies with micrognathia, a fish-mouth appearance, high-arched palate with dental abnormalities, epicanthal folds, ptosis, low-set or deformed ears, short neck with low hairline, webbing (i.e., pterygium colli), and recurrent otitis media, often leading to impaired hearing (25% of affected adults require hearing aids[562]). A broad, shieldlike chest leads to the appearance of widely spaced nipples, and the areolae are often hypoplastic. Skeletal defects include short fourth metacarpals and cubitus valgus (which may develop after birth), Madelung deformity of the wrist (in about 7%), genu valgum, and scoliosis. There are extensive pigmented nevi,[562] a tendency to keloid formation, and hypoplastic nails. Lymphatic obstruction leads to the infantile puffiness of extremities and pterygium colli and to a distinctive shape of the ears. Cardiovascular anomalies affect the left side of the heart and include coarctation of the aorta in about 10% (40% of these have associated webbing of the neck), aortic stenosis, and bicuspid aortic valves; the latter individuals are at risk for a dissecting aortic aneurysm. An echocardiogram of the cardiovascular system must be performed, and prophylactic

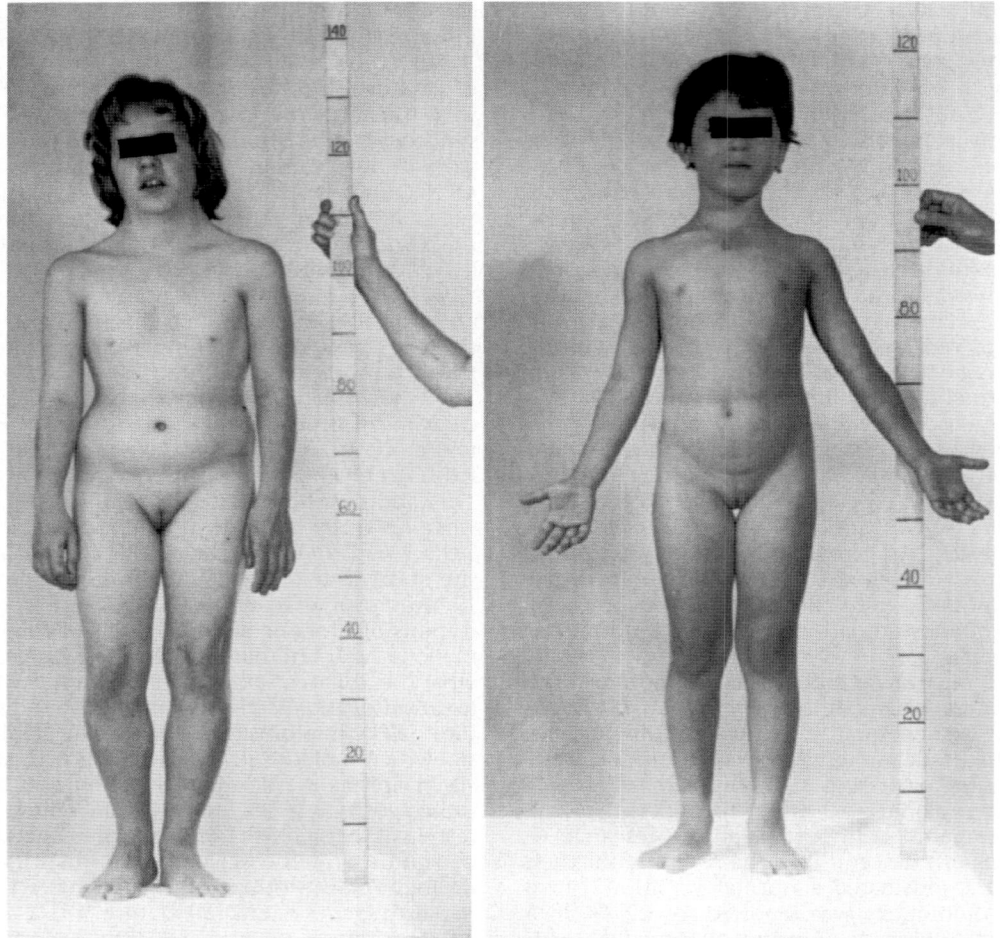

Figure 25-47 *Left*, A girl aged 14 years and 10 months with the typical form of the syndrome of gonadal dysgenesis (Turner syndrome). The X chromatin pattern was negative, and the karyotype was 45,X. She was short (height, 134.5 cm; height age, 9 years and 5 months) and sexually infantile except for the appearance of sparse pubic hair. She exhibited characteristic stigmata of the syndrome: a short, webbed neck; shield-like chest with widely separated nipples; bilateral metacarpal signs; puffiness over the dorsum of the fingers; cubitus valgus; increased number of pigmented nevi; characteristic facies; and low-set ears. The bone age was 13.5 years; the urinary 17-ketosteroid level was 5.1 mg/day; and the urinary gonadotropin level was greater than 100 mU/day. Vaginal smears and the urocytogram showed an immature pattern in which cornified squamous cells were absent. Female secondary sexual characteristics were induced with estrogen therapy, and the cyclic administration resulted in periodic estrogen withdrawal bleeding. *Right*, A 45,X girl aged 9 years and 11 months with Turner syndrome. Apart from short stature (height, 118 cm; height age, 6 years and 11 months), increased pigmented nevi, and subtle changes in the fingers and toes, she had few somatic anomalies. In contrast to the patient on the left, the main clinical feature was short stature.

antibiotics are indicated if an anatomic abnormality is demonstrated. Elevated values on the ambulatory arterial stiffness index (AASI) may be another risk factor for later serious cardiac disease.[606] Abnormal pelvocaliceal collecting systems, abnormal position or alignment of the kidneys, and an abnormal vascular supply to the kidney are encountered in 30% to 60% of patients. Recurrent urinary tract infections are common. Defects of the gastrointestinal system include intestinal telangiectasias and hemangiomatoses that rarely can lead to massive gastrointestinal bleeding. The prevalence of inflammatory bowel disease, chronic liver disease, and colon cancer is increased. Autoimmune diseases, such as Hashimoto thyroiditis (16-fold relative risk) and Graves disease, are common, and an association with juvenile rheumatoid arthritis and psoriatic arthritis has been described.

The age of diagnosis of Turner syndrome continues to be delayed, with the exception of newborns with the striking phenotype of the Bonnevie-Ullrich syndrome or those diagnosed on amniocentesis. It is recommended that all prepubertal age girls below −2.0 SD who have at least two somatic stigmata of the syndrome have a karyotype analysis; early diagnosis is key for optimal management of the growth failure and the detection of occult features of the syndrome.

Pelvic ultrasonography or MRI usually permits the detection of even a small, infantile uterus and reveals streak gonads. Ultrasensitive estrogen bioassays can confirm decreased ovarian function in girls with Turner syndrome because estradiol values are significantly lower than those found in average girls in puberty. Long-term follow-up of affected women previously treated with GH and estrogen demonstrated normal adult uterine length only in those with 45,X/46,XX karyotypes, whereas those with pure 45,X karyotypes had a smaller uterus length and volume.[607] The streak gonads result in sexual infantilism, but in about 10% of cases, puberty, menarche, and rarely, pregnancy may occur.[562] Women with some of the variants have been able to achieve fertility and deliver normal infants, although cardiovascular risks increase the danger. Affected adults can undergo hormone replacement to prepare the uterus to receive a donated embryo and proceed to delivery.

Unfortunately, some patients receiving a donated ovum have died because of dissection or rupture of the aorta, and caution should be used in recommending this technique.[601,608] Long-term regular follow-up of adults with Turner syndrome with echocardiography is recommended every 5 years in adulthood.[590]

Intrauterine growth retardation with a mean deficit in birth length of 2.6 cm (−1.24 SD) and a slow childhood growth rate result in a loss of about 8 to 9 cm (−3.0 SD) by age 3 years in girls with Turner syndrome.[609] A major portion of the height deficit occurs during the first 3 years of life. Decreased growth rate occurs at the time of expected puberty, and the pubertal growth spurt is absent in those without pubertal development. Untreated individuals with Turner syndrome in the United Kingdom and United States have a mean adult height of approximately 142 to 143 cm, which is about 20 cm less than the average height of typical women; the adult stature of these patients correlates with midparental height and with the height of unaffected women of the same ethnic group. Haploinsufficiency of the *SHOX* gene is estimated to contribute two thirds of the height deficit. It is postulated that a second gene on the short arm of the X chromosome that does not undergo X-chromosome inactivation contributes the other one third of the deficit. In girls with Turner syndrome with spontaneous puberty, pubertal height velocity was transiently higher than in girls with amenorrhea, but adult height was not different.[562] Specific growth curves are available for plotting the growth of affected children.[610]

GH treatment is approved by the FDA for Turner syndrome to increase growth and adult height. The addition of estrogen therapy at low doses in additon to GH has a modest additive effect on adult height; untreated height was 144.6 ± 5.5 cm, 140.8 ± 5.0 cm for estrogen treatment alone, 147.9 ± 7.2 cm for the GH treatment alone, and 149.3 ± 6.6 cm for GH and estradiol combined over an average 7.2 ± 2.5-year treatment/observation period.[611] The average height gain in various studies has varied from 4 to 16 cm, and a systematic review of the literature shows a 5-cm gain to be the most likely outcome.[612] This variability in gain in height is incompletely understood, but many factors have been implicated, including the age of initiation of therapy, dose duration, age (especially number of years from beginning hGH treatment) at the beginning of estrogen replacement, number of injections per week, compliance, and whether the last measured height represented the adult height. Early initiation of hGH therapy (e.g., 2 to 8 years of age) leads to greatest effect. GH treatment of Turner patients has been safe, and untoward events are no more common than in other conditions treated with GH. There is some degree of improvement of the abnormal body proportions of Turner syndrome with hGH treatment, but the disproportionate growth of the foot may dissuade some girls from continuing treatment to maximal benefit on height. Five-year follow-up of young adults with Turner syndrome demonstrated continued beneficial effects of GH on blood pressure, lipid levels, and increased adult height.[613]

A nationwide survey of 632 Danish girls with Turner syndrome demonstrated an increased prevalence of fractures, mainly in the forearm, compared with control subjects. The prevalence was higher still in the absence of ovarian function and in girls with family history of fractures and presumed familial disorders of bone density.[614] It appears that estrogen therapy is critical for the prevention and repair of osteoporosis, but for adolescents and adults, the optimal dose preparation and site of delivery for the prevention of osteoporosis are not known. GH treatment

of Turner syndrome for at least 1 year showed no difference in volumetric BMD, although LBM was higher and fat mass was lower than in the control subjects.[615]

About 50% of patients with Turner syndrome have a tendency toward impaired glucose tolerance without GH treatment; in some, this may be caused by associated obesity, and risk of type 2 diabetes mellitus is increased. Although glucose values do not change with GH therapy, insulin levels reversibly rise during treatment, indicating an additional degree of insulin resistance caused by the GH.[616] Turner syndrome patients as young as 11 years can already have elevated serum cholesterol concentrations before treatment with GH or estrogen.

The biphasic pattern of gonadotropin secretion in normal infancy and childhood is exaggerated in Turner syndrome[383] (see Fig. 25-27).

The appearance of pubic hair (i.e., pubarche) is often delayed in the syndrome of gonadal dysgenesis, even though adrenarche, as assessed by the increase in concentration of plasma DHEAS, occurs at the normal age.[402] Girls with ovarian failure demonstrate early adrenarche, and therefore higher serum values of DHEAS, but later pubarche, whereas those who demonstrate at least beginning breast development follow a course of adrenarche similar to that of unaffected girls. This suggests that ovarian function is necessary to convert DHEA to the active androgens responsible for the appearance of pubic hair in normal girls. The pubic hair of affected individuals is sparse, but estrogen therapy increases the growth of pubic hair despite a lack of increase in adrenal androgen secretion, and estrogen affects pubic hair appearance.

Behavior and Development of Turner Syndrome. Counseling and a peer support group are exceedingly important components of long-term management. Girls with Turner syndrome younger than 6 years did not perceive that they had a problem with height, but by 7 to 12 years and especially by 13 to 15 years, affected Turner girls have a strong desire for GH therapy and even unrealistic expectations of what GH therapy can accomplish in terms of adult height. GH therapy improved self-esteem even if there remained a significant difference in height between Turner girls and the normal range. Height gained with GH therapy did not affect quality of life, although cardiac defects and otologic complications did.[617] Girls who have discontinued GH therapy after reaching adult height showed no evidence of depression but still had remaining problems with self-perception and bodily attitude despite significant height gains. Psychological problems in Turner syndrome are not necessarily diminished with GH treatment and an increase in adult height.

Turner syndrome girls resemble normal girls in verbal and language skills, and IQ is normal when verbal ability, including comprehension and vocabulary, are considered, but visual-constructional or visual-perceptual spatiotemporal processing, visuomotor coordination, and mathematical ability (particularly in geometry) may be impaired, leading to a decrease in the performance of IQ tests due to mistakes on operation and alignment processes.[618] Girls with 45,X mosaicism associated with a 46,XX cell line, 45,X/46,XX, scored closer to normal than those with other types of mosaicisms. Only 3.3% of girls with Turner syndrome have developmental delay in the absence of a variant of Turner syndrome caused by a ring X chromosome. It is useful to monitor the patient's progress in high school mathematics. There are consistent MRI abnormalities in the right parietal lobe and the occipital lobes, and decreased volumes in these areas are implicated in defects in visual-spatial processing. These anatomic data relate to the difficulties in visual-spatial skills found in most studies of girls with Turner syndrome, because these difficulties are most closely linked to the right parietal region.

There is an increased risk of impaired social adjustment in Turner syndrome. Although there was evidence that the origin of the remaining X chromosome in classic Turner syndrome affected behavior due to imprinting, recent evidence could not support the effect of imprinting on social behavior.[619]

Transition of girls with Turner syndrome to adult care is best carried out by an experienced team, which is ideally composed of an endocrinologist; cardiologist; nephrologist; reproductive endocrinologist; audiologic physician; ear, nose, and throat surgeon; plastic surgeon; dentist; and psychologist because of the multiplicity of complications that affected individuals may encounter in the areas of growth failure, cardiovascular disease, gonadal failure, and learning disabilities.[618]

Sex Chromatin–Positive Variants of the Syndrome of Gonadal Dysgenesis. Mosaicism of 45,X/46,XX; 45,X/47,XXX; or 45,X/46,XX/47,XXX chromosomes is associated with a chromatin-positive buccal smear and usually with fewer manifestations of the syndrome of gonadal dysgenesis. Likewise, structural abnormalities of the X chromosome can be associated with fewer phenotypic features of the syndrome. Lack of genetic material on the long or the short arm of the second X chromosome can cause decreased gonadal function; loss of all or part of the short arm of the X leads to the physical findings of Turner syndrome.[562] Depending on the location and extent of the deletion on the short arm of the X chromosome, these patients may be more likely to have modest pubertal growth and some spontaneous pubertal development.

Sex Chromatin–Negative Variants of Gonadal Dysgenesis. These variants include 45,X/46,XY mosaicism and structural abnormalities of the Y chromosome. Affected individuals have phenotypes that vary from those of classic gonadal dysgenesis to those of ambiguous genitalia to phenotypic males.[562] Patients may present with short stature, delayed puberty, and a history of hypospadias repair. There is variable testicular differentiation, ranging from a streak gonad to functioning testes. Patients with mosaicism involving a Y cell line or abnormalities of the Y chromosome are at risk for neoplastic transformation of the dysgenetic testes. Gonadoblastomas, which are benign, nonmetastasizing tumors, may arise within the gonad and produce testosterone or estrogens. The neoplasm may become calcified sufficiently to be detected on an abdominal radiograph. The appearance of feminization or virilization in a patient with dysgenetic gonads and a Y cell line may indicate gonadoblastoma formation. Of greater significance is the increased prevalence of malignant germ cell tumors, arising within the dysgenetic gonad or gonadoblastoma. Examples are dysgerminomas, mature teratomas, and testicular intraepithelial neoplasia.[620] These tumors occur more often in postpubertal subjects and rarely in children.[562]

46,XX and 46,XY Gonadal Dysgenesis. The term *pure gonadal dysgenesis* refers to phenotypic females with sexual infantilism and a 46,XX or 46,XY karyotype without chromosomal abnormalities.[562]

Familial and Sporadic 46,XX Gonadal Dysgenesis and Its Variants. The usual phenotype of 46,XX gonadal dysgenesis includes normal stature, sexual infantilism, bilateral streak gonad, normal female internal and external genitalia, and primary amenorrhea. The streak gonad occasionally produces estrogens or androgens, but malignant transformation is rare. Incomplete forms of this condition may result in hypoplastic ovaries that produce enough estrogen to cause some breast development and a few menstrual periods, followed by secondary amenorrhea. This hetero-geneous syndrome occurs sporadically or with autosomal recessive inheritance,[562] and in some instances, it is associated with other congenital malformations. Some familial cases have been associated with sensorineural deafness (i.e., Perrault syndrome).

Familial and Sporadic 46,XY Gonadal Dysgenesis and Its Variants. A phenotype that includes female genitalia with or without clitoral enlargement, normal or tall stature, bilateral streak gonads, normal müllerian structures, sexual infantilism, and a eunuchoid habitus is typical of 46,XY gonadal dysgenesis. About 15% of the patients have a deletion or mutation in the sex-determining region Y (*SRY*) gene. If the dysgenetic testes produce significant amounts of testosterone, slight clitoral enlargement may occur at birth, and virilization may ensue at puberty. The incomplete form of 46,XY gonadal dysgenesis may involve any degree of ambiguity of the external genitalia and internal ducts. The risk of neoplastic transformation of the streak gonads or dysgenetic testes is increased, and gonadectomy is indicated. The disorder is usually transmitted as an X-linked or sex-limited autosomal dominant trait or less commonly as an autosomal recessive trait.[562]

All patients with dysgenetic gonads and a Y chromosome or an *SRY* gene are susceptible to neoplasia or carcinoma formation in the gonad. The evidence on optimal therapy is not supported by high-quality evidence, but gonadectomy is indicated at diagnosis, especially if the gonad cannot be palpated.[621]

Other Causes of Primary Ovarian Failure. The prevalence of primary ovarian failure is increasing as a consequence of the long-term effects of cytotoxic chemotherapy and radiation therapy as these agents prolong the lives of children and adolescents with cancer. The same pattern occurs for males with testes that have been treated with these modalities.

Radiation Therapy. Ovarian transposition, moving the ovaries out of the radiation field if they are not the target of therapy, before radiation therapy is compatible with normal menses, pubertal development, and pregnancy in the few cases reported.[622] The uterus may be affected by radiation and may not expand normally during pregnancy.

Chemotherapy. Successful treatment of childhood acute lymphoblastic leukemia has become commonplace. Chemotherapy and radiation therapy to the CNS or ovaries exert damage in a dose-dependent manner.[623] Attempts to protect the gonads by suppressing the pituitary-gonadal axis with gonadal steroids or GnRH agonists are probably ineffective.[624] Oncofertility is a new field of investigation that aims to preserve fertility in children and teenagers subject to cancer therapy and is leading to improved methods of preservation.[625] A major problem is lack of discussion of possible method of preservation by oncologists with the families. Careful endocrine follow-up of children and adolescents treated with chemotherapy or radiation therapy is essential.

Autoimmune Oophoritis. Premature menopause may occur at any age before the normal climacteric and has been reported in adolescent girls. Cessation of ovarian function usually manifests as secondary amenorrhea.[626] Autoimmune oophoritis can cause ovarian failure leading to primary amenorrhea, oligomenorrhea, arrest of puberty, and occasionally cystic enlargement of the ovaries. Most often, it is associated with other autoimmune endocrinopathies, especially autoimmune Addison disease, in which it may precede the onset of adrenal insufficiency, but it rarely occurs in isolated premature ovarian failure. Glucocorticoid therapy may improve, at least temporarily, ovarian function.

Type I autoimmune polyglandular insufficiency, also known as autoimmune polyendocrinopathy-candidiasis-ectodermal dystrophy (APECED), is a rare systemic autoimmune disorder with an array of clinical features, including hypoparathyroidism, adrenal insufficiency, gonadal failure, diabetes mellitus, pernicious anemia, hypothyroidism, chronic hepatitis, mucocutaneous candidiasis, dystrophic nail hypoplasia, vitiligo, alopecia, keratinopathy, and intestinal malabsorption. Thirty-six percent of women with APECED exhibited ovarian failure before age 20, whereas only 4% of affected men had testicular failure by that age. This autosomal recessive disorder is caused by more than 42 mutations in the *CDK14 (AIRE1)* gene at gene map locus 21q22.3.

Autoimmune oophoritis occurs in more than 20% of patients with autoimmune adrenal insufficiency. Various autoantibodies have been detected in autoimmune oophoritis, including autoantibodies to cytochrome P450 steroidogenic enzymes; some are organ specific, whereas others react with antigens in more than one tissue and more than one cell type.

Homozygous Galactosemia. Homozygous galactosemia due to mutation in the galactose-1-phosphate uridylyltransferase gene *(GALT)* is commonly associated with primary ovarian failure, from failure to develop puberty to primary or secondary amenorrhea and premature menopause, but puberty is usually normal in males, and the risk of testicular dysfunction is low; compound heterozygotes have normal onset of puberty. Dietary restriction programs have not prevented the ovarian failure, nor are other means of avoiding ovarian failure effective.[627] The pathogenesis of galactose-induced ovarian toxicity remains unclear but probably involves galactose itself and its metabolites, such as galactitol and uridine diphosphate galactose. Most cases are detected by newborn screening programs.

Haploinsufficiency of the FOXL2 Gene. A rare autosomal dominant disorder involving eyelid dysplasia and premature ovarian failure is caused by haploinsufficiency of the *FOXL2* gene, a member of the winged helix/forkhead family of transcription factors.[628] The eyelid abnormalities include small palpebral fissures, ptosis, and a small skinfold extending inward and upward from the lower lid (i.e., epicanthus inversus). The gene is expressed in the follicular cells, and the mutations that lead to haploinsufficiency are associated with an increased rate of follicular atresia. The degree of ovarian failure varies from primary amenorrhea to irregular menses and premature ovarian failure, with ultrasound findings ranging from normal-appearing ovaries to streak gonads with an inconsistent number of primordial follicles found on ovarian biopsy. The infertility component of the syndrome is limited to females. Animal studies provide insights into other genetic mutations that may cause premature ovarian failure in humans, including mutations of *BMP15, FMR1, POF1B,* and *FOXO3A.*[629]

Congential Disorders of Glycosylation-1: Carbohydrate-Deficient Glycoprotein Syndrome Type Ia. The congential disorders of glycosylation-1 (i.e., carbohydrate-deficient glycoprotein syndrome type Ia) include an autosomal recessive disorder associated with circulating glycoproteins deficient in their terminal carbohydrate moieties, including a wide range of glycoproteins, enzymes, binding proteins, and coagulation factors.[630] A typical isoform pattern of serum transferrin detected by isoelectric focusing is used as a diagnostic test. The dominant clinical feature is the neurologic manifestations of involvement of the central and peripheral nervous system. Among the other organ systems affected is the pituitary-gonadal system.

The hypergonadotropic-hypogonadism is more severe in females because males virilize at puberty. The ovary and the pituitary are affected. Affected girls have sexual infantilism; the ovaries are hypoplastic or atrophic. High serum FSH and LH levels exhibited normal electrophoretic isoform patterns, but they appeared to have decreased but not absent FSH bioactivity in an FSH bioassay.

Follicle-Stimulating Hormone Receptor Resistance: Gene Mutations and Hypergonadotropic Hypogonadism. The FSH receptor is a member of the G protein–linked receptor, seven-transmembrane superfamily. It has a large, extended extracellular ligand-binding domain. An autosomal recessive disorder due to a mutation in the extracellular ligand-binding domain of the FSH receptor in affected females in six Finnish families mainly from the north central region resulted in delayed (40%) or normal puberty but primary amenorrhea, elevated gonadotropin levels, and hypergonadotropic ovarian dysgenesis with arrest of ovarian follicular development at the primary follicle stage and continued atresia.[583] The clinical features are very similar to the findings in FSH-deficient mice generated by targeted disruption of the gene encoding the FSH β-subunit. This disorder likely is responsible for most cases of the resistant ovary syndrome. The FSH receptor gene contains nine small exons (1 through 9) that encode the extracellular ligand-binding domain and one large exon 10 that designates the remainder of the receptor, including the seven-transmembrane and intracellular domains. The Finnish mutation, an Ala1989Val substitution, is in the extracellular domain. Expression of the mutation in transfected cells indicated a small FSH effect on cAMP production, a striking reduction of FSH-binding capacity, but apparently normal binding affinity.

The FSH receptor mutation in the Finnish patients is not a null mutation. It remains to be determined whether the loss or complete inactivation of the FSH receptor leads to failure of puberty and sexual infantilism or to estrogen synthesis by the immature ovarian follicles described in the FSH β-subunit knockout mouse. Affected males in these families are normally masculinized at puberty but tend to have small testes. They have a variable degree of spermatogenic insufficiency, but not azoospermia, increased plasma concentrations of FSH and LH, decreased inhibin B levels, and normal plasma testosterone values.[631]

Luteinizing Hormone and Human Chorionic Gonadotropin Resistance. LH/hCG resistance due to mutations in the gene encoding the seven-transmembrane LHCGR is discussed in Chapter 23. In the affected XY individual, this autosomal recessive disorder leads to various degrees of male pseudohermaphroditism; the mildest form is represented by an isolated micropenis.[632] Less severe mutations of the *LHCGR* may be associated with delayed puberty. In affected females, LH/hCG resistance does not affect pubertal maturation but does lead to amenorrhea with high serum LH levels but normal FSH and estradiol concentrations.

Polycystic Ovary Syndrome. PCOS, or functional ovarian hyperandrogenism, does not delay the onset of puberty but often delays menarche or causes menstrual abnormalities.[633] It can have serious long-term metabolic consequences such as dyslipidemia and insulin resistance over and above androgen excess and reproductive difficulties.

Noonan Syndrome. Individuals with Noonan syndrome (i.e., pseudo-Turner syndrome, Ullrich syndrome) have webbed neck, ptosis, down-slanting palpebral fissures, low-set ears, short stature, cubitus valgus, and lymphedema, which explains why this phenotype has been called *pseudo-Turner syndrome.*[562] Features that differentiate these individuals from those with Turner syndrome include triangular facies, pectus excavatum, right-sided heart disease (e.g., pulmonary stenosis, often with valve dysplasia; atrial septal defect) compared with the left-sided heart disease in Turner syndrome, hypertrophic cardiomyopathy, varied blood clotting defects, and an increased incidence of mental retardation. Females with Noonan syndrome have normal ovarian function. Males have normal differentiation of external genitalia but may have undescended testes; germinal aplasia or hypoplasia and impaired Leydig cell function may be present. Puberty is often delayed as 35% of boys enter puberty after age 13.5 years and 44% of girls enter puberty after age 13 years.[634] Stature is decreased after normal birth length and weight, with a mean adult height of 162.5 cm (63.9 inches) for men and 152.7 cm (60.1 inches) for women, usually following the −2 SD curve. The pubertal growth spurt is often delayed or attenuated.

Noonan syndrome is inherited as an autosomal dominant trait.[562] A gene implicated in Noonan syndrome has been localized to the long arm of chromosome 12 (12q24.2-q24.31), and a mutation in *PTPN11* was identified, but at least three other gene mutations have been identified. Noonan syndrome is linked to the chromosomal band 12q24.1, and eight genes in the RAS-MAPK signaling pathway cause Noonan syndrome: *PTPN11, SOS1, KRAS, NRAS, RAF1, BRAF, SHOC2,* and *CBL.*[634] The incidence is estimated at 1 case in 1000 to 1 in 2500 people. One parent may have features of the syndrome in 40% to 60% of cases. About 50% of patients are thought to have new mutations.

Administration of hGH is approved by the FDA for use in Noonan syndrome. Response to GH is decreased with *PTN11* mutations in some but not all[635] reports, and there is an increase in risk for neoplasia in this genotype as well.[636] GH therapy can allow affected children to reach the lower normal range of stature.

Frasier Syndrome. Germline mutations in exon 8 or 9, coding for zinc fingers 2 or 3 of the Wilms tumor suppressor gene, *WT1*, leads to Denys-Drash syndrome, which includes Wilms tumor, male pseudohermaphroditism, and early nephrotic syndrome with diffuse mesangial sclerosis. Frasier syndrome includes male pseudohermaphroditism, nephrotic syndrome with focal and segmental glomerular sclerosis, and the development of gonadoblastoma and is associated with mutations in the second splice donor site in intron 9 leading to a decrease in the KTS+ isoforms. Although most patients with Frasier syndrome present with ambiguous genitalia, this diagnosis should be considered for any phenotypic female with end-stage renal disease (due to focal segmental glomerulosclerosis) and sexual infantilism. The karyotype may be 46,XY or 46,XX.

Diagnosis of Delayed Puberty and Sexual Infantilism

When girls remain prepubertal at 13 years or boys remain prepubertal at 14 years, the physician must make a clinical judgment about who are variants of the norm and who require extensive evaluation and treatment (Figs. 25-48

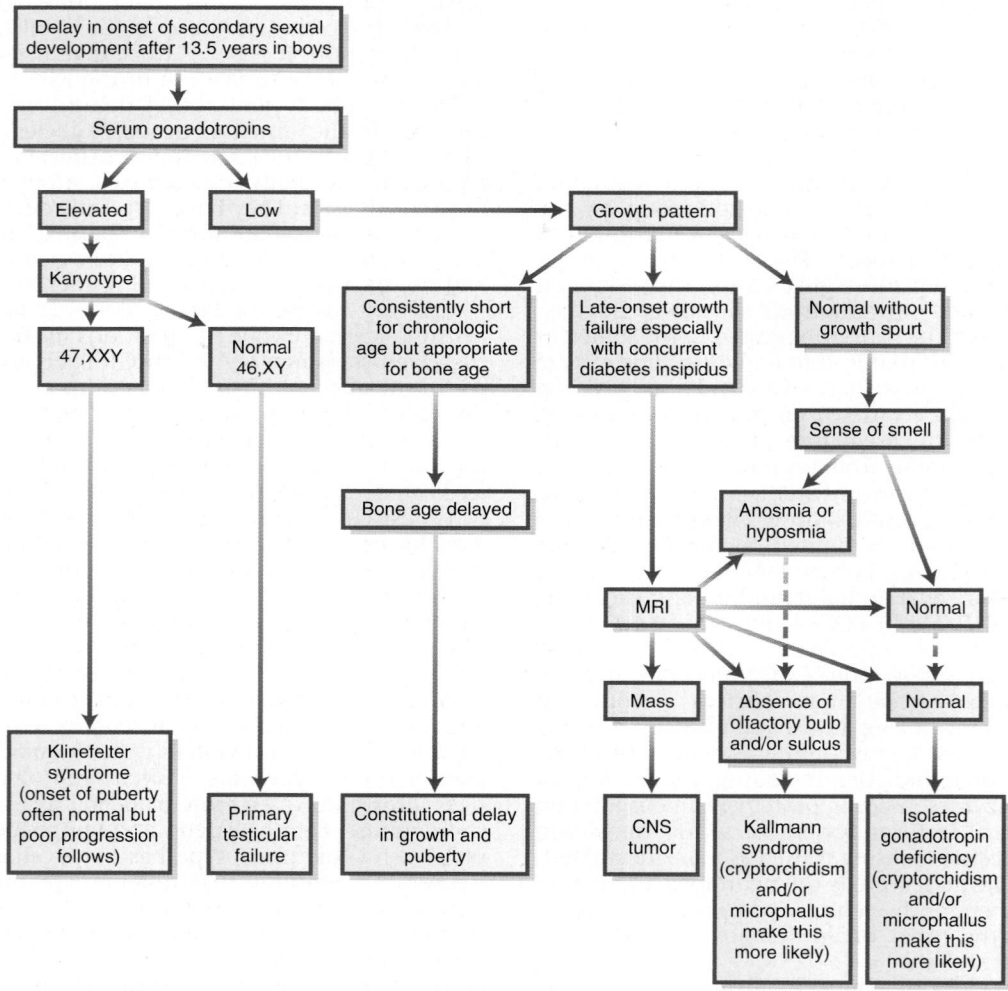

Figure 25-48 Flow chart for the evaluation of delayed puberty in boys. CNS, central nervous system; MRI, magnetic resonance imaging.

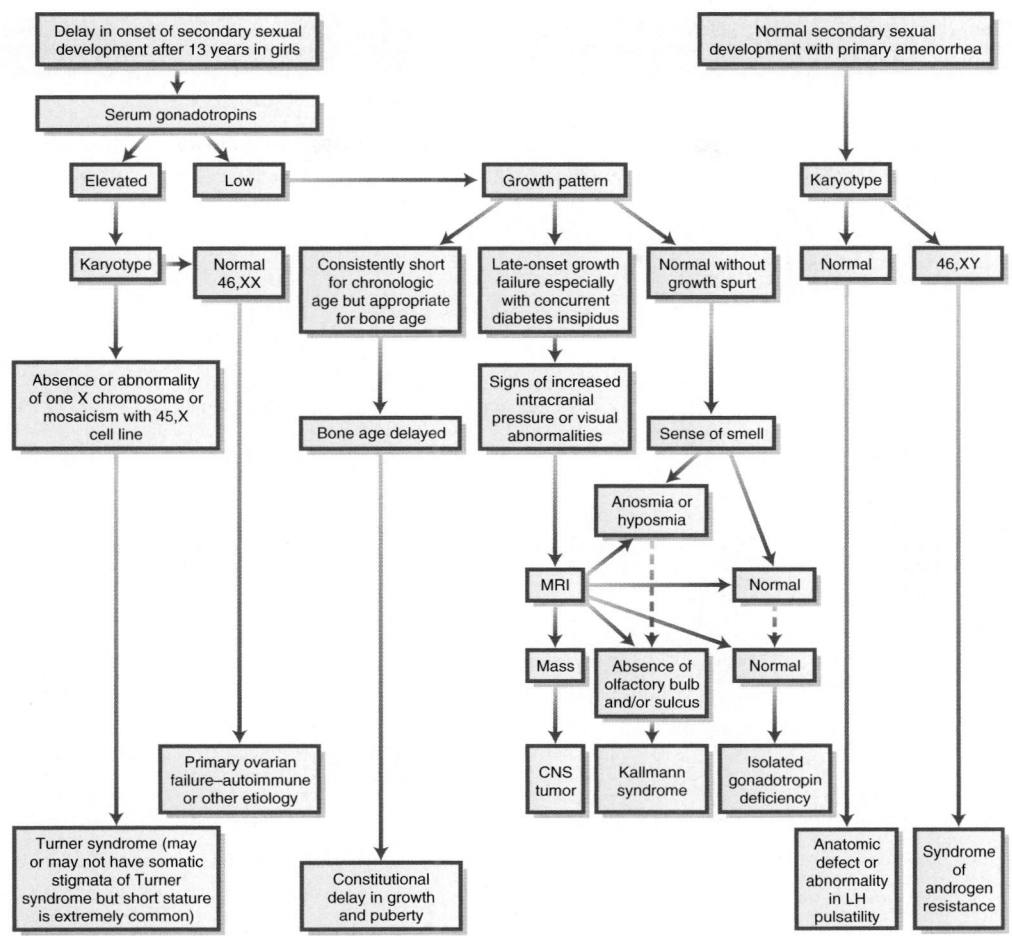

Figure 25-49 Flow chart for the evaluation of delayed puberty in girls. CNS, central nervous system; LH, luteinizing hormone; MRI, magnetic resonance imaging.

and 25-49; Tables 25-20 and 25-21). A boy who has not completed secondary sexual maturation within 4.5 years after onset of puberty or a girl who does not menstruate within 5 years after onset may have a hypothalamic, pituitary, or gonadal disorder. The diagnosis of hypergonadotropic hypogonadism is readily established by elevation of random plasma LH and FSH concentrations. However, differentiating the diagnosis of hypogonadotropic hypogonadism from constitutional delay in growth and adolescence remains difficult in spite of decades of study owing to the overlap in physical and laboratory findings for the two conditions (see Table 25-21). Most boys with pubertal delay have a self-limited variant in the tempo of growth and pubertal-onset CDP.

Medical history must elicit all symptoms of chronic or intermittent illnesses and all details pertaining to growth and development. Questions about the patient's sense of smell are essential. Has puberty failed to occur, or did it begin but failed to progress or even regress? Disorders of pregnancy, abnormalities of labor and delivery, and birth trauma, if part of the patient's history, suggest that a congenital or neonatal event may be related to the delay in puberty. Poor linear growth and poor nutritional status during the neonatal period and childhood may reflect long-standing abnormalities of development. Family history may reveal disorders of puberty or infertility, anosmia, or hyposmia in relatives and delay in the age at onset of puberty in parents or siblings. Recalled age of pubertal onset is relatively reliable in women but less often

accurate in men. A history of consanguinity is important in the detection of autosomal recessive disorders.

The physical examination starts with accurate determination of height, weight, and BMI. A growth chart is plotted to represent graphically growth velocity from birth (see Chapter 24). Late-onset growth failure usually indicates a serious condition requiring immediate evaluation. Weight is plotted to determine states of malnutrition. BMI should be calculated and plotted by age and gender in this era of epidemic obesity or to further determine nutritional status. The height velocity should be documented over a period of at least 6 months, preferably 12 months. The U/L segment ratio and the arm span are measured and compared with the height. The signs of puberty are assessed, and the stage of secondary sexual development is determined by physical examination according to the standards presented earlier (see Figs. 25-5, 25-6, and 25-10). Questionnaires with pictures are used to allow a child to determine his or her own stage of puberty in some studies but do not replace the physical examination, as there is a tendency to overestimate development early in puberty and underestimate it late in puberty. The length and width of the testes are measured in boys, or the volume is assessed using an orchidometer. The length and diameter of the gently stretched penis are determined in boys, and the diameter of glandular breast tissue and areolar size are determined in girls. The presence or absence of galactorrhea is documented. Obese boys often appear to have a small penis because of excessive adipose tissue surrounding

TABLE 25-20

Differential Diagnostic Features of Delayed Puberty and Sexual Infantilism

Condition	Stature	Plasma Gonadotropins	GnRH Test LH Response	Plasma Gonadal Steroids	Plasma DHEAS	Karyotype	Olfaction
Constitutional delay in growth and adolescence	Short for chron. age, usually appropriate for bone age	Prepubertal, later pubertal	Prepubertal, later pubertal	Low, later normal	Low for chron. age, appropriate for bone age	Normal	Normal
Hypogonadotropic Hypogonadism							
Isolated gonadotropin deficiency	Normal, absent pubertal growth spurt	Low	Prepubertal or no response	Low	Appropriate for chron. age	Normal	Normal
Kallmann syndrome	Normal, absent	Low	Prepubertal or no response	Low	Appropriate for chron. age	Normal	Anosmia; pubertal growth spurt or hyposmia
Idiopathic multiple pituitary hormone deficiencies	Short stature and poor growth since early childhood	Low	Prepubertal or no response	Low	Usually low	Normal	Normal
Hypothalamic-pituitary tumors	Late-onset decrease in growth velocity	Low	Prepubertal or no response	Low	Normal or low for chron. age	Normal	Normal
Primary Gonadal Failure							
Syndrome of gonadal dysgenesis (Turner syndrome) and variants	Short stature since childhood	High	Hyperresponse for age	Low	Normal for chron. age	45,X or variant	Normal
Klinefelter syndrome and variants	Normal to tall	High	Hyperresponse at puberty	Low or normal	Normal for chron. age	47,XXY or variant	Normal
Familial XX or XY gonadal dysgenesis	Normal for age	High	Hyperresponse	Low	Normal for chron. age	46,XX or 46,XY	Normal

chron., chronologic; DHEAS, dehydroepiandrosterone sulfate; GnRH, gonadotropin-releasing hormone; LH, luteinizing hormone.

TABLE 25-21

Endocrine Diagnosis of Constitutional Delayed Adolescence and Hypogonadotropic Hypogonadism

No single test reliably discriminates between the two diagnoses.
Onset of puberty in boys is indicated by
 Testes >2.5 cm in diameter
 Serum testosterone concentration >50 ng/dL
 Pubertal LH response to GnRH bolus
 Pubertal pattern of LH pulsatility

GnRH, gonadotropin-releasing hormone; LH, luteinizing hormone.

TABLE 25-22

Endocrine and Imaging Studies in Delayed Adolescence

Initial assessment
 Plasma testosterone or estradiol
 Plasma FSH and LH
 Plasma thyroxine (and prolactin)
 Bone age and lateral skull roentgenograph
 Test of olfaction
Follow-up studies
 Karyotype (short, phenotypic females)
 MRI with contrast enhancement
 Pelvic ultrasonography (females)
 GnRH test
 hCG test (males)
 Pattern of pulsatile LH secretion
 Visual acuity and visual fields

FSH, follicle-stimulating hormone; GnRH, gonadotropin-releasing hormone; hCG, human chorionic gonadotropin; LH, luteinizing hormone; MRI, magnetic resonance imaging.

the phallus; only when the fat is retracted can the full extent of phallic development be assessed. This is among the most common causes of inappropriate referral for hypogonadism. The extent of pubic and axillary hair is assessed, as is the degree of acne or comedones. The possibility of cryptorchidism or retractile testes should be determined if no testes are palpated in the scrotum. Neurologic examination, including examination of the optic discs and visual fields by frontal confrontation perimetry, may reveal findings, suggesting the presence of a CNS neoplasm or a developmental defect, and may suggest more accurate ophthalmologic evaluation is needed. Determination of olfaction is important because many patients with Kallmann syndrome wait years for the correct diagnosis to be made even in the presence of classic findings; physicians must remain alert to the possibility of this diagnosis and to the fact that congenital anosmia may not be noted by the patient or family for years. The stigmata of gonadal dysgenesis (i.e., Turner syndrome) or the small testes and

gynecomastia of Klinefelter syndrome may suggest a karyotypic abnormality. Complete physical examination, including the lungs, heart, kidney, and gastrointestinal tract, is important in the search for a chronic disorder that may delay puberty.

Laboratory studies (Table 25-22) include determination of plasma LH and FSH concentrations by sensitive third-generation assays in pediatric endocrine laboratories, measurement of the rise in the LH level after GnRH or GnRH agonist administration, and determination of testosterone concentrations in boys and estradiol levels in girls in pediatric endocrine laboratories using HPLC-MS/MS, all with pediatric standards for that laboratory. One of the few national endocrine laboratories should be used for determinations of the hormones of puberty, because most local laboratories are interested only in differentiating the normally higher adult values from inappropriately low levels, and they cannot determine the gradations of the low levels found in puberty.[235] Results of commercial immunochemiluminometric assays (ICMA) for LH and FSH are reported to be more sensitive for use in pediatrics than immunofluorometric assays (IFMA).[637] Several national laboratories began using liquid chromatography with tandem mass spectrometry methods for improved sensitivity and specificity and determinations in children (and women) for increased accuracy.[235] Newer ultrasensitive bioassays are not yet available commercially for the determination of low values of testosterone and estradiol or for total androgen or estrogen. Measurements of T_4 and TSH concentrations in boys and girls are usually necessary and prolactin is often useful as well.

Radiographic examination may include bone age determination and, if the history or physical examination is consistent with a CNS lesion, an MRI of the brain, with specific attention to the pituitary and hypothalamic area using contrast. T2-weighted coronal views will be useful in the diagnosis of Kallmann syndrome. MRI of the olfactory tract using CT can detect calcification, in contrast to MRI scans or plain radiographs, in most cases. Ultrasound evaluation of the uterus and ovaries provides useful information about the state of development of these structures but only if the ultrasonographer has experience with children and young adolescents. DXA evaluation of bone density should be considered in hypogonadotropic hypogonadism.

Assessment of karyotype should be considered for all undiagnosed short girls, even in the absence of somatic signs of Turner syndrome and especially if puberty is delayed or unexplained short stature is involved. Karyotype assessment should be performed for boys with suspected Klinefelter syndrome stigmata or behavior.

A presumptive diagnosis of constitutional delay in growth and adolescence is made if the history and growth chart reveal a history of short stature but a consistent growth rate for skeletal age (and no signs or symptoms of hypothalamic lesions), if the family history includes parents or siblings with delayed puberty, if the physical examination (including assessment of the olfactory threshold) is normal, if optic discs and visual fields are normal, and if the bone age is significantly delayed. In classic cases, MRI of the hypothalamic-pituitary region may not be necessary. The rate of growth in these patients is usually appropriate for bone age; a decrease in growth velocity occurs in some normal children just before the appearance of secondary sexual characteristics and may awaken concerns if such a pattern occurs in these subjects. The onset at puberty correlates better with bone age than with chronologic age, although bone age is not any better at estimating the onset of puberty in normal boys than is chronologic age and cannot be considered a highly accurate test.[138] Elevated concentrations of gonadotropins and gonadal steroids to early pubertal levels precede secondary sexual development by several months; measurements of serum LH, FSH, estradiol, or testosterone levels in appropriate assays may help to predict future development. The third-generation LH assays are sufficiently sensitive to allow in most boys the determination of the onset of endocrine puberty with a single blood sample, but a dynamic GnRH test is still often performed using GnRH agonists. The measurement of gonadotropins 1 hour (or 4 hours in some reports) after a subcutaneous injection of GnRH agonist is the current method of testing dynamic secretion of gonadotropins in the absence of native GnRH supplies.

Measurement of an 8 AM serum testosterone level provides an accurate indication of impending pubertal development; a value of greater than 0.7 nmol/L (20 ng/dL) predicts enlargement of testes to greater than 4 mL by 12 months in 77% of cases and in 15 months in 100% of cases, whereas of those with a value less than 0.7 nmol/L, only 12% entered puberty in 12 months and only 25% entered puberty in 15 months. This technique may help predict spontaneous pubertal development, but it still requires considerable watching and waiting.[415] A single inhibin B value over 35 pg/mL holds promise in eliminating CDP.[230] A recent report describes a reliable method of separating CDP from IHH: basal LH less than 0.3 IU/L, stimulated (100 μg of triptorelin acetate) LH (4 hour) less than 5.3 IU/L or inhibin B less than 111 pg/mL had 100% sensitivity for IHH, and basal LH less than 0.3 IU/L with inhibin B less than 111 pg/mL has a specificity of 98.1% for IHH.[638] Low AMH values are found in severe IHH.[245] These methods require continued evaluation before they become standard clinically. Watchful waiting may remain the procedure of choice when a patient does not fulfill the delineated criteria and does not fall into a diagnosable grouping.

The presence of red flags is suggested to be strong indication of gonadotropin deficiency rather than CDP. Thus, lack of prior minipuberty of infancy (such as cryptorchidism or micropenis), or the presence of congenital defects, including anosmia, deafness, mirror movements, renal agenesis, dental/digital anomalies, clefting or coloboma, or findings of CHARGE syndrome, make the diagnosis of gonadotropin deficiency more likely.[639] Genetic testing for many of the genes that cause Kallmann syndrome is available; it is suggested that priorities for such testing may be best focused upon subjects with synkinesia, dental agenesis, digital bony abnormalities, and hearing loss.[640] Genetic testing for *PROP* mutations is commercially available for combined hypopituitarism.

A typical patient with isolated gonadotropin deficiency is of average height for age and has eunuchoid proportions; has low plasma concentrations of gonadal steroids, LH, and FSH; and has no increase or a blunted response of LH after GnRH or GnRH agonist administration. The amplitude and usually the frequency of LH pulses are decreased when serial blood samples are studied over a 24-hour period. In some forms of Kallmann syndrome, the sense of smell is absent or impaired. However, as stated, differentiation of isolated gonadotropin deficiency in the absence of hyposmia or anosmia from CDP may be difficult at initial study. Gonadotropin-deficient patients may be as short as those with constitutional delay in growth and adolescence, and concentrations of LH and FSH in hypogonadotropic hypogonadism may be indistinguishable from those of normal prepubertal children or children with constitutional delay. Sometimes, years of observation are necessary to detect the appearance of spontaneous and progressive signs of secondary sexual development or to document rising concentrations of gonadotropins or gonadal steroids before the diagnosis is clear. There is a tendency for hypogonadotropic patients to undergo adrenarche at a normal age and to have higher DHEAS concentrations than those with constitutional delay in growth, and this pattern is helpful in making the differential diagnosis.[402] In most cases, absence of the first signs of sexual maturation or failure of a rise in gonadotropins or gonadal steroid levels by age 18 years in the presence of a normal concentration of serum DHEAS for chronologic age supports the diagnosis of isolated gonadotropin deficiency.

Patients with deficiency of gonadotropins combined with deficiency of other pituitary hormones require careful evaluation for a CNS neoplasm. Visual field or optic disc abnormalities support the diagnosis of CNS tumor; even if these tests are normal, cranial MRI should be done to evaluate the pituitary gland and stalk and the hypothalamic region. MRI appears superior to CT for detecting mass lesions and developmental abnormalities of the hypothalamic-pituitary region.

Treatment of Delayed Puberty and Sexual Infantilism

Patients with constitutional delay in growth and adolescence ultimately have spontaneous onset and progression through puberty. Often, reassurance and continued observation to ensure that the expected sexual maturation occurs are sufficient. However, the stigma of appearing less mature than one's peers can cause psychological stress. These individuals may be unable to participate in the dating activities their friends are starting; smaller size may lead them to avoid participation in athletics; immature appearance may lead to ridicule, especially in the locker room; and schoolwork may suffer because of their poor self-image. Some children feel such intense peer pressure and low self-esteem that only the appearance of signs of puberty can reassure them and enable them to participate in sports and social activities with their peers. Poor self-image in late-maturing boys may carry into adulthood, even after normal puberty ensues. Growth retardation appears more often responsible for most of the stress rather than the delay in pubertal development itself.

For psychological reasons, for boys 14 years old or older who show no signs of puberty, a 3- to 6-month course of testosterone enanthate, cypionate, or cyclopropionate (50-mg dose given intramuscularly every 4 weeks) may be helpful. Because starting with the higher dose of 100 mg can lead to priapism in treatment-naïve boys, care, lower dosage, and short-acting preparations are advisable. Decades of experience confirm no effect on adult height of low dosages in the short term.[641] The low dose of testosterone enanthate is considered to be safe but can raise apolipoprotein B (apoB) and decrease HDL-cholesterol and apoAI levels (estradiol increases HDL-cholesterol and decreases triglycerides, LDL-cholesterol, and apoB). Although the use of exogenous androgens may improve self-image and start the secondary sexual changes of puberty, low-dose androgen use does not improve final height.

Alkylated testosterone preparations should be avoided because of the risk of peliosis hepatis (i.e., hemorrhagic liver cysts), which is not related to dose or duration of treatment. Although regression is possible with discontinuation of testosterone treatment, progression to liver failure can occur.

A course of low-dose oxandrolone (2.5 mg/day orally) is sometimes used as an oral alternative to intramuscular testosterone enanthate; this agent increases growth through androgenic effects reflected by suppression of LH and FSH but does not stimulate GH secretion, because it is not aromatized to estrogen. The temporary increase in growth velocity found with oxandrolone does not affect adult height in most studies. Oral treatment with 2.5 mg of fluoxymesterone (Halotestin) for 6 to 60 months allows increased pubertal development without adverse effect on adult height, although the necessity to take a daily dose may decrease compliance. Testosterone undecanoate at 40 mg/day is likewise an effective but expensive treatment for those opting for an oral therapy (not FDA approved for this use). This treatment can increase the growth rate but does not result in a change in LH pulsatility; mean overnight LH, testosterone, or SHBG levels; or free androgen index, PSA, and testicular volume values.[642] There is a preparation of testosterone undecanoate, given every 6 to 9 weeks, available that induces puberty in IHH in adults but there is no published experience in teenagers.[643] Transdermal testosterone may be applied as a daily patch or a gel (not FDA approved for this use), although experience with these forms of androgen is more limited than with the other forms. Preliminary experience suggests that overnight (about 8 to 9 hours) or every-other-night use of a 2.5-mg Androderm patch can achieve physiologic testosterone levels, produce lower SHBG levels, promote growth and virilization, and increase BMD in hypogonadal teenagers without significant side effects. An overnight study of transdermal testosterone (5 mg of Virormone) applied overnight (8 to 12 hours) for 4-week periods in boys with delayed puberty and short stature raised salivary testosterone levels, stimulated leg growth measured by knemometry (i.e., sensitive short-term measurements of leg growth), and stimulated bone turnover, as reflected by increased serum alkaline phosphatase[644] levels.[641] Testosterone cream is approved for adults but is not approved for use in teenagers with delayed puberty.

The type and route of estrogen administration are being reconsidered. Many suggest the use of 17β-estradiol rather than ethinyl estradiol owing to more physiologic effects; there is evidence in the treatment of transgender individuals that the use of ethinyl estradiol or conjugated estrogen carries a higher risk for venous and arterial thrombosis.[639] For girls 13 years of age or older, transdermal estrogen has been used in clinical trials for decades in the treatment of delayed puberty or hypogonadism with beneficial results on physical development and bone density and is entering widespread use.[645] There is support for such therapy based on understanding the adverse effects of oral estrogen that enters the portal circulation initially at a high dose (first pass) stimulates the production of proteins such as C-reactive protein, angiotensin precursor, and activated protein C, which are involved in cardiac complications. This contrasts with dermal estrogen, which is administered in lower dosages and reaches its therapeutic targets relatively unchanged and in lower, more physiologic concentrations; there is no change in the listed proteins with dermal estrogen administration.[643,646] Estrogen patches are used in doses of 0.05 to 0.07 µg/kg up to 0.08 to 0.12 µg/kg, which is a fraction of an Evorel patch available in Europe given every night or ⅙ to ⅛ of a Vivelle-Dot patch available in the United States once or twice per week.[618] There is individual variation up to 10% in absorption, but in an individual similar plasma levels are achieved using 2 mg daily oral 17β-estradiol, 2 mg daily gel, and 100 mg patch.[639] However, these patches are not FDA approved for such use at this time.

If during the 3 to 6 months after discontinuing gonadal steroid therapy spontaneous puberty does not ensue or the concentrations of plasma gonadotropins and plasma testosterone in boys or plasma estradiol in girls do not increase, the treatment may be repeated. Only one or two courses of therapy usually are necessary. When treatment is discontinued after bone age has advanced, for example, to 12 to 13 years in girls or 13 or 14 years in boys, patients with constitutional delay usually continue pubertal development on their own, whereas those with gonadotropin deficiency do not progress and may regress.

Functional hypogonadotropic hypogonadism associated with chronic disease is treated by alleviating the underlying problem. Delayed puberty in this situation is usually a result of inadequate nutrition and low weight

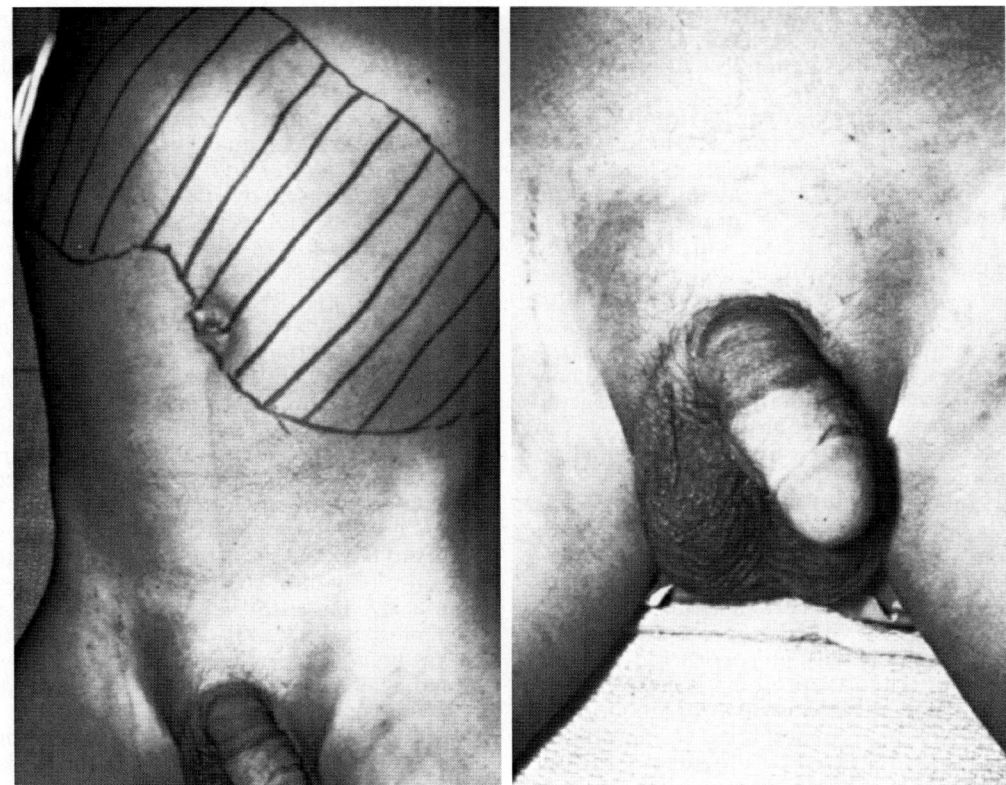

Figure 25-61 A boy aged 1 year and 5 months with a human chorionic gonadotropin (hCG)-secreting hepatoblastoma. Notice the outline of the large liver *(left)* and the penile enlargement *(right)*. The testes were 2 × 1 cm, and pubic hair was stage 2. The plasma hCG level was 50 mIU/mL; the plasma testosterone level was 168 ng/dL; and the plasma α-fetoprotein level was 160,000 ng/mL. Metastatic lesions in both lungs were seen on the chest radiograph. To convert testosterone values to SI units, see Figure 25-19. To convert hCG values to international units per liter, multiply by 1.0. To convert α-fetoprotein values to micrograms per liter, multiply by 1.0. (From Kaplan SL, Grumbach MM. Pathogenesis of sexual precocity. In: Grumbach MM, Sizonenko PC, Aubert ML, eds. *Control of the Onset of Puberty.* Baltimore, MD: Williams & Wilkins; 1990:620-660.)

survival time of only 3 months.[706] About 20% of mediastinal germ cell tumors occur in boys with 47,XXY or mosaic Klinefelter syndrome, a prevalence 30 to 50 times more common than in unaffected boys. Plasma α-fetoprotein is a useful additional marker for yolk sac (endodermal sinus) or mixed germ cell tumors; the cells in the tumor that secrete α-fetoprotein appear to differ from those that secrete hCG. Rarely, the germ cells contain enough aromatase activity to convert circulating C19 precursors (of adrenal origin after adrenarche) to estradiol, which in some instances is sufficient to induce breast development.[707]

Some teratomas, chorioepitheliomas, and mixed germ cell tumors in the hypothalamic region (or in the mediastinum, lungs, gonads, or retroperitoneum); certain pineal tumors (usually a germ cell tumor or mixed germ cell tumor); and, less commonly, a chorioepithelioma or its variants cause sexual precocity in boys by secreting hCG rather than by activating the pituitary gonadotropin-gonadal axis via the hypothalamic GnRH pulse generator.

Intracranial germ cell tumors account for 3% to 11% of malignant CNS tumors in children and adolescents, with a predominance in the Far East. Germ cell tumors of the hypothalamus or pineal region constitute fewer than 1% of primary CNS tumors in Western countries but account for 4.5% of such tumors in Japan. The prevalence of intracranial germ cell tumors is 2.6 times greater in males than in females, but germ cell tumors in the suprasellar-hypothalamic region do not exhibit a sex predominance and are generally associated with pituitary hormone deficiencies including diabetes insipidus and delayed puberty.[440] Germ cell tumors do not cause gonadotropin-induced ISP

in females because of the paucity of effects of hCG in prepubertal females. However, CPP may occur through disinhibition of the hypothalamic GnRH pulse generator by local mass effects. Calcification of the pineal is found in 8% to 11% of 8- to 11-year-old children and by itself is not indicative of a tumor.

Germ cell tumors that secrete hCG are rarely located in the thalamus and basal ganglia. In "true" pure CNS germ cell tumors (germinomas), hCG cannot be readily detected in the circulation but may be detected in the cerebrospinal fluid.[440] In mixed germ cell tumors, hCG is commonly found in the blood as well as in cerebrospinal fluid. Extremely elevated levels of hCG in a CNS tumor suggest a primary intracranial choriocarcinoma or germ cell tumor with a high risk of tumor hemorrhage during biopsy, and surgical removal or debulking rather than diagnostic biopsy may be the initial operative approach.[708]

Mixed germ cell tumors and especially pure germinomas are radiosensitive, and if the bone age is less than 11 years, sexual precocity may regress, only to progress later into normal puberty. Long-term survival is reported in 88% of patients with CNS germ cell tumors after appropriate therapy. However, testicular germ cell tumors are occasionally found years after successful therapy for CNS germ cell tumors, so long-term surveillance is always indicated.[444]

Pineal cysts are a rare cause of CPP.[709]

All pituitary adenomas, including gonadotropin-secreting pituitary adenomas, are exceedingly rare in children. An LH-secreting pituitary adenoma (basal serum LH of 900 IU/L with no rise after GnRH) and a prolactin-secreting pituitary adenoma (215 µg/L) caused sexual precocity in two boys with serum testosterone levels of 7 nmol/L (200 ng/dL).[710] Prepubertal values returned after removal of these chromophobe adenomas with suprasellar extension.

Precocious Androgen Secretion Caused by the Adrenal Gland

Virilizing Congenital Adrenal Hyperplasia. Virilizing CAH caused by a defect in 21-hydroxylation (CYP21 deficiency) leads to elevated androgen concentrations and masculinization and is a common cause of GISP in boys.[711] Approximately 75% of patients with CYP21 deficiency have salt loss resulting from impaired aldosterone secretion as well as low serum sodium and high serum potassium concentrations. Increased plasma concentrations of 17-hydroxyprogesterone, increased levels of urinary 17-ketosteroids and pregnanetriol, and advanced bone age and rapid growth are characteristic. Recent discovery of alternative steroidogenic pathways toward the production of virilizing androgens in this condition hold promise for new methods of evaluation of optimal treatment regimens.[712,713]

Treatment with glucocorticoids suppresses the abnormal androgen secretion and arrests virilization; treatment with mineralocorticoids, when necessary, corrects the electrolyte imbalance. Virilizing CAH accompanied by hypertension occurs in 11β-hydroxylase deficiency (CYP11B1 deficiency); the progressive virilization ceases and the blood pressure falls to normal with glucocorticoid therapy. All forms of CAH are inherited as autosomal recessive traits. Untreated virilizing CAH causes anovulatory amenorrhea in females and oligospermia in males; these conditions are reversible with treatment. Delayed treatment of virilizing CAH may reveal GnRH-dependent CPP (secondary CPP) as a consequence of the advanced somatic and hypothalamic maturation resulting from long exposure to adrenal androgen. Further difficulty is presented in the treatment of CAH during the pubertal years, when androgen secretion normally increases and increased clearance of glucocorticoids at puberty in girls may alter dosing requirements.

As with most chronic diseases originating in childhood, transition of care to adult providers during late teenage years is essential. Comprehensive care clinics are suggested to offer the best method to provide care to children and adults with CAH.[714]

Virilizing Adrenal Tumor. Virilizing adrenal carcinomas or adenomas secrete large amounts of DHEA and DHEAS and, on occasion, testosterone. Glucocorticoids do not suppress the increased secretion of adrenal androgens to the normal range for age in carcinoma, as they do in CAH. Cushing syndrome resulting from adrenal carcinoma may cause ISP and growth failure in boys. Rarely, an adrenal adenoma produces both testosterone and aldosterone, leading to sexual precocity and hypertension with hypokalemia.

Adrenal rests, or heterotopic adrenal tissue in the testes, are found in a over 90% of boys with CAH and may enlarge (sometimes to massive size) and may mimic bilateral or unilateral interstitial cell tumors. The size of these testicular adrenal rest tissues, or TART, were thought to be related to poor control of CAH during childhood and adolescence, but recent evidence shows no relationship between biochemical control or plasma ACTH concentration or growth patterns, raising the likelihood that other control mechanisms perhaps originating in fetal life determine the size of these tumors.[715] MRI sonography, including Doppler flow studies of the testes, is useful to define the extent and nature of the testicular masses. These tumors can significantly decrease fertility, but surgical management, including enucleation of the tumor or tumors, has been useful to prevent further damage to the testes and improve the potential for fertility in some but not all studies.

NROB1 (DAX1) Gene Mutations. Two cases of *NROB1* frameshift mutations demonstrated adrenal failure and GISP that was suppressible by glucocorticoid therapy but not by GnRH agonist. The exceedingly high ACTH levels, possibly acting through the human melanocortin 1 receptor present in human Leydig cells, may have been the underlying cause of the increased steroidogenesis and testosterone secretion that were reversed by glucocorticoid treatment. Because *NROB1* inhibits transactivation of SF1, a regulator of steroidogenic genes, loss of *NROB1* inhibition of SF1 transcriptional activity also may have had a role.[716,717]

Leydig Cell Tumor. Testicular tumors are rare in childhood, representing 1% to 2% of all pediatric solid tumors, and Leydig cell tumors make up only 1.5% of those.[718] Androgen-producing Leydig cell tumors rarely are malignant and are slow growing but must be treated or epiphyseal fusion will limit height and precocious puberty will affect social development. They derive from primordial mesenchyme, are classified as interstitial cell tumors, and occur most frequently around the age of 4 to 5 years. Unilateral enlargement (often nodular) of the testis usually occurs in boys with this neoplasm (although 5% to 10% of cases are bilateral); in contrast, both testes are usually of normal size (small) for chronologic age in boys with CAH or a virilizing adrenal tumor.[719] Although LH receptor–activating mutations were detected in several boys with sporadic Leydig cell adenomas,[695] no known mutations can be found in others.

Pituitary Gonadotropin–Independent Familial Premature Leydig Cell and Germ Cell Maturation: Familial or Sporadic Testotoxicosis.[300,695,720-732] Pituitary gonadotropin–independent familial premature Leydig cell and germ cell maturation, or testotoxicosis,[720,721,725] causes boys to develop secondary sexual characteristics with penile enlargement, which may be present at birth, and bilateral enlargement of testes to the early or midpubertal range, although the testes often are smaller than expected in relation to penile growth and pubertal maturation (Fig. 25-62). Premature maturation of Leydig and Sertoli cells and spermatogenesis occur. Leydig cell hyperplasia may occur; the Leydig cells in affected boys produce dimeric inhibin B as well as testosterone, and Leydig cells and spermatogonia stain positively for the α and β$_B$ segments of inhibin. The rate of linear growth is rapid, skeletal maturation is advanced, and muscular development is prominent. The presence of prepubertal basal and GnRH-stimulated gonadotropin concentrations, lack of a pubertal pattern of LH pulsatility (as measured by immunologic or bioassay techniques), and normal pubertal or adult testosterone levels and clearance of testosterone are characteristic (Table 25-37). The onset of adrenarche and its

---

TABLE 25-37

Testotoxicosis: Clinical and Laboratory Characteristics

Sex-limited autosomal dominant inheritance; activating mutation in the gene encoding the LH receptor

Early onset of sexual precocity in boys, with bilateral testicular enlargement

Prepubertal immunologic and biologic LH response to GnRH; prepubertal LH pulse secretory pattern

Concentration of plasma testosterone in pubertal range

Premature Leydig cell and seminiferous tubule maturation

No CNS, adrenal, or testicular abnormalities demonstrable by radiologic or hormonal studies

Lack of suppression of plasma testosterone or physical signs of puberty by GnRH agonist

CNS, central nervous system; GnRH, gonadotropin-releasing hormone; LH, luteinizing hormone.

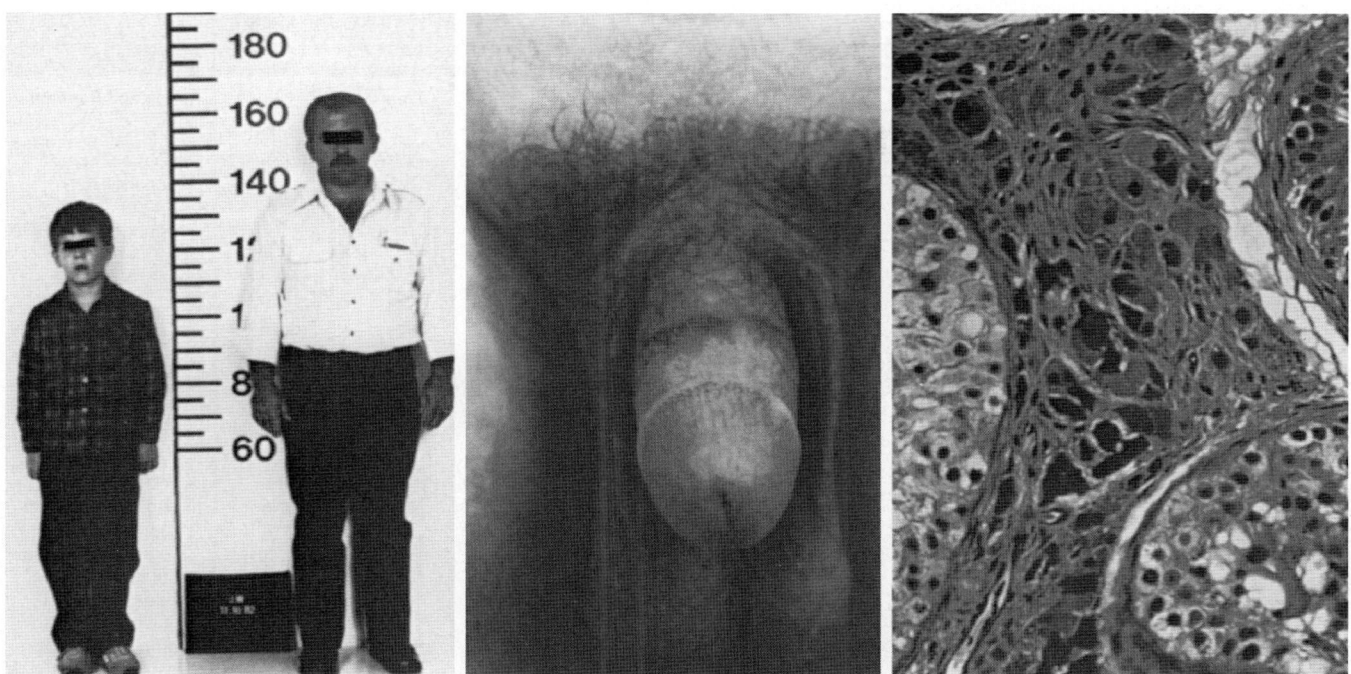

Figure 25-62 *Left*, A boy aged 5.5 years and his 28-year-old father with familial testotoxicosis. The boy exhibited signs of sexual precocity by 3 years of age. His height was 130.6 cm (+4.8 SD [standard deviation]), and his bone age was 12.5 years. The plasma testosterone level was 267 ng/dL; the dihydrotestosterone level was 46 ng/dL; and the dehydroepiandrosterone sulfate (DHEAS) level was 23 μg/dL. The plasma luteinizing hormone (LH) and follicle-stimulating hormone (FSH) levels were low, and neither rose after treatment. Pulsatile LH secretion was not demonstrable. Treatment with deslorelin, a gonadotropin-releasing hormone (GnRH) agonist, had no effect. The father had begun sexual maturation by 3 years of age and had reached a final height of 162.6 cm in his early teens. The plasma testosterone level was 294 ng/dL; the LH level was 0.5 ng/mL (LER-960); and the FSH level was 0.5 ng/mL (LER-869). The father had an adult-type LH and FSH response to GnRH; the LH level increased to 7.5 ng/mL, and the FSH level increased to 2 ng/mL. At least 28 male family members over nine generations are affected. To convert dihydrotestosterone values to nanomoles per liter, multiply by 0.03467. For other conversions to SI units, see Figures 25-19 and 25-20. *Center*, External genitalia of the 5.5-year-old boy. The penis measured 12 × 2.8 cm, the right testis was 4 × 2 cm, and the left testis was 3.5 × 2.5 cm. *Right*, Testis of the boy showed Leydig cell maturation without Reinke crystalloids and spermatogenesis (Mallory trichrome stain).

biochemical marker, serum DHEAS, correlate with bone age rather than chronologic age.

Treatment with an GnRH agonist does not suppress testicular function or maturation in the initial phase.[720] In late childhood or early adolescence, fertility is achieved and an adult pattern of LH secretion and response to GnRH is demonstrable[725]; secondary GnRH-dependent CPP may be superimposed on the substrate of testotoxicosis. In some adults, impaired spermatogenic function is associated with elevated concentrations of plasma FSH. Testotoxicosis may occur sporadically, probably as a consequence of a germline mutation or even a postzygotic one, but it is usually inherited as a sex-limited autosomal dominant trait. A kindred with nine generations of affected males has been reported; obligatory female carriers of the trait were unaffected, because constitutional activation of the LH receptor on the ovary causes no ill effects.[728]

Heterozygous activating mutations of the heterotrimeric G_s protein–coupled LHCGR that in concert transduce the LH/hCG signal to the main effector, adenyl cyclase, are the cause of testotoxicosis[733] (Fig. 25-63). The LH receptor cloned from the human is a glycoprotein of 80 to 90 kDa that belongs to a subfamily of the seven transmembrane–spanning, G protein–coupled receptors. The gene is localized to chromosome 2p21 (the same as for the FSH receptor); it spans at least 70 kilobases and contains 11 exons separated by 10 introns. The large glycosylated N-terminal extracellular hormone binding domain of the 701–amino acid LHCGR is encoded by exons 1 through 10. A single exon, the large exon 11, encodes the entire G protein–linked transmembrane domain with its seven α-helical segments connected by alternating extracellular and intra-

cellular loops, the intracellular domain, and the three untranslated regions—almost two thirds of the receptor.[727]

Fourteen constitutive activating heterozygous missense mutations are reported in more than 60 patients[733] (see Fig. 25-63). Nine mutations were located between amino acid residues 542 and 581, suggesting a mutation hot spot. There appears to be a limited repertoire of mutations in American boys, consistent with a founder effect. European pedigrees are more diverse. A model of the transmembrane domain of the receptor provides novel suggestions for the structural and functional effects of these activating mutations.[731] Transfected cultured cells with these mutations exhibited increased basal cAMP production in the absence of agonist, observations consistent with a constitutive activating mutation.[732] Various possibilities for the conformational changes in the LH receptor that lead to its constitutive activation have been considered. Inactivating mutations of the LHCGR and their clinical consequences are discussed earlier in this chapter.

Although affected boys do not respond to chronic administration of a GnRH agonist with suppression of testosterone secretion, testosterone secretion, height velocity and rate of bone maturation, and aggressive and hyperactive behavior have reportedly been decreased by treatment with oral medroxyprogesterone acetate[720] (Table 25-38).

Ketoconazole, an orally active substituted imidazole derivative, suppresses gonadal and adrenal biosynthesis by inhibiting the enzyme CYP17, which regulates both 17-hydroxylation and the scission (17,20-lyase) of 17α-hydroxypregnenolone (Δ5-17P) to DHEA (see "Nature and Regulation of Adrenal Androgens"). In the dosage used for treatment of testotoxicosis (200 mg every 8 to 12 hours,

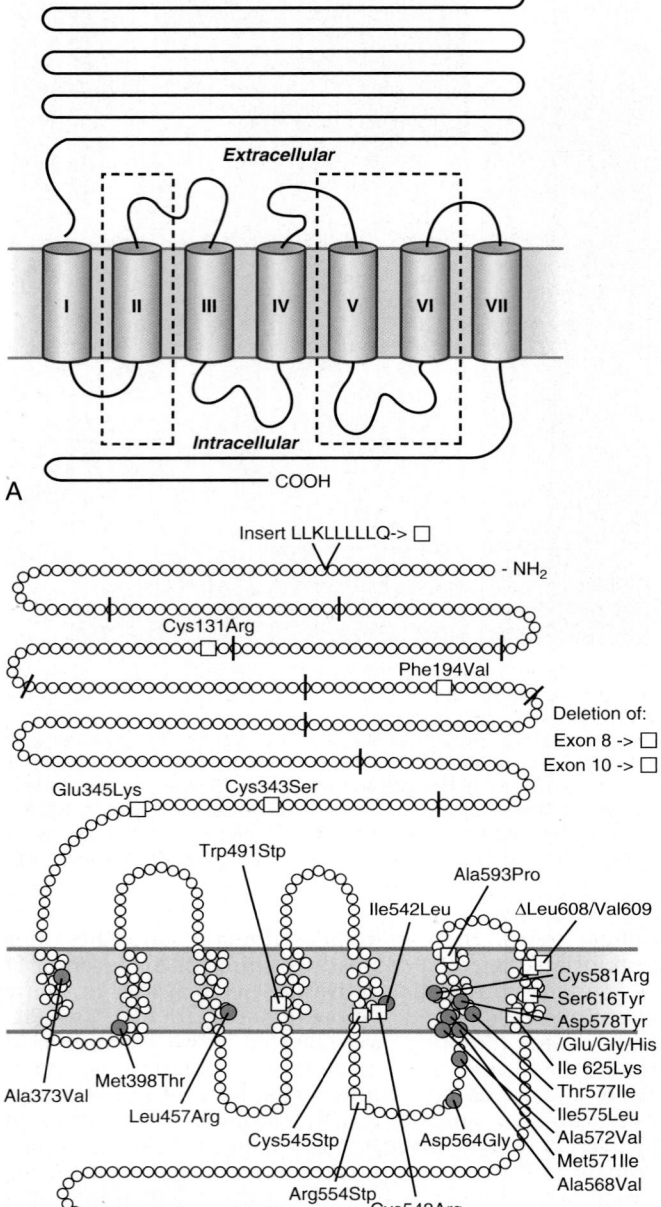

TABLE 25-38

Pharmacologic Therapy for Sexual Precocity

Disorder	Treatment	Action and Rationale
GnRH Dependent		
True or central precocious puberty	GnRH agonists	Desensitization of gonadotrophs; blocks action of endogenous GnRH
GnRH Independent		
Incomplete sexual precocity		
Girls		
Autonomous ovarian cysts	Medroxyprogesterone acetate	Inhibition of ovarian steroidogenesis; regression of cyst (inhibition of FSH release)
McCune-Albright syndrome	Medroxyprogesterone acetate*	Inhibition of ovarian steroidogenesis; regression of cyst (inhibition of FSH release)
	Third-generation aromatase inhibitor (e.g., letrozole)	Inhibition of P450 aromatase; blocks estrogen synthesis
Boys		
Familial testotoxicosis	Ketoconazole*	Inhibition of CYP17 (mainly 17,20-lyase activity)
	Flutamide or bicalutamide and letrozole or anastrozole	Antiandrogen Inhibition of aromatase; blocks estrogen synthesis
	Medroxyprogesterone acetate*	Inhibition of testicular steroidogenesis

*If true precocious puberty develops, an LHRH agonist can be added.
CYP17, cytochrome P450 17α-hydroxylase/17,20-lyase; FSH, follicle-stimulating hormone; GnRH, gonadotropin-releasing hormone; LHRH, luteinizing hormone–releasing hormone.
Modified from Grumbach MM, Kaplan SL. Recent advances in the diagnosis and management of sexual precocity. *Acta Paediatr Jpn.* 1988:30(Suppl): 155-175.

Figure 25-63 **A,** The serpentine, seven-transmembrane, G_s protein–coupled human luteinizing hormone/human chorionic gonadotropin (hLH/hCG) receptor with its large extracellular domain and the intracellular domain. The seven helical transmembrane domains are indicated by roman numerals. **B,** Mutations in the LH receptor protein are shown in the schematic structure of the LH receptor protein and localization of the inactivating *(open squares)* and activating *(blue-filled circles)* mutations in the human LH receptor. Notice the cluster of mutations in the VI transmembrane helix and third cytoplasmic loop. The Asx578Gly mutation is the most common activating mutation. The *short lines* across the amino acid chain separate the 11 exons. (A redrawn from Yano K, Kohn LD, Saji M, et al. A case of male limited precocious puberty caused by a point mutation in the second transmembrane domain of the luteinizing hormone choriogonadotropin receptor gene. *Biochem Biophys Res Commun.* 1996;220:1036-1042; B from Themmen APN, Huhtaniemi IT. Mutations of gonadotropins and gonadotropin receptors. *Endocr Rev.* 2000;21:551-583.)

given orally[734]), the agent produces a mild transient decrease in cortisol secretion and interferes with binding of testosterone to TeBG. Secondary CPP often occurs when the bone age advances to or has already reached the pubertal range (usually >11.5 years), at which time the addi-

tion of a GnRH agonist is appropriate.[734] Ketoconazole can cause hepatic injury, which is usually mild and reversible, but in rare cases hepatotoxicity is severe. Reversible renal injury, rash, and interstitial pneumonia were reported in a patient who tolerated lower doses, suggesting a dose-response effect. Nonetheless, five patients treated with ketoconazole experienced no side effects other than one mild and transient elevation of liver enzymes; they had appropriate age of onset of true puberty and reached an adult height almost identical to the target height (a mean increase of 8 cm over the initially predicted height), suggesting great benefit of this therapy in this condition.[735,736]

The antiandrogen (and antimineralocorticoid) spironolactone, in combination with testolactone, an inhibitor of aromatase (CYP19), the key enzyme in the conversion of androgens to estrogens, is also used to treat testotoxicosis.[737] The addition of a GnRH agonist is a useful step to suppress pituitary gonadotropin secretion and secondary CPP that may later develop.[731] More potent nonsteroidal antiandrogens (e.g., flutamide, nilutamide) and aromatase inhibitors (e.g., letrozole) inhibit the rate of skeletal maturation and linear growth by suppressing estradiol synthesis, potentially with greater therapeutic efficacy.[133,134] The combination of bicalutamide and anastrozole is proposed as another approach.[738] Table 25-38 lists the various agents used in the treatment of testotoxicosis; which of these agents or combination of agents will be effective and safe for long-term treatment remains to be determined.

A study of an untreated boy with testotoxicosis (GISP) had the expected pattern of rapid growth and early cessation, and the adult height of 174 cm was within target height range (171.5 to 188.5 cm), indicating the critical importance of individual approaches to affected boys when considering treatment to maximize height.[737]

Follow-up of boys with testotoxicosis indicates an increased risk of seminoma in adult life and Leydig cell adenoma in later childhood.[695,739] One boy with testotoxicosis developed nodular Leydig cell hyperplasia at 10 years of age.[740] These cases support a relationship between an activating mutation of the gene encoding the LH receptor and of Leydig cell tumors.[741]

Gonadotropin-Independent Sexual Precocity and Pseudohypoparathyroidism Type Ia. A mutation in $G_s\alpha$ can constitutively activate or inactivate adenyl cyclase.[742] Two boys who presented in infancy with classic pseudohypoparathyroidism type Ia (PHPIa), a disorder characterized by resistance to hormones whose action is mediated by cAMP, developed signs of sexual precocity with the hormonal characteristics of testotoxicosis (i.e., gonadotropin-independent sexual precocity) at about 24 months of age. Whereas the alanine residue is usually absolutely conserved in all heterotrimeric G proteins, both of these patients had a unique Ala366Ser mutation in one allele of the $G_s\alpha$ gene. PHPIa is caused by a wide variety of inactivating mutations in $G_s\alpha$ that lead to an approximately 50% reduction in $G_s\alpha$ activity in functional assays.

The paradox of a $G_s\alpha$ mutation causing both inactivation with PHP and constitutive activation with testotoxicosis was resolved by the in vitro demonstration that, unlike other activating mutations of $G_s\alpha$, which involve mutations inhibiting its intrinsic GTPase activity and decreasing the rate of hydrolysis of GTP to GDP, the mutation in these two boys caused accelerated dissociation of GDP at 33°C in transfected Leydig cells but was rapidly degraded at 37°C in a lymphoma cell line[743] and at 33°C and 37°C in skin fibroblasts transfected with the mutation. These observations explain the clinical consequences of increased $G_s\alpha$ activity in the testis, which are 3° to 5°C cooler than the body, and the tissue specificity and temperature dependency of the mutation. The mother of one patient appeared to be a mosaic for the $G_s\alpha$ mutation; in the other boy, a germline mutation was likely.

Girls. GISP in girls (see Table 25-25) is caused by autonomous estrogen secretion by an ovarian cyst or tumor or an adrenal neoplasm or by inadvertent exposure to estrogen. Girls harboring a teratoma or teratocarcinoma (or a CNS germ cell tumor) that secretes hCG have experienced sexual precocity caused by concurrent estrogen secretion by the tumor but no effect from the hCG alone; these girls also may have galactorrhea, especially if chorionic somatomammotropin (hCS or hPL) is also secreted.

Autonomous Ovarian Follicular Cysts. The most common childhood estrogen-secreting ovarian mass and ovarian cause of sexual precocity is the follicular cyst.[743] Antral follicles up to about 8 mm in diameter are common in the ovaries of normal prepubertal girls and may be seen in third trimester fetuses and newborn infants.[744] They may appear and regress spontaneously. Larger follicular cysts may be discovered because of the presence of an abdominal mass or abdominal pain, especially after torsion or as an unexpected finding on pelvic sonography performed for other reasons. Occasionally, the antral follicles secrete estrogen and may form large masses, or the follicular cysts may recur and cause recurrent signs of sexual precocity and acyclic vaginal bleeding. Enlarged antral follicles or cysts occur in premature thelarche, CPP, and transient or incomplete sexual precocity. In some patients with ovarian follicular cysts, the transient or recurrent sexual precocity is GnRH independent (Fig. 25-64). The concentration of

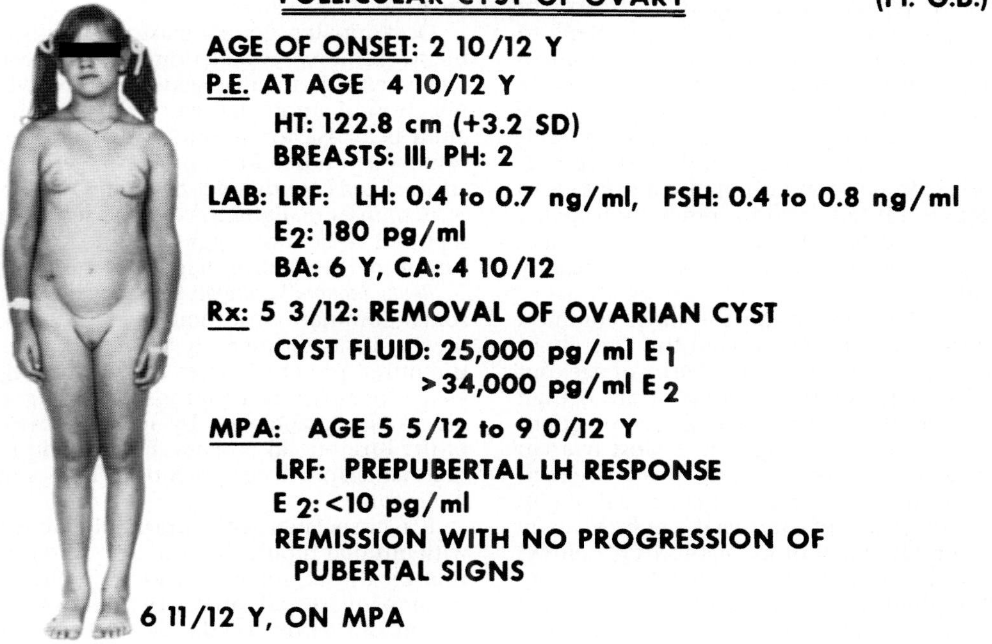

FOLLICULAR CYST OF OVARY   **(Pt. G.B.)**

<u>AGE OF ONSET</u>: 2 10/12 Y

<u>P.E. AT AGE</u> 4 10/12 Y

    HT: 122.8 cm (+3.2 SD)
    BREASTS: III, PH: 2

<u>LAB</u>: LRF: LH: 0.4 to 0.7 ng/ml, FSH: 0.4 to 0.8 ng/ml
    E_2: 180 pg/ml
    BA: 6 Y, CA: 4 10/12

<u>Rx</u>: 5 3/12: REMOVAL OF OVARIAN CYST
    CYST FLUID: 25,000 pg/ml E_1
                >34,000 pg/ml E_2

<u>MPA</u>: AGE 5 5/12 to 9 0/12 Y

    LRF: PREPUBERTAL LH RESPONSE
    E_2: <10 pg/ml
    REMISSION WITH NO PROGRESSION OF
      PUBERTAL SIGNS

6 11/12 Y, ON MPA

Figure 25-64 A girl aged 4 years and 10 months with recurrent, "autonomous" follicular cysts of the ovary. For conversion to SI units, see Figure 25-19. BA, bone age; CA, chronologic age; E_2, estradiol; FSH, follicle-stimulating hormone; LH, luteinizing hormone; LRF, luteinizing hormone-releasing factor; MPA, medroxyprogesterone acetate (oral); P.E., physical examination; Rx, treatment. (From Kaplan SL, Grumbach MM. Pathogenesis of sexual precocity. In: Grumbach MM, Sizonenko PC, Aubert ML, eds. *Control of the Onset of Puberty.* Baltimore, MD: Williams & Wilkins; 1990:620-660.)

estradiol fluctuates, usually correlating with changes in the size of the follicular cyst or cysts when monitored by pelvic sonography, and may increase to levels found in granulosa cell tumors, although values may also be in the pubertal range.

These patients do not have increased plasma granulosa cell tumor markers such as AMH or inhibin.[745] The concentration of LH is suppressed, a pubertal pattern of pulsatile LH secretion is absent, and the LH rise induced by GnRH is prepubertal. A constitutive activating mutation of the FSH receptor has not been described in a female, but a heterozygous mutation, Asp567Gly, was detected in the third intracellular loop of the FSH receptor in a hypophysectomized man who, despite the gonadotropin deficiency, was fertile and had normal-sized testes.[733] Accordingly, the possibility that some girls with recurrent ovarian cysts harbor an activating mutation of the FSH receptor seems worthy of study. The McCune-Albright syndrome may lead to recurrent ovarian cysts even in the apparent initial absence of other features of this disorder due to somatic activating mutations in the gene encoding the α-subunit of the heterotrimeric G_s protein. The luteinization of follicular cysts may be related to subtle elevations and increased pulses of plasma FSH. Ovarian cysts and sexual precocity have been associated with the fragile X syndrome in girls.[746]

Estradiol-secreting ovarian cysts occur in preterm infants born before 30 weeks' gestation; they are associated with edema of the labia majora and, in some instances, of the lower abdominal wall.[747] The LH and FSH response to GnRH in these patients suggests GnRH dependence, and treatment with medroxyprogesterone acetate is associated with regression of the cysts. A case of massive ovarian edema associated with ovarian cysts found in a 6-month-old with breast and pubic hair development has been reported.[748]

GnRH agonists are useful in the treatment of ovarian follicular cysts associated with CPP (GISP) but not of so-called autonomous cysts. However, autonomously functioning ovarian follicular cysts, whether recurrent or manifesting in an isolated episode, often respond to treatment with oral medroxyprogesterone acetate, which seems to prevent recurrence, to accelerate involution of the follicular cysts,[748] and to reduce the risk of torsion. The use of a potent aromatase inhibitor such as letrozole to reduce estradiol secretion is another potential approach to treatment and has been successfully used in girls with no stigmata of McCune-Albright syndrome other than autonomous ovarian cysts.[749] Surgical intervention is rarely indicated; a large or persistent cyst can be reduced by puncture at laparoscopy and the size of the cyst can be monitored readily by pelvic sonography.

Ovarian Tumors. Ovarian tumors are the most common genitourinary tumors of girls,[750,751] accounting for about 1% of all tumors in girls younger than 17 years of age, but they are rare in the prepubertal period. Most are benign according to most reports,[752] but a referral center might find a majority of tumors are malignant.[753] Most ovarian tumors arise from germ cells or sex cord–stromal cells in childhood with fewer than 20% being of epithelial origin, whereas in adults, most are of epithelial origin.[754] Early diagnosis of most childhood tumors of the ovary allows successful cure, unlike ovarian cancer in adult women. Most of these girls present with pain or an abdominal mass. Tumors smaller than 5 cm at diagnosis are more likely to be non-neoplastic, and those larger than 10 cm are more likely to be neoplastic.[743,755] Ultrasonography is helpful in evaluation but does not usually lead to the correct histologic diagnosis. The successful use of tumor markers for

diagnosis varies by cause. For example, in one series, cystic teratomas resulted in lactate dehydrogenase (LDH) elevation and an increased erythrocyte sedimentation rate; immature teratomas produced elevated levels of LDH, α-fetoprotein, and cancer antigen 125 (CA125); and granulosa cell tumors had elevated sex steroids (estradiol or testosterone[753] or both).[756]

Granulosa cell tumor of the ovary is rare in childhood, although theca cell tumors are even less common.[757] Because most produce estrogen, incomplete isosexual precocity occurs in the youngest girls affected. Characteristic histologic features of juvenile granulosa cell tumors include nodular architecture, follicle formation, abundant interstitial and intrafollicular acid mucopolysaccharide-rich fluid, irregular microcysts, individual cell necrosis, and high mitotic activity (mean activity, 11 mitotic figures per 10 high-power fields). Size can vary from 2.5 to 25 cm, with a mean diameter of 12 cm. The interstitial mucinous fluid consists predominantly of hyaluronic acid. Prognosis is good, the mortality rate being about 3%, but delay in treatment leads to substantial complications. In one series, girls who presented with ISP and were correctly diagnosed had no intra-abdominal spread and had Federation of Gynecology and Obstetrics (FIGO) stage IA disease, whereas those who presented with acute abdominal symptoms had 50% prevalence of intra-abdominal spread and two recurrences after surgery. When the diagnosis was made after normal puberty had begun, some girls experienced virilization or abdominal symptoms; 80% had intra-abdominal spread, and 30% had recurrence with FIGO stage IIC.

Approximately 80% of granulosa cell tumors can be palpated on bimanual examination, whereas fewer than 5% are bilateral or clinically malignant. The concentration of plasma estradiol may increase to high levels, and serum FSH and LH concentrations are usually suppressed. AMH and inhibin are sensitive tumor markers and are used to screen for metastases especially if elevated at diagnosis[758]; an elevated estradiol concentration in an affected patient younger than 9 years of age or an abnormal rise in concentration of plasma AMH or inhibin at any age suggests recurrence or metastasis.

Occasionally, gonadoblastomas in streak gonads, rare lipoid tumors, cystadenomas, and ovarian carcinomas secrete estrogens, androgens, or both. Even with successful resection of a gonadal sex steroid–secreting neoplasm, the child is at risk for secondary CPP in the future. Gonadal tumors composed of a mixture of germ cells and sex cord–stromal cells are distinct from gonadoblastoma. They may be benign or malignant, with the Sertoli-Leydig cell tumors reported to be most aggressive.[759] α-Fetoprotein and other tumor markers aid in diagnosis.

Peutz-Jeghers Syndrome. Peutz-Jeghers syndrome, an autosomal dominant syndrome, is usually caused by mutations in the gene located on 9p13.3 that encodes a serine/threonine protein kinase, STK11, leading to haploinsufficiency of this novel tumor-suppressing gene.[760] This condition is characterized by mucocutaneous pigmentation of the lips, buccal mucosa, fingers, and toes; gastrointestinal hamartomatous polyposis; and a predisposition to malignancy.

It is associated with a rare, distinctive sex cord tumor with annular tubules in both boys and girls. Estrogen secretion by the tumor may lead to feminization in girls and incomplete sexual precocity in boys. Less frequently, a feminizing Sertoli-Leydig cell tumor has been found in patients with Peutz-Jeghers syndrome. The rare feminizing large-cell calcifying Sertoli cell tumors of the testes present with gynecomastia in boys and are found in Peutz-Jeghers syndrome and Carney complex, the latter of which is most often caused by *PRKAR1A* mutations, the gene encoding regulatory subunit type 1 of protein kinase A.

Sex cord–stromal cell tumors derive from the celomic epithelium or mesenchymal cells of the embryonic gonads and are composed of granulosa, theca, Leydig, and Sertoli cells. Estrogen secretion from these tumors can cause ISP in girls, and androgen secretion can cause virilization. Inhibin A and B activin are produced, as is AMH; all serve as useful tumor markers. Sex cord–stromal cell tumors not associated with Peutz-Jeghers syndrome are malignant in 25% of cases; these tumors can grow quite large, but those associated with Peutz-Jeghers syndrome are often small and multiple, and they contain calcifications.[761]

Girls with this disorder should be examined at regular intervals for the presence of gonadal tumors by pelvic sonography. Peutz-Jeghers syndrome should be considered in boys with unexplained gynecomastia, expecially if in the prepubertal years.

Adrenal Adenomas. Adrenocortical tumors are rare in childhood (0.6% of all childhood tumors and 0.3% of all malignant childhood tumors), but most produce steroid hormones, whereas those in adults usually do not. The median age at diagnosis is 4 years, but 41% of these tumors manifest before 2 years and 71% before 5 years of age. Most cause virilization or Cushing syndrome, but adrenal tumors may produce estrogen as well as androgens and can cause sexual precocity in a girl or gynecomastia in a boy. One adrenal adenoma found in a 7-year-old girl expressed the gene for aromatase, demonstrating that the tumor could directly produce estrogen[762] to a level of 145 pg/mL, within the range found in adrenal carcinomas.

Boys and Girls

McCune-Albright Syndrome. McCune-Albright syndrome occurs about twice as often in girls than in boys; it is sporadic and is caused by somatic activating mutations (Cys or His to Arg201) in exon 8 of the gene (*GNAS1*) encoding the α-subunit of the trimeric GTP-binding protein ($G_s\alpha$) that stimulates adenyl cyclase.[763,764] This leads to a constitutive ligand-free activation of cellular function in a mosaic distribution, leading to a high variability of organ involvement and degree of severity.[429] It is characterized by the triad of irregularly edged hyperpigmented macules (café au lait spots of the coast of Maine type); a slowly progressive bone disorder, polyostotic fibrous dysplasia, that can involve any bone and is frequently associated with facial asymmetry and hyperostosis of the base of the skull; and, more commonly in girls, GISP (Fig. 25-65 and Table 25-39). At least two of the features must be present to consider the diagnosis.

Autonomous hyperfunction most commonly involves the ovary, but other endocrine involvement includes the thyroid gland (nodular hyperplasia with thyrotoxicosis or, remarkably, with euthyroid status); adrenal gland (multiple hyperplastic nodules with Cushing syndrome that may occur in the neonatal period and may be followed by adrenal insufficiency),[765] pituitary gland (adenoma or mammosomatotroph hyperplasia with gigantism, acromegaly, and hyperprolactinemia), and parathyroid glands (adenoma or hyperplasia with hyperparathyroidism).[766,767] Hypophosphatemic vitamin D–resistant rickets or osteomalacia occurs either because of overproduction of a phosphaturic factor, phosphatonin, that is secreted by the bone lesions or because of an intrinsic renal abnormality leading to the excess generation of nephrogenous cAMP in the proximal tubule and, as a result, decreased reabsorption of phosphate. Hepatocellular dysfunction may occur due to expression of the mutant activating gene in liver cells, which leads to jaundice associated with hepatobiliary disease, and pancreatitis. Another nonendocrine manifes-

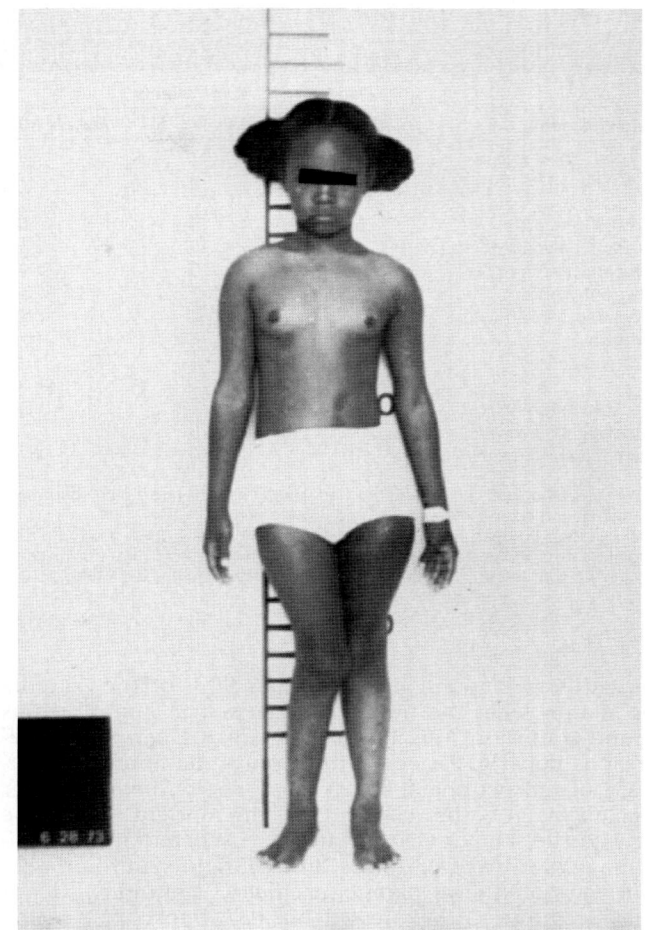

Figure 25-65 A girl aged 7 years and 4 months with gonadotropin-releasing hormone (GnRH)-independent sexual precocity associated with McCune-Albright syndrome. She had breast development since infancy, and it increased noticeably at about 3 years of age; 6 months later, episodes of recurrent vaginal bleeding began. Growth of pubic hair was noticed at about 4 to 5 years. At age 5.5 years, the bone age was 6 years and 11 months; height was +1 SD (standard deviation) above the mean value for age. By 6.5 years, when she was seen at the University of California, San Francisco, the bone age had advanced to 9 years, and height was at +1 SD. Breasts were at Tanner stage 4, and pubic hair at stage 3. Extensive, irregular café au lait macules cover the right side of the face, left lower abdomen and thigh, and both buttocks. A bone survey showed widespread involvement of the long bones with typical polyostotic fibrous dysplasia, the floor of the anterior fossa of the skull was sclerotic, and the diploetic space had widened. She has had two pathologic fractures through bone cysts in the right upper femur. Notice the osseous deformities. Plasma estradiol concentrations were consistently in the pubertal range; the luteinizing hormone (LH) response to GnRH was prepubertal. Results of thyroid function studies were normal, including the thyrotropin response to thyrotropin-releasing hormone administration, and antithyroid antibodies were not detected. Treatment with oral medroxyprogesterone acetate suppressed menses and arrested pubertal development but did not slow skeletal maturation. Her final height is 142 cm (−2.5 SD). Menstrual cycles are regular.

tation is cardiac disease, and patients carry the risk of cardiac arrhythmia and sudden death. This is a sporadic condition that can be concordant or discordant in monozygotic twins.

Considering children with at least one of the signs of McCune-Albright syndrome, 24% had the classic triad, 33% had two signs, and 40% had only one classic sign. The mutation was detected in 46% of blood samples from patients presenting the classic triad but in only 21% and 8% of samples from patients with two signs or one sign, respectively. If an affected tissue was available, the

TABLE 25-39

Clinical Manifestations of McCune-Albright Syndrome in 158 Reported Patients*

Manifestation	% of Patients Total (N = 158)	Male (n = 53)	Female (n = 105)	Mean Age at Diagnosis (yr) and Range	Comments
Fibrous dysplasia	97	51	103	7.7 (0-52)	Polystotic more common than monostotic
Café au lait lesion	85	49	86	7.7 (0-52)	Variable size and number of lesions, irregular border (coast of Maine)
Sexual precocity	52	8	74	4.9 (0.3-9)	Common initial manifestation
Acromegaly/gigantism	27	20	22	14.8 (0.2-42)	17/26 of patients with adenoma on MRI/CT
Hyperprolactinemia	15	9	14	16.0 (0.2-42)	23/42 of acromegalic patients with PRL
Hyperthyroidism	19	7	23	14.4 (0.5-37)	Euthyroid goiter is common
Hypercortisolism	5	4	5	4.4 (0.2-17)	All primary adrenal
Myxomas	5	3	5	34 (17-50)	Extremity myxomas
Osteosarcoma	2	1	2	36 (34-37)	At site of fibrous dysplasia, not related to prior radiation therapy
Rickets/osteomalacia	3	1	3	27.3 (8-52)	Responsive to phosphorus plus calcitriol
Cardiac abnormalities	11	8	9	(0.1-66)	Arrhythmias and CHF reported
Hepatic abnormalities	10	6	10	1.9 (0.3-4)	Neonatal icterus is most common

*Evaluations include clinical and biochemical data; other rarely described manifestations include metabolic acidosis, nephrocalcinosis, developmental delay, thymic and splenic hyperplasia, and colonic polyps.
CHF, congestive heart failure; CT, computed tomography; MRI, magnetic resonance imaging; PRL, prolactin.
Modified from Ringel MD, Schwindinger WF, Levine MA. Clinical implication of genetic defects in G proteins: the molecular basis of McCune-Albright syndrome and Albright hereditary osteodystrophy. *Medicine (Baltimore)*. 1996;75:171-184.

mutation was found in more than 90% of the patients no matter what the number of signs. The mutation was found in 33% of the 39 cases of isolated peripheral precocious puberty. Patients with monostotic fibrous dysplasia, isolated peripheral precocious puberty, neonatal liver cholestasis, or the classic McCune-Albright syndrome all had the same molecular defect.[768] Whereas most endocrine organs involved in McCune-Albright syndrome were not associated with parent specificity,[769] pituitary adenomas secreting GH expressed NESP55 transcripts, which are monoallelically expressed from the maternal alleles rather than from the exon 1A paternal allele. Mutation of *GNAS1* involving Arg201His replacement is associated with apparent premature or exaggerated thelarche and early menarche.[770,771]

Most patients have pigmented skin lesions in infancy which usually increase in size along with body growth.[772] The irregularly bordered, café au lait macules usually do not cross the midline, but they may; they often are located on the same side as the main bone lesions and have a segmented distribution.

The skeletal lesions in the cortex are dysplastic and are filled with spindle cells with poorly organized collagen support; they take the form of scattered cystic areas of rarefaction on radiography and often result in pathologic fractures and progressive deformities (Fig. 25-66). Technetium bone scintigraphy has been the most sensitive approach to the detection of bone lesions before they are visible radiographically. Fractures are most common between the sixth and the tenth years but decline thereafter, and they are more frequent if phosphaturia is present.[773] Patients referred for fibrous dysplasia of the bone in one or more locations are often found to have endocrine or dermatologic manifestations of McCune-Albright syndrome as well as *GNAS1* mutations, so suspicion should be kept high when evaluating fibrous lesions.[774] If the skull is involved, there may be entrapment and compression of optic or auditory nerve foramina, which can lead to blindness, deafness, facial asymmetry, and ptosis. Asymetria of the jaw is another manifestation of McCune-Albright syndrome. Fifty percent of affected children in one series manifested bone abnormalities by 8 years of age.[772] Increased serum GH levels occurs in up to 30% of cases and

have an adverse effect on the skull deformities, depending on the age at onset; somatostatin analogues have variable efficacy. Irradiation of the hypothalamic-pituitary area may be invoked, but it carries a risk of later occurrence of sarcoma. Rapid control of elevated GH can be achieved by the use of long-acting somatostatin agonists such as pegvisomant, which is often but not always successful.[775]

The sexual precocity often begins during the first 2 years of life and is frequently heralded by menstrual bleeding; the cause is autonomously functioning luteinized follicular cysts of the ovary in girls (Table 25-40).[764] The ovaries contain no corpora lutea and commonly exhibit asymmetric enlargement as a result of a large solitary follicular cyst that characteristically enlarges and then spontaneously regresses, only to recur (Fig. 25-67).[764] Serum estradiol is elevated (at times to extraordinary levels); in contrast, the LH response to GnRH is prepubertal, and the pubertal pattern of nighttime LH pulses is absent at the onset and during the initial years. Later in the course of the sexual precocity, when the bone age approaches 12 years, the GnRH pulse generator becomes operative and ovulatory cycles ensue.

An affected girl may progress from GnRH-independent puberty to GnRH-dependent puberty (see Table 25-40). GnRH agonists are not effective for treatment in the GnRH-independent stage. Testolactone, fadrozole, anastrozole, and letrozole have been equivocal or not effective.[429] After a single case report of treatment with tamoxifen, an antiestrogen, showed decreases in bone age advancement, growth rate, menses, and pubertal development, a multicenter trial demonstrated the utility of this agent in decreasing vaginal bleeding and decreasing the rate of bone age advancement and growth rate in affected girls.[776] However, ovarian and uterine volumes remained elevated.

Sexual precocity is rare in boys with McCune-Albright syndrome[764]; however, testicular disease occurs as frequently in affected boys as girls.[777] Affected boys may have asymmetric enlargement of the testes in addition to signs of sexual precocity. The histologic changes and hormonal findings are reminiscent of those observed in testotoxicosis: the seminiferous tubules are enlarged and exhibit spermatogenesis, and Leydig cells may be hyperplastic, the

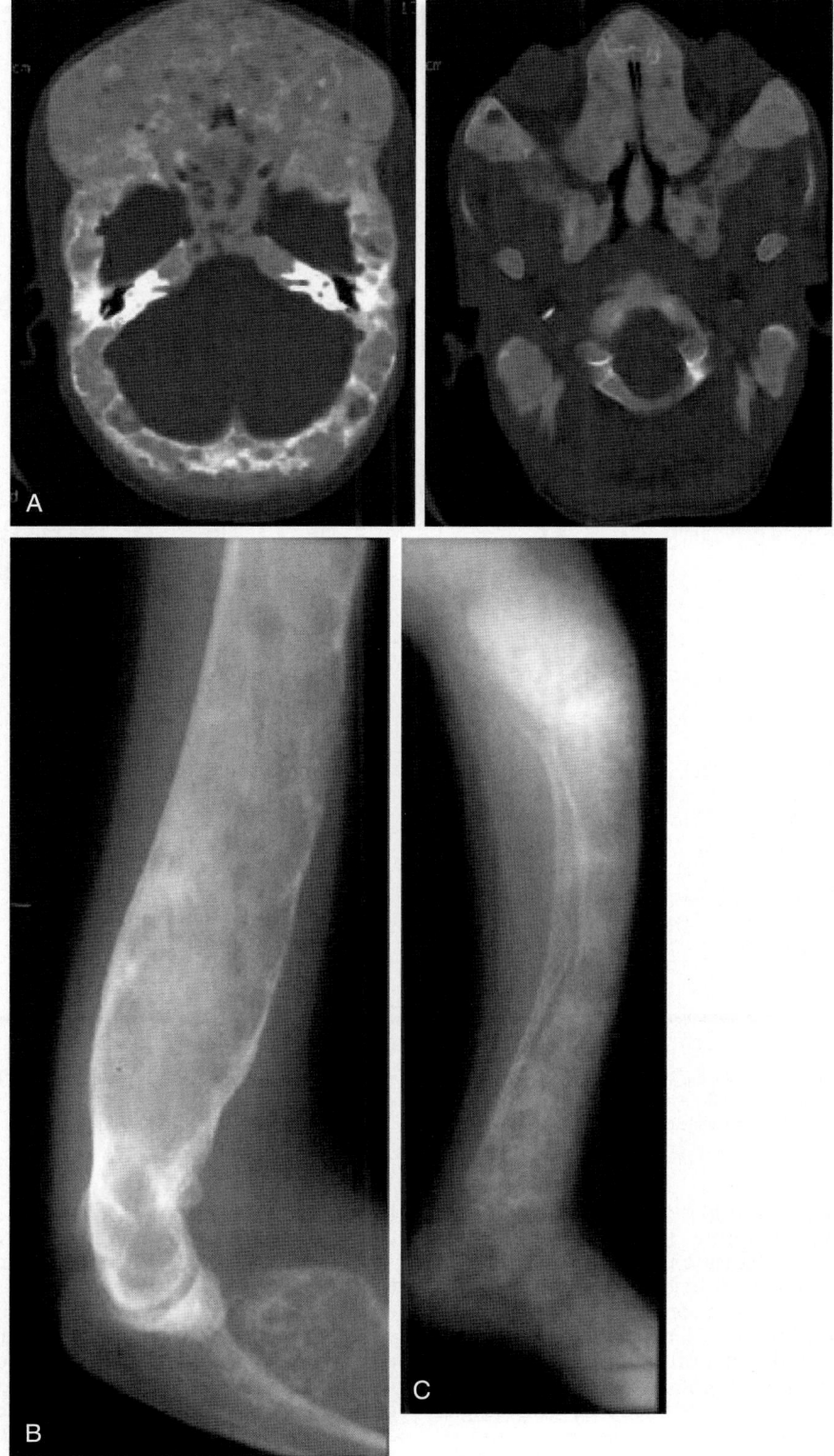

Figure 25-66 Bone lesions in McCune-Albright syndrome. **A,** The skull has severe thickening primarily at the base due to fibrous dysplasia. The auditory and optic nerves can be caught in narrowed foramina, but that is not the case in these patients. **B** and **C,** Distortions of the long bones can develop into a "shepherd's crook" appearance. Notice the multiple bone cysts.

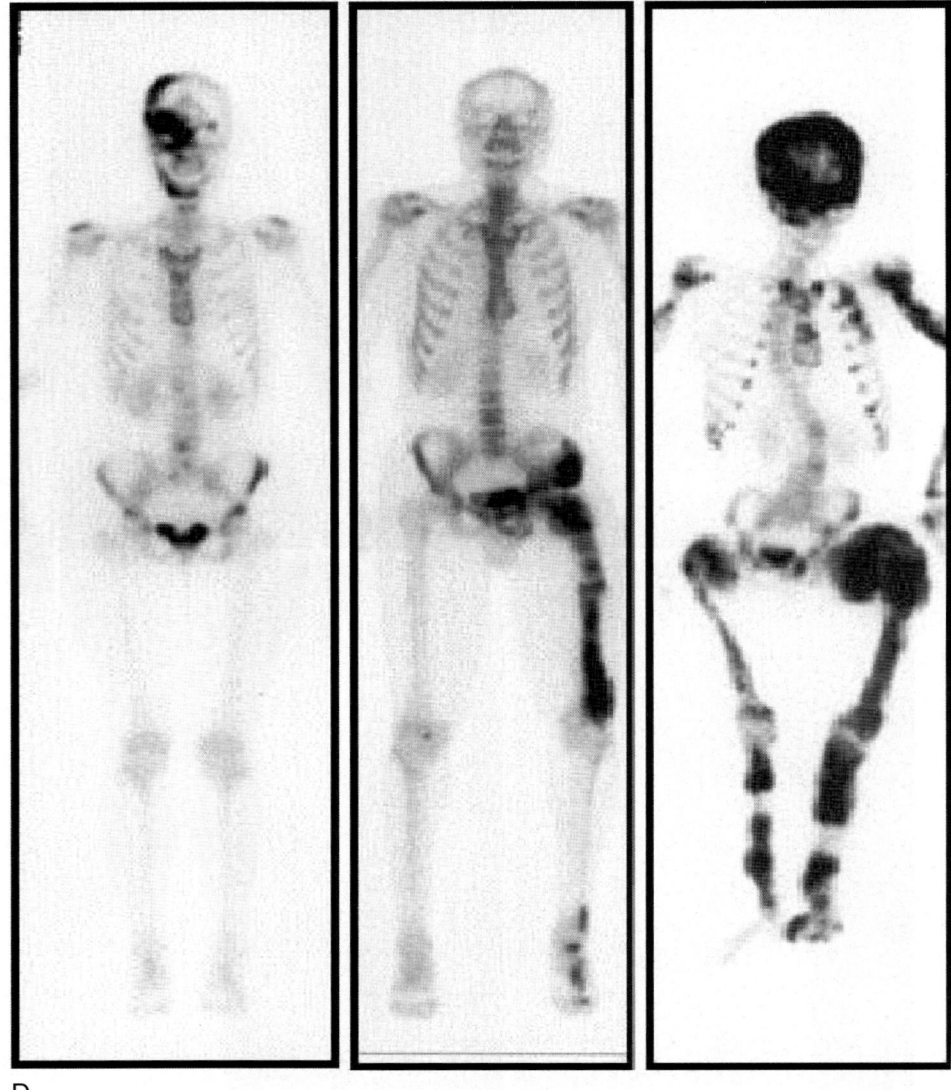

D

Figure 25-66, cont'd D, Bone scan shows the areas of remodeling that "light up," depending on the area affected in individual patients. There are examples of patients primarily affected in the craniofacial area or in the appendicular area, or both areas, and the axial skeleton. (Courtesy of Michael T. Collins, M.D., National Institutes of Health, Bethesda, MD, and Sandra Gorges, M.D., University of California, Davis, CA.)

most common histologic finding.[764,777] A 3.8-year-old boy with McCune-Albright syndrome (several café au lait lesions on the back and polyostotic fibrous dysplasia) had an Arg201His mutation detected in bone and testis tissue and the unusual feature of macroorchidism (right testis, 9 mL; left testis, 7 mL), but sexual precocity was absent. Basal and GnRH-stimulated gonadotropins and sex steroid levels were prepubertal, but serum inhibin B and AMH concentrations were strikingly elevated. On histologic examination of the testes, most of the seminiferous tubules were slightly increased in diameter and filled with Sertoli cells but lacked a lumen. The tubules stained intensively for inhibin β_B subunit; mature Leydig cells were absent.[778] An increased incidence of the rare condition testicular microlithiasis was described in boys with McCune-Albright syndrome evaluated by ultrasonography.[779,780]

McCune-Albright syndrome may occur concordantly or discordantly in monozygotic twins; familial cases have not been convincingly described. In 1986, Happle[781] posited that the disorder is caused by an autosomal dominant

lethal gene that results in loss of the zygote in utero and that cells bearing this mutation survive only in embryos mosaic for the lethal gene. Early somatic mutation would lead to a mosaic cell pattern of the distribution of cells containing the mutation. The severity of the disorder would depend on the proportion of mutant cells in various embryonic tissues. The description of somatic mutations in human endocrine tumors that convert the peptide chain of the G_s protein into a putative oncogene (referred to as a *gsp* mutation) raised the possibility of a similar defect in McCune-Albright syndrome that both affects a differentiated function such as a signaling pathway and mediates the regulation of proliferation. These hypotheses are now established, because mutations in the gene encoding the α-subunit of the stimulatory G protein for adenyl cyclase was identified in the tissues of children with the McCune-Albright syndrome.

The heterotrimeric guanine nucleotide–binding proteins (G proteins) are a subfamily within the large superfamily of GTP-binding proteins and serve to transduce

TABLE 25-40
A Patient with McCune-Albright Syndrome and Recurrent Ovarian Cysts

Chronologic Age (yr)	Bone Age (yr)	Height (cm)	Physical Signs	Basal and Post-LHRH (ng/mL)*†	Plasma Estradiol (pmol/L [pg/mL])	Radiography (Long Bones)
1⁴⁄₁₂	1³⁄₁₂	81.1	Café au lait pigmentation, B2, PH1 Vaginal bleeding (×2 mo)	LH 0.6-1.3 FSH 1.9-3.2 DHEAS <50 ng/mL (<0.14 mmol/L)	40 (11)	Normal
1⁸⁄₁₂			B1, PH1			
2⁶⁄₁₂	2⁶⁄₁₂	92.4	B2, PH2 Vaginal bleeding	LH 0.6-1.1 FSH 1.9-3.2 DHEAS <50 ng/mL (<0.14 mmol/L)	55-66 (15-18)	Normal
3⁷⁄₁₂		98.3	B1, PH1			
3¹⁰⁄₁₂	3¹⁰⁄₁₂		B2, PH1	LH 1.1-2.0 FSH 1-1.7	51-95 (14-26)	Normal
4³⁄₁₂			B1, PH1		7.3-7.3 (20-20)	Polyostotic fibrous dysplasia of femurs
5¹¹⁄₁₂	6	123.4	B3, PH2 Vaginal bleeding (×2 mo)	LH 1.1-4.3 FSH 1.0-2.0		
6⁶⁄₁₂	7¹⁰⁄₁₂	128.5	B3, PH2 Oral medroxyprogesterone acetate, 10 mg bid stated		<5	
7¹¹⁄₁₂	8¹⁰⁄₁₂	136.8				
8⁷⁄₁₂		142.2				

*Matched standard reagents were LER-960 for LH and LER-869 for FSH. To convert ng/mL to IU/L, multiply LH value by 3.8 and FSH value by 8.4.
†Note the prepubertal LH response to GnRH consistent with GnRH-independent sexual precocity until age 5¹¹⁄₁₂ yr, and the pubertal LH response at 5¹¹⁄₁₂ yr, consistent with the development of secondary true precocious puberty (GnRH-dependent). Note discrepancy between gonadarche and adrenarche as evidenced by preadrenarchal concentration of DHEAS.
B, breast stage; bid, twice a day; DHEAS, dehydroepiandrosterone sulfate; FSH, follicle-stimulating hormone; GnRH, gonadotropin-releasing hormone; LER, matched standard reagent; LH, luteinizing hormone; LHRH, luteinizing hormone–releasing hormone; PH, pubic hair stage.

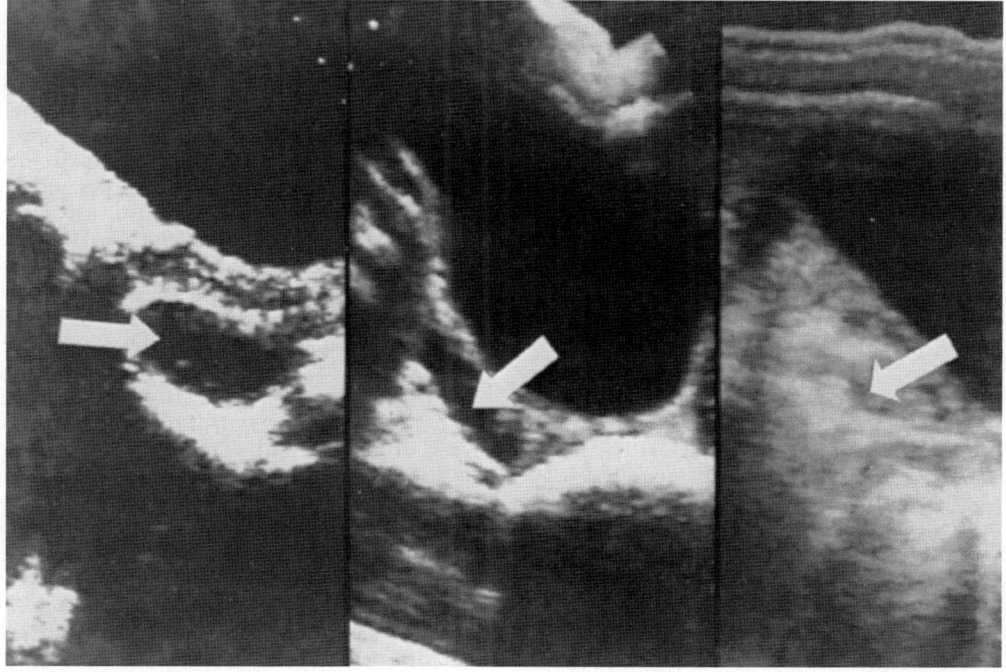

Figure 25-67 Serial pelvic ultrasonograms at 2-week intervals of a 6-year-old girl with McCune-Albright syndrome. Breast development and vaginal bleeding coincided with the enlargement of the ovarian cyst; *white arrows* denote the decreasing size of the cyst. With the spontaneous regression of the large ovarian cyst, the breasts regressed in size, and vaginal bleeding ceased. (From Kaplan SL, Grumbach MM. Pathogenesis of sexual precocity. In: Grumbach MM, Sizonenko PC, Aubert ML, eds. *Control of the Onset of Puberty*. Baltimore, MD: Williams & Wilkins; 1990:620-660.)

signals from a large number of cell surface receptors with a common structural motif of seven-transmembrane–spanning domains to their intracellular effector molecules, including enzymes and ion channels; in essence, they couple serpentine cell surface receptors to effectors (Fig. 25-68). For G_s, the stimulatory G protein, the effector is adenyl cyclase, which is controlled by G_s and an inhibitory G protein,[741] G_i. The heterotrimer is composed of an α-subunit (39 to 45 kDa) that binds GTP, has intrinsic GTPase activity, and converts GTP to GDP; a β-subunit (35

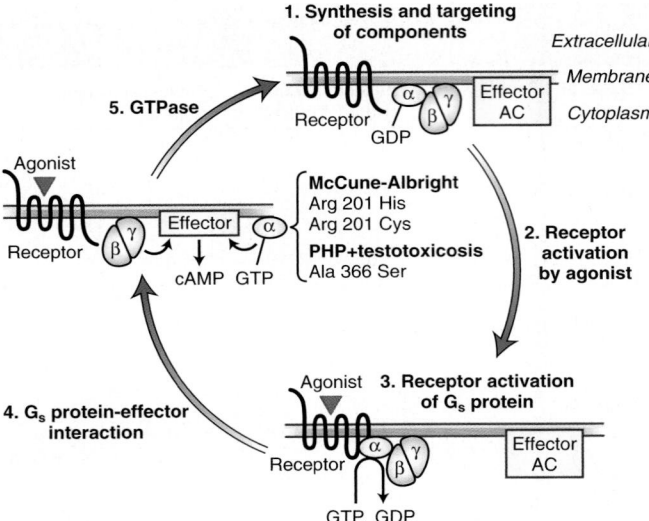

Figure 25-68 The G protein guanosine triphosphatase (GTPase) cycle. The heterotrimeric guanine nucleotide-binding proteins (G proteins), which are composed of three subunits (α, β, γ), couple cell surface receptors consisting of a single serpentine polypeptide having seven helical membrane-spanning domains with an effector. In this instance, adenylate cyclase (AC) catalyzes the transformation of adenosine triphosphate (ATP) to cyclic adenosine monophosphate (cAMP). The G protein stimulation subunit α (Gs) mediates the stimulation of cAMP generation. In the inactive, unstimulated state, the G protein is a heterotrimer, and guanosine diphosphate (GDP) is tightly bound to the α-subunit. When the cell surface receptor is activated by its cognate agonist, the receptor catalyzes the release of the tightly bound GDP, which enables GTP to bind to the α-subunit. The GTP-bound α-subunit (α-GTP) dissociates from the tightly bound βγ dimer, and both play a role in the G protein activation of the effector, adenylate cyclase. The intrinsic GTPase activity of the α-subunit ends the stimulation of the effector by converting the bound α-GTP to α-GDP; as a consequence, the α-subunit again returns to its inactive state and reassociates with high affinity with the βγ subunit, yielding the α, β, γ heterotrimer. Disorders of signal transduction can arise from germ cell or somatic mutations at any of the five stages of the cycle. The gain-of-function, activating somatic mutations in the *GNAS1* gene that encodes the G Gsα-subunit and leads to McCune-Albright syndrome (shown in the bracket), involves the highly conserved arginine 201 residue. These mutations inhibit the intrinsic GTPase activity of the α-subunit and therefore the conversion of the bound GTP to GDP. The Ala366Ser mutation (shown in the bracket) was detected in two boys, both of whom had pseudohypothyroidism 1a (PHP1a) and testotoxicosis. The mutant protein was constitutively activated in the Leydig cells at the scrotal temperature (32° to 33° C), leading to testotoxicosis, but it was rapidly degraded at body temperature, 37° C, which led to PHP1a. (Modified from Spiegel AM. Mutations in G proteins and G protein-coupled receptors in endocrine disease. *J Clin Endocrinol Metab.* 1996;81:2434-2442.)

to 36 kDa); and a smaller β-subunit (7 to 8 kDa). The latter two subunits are tightly but noncovalently associated with each other. Each of the subunits is encoded by a distinct gene. The G proteins function as conformational switches. The GDP-liganded α-subunit is bound to the βγ-subunits and is in an inactivated state. When the cell surface receptor is activated by its ligand or agonists, the GDP is catalytically released from the α-subunit, enabling GTP to bind. This leads to dissociation of the GTP-activated α-subunit from the bound βγ-subunits and activation of the effector, adenyl cyclase. When GTP is hydrolyzed by the intrinsic GTPase activity of Gsα, the α- and βγ-subunits reassociate, and the α-subunit is in the off or inactive conformation. The three-dimensional structure of the heterotrimeric G proteins has been determined.

Activating heterozygous mutations in the Gsα-subunit that occurred as an early postzygotic event are described in the McCune-Albright syndrome. The somatic constitutive activating mutation, which leads to excess cAMP production and, in some tissues, cAMP-induced hyperplasia, has

a mosaic pattern; the proportion of the hyperactive mutant compared with normal cells varies in different tissues, contributing, at least in part, to the varied clinical findings, the severity, the sporadic nature of the syndrome, and the discordant occurrence in monozygotic twins. A germline mutation is presumed to be lethal to the embryo. Two gain-of-function somatic missense mutations have been described in this disorder, both of which involve the arginine 201 residue of the α-subunit.[741] This is the site of covalent modification by cholera toxin: either a cysteine or a histidine is substituted for arginine 201 (see Fig. 25-68). The arginine 201 residue is critical for α-subunit GTPase activity, and each of these two mutations decreases the GTPase activity of the Gsα-subunit, leading to constitutive activation. These activating mutations have been found in all tissues affected by the syndrome, including bone lesions. There are reports of fertility in adults with McCune-Albright syndrome.

Juvenile Hypothyroidism. Long-standing untreated primary hypothyroidism, usually a consequence of Hashimoto thyroiditis, is an uncommon cause of incomplete ISP in both girls and boys and occurs in association with impaired growth and delayed skeletal maturation.[292] If the concentration of plasma prolactin is elevated, galactorrhea may be demonstrable, more commonly in affected girls than boys (Figs. 25-69 and 25-70). Girls have breast development, enlarged labia minora, and estrogenic changes in the vaginal smear, usually without the appearance of pubic hair; some girls have irregular vaginal bleeding that could proceed to metrorrhagia, and solitary or multiple ovarian cysts may be demonstrable by pelvic sonography or on physical examination.[782] It is important to recognize the condition to avoid unnecessary surgery for the ovarian cysts or the accompanying pituitary enlargement, which would be a tragic mistake in view of the success of medical management. In about 80% of boys with juvenile hypothyroidism, the testes are enlarged because of an increase in the size of the seminiferous tubules, but signs of virilization and Leydig cell maturation are absent, and the plasma concentration of testosterone is prepubertal. Enlargement of the sella turcica and the pituitary gland in the face of hypersecretion of TSH (see Fig. 25-70) as well as associated galactorrhea has led to the misdiagnosis of a pituitary neoplasm. The hypothyroidism, incomplete sexual maturation, galactorrhea, and pituitary enlargement are reversed or corrected by levothyroxine therapy within a few months.

In 1960, Van Wyk and Grumbach[292] suggested that the syndrome resulted from hormonal overlap in negative feedback regulation with increased secretion of gonadotropins, prolactin, and TSH as a consequence of the chronic hypothyroidism. With the advent of radioimmunoassays for pituitary hormones, increased prolactin secretion was documented in children and adults with primary hypothyroidism and in affected girls with the syndrome. GH release is usually decreased, as in uncomplicated primary hypothyroidism.

However, the explanation for the sexual maturation remains uncertain. Pubertal development in primary hypothyroidism is usually delayed and is only rarely advanced for chronologic age. By the use of radioimmunoassays or other methods for FSH and LH in which the cross-reaction with TSH is negligible, an increased (pubertal) concentration of plasma immunoreactive and bioactive FSH, but not LH, has been detected. Bioactive LH activity is also low. Increased FSH pulsatility, mainly at night, but not LH release was demonstrated in patients with the syndrome and in some children with primary hypothyroidism who did not exhibit premature sexual maturation. The increased FSH release and the high FSH/LH ratio (in contrast to

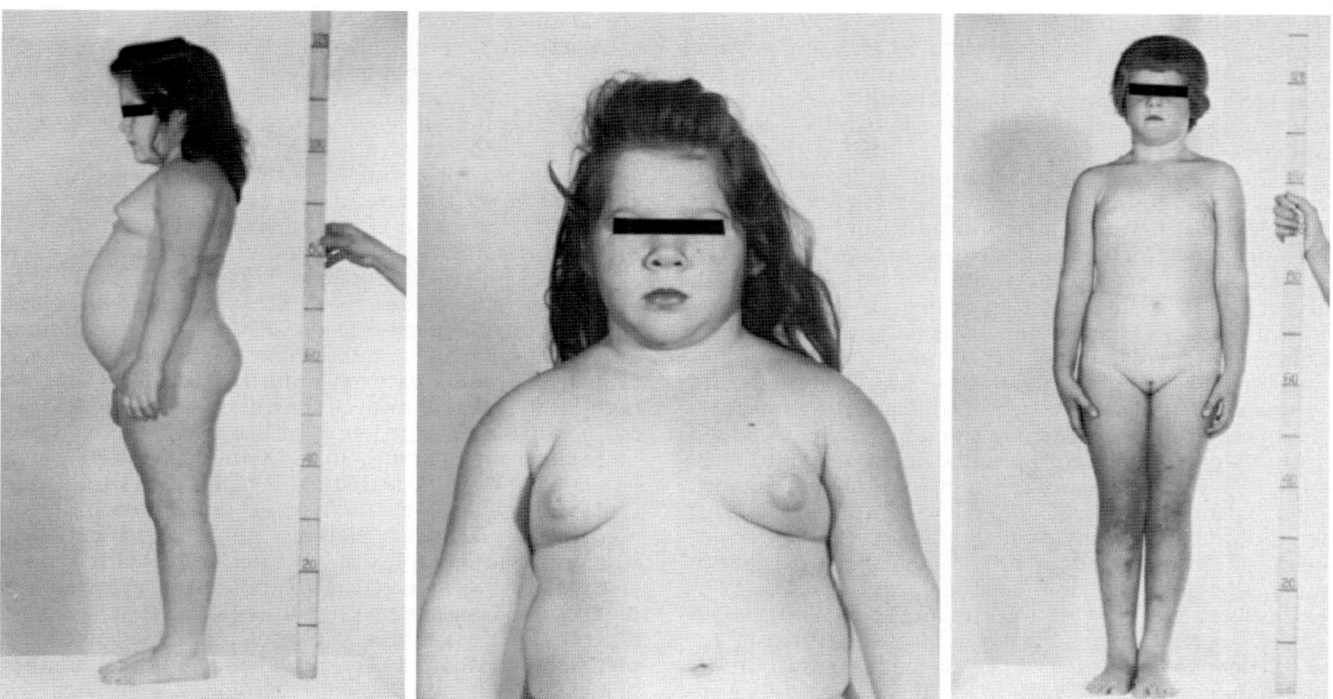

Figure 25-69 *Left* and *center*, Severe, chronic hypothyroidism of Hashimoto thyroiditis in a girl aged 7 years and 1 month with sexual precocity (without pubic or axillary hair), episodic vaginal bleeding, and galactorrhea. She had symptoms of hypothyroidism and a sharply decreased rate of growth over the previous 2 years (height, −1 SD [standard deviation]; bone age, 5 years and 3 months). Breast development was Tanner stage 3, the labia minora were enlarged, and the vaginal mucosa was dull pink, thickened, and rugated, with evidence of an estrogenic effect. No acne, seborrhea, or hirsutism was present. The uterus was of adolescent size, and the endometrial mucosa was in a proliferative phase. Urinary gonadotropins were barely detectable by bioassay. *Right*, Striking change in appearance after 8 months of thyroid hormone treatment. She had grown 7 cm in height and lost 8.1 kg in weight. The breasts had decreased in size, galactorrhea was no longer demonstrable, the labia minora had regressed, and the vaginal mucosa was pink and glistening (no estrogen effect). Ten weeks after the initiation of thyroid hormone replacement therapy, she developed a right slipped capital femoral epiphysis that was repaired surgically; recovery was uneventful.

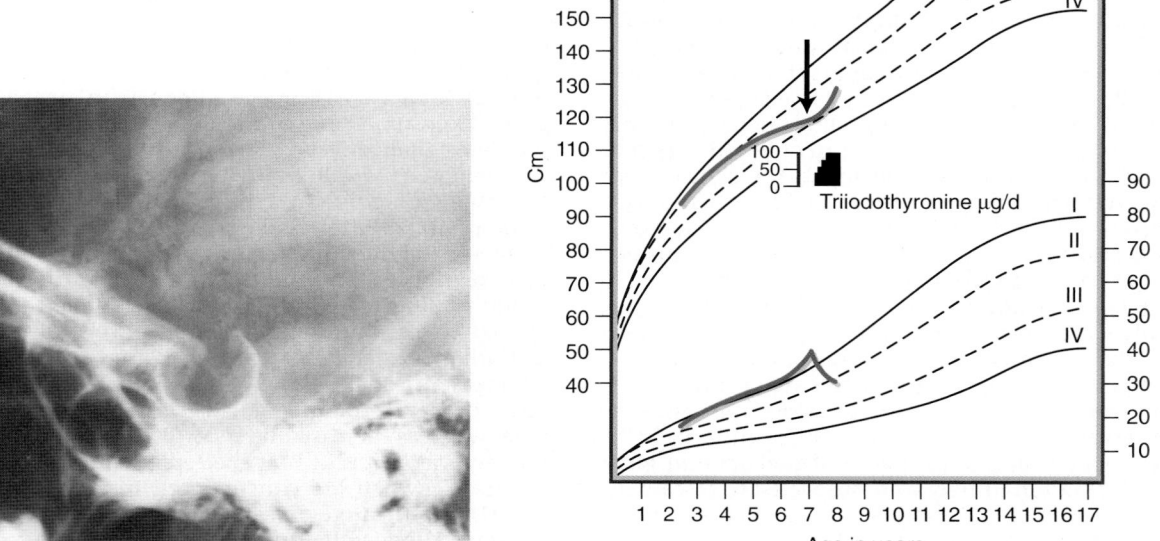

Figure 25-70 *Left*, Radiograph of the skull of a patient with hypothyroidism shows an enlarged pituitary fossa in the lateral view. The dorsum sellae was thin and demineralized, and the floor had a double contour line. The area of the sella turcica was 150 mm^2. Pneumoencephalography showed a suprasellar mass impinging on the cisterna chiasmatica. After thyroid hormone treatment for 8 months, the volume of the sella had decreased 30% to 100 mm^2, the dorsum sellae had remineralized, and the double floor was no longer evident. *Right*, Growth curve illustrates the decrease in growth rate despite sexual precocity and the catch-up growth induced by thyroid hormone therapy. (From Van Wyk JJ, Grumbach MM. Syndrome of precocious menstruation and galactorrhea in juvenile hypothyroidism: an example of hormonal overlap in pituitary feedback. *J Pediatr.* 1960;57:416-435.)

that observed in normal puberty) seem to account for the increased ovarian estrogen secretion in girls and for the enlarged testes without signs of virilization in affected boys; the suggestion here is that FSH-induced Sertoli cell proliferation is an important determinant of mature testis size.

A GnRH-independent mechanism is likely, because GnRH did not suppress the pubertal LH levels. Pulsatile TSH release is increased at night, and administration of TRH appears to increase FSH release in normal children (but not in adults). Moreover, the FSH response to TRH, but not GnRH, is augmented in primary hypothyroidism, and this response can occur in gonadotropin-secreting pituitary adenomas. If the latter observations are confirmed, it is likely that the incomplete sexual precocity and the increased prolactin secretion and galactorrhea are a consequence of the increased release of TRH, the increased sensitivity of the mammotrophs and gonadotroph to TRH, or both.[292] This mechanism, which has gained support, would explain the relatively rapid and complete reversal of the syndrome by levothyroxine treatment. Human recombinant TSH at a dose about 1000-fold greater than that of human FSH evoked a dose-dependent cAMP response in COS7 cells transfected with the human FSH receptor, which suggests another possible but less likely mechanism for the FSH-dependent (or FSH-like–dependent) but GnRH-independent sexual precocity.[783] A direct effect of severe hypothyroidism on the prepubertal testis that leads to overproliferation of Sertoli cells also has been advanced as an explication of the macroorchidism.

Iatrogenic Sexual Precocity and Endocrine Disruptors. Prepubertal children are remarkably sensitive to exogenous gonadal steroids and may show signs of sexual maturation resulting from overlooked sources of androgens or estrogens, such as ingested or absorbed tonics, lotions, or hair creams or hair straighteners that contain or are inadvertently contaminated with an estrogen.[784] Dermal exposure to estrogen may add up to more than 300 µg, far in excess of a therapeutic dose and possibly greater in infants and children exposed to estrogen dermal gel. Compounds containing tea tree and lavender oils were reported to cause gynecomastia in three prepuberal boys and demonstrated estrogenic activity in vitro.[785] A short course of application of estrogen cream is used to treat labial adhesions, but long courses may lead to breast development or even withdrawal bleeding. In addition to breast development, pigmentation of the areolae and the linea alba and the appearance of pubic hair may be seen in children exposed to dermal estrogen. Children who touch the skin or the towels of men using androgen gel therapy may themselves develop virilization.[786] The administration of hCG to boys with undescended testes may induce secretion of testosterone sufficient to cause incomplete sexual precocity.

FDA guidelines define a limit of not more than 1% of normal daily estrogen production in prepubertal children as a safe intake of estrogen[740]; this is equivalent to 0.43 ng/day for boys and 3.24 ng/day for girls, based on the most recent data from extremely sensitive estrogen assays, but food is still a suspected source of endocrine disruption.[784,787] Epidemics of gynecomastia in boys and thelarche in girls among schoolchildren in Italy were suspected to be caused by contaminated meat. During a 10-year period, more than 600 cases of gynecomastia in boys and premature thelarche or incomplete sexual precocity in girls were discovered in Puerto Rico; this is the highest prevalence reported in the world, about 10 to 15 times higher than that measured in a survey in Olmsted, Minnesota.[788,789] Maternal ovarian cysts were demonstrated in two thirds of affected Puerto Rican girls. The clandestine use of estrogen preparations in animals to stimulate weight gain, leading to ingestion of estrogen-contaminated meat from these animals, was raised as a possible cause, but this was neither confirmed nor excluded by selected analyses of meat, poultry, and milk in Puerto Rico by the U.S. Department of Agriculture.

There are rising concerns that endocrine-disrupting chemicals (EDCs), defined as "an exogenous substance that causes adverse health effects in an intact organism, or its progeny, secondary to changes in endocrine function" exert many effects on growth and development of children including pubertal development.[755] Far more conclusive evidence of an adverse effect of EDCs comes from animal, rather than human, studies, and some of the data on human beings derive from industrial accidents and very high-level exposure rather than the lower level exposures most individuals experience, so EDCs must be studied in more detail in human beings. Method of ascertainment, laboratory methods, activity and half-life of various molecules of interest, and the frequent difficulties in drawing conclusions from associations rather than controlled studies present complexities in interpreting data.

Girls who were breast-fed or exposed during intrauterine life to polybrominated biphenyls (PBBs) after an accidental exposure of their mothers in Michigan experienced early menarche (by about 1 year of age) and early appearance of pubic hair but not breast development, compared with girls who were not exposed or breast-fed, and the NHANES 2003-2004 data demonstrate a slighty lower age at menarche with higher serum polybrominated diphenyl ether (PBDE) concentrations.[790,791] Exposure to polychlorinated biphenyls (PCBs) in inner-city girls with reduced BMI values reportedly delayed thelarche.[50] There was a 9.56 increase in relative risk for precocious puberty treated by GnRH agonist in a localized area in Italy, compared with surrounding areas, suggesting the presence of an endocrine disruptor in the area.[792] Recent longitudinal studies demonstrate no effect in secondary sexual development in girls with a slight decrease in the age of puberty in boys related to levels of phthalate excretion in urine.[793]

Widespread exposure to 2,3,7,8-tetrachlorodibenzo-*p*-dioxin (TCDD), an extremely potent antiestrogenic xenobiotic, in Italy revealed that girls younger than 8 years of age at the time of exposure, who presumably had the highest dose per BMI compared with older girls, showed a tendency for a decrease in age at menarche, suggesting that age of exposure to environmental endocrine disruptors modulates their effects.[794] Follow-up of adolescents who were exposed to di-(2-ethylhexyl)-phthalate (DEHP), a component of polyvinyl chloride (PVC) that is used in plastic tubing and medical devices, when they underwent extracorporeal membrane oxygenation (ECMO) as neonates, demonstrated no effects on pubertal development despite findings of disruption of development in animals exposed to this substance, demonstrating difficulties in translating animal data to human beings.[795]

Increased lead levels in Mohawk girls living near the border of New York and Canada delayed the age of menarche, whereas increased levels of PCB promoted it[796]; surprisingly, variations in BMI exerted no effect of these toxic substances, which are concentrated in adipose tissue. In the NHANES III survey, a serum lead level of 0.7 to 2.0 µg/dL delayed menarche and pubic hair development, and African Americans exposed to 3 µg/dL also experienced delay in breast development.[797] A long-term study of puberty in Chapaevsk, Russia, an area highly contaminated with industrial waste, demonstrated 43% reduced odds of entering stage 2 genitalia among 8- to 9-year-old boys with serum lead levels equal to or greater than 5 µg/dL.[798]

There is a high frequency of reproductive problems among adult Danish men, including impaired semen quality, testicular cancer, and increased rate of infantile testicular cancer; these disorders occur in a pattern that is attributed to environmental disruptors, described in the testicular dysgenesis syndrome (TDS).[599] A higher rate of hypospadias in Danish newborns and smaller testes with lower serum inhibin B, compared with Finnish infants, suggested that environmental agents played a role. Phthalates were found in the breast milk of mothers from both countries, and although there was no relationship to the finding of hypospadias, there was an indication of altered reproductive hormones in the boys in a pattern suggesting effects on Leydig cells. There may be a genetic component to susceptibility to the TDS based upon GWAS analysis, indicating a gene X environment basis for the disorder.[751]

Longitudinal observation of girls in Copenhagen, Denmark, using physical examination of breast tissue, showed a significant decline in the age of Tanner stage 2 breast development (estimated mean age, 9.86 years in 2006-2008 vs. 10.88 years in 1991) and the age at menarche (13.13 vs. 13.42 years, respectively); there was no change in serum gonadotropins, but the serum estradiol concentration was decreased in 2006.[42] Changes in BMI did not occur in this study between the cohorts, leaving open the possibility of endocrine-disrupting chemicals as an explanation.

Boys exposed to PCBs and polychlorinated dibenzofurans (PCDFs) in utero from contamination of rice ingested by their mothers had decreased testosterone and defects in postpubertal sperm production in a preliminary study, as well as increased estrogen compared with control subjects, although there was no difference on physical examination or in age at onset of puberty.[799] Boys exposed to DDT in utero did not demonstrate any abnormalities in puberty in a study from Philadelphia, Pennsylvania.[756]

The complexities of the study of endocrine disruptors are complicated by type, amount, developmental age at exposure, and other factors are difficult to tease apart. In the United States, chemicals can enter the environment before their safety is proved, leading to an ever-expanding list of potential EDCs without data to prove their effects. Well-designed longitudinal studies are needed in this area.[800]

Diagnosis of Sexual Precocity

As with delayed puberty the majority of patients referred for precocious puberty will prove to have variations of normal development or to be inappropriately referred due to a misinterpretation of the normal ages of puberty by the referring physicians. However, precocious puberty can certainly be the outward sign of a serious condition. Thus, the separation of patients with self-limited benign disorders, such as premature adrenarche, premature thelarche, or normal but early puberty, from those with serious or even potentially fatal disorders is the first step in evaluation (Figs. 25-71 through 25-73 and Table 25-41). The history may reveal symptoms suggesting perinatal abnormalities or injuries, previous infections, adventitious ingestion of or exposure to gonadal steroids, or the presence of similar conditions in family members. Previous measurements should be plotted on a growth chart to determine height velocity and the age at onset of any increase in the rate of growth.

Important aspects of the physical examination include description of the secondary sexual development according to Tanner stages; measurement of the penis (length and width) and the testes in boys (greatest diameter without the epididymis) and of the breast tissue in girls (areolar and glandular diameters); and examination for comedones and acne, oily skin, facial and body hair, pubic and axillary hair development, axillary apocrine gland odor, muscular development, and galactorrhea. A careful examination of the external genitalia should be done with a nonrelated chaperone present. A thorough neurologic examination is indicated, with emphasis on assessment of the visual fields and optic discs in a search for signs of increased intracranial pressure; evaluation for skin lesions associated with the McCune-Albright syndrome or neurofibromatosis; and examination for abdominal, gonadal, or adnexal masses and for coexisting endocrine disease. Bone age is determined in all cases, although it is an imperfect measure. Dental development can be determined as an index of physical development but is rarely invoked clinically except in forensic cases.[801]

Ultrasonography of the ovary and uterus is exceedingly useful in the evaluation of affected girls, because standards are available for shape and volume of the uterus and the ovaries.[802] The largest measurements of uterine size by sonography in infants and children are found at puberty and in the neonatal period. The upper limit of uterine length in the prepubertal state is 3.5 cm. A uterine volume of greater than 1.8 mL is specific for the onset of puberty, but increased ovarian volume is less specific. Patients with premature thelarche were indistinguishable from age-matched control subjects when this sonographic standard was used.[104] The presence of microcysts and macrocysts of the ovary also can be detected on ultrasound examination. Cysts may be found in the ovaries in patients with CPP or GnRH-independent ISP; they usually are smaller than 9 mm in the former and larger than 9 mm in the latter[803] condition. Ovarian volume is reportedly the best indicator of precocious puberty, and uterine length was best for the differentiation of premature thelarche from premature puberty.[804] However, in the earliest stages of pubertal development ultrasonography of the pelvis may not differentiate the patient from the prepubertal state, although stimulated gonadotropin response will do so.[805] The presence of an endometrial stripe was indicative of precocious puberty.[104] Ultrasonography of the breast is suggested as a method of determining rapidly progressive versus slowly progressive or transient precocious puberty; accuracy is increased when breast ultrasound findings are added to those of uterine ultrasound and the other factors discussed previously.[806]

CPP in males usually begins with enlargement of the testes, followed by other signs of secondary sexual maturation. A Leydig cell tumor usually causes asymmetric enlargement of the testes, whereas an extragonadal hCG-secreting tumor is associated with less marked testicular enlargement than occurs at the same stage of masculinization in CPP. Testicular adrenal rest tissues (TARTs) may enlarge in boys with CAH and may be bilateral, although they are unlikely to closely mimic normal pubertal testicular development. An elevated hCG level with a prepubertal GnRH test indicates an ectopic, autonomous, gonadotropin-secreting tumor. If this tumor is in the CNS, abnormalities will be present on MRI or CT brain scans. Enlargement of the liver or a mediastinal, retroperitoneal mass in boys with sexual precocity suggests an hCG-producing hepatic or germ cell tumor; the possibility of Klinefelter syndrome needs to be considered in the latter case.

It is essential that laboratory tests for sex steroids and gonadotropin to be carried out by appropriate methods in the experienced laboratories. Simply ordering LH or FSH levels in a standard laboratory will usually lead to a determination of whether there are high levels with gonadal failure such as menopause or normal levels of adults but

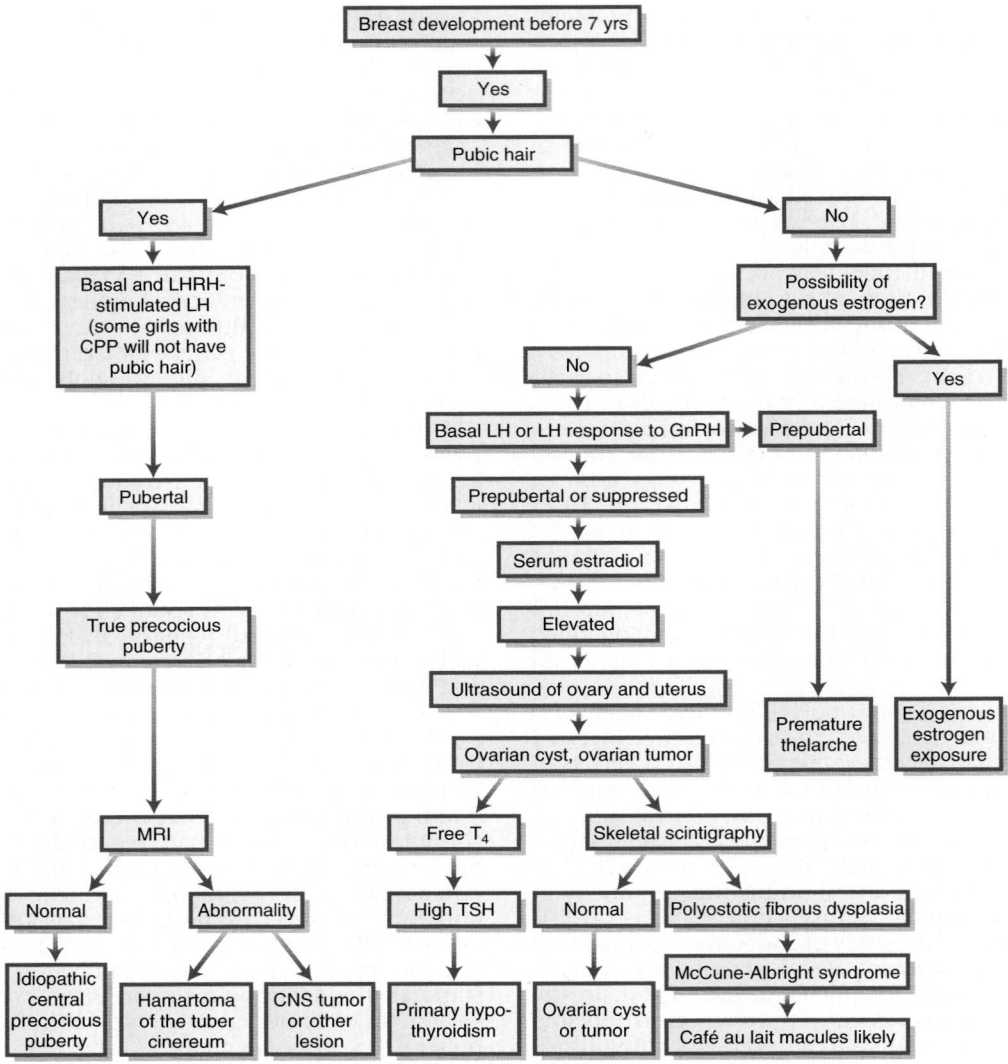

Figure 25-71 Flow chart for diagnosing sexual precocity in girls. CNS, central nervous system; CPP, central precocious puberty; FSH, follicle-stimulating hormone; GnRH, gonadotropin-releasing hormone; LH, luteinizing hormone; LHRH, LH-releasing hormone; MRI, magnetic resonance imaging; T_4, thyroxine; TSH, thyroid-stimulating hormone.

rarely can such an assay have the ability to determine subtle changes that are characteristic of childhood and adolescence. A highly sensitive third-generation assay with pediatric standards must be ordered. Further standard testosterone assays can differentiate between a normal male and one with gonadal failure but cannot determine the low levels characteristic of the preadult stages of puberty. For children and adolescents and indeed for women an HPLC-MS/MS method with pediatric standards is necessary; the same type of assay must be used for the determination of estradiol levels in girls.[235]

Measurements of basal plasma gonadotropin concentrations and the LH response to administration of GnRH (presently not available) or GnRH agonist or the amplitude and frequency of LH pulses, especially at night, using third-generation assays with pediatric standards, as well as measurements of the plasma concentration of testosterone in boys or of estradiol in girls using LC/MS-MS assays, are of primary importance in diagnosis. A recent report stated that patients with a basal LH level 0.3 IU/L or higher had subsequent pubertal progression, whereas 39 of 41 patients with a basal LH 0.2 IU/L or lower did not progress,

resulting in 100% specificity (95% CI 92% to 100%) and 90.5% sensitivity (69.6% to 98.8%).[230] Girls early in the course of CPP may have elevation of estradiol (this is not always noted, however) associated with increasing LH levels but not necessarily an increase in the concentration of FSH. Boys will have elevating values of testosterone as puberty commences. Pubertal concentrations of LH and FSH, a pubertal mode of pulsatile LH secretion (initially during sleep), or pubertal LH response to GnRH or GnRH agonist confirms the diagnosis of CPP (and in boys differentiates CPP from familial testotoxicosis). Determination of T_4 concentration (usually free T_4) is indicated when hypothyroidism as a cause of precocious puberty is suspected.

A CNS tumor must be considered as a potential cause of this premature activation of the hypothalamic GnRH pulse generator, especially in boys. The evaluation for a CNS tumor as a cause of CPP is similar to the investigation of an hCG-secreting tumor of the CNS. Although CT scanning is now a well-established procedure for determining the presence of a CNS abnormality, MRI with contrast is more sensitive for the detection of small tumors in the

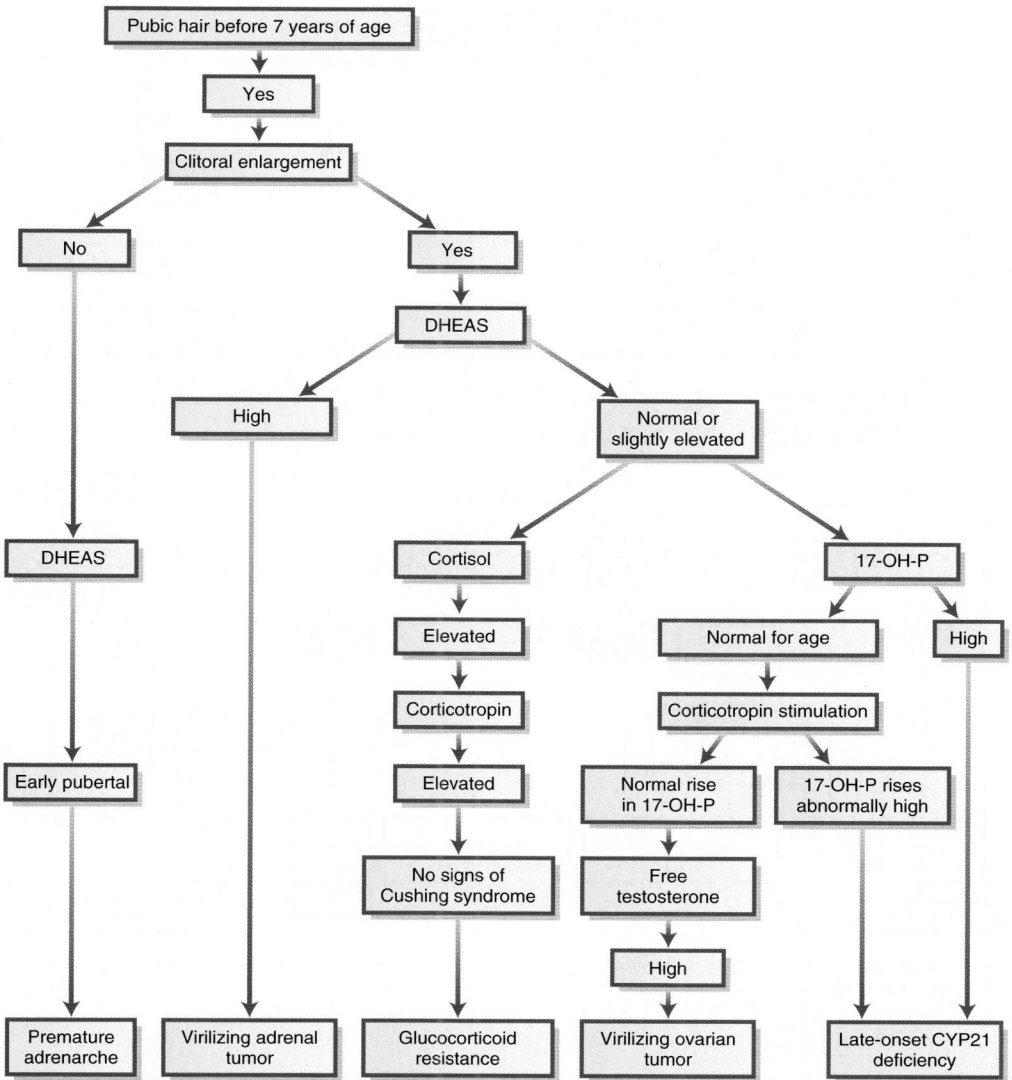

Figure 25-72 Flow chart for the evaluation of pubic hair in normal phenotypic girls before 7 years. DHEAS, dehydroepiandrosterone sulfate; 17-OH-P, 17-hydroxyprogesterone.

hypothalamus, such as a hamartoma of the tuber cinereum (see Fig. 25-55). The use of contrast adds to diagnostic certainty and is recommended for MRI of the CNS. All boys with CPP should have CNS MRI evaluation, but girls do not always receive the same recommendation, because a CNS tumor is less likely in girls than in boys to be the cause of CPP. However, studies using MRI or CT brain scans indicate that the hypothalamic hamartoma is more prevalent in both boys and girls with so-called idiopathic CPP than was previously suspected. An unselected group of girls with precocious puberty and no other symptoms underwent CNS MRI; 15% were found to have intracranial trauma, and the investigators found no clinical difference between those girls and the other 85% of girls studied, suggesting that CNS MRI is indicated for girls with precocious puberty.[807]

The height of the pituitary gland on MRI correlates with advancing age and with pubertal development[808]; patients with CPP had pituitary heights exceeding 6 mm on average, whereas those with precocious thelarche had lower heights. The shape of the pituitary gland is also of importance: a convex appearance rather than a flat top is associated with CPP of any cause.[674] Physiologic enlargement of the

pituitary gland characteristic of puberty is the source of many needless neurosurgery referrals.[809] The size and shape of the pituitary gland do not decrease with successful GnRH therapy.

T1-weighted images indicate a convex upper border of the pituitary gland in both normal patients and those with CPP, indicating the similarity in the physiologic changes in both conditions. Pituitary gland hyperplasia (height > 1 cm) is a rare finding reported in CPP. The empty sella syndrome is less frequently observed in patients with CPP than in patients with pituitary hypofunction. Empty sella is found in 10% of children who are imaged for suspected hypothalamic-pituitary disorders including hypogonadotropic hypogonadism.[810]

The premature appearance of pubic hair, phallic enlargement, and other signs of virilization in a male without enlargement of the testes or the liver suggests the diagnosis of congenital virilizing CAH, virilizing adrenal tumor, or, rarely, Cushing syndrome. Measurement of plasma 17-hydroxyprogesterone and DHEAS concentrations and their suppressibility with glucocorticoids will distinguish CAH from a virilizing adrenal tumor. If growth rate is suppressed, the possibility of primary hypothyroidism or Cushing

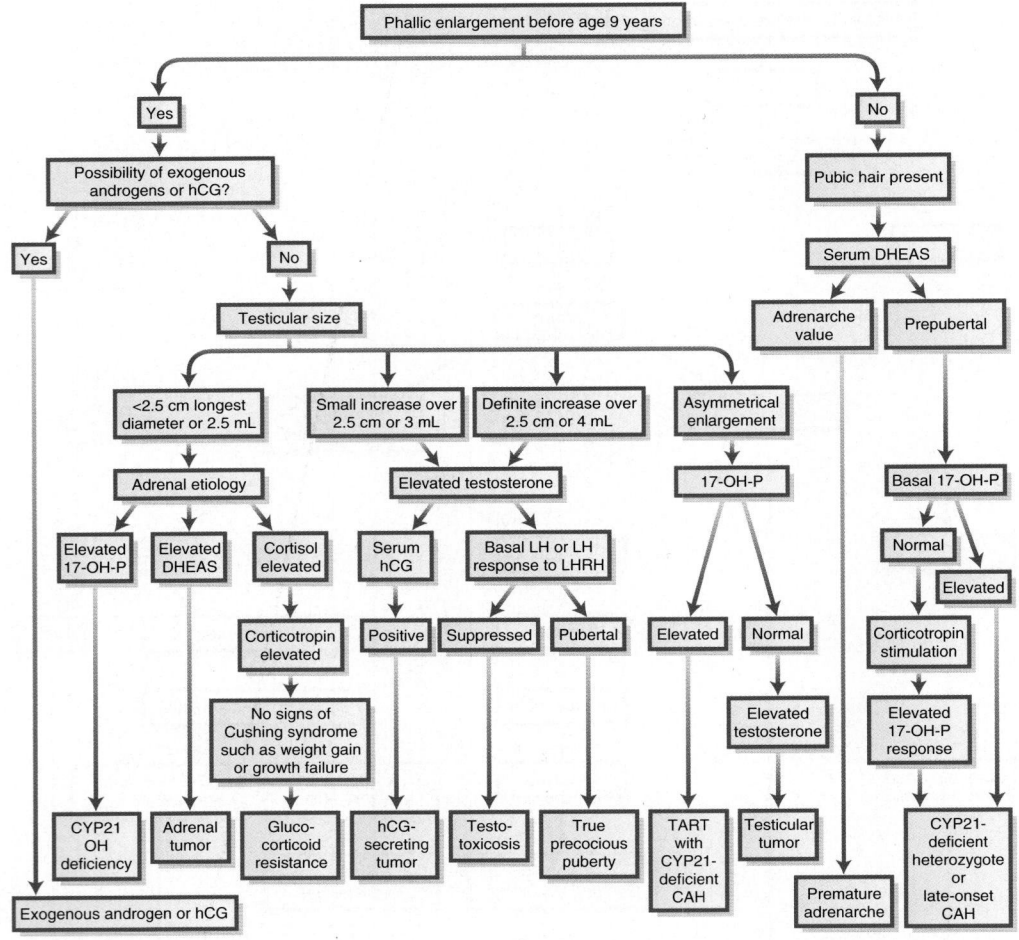

Figure 25-73 Flow chart for diagnosing sexual precocity in a phenotypic male. CAH, congenital adrenal hyperplasia; DHEAS, dehydroepiandrosterone sulfate; hCG, human chorionic gonadotropin; LH, luteinizing hormone; LHRH, LH-releasing hormone; 17-OH-P, 17-hydroxyprogesterone; TART, testicular adrenal rest tissue.

TABLE 25-41

Differential Diagnosis of Sexual Precocity

Disorder	Plasma Gonadotropins	LH Response to GnRH	Serum Sex Steroid Concentration	Gonadal Size	Miscellaneous
Gonadotropin-Dependent					
True precocious puberty	Prominent LH pulses (premature reactivation of GnRH pulse generator)	Pubertal LH response initially during sleep	Pubertal values of testosterone or estradiol	Normal pubertal testicular enlargement or ovarian and uterine enlargement	MRI of brain to rule out CNS tumor or other abnormality; skeletal survey for McCune-Albright syndrome (by US)
Incomplete Sexual Precocity (Pituitary Gonadotropin-Independent)					
Males					
Chorionic gonadotropin-secreting tumor in males	High hCG, low LH	Prepubertal LH response	Pubertal value of testosterone	Slight to moderate uniform enlargement of testes	Hepatomegaly suggests hepatoblastoma; CT scan of brain if chorionic gonadotropin-secreting CNS tumor suspected
Leydig cell tumor in males	Suppressed	No LH response	Very high testosterone	Irregular, asymmetric enlargement of testes	
Familial testotoxicosis	Suppressed	No LH response	Pubertal values of testosterone	Testes symmetric and >2.5 cm but smaller than expected for pubertal development; spermatogenesis occurs	Familial; probably sex-limited, autosomal dominant trait

TABLE 25-41

Differential Diagnosis of Sexual Precocity—cont'd

Disorder	Plasma Gonadotropins	LH Response to GnRH	Serum Sex Steroid Concentration	Gonadal Size	Miscellaneous
Virilizing congenital adrenal hyperplasia	Prepubertal	Prepubertal LH response	Elevated 17-OHP in CYP21 deficiency or elevated 11-deoxycortisol in CYP11B1 deficiency	Testes prepubertal	Autosomal recessive, may be congenital or late-onset form, may have salt loss in CYP21 deficiency or hypertension in CYP11B1 deficiency
Virilizing adrenal tumor	Prepubertal	Prepubertal LH response	High DHEAS and androstenedione values	Testes prepubertal	CT, MRI, or US of abdomen
Premature adrenarche	Prepubertal	Prepubertal LH response	Prepubertal testosterone, DHEAS, or urinary 17-ketosteroid values appropriate for pubic hair stage 2	Testes prepubertal	Onset usually after 6 yr of age; more frequent in CNS-injured children
Females					
Granulosa cell tumor (follicular cysts may present similarly)	Suppressed	Prepubertal LH response	Very high estradiol	Ovarian enlargement on physical examination, CT, or US	Tumor often palpable on physical examination
Follicular cyst	Suppressed	Prepubertal LH response	Prepubertal to very high estradiol	Ovarian enlargement on physical examination, CT, or US	Single or recurrent episodes of menses and/or breast development; exclude McCune-Albright syndrome
Feminizing adrenal tumor	Suppressed	Prepubertal LH response	High estradiol and DHEAS values	Ovaries prepubertal	Unilateral adrenal mass
Premature thelarche	Prepubertal	Prepubertal LH, pubertal	Prepubertal or early estradiol response	Ovaries prepubertal	Onset usually before 3 yr of age
Premature adrenarche	Prepubertal	Prepubertal LH response	Prepubertal estradiol; DHEAS or urinary 17-ketosteroid values appropriate for pubic hair stage 2	Ovaries prepubertal	Onset usually after 6 yr of age; more frequent in brain-injured children
Late-onset virilizing congenital adrenal hyperplasia	Prepubertal	Prepubertal LH response	Elevated 17-OHP in basal or corticotropin-stimulated state	Ovaries prepubertal	Autosomal recessive
In Both Sexes					
McCune-Albright syndrome	Suppressed	Suppressed	Sex steroid pubertal or higher	Ovarian (on US); slight testicular enlargement	Skeletal survey for polyostotic fibrous dysplasia and skin examination for café au lait spots
Primary hypothyroidism	LH prepubertal; FSH may be slightly elevated	Prepubertal FSH may be increased	Estradiol may be pubertal	Testicular enlargement; ovaries cystic	TSH and prolactin elevated; T$_4$ low

CNS, central nervous system; CT, computed tomography; CYP, P450 cytochrome isoenzyme; DHEAS, dehydroepiandrosterone sulfate; GnRH, gonadotropin-releasing hormone; hCG, human chorionic gonadotropin; LH, luteinizing hormone; MRI, magnetic resonance imaging; 17-OHP, 17-hydroxyprogesterone; T$_4$, thyroxine; TSH, thyrotropin; US, ultrasonography.

syndrome is raised; elevated plasma concentrations of cortisol, urinary free cortisol, 17-hydroxycorticosteroid, or salivary cortisol after suppression with dexamethasone confirm the latter diagnosis. The appearance in a girl of pubic hair and other signs of virilization, such as clitoral enlargement, acne, deepening voice, muscular development, or growth spurt, is caused by CAH, virilizing adrenal tumor, or virilizing ovarian tumor. Cushing syndrome caused by an adrenocortical carcinoma can result in virilization associated with growth failure, and a virilizing adrenocortical carcinoma can manifest with so much androgen effect that the Cushing syndrome is not apparent, as rapid growth and virilization are first noted; estradiol may be secreted by these tumors as well as androgens.

Virilizing ovarian tumors may be detected by pelvic ultrasonography.

The appearance of pubic hair without other signs of puberty in boys or girls is usually a result of premature adrenarche but may alternatively be the first sign of sexual precocity or of adrenal virilism from other causes.

In a girl, breast development associated with dulling and thickening of the vaginal mucosa and enlargement of the labia minora indicate significant estrogen secretion or iatrogenic exposure to estrogen. The differential diagnosis includes CPP, an estrogen-secreting neoplasm, and a cyst of the ovary. If the plasma concentrations of gonadotropins are in the pubertal range, if LH pulses of pubertal amplitude are detected, or if a pubertal LH response to

GnRH or GnRH agonist is elicited, CPP is present. In one report, a child had pubertal-level serum LH due to heterophile antibodies that interfered with the LH assay and fallaciously elevated the values in the basal and stimulated state; after addition of anti-mouse antibody, LH values decreased.[811] As always, clinical observation should be congruent with laboratory findings, and the assays should be highly sensitive and associated with valid pediatric standards.

Estradiol concentrations in girls early in normal puberty or CPP are in the prepubertal range for much of the day, and a single determination may be inadequate to reflect ovarian function.[134]

If the concentration of plasma estradiol is elevated but gonadotropin levels are low, an estrogen-secreting cyst or neoplasm is present or exogenous estrogens are the cause. Ovarian tumors of moderate size can be palpated by bimanual examination. Advances in pelvic sonography allow the delineation of ovarian cysts or tumors and the determination of uterine size and the size of the endometrial stripe.[104] An estrogen-secreting neoplasm of the ovary is usually accompanied by high estradiol concentrations, but some ovarian cysts are associated with concentrations of estradiol as high as those in granulosa cell tumors; the differential diagnosis between these cysts and ovarian neoplasms rarely requires exploratory laparotomy or laparoscopy and usually can be resolved by pelvic sonography and the use of tumor markers. Breast development in the absence of other estrogen effects is almost always a result of premature thelarche.

Contrasexual Precocity: Feminization in Boys and Virilization in Girls

Boys. Feminization in a boy before the age of puberty is rare. Rarely, an estrogen-secreting adrenal adenoma or a chorionepithelioma causes gynecomastia. Gynecomastia has been reported in a 1-year-old boy with 11β-hydroxylase deficiency and in boys with late-onset CAH.[812]

Aromatase Excess Syndrome. Gynecomastia in prepubertal boys can be caused by increased extraglandular aromatization of C19 steroids of adrenal origin, such as androstenedione, and subsequent increased extraglandular estrogen production in sporadic or familial cases. The autosomal dominant form leads to excess estrogen synthesis from C19 precursors due to aromatase overexpression, especially in fat and skin; it is a consequence of gain-of-function mutations of *CYP19*, the gene that encodes aromatase, resulting from a chromosome arrangement that gives rise to a cryptic promoter.[813] An autosomal dominant pattern of prepubertal gynecomastia and adult hypogonadism but not short stature in the presence of elevated serum estrone (with little or no elevation of estradiol) has been reported; the mutations in the *CYP19* gene in these patients appeared to be different from those in the families described earlier with gain-of-function mutations resulting from gene inversions.[814] In a Turkish kindred, there was a potential rearrangement between *CYP19* and *TRPM7* genes on chromosome 15q21.2 as a cause of aromatase excess syndrome.[815] Recent study indicates that aromatase excess syndrome is caused by duplications involving *CYP19A1* and simple and complex rearrangements generated by both recombination- and replication-mediated mechanisms, independent of the known rearrangement-inducing DNA features or late-replication timing.[816] This condition is suggested to offer a unique model for human genomic disorders.

Feminizing Testicular Tumors. Feminizing testicular tumors may cause gynecomastia in boys younger than 6 years of age who have the Peutz-Jeghers syndrome.[817] Aromatase is absent or is present in barely detectable amounts in prepubertal testes, but maximal amounts appear in late puberty. In normal testes, aromatase is predominantly present in the Leydig cells, but in testicular tumors of Sertoli cells or Leydig cells (e.g., associated with the Peutz-Jeghers syndrome), the Sertoli cells of the tumor express aromatase. Both testes may be enlarged, and the histologic examination indicates sex cord or Sertoli cell tumors that form annular tubules and often have areas of calcification; increased estradiol secretion is noted in the basal state, and a further rise occurs after hCG administration. Otherwise, feminizing Sertoli cell tumors are very rare in boys.[818] Sonography or MRI of the testes may be useful in making the diagnosis.

In one series, 5% of 581 boys referred for evaluation of gynecomastia were prepubertal at diagnosis (mean age, 9 years), and in 93% no underlying cause was identified.[819] Spontaneous resolution was recorded in 6 boys, no change in was found in 15, and further breast enlargement was found in 6. Prepubertal gynecomastia can also be caused by neurofibromatosis.

Girls

Adrenal Causes of Virilization. Virilization in a girl indicates organic disease except for premature adrenarche. CAH resulting from 21-hydroxylase or 11β-hydroxylase deficiency or from androgen-producing tumors of the adrenal can cause virilization (see earlier discussion of their occurrence in males). Nonclassic or late-onset forms of CAH do not demonstrate ambiguous genitalia, but there is evidence of androgen effect in prepuberty or the teenage years. 3β-HSD/Δ⁴,⁵-isomerase deficiency is a rare type of CAH characterized by elevated levels of Δ^5-17P, DHEA, and DHEAS, as well as decreased secretion of aldosterone and cortisol in the severe form. Severely affected patients have mineralocorticoid and glucocorticoid deficiencies and may die in infancy. Excess adrenal androgens lead to virilization in utero and to ambiguous external genitalia, including clitoral enlargement in females with continued virilization after birth. Milder forms of this disorder can cause hirsutism in women. Women with a 46,XY phenotype and incomplete forms of androgen resistance syndrome or 17β-HSD type 3 deficiency may have virilization as well as breast development at the time of expected puberty. Aromatase deficiency due to mutations in the *CYP19* gene, which encodes aromatase, is associated with intrauterine masculinization of the external genitalia in affected 46,XX individuals and with progressive virilization, lack of female secondary sex characteristics, multicystic ovaries at the age of puberty, tall stature, and osteopenia.[242,244,270,272]

Cushing syndrome resulting from adrenal carcinoma usually manifests as growth failure with or without virilization, obesity, and moon facies; striae may not appear until months to years later.

Syndrome of Glucocorticoid Resistance. The syndrome of glucocorticoid resistance has variable manifestations. Some patients demonstrate hyperandrogenic signs such as acne, hirsutism, male-type baldness, menstrual irregularities, and oligoanovulation and infertility.[820] Dexamethasone decreases the excessive adrenal androgen secretion, virilization, and advancing bone age found in general glucocorticoid resistance.

Virilizing Ovarian Tumors. Arrhenoblastoma, also called Sertoli tumor of the ovary, is the most common virilizing ovarian tumor, but it is rare in children.[771] Recently somatic missense mutations affecting the RNase IIIb domain of DICER1 that alter DICER1 function in a manner that perturbation of microRNA processing may be oncogenic are common in these nonepithelial ovarian tumors.[821]

Lipoid-cell tumors of the ovary and gonadoblastomas of the ovary are even more unusual sources of androgens.

Variations of Pubertal Development

Premature Thelarche. Unilateral or bilateral breast enlargement without other signs of sexual maturation (e.g., sexual hair, growth of the labia minora, growth of the uterus) is not uncommon in infancy and childhood and is termed *premature thelarche*. The disorder usually occurs by age 2 (>80% of cases) and rarely after age 4.[822] In a retrospective study in Minnesota, the incidence of premature thelarche was 21.2 per 100,000 patient-years, 60% of cases were identified in patients between 6 months and 2 years of age, and most cases regressed within 6 months to 6 years after diagnosis, although a few persisted until puberty. When 10- to 35-year follow-up was available, no untoward effects on later health, growth, or fertility were evident.[789] Breast enlargement usually regresses after a few months but occasionally persists for years or until the onset of normal puberty; in about half of affected girls, the breast development, which is characteristically cyclic, lasts 3 to 5 years; this is found with age of onset over 2 years.[823] Usually, significant nipple and areola development is absent, and estrogen-induced thickening and dulling of the vaginal mucosa is uncommon. Enlargement of the uterus on ultrasonography (volume >1.8 mL, length >36 mm) is rare. Measurement of the ellipsoid volume of the uterus (V = longitudinal diameter × anteroposterior diameter × transverse diameter × 0.523) is the most sensitive and specific discriminator between premature thelarche and early[104] CPP and provides better early discrimination than the LH response to GnRH or GnRH agonist. Growth in stature is normal.

This is a benign, self-limited disorder that is compatible with normal pubertal development at an appropriate age; usually, only reassurance and follow-up are necessary. However, the appearance of premature thelarche can be the harbinger of further sexual maturation in a minority of cases. Although onset occurring soon after birth and before 2 years of age carries a higher prognosis for regression, 14% of two large series did progress no matter the age of onset of premature thelarche.[823] Because the breast development may be unilateral, it is important to consider the condition in girls who have unilateral breast development so that needless worry about a breast neoplasm is not stimulated in the parents and no unnecessary surgical procedure is carried out. Removal of tissue in premature thelarche may leave the child with no possibility of future breast development. In selected instances, sonography of the breast is useful to distinguish unilateral premature thelarche from less benign conditions. The most common cause of a breast mass in a pubertal girl is fibroadenoma, and although metastatic disease may locate in the pubertal breast, breast carcinoma is exceedingly rare in young patients.

Plasma estradiol levels are prepubertal in most standard assays but were slightly higher for age in patients with premature thelarche determined by a highly sensitive estrogen bioassay.[824] However, there is usually no significant increase in plasma levels of TeBG or in thyroxine-binding globulin, which are indicators of estrogen action on circulating plasma proteins, although a modest increase of TeBG for age has been reported. The urocytogram often reveals an estrogen effect on squamous epithelial cells in the urine.[745,825]

The concentration of serum FSH may be in the pubertal range, nocturnal FSH pulsatility has been detected, and the rise in FSH elicited by administration of GnRH may be augmented for chronologic age, with an FSH/LH ratio higher in precocious thelarche than in normal individuals or in girls with CPP. However, the results overlap those in normal prepubertal girls.

As postulated for some recurrent ovarian cysts, premature thelarche appears to result from the ovarian response to transient increases in FSH levels and possibly from variations in ovarian sensitivity to FSH. The LH response to GnRH is prepubertal in all cases.[397,826] Plasma inhibin B and FSH levels are higher in girls with precocious thelarche than in control subjects, in a range similar to that observed in patients with precocious puberty. Activin concentrations have not been reported. The possible role of a paracrine-acting pituitary factor in stimulating FSH independent of GnRH is not known.

Sonograms of the ovary often show one or several cysts larger than 0.5 cm that disappear and reappear, usually correlating with changes in the size of the breasts, but the volume of the ovary and uterus is prepubertal.[104] In clinical practice, it is rare to find a cyst at the time of presentation and on ultrasonic study.

Exaggerated thelarche is described as premature thelarche with the added findings of advanced bone age and increased growth rate, which are estrogen effects. The endocrine measurements in the basal state are in the normal prepubertal range, but after GnRH agonist stimulation, the level of FSH (but not of LH) rose higher than in control subjects or in patients with CPP. Mutation of *GNAS1* involving Arg201His is associated with apparent premature or exaggerated thelarche and early menarche.[663]

Unfortunately there are no guidelines that can determine which girl will undergo progression from premature thelarche to precocious puberty. Clinical follow-up is essential to determine which course will occur.

Premature Isolated Menarche. Rarely, girls begin periodic vaginal bleeding at between 1 and 9 years of age without any other signs of secondary sexual development. The bleeding can recur for 1 to 6 years and then cease. At the normal age of puberty (3 to 11 years later), secondary sexual development and menses ensue and follow a normal pattern, as does stature. Fertility was later demonstrated after a normal onset of puberty in women with this variant of pubertal development. The cause is uncertain, but it may be a counterpart of premature thelarche. There is a predominance of FSH secretion, but the gonadotropin secretion pattern is not characteristic of CPP.[827] Isolated menarche may appear before other manifestations of sexual precocity in patients with the McCune-Albright syndrome and in those with the premature sexual maturation that can occur in juvenile hypothyroidism.

Before the diagnosis of premature menarche is accepted, all other causes of vaginal bleeding and precocious estrogen secretion and of exposure to exogenous estrogens should be excluded, including neoplasms, granulomas, infection of the vagina or cervix, and presence of a foreign body. A careful examination for trauma, such as that caused by sexual abuse, is indicated. Urethral prolapse may be misdiagnosed as vaginal bleeding.

Premature Adrenarche. Premature adrenarche (i.e., pubarche) is the precocious appearance of pubic hair or axillary hair or both and, less commonly, an apocrine odor, comedones, and acne, without other signs of puberty or virilization. It is characterized by premature and mild adrenal hyperandrogenism.[404,828] The term *premature adrenarche* refers to the rise in serum concentrations of adrenal androgens that cause the appearance of the pubic hair. In the past, this designation was assigned when these clinical features appeared before age 8 years in girls or 9 years in boys. Although in boys the 9 years still seems appropriate as a cutoff point, the age of 8 years can no longer be used for American girls, according to the results of the PROS study[14] described earlier (mean ages are shown in Table 25-1). We recommend that the diagnosis of premature pubarche should be limited to African-American girls younger than 6 years of age and white American girls younger than 7 years, which should affect the age at which laboratory studies are initiated unless there are other signs of virilization, such as clitoromegaly or rapid growth.

Premature adrenarche is about 10 times more common in girls than in boys.[258,829,830] The prevalence is increased in children with CNS abnormalities without a clear sex difference; the electroencephalogram may be abnormal in the absence of other neurologic findings. Familial transmission is uncommon. Premature adrenarche is commonly slowly progressive and does not have an untoward effect on either the onset or the normal progression of gonadarche or final adult height. Nonetheless, there is a relationship between reduced fetal growth leading to intrauterine growth retardation and subsequent SGA and the increased prevalence of premature adrenarche, hyperinsulinism, and ovarian hyperandrogenism in life, although the relationship may change among different ethnic groups.[831]

Plasma concentrations of DHEA, DHEAS, androstenedione, testosterone, 17-hydroxyprogesterone, and Δ^5-17P are comparable to values normally found in pubic hair stage 2. ACTH stimulation increases serum DHEA and DHEAS concentrations and the excretion of urinary 17-ketosteroids, but the concentrations of plasma 17-hydroxyprogesterone and Δ^5-17P do not increase to the levels found in individuals with virilizing forms of CAH.[780] Shorter *AR* gene CAG number, indicative of increased androgen sensitivity, is reported in some girls with precocious adrenarche, suggesting that increased sensitivity to low androgen levels may be the basis rather than high androgen values per se. As in CAH, dexamethasone suppresses adrenal androgen and androgen precursor secretion. Serum gonadotropin levels in the basal state and after GnRH are in the prepubertal range in patients with premature adrenarche.[397] Premature adrenarche occurs independently of gonadarche and results from some unknown factor other than increased secretion of GnRH or ACTH. Bone age, height, and weight gain are slightly advanced for chronologic age, but normal adult height is commonly achieved, except, rarely, in some individuals with unusually high levels of adrenal androgens, hirsutism, acne, and a bone age more than 2 years advanced or 2.5 SD above the mean value for chronologic age.[832] In a follow-up study of 20 girls, the functional adrenal hyperandrogenism in premature adrenarche was limited to childhood.

Premature adrenarche may be considered to be a developmentally regulated, normal variation in the differentiation, growth, and function of the zona reticularis of the adrenal cortex, marked biochemically by the precocious increase in the concentration of plasma DHEAS to more than 40 μg/dL.[259] The latter is probably related to the independent increase of 17,20-lyase activity in the developing zona reticularis, which is mediated by increased phosphorylation of serine and threonine residues on the CYP17 enzyme, and the increased abundance of cytochrome b_5 and of electron-donating redox partners such as cytochrome P450 oxidoreductase and cytochrome b_5, which are essential for the 17,20-lyase activity of this functional microsomal enzyme (see Fig. 25-36).[780] A rise in intra-adrenal cortisol may inhibit 3β-HSD activity, thereby increasing DHEA according to in vitro evidence.[828] Nonetheless, the factors stimulating development and function of the zona reticularis, independent of ACTH, remain elusive.

The appearance of premature pubarche can be a manifestation of nonclassic 21-hydroxylase deficiency CAH caused by homozygous or compound heterozygous missense mutations in the *CYP21* gene.[833] This condition can readily be detected by a plasma 17-hydroxyprogesterone response to ACTH that is at least 6 SD above the mean value. The prevalence of 21-hydroxylase deficiency in children apparently presenting with premature adrenarche is low except in some ethnic groups (e.g., Hispanics, Italians, Ashkenazi Jews), in which the prevalence may be as high as 20% to 30%.

The cause of the observed mild deficiency in 3β-HSD activity is unknown, but it may be multifactorial and may lead to a wide range in secretory capacity of the zona reticularis. A family constellation was described with a dominant pattern of inheritance of elevated adrenal androgens and androgen precursors that manifested as premature pubarche[829]; later-affected individuals developed hirsutism and anovulation. Several investigators joined to propose hormonal standards for the diagnosis of 3β-HSD deficiency in cases of apparent premature pubarche and stated that ACTH-stimulated Δ^5-17P values must exceed 294 nmol/L or 54 SD above the mean for Tanner stage 2 (17 ± 5 nmol/L) or the ratio of Δ^5-17P to cortisol (F) must be at least 363, which is 3.0 SD above the mean ratio of 20 ± 5. Studies relating genotype and hormonal analyses in basal and ACTH-stimulated conditions have confirmed that significant elevations of the Δ^5-17P-to-F ratio are necessary to prove true 3β-HSD deficiency in genetically proven disease and that this is a rare disorder in patients presenting with putative premature adrenarche.[834] However, patients with a constellation of findings indicating PCOS may have subtler elevations of these values and present a picture of adrenal impairment of 3β-HSD activity in the absence of mutations in the gene coding for the enzyme; these children presenting with premature pubarche are postulated to develop clinical PCOS at a later age.

The phenotype of premature pubarche is also associated with the rarer nonclassic 11β-hydroxylase deficiency. Mutation of *HSD3B2* or *HSD3B1* is an uncommon cause of premature pubarche, exaggerated adrenarche, and hirsutism in adolescent girls and women.

DHEA stimulates sebaceous gland activity,[835] and prepubertal acne or comedones may appear in association with elevated serum DHEAS concentrations in some children without the appearance of pubic hair, suggesting that a variant of premature adrenarche may manifest in this manner.[118] More significant androgen effects (e.g., clitoral or penile enlargement, rapid growth, hirsutism, deepening of the voice) exclude premature adrenarche and indicate a more severe form of hyperandrogenism.

Although premature adrenarche was usually considered to be a benign condition with no substantial long-term risk, accumulating observations indicate that girls with premature adrenarche are at increased risk of developing functional ovarian hyperandrogenism and PCOS, hyperinsulinism, acanthosis nigricans, and dyslipidemia in adolescence and adult life, especially if fetal growth was reduced and the birth weight was low.[830] Affected girls have BMI values similar to those of control subjects but differing distribution of fat; they are more likely to have increased waist circumference along with measures of insulin resistance.[836] The concept of exaggerated adrenarche was first advanced in relation to a postulated childhood antecedent of PCOS. It has been extended to include rare instances of premature adrenarche associated with excessive responses of Δ^5-17P, DHEAS, and androstenedione to ACTH found in women with functional adrenal hyperandrogenism.

A recent report of a patient with premature adrenarche, advanced bone age, excessive acne, hyperandrogenic anovulation, very low DHEAS levels, and increased androgen levels demonstrated a mutation in PAPSS2, an enzyme that generates the sulfate donor 3′-phosphoadenosine-5′-phosphosulfate (PAPS), which is required for conversion of DHEA to DHEAS by the enzyme SULT2A1. Although the child was described as having premature pubarche, the androgen effects were greater than those usually encountered in this condition. The DHEA level was not elevated for age, but androstenedione was high owing to inadequate formation of DHEAS that decreases the conversion of DHEA to androstenedione. This presentation would ordinarily suggest an ovarian cause of the virilization. This monogenetic defect must be added to the differential diagnosis of premature adrenarche.[260]

Polycystic Ovary Disease. PCOS is the most common endocrine disease; it is estimated to affect 10% of women.[837] The hallmarks of this condition are hyperandrogenism, hirsutism,[838] anovulation, amenorrhea or oligomenorrhea, and insulin resistance; there is compensatory hyperinsulinemia, with its attendant risk of major metabolic sequelae including type 2 diabetes mellitus, dyslipidemia, an increased propensity to coronary heart disease, and, in about 50% of affected women, obesity. PCOS is considered to be equivalent to the metabolic syndrome in its many manifestations in females. A 2013 review of diagnostic criteria supports the use of the Rotterdam criteria for diagnosis, noting the weakness of the method as well. Thus, diagnosis rests upon the presence of two of the following criteria: androgen excess, ovulatory dysfunction, or polycystic ovaries.[633] Some prefer *hyperinsulinemic androgen excess* as a term that is a better indicator of the basis of the disorder in view of the fact that polycystic ovaries are not required for diagnosis.[831] Indeed criteria for the diagnosis of polycystic ovary morphologic appearance may require a greater number of follicles (more than 25 on ultrasound) than recommended by the Rotterdam criteria, and standards may yet change.[839] The use of AMH in the diagnosis of PCOS is under consideration but remains controversial owing to differences in study criteria and in the assays used to report AMH values.[840] At least it can be said that AMH appears to correlate with polycystic appearance and androgen manifestations in many studies and in the future may become a diagnostic criterion.

Premature adrenarche in some populations is a risk factor for the later development of the PCOS and functional ovarian hyperandrogenism in adolescent and adult women; the magnitude of this risk is unknown, but it appears to be rare, except in girls with a history of SGA.[841] However, catch-up growth after SGA may be as important a factor in the development of PCOS, and even prematurity may be a risk. In an 880-member cohort of 8-year-olds, serum androstenedione and DHEAS levels were directly related to weight gain between 1 and 3 years and current weight and inversely related to birth weight.[842] However, a Dutch study could not confirm such a relationship between increase in premature adrenarche and SGA birth weight in 181 subjects born SGA compared with 170 subjects born with AGA.[843]

In certain ethnic groups, and especially in African-American and Hispanic girls, there is a greater association of premature adrenarche with the metabolic syndrome (obesity, hyperinsulinism, dyslipidemia, and other factors that increase the risk of later coronary heart disease) and the development of PCOS in late adolescence and early adulthood, especially if decreased insulin sensitivity and acanthosis nigricans accompany the premature adrenarche.[844]

As discussed earlier, hyperinsulinism is associated with many metabolic and endocrine conditions and functional ovarian hyperandrogenism that, in some cases, is heralded by premature adrenarche. Lifestyle modification is the primary approach to the treatment of PCOS and although success is achievable,[845] the failure rate is substantial. Oral contraceptives are often invoked but may be considered to treat the effects rather than the cause based on insulin resistance and excessive adiposity; nonetheless, the use of oral contraceptives with progestational and antiandrogen effects can regulate menstrual periods[831] although long-term studies of progestation-only contraceptives in teenagers with PCOS are lacking.[846] Therapeutic approaches to reduce insulin resistance, especially the use of insulin sensitizers, have been introduced into the therapy for PCOS. The most widely used drug is metformin because of its low prevalence of adverse effects and therapeutic efficacy. Substantial data support the safety and efficacy of its use in adolescents with insulin resistance,[831] although metformin is not FDA-approved for such use. Although flutamide in higher doses has caused hepatotoxicity, low-dose flutamide (1 mg/kg) is reportedly safe and effective in hirsute young women (but has not been proved to have such a safety profile in obesity or steatohepatitis)[847]; abstinence or contraception is essential when using this teratogenic agent. Thiazolidinediones are not recommened because of safety concerns.[633]

In a trial involving girls just past menarche who had a history of low birth weight and premature adrenarche and were therefore at risk for development of PCOS, metformin prevented this predicted course.[841] Treatment of 8-year-old girls who had similar risk factors appeared to diminish the risk during short-term studies. The beneficial effects on body composition, dyslipidemia, insulin resistance, and other parameters were present only during therapy; they reverted to increased risk factors after discontinuation of metformin. Weight loss is documented with the combination of metformin and oral contraceptives.[848]

Adolescent Gynecomastia. Normal boys, usually in the early stages of puberty, may have either unilateral breast enlargement (approximately 25% of boys)[849] or bilateral breast enlargement (approximately 50% to 65% of boys to varying degrees); this commonly occurs between chronologic ages 14 and 14.5 years or with pubic hair stages 3 and 4. In these boys, the plasma concentrations of testosterone and estrogen are normal for their stage of puberty. Some have suggested that the ratio of estrogen to androgen or an increase in the ratio of testosterone to dihydrotestosterone is a cause. In a prospective study, adolescent boys with gynecomastia had a lower mean free testosterone concentration, lower weight, higher plasma TeBG levels, and a tendency toward earlier onset of puberty and more rapid progression through puberty.[849] In one study, a significant decrease in the concentration ratio of plasma androstenedione to estrone and estradiol and a similarly low ratio of DHEAS to estrone and estradiol were described in boys with pubertal gynecomastia who had normal ratios of plasma estrone and estradiol to testosterone. It was postulated that decreased adrenal production of androgens or (more likely) increased peripheral conversion of adrenal androgens to estrogens was a factor in the development of pubertal gynecomastia.[850]

Trials of estrogen receptor antagonists (e.g., tamoxifen, raloxifene) show promise, but more study is required.[851] Exogenous androgen administration has had mixed results in gynecomastia. One study of boys (average age, 13 years) with gynecomastia involving a mean of 7 months of treatment with anastrozole demonstrated a substantial decrease in breast area (63%) and volume (53%), as measured manually and by ultrasonography, compared with watchful waiting[852]; however, larger studies are recommended to prove the utility of this approach because another study found no such result.

Pubertal gynecomastia usually resolves spontaneously within 1 to 2 years after onset, and reassurance and continued observation are often adequate treatment. Nevertheless, some boys have conspicuous gynecomastia, and if it lasts longer than 2 years (5-20% in various studies), it is likely to become permanent. These children may have sufficient psychological distress to warrant a reduction mammoplasty. Indeed the psychological stress appears unrelated to the duration or severity, and counseling should be considered in appropriate boys.[853] Liposuction is an alternative approach, but its efficacy in adolescent gynecomastia remains to be established. Untreated persistent gynecomastia persists into adulthood. The histologic examination of physiologic gynecomastia tissue rarely reveals carcinoma, so routine disease examination may be unnecessary.[854]

Gynecomastia is a component of Klinefelter syndrome, anorchia, primary and secondary hypogonadism, biosynthetic defects in testosterone synthesis, increased aromatase activity in adipose and other tissues (aromatase excess syndrome), Sertoli cell tumors, adventitious exposure to estrogens in meat or cosmetics, and variants of the androgen resistance syndromes, including Rosewater syndrome (familial hypogonadism and gynecomastia) and Reifenstein syndrome (hypospadias, hypogonadism, and gynecomastia). These disorders usually have characteristic findings or environmental circumstances that allow ready differentiation from the normal gynecomastia of puberty.[562] Gynecomastia has been described in association with the administration of drugs such as cimetidine, spironolactone, digitalis, and phenothiazines; with GH therapy; and with the use of marijuana. The aromatase excess syndrome was described earlier.

Macroorchidism. Macroorchidism is defined as testes twice the normal size for age without androgenization. It is a rare manifestation of the McCune-Albright syndrome[778] and an occasional finding in prepubertal boys with long-standing primary hypothyroidism. This form of testicular enlargement appears to result from increased FSH secretion, independent of a pubertal increase in LH secretion or a pubertal LH response to GnRH. Testicular adrenal rests in CAH can cause bilateral macroorchidism, as can lymphoma. In the McCune-Albright syndrome, an activating mutation in the $G_s\alpha$ gene primarily expressed in the Sertoli cells can cause macroorchidism due to Sertoli cell proliferation and hyperfunction with increased concentration of serum inhibin B and AMH but without increased testosterone levels due to Leydig cell hyperplasia, elevated gonadotropins, or signs of puberty.[295] Macroorchidism is a feature of severe aromatase deficiency in young male adults[272] and in men with an FSH-secreting pituitary macroadenoma. Bilateral megalotestis (testicular volume, 26 mL) in adults can occur as a normal variant.[855] One may speculate that some instances of bilateral macroorchidism are the result of a heterozygous constitutive activating mutation of the FSH receptor. As noted earlier, prepubertal enlargement of the testes was reported with a single-base-pair deletion at codon 434 (1301delT) of the *NR0B1/DAX1* gene and led to prepubertal testosterone and gonadotropin values.[717] Testes will enlarge during treatment with aromatase inhibitors.

The fragile X syndrome is associated with developmental delay, a long face and large prominent ears, and macroorchidism in 80% of affected pubertal boys. Macroorchidism may be evident only after careful measurements. The enlarged testes are caused by increased interstitial volume and excessive connective tissue, including increased peritubular collagen fibers, rather than by an increase in the seminiferous tubules. Enlargement of the testes is demonstrable in the prepubertal period in most patients with fragile X syndrome, but the onset of true macroorchidism (>4 cm) occurs only in the later prepubertal period.[856]

REFERENCES

1. Grumbach MM. Onset of puberty. In: Berenberg SR, ed. *Puberty, Biologic and Social Components.* Leiden, The Netherlands: H. E. Stenfert Kroese; 1975:1-21.
2. Bogin B. Childhood, adolescence, and longevity: a multilevel model of the evolution of reserve capacity in human life history. *Am J Hum Biol.* 2009;21(4):567-577.
3. Gluckman PD, Hanson MA. Changing times: the evolution of puberty. *Mol Cell Endocrinol.* 2006;254-255:26-31.
4. Gluckman PD, Bergstrom CT. Evolutionary biology within medicine: a perspective of growing value. *BMJ.* 2011;343:d7671.
5. Verkauskiene R, Petraitiene I, Albertsson Wikland K. Puberty in children born small for gestational age. *Horm Res Paediatr.* 2013;80(2):69-77.
6. Sloboda DM, Hart R, Doherty DA, et al. Age at menarche: influences of prenatal and postnatal growth. *J Clin Endocrinol Metab.* 2007;92(1):46-50.
7. Tam CS, de Zegher F, Garnett SP, et al. Opposing influences of prenatal and postnatal growth on the timing of menarche. *J Clin Endocrinol Metab.* 2006;91(11):4369-4373.
8. Ong KK, Emmett P, Northstone K, et al. Infancy weight gain predicts childhood body fat and age at menarche in girls. *J Clin Endocrinol Metab.* 2009;94(5):1527-1532.
9. Tanner JM. *A History of the Study of Human Growth.* Cambridge, UK: Cambridge University Press; 1981.
10. Wyshak G, Frisch RE. Evidence for a secular trend in age of menarche. *N Engl J Med.* 1982;306:1033-1035.
11. Biro FM, Huang B, Crawford PB, et al. Pubertal correlates in black and white girls. *J Pediatr.* 2006;148(2):234-240.
12. Must A, Phillips SM, Naumova EN, et al. Recall of early menstrual history and menarcheal body size: after 30 years, how well do women remember? *Am J Epidemiol.* 2002;155(7):672-679.
13. Artaria MD, Henneberg M. Why did they lie? Socio-economic bias in reporting menarcheal age. *Ann Hum Biol.* 2000;27(6):561-569.
14. Herman-Giddens ME, Slora EJ, Wasserman RC, et al. Secondary sexual characteristics and menses in young girls seen in office practice: a study from the Pediatric Research in Office Settings network. *Pediatrics.* 1997;99:505-512.
15. Coleman L, Coleman J. The measurement of puberty: a review. *J Adolesc.* 2002;25(5):535-550.
16. Rockett JC, Lynch CD, Buck GM. Biomarkers for assessing reproductive development and health: part 1—pubertal development. *Environ Health Perspect.* 2004;112(1):105-112.
17. Shirtcliff EA, Dahl RE, Pollak SD. Pubertal development: correspondence between hormonal and physical development. *Child Dev.* 2009;80(2):327-337.
18. Marshall WA, Tanner JM. Puberty. In: Falkner F, Tanner JM, eds. *Human Growth.* New York, NY: Plenum; 1986:171-209.
19. Parent AS, Teilmann G, Juul A, et al. The timing of normal puberty and the age limits of sexual precocity: variations around the world, secular trends, and changes after migration. *Endocr Rev.* 2003;24(5):668-693.
20. Ong KK, Ahmed ML, Dunger DB. Lessons from large population studies on timing and tempo of puberty (secular trends and relation to body size): the European trend. *Mol Cell Endocrinol.* 2006;254-255:8-12.
21. Freedman DS, Khan LK, Serdula MK, et al. Relation of age at menarche to race, time period, and anthropometric dimensions: the Bogalusa Heart Study. *Pediatrics.* 2002;110(1):e43.
22. Styne DM. Puberty, obesity and ethnicity. *Trends Endocrinol Metab.* 2004;15(10):472-478.
23. Chumlea WC, Schubert CM, Roche AF, et al. Age at menarche and racial comparisons in US girls. *Pediatrics.* 2003;111(1):110-113.
24. Himes JH. Examining the evidence for recent secular changes in the timing of puberty in US children in light of increases in the prevalence of obesity. *Mol Cell Endocrinol.* 2006;254-255:13-21.
25. Harlan WR, Harlan EA, Grillo GP. Secondary sex characteristics of girls 12 to 17 years of age: the U.S. Health Examination Survey. *J Pediatr.* 1980;96:1074-1078.
26. Biro FM, McMahon RP, Striegel-Moore R, et al. Impact of timing of pubertal maturation on growth in black and white female adolescents: the National Heart, Lung, and Blood Institute Growth and Health Study. *J Pediatr.* 2001;138(5):636-643.
27. Russell DL, Keil MF, Bonat SH, et al. The relation between skeletal maturation and adiposity in African American and Caucasian children. *J Pediatr.* 2001;139(6):844-848.

28. Krebs NF, Himes JH, Jacobson D, et al. Assessment of child and adolescent overweight and obesity. *Pediatrics*. 2007;120(Suppl 4): S193-S228.
29. August GP, Caprio S, Fennoy I, et al. Prevention and treatment of pediatric obesity: an Endocrine Society clinical practice guideline based on expert opinion. *J Clin Endocrinol Metab*. 2008;93(12):4576-4599.
30. Kaplowitz PB, Slora EJ, Wasserman RC, et al. Earlier onset of puberty in girls: relation to increased body mass index and race. *Pediatrics*. 2001;108(2):347-353.
31. Rosenfield RL, Lipton RB, Drum ML. Thelarche, pubarche, and menarche attainment in children with normal and elevated body mass index. *Pediatrics*. 2009;123(1):84-88.
32. Anderson SE, Dallal GE, Must A. Relative weight and race influence average age at menarche: results from two nationally representative surveys of US girls studied 25 years apart. *Pediatrics*. 2003;111(4 Pt 1): 844-850.
33. Himes JH, Obarzanek E, Baranowski T, et al. Early sexual maturation, body composition, and obesity in African-American girls. *Obes Res*. 2004;12(Suppl):64S-72S.
34. Herman-Giddens ME, Steffes J, Harris D, et al. Secondary sexual characteristics in boys: data from the Pediatric Research in Office Settings Network. *Pediatrics*. 2012;130(5):e1058-e1068.
35. Biro FM, Lucky AW, Simbartl LA, et al. Pubertal maturation in girls and the relationship to anthropometric changes: pathways through puberty. *J Pediatr*. 2003;142(6):643-646.
36. Schubert CM, Chumlea WC, Kulin HE, et al. Concordant and discordant sexual maturation among U.S. children in relation to body weight and BMI. *J Adolesc Health*. 2005;37(5):356-362.
37. Adair LS, Gordon-Larsen P. Maturational timing and overweight prevalence in US adolescent girls. *Am J Public Health*. 2001;91(4):642-644.
38. Davison KK, Susman EJ, Birch LL. Percent body fat at age 5 predicts earlier pubertal development among girls at age 9. *Pediatrics*. 2003;111(4 Pt 1):815-821.
39. Demerath EW, Towne B, Chumlea WC, et al. Recent decline in age at menarche: the Fels Longitudinal Study. *Am J Hum Biol*. 2004;16(4): 453-457.
40. van Hooff MH, Voorhorst FJ, Kaptein MB, et al. Insulin, androgen, and gonadotropin concentrations, body mass index, and waist to hip ratio in the first years after menarche in girls with regular menstrual cycles, irregular menstrual cycles, or oligomenorrhea. *J Clin Endocrinol Metab*. 2000;85(4):1394-1400.
41. He Q, Karlberg J. BMI in childhood and its association with height gain, timing of puberty, and final height. *Pediatr Res*. 2001;49(2): 244-251.
42. Aksglaede L, Sorensen K, Petersen JH, et al. Recent decline in age at breast development: the Copenhagen Puberty Study. *Pediatrics*. 2009; 123(5):e932-e939.
43. Ellis BJ. Timing of pubertal maturation in girls: an integrated life history approach. *Psychol Bull*. 2004;130(6):920-958.
44. Remer T, Shi L, Buyken AE. Prepubertal adrenarchal androgens and animal protein intake independently and differentially influence pubertal timing. *J Clin Endocrinol Metab*. 2010;95(6):3002-3009.
45. Rogers IS, Northstone K, Dunger DB, et al. Diet throughout childhood and age at menarche in a contemporary cohort of British girls. *Public Health Nutr*. 2010;13(12):2052-2063.
46. Koo MM, Rohan TE, Jain M, et al. A cohort study of dietary fibre intake and menarche. *Public Health Nutr*. 2002;5(2):353-360.
47. Cheng G, Remer T, Prinz-Langenohl R, et al. Relation of isoflavones and fiber intake in childhood to the timing of puberty. *Am J Clin Nutr*. 2010;92(3):556-564.
48. Rosell M, Appleby P, Key T. Height, age at menarche, body weight and body mass index in life-long vegetarians. *Public Health Nutr*. 2005; 8(7):870-875.
49. Dorgan JF, Hunsberger SA, McMahon RP, et al. Diet and sex hormones in girls: findings from a randomized controlled clinical trial. *J Natl Cancer Inst*. 2003;95(2):132-141.
50. Wolff MS, Britton JA, Boguski L, et al. Environmental exposures and puberty in inner-city girls. *Environ Res*. 2008;107(3):393-400.
51. Mervish NA, Gardiner EW, Galvez MP, et al. Dietary flavonol intake is associated with age of puberty in a longitudinal cohort of girls. *Nutr Res*. 2013;33(7):534-542.
52. Boynton-Jarrett R, Rich-Edwards J, Fredman L, et al. Gestational weight gain and daughter's age at menarche. *J Women's Health*. 2011; 20(8):1193-1200.
53. Fried PA, James DS, Watkinson B. Growth and pubertal milestones during adolescence in offspring prenatally exposed to cigarettes and marihuana. *Neurotoxicol Teratol*. 2001;23(5):431-436.
54. Colbert LH, Graubard BI, Michels KB, et al. Physical activity during pregnancy and age at menarche of the daughter. *Cancer Epidemiol Biomarkers Prev*. 2008;17(10):2656-2662.
55. Ellis BJ. The hypothalamic-pituitary-gonadal axis: a switch-controlled, condition-sensitive system in the regulation of life history strategies. *Horm Behav*. 2013;64(2):215-225.
56. Sloboda DM, Beedle AS, Cupido CL, et al. Impaired perinatal growth and longevity: a life history perspective. *Curr Gerontol Geriatr Res*. 2009;608-740.
57. Tither JM, Ellis BJ. Impact of fathers on daughters' age at menarche: a genetically and environmentally controlled sibling study. *Dev Psychol*. 2008;44(5):1409-1420.
58. Prebeg Z, Bralic I. Changes in menarcheal age in girls exposed to war conditions. *Am J Human Biol*. 2000;12(4):503-508.
59. Henrichs KL, McCauley HL, Miller E, et al. Early menarche and childhood adversities in a nationally representative sample. *Int J Pediatr Endocrinol*. 2014;2014(1):14.
60. Li L, Denholm R, Power C. Child maltreatment and household dysfunction: associations with pubertal development in a British birth cohort. *Int J Epidemiol*. 2014;43(4):1163-1173.
61. Matsuo N, Anzo M, Sato S, et al. Testicular volume in Japanese boys up to the age of 15 years. *Eur J Pediatr*. 2000;159(11):843-845.
62. Ersoy B, Balkan C, Gunay T, Egemen A. The factors affecting the relation between the menarcheal age of mother and daughter. *Child Care Health Dev*. 2005;31(3):303-308.
63. Eaves L, Silberg J, Foley D, et al. Genetic and environmental influences on the relative timing of pubertal change. *Twin Res*. 2004;7(5): 471-481.
64. Towne B, Czerwinski SA, Demerath EW, et al. Heritability of age at menarche in girls from the Fels Longitudinal Study. *Am J Phys Anthropol*. 2005;128(1):210-219.
65. He C, Kraft P, Chen C, et al. Genome-wide association studies identify loci associated with age at menarche and age at natural menopause. *Nat Genet*. 2009.
66. Sulem P, Gudbjartsson DF, Rafnar T, et al. Genome-wide association study identifies sequence variants on 6q21 associated with age at menarche. *Nat Genet*. 2009.
67. Perry JR, Stolk L, Franceschini N, et al. Meta-analysis of genome-wide association data identifies two loci influencing age at menarche. *Nat Genet*. 2009.
68. Cousminer DL, Berry DJ, Timpson NJ, et al. Genome-wide association and longitudinal analyses reveal genetic loci linking pubertal height growth, pubertal timing and childhood adiposity. *Hum Mol Genet*. 2013;22(13):2735-2747.
69. Sedlmeyer IL, Pearce CL, Trueman JA, et al. Determination of sequence variation and haplotype structure for the gonadotropin-releasing hormone (GnRH) and GnRH receptor genes: investigation of role in pubertal timing. *J Clin Endocrinol Metab*. 2005;90(2):1091-1099.
70. Comings DE, Gade R, Muhleman D, et al. The LEP gene and age of menarche: maternal age as a potential cause of hidden stratification in association studies. *Mol Genet Metab*. 2001;73(3):204-210.
71. Stavrou I, Zois C, Ioannidis JP, Tsatsoulis A. Association of polymorphisms of the oestrogen receptor alpha gene with the age of menarche. *Hum Reprod*. 2002;17(4):1101-1105.
72. Kadlubar FF, Berkowitz GS, Delongchamp RR, et al. The CYP3A4*1B variant is related to the onset of puberty, a known risk factor for the development of breast cancer. *Cancer Epidemiol Biomarkers Prev*. 2003;12(4):327-331.
73. Johnson N, Dudbridge F, Orr N, et al. Genetic variation at CYP3A is associated with age at menarche and breast cancer risk: a case-control study. *Breast Cancer Res*. 2014;16(3):R51.
74. Xita N, Tsatsoulis A, Stavrou I, Georgiou I. Association of SHBG gene polymorphism with menarche. *Mol Hum Reprod*. 2005;11(6): 459-462.
75. Matchock RL, Susman EJ, Brown FM. Seasonal rhythms of menarche in the United States: correlates to menarcheal age, birth age, and birth month. *Womens Health Issues*. 2004;14(6):184-192.
76. Collaborative Group on Hormonal Factors in Breast Cancer. Menarche, menopause, and breast cancer risk: individual participant meta-analysis, including 118 964 women with breast cancer from 117 epidemiological studies. *Lancet Oncol*. 2012;13(11):1141-1151.
77. Clavel-Chapelon F, Gerber M. Reproductive factors and breast cancer risk. Do they differ according to age at diagnosis? *Breast Cancer Res Treat*. 2002;72(2):107-115.
78. Hamilton AS, Mack TM. Puberty and genetic susceptibility to breast cancer in a case-control study in twins. *N Engl J Med*. 2003;348(23): 2313-2322.
79. De Stavola BL, dos Santos Silva I, McCormack V, et al. Childhood growth and breast cancer. *Am J Epidemiol*. 2004;159(7):671-682.
80. Ahlgren M, Melbye M, Wohlfahrt J, Sorensen TI. Growth patterns and the risk of breast cancer in women. *N Engl J Med*. 2004;351(16): 1619-1626.
81. Tehard B, Kaaks R, Clavel-Chapelon F. Body silhouette, menstrual function at adolescence and breast cancer risk in the E3N cohort study. *Br J Cancer*. 2005;92(11):2042-2048.
82. Hatch EE, Linet MS, Zhang J, et al. Reproductive and hormonal factors and risk of brain tumors in adult females. *Int J Cancer*. 2005;114(5): 797-805.
83. Zhang Y, Holford TR, Leaderer B, et al. Menstrual and reproductive factors and risk of non-Hodgkin's lymphoma among Connecticut women. *Am J Epidemiol*. 2004;160(8):766-773.
84. Remsberg KE, Demerath EW, Schubert CM, et al. Early menarche and the development of cardiovascular disease risk factors in adolescent girls: the Fels Longitudinal Study. *J Clin Endocrinol Metab*. 2005;90(5): 2718-2724.

85. Harlan WR, Grillo GP, Cornoni-Huntley J, Leaverton PE. Secondary sex characteristics of boys 12 to 17 years of age: the U.S. Health Examination Survey. *J Pediatr.* 1979;95:293-297.

86. Roche AF, Wellens R, Attie KM, Siervogel RM. The timing of sexual maturation in a group of U.S. white youths. *J Pediatr Endocrinol.* 1995;8:11-18.

87. Wu T, Mendola P, Buck GM. Ethnic differences in the presence of secondary sex characteristics and menarche among US girls: the Third National Health and Nutrition Examination Survey, 1988-1994. *Pediatrics.* 2002;110(4):752-757.

88. Sun SS, Schubert CM, Chumlea WC, et al. National estimates of the timing of sexual maturation and racial differences among US children. *Pediatrics.* 2002;110(5):911-919.

89. Marti-Henneberg C, Vizmanos B. The duration of puberty in girls is related to the timing of its onset. *J Pediatr.* 1997;131(4):618-621.

90. Lee PA, Guo SS, Kulin HE. Age of puberty: data from the United States of America. *APMIS.* 2001;109(2):81-88.

91. Kaplowitz PB, Oberfield SE. Reexamination of the age limit for defining when puberty is precocious in girls in the United States: implications for evaluation and treatment. Drug and Therapeutics and Executive Committees of the Lawson Wilkins Pediatric Endocrine Society. *Pediatrics.* 1999;104(4 Pt 1):936-941.

92. Midyett LK, Moore WV, Jacobson JD. Are pubertal changes in girls before age 8 benign? *Pediatrics.* 2003;111(1):47-51.

93. Kaplowitz P. Clinical characteristics of 104 children referred for evaluation of precocious puberty. *J Clin Endocrinol Metab.* 2004;89(8):3644-3650.

94. De Vries L, Phillip M. Children referred for signs of early puberty warrant endocrine evaluation and follow-up. *J Clin Endocrinol Metab.* 2005;90(1):593-594.

95. Chalumeau M, Hadjiathanasiou CG, Ng SM, et al. Selecting girls with precocious puberty for brain imaging: validation of European evidence-based diagnosis rule. *J Pediatr.* 2003;143(4):445-450.

96. Fenton SE. Endocrine-disrupting compounds and mammary gland development: early exposure and later life consequences. *Endocrinology.* 2006;147(6 Suppl):S18-S24.

97. McCartney CR, Prendergast KA, Blank SK, et al. Maturation of luteinizing hormone (gonadotropin-releasing hormone) secretion across puberty: evidence for altered regulation in obese peripubertal girls. *J Clin Endocrinol Metab.* 2009;94(1):56-66.

98. McCartney CR, Blank SK, Prendergast KA, et al. Obesity and sex steroid changes across puberty: evidence for marked hyperandrogenemia in pre- and early pubertal obese girls. *J Clin Endocrinol Metab.* 2007;92(2):430-436.

99. Rohn RD. Nipple (papilla) development in puberty: longitudinal observations in girls. *Pediatrics.* 1987;79:745-747.

100. Vargas SO, Kozakewich HP, Boyd TK, et al. Childhood asymmetric labium majus enlargement: mimicking a neoplasm. *Am J Surg Pathol.* 2005;29(8):1007-1016.

101. Smith P, Wilhelm D, Rodgers RJ. Development of mammalian ovary. *J Endocrinol.* 2014;221(3):R145-R161.

102. Grumbach MM, Gluckman PD. The human fetal hypothalamus and pituitary gland; the maturation of neuroendocrine mechanisms controlling the secretion of fetal pituitary growth hormone, prolactin, gonadotropin, and adrenocorticotropin-related peptides and thyrotropin. In: Tulchinsky D, Little AB, eds. *Maternal-Fetal Endocrinology.* 2nd ed. Philadelphia, PA: WB Saunders; 1994:193-261.

103. Hart R, Sloboda DM, Doherty DA, et al. Prenatal determinants of uterine volume and ovarian reserve in adolescence. *J Clin Endocrinol Metab.* 2009;94(12):4931-4937.

104. De Vries L, Horev G, Schwartz M, Phillip M. Ultrasonographic and clinical parameters for early differentiation between precocious puberty and premature thelarche. *EurJ Endocrinol.* 2006;154(6):891-898.

105. Battaglia C, Mancini F, Regnani G, et al. Pelvic ultrasound and color Doppler findings in different isosexual precocities. *Ultrasound Obstet Gynecol.* 2003;22(3):277-283.

106. Batt RE, Mitwally MF. Endometriosis from thelarche to midteens: pathogenesis and prognosis, prevention and pedagogy. *J Pediatr Adolesc Gynecol.* 2003;16(6):337-347.

107. Martin JA, Hamilton BE, Ventura SJ, et al. Births: final data for 2011. *Natl Vital Statistics Rep.* 2013;62(1):1-69, 72.

108. Taskinen S, Taavitsainen M, Wikstrom S. Measurement of testicular volume: comparison of 3 different methods. *J Urol.* 1996;155:930-933.

109. Zachmann M, Prader A, Kind HP, et al. Testicular volume during adolescence. Cross-sectional and longitudinal studies. *Helv Paediatr Acta.* 1974;29(1):61-72.

110. Biro FM, Lucky AW, Huster GA, Morrison JA. Pubertal staging in boys. *J Pediatr.* 1995;127:40-46.

111. Ankarberg-Lindgren C, Norjavaara E. Changes of diurnal rhythm and levels of total and free testosterone secretion from pre to late puberty in boys: testis size of 3 ml is a transition stage to puberty. *Eur J Endocrinol.* 2004;151(6):747-757.

112. Sutherland RS, Kogan BA, Baskin LS, et al. The effect of prepubertal androgen exposure on adult penile length. *J Urol.* 1996;156:783-787.

113. Gondos B, Kogan SJ. Testicular development during puberty. In: Grumbach MM, Sizonenko PC, Aubert ML, et al., eds. *Control of the Onset of Puberty.* Baltimore, MD: Williams & Wilkins; 1990:387-402.

114. Prince FP. The triphasic nature of Leydig cell development in humans, and comments on nomenclature. *J Endocrinol.* 2001;168(2):213-216.

115. Nysom K, Pedersen JL, Jorgensen M, et al. Spermaturia in two normal boys without other signs of puberty. *Acta Paediatr.* 1994;83:520-521.

116. Laron Z, Arad J, Gurewitz R, et al. Age at first conscious ejaculation: a milestone in male puberty. *Helv Paediatr Acta.* 1980;35:13-20.

117. Amir O, Biron-Shental T. The impact of hormonal fluctuations on female vocal folds. *Curr Opin Otolaryngol Head Neck Surg.* 2004;12(3):180-184.

118. Lucky AW, Biro FM, Simbartl LA, et al. Predictors of severity of acne vulgaris in young adolescent girls: results of a five-year longitudinal study. *J Pediatr.* 1997;130:30-39.

119. Adebamowo CA, Spiegelman D, Danby FW, et al. High school dietary dairy intake and teenage acne. *J Am Acad Dermatol.* 2005;52(2):207-214.

120. Cozza P, Stirpe G, Condo R, Donatelli M. Craniofacial and body growth: a cross-sectional anthropometric pilot study on children during prepubertal period. *Eur J Paediatr Dent.* 2005;6(2):90-96.

121. Boyanov MA, Temelkova NL, Popivanov PP. Determinants of thyroid volume in school children: fat-free mass versus body fat mass—a cross-sectional study. *Endocr Pract.* 2004;10(5):409-416.

122. Hero M, Wickman S, Hanhijarvi R, et al. Pubertal upregulation of erythropoiesis in boys is determined primarily by androgen. *J Pediatr.* 2005;146(2):245-252.

123. Duncan GJ, Kirkendall NJ, Citro CF, eds. *The National Children's Study 2014: An Assessment.* Washington, DC: The National Academies Press; 2014.

124. Veldhuis JD, Roemmich JN, Richmond EJ, et al. Endocrine control of body composition in infancy, childhood, and puberty. *EndocrRev.* 2005;26(1):114-146.

125. Tanner JM, Whitehouse RH, Marubini E, Resele LF. The adolescent growth spurt of boys and girls of the Harpenden growth study. *Ann Hum Biol.* 1976;3:109-126.

126. Iuliano-Burns S, Hopper J, Seeman E. The age of puberty determines sexual dimorphism in bone structure: a male/female co-twin control study. *J Clin Endocrinol Metab.* 2009;94(5):1638-1643.

127. Karlberg J, Kwan CW, Gelander L, Albertsson-Wikland K. Pubertal growth assessment. *Horm Res.* 2003;60(Suppl 1):27-35.

128. Tanner JM, Davies PSW. Clinical longitudinal standards for height and height velocity for North American children. *J Pediatr.* 1985;107:317-329.

129. Caino S, Kelmansky D, Lejarraga H, Adamo P. Short-term growth at adolescence in healthy girls. *Ann Hum Biol.* 2004;31(2):182-195.

130. Luo ZC, Cheung YB, He Q, et al. Growth in early life and its relation to pubertal growth. *Epidemiology.* 2003;14(1):65-73.

131. McKusick VA. *Heritable Disorders of Connective Tissue.* St. Louis, MO: Mosby; 1972.

132. Tanner JM. *Assessment of Skeletal Maturity and Prediction of Adult Height: TW 2 Method.* New York, NY: Academic Press; 1983.

133. Grumbach MM, Auchus RJ. Estrogen: consequences and implication of human mutations in synthesis and action. *J Clin Endocrinol Metab.* 1999;84:4677-4694.

134. Grumbach MM. Estrogen, bone, growth, and sex: a sea change in conventional wisdom. *J Pediatr Endocrinol Metab.* 2000;13(Suppl 6):1439-1455.

135. Rochira V, Balestrieri A, Faustini-Fustini M, Carani C. Role of estrogen on bone in the human male: insights from the natural models of congenital estrogen deficiency. *Mol Cell Endocrinol.* 2001;178(1-2):215-220.

136. Greulich WS, Pyle SI. *Radiographic Atlas of Skeletal Development of the Hand and Wrist.* Stanford, CA: Stanford University Press; 1959.

137. Tanner JM, Whitehouse RH, Marshall WA, et al. *Assessment of Skeletal Maturity and Prediction of Adult Height: TW 2 Method.* New York, NY: Academic Press; 1975.

138. Flor-Cisneros A, Roemmich JN, Rogol AD, Baron J. Bone age and onset of puberty in normal boys. *Mol Cell Endocrinol.* 2006;254-255:202-206.

139. Aicardi G, Vignolo M, Milani S, et al. Assessment of skeletal maturity of the hand-wrist and knee: a comparison among methods. *Am J Human Biol.* 2000;12(5):610-615.

140. Thodberg HH. Clinical review: an automated method for determination of bone age. *J Clin Endocrinol Metab.* 2009;94(7):2239-2244.

141. Roche AF. *Skeletal maturity of children 6-11 years: racial, geographic area of residence, socioeconomic differentials.* National Health Survey. DHEW Vital and Health Statistics Series 11, No. 149. Washington, DC: Government Printing Office; 1975.

142. Zhang A, Sayre JW, Vachon L, et al. Racial differences in growth patterns of children assessed on the basis of bone age. *Radiology.* 2009;250(1):228-235.

143. Bayley N, Pinneau SR. Tables for predicting adult height from skeletal age: revised for use with the Greulich-Pyle standards. *J Pediatr.* 1952;40:423-441.

144. Roche AF, Wainer H, Thissen D. The RWT method for the prediction of adult stature. *Pediatrics.* 1975;56(6):1027-1033.

145. Khamis HJ, Roche AF. Predicting adult stature without using skeletal age: the Khamis-Roche method. *Pediatrics.* 1994;94(4 Pt 1):504-507.
146. Tanner JM. *Assessment of Skeletal Maturity and Prediction of Adult Height: TW 3 Method.* Philadelphia, PA: WB Saunders; 2001.
147. Topor LS, Feldman HA, Bauchner H, Cohen LE. Variation in methods of predicting adult height for children with idiopathic short stature. *Pediatrics.* 2010;126(5):938-944.
148. Seeman E. Pathogenesis of bone fragility in women and men. *Lancet.* 2002;359(9320):1841-1850.
149. Seeman E. Periosteal bone formation: a neglected determinant of bone strength. *N Engl J Med.* 2003;349(4):320-323.
150. Bachrach LK. Acquisition of optimal bone mass in childhood and adolescence. *Trends Endocrinol Metab.* 2001;12(1):22-28.
151. Gafni RI, Baron J. Childhood bone mass acquisition and peak bone mass may not be important determinants of bone mass in late adulthood. *Pediatrics.* 2007;119(Suppl 2):S131-S136.
152. Bailey DA, Martin AD, McKay HA, et al. Calcium accretion in girls and boys during puberty: a longitudinal analysis. *J Bone Miner Res.* 2000; 15(11):2245-2250.
153. Bachrach LK, Hastie T, Wang M, et al. Bone mineral acquisition in healthy Asian, Hispanic, black and caucasian youth: a longitudinal study. *J Clin Endocrinol Metab.* 1999;84:4702-4712.
154. Adams JE, Engelke K, Zemel BS, Ward KA. Quantitative computer tomography in children and adolescents: the 2013 ISCD Pediatric Official Positions. *J Clin Densitom.* 2014;17(2):258-274.
155. Schonau E. The peak bone mass concept: is it still relevant? *Pediatr Nephrol.* 2004;19(8):825-831.
156. Bass S, Delmas PD, Pearce G, et al. The differing tempo of growth in bone size, mass, and density in girls is region-specific [see comments]. *J Clin Invest.* 1999;104(6):795-804.
157. Seeman E. Clinical review 137: sexual dimorphism in skeletal size, density, and strength. *J Clin Endocrinol Metab.* 2001;86(10):4576-4584.
158. Bradney M, Karlsson MK, Duan Y, et al. Heterogeneity in the growth of the axial and appendicular skeleton in boys: implications for the pathogenesis of bone fragility in men. *J Bone Miner Res.* 2000; 15(10):1871-1878.
159. Arabi A, Tamim H, Nabulsi M, et al. Sex differences in the effect of body-composition variables on bone mass in healthy children and adolescents. *Am J Clin Nutr.* 2004;80(5):1428-1435.
160. Crabtree NJ, Kibirige MS, Fordham JN, et al. The relationship between lean body mass and bone mineral content in paediatric health and disease. *Bone.* 2004;35(4):965-972.
161. Binkley TL, Specker BL, Wittig TA. Centile curves for bone densitometry measurements in healthy males and females ages 5-22 yr. *J Clin Densitom.* 2002;5(4):343-353.
162. Stanford University. Z-score for BMD or BMAD measurements at the lumbar spine (L2-4), hip, or whole body using the Hologic 1000W with respect to the age, gender, and ethnicity of the subject. Available at <https://jhuccs1.us/.../Bone%20Mineral%20Density%20Applet%20 Website>.
163. Baroncelli GI. Quantitative ultrasound methods to assess bone mineral status in children: technical characteristics, performance, and clinical application. *Pediatr Res.* 2008;63(3):220-228.
164. Wang Q, Alen M, Nicholson P, et al. Growth patterns at distal radius and tibial shaft in pubertal girls: a 2-year longitudinal study. *J Bone Miner Res.* 2005;20(6):954-961.
165. Saito T, Nakamura K, Okuda Y, et al. Weight gain in childhood and bone mass in female college students. *J Bone Miner Metab.* 2005; 23(1):69-75.
166. Loro ML, Sayre J, Roe TF, et al. Early identification of children predisposed to low peak bone mass and osteoporosis later in life. *J Clin Endocrinol Metab.* 2000;85(10):3908-3918.
167. Rauch F, Bailey DA, Baxter-Jones A, et al. The "muscle-bone unit" during the pubertal growth spurt. *Bone.* 2004;34(5):771-775.
168. Loud KJ, Gordon CM, Micheli LJ, Field AE. Correlates of stress fractures among preadolescent and adolescent girls. *Pediatrics.* 2005;115(4): e399-e406.
169. McKay HA, MacLean L, Petit M, et al. "Bounce at the bell": a novel program of short bouts of exercise improves proximal femur bone mass in early pubertal children. *Br J Sports Med.* 2005;39(8):521-526.
170. Laing EM, Wilson AR, Modlesky CM, et al. Initial years of recreational artistic gymnastics training improves lumbar spine bone mineral accrual in 4- to 8-year-old females. *J Bone Miner Res.* 2005;20(3): 509-519.
171. Goulding A, Rockell JE, Black RE, et al. Children who avoid drinking cow's milk are at increased risk for prepubertal bone fractures. *J Am Diet Assoc.* 2004;104(2):250-253.
172. Winzenberg TM, Shaw K, Fryer J, Jones G. Calcium supplementation for improving bone mineral density in children. *Cochrane Database Syst Rev.* 2006;(2):CD005119.
173. Chevalley T, Rizzoli R, Hans D, et al. Interaction between calcium intake and menarcheal age on bone mass gain: an eight-year follow-up study from prepuberty to postmenarche. *J Clin Endocrinol Metab.* 2005;90(1):44-51.
174. Cheng S, Tylavsky F, Kroger H, et al. Association of low 25-hydroxyvitamin D concentrations with elevated parathyroid hormone concentrations and low cortical bone density in early pubertal and prepubertal Finnish girls. *Am J Clin Nutr.* 2003;78(3):485-492.
175. Suuriniemi M, Mahonen A, Kovanen V, et al. Association between exercise and pubertal BMD is modulated by estrogen receptor alpha genotype. *J Bone Miner Res.* 2004;19(11):1758-1765.
176. Gustavsson A, Thorsen K, Nordstrom P. A 3-year longitudinal study of the effect of physical activity on the accrual of bone mineral density in healthy adolescent males. *Calcif Tissue Int.* 2003;73(2):108-114.
177. Chevalley T, Bonjour JP, Ferrari S, Rizzoli R. Influence of age at menarche on forearm bone microstructure in healthy young women. *J Clin Endocrinol Metab.* 2008;93(7):2594-2601.
178. Remer T, Manz F, Hartmann MF, et al. Prepubertal healthy children's urinary androstenediol predicts diaphyseal bone strength in late puberty. *J Clin Endocrinol Metab.* 2009;94(2):575-578.
179. Bollen AM. A prospective longitudinal study of urinary excretion of a bone resorption marker in adolescents. *Ann Hum Biol.* 2000;27(2): 199-211.
180. Calvo MS, Eyre DR, Gundberg CM. Molecular basis and clinical application of biologic markers of bone turnover. *Endocr Rev.* 1996;17: 333-368.
181. Loomba-Albrecht LA, Styne DM. Effect of puberty on body composition. *Curr Opin Endocrinol Diabetes Obes.* 2009;16(1):10-15.
182. Rogol AD. Sex steroids, growth hormone, leptin and the pubertal growth spurt. *Endocr Dev.* 2010;17:77-85.
183. He Q, Horlick M, Thornton J, et al. Sex-specific fat distribution is not linear across pubertal groups in a multiethnic study. *Obes Res.* 2004; 12(4):725-733.
184. Dore E, Martin R, Ratel S, et al. Gender differences in peak muscle performance during growth. *Int J Sports Med.* 2005;26(4):274-280.
185. Skinner AC, Skelton JA. Prevalence and trends in obesity and severe obesity among children in the United States, 1999-2012. *JAMA Pediatrics.* 2014;168(6):561-566.
186. Centers for Disease Control and Prevention. Clinical Growth Charts. Available at <www.CDC.gov/growthcharts/clinical_charts.htm>.
187. Taksali SE, Caprio S, Dziura J, et al. High visceral and low abdominal subcutaneous fat stores in the obese adolescent: a determinant of an adverse metabolic phenotype. *Diabetes.* 2008;57(2):367-371.
188. Liska D, Dufour S, Zern TL, et al. Interethnic differences in muscle, liver and abdominal fat partitioning in obese adolescents. *PLoS ONE.* 2007;2(6):e569.
189. Koren D, Marcus CL, Kim C, et al. Anthropometric predictors of visceral adiposity in normal-weight and obese adolescents. *Pediatr Diabetes.* 2013;14(8):575-584.
190. Franks PW, Hanson RL, Knowler WC, et al. Childhood obesity, other cardiovascular risk factors, and premature death. *N Engl J Med.* 2010; 362(6):485-493.
191. Morrison JA, Barton BA, Biro FM, Sprecher DL. Sex hormones and the changes in adolescent male lipids: longitudinal studies in a biracial cohort. *J Pediatr.* 2003;142(6):637-642.
192. Cook S, Kavey RE. Dyslipidemia and pediatric obesity. *Pediatr Clin North Am.* 2011;58(6):1363-1373, ix.
193. Lee S, Bacha F, Gungor N, Arslanian S. Comparison of different definitions of pediatric metabolic syndrome: relation to abdominal adiposity, insulin resistance, adiponectin, and inflammatory biomarkers. *J Pediatr.* 2008;152(2):177-184.
194. McGill HC, McMahan CA, Zieske AW, et al. Association of coronary heart disease risk factors with microscopic qualities of coronary atherosclerosis in youth. *Circulation.* 2000;102(4):374-379.
195. D'Adamo E, Santoro N, Caprio S. Metabolic syndrome in pediatrics: old concepts revised, new concepts discussed. *Curr Probl Pediatr Adolesc Health Care.* 2013;43(5):114-123.
196. Levy-Marchal C, Arslanian S, Cutfield W, et al. ESPE-LWPES-ISPAD-APPES-APEG-SLEP J; Insulin Resistance in Children Consensus Conference Group. Insulin resistance in children: consensus, perspective, and future directions. *J Clin Endocrinol Metab.* 2010;95(12): 5189-5198.
197. Goran MI, Bergman RN, Gower BA. Influence of total vs. visceral fat on insulin action and secretion in African American and white children. *Obes Res.* 2001;9(8):423-431.
198. Cruz ML, Weigensberg MJ, Huang TT, et al. The metabolic syndrome in overweight Hispanic youth and the role of insulin sensitivity. *J Clin Endocrinol Metab.* 2004;89(1):108-113.
199. Gungor N, Bacha F, Saad R, et al. Youth type 2 diabetes: insulin resistance, beta-cell failure, or both? *Diabetes Care.* 2005;28(3):638-644.
200. Vaxillaire M, Froguel P. Monogenic diabetes in the young, pharmacogenetics and relevance to multifactorial forms of type 2 diabetes. *Endocr Rev.* 2008;29(3):254-264.
201. Musso C, Cochran E, Moran SA, et al. Clinical course of genetic diseases of the insulin receptor (type A and Rabson-Mendenhall syndromes): a 30-year prospective. *Medicine (Baltimore).* 2004;83(4): 209-222.
202. Musso C, Cochran E, Javor E, et al. The long-term effect of recombinant methionyl human leptin therapy on hyperandrogenism and menstrual function in female and pituitary function in male and female hypoleptinemic lipodystrophic patients. *Metabolism.* 2005; 54(2):255-263.

203. The Fourth Report on the Diagnosis, Evaluation, and Treatment of High Blood Pressure in Children and Adolescents. *Pediatrics*. 2004;114:555. Available at: <http://pediatrics.aappublications.org/content/114/Supplement_2/555.full.html>.

204. Tu W, Eckert GJ, Saha C, Pratt JH. Synchronization of adolescent blood pressure and pubertal somatic growth. *J Clin Endocrinol Metab*. 2009; 94(12):5019-5022.

205. Lenroot RK, Giedd JN. Annual research review: developmental considerations of gene by environment interactions. *J Child Psychol Psychiatry*. 2011;52(4):429-441.

206. Sowell ER, Thompson PM, Toga AW. Mapping changes in the human cortex throughout the span of life. *Neuroscientist*. 2004;10(4):372-392.

207. Gogtay N, Giedd JN, Lusk L, et al. Dynamic mapping of human cortical development during childhood through early adulthood. *Proc Natl Acad Sci U S A*. 2004;101(21):8174-8179.

208. Thompson PM, Sowell ER, Gogtay N, et al. Structural MRI and brain development. *Int Rev Neurobiol*. 2005;67:285-323.

209. Peper JS, Brouwer RM, Schnack HG, et al. Sex steroids and brain structure in pubertal boys and girls. *Psychoneuroendocrinology*. 2009;34(3): 332-342.

210. Yun AJ, Bazar KA, Lee PY. Pineal attrition, loss of cognitive plasticity, and onset of puberty during the teen years: is it a modern maladaptation exposed by evolutionary displacement? *Med Hypotheses*. 2004;63(6):939-950.

211. Feinberg I, Higgins LM, Khaw WY, Campbell IG. The adolescent decline of NREM delta, an indicator of brain maturation, is linked to age and sex but not to pubertal stage. *Am J Physiol Regul Integr Comp Physiol*. 2006;291(6):R1724-R1729.

212. Hagenauer MH, Lee TM. The neuroendocrine control of the circadian system: adolescent chronotype. *Front Neuroendocrinol*. 2012;33(3): 211-229.

213. Knutson KL. The association between pubertal status and sleep duration and quality among a nationally representative sample of U.S. adolescents. *Am J Hum Biol*. 2005;17(4):418-424.

214. Dahl RE, Lewin DS. Pathways to adolescent health sleep regulation and behavior. *J Adolesc Health*. 2002;31(6 Suppl):175-184.

215. Roenneberg T, Kuehnle T, Pramstaller PP, et al. A marker for the end of adolescence. *Curr Biol*. 2004;14(24):R1038-R1039.

216. Remschmidt H. Psychosocial milestones in normal puberty and adolescence. *Horm Res*. 1994;41(Suppl 2):19-29.

217. Steinberg L, Morris AS. Adolescent development. *Annu Rev Psychol*. 2001;52:83-110.

218. Styne DM, Grumbach MM. Puberty in boys and girls. In: Pfaff DW, ed. *The Brain, Hormones and Behaviors*. New York, NY: Academic Press; 2002:661-716.

219. Offer D, Schonert-Reichl KA. Debunking the myths of adolescence: findings from recent research. *J Am Acad Child Adolesc Psychiatry*. 1992;31:1003-1014.

220. Patton GC, McMorris BJ, Toumbourou JW, et al. Puberty and the onset of substance use and abuse. *Pediatrics*. 2004;114(3):e300-e306.

221. Hamilton BH, Martin JA, Ventura SJ. Births: preliminary data for 2008. *Natl Vital Statistics Rep*. 2010;58:(16).

222. Mitamura R, Yano K, Suzuki N, et al. Diurnal rhythms of luteinizing hormone, follicle-stimulating hormone, and testosterone secretion before the onset of male puberty. *J Clin Endocrinol Metab*. 1999; 84(1):29-37.

223. Mitamura R, Yano K, Suzuki N, et al. Diurnal rhythms of luteinizing hormone, follicle-stimulating hormone, testosterone, and estradiol secretion before the onset of female puberty in short children. *J Clin Endocrinol Metab*. 2000;85(3):1074-1080.

224. Kaplan SL, Grumbach MM, Aubert ML. The ontogenesis of pituitary hormones and hypothalamic factors in the human fetus: maturation of central nervous system regulation of anterior pituitary function. *Recent Prog Horm Res*. 1976;32:161-243.

225. Veldhuis JD, Pincus SM, Mitamura R, et al. Developmentally delimited emergence of more orderly luteinizing hormone and testosterone secretion during late prepuberty in boys. *J Clin Endocrinol Metab*. 2001;86(1):80-89.

226. Grumbach MM, Roth JC, Kaplan SL, et al. Hypothalamic-pituitary regulation of puberty in man: evidence and concepts derived from clinical research. In: Grumbach MM, Grave GD, Mayer FE, eds. *Control of the Onset of Puberty*. New York, NY: John Wiley & Sons; 1974: 115-166.

227. Bhatia S, Neely EK, Wilson DM. Serum luteinizing hormone rises within minutes after depot leuprolide injection: implications for monitoring therapy. *Pediatrics*. 2002;109(2):E30.

228. Brito VN, Latronico AC, Arnhold IJ, Mendonca BB. A single luteinizing hormone determination 2 hours after depot leuprolide is useful for therapy monitoring of gonadotropin-dependent precocious puberty in girls. *J Clin Endocrinol Metab*. 2004;89(9):4338-4342.

229. Rosenfield RL, Bordini B, Yu C. Comparison of detection of normal puberty in boys by a hormonal sleep test and a gonadotropin-releasing hormone agonist test. *J Clin Endocrinol Metab*. 2012;97(12):4596-4604.

230. Harrington J, Palmert MR, Hamilton J. Use of local data to enhance uptake of published recommendations: an example from the diagnostic evaluation of precocious puberty. *Arch Dis Child*. 2014;99(1):15-20.

231. Demir A, Voutilainen R, Juul A, et al. Increase in first morning voided urinary luteinizing hormone levels precedes the physical onset of puberty. *J Clin Endocrinol Metab*. 1996;81:2963-2967.

232. Olivares A, Soderlund D, Castro-Fernandez C, et al. Basal and gonadotropin-releasing hormone-releasable serum follicle-stimulating hormone charge isoform distribution and in vitro biological-to-immunological ratio in male puberty. *Endocrine*. 2004;23(2-3):189-198.

233. Wang C, Catlin DH, Demers LM, et al. Measurement of total serum testosterone in adult men: comparison of current laboratory methods versus liquid chromatography-tandem mass spectrometry. *J Clin Endocrinol Metab*. 2004;89(2):534-543.

234. Taieb J, Mathian B, Millot F, et al. Testosterone measured by 10 immunoassays and by isotope-dilution gas chromatography-mass spectrometry in sera from 116 men, women, and children. *Clin Chem*. 2003; 49(8):1381-1395.

235. Albrecht L, Styne D. Laboratory testing of gonadal steroids in children. *Pediatr Endocrinol Rev*. 2007;5(Suppl 1):599-607.

236. Raivio T, Dunkel L, Wickman S, Janne OA. Serum androgen bioactivity in adolescence: a longitudinal study of boys with constitutional delay of puberty. *J Clin Endocrinol Metab*. 2004;89(3):1188-1192.

237. Chen J, Sowers MR, Moran FM, et al. Circulating bioactive androgens in mid-life women. *J Clin Endocrinol Metab*. 2006;91(11):4387-4394.

238. Klein KO, Martha PMJ, Blizzard RM, et al. A longitudinal assessment of hormonal and physical alterations during normal puberty in boys. II. Estrogen levels as determined by an ultrasensitive bioassay. *J Clin Endocrinol Metab*. 1996;81:3203-3207.

239. Paris F, Servant N, Terouanne B, et al. A new recombinant cell bioassay for ultrasensitive determination of serum estrogenic bioactivity in children. *J Clin Endocrinol Metab*. 2002;87(2):791-797.

240. Weise M, De Levi S, Barnes KM, et al. Effects of estrogen on growth plate senescence and epiphyseal fusion. *Proc Natl Acad Sci U S A*. 2001; 98(1):6871-6876.

241. Robertson DM, Hale GE, Jolley D, et al. Interrelationships between ovarian and pituitary hormones in ovulatory menstrual cycles across reproductive age. *J Clin Endocrinol Metab*. 2009;94(1):138-144.

242. Wallace E, Riley SM, Crossley JA, et al. Dimeric inhibins in amniotic fluid, maternal serum, and fetal serum in human pregnancy. *J Clin Endocrinol Metab*. 1997;82:218-222.

243. Majdic G, McNeilly AS, Sharpe R, et al. Testicular expression of inhibin and activin subunits and follistatin in the rat and human fetus and neonate and during postnatal development in the rat. *Endocrinology*. 1997;138:2136-2147.

244. Andersson A, Skakkebaek NE. Serum inhibin B levels during male childhood and puberty. *Mol Cell Endocrinol*. 2001;180(1-2):103-107.

245. Hero M, Tommiska J, Vaaralahti K, et al. Circulating antimullerian hormone levels in boys decline during early puberty and correlate with inhibin B. *Fertil Steril*. 2012;97(5):1242-1247.

246. Chada M, Prusa R, Bronsky J, et al. Inhibin B, follicle stimulating hormone, luteinizing hormone and testosterone during childhood and puberty in males: changes in serum concentrations in relation to age and stage of puberty. *Physiol Res*. 2003;52(1):45-51.

247. Chada M, Prusa R, Bronsky J, et al. Inhibin B, follicle stimulating hormone, luteinizing hormone, and estradiol and their relationship to the regulation of follicle development in girls during childhood and puberty. *Physiol Res*. 2003;52(3):341-346.

248. Foster CM, Olton PR, Padmanabhan V. Diurnal changes in FSH-regulatory peptides and their relationship to gonadotrophins in pubertal girls. *Hum Reprod*. 2005;20(2):543-548.

249. Crofton PM, Evans AE, Wallace AM, et al. Nocturnal secretory dynamics of inhibin B and testosterone in pre- and peripubertal boys. *J Clin Endocrinol Metab*. 2004;89(2):867-874.

250. Young J, Chanson P, Salenave S, et al. Testicular anti-mullerian hormone secretion is stimulated by recombinant human FSH in patients with congenital hypogonadotropic hypogonadism. *J Clin Endocrinol Metab*. 2005;90(2):724-728.

251. Elsholz DD, Padmanabhan V, Rosenfield RL, et al. GnRH agonist stimulation of the pituitary-gonadal axis in children: age and sex differences in circulating inhibin-B and activin-A. *Hum Reprod*. 2004;19(12): 2748-2758.

252. Foster CM, Olton PR, Racine MS, et al. Sex differences in FSH-regulatory peptides in pubertal age boys and girls and effects of sex steroid treatment. *Hum Reprod*. 2004;19(7):1668-1676.

253. Lee PA, Coughlin MT, Bellinger MF. No relationship of testicular size at orchiopexy with fertility in men who previously had unilateral cryptorchidism. *J Urol*. 2001;166(1):236-239.

254. Kubini K, Zachmann M, Albers N, et al. Basal inhibin B and the testosterone response to human chorionic gonadotropin correlate in prepubertal boys. *J Clin Endocrinol Metab*. 2000;85(1):134-138.

255. Josso N, Rey RA, Picard JY. Anti-mullerian hormone: a valuable addition to the toolbox of the pediatric endocrinologist. *Int J Endocrinol*. 2013;2013:674105.

256. Sir-Petermann T, Marquez L, Carcamo M, et al. Effects of birth weight on anti-müllerian hormone serum concentrations in infant girls. *J Clin Endocrinol Metab*. 2010;95:903-910.

257. Bergada I, Milani C, Bedecarras P, et al. Time course of the serum gonadotropin surge, inhibins, and anti-mullerian hormone in normal newborn males during the first month of life. *J Clin Endocrinol Metab.* 2006;91(10):4092-4098.

258. Lee MM, Donahoe PK, Silverman BL, et al. Measurements of serum mullerian inhibiting substance in the evaluation of children with nonpalpable gonads. *N Engl J Med.* 1997;336:1480-1486.

259. Grumbach MM, Richards GE, Conte FA, et al. Clinical disorders of adrenal function and puberty: an assessment of the role of the adrenal cortex in normal and abnormal puberty in man and evidence for an ACTH-like pituitary adrenal androgen stimulating hormone. In: James VHT, Serio M, Giusti G, et al, eds. *The Endocrine Function of the Human Adrenal Cortex, Serono Symposium.* New York, NY: Academic Press; 1977:583-612.

260. Noordam C, Dhir V, McNelis JC, et al. Inactivating PAPSS2 mutations in a patient with premature pubarche. *N Engl J Med.* 2009;360(22):2310-2318.

261. August GP, Tkachuk M, Grumbach MM. Plasma testosterone-binding affinity and testosterone in umbilical cord plasma, late pregnancy, prepubertal children and adults. *J Clin Endocrinol Metab.* 1969;29:891-899.

262. Aubert ML, Sizonenko PC, Kaplan SL, et al. The ontogenesis of human prolactin from fetal life to puberty. In: Crosignani PG, Robyn C, eds. *Prolactin and Human Reproduction.* New York, NY: Academic Press; 1977:9-20.

263. Park AS, Lawson MA, Chuan SS, et al. Serum anti-mullerian hormone concentrations are elevated in oligomenorrheic girls without evidence of hyperandrogenism. *J Clin Endocrinol Metab.* 2010;95(4):1786-1792.

264. Wikstrom AM, Bay K, Hero M, et al. Serum insulin-like factor 3 levels during puberty in healthy boys and boys with Klinefelter syndrome. *J Clin Endocrinol Metab.* 2006;91(11):4705-4708.

265. Trabado S, Maione L, Bry-Gauillard H, et al. Insulin-like peptide 3 (INSL3) in men with congenital hypogonadotropic hypogonadism/ Kallmann syndrome and effects of different modalities of hormonal treatment: a single-center study of 281 patients. *J Clin Endocrinol Metab.* 2014;99(2):E268-E275.

266. Randell EW, Diamandis EP, Ellis G. Serum prostate-specific antigen measured in children from birth to age 18 years. *Clin Chem.* 1996;42:420-423.

267. Vieira JG, Nishida SK, Pereira AB, et al. Serum levels of prostate-specific antigen in normal boys throughout puberty. *J Clin Endocrinol Metab.* 1994;78:1185-1187.

268. van der Eerden BC, Karperien M, Wit JM. Systemic and local regulation of the growth plate. *Endocr Rev.* 2003;24(6):782-801.

269. Attie KM, Ramirez NR, Conte FA, et al. The pubertal growth spurt in eight patients with true precocious puberty and growth hormone deficiency: evidence for a direct role of sex steroids. *J Clin Endocrinol Metab.* 1990;71:975-983.

270. Conte FA, Grumbach MM, Ito Y, et al. A syndrome of female pseudo-hermaphrodism, hypergonadotropic hypogonadism and multicystic ovaries associated with missence mutations in the gene encoding aromatase (P450 arom). *J Clin Endocrinol Metab.* 1994;78:1287-1292.

271. Smith EP, Boyd J, Frank GR, et al. Estrogen resistance caused by a mutation by the estrogen-receptor in a man. *N Engl J Med.* 1994;331:1056-1061.

272. Morishima A, Grumbach MM, Simpson ER, et al. Aromatase deficiency in male and female siblings caused by a novel mutation and the physiological role of estrogens. *J Clin Endocrinol Metab.* 1995;80:3689-3698.

273. Bilezikian JP, Morishima A, Bell J, Grumbach MM. Increased bone mass as a result of estrogen therapy in a man with aromatase deficiency. *N Engl J Med.* 1998;339(9):599-603.

274. Carani C, Qin K, Simoni M, et al. Effect of testosterone and estradiol in a man with aromatase deficiency. *N Engl J Med.* 1997;337(2):91-95.

275. Rochira V, Faustini-Fustini M, Balestrieri A, Carani C. Estrogen replacement therapy in a man with congenital aromatase deficiency: effects of different doses of transdermal estradiol on bone mineral density and hormonal parameters. *J Clin Endocrinol Metab.* 2000;85(5):1841-1845.

276. Stratakis CA, Vottero A, Brodie A, et al. The aromatase excess syndrome is associated with feminization of both sexes and autosomal dominant transmission of aberrant P450 aromatase gene transcription. *J Clin Endocrinol Metab.* 1998;83(4):1348-1357.

277. Weise M, Flor A, Barnes KM, et al. Determinants of growth during gonadotropin-releasing hormone analog therapy for precocious puberty. *J Clin Endocrinol Metab.* 2004;89(1):103-107.

278. Eastell R. Role of oestrogen in the regulation of bone turnover at the menarche. *J Endocrinol.* 2005;185(2):223-234.

279. Hogler W, Briody J, Moore B, et al. Importance of estrogen on bone health in Turner syndrome: a cross-sectional and longitudinal study using dual-energy X-ray absorptiometry. *J Clin Endocrinol Metab.* 2004;89(1):193-199.

280. Jarvinen TL, Kannus P, Sievanen H. Estrogen and bone: a reproductive and locomotive perspective. *J Bone Miner Res.* 2003;18(11):1921-1931.

281. Vanderschueren D, Vandenput L, Boonen S, et al. Androgens and bone. *Endocr Rev.* 2004;25(3):389-425.

282. Marcus R, Leary D, Schneider DL, et al. The contribution of testosterone to skeletal development and maintenance: lessons from the androgen insensitivity syndrome. *J Clin Endocrinol Metab.* 2000;85(3):1032-1037.

283. Veldhuis JD, Roemmich JN, Rogol AD. Gender and sexual maturation-dependent contrasts in the neuroregulation of growth hormone secretion in prepubertal and late adolescent males and females: a general clinical research center-based study. *J Clin Endocrinol Metab.* 2000;85(7):2385-2394.

284. Racine MS, Symons KV, Foster CM, Barkan AL. Augmentation of growth hormone secretion after testosterone treatment in boys with constitutional delay of growth and adolescence: evidence against an increase in hypothalamic secretion of growth hormone-releasing hormone. *J Clin Endocrinol Metab.* 2004;89(7):3326-3331.

285. Harris DA, Van Vliet G, Egli CA, et al. Somatomedin-C in normal puberty and in true precocious puberty before and after treatment with a potent luteinizing hormone-releasing hormone agonist. *J Clin Endocrinol Metab.* 1985;61:152-159.

286. Juul A, Fisker S, Scheike T, et al. Serum levels of growth hormone binding protein in children with normal and precocious puberty: relation to age, gender, body composition and gonadal steroids. *Clin Endocrinol.* 2000;52(2):165-172.

287. Lofqvist C, Andersson E, Gelander L, et al. Reference values for IGF-I throughout childhood and adolescence: a model that accounts simultaneously for the effect of gender, age, and puberty. *J Clin Endocrinol Metab.* 2001;86(12):5870-5876.

288. Lofqvist C, Andersson E, Gelander L, et al. Reference values for insulin-like growth factor-binding protein-3 (IGFBP-3) and the ratio of insulin-like growth factor-I to IGFBP-3 throughout childhood and adolescence. *J Clin Endocrinol Metab.* 2005;90(3):1420-1427.

289. Juul A, Dalgaard P, Blum WF, et al. Serum levels of insulin-like growth factor (IGF)-binding protein-3 (IGFBP-3) in healthy infants, children, and adolescents: the relation to IGF-I, IGF-II, IGFBP-1, IGFBP-2, age, sex, body mass index, and pubertal maturation. *J Clin Endocrinol Metab.* 1995;80:2534-2542.

290. Jorge AA, Souza SC, Arnhold IJ, Mendonca BB. The first homozygous mutation (S226I) in the highly-conserved WSXWS-like motif of the GH receptor causing Laron syndrome: suppression of GH secretion by GnRH analogue therapy not restored by dihydrotestosterone administration. *Clin Endocrinol (Oxf).* 2004;60(1):36-40.

291. Sjogren K, Liu JL, Blad K, et al. Liver-derived insulin-like growth factor I (IGF-I) is the principal source of IGF-I in blood but is not required for postnatal body growth in mice. *Proc Natl Acad Sci U S A.* 1999;96(12):7088-7092.

292. Van Wyk JJ, Grumbach MM. Syndrome of precocious menstruation and galactorrhea in juvenile hypothyroidism: an example of hormonal overlap in pituitary feedback. *J Pediatr.* 1960;57:416-435.

293. Auchus RJ. The physiology and biochemistry of adrenarche. *Endocr Dev.* 2011;20:20-27.

294. Grumbach MM, Kaplan SL. The neuroendocrinology of human puberty: an ontogenetic perspective. In: Grumbach MM, Sizonenko PC, Aubert ML, eds. *Control of the Onset of Puberty.* Baltimore, MD: Williams & Wilkins; 1990:1-68.

295. Grumbach MM. A window of opportunity: the diagnosis of gonadotropin deficiency in the male infant. *J Clin Endocrinol Metab.* 2005;90(5):3122-3127.

296. Plant TM. Hypothalamic control of the pituitary-gonadal axis in higher primates: key advances over the last two decades. *J Neuroendocrinol.* 2008;20(6):719-726.

297. Terasawa E, Kurian JR, Guerriero KA, et al. Recent discoveries on the control of gonadotrophin-releasing hormone neurones in nonhuman primates. *J Neuroendocrinol.* 2010;22(7):630-638.

298. Martinez de la Escalera G, Clapp C. Regulation of gonadotropin-releasing hormone secretion: insights from GT1 immortal GnRH neurons. *Arch Med Res.* 2001;32(6):486-498.

299. Shacham S, Harris D, Ben-Shlomo H, et al. Mechanism of GnRH receptor signaling on gonadotropin release and gene expression in pituitary gonadotrophs. *Vitam Horm.* 2001;63:63-90.

300. Themmen APN, Huhtaniemi IT. Mutations of gonadotropins and gonadotropin receptors: elucidating the physiology and pathophysiology of pituitary-gonadal function. *Endocr Rev.* 2000;21(5):551-583.

301. Pitteloud N, Dwyer AA, DeCruz S, et al. Inhibition of luteinizing hormone secretion by testosterone in men requires aromatization for its pituitary but not its hypothalamic effects: evidence from the tandem study of normal and gonadotropin-releasing hormone-deficient men. *J Clin Endocrinol Metab.* 2008;93(3):784-791.

302. Blackman BE, Yoshida H, Paruthiyil S, Weiner RI. Frequency of intrinsic pulsatile gonadotropin-releasing hormone secretion is regulated by the expression of cyclic nucleotide-gated channels in GT1 cells. *Endocrinology.* 2007;148(7):3299-3306.

303. Abe H, Terasawa E. Firing pattern and rapid modulation of activity by estrogen in primate luteinizing hormone releasing hormone-1 neurons. *Endocrinology.* 2005;146(10):4312-4320.

304. Knobil E. The neuroendocrine control of the menstrual cycle. *Recent Prog Horm Res.* 1980;36:53-88.

305. Grumbach MM. The neuroendocrinology of human puberty revisited. *Horm Res.* 2002;57(Suppl 2):2-14.

306. Mahachoklertwattana P, Black SM, Kaplan SL, et al. Nitric oxide synthesized by gonadotropin-releasing hormone neurons is a mediator of N-methyl-D-aspartate (NMDA)-induced GnRH secretion. *Endocrinology.* 1994;135:1709-1712.

307. Herde MK, Iremonger KJ, Constantin S, Herbison AE. GnRH neurons elaborate a long-range projection with shared axonal and dendritic functions. *J Neurosci.* 2013;33(31):12689-12697.

308. Ubuka T, Tsutsui K. Evolution of gonadotropin-inhibitory hormone receptor and its ligand. *Gen Comp Endocrinol.* 2014;209:148-161.

309. Clarke IJ, Parkington HC. Gonadotropin inhibitory hormone (GnIH) as a regulator of gonadotropes. *Mol Cell Endocrinol.* 2014;385(1-2):36-44.

310. Lima CJ, Cardoso SC, Lemos EF, et al. Mutational analysis of the genes encoding RFRP-3, the human ortholog of gonadotropin-inhibitory hormone, and its receptor (GPR147) in patients with GnRH-dependent pubertal disorders. *J Neuroendocrinol.* 2014;26(11):817-824.

311. Seminara SB, Crowley WF Jr. Kisspeptin and GPR54: discovery of a novel pathway in reproduction. *J Neuroendocrinol.* 2008;20(6):727-731.

312. Smith JT, Clifton DK, Steiner RA. Regulation of the neuroendocrine reproductive axis by kisspeptin-GPR54 signaling. *Reproduction.* 2006;131(4):623-630.

313. Muir AI, Chamberlain L, Elshourbagy NA, et al. AXOR12, a novel human G protein-coupled receptor, activated by the peptide KiSS-1. *J Biol Chem.* 2001;276(31):28969-28975.

314. Ohtaki T, Shintani Y, Honda S, et al. Metastasis suppressor gene KiSS-1 encodes peptide ligand of a G-protein-coupled receptor. *Nature.* 2001;411(6837):613-617.

315. Shahab M, Mastronardi C, Seminara SB, et al. Increased hypothalamic GPR54 signaling: a potential mechanism for initiation of puberty in primates. *Proc Natl Acad Sci U S A.* 2005;102(6):2129-2134.

316. Gottsch ML, Cunningham MJ, Smith JT, et al. A role for kisspeptins in the regulation of gonadotropin secretion in the mouse. *Endocrinology.* 2004;145(9):4073-4077.

317. Messager S, Chatzidaki EE, Ma D, et al. Kisspeptin directly stimulates gonadotropin-releasing hormone release via G protein-coupled receptor 54. *Proc Natl Acad Sci U S A.* 2005;102(5):1761-1766.

318. Han SK, Gottsch ML, Lee KJ, et al. Activation of gonadotropin-releasing hormone neurons by kisspeptin as a neuroendocrine switch for the onset of puberty. *J Neurosci.* 2005;25(49):11349-11356.

319. Nazian SJ. Role of metastin in the release of gonadotropin-releasing hormone from the hypothalamus of the male rat. *J Androl.* 2006;27(3):444-449.

320. Seminara SB, Messager S, Chatzidaki EE, et al. The GPR54 gene as a regulator of puberty. *N Engl J Med.* 2003;349(17):1614-1627.

321. Castellano JM, Navarro VM, Fernandez-Fernandez R, et al. Changes in hypothalamic KiSS-1 system and restoration of pubertal activation of the reproductive axis by kisspeptin in undernutrition. *Endocrinology.* 2005;146(9):3917-3925.

322. Patterson M, Murphy KG, Thompson EL, et al. Administration of kisspeptin-54 into discrete regions of the hypothalamus potently increases plasma luteinising hormone and testosterone in male adult rats. *J Neuroendocrinol.* 2006;18(5):349-354.

323. Navarro VM, Castellano JM, Fernandez-Fernandez R, et al. Characterization of the potent luteinizing hormone-releasing activity of KiSS-1 peptide, the natural ligand of GPR54. *Endocrinology.* 2005;146(1):156-163.

324. Navarro VM, Castellano JM, Fernandez-Fernandez R, et al. Effects of KiSS-1 peptide, the natural ligand of GPR54, on follicle-stimulating hormone secretion in the rat. *Endocrinology.* 2005;146(4):1689-1697.

325. Navarro VM, Castellano JM, Fernandez-Fernandez R, et al. Developmental and hormonally regulated messenger ribonucleic acid expression of KiSS-1 and its putative receptor, GPR54, in rat hypothalamus and potent luteinizing hormone-releasing activity of KiSS-1 peptide. *Endocrinology.* 2004;145(10):4565-4574.

326. Navarro VM, Fernandez-Fernandez R, Castellano JM, et al. Advanced vaginal opening and precocious activation of the reproductive axis by KiSS-1 peptide, the endogenous ligand of GPR54. *J Physiol.* 2004;561(Pt 2):379-386.

327. Matsui H, Takatsu Y, Kumano S, et al. Peripheral administration of metastin induces marked gonadotropin release and ovulation in the rat. *Biochem Biophys Res Commun.* 2004;320(2):383-388.

328. Plant TM, Ramaswamy S. Kisspeptin and the regulation of the hypothalamic-pituitary-gonadal axis in the rhesus monkey *(Macaca mulatta).* *Peptides.* 2009;30(1):67-75.

329. Ramaswamy S, Guerriero KA, Gibbs RB, Plant TM. Structural interactions between kisspeptin and GnRH neurons in the mediobasal hypothalamus of the male rhesus monkey *(Macaca mulatta)* as revealed by double immunofluorescence and confocal microscopy. *Endocrinology.* 2008;149(9):4387-4395.

330. Seminara SB, Dipietro MJ, Ramaswamy S, et al. Continuous human metastin 45-54 infusion desensitizes G protein-coupled receptor 54-induced gonadotropin-releasing hormone release monitored indirectly in the juvenile male Rhesus monkey *(Macaca mulatta):* a finding with therapeutic implications. *Endocrinology.* 2006;147(5):2122-2126.

331. Young J, George JT, Tello JA, et al. Kisspeptin restores pulsatile LH secretion in patients with neurokinin B signaling deficiencies: physiological, pathophysiological and therapeutic implications. *Neuroendocrinology.* 2013;97(2):193-202.

332. Shibata M, Friedman RL, Ramaswamy S, Plant TM. Evidence that down regulation of hypothalamic KiSS-1 expression is involved in the negative feedback action of testosterone to regulate luteinising hormone secretion in the adult male rhesus monkey *(Macaca mulatta).* *J Neuroendocrinol.* 2007;19(6):432-438.

333. Pompolo S, Pereira A, Estrada KM, Clarke IJ. Colocalization of kisspeptin and gonadotropin-releasing hormone in the ovine brain. *Endocrinology.* 2006;147(2):804-810.

334. Skorupskaite K, George JT, Anderson RA. The kisspeptin-GnRH pathway in human reproductive health and disease. *Hum Reprod Update.* 2014;20(4):485-500.

335. Jayasena CN, Nijher GM, Narayanaswamy S, et al. Age-dependent elevations in plasma kisspeptin are observed in boys and girls when compared with adults. *Ann Clin Biochem.* 2014;51(Pt 1):89-96.

336. Kumar D, Boehm U. Genetic dissection of puberty in mice. *Exp Physiol.* 2013;98(11):1528-1534.

337. Schwanzel-Fukuda M, Crossin KL, Pfaff DW, et al. Migration of luteinizing hormone-releasing hormone (LHRH) neurons in early human embryos. *J Comp Neurol.* 1996;366:547-557.

338. Tobet SA, Schwarting GA. Minireview: recent progress in gonadotropin-releasing hormone neuronal migration. *Endocrinology.* 2006;147(3):1159-1165.

339. Clarkson J, Herbison AE. Development of GABA and glutamate signaling at the GnRH neuron in relation to puberty. *Mol Cell Endocrinol.* 2006;254-255:32-38.

340. Schwanzel-Fukuda M, Bick D, Pfaff DW. Luteinizing hormone-releasing hormone (LHRH)-expressing cells do not migrate normally in an inherited hypogonadal (Kallmann) syndrome. *Mol Brain Res.* 1989;6:311-326.

341. Terasawa E. Postnatal remodeling of gonadotropin-releasing hormone I neurons: toward understanding the mechanism of the onset of puberty. *Endocrinology.* 2006;147(8):3650-3651.

342. Habert R, Lejeune H, Saez JM. Origin, differentiation and regulation of fetal and adult Leydig cells. *Mol Cell Endocrinol.* 2001;179(1-2):47-74.

343. Boukari K, Meduri G, Brailly-Tabard S, et al. Lack of androgen receptor expression in Sertoli cells accounts for the absence of anti-mullerian hormone repression during early human testis development. *J Clin Endocrinol Metab.* 2009;94(5):1818-1825.

344. Mesiano S, Hart CS, Heyer BW, et al. Hormone ontogeny in the ovine fetus XXVI. A sex difference in the effect of castration on the hypothalamic-pituitary gonadotropin unit in the ovine fetus. *Endocrinology.* 1991;129:3073-3079.

345. Cuttler L, Egli CA, Styne DM, et al. Hormone ontogeny in the ovine fetus. XVIII. The effect of an opioid antagonist on luteinizing hormone secretion. *Endocrinology.* 1985;116:1997-2002.

346. Bettendorf M, de Zegher F, Albers N, et al. Acute N-methyl-D,L-aspartate administration stimulates the luteinizing hormone releasing hormone pulse generator in the ovine fetus. *Horm Res.* 1999;51(1):25-30.

347. Albers N, Hart CS, Kaplan SL, et al. Hormone ontogeny in the ovine fetus. XXIV. Porcine follicular fluid "inhibins" selectively suppress plasma follicle-stimulating hormone in the ovine fetus. *Endocrinology.* 1989;125:675-678.

348. Corbier P, Dehenin L, Castanier M, et al. Sex differences in serum luteinizing hormone and testosterone in the human neonate during the first few hours after birth. *J Clin Endocrinol Metab.* 1990;71:1347-1348.

349. Lustig RH, Conte FA, Kogan BA, et al. Ontogeny of gonadotropin secretion in congenital anorchism: sexual dimorphism versus syndrome of gonadal dysgenesis and diagnostic considerations. *J Urol.* 1987;138:587-591.

350. Terasawa E, Fernandez DL. Neurobiological mechanisms of the onset of puberty in primates. *Endocr Rev.* 2001;22(1):111-151.

351. Sharpe RM, Fraser HM, Brougham MF, et al. Role of the neonatal period of pituitary-testicular activity in germ cell proliferation and differentiation in the primate testis. *Hum Reprod.* 2003;18(10):2110-2117.

352. Sharpe RM, McKinnell C, Kivlin C, Fisher JS. Proliferation and functional maturation of Sertoli cells, and their relevance to disorders of testis function in adulthood. *Reproduction.* 2003;125(6):769-784.

353. Salti R, Galluzzi F, Bindi G, et al. Nocturnal melatonin patterns in children. *J Clin Endocrinol Metab.* 2000;85(6):2137-2144.

354. Lomniczi A, Wright H, Castellano JM, et al. A system biology approach to identify regulatory pathways underlying the neuroendocrine control of female puberty in rats and nonhuman primates. *Horm Behav.* 2013;64(2):175-186.

355. Lomniczi A, Wright H, Ojeda SR. Epigenetic regulation of female puberty. *Front Neuroendocrinol.* 2015;36:90-107.

356. Gajdos ZK, Henderson KD, Hirschhorn JN, Palmert MR. Genetic determinants of pubertal timing in the general population. *Mol Cell Endocrinol.* 2010;324(1-2):21-29.

357. Johnston FE, Roche AF, Schell LM, et al. Critical weight at menarche. *Am J Dis Child*. 1975;129(1):19-23.
358. Vizmanos B, Marti-Henneberg C. Puberty begins with a characteristic subcutaneous body fat mass in each sex. *Eur J Clin Nutr*. 2000;54(3):203-208.
359. Buyken AE, Karaolis-Danckert N, Remer T. Association of prepubertal body composition in healthy girls and boys with the timing of early and late pubertal markers. *Am J Clin Nutr*. 2009;89(1):221-230.
360. Zhang Y, Proenca R, Maffei M, et al. Positional cloning of the mouse obese gene and its human analogue. *Nature*. 1994;372:425-432.
361. Spiegelman BM, Flier J. Adipogenesis and obesity: rounding out the big picture. *Cell*. 1996;87:377-389.
362. Tartaglia LA, Dembski M, Weng X, et al. Identification and expression cloning of a leptin receptor, OB-R. *Cell*. 1995;83:1263-1271.
363. Cheung CC, Thornton JE, Nurani SD, et al. A reassessment of leptin's role in triggering the onset of puberty in the rat and mouse. *Neuroendocrinology*. 2001;74(1):12-21.
364. Woller M, Tessmer S, Neff D, et al. Leptin stimulates gonadotropin releasing hormone release from cultured intact hemihypothalami and enzymatically dispersed neurons. *Exp Biol Med (Maywood)*. 2001;226(6):591-596.
365. Quennell JH, Mulligan AC, Tups A, et al. Leptin indirectly regulates gonadotropin-releasing hormone neuronal function. *Endocrinology*. 2009;150(6):2805-2812.
366. Donato J Jr, Cravo RM, Frazao R, et al. Leptin's effect on puberty in mice is relayed by the ventral premammillary nucleus and does not require signaling in Kiss1 neurons. *J Clin Invest*. 2011;121(1):355-368.
367. Ahima RS. No Kiss1ng by leptin during puberty? *J Clin Invest*. 2011;121(1):34-36.
368. Ahmed ML, Ong KK, Morrell DJ, et al. Longitudinal study of leptin concentrations during puberty: sex differences and relationship to changes in body composition. *J Clin Endocrinol Metab*. 1999;84(3):899-905.
369. Horlick MB, Rosenbaum M, Nicolson M, et al. Effect of puberty on the relationship between circulating leptin and body composition. *J Clin Endocrinol Metab*. 2000;85(7):2509-2518.
370. Palmert MR, Radovick S, Boepple PA. The impact of reversible gonadal sex steroid suppression on serum leptin concentrations in children with central precocious puberty [see comments]. *J Clin Endocrinol Metab*. 1998;83(4):1091-1096.
371. Clayton PE, Trueman JA. Leptin and puberty. *Arch Dis Child*. 2000;83(1):1-4.
372. Grasemann C, Wessels HT, Knauer-Fischer S, et al. Increase of serum leptin after short-term pulsatile GnRH administration in children with delayed puberty. *Eur J Endocrinol*. 2004;150(5):691-698.
373. Mann DR, Bhat GK, Ramaswamy S, et al. Regulation of circulating leptin and its soluble receptor during pubertal development in the male rhesus monkey *(Macaca mulatta)*. *Endocrine*. 2007;31(2):125-129.
374. Li HJ, Ji CY, Wang W, Hu YH. A twin study for serum leptin, soluble leptin receptor, and free insulin-like growth factor-I in pubertal females. *J Clin Endocrinol Metab*. 2005;90(6):3659-3664.
375. Banerjee I, Trueman JA, Hall CM, et al. Phenotypic variation in constitutional delay of growth and puberty: relationship to specific leptin and leptin receptor gene polymorphisms. *Eur J Endocrinol*. 2006;155(1):121-126.
376. Ozata M, Ozdemir IC, Licinio J. Human leptin deficiency caused by a missense mutation: multiple endocrine defects, decreased sympathetic tone, and immune system dysfunction indicate new targets for leptin action, greater central than peripheral resistance to the effects of leptin, and spontaneous correction of leptin-mediated defects. *J Clin Endocrinol Metab*. 1999;84(10):3686-3695.
377. Clement K, Vaisse C, Lahlou N, et al. A mutation in the human leptin receptor gene causes obesity and pituitary dysfunction. *Nature*. 1998;392(6674):398-401.
378. Farooqi IS, Jebb SA, Langmack G, et al. Effects of recombinant leptin therapy in a child with congenital leptin deficiency. *N Engl J Med*. 1999;341(12):879-884.
379. Andreelli F, Hanaire-Broutin H, Laville M, et al. Normal reproductive function in leptin-deficient patients with lipoatropic diabetes. *J Clin Endocrinol Metab*. 2000;85(2):715-719.
380. Fernandez-Fernandez R, Martini AC, Navarro VM, et al. Novel signals for the integration of energy balance and reproduction. *Mol Cell Endocrinol*. 2006;254-255:127-132.
381. Bottner A, Kratzsch J, Muller G, et al. Gender differences of adiponectin levels develop during the progression of puberty and are related to serum androgen levels. *J Clin Endocrinol Metab*. 2004;89(8):4053-4061.
382. Gerber M, Boettner A, Seidel B, et al. Serum resistin levels of obese and lean children and adolescents: biochemical analysis and clinical relevance. *J Clin Endocrinol Metab*. 2005;90(8):4503-4509.
383. Conte FA, Grumbach MM, Kaplan SL, Reiter EO. Correlation of luteinizing hormone-releasing factor-induced luteinizing hormone and follicle-stimulating hormone release from infancy to 19 years with the changing pattern of gonadotropin secretion in agonadal patients: relation to the restraint of puberty. *J Clin Endocrinol Metab*. 1980;50:163-168.
384. Comite F, Cassorla F, Barnes KM, et al. Luteinizing hormone releasing hormone analogue therapy for central precocious puberty. Long term effect on somatic growth, bone maturation, and predicted height. *JAMA*. 1986;255:2613-2616.
385. Judge DM, Kulin HE, Santen R, et al. Hypothalamic hamartoma: a source of luteinizing-hormone-releasing factor in precocious puberty. *N Engl J Med*. 1977;296:7-10.
386. Mahachoklertwattana P, Kaplan SL, Grumbach MM. The luteinizing hormone-releasing hormone-secreting hypothalamic hamartoma is a congenital malformation: natural history. *J Clin Endocrinol Metab*. 1993;77:118-124.
387. Abreu AP, Dauber A, Macedo DB, et al. Central precocious puberty caused by mutations in the imprinted gene MKRN3. *N Engl J Med*. 2013;368(26):2467-2475.
388. Hughes IA. Releasing the brake on puberty. *N Engl J Med*. 2013;368(26):2513-2515.
389. Macedo DB, Brito VN, Latronico AC. New causes of central precocious puberty: the role of the genetic factors. *Neuroendocrinology*. 2014;100(1):1-8.
390. Di Giorgio NP, Semaan SJ, Kim J, et al. Impaired GABAB receptor signaling dramatically up-regulates Kiss1 expression selectively in non-hypothalamic brain regions of adult but not prepubertal mice. *Endocrinology*. 2014;155(3):1033-1044.
391. Ganguly K, Schinder AF, Wong ST, Poo M. GABA itself promotes the developmental switch of neuronal GABAergic responses from excitation to inhibition. *Cell*. 2001;105(4):521-532.
392. Ottem EN, Godwin JG, Krishnan S, Petersen SL. Dual-phenotype GABA/glutamate neurons in adult preoptic area: sexual dimorphism and function. *J Neurosci*. 2004;24(37):8097-8105.
393. Ha CM, Choi J, Choi EJ, et al. NELL2, a neuron-specific EGF-like protein, is selectively expressed in glutamatergic neurons and contributes to the glutamatergic control of GnRH neurons at puberty. *Neuroendocrinology*. 2008;88(3):199-211.
394. Terasawa E, Luchansky LL, Kasuya E, Nyberg CL. An increase in glutamate release follows a decrease in gamma aminobutyric acid and the pubertal increase in luteinizing hormone releasing hormone release in the female rhesus monkeys. *J Neuroendocrinol*. 1999;11(4):275-282.
395. Mahachoklertwattana P, Sanchez J, Kaplan SL, Grumbach MM. N-methyl-D-aspartate (NMDA) receptors mediate the release of hormone (GnRH) by NMDA in a hypothalamic neuronal cell line (GT1-1). *Endocrinology*. 1994;134(3):1023-1030.
396. Blogowska A, Rzepka-Gorska I, Krzyzanowska-Swiniarska B. Is neuropeptide Y responsible for constitutional delay of puberty in girls? A preliminary report. *Gynecol Endocrinol*. 2004;19(1):22-25.
397. Reiter EO, Kaplan SL, Conte FA, Grumbach MM. Responsivity of pituitary gonadotropes to luteinizing hormone-releasing factor in idiopathic precocious puberty, precocious thelarche, precocious adrenarche, and in patients treated with medroxyprogesterone acetate. *Pediatr Res*. 1975;9:111-116.
398. Wildt L, Marshall G, Knobil E. Experimental induction of puberty in the infantile female rhesus monkey. *Science*. 1980;207:1373-1375.
399. Crowley WF Jr, McArthur JW. Stimulation of the normal menstrual cycle in Kallmann's syndrome by pulsatile administration of luteinizing hormone-releasing hormone (LHRH). *J Clin Endocrinol Metab*. 1980;51(1):173-175.
400. Hayes FJ, Seminara SB, DeCruz S, et al. Aromatase inhibition in the human male reveals a hypothalamic site of estrogen feedback. *J Clin Endocrinol Metab*. 2000;85(9):3027-3035.
401. Apter D, Vihko R. Serum pregnenolone, progesterone, 17-hydroxyprogesterone, testosterone and 5 alpha-dihydrotestosterone during female puberty. *J Clin Endocrinol Metab*. 1977;45:1039-1048.
402. Sklar CA, Kaplan SL, Grumbach MM. Evidence for dissociation between adrenarche and gonadarche: studies in patients with idiopathic precocious puberty, gonadal dysgenesis, isolated gonadotropin deficiency, and constitutionally delayed growth and adolescence. *J Clin Endocrinol Metab*. 1980;51:548-556.
403. Reiter EO, Fuldauer VG, Root AW. Secretion of the adrenal androgen, dehydroepiandrosterone sulfate, during normal infancy, childhood, and adolescence, in sick infants, and in children with endocrinologic abnormalities. *J Pediatr*. 1977;90:766-770.
404. Voutilainen R, Jaaskelainen J. Premature adrenarche: etiology, clinical findings, and consequences. *J Steroid Biochem Mol Biol*. 2015;145:226-236.
405. Campbell B. Adrenarche and the evolution of human life history. *Am J Hum Biol*. 2006;18(5):569-589.
406. Auchus RJ, Miller WL. Molecular modeling of human P450c17 (17alpha-hydroxylase/17,20-lyase): insights into reaction mechanisms and effects of mutations. *Mol Endocrinol*. 1999;13(7):1169-1182.
407. Karteris E, Randeva HS, Grammatopoulos DK, et al. Expression and coupling characteristics of the CRH and orexin type 2 receptors in human fetal adrenals. *J Clin Endocrinol Metab*. 2001;86(9):4512-4519.
408. Biason-Lauber A, Zachmann M, Schoenle EJ. Effect of leptin on CYP17 enzymatic activities in human adrenal cells: new insight in the onset of adrenarche. *Endocrinology*. 2000;141(4):1446-1454.

409. Remer T, Manz F. Role of nutritional status in the regulation of adrenarche. *J Clin Endocrinol Metab*. 1999;84(11):3936-3944.

410. Reiter EO, Grumbach MM, Kaplan SL, Conte FA. The response of pituitary gonadotropes to synthetic LRF in children with glucocorticoid-treated congenital adrenal hyperplasia: lack of effect of intrauterine and neonatal androgen excess. *J Clin Endocrinol Metab*. 1975;40(2):318-325.

411. Remer T, Manz F. The midgrowth spurt in healthy children is not caused by adrenarche. *J Clin Endocrinol Metab*. 2001;86(9):4183-4186.

412. Sedlmeyer IL, Palmert MR. Delayed puberty: analysis of a large case series from an academic center. *J Clin Endocrinol Metab*. 2002;87(4):1613-1620.

413. Sedlmeyer IL, Hirschhorn JN, Palmert MR. Pedigree analysis of constitutional delay of growth and maturation: determination of familial aggregation and inheritance patterns. *J Clin Endocrinol Metab*. 2002;87(12):5581-5586.

414. Han JC, Damaso L, Welch S, et al. Effects of growth hormone and nutritional therapy in boys with constitutional growth delay: a randomized controlled trial. *J Pediatr*. 2011;158(3):427-432.

415. Wu FC, Brown DC, Butler GE, et al. Early morning plasma testosterone is an accurate predictor of imminent pubertal development in prepubertal boys. *J Clin Endocrinol Metab*. 1993;76:26-31.

416. Du Caju MV, Op De Beeck L, Sys SU, et al. Progressive deceleration in growth as an early sign of delayed puberty in boys. *Horm Res*. 2000;54(3):126-130.

417. Wehkalampi K, Vangonen K, Laine T, Dunkel L. Progressive reduction of relative height in childhood predicts adult stature below target height in boys with constitutional delay of growth and puberty. *Horm Res*. 2007;68(2):99-104.

418. Wehkalampi K, Pakkila K, Laine T, Dunkel L. Adult height in girls with delayed pubertal growth. *Horm Res Paediatr*. 2011;76(2):130-135.

419. Yanovski JA, Rose SR, Municchi G, et al. Treatment with a luteinizing hormone-releasing hormone agonist in adolescents with short stature. *N Engl J Med*. 2003;348(10):908-917.

420. Carel JC, Ecosse E, Nicolino M, et al. Adult height after long term treatment with recombinant growth hormone for idiopathic isolated growth hormone deficiency: observational follow up study of the French population based registry. *BMJ*. 2002;325(7355):70.

421. Ranke MB, Lindberg A, Martin DD, et al. The mathematical model for total pubertal growth in idiopathic growth hormone (GH) deficiency suggests a moderate role of GH dose. *J Clin Endocrinol Metab*. 2003;88(10):4748-4753.

422. Reiter EO. A brief review of the addition of gonadotropin-releasing hormone agonists (GnRH-Ag) to growth hormone (GH) treatment of children with idiopathic growth hormone deficiency: Previously published studies from America. *Mol Cell Endocrinol*. 2006;254-255:221-225.

423. Carel JC, Eugster EA, Rogol A, et al. Consensus statement on the use of gonadotropin-releasing hormone analogs in children. *Pediatrics*. 2009;123(4):e752-e762.

424. Finkelstein BS, Imperiale TF, Speroff T, et al. Effect of growth hormone therapy on height in children with idiopathic short stature: a meta-analysis. *Arch Pediatr Adolesc Med*. 2002;156(3):230-240.

425. Bryant J, Baxter L, Cave CB, Milne R. Recombinant growth hormone for idiopathic short stature in children and adolescents. *Cochrane Database Syst Rev*. 2007;(3):CD004440.

426. Hero M, Toiviainen-Salo S, Wickman S, et al. Vertebral morphology in aromatase inhibitor treated males with idiopathic short stature or constitutional delay of puberty. *J Bone Miner Res*. 2010;25(7):1536-1543.

427. Mauras N, Gonzalez dP, Hsiang HY, et al. Anastrozole increases predicted adult height of short adolescent males treated with growth hormone: a randomized, placebo-controlled, multicenter trial for one to three years. *J Clin Endocrinol Metab*. 2008;93(3):823-831.

428. Dunkel L. Use of aromatase inhibitors to increase final height. *Mol Cell Endocrinol*. 2006;254-255:207-216.

429. Wit JM, Hero M, Nunez SB. Aromatase inhibitors in pediatrics. *Nat Rev Endocrinol*. 2012;8(3):135-147.

430. Lin L, Conway GS, Hill NR, et al. A homozygous R262Q mutation in the gonadotropin-releasing hormone receptor (GNRHR) presenting as constitutional delay of growth and puberty with subsequent borderline oligospermia. *J Clin Endocrinol Metab*. 2006;91(12):5117-5121.

431. Muller HL. Childhood craniopharyngioma. *Pituitary*. 2013;16(1):56-67.

432. Keil MF, Stratakis CA. Pituitary tumors in childhood: update of diagnosis, treatment and molecular genetics. *Expert Rev Neurother*. 2008;8(4):563-574.

433. Brastianos PK, Taylor-Weiner A, Manley PE, et al. Exome sequencing identifies BRAF mutations in papillary craniopharyngiomas. *Nat Genet*. 2014;46(2):161-165.

434. Holsken A, Buchfelder M, Fahlbusch R, et al. Tumour cell migration in adamantinomatous craniopharyngiomas is promoted by activated Wnt-signalling. *Acta Neuropathol*. 2010;119(5):631-639.

435. Bretault M, Boillot A, Muzard L, et al. Clinical review: bariatric surgery following treatment for craniopharyngioma: a systematic review and individual-level data meta-analysis. *J Clin Endocrinol Metab*. 2013;98(6):2239-2246.

436. Elowe-Gruau E, Beltrand J, Brauner R, et al. Childhood craniopharyngioma: hypothalamus-sparing surgery decreases the risk of obesity. *J Clin Endocrinol Metab*. 2013;98(6):2376-2382.

437. Muller HL, Handwerker G, Gebhardt U, et al. Melatonin treatment in obese patients with childhood craniopharyngioma and increased daytime sleepiness. *Cancer Causes Control*. 2006;17(4):583-589.

438. Cohan P, Foulad A, Esposito F, et al. Symptomatic Rathke's cleft cysts: a report of 24 cases. *J Endocrinol Invest*. 2004;27(10):943-948.

439. Schneider DT, Calaminus G, Koch S, et al. Epidemiologic analysis of 1,442 children and adolescents registered in the German germ cell tumor protocols. *Pediatr Blood Cancer*. 2004;42(2):169-175.

440. Mootha SL, Barkovich AJ, Grumbach MM, et al. Idiopathic hypothalamic diabetes insipidus, pituitary stalk thickening and the occult intracranial germinoma in children and adolescents. *J Clin Endocrinol Metab*. 1997;82(5):1362-1367.

441. Khatua S, Dhall G, O'Neil S, et al. Treatment of primary CNS germinomatous germ cell tumors with chemotherapy prior to reduced dose whole ventricular and local boost irradiation. *Pediatr Blood Cancer*. 2010;55(1):42-46.

442. da Silva NS, Cappellano AM, Diez B, et al. Primary chemotherapy for intracranial germ cell tumors: results of the third international CNS germ cell tumor study. *Pediatr Blood Cancer*. 2010;54(3):377-383.

443. Maity A, Shu HK, Judkins AR, et al. Testicular seminoma 16 years after treatment for CNS germinoma. *J Neurooncol*. 2004;70(1):83-85.

444. Rothman J, Greenberg RE, Jaffe WI. Nonseminomatous germ cell tumor of the testis 9 years after a germ cell tumor of the pineal gland: case report and review of the literature. *Can J Urol*. 2008;15(3):4122-4124.

445. Bowers DC, Nathan PC, Constine L, et al. Subsequent neoplasms of the CNS among survivors of childhood cancer: a systematic review. *Lancet Oncol*. 2013;14(8):e321-e328.

446. Chahal HS, Chapple JP, Frohman LA, et al. Clinical, genetic and molecular characterization of patients with familial isolated pituitary adenomas (FIPA). *Trends Endocrinol Metab*. 2010;21(7):419-427.

447. Freda PU, Beckers AM, Katznelson L, et al. Endocrine Society. Pituitary incidentaloma: an Endocrine Society clinical practice guideline. *J Clin Endocrinol Metab*. 2011;96(4):894-904.

448. Kars M, Souverein PC, Herings RM, et al. Estimated age- and sex-specific incidence and prevalence of dopamine agonist-treated hyperprolactinemia. *J Clin Endocrinol Metab*. 2009;94(8):2729-2734.

449. Fideleff HL, Boquete HR, Suarez MG, Azaretzky M. Prolactinoma in children and adolescents. *Horm Res*. 2009;72(4):197-205.

450. Knoepfelmacher M, Gomes MC, Melo ME, Mendonca BB. Pituitary apoplexy during therapy with cabergoline in an adolescent male with prolactin-secreting macroadenoma. *Pituitary*. 2004;7(2):83-87.

451. Colao A, Galderisi M, Di Sarno A, et al. Increased prevalence of tricuspid regurgitation in patients with prolactinomas chronically treated with cabergoline. *J Clin Endocrinol Metab*. 2008;93(10):3777-3784.

452. Fahie-Wilson M, Smith TP. Determination of prolactin: the macroprolactin problem. *Best Pract Res Clin Endocrinol Metab*. 2013;27(5):725-742.

453. Abla O, Egeler RM, Weitzman S. Langerhans cell histiocytosis: current concepts and treatments. *Cancer Treat Rev*. 2010;36(4):354-359.

454. Frisk P, Arvidson J, Gustafsson J, Lonnerholm G. Pubertal development and final height after autologous bone marrow transplantation for acute lymphoblastic leukemia. *Bone Marrow Transplant*. 2004;33(2):205-210.

455. Gurney JG, Kadan-Lottick NS, Packer RJ, et al. Endocrine and cardiovascular late effects among adult survivors of childhood brain tumors: Childhood Cancer Survivor Study. *Cancer*. 2003;97(3):663-673.

456. Byrne J, Fears TR, Mills JL, et al. Fertility in women treated with cranial radiotherapy for childhood acute lymphoblastic leukemia. *Pediatr Blood Cancer*. 2004;42(7):589-597.

457. Silveira LF, Latronico AC. Approach to the patient with hypogonadotropic hypogonadism. *J Clin Endocrinol Metab*. 2013;98(5):1781-1788.

458. Harrington J, Palmert MR. Clinical review: distinguishing constitutional delay of growth and puberty from isolated hypogonadotropic hypogonadism: critical appraisal of available diagnostic tests. *J Clin Endocrinol Metab*. 2012;97(9):3056-3067.

459. Van Dop C, Burstein S, Conte FA, et al. Isolated gonadotropin deficiency in boys: clinical characteristics and growth. *J Pediatr*. 1987;111:684-692.

460. Sidhoum VF, Chan YM, Lippincott MF, et al. Reversal and relapse of hypogonadotropic hypogonadism: resilience and fragility of the reproductive neuroendocrine system. *J Clin Endocrinol Metab*. 2014;99(3):861-870.

461. Kallmann F, Schonfeld WA, Barrera SW. Genetic aspects of primary eunuchoidism. *Am J Ment Defic*. 1944;48:203-236.

462. Pitteloud N, Hayes FJ, Boepple PA, et al. The role of prior pubertal development, biochemical markers of testicular maturation, and genetics in elucidating the phenotypic heterogeneity of idiopathic hypogonadotropic hypogonadism. *J Clin Endocrinol Metab*. 2002;87(1):152-160.

463. Manara R, Salvalaggio A, Favaro A, et al. Brain changes in Kallmann syndrome. *Am J Neuroradiol.* 2014;35(9):1700-1706.

464. Miraoui H, Dwyer AA, Sykiotis GP, et al. Mutations in FGF17, IL17RD, DUSP6, SPRY4, and FLRT3 are identified in individuals with congenital hypogonadotropic hypogonadism. *Am J Hum Genet.* 2013;92(5): 725-743.

465. Sato N, Katsumata N, Kagami M, et al. Clinical assessment and mutation analysis of Kallmann syndrome 1 (KAL1) and fibroblast growth factor receptor 1 (FGFR1, or KAL2) in five families and 18 sporadic patients. *J Clin Endocrinol Metab.* 2004;89(3):1079-1088.

466. Oliveira LM, Seminara SB, Beranova M, et al. The importance of autosomal genes in Kallmann syndrome: genotype- phenotype correlations and neuroendocrine characteristics. *J Clin Endocrinol Metab.* 2001; 86(4):1532-1538.

467. Dode C, Levilliers J, Dupont JM, et al. Loss-of-function mutations in FGFR1 cause autosomal dominant Kallmann syndrome. *Nat Genet.* 2003;33(4):463-465.

468. Pitteloud N, Acierno JS Jr, Meysing AU, et al. Reversible Kallmann syndrome, delayed puberty, and isolated anosmia occurring in a single family with a mutation in the fibroblast growth factor receptor 1 gene. *J Clin Endocrinol Metab.* 2005;90(3):1317-1322.

469. Chung WC, Moyle SS, Tsai PS. Fibroblast growth factor 8 signaling through fibroblast growth factor receptor 1 is required for the emergence of gonadotropin-releasing hormone neurons. *Endocrinology.* 2008;149(10):4997-5003.

470. Semple RK, Kemal TA. The recent genetics of hypogonadotrophic hypogonadism—novel insights and new questions. *Clin Endocrinol (Oxf).* 2010;72(4):427-435.

471. Delphine Z, Bretones P, Lambe C, et al. Paediatric phenotype of Kallmann syndrome due to mutations of fibroblast growth factor receptor 1 (FGFR1). *Mol Cell Endocrinol.* 2006;254-255:78-83.

472. Matsumoto S, Yamazaki C, Masumoto KH, et al. Abnormal development of the olfactory bulb and reproductive system in mice lacking prokineticin receptor PKR2. *Proc Natl Acad Sci U S A.* 2006;103(11): 4140-4145.

473. Pitteloud N, Zhang C, Pignatelli D, et al. Loss-of-function mutation in the prokineticin 2 gene causes Kallmann syndrome and normosmic idiopathic hypogonadotropic hypogonadism. *Proc Natl Acad Sci U S A.* 2007;104(44):17447-17452.

474. Xu N, Kim HG, Bhagavath B, et al. Nasal embryonic LHRH factor (NELF) mutations in patients with normosmic hypogonadotropic hypogonadism and Kallmann syndrome. *Fertil Steril.* 2011;95(5):1613-1620.e1611-1613-1620.e1617.

475. Hanchate NK, Giacobini P, Lhuillier P, et al. SEMA3A, a gene involved in axonal pathfinding, is mutated in patients with Kallmann syndrome. *PLoS Genet.* 2012;8(8):e1002896.

476. Pingault V, Bodereau V, Baral V, et al. Loss-of-function mutations in SOX10 cause Kallmann syndrome with deafness. *Am J Hum Genet.* 2013;92(5):707-724.

477. Tornberg J, Sykiotis GP, Keefe K, et al. Heparan sulfate 6-O-sulfotransferase 1, a gene involved in extracellular sugar modifications, is mutated in patients with idiopathic hypogonadotrophic hypogonadism. *Proc Natl Acad Sci U S A.* 2011;108(28):11524-11529.

478. Newbern K, Natrajan N, Kim HG, et al. Identification of HESX1 mutations in Kallmann syndrome. *Fertil Steril.* 2013;99(7):1831-1837.

479. Kotan LD, Hutchins BI, Ozkan Y, et al. Mutations in FEZF1 cause Kallmann syndrome. *Am J Hum Genet.* 2014;95(3):326-331.

480. Jongmans MC, Ravenswaaij-Arts CM, Pitteloud N, et al. CHD7 mutations in patients initially diagnosed with Kallmann syndrome—the clinical overlap with CHARGE syndrome. *Clin Genet.* 2009;75(1): 65-71.

481. Beier DR, Dluhy RG. Bench and bedside—the G protein-coupled receptor GPR54 and puberty. *N Engl J Med.* 2003;349(17):1589-1592.

482. Achermann JC, Weiss J, Lee EJ, Jameson JL. Inherited disorders of the gonadotropin hormones. *Mol Cell Endocrinol.* 2001;179(1-2):89-96.

483. de Roux N, Milgrom E. Inherited disorders of GnRH and gonadotropin receptors. *Mol Cell Endocrinol.* 2001;179(1-2):83-87.

484. Deleted in review.

485. Bouligand J, Ghervan C, Tello JA, et al. Isolated familial hypogonadotropic hypogonadism and a GNRH1 mutation. *N Engl J Med.* 2009; 360(26):2742-2748.

486. Chan YM, de Guillebon A, Lang-Muritano M, et al. GNRH1 mutations in patients with idiopathic hypogonadotropic hypogonadism. *Proc Natl Acad Sci U S A.* 2009;106(28):11703-11708.

487. Bedecarrats GY, Linher KD, Janovick JA, et al. Four naturally occurring mutations in the human GnRH receptor affect ligand binding and receptor function. *Mol Cell Endocrinol.* 2003;205(1-2):51-64.

488. Janovick JA, Maya-Nunez G, Conn PM. Rescue of hypogonadotropic hypogonadism-causing and manufactured GnRH receptor mutants by a specific protein-folding template: misrouted proteins as a novel disease etiology and therapeutic target. *J Clin Endocrinol Metab.* 2002; 87(7):3255-3262.

489. Maya-Nunez G, Janovick JA, Ulloa-Aguirre A, et al. Molecular basis of hypogonadotropic hypogonadism: restoration of mutant (E(90)K) GnRH receptor function by a deletion at a distant site. *J Clin Endocrinol Metab.* 2002;87(5):2144-2149.

490. Brothers SP, Cornea A, Janovick JA, Conn PM. Human loss-of-function gonadotropin-releasing hormone receptor mutants retain wild-type receptors in the endoplasmic reticulum: molecular basis of the dominant-negative effect. *Mol Endocrinol.* 2004;18(7):1787-1797.

491. Gianetti E, Hall JE, Au MG, et al. When genetic load does not correlate with phenotypic spectrum: lessons from the GnRH receptor (GNRHR). *J Clin Endocrinol Metab.* 2012;97(9):E1798-E1807.

492. Bin-Abbas B, Conte FA, Grumbach MM, Kaplan SL. Congenital hypogonadotropic hypogonadism and micropenis: effect of testosterone treatment on adult penile size why sex reversal is not indicated. *J Pediatr.* 1999;134(5):579-583.

493. Semple RK, Achermann JC, Ellery J, et al. Two novel missense mutations in G protein-coupled receptor 54 in a patient with hypogonadotropic hypogonadism. *J Clin Endocrinol Metab.* 2005;90(3):1849-1855.

494. de Roux N, Genin E, Carel JC, et al. Hypogonadotropic hypogonadism due to loss of function of the KiSS1-derived peptide receptor GPR54. *Proc Natl Acad Sci U S A.* 2003;100(19):10972-10976.

495. Wacker JL, Feller DB, Tang XB, et al. Disease-causing mutation in GPR54 reveals the importance of the second intracellular loop for class A G-protein-coupled receptor function. *J Biol Chem.* 2008;283(45): 31068-31078.

496. Jadhav U, Harris RM, Jameson JL. Hypogonadotropic hypogonadism in subjects with DAX1 mutations. *Mol Cell Endocrinol.* 2011;346(1-2): 65-73.

497. Merke DP, Tajima T, Baron J, Cutler GJ. Hypogonadotropic hypogonadism in a female caused by an X-linked recessive mutation in the DAX1 gene. *N Engl J Med.* 1999;340(16):1248-1252.

498. Seminara SB, Achermann JC, Genel M, et al. X-linked adrenal hypoplasia congenita: a mutation in DAX1 expands the phenotypic spectrum in males and females. *J Clin Endocrinol Metab.* 1999;84(4501):4509.

499. Tabarin A, Achermann JC, Recan D, et al. A novel mutation in DAX1 causes delayed-onset adrenal insufficiency and incomplete hypogonadotropic hypogonadism. *J Clin Invest.* 2000;105(3):321-328.

500. Talaban R, Sellick GS, Spendlove HE, et al. Inherited pericentric inversion (X)(p11.4q11.2) associated with delayed puberty and obesity in two brothers. *Cytogenet Genome Res.* 2005;109(4):480-484.

501. Topaloglu AK, Reimann F, Guclu M, et al. TAC3 and TACR3 mutations in familial hypogonadotropic hypogonadism reveal a key role for Neurokinin B in the central control of reproduction. *Nat Genet.* 2009; 41(3):354-358.

502. Young J, Bouligand J, Francou B, et al. TAC3 and TACR3 Defects cause hypothalamic congenital hypogonadotropic hypogonadism in humans. *J Clin Endocrinol Metab.* 2010;95(5):2287-2295.

503. Gianetti E, Tusset C, Noel SD, et al. *TAC3/TACR3* mutations reveal preferential activation of GnRH release by neurokinin B in neonatal life followed by reversal in adulthood. *J Clin Endocrinol Metab.* 2010; 95(6):2857-2867.

504. Jackson RS, Creemers JW, Farooqi IS, et al. Small-intestinal dysfunction accompanies the complex endocrinopathy of human proprotein convertase 1 deficiency. *J Clin Invest.* 2003;112(10):1550-1560.

505. Pitteloud N, Boepple PA, DeCruz S, et al. The fertile eunuch variant of idiopathic hypogonadotropic hypogonadism: spontaneous reversal associated with a homozygous mutation in the gonadotropin-releasing hormone receptor. *J Clin Endocrinol Metab.* 2001;86(6):2470-2475.

506. Siegel ET, Kim HG, Nishimoto HK, Layman LC. The molecular basis of impaired follicle-stimulating hormone action: evidence from human mutations and mouse models. *Reprod Sci (Thousand Oaks, Calif.).* 2013; 20(3):211-233.

507. Hanna CE, Mandel SH, LaFranchi SH. Puberty in the syndrome of septo-optic dysplasia. *Am J Dis Child.* 1989;143:186-189.

508. Kaplan SL, Grumbach MM, Hoyt WF. A syndrome of hypopituitary dwarfism, hypoplasia of optic nerves, and malformation of prosencephalon: report of 6 patients. *Pediatr Res.* 1970;4:480-481.

509. Birkebaek NH, Patel L, Wright NB, et al. Endocrine status in patients with optic nerve hypoplasia: relationship to midline central nervous system abnormalities and appearance of the hypothalamic-pituitary axis on magnetic resonance imaging. *J Clin Endocrinol Metab.* 2003; 88(11):5281-5286.

510. McCabe MJ, Alatzoglou KS, Dattani MT. Septo-optic dysplasia and other midline defects: the role of transcription factors: HESX1 and beyond. *Best Pract Res Clin Endocrinol Metab.* 2011;25(1):115-124.

511. Nanni L, Ming JE, Du Y, et al. SHH mutation is associated with solitary median maxillary central incisor: a study of 13 patients and review of the literature. *Am J Med Genet.* 2001;102(1):1-10.

512. Raivio T, Falardeau J, Dwyer A, et al. Reversal of idiopathic hypogonadotropic hypogonadism. *N Engl J Med.* 2007;357(9):863-873.

513. Netchine I, Sobrier ML, Krude H, et al. Mutations in LHX3 result in a new syndrome revealed by combined pituitary hormone deficiency. *Nat Genet.* 2000;25(2):182-186.

514. Davis SW, Castinetti F, Carvalho LR, et al. Molecular mechanisms of pituitary organogenesis: in search of novel regulatory genes. *Mol Cell Endocrinol.* 2010;323(1):4-19.

515. Reynaud R, Chadli-Chaieb M, Vallette-Kasic S, et al. A familial form of congenital hypopituitarism due to a PROP1 mutation in a large kindred: phenotypic and in vitro functional studies. *J Clin Endocrinol Metab.* 2004;89(11):5779-5786.

516. Colvin SC, Mullen RD, Pfaeffle RW, Rhodes SJ. LHX3 and LHX4 transcription factors in pituitary development and disease. *Pediatr Endocrinol Rev.* 2009;6(Suppl 2):283-290.

517. Takagi M, Ishii T, Inokuchi M, et al. Gradual loss of ACTH due to a novel mutation in LHX4: comprehensive mutation screening in Japanese patients with congenital hypopituitarism. *PLoS ONE.* 2012;7(9): e46008.

518. Franca MM, Jorge AA, Carvalho LR, et al. Novel heterozygous nonsense GLI2 mutations in patients with hypopituitarism and ectopic posterior pituitary lobe without holoprosencephaly. *J Clin Endocrinol Metab.* 2010;95(11):E384-E391.

519. Solomon NM, Ross SA, Morgan T, et al. Array comparative genomic hybridisation analysis of boys with X linked hypopituitarism identifies a 3.9 Mb duplicated critical region at Xq27 containing SOX3. *J Med Genet.* 2004;41(9):669-678.

520. Tziaferi V, Kelberman D, Dattani MT. The role of SOX2 in hypogonadotropic hypogonadism. *Sex Dev.* 2008;2(4-5):194-199.

521. Cassidy SB, Schwartz S, Miller JL, Driscoll DJ. Prader-Willi syndrome. *Genet Med.* 2012;14(1):10-26.

522. Crino A, Schiaffini R, Ciampalini P, et al. Hypogonadism and pubertal development in Prader-Willi syndrome. *Eur J Pediatr.* 2003;162(5): 327-333.

523. Hirsch HJ, Eldar-Geva T, Benarroch F, et al. Primary testicular dysfunction is a major contributor to abnormal pubertal development in males with Prader-Willi syndrome. *J Clin Endocrinol Metab.* 2009;94(7): 2262-2268.

524. Schmidt H, Pozza SB, Bonfig W, et al. Successful early dietary intervention avoids obesity in patients with Prader-Willi syndrome: a ten-year follow-up. *J Pediatr Endocrinol Metab.* 2008;21(7):651-655.

525. Carrel AL, Myers SE, Whitman BY, Allen DB. Sustained benefits of growth hormone on body composition, fat utilization, physical strength and agility, and growth in Prader-Willi syndrome are dose-dependent. *J Pediatr Endocrinol Metab.* 2001;14(8):1097-1105.

526. Zaglia F, Zaffanello M, Biban P. Unexpected death due to refractory metabolic acidosis and massive hemolysis in a young infant with Prader-Willi syndrome. *Am J Med Genet A.* 2005;132(2):219-221.

527. Fillion M, Deal C, Van Vliet G. Retrospective study of the potential benefits and adverse events during growth hormone treatment in children with Prader-Willi syndrome. *J Pediatr.* 2009;154(2):230-233.

528. Tauber M, Diene G, Mimoun E, et al. Prader-Willi syndrome as a model of human hyperphagia. *Front Horm Res.* 2014;42:93-106.

529. Forsythe E, Beales PL. Bardet-Biedl syndrome. *Eur J Hum Genet.* 2013;21(1):8-13.

530. Swenne I. Weight requirements for return of menstruations in teenage girls with eating disorders, weight loss and secondary amenorrhoea. *Acta Paediatr.* 2004;93(11):1449-1455.

531. Zhang Z, Lindstrom MJ, Lai HJ. Pubertal height velocity and associations with prepubertal and adult heights in cystic fibrosis. *J Pediatr.* 2013;163(2):376-382.

532. Arrigo T, De Luca F, Lucanto C, et al. Nutritional, glycometabolic and genetic factors affecting menarcheal age in cystic fibrosis. *Diabetes Nutr Metab.* 2004;17(2):114-119.

533. Zemel BS, Kawchak DA, Ohene-Frempong K, et al. Effects of delayed pubertal development, nutritional status, and disease severity on longitudinal patterns of growth failure in children with sickle cell disease. *Pediatr Res.* 2007;61(5 Pt 1):607-613.

534. Chatterjee R, Mukhopadhyay TN, Chandra S, Bajoria R. Sex steroid priming for induction of puberty in thalassemia patients with pulsatile reversible hypogonadotrophic hypogonadism. *Hemoglobin.* 2011; 35(5-6):659-664.

535. Caruso-Nicoletti M, De Sanctis V, Raiola G, et al. No difference in pubertal growth and final height between treated hypogonadal and non-hypogonadal thalassemic patients. *Horm Res.* 2004;62(1): 17-22.

536. Hovi L, Saarinen-Pihkala UM, Taskinen M, et al. Subnormal androgen levels in young female bone marrow transplant recipients with ovarian dysfunction, chronic GVHD and receiving glucocorticoid therapy. *Bone Marrow Transplant.* 2004;33(5):503-508.

537. Williams PL, Abzug MJ, Jacobson DL, et al. Pubertal onset in children with perinatal HIV infection in the era of combination antiretroviral treatment. *AIDS.* 2013;27(12):1959-1970.

538. Wikstrom AM, Hovi L, Dunkel L, Saarinen-Pihkala UM. Restoration of ovarian function after chemotherapy for osteosarcoma. *Arch Dis Child.* 2003;88(5):428-431.

539. Steffens M, Beauloye V, Brichard B, et al. Endocrine and metabolic disorders in young adult survivors of childhood acute lymphoblastic leukaemia (ALL) or non-Hodgkin lymphoma (NHL). *Clin Endocrinol (Oxf).* 2008;69(5):819-827.

540. Nottage KA, Ness KK, Li C, et al. Metabolic syndrome and cardiovascular risk among long-term survivors of acute lymphoblastic leukaemia—from the St. Jude Lifetime Cohort. *Br J Haematol.* 2014; 165(3):364-374.

541. Halmi KA. Anorexia nervosa: an increasing problem in children and adolescents. *Dialogues Clin Neurosci.* 2009;11(1):100-103.

542. Attia E, Roberto CA. Should amenorrhea be a diagnostic criterion for anorexia nervosa? *Int J Eat Disord.* 2009;42(7):581-589.

543. American Psychiatric Association. *Diagnostic and Statistical Manual of Mental Disorders.* 5th ed. Arlington, VA: American Psychiatric Publishing; 2013.

544. Arcelus J, Mitchell AJ, Wales J, Nielsen S. Mortality rates in patients with anorexia nervosa and other eating disorders. A meta-analysis of 36 studies. *Arch Gen Psychiatry.* 2011;68(7):724-731.

545. Misra M, Klibanski A. Neuroendocrine consequences of anorexia nervosa in adolescents. *Endocr Dev.* 2010;17:197-214.

546. Watson HJ, Bulik CM. Update on the treatment of anorexia nervosa: review of clinical trials, practice guidelines and emerging interventions. *Psychol Med.* 2013;43(12):2477-2500.

547. Caronia LM, Martin C, Welt CK, et al. A genetic basis for functional hypothalamic amenorrhea. *N Engl J Med.* 2011;364(3):215-225.

548. Kaye WH, Klump KL, Frank GK, Strober M. Anorexia and bulimia nervosa. *Annu Rev Med.* 2000;51:299-313.

549. Birmingham CL, Touyz S, Harbottle J. Are anorexia nervosa and bulimia nervosa separate disorders? Challenging the "transdiagnostic" theory of eating disorders. *Eur Eat Disord Rev.* 2009;17(1):2-13.

550. Torstveit MK, Sundgot-Borgen J. Participation in leanness sports but not training volume is associated with menstrual dysfunction: a national survey of 1276 elite athletes and controls. *Br J Sports Med.* 2005;39(3):141-147.

551. Claessens AL, Bourgois J, Beunen G, et al. Age at menarche in relation to anthropometric characteristics, competition level and boat category in elite junior rowers. *Ann Hum Biol.* 2003;30(2):148-159.

552. Markou KB, Mylonas P, Theodoropoulou A, et al. The influence of intensive physical exercise on bone acquisition in adolescent elite female and male artistic gymnasts. *J Clin Endocrinol Metab.* 2004; 89(9):4383-4387.

553. Theodoropoulou A, Markou KB, Vagenakis GA, et al. Delayed but normally progressed puberty is more pronounced in artistic compared with rhythmic elite gymnasts due to the intensity of training. *J Clin Endocrinol Metab.* 2005;90(11):6022-6027.

554. Klentrou P, Plyley M. Onset of puberty, menstrual frequency, and body fat in elite rhythmic gymnasts compared with normal controls. *Br J Sports Med.* 2003;37(6):490-494.

555. Malina RM, Baxter-Jones AD, Armstrong N, et al. Role of intensive training in the growth and maturation of artistic gymnasts. *Sports Med.* 2013;43(9):783-802.

556. Munoz MT, de la Piedra C, Barrios V, et al. Changes in bone density and bone markers in rhythmic gymnasts and ballet dancers: implications for puberty and leptin levels. *Eur J Endocrinol.* 2004;151(4): 491-496.

557. Fenichel RM, Warren MP. Anorexia, bulimia, and the athletic triad: evaluation and management. *Curr Osteoporos Rep.* 2007;5(4):160-164.

558. Georgopoulos NA, Theodoropoulou A, Leglise M, et al. Growth and skeletal maturation in male and female artistic gymnasts. *J Clin Endocrinol Metab.* 2004;89(9):4377-4382.

559. Kaplan P, Baris H, De Meirleir L, et al. Revised recommendations for the management of Gaucher disease in children. *Eur J Pediatr.* 2013; 172(4):447-458.

560. Picardi A, Cipponeri E, Bizzarri C, et al. Menarche in type 1 diabetes is still delayed despite good metabolic control. *Fertil Steril.* 2008; 90(5):1875-1877.

561. Dias J, Martins S, Carvalho S, et al. Mauriac syndrome still exists. *Endocrinol Nutr.* 2013;60(5):245-248.

562. Achermann JC, Hughes IA. Disorders of sex development. In: Melmed S, Polonsky KS, Larsen PR, Kronenberg HM, eds. *Williams Textbook of Endocrinology.* 12th ed. Philadelphia, PA: WB Saunders; 2011:868-934.

563. Klinefelter HF Jr, Reifenstein EC Jr, Albright F. Syndrome characterized by gynecomastia, aspermatogenesis without A-leydigism, and increased excretion of follicle-stimulating hormone. *J Clin Endocrinol.* 1942;2: 615-627.

564. Aksglaede L, Link K, Giwercman A, et al. 47,XXY Klinefelter syndrome: clinical characteristics and age-specific recommendations for medical management. *Am J Med Genet C Semin Med Genet.* 2013;163C(1):55-63.

565. Cabrol S, Ross JL, Fennoy I, et al. Assessment of Leydig and Sertoli cell functions in infants with nonmosaic Klinefelter syndrome: insulin-like peptide 3 levels are normal and positively correlated with LH levels. *J Clin Endocrinol Metab.* 2011;96(4):E746-E753.

566. Ross JL, Samango-Sprouse C, Lahlou N, et al. Early androgen deficiency in infants and young boys with 47,XXY Klinefelter syndrome. *Horm Res.* 2005;64(1):39-45.

567. Christiansen P, Andersson AM, Skakkebaek NE. Longitudinal studies of inhibin B levels in boys and young adults with Klinefelter syndrome. *J Clin Endocrinol Metab.* 2003;88(2):888-891.

568. Wikstrom AM, Painter JN, Raivio T, et al. Genetic features of the X chromosome affect pubertal development and testicular degeneration in adolescent boys with Klinefelter syndrome. *Clin Endocrinol (Oxf).* 2006;65(1):92-97.

569. Fullerton G, Hamilton M, Maheshwari A. Should non-mosaic Klinefelter syndrome men be labelled as infertile in 2009? *Hum Reprod.* 2010;25(3):588-597.

570. Van Saen D, Gies I, De Schepper J, et al. Can pubertal boys with Klinefelter syndrome benefit from spermatogonial stem cell banking? *Hum Reprod.* 2012;27(2):323-330.

571. Wikstrom AM, Dunkel L, Wickman S, et al. Are adolescent boys with Klinefelter syndrome androgen deficient? A longitudinal study of Finnish 47,XXY boys. *Pediatr Res.* 2006;59(6):854-859.

572. Zinn AR, Ramos P, Elder FF, et al. Androgen receptor CAGn repeat length influences phenotype of 47,XXY (Klinefelter) syndrome. *J Clin Endocrinol Metab.* 2005;90(9):5041-5046.

573. Zitzmann M, Depenbusch M, Gromoll J, Nieschlag E. X-chromosome inactivation patterns and androgen receptor functionality influence phenotype and social characteristics as well as pharmacogenetics of testosterone therapy in Klinefelter patients. *J Clin Endocrinol Metab.* 2004;89(12):6208-6217.

574. Groth KA, Skakkebaek A, Host C, et al. Clinical review: Klinefelter syndrome—a clinical update. *J Clin Endocrinol Metab.* 2013;98(1): 20-30.

575. Fennoy I. Testosterone and the child (0-12 years) with Klinefelter syndrome (47XXY): a review. *Acta Paediatr.* 2011;100(6):846-850.

576. Patterson BC, Wasilewski-Masker K, Ryerson AB, et al. Endocrine health problems detected in 519 patients evaluated in a pediatric cancer survivor program. *J Clin Endocrinol Metab.* 2012;97(3):810-818.

577. van den Berg H, Furstner F, van den Bos C, Behrendt H. Decreasing the number of MOPP courses reduces gonadal damage in survivors of childhood Hodgkin disease. *Pediatr Blood Cancer.* 2004;42(3):210-215.

578. Ginsberg JP, Carlson CA, Lin K, et al. An experimental protocol for fertility preservation in prepubertal boys recently diagnosed with cancer: a report of acceptability and safety. *Hum Reprod.* 2010; 25(1):37-41.

579. Auchus RJ. The genetics, pathophysiology, and management of human deficiencies of P450c17. *Endocrinol Metab Clin North Am.* 2001;30(1):101-119, vii.

580. Martin RM, Lin CJ, Costa EM, et al. P450c17 deficiency in Brazilian patients: biochemical diagnosis through progesterone levels confirmed by CYP17 genotyping. *J Clin Endocrinol Metab.* 2003;88(12):5739-5746.

581. Miller WL. Steroid hormone synthesis in mitochondria. *Mol Cell Endocrinol.* 2013;379(1-2):62-73.

582. Kaku U, Kameyama K, Izawa M, et al. Ovarian histological findings in an adult patient with the steroidogenic acute regulatory protein (StAR) deficiency reveal the impairment of steroidogenesis by lipoid deposition. *Endocr J.* 2008;55(6):1043-1049.

583. Huhtaniemi I, Alevizaki M. Gonadotrophin resistance. *Best Pract Res Clin Endocrinol Metab.* 2006;20(4):561-576.

584. Bay K, Main KM, Toppari J, Skakkebaek NE. Testicular descent: INSL3, testosterone, genes and the intrauterine milieu. *Nat Rev Urol.* 2011;8(4): 187-196.

585. Sijstermans K, Hack WW, Meijer RW, van der Voort-Doedens LM. The frequency of undescended testis from birth to adulthood: a review. *Int J Androl.* 2008;31(1):1-11.

586. Jensen MS, Toft G, Thulstrup AM, et al. Cryptorchidism concordance in monozygotic and dizygotic twin brothers, full brothers, and half-brothers. *Fertil Steril.* 2010;93(1):124-129.

587. Wood HM, Elder JS. Cryptorchidism and testicular cancer: separating fact from fiction. *J Urol.* 2009;181(2):452-461.

588. Grinspon RP, Ropelato MG, Bedecarras P, et al. Gonadotrophin secretion pattern in anorchid boys from birth to pubertal age: pathophysiological aspects and diagnostic usefulness. *Clin Endocrinol (Oxf).* 2012;76(5):698-705.

589. Grinspon RP, Loreti N, Braslavsky D, et al. Sertoli cell markers in the diagnosis of paediatric male hypogonadism. *J Pediatr Endocrinol Metab.* 2012;25(1-2):3-11.

590. Bondy CA. Care of girls and women with Turner syndrome: a guideline of the Turner Syndrome Study Group. *J Clin Endocrinol Metab.* 2007; 92(1):10-25.

591. Gatti JM, Ostlie DJ. The use of laparoscopy in the management of nonpalpable undescended testes. *Curr Opin Pediatr.* 2007;19(3): 349-353.

592. Shibata Y, Kojima Y, Mizuno K, et al. Optimal cutoff value of contralateral testicular size for prediction of absent testis in Japanese boys with nonpalpable testis. *Urology.* 2010;76(1):78-81.

593. Akre O, Pettersson A, Richiardi L. Risk of contralateral testicular cancer among men with unilaterally undescended testis: a meta analysis. *Int J Cancer.* 2009;124(3):687-689.

594. Bakker NE, Wolffenbuttel KP, Looijenga LH, Hokken-Koelega AC. Testes in infants with Prader-Willi syndrome: hCG treatment, surgery and histology. *J Urol.* 2015;193(1):291-298.

595. Thorup J, Petersen BL, Kvist K, Cortes D. Bilateral undescended testes classified according to preoperative and postoperative status of gonadotropins and inhibin B in relation to testicular histopathology at bilateral orchiopexy in infant boys. *J Urol.* 2012;188(4 Suppl): 1436-1442.

596. Lee PA, Coughlin MT. Fertility after bilateral cryptorchidism. Evaluation by paternity, hormone, and semen data. *Horm Res.* 2001;55(1): 28-32.

597. Giwercman A, Hansen LL, Skakkebaek NE. Initiation of sperm production after bilateral orchiopexy: clinical and biological implications. *J Urol.* 2000;163(4):1255-1256.

598. Moller H, Evans H. Epidemiology of gonadal germ cell cancer in males and females. *APMIS.* 2003;111(1):43-46.

599. Main KM, Skakkebaek NE, Toppari J. Cryptorchidism as part of the testicular dysgenesis syndrome: the environmental connection. *Endocr Dev.* 2009;14:167-173.

600. Thorup J, McLachlan R, Cortes D, et al. What is new in cryptorchidism and hypospadias—a critical review on the testicular dysgenesis hypothesis. *J Pediatr Surg.* 2010;45(10):2074-2086.

601. La Scala GC, Ein SH. Retractile testes: an outcome analysis on 150 patients. *J Pediatr Surg.* 2004;39(7):1014-1017.

602. Cicognani A, Alessandroni R, Pasini A, et al. Low birth weight for gestational age and subsequent male gonadal function. *J Pediatr.* 2002;141(3):376-379.

603. Allvin K, Ankarberg-Lindgren C, Fors H, Dahlgren J. Elevated serum levels of estradiol, dihydrotestosterone, and inhibin B in adult males born small for gestational age. *J Clin Endocrinol Metab.* 2008;93(4): 1464-1469.

604. Jensen RB, Vielwerth S, Larsen T, et al. Pituitary-gonadal function in adolescent males born appropriate or small for gestational age with or without intrauterine growth restriction. *J Clin Endocrinol Metab.* 2007;92(4):1353-1357.

605. Marchini A, Rappold G, Schneider KU. SHOX at a glance: from gene to protein. *Arch Physiol Biochem.* 2007;113(3):116-123.

606. Mortensen KH, Hansen KW, Erlandsen M, et al. Ambulatory arterial stiffness index in Turner syndrome: the impact of sex hormone replacement therapy. *Horm Res.* 2009;72(3):184-189.

607. Doerr HG, Bettendorf M, Hauffa BP, et al. Uterine size in women with Turner syndrome after induction of puberty with estrogens and long-term growth hormone therapy: results of the German IGLU Follow-up Study 2001. *Hum Reprod.* 2005;20(5):1418-1421.

608. Karnis MF, Zimon AE, Lalwani SI, et al. Risk of death in pregnancy achieved through oocyte donation in patients with Turner syndrome: a national survey. *Fertil Steril.* 2003;80(3):498-501.

609. Even L, Cohen A, Marbach N, et al. Longitudinal analysis of growth over the first 3 years of life in Turner's syndrome. *J Pediatr.* 2000; 137(4):460-464.

610. Ranke MB, Stubbe P, Majewski F, Bierich JR. Spontaneous growth in Turner's syndrome. *Acta Paediatr Scand Suppl.* 1988;343:22-30.

611. Ross JL, Quigley CA, Cao D, et al. Growth hormone plus childhood low-dose estrogen in Turner's syndrome. *N Engl J Med.* 2011;364(13): 1230-1242.

612. Cave CB, Bryant J, Milne R. Recombinant growth hormone in children and adolescents with Turner syndrome. *Cochrane Database Syst Rev.* 2003;(3):CD003887.

613. Bannink EM, van der Palen RL, Mulder PG, de Muinck Keizer-Schrama SM. Long-term follow-up of GH-treated girls with Turner syndrome: metabolic consequences. *Horm Res.* 2009;71(6):343-349.

614. Gravholt CH, Vestergaard P, Hermann AP, et al. Increased fracture rates in Turner's syndrome: a nationwide questionnaire survey. *Clin Endocrinol (Oxf).* 2003;59(1):89-96.

615. Ari M, Bakalov VK, Hill S, Bondy CA. The effects of GH treatment on bone mineral density and body composition in girls with Turner syndrome. *J Clin Endocrinol Metab.* 2006;91(11):4302-4305.

616. Sas TC, de Muinck Keizer-Schrama S, Stijnen T, et al. Carbohydrate metabolism during long-term growth hormone (GH) treatment and after discontinuation of GH treatment in girls with Turner syndrome participating in a randomized dose-response study. Dutch Advisory Group on Growth Hormone. *J Clin Endocrinol Metab.* 2000;85(2): 769-775.

617. Carel JC, Ecosse E, Bastie-Sigeac I, et al. Quality of life determinants in young women with Turner's syndrome after growth hormone treatment: results of the StaTur population-based cohort study. *J Clin Endocrinol Metab.* 2005;90(4):1992-1997.

618. Davenport ML. Approach to the patient with Turner syndrome. *J Clin Endocrinol Metab.* 2010;95(4):1487-1495.

619. Lepage JF, Hong DS, Hallmayer J, Reiss AL. Genomic imprinting effects on cognitive and social abilities in prepubertal girls with Turner syndrome. *J Clin Endocrinol Metab.* 2012;97(3):E460-E464.

620. Hoepffner W, Horn LC, Simon E, et al. Gonadoblastomas in 5 patients with 46,XY gonadal dysgenesis. *Exp Clin Endocrinol Diabetes.* 2005; 113(4):231-235.

621. McCann-Crosby B, Mansouri R, Dietrich JE, et al. State of the art review in gonadal dysgenesis: challenges in diagnosis and management. *Int J Pediatr Endocrinol.* 2014;2014(1):4.

622. Irtan S, Orbach D, Helfre S, Sarnacki S. Ovarian transposition in prepubescent and adolescent girls with cancer. *Lancet Oncol.* 2013;14(13): e601-e608.

623. Metzger ML, Meacham LR, Patterson B, et al. Female reproductive health after childhood, adolescent, and young adult cancers: guidelines for the assessment and management of female reproductive complications. *J Clin Oncol.* 2013;31(9):1239-1247.

624. Hughes EG, Neal MS. Ovulation suppression to protect against chemotherapy-induced ovarian toxicity: helpful or just hopeful? *Hum Reprod Update.* 2008;14(6):541-542.

625. Waimey KE, Duncan FE, Su HI, et al. Future directions in oncofertility and fertility preservation: a report from the 2011 Oncofertility Consortium Conference. *J Adolesc Young Adult Oncol.* 2013;2(1): 25-30.

626. Welt CK. Primary ovarian insufficiency: a more accurate term for premature ovarian failure. *Clin Endocrinol (Oxf).* 2008;68(4):499-509.
627. Rubio-Gozalbo ME, Gubbels CS, Bakker JA, et al. Gonadal function in male and female patients with classic galactosemia. *Hum Reprod Update.* 2010;16(2):177-188.
628. Crisponi L, Deiana M, Loi A, et al. The putative forkhead transcription factor FOXL2 is mutated in blepharophimosis/ptosis/epicanthus inversus syndrome. *Nat Genet.* 2001;27(2):159-166.
629. Skillern A, Rajkovic A. Recent developments in identifying genetic determinants of premature ovarian failure. *Sex Dev.* 2008;2(4-5):228-243.
630. Jaeken J, Matthijs G. Congenital disorders of glycosylation. *Annu Rev Genomics Hum Genet.* 2001;2:129-151.
631. Tapanainen JS, Aittomaki K, Min J, et al. Men homozygous for an inactivating mutation of the follicle-stimulating hormone (FSH) receptor gene present variable suppression of spermatogenesis and fertility. *Nat Genet.* 1997;15:205-206.
632. Latronico AC, Arnhold IJ. Inactivating mutations of the human luteinizing hormone receptor in both sexes. *Semin Reprod Med.* 2012;30(5):382-386.
633. Legro RS, Arslanian SA, Ehrmann DA, et al. Diagnosis and treatment of polycystic ovary syndrome: an Endocrine Society clinical practice guideline. *J Clin Endocrinol Metab.* 2013;98(12):4565-4592.
634. Roberts AE, Allanson JE, Tartaglia M, Gelb BD. Noonan syndrome. *Lancet.* 2013;381(9863):333-342.
635. Noordam C, Peer PG, Francois I, et al. Long-term GH treatment improves adult height in children with Noonan syndrome with and without mutations in protein tyrosine phosphatase, non-receptor-type 11. *Eur J Endocrinol.* 2008;159(3):203-208.
636. Binder G. Response to growth hormone in short children with Noonan syndrome: correlation to genotype. *Horm Res.* 2009;72(Suppl 2):52-56.
637. Resende EA, Lara BH, Reis JD, et al. Assessment of basal and gonadotropin-releasing hormone-stimulated gonadotropins by immunochemiluminometric and immunofluorometric assays in normal children. *J Clin Endocrinol Metab.* 2007;92(4):1424-1429.
638. Binder G, Schweizer R, Blumenstock G, Braun R. Inhibin B plus LH versus GnRH agonist test for distinguishing constitutional delay of growth and puberty from isolated hypogonadotropic hypogonadism in boys. *Clin Endocrinol (Oxf).* 2015;82(1):100-105.
639. Dunkel L, Quinton R. Transition in endocrinology: induction of puberty. *Eur J Endocrinol.* 2014;170(6):R229-R239.
640. Costa-Barbosa FA, Balasubramanian R, Keefe KW, et al. Prioritizing genetic testing in patients with Kallmann syndrome using clinical phenotypes. *J Clin Endocrinol Metab.* 2013;98(5):E943-E953.
641. Palmert MR, Dunkel L. Clinical practice. Delayed puberty. *N Engl J Med.* 2012;366(5):443-453.
642. Ahmed SF, Tucker P, Mayo A, et al. Randomized, crossover comparison study of the short-term effect of oral testosterone undecanoate and intramuscular testosterone depot on linear growth and serum bone alkaline phosphatase 4171. *J Pediatr Endocrinol Metab.* 2004;17(7):941-950.
643. Santhakumar A, Miller M, Quinton R. Pubertal induction in adult males with isolated hypogonadotropic hypogonadism using long-acting intramuscular testosterone undecanoate 1-g depot (Nebido). *Clin Endocrinol (Oxf).* 2014;80(1):155-157.
644. Mayo A, Macintyre H, Wallace AM, Ahmed SF. Transdermal testosterone application: pharmacokinetics and effects on pubertal status, short-term growth, and bone turnover. *J Clin Endocrinol Metab.* 2004;89(2):681-687.
645. Ankarberg-Lindgren C, Kristrom B, Norjavaara E. Physiological estrogen replacement therapy for puberty induction in girls: a clinical observational study. *Horm Res Paediatr.* 2014;81(4):239-244.
646. Turgeon JL, McDonnell DP, Martin KA, Wise PM. Hormone therapy: physiological complexity belies therapeutic simplicity. *Science.* 2004;304(5675):1269-1273.
647. Rosenfeld RG, Nicodemus BC. The transition from adolescence to adult life: physiology of the "transition" phase and its evolutionary basis. *Horm Res.* 2003;60(Suppl 1):74-77.
648. Lee PA, Houk CP. Outcome studies among men with micropenis. *J Pediatr Endocrinol Metab.* 2004;17(8):1043-1053.
649. Delemarre-van de Waal HA. Application of gonadotropin releasing hormone in hypogonadotropic hypogonadism—diagnostic and therapeutic aspects. *Eur J Endocrinol.* 2004;151(Suppl 3):U89-U94.
650. Kunz GJ, Klein KO, Clemons RD, et al. Virilization of young children after topical androgen use by their parents. *Pediatrics.* 2004;114(1):282-284.
651. Piippo S, Lenko H, Kainulainen P, Sipila I. Use of percutaneous estrogen gel for induction of puberty in girls with Turner syndrome. *J Clin Endocrinol Metab.* 2004;89(7):3241-3247.
652. Hindmarsh PC. How do you initiate oestrogen therapy in a girl who has not undergone puberty? *Clin Endocrinol (Oxf).* 2009;71(1):7-10.
653. Gussinye M, Terrades P, Yeste D, et al. Low areal bone mineral density values in adolescents and young adult Turner syndrome patients increase after long-term transdermal estradiol therapy. *Horm Res.* 2000;54(3):131-135.
654. Wit JM, Langenhorst VJ, Jansen M, et al. Dehydroepiandrosterone sulfate treatment for atrichia pubis. *Horm Res.* 2001;56(3-4):134-139.
655. Kaplan SL, Grumbach MM. Clinical review 14: pathophysiology and treatment of sexual precocity. *J Clin Endocrinol Metab.* 1990;71:785-789.
656. Thamdrup E. *Precocious Sexual Development: A Clinical Study of 100 Patients.* Springfield, IL: Charles C Thomas; 1961.
657. Paul D, Conte FA, Grumbach MM, Kaplan SL. Long-term effect of gonadotropin-releasing hormone agonist therapy on final and near-final height in 26 children with true precocious puberty treated at a median age of less than 5 years. *J Clin Endocrinol Metab.* 1995;80:546-551.
658. National High Blood Pressure Education Program Working Group on High Blood Pressure in Children and Adolescents. The fourth report on the diagnosis, evaluation, and treatment of high blood pressure in children and adolescents. *Pediatrics.* 2004;114(2 Suppl 4th Report):555-576.
659. De Vries L, Kauschansky A, Shohat M, Phillip M. Familial central precocious puberty suggests autosomal dominant inheritance. *J Clin Endocrinol Metab.* 2004;89(4):1794-1800.
660. Teles MG, Bianco SD, Brito VN, et al. A GPR54-activating mutation in a patient with central precocious puberty. *N Engl J Med.* 2008;358(7):709-715.
661. Silveira LG, Noel SD, Silveira-Neto AP, et al. Mutations of the KISS1 gene in disorders of puberty. *J Clin Endocrinol Metab.* 2010;95(5):2276-2280.
662. Palmert MR, Malin HV, Boepple PA. Unsustained or slowly progressive puberty in young girls: initial presentation and long-term follow-up of 20 untreated patients [see comments]. *J Clin Endocrinol Metab.* 1999;84(2):415-423.
663. Codner E, Roman R. Premature thelarche from phenotype to genotype. *Pediatr Endocrinol Rev.* 2008;5(3):760-765.
664. Bizzarri C, Spadoni GL, Bottaro G, et al. The response to gonadotropin releasing hormone (GnRH) stimulation test does not predict the progression to true precocious puberty in girls with onset of premature thelarche in the first three years of life. *J Clin Endocrinol Metab.* 2014;99(2):433-439.
665. Willemsen RH, Elleri D, Williams RM, et al. Pros and cons of GnRHa treatment for early puberty in girls. *Nat Rev Endocrinol.* 2014;10(6):352-363.
666. Palmert MR, Boepple PA. Variation in the timing of puberty: clinical spectrum and genetic investigation. *J Clin Endocrinol Metab.* 2001;86(6):2364-2368.
667. Lazar L, Meyerovitch J, de Vries L, et al. Treated and untreated women with idiopathic precocious puberty: long-term follow-up and reproductive outcome between the third and fifth decades. *Clin Endocrinol (Oxf).* 2014;80(4):570-576.
668. Armstrong GT, Whitton JA, Gajjar A, et al. Abnormal timing of menarche in survivors of central nervous system tumors: A report from the Childhood Cancer Survivor Study. *Cancer.* 2009;115(11):2562-2570.
669. Soriano-Guillen L, Corripio R, Labarta JI, et al. Central precocious puberty in children living in Spain: incidence, prevalence, and influence of adoption and immigration. *J Clin Endocrinol Metab.* 2010;95(9):4305-4313.
670. Erkula G, Jones KB, Sponseller PD, et al. Growth and maturation in Marfan syndrome. *Am J Med Genet.* 2002;109(2):100-115.
671. Sadeghi-Nejad A, Kaplan SL, Grumbach MM. The effect of medroxyprogesterone acetate on adrenocortical function in children with precocious puberty. *J Pediatr.* 1971;78:616-624.
672. Knobil E, Plant TM, Wildt L, et al. Control of the rhesus monkey menstrual cycle: permissive role of the hypothalamic gonadotropin-releasing hormone. *Science.* 1980;207:1371-1373.
673. Chan YM, Fenoglio-Simeone KA, Paraschos S, et al. Central precocious puberty due to hypothalamic hamartomas correlates with anatomic features but not with expression of GnRH, TGFalpha, or KISS1. *Horm Res Paediatr.* 2010;73(5):312-319.
674. Jung H, Parent AS, Ojeda SR. Hypothalamic hamartoma: a paradigm/model for studying the onset of puberty. *Endocr Dev.* 2005;8:81-93.
675. Styne DM, Harris DA, Egli CA, et al. Treatment of true precocious puberty with a potent luteinizing hormone-releasing factor agonist: effect on growth, sexual maturation, pelvic sonography, and the hypothalamic-pituitary-gonadal axis. *J Clin Endocrinol Metab.* 1985;61(1):142-151.
676. Jung H, Carmel P, Schwartz MS, et al. Some hypothalamic hamartomas contain transforming growth factor α, a puberty-inducing growth factor, not luteinizing hormone releasing hormone neurons. *J Clin Endocrinol Metab.* 1999;84:4695-4701.
677. Pescovitz OH, Comite F, Hench K, et al. The NIH experience with precocious puberty: diagnostic subgroups and response to short-term luteinizing hormone releasing hormone analogue therapy. *J Pediatr.* 1986;108:47-54.
678. Rosenfeld JV, Harvey AS, Wrennall J, et al. Transcallosal resection of hypothalamic hamartomas, with control of seizures, in children with gelastic epilepsy. *Neurosurgery.* 2001;48(1):108-118.

679. Brandberg G, Raininko R, Eeg-Olofsson O. Hypothalamic hamartoma with gelastic seizures in Swedish children and adolescents. *Eur J Paediatr Neurol.* 2004;8(1):35-44.

680. Fohlen M, Lellouch A, Delalande O. Hypothalamic hamartoma with refractory epilepsy: surgical procedures and results in 18 patients. *Epileptic Disord.* 2003;5(4):267-273.

681. Barajas MA, Ramirez-Guzman MG, Rodriguez-Vazquez C, et al. Gamma knife surgery for hypothalamic hamartomas accompanied by medically intractable epilepsy and precocious puberty: experience in Mexico. *J Neurosurg.* 2005;102(Suppl):53-55.

682. Freeman JL, Zacharin M, Rosenfeld JV, Harvey AS. The endocrinology of hypothalamic hamartoma surgery for intractable epilepsy. *Epileptic Disord.* 2003;5(4):239-247.

683. Mashour GA, Driever PH, Hartmann M, et al. Circulating growth factor levels are associated with tumorigenesis in neurofibromatosis type 1. *Clin Cancer Res.* 2004;10(17):5677-5683.

684. Neurofibromatosis. Conference statement. National Institutes of Health Consensus Development Conference. *Arch Neurol.* 1988;45(5):575-578.

685. Boulanger JM, Larbrisseau A. Neurofibromatosis type 1 in a pediatric population: Ste-Justine's experience. *Can J Neurol Sci.* 2005;32(2):225-231.

686. Clark SJ, Van Dop C, Conte FA, et al. Reversible true precocious puberty secondary to a congenital arachnoid cyst. *Am J Dis Child.* 1988;142:255-256.

687. Teilmann G, Petersen JH, Gormsen M, et al. Early puberty in internationally adopted girls: hormonal and clinical markers of puberty in 276 girls examined biannually over two years. *Horm Res.* 2009;72(4):236-246.

688. Lee PA, Klein K, Mauras N, et al. Efficacy and safety of leuprolide acetate 3-month depot 11.25 milligrams or 30 milligrams for the treatment of central precocious puberty. *J Clin Endocrinol Metab.* 2012;97(5):1572-1580.

689. Lewis KA, Goldyn AK, West KW, Eugster EA. A single histrelin implant is effective for 2 years for treatment of central precocious puberty. *J Pediatr.* 2013;163(4):1214-1216.

690. Boepple PA, Mansfield MJ, Wierman ME, et al. Use of a potent, long acting agonist of gonadotropin-releasing hormone in the treatment of precocious puberty. *Endocr Rev.* 1986;7:24-33.

691. Mouat F, Hofman PL, Jefferies C, et al. Initial growth deceleration during GnRH analogue therapy for precocious puberty. *Clin Endocrinol (Oxf).* 2009;70(5):751-756.

692. Sklar CA, Rothenberg S, Blumberg D, et al. Suppression of the pituitary-gonadal axis in children with central precocious puberty: effects on growth, growth hormone, insulin-like growth factor-I, and prolactin secretion. *J Clin Endocrinol Metab.* 1991;73:734-738.

693. Pasquino AM, Pucarelli I, Accardo F, et al. Long-term observation of 87 girls with idiopathic central precocious puberty treated with gonadotropin-releasing hormone analogs: impact on adult height, body mass index, bone mineral content, and reproductive function. *J Clin Endocrinol Metab.* 2008;93(1):190-195.

694. Tanaka T, Niimi H, Matsuo N, et al. Results of long-term follow-up after treatment of central precocious puberty with leuprorelin acetate: evaluation of effectiveness of treatment and recovery of gonadal function. The TAP-144-SR Japanese Study Group on Central Precocious Puberty. *J Clin Endocrinol Metab.* 2005;90(3):1371-1376.

695. Liu G, Duranteau L, Carel JC, et al. Leydig-cell tumors caused by an activating mutation of the gene encoding the luteinizing hormone receptor [see comments]. *N Engl J Med.* 1999;341(23):1731-1736.

696. Wu MH, Lin SJ, Wu LH, et al. Clinical suppression of precocious puberty with cetrorelix after failed treatment with GnRH agonist in a girl with gonadotrophin-independent precocious puberty. *Reprod Biomed Online.* 2005;11(1):18-21.

697. Arrigo T, De Luca F, Antoniazzi F, et al. Reduction of baseline body mass index under gonadotropin-suppressive therapy in girls with idiopathic precocious puberty. *Eur J Endocrinol.* 2004;150(4):533-537.

698. Verrotti A, Basciani F, Trotta D, et al. Serum leptin levels in girls with precocious puberty. *Diabetes NutrMetab.* 2003;16(2):125-129.

699. Lewis KA, Eugster EA. Random luteinizing hormone often remains pubertal in children treated with the histrelin implant for central precocious puberty. *J Pediatr.* 2013;162(3):562-565.

700. Feuillan PP, Jones JV, Barnes KM, et al. Boys with precocious puberty due to hypothalamic hamartoma: reproductive axis after discontinuation of gonadotropin-releasing hormone analog therapy. *J Clin Endocrinol Metab.* 2000;85(11):4036-4038.

701. Heger S, Muller M, Ranke M, et al. Long-term GnRH agonist treatment for female central precocious puberty does not impair reproductive function. *Mol Cell Endocrinol.* 2006;254-255:217-220.

702. Franceschi R, Gaudino R, Marcolongo A, et al. Prevalence of polycystic ovary syndrome in young women who had idiopathic central precocious puberty. *Fertil Steril.* 2010;93(4):1185-1191.

703. Cheng S, Volgyi E, Tylavsky FA, et al. Trait-specific tracking and determinants of body composition: a 7-year follow-up study of pubertal growth in girls. *BMC Med.* 2009;7:5.

704. van Puijenbroek E, Verhoef E, de Graaf L. Slipped capital femoral epiphyses associated with the withdrawal of a gonadotrophin releasing hormone. *BMJ.* 2004;328(7452):1353.

705. van der Hoef M, Niggli FK, Willi UV, Huisman TA. Solitary infantile choriocarcinoma of the liver: MRI findings. *Pediatr Radiol.* 2004;34(10):820-823.

706. Blohm ME, Gobel U. Unexplained anaemia and failure to thrive as initial symptoms of infantile choriocarcinoma: a review. *Eur J Pediatr.* 2004;163(1):1-6.

707. Starzyk J, Starzyk B, Bartnik-Mikuta A, et al. Gonadotropin releasing hormone-independent precocious puberty in a 5-year-old girl with suprasellar germ cell tumor secreting beta-hCG and alpha-fetoprotein. *J Pediatr Endocrinol Metab.* 2001;14(6):789-796.

708. Shinoda J, Sakai N, Yano H, et al. Prognostic factors and therapeutic problems of primary intracranial choriocarcinoma/germ-cell tumors with high levels of HCG. *J Neurooncol.* 2004;66(1-2):225-240.

709. Dickerman RD, Stevens QE, Steide JA, Schneider SJ. Precocious puberty associated with a pineal cyst: is it disinhibition of the hypothalamic-pituitary axis? *Neuro Endocrinol Lett.* 2004;25(3):173-175.

710. Ambrosi B, Bassetti M, Ferrario R, et al. Precocious puberty in a boy with a PRL-, LH- and FSH-secreting pituitary tumour: hormonal and immunocytochemical studies. *Acta Endocrinol (Copenh).* 1990;122:569-576.

711. Speiser PW, Azziz R, Baskin LS, et al. Congenital adrenal hyperplasia due to steroid 21-hydroxylase deficiency: an Endocrine Society clinical practice guideline. *J Clin Endocrinol Metab.* 2010;95(9):4133-4160.

712. Auchus RJ, Miller WL. Congenital adrenal hyperplasia—more dogma bites the dust. *J Clin Endocrinol Metab.* 2012;97(3):772-775.

713. Kamrath C, Hochberg Z, Hartmann MF, et al. Increased activation of the alternative "backdoor" pathway in patients with 21-hydroxylase deficiency: evidence from urinary steroid hormone analysis. *J Clin Endocrinol Metab.* 2012;97(3):E367-E375.

714. Auchus RJ, Witchel SF, Leight KR, et al. Guidelines for the Development of Comprehensive Care Centers for Congenital Adrenal Hyperplasia: guidance from the CARES Foundation Initiative. *Int J Pediatr Endocrinol.* 2010;275213:2010.

715. Reisch N, Rottenkolber M, Greifenstein A, et al. Testicular adrenal rest tumors develop independently of long-term disease control: a longitudinal analysis of 50 adult men with congenital adrenal hyperplasia due to classic 21-hydroxylase deficiency. *J Clin Endocrinol Metab.* 2013;98(11):E1820-E1826.

716. Domenice S, Latronico AC, Brito VN, et al. Adrenocorticotropin-dependent precocious puberty of testicular origin in a boy with X-linked adrenal hypoplasia congenita due to a novel mutation in the DAX1 gene. *J Clin Endocrinol Metab.* 2001;86(9):4068-4071.

717. Argente J, Ozisik G, Pozo J, et al. A novel single base deletion at codon 434 (1301delT) of the DAX1 gene associated with prepubertal testis enlargement. *Mol Genet Metab.* 2003;78(1):79-81.

718. Petkovic V, Salemi S, Vassella E, et al. Leydig-cell tumour in children: variable clinical presentation, diagnostic features, follow-up and genetic analysis of four cases. *Horm Res.* 2007;67(2):89-95.

719. Leung AC, Kogan SJ. Focal lobular spermatogenesis and pubertal acceleration associated with ipsilateral Leydig cell hyperplasia. *Urology.* 2000;56(3):508-509.

720. Rosenthal SM, Grumbach MM, Kaplan SL. Gonadotropin-independent familial sexual precocity with premature Leydig and germinal cell maturation (familial testotoxicosis): effects of a potent luteinizing hormone-releasing factor agonist and medroxyprogesterone acetate therapy in four cases. *J Clin Endocrinol Metab.* 1983;57:571-579.

721. Gondos B, Egli CA, Rosenthal SM, Grumbach MM. Testicular changes in gonadotropin-independent familial male sexual precocity. Familial testotoxicosis. *Arch Pathol Lab Med.* 1985;109:990-995.

722. Wierman ME, Beardsworth DE, Mansfield MJ, et al. Puberty without gonadotropins. A unique mechanism of sexual development. *N Engl J Med.* 1985;312:65-72.

723. Huhtaniemi I. The Parkes lecture. Mutations of gonadotrophin and gonadotrophin receptor genes: what do they teach us about reproductive physiology? *J Reprod Fertil.* 2000;119(2):173-186.

724. Soriano-Guillen L, Mitchell V, Carel JC, et al. Activating mutations in the luteinizing hormone receptor gene: a human model of non-follicle-stimulating hormone-dependent inhibin production and germ cell maturation. *J Clin Endocrinol Metab.* 2006;91(8):3041-3047.

725. Egli CA, Rosenthal SM, Grumbach MM, et al. Pituitary gonadotropin-independent male-limited autosomal dominant sexual precocity in nine generations: familial testotoxicosis. *J Pediatr.* 1985;106:33-40.

726. Rosenthal IM, Refetoff S, Rich B, et al. Response to challenge with gonadotropin-releasing hormone agonist in a mother and her two sons with a constitutively activating mutation of the luteinizing hormone receptor—a clinical research center study. *J Clin Endocrinol Metab.* 1996;81:3802-3806.

727. Dufau ML. The luteinizing hormone receptor. *Annu Rev Physiol.* 1998;60:461-496.

728. Shenker A, Laue L, Kosugi S, et al. A constitutively activating mutation of the luteinizing hormone receptor in familial male precocious puberty. *Nature.* 1993;365:652-654.

729. Latronico AC, Segaloff DL. Naturally occurring mutations of the luteinizing-hormone receptor: lessons learned about reproductive physiology and G protein-coupled receptors. *Am J Hum Genet.* 1999; 65(4):949-958.

730. Kremer H, Martens JW, van Reen M, et al. A limited repertoire of mutations of the luteinizing hormone (LH) receptor gene in familial and sporadic patients with male LH-independent precocious puberty. *J Clin Endocrinol Metab.* 1999;84(3):1136-1140.

731. Laue L, Chan WY, Hsueh AJ, et al. Genetic heterogeneity of constitutively activating mutations of the human luteinizing hormone receptor in familial male-limited precocious puberty. *Proc Natl Acad Sci U S A.* 1995;92:1906-1910.

732. Wu SM, Leschek EW, Rennert OM, Chan WY. Luteinizing hormone receptor mutations in disorders of sexual development and cancer. *Front Biosci.* 2000;5:D343-D352.

733. Ulloa-Aguirre A, Reiter E, Bousfield G, et al. Constitutive activity in gonadotropin receptors. *Adv Pharmacol (San Diego, Calif.).* 2014;70:37-80.

734. Holland FJ, Fishman L, Bailey JD, Fazekas AT. Ketoconazole in the management of precocious puberty not responsive to LHRH-analogue therapy. *N Engl J Med.* 1985;312(16):1023-1028.

735. Soriano-Guillen L, Lahlou N, Chauvet G, et al. Adult height after ketoconazole treatment in patients with familial male-limited precocious puberty. *J Clin Endocrinol Metab.* 2005;90(1):147-151.

736. Laue L, Kenigsberg D, Pescovitz OH, et al. Treatment of familial male precocious puberty with spironolactone and testolactone. *N Engl J Med.* 1989;320(8):496-502.

737. Partsch CJ, Krone N, Riepe FG, et al. Long-term follow-up of spontaneous development in a boy with familial male precocious puberty. *Horm Res.* 2004;62(4):177-181.

738. Lenz AM, Shulman D, Eugster EA, et al. Bicalutamide and third-generation aromatase inhibitors in testotoxicosis. *Pediatrics.* 2010; 126(3):e728-e733.

739. Leschek EW, Chan WY, Diamond DA, et al. Nodular Leydig cell hyperplasia in a boy with familial male-limited precocious puberty. *J Pediatr.* 2001;138(6):949-951.

740. Andersson AM, Skakkebaek NE. Exposure to exogenous estrogens in food: possible impact on human development and health. *Eur J Endocrinol.* 1999;140(6):477-485.

741. Spiegel AM. Mutations in G proteins and G protein-coupled receptors in endocrine disease. *J Clin Endocrinol Metab.* 1996;81:2434-2442.

742. Nakamoto JM, Zimmerman D, Jones EA, et al. Concurrent hormone resistance (pseudohypoparathyroidism type Ia) and hormone independence (testotoxicosis) caused by a unique mutation in the G alpha s gene. *Biochem Mol Med.* 1996;58:18-24.

743. de Silva KS, Kanumakala S, Grover SR, et al. Ovarian lesions in children and adolescents—an 11-year review. *J Pediatr Endocrinol Metab.* 2004; 17(7):951-957.

744. Arisaka O, Hosaka A, Shimura N, et al. Effect of neonatal ovarian cysts on infant growth. *Clin Pediatr Endocrinol.* 1995;4:155-162.

745. Jenner MR, Kelch RP, Kaplan SL, Grumbach MM. Hormonal changes in puberty. IV. Plasma estradiol, LH, and FSH in prepubertal children, pubertal females, and in precocious puberty, premature thelarche, hypogonadism, and in a child with a feminizing ovarian tumor. *J Clin Endocrinol Metab.* 1972;34:521-530.

746. Butler MG, Najjar JL. Do some patients with fragile X syndrome have precocious puberty. *Am J Med Genet.* 1988;31:779-781.

747. Natarajan A, Wales JK, Marven SS, Wright NP. Precocious puberty secondary to massive ovarian oedema in a 6-month-old girl. *Eur J Endocrinol.* 2004;150(2):119-123.

748. Richards GE, Kaplan SL, Grumbach MM. Sexual precocity associated with functional follicular cysts, prepubertal gonadotropins and LRF response and fluctuating estrogen levels. *Pediatr Res.* 1977;11:431.

749. Feuillan PP, Jones J, Oerter KE, et al. Luteinizing hormone-releasing hormone (LHRH)-independent precocious puberty unresponsive to LHRH agonist therapy in two girls lacking the features of the McCune-Albright syndrome. *J Clin Endocrinol Metab.* 1991;73:1370-1373.

750. Hassan E, Creatsas G, Michalas S. Genital tumors during childhood and adolescence. A clinical and pathological study of 71 cases. *Clin Exp Obstet Gynecol.* 1999;26(1):20-21.

751. Dalgaard MD, Weinhold N, Edsgard D, et al. A genome-wide association study of men with symptoms of testicular dysgenesis syndrome and its network biology interpretation. *J Med Genet.* 2012;49(1):58-65.

752. Sarnacki S, Brisse H. Surgery of ovarian tumors in children. *Horm Res Paediatr.* 2011;75(3):220-224.

753. Schultz KA, Sencer SF, Messinger Y, et al. Pediatric ovarian tumors: a review of 67 cases. *Pediatr Blood Cancer.* 2005;44(2):167-173.

754. Shankar KR, Wakhlu A, Kokai GK, et al. Ovarian adenocarcinoma in premenarchal girls. *J Pediatr Surg.* 2001;36(3):511-515.

755. Diamanti-Kandarakis E, Bourguignon JP, Giudice LC, et al. Endocrine-disrupting chemicals: an Endocrine Society scientific statement. *Endocr Rev.* 2009;30(4):293-342.

756. Gladen BC, Klebanoff MA, Hediger ML, et al. Prenatal DDT exposure in relation to anthropometric and pubertal measures in adolescent males. *Environ Health Perspect.* 2004;112(17):1761-1767.

757. Pectasides D, Pectasides E, Psyrri A. Granulosa cell tumor of the ovary. *Cancer Treat Rev.* 2008;34(1):1-12.

758. Geerts I, Vergote I, Neven P, Billen J. The role of inhibins B and anti-mullerian hormone for diagnosis and follow-up of granulosa cell tumors. *Int J Gynecol Cancer.* 2009;19(5):847-855.

759. Cecchetto G, Ferrari A, Bernini G, et al. Sex cord stromal tumors of the ovary in children: a clinicopathological report from the Italian TREP project. *Pediatr Blood Cancer.* 2011;56(7):1062-1067.

760. Abed AA, Gunther K, Kraus C, et al. Mutation screening at the RNA level of the STK11/LKB1 gene in Peutz-Jeghers syndrome reveals complex splicing abnormalities and a novel mRNA isoform (STK11 c.597598insIVS4). *Hum Mutat.* 2001;18(5):397-410.

761. Zumkeller W, Krause U, Holzhausen HJ, et al. Ovarian sex cord tumor with annular tubules associated with precocious puberty. *Med Pediatr Oncol.* 2000;35(2):144-146.

762. Phornphutkul C, Okubo T, Wu K, et al. Aromatase p450 expression in a feminizing adrenal adenoma presenting as isosexual precocious puberty. *J Clin Endocrinol Metab.* 2001;86(2):649-652.

763. Shenker A, Weinstein LS, Moran A, et al. Severe endocrine and non-endocrine manifestations of the McCune-Albright syndrome associated with activating mutations of stimulatory G protein Gs. *J Pediatr.* 1993;123:509-518.

764. Horvath A, Stratakis CA. Clinical and molecular genetics of acromegaly: MEN1, Carney complex, McCune-Albright syndrome, familial acromegaly and genetic defects in sporadic tumors. *Rev Endocr Metab Disord.* 2008;9(1):1-11.

765. Brown RJ, Kelly MH, Collins MT. Cushing syndrome in the McCune-Albright syndrome. *J Clin Endocrinol Metab.* 2010;95(4):1508-1515.

766. Dumitrescu CE, Collins MT. McCune-Albright syndrome. *Orphanet J Rare Dis.* 2008;3:12.

767. Paris F, Philibert P, Lumbroso S, et al. Isolated Cushing's syndrome: an unusual presentation of McCune-Albright syndrome in the neonatal period. *Horm Res.* 2009;72(5):315-319.

768. Lumbroso S, Paris F, Sultan C. Activating Gsalpha mutations: analysis of 113 patients with signs of McCune-Albright syndrome—a European Collaborative Study. *J Clin Endocrinol Metab.* 2004;89(5):2107-2113.

769. Mantovani G, Bondioni S, Lania AG, et al. Parental origin of Gsalpha mutations in the McCune-Albright syndrome and in isolated endocrine tumors. *J Clin Endocrinol Metab.* 2004;89(6):3007-3009.

770. Roman R, Johnson MC, Codner E, et al. Activating GNAS1 gene mutations in patients with premature thelarche. *J Pediatr.* 2004;145(2): 218-222.

771. Tavassoli FA, Norris HJ. Sertoli tumors of the ovary: a clinicopathologic study of 28 cases with ultrastructural observations. *Cancer.* 1980;46: 2282-2297.

772. De Sanctis C, Lala R, Matarazzo P, et al. McCune-Albright syndrome: a longitudinal clinical study of 32 patients. *J Pediatr Endocrinol Metab.* 1999;12(6):817-826.

773. Leet AI, Chebli C, Kushner H, et al. Fracture incidence in polyostotic fibrous dysplasia and the McCune-Albright syndrome. *J Bone Miner Res.* 2004;19(4):571-577.

774. Hannon TS, Noonan K, Steinmetz R, et al. Is McCune-Albright syndrome overlooked in subjects with fibrous dysplasia of bone? *J Pediatr.* 2003;142(5):532-538.

775. Salenave S, Boyce AM, Collins MT, Chanson P. Acromegaly and McCune-Albright syndrome. *J Clin Endocrinol Metab.* 2014;99(6): 1955-1969.

776. Eugster EA, Rubin SD, Reiter EO, et al. Tamoxifen treatment for precocious puberty in McCune-Albright syndrome: a multicenter trial. *J Pediatr.* 2003;143(1):60-66.

777. Boyce AM, Chong WH, Shawker TH, et al. Characterization and management of testicular pathology in McCune-Albright syndrome. *J Clin Endocrinol Metab.* 2012;97(9):E1782-E1790.

778. Coutant R, Lumbroso S, Rey R, et al. Macroorchidism due to autonomous hyperfunction of Sertoli cells and G(s)alpha gene mutation: an unusual expression of McCune-Albright syndrome in a prepubertal boy. *J Clin Endocrinol Metab.* 2001;86(4):1778-1781.

779. Wasniewska M, De Luca F, Bertelloni S, et al. Testicular microlithiasis: an unreported feature of McCune-Albright syndrome in males. *J Pediatr.* 2004;145(5):670-672.

780. Miller WL, Auchus RJ, Geller DH. The regulation of 17,20 lyase activity. *Steroids.* 1997;62:133-142.

781. Happle R. The McCune Albright syndrome: a lethal gene surviving by mosaicism. *Clin Genet.* 1986;29:321-324.

782. Chattopadhyay A, Kumar V, Marulaiah M. Polycystic ovaries, precocious puberty and acquired hypothyroidism: the Van Wyk and Grumbach syndrome. *J Pediatr Surg.* 2003;38(9):1390-1392.

783. Anasti JN, Flack MR, Froehlich J, et al. A potential novel mechanism for precocious puberty in juvenile hypothyroidism [see comments]. *J Clin Endocrinol Metab.* 1995;80:276-279.

784. Partsch CJ, Sippell WG. Pathogenesis and epidemiology of precocious puberty. Effects of exogenous oestrogens. *Hum Reprod Update.* 2001; 7(3):292-302.

785. Henley DV, Lipson N, Korach KS, Bloch CA. Prepubertal gynecomastia linked to lavender and tea tree oils. *N Engl J Med.* 2007;356(5):479-485.

786. Yu YM, Punyasavatsu N, Elder D, D'Ercole AJ. Sexual development in a two-year-old boy induced by topical exposure to testosterone. *Pediatrics.* 1999;104(2):e23.

787. Andersson AM, Skakkebaek NE. Exposure to exogenous estrogens in food: possible impact on human development and health. *Eur J Endocrinol.* 1999;140(6):477-485.

788. Larriuz-Serrano MC, Perez-Cardona CM, Ramos-Valencia G, Bourdony CJ. Natural history and incidence of premature thelarche in Puerto Rican girls aged 6 months to 8 years diagnosed between 1990 and 1995. *P R Health Sci J.* 2001;20(1):13-18.

789. Van Winter JT, Noller KL, Zimmerman D, Melton LJ 3rd. Natural history of premature thelarche in Olmsted County, Minnesota, 1940 to 1984. *J Pediatr.* 1990;116(2):278-280.

790. Blanck HM, Marcus M, Tolbert PE, et al. Age at menarche and Tanner stage in girls exposed in utero and postnatally to polybrominated biphenyl. *Epidemiology.* 2000;11(6):641-647.

791. Chen A, Chung E, DeFranco EA, et al. Serum PBDEs and age at menarche in adolescent girls: analysis of the National Health and Nutrition Examination Survey 2003-2004. *Environ Res.* 2011;111(6):831-837.

792. Massart F, Seppia P, Pardi D, et al. High incidence of central precocious puberty in a bounded geographic area of northwest Tuscany: an estrogen disrupter epidemic? *Gynecol Endocrinol.* 2005;20(2):92-98.

793. Mouritsen A, Frederiksen H, Sorensen K, et al. Urinary phthalates from 168 girls and boys measured twice a year during a 5-year period: associations with adrenal androgen levels and puberty. *J Clin Endocrinol Metab.* 2013;98(9):3755-3764.

794. Wolff MS, Britton JA, Russo JC. TCDD and puberty in girls. *Environ Health Perspect.* 2005;113(1):A17.

795. Rais-Bahrami K, Nunez S, Revenis ME, et al. Follow-up study of adolescents exposed to di(2-ethylhexyl) phthalate (DEHP) as neonates on extracorporeal membrane oxygenation (ECMO) support. *Environ Health Perspect.* 2004;112(13):1339-1340.

796. Denham M, Schell LM, Deane G, et al. Relationship of lead, mercury, mirex, dichlorodiphenyldichloroethylene, hexachlorobenzene, and polychlorinated biphenyls to timing of menarche among Akwesasne Mohawk girls. *Pediatrics.* 2005;115(2):e127-e134.

797. Wu T, Buck GM, Mendola P. Blood lead levels and sexual maturation in U.S. girls: the Third National Health and Nutrition Examination Survey, 1988-1994. *Environ Health Perspect.* 2003;111(5):737-741.

798. Hauser R, Sergeyev O, Korrick S, et al. Association of blood lead levels with onset of puberty in Russian boys. *Environ Health Perspect.* 2008; 116(7):976-980.

799. Hsu PC, Lai TJ, Guo NW, et al. Serum hormones in boys prenatally exposed to polychlorinated biphenyls and dibenzofurans. *J Toxicol Environ Health A.* 2005;68(17-18):1447-1456.

800. Buck Louis GM, Gray LE Jr, Marcus M, et al. Environmental factors and puberty timing: expert panel research needs. *Pediatrics.* 2008; 121(Suppl 3):S192-S207.

801. Maber M, Liversidge HM, Hector MP. Accuracy of age estimation of radiographic methods using developing teeth. *Forensic Sci Int.* 2006; 159(Suppl 1):S68-S73.

802. Badouraki M, Christoforidis A, Economou I, et al. Sonographic assessment of uterine and ovarian development in normal girls aged 1 to 12 years. *J Clin Ultrasound.* 2008;36(9):539-544.

803. Bridges NA, Cooke A, Healy MJ, et al. Ovaries in sexual precocity. *Clin Endocrinol (Oxf).* 1995;42:135-140.

804. Badouraki M, Christoforidis A, Economou I, et al. Evaluation of pelvic ultrasonography in the diagnosis and differentiation of various forms of sexual precocity in girls. *Ultrasound Obstet Gynecol.* 2008;32(6): 819-827.

805. Sathasivam A, Rosenberg HK, Shapiro S, et al. Pelvic ultrasonography in the evaluation of central precocious puberty: comparison with leuprolide stimulation test. *J Pediatr.* 2011;159(3):490-495.

806. Calcaterra V, Sampaolo P, Klersy C, et al. Utility of breast ultrasonography in the diagnostic work-up of precocious puberty and proposal of a prognostic index for identifying girls with rapidly progressive central precocious puberty. *Ultrasound Obstet Gynecol.* 2009;33(1): 85-91.

807. Ng SM, Kumar Y, Cody D, et al. Cranial MRI scans are indicated in all girls with central precocious puberty. *Arch Dis Child.* 2003;88(5): 414-418.

808. Wong AP, Pipitone J, Park MT, et al. Estimating volumes of the pituitary gland from T1-weighted magnetic-resonance images: effects of age, puberty, testosterone, and estradiol. *Neuroimage.* 2014;94: 216-221.

809. Aquilina K, Boop FA. Nonneoplastic enlargement of the pituitary gland in children. *J Neurosurg Pediatr.* 2011;7(5):510-515.

810. Cacciari E, Zucchini S, Ambrosetto P, et al. Empty sella in children and adolescents with possible hypothalamic-pituitary disorders. *J Clin Endocrinol Metab.* 1994;78:767-771.

811. Segal DG, DiMeglio LA, Ryder KW, et al. Assay interference leading to misdiagnosis of central precocious puberty. *Endocrine.* 2003;20(3): 195-199.

812. Wasniewska M, Raiola G, Galati MC, et al. Non-classical 21-hydroxylase deficiency in boys with prepubertal or pubertal gynecomastia. *Eur J Pediatr.* 2008;167(9):1083-1084.

813. Shozu M, Sebastian S, Takayama K, et al. Estrogen excess associated with novel gain-of-function mutations affecting the aromatase gene. *N Engl J Med.* 2003;348(19):1855-1865.

814. Binder G, Iliev DI, Dufke A, et al. Dominant transmission of prepubertal gynecomastia due to serum estrone excess: hormonal, biochemical, and genetic analysis in a large kindred. *J Clin Endocrinol Metab.* 2005; 90(1):484-492.

815. Tiulpakov A, Kalintchenko N, Semitcheva T, et al. A potential rearrangement between CYP19 and TRPM7 genes on chromosome 15q21.2 as a cause of aromatase excess syndrome. *J Clin Endocrinol Metab.* 2005;90(7):4184-4190.

816. Fukami M, Tsuchiya T, Vollbach H, et al. Genomic basis of aromatase excess syndrome: recombination- and replication-mediated rearrangements leading to CYP19A1 overexpression. *J Clin Endocrinol Metab.* 2013;98(12):E2013-E2021.

817. Coen P, Kulin H, Ballantine T, et al. An aromatase-producing sex-cord tumor resulting in prepubertal gynecomastia. *N Engl J Med.* 1991; 324(5):317-322.

818. Berensztein E, Belgorosky A, de Davila MT, Rivarola MA. Testicular steroid biosynthesis in a boy with a large cell calcifying Sertoli cell tumor producing prepubertal gynecomastia. *Steroids.* 1995;60: 220-225.

819. Harigopal M, Murray MP, Rosen PP, Shin SJ. Prepubertal gynecomastia with lobular differentiation. *Breast J.* 2005;11(1):48-51.

820. Charmandari E, Kino T, Chrousos GP. Primary generalized familial and sporadic glucocorticoid resistance (Chrousos syndrome) and hypersensitivity. *Endocr Dev.* 2013;24:67-85.

821. Heravi-Moussavi A, Anglesio MS, Cheng SW, et al. Recurrent somatic DICER1 mutations in nonepithelial ovarian cancers. *N Engl J Med.* 2012;366(3):234-242.

822. Volta C, Bernasconi S, Cisternino M, et al. Isolated premature thelarche and thelarche variant: clinical and auxological follow-up of 119 girls. *J Endocrinol Invest.* 1998;21(3):180-183.

823. de Vries L, Guz-Mark A, Lazar L, et al. Premature thelarche: age at presentation affects clinical course but not clinical characteristics or risk to progress to precocious puberty. *J Pediatr.* 2010;156(3):466-471.

824. Klein KO, Mericq V, Brown-Dawson JM, et al. Estrogen levels in girls with premature thelarche compared with normal prepubertal girls as determined by an ultrasensitive recombinant cell bioassay. *J Pediatr.* 1999;134(2):190-192.

825. Collett-Solberg PR, Grumbach MM. A simplified procedure for evaluating estrogenic effects and the sex chromatin pattern in exfoliated cells in urine: studies in premature thelarche and gynecomastia of adolescence. *J Pediatr.* 1965;66:883-890.

826. Pescovitz OH, Hench KD, Barnes KM, et al. Premature thelarche and central precocious puberty: the relationship between clinical presentation and the gonadotropin response to luteinizing hormone-releasing hormone. *J Clin Endocrinol Metab.* 1988;67:474-479.

827. Saggese G, Ghirri P, Del Vecchio A, et al. Gonadotropin pulsatile secretion in girls with premature menarche. *Horm Res.* 1990;33:5-10.

828. Williams RM, Ward CE, Hughes IA. Premature adrenarche. *Arch Dis Child.* 2012;97(3):250-254.

829. Lee PA, Migeon CJ, Bias WB, et al. Familial hypersecretion of adrenal androgens transmitted as a dominant, non-HLA linked trait. *Obstet Gynecol.* 1987;69(2):259-264.

830. Ibanez L, DiMartino-Nardi J, Potau N, Saenger P. Premature adrenarche—normal variant or forerunner of adult disease? *Endocr Rev.* 2000;21(6):671-696.

831. Ibanez L, Ong KK, Lopez-Bermejo A, et al. Hyperinsulinaemic androgen excess in adolescent girls. *Nat Rev Endocrinol.* 2014;10(8): 499-508.

832. Utriainen P, Voutilainen R, Jaaskelainen J. Girls with premature adrenarche have accelerated early childhood growth. *J Pediatr.* 2009;154(6): 882-887.

833. New MI, Abraham M, Gonzalez B, et al. Genotype-phenotype correlation in 1,507 families with congenital adrenal hyperplasia owing to 21-hydroxylase deficiency. *Proc Natl Acad Sci U S A.* 2013;110(7): 2611-2616.

834. Carbunaru G, Prasad P, Scoccia B, et al. The hormonal phenotype of nonclassic 3 beta-hydroxysteroid dehydrogenase (HSD3B) deficiency in hyperandrogenic females is associated with insulin-resistant polycystic ovary syndrome and is not a variant of inherited HSD3B2 deficiency. *J Clin Endocrinol Metab.* 2004;89(2):783-794.

835. Deplewski D, Rosenfield RL. Role of hormones in pilosebaceous unit development. *Endocr Rev.* 2000;21(4):363-392.

836. Ibanez L, Ong K, de Zegher F, et al. Fat distribution in non-obese girls with and without precocious pubarche: central adiposity related to insulinaemia and androgenaemia from prepuberty to postmenarche. *Clin Endocrinol (Oxf).* 2003;58(3):372-379.

837. Welt CK, Carmina E. Clinical review: lifecycle of polycystic ovary syndrome (PCOS): from in utero to menopause. *J Clin Endocrinol Metab.* 2013;98(12):4629-4638.

838. Ferriman D, Gallwey JD. Clinical assessment of body hair growth in women. *J Clin Endocrinol Metab.* 1961;21:1440-1447.

839. Dewailly D. Ultrasound definition of polycystic ovarian morphology: good news and bad news. *Fertil Steril.* 2014;101(1):49-50.

840. Dewailly D, Andersen CY, Balen A, et al. The physiology and clinical utility of anti-mullerian hormone in women. *Hum Reprod Update.* 2014;20(3):370-385.

841. Ibanez L, de Zegher F. Puberty and prenatal growth. *Mol Cell Endocrinol.* 2006;254-255:22-25.

842. Ong KK, Potau N, Petry CJ, et al. Opposing influences of prenatal and postnatal weight gain on adrenarche in normal boys and girls. *J Clin Endocrinol Metab.* 2004;89(6):2647-2651.

843. Boonstra VH, Mulder PG, De Jong FH, Hokken-Koelega AC. Serum dehydroepiandrosterone sulfate levels and pubarche in short children born small for gestational age before and during growth hormone treatment. *J Clin Endocrinol Metab.* 2004;89(2):712-717.

844. Vuguin P, Grinstein G, Freeman K, et al. Prediction models for insulin resistance in girls with premature adrenarche. The premature adrenarche insulin resistance score: PAIR score. *Horm Res.* 2006;65(4):185-191.

845. Lass N, Kleber M, Winkel K, et al. Effect of lifestyle intervention on features of polycystic ovarian syndrome, metabolic syndrome, and intima-media thickness in obese adolescent girls. *J Clin Endocrinol Metab.* 2011;96(11):3533-3540.

846. Gordon CM, Pitts SA. Approach to the adolescent requesting contraception. *J Clin Endocrinol Metab.* 2012;97(1):9-15.

847. de Zegher F, Ibanez L. Therapy: low-dose flutamide for hirsutism: into the limelight, at last. *Nat Rev Endocrinol.* 2010;6(8):421-422.

848. Glintborg D, Altinok ML, Mumm H, et al. Body composition is improved during 12 months' treatment with metformin alone or combined with oral contraceptives compared with treatment with oral contraceptives in polycystic ovary syndrome. *J Clin Endocrinol Metab.* 2014;99(7):2584-2591.

849. Biro FM, Lucky AW, Huster GA, Morrison JA. Hormonal studies and physical maturation in adolescent gynecomastia. *J Pediatr.* 1990;116:450-455.

850. Moore DC, Schlaepfer LV, Punier L, et al. Hormonal changes during puberty: V. Transient pubertal gynecomastia: abnormal androgen-estrogen ratios. *J Clin Endocrinol Metab.* 1997;58(3):492-499.

851. Lawrence SE, Faught KA, Vethamuthu J, Lawson ML. Beneficial effects of raloxifene and tamoxifen in the treatment of pubertal gynecomastia. *J Pediatr.* 2004;145(1):71-76.

852. Mauras N, Bishop K, Merinbaum D, et al. Pharmacokinetics and pharmacodynamics of anastrozole in pubertal boys with recent-onset gynecomastia. *J Clin Endocrinol Metab.* 2009;94(8):2975-2978.

853. Nuzzi LC, Cerrato FE, Erickson CR, et al. Psychosocial impact of adolescent gynecomastia: a prospective case-control study. *Plast Reconstr Surg.* 2013;131(4):890-896.

854. Koshy JC, Goldberg JS, Wolfswinkel EM, et al. Breast cancer incidence in adolescent males undergoing subcutaneous mastectomy for gynecomastia: is pathologic examination justified? A retrospective and literature review. *Plast Reconstr Surg.* 2011;127(1):1-7.

855. Meschede D, Behre HM, Nieschlag E. Endocrine and spermatologic characteristics of 135 patients with bilateral megalotestis. *Andrologia.* 1995;27(4):207-212.

856. Lachiewicz AM, Dawson DV, Spiridigliozzi GA. Physical characteristics of young boys with fragile X syndrome: reasons for difficulties in making a diagnosis in young males. *Am J Med Genet.* 2000;92(4):229-236.

CHAPTER 26

Hormones and Athletic Performance

FABIO LANFRANCO • EZIO GHIGO • CHRISTIAN J. STRASBURGER

KEY POINTS

- Physical activity exerts an important influence on the endocrine system, modulating synthesis and secretion of several hormones. Almost every organ and system in the body are affected by physical activity and exercise, mainly through the endocrine and neuroendocrine systems.
- Mode, intensity, and duration of the exercise bout; age, gender, and fitness level of the individual; and environmental and psychological factors may affect the endocrine response to physical activity.
- Several hormones are able to influence physical performance and body composition. Thus, a bidirectional interrelationship between exercise and hormones exists.
- In the past decades, hormone abuse has become a widespread habit among professional and recreational athletes. A substantial part of this chapter is devoted to the effects of exogenous hormones on physical performance. Anabolic steroids, growth hormone (GH) and GH secretagogues, insulin-like growth factor 1 (IGF-1), insulin, erythropoietin (EPO), and glucocorticosteroid (GC) properties, along with their use and misuse in sports, are widely described. Specific methods to detect hormone abuse are presented and discussed.
- The purpose of this chapter is to provide all professionals involved in sports medicine and endocrinology a state-of-the-art overview of the complex interactions between physical activity and the endocrine system and to focus on hormone abuse in sports at competitive and recreational levels, highlighting its negative consequences for long-term health.

EFFECT OF ATHLETIC PERFORMANCE ON HORMONAL SYSTEMS

Catecholamines

Norepinephrine and epinephrine are closely coupled in their actions and respond rapidly to exercise in order to redistribute blood flow to meet metabolic demands. Norepinephrine increases from a resting level of 1.2 to 3.0 nmol/L to levels as high as 12.0 nmol/L at maximal exercise. Resting concentrations of epinephrine are 380 to 655 pmol/L. With maximal exercise, epinephrine concentrations can increase to up to 3300 pmol/L. Both of these hormones progressively increase as workload increases.[1] Following exercise, plasma levels of cathecolamines return to resting levels in a matter of minutes.

Mild exercise produces little or no response in catecholamines, whereas at moderate exercise levels norepinephrine significantly increases with minimal change in circulating epinephrine. At intense or prolonged exercise levels both hormones increase significantly. Acute, short-duration maximal exercise can significantly increase norepinephrine and epinephrine levels. This rapid response suggests that the levels are primarily regulated via neural release mediated by activation of the sympathetic nervous system. Spillover from active muscle during exercise appears to be the primary contributor, but the kidneys are a possible other source.[1] Moreover, alteration in the ratio of norepinephrine to epinephrine, with a greater increase in the release of epinephrine from the adrenal medulla during exercise, suggests a possible hypothalamic mediation in the response to exercise.

Graded exercise produces a lower catecholamine response than continuous prolonged exercise. The responses are directly related to workload and oxygen uptake and are greater with small muscle groups than with large muscle groups.

Many studies report a higher adrenaline response to exercise in endurance-trained compared with untrained subjects in response to intense exercise at the same relative intensity as all-out exercise. This higher capacity to secrete adrenaline was observed in response to both physical exercise and other stimuli such as hypoglycemia and hypoxia.[2] For some authors, this phenomenon can partly explain the higher physical performance observed in trained compared with untrained subjects. More recently, these findings have also been reported in anaerobic-trained subjects in response to supramaximal exercise. Interestingly, studies in women remain scarce; the results are more conflicting than those in men, and the physical training type (aerobic or anaerobic) effects on catecholamine response remain to be specified.[2]

Epinephrine and norepinephrine are responsible for many adaptations both at rest and during exercise. These changes include cardiovascular and respiratory adjustments and substrate mobilization and use.[2] Redistribution of circulation to working muscles and to the skin for heat loss and sweating is mediated through changes in catecholamines directly or indirectly via other intermediate hormones. Moreover, catecholamines may mediate mental performance improvement that occurs through exercise.[2]

Fluid Homeostasis: Vasopressin and the Renin-Angiotensin-Aldosterone System

During physical exercise there is a considerable loss of water and electrolytes in sweat, which is necessary to maintain body temperature by dissipating heat generated from muscle use. The rate of fluid loss due to sweating may be as high as 1500 mL/hour. The loss of fluids is replaced by the subsequent ingestion of liquids, which is modulated by thirst. The replacement of electrolytes is the result of the normal intake of food. Renal function is the major mechanism by which electrolytes are conserved following exercise.

The maintenance of fluid and electrolyte homeostasis during physical exercise depends on the action of arginine vasopressin (AVP), natriuretic peptides, the renin-angiotensin-aldosterone (RAA) axis, and catecholamines. These hormonal systems are modified in response to exercise, with different patterns depending on the amount of relative work performed, the duration of exercise, and the training status. Other factors influencing the response of hormones to exercise include the mode of exercise, environmental factors, age and gender of the subjects, and several medical/physiologic conditions.[1] Hormones involved in the regulation of fluid and electrolyte homeostasis show a relatively consistent response among individuals.

AVP concentrations increase during exercise up to 24 pg/mL, and elevated levels persist for over 60 minutes following maximal exercise. The stimulus for the increase in AVP during exercise is the increase in plasma osmolality and reduction in blood volume.[3] Animal experiments have demonstrated an increase in activation of hypothalamic neurons, indicating an increased vasopressin content and performance above the anaerobic threshold.[4] Thus, the response of vasopressin appears to be associated with the onset of anaerobic metabolism, which is also related to increases in stress hormones such as cortisol and adrenocorticotropic hormone (ACTH).

Atrial natriuretic peptide (ANP) and brain natriuretic peptide (BNP), which may be altered by exercise,[1] also elicit a natriuretic effect. ANP is increased with exercise in a linear response. In case of prolonged exercise, ANP undergoes an initial increase, a subsequent fall, and then a re-elevation of levels, persisting until completion of the exercise.[1] The increase in ANP with exercise appears to be related to stretch of the atrium due to volume changes, neurologic inputs, and sodium intake.[1] BNP response to exercise is modulated by sodium intake and by the hydration status.[1] BNP is not consistently altered in normal subjects in response to acute exercise, whereas it increases with long-duration exercise such as a 100-km ultramarathon.[1]

The RAA system responds to exercise with a significant increase of activity. In fact, increased values of plasma renin activity (PRA) are reported following maximal exercise.[1] The increase in PRA occurs at submaximal workloads of more than 60% to 70%. With the increase in PRA during exercise, there is a concomitant increase in angiotensin II (A-II), which partially mediates the increase in circulating aldosterone concentrations up to 250 to 3300 pmol/L. Elevated levels of aldosterone may persist for days after the end of exercise, depending on water and sodium intake. The primary activator of the RAA system during exercise is

the sympathetic nervous system. Stimulation of the release of renin is modulated by changes in renal sympathetic nerve activity resulting in an increase in local norepinephrine. The increase in aldosterone with exercise is assumed to be mediated by the increase in A-II in response to activation of the RAA system. However, inhibition of angiotensin-converting enzyme does not attenuate the increase in aldosterone with maximal exercise in healthy subjects.[5] Other factors involved in the activation of aldosterone production include sodium intake, potassium balance, and levels of ACTH. Elevated levels of aldosterone may persist for days after the end of exercise, depending on water and sodium intake.[1] The persistent increase of aldosterone long after the end of exercise may be associated with reductions in plasma osmolality and sodium concentrations due to ingestion of water to replace total body water losses.[1] Thus, the interaction of a number of regulating factors is involved in mediating the response of aldosterone.

Hypothalamic-Pituitary-Adrenal Axis
Glucocorticoids

Since the pioneering studies of Davies and Few, it has been known that exercise of an appropriate intensity is a potent stimulus for cortisol secretion.[6] Glucocorticoids exert many beneficial effects in exercising humans, increasing the availability of metabolic substrates for the need of energy of muscles, maintaining normal vascular integrity and responsiveness, and protecting the organism from an overreaction of the immune system in the face of exercise-induced muscle damage.[7]

During acute exercise, the hypothalamic-pituitary-adrenal (HPA) axis responds to numerous stimuli demonstrating the regulatory and integrative functions of the HPA axis: neuronal homeostatic signals (chemoreceptor, baroreceptor, and osmoreceptor stimulation), circulating homeostatic signals (glucose, leptin, atrial natriuretic petide), and inflammatory signals such as interleukin 1 (IL-1), IL-6, and tumor necrosis factor-α (TNF-α).[8,9]

A number of individual and environmental factors modulate the response of the HPA axis to physical activity. The response of the HPA axis to exercise is independent of age and gender[10,11] and depends on the duration and the type of the physical activity.[9]

Cortisol response is dependent on the relative exercise workload for both aerobic and strength exercise, and the rise of plasma cortisol is associated with an increase in ACTH concentration.[12] Moderate- to high-intensity exercise (60% and 80% of maximal oxygen consumption [Vo_2max]) has been shown to provoke increases in circulating cortisol levels, which seemed due to a combination of hemoconcentration and HPA axis stimulus (ACTH). In contrast, low-intensity exercise (40%) did not result in significant increases in cortisol levels.[13]

In contrast to sustained aerobic activity, intermittent exercise of varying intensities, such as matchplay tennis, does not appear to induce activation of the HPA axis.[14] Isometric exercise induces activation of the HPA axis, which is intensity dependent.[15] Anaerobic exercise induces a greater increase in plasma cortisol than aerobic exercise of the same total work output.[16]

A number of other factors modify the response of the HPA axis to physical activity. The cortisol response to exercise is modulated by hypohydration, meals, and time of day. Independently of external thermal stress, hypohydration (up to 4.8% body mass loss) greatly amplifies the exercise-induced responses of cortisol to exercise. This enhancement probably results from an increased core temperature and cardiovascular demand concurrent with decreased plasma volume.[17] Meals also regulate cortisol release in humans. Exercise performed immediately after food ingestion results in a blunted cortisol response to the exercise stimulus. Finally, the cortisol response to exercise is significantly modulated by time of day. In fact, the incremental response of cortisol to exercise is enhanced during the evening compared to morning exercise.[18]

Endurance training has been compared with chronic stress in humans. When the HPA axis is repeatedly challenged by exercise, humans demonstrate modifications in the activity of the HPA axis, suggesting an adapting process to endurance training. Several studies have shown that in endurance-trained subjects, the HPA axis activity in resting conditions is similar to that of healthy sedentary subjects.[18,19] However, when the HPA axis is challenged, endurance-trained subjects demonstrate a decreased pituitary sensitivity to the negative feedback of glucocorticoids that explains their capacity to successfully achieve a second bout of exercise after a short rest period.[18] Different mechanisms can be involved in this adaptation. At the central nervous system level, neuropeptides and corticosteroid receptors (glucocorticoid receptors, mineralocorticoid receptors) in the brain and anterior pituitary play a major role in the regulation of circulating cortisol levels. At the peripheral level, tissue sensitivity to glucocorticoids may also be different between endurance-trained and sedentary subjects.[20] Altogether, these adaptation processes are finalized to protect the body from the severe metabolic and immune consequences of increased cortisol levels.

Mineralocorticoids

The RAA system is closely coupled and responds to exercise. PRA values increase following maximal exercise. Progressively higher increases in aldosterone levels have been observed with increasing degrees of exertion. Elevated levels of aldosterone may persist for days after the end of exercise, depending on water and sodium intake.[1] The interaction of a number of regulating factors is involved in mediating the response of aldosterone. These regulators include the sympathetic nervous system, renin activity, A-II, sodium intake, potassium balance, blood volume reductions, and levels of ACTH.[1]

Endorphins

Exercise is able to influence the release of β-endorphins depending on intensity and duration of the physical activity. If a threshold intensity is exceeded, endogenous opiate levels start to increase. Incremental graded exercise tests elevate β-endorphin levels 1.5- to 7-fold.[21] Several studies suggest that circulating β-endorphins can increase with an appropriate minimal intensity of exercise (>60% $\dot{V}o_2$max), but this is not always the case.[21] Instead of a critical intensity related to aerobic capacity, other studies related the increase in β-endorphins to the lactate threshold.[21] Moreover, other factors such as diet, training status, and immune function can influence the β-endorphin response.

Very little is known about the influence of training status on the release of β-endorphins and study results are often inconsistent. Interestingly, the psychological and physiologic stress related to competitive practice has been proposed to stimulate the secretion of endorphins in order to counter the negative effects of competitive stress.[22] A physiologic purpose of endogenous opiate increase in athletes can be the modulation of pain and the improvement of mood.[23] Altogether, the action of endogenous opiates can be described as a rewarding system that causes the athlete to continue physical activity.

Hypothalamic-Pituitary-Gonadal Axis
Male Gonadal Axis

The effects of physical activity on the male gonadal axis vary with the intensity and duration of the activity, the fitness level of the individual, and his nutritional-metabolic status. Relatively short, intense exercise usually increases serum testosterone levels but more prolonged exercise usually decreases them.[24-26] Increased serum testosterone levels have been reported during relatively strenuous free and treadmill running, weight training, rock climbing, and ergometer cycling.[27]

The testosterone response increases with increased exercise load.[28] Similar workloads produce similar responses, regardless of whether the load is aerobic or anaerobic.[16] Increased and decreased ambient temperature, altitude, and dehydration have no effect on testosterone response to intense exercise.[30] Acute exercise-induced testosterone increments are also seen in older men, despite their different hormonal milieu.[31]

The exercise-associated increment in circulating testosterone is considered not to be mediated by luteinizing hormone (LH), due to the inconsistent LH response and to the evidence that testosterone levels increase more quickly than LH in response to exercise. Possible mechanisms such as hemoconcentration, reduced clearance, and increased testosterone synthesis may be involved.[27] However, the timing of testosterone response differs from that of other circulating steroids (e.g., androstenedione and dehydroepiandrosterone [DHEA] increase simultaneously with cortisol), thus suggesting that specific testicular mechanisms are involved.[32] These mechanisms may include the activation of the sympathetic system, which stimulates testicular testosterone production during exercise via a direct neural pathway in some species.

In contrast to the short-term testosterone increment, a suppression of serum testosterone levels occurs during and subsequent to more prolonged exercise and to some extent in the hours following intense short-term exercise. The effects of endurance exercise training on the male reproductive system have been investigated beginning in the 1980s. Research in exercising men demonstrates the existence of a select group who, through chronic exposure to endurance exercise training, have developed alterations in their reproductive hormonal profile, meaning persistently low basal resting testosterone concentrations.[33] In particular, the majority of these men exhibits clinically "normal" testosterone concentrations, but these concentrations are at the low end of normal range or even reach subclinical status. The health consequences of such hormonal changes are increased risk of abnormal spermatogenesis, male infertility problems, and compromised bone mineralization.[33] The prevalence of such health problems seems low, but investigative studies examining this condition and its consequences are few in number.[33] The specific terminology used to refer to this condition has not been universally agreed upon. In 2005, Hackney and associates proposed the use of the phrase "the exercise-hypogonadal male" as a label for this condition.[34]

A variety of systems could influence the decrease of testosterone synthesis during and subsequent to prolonged exercise. Exercise-hypogonadal men frequently display a lack of significant elevation in basal LH corresponding with the reduced testosterone concentration, reflecting hypogonadotrophic-hypogonadism characteristics.[33] Moreover, exercise-hypogonadal men have been shown to have altered basal prolactin.[33] At either excessively low or high circulating levels, prolactin can result in suppression of testosterone levels in men.

Leptin and ghrelin levels, which may be influenced by physical exercise, have been suggested to be altered in exercise-hypogonadal men. Leptin is an adipocyte-released hormone associated in part with communicating to the hypothalamus satiety and energy reserve status.[35] It is also linked to reproductive function both in women and in men. Acute and chronic exercise can impact upon resting leptin concentrations, independent of changes in body adiposity.[36] However, to date no research studies have examined whether leptin concentrations are altered in exercise-hypogonadal men.

Ghrelin is another hormone associated with appetite regulation. Evidence from several experimental studies in animals and in humans suggests that ghrelin may function as a metabolic modulator of the gonadotropic axis, with predominant inhibitory effects in line with its role as a signal of energy deficit.[37,38] Acute and chronic exercise has been shown to influence ghrelin concentration levels.[39] However, no research has yet examined whether ghrelin levels in exercise-hypogonadal men are normal.

Another potential disruptive hormone to the gonadal axis is cortisol. Cumming and associates[40] have demonstrated that the direct infusion of cortisol in men results in concurrent declines in testosterone levels. However, in the hormonal profile studies reporting the existence of low testosterone in trained men, none has reported elevated resting cortisol levels.[27] Thus, at this time the role of cortisol in the changes found in the gonadal axis of trained men is in need of further study.

Female Gonadal Axis

The endocrine equilibrium that regulates the reproductive function in women can be affected by physical and psychological factors. Women who engage in regular high-intensity exercise may be at risk of developing menstrual disturbances such as delayed menarche, oligomenorrhea, amenorrhea, and luteal phase defects.[41]

Although factors such as the physical and psychological stress of competition have been postulated to underlie the exercise-induced reproductive disorder, evidence accumulated to date indicates that negative energy balance is the primary cause of the impairment of normal reproductive function commonly observed in female athletes.[42,43] In 1939 Hans Selye reported that "the ovaries undergo atrophy and more or less permanent anestrus ensues" when young female rats were forced to exercise for prolonged periods.[44] Selye observed a *general adaptation syndrome* also involving hypertrophy of the adrenal glands, cessation of growth and lactation, shrinkage of the liver, loss of muscular tone, a fall in body temperature, and the disappearance of adipose tissue.[45] In 1980, Warren was the first to suggest that menstrual disorders in dancers are caused by an "energy drain."[42] In 1984, Winterer and colleagues hypothesized that lack of sufficient metabolic fuels to meet the energy requirements of the brain causes an alteration in brain function that disrupts the gonadotropin-releasing hormone (GnRH) pulse generator, although the mechanism of this alteration was unknown.[46] The energy availability hypothesis is supported by endocrine observations of athletes. Amenorrheic athletes display low 24-hour blood glucose levels, low 24-hour insulin levels, high 24-hour levels of IGF-binding protein 1 (IGFBP-1),[47] loss of the leptin diurnal rhythm,[48] and low triiodothyronine (T_3) levels in the morning.[49] Loucks and coworkers[50] found that low energy availability reduced LH pulse frequency and increased LH pulse amplitude and that exercise stress had no suppressive effect on LH pulsatility beyond the impact of the energy cost of exercise on energy availability. LH pulsatility was

disrupted regardless of whether energy availability was reduced by extreme energy restriction alone, by extreme exercise energy expenditure alone, or by a combination of moderate dietary energy restriction and moderate exercise energy expenditure. Dietary supplementation prevented the suppression of LH pulsatility by exercise energy expenditure.

To investigate the dose-response relationship between energy availability and LH pulsatility in exercising women, Loucks and Thuma[51] administered balanced energy intake or one of three low-energy availabilities (45 and either 10, 20, or 30 kcal/kg fat-free mass [FFM] per day) to healthy, habitually sedentary, regularly menstruating, older adolescent women for 5 days. LH pulsatility was disrupted only below 30 kcal/kg FFM per day. This finding was consistent with the results of many studies of amenorrheic runners, all of which indicated similar results with energy availabilities less than 30 kcal/kg FFM per day,[52] and with the only prospective study of the refeeding of amenorrheic athletes, in which menstrual cycles were restored in runners by increasing energy availability from 25 to 31 kcal/kg FFM per day.[53]

The discovery of leptin in 1994 was fundamental in clarifying the relationship between negative energy balance and reproductive dysfunction. Various sets of data suggest that leptin may serve as a signal to the central nervous system with information on the critical amount of adipose tissue stores that is necessary for GnRH secretion and pubertal activation of the hypothalamic-pituitary-gonadal axis. Several unfavorable metabolic situations are associated with low plasma leptin, increased secretion of hypothalamic neuropeptide Y (NPY), and hypogonadism, and a causal relationship has been evoked. Severe dietary restriction in juvenile female rats is associated with low plasma leptin and sexual immaturity. Cessation of food restriction leads to an immediate increase in plasma leptin followed by sexual maturation.[54] Leptin administration for the relative leptin deficiency in women with hypothalamic amenorrhea improves reproductive, thyroid, and GH axes and markers of bone formation, confirming that leptin is required for normal reproductive and neuroendocrine function.[55]

In 2007, the American College of Sports Medicine (ACSM) published a revised position stand on the female athlete triad,[56] correcting the former misunderstanding of the triad as a narrow syndrome consisting of disordered eating, amenorrhea, and osteoporosis by describing the triad more broadly as the harmful effects of low energy availability on menstrual function and bone mineral density.[43]

Impaired production of gonadotropins, which leads to luteal phase deficiency and anovulation, is a common hormonal finding with exercise-induced menstrual disturbances, but several other hormones may show significant alterations.

The HPA axis activation may be involved in the gonadal axis functional disruption during physical exercise. The so-called stress hypothesis holds that exercise activates the HPA axis, which disrupts the GnRH pulse generator by another unknown mechanism. Amenorrheic athletes may display mildly elevated cortisol levels, and this observation is the basis for attributing their amenorrhea to stress. However, because cortisol is a glucoregulatory hormone activated by low blood glucose levels, the mild hypercortisolism observed in amenorrheic athletes may reflect a chronic energy deficiency rather than exercise stress.[43]

The involvement of endogenous opioid peptides and catecholestrogens in provoking menstrual irregularities in women athletes has been also suggested.[57] In basal circumstances β-endorphins may decrease LH levels by suppressing hypothalamic GnRH; some catecholestrogens may suppress LH levels, yet others seem to potentiate and induce LH surge. The activities of both β-endorphins and catecholestrogens depend on the essential presence of a sufficiently estrogenic environment. In addition, both endogenous opioid peptides and some of the catecholestrogens appear to be able to suppress prolactin release, probably by interfering with its inhibiting factor dopamine. The increased plasma concentrations of β-endorphin, which are found after physical exercise, give rise to speculations as to their involvement in the frequently appearing menstrual irregularities in women athletes.[57]

Hyperandrogenism has been suggested as a possible alternative mechanism underlying oligomenorrhea or amenorrhea in some female athletes with menstrual disturbances.[58] Sports that emphasize strength over leanness, such as swimming and rowing, are not associated with low weight and restrictive eating patterns, yet athletes engaged in these sports are vulnerable to menstrual irregularities as well. The endocrine profile of athletes engaged in these sports is characterized by mildly elevated LH levels, elevated LH/FSH (follicle-stimulating hormone) ratios, and mild hyperandrogenism rather than hypoestrogenism. Interestingly, hyperandrogenic female athletes have a more anabolic body composition and higher Vo_2max and performance values in comparison with female athletes with menstrual disturbances but normal androgen concentrations.[58]

Prolactin

Blood prolactin levels increase during exercise, and this response appears proportional to the exercise intensity.[59] Provided that the intensity is adequate, the increase in prolactin is quite rapid. Nonetheless, short-term graded exercise may result in a peak hormonal response after the exercise ends. As for prolonged exercise, the prolactin response is proportional to the intensity at which it is performed. However, extending the duration of exercise can augment the magnitude of the prolactin response.[59]

The chronic effects of exercise training on basal resting prolactin levels are yet unclear and in need of further research. Studies have found increases in resting levels, but others have found decreased levels.[59] These contradictions seem to be related to differences in training protocols (intensity, frequency, and duration of training sessions).

The mechanisms by which prolactin increases with exercise are unclear. Prolactin levels may increase when the anaerobic threshold is reached, perhaps concomitantly with a GH increase.[60] Even prolonged (90 minutes) exercise below this threshold fails to elicit any response.[61] Prolactin increments with exercise appear to be correlated with pro-opiomelanocortin derivatives, ACTH, and β-endorphins.[62] Moreover, the prolactin increase may be related to changes in body temperature and dehydration, is exaggerated by stress, is reduced with habituation and hypoxia, and is unresponsive to metabolic events.[63]

Growth Hormone and the Insulin-like Growth Factor 1 Axis

In 1963 Roth and associates[64] demonstrated that plasma levels of GH increase during exercise, and it was later shown that exercise is the most potent physiologic stimulus to GH release.[65] The vast majority of the current knowledge regarding the GH response to exercise is based on studies of the effect of aerobic-type exercise.

The GH response to exercise is dependent on the duration and intensity of the exercise bout, the fitness level of the exercising subject, the refractoriness of pituitary somatotroph cells to the exercise stimuli, and other environmental factors.[66] Lactate and nitric oxide are suggested to be afferent stimulation for the exercise-induced GH response.[67] A linear dose-response relationship between exercise intensity and the GH secretory response was demonstrated, with escalating GH release across the range of exercise intensities (25% to 175% of lactate threshold).

The exercise duration should be at least 10 minutes, because exercise of shorter duration both below and above the lactate threshold was not accompanied by increases in circulating GH levels.[66] Exercise-induced GH peak occurs 25 to 30 minutes after the start of exercise, irrespective of the exercise duration.[66] Thus, when the task is brief a peak may be reached after its cessation, but when the task is long (e.g., 45 minutes) the GH peak occurs while the individual is still exercising.

The nature of the exercise may also influence the GH response. Although the continuous exercise protocols may be comparable to competition events, the endurance-type training undertaken by many athletes involves intermittent or interval exertion. Comparing exercise at equivalent total workloads, GH levels are lower with continuous (40-45% $\dot{V}o_2$max) as opposed to interval protocols, with twice the work rate for half the time, reflecting the greater metabolic stress and lactate levels in the latter.[68] With resistance exercise, incremental GH responses have also been described.[69] The important determinants appear to be the relationship between load and frequency of individual repetitions. Greater GH increments have been reported following "hypertrophy" protocols (moderate loads, high number of repetitions) than "strength" protocols (heavy loads, low repetitions) in both men and women.[70]

There is conflicting evidence regarding the neuroendocrine pathways that regulate GH secretion during exercise. Mechanisms involving cholinergic, serotoninergic, α-adrenergic, dopaminergic, and opioidergic pathways have been proposed.[71] There may be interactions among the pathways and they may operate at different exercise intensities. In young males regular but not acute exercise is associated with higher GH production and also augments GH stimulation of GH release by growth hormone–releasing hormone (GHRH).[72] It has been hypothesized that this is due to decreased hypothalamic somatostatinergic activity and higher GH pulsatility.

The GH response to exercise is greater in women than in men—as is the unstimulated GH output over time—and declines with aging.[71] In fact, even in early middle age (mean age, 42 years), the GH response to exhaustive exercise is greatly attenuated compared with younger (mean age, 21 years) subjects.[73] However, it is difficult to separate the effects of aging from changes in body composition, because body fat increases with aging and GH secretory rates are reduced in overweight subjects.[74]

Environmental and nutritional factors as well as some pathologic states may interfere with the GH response to exercise. Cappon and colleagues[75] showed that a high-fat meal could inhibit the magnitude of GH response to exercise, the inhibition of the exercise-induced GH response being correlated with circulating levels of somatostatin. High ambient temperature may in itself increase circulating GH levels,[76] whereas low temperature attenuates GH release.[77] Obesity and polycystic ovary syndrome are characterized by attenuated GH response to exercise.[78]

Exercise exerts acute effects on other components of the GH/IGF-1 axis. The effect of exercise on circulating IGF-1 has been examined by several investigators with differing results depending on the intensity, duration, and type of the exercise performed. Schwarz and coworkers[79] demonstrated IGF-1 increases following 10 minutes of exercise at both below and above the lactate/anaerobic threshold (LAT). This study suggests that the increase in IGF-1 accompanying exercise is not related to GH.

The transient nature of IGF increases suggests that hemodynamic or metabolic effects of exercise per se might play a role. Exercise in humans is accompanied by the rapid "hemotransfusion" of hemoconcentrated blood from the spleen into the circulation by increased blood flow to the exercising muscle and by loss of plasma water. These phenomena might explain, at least in part, an increased IGF concentration by changes in IGF flux and volume of distribution.

Longer periods of exercise training, however, are able to stimulate *IGF1* gene expression both in the central neuroendocrine and in the local tissue components of the GH/IGF-1 system. Eliakim and associates[80] showed that muscle IGF-1 protein concentrations in rats can increase with endurance training despite the lack of change in muscle IGF-1 mRNA (messenger RNA) or serum IGF-1.

Few studies have investigated the response of IGFBPs to exercise. IGFBP-1 levels have been shown not to change during 30 minutes of moderate exercise,[70] but to increase transiently after acute exercise.[81] The physiologic role of the postexercise increase in IGFBP-1, given IGFBP-1 inhibition of IGF-1 metabolic actions, may be to prevent late hypoglycemia.

Schwarz and coworkers[79] have demonstrated that IGFBP-3 levels increased with both low- and high-intensity exercise and that high-intensity exercise increased IGFBP-3 proteolysis. A transient increase in IGFBP-3 levels in response to acute exercise has been confirmed also by Wallace and colleagues[81] who described an acute increase of all components of the ternary complex, IGF-1, IGFBP-3, and acid-labile subunit (ALS).

Eliakim and associates[82] have described that functional and structural indices of fitness were correlated with mean overnight GH levels, growth hormone–binding protein (GHBP), and serum IGF-1 levels in late pubertal adolescent girls. Moreover, thigh muscle volume was inversely correlated with IGFBP-2 and IGFBP-4.

The acute increase in serum GHBP in response to acute exercise has been described also by Wallace and colleagues[81]; because GHBP at rest acts as a damper on GH oscillation, these authors speculate that the postexercise GHBP increase may prolong the GH signal, increasing the GH-mediated signal for postexercise protein synthesis, tissue repair, and muscle glycogen replenishment. The increment in the serum GHBP concentration may represent either increased synthesis from the liver or reduced clearance.[81]

Hypothalamic-Pituitary-Thyroid Axis

Exercise has effects on thyroid function, which can be viewed as an adaptive mechanism associated with enhanced performance possibly serving to provide a better balance between energy consumption and expenditure.[83] Short-term incremental exercise (≤20 minutes) increases blood TSH (thyroid-stimulating hormone, or thyrotropin) levels, with a critical intensity threshold of approximately 50% or more of $\dot{V}O_2$max necessary to induce significant changes.[59] Even though TSH is elevated, most research involving short-term exercise indicates total and free thyroxine (T_4) and T_3 are not immediately affected.[59] On the other hand, total T_4 and T_3 levels can increase following such exercise, although these findings appear primarily due to exercise-induced hemoconcentration.[84]

The influence of more prolonged submaximal exercise (approaching 60 minutes) on thyroid hormones is controversial. Some investigations report no effect on blood TSH levels, but others have found TSH and free T_3 (fT_3) to increase progressively with high-intensity steady-state workloads.[59] These divergent findings are difficult to interpret due to the highly variable exercise sessions (i.e., different durations and intensities of exercise) and the varying blood sampling protocol employed.[85]

Energy balance plays an important role in the body thyroid hormone response to exercise. Loucks and Heath[86] found a decrease in T_3 and fT_3 along with an increase in reverse T_3 (rT_3) in healthy women undergoing aerobic exercise testing with low caloric intake. This "low T_3 syndrome" was not seen in individuals receiving a higher caloric diet. An increase in rT_3 concentrations has been described as one of the more consistent findings, particularly when a caloric energy deficiency is associated with exercise.[83]

Insulin and Glucose Metabolism

Physical activity affects the metabolism of glucose and other intermediate substrates in normal subjects and in subjects with diabetes. The effects of exercise on carbohydrate metabolism are complex and involve type, intensity, and duration of exercise, changes in body composition, alterations in other behaviors, such as food intake, degree of insulin deficiency, and a complex time course of the glucose-insulin response.[87]

In normal individuals, no major alterations in blood glucose levels are usually seen during exercise, despite the increase in glucose use by skeletal muscle. With the onset of activity, activation of the α-adrenergic system results in inhibition of insulin release from the pancreas. This results in an increased rate of lipolysis in the periphery as well as a stimulation of hepatic glucose output. As glucose levels begin to fall, glucagon levels rise, further stimulating hepatic glucose output. Finally, as plasma glucose drops toward hypoglycemic levels, epinephrine is released, further stimulating hepatic glucose production and increasing lipolysis in the periphery. The increased availability of free fatty acid (FFA) for muscle metabolism helps to restrain the rate of glucose use. It has been shown that when one of these mechanisms fails, the others can largely compensate, avoiding hypoglycemia.[87]

Training induces a reduction in basal insulin levels and in the exercise-associated changes in glucagon and insulin, increases insulin sensitivity at rest and in response to a glucose load, and reduces insulin decline during acute exercise.[88] Regular exercise has become an integral part of the treatment recommendations for type 2 diabetic patients because it improves insulin sensitivity and reduces average blood glucose concentrations.[87] Physical training results in an increase in insulin-stimulated glucose disposal and improves glucose control in type 2 diabetes. However, the increase in insulin sensitivity is rapidly lost if exercise is not performed on a regular basis. Exercise may also be effective in delaying or preventing the development of type 2 diabetes.[89]

PERFORMANCE-ENHANCING (AB)USE OF HORMONES

Anabolic Androgenic Steroids

The use of ergogenic substances by professional and recreational athletes continues to be a growing problem, and androgens are among the most frequently abused drugs.[90] Anabolic androgenic steroids (AAS) are chemically modified analogues of testosterone that have been used in sport for over 70 years. The International Olympic Committee (IOC) introduced antidoping regulations for the first time in 1967 and performed the first antidoping testing in the 1972 Munich Olympics. In 1976 androgens were placed on the IOC doping list.[90]

The exact prevalence of androgen abuse is difficult to determine and surveys of androgen abuse depend mainly on self-report. An estimated 1 million Americans had used androgens at some time in their lives, accounting for approximately 1% of the U.S. population.[91]

Interestingly, an early and comprehensive review of previous results concluded that there was little evidence for supraphysiologic doses of testosterone or synthetic AAS having any appreciable effect on muscle size or strength in healthy men.[92] However, many of the studies reviewed had a lack of adequate control and standardization. Conclusions from more recent reviews suggested that the administration of AAS could consistently result in significant increases in strength if male athletes satisfied certain criteria, including the timing of doses and dietary factors.[93,94] Then, in 1996 Bhasin and coworkers[95] demonstrated that the administration of supraphysiologic doses of testosterone in combination with exercise in male weight lifters induced a greater increase in muscle size and strength compared with exercise alone or testosterone treatment alone, concluding that the effects of combining supraphysiologic doses of testosterone with exercise are additive. Subsequent work showed that increases in FFM, muscle size, strength, and power are highly dose-dependent and correlated with serum testosterone concentrations.[96,97]

The anabolic effect of testosterone is dose dependent, and significant increases in muscle size and strength occur only with doses of 300 mg per week and higher.[96] The increase in muscle size is due to a hypertrophy that results from an increase in cross-sectional areas of both type I and type II muscle fibers and an increase in myonuclear number.[98]

The anabolic effects of androgens are primarily mediated through the androgen receptor signaling. Androgen receptors are expressed in the satellite cells and other stem-like cells in the interstitium of the skeletal muscle fibers.[99] A growing body of evidence supports the hypothesis that testosterone and dihydrotestosterone promote myogenic differentiation of mesenchymal, multipotent stem cells and inhibit their differentiation into the adipogenic lineage.[100,101]

The AAS used for nontherapeutic purposes are endogenous androgens (e.g., androstenedione, DHEA); 17β-esters of testosterone (e.g., cypionate, enanthate, heptylate, propionate, undecanoate, bucyclate); 17α-alkyl derivatives of testosterone (e.g., methyltestosterone, fluoxymesterone, oxandrolone, stanozol); 19-nortestosterone (nandrolone); 17β-esters of 19-nortestosterone (e.g., decanoate, phenpropionate); 19-norandrostenedione and 19-norandrostenediol; and tetrahydrogestrinone. More than 100 different AAS have been developed, with most of them being used illegally, synthesized in clandestine laboratories, commercialized without medical prescription or safety controls, and sometimes unknown to the scientific world[102] (Table 26-1). The updated list of AAS is available on the World Anti-Doping Agency (WADA) website: http://list.wada-ama.org/.[103]

Intramuscular injections are used far more frequently than oral formulations. The dose of AAS used by athletes varies considerably and is often thought to exceed 10 to 40 times the recommended therapeutic dose. Also,

TABLE 26-1
Performance-Enhancing Hormones

Anabolic Androgenic Steroids

17β-Esters of testosterone (cypionate, enanthate, heptylate, propinate, undecanoate, bucyclate)
17α-Alkyl derivatives of testosterone (methyltestosterone, fluoxymesterone, oxandrolone, stanozolol)
19-Nortestosterone (nandrolone)
17β-Esters of 19-nortestosterone (decanoate, phenpropionate)
19-Norandrostenedione
19-Norandrostenediol
Tetrahydrogestrinone

Peptide Hormones

Growth hormone (GH)
Insulin-like growth factor 1 (IGF-1)
Insulin
Erythropoietin

combinations of androgens are used more frequently than single agents.[104] Multiple androgens may be combined in a practice known as "stacking," in which two or more androgens are added in progressively increasing doses over a period of several weeks. Athletes also often use a practice called "cycling," in which weeks of androgen use are followed by periods of drug holiday; this routine is based on the unproven premise that cycling prevents desensitization to massive doses of androgen. Building a pyramid refers to the progressive increase in the doses of androgens during a cycle. Toward the end of a cycle, athletes may reduce the doses of androgens or switch to other drugs, such as human chorionic gonadotropin (hCG) or aromatase inhibitors or estrogen antagonists, that they believe will reduce the likelihood of testicular suppression.[104] In most surveys, the duration of steroid administration or steroid cycle lasts between 4 and 12 weeks.[105]

Adverse Effects

The side effects associated with AAS use are numerous and involve multiple organ systems[100,102] (Table 26-2). Systematic investigations of the adverse effects of androgens in athletes and recreational body builders have been difficult for many reasons. With the exception of the association between hepatic dysfunction and the use of some oral AAS, many of the reports of serious side effects in otherwise healthy individuals have come from anecdotal case studies or small retrospective studies based largely on self-reported data.[100,104] Confounding factors, such as undiagnosed pre-existing conditions, family history, and concurrent use of other drugs, further dampen the credibility of case reports. Moreover, because most anabolic steroids are obtained on the black market and are of dubious quality, there is potential for adverse medical events to occur independent of steroid use. However, data from larger observational studies suggest that the majority (88-96%) of AAS users experience at least one minor subjective side effect, including acne (40-54%), testicular atrophy (40-51%), gynecomastia (10-34%), cutaneous striae (34%), and injection site pain (36%).[106]

AAS may also induce dyslipidemia, cardiovascular disease, insulin resistance, glucose intolerance, diabetes mellitus, and liver disease.[100] In general, the ingestion of oral C17α-alkylated anabolic steroids causes an average 30% decrease in high-density lipoprotein (HDL) and an average 30% increase in low-density lipoprotein (LDL).[107] The mechanisms for this effect are unknown but

TABLE 26-2
Adverse Effects of Anabolic Androgenic Steroids

Cardiovascular

Cardiomyopathy
Lipid disorders (decreased HDL, increased LDL)
Increased platelet aggregation
Increased hematocrit
Elevated blood pressure

Cosmetic

Gynecomastia
Acne
Hair loss
Cutaneous striae

Reproductive-Endocrine

Libido changes
Subfertility

In Males:
Testicular atrophy
Impaired spermatogenesis
Erectile dysfunction
Prostate diseases

In Females:
Hirsutism
Breast atrophy
Voice deepening
Virilization (clitoromegaly)
Menstrual disturbances

Hepatic

Cholestasis
Steatosis
Tumors
    Hepatocellular adenoma and carcinoma
    Hepatic angiosarcoma and cholangiocarcinoma

Psychological

Aggression
Mood swings
Anxiety
Psychosis
Irritability
Dependence
Withdrawal
Depression

Injection Related

Infection
Bruising
Fibrosis
Injection site pain

HDL, high-density lipoprotein; LDL, low-density lipoprotein.

apparently include an increase in the activity of hepatic triglyceride lipase that catabolizes HDL particles. Most studies indicate that injectable non–C17α-alkylated anabolic steroids, such as testosterone and nandrolone esters, exert minimal adverse effects on blood lipids.[105,107] It is unclear if the adverse changes in blood lipids as a function of testosterone use actually lead to an increase in the incidence of coronary artery disease.

AAS may also adversely influence platelet aggregation and the myocardium, although the relationship between these effects and cardiovascular disease is unclear. Occasional reports of cardiomyopathies and arrhythmias associated with steroid use have been published, and several mechanisms have been proposed.[108]

Liver disease is a well-documented side effect of most, but not all, C17α-alkylated AAS, the exception being oxan-

drolone. In contrast, most non–C17α-alkylated steroids exert minimal hepatotoxicity. Liver diseases associated with anabolic steroids include cholestasis, peliosis hepatis, hepatocellular adenoma and carcinoma, and hepatic angiosarcoma and cholangiocarcinoma.[105]

Potential effects on the reproductive system include infertility and testicular atrophy in men and menstrual and genital tract alterations and infertility in women.[105] Although all AAS suppress the hypothalamic-pituitary axis to some extent, the resulting infertility in males is generally reversible.

The effects of AAS use on fertility in women are unknown. High doses of androgens decrease circulating FSH and sex hormone–binding globulin (SHBG) concentrations in eugonadal women, whereas no changes are observed in mean nadir and LH pulse amplitude and in circulating concentrations of estradiol, estrone, and adrenal steroids.[109] Menstruation is either diminished or absent in steroid users, but ovulation may occur.[110]

Balding is common in those who use AAS undergoing 5α reduction to potent androgens. In some male steroid users, gynecomastia may be caused by increased circulating estrogen associated with the use of aromatizable androgens or hCG, with decreased clearance of circulating estrogens as a result of impaired hepatic function, or with a temporary state of hypotestosteronemia following AAS withdrawal.[105]

Several studies have suggested that AAS use may lead to significant psychological morbidity. Anxiety, psychosis, irritability, increased aggression, and antisocial and violent behavior have been described to be associated with AAS use. In addition, dependence, withdrawal symptoms, and depression may accompany or follow the nonmedical use of AAS.[111]

Finally, there are concerns about potential effects of androgens on the risk of prostate disease, although the long-term effects of supraphysiologic doses of androgens on the risk of prostate cancer, benign prostatic hypertrophy, and lower urinary tract symptoms are still unknown.[112]

Detection

All known AAS can be detected via urinalysis for a period of time following the last dose. Detection of the misuse of exogenous substances is preferably done using gas chromatography/mass spectrometry (GC-MS) complemented by liquid chromatography/tandem mass spectrometry (LC-MS/MS). To improve the selectivity and sensitivity, traditional GC-MS methods are accompanied by high-resolution mass spectrometry (HRMS) or MS/MS techniques.[113]

Endogenous androgens and their metabolites occur naturally in the human body; thus, specific indicators for the detection of the exogenous administration of these steroids are required.[113] For screening purposes a set of urinary concentrations of several endogenous steroids or metabolites is determined by the GC-MS method used for the detection of steroid abuse. The method of steroid profiling was first introduced into routine doping control by Donike and colleagues in 1983 (testosterone to epitestosterone [T/E] ratio). The most important steroid profile parameters in doping control are the ratios of T/E, androsterone/etiocholanolone, androstane/testosterone, and the 5α/5β forms of androstane-3,17-diol. The administration of steroids such as testosterone or its precursors (e.g., androstenediol, androstenedione, or DHEA) or metabolites (e.g., dihydrotestosterone or epitestosterone), has been proved to alter one or more of the parameters of the urinary steroid profile.[114] Consequently, monitoring the urinary steroid profile parameters allows screening for potential misuse.

Growth Hormone

GH has been used as a drug of abuse in sports since the early 1980s, although the first scientific studies demonstrating a clear-cut physiologic role for GH in adults were only published in the peer-reviewed medical literature in 1989.[115,116]

GH functions as a major metabolic hormone in the adult by optimizing body composition and physical function and regulating energy and substrate metabolism. GH causes nitrogen retention and promotes positive protein balance in skeletal muscle by increasing protein anabolism and possibly by decreasing protein catabolism.[117,118]

In 2008 Liu and coworkers completed a systematic review of 44 randomized controlled trials that compared GH treatment to no GH treatment in healthy adults. Their review suggests that although GH administration may increase FFM, strength and exercise performance did not improve with GH, and edema and fatigue were more common in the GH-treated subjects. The authors concluded that claims that GH improves athletic performance are not supported by the available scientific literature.[119]

On the other hand, Graham and associates[120] performed a very well-controlled study that showed an effect on strength in a group of well-defined abstinent steroid abusers using recombinant human GH (rhGH). Finally, a recent study in recreational athletes demonstrated that, in the short term, GH significantly increased lean body mass, reduced fat mass, and improved sprint capacity but not strength, power, or endurance.[121]

Because GH is a banned substance, the doses that athletes use are difficult to evaluate. It has been suggested that athletes abusing GH take rhGH three to four times per week at a dose of 10 to 25 IU/day to increase their lean body mass.[122]

GH abuse extends beyond professional sports and is also present among adolescents engaged in sports in schools. This widespread use presents a public health problem because GH use is accompanied by adverse effects, and long-term use can lead to serious morbidity.[123]

Adverse Effects

The side effects of GH treatment in GH-deficient adults are well documented and include edema, arthralgias, myalgias, sweating, fatigue, and dizziness.[124] Athletes typically take pharmacologic doses that are likely 10 or more times greater than typical replacement doses. Although the long-term adverse effects of these megadoses are not known at present, some insight may be obtained from patients with acromegaly. Acromegalic patients have an increased risk of insulin resistance and diabetes, hypertension, cardiomyopathy, and certain forms of cancers (colorectal, thyroid, breast, and prostate).[117]

Finally, the risk of infections such as human immunodeficiency virus/acquired immunodeficiency syndrome (HIV/AIDS) or hepatitis due to the use of nonsterile or contaminated syringes[122] as well as the availability on the black market of GH that comes from extracts of human pituitary glands and represents a source for Creutzfeldt-Jakob disease must be taken into account.

Detection

Two different strategies have been proposed to detect GH doping in sports.[125] For the marker method "pharmacody-namic endpoints of GH-use" the consortium GH-2000 identified biochemical parameters of the IGF system such as IGF-1, IGFBP-3, and the ALS as suitable markers of GH use in combination with procollagen cleavage products, which also show a clear-cut increase following GH use. The combination of IGF-1 and the procollagen III amino-terminal extension peptide (PIIIP) is proposed to provide a set of markers that allow the detection of GH abuse in athletes for up to 2 weeks after the last application.

The "GH isoform method" exploits the difference in isoform composition between recombinant GH, consisting mostly of monomeric 22-kilodalton (kDa) hGH, and a variety of GH isoforms secreted by the pituitary, including a 20-kDa form lacking 14 amino acids as well as amidated and acylated isoforms. After peripheral injection of recombinant 22-kDa hGH, the pituitary's production of GH isoforms is reduced by negative feedback via IGF-1. Serum samples are subjected to two immunoassay analyses: one is specific for 22-kDa monomeric hGH and the other recognizes the majority of isoforms released from the pituitary, allowing the calculation of an isoform ratio (Fig. 26-1).

The isoform test is an excellent strategy to detect GH doping, provided it is administered shortly after the last GH dose (within 24-36 hours, depending on the dose),[126] realistically probably within 12 to 24 hours.[123] Because of this short window of opportunity the test is not well suited for in-competition testing. Its use in unannounced out-of-competition testing, however, should be more successful in catching GH abusers, and recently it has been used mostly in that setting.[123]

Growth Hormone Secretagogues

GH secretagogues are peptides or nonpeptidic agents that act to release GH from the pituitary. There is evidence that they are being used by athletes as an indirect method for GH doping. Secretagogues include GHRH and its analogues, ghrelin analogues (known as GH-releasing peptides) or GHS (GH secretagogues in a narrower sense), and amino acids (e.g., arginine or ornithine). GH secretagogues have short-lived effects and provide a relatively weak boost in GH exposure compared with what can be achieved by direct GH administration.[123] Nevertheless, GH secretagogues may be attractive to athletes who want to avoid detection because the GH released is endogenous and therefore not detectable by the GH isoform test.[123]

Currently there is no published method to detect use of these GHRH analogues, but because they differ structurally from native GHRH, unequivocal detection methods should be feasible if sufficient sensitivity can be achieved.[123]

Insulin-like Growth Factor-1

Recombinant human IGF-1 (rhIGF-1) is used in clinical practice, but a variety of IGF-1 compounds and IGF-1 analogues are also advertised on the Internet, and many have been available on the black market for several years.[127] The rationale for using rhIGF-1 as an ergogenic aid differs little from that for using rhGH. The potential benefits include increased muscle protein synthesis, increased glycogen synthesis, and FFA availability.[118]

Abuse of IGF-1 is more recent than that of rhGH. In fact, until recently, IGF-1 was only available in limited supply, partly because there is no natural source for this hormone and partly because there were no pharmaceutical preparations. This situation has changed recently with the development of two compounds, mecasermin (Increlex) by Tercica (Brisbane, CA) and mecasermin rinfabate (iPlex) by

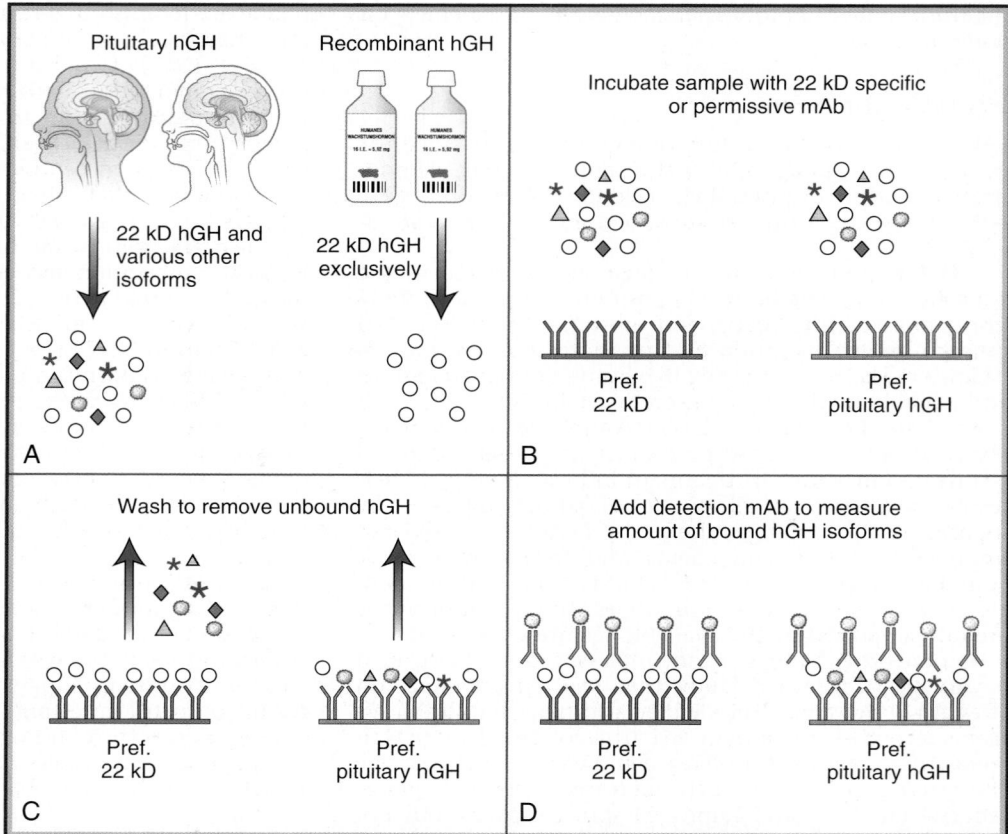

Figure 26-1 Distinguishing immunoassays for growth hormone isoform composition. hGH, human growth hormone; mAb, monoclonal antibody.

Insmed (Richmond, VA). Both preparations have received U.S. Food and Drug Administration (FDA) approval for clinical use in the treatment of growth failure in children with severe primary IGF-1 deficiency or with GH gene deletion who have developed neutralizing GH antibodies.[128] Although there are no confirmed cases of IGF-1 misuse by athletes, the drug seems to be already popular among amateur bodybuilders. IGF-1 is extensively discussed on Internet bodybuilding forums. The purported benefits include increases in muscle size and strength, improvements in energy and endurance, benefits to the immune system, and increased bone density.[127] However, although a positive correlation between circulating IGF-1 concentration and physical fitness has been observed,[82] it has not yet been proved that administering rhIGF-1 to healthy athletes will improve physical performance or alter body composition.

Adverse Effects

The adverse effects that have been reported with Increlex include hypoglycemia, jaw pain, headache, myalgias, and fluid retention.[130] The most common adverse effects observed so far with the use of mecasermin rinfabate include local injection site erythema and lipohypertrophy, although headaches, increased liver and kidney size, and altered liver function tests have also been reported.[128] It also seems reasonable to hypothesize that IGF-1 could result in adverse effects that are similar to acromegaly.[118]

Detection

At present there is no specific test to detect IGF-1 abuse, and detection of this form of doping poses many chal-

lenges. IGF-1 is excreted in urine at low concentrations, and methods for measuring urinary IGF-1 are complex and time-consuming. Several factors contribute to renal clearance of IGF-1: a significant increase in urinary IGF-1 concentration is observed as part of the proteinuria that occurs in response to exercise. Blood sample collection, rather than urine, will thus be required for IGF-1 doping tests.[127]

The GH-2004 research group has been investigating methods for detection of IGF-1 misuse, and a test is being developed on the basis of the principles of the successful GH-2000 marker method. Commercial immunoassays for these markers have been validated for antidoping purposes, but new methods, including IGF-1 measurement by use of mass spectrometry, should improve the performance of the tests and help in the detection of athletes who are doping with these peptide hormones.[127,131]

Insulin

Insulin stimulates the uptake of glucose into muscle and fat by making available an increased number of glucose transporters (e.g., GLUT4) at the cell membrane. However, its main effect is inhibitory to lipolysis, glycolysis, gluconeogenesis, ketogenesis, and proteolysis.[132]

Insulin regulates hepatic glucose output by inhibiting gluconeogenesis and promoting glycogen storage. Similarly, in muscle cells, insulin-mediated glucose uptake enables glycogen to be synthesized and stored and for carbohydrates, rather than fatty acids or amino acids, to be used as the immediately available energy source for muscle contraction. Although insulin stimulates the uptake of amino acids into cells and promotes protein synthesis in a range of tissues at high insulin concentrations, the major action of insulin is to inhibit proteolysis, which occurs at lower insulin concentrations.[118]

The theoretical performance benefits of insulin are mediated by an increase in muscle glycogen storage and the inhibition of proteolysis but have not been demonstrated in clinical or scientific trials.[118] The first suggestions of insulin as an anabolic agent were published in two bodybuilding magazines in 1996, which were commented on in the *British Journal of Sports Medicine* in 1997.[133] At the Winter Olympic Games in Nagano in 1998, a Russian medical officer inquired whether the use of insulin was restricted to type 1 diabetes.[134] This drew attention to its role as a potential performance-enhancing drug and led to its ban in 1999 by the IOC.[128]

An extensive literature search identified very few cases of insulin abuse.[135] However, from the few cases that have been published, it is apparent that the problem of insulin abuse may be much more widespread than these few isolated cases.

Adverse Effects

The most common adverse effect of insulin use is hypoglycemia. Most athletes who abuse insulin usually balance the ingestion of carbohydrate when injecting rapid-acting insulin analogues. Another problem associated with insulin is weight gain, although most competitive athletes are accustomed to diet restrictions and follow training regimens that allow them to have strict control over weight gain.[118,128]

Detection

So far, no screening tool is available providing fast and reliable information on possible insulin misuse. Only sophisticated procedures including immunoaffinity purification followed by liquid chromatography and tandem mass spectrometry have enabled the detection of synthetic insulins in doping control blood or urine samples.[136] Insulin analogues have been designed to alter their pharmacokinetics by genetic substitutions of one or two amino acids from human insulin. These small differences can be used to differentiate between native and exogenous insulin.[128]

Erythropoietin and the Erythropoietin System

EPO, a glycoprotein hormone naturally produced in the kidney and the liver, is an essential growth factor for the erythrocytic progenitors in the bone marrow. Tissue hypoxia is the physiologic stimulus for EPO expression and erythropoiesis. Once released, it serves to stimulate an increase in hemoglobin. In this way, it increases the oxygen-carrying capacity of the blood.[137]

Successful cloning of the human *EPO* gene allowed for the production of recombinant human EPO (rhEPO) and later the approval to treat patients with anemia. More recently, several newer generations of EPO analogues have been produced.[138]

Unfortunately, some athletes and their coaches were eager to abuse rhEPO because it increases the O_2 supply to the muscles and boosts performance in endurance sports such as skiing, running, and cycling.[139] In theory, the rise in hemoglobin mass should be particularly effective during bouts of exercise, such as during sprints and mountain riding in bicycle races. Reportedly, however, the prolonged administration of rhEPO improves submaximal performance more than the aerobic capacity.[140]

Apart from rhEPO, several other erythropoiesis-stimulating agents (ESAs) have been developed. Darbepoetin alfa is an rhEPO glycosylation analogue that was approved for use in 2002-2003 in the European Union and United States. It has the same mechanism of action as rhEPO, binding and activation of the EPO receptor, but it has a longer serum half-life and an increased in vivo potency. Additional ESAs are in various stages of clinical development and may appear in the athletic arena. These agents include polyethylene glycol (PEG)-conjugated epoetin beta and an EPO mimetic peptide, Hematide. PEG epoetin beta was recently approved by regulators in the European Union. Other ESAs have been described, including EPO fusion proteins (rhEPO-IL3, EPO-albumin, rhEPO-PAI1, rhEPO-Fc, and rhEPO dimers).[137,139]

The expression of the *EPO* gene (chromosome 7q22) is under the control of several transcription factors, including GATA-2 binding protein, which inhibits *EPO* expression. Under development are GATA inhibitors that can be taken orally and will prevent GATA-2 from suppressing the *EPO* promoter.[141] GATA inhibitors may be misused in sports, because they have been shown to increase EPO concentrations, hemoglobin levels, and endurance performance in mice.[137]

Adverse Effects

Artificially raising hemoglobin levels can have dangerous consequences. In contrast to the effect of endurance training, which results in an increased plasma volume, the administration of rhEPO produces a selective increase in red blood cell mass. If hematocrit exceeds 0.50, blood viscosity and cardiac afterload increase significantly. The main risks of erythrocytosis with hematocrit greater than 0.55 include heart failure, myocardial infarction, seizures, peripheral thromboembolic events, and pulmonary embolism.[142] Moreover, EPO withdrawal may be implicated in neocytolysis, that is, the hemolysis of young red blood cells in the presence of increased hematocrit.[143]

Detection

The authorities of sports forbade the use of EPO in 1990, and now any analogue or mimetic is also included in the list of prohibited substances of the World Anti-Doping Agency.[103] The challenge of detecting the misuse of EPO has given strength to the proposal of several strategies.[144] The marker methods rely on the measurement of some hematologic and serum parameters and their comparison with population or individual limit values.[145] An indirect test based on the measurement of five blood parameters—reticulocyte hematocrit, serum EPO, hematocrit, soluble transferrin receptor, and the percentage of macrocytes—was developed by Parisotto and coworkers.[146] Two models were developed. The "on" model used all parameters to detect recent use of EPO. The "off" model used three parameters to detect EPO use more retrospective.[145] An advantage of indirect methods to detect rhEPO is its universal coverage of different types of analogues and mimetics, a field in clear expansion.

The most powerful way to directly discriminate between endogenous and rhEPO is probably based on the glycosylation differences existing between both types of molecules.[147] In 1995, Wide and colleagues proposed for the first time a method able to separate both types of molecules in blood and urine.[148] This technique was reliable, as it allowed clear identification of the presence of rhEPO in urine and blood. The proposed method was powerful as long as the biologic samples were collected within 24 hours after the last rhEPO injection, but it appeared to be far less sensitive on samples that had been collected later after injection.

In June 2000—a few weeks before the Sydney Olympic games—Lasne and de Ceaurriz presented in *Nature*[149] an innovative test based on the isoelectric separation of urinary EPO isoforms on a polyacrylamide gel followed by a double blotting process.[150] In the past 10 years this test has been adapted to several recombinant EPO forms, such as darbepoetin-α, whose isoforms are located in the most acidic part of the gel, epoetin-δ, or more recently, generic (biosimilar) or "copy" EPOs.

Glucocorticosteroids

GCs were first purified and manufactured in the 1930s and 1940s following the discovery of their potent anti-inflammatory actions.[151] GCs are widely used in medicine and have shown unchallenged therapeutic potential in several chronic inflammatory and other diseases. GCs are also widely used in sports medicine for the treatment of conditions such as asthma and acute injuries. Nevertheless, their beneficial effect in certain conditions in sports, when inflammation is only a secondary reaction, remains to be validated.[152]

According to the World Anti-Doping Code, all orally, rectally, intravenously, and intramuscularly administered GCs are prohibited, and their medical use requires a standard therapeutic use exemption (TUE). Administration of GCs by all other routes requires an abbreviated TUE, except dermatologic preparations, which are not prohibited.[152] Because of the complexity of GCs, determining the boundaries between their medical use and abuse is a constant challenge for antidoping organizations.

The first use of GCs as performance-enhancing drugs has been described in the 1960s.[151] With regard to athletes, the most interesting systemic effect of the GCs is energy production by stimulation of gluconeogenesis and mobilization of amino acids and fatty acids. A possible increase in cardiovascular performance is a matter of debate as there is no evidence for such effects. As a consequence, systemic GCs have been misused for decades to enhance performance, and they once belonged to the group of most commonly used doping substances in sports.[152] Indeed, the expected effects of the use and abuse of GCs are numerous: neurostimulatory effects at cerebral GC receptors could attenuate central impressions of fatigue, and anti-inflammatory and analgesic effects could inhibit sensations of muscle pain on effort and raise the fatigue threshold.[153]

Few studies have examined the effects of GCs on exercise performance. An extensive review of the scientific literature performed by Duclos[154] showed two types of results: studies supporting the hypothesis that there is no relationship between performance and corticosteroid use in humans (negative studies) and studies supporting the hypothesis that there are relationships between performance and corticosteroid use in humans (positive studies).

Inconsistencies found regarding the ergogenic effects of GC administration in humans may be attributed to (1) the GC administration dosage, route, and mode (acute or short term); (2) the type, duration, and intensity (submaximal, maximal) of exercise tested; (3) the participants (highly trained or professional vs. recreational trained); (4) the differences in diet, such as whether or not experiments are food-controlled and whether or not subjects fasted; and (5) GC intake coupled or not with intensive training.[154]

It is noteworthy that data reported by the "negative studies" mainly derived from acute administration of GCs. Animal and human studies performed using higher doses of GCs or longer periods of administration (positive studies) clarified the effects of GC based on scientific evidence and clearly demonstrated that GCs have ergogenic effects (performance-enhancing effects) both in animals and in humans.[154]

Adverse Effects

GCs have pleiotropic effects, causing several adverse effects, especially at higher doses and for long periods, such as osteoporosis, insulin resistance, and cardiovascular effects (hypertension and atherosclerosis).[155] Moreover, a major (possibly life-threatening) complication can arise on the withdrawal of GCs: acute adrenal insufficiency.

Detection

The detection of the administration of GCs is complicated by the fact that the human body produces these steroids naturally. Several groups have described protocols and screening methods for the analysis of endogenous GC urinary metabolites using liquid chromatography/mass spectrometry. Some methods allow for the analysis of a large number of analytes from most of the classes in the WADA Prohibited List, including anabolic agents, β2-agonists, hormone antagonists and modulators, diuretics, stimulants, narcotics, glucocorticoids, and beta blockers, and do so while meeting the WADA sensitivity requirements.[103,156]

REFERENCES

1. Wade CE. Hormonal regulation of fluid and electrolyte homeostasis during exercise. In: Constantini N, Hackney AC, eds. *Contemporary Endocrinology: Endocrinology of Physical Activity and Sport.* 2nd ed. New York, NY: Springer; 2013:221-244.
2. Zouhal H, Jacob C, Delamarche P, Gratas-Delamarche A. Catecholamines and the effects of exercise, training and gender. *Sports Med.* 2008;38:401-423.
3. Wade CE, Claybaugh J. Renin activity, vasopressin concentration, and urinary excretory responses to exercise in men. *J Appl Physiol.* 1980; 49:930-936.
4. Saito T, Soya H. Delineation of responsive AVP-containing neurons to running stress in the hypothalamus. *Am J Physiol Regul Integr Comp Physiol.* 2004;286:R484-R490.
5. Wade CE, Ramee SR, Hunt MM, White CJ. Hormonal and renal responses to converting enzyme inhibition during maximal exercise. *J Appl Physiol.* 1987;63:1796-1800.
6. Davies CT, Few JD. Effects of exercise on adrenocortical function. *J Appl Physiol.* 1973;35:887-891.
7. Duclos M, Guinot M, Le Bouc Y. Cortisol and GH: odd and controversial ideas. *Appl Physiol Nutr Metab.* 2007;32:895-903.
8. Sapolsky RM, Romero M, Munck AU. How do glucocorticoids influence stress responses? Integrating permissive, suppressive, stimulatory, and preparative actions. *Endocr Rev.* 2000;21:55-89.
9. St-Pierre DH, Richard D. The effect of exercise on the hypothalamic-pituitary-adrenal axis. In: Constantini N, Hackney AC, eds. *Contemporary Endocrinology: Endocrinology of Physical Activity and Sport.* 2nd ed. New York, NY: Springer; 2013:37-47.
10. Silverman HG, Mazzeo RS. Hormonal responses to maximal and submaximal exercise in trained and untrained men of various ages. *J Gerontol A Biol Sci Med Sci.* 1996;51:B30-B37.
11. Davis SN, Galassetti P, Wasserman DH, Tate D. Effects of gender on neuroendocrine and metabolic counterregulatory responses to exercise in normal man. *J Clin Endocrinol Metab.* 2000;85:224-230.
12. Raastad T, Bjoro T, Hallen J. Hormonal responses to high- and moderate-intensity strength exercise. *Eur J Appl Physiol.* 2000;82: 121-128.
13. Hill EE, Zack E, Battaglini C, et al. Exercise and circulating cortisol levels: the intensity threshold effect. *J Endocrinol Invest.* 2008;31: 587-591.
14. Bergeron MF, Maresh CM, Kraemer WJ, et al. Tennis: a physiological profile during match play. *Int J Sports Med.* 1991;12:474-479.
15. Häkkinen K, Pakarinen A. Acute hormonal responses to two different fatiguing heavy-resistance protocols in male athletes. *J Appl Physiol.* 1993;74:882-887.
16. Hackney AC, Premo MC, McMurray RG. Influence of aerobic versus anaerobic exercise on the relationship between reproductive hormones in men. *J Sports Sci.* 1995;13:305-311.

17. Judelson DA, Maresh CM, Yamamoto LM, et al. Effect of hydration state on resistance exercise-induced endocrine markers of anabolism, catabolism, and metabolism. *J Appl Physiol.* 2008;105:816-824.

18. Duclos M, Corcuff J-B, Rashedi M, et al. Trained versus untrained men: different immediate post-exercise responses of pituitary-adrenal axis. A preliminary study. *Eur J Appl Physiol.* 1997;75:343-350.

19. Gouarne C, Groussard C, Duclos M. Overnight urinary cortisol and cortisone add new insights into adaptation to training. *Med Sci Sports Exerc.* 2005;37:1157-1167.

20. Duclos M, Gouarne C, Bonnemaison D. Acute and chronic effects of exercise on tissue sensitivity to glucocorticoids. *J Appl Physiol.* 2003;94: 869-875.

21. Goldfarb AH. Exercise and endogenous opiates. In: Constantini N, Hackney AC, eds. *Contemporary Endocrinology: Endocrinology of Physical Activity and Sport.* 2nd ed. New York, NY: Springer; 2013:21-36.

22. Carrasco L, Villaverde C, Oltras CM. Endorphin responses to stress induced by competitive swimming event. *J Sports Med Phys Fitness.* 2007;47:239-245.

23. Allen M. Activity-generated endorphins: a review of their role in sports science. *Can J Appl Sport Sci.* 1983;8:115-133.

24. Cumming DC, Wheeler GD, McColl EM. The effects of exercise on reproductive function in men. *Sports Med.* 1989;7:1-17.

25. Vingren JL, Kraemer WJ, Ratamess NA, et al. Testosterone physiology in resistance exercise and training: the up-stream regulatory elements. *Sports Med.* 2010;40:1037-1053.

26. Zitzmann M. Exercise, training, and the hypothalamic-pituitary-gonadal axis in men. In: Ghigo E, Lanfranco F, Strasburger CJ, eds. *Hormone Use and Abuse by Athletes.* New York, NY: Springer; 2011: 25-30.

27. Lanfranco F, Minetto MA. The male reproductive system, exercise, and training: endocrine adaptations. In: Constantini N, Hackney AC, eds. *Contemporary Endocrinology: Endocrinology of Physical Activity and Sport.* 2nd ed. New York, NY: Springer; 2013:121-132.

28. Gotshalk LA, Loebel CC, Nindl BC, et al. Hormonal responses of multiset versus single-set heavy-resistance exercise protocols. *Can J Appl Physiol.* 1997;22:244-255.

29. Reference deleted in proofs.

30. Hoffman JR, Falk B, Radom-Isaac S, et al. The effect of environmental temperature on testosterone and cortisol responses to high intensity, intermittent exercise in humans. *Eur J Appl Physiol Occup Physiol.* 1997; 75:83-87.

31. Häkkinen K, Pakarinen A. Acute hormonal responses to heavy resistance exercise in men and women at different ages. *Int J Sports Med.* 1995;16:507-513.

32. Cumming DC, Brunsting LA 3rd, Strich G, et al. Reproductive hormone increases in response to acute exercise in men. *Med Sci Sports Exerc.* 1986;18:369-373.

33. Hackney AC. Effects of endurance exercise on the reproductive system of men: the "exercise-hypogonadal male condition." *J Endocrinol Invest.* 2008;31:932-938.

34. Hackney AC, Moore AW, Brownlee KK. Testosterone and endurance exercise: development of the "exercise-hypogonadal male condition." *Acta Physiol Hung.* 2005;92:121-137.

35. Blueher S, Mantzoros CS. Leptin in reproduction. *Curr Opin Endocrinol Diabetes Obes.* 2007;14:458-464.

36. Baylor LS, Hackney AC. Resting thyroid and leptin hormone changes in women following intense, prolonged exercise training. *Eur J Appl Physiol.* 2003;88:480-484.

37. Lanfranco F, Bonelli L, Baldi M, et al. Acylated ghrelin inhibits spontaneous LH pulsatility and responsiveness to naloxone, but not that to GnRH in young men: evidence for a central inhibitory action of ghrelin on the gonadal axis. *J Clin Endocrinol Metab.* 2008;93: 3633-3639.

38. Tena-Sempere M. Ghrelin and reproduction: ghrelin as novel regulator of the gonadotropic axis. *Vitam Horm.* 2008;77:285-300.

39. Jürimäe J, Cicchella A, Jürimäe T, et al. Regular physical activity influences plasma ghrelin concentration in adolescent girls. *Med Sci Sports Exerc.* 2007;39:1736-1741.

40. Cumming DC, Quigley ME, Yen SS. Acute suppression of circulating testosterone levels by cortisol in men. *J Clin Endocrinol Metab.* 1983; 57:671-673.

41. Loucks AB, Vaitukaitis J, Cameron JL, et al. The reproductive system and exercise in women. *Med Sci Sports Exerc.* 1992;24:288-293.

42. Warren MP. The effects of exercise on pubertal progression and reproductive function in girls. *J Clin Endocrinol Metab.* 1980;51: 1150-1157.

43. Loucks AB. Exercise training in the normal female: effects of low energy availability on reproductive function. In: Constantini N, Hackney AC, eds. *Contemporary Endocrinology: Endocrinology of Physical Activity and Sport.* 2nd ed. New York, NY: Springer; 2013:185-205.

44. Selye H. The effect of adaptation to various damaging agents on the female sex organs in the rat. *Endocrinology.* 1939;25:615-624.

45. Selye H. A syndrome produced by diverse nocuous agents. *Nature.* 1936;138:32.

46. Winterer J, Cutler GB Jr, Loriaux DL. Caloric balance, brain to body ratio, and the timing of menarche. *Med Hypotheses.* 1984;15:87-91.

47. Laughlin GA, Yen SS. Nutritional and endocrine-metabolic aberrations in amenorrheic athletes. *J Clin Endocrinol Metab.* 1996;81:4301-4309.

48. Laughlin GA, Yen SS. Hypoleptinemia in women athletes: absence of a diurnal rhythm with amenorrhea. *J Clin Endocrinol Metab.* 1997;82: 318-321.

49. Loucks AB, Laughlin GA, Mortola JF, et al. Hypothalamic-pituitary-thyroidal function in eumenorrheic and amenorrheic athletes. *J Clin Endocrinol Metab.* 1992;75:514-518.

50. Loucks AB, Verdun M, Heath EM. Low energy availability, not stress of exercise, alters LH pulsatility in exercising women. *J Appl Physiol.* 1998;84:37-46.

51. Loucks AB, Thuma JR. Luteinizing hormone pulsatility is disrupted at a threshold of energy availability in regularly menstruating women. *J Clin Endocrinol Metab.* 2003;88:297-311.

52. Loucks AB. Low energy availability in the marathon and other endurance sports. *Sports Med.* 2007;37:348-352.

53. Kopp-Woodroffe SA, Manore MM, Dueck CA, et al. Energy and nutrient status of amenorrheic athletes participating in a diet and exercise training intervention program. *Int J Sport Nutr.* 1999;9:70-88.

54. Aubert ML, Pierroz DD, Gruaz NM, et al. Metabolic control of sexual function and growth: role of neuropeptide Y and leptin. *Mol Cell Endocrinol.* 1998;140:107-113.

55. Chan JL, Mantzoros CS. Role of leptin in energy-deprivation states: normal human physiology and clinical implications for hypothalamic amenorrhoea and anorexia nervosa. *Lancet.* 2005;366:74-85.

56. Nattiv A, Loucks AB, Manore MM, et al. American College of Sports Medicine. American College of Sports Medicine position stand. The female athlete triad. *Med Sci Sports Exerc.* 2007;39:1867-1882.

57. De Cree C. The possible involvement of endogenous opioid peptides and catecholestrogens in provoking menstrual irregularities in women athletes. *Int J Sports Med.* 1990;11:329-348.

58. Rickenlund A, Carlstrom K, Ekblom B, et al. Hyperandrogenicity is an alternative mechanism underlying oligomenorrhea or amenorrhea in female athletes and may improve physical performance. *Fertil Steril.* 2003;79:947-955.

59. Hackney AC. Thyroid axis, prolactin and exercise. In: Ghigo E, Lanfranco F, Strasburger CJ, eds. *Hormone Use and Abuse by Athletes.* New York, NY: Springer; 2011:17-24.

60. De Meirleir KL, Baeyens L, L'Hermite-Baleriaux M, et al. Exercise-induced prolactin release is related to anaerobiosis. *J Clin Endocrinol Metab.* 1985;60:1250-1252.

61. Mastrogiacomo I, Toderini D, Bonanni G, Bordin D. Gonadotropin decrease induced by prolonged exercise at about 55% of the VO_2max in different phases of the menstrual cycle. *Int J Sports Med.* 1990;11: 198-203.

62. Oleshansky MA, Zoltick JM, Herman RH, et al. The influence of fitness on neuroendocrine responses to exhaustive treadmill exercise. *Eur J Appl Physiol Occup Physiol.* 1990;59:405-410.

63. Benso A, Broglio F, Aimaretti G, et al. Endocrine and metabolic responses to extreme altitude and physical exercise in climbers. *Eur J Endocrinol.* 2007;157:733-740.

64. Roth J, Glick SM, Yalow RS. Hypoglycemia: a potent stimulus to the secretion of growth hormone. *Science.* 1963;140:987-988.

65. Sutton JR, Lazarus L. Growth hormone and exercise comparison of physiological and pharmacological stimuli. *J Appl Physiol.* 1976;41: 523-527.

66. Eliakim A, Nemet D. Exercise and the GH-IGF-I axis. In: Constantini N, Hackney AC, eds. *Contemporary Endocrinology: Endocrinology of Physical Activity and Sport.* 2nd ed. New York, NY: Springer; 2013:69-83.

67. Godfrey R, Madgwick Z, Whyte G. The exercise-induced growth hormone response in athletes. *Sports Med.* 2003;33:599-613.

68. Karagiorgos A, Garcia JF, Brooks GA. Growth hormone response to continuous and intermittent exercise. *Med Sci Sports.* 1979;11: 302-307.

69. Häkkinen K, Pakarinen A, Alen M, et al. Neuromuscular and hormonal responses in elite athletes to two successive strength training sessions in one day. *Eur J Appl Physiol.* 1988;57:133-139.

70. Cuneo RC, Wallace JD. Growth hormone, insulin-like growth factors and sport. *J Clin Endocrinol Metab.* 1994;1:3-13.

71. Wideman L, Weltman JY, Hartman ML, et al. Growth hormone release during acute and chronic aerobic and resistance exercise: recent findings. *Sports Med.* 2002;32:987-1004.

72. Kanaley JA, Weltman JY, Veldhuis JD, et al. Human growth hormone response to repeated bouts of aerobic exercise. *J Appl Physiol.* 1997;83: 1756-1761.

73. Zaccaria M, Varnier M, Piazza P, et al. Blunted growth hormone response to maximal exercise in middleaged versus young subjects and no effect of endurance training. *J Clin Endocrinol Metab.* 1999;84: 2303-2307.

74. Veldhuis JD, Liem AY, South S, et al. Differential impact of age, sex steroid hormones, and obesity on basal versus pulsatile growth hormone secretion in men as assessed in an ultrasensitive chemiluminescence assay. *J Clin Endocrinol Metab.* 1995;80:3209-3222.

75. Cappon JP, Ipp E, Brasel JA, Cooper DM. Acute effect of high-fat and high-glucose meals on the growth hormone response to exercise. *J Clin Endocrinol Metab.* 1993;76:1418-1422.

76. Okada Y, Hikita T, Ishitobi K, et al. Human growth hormone secretion during exposure to hot air in normal adult male subjects. *J Clin Endocrinol Metab.* 1972;34:759-763.

77. Christensen SE, Jorgensen OL, Moller N, Orskov H. Characterization of growth hormone release in response to external heating. Comparison to exercise induced release. *Acta Endocrinol (Copenh).* 1984;107:295-301.

78. Wilkinson PW, Parkin JM. Growth hormone response to exercise in obese children. *Lancet.* 1974;2:55.

79. Schwarz AJ, Brasel JA, Hintz RL, et al. Acute effect of brief low- and high-intensity exercise on circulating IGF-1, II, and IGF binding protein-3 and its proteolysis in young healthy men. *J Clin Endocrinol Metab.* 1996;81:3492-3497.

80. Eliakim A, Moromisato M, Moromisato D, et al. Increase in muscle IGF-I protein but not IGF-I mRNA after 5 days of endurance training in young rats. *J Appl Physiol.* 1997;42:1557-1561.

81. Wallace JD, Cuneo RD, Baxter R, et al. Responses of the growth hormone (GH) and insulin-like growth factor axis to exercise, GH administration, and GH withdrawal in trained adult males: a potential test for GH abuse in sport. *J Clin Endocrinol Metab.* 1999;84:3591-3601.

82. Eliakim A, Brasel JA, Mohan S, et al. Physical fitness, endurance training, and the GH-IGF-1 system in adolescent females. *J Clin Endocrinol Metab.* 1996;81:3986-3992.

83. Klubo-Gwiezdzinska J, Bernet VJ, Wartofsky L. Exercise and thyroid function. In: Constantini N, Hackney AC, eds. *Contemporary Endocrinology: Endocrinology of Physical Activity and Sport.* 2nd ed. New York, NY: Springer; 2013:85-119.

84. McMurray RG, Eubanks TE, Hackney AC. Nocturnal hormonal responses to weight training exercise. *Eur J Appl Physiol.* 1995;72:121-126.

85. Hackney AC, Viru A. Research methodology: issues with endocrinological measurements in exercise science and sport medicine. *J Athl Train.* 2008;43:631-639.

86. Loucks AB, Heath EM. Induction of low-T3 syndrome in exercising women occurs at a threshold of energy availability. *Am J Physiol.* 1994;266:R817-R823.

87. De Feo P, Fatone C, Mazzeschi C, Battistini D. Diabetes and exercise. In: Constantini N, Hackney AC, eds. *Contemporary Endocrinology: Endocrinology of Physical Activity and Sport.* 2nd ed. New York, NY: Springer; 2013:501-511.

88. O'Rahilly SO, Hosker JP, Rudenski AS, et al. The glucose stimulus-response curve of the beta-cell in physically trained humans, assessed by hyperglycemic clamps. *Metabolism.* 1988;37:919-923.

89. Roberts CK, Barnard RJ. Effects of exercise and diet on chronic disease. *J Appl Physiol.* 2005;98:3-30.

90. Choong K, Jasuja R, Basaria S, et al. Androgen abuse. In: Ghigo E, Lanfranco F, Strasburger CJ, eds. *Hormone Use and Abuse by Athletes.* New York, NY: Springer; 2011:43-49.

91. Yamaguchi R, Johnston LD, O'Malley PM. Relationship between student illicit drug use and school drug-testing policies. *J Sch Health.* 2003;73:59-164.

92. Ryan AJ. Athletics. In: Kochakian CD, ed. *Anabolic-Androgenic Steroids,* Vol. 43. Berlin: Springer-Verlag; 1976:515-534.

93. Haupt HA, Rovere GD. Anabolic steroids: a review of the literature. *Am J Sports Med.* 1984;12:469-484.

94. Strauss RH, Yesalis CE. Anabolic steroids in the athlete. *Annu Rev Med.* 1991;42:449-457.

95. Bhasin S, Storer TW, Berman N, et al. The effects of supraphysiological doses of testosterone on muscle size and strength in normal men. *N Engl J Med.* 1996;335:1-7.

96. Bhasin S, Woodhouse L, Casaburi R, et al. Testosterone dose-response relationships in healthy young men. *Am J Physiol Endocrinol Metab.* 2001;281:E1172-E1181.

97. Woodhouse LJ, Reisz-Porszasz S, Javanbakht M, et al. Development of models to predict anabolic response to testosterone administration in healthy young men. *Am J Physiol Endocrinol Metab.* 2003;284:E1009-E1017.

98. Sinha-Hikim I, Artaza J, Woodhouse L, et al. Testosterone-induced increase in muscle size in healthy young men is associated with muscle fiber hypertrophy. *Am J Physiol Endocrinol Metab.* 2002;283:E154-E164.

99. Sinha-Hikim I, Taylor WE, Gonzalez-Cadavid NF, et al. Androgen receptor in human skeletal muscle and cultured muscle satellite cells: up-regulation by androgen treatment. *J Clin Endocrinol Metab.* 2004;89:5245-5255.

100. Singh R, Artaza JN, Taylor WE, et al. Androgens stimulate myogenic differentiation and inhibit adipogenesis in C3H 10T1/2 pluripotent cells through an androgen receptor-mediated pathway. *Endocrinology.* 2003;144:5081-5088.

101. Singh R, Bhasin S, Braga M, et al. Regulation of myogenic differentiation by androgens: cross talk between androgen receptor/ beta-catenin and follistatin/transforming growth factor-beta signaling pathways. *Endocrinology.* 2009;150:1259-1268.

102. Di Luigi L, Romanelli F, Lenzi A. Androgenic-anabolic steroids abuse in males. *J Endocrinol Invest.* 2005;28:81-84.

103. WADA. The World Anti-Doping Code: The 2015 Prohibited List International Standard. Available at: http:www//wada-ama.org/ (accessed 22 February 2015).

104. Hoffman JR, Kraemer WJ, Bhasin S, et al. Position stand on androgen and human growth hormone use. *J Strength Cond Res.* 2009;23:S1-S59.

105. Evans NA. Current concepts in anabolic-androgenic steroids. *Am J Sports Med.* 2004;32:534-542.

106. Kicman AT. Pharmacology of anabolic steroids. *Br J Pharmacol.* 2008;154:502-521.

107. Thompson PD, Cullinane EM, Sady SP, et al. Contrasting effects of testosterone and stanozolol on serum lipoprotein levels. *JAMA.* 1989;261:1165-1168.

108. Parssinen M, Seppala T. Steroid use and long term health risks in former athletes. *Sports Med.* 2002;32:83-94.

109. Spinder T, Spijkstra JJ, Van Den Tweel JG, et al. The effects of long term testosterone administration on pulsatile luteinizing hormone secretion and on ovarian histology in eugonadal female to male transsexual subjects. *J Clin Endocrinol Metab.* 1989;69:151-157.

110. Strauss RH, Liggett M, Lanese RR. Anabolic steroid use and perceived effects in ten weight-trained women athletes. *JAMA.* 1985;253:2871-2873.

111. Evans NA. Gym & tonic: a profile of 100 male steroid users. *Br J Sports Med.* 1997;31:54-58.

112. Bhasin S, Calof O, Storer TW, et al. Drug insight: testosterone and selective androgen receptor modulators as anabolic therapies for chronic illness and aging. *Nat Clin Pract Endocrinol Metab.* 2006;2:146-159.

113. Parr MK, Flenker U, Schaenzer W. The assay of endogenous and exogenous anabolic androgenic steroids. In: Ghigo E, Lanfranco F, Strasburger CJ, eds. *Hormone Use and Abuse by Athletes.* New York, NY: Springer; 2011:121-130.

114. Donike M, Barwald KR, Klostermann K, et al. The detection of exogenous testosterone. *Int J Sports Med.* 1983;4:68.

115. Jorgensen JOL, Pedersen SA, Thuesen L, et al. Beneficial effects of growth hormone treatment in GH deficient adults. *Lancet.* 1989;1:1221-1225.

116. Cuneo RC, Salomon F, Wiles CM, Sönksen PH. Skeletal muscle performance in adults with growth hormone deficiency. *Horm Res.* 1990;33:55-60.

117. Weltman A. Growth hormone. In: Ghigo E, Lanfranco F, Strasburger CJ, eds. *Hormone Use and Abuse by Athletes.* New York, NY: Springer; 2011:89-98.

118. Richmond EJ, Rogol AD. Hormones as performance enhancing agents. In: Constantini N, Hackney AC, eds. *Contemporary Endocrinology: Endocrinology of Physical Activity and Sport.* 2nd ed. New York, NY: Springer; 2013:535-546.

119. Liu H, Bravata DM, Olkin I, et al. Systematic review: the effects of growth hormone on athletic performance. *Ann Intern Med.* 2008;148:747-758.

120. Graham MR, Baker JS, Evans P, et al. Physical effects of short-term recombinant human growth hormone administration in abstinent steroid dependency. *Horm Res.* 2008;69:343-354.

121. Meinhardt U, Nelson AE, Hansen JL, et al. The effects of growth hormone on body composition and physical performance in recreational athletes: a randomized trial. *Ann Intern Med.* 2010;152:568-577.

122. Saugy M, Robinson N, Saudan C, et al. Human growth hormone doping in sport. *Br J Sports Med.* 2006;40:i35-i39.

123. Baumann GP. Growth hormone doping in sports: a critical review of use and detection strategies. *Endocr Rev.* 2012;33:155-186.

124. Giustina A, Barkan A, Chanson P, et al. Guidelines for the treatment of growth hormone excess and growth hormone deficiency is adults. *J Endocrinol Invest.* 2008;31:820-838.

125. Bidlingmaier M. New detection methods for growth hormone and growth factors. *Endocr Dev.* 2012;23:52-59.

126. Bidlingmaier M, Suhr J, Ernst A, et al. High-sensitivity chemiluminescence immunoassays for detection of growth hormone doping in sports. *Clin Chem.* 2009;55:445-453.

127. Guha N, Cowan DA, Sonksen P, Holt RIG. Insulin-like growth factor-I (IGF-I) misuse in athletes and potential methods for detection. *Ann Bioanal Chem.* 2013;405:9669-9683.

128. Erotokritou-Mulligan I, Holt RIG. Insulin-like growth factor I and insulin and their abuse in sport. *Endocrinol Metab Clin North Am.* 2010;39:33-43.

129. Reference deleted in proofs.

130. Williams RM, McDonald A, O'Savage M, et al. Mecasermin rinfabate: rhIGF-I/rhIGFBP-3 complex: iPLEX. *Expert Opin Drug Metab Toxicol.* 2008;4:311-324.

131. Guha N, Erotokritou-Mulligan I, Bartlett C, et al. Biochemical markers of insulin-like growth factor-I misuse in athletes: the response of serum IGF-I, procollagen type III amino-terminal propeptide, and the GH-2000 score to the administration of rhIGF-I/rhIGF binding protein-3 complex. *J Clin Endocrinol Metab.* 2014;99:2259-2268.

132. Ho RC, Alcazar O, Goodyer LJ. Exercise regulation of insulin action in skeletal muscle. In: Kraemer WJ, Rogol AD, eds. *The Endocrine System*

in Sports and Exercise, in Collaboration with the International Federation of Sports Medicine. Oxford: Blackwell Publishing; 2005:388-407.

133. Dawson RT, Harrison MW. Use of insulin as an anabolic agent. *Br J Sports Med.* 1997;31:259.

134. Sonksen PH. Insulin, growth hormone and sport. *J Endocrinol.* 2001; 170:13-25.

135. Evans PJ, Lynch RM. Insulin as a drug of abuse in body building. *Br J Sports Med.* 2003;37:356-357.

136. Thevis M, Thomas A, Schaenzer W. Insulin. *Handb Exp Pharmacol.* 2010;195:209-226.

137. Jelkmann W. Erythropoietin. In: Ghigo E, Lanfranco F, Strasburger CJ, eds. *Hormone Use and Abuse by Athletes.* New York, NY: Springer; 2011: 99-109.

138. Lamon S, Robinson N, Saugy M. Procedures for monitoring recombinant erythropoietin and analogs in doping. *Endocrinol Metab Clin North Am.* 2010;39:141-154.

139. Elliott S. Erythropoiesis-stimulating agents and other methods to enhance oxygen transport. *Br J Pharmacol.* 2008;154:529-541.

140. Thomsen JJ, Rentsch RL, Robach P, et al. Prolonged administration of recombinant human erythropoietin increases submaximal performance more than maximal aerobic capacity. *Eur J Appl Physiol.* 2007; 101:481-486.

141. Nakano Y, Imagawa S, Matsumoto K, et al. Oral administration of K-11706 inhibits GATA binding activity, enhances hypoxia-inducible factor 1 binding activity, and restores indicators in an in vivo mouse model of anemia of chronic disease. *Blood.* 2004;104:4300-4307.

142. Eichner ER. Blood doping: infusions, erythropoietin and artificial blood. *Sports Med.* 2007;37:389-391.

143. Trial J, Rice L, Alfrey CP. Erythropoietin withdrawal alters interactions between young red blood cells, splenic endothelial cells, and macrophages: an in vitro model of neocytolysis. *J Investig Med.* 2001;49: 335-345.

144. Leuenberger N, Reichel C, Lasne F. Detection of erythropoiesis-stimulating agents in human anti-doping control: past, present and future. *Bioanalysis.* 2012;4:1565-1575.

145. Segura J, Zorzoli M. Distinction between endogenous and exogenous erythropoietin: marker methods. In: Ghigo E, Lanfranco F, Strasburger CJ, eds. *Hormone Use and Abuse by Athletes.* New York, NY: Springer; 2011:151-161.

146. Parisotto R, Gore CJ, Emslie KR, et al. A novel method utilising markers of altered erythropoiesis for the detection of recombinant human erythropoietin abuse in athletes. *Haematologica.* 2000;85:564-572.

147. Choi D, Kim M, Park J. Erythropoietin: physico- and biochemical analysis. *J Chromatogr B Biomed Appl.* 1996;687:189-199.

148. Wide L, Bengtsson C, Berglund B, Ekblom B. Detection in blood and urine of recombinant erythropoietin administered to healthy men. *Med Sci Sports Exerc.* 1995;27:1569-1576.

149. Lasne J, de Ceaurriz J. Recombinant erythropoietin in urine. *Nature.* 2000;405:635.

150. Lasne F. Double-blotting: a solution to the problem of nonspecific binding of secondary antibodies in immunoblotting procedures. *J Immunol Methods.* 2003;276:223-226.

151. Nichols AW. Complications associated with the use of corticosteroids in the treatment of athletic injuries. *Clin J Sport Med.* 2005;15: 370-375.

152. Dvorak J, Feddermann N, Grimm K. Glucocorticosteroids in football: use and misuse. *Br J Sports Med.* 2006;40:i48-i54.

153. Duclos M. Glucocorticoids: a doping agent? *Endocrinol Metab Clin North Am.* 2010;39:107-126.

154. Duclos M. Evidence on ergogenic action of glucocorticoids as a doping agent risk. *Phys Sportsmed.* 2010;38:121-127.

155. Buttgereit F, Burmester GR, Lipworth BJ. Optimised glucocorticoid therapy: the sharpening of an old spear. *Lancet.* 2005;365:801-803.

156. Musenga A, Cowan DA. Use of ultra-high pressure liquid chromatography coupled to high resolution mass spectrometry for fast screening in high throughput doping control. *J Chromatogr A.* 2013;1288: 82-95.

CHAPTER 27

Endocrinology and Aging

STEVEN W. J. LAMBERTS • ANNEWIEKE W. VAN DEN BELD

KEY POINTS

- Treatment of subclinical hypothyroidism is associated with fewer ischemic heart disease events in younger individuals, but this is not evident in older people (>70 years).
- Subclinical hyperthyroidism is associated with an increased risk of total and ischemic heart disease mortality, and incident atrial fibrillation. Currently, treating subclinical hyperthyroidism is recommended when the confirmed TSH (thyroid-stimulating hormone, thyrotropin) level is less than 0.1 mU/L in individuals 65 years of age or older, in postmenopausal women not on bisphosphonates or estrogen, and in patients with cardiac risk factors, heart disease, or osteoporosis. At a TSH level between 0.1 and 0.5 mU/L, treatment should be considered only for individuals 65 years of age or older and in patients with cardiac disease or hyperthyroid symptoms.
- Aging is associated with late-day and evening increases in cortisol levels, earlier morning cortisol maximum (phase advance)—for example, 6:30 AM (older) versus 9:00 AM (younger)—lower circadian amplitude, and more irregular cortisol secretion patterns.
- Estrogen hormone therapy (HT) is currently recommended only in the perimenopausal period in those women suffering from menopausal symptoms. HT is not indicated for cardioprotection for women in their 70s.
- The current recommendation is not to replace testosterone in asymptomatic older men with age-related decline in testosterone levels. Clinicians can consider offering testosterone therapy on an individualized basis to older men with low testosterone levels and clinically significant symptoms of androgen deficiency. Control of prostate size, prostate-specific antigen (PSA) levels, and hematocrit is mandatory.
- During the aging process, growth hormone–insulin-like growth factor 1 (GH–IGF-1) axis activity declines. At present, there is no evidence to recommend medical intervention in the GH–IGF-1 axis as an antiaging effort, to prolong life, or to rejuvenate healthy elderly people.

Life expectancy at birth in high-income countries is currently 75.8 years for men and 82 years for women.[1] Average global life expectancy at birth is predicted to increase by 7 years during the period 1998-2025, and life expectancy at birth will be above 80 years in 26 countries.[2] Between 1950 and 2050, the number of people in the world aged over 80 years is expected to increase from 14.5 million to 394.7 million.[3]

It is not clear, however, whether these additional years will be satisfactory. Healthy life expectancy in high-income countries at birth in 2012 for males and females combined was 69.8 years, 8.9 years lower than total life expectancy at birth.[1] Most data indicate a modest gain in the number of healthy years lived but a far greater increase in years of compromised physical, mental, and social function.[4] The number of days with restricted activity and admissions to hospitals and nursing homes increases sharply after 70 years of age.[5] The compression-of-morbidity hypothesis[6] suggests that it may be possible to reduce cumulative lifetime morbidity. Because chronic illness and disability usually occur late in life, cumulative lifetime disability could be reduced if primary prevention measures postponed the onset of chronic illness. Indeed, smoking, body mass index, and exercise patterns in midlife and late adulthood are important predictors of subsequent disability.[7] Not only do persons with better health habits live longer, but in such persons, disability is postponed and compressed into fewer years at the end of life.

AGING AND PHYSICAL FRAILTY

Throughout adult life, all physiologic functions start to decline gradually.[8] There is a diminished capacity for cellular protein synthesis, a decline in immune function, an increase in fat mass, a loss of muscle mass and strength, and a decrease in bone mineral density.[8] Most older adults die of atherosclerosis, cancer, or dementia, but in an increasing number of the "healthy" oldest old, loss of muscle strength is the limiting factor that determines their chances of an independent life until death.

Age-related disability is characterized by generalized weakness, impaired mobility and balance, and poor endurance. In the oldest old, this state is termed *physical frailty*, defined as "a state of reduced physiological reserves associated with increased susceptibility to disability."[9] Clinical correlates of physical frailty include falls, fractures, impairment in activities of daily living, and loss of independence. Falls contribute to 40% of admissions to nursing homes.[10]

Loss of muscle strength is an important factor in the development of frailty. Muscle weakness can be caused by aging of muscle fibers and their innervation, osteoarthritis, and chronic debilitating diseases.[11] A sedentary lifestyle, decreased physical activity, and disuse, however, are also important determinants of the decline in muscle strength.

In a study of 100 frail nursing home residents (average age, 87 years), lower extremity muscle mass and strength were closely related.[12] Supervised resistance exercise training (45 minutes three times a week for 10 weeks) doubled muscle strength and significantly increased gait velocity and stair-climbing power. This finding demonstrates that frailty in the elderly population is not an irreversible effect of aging and disease but can be influenced and perhaps even prevented.[12] Further, in nondisabled elderly persons living in the community, objective measures of lower extremity function are highly predictive of subsequent disability.[13] Prevention of frailty may be achieved by caloric and protein support, vitamin D supplementation, reduction in polypharmacy, and working (training).[14] However, exercise is difficult to implement in the daily routine of the aging population, and the number of dropouts from exercise programs is very high.

Part of the aging process involving body composition (i.e., loss of muscle [strength] and bone, increase in fat mass) might also be related to changes in the endocrine system.[15] Current knowledge has shed light on the effects of long-term hormonal replacement therapy on body composition as well as on atherosclerosis, cancer formation, and cognitive function.

THE ENDOCRINOLOGY OF AGING

The two most important clinical changes in endocrine activity during aging involve the pancreas and the thyroid gland. Approximately 40% of individuals aged 65 to 74 years and 50% of those older than 80 years have impaired glucose tolerance or diabetes mellitus, and in nearly 50% of elderly adults with diabetes the disease is undiagnosed.[16] These adults are at risk for development of secondary, mainly macrovascular, complications at an accelerated rate. Pancreatic, insulin receptor, and postreceptor changes associated with aging are critical components of the endocrinology of aging. Apart from decreased (relative) insulin secretion by the beta cells, peripheral insulin resistance related to poor diet, physical inactivity, increased abdominal fat mass, and decreased lean body mass contribute to the deterioration of glucose metabolism.[16] Dietary management, exercise, oral hypoglycemic agents, and insulin are the four components of treatment for these patients, whose medical care is costly and intensive (see Chapter 31).

Age-related thyroid dysfunction is also common.[17] Lowered plasma thyroxine (T_4) and increased TSH concentrations occur in 5% to 10% of elderly women.[17] These abnormalities are primarily caused by autoimmunity and are thus an expression of age-associated disease rather than a consequence of the aging process. Normal aging is accompanied by an increase in serum TSH levels in iodine-sufficient areas but not in a population with borderline iodine intake.[18-20] Serum free T_4 levels remain largely unaffected during aging, but decreased peripheral degradation of T_4 results in a gradual age-dependent decline in serum triiodothyronine (T_3) concentrations.[17] This slight decrease in plasma T_3 concentrations occurs largely within the broad normal range of the healthy elderly population and has not been convincingly related to functional changes during the aging process. It remains to be clarified why serum TSH levels increase with advancing age. Several mechanisms, like a changed pituitary sensitivity or affected TSH glycosylation and thus TSH bioactivity, have been proposed.[19] The detrimental effects of overt thyroid dysfunction in elderly individuals are clearly recognized;

however, the clinical relevance of mild forms of hypo- and hyperthyroidism are a matter of debate. Subclinical hypothyroidism is present in about 4% to 8.5% of adults in the United States without known thyroid disease.[21] Subtle thyroid dysfunction in the oldest-old fraction of the elderly population (i.e., those >85 years) is often present. Although subclinical hypothyroidism in younger individuals is associated with an increased risk of atherosclerosis[22] in elderly subjects above 65 years of age, such an association is not present.[23,24] In addition, an observational study of real-life practice performed from data obtained from the United Kingdom General Practitioners Research Database showed that treatment of subclinical hypothyroidism with levothyroxine was associated with fewer ischemic heart disease events in younger individuals, but this was not evident in older people (>70 years).[23] In fact, in 85-year-old "healthy" individuals hypothyroidism was, in the subsequent 4 years, accompanied by lower all-cause and cardiovascular mortality rates when compared with euthyroid individuals.[25] In a group of 400 males with a mean age of 78 years, van den Beld and associates[26] showed that low serum free T_4 and T_3 (with normal reverse T_3 [rT_3]) concentrations were associated with a better physical performance and 4-year survival, whereas subjects with low serum T_3 and high rT_3 concentrations (i.e., fulfilling the criteria for the "low T_3 syndrome") did not show a survival advantage and had lower physical activity (Fig. 27-1). These last studies support the concept that some degree of physiologically decreased thyroid activity at the tissue level might even have favorable effects in the oldest-old subjects, but caution should be exercised when interpreting the predictive value of thyroid dysfunction in old subjects, which may give a double-faced "Janus response" if not considered in the appropriate context.[27,28] Subclinical hyperthyroidism seems to be associated with an increased risk of total and ischemic heart disease mortality, and incident atrial fibrillation, as was concluded by recently pooled individual data from 10 prospective cohort studies.[29] Controversy persists about whether treatment is warranted. A recent consensus guideline recommends treating subclinical hyperthyroidism, after diagnosing the underlying disorder, based on the level of TSH suppression. When the TSH is less than 0.1 mU/L and confirmed after a 3- to 6-month period, treatment is advised in individuals with hyperthyroid symptoms, all individuals 65 years of age or older, postmenopausal women not on bisphosphonates or estrogen, and patients with cardiac risk factors, heart disease, or osteoporosis. At a TSH level between 0.1 and 0.5 mU/L, treatment should be considered only for individuals 65 years of age or older and in patients with cardiac disease or hyperthyroid symptoms.[30] Furthermore, a recent systematic review concluded that there is a substantial body of evidence to support the association between subclinical hyperthyroidism and cognitive impairment. There is, however, so far also lack of evidence to suggest that antithyroid treatment might ameliorate dementia.[31]

Also, cortisol homeostasis is influenced by age, mostly via unknown mechanisms. Most clinical studies show circadian cortisol changes with age (reviewed by Veldhuis and colleagues[32]). Aging is associated with late-day and evening increases in cortisol levels, earlier morning cortisol maximum (phase advance)—for example, 6:30 AM (older) versus 9:00 AM (young)—lower circadian amplitude (24-hour decrement for peak minus nadir or attenuated wake-evening slopes), and more irregular (less orderly) cortisol secretion patterns.

The question remains as to which degree these alterations reflect or cause aging-associated changes in functional ability, cognition, and possibly depression. A recent

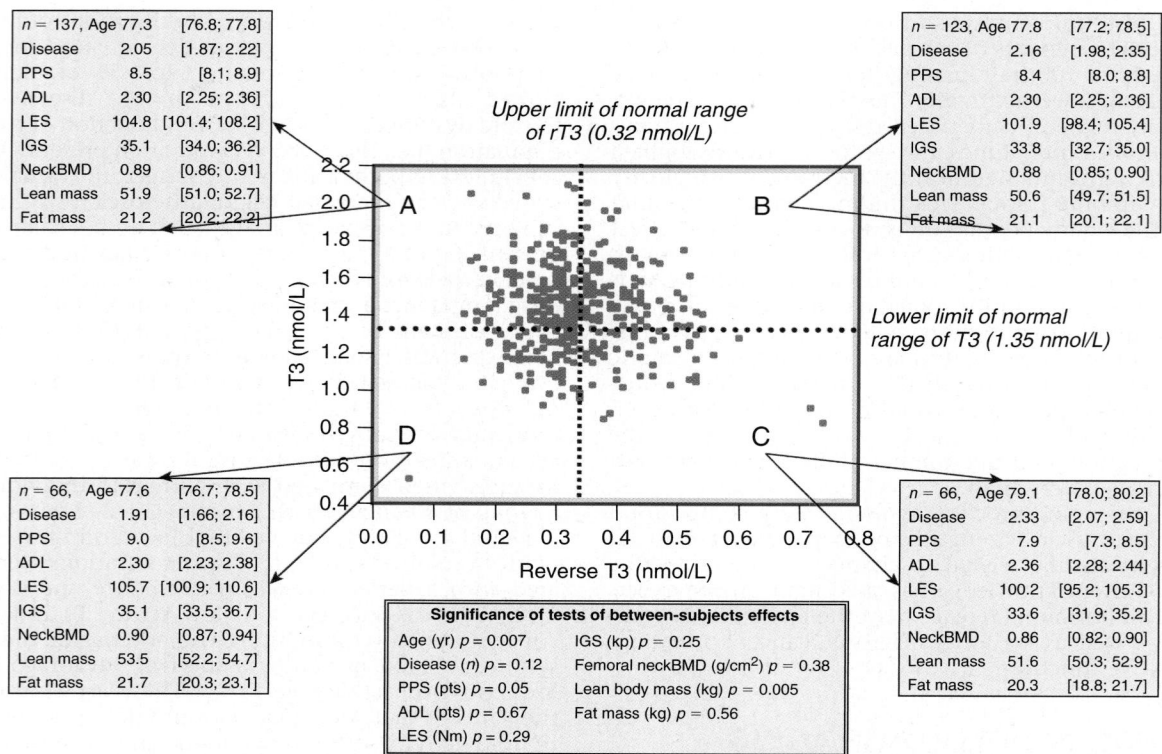

n = 137, Age 77.3	[76.8; 77.8]
Disease	2.05	[1.87; 2.22]
PPS	8.5	[8.1; 8.9]
ADL	2.30	[2.25; 2.36]
LES	104.8	[101.4; 108.2]
IGS	35.1	[34.0; 36.2]
NeckBMD	0.89	[0.86; 0.91]
Lean mass	51.9	[51.0; 52.7]
Fat mass	21.2	[20.2; 22.2]

n = 123, Age 77.8	[77.2; 78.5]
Disease	2.16	[1.98; 2.35]
PPS	8.4	[8.0; 8.8]
ADL	2.30	[2.25; 2.36]
LES	101.9	[98.4; 105.4]
IGS	33.8	[32.7; 35.0]
NeckBMD	0.88	[0.85; 0.90]
Lean mass	50.6	[49.7; 51.5]
Fat mass	21.1	[20.1; 22.1]

n = 66, Age 77.6	[76.7; 78.5]
Disease	1.91	[1.66; 2.16]
PPS	9.0	[8.5; 9.6]
ADL	2.30	[2.23; 2.38]
LES	105.7	[100.9; 110.6]
IGS	35.1	[33.5; 36.7]
NeckBMD	0.90	[0.87; 0.94]
Lean mass	53.5	[52.2; 54.7]
Fat mass	21.7	[20.3; 23.1]

n = 66, Age 79.1	[78.0; 80.2]
Disease	2.33	[2.07; 2.59]
PPS	7.9	[7.3; 8.5]
ADL	2.36	[2.28; 2.44]
LES	100.2	[95.2; 105.3]
IGS	33.6	[31.9; 35.2]
NeckBMD	0.86	[0.82; 0.90]
Lean mass	51.6	[50.3; 52.9]
Fat mass	20.3	[18.8; 21.7]

Significance of tests of between-subjects effects

Age (yr) $p = 0.007$		IGS (kp) $p = 0.25$	
Disease (n) $p = 0.12$		Femoral neckBMD (g/cm^2) $p = 0.38$	
PPS (pts) $p = 0.05$		Lean body mass (kg) $p = 0.005$	
ADL (pts) $p = 0.67$		Fat mass (kg) $p = 0.56$	
LES (Nm) $p = 0.29$			

Figure 27-1 Overview of the values of triiodothyronine (T$_3$) and reverse T$_3$ (rT$_3$) within a population of 403 elderly men. The *spotted lines* indicate the normal values of T$_3$ and rT$_3$. ADL, activities of daily living; BMD, bone mineral density; IGS, isometric grip strength; LES, leg extensor strength; PPS, physical performance score. (From van den Beld AW, Visser TJ, Feelders RA, et al. Thyroid hormone concentrations, disease, physical function, and mortality in elderly men. *J Clin Endocrinol Metab.* 2005;90:6403-6409.)

meta-analysis indicated that a more dynamic activity of the hypothalamic-pituitary-adrenal axis (i.e., a greater diurnal decline) was associated with a better physical performance in later life.[33] Further, data from a prospective cohort study among more than 400 men and women, with a mean age of 61 years, demonstrated that a flatter scope in cortisol levels across the day was associated with increased risk of all-cause 6-year mortality.[34] In addition, results from the Longitudinal Amsterdam Study of Aging showed that higher morning salivary cortisol levels were associated with increased mortality rate in men and that higher night-time salivary cortisol levels were associated with increased mortality rate in women.[35] Future clinical research is necessary to determine whether diurnal cortisol measures are relevant in identifying those who might benefit from intervention therapies.

Three other hormonal systems exhibit lowered circulating hormone concentrations during normal aging, and these changes have thus far been considered mainly physiologic (Figs. 27-2 and 27-3). Hormone replacement strategies have been developed, but many aspects remain controversial, and replenishing hormone blood levels to those found in 30- to 50-year-old patients has not yet uniformly proved beneficial and safe.

The most dramatic and rapidly occurring change in women around age 50 years is *menopause*.[36] Cycling estradiol production during the reproductive years is replaced by very low, constant estradiol levels. For many years, the prevailing view was that menopause resulted from exhaustion of ovarian follicles. An alternative perspective is that age-related changes in the central nervous system and the hypothalamic-pituitary unit initiate the menopausal transition. The evidence that both the ovary and the brain are key pacemakers in menopause is compelling.[36]

Changes in the activity of the hypothalamic-pituitary-gonadal axis in men are slower and more subtle. During aging, a gradual decline in serum total and free testosterone levels occurs.[37] *Andropause* is characterized by a decrease in testicular Leydig cell numbers and their secretory capacity as well as by an age-related decrease in episodic and stimulated gonadotropin secretion.[38,39] The primary site of the aging effect appears to be the Leydig cell's ability to respond to luteinizing hormone with increased testosterone production.

The second hormonal system demonstrating age-related changes is *adrenopause*, a term that describes the gradual decline in circulating levels of dehydroepiandrosterone (DHEA) and its sulfate (DHEAS).[40,41] Adrenal secretion of DHEA gradually decreases over time, while corticotropin secretion, which is physiologically linked to plasma cortisol levels, remains largely unchanged. The decline in DHEA and DHEAS levels in both sexes, therefore, contrasts with the maintenance of plasma cortisol levels and seems to be caused by a selective decrease in the number of functional zona reticularis cells in the adrenal cortex instead of being regulated by a central (hypothalamic) pacemaker of aging.[42]

The third endocrine system that gradually declines in activity during aging is the GH–IGF-1 axis (see Fig. 27-3).[43] Mean pulse amplitude and duration and fraction of GH secreted, but not pulse frequency, gradually decrease during aging. In parallel, a progressive drop in circulating IGF-1 levels occurs in both sexes.[43,44] There is no evidence for a peripheral factor in this process of *somatopause*, and its triggering pacemaker seems mainly localized in the hypothalamus because pituitary somatotropes, even of the oldest old, can be restored to their youthful secretory capacity by treatment with GH-releasing peptides (see later discussion).

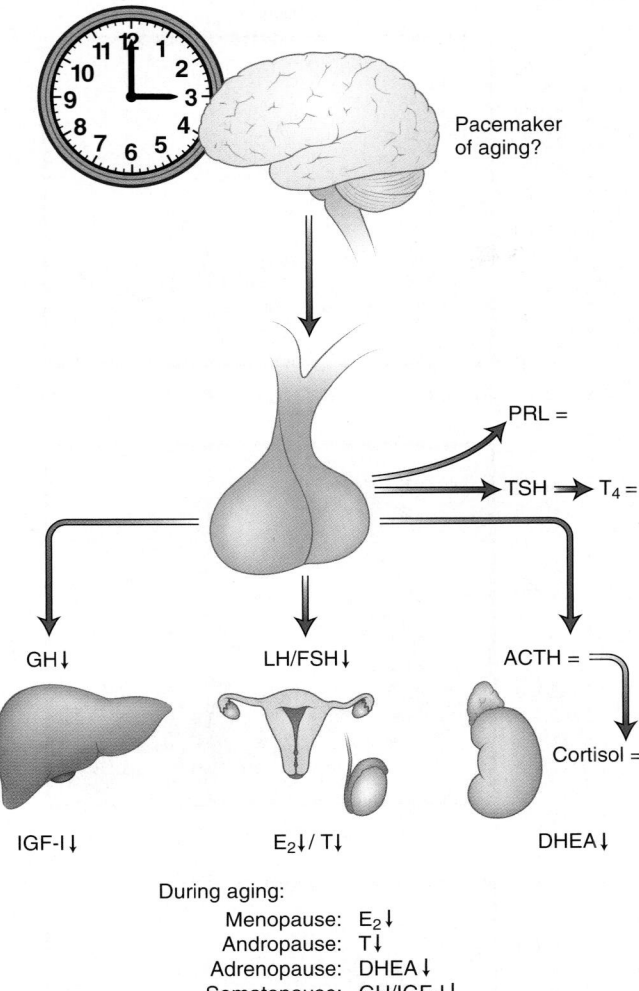

Figure 27-2 During aging, declines in the activities of a number of hormonal systems occur. *Left*, A decrease in growth hormone (GH) release by the pituitary gland causes a decrease in the production of insulin-like growth factor 1 (IGF-1) by the liver and other organs (somatopause). *Middle*, A decrease in release of gonadotropin luteinizing hormone (LH) and follicle-stimulating hormone (FSH) and decreased secretion at the gonadal level (from the ovaries, decreased estradiol [E_2]; from the testicle, decreased testosterone [T]) cause menopause and andropause, respectively. (Immediately after the initiation of menopause, serum LH and FSH levels increase sharply.) *Right*, The adrenocortical cells responsible for the production of dehydroepiandrosterone (DHEA) decrease in activity (adrenopause) without clinically evident changes in corticotropin (adrenocorticotropic hormone, ACTH) and cortisol secretion. A central pacemaker in the hypothalamus or higher brain areas (or both) is hypothesized, which together with changes in the peripheral organs (the ovaries, testicles, and adrenal cortex) regulates the aging process of these endocrine axes. PRL, prolactin; T_4, thyroxine; TSH, thyrotropin.

It is unclear whether changes in gonadal function (menopause, andropause) are interrelated with the processes of adrenopause and somatopause, which occur in both men and women. Also, functional correlates (decrease in muscle size and function and bone mass, progression of atherosclerosis, and decline of cognitive function) have not been demonstrated to be directly causally related to these changes in endocrine activity. However, a number of effects of normal aging closely resemble features of (isolated) hormonal deficiency (hypogonadism, GH deficiency), which in subjects in middle adulthood are successfully reversed by replacement of the appropriate hormone.[45,46] Although aging does not simply result from a variety of hormone

deficiency states, medical intervention in the processes of menopause, andropause, adrenopause, or somatopause might prevent or delay some aspects of the aging process.

MENOPAUSE

Menopause is the permanent cessation of menstruation resulting from the loss of ovarian follicular function and is diagnosed retrospectively after 12 months of amenorrhea. In most women, vasomotor reactions, depressed mood, and urogenital complaints accompany this period of estrogen decline. In the subsequent years, the loss of estrogens is followed by a high incidence of cardiovascular disease (CVD), loss of bone mass, and cognitive impairment. The average age of menopause (51.4 years) has not changed over time and seems to be largely determined by genetic factors.

In the past decade, anti-müllerian hormone (AMH) has been proposed as a marker to predict age at natural menopause. In women, AMH is exclusively produced by granulosa cells of ovarian follicles during the early stages of follicle development. After an initial increase until early adulthood, AMH concentrations slowly decrease with increasing age until becoming undetectable approximately 5 years before menopause when the stock of primordial follicles is exhausted.[47] In a long-term follow-up study, 257 women were followed for 11 years. It was demonstrated that using age and AMH, the age range in which menopause will subsequently occur can be individually calculated.[48,49] A study among 401 women participating in the Penn Ovarian Aging Study demonstrated that among women with a baseline AMH level below 0.20 ng/mL, the median time to menopause was 5.99 years (95% confidence interval [CI], 4.20-6.33) in the 45- to 48-year age group and 9.94 years (95% CI, 3.31-12.73) in the 35- to 39-year age group. With higher baseline AMH levels above 1.50 ng/mL, the median time to menopause was 6.23 years in the oldest age group and more than 13.01 years in the youngest age group. Smoking significantly reduced the time to menopause.[50]

Perimenopausal Use of Hormone Therapy

Typical symptoms that result from the sudden decrease in estrogen production around menopause are menstrual cycle disorders, vasomotor changes (hot flushes, night sweats), and urogenital complications (atrophic vaginal irritation and dryness, dyspareunia, atrophic urethral epithelium leading to micturition disorders). Additional symptoms are irritability, mood swings, joint pain, and sleep disturbances. Frequency, severity, onset, and duration of symptoms vary widely among individuals and among ethnic groups. About 75% of women in Western societies experience so few troublesome symptoms during the menopausal transition that HT is not needed or requested.[51] HT rapidly alleviates the symptoms of menopause. Hot flushes and vasomotor instability as well as symptoms of urogenital atrophy rapidly disappear upon the start of HT.

Long-Term Hormone Replacement Therapy

Because life expectancy is increasing, the time a woman spends after menopause constitutes more than one third of her life. Until recently long-term use of HT (5 to 10 years) was considered to offer advantages with regard to the prevention of the three chronic disorders most common in the elderly: CVDs, osteoporosis, and dementia. In the early 1990s a number of cross-sectional and prospective

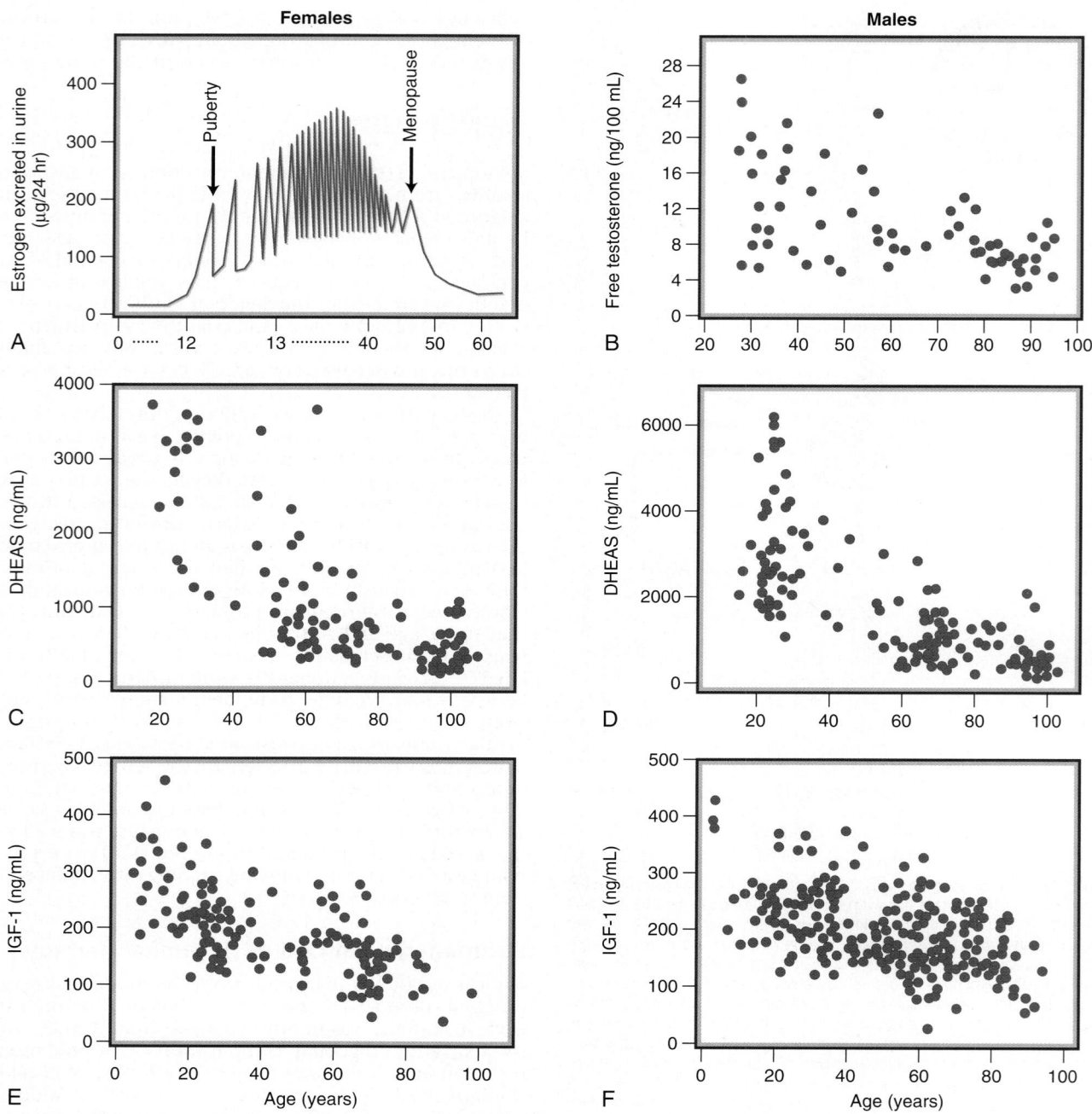

Figure 27-3 Changes in the hormone levels of normal women *(left)* and men *(right)* during the aging process. **A** and **B,** Estrogen secretion throughout an individual normal woman's life (expressed as urinary estrogen excretion) (**A**) and mean free testosterone (T) index (the ratio of serum total T to sex hormone–binding globulin levels) during the life span of healthy men (**B**). **C** and **D,** Serum dehydroepiandrosterone sulfate (DHEAS) concentrations in 114 healthy women (**C**) and 163 healthy men (**D**). **E** and **F,** The course of serum insulin-like growth factor 1 (IGF-1) concentrations in 131 healthy women (**E**) and 223 healthy men (**F**) during aging. Note the difference in the distribution of ages in the different panels. (**A** and **B,** From Guyton A. *Textbook of Medical Physiology*, 8th ed. Philadelphia, PA: Saunders; 1991:899. **C** and **D,** Adapted from Ravaglia G, Forti P, Maioli F, et al. The relationship of dehydroepiandrosterone sulfate (DHEAS) to endocrine-metabolic parameters and functional status in the oldest-old. Results from an Italian study on healthy free-living over-ninety-year-olds. *J Clin Endocrinol Metab.* 1996;81:1173-1178. **E** and **F,** Adapted from Corpas E, Harman SM, Blackman MR. Human growth hormone and human aging. *Endocr Rev.* 1993;14:20-39.)

studies demonstrated a statistically significant reduction in coronary heart disease in menopausal women taking HT. Grady and coworkers[52] presented a meta-analysis of published observational studies and reported that HT was associated with a reduction in fatal coronary heart disease by one third. A meta-analysis of 25 observational studies conducted between 1976 and 1996 showed that the relative risk for coronary heart disease in women who ever used HT compared with those who never used HT was 0.70.[53]

The Nurse's Health Study was a comprehensive investigation conducted in 121,700 female nurses aged 30 to 55 years. In the latest report, compiled with data from 70,533 postmenopausal nurses followed for 20 years, the overall risk of coronary heart disease in current users of HT was reduced, with a relative risk of 0.61.[54]

Since the turn of the new century, however, findings from a number of prospective randomized controlled trials have fully changed the attitudes concerning benefits and harms of HT. The Women's Health Initiative (WHI) trial comprised two large, randomized, placebo-controlled clinical trials, including estrogen-only and combined estrogen-progestin studies in more than 161,000 "healthy" postmenopausal women, aged 50 to 79 years.[55] It was expected that the WHI trial would definitively answer whether or not estrogen is cardioprotective. However, the estrogen-progestin versus placebo trial, which involved more than 16,000 women, was discontinued early because of an increase in cardiovascular complications (coronary heart disease, stroke, and venous thromboembolism) as well as an increased incidence of breast cancer in the treatment group.[55] Although important benefits were also seen (risk reduction for fractures and colon cancer), there was concern that the risks of combined estrogen-progestin outweighed the benefits. The estrogen-only versus placebo trial included nearly 11,000 women who had undergone hysterectomy and therefore did not require a progestin. This trial was also stopped early because a small increase in breast cancer and coronary heart disease risk was seen, although hip fracture risk was reduced.[56]

Three other randomized controlled trials supported the absence of benefit of HT for prevention of coronary heart disease and ischemic stroke.[57,58] These studies were carried out in postmenopausal women with documented ischemic stroke or transient ischemic attack,[59] in women after documented myocardial infarction,[57] and in women with documented coronary heart disease.[58]

Taken together, the WHI trial, which studied women presumed healthy at recruitment, and the three other trials carried out in women with documented cardiovascular disorders argue strongly against the earlier assumptions made on the basis of observational studies that estrogen users had a 30% to 40% reduced risk of coronary heart disease mortality and morbidity relative to nonusers.

A series of commentaries has addressed the differences in outcome between the observational studies and the randomized trials.[60,61] Healthy user bias, the age at which study participants started HT, and the different estrogen and progestin preparations and doses all have been mentioned as possible confounders.

Subsequently, reassessment of the data from the WHI and other studies has led to a different interpretation of the data, in that groups of perimenopausal and early postmenopausal women may in fact derive cardiovascular benefits from HT. In this regard much interest has focused on the "timing hypothesis," which states that estrogens are atheroprotective if used in an early phase of atherosclerosis development. In an arm of the WHI trial, in which 50- to 59-year-old women were treated with conjugated estrogens, only coronary artery calcium scores were slightly but significantly lower.[62] The "timing hypothesis" is also supported by a recent Danish study in which it was shown that participants who were assigned to HT and were aged less than 50 years at baseline had a 65% lower risk of a combined outcome of all-cause mortality, heart failure, or myocardial infarction. Unfortunately, there was no placebo and the trial was not blinded.[63] Further, an independent subanalysis from the WHI also supported the "timing hypothesis." In addition, this study also demonstrated that the duration of treatment is of importance. Comparison of the rate ratios for years 1 to 6 versus 7 to 8 showed a statistically significant ($p < 0.003$) reduction in CVD risk after more than 6 years of use of conjugated equine estrogens (CEE) versus placebo.[64] In summary, the majority of long-term large observational studies and a number of small randomized controlled trials (RCTs) strongly suggest that menopausal HT should be protective against atherosclerosis if initiated early but is potentially harmful if administered to women who already have mature at-risk plaque.[65]

Subsequently a number of studies have confirmed the risk of breast cancer, which increases with longer duration of HT.[66-68] In the Million Women Study, current users of estrogen had an increased risk of incident invasive breast cancer of 30%, and in women using estrogen plus progestin this risk had doubled. Breast cancer risk was unchanged in both the older and younger women with a prior hysterectomy treated with estrogen only. Past users of HT also had no increased risk.[69]

Also the earlier expectations from observational studies that estrogen use might prevent cognitive decline were not confirmed by randomized placebo-controlled trials. Estrogen therapy alone did not reduce dementia or mild cognitive impairment in women 65 years of age or older, but the estrogen-progestin combination resulted in slightly increased risks for both end points.[70]

The efficacy of HT in the prevention of osteoporotic fractures remains indisputed with regard to hip as well as other fractures (Table 27-1).[71]

The findings of the WHI trial are so important and have been so broadly publicized that they have created the perception that HT, in general, always carries risks that exceed its benefits. Given the noted uncertainties, HT is currently only recommended in the perimenopausal period in those women suffering from menopausal symptoms. HT is highly effective in alleviating hot flashes and night sweats. An association between endometrial cancer and estrogen use was observed many years ago. Ten years of unopposed

TABLE 27-1

Absolute Risks and Benefits of Clinical Events With Estrogen-Progestin and Estrogen-Only Therapy Compared With Placebo in the Women's Health Initiative Trial*

Health Event	Estrogen-Progestin Therapy		Estrogen Therapy	
	Absolute Risk (per 10,000 women/yr)	Absolute Benefit (per 10,000 women/yr)	Absolute Risk (per 10,000 women/yr)	Absolute Benefit (per 10,000 women/yr)
Coronary heart disease	8	—	—	3
Stroke	8	—	11	—
Breast cancer	8	—	—	8
Venous thromboembolism	18	—	8	—
Colorectal cancer	—	7	1	—
Hip fracture	—	5	—	6
Any fracture	—	47	—	56
New-onset diabetes	—	15	—	14

*For overall hazard ratio, 95% confidence interval, and adjustments, see original paper.

Adapted from Hodis HN. Assessing benefits and risks of hormone therapy in 2008: new evidence, especially with regard to the heart. *Cleve Clin J Med.* 2008;75(Suppl 4):S3-12.

estrogen use increases the risk for endometrial cancer 10-fold.[52] For this reason, the HT regimens were supplemented with progestagens, which almost completely prevented this excess risk for endometrial cancer.

Presently advised doses of estrogen were originally designed to prevent bone loss, and progestagen regimens were opposed to prevent endometrial cancer. Several estrogen and progestagen preparations are available for HT.[51] Components of available preparations vary in their effects on different target tissues. Commercial preparations differ in their clinical effect by design, and individual women differ in their responses. HT can be administered orally, transdermally, topically, intranasally, or subcutaneously through implants.

Although HT in the perimenopausal state can cause some symptoms (e.g., vaginal discharge, uterine bleeding, and breast tenderness), it relieves many others including hot flashes and the severity of night sweats.[72] Grady and coworkers[52] have estimated that about one serious adverse event will occur among every 1000 50-year-old women using HT for 1 year. The HT regimen used in the WHI trial combined 0.625 mg/day CEE and 2.5 mg/day medroxyprogesterone acetate. The dose of estrogen necessary to diminish perimenopausal symptoms, however, can be lower in many women. A dose of 0.3 or 0.45 mg/day CEE is effective at diminishing the number and the intensity of hot flushes as well.[73]

Selective Estrogen Receptor Modulators

In the search for optimal HT during menopause, it was observed that tamoxifen has variable antiestrogenic and estrogenic actions in different tissues.[74,75] Tamoxifen suppresses the growth of estrogen receptor–positive breast cancer cells. Long-term treatment of menopausal patients with breast cancer with tamoxifen also lowered the incidence of new (contralateral) breast cancer by 40%. In addition, the number of cardiovascular incidents decreased by 70%, and the age-related decrease in bone mineral density was partially prevented.[76]

These initially puzzling observations were explained by the fact that tamoxifen and other compounds such as raloxifene have selective estrogen receptor–modulating effects, exerting antiestrogenic actions on normal and cancerous breast tissue but agonistic actions on bone, lipids, and the blood vessel walls.[77] These effects of tamoxifen and raloxifene may be explained by differential stabilization of the conformation of the estrogen receptor, which facilitates interactions with coactivator or corepressor proteins, and subsequently initiates or suppresses transcription of target genes. These specific interactions in the target cell lead to tissue selective actions.[78] A number of other selective estrogen receptor modulators (SERMs) have been evaluated for the treatment of breast cancer, osteoporosis, and menopausal symptoms.[79] Two of the third-generation SERMs, lasofoxifene and bazedoxifene, are approved in the European Union for the treatment of postmenopausal osteoporosis in women at increased risk of fracture.[80]

The efficacy and safety of raloxifene for the prevention of osteoporosis in postmenopausal women were demonstrated in a study that found a 2.5% increase in bone mineral density in the lumbar spine and hip in a group of postmenopausal nonosteoporotic women treated with raloxifene for 2 years.[81] A significant reduction of vertebral fracture risk by raloxifene was subsequently demonstrated[82] in a study of 7705 postmenopausal women with existing osteoporosis. After 36 months, bone mineral density at the hip and spine increased in the women treated with 60 mg of raloxifene by 2.1% and 2.6%, respectively, compared

with those receiving placebo. At 36 months, 7.4% of women had at least one new vertebral fracture, including 10.1% of women receiving placebo and 6.6% of those receiving raloxifene at 60 mg/day. Compared with the placebo group, those receiving 60 mg of raloxifene had a relative risk for fracture of 0.7 ($p < 0.001$). Forty-six subjects needed raloxifene at 60 mg for 3 years to prevent one vertebral fracture in menopausal women without an existing fracture; for those with an existing fracture, 16 subjects required treatment. A recent meta-analysis confirmed the effects of raloxifene treatment on reduction of vertebral fracture risk in postmenopausal women without an effect on nonvertebral fracture risk.[83]

In a placebo-controlled clinical trial of 10,000 postmenopausal women with an increased risk of coronary heart disease followed for 5 to 6 years, raloxifene had an overall neutral effect on the incidence of cardiovascular events.[84] The incidence of all strokes did not differ between the raloxifene- and placebo-treated participants. However, in the raloxifene-treated individuals there was a higher incidence of fatal stroke, especially in smokers, as well as venous thromboembolic events (incidence rates per 100 women-years 0.22 vs. 0.15 [$p < 0.0499$] and 0.39 vs. 0.27 [$p = 0.02$], respectively).[85]

Raloxifene, in contrast to tamoxifen and estrogen, does not stimulate endometrial thickness or vaginal bleeding.[81] With regard to side effects, raloxifene causes an increased incidence of leg cramps and hot flushes.[86]

Endocrine approaches to breast cancer prevention have been increasingly successful in recent years. Four trials of tamoxifen administration for 5 years or longer in women at increased risk of breast cancer showed an approximately 50% reduction in breast cancer, but only for estrogen receptor–positive disease[87] (Fig. 27-4). Follow-up indicates that there was a carryover effect of tamoxifen after the completion of treatment at 5 years so that the preventive effect at 10 years is significantly greater than at 5 years.

Raloxifene has been compared with placebo in three trials—one in women with osteoporosis,[82,88] one in women with or at risk for cardiac disease,[84] and one in which raloxifene was compared with tamoxifen in women at high risk of breast cancer[89]—and reductions of 66%, 44%, and 50% in breast cancer risk were noted after 4 to 5 years of raloxifene therapy, respectively. The last trial showed that raloxifene was as effective as tamoxifen.[89] As with the

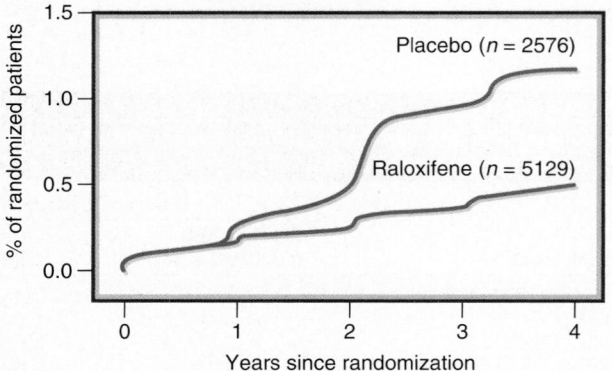

Figure 27-4 Effect of raloxifene administration (60 to 120 mg/day) on the cumulative incidence of breast cancer in 7705 postmenopausal women (mean age, 66.5 years) with osteoporosis. Statistical significance of the difference between the groups was $p < 0.001$. (From Cummings SR, Eckert S, Krueger KA, et al. The effect of raloxifene on risk of breast cancer in postmenopausal women: results from the MORE randomized trial. Multiple outcomes of raloxifene evaluation. *JAMA.* 1999;281:2189-2197.)

previous tamoxifen studies, raloxifene was only reducing the risk of estrogen receptor α–positive tumors.

In the United States, the 60-mg dose of raloxifene is now indicated for the treatment and prevention of osteoporosis in postmenopausal women, for reduction in risk of invasive breast cancer in postmenopausal women with osteoporosis, and in postmenopausal women at high risk for invasive breast cancer.[90,91] Although approved for use in the European Union for the prevention of vertebral fractures, lasofoxifene was never marketed. Also bazedoxifene is approved for use in the European Union. In a 3-year randomized controlled trial with an extension to 5 and 7 years among nearly 7000 postmenopausal women, bazedoxifene decreased the incidence of new vertebral fractures (2.3% with 20 mg bazedoxifene daily vs. 4.1% using placebo). Bazedozifene treatment was not associated with an increased risk of breast cancer or with increases in endometrial thickness or carcinoma.[92-94]

Tibolone is a compound that also regulates estrogen activity selectively at different tissues. It has a high efficacy in the treatment of climacteric symptoms and the prevention of bone loss. The compound is approved in many countries but not in the United States. In a 5-year trial tibolone (2.5 mg/day) was associated with a 45% decrease in vertebral fractures, a 26% decrease in nonvertebral fractures, a 68% decrease in invasive breast cancer, and a 69% decreased risk of colon cancer.[95] However, the tibolone-treated group had an increased risk of stroke (relative hazard 2.19 (p = 0.02).

Androgen Replacement

In premenopausal women androgen production originates equally from the adrenal glands and the ovaries. Androgen production in women declines with age. After menopause, circulating androgen levels decrease by more than 50%.

At present there is increasing awareness of the impact of low androgen levels on emotional and sexual well-being in perimenopausal women. No single androgen level is predictive of low female sexual function, and in one study the majority of 1423 women aged 18 to 75 years with low DHEAS levels had normal sexual function.[96]

The efficacy and safety of testosterone treatment for hypoactive sexual desire disorder in postmenopausal women were recently studied in a double-blind, placebo-controlled, 52-week trial in which over 800 women participated.[97] Treatment with a patch delivering 300 µg of testosterone per day resulted in a modest but meaningful improvement in sexual function. Similar results were found in a smaller study among 272 women treated with a testosterone patch for 6 months.[98] The long-term effects of testosterone, including effects on the breast, remain uncertain.

Hormone Therapy, Selective Estrogen Receptor Modulators, or No Treatment?

The issue of HT in postmenopausal women is controversial, and many aspects remain unresolved. The idea that HT is a global risk reduction strategy has been abandoned. Although the general benefits of HT in the short term during and after the menopausal transition are evident in women suffering from estrogen-withdrawal symptoms, the balance of the effects of long-term HT after menopause points in general to a negative outcome, with more harm than benefits. The evolution of the association of HT and cardiovascular risk from protection to harm and now to possible protection again has resulted in controversy and confusion.[99,100]

HT is usually prescribed for women aged 45 to 60 years who are experiencing vasomotor symptoms. HT is not indicated for cardioprotection for women in their 70s or for women who do not suffer from vasomotor symptoms or urogenital atrophy. Data clearly demonstrate, however, that clinicians can prescribe and women can use low-dose HT confidently during the time when therapy is most needed. The debate regarding the potential benefits of HT on cardiovascular risk and mortality for women who start therapy in proximity to the menopausal transition is not resolved. The benefit and risk of any therapy, including HT, should be reassessed periodically in each individual based on future scientific evidence.[100]

Currently, a vast armamentarium of other pharmacologic treatments to reduce cardiovascular and bone risks is available; these agents include cholesterol-lowering statins, beta blockers, SERMs, and bisphosphonates. An optimal choice of these different lifestyle drugs for menopausal women requires individualization of the treatment decision. Coronary artery disease, for example, is a complex disorder, resulting from an interaction of genetic predisposition and environmental factors. Risk factor modification (diet, smoking, physical activity) should be advised. Secondary prevention of coronary artery disease and atherosclerosis includes lipid-lowering drugs, aspirin, nitrates, and beta blockers.[101] For women with existing osteoporosis, HT is effective. However, SERMs and especially bisphosphonates come close or are better in their fracture-reducing effects. Recognition of an increased risk for breast cancer in menopausal women is an important consideration in the choice for SERMs. Chemoprevention of breast cancer with raloxifene has become a major consideration in the pharmacologic choice for risk reduction in the long-term preventive treatment of postmenopausal women.

ANDROPAUSE VERSUS LATE-ONSET HYPOGONADISM

Role of Testosterone During Aging

Age-associated hypogonadism does not develop as clearly in men at andropause as in women at menopause. The key difference is the gradual, often subtle, change in androgen levels in men versus the precipitate fall of estrogen production in women. It is generally agreed that as men age, there is a decline in serum total testosterone concentration that begins after the age of 40 years. In cross-sectional studies, the annual decline in total and free testosterone is 1.0%, and 1.2%, respectively. The higher decline in free testosterone levels is related to the increase in sex hormone–binding globulin (SHBG) levels with age.[37,102] However, it was also recently reported that serum testosterone was stable across age strata among men self-reporting very good health.[103] It remains unclear whether the well-known biologic changes occurring during aging in men (e.g., reduced sexual activity, muscle mass and strength, and skeletal mineralization) are causally related to these changes in testosterone bioactivity. The gradual decline in testosterone levels is called late-onset hypogonadism (LOH). In recent years there has been major disagreement on how to define androgen deficiency in the elderly male. According to practice guidelines,[104,105] the diagnosis of androgen deficiency in the elderly or LOH, for which testosterone treatment might be considered, should be based on the concurrent presence of consistent symptoms of hypogonadism and unequivocally low serum (free) testosterone.

The biochemical part consists of measuring morning serum total testosterone levels (two times) or determining a "free" testosterone concentration by additionally measuring SHBG levels. Most elderly men have testosterone levels within the normal range, with prevalence estimates of "low" (e.g., <10.4 nmol/L or <300 ng/dL) serum testosterone concentrations generally between 10% and 25%.[106,107] Most of these men with low testosterone levels will not come to clinical attention because testosterone levels are not routinely measured in clinical practice.[108] An important problem with a biochemical approach of the diagnosis of LOH in elderly men is also that men with low testosterone may not exhibit clinically significant symptoms, raising the possibility that large numbers of men, simply by virtue of falling below an arbitrary threshold, are diagnosed as needing testosterone replacement therapy.

Also, the clinical part to the diagnosis of androgen deficiency of the aging male has important drawbacks.[109] All symptoms and signs of androgen deficiency are nonspecific and readily accounted for or modified by several comorbid conditions and medications. Lethargy, reduced concentration, sleep disturbance, irritability, and depressed mood may relate to physical illness (and side effects of treatment), obesity, and lack of physical exercise and other lifestyle issues (such as alcohol or drug use), relationship difficulties, and occupational or financial stresses. Indeed, existing screening tools for androgen deficiency lack adequate specificity and sensitivity to be reliably employed in directing clinical diagnosis and treatment.

Araujo and associates[108] defined the prevalence of symptomatic androgen deficiency in men by studying the association between symptoms of androgen deficiency (low libido, erectile dysfunction, osteoporosis or fracture, or two of the following symptoms: sleep disturbance, depressed mood, lethargy, and diminished physical performance) and low serum total testosterone (<10.4 nmol/L = <300 ng/dL) and free testosterone (<0.17 nmol/L = <5 ng/dL) concentrations. In nearly 1500 men (aged 30-79 years), they found 24% with total testosterone levels less than 10.4 nmol/L and 11% with free testosterone levels below 0.17 nmol/L. The prevalence of symptoms was as follows: low libido (12%), erectile dysfunction (16%), osteoporosis/fracture (1%), and two or more of the nonspecific symptoms (20%). Although low testosterone levels were associated with symptoms, many men with low testosterone levels were asymptomatic (e.g., in men over 50 years: 47.6%). In Figure 27-5 the interrelationships are shown: symptomatic androgen deficiency with low serum testosterone levels (<10.4 nmol/L) was observed in 4.2% of men younger than 50 years and 8.4% of men older than 50 years. This prevalence rapidly increases with age, amounting to 18.4% among 70-year-olds.

Wu and coworkers tried to better identify those with LOH.[110] They surveyed a random population sample of 3369 men between the ages of 40 and 79 years (the European Male Aging Study, EMAS) and proposed minimal diagnostic criteria, consisting of the "syndromic" simultaneous presence of three sexual symptoms (i.e., poor morning erections, decreased sexual interest, and erectile dysfunction), together with a serum total testosterone level of 11 nmol/L (320 ng/dL) and free testosterone level of 220 pmol/L (6.4 ng/dL). Men fulfilling these criteria with serum total testosterone level at or below 8 nmol/L (230 ng/dL) are considered as having severe LOH. Prevalence of such defined LOH in the EMAS population increased with age, body mass index (BMI), and number of coexisting illnesses and was 5.1% in men 70 to 79 years old.[110] The men with LOH had a lower hemoglobin level, less muscle and bone mass, and poorer physical performance and general

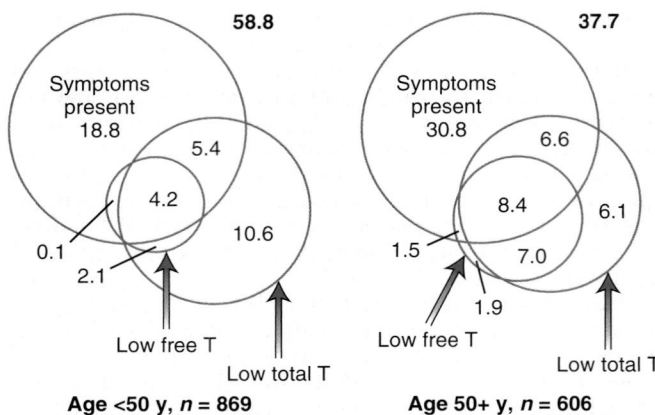

Figure 27-5 Venn diagrams showing the interrelationships among symptoms, low total testosterone (<10.4 nmol/L or <300 ng/dL), and low free testosterone (<0.17 nmol/L or <5 ng/dL) among men younger than 50 years *(left)* and men age 50 years or older *(right)*. Numbers displayed are percentages within each area. Positive symptom reports and low total and free testosterone were more common among older men. The presence of symptoms was related more strongly to testosterone levels in older as compared with younger men as indicated by a greater degree of overlap between symptom presence and low total and free testosterone among older (52.4% of men with low total or free testosterone had symptoms) compared with younger (43.1% of men with low total or free testosterone had symptoms) men. The intersection of symptoms and low total and free testosterone levels was more common in older men (prevalence of symptomatic androgen deficiency was 4.2% among men younger than 50 years of age and 8.4% among men age 50 years or older). *Note:* Circles for the Venn diagrams are proportional within age strata. T, testosterone. (From Araujo AB, Esche GR, Kupelian V, et al. Prevalence of symptomatic androgen deficiency in men. *J Clin Endocrinol Metab.* 2007;92:4241-4247.)

health compared with their peers; men with low testosterone only, irrespective of sexual symptoms, showed lesser magnitudes of associations with the same end points.[111]

In recent years it has become clear that an association exists between LOH and adverse metabolic conditions, such as obesity, metabolic syndrome (MetS), and type 2 diabetes mellitus.[112-114] An obesity-induced estrogen increase seems to play a major role in determining the negative feedback at the pituitary level, therefore inducing hypogonadotropic hypogonadism with low, or inappropriately normal, gonadotropin levels. Also, insulin resistance may contribute to the low testosterone levels seen in obese men.[112] Comorbid conditions were also associated with a lower total testosterone level. Three independent meta-analyses published in 2011, as well as a recent large observational study among nearly 2600 men participating in the EMAS, demonstrated an association between hypogonadism and overall and cardiovascular mortality rates, but they failed to find any statistical association with incident cardiovascular events.[114-117] These findings support the concept that cardiovascular frailty is associated with male hypogonadism.

Testosterone Replacement Therapy

Many persuasive reports in the literature demonstrate that testosterone replacement in men of all ages (young, adult, and old) with clear clinical and severe biochemical hypogonadism instantly reverses vasomotor activity (flushes and sweats); improves libido, sexual activity, and mood; increases muscle mass, strength, and bone mineralization; prevents fractures; decreases fat mass; and decreases fatigue and poor concentration.[46,102,118] Also, the treatment of normal adult men with supraphysiologic doses of testosterone, especially when combined with resistance exercise training, increased fat-free mass and muscle size and strength.[119]

Most studies reporting the results of androgen therapy in older men were small, short-term, noncontrolled, and without uniform end points. The results of a large randomized study in healthy elderly men seem representative for effects expected of androgen therapy.[120,121] Ninety-six men (mean age 73 years) wore a testosterone patch on the scrotum (6 mg of testosterone per 24 hours) or a placebo patch for 36 months. Mean serum testosterone concentrations in the men treated with testosterone increased from 12.7 ± 2.9 nmol/L (367 ± 7.9 ng/dL) before treatment to 21.7 ± 8.6 nmol/L (625 ± 249 ng/dL; $p < 0.001$) at 6 months of treatment and remained at that level for the duration of the study. The decrease in fat mass (-3.0 ± 0.5 kg) in the testosterone-treated men during the 36 months of treatment was significantly different from the decrease (-0.7 ± 0.5 kg) in the placebo-treated men ($p < 0.001$) (Fig. 27-6). The increase in lean mass (1.9 ± 0.3 kg) in the testosterone-treated men was significantly different from that in the placebo-treated men (0.2 ± 0.2 kg; $p < 0.001$).

Changes in knee extension and flexion strength, hand grip, walking speed, and other parameters of muscle strength and function were not significantly different in the two groups. Bone mineral density in the lumbar spine increased in both the testosterone-treated ($4.2\% \pm 0.8\%$) and placebo-treated ($2.5\% \pm 0.6\%$) groups, but mean changes did not differ between groups (see Fig. 27-6). However, the lower the pretreatment serum testosterone concentration, the greater the effects of testosterone treatment on lumbar spine bone density after 36 months ($p = 0.02$). A minimal effect ($0.9 \pm 1.0\%$) of testosterone treatment on bone mineral density was observed in men with a pretreatment serum testosterone concentration of 13.9 nmol/L (400 ng/dL), but an increase of $5.9\% \pm 2.2\%$ was found in men with a pretreatment testosterone concentration of 6.9 nmol/L (200 ng/dL).

The subjective perception of physical functioning decreased significantly during the 36 months of treatment in the placebo-treated group ($p < 0.001$) but not in the testosterone-treated group. Interestingly, the effect of testosterone treatment on the perception of physical functioning varied inversely with the pretreatment serum testosterone concentration ($p < 0.01$). There was no significant difference between the two treatment groups with regard to the subjective perception of energy or sexual functions.

With regard to the potential adverse effects of testosterone treatment in healthy elderly men, again the study by Snyder and colleagues[121] seems representative. The mean serum PSA concentration did not change during the 36 months of treatment in the placebo-treated group but increased by a relatively small but statistically significant ($p < 0.001$) amount by 6 months of treatment in the testosterone-treated group and remained relatively stable for the remainder of the study. The urine flow rate, volume of urine in the bladder after voiding, and number of clinically significant prostate events during the 3 years of the study were similar in the two groups. Hemoglobin and hematocrit did not change in the placebo-treated group during treatment, but both increased significantly ($p < 0.001$) in the testosterone-treated group within 6 months and remained relatively stable for the remainder of the study. Three men treated with testosterone developed persistent erythrocytosis (hemoglobin > 17.5 g/dL; hematocrit > 52%) during treatment.

Numerous studies of large populations of healthy men have shown a marked rise in the incidence of impotence to over 50% in men 60 to 70 years old.[122] Although this increased rate occurs in the same age group who show a clear decline in serum (free) testosterone levels, no causal

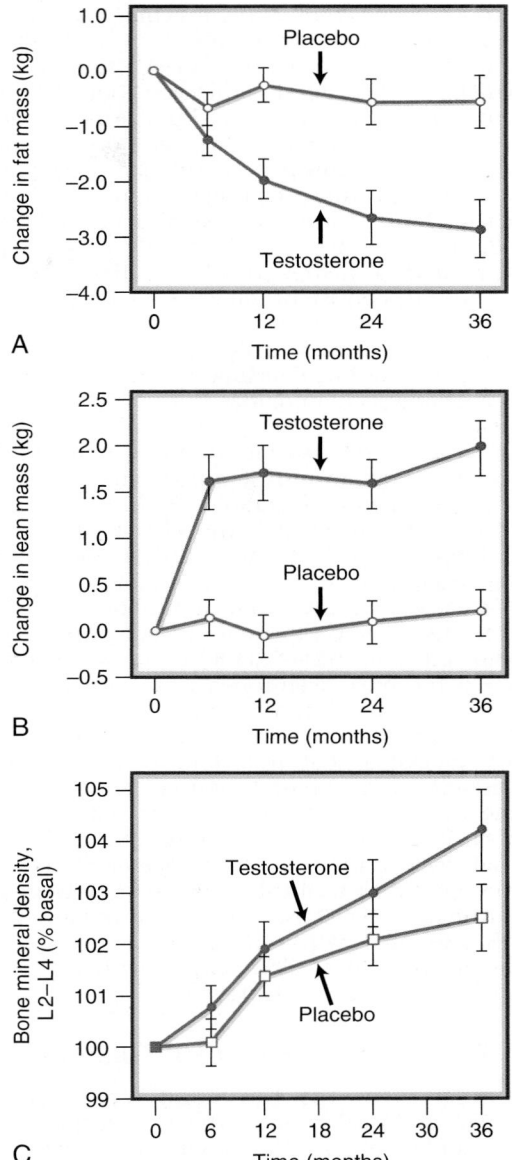

Figure 27-6 A to **C,** Mean ($\pm$ standard error) change from baseline in fat mass, lean mass, and bone mineral density of the lumbar spine (L2 to L4) as determined by dual-energy x-ray absorptiometry in 108 men older than 65 years who were treated with either testosterone or placebo (54 men each). The decrease in fat mass ($p < 0.005$) and the increase in lean mass ($p < 0.01$) in the testosterone-treated subjects were significantly different from those in placebo-treated subjects at 36 months. Bone mineral density increased significantly in both groups. (**A** and **B,** From Snyder PJ, Peachey H, Hannoush P, et al. Effect of testosterone treatment on body composition and muscle strength in men over 65 years of age. *J Clin Endocrinol Metab.* 1999;84:2647-2653. **C,** From Snyder PJ, Peachey H, Hannoush P, et al. Effect of testosterone treatment on bone mineral density in men over 65 years of age. *J Clin Endocrinol Metab.* 1999;84:1966-1972.)

relationships have been demonstrated. A systematic review and meta-analysis of randomized placebo-controlled trials concluded that testosterone use in normal men is associated with a small improvement in satisfaction with erectile function and moderate improvements in libido.[123] Other factors, such as atherosclerosis, alcohol consumption, smoking, and the quality of personal relationships, seem to be more important.[124,125] Only in the case of clear hypogonadism is the decrease in libido and potency restored by testosterone therapy.[105,118] The Endocrine Society Clinical Practice Guideline on testosterone therapy in adult men with androgen deficiency syndromes[104] summarized the observed effects of randomized placebo-controlled trials of testosterone administration over 1 to 3 years in older men with low-normal to low testosterone concentrations: a moderate effect on lumbar bone mineral density, but no reports on bone fracture rate; a significant increase in lean body mass (+2.7 kg on the average) and a reduction in fat mass (–2.0 kg) without a change in body weight; a greater improvement in grip strength (3.3 kg) than the placebo group, without consistent effects on lower extremity muscle strength and unequivocal effects on physical function; and inconsistent or insignificant effects on sexual function, quality of life, depression, and cognition.

The Guideline also summarized all reported adverse outcomes with testosterone therapy in elderly men.[104] It concluded that the combined rate of all prostate events was significantly greater in testosterone-treated men than in placebo-treated men (odds ratio 1.78; 95% CI, 1.07-2.95). Rates of prostate cancer, PSA greater than 4 ng/mL, and prostate biopsies were not significantly higher in the testosterone group than in the placebo group. Testosterone-treated men were nearly four times more likely than placebo-treated men to experience hematocrit greater than 50% (odds ratio 3.69; 95% CI, 1.82-7.51). The frequency of cardiovascular events, sleep apnea, and death did not differ significantly among groups. No significant changes in lipids were observed. A recently updated meta-analysis, however, suggested that testosterone therapy increases cardiovascular-related events among men. The risk of testosterone therapy was particularly marked in trials not funded by the pharmaceutical industry.[126] Cardiovascular-related adverse events should be adequately assessed in large randomized clinical trials involving older men with androgen deficiency. Thus, testosterone therapy of older men was associated with a higher risk of prostate events and hematocrit above 50% and potentially increased cardiovascular-related events.

Which Elderly Men Should Be Treated?

A key lesson from the Heart and Estrogen/Progestin Replacement and WHI studies is that conventional medical practice should not precede substantiation with reliable clinical evidence of safety and efficacy.[127] Androgen replacement in older men is the male counterpart of HT in postmenopausal women but differs crucially in that a clear syndrome of androgen deficiency is lacking. On the basis of a number of suggestive clinical features collected from the history, symptoms, or signs of an elderly man, the biochemical confirmation of androgen deficiency is sought. In previous discussions of testosterone replacement in older men,[124,128] it was suggested that the biochemical diagnosis of "true" hypogonadism seems certain if the serum total testosterone concentration is less than 6.9 nmol/L (200 ng/dL). This cutoff remains arbitrary and does not answer the question whether healthy elderly men with testosterone levels between 6.9 and 10.4 nmol/L are hypogonadal or whether such men would benefit from replacement therapy with testosterone. Also, it has been demonstrated that intercurrent diseases frequently result in a transient, sharp drop in serum testosterone concentrations,[129] whereas frail, elderly men in general tend to have testosterone levels 10% to 15% lower than those of healthy, age-matched control subjects.[130]

The current recommendation[104] is not to treat asymptomatic older men with age-related decline in testosterone levels. The latest Guideline suggests that clinicians con-

sider offering testosterone therapy on an individualized basis to older men with low testosterone levels on more than one occasion and clinically significant symptoms of androgen deficiency, after explicit discussion of uncertainty about the risks and benefits of testosterone therapy. Among experts there is disagreement on serum levels below which testosterone therapy should be offered to older men with symptoms. When a serum testosterone concentration is found to be low, an additional evaluation with measurements of serum gonadotropins and prolactin is mandatory in order to exclude pituitary disease.

If one decides to start testosterone replacement, the Guideline suggests that clinicians aim at achieving total testosterone levels in the lower part of the normal range of young men (400-500 ng/dL [14.0-17.5 nmol/L 0]). The dose should thus be titrated according to serum levels. Considerations concerning the choice of testosterone preparation as well as the route of administration (oral, injectable, implantable, or transdermal) are discussed in Chapter 20.

At present, the duration of testosterone administration is uncertain. Control of prostate size, PSA levels, and hematocrit is mandatory. The identification of elderly men who might benefit most from testosterone treatment remains uncertain, and the risks to the prostate and increased blood viscosity require further study.

ADRENOPAUSE

Role of Dehydroepiandrosterone During Aging

Humans are unique among primates and rodents because the human adrenal cortex secretes large amounts of the steroid precursor DHEA and its sulfate derivative DHEAS.[131] Serum DHEAS concentrations in adult men and women are 100 to 500 times higher than those of testosterone and 1000 to 10,000 times higher than those of estradiol. In normal subjects, serum concentrations of DHEA and DHEAS are highest in the third decade of life, after which the concentrations of both gradually decrease, so that by the age of 70 to 80 years, the values are about 20% of peak values in men and 30% of peak values in women (see Fig. 27-3).[41]

DHEA and DHEAS seem to be inactive precursors that are transformed within human tissues by a complicated network of enzymes into androgens or estrogens, or both (Fig. 27-7). The key enzymes are aromatase, steroid sulfatase, 3β-hydroxysteroid dehydrogenases (3β-HSD-1 and 3β-HSD-2), and at least seven organ-specific 17β-hydroxysteroid dehydrogenases (17β-HSD-1 to 17β-HSD-7). Labrie and coworkers[131] introduced the term *intracrinology* to describe this synthesis of active steroids in peripheral target tissues in which the action is exerted in the same cells in which synthesis takes place, without release into the extracellular space and general circulation.

In postmenopausal women, nearly 100% of sex steroids are synthesized in peripheral tissues from precursors of adrenal origin except for a small contribution from ovarian or adrenal testosterone and androstenedione. Thus, in postmenopausal women, virtually all active sex steroids are made in target tissues by an intracrine mechanism. In elderly men, the intracrine production of androgens is also important; less than 50% of the androgen supply is derived from testicular production.

The high secretion rate of adrenal precursor sex steroids in men and women differs from that in laboratory animal models, in which the secretion of sex steroids occurs

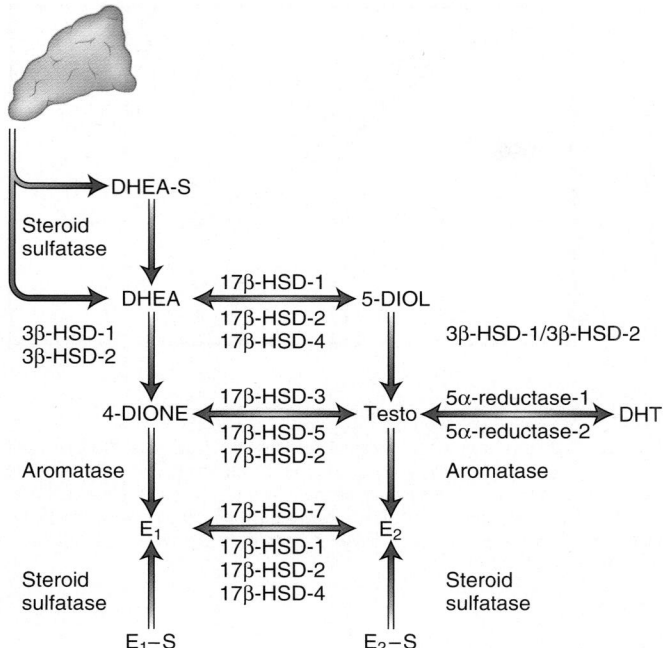

Figure 27-7 Human steroidogenic enzymes in peripheral intracrine tissues. DHEA, dehydroepiandrosterone; DHEAS, DHEA sulfate; DHT, dihydrotestosterone; 5-DIOL, androsterone-5-ene-3β,17β-diol; 4-DIONE, androstenedione; E_1, estrone; E_2, estradiol; 3β-HSD, 3β-hydroxysteroid dehydrogenase; 17β-HSD, 17β-hydroxysteroid dehydrogenase; Testo, testosterone. (Modified from Labrie F, Luu-The V, Lin SX, et al. Intracrinology: role of the family of 17 beta-hydroxysteroid dehydrogenases in human physiology and disease. *J Mol Endocrinol.* 2000;25:1-16.)

exclusively in the gonads. In rats and mice, long-term administration of DHEA prevented obesity, diabetes mellitus, cancer, and heart disease and enhanced immune function.[40,42,132]

These experimental animal data have been used to argue that DHEA administration in adult or elderly individuals prolongs life span and might be an "elixir of youth." Supportive data in humans are few, however, and highly controversial (see later). Epidemiologic studies indeed point to a mild cardioprotective effect of higher DHEAS levels in both men and women.[133] Functional parameters of activities of daily living in men older than 90 years were lowest in those with the lowest serum DHEAS concentrations,[41] and in healthy elderly individuals there was an association between the ratio of cortisol to DHEAS levels and cognitive impairment.[134]

CYP3A7, expressed in the human fetal liver and normally silenced after birth, plays a major role in the 16α-hydroxylation of DHEA, DHEAS, and estron. A common polymorphism in the *CYP3A7* gene *(CYP3A7*1C)* causes persistence of the enzymatic activity of the gene during adult life. Between 6% and 8% of the population are heterozygous carriers of this polymorphism, resulting in almost 50% lower DHEAS levels compared with homozygous carriers of the reference allele.[135] Interestingly, no evidence was found that such lowered levels are associated with an acceleration of the aging process.

Dehydroepiandrosterone Replacement Therapy

A physiologic functional role of DHEA in women has been ascertained in a careful double-blind study. In women with adrenal insufficiency,[136] DHEA administration (50 mg/day)

normalized serum concentrations of DHEA, DHEAS, androstenedione, and testosterone. DHEA significantly improved overall well-being as well as scores for depression and anxiety, the frequency of sexual thoughts, sexual interest, and satisfaction with both mental and physical aspects of sexuality.

A number of short controlled trials with DHEA in small groups of elderly individuals provided ambiguous results.[137,138] A 2-year placebo-controlled trial showed no effect of the oral administration of DHEA (at a dose of 75 mg/day in men and 50 mg/day in women) on body composition, muscle strength, or insulin sensitivity, as compared with placebo.[139] In this study involving 87 elderly men with low levels of DHEAS and bioavailable testosterone and 57 elderly women with low levels of DHEAS, DHEA levels increased in both sexes during DHEA administration by about 9.5 μmol/L.

These results are in line with a previous study[140] in 280 healthy subjects aged 60 to 79, in which 50 mg DHEA daily for 1 year did not improve body composition or muscle strength, although in women an increase in libido was noted. Also, a double-blind randomized controlled trial with 50 mg DHEA daily for 36 weeks in 50 elderly men, aged 70 or over, with low scores on muscle strength tests did not improve isometric grip strength, leg extensor power, and physical performance.[141]

With regard to one beneficial effect of DHEA administration the results seem rather consistently positive: increases in bone mineral density in women were repeatedly reported.[139,140,142,143] These positive effects, however, were very small and not more than approximately half the results observed with current osteoporosis therapies, such as with estrogens and bisphosphonates; therefore, they are unlikely to have a significant effect on the risk of fracture.[139] Review of placebo-controlled RCTs does not show benefits of oral DHEA in postmenopausal women for impaired sexual function, well-being, and cognitive performance or effects on lipid and carbohydrate metabolism.[144] A study from Weiss and colleagues, however, in both elderly men (*n* = 92) and women (*n* = 51) showed that DHEA supplementation in a dosage of 50 mg/day with a follow-up period of 12 months reduces arterial stiffness.[145]

Results from a recent meta-analysis showed that among the 644 elderly men enrolled in 8 RCTs measuring bone parameters, DHEA supplementation with a mean follow-up period of 52 weeks did not improve lumbar or femoral bone mineral density or formation or resorption of bone turnover markers.[146] The same meta-analysis, including a total of 25 RCTs with 1353 elderly men and a mean follow-up of 36 weeks, showed that DHEA supplementation of 50 to 100 mg/day was associated with a reduction of fat mass. No effect was observed for lipid and glycemic metabolism, sexual function, or quality of life.

Conclusions

DHEAS is a universal precursor for the peripheral local production and action of estrogens and androgens in target tissues such as brain, bone, skin, and adipose tissue. However, the importance of these pathways remains undefined, particularly in men, who have a relatively much higher production of testosterone from testicular origin. DHEA administration in the elderly, compared with placebo, increases serum DHEAS, testosterone, free testosterone, estrone, estradiol, and IGF-1 concentrations and lowers SHBG levels.[139,141,142] It is not known whether this increase in sex steroid levels induced by DHEA administration in the long term is safe with regard to the development or growth of ovarian, prostate, or other types of steroid-dependent cancers. The addition of DHEA (50 mg/day) to the existing large pool of DHEA and DHEAS in elderly individuals, even if they have been selected on the basis of low(ered) circulating levels of these steroids, has very limited clinically meaningful effects, if any.

DHEA, which is currently available as a dietary supplement, is widely used within the United States as an unapproved preventive treatment against aging. There are no convincing arguments at present to recommend the (routine) use of DHEA for delaying or preventing the physiologic consequences of aging, and its safety is unknown.[147,148]

SOMATOPAUSE

Role of Growth Hormone and Insulin-Like Growth Factor 1 During Aging

Elderly men and women secrete GH less frequently and at lower amplitude than do young people.[24] In fact, GH secretion declines approximately 14% per decade in normal individuals.[149,150] In parallel, serum levels of IGF-1 (see Fig. 27-3) are 20% to 80% lower in healthy elderly individuals than in healthy young adults.[151] However, whether this decline has adverse or beneficial effects is controversial. In invertebrates and rodents an attenuation of the insulin/IGF signaling pathway has led to an extension of life span.[152] Also, in humans, genetic defects in the somatotropic axis resulting in lower or decreased IGF-1 signaling may be associated with increased survival time.[153] Paradoxically, low IGF-1 concentrations in humans have been associated with increased risk for CVD, stroke, type 2 diabetes mellitus, and osteoporosis. A large number of studies over the last decade have looked for associations between IGF-1 levels and mortality risk. Some have found no association,[154-156] whereas other studies have found that lower levels of serum IGF-1[157,158] or serum IGF-1 bioactivity[159] were associated with greater all-cause mortality risk, and others found that low IGF-1 levels were predictive of extended survival.[160] One study found that higher IGF-1 levels were associated with a higher mortality risk,[161] and two studies found a higher risk in subjects with both high and low IGF-1 levels.[162,163] A recent meta-analysis indicated that both high and low IGF-1 concentrations are associated with increased cancer and cardiovascular-related mortality rates in the general population.[164]

IGF-1 and IGF-2 actions can be modulated by IGF binding proteins (IGFBP). IGFBP-2 is the second most abundant IGFBP in the circulation. This protein has received a lot of attention since the turn of the new century because of its potential role in the metabolic syndrome and several forms of cancer. IGFBP-2 levels increase with increasing age and decrease with increasing BMI.[165,166] A strong association between low IGFBP-2 levels and metabolic syndrome and low insulin sensitivity has been identified.[166-169] Surprisingly, however, although it was found that higher IGFBP-2 was associated with favorable risk factors, including lower fasting glucose and lower fasting insulin, recently, two studies found a strong association between higher IGFBP-2 and mortality rate in older adults (Fig. 27-8).[166,167] In both studies, the association appeared to be independent of acute-phase reactants (C-reactive protein and interleukin 6). Earlier, it was published that high serum IGFBP-2 concentrations are associated with a diminished physical function, lower muscle mass, and lower bone density in a population of elderly men.[170] The association of high IGFBP-2 concentrations

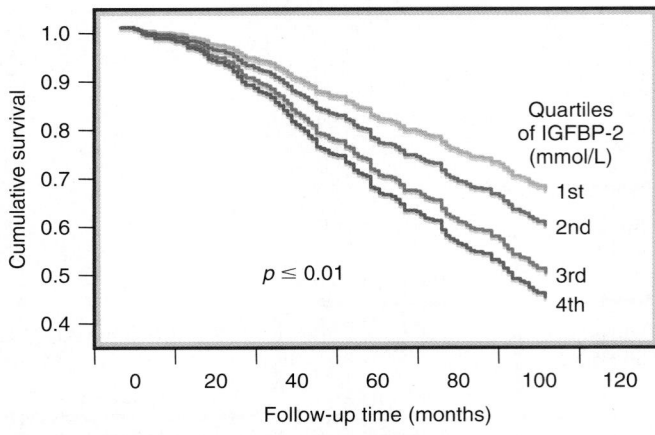

Figure 27-8 Survival curves showing the relationship between overall survival and insulin-like growth factor binding protein 2 (IGFBP-2) concentrations. *P* value denotes the significance between the first and the fourth quartiles. (From van den Beld AW, Blum WF, Brugts MP, et al. High IGFBP2 levels are not only associated with a better metabolic risk profile but also with increased mortality in elderly men. *Eur J Endocrinol.* 2012;167:111-117.)

and increased 8-year mortality rate was independent of the physical function. The clinical features of subjects with high IGFBP-2 levels are similar to those of subjects with protein energy malnutrition. Interestingly, these associations were, however, present in a population with a normal BMI and in subjects who lived independently.

IGFBP-2 concentrations are overexpressed in several forms of malignancies.[171] It is so far unclear what role IGFBP-2 plays in the development and progression of human cancers.[171] In the abovementioned studies, the associations between high IGFBP-2 levels and increased mortality rate were independent of the presence of malignancy. The role of IGFBP-2 in the aging process remains to be elucidated. The concept that this decline in GH and IGF-1 secretion contributes to the decline of functional capacity in elderly people (somatopause) is mainly derived from studies in which GH replacement therapy in GH-deficient adults was shown to increase muscle mass, muscle strength, bone mass, and the quality of life. A beneficial effect on the lipid profile and an important decrease in fat mass were also observed in these patients.[45,172,173] As in hypogonadal individuals, adult GH deficiency can thus be considered a model of normal aging because a number of catabolic processes that are central in the biology of aging can be reversed by GH replacement.

Growth Hormone Replacement Therapy

Rudman and colleagues,[174] after a ground-breaking randomized controlled trial in healthy men 61 to 81 years old with serum IGF-1 concentrations in the lower third for their age, reported in 1990 that GH treatment (30 mg/kg three times weekly for 6 months) restored the men's IGF-1 levels to "normal." In the treatment group, lean body mass rose by 8.8% and lumbar vertebral density increased by 1.6%. The magnitudes of these initial changes were equivalent to a reversal of the age-related changes by 10 to 20 years. However, during continuation of this study to 12 months, the significant positive effect on bone mineral density at any site was lost.[175]

In the subsequent years, it became clear that GH administration in healthy elderly individuals frequently caused acute adverse effects, such as carpal tunnel syndrome, gynecomastia, fluid retention, and hyperglycemia, which

TABLE 27-2

Effects of Growth Hormone Administration in Healthy Older Men*

Parameter	Mean Change in Variable		
	GH (n = 26)	Placebo (n = 26)	p Value
IGF-1 (ng/mL)	119.2	7.6	<.0001
Body Weight and Composition			
Weight, kg	0.5	1.0	>.2
Lean mass, %	4.3	−0.1	<.001
Fat mass, %	−13.1	−0.3	<.001
Bone mineral content, %	0.9	−0.1	.05
Skin thickness, %	13.4	1.1	.09
Muscle Strength, %			
Knee extension	3.8	1.3	>.2
Knee flexion	10.0	8.2	>.2
Hand grip	−1.5	3.8	.11
Maximal Oxygen Consumption, %	2.5	−2.0	>.2

*GH, 30 µg/kg three times a week, was administered for 6 months to 52 healthy 69-year-old men with well-preserved functional ability but low levels of IGF-1.
GH, growth hormone; IGF-1, insulin-like growth factor 1.
From Papadakis MA, Grady D, Black D, et al. Growth hormone replacement in healthy older men improves body composition but not functional ability. *Ann Intern Med.* 1996;124:708-716.

were severe enough for an appreciable number of individuals to drop out of these studies. The most disappointing aspect, however, was that no positive effects of GH administration were observed on muscle strength, maximal oxygen consumption, or functional capacity. In contrast, when GH was administered in combination with resistance exercise training, a significant positive effect on muscle mass and muscle strength was recorded that did not differ from that seen with placebo treatment, which suggests that GH does not add to the beneficial effects of exercise.[176,177] A representative example of a well-controlled study[178] of GH administration in unselected elderly men is given in Table 27-2.

In a systematic study of 31 articles describing 18 unique well-defined study populations the safety and efficacy of GH in the healthy elderly were reviewed.[179] A total of 220 participants who received GH for 107 person-years completed their studies. Their mean age was 69 years and they were overweight (mean BMI 28 kg/m²). Initial daily GH dose (mean 14 µg/kg body weight) and treatment duration (mean 27 weeks) varied. Overall fat mass decreased by 2.1 kg, and lean body mass increased by 2.1 kg in those treated with GH, and total cholesterol levels decreased by 0.29 mmol/L. Disappointingly, no consistent changes in muscle strength, physical activity, or psychosocial outcomes were observed.

GH is associated with substantial adverse effects.[179] In order to obtain insights into what can be expected the details of one particularly well-carried-out placebo-controlled study in healthy women (n = 57) and men (n = 74) aged 65 to 88 years is presented[180]: GH administered subcutaneously at an initial dose of 30 µg/kg, three times per week, then reduced to 20 µg/kg for 26 weeks, was associated with carpal tunnel syndrome in 38% of women versus 7% of those taking placebo and in 24% of men versus 0% of those taking placebo; edema in 39% of women (0% for placebo) and 30% of men (12% for placebo); and arthralgias in 46% of women (7% for placebo) and 41% of men (0% for placebo). Troublesome was the report that 18 men treated with GH developed glucose intolerance or

diabetes compared with 7 men in the nontreatment group.[180]

In a randomized controlled trial, Blackman and associates[180] studied the effects of a combination of GH and sex steroids in healthy elderly women and men. A slight increase in lean body mass and muscle strength was observed in elderly men treated with GH and testosterone but not in women who received GH and estrogen. In a study in healthy elderly men coadministration of low-dose GH with testosterone resulted also in slightly beneficial changes (muscle strength, quality of life) compared to GH or testosterone alone.[181] In a partially placebo-controlled trial among 112 older men, testosterone and recombinant human GH administration appeared not to worsen cardiometabolic risk in healthy older men after 4 months.[182] Earlier studies demonstrated that pharmacologic doses of GH prevent the *autocannibalistic* effects of acute diseases on muscle mass.[183] Confirmation is needed, however, before GH can gain a place in the treatment of acute catabolic states in frail elderly people.

Other components in the regulation of the GH–IGF-1 axis are effective in activating GH and IGF-1 secretion. Long-acting derivatives of the hypothalamic peptide growth hormone–releasing hormone, given twice daily subcutaneously for 14 days to healthy 70-year-old men, increased GH and IGF-1 levels to those encountered in 35-year-olds.[43] These studies suggest that somatopause is driven primarily by the hypothalamus and that pituitary somatotropes retain their capacity to synthesize and secrete high levels of GH.

Two ghrelin-mimetic GH secretagogues (GHSs) have also been demonstrated to be able to restore levels of GH and IGF-1 in elderly individuals to those of young adults.[184] Ghrelin, an octanoylated 28–amino acid peptide, stimulates GH secretion via a distinct, endogenous GHS receptor but also has appetite-stimulating activity.[185] These GHSs slightly increased fat-free mass without changing fat mass, muscle strength and function, or quality of life[186] and changed body composition and increased appetite, which was accompanied by small but significant improvements in some measures of physical function[187] in older adults.

The long-term safety of activating GH and IGF-1 levels in older people has become a concern because of reports of an association between serum IGF-1 concentrations and cancer risk. Individuals with high IGF-1 levels (or low IGFBP-3 levels) within the broad normal range have an increased risk of prostate, colon, and breast cancer.[188-190] These epidemiologic studies, together with experimental data, suggest that the IGF-1 system is involved in tumor development and progression. However, no causal relationship between IGF-1 levels and cancer risk has yet been established, and possible medical intervention directed at increasing IGF-1 bioactivity in elderly people will in most instances be given toward the end of life, presumably not allowing enough time to affect tumor development or progression.

Conclusions

During the aging process, GH–IGF-1 axis activity declines. It is unclear whether changes in body composition and functional capacity are directly related. GH administration in older adults causes an increase in lean body mass and an appreciable loss of fat mass. However, GH treatment does not improve muscle strength and functional capacity in elderly people, despite restoration of circulating IGF-1 concentrations to young adult levels. Furthermore, most dose regimens of GH cause appreciable adverse effects, and long-term safety with regard to tumor development and progression remains uncertain. Oral ghrelin-mimetics are also capable of restoring GH and IGF-1 levels in the elderly population, together with an increase in appetite. Modest functional improvement was observed in one study after 2 years of administration.

In the near future, clinical trials with such orally active molecules in frail elderly people or in elderly individuals with clearly lowered IGF-1 levels, or both, should be able to delineate the precise role of the GH–IGF-1 axis in the aging process. In such trials, much emphasis must be given to safety aspects. At present, there is no evidence to recommend medical intervention in the GH–IGF-1 axis as an antiaging effort, to prolong life, or to rejuvenate healthy elderly people.[191,192] Only elderly patients with GH deficiency caused by organic diseases, such as pituitary adenomas, clearly benefit from GH replacement therapy.[193]

THE CONCEPT OF SUCCESSFUL AGING

There is considerable variation in the effects of aging on healthy individuals, with some people exhibiting greater and others evidencing few or no age-related alterations in physiologic functions. It has been suggested that it might be useful to distinguish between usual and successful patterns of aging.[194] Genetic factors, lifestyle, and societal investments in a safe and healthful environment are important aspects of successful aging.[195] Traditionally, the aging process, including the development of physical frailty toward the end of life, has been considered physiologic and unavoidable.

It has recently become evident, however, that it might not be necessary to accept the grim stereotype of aging as an unalterable process of decline and loss.[194] As life expectancy rises further in the coming decades, the overarching goal should be "an increase in years of healthy life with a full range of functional capacity at each stage of life."[196] Such a compression of morbidity can be achieved by adapting lifestyle measures, but a number of aspects of the aging process of the endocrine system invite the development of routine medical intervention programs offering long-term replacement therapy with one or more hormones in order to delay the aging process and to allow humans to live for a longer period in a relatively intact state.[197] However, unfortunately, it should be concluded at present that hormonal interventions with sex steroids, DHEA, GH, and oral ghrelin agonists have very limited effects on physical capacity in elderly individuals but that adverse effects are often considerable.

REFERENCES

1. *WHO Methods for Life Expectancy and Healthy Life Expectancy*. Geneva, Switzerland: Department of Health Statistics and Information Systems (WHO); 2014.
2. *WHO World Health Report 2008: Primary Health Care Now More Than Ever*. Geneva, Switzerland: World Health Organization (WHO); 2008.
3. Department of Economic and Social Affairs (DESA). *World Population Aging 2009*. New York, NY: United Nations; 2009.
4. Campion EW. The oldest old. *N Engl J Med*. 1994;330:1819-1820.
5. Kosorok MR, Omenn GS, Diehr P, et al. Restricted activity days among older adults. *Am J Public Health*. 1992;82:1263-1267.
6. Fries JF. Aging, natural death, and the compression of morbidity. *N Engl J Med*. 1980;303:130-135.
7. Vita AJ, Terry RB, Hubert HB, Fries JF. Aging, health risks, and cumulative disability. *N Engl J Med*. 1998;338:1035-1041.
8. Rudman D, Rao MP. Serum insulin-like growth factor in healthy older men in relation to physical activity. In: Morley JE, Korenman SG, eds. *Endocrinology and Metabolism in the Elderly*. Oxford: Blackwell Scientific; 1992:50.
9. Buchner DM, Wagner EH. Preventing frail health. *Clin Geriatr Med*. 1992;8:1-17.
10. Tinetti ME, Speechley M, Ginter SF. Risk factors for falls among elderly persons living in the community. *N Engl J Med*. 1988;319:1701-1707.
11. Kallman DA, Plato CC, Tobin JD. The role of muscle loss in the age-related decline of grip strength: cross-sectional and longitudinal perspectives. *J Gerontol*. 1990;45:M82-M88.
12. Fiatarone MA, O'Neill EF, Ryan ND, et al. Exercise training and nutritional supplementation for physical frailty in very elderly people. *N Engl J Med*. 1994;330:1769-1775.
13. Guralnik JM, Ferrucci L, Simonsick EM, et al. Lower-extremity function in persons over the age of 70 years as a predictor of subsequent disability. *N Engl J Med*. 1995;332:556-561.
14. Morley JE. Pathophysiology of the anorexia of aging. *Curr Opin Clin Nutr Metab Care*. 2013;16:27-32.
15. Rudman WJ, Hagiwara AF. Sexual exploitation in advertising health and wellness products. *Women Health*. 1992;18:77-89.
16. Petersen RC, Smith GE, Waring SC, et al. Aging, memory, and mild cognitive impairment. *Int Psychogeriatr*. 1997;9(Suppl 1):65-69.
17. Mariotti S, Franceschi C, Cossarizza A, Pinchera A. The aging thyroid. *Endocr Rev*. 1995;16:686-715.
18. Hollowell JG, Staehling NW, Flanders WD, et al. Serum TSH, T(4), and thyroid antibodies in the United States population (1988 to 1994): National Health and Nutrition Examination Survey (NHANES III). *J Clin Endocrinol Metab*. 2002;87:489-499.
19. Bremner AP, Feddema P, Leedman PJ, et al. Age-related changes in thyroid function: a longitudinal study of a community-based cohort. *J Clin Endocrinol Metab*. 2012;97:1554-1562.
20. Waring AC, Arnold AM, Newman AB, et al. Longitudinal changes in thyroid function in the oldest old and survival: the cardiovascular health study all-stars study. *J Clin Endocrinol Metab*. 2012;97:3944-3950.
21. Surks MI, Ortiz E, Daniels GH, et al. Subclinical thyroid disease: scientific review and guidelines for diagnosis and management. *JAMA*. 2004;291:228-238.
22. Biondi B, Palmieri EA, Lombardi G, Fazio S. Effects of subclinical thyroid dysfunction on the heart. *Ann Intern Med*. 2002;137:904-914.
23. Razvi S, Shakoor A, Vanderpump M, et al. The influence of age on the relationship between subclinical hypothyroidism and ischemic heart disease: a metaanalysis. *J Clin Endocrinol Metab*. 2008;93:2998-3007.
24. Hyland KA, Arnold AM, Lee JS, Cappola AR. Persistent subclinical hypothyroidism and cardiovascular risk in the elderly: the cardiovascular health study. *J Clin Endocrinol Metab*. 2013;98:533-540.
25. Gussekloo J, van Exel E, de Craen AJ, et al. Thyroid status, disability and cognitive function, and survival in old age. *JAMA*. 2004;292:2591-2599.
26. van den Beld AW, Visser TJ, Feelders RA, et al. Thyroid hormone concentrations, disease, physical function, and mortality in elderly men. *J Clin Endocrinol Metab*. 2005;90:6403-6409.
27. Mariotti S. Thyroid function and aging: do serum 3,5,3'-triiodothyronine and thyroid-stimulating hormone concentrations give the Janus response? *J Clin Endocrinol Metab*. 2005;90:6735-6737.
28. Mariotti S. Mild hypothyroidism and ischemic heart disease: is age the answer? *J Clin Endocrinol Metab*. 2008;93:2969-2971.
29. Collet TH, Gussekloo J, Bauer DC, et al. Subclinical hyperthyroidism and the risk of coronary heart disease and mortality. *Arch Intern Med*. 2012;172:799-809.
30. Bahn RS, Burch HB, Cooper DS, et al. Hyperthyroidism and other causes of thyrotoxicosis: management guidelines of the American Thyroid Association and American Association of Clinical Endocrinologists. *Endocr Pract*. 2011;17:456-520.
31. Gan EH, Pearce SH. Clinical review: the thyroid in mind: cognitive function and low thyrotropin in older people. *J Clin Endocrinol Metab*. 2012;97:3438-3449.
32. Veldhuis JD, Sharma A, Roelfsema F. Age-dependent and gender-dependent regulation of hypothalamic-adrenocorticotropic-adrenal axis. *Endocrinol Metab Clin North Am*. 2013;42:201-225.
33. Gardner MP, Lightman S, Sayer AA, et al. Dysregulation of the hypothalamic pituitary adrenal (HPA) axis and physical performance at older ages: an individual participant meta-analysis. *Psychoneuroendocrinology*. 2013;38:40-49.
34. Kumari M, Shipley M, Stafford M, Kivimaki M. Association of diurnal patterns in salivary cortisol with all-cause and cardiovascular mortality: findings from the Whitehall II study. *J Clin Endocrinol Metab*. 2011;96:1478-1485.
35. Schoorlemmer RM, Peeters GM, van Schoor NM, Lips P. Relationships between cortisol level, mortality and chronic diseases in older persons. *Clin Endocrinol (Oxf)*. 2009;71:779-786.
36. Wise PM, Krajnak KM, Kashon ML. Menopause: the aging of multiple pacemakers. *Science*. 1996;273:67-70.
37. Vermeulen A. Clinical review 24: androgens in the aging male. *J Clin Endocrinol Metab*. 1991;73:221-224.
38. Harman SM, Tsitouras PD. Reproductive hormones in aging men. I. Measurement of sex steroids, basal luteinizing hormone, and Leydig cell response to human chorionic gonadotropin. *J Clin Endocrinol Metab*. 1980;51:35-40.
39. Harman SM, Tsitouras PD, Costa PT, Blackman MR. Reproductive hormones in aging men. II. Basal pituitary gonadotropins and

gonadotropin responses to luteinizing hormone-releasing hormone. *J Clin Endocrinol Metab.* 1982;54:547-551.

40. Herbert J. The age of dehydroepiandrosterone. *Lancet.* 1995;345: 1193-1194.

41. Ravaglia G, Forti P, Maioli F, et al. The relationship of dehydroepi-androsterone sulfate (DHEAS) to endocrine-metabolic parameters and functional status in the oldest-old. Results from an Italian study on healthy free-living over-ninety-year-olds. *J Clin Endocrinol Metab.* 1996;81:1173-1178.

42. Hornsby PJ. Biosynthesis of DHEAS by the human adrenal cortex and its age-related decline. *Ann N Y Acad Sci.* 1995;774:29-46.

43. Corpas E, Harman SM, Pineyro MA, et al. Growth hormone (GH)-releasing hormone-(1-29) twice daily reverses the decreased GH and insulin-like growth factor-I levels in old men. *J Clin Endocrinol Metab.* 1992;75:530-535.

44. Blackman MR. Pituitary hormones and aging. *Endocrinol Metab Clin North Am.* 1987;16:981-994.

45. Attanasio AF, Lamberts SW, Matranga AM, et al. Adult growth hormone (GH)-deficient patients demonstrate heterogeneity between childhood onset and adult onset before and during human GH treatment. Adult Growth Hormone Deficiency Study Group. *J Clin Endocrinol Metab.* 1997;82:82-88.

46. Wang C, Swerdloff RS, Iranmanesh A, et al. Transdermal testosterone gel improves sexual function, mood, muscle strength, and body composition parameters in hypogonadal men. *J Clin Endocrinol Metab.* 2000;85:2839-2853.

47. Broer SL, Broekmans FJ, Laven JS, Fauser BC. Anti-mullerian hormone: ovarian reserve testing and its potential clinical implications. *Hum Reprod Update.* 2014;20(5):688-701.

48. Broer SL, Eijkemans MJ, Scheffer GJ, et al. Anti-mullerian hormone predicts menopause: a long-term follow-up study in normoovulatory women. *J Clin Endocrinol Metab.* 2011;96:2532-2539.

49. Tehrani FR, Shakeri N, Solaymani-Dodaran M, Azizi F. Predicting age at menopause from serum antimullerian hormone concentration. *Menopause.* 2011;18:766-770.

50. Freeman EW, Sammel MD, Lin H, Gracia CR. Anti-mullerian hormone as a predictor of time to menopause in late reproductive age women. *J Clin Endocrinol Metab.* 2012;97:1673-1680.

51. Barrett-Connor E. Hormone replacement therapy. *BMJ.* 1998;317: 457-461.

52. Grady D, Rubin SM, Petitti DB, et al. Hormone therapy to prevent disease and prolong life in postmenopausal women. *Ann Intern Med.* 1992;117:1016-1037.

53. Barrett-Connor E, Grady D. Hormone replacement therapy, heart disease, and other considerations. *Annu Rev Public Health.* 1998;19: 55-72.

54. Grodstein F, Manson JE, Colditz GA, et al. A prospective, observational study of postmenopausal hormone therapy and primary prevention of cardiovascular disease. *Ann Intern Med.* 2000;133:933-941.

55. Rossouw JE, Anderson GL, Prentice RL, et al. Risks and benefits of estrogen plus progestin in healthy postmenopausal women: principal results from the Women's Health Initiative randomized controlled trial. *JAMA.* 2002;288:321-333.

56. Anderson GL, Limacher M, Assaf AR, et al. Effects of conjugated equine estrogen in postmenopausal women with hysterectomy: the Women's Health Initiative randomized controlled trial. *JAMA.* 2004; 291:1701-1712.

57. Cherry N, Gilmour K, Hannaford P, et al. Oestrogen therapy for prevention of reinfarction in postmenopausal women: a randomised placebo controlled trial. *Lancet.* 2002;360:2001-2008.

58. Hulley S, Grady D, Bush T, et al. Randomized trial of estrogen plus progestin for secondary prevention of coronary heart disease in postmenopausal women. Heart and Estrogen/progestin Replacement Study (HERS) Research Group. *JAMA.* 1998;280:605-613.

59. Viscoli CM, Brass LM, Kernan WN, et al. A clinical trial of estrogen-replacement therapy after ischemic stroke. *N Engl J Med.* 2001;345: 1243-1249.

60. Dubey RK, Imthurn B, Zacharia LC, Jackson EK. Hormone replacement therapy and cardiovascular disease: what went wrong and where do we go from here? *Hypertension.* 2004;44:789-795.

61. Peterson HB, Thacker SB, Corso PS, et al. Hormone therapy: making decisions in the face of uncertainty. *Arch Intern Med.* 2004;164: 2308-2312.

62. Manson JE, Allison MA, Rossouw JE, et al. Estrogen therapy and coronary-artery calcification. *N Engl J Med.* 2007;356:2591-2602.

63. Schierbeck LL, Rejnmark L, Tofteng CL, et al. Effect of hormone replacement therapy on cardiovascular events in recently postmeno-pausal women: randomised trial. *BMJ.* 2012;345:e6409.

64. Harman SM, Vittinghoff E, Brinton EA, et al. Timing and duration of menopausal hormone treatment may affect cardiovascular outcomes. *Am J Med.* 2011;124:199-205.

65. Harman SM. Menopausal hormone treatment cardiovascular disease: another look at an unresolved conundrum. *Fertil Steril.* 2014;101: 887-897.

66. Chlebowski RT, Hendrix SL, Langer RD, et al. Influence of estrogen plus progestin on breast cancer and mammography in healthy post-menopausal women: the Women's Health Initiative Randomized Trial. *JAMA.* 2003;289:3243-3253.

67. Li CI, Malone KE, Porter PL, et al. Relationship between long durations and different regimens of hormone therapy and risk of breast cancer. *JAMA.* 2003;289:3254-3263.

68. Weiss LK, Burkman RT, Cushing-Haugen KL, et al. Hormone replace-ment therapy regimens and breast cancer risk (1). *Obstet Gynecol.* 2002;100:1148-1158.

69. Beral V. Breast cancer and hormone-replacement therapy in the Million Women Study. *Lancet.* 2003;362:419-427.

70. Shumaker SA, Legault C, Kuller L, et al. Conjugated equine estrogens and incidence of probable dementia and mild cognitive impairment in postmenopausal women: Women's Health Initiative Memory Study. *JAMA.* 2004;291:2947-2958.

71. Hodis HN. Assessing benefits and risks of hormone therapy in 2008: new evidence, especially with regard to the heart. *Cleve Clin J Med.* 2008;75(Suppl 4):S3-S12.

72. Hays J, Ockene JK, Brunner RL, et al. Effects of estrogen plus progestin on health-related quality of life. *N Engl J Med.* 2003;348:1839-1854.

73. Utian WH, Shoupe D, Bachmann G, et al. Relief of vasomotor symp-toms and vaginal atrophy with lower doses of conjugated equine estrogens and medroxyprogesterone acetate. *Fertil Steril.* 2001;75: 1065-1079.

74. Santen RJ. Long-term tamoxifen therapy: can an antagonist become an agonist? *J Clin Endocrinol Metab.* 1996;81:2027-2029.

75. Grainger DJ, Metcalfe JC. Tamoxifen: teaching an old drug new tricks? *Nat Med.* 1996;2:381-385.

76. Grey AB, Stapleton JP, Evans MC, et al. The effect of the antiestrogen tamoxifen on bone mineral density in normal late postmenopausal women. *Am J Med.* 1995;99:636-641.

77. Draper MW, Flowers DE, Huster WJ, et al. A controlled trial of raloxi-fene (LY139481) HCl: impact on bone turnover and serum lipid profile in healthy postmenopausal women. *J Bone Miner Res.* 1996;11: 835-842.

78. Palacios S. The future of the new selective estrogen receptor modula-tors. *Menopause Int.* 2007;13:27-34.

79. Komm BS, Mirkin S. An overview of current and emerging SERMs. *J Steroid Biochem Mol Biol.* 2014;143:207-222.

80. Hadji P. The evolution of selective estrogen receptor modulators in osteoporosis therapy. *Climacteric.* 2012;15:513-523.

81. Delmas PD, Bjarnason NH, Mitlak BH, et al. Effects of raloxifene on bone mineral density, serum cholesterol concentrations, and uterine endometrium in postmenopausal women. *N Engl J Med.* 1997;337: 1641-1647.

82. Ettinger B, Black DM, Mitlak BH, et al. Reduction of vertebral fracture risk in postmenopausal women with osteoporosis treated with raloxi-fene: results from a 3-year randomized clinical trial. Multiple Out-comes of Raloxifene Evaluation (MORE) Investigators. *JAMA.* 1999; 282:637-645.

83. Seeman E, Crans GG, Diez-Perez A, et al. Anti-vertebral fracture effi-cacy of raloxifene: a meta-analysis. *Osteoporos Int.* 2006;17:313-316.

84. Barrett-Connor E, Mosca L, Collins P, et al. Effects of raloxifene on cardiovascular events and breast cancer in postmenopausal women. *N Engl J Med.* 2006;355:125-137.

85. Mosca L, Grady D, Barrett-Connor E, et al. Effect of raloxifene on stroke and venous thromboembolism according to subgroups in post-menopausal women at increased risk of coronary heart disease. *Stroke.* 2009;40:147-155.

86. Davies GC, Huster WJ, Lu Y, et al. Adverse events reported by post-menopausal women in controlled trials with raloxifene. *Obstet Gynecol.* 1999;93:558-565.

87. Howell A. The endocrine prevention of breast cancer. *Best Pract Res Clin Endocrinol Metab.* 2008;22:615-623.

88. Martino S, Cauley JA, Barrett-Connor E, et al. Continuing outcomes relevant to Evista: breast cancer incidence in postmenopausal osteo-porotic women in a randomized trial of raloxifene. *J Natl Cancer Inst.* 2004;96:1751-1761.

89. Vogel VG, Costantino JP, Wickerham DL, et al. Effects of tamoxifen vs raloxifene on the risk of developing invasive breast cancer and other disease outcomes: the NSABP Study of Tamoxifen and Raloxifene (STAR) P-2 trial. *JAMA.* 2006;295:2727-2741.

90. Moen MD, Keating GM. Raloxifene: a review of its use in the preven-tion of invasive breast cancer. *Drugs.* 2008;68:2059-2083.

91. Shelly W, Draper MW, Krishnan V, et al. Selective estrogen receptor modulators: an update on recent clinical findings. *Obstet Gynecol Surv.* 2008;63:163-181.

92. Silverman SL, Chines AA, Kendler DL, et al. Sustained efficacy and safety of bazedoxifene in preventing fractures in postmenopausal women with osteoporosis: results of a 5-year, randomized, placebo-controlled study. *Osteoporos Int.* 2012;23:351-363.

93. Silverman SL, Christiansen C, Genant HK, et al. Efficacy of bazedoxi-fene in reducing new vertebral fracture risk in postmenopausal women with osteoporosis: results from a 3-year, randomized, placebo-, and active-controlled clinical trial. *J Bone Miner Res.* 2008;23:1923-1934.

94. Palacios S, de Villiers TJ, Nardone Fde C, et al. Assessment of the safety of long-term bazedoxifene treatment on the reproductive tract in

postmenopausal women with osteoporosis: results of a 7-year, randomized, placebo-controlled, phase 3 study. *Maturitas.* 2013;76:81-87.

95. Cummings SR, Ettinger B, Delmas PD, et al. The effects of tibolone in older postmenopausal women. *N Engl J Med.* 2008;359:697-708.

96. Davis SR, Davison SL, Donath S, Bell RJ. Circulating androgen levels and self-reported sexual function in women. *JAMA.* 2005;294:91-96.

97. Davis SR, Moreau M, Kroll R, et al. Testosterone for low libido in postmenopausal women not taking estrogen. *N Engl J Med.* 2008;359: 2005-2017.

98. Panay N, Al-Azzawi F, Bouchard C, et al. Testosterone treatment of HSDD in naturally menopausal women: the ADORE study. *Climacteric.* 2010;13:121-131.

99. Rossouw JE. Postmenopausal hormone therapy for disease prevention: have we learned any lessons from the past? *Clin Pharmacol Ther.* 2008;83:14-16.

100. Tannen RL, Weiner MG, Xie D, Barnhart K. Perspectives on hormone replacement therapy: the Women's Health Initiative and new observational studies sampling the overall population. *Fertil Steril.* 2008;90: 258-264.

101. Nabel EG. Coronary heart disease in women—an ounce of prevention. *N Engl J Med.* 2000;343:572-574.

102. Tenover JS. Androgen administration to aging men. *Endocrinol Metab Clin North Am.* 1994;23:877-892.

103. Sartorius G, Spasevska S, Idan A, et al. Serum testosterone, dihydrotestosterone and estradiol concentrations in older men self-reporting very good health: the healthy man study. *Clin Endocrinol (Oxf).* 2012;77: 755-763.

104. Bhasin S, Cunningham GR, Hayes FJ, et al. Testosterone therapy in men with androgen deficiency syndromes: an Endocrine Society Clinical Practice Guideline. *J Clin Endocrinol Metab.* 2010;95:2536-2559.

105. Wang C, Nieschlag E, Swerdloff R, et al. Investigation, treatment and monitoring of late-onset hypogonadism in males: ISA, ISSAM, EAU, EAA and ASA recommendations. *Eur J Endocrinol.* 2008;159:507-514.

106. Vermeulen A, Kaufman JM. Diagnosis of hypogonadism in the aging male. *Aging Male.* 2002;5:170-176.

107. Harman SM, Metter EJ, Tobin JD, et al. Longitudinal effects of aging on serum total and free testosterone levels in healthy men. Baltimore Longitudinal Study of Aging. *J Clin Endocrinol Metab.* 2001; 86:724-731.

108. Araujo AB, Esche GR, Kupelian V, et al. Prevalence of symptomatic androgen deficiency in men. *J Clin Endocrinol Metab.* 2007;92:4241-4247.

109. McLachlan RI, Allan CA. Defining the prevalence and incidence of androgen deficiency in aging men: where are the goal posts? *J Clin Endocrinol Metab.* 2004;89:5916-5919.

110. Wu FC, Tajar A, Beynon JM, et al. Identification of late-onset hypogonadism in middle-aged and elderly men. *N Engl J Med.* 2010;363: 123-135.

111. Tajar A, Huhtaniemi IT, O'Neill TW, et al. Characteristics of androgen deficiency in late-onset hypogonadism: results from the European Male Aging Study (EMAS). *J Clin Endocrinol Metab.* 2012;97: 1508-1516.

112. Wu FC, Tajar A, Pye SR, et al. Hypothalamic-pituitary-testicular axis disruptions in older men are differentially linked to age and modifiable risk factors: the European Male Aging Study. *J Clin Endocrinol Metab.* 2008;93:2737-2745.

113. Corona G, Monami M, Rastrelli G, et al. Type 2 diabetes mellitus and testosterone: a meta-analysis study. *Int J Androl.* 2011;34:528-540.

114. Corona G, Monami M, Rastrelli G, et al. Testosterone and metabolic syndrome: a meta-analysis study. *J Sex Med.* 2011;8:272-283.

115. Araujo AB, Dixon JM, Suarez EA, et al. Clinical review: endogenous testosterone and mortality in men: a systematic review and meta-analysis. *J Clin Endocrinol Metab.* 2011;96:3007-3019.

116. Ruige JB, Mahmoud AM, De Bacquer D, Kaufman JM. Endogenous testosterone and cardiovascular disease in healthy men: a meta-analysis. *Heart.* 2011;97:870-875.

117. Pye SR, Huhtaniemi IT, Finn JD, et al. Late-onset hypogonadism and mortality in aging men. *J Clin Endocrinol Metab.* 2014;99:1357-1366.

118. Wang C, Eyre DR, Clark R, et al. Sublingual testosterone replacement improves muscle mass and strength, decreases bone resorption, and increases bone formation markers in hypogonadal men—a clinical research center study. *J Clin Endocrinol Metab.* 1996;81:3654-3662.

119. Bhasin S, Storer TW, Berman N, et al. The effects of supraphysiologic doses of testosterone on muscle size and strength in normal men. *N Engl J Med.* 1996;335:1-7.

120. Snyder PJ, Peachey H, Hannoush P, et al. Effect of testosterone treatment on body composition and muscle strength in men over 65 years of age. *J Clin Endocrinol Metab.* 1999;84:2647-2653.

121. Snyder PJ, Peachey H, Hannoush P, et al. Effect of testosterone treatment on bone mineral density in men over 65 years of age. *J Clin Endocrinol Metab.* 1999;84:1966-1972.

122. Pearlman CK, Kobashi LI. Frequency of intercourse in men. *J Urol.* 1972;107:298-301.

123. Bolona ER, Uraga MV, Haddad RM, et al. Testosterone use in men with sexual dysfunction: a systematic review and meta-analysis of randomized placebo-controlled trials. *Mayo Clin Proc.* 2007;82:20-28.

124. Bhasin S, Bremner WJ. Clinical review 85: emerging issues in androgen replacement therapy. *J Clin Endocrinol Metab.* 1997;82:3-8.

125. Bagatell CJ, Bremner WJ. Androgens in men—uses and abuses. *N Engl J Med.* 1996;334:707-714.

126. Xu L, Freeman G, Cowling BJ, Schooling CM. Testosterone therapy and cardiovascular events among men: a systematic review and meta-analysis of placebo-controlled randomized trials. *BMC Med.* 2013;11: 108.

127. Liu PY, Swerdloff RS, Veldhuis JD. Clinical review 171: the rationale, efficacy and safety of androgen therapy in older men: future research and current practice recommendations. *J Clin Endocrinol Metab.* 2004;89:4789-4796.

128. Bhasin S, Bagatell CJ, Bremner WJ, et al. Issues in testosterone replacement in older men. *J Clin Endocrinol Metab.* 1998;83:3435-3448.

129. Morley JE, Melmed S. Gonadal dysfunction in systemic disorders. *Metabolism.* 1979;28:1051-1073.

130. Gray A, Feldman HA, McKinlay JB, Longcope C. Age, disease, and changing sex hormone levels in middle-aged men: results of the Massachusetts Male Aging Study. *J Clin Endocrinol Metab.* 1991;73: 1016-1025.

131. Labrie F, Luu-The V, Lin SX, et al. Intracrinology: role of the family of 17 beta-hydroxysteroid dehydrogenases in human physiology and disease. *J Mol Endocrinol.* 2000;25:1-16.

132. Labrie F, Belanger A, Simard J, et al. DHEA and peripheral androgen and estrogen formation: intracinology. *Ann N Y Acad Sci.* 1995;774: 16-28.

133. Barrett-Connor E, Goodman-Gruen D. The epidemiology of DHEAS and cardiovascular disease. *Ann N Y Acad Sci.* 1995;774:259-270.

134. Kalmijn S, Launer LJ, Stolk RP, et al. A prospective study on cortisol, dehydroepiandrosterone sulfate, and cognitive function in the elderly. *J Clin Endocrinol Metab.* 1998;83:3487-3492.

135. Smit P, van Schaik RH, van der Werf M, et al. A common polymorphism in the CYP3A7 gene is associated with a nearly 50% reduction in serum dehydroepiandrosterone sulfate levels. *J Clin Endocrinol Metab.* 2005;90:5313-5316.

136. Arlt W, Callies F, van Vlijmen JC, et al. Dehydroepiandrosterone replacement in women with adrenal insufficiency. *N Engl J Med.* 1999;341:1013-1020.

137. Morales AJ, Nolan JJ, Nelson JC, Yen SS. Effects of replacement dose of dehydroepiandrosterone in men and women of advancing age. *J Clin Endocrinol Metab.* 1994;78:1360-1367.

138. Yen SS, Morales AJ, Khorram O. Replacement of DHEA in aging men and women. Potential remedial effects. *Ann N Y Acad Sci.* 1995;774: 128-142.

139. Nair KS, Rizza RA, O'Brien P, et al. DHEA in elderly women and DHEA or testosterone in elderly men. *N Engl J Med.* 2006;355:1647-1659.

140. Baulieu EE, Thomas G, Legrain S, et al. Dehydroepiandrosterone (DHEA), DHEA sulfate, and aging: contribution of the DHEAge Study to a sociobiomedical issue. *Proc Natl Acad Sci U S A.* 2000;97:4279-4284.

141. Muller M, van den Beld AW, van der Schouw YT, et al. Effects of dehydroepiandrosterone and atamestane supplementation on frailty in elderly men. *J Clin Endocrinol Metab.* 2006;91:3988-3991.

142. Jankowski CM, Gozansky WS, Kittelson JM, et al. Increases in bone mineral density in response to oral dehydroepiandrosterone replacement in older adults appear to be mediated by serum estrogens. *J Clin Endocrinol Metab.* 2008;93:4767-4773.

143. Weiss EP, Shah K, Fontana L, et al. Dehydroepiandrosterone replacement therapy in older adults: 1- and 2-y effects on bone. *Am J Clin Nutr.* 2009;89:1459-1467.

144. Davis SR, Panjari M, Stanczyk FZ. Clinical review: DHEA replacement for postmenopausal women. *J Clin Endocrinol Metab.* 2011;96:1642-1653.

145. Weiss EP, Villareal DT, Ehsani AA, et al. Dehydroepiandrosterone replacement therapy in older adults improves indices of arterial stiffness. *Aging Cell.* 2012;11:876-884.

146. Corona G, Rastrelli G, Giagulli VA, et al. Dehydroepiandrosterone supplementation in elderly men: a meta-analysis study of placebo-controlled trials. *J Clin Endocrinol Metab.* 2013;98:3615-3626.

147. Skolnick AA. Scientific verdict still out on DHEA. *JAMA.* 1996;276: 1365-1367.

148. Stewart PM. Aging and fountain-of-youth hormones. *N Engl J Med.* 2006;355:1724-1726.

149. Toogood AA, Jones J, O'Neill PA, et al. The diagnosis of severe growth hormone deficiency in elderly patients with hypothalamic-pituitary disease. *Clin Endocrinol (Oxf).* 1998;48:569-576.

150. Toogood AA, O'Neill PA, Shalet SM. Beyond the somatopause: growth hormone deficiency in adults over the age of 60 years. *J Clin Endocrinol Metab.* 1996;81:460-465.

151. Borst SE, Millard WJ, Lowenthal DT. Growth hormone, exercise, and aging: the future of therapy for the frail elderly. *J Am Geriatr Soc.* 1994;42:528-535.

152. Tatar M, Bartke A, Antebi A. The endocrine regulation of aging by insulin-like signals. *Science.* 2003;299:1346-1351.

153. Laron Z. Do deficiencies in growth hormone and insulin-like growth factor-1 (IGF-1) shorten or prolong longevity? *Mech Ageing Dev.* 2005; 126:305-307.

154. Kaplan RC, McGinn AP, Pollak MN, et al. High insulinlike growth factor binding protein 1 level predicts incident congestive heart failure in the elderly. *Am Heart J.* 2008;155:1006-1012.

155. Saydah S, Graubard B, Ballard-Barbash R, Berrigan D. Insulin-like growth factors and subsequent risk of mortality in the United States. *Am J Epidemiol.* 2007;166:518-526.

156. Laughlin GA, Barrett-Connor E, Criqui MH, Kritz-Silverstein D. The prospective association of serum insulin-like growth factor I (IGF-I) and IGF-binding protein-1 levels with all cause and cardiovascular disease mortality in older adults: the Rancho Bernardo Study. *J Clin Endocrinol Metab.* 2004;89:114-120.

157. Cappola AR, Xue QL, Ferrucci L, et al. Insulin-like growth factor I and interleukin-6 contribute synergistically to disability and mortality in older women. *J Clin Endocrinol Metab.* 2003;88:2019-2025.

158. Friedrich N, Haring R, Nauck M, et al. Mortality and serum insulin-like growth factor (IGF)-I and IGF binding protein 3 concentrations. *J Clin Endocrinol Metab.* 2009;94:1732-1739.

159. Brugts MP, Ranke MB, Hofland LJ, et al. Normal values of circulating insulin-like growth factor-I bioactivity in the healthy population: comparison with five widely used IGF-I immunoassays. *J Clin Endocrinol Metab.* 2008;93:2539-2545.

160. Milman S, Atzmon G, Huffman DM, et al. Low insulin-like growth factor-1 level predicts survival in humans with exceptional longevity. *Aging Cell.* 2014;13(4):769-771.

161. Andreassen M, Kistorp C, Raymond I, et al. Plasma insulin-like growth factor I as predictor of progression and all cause mortality in chronic heart failure. *Growth Horm IGF Res.* 2009;19:486-490.

162. Friedrich N, Schneider H, Dorr M, et al. All-cause mortality and serum insulin-like growth factor I in primary care patients. *Growth Horm IGF Res.* 2011;21:102-106.

163. van Bunderen CC, van Nieuwpoort IC, van Schoor NM, et al. The association of serum insulin-like growth factor-I with mortality, cardiovascular disease, and cancer in the elderly: a population-based study. *J Clin Endocrinol Metab.* 2010;95:4616-4624.

164. Burgers AM, Biermasz NR, Schoones JW, et al. Meta-analysis and dose-response metaregression: circulating insulin-like growth factor I (IGF-I) and mortality. *J Clin Endocrinol Metab.* 2011;96:2912-2920.

165. Mattsson A, Svensson D, Schuett B, et al. Multidimensional reference regions for IGF-I, IGFBP-2 and IGFBP-3 concentrations in serum of healthy adults. *Growth Horm IGF Res.* 2008;18:506-516.

166. van den Beld AW, Blum WF, Brugts MP, et al. High IGFBP2 levels are not only associated with a better metabolic risk profile but also with increased mortality in elderly men. *Eur J Endocrinol.* 2012;167: 111-117.

167. Hu D, Pawlikowska L, Kanaya A, et al. Serum insulin-like growth factor-1 binding proteins 1 and 2 and mortality in older adults: the Health, Aging, and Body Composition Study. *J Am Geriatr Soc.* 2009; 57:1213-1218.

168. Arafat AM, Weickert MO, Frystyk J, et al. The role of insulin-like growth factor (IGF) binding protein-2 in the insulin-mediated decrease in IGF-I bioactivity. *J Clin Endocrinol Metab.* 2009;94:5093-5101.

169. Heald AH, Kaushal K, Siddals KW, et al. Insulin-like growth factor binding protein-2 (IGFBP-2) is a marker for the metabolic syndrome. *Exp Clin Endocrinol Diabetes.* 2006;114:371-376.

170. van den Beld AW, Blum WF, Pols HA, et al. Serum insulin-like growth factor binding protein-2 levels as an indicator of functional ability in elderly men. *Eur J Endocrinol.* 2003;148:627-634.

171. Hoeflich A, Reisinger R, Lahm H, et al. Insulin-like growth factor-binding protein 2 in tumorigenesis: protector or promoter? *Cancer Res.* 2001;61:8601-8610.

172. Nass R, Huber RM, Klauss V, et al. Effect of growth hormone (hGH) replacement therapy on physical work capacity and cardiac and pulmonary function in patients with hGH deficiency acquired in adulthood. *J Clin Endocrinol Metab.* 1995;80:552-557.

173. Salomon F, Cuneo RC, Hesp R, Sonksen PH. The effects of treatment with recombinant human growth hormone on body composition and metabolism in adults with growth hormone deficiency. *N Engl J Med.* 1989;321:1797-1803.

174. Rudman D, Feller AG, Nagraj HS, et al. Effects of human growth hormone in men over 60 years old. *N Engl J Med.* 1990;323:1-6.

175. Rudman D, Feller AG, Cohn L, et al. Effects of human growth hormone on body composition in elderly men. *Horm Res.* 1991;36(Suppl 1): 73-81.

176. Taaffe DR, Pruitt L, Reim J, et al. Effect of recombinant human growth hormone on the muscle strength response to resistance exercise in elderly men. *J Clin Endocrinol Metab.* 1994;79:1361-1366.

177. Yarasheski KE, Zachwieja JJ, Campbell JA, Bier DM. Effect of growth hormone and resistance exercise on muscle growth and strength in older men. *Am J Physiol.* 1995;268:E268-E276.

178. Papadakis MA, Grady D, Black D, et al. Growth hormone replacement in healthy older men improves body composition but not functional ability. *Ann Intern Med.* 1996;124:708-716.

179. Liu H, Bravata DM, Olkin I, et al. Systematic review: the safety and efficacy of growth hormone in the healthy elderly. *Ann Intern Med.* 2007;146:104-115.

180. Blackman MR, Sorkin JD, Munzer T, et al. Growth hormone and sex steroid administration in healthy aged women and men: a randomized controlled trial. *JAMA.* 2002;288:2282-2292.

181. Giannoulis MG, Sonksen PH, Umpleby M, et al. The effects of growth hormone and/or testosterone in healthy elderly men: a randomized controlled trial. *J Clin Endocrinol Metab.* 2006;91:477-484.

182. He J, Bhasin S, Binder EF, et al. Cardiometabolic risks during anabolic hormone supplementation in older men. *Obesity (Silver Spring).* 2013;21:968-975.

183. Herndon DN, Barrow RE, Kunkel KR, et al. Effects of recombinant human growth hormone on donor-site healing in severely burned children. *Ann Surg.* 1990;212:424-429, discussion 430-421.

184. Chapman IM, Hartman ML, Pezzoli SS, Thorner MO. Enhancement of pulsatile growth hormone secretion by continuous infusion of a growth hormone-releasing peptide mimetic, L-692,429, in older adults—a clinical research center study. *J Clin Endocrinol Metab.* 1996;81:2874-2880.

185. Smith RG, Jiang H, Sun Y. Developments in ghrelin biology and potential clinical relevance. *Trends Endocrinol Metab.* 2005;16:436-442.

186. Nass R, Pezzoli SS, Oliveri MC, et al. Effects of an oral ghrelin mimetic on body composition and clinical outcomes in healthy older adults: a randomized trial. *Ann Intern Med.* 2008;149:601-611.

187. White HK, Petrie CD, Landschulz W, et al. Effects of an oral growth hormone secretagogue in older adults. *J Clin Endocrinol Metab.* 2009;94: 1198-1206.

188. Chan JM, Stampfer MJ, Giovannucci E, et al. Plasma insulin-like growth factor-I and prostate cancer risk: a prospective study. *Science.* 1998;279:563-566.

189. Hankinson SE, Willett WC, Colditz GA, et al. Circulating concentrations of insulin-like growth factor-I and risk of breast cancer. *Lancet.* 1998;351:1393-1396.

190. Ma J, Giovannucci E, Pollak M, Stampfer M. RESPONSE: Re: Prospective study of colorectal cancer risk in men and plasma levels of insulin-like growth factor (IGF)-I and IGF-binding protein-3. *J Natl Cancer Inst.* 1999;91:2052.

191. Olshansky SJ, Perls TT. New developments in the illegal provision of growth hormone for "anti-aging" and bodybuilding. *JAMA.* 2008; 299:2792-2794.

192. Perls TT, Reisman NR, Olshansky SJ. Provision or distribution of growth hormone for "antiaging": clinical and legal issues. *JAMA.* 2005;294:2086-2090.

193. Shalet SM. GH deficiency in the elderly: the case for GH replacement. *Clin Endocrinol (Oxf).* 2000;53:279-280.

194. Rowe JW, Kahn RL. Human aging: usual and successful. *Science.* 1987;237:143-149.

195. Hazzard WR. Weight control and exercise. Cardinal features of successful preventive gerontology. *JAMA.* 1995;274:1964-1965.

196. *National and Health Promotion and Disease Prevention Objectives.* Washington, DC: Government Printing Office; 1991.

197. Lamberts SW, van den Beld AW, van der Lely AJ. The endocrinology of aging. *Science.* 1997;278:419-424.

Section VII

Mineral Metabolism

CHAPTER 28

Hormones and Disorders of Mineral Metabolism

F. RICHARD BRINGHURST • MARIE B. DEMAY • HENRY M. KRONENBERG

KEY POINTS

- Parathyroid hormone (PTH), vitamin D, and fibroblast growth factor 23 (FGF23) together regulate the levels of calcium and phosphorus in the bloodstream to keep them relatively constant and slightly above the inherent solubility product of calcium and phosphate. These hormones act largely on cells in intestine, kidney, bone, and parathyroid gland.
- Primary hyperparathyroidism and malignant hypercalcemia are the commonest causes of hypercalcemia. All causes of hypercalcemia can be grouped as either PTH-dependent or PTH-independent.
- Hypocalcemic disorders can be usefully organized as PTH-related, vitamin D-related, or miscellaneous disorders.
- Disorders associated with abnormal levels of phosphate in the blood are usually caused by diseases of the kidney.
- Magnesium disorders usually reflect abnormalities of influx of magnesium across the intestine, excretion of magnesium by the kidney, or shifts among the intracellular and extracellular compartments.

BASIC BIOLOGY OF MINERAL METABOLISM: ROLES OF THE MINERAL IONS

Calcium (Ca) and phosphorus (P) are the principal constituents of bone, and together they compose 65% of its weight. Bone, in turn, contains nearly all of the calcium and phosphorus and over half of the magnesium in the human body. The quantitatively minor amounts of each of these ions in the extracellular fluid and within cells play crucial roles in normal physiology (Fig. 28-1).

Ninety-nine percent of total body calcium resides in bone, of which 99% is located within the crystal structure of the mineral phase. The remaining 1% of bone calcium is rapidly exchangeable with extracellular calcium; this calcium is equally distributed between the intracellular and extracellular fluids. Extracellular calcium is the principal substrate for the mineralization of cartilage and bone, but it also serves as a cofactor for many extracellular enzymes, most notably the enzymes of the coagulation cascade, and as a source of calcium ions that serve as signaling molecules for a great diversity of intracellular processes. These processes include automaticity of nerve and muscle; contraction of cardiac, skeletal, and smooth muscle; neurotransmitter release; and various forms of endocrine and exocrine secretion.

In blood, approximately 50% of total calcium is bound to proteins, mainly albumin and globulins. The ionized calcium concentration in serum is approximately 1.2 mmol/L (5 mg/dL), and it is this ionized fraction that is biologically active and that is tightly controlled by hormonal mechanisms. Because intracellular cytosolic free calcium concentrations typically are in the range of only 100 nM, a very large chemical gradient (i.e., $10,000:1$), augmented by the large negative electrical potential, favors calcium entry into cells through calcium channels. This gradient is maintained by the limited conductance of resting calcium channels and by the energy-dependent extrusion of calcium into the extracellular fluid via high-affinity Ca^{2+}- and H^+-adenosine triphosphatases (ATPases) and low-affinity sodium-calcium (Na^+-Ca^{2+}) exchangers.

More than 99% of intracellular calcium exists in the form of complexes within the mitochondrial compartment, bound to the inner plasma membrane, or associated with the inner membranes of the endoplasmic reticulum and other compartments. Release of calcium from membrane-bound compartments transduces cellular signals and is tightly regulated. The mechanisms responsible for translocations of intracellular calcium between the cytosol and these sequestered regions have become better understood with the identification of specific receptors for calciotropic signaling molecules such as the inositol triphosphate (IP_3) receptor and ryanodine receptors.

Phosphate is more widely distributed to nonosseous tissues than is calcium. Eighty-five percent of body

	Calcium ions	Phosphate ions
Extracellular		
Concentration		
total, in serum	2.5×10^{-3} M	1.00×10^{-3} M
free	1.2×10^{-3} M	0.85×10^{-3} M
Functions	Bone mineral Blood coagulation Membrane excitability	Bone mineral
Intracellular		
Concentration	10^{-7} M	$1-2 \times 10^{-3}$ M
Functions	**Signal for:** • Neuron activation • Hormone secretion • Muscle contraction	• Structural role • High energy bonds • Regulation of proteins by phosphorylation

Figure 28-1 Distribution and function of calcium and phosphate. Note the dramatic differences between intracellular and extracellular concentrations of calcium ion and the dramatically different functions of calcium and phosphate inside cells.

phosphate is in the mineral phase of bone, and the remainder is located in inorganic or organic form throughout the extracellular and intracellular compartments. In human serum, inorganic phosphate (P_i) is present at a concentration of approximately 1 mmol/L and exists almost entirely in ionized form as either $H_2PO_4^-$ or HPO_4^{2-}. Only 12% of serum phosphate is protein-bound, and an additional small fraction is loosely complexed with calcium, magnesium, and other cations. Intracellular free phosphate concentrations are generally comparable to those in the extracellular fluid (i.e., 1-2 mmol/L), although the inside-negative electrical potential of the cell creates a significant energy requirement for translocation of phosphate into cells. This process generally is accomplished through sodium-phosphate cotransport driven by the transmembrane sodium gradient. A number of sodium-phosphate cotransporters have been cloned; various cells and tissues employ different species of such transporters with distinctive regulatory characteristics.

Organic phosphate is a key component of virtually all classes of structural, informational, and effector molecules that are essential for normal genetic, developmental, and physiologic processes. Phosphate is an integral constituent of nucleic acids; phospholipids; complex carbohydrates; glycolytic intermediates; structural, signaling, and enzymatic phosphoproteins; and nucleotide cofactors for enzymes and G proteins. The need for the large amounts of phosphate incorporated into cellular constituents during cell proliferation explains why phosphate levels in the blood are regulated by insulin-like growth factor 1, in addition to regulation by hormones of bone mineralization. Of particular importance are the high-energy phosphate ester bonds present in molecules such as adenosine triphosphate (ATP), diphosphoglycerate, and creatine phosphate that store chemical energy. Phosphate plays a particularly prominent role as the key substrate or recognition site in numerous kinase and phosphatase regulatory cascades. Cytosolic phosphate per se also directly regulates a number of crucial intracellular reactions, including those involved in glucose transport, lactate production, and synthesis of ATP. In light of these diverse roles, it is not surprising that disorders of phosphate homeostasis associated with severe depletion of intracellular phosphate lead to profound and global impairment of organ function. Note that none of these roles for intracellular phosphate involves actions of intracellular calcium; the reason we are discussing these

together results solely from their intimate relationship in regulating bone mineralization outside cells.

Magnesium is the fourth most abundant cation in the body. Roughly half is found in bone and half in muscle and other soft tissues. As much as half of the magnesium in bone is not sequestered in the mineral phase but is freely exchangeable with the extracellular fluid and, therefore, may serve as a buffer against changes in extracellular magnesium concentration. Less than 1% of all magnesium in the body is present in the extracellular fluid, where the magnesium concentration is approximately 0.5 mmol/L. The concentration of magnesium in serum normally is 0.7 to 1.0 mmol/L, of which roughly one third is protein bound, 15% is loosely complexed with phosphate or other anions, and 55% is present as the free ion. Over 95% of intracellular magnesium is bound to other molecules, most notably ATP, the concentration of which is approximately 5 mmol/L. The intracellular cytosolic free magnesium concentration is approximately 0.5 mmol/L (i.e., 1000-fold higher than that of calcium) and is maintained by an active sodium-magnesium antiporter. The mechanism(s) whereby magnesium enters cells, presumably down a favorable electrochemical gradient, is unknown, although some evidence for regulated channels has been obtained.[1]

Intracellular magnesium, like phosphate, is necessary for a wide range of cellular functions. It is an essential cofactor in enzymatic reactions, including most of the same glycolytic, kinase, and phosphatase pathways that also involve phosphate. Magnesium serves to directly stabilize the structures of a variety of macromolecules and complexes, including deoxyribonucleic acid (DNA), ribonucleic acid (RNA), and ribosomes; is a key activator of the many ATPase-coupled ion transporters; and plays a direct role in mitochondrial oxidative metabolism. As a result, magnesium is critical for energy metabolism and the maintenance of a normal intracellular environment. Extracellular magnesium is crucial for normal neuromuscular excitability and nerve conduction, and many of the clinical consequences of magnesium deficiency or excess reflect abnormalities in this sphere.

The levels of extracellular calcium and phosphate are regulated in a coordinated way that reflects the roles of calcium and phosphate in mineralization of bone. The concentrations of these ions in body fluids are together close to the concentrations that could lead to spontaneous precipitation in soft tissues. In fact, elaborate mechanisms, most poorly understood, have evolved to prevent calcium phosphate precipitation in tissues and yet to allow the controlled deposition of calcium and phosphate in bone.[2] The importance of the mineral ions for normal cellular physiology as well as skeletal integrity is reflected in the powerful endocrine control mechanisms that have evolved to maintain their extracellular concentrations within relatively narrow limits. The following sections describe the structures, secretory controls, actions, and interactions of parathyroid hormone, calcitonin, 1,25-dihydroxyvitamin D (1,25[OH]₂D₃ or calcitriol), and fibroblast growth factor 23 (FGF23)—the major hormones involved in mineral ion homeostasis. Subsequent sections cover the wide variety of clinical disorders that accompany abnormalities in this hormonal network.

PARATHYROID HORMONE

Parathyroid hormone (PTH) is the peptide hormone that controls the minute-to-minute level of ionized calcium in the blood and extracellular fluids. PTH binds to cell surface receptors in bone and kidney, thereby triggering responses

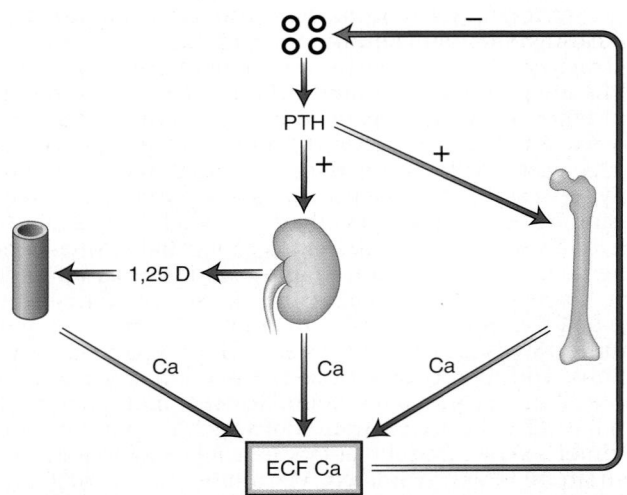

Figure 28-2 Parathyroid hormone (PTH)-calcium feedback loop that controls calcium homeostasis. Four organs—the parathyroid glands, intestine, kidney, and bone—together determine the parameters of calcium homeostasis. ECF, extracellular fluid; 1,25 D, 1,25-hydroxyvitamin D; –, negative effect; +, positive effect.

that increase blood calcium (Fig. 28-2). PTH also increases renal synthesis of $1,25(OH)_2D_3$, the hormonally active form of vitamin D, which then acts on the intestine to augment absorption of dietary calcium, in addition to promoting calcium fluxes into blood from bone and kidney. The resulting increase in blood calcium (and in $1,25[OH]_2D_3$) feeds back on the parathyroid glands to decrease the secretion of PTH. The parathyroid glands, bones, kidney, and gut are thus the crucial organs that participate in PTH-mediated calcium homeostasis.

Parathyroid Gland Biology

Parathyroid glands first appeared in evolutionary history with the exit of amphibians from the sea and a switch from dependence on gills to sole dependence on bone, intestine, and kidney to maintain extracellular calcium homeostasis. Reptiles, birds, and mammals all have parathyroid glands that develop as epithelial specializations from the endoderm of the pharyngeal pouches. Though fish have no discrete parathyroid glands, they do synthesize PTH.[3] The physiologic role of this PTH in fish is not yet defined.

Parathyroid chief cells have three properties vital to their homeostatic function: First, they rapidly secrete PTH in response to changes in blood calcium. Second, they can synthesize, process, and store large amounts of PTH in a regulated manner. Third, parathyroid cells replicate when chronically stimulated. These functional attributes allow for short-term, intermediate-term, and long-term adaptation, respectively, to changes in calcium availability.

Parathyroid Hormone Biosynthesis

PTH, a protein of 84 amino acids in mammals, is synthesized as a larger precursor, pre-proparathyroid hormone (pre-pro-PTH); with the explosion of genome sequencing in the past decade, the gene has been sequenced in a large number of species (see sequences in Genbank: http://www.ncbi.nlm.nih.gov/gene/5741) from fish to humans (reviewed in Pinheiro and associates[4]). Figure 28-3 illustrates representative pre-pro-PTH sequences. These pre-pro-PTH sequences share a 25-residue "pre" or signal sequence and a 6-residue "pro" sequence. The signal sequence, along with the short pro sequence, functions to direct the protein

```
            PRE              ↓ PRO ↓      PTH
         -31                   -6  +1       +10
Human    MIPAKDMAKVMIVMLAICFLTKSDG KSVKKR SVSEIQLMHN
Bovine   MMSAKDMVKVMIVMLAICFLARSDG KSVKKR AVSEIQFMHN
Porcine  MMSAKDTVKVMVVMLAICFLARSDG KPIKKR SVSEIQFMHN
Rat      MMSASTMAKVMILMLAVCFLTQADG KPVKKR AVSEIQLMHN
Canine   MMSAKDMVKVMIVMFAICFLAKSDG KPVKKR SVSEIQFMHN
Chicken  MTSTKNLAKAIVILYAICFFTNSDG RPMMKR SVSEMQLMHN

            +20       +30       +40       +50
Human    LGKHLNSMERVEWLRKKLQDVHNFVALGAPLAPRDAGSQRPRK
Bovine   LGKHLSSMERVEWLRKKLQDVHNFVALGASIAYRDGSSQRPRK
Porcine  LGKHLSSLERVEWLRKKLQDVHNFVALGASIVHRDGGSQRPRK
Rat      LGKHLASVERMQWLRKKLQDVHNFVSLGVQMAAREGSYQRPTK
Canine   LGKHLSSMERVEWLRKKLQDVHNFVALGAPIAHRDGSSQRPLK
Chicken  LGEHRHTVERQDWLQMKLQDVH..SALE......DARTQRPRN

            +60       +70                 +80
Human    KEDNVLVE...SHEKSLGEA..........DKADVNVLTKAKSQ
Bovine   KEDNVLVE...SHQKSLGEA..........DKADVDVLIKAKPQ
Porcine  KEDNVLVE...SHQKSLGEA..........DKAAVDVLIKAKPQ
Rat      KEENVLVD...GNSKSLGEG..........DKADVDVLVKAKSQ
Canine   KEDNVLVE...SYQKSLGEA..........DKADVDVLTKAKSQ
Chicken  KEDIVLGEIRNRRLLPEHLRAAVQKKSIDLDKAYMNVLFKTKP.
```

Figure 28-3 Sequences of pre-proparathyroid hormone from six species. Completely conserved residues are in boldface. Arrows indicate the sites of signal sequence ("pre") and "pro" sequence cleavage. Numbers start at residue +1 of mature parathyroid hormone (PTH); because of gaps, the numbers correspond only to the mammalian and not to the chicken sequence. Amino acids are indicated by the single-letter code: A, Ala; R, Arg; N, Asn; D, Asp; C, Cys; Q, Gln; E, Glu; G, Gly; H, His; I, Ile, L, Leu; K, Lys; M, Met; F, Phe; P, Pro; S, Ser; T, Thr; W, Trp; Y, Tyr; V, Val.

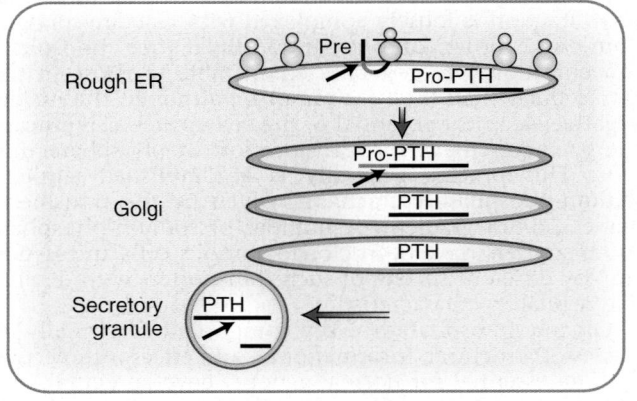

Figure 28-4 Intracellular processing of pre-proparathyroid hormone (pre-pro-PTH). *Diagonal arrows* indicate sites of cleavage by enzymes that generate pro-PTH in the rough endoplasmic reticulum (ER), PTH in the Golgi, and carboxy-terminal fragments of PTH in the secretory granule.

into the secretory pathway (Fig. 28-4). During transit across the membrane of the endoplasmic reticulum, the signal sequence is cleaved off and rapidly degraded. The importance of the signal sequence for normal secretion of PTH is illustrated by the hypoparathyroidism inherited in families carrying mutations in the signal sequence of pre-pro-PTH.[5,6]

The role of the short pro sequence is not completely understood; it may help the signal sequence work efficiently and ensure accurate cleavage of the precursor.[7] After cleavage of the pro sequence, the mature PTH(1–84) is concentrated in secretory vesicles and granules. One morphologically distinct subtype of granule contains both PTH and the proteases cathepsin B and cathepsin H. This co-localization of proteases and PTH in secretory granules probably explains the observation that a portion of the PTH secreted from parathyroid glands consists of carboxy-terminal PTH fragments. No amino-terminal fragments of

PTH are secreted. Although the possible functions of carboxy-terminal fragments of PTH are still poorly characterized, these fragments do not activate the PTH/PTHrP (PTH-related protein) receptor and may even block bone resorption[8] (see later discussion). The intracellular degradation of newly synthesized PTH thus may provide an important regulatory mechanism. Under conditions of hypercalcemia, the secretion of PTH is substantially decreased, and most of what is secreted consists of carboxy-terminal fragments.[9]

Parathyroid Hormone Secretion

Although catecholamines, magnesium, and other stimuli can affect PTH secretion, the major regulator of PTH secretion is the concentration of ionized calcium in blood. Increased serum ionized calcium leads to a decrease in PTH secretion (Fig. 28-5A). The shape of the dose-response curve is sigmoid. Properties of the parathyroid cell determine the conformation of the sigmoid curve but do not alone determine the point on the curve that represents a physiologic steady state for an individual. This point, usually between the midpoint and the bottom of the curve, is determined by how vigorously target organs respond to PTH.[10] Figure 28-5C *(solid line)* shows how an individual's calcium level rises in response to increases in PTH; the parathyroid gland's sigmoid curve is the *dotted line.* In the steady state, an individual's blood levels of PTH and calcium represent the intersection of the two lines.

The sigmoid curve reveals several important physiologic properties of the parathyroid gland. The minimal secretory rate is low, but not zero. The maximal secretory rate represents the reserve of the parathyroid's capacity to respond to hypocalcemia. Because values from normal persons in the steady state are located in the lower portion of the sigmoid curve, the system seems designed to respond more dramatically to hypocalcemia than to hypercalcemia.

Physiologic studies in humans confirmed this sigmoid relationship and have also revealed that the parathyroid cell responds both to the absolute level of blood calcium

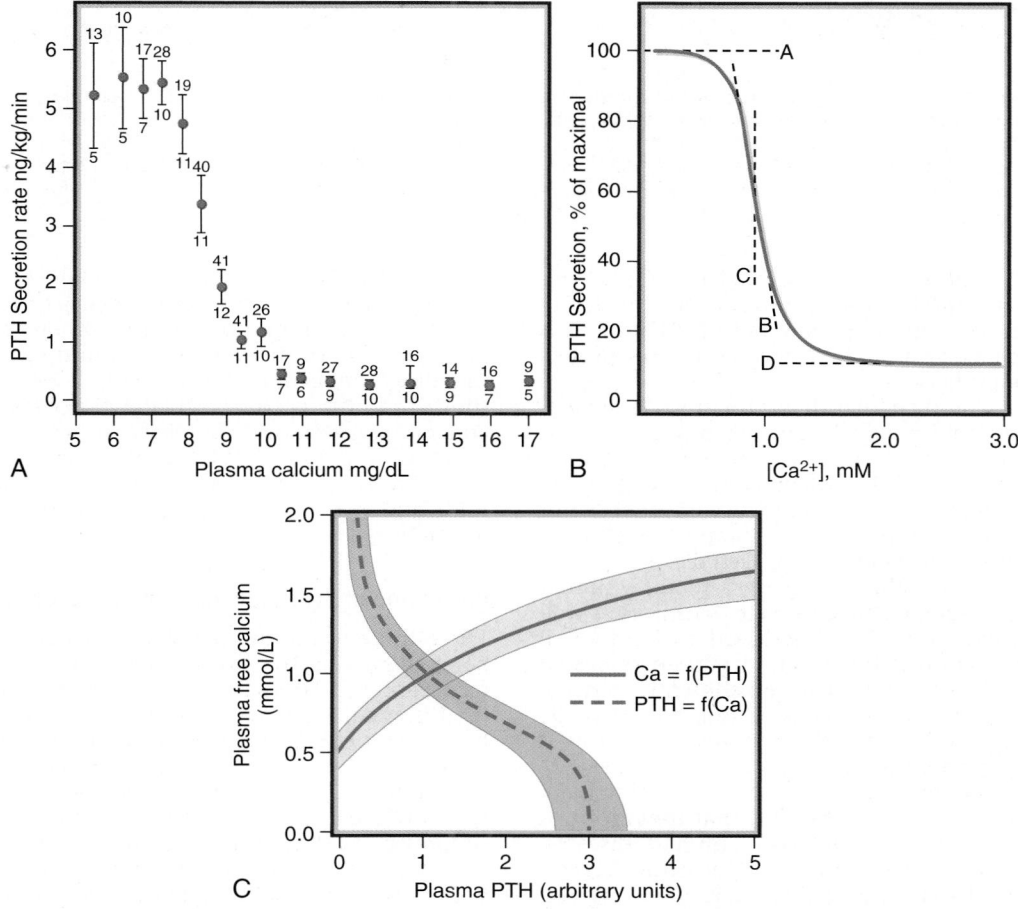

Figure 28-5 Parathyroid hormone (PTH) secretion. **A,** Secretory response of bovine parathyroid glands to induced alterations of plasma calcium concentration. Calves were infused with calcium chloride or ethylenediaminetetra-acetic acid (EDTA), and PTH secretion was assessed by measuring PTH levels in the parathyroid venous effluent. The symbols and *vertical bars* indicate the secretory rate (mean ± SE) in calcium concentration ranges of 1.0 or 0.5 mg/100 mL. The number of calves and samples are indicated, respectively, by numbers below and above the bars. **B,** Sigmoidal curve generated by the equation $Y = \{[A - D]/[1 + (X/C)^s]\} + D$. Such a curve can be defined by four parameters: the maximal secretory rate *(A)*, the slope of the curve at its midpoint *(B)*, the level of calcium at the midpoint (often called the set-point) *(C)*, and the minimal secretory rate *(D)*; the significance of *A, B, C,* and *D* is described in the text. **C,** Relationships between calcium and PTH levels when each in turn is treated as an independent variable. The *dashed line* represents the sigmoidal relationship between calcium and PTH, when calcium is the independent variable. This curve is the same as that in **A** and **B**, but it is turned on its side, because the axes are reversed. The *solid line* represents the relationship between calcium and PTH when PTH is considered the independent variable; values for this curve result from measurements made during PTH infusion into parathyroidectomized animals. Actual data are limited; thus, the curves should be viewed as illustrative. (A from Mayer GP, Hurst JG. Sigmoidal relationship between parathyroid hormone secretion rate and plasma calcium concentration in calves. *Endocrinology.* 1978;10:1037-1042; B modified from Brown EM. Four-parameter model of the sigmoidal relationship between parathyroid hormone release and extracellular calcium concentration in normal and abnormal parathyroid tissue. *J Clin Endocrinol Metab.* 1983;56:572-581; C from Parfitt AM. Calcium homeostasis. In: Mundy GR, Martin TJ, eds. *Physiology and Pharmacology of Bone.* Berlin: Springer-Verlag; 1993.)

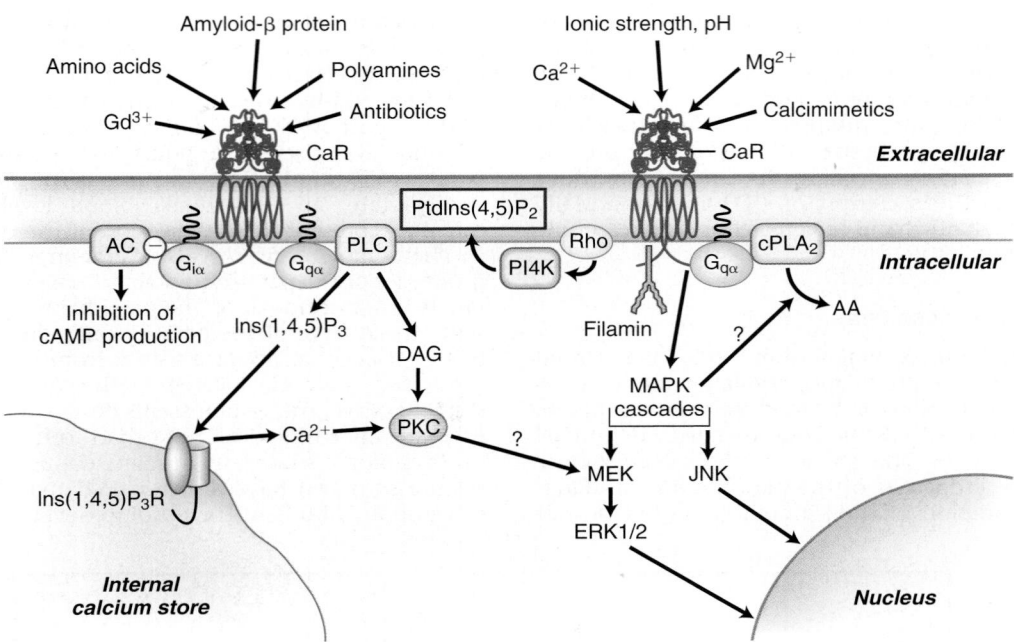

Figure 28-6 Signaling by the calcium-sensing receptor. Numerous agonists activate the calcium-sensing receptor (CaR) and trigger intracellular pathways. AA, arachidonic acid; AC, adenylate cyclase; cAMP, cyclic adenosine monophosphate; cPLA$_2$, cytosolic phospholipase A$_2$; DAG, diacylglycerol; ERK, extracellular signal–regulated kinase; G$_{i\alpha}$ and G$_{q\alpha}$, α-subunits of the i- and q-type heterotrimeric G proteins, respectively; Ins(1,4,5)P$_3$, inositol-1,4,5-trisphosphate; Ins(1,4,5)P$_3$R, inositol-1,4,5-trisphosphate receptor; JNK, Jun amino-terminal kinase; MAPK, mitogen-activated protein kinase; MEK, MAPK kinase; PI4K, phosphatidylinositol 4-kinase; PKC, protein kinase C; PLC, phospholipase C; PtdIns(4,5)P$_2$, phosphatidylinositol-4,5-bisphosphate. (From Hofer AM, Brown EM. Extracellular calcium sensing and signaling. *Nat Rev Mol Cell Biol.* 2003;4:530-538.)

and to the rate of fall of calcium level. Thus, PTH levels briefly rise higher during a sudden drop in blood calcium than they do during a more gradual fall in calcium. This property of the parathyroid cell offers an additional protection against sudden hypocalcemia.

The biochemical and cellular determinants of the parathyroid gland's sigmoid response curve are beginning to be defined. A parathyroid calcium-sensing receptor (CaSR) on the parathyroid cell surface is a member of the G protein–coupled family of receptors.[11] The sequence of the receptor suggests that it spans the plasma membrane seven times, like other receptors in the G protein–linked receptor family (Fig. 28-6). A large extracellular domain resembles similar domains in brain metabotropic glutamate receptors as well as bacterial periplasmic proteins designed to bind small ligands, including cations. The receptor has been expressed in a number of cell types and has been shown to activate phospholipase C (PLC) and to block stimulation of cyclic adenosine monophosphate (cAMP) production, just as it does in normal parathyroid cells.

The most convincing proof of the identity of the parathyroid CaSR has been the observation that mutations in the receptor gene cause characteristic human diseases. Inactivating mutations cause familial hypocalciuric hypercalcemia (FHH), a disease of defective calcium sensing (see later discussion),[12] whereas activating mutations cause familial hypoparathyroidism with hypercalciuria.[13] Furthermore, mice genetically engineered to have only one functioning copy of the *CASR* gene also have the expected defects in parathyroid calcium sensing.[14] Of importance, calcimimetic compounds that activate the cloned CaSR have been shown to inhibit PTH secretion in humans and are useful in the treatment of secondary hyperparathyroidism.[15,16] Despite the enormous increase in understanding of how extracellular calcium activates the parathyroid CaSR, the mechanism whereby this activation leads to a decrease in PTH secretion is poorly understood.

The CaSR is expressed widely. Expression in the renal tubules and calcitonin-producing cells of the thyroid contributes to calcium homeostasis, whereas expression in organs such as the brain points to multiple roles for calcium signaling. Knockout of the CaSR in osteoblasts of mice shows that this receptor regulates osteoblast differentiation and mineralization.[17] The observation that the CaSR also responds to physiologic levels of certain amino acids[18] suggests that the expression of the CaSR in the gut, parathyroid, and other sites may facilitate the assimilation of multiple nutrients.

Regulation of the Parathyroid Hormone Gene

The minute-to-minute regulation of PTH blood levels can be explained by the two mechanisms already discussed—regulation of PTH secretion by the CaSR and amplification of this regulation by intracellular degradation of stored hormone. Over a longer time frame, the parathyroid cell regulates the expression of the PTH gene as well.

Although 1,25(OH)$_2$D$_3$—the active form of vitamin D—has no direct effect on PTH secretion, it dramatically suppresses PTH gene transcription.[19] This suppression of transcription does not occur when 1,25(OH)$_2$D$_3$ is administered to chronically hypocalcemic animals, however, perhaps because hypocalcemia leads to a fall in parathyroid cell vitamin D receptors (VDRs) or because hypocalcemia increases the expression of calreticulin in the parathyroid.[20] The capability of hypocalcemia to override the effects of high levels of 1,25(OH)$_2$D$_3$ represents an important defense, because it provides a way for the parathyroid cell to synthesize large amounts of PTH and 1,25(OH)$_2$D$_3$ at the same time, when both are needed.

Calcium also regulates the biosynthesis of PTH. In vivo studies show that acute hypocalcemia in rats leads, within an hour, to an increase in PTH messenger RNA (mRNA). In contrast, hypercalcemia leads to little or no change in PTH mRNA. Thus, under normal conditions, the inhibition by calcium of PTH biosynthesis already is nearly maximal, just as it is for PTH secretion. The parathyroid gland is poised to respond to a fall in calcium much more readily than to a rise. The mechanism for the increase in PTH mRNA in response to hypocalcemia is uncertain; differing experimental paradigms suggest regulation at the levels of gene transcription, mRNA translation, and mRNA stability. The latter mechanism is the one best understood at the molecular level.[21] In the parathyroid cell, peptidyl-prolyl isomerase Pin1 binds to and leads to the activation of K-homology splicing regulator protein (KSRP), an RNA binding protein that destabilizes PTH mRNA. Mice without Pin1 have high PTH and PTH mRNA levels, and hypocalcemic rats and rats with chronic kidney disease have low Pin1 levels. Thus, Pin1 and KSRP regulate PTH mRNA levels in normal physiology and disease and mediate the effects of calcium and phosphate on PTH mRNA stability.[22]

For decades it has been known that phosphate elevation stimulates PTH secretion largely by lowering blood calcium and $1,25(OH)_2D_3$ levels. More recently, a series of studies in vitro[23,24] and in vivo[25] have demonstrated that phosphate can increase PTH secretion directly, independent of effects on blood calcium and $1,25(OH)_2D_3$. Phosphate increases PTH secretion acutely only after a delay and probably works largely through regulation of PTH mRNA levels. The mechanisms that phosphate uses to regulate parathyroid cells are unknown. FGF23, an important phosphate-regulating hormone (see later), activates FGF receptor 1 and its co-receptor, Klotho, on parathyroid cells and thereby suppresses PTH synthesis.[26] Whether this regulation by FGF23 is involved in the regulation of parathyroid function by phosphate is unknown. Even in the absence of Klotho in parathyroid cells, FGF23 can still suppress PTH synthesis through a calcineurin-sensitive pathway.[27] The regulation of the PTH gene has particular clinical relevance in patients with renal failure. Hypocalcemia, low levels of $1,25(OH)_2D_3$, hyperphosphatemia, FGF23 (see later in this chapter), and possibly, uremic toxins disrupt normal calcium homeostasis in this setting. Therapy with $1,25(OH)_2D_3$ and calcium increases calcium absorption and also inhibits PTH synthesis by direct effects on the parathyroid gland. Cinacalcet, an activator of the CaSR, lowers PTH secretion and thereby lowers both calcium and phosphorus levels.[15] (In renal failure, the role of PTH to increase release of phosphorus from bone dominates over any action of PTH to increase phosphaturia.) Prevention of hyperphosphatemia avoids the direct and indirect actions of phosphate to stimulate PTH secretion.

Regulation of Parathyroid Cell Number

Parathyroid cells divide during the growth of young animals but replicate little in adulthood.[28] Parathyroid cell number can dramatically increase, however, in the setting of hypocalcemia, low levels of $1,25(OH)_2D_3$, hyperphosphatemia, or uremia, or during neoplastic growth.

Calcium, acting through the parathyroid CaSR, restrains parathyroid proliferation. This effect has been demonstrated clinically in patients who lack both copies of the *CASR* gene. These neonates exhibit severe primary hyperparathyroidism with large, diffusely hyperplastic glands that presumably have developed because of insufficient activation of the parathyroid CaSR by extracellular calcium. Furthermore, administration of the calcimimetic compound NPS R-568, which activates the CaSR directly, prevents parathyroid cell proliferation in experimental uremia.

The role of $1,25(OH)_2D_3$, independent of blood calcium, in regulating parathyroid cell proliferation is less well established than that of calcium. That $1,25(OH)_2D_3$ can dramatically affect parathyroid cell number has been shown in vivo in many settings, but such studies cannot rigorously eliminate effects of transient changes in blood calcium. The suppression of proliferation of cultured parathyroid cells by $1,25(OH)_2D_3$[29] suggests that $1,25(OH)_2D_3$ can directly inhibit parathyroid cell replication. In experimental renal failure, the action of $1,25(OH)_2D_3$ to suppress the increase in parathyroid cell transforming growth factor-α (TGF-α) and epidermal growth factor (EGF) receptor expression that otherwise would occur may partly explain the dampening of parathyroid cell proliferation.[30] Nevertheless, vitamin D action through the VDR is not essential for control of parathyroid cell number, because calcium alone can prevent parathyroid cell hyperplasia in mice engineered to lack VDRs.[31]

Although the ability to increase parathyroid cell number in response to physiologic challenge represents an important defense against hypocalcemia, it is a slow response that is not easily reversible. When the need for an increased number of parathyroid cells disappears (e.g., after renal transplantation for uremia), persistent hyperparathyroidism can cause vexing clinical problems for months and years thereafter. The mechanisms for decreasing parathyroid cell number, if they exist, are poorly understood. Apoptosis of normal parathyroid cells in response to experimental manipulation has not been demonstrated.

Parathyroid Gland Development

Genes involved in making parathyroid cells during development may also regulate PTH synthesis and parathyroid cell number throughout life and may be mutated in human inherited hypoparathyroidism[32]; thus, an understanding of parathyroid cell development may have broad clinical implications. Although the genetic mechanisms used to generate parathyroid chief cells during development are largely unknown, the importance of several specific genes has become clear. Studies of gene knockout mice have shown that the hoxa3,[33] pax1,[34] pax9,[35] and Eya1[36] transcription factors are needed to form parathyroid glands as well as many other pharyngeal pouch derivatives, such as the thymus (reviewed in Liu and associates[37]). Another transcription factor, Tbx1, regulated by the developmental paracrine factor, sonic hedgehog, is expressed early in parathyroid development and is essential for parathyroid cell development. In humans and mice, haploinsufficiency for the transcription factor Tbx1 is likely to be responsible for many of the abnormalities found in DiGeorge syndrome, including hypoparathyroidism.[38] Even though these transcription factors together are essential for the early generation of parathyroid cells, another transcription factor, gcm2 in mice and GCMB in humans, is needed for the continued survival of parathyroid cells.[37] Furthermore, mice or humans[39] missing the *gcm2* and *GCMB* genes, respectively, have no parathyroid glands. In both species, the deletion of *gcm2* or *GCMB* (the human equivalent) is very specific for controlling parathyroid development because no abnormalities in other tissues have been noted. Studies of human hypoparathyroidism have led to the discovery of the likely roles of other transcription factors in parathyroid development. Sox3 is a transcription factor expressed in the pharyngeal pouches that give rise to parathyroid cells. Humans with X-linked hypoparathyroidism manifest a deletion-insertion near the end of the *SOX3* gene, a finding that suggests an important role for Sox3 in parathyroid development.[40] People with mutations in the gene encoding the transcription factor GATA3 exhibit a syndrome of hypoparathyroidism, sensorineural deafness, and renal anomalies when only one copy of the gene is mutated.[41]

Metabolism of Parathyroid Hormone

The earliest radioimmunoassays for PTH demonstrated that the molecular forms of PTH in the circulation differ from those in the parathyroid gland. Characterization of the metabolism of PTH and its fragments has clarified the origins and significance of immunoreactive PTH (iPTH) molecules in the bloodstream.[42] As noted previously, both PTH(1-84) and carboxy-terminal fragments of PTH are secreted from the parathyroid gland; the ratio of inactive PTH to active PTH secretion increases with increasing blood calcium. Secreted intact PTH(1-84) is extensively metabolized by liver (70%) and kidney (20%) and disappears from the circulation with a half-life of 2 minutes. This rapid peripheral metabolism of PTH is unaffected by widely varying levels of blood calcium or $1,25(OH)_2D_3$. Less than 1% of the secreted hormone finds its way to PTH receptors on physiologic target organs. These features of PTH metabolism ensure that the blood level of PTH is determined principally by the activity of the parathyroid glands and that the PTH level can respond rapidly to small changes in the rate of secretion of the hormone.

In the liver, a small amount of PTH binds to physiologically relevant PTH receptors, but most of the intact PTH is cleaved, initially after residues 33 and 36, probably by cathepsins. In the kidney, a small amount of intact PTH binds to physiologic PTH receptors, but most of the intact PTH is filtered at the glomerulus and subsequently bound by a large, membrane-bound luminal protein, megalin[43]; this binding leads to internalization and degradation of PTH by the tubules.[44] Carboxy-terminal fragments are also cleared efficiently by glomerular filtration. In fact, the kidney is the only known site of clearance of carboxy-terminal PTH fragments; these fragments thus accumulate dramatically when the glomerular filtration rate (GFR) falls. Even in the presence of normal renal function, the half-life of carboxy-terminal fragments of PTH exceeds that of PTH(1-84) by severalfold. Consequently, the concentration of carboxy-terminal fragments in the circulation exceeds that of intact PTH, even though intact PTH usually is the major form of PTH secreted from the parathyroid gland.

Careful analysis of PTH fragments using high-performance liquid chromatography (HPLC) and immunologic methods has revealed almost full-length PTH fragments missing the first several amino acids of the hormone, but containing most or all of the remaining hormone sequence.[45] These still incompletely characterized fragments are both secreted from the parathyroid gland and generated by peripheral metabolism of the hormone. Because they are missing the amino-terminal portion of PTH, they cannot stimulate cAMP production by the PTH/PTHrP receptor, and except in renal failure, they circulate in small amounts. Nevertheless, the possible biologic activity of these and other PTH fragments, possibly through novel receptors, remains an area of active investigation. Experiments with PTH(7-84) suggest that such extended carboxy-terminal fragments may exert potent effects in vivo, opposing those of intact PTH (see later discussion).[8,46,47]

Actions of Parathyroid Hormone

Actions of Parathyroid Hormone on the Kidney

Stimulation of Calcium Reabsorption. Almost all of the calcium in the initial glomerular filtrate is reabsorbed by the renal tubules. Sixty-five percent or more is reabsorbed by the proximal convoluted and straight tubules via a passive, paracellular route.[48] Changes in the transepithelial voltage gradient, determined largely by the rate of sodium reabsorption, control the rate of calcium transport in the proximal tubule, and PTH does little to affect calcium flux in this region. The remaining calcium is largely reabsorbed more distally—20% of the initial filtrate in the cortical thick ascending limb (cTAL) of Henle's loop and 10% in the distal convoluted and connecting tubules. In the cTAL, calcium reabsorption also is mainly passive and paracellular, although some transcellular, active calcium transport may occur as well. Efficient paracellular calcium and magnesium movement requires expression of a unique tight-junction protein, paracellin-1, also called claudin-16; mutant paracellin-1 genes underlie a rare renal calcium- and magnesium-wasting disorder.[49] Because paracellular cation transport in the cTAL is driven by the lumen-positive transepithelial voltage gradient that is established by active Na-K-Cl2 reabsorption, calcium reabsorption there is strongly inhibited by loop diuretics such as furosemide. The CaSR, initially characterized in the parathyroid, also is expressed in the cTAL. When activated by high blood calcium or magnesium, this receptor inhibits Na-K-Cl2 reabsorption in the cTAL and, thereby, paracellular calcium reabsorption as well. This provides a parathyroid-independent mechanism for controlling renal calcium handling in direct response to changes in blood calcium concentration.

Although PTH modestly stimulates paracellular calcium reabsorption in the cTAL, the primary site for hormonal regulation of renal calcium reabsorption is the distal nephron, which normally reabsorbs nearly all of the remaining 10% of filtered calcium by a unique transcellular active transport mechanism. As depicted in Figure 28-1, the intracellular level of calcium is extremely low, about 150 nM, compared with the millimolar levels in the glomerular filtrate and the blood. Calcium enters distal tubular cells from the tubular lumen down a highly favorable electrochemical gradient via selective channels (TRPV5 and TRPV6) present on the apical membrane of cells in the distal convoluted tubule (DCT) and connecting tubule (CNT). Intracellular calcium inhibits the activity of these channels, but this is minimized by the avid binding of calcium to calbindin-D28K, which effectively buffers cytosolic calcium and transports it to the basolateral membrane. There, calcium is ejected via active processes involving mainly the sodium-calcium exchanger NCX1 and an ATP-driven calcium pump (PMCA).[50] PTH stimulates DCT and CNT active calcium transport by upregulating several of these components, including TRPV5, calbindin-D28K, and NCX1, both directly and indirectly, via increased synthesis of $1,25(OH)_2D$.[50] PTH acutely increases the flux of calcium through TRPV5 by leading to protein kinase A (PKA) phosphorylation of a residue of TRPV5 that otherwise would bind calmodulin and thereby close the channel.[51]

The amount of calcium in the final urine reflects all of the tubular reabsorption processes just enumerated but also depends crucially on the initial filtered load of calcium. All of PTH's actions serve to raise the blood calcium level so that the filtered load of calcium is high in states of PTH excess. In that setting, even though the rate of distal tubular calcium reabsorption is increased by PTH, the total amount of calcium in the final urine is likely to be high, because of the high initial filtered load.

Inhibition of Phosphate Transport. Phosphate reabsorption occurs mainly in the proximal renal tubules, which reclaim roughly 80% of the filtered load. Some additional phosphate (8% to 10%) is reabsorbed in the distal tubule (but

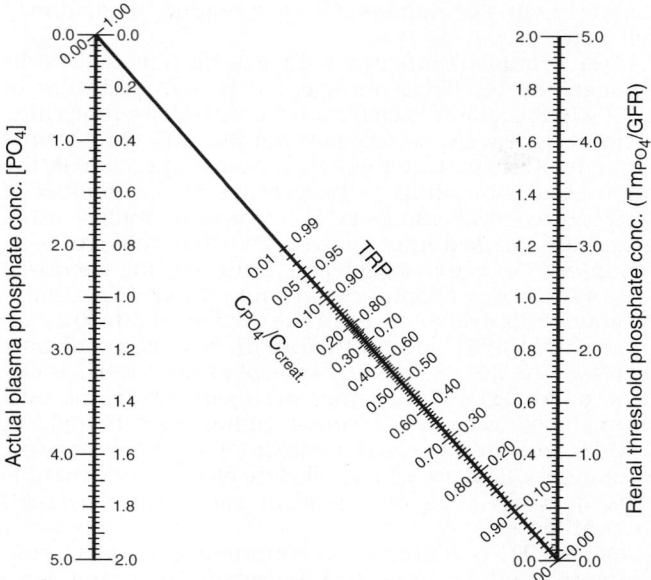

Figure 28-7 Nomogram for determining renal threshold phosphate concentration (Tm_{PO4}/GFR) from the plasma phosphate concentration and the fractional reabsorption of filtered phosphate (TRP) or fractional excretion of filtered phosphate (1 − TRP, or C_{PO4}/C_{creat}). Because the blood level of phosphate influences the renal handling of phosphate, the renal threshold phosphate concentration best separates normal from abnormal renal phosphate handling. C, clearance; creat, creatinine; GFR, glomerular filtration rate; TRP, tubular resorption of phosphate. (From Walton RJ, Bijvoet OLM. Nomogram of derivation of renal threshold phosphate concentration. *Lancet.* 1975; 2:309-310.)

not in Henle's loop), leaving about 10% to 12% for excretion in the urine. The normal overall fractional tubular reabsorption of phosphate (TRP), therefore, is about 90%, although a more reliable measure of renal phosphate handling is the *phosphate threshold* (TmP/GFR), which can be derived from the TRP through the use of a nomogram (Fig. 28-7) based on studies of experimental phosphate infusions in healthy persons and in patients with a variety of diseases that affect phosphate excretion.[52]

Phosphate reabsorption in both proximal and distal tubules is strongly inhibited by PTH, although the proximal effect is quantitatively most important. Phosphate is reabsorbed by a transepithelial route. Transport from the glomerular filtrate into the cell is mediated by specific sodium phosphate (NaPi) cotransporters, several types of which have been cloned and extensively characterized.[53] The low level of sodium within the cell drives the cotransport of sodium and phosphate, even though the phosphate travels up an electrochemical gradient. In response to PTH, the maximum velocity (V_{max}) for sodium phosphate cotransport decreases because NaPi cotransporters (both NaPi-IIa and NaPi-IIc) are rapidly (in 15 minutes) sequestered within subapical endocytic vesicles, after which they are delivered to lysosomes and undergo proteolysis.[54] cAMP and PKA mediate the rapid decrease in phosphate transport in response to PTH, though PLC activation by the PTH receptor is also required for prolonged suppression of phosphate transport by PTH.[55] This response to PTH is dependent upon Na+/H+ exchange regulatory factors (NHERFs), which physically interact with both the PTH/PTHrP receptor and the NaPi-II transporters and control the pattern of PTH receptor signaling.[56,57] Conversely, in hypoparathyroidism expression of NaPi protein and mRNA is strongly upregulated.

Dietary intake of phosphate also reciprocally regulates the expression and activity of NaPi cotransporters and, thus, the proximal tubular absorption of phosphate by a mechanism that is independent of PTH. Dietary deprivation of phosphate, for example, leads to a stimulation of phosphate reabsorption that can override the effects of PTH on the proximal tubule. It is likely that this dietary regulation of NaPi expression is mediated by FGF23[58] (see later discussion).

Other Renal Effects of Parathyroid Hormone. PTH stimulates the synthesis of 1,25(OH)₂D in the proximal tubule by rapidly inducing transcription of the 25-hydroxyvitamin D (25[OH]D) 1α-hydroxylase gene, an effect that can be overridden by hypercalcemia or by 1,25(OH)₂D. The interactions of 1,25(OH)₂D and PTH in regulating the 25(OH)D 1α-hydroxylase gene involve both PKA-mediated phosphorylation of an activating transcription factor and protein kinase C–mediated demethylation of DNA upstream of the 25(OH)D 1α-hydroxylase gene.[59] PTH inhibits proximal tubular transcription of the 25(OH)D 24-hydroxylase gene and antagonizes the upregulation of 24-hydroxylase activity by 1,25(OH)₂D. (See discussion under "Metabolism of Vitamin D.") PTH inhibits proximal tubular sodium, water, and bicarbonate reabsorption, mainly via inhibition of the apical Na+/H+ exchanger (NHE3) and the basolateral Na+/K+-ATPase. PTH also stimulates proximal tubular gluconeogenesis and acts directly on glomerular podocytes to decrease both single nephron and whole kidney GFR.

Actions of Parathyroid Hormone on Bone

The actions of PTH on bone are complicated because PTH acts on a number of cell types both directly and indirectly. For years, the release of calcium from bone through stimulation of bone resorption has been considered to be the major action of PTH on bone. This is only part of the story, however. In fact, PTH administration by any route increases both bone resorption by increasing osteoclast number and bone formation by increasing osteoblast number. Which action dominates depends on the dose of PTH and the route of administration. When PTH is administered continuously, the effect of PTH on bone resorption dominates, and the net result is release of calcium from bone and a decrease in bone mass. This action of PTH thus contributes to the increase in blood calcium seen in the disease, primary hyperparathyroidism. In similar fashion, administration of a soluble form of receptor activator for nuclear factor κB (RANK) ligand (RANKL), a major mediator of PTH's increase in osteoclastic bone resorption (Fig. 28-8), also increases osteoclast number. But RANKL administration causes even lower bone mass than PTH because continuously administered PTH increases osteoblast number more vigorously than RANKL does.[60] This finding suggests that one teleologic reason for PTH to increase bone formation is that this separate action of PTH might help preserve bone mass during prolonged requirements for PTH action.

PTH Increases Bone Formation. Administration of low doses of PTH or active amino-terminal fragments of PTH by once-daily subcutaneous injection leads to a net increase in bone mass, with only transient effects on blood calcium. Mechanisms for these divergent effects of PTH are incompletely understood but certainly reflect the variety of cell types in bone that respond directly to PTH, the varying time courses of these responses, and the indirect effects of PTH caused by autocrine and paracrine responses to PTH.[61]

Figure 28-9 illustrates the cells of the osteoblast lineage (see also Chapter 29). Osteoblasts are probably derived from pluripotent mesenchymal stem cells that, at least in vitro, can differentiate into chondrocytes, adipocytes,

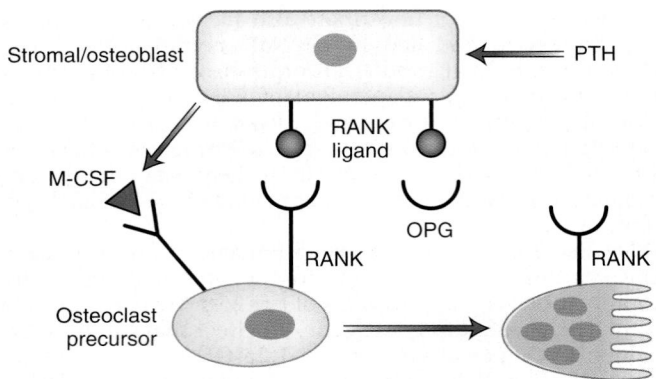

Figure 28-8 Osteoblast lineage cell control of osteoclastogenesis and osteoclast activity. Parathyroid hormone (PTH) acts on PTH/PTH-related protein (PTHrP) receptors on precursors of osteoblasts to increase the production of macrophage colony-stimulating factor (M-CSF) and receptor activator for nuclear factor κB (RANK) ligand and to decrease the production of osteoprotegerin (OPG). M-CSF and RANK ligand stimulate the production of osteoclasts and increase the activity of mature osteoclasts by binding to the receptor RANK. OPG blocks the interaction of RANK ligand and RANK.

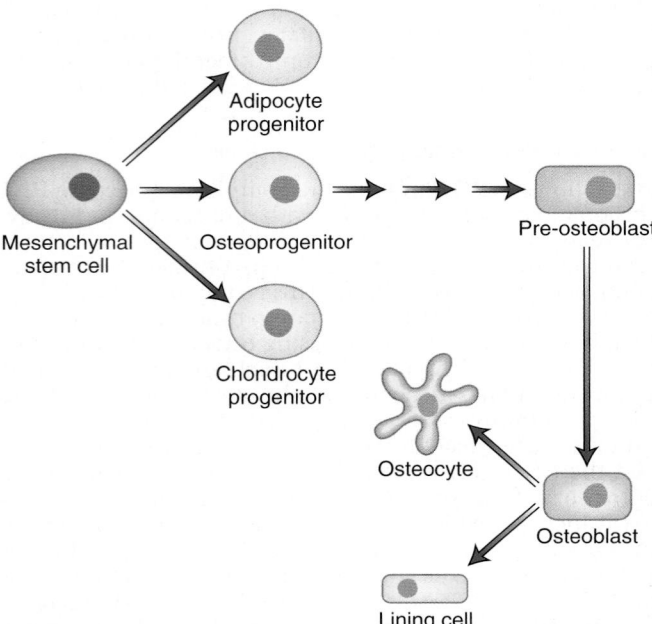

Figure 28-9 Osteoblast lineage. All precursors of osteoblasts can proliferate; osteoblasts are transformed to osteocytes and lining cells without further proliferation. Lining cells can revert to osteoblast function after parathyroid hormone stimulation. At each stage in the lineage, apoptotic cell death is probably an alternative fate.

osteoblasts, and other cell types.[62] Perivascular cells within human bone can reconstitute bone that supports hematopoiesis after subcutaneous transplantation in mice[63]; these cells may well represent one group of osteoblast stem cells in vivo. Within the osteoblast lineage, committed osteoprogenitor cells divide, become preosteoblastic stromal cells (which can divide further), and then become osteoblasts. Osteoblasts no longer divide and are cuboidal cells found on the bone surface actively laying down new bone. These cells can surround themselves with newly formed bone matrix and extend large numbers of dendritic processes, becoming osteocytes. Alternatively, osteoblasts can stop synthesizing matrix and remain on the bone surface as bone lining cells. Not all preosteoblasts and osteoblasts

mature; a variable number die by apoptotic, programmed cell death.[64]

PTH administration can influence movement of cells through the osteoblast lineage.[61] PTH administration in vivo, whether administered continuously or intermittently, increases osteoblast surface and number and bone formation rate. With intermittent PTH administration to rats, the number of bone lining cells decreases as the number of active osteoblasts increases[65]: subsequent studies using genetically marked mice showed that PTH converts bone lining cells to active osteoblasts.[66] Further, the decreased rate of osteoblast apoptosis after intermittent PTH administration leads to an increase in the number of osteoblasts.[64] Intermittent PTH administration in vivo also probably increases the number of early osteoblast precursors, as evidenced, for example, by the increased number of total stromal cell colonies (colony-forming unit fibroblasts, CFU-F) and an increased number of CFU-F expressing alkaline phosphatase generated after plating bone marrow cells in vitro after treatment of rats with PTH(1-34) intermittently.[67]

When PTH is administered continuously to rats, mimicking the findings in primary hyperparathyroidism, large numbers of proliferating, alkaline phosphatase–positive fibroblastic cells accumulate in the marrow, perhaps mimicking the findings of osteitis fibrosa in primary hyperparathyroidism. When the infusion of PTH was stopped, the fibroblastic cells disappeared and recently proliferated osteoblasts appeared, suggesting that many of the fibroblastic cells were osteoblast precursors.[68]

In addition to changing osteoblast numbers, PTH changes the activity of mature osteoblasts by a variety of mechanisms. When PTH is added to calvariae in vitro, the osteoblasts decrease their synthesis of collagen I and other matrix proteins. This action may reflect, in part, the action of PTH to steer the essential osteoblast transcription factor Runx2 toward proteosomal destruction.[69] In vivo, however, the most obvious effects of PTH are to increase bone formation by osteoblasts, probably by indirect actions of PTH on autocrine and paracrine pathways. PTH stimulation of osteoblastic cells leads to release of growth factors such as insulin-like growth factor 1, FGF2, and amphiregulin from these cells.[70] PTH also decreases the synthesis of dickkopf-1[71] and sclerostin,[72] inhibitors of Wnt signaling[73]; these actions are expected to increase the anabolic actions of Wnt proteins on osteoblasts. Further, because bone matrix is a rich source of osteoblast growth factors, the release of these growth factors from this matrix following PTH-induced bone resorption may increase bone formation and bring osteoblastic cells to sites of bone formation.[74] Thus, a variety of both direct and indirect actions of PTH can lead to the increased production of bone.

PTH Increases Bone Resorption. Surprisingly, osteoclasts, the bone-resorbing cells derived from hematopoietic precursors, have no PTH receptors on their surfaces. Instead, cells of the osteoblast lineage, including preosteoblasts, osteoblasts, and osteocytes, signal to osteoclast precursors to cause them to fuse and form mature osteoclasts. This signaling also serves to stimulate mature osteoclasts to resorb bone and to avoid apoptosis (see Fig. 28-8). Two cell surface proteins, macrophage colony-stimulating factor (M-CSF) and RANKL, are essential for stimulation of osteoclastogenesis,[75] and RANKL is essential for the activation of mature osteoclasts. The growth factor M-CSF (or CSF1) is expressed both as a secreted protein and as a cell surface protein; the production of both forms is stimulated by PTH.[76] RANKL—also named osteoprotegerin ligand (OPGL), osteoclast-differentiating factor (ODF), and TRANCE—is a membrane-bound member of the tumor necrosis factor

(TNF) family; its synthesis is also increased by PTH. RANKL binds to its receptor, RANK, a member of the TNF receptor family. RANK is found both on osteoclast precursors and on mature osteoclasts. The binding of RANKL to RANK can be blocked by osteoprotegerin (OPG), another member of the TNF receptor family. OPG (also called OCIF and TR1) circulates and is also secreted by cells of the osteoblastic lineage. PTH decreases the synthesis and secretion of OPG from these cells. Thus, PTH, by increasing RANK and decreasing OPG locally in bone, serves to increase bone resorption.

Activation of PTH receptors also causes release of calcium from bone by a less understood mechanism called osteocytic osteolysis. Osteocytes can directly release mineral from the matrix immediately surrounding them. For example, during lactation in mice, lacunae surrounding osteocytes release calcium; this release depends upon those osteocytes expressing PTH/PTHrP receptors.[77] Little is known about the quantitative importance of osteocytic osteolysis versus osteoclastic bone resorption in various settings.

Molecular Basis of Parathyroid Hormone Action

Ever since the discovery that PTH stimulates the secretion of cAMP into the urine,[78] PTH has been thought to act by triggering a cascade of intracellular second messengers. This guiding hypothesis, in its current form, postulates that all of the actions of PTH result from the binding of the hormone to a receptor on the plasma membrane of target tissues. This receptor is a member of a large family of G protein–linked receptors that span the plasma membrane seven times (Fig. 28-10). The binding of hormone on the outside of the membrane causes conformational changes in the disposition of the seven transmembrane helices that activate the receptor's ability to release guanosine diphosphate (GDP) from the α-subunit of a G protein bound to the receptor. The G protein then binds guanosine triphosphate (GTP) in place of GDP. The GTP-binding α-subunit of the G protein then separates from the βγ-subunits, and the separate subunits of the G protein then modulate the activity of enzymes and channels. The activity of these

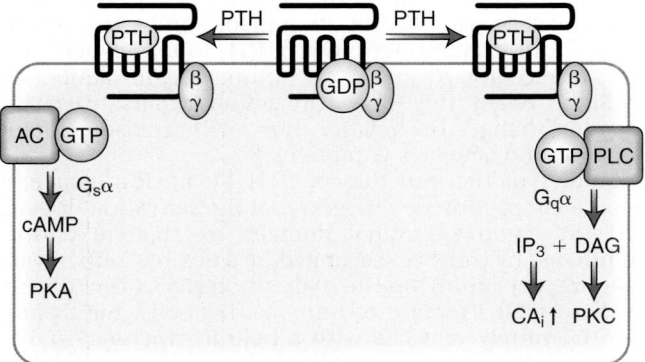

Figure 28-10 Parathyroid hormone (PTH)/PTH-related protein (PTHrP) receptors act as nucleotide exchangers. PTH binding to the receptor leads to exchange of guanosine triphosphate (GTP) for guanosine diphosphate (GDP) bound to G protein (G_s) α-subunits. G_s α-subunits bound to GTP are released from the receptor and from the βγ-subunits and then activate effectors. $G_s\alpha$ activates adenylate cyclase (AC), leading to the formation of cyclic adenosine monophosphate (cAMP), which then activates protein kinase A (PKA). $G_q\alpha$ and related α-subunits activate phospholipase C (PLC). PLC hydrolyzes phosphatidylinositol 1,4,5-trisphosphate to generate diacylglycerol (DAG) and inositol 1,4,5-trisphosphate (IP_3). The DAG then activates protein kinase C (PKC), and the IP_3 activates a receptor on microsomal vesicles that directs the movement of calcium (CA_i) from microsomal vesicles into the cytosol.

enzymes and channels then affects proteins farther downstream, eventually leading to the physiologic responses of bone and kidney cells.

Parathyroid Hormone and Parathyroid Hormone–Related Protein Receptors. DNA encoding a PTH/PTHrP receptor has been isolated from tissues of many species, including rat, opossum, human, pig, *Xenopus* (toad), and zebrafish,[79] and even some insects.[80] The receptor mediates actions of both PTH and PTHrP (see later discussion of PTHrP). The predicted amino acid sequence of the receptor and direct mapping of inserted epitopes suggest that the receptor spans the plasma membrane seven times, but the sequence does not closely resemble the sequences of most known G protein–linked receptors. Instead, it is a member of a distinct subfamily of closely related receptors called family B. Most of these receptors bind peptides of 30 to 40 amino acids in length. Known members include receptors for the secretin family of peptides (secretin, vasoactive intestinal peptide [VIP], glucagon, glucagon-like peptide, growth hormone–releasing hormone, pituitary adenylate cyclase–activating peptide, gastric inhibitory peptide), corticotropin-releasing hormone, calcitonin, and insect diuretic hormones related to corticotropin-releasing hormone. The PTH/PTHrP receptor most closely resembles receptors of the secretin group. The gene encoding the PTH/PTHrP receptor has a complicated structure, with 13 introns interrupting the coding sequence.

The cloned PTH/PTHrP receptor binds amino-terminal fragments of PTH and PTHrP with equal affinity. The receptor is expressed at high levels in kidney and in osteoblasts of bone but is also expressed in a wide variety of tissues, such as smooth muscle, brain, and a variety of fetal tissues, which are thought to be target tissues more for PTHrP than for PTH. The binding sites on the PTH/PTHrP receptor for PTH and PTHrP overlap, and some are distinct[81]; presumably, these differences explain ways that PTH and PTHrP actions can differ. For example, after binding to the receptor, PTH continues to interact with the receptor for much longer times than does PTHrP.[82] This more stable binding mode of PTH involves interactions with the receptor that allow the ligand to remain receptor bound even when G molecules are not interacting with the receptor. This more stable binding leads PTH to have a different intracellular fate from that of PTHrP and leads to more prolonged activation of the receptor by PTH.[83,84] In response to binding of PTH or PTHrP, the receptor activates several G proteins, including G_s, G_q, G_{11}, G_i, G_{12}, and G_{13}.

The PTH/PTHrP receptor mediates many of the actions of both PTH and PTHrP. The ligand-binding and signaling properties of the receptor in cultured cells, the pattern of expression of the receptor in tissues, and the functional consequences of mutation of the receptor sequence (see later) are persuasive evidence in this regard. Nevertheless, the scheme of PTH action illustrated in Figure 28-10 should be considered a simplified outline. It is unlikely that all of the actions of PTH can be explained by interactions with the cloned PTH/PTHrP receptor: Fragments of PTH that seem not to bind the receptor may be biologically active.[85] Furthermore, the carboxy-terminal portion of PTH(1-84) binds a cell surface protein distinct from the PTH/PTHrP receptor.

A second PTH receptor, which can be activated by PTH but not by PTHrP, called the PTH2 receptor (PTH2R), has been cloned. This receptor is expressed in multiple tissues, including brain, vascular endothelium and smooth muscle, endocrine cells of the gastrointestinal tract, and sperm. Expression is not seen in osteoblasts or renal tubules, however. Although PTH activates the human PTH2R well, PTH only poorly activates the PTH2R in rats and other species. Furthermore, a novel ligand called TIP39 (tubero-infundibular peptide of 39 residues) has been characterized and shown to be a potent activator of PTH2R. TIP39 bears only a weak resemblance to PTH or PTHrP and is likely to be a physiologically relevant activator of the PTH2. The functional role of the PTH2R is unknown, but it appears to mediate many actions of TIP39 in the brain and testis; studies of knockout mice implicate TIP39 in regulation of responses to stress[86] and germ cell development.[87] The two cloned PTHRs, as well as distinct receptors for fragments of PTHrP (see later), probably are part of a complex network of ligands and receptors (Fig. 28-11).

Functional Implications of Parathyroid Hormone Structure. Amino-terminal fragments of PTH as short as PTH(1-34) have potency at least as great as that of the full-length PTH(1-84).[79] Several discrete portions of the PTH(1-34) peptide interact with the receptor (Fig. 28-12). The first

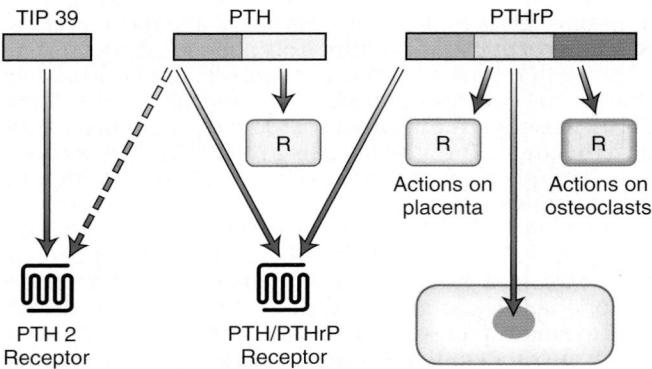

Figure 28-11 Network of parathyroid hormone (PTH) ligands and receptors (R). PTH and PTH-related protein (PTHrP) closely resemble each other at the amino-terminal region; TIP 39 (tubero-infundibular peptide of 39 residues) is more distantly related. Although only the PTH/PTHrP receptor and the PTH2 receptors have been cloned, biologic actions suggest that there are receptors specific for the carboxy-terminal portion of PTH, as well as distinct receptors for the midregion of PTHrP and for a more distal region of PTHrP. PTHrP is also found in nuclei and may act directly there.

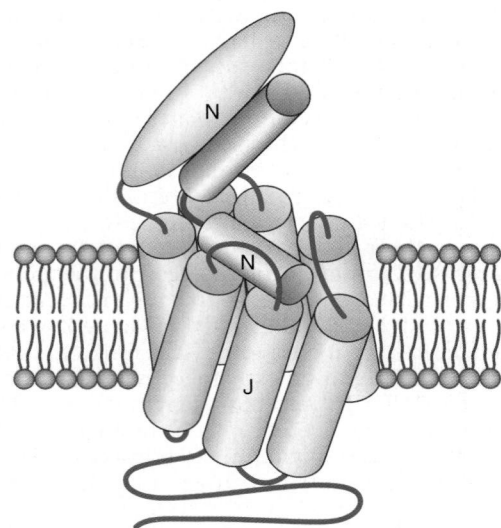

Figure 28-12 Binding of PTH(1-34) peptide of the parathyroid hormone (PTH) to the PTH/PTH-related protein (PTHrP) receptor. The amino-terminal (N) extracellular domain of the receptor (in green) binds rapidly to the carboxy-terminal portion of the ligand. The J domain of the receptor, containing the transmembrane domains and associated loops, binds to the amino-terminal domain of the ligand (red cylinder marked N). This binding is slower and may require conformational changes in both the ligand and receptor. These conformational changes then trigger G protein activation, receptor internalization, and other actions. (Courtesy of Tom Gardella.)

several residues of PTH are particularly important for triggering the conformational change in the receptor that results in activation of G_s and adenylate cyclase. Sequences responsible for transmembrane activation of G_s make up most of the first 13 residues of PTH; these are the residues that are highly conserved between PTH and PTHrP. At high concentrations, PTH(1-14) by itself can activate the PTH/PTHrP receptor. This activation domain interacts with the receptor's transmembrane domains and extracellular loops. When the first nine residues of PTH are covalently linked to the receptor's transmembrane domains and extracellular loops, they can activate the receptor. An analogue of PTH(1-14) can trigger G_q activation, thus activating PLC.[88] These data, plus the observation that a PTH analogue modified at position 1 selectively loses its ability to activate PLC,[89] demonstrate that the amino-terminal portion of PTH is essential for activation of both G_s and G_q. More distal regions of PTH(1-34) can activate protein kinase C and can raise intracellular calcium levels by mechanisms that have not been fully clarified. Remarkably, a PTH analogue that is missing the first 6 residues and that cannot activate G proteins can still activate the PTH/PTHrP receptor and increase bone mass in vivo.[90] This analogue can activate mitogen-activated protein (MAP) kinase signaling through interactions of the receptor with β-arrestin; these studies illustrate how the PTH/PTHrP receptor can signal intracellularly without activating G proteins.

The more carboxy-terminal portions of PTH(1-34) contribute importantly to the specificity and tight binding of PTH to the PTH/PTHrP receptor, at least partly through interactions with the receptor's amino-terminal extracellular domain (see Fig. 28-12). A variety of studies of genetically altered receptors, and biochemical studies using photoactivated cross-links between PTH and the receptor, and studies of co-crystals of the receptor's amino-terminal domain and PTH/PTHrP fragments,[81,91] have reinforced each other and show that the carboxy-terminal portion of PTH makes multiple contacts with the amino-terminal extension of the receptor and with its extracellular loops. This interaction of PTH with the amino-terminal portion of the receptor occurs extremely rapidly, with a time constant of 140 ms.[92] In contrast, the subsequent interaction of the amino-terminal portion of PTH with the so-called J domain of the receptor (the transmembrane domains and associated extracellular loops) occurs more slowly, with a time constant of 1 second. Presumably, this extra time is needed for the amino-terminus of PTH to form a helix and for the receptor to attain an optimal conformation for binding. When this slow interaction occurs, then the receptor changes the relationships of its transmembrane domains and activates G proteins.[93]

Studies of the structure of PTH by nuclear magnetic resonance spectroscopy suggest that the activation domain and the carboxy-terminal domain are discrete entities dominated by α-helices separated by a flexible loop of variable size, depending on the hydrophobicity of the solvent. In the crystal structure of human PTH(1-34), the flexible loop is entirely replaced with a helical structure.[94] Taken together, these studies suggest that the carboxy-terminal portion of PTH(1-34) makes multiple contacts with the receptor that allow high-affinity binding and position the amino-terminal portion of PTH to activate the receptor through contacts with transmembrane domains and associated loops.

Activation of Second Messengers. Precisely how binding of PTH to the extracellular domains of the PTH/PTHrP receptor leads to activation of G proteins is not understood. The crystal structures of the transmembrane portions of the glucagon receptor and the corticotropin-releasing factor receptor 1 receptors have been determined and, because they resemble each other, presumably have lessons for understanding the structure of the related PTH/PTHrP receptor.[95] The structures of these receptors resemble those of the more extensively studied rhodopsin family A receptors, but differ in that the potential pocket expected to bind the peptide ligands is larger, forming a V when seen from the side, with transmembrane domains (TMDs) 1, 6, and 7 forming one arm of the V and TMDs 2 to 5 forming the other. This proposed structure, with TMD 1 adjacent to TMDs 6 and 7, is consistent with the behavior of certain mutant PTH/PTHrP receptors.[96,97] Presumably, binding of PTH to several different regions of the receptor changes the relationships of the transmembrane domains[93] such that the receptor's three intracellular loops and carboxy-terminal tail interact with G proteins in an altered way.

Receptors with certain point mutations in the second, sixth, and seventh transmembrane domains can activate G_s even without stimulation by hormone. These mutant receptors were discovered by analyzing the PTH/PTHrP receptors in patients with Jansen metaphyseal chondrodystrophy.[98] Patients with this disorder have signs of parathyroid overactivity (hypercalcemia, hypophosphatemia, and high levels of 1,25[OH]$_2$D$_3$ and urinary cAMP) but low PTH and PTHrP levels. The mutations, all near the bottom of the predicted V-shaped structure of the transmembrane domains,[95] must change the conformation of the intracellular portion of the receptor in a way that resembles the effect of binding of PTH to the normal receptor. The observation that inappropriate activation of the PTH/PTHrP receptor in Jansen chondrodystrophy leads to all of the metabolic abnormalities found in primary hyperparathyroidism is one of the most persuasive pieces of evidence that the cloned PTH/PTHrP receptor does, in fact, mediate the actions of PTH in bone and kidney in humans in vivo.

Second Messengers and Distal Effects of Parathyroid Hormone. The activation of multiple G proteins by PTH raises questions about the individual roles of each second messenger and their possible interactions. The importance of cAMP as a mediator of the physiologic actions of PTH has been demonstrated by studies in vivo[78] and in vitro.[99] Furthermore, patients with pseudohypoparathyroidism type I, who cannot increase urinary cAMP levels in response to PTH, show clear renal resistance to PTH (see later).

Activation of PLC, with concomitant activation of protein kinase C and synthesis of IP$_3$, may contribute to physiologic actions of PTH as well, such as inhibition of sodium-phosphate cotransport[100] and stimulation of the renal 25(OH)D 1α-hydroxylase.[101] Mice with mutant PTH/PTHrP receptors that cannot activate PLC have a mild delay in bone development,[102] growth plate abnormalities manifest when G_s is also defective in the growth plates,[103] and abnormalities of phosphate handling by the kidney when challenged with a low-calcium diet.[104] When these mutant mice are challenged with infusions of PTH peptides, their phosphate response in normal at first, but a defect in phosphate handling occurs during prolonged infusion.[55] When these same mutant mice are infused with high levels of PTH, they also exhibit a defect in generation of the expected accumulation of stromal cells in the marrow (osteitis fibrosa) that normal mice exhibit after prolonged PTH infusion.[105] Thus, the actions of PTH on bone and kidney that require PLC activation are most clearly seen with high levels of PTH sustained for some time.

The stimulation of one G protein or another by the PTH/PTHrP receptor can vary in different types of cells and even in differing regions of the same cell.[100] In some settings, this choice may be influenced by the interactions of the PTH/PTHrP receptor with intracellular scaffolding proteins, such as NHERF1 and NHERF2 (Na$^+$/H$^+$ exchanger regulatory factor). Binding of the PTH/PTHrP receptor to NHERFs is directed by the last four amino acids in the receptor sequence. This binding, particularly prominent at the apical surface of the proximal tubular cells of the kidney, for example, may change the G protein activated by the PTH/PTHrP receptor from predominantly G_s to predominantly G_i.[106]

Target Cell Responsiveness to Parathyroid Hormone. Physiologic responses to PTH depend not only on the concentration of PTH in blood but also on the responsiveness of target cells to PTH. This responsiveness can be modified by previous exposure to PTH or by exposure to a variety of other hormones and paracrine factors. Responsiveness can be changed by alterations at virtually every step in the cellular response to PTH.

Major regulators of PTH/PTHrP receptor gene expression include, not surprisingly, PTH and 1,25(OH)$_2$D$_3$, both of which can decrease PTH/PTHrP receptor mRNA in certain target cells. In some settings, PTH decreases the amount of immunoreactive and functional receptor on the cell surface without changing the levels of PTH/PTHrP mRNA. This decrease reflects ligand-induced internalization and degradation of receptors. Internalization of receptor is stimulated by PTH binding, which leads to phosphorylation of specific serines found in the receptor's cytoplasmic tail and subsequent internalization directed by binding of arrestin to the receptor.[107,108] Even without change in receptor number, the binding of arrestin to the PTH/PTHrP receptor decreases the efficiency of activation of G proteins (desensitization). Nevertheless, certain analogues of PTH designed to bind particularly tightly to the PTH/PTHrP receptor can continue activating adenylate cyclase even after internalization of the ligand-receptor complex in vesicles, leading to prolonged action of these analogues.[84]

Parathyroid Hormone–Related Protein

PTHrP was discovered because the secretion of PTHrP by a wide variety of tumors contributes to the humoral hypercalcemia of malignancy. For this reason, the initial studies of PTHrP in humans and animals stressed the PTH-like structure and properties of the molecule. Subsequent studies soon showed, however, that PTHrP, unlike PTH, is made by a wide variety of tissues, in which it acts locally in ways that may have little relevance to the control of blood calcium.

Gene and Protein Structure

PTHrP sequences in several species, ranging from fish to humans, have been identified[109,110] (Fig. 28-13). In humans, alternative RNA splicing yields transcripts that encode three distinct proteins of 139, 141, and 173 residues that differ only after residue 139.

Inspection of these sequences suggests that PTHrP has several functionally distinct domains. Eight or nine of the first 13 residues of PTHrP are identical to those in known mammalian PTH sequences. These sequences encompass the known "activation" domain of PTH (see earlier) and are instrumental in the ability of PTHrP to activate PTH/PTHrP receptors. The conserved histidine at position 5 of all PTHrP molecules, except those of fish, differs from the hydrophobic residue found at the corresponding position of all PTHs and allows PTHrP to activate the PTH/PTHrP receptor but not the PTH2 receptor.

The sequences in PTHrP(14-34) are also highly conserved. Although these sequences little resemble the corresponding region of PTH, they can displace PTH from the

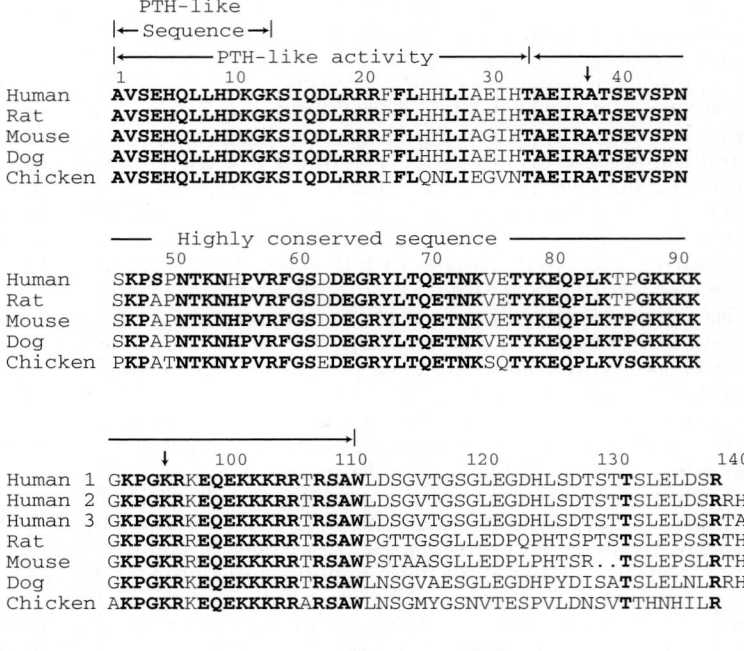

```
                              PTH-like
                              |← Sequence →|
                              |←————————PTH-like activity————————→|←————|
                              1        10        20        30    ↓   40
         Human  AVSEHQLLHDKGKSIQDLRRRFFLHHLIAEIHTAEIRATSEVSPN
         Rat    AVSEHQLLHDKGKSIQDLRRRFFLHHLIAEIHTAEIRATSEVSPN
         Mouse  AVSEHQLLHDKGKSIQDLRRRFFLHHLIAGIHTAEIRATSEVSPN
         Dog    AVSEHQLLHDKGKSIQDLRRRFFLHHLIAEIHTAEIRATSEVSPN
         Chicken AVSEHQLLHDKGKSIQDLRRRIFLQNLIEGVNTAEIRATSEVSPN


                ———— Highly conserved sequence ————
                      50        60        70        80        90
         Human  SKPSPNTKNHPVRFGSDDEGRYLTQETNKVETYKEQPLKTPGKKKK
         Rat    SKPAPNTKNHPVRFGSDDEGRYLTQETNKVETYKEQPLKTPGKKKK
         Mouse  SKPAPNTKNHPVRFGSDDEGRYLTQETNKVETYKEQPLKTPGKKKK
         Dog    SKPAPNTKNHPVRFGSDDEGRYLTQETNKVETYKEQPLKTPGKKKK
         Chicken PKPATNTKNYPVRFGSEDEGRYLTQETNKSQTYKEQPLKVSGKKKK


                ————————————————————————→|
                      ↓   100       110       120       130       140
         Human 1 GKPGKRKEQEKKKRRTRSAWLDSGVTGSGLEGDHLSDTSTTSLELDSR
         Human 2 GKPGKRKEQEKKKRRTRSAWLDSGVTGSGLEGDHLSDTSTTSLELDSRRH
         Human 3 GKPGKRKEQEKKKRRTRSAWLDSGVTGSGLEGDHLSDTSTTSLELDSRTA
         Rat     GKPGKRKEQEKKKRRTRSAWPGTTGSGLLEDPQPHTSPTSTSLEPSSRTH
         Mouse   GKPGKRKEQEKKKRRTRSAWPSTAASGLLEDPLPHTSR..TSLEPSLRTH
         Dog     GKPGKRKEQEKKKRRTRSAWLNSGVAESGLEGDHPYDISATSLELNLRRH
         Chicken AKPGKRKEQEKKKRRARSAWLNSGMYGSNVTESPVLDNSVTTHNHILR


                      150       160       170
         Human 3 LLWGLKKKKENNRRTHHMQLMISLFKSPLLLL
```

Figure 28-13 Sequences of parathyroid hormone–related protein (PTHrP) from five species. Completely conserved residues are in boldface; note the high level of conservation through residue 111. *Arrows* indicate sites of internal cleavage after residues 37 and 95, which lead to generation of PTHrP(38-94) amide and PTHrP(38-95). Another site of cleavage, generating PTHrP(38-101) and, perhaps, PTHrP(107-139), is not shown.[110] The three human sequences represent proteins synthesized from alternatively spliced messenger RNAs and differ only after residue 139. Amino acids are indicated by the single-letter code (see Fig. 28-3).

PTH/PTHrP receptor and, in the crystal structure of the amino-terminal domain of the PTH/PTHrP receptor, bind to overlapping but distinct contact sites.[81] Studies of the secondary and tertiary structures of PTHrP(1-34) and PTH(1-37) suggest that they have similar structures dominated by α-helices connected by a flexible hinge.

The remaining portion of the PTHrP molecule bears no resemblance to corresponding sequences in PTH. Nevertheless, residues 35 to 111 of PTHrP are strikingly well conserved, with only nine residues differing between mammalian and chicken PTHrP sequences. This sequence conservation is considerably greater than that found in the carboxy-terminal portion of PTH, suggesting that this region of PTHrP has unique and important functions. This region also includes a nuclear localization signal that has been demonstrated to be functional in cultured cells.[111] After residue 111, the PTHrP sequences vary considerably from species to species.

Interspersed within the PTHrP sequences are multiple sites containing one or several basic residues that might serve as post-translational cleavage sites (see Fig. 28-13). Extensive analysis of PTHrP fragments in tumors, cell lines, and transfected cells has shown that several of these sites are, in fact, functional cleavage signals. PTHrP is cleaved after the arginine at residue 37; this cleavage, followed by carboxypeptidase cleavage, generates a PTH-like PTHrP (1-36) fragment as well as the fragments PTHrP(38-94) amide, PTHrP(38-95), and PTHrP(38-101).[112] More carboxy-terminal fragments of PTHrP have been detected in cells as well. Fragments such as PTHrP(107-139) and PTHrP(107-111) can trigger intracellular kinase cascades and affect bone mass in vivo,[113] though the physiologic roles of any of the carboxy-terminal fragments of PTHrP have not yet been established.

In the blood of patients with humoral hypercalcemia of malignancy, multiple immunoreactive species of PTHrP have been found that may well correspond to the fragments of PTHrP in cells and tissue culture media, although precise characterization of these various immunoreactive species is incomplete (see later). Full-length PTHrP may

well not circulate, because an amino-terminal–specific immunoaffinity column was unable to extract carboxy-terminal immunoreactivity from the serum of patients with malignant hypercalcemia.[114]

Functions of Parathyroid Hormone–Related Protein

The first actions of PTHrP to be defined were the PTH-like actions associated with the humoral hypercalcemia of malignancy. In this pathologic entity, PTHrP acts as a hormone; it is secreted from the tumor into the bloodstream and then acts on bone and kidney to raise calcium level (see discussion under "Hypercalcemia of Malignancy" later).[115] Whether or not PTHrP circulates at high enough levels in normal adults to contribute to normal calcium homeostasis is an unanswered question. With metastases of breast cancer to bone, locally produced PTHrP can raise serum calcium without necessarily raising blood levels of PTHrP. PTHrP expression by tumors also contributes to the cachexia seen in cancer patients and stimulates the "browning" of adipocytes in tumor models.[116]

PTHrP acts as a calciotropic hormone during fetal life and in lactation. Fetal mice missing the PTHrP gene transport calcium-45 (^{45}Ca) across the placenta inefficiently. This action of PTHrP requires only the mid-region of PTHrP and probably involves a receptor distinct from the PTH/PTHrP receptor. Amino-terminal portions of PTHrP and PTH may also be able to increase placental calcium transport, because PTH(1-84) can also increase placental calcium transport in mice missing the PTH gene.[117]

The second setting for humoral actions of PTHrP is lactation. In mice, secretion of PTHrP from the breast into the bloodstream leads to an increase in bone resorption.[118] Calcium then activates the CaSR in breast tissue, increases the movement of calcium into milk, and downregulates expression of PTHrP in the breast.[119] PTHrP, therefore, probably contributes to the dramatic but largely reversible bone loss during lactation in humans, which is only minimally affected by calcium supplementation.[120] An exaggeration of this lactational role of PTHrP may explain the rare presentation of hypercalcemia and high PTHrP levels in pregnant and lactating women.[121] Large amounts of PTHrP are also secreted into breast milk, although the role of PTHrP in milk is unknown.

Most of the actions of PTHrP are likely to be paracrine or autocrine.[122] PTHrP is synthesized at one time or another during fetal life in virtually every tissue. Its role in the development of fetal bone has been demonstrated through the striking abnormalities found in genetically engineered mice missing the PTHrP gene. These abnormalities suggest that PTHrP normally keeps chondrocytes proliferating in orderly columns, thereby delaying chondrocyte differentiation.[123] PTHrP blocks the actions of Mef2 and Runx2 transcription factors to activate chondrocyte differentiation by driving class IIa histone deacetylases into the nucleus.[124] The role of PTHrP in many other fetal tissues may analogously involve regulation of proliferation and differentiation. The widespread expression of the PTHrP in fetal life probably underlies the expression of PTHrP in a wide variety of malignancies. As is often the case in malignancy, the expression of PTHrP represents the reinitiation of a fetal pattern of gene expression.

PTHrP is synthesized by many adult tissues. In tissues such as skin, hair, and breast, it is likely that PTHrP regulates cell proliferation and differentiation. PTHrP is also synthesized in response to stretch in the smooth muscle of blood vessels and of the gastrointestinal tract, uterus, and bladder and acts in an autocrine fashion to relax the smooth muscle.[125] PTHrP is also widely expressed in neurons of the central nervous system; its function in the brain is unknown, but it may protect neurons from excitotoxicity by decreasing flux through voltage-gated calcium channels; an analogous mechanism may explain the role of PTHrP in smooth muscle relaxation.

Many of the actions of PTHrP are mediated by the PTH/PTHrP receptor. Others, such as the activation of placental calcium transport, are probably mediated in part by a distinct receptor, and other actions on bone cells probably involve yet another receptor responsive to more distal portions of PTHrP. Increasing evidence suggests, furthermore, that some actions of PTHrP involve direct nuclear actions of PTHrP.[126] Thus, both PTH and PTHrP are likely to use multiple mechanisms to stimulate cells (see Fig. 28-11).

CALCITONIN

Calcitonin has an important role in regulating blood calcium in fish and a demonstrable role in rodents; however, the importance of calcitonin in human calcium homeostasis remains uncertain.

The existence of a second calcium-regulating hormone, in addition to PTH, was first demonstrated during perfusion studies of the thyroid/parathyroid glands of dogs.[127] High calcium perfusion resulted in a rapid decrease in plasma calcium, even more rapid than after parathyroidectomy. This suggested that calcium had stimulated the secretion of a hormone that lowered blood calcium. It was subsequently demonstrated that this missing hormone, named calcitonin for its role in regulating the "tone" or level of calcium, was elaborated by the thyroid gland, not the parathyroids. Calcitonin is found in the nonfollicular cells of the thyroid, called C cells, which originate from the neural crest.[128] In fish, the location of the C cells in discrete organs led to the rapid isolation of calcitonin from these ultimobranchial bodies in dogfish, salmon, and several other species. The identification of the glandular origin of calcitonin enabled the isolation of sufficient quantities of calcitonin for sequence analysis[129] and studies of its structure and biologic function.

Synthesis and Secretion

Calcitonin consists of a 32–amino acid polypeptide with an intrachain disulfide bond provided by the cysteines at positions 1 and 7 (Fig. 28-14). These two cysteine residues, along with the carboxy-terminal proline amide and six additional residues, are the only amino acids conserved among the calcitonins isolated from various species. The disulfide linkage and proline amide residues are important for the function of the molecule, although biologically active analogues lacking disulfide bonds have been developed. Interestingly, fish calcitonin is more potent in mammals than is the mammalian hormone. The mature peptide is derived from the middle of a 136–amino acid precursor. The human calcitonin gene, located on the short arm of chromosome 11, contains 6 exons, which are alternatively spliced in a tissue-specific manner to yield the mRNAs encoding calcitonin or calcitonin gene-related peptide (CGRP) (see Fig. 28-14). The mRNA encoding calcitonin is derived by splicing together the first four exons[130] and represents over 95% of mature transcripts in the thyroid C cells. The splicing of the first three exons to exons 5 and 6 results in an mRNA that encodes the 37-amino acid α-CGRP peptide. The mRNA encoding α-CGRP is expressed in multiple tissues and is the only mature transcript of the calcitonin gene detected in neural tissue. A second CGRP gene encodes the closely related

Peptide	Species	Sequence	
CT	Human	**C**GNLST**C**MLGTYTQDFNKFHTFPQTAIGVGAP	-NH2
	Salmon-1	**C**S----**C**V--KLS-ELH-LQTY-R-NT-SGT-	-NH2
	Salmon-2	**C**S----**C**V--KLS-DLH-LQTF-R-NT-AGV-	-NH2
	Salmon-3	**C**S----**C**M--KLS-DLH-LQTF-R-NT-AGV-	-NH2
CGRP	Human α	A**C**DTAT**C**VTHRLAGLLSRSGGVVKNNFVPTNVGSKAF	-NH2
	Human β	-**C**N---**C**----------------S------------	-NH2
	Salmon	-**C**N---**C**------DF-N-----GNS-----------	-NH2
Amylin	Human	A**C**DTAT**C**VTHRLAGLLSRSGGVVKNNFVPTNVGSKAF	-NH2
ADM	Human	YRQSMNNFQGLRSFG**C**RFGT**C**TVQKLAHQIYQFTDKDKDNVAPRSKISPQGY	-NH2
IMD	Human	TQAQLLRVG**C**VLGT**C**QVQNLSHRLWQLMGPAGRQDSAPVDPSSPHSYG	-NH2
CRSP-1	Porcine	S**C**NTAT**C**MTHRLVGLLSRSGSMVRSNLLPTKMGFKVFG	-NH2
CRSP-2	Porcine	-**C**---S**C**V--KMT-W------VAKN-FM--NVDS-IL	-NH2
CRSP-3	Porcine	-**C**---I**C**V--KMA-W------V-KN-FM-IN--S-VL	-NH2

Figure 28-14 The amino acid sequences of calcitonin (CT), calcitonin gene–related peptide (CGRP), amylin, adrenomedullin (ADM), intermedin (IMD), and calcitonin receptor–stimulating proteins (CSRP) from selected species. The bold Cs represent the cysteine residues that form the disulfide linkages critical for the secondary structure of these peptides. The other conserved residues are indicated by a *dashed line* (see Fig. 28-3 for the single-letter amino acid codes).

β-CGRP. In humans, the predicted sequence of the mature peptide differs from that of α-CGRP by only three amino acids (see Fig. 28-14). The β-CGRP gene is also found on chromosome 11; its tissue distribution is the same as that of α-CGRP.

The synthesis and secretion of calcitonin are tightly regulated. Studies in a porcine model reveal a linear relationship between the secretion of calcitonin and ambient calcium levels.[131] Cell culture studies with calcium ionophores and calcium channel blockers demonstrate that the calcium ion concentration within the C cell determines this secretion rate.[132] The CaSR cloned from parathyroid cells is also expressed in C cells and contributes to the regulation of calcitonin secretion.[133] Other calcitonin secretagogues include glucocorticoids, CGRP, glucagon, enteroglucagon, gastrin, pentagastrin, pancreozymin, and β-adrenergic agents.[134] The physiologic role of the gastrointestinal hormones in regulating calcitonin remains unclear; however, they have been postulated to play a role in the regulation of postprandial hypercalcemia. The secretion of calcitonin is inhibited by somatostatin, which is also secreted by the thyroidal C cells. In vivo[135] and in vitro[136] studies have demonstrated that $1,25(OH)_2D_3$ decreases calcitonin mRNA levels by a transcriptional mechanism.

Calcitonin, when administered acutely, decreases tubular resorption of calcium[137] and impairs osteoclast-mediated bone resorption by a direct action on osteoclasts.[138] In rodents, calcitonin has been shown to play a role in the regulation of postprandial hypercalcemia[139] and the skeletal response to lactation.[140] Studies in calcitonin knockout mice reveal a doubling of bone formation rate in the absence of hormone, accompanied by resistance to ovariectomy-induced bone loss.[141] A similar increase in bone formation is found in mice heterozygous for ablation of the calcitonin receptor.[142] The mechanism of this apparent effect of calcitonin on bone formation is not understood.

The physiologic role of calcitonin in humans, however, remains elusive. The effect of calcitonin on bone density was examined in patients with long-term hypercalcitoninemia secondary to medullary carcinoma of the thyroid (MCT) and in patients with subtotal thyroidectomy resulting in lack of calcitonin secretory reserve.[143] The abnormal calcitonin levels had no influence on the bone density at the lumbar spine and distal radius. Furthermore, long-term, high-dose administration of exogenous calcitonin caused no physiologic abnormalities.[144]

Many of the effects of calcitonin are mediated by a G protein–coupled cell surface receptor in the PTH/secretin receptor family.[145,146] The mRNA encoding this receptor has been found in multiple tissues including kidney, brain, and osteoclasts. The coupling of this receptor to different G proteins results in the activation of either adenylate cyclase or PLC; in some settings, this is cell cycle dependent.[147]

Calcitonin Family: Calcitonin Gene-Related Peptide, Amylin, Adrenomedullin, Calcitonin Receptor-Stimulating Peptides, and Intermedin

CGRP, amylin, adrenomedullin, calcitonin receptor-stimulating peptide 1 (CRSP-1), and intermedin have all been shown to have high-affinity binding sites on cell membranes, and displacement studies suggest that several receptor subtypes for these related ligands are present. However, cloning of specific receptors for these ligands proved difficult, because the functional receptors consist of heterodimers between G protein–coupled receptors and single transmembrane proteins of the RAMP (receptor activity modifying proteins) family.[148,149] Interaction of the calcitonin receptor-like receptor, a relative of the calcitonin receptor, with RAMP1 results in a CGRP receptor, whereas RAMP2 and RAMP3 interactions with the same calcitonin receptor-like receptor generate adrenomedullin receptors. Interaction of RAMP1 with the calcitonin receptor generates an amylin receptor.[150]

CGRP is thought to act as a neurotransmitter and vasodilator rather than as a hormone. In support of this hypothesis, mice lacking α-CGRP have been shown to have an increase in mean arterial pressure.[151] Immunohistochemical studies of CGRP in the brain and peripheral nervous system suggest that this neuropeptide also plays an important role in sensory and integrative motor functions.

Three structurally related peptides have been isolated from porcine brain (see Fig. 28-14). These calcitonin receptor-stimulating peptides (CRSPs) are also expressed in the thyroid gland. CRSP-1, which is 60% homologous to α-CGRP at the amino acid level, binds to the calcitonin receptor, dose-dependently stimulates cAMP production, and inhibits osteoclastogenesis.[152] Consistent with this observation, administration of CRSP-1, like that of calcitonin, results in a decrease in serum calcium. The receptors for CRSP-2 and CRSP-3 have not been identified.[153]

Amylin is highly homologous to CGRP and calcitonin (see Fig. 28-14). Although amylin has been shown to have skeletal actions, the presence of amylin in the pancreas of patients with type 2 diabetes mellitus suggests an etiologic role for this peptide in this disorder.[154] Because amylin slows gastric emptying, promoting satiety and attenuating the postprandial rise in glucagon, analogues of this peptide are currently being used as therapeutic agents for type 2 diabetes. Amylin administration inhibits bone loss associated with ovariectomy and streptozotocin-induced diabetes mellitus in rats.[155,156] Targeted ablation of amylin in mice results in low bone mass due to an increase in bone resorption.[142] Amylin has also been shown to decrease food intake and inhibit gastric acid secretion, protecting against ulcer development in numerous models.[157]

Adrenomedullin (see Fig. 28-14) has vasodilatory effects similar to those of CGRP. In addition to activating CGRP receptors, adrenomedullin binds to specific receptors in the vascular system.[158] Mice missing DNA coding adrenomedullin die in midgestation.[159] Haploinsufficiency of RAMP2, which regulates binding of adrenomedullin to the calcitonin receptor, results in hyperprolactinemia, delayed bone development, and decreased bone mineral density.[160] Unlike other family members, adrenomedullin does not inhibit osteoclast activity or formation.[152] The physiologic role of adrenomedullin in the skeleton remains to be clarified.

Intermedin (adrenomedullin-2), the newest member of this family (see Fig. 28-14), was identified by homology screening of expressed sequence tags. It is expressed primarily in the pituitary and the gastrointestinal tract. Intermedin is able to signal through CGRP receptors and competes with CGRP for receptor binding.[161] However, unlike CGRP and adrenomedullin, intermedin is a nonselective agonist for the RAMP co-receptors.

Calcitonin in Human Disease

Calcitonin is secreted by several endocrine malignancies and, therefore, can serve as a tumor marker. Basal and pentagastrin-stimulated calcitonin levels have been used to identify and follow those at risk for, or affected by, medullary carcinoma of the thyroid (see Chapter 39), although abnormal basal and stimulated levels may be observed in patients on chronic hemodialysis.[162] Calcitonin may also be ectopically secreted by other tumors, including insulinomas, VIPomas, and lung cancers. Severely ill patients, including those with burn inhalation injury,[163] toxic shock syndrome,[164] and pancreatitis,[165] may also have elevated calcitonin levels.

Therapeutic Uses

The observation that calcitonin inhibits osteoclastic bone resorption has led to its therapeutic use for the treatment of several disorders associated with excess bone resorption, including osteoporosis and Paget disease (see Chapter 29). Calcitonin has also been used for its analgesic effect, in the treatment of patients with vertebral crush fractures, osteolytic metastases, or phantom limb.[166,167] Based on a potential increased risk of malignancy in those being treated with salmon calcitonin and the marginal efficacy of the drug, it is no longer recommended for treatment of osteoporosis.[168]

VITAMIN D

Metabolism of Vitamin D

Vitamin D is not a true vitamin, because nutritional supplementation is not required in humans who have adequate sun exposure. When exposed to ultraviolet irradiation, the cutaneous precursor of vitamin D, 7-dehydrocholesterol, undergoes photochemical cleavage of the carbon bond between carbons 9 and 10 of the steroid ring (Fig. 28-15). The resultant product, previtamin D, is thermally labile and over a period of 48 hours undergoes a temperature-dependent molecular rearrangement that results in the production of vitamin D. Alternatively, this thermally labile product can isomerize to two biologically inert products, luminosterol and tachysterol. This alternative photoisomerization prevents production of excessive amounts of vitamin D with prolonged sun exposure. The degree of skin pigmentation, which increases in response to solar exposure, also regulates the conversion of 7-dehydrocholesterol to vitamin D by blocking the penetration of ultraviolet rays.

The alternative source of vitamin D is dietary. The elderly, the institutionalized, and those living in northern climates likely obtain most of their vitamin D from dietary sources. However, with increasing avoidance of sun exposure by the general population, ensuring adequate dietary intake of vitamin D has become important for the population at large. Vitamin D deficiency is prevalent and has been shown to contribute significantly to osteopenia and fracture risk. The major dietary sources of vitamin D are fortified dairy products, although the lack of monitoring of this supplementation results in marked variation in the amount of vitamin D provided.[169] Other dietary sources include egg yolks, fish oils, and fortified cereal products. Vitamin D provided by plant sources is in the form of vitamin D_2, whereas that provided by animal sources is in the form of vitamin D_3 (see Fig. 28-15). These two forms have equivalent biologic potencies and are activated equally efficiently by the hydroxylases in humans; however, vitamin D_3 may be more effective at increasing 25-hydroxyvitamin D levels.[170] This difference may be due to the population studied, because the modest increase in the half-life of 25-hydroxyvitamin D_2 versus 25-hydroxyvitamin D_3 is influenced by vitamin D–binding protein (VDBP) concentration and genotype.[171]

Vitamin D is absorbed into the lymphatics and enters the circulation bound primarily to VDBP, although a

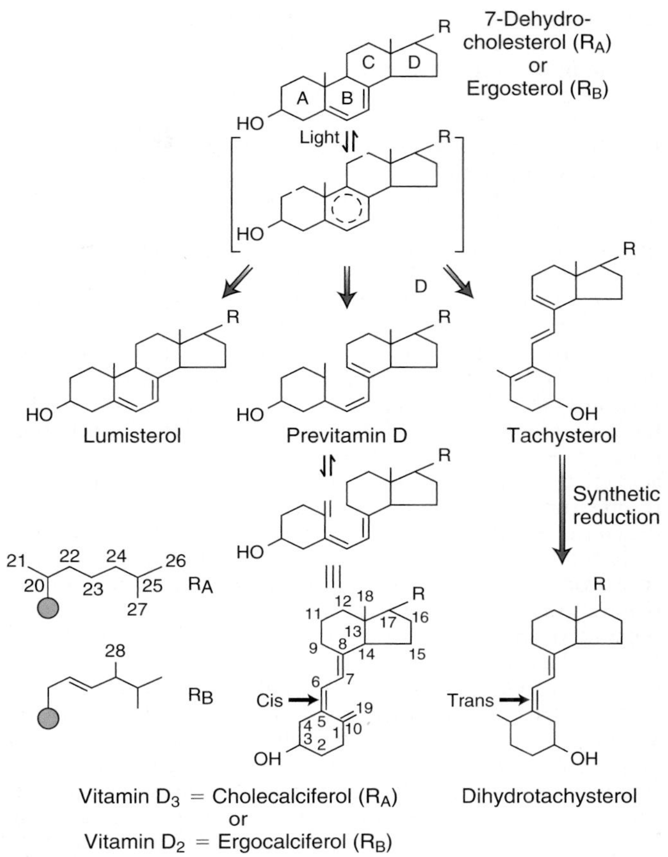

Figure 28-15 Vitamin D precursors and alternative reaction products. The numbering system for vitamin D carbons and the distinct structures of vitamin D_2 (ergocalciferol) and D_3 (cholecalciferol) are noted, as is the structure of dihydrotachysterol, a synthetic product not produced in vivo. Note that the 3-hydroxyl group of dihydrotachysterol is in a pseudo-1-hydroxyl configuration. This may explain the relatively high potency of dihydrotachysterol in conditions associated with low 1α-hydroxylase activity.

fraction of vitamin D circulates bound to albumin. The human VDBP is a 52-KDa α-globulin synthesized in the liver. The protein has a high affinity for 25(OH)D but also binds vitamin D and 1,25(OH)$_2$D. Approximately 88% of 25(OH)D circulates bound to the VDBP, 0.03% is free, and the rest circulates bound to albumin. In contrast, 85% of the circulating 1,25(OH)$_2$D$_3$ binds to the VDBP, 0.4% is free, and the rest binds to albumin. Mice lacking VDBP have increased susceptibility to 1,25(OH)$_2$D$_3$ toxicity as well as to dietary vitamin D deficiency.[172] Thus, the role of VDBP is to maintain a serum reservoir and to modulate the activity of vitamin D metabolites. Studies in megalin null mice suggest that VDBP is filtered by the glomerulus and reabsorbed by a megalin-dependent pathway in the proximal renal tubule.[173] Further investigations will be required to determine the importance of this pathway in vitamin D metabolism and the tissues in which megalin-dependent endocytosis plays an important role.[174]

In the liver, vitamin D undergoes 25-hydroxylation by a cytochrome P450–like enzyme present in the mitochondria and microsomes. The half-life of 25(OH)D is approximately 2 to 3 weeks. The 25-hydroxylation of vitamin D is not tightly regulated; therefore, the blood levels of 25(OH)D reflect the amount of vitamin D entering the circulation. When levels of VDBP are low, such as in nephrotic syndrome, circulating levels of 25(OH)D are also reduced. The half-life of 25(OH)D is shortened by increases in levels of its active metabolite, $1,25(OH)_2D_3$.

The final step in the production of the active hormone is the renal 1α-hydroxylation of 25(OH)D to $1,25(OH)_2D_3$. The half-life of this hormone is approximately 6 to 8 hours. Like the 25-hydroxylase, the 1α-hydroxylase in the proximal convoluted tubule is a cytochrome P450–like mixed function oxidase, but unlike the 25-hydroxylase, the 1α-hydroxylase is tightly regulated. PTH and hypophosphatemia are the major inducers of this microsomal enzyme, whereas calcium, $1,25(OH)_2D$, and FGF23 repress it.[175,176] Analogous to mice lacking FGF23, mice with inactivating mutations of the FGF23 co-receptor, α-Klotho, a type I membrane protein with homology to β-glycosidases, develop hypercalcemia as a result of increased levels of $1,25(OH)_2D_3$. Like the FGF23 null mice, Klotho null mice have increased levels of the 1α-hydroxylase[177] and their phenotype is ameliorated by impairment of $1,25(OH)_2D_3$ action. In animal models and in vitro studies, other hormones such as estrogen, calcitonin, growth hormone, and prolactin have been shown to increase 1α-hydroxylase activity; however, the clinical importance of these observations has not been established. Ketoconazole has been shown to decrease levels of $1,25(OH)_2D_3$ in a dose-dependent manner, presumably by interfering with 1α-hydroxylase activity.

The 1α-hydroxylase enzyme is also expressed in keratinocytes, the trophoblastic layer of the placenta, and the activated macrophages in granulomas, including sarcoid granulomas, among many other tissues. In granulomatous tissue, the 1α-hydroxylase gene that is expressed is identical to that expressed in the kidney but is not regulated by PTH, phosphate, calcium, or vitamin D metabolites in these cells. Activation of macrophages with interferon-γ[178] or with ligands that activate the heterodimer of toll-like receptors 1 and 2,[179] however, increases the expression of the 1α-hydroxylase in macrophages, whereas treatment of sarcoidosis-associated hypercalcemia with glucocorticoids,[180] ketoconazole,[180] or chloroquine[181] has been shown to lower serum $1,25(OH)_2D_3$ levels. Activation of the VDR in human macrophages induces the antimicrobial peptide cathelicidin and increases killing of intracellular *Mycobacterium*

tuberculosis.[179] Thus, the pathologic excess of $1,25(OH)_2D_3$ in sarcoidosis may represent an exaggeration of a healthy paracrine response of tissue macrophages. This action can be viewed as a paradigm for many other actions of vitamin D that are mediated more by the local production of $1,25(OH)_2D_3$ than by circulating $1,25(OH)_2D_3$.

25(OH)D and $1,25(OH)_2D_3$ can also be hydroxylated by vitamin D 24-hydroxylase, which is present in most tissues including kidney, cartilage, and intestine. $1,25(OH)_2D_3$ increases the activity of the 24-hydroxylase, thereby inducing its own metabolism. The 24-hydroxylated vitamin D metabolites, $24,25(OH)_2D_3$ and $1,24,25(OH)_3D_3$, are not thought to play major biologic roles other than inactivation of $1,25(OH)_2D_3$. Mice null for the 24-hydroxylase gene demonstrate hypercalcemia, hypercalciuria, and nephrocalcinosis due to vitamin D toxicity.[182] Although $24,25(OH)_2D_3$ has been shown to have unique actions in a number of biologic systems,[183] no unique receptor for this metabolite has been identified and the physiologic role of $24,25(OH)_2D_3$ is unclear.

$1,25(OH)_2D_3$ is also metabolized to several inactive products by 23- or 26-hydroxylation and side chain oxidation and cleavage. This latter side chain cleavage, resulting in the formation of calcitroic acid, occurs in the liver and intestine, whereas inactivation of $1,25(OH)_2D_3$ in a wide variety of target tissues occurs by 24-hydroxylation. In addition, polar metabolites of $1,25(OH)_2D_3$ are excreted in the bile. Some of these metabolites are deconjugated in the intestine and reabsorbed into the enterohepatic circulation.

Actions of Vitamin D

Vitamin D Receptors

$1,25(OH)_2D_3$ exerts its biologic functions by binding to a nuclear receptor, which then regulates transcription of DNA into RNA. Among the other nuclear receptors, the VDR most closely resembles the retinoic acid, triiodothyronine, and retinoid X receptors (RXRs). The affinity of the receptor for $1,25(OH)_2D_3$ is approximately three orders of magnitude higher than that for other vitamin D metabolites (Fig. 28-16). Although $25(OH)D_3$ is less potent on a

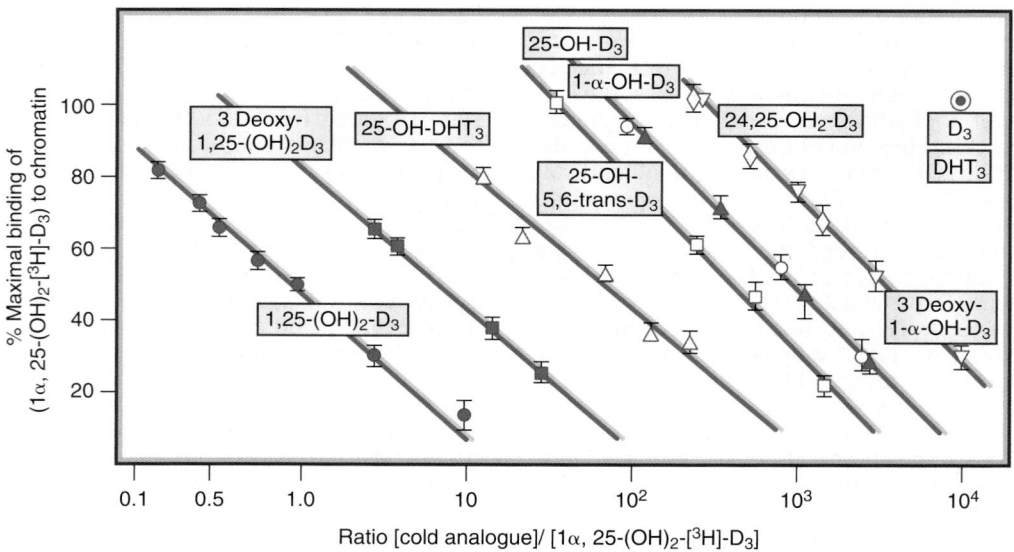

Figure 28-16 Relative potency of analogues of $1,25(OH)_2D_3$ (1,25-dihydroxyvitamin D_3) in competitive binding to vitamin D receptors of chick intestinal mucosa. Slopes are plotted for *(left to right)* $1,25$-$(OH)_2$-D_3 (1,25-dihydroxyvitamin D_3); 3 deoxy-$1,25(OH)_2D_3$ (3 deoxy-1,25-dihydroxyvitamin D_3); 25-OH-DHT_3 (25-hydroxydihydrotachysterol); 25-OH-5,6-trans-D_3 (25-hydroxy-5,6-transvitamin D_3); 25-OH-D_3 (25-hydroxyvitamin D_3); 1-α-OH-D_3 (1α-hydroxyvitamin D_3); $24,25$-OH_2-D_3 (24,25-dihydroxyvitamin D_3); 3 deoxy-1-α-OH-D_3 (3-deoxy-1α-hydroxyvitamin D_3); D_3 (vitamin D_3); DHT_3 (dihydrotachysterol). (From Proscal DA, Okamura WH, Norman AW. Structural requirements for the interaction of 1α,25-$(OH)_2$-vitamin D_3 with its chick intestinal system. *J Biol Chem*. 1975;250:8382-8388.)

molar basis, its concentration in the serum is approximately three orders of magnitude higher than that of $1,25(OH)_2D$. However, its free concentration is only two orders of magnitude greater than that of $1,25(OH)_2D_3$. Therefore, under normal circumstances it is unlikely that $25(OH)D_3$ contributes importantly to calcium homeostasis. As a substrate for local 1α-hydroxylases in many tissues, however, $25(OH)D_3$ may contribute to local tissue homeostasis.

Because the affinity of the VDBP for $25(OH)D_3$ is greater than that for $1,25(OH)_2D_3$, in states of vitamin D intoxication (with its associated high levels of $25[OH]D_3$), the free levels of $1,25(OH)_2D_3$ increase[184] because $25(OH)D$ displaces it from the VDBP. $25(OH)D_3$ may, therefore, play a role in the clinical syndrome of vitamin D intoxication both by its direct biologic effects, when present at toxic levels, as well as by increasing free levels of $1,25(OH)_2D_3$. Under normal circumstances $25(OH)D$ is not thought to play a role in mineral ion homeostasis; however, local activation of this prohormone may contribute to host immune response and barrier function.

The VDR acts by forming a heterodimer with the RXR, binding to DNA elements, and recruiting coactivators in a ligand-dependent fashion. These coactivators link the receptor complex to the basal transcription apparatus, thereby regulating transcription of target genes. In most cases, the upregulatory response elements for vitamin D contain hexameric repeats separated by three bases (Fig. 28-17).[185] However, vitamin D also promotes the DNA-protein interactions of other transcription factors, such as SP1 and NF-Y, in genes lacking classical response elements, by uncertain mechanisms.[186] The mechanism of transcriptional repression by vitamin D is varied. For example, VDR-RXR heterodimers repress the 1α-hydroxylase and renin genes by blocking the function of other transcription factors,[187,188] and interaction of the VDR with the Ku antigen, acting as a transcription factor, is required for transcriptional repression of the hPTHrP gene.[189]

Glucocorticoids have been shown to decrease the expression of the VDR gene in osteosarcoma cell lines, whereas $1,25(OH)_2D_3$ increases its expression in many cell types. In the renal proximal convoluted tubule, however, $1,25(OH)_2D_3$ decreases the levels of VDRs. This decrease has been postulated to lead to decreased activation of the renal 24-hydroxylase by $1,25(OH)_2D_3$ and, thereby, protect the newly synthesized $1,25(OH)_2D$ from local inactivation.[190]

$1,25(OH)_2D_3$ also has some biologic effects that occur too rapidly for transcriptional mechanisms to be implicated. These "nongenomic actions," including a rapid increase in intracellular calcium, activation of PLC, and opening of calcium channels, are observed in several cell types within minutes of exposure to $1,25(OH)_2D_3$. Additional data supporting the hypothesis that "nongenomic actions" are not dependent on the classical receptor include

the identification of specific binding sites for $1,25(OH)_2D_3$ on the antiluminal surface of intestinal cells[191] and a disparity between the affinity of the various vitamin D analogues for the nuclear receptor and their potency in these nongenomic actions. However, both the rapid intracellular accumulation of cGMP in association with the VDR and the rapid increase in intracellular calcium in response to $1,25(OH)_2D$ are dependent upon the presence of an intact nuclear receptor, because these effects are not observed in cells derived from patients and mice with VDR mutations.[192] The physiologic importance of the nongenomic actions of vitamin D metabolites[193] has not yet been established.

The VDR is expressed in most tissues and has been shown to regulate cellular differentiation and function in many cell types. Nevertheless, the most dramatic physiologic effects of vitamin D, acting through the VDR, involve regulation of intestinal calcium transport. This is most clearly demonstrated by the phenotype of patients and mice with mutant VDRs (hereditary vitamin D–resistant rickets)[31,194]: dramatic abnormalities in bone mineralization can be reversed by bypassing the defect in intestinal calcium absorption.[195-197]

Intestinal Calcium Absorption

Under normal dietary conditions, calcium intake is in the range of 700 to 900 mg daily. Approximately 30% to 35% of this calcium is absorbed; however, losses from intestinal secretion of calcium lead to a net daily uptake of approximately 200 mg. Studies in mice lacking the VDR confirm a critical role for this receptor in intestinal calcium absorption.[198-200] Though vitamin D is the major hormonal determinant of intestinal calcium absorption, the bioavailability of mineral ions in the intestinal lumen may be affected by a number of local factors and dietary constituents. Absorption of calcium and magnesium is impaired by bile salt deficiency, unabsorbed free fatty acids in steatorrheic states, and high dietary content of fiber or phytate. Gastric acid is needed to promote dissociation of calcium from anionic components of food or therapeutic preparations of calcium salts. Administration of calcium salts with meals, especially in achlorhydrics, and use of divided doses or more soluble salts such as calcium citrate are commonly employed strategies to increase calcium bioavailability.

Calcium is thought to be absorbed by two pathways: a saturable transcellular pathway and a nonsaturable paracellular route. The transcellular pathway is dependent on $1,25(OH)_2D_3$. Although the necessity of vitamin D for paracellular calcium absorption remains controversial, substantial evidence exists that the hormone enhances this pathway as well.[201] Notably, $1,25(OH)_2D_3$ induces the expression of claudin-2 and claudin-12, which contribute to intestinal calcium absorption and are thought to form paracellular channels between neighboring cells.[202]

The most extensively studied mechanism of intestinal calcium absorption involves the transcellular route. This pathway is thought to involve three steps: entry of calcium into the enterocyte (which is the rate-limiting step), transport across the cell, and extrusion across the basolateral membrane.

Entry into the Enterocyte. $1,25(OH)_2D_3$ induces synthesis of a number of brush border proteins, including the intestinal membrane calcium-binding protein, brush border alkaline phosphatase, and low-affinity Ca^{2+}/Mg^{2+}-ATPase. The activity of these proteins correlates with active calcium transport; however, a causal relationship remains to be established. Two calcium channels, TRPV5 and TRPV6, members of the transient receptor potential vanilloid

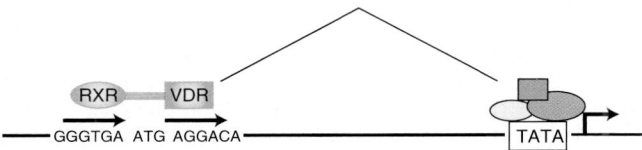

Figure 28-17 Transcriptional activation by 1,25-dihydroxyvitamin D_3 (1,25(OH)$_2$D$_3$). A heterodimer of retinoid X receptor (RXR) and vitamin D receptor (VDR) binds to a pair of hexameric sequences separated by three intervening bases (ATG). *Arrows* indicate that the hexamers found in the upregulated rat osteocalcin gene are variants of a consensus sequence, repeated here with identical orientations (direct repeats). Upon binding to DNA, the RXR-VDR heterodimer facilitates formation of a transcription initiation complex, which binds to DNA at and near the TATA sequence.

receptor subfamily containing six membrane-spanning domains, are expressed in the duodenum, the jejunum, and the kidney as well as in other tissues. TRPV6 is thought to play a critical role in intestinal calcium absorption, and $1,25(OH)_2D_3$ increases its expression, as well as that of TRP5.[203] Studies in mice lacking TRPV5 demonstrate that this channel is primarily responsible for renal calcium reabsorption, because mice lacking TRPV5 have enhanced, rather than impaired, intestinal calcium absorption owing to their high circulating levels of $1,25(OH)_2D$.[204] In contrast, mice missing TRPV6 do exhibit a decrease in intestinal calcium transport and the stimulation of this transport by vitamin D. Nevertheless, these knockout mice retain some responsiveness of intestinal calcium transport to $1,25(OH)_2D_3$, emphasizing our still incomplete understanding of this process.[205] Upon entering the enterocyte, calcium binds to components of the brush border complex subjacent to the plasma membrane. Calmodulin is redistributed to the brush border in response to $1,25(OH)_2D_3$ and may play a role in this process, as may the $1,25(OH)_2D_3$-inducible calcium-binding protein, calbindin-9K.

Transcellular Transport. The best studied effect of vitamin D on the enterocyte is the induction of synthesis of the intestinal calcium-binding protein, calbindin-9K. This protein has an EF hand structure that permits the binding of two calcium ions per molecule. The affinity of calbindin for calcium is approximately four times that of the brush border calcium-binding components, so calcium is preferentially transferred to calbindin. Calbindin serves to buffer the intracellular free calcium concentration during calcium absorption. It associates with microtubules and may play a role in the transport of calcium across the enterocyte. Nevertheless, mice without calbindin-9K exhibit normal vitamin D–mediated intestinal calcium transport; this demonstrates that the role of calbindin-9K is not rate-limiting for this activity.[205] Organelles such as the mitochondria, Golgi apparatus, and endoplasmic reticulum also serve as repositories for intracellular calcium.

Exit from the Enterocyte. The transport of calcium across the antiluminal surface of the enterocyte, the final process involved in intestinal calcium absorption, is dependent on $1,25(OH)_2D_3$. The main mechanism of calcium extrusion is the $1,25(OH)_2D_3$-inducible ATP-dependent Ca^{2+} pump (PMCA1b). The affinity of the pump for calcium is approximately 2.5 times that of calbindin. With high calcium intake, a $1,25(OH)_2D_3$-independent Na^+/Ca^{2+} exchanger may play a role in the transfer of calcium across the basolateral membrane as well.

Actions on the Parathyroid Gland

$1,25(OH)_2D_3$ has been shown to regulate gene transcription and cell proliferation in the parathyroids. The hormone also inhibits the proliferation of dispersed parathyroid cells in culture, although the relative contribution of calcium and $1,25(OH)_2D_3$ in the regulation of parathyroid cell proliferation in vivo has not been established. Normocalcemic mice lacking functional VDRs have normal serum PTH levels and normal-sized parathyroid glands, demonstrating that the genomic actions of $1,25(OH)_2D_3$ are not essential for parathyroid cellular homeostasis.[197] $1,25(OH)_2D_3$ has, however, been shown to decrease the transcription of the PTH gene both in vivo and in vitro. This action has been exploited in the use of $1,25(OH)_2D_3$ for the treatment of the secondary hyperparathyroidism associated with chronic renal failure (see discussions under "Parathyroid Hormone Biosynthesis" and "Vitamin D Deficiency"). Nevertheless, the VDR in parathyroid cells has a modest role in normal physiology. When the receptor is removed specifically from parathyroid cells in genetically manipulated mice, the resultant mice have modest decreases in the levels of CaSRs in their parathyroids, accompanied by modest elevations of blood PTH levels and evidence of increased resorption of bone.[206]

Actions on Bone

The effects of $1,25(OH)_2D_3$ on bone are numerous. $1,25(OH)_2D_3$ is a major transcriptional regulator of the two most abundant bone matrix proteins: it represses the synthesis of type I collagen and induces the synthesis of osteocalcin. $1,25(OH)_2D_3$ promotes the differentiation of osteoclasts from monocyte-macrophage stem cell precursors in vitro and increases osteoclastic bone resorption in high doses in vivo by stimulating production of RANKL (also called osteoclast differentiating factor) by osteoblasts.[207] Despite the multiple effects of $1,25(OH)_2D_3$ on the biology of bone in vitro, in vivo studies in $1,25(OH)_2D_3$-deficient rats and in mice lacking functional VDRs[31,195] suggest that the major osseous consequences of hormone and receptor deficiency can be reversed when mineral ion homeostasis is normalized. In addition, parenteral calcium infusions have been shown to heal the osteomalacic lesions in children with mutant VDRs.[196] These observations suggest that the major role of $1,25(OH)_2D_3$ in bone is to provide the proper microenvironment for bone mineralization through stimulation of the intestinal absorption of calcium and phosphate. Studies in mice with intestine-specific VDR ablation demonstrate that high levels of $1,25(OH)_2D_3$ impair bone mineralization by increasing inhibitors of mineralization.[198] This finding may represent a homeostatic response aimed at preserving serum calcium levels when intestinal calcium absorption is impaired.

Other Actions of Vitamin D

The effects of $1,25(OH)_2D_3$ on phosphate transport are less well studied than those on calcium transport; however, vitamin D has been shown to promote the already efficient intestinal phosphate absorption. Importantly, $1,25(OH)_2D_3$ also induces the expression of the phosphaturic hormone, FGF23.[58]

One of the striking, but poorly understood, clinical features of profound vitamin D deficiency is the severe proximal myopathy. Muscle cells express VDRs and $1,25(OH)_2D_3$ has nongenomic effects on muscle. Further, $1,25(OH)_2D_3$ increases amino acid uptake and alters phospholipid metabolism in vitro in muscle cells. Vitamin D administration has been shown to increase the concentration of troponin C, a calcium-binding protein in muscle that plays a role in excitation coupling and increases the rate of uptake of calcium by the sarcoplasmic reticulum. VDR knockout mice demonstrate a delay in myoblast differentiation[208]; however, little is known regarding the direct role of vitamin D in normal muscle physiology. The myopathy that accompanies vitamin D deficiency is characterized by normal creatine phosphokinase levels, a myopathic electromyogram, and biopsy findings of loss of myofibrils, fatty infiltration, and interstitial fibrosis. The myopathy resolves within days to weeks of vitamin D replacement and does not correlate with normalization of mineral ion homeostasis.

Vitamin D Analogues

The recognition that $1,25(OH)_2D_3$ promotes cellular differentiation and inhibits cellular proliferation has led to efforts directed at producing new analogues that retain these effects but do not cause hypercalcemia. Several analogues have been shown to have antiproliferative effects on normal cells as well as on malignant cells in vitro and in xenografts in immunosuppressed mice.[209] In addition, analogues of vitamin D have been shown to synergize with cyclosporine in preventing rejection of transplanted islet cells in a murine model.[210] One "nonhypercalcemic" analogue, 22-oxacalcitriol, has been shown to suppress PTH synthesis and secretion in rats,[211] at doses that stimulate intestinal calcium absorption less than $1,25(OH)_2D_3$ does. This suggests that such analogues may be useful in the prevention and treatment of hyperparathyroidism. The antiproliferative effects of vitamin D have been exploited clinically in the treatment of psoriasis.[212] Although analogues with reduced calcemic activity are predominantly used, hypercalcemic crisis after excessive topical use of such compounds can occur.

The physiology underlying the differential biologic effects of these analogues is not completely understood. Altered affinity for the VDBP, metabolism by target tissues,[213] and effects on recruitment of coactivators by the VDR may contribute to the unique properties of vitamin D analogues.[214]

FIBROBLAST GROWTH FACTOR 23

FGF23 in Human Disease

A new era in our understanding of phosphate metabolism was ushered in with the identification of the molecular basis for the human disorder, autosomal dominant hypophosphatemic rickets (ADHR).[215] Linkage analyses of affected kindreds identified mutation of the gene encoding FGF23 as the basis for ADHR. The mutation in affected individuals abolishes an RXXR protease recognition motif that is thought to be responsible for the cleavage and inactivation of FGF23.[216,217] The complementary DNA encoding FGF23 predicts a peptide of 251 amino acids, the first 24 of which compose a signal peptide. Studies using recombinant FGF23 demonstrate that the full-length mature peptide is required for its biologic activity and that the cleavage site mutated in the ADHR patients is responsible for its inactivation. Cleavage of FGF23 is blocked by furin inhibition, suggesting that the enzyme responsible is a subtilisin-like proprotein convertase.

Analyses of tumors isolated from patients with tumor-induced osteomalacia (TIO) revealed a dramatic increase in levels of mRNA encoding FGF23.[218] Serum levels of FGF23 were elevated in patients with TIO and have been shown to normalize after removal of the tumor, correlating with resolution of the hypophosphatemia that characterizes this disorder.[219-221] Conversely, patients with the rare syndrome tumoral calcinosis present with hyperphosphatemia and soft tissue calcium phosphate deposits. Some of these patients have point mutations in the FGF23 gene that cause abnormal processing of the protein, with low levels of the active hormone in the blood and high levels of inactive fragments.[222-224] Yet others have mutations in the FGF23 co-receptor Klotho or in GALNT 3, which normally O-glycosylates FGF23.[225,226] Thus, human diseases of both increased and decreased FGF23 activity suggest that this "new" factor represents an important regulator of phosphate metabolism.

Actions of FGF23

Evidence that FGF23 is a novel hormone that plays a key role in normal phosphate homeostasis has been obtained in murine models of overexpression and ablation. Overexpression of FGF23 or administration of FGF23 to animals results in the development of hypophosphatemia[217] and impaired 1α-hydroxylation of 25(OH)D,[176,227] recapitulating the findings observed in patients affected by TIO. Investigations in mice with targeted ablation of FGF23 have proved that endogenous production of this hormone is critical for normal phosphate homeostasis and the regulation of vitamin D metabolism.[228,229] Absence of FGF23 results in impaired renal phosphate excretion, leading to the development of hyperphosphatemia within the first 2 weeks of life. Affected mice also develop hypercalcemia due to high levels of $1,25(OH)_2D$, a result of the lack of the normal suppressive effect of FGF23 on the renal 25(OH)D 1α-hydroxylase.[176] Ablation of FGF23 results in premature death associated with ectopic mineralization of soft tissues, including the kidney. Impairing $1,25(OH)_2D$ action in these animals prevents the development of hypercalcemia and improves survival, suggesting that the premature death is a direct consequence of impaired mineral ion homeostasis rather than a specific developmental or maturational effect of FGF23.[230]

FGF23 impairs Na^+-dependent phosphate transport in both intestinal and renal brush border membrane vesicles.[231] It has been shown to decrease the levels of the types IIa, IIb, and IIc Na^+-dependent phosphate transporters, thereby regulating both intestinal and renal phosphate transport.[232-234] FGF23 decreases circulating levels of $1,25(OH)_2D$, both by decreasing mRNA levels for the renal 25(OH)D 1α-hydroxylase as well as by increasing expression of the 24-hydroxylase, the key enzyme involved in inactivation of $1,25(OH)_2D$.[176] FGF23 activates FGF receptor 1 in the presence of Klotho, a single-pass transmembrane protein that acts as a co-receptor.[235] Klotho knockout mice exhibit the same hyperphosphatemia and high $1,25(OH)_2D_3$ levels seen in the FGF23 knockout mouse,[177] demonstrating that it plays a critical role in mediating the actions of FGF23. In the proximal tubule, FGF23 activates FGF receptor/Klotho to, in turn, activate extracellular signal–regulated kinases (ERKs), which activate serum and glucocorticoid-regulated kinase 1 (SGK1), which then phosphorylates NHERF1, thereby releasing NaPi-IIa from the plasma membrane.[236]

The physiologic actions of FGF23 on the proximal tubule, which include suppression of phosphate transport and 25(OH)D 1α-hydroxylation, are the best understood actions of FGF23. In the proximal tubule, FGF23 binds to FGF receptor/Klotho leading to ERK phosphorylation and activation of SGK1 kinase. NHERF1 phosphorylation by SGK1 releases NaPi-IIa from the plasma membrane, leading to renal phosphate loss.[236] In the distal tubule, FGF23 increases calcium and sodium reabsorption by increasing the abundance of the TRPV5 calcium channel[237] and the Na^+/Cl^- cotransporter, NCC.[238] As in the proximal tubule, these actions require activation of the FGF receptor/Klotho complex, followed by ERK and SGK1 kinase activation.

Regulation of FGF23

Circulating FGF23 levels are increased by dietary phosphorus, serum phosphorus, and 1,25-dihydroxyvitamin D.[58,239,240] Iron deficiency has also been shown to increase expression of FGF23 in bone through a hypoxia-inducible factor (HIF)-1α–dependent mechanism.[241] However, iron deficiency does not lead to increased FGF23 activity in unaffected individuals because inactivation of FGF23 by cleavage balances the increased production.[242] Interestingly, mice with chondrocyte-specific ablation of the VDR have increased circulating FGF23, suggesting that chondrocytes express a vitamin D–regulated repressor of FGF23 production.[243]

Studies in mice with mutations in the *Phex* or *Dmp1* genes suggest that these genes are upstream of FGF23 and suppress its expression.[229,244] These genes, as well as FGF23 itself, are synthesized primarily by osteocytes embedded in the bone matrix. ENPP-1 (ectonucleotide pyrophosphatase-1), which generates pyrophosphate from its substrate, ATP[245], also suppresses expression of FGF23 by an uncertain mechanism.

During or after its synthesis, FGF23 is targeted by a series of enzymes at a furin-like protease cleavage site, R176XXR179/S180. Threonine-178 is *O*-glycosylated by polypeptide *N*-acetylgalactosaminyltransferase 3 (GalNAc-T3); this glycosylation protects FGF23 from cleavage. The furin-like cleavage also requires phosphorylation at serine-180 by the secreted kinase, FAM20C.[246,247] Thus inactivating mutations in GalNAc-T3 lead to increased cleavage of FGF23, and mutations of FAM20C lead to decreased cleavage of FGF23, leading to the diseases tumoral calcinosis and hypophosphatemic rickets, respectively (see later discussions under "Hyperphosphatemia" and "Hypophosphatemia").

In patients with chronic renal failure, an increase in FGF23 levels has been shown to antedate the development of secondary hyperparathyroidism and thus may be beneficial in predicting which individuals will develop this disorder.[248] FGF23 levels have been shown to be strong predictors of fatality in humans with chronic renal failure.[249] Direct effects of FGF23 on the heart,[250] compounding the effects of FGF23 to raise blood pressure,[238] might contribute to this increased mortality risk, independent of correlations with blood phosphate level. These studies suggest that lowering FGF23 levels in renal failure might be advantageous, though the use of a monoclonal antibody to FGF23 in one rat model of chronic renal failure, in fact, increased mortality risk.[251] Thus, the role of FGF23 and the effects of modifying levels of FGF23 in renal failure are currently incompletely understood.

CALCIUM AND PHOSPHATE HOMEOSTASIS

The cytosolic concentrations of intracellular calcium, phosphorus, and magnesium differ markedly, as reviewed previously, and their physiologic roles within cells are diverse and largely unrelated (see Fig. 28-1). In contrast, the concentrations of these mineral ions in extracellular fluid are quite comparable (i.e., 1-2 mmol/L), and it is here that they exert important interactions, both with cells and with one another, that are critical for bone mineralization, neuromuscular function, and normal mineral ion homeostasis. Extracellular calcium and phosphate, in particular, exist so close to the limits of their mutual solubility that stringent regulation of their concentrations is required to avoid diffuse precipitation of calcium phosphate crystals in tissues.

Serum concentrations and total body balances of the mineral ions are maintained within narrow limits by powerful, interactive homeostatic mechanisms. PTH, 1,25(OH)₂D, and FGF23 regulate mineral ion levels; mineral ion levels, in turn, regulate PTH, 1,25(OH)₂D, and FGF23 secretion; and these hormones may regulate the production of one another. Calcium sensors in the parathyroid glands control PTH secretion by monitoring the blood concentration of ionized calcium, and those in the kidney act to adjust tubular calcium reabsorption, independently of PTH or 1,25(OH)₂D. In contrast, the mechanisms of the phosphate sensing needed for normal homeostasis are not understood. The operation of these homeostatic mechanisms can be appreciated by considering the following examples of how the organism adapts to changes in calcium loads (Fig. 28-18).

Dietary calcium restriction, for example, is followed by an increase in the efficiency of intestinal calcium absorption. This increased efficiency results from a sequence of homeostatic responses in which lowered blood ionized calcium activates secretion of PTH, PTH augments synthesis of 1,25(OH)₂D₃ by the proximal tubules of the kidney, and 1,25(OH)₂D₃ then acts directly upon enterocytes to increase active transcellular transport of calcium. Enhanced intestinal calcium absorption is quantitatively the most important response to calcium deprivation, but a series of other homeostatic events also occur that limit the impact of this stress. Renal tubular calcium reabsorption is increased by PTH, an effect that is enhanced by increased 1,25(OH)₂D₃-stimulated expression of calbindin-D28K in the distal tubules. Calcium reabsorption is also enhanced directly by any tendency to hypocalcemia, which is detected by CaSRs in Henle's loop (and possibly also in the distal nephron) that control transepithelial calcium movements independent of PTH or 1,25(OH)₂D₃.

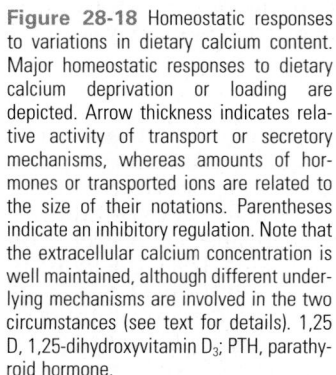

Figure 28-18 Homeostatic responses to variations in dietary calcium content. Major homeostatic responses to dietary calcium deprivation or loading are depicted. Arrow thickness indicates relative activity of transport or secretory mechanisms, whereas amounts of hormones or transported ions are related to the size of their notations. Parentheses indicate an inhibitory regulation. Note that the extracellular calcium concentration is well maintained, although different underlying mechanisms are involved in the two circumstances (see text for details). 1,25 D, 1,25-dihydroxyvitamin D₃; PTH, parathyroid hormone.

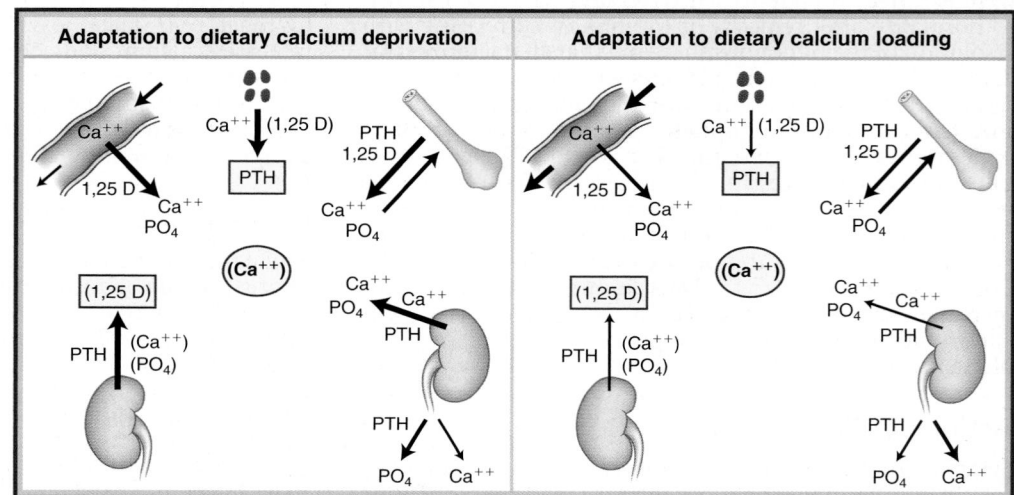

The impact of dietary calcium deprivation is reduced by approximately 15% through release of calcium from bone in response to PTH and $1,25(OH)_2D_3$. The concomitant increase in net bone resorption causes release of phosphate as well as calcium into the extracellular fluid. Intestinal phosphate absorption also is increased by $1,25(OH)_2D_3$. These phosphate loads are problematic, in that phosphate directly lowers ionized calcium in extracellular fluid, suppresses renal synthesis of $1,25(OH)_2D_3$, and directly inhibits bone resorption. These potentially negative effects of phosphate are obviated by the powerful phosphaturic action of PTH and of FGF23, the secretion of which is promoted by phosphate, calcium, and $1,25(OH)_2D$.

Finally, the possibility of unrestrained secretion of PTH, leading to excessive bone resorption and severe hypophosphatemia, is prevented by the effects of calcium on PTH secretion and by the direct suppressive effect of $1,25(OH)_2D_3$ on the synthesis of PTH and of PTH receptors. As a result of these homeostatic responses, calcium-deprived people maintain near-normal serum calcium and phosphate concentrations but display increased intestinal calcium absorption, increased bone resorption and progressive osteopenia, increased renal tubular calcium reabsorption, decreased renal tubular phosphate reabsorption, low urinary calcium excretion, elevated urinary phosphate excretion, and high serum concentrations of PTH and $1,25(OH)_2D_3$.

Calcium loads induce an opposite series of adaptations: parathyroid suppression, inhibition of renal $1,25(OH)_2D_3$ synthesis, decreased intestinal active transport of calcium, increased renal excretion of calcium and decreased renal excretion of phosphate (secondary to functional hypoparathyroidism), and a decrease in bone resorption sufficient to allow positive skeletal calcium balance. The decline in intestinal calcium absorption is the major safeguard against calcium overload, although this mechanism may be overridden with extraordinarily high intakes of calcium because of the persistence of the passive, non–vitamin D–dependent mode of calcium absorption. Moreover, nonenteral sources of calcium, such as intravenous calcium infusion or excessive net bone resorption (as from immobilization or malignancy), may readily overwhelm the limited homeostatic adaptations that remain once suppressed intestinal calcium absorption is bypassed. In such situations, the kidney rather than the intestine becomes the principal defense against hypercalcemia, and calcium homeostasis becomes critically dependent on adequate renal function. If renal function is impaired in these settings, as frequently occurs clinically, severe hypercalcemia and pathologic calcium deposition in extraskeletal sites may ensue.

LABORATORY ASSESSMENT OF MINERAL METABOLISM

Parathyroid Hormone

The major challenges in the measurement of blood PTH have been the low levels of circulating PTH and the presence of inactive PTH fragments in far greater abundance than for the intact, biologically active PTH molecule. The measurement of inactive fragments would not be a concern if the ratio of inactive to active PTH molecules remained constant. However, this ratio does change in response to changes in GFR and in parathyroid gland secretory activity (see earlier discussions under "Parathyroid Hormone Secretion" and "Metabolism of Parathyroid Hormone"). Consequently, radioimmunoassays of PTH have suffered from

lack of sensitivity and from the inability to measure the biologically active hormone directly.

For these reasons, two-site assays that require the presence of amino-terminal and carboxy-terminal sequences of full-length PTH(1-84) on the same molecule have replaced older radioimmunoassay.[252] The assays are sensitive enough to detect PTH in all normal persons. The assays have demonstrated modest circadian variation in PTH levels and some pulsatility in PTH secretion, but these variations have not interfered with the diagnostic usefulness of randomly drawn PTH measurements. Some studies have reported modest increases of PTH levels with age, although others have not. Unlike older radioimmunoassays, the two-site assays demonstrate virtually no overlap in PTH levels between patients with primary hyperparathyroidism and those with nonparathyroid hypercalcemia (Fig. 28-19). Because this distinction represents the most important challenge in the clinical setting, the use of the two-site assay has dramatically facilitated the clinician's task.

This straightforward picture has been complicated by the realization that most two-site assays detect small amounts of PTH fragments that are large but do not extend to the hormone's amino-terminus.[253] These fragments accumulate in significant amounts in patients with renal failure. These observations have prompted the development of two-site PTH assays that use antibodies specific for the first four amino acids of PTH and thus do not detect large fragments of PTH. Although it seems plausible that such assays might prove particularly useful in some clinical situations, their role is presently unclear. They offer no advantage over older two-site assays, for example, in diagnosing primary hyperparathyroidism.[254] These assays do detect a minor peak of PTH immunoreactivity that is also recognized by antibodies directed to the carboxy-terminus

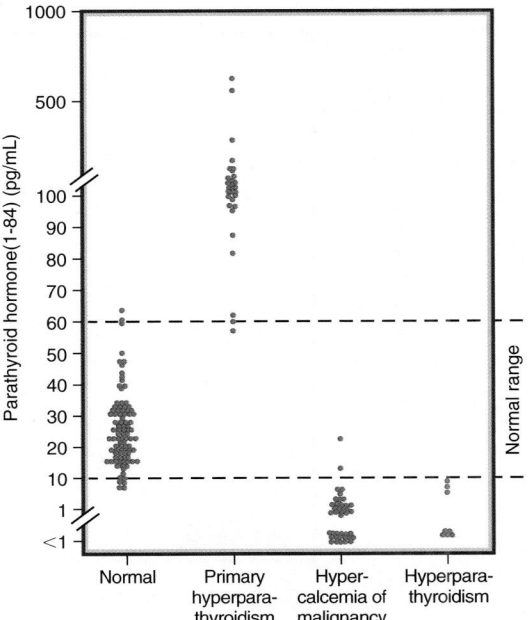

Figure 28-19 Intact immunoreactive parathyroid hormone (PTH) determined using a two-site immunoradiometric assay in normal subjects and in three different patient groups. Note some overlap between normal people and patients with primary hyperparathyroidism, but no overlap between hypercalcemic patients with primary hyperparathyroidism and those with hypercalcemia of malignancy. (From Segre GV. Advances in techniques for measurement of parathyroid hormone: current applications in clinical medicine and directions for future research. *Trends Endocrinol Metab.* 1990;1:243-247.)

of PTH and yet is not recognized by the usual "intact" PTH assays, perhaps because of a post-translational modification of PTH in the PTH(15-20) region.[255] Perhaps because of detection of this unusual form of PTH, the PTH immunoreactivity recognized using the antibody to PTH(1-4) is particularly high in patients with parathyroid cancer when compared to patients with benign primary hyperparathyroidism.[256]

Parathyroid Hormone–Related Protein

The measurement of PTHrP in serum presents a series of challenges. The concentration of PTHrP in the bloodstream, even in some patients with PTHrP-mediated malignant hypercalcemia, is not high, and the molecular definition of circulating, biologically active fragments is incomplete. Despite these problems, several groups of investigators have developed assays for PTHrP that can be helpful in the evaluation of a subset of hypercalcemic patients. Radioimmunoassays for amino-terminal portions of PTHrP and two-site assays for amino-terminal and mid-region PTHrP[114] separate healthy persons and patients with nonmalignant hypercalcemia from most patients with the humoral hypercalcemia of malignancy (Fig. 28-20). When measured with the most recently developed assays, PTHrP levels are elevated in almost all patients with malignant hypercalcemia without bone metastases and in most patients with hypercalcemia and bone metastases.

In occasional patients, the PTHrP assay has helped distinguish an occult malignancy from other causes of non–PTH-dependent hypercalcemia. Nevertheless, because the diagnosis of malignancy as the cause of hypercalcemia is usually clinically obvious, and the PTH assay can be used to diagnose primary hyperparathyroidism, the role of PTHrP assays in clinical practice is limited.[257]

Calcitonin

Several assays for measuring serum calcitonin are commercially available. The measurements are based on single or double antibody radioimmunoassays or enzyme immunoassays, several of which are sufficiently sensitive to detect calcitonin deficiency.[258] The calcitonin monomer is thought to be the biologically active molecule; therefore, some investigators feel that extraction of the multimeric forms prior to radioimmunoassay provides a more sensitive and specific measurement of serum calcitonin levels. However, the double antibody assays are thought to provide the same information with less sample manipulation. The only clinical use of the calcitonin assay is as a tumor marker, primarily in medullary carcinoma of the thyroid.

Vitamin D Metabolites

The radioligand assays for determining the levels of vitamin D metabolites require fractionation and extraction of the hormone from serum proteins by HPLC or silica cartridges. These assays are sufficiently sensitive to detect subnormal values. Because the assays measure both protein-bound and unbound vitamin D metabolites, results may not always reflect the levels of biologically relevant ("free") metabolites. This limitation may lead to misleading results in patients with nephrotic syndrome and vitamin D intoxication. With the move away from using radioligand-based assays, other methods for measuring vitamin D metabolites, including chemiluminescent assays, have been pioneered.[259] Although these assays have not withstood the test of time, they have proved to be as accurate as the currently available radioimmunoassay. Mass spectrometry is being increasingly used for measuring 25(OH)D levels. Regardless of the method used, it has been recognized that

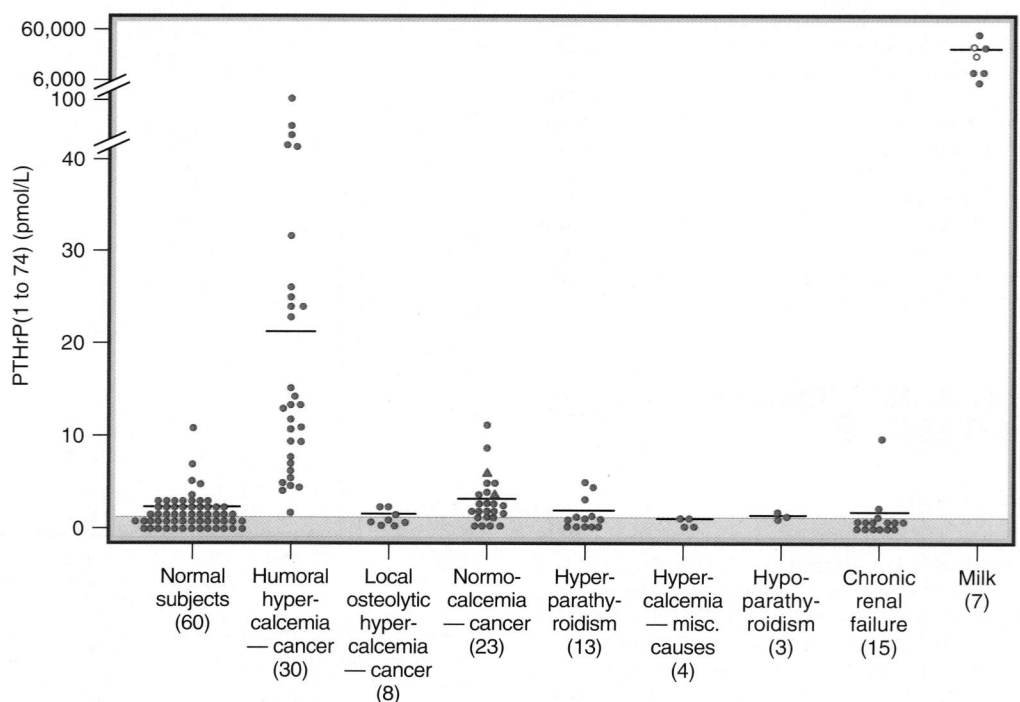

Figure 28-20 Plasma PTHrP(1-74) determined by two-site immunoradiometric assay in selected patient groups and normal subjects. Also shown are concentrations of PTHrP in human milk *(filled circles)* and in bovine milk *(open circles)*. Two normocalcemic patients with cancer *(filled triangles)* subsequently became hypercalcemic. *Shaded area* denotes levels too low to detect with this assay. PTHrP, parathyroid hormone–related protein. (Adapted from Burtis WJ, Brady TG, Orloff JJ, et al. Immunochemical characterization of circulating parathyroid hormone–related protein in patients with humoral hypercalcemia of cancer. *N Engl J Med.* 1990;322:1106-1112.)

a central repository for uniform standards is required for validation of these assays and of the laboratories performing them. The National Institute of Standards and Technology in the United States has developed standard reference materials for this purpose.[260]

The levels of 25(OH)D correlate better with the clinical signs and symptoms of vitamin D deficiency than do the levels of 1,25(OH)$_2$D$_3$. Because the 25-hydroxylation of vitamin D is not tightly regulated, measurements of 25(OH) D more accurately reflect body stores of vitamin D. Measurement of this metabolite should, therefore, be performed when vitamin D deficiency is suspected.

Measurements of 1,25(OH)$_2$D$_3$ should be reserved for cases in which excessive or impaired 1α-hydroxylation is suspected. High 1,25(OH)$_2$D$_3$ levels can be seen in sarcoidosis, lymphomas, Williams syndrome, and intoxication with 1α-hydroxylated metabolites (see "Parathyroid-Independent Hypercalcemia"). Impaired 1α-hydroxylation can contribute to the hypocalcemia of patients with renal dysfunction, oncogenic osteomalacia, and hereditary defects of vitamin D metabolism (see "Hypocalcemic Disorders").

Fibroblast Growth Factor 23

Currently two types of immunoassays are available for the measurement of serum FGF23 in humans. An assay using two polyclonal antibodies directed against C-terminal epitopes[261] detects most, if not all, circulating forms of FGF23 but does not discriminate between the intact active hormone and the cleaved fragment, which is not thought to have biologic activity. An assay for the intact hormone is a classic sandwich assay with antibodies directed against both the N- and C-terminus of the hormone.[262] This latter assay has been shown to be more useful for studying the effects of dietary phosphate on FGF23 levels in humans, and thus it is thought to provide a more precise determination of the biologically active levels of the hormone in the circulation, particularly when such levels may be changing.[263] Increased cleavage of FGF23 does occur in certain settings, such as in fibrous dysplasia[264] (see "Hypophosphatemia" later) and some forms of tumoral calcinosis[265] (see "Hyperphosphatemia" later), so in those settings assessment of both intact and cleaved FGF23 can be useful.

HYPERCALCEMIC DISORDERS

Parathyroid-Dependent Hypercalcemia

It is useful to delineate two categories of hypercalcemia: (1) that associated with dysfunction of the parathyroid cell and (2) that in which hypercalcemia occurs despite appropriate parathyroid suppression. This distinction is particularly useful clinically because it emphasizes the centrality of the PTH assay in the diagnostic approach to the hypercalcemic patient. Abnormal parathyroid glands are associated with hypercalcemia in three settings: (1) primary hyperparathyroidism, (2) familial hypocalciuric hypercalcemia (FHH), and (3) lithium-induced hypercalcemia.

Primary Hyperparathyroidism

In primary hyperparathyroidism, a primary abnormality of parathyroid tissue leads to inappropriate secretion of PTH. In contrast, increased secretion of PTH that is an appropriate response to hypocalcemia is called secondary hyperparathyroidism. The inappropriately high serum concentration of PTH in primary hyperparathyroidism, in turn, sustains excessive renal calcium reabsorption, phosphaturia, and 1,25(OH)$_2$D synthesis, as well as increased bone resorption. These actions of PTH produce the characteristic biochemical phenotype of hypercalcemia and hypophosphatemia, loss of cortical bone, hypercalciuria, and the various clinical sequelae of chronic hypercalcemia. Primary hyperparathyroidism results most often (75-80%) from the occurrence of one or more adenomas in previously normal parathyroid glands, although in 20% of cases diffuse hyperplasia of all parathyroid glands may be present or, rarely, parathyroid carcinoma may be found (less than 1-2%).[266-269]

Classical Primary Hyperparathyroidism. The bone disease "osteitis fibrosa cystica" first was described by von Recklinghausen in 1891, but the etiologic link between this disease and parathyroid neoplasms was not established until 1925, when Mandl observed clinical improvement following removal of a parathyroid adenoma from a young male with severe bone disease. In early clinical descriptions of primary hyperparathyroidism, the disease emerged as a distinctly uncommon disorder with significant morbidity and mortality rates, in which nearly all affected patients manifested radiographically significant or symptomatic skeletal or renal involvement, or both.

The skeletal involvement in "classical" primary hyperparathyroidism reflects a striking and generalized increase in osteoclastic bone resorption, which is accompanied by fibrovascular marrow replacement and increased osteoblastic activity. The radiographic appearance (Fig. 28-21)

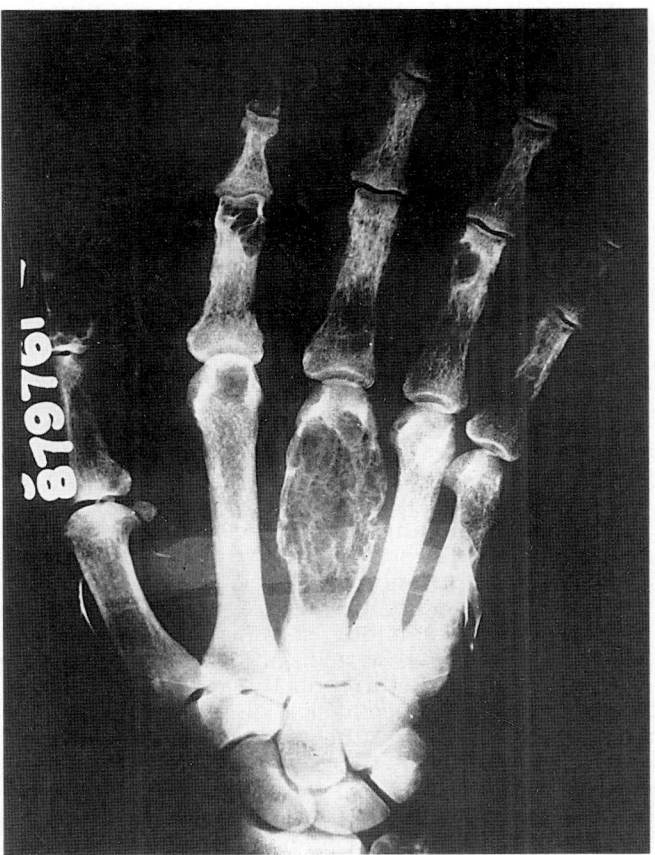

Figure 28-21 Radiograph of the hand of a patient with severe primary hyperparathyroidism. Note the dramatic remodeling associated with the intense region of high bone turnover in the third metacarpal in addition to widespread evidence of subperiosteal, endosteal, and trabecular resorption. (Courtesy of Fuller Albright Collection, Massachusetts General Hospital, Boston, MA.)

features *generalized demineralization* of bone, with coarsening of the trabecular pattern (due to osteoclastic resorption of the smaller trabeculae); characteristic *subperiosteal resorption*, often most evident in the phalanges of the hands, which gives an irregular, serrated appearance to the outer, subperiosteal cortex and may progress to extensive cortical resorption; *bone cysts*, usually multiple, which contain a brownish serous or mucoid fluid, tend to occur in the central medullary portions of the shafts of the metacarpals, ribs, or pelvis, and may expand into and disrupt the overlying cortex; *osteoclastomas*, or *brown tumors*, composed of numerous multinucleated osteoclasts ("giant cells") admixed with stromal cells and matrix, which are found most often in trabecular portions of the jaw, long bones, and ribs; and pathologic *fractures*.

The skull may exhibit a finely mottled, "salt-and-pepper" radiographic appearance, with loss of definition of the inner and outer cortices. Dental radiographs typically show erosion or disappearance of the lamina dura due to subperiosteal resorption, often with extension into the adjacent mandibular bone. The erosion and demineralization of cortical bone may lead to radiographic disappearance of some bones, most notably the tufts of the distal phalanges of the hands, the inferolateral cortex of the distal third of the clavicles, the distal ulna, the inferior margin of the femoral neck and pubis, and the medial aspect of the proximal tibia. The clinical correlates of these changes may include aching bone pain and tenderness, "bowing" of the shoulders, kyphosis and loss of height, and collapse of lateral ribs and pelvis with "pigeon breast" and triradiate deformities, respectively.

The renal manifestations of classical severe primary hyperparathyroidism include recurrent calcium nephrolithiasis, nephrocalcinosis, and renal functional abnormalities that range from impaired concentrating ability to end-stage renal failure. Associated signs and symptoms include recurrent flank pain, polyuria, and polydipsia. No unique features of the stone disease in primary hyperparathyroidism serve to distinguish it from that associated with other, more common causes of calcium kidney stones. The stone disease more often may be recurrent and severe, and in some patients, the stones may be composed entirely of calcium phosphate, instead of the pure oxalate or mixtures of oxalate and phosphate more commonly encountered in other disorders. In patients diagnosed before 1965, the frequency with which nephrolithiasis complicated primary hyperparathyroidism was as high as 60% to 80% (the frequency is currently less than 25%), yet in studies of unselected patients conducted throughout the past 50 years, primary hyperparathyroidism has accounted for fewer than 5% of all calcium kidney stones.

Other clinical features that have been reported in association with classical severe primary hyperparathyroidism are conjunctival calcifications, band keratopathy, hypertension (50%), gastrointestinal signs and symptoms (anorexia, nausea, vomiting, constipation, or abdominal pain), peptic ulcer disease, and acute or chronic pancreatitis. The issue of whether primary hyperparathyroidism increases the risk for peptic ulcer disease and pancreatitis remains controversial. Although hyperparathyroidism is associated with a higher risk of hypertension, successful parathyroidectomy has not been shown to correct the hypertension.

Signs and symptoms in primary hyperparathyroidism may result from the involvement of bone (fracture, bone pain) or kidneys (renal colic, renal failure), peptic ulcer disease, pancreatitis, or hypercalcemia per se (weakness, apathy, depression, polyuria, constipation, coma). The presence and severity of neuropsychiatric symptoms, in particular, correlate poorly with the serum calcium concentration, although few patients with severe hypercalcemia are entirely asymptomatic. Elderly persons are most likely to exhibit such symptoms. A peculiar neuromuscular syndrome, first described in 1949 but rarely encountered now, includes symmetric proximal weakness and gait disturbance, with muscle atrophy, characteristic electromyographic abnormalities, generalized hyperreflexia, and tongue fasciculations.[270]

Contemporary Primary Hyperparathyroidism. The clinical spectrum of primary hyperparathyroidism was changed dramatically in the early 1970s by the introduction of routine multichannel serum chemistry screening, which unearthed a large population of patients with previously unsuspected, asymptomatic disease. In Rochester, Minnesota, for example, the annual incidence of the disease increased abruptly from 0.15 to 1.12 per 1000 persons between the prescreening era (1965-1974) and 1975, the year after routine screening was introduced.[271] The peak incidence occurs in the sixth decade of life, and the disease rarely is encountered in patients below age 15. It is two to three times more common in women, who are slightly older at diagnosis than are men. Subsequently, the incidence of primary hyperparathyroidism has fallen; this decreased incidence may not simply be a residual effect of "sweeping the population," because it remained low when serially checked in Rochester, Minnesota, most recently from 1992 to 2001, when the incidence was 0.21 per 1000.[272]

Ascertainment of mild or asymptomatic disease may decline even further in the future because of prevalent economic disincentives to routine serum chemistry screening in the primary care setting. On the other hand, insistence upon overt hypercalcemia as a diagnostic criterion may underestimate the true incidence of the disease. For example, when serum calcium and iPTH were measured in a large population of Swedish women undergoing routine mammographic screening, the prevalence of unsuspected primary hyperparathyroidism, defined by criteria that included the combination of high-normal serum calcium plus elevated or high-normal iPTH, was 2.1%.[273] Two thirds of these women (72/109) were normocalcemic (10.0-10.4 mg/dL), yet bone density was reduced in the group as a whole and the disease was confirmed histologically in 98% of the 61 who had surgery. Further, the widespread practice of evaluating PTH levels in patients with osteoporosis has led to the identification of patients with high PTH levels and normocalcemia.[274] Many of these patients become hypercalcemic during follow-up.

Not surprisingly, given that primary hyperparathyroidism now usually is diagnosed incidentally, few patients are found to have overt signs or symptoms of the classical disease and thus are considered to be "asymptomatic." For example, only 2% of patients with primary hyperparathyroidism residing in Olmsted County, Minnesota, and only 17% of 121 patients studied at an academic referral center in New York City had classical disease symptoms.[271,275] In most of them, the relevant symptom was urolithiasis. Many clinicians argue, however, that most patients regarded as having "asymptomatic" primary hyperparathyroidism and only minimally elevated serum calcium actually suffer from various neuropsychiatric or other symptoms that may improve following curative surgery.[276] These symptoms, however, which include fatigability, weakness, forgetfulness, depression, somatization, polydipsia, polyuria, and bone and joint pain, are common in otherwise normal persons. In the small randomized studies of surgery for primary hyperparathyroidism (see later), the effects of surgery on measures of quality of life have been conflicting.[274,277-279] This remains a critical issue, as the advent of less invasive operative approaches and concerns regarding fracture, cancer, and mortality risk have lowered the threshold for consideration of surgery in many patients with the disease (see later). Throughout this chapter, "asymptomatic primary hyperparathyroidism" refers to patients who lack signs or symptoms of the classical disease, whether or not they experience any of the subtle symptoms mentioned earlier.

The natural history of untreated asymptomatic primary hyperparathyroidism, as currently detected, remains incompletely understood. Few patients seem to experience progression of disease, as measured by extreme elevations of serum or urinary calcium, appearance of renal dysfunction or nephrocalcinosis or worsening osteopenia, over many years of observation.[275] On the other hand, late cortical bone loss observed at the femoral neck and distal radius in a small number of patients followed without surgery for 15 years points to the potential importance of continued monitoring in such patients.[280] Also, an excess risk of mortality, mainly from cardiovascular disease, has been noted during extended follow-up of large cohorts of patients with chronic hypercalcemia (and presumed primary hyperparathyroidism) identified by population health screening in Sweden,[281] and similar observations have been made during extended follow-up of postsurgical patients with hyperparathyroidism.[276] Associations of hypertension, hyperuricemia, and glucose intolerance with primary hyperparathyroidism have been implicated, together with hypercalcemia per se, as contributors to this elevated risk.[275] Abnormal cardiac calcification and left ventricular hypertrophy (reversible by successful parathyroidectomy) have been reported in primary hyperparathyroidism as well.[282] Increased cardiovascular mortality risk may be a feature only of severe hyperparathyroidism, as it was restricted to those in the highest quartile of serum calcium in the Olmsted County study, which otherwise showed an overall decreased risk of death.[283] A 40% excess risk of malignancy

also was reported among 4163 Swedish patients who had undergone surgery more than a year earlier for (presumably symptomatic) primary hyperparathyroidism.[284] It has been argued that these increased risks for mortality and malignancy, even if confirmed, may apply only to those with primary hyperparathyroidism that is more severe than the "asymptomatic" version typically encountered today.[275]

Abnormalities of bone in modern, mild primary hyperparathyroidism are far subtler than those associated with the classical disease. Histologically, the rate at which new bone remodeling cycles are activated is increased. Because the phase of restorative bone formation at each remodeling site takes much more time than does the initial resorptive phase, such an increase in remodeling rate inevitably increases the ambient volume of the "remodeling space" and, thus, the porosity of bone. Depending upon the rate and extent of the accompanying increase in osteoblastic activity and the resulting local balance between net bone formation and resorption, mineralized bone volume may decrease further, remain stable, or even increase (despite an increased remodeling space). For reasons not yet understood, the balance achieved between increased resorption and formation of bone in primary hyperparathyroidism depends not only upon the severity of the hyperparathyroidism but also upon skeletal location. Thus, net resorption of endosteal bone may predominate in cortical sites, whereas net apposition of mineral may occur in trabecular bone, when measured through biopsy of the iliac crest[285,286] (Fig. 28-22). Thus, bone mineral density may be reduced, particularly at sites of predominantly cortical bone such as the mid-radius, by as much as 10% to 20%.[287] In contrast, studies using dual energy x-ray absorptiometry (DXA) demonstrate relative preservation of vertebral bone mass in primary hyperparathyroidism.[288] Despite this evidence of preserved trabecular bone mass in primary hyperparathyroidism, the incidence of vertebral fracture is increased.[289,290] The explanation for this paradox appears to

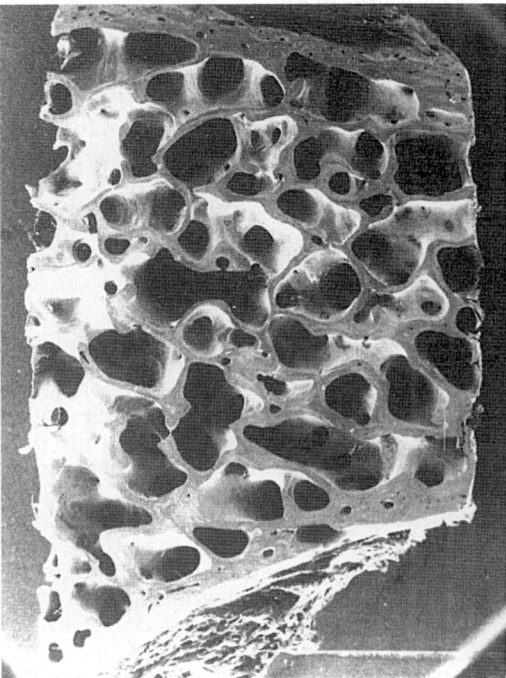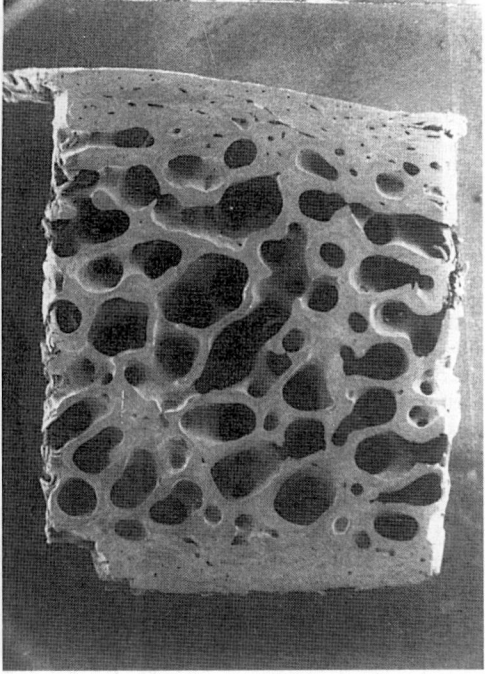

Figure 28-22 Iliac crest biopsy specimens from a patient with primary hyperparathyroidism *(left)* and a normal control subject *(right)*, viewed by scanning electron microscopy. Note the thin cortices and contrasting maintenance of trabecular bone in the patient. (From Parisien M, Silverberg SJ, Shane E, et al. The histomorphometry of bone in primary hyperparathyroidism: preservation of cancellous bone structure. *J Clin Endocrinol Metab.* 1990;70:930-938.)

relate to abnormalities in trabecular (and cortical) micro-architecture that can be detected using high-resolution peripheral quantitative computed tomography (CT) or by evaluating the trabecular bone score during DXA measurements.[291,292] These abnormalities reflect shifts from plate- to rod-like microstructure that weaken the bone and presumably account for the elevated risk of vertebral fracture. These defects are improved following successful parathyroidectomy.[293]

Kidney stones now are reported in only 10% to 25% of patients with primary hyperparathyroidism, although some degree of renal dysfunction, either a significant reduction in creatinine clearance or impaired concentrating or acidifying ability, may be found in up to one third of those with asymptomatic disease. These renal abnormalities are not progressive in the majority of affected patients.[275,294] No parameters of disease severity predict a lower estimated GFR.[295] The association of kidney stones with primary hyperparathyroidism generally is viewed as an indication for parathyroidectomy, however, because successful surgery usually prevents further symptomatic stone disease.[275,276] On the other hand, it is not possible at present to confidently predict, from biochemical measurements in blood or urine, which asymptomatic patients with hyperparathyroidism will go on to develop new stone disease. Stone-formers are more likely to be hypercalciuric than not, but less than one third of hypercalciuric patients with hyperparathyroidism actually develop stones.

Etiology and Pathogenesis. Parathyroid adenomas are caused by mutations in the DNA of parathyroid cells; these mutations confer a proliferative or survival advantage for affected cells over their normal neighbors.[296,297] As a consequence of this advantage, the descendants of one particular parathyroid cell, a clone of cells, undergo clonal expansion to produce an adenoma.

Multiple chromosomal regions are missing in the parathyroid cells of individual parathyroid adenomas. These genetic deletions probably reflect the deletion of tumor suppressor genes. These chromosomal loci include portions of chromosome 1p–pter (in 40% of adenomas), 6q (in 32% of adenomas), 15q (in 30% of adenomas), and 11q (in 25% to 30% of adenomas). Many of the 11q deletions are associated, in the undeleted chromosome 11, with mutations in the gene encoding the transcription factor menin, the gene mutated in multiple endocrine neoplasia type 1 (MEN1). Thus, this gene is also involved commonly in somatic mutations in patients with sporadic parathyroid adenomas. Somatic mutations have also been found in the mitochondrial genomes of a fraction of chief cell adenomas and have been found even more frequently in so-called oxyphil adenomas, known to exhibit mitochondria with abnormal morphologic appearance.[298] The widespread presence of somatic mutations in sporadic parathyroid adenomas, which are detectable only because large numbers of cells in any one tumor contain the same deletion, constitutes the strongest evidence that parathyroid adenomas are clonal expansions of mutant cells.

One parathyroid proto-oncogene, the PRAD1 or cyclin D1 gene, has been identified.[299] This gene was discovered at the breakpoint of an inversion on chromosome 11 in a parathyroid adenoma. This inversion led to the juxtaposition of the PTH gene's regulatory region and the DNA encoding cyclin D1. As a consequence, the cyclin D1 gene was overexpressed. Cyclin D1 is an important regulator of the transition from the G_1 phase of the cell cycle (which follows mitosis) to the S phase (associated with DNA synthesis) and is mutated or amplified in a wide variety of malignancies. Cyclin D1 is overexpressed in about 20% of parathyroid adenomas, though cyclin D1 gene rearrange-ments have been documented in only 5% of adenomas. Overexpression of cyclin D1 in the parathyroids of transgenic mice leads to formation of parathyroid adenomas and hypercalcemia over many months.[300] The phenotype of these mice demonstrates that cyclin D1 overexpression can cause primary hyperparathyroidism.

Improvements in DNA sequencing technology have allowed the sequencing of virtually all the exons in the human genome, and this sort of "whole exome" sequencing has been performed by two groups.[301,302] The most striking finding of these studies (sequencing 24 tumors between them) was that these tumors averaged roughly 7 exome mutations per tumor (with the exception of one tumor with 110 mutations in association with a mutation in the protection of telomeres 1 gene [POT1] known to increase genetic instability). This number is considerably lower than the number of mutations typically found in cancers that have been sequenced. In both studies 35% of the tumors harbored mutations in the MEN1 gene, usually in association with deletion of the second MEN1 gene. No other gene was mutated frequently in these series, though mutation in a known oncogene, an activating mutation in EZH2, was found a second time when a larger series of tumors was tested for that mutation.[301] Whole genome sequencing is not designed to detect chromosomal rearrangements or gene amplification.

As expected for a disease caused by mutations in DNA, parathyroid adenomas occur more frequently in patients who underwent neck irradiation decades earlier, with greater radiation exposure leading to higher risk. Most patients have no definite history of exposure to specific mutagens, however. An intriguing clue that abnormalities of vitamin D physiology may predispose to primary hyperparathyroidism has come from the observation that patients with parathyroid adenomas are more likely than others to inherit a particular allele of the VDR gene.[303] These patients have tumors with particularly low levels of mRNA encoding the VDR. Nevertheless, no mutations in the coding regions of the gene encoding the VDR have been found in parathyroid adenomas.[304]

The cause of sporadic primary parathyroid hyperplasia is unknown. The known stimulus for parathyroid cell proliferation—low levels of blood calcium or $1,25(OH)_2D_3$—is not present in this disease. Presumably, some other stimulus outside the parathyroid glands or a genetic abnormality present in all four parathyroid glands leads to inappropriate cell proliferation. Such abnormalities have been found in several inherited forms of parathyroid hyperplasia (see later), but most cases of parathyroid hyperplasia are not found in familial clusters.

The theoretical distinction between adenoma as a clonal proliferation and hyperplasia as a polyclonal growth is clear-cut. In some settings, however, clonal expansion can occur in the context of preexisting nonclonal proliferation. The clearest example of this complication has been found in the large glands associated with severe renal failure. In many such glands removed surgically because of hypercalcemia or severe parathyroid-dependent bone disease, evidence for clonal proliferation complicating secondary hyperplasia has been found. Interestingly, the pattern of chromosomal abnormalities in these clonal tumors differs from that found in parathyroid adenomas in the absence of renal failure.[305] Analogous mechanisms may be operative in a number of settings associated with stimuli to parathyroid cell proliferation, such as X-linked hypophosphatemia and long-term lithium therapy. Furthermore, just as clonal tumors can arise in the setting of *secondary* parathyroid hyperplasia, they can also arise in the setting of sporadic *primary* parathyroid hyperplasia[306] and in MEN1.[307]

The distinction between adenoma and hyperplasia is clinically important, because removal of the one abnormal gland can be expected to cure a parathyroid adenoma, whereas removal of multiple glands is required to successfully treat parathyroid hyperplasia. Unfortunately, differentiating adenoma from hyperplasia from normal parathyroid tissue at pathologic examination is not straightforward. Pathologists distinguish normal from abnormal parathyroid glands by the increase in size and the paucity of fat in abnormal glands. Attempts have been made to distinguish an adenoma from an individual hyperplastic gland on the basis of morphologic features, but no criteria have proved completely reliable.[308] The formation of clonal neoplasms in originally hyperplastic tumors may explain some of the difficulty in pathologic diagnosis.

An increase in cell number is not the only abnormality in primary hyperparathyroidism. The ability of the normal parathyroid cell to suppress PTH secretion in response to hypercalcemia might be expected to protect the individual from sustained hypercalcemia, even if the number of parathyroid cells increased moderately. Unfortunately, parathyroid cells in parathyroid adenomas usually demonstrate abnormalities in their responsiveness to calcium, with a shift in set point to the right (Fig. 28-23). This set-point shift, combined with the nonsuppressible component of PTH secretion, leads to a new steady state in which both the PTH level and the blood calcium level are higher than normal. The molecular underpinning of the abnormal parathyroid cell responsiveness is beginning to be understood. Parathyroid cells from adenomas respond to changes in extracellular calcium with smaller than normal increases in intracellular calcium, and the amount of CaSR protein on the cell surface is reduced.[309] Perhaps surprisingly, no mutations in the gene encoding the CaSR have been found in parathyroid adenomas. In the experimental model in which overexpression of cyclin D1 results in primary hyperparathyroidism,[300] reduced expression of the CaSR occurs only after cell proliferation has been increased for some time. Thus, the decreased expression of the CaSR in parathyroid adenomas is likely to be a secondary response that occurs during tumor formation. One demonstrated regulator of expression of the *CASR* gene in parathyroid cells is the developmental regulator, *gcm2*.[310]

Inherited Primary Hyperparathyroidism. Although uncommon, inherited forms of primary hyperparathyroidism are clinically important for several reasons. The management of the parathyroid tumors found in familial parathyroid syndromes often differs from that of sporadic primary hyperparathyroidism. Furthermore, extraparathyroidal manifestations of inherited syndromes may need treatment, and awareness of familial clustering should prompt systematic family screening.

Multiple Endocrine Neoplasia Type 1 (see also Chapter 39). MEN1 is caused by inactivating mutations in the tumor suppressor gene encoding menin.[311] Menin is a ubiquitously expressed transcription factor that is part of a complex that targets histone H_3 for methylation,[312] and thereby leads to expression of cell cyle inhibitors in pancreatic islets and other tissues.[313] Menin interacts with many nuclear proteins and it is not known which interactions are central to the pathogenesis of MEN1.[314] Rarely, mutations in genes encoding cyclin-dependent kinase inhibitors, such as p27, are found in MEN1 patients without menin mutations[315]; some have termed this variant, which presents primarily with parathyroid and pituitary tumors, *MEN4*.[316] Although MEN1 includes tumors of the parathyroid, anterior pituitary, and pancreatic islets, the parathyroid tumors are far more prevalent than the others; 95% of affected patients eventually develop hyperparathyroidism. Most of the parathyroid tumors harbor mutations in both copies of the menin gene; one mutation is inherited and the second occurs in the parathyroid cell whose progeny form the tumor.

The onset of hypercalcemia occurs in the second and third decades of life, though occasional patients present in the first decade. Hypercalcemia never presents at birth or in infancy. The disease involves all four parathyroid glands, although the involvement can be asymmetric and apparently asynchronous. Apart from the earlier age at diagnosis, the presenting clinical picture generally resembles that of sporadic primary hyperparathyroidism, perhaps with somewhat greater loss of bone density.[317] One common complicating feature is that hypercalcemia can dramatically increase the gastrin levels and symptomatology of patients who also have gastrinomas. Treatment of the parathyroid disease in this setting can greatly simplify the management of the gastric hyperacidity. After parathyroid surgery, hypoparathyroidism and recurrent hyperparathyroidism are more common than in other forms of hyperparathyroidism.[318] The timing and type of surgery are therefore more complicated issues than in sporadic primary hyperparathyroidism. Most authorities agree that parathyroid disease recurs eventually, particularly if fewer than three glands are removed. Some surgeons prefer subtotal parathyroidectomy, whereas others prefer total

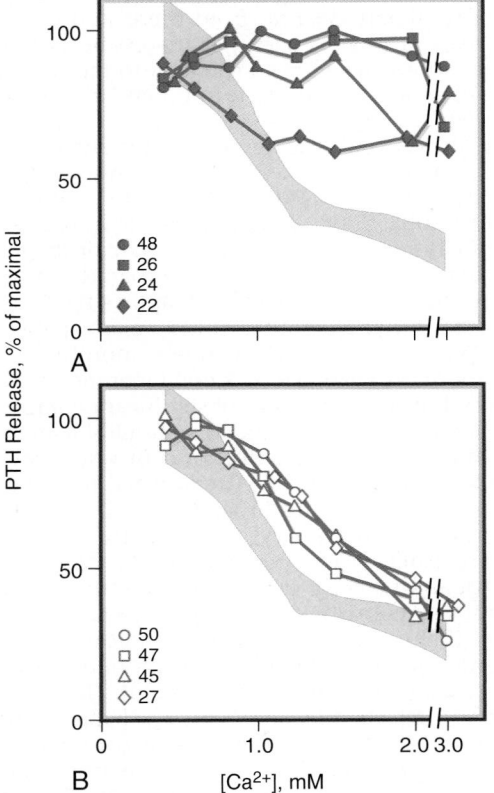

Figure 28-23 Abnormal patterns of parathyroid hormone (PTH) secretion from cells prepared from adenomatous glands and stimulated with varying levels of calcium in tissue culture. The *shaded area* shows the pattern of PTH release (±1 SD) from normal human parathyroid cells. Panel **A** illustrates the pattern from four patients with little suppression of PTH secretion by calcium. Panel **B** illustrates the pattern from four patients with relatively intact mechanism of suppression of PTH secretion by calcium. Even in this group the set point for calcium suppression is shifted to the right. (From Brown, EM. Calcium-regulated parathyroid hormone release in primary hyperparathyroidism: studies in vitro with dispersed parathyroid cells. *Am J Med.* 1979;66: 923-931.)

parathyroidectomy with forearm implantation of a small amount of parathyroid tissue.

Multiple Endocrine Neoplasia Type 2a (see also Chapter 39). Parathyroid disease is a usually late and infrequent (5% to 20%) occurrence in MEN2a, a disease defined by the clustering of medullary carcinoma of the thyroid, pheochromocytoma, and hyperparathyroidism. In some families, hyperparathyroidism is more common; however, these families have the same mutations in the *RET* gene that are found in families without frequent hyperparathyroidism. Both parathyroid hyperplasia and adenoma have been noted at surgery. Because asymptomatic parathyroid hyperplasia has been noted at the time of thyroid surgery, a progression from hyperplasia to adenoma in MEN2a has been suggested. The approach to diagnosis and treatment of hyperparathyroidism is similar to that in sporadic primary hyperparathyroidism, but hyperplasia is more frequently the underlying disorder. The pathogenesis of the hyperparathyroidism is uncertain, but the *RET* gene, mutated in virtually all cases of MEN2a, is expressed in parathyroid cells,[319] so abnormal *RET* expression in parathyroid cells may directly cause parathyroid tumor formation. Hyperparathyroidism does not occur in MEN2b, the variant associated with mucosal neuromas.

Hyperparathyroidism–Jaw Tumor Syndrome. Patients with hereditary hyperparathyroidism–jaw tumor syndrome[320] present with parathyroid adenomas that can be multiple and that are usually cystic. These tumors are often but not invariably associated with fibrous jaw tumors that are unrelated to the hyperparathyroidism. Importantly, the parathyroid tumors are frequently malignant, in contrast to the findings in MEN1 and 2. Wilms tumor and polycystic renal disease also have occurred in affected families. The gene mutated in this syndrome, called *CDC73* or *HRPT2*, encodes the nuclear protein, parafibromin.[321] Parafibromin is part of the evolutionarily highly conserved PAF complex that binds RNA polymerase II, regulates chromatin structure, and regulates gene expression.[322-324] Parafibromin binds β-catenin and can mediate Wnt pathway signaling and notch signaling, though whether these properties of parafibromin are related to its tumor suppressor function is unknown.[325] Inactivating mutations in parafibromin are found in a high number of patients with apparently sporadic parathyroid cancer.[326] Because some of these patients have subsequently proved to be members of families with inherited *CDC73* mutations, perhaps all patients with parathyroid cancer should be screened for germ-line mutations in *CDC73*.

Management of Primary Hyperparathyroidism. The strategy for management of primary hyperparathyroidism has evolved in parallel with the changing presentation of the disease. The only opportunity for permanent cure is surgical removal of the abnormal gland(s), an approach that clearly was appropriate for virtually all patients in whom the classical, severe form of the disease was diagnosed many decades ago and which still is the treatment of choice for those patients who do present with recurrent kidney stones, nephrocalcinosis, clinically overt bone disease, or severe hypercalcemia.

In contrast, the choice of surgical versus medical management for patients with asymptomatic primary hyperparathyroidism remains an open and hotly debated question. Those who favor surgery point to the expected improvement in bone mineral density (at the hip and spine) and left ventricular hypertrophy following successful surgical intervention; evidence of increased risk for fracture, cardiovascular mortality, malignancy, and neuropsychiatric symptoms associated with primary hyperparathyroidism; and the recent successful development of

effective minimally invasive surgical procedures (see later). Those who favor an observational approach emphasize the evidence for lack of disease progression in most asymptomatic patients; the small but finite risk of surgical failure and postoperative complications; the probability that excess mortality and cancer risks documented in patients with relatively severe disease may not apply to those with mild, asymptomatic primary hyperparathyroidism; the difficulty in assigning vague neuropsychiatric symptoms to the parathyroid disorder; the lack of evidence (or negative evidence) that hypertension and increased risk of cancer, fracture, or cardiovascular mortality, even if present, are improved by successful parathyroidectomy; and the availability of sensitive techniques for monitoring disease status in nonoperated patients.[275]

Unfortunately, no large prospective studies powered to compare clinical outcomes in patients with asymptomatic primary hyperparathyroidism randomly assigned to surgery versus medical management have been conducted. Nevertheless, three valuable smaller, randomized controlled trials of surgery versus observation have been conducted that allow some conclusions about surrogate markers of disease.[277-279] All three trials demonstrated increases in bone density in the spine and hip in the surgical group; these increases were similar to those produced with bisphosphonate therapy in primary hyperparathyroidism (see later). Two of the three studies showed modest improvements in some quality of life measures, though the unblinded nature of the studies limits interpretation of these findings. All of the findings reported so far from these studies have been after 2 years or less. As useful as these studies have been, their limitations have forced the field to tap observational studies to draw tentative recommendations based on limited data.

Such provisional recommendations have emanated from a series of conferences: an NIH-sponsored Consensus Conference held in 1990, followed by more informal updates in 2002, 2008, and most recently, in 2014.[327] The major conclusion of that group was that, although surgery is indicated for symptomatic hyperparathyroidism and always should be considered an appropriate option in asymptomatic hyperparathyroidism, many patients with asymptomatic disease can be safely monitored without surgery for many years. Those suitable for medical observation should have no evidence of significant compromise of skeletal integrity or renal function, should have no history of urolithiasis or gastrointestinal or neuropsychiatric symptoms, and should meet the criteria listed in Table 28-1.[328] Such patients account for at least 50% of those who currently present with primary hyperparathyroidism.

On the other hand, surgery could be preferable if the patient desired surgery even when asymptomatic, if the probability of consistent monitoring seemed low, if concomitant illness seemed likely to complicate management or obscure significant disease progression, or if the patient was relatively young (under 50 years old). The latter recommendation reflects the absence of reliable information about the natural history of the disease over many decades of follow-up; the cumulative cost of medical monitoring, which begins to exceed that of surgery by 5 to 10 years; and some data suggesting that young people are more likely than others to have progressive disease.[329] On the other hand, age alone was not viewed as a contraindication to parathyroidectomy, as the procedure has been accomplished with excellent results, with a perioperative mortality rate of 1% to 3%, in large numbers of appropriately selected patients over the age of 75 years. Because hypertension is not thought to be a feature of mild primary hyperparathyroidism, and because hypertension generally

TABLE 28-1

Indications for Surgery in Primary Hyperparathyroidism

Overt clinical manifestations of disease
    Kidney stones or nephrocalcinosis
    Fractures or classical radiographic findings of osteitis fibrosa
    Classical neuromuscular disease
    Symptomatic or life-threatening hypercalcemia
Serum calcium > 1 mg/dL above upper limit of normal
Creatinine clearance < 60 mL/min, presence of stone(s) by radiograph, CT, or ultrasound
Urinary calcium > 400 mg/day plus other urinary biochemical indices of stone risk
Bone mineral density low (T score ≤ –2.5) at any site*
Presence of vertebral fracture by radiograph or by vertebral fracture analysis on DXA
History of fragility fracture
Young age (<50 years)
Uncertain prospects for adequate medical monitoring

*Z score ≤ –2.5 in premenopausal women and in men < 50 years old.
CT, computed tomography; DXA, dual-energy x-ray absorptiometry.
Modified from Bilezikian JP, Khan AA, Potts JT Jr, Third International Workshop on the Management of Asymptomatic Primary H. Guidelines for the management of asymptomatic primary hyperparathyroidism: summary statement from the Third International Workshop. *J Clin Endocrinol Metab.* 2009;94(2):335-339. Based upon recommendations of the 2014 NIH-sponsored "Workshop on the Management of Asymptomatic Primary Hyperparathyroidism."

is not improved by parathyroidectomy, hypertension was not viewed as an indication for surgery.

Although the Consensus Conference recommendations and subsequent modifications provide a useful framework for decision making, supporting data from large clinical trials are lacking. In a series of 52 asymptomatic patients selected for nonoperative management mainly on the basis of the 1990 Consensus Conference criteria and whose course was followed for 10 years, approximately 25% developed one or more new indications for surgery.[275] Patients who do not meet the Consensus Conference criteria for surgery may nevertheless experience the same postsurgical increase in bone density as those who do.[330] Some have emphasized that evidence of baseline vertebral osteopenia, an unusual finding in primary hyperparathyroidism, should be considered among the criteria for surgery[331] and that surgery also should be considered for postmenopausal women who exhibit vertebral bone loss in the setting of primary hyperparathyroidism.[275]

A common dilemma is the inability to ascertain whether vague but troublesome symptoms such as fatigue, lethargy, weakness (without objective muscle weakness), and depression are due to hyperparathyroidism and thus qualify as "significant" in the context of considering the decision for surgery. Most clinicians do not routinely recommend parathyroidectomy on the basis of such symptoms alone, although dramatic responses to surgery are occasionally seen. With the availability of improved, minimally invasive surgical approaches, the threshold for considering surgery in patients who are significantly disabled by such symptoms clearly is lower now than in the past. Some have advocated, in selected cases, a limited trial of medical therapy to reduce serum calcium (i.e., calcimimetics—see later) and thereby attempt to predict the symptomatic response to surgical cure.

Medical Monitoring of Primary Hyperparathyroidism. The updated NIH Consensus Conference recommendations suggest that patients not treated surgically should be followed carefully, with annual measurement of serum calcium and calculated creatinine clearance and serial determination of bone mineral density at 1- to 2-year

intervals. The most appropriate bone densitometric site is considered to be one that reflects mainly changes in cortical bone (i.e., distal forearm), although the importance of following vertebral bone density as well has been emphasized,[275] and current criteria acknowledge the importance of significant bone loss at any site.[328]

Patients undergoing nonoperative medical management must be cautioned to maintain adequate hydration, to avoid diuretics and prolonged immobilization, and to seek prompt medical attention in the event of illnesses accompanied by significant vomiting or diarrhea. Dietary calcium should not be restricted.

The goal of an effective pharmacologic therapy for primary hyperparathyroidism remains elusive, though studies of sex hormones and selective estrogen receptor modulators, bisphosphonates, and calcimimetics continue. Estrogens and progestins may reduce serum calcium and phosphorus, urinary calcium and hydroxyproline, and histologic evidence of active bone resorption in women with primary hyperparathyroidism, although safety concerns have limited these therapeutic options in postmenopausal women.

Intravenous bisphosphonates have been employed successfully in the urgent therapy of hypercalcemia due to primary hyperparathyroidism, and several trials have shown that treatment with oral alendronate for a year or more improves bone density at the spine and hip, with only transient effects on serum calcium and PTH.[332,333] The calcimimetics represent a new class of agents that, by sensitizing the CaSR to extracellular calcium, can reduce PTH secretion. Cinacalcet, the first calcimimetic approved for control of secondary hyperparathyroidism in renal disease, was shown to lower serum calcium and PTH in primary hyperparathyroidism (and in some patients with parathyroid carcinoma), although improvement on bone density has not been documented in this population.[334]

Thus, in patients for whom surgery for ayymptomatic primary hyperparathyroidism is not an option, therapy with oral bisphosphonates can improve bone density without worsening other features of the disease, at least over 2 years of follow-up, and cinacalcet can control blood calcium. Whether these agents or any other medical therapy offers a beneficial long-term alternative to surgery is unknown.

Surgical Treatment of Primary Hyperparathyroidism. Parathyroidectomy is a safe and highly effective approach to definitive treatment of primary hyperparathyroidism. The most serious potential complications of parathyroid surgery—vocal cord paralysis and permanent hypoparathyroidism—occur after fewer than 1% and 4%, respectively, of procedures performed by highly skilled surgeons, although these rates can be much higher in less experienced hands. Such complications occur most often in patients who require subtotal parathyroid resections for hyperplasia or resection of carcinoma. The surgical cure rate for primary hyperparathyroidism in the best hands is at least 95%.[335,336] Apart from operator inexperience, the usual cause of initial surgical failure ("persistent disease") is the presence of either unrecognized (often very asymmetric) parathyroid hyperplasia or ectopic parathyroid tissue (i.e., intrathyroidal, undescended, retroesophageal, or mediastinal glands)[337] (Fig. 28-24). Up to one in five parathyroid glands may be located ectopically, and this is especially true of supernumerary glands. Recurrent disease, defined as that occurring after an interval of at least 6 to 12 months of normocalcemia, varies in incidence from 2% to 16%. Recurrent hyperparathyroidism usually arises in unresected hyperplastic glands, but rarely it may be due to parathyroid carcinoma, to a second adenoma, or to a multicentric or miliary

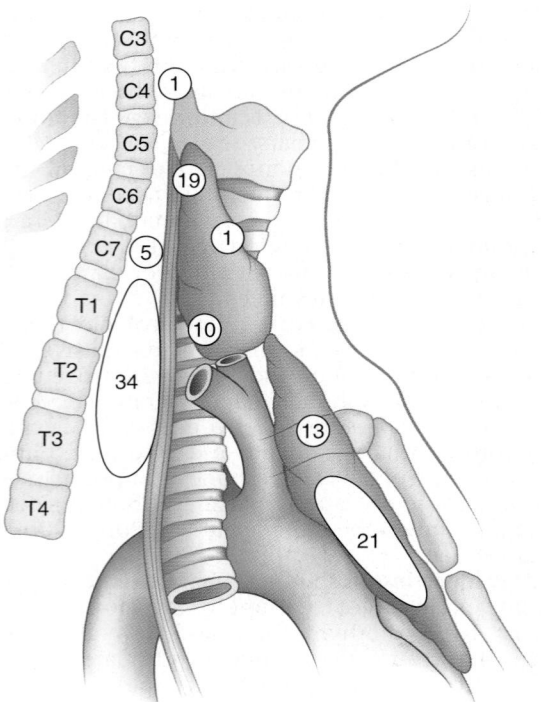

"parathyromatosis" engendered by inadvertent local seeding of parathyroid tissue (usually hyperplastic) into the neck during previous parathyroid surgery.[266,338]

In the past, there was broad agreement that the best approach is a bilateral neck exploration in which all four parathyroids are identified and all enlarged glands removed. With this procedure, preoperative parathyroid localization studies prior to initial cervical exploration are superfluous, as the positive predictive value of even the best technique (^{99m}Tc-sestamibi scanning) falls well short of the success rate of experienced surgeons unaided by prior imaging.[266,339]

With the advent of preoperative ^{99m}Tc-sestamibi scanning, which can accurately localize 80% to 90% of the single adenomas that account for 75% to 85% of cases, there has been renewed interest in performance of directed unilateral explorations, which reduce operative and recovery-room time, minimize the number of frozen sections required, are associated with significantly fewer postoperative complications, and can more readily be performed using minimally invasive techniques (including local anesthesia and intravenous sedation) that enable same-day discharge.[340] Sestamibi scanning also can identify the occasional mediastinal adenoma and thereby allow the avoidance of an unnecessary neck exploration. On the other hand, the sensitivity and positive predictive value of sestamibi scanning is poor (<50%) in the presence of multiglandular disease (hyperplasia or double adenomas), and thus, the test may frequently miss the presence of bilateral disease.[336] To reduce this failure rate, which is unacceptably high in comparison to bilateral exploration, supplemental preoperative ultrasonic imaging or high-resolution CT with dynamic contrast administration (four-dimensional CT [4D-CT])[341] is often employed (with or without needle biopsy), and rapid intraoperative PTH assays have been developed to verify successful excision.[342] Because the half-life of intact PTH in blood is very short (<2 minutes), a

decline of 50% or more from baseline within 10 minutes or so can signal successful removal of all hyperfunctioning parathyroid tissue. This approach has functioned well in patients with single adenomas, but can be misleading in those with multiglandular disease unless more stringent criteria for cure are applied (i.e., >90% decline, or even normalization, of iPTH).[343]

At present, preoperative imaging enables consideration of a minimally invasive unilateral parathyroidectomy in approximately 70% of those patients thought preoperatively to have sporadic primary hyperparathyroidism due to a solitary adenoma. Surgical cure rates in appropriately selected patients are comparable to those after bilateral neck exploration (i.e., 95-97%),[336] although a recent study in which all patients selected for minimally invasive surgery were also subjected to immediate bilateral neck dissection demonstrated a failure to recognize multiglandular disease in 16% of these subjects.[344] Patients known or suspected to have muliglandular disease, such as those with MEN1 and those younger than 30 years of age, should undergo bilateral neck exploration.[345] Options for patients with hyperplasia include resection limited to visibly abnormal glands, subtotal parathyroidectomy with cryopreservation of tissue, and total parathyroidectomy with immediate autotransplantation (i.e., in the forearm) of some excised tissue. In patients with MEN1, considerations of recurrence rates (30-50% or higher with long-term follow-up) and the timing thereof versus the potential morbidity of surgical hypoparathyroidism tend to favor subtotal parathyroidectomy as the preferred approach at present.

The incidence of parathyroid carcinoma in primary hyperparathyroidism is less than 1%,[269] but this possibility should be strongly considered in patients with unusually severe hyperparathyroidism, a palpable neck mass, hoarseness, evidence of local invasion at surgery, or recurrent hypercalcemia.[346] Even so, parathyroid carcinoma rarely is suspected preoperatively and often eludes diagnosis at the time of initial surgery. When the disease is recognized, vigorous attempts should be made to remove the tumor en bloc. The incidence of local recurrence approaches 50%, however, and distant metastases, particularly to lung, may be heralded by recurrent, severe hyperparathyroidism.[347] Because apparently sporadic and isolated parathyroid cancer can occur in families with parafibromin mutations, a search for such mutations in all patients with parathyroid cancer can facilitate family counseling.[326]

The immediate postoperative management of parathyroidectomy focuses on establishing the success of the surgery and monitoring the patient closely for symptomatic hypocalcemia and for uncommon but potentially serious acute complications such as bleeding, vocal cord paralysis, or laryngospasm. After successful resection of a parathyroid adenoma, serum intact PTH levels decline rapidly, often to undetectable concentrations, with a disappearance half-time of about 2 minutes, whereas serum calcium typically reaches a nadir between 24 and 36 hours. Serum PTH returns to the normal range within 30 hours, although measurements of the parathyroid secretory response to hypocalcemia suggest that it does not fully normalize for at least several weeks.[348]

In the past, patients generally were maintained on a low-calcium diet until normalization of serum calcium was clearly documented, ampoules of injectable calcium and other seizure precautions were maintained at the bedside, serum calcium was measured at least every 12 hours until stable, and symptomatic hypocalcemia was promptly treated with calcium, either intravenously (90-mg bolus, 50-100 mg/hour) or orally (1.5-3.0 g/day). This approach is no longer appropriate for most patients, who are discharged within a few hours after limited surgery. Instead, oral calcium supplements routinely are provided as soon as oral intake is reestablished, and moderate doses of $1,25(OH)_2D$ (0.5-1.0 µg daily) are added for those with large adenomas and severe hyperparathyroidism or for those in whom alkaline phosphatase had been elevated properatively—i.e., patients in whom an impressive calcium requirement can be anticipated, often for many weeks postoperatively, as they remineralize their skeletons. This "hungry bone" syndrome is associated with hypocalcemia, hypophosphatemia, and low urinary calcium excretion.

Serum calcium should be checked at intervals of several days initially to guide adjustment of calcium and vitamin D therapy as needed to achieve a stable result. In those in whom hypocalcemia persists for more than several days, serum PTH should be measured to exclude the possibility of postoperative hypoparathyroidism. Given evidence that bone mineral density continues to increase for at least a year after successful parathyroidectomy,[275] it is prudent to continue calcium supplementation for at least that long.

The approach to patients with persistent or recurrent hyperparathyroidism is informed by the recognition that parathyroid hyperplasia or carcinoma, ectopic or supernumerary parathyroid tissue, and postoperative hypoparathyroidism and other complications of further surgery all are more common in this population.[337,339] The first issue to address is whether surgery is indicated. When a presumed adenoma had not been identified initially, the original indications for surgery generally still exist, although some patients may not be suitable candidates for more extensive surgery, such as a median sternotomy, because of concurrent medical illness. Patients with parathyroid hyperplasia may have experienced significant clinical improvement, even after incomplete parathyroidectomy, although those with MEN1 are very likely to experience further progression of their disease.

Preoperative localization studies are recommended for patients with persistent or recurrent disease after a first operation. Scanning with ^{99m}Tc-sestamibi offers the highest sensitivity and acccuracy, although other studies (ultrasonography, CT, magnetic resonance imaging) may provide additional or confirmatory information.[349] Sestamibi does localize to thyroid nodules, which may accompany parathyroid disease in 20% to 40% of patients, although it tends to wash out of thyroid tissue much more rapidly than from parathyroids. ^{99m}Tc-sestamibi can be combined with ^{123}I scanning to improve distinction of parathyroids from thyroid nodules or with single photon emission CT (SPECT) imaging to achieve accuracy in localization not possible with planar imaging (Fig. 28-25). On the other hand, sestamibi scanning may fail to reveal small glands (uptake is related to gland size and PTH levels[350]) or to demonstrate multiple abnormal glands in cases of parathyroid hyperplasia, the most common cause of persistent postoperative hyperparathyroidism.[336,351] Use of 4D-CT with synchronous contrast-enhanced multiplanar anatomic reconstruction has been shown to provide sensitivity superior to sestimibi scanning alone for localizing functioning parathyroid tissue in candidates for reoperation.[352]

More invasive techniques have been employed as well, including angiography and selective venous sampling for measurement of PTH.[353,354] Ultrasound- or CT-guided fine-needle aspiration of suspected parathyroid tissue may be used to obtain cytologic or immunochemical confirmation prior to surgery, and intraoperative ultrasonography has been useful in some cases to locate cervical or intrathyroidal glands.[339] Success with video-assisted thoracoscopic resection of documented mediastinal lesions[326,355] offers a

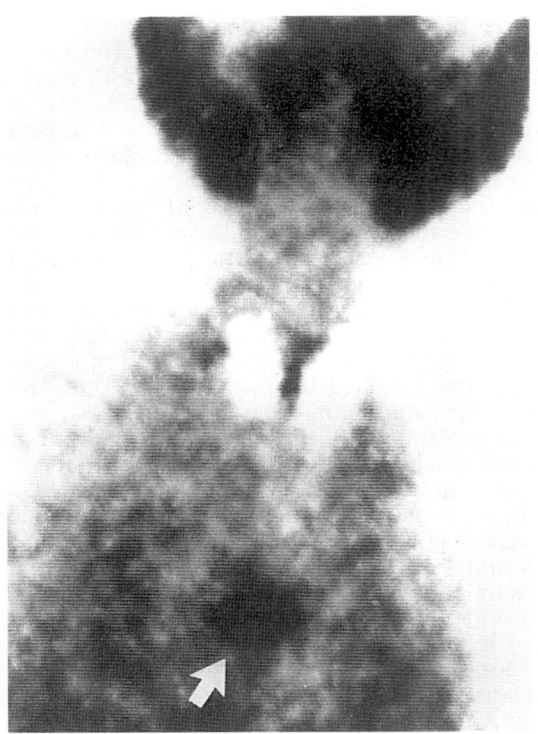

Figure 28-25 Technetium-99m (^{99m}Tc) sestamibi, iodine-123 (^{123}I) subtraction scanning of a patient with persistent hyperparathyroidism after two previous unsuccessful operations. *Arrow* points to parathyroid adenoma, shown as increased tracer uptake in the aortopulmonary window. (From Thule P, Thakore K, Vansant J, et al. Preoperative localization of parathyroid tissue with technetium-99m sestamibi^{123}I subtraction scanning. *J Clin Endocrinol Metab.* 1994;78:77-82.)

less invasive alternative to median sternotomy for this relatively common cause of persistent hyperparathyroidism.

The need for these procedures depends on the experience of the original surgeon and the confidence that the neck was adequately explored initially. For example, among reoperations at one center, over half of the "missed" hyperplastic parathyroid glands in those cases previously explored by a highly experienced parathyroid surgeon were found in the mediastinum or another ectopic location, whereas over 90% of those referred by less experienced surgeons were discovered in a normal anatomic location in the neck.[266]

Following successful surgery for primary hyperparathyroidism, bone mass generally improves by as much as 5% to 10% in the first year at sites rich in trabecular bone (spine, femoral neck), whereas improvement at cortical sites (distal radius) is less predictable.[356,357] Increases at trabecular sites may continue for several years, to as much as 12% to 15% after 10 years, although normal bone mineral density may not be achieved. This improvement, which is most apparent in those with the greatest preoperative reductions in bone mass, may be related in part to rapid remineralization of the previously enlarged bone remodeling volume,[330] but the continued improvement over years suggests a more sustained increase in net bone formation and total bone volume as well.[275]

Familial Hypocalciuric Hypercalcemia

FHH, also appropriately called *familial benign hypercalcemia*, is, in most families, a disorder of autosomal dominant inheritance caused most often by mutations of the *CASR* gene found in parathyroid glands, kidney, and other organs (see earlier discussion of calcium sensing). The mutations, which cause complete or partial loss of function of the CaSR, lead to a shift in the parathyroid cell's set point for calcium.[358] As a consequence, higher than normal levels of blood calcium are needed to suppress PTH secretion. Furthermore, abnormal function of the CaSR in the renal thick ascending limb leads to increased, PTH-independent calcium reabsorption and consequent hypocalciuria. In a minority of patients, mutations in two other genes in the signaling pathway activated by the CaSR have been found. One encodes the α-subunit of the G11 heterotrimeric G protein[359] known to participate in responding to the activation of the CaSR, and the other is in the *AP2S1* gene that encodes the α-subunit of adapter protein complex 2, a scaffolding protein needed for formation of clathrin-coated pits needed to internalize the CaSR.[360] The clinical presentation of patients with either of these two mutations is identical to that seen in FHH.

The presence of one normal sensing receptor gene with the abnormal one usually leads to a very mild clinical disorder, although the receptor functions as a dimer, and certain mutations can worsen the function of the normal allele. Rare patients who inherit mutant *CASR* genes from both parents present at birth with severe, life-threatening, primary hyperparathyroidism and almost always require immediate parathyroid surgery. In another genetic variation, a familial form of CaSR–dependent hypercalcemia has been described in association with other autoimmune disorders such as Hashimoto hypothyroidism and celiac sprue, in which autoantibodies directed against the sensor apparently antagonize calcium recognition by the parathyroids and renal tubules.[361,362]

FHH is manifested at birth by hypercalcemia. Although some controversy exists, most observers note that the condition is asymptomatic and that apparent symptoms represent ascertainment bias. Possible exceptions include the occurrence of chondrocalcinosis and perhaps pancreatitis. The blood calcium level is usually less than 12 mg/dL but can be higher. Phosphate measurements are low, as in primary hyperparathyroidism. Blood magnesium levels are high-normal or slightly elevated. PTH levels are inappropriately normal for the degree of hypercalcemia and are occasionally modestly elevated. Urine calcium is usually low, though one novel mutation in the receptor's intracellular tail has been associated with hypercalciuria, possibly because of only mild dysfunction in the kidney.[363]

When patients present as adults, the distinction from mild primary hyperparathyroidism can be difficult. The distinction between FHH and primary hyperparathyroidism is a crucial one, however. Young patients with primary hyperparathyroidism are usually treated surgically and cured. In contrast, hypercalcemia always recurs after surgery for FHH, unless the patient is rendered hypoparathyroid by the removal of all parathyroid tissue. Therefore, surgery is contraindicated as therapy for FHH, except in the very rare patient with severe, symptomatic hypercalcemia. No blood or urine measurements are completely reliable for distinguishing between the two conditions, though the ratio of calcium clearance to creatinine clearance distinguishes most patients with FHH from those with primary hyperparathyroidism.[364] Figure 28-26 shows, however, that this ratio separates the two groups, with modest overlap between the groups. However, because primary hyperparathyroidism is much more common than FHH, most patients with values near the "cut-off" value of 0.01 for the ratio of calcium clearance to creatinine clearance will have primary hyperparathyroidism and not FHH. Consequently, a case can be made[365] that many of such patients, particularly before parathyroid surgery, should undergo sequencing of

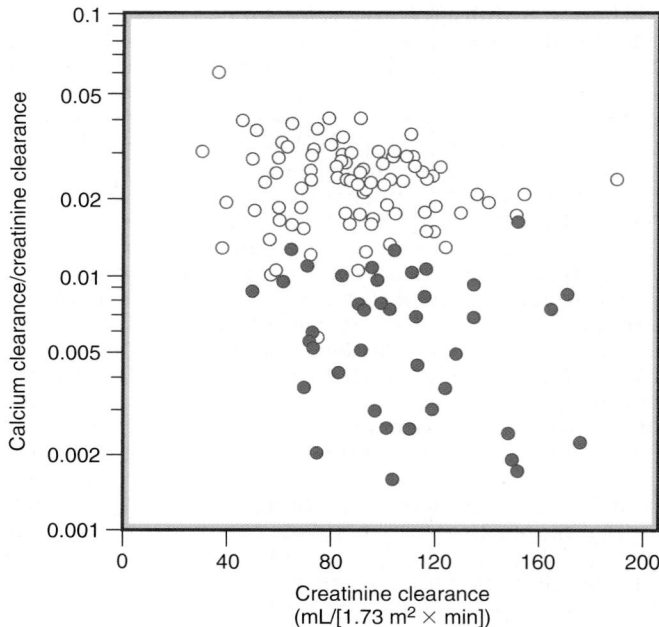

Figure 28-26 Index of urinary excretion rate for calcium as a function of creatinine clearance. Each point represents the mean of multiple determinations for a hypercalcemic patient with familial hypocalciuric hypercalcemia *(filled circles)* or with typical primary hyperparathyroidism *(open circles)*. The data are based on average 24-hour urinary excretion values and average fasting serum samples. (From Marx SJ, Attie MF, Levine M, et al. The hypocalciuric or benign variant of familial hypercalcemia: clinical and biochemical features in fifteen kindreds. *Medicine*. 1981;60:397-412.)

their *CASR* gene, now available commercially. The most helpful diagnostic information is the presence of hypercalcemia in an infant relative; such early hypercalcemia does not occur in MEN1. Furthermore, a past history of clearly normal blood calcium, considerably lower than current measurements, makes FHH unlikely if no other reason, such as severe vitamin D deficiency, for a change in blood calcium exists.

Lithium Toxicity

Treatment of bipolar affective disorders with lithium commonly leads to mild, persistent increases in blood calcium,[366] occasionally out of the normal range, in affected persons. Measurement of ionized calcium has shown that ionized calcium is a more sensitive index of lithium effect and was elevated in 24% of consecutive patients in a cross-sectional study.[367] After several years of therapy, clear elevations of PTH levels and modest increases in parathyroid gland size, detected by ultrasonography, often occur. Usually, when lithium therapy is stopped, the blood calcium and PTH normalize within several months. Uncommonly, substantial hypercalcemia and clear hyperparathyroidism ensue. At surgery, both single-gland and multigland disease are found, with a higher fraction of multigland disease than found in primary hyperparathyroidism not associated with lithium therapy.[368,369]

The management of patients with mild lithium-induced hypercalcemia is somewhat complicated. Like patients with mild primary hyperparathyroidism, patients taking lithium usually tolerate mild hypercalcemia without obvious symptoms. These patients can be monitored with protocols similar to those for patients with asymptomatic primary hyperparathyroidism. Close attention must be paid to urine-concentrating ability in these patients, however, because the nephrogenic diabetes insipidus associated with lithium therapy can lead to dehydration and sudden worsening of hypercalcemia. Substantial hypercalcemia should lead to withdrawal of lithium therapy, if possible, with substitution of newer psychopharmacologic agents. If hypercalcemia persists after withdrawal of lithium, decisions about surgery follow the same guidelines as those for patients with primary hyperparathyroidism.

Lithium increases the set point for PTH secretion when it is added to isolated parathyroid cells in vitro. The set point for PTH secretion in vivo is shifted to the right in patients who have received lithium for several years as well. A corresponding shift in the concentration of extracellular calcium needed to raise intracellular calcium levels[370] suggests that lithium interferes with the action of the parathyroid CaSR.

Parathyroid-Independent Hypercalcemia

In parathyroid-independent hypercalcemia, PTH secretion is appropriately suppressed. PTH levels, measured using two-site assays, are invariably lower than 25 pg/mL and are usually lower than normal or undetectable. Most affected patients have malignant hypercalcemia, although parathyroid-independent hypercalcemia occurs in a number of other settings as well.[371]

Hypercalcemia of Malignancy

The diagnosis of malignant hypercalcemia is seldom a subtle one.[115] Most malignancies produce hypercalcemia only when they are far advanced; the diagnosis becomes evident after routine studies, guided by the history and physical examination. Patients with malignant hypercalcemia usually die a month or two after hypercalcemia is discovered. Patients present with the classic signs and symptoms of hypercalcemia: confusion, polydipsia, polyuria, constipation, nausea, and vomiting. Perhaps because of the acuteness of the hypercalcemia and the elderly patient population involved, dramatic changes in mental status, culminating in coma, are relatively common. The diagnosis can be missed because the manifestations often overlap those of the underlying malignancy and because low blood albumin may lead to an apparently normal total blood calcium, despite an elevated blood ionized calcium. Even though the overall prognosis is grim, the diagnosis of malignant hypercalcemia is important to make.

Treatment is usually simple and effective in the short term; such treatment can importantly reverse the patient's symptoms for several weeks and even provide time for a fundamental attack on the underlying tumor, if it is treatable. Treatment consists of restoration of volume, followed by intravenous bisphosphonate or denosumab (see "Management of Severe Hypercalcemia"). Only effective treatment of the underlying neoplasm can significantly influence the long-term prognosis for patients with malignant hypercalcemia.

Although mechanisms in a given patient may be multiple, it is still useful to distinguish hypercalcemia associated with local involvement of bone from that caused by humoral mechanisms. In all cases, resorption of bone plays a pivotal role in the pathogenesis.

Local Osteolytic Hypercalcemia. Hypercalcemia resulting from tumors invading bone occurs most clearly in multiple myeloma and some patients with breast cancer. There is little evidence that the tumor cells themselves resorb bone. Instead, active osteoclasts found near the tumor cells are thought to be the proximate mediators of bone resorption.[372] Myeloma cells and marrow cells associated with

myeloma cells secrete numerous cytokines and chemokines capable of stimulating bone resorption, including macrophage inflammatory protein 1 (MIP-1), lymphotoxin (tumor necrosis factor-β), and interleukins 1β, 3, and 6. These factors lead to increased expression of RANKL (see Fig. 28-8) on the surface of marrow stromal cells and stimulation of osteoclast formation and activity. RANKL is also found on the surface of myeloma cells and therefore these cells may directly stimulate the production and activity of osteoclasts. The increased bone resorption not only releases calcium into the circulation but also weakens the bone structurally. Bone is further weakened by the suppression of bone formation by the secretion of dickkopf-1, an inhibitor of Wnt signaling, by myeloma cells.[373,374] In patients with myeloma, treatment with intermittent intravenous bisphosphonates inhibits bone resorption and reduces the incidence of bone pain, fracture, and hypercalcemia.

The pathogenesis of hypercalcemia in breast cancer is not completely understood. Extensive metastases to bone are detected in most patients with hypercalcemia and breast cancer; this finding suggests that factors produced in bone by the metastatic tumor cells may be important. Breast cancer cells make a host of cytokines capable of resorbing bone. The role of tumor-produced PTHrP may be particularly important.[374] A majority of breast cancer patients with hypercalcemia have elevated blood levels of PTHrP. This circulating PTHrP, as well as PTHrP produced in bone by metastatic tumor cells, may generate the hypercalcemia. Primary breast tumors that stain for PTHrP are more likely to result in bone metastases than are those that do not stain for PTHrP; this PTHrP may be instrumental in the establishment of lytic metastases. Animal models indicate that transforming growth factor-β (TGF-β), released from bone matrix by PTHrP-stimulated osteoclastic resorption, may further augment PTHrP secretion by the tumor cells. The latter may be further promoted by estrogen, which may explain the occasional occurrence of hypercalcemia following institution of estrogen or tamoxifen therapy in this disease.[375]

Humoral Hypercalcemia of Malignancy. Albright, in 1941, was the first to propose that a PTH-like humoral factor caused the hypercalcemia in patients with malignancy but few or no bone metastases.[376] Four decades later biochemical analysis demonstrated that such patients have high blood calcium levels, low blood phosphate levels, and high urinary cAMP levels like those found in primary hyperparathyroidism, but no elevation in iPTH levels.[377] The stimulation of cAMP production was used as an assay to eventually purify PTHrP from human tumors associated with the humoral hypercalcemia of malignancy.[378]

The evidence that PTHrP mediates the humoral hypercalcemia of malignancy in most patients is substantial. As noted previously, PTHrP binds to the PTH/PTHrP receptor and mimics all of the actions of amino-terminal fragments of PTH. Blood levels of PTHrP are elevated in most patients with solid tumors and hypercalcemia. In animal models of the humoral hypercalcemia of malignancy, antibodies against PTHrP can reverse the hypercalcemia.[379]

The acute actions of PTHrP cannot explain all of the findings in patients with the hypercalcemia of malignancy, however. Acutely administered PTHrP increases blood levels of $1,25(OH)_2D_3$ by stimulating the renal 1α-hydroxylase, though the stimulation is less than that induced by PTH.[380] Nevertheless, patients with the humoral hypercalcemia of malignancy usually have low levels of $1,25(OH)_2D_3$.[377] This finding is particularly puzzling, because human tumors from patients with elevated calcium and PTHrP but with low $1,25(OH)_2D_3$ levels stimulate $1,25(OH)_2D_3$ synthesis after they are transplanted into nude mice.[381] Possible explanations for the low $1,25(OH)_2D_3$ levels in patients include the weak activation of the renal 1α-hydroxylase in humans by PTHrP, combined with the inhibition of the 1α-hydroxylase by hypercalcemia[382] or by tumor products.

A second disparity between the acute actions of PTHrP and the findings in patients with malignant hypercalcemia involves the rate of bone formation. Acutely, PTHrP infusions in rats, like PTH, leads to increased bone formation.[383] Nevertheless, in patients with malignant hypercalcemia, bone formation is markedly lower than normal. The explanation for this effect may well lie in the action of other cytokines, immobilization, or particular fragments of PTHrP with novel properties.

The tumors most commonly associated with humoral hypercalcemia include squamous cell cancers of the lung, head and neck, esophagus, cervix, vulva, and skin; breast cancer; renal cell cancer; and bladder cancer. Benign or malignant pheochromocytomas, islet cell tumors, and carcinoids can also overproduce PTHrP, causing hypercalcemia. The aggressive T-cell lymphoma associated with human T-cell lymphotropic virus type 1 (HTLV-1) infection is the only hematologic malignancy commonly associated with PTHrP overproduction and hypercalcemia.

Cachexia often accompanies the hypercalcemia of malignancy. In experimental models, administration of a monoclonal antibody to PTHrP ameliorates the cachexia, not simply by lowering blood calcium but also by blocking the ability of PTHrP to convert white adipose tissue to brown, heat-generating adipose tissue.[116]

It is unlikely that PTHrP is the sole cause of the humoral hypercalcemia of malignancy. As noted previously, many cytokines produced by tumors can stimulate bone resorption. The actions of these cytokines have been shown to synergize with those of PTHrP in a number of experimental models. Furthermore, in hypercalcemic patients with non-Hodgkin lymphoma, blood levels of $1,25(OH)_2D_3$ were found to be higher than otherwise expected,[384] and such patients show abnormal sensitivity to 25-hydroxyvitamin D administration.[385] In these hypercalcemic patients, the relative importance of $1,25(OH)_2D_3$ cytokines, PTHrP, and immobilization needs to be clarified.

In a few reported cases, malignant tumors secrete PTH and not PTHrP.[115] Although this phenomenon has now been well documented, it should be stressed that in almost all patients with cancer and high PTH levels, concurrent primary hyperparathyroidism, not ectopic PTH production, is the cause of the hyperparathyroidism.

Vitamin D Intoxication

Because the synthesis of $1,25(OH)_2D_3$ is so tightly regulated, extremely large doses of vitamin D, on the order of 100,000 units per day, are required to cause hypercalcemia. Such doses are available in the United States only by prescription; therefore, most cases of vitamin D intoxication are iatrogenic. Occasionally, inadvertent ingestion occurs. Patients present with nausea, vomiting, weakness, and altered level of consciousness. Hypercalcemia can be severe and prolonged, because of the storage of vitamin D in fat. As expected, PTH levels are suppressed, and levels of 25(OH)D, which are poorly regulated and reflect levels of ingested vitamin D, are dramatically elevated. In contrast, the levels of $1,25(OH)_2D_3$ are only modestly elevated or can be normal or even low. The modest changes in $1,25(OH)_2D_3$ levels result from the downregulation of the renal 1α-hydroxylase by low levels of PTH and high levels of phosphate, calcium, FGF23, and $1,25(OH)_2D_3$ itself. The cause of the hypercalcemia, when it occurs in the face of

normal levels of $1,25(OH)_2D_3$, is uncertain but may reflect the direct action of 25(OH)D and possibly other vitamin D metabolites, which are capable of binding the $1,25(OH)_2D_3$ receptor weakly or which may be locally 1α-hydroxylated by nonrenal 1α-hydroxylases. Of note, vitamin D causes hypercalcemia with identical effectiveness in normal mice and in those missing the 1α-hydroxylase gene,[386] arguing that 25(OH)D and other metabolites, when present in large amounts, are sufficient to cause hypercalcemia. Also, the weaker vitamin D metabolites may displace $1,25(OH)_2D_3$ from the circulating VDBP and increase the concentration of active, free $1,25(OH)_2D_3$.[184,387]

The hypercalcemia of vitamin D intoxication results both from increased intestinal absorption of calcium and from the direct effect of $1,25(OH)_2D_3$ to increase resorption of bone. In severe cases, therefore, bisphosphonate therapy can be usefully added to the therapeutic regimen of hydration and omission of dietary calcium.

Sarcoidosis and Other Granulomatous Diseases

Sarcoidosis may be associated with hypercalcemia and, even more commonly, hypercalciuria.[388] Hypercalcemic patients have high levels of $1,25(OH)_2D_3$; the high level of $1,25(OH)_2D_3$ probably causes the hypercalcemia, although overproduction of bone-resorbing cytokines and PTHrP may contribute in some patients. As expected in $1,25(OH)_2D_3$-dependent hypercalcemia, intestinal absorption of calcium is increased and PTH levels are suppressed. Furthermore, the hypercalcemia and high levels of $1,25(OH)_2D_3$ fall upon treatment with glucocorticoids. The unregulated synthesis of $1,25(OH)_2D_3$, found even in an anephric patient, occurs not in the kidney but rather in the sarcoid granulomas. Removal of a large amount of granulomatous tissue can reverse hypercalcemia. Furthermore, isolated sarcoid macrophages can synthesize $1,25(OH)_2D_3$ from 25(OH)D, as can normal macrophages stimulated with interferon-γ or after activation of toll-like receptors. Such macrophages express the gene encoding the identical 25(OH)D 1α-hydroxylase found in the kidney. The local synthesis of $1,25(OH)_2D_3$ by activated macrophages and activation of VDRs in those cells is a paracrine system that activates antibacterial mechanisms as part of the normal action of macrophages.[179]

The unusual increase in the numbers of activated macrophages in sarcoidosis leads, however, to elevations of blood calcium in these patients. These patients have unusual sensitivity to vitamin D and can become hypercalcemic in response to ultraviolet radiation or oral vitamin D intake. Abnormalities in calcium metabolism are usually found only in patients with active disease and large, clinically obvious total-body burdens of granulomas. Nevertheless, hypercalcemia can present in patients without obvious pulmonary disease. Furthermore, subtle abnormalities of vitamin D metabolism can be demonstrated even in patients with mildly active sarcoidosis.

Hypercalcemia is also associated with other granulomatous diseases, such as tuberculosis, fungal infections, and berylliosis and has been reported in Wegener granulomatosis, in acquired immunodeficiency syndrome (AIDS)-related *Pneumocystis jirovecii* infection, fat necrosis of the newborn,[389] and even in association with extensive granulomatous foreign body reactions.[371] Patients with Crohn disease occasionally have hypercalcemia with elevations of $1,25(OH)_2D_3$ levels but often have elevated $1,25(OH)_2D_3$ levels with normal calcium levels and low bone mass, associated with increased production of $1,25(OH)_2D_3$ in intestinal macrophages.[390] In an analysis of 101 patients with hypercalcemia and high levels of $1,25(OH)_2D_3$ in

Australia, half the patients had sarcoidosis and the others had hematologic malignancies, other infections, or other causes.[391]

Hyperthyroidism

Mild hypercalcemia can result from thyrotoxicosis.[392] Blood calcium levels seldom exceed 11 mg/dL, but mild elevations are found in a quarter of patients. Patients have low PTH levels, low $1,25(OH)_2D_3$ levels, and hypercalciuria. The hypercalcemia is caused by a direct action of thyroid hormone to stimulate bone resorption.[393] β-Adrenergic blocking agents can reverse the hypercalcemia.[394]

Vitamin A Intoxication

Excess ingestion of vitamin A (retinol) results in a syndrome of dry skin, pruritus, headache from pseudotumor cerebri, bone pain, and, occasionally, hypercalcemia. Hypercalcemia occurs only with the ingestion of 10 times the Recommended Dietary Allowance (RDA) (5000 IU/day). The identical syndrome can result from ingestion of the vitamin A derivatives isotretinoin (13-*cis*-retinoic acid [Accutane]) and tretinoin (all-*trans*-retinoic acid [Retin-A]), used to treat acne and acute promyelocytic leukemia.[395,396] Bones can show characteristic periosteal calcification on radiographs. The hypercalcemia is probably caused by the action of retinoids to stimulate bone resorption. The diagnosis is made by the association of a history of excess ingestion of retinoids with the characteristic syndrome and abnormal results of liver function tests; elevated vitamin A levels confirm the diagnosis. Treatment involves hydration and, if necessary, glucocorticoids or bisphosphonates.

Adrenal Insufficiency

Hypercalcemia occurs in the setting of adrenal insufficiency. Blood calcium is elevated partly as a result of hemoconcentration and increased albumin levels, but the level of ionized calcium can be increased as well.[397] PTH and $1,25(OH)_2D_3$ levels are low to low-normal.[398] The hypercalcemia in this study resulted from a combination of influx of calcium into the vascular space, probably from bone, combined with low renal clearance.

Thiazide Diuretics

Thiazide diuretics do not cause hypercalcemia by themselves, but they can exacerbate the hypercalcemia of primary hyperparathyroidism or any other cause of increased input of calcium into the bloodstream that is not suppressed by hypercalcemia. The mechanism of the hypercalcemia may involve the action of thiazide diuretics to increase proximal tubular calcium reabsorption as a secondary consequence of direct action of thiazides on the distal tubule.[399,400] Decreased renal clearance of calcium alone would be expected to raise blood calcium in the normal human only transiently because the transient hypercalcemia would be expected to suppress PTH secretion and lead to return of the blood calcium to normal. However, in the presence of primary hyperparathyroidism, sarcoidosis, excess calcium intake, or any other cause of high, fixed calcium load, thiazide administration will increase the level of calcium in blood.

As predicted by this model, thiazide administration leads to chronic hypercalcemia in patients with abnormal parathyroid physiology but not in normal subjects.[401] In primary hyperparathyroidism, thiazide administration exacerbates the hypercalcemia, and in hypoparathyroidism, thiazide administration facilitates the maintenance of normocalcemia when given in conjunction with $1,25(OH)_2D_3$ and calcium.

Milk-Alkali Syndrome

The triad of hypercalcemia, metabolic alkalosis, and renal failure can be the consequence of massive ingestion of calcium and absorbable alkali. This syndrome was first described when milk and sodium bicarbonate were used in large amounts to treat peptic ulcer disease. With the change in ulcer treatment to nonabsorbable antacids and suppression of acid secretion, milk-alkali syndrome became rare. In the last several years, however, the increased use of calcium carbonate to treat dyspepsia and osteoporosis has led to the reappearance of milk-alkali syndrome.[402] In most cases, a history of ingestion of several grams per day of calcium in the form of calcium carbonate can be elicited. Some reports suggest that less than 4 g of calcium daily can cause milk-alkali syndrome, fewer than previously estimated, perhaps because of greater ingestion of vitamin D than in the past.[403] The pathogenesis of the syndrome is not understood in detail but may well involve a vicious circle in which alkalosis decreases renal calcium clearance and hypercalcemia helps maintain alkalosis. Nephrocalcinosis, nephrogenic diabetes insipidus, decrease in GFR associated with hypercalcemia, and hypovolemia from vomiting all lead to renal failure, which can be severe. PTH levels, measured with currently available two-site assays, are invariably low in hypercalcemic patients, as are levels of $1,25(OH)_2D_3$. After clearance of the calcium by hydration or dialysis, if necessary, renal function generally returns to normal, unless the disorder has been severe and long-standing.

Immobilization

Immobilization can lead to bone resorption sufficient to cause hypercalcemia. The immobilization is usually caused by spinal cord injury or extensive casting after fractures, though it can occur in settings such as Parkinson disease.[399] Hypercalcemia after trauma requiring immobilization is common, when studied prospectively, and is usually asymptomatic.[404] Hypercalcemia of immobilization occurs predominantly in the young or in patients with other reasons for a high rate of bone turnover, such as Paget disease or extensive fractures. Hypercalciuria and substantial bone loss are more common than hypercalcemia. After spinal cord injury, the hypercalciuria is maximal at 4 months and can persist for more than a year. PTH and $1,25(OH)_2D_3$ levels are suppressed; bone biopsies show increased resorption and decreased formation of bone. Bisphosphonates and denosumab have been used to reverse the hypercalcemia and hypercalciuria of immobilization.

Renal Failure

Following rhabdomyolysis, during the oliguric phase of acute renal failure, severe hypocalcemia can result from acute hyperphosphatemia and calcium deposition in muscle.[405] PTH levels are high, in response to the hypocalcemia. In the diuretic phase that follows, hypercalcemia can occur. The hypercalcemia results from the mobilization of the calcium deposits and, in a fraction of patients, from associated high $1,25(OH)_2D_3$ levels sometimes seen.[406]

In chronic renal failure, hypercalcemia can result from tertiary hyperparathyroidism or may appear during therapy of aplastic bone disease associated with low PTH levels and sometimes with aluminum toxicity.

Williams Syndrome

Williams syndrome is a developmental disorder in which supravalvular aortic stenosis is associated with elfin facies and mental retardation.[407] Hypercalcemia can occur transiently in the first 4 years of life. Affected hypercalcemic infants have been found to have increased intestinal absorption of calcium and associated elevations of $1,25(OH)_2D_3$ that fall to normal as the blood calcium normalizes.[408] Levels of $25(OH)D$ are normal. The hypercalcemia can generally be controlled by dietary manipulation and, if needed, bisphosphonates.[409]

Molecular analysis has clarified the origin of the connective tissue component of Williams syndrome. Williams syndrome is a contiguous gene syndrome with deletions of one or several genes. Isolated supravalvular aortic stenosis is associated with deletion or translocation of the distal portion of the elastin gene. Williams syndrome, with more protean connective tissue abnormalities and mental retardation, is associated with large deletions that include the elastin gene and a gene encoding the protein kinase LIM-kinase 1. A gene within the Willams syndrome deletion region encodes a nuclear protein, Williams syndrome transcription factor, that is part of a large chromatin remodeling complex that can bind the VDR and influence the transcription of VDR-responsive genes.[410] For this reason, this gene is a strong candidate for the gene associated with transient hypercalcemia in this disorder. Genetic proof that this gene is responsible for the hypercalcemia and a connection between the gene and hypercalcemia, however, is lacking.

Jansen Metaphyseal Chondrodysplasia

Jansen metaphyseal chondrodysplasia is a rare disease in which affected persons present in childhood with short stature and hypercalcemia (Fig. 28-27). Blood chemistry studies suggest hyperparathyroidism, with high calcium, low-normal phosphate, high $1,25(OH)_2D_3$, high alkaline phosphatase, and high urinary hydroxyproline levels, but PTH levels are suppressed.[411] A generalized defect in endochondral bone formation results from abnormally organized chondrocytes in growth plates. Metaphyses appear disordered and rachitic on radiographs. The bones may show signs of osteitis fibrosa cystica. Constitutive activation of the PTH/PTHrP receptor, caused by point mutations in the transmembrane domains of the receptor, explains the findings in this disorder.[98,412] The abnormalities on serum chemistry studies result from PTH-like actions of the receptor in bone and kidney; one patient has been noted to have increased blood levels of FGF23.[413] The growth plate disorder results from PTHrP-like actions of the receptor on the growth plate.

Approach to the Hypercalcemic Patient

The diagnostic approach to the hypercalcemic patient is strongly influenced by the clinical setting and the knowledge that primary hyperparathyroidism is at least twice as common as all other causes combined (Table 28-2). These considerations are particularly significant in the patient who seems otherwise well and in whom the hypercalcemia is detected incidentally or is mild, stable, or known to be of long duration (i.e., years). Among outpatients referred to endocrinologists for evaluation of hypercalcemia, for example, more than 90% are found to have primary hyperparathyroidism. In ill or hospitalized patients, malignant disease is the cause in more than 50% of cases. The differential diagnosis is seldom complicated, however, because malignant hypercalcemia usually presents in the context of advanced, clinically obvious disease.

Because hypercalcemia usually is first detected as an elevation of total serum calcium, it is important to distinguish hemoconcentration or rare instances of calcium-binding paraproteinemia or thrombocythemia-associated hypercalcemia (due to release of intracellular calcium in

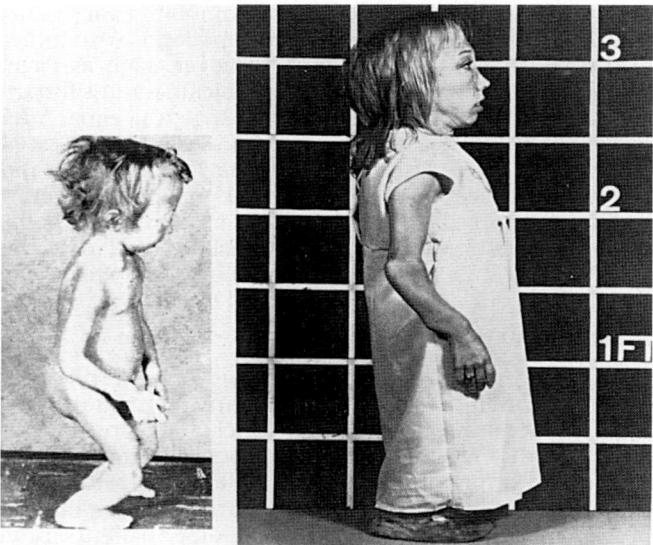

Figure 28-27 A patient with Jansen metaphyseal chondrodysplasia at ages 5 years and 22 years. Note the short stature, characteristic facies, and misshapen metaphyseal region of long bones. (From Frame B, Poznanski AK. Conditions that may be confused with rickets. In DeLuca HF, Anastas CS, eds. *Pediatric Diseases Related to Calcium.* New York, NY: Elsevier; 1980:269-289.)

TABLE 28-2
Causes of Hypercalcemia

Parathyroid-Dependent Hypercalcemia
Primary hyperparathyroidism
Tertiary hyperparathyroidism
Familial hypocalciuric hypercalcemia
Lithium-associated hypercalcemia
Antagonistic autoantibodies to the calcium-sensing receptor

Parathyroid-Independent Hypercalcemia
Neoplasms
PTHrP-dependent
Other humoral syndromes
Local osteolytic disease (including metastases)
PTHrP excess (non-neoplastic)
Excess vitamin D action
Ingestion of excess vitamin D or vitamin D analogues
Topical vitamin D analogues
Granulomatous disease
Williams syndrome
Thyrotoxicosis
Adrenal insufficiency
Renal failure
Acute renal failure
Chronic renal failure with aplastic bone disease
Immobilization
Jansen disease
Drugs
Vitamin A intoxication
Milk-alkali syndrome
Thiazide diuretics
Theophylline

PTHrP, parathyroid hormone–related protein.

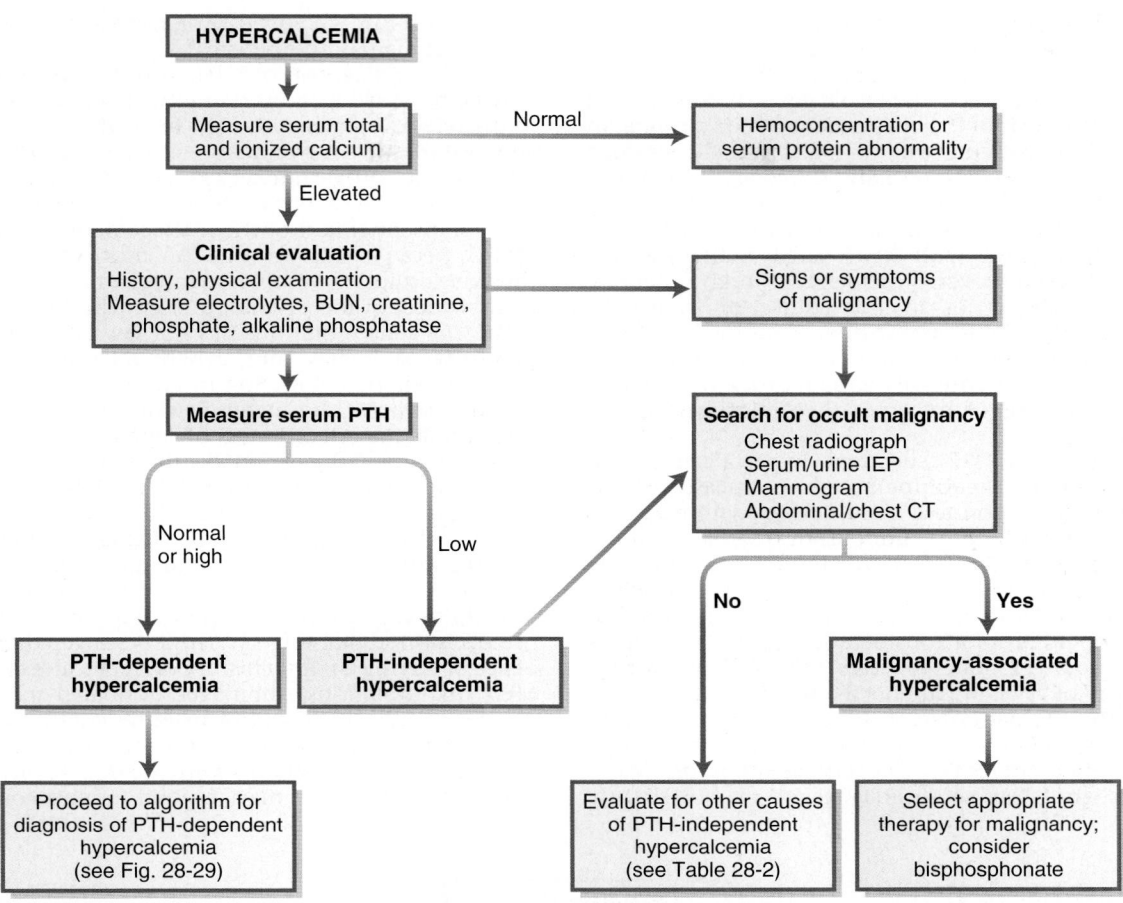

Figure 28-28 Approach to the management of the hypercalcemic patient. BUN, blood urea nitrogen; CT, computed tomography; IEP, immunoelectrophoresis; PTH, parathyroid hormone.

vitro) from a true increase in serum ionized calcium (Fig. 28-28). The presence of hypercalcemia should be confirmed by direct measurement of ionized calcium, and total calcium should be repeated, together with albumin, globulin electrolytes, blood urea nitrogen, creatinine, and phosphate. Especially when hypercalcemia is mild, it is prudent to repeat the serum total or ionized calcium measurement at least twice, preferably fasting and without venous occlusion, before proceeding with more costly studies directed at its cause.

A careful history and physical examination, combined with efforts to assess chronicity by seeking prior results of routine multichannel serum chemistry determinations, most often will point to the likely diagnosis. Serum phosphate often is low in hyperparathyroidism, but as this often is true also of PTHrP-secreting malignancies, the presence of hypophosphatemia is not helpful in distinguishing these possibilities. When serum phosphate is normal or high despite correction of dehydration, the possibility of PTH- or PTHrP-independent hypercalcemia should be considered more strongly, however. Elevations in serum chloride and alkaline phosphatase, often observed in primary hyperparathyroidism, cannot be reliably employed in the differential diagnosis of hypercalcemia. Important elements of the medical history of hypercalcemic patients include inquiries about kidney stones or fractures; weight loss; back or bone pain; fatigue or weakness; cough or dyspnea; ulcer disease or pancreatitis; ingestion of vitamins, calcium preparations, lithium, or thiazides; dates of most recent mammograms and chest radiographs; and a family history of hypercalcemia, kidney stones, ulcer disease, endocrinopathy, or tumors of the head or neck. Because malignancy is a common cause of hypercalcemia and may occur concomitantly with primary hyperparathyroidism, clinical findings strongly suggestive of malignancy should be acted upon by proceeding directly to a search for an underlying tumor, regardless of serum PTH.

The single most important test in the differential diagnosis of hypercalcemia is the measurement of serum PTH, preferably in a two-site assay specific for the intact, biologically active molecule (see Fig. 28-19). New PTH assays have been introduced that ignore long circulating fragments of the hormone, which lack the amino-terminal residues required for activity at the PTH/PTHrP receptor, but whether these new assays will be more useful than standard "intact PTH" assays remains to be established.[414,415] A consistently elevated serum PTH in the presence of true hypercalcemia always is abnormal and almost always indicates the presence of primary hyperparathyroidism. The exceptions that also can be associated with elevated PTH levels are FHH, autonomous parathyroid secretion complicating secondary hyperparathyroidism (tertiary hyperparathyroidism), lithium-associated hyperparathyroidism, and, very rarely, ectopic PTH secretion by a malignant neoplasm or antagonizing autoantibodies directed against the CaSR in patients with other autoimmune disease(s)—an acquired condition that mimics FHH.[361,362]

Diagnosis of primary hyperparathyroidism is complicated, however, by the fact that some patients fail to exhibit both hypercalcemia and elevated iPTH. In up to 10% of patients with hypercalcemia and primary hyperparathyroidism, PTH levels may fall within the normal range (high normal) with current PTH assays. Such PTH levels are inappropriate in the face of hypercalcemia, however, and support the diagnosis of PTH-dependent hypercalcemia. In fact, many such patients will manifest frankly elevated serum PTH if retested, especially if dietary calcium is restricted beforehand. As noted earlier, some patients may present with serum calcium in the high-normal range (>10.0 mg/dL) together with an elevated or high-normal PTH. This may be discovered incidentally in an otherwise asymptomatic subject or in the course of evaluating recurrent urolithiasis or osteopenia. Those with persistently high-normal serum calcium and high-normal iPTH should be retested at intervals and, meanwhile, given a provisional diagnosis of hyperparathyroidism and evaluated accordingly.

In patients with PTH-dependent hypercalcemia (Fig. 28-29), calcium and creatinine should be measured in a 24-hour urine collection and simultaneous serum sample to measure total urinary calcium output (mg/day) and the clearance ratio of calcium (Ca)/creatinine (Creat) in urine (U) and serum (S): $U_{Ca}/S_{Ca} \times S_{Creat}/U_{Creat}$. A daily calcium excretion of less than 100 mg/day, or a clearance ratio less than 0.01, should prompt consideration of FHH, especially in patients younger than 40 years old, or those with a family history of FHH, or patients whose serum iPTH levels are within the normal range. A urinary calcium excretion greater than 4 mg/kg/day or clearance ratio greater than 0.02 effectively excludes FHH. In FHH, serum phosphate is normal or slightly low, serum magnesium may be slightly high, and serum $1,25(OH)_2D_3$ is normal or low (unlike in primary hyperparathyroidism).

A definite diagnosis of FHH, as in the MEN syndromes, may be provided by confirming the presence of mutations in the relevant genes, although such studies are not invariably informative (presumably because of mutations in introns and other unchecked regions) and usually are unnecessary. The identification of *RET* gene mutations is now an essential part of the management of families with MEN2, because this information most effectively guides the decision for preventive thyroidectomy to prevent medullary cancer of the thyroid. In contrast, the identification of *MENIN* gene mutations has not yet led to any effective preventive strategies; thus, genetic analysis may be useful only for genetic counseling in families with MEN1. Even for this purpose, the incomplete ascertainment of mutations limits the effectiveness of such analysis.

In patients with suspected lithium-induced hyperparathyroidism, a trial off lithium, if feasible clinically, may confirm the diagnosis or indicate the presence of persistant primary hyperparathyroidism. Patients with primary hyperparathyroidism should undergo bone densitometry, preferably at sites rich in cortical and trabecular bone (i.e., forearm or hip and lumbar spine, respectively) to assist in the decision about surgery. Those younger than 40 years of age or having a family history of hypercalcemia (or other MEN manifestations) should be evaluated for these syndromes as well. Patients not meeting criteria for parathyroidectomy should be followed medically, as should those with FHH. In rare patients with CaSR-blocking autoantibodies, hypercalcemia may respond to glucocorticoids.[362]

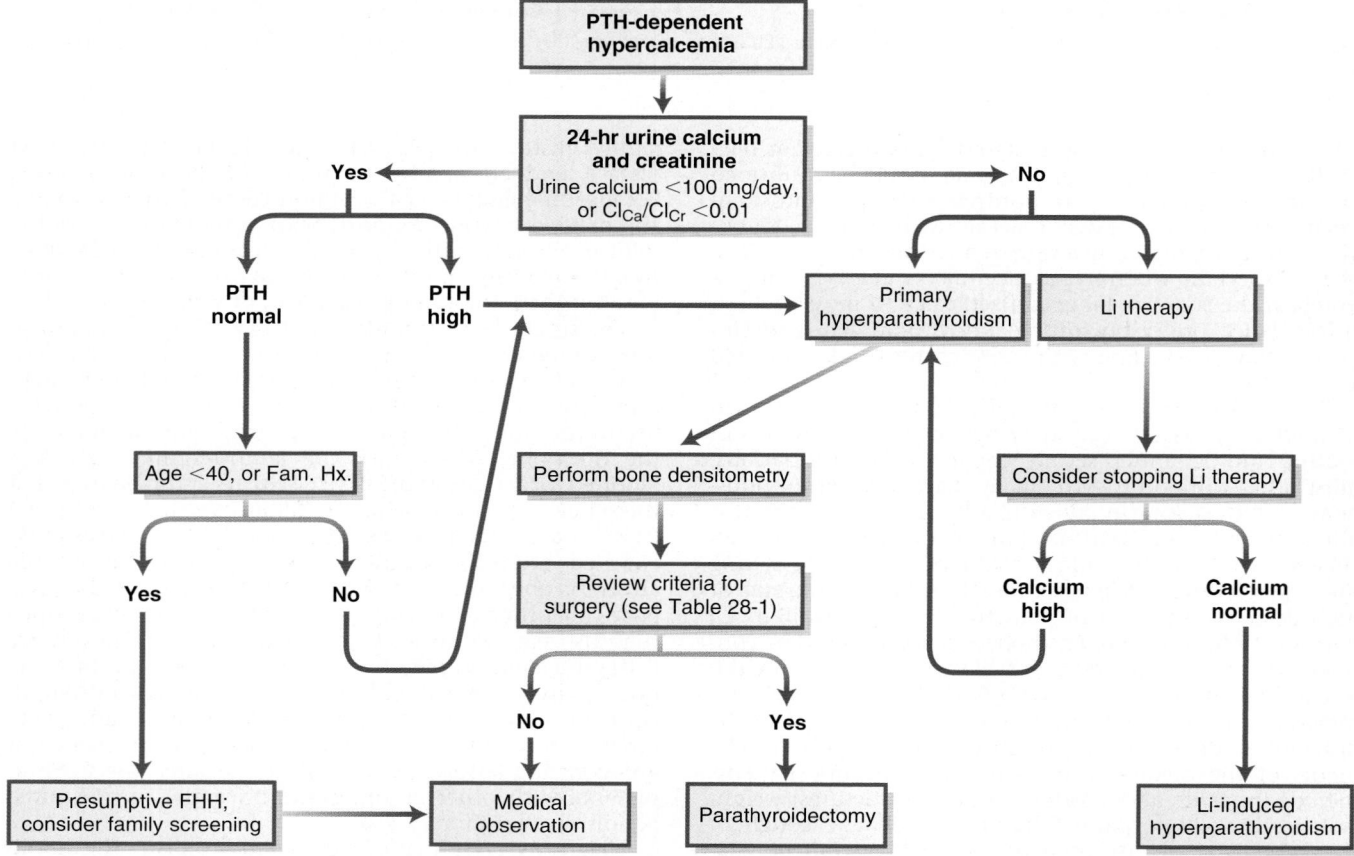

Figure 28-29 Approach to the management of the hypercalcemic patient with parathyroid hormone–dependent hypercalcemia. Cl, clearance; Fam. Hx., family history; FHH, familial hypocalciuric hypercalcemia; Li, lithium; PTH, parathyroid hormone.

A low or undetectable serum PTH level signifies the presence of nonparathyroid hypercalcemia and should prompt a detailed evaluation for malignancy or other causes of PTH-independent hypercalcemia (see Table 28-2). Breast and lung cancers alone account for over 50% of all malignancy-associated hypercalcemias. Mammography, chest radiography with or without CT, abdominal CT, and serum and urinary immunoelectrophoresis are among the more useful tests for detecting the cause of nonparathyroid hypercalcemia. Although humoral mechanisms, especially secretion of PTHrP, are implicated in the pathogenesis of most cancer-associated hypercalcemias, bone metastases are common, particularly in breast cancer. Technetium-99m bone scanning, therefore, generally is useful for detecting this syndrome and identifying bones vulnerable to fracture. The utility of serum PTHrP measurements probably is limited to the unusual situation in which serum PTH is suppressed but an underlying malignancy cannot readily be demonstrated. PTHrP-associated hypercalcemia can occur rarely during pregnancy and lactation, via secretion from benign neoplasms or in association with lymphoid hyperplasia in lupus erythematosus or HIV.[371]

In the absence of evident malignancy, unusual causes of hypercalcemia should be sought.[371] Vitamin D and vitamin A intoxication can be excluded by measurement of serum 25(OH)D and retinoids, respectively. Elevated $1,25(OH)_2D_3$ and hypercalcemia may occur in several settings, including sarcoidosis and other granulomatous diseases, B-cell and T-cell lymphomas (including AIDS-associated lymphomas), and uncommonly, in Crohn disease, in neonatal subcutaneous fat necrosis syndrome, or in epithelial neoplasms such as lung cancer. Very rarely, patients with severe idiopathic hypercalciuria and excessive absorption of dietary calcium may manifest mild, dietary-dependent hypercalcemia. Overtreatment of hypoparathyroidism or other conditions with oral $1,25(OH)_2D_3$ or topical use of analogues of the active metabolite in psoriasis should be obvious from the history. Because hypercalcemia and hypercalciuria are observed in up to 10% and 30%, respectively, of patients with thyrotoxicosis, measurement of serum thyroid-stimulating hormone (TSH) may be helpful, especially in older patients who may be less overtly symptomatic. Adrenal insufficiency and pheochromocytoma usually are accompanied by characteristic clinical features, but a definite diagnosis may be sought with appropriate studies. Granulomatous diseases are among the more common disorders that underlie initially unexplained hypercalcemia.

Causes of Severe Hypercalcemia

The need for urgent therapy of acute, severe hypercalcemia, usually defined as a serum calcium concentration greater than 14 mg/dL (3.5 mmol/L), is unusual. This is because most patients with hypercalcemia have primary hyperparathyroidism, in which hypercalcemia is typically chronic and mild. Episodes of acute, severe hypercalcemia may occur occasionally in primary hyperparathyroidism (parathyroid crisis), usually in patients with large parathyroid adenomas and very high PTH levels. The severe hypercalcemia in this setting may be triggered by dehydration due to diarrheal illness, protracted vomiting or diuretic therapy, recovery from major surgery, immobilization, ingestion of large amounts of oral calcium salts, hemorrhage or rupture of a cystic parathyroid neoplasm, or parathyroid carcinoma.

Most often, acute, severe hypercalcemia is encountered in patients with underlying malignancy, in whom accelerated bone resorption dramatically increases the filtered load of calcium. The ensuing profound hypercalciuria

impairs renal tubular sodium reabsorption, which induces progressive extracellular volume depletion, reduces GFR, impairs renal calcium clearance, and further aggravates the hypercalcemia. In many such patients, elevated circulating levels of PTHrP compound the problem by mimicking the action of PTH to enhance distal tubular calcium reabsorption.

Clinical Features of Severe Hypercalcemia

The indications for urgent therapy of hypercalcemia usually relate more to the presence of clinical symptoms of hypercalcemia than to the absolute level of serum calcium, although few clinicians would hesitate to treat patients in whom total serum calcium exceeded 14 mg/dL (3.5 mmol/L). Many patients with previously mild hypercalcemia become symptomatic when serum calcium concentrations exceed 12 mg/dL (3.0 mmol/L). It is important to remember that hypoalbuminemia may mask significant elevations of ionized calcium. The most common symptoms of severe hypercalcemia are referable to disturbances of nervous system and gastrointestinal function—fatigue, weakness, lethargy, confusion, coma (rarely), anorexia, nausea, abdominal pain (rarely due to pancreatitis), and constipation. Polyuria, nocturia, and polydipsia commonly are present also.

Bone pain is often present but is usually due to underlying metastatic disease. Cardiac arrhythmias may occur, particularly bradyarrhythmias or heart block; digitalis toxicity may be potentiated; and ST-segment elevation responsive to treatment of the hypercalcemia may be seen. Patients who suffer a fatal outcome from acute severe hypercalcemia may manifest coma, hypotension, acute pancreatitis, acute renal failure, widespread soft tissue calcification, heart failure, or venous thrombosis, particularly of the renal veins.

Management of Severe Hypercalcemia

The first decision to be made in the management of acute, severe hypercalcemia is whether or not to treat the problem at all. This may become an issue for the patient with an untreatable, widely disseminated malignancy, when all other approaches to controlling the neoplasm have been exhausted, and the patient has chosen not to have complications treated. Otherwise, as noted earlier, patients who are symptomatic or have serum calcium levels above 14 mg/dL ordinarily should be treated aggressively. Treatment most often entails rehydration and administration of a bisphosphonate intravenously (Table 28-3). Calcitonin can be useful as a temporary measure early in therapy, and glucocorticoids or dialysis may be indicated in some patients.[115]

TABLE 28-3

Treatment of Severe Hypercalcemia

Type of Therapy	Usual Dose	Frequency
Rehydration	2-4 L/day of 0.9% NaCl IV	qd × 1-5 days
Furosemide	20-40 mg IV (after rehydration)	q12-24 hr
Pamidronate	60-90 mg IV over 2-4 hr	Once
Zoledronate	4 mg IV over 15-30 min	Once
Denosumab	60 mg SC	Weekly
Calcitonin	4-8 IU/kg SC	q12-24 hr
Gallium nitrate	200 mg/m² IV over 24 hr	qd × 5 days
Glucocorticoids	200-300 mg hydrocortisone IV	qd × 3-5 days
	40-60 mg prednisone PO	qd × 3-5 days
Dialysis		

IV, intravenous; PO, orally; q, every; qd, every day; SC, subcutaneous.

Volume Repletion

When treatment is indicated, the first priority is to correct the extracellular volume depletion that almost invariably is present, usually by infusing isotonic saline at a rate of 2 to 4 L/day. The aggressiveness with which the individual patient is rehydrated must be considered in relation to both the patient's volume status and the risk of precipitating or aggravating congestive heart failure or ascites. Diuretics, particularly thiazides, should be discontinued. The use of furosemide or other potent "loop" diuretics to promote calciuresis may exacerbate extracellular volume depletion if used too early in the course of treatment. In light of the availability of highly effective alternatives for the therapy of hypercalcemia, such drugs probably are best avoided, except in circumstances in which vigorous rehydration fails to improve severe hypercalcemia or might precipitate congestive heart failure. In any case, prolonged use of saline-induced calciuresis without the early introduction of an effective antiresorptive agent is ill-advised and ultimately futile.

Bisphosphonates

Intravenous bisphosphonates rapidly inhibit bone resorption and currently are the agents of first choice in managing severe hypercalcemia that is known or suspected to be driven mainly by osteoclastic bone resorption.[115] Bisphosphonates should not be used in patients with milk-alkali syndrome, for example, in whom they are likely to induce posttreatment hypocalcemia.[416] Pamidronate and zoledronate are approved by the Food and Drug Administration (FDA) for treatment of hypercalcemia of malignancy and are the most widely used agents in the United States, although ibandronate and clodronate have been successfully deployed elsewhere. These drugs generally are well tolerated, although local pain or swelling at the infusion site, low-grade fever 1 to 2 days after the infusion, transient lymphopenia, and mild hypophosphatemia or hypomagnesemia may occur. Serum calcium usually declines within 24 hours and reaches a nadir within a week following a single infusion, at which point calcium levels may be normal in 70% to 90% of treated patients. Intravenous bisphosphonates may be nephrotoxic, but clinical data to guide their use in patients with renal insufficiency are not yet available. Most clinicians will employ the standard dose (see Table 28-3)—perhaps at half or less of the usual rate of administration—in patients with moderate renal insufficiency (GFR >30 mL/minute), which is common in the setting of severe hypercalcemia. In patients with more severe renal insufficiency, bisphosphonates probably are best avoided and dialysis may be a more appropriate alternative (see later). The duration of the response to intravenous bisphosphonate treatment is quite variable, ranging from 1 or 2 weeks to several months. Depending on clinical circumstances, repeated courses of therapy may be indicated and effective.

Denosumab

Denosumab, a monoclonal antibody directed against RANKL, has been shown to be effective in managing malignancy-associated hypercalcemia, including patients refractory to bisphosphonates.[417] Denosumab offers an alternative to intravenous bisphosphonates in patients with renal failure, but like bisphosphonates, denosumab carries a small risk of osteonecrosis of the jaw. Typical dosage is 60 mg given subcutaneously every week for a month, followed by 60 mg per month.

Calcitonin

Calcitonin, which directly inhibits osteoclast function, may be used with other antiresorptive agents to achieve more rapid control of severe hypercalcemia. Calcitonin rarely produces a decline in serum calcium of more than 1 to 2 mg/dL; however, and its efficacy typically is limited to a few days at most, possibly because of receptor downregulation in target cells of bone and kidney. Its major advantages are a more rapid onset of action than bisphosphonates (several hours) and its potential to augment renal calcium excretion directly. Calcitonin generally is well tolerated, although transient nausea, vomiting, abdominal cramps, flushing, and local skin reactions may occur.

Other Approaches to Treatment of Severe Hypercalcemia

Because of their potential toxicity, other antiresorptives such as gallium nitrate, plicamycin (mithramycin), and intravenous phosphate (in patients with severe hypophosphatemia) have largely been abandoned in the treatment of severe hypercalcemia, although a randomized trial demonstrated that gallium nitrate may be more effective than bisphosphonate in controlling hypercalcemia of malignancy.[418] Oral or enteral phosphate repletion is appropriate for patients with significant hypophosphatemia (<2.5 mg/dL), provided that serum phosphate and renal function are closely monitored. Intravenous or oral glucocorticoids should be considered early in patients with suspected vitamin D–dependent hypercalcemia, including those with lymphoma or granulomatous disease. The response to glucocorticoids may be more delayed than that to bisphosphonates. Successful treatment of hypercalcemia in Crohn disease with infliximab has been reported.[419]

In patients with severe renal insufficiency, with or without complicating heart disease, in whom saline rehydration and associated calciuresis may not be feasible and bisphosphonates probably are best avoided, dialytic therapy against a low- or zero-calcium dialysate may be the most appropriate tactic. In patients with known primary hyperparathyroidism and intercurrent severe hypercalcemia (parathyroid storm), urgent parathyroidectomy (following initial medical stabilization) should be considered.

Novel approaches to the treatment of severe hypercalcemia currently are in development. One available therapy for parathyroid carcinoma is the calcimimetic cinacalcet, which may be effective in some patients,[420] and monoclonal antibodies directed against PTHrP could prove useful in controlling PTHrP-dependent hypercalcemia.[421]

HYPOCALCEMIC DISORDERS

Clinical Presentation

The predominant clinical symptoms and signs of hypocalcemia are those of neuromuscular irritability, including perioral paresthesias, tingling of the fingers and toes, and spontaneous or latent tetany. Tetany can be elicited by percussion of the facial nerve below the zygoma, resulting in ispilateral contractions of the facial muscle (Chvostek sign) or by 3 minutes of occlusive pressure with a blood pressure cuff resulting in carpal spasm, which, on occasion, can be very painful (Trousseau sign) (Fig. 28-30). The usefulness of these signs in diagnosing hypocalcemia and in following therapeutic responses cannot be overemphasized.

Electrocardiographic abnormalities also result from hypocalcemia, including prolonged QT intervals and

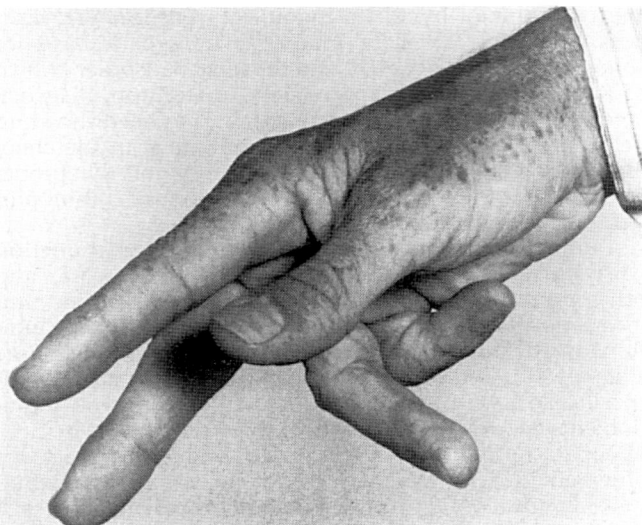

Figure 28-30 Trousseau sign. (From Burnside JW, McGlynn TJ. *Physical Diagnosis*, 17th ed. Baltimore, MD: Williams & Wilkins; 1987:63.)

marked QRS complex and ST-segment changes that may mimic acute myocardial infarction or conduction abnormalities. Ventricular arrhythmias are a rare complication of hypocalcemia, although congestive heart failure, corrected by normalization of serum calcium, has been reported.

In profound hypocalcemia or during acute falls in serum calcium, grand mal seizures or laryngospasm also may be observed. Chronic hypocalcemia is associated with milder symptoms and signs of neuromuscular irritability and may even be asymptomatic. Long-standing hypocalcemia associated with hyperphosphatemia (observed with PTH deficiency or resistance) may lead to calcification of the basal ganglia and occasional extrapyramidal disorders. In addition, mineral ion deposits in the lens may lead to cataract formation.

Chronic hypocalcemia, particularly when associated with hypophosphatemia, as in vitamin D deficiency, is associated with growth plate abnormalities in children (rickets) and defects in the mineralization of new bone (osteomalacia) (see Chapter 29). Severe symptomatic hypocalcemia constitutes an emergency that requires immediate attention to prevent seizures and death from laryngospasm or cardiac causes.

Total calcium in serum includes both the free (biologically active) and protein-bound components; the major binding protein is albumin (discussed earlier). Therefore, measurements of total calcium cannot be interpreted without concurrent measurement of albumin. Studies of hypoalbuminemic patients with cirrhosis have led to a formula for correction of total calcium based on concurrent albumin levels (a decrease in calcium of 0.8 mg/dL for every 1-g/dL decrease in albumin). No formula has proved to be accurate, however, for assessment of calcium in acutely ill patients. This probably relates to the variety of factors that may increase protein binding and decrease the fraction of total calcium present as the free ion, including alkalosis, elevated circulating free fatty acids, and lipid infusions. Consequently, ionized calcium should be measured when the diagnosis of hypocalcemia is considered in the setting of acute illness and severe hypoalbuminemia.

Chronic hypocalcemia is most often due to deficiency of PTH or $1,25(OH)_2D_3$ or to resistance to the biologic effects of these calcium-regulating hormones (Table 28-4).

TABLE 28-4

Causes of Hypocalcemia

Parathyroid-Related Disorders

Absence of the Parathyroid Glands or of PTH
Congenital
    DiGeorge syndrome
    X-linked or autosomally inherited hypoparathyroidism
    Autoimmune polyglandular syndrome type I
    PTH gene mutations
Postsurgical hypoparathyroidism
Infiltrative disorders
    Hemochromatosis
    Wilson disease
    Metastases
Hypoparathyroidism following radioactive iodine thyroid ablation

Impaired Secretion of PTH
Hypomagnesemia
Respiratory alkalosis
Activating mutations of the calcium sensor

Target Organ Resistance
Hypomagnesemia
Pseudohypoparathyroidism
    Type 1
    Type 2

Vitamin D–Related Disorders

Vitamin D deficiency
    Dietary absence
    Malabsorption
Accelerated loss
    Impaired enterohepatic recirculation
    Anticonvulsant medications
Impaired 25-hydroxylation
    Liver disease
    Isoniazid
    CYP2R1 mutation
Impaired 1α-hydroxylation
    Renal failure
Vitamin D–dependent rickets, type I
Oncogenic osteomalacia
Target organ resistance
    Vitamin D–dependent rickets, type II
    Phenytoin

Other Causes

Excessive deposition into the skeleton
    Osteoblastic malignancies
    Hungry bone syndrome
Impaired bone resorption
    Vitamin D deficiency
    Bisphosphonates
    RANKL inhibition
Chelation
    Foscarnet
    Phosphate infusion
    Infusion of citrated blood products
    Infusion of EDTA-containing contrast reagents
    Fluoride
Neonatal hypocalcemia
    Prematurity
    Asphyxia
    Diabetic mother
    Hyperparathyroid mother
HIV infection
    Drug therapy
    Vitamin D deficiency
    Hypomagnesemia
    Impaired PTH responsiveness
Critical illness
    Pancreatitis
    Toxic shock syndrome
    Intensive care unit patients

EDTA, ethylenediaminetetra-acetic acid; HIV, human immunodeficiency virus; PTH, parathyroid hormone; RANKL, receptor activator for nuclear factor κB ligand.

Parathyroid-Related Disorders

Hypocalcemia associated with parathyroid dysfunction can be differentiated from other causes of hypocalcemia by routine laboratory tests. Serum calcium is low owing to lack of PTH-mediated bone resorption and urinary calcium reabsorption. Serum phosphate is increased owing to impaired renal clearance. Serum $1,25(OH)_2D_3$ is low because PTH and hypophosphatemia stimulate the renal $25(OH)D$ 1α-hydroxylase. Consequently, $1,25(OH)_2D_3$-mediated intestinal calcium absorption is markedly decreased, further exacerbating the hypocalcemia. PTH levels measured using sensitive two-site PTH assays (see Fig. 28-19) are usually low or undetectable but may be inappropriately normal if some degree of PTH production is preserved. Elevated levels of PTH are found in syndromes associated with resistance to the biologic effects of PTH.

Congenital or Inherited Parathyroid Disorders

Several rare syndromes associated with congenital or inherited hypoparathyroidism appear sporadically or in a variety of inheritance patterns, suggesting multiple causes. Mutation of a parathyroid-specific transcription factor, glial cells missing homolog B (GCMB) (chromosome 6p23), which is expressed in the PTH-secreting cells of the developing parathyroids, has been shown to be a cause of familial hypoparathyroidism in humans and mice.[39] Although usually inherited in an autosomal recessive fashion, GCMB-associated hypoparathyroidism can be autosomal dominant through expression of a dominant-negative mutant GCMB.[422] The genetic abnormality responsible for X-linked, recessive hypoparathyroidism has been identified as a deletion/insertion of DNA near the *SOX3* gene at Xq26-Xq27.[40]

In a number of diseases, hypoparathyroidism is associated with multiple abnormalities in embryonic development in the neck/chest region. DiGeorge syndrome occurs sporadically and is associated with an embryologic defect in the formation of the third, fourth, and fifth branchial pouches, resulting in the absence of parathyroid glands. DiGeorge syndrome may, in fact, be a neurocrestopathy, because ablation of the premigratory cephalic neural crest in chick embryos produces the same phenotype.[423] The contribution of homeobox genes to parathyroid development and their potential relationship to DiGeorge syndrome also has been demonstrated by the absence of thymic and parathyroid tissue, accompanied by cardiac and craniofacial abnormalities, in mice lacking the homeobox gene *hoxa3*.[424] DiGeorge syndrome is often associated with other congenital abnormalities in a syndrome referred to by the acronym CATCH 22 (*c*ardiac defect, *a*bnormal facies, *t*hymic hypoplasia, *c*left palate, *h*ypocalcemia, and 22q11 deletions).[425] Microdeletion of 22q11.21-q11.23[426] and a t(2;22)(q14;q11) balanced translocation suggest that a gene at chromosome 22q11 may be pathogenetic in this syndrome.[427] Hypoparathyroidism also has been reported in two patients with a 22q11 deletion.[428] The *TBX1* gene is the relevant locus, because point mutations in this gene result in DiGeorge syndrome.[429] A number of cases of DiGeorge and velocardiofacial syndromes have been shown to have no detectable abnormality at 22q11, but rather terminal 10p deletions or interstitial 10p13/10p14 deletions, suggesting that two loci may be critical for development of branchial pouch structures.[430] Terminal deletions of 10p accompanied by hypoparathyroidism can be further subdivided into DiGeorge critical region II (10p13-14) and a more telomeric region (10p14-10pter), wherein mutation of the transcription factor GATA3 causes the syndrome of hypoparathyroidism, sensorineural deafness, and renal anomaly (HDR).[431] The genetic basis for some individuals with HDR and the related disorder known as Kenny-Caffey syndrome, which, in addition, is associated with recurrent bacterial infections, has been shown to be linked to 1q43-44 and involve mutations in the chaperone protein, TBCE, which is required for the proper folding of α-tubulin and the formation of $\alpha\beta$-tubulin heterodimers.[432]

Familial hypoparathyroidism is seen in conjunction with mucocutaneous candidiasis, Addison disease, and other immune disorders in autosomal recessive autoimmune polyglandular syndrome, type I, caused by mutations in the autoimmune regulatory gene *(AIRE)*[433,434] (see Chapter 40). NALP5 has been identified as a parathyroid-specific antigen in affected patients.[435] *AIRE* gene mutations have also been found in young women with isolated hypoparathyroidism.[436] Hypoparathyroidism may also be observed in association with mitochondrial myopathies such as mitochondrial trifunctional protein deficiency[437] and the Kearns-Sayre syndrome.[438] Other inherited forms of hypoparathyroidism may be observed as an isolated defect[439] or may present with other features such as lymphedema, dysmorphism, and renal and cardiac abnormalities.[440,441]

Abnormalities in the Parathyroid Hormone Gene

Specific defects have been found in the PTH gene in a small number of kindreds affected by congenital hypoparathyroidism. These include point mutations in the signal peptide[5,6] and in an intron border, leading to aberrant splicing[442] as well as a homozygous mutation in exon 2 of the PTH gene, leading to premature termination of the transcript.[443]

Destruction of the Parathyroid Glands

The most common cause of chronic hypocalcemia is post-surgical hypoparathyroidism. This may occur after removal of all parathyroid tissue during thyroidectomy and radical neck dissection for malignancies or after inadvertent interruption of the blood supply to the parathyroid glands during head and neck surgery. Transient hypoparathyroidism, attributed to reversible damage to the remaining normal glands, is common after parathyroidectomy; permanent hypoparathyroidism may occur after vascular or surgical injury or inadvertent removal of all parathyroid tissue. Rarely, transient hypoparathyroidism may follow spontaneous infarction of autonomous tissue in primary hyperparathyroidism.[444] Hypoparathyroidism is a rare complication of radioactive iodine ablation of the thyroid gland for Graves disease.[445]

Hypoparathyroidism also can occur as a result of infiltrative diseases of the parathyroids. This is seen in diseases of iron overload such as hemochromatosis and in patients with thalassemia major who have been heavily transfused.[446] Copper deposition in Wilson disease[447] may also cause parathyroid dysfunction. Metastatic disease to the parathyroids can cause hypoparathyroidism, but rarely, presumably because of the need for four-gland involvement before significant hypoparathyroidism is observed.

Impaired Parathyroid Hormone Secretion

Impaired secretion of PTH from the parathyroid glands can lead to functional hypoparathyroidism. This is commonly seen in profound hypomagnesemia,[448] in which target organ resistance to PTH can also occur. Both of these

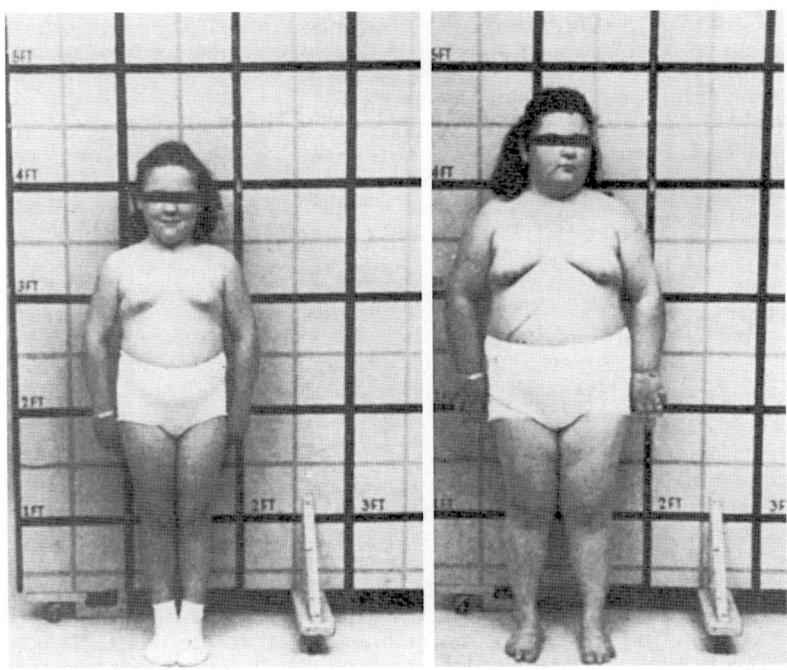

Figure 28-31 Daughter *(left)* and mother *(right)* with pseudohypoparathyroidism and Albright hereditary osteodystrophy.

abnormalities are reversible upon magnesium repletion[449,450] (see "Disorders of Magnesium Metabolism").

Chronic respiratory alkalosis leads to hyperphosphatemia and decreased ionized calcium levels accompanied by impaired renal calcium resorption and inappropriately normal PTH levels.[451] This biochemical phenotype suggests both an abnormality of PTH secretion and renal resistance to PTH. Acute alkalosis in dogs also suppresses PTH secretion.[452]

Activating mutations in the CaSR cause autosomal dominant hypocalcemia type 1 (ADH1) associated with inappropriately normal PTH levels. This syndrome can also be seen in patients with activating antibodies directed against this receptor.[453] Gain of function mutations of the α-subunit of the G protein, G11 (GNA11), cause a second form of autosomal dominant hypocalcemia (ADH2).[359]

The clinical syndrome in ADH1 is variable; patients present with hypocalcemia and seizures, whereas their affected relatives may be only subsequently diagnosed with asymptomatic hypocalcemia.[13] Unlike patients with inactivating mutations of the calcium sensor, homozygously affected individuals do not appear to have a more severe phenotype. The presence of hypercalciuria in these patients makes medical management uniquely challenging. Treatment with vitamin D metabolites often results in a marked increase in renal calcium excretion, associated with renal calcification and resultant renal impairment. Based on these observations, it has been suggested that asymptomatic individuals be left untreated and that the goal of therapy in individuals with symptomatic hypocalcemia be solely to relieve symptoms, not to achieve normocalcemia. Treatment with calcium and vitamin D metabolites should be accompanied by the use of thiazide diuretics to decrease urinary calcium excretion as well as ensuring adequate urinary volume to decrease urinary calcium concentration.

Pseudohypoparathyroidism

The idiopathic and inherited forms of PTH resistance are referred to as pseudohypoparathyroidism (PHP). There are two main types of PHP: type 1, which is characterized by impaired cAMP and phosphaturic responses to PTH, and type 2, in which the cAMP response to PTH is preserved, but the phosphaturic response is not. Albright described the first cases of documented PTH resistance in 1942.[454] These patients were hypocalcemic and hyperphosphatemic, and they exhibited a number of features that are now called Albright hereditary osteodystrophy (AHO). These features include short stature, rounded face, foreshortened fourth and other metacarpals, obesity, and subcutaneous calcifications (Figs. 28-31 and 28-32).

PTH administration to these patients failed to provoke a phosphate diuresis or an increase in serum calcium. It was subsequently demonstrated that hypocalcemic patients with features of AHO had elevated PTH levels and that PTH infusions failed to stimulate renal production of cAMP. Failure of stimulation of cAMP production suggested a defect in the PTH receptor or in its cAMP-mediated signal transduction.[455] The measurement of cAMP in the urine following an infusion of synthetic PTH(1-34) is now used to establish the diagnosis of PTH resistance.[456]

The variable presence of AHO and renal resistance to PTH in PHP has led to the subclassification of PHP (Table 28-5). Type 1a is characterized by AHO and diminished $G_s\alpha$ activity (approximately 50% of normal). These patients usually have mutations that inactivate one allele of the $G_s\alpha$ coding region through a variety of mechanisms (missense mutations, chain-terminating mutations, changes that induce abnormal splicing, small insertions, deletions, or inversions).[457] The resultant diminished $G_s\alpha$ activity has been demonstrated in several tissues, including kidney, fibroblasts, transformed lymphocytes, platelets, and erythrocytes. Though abnormalities of imprinting in the genetic locus encoding $G_s\alpha$ usually cause PHP type 1b (see later), occasionally similar imprinting abnormalities can result in PHP 1a. In a series of 40 patients without identified *GNAS* mutations, 24 were found to have *GNAS* cluster imprinting defects.[458] This finding was not associated with any difference in AHO phenotype or severity from patients with inactivating mutations of $G_s\alpha$.

TABLE 28-5

Types of Pseudohypoparathyroidism

Disorder	Urinary cAMP Response to PTH	Urinary PO₄ Response to PTH	Other Hormonal Resistance	AHO	Pathophysiology
Pseudohypoparathyroidism 1a	Decreased	Decreased	Yes	Yes	G$_s$α mutation or imprinting abnormality
Pseudo-pseudohypoparathyroidism	Normal	Normal	No	Yes	G$_s$α mutation
Pseudohypoparathyroidism 1b	Decreased	Decreased	Rare	No	*GNAS1* locus imprinting abnormality
Pseudohypoparathyroidism 1c	Decreased	Decreased	Yes	Yes	G$_s$α function normal, imprinting abnormality
Pseudohypoparathyroidism 2	Normal	Decreased *PRKAR1A* mutation with AHO	No	Rare	Vitamin D deficiency or myotonic dystrophy

AHO, Albright hereditary osteodystrophy; cAMP, cyclic adenosine monophosphate; *GNAS1,* portion of the *GNAS* complex locus encoding G$_s$α; G$_s$α, α-subunit of the stimulatory G protein; PO₄, phosphate; PTH, parathyroid hormone.

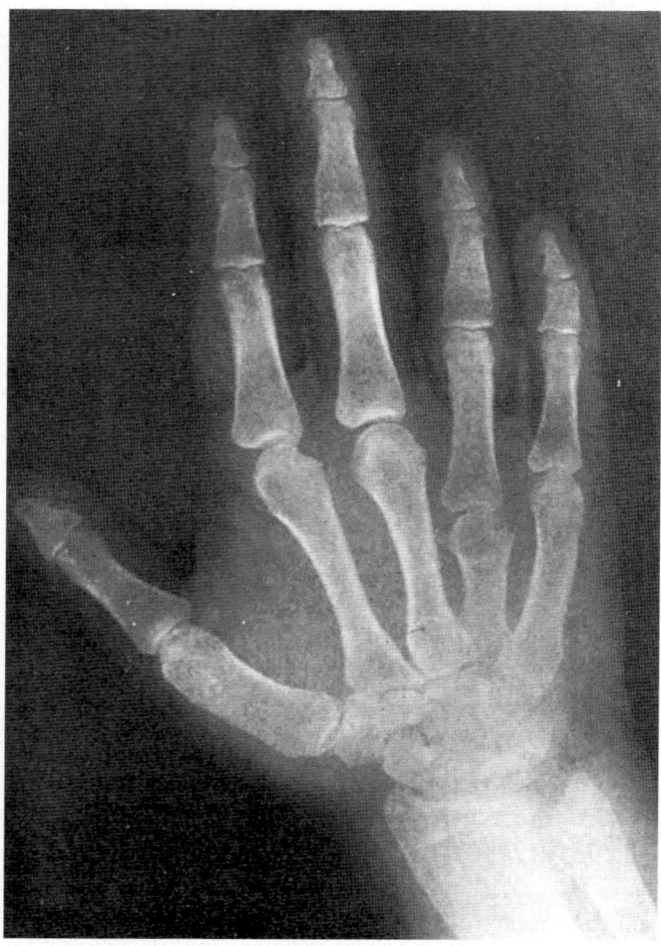

Figure 28-32 Radiograph of the hand from a patient with pseudohypoparathyroidism and Albright hereditary osteodystrophy. Note the shortened fourth metacarpal.

Impaired mentation is seen in approximately half of the patients with PHP 1a and appears to be related to the G$_s$α deficiency rather than to chronic hypocalcemia, because patients with other forms of PHP and hypocalcemia have normal mentation. The G$_s$α deficiency in PHP 1a may be associated not only with PTH resistance but also with resistance to other hormones such as TSH, glucagon, and gonadotropins, resulting in thyroidal and gonadal dysfunction. Paradoxically, two unrelated males with both PHP 1a and gonadotropin-independent precocious puberty have

been described. The G$_s$α point mutation found in these individuals is thought to lead to a protein that is unstable at 37° C and, therefore, to confer renal resistance to PTH. At the lower temperature of the testes, however, the protein is not degraded. In this setting, the stable but mutated protein is constitutively active and stimulates the Leydig cell in a manner similar to the skeletal effects of the G$_s$ mutations in McCune-Albright syndrome (see Chapter 25).[459]

Pseudo-pseudohypoparathyroidism (pseudo-PHP) is a term coined by Albright to refer to individuals with the phenotype of AHO but without evidence of PTH resistance. Patients with pseudo-PHP often are found in the same kindreds as those with PHP 1a, and they invariably inherit the same abnormal G$_s$α gene found in their PTH-resistant relatives.[460] When patients inherit the mutant G$_s$α gene from their fathers, they exhibit pseudo-PHP; when they inherit the mutant G$_s$α gene from their mothers, they exhibit PHP.[461,462] This pattern, in which the renal hormone resistance phenotype depends on the parent of origin, is termed a form of tissue-specific genetic imprinting; mice with targeted ablation of the G$_s$α gene *(Gnas1)* also display such imprinting.[463] In addition to the AHO phenotype, inheritance of paternal *GNAS* mutations leads to severe intrauterine growth retardation, suggesting a role for paternally imprinted genes in fetal growth and development.[464] Further, although subcutaneous ossification is seen in patients with both PHP 1a and pseudo-PHP, extension of this ossification deep into muscle (called progressive osseous heteroplasia) is seen virtually exclusively in patients with pseudo-PHP.[465]

The observation of a phenotype in a heterozygous "loss-of-function" mutation in G$_s$α is in contrast to the findings in mice with targeted deletions of the other Gα genes (G$_{i2}$α, G$_o$α, G$_q$α, G$_{13}$α), in which a phenotype is observed only in the homozygous state.[466] The fact that the *GNAS1* gene is imprinted has partly resolved the dilemma of this dominant phenotype. Studies in mice have shown that only the allele of G$_s$α inherited from the mother is expressed in the renal proximal tubule. Consequently, mice with targeted ablation of the maternally inherited *Gnas1* gene fail to express G$_s$α mRNA in the renal cortex but have normal expression in the cortex when the mutant gene is inherited from the father. No such imprinting pattern is seen in the inner medulla; this correlates with the mice (and human patients) exhibiting PTH, but not vasopressin, resistance.[463]

PHP type 1b presents with hypocalcemia, high PTH levels, and failure of PTH infusions to increase urinary cAMP production. However, PHP 1b is usually not accompanied by any of the clinical features of AHO, nor is it

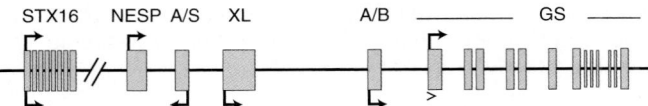

Figure 28-33 The *GNAS* locus. A schematic representation of the *GNAS* locus is shown, with the boxes indicating exons for syntaxin (STX-16), neuroendocrine secretory protein 55 (NESP), the antisense (A/S) NESP55 transcript, the $G_s\alpha$ isoforms $XL\alpha s$ (XL), loss-of-methylation locus A/B, and $G_s\alpha$ (GS). The start site of and direction (sense versus antisense) of transcription are indicated by the arrows. Genes that are maternally transcribed are indicated by arrows above the relevant genes, whereas those that are paternally transcribed are indicated below. The expression of $XL\alpha s$, A/B, and A/S is from the paternal allele, whereas the maternal NESP55 transcript is expressed. Expression of STX-16 is biallelic. The arrowhead below the $G_s\alpha$ locus indicates that only the maternal allele is expressed in the renal tubules.

associated with abnormal $G_s\alpha$ levels in fibroblasts. As in PHP 1a, mild TSH resistance has been reported.[467-469] The PTH target organ manifestations of PHP 1b are variable, with some affected individuals having manifestations of PTH overactivity in bone and PTH resistance in kidney, a pattern that resembles that of PHP 1a. Cultured osteoblast-like cells from a patient with PHP 1b demonstrated normal cAMP responsiveness to PTH, despite the lack of renal responsiveness.[470]

When inherited, PHP 1b has been found to map to chromosome 20q13.3,[471] the same region that contains the *GNAS1* gene, encoding $G_s\alpha$. The disease is inherited with the imprinting characteristic of PHP 1a, but sequencing studies and analysis of DNA methylation suggest that the disease-causing mutations are close to but distinct from the $G_s\alpha$ coding region. The mutations in these patients cause imprinting abnormalities of the *GNAS* locus.[467,472,473]

The *GNAS* locus gives rise to multiple transcripts (Fig. 28-33), including $G_s\alpha$. $G_s\alpha$ is biallelically expressed in most tissues, but only the maternal transcript is expressed in the renal proximal tubules and, to a variable extent, in the thyroid, gonads, and pituitary. In contrast, expression of the $XL\alpha s$, A/B, and antisense (A/S) transcripts are paternally expressed whereas the NESP55 (neuroendocrine secretory protein 55) transcript is maternally expressed; these patterns of expression are associated with differential methylation of DNA sequences associated with each transcript. All patients with PHP 1b exhibit loss of methylation at exon A/B, which results in biallelic expression of the transcript. This abnormality is thought to play a role in the suppression of $G_s\alpha$ expression in the proximal tubule and consequent hormone resistance.[473] The methylation defect in exon A/B, when found in families with PHP 1b, is most often caused by 3-kilobase deletions of DNA not in exon A/B but instead 200 kilobases upstream of GNAS.[474,475] How this and other deletions lead to methylation abnormalities in exon A/B is unknown. In sporadic cases of PHP 1b, deletions within GNAS also cause abnormal methylation of exon A/B and an abnormal expression pattern of $G_s\alpha$.

Several patients with AHO and PTH resistance have been found to have normal $G_s\alpha$ activity; this subgroup has been designated PHP 1c. Biochemical characterization in one case[476] revealed a significant decrease in the manganese-stimulated adenylate cyclase activity in fibroblast membranes of the affected individual, raising the possibility that a second defect in the cAMP pathway may lead to the phenotype of PHP 1c. Another PHP 1c patient, studied after $G_s\alpha$ sequencing became easier, was found to have a short deletion at the carboxy-terminus of G_s, leading to normal levels of G_s activity when assayed in erythrocytes but defective activation by receptors.[477]

In PHP type 2, PTH infusions increase urinary cAMP normally; however, PTH does not elicit a phosphaturic response.[478] This syndrome, like PHP 1b, lacks signs of AHO or resistance to other hormones and is not familial in origin. The age of onset of patients with this disorder is variable, ranging from infancy to senescence, suggesting that it is an acquired defect or that the biochemical phenotype may be unmasked by intercurrent abnormalities. A subset of patients with myotonic dystrophy display the biochemical features of PHP 2, the degree of PTH resistance correlating with the degree of expansion of the pathogenetic CTG repeats in the myotonin protein kinase gene. A similar biochemical phenotype can also be observed in vitamin D deficiency,[479] and some authors have suggested that PHP 2 is a manifestation of vitamin D deficiency rather than a distinct clinical entity.[480] Minagawa and colleagues reported cases of three neonates with no signs of rickets and with normal levels of vitamin D who presented with transient PHP 2 that resolved at about 6 months of age.[481] They postulated that PTH responsiveness is subject to maturation during fetal and neonatal development. PHP 2, therefore, seems to reflect a heterogeneous clinical disorder associated with defects in PTH responsiveness distal to cAMP or involving a separate signal transduction pathway.[482]

The selectivity of PTH resistance for the proximal tubule has implications for the management of patients with PHP. Because bone is not resistant to PTH, hyperparathyroid bone disease may occur.[483,484] Patients with PHP have lower bone density than normal and hypoparathyroid control subjects. Basal urinary hydroxyproline excretion in patients with PHP is twice that of hypoparathyroid control subjects, and they have similar increases in response to parathyroid extract.[485] Further, the renal resistance to PTH is limited to the proximal tubule, where the 1α-hydroxylase activates 25(OH)D. Consequently, the normal distal tubular reabsorption of calcium keeps the urinary calcium excretion low in comparison to those with primary hypoparathyroidism.[486] Therefore, therapy with $1,25(OH)_2D_3$ can be used with the goal of normalizing PTH levels to avoid bone disease, with less concern than otherwise that urinary calcium excretion might be excessive.

Vitamin D–Related Disorders

Hypocalcemia secondary to vitamin D deficiency or resistance to the biologic effects of $1,25(OH)_2D_3$ is easily differentiated from the hypocalcemia of hypoparathyroidism by routine clinical and laboratory evaluation. The primary cause of hypocalcemia in vitamin D deficiency is decreased intestinal absorption of calcium. In the setting of normal renal function, the hypocalcemia of vitamin D deficiency, unlike that of hypoparathyroidism, is accompanied by hypophosphatemia and increased renal phosphate clearance. This increase in phosphate clearance is a direct result of compensatory (secondary) hyperparathyroidism. The hyperparathyroidism is a consequence of the hypocalcemic stimulus to PTH secretion and the stimulation of PTH gene expression and parathyroid cell proliferation caused by hypocalcemia (see "Parathyroid Hormone Biosynthesis" earlier). Therefore, measurement of serum phosphate and PTH are very useful in distinguishing these disorders from hypoparathyroidism. The secondary hyperparathyroidism results in increased calcium mobilization from the skeleton, increased renal reabsorption of calcium, and increased renal 1α-hydroxylation of 25(OH)D. In severe vitamin D deficiency, the increased levels of PTH no longer lead to increased bone resorption, perhaps because osteoclasts appear not to resorb unmineralized osteoid.

In profound vitamin D deficiency, the level of $1,25(OH)_2D_3$ is usually low; in moderate vitamin D deficiency, the stimulation of the renal 1α-hydroxylase by PTH can result in a normal or even elevated 1,25(OH)$_2$D$_3$ level. These high levels of 1,25(OH)$_2$D$_3$ reflect the action of PTH on the renal 1α-hydroxylase. The ineffectiveness of the high levels of total 1,25(OH)$_2$D$_3$ to normalize serum calcium may be explained by increased binding of this metabolite to VDBP when the levels of 25(OH)D are very low.

Vitamin D Deficiency

Because the two sources of vitamin D are the diet and cutaneous synthesis after ultraviolet irradiation, lack of solar irradiation and decreased intake or impaired absorption of vitamin D can lead to vitamin D deficiency. As the population has become increasingly educated about the risks of skin cancer from solar irradiation, the avoidance of long periods of intense sun exposure and the use of high SPF (solar protective factor) sun blocks have resulted in increased reliance on dietary sources of vitamin D. The recommended dietary allowance for vitamin D is 200 IU; however, in the absence of solar exposure, 400-600 IU of vitamin D are required to prevent vitamin D deficiency.[487] Vitamin D is present in many food sources, both vegetable and animal. In addition, many prepared foods, especially cereal products, are fortified with vitamin D. Although dairy products have been fortified with vitamin D as well, the actual amount of vitamin D provided does not correlate well with the purported content.[169] The vitamin D derived from vegetable sources is vitamin D$_2$ and that from animal sources is vitamin D$_3$. These two forms of vitamin D are metabolized identically and have been used to fortify foods. Although it is thought that their ability to raise 25-hydroxyvitamin D levels is equivalent, this premise remains controversial.[488] The more beneficial effect of vitamin D$_3$ reported by some may be due to the population studied, because the modest increase in the half-life of 25-hydroxyvitamin D$_2$ versus 25-hydroxyvitamin D$_3$ is influenced by VDBP concentration and genotype.[171]

The Institute of Medicine has defined vitamin D "sufficiency" as a level higher than 50 nmol/L (>20 ng/mL); however, higher levels may be required to optimize intestinal calcium absorption in those with disorders such as intestinal disease, short bowel syndrome, and obesity as well as in the elderly. Although elderly, homebound individuals are at high risk, several studies have demonstrated that vitamin D deficiency is prevalent in the general population (reviewed by Thomas and coworkers[489]). The clinical relevance of this vitamin D deficiency has been confirmed by a study demonstrating that vitamin D administration (800 IU/day) to an ambulatory elderly population decreases serum PTH levels as well as the incidence of hip fracture.[490] Malabsorption also remains an important cause of vitamin D deficiency in all age groups. Because vitamin D is a fat-soluble vitamin, its absorption is dependent upon emulsification by bile acids. Any cause of fat malabsorption or short bowel syndrome can result in vitamin D deficiency; therefore, malabsorption should be ruled out in patients with very low 25(OH)D levels (<8 ng/dL).

Accelerated Loss of Vitamin D

25(OH)D and 1,25(OH)$_2$D$_3$ are secreted with bile salts and undergo enterohepatic circulation; therefore, intestinal disease may also result in vitamin D deficiency due to excessive losses. Increased metabolism of vitamin D, leading to low blood levels of 25(OH)D, is seen in individuals given anticonvulsant medications and antituberculosis therapy. Phenobarbital, primidone, phenytoin,[491] rifampin, and glutethimide[492] have all been reported to accelerate the hepatic inactivation of vitamin D.

Impaired 25-Hydroxylation of Vitamin D

The vitamin D that is absorbed undergoes 25-hydroxylation in the liver; therefore, severe hepatic parenchymal damage can result in 25(OH)D deficiency. Clinically, severe vitamin D deficiency as a consequence of liver disease is rare, because the degree of hepatic destruction necessary to impair 25-hydroxylation is incompatible with long-term survival. However, isoniazid has been shown to decrease the 25-hydroxylation of vitamin D.[493] Kindreds have been described in whom the clinical and biochemical presentations and therapeutic responses suggest an inherited 25-hydroxylation defect.[494,495] A homozygous mutation in the *CYP2R1* gene that encodes a hepatic microsomal vitamin D 25-hydroxylase has been found in these kindreds,[495,496]; however, genetic analysis of a nonrelated individual with a similar phenotype characterized by autosomal dominant inheritance failed to find mutations in either the coding region or splice junctions of *CYP2R1*.[497] These findings, combined with the observation that ablation of *Cyp2r1* in mice leads to only a 50% reduction in 25-OH(D) levels, suggest that there is more than one enzyme capable of 25-hydroxylation of vitamin D.[498]

Impaired 1α-Hydroxylation of 25-Hydroxyvitamin D

The final step in the activation of vitamin D is the hydroxylation of 25(OH)D by the renal 1α-hydroxylase to yield 1,25(OH)$_2$D$_3$. Renal parenchymal damage, therefore, can result in deficiency of the active metabolite of vitamin D. Impaired 1α-hydroxylation is observed once creatinine clearance decreases to approximately 30 to 40 mL/minute. Unlike with liver failure, with renal failure, dialysis permits long-term survival; therefore, deficiency of 1,25(OH)$_2$D$_3$ as a result of impaired renal 1α-hydroxylation is a common and important clinical entity. The metabolic consequences of chronic renal failure on the parathyroid glands and the skeleton are complex (see Chapter 29). Impaired renal 1α-hydroxylation leads to decreased intestinal absorption of calcium, resulting in hypocalcemia. The diminished phosphate clearance associated with renal failure leads to elevated levels of blood phosphate and consequently increases in circulating FGF23; this, in turn, further lowers levels of 1,25(OH)$_2$D$_3$ and calcium. The resultant secondary hyperparathyroidism increases release of calcium and phosphate from bone; however, because of the renal insufficiency, PTH has a blunted phosphaturic effect. As a result, the increased serum phosphate rises further. Oral phosphate binders are used to lower blood phosphate. Calcium-containing antacids, which replaced the more toxic aluminum-containing antacids (see Chapter 29), are being supplemented or replaced with the phosphate-binding exchange resin sevelamer. Calcium administration also attenuates the hypocalcemic stimulus to parathyroid secretion. 1,25(OH)$_2$D$_3$ therapy is critical for the absorption of this calcium and should be administered early in the course of renal failure (when the creatinine clearance falls below 30-40 mL/minute) to avoid the development of secondary hyperparathyroidism, with careful monitoring to avoid hypercalcemia. Once secondary hyperparathyroidism has developed, pharmacologic doses of 1,25(OH)$_2$D$_3$, delivered intravenously or orally, or calcimimetics[499] may be required to suppress PTH gene transcription and parathyroid cellular proliferation. Efforts are currently under way to develop nonhypercalcemic analogues of 1,25(OH)$_2$D$_3$ that maintain their PTH-suppressing and antiproliferative effects. Such analogues would be invaluable for the prevention and treatment of secondary hyperparathyroidism in the setting of chronic renal failure and perhaps in the treatment of malignancies whose proliferation is inhibited by pharmacologic doses of $1,25(OH)_2D_3$.

Decreased levels of $1,25(OH)_2D_3$ may also be observed in patients taking ketoconazole[180] and in those with X-linked hypophosphatemia and TIO, diseases associated with high FGF23 levels (see Chapter 29).[176]

Rarely, mutations in both alleles of the gene encoding the 1α-hydroxylase can cause resistance to vitamin D. Biochemically, this disease, called pseudo–vitamin D deficiency rickets (PDDR) is characterized by hypocalcemia and secondary hyperparathyroidism. The only metabolic abnormalities that differentiate it from dietary vitamin D deficiency are the presence of normal or elevated levels of vitamin D and 25(OH)D accompanied by low levels of $1,25(OH)_2D_3$.[500,501] The disease is inherited in an autosomal recessive fashion and presents in infancy with rickets, osteomalacia, and seizures.[502] Administration of physiologic replacement doses of 1α-hydroxylated metabolites of vitamin D results in clinical remission.[503]

Target Organ Resistance to 1,25-Dihydroxyvitamin D₃

Mutations in the VDR cause a second rare inherited disorder, characterized by resistance to the biologic actions of $1,25(OH)_2D_3$. This disorder, referred to as hereditary vitamin D–resistant rickets (HVDRR), is also characterized by autosomal recessive inheritance. Its biochemical presentation, with hypocalcemia, hypophosphatemia, and secondary hyperparathyroidism, resembles that of vitamin D deficiency, but it is accompanied by elevated levels of $1,25(OH)_2D_3$. The molecular basis for this disease is mutation of the VDR gene, resulting in impaired target organ responsiveness. Most of the mutations that have been described involve the DNA binding domain of the receptor. These mutations result in a decreased affinity of the receptor for its response elements on target genes leading to impaired regulation of these genes. Mutations in the hormone binding and nuclear receptor coactivator binding domains of the receptor have also been described in kindreds with HVDRR.[504]

The clinical presentation of HVDRR is variable; however, most patients present in infancy with rickets, hypophosphatemia, and seizures, although presentation in late adolescence has also been described. Alopecia totalis, developing in the first 2 years of life, is present in some kindreds.[505] The finding of alopecia in mice with VDR mutations[31,192] confirms the association of alopecia with disruption of the VDR gene.

Because of the target organ resistance to the active metabolite of vitamin D, there is no ideal treatment for HVDRR. Pharmacologic doses of vitamin D, 25(OH)D, 24,25(OH)D, and $1,25(OH)_2D_3$ have been administered in an attempt to overcome this target organ resistance,[506] with variable effects. In those patients in whom the hypocalcemia and osteomalacia are resistant to such therapeutic interventions, parenteral calcium infusions have been used to heal osteomalacic lesions.[196] Studies in VDR-ablated mice have demonstrated that maintenance of normal mineral ion homeostasis prevents all the complications of VDR ablation except alopecia.[195,197] Based on these observations, patients with VDR mutations should be treated early and aggressively to prevent skeletal abnormalities and parathyroid hyperplasia. Lifelong therapy is usually required, although spontaneous remissions off therapy have been described.[507] The pathophysiology of the spontaneous remissions is not well understood, because the underlying genetic defect still exists. It is likely that these "remissions" reflect compensated calcium homeostasis once the needs of the growing skeleton are met. In support of this hypothesis is a report of a relapse in a pregnant woman, followed by a remission post partum.[508]

Phenytoin causes target organ resistance to the biologic effects of $1,25(OH)_2D_3$, in addition to its acceleration of the hepatic catabolism of vitamin D metabolites. Phenytoin has been shown to impair intestinal calcium absorption in vivo in rats[509] and impair PTH and $1,25(OH)_2D_3$-mediated bone resorption in vitro. Combination chemotherapy with 5-fluorouracil and low-dose leucovorin has been reported to cause hypocalcemia in 65% of patients, associated with an acute decrease in plasma $1,25(OH)_2D_3$ levels.[510]

Other Causes of Hypocalcemia
Excessive Deposition into the Skeleton

Excessive deposition of calcium into the skeleton can occur in association with osteoblastic metastases, with chondrosarcomas,[511] or in the hungry bone syndrome. This syndrome presents as prolonged hypocalcemia, hypocalciuria, and hypophosphatemia following parathyroidectomy for primary hyperparathyroidism (see "Primary Hyperparathyroidism"). The hypocalcemia is a consequence of remineralization of a skeleton that has been subjected to the bone-resorbing effects of PTH over a prolonged period. Hungry bone syndrome can also be observed after treatment of other diseases that are associated with excessive bone resorption. It has been described following radioactive iodine treatment of a patient with Graves disease.[512]

Chelation

Decreases in ionized calcium have been reported with foscarnet, a pyrophosphate analogue that is used as an antiviral agent,[513] perhaps because of complex formation between ionized calcium and the drug.

Hyperphosphatemia, due to phosphate administration or rapid destruction of soft tissue (i.e., rhabdomyolysis, chemotherapy of hematologic malignancies), may produce profound hypocalcemia by directly complexing and precipitating calcium in bone or soft tissues, by inhibiting bone resorption, and by blocking renal synthesis of $1,25(OH)_2D_3$ (see "Hyperphosphatemia").

Massive infusions of citrated blood products may cause hypocalcemia, presumably because citrate complexes calcium in the recipient's plasma.[514] Large doses of ethylenediaminetetra-acetic acid (EDTA)-containing radiographic contrast dyes have also been reported to cause hypocalcemia. Hypocalcemia due to complexes of calcium and fluoride has been reported with hydrofluoric acid burns[515] or ingestion.[516]

Neonatal Hypocalcemia

Neonatal hypocalcemia is seen in infants of hyperparathyroid mothers, infants of diabetic mothers, in premature infants, and in infants with birth asphyxia. The cause of hypocalcemia in infants of diabetic mothers is likely multifactorial. Prematurity per se does not account for the higher incidence.[517] The response of premature infants and infants of diabetic mothers to exogenous PTH suggests that functional hypoparathyroidism may, in part, account for the increased hypocalcemia in these two populations.[517,518] The hypocalcemia in infants of hyperparathyroid mothers is presumably secondary to the maternal hypercalcemia that, in turn, suppresses fetal parathyroid function.[519]

Human Immunodeficiency Virus Infection

Hypocalcemia is sixfold more prevalent in HIV-infected patients than in the general population.[520] Although hypocalcemia is often a consequence of antiretroviral and antibiotic/antimycotic therapy, vitamin D deficiency and hypomagnesemia are also common in patients with AIDS. Impaired parathyroid responsiveness to hypocalcemia has also been documented (see Chapter 41, "Endocrinology of HIV/AIDS").

Critical Illness

Hypocalcemia is commonly seen in critically ill patients and is thought to be a reflection of parathyroid gland suppression, failure to activate vitamin D, calcium chelation or sequestration, hypomagnesemia, or some combination of these disorders. However, an increased basal level and secretory response of PTH to lowering of serum calcium has been observed in some septic and nonseptic intensive care patients, emphasizing the multifactorial origin of the hypocalcemia.[521] There was a correlation between cytokine levels and hypocalcemia in this and other studies, suggesting that these inflammatory agents may play a role in redistribution of calcium to the intracellular or other pools. Interleukins 1 and 6 have been shown to increase the expression of the CaSR on parathyroid cells and lower PTH secretion and blood calcium in rats injected with the cytokine.[522,523] Severe acute pancreatitis is often associated with hypocalcemia and this association is a negative prognostic indicator. The hypocalcemia occurs shortly after the onset of the pancreatitis and is associated with an increase in PTH levels, suggesting that parathyroid function is normal. It has long been thought that this hypocalcemia is secondary to deposition of "calcium soaps" consisting of calcium and fatty acids. Supporting this hypothesis, studies in a patient with a pancreatic fistula have demonstrated hypocalcemia (4.3 mg/dL) in the setting of high levels of calcium (26 mg/dL) and fatty acids in ascitic fluid.[524] Subsequent studies in a rat model have supported this finding and demonstrated that oleate has a high binding capacity for calcium.[525] However, other investigations in a porcine model of experimental pancreatitis have demonstrated that hypocalcemia does not occur if the animals are subjected to thyroidectomy prior to the induction of pancreatitis.[526] This finding suggests a role for calcitonin in the development of hypocalcemia with acute pancreatitis, although several clinical studies have documented normal calcitonin levels in hypocalcemic individuals with pancreatitis.[527] Severe hypocalcemia with hypercalcitoninemia and hypophosphatemia has been reported in the patients with toxic shock syndrome, in those with sepsis, and in critically ill patients.[528] As in acute pancreatitis, this hypocalcemia is usually accompanied by increases in serum levels of PTH, and the degree of hypocalcemia is a negative prognostic indicator. The mechanism of hypocalcemia in these patients is likely to be heterogeneous and has not been clearly defined.

Treatment of Hypocalcemia

Acute hypocalcemia is an emergency that requires prompt attention. If symptoms of neuromuscular irritability are present and carpopedal spasm is elicited on physical examination, treatment with intravenous calcium is indicated until the signs and symptoms of hypocalcemia subside. Approximately 100 mg of elemental calcium should be infused over a period of 10 to 20 minutes (Table 28-6). If

TABLE 28-6
Therapeutic Mineral Ion Preparations

Compound	MW*	Mineral Ion Content mg/g	Mineral Ion Content mmol/g	Oral Preparations Compound	Oral Mineral Ion Content mg/g	Oral Mineral Ion Content mmol/g	Parenteral Compound	Parenteral Mineral Ion Content mg/g	Parenteral Mineral Ion Content mmol/g
Calcium									
Ca carbonate	100	400	10.0	1250 mg[†]	500 mg	12.5 mmol			
Ca phosphate	310	383	9.6	1565 mg	600 mg	15.0 mmol			
Ca acetate	158	253	6.3	668 mg[†]	167 mg	4.2 mmol			
Ca citrate	498	210	6.0	950 mg[†]	200 mg	5.0 mmol			
Ca lactate	218	130	4.6	650 mg[†]	84 mg	2.1 mmol			
Ca glubionate		64	1.7	5 mL	115 mg	2.0 mmol			
Ca gluconate	430	93	2.3	1000 mg[†]	93 mg	2.3 mmol	10% soln	93 mg/10 mL	2.3 mmol/10 mL
Ca gluceptate	488	82	2.0				22% soln	90 mg/5 mL	2.3 mmol/10 mL
Ca chloride	147	273	6.8				10% soln	273 mg/10 mL	11.2 mmol/mL
Magnesium									
Mg oxide	40	603	24.8	400 mg[†]	241 mg	9.9 mmol			
Mg gluconate	450	54	2.2	500 mg	27 mg	1.1 mmol			
Mg chloride	203	120	4.9	535 mg	64 mg	2.6 mmol	20% soln	24 mg/mL	1.0 mmol/mL
Mg sulfate	246	99	4.1				50% soln[†]	49 mg/mL	2.0 mmol/mL
Phosphorus[‡]									
Na/K phosphate (neutral)				Capsule	250 mg	8.1 mmol			
K phosphate (neutral)				Capsule	250 mg	8.1 mmol	soln	94 mg/mL	3.0 mmol/mL
Na phosphate (neutral)							soln	94 mg/mL	3.0 mmol/mL

*Molecular weights (MW) shown are for the usual chemical form, including water molecules (e.g., $MgSO_4 \cdot 7 H_2O$).
[†]Other formulations exist. Those shown are among those approved in the United States.
[‡]Phosphate preparations contain buffered mixtures of monobasic ($H_2PO_4^-$) and dibasic (HPO_4^-) ions; the phosphorus content therefore is specified in millimoles.
  Oral phosphates contain 7 mEq sodium and potassium per capsule (Na/K form) or 14 mEq potassium per capsule (K form). Parenteral solutions typically contain 4 mEq of sodium or potassium per milliliter.
MW, molecular weight; soln, solution.
Data from *Drug Facts and Comparisons*. St. Louis, MO: Facts and Comparisons; 1995.

this amount is not sufficient to alleviate the clinical findings of hypocalcemia, an infusion of 100 mg/hour can be given to adults for several hours with close monitoring of calcium levels. In hypocalcemia associated with hypomagnesemia, magnesium replacement also is required. Magnesium should be given intravenously, 100 mEq over 24 hours in the acute setting. Because most of the parenteral magnesium is excreted in the urine, oral magnesium oxide should be instituted as soon as possible to replete body stores. Special caution and reduced doses are necessary when administering magnesium to patients in renal failure (see "Disorders of Magnesium Metabolism").

The treatment of hypocalcemia should be directed at the underlying disorder. In all cases, replacement with exogenous calcium (1 to 3 g of elemental calcium daily, given orally) should be instituted. Calcium carbonate is the least expensive formulation but requires acidification for efficient absorption. This feature becomes important in patients with achlorhydria and those in whom gastric acid production is being suppressed with pharmacologic agents. Notable in this respect is the acid-buffering capacity of calcium carbonate. Because of this, it is recommended that patients take calcium carbonate supplements in divided doses of 1 g or less. In these cases, the calcium should be taken with food or citrus drinks to promote maximal absorption.

In cases of vitamin D deficiency or resistance, the metabolite of vitamin D chosen depends on the underlying disorder. If impaired renal 1α-hydroxylation is present, such as in renal failure, hypoparathyroidism (or PTH resistance), or the vitamin D–dependent rickets syndromes, metabolites that do not require this modification should be administered (calcitriol 0.25 to 1 μg/day or dihydrotachysterol 0.2 to 1 mg/day). If decreased intake or increased losses are the problem, vitamin D should be administered and the treatment directed at the underlying disorder. Initial repletion of stores can be undertaken with 50,000 IU of vitamin D daily for 2 to 3 weeks, followed by weekly or bimonthly administration until the underlying disorder has been treated. In patients with resistance to vitamin D, such as those on phenytoin, high doses (50,000 IU one to three times weekly) should be used as maintenance therapy. In other patients, once treatment of the underlying disorder and repletion of body stores have been addressed, two multivitamins (800 IU) should provide sufficient maintenance therapy. In cases of severe malabsorption, vitamin D can be administered parenterally.

Patients should be monitored closely to assess both response to therapy and to prevent therapeutic complications. Serum calcium should be monitored frequently (daily in profound hypocalcemia, weekly in moderate hypocalcemia) for the first month of therapy. Concomitant with resolution of hypocalcemia, one should observe a decline in the serum PTH level as the secondary hyperparathyroidism resolves. Measurement of serum PTH and assessment of 24-hour urinary calcium excretion should be performed within 2 to 4 weeks of institution of therapy. The urinary calcium measurement reflects the effect of therapy on the patient's ability to absorb calcium and the net uptake of calcium by bone. A low urine calcium concentration indicates poor adherence to a regimen, poor absorption of calcium, or increased uptake by bone. In addition, the urine calcium level provides important information on which to base therapeutic modifications to avoid nephrolithiasis.

Once normalization of serum and urinary calcium levels and a decrease in PTH levels are observed, a transition from aggressive replacement therapy to maintenance therapy should be undertaken to prevent hypercalcemia and nephrolithiasis. These same parameters should be monitored 1 and 3 months after a dose change to assess the effect of the therapeutic intervention. Monitoring of the alkaline phosphatase can also be performed at this time. Alkaline phosphatase levels may actually increase soon after starting treatment because of healing of the osteomalacic lesions; however, by 3 to 4 months after institution of therapy, a clear downward trend should be observed. Alkaline phosphatase and PTH values may remain elevated for 6 to 12 months after institution of therapy and should not be a cause for alarm, provided that they are declining and that the other parameters suggest that therapy is effective.

The treatment of hypoparathyroidism is similar to that of vitamin D deficiency with the exception that these patients have impaired renal 1α-hydroxylation of 25(OH)D and, therefore, require treatment with 1α-hydroxylated metabolites. PTH has been used experimentally for the treatment of hypoparathyroidism, with twice-daily injections providing a better result than once daily.[529] This therapy controls hypocalcemia with lower urine calcium excretion than with calcium and calcitriol therapy, but it is expensive and requires parenteral administration. Oral calcium and 1α-hydroxylated vitamin D metabolites, therefore, remain the mainstay of therapy. Monitoring of serum and urinary calcium should be performed as in the treatment of vitamin D deficiency. Therapy in these patients is lifelong; therefore, careful monitoring is required to avoid renal or hypercalcemic complications. The aim of therapy should be to maintain serum calcium in the low normal range without causing frank hypercalciuria to avoid nephrolithiasis and decrease in GFR. Because PTH plays an important role in renal calcium reabsorption, difficulties are often encountered in attaining these therapeutic goals. In such cases, renal calcium losses can be minimized by the addition of a thiazide diuretic to the treatment regimen. As noted earlier, in patients with PHP, the intact distal tubular reabsorption of calcium leads less often to hypercalciuria and allows more aggressive treatment aimed at normalizing PTH levels to protect bones from the hyperparathyroid bone disease sometimes seen in PHP.

One of the frustrations often encountered in treating patients with hypoparathyroidism is the fluctuating response to a seemingly stable therapeutic regimen. Episodes of hypercalcemia are occasionally observed without any discernible cause. Because of this, serum calcium should be monitored every 3 months to permit temporary withdrawal of 1,25(OH)$_2$D$_3$, should a hypercalcemic trend be observed. Fortunately the half-life of this metabolite is short, so that discontinuation for a few days to a week with resumption of a lower dose is usually efficacious. Though the therapeutic principles for treating hypoparathyroidism with calcium and 1,25(OH)$_2$D$_3$ appear straightforward, these patients frequently experience diminished renal function, episodes of hyper- and hypocalcemia, and nephrocalcinosis/nephrolithiasis.[530]

All patients receiving vitamin D metabolites and calcium need to be aware of potential therapeutic complications. Importantly, the mild symptoms of hypercalcemia should be emphasized to the patient. It is essential that these patients be aware that their calcium should be monitored more frequently during intercurrent illnesses that may affect the absorption of calcium or their hydration status, and upon introduction of drugs such as thiazides or loop diuretics that might change required dosing, to prevent the development of hypocalcemia or severe hypercalcemia.

DISORDERS OF PHOSPHATE METABOLISM

Hyperphosphatemia

Serum phosphate levels are controlled primarily by the rate of proximal renal tubular phosphate reabsorption, which is due, in turn, to the integrated activity of the major sodium-dependent cotransporters (NaPi-IIa and NaPi-IIc). The latter are strongly downregulated by parathyroid hormone and FGF23, both of which are stimulated by phosphate. Thus, absent extraordinary filtered loads of phosphate, the capacity of normal kidneys to excrete phosphate is not easily exceeded. Consequently, the occurrence of hyperphosphatemia usually signifies impaired renal functon, hypoparathyroidism, defective FGF23 action, a huge flux of phosphate into the extracellular fluid, or some combination of these factors (Table 28-7).

The most common cause of hyperphosphatemia is acute or chronic renal failure in which GFR is so reduced that the usual daily load of phosphate cannot be excreted at a normal level of serum phosphate, despite maximal inhibition of phosphate reabsorption in the remaining functional nephrons. In hypoparathyroidism (or PHP), serum phosphate may rise to levels as high as 6 to 8 mg/dL because of loss of the tonic inhibitory effect of PTH on phosphate reabsorption, although elevated FGF23 levels may prevent even further increases in serum phosphate.[531] The hyperphosphatemia of hypoparathyroidism is only partly due to the absence of PTH per se. Hypocalcemia may further impair phosphate clearance in this setting, and correction of hypocalcemia by treatment with vitamin D metabolites and oral calcium may reduce serum phosphate, for example, even though PTH levels remain low.[532]

Other circumstances in which renal tubular phosphate excretion is decreased, in the absence of renal failure, include acromegaly,[533] chronic therapy with heparin, and familial tumoral calcinosis.[534] Familial tumoral calcinosis can result from inactivating mutations in either FGF23 or the O-linked glycosyl transferase GalNAc-T3, which glycosylates FGF23 at its cleavage site targeted by furin-like proteases, thereby suppressing this cleavage.[247] In the absence of GalNAc-T3, FGF23 is cleaved at an accelerated rate.[265,535,536] The choice of FGF23 assay is important, therefore, for diagnosing tumoral calcinosis. The responsible FGF23 and GalNac-T3 mutations may render the molecule more susceptible to proteolyic degradation, such that the blood levels of (inactive) carboxyl fragments may be quite high in contrast to low levels of (bioactive) intact FGF23.[535] Affected patients may display focal hyperostosis; large, lobulated periarticular ectopic calcifications, especially around shoulders or hips; hyperphosphatemia due to increased renal tubular reabsorption of phosphate; increased serum 1,25(OH)$_2$D despite normal or low serum PTH; and increased intestinal calcium absorption, consistent with the elevated serum 1,25(OH)$_2$D concentration. The disorder may present in childhood or adulthood, is more common in blacks, and is lifelong, with a tendency for the tumoral calcifications to progress at affected sites. In contrast to the elevated serum 1,25(OH)$_2$D, hyperphosphatemia is not a constant feature of tumoral calcinosis, although it tends to be most severe in those with prominent calcifications. Despite their chronic hyperphosphatemia, secondary hyperparathyroidism does not develop in these patients, presumably because of the high 1,25(OH)$_2$D levels and intestinal hyperabsorption of calcium. Treatment is problematic, although some success has been reported with phosphate-binding antacids, calcium deprivation, calcitonin, and acetazolamide therapy.[537]

Hyperphosphatemia may result from overly rapid administration of therapeutic phosphate preparations or phosphate-rich drugs (fosphenytoin, liposomal amphotericin B), especially if renal function is compromised[538] or from rapid shifts of phosphate out of cells, most often provoked by mechanical injury or metabolic insult. Most cases of hyperphosphatemia associated with intestinal phosphate loads have involved children who received phosphate-containing laxatives or enemas or older adults with impaired renal function receiving phosphate-based cathartics in preparation for colonoscopy.[539] Hyperphosphatemia due to cytolytic release of intracellular phosphate can be quite dramatic, with serum phosphate concentrations up to or exceeding 20 mg/dL. This disorder was described initially as a complication of rapid induction chemotherapy for certain hematologic malignancies (tumor lysis syndrome), although it also may occur from cellular injury associated with trauma, hyperthermia, overwhelming infection, hemolysis, rhabdomyolysis, or metabolic acidosis.[540] Rarely, apparent hyperphosphatemia may reflect measurement artifact caused by paraproteins in myeloma.[541]

Most often, hyperphosphatemia is mild and asymptomatic, although chronic hyperphosphatemia is an important factor in the development of secondary hyperparathyroidism in progressive renal failure. The clinical manifestations of acute, severe hyperphosphatemia are related mainly to those of the accompanying hypocalcemia, caused by formation of insoluble calcium phosphate precipitates. Thus, tetany, muscle cramps, paresthesias, and seizures may occur, and they may be compounded by other metabolic disturbances (hyperkalemia, acidosis, hyperuricemia) that frequently coexist. Generalized precipitation of calcium phosphate into soft tissues may produce organ dysfunction, notably renal failure.[539]

TABLE 28-7

Causes of Hyperphosphatemia

Impaired Renal Phosphate Excretion

Renal insufficiency
Familial tumoral calcinosis
Endocrinopathies
   Acromegaly
   Hypoparathyroidism
   Pseudohypoparathyroidism
Heparin

Increased Extracellular Phosphate

Rapid Administration of Phosphate (Intravenous, Oral, Rectal)
Phosphate salts
Fosphenytoin
Liposomal amphotericin B

Rapid Cellular Catabolism or Lysis
Catabolic states
Tissue injury
   Hyperthermia
   Crush injuries
   Fulminant hepatitis
Cellular lysis
   Hemolytic anemia
   Rhabdomyolysis
   Tumor lysis syndrome

Transcellular Shifts of Phosphate
Metabolic acidosis
Respiratory acidosis

Therapeutic options for hyperphosphatemia are limited. Volume expansion may be helpful to improve GFR in acute syndromes. Identification and removal of any exogenous sources of phosphate are important, and phosphate-binding aluminum hydroxide antacids may be useful in limiting intestinal phosphate absorption and chelating phosphate secreted into the intestine. Hemodialysis is the most effective approach and should be considered early in severe hyperphosphatemia, especially in the tumor lysis syndrome and particularly if symptomatic hypocalcemia cannot be adequately treated for fear of inducing widespread soft tissue calcification.

Hypophosphatemia

Etiology

Hypophosphatemia may result from one or more of three general mechanisms (Table 28-8): increased urinary losses due to decreased net renal tubular phosphate reabsorption; rapid shifts of phosphate from extracellular fluid into the intracellular space or the mineral phase of bone; or rarely, severe and selective deprivation of dietary phosphate, as may occur with chronic ingestion of large amounts of nonabsorbable aluminum-containing antacids. Fasting or starvation does not lead directly to hypophosphatemia, apparently because phosphate is mobilized from catabolized bone and soft tissue in amounts sufficient to maintain serum phosphate, even during prolonged caloric deprivation.[542] Starvation does induce phosphate deficiency and, therefore, predisposes to subsequent hypophosphatemia upon refeeding.[543]

Chronic hypophosphatemia usually can be traced to ongoing renal phosphate wasting. Elevation of serum PTH for any reason (other than renal failure), as in primary hyperparathyroidism or secondary hyperparathyroidism due to vitamin D or calcium deficiency, results in inhibition of tubular phosphate reabsorption and fasting hypophosphatemia. Phosphate clearance also is increased in PTHrP-associated hypercalcemia of malignancy, although when such patients develop severe hypercalcemia, hypophosphatemia may be masked initially by underlying volume depletion and compromised GFR. Therapy with the tyrosine kinase inhibitors imatinib and nilotinib appears to cause hypophosphatemia, at least in part, by inhibiting both osteoblast and osteoclast formation, lowering serum calcium and stimulating secondary hyperparathyroidism.[544-546] When PTH secretion is compromised by severe hypomagnesemia, rapid intravenous administration of magnesium alone, without concurrent attention to coexisting hypocalcemia, can provoke massive phosphaturia and hypophosphatemia in patients with underlying phosphate depletion.

The discovery that gain-of-function mutations in FGF23 cause autosomal dominant hypophosphatemic rickets (ADHR) inaugurated a new era in understanding of phosphate homeostasis.[547-549] Elevated FGF23 also occurs in autosomal recessive hypophosphatemia (ARHP), which is caused by mutations in the genes encoding dentin matrix protein-1 (DMP1) and FAM20C. DMP1 is expressed in osteocytes and presumably regulates local production of FGF23.[550] FAM20C is a secreted kinase that phosphorylates FGF23 near the furin cleavage site; this phosphorylation is required for inactivating cleavage by a furin-like protease. Immunoassays for FGF23[551] have pointed to elevated circulating FGF23 as at least one "phosphatonin" responsible for reduction of phosphate reabsorption and serum 1,25(OH)$_2$D levels in the more common disorder, X-linked hypophosphatemic rickets (XLH), in the rare but distinctive TIO and epidermal nevus syndromes, and in the

TABLE 28-8

Causes of Hypophosphatemia

Reduced Renal Tubular Phosphate Reabsorption

Excess PTH or PTHrP
Primary hyperparathyroidism
PTHrP-dependent hypercalcemia of malignancy
Secondary hyperparathyroidism
    Vitamin D deficiency/resistance
    Calcium starvation or malabsorption
    Imatinib
    Rapid, selective correction of severe hypomagnesemia

Excess FGF23 or Other "Phosphatonins"
Familial hypophosphatemic rickets (XLH)
Autosomal dominant hypophosphatemic rickets (ADHR)
Autosomal recessive hypophosphatemia (ARHP)
Tumor-induced osteomalacia syndrome (TIO)
McCune-Albright syndrome (fibrous dysplasia)
Epidermal nevus syndrome
Following renal or hepatic transplantation
Idiopathic hypercalciuria

Intrinsic Renal Disease
Fanconi syndrome(s), other renal tubular disorders

Cystinosis	Wilson disease
Amyloidosis	Multiple myeloma
Hemolytic uremic syndrome	Heavy metal toxicity
Magnesium deficiency	Rewarming or hyperthermia

NaPi-IIa mutations
NaPi-II2c mutations (HHRH)

Other
Poorly controlled diabetes, alcoholism
Hyperaldosteronism
Folowing partial hepatectomy
Following renal transplantation
Drugs or toxins

Ethanol	High-dose estrogens
Acetazolamide, other diuretics	Ifosfamide
High-dose glucocorticoids	Cisplatin
Bicarbonate	Suramin
Toluene	Foscarnet
Heavy metals (Pb, Cd)	*N*-methylformamide
Calcitonin	Bisphosphonates
Tenofovir	Paraquat

Shifts of Extracellular Phosphate into Cells or Bone

Acute Intracellular Shifts
Intravenous glucose, fructose, glycerol
Insulin therapy for hyperglycemia, diabetic ketoacidosis
Catecholamines (epinephrine, albuterol, terbutaline, dopamine)
Thyrotoxic periodic paralysis
Acute respiratory alkalosis, salicylate intoxication, acute gout
Gram-negative sepsis, toxic shock syndrome
Recovery from acidosis, starvation, anorexia nervosa, hepatic failure
Rapid cellular proliferation
    Leukemic blast crisis
    Intensive erythropoietin, G-CSF therapy

Accelerated Net Bone Formation
Following parathyroidectomy
Osteoblastic metastases
Treatment of vitamin D deficiency
Antiresorptive therapy of severe Paget disease

Impaired Intestinal Phosphate Absorption

Aluminum-containing antacids

FGF23, fibroblast growth factor 23; G-CSF, granulocyte colony-stimulating factor; HHRH, hereditary hypophosphatemic rickets with hypercalciuria; PTH, parathyroid hormone; PTHrP, parathyroid hormone–related hormone.

approximately 50% of patients with McCune-Albright syndrome (fibrous dysplasia of bone) who manifest hypophosphatemia.[547-549,552-554] These disorders share a common biochemical phenotype, which may include a more generalized proximal tubular dysfunction, with modest proteinuria and aminoaciduria. Serum calcium usually is normal or low-normal, urinary calcium often is low, PTH is normal or only slightly elevated, and $1,25(OH)_2D$ is inappropriately normal. The clinical picture is dominated by weakness, bone pain, and other features attributable to the associated rickets or osteomalacia (see Chapter 29). Increased FGF23 also may play a role in impaired phosphate reabsorption seen in the 20% or so of patients with calcium kidney stones and idiopathic hypercalciuria who exhibit fasting hypophosphatemia,[555] although a few such patients may harbor mutations in the NaPi-IIa sodium phosphate cotransporter.[556]

Renal phosphate clearance may be impaired in the context of a more generalized renal tubular disorder such as Fanconi syndrome(s) or others associated with systemic diseases such as amyloidosis, Wilson disease, or cystinosis (see Table 28-8). In addition to NaPi-IIa mutations, inactivating mutations in the NaPi-IIc cotransporter, also expressed in the proximal tubule and known to be regulated by both PTH and FGF23, have been shown to account for the rare disorder, known as hereditary hypophosphatemic rickets with hypercalciuria, in which primary renal tubular phosphate wasting causes appropriate elevation of serum $1,25(OH)_2D$ and resulting hypercalciuria.[557,558] Other causes of impaired renal tubular phosphate reabsorption include the osmotic diuresis associated with poorly controlled diabetes, alcoholism, hyperaldosteronism, and exposure to any of a wide variety of drugs or toxins (see Table 28-8). The pathogenesis of phosphate wasting that often follows partial hepatectomy or renal transplantation remains unclear, but humoral mechanisms seem to be involved.[559,560]

Rapid egress of extracellular phosphate into cells is the cause of hypophosphatemia that develops acutely during administration of intravenous glucose, insulin therapy for hyperglycemia, administration of catecholamines (pressors or bronchodilators), thyrotoxic periodic paralysis, profound respiratory alkalosis, refeeding syndrome in the wake of severe acidosis or starvation, recovery from acute hepatic failure (in which hypophosphatemia is a recognized favorable prognostic factor[561]), or other circumstances involving rapid cellular proliferation such as leukemic blast crisis or responsiveness to hematopoietic growth factors. Hypophosphatemia in these situations is most pronounced when there is underlying phosphate depletion, as in hyperparathyroidism or vitamin D deficiency, or following prolonged malnutrition, alcoholism, or glycosuria. Accelerated uptake of phosphate into cells is particularly common in postsurgical, burn, or trauma patients, in whom it may be promoted by high levels of circulating catecholamines and exacerbated by concurrent respiratory alkalosis, fever, volume expansion, sepsis, and hypokalemia. Situations of greatly accelerated net bone formation, such as hungry bone syndrome occurring immediately following parathyroidectomy for primary or tertiary hyperparathyroidism, during initial treatment of severe vitamin D deficiency or Paget disease, or in occasional patients with extensive osteoblastic bone metastases, may manifest hypophosphatemia as well as hypocalcemia.

Clinical Features

The clinical significance of hypophosphatemia depends on the presence and severity of underlying phosphate depletion. Unfortunately, the status of the total-body phosphorus pool, and more particularly the critical intracellular pool, is reflected only indirectly by the concentration of phosphate in the extracellular fluid, which contains less than 0.5% of body phosphorus. Thus, although serum phosphate concentrations generally are used to characterize hypophosphatemia as severe (<1-1.5 mg/dL, or <0.3-0.5 mmol/L), moderate (1.5-2.2 mg/dL, 0.5-0.7 mmol/L), or mild (2.2-3.0 mg/dL, 0.75-1.0 mmol/L), serum phosphate may be normal or even high (depending on renal function) in the presence of profound intracellular phosphate deficiency. Conversely, it may be low when intracellular phosphate is relatively normal, such as following a sudden movement of extracellular phosphate into cells.

The prevalence of severe hypophosphatemia among hospitalized patients overall is less than 1%, whereas mild or moderate hypophosphatemia may be detected in 2% to 5%.[562] Hypophosphatemia is recognized most often in critically ill patients, alcoholics or other malnourished individuals, decompensated diabetics, and those with acute infectious or pulmonary disorders.[562]

The clinical manifestations of severe hypophosphatemia are protean. Among the most common are various neuromuscular symptoms, ranging from progressive lethargy, muscle weakness, and paresthesias to paralysis, coma, and even death, depending on the severity of the phosphate depletion. Confusion, profound weakness, paralysis, seizures, and other major sequelae generally are limited to those with serum phosphate concentrations below 0.8 to 1.0 mg/dL.[563] Biochemical evidence of muscle injury is observed within 1 to 2 days in over one third of patients whose serum phosphate concentrations fall to less than 2 mg/dL.[564] Overt rhabdomyolysis also may occur, especially in the setting of chronic alcoholism with underlying malnutrition and phosphate depletion.[565,566] However, by the time this is recognized the serum phosphate often has been raised by the large amounts of cellular phosphate released from damaged muscle. Reversible respiratory failure due to respiratory muscle weakness may preclude successful weaning from ventilatory support.[567,568] Left ventricular dysfunction, heart failure, and ventricular arrhythmias may result from profound hypophosphatemia but may not be significant if serum phosphate is greater than 1.5 mg/dL.[569] Correction of moderate hypophosphatemia (<2 mg/dL) in patients with septic shock led to a significant increase in blood pressure as well as left ventricular function and arterial pH.[569] Hematologic sequelae of severe hypophosphatemia include hemolysis, platelet dysfunction with bleeding, and impaired leukocyte function (phagocytosis and killing).[570] Erythrocytes demonstrate increased fragility; altered membrane composition, rigidity, and microspherocytosis; and reduced levels of ATP and 2,3-diphosphoglycerate (2,3-DPG).[570] The reduction in erythrocyte 2,3-DPG impairs oxyhemoglobin dissociation and thereby may reduce oxygen delivery to tissues. This problem, together with accelerated hemolysis, may provoke a substantial increase in cardiac output. The blockade in cellular glycolysis becomes demonstrable at levels of serum phosphate between 1 and 2 mg/dL.[571] Glucose intolerance and insulin resistance also have been demonstrable in these patients.[572]

Treatment

Hypophosphatemia appears most often in acutely or critically ill individuals. Accordingly, it often is difficult to discern whether hypophosphatemia is responsible for features of the multiple organ dysfunction commonly encountered in this population. For example, although depression of intracellular high-energy organophosphates has been demonstrated during treatment of diabetic keto-acidosis and phosphate repletion leads to more rapid recovery of erythrocyte 2,3-DPG concentrations, opinion is divided as to whether phosphate therapy in this setting hastens recovery, prevents complications, or reduces mortality rate.[573,574] Nevertheless, because severe hypophosphatemia has been associated, in a variety of clinical settings, with serious neuromuscular, cardiovascular, and hematologic dysfunction that is at least partially reversible with phosphate repletion, most now agree that one should adopt a relatively low threshold for treatment.[569]

The decision to correct hypophosphatemia urgently should be guided by the estimated severity of the cellular phosphate deficit, the presence of signs or symptoms suggestive of phosphate depletion, and the overall clinical status of the patient. The presence of renal insufficiency (a risk for iatrogenic hyperphosphatemia), concomitant administration of intravenous glucose (alone or as a component of hyperalimentation solutions), and the potential for aggravating coexistent hypocalcemia also should be considered.

Limited data are available from clinical trials to predict the appropriate dose and rate of phosphate administration. In patients without severe renal insufficiency or hypocalcemia, administration of intravenous phosphate at rates of 2 to 8 mmol/hour of elemental phosphorus over 4 to 8 hours frequently corrects hypophosphatemia without provoking hyperphosphatemia or hypocalcemia.[562,575-577] Suggested guidelines based on serum phosphate are shown in Table 28-9. It is essential that serum calcium and phosphate be monitored every 6 to 12 hours during and after phosphate therapy, both to detect untoward consequences and because many patients require additional infusions for recurrent hypophosphatemia within 24 to 48 hours of apparently successful repletion.[576] Less acute or severe hypophosphatemia should be managed with oral (or enteral) phosphate supplements if possible, generally given as a total of 1.0 to 2.0 g/day (as elemental phosphate) of neutral sodium or potassium phosphate in divided doses three to four times a day (see Table 28-6). In many patients, however, oral phosphate therapy is limited by gastrointestinal symptoms such as nausea or diarrhea.

DISORDERS OF MAGNESIUM METABOLISM

The fourth most abundant extracellular cation, magnesium, like calcium, plays a critical physiologic role, particularly in neuromuscular function but also as a component of the mineral phase of bone. Intracellular magnesium is crucial for normal energy metabolism, as a cofactor for ATP and numerous enzymes and transporters, which is reflected in the rather global clinical effects that accompany disorders of magnesium homeostasis. Hypomagnesemia and hypermagnesemia are among the most common electrolyte disturbances; one or the other of these abnormalities is observed in as many as 20% of hospitalized patients and even more frequently (i.e., 30-40%) among those admitted to intensive care units.[578]

Hypermagnesemia

Magnesium homeostasis is achieved mainly through highly efficient regulation of tubular magnesium reabsorption in the loop of Henle.[1] Because normal kidneys can readily excrete even large amounts of magnesium (i.e., 500 mEq/day), high filtered loads of magnesium rarely cause hypermagnesemia except in patients with significant renal insufficiency.[579] Increased magnesium loads in such cases may arise from ingestion of large amounts of oral magnesium salts, typically given as cathartics or antacids, or from extensive soft tissue ischemia or necrosis in patients with trauma, sepsis, cardiopulmonary arrest, burns, or shock[579] (Table 28-10). Hypermagnesemia may result from parenteral administration of magnesium salts, such as when magnesium is used to treat preeclampsia or as a tocolytic.[580] The infants of such hypermagnesemic mothers may manifest transient hypermagnesemia as well, along with parathyroid suppression and neurobehavioral symptoms.[581,582] The use of oral magnesium preparations as laxatives may lead to hypermagnesemia if absorption is increased by intestinal ileus, obstruction, or perforation.[583]

The most prominent clinical manifestations of hypermagnesemia are vasodilatation and neuromuscular blockade, which may involve both pre- and postsynaptic

---

TABLE 28-9

Urgent Therapy of Hypophosphatemia*

Factors to Consider

Severity of hypophosphatemia
Likelihood of underlying phosphate depletion
Clinical condition of the patient
Renal function
Serum calcium
Concurrent parenteral therapy (glucose, hyperalimentation)

Guidelines

Serum PO$_4$ (mg/dL)	Rate of Infusion (mmol/hr)	Duration (hr)	Total PO$_4$ (mmol)
<2.5	2.0	6	12
<1.5	4.0	6	24
<1.0	8.0	6	48

*Rates shown are normalized for a 70-kg person. Most formulations available in the United States provide 3 mmol/mL of sodium or potassium phosphate.
PO$_4$, phosphate.

TABLE 28-10

Causes of Hypermagnesemia

Excessive Magnesium Intake

Cathartics, antacids, enemas
Dead Sea drowning
Parenteral magnesium administration
Magnesium-rich urologic irrigants
Intestinal obstruction or perforation following magnesium ingestion

Rapid Mobilization from Soft Tissues

Trauma
Shock, sepsis
Cardiac arrest
Burns

Impaired Magnesium Excretion

Renal failure
Familial hypocalciuric hypercalcemia

Other

Adrenal insufficiency
Hypothyroidism
Hypothermia

inhibition of neuromuscular transmission.[584] Signs and symptoms generally do not appear unless the serum magnesium exceeds 4 mEq/L.[579] Hypotension, often refractory to pressors and volume expansion, may be one of the earliest signs of progressive hypermagnesemia.[584,585] Lethargy, nausea, and weakness, accompanied by reduction or loss of deep tendon reflexes, may progress to stupor or coma with respiratory insufficiency or quadriparesis at serum concentrations in excess of 8 to 10 mEq/L. Gastrointestinal hypomotility or ileus is common. Facial flushing and pupillary dilatation may be observed. Hypotension may be complicated by a paradoxical relative bradycardia, and other cardiac effects may be evident, including prolongation of the PR, QRS, and QTc intervals, appearance of heart block, and ultimately, asystole as serum concentrations approach 20 mEq/L.

Hypermagnesemia activates CaSRs in the parathyroids, thereby suppressing PTH secretion,[586] and in the renal distal tubules, thereby reducing tubular calcium and magnesium reabsorption. Severe hypocalcemia opposes the effect of hypermagnesemia on PTH secretion, so that serum PTH may remain within the normal range but still inappropriate for the level of serum calcium.[587]

Successful treatment of hypermagnesemia requires identification and interruption of the source of magnesium, together with measures to increase clearance of magnesium from the extracellular fluid. Use of magnesium-free cathartics or enemas to accelerate clearance of ingested magnesium from the gastrointestinal tract, together with vigorous intravenous hydration, generally have been successful in reversing hypermagnesemia. Refractory cases, especially those with advanced renal insufficiency, may require hemodialysis. Intravenous calcium (100-200 mg) infusions have been advocated as an effective antidote to hypermagnesemia, and there are examples in which this approach has apparently been successful, at least temporarily.[579,584,588]

Hypomagnesemia

Hypomagnesemia may occur because of impaired intestinal magnesium absorption or, more commonly, because of excessive gastrointestinal losses due to diarrhea, preprocedural bowel preparation, or prolonged drainage. Most often, hypomagnesemia reflects defective renal tubular reabsorption of magnesium, although rapid shifts into cells, other extrarenal losses, or incorporation into new bone may occur (Table 28-11). Because only 1% of the body's magnesium content is present in extracellular fluid, measurements of serum total or ionized magnesium concentration may not adequately reflect total-body magnesium or the magnesium status of the intracellular compartment in critical tissues such as muscle.[589] Thus, patients with deficiency of tissue magnesium may fail to manifest overt hypomagnesemia[590] but may exhibit abnormal retention (i.e., >50% in 24 hours) of infused magnesium, a maneuver that may be employed to assess magnesium status.[591]

Etiology

Intestinal Causes of Hypomagnesemia. Selective dietary magnesium deficiency does not occur, and it is remarkably difficult, in fact, to induce magnesium depletion experimentally by feeding magnesium-deficient diets, probably because renal magnesium conservation is so efficient. Large amounts of magnesium may be lost in chronic diarrheal states (this fluid may contain more than 10 mEq/L of magnesium) or via intestinal fistulas or prolonged gastrointestinal drainage.[592] More commonly, magnesium becomes

TABLE 28-11

Causes of Hypomagnesemia

Impaired Intestinal Magnesium Absorption

Hypomagnesemia with secondary hypocalcemia
Malabsorption syndromes

Increased Intestinal Magnesium Losses

Protracted vomiting or diarrhea
Bowel preparation (procedures, surgery)
Intestinal drainage or fistulas

Impaired Renal Tubular Magnesium Reabsorption

Genetic Magnesium-Wasting Syndromes
Bartter syndrome(s)
Familial hypomagnesemia with hypercalciuria and nephrocalcinosis
Autosomal dominant hypocalcemia
Gitelman syndrome
Isolated renal magnesium wasting
Hypomagnesmia with hypertension and hypercholesterolemia
Hypomagnesemia with secondary hypocalcemia

Acquired Renal Disease
Tubulointerstitial disease
Postobstruction, acute tubular necrosis (diuretic phase)
Renal transplantation

Drugs and Toxins
Ethanol
Digoxin
Diuretics (loop, thiazide, osmotic)
cis-Platinum
Cyclosporine
Tacrolimus
Cetuximab
Interleukin 2
Pentamidine
Aminoglycosides
Foscarnet
Amphotericin B

Endocrine and Metabolic Abnormalities
Extracellular fluid volume expansion
Hyperaldosteronism (primary, secondary)
Inappropriate antidiuretic hormone secretion
Diabetes mellitus
Hypercalcemia
Phosphate depletion
Metabolic acidosis
Hyperthyroidism

Other
Hypothermia
Sézary syndrome
Acute brain injury
Hydrogen fluoride burns

Rapid Shifts of Magnesium Out of Extracellular Fluid

Intracellular Redistribution
Recovery from diabetic ketoacidosis
Refeeding syndrome
Correction of respiratory acidosis
Catecholamines
Thyrotoxic periodic paralysis

Accelerated Net Bone Formation
Following parathyroidectomy
Osteoblastic metastases
Treatment of vitamin D deficiency
Calcitonin therapy

Other Losses
Pancreatitis
Blood transfusions
Extensive burns
Excessive sweating
Pregnancy (third trimester) and lactation

trapped within fatty acid soaps in disorders associated with chronic malabsorption.[593] Investigation of a rare autosomal recessive disorder, hypomagnesmia with secondary hypocalcemia (HSH) led to the identification of the transient receptor potential channel protein TRPM6, in the form of a hetero-oligomer with the closely related channel protein TRPM7, as a key molecular mediator of intestinal (and renal tubular) transepithelial magnesium transport.[594]

Renal Causes of Hypomagnesemia. Roughly 60% of renal magnesium reabsorption occurs in the thick ascending limb of Henle's loop, and another 5% to 10% is reabsorbed in the distal tubules.[1] Investigation of the pathogenesis of several genetic disorders associated with renal magnesium wasting have identified key pathways of magnesium reabsorption at these sites (see Table 28-11). Thus, in familial hypomagnesemia with hypercalciuria and nephrocalcinosis, loss-of-function mutations in the claudin 16 gene encoding the paracellin-1 protein (or in the related gene claudin 19), a component of the tight junctions between adjacent epithelial cells, selectively impair paracellular magnesium (and calcium) reabsorption in response to the (lumen-positive) transepithelial voltage gradient.[49,595]

In Bartter syndrome(s), inactivating mutations in any of several transporters involved in sodium chloride reabsorption in the ascending limb cause salt wasting, compromise the voltage gradient, and similarly impair paracellular magnesium and calcium reabsorption.[596-598] In autosomal dominant hypocalcemia, mutations causing increased sensitivity of CaSRs to cationic agonists cause hypomagnesemia, as well as hypocalcemia, through inappropriate CaSR-dependent suppression of PTH secretion and of renal tubular cation reabsorption.[599]

In Gitelman syndrome, inactivating mutations in the luminal thiazide-sensitive NaCl cotransporter (NCC) expressed in the distal convoluted tubules lead to sodium chloride and magnesium wasting, in this case with hypocalciuria.[596-598,600] The manner whereby impaired NCC activity compromises (transcellular) magnesium reabsorption in this segment is unclear, although NCC-knockout mice (or normal mice treated with thiazides) display reduced distal tubular expression of the TRPM6 channel protein required for normal magnesium transport across the apical membrane.[399]

Mutations in the FXYD2 γ-subunit of the distal tubular basolateral Na+/K+-ATPase similarly impair salt and magnesium reabsorption at that site and account for some, but not all, cases of isolated renal magnesium wasting.[601,602] An autosomal recessive form of renal hypomagnesemia is caused by inactivating mutations in the EGF gene, which likely also explains why hypomagnesemia may complicate use of cetuximab, a monoclonal antibody directed against the EGF receptor.[603] Another genetic syndrome featuring renal magnesium wasting and hypocalciuria (as in Gitelman syndrome), and thus presumably involving a defect in distal tubular function as well, in association with hypertension and hypercholesterolemia, is linked to a mutation in mitochondrial tRNA DNA.[604] Other rare genetic causes of distal tubular magnesium wasting involve mutations in K channels (Kv1.1 or Kir4.1) that disrupt voltage gradients needed for efficient magnesium reabsorption.[605]

Most often, renal magnesium wasting is attributable to an acquired abnormality in tubular magnesium reabsorption. In normal subjects, magnesium reabsorption is virtually complete within several days of instituting experimental dietary magnesium deficiency, even before serum magnesium has declined substantially.[606] Thus, the finding of more than 1 mEq/day of urinary magnesium in a frankly hypomagnesemic patient indicates a defect in renal tubular

magnesium reabsorption. The causes of acquired primary tubular magnesium wasting include various tubulointerstitial disorders, recovery from acute tubular necrosis or obstruction, renal transplantation, various endocrinopathies, alcoholism, and exposure to certain drugs (see Table 28-11).

Hypomagnesemia or magnesium depletion due to subnormal renal reabsorption may complicate a variety of endocrinopathies, including hyperaldosteronism, hyperthyroidism, and disorders associated with hypercalcemia, hypercalciuria, or phosphate depletion.[591] In primary hyperparathyroidism, PTH stimulates increased tubular magnesium reabsorption, but this action is opposed by a direct tubular effect of hypercalcemia. As a result, serum magnesium in primary hyperparathyroidism generally is normal or only slightly reduced.[607] In hypoparathyroidism, serum and urinary magnesium are low. The magnesium depletion in hypoparathyroidism is consistent with loss of both the magnesium-retaining renal action of PTH and the stimulatory effect of 1,25(OH)$_2$D on intestinal magnesium absorption.[608]

Diabetes is among the most common disorders associated with hypomagnesemia.[609,610] The severity of the hypomagnesemia in diabetics correlates with indices of glycosuria and poor glycemic control,[611] suggesting that urinary losses of magnesium on the basis of glycosuria may partly explain the magnesium depletion. Rapid correction of hyperglycemia with insulin therapy causes magnesium to enter cells and may further lower the extracellular magnesium concentration during treatment.

Alcoholism is another very common clinical setting in which hypomagnesemia occurs. Magnesium depletion in alcoholism may result in part from nutritional deficiency of magnesium, overall caloric starvation and ketosis, and gastrointestinal losses due to vomiting or diarrhea, but an acute magnesuric effect of alcohol ingestion likely plays the major role.[612] This effect of alcohol is most evident during the rising limb of the blood ethanol curve and may be related to transient suppression of PTH secretion.[612] Other factors that may contribute to hypomagnesemia in alcoholism include pancreatitis, malabsorption, secondary hyperaldosteronism, respiratory alkalosis, and elevated plasma catecholamines, which increase intracellular sequestration of magnesium.[591]

A number of drugs have been identified as causes of defective renal tubular magnesium reabsorption and hypomagnesemia.[591] These drugs include diuretics (especially loop diuretics), digoxin, cisplatin, cetuximab, pentamidine, cyclosporine, tacrolimus, interleukin 2, aminoglycosides, foscarnet, and amphotericin B. Most often, drug-induced hypomagnesemia is mild and reversible, particularly when it is associated with diuretic therapy. In over half of patients treated with cisplatin, hypomagnesemia occurs within days or weeks, and roughly half of those who develop it exhibit persistent hypomagnesemia many months or even years later. The median duration of hypomagnesemia in cisplatin-treated patients is about 2 months, but recovery has been observed for up to 2 years after treatment.[613] Cisplatin may induce a more global nephropathy and azotemic renal failure, but the magnesium wasting appears to be an isolated functional abnormality.

Other Causes of Hypomagnesemia. Magnesium, like phosphate, is a major intracellular ion, and significant shifts of magnesium from the extracellular compartment therefore may occur during recovery from chronic respiratory acidosis or acute ketoacidosis, after refeeding, following administration of hyperalimentation solutions, and in response to elevations of circulating catecholamines.[591] Other rapid losses of extracellular magnesium may occur during periods of greatly accelerated net bone formation (after parathy-roidectomy, during recovery from vitamin D deficiency, with osteoblastic metastases) or with large losses due to pancreatitis, cardiopulmonary bypass surgery,[614] massive transfusion,[615] extensive burns, excessive sweating, preg-nancy, or lactation.

Consequences of Hypomagnesemia

Most of the signs and symptoms of hypomagnesemia reflect alterations in neuromuscular function: tetany, hyperreflexia, positive Chvostek and Trousseau signs, tremors, fasciculations, seizures, ataxia, nystagmus, vertigo, choreoathetosis, muscle weakness, apathy, depression, irri-tability, delirium, and psychosis.[591] Patients usually are not symptomatic unless serum magnesium falls below 1 mEq/L, although occurrence of symptoms, like intracellular mag-nesium, may not correlate well with serum magnesium. Atrial or ventricular arrhythmias may occur, as may various electrocardiographic abnormalities—prolonged PR or QT intervals, T-wave flattening or inversion, or ST-segment straightening.[591] Hypomagnesemia also increases myocar-dial sensitivity to digitalis intoxication.[616]

Hypomagnesemia evokes important alterations in mineral ion and potassium homeostasis that frequently aggravate the clinical syndrome. Magnesium-deprived humans or animals develop hypocalcemia, hypocalciuria, hypokalemia (due to impaired tubular reabsorption of potassium), and positive calcium and sodium balance.[606,617] Sustained correction of hypocalcemia or hypokalemia cannot be achieved by administration of calcium or potas-sium alone, respectively, whereas both abnormalities respond to administration of magnesium.[593,618]

The mechanism of hypocalcemia in this setting may be multifactorial. Inappropriately normal or low serum PTH, despite hypocalcemia, is common and indicates a defect in PTH secretion,[619] which is due to augmented signaling by CaSR-associated G proteins, normally inhibited by magne-sium, within the parathroid cell.[620] Other evidence indi-cates that hypomagnesemia also may impair PTH action on target cells in bone and kidney, although some have observed normal responsiveness and the issue remains controversial.[448,449,618,619,621]

Vitamin D resistance also is a feature of hypomagnese-mic states.[622,623] This disorder appears to be due mainly to impaired renal 1α-hydroxylation of 25(OH)D, although tissue resistance to 1,25(OH)$_2$D also may play a role.[608,624] The serum 1,25(OH)$_2$D concentration usually is low during hypomagnesemia, which may result from magnesium depletion per se, parathyroid insufficiency, or coexistent vitamin D deficiency.[625-627] Deficiency of 1,25(OH)$_2$D prob-ably is not the main cause of hypocalcemia in these patients, however, because hypocalcemia can be rapidly corrected (within hours to days) by magnesium therapy alone, well in advance of any increase in the serum 1,25(OH)$_2$D concentration.[625,626]

Therapy of Hypomagnesemia

Patients with mild, asymptomatic hypomagnesemia may be treated with oral magnesium salts (i.e., MgCl$_2$, MgO, Mg[OH]$_2$), usually given in divided doses totaling 40 to 60 mEq (480-720 mg) per day (see Table 28-6). Diarrhea sometimes occurs with larger doses but generally is not a problem. The gluconate form (54 mg magnesium per gram) is said to cause less diarrhea.[591] Patients with malabsorption or ongoing urinary magnesium losses may require chronic oral therapy to avoid recurrent magnesium depletion. Although intestinal magnesium absorption is severely

impaired in renal failure,[628] oral magnesium must be administered with great caution in this setting, especially in patients receiving concomitant therapy with 1,25(OH)$_2$D.

Symptomatic or severe (<1 mEq/L) hypomagnesemia, especially if complicated by hypocalcemia, usually signifies magnesium deficits of at least 1 to 2 mEq/kg and is best treated promptly with parenteral magnesium salts. The use of intramuscular MgSO$_4$ is to be discouraged, as the injec-tions are painful and provide relatively little magnesium (2 mL of 50% MgSO$_4$ supplies only 8 mEq of magnesium, compared with typical magnesium deficits in excess of 100 mEq). Moreover, because unretained sulfate ions also may increase urinary calcium excretion, intravenous mag-nesium chloride or gluconate probably is the most logical approach to initial parenteral therapy for patients who also may be hypocalcemic. In adult hypomagnesemic patients with normal renal function, rates of infusion of 2-4 mEq/hour (i.e., 50-100 mEq/day) generally are needed to main-tain serum magnesium in the range of 2 to 3 mEq/L.[587,619,623] Up to 100 mEq/day for 2 days can be safely administered without elevating serum magnesium above 4 mEq/L, whereas doses of 200 mEq/day may increase serum mag-nesium to 4.5 to 5.5 mEq/L and thus are excessive.[629] In patients with active seizures or other urgent indications, the infusion may be preceded by a slowly administered bolus of 10 to 20 mEq, followed by a higher rate of infusion (i.e., 10-15 mEq/hour) for the first 1 to 2 hours only. Patients with normal renal function can readily excrete over 400 mEq/day of magnesium in the urine without becoming hypermagnesemic, but even mild renal failure may greatly limit magnesium excretion. Therefore, doses of magnesium supplements should be reduced twofold to threefold and careful serial monitoring of serum magne-sium performed in patients with compromised renal function.

It is important to appreciate that a large fraction of parenterally administered magnesium may be excreted in the urine, even in patients with profound magnesium defi-ciency. Many such patients will excrete as much as 50% to 75% of infused magnesium, whereas in normal subjects this approaches 100%.[593] Moreover, because equilibration of the intracellular and extracellular magnesium pools is relatively slow, it is generally necessary to continue mag-nesium therapy for 3 to 5 days to achieve adequate reple-tion of the typical 1- to 2-mEq/kg deficit. Because serum magnesium may become normal well before tissue stores are repleted, monitoring of urinary magnesium excretion is a more reliable measure of the approach to full repletion, especially after patients are switched to oral therapy.

The need for calcium, potassium, and phosphate supple-mentation should be considered in the usual clinical setting of hypomagnesemia. Vitamin D deficiency also fre-quently coexists and should be treated with oral or paren-teral vitamin D or 25(OH)D. Use of 1,25(OH)$_2$D is not necessary, does not hasten recovery, and may actually worsen hypomagnesemia by suppressing PTH secretion and thereby promoting renal magnesium excretion.[630] Initial parenteral magnesium therapy in hypocalcemic patients may produce dramatic hypophosphatemia via the rapid stimulation of PTH secretion. This is most likely to be problematic in those with underlying phosphate deple-tion (malabsorption, alcoholism, diabetes), in whom it may provoke acute neuromuscular dysfunction, and it may be avoided by concomitant intravenous calcium therapy.

REFERENCES

1. de Rouffignac C, Quamme G. Renal magnesium handling and its hormonal control. *Physiol Rev.* 1994;74(2):305-322.

2. Murshed M, Harmey D, Millan JL, et al. Unique coexpression in osteoblasts of broadly expressed genes accounts for the spatial restriction of ECM mineralization to bone. *Genes Dev.* 2005;19(9):1093-1104.
3. Guerreiro PM, Renfro JL, Power DM, Canario AV. The parathyroid hormone family of peptides: structure, tissue distribution, regulation, and potential functional roles in calcium and phosphate balance in fish. *Am J Physiol Regul Integr Comp Physiol.* 2007;292(2):R679-R696.
4. Pinheiro PL, Cardoso JC, Gomes AS, et al. Gene structure, transcripts and calciotropic effects of the PTH family of peptides in *Xenopus* and chicken. *BMC Evol Biol.* 2010;10:373.
5. Arnold A, Horst SA, Gardella TJ, et al. Mutation of the signal peptide-encoding region of the preproparathyroid hormone gene in familial isolated hypoparathyroidism. *J Clin Invest.* 1990;86(4):1084-1087.
6. Sunthornthepvarakul T, Churesigaew S, Ngowngarmratana S. A novel mutation of the signal peptide of the preproparathyroid hormone gene associated with autosomal recessive familial isolated hypoparathyroidism. *J Clin Endocrinol Metab.* 1999;84(10):3792-3796.
7. Wiren KM, Potts JT Jr, Kronenberg HM. Importance of the propeptide sequence of human preproparathyroid hormone for signal sequence function. *J Biol Chem.* 1988;263(36):19771-19777.
8. Divieti P, John MR, Juppner H, Bringhurst FR. Human PTH-(7-84) inhibits bone resorption in vitro via actions independent of the type 1 PTH/PTHrP receptor. *Endocrinology.* 2002;143(1):171-176.
9. D'Amour P, Rakel A, Brossard JH, et al. Acute regulation of circulating parathyroid hormone (PTH) molecular forms by calcium: utility of PTH fragments/PTH(1-84) ratios derived from three generations of PTH assays. *J Clin Endocrinol Metab.* 2006;91(1):283-289.
10. Parfitt AM. Calcium homeostasis. In: Mundy GR, Martin TJ, eds. *Physiology and Pharmacology of Bone.* Berlin: Springer-Verlag; 1993:1-65.
11. Brown EM. Role of the calcium-sensing receptor in extracellular calcium homeostasis. *Best Pract Res Clin Endocrinol Metab.* 2013;27(3):333-343.
12. Pollak MR, Brown EM, Chou YH, et al. Mutations in the human Ca²⁺-sensing receptor gene cause familial hypocalciuric hypercalcemia and neonatal severe hyperparathyroidism. *Cell.* 1993;75:1297-1303.
13. Pearce SHS, Williamson C, Kifor O, et al. A familial syndrome of hypocalcemia with hypercalciuria due to mutations in the calcium-sensing receptor. *N Engl J Med.* 1996;335(15):1115-1122.
14. Ho C, Conner DA, Pollack MR, et al. A mouse model of human familial hypocalciuric hypercalcemia and neonatal severe hyperparathyroidism. *Nat Genet.* 1995;11:389-394.
15. Drueke TB, Ritz E. Treatment of secondary hyperparathyroidism in CKD patients with cinacalcet and/or vitamin D derivatives. *Clin J Am Soc Nephrol.* 2009;4(1):234-241.
16. Moe SM, Cunningham J, Bommer J, et al. Long-term treatment of secondary hyperparathyroidism with the calcimimetic cinacalcet HCl. *Nephrol Dial Transplant.* 2005;20(10):2186-2193.
17. Dvorak-Ewell MM, Chen TH, Liang N, et al. Osteoblast extracellular Ca²⁺-sensing receptor regulates bone development, mineralization, and turnover. *J Bone Miner Res.* 2011;26(12):2935-2947.
18. Conigrave AD, Mun HC, Delbridge L, et al. L-amino acids regulate parathyroid hormone secretion. *J Biol Chem.* 2004;279(37):38151-38159.
19. Silver J, Naveh-Many T, Mayer H, et al. Regulation by vitamin D metabolites of parathyroid hormone gene transcription in vivo in the rat. *J Clin Invest.* 1986;78(5):1296-1301.
20. Sela-Brown A, Russell J, Koszewski NJ, et al. Calreticulin inhibits vitamin D's action on the PTH gene *in vitro* and may prevent vitamin D's effect *in vivo* in hypocalcemic rats. *Mol Endocrinol.* 1998;12:1193-1200.
21. Nechama M, Uchida T, Mor Yosef-Levi I, et al. The peptidyl-prolyl isomerase Pin1 determines parathyroid hormone mRNA levels and stability in rat models of secondary hyperparathyroidism. *J Clin Invest.* 2009;119(10):3102-3114.
22. Naveh-Many T. Minireview: the play of proteins on the parathyroid hormone messenger ribonucleic acid regulates its expression. *Endocrinology.* 2010;151(4):1398-1402.
23. Almaden Y, Canalejo A, Hernandez A, et al. Direct effect of phosphorus on PTH secretion from whole rat parathyroid glands in vitro. *J Bone Miner Res.* 1996;11(7):970-976.
24. Slatopolsky E, Finch J, Denda M, et al. Phosphorus restriction prevents parathyroid gland growth. *J Clin Invest.* 1996;97(11):2534-2540.
25. Kilav R, Silver J, Naveh-Many T. Parathyroid hormone gene expression in hypophosphatemic rats. *J Clin Invest.* 1995;96:327-333.
26. Silver J, Naveh-Many T. FGF23 and the parathyroid. *Adv Exp Med Biol.* 2012;728:92-99.
27. Olauson H, Lindberg K, Amin R, et al. Parathyroid-specific deletion of Klotho unravels a novel calcineurin-dependent FGF23 signaling pathway that regulates PTH secretion. *PLoS Genet.* 2013;9(12):e1003975.
28. Parfitt AM. Parathyroid growth: normal and abnormal. In: Bilezikian JP, ed. *The Parathyroids.* 2nd ed. San Diego: Academic Press; 2001:293-329.
29. Kremer R, Bolivar I, Goltzman D, Hendy GN. Influence of calcium and 1,25-dihydroxycholecalciferol on proliferation and proto-oncogene expression in primary cultures of bovine parathyroid cells. *Endocrinology.* 1989;125:935-941.
30. Dusso A, Cozzolino M, Lu Y, et al. 1,25-Dihydroxyvitamin D down-regulation of TGFalpha/EGFR expression and growth signaling: a mechanism for the antiproliferative actions of the sterol in parathyroid hyperplasia of renal failure. *J Steroid Biochem Mol Biol.* 2004;89-90(1-5):507-511.
31. Li YC, Pirro AE, Amling M, et al. Targeted ablation of the vitamin D receptor: an animal model of vitamin D-dependent rickets type II with alopecia. *Proc Natl Acad Sci U S A.* 1997;94(18):9831-9835.
32. Grigorieva IV, Thakker RV. Transcription factors in parathyroid development: lessons from hypoparathyroid disorders. *Ann N Y Acad Sci.* 2011;1237:24-38.
33. Manley NR, Capecchi MR. Hox group 3 paralogs regulate the development and migration of the thymus, thyroid, and parathyroid glands. *Dev Biol.* 1998;195(1):1-15.
34. Su D, Ellis S, Napier A, et al. Hoxa3 and pax1 regulate epithelial cell death and proliferation during thymus and parathyroid organogenesis. *Dev Biol.* 2001;236(2):316-329.
35. Peters H, Neubuser A, Kratochwil K, Balling R. Pax9-deficient mice lack pharyngeal pouch derivatives and teeth and exhibit craniofacial and limb abnormalities. *Genes Dev.* 1998;12(17):2735-2747.
36. Xu PX, Zheng W, Laclef C, et al. Eya1 is required for the morphogenesis of mammalian thymus, parathyroid and thyroid. *Development.* 2002;129(13):3033-3044.
37. Liu Z, Yu S, Manley NR. Gcm2 is required for the differentiation and survival of parathyroid precursor cells in the parathyroid/thymus primordia. *Dev Biol.* 2007;305(1):333-346.
38. Baldini A. Dissecting contiguous gene defects: TBX1. *Curr Opin Genet Dev.* 2005;15(3):279-284.
39. Ding C, Buckingham B, Levine MA. Familial isolated hypoparathyroidism caused by a mutation in the gene for the transcription factor GCMB. *J Clin Invest.* 2001;108(8):1215-1220.
40. Bowl MR, Nesbit MA, Harding B, et al. An interstitial deletion-insertion involving chromosomes 2p25.3 and Xq27.1, near SOX3, causes X-linked recessive hypoparathyroidism. *J Clin Invest.* 2005;115(10):2822-2831.
41. Ali A, Christie PT, Grigorieva IV, et al. Functional characterization of GATA3 mutations causing the hypoparathyroidism-deafness-renal (HDR) dysplasia syndrome: insight into mechanisms of DNA binding by the GATA3 transcription factor. *Hum Mol Genet.* 2007;16(3):265-275.
42. Bringhurst FR. Circulating forms of parathyroid hormone: peeling back the onion. *Clin Chem.* 2003;49(12):1973-1975.
43. Hilpert J, Nykjaer A, Jacobsen C, et al. Megalin antagonizes activation of the parathyroid hormone receptor. *J Biol Chem.* 1999;274(9):5620-5625.
44. Martin KJ, Hruska KA, Freitag JJ, et al. The peripheral metabolism of parathyroid hormone. *N Engl J Med.* 1979;301(20):1092-1098.
45. D'Amour P, Brossard JH, Rousseau L, et al. Structure of non-(1-84) PTH fragments secreted by parathyroid glands in primary and secondary hyperparathyroidism. *Kidney Int.* 2005;68(3):998-1007.
46. Slatopolsky E, Finch J, Clay P, et al. A novel mechanism for skeletal resistance in uremia. *Kidney Int.* 2000;58(2):753-761.
47. D'Amour P, Brossard JH. Carboxyl-terminal parathyroid hormone fragments: role in parathyroid hormone physiopathology. *Curr Opin Nephrol Hypertens.* 2005;14(4):330-336.
48. Friedman PA, Gesek FA. Calcium transport in renal epithelial cells. *Am J Physiol.* 1993;264:F181-F198.
49. Simon DB, Lu Y, Choate KA, et al. Paracellin-1, a renal tight junction protein required for paracellular Mg²⁺ resorption. *Science.* 1999;285(5424):103-106.
50. Hoenderop JG, Nilius B, Bindels RJ. Calcium absorption across epithelia. *Physiol Rev.* 2005;85(1):373-422.
51. de Groot T, Kovalevskaya NV, Verkaart S, et al. Molecular mechanisms of calmodulin action on TRPV5 and modulation by parathyroid hormone. *Mol Cell Biol.* 2011;31(14):2845-2853.
52. Walton RJ, Bijvoet OL. Nomogram for derivation of renal threshold phosphate concentration. *Lancet.* 1975;2(7929):309-310.
53. Murer H, Forster I, Biber J. The sodium phosphate cotransporter family SLC34. *Pflugers Arch.* 2004;447(5):763-767.
54. Segawa H, Yamanaka S, Onitsuka A, et al. Parathyroid hormone-dependent endocytosis of renal type IIc Na-Pi cotransporter. *Am J Physiol Renal Physiol.* 2007;292(1):F395-F403.
55. Guo J, Song L, Liu M, et al. Activation of a non-cAMP/PKA signaling pathway downstream of the PTH/PTHrP receptor is essential for a sustained hypophosphatemic response to PTH infusion in male mice. *Endocrinology.* 2013;154(5):1680-1689.
56. Capuano P, Bacic D, Roos M, et al. Defective coupling of apical PTH receptors to phospholipase C prevents internalization of the Na⁺-phosphate cotransporter NaPi-IIa in Nherf1-deficient mice. *Am J Physiol Cell Physiol.* 2007;292(2):C927-C934.
57. Weinman EJ, Lederer ED. NHERF-1 and the regulation of renal phosphate reabsorption: a tale of three hormones. *Am J Physiol Renal Physiol.* 2012;303(3):F321-F327.
58. Saito H, Maeda A, Ohtomo S, et al. Circulating FGF-23 is regulated by 1alpha,25-dihydroxyvitamin D3 and phosphorus in vivo. *J Biol Chem.* 2005;280(4):2543-2549.

59. Kim MS, Kondo T, Takada I, et al. DNA demethylation in hormone-induced transcriptional derepression. *Nature*. 2009;461(7266):1007-1012.

60. Jilka RL, O'Brien CA, Bartell SM, et al. Continuous elevation of PTH increases the number of osteoblasts via both osteoclast-dependent and -independent mechanisms. *J Bone Miner Res*. 2010;25(11):2427-2437.

61. Jilka RL. Molecular and cellular mechanisms of the anabolic effect of intermittent PTH. *Bone*. 2007;40(6):1434-1446.

62. Aubin J. Mesenchymal stem cells and osteoblast differentiation. In: Bilezikian J, Raisz L, Martin T, eds. *Principles of Bone Biology*. 3rd ed. Amsterdam: Elsevier; 2008:85-108.

63. Sacchetti B, Funari A, Michienzi S, et al. Self-renewing osteoprogenitors in bone marrow sinusoids can organize a hematopoietic microenvironment. *Cell*. 2007;131(2):324-336.

64. Jilka RL, Weinstein RS, Parfitt AM, Manolagas SC. Quantifying osteoblast and osteocyte apoptosis: challenges and rewards. *J Bone Miner Res*. 2007;22(10):1492-1501.

65. Dobnig H, Turner RT. Evidence that intermittent treatment with parathyroid hormone increases bone formation in adult rats by activation of bone lining cells. *Endocrinology*. 1995;136(8):3632-3638.

66. Kim SW, Pajevic PD, Selig M, et al. Intermittent parathyroid hormone administration converts quiescent lining cells to active osteoblasts. *J Bone Miner Res*. 2012;27(10):2075-2084.

67. Nishida S, Yamaguchi A, Tanizawa T, et al. Increased bone formation by intermittent parathyroid hormone administration is due to the stimulation of proliferation and differentiation of osteoprogenitor cells in bone marrow. *Bone*. 1994;15:717-723.

68. Lotinun S, Sibonga JD, Turner RT. Evidence that the cells responsible for marrow fibrosis in a rat model for hyperparathyroidism are pre-osteoblasts. *Endocrinology*. 2005;146(9):4074-4081.

69. Bellido T, Ali AA, Plotkin LI, et al. Proteasomal degradation of Runx2 shortens parathyroid hormone-induced anti-apoptotic signaling in osteoblasts. A putative explanation for why intermittent administration is needed for bone anabolism. *J Biol Chem*. 2003;278(50):50259-50272.

70. Qin L, Tamasi J, Raggatt L, et al. Amphiregulin is a novel growth factor involved in normal bone development and in the cellular response to parathyroid hormone stimulation. *J Biol Chem*. 2005;280(5):3974-3981.

71. Kulkarni NH, Halladay DL, Miles RR, et al. Effects of parathyroid hormone on Wnt signaling pathway in bone. *J Cell Biochem*. 2005;95(6):1178-1190.

72. Bellido T, Ali AA, Gubrij I, et al. Chronic elevation of parathyroid hormone in mice reduces expression of sclerostin by osteocytes: a novel mechanism for hormonal control of osteoblastogenesis. *Endocrinology*. 2005;146(11):4577-4583.

73. Semenov M, Tamai K, He X. SOST is a ligand for LRP5/LRP6 and a Wnt signaling inhibitor. *J Biol Chem*. 2005;280(29):26770-26775.

74. Tang Y, Wu X, Lei W, et al. TGF-beta1-induced migration of bone mesenchymal stem cells couples bone resorption with formation. *Nat Med*. 2009;15(7):757-765.

75. Teitelbaum SL, Ross FP. Genetic regulation of osteoclast development and function. *Nat Rev Genet*. 2003;4(8):638-649.

76. Yao GQ, Sun B, Hammond EE, et al. The cell-surface form of colony-stimulating factor-1 is regulated by osteotropic agents and supports formation of multinucleated osteoclast-like cells. *J Biol Chem*. 1998;273(7):4119-4128.

77. Qing H, Ardeshirpour L, Pajevic PD, et al. Demonstration of osteocytic perilacunar/canalicular remodeling in mice during lactation. *J Bone Miner Res*. 2012;27(5):1018-1029.

78. Chase LR, Aurbach GD. Parathyroid function and the renal excretion of 3'5'-adenylic acid. *Proc Natl Acad Sci U S A*. 1967;58(2):518-525.

79. Gensure RC, Gardella TJ, Juppner H. Parathyroid hormone and parathyroid hormone-related peptide, and their receptors. *Biochem Biophys Res Commun*. 2005;328(3):666-678.

80. Li C, Chen M, Sang M, et al. Comparative genomic analysis and evolution of family-B G protein-coupled receptors from six model insect species. *Gene*. 2013;519(1):1-12.

81. Pioszak AA, Parker NR, Gardella TJ, Xu HE. Structural basis for parathyroid hormone-related protein binding to the parathyroid hormone receptor and design of conformation-selective peptides. *J Biol Chem*. 2009;284(41):28382-28391.

82. Okazaki M, Ferrandon S, Vilardaga JP, et al. Prolonged signaling at the parathyroid hormone receptor by peptide ligands targeted to a specific receptor conformation. *Proc Natl Acad Sci U S A*. 2008;105(43):16525-16530.

83. Ferrandon S, Feinstein TN, Castro M, et al. Sustained cyclic AMP production by parathyroid hormone receptor endocytosis. *Nat Chem Biol*. 2009;5(10):734-742.

84. Vilardaga JP, Gardella TJ, Wehbi VL, Feinstein TN. Non-canonical signaling of the PTH receptor. *Trends Pharmacol Sci*. 2012;33(8):423-431.

85. Murray TM, Rao LG, Divieti P, Bringhurst FR. Parathyroid hormone secretion and action: evidence for discrete receptors for the carboxyl-terminal region and related biological actions of carboxyl-terminal ligands. *Endocr Rev*. 2005;26(1):78-113.

86. Dobolyi A, Dimitrov E, Palkovits M, Usdin TB. The neuroendocrine functions of the parathyroid hormone 2 receptor. *Front Endocrinol*. 2012;3:121.

87. Usdin TB, Paciga M, Riordan T, et al. Tuberoinfundibular peptide of 39 residues is required for germ cell development. *Endocrinology*. 2008;149(9):4292-4300.

88. Shimizu M, Potts JT Jr, Gardella TJ. Minimization of parathyroid hormone. *J Biol Chem*. 2000;275(29):21836-21843.

89. Takasu H, Gardella TJ, Luck MD, et al. Amino-terminal modifications of human parathyroid hormone (PTH) selectively alter phospholipase C signaling via the type 1 PTH receptor: implications for design of signal-specific PTH ligands. *Biochemistry*. 1999;38(41):13453-13460.

90. Gesty-Palmer D, Flannery P, Yuan L, et al. A b-arrestin–biased agonist of the parathyroid hormone receptor (PTH1R) promotes bone formation independent of G protein activation. *Sci Transl Med*. 2009;1(1):1ra.

91. Pioszak AA, Xu HE. Molecular recognition of parathyroid hormone by its G protein-coupled receptor. *Proc Natl Acad Sci U S A*. 2008;105(13):5034-5039.

92. Castro M, Nikolaev VO, Palm D, et al. Turn-on switch in parathyroid hormone receptor by a two-step parathyroid hormone binding mechanism. *Proc Natl Acad Sci U S A*. 2005;102(44):16084-16089.

93. Vilardaga JP, Bunemann M, Krasel C, et al. Measurement of the millisecond activation switch of G protein-coupled receptors in living cells. *Nat Biotechnol*. 2003;21(7):807-812.

94. Jin L, Briggs SL, Chandrasekhar S, et al. Crystal structure of human parathyroid hormone 1-34 at 0.9-A resolution. *J Biol Chem*. 2000;275(35):27238-27244.

95. Hollenstein K, de Graaf C, Bortolato A, et al. Insights into the structure of class B GPCRs. *Trends Pharmacol Sci*. 2014;35(1):12-22.

96. Gardella TJ, Luck MD, Fan MH, Lee C. Transmembrane residues of the parathyroid hormone (PTH)/PTH-related peptide receptor that specifically affect binding and signaling by agonist ligands. *J Biol Chem*. 1996;271(22):12820-12825.

97. Sheikh SP, Vilardarga JP, Baranski TJ, et al. Similar structures and shared switch mechanisms of the beta2-adrenoceptor and the parathyroid hormone receptor. Zn(II) bridges between helices III and VI block activation. *J Biol Chem*. 1999;274(24):17033-17041.

98. Bastepe M, Raas-Rothschild A, Silver J, et al. A form of Jansen's metaphyseal chondrodysplasia with limited metabolic and skeletal abnormalities is caused by a novel activating parathyroid hormone (PTH)/PTH-related peptide receptor mutation. *J Clin Endocrinol Metab*. 2004;89(7):3595-3600.

99. Bringhurst FR, Zajac JD, Daggett AS, et al. Inhibition of parathyroid hormone responsiveness in clonal osteoblastic cells expressing a mutant form of 3',5'-cyclic adenosine monophosphate-dependent protein kinase. *Mol Endocrinol*. 1989;3:60-67.

100. Traebert M, Volkl H, Biber J, et al. Luminal and contraluminal action of 1-34 and 3-34 PTH peptides on renal type IIa Na-P(i) cotransporter. *Am J Physiol Renal Physiol*. 2000;278(5):F792-F798.

101. Janulis M, Tembe V, Favus MJ. Role of protein kinase C in parathyroid hormone stimulation of renal 1,25-dihydroxyvitamin D3 secretion. *J Clin Invest*. 1992;90(6):2278-2283.

102. Guo J, Chung UI, Kondo H, et al. The PTH/PTHrP receptor can delay chondrocyte hypertrophy in vivo without activating phospholipase C. *Dev Cell*. 2002;3(2):183-194.

103. Chagin AS, Vuppalapati KK, Kobayashi T, et al. G-protein stimulatory subunit alpha and Gq/11alpha G-proteins are both required to maintain quiescent stem-like chondrocytes. *Nat Commun*. 2014;5:3673.

104. Guo J, Liu M, Thomas CC, et al. Phospholipase C signaling via the PTH/PTHrP receptor is essential for normal full response to PTH in both bone and kidney. *J Bone Miner Res*. 2007;22(Suppl):1119 (Abstract).

105. Guo J, Liu M, Yang D, et al. Phospholipase C signaling via the parathyroid hormone (PTH)/PTH-related peptide receptor is essential for normal bone responses to PTH. *Endocrinology*. 2010;151(8):3502-3513.

106. Mahon MJ, Segre GV. Stimulation by parathyroid hormone of a NHERF-1-assembled complex consisting of the parathyroid hormone I receptor, phospholipase C{beta}, and actin increases intracellular calcium in opossum kidney cells. *J Biol Chem*. 2004;279(22):23550-23558.

107. Vilardaga JP, Krasel C, Chauvin S, et al. Internalization determinants of the parathyroid hormone receptor differentially regulate beta-arrestin/receptor association. *J Biol Chem*. 2002;277(10):8121-8129.

108. Tawfeek HA, Qian F, Abou-Samra AB. Phosphorylation of the receptor for PTH and PTHrP is required for internalization and regulates receptor signaling. *Mol Endocrinol*. 2002;16(1):1-13.

109. Canario AV, Rotllant J, Fuentes J, et al. Novel bioactive parathyroid hormone and related peptides in teleost fish. *FEBS Lett*. 2006;580(1):291-299.

110. Orloff JJ, Reddy D, de Papp AE, et al. Parathyroid hormone-related protein as a prohormone: posttranslational processing and receptor interactions. *Endocr Rev*. 1994;15(1):40-60.

111. Lam MH, Briggs LJ, Hu W, et al. Importin beta recognizes parathyroid hormone-related protein with high affinity and mediates its nuclear import in the absence of importin alpha. *J Biol Chem*. 1999;274(11):7391-7398.

112. Wu TL, Vasavada RC, Yang KH, et al. Structural and physiologic characterization of the mid-region secretory species of parathyroid hormone-related protein. *J Biol Chem.* 1996;271(40):24371-24381.
113. Garcia-Martin A, Acitores A, Maycas M, et al. Src kinases mediate VEGFR2 transactivation by the osteostatin domain of PTHrP to modulate osteoblastic function. *J Cell Biochem.* 2013;114(6):1404-1413.
114. Burtis WJ, Brady TG, Orloff JJ, et al. Immunochemical characterization of circulating parathyroid hormone related protein in patients with humoral hypercalcemia of cancer. *N Engl J Med.* 1990;322:1106-1112.
115. Stewart AF. Clinical practice. Hypercalcemia associated with cancer. *N Engl J Med.* 2005;352(4):373-379.
116. Kir S, White JP, Kleiner S, et al. Tumour-derived PTH-related protein triggers adipose tissue browning and cancer cachexia. *Nature.* 2014;513(7516):100-104.
117. Simmonds CS, Karsenty G, Karaplis AC, Kovacs CS. Parathyroid hormone regulates fetal-placental mineral homeostasis. *J Bone Miner Res.* 2010;25(3):594-605.
118. VanHouten JN, Dann P, Stewart AF, et al. Mammary-specific deletion of parathyroid hormone-related protein preserves bone mass during lactation. *J Clin Invest.* 2003;112(9):1429-1436.
119. VanHouten J, Dann P, McGeoch G, et al. The calcium-sensing receptor regulates mammary gland parathyroid hormone-related protein production and calcium transport. *J Clin Invest.* 2004;113(4):598-608.
120. Kalkwarf HJ, Specker BL, Ho M. Effects of calcium supplementation on calcium homeostasis and bone turnover in lactating women. *J Clin Endocrinol Metab.* 1999;84(2):464-470.
121. Khosla S, Johansen KL, Ory SJ, et al. Parathyroid hormone-related peptide in lactation and in umbilical cord blood. *Mayo Clin Proc.* 1990;65:1408-1414.
122. Strewler G. The physiology of parathyroid hormone-related protein. *N Engl J Med.* 2000;342:177-185.
123. Kronenberg HM. Developmental regulation of the growth plate. *Nature.* 2003;423(6937):332-336.
124. Kozhemyakina E, Cohen T, Yao TP, Lassar AB. Parathyroid hormone-related peptide represses chondrocyte hypertrophy through a protein phosphatase 2A/histone deacetylase 4/MEF2 pathway. *Mol Cell Biol.* 2009;29(21):5751-5762.
125. Maeda S, Sutliff RL, Qian J, et al. Targeted overexpression of parathyroid hormone-related protein (PTHrP) to vascular smooth muscle in transgenic mice lowers blood pressure and alters vascular contractility. *Endocrinology.* 1999;140(4):1815-1825.
126. Miao D, Su H, He B, et al. Severe growth retardation and early lethality in mice lacking the nuclear localization sequence and C-terminus of PTH-related protein. *Proc Natl Acad Sci U S A.* 2008;105(51):20309-20314.
127. Copp DH, Cameron EC, Cheney B, et al. Evidence for calcitonin—a new hormone from the parathyroid that lowers blood calcium. *Endocrinology.* 1962;70:638-649.
128. Pearse AGE. The cytochemistry of the thyroid C cells and their relationship to calcitonin. *Proc Roy Soc London.* 1966;170:71-80.
129. Potts JT, Niall HD, Keutmann HT, et al. The amino acid sequence of procine thyrocalcitonin. *Proc Natl Acad Sci U S A.* 1968;59:1321-1328.
130. Amara SG, Jones V, Rosenfeld MG, et al. Alternative RNA processing in calcitonin gene expression generates mRNAs encoding different polypeptide products. *Nature.* 1982;298:240-244.
131. Care AD, Cooper CW, Duncan T, Orimo H. A study of thyrocalcitonin secretion by direct measurement of in vivo secretion rates in pigs. *Endocrinology.* 1968;83:161-169.
132. Cooper CW, Borosky SA, Farrell PE, Steinsland OS. Effects of the calcium channel activator BAY-K-8644 on in vitro secretion of calcitonin and parathyroid hormone. *Endocrinology.* 1986;118:545-549.
133. Garrett JE, Tamir H, Kifor O, et al. Calcitonin-secreting cells of the thyroid express and extracellular calcium receptor gene. *Endocrinology.* 1995;136(11):5202-5211.
134. Care AD. The regulation of the secretion of calcitonin. *Bone Miner.* 1992;16:182-185.
135. Naveh-Many T, Raue F, Grauer A, Silver J. Regulation of calcitonin gene expression by hypocalcemia, hypercalcemia, and vitamin D in the rat. *J Bone Miner Res.* 1992;7:1233-1237.
136. Peleg S, Abruzzese RV, Cooper CW, Gagel RF. Down-regulation of calcitonin gene transcription by vitamin D requires two widely separated enhancer sequences. *Mol Endocrinol.* 1993;7:999-1008.
137. Friedman PA, Gesek FA. Cellular calcium transport in renal epithelial: measurement, mechanisms and regulation. *Physiol Rev.* 1995;75(3):429-471.
138. Chambers TJ, McSheehy PM, Thomson BM, Fuller K. The effect of calcium-regulating hormones and prostaglandins on bone resorption by osteoclasts disaggregated from neonatal rabbit bones. *Endocrinology.* 1985;116(1):234-239.
139. Talmage RV, Vanderwiel CJ, Decker SA, Grubb SA. Changes produced in postprandial urinary calcium excretion by thyroidectomy and calcitonin administration in rats on different calcium regimes. *Endocrinology.* 1979;105:459-464.
140. Woodrow JP, Sharpe CJ, Fudge NJ, et al. Calcitonin plays a critical role in regulating skeletal mineral metabolism during lactation. *Endocrinology.* 2006;147(9):4010-4021.
141. Hoff A, Catalia-Lehnen P, Thomas P, et al. Increased bone mass is an unexpected phenotype associated with deletion of the calcitonin gene. *J Clin Invest.* 2002;110:1849-1857.
142. Dacquin R, Davey RA, Laplace C, et al. Amylin inhibits bone resorption while the calcitonin receptor controls bone formation in vivo. *J Cell Biol.* 2004;164(4):509-514.
143. Hurley DL, Tiegs RD, Wahner HW, Heath H. Axial and appendicular bone mineral density in patients with long-term deficiency or excess of calcitonin. *N Engl J Med.* 1987;317:537-541.
144. Wimalawansa SJ. Long- and short-term side effects and safety of calcitonin in man: a prospective study. *Calcif Tissue Int.* 1993;52:90-93.
145. Lin HY, Harris TL, Flannery MS, et al. Expression cloning of an adenylate cyclase-coupled calcitonin receptor. *Science.* 1991;254:1022-1024.
146. Purdue BW, Tilakaratne N, Sexton PM. Molecular pharmacology of the calcitonin receptor. *Receptors Channels.* 2002;8(3-4):243-255.
147. Chakraborty M, Chatterjee D, Kellokumpu S, et al. Cell cycle-dependent coupling of the calcitonin receptor to different G proteins. *Science.* 1991;251:1078-1082.
148. McLatchie L, Fraser N, Main M, et al. RAMPS regulate the transport and ligand specificity of the calcitonin-receptor like receptor. *Nature.* 1998;393:333-339.
149. Udawela M, Hay DL, Sexton PM. The receptor activity modifying protein family of G protein coupled receptor accessory proteins. *Semin Cell Dev Biol.* 2004;15(3):299-308.
150. Zumpe ET, Tilakaratne N, Fraser NJ, et al. Multiple ramp domains are required for generation of amylin receptor phenotype from the calcitonin receptor gene product. *Biochem Biophys Res Commun.* 2000;267(1):368-372.
151. Gangula PR, Zhao H, Supowit SC, et al. Increased blood pressure in alpha-calcitonin gene-related peptide/calcitonin gene knockout mice. *Hypertension.* 2000;35(1 Pt 2):470-475.
152. Granholm S, Henning P, Lerner UH. Comparisons between the effects of calcitonin receptor-stimulating peptide and intermedin and other peptides in the calcitonin family on bone resorption and osteoclastogenesis. *J Cell Biochem.* 2011;112(11):3300-3312.
153. Katafuchi T, Minamino N. Structure and biological properties of three calcitonin receptor-stimulating peptides, novel members of the calcitonin gene-related peptide family. *Peptides.* 2004;25(11):2039-2045.
154. Lorenzo A, Razzaboni B, Weir GC, Yankner BA. Pancreatic islet cell toxicity of amylin associated with type-2 diabetes mellitus. *Nature.* 1994;368:756-757.
155. Horcajada-Molteni MN, Chanteranne B, Lebecque P, et al. Amylin and bone metabolism in streptozotocin-induced diabetic rats. *J Bone Miner Res.* 2001;16(5):958-965.
156. Horcajada-Molteni MN, Davicco MJ, Lebecque P, et al. Amylin inhibits ovariectomy-induced bone loss in rats. *J Endocrinol.* 2000;165(3):663-668.
157. Samonina GE, Kopylova GN, Lukjanzeva GV, et al. Antiulcer effects of amylin: a review. *Pathophysiology.* 2004;11(1):1-6.
158. Hinson JP, Kapas S, Smith DM. Adrenomedullin, a multifunctional regulatory peptide. *Endocr Rev.* 2000;21(2):138-167.
159. Shimosawa T, Shibagaki Y, Ishibashi K, et al. Adrenomedullin, an endogenous peptide, counteracts cardiovascular damage. *Circulation.* 2002;105(1):106-111.
160. Kadmiel M, Fritz-Six K, Pacharne S, et al. Research resource: haploinsufficiency of receptor activity-modifying protein-2 (RAMP2) causes reduced fertility, hyperprolactinemia, skeletal abnormalities, and endocrine dysfunction in mice. *Mol Endocrinol.* 2011;25(7):1244-1253.
161. Roh J, Chang CL, Bhalla A, et al. Intermedin is a calcitonin/calcitonin gene-related peptide family peptide acting through the calcitonin receptor-like receptor/receptor activity-modifying protein receptor complexes. *J Biol Chem.* 2004;279(8):7264-7274.
162. Niccoli P, Brunet P, Roubicek C, et al. Abnormal calcitonin basal levels and pentagastrin response in patients with chronic renal failure on maintenance hemodialysis. *Eur J Endocrinol.* 1995;132:75-81.
163. O'Neill WJ, Jordan MH, Lewis MS, et al. Serum calcitonin may be a marker for inhalation injury in burns. *J Burn Care Rehabil.* 1992;13:605-616.
164. Sperber SJ, Blevins DD, Francis JB. Hypercalcitoninemia, hypocalcemia, and toxic shock syndrome. *Rev Infect Dis.* 1990;12:736-739.
165. Canale DD, Donabedian RK. Hypercalcitoninemia in acute pancreatitis. *J Clin Endocrinol Metab.* 1975;40:738-741.
166. Szanto J, Ady N, Jozsef S. Pain killing with calcitonin nasal spray in patients with malignant tumors. *Oncology.* 1992;49:180-182.
167. Jaeger H, Maier C. Calcitonin in phantom limb pain: a double-blind study. *Pain.* 1992;48:21-27.
168. Overman RA, Borse M, Gourlay ML. Salmon calcitonin use and associated cancer risk. *Ann Pharmacother.* 2013;47(12):1675-1684.
169. Holick MF, Shao Q, Liu WW, Chen TC. The vitamin D content of fortified milk and infant formula. *N Engl J Med.* 1992;326:1178-1181.
170. Lehmann U, Hirche F, Stangl GI, et al. Bioavailability of vitamin D(2) and D(3) in healthy volunteers, a randomized placebo-controlled trial. *J Clin Endocrinol Metab.* 2013;98(11):4339-4345.
171. Jones KS, Assar S, Harnpanich D, et al. 25(OH)D2 half-life is shorter than 25(OH)D3 half-life and is influenced by DBP concentration and genotype. *J Clin Endocrinol Metab.* 2014;99(9):3373-3381.

172. Safadi FF, Thornton P, Magiera H, et al. Osteopathy and resistance to vitamin D toxicity in mice null for vitamin D binding protein. *J Clin Invest.* 1999;103(2):239-251.

173. Nykjaer A, Dragun D, Walther D, et al. An endocytic pathway essential for renal uptake and activation of the steroid 25-(OH) vitamin D3. *Cell.* 1999;96(4):507-515.

174. Saito A, Iino N, Takeda T, Gejyo F. Role of megalin, a proximal tubular endocytic receptor, in calcium and phosphate homeostasis. *Ther Apher Dial.* 2007;11(Suppl 1):S23-S26.

175. Murayama A, Takeyama K, Kitanaka S, et al. Positive and negative regulations of the renal 25-hydroxyvitamin D3 1alpha-hydroxylase gene by parathyroid hormone, calcitonin, and 1alpha,25(OH)2D3 in intact animals. *Endocrinology.* 1999;140(5):2224-2231.

176. Shimada T, Hasegawa H, Yamazaki Y, et al. FGF-23 is a potent regulator of vitamin D metabolism and phosphate homeostasis. *J Bone Miner Res.* 2004;19(3):429-435.

177. Yoshida T, Fujimori T, Nabeshima Y. Mediation of unusually high concentrations of 1,25-dihydroxyvitamin D in homozygous klotho mutant mice by increased expression of renal 1alpha-hydroxylase gene. *Endocrinology.* 2002;143(2):683-689.

178. Overbergh L, Decallonne B, Valckx D, et al. Identification and immune regulation of 25-hydroxyvitamin D-1-alpha-hydroxylase in murine macrophages. *Clin Exp Immunol.* 2000;120(1):139-146.

179. Liu PT, Stenger S, Li H, et al. Toll-like receptor triggering of a vitamin D-mediated human antimicrobial response. *Science.* 2006;311(5768):1770-1773.

180. Adams JS, Sharma OP, Diz MM, Endres DB. Ketoconazole decreases the serum 1,25-dihydroxyvitamin D and calcium concentration in sarcoidosis-associated hypercalcemia. *J Clin Endocrinol Metab.* 1990;70:1090-1095.

181. Adams JS, Diz MM, Sharma OP. Effective reduction in the serum 1,25-dihydroxyvitamin D and calcium concentration in sarcoidosis-associated hypercalcemia with short-course chloroquine therapy. *Ann Intern Med.* 1989;111:437-438.

182. St-Arnaud R, Arabian A, Travers R, et al. Deficient mineralization of intramembranous bone in vitamin D-24-hydroxylase-ablated mice is due to elevated 1,25-dihydroxyvitamin D and not to the absence of 24,25-dihydroxyvitamin D. *Endocrinology.* 2000;141(7):2658-2666.

183. Schwartz Z, Brooks B, Swain L, et al. Production of 1,25-dihydroxyvitamin D$_3$ and 24,25-dihydroxyvitamin D$_3$ by growth zone and resting zone chondrocytes is dependent on cell maturation and is regulated by hormones and growth factors. *Endocrinology.* 1992;130:2495-2504.

184. Pettifor JM, Bikle DD, Cavaleros M, et al. Serum levels of free 1,25-dihydroxyvitamin D in vitamin D toxicity. *Ann Intern Med.* 1995;122:511-513.

185. Meyer MB, Benkusky NA, Lee CH, Pike JW. Genomic determinants of gene regulation by 1,25-dihydroxyvitamin D3 during osteoblast-lineage cell differentiation. *J Biol Chem.* 2014;289(28):19539-19554.

186. Inoue T, Kamiyama J, Sakai T. Sp1 and NF-Y synergistically mediate the effect of vitamin D(3) in the p27(Kip1) gene promoter that lacks vitamin D response elements. *J Biol Chem.* 1999;274(45):32309-32317.

187. Kim MS, Fujiki R, Murayama A, et al. 1Alpha,25(OH)2D3-induced transrepression by vitamin D receptor through E-box-type elements in the human parathyroid hormone gene promoter. *Mol Endocrinol.* 2007;21(2):334-342.

188. Yuan W, Pan W, Kong J, et al. 1,25-dihydroxyvitamin D3 suppresses renin gene transcription by blocking the activity of the cyclic AMP response element in the renin gene promoter. *J Biol Chem.* 2007;282(41):29821-29830.

189. Nishishita T, Okazaki T, Ishikawa T, et al. A negative vitamin D response DNA element in the human parathyroid hormone-related peptide gene binds to vitamin D receptor along with Ku antigen to mediate negative gene regulation by vitamin D. *J Biol Chem.* 1998;273(18):10901-10907.

190. Iida K, Shinki T, Yamaguchi A, et al. A possible role of vitamin D receptors in regulating vitamin D activation in the kidney. *Proc Natl Acad Sci U S A.* 1995;92:6112-6116.

191. Nemere I, Dormanen MC, Hammond MW, et al. Identification of a specific binding protein for 1a,25-dihydroxyvitamin D$_3$ in basal-lateral membranes of chick intestinal epithelium and relationship to trans-caltachia. *J Biol Chem.* 1994;269:23750-23756.

192. Erben RG, Soegiarto DW, Weber K, et al. Deletion of deoxyribonucleic acid binding domain of the vitamin D receptor abrogates genomic and nongenomic functions of vitamin D. *Mol Endocrinol.* 2002;16(7):1524-1537.

193. Buitrago C, Pardo VG, Boland R. Role of VDR in 1alpha,25-dihydroxyvitamin D3-dependent non-genomic activation of MAPKs, Src and Akt in skeletal muscle cells. *J Steroid Biochem Mol Biol.* 2013;136:125-130.

194. Hughes MR, Malloy PJ, Kieback DG, et al. Point mutations in the human vitamin D receptor gene associated with hypocalcemic rickets. *Science.* 1988;242:1702-1705.

195. Amling M, Priemel M, Holzmann T, et al. Rescue of the skeletal phenotype of vitamin D receptor-ablated mice in the setting of normal mineral ion homeostasis: formal histomorphometric and biomechanical analyses. *Endocrinology.* 1999;140(11):4982-4987.

196. Balsan S, Garabedian M, Larchet M, et al. Long-term nocturnal calcium infusions can cure rickets and promote normal mineralization in hereditary resistance to 1,25-dihydroxyvitamin D. *J Clin Invest.* 1986;77:1661-1667.

197. Li YC, Amling M, Pirro A, et al. Normalization of mineral ion homeostasis by dietary means prevents hyperparathyroidism, rickets, and osteomalacia, but not alopecia in vitamin D receptor-ablated mice. *Endocrinology.* 1998;139:4391-4396.

198. Lieben L, Masuyama R, Torrekens S, et al. Normocalcemia is maintained in mice under conditions of calcium malabsorption by vitamin D-induced inhibition of bone mineralization. *J Clin Invest.* 2012;122(5):1803-1815.

199. Van Cromphaut SJ, Dewerchin M, Hoenderop JG, et al. Duodenal calcium absorption in vitamin D receptor-knockout mice: functional and molecular aspects. *Proc Natl Acad Sci U S A.* 2001;98(23):13324-13329.

200. Xue Y, Fleet JC. Intestinal vitamin D receptor is required for normal calcium and bone metabolism in mice. *Gastroenterology.* 2009;136(4):1317-1327, e1-2.

201. Karbach U. Paracellular calcium transport across the small intestine. *J Nutr.* 1992;122:672-677.

202. Fujita H, Sugimoto K, Inatomi S, et al. Tight junction proteins claudin-2 and -12 are critical for vitamin D-dependent Ca2+ absorption between enterocytes. *Mol Biol Cell.* 2008;19(5):1912-1921.

203. van de Graaf SF, Boullart I, Hoenderop JG, Bindels RJ. Regulation of the epithelial Ca2+ channels TRPV5 and TRPV6 by 1alpha,25-dihydroxy vitamin D3 and dietary Ca2+. *J Steroid Biochem Mol Biol.* 2004;89-90(1–5):303-308.

204. Hoenderop JG, van Leeuwen JP, van der Eerden BC, et al. Renal Ca2+ wasting, hyperabsorption, and reduced bone thickness in mice lacking TRPV5. *J Clin Invest.* 2003;112(12):1906-1914.

205. Benn BS, Ajibade D, Porta A, et al. Active intestinal calcium transport in the absence of transient receptor potential vanilloid type 6 and calbindin-D9k. *Endocrinology.* 2008;149(6):3196-3205.

206. Meir T, Levi R, Lieben L, et al. Deletion of the vitamin D receptor specifically in the parathyroid demonstrates a limited role for the receptor in parathyroid physiology. *Am J Physiol Renal Physiol.* 2009;297(5):F1192-F1198.

207. Yasuda H, Shima N, Nakagawa N, et al. Osteoclast differentiation factor is a ligand for osteoprotegerin/osteoclastogenesis-inhibitory factor and is identical to TRANCE/RANKL. *Proc Natl Acad Sci U S A.* 1998;95(7):3597-3602.

208. Endo I, Inoue D, Mitsui T, et al. Deletion of vitamin D receptor gene in mice results in abnormal skeletal muscle development with deregulated expression of myoregulatory transcription factors. *Endocrinology.* 2003;144(12):5138-5144.

209. Zhou JY, Norman AW, Chen DL, et al. 1,25-Dihydroxy-16-ene-23-yne-vitamin D$_3$ prolongs survival time of leukemic mice. *Proc Natl Acad Sci U S A.* 1990;87:3929-3932.

210. Mathieu C, Laureys J, Waer M, Bouillon R. Prevention of autoimmune destruction of transplanted islets in spontaneously diabetic NOD mice by KH1060, a 20-epi analog of vitamin D: synergy with cyclosporine. *Transplant Proc.* 1994;26(6):3128-3129.

211. Brown AJ, Ritter CR, Finch JL, et al. The noncalcemic analogue of vitamin D, 22-oxacalcitriol, suppresses parathyroid hormone synthesis and secretion. *J Clin Invest.* 1989;84:728-732.

212. Holick MF, Smith E, Pincus S. Skin as the site of vitamin D synthesis and target tissue for 1,25-dihydroxyvitamin D$_3$. Use of calcitriol (1,25-dihydroxyvitamin D$_3$) for treatment of psoriasis. *Arch Dermatol.* 1987;123:1677-1683.

213. Kamimura S, Gallieni M, Kubodera N, et al. Differential catabolism of 22-oxacalcitriol and 1,25-dihydroxyvitamin D$_3$ by normal human peripheral monocytes. *Endocrinology.* 1993;133:2719-2722.

214. Peleg S, Sastry M, Collins ED, et al. Distinct conformational changes induced by 20-epi analogues of 1a,25-dihydroxyvitamin D$_3$ are associated with enhanced activation of the vitamin D receptor. *J Biol Chem.* 1995;270:10551-10558.

215. ADHR Consortium. Autosomal dominant hypophosphataemic rickets is associated with mutations in FGF23. *Nat Genet.* 2000;26(3):345-348.

216. White KE, Carn G, Lorenz-Depiereux B, et al. Autosomal-dominant hypophosphatemic rickets (ADHR) mutations stabilize FGF-23. *Kidney Int.* 2001;60(6):2079-2086.

217. Shimada T, Muto T, Urakawa I, et al. Mutant FGF-23 responsible for autosomal dominant hypophosphatemic rickets is resistant to proteolytic cleavage and causes hypophosphatemia in vivo. *Endocrinology.* 2002;143(8):3179-3182.

218. Shimada T, Mizutani S, Muto T, et al. Cloning and characterization of FGF23 as a causative factor of tumor-induced osteomalacia. *Proc Natl Acad Sci U S A.* 2001;98(11):6500-6505.

219. White KE, Jonsson KB, Carn G, et al. The autosomal dominant hypophosphatemic rickets (ADHR) gene is a secreted polypeptide overexpressed by tumors that cause phosphate wasting. *J Clin Endocrinol Metab.* 2001;86(2):497-500.

220. Ward LM, Rauch F, White KE, et al. Resolution of severe, adolescent-onset hypophosphatemic rickets following resection of an FGF-23-producing tumour of the distal ulna. *Bone.* 2004;34(5):905-911.

221. Endo I, Fukumoto S, Ozono K, et al. Clinical usefulness of measurement of fibroblast growth factor 23 (FGF23) in hypophosphatemic patients: proposal of diagnostic criteria using FGF23 measurement. *Bone.* 2008;42(6):1235-1239.

222. Araya K, Fukumoto S, Backenroth R, et al. A novel mutation in fibroblast growth factor 23 gene as a cause of tumoral calcinosis. *J Clin Endocrinol Metab.* 2005;90(10):5523-5527.

223. Chefetz I, Heller R, Galli-Tsinopoulou A, et al. A novel homozygous missense mutation in FGF23 causes familial tumoral calcinosis associated with disseminated visceral calcification. *Hum Genet.* 2005;118(2):261-266.

224. Larsson T, Yu X, Davis SI, et al. A novel recessive mutation in fibroblast growth factor-23 causes familial tumoral calcinosis. *J Clin Endocrinol Metab.* 2005;90(4):2424-2427.

225. Garringer HJ, Fisher C, Larsson TE, et al. The role of mutant UDP-N-acetyl-alpha-D-galactosamine-polypeptide N-acetylgalactosaminyltransferase 3 in regulating serum intact fibroblast growth factor 23 and matrix extracellular phosphoglycoprotein in heritable tumoral calcinosis. *J Clin Endocrinol Metab.* 2006;91(10):4037-4042.

226. Ichikawa S, Imel EA, Kreiter ML, et al. A homozygous missense mutation in human KLOTHO causes severe tumoral calcinosis. *J Clin Invest.* 2007;117(9):2684-2691.

227. Larsson T, Marsell R, Schipani E, et al. Transgenic mice expressing fibroblast growth factor 23 under the control of the alpha1(I) collagen promoter exhibit growth retardation, osteomalacia, and disturbed phosphate homeostasis. *Endocrinology.* 2004;145(7):3087-3094.

228. Shimada T, Kakitani M, Yamazaki Y, et al. Targeted ablation of Fgf23 demonstrates an essential physiological role of FGF23 in phosphate and vitamin D metabolism. *J Clin Invest.* 2004;113(4):561-568.

229. Sitara D, Razzaque MS, Hesse M, et al. Homozygous ablation of fibroblast growth factor-23 results in hyperphosphatemia and impaired skeletogenesis, and reverses hypophosphatemia in Phex-deficient mice. *Matrix Biol.* 2004;23(7):421-432.

230. Razzaque MS, Lanske B. Hypervitaminosis D and premature aging: lessons learned from Fgf23 and Klotho mutant mice. *Trends Mol Med.* 2006;12(7):298-305.

231. Saito H, Kusano K, Kinosaki M, et al. Human fibroblast growth factor-23 mutants suppress Na+-dependent phosphate co-transport activity and 1alpha,25-dihydroxyvitamin D3 production. *J Biol Chem.* 2003;278(4):2206-2211.

232. Segawa H, Kawakami E, Kaneko I, et al. Effect of hydrolysis-resistant FGF23-R179Q on dietary phosphate regulation of the renal type-II Na/Pi transporter. *Pflugers Arch.* 2003;446(5):585-592.

233. Yan X, Yokote H, Jing X, et al. Fibroblast growth factor 23 reduces expression of type IIa Na+/Pi co-transporter by signaling through a receptor functionally distinct from the known FGFRs in opossum kidney cells. *Genes Cells.* 2005;10(5):489-502.

234. Miyamoto K, Ito M, Kuwahata M, et al. Inhibition of intestinal sodium-dependent inorganic phosphate transport by fibroblast growth factor 23. *Ther Apher Dial.* 2005;9(4):331-335.

235. Kurosu H, Ogawa Y, Miyoshi M, et al. Regulation of fibroblast growth factor-23 signaling by klotho. *J Biol Chem.* 2006;281(10):6120-6123.

236. Andrukhova O, Zeitz U, Goetz R, et al. FGF23 acts directly on renal proximal tubules to induce phosphaturia through activation of the ERK1/2-SGK1 signaling pathway. *Bone.* 2012;51(3):621-628.

237. Andrukhova O, Smorodchenko A, Egerbacher M, et al. FGF23 promotes renal calcium reabsorption through the TRPV5 channel. *EMBO J.* 2014;33(3):229-246.

238. Andrukhova O, Slavic S, Smorodchenko A, et al. FGF23 regulates renal sodium handling and blood pressure. *EMBO Mol Med.* 2014;6(6):744-759.

239. Yu X, Sabbagh Y, Davis SI, et al. Genetic dissection of phosphate- and vitamin D-mediated regulation of circulating Fgf23 concentrations. *Bone.* 2005;36(6):971-977.

240. Perwad F, Azam N, Zhang MY, et al. Dietary and serum phosphorus regulate fibroblast growth factor 23 expression and 1,25-dihydroxyvitamin D metabolism in mice. *Endocrinology.* 2005;146(12):5358-5364.

241. Farrow EG, Yu X, Summers LJ, et al. Iron deficiency drives an autosomal dominant hypophosphatemic rickets (ADHR) phenotype in fibroblast growth factor-23 (Fgf23) knock-in mice. *Proc Natl Acad Sci U S A.* 2011;108(46):E1146-E1155.

242. Wolf M, White KE. Coupling fibroblast growth factor 23 production and cleavage: iron deficiency, rickets, and kidney disease. *Curr Opin Nephrol Hypertens.* 2014;23(4):411-419.

243. Masuyama R, Stockmans I, Torrekens S, et al. Vitamin D receptor in chondrocytes promotes osteoclastogenesis and regulates FGF23 production in osteoblasts. *J Clin Invest.* 2006;116(12):3150-3159.

244. Ye L, Mishina Y, Chen D, et al. Dmp1-deficient mice display severe defects in cartilage formation responsible for a chondrodysplasia-like phenotype. *J Biol Chem.* 2005;280(7):6197-6203.

245. Mackenzie NC, Huesa C, Rutsch F, MacRae VE. New insights into NPP1 function: lessons from clinical and animal studies. *Bone.* 2012;51(5):961-968.

246. Rafaelsen SH, Raeder H, Fagerheim AK, et al. Exome sequencing reveals FAM20c mutations associated with fibroblast growth factor 23-related

247. Tagliabracci VS, Engel JL, Wiley SE, et al. Dynamic regulation of FGF23 by Fam20C phosphorylation, GalNAc-T3 glycosylation, and furin proteolysis. *Proc Natl Acad Sci U S A.* 2014;111(15):5520-5525.

248. Nakanishi S, Kazama JJ, Nii-Kono T, et al. Serum fibroblast growth factor-23 levels predict the future refractory hyperparathyroidism in dialysis patients. *Kidney Int.* 2005;67(3):1171-1178.

249. Gutierrez OM, Mannstadt M, Isakova T, et al. Fibroblast growth factor 23 and mortality among patients undergoing hemodialysis. *N Engl J Med.* 2008;359(6):584-592.

250. Faul C, Amaral AP, Oskouei B, et al. FGF23 induces left ventricular hypertrophy. *J Clin Invest.* 2011;121(11):4393-4408.

251. Shalhoub V, Shatzen EM, Ward SC, et al. FGF23 neutralization improves chronic kidney disease-associated hyperparathyroidism yet increases mortality. *J Clin Invest.* 2012;122(7):2543-2553.

252. Nussbaum SR, Zahradnik RJ, Lavigne JR, et al. Highly sensitive two-site immunoradiometric assay of parathyrin and its clinical utility in evaluating patients with hypercalcemia. *Clin Chem.* 1987;33:1364-1367.

253. Gao P, D'Amour P. Evolution of the parathyroid hormone (PTH) assay: importance of circulating PTH immunoheterogeneity and of its regulation. *Clin Lab.* 2005;51(1-2):21-29.

254. Boudou P, Ibrahim F, Cormier C, et al. Third- or second-generation parathyroid hormone assays: a remaining debate in the diagnosis of primary hyperparathyroidism. *J Clin Endocrinol Metab.* 2005;90(12):6370-6372.

255. D'Amour P, Brossard JH, Rousseau L, et al. Amino-terminal form of parathyroid hormone (PTH) with immunologic similarities to hPTH(1-84) is overproduced in primary and secondary hyperparathyroidism. *Clin Chem.* 2003;49(12):2037-2044.

256. Cavalier E, Betea D, Schleck ML, et al. The third/second generation PTH assay ratio as a marker for parathyroid carcinoma: evaluation using an automated platform. *J Clin Endocrinol Metab.* 2014;99(3):E453-E457.

257. Fritchie K, Zedek D, Grenache DG. The clinical utility of parathyroid hormone-related peptide in the assessment of hypercalcemia. *Clin Chim Acta.* 2009;402(1-2):146-149.

258. Machens A, Lorenz K, Dralle H. Utility of serum procalcitonin for screening and risk stratification of medullary thyroid cancer. *J Clin Endocrinol Metab.* 2014;99(8):2986-2994.

259. Ersfeld DL, Rao DS, Body JJ, et al. Analytical and clinical validation of the 25 OH vitamin D assay for the LIAISON automated analyzer. *Clin Biochem.* 2004;37(10):867-874.

260. Phinney KW. Development of a standard reference material for vitamin D in serum. *Am J Clin Nutr.* 2008;88(2):511S-512S.

261. Jonsson KB, Zahradnik R, Larsson T, et al. Fibroblast growth factor 23 in oncogenic osteomalacia and X-linked hypophosphatemia. *N Engl J Med.* 2003;348(17):1656-1663.

262. Yamazaki Y, Okazaki R, Shibata M, et al. Increased circulatory level of biologically active full-length FGF-23 in patients with hypophosphatemic rickets/osteomalacia. *J Clin Endocrinol Metab.* 2002;87(11):4957-4960.

263. Burnett SM, Gunawardene SC, Bringhurst FR, et al. Regulation of C-terminal and intact FGF-23 by dietary phosphate in men and women. *J Bone Miner Res.* 2006;21(8):1187-1196.

264. Bhattacharyya N, Wiench M, Dumitrescu C, et al. Mechanism of FGF23 processing in fibrous dysplasia. *J Bone Miner Res.* 2012;27(5):1132-1141.

265. Kato K, Jeanneau C, Tarp MA, et al. Polypeptide GalNAc-transferase T3 and familial tumoral calcinosis. Secretion of fibroblast growth factor 23 requires O-glycosylation. *J Biol Chem.* 2006;281(27):18370-18377.

266. Weber CJ, Sewell CW, McGarity WC. Persistent and recurrent sporadic primary hyperparathyroidism: histopathology, complications, and results of reoperation. *Surgery.* 1994;116(6):991-998.

267. LiVolsi VA. Embryology, anatomy, and pathology of the parathyroids. In: Bilezikian JP, ed. *The Parathyroids.* New York: Raven Press; 1994:1-14.

268. Rosen IB, Young JEM, Archibald SD, et al. Parathyroid cancer: clinical variations and relationships to autotransplantation. *Can J Cancer.* 1994;37:465-469.

269. Shane E, Bilezikian JP. Parathyroid carcinoma: a review of 62 patients. *Endocr Rev.* 1982;3:218-226.

270. Patten BM, Bilezikian JP, Mallette LE, et al. Neuromuscular disease in hyperparathyroidism. *Ann Intern Med.* 1974;80:182-193.

271. Wermers RA, Khosla S, Atkinson EJ, et al. The rise and fall of primary hyperparathyroidism: a population-based study in Rochester, Minnesota, 1965-1992. *Ann Intern Med.* 1997;126(6):433-440.

272. Wermers RA, Khosla S, Atkinson EJ, et al. Incidence of primary hyperparathyroidism in Rochester, Minnesota, 1993-2001: an update on the changing epidemiology of the disease. *J Bone Miner Res.* 2006;21(1):171-177.

273. Lundgren E, Rastad J, Thrufjell E, et al. Population-based screening for primary hyperparathyroidism with serum calcium and parathyroid hormone values in menopausal women. *Surgery.* 1997;121(3):287-294.

hypophosphatemia, dental anomalies, and ectopic calcification. *J Bone Miner Res.* 2013;28(6):1378-1385.

274. Lowe H, McMahon DJ, Rubin MR, et al. Normocalcemic primary hyperparathyroidism: further characterization of a new clinical phenotype. *J Clin Endocrinol Metab.* 2007;92(8):3001-3005.

275. Silverberg SJ, Shane E, Jacobs TP, et al. A 10-year prospective study of primary hyperparathyroidism with or without parathyroid surgery. *N Engl J Med.* 1999;341(17):1249-1255.

276. Walgenbach S, Hommel G, Junginger T. Outcome after surgery for primary hyperparathyroidism: ten-year prospective follow-up study. *World J Surg.* 2000;24(5):564-569, discussion 569-570.

277. Rao DS, Phillips ER, Divine GW, Talpos GB. Randomized controlled clinical trial of surgery versus no surgery in patients with mild asymptomatic primary hyperparathyroidism. *J Clin Endocrinol Metab.* 2004;89(11):5415-5422.

278. Ambrogini E, Cetani F, Cianferotti L, et al. Surgery or surveillance for mild asymptomatic primary hyperparathyroidism: a prospective, randomized clinical trial. *J Clin Endocrinol Metab.* 2007;92(8):3114-3121.

279. Bollerslev J, Jansson S, Mollerup CL, et al. Medical observation, compared with parathyroidectomy, for asymptomatic primary hyperparathyroidism: a prospective, randomized trial. *J Clin Endocrinol Metab.* 2007;92(5):1687-1692.

280. Rubin MR, Bilezikian JP, McMahon DJ, et al. The natural history of primary hyperparathyroidism with or without parathyroid surgery after 15 years. *J Clin Endocrinol Metab.* 2008;93(9):3462-3470.

281. Palmer M, Adami HO, Bergstrom R, et al. Mortality after surgery for primary hyperparathyroidism: a followup of 441 patients operated on from 1956-1979. *Surgery.* 1987;102:1-7.

282. Stefenelli T, Abela C, Frank H, et al. Cardiac abnormalities in patients with primary hyperparathyroidism: implications for follow-up. *J Clin Endocrinol Metab.* 1997;82(1):106-112.

283. Wermers RA, Khosla S, Atkinson EJ, et al. Survival after the diagnosis of hyperparathyroidism: a population-based study. *Am J Med.* 1998;104(2):115-122.

284. Palmer M, Adami HO, Krusemo UB, Ljunghall S. Increased risk of malignant diseases after surgery for primary hyperparathyroidism. A nationwide cohort study. *Am J Epidemiol.* 1988;127:1031-1040.

285. Parisien M, Silverberg SJ, Shane E, et al. The histomorphometry of bone in primary hyperparathyroidism: preservation of cancellous bone structure. *J Clin Endocrinol Metab.* 1990;70:930-938.

286. Dempster DW, Muller R, Zhou H, et al. Preserved three-dimensional cancellous bone structure in mild primary hyperparathyroidism. *Bone.* 2007;41(1):19-24.

287. Silverberg SJ, Gartenberg F, Jacobs TP, et al. Longitudinal measurements of bone density and biochemical indices in untreated primary hyperparathyroidism. *J Clin Endocrinol Metab.* 1995;80(3):723-728.

288. Bilezikian JP, Silverberg SJ, Shane E, et al. Characterization and evaluation of asymptomatic primary hyperparathyroidism. *J Bone Miner Res.* 1991;6(Suppl 2):S85-S89, discussion S121-S124.

289. Khosla S, Melton LJ 3rd, Wermers RA, et al. Primary hyperparathyroidism and the risk of fracture: a population-based study. *J Bone Miner Res.* 1999;14(10):1700-1707.

290. Vignali E, Viccica G, Diacinti D, et al. Morphometric vertebral fractures in postmenopausal women with primary hyperparathyroidism. *J Clin Endocrinol Metab.* 2009;94(7):2306-2312.

291. Stein EM, Silva BC, Boutroy S, et al. Primary hyperparathyroidism is associated with abnormal cortical and trabecular microstructure and reduced bone stiffness in postmenopausal women. *J Bone Miner Res.* 2013;28(5):1029-1040.

292. Vu TD, Wang XF, Wang Q, et al. New insights into the effects of primary hyperparathyroidism on the cortical and trabecular compartments of bone. *Bone.* 2013;55(1):57-63.

293. Hansen S, Hauge EM, Rasmussen L, et al. Parathyroidectomy improves bone geometry and microarchitecture in female patients with primary hyperparathyroidism: a one-year prospective controlled study using high-resolution peripheral quantitative computed tomography. *J Bone Miner Res.* 2012;27(5):1150-1158.

294. Rao DS, Wilson RJ, Kleerekoper M, Parfitt AM. Lack of biochemical progression or continuation of accelerated bone loss in mild asymptomatic primary hyperparathyroidism: evidence for biphasic disease course. *J Clin Endocrinol Metab.* 1988;67:1294-1298.

295. Walker MD, Nickolas T, Kepley A, et al. Predictors of renal function in primary hyperparathyroidism. *J Clin Endocrinol Metab.* 2014;99(5):1885-1892.

296. Arnold A, Staunton CE, Kim HG, et al. Monoclonality and abnormal parathyroid hormone genes in parathyroid adenomas. *N Engl J Med.* 1988;318:658-662.

297. Arnold A, Shattuck TM, Mallya SM, et al. Molecular pathogenesis of primary hyperparathyroidism. *J Bone Miner Res.* 2002;17(Suppl 2):N30-N36.

298. Costa-Guda J, Tokura T, Roth SI, Arnold A. Mitochondrial DNA mutations in oxyphilic and chief cell parathyroid adenomas. *BMC Endocr Disord.* 2007;7:8.

299. Motokura T, Bloom T, Kim HG, et al. A BCL1-linked candidate oncogene which is rearranged in parathyroid tumors encodes a novel cyclin. *Nature.* 1991;350:512-515.

300. Mallya SM, Gallagher JJ, Wild YK, et al. Abnormal parathyroid cell proliferation precedes biochemical abnormalities in a mouse model of primary hyperparathyroidism. *Mol Endocrinol.* 2005;19(10):2603-2609.

301. Cromer MK, Starker LF, Choi M, et al. Identification of somatic mutations in parathyroid tumors using whole-exome sequencing. *J Clin Endocrinol Metab.* 2012;97(9):E1774-E1781.

302. Newey PJ, Nesbit MA, Rimmer AJ, et al. Whole-exome sequencing studies of nonhereditary (sporadic) parathyroid adenomas. *J Clin Endocrinol Metab.* 2012;97(10):E1995-E2005.

303. Carling T. Molecular pathology of parathyroid tumors. *Trends Endocrinol Metab.* 2001;12(2):53-58.

304. Samander EH, Arnold A. Mutational analysis of the vitamin D receptor does not support its candidacy as a tumor suppressor gene in parathyroid adenomas. *J Clin Endocrinol Metab.* 2006;91(12):5019-5021.

305. Imanishi Y, Tahara H, Palanisamy N, et al. Clonal chromosomal defects in the molecular pathogenesis of refractory hyperparathyroidism of uremia. *J Am Soc Nephrol.* 2002;13(6):1490-1498.

306. Arnold A, Brown MF, Urena P, et al. Monoclonality of parathyroid tumors in chronic renal failure and in primary parathyroid hyperplasia. *J Clin Invest.* 1995;95:2047-2053.

307. Friedman E, Sakaguchi K, Bale AE, et al. Clonality of parathyroid tumors in familial multiple endocrine neoplasia type I. *N Engl J Med.* 1989;321:213-218.

308. Livolsi V. Parathyroids: morphology and pathology. In: Bilezikian J, ed. *The Parathyroids: Basic and Clinical Concepts.* 2nd ed. San Diego: Academic Press; 2001:1-16.

309. Kifor O, Moore FD, Wang P, et al. Reduced immunostaining for the extracellular Ca2+-sensing receptor in primary and uremic secondary hyperparathyroidism. *J Clin Endocrinol Metab.* 1996;81(4):1598-1606.

310. Mizobuchi M, Ritter CS, Krits I, et al. Calcium-sensing receptor expression is regulated by glial cells missing-2 in human parathyroid cells. *J Bone Miner Res.* 2009;24(7):1173-1179.

311. Marx SJ. Molecular genetics of multiple endocrine neoplasia types 1 and 2. *Nat Rev Cancer.* 2005;5(5):367-375.

312. Hughes CM, Rozenblatt-Rosen O, Milne TA, et al. Menin associates with a trithorax family histone methyltransferase complex and with the hoxc8 locus. *Mol Cell.* 2004;13(4):587-597.

313. Karnik SK, Hughes CM, Gu X, et al. Menin regulates pancreatic islet growth by promoting histone methylation and expression of genes encoding p27Kip1 and p18INK4c. *Proc Natl Acad Sci U S A.* 2005;102(41):14659-14664.

314. Matkar S, Thiel A, Hua X. Menin: a scaffold protein that controls gene expression and cell signaling. *Trends Biochem Sci.* 2013;38(8):394-402.

315. Agarwal SK, Mateo CM, Marx SJ. Rare germline mutations in cyclin-dependent kinase inhibitor genes in multiple endocrine neoplasia type 1 and related states. *J Clin Endocrinol Metab.* 2009;94(5):1826-1834.

316. Lee M, Pellegata NS. Multiple endocrine neoplasia type 4. *Front Horm Res.* 2013;41:63-78.

317. Eller-Vainicher C, Chiodini I, Battista C, et al. Sporadic and MEN1-related primary hyperparathyroidism: differences in clinical expression and severity. *J Bone Miner Res.* 2009;24(8):1404-1410.

318. Norton JA, Venzon DJ, Berna MJ, et al. Prospective study of surgery for primary hyperparathyroidism (HPT) in multiple endocrine neoplasia-type 1 and Zollinger-Ellison syndrome: long-term outcome of a more virulent form of HPT. *Ann Surg.* 2008;247(3):501-510.

319. Pausova Z, Soliman E, Amizuka N, et al. Role of the RET proto-oncogene in sporadic hyperparathyroidism and in hyperparathyroidism of multiple endocrine neoplasia type 2. *J Clin Endocrinol Metab.* 1996;81(7):2711-2718.

320. Haven CJ, Wong FK, van Dam EW, et al. A genotypic and histopathological study of a large Dutch kindred with hyperparathyroidism-jaw tumor syndrome. *J Clin Endocrinol Metab.* 2000;85(4):1449-1454.

321. Carpten JD, Robbins CM, Villablanca A, et al. HRPT2, encoding parafibromin, is mutated in hyperparathyroidism-jaw tumor syndrome. *Nat Genet.* 2002;32(4):676-680.

322. Rozenblatt-Rosen O, Hughes CM, Nannepaga SJ, et al. The parafibromin tumor suppressor protein is part of a human Paf1 complex. *Mol Cell Biol.* 2005;25(2):612-620.

323. Yart A, Gstaiger M, Wirbelauer C, et al. The HRPT2 tumor suppressor gene product parafibromin associates with human PAF1 and RNA polymerase II. *Mol Cell Biol.* 2005;25(12):5052-5060.

324. Newey PJ, Bowl MR, Thakker RV. Parafibromin: functional insights. *J Intern Med.* 2009;266(1):84-98.

325. Mosimann C, Hausmann G, Basler K. Parafibromin/Hyrax activates Wnt/Wg target gene transcription by direct association with beta-catenin/Armadillo. *Cell.* 2006;125(2):327-341.

326. Shattuck TM, Valimaki S, Obara T, et al. Somatic and germ-line mutations of the HRPT2 gene in sporadic parathyroid carcinoma. *N Engl J Med.* 2003;349(18):1722-1729.

327. Bilezikian JP, Brandi ML, Eastell R, et al. Guidelines for the management of asymptomatic primary hyperparathyroidism: summary statement from the fourth international workshop. *J Clin Endoc Metabolism.* 2014;99:(in press).

328. Bilezikian JP, Khan AA, Potts JT Jr. Third International Workshop on the Management of Asymptomatic Primary H. Guidelines for the management of asymptomatic primary hyperparathyroidism: summary

statement from the third international workshop. *J Clin Endocrinol Metab.* 2009;94(2):335-339.

329. Silverberg SJ, Brown I, Bilezikian JP. Age as a criterion for surgery in primary hyperparathyroidism. *Am J Med.* 2002;113(8):681-684.

330. Nakaoka D, Sugimoto T, Kobayashi T, et al. Prediction of bone mass change after parathyroidectomy in patients with primary hyperparathyroidism. *J Clin Endocrinol Metab.* 2000;85(5):1901-1907.

331. Silverberg SJ, Locker FG, Bilezikian JP. Vertebral osteopenia: a new indication for surgery in primary hyperparathyroidism. *J Clin Endocrinol Metab.* 1996;81(11):4007-4012.

332. Khan AA, Bilezikian JP, Kung AW, et al. Alendronate in primary hyperparathyroidism: a double-blind, randomized, placebo-controlled trial. *J Clin Endocrinol Metab.* 2004;89(7):3319-3325.

333. Chow CC, Chan WB, Li JK, et al. Oral alendronate increases bone mineral density in postmenopausal women with primary hyperparathyroidism. *J Clin Endocrinol Metab.* 2003;88(2):581-587.

334. Peacock M, Bolognese MA, Borofsky M, et al. Cinacalcet treatment of primary hyperparathyroidism: biochemical and bone densitometric outcomes in a five-year study. *J Clin Endocrinol Metab.* 2009;94(12):4860-4867.

335. Grant CS, Thompson G, Farley D, van Heerden J. Primary hyperparathyroidism surgical management since the introduction of minimally invasive parathyroidectomy: Mayo Clinic experience. *Arch Surg.* 2005;140(5):472-478, discussion 478-479.

336. Ruda JM, Hollenbeak CS, Stack BC Jr. A systematic review of the diagnosis and treatment of primary hyperparathyroidism from 1995 to 2003. *Otolaryngol Head Neck Surg.* 2005;132(3):359-372.

337. Akerstrom G, Rundberg C, Grimelius L, et al. Causes of failed primary exploration and technical aspects of reoperation in primary hyperparathyroidism. *World J Surg.* 1992;16:562-569.

338. Kollmorgen CF, Aust MR, Ferreiro JA, et al. Parathyromatosis: a rare yet important cause of persistent or recurrent hyperparathyroidism. *Surgery.* 1994;116(1):111-115.

339. Mitchell BK, Merrell RC, Kinder BK. Localization studies in patients with hyperparathyroidism. *Surg Clin North Am.* 1995;75(3):483-498.

340. Udelsman R, Donovan PI. Open minimally invasive parathyroid surgery. *World J Surg.* 2004;28(12):1224-1226.

341. Kelly HR, Hamberg LM, Hunter GJ. 4D-CT for preoperative localization of abnormal parathyroid glands in patients with hyperparathyroidism: accuracy and ability to stratify patients by unilateral versus bilateral disease in surgery-naive and re-exploration patients. *Am J Neuroradiol.* 2014;35(1):176-181.

342. Inabnet WB. Intraoperative parathyroid hormone monitoring. *World J Surg.* 2004;28(12):1212-1215.

343. Weber KJ, Misra S, Lee JK, et al. Intraoperative PTH monitoring in parathyroid hyperplasia requires stricter criteria for success. *Surgery.* 2004;136(6):1154-1159.

344. Siperstein A, Berber E, Barbosa GF, et al. Predicting the success of limited exploration for primary hyperparathyroidism using ultrasound, sestamibi, and intraoperative parathyroid hormone: analysis of 1158 cases. *Ann Surg.* 2008;248(3):420-428.

345. Lambert LA, Shapiro SE, Lee JE, et al. Surgical treatment of hyperparathyroidism in patients with multiple endocrine neoplasia type 1. *Arch Surg.* 2005;140(4):374-382.

346. Marcocci C, Cetani F, Rubin MR, et al. Parathyroid carcinoma. *J Bone Miner Res.* 2008;23(12):1869-1880.

347. Oertli D, Richter M, Kraenzlin M, et al. Parathyroidectomy in primary hyperparathyroidism: preoperative localization and routine biopsy of unaltered glands are not necessary. *Surgery.* 1995;117(4):392-396.

348. Bergenfelz A, Valdermarsson S, Ahren B. Functional recovery of the parathyroid glands after surgery for primary hyperparathyroidism. *Surgery.* 1994;116(5):827-836.

349. Gross ND, Weissman JL, Veenker E, Cohen JI. The diagnostic utility of computed tomography for preoperative localization in surgery for hyperparathyroidism. *Laryngoscope.* 2004;114(2):227-231.

350. Biertho LD, Kim C, Wu HS, et al. Relationship between sestamibi uptake, parathyroid hormone assay, and nuclear morphology in primary hyperparathyroidism. *J Am Coll Surg.* 2004;199(2):229-233.

351. Milas M, Wagner K, Easley KA, et al. Double adenomas revisited: non-uniform distribution favors enlarged superior parathyroids (fourth pouch disease). *Surgery.* 2003;134(6):995-1003, discussion 1003-1004.

352. Mortenson MM, Evans DB, Lee JE, et al. Parathyroid exploration in the reoperative neck: improved preoperative localization with 4D-computed tomography. *J Am Coll Surg.* 2008;206(5):888-895, discussion 895-896.

353. Estella E, Leong MS, Bennett I, et al. Parathyroid hormone venous sampling prior to reoperation for primary hyperparathyroidism. *ANZ J Surg.* 2003;73(10):800-805.

354. Chaffanjon PC, Voirin D, Vasdev A, et al. Selective venous sampling in recurrent and persistent hyperparathyroidism: indication, technique, and results. *World J Surg.* 2004;28(10):958-961.

355. Smythe WR, Bavaria JE, Hall RA, et al. Thoracoscopic removal of mediastinal parathyroid adenoma. *Ann Thorac Surg.* 1995;59(1):236-238.

356. Silverberg SJ, Shane E, Dempster DW, Bilezikian JP. The effects of vitamin D insufficiency in patients with primary hyperparathyroidism. *Am J Med.* 1999;107(6):561-567.

357. Nomura R, Sugimoto T, Tsukamoto T, et al. Marked and sustained increase in bone mineral density after parathyroidectomy in patients with primary hyperparathyroidism; a six-year longitudinal study with or without parathyroidectomy in a Japanese population. *Clin Endocrinol.* 2004;60(3):335-342.

358. Khosla S, Ebeling PR, Firek AF, et al. Calcium infusion suggests a "set-point" abnormality of parathyroid gland function in familial benign hypercalcemia and more complex disturbances in primary hyperparathyroidism. *J Clin Endocrinol Metab.* 1993;76:715-720.

359. Nesbit MA, Hannan FM, Howles SA, et al. Mutations affecting G-protein subunit alpha11 in hypercalcemia and hypocalcemia. *N Engl J Med.* 2013;368(26):2476-2486.

360. Nesbit MA, Hannan FM, Howles SA, et al. Mutations in AP2S1 cause familial hypocalciuric hypercalcemia type 3. *Nat Genet.* 2013;45(1):93-97.

361. Kifor O, Moore FD Jr, Delaney M, et al. A syndrome of hypocalciuric hypercalcemia caused by autoantibodies directed at the calcium-sensing receptor. *J Clin Endocrinol Metab.* 2003;88(1):60-72.

362. Pallais JC, Kifor O, Chen YB, et al. Acquired hypocalciuric hypercalcemia due to autoantibodies against the calcium-sensing receptor. *N Engl J Med.* 2004;351(4):362-369.

363. Carling T, Szao E, Bai M, et al. Familial hypercalcemia and hypercalciuria caused by a novel mutation in the cytoplasmic tail of the calcium receptor. *J Clin Endoc Metab.* 2000;85(5):2042-2047.

364. Marx SJ, Attie MF, Levine MA, et al. The hypocalciuric or benign variant of familial hypercalcemia: clinical and biochemical features in fifteen kindreds. *Medicine (Baltimore).* 1981;60(6):397-412.

365. Christensen SE, Nissen PH, Vestergaard P, et al. Discriminative power of three indices of renal calcium excretion for the distinction between familial hypocalciuric hypercalcaemia and primary hyperparathyroidism: a follow-up study on methods. *Clin Endocrinol.* 2008;69(5):713-720.

366. Mallette LE, Khouri K, Zengotita H, et al. Lithium treatment increases intact and midregion parathyroid hormone and parathyroid volume. *J Clin Endocrinol Metab.* 1989;68(3):654-660.

367. Albert U, De Cori D, Aguglia A, et al. Lithium-associated hyperparathyroidism and hypercalcaemia: a case-control cross-sectional study. *J Affect Disord.* 2013;151(2):786-790.

368. Saunders BD, Saunders EF, Gauger PG. Lithium therapy and hyperparathyroidism: an evidence-based assessment. *World J Surg.* 2009;33(11):2314-2323.

369. Marti JL, Yang CS, Carling T, et al. Surgical approach and outcomes in patients with lithium-associated hyperparathyroidism. *Ann Surg Oncol.* 2012;19(11):3465-3471.

370. McHenry CR, Racke F, Meister M, et al. Lithium effects on dispersed bovine parathyroid cells grown in tissue culture. *Surgery.* 1991;110(6):1061-1066.

371. Jacobs TP, Bilezikian JP. Clinical review: rare causes of hypercalcemia. *J Clin Endocrinol Metab.* 2005;90(11):6316-6322.

372. Ehrlich LA, Roodman GD. The role of immune cells and inflammatory cytokines in Paget's disease and multiple myeloma. *Immunol Rev.* 2005;208:252-266.

373. Tian E, Zhan F, Walker R, et al. The role of the Wnt-signaling antagonist DKK1 in the development of osteolytic lesions in multiple myeloma. *N Engl J Med.* 2003;349(26):2483-2494.

374. Gavriatopoulou M, Dimopoulos MA, Christoulas D, et al. Dickkopf-1: a suitable target for the management of myeloma bone disease. *Expert Opin Ther Targets.* 2009;13(7):839-848.

375. Guise TA. Molecular mechanisms of osteolytic bone metastases. *Cancer.* 2000;88(Suppl 12):2892-2898.

376. Albright F. Case records of the Massachusetts General Hospital (case 27461). *N Engl J Med.* 1941;225:789-791.

377. Stewart AF, Horst R, Deftos LJ, et al. Biochemical evaluation of patients with cancer-associated hypercalcemia: evidence for humoral and non-humoral groups. *N Engl J Med.* 1980;303(24):1377-1383.

378. Suva LJ, Winslow GA, Wettenhall RE, et al. A parathyroid hormone-related protein implicated in malignant hypercalcemia: cloning and expression. *Science.* 1987;237(4817):893-896.

379. Kukreja SC, Shevrin DH, Wimbiscus SA, et al. Antibodies to parathyroid hormone-related protein lower serum calcium in athymic mouse models of malignancy-associated hypercalcemia due to human tumors. *J Clin Invest.* 1988;82:1798-1802.

380. Horwitz MJ, Tedesco MB, Sereika SM, et al. Continuous PTH and PTHrP infusion causes suppression of bone formation and discordant effects on 1,25(OH)2 vitamin D. *J Bone Miner Res.* 2005;20(10):1792-1803.

381. Strewler GJ, Wronski TJ, Halloran BP. Pathogenesis of hypercalcemia in nude mice bearing a human renal carcinoma. *Endocrinology.* 1986;119:303-309.

382. Bushinsky DA, Riera GS, Favus MJ, Coe FL. Evidence that blood ionized calcium can regulate serum $1,25(OH)_2D_3$ independently of parathyroid hormone and phosphorus in the rat. *J Clin Invest.* 1985;76:1599-1604.

383. Kitazawa R, Imai Y, Fukase M, Fujita T. Effects of continuous infusion of parathyroid hormone and parathyroid hormone-related peptide on rat bone in vivo: comparative study by histomorphometry. *Bone Miner.* 1991;12(3):157-166.

384. Seymour JF, Gagel RF, Hagemeister FB, et al. Calcitriol production in hypercalcemic and normocalcemic patients with non-Hodgkin lymphoma. *Ann Intern Med.* 1994;121:633-640.
385. Davies M, Hayes ME, Yin JA, et al. Abnormal synthesis of 1,25-dihydroxyvitamin D in patients with malignant lymphoma. *J Clin Endocrinol Metab.* 1994;78(5):1202-1207.
386. Deluca HF, Prahl JM, Plum LA. 1,25-Dihydroxyvitamin D is not responsible for toxicity caused by vitamin D or 25-hydroxyvitamin D. *Arch Biochem Biophys.* 2011;505(2):226-230.
387. Jones G. Pharmacokinetics of vitamin D toxicity. *Am J Clin Nutr.* 2008;88(2):582S-586S.
388. Conron M, Young C, Beynon HL. Calcium metabolism in sarcoidosis and its clinical implications. *Rheumatology (Oxford).* 2000;39(7):707-713.
389. Farooque A, Moss C, Zehnder D, et al. Expression of 25-hydroxyvitamin D3-1alpha-hydroxylase in subcutaneous fat necrosis. *Br J Dermatol.* 2009;160(2):423-425.
390. Abreu MT, Kantorovich V, Vasiliauskas EA, et al. Measurement of vitamin D levels in inflammatory bowel disease patients reveals a subset of Crohn's disease patients with elevated 1,25-dihydroxyvitamin D and low bone mineral density. *Gut.* 2004;53(8):1129-1136.
391. Donovan PJ, Sundac L, Pretorius CJ, et al. Calcitriol-mediated hypercalcemia: causes and course in 101 patients. *J Clin Endocrinol Metab.* 2013;98(10):4023-4029.
392. Auwerx J, Bouillon R. Mineral and bone metabolism in thyroid disease: a review. *Q J Med.* 1986;60:737-752.
393. Bassett JH, Williams GR. The molecular actions of thyroid hormone in bone. *Trends Endocrinol Metab.* 2003;14(8):356-364.
394. Mallette LE, Rubenfeld S, Silverman V. A controlled study of the effects of thyrotoxicosis and propranolol treatment on mineral metabolism and parathyroid hormone immunoreactivity. *Metabolism.* 1985;34:999-1006.
395. Valentic JP, Elias AN, Weinstein GD. Hypercalcemia associated with oral isotretinoin in the treatment of severe acne. *J Am Med Assoc.* 1986;250:1899-1900.
396. Bennett MT, Sirrs S, Yeung JK, Smith CA. Hypercalcemia due to all trans retinoic acid in the treatment of acute promyelocytic leukemia potentiated by voriconazole. *Leuk Lymphoma.* 2005;46(12):1829-1831.
397. Muls E, Bouillon R, Boelaert J, et al. Etiology of hypercalcemia in a patient with Addison's disease. *Calcif Tissue Int.* 1982;34:523-526.
398. Katahira M, Yamada T, Kawai M. A case of Cushing syndrome with both secondary hypothyroidism and hypercalcemia due to postoperative adrenal insufficiency. *Endocr J.* 2004;51(1):105-113.
399. Nijenhuis T, Vallon V, van der Kemp AW, et al. Enhanced passive Ca2+ reabsorption and reduced Mg2+ channel abundance explains thiazide-induced hypocalciuria and hypomagnesemia. *J Clin Invest.* 2005;115(6):1651-1658.
400. Bergsland KJ, Worcester EM, Coe FL. Role of proximal tubule in the hypocalciuric response to thiazide of patients with idiopathic hypercalciuria. *Am J Physiol Renal Physiol.* 2013;305(4):F592-F599.
401. Wermers RA, Kearns AE, Jenkins GD, Melton LJ 3rd. Incidence and clinical spectrum of thiazide-associated hypercalcemia. *Am J Med.* 2007;120(10):911, e9-15.
402. Medarov BI. Milk-alkali syndrome. *Mayo Clin Proc.* 2009;84(3):261-267.
403. Patel AM, Adeseun GA, Goldfarb S. Calcium-alkali syndrome in the modern era. *Nutrients.* 2013;5(12):4880-4893.
404. Yusuf MB, Ikem IC, Oginni LM, et al. Comparison of serum and urinary calcium profile of immobilized and ambulant trauma patients. *Bone.* 2013;57(2):361-366.
405. Llach F, Felsenfeld AJ, Haussler MR. The pathophysiology of altered calcium metabolism in rhabdomyolysis-induced acute renal failure. *N Engl J Med.* 1981;305:117-123.
406. Shrestha SM, Berry JL, Davies M, et al. Biphasic hypercalcemia in severe rhabdomyolysis: serial analysis of PTH and vitamin D metabolites. A case report and literature review. *Am J Kidney Dis.* 2004;43:e31-e35.
407. Williams JCP, Barratt-Boyes BG, Lowe JB. Supravalvular aortic stenosis. *Circulation.* 1961;24:1311-1318.
408. Garabedian M, Jacqz E, Guillozo H, et al. Elevated plasma 1,25-dihydroxyvitamin D concentrations in infants with hypercalcemia and an elfin facies. *N Engl J Med.* 1985;312:948-952.
409. Cagle AP, Waguespack SG, Buckingham BA, et al. Severe infantile hypercalcemia associated with Williams syndrome successfully treated with intravenously administered pamidronate. *Pediatrics.* 2004;114(4):1091-1095.
410. Kitagawa H, Fujiki R, Yoshimura K, et al. The chromatin-remodeling complex WINAC targets a nuclear receptor to promoters and is impaired in Williams syndrome. *Cell.* 2003;113(7):905-917.
411. Kruse K, Schutz C. Calcium metabolism in the Jansen type of metaphyseal dysplasia. *Eur J Pediatr.* 1993;152(11):912-915.
412. Schipani E, Kruse K, Juppner H. A constitutively active mutant PTH-PTHrP receptor in Jansen-type metaphyseal chondrodysplasia. *Science.* 1995;268(5207):98-100.
413. Brown WW, Juppner H, Langman CB, et al. Hypophosphatemia with elevations in serum fibroblast growth factor 23 in a child with Jansen's metaphyseal chondrodysplasia. *J Clin Endocrinol Metab.* 2009;94(1):17-20.
414. Silverberg SJ, Gao P, Brown I, et al. Clinical utility of an immunoradiometric assay for parathyroid hormone (1-84) in primary hyperparathyroidism. *J Clin Endocrinol Metab.* 2003;88(10):4725-4730.
415. Carnevale V, Dionisi S, Nofroni I, et al. Potential clinical utility of a new IRMA for parathyroid hormone in postmenopausal patients with primary hyperparathyroidism. *Clin Chem.* 2004;50(3):626-631.
416. Picolos MK, Lavis VR, Orlander PR. Milk-alkali syndrome is a major cause of hypercalcaemia among non-end-stage renal disease (non-ESRD) inpatients. *Clin Endocrinol.* 2005;63(5):566-576.
417. Hu MI, Glezerman I, Lebonlleux S, et al. Denosumab for patients with persistent or relapsed hypercalcemia of malignancy despite recent bisphosphonate treatment. *J Natl Cancer Inst.* 2013;105(18):1417-1420.
418. Cvitkovic F, Armand JP, Tubiana-Hulin M, et al. Randomized, double-blind, phase II trial of gallium nitrate compared with pamidronate for acute control of cancer-related hypercalcemia. *Cancer J.* 2006;12(1):47-53.
419. Ioachimescu AG, Bauer TW, Licata A. Active Crohn disease and hypercalcemia treated with infliximab: case report and literature review. *Endocr Pract.* 2008;14(1):87-92.
420. Barman Balfour JA, Scott LJ. Cinacalcet hydrochloride. *Drugs.* 2005;65(2):271-281.
421. Onuma E, Sato K, Saito H, et al. Generation of a humanized monoclonal antibody against human parathyroid hormone-related protein and its efficacy against humoral hypercalcemia of malignancy. *Anticancer Res.* 2004;24(5A):2665-2673.
422. Mannstadt M, Bertrand G, Muresan M, et al. Dominant-negative GCMB mutations cause an autosomal dominant form of hypoparathyroidism. *J Clin Endocrinol Metab.* 2008;93:3568-3576.
423. Bockman DE, Kriby ML. Dependence of thymus development on derivatives of the neural crest. *Science.* 1984;223:498-500.
424. Chisaka O, Capecchi MR. Regionally restricted developmental defects resulting from targeted disruption of the mouse homeobox gene hox-1.5. *Nature.* 1991;350:473-479.
425. Garabedian M. Hypocalcemia and chromosome 22q11 microdeletion. *Genet Couns.* 1999;10(4):389-394.
426. Karayiorgou M, Morris MA, Morrow B, et al. Schizophrenia susceptibility associated with interstitial deletions of chromosome 22q11. *Proc Natl Acad Sci U S A.* 1995;92:7612-7616.
427. Budarf ML, Collins J, Gong W, et al. Cloning a balanced translocation associated with DiGeorge syndrome and identfication of a disrupted candidate gene. *Nat Genet.* 1995;10:269-278.
428. Scire G, Dallapiccola B, Iannetti P, et al. Hypoparathyroidism as the major manifestation in two patients with 22q11 deletions. *Am J Med Genet.* 1994;52:478-482.
429. Yagi H, Furutani Y, Hamada H, et al. Role of TBX1 in human del22q11.2 syndrome. *Lancet.* 2003;362(9393):1366-1373.
430. Daw SC, Taylor C, Kraman M, et al. A common region of 10p deleted in DiGeorge and velocardiofacial syndromes. *Nat Genet.* 1996;13(4):458-460.
431. Van Esch H, Groenen P, Nesbit MA, et al. GATA3 haplo-insufficiency causes human HDR syndrome. *Nature.* 2000;406(6794):419-422.
432. Parvari R, Hershkovitz E, Grossman N, et al. Mutation of TBCE causes hypoparathyroidism-retardation-dysmorphism and autosomal recessive Kenny-Caffey syndrome. *Nat Genet.* 2002;32(3):448-452.
433. Su MA, Anderson MS. Aire: an update. *Curr Opin Immunol.* 2004;16(6):746-752.
434. Gardner JM, Fletcher AL, Anderson MS, Turley SJ. AIRE in the thymus and beyond. *Curr Opin Immunol.* 2009;21(6):582-589.
435. Alimohammadi M, Bjorklund P, Hallgren A, et al. Autoimmune polyendocrine syndrome type 1 and NALP5, a parathyroid autoantigen. *N Engl J Med.* 2008;358(10):1018-1028.
436. Cervato S, Morlin L, Albergoni MP, et al. AIRE gene mutations and autoantibodies to interferon omega in patients with chronic hypoparathyroidism without APECED. *Clin Endocrinol (Oxf).* 2010;73(5):630-636.
437. Dionisi-Vici C, Garavaglia B, Burlina AB, et al. Hypoparathyroidism in mitochondrial trifunctional protein deficiency. *J Pediatr.* 1996;129(1):159-162.
438. Papadimitriou A, Hadjigeorgiou GM, Divari R, et al. The influence of coenzyme Q10 on total serum calcium concentration in two patients with Kearns-Sayre syndrome and hypoparathyroidism. *Neuromuscul Disord.* 1996;6(1):49-53.
439. Ahn TG, Antonarakis SE, Kronenberg HM, et al. Familial isolated hypoparathyroidism: a molecular genetic analysis of 8 families with 23 affected persons. *Medicine.* 1986;65:73-81.
440. Baldellou A, Bone J, Tamparillas M, et al. Congenital hypoparathyroidism, ocular colobomata, unilateral renal agenesis and dysmorphic features. *Genet Couns.* 1991;2:245-247.
441. Dahlberg PJ, Borer WZ, Newcomer KL, Yutuc WR. Autosomal or X-linked recessive syndrome of congenital lymphedema, hypoparathyroidism, nephropathy, prolapsing mitral valve, and brachytelephalangy. *Am J Med Genet.* 1983;16:99-104.

442. Parkinson DB, Thakker RV. A donor splice site mutation in the parathyroid hormone gene is associated with autosomal recessive hypoparathyroidism. *Nat Genet.* 1992;2:149-152.
443. Ertl DA, Stary S, Streubel B, et al. A novel homozygous mutation in the parathyroid hormone gene (PTH) in a girl with isolated hypoparathyroidism. *Bone.* 2012;51(3):629-632.
444. Hammes M, DeMory A, Sprague SM. Hypocalcemia in end-stage renal disease: a consequence of spontaneous parathyroid gland infarction. *Am J Kidney Dis.* 1994;24:519-522.
445. Burch WM, Posillico JT. Hypoparathyroidism after I-131 therapy with subsequent return of parathyroid function. *J Clin Endocrinol Metab.* 1983;57:398-401.
446. Gertner JM, Broadus AE, Anast CS, et al. Impaired parathyroid response to induced hypocalcemia in thalassemia major. *J Pediatr.* 1979;95:210-213.
447. Carpenter TO, Carnes DL, Anast CS. Hypoparathyroidism in Wilson's disease. *N Engl J Med.* 1983;309:873-877.
448. Suh SM, Tashjian AH, Matsuo N, et al. Pathogenesis of hypocalcemia in primary hypomagnesemia: normal end-organ responsiveness to parathyroid hormone, impaired parathyroid gland function. *J Clin Invest.* 1973;52:153-160.
449. Estep H, Shaw WA, Watlington C, et al. Hypocalcemia due to hypomagnesemia and reversible parathyroid hormone unresponsiveness. *J Clin Endocrinol Metab.* 1969;29:842-848.
450. Rude RK, Oldham SB, Singer FR. Functional hypoparathyroidism and parathyroid hormone end-organ resistance in human magnesium deficiency. *Clin Endocrinol.* 1976;5:209-224.
451. Krapf R, Jaeger P, Hulter HN, et al. Chronic respiratory alkalosis induces renal PTH-resistance, hyperphosphatemia and hypocalcemia in humans. *Kidney Int.* 1992;42:727-734.
452. Lopez I, Rodriguez M, Felsenfeld AJ, et al. Direct suppressive effect of acute metabolic and respiratory alkalosis on parathyroid hormone secretion in the dog. *J Bone Miner Res.* 2003;18(8):1478-1485.
453. Kifor O, McElduff A, LeBoff MS, et al. Activating antibodies to the calcium-sensing receptor in two patients with autoimmune hypoparathyroidism. *J Clin Endocrinol Metab.* 2004;89(2):548-556.
454. Albright F, Aub J, Bauer W. Hyperparathyroidism. A common and polymorphic condition as illustrated by seventeen proved cases from one clinic. *J Am Med Assoc.* 1934;102:1276-1287.
455. Chase LR, Melson GL, Aurbach GD. Pseudohypoparathyroidism: defective excretion of 3',5'-AMP in response to parathyroid hormone. *J Clin Invest.* 1969;48:1832-1844.
456. Mallette LE, Kirkland JL, Gagel RF, et al. Synthetic human parathyroid hormone-(1-34) for the study of pseudohypoparathyroidism. *J Clin Endocrinol Metab.* 1988;67:964-972.
457. Bastepe M. The GNAS locus and pseudohypoparathyroidism. *Adv Exp Med Biol.* 2008;626:27-40.
458. Mantovani G, de Sanctis L, Barbieri AM, et al. Pseudohypoparathyroidism and GNAS epigenetic defects: clinical evaluation of Albright hereditary osteodystrophy and molecular analysis in 40 patients. *J Clin Endocrinol Metab.* 2010;95(2):651-658.
459. Iiri T, Herzmark P, Nakamoto JM, et al. Rapid GDP release from Gsa in patients with gain and loss of endocrine function. *Nature.* 1994;371:164-168.
460. Levine MA, Ahn TG, Klupt SF, et al. Genetic deficiency of the a subunit of the guanine nucleotide-binding protein Gs as the molecular basis for Albright hereditary osteodystrophy. *Proc Natl Acad Sci U S A.* 1988;85:617-621.
461. Davies SJ, Hughes HE. Imprinting in Albright's hereditary osteodystrophy. *J Med Genet.* 1993;30:101-103.
462. Wilson LC, Oude Luttikhuis ME, Clayton PT, et al. Parental origin of Gs alpha gene mutations in Albright's hereditary osteodystrophy. *J Med Genet.* 1994;31:835-839.
463. Yu S, Yu D, Lee E, et al. Variable and tissue-specific hormone resistance in heterotrimeric Gs protein alpha-subunit (Gsalpha) knockout mice is due to tissue-specific imprinting of the Gsalpha gene. *Proc Natl Acad Sci U S A.* 1998;95(15):8715-8720.
464. Richard N, Molin A, Coudray N, et al. Paternal GNAS mutations lead to severe intrauterine growth retardation (IUGR) and provide evidence for a role of XLalphas in fetal development. *J Clin Endocrinol Metab.* 2013;98(9):E1549-E1556.
465. Adegbite NS, Xu M, Kaplan FS, et al. Diagnostic and mutational spectrum of progressive osseous heteroplasia (POH) and other forms of GNAS-based heterotopic ossification. *Am J Med Genet A.* 2008;146A(14):1788-1796.
466. Farfel Z, Bourne HR, Iiri T. The expanding spectrum of G protein diseases. *N Engl J Med.* 1999;340(13):1012-1020.
467. Bastepe M, Lane AH, Juppner H. Paternal uniparental isodisomy of chromosome 20q—and the resulting changes in GNAS1 methylation—as a plausible cause of pseudohypoparathyroidism. *Am J Hum Genet.* 2001;68(5):1283-1289.
468. Bastepe M, Pincus JE, Sugimoto T, et al. Positional dissociation between the genetic mutation responsible for pseudohypoparathyroidism type Ib and the associated methylation defect at exon A/B: evidence for a long-range regulatory element within the imprinted GNAS1 locus. *Hum Mol Genet.* 2001;10(12):1231-1241.
469. Liu J, Erlichman B, Weinstein LS. The stimulatory G protein alpha-subunit Gs alpha is imprinted in human thyroid glands: implications for thyroid function in pseudohypoparathyroidism types 1A and 1B. *J Clin Endocrinol Metab.* 2003;88(9):4336-4341.
470. Murray TM, Rao LG, Wong MM, et al. Pseudohypoparathyroidism with osteitis fibrosa cystica: direct demonstration of skeletal responsiveness to parathyroid hormone in cells cultured from bone. *J Bone Miner Res.* 1993;8:83-91.
471. Jüppner H, Schipani E, Bastepe M, et al. The gene responsible for pseudohypoparathyroidism type Ib is paternally imprinted and maps in four unrelated kindreds to chromosome 20q13.3. *Proc Natl Acad Sci U S A.* 1998;95:11798-11803.
472. Jan de Beur S, Ding C, Germain-Lee E, et al. Discordance between genetic and epigenetic defects in pseudohypoparathyroidism type 1b revealed by inconsistent loss of maternal imprinting at GNAS1. *Am J Hum Genet.* 2003;73(2):314-322.
473. Liu J, Litman D, Rosenberg MJ, et al. A GNAS1 imprinting defect in pseudohypoparathyroidism type IB. *J Clin Invest.* 2000;106(9):1167-1174.
474. Bastepe M, Frohlich LF, Hendy GN, et al. Autosomal dominant pseudohypoparathyroidism type Ib is associated with a heterozygous microdeletion that likely disrupts a putative imprinting control element of GNAS. *J Clin Invest.* 2003;112(8):1255-1263.
475. Linglart A, Gensure RC, Olney RC, et al. A novel STX16 deletion in autosomal dominant pseudohypoparathyroidism type Ib redefines the boundaries of a cis-acting imprinting control element of GNAS. *Am J Hum Genet.* 2005;76(5):804-814.
476. Barrett D, Breslau NA, Wax MB, et al. New form of pseudohypoparathyroidism with abnormal catalytic adenylate cyclase. *Am J Physiol.* 1989;257:E277-E283.
477. Linglart A, Carel JC, Garabedian M, et al. GNAS1 lesions in pseudohypoparathyroidism Ia and Ic: genotype phenotype relationship and evidence of the maternal transmission of the hormonal resistance. *J Clin Endocrinol Metab.* 2002;87(1):189-197.
478. Drezner M, Neelon FA, Lebovitz HE. Pseudohypoparathyroidism type II: a possible defect in the reception of the cyclic AMP signal. *N Engl J Med.* 1973;289:1056-1060.
479. Rao DS, Parfitt AM, Kleerekoper M, et al. Dissociation between the effects of endogenous parathyroid hormone on adenosine 3',5'-monophosphate generation and phosphate reabsorption in hypocalcemia due to vitamin D depletion: an acquired disorder resembling pseudohypoparathyroidism type II. *J Clin Endocrinol Metab.* 1985;61(2):285-290.
480. Koo BB, Schwindinger WF, Levine MA. Characterization of Albright hereditary osteodystrophy and related disorders. *Acta Pediatr Sin.* 1995;36:3-13.
481. Minagawa M, Yasuda T, Kobayashi Y, Niimi H. Transient pseudohypoparathyroidism of the neonate. *Eur J Endocrinol.* 1995;133:151-155.
482. Silve C. Pseudohypoparathyroidism syndromes: the many faces of parathyroid hormone resistance. *Eur J Endocrinol.* 1995;133:145-146.
483. Kidd GS, Schaaf M, Adler RA, et al. Skeletal responsiveness in pseudohypoparathyroidism. *Am J Med.* 1980;68:772-781.
484. Kruse K, Kracht U, Wohlfart K, Kruse U. Biochemical markers of bone turnover, intact serum parathyroid hormone and renal calcium excretion in patients with pseudohypoparathyroidism and hypoparathyroidism before and during vitamin D treatment. *Eur J Pediatr.* 1989;148:535-539.
485. Breslau NA, Moses AM, Pak CYC. Evidence for bone remodeling but lack of calcium mobilization response to parathyroid hormone in pseudohypoparathyroidism. *J Clin Endocrinol Metab.* 1983;57:638-644.
486. Yamamoto M, Takuwa Y, Masuko S, Ogata E. Effects of endogenous and exogenous parathyroid hormone on tubular reabsorption of calcium in pseudohypoparathyroidism. *J Clin Endocrinol Metab.* 1988;66(3):618-625.
487. Thomas MK, Lloyd-Jones DM, Thadhani RI, et al. Hypovitaminosis D in medical inpatients. *N Engl J Med.* 1998;338(12):777-783.
488. Tripkovic L, Lambert H, Hart K, et al. Comparison of vitamin D2 and vitamin D3 supplementation in raising serum 25-hydroxyvitamin D status: a systematic review and meta-analysis. *Am J Clin Nutr.* 2012;95(6):1357-1364.
489. Thomas MK, Demay MB. Vitamin D deficiency and disorders of vitamin D metabolism. *Endocrinol Metab Clin North Am.* 2000;29(3):611-627.
490. Chapuy MC, Arlot ME, Duboeuf F, et al. Vitamin D3 and calcium to prevent hip fractures in elderly women. *N Engl J Med.* 1992;327:1637-1642.
491. Hahn TJ, Hendin BA, Scharp CR, Haddad JG. Effect of chronic anticonvulsant therapy on serum 25-hydroxycalciferol levels in adults. *N Engl J Med.* 1972;287:900-904.
492. Greenwood RH, Pruntz FTG, Silver J. Osteomalacia after prolonged glutethimide administration. *Br Med J.* 1973;1:643-645.
493. Brodie MJ, Boobis AR, Hillyard CJ, et al. Effect of rifampicin and isoniazid on vitamin D metabolism. *Clin Pharmacol Ther.* 1982;32:525-530.
494. Casella SJ, Reiner BJ, Chen TC, et al. A possible genetic defect in 25-hydroxylation as a cause of rickets. *J Pediatr.* 1994;124:929-932.

495. Al Mutair AN, Nasrat GH, Russell DW. Mutation of the CYP2R1 vitamin D 25-hydroxylase in a Saudi Arabian family with severe vitamin D deficiency. *J Clin Endocrinol Metab.* 2012;97(10): E2022-E2025.

496. Cheng JB, Levine MA, Bell NH, et al. Genetic evidence that the human CYP2R1 enzyme is a key vitamin D 25-hydroxylase. *Proc Natl Acad Sci U S A.* 2004;101(20):7711-7715.

497. Tosson H, Rose SR. Absence of mutation in coding regions of CYP2R1 gene in apparent autosomal dominant vitamin D 25-hydroxylase deficiency rickets. *J Clin Endocrinol Metab.* 2012; 97(5):E796-E801.

498. Zhu JG, Ochalek JT, Kaufmann M, et al. CYP2R1 is a major, but not exclusive, contributor to 25-hydroxyvitamin D production in vivo. *Proc Natl Acad Sci U S A.* 2013;110(39):15650-15655.

499. Goodman WG. Calcimimetic agents for the treatment of secondary hyperparathyroidism. *Semin Nephrol.* 2004;24(5):460-463.

500. Delvin EE, Glorieux FH, Marie PJ, Pettifor JM. Vitamin D dependency: replacement therapy with calcitriol. *Pediatrics.* 1981;99:26-34.

501. Scriver CR, Reade TM, DeLuca HF, Hamstra AJ. Serum 1,25-dihydroxyvitamin D levels in normal subjects and in patients with hereditary rickets or bone disease. *N Engl J Med.* 1978;299: 976-979.

502. Fraser D, Kooh SW, Kind HP, et al. Pathogenesis of hereditary vitamin-D-dependent rickets: an inborn error of vitamin D metabolism involving defective conversion of 25-hydroxyvitamin D to 1a,25-dihydroxyvitamin D. *N Engl J Med.* 1973;289:817-822.

503. Glorieux FH. Calcitriol treatment in vitamin D-dependent and vitamin D-resistant rickets. *Metabolism.* 1990;39:10-12.

504. Malloy PJ, Pike JW, Feldman D. The vitamin D receptor and the syndrome of hereditary 1,25-dihydroxyvitamin D-resistant rickets. *Endocr Rev.* 1999;20(2):156-188.

505. Fraher LJ, Karmali R, Hinde FRJ, et al. Vitamin D-dependent rickets type II: extreme end organ resistance to 1,25-dihydroxy vitamin D$_3$ in a patient without alopecia. *Eur J Pediatr.* 1986;145:389-395.

506. Bell NH. Vitamin D-dependent rickets type II. *Calcif Tissue Int.* 1980;31:89-91.

507. Takeda E, Yokota I, Kawakami I, et al. Two siblings with vitamin-D-dependent rickets type II: no recurrence of rickets for 14 years after cessation of therapy. *Eur J Pediatr.* 1989;149:54-57.

508. Marx SJ, Liberman UA, Eil C, et al. Hereditary resistance to 1,25-dihydroxyvitamin D. *Recent Prog Horm Res.* 1984;40:589-615.

509. Harrison HC, Harrison HE. Inhibition of vitamin D-stimulated active transport of calcium of rat intestine by diphenylhydantoin-phenobarbital treatment. *Proc Soc Exp Biol Med.* 1976;153:220-224.

510. Kido Y, Okamura T, Tomikawa M, et al. Hypocalcemia associated with 5-fluorouracil and low dose leucovorin in patients with advanced colorectal or gastric carcinomas. *Cancer.* 1996;78(8):1794-1797.

511. Relkin R. Hypocalcemia resulting from calcium accretion by a chondrosarcoma. *Cancer.* 1974;34:1834-1837.

512. Dembinski TC, Yatscoff RW, Blandford DE. Thyrotoxicosis and hungry bone syndrome—a cause of posttreatment hypocalcemia. *Clin Biochem.* 1994;27:69-74.

513. Jacobson MA, Gambertoglio JG, Aweeka FT, et al. Foscarnet-induced hypocalcemia and effects of foscarnet on calcium metabolism. *J Clin Endocrinol Metab.* 1991;72:1130-1135.

514. Aggeler PM, Perkins HA, Watkins HB. Hypocalcemia and defective hemostasis after massive blood transfusion. Report of a case. *Transfusion.* 1967;7:35-39.

515. Greco RJ, Hartford CE, Haith LR, Patton ML. Hydrofluoric acid-induced hypocalcemia. *J Trauma.* 1988;28:1593-1596.

516. Kao WF, Dart RC, Kuffner E, Bogdan G. Ingestion of low-concentration hydrofluoric acid: an insidious and potentially fatal poisoning. *Ann Emerg Med.* 1999;34(1):35-41.

517. Tsang RC, Kleinman LI, Sutherland JM, Light IJ. Hypocalcemia in infants of diabetic mothers. *J Pediatr.* 1972;80:384-395.

518. Tsang RC, Light IJ, Sutherland JM, Kleinman LI. Possible pathogenetic factors in neonatal hypocalcemia of prematurity. *J Pediatr.* 1973;82: 423-429.

519. Kaplan EL, Burrington JD, Klementschitsch P, et al. Primary hyperparathyroidism, pregnancy and neonatal hypocalcemia. *Surgery.* 1984;96: 717-722.

520. Kuehn EW, Anders HJ, Bogner JR, et al. Hypocalcaemia in HIV infection and AIDS. *J Intern Med.* 1999;245(1):69-73.

521. Lind L, Carlstedt F, Rastad J, et al. Hypocalcemia and parathyroid hormone secretion in critically ill patients. *Crit Care Med.* 2000;28(1): 93-99.

522. Canaff L, Hendy GN. Calcium-sensing receptor gene transcription is up-regulated by the proinflammatory cytokine, interleukin-1beta. Role of the NF-kappaB PATHWAY and kappaB elements. *J Biol Chem.* 2005; 280(14):14177-14188.

523. Canaff L, Zhou X, Hendy GN. The proinflammatory cytokine, interleukin-6, up-regulates calcium-sensing receptor gene transcription via Stat1/3 and Sp1/3. *J Biol Chem.* 2008;283(20):13586-13600.

524. Stewart AF, Longo W, Kreutter D, et al. Hypocalcemia associated with calcium-soap formation in a patient with a pancreatic fistula. *N Engl J Med.* 1986;315:496-498.

525. Dettelbach MA, Deftos LJ, Stewart AF. Intraperitoneal free fatty acids induce severe hypocalcemia in rats: a model for the hypocalcemia of pancreatitis. *J Bone Miner Res.* 1990;5:1249-1255.

526. Norberg HP, DeRoos J, Kaplan EL. Increased parathyroid hormone secretion and hypocalcemia in experimental pancreatitis: necessity for an intact thyroid gland. *Surgery.* 1975;77:773-779.

527. Weir GC, Lesser PB, Drop LJ, et al. The hypocalcemia of acute pancreatitis. *Ann Intern Med.* 1975;83:185-189.

528. Desai TK, Carlson RW, Geheb MA. Prevalence and clinical implications of hypocalcemia in acutely ill patients in a medical intensive care setting. *Am J Med.* 1988;84:209-214.

529. Winer KK, Sinaii N, Peterson D, et al. Effects of once versus twice-daily parathyroid hormone 1-34 therapy in children with hypoparathyroidism. *J Clin Endocrinol Metab.* 2008;93(9):3389-3395.

530. Mitchell DM, Regan S, Cooley MR, et al. Long-term follow-up of patients with hypoparathyroidism. *J Clin Endocrinol Metab.* 2012; 97(12):4507-4514.

531. Gupta A, Winer K, Econs MJ, et al. FGF-23 is elevated by chronic hyperphosphatemia. *J Clin Endocrinol Metab.* 2004;89(9):4489-4492.

532. Okano K, Furukawa Y, Hirotoshi M, Fujita T. Comparative efficacy of various vitamin D metabolites in the treatment of various types of hypoparathyroidism. *J Clin Endocrinol Metab.* 1982;55:238-242.

533. Corvilain J, Abramow M. Growth and renal control of plasma phosphate. *J Clin Endocrinol Metab.* 1972;34:452-459.

534. Lyles KW, Halsey DL, Friedman NE, Lobaugh B. Correlations of serum concentrations of 1,25-dihydroxyvitamin D, phosphorus, and parathyroid hormone in tumoral calcinosis. *J Clin Endocrinol Metab.* 1988; 67(1):88-92.

535. Larsson T, Davis SI, Garringer HJ, et al. Fibroblast growth factor-23 mutants causing familial tumoral calcinosis are differentially processed. *Endocrinology.* 2005;146(9):3883-3891.

536. Topaz O, Shurman DL, Bergman R, et al. Mutations in GALNT3, encoding a protein involved in O-linked glycosylation, cause familial tumoral calcinosis. *Nat Genet.* 2004;36(6):579-581.

537. Finer G, Price HE, Shore RM, et al. Hyperphosphatemic familial tumoral calcinosis: response to acetazolamide and postulated mechanisms. *Am J Med Genet A.* 2014;164A(6):1545-1549.

538. McBryde KD, Wilcox J, Kher KK. Hyperphosphatemia due to fosphenytoin in a pediatric ESRD patient. *Pediatr Nephrol.* 2005;20(8): 1182-1185.

539. Markowitz GS, Stokes MB, Radhakrishnan J, D'Agati VD. Acute phosphate nephropathy following oral sodium phosphate bowel purgative: an underrecognized cause of chronic renal failure. *J Am Soc Nephrol.* 2005;16(11):3389-3396.

540. Miller PD, Heinig RE, Waterhouse C. Treatment of alcoholic ketoacidosis. *Arch Intern Med.* 1978;138:57-72.

541. Marcu CB, Hotchkiss M. Pseudohyperphosphatemia in a patient with multiple myeloma. *Conn Med.* 2004;68(2):71-72.

542. Spencer H, Lewin I, Samachson J, Lazlo J. Changes in metabolism in obese persons during starvation. *Am J Med.* 1966;40:27-37.

543. Silvis SE, Paragas PU Jr. Paresthesias, weakness, seizures and hypophosphatemia in patients receiving hyperalimentation. *Gastroenterology.* 1972;62:513-520.

544. Berman E, Nicolaides M, Maki RG, et al. Altered bone and mineral metabolism in patients receiving imatinib mesylate. *N Engl J Med.* 2006;354(19):2006-2013.

545. Vandyke K, Fitter S, Dewar AL, et al. Dysregulation of bone remodeling by imatinib mesylate. *Blood.* 2010;115(4):766-774.

546. O'Sullivan S, Lin JM, Watson M, et al. The skeletal effects of the tyrosine kinase inhibitor nilotinib. *Bone.* 2011;49(2):281-289.

547. Quarles LD. FGF23, PHEX, and MEPE regulation of phosphate homeostasis and skeletal mineralization. *Am J Physiol Endocrinol Metab.* 2003; 285(1):E1-E9.

548. Schiavi SC, Kumar R. The phosphatonin pathway: new insights in phosphate homeostasis. *Kidney Int.* 2004;65(1):1-14.

549. Berndt TJ, Schiavi S, Kumar R. Phosphatonins and the regulation of phosphorus homeostasis. *Am J Physiol Renal Physiol.* 2005;289(6): F1170-F1182.

550. Lorenz-Depiereux B, Bastepe M, Benet-Pages A, et al. DMP1 mutations in autosomal recessive hypophosphatemia implicate a bone matrix protein in the regulation of phosphate homeostasis. *Nat Genet.* 2006; 38(11):1248-1250.

551. Ito N, Fukumoto S, Takeuchi Y, et al. Comparison of two assays for fibroblast growth factor (FGF)-23. *J Bone Miner Metab.* 2005;23:435-440.

552. Yamamoto T, Imanishi Y, Kinoshita E, et al. The role of fibroblast growth factor 23 for hypophosphatemia and abnormal regulation of vitamin D metabolism in patients with McCune-Albright syndrome. *J Bone Miner Metab.* 2005;23:231-237.

553. Riminucci M, Collins MT, Fedarko NS, et al. FGF-23 in fibrous dysplasia of bone and its relationship to renal phosphate wasting [see comment]. *J Clin Invest.* 2003;112:683-692.

554. Hoffman WH, Jueppner HW, Deyoung BR, et al. Elevated fibroblast growth factor-23 in hypophosphatemic linear nevus sebaceous syndrome. *Am J Med Genet.* 2005;134:233-236.

555. Rendina D, Mossetti G, De Filippo G, et al. Fibroblast growth factor 23 is increased in calcium nephrolithiasis with hypophosphatemia

and renal phosphate leak. *J Clin Endocrinol Metab.* 2006;91(3): 959-963.

556. Prié D, Huart V, Bakouh N, et al. Nephrolithiasis and osteoporosis associated with hypophosphatemia caused by mutations in the type 2a sodium phosphate cotransporter. *N Engl J Med.* 2002;347(13): 983-991.

557. Bergwitz C, Roslin NM, Tieder M, et al. SLC34A3 mutations in patients with hereditary hypophosphatemic rickets with hypercalciuria predict a key role for the sodium-phosphate cotransporter NaPi-IIc in maintaining phosphate homeostasis. *Am J Hum Genet.* 2006;78(2): 179-192.

558. Lorenz-Depiereux B, Benet-Pages A, Eckstein G, et al. Hereditary hypophosphatemic rickets with hypercalciuria is caused by mutations in the sodium-phosphate cotransporter gene SLC34A3. *Am J Hum Genet.* 2006;78(2):193-201.

559. Green J, Debby H, Lederer E, et al. Evidence for a PTH-independent humoral mechanism in post-transplant hypophosphatemia and phosphaturia. *Kidney Int.* 2001;60(3):1182-1196.

560. Salem RR, Tray K. Hepatic resection-related hypophosphatemia is of renal origin as manifested by isolated hyperphosphaturia. *Ann Surg.* 2005;241(2):343-348.

561. Chung PY, Sitrin MD, Te HS. Serum phosphorus levels predict clinical outcome in fulminant hepatic failure. *Liver Transplant.* 2003;9(3): 248-253.

562. Daily WH, Tonnesen AS, Allen SJ. Hypophosphatemia. Incidence, etiology and prevention in the trauma patient. *Crit Care Med.* 1990; 18:1210-1214.

563. Vanneste J, Hage J. Acute severe hypophosphatemia mimicking Wernicke's encephalopathy. *Lancet.* 1986;1:44.

564. Singhal PC, Kumar A, Desroches L, et al. Prevalence and predictors of rhabdomyolysis in patients with hypophosphatemia. *Am J Med.* 1992; 92:458-464.

565. Gabow PA, Kaehny WD, Kelleher SP. The spectrum of rhabdomyolysis. *Medicine.* 1982;61:141-152.

566. Knochel JR, Bilbrey GL, Fuller TJ, Carter NW. The muscle cell in chronic alcoholism: the possible role of phosphate depletion in alcoholic myopathy. *Ann N Y Acad Sci.* 1975;252:274-286.

567. Agusti AG, Torres A, Estopa R, Agusti-Vidal A. Hypophosphatemia as a cause of failed weaning: the importance of metanolic factors. *Crit Care Med.* 1984;12:142-143.

568. Aubier M, Murciano D, Lecocguic Y, et al. Effect of hypophosphatemia on diaphragmatic contractility in patients with acute respiratory failure. *N Engl J Med.* 1985;3131:420-424.

569. Bollaert PE, Levy B, Nace L, et al. Hemodynamic and metabolic effects of rapid correction of hypophosphatemia in patients with septic shock. *Chest.* 1995;107(6):1698-1701.

570. Lichtman MA, Miller DR, Cohen J, Waterhouse C. Reduced red cell glycolysis, 2,3-diphosphoglycerate and adenosine triphosphate concentration and increased hemoglobin oxygen affinity caused by hypophosphatemia. *Ann Intern Med.* 1971;74:562-568.

571. Travis SF, Sugerman HJ. Alterations in red-cell glycolytic intermediates and oxygen transport as a consequence of hypophosphatemia in patients receiving intravenous hyperalimentation. *N Engl J Med.* 1971; 285:763-768.

572. DeFronzo RA, Lang R. Hypophosphatemia and glucose interolerance: evidence for tissue insensitivity to insulin. *N Engl J Med.* 1980; 202:1259-1263.

573. Wilson HK, Keuer SP, Lea AS, et al. Phosphate therapy in diabetic ketoacidosis. *Arch Intern Med.* 1982;142:517-520.

574. Keller U, Berger W. Prevention of hypophosphatemia by phosphate infusion during treatment of diabetic ketoacidosis and hyperosmolar coma. *Diabetes.* 1980;29:87-95.

575. Rosen GH, Boullata JI, O'Rangers EA, et al. Intravenous phosphate repletion regimen for critically ill patients with moderate hypophosphatemia. *Crit Care Med.* 1995;23(7):1204-1210.

576. Charron T, Bernard F, Skrobik Y, et al. Intravenous phosphate in the intensive care unit: more aggressive repletion regimens for moderate and severe hypophosphatemia. *Intensive Care Med.* 2003;29(8): 1273-1278.

577. Taylor BE, Huey WY, Buchman TG, et al. Treatment of hypophosphatemia using a protocol based on patient weight and serum phosphorus level in a surgical intensive care unit. *J Am Coll Surg.* 2004; 198(2):198-204.

578. Broner CW, Stidham GL, Westenkirchner DF, Tolley EA. Hypermagnesemia and hypocalcemia as predictors of high mortality in critically ill pediatric patients. *Crit Care Med.* 1990;18(9):921-928.

579. Mordes JP, Wacker WE. Excess magnesium. *Pharmacol Rev.* 1978;29: 273-300.

580. Cao Z, Bideau R, Valdes R Jr, Elin RJ. Acute hypermagnesemia and respiratory arrest following infusion of MgSO$_4$ for tocolysis. *Clin Chim Acta.* 1999;285(1–2):191-193.

581. Rasch DK, Huber PA, Richardson CJ, et al. Neurobehavioral effects of neonatal hypermagnesemia. *J Pediatr.* 1982;100(2):272-276.

582. Donovan EF, Tsang RC, Steichen JJ, et al. Neonatal hypermagnesemia: effect on parathyroid hormone and calcium homeostasis. *J Pediatr.* 1980;96(2):305-310.

583. Brand JM, Greer FR. Hypermagnesemia and intestinal perforation following antacid administration in a premature infant [see comments]. *Pediatrics.* 1990;85(1):121-124.

584. Mordes JP, Swartz R, Arky RA. Extreme hypermagnesemia as a cause of refractory hypotension. *Ann Intern Med.* 1975;83(5):657-658.

585. Ferdinandus J, Pederson JA, Whang R. Hypermagnesemia as a cause of refractory hypotension, respiratory depression, and coma. *Arch Intern Med.* 1981;141(5):669-670.

586. Cholst IN, Steinberg SF, Tropper PJ, et al. The influence of hypermagnesemia on serum calcium and parathyroid hormone levels in human subjects. *N Engl J Med.* 1984;310:1221-1225.

587. Cruikshank DP, Pitkin RM, Donnelly E, Reynolds WA. Urinary magnesium, calcium, and phosphate excretion during the magnesium sulfate infusion. *Obstet Gynecol.* 1981;58:430-434.

588. Fassler CA, Rodriguez RM, Badesch DB, et al. Magnesium toxicity as a cause of hypotension and hypoventilation. Occurrence in patients with normal renal function. *Arch Intern Med.* 1985;145(9):1604-1606.

589. Alfrey AC, Miller NL, Butkus D. Evaluation of body magnesium stores. *J Lab Clin Med.* 1974;84:153-162.

590. Lim P, Jacob E. Magnesium status of alcoholic patients. *Metabolism.* 1972;21:1045-1051.

591. Al-Ghamdi SMG, Cameron EC, Sutton RAL. Magnesium deficiency: pathophysiologic and clinical overview. [Review]. *Am J Kidney Dis.* 1994;24(5):737-752.

592. Barnes BA. Magnesium conservation: a study of surgical patients. *Ann N Y Acad Sci.* 1969;162:786-801.

593. Rude RK, Singer FR. Magnesium deficiency and excess. *Ann Rev Med.* 1981;32:245-259.

594. Schmitz C, Perraud AL, Fleig A, Scharenberg AM. Dual-function ion channel/protein kinases: novel components of vertebrate magnesium regulatory mechanisms. *Pediatr Res.* 2004;55(5):734-737.

595. Konrad M, Schaller A, Seelow D, et al. Mutations in the tight-junction gene claudin 19 (CLDN19) are associated with renal magnesium wasting, renal failure, and severe ocular involvement. *Am J Hum Genet.* 2006;79(5):949-957.

596. Ellison DH. Divalent cation transport by the distal nephron: insights from Bartter's and Gitelman's syndromes. *Am J Physiol Renal Physiol.* 2000;279(4):F616-F625.

597. Konrad M, Schlingmann KP, Gudermann T. Insights into the molecular nature of magnesium homeostasis. *Am J Physiol Renal Physiol.* 2004; 286(4):F599-F605.

598. Schlingmann KP, Konrad M, Seyberth HW. Genetics of hereditary disorders of magnesium homeostasis. *Pediatr Nephrol.* 2004;19(1): 13-25.

599. Nagase T, Murakami T, Tsukada T, et al. A family of autosomal dominant hypocalcemia with a positive correlation between serum calcium and magnesium: identification of a novel gain of function mutation (Ser(820)Phe) in the calcium-sensing receptor. *J Clin Endocrinol Metab.* 2002;87(6):2681-2687.

600. Simon DB, Nelson-Williams C, Bia MJ, et al. Gitelman's variant of Bartter's syndrome, inherited hypokalaemic alkalosis, is caused by mutations in the thiazide-sensitive Na-Cl cotransporter. *Nat Genet.* 1996;12(1):24-30.

601. Meij IC, Koenderink JB, De Jong JC, et al. Dominant isolated renal magnesium loss is caused by misrouting of the Na+,K+-ATPase gamma-subunit. *Ann N Y Acad Sci.* 2003;986:437-443.

602. Kantorovich V, Adams JS, Gaines JE, et al. Genetic heterogeneity in familial renal magnesium wasting. *J Clin Endocrinol Metab.* 2002;87(2): 612-617.

603. Groenestege WM, Thebault S, van der Wijst J, et al. Impaired basolateral sorting of pro-EGF causes isolated recessive renal hypomagnesemia. *J Clin Invest.* 2007;117(8):2260-2267.

604. Wilson FH, Hariri A, Farhi A, et al. A cluster of metabolic defects caused by mutation in a mitochondrial tRNA. *Science.* 2004;306(5699): 1190-1194.

605. Glaudemans B, Knoers NV, Hoenderop JG, Bindels RJ. New molecular players facilitating Mg(2+) reabsorption in the distal convoluted tubule. *Kidney Int.* 2010;77(1):17-22.

606. Shils ME. Experimental human magnesium depletion. *Medicine.* 1969;48:61-85.

607. King RG, Stanbury SW. Magnesium metabolism in primary hyperparathyroidism. *Clin Sci.* 1970;39:281-303.

608. Jones KH, Fourman P. Effects of infusions of magnesium and of calcium in parathyroid insufficiency. *Clin Sci.* 1966;30:139-150.

609. Jackson CE, Meier DW. Routine serum magnesium analysis. *Ann Intern Med.* 1968;69:743-748.

610. Mather HM, Nisbet JA, Burton GH, et al. Hypomagnesemia in diabetes. *Clin Chim Acta.* 1979;95:235-242.

611. Martin HE. Clinical magnesium deficiency. *Ann N Y Acad Sci.* 1969;162: 891-900.

612. Laitinen K, Lamberg-Allardt C, Tunninen R, et al. Transient hypoparathyroidism during acute alcohol intoxication. *N Engl J Med.* 1991;324: 721-727.

613. Schilsky RI, Anderson T. Hypomagnesemia and renal magnesium wasting in patients receiving cisplatin. *Ann Intern Med.* 1979;90: 929-931.

614. England MR, Gordon G, Salem M, Chernow B. Magnesium administration and dysrhythmias after cardiac surgery. A placebo-controlled, double-blind, randomized trial [see comments]. *J Am Med Assoc.* 1992; 268(17):2395-2402.

615. McLellan BA, Reid SR, Lane PL. Massive blood transfusion causing hypomagnesemia. *Crit Care Med.* 1984;12:146-147.

616. Beller GA, Hood DB, Smith TW, et al. Correlation of serum magnesium levels and cardiac digitalis intoxication. *Am J Cardiol.* 1974;33: 225-229.

617. Whang R, Morosi HJ, Rodgers D, Reyes R. The influence of sustained magnesium deficiency on muscle potassium repletion. *J Lab Clin Med.* 1967;70:895-902.

618. Muldowney FP, McKenna TJ, Kyle LH, et al. Parathormone-like effect of magnesium replenishment in steatorrhea. *N Engl J Med.* 1970;281: 61-68.

619. Allgrove J, Adami S, Fraher L, et al. Hypomagnesemia: studies of parathyroid hormone secretion and function. *Clin Endocrinol.* 1984;21: 435-449.

620. Quitterer U, Hoffmann M, Freichel M, Lohse MJ. Paradoxical block of parathormone secretion is mediated by increased activity of G alpha subunits. *J Biol Chem.* 2001;276(9):6763-6769.

621. Johannesson AJ, Raisz LG. Effects of low media magnesium concentration on bone resorption in response to parathyroid hormone and 1,25-dihydroxyvitamin D in organ culture. *Endocrinology.* 1983;113: 2294-2298.

622. Medalle R, Waterhouse C, Hahn TJ. Vitamin D resistance in magnesium deficiency. *Am J Clin Nutr.* 1976;29:854-858.

623. Heaton FW, Fourman P. Magnesium deficiency and hypocalcaemia in intestinal malabsorption. *Lancet.* 1965;2:50-52.

624. Rosler A, Rabinowitz D. Magnesium induced reversal of vitamin D resistance in hypoparathyroidism. *Lancet.* 1973;1:803-805.

625. Rude RK, Adams JS, Ryzen E, et al. Low serum concentrations of 1,25-dihydroxyvitamin D in human magnesium deficiency. *J Clin Endocrinol Metab.* 1985;61:933-940.

626. Fuss M, Cogan E, Gillet C, et al. Magnesium administration reverses the hypocalcemia secondary to hypomagnesemia despite low circulating levels of 25-hydroxyvitamin D and 1,25-dihydroxyvitamin D. *Clin Endocrinol.* 1985;22:807-815.

627. Fuss M, Bergmann P, Bergans A, et al. Correction of low circulating levels of 1,25-dihydroxyvitamin D by 25-hydroxyvitamin D during reversal of hypomagnesaemia. *Clin Endocrinol.* 1989;31:31-38.

628. Brannan PG, Vergne-Marini P, Pak CYC, et al. Magnesium absorption in the human small intestine. *J Clin Invest.* 1976;57:1412-1418.

629. Flink EB. Therapy of magnesium deficiency. *Ann N Y Acad Sci.* 1969; 162:901-905.

630. Sutton RAL, Walker VR, Halabe A, et al. Chronic hypomagnesemia caused by cisplatin: effect of calcitriol. *J Lab Clin Med.* 1991;117: 40-43.

CHAPTER 29

Osteoporosis and Bone Biology

FRANCISCO J. A. DE PAULA • DENNIS M. BLACK • CLIFFORD J. ROSEN

KEY POINTS

- The functional significance of bone has been completely reexamined in light of recent discoveries. For example, in addition to the obvious mechanical support and storage of mineral that have been considered the classic roles of the skeleton, the mineralized mesenchymal tissue also exports peptides critical for the regulation of circulating phosphate, whole-body energy metabolism, and insulin sensitivity. Thus, we now have a much more complete picture of the skeleton and its role in maintaining mineral and metabolic homeostasis.

- Osteoporosis, the most frequent metabolic disorder of bone, has a great impact on quality of life and mortality because of its negative impact on bone strength. In the past 3 decades the risk factors for fractures have been exhaustively scrutinized. In parallel, biochemical markers of bone remodeling and radiologic examinations to evaluate bone metabolism and structure, respectively, are now employed for the early recognition of fracture susceptibility.

- As a result of rapid advances in our knowledge of the mechanisms driving bone loss, the development of cost-effective drugs for the prevention of fractures has accelerated. Moreover, ongoing studies point to additional and more effective drugs for osteoporosis.

- This chapter focuses on the metabolic aspects of the bone remodeling unit and its response to hormonal, genetic, and environmental changes as well as its importance for tissue homeostasis. Unlike the therapeutic options for other chronic disorders, osteoporosis therapy is in a unique position in that weekly, monthly, biannual, or even annual dosing may be sufficient to accomplish successful treatment. The current challenge in osteoporosis medicine is defining those women (and sometimes men) who are at risk for early skeletal failure.

HISTORICAL CONTEXT

Osteoporosis is a disorder characterized by reduced bone mass, impaired bone quality, and a propensity to fracture in both men and women. Previously, this disease was considered within the context of a syndrome identified by back pain, vertebral fractures, and reduced mineralization on plain radiographs. In the past, the approach to patients with these features focused on identifying secondary causes of low bone mass and treating fractures with orthopedic intervention and pain management.[1] However, with the advent of bone density measurements, the development of new treatment options, and greater public awareness, osteoporosis emerged as a primary disease manifested in multiple ways and managed by aggressive prevention as well as intervention. During this period, significant progress was also made in understanding the complex pathogenesis of the disease.[2-5] Furthermore, there have been tremendous advances in delineating the role of bone remodeling in normal physiology particularly in defining the process of peak bone acquisition.[6,7] Unexpectedly, the skeleton was also found to be an endocrine organ regulating metabolic homeostasis through the release of bone-specific peptides that modulate glucose transport, phosphate balance, and muscle function.

In addition to these developments, a consensus began to emerge concerning the strength of the association between low bone mineral density (BMD) and fracture risk and about the importance of qualitative aspects of the skeleton as additional risk determinants of fractures.[8,9] Newer imaging technology provided a window into the microstructural world of bone, and these advances now allow investigators to better understand the many diseases and drugs associated with skeletal fragility.[10-12] Great strides have also been accomplished in understanding the epidemiology of this disease and the socioeconomic impact of fractures on patients as well as society. The picture that has emerged is that osteoporosis is a disease with a significant degree of morbidity and mortality risks.[13-15] Thus, a systematic approach to understanding and treating this disease lies in appreciating the physiology of skeletal remodeling and the processes by which the basic skeletal unit becomes disordered.

SKELETAL BIOLOGY

Structure and Function of the Skeleton

The skeleton is one of the largest organ systems in the body, consisting of a mineralized matrix and a highly active cellular remodeling unit, composed of osteoblasts, osteoclasts, osteocytes, and lining cells. The most apparent function of the skeleton is to provide structural integrity for the organism while maintaining a degree of elasticity that allows for a range of locomotor activity. In addition to its structural function, the skeleton also serves as a mineral depot ensuring the maintenance of serum calcium and phosphate levels through normal remodeling processes and by secretion of bone-specific factors, such as fibroblast growth factor 23 (FGF23). Just as important, the skeleton is the home for hematopoiesis, maintaining a niche within trabecular bone elements that consists of osteoblasts, adipocytes, reticuloendothelial cells, sinusoids, and mesenchymal stromal and stem cells in a hypoxic environment. That niche provides progenitors that can respond to injuries at any site in the body for critical repair processes. Remarkably, the adult skeleton also harbors a huge adipose depot, composing 10% to 15% of all fat tissues in the body. Thus, it is clear that alterations in either the structural or metabolic functions of the skeleton have tremendous implications for the overall health of the organism.[16]

Embryology and Anatomy

Skeletal development begins early in embryonic life. The process begins with the condensation of mesenchymal cells that differentiate into a cartilaginous structure. Bone formation can then take place through one of two mechanisms: endochondral (i.e., through use of a cartilage framework and involving osteoblasts laying down true bone matrix on top of the cartilaginous matrix, followed by osteoclast-driven turnover of matrix and cells) or intramembranous bone formation in which the mesenchymal precursors differentiate into bone-forming osteoblasts and lay down bone matrix without a cartilage template.[17] The growth of long bones and vertebrae involves endochondral bone formation. The cartilage cells in the growth plate proliferate and undergo hypertrophy; the hypertrophic chondrocytes then direct the mineralization of their matrix and, along with the action of osteoclasts, partly degrade their matrix. The cartilage is invaded by vessels, and the spicules of mineralized cartilage are covered by osteoblasts to form a cancellous or trabecular bone often called the *primary spongiosa*. These structures are resorbed and replaced by trabecular plates made up entirely of bone, called *secondary spongiosa* (Fig. 29-1). This process occurs at the ends of the long bones and in the bodies of the vertebrae.

Intramembranous bone formation occurs next to the cartilage template in flat bones, such as the skull, scapula, and ileum, and on the outer surfaces of long bones, leading to periosteal apposition and expansion. Woven bone, with disordered fibrils of collagen I and a disorganized osteocyte network, is formed during the early stages of intramembranous acquisition but then becomes more organized, as lamellar bone is produced by oriented layers of osteoblasts. As noted previously, the main difference between endochondral and intramembranous bone formation is that the latter does not use calcified cartilage as a direct template for osteoblasts.

Cortical bone is dense bone found in the shafts of long bones. It makes up 80% of the mass of the skeleton, determines its shape, and provides much of its strength. During longitudinal skeletal growth, endochondral and periosteal appositional bone formation determine the length and width of the bones.[18] New cortical bone is shaped by a process called *modeling*, in which osteoblast activity occurs uncoupled to osteoclastic bone resorption. Modeling leads to skeletal shape changes, which are critical for defining the strength of bone. Importantly, modeling is influenced by mechanical forces and is increased during the adolescent growth spurt.[19] As bones elongate, the wide cortex formed just below the growth plate must be sculpted by the modeling/resorption process to allow these bones to

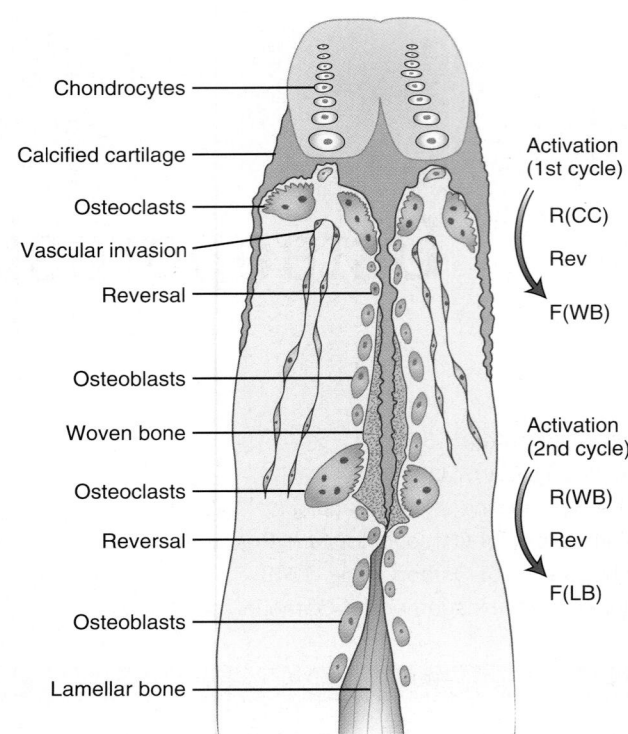

Figure 29-1 Steps in endochondral bone formation. CC, calcified cartilage; F, formation; LB, lamellar bone; R, resorption; Rev, reversal; WB, woven bone. (Redrawn from Baron R. Anatomy and ultrastructure of bone. In: Favus MJ, ed. *Primer on the Metabolic Bone Diseases and Disorders of Mineral Metabolism*, 2nd ed. New York, NY: Lippincott-Raven; 1993:3-9. Copyright 1993, American Society for Bone and Mineral Research.)

elongate while maintaining and extending the narrow tubular structure of the diaphysis.

Bone remodeling is an essential element of skeletal activity that provides skeletal stability and elasticity. It is the process that defines adult bone mass and maintenance (Fig. 29-2). Remodeling is temporally orchestrated to maintain a balance between the amount of bone formed and the amount resorbed. Basic multicellular units (BMUs) carry out bone remodeling and consist of osteoblasts, osteoclasts, bone lining cells, and osteocytes. Remodeling is more active in cancellous or trabecular bone than in cortical bone.[20] In smaller animals, such as rodents, cortical bone can remain lamellar. In large animals and humans, lamellar cortical bone is gradually replaced through haversian remodeling to form cylindrical osteons. The initiation of bone remodeling is directed by endocrine, paracrine, and autocrine factors. The osteocyte, communicating by release of factors through tiny canaliculi, is thought to initiate the remodeling process, providing signals to the lining cell as well as the osteoblast.[21,22] These cells can then signal to attract the osteoclast to the remodeling site where bone resorption occurs. This is followed by the release of matrix proteins that, in combination with osteoclast-derived factors, direct osteoblast differentiation, collagen synthesis, and ultimately matrix mineralization.

Bone Matrix and Mineral

The bone matrix consists of fibers of type I collagen laid down in layers that have various orientations, a portion of which in the mammalian skeleton may be disordered but

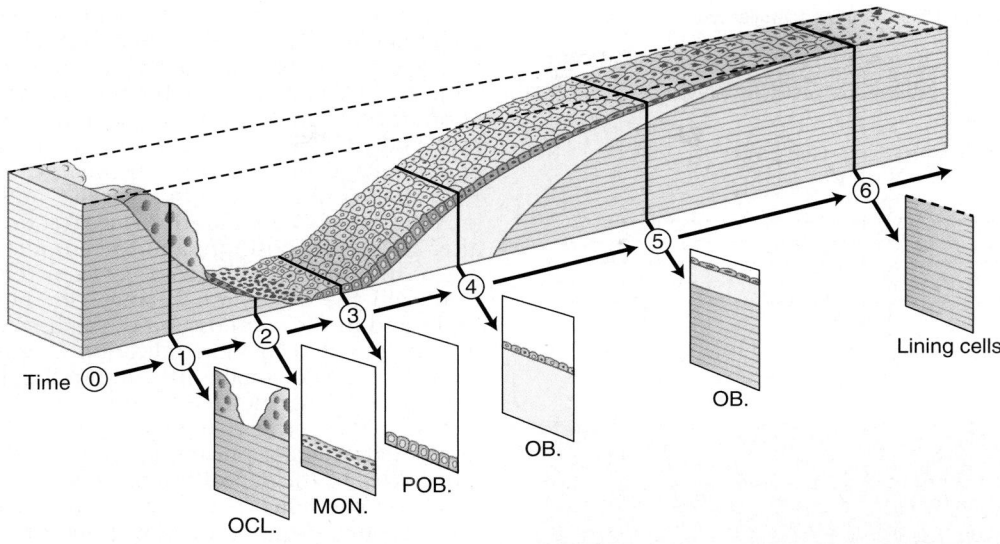

Figure 29-2 Three-dimensional reconstruction of the remodeling sequence in human trabecular bone. *1*, Early bone resorption with osteoclasts (OCL); *2*, late bone resorption with mononuclear cells (MON); *3*, reversal phase with preosteoblasts (POB); *4*, early matrix formation by osteoblasts (OB); *5*, late bone formation with mineralization; *6*, completed remodeling cycle with reversion to lining cells. (From Eriksen EF. Normal and pathological remodeling of human trabecular bone: three dimensional reconstruction of the remodeling sequence in normals and in metabolic bone disease. *Endocr Rev.* 1986;7:379-408. Copyright 1986 by The Endocrine Society.)

still adds to the strength of the matrix (Figs. 29-3 and 29-4). The matrix contains several additional proteins, including other collagen types that may be important in the interaction of type I collagen with noncollagen proteins within the matrix. The noncollagen proteins, such as osteocalcin and several proteoglycans, represent about 10% of the total protein in bone and may direct the formation of fibers, mineralize bone, regulate the attachment of bone cells to its matrix, and play a role in the function of bone-forming and resorbing cells.

Protein composition of the matrix may vary, particularly between woven and lamellar bone.[23] These proteins range from the large cell-attachment proteins (e.g., thrombospondin, fibronectin), which have molecular masses higher than 400 kDa, to the small, vitamin K–dependent γ-carboxylated proteins (e.g., matrix Gla protein and osteocalcin), which are 6-kDa calcium-binding proteins. Osteocalcin can be incompletely or totally carboxylated depending on the number of glutamic acid sites within the molecule that are changed to γ-carboxylated glutamic acid by vitamin K–dependent enzymes; incomplete γ-carboxylation may represent the action of inhibitors such as warfarin or the action of decarboxylating processes. Undercarboxylated osteocalcin (GLU13-OCN) is released from the skeletal matrix during bone resorption (see later). Some noncollagen proteins (e.g., biglycan, decorin, bone sialoprotein, osteopontin, osteoadherin) are highly acidic and play an important role in both signaling and in the matrix of the hematopoietic niche. In addition to cell-attachment sequences, these proteins contain various amounts of carbohydrate and are called *glycoproteins* or *proteoglycans*. Noncollagen proteins of bone are often highly phosphorylated, which enables them to bind calcium, and thus may regulate mineralization. Genetic manipulations in experimental mouse models have provided important information on the function of noncollagenous proteins. For example, null mutations of the osteonectin gene lead to osteopenia in some studies, indicating that this matrix protein may be important for the maintenance of a normal bone structure.[24] On the other hand, deletion of the osteocalcin gene increased bone mass.[25]

The osteocalcin null mice also have a striking body composition and insulin sensitivity phenotype.[26] Studies principally from the Karsenty laboratory but now validated by other groups have shown that GLU13-OCN is released from the skeletal matrix and can bind to a G protein–coupled receptor on the surface of beta cells and adipocytes.[27] This results in enhanced insulin production and greater glucose transport in adipocytes. Moreover, insulin itself can stimulate release of matrix GLU13-OCN. This activity requires the coparticipation of osteoclasts, integrating bone remodeling in the regulation of insulin sensitivity. Insulin signaling in osteoblasts downregulates osteoprotegerin (OPG) via the forkhead box protein O1 (FOXO1), thereby enhancing osteoclastogenesis and ultimately greater bone resorption. The resultant increased osteoclastic activity creates the conditions necessary for acid-mediated decarboxylation of γ-carboxyglutamate residues (Fig. 29-5).[28,29] This was the first of several remarkable studies demonstrating the endocrine nature of the skeleton, in this case due to release of matrix proteins. Importantly, this finding led to even greater insights into the role of the skeleton in modulating energy metabolism.

Collagen Synthesis

Type I collagen is the most abundant protein of the bone matrix. It is a rigid, rod-like, insoluble molecule composed of two α1 chains and one α2 chain (see Fig. 29-4).[30,31] Collagen chains consist of repeating triplets of amino acids, with glycine in every third position and a high content of proline and lysine. The two α1 and the α2 collagen chains form a triple helix that is stabilized by the hydroxylation of proline and lysine residues and requires ascorbic acid. Collagen is synthesized as a soluble proprotein with large nonhelical extensions at the carboxy (C)- and amino (N)-terminal ends. Procollagen also contains C-terminal interchain disulfide bonds that help to initiate formation of the triple helical structure. Procollagen is released into the cisternae of the rough endoplasmic reticulum, packaged in the Golgi vesicles, and secreted extracellularly. The procollagen peptide ends are then removed by specific peptidases to produce mature insoluble collagen molecules, which are

Type I collagen monomeric and fibrillar structure

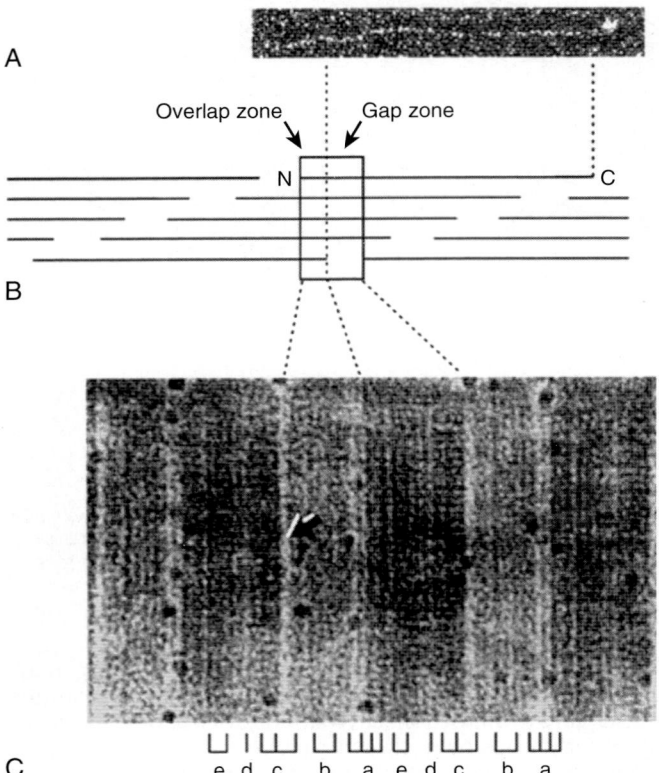

Figure 29-3 Type I collagen monomeric and fibrillar structure. **A,** By rotary shadowing electron microscopy, procollagen (≅300 nm long) appears as a rope-like triple helix to which globular carboxy (C)-terminal (to the right) and amino (N)-terminal domains are attached. **B,** Chapman's model of the collagen fibril. Diagram showing the arrangement of tropocollagen monomers within the collagen fibril, relative to the location of the overlap and gap zone fibril staining pattern. Tropocollagen molecules are shown as horizontal rods, and the polarity of all monomers in the fibril is indicated by N (NH2 terminus) and C (COOH terminus) markings on one monomer. **C,** Electron micrograph of glutaraldehyde-fixed, heparin-gold type I collagen fibril complexes, in fibrils visualized by uranyl acetate staining. Letters below micrograph show positions of positively stained fibril bands, following the accepted notation. Dotted lines between molecular model in **B** and the electron micrograph show corresponding overlap and gap zones. The location of heparin-gold particles relative to the molecular structure of the fibril can be measured within each 67-nm period, beginning at the center of the left border of the overlap zone (origin, *arrow*), and extending to the center of the right border of the gap zone. Heparin-gold particles appear as circular dark objects present mainly in the "a" bands region of the fibrils. (From San Antonio JD, Lander AD, Karnovsky MJ, Slayter HS. Mapping the heparin-binding sites on type I collagen monomers and fibrils. *J Cell Biol.* 1994;125:1179-1188 by copyright permission of The Rockefeller University Press.)

further stabilized by intramolecular and intermolecular cross-links. The major collagen cross-links are formed by lysine and hydroxylysine residues that ultimately form pyridinium ring structures (Fig. 29-6).

Mineralization

Bone mineral is formed by small, imperfect hydroxyapatite crystals, which contain carbonate, magnesium, sodium, and potassium in addition to calcium and phosphate. Mineralization occurs by two distinct mechanisms, one outside the cell and catalyzed by alkaline phosphatase, and one in matrix vesicles that is accelerated by the enzyme phospho1.[32] Both enzymes are critical for adequate mineralization, the former acting to enhance the breakdown of pyrophosphate, an inhibitor of calcium-phosphate precipitation, and the latter to accelerate phosphate availability within

the matrix by acting on phosphocholine and phosphoethanolamine. The initial mineralization of calcified cartilage and woven bone probably occurs by means of matrix vesicles.[33] These membrane-bound bodies are released from chondrocytes and osteoblasts, contain alkaline phosphatase, and can form a nidus for crystallization in the presence of adequate phosphate. In contrast, in lamellar bone, the collagen fibers are tightly packed, and matrix vesicles are rarely seen. Mineralization does not occur immediately after collagen deposition, and there is a layer of 10 to 100 μm of unmineralized osteoid between the mineralization front and the osteoblast. Changes in the packing of the fibrils and in the composition of the noncollagen proteins may be required for mineralization. A group of proteins, named SIBLINGs (small, integrin-binding ligand, N-linked glycoprotein), synthesized in osteocytes (i.e., osteopontin, dentin matrix protein-1 [DMP1], bone sialoprotein, and matrix extracellular phosphoglycoprotein [MEPE]), have a crucial role in the deposition of calcium into bone matrix. SIBLINGs combined with several endopeptidases, including phosphate-regulating endopeptidase homolog, X-linked (PHEX) modulate phosphate metabolism through the regulation of FGF23 synthesis, but also affect osteoclastogenesis and energy metabolism.[34,35] Mineralization of collagen fibrils begins in the *hole zones* of the calcium fibrils, where there is more room for inorganic ions to accumulate (see Fig. 29-3). Mineralization requires calcium, phosphate, and alkaline phosphatase. This process is impaired in circumstances of vitamin D deficiency, very low calcium intake, hypophosphatemia, mutation in the gene encoding alkaline phosphatase, and importantly by the mineralization inhibitor pyrophosphate.[35-37] The characteristic feature of undermineralization on bone biopsy is greater osteoid (i.e., newly synthesized, nonmineralized collagen at the bone surface), and the most dramatic undermineralization occurs in the syndrome of hypophosphatasia, which is due to an absence of total nonspecific alkaline phosphatase. Recent work using a recombinant form of alkaline phosphatase has shown promising results by promoting complete mineralization of the skeleton and improvement in quality of life of patients with hypophosphatasia.[38]

Collagen Degradation by Osteoblasts and Osteocytes

As part of the bone remodeling process, collagen is cleaved and degraded by a group of proteases called *collagenases*. They are matrix metalloproteases (MMPs) that can initiate cleavage of collagen fibrils at neutral pH, and they are central to the process of collagen degradation, matrix breakdown, and bone remodeling. Three collagenases have been described: collagenase 1 (MMP1), 2 (MMP8), and 3 (MMP13).[39] Human osteoblasts express the collagenase 1 and 3 genes (*MMP1* and *MMP13*). Resting osteoblasts secrete limited amounts of collagenase, and changes in the synthesis of collagenase correlate with changes in bone resorption. Collagenase plays a critical function in bone remodeling. Mice with deletions of the collagenase 3 gene or mutations of the α1[16] type I collagen gene have resistance to collagenase 3 cleavage and fail to resorb bone after exposure to parathyroid hormone (PTH).[40] The synthesis of collagenase by osteoblasts is regulated by hormones and by cytokines in the bone microenvironment that act by transcriptional and post-transcriptional mechanisms.[41] It should be noted that, although cleavage by collagenase is an early and obligatory event, most degradation of collagen during remodeling is accomplished by osteoclasts that secrete protons and enzymes (e.g., cathepsin K) that solubilize mineral and degrade the matrix. Cleavage of collagen fragments leads to their excretion in the urine, in which

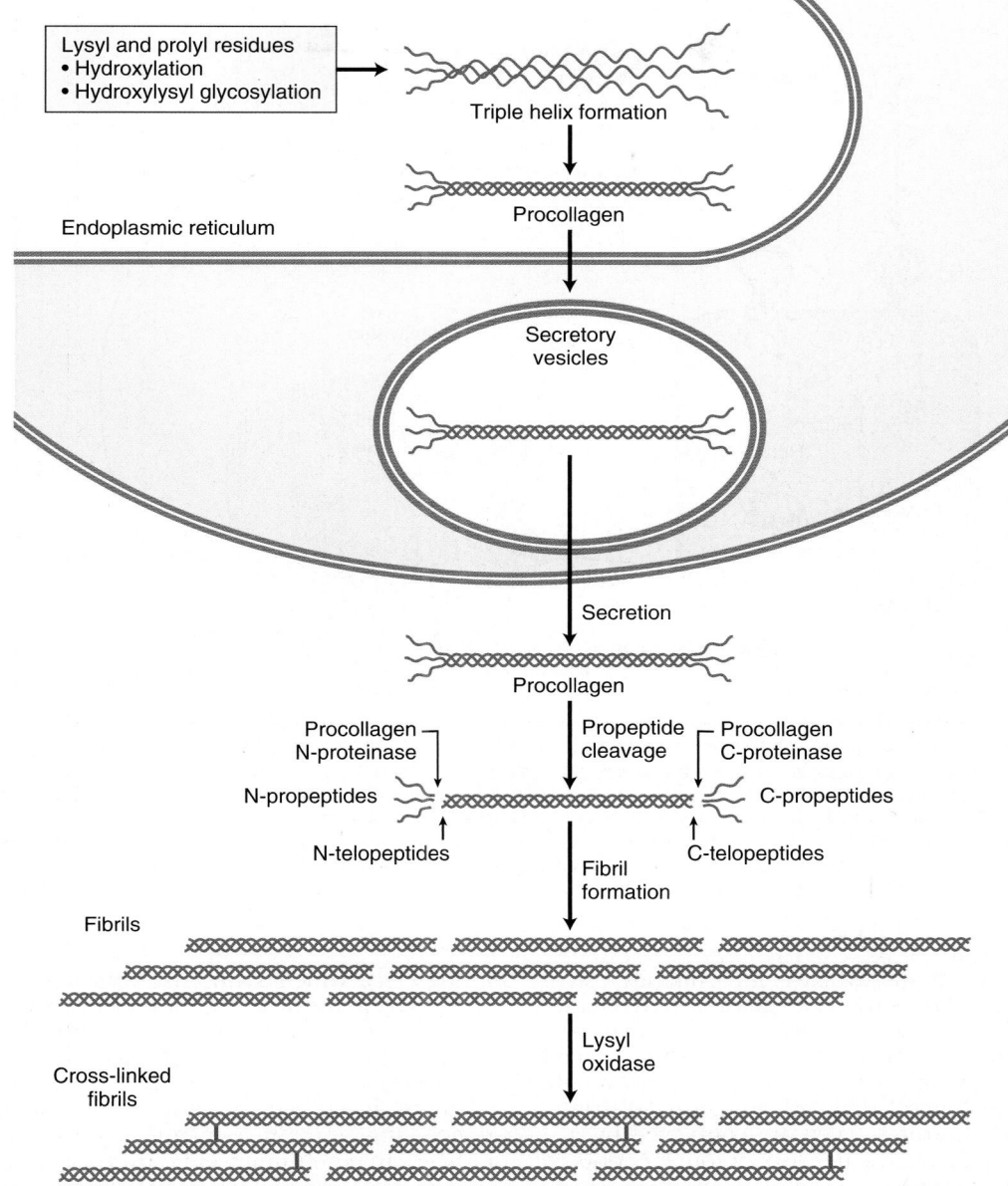

Figure 29-4 Schematic diagram showing the different post-translational modifications and assembly of type I collagen into fibrils. (Modified from Myllyharju J, Kivirikko KI. Collagens, modifying enzymes and their mutations in humans, flies and worms. *Trends Genet.* 2004;20:33-43 and Viguet-Carrin S, Garnero P, Delmas PD. The role of collagen in bone strength. *Osteoporos Int.* 2006;17:319-336, with permission.)

sensitive assays can detect the N-terminal or C-terminal fragments (see later).

Recent evidence points to the participation of osteocytes in aspects of remodeling. Osteocytes are terminally differentiated osteoblasts that are buried within the matrix of the skeleton but possess receptors for PTH and have metabolic activity. These cells are arranged in a functional unit termed the *osteon* that includes an elaborate dendritic network that communicates with the bone surface and probably participates in mechanical sensing. Osteocytes also are a rich source of receptor activator for nuclear factor κB ligand (RANKL), which enhances osteoclast differentiation, particularly during states of increased calcium demand, such as lactation, or immediately following estrogen deficiency. Moreover, osteocytes can secrete enzymes that directly degrade bone matrix in a process called *osteocytic osteolysis*, likely through elaboration of acid phospha-

tase and collagenases. Whether osteocytes also secrete alkaline phosphatase and participate in normal skeletal remodeling per se is still open to debate.

Bone Lining Cells, Osteoblasts, and Osteocytes

Bone is formed by *osteoblasts*, which are terminally differentiated cells that do not undergo mitosis and have many unique features (Fig. 29-7).[42] Osteoblasts are derived from mesenchymal cells in the skeletal microenvironment.[43] Some osteogenic precursors may appear in the circulation, particularly during growth or following injury; they originate from skeletal tissue, and their contribution to bone formation is not certain. Osteoprogenitor cells, or preosteoblasts, replicate and differentiate into active osteoblasts that exhibit various phenotypic characteristics.[42] For example, osteoblasts in early development and during

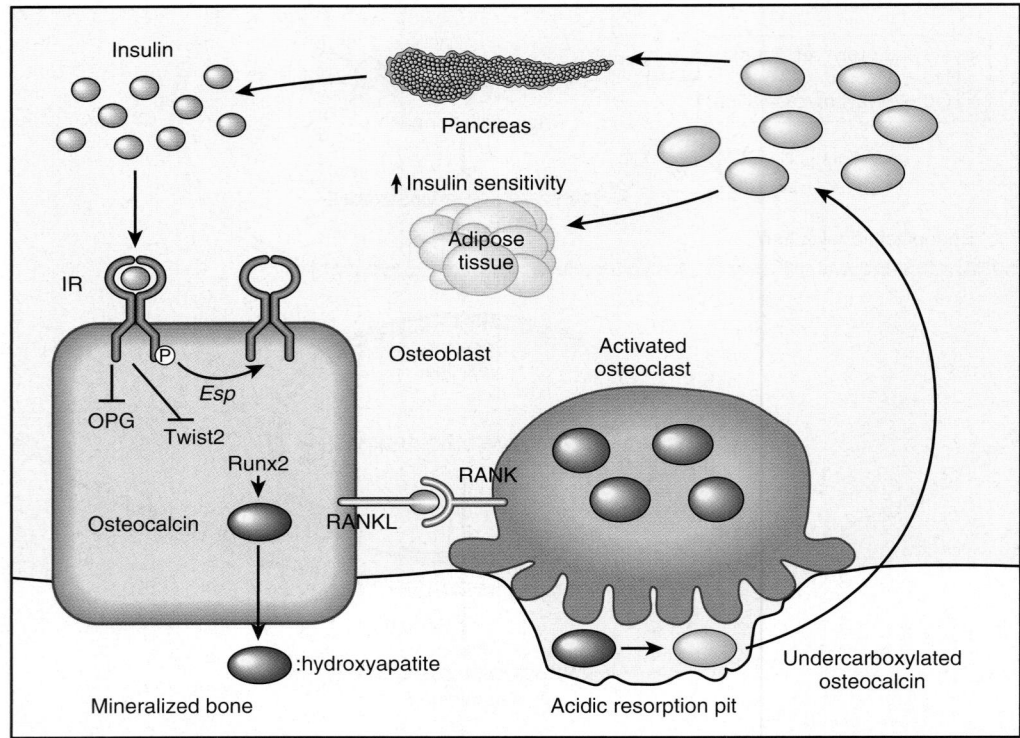

Figure 29-5 Energy regulation and bone turnover by the insulin/osteocalcin axis. A putative feed-forward regulatory loop ties bone turnover to energy regulation as proposed by Ferron and associates[29] and Fulzele and colleagues.[28] Insulin activates skeletal remodeling (i.e., increases bone formation by osteoblasts and resorption by osteoclasts), which in turn releases uncarboxylated osteocalcin from the skeletal matrix into the circulation. This enhances insulin secretion and increases the insulin sensitivity of adipocytes. A tyrosine phosphatase OST-PTP, which is encoded by the *Esp* gene, binds the insulin receptor (IR) and suppresses its activation through dephosphorylation. The transcription factor Twist2 is a critical downstream suppressor of osteoblast differentiation. Osteoprotegerin (OPG) is an osteoblast-specific inhibitor of receptor activator for nuclear factor κB ligand (RANKL), acting as a decoy receptor to block bone resorption. Hydroxyapatite is the mineral component of bone. (From Rosen CJ, Motyl KJ. No bones about it: insulin modulates skeletal remodeling. *Cell.* 2010;142(2):198-200.)

repair produce woven bone, whereas more mature osteo-blasts produce lamellar bone. Osteoblast activity varies during bone formation. Some cells are tall and closely packed and produce a large amount of matrix in a small area; others are flatter and produce matrix at a slower rate over a larger area. Nevertheless, all differentiated osteo-blasts share certain features. They are connected by gap junctions and contain a dense network of rough endoplas-mic reticulum and a large Golgi complex, and they secrete collagen and noncollagen proteins in an oriented fashion. Some products, such as osteocalcin, are synthesized almost uniquely by osteoblasts and osteocytes. A large proportion of the osteocalcin originating from osteoblasts is deposited in the matrix and subsequently released during bone remodeling. Hence, changes in serum levels of osteocalcin reflect bone turnover rather than bone formation per se. As noted previously, GLU13-OCN may serve as an endo-crine hormone prompting insulin secretion and enhancing insulin sensitivity in peripheral tissues.

Mature osteoblasts have a finite capacity to produce matrix, and bone formation is sustained by the arrival of new populations of cells at the bone surface. The number and the function of osteoblasts are determined by hor-mones, local growth factors, and cytokines. Some act as classic cell mitogens and increase the population of pre-osteoblastic cells, some determine their differentiation into mature osteoblasts, and others modify the function of mature cells or enhance osteocytic formation.[44] The ulti-mate fate of mature osteoblasts varies. They may die by apoptosis, they may become embedded in the matrix and become osteocytes, or they may be converted to flattened

lining cells, which synthesize little protein and cover a large percentage of the surface of bone with a thin cyto-plasmic layer (i.e., the bone lining cell) (see Fig. 29-7).

The bone lining cells are flattened and have a fibroblastic-like appearance. Recent work has begun to clarify the role of these lining cells as more active participants in the remodeling unit, in a manner similar to the osteocyte rather than purely quiescent cells. For example, bone lining cells express *osterix* (Sp7) a major transcription factor for osteoblast differentiation. In addition, these cells are in communication through small canaliculi with osteocytes buried within the matrix and express similar markers of differentiation. In response to PTH, a bone remodeling stimulant, bone lining cells differentiate into osteoblasts and thus become a pool of reserve cells necessary during accelerated turnover within the remodeling unit.[45]

Bone marrow stroma contain pluripotent cells that can differentiate into diverse cells of mesenchymal lineage, including osteoblasts, chondrocytes, and adipocytes (Fig. 29-8).[43] The ultimate cellular phenotype depends on factors present in the cellular microenvironment, the degree of hypoxia, the biochemical and metabolic signature of these cells, and their effects on intracellular signals and gene expression. The types and numbers of transcription factors are nuclear proteins that bind to DNA to regulate gene transcription. Some can determine the fate of undifferenti-ated cells, although the process is complex and includes metabolic determinants such as sufficient mitochondrial and glycolytic machinery.[46]

CCAAT/enhancer binding proteins (C/EBPs) β and δ and peroxisome proliferator-activated receptor-γ (PPARG)

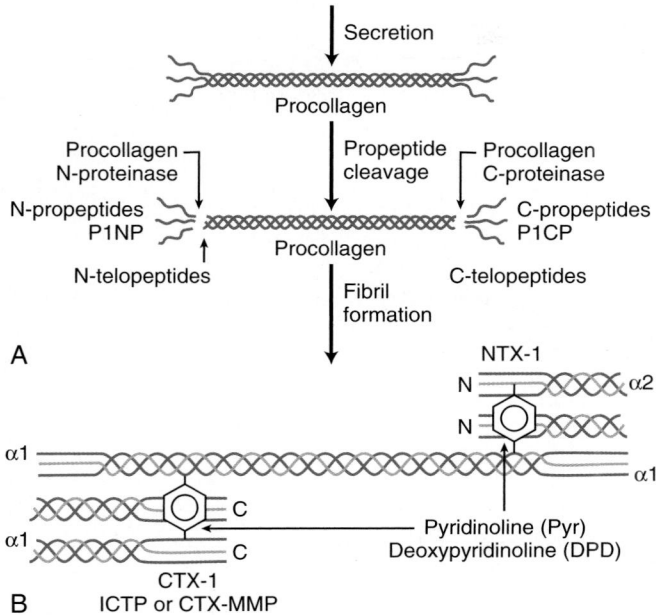

play an essential role in the differentiation of cells toward adipocytes, whereas runt-related transcription factor 2 (RUNX2) plays a central role in the differentiation of cells toward osteoblasts.[47,48] Targeted disruption of the *RUNX2* gene results in disorganized chondrocyte maturation and a complete lack of bone formation due to an arrest of osteoblast development.[49]

Osterix (Sp7) is another transcription factor that is required for endochondral and intramembranous bone formation. It is regulated by RUNX2 and thought to be the next stage in osteoblast differentiation. *Osterix*-null mice fail to develop a mineralized skeleton because of an arrest of late stages of osteoblast differentiation. Interactions between nuclear factors are common steps in the regulation of transcription and differentiation.[50] Osterix associates and acts cooperatively with nuclear factor of activated T cells (NFAT), a transcription factor that regulates osteoblastogenesis and osteoclastogenesis.[51] C/EBPs can interact with RUNX2 and with the activating transcription factor (ATF)/cyclic adenosine monophosphate (cAMP) response element–binding protein (CREB) family of proteins. ATF4 plays a central role in osteoblastic function, and its activity is regulated by a nuclear matrix attachment region binding protein, SATB2, which interacts with ATF4 and RUNX2 to regulate osteoblast differentiation.[52]

The conversion of osteoblasts to osteocytes involves a change in metabolic activity and the development of an extensive network of dendrite-like processes that communicate with those on adjacent osteocytes and cells of the bone surface (Fig. 29-9).[53] Both osteoblasts and bone lining cells contain cell processes that are connected to underlying osteocytes through small canaliculi. After mineralization is complete and the osteocyte is encased in mineralized

Figure 29-6 A, During bone formation, the type I collagen molecule is synthesized as procollagen, and then amino (N)-terminal and carboxy (C)-terminal propeptides (P1NP and P1CP, respectively) are cleaved. The central part of the molecule, triple helix of collagen, is incorporated into bone matrix. **B,** During bone resorption, different products of the breakdown of type I collagen are produced: cross-linked molecules (pyridinoline [Pyr], deoxypyridinoline [DPD]), C-terminal and N-terminal cross-linked telopeptides generated by cathepsin K (CTX-I and NTX-I, respectively), and C-terminal telopeptide generated by metalloproteinases (ICTP or CTX-MMP). (Redrawn from Szulc P, Kaufman JM, Delmas PD. Biochemical assessment of bone turnover and bone fragility in men. *Osteoporos Int.* 2007;18:1451-1461.)

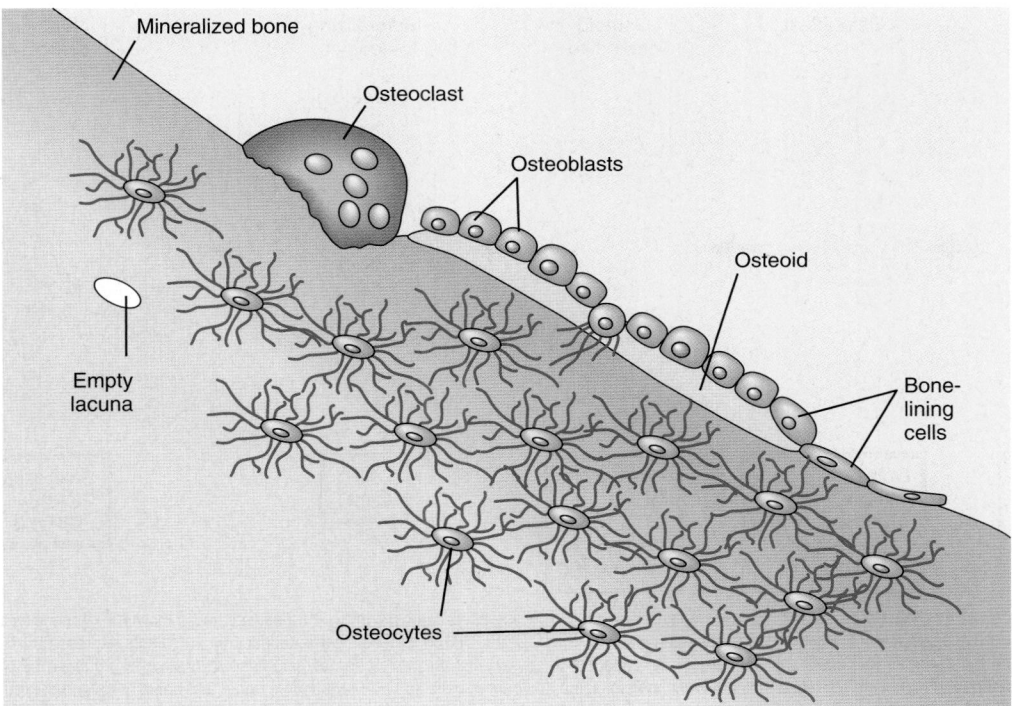

Figure 29-7 Microstructure of an actively remodeling trabecular bone surface. The osteoclast initiates the remodeling cycle by resorbing an area of bone matrix, immediately followed by osteoblast differentiation and osteoid (unmineralized bone matrix) production to replace the resorbed bone. During this process, a small fraction of osteoblasts differentiate further to become osteocytes, encasing themselves within the mineralizing bone matrix and joining the osteocyte network. Mature bone surfaces are populated with bone-lining cells, whose origin and function remain unclear. (From DiGirolamo DJ, Clemens TL, Kousteni S. The skeleton as an endocrine organ. *Nat Rev Rheumatol.* 2012;8(11):674-683.)

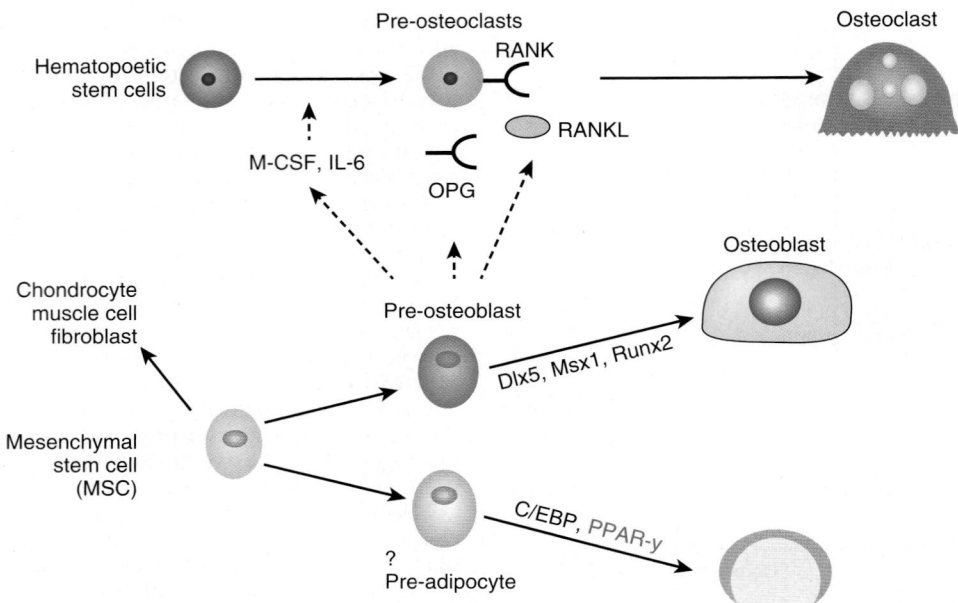

Figure 29-8 For a mesenchymal stem cell to become an osteoblast, activation of several key factors such as runt-related transcription factor 2, bone morphogenetic protein 2, transforming growth factor-β, and transcription factor Sp7 (osterix), are necessary, although the precise sequence of events in this cascade has not been fully clarified. In contrast, to achieve full adipocytic differentiation, there are two groups of critical factors already present in mesenchymal stem cells that need to be activated: CCAAT/enhancer binding proteins α, β, and δ, and peroxisome proliferative activated receptors α, γ2, and δ. Peroxisome proliferative activated receptor γ2 activation by endogenous (e.g., prostaglandin J_2, long-chain and oxidized fatty acids) or exogenous (e.g., rosiglitazone) ligands dramatically shifts allocation of mesenchymal stem cells toward the adipocytic pathway and away from the osteoblast lineage. In vitro, this shift is characterized as an *either/or* allocation: *either* the cell becomes a fat cell *or* it becomes a bone cell, but not both. Inflammatory cytokines can be released from adipocytes, and circulating hormones such as leptin, adipsin, adiponectin, and resistin are also produced by fat cells. The solid arrows represent confirmed networks for regulation and the dashed arrows represent potential regulatory pathways. BMP, bone morphogenetic protein; C/EBP, CCAAT/ enhancer binding proteins; Dlx5, distal-less homeobox 5; HSC, hematopoietic stem cell; IGF, insulin-like growth factor; IGFR, insulin-like growth factor receptor; IL, interleukin; M-CSF, macrophage colony-stimulating factor; Msx1, MSH homeobox homolog 1; OPG, osteoprotegerin (tumor necrosis factor ligand superfamily, member 11); PPAR, peroxisome proliferative activated receptors; RANK, receptor activator of nuclear transcription factor κB (tumor necrosis factor receptor superfamily, member 11a); RANKL, receptor activator of nuclear transcription factor κB ligand (tumor necrosis factor receptor superfamily, member 11); Runx2, runt-related transcription factor 2; TGF, transforming growth factor. (From Rosen CJ, Bouxsein ML. Mechanisms of disease: is osteoporosis the obesity of bone? *Nat Clin Pract Rheumatol.* 2006;2(1):35-43.)

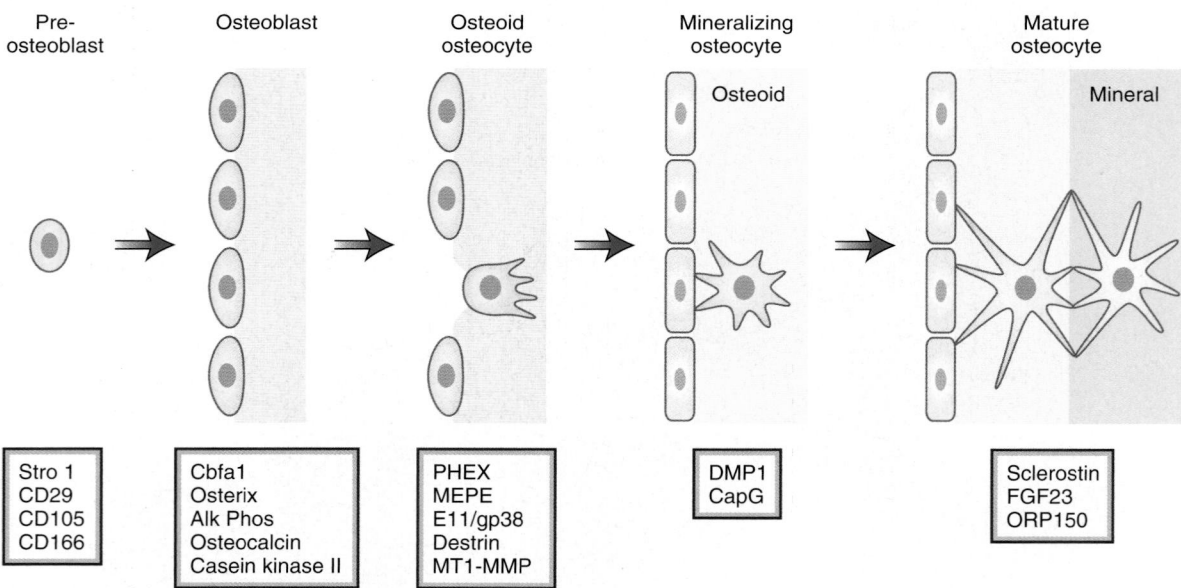

Figure 29-9 Expression of markers during osteoblast-to-osteocyte ontogeny. The osteocyte appears to be the descendant of the matrix-producing osteoblast, which is a descendant of the mesenchymal stem cell known to express markers such as Stro1, CD29, CD105, CD166. Matrix-producing osteoblasts express Cbfa1 and osterix, necessary for osteoblast differentiation, followed by alkaline phosphatase and collagen, necessary for the production of osteoid. Osteocalcin is produced by the late osteoblast and continues to be expressed by the osteocyte. By some unknown mechanism, some designated cells begin to embed in osteoid and begin to extend dendritic projections, keeping connections with already embedded cells and cells on the bone surface. Molecules such as E11/gp38 and MT1-MMP appear to play a role in dendrite/canaliculi formation, whereas molecules such as destrin and CapG regulate the cytoskeleton. Phosphate-regulating endopeptidase homolog, X-linked (PHEX), matrix extracellular phosphoglycoprotein (MEPE), and dentin matrix protein-1 (DMP1) regulate biomineralization and mineral metabolism, and fibroblast growth factor 23 (FGF23) regulates renal phosphate excretion. FGF23 is elevated not only in osteocytes from hypophosphatemic animals but also in those of normal rats. Sclerostin is a marker of the mature osteocyte and is a negative regulator of bone formation. ORP150 may preserve viability of this cell in a hypoxic environment. (Redrawn from Bonewald LF. The amazing osteocyte. *J Bone Miner Res.* 2011; 26(2):229-238.)

bone, these processes maintain connections among osteocytes and allow for at least two important features that are essential for the multicellular unit. First, the extended syncytium with its extensive canalicular network that allows rapid diffusion of small molecules from the marrow space, along with cell-cell junctions that allow transport from the cytoplasm of one osteocyte directly to that of another, is important for supporting the viability of the osteocytes. Second, it allows a constant exchange of information in the form of secreted factors between the endocortical surface and the matrix to regulate remodeling as well as potential recruitment of precursors such as the bone lining cells (Figs. 29-9 and 29-10).

Initially, osteocytes may continue to synthesize collagen and play a role in mineralization. Later, the major role of the osteocyte-osteoblast syncytium may be to sense mechanical forces.[54] Osteocytes probably sense bone defor-mation as well as fluid shifts and provide signals for the adaptive remodeling of bone size and shape.[55] One hypothesis is that small strains produce fluid shear stress in the canaliculi between osteocytes. This effect may result in intracellular signaling through changes in ion channels or in the production of biologically active molecules. Regions of bone microdamage contain apoptotic osteocytes, which may provide signals for the initiation of bone remodeling by osteoclasts and the consequent removal of damaged bone.[30]

Cells of the osteoblastic lineage are important for forming bone and for initiating bone resorption. Both mature osteoblasts and osteocytes may play a role in activating resorption. Most of the hormonal factors that stimulate bone resorption act on cells of the osteoblastic lineage. They stimulate the synthesis and perhaps release of RANKL and colony-stimulating factor 1 (CSF1), which are essential

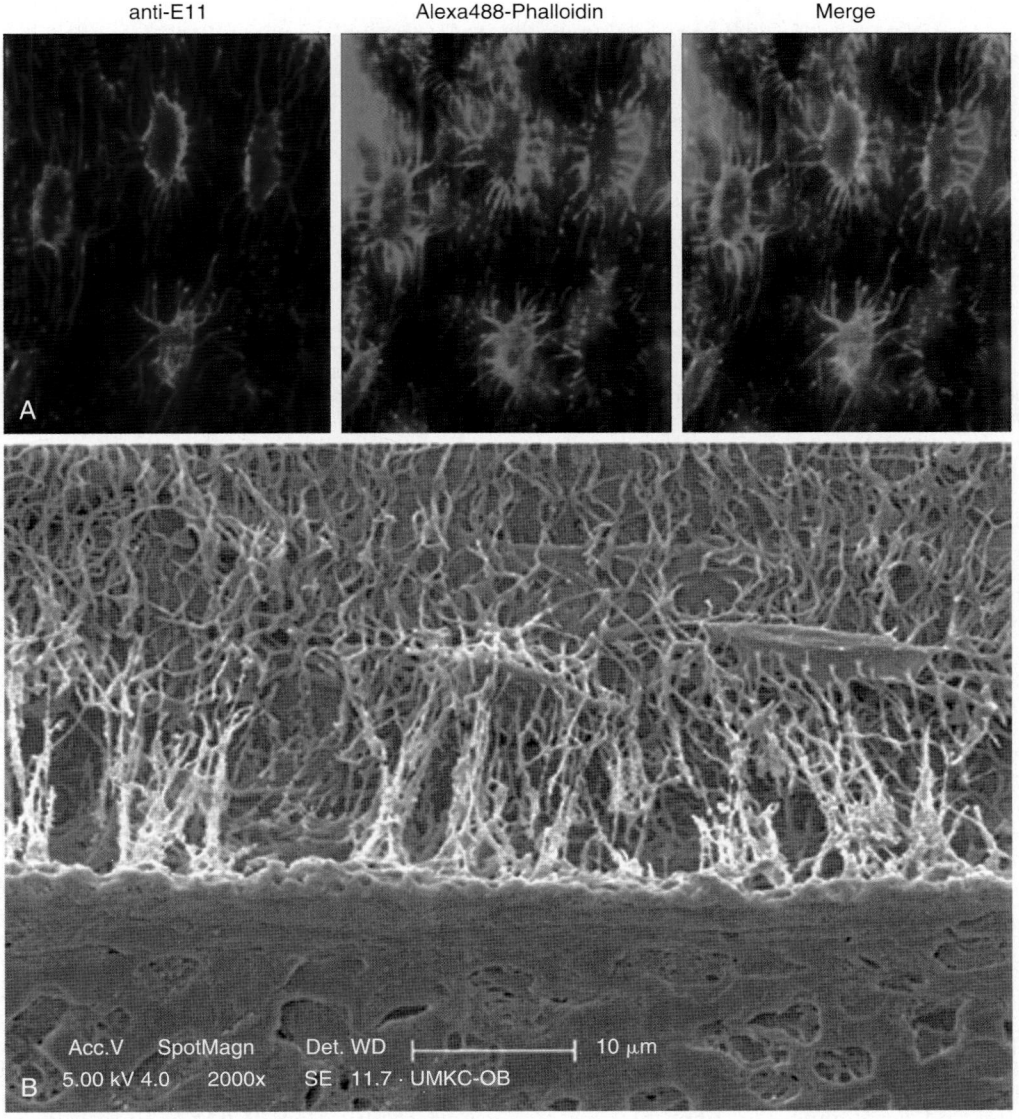

Figure 29-10 A, Visualization of early, embedding osteocytes. Using anti-E11 immunostaining and visualization of the actin cytoskeleton by alexa488 staining for phalloidin, one can visualize the embedding osteocyte and the early osteocyte in 12-day murine calvaria. The merged image shows that the majority of the E11 is on the cell surface and along the dendritic processes. Also, if one looks closely, the dendrites that end on the cell surface have a bulbous tip of unknown function. This structure must interface with the cells on the bone surface. **B,** An acid-etched resin-embedded murine sample showing an osteocyte lacuna sending canaliculi to the bone surface. Note the rough surfaces of canaliculi toward the bone surface and the smooth surface of canaliculi that project away from the bone surface, suggesting a difference between forming and formed canaliculi. Both sets of images demonstrate the complexity of this network and the interface of osteocytes with the bone surface. (The images in **A** are provided by Dr. Sarah Dallas, University of Missouri at Kansas City, MO; **B,** From Bonewald LF. The amazing osteocyte. *J Bone Miner Res.* 2011;26(2):229-238.)

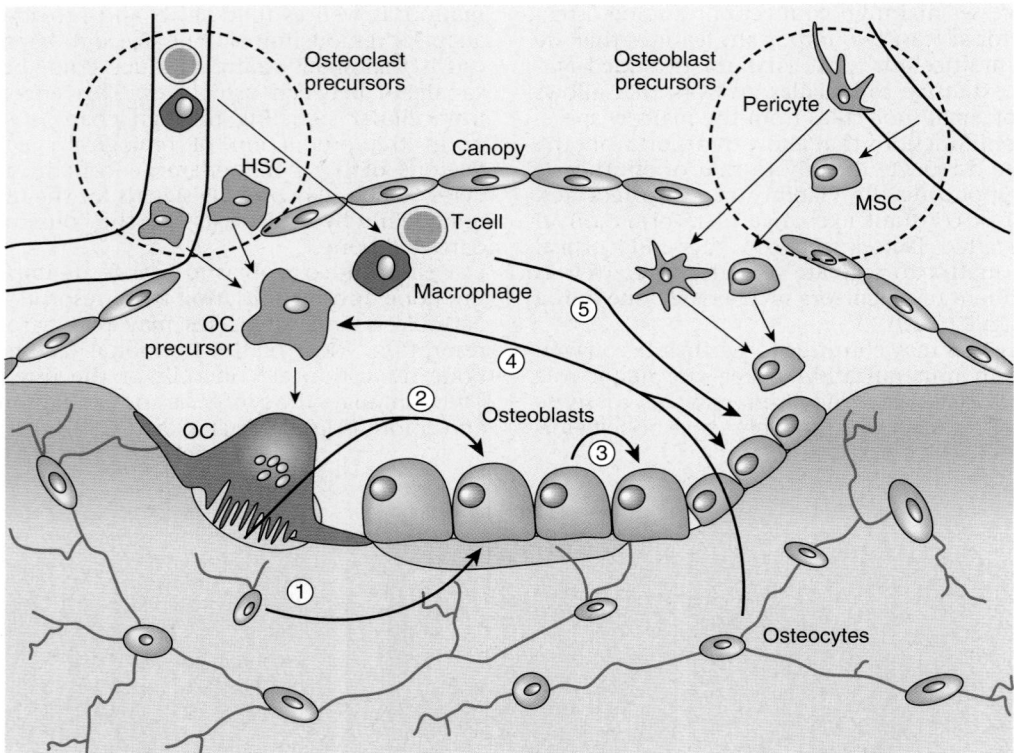

Figure 29-11 Intercellular communication pathways within the basic multicellular unit (BMU) that comprise all steps of the bone remodeling process. *1,* Stimulatory and inhibitory signals from osteocytes to osteoblasts (e.g., Oncostatin M [OSM], parathyroid hormone-related peptide [PTHrP], and sclerostin). *2,* Stimulatory and inhibitory signals from osteoclasts to osteoblasts (e.g., matrix-derived transforming growth factor-β [TGF-β] and insulin-like growth factor 1 [IGF-1], secreted CT-1, Sema4D, and S1P). *3,* Signaling within the osteoblast lineage (e.g., ephrinB2 and EphB4, Sema3a, PTHrP, OSM). *4,* Stimulatory and inhibitory signals between the osteoblast and osteoclast lineages (e.g., receptor activator for nuclear factor κB ligand [RANKL], Sema3B, Wnt5a, and osteoprotegerin [OPG]). *5,* Marrow cell signals to osteoblasts (e.g., macrophage-derived OSM, T-cell–derived interleukins, and RANKL). HSC, hematopoietic stem cell; MSC, mesenchymal stem cell; OC, osteoclast. (From Sims NA, Martin TJ. Coupling the activities of bone formation and resorption: a multitude of signals within the basic multicellular unit. *Bonekey Rep.* 2014;3:481.)

for osteoclastogenesis.[3,56] Osteoblasts also produce additional factors that regulate bone resorption, including cytokines, prostaglandins, and local growth factors. In cell culture, contact between osteoblastic cells and hematopoietic cells appears to be necessary for osteoclast formation (Fig. 29-11). Osteoblasts, as noted earlier, may also play a role in initiating bone resorption by releasing collagenases, other metalloproteinases, and plasminogen activator. These enzymes may remove the surface proteins of bone, which prevent the access of osteoclasts to the mineralized matrix. Osteoblasts also influence the development and maintenance of the marrow through their production of growth factors, cytokines, and chemokines that regulate the growth and development of hematopoietic cells.

Osteoclast Differentiation and Function

Osteoclasts are derived from hematopoietic progenitors and are myeloid in origin. Hematopoietic stem cells under the direction of cytokines and possibly cell-cell interactions express transcription factors that define their commitment to the osteoclast lineage. CSF1 (i.e., macrophage colony-stimulating factor [M-CSF]) is the major cytokine regulating the replication and development in bone marrow of progenitor cells that are capable of differentiating into osteoclasts. Expression of the transcription factor SPI1 (formerly called PU.1) is also necessary for the osteoclast precursor cell to develop.[57] In bone marrow the osteoclast precursor cell is multipotent and can differentiate into monocyte-macrophages, dendritic cells, or preosteoclasts.[58]

The latter fuse to form highly differentiated, multinucleated osteoclasts that resorb bone (Fig. 29-12). Progression through the osteoclast pathway is influenced by multiple local and systemic hormones that may include 1,25-dihydroxyvitamin D [1,25(OH)$_2$D], prostaglandins, and the cytokines interleukin 1 (IL-1), IL-6, and tumor necrosis factor (TNF). Osteomacs are macrophages in the bone remodeling unit and may be important for development of a canopy over the remodeling unit and clearance of degraded proteins as well as antigen presentation.

The nature of the osteoblast-lineage cell products, which directly regulate osteoclast formation and function, has been clarified.[56] The principal stimulator of osteoclast formation is the RANKL, a member of the TNF protein superfamily. This protein was originally identified as a product of activated T lymphocytes, but it is also recognized as a critical stimulator of osteoclastogenesis from mesenchymal stromal cells, preosteoblasts, osteocytes, and hypertrophic chondrocytes. Production of RANKL in osteoblast-lineage cells is stimulated by essentially all agents that enhance osteoclast formation, including PTH, 1,25(OH)$_2$D, prostaglandins, and many cytokines. Mice that are deficient in RANKL do not form osteoclasts and have osteopetrosis. In contrast, injection of RANKL into mice stimulates osteoclast formation and bone resorption but may also be associated with increases in marrow adiposity. RANKL is produced as a membrane protein; in activated T lymphocytes, RANKL is cleaved from the cell membrane and is released as a soluble factor.[59] It is unclear whether similar events occur in osteoblast-lineage cells, although there is some evidence

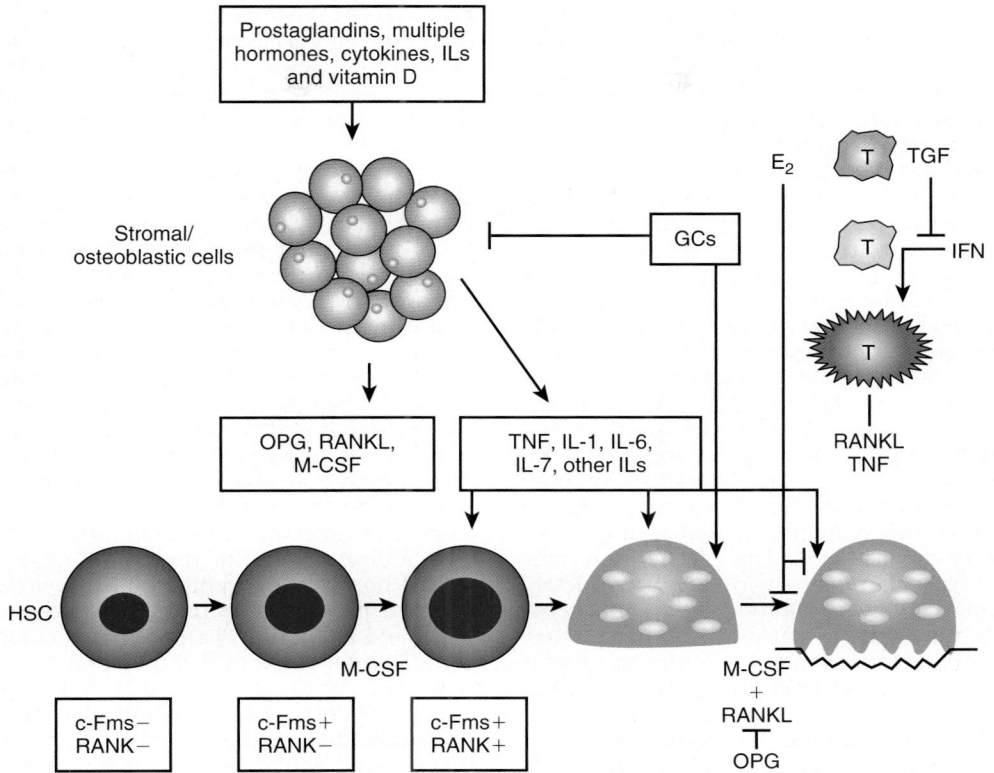

Figure 29-12 Role of cytokines, hormones, steroids, and prostaglandins in osteoclast formation. Under the influence of other cytokines (data not shown), hematopoietic stem cells (HSCs) commit to the myeloid lineage, express c-Fms and receptor activator for nuclear factor κB (RANK), the receptors for macrophage colony-stimulating factor (M-CSF) and RANK ligand (RANKL), respectively, and differentiate into osteoclasts. Mesenchymal cells in the marrow respond to a range of stimuli, secreting a mixture of pro- and anti-osteoclastogenic proteins, the latter primarily osteoprotegerin (OPG). Glucocorticoids (GCs) suppress bone resorption indirectly but possibly also target osteoclasts and their precursors. Estrogen (E_2), by a complex mechanism, inhibits activation of T cells, decreasing their secretion of RANKL and tumor necrosis factor-α (TNF-α); the sex steroid also inhibits osteoblast and osteoclast differentiation and lifespan. A key factor regulating bone resorption is the RANKL/OPG ratio. IFN, interferon; IL, interleukin; M-CSF, macrophage colony-stimulating factor; TGF, transforming growth factor. (From Rosen CJ, ed. *Primer on the Metabolic Bone Diseases and Disorders of Mineral Metabolism*, 8th ed. Ames, IA: Wiley-Blackwell; 2013:2-33, Copyright 2013, American Society for Bone and Mineral Research.).

that cleavage and release of soluble RANKL occurs in malignant cells that metastasize to bone.

OPG is a native inhibitor of osteoclastogenesis; it is a soluble receptor for RANKL that binds this ligand and prevents interaction of RANKL with its cognate receptor, RANK. OPG is produced widely. In bone marrow cultures, a number of stimulators of resorption, including PTH, $1,25(OH)_2D$, and prostaglandin E_2 (PGE_2), inhibit OPG production. For these factors, there is a reciprocal relationship between RANKL stimulation and OPG inhibition that causes activation of osteoclastogenesis and enhanced resorption. Mice that are deficient in OPG have osteoporosis, whereas mice that overexpress OPG have increased bone mass. These results, together with those for RANKL-deficient mice and mice injected with RANKL, demonstrate that osteoclast-mediated bone resorption is tightly regulated by the combined actions of RANKL and OPG.

The active receptor for RANKL is RANK, a member of the TNF receptor superfamily. Osteoclasts and their immediate precursor cells express RANK, and this expression is induced by M-CSF.[60] Binding of RANKL to RANK activates a series of intracellular pathways that activate NF-κB and mitogen-activated protein (MAP) kinases, as well as NFAT and the activator protein-1 (AP1) family of transcription factors. The TNF receptor-associated factors (TRAFs), and particularly TRAF-6, are ubiquitin E3 ligases that bind RANK intracellularly and are involved in RANK responses. Mice deficient in TRAF-6, like those deficient in RANK, develop osteopetrosis. In addition to its effects on bone,

the RANKL/RANK system is involved in lymphocyte function, barrier functions in the skin, and breast and lymph node development. Mature osteoclasts express RANK, and treatment of these cells with RANKL inhibits apoptosis and stimulates resorptive activity.[61]

In addition to RANKL, M-CSF is essential for osteoclast formation. Mice that are deficient in M-CSF have osteopetrosis and few osteoclasts.[62] In cultures of isolated osteoclast precursor cells, both M-CSF and RANKL must be present to form mature osteoclasts. M-CSF enhances RANK production in osteoclast precursors and inhibits apoptosis of osteoclast precursors and mature osteoclasts. The receptor for M-CSF, CSF1 receptor (CSF1R) (formerly designated C-FMS), is present on osteoclast precursors and mature osteoclasts.[60,63] Binding of CSF1R by M-CSF activates tyrosine kinase activity in the receptor, which initiates a series of intracellular downstream events.

A series of coactivator molecules is critical for osteoclast development. These molecules include members of the cytoplasmic immunoreceptor tyrosine-based activation motif (ITAM) family, namely, Fc-receptor γ-subunit (FcRγ) and DNAX activation protein 12 (DAP12). ITAM proteins interact with receptor proteins in the cell membrane of osteoclast precursor cells. The search for receptors associated with these ITAM adaptors in myeloid cells has identified at least two candidates that associate with FcRγ—osteoclast-associated receptor (OSCAR) and paired immunoglobulin-like receptor (PIR)—and two that associate with DAP12—the triggering receptor expressed by myeloid cells-2 (TREM2) and the signal regulatory protein-β1 (SIRPB1). Mice that are deficient in FcRγ and DAP12 have osteopetrosis and deficient osteoclast formation despite their ability to express RANKL, RANK, M-CSF, and CSF1R.[51,64] This signaling pathway responds to ligands that have not yet been established genetically; together with RANK, it stimulates the accumulation of intracellular calcium, which is required for dephosphorylation of NFAT; this allows the transport of NFAT into the nucleus, where it acts as a transcription factor.

The formation of multinucleated osteoclast-like cells in vitro requires hematopoietic precursors and cells of the mesenchymal/osteoblast lineage present within the niche.[65,66] In vivo and in cultures with devitalized bone, mononuclear preosteoclasts attach to the bone surface and form multinucleated osteoclasts by fusion.[67] The accumulation of additional nuclei into osteoclasts by fusion probably continues while the cell is actively resorbing. The life span of the osteoclast is limited. As osteoclasts become inactive, they die by apoptosis. Hormones that enhance bone resorption may delay apoptosis, and inhibitors of resorption probably accelerate it. The mechanisms that limit the extent of osteoclastic resorption are incompletely understood and may involve inhibition by calcium ions, which accumulate under the osteoclast resorbing surface, or by local inhibitory factors, such as transforming growth factor-β (TGF-β), which are released and activated during resorption.

The mature osteoclast is a unique and highly specialized cell (Fig. 29-13). It usually contains 10 to 20 nuclei, but giant osteoclasts with up to 100 nuclei can be seen in Paget disease and in giant cell tumors of bone. The large size of osteoclasts is probably essential for their resorptive function. The best evidence for this comes from studies of dendritic cell–specific transmembrane protein (DC-STAMP), because inhibition of this protein or its complete deficiency in mouse models results in the generation of only mononuclear osteoclasts that have impaired resorptive activity.[68,69]

The capacity of osteoclasts to resorb bone depends on their ability to isolate a region of the bone surface from the extracellular fluid and produce a local environment that can dissolve bone mineral and degrade matrix. The osteoclast must polarize and produce a basolateral membrane opposite the resorption space, which facilitates the excretion of resorption products (see Fig. 29-13). The resorbing apparatus consists of a central ruffled border area, which secretes hydrogen ions and proteolytic enzymes, surrounded by a clear or sealing zone in a structure called the *podosome*. The podosome contains filamentous actin linked to $\alpha_v\beta_3$ integrin, and it anchors the cell to the bone surface. The osteoclast attaches to bone through the interaction of integrins in the podosome with noncollagenous proteins such as vitronectin and osteopontin in the matrix.

Acidification of the resorption space adjacent to the ruffled border membrane requires that osteoclasts have a vacuolar proton pump (H^+-ATPase [adenosine triphosphatase]) and a chloride channel that is charge coupled to H^+ secretion across the ruffled membrane to preserve electron neutrality.[70,71] These osteoclast H^+-ATPase pumps are similar to the vacuolar proton pumps that acidify intracellular organelles, but in the osteoclast they are exteriorized to increase the extracellular hydrogen ion concentration in the resorption space. The hydrogen ions dissociate from carbonic acid, which is synthesized by carbonic anhydrase II; the bicarbonate generated by this dissociation is removed

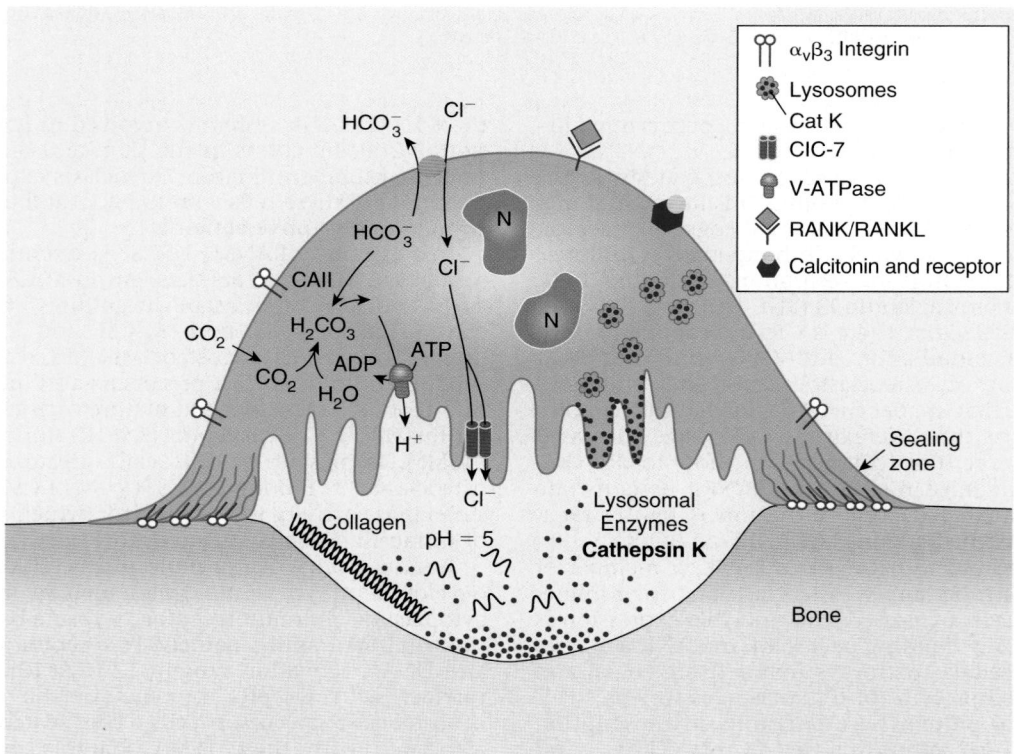

Figure 29-13 Schematic representation of a resorbing osteoclast. The osteoclast acidifies the resorption lacunae by secreting H^+ and Cl^- ions for demineralization, and lysosomal cathepsin K for degradation of type I collagen. ADP, adenosine diphosphate; ATP, adenosine triphosphate; ATPase, adenosine triphosphatase; CLC-7, chloride channel 7; RANK, receptor activator of nuclear transcription factor κB; RANKL, RANK ligand. (From Rodan SB, Duong LT (2008). Cathepsin K—a new molecular target for osteoporosis. *IBMS Bonekey.* 2008;5:16-24.)

from the cell by chloride-bicarbonate exchange at the basolateral membrane of the osteoclast. Ion pumps can transport the dissolved calcium from the bone surface through the cell to the extracellular fluid (see Fig. 29-13).

However, calcium can also reach the extracellular fluid directly if the sealing zone is disrupted. The proteolytic enzymes produced by the osteoclast include lysosomal enzymes and metalloproteinases.[72] Lysosomal proteases can degrade collagen at the low pH present in the ruffled border area. Cathepsin K is probably the most important of these.[73] Metalloproteinases, which are active at neutral pH, have also been detected at the resorption site.[74] The products of resorption are transported across the ruffled border membrane and excreted through the basolateral membrane of the osteoclast by a process called *transcytosis*.[75] In trabecular bone, osteoclasts characteristically resorb to a limited depth and then move laterally to produce irregular, platelike resorption areas called *Howship lacunae*. In cortical remodeling, the path of directed resorption is longer, possibly because of renewal of osteoclasts from hematopoietic cells brought to the site through the haversian canal.

BONE REMODELING AND ITS REGULATION

Overview of Remodeling

Adult bone mass is determined by two processes: acquisition of peak bone mass during adolescence and the subsequent bone loss after maturity. Changes in bone mass result from physiologic and pathophysiologic processes in the bone remodeling cycle, and ultimately this can lead to skeletal fragility.[76] The most vulnerable periods in women are during accelerated linear growth in adolescence (ages 10 to 16) and later in life, usually immediately after menopause (ages 45 to 60). Male bone loss is much more gradual but is also determined by peak acquisition and age-related loss.

The bone remodeling cycle is a tightly coupled process whereby bone is resorbed at approximately the same rate as new bone is formed. BMUs comprise the remodeling unit of bone and as noted previously include osteoclasts, osteoblasts, osteocytes, and bone lining cells.[18] The bone marrow niche includes these cells plus hematopoietic elements, adipocytes, reticuloendothelial cells lining the sinusoids, and mesenchymal stromal cells (see Fig. 29-11). Activation of the remodeling cycle serves two functions in the adult skeleton: (1) to supply calcium acutely, as well as chronically, to the extracellular space, and (2) to provide elasticity and strength to the skeleton. When the remodeling process is uncoupled so that resorption exceeds formation, bone is lost. On the other hand, during peak bone acquisition, formation exceeds resorption, resulting in a net gain of bone. Remodeling is more pronounced in the trabecular skeleton (e.g., spine, calcaneus, and proximal femur), the most metabolically active compartment of bone. The trabecular elements are likely surrounded by a canopy that encloses the BMU and contains a capillary network for nutrient supply as well as cells that can be identified as osteomacs. Although trabecular bone remodels more frequently than cortical bone, it is also extremely vulnerable to perturbations by local or systemic factors that can cause significant imbalances in bone turnover.

The bone remodeling cycle begins with activation of resting osteoblasts on the surface of bone, as well as the bone lining cells (see Fig. 29-11). The initial signal for remodeling has been actively debated, as has been the source of that signal (i.e., systemic or local). Microdamage or force changes sensed by the osteocyte may initiate the remodeling signal, although it is likely that local factors secreted by osteoblasts, osteoclasts, or lining cells could also begin the process. That initiating signal is followed by a series of secretory products originating from activated osteoblasts, to osteoclasts and their precursors. These intercellular signals recruit and differentiate multinucleated cells from hematopoietic stem cells.[77] After osteoclast-induced bone resorption, matrix components such as TGF-β and insulin-like growth factor 1 (IGF-1), as well as collagen, osteocalcin, calcium, and other protein and mineral components, are released into the microenvironment. Growth factors released by resorption contribute to the recruitment of new osteoblasts to the bone surface, which begin the process of collagen synthesis and biomineralization. In addition, cytokines released by activated osteoclasts such as bone morphogenetic protein (BMP) 7, Wnt 10b, and sphingosine 1-phosphate can stimulate osteoblastogenesis in reverse sequence.[78] Ephrins serving as both ligands and receptors also contribute to this bidirectional signaling mechanism (Fig. 29-14).[79] In healthy adults as many as 2 million remodeling sites may be active at any given time, and it is estimated that nearly one fourth of all trabecular bone is remodeled each year. In general, resorption takes only 10 to 13 days, whereas formation is much more deliberate and can take upward of 3 months (see Fig. 29-2). Under ideal circumstances, by the end of the cycle, the amount of bone resorbed equals the amount re-formed.

Although 80% of skeletal mass is cortical bone, the surface area of cortical bone is only about one fifth that of cancellous bone. Moreover, more osteoclast precursor cells are available in cancellous bone and on the endosteal surfaces of cortical bone. Consequently, turnover is greater on these surfaces than on periosteal bone, which normally undergoes little remodeling. However, subperiosteal resorption can be activated in hyperparathyroidism, and the periosteal surface contains preosteoblasts that may become active late in life and cause an age-related increase in the periosteal diameter of long bones.[80] This periosteal expansion may maintain bone strength and compensate for losses at the endosteal surfaces and in cancellous bone.

Several key components of the remodeling cycle are susceptible to systemic and local alterations, which can lead to deleterious changes in bone mass. In particular, activation of remodeling via the osteoblast and recruitment of osteoclasts represent the two most vulnerable sites in the cycle. Often, with systemic changes in circulating hormones such as estrogen deficiency, chronic PTH excess, or hyperthyroidism, the remodeling cycle is stressed such that coupling of the two processes cannot be maintained. This failure is due to the difference in timing between resorption, which generally occurs within a BMU over about 2 weeks, and formation, which can take upward of 12 weeks to fully mineralize newly synthesized matrix. Not surprisingly, a third cell altered in disease states is the osteocyte. Remodeling of the skeleton implies coupling of resorption to formation, and therefore no net change in bone mass. Because the osteocyte responds to mechanical loading or stress by communicating with bone lining cells and osteoblasts, these cells could also become damaged (see Fig. 29-11).[81] Indeed, osteocyte apoptosis may contribute to age-related osteoporosis either directly or through the elaboration of systemic peptides. Interestingly, remodeling may end with the osteocyte as well, because it produces the protein *sclerostin*, which inhibits osteoblast activity by antagonizing the Wnt/lipoprotein receptor–related protein (LRP) 5 and BMP pathways.[22]

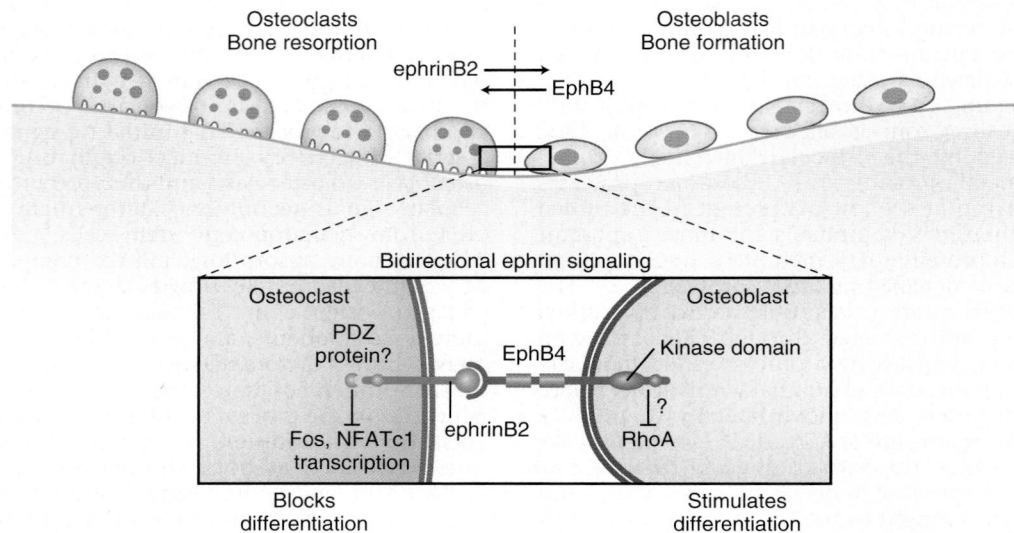

Figure 29-14 Ephrin-Eph signaling and bone homeostasis. Osteoclasts are responsible for the resorption of a localized packet of bone, and when they cease their activity, a team of osteoblasts is attracted to the resorption site, where they proliferate, differentiate, and then re-form the packet of bone. **Inset,** Ephrin-Eph forward signaling from osteoclasts to osteoblasts may be responsible for driving the formation of the new bone packet, and ephrin-Eph reverse signaling may be responsible for the cessation of continued bone resorption by osteoclasts. (Redrawn from Mundy GR, Elefteriou F. Boning up on ephrin signaling. *Cell.* 2006;126(3):441-443.)

Monoclonal antibodies that bind to sclerostin have been developed, and at least one is currently in phase III trials as a means of reducing the inhibitory effect of this protein on osteoblast differentiation and thereby increasing bone mass.[82,83]

As noted, uncoupled remodeling occurs during menopause because of estrogen deprivation or in response to endogenous PTH fluxes, cytokine stimulation, growth hormone surges, glucocorticoid excess, or changes in serum calcium. For the most part, estrogen deprivation remains one of the most common and critical elements in shifting resorption rates to a higher set-point. Although bone formation initially can "catch up," the length of time for each component of the remodeling cycle clearly favors resorption over formation as the process of laying down new bone requires the interaction of several processes (see Fig. 29-2).[81] However, it is still unclear why falling estrogen levels, which is a universal event during the menopausal years, causes rapid bone loss in a relatively small percentage of women, although insidious bone loss has been clearly demonstrated for most if not all women who enter menopause.[84] Other factors such as peripheral conversion of testosterone to estradiol, which occurs to a greater degree in obese individuals, higher adrenal androgen production, and/or genetic determinants, as well as other local signals, may be important. Although the genetic causes of rapid bone loss have not been identified in humans, mice have strong heritable determinants that affect the rate of age-related and estrogen-deficient bone loss.[85,86]

The nature of the osteocyte-osteoblast-osteoclast interaction has been one of the most active areas of investigation (see Fig. 29-11). External signals (such as PTH, growth hormone, IL-1, estrogen deprivation) to resting osteoblasts and stromal cells cause these cells to release cytokines (i.e., interleukins such as IL-1, IL-6, and IL-11 as well as M-CSF, TNF, and TGF-β) that enhance the recruitment and differentiated function of multinucleated giant cells destined to become bone-resorbing cells.[3] However, one of the most critical pathways in the osteoblast-osteoclast interaction scheme is the RANKL-OPG relationship.[56]

The OPG, RANKL, and RANK system, which affects osteoclast differentiation, in addition to the effects of

M-CSF on osteoclast proliferation, provides the critical link between osteoclasts and osteoblasts. It has also led to the synthesis of RANKL antibodies that, after successful human trials, have become therapeutic agents to inhibit bone resorption. Denosumab (Prolia) is the first monoclonal antibody against RANKL and was approved by the U.S. Food and Drug Administration (FDA), European regulatory agencies, and Endocrinologic and Metabolic Drugs Advisory Committee (EMDAC) for the treatment of postmenopausal osteoporosis, as well as for metastatic bone diseases, owing to its strong efficacy in reducing spine and hip fractures.[87] It is administered once every 6 months and it suppresses bone resorption by 80% to 90%. Long-term follow-up of the original phase III trials reveals significant improvement in bone mass at both the spine and hip out to 8 years, with maintenance of antifracture efficacy and few if any adverse events. Denosumab has also been approved for the treatment of women with breast cancer and skeletal metastases and is the only agent shown to reduce fractures in men undergoing androgen deprivation therapy for prostate cancer.[88,89]

The osteoblast functions not only to signal osteoclasts during remodeling but also to lay down collagen and orchestrate mineralization of previously resorbed lacunae in the skeletal matrix. These complex functions are tied to differentiation of mesenchymal stromal cells and bone lining cells, which become osteoblasts and rest on the surface of the remodeling space.[90] Recruitment of stromal cells into osteoblasts, rather than adipocytes, is a critical step in bone formation and requires a series of factors that enhance differentiation (see Fig. 29-8). One of the most important drivers of this process is RUNX2, a transcription factor that is essential for the early differentiative pathway of stromal cells toward bone and away from adipogenesis.[91,92] Regulation of RUNX2 and its downstream effects has become a major focus of work as investigators have begun to consider novel ways to enhance bone formation and reduce marrow adipogenesis. However, within that context it is clear that preadipocytes or preosteoblasts may have significant plasticity such that the older paradigm illustrated in Figure 29-8 may not truly represent the status of mesenchymal cells within the marrow niche.

During activation of resting osteoblasts, the mature cells synthesize collagen I, several minor collagens, the noncollagenous matrix proteins, and a series of growth factors such as IGF-1, IGF-2, and TGF-β. These, in turn, are necessary for further recruitment of bone-forming cells.[93] In addition, osteoblasts deposit growth factors in the skeletal matrix, where they are stored in latent forms (e.g., TGF-β, IGF-1 and -2) and released during subsequent remodeling cycles. Osteoblast fate is determined within the remodeling sequence by a number of different systemic and local factors. Osteoblasts can further differentiate into osteocytes, become quiescent lining cells on the bone surface, or die through apoptosis.[94] As noted earlier, osteocytes may participate in bone resorption of the cortex by secreting RANKL to stimulate osteoclastogenesis and can also participate in osteocytic osteolysis, which may occur during lactation and other states of high calcium demand.[95]

The Wnt/β-catenin signaling pathway has emerged as a major regulator of bone formation and a potential mediator of the mechanostat. Wnts belong to a large family of proteins that bind to frizzled receptors and activate multiple pathways within the cell. When Wnts also bind to several coreceptors LRP5, LRP6, and probably LRP4, a so-called canonical signaling pathway is triggered.[2] Activation of this pathway occurs through a complex intracellular signaling pathway mediated by β-catenin, which translocates to the nucleus and stimulates the transcription of genes through cooperative interactions with TCF/Lef transcription factors. Sclerostin (the product of the *SOST* gene), the osteocyte-specific protein that inhibits bone formation and another important Wnt inhibitor, dickkopf-1 (Dkk1), work by binding to LRP5 and LRP6, thereby blocking Wnt signaling.[96]

Local Regulators of Remodeling

Characterization of local regulators produced within the bone itself represents a major advance in bone biology.[97,98] These local factors can be synthesized by bone cells or by adjacent hematopoietic cells and can interact with each other and with systemic hormones. They are critical in the repair of skeletal damage and in the response to mechanical forces.

Cytokines

The proinflammatory cytokines IL-1α, IL-1β, TNF-α, and TNF-β are potent stimulators of bone resorption and inhibitors of bone formation; thus, they may play a role in the bone loss after estrogen withdrawal.[99,100] IL-6 increases osteoclastogenesis in cell cultures and may mediate some of the resorbing activity of PTH. IL-6 is synthesized by osteoblasts and immune cells, and its production is stimulated by PTH,[101] PGE2, and other factors that increase bone resorption.

IL-11, another member of the IL-6 cytokine family, also stimulates resorption. LIF, also a member of the IL-6 family, increases proliferation of osteoblast precursors but then slows their subsequent differentiation into mineralizing osteoblasts.[102] Inflammatory cytokines such as IL-7, IL-15, and IL-17 stimulate bone resorption, whereas IL-4, IL-13, IL-10, and IL-18 inhibit bone resorption.[103-106] Interferon-β and interferon-γ inhibit resorption by blocking RANK signaling pathways.[107] IL-10 is an inhibitor of osteoclastogenesis and bone resorption.[105] IL-15 and IL-17 stimulate resorption, whereas IL-18 is inhibitory through its ability to increase production of granulocyte-macrophage colony-stimulating factor (GM-CSF).[106] Interferon-β and interferon-γ inhibit resorption by blocking RANK signaling pathways.[107]

In addition to direct effects, responses to cytokines can be blocked by inhibitors, such as the IL-1 receptor antagonist and the soluble TNF receptor, or they can be enhanced by activators such as the soluble IL-6 receptor.

Transforming Growth Factor-α and Epidermal Growth Factor

These peptides stimulate bone resorption through the same receptor and act by prostaglandin-dependent and prostaglandin-independent pathways. TGF-α and epidermal growth factor (EGF) are potent mitogens in bone that probably act on mesenchymal and hematopoietic precursors.[108,109] The EGF family of peptides regulates cell migration and adhesion, playing an important role in the early recruitment of osteoblast progenitors to the remodeling site. Signaling in preosteoblasts by the EGFs is via the Cdc42/Rac network.[110] TGF-α is produced by neoplasms and may play a role in the increased bone resorption that occurs in certain malignancies.

Prostaglandins

Prostaglandins are potent regulators of bone cell metabolism and are synthesized by many cell types in the skeleton.[111] Prostaglandin production in bone is regulated by effects of local and systemic hormones and mechanical forces on the inducible cyclooxygenase 2 (COX2). Increased prostaglandin production may contribute to the increase in bone resorption that occurs with immobilization, the enhanced bone formation seen with impact loading, and the bone loss after estrogen withdrawal. Many of the hormones, cytokines, and growth factors that stimulate bone resorption also increase prostaglandin production. Prostaglandins have biphasic effects on bone formation. Stimulation of bone formation is seen in vivo, and inhibition of collagen synthesis occurs in osteoblast cultures. Bone cells produce PGE2, PGF2α, prostacyclin, and lipoxygenase products (e.g., leukotriene B4), which may also stimulate bone resorption.

Peptide Growth Factors

Skeletal cells synthesize a variety of growth factors that regulate the replication, differentiation, and function of bone cells. These growth factors are not synthesized only by skeletal cells, and some are present in the systemic circulation and can act as local and systemic regulators of bone remodeling. Skeletal cells also synthesize growth factor binding proteins, which regulate the activity and storage of specific factors and their interactions with other proteins in the extracellular matrix.[97]

Fibroblast Growth Factors. Fibroblast growth factors (FGFs) form a large family of polypeptides characterized by their affinity to glycosaminoglycan heparin binding sites.[112] FGF1 and FGF2, which have been studied extensively, have mitogenic properties for cells of the osteoblastic lineage, although eventual differentiation into mature osteoblasts does not occur in the presence of the FGF family of peptides.[113] In fact, FGF2 inhibits Wnt signaling and the synthesis of IGF-1, which results in a decrease in osteoblastogenesis and in osteoblastic function.[114,115] In vivo experiments have confirmed this action of FGF, and mice overexpressing FGF2 are osteopenic.[116] However, studies in *Fgf2*-null mice indicate that FGF is necessary for osteoblast formation, possibly because of its early effects on cell replication.[117] FGF can stimulate bone resorption by prostaglandin-dependent and -independent pathways.[118] The FGFs bind to a series of four FGF receptors that have intrinsic tyrosine kinase activity. In vertebrates, the 22 members of the FGF family range in molecular mass from 17 to 34 kDa and share 13% to 71% amino acid identity. Among vertebrate species, FGFs are highly conserved in both gene structure and amino acid sequence. FGFs have a high affinity for heparan sulfate proteoglycans and require heparan sulfate to activate one of four cell-surface FGF receptors. During embryonic development, FGFs have diverse roles in regulating cell proliferation, migration, and differentiation. In the adult organism, FGFs are homeostatic factors and function in tissue repair and response to injury. When inappropriately expressed, some FGFs can contribute to the pathogenesis of cancer.

FGF19, FGF21, and FGF23 are unique in that they bind to FGF receptors that heterodimerize with alpha- or beta-Klotho. FGF23 is secreted by osteocytes and has been shown to regulate phosphate homeostasis by inhibiting vitamin D 1α-hydroxylase activity in the kidney, thereby suppressing the production of $1,25(OH)_2D$. In addition, FGF23 promotes phosphate loss in the renal tubule, acting as an endocrine hormone produced by bone cells. Disorders in FGF23, including excess production or impaired degradation, result in several syndromes that are characterized by hypophosphatemia and osteomalacia. FGF21 is produced in the liver and in adipocytes. It is an important counterregulatory hormone that stimulates PPARα and oxidation of fatty acids.[119] FGF21 is high during calorie restriction, malnutrition, and lactation. It can potentially cause browning of white adipocytes but in mice has been shown to stimulate bone resorption. Recently FGF21 has been shown to induce significant bone resorption, and the FGF21 null mice have very high bone mass.[120]

Platelet-Derived Growth Factors, Vascular Endothelial Growth Factors, Hypoxia-Inducible Factors, and Reactive Oxygen Species. Platelet-derived growth factor (PDGF) was originally isolated from human platelets, and four members of the *PDGF* gene family have been identified: *PDGFA, PDGFB, PDGFC,* and *PDGFD*.[121] These peptides signal through the PDGFR family of receptors. Vascular endothelial growth factor (VEGF) shares a high degree of sequence homology with PDGF, and these factors are often referred to as members of the PDGF/VEGF family.[122]

PDGFs must form homodimers or heterodimers to exhibit activity. PDGF-AA, -AB, and -BB are the isoforms studied more extensively in skeletal cells, and they exert similar biologic actions. The primary function of PDGF in bone is the stimulation of cell replication, and PDGF impairs osteoblast differentiation and function.[123] PDGF also stimulates bone resorption. In mice, null mutations of *Pdfga* or *Pdfgb* and their receptors cause embryonic lethality or perinatal death, not allowing the study of the function of PDGF in the postnatal skeleton.[124] Although skeletal cells express products of the *Pdfga, Pdfgb,* and *Pdfgc* genes, the major source of PDGF is the systemic circulation, and skeletal cells become exposed to PDGF after platelet aggregation. The PDGF receptor 1a (PDGFR1a) is expressed on numerous progenitor cells in the hematopoietic niche including early osteoblasts and adipocytes.

Vascular endothelial growth factor A (VEGFA) is essential for angiogenesis, and *VEGFA* and VEGF receptor genes are expressed by chondrocytes and osteoblasts.[125] VEGFA is essential for blood vessel formation and vessel invasion into cartilage during the process of endochondral bone formation and for chondrocyte survival during skeletal development.[126] Importantly, VEGFA is also required for intramembranous bone formation and osteoblastic maturation.[127] Osteoblast expression of PDGF and VEGF is regulated by other locally derived growth factors.

Hypoxia-inducible factors (HIFs) are produced locally in response to low oxygen tension in the hematopoietic niche

and are transcription factors that mediate pathways that lead to angiogenesis, including production of VEGF. HIFs also induce genes essential for glycolysis, an essential biochemical pathway for ATP generation in the niche. During fracture repair, it has been demonstrated that more bone is produced in a mouse model with constitutively active HIF-1α in osteoblasts. Conversely, mice deficient in HIF-1α in osteoblasts had defective bone healing.[128]

Reactive oxygen species (ROS), which are free radicals that include peroxides, are products of cell metabolism, particularly oxidative phosphorylation. These products are inactivated by several enzymes that serve to prevent mitochondrial and cell damage. In several mouse models of aging, changes that occur in bone turnover and cell metabolism were associated with increases in ROS in bone cells.[129] Suppressing ROS through antioxidant therapy can reverse some of the effects on bone from the loss of sex steroids. However, ROS generation may be important to maintain a certain level of metabolic activity, and differences in ROS production may be critical to determining the fate switch between osteoblasts and adipocytes.

Insulin-like Growth Factors. IGFs are mitogens that also can increase the differentiated function of the osteoblast, supporting mineralization and bone formation.[130] Mouse models have demonstrated that both systemic and locally synthesized IGF-1 contribute to bone formation.[131] Transgenic mice overexpressing IGF-1 have increased bone mass, whereas *Igf1*-null mice exhibit decreased bone formation, reduced mineralization, and decreased cortical bone.[132] IGF-1 stimulates bone turnover by increasing osteoclastogenesis and bone remodeling.[133] Both IGF-1 and IGF-2 are synthesized by bone cells and are stored in the bone matrix, but IGF-1 is a more potent stimulator of osteoblastic function.[130] Six IGF-binding proteins have been identified in bone and in the circulation (e.g., IGFBP1 through IGFBP6). IGFBPs can inhibit or enhance IGF responses, depending on their local concentration relative to IGFs and the presence of proteases that can cleave the IGFBPs. IGFBP2 has been shown to be synergistic in its actions on osteoblasts with IGF-1 via signaling through the pleiotropin receptor that phosphorylates PTEN (phosphatase and tensin homolog).[134] PTH and PGE_2 are major inducers of skeletal IGF-1 and IGFBP2 synthesis, and glucocorticoids suppress IGF-1 transcription.[130] Thus IGFs can mediate selected effects of these hormones on bone formation.

Transforming Growth Factor-β. TGF-β belongs to a family of closely related polypeptides with various degrees of structural homology and important effects on cell function.[135] Skeletal cells express TGF-β1, TGF-β2, and TGF-β3. TGF-β has complex and somewhat contradictory actions in bone cells. TGF-β can stimulate osteoblastic cell replication and bone formation, but it does not favor osteoblastic differentiation.[136,137] The effects of TGF-β depend on the target cell and experimental conditions. The actions of TGF-β on bone resorption have been a source of controversy. TGF-β has a biphasic effect on osteoclastogenesis, but it decreases bone resorption.[138] Targeted disruption of the mouse *Tgfb1* gene is lethal but does not result in abnormal skeletal development.[139] TGF-β is secreted as a latent high-molecular-weight complex consisting of the C-terminal remnant of the TGF-β precursor and a TGF-β-binding protein.[140] The biologically active levels of TGF-β depend on changes in its synthesis and in its activation from its latent form.

Bone Morphogenetic Proteins and Wnt Proteins. BMPs are members of the TGF-β superfamily of polypeptides, and they were originally identified because of their ability to induce endochondral bone formation. BMPs are expressed by osteoblasts and play an autocrine role in osteoblastic differentiation and function.[97] The fundamental function of BMPs is the induction of osteoblastic cell differentiation, endochondral ossification, and chondrogenesis.[97,141] The genesis and differentiation of osteoblasts and osteoclasts are coordinated events, and BMPs also induce osteoclastogenesis and osteoclast survival.[142]

BMP activity is regulated by a large group of secreted polypeptides that bind and limit BMP action. These extracellular BMP antagonists prevent BMP signaling. Extracellular BMP antagonists include noggin, follistatin, myostatin, twisted gastrulation, the chordin family, and the Dan/Cerberus family of proteins.[97] These molecules can also bind to one or two activin receptors, ACVR2A and ACVR2B. Myostatin, a TGF-β superfamily member, is a negative regulator of muscle growth acting through ACVR2B. Inhibitors of these signaling peptides and their receptors may result in enhanced muscle mass and in some cases increased bone mass.[143]

The Wnt family of secreted glycoproteins, like BMPs, plays a critical role in directing osteoblastogenesis. In skeletal cells, many Wnt family members use the canonical Wnt/β-catenin signaling pathway.[144] In the absence of Wnt, the proteins axin, adenomatous polyposis coli (APC), and β-catenin form a complex that facilitates the phosphorylation and degradation of β-catenin. Binding of Wnt family proteins to specific frizzled membrane receptors and their coreceptors (LRP5 and LRP6) leads to the stabilization of β-catenin. This allows β-catenin to be translocated to the nucleus, where it can regulate the transcription of target genes. The Wnt/β-catenin signaling pathway is central to osteoblastogenesis and bone formation, and Wnt and BMPs act in concert to regulate cell differentiation. Deletions of Wnt or β-catenin genes result in the absence of osteogenesis and of skeletal tissue, and inactivating mutations of Wnt coreceptors result in osteopenia.[145] Wnt/β-catenin signaling induces OPG, and through this mechanism, Wnts are negative regulators of osteoclastogenesis.[146,147] Wnt activity, like that of BMPs, is controlled by extracellular antagonists and intracellular signaling proteins.[98] Extracellular antagonists such as sclerostin and Dkk1 prevent interactions between Wnt family members and coreceptors, although others, like soluble frizzled-related proteins, bind Wnts directly and block their actions. These antagonists limit Wnt signaling, which decreases osteoblast function and bone mass.[144,148] Conversely, deletion of sclerostin in mice produces a high bone mass phenotype.[149] Sclerostin, made predominantly by osteocytes, is regulated by systemic factors such as PTH and by mechanical forces on bone. Precisely how circulating versus local sclerostin regulates bone formation and resorption is an important unanswered question, particularly because circulating sclerostin levels have been shown to have a negative or positive relationship to bone mass and fractures in normal individuals and patients with type II diabetes mellitus.[150,151]

Systemic Hormones and Bone Remodeling

Remodeling is activated by systemic as well as local factors. Changes in mechanical force can activate remodeling to improve skeletal strength, and remodeling removes and repairs bone that has undergone microdamage. This occurs particularly in cortical bone and may explain the fact that remodeling is sustained in the aging skeleton.[152] However, loss of osteocytes with age may impair this response.[153] Systemic hormones influence bone remodeling to regulate the movement of mineral from bone to the extracellular fluid to maintain serum calcium levels and to sustain linear growth. During pubertal growth, bone modeling and

remodeling intensify and correlate with serum levels of IGF-1, supporting the role of growth hormone as a major mediator of skeletal formation.[19] In addition to the GH/IGF-1 axis it is now apparent that testosterone and estradiol must be present during peak acquisition to attain the highest possible BMD. Mineralization of newly formed bone is assured by activation of vitamin D 1α-hydroxylase in the kidney leading to greater calcium absorption and higher 1,25(OH)$_2$D levels. Hence, modeling and epiphyseal closure are both modulated by systemic hormones that are both calcium regulating and growth centric.

Calcium-Regulating Hormones

Parathyroid Hormone. PTH acts on bone to stimulate resorption but does not act on osteoclasts in the absence of cells of the osteoblastic lineage. PTH receptors are abundant on osteoblasts, bone lining cells, and osteocytes but not on osteoclasts.[154] PTH acts on osteoblasts to cause cell contraction; to induce immediate-early response genes, including c-Fos and the inducible form of prostaglandin G/H synthase (i.e., COX), and to increase the synthesis of local mediators, IGF-1 and IL-6.[154,155] High concentrations of PTH in vitro inhibit the expression of type I collagen, but intermittent administration of PTH in vivo or in vitro can stimulate bone formation.[155] PTH induces the production of RANKL and inhibits the production of OPG by cells of the osteoblast lineage, thereby increasing osteoclastogenesis and thus bone resorption. In some circumstances, PTH increases proliferation of cells of the osteoblast lineage and decreases their death by apoptosis.[156] PTH also induces 1α-hydroxylase activity in the kidney, thereby enhancing the active form of vitamin D (see later). In osteocytes, PTH not only stimulates production of RANKL but also inhibits production of sclerostin and increases synthesis of FGF23. In this way, PTH uses osteocytes to regulate bone remodeling and systemic calcium/phosphate homeostasis.

Vitamin D. The hormonal form of vitamin D, 1,25(OH)$_2$D$_3$, is necessary for intestinal calcium and phosphorus absorption and therefore for mineralization. This form of vitamin D also has effects on the skeleton, but its physiologic role in bone remodeling is not clear.[157] By increasing RANKL production on osteoblasts or osteoblast progenitor cells, vitamin D is a potent stimulator of osteoclast formation in cell culture. High concentrations increase osteocalcin synthesis by osteoblasts and inhibit collagen synthesis and mineralization in vitro (Fig. 29-15).[36] Lower concentrations may increase bone formation, although not to the extent seen with intermittent administration of PTH. Recent studies using conditional deletions of the vitamin D receptor (VDR) in bone and intestine provide further insight into the physiologic role of vitamin D on the bone remodeling unit. Intestinal deletion of the VDR mimics a low-calcium diet and is associated with bone loss related to increased bone resorption and decreased bone formation. However, serum calcium is preserved.[36] On the other hand, in the osteocyte and mature osteoblast-specific VDR null mice there is no alteration in circulatory levels of calcium, phosphorus, PTH, and 1,25(OH)$_2$D as well as no bone phenotype. Moreover, mice missing the VDR only in the intestine have a delay in mineralization through the actions of high levels of 1,25(OH)$_2$D$_3$ on osteoblastic cells.[36] These data provide a strong mechanistic rationale for active vitamin D action on remodeling: high 1,25(OH)$_2$D levels due to increased 1,25(OH)$_2$D bind to the VDR on osteoblasts and stimulate RANKL production leading to increased bone resorption as a way to protect the body against low serum calcium. It further slows entry of calcium into the skeleton by suppressing mineralization in vitro and in

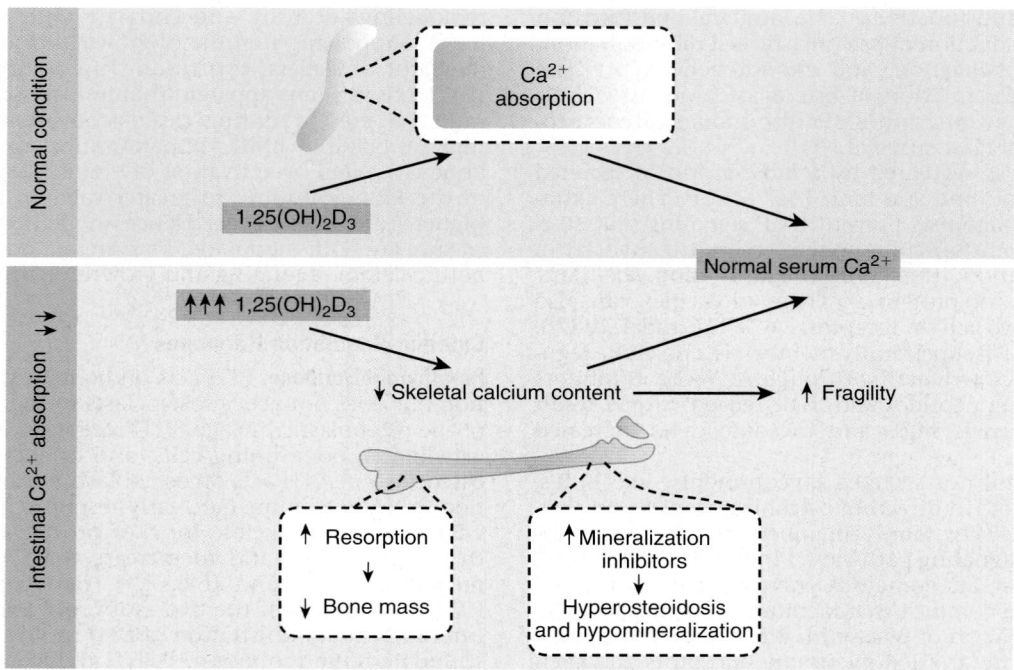

Figure 29-15 Vitamin D₃ (1,25[OH]₂D₃) induces skeletal hypomineralization and osteopenia to preserve serum calcium. (From Lieben L, Masuyama R, Torrekens S, et al. Normocalcemia is maintained in mice under conditions of calcium malabsorption by vitamin D–induced inhibition of bone mineralization. *J Clin Invest.* 2012;122:1803-1815.)

vivo, thereby preserving essential functions of the mammal (see Fig. 29-15).

Calcitonin. Calcitonin inhibits bone resorption by acting directly on the osteoclast, but it appears to play a smaller role in the regulation of bone turnover in adults.[158] Bone mass is not greatly altered in patients with medullary thyroid carcinoma, who have an excess of calcitonin production, or in athyreotic patients receiving adequate thyroid hormone replacement, who have low calcitonin levels.[159,160] Bone turnover is increased in patients with medullary thyroid carcinoma.[161] Mice with a deletion of the gene for calcitonin/calcitonin-related polypeptide-α (*CALCA*), which is responsible for the production of calcitonin and its alternate transcript calcitonin gene–related peptide, have increased bone mass and enhanced rates of bone formation.[162] In contrast, mice with a deletion of only the calcitonin gene–related peptide have decreased bone mass.[163] These results imply that calcitonin influences both bone formation and bone resorption. However, the mechanisms by which calcitonin affects bone formation remain unknown.

Other Systemic Hormones That Influence Remodeling

Growth Hormone. Deficiency and excess of growth hormone have marked effects on skeletal growth, as noted previously.[164,165] Growth hormone increases circulating and local levels of IGF-1, which mediates many of the skeletal effects of growth hormone. Exogenous growth hormone and IGF-1 increase bone remodeling presumably by directly acting on osteoblasts, although IGF-1 is also present on osteoclasts, and recombinant IGF-1 stimulates bone resorption. Osteocytes also possess IGF-1, and one can speculate that it might play an important role in regulating phosphate homeostasis via FGF23 during critical growth phases. Growth hormone stimulates cartilage growth, probably through an increase in local and systemic IGF-1 production and possibly by direct stimulation of cartilage

cell proliferation, because low levels of growth hormone receptors are present in chondrocytes.

Glucocorticoids. Glucocorticoids exert profound effects on bone remodeling.[166] Glucocorticoids decrease the intestinal absorption of calcium and have the potential to induce osteoclastogenesis and bone resorption because they increase the expression of RANKL and CSF1 in osteoblasts.[167] However, the most significant effect of glucocorticoids is their ability to suppress bone remodeling through depletion of the osteoblastic cell population.[168] Glucocorticoids inhibit the replication of osteoblast precursors and their differentiation into mature osteoblasts. This effect occurs in part because they suppress Wnt signaling and factors necessary for osteoblastic differentiation.[169] In a recent study it was observed in humans that glucocorticoids have diverse effects in the serum levels of two Wnt signaling antagonists: a progressive decrease in Dkk1 with a significant increase in circulatory levels of sclerostin.[170] Glucocorticoids induce the apoptosis of osteoblasts and osteocytes, contributing to the decrease in bone-forming cells.[171] Glucocorticoids inhibit the differentiated function of the osteoblast and bone formation. This results from direct effects of glucocorticoids on the osteoblast and suppression of IGF-1 transcription.[172]

Thyroid Hormones. Thyroid hormone signaling is mediated by thyroid hormone receptor (TR), a ligand-dependent transcription regulator molecule. TR is encoded by the thyroid hormone receptor alpha (*THRA* or c-erbAα) and beta (*THRB* or c-erbAβ) genes, which have different isoforms for which distribution is tissue- and age-dependent.[173,174] The TRβ1 and TRα1 isoforms are expressed in bone, but previous studies suggested that TRα1 is the major mediator of thyroid hormone effects in the skeleton.[175] However, the net effect of thyroid hormone is complex and it depends on the circumstances.[176] In children, hyperthyroidism is associated with increased bone mineralization and epiphyseal maturation, and hypothyroidism results in decreased growth.[177] On the other hand, in adults, hyperthyroidism is associated with bone loss. Thyroid hormones are crucial for cartilage growth and differentiation and enhance the response to growth hormone. Thyroid hormones increase bone resorption and turnover, although their effects on bone formation are less clear.[178] Coupled with their effects on bone resorption, thyroid hormones increase the transcription of collagenase and gelatinase by osteoblasts.[179] As thyroid hormones increase bone remodeling, thyroxine (T_4) may also increase bone formation. Thyroid hormones also have indirect effects on skeletal metabolism by suppressing the synthesis of thyroid-stimulating hormone (TSH, or thyrotropin), which can inhibit osteoclast formation and survival and as a consequence suppressed bone resorption.[180,181] Whether TSH has direct effects on osteoblasts and osteoclasts is still debated, however.

Insulin. Normal skeletal growth depends on an adequate amount of insulin.[182] Excess insulin production by the fetuses of mothers with uncontrolled diabetes results in excessive growth of the skeleton and other tissues, possibly through its actions on IGF-1. Poorly controlled diabetes mellitus leads to impaired skeletal growth and mineralization. Children and adolescents with type 1 diabetes are at increased risk for decreased bone mineral acquisition and accumulation of advanced glycosylated end products (AGEs).[183] Type 2 diabetes is associated with normal bone mass but increased skeletal fragility in part due to enhanced cortical porosity and increased AGEs in the matrix. In vitro, insulin at physiologic concentrations selectively stimulates osteoblastic collagen synthesis by a pretranslational mechanism. Insulin can mimic the effects of IGF-1, although only at supraphysiologic levels.[113] Mice deficient in insulin receptor substrate 1, a major substrate of insulin and IGF-1 receptor tyrosine kinases, exhibit impaired differentiative osteoblast function, low-turnover osteopenia, and an impaired response to PTH, documenting the central role of insulin and IGF-1 signaling in the maintenance of bone remodeling.[184] More recently, insulin has been shown to stimulate osteoblastic function and bone resorption leading to greater release of GLU13-OCN (see Fig. 29-5), which in turn causes greater insulin sensitivity and enhanced insulin synthesis in the islet cells. The effect of insulin on glucose transport in osteoblasts is still controversial, although deletion of the insulin receptor in osteoblasts, using the osteocalcin Cre promoter, results in low bone mass, obesity, and insulin resistance. Moreover, insulin deficiency and insulin resistance are associated with excessive formation of AGEs, which are involved in the development of classic diabetic micro- and macroangiopathy. AGEs may also impact bone microarchitecture through effects on collagen cross-linking, major post-translational modifications of collagen that influence bone strength. Collagen cross-links can be formed not only by lysyl hydroxylase and lysyloxidase-mediated enzymatic immature divalent cross-links and mature trivalent pyridinoline and pyrrole cross-links, but cross-links also can be produced by glycation- or oxidation-induced nonenzymatic cross-links (AGEs), such as glucosepane and pentosidine. The last may impair mineralization and the capacity of bone to repair itself from microdamage. This mechanism can be a common link to bone fragility, which is common in both type 1 and type 2 diabetic patients.[185,186]

Gonadal Hormones. Estrogens and androgens are critical for skeletal development and maintenance. Bone cells contain estrogen and androgen receptors, but it has been difficult to demonstrate direct effects of gonadal steroids on bone formation or resorption in cell and organ culture. Gonadal hormones are crucial for the pubertal growth spurt, and estrogen is necessary for epiphyseal closure.[187] Deficiency of estrogen or androgen increases bone resorption in vivo, partly by increasing the local synthesis or sensitivity to cytokines, such as IL-1 and IL-6 or TNF-α; to prostaglandins; and through direct actions on estrogen receptors in osteoclasts. Androgens can increase bone formation in vivo.[188] The effect of estrogens on bone formation is less clear, depending on the animal model and the dose of estrogen. The absolute rate of bone formation is increased in estrogen deficiency states because of an increase in bone remodeling. However, estrogen deficiency causes bone loss, implying a relative deficiency in bone formation. In other words, in the condition of hypoestrogenism, the increase in bone formation is not of the same magnitude as the enhancement in bone resorption.

EPIDEMIOLOGY OF OSTEOPOROSIS AND FRACTURES

Over the past 25 years, our understanding of fractures and their causes has significantly evolved and along with it, the definition of the disease osteoporosis. Its current definition was developed by an international Consensus Development Committee in 1993 as "a disease characterized by low bone mass and microarchitectural deterioration of bone tissue, leading to enhanced bone fragility and a consequent increase in fracture risk."[189] This definition reflects our understanding of the link between low bone quantity, compromised bone quality, and increased fracture risk. Although hip, vertebral, and wrist fractures are most commonly associated with osteoporosis, risk of other fractures is also increased.

Fractures

Hip Fractures

Proximal femur fractures are a major cause of morbidity and fatality and occur much more frequently in older people, increasing the costs of osteoporosis. Most commonly, these fractures occur in the femoral neck or intertrochanteric regions and require surgical repair. Increased risk of falls together with decreases in bone strength account for the increased risk with increasing age. Morbidity and mortality rates associated with hip fractures are substantial. The mortality rate within 1 year of the fracture is between 5% and 20%.[190] They are a major source of disability and loss of independence. For example, it is estimated that of those living independently before a hip fracture, only 50% are able to do so 1 year after the hip fracture.[13] After a hip fracture, there is also a substantial risk of other fractures, including a second hip fracture, and it is therefore important that further assessment and possible treatment be considered in patients with fractures at the hip (and other sites).[191,192]

Vertebral Fractures

Vertebral fractures are the most common manifestation of osteoporosis.[193] These fractures occur in a range of severities. Mild fractures, only some of which may be symptomatic, may only be apparent via radiographic or other types of imaging but are still, in aggregate, associated with clinical symptoms.[194,195] On the other hand, severe vertebral fractures can be accompanied by significant acute back pain that may persist for many weeks or indefinitely. Long-term consequences of vertebral fractures, particularly accumulation of multiple vertebral fractures, are substantial, leading to height loss, kyphosis, increased disability, decreased pulmonary function, substantial chronic back pain, and diminished overall quality of life.[196] There is also increased fatality associated with vertebral fractures.[197] Severity of these consequences increases with increasing severity and number of these fractures. Although they can be caused by trauma, they are often associated with little or no trauma.

Vertebral fractures have often been called the hallmarks of osteoporosis and tend to occur at younger ages than other fractures. Vertebral fractures increase the future risk of additional vertebral fractures by 5 to 10 times and are associated with a much higher risk of nonvertebral fractures, including hip fractures.[198,199] Therefore, like hip fractures, they should lead to further assessment (e.g., dual-energy x-ray absorptiometry [DXA]) and consideration of osteoporosis prevention and treatment. This is particularly true of incidental findings noted on chest and lumbar radiographs for other reasons. Often, vertebral fractures reported on radiographs are asymptomatic, and a history of trauma cannot be ascertained. This does not diminish the importance of the fracture with respect to future risk or associated morbidity.

Wrist Fractures

Fractures of the distal radius are common in postmenopausal women and are associated with osteoporosis. However, in general they have less morbidity and fewer costs than hip or spine fractures. Their incidence rises in women at menopausal age but then rises no further with increasing age. This pattern may be explained by different reactions to falling with age. Men have a much lower incidence of wrist fracture.

Other Types of Fractures

In addition to hip, spine, and wrist fractures, a large number of other fracture sites such as the arm, lower leg, humerus, and ribs are common and have been shown to have significant morbidity and mortality risks.[200] Furthermore, there is increasing evidence that the risk of most, if not all, of these fracture types are increased in those with low BMD or osteoporosis[201] and can be reduced by osteoporosis treatment.[192,202-204]

Clinical Assessments of Osteoporosis
Dual-Energy X-Ray Absorptiometry

DXA is the standard method for assessing the presence and extent of osteoporosis. DXA is most often performed at the spine and hip, although other sites (whole body, distal radius) can also be assessed. Although not a true density, it provides an areal density of mass per area in units of g/cm². The International Osteoporosis Foundation (IOF) and other organizations have developed a classification system for DXA values called T-scores that classify the measurement (Table 29-1). T-scores are calculated by comparing a specific value to a normative reference range for patients of the same gender and ethnicity. The T-score is the number of standard deviations (SD) below young normal values. A value below −2.5 SD is usually considered osteoporotic. Clinically, usually three regions are used for diagnosis: BMD at the total hip, the femoral neck, and the lumbar spine.

DXA values at the hip generally peak at about age 30 to 40 and then begin to decline (Fig. 29-16). The decline is somewhat accelerated at menopause for a few years and then becomes accelerated again after about age 65 or 70 in women.[205] Spine BMD measurements can be useful but in older women and especially men can be confounded by osteophytes, aortic calcification, degenerative disease, and other conditions that increase the apparent spinal BMD and therefore are less reliable in those over age 65 to 70.

A large number of studies (many of them prospective) have consistently shown that DXA BMD is strongly predictive of future risk of fracture. Hip BMD is predictive of various types of nonvertebral as well as vertebral fracture but is particularly strongly predictive of hip fractures. Although the risk of fracture increases significantly with

TABLE 29-1	
Diagnostic Categories for Osteoporosis Based on Measurements of Bone Mineral Density and Bone Mineral Content	
Category	**Definition**
Normal	BMD ± 1 SD of the young adult reference mean
Low bone mass (osteopenia)	BMD > 1 SD and < 2.5 SD lower than the young adult mean
Osteoporosis	BMD > 2.5 SD lower than the young adult mean
Severe osteoporosis (established osteoporosis)	BMD > 2.5 SD lower than the young adult mean in the presence of one or more fragility fractures

BMC, bone mineral content; BMD, bone mineral density; SD, standard deviation.

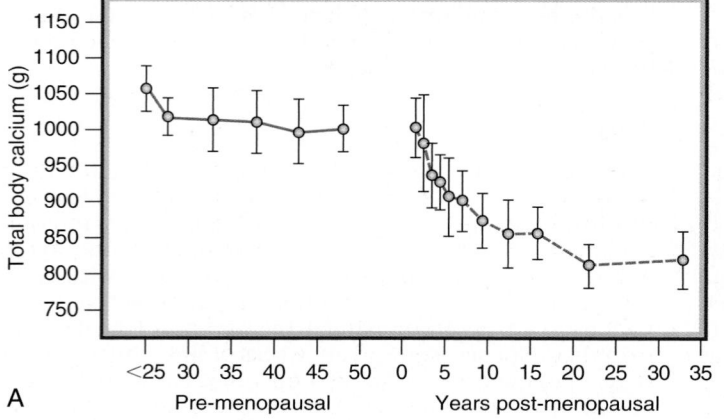

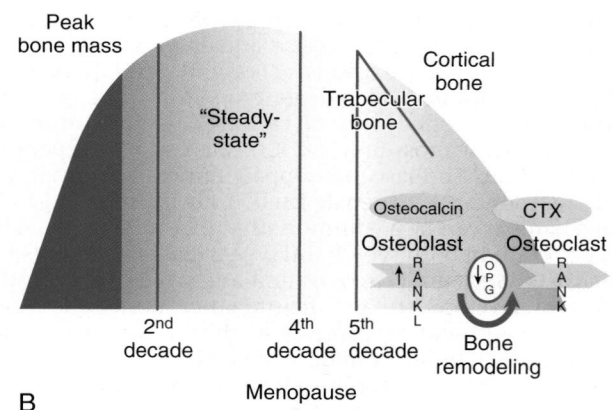

Figure 29-16 A, Bone mass development, maintenance, and loss: trabecular bone loss starts earlier and is more intense than in cortical bone. **B,** The decline of total body calcium with years since menopause. CTX, cross-linked telopeptide of type I collagen; OPG, osteoprotegerin; RANK, receptor activator of nuclear transcription factor κB. (Redrawn from Tella SH, Gallagher JC. Prevention and treatment of postmenopausal osteoporosis. *J Steroid Biochem Mol Biol.* 2014;142:155-170.)

decreasing BMD, several studies verified that osteoporotic fractures occur across a wide spectrum of BMDs. Most likely, these events are related to bone quality, a component not captured by DXA measurements. The World Health Organization (WHO) definition is a guideline for interpreting DXA results, not a definitive way of diagnosing osteoporosis. Therefore, DXA is the primary imaging tool used in diagnosing and treating osteoporosis. It can be used in conjunction with other risk assessment tools that combine other risk factors with DXA (see later). DXA measurements have been somewhat standardized across different types of scanners, although follow-up measures to assess change should be performed on the same scanner if at all possible.

Quantitative Computed Tomography

Other imaging modalities have been studied and may be used for osteoporosis assessment, although DXA remains the preferred method when available. Quantitive computed tomography (QCT) can be performed at the hip and spine, and studies have shown that it can predict fracture risk.[204,206,207] Several versions of software[208,209] are commercially available for analysis of QCT scans. One advantage of QCT is that it can provide specific measurements of trabecular and cortical BMD. However, QCT has the disadvantages (compared to DXA) of higher radiation exposure, less standardization across CT scanners, and higher cost. Peripheral QCT (pQCT) and high-resolution pQCT (HRpQCT) have been developed and can currently measure bone density and bone microarchitechture (in the case of HRpQCT) in the radius and tibia. Although these measurements can be helpful in the research context to help understand the impact of diseases such as diabetes and medications such as biphosphonates on bone microarchitecture and quality, there is little evidence that they have advantages in clinical practice for predicting fracture risk compared to DXA (examples of such measurements are shown in Fig. 29-17).

Other measurement tools to assess risk include ultrasound of the fingers, calcaneus, and distal extremities and magnetic resonance imaging (MRI) of the radius. Ultrasound has predictive value for fracture risk, but longitudinal assessments have not proved helpful clinically.[210] MRI provides significant insight into trabecular and cortical microstructure but is basically a research tool because of expense and time on the machines.

Bone Turnover Markers

The balance between bone resorption and formation is an important contributor to bone loss and osteoporosis. Bone turnover markers (BTMs) can provide an assessment of resorption and formation and might therefore be useful in understanding these imbalances within individual patients, prediction of fracture risk, and the effect of treatment. Bone formation can be assessed by a number of biochemical markers including bone-specific alkaline phosphatase (BSAP), total procollagen type 1 N-terminal propeptide (P1NP), and osteocalcin. Bone resorption has traditionally been assessed with urinary N-terminal cross-linked telopeptide (NTX) but is now more commonly assessed by serum C-terminal cross-linked telopeptide (CTX), both being collagen cross-linked peptides assessed with antibodies (Table 29-2).

There are a number of potential clinical applications of BTMs. However, all of them must take into account the high analytic variability (both within individual and between assays and laboratories) for these markers.[211] Important sources of variation within individuals include circadian variation, food intake, exercise, seasonal variation, diseases such as renal impairment, and recent fractures. For predicting fracture risk, there is controversy about whether BTMs predict fracture independently of BMD and other risk factors, with some studies showing a positive relationship, whereas others have not shown that BTMs independently predict fracture.[212-214] Because BTMs change dramatically and quickly with antiresorptive, as well as anabolic, treatment, it has been suggested that they may be of some use in monitoring therapy. Although the value of this application is controversial, they could have some value for a clinician with patients whose self-reported compliance may be unreliable.[215-217] They are more commonly used in specialty practices where they can be helpful

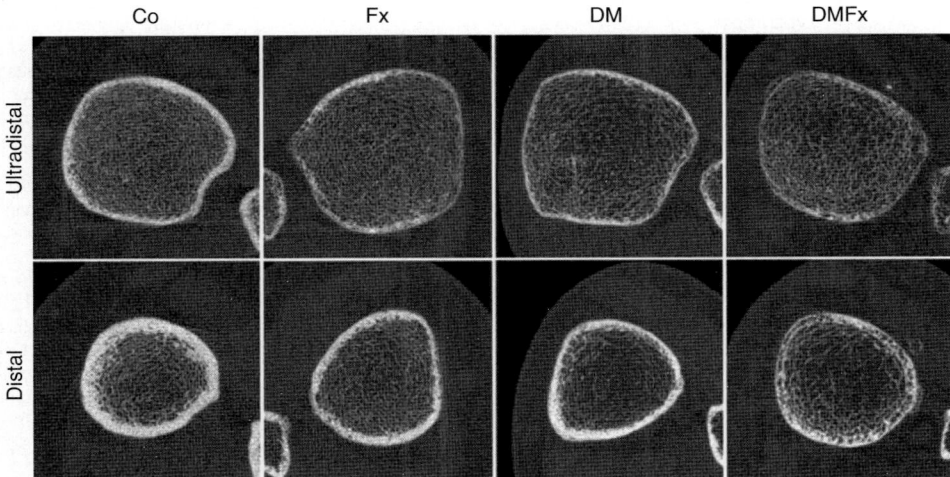

Figure 29-17 Representative high-resolution peripheral quantitative computed tomography (HR-pQCT) images of the ultradistal *(above)* and distal *(below)* tibia: shown are the mid-stack tomograms for the Co *(left)*, Fx *(left-center)*, DM *(right-center)*, and DMFx *(right)* groups. Major cortical porosity can be seen in DMFx *(right)*. Co, controls; Fx, nondiabetic fracture patients; DM, diabetic patients without fractures; DMFx, diabetic patients with fractures. (From Patsch JM, Burghardt AJ, Yap SP, et al. Increased cortical porosity in type 2 diabetic postmenopausal women with fragility fractures. *J Bone Miner Res.* 2013;28(2):313-324.)

TABLE 29-2

Markers of Bone Turnover

Marker	Tissue of Origin	Specimen	Analytic Method	Remarks
Bone Formation				
Bone-specific alkaline phosphatase (BAP)	Bone	Serum	Electrophoresis, precipitation, IRMA, EIA, ECMA	Specific product of osteoblasts; some assays show up to 20% cross-reactivity with the liver isoenzyme (LAP)
Osteocalcin (OC)	Bone, platelets	Serum	RIA, IRMA, EIA	Specific product of osteoblasts; many immunoreactive forms in blood; some may be derived from bone resorption
C-terminal propeptide of type I procollagen (PICP)	Bone, soft tissue skin	Serum	RIA, EIA	Specific product of proliferating osteoblasts and fibroblasts
N-terminal propeptide of type I procollagen (PINP)	Bone, soft tissue skin	Serum	RIA, EIA	Specific product of proliferating osteoblast and fibroblasts; partly incorporated into bone extracellular matrix
Markers of Bone Resorption				
Collagen-Related Markers				
Hydroxyproline, total and dialyzable (Hyp)	Bone, cartilage, soft tissue, skin	Urine	Colorimetry HPLC	Present in all fibrillar collagens and partly in collagenous proteins, including C1q and elastin. Present in newly synthesized and mature collagen, i.e., both collagen synthesis and tissue breakdown contribute to urinary hydroxyproline
Hydroxylysine-glycosides	Bone, soft tissue, skin, serum complement	Urine, serum	HPLC, EIA	Hydroxylysine in collagen is glycosylated to varying degrees, depending on tissue type. Glycosylgalactosyl-OH-Lys in high proportion in collagens of soft tissues, and C1q. Galactosyl-OH-Lys in high proportion in skeletal collagens
Pyridinoline (PYD)	Bone, tendon, cartilage, blood vessels	Urine, serum	HPLC, EIA	Collagens, with highest concentrations in cartilage and bone; absent from skin; present in mature collagen only
Deoxypyridinoline (DPD)	Bone, dentin	Urine, serum	HPLC, EIA	Collagens, with highest concentration in bone; absent from cartilage or skin; present in mature collagen only
C-terminal cross-linked telopeptide of type I collagen (ICTP, CTX-MMP)	Bone, skin	Serum	RIA, EIA	Collagen type I, with highest contribution probably from bone; may be derived from newly synthesized collagen
C-terminal cross-linked telopeptide of type I collagen (CTX-I)	All tissues containing type I collagen	Urine (α/β), serum (β only)	EIA, RIA	Collagen type I, with highest contribution probably from bone; isomerization of aspartyl to β-aspartyl occurs with aging of collagen molecule
N-terminal cross-linked telopeptide of type I collagen (NTX-I)	All tissues containing type I collagen	Urine, serum	EIA, RIA, CLIA	Collagen type I, with highest contribution from bone
Collagen I alpha 1 helicoidal peptide (HELP)	All tissues containing type I collagen	Urine	EIA	Degradation fragment derived from the helical part of type I collagen, α1 chain, AA (620-633); correlates highly with other markers of collagen degradation, no specific advantage or difference in regard to clinical outcomes
Noncollagenous Proteins				
Bone sialoprotein (BSP)	Bone, dentin, hypertrophic cartilage	Serum	RIA, EIA	Acidic, phosphorylated glycoprotein, synthesized by osteoblasts and osteoclastlike cells, laid down in bone extracellular matrix; appears to be associated with osteoclast function
Osteocalcin fragments (uf-OC, U-Mid-OC, U-Long-OC)	Bone	Urine	EIA	Certain age-modified fragments are released during osteoclastic bone resorption and may be considered an index of bone resorption
Osteoclast Enzymes				
Tartrate-resistant acid phosphatase (TRAcP)	Bone	Blood plasma	Serum colorimetry, RIA, ELISA	Six isoenzymes found in human tissues (osteoclasts, platelets, erythrocytes); band 5b predominant in bone (osteoclasts)
Cathepsins (e.g., K, L)	K: Primarily in osteoclasts; L: macrophage, osteoclasts	Plasma, serum	ELISA	Cathepsin K, a cysteine protease, plays an essential role in osteoclast-mediated bone matrix degradation by cleaving helical and telopeptide regions of collagen type I; Cathepsin K and L cleave the loop domain of TRAP and activate the latent enzyme; Cathepsin L has a similar function in macrophages; tests for measurement of Cathepsins in blood are presently under evaluation

BAP or Bone ALP, serum bone alkaline phosphatase; BMD, bone mineral density; BSP, bone sialoprotein; β-CTX-I, epitope of C-terminal cross-linked telopeptide of collagen type I; CLIA, chemiluminescent immunoassay; C-terminal, carboxy-terminal; CTX-MMP, C-terminal cross-linking telopeptide of type I collagen generated by matrix metalloproteinases; DPD, deoxypyridinoline; ECMA, electrometric immunoassay; EIA, enzyme immunoassay; HPLC, high-performance liquid chromatography; ICTP, carboxyterminal type I collagen telopeptide; IRMA, immunoradiometric assay; N-terminal, amino-terminal; NTX-I, N-terminal cross-linked telopeptide of collagen type I; PICP, C-terminal propeptide of procollagen type I; PINP, N-terminal propeptide of procollagen type I; PTH, parathyroid hormone; PTHrP, parathyroid hormone-related peptide; PYD, pyridinoline; RIA, radioimmunoassay; TAP, serum total alkaline phosphatase; TRAP or TRAcP, tartrate-resistant acid phosphatase; ufOC, urinary fragments of osteocalcin; U-long-OC, long N-terminal fragment; U-Mid-OC, midmolecule epitope of the OC.

Adapted from Seibel MJ. Biochemical markers of bone turnover: part I: biochemistry and variability. *Clin Biochem Rev.* 2005;26(4):97-122.

in defining secondary causes of osteoporosis. BTMs are particularly useful when measured in groups of patients during the development of new medications. In the research setting these measurements can provide early assessments of potency of drugs, their effects over time, and determining optimal doses.[218,219]

Bone Biopsy

Bone biopsy is used clinically to assess dynamic and static indices related to bone remodeling. It is rarely used clinically to diagnose osteoporosis but can be useful to assess the degree of mineralization (e.g., to exclude osteomalacia), rates of bone formation or resorption, and the overall status of remodeling (e.g., to exclude adynamic renal bone disease). Universal criteria can then be applied to the indices obtained after labeling bone by timed tetracycline administration.[220] Transiliac biopsies can be performed by physicians who specialize in osteoporosis medicine or by orthopedic surgeons and requires local anesthetic for a core biopsy, which generally requires a 7.5-mm trephine core for bone histologic diagnosis and histomorphometry. Mineral apposition rate, mineralizing surface, bone formation rate, eroded surfaces, number of osteoblasts and osteoclasts, and osteoid volume/bone volume all can be determined from a single biopsy but only after serial tetracyclin labeling, which is required to measure the distance between two mineralization fronts. Labeling intervals vary somewhat but generally are for 3 days at the beginning (days 1-3) and for 3 days 21 days later, using demeclocycline 200 mg three times day. Several commercial laboratories provide analysis of biopsies, although turnaround time can vary from 1 to several months. Not infrequently, however, bone biopsies in age-related or postmenopausal osteoporosis are normal, and hence the diagnostic specificity is low.

Fracture Epidemiology

Some of the central features of the epidemiology of fractures for the three primary osteoporotic fractures are illustrated in Figure 29-18. These data show very clearly the exponential increase in women in hip and spine fractures. For example, an average Caucasian woman at age 50 has about a 15% to 20% annual risk of hip fracture that increases still further beyond age 80. Wrist fractures show a different pattern in women with an increase at the time of menopause but then no further increase with time. In men, the exponential increase in hip and spine fractures with age is parallel to that for women. However, importantly, the age-specific risk of hip and spine fractures in men is much lower than that in women (approximately 50%), highlighting the key role of gender in the epidemiology of osteoporotic fractures. Wrist fracture incidence in men is much lower than in women at all ages.

Ethnicity and culture also play a key role in the epidemiology of osteoporosis (Fig. 29-19). For hip fractures, those of Caucasian ethnicity are at higher risk, Hispanics and Asians are at medium risk, and African Americans are at lowest risk. However, these general relationships can often be more subtle: for example, in Asians, there is evidence that rates are very low in areas with traditional lifestyles and that they increase substantially with increasing urbanization and adoption of Western lifestyles.[221] Rates of spine fractures are more challenging to assess, but many studies suggest that these rates vary less geographically than do rates of hip fracture.

Another key epidemiologic factor that interacts with age, gender, and ethnicity is weight or body mass index (BMI). In general, higher BMI individuals are at lower risk of hip and spine fractures, owing to several factors, including a larger number of fat cells that produce greater amounts of estrogen, which is protective, and the higher amount of padding in higher BMI patients, which produces a larger distribution of the forces in the event of a fall. Although some data suggest that obese individuals have a higher risk of fractures, most studies support the tenet that a higher BMI is protective for most types of fractures, the exception possibly being lower limb fractures. Very importantly, those at low BMI are at particularly high risk of hip fracture for several reasons, one of which may be that low BMI, particularly in the elderly, may be a sign of frailty.[222,223]

Clinical Risk Factors and Their Combination With Bone Mineral Density

A number of other clinical risk factors (in addition to BMD, age, gender, and race) have been consistently associated with fracture risk (Fig. 29-20). Most important of these is a history of fracture since age 50 or a mother's (or father's) history of hip fracture.[224] Other risk factors including cigarette smoking, excessive alcohol consumption (more than two drinks per day), rheumatoid arthritis, and glucocorticoid use also have some association with risk.[223,225] Compromised neurologic or muscular function is a strong risk factor, probably through an increased likelihood of falls. There is also a growing awareness that diabetics, despite a generally high BMI, are at higher risk of fracture and that this risk at the same BMD is higher than that for nondiabetics.[226] Surprisingly, some recent studies have suggested that obesity may be a risk factor for fracture in some settings: in the MrOS (osteoporotic fractures in men) study, it was suggested at the same BMD, elderly men who were obese were at higher risk than those who were not obese.[227]

There is a growing appreciation that fracture risk, like heart disease risk, is multifactorial and that these risk factors work in combination to increase risk.[223,225] More recently, risk assessment tools predicting 5- or 10-year risk of fracture from combinations of BMD and risk factors together have been developed. Most widely used and available is the FRAX fracture risk assessment tool, which includes the risk factors in Table 29-3 and has been implemented with country-specific versions[228] for predicting risk of hip and major osteoporotic fractures. Other risk assessment tools have also been proposed and include different

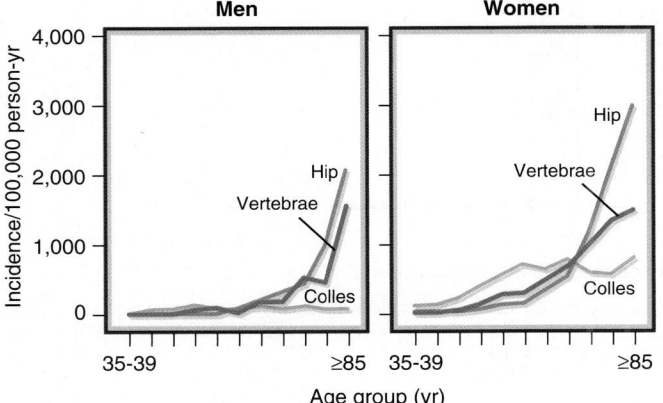

Figure 29-18 Age-specific incidence rates for hip, vertebral, and Colles fractures in Rochester, Minnesota. (From Cooper C, Melton LJ. Epidemiology of osteoporosis. *Trends Endocrinol Metab.* 1992;3:224. Copyright 1992 by Elsevier Science, Inc.)

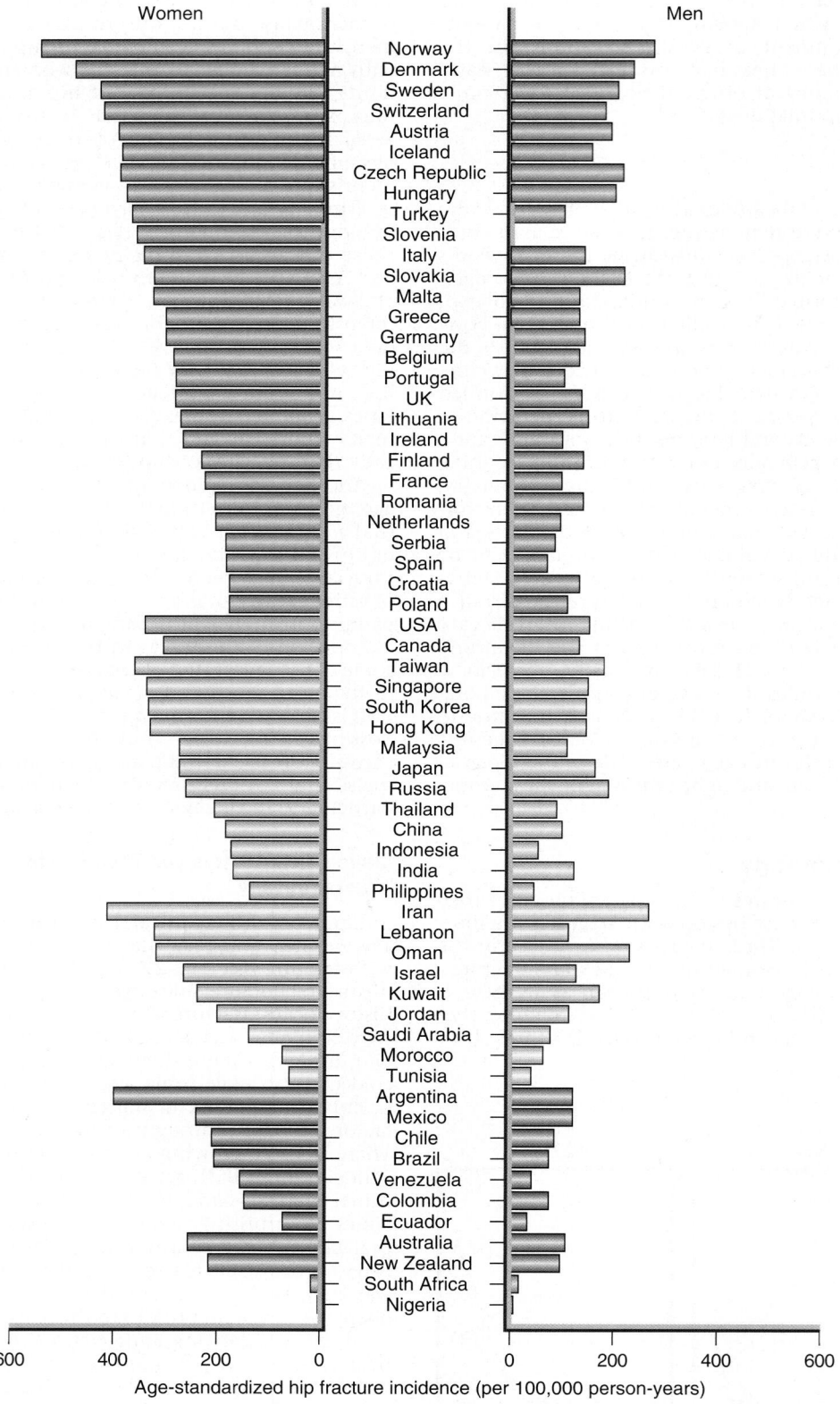

Figure 29-19 Age-standardized hip fracture incidence rates in women and men according to country. Countries are organized by continent or geographic region: Europe *(dark pink)*; North America *(green)*; Asia *(light blue)*; Middle East *(yellow)*; South America *(purple)*; Oceania *(dark blue)*; Africa *(red)*. (Redrawn from Cauley JA, Chalhoub D, Kassem AM, Fuleihan Gel-H. Geographic and ethnic disparities in osteoporotic fractures. *Nat. Rev. Endocrinol.* 2014;10(6):338-351.)

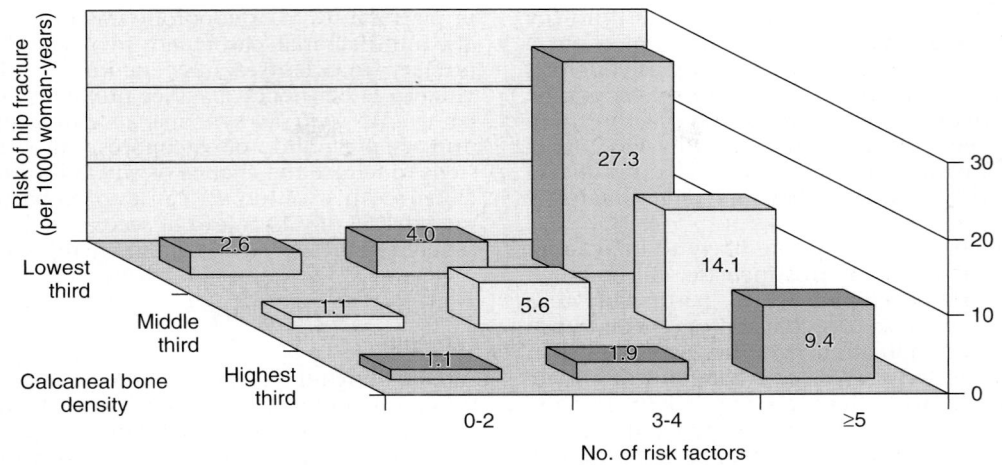

Figure 29-20 Annual risk of hip fracture according to the number of risk factors and the age-specific calcaneal bone density. (Redrawn from Cummings SR, Nevitt MC, Browner WS, et al. Risk factors for hip fracture in white women. Study of Osteoporotic Fractures Research Group. *N Engl J Med.* 1995;332:767-773. Copyright © 1995 Massachusetts Medical Society. Reprinted with permission.)

TABLE 29-3

Different Combinations of Relevant Fracture Risk Factors Used to Calculate an Individual's Probability of Fracture in 10 Years

FRAX	Q-Fracture Score	Garvan
Age	Age	Age
Sex	Sex	Sex
Weight	Weight	
Personal history of fracture (vertebral inclusive)		Personal history of fracture
Parental history of hip fracture	Parental history of hip fracture	
Current smoking	Current smoking (graded)	
Glucocorticoid (prednisolone equivalent 5 mg for ≥3 months)	At least two prescriptions for systemic corticosteroids in the 6 months before baseline	
Rheumatoid arthritis	Rheumatoid arthritis	
Secondary osteoporosis, type 1 diabetes mellitus, osteogenesis imperfecta in adults, hyperthyroidism, hypogonadism, chronic malnutrition, and liver disease	Secondary osteoporosis, cardiovascular disease, type 2 diabetes mellitus, asthma, chronic liver disease, gastrointestinal conditions likely to result in malabsorption (such as Crohn disease, ulcerative colitis, celiac disease, steatorrhea, blind loop syndrome), thyrotoxicosis, primary or secondary hyperparathyroidism, Cushing syndrome	
Alcohol ingestion (>3 units/day)	Alcohol ingestion (>3 units/day)	
	At least two prescriptions for tricyclic antidepressants in the 6 months before baseline	
	At least two prescriptions for hormone replacement therapy (in women) in the 6 months before baseline	
	History of falls before baseline	History of falls
BMD (optional)		BMD

or fewer risk factors.[229] Clinical guidelines for treatment have been developed incorporating these tools (discussed later) (see Table 29-3).

Prevalence of Osteoporosis and Incidence of Fractures in the Population

Estimates of the prevalence of osteoporosis have depended on the working definition of this disease and the appropriate diagnostic criteria and have been based either on the prevalence of low BMD or on fracture incidence.[9,14,230] Basing a definition solely on BMD became increasingly possible after the development and clinical availability of DXA. In 1992, the WHO set a cutoff point of 2.5 SD below a young normal mean value for BMD as a tool for estimating osteoporosis prevalence and comparing across populations (see Table 29-1).[231] The use of DXA in larger epidemiologic studies in women, such as the Study of

Osteoporotic Fractures (SOF), and men (MrOs) and particularly in population-based samples such as the National Health and Nutrition Examination Study (NHANES) have provided estimates of the proportion of people with osteoporosis by BMD.[232-234] Estimates of overall prevalence of osteoporosis vary greatly but place the number close to 40 million Americans.[9,235]

Based on fracture incidence, currently most estimates suggest that there are approximately 0.3 million hip fractures per annum in the United States and 0.6 million hip fractures in Europe.[14,230] Best estimates are that more than a million American postmenopausal women will suffer a spine fracture in the course of a single year.[9,235] Considering the importance of fracture from an individual's point of view, a 50-year-old Caucasian woman has approximately a 15% to 20% lifetime risk of hip fracture, a similar lifetime risk of wrist fracture, about a 16% lifetime risk of clinical spine fracture, and approximately a 50% risk of at least one osteoporotic fracture.[236-238] Men have about one third the lifetime risk of hip and spine fractures as women but a much lower risk of wrist fracture. Combining osteoporosis prevalence based on either the presence of osteoporotic fractures (i.e., vertebral compressions, wrist fractures, hip fractures, or humerus/tibial fractures) or low BMD, it is estimated that more than 40 million Americans are afflicted with osteoporosis.[239] Worldwide there are approximately 9 million fractures a year.[240]

Although numbers of fractures are likely to increase in the United States and Europe, this increase will be much more striking in the developing world, particularly Asia and Latin America, because of a collision of several trends including increasing population size, increasing life span (into the high–fracture-risk ages), and adoption of a more Western lifestyle (particularly decreasing activity in daily living). This increase will result in a consequent increase in need for health care resources. Interestingly, although hip fractures are the most costly individual fractures, the overall costs of other types of fractures together may be greater than that for hip fractures.[241]

PATHOGENESIS OF OSTEOPOROSIS

Osteoporosis is a complex disease with a multifactorial origin (Fig. 29-21). The cardinal feature of this disease is fractures usually accompanied by enhanced skeletal fragility. Although the primary focus of this chapter is on the endocrine and metabolic aspects of this disease, it should be noted that falls cause fractures and that one of the

primary causes of osteoporotic fractures is falling. Falls are also multifactorial, particularly in older individuals, because primary muscle weakness, neurologic disorders, drugs, vitamin D deficiency, balance problems, and cardiovascular events such as syncope all can cause falls. Hence, primary prevention of osteoporosis also mandates specific steps to reduce the chance of any fall for whatever reason. Noted in this section are causes of imbalance in the bone remodeling unit that lead to secondary bone loss and subsequent reduction in BMD, enhancing skeletal fragility.

Gonadal Deficiency

Estrogen

Altered bone remodeling is at the heart of the osteoporosis syndrome and can take many forms. Historically, the importance of estrogen in maintaining calcium homeostasis via coupled remodeling in the postmenopausal woman was first established by Fuller Albright in 1947.[242] Since that time much evidence has accumulated from randomized intervention trials demonstrating that gonadal steroid replacement (estrogen with or without progesterone) reduces bone turnover and increases bone mass, thus protecting the skeleton from fractures.[188,243] However, these data provide only indirect evidence that estrogen levels are important as pathogenic components of the osteoporosis syndrome. More recent studies provide stronger evidence of the association between low estradiol concentrations and low bone mass. Several investigators have demonstrated that the lowest estradiol levels in postmenopausal women (i.e., <5 pg/mL) are associated with the lowest BMD and

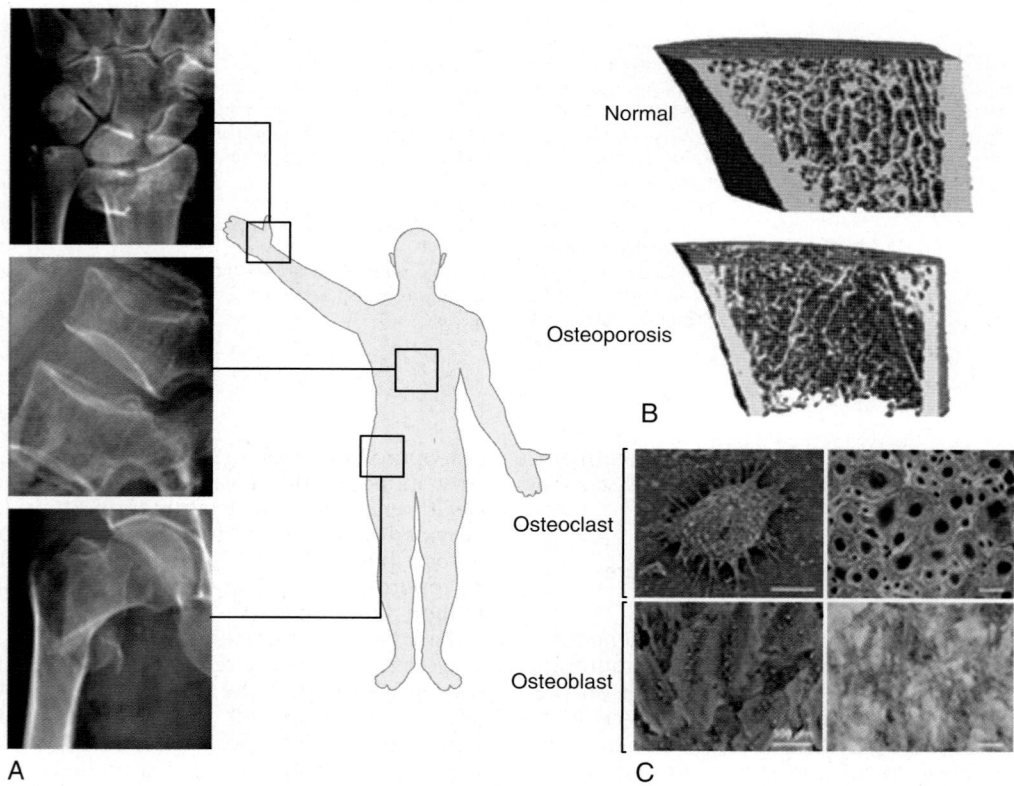

Figure 29-21 Osteoporosis at a glance. Osteoporosis is a systemic skeletal disease in which bone resorption exceeds bone formation and results in microarchitectural changes. **A,** Fragility fractures typically involve wrist, vertebrae, and hip. **B,** Microcomputed tomography shows marked trabecular thinning of osteoporotic bone compared with normal bone. **C,** Microscopic views of bone-resorbing osteoclasts and bone-forming osteoblasts: *1,* osteoclast with its distinctive morphologic appearance; *2,* tartrate-resistant acidic phosphatase staining of multinucleated osteoclasts; *3,* multiple osteoblasts on mineralized matrix; *4,* alkaline phosphatase staining of osteoblasts. (From Rachner TD, Khosla S, Hofbauer LC. Osteoporosis: now and the future. *Lancet.* 2011;377(9773):1276-1287.)

the greatest likelihood of fracture.[244] In addition, several studies have shown that males with osteoporosis have lower serum levels of estradiol than do age-matched men who do not have low bone mass.[245] Moreover, there are now several case reports describing mutations in genes encoding either aromatase or the estrogen receptor, producing a phenotype of severe osteoporosis in men.[246,247] In the former case, estrogen replacement therapy in those men resulted in a marked increase in spine and hip BMD. In both situations the lack of functional estrogen, despite normal to high levels of testosterone, resulted in severely low BMD.[187]

Although declining estradiol levels contribute to the osteoporosis syndrome, the precise molecular events or sequences that result from changes in ambient hormonal concentrations are not clear. In some animal models, estrogen deprivation is associated with a marked increase in IL-6 synthesis from stromal and osteoblastic cells. This is consistent with experimental findings that demonstrate that estrogen regulates the transcriptional activity of the IL-6 promoter.[248] However, results in other studies are conflicting. In other experimental paradigms, changes in TNF, IL-11, and IL-1 can be associated with increased bone resorption.[249-251] RANKL has been identified as a major regulator of osteoclast differentiation, and increases both locally and systemically likely contribute to the rapid increase in osteoclastogenesis after estrogen withdrawal. Thus, it seems likely that several cytokines, working in concert with RANKL, are active during estrogen deprivation, and each can accelerate the process of bone resorption. Osteoclasts express estrogen receptors and some evidence suggests that direct actions of estrogen on osteoclasts are important as well. Enhanced bone resorption eventually leads to bone loss from estrogen deprivation because bone formation rates cannot keep up with the high rates of bone resorption (see Fig. 29-16A).[3]

Androgens

In contrast to the plethora of studies on uncoupled bone remodeling and bone loss with low estradiol levels, there are fewer studies relating androgen deprivation to bone loss in both men and women. Androgen receptors are present on osteoblasts, and testosterone and dihydroxytestosterone both stimulate osteoblast differentiation.[252] Testosterone may also increase skeletal and circulating IGF-1. However, both in vitro and in vivo studies in men have yielded conflicting results with respect to bone resorption. Like estrogen, androgens can regulate the IL-6 promoter and in experimental animals, orchiectomy has been associated with increased IL-6 production and bone loss.[253] Men who undergo androgen deprivation therapy after prostate cancer lose bone rapidly as a result of increased bone resorption. Similarly, hypogonadal men, either due to primary or secondary insufficiency, have lower bone density values than control men. Because unlike estradiol, testosterone can stimulate bone formation, this may be an additional factor that contributes to bone loss when absent in men.[254]

Low testosterone levels that are found in postmenopausal women have not been causally associated with rapid bone loss, but women with greater body weight have greater capacity to enzymatically convert testosterone to estradiol, which may contribute to the protective effect of obesity on bone mass, at least in women. Notwithstanding, because in men chronically low androgen levels have been associated with low bone mass, testosterone replacement can be used to enhance BMD as well as to increase lean body mass.[254] However, as noted, estradiol levels in men

may be a more important risk factor for fracture than androgen levels. In sum, the combination of both estrogen and androgens probably determines peak bone mass and maintenance of BMD in both men and women. In elderly males, estradiol levels may be essential for maintaining trabecular bone mass. To underline that tenet, in one randomized trial using a GnRH analogue (to suppress gonadotropins) with and without an aromatase inhibitor in men, changing estrogen levels were associated with protection of the trabecular skeleton from bone resorption, whereas circulating androgen levels were more related to markers of bone formation than those of resorption.[188] In another study, Almeida and colleagues found that in rodents that protection of cortical bone mass by estrogens is mediated via ERα.[255] By contrast, the androgen receptor of mature osteoblasts was indispensable for the maintenance of trabecular bone mass in male mammals but was not required for the anabolic effects of androgens on cortical bone.[252,256]

In men, conditions other than hypogonadism can contribute to bone loss and fractures. These states include chronic alcoholism, glucocorticoid excess, and idiopathic hypercalcuria. In the first two cases, low testosterone levels probably contribute to the pathogenic features of osteoporosis syndrome, whereas hypercalcuria due to renal loss probably causes bone loss through secondary hyperparathyroidism. Less frequent but still important secondary causes of osteoporosis in men must also be considered independent of androgen levels, and these include gluten enteropathy, primary hyperparathyroidism, thyrotoxicosis, multiple myeloma, lymphomas, or granulomatous diseases, all of which can present with multiple fractures and low bone mass (see Table 29-3).[257]

Age-Related Bone Loss

In women, bone loss is accelerated immediately after menopause. However, recent studies demonstrate that markers of bone resorption are also very high later in life. In particular, women in their 80s and 90s have been noted to lose bone at a rate of greater than 1% per year from the spine and hip (see Fig. 29-16).[205] Contrary to earlier studies, it is now evident that the older woman who is not as physically active, and is not taking estrogen, is at extremely high risk of bone loss and subsequent fractures. The pathogenesis of this process is multifactorial, although dietary calcium deficiency, leading to secondary hyperparathyroidism, certainly plays some role. The average calcium intake of women in their eighth and ninth decades of life is now estimated to be between 800 and 1000 mg/day. If vitamin D intake is also suboptimal and serum levels of 25-hydroxyvitamin D are less than 20 ng/mL, or 50 nmol/L, secondary hyperparathyroidism may occur, although there are other causes in the elderly for increases in PTH, including a low glomerular filtration rate and low calcium intake.[258] PTH stimulates osteoblasts and provokes the remodeling sequence including the elaboration of several cytokines that accelerate bone resorption. Unfortunately, in most elders, bone formation is not enhanced, although the reasons for this are not entirely clear. Overall, the secondary hyperparathyroidism coupled with high $1,25(OH)_2D$ (see later discussion under "Vitamin D") leads to further uncoupling in the bone remodeling cycle and significant bone loss. Furthermore, among elders with poor calcium intake who live in northern latitudes, seasonal changes in vitamin D levels, lowering levels below 20 ng/mL, might aggravate bone loss.[258,259] Whether increased bone loss is an independent risk factor for future fractures in the elderly remains somewhat controversial, necessitating further studies to define such a risk.

Many older individuals already have established osteoporosis, so coincidental vitamin D deficiency due to poor intake, absent sunlight exposure, or impaired conversion of vitamin D to its active metabolite can result in osteomalacia as well as aggravating preexistent osteoporosis.[260] Osteomalacia can lead to dramatic changes in skeletal microarchitecture, as recently demonstrated in a cohort from Germany. Trabecular and cortical changes seen in that study led to microcracks and greater skeletal fragility. Priemel and associates reported that more than 50% of elders who presented with a hip fracture were vitamin D deficient.[261] Combining vitamin D deficiency with inadequate calcium intake enhances the likelihood of rapid bone loss in a very susceptible population. Despite these findings, elevated PTH levels in older women have been associated with bone loss in some studies but not in other studies. In elderly individuals, it has been reported that PTH levels are closely correlated with increased synthesis of IGFBP4, which suppresses IGF action on bone cells and may increase sclerostin secretion.[262,263] Because IGF-1 is an important growth factor for osteoblasts, it is conceivable that PTH downregulates IGF activity during states of relative calcium or vitamin D deficiency. This would shift the remodeling balance toward preserving intravascular calcium concentrations while inhibiting new calcium incorporation into the skeletal matrix. This response makes teleologic sense, although further studies are needed to assess whether serum IGFBP4 is a reliable marker of calcium deficiency in older individuals.[263] In sum, there is little doubt that calcium and vitamin D insufficiency can cause accelerated bone loss in the elderly, although the threshold for low vitamin D and poor calcium intake is still actively debated. Other concomitants of aging, such as accumulation of ROS (seen in aged mice) and other causes of damage to bone cells appear likely to contribute to age-associated osteoporosis as well.[264]

Secondary Osteoporosis

The division of osteoporosis into primary and secondary forms is somewhat arbitrary. For example, patients with diseases that lead to hypogonadism early in life are considered to have secondary osteoporosis, whereas osteoporosis in women with natural menopause and older men with low sex hormone levels is called primary. Moreover, patients may have a combination of primary and secondary forms. Although most postmenopausal women and older men do not have a definable secondary cause, those who do can be treated more effectively. This possibility should be considered for every patient. There are many causes of secondary osteoporosis (Table 29-4), only a few of which are discussed here.

Glucocorticoid-Induced Bone Loss

The most common cause of secondary osteoporosis is glucocorticoid-induced bone loss, which is often a result of pharmacologic doses of steroids used to treat inflammatory

TABLE 29-4
Causes of Secondary Osteoporosis

Endocrine Disorders	Mental Illness
Diabetes mellitus	Depression
Hyperparathyroidism	Eating disorders
Hyperthyroidism	**Cancer**
Cushing syndrome	
Hypogonadism	Breast
Menstrual irregularity (even athletes)	Prostate
Premature menopause	**Conective Tissue Disorders**
Low testosterone and estradiol levels in men	
Hyperprolactinemia	Osteogenesis imperfecta
Pregnancy and lactation	Ehlers-Danlos syndrome
Autoimmune Disorders	Marfan syndorme
	Menkes syndrome
Rheumatoid arthritis	**Drug-Induced Disorders**
Inflammatory bowel disease	
Lupus erythematosus	Glucocorticoids
Multiple sclerosis	Heparin
Ankylosing spondylitis	Anticonvulsants
Digestive and Gastrointestinal Disorders	Methotrexate, cyclosporine
	Luteinizing hormone-releasing hormone (LHRH) agonist or antagonist therapy
Celiac disease	Proton pump inhibitors
Inflammatory bowel disease	Aluminum-containing antacids
Weight loss surgery	**Other Diseases and Conditions**
Gastrectomy	
Hematologic/Blood Disorders	AIDS/HIV
	Chronic obstructive pulmonary disease
Leukemia and lymphoma	Female athlete triad
Multiple myeloma	Kidney disease
Sickle cell disease	Liver disease
Blood and bone marrow disorders	Organ transplant
Plasma cell dyscrasias: multiple myeloma and macroglobulinemia	Poliomyelitis and post-polio syndrome
Myeloproliferative disorders: polycythemia	Poor diet, including malnutrition
Thalassemia	Weight loss
Neurologic/Nervous System Disorders	Lipidoses: Gaucher disease
	Scurvy
Stroke, Parkinson disease, and multiple sclerosis	
Spinal cord injuries	

AIDS, acquired immunodeficiency syndrome; HIV, human immunodeficiency virus.

or autoimmune disorders. Generally, it is considered that glucocorticoids have a dose-dependent effect on the skeleton, such that longer duration and higher doses of steroids are most likely to cause bone loss and fractures. However, there clearly are subsets of individuals who are more or less sensitive to the skeletal effects of high doses of glucocorticoids. As a clinical rule, those individuals with a cushingoid appearance and fat redistribution phenotypes almost always have low bone mass and fractures. Notwithstanding, BMD measurements are indicated in patients on long-term glucocorticoids both for preventive approaches as well as treatment decisions.[265,266]

As noted previously, high circulating levels of glucocorticoids have a significant impact on bone acquisition and maintenance. In 1932 Harvey Cushing recognized the syndrome of endogenous steroid excess, which included marked osteopenia and fractures.[267,268] Long-term exposure to pharmacologic doses of glucocorticoids results in significant bone loss and enhanced marrow adipogenesis as marrow stromal cells differentiate down the fat lineage. In addition to having direct effects on the osteoclast and osteoblast, glucocorticoids also induce secondary hypogonadism and hyperparathyroidism, impaired vitamin D metabolism, muscle atrophy, and hypercalcuria. All these factors contribute to a rapid and sustained loss of bone during the first few months of steroid therapy.[92,166] The addition of other immunosuppressants such as cyclosporine has been shown to aggravate bone loss by further increasing bone resorption. Because the number of organ transplants has increased exponentially over the past decade, the prevalence of post-transplantation osteoporosis has risen substantially. Steroid-induced osteoporosis is now considered the second most common cause of low bone mass in the general population and one of the most common causes of osteoporotic fractures.[269]

The effects of glucocorticoids on the skeleton are multifaceted and are particularly devastating because these agents cause uncoupling in the remodeling unit. Besides the indirect suppressive effects of glucocorticoids on the hypothalamic-gonadal axis, and inhibition of calcium absorption in the gut due to impaired $1,25(OH)_2D$ production, high doses of steroids can stimulate osteoclastogenesis, increase RANKL production, and decrease OPG. This situation results in higher rates of bone resorption. Additionally, glucocorticoids also have a strong negative effect on bone formation by suppressing expression of IGF-1 in bone cells and by shifting marrow stromal cells into the fat lineage, rather than down the osteoblast differentiation pathway. It is presumed that just as fat redistribution is a clinical hallmark of Cushing syndrome in the supraclavicular and mediastinal area, enhanced adiposity in the bone marrow is a characteristic feature of steroid-induced bone disease, almost certainly as a function of increased stromal cell differentiation into adipocytes.[92] Bone strength is markedly compromised by dramatic uncoupling in remodeling, and bone loss can be rapid over a short period, particularly with high doses of glucocorticoids. Although there is no true dose-dependent effect on bone resorption, it is thought that prednisone doses as low as 5 mg/day may increase fracture risk.[270] Indeed, in this syndrome, baseline BMD is not predictive of fractures and can often be normal even in the presence of ongoing resorption and recurrent fractures.[266] Trabecular bone suffers the most in this syndrome, and spine DXA is the most sensitive indicator of bone loss. Markers of bone turnover are not helpful in the management of these patients.

Therapy for steroid-induced bone loss centers on treating the underlying disease and reducing the dose of glucocorticoids to the lowest possible regimen. Barring that, several interventions have been shown to retard bone loss and prevent fractures. Adequate calcium and vitamin D intake is critical for every patient receiving glucocorticoids. However, these measures alone are not sufficient. Regulatory approval for the prevention and treatment of glucocorticoid-induced osteoporosis has been consistent for the group of bisphosphonates, including alendronate, risedronate, and zoledronic acid.[271-274] These drugs are administered either weekly or cyclically to prevent bone loss and to reduce the risk of fractures. Some anecdotal data support the use of gonadal steroids in this condition, but clearly the bisphosphonates are superior. In a randomized trial PTH (teriparatide, 20 µg daily subcutaneously for 18 months) significantly increased hip and spine bone mass density and reduced the number of new vertebral fractures (7.2% to 3.4%) but not other fractures compared with alendronate.[275] More studies are needed to establish its long-term efficacy in this disease, particularly because secondary hyperparathyroidism is a frequent accompaniment of steroid-induced osteoporosis.

Factors That Impair Peak Bone Acquisition

Peak bone mass is acquired between the ages of 10 to 16 years. It is the zenith of bone acquisition and represents the sum of several processes including a marked increase in bone formation.[276] Boys tend to peak 2 years later than girls, and their BMD is higher than women at all skeletal sites. In part this difference relates to a greater cross-sectional bone area in males than females.[276] Peak bone mass results from linear growth and consolidation of cortical and trabecular components. Acquisition is most rapid during the latter stages of puberty and coincides with maximum growth hormone secretion, high serum IGF-1 levels, and rising levels of estradiol and testosterone. In addition, calcium absorption is maximum and skeletal accretion is optimal owing to higher levels of $1,25(OH)_2D$. These processes coalesce over a relatively short period to produce a bone mass that subsequently plateaus and then falls during later life. It is estimated that more than 60% of adult bone mass can be related to peak acquisition.[277] Hence, understanding the mechanisms responsible for low bone mass must include perturbations in peak bone acquisition.

There are several hormonal, environmental, and heritable determinants of peak bone mass, including estrogen/testosterone, growth hormone/IGF-1, calcium/vitamin D, and unknown genetic factors. If any is perturbed, dramatic alterations in peak bone mass may occur, setting the stage for low bone density throughout life. Not surprisingly gonadal steroids are essential not only to bone maintenance but also to acquisition. During puberty, estrogen and testosterone levels rise and contribute to consolidation of bone mass. Estrogen is also necessary for epiphyseal closure. Studies of males with an estrogen receptor mutation and men with an aromatase deficiency have established that estradiol is critical for bone acquisition.[187,246,247] These young men share several phenotypic characteristics including tall stature, unfused epiphysis, and very low bone mass. Hence, there must be a threshold effect for estradiol in men, and this effect must be time dependent. Similar conclusions can be drawn from studies in women. Acquired deficiencies in estrogen, such as occur with anorexia nervosa or chemotherapy-induced ovarian dysfunction, result in low peak bone mass and lead to subsequent risk for osteoporosis.[278,279] Similar findings have been noted in patients with untreated Turner syndrome and in men with Klinefelter syndrome.[280,281]

The timing of gonadal steroid surges is critical for bone acquisition because there is a relatively short window of time in which bone formation is favored and matrix synthesis is markedly enhanced. That time window is likely to be less than 3 years and earlier in girls than boys. Probably the best study that addressed this issue comes from a retrospective analysis of men in their 30s who underwent late onset of puberty (i.e., at the age of 17 or 18) but were otherwise normal by full endocrine testing.[282] These men had significantly lower BMD than age-matched men who went through puberty at the normal time. These data suggest that timing as well as quantity of gonadal steroids is critical for bone acquisition.

Pubertal surges of estrogen and androgens are also important for priming the growth hormone/IGF-1 axis. Rising levels of both contribute to growth hormone surges that lead to increases in circulating and tissue expression of IGF-1, an essential growth factor for chondrocyte hypertrophy and expansion. IGF-1 may also be critical in defining the cross-sectional size of bone, a potentially important determinant of bone strength.[283] Once again, studies in growth hormone–deficient, or growth hormone–resistant, individuals have established that low levels of circulating IGF-1, especially during puberty, are associated with reduced bone mass.[165,284] In addition, recombinant human growth hormone (rhGH) replacement has been shown to restore linear growth and improve peak bone mass acquisition. Several studies in experimental animals, including inbred strains of mice, have established that IGF-1 is important for bone acquisition and that the timing of IGF-1 peaks coincides with maximal rates of bone formation.[285] Impairment in production of IGF-1 due to acquired disorders (such as anorexia nervosa), malnutrition, delayed puberty, or diabetes mellitus can also impede peak bone acquisition.[286]

Hormonal abnormalities can not only enhance bone resorption in older individuals but may also blunt the capacity of bone cells to maximize bone formation during adolescence. Clearly, hypogonadal boys and girls have impaired peak bone mass, resulting in low adult BMD.[280,281] One form of contraception, Depo-Provera, may reduce estrogen concentrations enough in the teenage girl to reduce her capacity to acquire peak bone mass.[287] Similarly, it seems likely, although not yet proved, that smoking during the teen years could impair osteoblast activity and flatten projected trajectories for peak bone acquisition.

In order to mineralize newly synthesized bone, calcium must become bioavailable to the skeletal matrix. In experimental studies in rodents and humans, it is clear that the several pools of available calcium are markedly enhanced during puberty. These sources include calcium efflux from the gastrointestinal tract and the calcium pool available for incorporation in the matrix. It is no coincidence that growth hormone surges not only increase IGF-1 (thereby enhancing skeletal growth and matrix biosynthesis) but also result in increases in $1,25(OH)_2D$ (possibly via IGF-1 induction of 1α-hydroxylase activity), the active metabolite of vitamin D, which markedly enhances calcium absorption from the gut.[288-290] Although there are no longitudinal studies in pubertal individuals with prolonged calcium deficiency, several randomized placebo-controlled trials (RPCTs) in pubertal and prepubertal girls and boys have established that supplemental calcium can enhance BMD.[291,292] In a twin study in which one twin received calcium supplementation and one received placebo radial BMD increased by as much as 5% after 3 years in the twins given calcium when compared to those given placebo.[292] This study suggests that there is significant gene-environmental interaction and that, even in those individuals with heritable determinants of low peak bone mass, calcium supplementation may provide an important and relatively simple means of protecting individuals from future osteoporotic fractures.

Genetic Factors That Determine Peak Bone Mass

Probably the most important determinant of peak bone mass, albeit one that has lacked clear definition, is the genetic contribution. As noted earlier, low peak bone mass may be the most important pathogenic factor in the osteoporosis syndrome of later life. Further, it appears that at least 50% of peak bone mass is determined by genetic factors.[293-295] Efforts to define heritable determinants of peak bone mass have been plagued by a number of issues that are also common to other complex diseases. They include the following: (1) a quantifiable phenotype; (2) heterogeneity within a given population under study; (3) the polygenic nature of the disorder; and (4) In the postgenomic era it has become clear that complex diseases, such as osteoporosis, cannot be settled by single nucleotide polymorphisms (SNPs). Instead, they are originated by a confluence of multiple genetic variations. Naturally, the interest has been driven to assess epistasis to unveil the complex network involved within multiple SNP interactions, as well as the influence of environmental factor into gene expression. Notwithstanding these barriers, it is now clear that BMD is an acceptable phenotype for defining heritable determinants. In addition, BMD is fully quantifiable and therefore is amenable to complex trait analysis. Moreover, BMD in the population is distributed in a gaussian manner, thereby allowing analyses at the extremes (<–2.0 SD or >2.0 SD) of the density distribution. Large homogeneous and heterogeneous populations are now being studied to ascertain genetic determinants of bone density in humans. Candidate genes identified by whole genome studies include RANKL, OPG, the VDR, collagen IA1, the estrogen receptor IL-1, IGF-1, and others. Depending on the cohort, the phenotype, and the number of individuals studied, there are likely to be hundreds of genes that contribute to individual variation in bone mass.[295] Indeed, in most large genome-wide association studies (GWAS) using validation cohorts to confirm candidate genes, the effect size of most noncoding single nucleotide polymorphisms is at best 1%. Notwithstanding, there has been a major effort to consolidate studies from around the world to increase power and detect rare variants that might provide even greater insight into genetic determinants, and importantly shed greater light on the biology of low bone mass. Twin studies examining discordant or concordant phenotypes are also helpful, as are sibling-pair studies, although the results have been disappointing.[85,295,296]

Originally, Johnson and colleagues identified an extended family with very high bone density and fine-mapped the locus to a region in chromosome 11.[297] After several years of intense high-throughput analysis, the high–bone-density gene that was mutated in this family was identified as *LRP5*.[298] This member of the lipoprotein receptor family is important for binding Wnts, ligands critical for cell differentiation in several organisms. One year earlier, Gong and colleagues had identified mutations in the *LRP5* gene in several children with osteoporosis-pseudoglioma syndrome.[299] The potential pathways that direct osteoblast function and mineralization through LRP5, a coreceptor for the Wnt receptor, frizzled, have opened up new areas of investigation (Fig. 29-22). Moreover, natural antagonists to the Wnt/LRP5 signaling system, including sclerostin and Dkk1, have been studied using

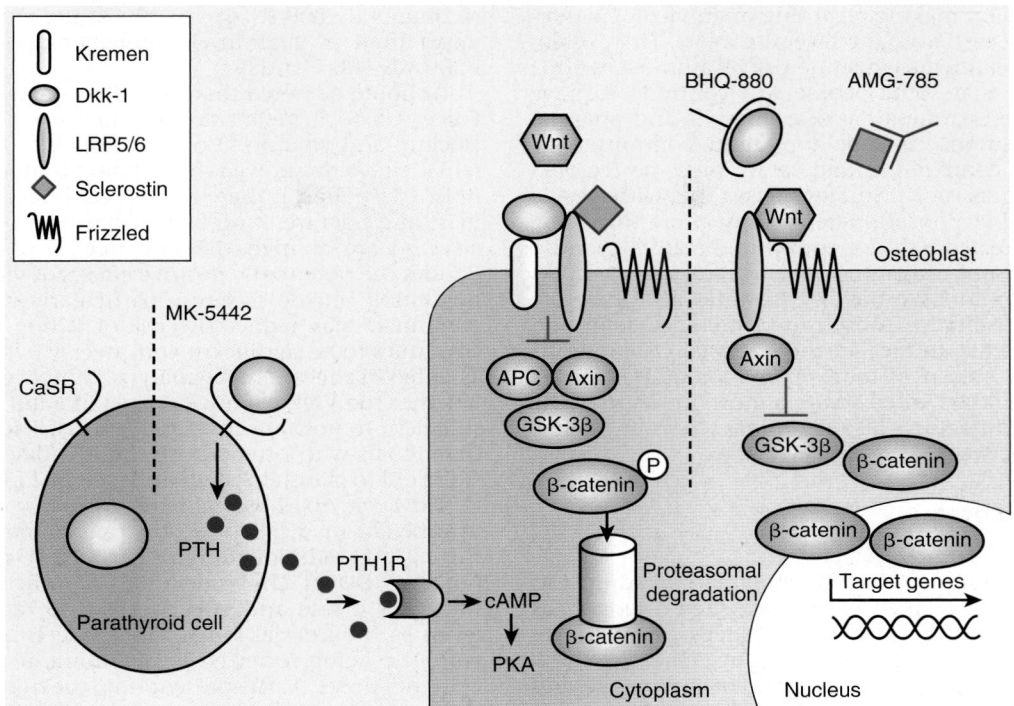

Figure 29-22 Osteoblast physiology and potential therapeutic targets: Calcium-sensing receptor is antagonized by MK-5442 and triggers short bursts of PTH secretion. Binding of PTH to its receptor enhances osteoblast functions and bone formation. Presence of Wnt antagonists Dkk-1 and sclerostin inhibits Wnt signaling. Dkk-1 needs to form complex with Kremen to bind LRP5/6, whereas sclerostin binds LRP5/6 directly. BHQ-880 and AMG-785 are antibodies for Dkk-1 and sclerostin, respectively. After neutralizing Dkk-1 and sclerostin, Wnt can bind to LRP5/6, which results in degradation GSK-3β. As a consequence, β-catenin is stabilized, accumulates, and translocates into the nucleus where it regulates transcription of osteoblastic genes. APC, adenomatosis polyposis coli; cAMP, cyclic adenosine monophosphate; CaSR, calcium-sensing receptor; Dkk-1, dickkopf-1; GSK, glycogen synthase kinase 3; LRP, lipoprotein receptor–related protein; PKA, protein kinase A; PTH, parathyroid hormone; PTH1R, PTH 1 receptor. (From Rachner TD, Khosla S, Hofbauer LC. Osteoporosis: now and the future. *Lancet.* 2011;377(9773):1276-1287.)

genetic engineering in mice. In the past 5 years, LRP5 has been studied extensively both in its function and its allelic effects through GWAS as well as in translational bench work. Importantly, LRP5 polymorphisms have been strongly associated with BMD and fractures in large cohort studies, consistent with its central role in human skeletal biology. Hence, this pathway must be important in defining peak bone mass. But, it is also clear that because BMD is a polygenic trait, other genes are soon to be discovered.

In addition to the search for osteoporosis genes, intervention studies in adolescents have provided insight into the environmental impact on genetic determinants.[295] In another twin study from the Indiana group, the investigators found that as long as calcium supplementation continued during puberty, young boys could enhance their peak bone mass.[300] In a Swiss study, younger prepubertal girls supplemented with a protein product had a significant increase in spine bone density, as did a cohort of pubertal girls receiving a milk powder in England.[301] Remarkably, in the latter cohort, serum IGF-1 levels also rose dramatically, providing further indirect evidence of a link between pubertal status, bone mass, and the growth hormone/IGF-1 axis.[301]

APPROACH TO MANAGEMENT OF OSTEOPOROSIS

A comprehensive management plan for osteoporosis includes diagnosing those at highest risk, excluding second-ary causes of low BMD, and selecting appropriate treatment. Screening by DXA to assess BMD at the hip and spine has been commonly recommended in most women over age 65 and men over age 70,[302,303] and many, but not all, have this assessment. In addition, there is a growing appreciation that occurrence of a fracture, particularly one due to minimal trauma, should be a signal for more comprehensive risk assessment including BMD and has led to the explosion in development of fracture liaison services over the past 5 years and the emphasis on their importance by many groups.[240,302,304]

With increasing recognition of the importance of risk factors in addition to BMD, an assessment of risk should include BMD as well as risk factors. These factors can be easily combined in the FRAX algorithm to attain an overall risk of fracture, which may be helpful, in addition to BMD alone, in making clinical decisions. FRAX scores are available online and have now been implemented within the software for most DXA scanners so that primary care physicians can easily obtain relevant diagnostic information in one report.

One commonly used algorithm in the United States is within the guidelines developed by the National Osteoporosis Foundation[302] (see Table 29-3), which strongly emphasize that patients with BMD T-score below −2.5 or a history of hip or spine fracture be considered for treatment. In these guidelines, FRAX is used for patients with BMD that is low but not in the osteoporotic range. In other countries treatment decisions are based solely on risk, but consideration of treatment of those with BMD T-scores below −2.5, regardless of other risk, is well justified by many clinical trial results.[305-307]

Clinical decision making regarding pharmacologic therapy should take into account several caveats. First, osteoporosis therapy can reduce fracture risk by as much as 50%, but this means that some people will continue to have fractures despite treatment. Second, lifestyle and pharmacologic interventions may be long-term commitments, such that cost, compliance, and safety must be factored into therapeutic decisions. Studies suggest that with weekly or monthly oral bisphosphonate therapy, more than 40% of individuals treated will not continue therapy beyond 1 year. Third, it is not uncommon for women with T-scores higher than −2.5 to have fragility fractures and therefore have osteoporosis by the Consensus Conference definition mentioned earlier.[186] In fact, in the National Osteoporosis Risk Assessment cohort of more than 140,000 postmenopausal women in the United States, almost one third of the women who had fractures also had BMD scores in the low BMD (T-score between −1 and −2.5) range.

General Measures

Diet

Calcium. Calcium supplementation should be an adjunct to drug treatments for women with established osteoporosis and must be part of any prevention strategy to ameliorate bone loss. Increased calcium intake reduces the secondary hyperparathyroidism often seen with advancing age and can enhance mineralization of newly formed bone. Evidence that calcium and vitamin D together or individually reduce fracture risk in the osteoporotic individual remains somewhat controversial. However, a recent meta-analysis of calcium and vitamin D intervention trials demonstrated a consistent albeit small increase in BMD and a reduction in nonvertebral fractures when 1200 mg of calcium is combined with more than 800 units of vitamin D.[308] Calcium supplementation alone has not been shown to reduce the incidence of nonvertebral fractures in high-risk women. Recently, a very large calcium intervention trial from the Women's Health Initiative (WHI) did not demonstrate hip fracture reduction with daily calcium supplements and 400 IU of vitamin D for all postmenopausal women, but for those over age 60 the risk reduction was statistically significant.[309] Interestingly, calcium supplementation in this cohort was associated with a 17% greater risk of kidney stones. Currently, an average total calcium intake of 1200 mg/day is still recommended by the National Institute of Medicine for all postmenopausal women. Certainly with intakes greater than 2000 mg/day, the risk of nephrocalcinosis increases.

Vitamin D. Vitamin D is essential for skeletal maintenance and for enhancement of calcium absorption. Insufficiency of this vitamin is a growing problem; as many as two thirds of all patients who have hip fractures are classified as vitamin D deficient. Elderly people in chronic care living situations are particularly vulnerable. One large RPCT demonstrated a 43% reduction in hip fractures for nursing home residents, aged 84 years, who received calcium and vitamin D compared with those receiving placebo.[310] However, those subjects had significantly suppressed 25(OH)D levels and hence were likely to also have osteomalacia. In a large population-based study with calcium and vitamin D, supplementation had no effect on nonvertebral fractures,[309] although compliance and assessment of vitamin D levels were not sufficiently well documented to exclude an effect. At least one meta-analysis suggests that 800 IU/day of vitamin D plus 1200 mg of calcium per day is needed to reduce hip fractures by about 10%.[308] The IOM recommends an average intake of 600 IU/day except for men and women older than age 70, for which the IOM recommends 800 IU of vitamin D per day. The tolerable upper limit of vitamin D supplementation noted by the IOM was 4000 IU/day.

It should be noted that the U.S. Preventive Services Task Force (USPSTF) meta-analysis failed to show an effect of calcium and vitamin D on fracture risk.[311] And three systematic reviews showed that vitamin D alone did not affect BMD.[312-314] Thus, if there is an effect of vitamin D on bone mass and fracture, it probably is limited to older individuals who are at high risk and have low calcium intake. Besides the potentially positive effects of vitamin D supplementation on the skeleton, particularly in older women, vitamin D may reduce the risk of falling, although there continues to be significant controversy over the effect size, as noted in a recent meta-analysis. Moreover, it is uncertain whether the VDR expression level in adult muscle tissue is sufficient to mediate any direct effects. Therefore, for most individuals with osteoporosis, 800 IU/day of vitamin D is sufficient to maintain adequate levels of 25-hydroxyvitamin D. However, in those patients with low bone mass and insufficient or deficient 25-hydroxyvitamin D levels (i.e., <20 ng/mL), administration of 50,000 IU of ergocalciferol (vitamin D_2) or cholecalciferol (vitamin D_3) given once weekly is a safe and effective way to restore vitamin D levels to the normal range. Upper levels of vitamin D are currently being reviewed to determine if there is toxicity at higher doses. At the present time the upper limit of tolerability is set at 4000 IU per day. The USPSTF did not recommend screening of normal individuals for adequacy of vitamin D levels; however, among osteoporotic patients measurement of at least one serum 25(OH)D level is considered standard of care, particularly for those individuals starting bisphosphonate therapy.

Vitamin D analogues have been used in the treatment of osteoporosis since the early 1980s. However, this remains a controversial area. High doses of $1,25(OH)_2D$ increase bone mass, but many patients develop hypercalciuria or hypercalcemia. At doses of 0.5 µg/day, $1,25(OH)_2D$ reduced the rate of both vertebral and nonvertebral fractures, and it increased bone density, but this finding was made in a very small randomized trial. Other studies have found little benefit with a narrow therapeutic window, particularly in relation to renal function and hypercalcemia. Currently vitamin D analogues are not recommended for the routine treatment of osteoporosis. A subset of patients with renal insufficiency (CKD ≥ 3 and high PTH levels) may benefit from supplementation with rocaltriol, with very careful monitoring of serum PTH.

Physical Activity

Bed rest or immobility, particularly in elderly persons, can result in rapid bone loss. Moreover, the number of falls increases with age, and the number of falls that result in fractures also rises. A meta-analysis by the Cochrane Review Group demonstrated that muscle strengthening, balance retraining, home hazard assessment, withdrawal of psychotropic medications, and use of a multidisciplinary risk factor assessment program are beneficial in protecting against falls.[315] An alternative approach is to reduce loads applied to the hip during a fall by padding. Hip protectors have been shown to reduce the risk of hip fractures in at least one population, although compliance is generally poor. A more recent study failed to demonstrate the efficacy of these devices in older women in an assisted living facility.[314a] Regular physical activity, including aerobic, weight-bearing, and resistant exercises, is effective in increasing spine BMD and in strengthening muscle mass in postmenopausal women, but no large-scale studies have established whether these interventions reduce fracture risk.

Lifestyle

Other interventions including smoking cessation and reduction of alcohol intake should be considered within the framework of an individual's preventive health strategy. However, studies to date have been inconclusive with respect to understanding how changes in these lifestyles affect overall fracture risk. Notwithstanding, some promising data support the use of Tai Chi to enhance balance and reduce falls and fractures.[315] The data on cigarette smoking and fractures are somewhat conflicted, although most investigators support the notion that smoking may impair peak bone acquisition in adolescence and could contribute to postmenopausal bone loss directly or via the development of chronic obstructive lung disease with hypoxia and hypercarbia.[316] Lifestyle also includes tools to manage activities of daily life with a particular focus on avoiding falls and eliminating barriers to ambulation.

Pharmacologic Approaches to the Treatment of Osteoporosis

Abundant evidence indicates that an aggressive intervention program can be successful in reducing fracture risk and in improving quality of life among postmenopausal women with preexisting osteoporosis. Several pharmacologic options are available, and they can be classified by their mechanism of action. The two major classes of osteoporosis drugs are (1) *antiresorptives* (i.e., agents that block bone resorption by inhibiting osteoclasts) and (2) *anabolics* (i.e., drugs that stimulate bone formation by primarily acting on osteoblasts).

Antiresorptive Agents

Antiresorptives inhibit bone resorption by suppressing osteoclast activity. Slowing the remodeling cycle allows bone formation to catch up to resorption, thereby enhancing matrix mineralization and stabilizing trabecular microarchitecture. The antiresorptives increase BMD and reduce fracture risk, but their efficacy varies.

Estrogen. Estrogen replacement therapy was long considered the cornerstone of therapy for postmenopausal women with osteoporosis. Studies in vitro and in vitro have supported the hypothesis that this hormone works by slowing bone resorption through inhibition of cytokine signaling from the osteoblast to the osteoclast, thereby increasing BMD. However, there is also compelling evidence from at least two groups that osteoclasts have estrogen receptors and that estrogen blocks apoptosis of osteoclasts.[317,318]

Estrogen treatment inhibits both cortical and trabecular bone loss, and BMD generally increases by 3% to 5% after 3 years.[319] There does not appear to be an additive effect from progesterone on bone mass in women also receiving estrogen. Conversely, progesterone is a necessary part of hormone replacement therapy in women with a uterus because it prevents the development of endometrial hyperplasia and carcinoma. In the WHI, estrogen and progesterone lowered hip fracture risk by one third.[243] Low-dose conjugated estrogens (0.3 or 0.45 mg/day) and ultra low-dose estradiol increase BMD and have been approved for the prevention of bone loss, but antifracture efficacy for these preparations has not been established. Discontinuation of estrogen results in measurable bone loss (3-5% in the first year), although controversy exists as to whether that translates into a greater fracture risk.

Significant concern has been noted about the nonskeletal risks associated with long-term estrogen and estrogen in combination with progesterone. Particularly troublesome is the increased risk of breast cancer with the long-term use of estrogen and progesterone. In the WHI, there was a 26% increase in risk of invasive breast cancer over a 5.2-year period of follow-up.[243] Hence, estrogen replacement is contraindicated in any woman with a history of breast cancer; yearly mammograms are indicated in all women receiving hormone replacement therapy. Previous case-control and retrospective studies suggested that estrogen could reduce the risk of coronary artery disease; however, in the WHI, the risk of myocardial infarction or death from coronary artery disease was 29% higher in women receiving combination therapy.[243] Thromboembolic disease is also increased more than threefold by hormone replacement therapy.[243] Hence, the use of estrogen or estrogen in combination with progestins for the prevention and treatment of osteoporosis has fallen dramatically. Moreover, the availability of newer and effective antiresorptive drugs for the treatment of osteoporosis has lessened enthusiasm for primary hormonal therapy in osteoporotic women.

Selective Estrogen Receptor Modulators. Selective estrogen receptor modulators such as tamoxifen and raloxifene also inhibit bone resorption by the same mechanisms used by estradiol. Both have been shown to reduce bone loss in postmenopausal women with breast cancer, but only raloxifene is approved by the FDA for the prevention and treatment of osteoporosis.

Both these agents block the actions of estrogen on the breast but act like an estrogen agonist in bone; tamoxifen, but not raloxifene, has estrogen agonistic properties on the uterus and is associated with a greater risk of endometrial carcinoma with long-term use.[320] Both agents have been associated with a reduction in new cases of breast cancer when they are administered as prophylaxis for high-risk patients.[321] Low-density lipoprotein cholesterol levels are also reduced in patients receiving these selective estrogen receptor modulators. Raloxifene increases spine BMD slightly (as does tamoxifen) and lowers the risk of vertebral fracture by 40%, although it has no effect on nonvertebral fracture risk.[322] Hot flashes, leg cramps, and a greater risk of deep venous thrombosis can occur with raloxifene therapy. The recommended dose of raloxifene is 60 mg once daily.

Tissue selectivity with these selective estrogen receptor modulators and others being investigated is a subject of great scientific interest. Raloxifene and estradiol both bind to the same region of the estrogen receptor, but they induce different conformational changes in that receptor. Differing coactivating and corepressing proteins are recruited to these receptor-ligand complexes, and it is thought that these coactivators and corepressors ultimately determine the activity of the nuclear complexes. Because recruitment also depends on cell type, it is highly likely that significant tissue selectivity exists for these partners. Newer agents have been designed to facilitate particular complexes and rearrangements within the nucleus; they are being studied at both the preclinical and the clinical levels.

Bisphosphonates. The bisphosphonates are the most widely prescribed antiresorptives and are often considered first-line therapy for the treatment of severe postmenopausal osteoporosis. These drugs are carbon-substituted analogues of pyrophosphate that bind tightly to hydroxyapatite crystals. It is thought that these agents directly suppress resorption by inhibiting osteoclast attachment and enhancing programmed cell death. The first-generation bisphosphonates include etidronate and clodronate. Neither is approved for the treatment of osteoporosis in the United States, although etidronate is used off label and in Europe. The dose of etidronate is 400 mg/day for 2 weeks every 3 months. The drug has few gastrointestinal side effects, and vertebral fracture risk reduction is significant with this agent. Alendronate and risedronate, two second-generation nitrogen-containing bisphosphonates, are effective in suppressing bone resorption and increasing BMD. In RPCTs of postmenopausal women with established osteoporosis, alendronate and risedronate reduced vertebral, hip, and nonvertebral fractures by nearly 50%, particularly during the first year of treatment.[204,323] As with other antiresorptive drugs, increases in BMD with alendronate or risedronate account for a small fraction of their antifracture efficacy. Hence, follow-up DXA measurements may significantly underestimate fracture risk reduction. Recent clinical trials have shown that these drugs can be safely administered for at least 5 years without adversely affecting bone strength. Moreover, discontinuation of alendronate after 5 years results in minimal bone loss over the ensuing 5 years without a significant increase in fracture risk.[324] Both drugs have excellent safety profiles, although erosive esophagitis is a serious complication of all oral nitrogen-containing bisphosphonates. Once-weekly administration of alendronate has been shown to reduce the prevalence of drug-induced esophagitis, and currently both alendronate and risedronate are marketed as once-weekly treatments.

Two other bisphosphonates have been approved by the FDA and have reached the market since 2007: ibandronate and zoledronate. The former is given orally in a single monthly dose (150 mg) or intravenously every 3 months (3 mg).[325,326] Ibandronate suppresses bone resorption and reduces the rate of spine fractures by nearly 50%,[306,327] but its efficacy in nonspine fractures is somewhat less than that of alendronate or risedronate. Compliance with the once-monthly regimen is higher than with the weekly dosing, although long-term data are not encouraging that this effect persists. First-dose hypersensitivity can occur with ibandronate, and because it is a nitrogen-containing bisphosphonate, it is also associated with esophageal reflux. Zoledronate is also approved for the prevention and treatment of osteoporosis. It is administered as a single intravenous infusion over 15 minutes (5 mg) once yearly. Large randomized controlled trials have unequivocally established antifracture efficacy for hip, spine, and other nonspine fractures.[328] Recently, the FDA approved the use of zoledronate for prevention of osteoporosis by administration of the drug once every 2 years. Both newer bisphosphonates can cause side effects with the first dose, including joint pain, stiffness, and low-grade fevers. Generally these do not persist with recurrent administration of the drug. However, the FDA has cautioned that zoledronic acid should be administered over an hour rather than 15 minutes to lessen any risk, albeit small, of renal damage. In addition, it should not be used in patients with a reduced glomerular filtration rate (GFR < 30 mL/minute) and used with caution in the elderly. Intravenous zoledronate has been approved for the treatment of malignant hypercalcemia, multiple myeloma, and skeletal metastases.

Other bisphosphonates are available for off-label use or are being studied for the treatment of osteoporosis. Intravenous pamidronate has been available since the mid-1990s for the treatment of Paget disease and malignant hypercalcemia. It is currently also used to treat osteoporotic women who cannot tolerate oral bisphosphonates, although it has not been formally approved by the FDA, and its antifracture efficacy has not been established. The dose ranges from 30 to 90 mg given every 3 to 9 months. Acute and delayed-type hypersensitivity reactions can

occur with this drug, and its use is contraindicated in patients who are vitamin D deficient because it can precipitously drop serum calcium, a concern that also applies to use of zoledronic acid and denosumab.

With widespread use of the bisphosphonates for both prevention and treatment, two uncommon but serious adverse events have been associated with administration of this class of agents: subtrochanteric, or atypical, femur fracture (AFF) and osteonecrosis of the jaw (ONJ).[329,330] With respect to the former, AFFs were found in some but not all studies to be associated with duration of bisphosphonate use and generally were noted in younger individuals relative to those affected by other types of hip fractures. Prodromal symptoms of hip or thigh pain and associated cortical thickening or beaking in the shaft of the proximal femur are risk indicators of these fractures, which with minimal trauma can have devastating consequences in terms of quality of life and mobility. Some guidelines recommend prophylactic rod placement to prevent fractures in high-risk individuals in the ipsilateral and contralateral femora. At the present time, the prevalence of this fracture is not well established, although meta-analyses suggest that there is a causal association with bisphosphonate use.

The prevalence of ONJ is very low when bisphosphonates are used in the doses used to treat osteoporosis. When much higher doses are used to prevent the skeletal complications of cancer, ONJ is a substantial concern. However, in osteoporosis patients, the prevalence is estimated to be less than 1 in 100,000 patients exposed to oral or intravenous bisphosphonates who are otherwise healthy. ONJ has devastating effects on the mandible and can require prolonged antibiotic treatment and local oral care. Patients with dental procedures that invade bone, such as tooth implantation and tooth extraction, are at increased risk. Concomitant treatment with glucocorticoids likely enhances the risk, and infection often accompanies the necrosis.

Calcitonin. Calcitonin is a 32–amino acid peptide normally produced by the thyroid C cells. Osteoclasts have calcitonin receptors, and calcitonin can rapidly inhibit bone resorption. Salmon calcitonin is more potent than human and is the preferred treatment choice. Nasal and subcutaneous calcitonin are both approved for the treatment of postmenopausal osteoporosis. However, the evidence favoring a strong effect from this hormone on either bone loss or fracture efficacy is lacking. In an RPCT of women with postmenopausal osteoporosis, 200 IU/day of nasal calcitonin reduced vertebral fracture incidence by one third.[331] However, methodologic flaws in that trial have limited enthusiasm for this agent as a primary treatment for osteoporosis. In at least one placebo-controlled study, nasal calcitonin reduced the pain associated with new spine fractures. The recommended dose of nasal calcitonin is 200 IU/day, and that of subcutaneous calcitonin is 100 IU/day. Side effects are uncommon with intranasal calcitonin and include nasal stuffiness and flushing. With subcutaneous administration, nausea is not infrequent.

Strontium Ranelate. Strontium ranelate is orally administered and stimulates calcium uptake in bone while it inhibits bone resorption. It is thought to have some anabolic activity, although the precise mechanism of action in the skeleton, where it is incorporated, is not known. In an RPCT of postmenopausal women with established disease, daily strontium reduced the risk of vertebral fractures by 40%.[332] However, a statistically significant effect on nonvertebral fractures was limited to a small subset of women in a post hoc analysis.[333] Recent data raised the safety issue of an increase in cardiovascular events among strontium users.[334] This drug is approved by European regulatory agencies but not by the FDA.

Denosumab. Denosumab is a fully human monoclonal antibody to the RANKL, the essential osteoclast-differentiating factor. The antibody inhibits osteoclast formation, decreases bone resorption, increases BMD, and reduces the risk of fracture. As noted previously, RANKL is a member of the TNF superfamily of ligands that is essential for the function of bone-resorbing osteoclasts. RANKL interacts with its receptor (RANK) on both osteoclast precursors and mature osteoclasts, and the RANKL-RANK interaction results in activation, migration, differentiation, and fusion of hematopoietic cells of the osteoclast lineage to begin the process of bone resorption. Denosumab blocks that activation by binding directly to RANKL. Unlike the bisphosphonates, denosumab does not persist in the skeleton and hence needs to be administered once every 6 months to maintain its efficacy. In fact, discontinuation of denosumab can lead to a rebound increase in bone resorption but no increase in fractures.[335]

Clinical trials with denosumab, 60 mg once every 6 months, included the very large (>7000 postmenopausal women with low bone mass and fractures) FREEDOM (Fracture Reduction Evaluation of Denosumab in Osteoporosis Every 6 Months) trial. This trial, which was used for registration of the agent with the FDA, demonstrated that after 3 years, denosumab improved BMD of the spine and hip compared with placebo (9.2% vs. 0% and 4.0% vs. −2.0%, respectively).[87] In addition, biochemical markers of bone turnover were significantly reduced in patients taking denosumab. Importantly, fractures of spine were reduced by 70%, and nonvertebral fractures, including hip fractures, were also significantly reduced. The long-term extension of the FREEDOM trial revealed that at 6 years, BMD continued to improve and fracture risk remained low.[336] In males undergoing androgen deprivation therapy, denosumab reduced bone loss and prevented fractures. Denosumab was the first biologic approved by the FDA for the treatment of osteoporosis in both men and women. Surprisingly, long-term studies (in 2015, out to 8 years in the extension trial) have failed to show significant adverse events for this agent, though atypical femoral fractures occur.

Cathepsin K Inhibitors. Cathepsin K is a proteinase that is secreted by osteoclasts and results in bone degradation, primarily of type I collagen (see Fig. 29-4). In addition, it is also produced by cancer cells that metastasize to bone. Odanacatib, one cathepsin K inhibitor, has been tested in postmenopausal women with osteoporosis and shown to be an effective suppressor of bone resorption. In addition, women receiving this agent in a large phase III registration trial showed significant increases in BMD of the spine and hip, as well as a reduction in spine and nonvertebral fractures, prompting premature discontinuation of the trial due to enhanced efficacy.[337] However, the safety profile for odanacatib is still not clearly defined, and the FDA has not yet approved this agent for use. Interestingly, women treated with odanacatib have suppressed bone resorption but no change or a slight increase in bone formation. This may be due to the finding that this agent blocks breakdown of collagen but does not kill osteoclasts; hence, signals from osteoclasts to osteoblasts may be maintained, thereby preserving bone formation. If correct, this is one of the first drugs for osteoporosis that can uncouple remodeling in a positive manner. A correlative study examining the effect of odanacatib in the setting of bony metastases from breast cancer demonstrated that it suppressed a biochemical marker of bone resorption, N-terminal telopeptide, in much the way that zoledronic acid did.[338]

Anabolic Agents

A new class of antiosteoporosis drugs was introduced in 2002. These so-called anabolic agents stimulate bone formation more than bone resorption. As such, these agents can enhance bone remodeling and contrast sharply with the antiresorptives, which slow bone turnover. PTH(1-34) (teriparatide) was the first of this class of drugs to be approved by the FDA. Previously the prototypical anabolic drug was sodium fluoride, which saw widespread use in the 1970s and 1980s because of its ability to stimulate new bone formation. However, an RPCT in 1990 established that although there were dramatic increases in BMD, nonvertebral fracture risk actually increased.

Parathyroid Hormone. It has been known for several decades that PTH, when given intermittently, increases bone formation and bone mass in mammals.[339] The increase in bone turnover begins with a dramatic increase in bone formation followed later by a marked rise in bone resorption, maintaining the coupling in the multicellular unit. On the other hand, chronically high levels of PTH cause bone loss in the cortical compartment as noted for primary and secondary hyperparathyroidism.[340] The development of PTH as an anabolic agent centered on defining the intermittent nature of administration, which for teriparatide (human PTH[1-34]) was by daily subcutaneous injections. Teriparatide has been approved in virtually every country for the treatment of postmenopausal osteoporosis because it not only increases bone mass but also reduces fractures. In the largest RPCT using teriparatide in postmenopausal women with severe osteoporosis, 20 μg/day of PTH, administered subcutaneously, reduced spinal and nonvertebral fractures by more than 50% while it substantially increased (i.e., 8%/year) lumbar BMD.[341] Similar findings were noted in men with osteoporosis who were treated for 11 months.[342] Unfortunately, the PTH trial in postmenopausal women was stopped after 20 months because of concerns related to the development of osteosarcoma in rats treated with high doses of PTH(1-34). However, retrospective studies have found no association between osteosarcoma and primary or secondary hyperparathyroidism, and only one case of osteosarcoma in PTH-treated patients has been reported from more than a million users. More recently recombinant human PTH(1-84) has shown similar benefits and is approved for the treatment of hypoparathyroidism in the United States.[343] In Europe and Asia, but not in the United States, PTH(1-84) is approved for the treatment of postmenopausal osteoporosis. Currently, it is recommended that PTH therapy be limited to those individuals with moderate to severe osteoporosis and then given for only 2 years, based on a long-term toxicity study in rats demonstrating an increased risk of osteosarcoma.

Despite the appeal of using an anabolic with an antiresorptive, most evidence indicates that combinations of classes of drugs are not additive or synergistic. PTH plus the bisphosphonates initiated together do not raise BMD more than PTH alone in either men or women.[344,345] However, PTH plus denosumab has been shown to increase BMD in the spine to 13% after just 1 year, a greater increase than that seen with other drugs.[346] That difference is maintained even after 2 years of combination therapy. Unlike with discontinuation of the bisphosphonates, discontinuation of PTH can result in bone loss of 3% to 4% in the first year after PTH cessation. This posttreatment effect is prevented by adding an antiresorptive agent once PTH is stopped. In general, PTH is well tolerated, although nausea, flushing, hypotension, and mild but asymptomatic hypercalcemia (i.e., serum calcium <11 mg/dL) can occur. Cost and compliance have been limiting factors.

Future Anabolic Agents. There is a significant appeal to the use of anabolic agents for the treatment of low bone mass and fractures in severely affected individuals (see Fig. 29-22). However, since teriparatide was approved in 2002 for use in the United States and around the world, no agent has come close to approval, or for that matter entered phase III trials, except for an N-terminal fragment of PTH-related peptide (PTHrP) and a monoclonal antibody to sclerostin.[347] The former, PTHrP, has been shown to work via the PTH receptor on osteoblasts to stimulate new bone formation in a manner analogous to PTH. PTHrP acts primarily as a paracrine growth/differentiation factor but also functions as a hormone during normal lactation and in the hypercalcemia of malignancy. However, when administered intermittently, PTHrP(1-36) increases BMD without significant hypercalcemia, again similar to PTH. Phase III trials with PTHrP(1-36) have been completed in Europe and show a significant reduction in both vertebral and nonvertebral fractures (including hip fractures), but whether it gains approval by regulatory agencies remains to be determined.

Monoclonal Antibodies to Sclerostin. As noted previously, sclerostin is produced by osteocytes and inhibits bone formation by blocking canonical Wnt signaling. Sclerostin-null mice have increased bone formation and high bone mass. It follows, therefore, that inhibition of sclerostin should enhance osteoblast function and improve bone mass. In animal models and in a phase I trial in healthy adults, administration of a sclerostin monoclonal antibody does increase bone mass. Similarly, in a phase 2 trial in postmenopausal women, all doses of a monoclonal anti-sclerostin antibody (romosozumab) increased bone density at the lumbar spine, total hip, and femoral neck.[82] In this 1-year trial, 419 postmenopausal women with low bone mass (T-score between −2.0 and −3.5 at the lumbar spine, total hip, or femoral neck) were randomly assigned to subcutaneous romosozumab (variable dosing once monthly or once every 3 months), an active comparator, versus alendronate 70 mg weekly, or subcutaneous teriparatide 20 µg daily, or placebo injections. The greatest increase in BMD was seen in the group receiving romosozumab, 210 mg monthly (11.3% compared with 4.1% and 7.1% in the alendronate and teriparatide groups, respectively).[82] Interestingly, there was a transient increase in bone formation markers and a more sustained decrease in bone resorption markers, a pattern that has not been seen among available osteoporosis therapies, again suggesting that it is possible to uncouple remodeling toward a more favorable balance. The suppression in bone resorption is most likely a function of reduced RANKL production due to inhibition of the Wnt/LRP5/6 signaling pathway. Safety studies and completion of the phase III trial will determine the place of this agent in treating osteoporosis.

REFERENCES

1. Marcus R. Clinical review 76: the nature of osteoporosis. *J Clin Endocrinol Metab.* 1996;81:1-5.
2. Manolagas SC. Wnt signaling and osteoporosis. *Maturitas.* 2014;78(3):233-237.
3. Raisz LG. Pathogenesis of osteoporosis: concepts, conflicts, and prospects. *J Clin Invest.* 2005;115:3318-3325.
4. Fazeli PK, Horowitz MC, MacDougald OA, et al. Marrow fat and bone—new perspectives. *J Clin Endocrinol Metab.* 2013;98(3):935-945.
5. Brotto M, Johnson ML. Endocrine crosstalk between muscle and bone. *Curr Osteoporos Rep.* 2014;12(2):135-141.
6. Teti A. Mechanisms of osteoclast-dependent bone formation. *Bonekey Rep.* 2013;2:449.
7. Harvey N, Dennison E, Cooper C. Osteoporosis: a lifecourse approach. *J Bone Miner Res.* 2014;29(9):1917-1925.
8. Khosla S, Melton LJ 3rd. Clinical practice. Osteopenia. *N Engl J Med.* 2007;356:2293-2300.
9. NIH Consensus Development Panel on Osteoporosis Prevention, Diagnosis, and Therapy. Osteoporosis prevention, diagnosis, and therapy. *JAMA.* 2001;285(6):785-795.
10. Silva BC, Leslie WD, Resch H, et al. Trabecular bone score: a noninvasive analytical method based upon the DXA image. *J Bone Miner Res.* 2014;29:518-530.
11. Boutroy S, Bouxsein ML, Munoz F, Delmas PD. In vivo assessment of trabecular bone microarchitecture by high-resolution peripheral quantitative computed tomography. *J Clin Endocrinol Metab.* 2005;90:6508-6515.
12. Chang G, Honig S, Brown R, et al. Finite element analysis applied to 3-T MR imaging of proximal femur microarchitecture: lower bone strength in patients with fragility fractures compared with control subjects. *Radiology.* 2014;272(2):464-474.
13. Cooper C. The crippling consequences of fractures and their impact on quality of life. *Am J Med.* 1997;103:12S-17S, discussion 17S-19S.
14. Hernlund E, Svedbom A, Ivergard M, et al. Osteoporosis in the European Union: medical management, epidemiology and economic burden. A report prepared in collaboration with the International Osteoporosis Foundation (IOF) and the European Federation of Pharmaceutical Industry Associations (EFPIA). *Arch Osteoporos.* 2013;8:136.
15. NIH Consensus Development Panel on Osteoporosis Prevention, Diagnosis, and Therapy, March 7-29, 2000: highlights of the conference. *South Med J.* 2001;94(6):569-573.
16. Raisz L, Shoukri K. *Pathogeneis of Osteoporosis in Physiology and Pharmacology of Bone.* New York, NY: Springer-Verlag; 1993.
17. Baron R. *Anatomy and Ultrastructure of Bone.* New York, NY: Lippincott Williams & Wilkins; 1999.
18. Parfitt AM. The mechanism of coupling: a role for the vasculature. *Bone.* 2000;26:319-323.
19. Canalis E. The fate of circulating osteoblasts. *N Engl J Med.* 2005;352:2014-2016.
20. Parfitt AM. The bone remodeling compartment: a circulatory function for bone lining cells. *J Bone Miner Res.* 2001;16:1583-1585.
21. Lau KH, Baylink DJ, Zhou XD, et al. Osteocyte-derived insulin-like growth factor I is essential for determining bone mechanosensitivity. *Am J Physiol.* 2013;305:E271-E281.
22. Dallas SL, Prideaux M, Bonewald LF. The osteocyte: an endocrine cell . . . and more. *Endocr Rev.* 2013;34:658-690.
23. Gorski JP. Is all bone the same? Distinctive distributions and properties of non-collagenous matrix proteins in lamellar vs. woven bone imply the existence of different underlying osteogenic mechanisms. *Crit Rev Oral Biol Med.* 1998;9:201-223.
24. Delany AM, Amling M, Priemel M, et al. Osteopenia and decreased bone formation in osteonectin-deficient mice. *J Clin Invest.* 2000;105:1325.
25. Ducy P, Desbois C, Boyce B, et al. Increased bone formation in osteocalcin-deficient mice. *Nature.* 1996;382:448-452.
26. Lee NK, Sowa H, Hinoi E, et al. Endocrine regulation of energy metabolism by the skeleton. *Cell.* 2007;130:456-469.
27. Wei J, Hanna T, Suda N, et al. Osteocalcin promotes beta-cell proliferation during development and adulthood through Gprc6a. *Diabetes.* 2014;63:1021-1031.
28. Fulzele K, Riddle RC, DiGirolamo DJ, et al. Insulin receptor signaling in osteoblasts regulates postnatal bone acquisition and body composition. *Cell.* 2010;142:309-319.
29. Ferron M, Wei J, Yoshizawa T, et al. Insulin signaling in osteoblasts integrates bone remodeling and energy metabolism. *Cell.* 2010;142:296-308.
30. Seeman E, Delmas PD. Bone quality—the material and structural basis of bone strength and fragility. *N Engl J Med.* 2006;354:2250-2261.
31. Viguet-Carrin S, Garnero P, Delmas PD. The role of collagen in bone strength. *Osteoporos Int.* 2006;17:319-336.
32. Millan JL. The role of phosphatases in the initiation of skeletal mineralization. *Calcif Tissue Int.* 2013;93:299-306.
33. Anderson HC. Molecular biology of matrix vesicles. *Clin Orthop Relat Res.* 1995;314:266-280.
34. Rowe PS. Regulation of bone-renal mineral and energy metabolism: the PHEX, FGF23, DMP1, MEPE ASARM pathway. *Crit Rev Eukaryot Gene Expr.* 2012;22(1):61-86.
35. Whyte M. Enzyme defects and the skeleton. In: Rosen CJ, ed. *Primer on the Metabolic Bone Diseases and Disorders of Mineral Metabolism.* 8th ed. Ames, IA: Wiley-Blackwell; 2013:838-840.
36. Lieben L, Masuyama R, Torrekens S, et al. Normocalcemia is maintained in mice under conditions of calcium malabsorption by vitamin D-induced inhibition of bone mineralization. *J Clin Invest.* 2012;122:1803-1815.
37. Lieben L, Carmeliet G. Vitamin D signaling in osteocytes: effects on bone and mineral homeostasis. *Bone.* 2013;54:237-243.
38. Whyte MP, Greenberg CR, Salman NJ, et al. Enzyme-replacement therapy in life-threatening hypophosphatasia. *N Engl J Med.* 2012;366:904-913.
39. Mauviel A. Cytokine regulation of metalloproteinase gene expression. *J Cell Biochem.* 1993;53:288-295.

40. Zhao W, Byrne MH, Boyce BF, Krane SM. Bone resorption induced by parathyroid hormone is strikingly diminished in collagenase-resistant mutant mice. *J Clin Invest.* 1999;103:517-524.

41. Rydziel S, Delany AM, Canalis E. AU-rich elements in the collagenase 3 mRNA mediate stabilization of the transcript by cortisol in osteoblasts. *J Biol Chem.* 2004;279:5397-5404.

42. Liu F, Malaval L, Aubin JE. The mature osteoblast phenotype is characterized by extensive plasticity. *Exp Cell Res.* 1997;232:97-105.

43. Bianco P, Gehron Robey P. Marrow stromal stem cells. *J Clin Invest.* 2000;105:1663-1668.

44. Canalis E, Deregowski V, Pereira RC, Gazzerro E. Signals that determine the fate of osteoblastic cells. *J Endocrinol Invest.* 2005;28:3-7.

45. Leaffer D, Sweeney M, Kellerman LA, et al. Modulation of osteogenic cell ultrastructure by RS-23581, an analog of human parathyroid hormone (PTH)-related peptide-(1-34), and bovine PTH-(1-34). *Endocrinology.* 1995;136:3624-3631.

46. Wang A, Midura RJ, Vasanji A, et al. Hyperglycemia diverts dividing osteoblastic precursor cells to an adipogenic pathway and induces synthesis of a hyaluronan matrix that is adhesive for monocytes. *J Biol Chem.* 2014;289:11410-11420.

47. Karsenty G. Minireview: transcriptional control of osteoblast differentiation. *Endocrinology.* 2001;142:2731-2733.

48. Tanaka T, Yoshida N, Kishimoto T, Akira S. Defective adipocyte differentiation in mice lacking the C/EBPbeta and/or C/EBPdelta gene. *EMBO J.* 1997;16:7432-7443.

49. Ducy P, Zhang R, Geoffroy V, et al. Osf2/Cbfa1: a transcriptional activator of osteoblast differentiation. *Cell.* 1997;89:747-754.

50. Nakashima K, Zhou X, Kunkel G, et al. The novel zinc finger-containing transcription factor osterix is required for osteoblast differentiation and bone formation. *Cell.* 2002;108:17-29.

51. Koga T, Inui M, Inoue K, et al. Costimulatory signals mediated by the ITAM motif cooperate with RANKL for bone homeostasis. *Nature.* 2004;428:758-763.

52. Tominaga H, Maeda S, Hayashi M, et al. CCAAT/enhancer-binding protein beta promotes osteoblast differentiation by enhancing Runx2 activity with ATF4. *Mol Biol Cell.* 2008;19:5373-5386.

53. Aarden EM, Burger EH, Nijweide PJ. Function of osteocytes in bone. *J Cell Biochem.* 1994;55:287-299.

54. Burger EH, Klein-Nulend J. Mechanotransduction in bone—role of the lacuno-canalicular network. *FASEB J.* 1999;13(Suppl):S101-S112.

55. Han Y, Cowin SC, Schaffler MB, Weinbaum S. Mechanotransduction and strain amplification in osteocyte cell processes. *Proc Natl Acad Sci U S A.* 2004;101:16689-16694.

56. Suda T, Takahashi N, Udagawa N, et al. Modulation of osteoclast differentiation and function by the new members of the tumor necrosis factor receptor and ligand families. *Endocr Rev.* 1999;20:345-357.

57. Tondravi MM, McKercher SR, Anderson K, et al. Osteopetrosis in mice lacking haematopoietic transcription factor PU.1. *Nature.* 1997; 386(6620):81-84.

58. Miyamoto T, Ohneda O, Arai F, et al. Bifurcation of osteoclasts and dendritic cells from common progenitors. *Blood.* 2001;98:2544-2554.

59. Lorenzo J. Interactions between immune and bone cells: new insights with many remaining questions. *J Clin Invest.* 2000;106:749-752.

60. Arai F, Miyamoto T, Ohneda O, et al. Commitment and differentiation of osteoclast precursor cells by the sequential expression of c-Fms and receptor activator of nuclear factor kappaB (RANK) receptors. *J Exp Med.* 1999;190:1741-1754.

61. Lacey DL, Tan HL, Lu J, et al. Osteoprotegerin ligand modulates murine osteoclast survival in vitro and in vivo. *Am J Pathol.* 2000;157:435-448.

62. Yoshida H, Hayashi S, Kunisada T, et al. The murine mutation osteopetrosis is in the coding region of the macrophage colony stimulating factor gene. *Nature.* 1990;345:442-444.

63. Hofstetter W, Wetterwald A, Cecchini MG, et al. Detection of transcripts and binding sites for colony-stimulating factor-1 during bone development. *Bone.* 1995;17:145-151.

64. Mocsai A, Humphrey MB, Van Ziffle JA, et al. The immunomodulatory adapter proteins DAP12 and Fc receptor gamma-chain (FcRgamma) regulate development of functional osteoclasts through the Syk tyrosine kinase. *Proc Natl Acad Sci U S A.* 2004;101:6158-6163.

65. Kurihara N, Gluck S, Roodman GD. Sequential expression of phenotype markers for osteoclasts during differentiation of precursors for multinucleated cells formed in long-term human marrow cultures. *Endocrinology.* 1990;127:3215-3221.

66. Kurihara N, Chenu C, Miller M, et al. Identification of committed mononuclear precursors for osteoclast-like cells formed in long term human marrow cultures. *Endocrinology.* 1990;126:2733-2741.

67. de la Mata J, Uy HL, Guise TA, et al. Interleukin-6 enhances hypercalcemia and bone resorption mediated by parathyroid hormone-related protein in vivo. *J Clin Invest.* 1995;95:2846-2852.

68. Kukita T, Wada N, Kukita A, et al. RANKL-induced DC-STAMP is essential for osteoclastogenesis. *J Exp Med.* 2004;200:941-946.

69. Yagi M, Miyamoto T, Sawatani Y, et al. DC-STAMP is essential for cell-cell fusion in osteoclasts and foreign body giant cells. *J Exp Med.* 2005; 202:345-351.

70. Blair HC, Teitelbaum SL, Ghiselli R, Gluck S. Osteoclastic bone resorption by a polarized vacuolar proton pump. *Science.* 1989;245(4920): 855-857.

71. Chatterjee D, Chakraborty M, Leit M, et al. Sensitivity to vanadate and isoforms of subunits A and B distinguish the osteoclast proton pump from other vacuolar H+ ATPases. *Proc Natl Acad Sci U S A.* 1992;89: 6257-6261.

72. Blair HC, Kahn AJ, Crouch EC, et al. Isolated osteoclasts resorb the organic and inorganic components of bone. *J Cell Biol.* 1986;102: 1164-1172.

73. Blair HC, Sidonio RF, Friedberg RC, et al. Proteinase expression during differentiation of human osteoclasts in vitro. *J Cell Biochem.* 2000;78: 627-637.

74. Delaisse JM, Eeckhout Y, Neff L, et al. (Pro)collagenase (matrix metalloproteinase-1) is present in rodent osteoclasts and in the underlying bone-resorbing compartment. *J Cell Sci.* 1993;106(Pt 4): 1071-1082.

75. Salo J, Lehenkari P, Mulari M, et al. Removal of osteoclast bone resorption products by transcytosis. *Science.* 1997;276:270-273.

76. Eghbali-Fatourechi GZ, Lamsam J, Fraser D, et al. Circulating osteoblast-lineage cells in humans. *N Engl J Med.* 2005;352:1959-1966.

77. Edwards JR, Mundy GR. Advances in osteoclast biology: old findings and new insights from mouse models. *Nat Rev.* 2011;7:235-243.

78. Pederson L, Ruan M, Westendorf JJ, et al. Regulation of bone formation by osteoclasts involves Wnt/BMP signaling and the chemokine sphingosine-1-phosphate. *Proc Natl Acad Sci U S A.* 2008;105:20764-20769.

79. Zhao C, Irie N, Takada Y, et al. Bidirectional ephrinB2-EphB4 signaling controls bone homeostasis. *Cell Metab.* 2006;4:111-121.

80. Christiansen P. The skeleton in primary hyperparathyroidism: a review focusing on bone remodeling, structure, mass, and fracture. *APMIS Suppl.* 2001;102:1-52.

81. Khosla S, Oursler MJ, Monroe DG. Estrogen and the skeleton. *Trends Endocrinol Metab.* 2012;23:576-581.

82. McClung MR, Grauer A, Boonen S, et al. Romosozumab in postmenopausal women with low bone mineral density. *N Engl J Med.* 2014;370: 412-420.

83. McColm J, Hu L, Womack T, et al. Single- and multiple-dose randomized studies of blosozumab, a monoclonal antibody against sclerostin, in healthy postmenopausal women. *J Bone Miner Res.* 2014;29:935-943.

84. Bouxsein ML, Myers KS, Shultz KL, et al. Ovariectomy-induced bone loss varies among inbred strains of mice. *J Bone Miner Res.* 2005;20: 1085-1092.

85. Rosen CJ, Beamer WG, Donahue LR. Defining the genetics of osteoporosis: using the mouse to understand man. *Osteoporos Int.* 2001;12: 803-810.

86. Richards JB, Zheng HF, Spector TD. Genetics of osteoporosis from genome-wide association studies: advances and challenges. *Nat Rev Genet.* 2012;13:576-588.

87. Cummings SR, San Martin J, McClung MR, et al. Denosumab for prevention of fractures in postmenopausal women with osteoporosis. *N Engl J Med.* 2009;361:756-765.

88. Vij R, Horvath N, Spencer A, et al. An open-label, phase 2 trial of denosumab in the treatment of relapsed or plateau-phase multiple myeloma. *Am J Hematol.* 2009;84:650-656.

89. Smith MR, Egerdie B, Hernandez Toriz N, et al. Denosumab in men receiving androgen-deprivation therapy for prostate cancer. *N Engl J Med.* 2009;361:745-755.

90. Jilka RL, Weinstein RS, Parfitt AM, Manolagas SC. Quantifying osteoblast and osteocyte apoptosis: challenges and rewards. *J Bone Miner Res.* 2007;22:1492-1501.

91. Kawai M, de Paula FJ, Rosen CJ. New insights into osteoporosis: the bone-fat connection. *J Intern Med.* 2012;272:317-329.

92. Rosen CJ, Bouxsein ML. Mechanisms of disease: is osteoporosis the obesity of bone? *Nat Clin Pract.* 2006;2:35-43.

93. Crane JL, Cao X. Bone marrow mesenchymal stem cells and TGF-beta signaling in bone remodeling. *J Clin Invest.* 2014;124:466-472.

94. Kim SW, Pajevic PD, Selig M, et al. Intermittent parathyroid hormone administration converts quiescent lining cells to active osteoblasts. *J Bone Miner Res.* 2012;27:2075-2084.

95. Wysolmerski JJ. Osteocytic osteolysis: time for a second look? *Bonekey Rep.* 2012;1:229.

96. Armstrong VJ, Muzylak M, Sunters A, et al. Wnt/beta-catenin signaling is a component of osteoblastic bone cell early responses to load-bearing and requires estrogen receptor alpha. *J Biol Chem.* 2007;282: 20715-20727.

97. Canalis E, Economides AN, Gazzerro E. Bone morphogenetic proteins, their antagonists, and the skeleton. *Endocr Rev.* 2003;24:218-235.

98. Canalis E, Giustina A, Bilezikian JP. Mechanisms of anabolic therapies for osteoporosis. *N Engl J Med.* 2007;357:905-916.

99. Lorenzo JA. The role of cytokines in the regulation of local bone resorption. *Crit Rev Immunol.* 1991;11:195-213.

100. Pacifici R. Cytokines, estrogen, and postmenopausal osteoporosis—the second decade. *Endocrinology.* 1998;139(6):2659-2661.

101. Grey A, Mitnick MA, Masiukiewicz U, et al. A role for interleukin-6 in parathyroid hormone-induced bone resorption in vivo. *Endocrinology.* 1999;140:4683-4690.
102. Sims NA, Johnson RW. Leukemia inhibitory factor: a paracrine mediator of bone metabolism. *Growth Factors.* 2012;30(2):76-87.
103. Onoe Y, Miyaura C, Kaminakayashiki T, et al. IL-13 and IL-4 inhibit bone resorption by suppressing cyclooxygenase-2-dependent prostaglandin synthesis in osteoblasts. *J Immunol.* 1996;156:758-764.
104. Miyaura C, Onoe Y, Inada M, et al. Increased B-lymphopoiesis by interleukin 7 induces bone loss in mice with intact ovarian function: similarity to estrogen deficiency. *Proc Natl Acad Sci U S A.* 1997;94: 9360-9365.
105. Owens JM, Gallagher AC, Chambers TJ. IL-10 modulates formation of osteoclasts in murine hemopoietic cultures. *J Immunol.* 1996;157: 936-940.
106. Horwood NJ, Udagawa N, Elliott J, et al. Interleukin 18 inhibits osteoclast formation via T cell production of granulocyte macrophage colony-stimulating factor. *J Clin Invest.* 1998;101:595-603.
107. Takayanagi H, Ogasawara K, Hida S, et al. T-cell-mediated regulation of osteoclastogenesis by signalling cross-talk between RANKL and IFN-gamma. *Nature.* 2000;408:600-605.
108. Guise TA, Yoneda T, Yates AJ, Mundy GR. The combined effect of tumor-produced parathyroid hormone-related protein and transforming growth factor-alpha enhance hypercalcemia in vivo and bone resorption in vitro. *J Clin Endocrinol Metab.* 1993;77:40-45.
109. Lorenzo JA, Quinton J, Sousa S, Raisz LG. Effects of DNA and prostaglandin synthesis inhibitors on the stimulation of bone resorption by epidermal growth factor in fetal rat long-bone cultures. *J Clin Invest.* 1986;77:1897-1902.
110. Fukuda A, Hikita A, Wakeyama H, et al. Regulation of osteoclast apoptosis and motility by small GTPase binding protein Rac1. *J Bone Miner Res.* 2005;20:2245-2253.
111. Pilbeam CC, Wastell HJ, Raisz LG. Prostaglandins and bone metabolism. In: Bilezikian JP, Raisz L, Rodan GA, eds. *Principles of Bone Biology.* San Diego, CA: Academic Press; 1997:715-728.
112. Itoh N, Ornitz DM. Evolution of the Fgf and Fgfr gene families. *Trends Genet.* 2004;20:563-569.
113. Canalis E. Effect of insulinlike growth factor I on DNA and protein synthesis in cultured rat calvaria. *J Clin Invest.* 1980;66:709-719.
114. Mansukhani A, Ambrosetti D, Holmes G, et al. Sox2 induction by FGF and FGFR2 activating mutations inhibits Wnt signaling and osteoblast differentiation. *J Cell Biol.* 2005;168:1065-1076.
115. Ambrosetti D, Holmes G, Mansukhani A, Basilico C. Fibroblast growth factor signaling uses multiple mechanisms to inhibit Wnt-induced transcription in osteoblasts. *Mol Cell Biol.* 2008;28:4759-4771.
116. Sobue T, Naganawa T, Xiao L, et al. Over-expression of fibroblast growth factor-2 causes defective bone mineralization and osteopenia in transgenic mice. *J Cell Biochem.* 2005;95:83-94.
117. Montero A, Okada Y, Tomita M, et al. Disruption of the fibroblast growth factor-2 gene results in decreased bone mass and bone formation. *J Clin Invest.* 2000;105:1085-1093.
118. Okada Y, Montero A, Zhang X, et al. Impaired osteoclast formation in bone marrow cultures of Fgf2 null mice in response to parathyroid hormone. *J Biol Chem.* 2003;278:21258-21266.
119. So WY, Cheng Q, Chen L, et al. High glucose represses beta-klotho expression and impairs fibroblast growth factor 21 action in mouse pancreatic islets: involvement of peroxisome proliferator-activated receptor gamma signaling. *Diabetes.* 2013;62:3751-3759.
120. Wei W, Dutchak PA, Wang X, et al. Fibroblast growth factor 21 promotes bone loss by potentiating the effects of peroxisome proliferator-activated receptor gamma. *Proc Natl Acad Sci U S A.* 2012;109:3143-3148.
121. Fredriksson L, Li H, Eriksson U. The PDGF family: four gene products form five dimeric isoforms. *Cytokine Growth Factor Rev.* 2004;15(4): 197-204.
122. Ferrara N, Davis-Smyth T. The biology of vascular endothelial growth factor. *Endocr Rev.* 1997;18:4-25.
123. Hock JM, Canalis E. Platelet-derived growth factor enhances bone cell replication, but not differentiated function of osteoblasts. *Endocrinology.* 1994;134:1423-1428.
124. Betsholtz C. Insight into the physiological functions of PDGF through genetic studies in mice. *Cytokine Growth Factor Rev.* 2004;15:215-228.
125. Zelzer E, Olsen BR. Multiple roles of vascular endothelial growth factor (VEGF) in skeletal development, growth, and repair. *Curr Top Dev Biol.* 2005;65:169-187.
126. Gerber HP, Vu TH, Ryan AM, et al. VEGF couples hypertrophic cartilage remodeling, ossification and angiogenesis during endochondral bone formation. *Nat Med.* 1999;5:623-628.
127. Street J, Bao M, deGuzman L, et al. Vascular endothelial growth factor stimulates bone repair by promoting angiogenesis and bone turnover. *Proc Natl Acad Sci U S A.* 2002;99:9656-9661.
128. Wan C, Gilbert SR, Wang Y, et al. Activation of the hypoxia-inducible factor-1alpha pathway accelerates bone regeneration. *Proc Natl Acad Sci U S A.* 2008;105:686-691.
129. Almeida M, Han L, Martin-Millan M, et al. Skeletal involution by age-associated oxidative stress and its acceleration by loss of sex steroids. *J Biol Chem.* 2007;282:27285-27297.
130. Yakar S, Rosen CJ. From mouse to man: redefining the role of insulin-like growth factor-I in the acquisition of bone mass. *Exp Biol Med (Maywood, NJ).* 2003;228(3):245-252.
131. Yakar S, Bouxsein ML, Canalis E, et al. The ternary IGF complex influences postnatal bone acquisition and the skeletal response to intermittent parathyroid hormone. *J Endocrinol.* 2006;189:289-299.
132. Bikle D, Majumdar S, Laib A, et al. The skeletal structure of insulin-like growth factor I-deficient mice. *J Bone Miner Res.* 2001;16:2320-2329.
133. Hill PA, Reynolds JJ, Meikle MC. Osteoblasts mediate insulin-like growth factor-I and -II stimulation of osteoclast formation and function. *Endocrinology.* 1995;136:124-131.
134. Kawai M, Breggia AC, DeMambro VE, et al. The heparin-binding domain of IGFBP-2 has insulin-like growth factor binding-independent biologic activity in the growing skeleton. *J Biol Chem.* 2011;286: 14670-14680.
135. Barnard JA, Lyons RM, Moses HL. The cell biology of transforming growth factor beta. *Biochim Biophys Acta.* 1990;1032:79-87.
136. Hock JM, Canalis E, Centrella M. Transforming growth factor-beta stimulates bone matrix apposition and bone cell replication in cultured fetal rat calvariae. *Endocrinology.* 1990;126:421-426.
137. Spinella-Jaegle S, Roman-Roman S, Faucheu C, et al. Opposite effects of bone morphogenetic protein-2 and transforming growth factor-beta1 on osteoblast differentiation. *Bone.* 2001;29:323-330.
138. Pfeilschifter J, Seyedin SM, Mundy GR. Transforming growth factor beta inhibits bone resorption in fetal rat long bone cultures. *J Clin Invest.* 1988;82:680-685.
139. Shull MM, Ormsby I, Kier AB, et al. Targeted disruption of the mouse transforming growth factor-beta 1 gene results in multifocal inflammatory disease. *Nature.* 1992;359:693-699.
140. Centrella M, McCarthy TL, Canalis E. Transforming growth factor-beta and remodeling of bone. *J Bone Joint Surg.* 1991;73:1418-1428.
141. Leboy P, Grasso-Knight G, D'Angelo M, et al. Smad-Runx interactions during chondrocyte maturation. *J Bone Joint Surg Am.* 2001;83-A (Suppl 1 Pt 1):S15-S22.
142. Kaneko H, Arakawa T, Mano H, et al. Direct stimulation of osteoclastic bone resorption by bone morphogenetic protein (BMP)-2 and expression of BMP receptors in mature osteoclasts. *Bone.* 2000;27:479-486.
143. Lee SJ, Huynh TV, Lee YS, et al. Role of satellite cells versus myofibers in muscle hypertrophy induced by inhibition of the myostatin/activin signaling pathway. *Proc Natl Acad Sci U S A.* 2012;109:E2353-E2360.
144. Johnson ML, Harnish K, Nusse R, Van Hul W. LRP5 and Wnt signaling: a union made for bone. *J Bone Miner Res.* 2004;19:1749-1757.
145. Glass DA 2nd, Karsenty G. Molecular bases of the regulation of bone remodeling by the canonical Wnt signaling pathway. *Curr Top Dev Biol.* 2006;73:43-84.
146. Glass DA 2nd, Karsenty G. Canonical Wnt signaling in osteoblasts is required for osteoclast differentiation. *Ann N Y Acad Sci.* 2006;1068: 117-130.
147. Holmen SL, Zylstra CR, Mukherjee A, et al. Essential role of beta-catenin in postnatal bone acquisition. *J Biol Chem.* 2005;280:21162-21168.
148. Baron R, Rawadi G. Targeting the Wnt/beta-catenin pathway to regulate bone formation in the adult skeleton. *Endocrinology.* 2007;148: 2635-2643.
149. Diederichs G, Link T, Marie K, et al. Feasibility of measuring trabecular bone structure of the proximal femur using 64-slice multidetector computed tomography in a clinical setting. *Calcif Tissue Int.* 2008;83: 332-341.
150. Gaudio A, Privitera F, Battaglia K, et al. Sclerostin levels associated with inhibition of the Wnt/beta-catenin signaling and reduced bone turnover in type 2 diabetes mellitus. *J Clin Endocrinol Metab.* 2012;97(10): 3744-3750.
151. Clarke BL, Drake MT. Clinical utility of serum sclerostin measurements. *Bonekey Rep.* 2013;2:361.
152. Hirano T, Turner CH, Forwood MR, et al. Does suppression of bone turnover impair mechanical properties by allowing microdamage accumulation? *Bone.* 2000;27:13-20.
153. Verborgt O, Gibson GJ, Schaffler MB. Loss of osteocyte integrity in association with microdamage and bone remodeling after fatigue in vivo. *J Bone Miner Res.* 2000;15:60-67.
154. Dempster DW, Cosman F, Parisien M, et al. Anabolic actions of parathyroid hormone on bone. *Endocr Rev.* 1993;14:690-709.
155. Canalis E, Centrella M, Burch W, McCarthy TL. Insulin-like growth factor I mediates selective anabolic effects of parathyroid hormone in bone cultures. *J Clin Invest.* 1989;83:60-65.
156. Manolagas SC. Birth and death of bone cells: basic regulatory mechanisms and implications for the pathogenesis and treatment of osteoporosis. *Endocr Rev.* 2000;21:115-137.
157. Shiraishi A, Takeda S, Masaki T, et al. Alfacalcidol inhibits bone resorption and stimulates formation in an ovariectomized rat model of osteoporosis: distinct actions from estrogen. *J Bone Miner Res.* 2000;15: 770-779.
158. de Paula FJ, Rosen CJ. Back to the future: revisiting parathyroid hormone and calcitonin control of bone remodeling. *Horm Metab Res.* 2010;42(5):299-306.

159. Hurley DL, Tiegs RD, Wahner HW, Heath H 3rd. Axial and appendicular bone mineral density in patients with long-term deficiency or excess of calcitonin. *N Engl J Med.* 1987;317:537-541.

160. Daripa M, Paula FJ, Rufino AC, Foss MC. Impact of congenital calcitonin deficiency due to dysgenetic hypothyroidism on bone mineral density. *Braz J Med Biol Res.* 2004;37:61-68.

161. Eriksen EF, Kudsk H, Emmertsen K, et al. Bone remodeling during calcitonin excess: reconstruction of the remodeling sequence in medullary thyroid carcinoma. *Bone.* 1993;14:399-401.

162. Hoff AO, Catala-Lehnen P, Thomas PM, et al. Increased bone mass is an unexpected phenotype associated with deletion of the calcitonin gene. *J Clin Invest.* 2002;110:1849-1857.

163. Schinke T, Liese S, Priemel M, et al. Decreased bone formation and osteopenia in mice lacking alpha-calcitonin gene-related peptide. *J Bone Miner Res.* 2004;19:2049-2056.

164. Giustina A, Mazziotti G, Canalis E. Growth hormone, insulin-like growth factors, and the skeleton. *Endocr Rev.* 2008;29:535-559.

165. de Paula FJ, Gois-Junior MB, Aguiar-Oliveira MH, et al. Consequences of lifetime isolated growth hormone (GH) deficiency and effects of short-term GH treatment on bone in adults with a mutation in the GHRH-receptor gene. *Clin Endocrinol.* 2009;70:35-40.

166. Canalis E, Mazziotti G, Giustina A, Bilezikian JP. Glucocorticoid-induced osteoporosis: pathophysiology and therapy. *Osteoporos Int.* 2007;18:1319-1328.

167. Hofbauer LC, Gori F, Riggs BL, et al. Stimulation of osteoprotegerin ligand and inhibition of osteoprotegerin production by glucocorticoids in human osteoblastic lineage cells: potential paracrine mechanisms of glucocorticoid-induced osteoporosis. *Endocrinology.* 1999;140:4382-4389.

168. Canalis E, Bilezikian JP, Angeli A, Giustina A. Perspectives on glucocorticoid-induced osteoporosis. *Bone.* 2004;34:593-598.

169. Smith E, Frenkel B. Glucocorticoids inhibit the transcriptional activity of LEF/TCF in differentiating osteoblasts in a glycogen synthase kinase-3beta-dependent and -independent manner. *J Biol Chem.* 2005;280:2388-2394.

170. Gifre L, Ruiz-Gaspa S, Monegal A, et al. Effect of glucocorticoid treatment on Wnt signalling antagonists (sclerostin and Dkk-1) and their relationship with bone turnover. *Bone.* 2013;57:272-276.

171. Weinstein RS, Jilka RL, Parfitt AM, Manolagas SC. Inhibition of osteoblastogenesis and promotion of apoptosis of osteoblasts and osteocytes by glucocorticoids. Potential mechanisms of their deleterious effects on bone. *J Clin Invest.* 1998;102:274-282.

172. Delany AM, Durant D, Canalis E. Glucocorticoid suppression of IGF I transcription in osteoblasts. *Mol Endocrinol (Baltimore, MD).* 2001;15:1781-1789.

173. Forrest D, Sjoberg M, Vennstrom B. Contrasting developmental and tissue-specific expression of alpha and beta thyroid hormone receptor genes. *EMBO J.* 1990;9:1519-1528.

174. Williams GR. Cloning and characterization of two novel thyroid hormone receptor beta isoforms. *Mol Cell Biol.* 2000;20:8329-8342.

175. Freitas FR, Moriscot AS, Jorgetti V, et al. Spared bone mass in rats treated with thyroid hormone receptor TR beta-selective compound GC-1. *Am J Physiol.* 2003;285:E1135-E1141.

176. Cardoso LF, de Paula FJ, Maciel LM. Resistance to thyroid hormone due to mutations in the THRB gene impairs bone mass and affects calcium and phosphorus homeostasis. *Bone.* 2014;67:222-227.

177. Greenspan SL, Greenspan FS. The effect of thyroid hormone on skeletal integrity. *Ann Intern Med.* 1999;130:750-758.

178. Engler H, Oettli RE, Riesen WF. Biochemical markers of bone turnover in patients with thyroid dysfunctions and in euthyroid controls: a cross-sectional study. *Clin Chim Acta.* 1999;289(1-2):159-172.

179. Pereira RC, Jorgetti V, Canalis E. Triiodothyronine induces collagenase-3 and gelatinase B expression in murine osteoblasts. *Am J Physiol.* 1999;277:E496-E504.

180. Abe E, Marians RC, Yu W, et al. TSH is a negative regulator of skeletal remodeling. *Cell.* 2003;115:151-162.

181. Sun L, Vukicevic S, Baliram R, et al. Intermittent recombinant TSH injections prevent ovariectomy-induced bone loss. *Proc Natl Acad Sci U S A.* 2008;105:4289-4294.

182. Bex M, Bouillon R. Growth hormone and bone health. *Horm Res.* 2003;60(Suppl 3):80-86.

183. Moyer-Mileur LJ, Slater H, Jordan KC, Murray MA. IGF-1 and IGF-binding proteins and bone mass, geometry, and strength: relation to metabolic control in adolescent girls with type 1 diabetes. *J Bone Miner Res.* 2008;23:1884-1891.

184. Ogata N, Chikazu D, Kubota N, et al. Insulin receptor substrate-1 in osteoblast is indispensable for maintaining bone turnover. *J Clin Invest.* 2000;105:935-943.

185. de Paula FJ, Horowitz MC, Rosen CJ. Novel insights into the relationship between diabetes and osteoporosis. *Diabetes Metab Res Rev.* 2010;26(8):622-630.

186. Saito M, Fujii K, Soshi S, Tanaka T. Reductions in degree of mineralization and enzymatic collagen cross-links and increases in glycation-induced pentosidine in the femoral neck cortex in cases of femoral neck fracture. *Osteoporos Int.* 2006;17:986-995.

187. Bilezikian JP, Morishima A, Bell J, Grumbach MM. Increased bone mass as a result of estrogen therapy in a man with aromatase deficiency. *N Engl J Med.* 1998;339:599-603.

188. Falahati-Nini A, Riggs BL, Atkinson EJ, et al. Relative contributions of testosterone and estrogen in regulating bone resorption and formation in normal elderly men. *J Clin Invest.* 2000;106:1553-1560.

189. Consensus development conference: diagnosis, prophylaxis, and treatment of osteoporosis. *Am J Med.* 1993;94(6):646-650.

190. Cooper C, Atkinson EJ, Jacobsen SJ, et al. Population-based study of survival after osteoporotic fractures. *Am J Epidemiol.* 1993;137:1001-1005.

191. Colon-Emeric C, Kuchibhatla M, Pieper C, et al. The contribution of hip fracture to risk of subsequent fractures: data from two longitudinal studies. *Osteoporos Int.* 2003;14:879-883.

192. Lyles KW, Colon-Emeric CS, Magaziner JS, et al. Zoledronic acid in reducing clinical fracture and mortality after hip fracture. *N Engl J Med.* 2007;357:40967.

193. Cooper C, Melton LJ. Vertebral fractures. *BMJ.* 1992;304(6830):793-794.

194. Ettinger B, Black DM, Nevitt MC, et al. Contribution of vertebral deformities to chronic back pain and disability. The Study of Osteoporotic Fractures Research Group. *J Bone Miner Res.* 1992;7:449-456.

195. Cooper C, Atkinson EJ, O'Fallon WM, Melton LJ 3rd. Incidence of clinically diagnosed vertebral fractures: a population-based study in Rochester, Minnesota, 1985-1989. *J Bone Miner Res.* 1992;7:221-227.

196. Oleksik A, Lips P, Dawson A, et al. Health-related quality of life in postmenopausal women with low BMD with or without prevalent vertebral fractures. *J Bone Miner Res.* 2000;15:1384-1392.

197. Yun H, Delzell E, Saag KG, et al. Fractures and mortality in relation to different osteoporosis treatments. *Clin Exp Rheumatol.* 2015;33(3):302-309.

198. Black DM, Arden NK, Palermo L, et al. Prevalent vertebral deformities predict hip fractures and new vertebral deformities but not wrist fractures. Study of Osteoporotic Fractures Research Group. *J Bone Miner Res.* 1999;14:821-828.

199. Wustrack R, Seeman E, Bucci-Rechtweg C, et al. Predictors of new and severe vertebral fractures: results from the HORIZON Pivotal Fracture Trial. *Osteoporos Int.* 2011;23:53-58.

200. Hagino H. Other non-vertebral fractures. *Best Pract Res.* 2013;27:731-741.

201. Seeley DG, Browner WS, Nevitt MC, et al. Which fractures are associated with low appendicular bone mass in elderly women? The Study of Osteoporotic Fractures Research Group. *Ann Intern Med.* 1991;115:837-842.

202. Black DM, Thompson DE, Bauer DC, et al. Fracture risk reduction with alendronate in women with osteoporosis: the Fracture Intervention Trial. FIT Research Group. *J Clin Endocrinol Metab.* 2000;85:4118-4124.

203. Harris ST, Watts NB, Genant HK, et al. Effects of risedronate treatment on vertebral and nonvertebral fractures in women with postmenopausal osteoporosis: a randomized controlled trial. Vertebral Efficacy with Risedronate Therapy (VERT) Study Group. *JAMA.* 1999;282:1344-1352.

204. Orwoll ES, Marshall LM, Nielson CM, et al. Finite element analysis of the proximal femur and hip fracture risk in older men. *J Bone Miner Res.* 2009;24:475-483.

205. Ensrud KE, Palermo L, Black DM, et al. Hip and calcaneal bone loss increase with advancing age: longitudinal results from the study of osteoporotic fractures. *J Bone Miner Res.* 1995;10:1778-1787.

206. Carpenter RD, Beaupre GS, Lang TF, et al. New QCT analysis approach shows the importance of fall orientation on femoral neck strength. *J Bone Miner Res.* 2005;20:1533-1542.

207. Black DM, Bouxsein ML, Marshall LM, et al. Proximal femoral structure and the prediction of hip fracture in men: a large prospective study using QCT. *J Bone Miner Res.* 2008;23:1326-1333.

208. Schafer AL, Sellmeyer DE, Palermo L, et al. Six months of parathyroid hormone (1-84) administered concurrently versus sequentially with monthly ibandronate over two years: the PTH and ibandronate combination study (PICS) randomized trial. *J Clin Endocrinol Metab.* 2012;97:3522-3529.

209. Lang TF, Keyak JH, Heitz MW, et al. Volumetric quantitative computed tomography of the proximal femur: precision and relation to bone strength. *Bone.* 1997;21:101-108.

210. Moayyeri A, Adams JE, Adler RA, et al. Quantitative ultrasound of the heel and fracture risk assessment: an updated meta-analysis. *Osteoporos Int.* 2012;23:143-153.

211. Schafer AL, Vittinghoff E, Ramachandran R, et al. Laboratory reproducibility of biochemical markers of bone turnover in clinical practice. *Osteoporos Int.* 2010;21:439-445.

212. Bauer DC, Garnero P, Harrison SL, et al. Biochemical markers of bone turnover, hip bone loss, and fracture in older men: the MrOS study. *J Bone Miner Res.* 2009;24:2032-2038.

213. Bauer DC, Schwartz A, Palermo L, et al. Fracture prediction after discontinuation of 4 to 5 years of alendronate therapy: the FLEX study. *JAMA Intern Med.* 2014;174(7):1126-1134.

214. Garnero P. Markers of bone turnover for the prediction of fracture risk. *Osteoporos Int.* 2000;11(Suppl 6):S55-S65.

215. Eastell R, Vrijens B, Cahall DL, et al. Bone turnover markers and bone mineral density response with risedronate therapy: relationship with fracture risk and patient adherence. *J Bone Miner Res.* 2011;26:1662-1669.

216. Burch J, Rice S, Yang H, et al. Systematic review of the use of bone turnover markers for monitoring the response to osteoporosis treatment: the secondary prevention of fractures, and primary prevention of fractures in high-risk groups. *Health Technol Assess (Winchester, England).* 2014;18(11):1-180.

217. Delmas PD, Vrijens B, Eastell R, et al. Effect of monitoring bone turnover markers on persistence with risedronate treatment of postmenopausal osteoporosis. *J Clin Endocrinol Metab.* 2007;92:1296-1304.

218. Reid IR, Brown JP, Burckhardt P, et al. Intravenous zoledronic acid in postmenopausal women with low bone mineral density. *N Engl J Med.* 2002;346:653-661.

219. Bone HG, Downs RW Jr, Tucci JR, et al. Dose-response relationships for alendronate treatment in osteoporotic elderly women. Alendronate Elderly Osteoporosis Study Centers. *J Clin Endocrinol Metab.* 1997;82:265-274.

220. Dempster DW, Compston JE, Drezner MK, et al. Standardized nomenclature, symbols, and units for bone histomorphometry: a 2012 update of the report of the ASBMR Histomorphometry Nomenclature Committee. *J Bone Miner Res.* 2013;28:2-17.

221. Lau EM, Suriwongpaisal P, Lee JK, et al. Risk factors for hip fracture in Asian men and women: the Asian osteoporosis study. *J Bone Miner Res.* 2001;16:572-580.

222. Kennedy CC, Ioannidis G, Rockwood K, et al. A Frailty Index predicts 10-year fracture risk in adults age 25 years and older: results from the Canadian Multicentre Osteoporosis Study (CaMos). *Osteoporos Int.* 2014;25(12):2825-2832.

223. Cummings SR, Nevitt MC, Browner WS, et al. Risk factors for hip fracture in white women. Study of Osteoporotic Fractures Research Group. *N Engl J Med.* 1995;332:767-773.

224. Kanis JA, Johnell O, De Laet C, et al. A meta-analysis of previous fracture and subsequent fracture risk. *Bone.* 2004;35:375-382.

225. Kanis JA, Oden A, Johnell O, et al. The use of clinical risk factors enhances the performance of BMD in the prediction of hip and osteoporotic fractures in men and women. *Osteoporos Int.* 2007;18:1033-1046.

226. Schwartz AV, Vittinghoff E, Bauer DC, et al. Association of BMD and FRAX score with risk of fracture in older adults with type 2 diabetes. *JAMA.* 2011;305:2184-2192.

227. Nielson CM, Marshall LM, Adams AL, et al. BMI and fracture risk in older men: the osteoporotic fractures in men study (MrOS). *J Bone Miner Res.* 2011;26:496-502.

228. FRAX. WHO Fracture Risk Assessment Tool. UK: World Health Organization Collaborating Centre for Metabolic Bone Diseases, University of Sheffield, UK. Available at: <http://www.shef.ac.uk/FRAX/>.

229. Nguyen ND, Pongchaiyakul C, Center JR, et al. Identification of high-risk individuals for hip fracture: a 14-year prospective study. *J Bone Miner Res.* 2005;20:1921-1928.

230. Harvey N, Dennison E, Cooper C. The epidemiology of osteoporotic fractures. In: Rosen CJ, ed. *Primer on the Metabolic Bone Diseases and Disorders of Mineral Metabolism.* 8th ed. Ames, IA: Wiley-Blackwell; 2013:348-356.

231. Assessment of fracture risk and its application to screening for postmenopausal osteoporosis. Report of a WHO Study Group. *World Health Organ Tech Rep Ser.* 1994;843:1-129.

232. Black DM, Palermo L, Nevitt MC, et al. Comparison of methods for defining prevalent vertebral deformities: the Study of Osteoporotic Fractures. *J Bone Miner Res.* 1995;10:890-902.

233. Cummings SR, Cawthon PM, Ensrud KE, et al. BMD and risk of hip and nonvertebral fractures in older men: a prospective study and comparison with older women. *J Bone Miner Res.* 2006;21:1550-1556.

234. Looker AC, Johnston CC Jr, Wahner HW, et al. Prevalence of low femoral bone density in older U.S. women from NHANES III. *J Bone Miner Res.* 1995;10:796-802.

235. Cummings SR, Melton LJ. Epidemiology and outcomes of osteoporotic fractures. *Lancet.* 2002;359:1761-1767.

236. Cummings SR, Black DM, Rubin SM. Lifetime risks of hip, Colles', or vertebral fracture and coronary heart disease among white postmenopausal women. *Arch Intern Med.* 1989;149:2445-2448.

237. Melton LJ 3rd, Kan SH, Wahner HW, Riggs BL. Lifetime fracture risk: an approach to hip fracture risk assessment based on bone mineral density and age. *J Clin Epidemiol.* 1988;41:985-994.

238. Melton LR. Lifetime risk of a hip fracture. *Am J Public Health.* 1990;80:501.

239. National Institute of Arthritis and Musculoskeletal and Skin Diseases (NIAMS). *What Is Osteoporosis? Fast Facts: An Easy-to-Read Series of Publications for the Public.* Bethesda, MD: National Institutes of Health; 2011. Available at: <http://www.niams.nih.gov/Health_Info/Bone/Osteoporosis/osteoporosis_hoh.asp>.

240. International Osteoporosis Foundation. Women over 50 will experience osteoporotic fractures, as will men: facts and statistics. Available at: <www.iofbonehealth.org/facts-statistics>.

241. Pike C, Birnbaum HG, Schiller M, et al. Economic burden of privately insured non-vertebral fracture patients with osteoporosis over a 2-year period in the US. *Osteoporos Int.* 2011;22:47-56.

242. Reifenstein EC Jr, Albright F. The metabolic effects of steroid hormones in osteoporosis. *J Clin Invest.* 1947;26:24-56.

243. Rossouw JE, Anderson GL, Prentice RL, et al. Risks and benefits of estrogen plus progestin in healthy postmenopausal women: principal results from the Women's Health Initiative randomized controlled trial. *JAMA.* 2002;288:321-333.

244. Riis BJ, Rodbro P, Christiansen C. The role of serum concentrations of sex steroids and bone turnover in the development and occurrence of postmenopausal osteoporosis. *Calcif Tissue Int.* 1986;38:318-322.

245. Slemenda CW, Longcope C, Zhou L, et al. Sex steroids and bone mass in older men. Positive associations with serum estrogens and negative associations with androgens. *J Clin Invest.* 1997;100:1755-1759.

246. Smith EP, Boyd J, Frank GR, et al. Estrogen resistance caused by a mutation in the estrogen-receptor gene in a man. *N Engl J Med.* 1994;331:1056-1061.

247. Carani C, Qin K, Simoni M, et al. Effect of testosterone and estradiol in a man with aromatase deficiency. *N Engl J Med.* 1997;337:91-95.

248. Sun WH, Keller ET, Stebler BS, Ershler WB. Estrogen inhibits phorbol ester-induced I kappa B alpha transcription and protein degradation. *Biochem Biophys Res Commun.* 1998;244:691-695.

249. Vargas SJ, Naprta A, Lee SK, et al. Lack of evidence for an increase in interleukin-6 expression in adult murine bone, bone marrow, and marrow stromal cell cultures after ovariectomy. *J Bone Miner Res.* 1996;11:1926-1934.

250. Rosen CJ, Verault D, Steffens C, et al. Effects of age and estrogen status on the skeletal IGF regulatory system. Studies with human marrow. *Endocrine.* 1997;7:77-80.

251. Yang N, Wang G, Hu C, et al. Tumor necrosis factor alpha suppresses the mesenchymal stem cell osteogenesis promoter miR-21 in estrogen deficiency-induced osteoporosis. *J Bone Miner Res.* 2013;28:559-573.

252. Manolagas SC, O'Brien CA, Almeida M. The role of estrogen and androgen receptors in bone health and disease. *Nat Rev Endocrinol.* 2013;9:699-712.

253. Zhang J, Pugh TD, Stebler B, et al. Orchiectomy increases bone marrow interleukin-6 levels in mice. *Calcif Tissue Int.* 1998;62:219-226.

254. Vanderschueren D, Vandenput L, Boonen S, et al. Androgens and bone. *Endocr Rev.* 2004;25:389-425.

255. Almeida M, Iyer S, Martin-Millan M, et al. Estrogen receptor-alpha signaling in osteoblast progenitors stimulates cortical bone accrual. *J Clin Invest.* 2013;123:394-404.

256. Notini AJ, McManus JF, Moore A, et al. Osteoblast deletion of exon 3 of the androgen receptor gene results in trabecular bone loss in adult male mice. *J Bone Miner Res.* 2007;22:347-356.

257. Watts NB, Adler RA, Bilezikian JP, et al. Osteoporosis in men: an Endocrine Society clinical practice guideline. *J Clin Endocrinol Metab.* 2012;97(6):1802-1822.

258. Heaney R. Nutrition and risk of osteoporosis. In: Marcus R, Feldman D, Dempster DW, et al., eds. *Osteoporosis.* 4th ed. Waltham, MA: Academic Press; 2013:645-681.

259. Ross AC, Manson JE, Abrams SA, et al. The 2011 report on dietary reference intakes for calcium and vitamin D from the Institute of Medicine: what clinicians need to know. *J Clin Endocrinol Metab.* 2011;96:53-58.

260. National Academies Press. *Dietary Reference Intakes for Calcium and Vitamin D.* Washington, DC: Institute of Medicine (IOM); 2011.

261. Priemel M, von Domarus C, Klatte TO, et al. Bone mineralization defects and vitamin D deficiency: histomorphometric analysis of iliac crest bone biopsies and circulating 25-hydroxyvitamin D in 675 patients. *J Bone Miner Res.* 2010;25:305-312.

262. Mohan S, Farley JR, Baylink DJ. Age-related changes in IGFBP-4 and IGFBP-5 levels in human serum and bone: implications for bone loss with aging. *Prog Growth Factor Res.* 1995;6:465-473.

263. Rosen C, Donahue LR, Hunter S, et al. The 24/25-kDa serum insulin-like growth factor-binding protein is increased in elderly women with hip and spine fractures. *J Clin Endocrinol Metab.* 1992;74:24-27.

264. Manolagas SC. From estrogen-centric to aging and oxidative stress: a revised perspective of the pathogenesis of osteoporosis. *Endocr Rev.* 2010;31:266-300.

265. Overman RA, Toliver JC, Yeh JY, et al. U.S. adults meeting 2010 American College of Rheumatology criteria for treatment and prevention of glucocorticoid-induced osteoporosis. *Arthritis Care Res (Hoboken).* 2014;66(11):1644-1652.

266. Compston J. Management of glucocorticoid-induced osteoporosis. *Nat Rev.* 2010;6:82-88.

267. Cushing H. The basophil adenomans of the pituitary body and their clinical manifestations. *Bull Johns Hopkins Hosp.* 1932;1:137-195.

268. Hermus AR, Smals AG, Swinkels LM, et al. Bone mineral density and bone turnover before and after surgical cure of Cushing's syndrome. *J Clin Endocrinol Metab.* 1995;80:2859-2865.

269. van Staa TP. The pathogenesis, epidemiology and management of glucocorticoid-induced osteoporosis. *Calcif Tissue Int.* 2006;79:129-137.

270. van Staa TP, Leufkens HG, Cooper C. The epidemiology of corticosteroid-induced osteoporosis: a meta-analysis. *Osteoporos Int.* 2002;13:777-787.

271. Homik JE, Cranney A, Shea B, et al. A metaanalysis on the use of bisphosphonates in corticosteroid induced osteoporosis. *J Rheumatol.* 1999;26:1148-1157.

272. Adachi JD, Saag KG, Delmas PD, et al. Two-year effects of alendronate on bone mineral density and vertebral fracture in patients receiving glucocorticoids: a randomized, double-blind, placebo-controlled extension trial. *Arthritis Rheum.* 2001;44(1):202-211.

273. Cohen S, Levy RM, Keller M, et al. Risedronate therapy prevents corticosteroid-induced bone loss: a twelve-month, multicenter, randomized, double-blind, placebo-controlled, parallel-group study. *Arthritis Rheum.* 1999;42:2309-2318.

274. Reid DM, Devogelaer JP, Saag K, et al. Zoledronic acid and risedronate in the prevention and treatment of glucocorticoid-induced osteoporosis (HORIZON): a multicentre, double-blind, double-dummy, randomised controlled trial. *Lancet.* 2009;373:1253-1263.

275. Saag KG, Shane E, Boonen S, et al. Teriparatide or alendronate in glucocorticoid-induced osteoporosis. *N Engl J Med.* 2007;357:2028-2039.

276. Parfitt AM. The two faces of growth: benefits and risks to bone integrity. *Osteoporos Int.* 1994;4:382-398.

277. Parfitt AM. Genetic effects on bone mass and turnover-relevance to black/white differences. *J Am Coll Nutr.* 1997;16:325-333.

278. Fazeli PK, Bredella MA, Misra M, et al. Preadipocyte factor-1 is associated with marrow adiposity and bone mineral density in women with anorexia nervosa. *J Clin Endocrinol Metab.* 2010;95:407-413.

279. Vehmanen LK, Elomaa I, Blomqvist CP, Saarto T. The effect of ovarian dysfunction on bone mineral density in breast cancer patients 10 years after adjuvant chemotherapy. *Acta Oncol (Stockholm, Sweden).* 2014;53:75-79.

280. Rubin K. Turner syndrome and osteoporosis: mechanisms and prognosis. *Pediatrics.* 1998;102:481-485.

281. Ferlin A, Schipilliti M, Di Mambro A, et al. Osteoporosis in Klinefelter's syndrome. *Mol Hum Reprod.* 2010;16:402-410.

282. Finkelstein JS, Klibanski A, Neer RM. A longitudinal evaluation of bone mineral density in adult men with histories of delayed puberty. *J Clin Endocrinol Metab.* 1996;81:1152-1155.

283. Yakar S, Canalis E, Sun H, et al. Serum IGF-1 determines skeletal strength by regulating subperiosteal expansion and trait interactions. *J Bone Miner Res.* 2009;24:1481-1492.

284. Heinrichs C, Vis HL, Bergmann P, et al. Effects of 17 months treatment using recombinant insulin-like growth factor-I in two children with growth hormone insensitivity (Laron) syndrome. *Clin Endocrinol.* 1993;38:647-651.

285. Yakar S, Rosen CJ, Beamer WG, et al. Circulating levels of IGF-1 directly regulate bone growth and density. *J Clin Invest.* 2002;110:771-781.

286. Canalis E. Skeletal growth factors. In: Marcus R, Feldman D, Dempster DW, et al., eds. *Osteoporosis.* Waltham, MA: Academic Press; 2013:391-410.

287. Committee Opinion No. 602: depot medroxyprogesterone acetate and bone effects. *Obstet Gynecol.* 2014;123(6):1398-1402.

288. Gray RW, Garthwaite TL. Activation of renal 1,25-dihydroxyvitamin D3 synthesis by phosphate deprivation: evidence for a role for growth hormone. *Endocrinology.* 1985;116:189-193.

289. Gray RW. Evidence that somatomedins mediate the effect of hypophosphatemia to increase serum 1,25-dihydroxyvitamin D3 levels in rats. *Endocrinology.* 1987;121:504-512.

290. Caverzasio J, Montessuit C, Bonjour JP. Stimulatory effect of insulin-like growth factor-1 on renal Pi transport and plasma 1,25-dihydroxyvitamin D3. *Endocrinology.* 1990;127:453-459.

291. Cameron MA, Paton LM, Nowson CA, et al. The effect of calcium supplementation on bone density in premenarcheal females: a co-twin approach. *J Clin Endocrinol Metab.* 2004;89:4916-4922.

292. Johnston CC Jr, Miller JZ, Slemenda CW, et al. Calcium supplementation and increases in bone mineral density in children. *N Engl J Med.* 1992;327:82-87.

293. Smith DM, Nance WE, Kang KW, et al. Genetic factors in determining bone mass. *J Clin Invest.* 1973;52:2800-2808.

294. Naganathan V, MacGregor AJ, Sambrook PN. The role of gene-environment interaction in determining bone mineral density in a twin population. *Twin Res Hum Genet.* 2007;10:191-197.

295. Eisman JA. Genetics of osteoporosis. *Endocr Rev.* 1999;20:788-804.

296. Hopper JL, Green RM, Nowson CA, et al. Genetic, common environment, and individual specific components of variance for bone mineral density in 10- to 26-year-old females: a twin study. *Am J Epidemiol.* 1998;147:17-29.

297. Johnson ML, Gong G, Kimberling W, et al. Linkage of a gene causing high bone mass to human chromosome 11 (11q12-13). *Am J Hum Genet.* 1997;60:1326-1332.

298. Boyden LM, Mao J, Belsky J, et al. High bone density due to a mutation in LDL-receptor-related protein 5. *N Engl J Med.* 2002;346:1513-1521.

299. Gong Y, Slee RB, Fukai N, et al. LDL receptor-related protein 5 (LRP5) affects bone accrual and eye development. *Cell.* 2001;107:513-523.

300. Slemenda CW, Peacock M, Hui S, et al. Reduced rates of skeletal remodeling are associated with increased bone mineral density during the development of peak skeletal mass. *J Bone Miner Res.* 1997;12:676-682.

301. Rizzoli R. Nutritional aspects of bone health. *Best Pract Res Clin Endocrinol Metab.* 2014;28(6):795-808.

302. National Osteoporosis Foundation (NOF). *Clinician's Guide to Prevention and Treatment of Osteoporosis.* Washington, DC: NOF; 2010. Also available at: <nof.org/files/nof/public/content/file/344/upload/159.pdf>.

303. Department of Health and Human Services, Office of the Surgeon General. *The Surgeon General's Report on Bone Health and Osteoporosis.* Rockville, MD: USDHHS; 2004. Also available at: <http://www.ncbi.nlm.nih.gov/books/NBK45513/>.

304. Huntjens KM, van Geel TA, van den Bergh JP, et al. Fracture liaison service: impact on subsequent nonvertebral fracture incidence and mortality. *J Bone Joint Surg.* 2014;96:e29.

305. McClung MR, Boonen S, Torring O, et al. Effect of denosumab treatment on the risk of fractures in subgroups of women with postmenopausal osteoporosis. *J Bone Miner Res.* 2012;27:211-218.

306. Chesnut IC, Skag A, Christiansen C, et al. Effects of oral ibandronate administered daily or intermittently on fracture risk in postmenopausal osteoporosis. *J Bone Miner Res.* 2004;19:1241-1249.

307. Compston J, Bowring C, Cooper A, et al. Diagnosis and management of osteoporosis in postmenopausal women and older men in the UK: National Osteoporosis Guideline Group (NOGG) update 2013. *Maturitas.* 2013;75(4):392-396.

308. Tang BM, Eslick GD, Nowson C, et al. Use of calcium or calcium in combination with vitamin D supplementation to prevent fractures and bone loss in people aged 50 years and older: a meta-analysis. *Lancet.* 2007;370:657-666.

309. Jackson RD, LaCroix AZ, Gass M, et al. Calcium plus vitamin D supplementation and the risk of fractures. *N Engl J Med.* 2006;354:669-683.

310. Chapuy MC, Arlot ME, Duboeuf F, et al. Vitamin D3 and calcium to prevent hip fractures in the elderly women. *N Engl J Med.* 1992;327:1637-1642.

311. Moyer VA. Vitamin D and calcium supplementation to prevent fractures in adults: U.S. Preventive Services Task Force recommendation statement. *Ann Intern Med.* 2012;158:691-696.

312. Reid IR, Bolland MJ, Grey A. Effects of vitamin D supplements on bone mineral density: a systematic review and meta-analysis. *Lancet.* 2014;383:146-155.

313. DIPART (Vitamin D Individual Patient Analysis of Randomized Trials) Group. Patient level pooled analysis of 68 500 patients from seven major vitamin D fracture trials in US and Europe. *BMJ.* 2010;340:b5463.

314. Avenell A, Gillespie WJ, Gillespie LD, O'Connell D. Vitamin D and vitamin D analogues for preventing fractures associated with involutional and post-menopausal osteoporosis. *Cochrane Database Syst Rev.* 2009;(2):CD000227.

314a. Santesso N, Carrasco-Labra A, Brignardello-Petersen R. Hip protectors for preventing hip fractures in older people. *Cochrane Database Syst Rev.* 2014;(3):CD001255. doi: 10.1002/14651858.CD001255.pub5.

315. Gillespie LD, Robertson MC, Gillespie WJ, et al. Interventions for preventing falls in older people living in the community. *Cochrane Database Syst Rev.* 2012;(9):CD007146.

316. Winther A, Dennison E, Ahmed LA, et al. The Tromso Study: fit futures: a study of Norwegian adolescents' lifestyle and bone health. *Arch Osteoporos.* 2014;9:185.

317. Shevde NK, Bendixen AC, Dienger KM, Pike JW. Estrogens suppress RANK ligand-induced osteoclast differentiation via a stromal cell independent mechanism involving c-Jun repression. *Proc Natl Acad Sci U S A.* 2000;97:7829-7834.

318. Nakamura T, Imai Y, Matsumoto T, et al. Estrogen prevents bone loss via estrogen receptor alpha and induction of Fas ligand in osteoclasts. *Cell.* 2007;130:811-823.

319. Effects of hormone therapy on bone mineral density: results from the postmenopausal estrogen/progestin interventions (PEPI) trial. The Writing Group for the PEPI. *JAMA.* 1996;276(17):1389-1396.

320. Fisher B, Costantino JP, Wickerham DL, et al. Tamoxifen for prevention of breast cancer: report of the National Surgical Adjuvant Breast and Bowel Project P-1 Study. *J Natl Cancer Inst.* 1998;90(18):1371-1388.

321. Vogel VG, Costantino JP, Wickerham DL, et al. Effects of tamoxifen vs raloxifene on the risk of developing invasive breast cancer and other disease outcomes: the NSABP Study of Tamoxifen and Raloxifene (STAR) P-2 trial. *JAMA.* 2006;295:2727-2741.

322. Ettinger B, Black DM, Mitlak BH, et al. Reduction of vertebral fracture risk in postmenopausal women with osteoporosis treated with raloxifene: results from a 3-year randomized clinical trial. Multiple Outcomes of Raloxifene Evaluation (MORE) Investigators. *JAMA.* 1999;282:637-645.

323. Black DM, Cummings SR, Karpf DB, et al. Randomised trial of effect of alendronate on risk of fracture in women with existing vertebral fractures. Fracture Intervention Trial Research Group. *Lancet.* 1996; 348:1535-1541.

324. Black DM, Schwartz AV, Ensrud KE, et al. Effects of continuing or stopping alendronate after 5 years of treatment: the Fracture Intervention Trial Long-term Extension (FLEX): a randomized trial. *JAMA.* 2006;296: 2927-2938.

325. Reginster JY, Adami S, Lakatos P, et al. Efficacy and tolerability of once-monthly oral ibandronate in postmenopausal osteoporosis: 2 year results from the MOBILE study. *Ann Rheum Dis.* 2006;65:654-661.

326. Delmas PD, Adami S, Strugala C, et al. Intravenous ibandronate injections in postmenopausal women with osteoporosis: one-year results from the dosing intravenous administration study. *Arthritis Rheum.* 2006;54:1838-1846.

327. Rossini M, Orsolini G, Adami S, et al. Osteoporosis treatment: why ibandronic acid? *Expert Opin Pharmacother.* 2013;14:1371-1381.

328. Black DM, Delmas PD, Eastell R, et al. Once-yearly zoledronic acid for treatment of postmenopausal osteoporosis. *N Engl J Med.* 2007;356: 1809-1822.

329. Shane E, Burr D, Abrahamsen B, et al. Atypical subtrochanteric and diaphyseal femoral fractures: second report of a task force of the American Society for Bone and Mineral Research. *J Bone Miner Res.* 2014;29:1-23.

330. Khan AA, Morrison A, Hanley DA, et al. Diagnosis and management of osteonecrosis of the jaw: a systematic review and international consensus. *J Bone Miner Res.* 2015;30:3-23.

331. Chesnut CH 3rd, Silverman S, Andriano K, et al. A randomized trial of nasal spray salmon calcitonin in postmenopausal women with established osteoporosis: the prevent recurrence of osteoporotic fractures study. PROOF Study Group. *Am J Med.* 2000;109:267-276.

332. Meunier PJ, Roux C, Seeman E, et al. The effects of strontium ranelate on the risk of vertebral fracture in women with postmenopausal osteoporosis. *N Eng J Med.* 2004;350:459-468.

333. Reginster JY, Seeman E, De Vernejoul MC, et al. Strontium ranelate reduces the risk of nonvertebral fractures in postmenopausal women with osteoporosis: Treatment of Peripheral Osteoporosis (TROPOS) study. *J Clin Endocrinol Metab.* 2005;90:2816-2822.

334. Donneau AF, Reginster JY. Cardiovascular safety of strontium ranelate: real-life assessment in clinical practice. *Osteoporos Int.* 2014;25: 397-398.

335. Bone HG, Bolognese MA, Yuen CK, et al. Effects of denosumab treatment and discontinuation on bone mineral density and bone turnover markers in postmenopausal women with low bone mass. *J Clin Endocrinol Metab.* 2011;96:972-980.

336. Bone HG, Chapurlat R, Brandi ML, et al. The effect of three or six years of denosumab exposure in women with postmenopausal osteoporosis: results from the FREEDOM extension. *J Clin Endocrinol Metab.* 2013;98: 4483-4492.

337. Engelke K, Fuerst T, Dardzinski B, et al. Odanacatib treatment affects trabecular and cortical bone in the femur of postmenopausal women: results of a 2-year placebo-controlled trial. *J Bone Miner Res.* 2015; 30(1):30-38.

338. Jensen AB, Wynne C, Ramirez G, et al. The cathepsin K inhibitor odanacatib suppresses bone resorption in women with breast cancer and established bone metastases: results of a 4-week, double-blind, randomized, controlled trial. *Clin Breast Cancer.* 2010;10:452-458.

339. Tam CS, Heersche JN, Murray TM, Parsons JA. Parathyroid hormone stimulates the bone apposition rate independently of its resorptive action: differential effects of intermittent and continuous administration. *Endocrinology.* 1982;110:506-512.

340. Parisien M, Mellish RW, Silverberg SJ, et al. Maintenance of cancellous bone connectivity in primary hyperparathyroidism: trabecular strut analysis. *J Bone Miner Res.* 1992;7:913-919.

341. Neer RM, Arnaud CD, Zanchetta JR, et al. Effect of parathyroid hormone (1-34) on fractures and bone mineral density in postmenopausal women with osteoporosis. *N Engl J Med.* 2001;344:1434-1441.

342. Orwoll ES, Scheele WH, Paul S, et al. The effect of teriparatide [human parathyroid hormone (1-34)] therapy on bone density in men with osteoporosis. *J Bone Miner Res.* 2003;18:9-17.

343. Clarke BL, Kay Berg J, Fox J, et al. Pharmacokinetics and pharmacodynamics of subcutaneous recombinant parathyroid hormone (1-84) in patients with hypoparathyroidism: an open-label, single-dose, phase I study. *Clin Ther.* 2014;36:722-736.

344. Finkelstein JS, Hayes A, Hunzelman JL, et al. The effects of parathyroid hormone, alendronate, or both in men with osteoporosis. *N Engl J Med.* 2003;349:1216-1226.

345. Finkelstein JS, Wyland JJ, Lee H, Neer RM. Effects of teriparatide, alendronate, or both in women with postmenopausal osteoporosis. *J Clin Endocrinol Metab.* 2010;95:1838-1845.

346. Tsai JN, Uihlein AV, Lee H, et al. Teriparatide and denosumab, alone or combined, in women with postmenopausal osteoporosis: the DATA study randomised trial. *Lancet.* 2013;382:50-56.

347. Horwitz MJ, Tedesco MB, Garcia-Ocana A, et al. Parathyroid hormone-related protein for the treatment of postmenopausal osteoporosis: defining the maximal tolerable dose. *J Clin Endocrinol Metab.* 2010;95: 1279-1287.

CHAPTER 30

Kidney Stones

ANIRBAN BOSE • REBECA D. MONK • DAVID A. BUSHINSKY

KEY POINTS

- Numerous factors, including sex, age, race and the patient's geographic location, determine the prevalence of kidney stones
- Kidney stones form when urine becomes supersaturated with respect to the specific components of the stone's constituents
- A multitude of monogenic hereditary disorders that result in changes of either calcium handling at the level of kidney, bone and gut, or calcium sensing at the calcium-sensing receptor on the parathyroid glands and renal tubular cells, can lead to hypercalciuria and stone formation.
- All patients, even those with a single stone, should undergo at least a basic evaluation in order to rule out a systemic etiology of stone formation.
- Increasing fluid intake is a simple measure that has considerable impact on reducing stone growth and new stone formation.

Nephrolithiasis is a common disorder with an incidence greater than 1 case per 1000 patients per year. In the year 2000, this resulted in nearly 2 million physician office visits with an estimated annual cost between $2 billion and $5.5 billion in the United States alone.[1,2] The prevalence in industrialized nations is approximately 6% in women and 12% in men and appears to be rising over time.[3] Its incidence peaks when patients are in their 30s and 40s. The prevalence increases with age until about the seventh decade of life.[3-6]

Stones may be composed of calcium oxalate, calcium phosphate, uric acid, magnesium ammonium phosphate (struvite), or cystine, alone or in combination. A variety of pathogenic mechanisms determine the type of stone formed. Symptomatic stones tend to localize in the renal tubules and collecting system but are also commonly found within the ureters and bladder.[7] The recurrence rate of calcium oxalate stones is about 50% at 5 to 10 years and higher for cystine, uric acid, and struvite stones.[8]

Kidney stones result in substantial morbidity. The severe pain of renal colic can lead to frequent hospitalization, shock wave lithotripsy, or invasive surgical procedures. Though rarely a cause of end-stage renal disease (ESRD), nephrolithiasis has been associated with chronic kidney disease (CKD) in various populations,[9-13] and even mild CKD is associated with significant adverse cardiovascular events.[14-16] Insight into the mechanisms involved in stone formation can help direct appropriate therapy, which is known to significantly decrease the incidence of stone formation and its associated morbidity. If this morbidity also includes cardiovascular disease, then stone prevention may have more significant overall health benefits for patients than merely controlling the pain and consequences of renal colic.

EPIDEMIOLOGY OF STONE FORMATION

Numerous factors determine the prevalence of stones, including sex, age, race, and geographic distribution. Men are two to four times as likely to get nephrolithiasis as women.[3-6,17] In the United States, blacks, Hispanics, and Asian Americans are much less likely to have stones than whites. Geography also appears to influence stone formation in the United States, with a decreasing prevalence from south to north and, to some degree, from east to west.[17] The greater exposure to sunlight in the southeastern United States may be responsible for the increased rates of nephrolithiasis in that area. Sun exposure can lead to more concentrated urine by increasing insensible fluid losses due to sweating.[18,19] Although increased sun exposure should increase levels of serum 25(OH)D (25-hydroxyvitamin D), there is no evidence for a subsequent increase in the level of 1,25(OH)$_2$D (1,25-dihydroxyvitamin D), nor is there any evidence that hypercalciuria will worsen.

Along with geography, genetic predisposition can influence the type of stone formed.[18,20] For example, uric acid stones are seen in up to 75% of all cases in Mediterranean and Middle Eastern countries but constitute fewer than 10% of cases in the United States. By contrast, more than 70% of stones formed in the United States are calcium-based. Less common are magnesium ammonium phosphate (struvite or infection) stones, which account for about 10% to 25% of stones formed, and cystine stones, which are due to an autosomal recessive disorder and constitute only about 2% of all stones formed (Fig. 30-1).[4,21,22]

Diet and pharmacologic agents can also significantly impact stone formation. In a dramatic example, an outbreak of nephrolithiasis in Chinese infants was attributed to ingestion of melamine in infant formulas and milk powder. Melamine, intentionally added to raise the apparent protein content of the concentrates, led to the formation of large particles in the kidney and resulted in many cases of nephrolithiasis and renal failure due to obstructive uropathy.[23-25] A variety of other dietary factors can have a significant impact on both the formation and prevention of kidney stones (see later discussion).

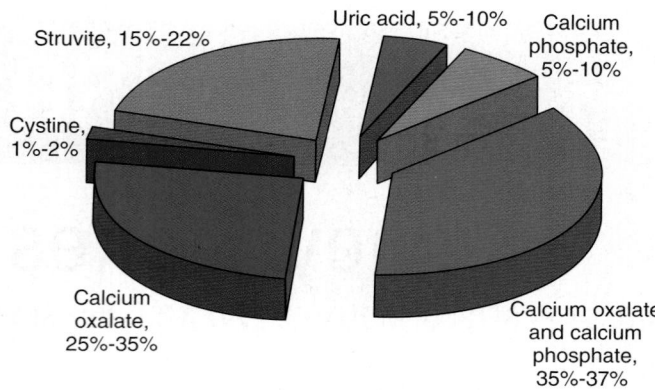

Figure 30-1 Frequency of different types of kidney stones.

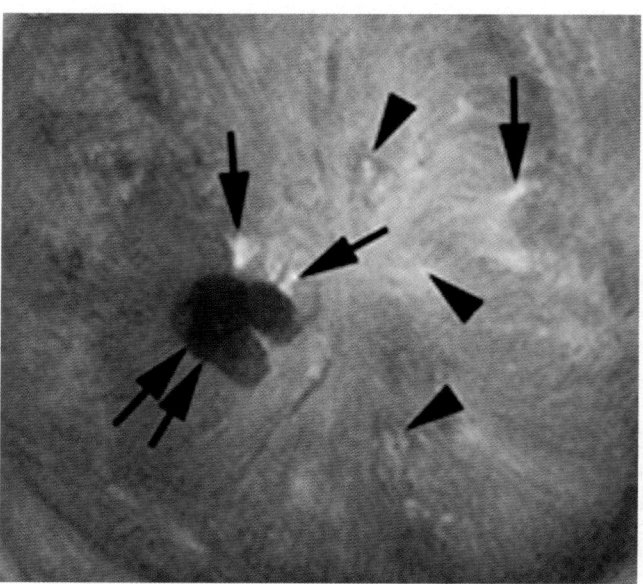

Figure 30-2 An attached stone *(paired arrows)* is seen resting on a region of white plaque *(single arrows)* and intermixed with small areas of white *(single arrow)* and yellow plaques *(arrowheads)*. (From Evan AP, Lingeman JE, Worcester EM, et al. Renal histopathology and crystal deposits in patients with small bowel resection and calcium oxalate stone disease. *Kidney Int.* 2010;78:310-317.)

PATHOGENESIS OF STONE FORMATION

Physiology

Kidney stones form when urine becomes supersaturated with respect to the specific components of the stone. Saturation is dependent on chemical free ion activities of the stone constituents. Factors that affect chemical free ion activity include urinary ion concentration, pH, and the combination of the constituent ion with other substances. For example, an increase in the urinary calcium concentration or a decrease in urine volume increases the free ion activity of calcium ions in the urine. Urinary pH can also modify chemical free ion activity. A low urinary pH increases the free ion activity of uric acid ions. However, a high urine pH promotes the complexation of calcium with phosphorus, which decreases the free ion activity of both calcium and phosphorus. Citrate combines with calcium ions to form soluble complexes and will decrease the free ion activity of unbound citrate and calcium. When the chemical free ion activities are increased, the urine becomes supersaturated (also termed *oversaturated*). In this setting, new stones may form and established stones may grow. In the event of decreased free ion activity, urine becomes undersaturated, and stones do not grow and can even dissolve. The *equilibrium solubility product* is the chemical free ion activity of the stone components in a solution at which the stone neither grows nor dissolves.

Stones form through the processes of homogeneous or heterogeneous nucleation. In *homogeneous nucleation*, progressive supersaturation eventually results in formation of small clusters secondary to the aggregation of identical molecules. These clusters grow to form a permanent solid phase, or crystals. *Heterogeneous nucleation* refers to crystal formation on the surface of a different crystal type or on other dissimilar substances, such as cells. In vivo, this type of nucleation is more common than homogeneous nucleation because crystals form at a lower level of supersaturation in the presence of a solid phase.

The small crystals may then aggregate into larger clinically significant stones. Crystals generally anchor to renal tubular epithelium; this allows more time for growth. This anchoring of crystals occurs at the renal papillae, over areas of interstitial calcium phosphate present in the form of apatite termed *Randall plaques* (Fig. 30-2).[26-28] The apatite crystals appear to originate at the basement membrane of tubular cells in the thin loop of Henle and extend into the interstitium without damaging the cells themselves or filling the tubular lumens. A combination of apatite crystal and organic material extends from the loop of Henle tubular basement membrane to the papillary uroepithelial surface, where calcium oxalate crystals or other crystals can adhere and form stones. If the stone breaks this anchor to the urothelial surface, it will then be carried by the urine through the ureter and into the bladder. If the stone is small (generally ≤5 mm in diameter) it may pass with only minor discomfort; however, if it has grown sufficiently, this migration may be extremely painful, and if the stone is of sufficient size, it may even completely obstruct the ureter, leading to nonfunction of the unilateral kidney.

An important factor in the development of kidney stones may be the absence of adequate levels or activity of crystallization inhibitors in the urine. Uropontin, pyrophosphate, citrate, and nephrocalcin are endogenously produced substances that have been shown to inhibit calcium crystallization. Differences in the amount or activity of inhibitors are thought to account for the variability in stone formation among people with similar degrees of urinary supersaturation.[22,29]

Clinically, most physicians evaluate the lithogenic potential of the urine from stone formers by measuring the rate of excretion of the principal stone-forming elements in mass per unit time (e.g., milligrams or millimoles per 24 hours). It is clear, however, that the lithogenic potential of urine is better determined by the degree of supersaturation. Computer programs that calculate saturation from concentrations of various elements in the urine and the urinary pH are now available (e.g., both Quest Diagnostics and Litholink are commercial laboratories that measure urine ion excretion and calculate supersaturation) and more accurately determine the risk of stone formation. Any calculation of mean saturation underestimates the maximum supersaturation, which may drive stone formation, because of hourly variations in water and solute excretion throughout the day.

Diet

Dietary factors have a great influence on the concentration of excreted ions. Simply instructing patients to increase fluid intake appears to have a considerable impact on reducing stone growth and formation.[30-32] Renal calcium excretion is augmented by increased sodium excretion,[33] and hypercalciuric patients tend to have a greater calciuric response to a sodium load than control subjects.[34] Dietary sodium restriction with the consequent decrease in urinary sodium excretion reduces calcium excretion and lowers supersaturation with respect to calcium-containing kidney stones. Patients are counseled to limit their daily sodium intake to a maximum of 3000 mg (~130 mEq) to reduce hypercalciuria.[4,33,35]

A moderate reduction in animal protein (~1.0 mg/kg per day) is known to be beneficial in patients with nephrolithiasis. Animal protein contributes to stone formation via multiple mechanisms.[35] A mild metabolic acidosis develops when animal proteins are metabolized. In order to buffer the excess hydrogen ions, calcium is resorbed from bone, which leads to an increased filtered load of calcium.[36] Metabolic acidosis also directly decreases renal tubular calcium reabsorption, which further enhances hypercalciuria.[36] In addition, metabolism of amino acids contained in animal protein generates sulfate ions, which couple with calcium ions to form insoluble complexes.[36,37] Citrate, a base, acts as a urinary inhibitor of stone formation. Citrate forms soluble complexes with calcium and lowers calcium oxalate and calcium phosphate supersaturation. During metabolic acidosis, citrate is reabsorbed proximally, reducing the amount excreted in the urine.[38] Hypokalemia can also lead to reduced citrate excretion. An animal protein–induced reduction in urinary citrate can promote formation of both calcium oxalate and uric acid stones.[34,39]

Fructose has become a ubiquitous sweetener in American processed foods. In large food questionnaire studies this sugar has been associated with a significant risk of developing nephrolithiasis. Though the mechanism is not known, fructose is the only carbohydrate that can increase uric acid production, and fructose metabolism may increase stone formation.[40]

Several studies have demonstrated the benefits of a diet containing an age- and gender-appropriate amount of calcium in patients with kidney stones.[31,35,41,42] Ingested calcium binds intestinal oxalate, reducing its absorption and consequent renal excretion.[31] In a long-term prospective trial, Borghi and colleagues randomized hypercalciuric male stone formers to either a low-calcium diet or to a diet with a normal amount of calcium but low in sodium and animal protein.[35] Both groups of men were instructed to restrict oxalate intake and drink 2 to 3 L of water daily. The group of men on a normal-calcium, low-sodium, and low–animal protein diet had a significantly lower recurrence of nephrolithiasis and a greater reduction in oxalate excretion and calcium oxalate supersaturation compared with the men on the low-calcium diet.[35]

Thus, patients should be maintained on an age- and gender-appropriate intake of calcium.[42] Dietary calcium restriction should be strongly discouraged because it not only increases risk of recurrent stone formation but also engenders a significant risk of bone demineralization and development of osteoporosis.[43,44] Note that although *dietary* calcium intake has been associated with a reduced incidence of kidney stones, calcium intake in the form of *supplements* can exacerbate stone formation in older women. The recommended dietary intake for men and women is 1000 mg of elemental calcium from ages 19 through 50 years and 1200 mg of calcium thereafter.[45] Teenagers should consume 1300 mg of calcium per day. Excess calcium should be avoided, because the combination of calcium and vitamin D supplementation has recently been shown to significantly increase the risk of kidney stones in postmenopausal women.[46]

Pathogenesis of Idiopathic Hypercalciuria

Idiopathic hypercalciuria (IH) is defined as excessive urinary calcium excretion in the setting of normocalcemia and the absence of secondary causes of hypercalciuria. IH is the most common cause of calcium-containing kidney stones. The disorder is familial; it was initially thought to exhibit an autosomal dominant pattern of inheritance but is almost certainly polygenic.[47]

The mechanism by which IH leads to hypercalciuria is not known. It has been postulated that IH comprises three distinct disorders: excessive intestinal calcium absorption, decreased renal tubular calcium reabsorption, and enhanced bone demineralization. In a genetic strain of hypercalciuric stone-forming rats, hypercalciuria appears to be due to an excessive number of enteric vitamin D receptors leading to a generalized disorder of calcium transport at all sites of calcium transport including the kidney, intestine, and bone.[48] In humans, recent observations also suggest that IH may be a systemic disorder of calcium homeostasis with dysregulation of calcium transport.[49] An understanding of calcium homeostasis helps elucidate the potential mechanisms involved in IH.

Calcium Homeostasis (Also See Chapter 28)

Urinary calcium homeostasis is regulated in the gastrointestinal (GI) tract, the kidneys, and bone by parathyroid hormone (PTH) and $1,25(OH)_2D$. Approximately 99% of the calcium in the body is contained within the bone mineral. Daily bone resorption and bone formation, which in healthy, nonpregnant, nonosteoporotic adults should be equal, allow less than 1% of bone calcium to be exchanged with that in the extracellular fluid.

Both PTH and $1,25(OH)_2D$ at high concentrations stimulate release of calcium from the bone mineral through osteoclast-mediated bone resorption. Net calcium influx into the extracellular fluid is achieved by absorption from the GI tract, which occurs through $1,25(OH)_2D$-dependent and -independent mechanisms. Although PTH appears to have no direct effect on GI calcium absorption, increased levels of the hormone stimulate production of $1,25(OH)_2D$, which in turn leads to enhanced absorption. Increased serum levels of calcium and $1,25(OH)_2D$ provide negative feedback to the parathyroid glands, resulting in reduced PTH secretion.

The roughly 60% of calcium in the extracellular fluid is not protein bound and is freely filtered by the renal glomeruli. Approximately 80% to 85% of this amount is passively reabsorbed in the proximal tubule. Most of the remaining calcium is reabsorbed in the thick ascending limb (TAL) of Henle and distal cortical tubules under PTH stimulation. Ultimately, these reabsorptive mechanisms result in a urinary calcium excretion that is less than 2% of the daily filtered load of calcium.[50] Except during pregnancy and lactation, in healthy, nonosteoporotic adults, urinary calcium excretion (and any calcium lost in sweat) precisely equals net intestinal calcium absorption.

Potential Mechanisms for the Development of Idiopathic Hypercalciuria

Dysregulation of calcium transport in the intestine, kidney, or bone can lead to hypercalciuria. For example, excessive calcium absorption by the GI tract leads to a transient increase in the serum calcium. This increase in serum calcium suppresses secretion of PTH that, along with the increased filtered load of calcium to the kidneys, results in hypercalciuria. Excessive $1,25(OH)_2D$ has a similar effect of increasing intestinal calcium absorption but also results in an influx of calcium into the extracellular fluid because of enhanced bone resorption. The result is hypercalciuria even in the setting of a low-calcium diet or an overnight fast. The excess $1,25(OH)_2D$ also suppresses PTH secretion, thereby further reducing renal tubular reabsorption of calcium.

If a primary defect in renal calcium reabsorption leads to hypercalciuria, there is a fall in the serum calcium concentration that stimulates synthesis of PTH and $1,25(OH)_2D$. Increased $1,25(OH)_2D$ results in enhanced intestinal calcium absorption and bone resorption. The renal loss of calcium persists even with a low-calcium diet or overnight fast.

Hypercalciuria can also develop as a result of a defect in renal phosphate reabsorption. The resultant hypophosphatemia leads to enhanced $1,25(OH)_2D$ production, which stimulates intestinal absorption of phosphorus and calcium. The increased serum calcium and $1,25(OH)_2D$ suppresses PTH synthesis and release. The increased filtered load of calcium in the setting of suppressed PTH leads to hypercalciuria. Enhanced bone resorption due to excessive $1,25(OH)_2D$ increases the serum calcium concentration, which in turn suppresses PTH production further. The increase in the filtered load of calcium in this setting results in hypercalciuria.

Thus, there are several potential mechanisms for hypercalciuria.[49] Do human or animal data support one mechanism above all others? From a clinical therapeutic standpoint, is it worth differentiating among the various potential mechanisms in each patient with suspected IH?

Human Data

Lemann[51] compiled the results of numerous calcium balance studies on patients with IH and normocalciuric control subjects and normalized the results for calcium intake. He found that intestinal calcium absorption was significantly higher in the subjects with IH.

Coe and colleagues, also collecting data from published metabolic balance studies, compared net intestinal calcium absorption and urinary calcium excretion in hypercalciuric and normocalciuric adults.[52] They also noted an increase in intestinal calcium absorption in subjects with IH but found that urinary excretion of calcium was increased to an even greater degree, thus placing many of these patients in net negative calcium balance. Although these data confirm that enhanced intestinal absorption of calcium probably plays a role in the pathogenesis of IH, the investigators could not clarify whether this is the primary defect or if it is secondary to another lesion, such as a primary dysregulation of renal tubular calcium reabsorption. Others suggested that the increase in intestinal calcium absorption, in combination with a decrease in renal calcium reabsorption, indicated a more generalized defect in calcium homeostasis. Nonetheless, the finding of enhanced calcium absorption makes enhanced bone resorption an unlikely primary mechanism of IH, because the increase in serum calcium concentration resulting from bone resorption would suppress $1,25(OH)_2D$-mediated intestinal calcium absorption.

In most published studies, patients with IH have higher serum levels of $1,25(OH)_2D$ than normocalciuric control subjects.[7,49,53] Kaplan and colleagues[53] determined that $1,25(OH)_2D$ levels were higher than control values in approximately one third of patients with IH and that intestinal calcium absorption was inappropriately high for the level of $1,25(OH)_2D$. These studies support either $1,25(OH)_2D$-mediated intestinal calcium absorption or a primary defect in renal tubular calcium reabsorption as a primary mechanism of hypercalciuria in IH.

PTH levels in patients with IH have been reported as normal or slightly lower than those in control subjects.[39,43] This finding argues against a reduction in renal tubular calcium reabsorption as the primary defect in IH, because with this mechanism the hypercalciuria would lead to low serum calcium levels and stimulation of PTH secretion. This finding also does not support the hypothesis that an elevated level of PTH is the stimulus for the increased levels of serum $1,25(OH)_2D$ observed in many studies. It is, however, consistent with the other potential mechanisms for IH.

Bone mass in patients with IH has been assessed by a number of methods, including radiologic densitometry, quantitative computed tomography (CT), dual-energy x-ray absorptiometry (DXA), single-photon absorptiometry, and others. Studies of patients with IH have generally shown a mild reduction of bone mineral density compared with values in control subjects.[39,43,54] The studies were unable to reveal a unifying mechanism for the mild reduction in bone mineral density. Altered $1,25(OH)_2D$ regulation would be consistent with this finding because the effects of $1,25(OH)_2D$ on bone resorption would be mitigated by the increased intestinal calcium absorption stimulated by the hormone.

Previously it was considered essential to determine whether a patient with IH tended to have excessive GI calcium absorption (absorptive hypercalciuria) or excessive renal excretion (renal leak).[55,56] Patients with excessive renal calcium excretion were prescribed thiazide diuretics, and those thought to have a predominantly absorptive defect were prescribed a low-calcium diet. Coe and colleagues[43] undermined the validity of this approach in a study in which 24 patients with IH and 9 control subjects were given a low-calcium diet (2 mg/kg/day) for more than 1 week. Urine and blood tests revealed normal serum calcium levels, a mild decrease in PTH levels in the patients with IH, and no difference in $1,25(OH)_2D$ levels. The striking finding was that, whereas all the normocalciuric subjects excreted less calcium than they ingested on the low-calcium diet, 16 of the 24 subjects with IH had urinary calcium excretion that exceeded their intake. Thus, most of the patients with IH receiving a low-calcium diet were in net negative calcium balance. There was no clear demarcation between the patients who excreted excessive amounts of calcium and those who did not. Instead, there was a smooth continuum of urinary calcium excretion among patients with and without IH that appeared not to be influenced by calcemic hormones. From a therapeutic standpoint, these findings have rendered obsolete both the need to clinically distinguish IH mechanisms in humans and the prescription of a low-calcium diet in any of these patients. This approach to diet is important because a low-calcium diet can result in a dangerous reduction in bone mineral density, especially in women.[43,44,49,54] As mentioned earlier (see "Pathogenesis of Stone Formation"), a low-calcium diet also appears to increase recurrent stone formation.[31,35] Thus, there is no benefit, and a number of well-documented risks, to advising a low-calcium diet to prevent recurrent stone formation in patients with IH.

Genetic Hypercalciuric Stone-Forming Rats

To explain more fully the mechanism of IH in humans, we have developed an animal model of this disorder.[48,57-61] Through more than 100 generations of successive inbreeding of the most hypercalciuric progeny of hypercalciuric Sprague-Dawley rats, we have established a strain of rats

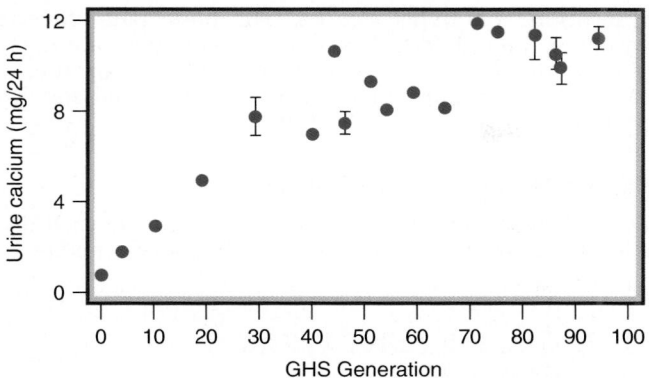

All data from published studies.

Figure 30-3 Hypercalciuria in subsequent generations of genetic hypercalciuric stone-forming (GHS) rats.

that excrete 8 to 10 times as much urinary calcium as control Sprague-Dawley rats (Fig. 30-3).

Compared with control Sprague-Dawley rats, the genetic hypercalciuric rats absorb far more calcium at lower dietary levels of $1,25(OH)_2D$.[48,62] When these hypercalciuric rats were fed a diet very low in calcium, their urinary calcium excretion remained elevated compared with that of similarly treated control rats, indicating a defect in renal calcium reabsorption or an increase in bone resorption, or both,[63] again similar to observations in humans.[43,64] Bone from these hypercalciuric rats released more calcium than the bone of control rats when exposed to increasing amounts of $1,25(OH)_2D$,[65] and their bone mineral densities were lower than those of control rats.[66] The administration of a bisphosphonate to the genetic hypercalciuric rats fed a low-calcium diet significantly reduced urinary calcium excretion.[67] In addition, a primary defect in renal calcium reabsorption was observed during clearance studies.[68] We have shown that besides the intestine, both the bone and kidney of the hypercalciuric rats have an increased number of vitamin D receptors and calcium receptors.[57,61,65,69,70]

Thus, hypercalciuric rats appear to have a systemic abnormality in calcium homeostasis. They absorb more intestinal calcium, they resorb more bone, and they do not adequately reabsorb filtered calcium. Because every one of the hypercalciuric rats forms renal stones, we have described them as genetic hypercalciuric stone-forming (GHS) rats.[48,59] These studies suggest that an increased number of vitamin D and calcium receptors may be the underlying mechanism for hypercalciuria in these rats[70] and perhaps in humans as well.[48,59,69] Circulating monocytes from humans with IH have been shown to have an increased number of vitamin D receptors.[71]

Genetics of Idiopathic Hypercalciuria in Humans

The difficulty in ascertaining the genetics of IH arises, in part, from the numerous other factors that influence stone formation, such as diet, environment, and gender. Because half of patients with IH report a family history of stones and male patients often have fathers or sons with the disorder, inheritance is not believed to be recessive or X-linked. A multitude of monogenic hereditary disorders (see later discussion) can lead to hypercalciuria because they are caused by a variety of mutations resulting in changes in calcium handling at the level of kidney, bone, gut, and the calcium-sensing receptor in the kidneys and parathyroid glands. Given the evidence that IH is a complex trait with

multiple pathways for developing the hypercalciuria phenotype, it is most likely a polygenic disorder, with heterogeneity of loci and possibly polygenic modifiers. Although attempts to diagnose the exact cause of IH in a particular patient might not be critical from a therapeutic standpoint, determining the cause of IH in a particular family is essential for researchers attempting to clarify the genetics of IH.[19,27,47,72] Recently a team of investigators using the technique of genome-wide association studies have found that a member of the claudin family, claudin 14, is associated with stone formation in Iceland.[73] Whether this association will be found in other populations, thus supporting its link to stone formation, remains to be determined.

Other Genetic Causes of Stones and Nephrocalcinosis

Numerous monogenic disorders cause hypercalciuria that leads to nephrolithiasis or nephrocalcinosis.[19,27,47,72,74-76] Disorders that lead to hypercalciuria by augmenting bone resorption include osteogenesis imperfecta type 1, multiple endocrine neoplasia type 1 (MEN1) syndrome with hyperparathyroidism, McCune-Albright syndrome, and infantile hypophosphatemia. Disorders that result in hypercalciuria because of excessive intestinal absorption of calcium include hereditary hypophosphatemic rickets due to disordered sodium phosphate cotransporter SCL34A3, Down syndrome, and congenital lactate deficiency. Others include autosomal dominant hypocalcemia (which is caused by an activating mutation of the calcium-sensing receptor), Lowe oculocerebrorenal syndrome, and Wilson disease. Next, we describe in more detail several disorders that result in hypercalciuria via their effect on genes expressed in the kidney.

X-Linked Hypercalciuric Nephrolithiasis (Dent Disease and Others)

Several families around the world were discovered to have a variable combination of disorders including hypercalciuria, low-molecular-weight proteinuria, nephrocalcinosis or stones, hypophosphatemic rickets, and renal failure.[74,75] Some affected persons demonstrate evidence of defects in proximal tubular reabsorption of amino acids, glucose, or phosphate. PTH tends to be quite low and $1,25(OH)_2D$ high in the majority of patients. The abnormalities completely resolve in the patients who receive renal transplants, a finding that suggests a renal tubular disorder rather than a systemic process. In all families, the pattern of inheritance is consistent with an X-linked recessive disorder, with male patients affected to a greater extent than female patients. The latter are often minimally affected but transmit the disorder to half of their male offspring.

Over time, the various disorders—X-linked recessive nephrolithiasis in the United States, Dent disease in the United Kingdom, X-linked recessive hypophosphatemic rickets in Italy, and low-molecular-weight proteinuria with hypercalciuria and nephrocalcinosis in Japan—have all been linked to mutations affecting the CLCN5 gene on the Xp11.22 locus of the X chromosome.[77] This gene encodes the CLC-5 protein, which is one of the nine members of the CLC family of voltage-gated hydrogen chloride exchangers. How defects in this channel lead to the array of disorders listed here, including hypercalciuria, stones, and renal failure, is not yet understood.

Bartter Syndrome

Bartter syndrome is caused by at least five genetic mutations, predominantly autosomal recessive, that lead to sodium chloride wasting at the TAL of the loop of Henle.[27,28,47,76,78] Defects can arise in NKCC2 (sodium potassium chloride cotransporter), ROMK (renal outer medullary potassium channel), the CLC-Kb (basolateral chloride channel), or in a chloride channel subunit known as *barttin*. These genes, all expressed in the TAL, cause a defect in sodium transport that leads to a reduction in the transtubular potential difference, resulting in a decrease in paracellular calcium reabsorption in the TAL. The ensuing reduction in intravascular volume also induces an aldosterone-mediated metabolic alkalosis. Bartter syndrome, therefore, resembles high-dose furosemide administration (that targets NKCC2) and differs from Gitelman syndrome in that hypercalciuria, nephrocalcinosis, and nephrolithiasis are seen with Bartter but not with Gitelman. An autosomal dominant form of Bartter syndrome results from a gain-of-function mutation in the calcium-sensing receptor in renal tubular cells. This mutation leads to reduced calcium reabsorption and hypocalcemia caused by low PTH levels. Therapy with vitamin D and calcium supplementation can exacerbate stone disease in this disorder.

Familial Hypomagnesemia With Hypercalciuria and Nephrocalcinosis

Familial hypomagnesemia with hypercalciuria and nephrocalcinosis (FHHNC) is an autosomal recessive disorder that results in hypomagnesemia, hypercalciuria, nephrolithiasis, and distal renal tubular acidosis (dRTA). Polyuria and severe nephrocalcinosis also ensue, and progressive renal failure is common by late childhood.[27,28] The genetic disorder results in defective production of either of the tight junction proteins, claudin 16 and claudin 19, that bind together to facilitate paracellular calcium and magnesium transport in the TAL as well as renal sodium reabsorption.[79,80]

Distal Renal Tubular Acidosis

dRTA is caused by dysfunctional α-intercalated cells, resulting in defective acid excretion.[27,28,47,72,81] This inability to adequately acidify the urine results in metabolic acidosis, hypocitraturia, hypokalemia, hypercalciuria, nephrocalcinosis, and stones. The metabolic acidosis leads to resorption of both calcium and phosphate from bone. The increased filtered load of calcium and phosphate, along with the elevated urine pH and hypocitraturia, results in favorable conditions for calcium phosphate stone formation. Although there are secondary causes of dRTA such as Sjögren syndrome and use of carbonic anhydrase inhibitors (e.g., acetazolamide), there are also a number of hereditary causes of dRTA.[82] Some are autosomal recessive and can also result in hearing loss; others are autosomal dominant. One form of dRTA that targets carbonic anhydrase II results in osteopetrosis and brain calcifications.[82] Patients with dRTA fail to lower their urine pH below 5.5 following ingestion of an acid load. Their urine citrate is extremely low despite mildly reduced or even normal serum bicarbonate levels.

Hereditary Hypophosphatemic Rickets With Hypercalciuria

Hereditary hypophosphatemic rickets with hypercalciuria is an autosomal form of hypophosphatemic rickets that is manifested clinically by hypophosphatemia secondary to renal phosphate wasting.[83,84] These patients have a hypophosphatemia-induced increase in levels of $1,25(OH)_2D$, which leads to increased intestinal calcium absorption and hypercalciuria. The bone pain, muscle weakness, limb deformities, and rickets remit completely with administration of oral phosphate. This disorder is caused by mutations in the gene for the renal sodium phosphate cotransporter, NaPi-IIc.

Primary Hyperoxaluria and Cystinuria

Primary hyperoxaluria (PHO) and cystinuria are each discussed later in their respective sections under "Therapy."

CLINICAL PRESENTATION AND EVALUATION

Kidney stones vary in clinical presentation from those discovered asymptomatically on routine imaging, to their painful passage through the ureters, to large, obstructing staghorn calculi that can significantly impair renal function and even lead to ESRD.[6,85] The severity of stone disease depends on the pathogenic factors contributing to the rate of stone formation as well as the stone type, size, and location.

In its most classic form, nephrolithiasis manifests as renal colic. This discomfort of abrupt onset intensifies over time into excruciating, severe flank pain that resolves only with stone passage or removal. The pain often migrates anteriorly along the abdomen and inferiorly to the groin, testicles, or labia majora as the stone moves toward the ureterovesical junction. Gross hematuria, urinary urgency and frequency, nausea, and vomiting may be present. Nephrolithiasis can also result in a dull, poorly localizing abdominal pain. The probability of passing a stone without intervention depends on its size and varies from 97% for stones less than 2 mm, to 50% for stones 4 to 6 mm, and less than 1% for stones larger than 6 mm.[86,87]

There is increasing evidence that nephrolithiasis is associated with a twofold increase in CKD that is independent of other risk factors, such as diabetes and hypertension found in stone formers.[88-90] A French study estimated the incidence rate of ESRD caused by nephrolithiasis to be about 3.1 cases per 1 million population per year,[91] and a Canadian study demonstrated that although only 0.8% of patients with ESRD had nephrolithiasis, any stone episode previously was associated with a increased risk of ESRD (hazard ratio 2.16).[92] The common reasons for loss of a single kidney in stone formers were staghorn calculi, high stone burden, infection, and ureteral obstruction.[93]

The development of CKD from stone disease is thought to be from ureteral obstruction leading to parenchymal damage.[88] Most data are derived from animal models and suggest that unilateral ureteral obstruction causes intense renal vasoconstriction that reduces renal blood flow and glomerular filtration rate (GFR).[94] Brushite ($CaHPO_4$) stone formers have an increased risk of cortical fibrosis,[95] and the formation of Randall plaques in such patients was associated with duct plugging, collecting duct cell death, and inflammation.[96] Renal biopsy specimens in patients with staghorn calculi demonstrate extensive inflammation and macrophage infiltration.[97] Other stone-forming diseases such as PHO, cystinuria, and Dent disease have all been associated with crystal formation in the renal parenchyma that presumably triggers subsequent inflammation and CKD.[98]

Certain disorders can lead to diffuse renal parenchymal calcifications termed *nephrocalcinosis*.[6,28,81,99] The calcifications, usually calcium phosphate or calcium oxalate, may be present in the cortex or medulla. Among the most common causes of stone-related nephrocalcinosis are PHO and medullary sponge kidney.

Metabolic Evaluation of Stone Formers

Although it is uniformly accepted that patients with multiple stones merit a thorough investigation into the cause of nephrolithiasis, the need for evaluation of the patient with a single stone is controversial. This is probably due to the difficulty in determining the cost-to-benefit ratio of stone evaluations and wide differences in reported rates of stone recurrence.

The National Institutes of Health has convened several consensus conferences to resolve such issues related to the prevention and treatment of kidney stones.[5] These panels determined that all patients, even those with a single stone, should undergo at least a basic evaluation in order to rule out a systemic etiologic mechanism. Patients with an increase in number or size of stones (metabolically active stones), all children, all noncalcium oxalate stone formers, and those in demographic groups not typically susceptible to stone formation warrant a more complete metabolic evaluation.[5]

The Basic Evaluation

Elements of the basic evaluation are listed in Table 30-1.

History

In addition to the medical history typically obtained from new patients, the evaluation of the stone former includes a stone history and a thorough review of diet, fluid intake, and lifestyle. Specific laboratory studies and radiographic tests are also required.

Stone History. The stone history begins with a chronologic account of stone events: age of incidence of first stone, size and number of stones formed, frequency of passage, stone type if known, and whether the stones occur equally in both kidneys or unilaterally. Also helpful is a report of the patient's symptoms with each episode as well as the need for and response to surgical intervention.

This information is useful to judge not only the severity of the stone disease but also clues to the origin of the patient's nephrolithiasis. For example, nephrolithiasis that begins at a young age may be attributable to an inherited metabolic disorder such as PHO or cystinuria. Large staghorn calculi that are difficult to eradicate and tend to recur despite frequent surgical intervention are more likely to be composed of struvite ($NH_4MgPO_4 \cdot 6H_2O$) instead of calcium oxalate. Cystine stones are not disintegrated thoroughly with the use of lithotripsy, and alternative surgical modalities are generally required for stone removal. In patients who tend to form stones in only one kidney, the possibility of congenital abnormalities of that kidney, such as megacalyx or medullary sponge kidney, should be explored.

Medical History. Systemic disorders that can contribute to nephrolithiasis are sought in the medical history. For example, any disorder that can result in hypercalcemia, such as sarcoidosis or certain malignancies, may also lead to hypercalciuria. A variety of GI disorders associated with malabsorption (e.g., sprue, Crohn disease) can cause calcium oxalate nephrolithiasis on the basis of enteric hyperoxaluria. Patients with gout or insulin resistance are more likely to have uric acid stones[19,20] (Tables 30-2 and 30-3).

TABLE 30-1

The Basic Evaluation of Stone Formers

History
    Stone history
    Medical history
    Family history
Medications
Occupation and lifestyle
Diet and fluid intake
Physical examination
Laboratory tests
    Urinalysis
    Urine culture and sensitivity
    Cystine screening
Blood tests
    Sodium, potassium, chloride, bicarbonate
    Calcium, phosphorus, uric acid, creatinine
    Intact parathyroid hormone if calcium is elevated or at upper limit
        of normal
    Tetrahydrodeoxycortisol, urinary free cortisol, and 25(OH)D levels
        as appropriate
Stone analysis
Radiology (choose appropriate study as indicated; see text)
    Unenhanced helical (spiral) computed tomography
    Kidneys, ureter, and bladder examination
    Intravenous pyelography
    Ultrasonography

Data from Monk RD. Clinical approach to adults. *Semin Nephrol.* 1996;16: 375-388; Monk RD, Bushinsky DA. Nephrolithiasis and nephrocalcinosis. In: Frehally J, Floege J, Johnson RJ, eds. *Comprehensive Clinical Nephrology*, 3rd ed. London, UK: Mosby; 2007:641-655.

TABLE 30-2

Causes of Calcium Stone Formation

Hypercalciuria
    Cushing syndrome
    Granulomatous diseases
    Hypercalcemic disorders
    Idiopathic hypercalciuria
    Immobilization
    Malignancy
    Milk-alkali syndrome
    Primary hyperparathyroidism
    Sarcoid
    Thyrotoxicosis
Medications (see Table 30-4)
Hyperoxaluria
    Biliary obstruction
    Chronic pancreatitis
    Crohn disease
    Dietary hyperoxaluria (urine oxalate secretion 40-60 mg/day)
    Enteric oxaluria (urine oxalate 60-100 mg/day)
    Jejunoileal bypass
    Malabsorptive disorders
    Primary hyperoxaluria types 1 and 2 (oxalate 80-300 mg/day)
    Sprue (celiac disease)
Hyperuricosuria (see Table 30-3)
Hypocitraturia
    Androgens
    Exercise
    Hypokalemia
    Hypomagnesemia
    Infection
    Metabolic acidosis
    Starvation
Renal tubular acidosis (distal, type 1)
Anatomic genitourinary tract abnormalities
    Congenital megacalyx
    Medullary sponge kidney
    Tubular ectasia

Data from Monk RD. Clinical approach to adults. *Semin Nephrol.* 1996;16: 375-388; Monk RD, Bushinsky DA. Nephrolithiasis and nephrocalcinosis. In: Frehally J, Floege J, Johnson RJ, eds. *Comprehensive Clinical Nephrology*, 3rd ed. London, UK: Mosby; 2007:641-655; Bushinsky DA, Monk RD. Calcium. *Lancet.* 1998;352:306-311.

TABLE 30-3

Factors Associated With Noncalcium Stone Formation

Uric Acid Stones

Cushing syndrome
Diarrhea
Diet high in animal protein
Excessive dietary purine
Excessive insensible losses
Genetic predisposition
Glucose-6-phosphatase deficiency
Gout
Hemolytic anemia
Hyperuricemia
Hyperuricosuria
Inadequate fluid intake
Inborn errors of metabolism
Insulin resistance
Intracellular to extracellular uric acid shift
Lesch-Nyhan syndrome
Low urine pH (<5.5)
Low urine volume
Malabsorptive disorders
Medications (see Table 30-4)
Metabolic syndrome
Myeloproliferative disorders
Obesity
Tumor lysis

Struvite Stones

Urease-producing bacteria
  Proteus, Pseudomonas, Haemophilus, Yersinia, Ureaplasma, Klebsiella,
    Corynebacterium, Serratia, Citrobacter, Staphylococcus, and others
Never *Escherichia coli*—not a urease producer
High urine pH (~6.5)
Indwelling urinary catheter
Neurogenic bladder

Cystine Stones

Autosomal recessive trait
Excessive excretion of cystine, ornithine, lysine, and arginine
Low solubility of cystine (<250 mg/L)

Data from Monk RD. Clinical approach to adults. *Semin Nephrol.* 1996;16:
  375-388; Monk RD, Bushinsky DA. Nephrolithiasis and nephrocalcinosis.
  In: Frehally J, Floege J, Johnson RJ, eds. *Comprehensive Clinical
  Nephrology*, 3rd ed. London, UK: Mosby; 2007:641-655.

TABLE 30-4

**Medications Associated With Renal Lithiasis
and Nephrocalcinosis**

Medications That Promote Calcium Stone Formation

Acetazolamide
Amphotericin B
Antacids (calcium and noncalcium antacids)
Calcium supplements
Glucocorticoids
Loop diuretics
Theophylline
Vitamin C?
Vitamin D

Medications That Promote Uric Acid Lithiasis

Allopurinol (associated with xanthene stones)
Probenecid
Salicylates

Medications That Can Precipitate Into Stones or Crystals

Acyclovir (when infused rapidly intravenously)
Indinavir
Nelfinavir
Sulfonamides
Triamterene

Data from Monk RD. Clinical approach to adults. *Semin Nephrol.* 1996;16:
  375-388; Monk RD, Bushinsky DA. Nephrolithiasis and nephrocalcinosis.
  In: Frehally J, Floege J, Johnson RJ, eds. *Comprehensive Clinical
  Nephrology*, 3rd ed. London, UK: Mosby; 2007:641-655.

acidosis and alkaline urine, favorable conditions for the development of calcium phosphate stones. Other uricosuric medications, such as salicylates and probenecid, have been implicated in uric acid lithiasis.[105]

Certain crystals or stones can consist completely of precipitated medication. Such medications include intravenously administered acyclovir, triamterene, indinavir, and various sulfonamides, such as sulfadiazine. Oxalate is a metabolic end product of vitamin C, and large doses increase oxalate excretion and may predispose to stone formation (Table 30-4).[106,107]

Lifestyle and Diet

Occupation and lifestyle are aspects of the social history that can be relevant to stone formation. Surgeons and traveling salespeople, for example, tend to minimize fluid intake in order to avoid frequent micturition throughout the day. Insensible losses of fluid can also exacerbate nephrolithiasis and may be related to employment (e.g., construction work) or hobbies (running, gardening).

The evaluation proceeds with a thorough review of the patient's diet and fluid intake. Patients are asked to review what they eat at all meals and snacks. Particular attention is paid to ingestion of foods high in sodium (fast foods, canned foods, added salt, or soy sauce) and the quantity of animal protein consumed (see later discussion). Patients are also asked to list four or five favorite foods or snacks to assess whether they may be consuming foods high in oxalate or purine as well. Many patients are erroneously counseled by physicians to avoid calcium-containing foods. As noted earlier, doing so is not only associated with increased risk of stone formation but it may also result in bone demineralization, a grave concern in women with stones.[31,35,41]

Physical Examination

For most patients with nephrolithiasis, physical findings are normal. In some patients, however, the findings may

Family History. As noted earlier, a number of stone disorders are inherited, making the family history an important component of the basic evaluation. IH appears to be a familial disorder. Although the exact chromosomes and genes have not yet been identified, the pattern of inheritance is almost certainly polygenic.

Stones arising in childhood or young adulthood can be related to autosomal recessive disorders such as cystinuria and primary oxaluria. These genetic disorders are reviewed later in the sections on treatment of cystine and oxalate stones.

The high prevalence of uric acid stones in certain areas of the world is suggestive of genetic as well as environmental risk factors. Genes that cause either excessively acidic urine or hyperuricosuria have been implicated.[4,6,20,27,99-102]

Medications

Medications can contribute to stone formation in several ways. Calcium-containing supplements, for example, can increase the amount of calcium absorbed and subsequently excreted.[46] Loop diuretics can directly promote renal tubular excretion of calcium and are associated with nephrocalcinosis in neonates who have received the drug.[103,104] Acetazolamide, a weak diuretic, induces a mild metabolic

reveal a systemic disorder related to the stone disease. An enterocutaneous fistula, for example, may be associated with Crohn disease, a common cause of enteric hyperoxaluria. A paraplegic patient with an indwelling catheter may be susceptible to frequent urinary tract infections with urease-producing organisms and consequent struvite stone formation. Hyperuricosuria and uric acid stone formation may be seen in patients with tophi related to gout.[4,6]

Laboratory Tests

Although valuable information is gleaned from the history and physical examination, it is often difficult to determine the metabolic cause of a patient's nephrolithiasis without laboratory data. The urinalysis is an easy and inexpensive test that provides a great deal of information. Often, the presence of different kinds of crystals can suggest the type of underlying stone (Fig. 30-4). Uric acid and calcium oxalate stones, for example, grow more favorably at an acidic pH, and a consistently high urinary pH may suggest calcium phosphate or struvite nephrolithiasis. The specific gravity, if high, can confirm suspicions of inadequate fluid intake.

Hematuria is often present in active stone disease. Microscopic examination of the urine in this case might reveal characteristic crystals. Bacteria and pyuria noted in conjunction with a high urinary pH (~6.5) are characteristic of struvite stone disease. Urine specimens for culture should be obtained in this setting. Because enough urease may be produced to form struvite stones even when colony counts are low (~50,000 colony-forming units), the microbiology laboratory should be instructed specifically to identify the organism and to check for urease-producing bacteria despite low colony counts.[108]

Qualitative cystine screening should be performed on a urine specimen. Urine turns purple-red when sodium nitroprusside is added to a specimen containing cystine at a concentration greater than 75 mg/L.[100]

Recommended blood tests in the basic evaluation include electrolytes (sodium, potassium, chloride, bicarbonate), uric acid, calcium, phosphorus, and serum creatinine to determine renal function.[4,5] If the serum calcium level is elevated or at the upper limit of normal or if the serum phosphorus level is reduced or at the lower limit of normal, a serum intact PTH level is also determined to rule out primary hyperparathyroidism. Low serum bicarbonate levels suggest a hypocitraturic disorder such as RTA or acetazolamide ingestion.

Stone Analysis

Stone analysis should be performed, whenever possible, in patients with a new history of nephrolithiasis or in patients with long-standing stone disease who note a difference in

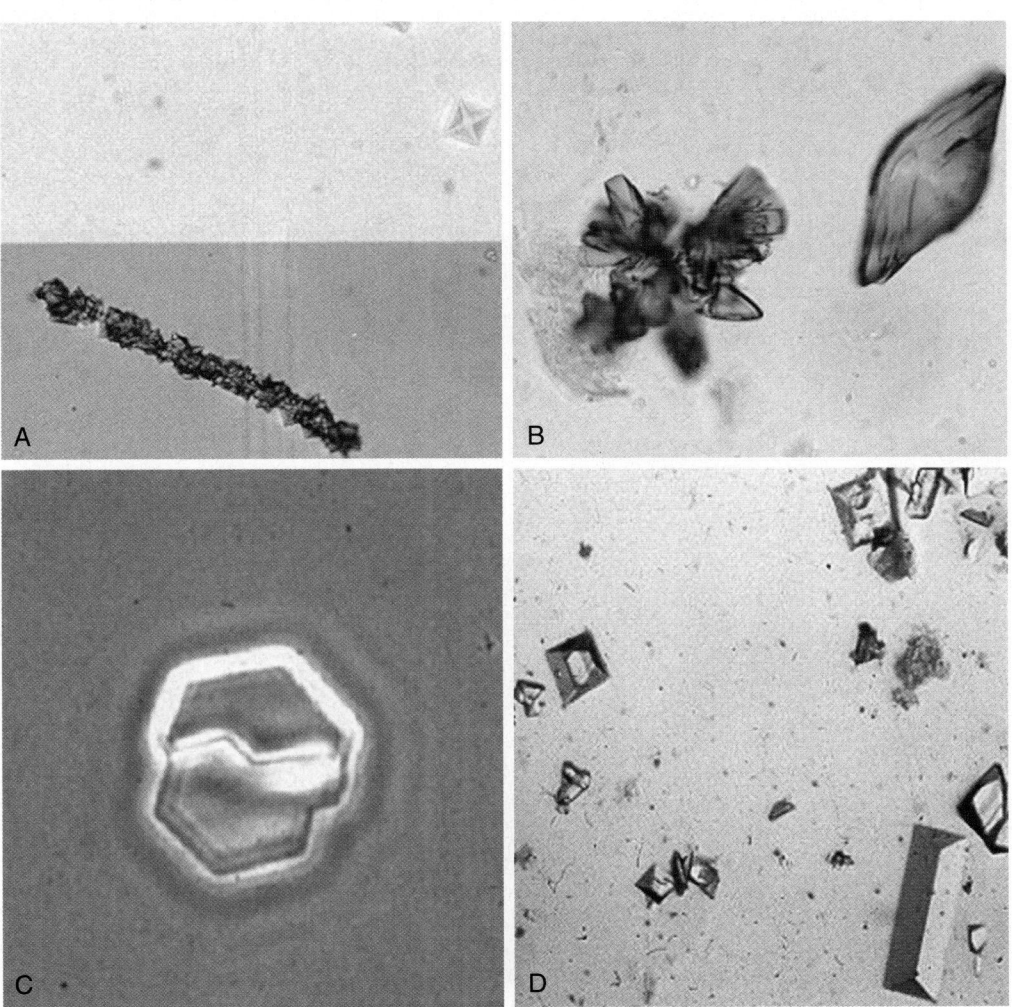

Figure 30-4 Crystals seen in urine of stone formers. **A,** Calcium oxalate. **B,** Urate. **C,** Cystine. **D,** Struvite.

clinical presentation or in the color, shape, or texture of any stone passed. Knowing the constituents of a stone can help the physician target certain elements of the medical history and specific urine studies. In most cases, the stone must be sent to an outside laboratory for examination. X-ray diffraction crystallography and infrared spectroscopy are currently the most accurate methods available for stone analysis.[109]

Radiologic Evaluation

Various radiologic tests can help determine the location and extent of the stone burden and might elucidate genitourinary abnormalities contributing to stone formation (Table 30-5). For acute renal colic, spiral (or helical) CT without contrast (unenhanced) has replaced intravenous pyelogram (IVP) as the optimal test for detection and localization of kidney stones. Helical CT has proved to be at least as sensitive and specific as IVP in detecting stones of all types in both the kidneys and ureters. In addition, it can more accurately reveal causes of flank pain and hematuria not related to stones and circumvents the use of intravenous contrast material. Radiation exposure is a disadvantage of both CT and IVP, and the exposure to patients undergoing helical CT may be triple that of IVP. As such, it should be used judiciously, especially in young patients with frequent episodes of renal colic. Helical CT takes less time to perform, a potential advantage in an emergency department setting, but it tends to be more expensive.[85,110-112]

CT should be followed by a plain film (radiograph) of the abdomen that includes the kidneys, ureter, and bladder (KUB). Plain films can assist in determining stone composition. Stones composed of calcium, cystine, and struvite are radiopaque and visible on KUB, whereas radiolucent stones, such as those composed of uric acid and xanthine, are not (Fig. 30-5).

IVPs are useful in detecting certain genitourinary abnormalities that can predispose to nephrolithiasis, such as medullary sponge kidney and caliceal abnormalities. Another advantage of IVP is that the osmotic diuresis generated by the administered contrast agent may aid in excretion of the offending stone during an episode of acute renal colic. A major disadvantage of IVP is exposure to

TABLE 30-5
Radiologic Evaluation of Nephrolithiasis

Procedure	Advantage	Disadvantage
Abdominal radiograph	Simple, easily available	Low sensitivity (45-59%) and specificity (71-77%)
Intravenous pyelography	More sensitive (64-87%) and specific (92-94%)	Can miss nonobstructing stones
	May even help stone move along ureter because of strong osmotic effect	Risk of contrast in patients with chronic kidney disease
		Radiation exposure
		Often reimaging is needed for high-grade obstruction because of inadequate contrast concentration
Ultrasound	Easily performed	Poor sensitivity, especially for ureteral stone (19%)
	No radiation	
	Very sensitive in detecting obstruction	
	Safe in pregnant women	
Noncontrast helical computed tomography	Very sensitive (95-98%) and specific (98%)	Radiation exposure is significantly higher
	Based on radiologic characteristic the type of stone can be diagnosed	More expensive
	Can assess for other causes of abdominal pain at the same time	

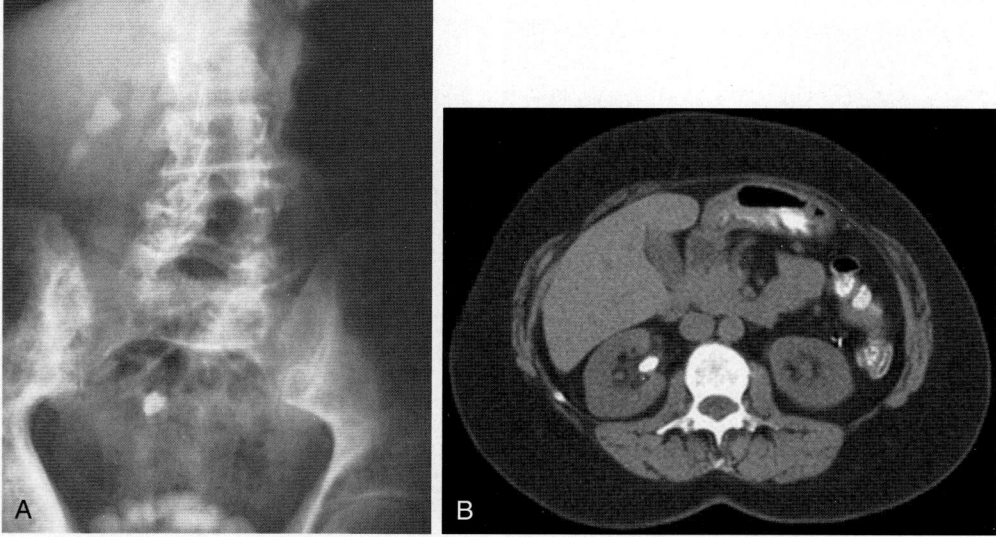

Figure 30-5 Renal stones on abdominal radiograph and computed tomography scan. **A,** Radiolucent kidney stone can be seen on the KUB (kidneys, ureter, and bladder) radiograph at the ureterovesical junction. **B,** Large stone is seen in the renal pelvis of the right kidney.

radiographic contrast material. Administration of contrast agent should be avoided in patients who are at high risk for developing nephrotoxicity from the contrast material, such as the elderly; those with diabetes mellitus, proteinuria, or preexisting kidney disease; and patients with significant intravascular volume depletion.

Renal ultrasound is a useful test for patients who must avoid exposure to radiation or contrast agent, such as pregnant women and children. It is fairly specific, but not as sensitive as spiral CT for detecting stones within the kidney. Ureteral stones are very difficult to visualize on ultrasound.

Once a patient is known to have a certain type of stone, specific tests may be used in follow-up. For example, a patient known to have asymptomatic calcium stones can have a KUB test 6 to 12 months later to assess for any increase in stone size or number.[4,6] However, because of the radiation exposure, reimaging should be limited to patients in whom the results of the test will alter treatment. Little is gained in asymptomatic patients by checking for stone growth or movement if maximal dietary and pharmacologic therapy is already being prescribed.

The Complete Evaluation

The complete evaluation comprises the entire basic examination as well as a 24-hour urine collection to determine volume and levels of calcium, oxalate, citrate, sodium, urate, phosphorus, creatinine, and urinary supersaturation with respect to the common solid-phase components (Table 30-6). Creatinine is used to assess the adequacy of the collection: men should excrete approximately 15 to 20 mg/kg of creatinine per day, but women should excrete 10 to 15 mg/kg of creatinine per day. Cystine should also be measured in patients known to have cystine stones or in whom prior urine studies have not determined if there is excessive excretion of this amino acid.

Patients should be instructed to collect their urine on a day when they perform usual activities and have their typical fluid and dietary intake. The first morning's urine specimen is discarded; following this, all urine for the next 24 hours (including the next morning's specimen) is

TABLE 30-6
Optimal 24-Hour Urine Values in Patients With Nephrolithiasis

Parameter	Value
Volume	>2-2.5 L
pH	>5.5, <7.0 (24-h specimen not required)
Calcium	<300 mg or <3.5-4.0 mg/kg in men
	<250 mg or <3.5-4.0 mg/kg in women
Oxalate	<40 mg
Sodium	<3000 mg or <130 mEq
Uric acid	<800 mg in men
	<750 mg in women
Phosphorus	<1100 mg
Citrate	>320 mg
Creatinine	~15 mg/kg in men
	~10 mg/kg in women in order to ensure adequacy of collection
Supersaturation of calcium oxalate	<5
Supersaturation of calcium phosphate	0.5-2* (ideally <1)
Supersaturation of uric acid	0-1*

*Ideal values can vary among laboratories that perform supersaturation analysis.

collected in the container. The ideal 24-hour urine collection includes measurement and reporting of the daily excretion of the constituents listed in Table 30-6 and also reports supersaturation of calcium oxalate, calcium phosphate, and uric acid. Patients should be instructed to discontinue multivitamins approximately 5 days before the collection to prevent any antioxidant effect of the vitamins on the urine sample. In most cases, an acid or antibiotic is included in the collection container or added with the first urine sample as a preservative. Certain laboratories require various preservatives for the different factors measured. Physicians should ask their laboratory how many 24-hour urine collections and which preservatives are required for the complete evaluation. Simplifying this process to a single urine collection in which all of the measurements are performed and resultant supersaturation calculated, which is available from several national laboratories, almost certainly improves adherence and perhaps accuracy of the calculation of supersaturation.[4,113]

Patients who require the complete evaluation are as follows: all children, nonwhite patients (demographic groups not typically prone to nephrolithiasis in the United States), noncalcium stone formers, and patients with metabolically active stone disease (metabolically active stones are those that grow in size or number within 1 year).[4-6]

THERAPY

Surgical Treatment

Treatment of an acute episode of renal colic often involves surgical management for large stones that do not pass spontaneously. Stones smaller than 5 mm have a 68% chance of passing spontaneously, whereas those larger than 5 mm but smaller than 10 mm have a spontaneous stone passage rate less than 50%.[114] Most stones larger than 10 mm, and many larger than 5 mm, require surgical intervention for relief of renal colic, ureteral obstruction, or other symptoms of clinically active stone disease. With the advent of newer, less invasive urologic therapies, open surgical stone extraction is rarely performed. Current urologic therapy includes extracorporeal shock-wave lithotripsy (ESWL), ureteroscopic extraction (URS), and percutaneous nephrolithotomy (PN). The exact procedure used varies according to stone location in the kidney or ureter, size, composition, various patient factors, and surgical expertise.[114-117]

ESWL involves focusing sound waves from a lithotripter outside the body onto the kidney stone. The impulses fragment the stone into smaller stones, or "gravel," that can more easily be passed spontaneously. Newer generation lithotripters do not require a water bath and often require less analgesia.[118] Kidney stones less than about 15 mm, proximal ureteral stones, upper and middle pole kidney stones, and those not composed of cystine or calcium oxalate monohydrate respond best to ESWL.[114,116-118] Because fluoroscopy is typically used to visualize radiopaque stones during the procedure, ESWL may be more complicated in patients with uric acid lithiasis. ESWL is relatively contraindicated in patients with coagulopathy and in pregnant women. It may be less successful in patients with a higher body mass index, as a low skin-to-stone distance is necessary to achieve optimal success.[117,118]

Ureteroscopy, the passage of a semirigid or flexible scope through the bladder and into the ureter, has become a mainstay of surgical stone extraction for most ureteral stones, especially distal ureteral stones, and larger proximal stones. Endocorporeal lithotripsy can be added to URS to directly fragment visualized stones. One of the more commonly used devices is the holmium:yttrium-aluminum-garnet (YAG) laser lithotripter, which combines both pneumatic and ultrasound lithotripsy to fragment stones. This procedure results in high stone-free rates following the procedure.[115,119] Complications of ESWL and URS include urinary tract infection, sepsis, ureteral stricture, ureteral injury, and steinstrasse (stone street), the linear accumulation of small stones blocking a ureter following fragmentation of a larger stone.

PN involves placement of a large needle through the flank into the renal collecting system. The tract is dilated and instruments are used to rupture and remove the stone. Although more invasive than ESWL and URS, PN is more effective in removing large (>2 cm) or staghorn calculi and stones that do not fragment well with lithotripsy. Large, infected stones such as struvite stones, in which complete removal is desired, are best treated with PN.[116,117]

Medical Expulsive Therapy

Another form of therapy that has been shown to reduce the time to stone passage is medical expulsive therapy (MET). Several medications have shown benefit in reducing the time to stone passage and in assisting with passage of larger stones.[120] Most of these, such as the calcium-channel blocker nifedipine (extended-release formulation, 30 mg daily or twice daily) and α-adrenergic receptor blockers, such as tamsulosin (0.4 mg daily orally), terazosin, and doxasosin, act by reducing spasm of the ureteral smooth muscle and allowing ureteral peristalsis to more effectively move the stone through. The addition of corticosteroids may also assist with stone passage by reducing ureteral inflammation and swelling in the ureter where the stone is lodged. In several prospective, randomized controlled trials, calcium channel blockers and α-adrenergic blockers have shown significant benefit in both rates of successful stone passage and time to passage. In the controlled studies these therapies were compared with control groups involving placebo[121] or standard therapy such as antispasmodic therapy, nonsteroidal anti-inflammatory agents, or analgesics. In studies comparing α-adrenergic receptor blockers to calcium channel blockers, the α-adrenergic blocker tamsulosin was found in a few studies to result in higher stone passage rates and more rapid stone expulsion than nifedipine.[120,122,123] Both agents were generally well tolerated, though perhaps with less hypotension in the tamsulosin groups. MET may be cautiously attempted for up to 4 weeks as long as pain is well controlled and the patient has normal, stable kidney function, no urinary tract infection, and no bilateral obstruction or obstruction of a solitary kidney. Frequent follow-up and occasional imaging with ultrasound are recommended to ensure that the patient remains free of complications while awaiting stone passage.

Medical Preventive Therapy

Medical preventive therapy is the mainstay of medical management, and the remainder of the chapter will focus on prevention of stone recurrence.

Nonspecific Preventive Therapy

Most patients, irrespective of stone type, are given general advice about fluid and dietary modification to prevent further stone formation. These nonpharmacologic interventions, which include an increase in fluid intake as well as restriction of dietary sodium and animal protein, can reduce the incidence of stone formation, a result termed the *stone clinic effect.*[31,32,124] In one study, such interventions resulted in a 40% decrease in stone recurrence over 5 years.[30]

The mainstay of nonspecific therapy involves dietary measures (see "Diet" under "Pathogenesis of Stone Formation"): increased fluid intake to raise urine volume to approximately 2 to 2.5 L, a reduction in sodium intake to less than 3000 mg/day (130 mEq), moderate reduction in animal protein ingestion to approximately 1.0 mg/kg per day, and perhaps eating certain fruits or juices high in citrate.[4,33,31,32,124-126]

Dietary calcium restriction is no longer recommended because it not only can lead to a reduction in bone mineral content but also increases the rate of stone recurrence, presumably by decreasing intestinal calcium oxalate absorption and increasing urinary oxalate excretion.[31] In retrospective studies of dietary intake, both women and men have been found to have reduced stone formation with increased dietary calcium ingestion. Calcium supplements, however, were associated with an increased risk of stones in women. Patients should therefore be advised to maintain an age- and gender-appropriate intake of dietary calcium, preferably without supplements.[31,35,41,46,127]

Specific Therapy Matched to Specific Pathogenesis

The optimal therapy for a patient with metabolically active stone disease is directed at the patient's particular metabolic abnormality. Before medications for nephrolithiasis are prescribed, all patients should be treated with the nonspecific measures as previously noted. Prior to any therapeutic intervention, some clinicians assess the patient's existing stone burden with a radiologic examination (KUB, spiral CT, IVP, or ultrasonography). If stones are present, any subsequent passage of stones would not necessarily indicate therapeutic failure as the patient may simply be passing the stones formed prior to therapy. However, this approach must be weighed against the expense and the radiation exposure associated with the radiologic examination. Our personal opinion is to not obtain baseline radiographs in asymptomatic patients unless the results will alter subsequent therapy. The basic and complete evaluations help direct the clinician to the specific treatments discussed here.

Calcium Stones. Most kidney stones (~70%) contain calcium (see Fig. 30-1). More than one third of these are composed of calcium oxalate alone, and another 7% are composed of calcium phosphate alone. The rest are composed of a combination of calcium oxalate with either urate or calcium phosphate. The stones tend to be gray, brown, or tan and rarely grow larger than 1 to 2 cm.[4,29,109]

The main causes of calcium stone formation are hypercalciuria (excessive urinary calcium excretion), hyperoxaluria (excessive oxalate excretion), hyperuricosuria (excessive uric acid excretion), hypocitraturia (insufficient citrate excretion), RTA, congenital abnormalities of the genitourinary tract, and certain medications (see Tables 30-2 and 30-3).

Hypercalciuria. Patients with persistent hypercalciuria often benefit from a thiazide diuretic. This class of drugs is inexpensive and extremely effective at reducing urinary calcium excretion and stone formation.[4,128] To maximize the efficacy of thiazides, patients must consume a sodium-restricted diet. Urinary calcium excretion parallels sodium excretion (Fig. 30-6), and reducing sodium consumption is essential to reducing hypercalciuria. Whereas hydrochlorothiazide is commonly used for hypertension, chlorthalidone is favored for treating hypercalciuria because it has a longer half-life and requires only once-daily dosing. The

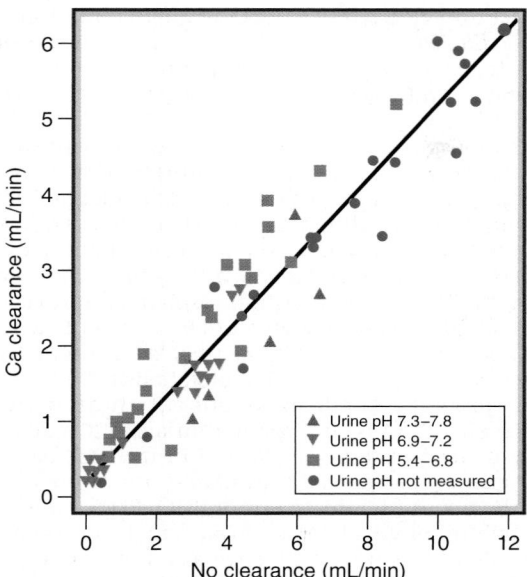

Figure 30-6 Relationship between urinary calcium and sodium excretion. This study shows how urinary calcium excretion parallels urinary sodium excretion. There is almost a linear relationship between the urinary excretion of calcium and sodium, making sodium restriction in diet imperative in the treatment of hypercalciuria. (From Walser M. Calcium clearance as a function of sodium clearance in the dog. *Am J Physiol.* 1961;200:1099-1104.)

starting dose is 25 mg and can be increased to 50 mg. In petite patients or those with low blood pressure, therapy can be initiated with 12.5 mg.

Side effects of thiazides include an increase in serum lipid levels and hyperglycemia. For patients in whom this is a concern, such as those with hypercholesterolemia, other cardiac risk factors, or elevated blood glucose levels, indapamide (1.25 to 2.5 mg) is an effective alternative.[129] This agent has less of an effect on serum lipids and blood sugar than thiazides.

Hypokalemia is another common side effect of thiazide therapy. Patients should be advised to increase their dietary intake of potassium-rich foods, and the potassium level should be checked 7 to 10 days after starting the medication. Hypokalemia can result not only in cardiac and neuromuscular problems but also in hypocitraturia, another risk factor for stone formation. The supplement of choice is potassium with a base, such as citrate or bicarbonate, as the accompanying anion. Potassium citrate is available as a liquid or as a wax-matrix tablet. The wax-matrix form is preferable because many patients find the liquid unpalatable. Patients with malabsorption disorders, however, may absorb potassium citrate better in the liquid form. Potassium citrate in the wax matrix formulation is available as 5- and 10-mEq tablets; 20 to 40 mEq/day in single or divided doses is usually adequate supplementation. Determination of follow-up potassium and bicarbonate levels may be required for further dose adjustment. Because citrate is a base, metabolic alkalosis can result with this medication, especially when given with a thiazide diuretic. In such a situation an alternative potassium supplement (e.g., potassium chloride) may be necessary. If hypokalemia persists or if large doses of supplemental medication are required, the patient might benefit from the addition of a potassium-sparing diuretic. Triamterene is generally avoided because it can precipitate into stones. Amiloride may be initiated at a starting dose of 5 mg or in a combination tablet with thiazide.

After 4 weeks of therapy with the new medication, the 24-hour urine collection should be repeated to assess the efficacy of therapy in reducing calcium levels. The 24-hour urinary sodium and citrate levels should also be measured. The thiazide dose may need to be increased to decrease calcium excretion to less than 3 to 4 mg/kg per day. If sodium excretion remains high in conjunction with elevated urinary calcium excretion, further dietary counseling aimed at reducing dietary sodium may be required. Additional potassium citrate may be required if urinary citrate or serum potassium levels remain low.[4,130]

Hyperoxaluria. Oxalate is produced predominantly by endogenous metabolism of glyoxylate and, to a lesser extent, by ascorbic acid. Some urinary oxalate is derived from dietary sources, such as rhubarb, cocoa, nuts, tea, and certain leafy green vegetables. Absorbed oxalate is excreted unchanged in the urine and raises urinary supersaturation with respect to calcium oxalate.[7,99,131,132] Hyperoxaluria, as the sole metabolic abnormality, accounts for the formation of only approximately 5% of all calcium-based stones, even though it is often present with other urinary abnormalities that lead to an increase in supersaturation.[27,133,134]

The three main causes of hyperoxaluria are excessive oxalate ingestion (dietary oxaluria), malabsorptive GI disorders (enteric oxaluria), and excessive endogenous production of oxalate related to a hepatic enzyme deficiency (PHO).

Because ethylene glycol (used as antifreeze in automobiles) is metabolized to oxalate, nephrolithiasis, in conjunction with severe metabolic acidosis and renal failure, is often observed in patients after ingestion of ethylene glycol.

Dietary Oxaluria. Dietary oxaluria results in urinary oxalate levels that are mildly elevated (40 to 60 mg/day). Many high oxalate foods are fruits, vegetables, and nuts that are generally considered beneficial in most diets. In a retrospective analysis, patients consuming diets similar to the Dietary Approaches to Stop Hypertension (DASH) diet have fewer stones than those who consume diets that are markedly different despite the DASH diet being high in oxalate.[135] The diet is also high in potassium and calcium and low in sodium, factors that may be more preventive in stone formation than oxalate is detrimental. Patients with dietary hyperoxaluria should be provided with a detailed list of high-oxalate foods to review (Table 30-7). How restrictive patients need to be with regard to the list is guided by urinary supersaturation and common sense, especially as many patients with stones may also have hypertension and diabetes mellitus and benefit from a diet high in fruits and vegetables. Patients should be instructed to ingest calcium-containing foods, such as a glass of milk, when eating foods high in oxalate. The calcium in milk binds the dietary oxalate and may prevent its absorption.[27,31] In patients who have severe dietary hyperoxaluria with active stone disease, 2 or 3 calcium carbonate tablets (500 to 650 mg/tablet) may be prescribed with high-oxalate meals. However, this should be done cautiously given the association between calcium supplements and kidney stones in women in the general population (see "Nonspecific Preventive Therapy," earlier).

Enteric Oxaluria. Enteric oxaluria results in higher urinary oxalate levels (60 to 100 mg/day) than dietary hyperoxaluria. GI malabsorptive conditions associated with normal colonic function, such as Crohn disease, celiac sprue, jejunoileal bypass, chronic pancreatitis, and biliary obstruction, can lead to enteric oxaluria. In these disorders, malabsorbed fatty acids bind calcium in the intestinal lumen, making more free oxalate available for absorption in the colon. In addition, the colonic mucosa becomes

TABLE 30-7

Foods High in Oxalate

Beans (green and dried)
Beer (draft, stout, lager, pilsner)
Beets
Berries (blackberries, blueberries, raspberries, strawberries, juice made
  from berries)
Black tea
Black pepper
Celery
Chocolate, cocoa
Eggplant
Figs, dried
Greens (collard greens, dandelion greens, endive, escarole, kale, leeks,
  mustard greens, parsley, sorrel, spinach, Swiss chard, watercress)
Green peppers
Lemon, lime, and orange peel
Nuts
Pecans, peanuts, peanut butter
Okra
Rhubarb
Sweet potato
Tofu

Data from Monk RD, Bushinsky DA. Nephrolithiasis and nephrocalcinosis.
In: Frehally J, Floege J, Johnson RJ, eds. *Comprehensive Clinical
Nephrology*, 3rd ed. London, UK: Mosby; 2007:641-655; Wainer L,
Resnik BA, Resnik MI. *Nutritional Aspects of Stone Disease*. Boston,
MA: Martinus Nijhoff; 1987.

more permeable to oxalate as a result of exposure to malabsorbed bile salts.[136-138]

The mainstay of treatment, whenever possible, is therapy for the underlying disorder. A gluten-free diet, for example, can significantly reduce hyperoxaluria associated with sprue. For other conditions (e.g., surgical short-bowel syndrome), no specific therapy is feasible. In such cases, reduction of malabsorption and oxalate absorption may be achieved by instituting general therapy for steatorrhea, such as a low-fat diet, cholestyramine and medium-chain triglycerides. As in patients with dietary oxaluria, an oxalate-restricted diet and calcium carbonate with meals should be prescribed.[31,139] Because of chronic diarrhea, these patients are at substantial risk for low urine volumes, hypocitraturia, hypokalemia, and hypomagnesuria. The acidic, concentrated urine also predisposes to development of uric acid stones.[140,141] Additional fluid intake must be stressed, and potassium citrate (the liquid form is generally better absorbed, though poorly tolerated in these patients) and magnesium supplementation are often prescribed. Magnesium appears to be an inhibitor of stone formation and is supplied as magnesium oxide at 400 mg by mouth twice a day or magnesium gluconate at 0.5 to 1 g by mouth three times a day.[142]

Primary Hyperoxaluria. PHO leads to nephrolithiasis because of hepatic enzyme deficiencies that lead to massive endogenous oxalate production and excretion in these patients.[99,101,143] PHO results not only in severe hyperoxaluria (80 to 300 mg/day) but also in widespread deposition of oxalate in numerous organs and tissues such as the heart, bone marrow, muscle, and renal parenchyma at a young age. Cardiomyopathy, bone marrow suppression, and renal failure can ensue. In type 1 PHO (80% of the cases), the deficient hepatic enzyme is alanine glyoxylate aminotransferase (AGT), and deficiency is caused by one of several mutations found in the AGT gene, *AGXT*. In some patients with type 1 PHO, pyridoxine (vitamin B$_6$) can increase enzyme activity, thereby reducing oxalate production. In type 2 PHO (10% of cases) patients lack D-glycerate

reductase and glyoxylate reductase due to mutations in the gene *GRHPR*. PHO type 3 is due to a defect in the *HOGA1* gene that encodes for mitochondrial 4-hydroxy-2-oxoglutarate aldolase and makes up the remaining cases of PHO.[144]

All patients with PHO should be treated with measures that reduce calcium oxalate supersaturation, such as ample fluid supplementation, potassium citrate, magnesium, and orthophosphate. Orthophosphate is an effective inhibitor of calcium oxalate crystallization but should be avoided in patients with a GFR less than 50 mL/minute. The combination of pyridoxine and orthophosphate improved renal survival at 20 years from 20% to 74% in patients with PHO type 1 and 2.[145] *Oxalobacter formigenes* is an enteric bacteria that relies on oxalate for its metabolism.[40,146] In small studies, probiotic supplementation of these bacteria to patients with PHO type 1 resulted in a slight reduction in urinary oxalate excretion.[40] Provision of these bacteria, if they become commercially available, may provide additional therapy in the treatment of PHO. PHO patients with renal failure might benefit from renal transplantation because dialysis is not as effective as a functioning kidney in oxalate removal. The general measures to treat PHO should be continued after renal transplantation to prevent rapid loss of the allograft caused by calcium oxalate deposition. Ultimately, for patients with type 1 PHO, liver transplantation can supply the missing AGT and is curative, especially if it is performed before the development of end-stage renal failure. Some patients require combined liver and kidney transplantation.[99,101,147]

Hyperuricosuria. Up to 15% of patients with hyperuricosuria have calcium stones. In contrast to patients with pure calcium oxalate stones, these patients typically have elevated urinary uric acid levels but normal urinary calcium and oxalate levels.[148,149] They also differ from patients with pure uric acid stones in that they tend to have a higher urinary pH.

The mechanism by which uric acid promotes calcium stone formation is unclear. The terms *heterogeneous nucleation* or *epitaxy* are used to describe the preferential formation of calcium oxalate crystals around a lattice of uric acid crystals present in the urine.[7,150,151] More recently this mechanism has come into question. Grover and associates have shown that the addition of sodium urate to urine or similar solutions increases calcium oxalate crystallization, with denser, more aggregated deposits, without the presence of urate crystals, and with no increase in calcium oxalate supersaturation. They attribute this to salting out, a process in which the solubility of electrolytes (or salts) in a solution is reduced (or the ion activity increased) by the addition of different electrolytes/salts. As such, the activity coefficient of calcium and oxalate would be increased not only by the concentrations of calcium and oxalate in the urine but also by the urate concentration.[152,153] This theory would explain why allopurinol is often an effective therapy for recalcitrant calcium oxalate nephrolithiasis, even in the absence of hyperuricosuria.[154,155] Another potential mechanism (but not borne out by studies) is that urate may reduce the concentration or the activity of urinary stone inhibitors.[156-158]

Whatever the mechanism, uric acid in the form of sodium urate is important in calcium oxalate crystal formation. Therapy has generally consisted of dietary purine restriction and increased fluid intake. If urinary uric acid levels remain uncontrolled with these measures, allopurinol, 100 to 300 mg/day, may be added.[148,149]

Hypocitraturia. Citrate, by combining with calcium to form a soluble complex, reduces calcium oxalate and calcium phosphate precipitation, thus acting as the most important inhibitor of calcium crystallization in urine.[7] In some patients, hypocitraturia is the principal metabolic abnormality found in the 24-hour urine collection. Risk factors for hypocitraturia include high protein intake, hypokalemia, metabolic acidosis, exercise, infection, starvation, and therapy with androgens or acetazolamide. Men tend to have lower urinary citrate concentrations than women, which may be responsible for the higher incidence of stone formation in men. Furthermore, women with nephrolithiasis have lower urinary citrate concentrations than non–stone-forming women.[159] Although citrate excretion below 320 mg/L per day of urine is defined as hypocitraturia, the risk of nephrolithiasis is a continuous function of urinary citrate concentration.[160]

Along with therapy for the underlying condition, such as moderating dietary protein intake, potassium citrate or potassium-magnesium citrate is prescribed, and both formulations are effective in preventing calcium stones, even in patients who are not hypocitraturic.[161] The potassium salt is preferable to sodium citrate because sodium excretion promotes calcium excretion in parallel and leads to hypercalciuria. Again, potassium citrate in the wax-matrix formulation is preferred to the liquid preparation because of increased palatability. Large amounts may be required (30 to 75 mEq/day) in divided doses in order to raise the urinary citrate concentration to more than 320 mg/day. Potassium and bicarbonate levels should be closely monitored, especially in patients with CKD. If metabolic alkalosis or hyperkalemia ensues, reduction of the dose may be necessary.[130,162]

Renal Tubular Acidosis. dRTA (type 1) is a disorder in which distal tubular hydrogen ion excretion is impaired, resulting in a non–anion gap metabolic acidosis and a persistently alkaline urine. The acidosis leads to calcium and phosphate release from bone as well as enhanced proximal tubular reabsorption of citrate and diminished tubular reabsorption of calcium. The net result is an increased filtered load and excretion of calcium and phosphate, severe hypocitraturia and an elevated urinary pH, all of which promote calcium phosphate precipitation. Nephrocalcinosis, or renal parenchymal calcification, is frequently seen in this setting.

The 24-hour urinary citrate levels are commonly lower than 100 mg in patients with dRTA. Therapy consists of potassium citrate or potassium bicarbonate supplementation in order to treat both the metabolic acidosis and hypocitraturia. Large doses of these medications are often required: 1 to 3 mEq/kg per day in two or three divided doses.[29,101,148]

Nephrocalcinosis. Nephrocalcinosis is a process in which calcium is deposited in the renal parenchyma. There are two forms: dystrophic calcification and metastatic calcification. In dystrophic calcification, calcium deposition arises from tissue necrosis secondary to neoplasm, infarction, or infection. It may be seen in the setting of renal transplant rejection, renal cortical necrosis, chronic glomerulonephritis, ethylene glycol toxicity, acquired immunodeficiency syndrome (AIDS)-related infections, and Alport syndrome. In general, in dystrophic calcification, serum calcium and phosphorus levels are normal and calcium phosphate deposition occurs predominantly in the renal cortex.

In metastatic calcification, patients often have elevated serum calcium and phosphate levels or an elevated urinary pH. Calcification in this setting occurs more commonly in the renal medulla. Common causes include RTA, primary hyperparathyroidism (or any disorder resulting in elevated serum calcium levels), medullary sponge kidney, papillary necrosis, PHO, and administration of acetazolamide, amphotericin B, oral sodium phosphate bowel prepara-

tions, and triamterene. PHO can result in both medullary and cortical calcifications.

Both medullary and cortical parenchymal calcifications are easily noted with ultrasonography and CT scanning, even before they can be detected on plain radiographs. Therapy consists of treating the underlying disorder whenever possible. Otherwise, measures aimed at reducing hypercalcemia, oxalosis, and hyperphosphatemia should be attempted.[28,47,163]

Uric Acid Stones. Uric acid lithiasis is far more common in Mediterranean countries than in the United States. However, the incidence of uric acid stones in the United States appears to be rising in parallel with the epidemic of obesity. Obesity and the metabolic syndrome are associated with insulin resistance, which results in a very low urine pH.[20,21] Uric acid stones tend to be round, smooth, and yellow-orange. Because they are radiolucent, they are not visible on plain films but can be detected by ultrasonography or CT or as filling defects on IVP. Uric acid is a purine metabolite and is also found in large quantities within cells. Most patients with uric acid stones have a reduced urinary pH, whereas other less common causes are low urine volume or elevated urinary uric acid levels. Factors associated with uric acid stones are listed in Table 30-3.

A low urine pH is the major cause of uric acid nephropathy. The solubility of uric acid increases sixfold with an increase in urine pH from 5.3 to 6.5 (Fig. 30-7).[20,149] Thus, conditions that lower urine pH tend to predispose patients to uric acid lithiasis. Loss of bicarbonate during chronic diarrheal diseases and the higher acid load of diets rich in animal protein lead to acidemia and contribute to an acidic urinary pH. In four studies, every patient with uric acid stones had a urine pH less than 6.[164-167] A low urinary pH leads to the formation of poorly soluble uric acid as opposed to the more soluble urate anion, thus predisposing to uric acid lithiasis, even when the total amount of uric acid being excreted is not above normal.[168]

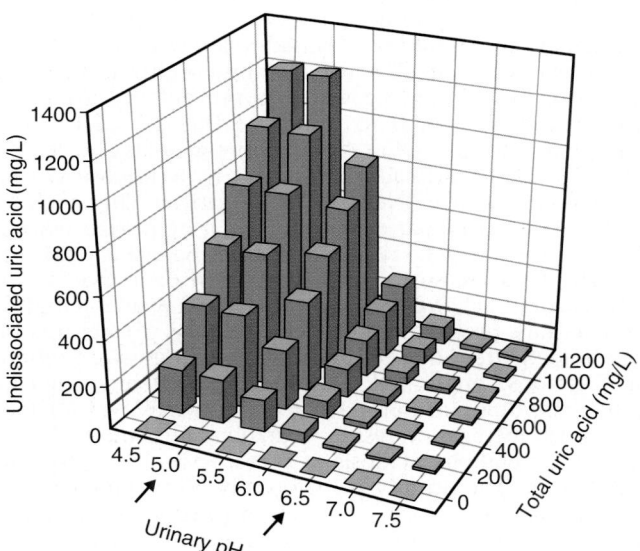

Figure 30-7 pH and solubility of uric acid. Relationship between undissociated uric acid, total uric acid, and urinary pH. The limit of solubility of undissociated uric acid is depicted by the colored line (~100 mg/L). Two hypothetical urine pHs are considered *(two arrows)*. At low urinary pH (e.g., 5.0), even a modest amount of total urinary uric acid will exceed its solubility. At high urine pH (e.g., 6.5), even massive hyperuricosuria is well tolerated. (From Maalouf NM, Cameron MA, Moe OW, Sakhaee K. Novel insights into the pathogenesis of uric acid nephrolithiasis. *Curr Opin Nephrol Hypertens.* 2004;13:181-189.)

Uric acid stone formers often have greater body weight and a higher incidence of insulin resistance and type 2 diabetes mellitus. The vast majority of these patients have significantly lower urinary pH compared with non–uric acid stone formers. It is thought that insulin resistance leads to impaired ammoniagenesis and ammonium excretion, resulting in excretion of more urinary hydrogen ions with anions other than ammonia and at a lower urinary pH.[19-21,165]

Hyperuricosuria may be evident in patients who ingest large quantities of dietary purine or animal protein. Foods high in purine include organ meats, shellfish, certain fish, meat extracts, yeast, gravy, and stock (Table 30-8). Hyperuricemic disorders such as gout, myeloproliferative disorders, tumor lysis syndrome, and certain inborn errors of metabolism (e.g., glucose-6-phosphatase deficiency, Lesch-Nyhan syndrome) can also contribute to an increased urinary filtered load of uric acid. Certain medications such as salicylates and probenecid are hyperuricosuric as well and can predispose patients to uric acid lithiasis.[6,20,106]

Therapy for patients with uric acid stones begins with nonspecific measures such as increasing fluid intake to maintain urine volume at about 3 L/day. A lowered animal protein diet is generally beneficial because the decreased endogenous acid production raises urinary pH.[36] Ideally, the urinary pH should be elevated to approximately 6.5 to 7.0, a level that can dissolve existing crystals and stones. However, care should be taken to prevent the urine pH from rising above 7.0 to minimize the risk of calcium phosphate lithiasis. A low-fructose diet may also be beneficial in reducing uric acid levels and hyperuricosuria (see discussion earlier in "Nonspecific Preventive Therapy").[40]

Potassium citrate at doses of 30 mEq by mouth twice a day or greater may be required to raise the urinary pH sufficiently to decrease the supersaturation of uric acid (see "Hypercalciuria" and "Hypocitraturia" on available potassium citrate preparations). If the urinary pH cannot be raised adequately despite high doses of potassium citrate or if the dose prescribed results in hyperkalemia, the carbonic anhydrase inhibitor acetazolamide may be initiated. Use of this medication results in an alkaline urine and mild systemic metabolic acidosis, a pattern similar to that in type 1 RTA. The urinary pH should be maintained at less than 7.0 in order to avoid calcium phosphate precipitation.[148] Prescription of nitrazine paper allows patients to monitor the urinary pH at various times of day and adjust their potassium citrate intake accordingly.

Patients with hyperuricemia are prescribed a low-purine diet to decrease uric acid production. Despite dietary intervention, hyperuricemia often persists, especially in patients with disorders of cellular metabolism. In this setting, allopurinol should be prescribed at a starting dose of 100 mg/day, increasing to 300 mg/day as needed.[7,169]

Although sodium bicarbonate can effectively alkalinize the urine, it should be avoided because the additional sodium excretion encourages sodium urate formation, which may result in further crystal formation (see "Hyperuricosuria" earlier).

Struvite Stones. Struvite stones are also called *triple phosphate stones, magnesium ammonium phosphate stones,* and *infection stones.* Although they make up only about 10% to 15% of all stones formed, most staghorn calculi (large stones that extend beyond a single renal calyx) are composed of struvite. The propensity of these stones to grow rapidly to a large size, to recur despite therapy, and to result in significant morbidity (and potential fatality) has also led to the apellation *stone cancer.* Infection with urease-producing bacteria must be present for these stones to form, and therefore severe renal infections as well as sepsis and loss of renal function can develop. Factors associated with struvite stones are listed in Table 30-3.

In contrast to other stone types, struvite stones occur with a higher incidence in women than in men, largely because of the increased susceptibility of women to urinary tract infections. Other groups at risk for development of struvite stones because of urinary stasis or infection include elderly people and patients with neurogenic bladders, indwelling urinary catheters, spinal cord lesions, or genitourinary abnormalities. Even without a stone analysis, struvite stones should be suspected in patients with large stones, an alkaline urinary pH (~7), and the presence of urease-producing urinary bacteria. Early detection and therapy are essential to prevent great potential morbidity.[108]

Urease-Producing Bacteria. The formation of struvite stones depends on the presence of both ammonium ions and an alkaline urinary pH; these conditions are met clinically only through the actions of urease-producing bacteria. Ammonium, magnesium, and carbonate apatite ($Ca_{10}[PO_4]_6CO_3$) in the urine combine with phosphate, which is present in its trivalent form in this setting.

Numerous bacteria, both gram-negative and gram-positive, as well as *Mycoplasma* and yeast species, have been implicated in urease production. Bacteria species in which urease is frequently isolated include *Proteus, Haemophilus, Corynebacterium,* and *Ureaplasma. Escherichia coli,* despite its frequent role as a urinary tract pathogen, has not been shown to produce urease and thus is not implicated in the genesis of struvite stones. Urease production adequate to stimulate stone formation may be present despite low bacterial colony counts. For this reason, the microbiology laboratory should be asked specifically to perform identification of bacteria and determine sensitivities even if colony counts are lower than 100,000 colony-forming units. If no bacteria are isolated but a urease producer is suspected, special cultures should be ordered for *Ureaplasma urealyticum,* a mycobacterium that tends to be a fastidious grower on regular culture media.[170]

Therapy for Struvite Stones. To eradicate struvite stones, early and aggressive medical and urologic management is required. Appropriate antibiotic therapy is essential but must be combined with long-term bacterial suppression and complete surgical or medical stone removal. ESWL is often adequate for fragmentation of stones smaller than 2 cm, but percutaneous nephrostolithotomy or a combination of the two procedures is usually required for larger stones.[171] Antibiotics should be continued on the basis of cultures of any stone fragments retrieved. After approximately 2 weeks of antibiotic therapy, when the urine culture is sterile, the dose of antibiotic should be halved. Suppressive antibiotics should continue at this dose until monthly surveillance cultures remain sterile for 3 consecutive months. At this point, antibiotics may be discontinued as long as surveillance urine cultures are obtained monthly for 1 year.[170,172]

In addition to antimicrobial therapy, medical treatment may involve urease inhibition and chemolysis. In chemolysis, the kidney is irrigated with an acidic solution through a nephrostomy tube or ureteral catheter. Although rarely used today with the advent of less invasive surgical techniques, this procedure may be useful in the dissolution of residual stone fragments. Ten percent hemiacidrin, the solution most commonly used, is composed of carbonic acid, citric acid, D-gluconic acid, and magnesium at a pH of 3.9. The use of chemolysis has been controversial because high mortality rates have been reported in the past.[173,174] The morbidity and mortality rates were mainly due to sepsis from instrumentation, local bacterial or fungal infections, and uroepithelial irritation rather than toxicity from the agents. When used as an adjuvant to surgical removal, chemolysis leads to lowered stone and infection recurrence rates.[173,175,176] The safety of the procedure remains in question due to the variety of techniques, stone burden, and comorbid conditions reported in older literature, but with close monitoring of serum magnesium levels, intrapelvic pressures, infection, and obstruction to flow, it may have a supporting role in the treatment of large struvite stones.[170,173,177]

Urease inhibition has been shown to retard stone growth and to prevent new stone formation.[178,179] It does not decrease bacterial counts and cannot eradicate existing stones. Combined with antimicrobial therapy, it serves primarily as palliative care for patients who cannot undergo definitive surgical management. The most common urease inhibitor is acetohydroxamic acid (AHA), which requires adequate renal clearance for therapeutic efficacy and is contraindicated in patients with a GFR less than 60 mL/minute. CKD increases the incidence of side effects of these medications, which are numerous and limit their use. Side effects that result in discontinuation of the drug include neurologic symptoms, GI upset, hair loss, hemolytic anemia, and rash. Fortunately, the side effects all resolve with discontinuation of the drug. AHA is also teratogenic. The starting dose of AHA is 250 mg by mouth twice a day. If it is well tolerated for about 1 month, the dose is increased to 250 mg by mouth three times a day.[170]

Cystine Stones. Cystinuria, not to be confused with the more serious and debilitating disorder cystinosis that results in extensive intracellular cystine accumulation, is an autosomal disorder that may be recessive or dominant with incomplete penetrance.[180] The disorder is due to mutations of the *SL3A1* gene on chromosome 2 or to mutations of the *SCLC7A9* gene on chromosome 19, both resulting in decreased renal tubular reabsorption and excessive urinary excretion of the dibasic amino acids cystine, ornithine, lysine, and arginine. The genetic defect would probably go unnoticed were it not for the low solubility of cystine of approximately 300 mg/L. Factors associated with cystine stones are listed in Table 30-3.

People with no tubular defect in cystine transport excrete approximately 30 to 50 mg of cystine per day that dissolves in the normal daily urine volume. Patients heterozygous for this condition excrete about 400 mg/day, whereas homozygotes often excrete more than 600 mg/day.[100] Even though the solubility of cystine increases significantly when urine pH is greater than 6.5, the excessive amounts produced in this condition lead to cystine crystals precipitating and aggregating as cystine stones.

Stones usually develop in patients within the second or third decade of life. The stones can grow to a large size and can appear as staghorn calculi or multiple stones. They are radiopaque because of the sulfur content of cystine. The disease should be suspected in any patient with stone onset in childhood, frequent recurrence of nephrolithiasis, and a strong family history of the disease. The presence of the classic hexagonal cystine crystals in the urine can verify the diagnosis. Because these crystals might not be evident in dilute or alkaline urine, qualitative screening with the sodium nitroprusside test better confirms the presence of cystinuria at a concentration greater than 75 mg/L. Quantitative cystine measures with a 24-hour urine sample should follow to determine the risk of stone formation and to guide therapy.

Therapy for Cystine Stones. The aim of treatment is to lower the urinary cystine concentration below the limits of solubility (~300 mg/L). Patients are advised to drink large quantities of fluids. A patient with a cystine excretion of 750 mg/day, for example, should ideally drink enough fluid to increase urine output to more than 3 L/day. Large quantities of milk should be avoided because dairy products and foods high in protein contain large amounts of methionine, an essential amino acid that is a precursor of cystine.[181] Because cystine is more soluble at a higher pH, juices are encouraged because they tend to alkalinize the urine. Potassium citrate (see "Hypercalciuria" and "Hypocitraturia" for details) is also prescribed to maintain the urinary pH between 6.5 and 7.0.

Approximately 50% of cystine stones are mixed stones. Patients with cystinuria often have other metabolic defects such as hypercalciuria, hypocitraturia, and hyperuricosuria. Therefore, a complete 24-hour urine collection for all stone-forming elements is necessary to treat nephrolithiasis fully in this setting. Restricting dietary sodium is also beneficial.[182]

If these measures are inadequate in controlling stone formation or if the urinary cystine concentration is too high to make adequate fluid intake practical, chelating agents called cystine-binding thiol drugs (CBTDs) may be added. D-Penicillamine is a CBTD that reduces the cystine concentration by forming a more soluble compound with cystine.[183] However, this medication is associated with numerous serious side effects that limit its use. Other CBTDs such as tiopronin, α-mercaptoproprionylglycine, and bucillamine are now available that reduce the cystine concentration with fewer side effects.[100,184-186]

REFERENCES

1. Brener ZZ, Winchester JF, Salman H, Bergman M. Nephrolithiasis: evaluation and management. *South Med J.* 2011;104:133-139.
2. Saigal CS, Joyce G, Timilsina AR. Direct and indirect costs of nephrolithiasis in an employed population: opportunity for disease management? *Kidney Int.* 2005;68:1808-1814.
3. Stamatelou KK, Francis ME, Jones CA. Time trends in reported prevalence of kidney stones in the United States: 1976-1994. *Kidney Int.* 2003;63(5):1817-1823.
4. Monk RD. Clinical approach to adults. *Semin Nephrol.* 1996;16:375-388.
5. Consensus Conference. Prevention and treatment of kidney stones. *JAMA.* 1988;260:977-981.
6. Monk RD, Bushinsky DA. Nephrolithiasis and nephrocalcinosis. In: Frehally J, Floege J, Johnson RJ, eds. *Comprehensive Clinical Nephrology.* 3rd ed. London, UK: Mosby; 2007:641-655.
7. Bushinsky DA, Coe FL, Moe OW. Nephrolithiasis. In: Brenner BM, ed. *The Kidney.* Philadelphia, PA: WB Saunders; 2008:1299-1349.
8. Coe FL. Recurrence of renal stones. *Lancet.* 1980;1:651.
9. Gillen DL, Worcester EM, Coe FL. Decreased renal function among adults with a history of nephrolithiasis: a study of NHANES III. *Kidney Int.* 2005;67:685-690.
10. Rule AD, Bergstralh EJ, Melton LJ III, et al. Kidney stones and the risk for chronic kidney disease. *Clin J Am Soc Nephrol.* 2009;4:804-811.
11. Chen N, Wang W, Huang Y, et al. Community-based study on CKD subjects and the associated risk factors. *Nephrol Dial Transplant.* 2009;24:2117-2123.

12. Stankus N, Hammes M, Gillen D, Worcester E. African American ESRD patients have a high pre-dialysis prevalence of kidney stones compared to NHANES III. *Urol Res.* 2007;35:83-87.
13. Sakhaee K. Nephrolithiasis as a systemic disorder. *Curr Opin Nephrol Hypertens.* 2008;17:304-309.
14. Anavekar NS, McMurray JJ, Velazquez EJ, et al. Relation between renal dysfunction and cardiovascular outcomes after myocardial infarction. *N Engl J Med.* 2004;351:1285-1295.
15. Go AS, Chertow GM, Fan D, et al. Chronic kidney disease and the risks of death, cardiovascular events, and hospitalization. *N Engl J Med.* 2004;351:1296-1305.
16. Weiner DE, Tighiouart H, Amin MG, et al. Chronic kidney disease as a risk factor for cardiovascular disease and all-cause mortality: a pooled analysis of community-based studies. *J Am Soc Nephrol.* 2004;15: 1307-1315.
17. Soucie JM, Coates RJ, McClellan W, et al. Relation between geographic variability in kidney stones: prevalence and risk factors for stones. *Am J Epidemiol.* 1996;143:487-495.
18. Soucie JM, Thun MJ, Coates RJ. Demographic and geographic variability of kidney stones in the United States. *Kidney Int.* 1994; 46:893-899.
19. Moe OW. Kidney stones: pathophysiology and medical management. *Lancet.* 2006;367:333-344.
20. Maalouf NM, Cameron MA, Moe OW, Sakhaee K. Novel insights into the pathogenesis of uric acid nephrolithiasis. *Curr Opin Nephrol Hypertens.* 2004;13:181-189.
21. Maalouf NM, Sakhaee K, Parks JH, et al. Association of urinary pH with body weight in nephrolithiasis. *Kidney Int.* 2004;65:1422-1425.
22. Mandel N. Mechanism of stone formation. *Semin Nephrol.* 1996; 16:364-374.
23. Hau AK, Kwan TH, Li PK. Melamine toxicity and the kidney. *J Am Soc Nephrol.* 2009;20:245-250.
24. Guan N, Fan Q, Ding J, et al. Melamine-contaminated powdered formula and urolithiasis in young children. *N Engl J Med.* 2009; 360:1067-1074.
25. Bhalla V, Grimm PC, Chertow GM, Pao AC. Melamine nephrotoxicity: an emerging epidemic in an era of globalization. *Kidney Int.* 2009; 75:774-779.
26. Evan AP, Lingeman JE, Coe FL, et al. Randall's plaque of patients with nephrolithiasis begins in basement membranes of thin loops of Henle. *J Clin Invest.* 2003;111:607-616.
27. Coe FL, Evan A, Worcester E. Kidney stone disease. *J Clin Invest.* 2005;115:2598-2608.
28. Sayer JA, Carr G, Simmons NL. Nephrocalcinosis: molecular insights into calcium precipitation within the kidney. *Clin Sci (Lond).* 2004; 106:549-561.
29. Bushinsky DA. Renal lithiasis. In: Humes HD, ed. *Kelly's Textbook of Medicine.* New York, NY: Lippincott Williams & Wilkins; 2000: 1243-1248.
30. Borghi L, Meschi T, Amato F, et al. Urinary volume, water and recurrences in idiopathic calcium nephrolithiasis: a 5-year randomized prospective study. *J Urol.* 1996;155:839-843.
31. Lemann J Jr, Pleuss JA, Worcester EA, et al. Urinary oxalate excretion increases with body size and decreases with increasing dietary calcium intake among healthy adults. *Kidney Int.* 1996;49:200-208. [Erratum in *Kidney Int.* 1996;50(1):341.]
32. Hosking DH, Erickson SB, Van den Berg CJ, et al. The stone clinic effect in patients with idiopathic calcium urolithiasis. *J Urol.* 1983;130(6): 1115-1118.
33. Muldowney FP, Freaney R, Moloney MF. Importance of dietary sodium in the hypercalciuria syndrome. *Kidney Int.* 1982;22:292-296.
34. Lemann J Jr, Worcester EA, Gray RW. Hypercalciuria and stones. *Am J Kidney Dis.* 1991;17:386-391.
35. Borghi L, Schianchi T, Meschi T, et al. Comparison of two diets for the prevention of recurrent stones in idiopathic hypercalciuria. *N Engl J Med.* 2002;346:77-84.
36. Lemann J Jr, Bushinsky DA, Hamm LL. Bone buffering of acid and base in humans. *Am J Physiol Renal Physiol.* 2003;285:F811-F832.
37. Bushinsky DA. Acid-base balance and bone health. In: Holick MF, Dawson-Hughes B, eds. *Nutrition and Bone Health.* Totowa, NJ: Humana Press; 2004:279-304.
38. Hamm LL. Renal handling of citrate. *Kidney Int.* 1990;38:728-735.
39. Bataille P, Achard JM, Fournier A, et al. Diet, vitamin D and vertebral mineral density in hypercalciuric calcium stone formers. *Kidney Int.* 1991;39:1193-1205.
40. Taylor EN, Curhan GC. Fructose consumption and the risk of kidney stones. *Kidney Int.* 2008;73:207-212.
41. Curhan GC, Willett WC, Rimm EB, Stampfer MJ. A prospective study of dietary calcium and other nutrients and the risk of symptomatic kidney stones. *N Engl J Med.* 1993;328:833-838.
42. Bushinsky DA. Recurrent hypercalciuric nephrolithiasis: does diet help? *N Engl J Med.* 2002;346:124-125.
43. Coe FL, Favus MJ, Crockett T, et al. Effects of low-calcium diet on urine calcium excretion, parathyroid function and serum 1,25(OH)2D3 levels in patients with idiopathic hypercalciuria and in normal subjects. *Am J Med.* 1982;72:25-32.
44. Freundlich M, Alonzo E, Bellorin-Font E, Weisinger JR. Reduced bone mass in children with idiopathic hypercalciuria and in their asymptomatic mothers. *Nephrol Dial Transplant.* 2002;17:1396-1401.
45. Standing Committee on the Scientific Evaluation of Dietary Reference Intakes, Food and Nutrition Board, Institute of Medicine. *Dietary Reference for Calcium, Phosphorus, Magnesium, Vitamin D, and Fluoride.* Washington, DC: National Academy Press; 1997.
46. Jackson RD, LaCroix AZ, Gass M, et al. Calcium plus vitamin D supplementation and the risk of fractures. *N Engl J Med.* 2006;354: 669-683.
47. Moe OW, Bonny O. Genetic hypercalciuria. *J Am Soc Nephrol.* 2005;16:729-745.
48. Bushinsky DA, Frick KK, Nehrke K. Genetic hypercalciuric stone-forming rats. *Curr Opin Nephrol Hypertens.* 2006;15:403-418.
49. Monk RD, Bushinsky DA, et al. Pathogenesis of idiopathic hypercalciuria. In: Coe F, Favus M, Pak C, eds. *Kidney Stones: Medical and Surgical Management.* Philadelphia, PA: Lippincott-Raven; 1996:759-772.
50. Bushinsky DA, Monk RD. Electrolyte quintet: calcium. *Lancet.* 1998;352:306-311.
51. Lemann J Jr. Pathogenesis of idiopathic hypercalciuria and nephrolithiasis. In: Coe FL, Favus M, eds. *Disorders of Bone and Mineral Metabolism.* New York, NY: Raven Press; 1992:685-706.
52. Coe FL, Favus MJ, Asplin JR. Nephrolithiasis. In: Brenner BM, Rector FC Jr, eds. *The Kidney.* Philadelphia, PA: WB Saunders; 2004: 1819-1866.
53. Kaplan RA, Haussler MR, Deftos LJ, et al. The role of 1 alpha, 25-dihydroxyvitamin D in the mediation of intestinal hyperabsorption of calcium in primary hyperparathyroidism and absorptive hypercalciuria. *J Clin Invest.* 1977;59:756-760.
54. Asplin JR, Bauer KA, Kinder J, et al. Bone mineral density and urine calcium excretion among subjects with and without nephrolithiasis. *Kidney Int.* 2003;63:662-669.
55. Pak CY, Odvina CV, Pearle MS, et al. Effect of dietary modification on urinary stone risk factors. *Kidney Int.* 2005;68:2264-2273.
56. Pak CY, Oata M, Lawrence EC, Snyder W. The hypercalciurias. Causes, parathyroid functions, and diagnostic criteria. *J Clin Invest.* 1974;54: 387-400.
57. Yao JJ, Bai S, Karnauskas AJ, et al. Regulation of renal calcium receptor gene expression by 1,25-dihydroxyvitamin D3 in genetic hypercalciuric stone-forming rats. *J Am Soc Nephrol.* 2005;16:1300-1308.
58. Bushinsky DA, Asplin JR. Thiazides reduce brushite, but not calcium oxalate, supersaturation, and stone formation in genetic hypercalciuric stone-forming rats. *J Am Soc Nephrol.* 2005;16:417-424.
59. Bushinsky DA, Parker WR, Asplin JR. Calcium phosphate supersaturation regulates stone formation in genetic hypercalciuric stone-forming rats. *Kidney Int.* 2000;57:550-560.
60. Bushinsky DA, Asplin JR, Grynpas MD, et al. Calcium oxalate stone formation in genetic hypercalciuric stone-forming rats. *Kidney Int.* 2002;61:975-987.
61. Hoopes RR Jr, Middleton FA, Sen S, et al. Isolation and confirmation of a calcium excretion quantitative trait locus on chromosome 1 in genetic hypercalciuric stone-forming congenic rats. *J Am Soc Nephrol.* 2006;17:1292-1304.
62. Bushinsky DA, Favus MJ. Mechanism of hypercalciuria in genetic hypercalciuric rats. Inherited defect in intestinal calcium transport. *J Clin Invest.* 1988;82:1585-1591.
63. Kim M, Sessler NE, Tembe V, et al. Response of genetic hypercalciuric rats to a low calcium diet. *Kidney Int.* 1993;43:189-196.
64. Pak CY. Nephrolithiasis. *Curr Ther Endocrinol Metab.* 1997;6:572-576.
65. Krieger NS, Stathopoulos VM, Bushinsky DA. Increased sensitivity to 1,25(OH)2D3 in bone from genetic hypercalciuric rats. *Am J Physiol.* 1996;271:C130-C135.
66. Grynpas M, Waldman S, Holmyard D, Bushinsky DA. Genetic hypercalciuric stone-forming rats have a primary decrease in BMD and strength. *J Bone Miner Res.* 2009;24:1420-1426.
67. Bushinsky DA, Neumann KJ, Asplin J, Krieger NS. Alendronate decreases urine calcium and supersaturation in genetic hypercalciuric rats. *Kidney Int.* 1999;55:234-243.
68. Tsuruoka S, Bushinsky DA, Schwartz GJ. Defective renal calcium reabsorption in genetic hypercalciuric rats. *Kidney Int.* 1997;51: 1540-1547.
69. Karnauskas AJ, van Leeuwen JP, van den Bemd GJ, et al. Mechanism and function of high vitamin D receptor levels in genetic hypercalciuric stone-forming rats. *J Bone Miner Res.* 2005;20:447-454.
70. Li XQ, Tembe V, Horwitz GM, et al. Increased intestinal vitamin D receptor in genetic hypercalciuric rats. A cause of intestinal calcium hyperabsorption. *J Clin Invest.* 1993;91:661-667.
71. Favus MJ, Karnauskas AJ, Parks JH, Coe FL. Peripheral blood monocyte vitamin D receptor levels are elevated in patients with idiopathic hypercalciuria. *J Clin Endocrinol Metab.* 2004;89:4937-4943.
72. Gambaro G, Vezzoli G, Casari G, et al. Genetics of hypercalciuria and calcium nephrolithiasis: from the rare monogenic to the common polygenic forms. *Am J Kidney Dis.* 2004;44:963-986.
73. Thorleifsson G, Holm H, Edvardsson V, et al. Sequence variants in the CLDN14 gene associate with kidney stones and bone mineral density. *Nat Genet.* 2009;41:926-930.

74. Scheinman SJ, Guay-Woodford LM, Thakker RV, Warnock DG. Genetic disorders of renal electrolyte transport. *N Engl J Med.* 1999;340: 1177-1187.

75. Lloyd SE, Pearce SH, Fisher SE, et al. A common molecular basis for three inherited kidney stone diseases. *Nature.* 1996;379:445-449.

76. Frick KK, Bushinsky DA. Molecular mechanisms of primary hypercalciuria. *J Am Soc Nephrol.* 2003;14:1082-1095.

77. Akuta N, Lloyd SE, Igarashi T, et al. Mutations of CLCN5 in Japanese children with idiopathic low molecular weight proteinuria, hypercalciuria and nephrocalcinosis. *Kidney Int.* 1997;52:911-916.

78. Naesens M, Steels P, Verberckmoes R, et al. Bartter's and Gitelman's syndromes: from gene to clinic. *Nephron Physiol.* 2004;96:65-78.

79. Hou J, Renigunta A, Konrad M, et al. Claudin-16 and claudin-19 interact and form a cation-selective tight junction complex. *J Clin Invest.* 2008;118:619-628.

80. Hou J, Renigunta A, Gomes AS, et al. Claudin-16 and claudin-19 interaction is required for their assembly into tight junctions and for renal reabsorption of magnesium. *Proc Natl Acad Sci U S A.* 2009;106: 15350-15355.

81. Nicoletta JA, Schwartz GJ. Distal renal tubular acidosis. *Curr Opin Pediatr.* 2004;16:194-198.

82. Batlle D, Haque SK. Genetic causes and mechanisms of distal renal tubular acidosis. *Nephrol Dial Transplant.* 2012;27:3691-3704.

83. Bergwitz C, Roslin NM, Tieder M, et al. SLC34A3 mutations in patients with hereditary hypophosphatemic rickets with hypercalciuria predict a key role for the sodium-phosphate cotransporter NaPi-IIc in maintaining phosphate homeostasis. *Am J Hum Genet.* 2006;78:179-192.

84. Levi M, Blaine J, Breusegem S, et al. Renal phosphate-wasting disorders. *Adv Chronic Kidney Dis.* 2006;13:155-165.

85. Teichman JMH. Clinical practice. Acute renal colic from ureteral calculus. *N Engl J Med.* 2004;350:684-693.

86. Ueno A, Kawamura T, Ogawa A, Takayasu H. Relation of spontaneous passage of ureteral calculi to size. *Urology.* 1977;10:544-546.

87. Segura JW, Patterson DE, LeRoy AJ, et al. Percutaneous removal of kidney stones: review of 1,000 cases. *J Urol.* 1985;134:1077-1081.

88. Keddis MT, Rule AD. Nephrolithiasis and loss of kidney function. *Curr Opin Nephrol Hypertens.* 2013;22:390-396.

89. Vupputuri S, Soucie JM, McClellan W, Sandler DP. History of kidney stones as a possible risk factor for chronic kidney disease. *Ann Epidemiol.* 2004;14:222-228.

90. El-Zoghby ZM, Lieske JC, Foley RN, et al. Urolithiasis and the risk of ESRD. *Clin J Am Soc Nephrol.* 2012;7:1409-1415.

91. Jungers P, Joly D, Barbey F, et al. [Nephrolithiasis-induced ESRD: frequency, causes and prevention]. *Nephrol Ther.* 2005;1(5):301-310.

92. Alexander RT, Hemmelgarn BR, Wiebe N, et al., Alberta Kidney Disease Network. Kidney stones and kidney function loss: a cohort study. *BMJ.* 2012;345:e5287.

93. Worcester E, Parks JH, Josephson MA, et al. Causes and consequences of kidney loss in patients with nephrolithiasis. *Kidney Int.* 2003;64: 2204-2213.

94. Gaudio KM, Siegel NJ, Hayslett JP, Kashgarian M. Renal perfusion and intratubular pressures during ureteral occlusion in rat. *Am J Physiol.* 1980;238(3):F205-F209.

95. Evan AP, Lingeman JE, Coe FL, et al. Crystal-associated nephropathy in patients with brushite nephrolithiasis. *Kidney Int.* 2005;67: 576-591.

96. Evan A, Lingeman J, Coe FL, Worcester E. Randall's plaque: pathogenesis and role in calcium oxalate nephrolithiasis. *Kidney Int.* 2006; 69:1313-1318.

97. Boonla C, Krieglstein K, Bovornpadungkitti S, et al. Fibrosis and evidence for epithelial-mesenchymal transition in the kidneys of patients with staghorn calculi. *BJU Int.* 2011;108:1336-1345.

98. Evan AP, Coe FL, Lingeman JE, et al. Renal crystal deposits and histopathology in patients with cystine stones. *Kidney Int.* 2006;69: 2227-2235.

99. Milliner DS. The primary hyperoxalurias: an algorithm for diagnosis. *Am J Nephrol.* 2005;25:154-160.

100. Sakhaee K. Pathogenesis and medical management of cystinuria. *Semin Nephrol.* 1996;16:435-447.

101. Danpure CJ. Molecular etiology of primary hyperoxaluria type 1: new directions for treatment. *Am J Nephrol.* 2005;25:303-310.

102. Nehrke K, Arreola J, Nguyen HV, et al. Loss of hyperpolarization-activated Cl(-) current in salivary acinar cells from Clcn2 knockout mice. *J Biol Chem.* 2002;277(26):23604-23611.

103. Gimpel C, Krause A, Franck P, et al. Exposure to furosemide as the strongest risk factor for nephrocalcinosis in preterm infants. *Pediatr Int.* 2010;52:51-56.

104. Schell-Feith EA, Kist-van Holthe JE, Conneman N, et al. Etiology of nephrocalcinosis in preterm neonates: association of nutritional intake and urinary parameters. *Kidney Int.* 2000;58:2102-2110.

105. Keith MP, Gilliland WR. Updates in the management of gout. *Am J Med.* 2007;120:221-224.

106. Daudon M, Jungers P. Drug-induced renal calculi: epidemiology, prevention and management. *Drugs.* 2004;64:245-275.

107. Taylor EN, Curhan GC. Determinants of 24-hour urinary oxalate excretion. *Clin J Am Soc Nephrol.* 2008;3:1453-1460.

108. Rodman JS. Struvite stones. *Nephron.* 1999;81(Suppl 1):50-59.

109. Mandel GS, Mandel N. Analysis of stones. In: Coe FL, Favus MJ, Pak CYC, et al, eds. *Kidney Stones: Medical and Surgical Management.* Philadelphia, PA: Lippincott-Raven; 1996:323-335.

110. Denton ER, Mackenzie A, Greenwell T, et al. Unenhanced helical CT for renal colic: is the radiation dose justifiable? *Clin Radiol.* 1999;54: 444-447.

111. Smith RC, Coll DM. Helical computed tomography in the diagnosis of ureteric colic. *BJU Int.* 2000;86(Suppl 1):33-41.

112. Nakada SY, Hoff DG, Attai S, et al. Determination of stone composition by noncontrast spiral computed tomography in the clinical setting. *Urology.* 2000;55:816-819.

113. Parks JH, Coward M, Coe FL. Correspondence between stone composition and urine supersaturation in nephrolithiasis. *Kidney Int.* 1997;51: 894-900.

114. Preminger GM, Tiselius HG, Assimos DG, et al. 2007 guideline for the management of ureteral calculi. *J Urol.* 2007;178:2418-2434.

115. Sofer M, Watterson JD, Wollin TA, et al. Holmium:YAG laser lithotripsy for upper urinary tract calculi in 598 patients. *J Urol.* 2002; 167:31-34.

116. Wignall GR, Canales BK, Denstedt JD, Monga M. Minimally invasive approaches to upper urinary tract urolithiasis. *Urol Clin North Am.* 2008;35:441-454.

117. Samplaski MK, Irwin BH, Desai M. Less-invasive ways to remove stones from the kidneys and ureters. *Cleve Clin J Med.* 2009;76:592-598.

118. Putman SS, Hamilton BD, Johnson DB. The use of shock wave lithotripsy for renal calculi. *Curr Opin Urol.* 2004;14:117-121.

119. Leveillee RJ, Lobik L. Intracorporeal lithotripsy: which modality is best? *Curr Opin Urol.* 2003;13:249-253.

120. Beach MA, Mauro LS. Pharmacologic expulsive treatment of ureteral calculi. *Ann Pharmacother.* 2006;40:1361-1368.

121. Borghi L, Meschi T, Amato F, et al. Nifedipine and methylprednisolone in facilitating ureteral stone passage: a randomized, double-blind, placebo-controlled study. *J Urol.* 1994;152:1095-1098.

122. Porpiglia F, Ghignone G, Fiori C, et al. Nifedipine versus tamsulosin for the management of lower ureteral stones. *J Urol.* 2004;172: 568-571.

123. Dellabella M, Milanese G, Muzzonigro G. Randomized trial of the efficacy of tamsulosin, nifedipine and phloroglucinol in medical expulsive therapy for distal ureteral calculi. *J Urol.* 2005;174:167-172.

124. Uribarri J, Oh MS, Carroll HJ. The first kidney stone. *Ann Intern Med.* 1989;111(12):1006-1009.

125. Meschi T, Maggiore U, Fiaccadori E, et al. The effect of fruits and vegetables on urinary stone risk factors. *Kidney Int.* 2004;66: 2402-2410.

126. Meschi T, Schianchi T, Ridolo E, et al. Body weight, diet and water intake in preventing stone disease. *Urol Int.* 2004;72:29-33.

127. Curhan GC, Willett WC, Speizer FE, et al. Comparison of dietary calcium with supplemental calcium and other nutrients as factors affecting the risk for kidney stones in women. *Ann Intern Med.* 1997;126:497-504.

128. Coe FL, Parks JH, Bushinsky DA, et al. Chlorthalidone promotes mineral retention in patients with idiopathic hypercalciuria. *Kidney Int.* 1988;33:1140-1146.

129. Borghi L, Meschi T, Guerra A, Novarini A. Randomized prospective-study of a nonthiazide diuretic, indapamide, in preventing calcium stone recurrences. *J Cardiovasc Pharmacol.* 1993;22:S78-S86.

130. Pak CY, Fuller C, Sakhaee K, et al. Long-term treatment of calcium nephrolithiasis with potassium citrate. *J Urol.* 1985;134:11-19.

131. Hatch M, Freel RW. Intestinal transport of an obdurate anion: oxalate. *Urol Res.* 2005;33:1-16.

132. Jaeger P, Robertson WG. Role of dietary intake and intestinal absorption of oxalate in calcium stone formation. *Nephron Physiol.* 2004; 98:64-71.

133. Holmes RP, Goodman HO, Assimos DG. Contribution of dietary oxalate to urinary oxalate excretion. *Kidney Int.* 2001;59:270-276.

134. Coe FL, Evan AP, Worcester EM, Lingeman JE. Three pathways for human kidney stone formation. *Urol Res.* 2010;38:147-160.

135. McIntyre CW. Calcium balance during hemodialysis. *Semin Dial.* 2008;21:38-42.

136. Barilla DE, Notz C, Kennedy D, Pak CY. Renal oxalate excretion following oral oxalate loads in patients with ileal disease and with renal and absorptive hypercalciurias. Effect of calcium and magnesium. *Am J Med.* 1978;64:579-585.

137. Hatch M, Freel RW, Goldner AM, Earnest DL. Comparison of effects of low concentrations of ricinoleate and taurochenodeoxycholate on colonic oxalate and chloride absorption. *Gastroenterology.* 1983;84: 1181.

138. Freel RW, Hatch M, Earnest DL, Goldner AM. Dihydroxy bile salt-induced alterations in NaCl transport across the rabbit colon. *Am J Physiol.* 1983;245:808-815.

139. Nordenvall B, Backman L, Larsson L, Tiselius HG. Effects of calcium, aluminium, magnesium and cholestyramine on hyperoxaluria in patients with jejunoileal bypass. *Acta Chir Scand.* 1983;149:93-98.

140. Clarke AM, McKenzie RG. Ileostomy and the risk of urinary uric acid stones. *Lancet.* 1969;2:395-397.

141. Rudman D, Dedonis JL, Fountain MT, et al. Hypocitraturia in patients with gastrointestinal malabsorption. *N Engl J Med.* 1980;303:657-661.

142. Worcester EM. Stones due to bowel disease. In: Coe FL, Favus MJ, Pak CYC, et al, eds. *Kidney Stones: Medical and Surgical Management.* Philadelphia, PA: Lippincott-Raven; 1996:883-903.

143. Petrarulo M, Vitale C, Facchini P, Marangella M. Biochemical approach to diagnosis and differentiation of primary hyperoxalurias: an update. *J Nephrol.* 1998;11(Suppl 1):23-28.

144. Cochat P, Rumsby G. Primary hyperoxaluria. *N Engl J Med.* 2013;369:649-658.

145. Milliner DS, Eickholt JT, Bergstralh EJ, et al. Results of long-term treatment with orthophosphate and pyridoxine in patients with primary hyperoxaluria. *N Engl J Med.* 1994;331:1553-1558.

146. Kwak C, Kim HK, Kim EC, et al. Urinary oxalate levels and the enteric bacterium *Oxalobacter formigenes* in patients with calcium oxalate urolithiasis. *Eur Urol.* 2003;44:475-481.

147. Watts RW, Danpure CJ, De Pauw L, Toussaint. Combined liver-kidney and isolated liver transplantations for primary hyperoxaluria type 1: the European experience. The European Study Group on Transplantation in Hyperoxaluria Type 1. *Nephrol Dial Transplant.* 1991;6(7):502-511.

148. Coe FL, Parks JH, Asplin JR. The pathogenesis and treatment of kidney stones. *N Engl J Med.* 1992;327:1141-1152.

149. Millman S, Strauss AL, Parks JH, Coe FL. Pathogenesis and clinical course of mixed calcium oxalate and uric acid nephrolithiasis. *Kidney Int.* 1982;22:366-370.

150. Grases F, Sanchis P, Isern B, et al. Uric acid as inducer of calcium oxalate crystal development. *Scand J Urol Nephrol.* 2007;41:26-31.

151. Pak CY, Arnold LH. Heterogeneous nucleation of calcium oxalate by seeds of monosodium urate. *Proc Soc Exp Biol Med.* 1975;149:930-932.

152. Grover PK, Ryall RL, Marshall VR. Dissolved urate promotes calcium oxalate crystallization: epitaxy is not the cause. *Clin Sci (Lond).* 1993;85:303-307.

153. Grover PK, Marshall VR, Ryall RL. Dissolved urate salts out calcium oxalate in undiluted human urine in vitro: implications for calcium oxalate stone genesis. *Chem Biol.* 2003;10:271-278.

154. Grover PK, Ryall RL. Allopurinol for stones: right drug—wrong reasons. *Am J Med.* 2007;120:380.

155. Coe FL. Treated and untreated recurrent calcium nephrolithiasis in patients with idiopathic hypercalciuria, hyperuricosuria, or no metabolic disorder. *Ann Intern Med.* 1977;87:404-410.

156. Zerwekh JE, Holt K, Pak CY. Natural urinary macromolecular inhibitors: attenuation of inhibitory activity by urate salts. *Kidney Int.* 1983;23:838-841.

157. Grover PK, Ryall RL, Marshall VR. Calcium oxalate crystallization in urine: role of urate and glycosaminoglycans. *Kidney Int.* 1992;41:149-154.

158. Ryall RL, Hibberd CM, Marshall VR. The effect of crystalline monosodium urate on the crystallisation of calcium oxalate in whole human urine. *Urol Res.* 1986;14:63-65.

159. Pak CY. Citrate and renal calculi: an update. *Miner Electrolyte Metab.* 1994;20:371-377.

160. Curhan GC, Taylor EN. 24-h uric acid excretion and the risk of kidney stones. *J Urol.* 2009;181:1721.

161. Ettinger B, Pak CY, Citron JT, et al. Potassium-magnesium citrate is an effective prophylaxis against recurrent calcium oxalate nephrolithiasis. *J Urol.* 1997;158:2069-2073.

162. Pak CYC, Fuller C. Idiopathic hypocitraturic calcium oxalate nephrolithiasis successfully treated with potassium citrate. *Ann Intern Med.* 1986;104:33-37.

163. Ramchandani P, Pollack HM. Radiologic evaluation of patients with urolithiasis. In: Coe FL, Favus MJ, Pak CYC, eds. *Kidney Stones: Medical and Surgical Management.* Philadelphia, PA: Lippincott-Raven; 1996:369-435.

164. Pak CY, Sakhaee K, Peterson RD, et al. Biochemical profile of idiopathic uric acid nephrolithiasis. *Kidney Int.* 2001;60:757-761.

165. Sakhaee K, Adams-Huet B, Moe OW, Pak CY. Pathophysiologic basis for normouricosuric uric acid nephrolithiasis. *Kidney Int.* 2002;62:971-979.

166. Negri AL, Spivacow R, Del Valle E, et al. Clinical and biochemical profile of patients with "pure" uric acid nephrolithiasis compared with "pure" calcium oxalate stone formers. *Urol Res.* 2007;35:247-251.

167. Pak CYC, Poindexter JR, Peterson RD, et al. Biochemical distinction between hyperuricosuric calcium urolithiasis and gouty diathesis. *Urology.* 2002;60:789-794.

168. Coe FL. Uric acid and calcium oxalate nephrolithiasis. *Kidney Int.* 1983;24:392-403.

169. Ettinger B, Tang A, Citron JT, et al. Randomized trial of allopurinol in the prevention of calcium oxalate calculi. *N Engl J Med.* 1986;315:1386-1389.

170. Wong HY, Riedl CR, Griffith DP. Medical management and prevention of struvite stones. In: Coe FL, Favus MJ, Pak CYC, eds. *Kidney Stones: Medical and Surgical Management.* Philadelphia, PA: Lippincott-Raven; 1996:941-950.

171. Preminger GM, Assimos DG, Lingeman JE, et al. Chapter 1: AUA guideline on management of staghorn calculi: diagnosis and treatment recommendations. *J Urol.* 2005;173:1991-2000.

172. Michaels EK. Surgical management of struvite stones. In: Coe FL, Favus MJ, Pak CYC, eds. *Kidney Stones: Medical and Surgical Management.* Philadelphia, PA: Lippincott-Raven; 1996:951-970.

173. Bernardo NO, Smith AD. Chemolysis of urinary calculi. *Urol Clin North Am.* 2000;27:355-365.

174. Dormia E, Dormia G, Malagola G, Minervini S. Experience with instrumental chemolysis for urolithiasis. *J Urol.* 2003;170:1105-1110.

175. Silverman DE, Stamey TA. Management of infection stones: the Stanford experience. *Medicine (Baltimore).* 1983;62:44-51.

176. Griffith DP, Moskowitz PA, Carlton CE. Adjunctive chemotherapy of infection-induced staghorn calculi. *J Urol.* 1979;121:711-715.

177. Sant GR, Blaivas JG, Meares EM. Hemiacidrin irrigation in the management of struvite calculi: long-term results. *J Urol.* 1983;130:1048-1050.

178. Griffith DP, Gleeson MJ, Lee H, et al. Randomized, double-blind trial of Lithostat (acetohydroxamic acid) in the palliative treatment of infection-induced urinary calculi. *Eur Urol.* 1991;20:243-247.

179. Williams JJ, Rodman JS, Peterson CM. A randomized double-blind study of acetohydroxamic acid in struvite nephrolithiasis. *N Engl J Med.* 1984;311:760-764.

180. Font-Llitjos M, Jimenez-Vidal M, Bisceglia L, et al. New insights into cystinuria: 40 new mutations, genotype-phenotype correlation, and digenic inheritance causing partial phenotype. *J Med Genet.* 2005;42:58-68.

181. Kolb FO, Earll JM, Harper HA. "Disappearance" of cystinuria in a patient treated with prolonged low methionine diet. *Metabolism.* 1967;16:378-381.

182. Jaeger P, Portmann L, Saunders A, et al. Anticystinuric effects of glutamine and of dietary-sodium restriction. *N Engl J Med.* 1986;315:1120-1123.

183. Singer A, Das S. Cystinuria: a review of the pathophysiology and management. *J Urol.* 1989;142:669-673.

184. Pak CYC. Prevention of recurrent nephrolithiasis. In: Pak CYC, Favus C, eds. *Renal Stone Disease: Pathogenesis, Prevention, and Treatment.* Boston, MA: Martinus-Njhoff; 1987:165-199.

185. Pak CYC. Cystine lithiasis. In: Resnick MI, Pak CYC, eds. *Urolithiasis: a Medical and Surgical Reference.* Philadelphia, PA: WB Saunders; 1990:133-143.

186. Lindell A, Denneberg T, Hellgren E, et al. Clinical course and cystine stone formation during tiopronin treatment. *Urol Res.* 1995;23:111-117.

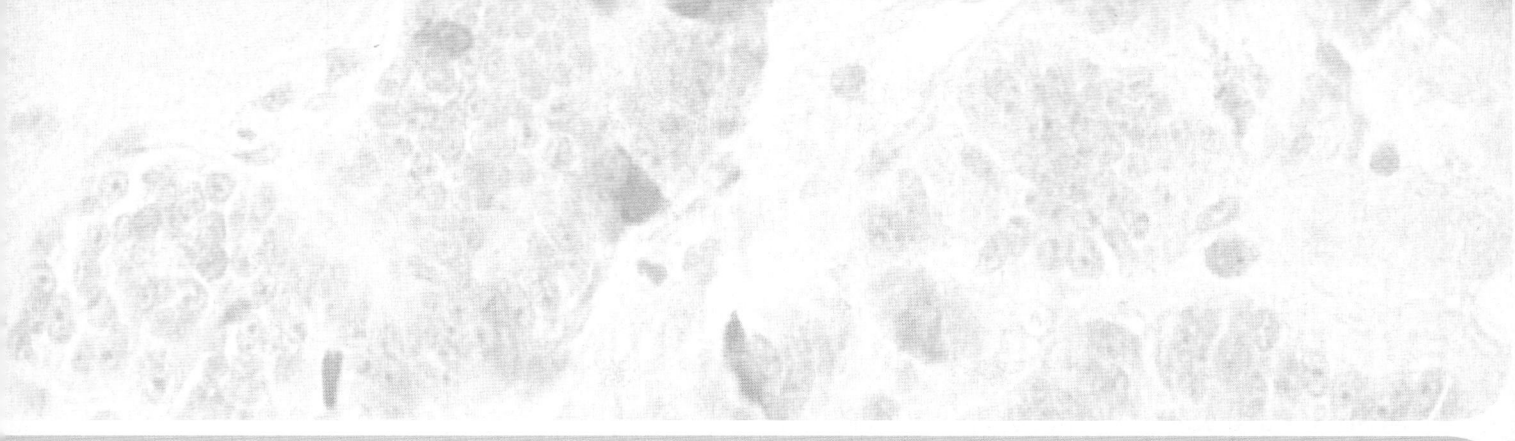

Section VIII

Disorders of Carbohydrate and Fat Metabolism

CHAPTER 31

Type 2 Diabetes Mellitus

KENNETH S. POLONSKY • CHARLES F. BURANT*

KEY POINTS

- Type 2 diabetes mellitus (T2DM) is one of the most common health problems facing mankind and is a major public health problem. The International Diabetes Federation (IDF) estimated in 2014 that 387 million people have diabetes worldwide and that by 2035 this number will rise to 592 million.
- T2DM is the predominant form of diabetes worldwide, accounting for 90% of cases globally.
- The pathogenesis of T2DM is complex and involves the interaction of genetic and environmental factors.
- A number of environmental factors have been shown to play a critical role in the development of the disease, particularly excessive caloric intake leading to obesity and a sedentary lifestyle.
- The clinical presentation is also heterogeneous, with a wide range in age at onset, severity of associated hyperglycemia, and degree of obesity.
- From a pathophysiologic standpoint, persons with T2DM consistently demonstrate three cardinal abnormalities:
  - Resistance to the action of insulin in peripheral tissues, particularly muscle and fat but also liver
  - Defective insulin secretion, particularly in response to a glucose stimulus
  - Increased glucose production by the liver
- Genetically, T2DM consists of monogenic and polygenic forms.
- A number of genes have been identified as causing monogenic diabetes.
- Close to 100 genetic variants have been demonstrated to be associated with risk for T2DM; collectively, these variants account for 5% to 10% of the overall genetic risk for T2DM.

- Significant advances have been made in the treatment of patients with T2DM over the past 10 to 15 years, and a large number of treatment options are available.
- A growing body of experience suggests that the use of metformin as initial therapy in combination with diet, exercise, and a comprehensive diabetes education program can provide impressive lowering of glucose with essentially no risk of hypoglycemia. If the response is judged to be inadequate over 3 months, essentially any other agent can be added. There are six recommended second-line therapies: sulfonylurea, thiazolidinedione, dipeptidyl peptidase 4 (DPP4) inhibitor, sodium-glucose cotransporter 2 (SGLT2) inhibitor, glucagon-like peptide-1 (GLP-1) receptor agonist, and basal insulin. Each has its advantages and disadvantages. If hemoglobin A_{1c} levels above target persist for an additional 3 months, adding virtually any agent not yet prescribed is acceptable.

EPIDEMIOLOGY AND DIAGNOSIS

Epidemiology

Type 2 diabetes mellitus is the predominant form of diabetes worldwide, accounting for 90% of cases globally. An epidemic of T2DM is under way in both developed and developing countries, although the brunt of the disorder is felt disproportionately in non-European populations. In the Pacific island of Nauru, diabetes was virtually unknown 50 years ago and is now present in approximately 40% of adults. The IDF estimated in 2014 that 387 million people have diabetes worldwide and that by 2035 this number will rise to 592 million. Of those with diabetes currently, 77% live in low- and middle-income countries and 179 million are undiagnosed. These estimates are substantially greater than predicted even a decade ago, suggesting that the global epidemic is still progressing. In the United States, the Centers for Disease Control and Prevention (CDC) estimated in 2014 that 29.1 million people, or 9.3% of the population, had diabetes and that 8.1 million of them (27.8%) were undiagnosed. In 2012, they estimated based on fasting glucose or hemoglobin A_{1c} levels that 86 million people (37% of adults over age 20) had prediabetes and thus were at high risk of developing diabetes.[1-4]

The economic burden of diabetes is enormous. The IDF estimates that in 2014 diabetes-related health expenditures amounted to 11% of total health spending on adults.[3] The CDC suggests that diabetes costs in the United States were $245 billion with average expenditures per person, adjusted for age and gender, 2.3-fold higher than in the nondiabetic

*John Buse was a coauthor of this chapter but has chosen to withdraw his name owing to his disagreement with Reed Elsevier's handling of "An open letter for the people in Gaza" (Manduca P, Chalmers I, Summerfield D, Gilbert M, Ang S. An open letter for the people in Gaza. *Lancet*. 2014;384(9941):397-398).

population.[4] The increases in cost are driven by complications, comorbid conditions, and increasing complexity of care driving prescription costs and the frequency of visits.[5]

Considerable information is available on the factors that are responsible for the development of T2DM, and these determinants are summarized in Table 31-1.[1] T2DM is thought to occur in genetically predisposed persons who are exposed to a series of environmental influences that precipitate the onset of clinical disease. The genetic basis of T2DM is discussed in detail later in this chapter, but the syndrome consists of monogenic and polygenic forms that can be differentiated both on clinical grounds and in terms of the genes that are involved in the pathogenesis of these disorders. Sex, age, and ethnic background are important factors in determining the risk of developing T2DM. The disorder is more common in women, and the increased prevalence in certain racial and ethnic groups has already been alluded to. Age is also a critical factor. T2DM has been viewed in the past as a disorder of aging, and this remains true today. However, the prevalence of obesity and T2DM in children has risen dramatically. In the past, it was believed that the overwhelming majority of children with diabetes had type 1 diabetes mellitus (T1DM), and only 1% to 2% of diabetic children were considered to have T2DM or other rare forms of diabetes. More recent reports suggest that as many as 20% to 25% of children in the United States with newly diagnosed diabetes have non–immune-mediated forms of the disease. Most of these children have T2DM, but other types are being increasingly identified. Nevertheless, T2DM in children remains relatively rare, with an estimated prevalence of 5 cases per 10,000 children.[4,6]

Diagnostic Criteria

The diagnosis of diabetes rests on the measurement of glycemia. Current criteria for the diagnosis of diabetes and various categories of prediabetes or high risk for diabetes are shown in Table 31-2.[7]

Because plasma glucose concentrations range as a continuum, the criteria are based on estimates of the threshold for the complications of diabetes. The primary end point used to evaluate the relationship between glucose levels and complications is retinopathy. All three tests—fasting plasma glucose (FPG), 2-hour plasma glucose (2-hour PG), and glycosylated hemoglobin A_{1c} (HbA_{1c})—are able to predict the presence of retinopathy and, by inference, glucose levels that are diagnostic of diabetes[8] (Fig. 31-1). Furthermore, there is a relationship between elevated levels of all three markers and cardiovascular disease, although the relationship is generally stronger for HbA_{1c}. Whereas previously HbA_{1c} was specifically not recommended for the diagnosis of diabetes and states of high diabetes risk based on poor standardization of assays, the current HbA_{1c} assay has several technical (preanalytic and analytic) advantages over the currently used laboratory measurements of glucose. Furthermore, measures of fasting and postchallenge glucose concentrations in the same individual over time are less reproducible than those for the HbA_{1c}. The intra-individual coefficient of variation in one study was 6.4% for the FPG and 16.7% for the 2-hour PG value, compared with less than 2% for HbA_{1c}.[8]

Although the oral glucose tolerance test (OGTT) is an invaluable tool in research, it is not recommended for routine use in diagnosing diabetes. It is inconvenient for patients, and in most cases the diagnosis can be made on the basis of either an elevated FPG concentration or an elevated random glucose determination in the presence of hyperglycemic symptoms.

Screening

Undiagnosed T2DM is common. Subjects at high risk for diabetes and with undiagnosed T2DM are at significantly

---

TABLE 31-1

Epidemiologic Determinants and Risk Factors of Type 2 Diabetes Mellitus

Genetic Factors

Genetic markers
Family history
"Thrifty genes"

Demographic Characteristics

Sex
Age
Ethnicity

Behavioral and Lifestyle-Related Risk Factors

Obesity (including distribution of obesity and duration)
Physical inactivity
Diet
Stress
Westernization, urbanization, modernization

Metabolic Determinants and Intermediate-Risk Categories of Type 2 Diabetes

Impaired glucose tolerance
Insulin resistance
Pregnancy-related determinants
Parity
Gestational diabetes
Diabetes in offspring of women with diabetes during pregnancy
Intrauterine malnutrition or overnutrition

From Zimmer P, Alberti KG, Shaw J. Global and societal implications of the diabetes epidemic. *Nature.* 2001;414:782-787.

TABLE 31-2

Criteria for the Diagnosis of Diabetes*

Test	Normoglycemia	Increased Risk*		High Risk	Diabetes[†]
		Impaired Fasting Glucose	Impaired Glucose Tolerance		
PG, fasting (mg/dL)	<100	100-125			≥126
PG, 2-hour (mg/dL)	<140		140-199		≥200
Hemoglobin A_{1c} (%)				5.7-6.4	≥6.5
PG, casual (mg/dL)					≥200 plus classical symptoms of diabetes or hyperglycemic crisis

*Risk for diabetes is continuous, extending below the lower limit and becoming disproportionately greater at the higher end of the ranges shown.
[†]In the absence of unequivocal hyperglycemia, a diagnostic result should be confirmed by repeat testing.
PG, plasma glucose.
Modified from American Diabetes Association. Standards of medical care in diabetes—2010. *Diabetes Care.* 2010;29:s11-s61.

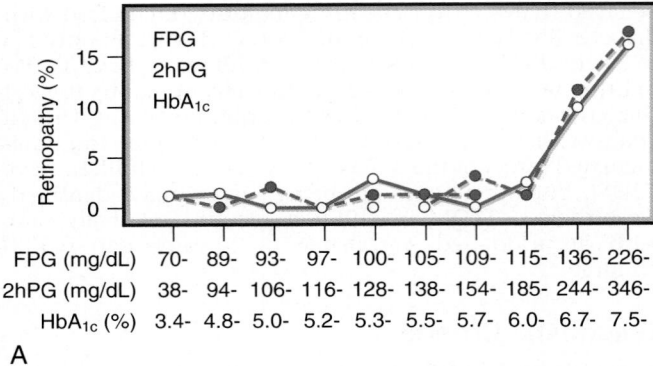

FPG (mg/dL) 70- 89- 93- 97- 100- 105- 109- 115- 136- 226-
2hPG (mg/dL) 38- 94- 106- 116- 128- 138- 154- 185- 244- 346-
HbA1c (%) 3.4- 4.8- 5.0- 5.2- 5.3- 5.5- 5.7- 6.0- 6.7- 7.5-

A

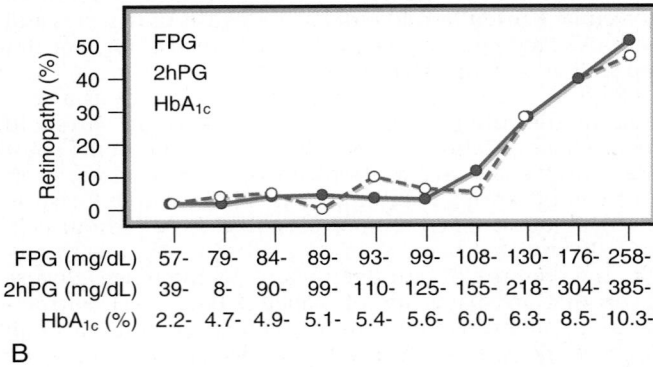

FPG (mg/dL) 57- 79- 84- 89- 93- 99- 108- 130- 176- 258-
2hPG (mg/dL) 39- 8- 90- 99- 110- 125- 155- 218- 304- 385-
HbA1c (%) 2.2- 4.7- 4.9- 5.1- 5.4- 5.6- 6.0- 6.3- 8.5- 10.3-

B

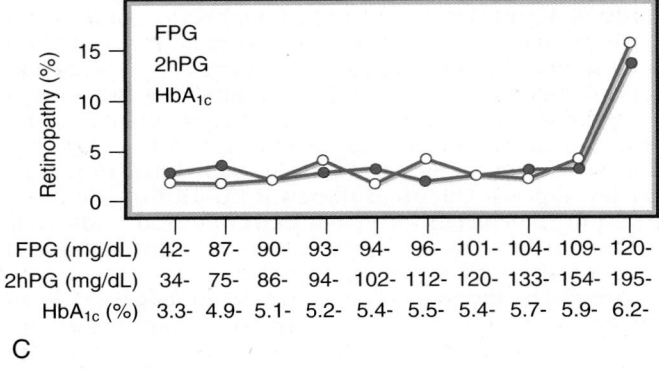

FPG (mg/dL) 42- 87- 90- 93- 94- 96- 101- 104- 109- 120-
2hPG (mg/dL) 34- 75- 86- 94- 102- 112- 120- 133- 154- 195-
HbA1c (%) 3.3- 4.9- 5.1- 5.2- 5.4- 5.5- 5.4- 5.7- 5.9- 6.2-

C

Figure 31-1 Prediction of retinopathy by parameters of glucose control by standard tests. (American Diabetes Association consensus): **A,** Fasting plasma glucose (FPG); **B,** 2-hour plasma glucose (2hPG); **C,** glycosylated hemoglobin (HbA1c).

TABLE 31-3
Major Risk Factors for Type 2 Diabetes

- Overweight (BMI ≥25 kg/m^2 or ≥23 kg/m^2 in Asian Americans)
- Physical inactivity
- First-degree relative with diabetes
- Member of a high-risk ethnic population (e.g., African American, Latino, Native American, Asian American, Pacific Islander)
- Female with a history of delivering a baby weighing >9 lb or prior diagnosis of GDM
- Hypertension (≥140/90 mm Hg or on therapy for hypertension)
- HDL cholesterol level <35 mg/dL (0.90 mmol/L) or triglyceride level >250 mg/dL (2.82 mmol/L) or both
- Female with polycystic ovary syndrome
- Hemoglobin A1c ≥5.7%, impaired glucose tolerance, or impaired fasting glucose on previous testing
- Other clinical conditions associated with insulin resistance (e.g., severe obesity, acanthosis nigricans)
- History of cardiovascular disease
- Age over 45 years

BMI, body mass index; GDM, gestational diabetes mellitus; HDL, high-density lipoprotein.
Modified from American Diabetes Association. Standards of medical care in diabetes—2015. *Diabetes Care.* 2015;38:s1-s93.

TABLE 31-4
Summary of Major Recommendations for Screening for Type 2 Diabetes Mellitus

- Testing to detect T2DM and to assess risk for future diabetes should be considered in asymptomatic adults of any age who are overweight or obese (BMI ≥25 kg/m^2 or ≥23 kg/m^2 in Asian Americans) and who have one or more additional risk factors for diabetes (see Table 31-3).
- In those without risk factors for T2DM, testing should begin at age 30-45 yr.
- If test results are normal, repeat testing should be carried out at 3- to 5-yr intervals.
- Any of the following tests is appropriate: HbA1c, FPG, 2-hr 75-g OGTT.
- In those found to have increased risk for future diabetes, identify and, if appropriate, treat other CVD risk factors.

BMI, body mass index; CVD, cardiovascular disease; FPG, fasting plasma glucose; HbA1c, glycosylated hemoglobin; OGTT, oral glucose tolerance test; T2DM, type 2 diabetes mellitus.
Modified from references American Diabetes Association. Standards of medical care in diabetes—2015. *Diabetes Care.* 2015;38:s1-s93; and Kahn R, Alperin P, Eddy D, et al. Age at initiation and frequency of screening to detect type 2 diabetes: a cost-effectiveness analysis. *Lancet.* 2010;375: 1365-1374.

increased risk for coronary heart disease, stroke, and peripheral vascular disease. Delay in the diagnosis of T2DM causes an increase in microvascular and macrovascular disease. In addition, affected individuals have a greater likelihood of having dyslipidemia, hypertension, and obesity. Therefore, it is important for the clinician to screen for diabetes in a cost-effective manner in subjects who demonstrate major risk factors for diabetes as summarized in Table 31-3. Recent modeling studies based on the U.S. population suggest that universal screening programs coupled with guideline-based therapy for T2DM is cost-effective when initiated between the ages of 30 and 45 and subsequently conducted every 3 to 5 years.[9] In a systematic review of 16 studies, for people with an HbA1c 6.0% to 6.5%, the 5-year risk of developing diabetes is 25% to 50%, a 20-fold excess risk compared to those with an HbA1c of 5%.[10] Recommendations for screening are summarized in Table 31-4. The pivotal role of screening to identify individuals at high risk in prevention strategies for T2DM is discussed at the end of this chapter.

PATHOGENESIS

The pathogenesis of T2DM is complex and involves the interaction of genetic and environmental factors. A number of environmental factors have been shown to play a critical role in the development of the disease, particularly excessive caloric intake leading to obesity and a sedentary lifestyle. The clinical presentation is also heterogeneous, with a wide range in age at onset, severity of associated hyperglycemia, and degree of obesity. From a pathophysiologic standpoint, persons with T2DM consistently demonstrate three cardinal abnormalities:

- Resistance to the action of insulin in peripheral tissues, particularly muscle and fat but also liver
- Defective insulin secretion, particularly in response to a glucose stimulus
- Increased glucose production by the liver

It has been suggested that the list of cardinal abnormalities in diabetes should be expanded to eight, adding accelerated lipolysis in the fat cell, incretin hormone deficiency and resistance, hyperglucagonemia, increased renal tubular reabsorption, and the role of the central nervous system (CNS) in metabolic regulation.[11]

Although the precise way in which genetic, environmental, and pathophysiologic factors interact to lead to the clinical onset of T2DM is not known, understanding of these processes has increased substantially. With the exception of specific monogenic forms of the disease that might result from defects largely confined to the pathways that regulate insulin action in muscle, liver, and fat or defects in insulin secretory function in the pancreatic beta cell, it is currently believed that the common forms of T2DM are polygenic in nature and are caused by a combination of insulin resistance, abnormal insulin secretion, and other factors.

From a pathophysiologic standpoint, it is the inability of the pancreatic beta cell to adapt to the reductions in insulin sensitivity that occur over a lifetime that precipitates the onset of T2DM. The most common factors that place an increased secretory burden on the beta cell are puberty, pregnancy, a sedentary lifestyle, and overeating leading to weight gain. An underlying genetic predisposition appears to be a critical factor in determining the frequency with which beta cell failure occurs.

Genetic Factors in the Development of Type 2 Diabetes Mellitus

Genetically, T2DM consists of monogenic and polygenic forms.[12,13] The monogenic forms, although relatively uncommon, are nevertheless important, and a number of the genes involved have been identified and characterized. The genes involved in the common polygenic forms of the disorder have been far more difficult to identify and characterize.

Monogenic Forms of Diabetes

In the monogenic forms of diabetes, the gene involved is both necessary and sufficient to cause disease. In other words, environmental factors play little or no role in determining whether a genetically predisposed person develops clinical diabetes. The monogenic forms of diabetes usually are diagnosed in younger patients, often in the first 2 to 3 decades of life; however, if only mild, asymptomatic elevations in blood glucose occur, the diagnosis may be missed until later in life.

The monogenic forms of diabetes are summarized in Table 31-5 and can be divided into those in which the mechanism is a defect in insulin secretion and those that involve defective responses to insulin or insulin resistance.

Monogenic Forms of Diabetes Associated With Insulin Resistance

Mutations in the Insulin Receptor. Numerous mutations have been identified in the insulin receptor gene in various insulin-resistant patients.[14] At least three clinical syndromes are caused by mutations in the insulin receptor gene. *Type A insulin resistance* is defined by the presence of insulin resistance, acanthosis nigricans, and hyperandrogenism.[15] Patients with *leprechaunism* have multiple abnormalities, including intrauterine growth retardation, fasting hypoglycemia, and death within the first 1 to 2 years of life.[16-18] The *Rabson-Mendenhall syndrome* is associ-

TABLE 31-5
Monogenic Forms of Diabetes

Forms Associated With Insulin Resistance

Mutations in the insulin receptor gene
Type A insulin resistance
Leprechaunism
Rabson-Mendenhall syndrome
Lipoatrophic diabetes
Mutations in the PPARγ gene

Forms Associated With Defective Insulin Secretion

Mutations in insulin or proinsulin genes
Mitochondrial gene mutations
Maturity-onset diabetes of the young (MODY)
  HNF-4α (MODY 1)
  Glucokinase (MODY 2)
  HNF-1α (MODY 3)
  IPF1 (MODY 4)
  HNF-1β (MODY 5)
  NeuroD1/BETA2 (MODY 6)

HNF, hepatocyte nuclear factor; IPF, insulin promoter factor; NeuroD1/BETA2, neurogenic differentiation 1/beta cell E-box *trans*-activator 2; PPAR, peroxisome proliferator-activated receptor.

ated with short stature, protuberant abdomen, and abnormalities of teeth and nails; pineal hyperplasia was a characteristic in the original description of this syndrome.[19]

These mutations impair receptor function by a number of different mechanisms, including decreasing the number of receptors expressed on the cell surface, such as by decreasing the rate of receptor biosynthesis (class 1), accelerating the rate of receptor degradation (class 5), or inhibiting the transport of receptors to the plasma membrane (class 2). The intrinsic function of the receptor may be abnormal if the affinity of insulin binding is reduced (class 3) or if receptor tyrosine kinase is inactivated (class 4). The insulin resistance that is associated with insulin receptor mutations can be severe, manifesting in the neonatal period (e.g., leprechaunism and Rabson-Mendenhall syndrome), or it can occur in a milder form in adulthood, leading to insulin-resistant diabetes with marked hyperinsulinemia, acanthosis nigricans, and hyperandrogenism.

Lipoatrophic Diabetes. In another monogenic form of diabetes, lipoatrophic diabetes, severe insulin resistance is associated with lipoatrophy and lipodystrophy. This form of diabetes is characterized by a paucity of fat, insulin resistance, and hypertriglyceridemia.[20] The disease has several genetic forms, including face-sparing partial lipoatrophy (the Dunnigan or Koberling-Dunnigan syndrome), an autosomal dominant form caused by mutations in the lamin A/C gene,[21] and congenital generalized lipoatrophy (the Seip-Berardinelli syndrome), an autosomal recessive form that appears to be due to mutations in either 1-acyl-*sn*-glycerol-3-phosphate acyltransferase-2 (AGPAT2) or in the seipin gene product.[22,23]

Mutations in Peroxisome Proliferator-Activated Receptor-γ. It has been demonstrated that mutations in the transcription factor peroxisome proliferator-activated receptor-γ (PPARγ) can cause T2DM of early onset (familial lipodystrophy type 3).[24] Two different heterozygous mutations were identified in the ligand-binding domain of PPARγ in three subjects with severe insulin resistance. In the PPARγ crystal structure, the mutations destabilize helix 12, which mediates *trans*-activation. Both receptor mutants showed markedly decreased transcriptional activation and inhibited the action of coexpressed wild-type PPARγ in a dominant negative manner. A Dutch kindred with a 14A → G mutation within the promoter of the PPARγ4 isoform, which results in decreased expression but no qualitative protein abnormalities, has been described.[25]

A common amino acid polymorphism (Pro12Ala) in PPARγ has been associated with T2DM. People homozygous for the Pro12 allele are more insulin resistant than those with one Ala12 allele and have a 1.25-fold increased risk of diabetes. There is also evidence for interaction between this polymorphism and fatty acids, linking this locus with diet. A second polymorphism, C161 → T, has been linked to insulin resistance in Hispanic and non-Hispanic white women.[26]

Neonatal Diabetes. Newborns may have permanent or transient neonatal diabetes. The prevalence of all causes of neonatal diabetes has been estimated to be between 1 in 100,000 and 1 in 300,000 live births. Transient neonatal diabetes usually resolves between 6 and 12 months of life. If the onset is before 6 months of age, a genetic reason is the most likely underlying cause. The presence of hyperglycemia is often undetected, and the diagnosis is then made when the clinical condition deteriorates due to marked hyperglycemia with or without ketoacidosis. The morbidity rate is high. Associated features include low birth weight below the 10th percentile (especially in the absence of maternal diabetes), developmental delay, learning disorders, speech disorders, muscle weakness especially with climbing stairs, and seizures. Some children have been diagnosed with attention deficit disorder (ADD) as well. Occasionally, multiple family members are also found to have early-onset, relapsing, or nonobese young adult appearance of diabetes, but most cases are sporadic.

Etiology. The most common cause of relapsing transient neonatal diabetes is the uniparental disomy 6 chromosome abnormality (UPD6), which can also be caused by methylation defects in this region of the chromosome. Mutations in the *ABCC8* gene or, less commonly, in *KCNJ11*, both components of the adenosine triphosphate (ATP)-sensitive potassium channel (K_{ATP} channel), may also be responsible. The K_{ATP} channel is well described as a key molecular switch in the beta cell that closes in response to generation of ATP after glucose metabolism. If the channel does not close at physiologic levels of glucose, hypoinsulinism and hyperglycemia result. This causes severe diabetes with low or negative C-peptide and ketosis in the first few weeks of life.

Permanent neonatal diabetes is most often caused by mutations in *KCNJ11* and less often by mutations in *ABCC8*. The K_{ATP} channel, composed of the beta-cell protein sulfonylurea receptor (SUR1) and inward-rectifying potassium channel subunit Kir6.2, is a key regulator of insulin release. It is inhibited by the binding of adenine nucleotides to subunit Kir6.2, which closes the channel, and it is activated by nucleotide binding or hydrolysis on SUR1, which opens the channel. The balance of these opposing actions determines the low open-channel probability, P_O, which controls the excitability of pancreatic beta cells.[27] It has been hypothesized that activating mutations in *ABCC8*, which encodes SUR1, can cause neonatal diabetes. Mutations in these genes that cause the opposite condition, decreased channel function, are a cause of familial hyperinsulinemia with hypoglycemia.[1,19,20]

After *KCNJ11* mutations, the second most common group of causes of permanent neonatal diabetes is mutations in the insulin gene *(INS)* itself. These mutations are also rare causes of young adult–onset T2DM and ketosis-prone type 1b diabetes, usually with negative diabetes-associated autoantibodies.[8] More than 200 cases have been identified worldwide. Rarely, homozygous gene mutations in glucokinase *(GCK)* and transcription factor genes lead to insulin insufficiency or failure of development of the endocrine pancreas or of the entire pancreas.

Therapy. Many of the mutations in *KCNJ11* and *ABCC8* can be treated with a relatively high dose of sulfonylureas. However, it is critical that this be done after a mutation has been documented, because the protocol involves high doses of sulfonylureas (administered in divided doses and off-label in the United States for children) and simultaneous aggressive insulin withdrawal. Collaboration with or referral to a center with experience in this treatment is highly encouraged because of potential side effects and other adverse effects. There is no therapy at this time for either UPD6 or *INS* mutations other than insulin replacement in the manner used for the treatment of T1DM.

Most of these mutations are heterozygous and dominant (i.e., each child of an affected individual has a 50% chance of having the disease). In the case of unaffected parents with one affected child, several studies have reported germline mosaicism as a known or possible cause of the presence of the syndrome in several siblings in one family. Therefore, the risk that each subsequent child will have neonatal diabetes can range from less than 10% to 50%, depending on the presence of mosaicism in the gametes.

Monogenic Forms of Diabetes Associated With Defects in Insulin Secretion

Mutant Insulin Syndromes. The first syndrome associated with diabetes to be characterized in terms of the clinical picture, genetic mechanisms, and clinical pathophysiology was that associated with mutant insulin or proinsulin.[28] Persons with this disorder present clinically with a mild, non–insulin-dependent form of diabetes. Affected persons characteristically have marked hyperinsulinemia on routine insulin assays. Increases in the concentration of insulin in association with diabetes usually indicate insulin resistance, but in this syndrome, insulin resistance can be easily excluded because the patients respond normally to administration of exogenous insulin. Characterization of the insulin by high-performance liquid chromatography (HPLC) reveals that the hyperinsulinemia results from the presence of the abnormal insulin or proinsulin and related breakdown products. The increased concentrations of insulin appear to be related to the presence of mutations in regions of the insulin molecule that are important for receptor binding, particularly the carboxy-terminus of the insulin B chain.

Because the liver is the major site of insulin clearance and first-pass hepatic insulin uptake and degradation are mediated by the insulin receptor, mutant forms of insulin with diminished insulin receptor binding ability are cleared more slowly from the circulation, and this reduction in insulin clearance leads to hyperinsulinemia. Alternatively, mutations in proinsulin can reduce the conversion of proinsulin to insulin, leading to accumulation of proinsulin.[29,30] Because proinsulin is cleared more slowly from the circulation than insulin, proinsulin levels increase. Proinsulin cross-reacts in most commercially available assays, and this insulin-like immunoreactivity can be characterized as being related to the presence of proinsulin (rather than insulin only) by HPLC or by the use of assays that are specific for insulin and proinsulin.

A patient with a mutation in prohormone convertase 1, one of the enzymes responsible for the conversion of proinsulin to insulin, has been described.[31]

Mitochondrial Diabetes. An A-to-G transition in the mitochondrial transfer RNA Leu(UUR) gene at base pair 3243 has been shown to be associated with maternally transmitted diabetes and sensorineural hearing loss.[32] In other subjects, this mutation is associated with diabetes and the syndrome of mitochondrial myopathy, encephalopathy, lactic acidosis, and stroke-like episodes (MELAS syndrome). The mitochondrion plays a key role in the regulation of insulin secretion, particularly in response to glucose. Abnormal insulin secretion may be seen in subjects with this mitochondrial mutation, even if diabetes has not yet developed and glucose tolerance is normal or impaired.[33]

Maturity-Onset Diabetes of the Young. Maturity-onset diabetes of the young (MODY) is a genetically and clinically heterogeneous group of disorders characterized by nonketotic diabetes mellitus, an autosomal dominant mode of inheritance, onset usually before 25 years of age and often in childhood or adolescence, and a primary defect in pancreatic beta-cell function. MODY has been reviewed[34,35] and the information contained in those reviews is summarized here.

Etiology and Clinical Presentation. MODY can result from mutations in any one of at least six different genes. One of these genes *(GCK)* encodes the glycolytic enzyme glucokinase; mutations in this gene cause MODY2.[36] The other five genes encode transcription factors. MODY1 is associated with mutations in the gene for hepatocyte nuclear factor-4α *(HNF4A)*[37]; MODY3 with mutations in *HNF1A*[38]; MODY4 with mutations in pancreatic and duodenal homeobox 1 *(PDX1)*, which encodes insulin promoter factor 1 (IPF1)[39]; MODY5 with mutations in *HNF1B*[40]; and MODY6 with mutations in *NEUROD1*, which encodes the neurogenic differentiation 1/beta cell E-box *trans*-activator 2 (NeuroD1/BETA2).[41] All of these genes are expressed in the insulin-producing pancreatic beta cell, and heterozygous mutations cause diabetes related to beta-cell dysfunction. Abnormalities in liver and kidney function occur in some forms of MODY, reflecting expression of the transcription factors in these tissues. Nongenetic factors that affect insulin sensitivity (infection, puberty, pregnancy, and rarely obesity) can trigger diabetes onset and affect the severity of hyperglycemia in MODY but do not play a significant role in the development of MODY.

The most common clinical presentation of MODY is a mild, asymptomatic increase in blood glucose in a child, adolescent, or young adult with a prominent family history of diabetes, often in successive generations, that suggests an autosomal dominant mode of inheritance. Some patients have mild hyperglycemia for many years, whereas others have varying degrees of impaired glucose tolerance (IGT) for several years before the onset of persistent hyperglycemia.[34] The diagnosis may not be made until adulthood even though the elevation in plasma glucose has been present for many years. Prospective testing indicates that in most patients the disease onset occurs in childhood or adolescence. In some patients, there may be a rapid progression to overt asymptomatic or symptomatic hyperglycemia, necessitating therapy with an oral hypoglycemic drug or insulin. The presence of persistently normal plasma glucose levels in subjects with mutations in any of the known MODY genes is unusual, and most eventually experience diabetes (with the exception of many patients with glucokinase mutations; see later discussion).

Although the exact prevalence of MODY is not known, current estimates suggest that MODY might account for 1% to 5% of all cases of diabetes in the United States and other industrialized countries.[34] Several clinical characteristics distinguish patients with MODY from those with T2DM, including a prominent family history of diabetes in three or more generations, young age at presentation, and absence of obesity.

Functional Effects of MODY Genes. The identification of several genes associated with diabetes has provided a unique opportunity to characterize the pathophysiologic mecha-

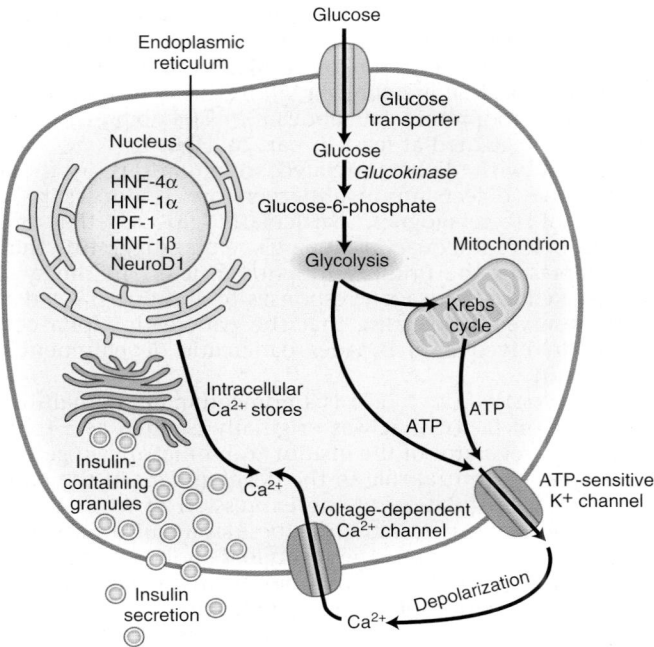

Figure 31-2 Model of a pancreatic beta cell and the proteins implicated in maturity-onset diabetes of the young. ATP, adenosine triphosphate; HNF, hepatocyte nuclear factor; IPF, insulin promoter factor; NeuroD1, neurogenic differentiation 1. (From Fajans SS, Bell GI, Polonsky KS. Molecular mechanisms and clinical pathophysiology of maturity-onset diabetes of the young. *N Engl J Med.* 2001;345:971.)

nisms by which genetic mutations can lead to an increase in the plasma glucose concentration. All the susceptibility genes identified to date cause impaired insulin secretory responses to glucose, although the mechanisms differ.

Glucokinase. Glucokinase is expressed at its highest levels in the pancreatic beta cell and the liver. It catalyzes the transfer of phosphate from ATP to glucose to generate glucose 6-phosphate (Fig. 31-2). This reaction is the first rate-limiting step in glucose metabolism. Glucokinase functions as the glucose sensor in the beta cell by controlling the rate of entry of glucose into the glycolytic pathway (glucose phosphorylation) and its subsequent metabolism. In the liver, glucokinase plays a key role in the ability to store glucose as glycogen, particularly in the postprandial state.

Heterozygous mutations leading to partial deficiency of glucokinase are associated with MODY, and homozygous mutations resulting in complete deficiency of this enzyme lead to permanent neonatal diabetes mellitus.[42] As predicted by the physiologic functions of glucokinase, the increase in plasma glucose concentrations in patients with this form of diabetes results from a combination of reduced glucose-induced insulin secretion from the pancreatic beta cell and reduced glycogen storage in the liver after glucose ingestion.

Liver-Enriched Transcription Factors. The transcription factors HNF-1α, HNF-1β, and HNF-4α play a key role in the tissue-specific regulation of gene expression in the liver[43] and are also expressed in other tissues, including pancreatic islets, kidney, and genital tissues. HNF-1α and HNF-1β are members of the homeodomain-containing family of transcription factors, and HNF-4α is an orphan nuclear receptor.[43,44]

HNF-1α, HNF-1β, and HNF-4α make up part of an interacting network of transcription factors that function together to control gene expression during embryonic development and in adult tissues in which they are coexpressed. In the pancreatic beta cell, these transcription factors regulate the expression of the insulin gene as well as proteins involved in glucose transport and metabolism and mitochondrial metabolism (all linked to insulin secretion) and lipoprotein metabolism.[45] The expression of HNF-1α is regulated at least in part by HNF-4α.

Persons with diabetes related to mutations in these genes have defects in insulin secretory responses to a variety of secretagogues, particularly glucose, that are present before the onset of hyperglycemia, suggesting that they represent the primary functional defect in the syndrome. Reduced glucagon responses to arginine have also been observed, suggesting that the pancreatic alpha cell is also involved in a broader pancreatic developmental abnormality.

Insulin Promoter Factor 1. IPF1 is a homeodomain-containing transcription factor that was originally isolated as a transcriptional regulator of the insulin and somatostatin genes. It also plays a central role in the development of the pancreas and in regulation of the expression of a variety of pancreatic islet genes, including (besides insulin) the genes encoding glucokinase, islet amyloid polypeptide, and glucose transporter 2. IPF1 also appears to mediate glucose-induced stimulation of insulin gene transcription.[46]

A child born with pancreatic agenesis was shown to have a mutation in IPF1 that lacked the homeodomain required for DNA binding and nuclear localization. Heterozygous carriers of an IPF1 mutation from the same kindred developed an early-onset autosomal dominant form of diabetes (i.e., MODY) caused by dominant negative inhibition of transcription of the insulin gene and other beta cell–specific genes regulated by the mutant IPF1.[47] Additional IPF1 mutations have been discovered in pedigrees with late-onset T2DM.[48] Therefore, mutations in IPF1 can cause a range of phenotypic manifestations, depending on whether the subjects have homozygous or heterozygous mutations and the severity of the functional effects.

Neurogenic Differentiation-1 Transcription Factor. The basic helix-loop-helix transcription factor NeuroD1/BETA2 was isolated on the basis of its ability to activate transcription of the insulin gene, and it is required for normal pancreatic islet development. Heterozygous mutations in NeuroD1 have been described in patients with diabetes.[41,49] It appears that mutations in NeuroD1 are a rare cause of MODY because studies in different populations have failed to detect mutations in NeuroD1 even in subjects with a MODY phenotype.

Genetics of the Polygenic Forms of Type 2 Diabetes Mellitus

The common polygenic form of T2DM has complex pathophysiology, and genetic and environmental factors play a major role. The phenotypic manifestations of the disease are also complex and include resistance to the action of insulin in muscle, fat, and liver; defects in insulin secretory responses from the pancreatic beta cell; and increases in hepatic glucose production. However, the primary defect or defects responsible for the development of the syndrome remain elusive and are not likely to be defined until more is known about the genes responsible for diabetes and the nature of the gene-environment interactions that are ultimately responsible for development of the disorder in predisposed persons.

Insulin resistance is present in persons predisposed to T2DM before the onset of hyperglycemia, and this finding has been interpreted by some to indicate that insulin resistance is the primary abnormality that is responsible for the development of T2DM. However, defective beta-cell function is also present before the onset of T2DM when IGT is present and in first-degree relatives of persons with T2DM who have completely normal plasma glucose concentrations. Therefore, although there is still controversy about whether insulin resistance or abnormal insulin secretion represents the primary defect in T2DM, there is general consensus that both defects are present in essentially all subjects with the disorder, often from an early preclinical stage.

In recent years, and particularly since 2007, there have been dramatic advances in understanding of the genetic basis of T2DM. Earlier genetic studies relied either on the candidate gene approach, in which the search for diabetes genes was dictated by the prevailing understanding of the pathways involved in glucose regulation, or on linkage studies. Linkage studies involve defining regions of chromosomal DNA that are shared to excess by affected family members. Parents are genotyped at a particular marker, and the offspring are scored for sharing of zero, one, or two alleles inherited from their parents. Markers are genotyped in family members in the regions of polymorphic repeats called *microsatellites* or *simple tandem repeats*.

Although these two approaches did identify important diabetes genes, the application of genome-wide association studies (GWAS) has led to a dramatic increase in the number of diabetes genes that have been identified. GWAS use an unbiased interrogation of the entire genome in cases and controls to determine which single-nucleotide polymorphisms (SNPs) are associated with disease. The development of this approach depended on a number of factors including the completion of the Human Genome Project, the genotyping of 3.8 million SNPs and identification of haplotype-tagged SNPs by the International HapMap Project, the development of affordable, high-throughput genotyping technologies, and the availability of multiple analytic tools for the cleaning,[50] mining, and interpretation of very large datasets. The genes that have been implicated in the pathogenesis of T2DM have been summarized in an excellent review by Grarup and associates[51] and are depicted in Figure 31-3. This is a rapidly changing field, and it is certain that the list of diabetes genes will increase. The following sections provide a brief summary of the genes that have been implicated in the pathogenesis of T2DM.[52-54]

Calpain-10 Gene

The linkage between calpain-10 and T2DM first observed by a group headed by Graeme Bell[55] was completely unexpected and was based purely on the application of sophisticated methods of analysis in a genetic study rather than on any novel physiologic insights. A number of studies have corroborated the initial observation that genetic variation in *CAPN10*, the calpain-10 gene, increases the risk of T2DM, but others have not. However, two meta-analyses of all the published data supported a role for this gene in diabetes susceptibility. Song and colleagues,[56] after analyzing 11 studies, showed an odds ratio for T2DM of 1.19 comparing persons with the G/G genotype of UCSNP43 in *CAPN10* with all carriers of the A allele. Weedon's group[57] calculated an odds ratio of 1.17 for UCSNP44.

Calpains are Ca^{2+}-dependent cysteine proteases.[58] The precise physiologic mechanisms by which genetic variation in *CAPN10* leads to altered susceptibility to diabetes are still being characterized. Pharmacologic inhibition of calpain activity results in insulin resistance and impaired insulin secretion.[59,60] Studies in mice have led to similar conclusions.[61,62] Therefore, calpains play a role in regulating insulin secretion and insulin action.

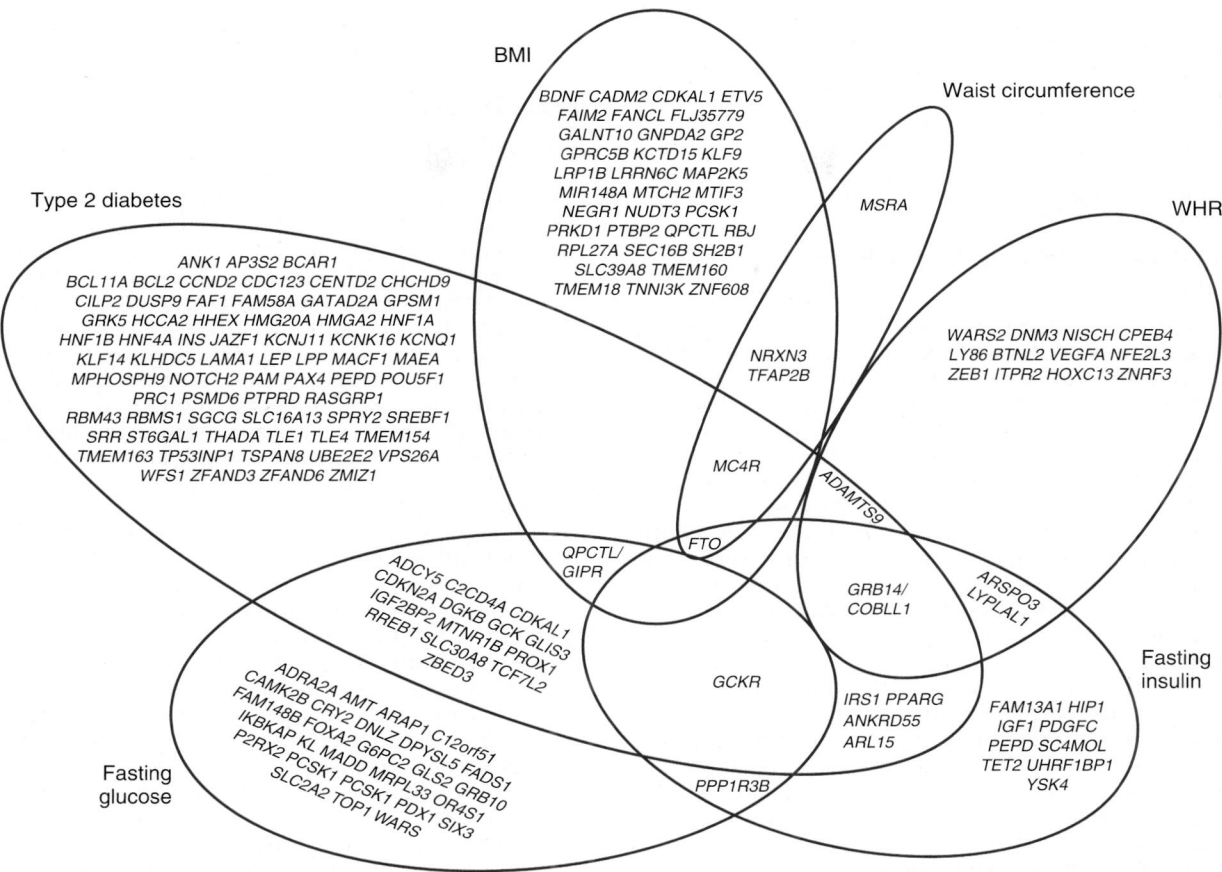

Figure 31-3 Venn diagram of intersection between loci associated at genome-wide significance with type 2 diabetes, measures of adiposity and glucose homeostasis. Genome-wide significant associations for six metabolic traits are shown. Gene symbols shown in the plot are by convention the closest gene and not necessarily the functional gene. BMI, body mass index; WHR, waist-to-hip ratio. (Redrawn from Grarup N, Sandholt CH, Hansen T, Pedersen O. Genetic susceptibility to type 2 diabetes and obesity: from genome wide association studies to rare variants and beyond. *Diabetologia.* 2014;57:1528-1541.)

Kir6.2 Gene

The beta-cell K_{ATP} channel is composed of two subunits, SUR1 and Kir6.2, as discussed earlier.[63] The missense mutation Glu23Lys (E23K) in *KCNJ11*, the gene encoding Kir6.2, has been associated with increased risk of T2DM in some but not all studies,[57,64-66] similar to what was observed with *CAPN10*. Meta-analyses have shown that the E23K variant affects diabetes risk.[57,67] The study by Love-Gregory and coworkers[67] suggested that the K allele of the E23K polymorphism increases the risk of T2DM by an average of 13% and that the KK homozygote is at greatest risk (relative risk, 1.28). 't Hart and colleagues examined the influence of the E23K variant of Kir6.2 on the insulin secretory responses to glucose and found no effect. However, they did not consider the confounding effect of insulin resistance.[68]

Peroxisome Proliferator-Activated Receptor-γ Gene

PPARγ is a member of the PPAR subfamily of nuclear receptors. It is an important regulator of lipid and glucose homeostasis and cellular differentiation. Although PPARγ is most abundantly expressed in adipose tissue, it is also expressed in the pancreatic beta cell, and targeted elimination of the receptor in the beta cell leads to a blunting of the normal increase in beta-cell mass that occurs on a high-fat diet.[69] Meta-analyses of all published studies performed by Altshuler and colleagues[70] in 2000 showed that the missense mutation Pro12Ala (P12A) in *PPARG* (the gene encoding PPARγ2) is associated with decreased risk for T2DM (estimated risk ratio for the alanine allele, 0.79).

Hepatocyte Nuclear Factor-4α Gene

The role of HNF-4α in the development of MODY has been clearly documented. Mutations in this gene lead to abnormalities in insulin secretion. Studies involving various populations[71-73] have demonstrated that genetic variation in the region of an alternative promoter for the *HNF4A* gene is associated with increased risk of T2DM. It is likely that these at-risk polymorphisms alter expression of *HNF4A*, thereby causing increased susceptibility to T2DM.

Transcription Factor 7–like 2 Gene

Grant and colleagues[74] genotyped 228 microsatellite markers in Icelandic patients with T2DM and in control subjects. A microsatellite, DG10S478, within intron 3 of the transcription factor 7–like 2 gene (*TCF7L2*; formerly *TCF4*) was associated with T2DM. This was replicated in a Danish cohort and in a U.S. cohort. Compared with non-carriers, heterozygous and homozygous carriers of the at-risk alleles (38% and 7% of the population, respectively) have relative risks of 1.45 and 2.41. This corresponds to a population attributable risk of 21%. The *TCF7L2* gene product is a high-mobility group box containing transcription factors previously implicated in blood glucose homeostasis. It is thought to act through regulation of proglucagon gene expression in enteroendocrine cells via the Wnt signaling pathway. Of the common variants that determine diabetes risk, variants at the *TCF7L2* locus still have the greatest impact.

In a follow-up study, Florez and colleagues[75] observed that specific polymorphisms in *TCF7L2* increase the risk of progression from IGT to T2DM, and this effect is mediated through a reduction of glucose-induced insulin secretion.

Diabetes Genes Identified by Genome-Wide Association Studies

GWAS continue to identify variants that determine genetic risk of T2DM and to define the genetic architecture of the disease. Grarup and associates[51] have summarized the current state of the field. As of the beginning of 2014, 90 genetic loci have been established as associated with risk of T2DM or associated with metabolic traits strongly associated with T2DM. Figure 31-3 depicts the intersection between loci associated at genome-wide significance with T2DM and five metabolic traits strongly associated with T2DM including body mass index (BMI), waist circumference, waist-to-hip ratio, fasting insulin, and fasting glucose. The figure demonstrates that there is substantial but not complete overlap in the loci significantly associated with these traits.

Based on these advances, the following general comments can be made regarding the genetics of T2DM:

1. A large number of genes are associated with increased susceptibility to this disease. Surprisingly, although the total number of loci identified to date is large in the aggregate, they account for a small proportion (estimated at no more than 5% to 10%) of the total genetic risk for diabetes in the population. In the search for this missing heritability increasing attention is being given to the *rare variant hypothesis*, which states that common diseases are due to variants in rare alleles with large effects.
2. The genes identified to date individually lead to a modest increase in the risk of diabetes. Persons with these individual polymorphisms have odds ratios between 1.10 and 1.45 when compared with individuals who do not have the at-risk polymorphisms.
3. The presence of multiple at-risk polymorphisms in a single individual substantially increases the risk of developing diabetes.
4. In the initial GWAS a substantial proportion of the genetic variants associated with increased risk for diabetes appear to do so by inhibiting insulin secretion. Few variants were shown to have an effect on insulin sensitivity.[76,77] In recent studies with larger sample sizes the number of SNPs associated with increased insulin sensitivity has increased and at least some of these effects on insulin sensitivity are not mediated by obesity.[78,79]
5. The majority of the SNPs associated with risk of T2DM appear to reside in noncoding regions of the chromatin. Studies have shown that these allelic variations exist in open chromatin regions alternatively called *stretch enhancers*,[80] which appear to be bound by proteins. Stretch enhancers across the genome are cell type specific and are located near and associated with increased expression of genes involved in cell-specific (as opposed to housekeeping) processes. Importantly, the allelic variations associated with T2DM are in stretch enhancer regions, which are highly enriched in pancreatic islets, consistent with the observation that the SNPs associated with T2DM affect insulin secretion.

The application of additional techniques of exomic and whole genome sequencing will certainly provide additional insights into the genetic architecture of T2DM. Such studies are under way at a number of centers.

Insulin Signaling

Insulin signaling is initiated through binding and activation of its cell-surface receptor and initiates a cascade of phosphorylation and dephosphorylation events, second-messenger generation, and protein-protein interactions that result in diverse metabolic events in almost every tissue (Fig. 31-4). The insulin receptor consists of two insulin-binding α-subunits and two catalytically active β-subunits that are disulfide linked into an $\alpha_2\beta_2$ heterotetrameric complex. Insulin binds to the extracellular α-subunits, activating the intracellular tyrosine kinase domain of the β-subunit.[81] One receptor β-subunit phosphorylates its partner on specific tyrosine residues that may have distinct functions such as stimulation of intermolecular association of signaling molecules such as Shc and Grb, IRS1 through IRS4, Shc adapter protein isoforms, and SIRP (signal regulatory protein) family members Gab-1, Cbl, CAP, and APS[82,83]; stimulation of mitogenesis[84]; and receptor internalization.[85]

The insulin receptor β-subunit has also been shown to undergo serine/threonine phosphorylation, which might decrease the ability of the receptor to autophosphorylate. The activities of a number of protein kinase C (PKC) isoforms that catalyze the serine or threonine phosphorylation of the insulin receptor are elevated in animal models of insulin resistance and in insulin-resistant humans.[86,87] Interventions that decrease serine phosphorylation of the insulin receptor result in increased insulin signaling.[88] Termination of the insulin-signaling event occurs when the receptor is internalized and dephosphorylated by protein tyrosine phosphatases. Increased activity of protein tyrosine phosphatase can attenuate insulin signaling while inhibition of the phosphatase maintains the activation state. Two protein tyrosine phosphatases that have been shown to negatively regulate insulin signaling, PTP1B and LAR (leukocyte antigen–related), have been reported to be elevated in insulin-resistant patients.[89,90] Conversely, disruption of PTB1B in mice resulted in a marked increase in insulin sensitivity and resistance to diet-induced obesity.[91]

Mutations in the insulin receptor are associated with rare forms of insulin resistance. These mutations affect insulin receptor number, splicing, trafficking, binding, and phosphorylation. The affected patients demonstrate severe insulin resistance, manifest as clinically diverse syndromes including the type A syndrome, leprechaunism, Rabson-Mendenhall syndrome, and lipoatrophic diabetes.[92,93]

Downstream Events After Insulin Receptor Phosphorylation

The insulin receptor substrates (IRSs) act as multifunctional docking proteins activated by tyrosine phosphorylation.[94] The IRS proteins have multiple functional domains—including pleckstrin homology (PH) and phosphotyrosine binding (PTB)—and Src homology (SH) domains that interact with other proteins to mediate the insulin-signaling events. Disruption of IRS1 in mice resulted in mild insulin resistance and growth retardation, whereas disruption of IRS2 resulted in beta-cell failure and secondary insulin resistance.[95] Serine phosphorylation of IRS proteins is an especially important target for reducing insulin signaling and is mediated by a variety of kinases, including PKC isoforms and mammalian target of rapamycin (mTOR)/S6 kinase (S6K). Serine phosphorylation on appropriate residues might increase ubiquitination and downregulation of

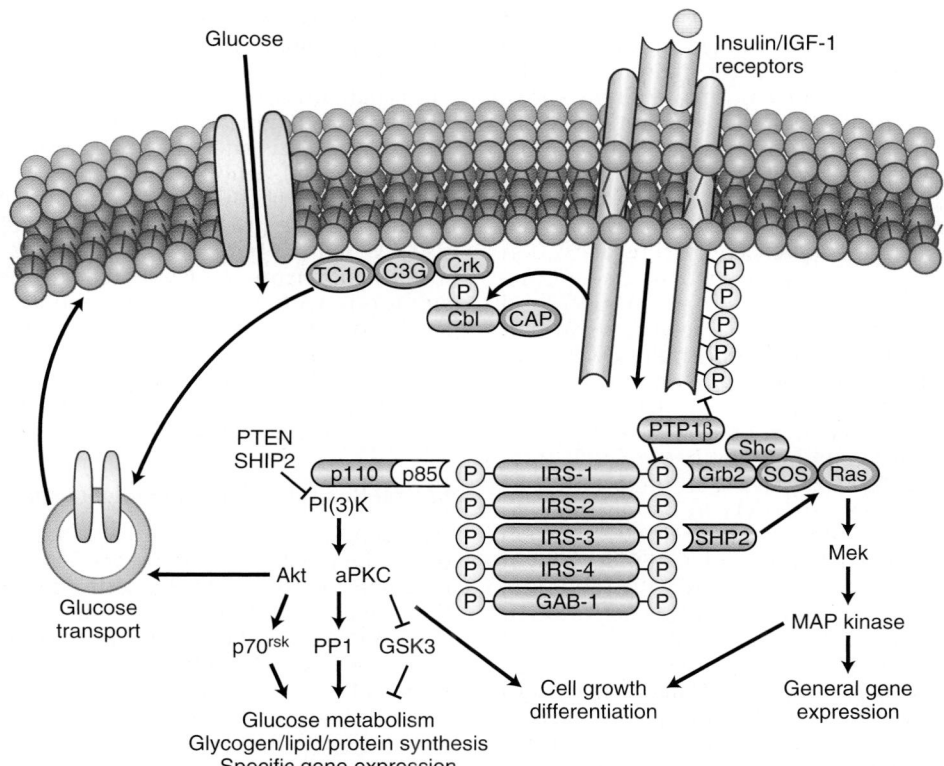

Figure 31-4 Insulin signaling. The insulin receptor is autophosphorylated on multiple tyrosine residues, allowing the docking and activation of multiple signaling molecules that mediate the increases in glucose uptake and metabolism as well as changes in protein and lipid metabolism. aPKC, atypical protein kinase C; C3G, guanine nucleotide exchange factor C3G; CAP, Cbl-associated protein; Cbl, Cas-Br-M (murine) ecotropic retroviral transforming sequence; Crk, CT10-related kinase; GAB, Grb2-associated binding protein; Grb2, growth factor receptor-bound protein 2; GSK3, glycogen synthase kinase-3; IGF, insulin-like growth factor; IRS, insulin receptor substrate; MAP, mitogen-activated protein; Mek, MAPK/ERK kinases; P, phosphate; PI(3)K, phosphatidylinositol-3-kinase; PP1, protein phosphatase I; PTEN, phosphatase and tensin homolog deleted on chromosome 10; PTP, protein tyrosine phosphatase; RAS, rat sarcoma oncogene; Shc, SH3-containing protein; SHIP2, SH2 domain–containing inositol 5-phosphatase; SHP2, SH2 domain–containing protein-tyrosine phosphatase (now called PTPN11); SOS, son of sevenless; TC10, small GTP binding protein TC10. (From Saltiel AR, Kahn CR. Insulin signalling and the regulation of glucose and lipid metabolism. *Nature.* 2001;414:799-806.)

the protein, which would result in decreased downstream signaling.[96]

Phosphoinositide 3-kinase (PI3K), which is regulated by interaction with IRS proteins, is necessary but not sufficient for stimulation of glucose transporter 4 (GLUT4)-mediated increase in glucose transport in insulin-sensitive tissues.[97] In addition, inhibition of PI3K activity with the fungal inhibitor wortmannin inhibited insulin-stimulated glucose uptake, glycogen synthesis, triglyceride accumulation, protein synthesis, and modulation of gene expression.[98] PI3K generates 3,4,5-phosphoinositol, which activates several phosphatidylinositol 3,4,5-triphosphate (PIP3)-dependent serine-threonine kinases, such as PI-dependent protein kinases 1 and 2 (PDK1 and PDK2), which in turn activate Akt, salt- and glucocorticoid-induced kinases,[99] PKC, wortmannin-sensitive and insulin-stimulated serine kinase, and others.

Akt kinase (also known as protein kinase B) exists as three distinct isoforms that are activated by phosphorylation on specific threonine and serine residues.[100,101] Full activation of Akt requires PDK1-directed phosphorylation at threonine 308 (T308) in the kinase domain (KD) followed by phosphorylation at serine 473 (S473) in the hydrophobic motif (HM) of Akt by the rictor-containing complex, mTOR complex 2 (mTORC2).[101] Activated Akt has the ability to phosphorylate proteins that regulate lipid synthesis, glycogen synthesis, protein synthesis, and apoptosis. Disruption of Akt2 results in insulin resistance and

diabetes in mice.[102] Several investigators have examined the role of PI3K and Akt in persons with insulin resistance. Studies have shown a decrease in IRS-associated PI3K[103] and Akt[104] activity in insulin-resistant skeletal muscle; however, in some patients with reduced PI3K activity, there was normal activation of Akt.[105]

A primary effect of insulin is to stimulate translocation of GLUT4 from an intracellular pool to the surface of cells, primarily in skeletal muscle, adipose tissue, and heart.[106] Akt substrate of 160 kDa (AS160) and TBC1D1 are paralog Rab family guanosine triphosphatase (GTPase)-activating proteins that have been proposed to inhibit the translocation of GLUT4 to the plasma membrane through interaction with insulin-responsive aminopeptidase (IRAP).[107] TBC1D1 appears to play a key role in exercise-regulated increase in glucose uptake.[108] Upon phosphorylation, the inhibition is relieved, contributing to the increased translocation. Although the composition and signaling pathways that converge on the intracellular GLUT4-containing vesicles to cause GLUT4 translocation are still not well understood, it appears that the number of glucose transporters in skeletal muscle of insulin-resistant persons is not changed, but the ability of insulin to effect this translocation is disrupted.[109-111]

The production of glucose by the liver is regulated primarily by the relative actions of glucagon and insulin to activate or suppress glucose production, respectively, although the nervous system[112] and glucose autoregulation of hepatic glucose production probably play less important roles.[113] The ability of insulin to reduce hepatic glucose output is an important mechanism for maintaining normal glucose tolerance.[114,115] Under normal circumstances, insulin suppresses up to 85% of glucose production in normal persons by directly inhibiting glycogenolysis, especially at lower insulin concentrations.[116] When glycogenolysis is enhanced by glucagon, the effects of insulin in suppressing hepatic glucose production may be even greater.[117] Glucagon increases glycogenolysis by activation of the classic protein kinase cascade involving adenosine monophosphate-activated protein kinase (AMPK) and phosphorylase and also increases gluconeogenesis in part by increasing transcription of phosphoenolpyruvate carboxykinase by means of the binding protein cyclic AMP (cAMP) response element–binding protein (CREB).[115,118,119]

Data suggest that the regulatory mechanisms triggered by cAMP are much more complex, with the CREB transcriptional coactivator, TORC2, playing an important role. TORC2 is specifically dephosphorylated in response to cAMP; this results in translocation of the TORC2 protein to the nucleus, allowing activation of CREB-dependent transcription of gluconeogenic enzymes.[120] In addition, CREB may increase transcription of PPARγ coactivator-1α (PGC-1α), which serves as a critical coactivator of the transcription factor forkhead box protein O1 (FOXO1), which also plays a role in the transcriptional activation of various genes associated with gluconeogenesis.[118] Recent data suggest that the nicotinamide adenine dinucleotide (NAD^+)-dependent protein deacetylase, SIRT1, can regulate gluconeogenesis. SIRT1 deacetylates PGC-1α and FOXO1, increasing their nuclear interaction with HNF4A. The PGC-1α/FOXO1/HNF4A complex is a potent activator of gluconeogenic gene transcription.[118]

Insulin decreases endogenous glucose production by direct and indirect mechanisms (Fig. 31-5).[121] In its direct action, portal insulin suppresses glucose production by inhibiting glycogenolysis through an increase in phosphodiesterase activity[122,123] or changes in the assembly of protein phosphatase complexes.[124,125] Insulin can also directly suppress gluconeogenesis by inhibiting the activation of phosphoenolpyruvate carboxykinase transcription through insulin-dependent phosphorylation of FOXO1 (and perhaps FOXA2), sequestering it in the cytoplasm.[126-129]

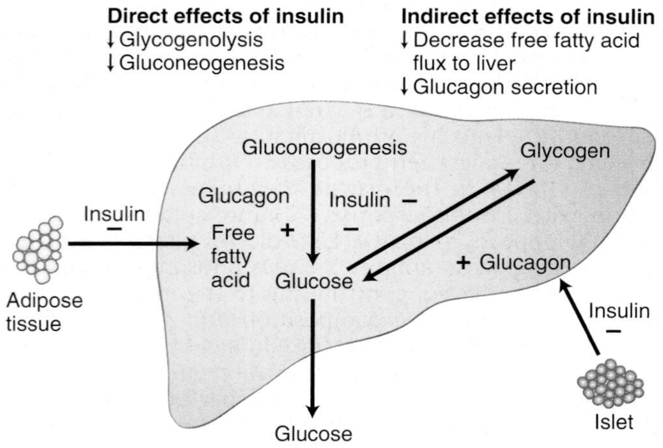

The indirect or peripheral effect of insulin in controlling glucose production by the liver is twofold. First, insulin profoundly decreases glucagon secretion by the alpha cell of the pancreas through systemic and paracrine effects.[130,131] The decrease in glucagon secretion decreases the activation of glycogenolysis and gluconeogenesis. The second important peripheral action of insulin is to decrease free fatty acid (FFA) levels by suppressing lipolysis. FFAs increase hepatic glucose production by stimulating gluconeogenesis.[132] When the reduction in plasma FFAs during a hyperinsulinemic clamp was prevented by infusion of triglyceride emulsions with heparin (which produces increased FFA levels through activation of lipoprotein lipase), insulin-mediated suppression of hepatic glucose output was reduced.[133,134] The suppression of glucagon secretion and the decrease in FFA delivery to the liver are additive in reducing liver glucose production.[135]

Central Control of Glucose Metabolism

The hypothalamus and perhaps other brain regions can sense metabolic requirements and change peripheral metabolism. Studies by Rossetti and colleagues suggested that uptake of fatty acids by the mediobasal hypothalamus decreases feeding behavior and decreases hepatic glucose production via CNS efferents.[136] Inhibition of central fatty acid oxidation results in decreased food intake and reduced glucose production, suggesting that buildup of long-chain fatty acids or their derivatives changes feeding and hepatic glucose production.

AMPK may also play a role in integrating CNS nutrient supply. AMPK is activated by cellular AMP levels and therefore is a sensor of energy supply.[137] Higher cellular energy, resulting from glucose or fatty acid surfeit, would lead to decreased activation of AMPK and its downstream target, acetyl-CoA carboxylase (ACC). ACC generates malonyl-CoA (an allosteric inhibitor of CPT1), which decreases the entry of long-chain fatty acids into the mitochondria, resulting in their buildup in the cytoplasm.

Insulin Resistance and the Risk of Type 2 Diabetes Mellitus

Insulin Resistance

The term *insulin resistance* indicates the presence of an impaired biologic response to either exogenously administered or endogenously secreted insulin. Insulin resistance is primarily manifested by decreased insulin-stimulated glucose transport and metabolism in adipocytes and skeletal muscle and impaired insulin suppression of adipocyte lipolysis and hepatic glucose output. However, it is clear that disorders of multiple metabolic pathways involving amino acids, glucose, and lipid metabolism are present in the insulin-resistant individual.

Insulin sensitivity is influenced by a number of factors, including age,[138] weight, ethnicity, body fat (especially abdominal), physical activity, and medications. Substantial data indicate that insulin resistance plays a major role in the development of IGT and diabetes. Insulin resistance is a consistent finding in patients with T2DM, and resistance is present years before the onset of diabetes.[139-144] Prospective studies have shown that insulin resistance predicts the onset of diabetes.[140,141,145] Although insulin resistance is associated with the progression to T2DM, diabetes is rarely seen in insulin-resistant persons without some degree of beta-cell dysfunction.[144] First-degree relatives of type 2 diabetics have insulin resistance even if they are not obese, implying a strong genetic component in the development of insulin resistance.[140,145,146] There is also a strong influence

Direct effects of insulin
↓ Glycogenolysis
↓ Gluconeogenesis

Indirect effects of insulin
↓ Decrease free fatty acid flux to liver
↓ Glucagon secretion

Figure 31-5 Insulin suppresses hepatic glucose production by direct and indirect mechanisms. In insulin resistance, the ability of insulin to suppress lipolysis in adipose tissue and glucagon secretion by alpha cells in the islet results in increased gluconeogenesis. In addition, insulin inhibition of glycogenolysis is impaired. Therefore, both hepatic and peripheral insulin resistance result in abnormal glucose production by the liver.

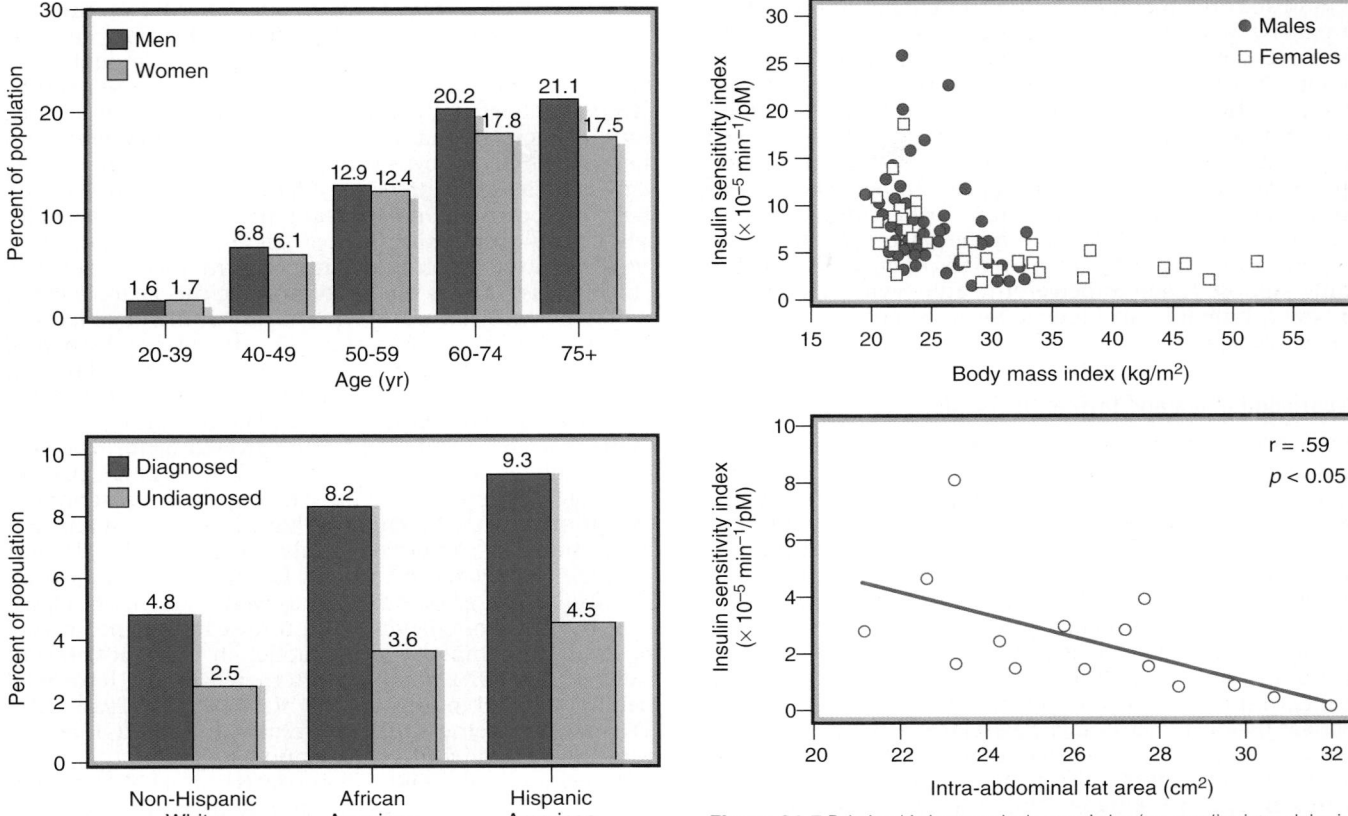

Figure 31-6 Prevalence of diabetes by age *(top panel)* and by ethnicity *(bottom panel)*. (From Harris MI, Flegal KM, Cowie CC, et al. Prevalence of diabetes, impaired fasting glucose, and impaired glucose tolerance in U.S. adults. The Third National Health and Nutrition Examination Survey, 1988-1994. *Diabetes Care.* 1998;21: 518-524.)

Figure 31-7 Relationship between body mass index *(top panel)* or intra-abdominal fat *(bottom panel)* and insulin sensitivity. (*Top* from Fujimoto WY, Bergstrom RW, Boyko EJ, et al. Susceptibility to development of central adiposity among populations. *Obesity Res.* 1995;3(Suppl 2):179S-186S; *bottom* from Kahn SE, Prigeon RL, McCulloch DK, et al. Quantification of the relationship between insulin sensitivity and beta-cell function in human subjects: evidence for a hyperbolic function. *Diabetes.* 1993;42: 1663-1672.)

of environmental factors on the genetic predisposition to insulin resistance and therefore to diabetes.[147,148]

Obesity and Type 2 Diabetes Mellitus

The association of obesity with T2DM has been recognized for decades. A close association between obesity and insulin resistance is seen in all ethnic groups and is found across the full range of body weights, across all ages, and in both sexes (Fig. 31-6).[149-151] A number of large epidemiologic studies have shown that the risk of diabetes, and presumably that of insulin resistance, rises as body fat content increases from the very lean to the very obese, implying that the absolute amount of body fat has an effect on insulin sensitivity across a broad range (Fig. 31-7).[152-154] There is a strong sexual dimorphism in the distribution of fat, with women having a greater percentage of fat below the waist than men.[155] It is important to point out that up to 30% of individuals with significant obesity have minimal metabolic abnormalities[156] though they still may be at risk for diabetes and cardiovascular diseases.[155,157]

Central (intra-abdominal) adiposity is more strongly linked to insulin resistance (see Fig. 31-7) and to a number of important metabolic variables, including plasma glucose, insulin, total plasma cholesterol and triglyceride concentrations, and decreased plasma high-density lipoprotein (HDL) cholesterol concentration, than is total adiposity.[158-164] In contrast, some studies have suggested that subcutaneous

fat is protective against insulin resistance.[165] The association between abdominal fat and glucose tolerance is independent of total adiposity.[166,167] The reason for the relationship between intra-abdominal fat and abnormal metabolism is not clearly defined, but a number of hypotheses, which are not mutually exclusive, have been proposed. First, abdominal fat is more lipolytically active than subcutaneous fat, perhaps because of its greater complement of adrenergic receptors.[168,169] In addition, the abdominal adipose store is resistant to the antilipolytic effects of insulin,[170] including alterations in lipoprotein lipase activity; this leads to increased lipase activity and a greater flux of fatty acids into the circulation, with the portal circulation receiving the greatest fatty acid load. Finally, the high levels of 11β-hydroxysteroid dehydrogenase type 1 (HSD11B1) in mesenteric fat could result in enhanced conversion of inactive cortisone to active cortisol, resulting in increased local cortisol production. This might change adipocytes to increase lipolysis and alter the production of adipokines, which may directly modulate glucose metabolism.

Brown adipose tissue has a distinct thermogenic ability to uncouple electron transport in the mitochondria via the expression of the uncoupling protein 1 (UCP1). Brown adipose tissue is activated by the sympathetic nervous system, which increases the mobilization and oxidation of fatty acids.[171] In humans, prolonged or repeated cold exposure can increase the mass and activity of intrascapular deposits of brown adipose tissue, as defined by the uptake of glucose, and can improve glucose homeostasis.[172] It has been recognized that rodents and humans also have fat depots of so-called beige or brite (brown in white) adipocytes,[173] which appear in white adipose tissue following cold and hormonal stimuli.[173] A defining feature of beige adipocytes is the expression of UCP1; however, the developmental origin of these cells appears to be distinct from brown adipose tissue. It continues to be controversial if these cells are formed de novo from precursor cells in the adipose tissue or arise by *transdifferentiation* of existing white adipose tissue to beige/brite adipocytes. The degree in which humans can increase beige adipocytes and how it may impact metabolism remains to be determined.

Hyperinsulinemia and Insulin Resistance

Hyperinsulinemia per se has been proposed to cause insulin resistance. Elevated concentrations of insulin can cause insulin resistance by downregulating insulin receptors and desensitizing postreceptor pathways.[174] Del Prato and associates showed that 24 and 72 hours of sustained physiologic hyperinsulinemia in normal persons specifically inhibited the ability of insulin to increase nonoxidative glucose disposal in association with an impaired ability of insulin to stimulate glycogen synthase activity.[175] Suppression of insulin secretion in obese, insulin-resistant persons results in increased insulin sensitivity.[176,177]

Nutrient Overload and Insulin Resistance. Cells have developed a number of ways to sense incoming nutrients, including direct and indirect activation of transcription factors and protein kinases. These pathways integrate with incoming hormonal signals to modulate cellular metabolism, increasing anabolic reactions in times of nutrient surfeit and catabolic reactions in postprandial or nutrient-deficient states. In a sense, the reaction of different tissues to obesity may be a relatively normal physiologic response to excess nutrient delivery, with prolonged activation leading to unintended and pathologic states that result in insulin resistance, inflammation, and even cell death. A variety of interacting factors functioning within and between tissues will determine the final phenotypic response of a person to continued nutrient overload. An individual can be obese with normal objective findings related to glucose and lipid homeostasis or other cardiovascular risk factors, whereas another person can be only slightly above normal weight and yet harbor a distinctly abnormal physiology. Clearly, genetics plays a role in these responses, as demonstrated by the increased burden of metabolic dysfunction in Asians at a much lower BMI than in Caucasians or other ethnic groups.[178]

Adipose Tissue and Insulin Resistance. To maintain metabolic homeostasis, nutrient intake exceeding expenditure must be converted to biologic precursors to increase cellular mass or it must be stored. Most excess nutrients, whether carbohydrate, protein, or lipid, are ultimately stored as triglyceride in adipose tissue. This storage segregates the excess nutrients in a form that is dense and can be easily mobilized in times of energy deficit. If the storage capacity of adipose tissue is exceeded, lipids and other nutrients enter nonstorage tissues, such as myocytes, hepatocytes, vascular cells, and beta cells, and trigger a variety of adaptive and nonadaptive cellular responses that lead to insulin resistance and cellular dysfunction. Indeed, some data suggest that the inability to expand fat mass in response to overeating may be a more important factor in the development of insulin resistance.[157]

Adipocytes are more than storage cells. They regulate the uptake and release of fatty acids; participate in the glycerol FFA cycle; release leptin and other hormones that signal the energy status of the body; and secrete an ever-expanding number of cytokines that have hormonal, paracrine, and autocrine actions.[179] The adipocyte itself can be adversely affected by accumulation of excess nutrients, leading to events that can have adverse consequences on the body. As adipocyte surface area increases in obesity, there is increased expression of leptin, interleukin 6 (IL-6), IL-8, monocyte chemoattractant protein-1, and granulocyte colony-stimulating factor. These and possibly other cytokines attract proinflammatory macrophages (M1 type), which release factors such as tumor necrosis factor-α (TNF-α) that may have local and systemic inflammatory effects.[180]

Mammalian Target of Rapamycin. The mTOR may be part of the integration of excess nutrient accumulation and insulin resistance. mTOR is part of a multisubunit serine/threonine protein kinase complex, called TORC, that integrates signaling from the insulin and other growth factor receptors and regulates many cell processes including growth, autophagy, apoptosis, protein synthesis, and transcription. Two primary mTOR complexes have been recognized that likely subserve different cellular actions. The TORC1 complex is activated by growth factors, including insulin and insulin-like growth factors, as well as nutrients, classically by the branched-chain amino acid leucine. mTOR regulation is complex. In one model, in nutrient-deficient states, the mTOR1 complex is tethered to the lysosomal membrane by binding to the Ras-related GTPase (Rag GTPase). Increasing nutrients results in mTORC1 release from the lysosomal membrane and activation.

Activation of TORC1 propagates anabolic signals through several downstream targets including S6K and inhibition of 4E-BP, resulting in activation of ribosomal translation, activation of lipogenesis through the activation of the sterol regulatory element–binding protein 1 (SREBP1), and increases in nucleotide synthesis by promoting flux through the pentose phosphate pathway.[181] As part of a feedback loop, S6K can phosphorylate IRS1 on serine and inhibit its activity, resulting in downregulation of insulin signaling.[182] Cells harboring tuberous sclerosis complex (TSC) mutations have high levels of IRS1 serine phosphorylation and are extremely insulin resistant. Conversely, mice with ablation of S6K-1 are protected from developing obesity and insulin resistance when given a high-fat diet, indicating a critical role in both growth and insulin resistance.[183]

Unfolded Protein Response. The endoplasmic reticulum (ER) functions in the post-translational processing of protein, including protein folding, maturation, quality control, and trafficking to other cellular compartments. As part of its quality control machinery, when the ER accumulates excess levels of unfolded or malfolded proteins, a distinct series of reactions occurs that slows overall protein synthesis while increasing the production of chaperones and other proteins that increase the fidelity of protein processing. The RNA-dependent protein kinase (PKR)-like eukaryotic initiation factor 2α (eIF2α) kinase known as PKR-like endoplasmic reticulum kinase (PERK), the inositol-requiring enzyme 1 (IRE1), and the activating transcription factor 6 (ATF6) are ER membrane–associated proteins that are normally complexed to the ER protein BiP/GRP78. Accumulation of unfolded proteins results in dissociation of these proteins from BiP/GRP78. PERK phosphorylates eukaryotic translation initiation factor 2 eIF2α, resulting in inhibition of most protein synthesis and alleviating ER workload. IRE1 is also phosphorylated, which activates cleavage of X-box binding protein 1 (XBP1), forming a messenger ribonucleic acid (mRNA) translated into the active transcription factor, which, in combination with

ATF6α, activates transcription to produce chaperones and proteins involved in ER biogenesis, phospholipid synthesis, ER-associated protein degradation (ERAD), and secretion.[184]

In states of overfeeding and obesity, evidence for activation of this unfolded protein response (UPR) can be seen in liver, adipose tissue, pancreatic beta cells, and muscle other tissues. The UPR to overnutrition is thought to have several effects, including activation of the Janus kinase (Jak) and nuclear factor-κB (NF-κB)/inhibitor of κB kinase (IKK) pathways leading to decreased IRS1 activity, increased levels of endogenous inflammatory mediators, alteration in SREBP1-mediated transcription, reduction in hepatic gluconeogenesis, and after prolonged activation, cellular dysfunction and apoptosis.[185]

Innate Immunity. The innate immune system was originally thought to be a cellular system that allowed discrimination of self and nonself so as to adapt cellular metabolism to fight microbial pathogens. However, this system is now recognized as a general response to cellular stress that activates the inflammation and cellular repair systems. The innate immune system contains a series of pattern-recognition receptor (PRR) proteins to detect microbial motifs. These proteins, including toll-like receptors (TLRs) and C-type lectins (CTLs), are expressed on a variety of cell types, including macrophages, monocytes, dendritic cells, neutrophils, and epithelial cells and cells of the adaptive immune system. The PRRs detect extracellular and intracellular pathogen-related molecules, including lipids and nucleic acids, and initiate a stereotypical response, including NF-κB activation and activator protein-1 (AP1) transcription, which increases expression of cytokines and chemokines.

Activation of the innate pathway also increases the production of so-called inflammasomes—large, multisubunit protein complexes that are important in the control of caspase 1–mediated, post-translational maturation and secretion of interleukins, primarily IL-1β, that have potent proinflammatory responses and are a risk factor for development of T2DM, perhaps through disruption of beta-cell function.[186]

Activation of the innate immune system in acute infection is associated with significant insulin resistance and likely plays a role in the insulin resistance seen in obesity, mediated by elevated levels of FFAs. TLRs, especially TLR2 and TLR4, which respond to bacterial cell wall lipids and induce the innate inflammatory response, are activated by saturated fatty acids, whereas polyunsaturated fatty acids inhibit TLR signaling. Activation of TLRs in cells results in insulin resistance, whereas genetic disruption of the TLR4 receptor in mice is protective against fatty acid–induced insulin resistance.[187]

Several pathways that modulate the inflammatory response are under investigation for the treatment of diabetics. They include targeting IKKb-NF-κB (salicylates, salsalate), TNF-α (etanercept, infliximab, adalimumab), IL-1β (anakinra, canakinumab) and IL-6 (tocilizumab), AMP-activated protein kinase activators, sirtuin-1 activators, mTOR inhibitors, and C-C motif chemokine receptor 2 antagonists.[188]

Circadian Rhythms, Obesity, and Insulin Resistance. Almost all mammals have a well-developed circadian cycle that is controlled by a complex, integrated network of transcription-translation feedback loops that work in a 24-hour cycle. A defined set of genes establishes the circadian cycle, which sets behavioral and physiologic functions, including sleep-wake cycles, feeding behaviors, hormone secretion, and metabolism. Oscillations in circulating blood glucose levels persist during forced dyssychrony when subjects are exposed to contiguous 20- or 28-hour days, showing that rhythms of carbohydrate metabolism are not secondary to alterations in physical activity or food intake during the day.[189] Evidence suggests that at least some of the 24-hour rhythms are driven by a cell autonomous 24-hour clock. In mammals, the clock is driven by two transcription factors, circadian locomotor output cycles kaput (CLOCK) and brain and muscle arylhydrocarbon receptor nuclear translocator (ARNT)-like 1 (BMAL1).[190,191] CLOCK and BMAL1 dimerize and bind the promoter region of target genes, including multiple period (PER) and cryptochrome (CRY) isoforms. The increased levels of these proteins promote heterodimerization and translocation to the nucleus, suppressing transcriptional activity of CLOCK-BMAL1. In a second negative feedback loop CLOCK-BMAL1 induces REV-ERBα (encoded by the nuclear receptor subfamily 1, group D, member 1 gene, NR1D1), which in turn influences BMAL1 transcription. Additional modulation of the activity and stability of these proteins is provided by post-translational modifications such as phosphorylation and ubiquitination.

There are significant epidemiologic associations in humans between reduction of sleep and increased obesity and other metabolic disturbances, including T2DM.[192,193] Obstructive sleep apnea, which combines sleep fragmentation and hypoxemia, is a major risk factor for insulin resistance and possibly diabetes. It is not yet clear whether glucose control in patients with T2DM patients can be improved by treating sleep apnea. Recently, sleep disturbances during pregnancy have been implicated as factors in the pathogenesis of gestational diabetes. Experimental sleep disruption can directly impair insulin action, alter secretion of leptin and ghrelin with stimulation of appetite, increase inflammatory cytokine production, and create alterations in other cardiovascular risk factors. Alterations in normal feeding patterns that are attuned to the circadian metabolism can change the relationship between nutrient appearance and nutrient-metabolizing enzymes. For instance, alterations in fatty acid appearance and lipoprotein lipase activity could lead to altered partitioning of lipids to vulnerable tissues, leading to lipotoxicity and decreased secretion of leptin, increasing appetite.[194] These disturbances can be exacerbated by obesity-related sleep apnea. Although the cognitive improvements associated with successful treatment of sleep apnea are clear, the metabolic benefits continue to be debated.[195]

Skeletal Muscle Insulin Resistance

The primary site of glucose disposal after a meal is skeletal muscle, and the primary mechanism of glucose storage is through its conversion to glycogen.[196] Given the relatively limited nutrient storage capacity of skeletal muscle, it is not surprising that, in obesity, insulin resistance in skeletal muscle is manifested before abnormalities in insulin signaling in adipose tissue and liver. Studies using the hyperinsulinemic-euglycemic clamp technique have demonstrated that in insulin-resistant people (with and without T2DM), there is a deficiency in the nonoxidative disposal of glucose related primarily to a defect in glycogen synthesis (Fig. 31-8).[197,198]

Elevated FFAs predict the progression from IGT to diabetes.[199,200] In the periphery, FFAs might not be markedly elevated because of efficient extraction by the liver and skeletal muscle. Therefore, normal or minimally elevated FFA levels might not reflect the true exposure of fatty acids to peripheral tissues. Increased fatty acid flux to skeletal muscle related to increased visceral lipolysis has been implicated in the inhibition of muscle glucose uptake.

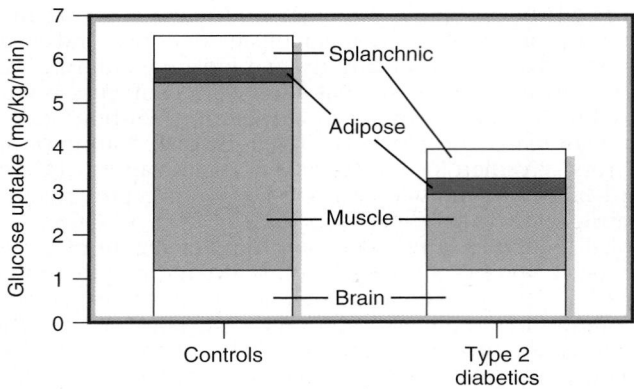

Figure 31-8 Tissue uptake of glucose in nondiabetic and insulin-resistant diabetic subjects during a hyperinsulinemic-euglycemic clamp. (From DeFronzo RA. The triumvirate: beta-cell, muscle, liver—a collusion responsible for NIDDM. Lilly Lecture 1987. *Diabetes.* 1988;37:667-687.)

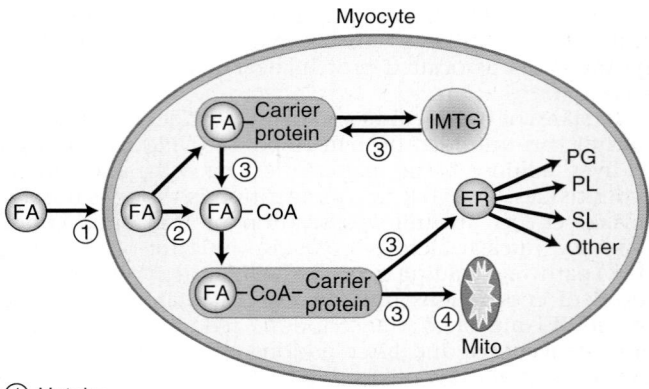

① Uptake
② Activation
③ Intracellular trafficking and distribution
④ Mitochondrial transport and oxidation

Figure 31-9 Simplified schematic diagram demonstrating fatty acid (FA) uptake, activation (formation of FA-CoA [coenzyme A]), and intracellular transport to organelles within a muscle cell. ER, endoplasmic reticulum; IMTG, intramuscular triglyceride; Mito, mitochondrion; PG, prostaglandin; PL, phospholipid; SL, sphingolipid.

The Randle hypothesis, or the glucose–fatty acid cycle, was originally proposed to account for the ability of FFAs to inhibit muscle glucose utilization. Randle's group[201] demonstrated that fatty acids compete with glucose for substrate oxidation in isolated muscle. The increase in fatty acid metabolism leads to an increase in the intramitochondrial acetyl coenzyme A (acetyl-CoA)/CoA and reduced nicotinamide adenine dinucleotide (NADH/NAD⁺) ratios, with subsequent inhibition of pyruvate dehydrogenase. The resulting increased intracellular mitochondrial (and cytosolic) citrate concentrations result in allosteric inhibition of phosphofructokinase, the key rate-controlling enzyme in glycolysis. Subsequent accumulation of glucose 6-phosphate inhibits hexokinase II activity, resulting in an increase in intracellular glucose concentrations and decreased glucose uptake.

Studies in vivo in humans suggest that the primary effect of fatty acids, at least in the presence of elevated insulin levels, is a decrease in glucose transport, as measured by a reduction in the rate of accumulation of intracellular glucose and glycogen using ¹³C and ³¹P nuclear magnetic resonance (NMR) spectroscopy. In normal subjects, elevated fatty acids, achieved by infusion of triglyceride emulsions and heparin (to activate lipoprotein lipase resulting in a spill of fatty acids into the circulation), resulted in a fall in intracellular glucose and glucose 6-phosphate concentrations that preceded the fall in glycogen accumulation.[202,203] These results challenge the Randle hypothesis (which predicts a rise in intracellular glucose 6-phosphate concentrations) as the basis of the reduction in insulin sensitivity seen with elevated fatty acids. Similar decreases in glucose transport have been seen in patients with T2DM[204] and in lean, normoglycemic, insulin-resistant offspring of type 2 diabetics.[205,206] These studies also found decreased activity of PI3K and increased protein kinase C-θ activity that might, in part, mediate the effect of elevated FFAs.[207,208]

Studies also suggest that PKC-mediated serine phosphorylation of the IKKβ subunit, leading to its degradation and the unregulated translocation of NF-κB into the nucleus, might also be important to fatty acid–induced insulin resistance.[209] This is the mechanism by which high-dose aspirin therapy improves glucose metabolism in T2DM.[209] Disruption of the IKKβ inflammatory pathway by high-dose aspirin therapy in a small human trial resulted in an improvement in insulin sensitivity.

Intramuscular Triglycerides. Insulin-stimulated glucose uptake is inversely related to the amount of intramuscular triglycerides. A strong correlation between intramuscular triglyceride concentration and insulin resistance was demonstrated by evaluation of intramuscular triglyceride with biopsy,[210] computed tomography,[211] and magnetic resonance imaging (MRI).[212] MRI has been a valuable addition because the magnetic resonance signal can distinguish intramyocellular from extramyocellular fat and demonstrates the increased triglyceride accumulation within the myofiber itself.[213] First-degree relatives of type 2 diabetics have an increase in intramyocellular fat, and in this group there is also a correlation with insulin resistance.[212]

The mechanism for accumulation of triglyceride in the skeletal muscle of obese and insulin-resistant persons is probably related to mismatching of FFA uptake and oxidation. During resting postabsorptive conditions, about 30% of fatty acid flux in the plasma pool is accounted for by oxidation, and the remaining 70% of flux is recycled into triglyceride, indicating a physiologic reserve that exceeds immediate tissue needs for oxidative substrates. The equilibrium between oxidation and reesterification within muscle is paramount in determining fatty acid storage within tissue. The uptake, transport, and metabolism of fatty acids are highly regulated processes (Fig. 31-9), and alteration of the balance between uptake and oxidation in skeletal muscle leads to increased intramyocellular triglycerides. The increased lipolysis associated with obesity provides an increased amount of FFA presented to muscle.

Increased muscle triglyceride content is not invariably linked to insulin resistance, because exercise training is associated with increased muscle triglyceride content,[214] and chronic exercise increases insulin sensitivity as well as the capacity for fatty acid oxidation.[215-219] Studies suggest that acute exercise increases intramyocellular triglyceride synthesis, reducing fatty acid oxidation and preventing fatty acid–induced insulin resistance.[220]

Fatty Acid Metabolism in Skeletal Muscle. The uptake of fatty acid from the serum, where it is mostly bound to albumin, is mediated by at least three families of proteins: fatty acid translocase, plasma membrane fatty acid–binding proteins (FABPs), and fatty acid transport proteins.[221-223] The levels of the putative transport proteins are regulated by exercise,[99] are correlated with body weight (at least in women), and can be modulated by insulin infusion.[224]

FABPs are capable of binding multiple hydrophobic ligands, including fatty acids, eicosanoids, and retinoids, with high affinity.[225] FABPs are thought to facilitate uptake of fatty acids and to promote subsequent intracellular transport to subcellular organelles.[226] There is a direct correlation between heart-type FABP content and oxidative capacity observed during development and among different muscle types.[227,228] In mice that have a disruption of the heart isoform[229] or the adipocyte isoform[230] of FABP, plasma fatty acid concentrations were significantly elevated and plasma glucose was decreased, suggesting a key role in normal regulation of fatty acid oxidation. Some,[230] but not all,[231] studies have shown a decrease in heart-type FABP in insulin-resistant humans.

Carnitine palmitoyltransferase 1 (CPT1) has been the subject of intense scrutiny for many years because of its central role in the balance between mitochondrial glucose and fatty acid metabolism, and primarily because of inhibition of mitochondrial fatty acid uptake by malonyl-CoA.[232,233] A specific isoform contributes 97% of the CPT1 in muscle and has 100-fold lower sensitivity to inhibition by malonyl-CoA.[234] This lower sensitivity to malonyl-CoA inhibition suggests that the level of CPT1 itself may be important in the balance of uptake and oxidation of fatty acids. Evidence for this in skeletal muscle stems from the finding that, as with other fatty acid–oxidizing enzymes, muscle CPT1 mRNA is regulated by PPARα activators, fat feeding, and exercise in rodents and is inversely correlated with obesity in humans.[235-238]

Long-chain fatty acids, after passing through the inner mitochondrial membrane as acylcarnitines, are metabolized at the surface of the inner mitochondrial membrane by CPT2 and the long chain–specific oxidation system consisting of very long chain acyl-CoA dehydrogenase (VLCAD) and the trifunctional protein (TFP) oxidation complex (Fig. 31-10). Transfer of the acyl chain from carnitine to CoA, catalyzed by CPT2, is followed by one cycle of oxidation catalyzed by VLCAD and TFP to yield a chain-shortened acyl-CoA that can recycle through the same oxidation system.[239] In actuality, four different acyl-CoA dehydrogenase enzymes catalyze the initial dehydrogenation of straight-chain fatty acids in mitochondria. Three of them—short-chain acyl-CoA dehydrogenase (SCAD), medium-chain acyl-CoA dehydrogenase (MCAD), and long-chain acyl-CoA dehydrogenase (LCAD)—are soluble enzymes located in the mitochondrial matrix as homotetramers. A fourth, VLCAD, is attached to the inner membrane as a homodimer. Their names derive from the length of the fatty acids that they process. VLCAD and LCAD shorten the long-chain fatty acids into medium-chain fatty acids that can then be processed by MCAD and SCAD.[240] The SCAD, MCAD, and LCAD monomers share a high degree of homology but do not share homology with VLCAD. At least some of these enzymes can be regulated in humans during exercise training.[241]

UCP1 is clearly related to the uncoupling of oxidative phosphorylation in brown adipose tissue.[204] UCP2 and UCP3 have structural similarities to UCP1, but it is not clear that they are actually uncouplers of oxidative phosphorylation.[242] Newer members of the family, such as brain mitochondrial carrier protein 1 (BMCP1) and UCP4, have an even more distant sequence relationship.[243] BMCP1 and UCP4 are predominantly expressed in neural tissues—namely, the brain. UCP3 mRNA is found primarily in skeletal muscle and in brown adipose tissue. UCP2 has a ubiquitous tissue distribution. UCP2 and UCP3 mRNA levels have been correlated with different physiologic states, and numerous studies indicate that expression of UCP2 and UCP3 is stimulated by thyroid hormones and in the presence of high levels of fatty acids.[244] In humans, the levels of UCP2 and UCP3 mRNAs were upregulated by a high-fat diet, and the upregulation was more pronounced in humans with high percentages of type IIA muscle fibers.[245] In a small study, exercise training in humans increased mitochondrial oxidative capacity but did not change UCP2 or UCP3 levels.[246] Obesity itself was shown to be positively correlated with a splice isoform of UCP3.[247]

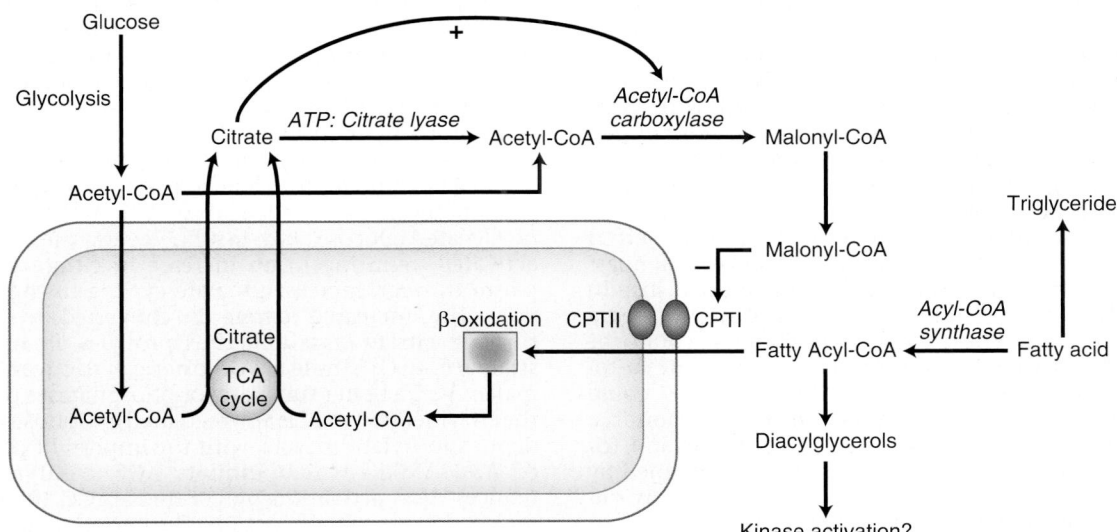

Figure 31-10 Glucose effect on triglyceride metabolism. Increased uptake of glucose results in increased production of acetyl coenzyme A (acetyl-CoA) as a product of glycolysis. The increased tricarboxylic acid (TCA) cycle activity associated with oxidation of triglycerides and glucose increases the production of citrate, which is shuttled to the cytoplasm, activates the enzyme acetyl-CoA carboxylase (ACC) by allosteric mechanisms, and increases the susceptibility of ACC to phosphatases. This leads to increased ACC activity, converting acetyl-CoA to malonyl-CoA. Malonyl-CoA is a potent inhibitor of carnitine palmitoyltransferase (CPT) I on the outer mitochondrial membrane, which leads to accumulation of fatty acyl-CoAs in the cytoplasm. This may result in the production of signaling molecules that can increase the activity of kinases and other enzymes and lead to insulin resistance. ATP, adenosine triphosphate.

A unique polymorphism in the promoter region of UCP3 correlated with expression of UCP3 in skeletal muscle.[248]

Mitochondrial Abnormalities and Insulin Resistance

A decrease in oxidative capacity is seen in both humans and animals with insulin resistance, obesity, and T2DM.[249,250] Studies have suggested that increases in intramyocellular fat content in skeletal muscle associated with insulin resistance (see earlier discussion) may be caused by alterations in mitochondrial mass. In one study, young insulin-resistant offspring of parents with T2DM demonstrated a 60% reduction in insulin-stimulated skeletal muscle glucose uptake compared with control subjects, and this reduction correlated with an increase of approximately 80% in intramyocellular lipid content.[251] The elevated intramyocellular lipid content was attributable to the 30% reduction in mitochondrial oxidative capacity. The insulin-resistant subjects showed a lower ratio of type I to type II muscle fibers. Type I fibers are mostly oxidative and contain more mitochondria than type II muscle fibers, which are more glycolytic.

Decreased expression of nuclear-encoded genes that regulate mitochondrial biogenesis, such as PPARγ coactivators-1α and -1β (PGC-1α and PGC-1β, respectively), have been shown to be important for mitochondrial biogenesis and for fiber type selection during development.[252] PGC-1α transcriptionally activates the nuclear respiratory factors NRF1 and NRF2, which are known to be important for mitochondrial biogenesis.[253] PGC-1α–responsive genes were found to be downregulated in obese white patients with IGT and T2DM.[254,255] In obese diabetic and nondiabetic Mexican Americans, PGC-1α and PGC-1β expression levels were reduced compared with levels in nonobese persons.[256] The activity of the electron transport chain is reduced and intramyofibrillar mitochondria are smaller in patients with T2DM, and both the size of intramyofibrillar mitochondria and electron transport chain activity in muscle homogenates correlate with severity of insulin resistance.[257]

In one study, rats bred for differences in oxidative capacity (determined by their intrinsic ability to run) were described.[258] The skeletal muscle of the animals with a low capacity for aerobic exercise showed a reduction in mitochondrial gene expression and PGC-1α, similar to that seen in humans. When multiple metabolic parameters were assessed, it was determined that the group with poor aerobic capacity had several significant abnormalities, including obesity, insulin resistance, hypertension, and dyslipidemia, suggesting that the defects found in humans could have a genetic basis.

More recent studies have questioned the cause-effect relationship between alterations in mitochondrial mass and mitochondrial function and skeletal muscle insulin resistance. Rather than mitochondrial insufficiency being an inherited trait, these observed changes could be acquired. First, because insulin itself can upregulate mitochondrial biogenesis, muscle insulin resistance could provide a mechanism for the reduction in mitochondria. Second, the observed reduction in ATP synthesis and tricarboxylic acid (TCA) cycle activity could be explained by reduced turnover of ATP in relatively sedentary individuals. Persistent delivery of fatty acids to skeletal muscle, seen in obesity and after high-fat feeding, increases fatty acid β-oxidation. In the absence of energy demand (e.g., exercise), the reduction in the adenosine diphosphate (ADP)/ATP ratio would impair electron transport in the mitochondria, increasing NADH levels, which would impair TCA cycle activity. This would result in the generation of reactive oxygen species due to elevated reducing pressure in the mitochondria.[259] Indicative of impaired oxidation in the mitochondria, mice fed a high-fat diet show a reduction in TCA cycle intermediates and an impairment of adequate β-oxidation of fatty acids marked by increases in even-chained acyl-carnitine levels.

Increases in plasma acyl-carnitines are found in obese, insulin-resistant individuals.[260] Longer chain acyl-carnitines arise from the mitochondria and plasma levels likely reflect the rate of uptake into the mitochondrial of muscle and liver. The medium-chain acyl-carnitines (from C6-C12) likely reflect the conversion of acyl-CoA intermediates to their cognate acyl-carnitines that build up in the mitochondrial in these tissues. A slowing of electron transport chain activity would result in accumulation of these intermediates. In addition, shorter chain acyl-carnitines (C3-C5) that arise from branched chain and other amino acids also accumulate in the plasma of insulin-resistant individuals, again likely reflecting reduced capacity of mitochondrial oxidation of the cognate CoAs. Although there has been some suggestion that these intermediates play a role in insulin resistance, it appears more likely that they are sensitive markers of resistance.[261]

It has been proposed that reversing the observed mitochondrial mass in muscle of type 2 diabetics may be a way to improve their metabolism. The potential beneficial effect of increasing mitochondrial mass by activation of PGC-1α activity has been dampened by the finding that overexpression of PGC-1α in mouse skeletal muscle does not improve metabolic status following a high-fat diet.[262]

Glucose Influence on Skeletal Muscle Fatty Acid Metabolism

An emerging concept that could couple increased fatty acid flux into skeletal muscle with impaired insulin action is the central role of malonyl-CoA in regulating fatty acid and glucose oxidation (see Fig. 31-10).[263] Malonyl-CoA is an allosteric inhibitor of CPT1, the enzyme that controls the transfer of long-chain fatty acyl-CoAs into the mitochondria.[232,264,265] Even in insulin-resistant skeletal muscle, glucose uptake into the skeletal muscle is higher than normal, especially at the elevated levels of glucose found in T2DM.[266,267] The glucose is shunted toward the glycolytic pathway, generating acetyl-CoA that can be converted to malonyl-CoA in the cytoplasm by the action of the highly regulated enzyme ACC.

In humans, an infusion of insulin and glucose at a high rate leads to increases in the concentration of malonyl-CoA in skeletal muscle and to decreases in whole-body and, presumably, muscle fatty acid oxidation.[268] In the presence of elevated glucose and insulin levels, the TCA cycle is activated, resulting in an increase in citrate in the cytoplasm through increased malate cycling in the mitochondria. The increased citrate is converted to acetyl-CoA through citrate lyase and thus provides an indirect substrate for ACC. Citrate also allosterically activates ACC and makes ACC a better substrate for phosphatases that activate the enzyme.[269,270] ACC is also regulated by a phosphorylation-dephosphorylation cycle, with the important participation of AMP-AMPK, which inhibits ACC basal activity and reduces ACC activation by citrate.[271] ACC then generates malonyl-CoA, which in turn allosterically inhibits CPT1 residing on the outer mitochondrial membrane, inhibiting uptake of acyl-CoA. The resulting buildup of LCADs and diacylglycerols is proposed to activate one or more PKC isoforms or other lipid-activated proteins, resulting in insulin resistance.[263] Support for this hypothesis is the finding that exercise, which activates AMPK, inactivates

ACC, lowers intracellular LCAD levels, and has an acute insulin-sensitizing effect.[272]

The recognition that post-translational modification of mitochondrial proteins by acetylation of up to dozens of lysine residues on each protein has a marked effect to alter their activity provides a potentially important mechanism for control of mitochondrial flux and insulin resistance.[273] In general, acetylation reduces mitochondrial enzyme activity and appears to occur through a pH-dependent chemical reaction wherein acetyl-CoA is the acetyl donor to exposed lysine residues. An increase in flux of nutrients in the mitochondria is expected to increase acetylation proportional to the steady-state levels of acetylation. An imbalance of formation to utilization, which occurs in overnutrition, would therefore be expected to brake further fuel utilization. The mitochondrial sirtuin, Sirt3, appears to be the primary deacetylase of the mitochondria[274] that is activated by NAD+. As ATP use increased, such as with exercise,[275] increased electron flow from NADH to support oxidative phosphorylation will result in increased intramitochondrial NAD+ leading to Sirt3-mediated protein deacetylation and increased mitochondrial capacity for substrate utilization.

Increased Hepatic Glucose Production in Diabetes Mellitus

The disposal of glucose after meals depends on the ability of insulin to increase peripheral glucose uptake and to simultaneously decrease endogenous glucose production. Although studies have suggested that the kidney can contribute up to 25% of endogenous glucose production,[276,277] the defect in T2DM is primarily in defective regulation of glucose production from the liver (hepatic glucose output). Two routes of glucose production by the liver are glycogenolysis of stored glycogen and gluconeogenesis from two- and three-carbon substrates derived primarily from skeletal muscle.[133,278] Under different conditions and at different times postprandially, the contribution of each of these mechanisms to maintenance of glucose levels varies. In studies using ^{13}C NMR spectroscopy combined with measurement of whole-body glucose production in normal human subjects at different intervals after fasting, it was found that gluconeogenesis accounted for 50% to 96% of glucose production, and the percentage increased with increasing duration of fasting.[279,280]

Hepatic insulin resistance plays an important role in the hyperglycemia of T2DM,[281-284] and the impaired suppression of hepatic glucose output appears to be quantitatively similar to, or even larger than, the defect in stimulation of peripheral glucose disposal.[282,285] There is a direct relationship between increased hepatic glucose output and fasting hyperglycemia[144] (Fig. 31-11). Insulin-mediated suppression of hepatic glucose output is impaired at both low and high plasma insulin levels in T2DM[285-288]; hepatic glucose production is elevated early in the course of the disease[289] but may be normal in lean, relatively insulin-sensitive type 2 diabetics.[288] Treatment of patients with metformin, which suppresses hepatic glucose production, results in improved glucose tolerance.[290]

Alterations in the direct and indirect effects of insulin in T2DM appear to play a role in the elevation of hepatic glucose production. Defects in the direct effect of insulin to suppress hepatic glucose production that have been demonstrated in humans[291] appear to be caused by a large rightward shift in the steep dose-response curve for insulin's inhibition of glycogenolysis.[292] However, peripheral insulin resistance may play the bigger role in elevated hepatic glucose production in T2DM. The resistance of adipose tissue, especially visceral fat, to suppression of

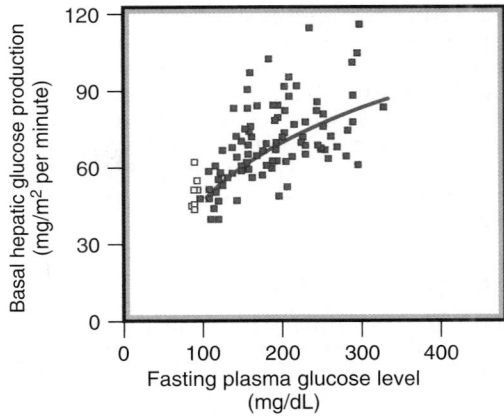

Figure 31-11 Relationship between fasting hepatic glucose output and fasting plasma glucose levels. *Open squares* represent nondiabetic control subjects; *closed squares* represent diabetic subjects. (From Maggs DG, Buchanan TA, Burant CF, et al. Metabolic effects of troglitazone monotherapy in type 2 diabetes mellitus: a randomized, double-blind, placebo-controlled trial. *Ann Intern Med.* 1998;128:176-185. © American College of Physicians, used with permission.)

lipolysis by insulin is responsible for part of insulin's inability to suppress hepatic glucose production by the indirect route, resulting in enhanced gluconeogenesis.[293,294] In addition, the suppression of glucagon levels in humans with insulin resistance may be impaired, again leading to an increase in endogenous glucose production.[295]

Glucocorticoid-Induced Insulin Resistance

Cushing syndrome and exogenous glucocorticoid treatment have long been known to induce significant insulin resistance in humans. Over 80% of individuals with rheumatoid arthritis treated with greater than 30 mg/day of prednisone who previously did not have diabetes had an increase in their HbA$_{1c}$. The exact mechanism is unknown; there are rapid effects that are related to increasing hepatic glucose production via activation of gluconeogenesis as well as acute insulin resistance in skeletal muscle, perhaps through the downregulation of IRS1.[296] Long-term treatment has profound effects, resulting in redistribution of fat from the periphery to the central compartment, increased lipolysis and elevations in triglyceride and FFA, increased muscle protein breakdown (leading to muscle atrophy), alterations in skin integrity, and reduction in insulin secretion. These effects are likely due to a combination of direct modulation of transcriptional events by glucocorticoids and through the profound inhibition of insulin and other growth factor signaling.

Tumor Necrosis Factor-α

Studies in humans and in animal models of obesity have identified changes in the expression and activity of key molecules involved in the insulin-signaling pathway. Decreases in the number and the kinase activity of insulin receptors[297] and impairment in the activation of IRS1,[298] PI3K,[299,300] and protein kinase B[301] have been observed. Although the basis for the changes is generally unknown, a TNF-α–mediated mechanism for the decreased activity in the initial steps of the insulin-signaling cascade has been proposed. TNF-α, made and secreted by adipocytes, is elevated in a variety of experimental models of obesity.[302] The kinase activity of the insulin receptor in rats[303] or in 3T3-L1 adipocytes[302] treated with TNF-α was reduced, possibly by increased serine phosphorylation.[304] Fat-fed mice with genetic ablation of TNF-α production had increased kinase activity of the insulin receptor compared with control mice and demonstrated increased insulin sensitivity.[305] In addition, rats treated with neutralizing antisera or soluble TNF receptors demonstrated an amelioration of their insulin resistance. As described later, other interventions to decrease TNF-α action result in increased insulin sensitivity.

Glucotoxicity, Glucosamine

Hyperglycemia is a primary factor in the development of diabetes complications, and decreases in average blood glucose have a profound effect to prevent complications in both T1DM[306] and T2DM.[307] Hyperglycemia itself can cause insulin resistance. In Pima Indians, the level of fasting glycemia is the primary determinant of insulin sensitivity.[308] The defect is primarily in skeletal muscle[309] and is related to the degree of hyperglycemia.

Entry of glucose into the cell results in its phosphorylation to glucose 6-phosphate, which has multiple metabolic fates. The hexosamine pathway is a relatively minor branch of the glycolytic pathway, encompassing less than 3% of total glucose used. The first and rate-limiting enzyme glutamine–fructose-6-phosphate (F6P) amidotransferase (GFAT), converts F6P and glutamine to glucosamine 6-phosphate (GlcN6P) and glutamate. Subsequent steps metabolize GlcN6P to uridine diphosphate-N-acetylglucosamine (UDP-GlcNAc), UDP-N-acetylgalactosamine (UDP-GalNAc), and cytidine monophosphate (CMP)-sialic acid, essential building blocks of the glycosyl side chains of glycoproteins, glycolipids, proteoglycans, and gangliosides.[310] Evidence suggests that the hexosamine pathway underlies the defect in glucose utilization associated with hyperglycemia. Increased flux through the hexosamine pathway appears to be required for some of the metabolic effects of sustained increased glucose flux, which promotes the complications of diabetes including diminished expression of sarcoplasmic reticulum Ca^{2+}-ATPase in cardiomyocytes and induction of transforming growth factor-β and plasminogen activator inhibitor 1 (PAI-1) in vascular smooth muscle cells, mesangial cells, and aortic endothelial cells.[311]

Hexosamines, such as glucosamine, when incubated with adipose tissue, induce insulin resistance in fat cells[312] and in skeletal muscle.[313] Infusion of glucosamine into rats resulted in a dose-dependent increase in insulin resistance of skeletal muscle,[313] and transgenic mice that overexpress GFAT specifically in skeletal muscle acquired severe insulin resistance.[314] By a pathway that is unclear, glucosamine overproduction resulted in a disruption of the ability of insulin to cause translocation of GLUT4 to the cell surface.[315] Through its anti-insulin action, the hexosamine pathway has been hypothesized to be a glucose sensor that allows the cell to sense and adapt to the prevailing level of glucose.[309]

Insulin Resistance and Lipodystrophy Associated With Human Immunodeficiency Virus Infection

A syndrome with many of the clinical and metabolic features of insulin resistance is increasingly being recognized in patients with human immunodeficiency virus (HIV) infection.[316] A cohort study of over 3800 patients showed nearly a doubling in the prevalence of T2DM in HIV versus non-HIV patients, and a significant portion of the increase

may be related to protease inhibitor treatment used to treat chronic HIV. Moreover, the HIV-infected patients had a 75% increase in the risk for acute myocardial infarction (MI) compared with noninfected patients, again related to protease inhibitor use. Other contributing factors to cardiometabolic risk are male sex, diagnosis of the acquired immunodeficiency syndrome (AIDS), responsiveness to antiretroviral treatment, and increases in CD4 T-cell counts.[317]

An unusual form of lipodystrophy is observed in these patients in whom there is significant fat redistribution from the extremities and face to the torso with accumulation of intra-abdominal and intrascapular fat. This form of lipodystrophy is associated with significant insulin resistance and T2DM, dyslipidemia with elevated total and low-density lipoprotein (LDL) cholesterol and suppressed HDL-cholesterol concentrations and a susceptibility to lactic acidemia.[318] Administration of ritonavir to normal subjects caused increases in plasma triglyceride and very low density lipoprotein (VLDL) cholesterol and decreased plasma HDL-cholesterol levels.[319] Indinavir administration for 4 weeks resulted in small increases in serum glucose and insulin levels and decreased insulin-mediated glucose disposal as assessed with a hyperinsulinemic euglycemic clamp; there were no changes in lipoprotein, triglyceride, or FFA levels.[320]

The molecular basis of the metabolic syndrome is not clear. A number of protease inhibitors can inhibit glucose transport in vitro and in vivo, and there is evidence for a direct interaction with GLUT4[321] that could inhibit glucose uptake specifically in insulin-responsive tissue. Mitochondrial abnormalities have been described in subcutaneous adipose tissue biopsy specimens obtained from HIV-infected patients with lipodystrophy compared with specimens from patients without the syndrome.[322] A direct effect of protease inhibitors on differentiation of adipocytes has also been described.[323-325] Additionally, reductions in mitochondrial number and oxidative function have been described in adipocytes from subcutaneous biopsies obtained from patients treated with highly active antiretroviral therapy (HAART).[326] The precise mechanism for the lipodystrophy associated with HIV infection is not known.

Treatment of HIV-associated lipodystrophy continues to be inadequate. Use of newer protease inhibitors might improve metabolic abnormalities, particularly those induced or increased by protease inhibitor therapy. However, changing protease inhibitors has little impact on body fat. Switching thymidine analogues has been the only intervention to improve lipoatrophy in independent studies.[327] Insulin-sensitizing thiazolidinediones have shown mixed results, with improvement in insulin sensitivity but little alteration in fat distribution.[328] More than 75% of patients with HIV who have acute MI are older than 55 years of age. Because of the increased risk of cardiovascular disease, treatment of hyperlipidemia is essential in these patients, with 3-hydroxy-3-methylglutaryl (HMG)-CoA reductase inhibitors and fibrates, alone or in combination, as first-line drugs.[329,330]

MEASURES TO IMPROVE INSULIN SENSITIVITY

Mechanisms of Reducing Insulin Resistance

The most effective measures to improve insulin sensitivity are weight loss and exercise. Both modalities are effective and can be additive in their ability to improve insulin action. Later in this chapter, the roles of these interventions in the treatment of patients with T2DM are discussed. The scientific basis and molecular mechanisms responsible for the improvements in insulin sensitivity seen with these interventions are summarized in the following paragraphs.

Mechanisms for Improved Insulin Sensitivity With Weight Loss

Weight loss can be a highly effective treatment for overweight patients with T2DM and other cardiovascular risk factors, and it is advocated as the first line of therapy. Weight loss also plays an important role in preventing T2DM.[152,331] In overweight patients with T2DM, weight loss can reduce hepatic glucose production, insulin resistance, and fasting hyperinsulinemia and can improve glycemic control. Weight loss in T2DM is also associated with a reduction in blood pressure and an improvement in the lipid profile. These benefits can occur with as little as 5% to 10% weight loss.[332-334] Moreover, preventing obesity in primates with long-term caloric restriction attenuates the development of insulin resistance.

The likely mechanism for improvements in insulin sensitivity through weight loss is the reduction in nutrient flux into tissues, reversing many of the cellular mechanisms that are triggered that protect individual cells from nutrient excess. Restriction of calories has a profound and immediate effect on improvement in insulin sensitivity even before change in weight.[335] There are clearly effects on the pattern of muscle fatty acid metabolism and the accumulation of lipid within muscle following weight loss.[263,264] Hepatic glucose production is markedly reduced,[336] as is adipose tissue lipolysis.[337] The improvement in insulin resistance and the reversal of T2DM following bariatric surgery are gaining interest because of the long-term success of the intervention. Although some have speculated that the improvement in insulin action and insulin secretion following bariatric surgery may be through overlapping, but distinct, mechanisms,[338] there is evidence that the effects may be similar, at least in the short term, mediated entirely by reduction in caloric intake.[339] The remission of T2DM is sustained for a longer period of time with surgery than medically induced weight loss, but this effect is likely to be due to sustained reduction in weight.

Mechanisms for Improved Insulin Sensitivity With Exercise

Exercise is clearly effective in increasing insulin sensitivity in animals and humans. There appear to be two separate but related effects of exercise on insulin action. A single bout of exercise can result in an acute increase in insulin-independent glucose transport that is measurable during and for a relatively short period after exercise.[340-344] Like insulin, exercise and muscle contractions increase glucose transport by translocation of intracellular GLUT4 to the cell surface and promote storage as glycogen.[345-347]

Acute Exercise

The signaling pathway leading to the exercise-induced increase in glucose transporter translocation and glucose transport is unknown, although there is ample evidence that the pathway is independent of the insulin-stimulated, receptor-mediated pathway. The effect of exercise and contractions on translocation and transport is additive to the maximal effect of insulin.[340,347-350] Insulin-stimulated glucose transport in muscle is inhibited by specific inhibitors of PI3K, such as wortmannin, whereas transport or translocation stimulated by muscle contractions is insensitive to these inhibitors.[347-352] Stimulation of muscle contractions in situ and exercise do not increase insulin receptor phosphorylation, tyrosine kinase activity, IRS phosphorylation, or PI3K activity.[346,353] In addition, in many insulin-resistant states, the acute exercise–stimulated (but not insulin-stimulated) glucose transport and GLUT4 translocation are normal. This has been demonstrated in the obese, insulin-resistant Zucker rat[354] and in patients with T2DM.[111] Finally, hypoxia, a stimulus for glucose transport that is also independent of the insulin receptor–mediated pathway, is effective in increasing glucose transport in muscle strips from obese, insulin-resistant patients and in patients with T2DM.[355]

The acute effect of exercise and hypoxia may be mediated by AMPK. AMPK is thought to be a sensor of intracellular energy stores and is activated by increases in intracellular AMP. A stable AMP analogue, 5-amino-4-imidazole carboxamide ribotide (ZMP), can be generated intracellularly from 5-aminoimidazole-4-carboxamide ribonucleoside (AICAR) and can activate AMPK in cells, leading to increased phosphorylation of known substrates for AMPK, including HMG-CoA reductase, acyl-CoA carboxylase, and creatine kinase.[356] Treatment of incubated skeletal muscle with AICAR resulted in increased glucose uptake and glucose transporter translocation.[357] Similarly, the inclusion of 2 mmol/L of AICAR in the perfusate of the rat hindlimb resulted in inactivation of ACC, decreases in malonyl-CoA levels, and a twofold increase in glucose uptake.[358,359]

The euglycemic clamp technique was used in conscious rats to demonstrate that infusion of AICAR results in a greater than twofold increase in glucose utilization.[360] Uptake of the glucose analogue 2-deoxyglucose was also increased twofold in vivo in soleus and gastrocnemius muscles. As with previous studies, this uptake was not associated with PI3K activation, again indicating a separate pathway from that of insulin.

A second effect of exercise, which becomes evident as the acute effect on glucose transport reverses, is a large increase in the sensitivity of glucose transport to stimulation by insulin.[361-364] This effect is due to translocation of a greater amount of GLUT4 to the cell surface for any given dose of insulin.[365,366] As with the acute stimulation of transport by exercise, the cellular mechanisms leading to enhanced translocation in response to submaximally effective stimuli are unknown. However, several studies have shown that steps in the insulin-signaling cascade leading to activation of PI3K are not enhanced after a bout of exercise. There is no change in insulin binding to its receptor,[353,367] insulin stimulation of receptor tyrosine kinase activity,[353,368] increased insulin-stimulated tyrosine phosphorylation of IRS1,[365] or PI3K activity associated with IRS1.[346,368]

Exercise Training

Exercise training also results in increases in insulin sensitivity[369,370] and can delay or prevent the onset of T2DM in those at high risk.[371] Using the hyperinsulinemic-euglycemic clamp, Perseghin and coworkers[372] compared exercise training for 45 minutes on a stair-climbing machine 4 days per week for 6 weeks in normal insulin-sensitive subjects and a group of high-risk, insulin-resistant relatives of T2DM. A 100% increase in insulin sensitivity was seen in both groups without a significant change in body weight. The higher basal and glucose-stimulated insulin release seen in the insulin-resistant subjects was not altered after exercise training. The effect of exercise training on insulin sensitivity has been proposed to be caused by upregulation.

Primary effects of exercise training include increased glucose transporter number, changes in capillary density, increased number of red glycolytic (type IIa) fibers, and increased density of mitochondria.[373,374] A reduction in mitochondrial oxidative capacity could underlie the dysregulation of lipid metabolism that results in reduced skeletal muscle glucose metabolism. Expression of nuclear-encoded genes that regulate mitochondrial biogenesis, such as the NRFs, PGC-1α, and PGC-1β, have been shown to be important for both mitochondrial biogenesis and fiber-type selection during development.[252,375] In muscle-specific transgenic mice, PGC-1α promotes muscle fiber-type switching from fast-twitch glycolytic fibers (types IIa and IIb) to slow-twitch oxidative fibers (type I), increases mitochondrial density, and improves oxidative capacity.[376] These changes are also observed after exercise training.

Many of the changes observed after exercise are likely to be mediated in part through PGC-1α levels and activity. Exercise-induced expression of PGC-1α in skeletal muscle is thought to be mediated by myocyte enhancer factor 2 (MEF2),[377] possibly through its interaction with MEF2C[378] and CREB.[377] PGC-1α regulates its own promoter activity in a positive autoregulation loop. Activation of estrogen-related receptor α (ERRα) and GA repeat–binding protein-α (Gabpa) by PGC-1α appears to mediate much of the effect to increase oxidative phosphorylation gene expression in muscle.[254] Nitric oxide produced by endothelial nitric oxide synthase controls mitochondrial biogenesis,[379] possibly through increased expression of PGC-1α and other transcription factors. This process is mediated by cyclic guanosine 3',5'-phosphate, resulting from activation of soluble guanylate cyclase.

The pathway from exercise to activation of PGC-1α has been partially elucidated. Increases in calcium levels activate calcium/calmodulin-dependent kinase IV (CaMKIV) and calcineurin. Activated CaMKIV phosphorylates CREB, which increases transcription at CREB-responsive elements in the PGC-1α promoter.[380] Exercise also increases PGC-1α activity via phosphorylation through p38 mitogen-activated protein kinase.[381,382] AMPK, which is activated by exercise-induced changes in AMP levels, also increases mitochondrial biogenesis and PGC-1α activity in skeletal muscle,[383-385] but at present there is no evidence that PGC-1α is an AMPK substrate. Other conditions that induce mitochondrial biogenesis also increase PGC-1α promoter activity.

MECHANISMS THAT LINK CARDIOVASCULAR DISEASE AND INSULIN RESISTANCE

The Metabolic Syndrome

MI, stroke, or nonischemic cardiovascular disease is the cause of death in up to 80% of patients with T2DM. Independent of other risk factors, T2DM increases the risk of cardiovascular morbidity and fatality but also provides a synergistic interaction with other risk factors such as smoking, hypertension, and dyslipidemia.[386] In a Finnish population, diabetes increased the risk of MI fivefold,[387] and insulin resistance, as measured by elevated fasting insulin levels, increased the risk of death from heart disease.[388] Women are particularly vulnerable to the cardiovascular effects of T2DM because they appear to lose the

protective effects of estrogen in the premenopausal period.[389,390]

A constellation of metabolic derangements often seen in patients with insulin resistance and T2DM are individually associated with an increased risk of cardiovascular disease. These metabolic derangements have been variously designated *syndrome X*; the *dysmetabolic syndrome*; hypertension, obesity, non–insulin-dependent diabetes mellitus (NIDDM), dyslipidemia, and atherosclerotic cardiovascular disease *(HONDA)*; and the *deadly quartet*.[391,392] The syndrome has also been associated with easily oxidized, small LDL particles; heightened blood-clotting activity (e.g., increased PAI-1); and elevated serum uric acid concentrations. The proposed central abnormality associated with the metabolic syndrome is insulin resistance. Some of the abnormalities themselves have also been proposed to contribute to insulin resistance.

Controversy surrounding the metabolic syndrome has called attention to the question the clustering of cardiovascular risk factors such as central obesity, dyslipidemia, and hypertension and the association of this clustering with the risk of developing diabetes and cardiovascular disease. The controversy largely focuses on the cause of the syndrome, how best to define its presence, how clinical decision making should be modified based on those definitions, and whether there are not more effective ways to screen for diabetes and cardiovascular risk.[393]

Perhaps the overriding risk factor for coronary artery disease in insulin resistance and T2DM is the associated dyslipidemia. The profile includes hypertriglyceridemia, low plasma HDL, and small, dense LDL particle concentrations. The percentage of men with T2DM who have abnormal cholesterol levels is not different from that of nondiabetic men. However, diabetic women, compared with nondiabetic women, have almost double the rate of hypercholesterolemia[394] and greater changes in other lipid parameters that increase the risk of cardiovascular disease (Fig. 31-12). The physiologic basis for this abnormal lipid

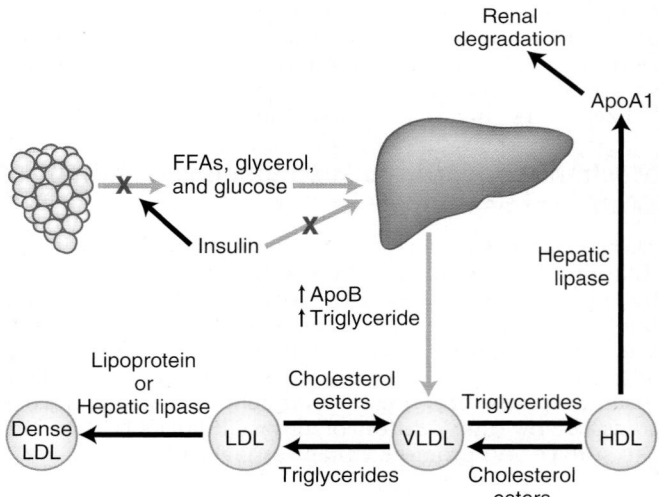

Figure 31-12 Insulin resistance and dyslipidemia. The suppression of lipoprotein lipase and very low density lipoprotein (VLDL) production by insulin is defective in insulin resistance, leading to increased flux of free fatty acids (FFAs) to the liver and increased VLDL production, which results in increased circulating triglyceride concentrations. The triglycerides are transferred to low-density lipoprotein (LDL) and high-density lipoprotein (HDL), and the VLDL particles gain cholesterol esters by the action of the cholesterol ester transfer protein (CETP). This leads to increased catabolism of HDL particles by the liver and loss of apolipoprotein (Apo) A, resulting in low HDL concentrations. The triglyceride-rich LDL particle is stripped of its triglycerides, resulting in the accumulation of atherogenic small, dense LDL particles.

profile appears to be overproduction of apolipoprotein B–containing VLDL particles. Production of apolipoprotein B by the liver is primarily post-translational[395] and is augmented by insulin and by the increased availability of FFAs in the portal circulation,[396-400] probably as a result of increased lipolysis in the visceral adipose tissue.[401-403] Part of the post-translational regulation may be due to insulin– and fatty acid–mediated increases in microsomal triglyceride transfer protein levels that catalyze the transfer of lipids to apolipoprotein B and decrease the ubiquitination-dependent degradation of apolipoprotein B.[404-406]

The overproduction of VLDL triglyceride results in increased transfer of VLDL triglyceride to HDL particles in exchange for HDL-cholesterol esters mediated by the cholesterol ester transfer protein.[407] The triglyceride-rich HDL is hydrolyzed by hepatic lipase; this leads to the generation of small HDL, which is degraded more readily by the kidney, resulting in low HDL levels in serum. Cholesterol ester transfer protein–mediated exchange of VLDL triglyceride for LDL-cholesterol esters and subsequent triglyceride hydrolysis by hepatic lipase probably result in generation of the small, dense LDL particles found in insulin-resistant subjects.[408-411]

The increased risk of heart disease in patients with diabetes has prompted the recommendation that persons with diabetes be treated for their dyslipidemia as aggressively as persons who have had a previous MI. In addition, patients with the metabolic syndrome of insulin resistance and obesity are considered to be in a higher risk category and should also be aggressively treated to lower lipids.[412]

The presence of hypertension and overt diabetes doubles the risk of cardiovascular disease. Defects in vasodilation and alterations in blood flow may provide a link to hypertension in insulin-resistant subjects. The normal vasodilative response of insulin is disrupted in obese, insulin-resistant, and diabetic persons,[413] perhaps through insulin's inability to increase the production of the potent vasodilator nitric oxide by endothelial cells.[414,415] The defect may be magnified by increases in plasma FFAs.[416] Other proposed mechanisms for insulin resistance leading to hypertension are activation of the sympathetic nervous system by insulin[417-419] and the intrinsic ability of insulin to cause salt and water resorption in the kidney, resulting in expanded plasma volume.[420-422]

Hypertension itself, independent of other risk factors, has been associated with the propensity to become diabetic.[423] A prospective cohort study found that T2DM was almost 2.5 times more likely to develop in subjects with hypertension than in subjects with normal blood pressure.[424] A possible mechanism is that an intrinsic defect in vasodilation might contribute to insulin resistance by decreasing the surface area of the vasculature perfusing skeletal muscle, decreasing the efficiency of glucose uptake.[416] Conversely, vasodilative agents might improve glucose uptake and might even prevent the onset of diabetes, as has been observed with angiotensin-converting enzyme (ACE) inhibitor therapy.[425]

Several factors involved in clotting and fibrinolysis, including fibrinogen, factor VII, and PAI-1, have been shown to be increased in persons with insulin resistance.[426-431] PAI-1 has been extensively studied, and there is a clear relationship between elevated PAI-1 levels and risk of coronary artery disease.[432] Insulin increased PAI-1 expression in hepatocytes, endothelial cells, and abdominal adipose tissue,[433-435] and insulin-sensitizing thiazolidinediones decreased PAI-1 activity.[436]

Upper-body rather than lower-body obesity (the apple rather than the pear shape) is highly correlated with insulin resistance and risk for T2DM. Therefore, the anatomic distribution of fat, rather than the overall degree of obesity, appears to determine risk for the metabolic syndrome. The reported association between increased abdominal (upper-body) fat and an increased risk of coronary heart disease is related to visceral fat, for which the waist-to-hip ratio is a convenient index. A waist-to-hip ratio greater than 1.0 in men or greater than 0.8 in women indicates abdominal obesity.[437] The National Cholesterol Education Program (NCEP) has suggested that a waist circumference greater than 40 inches (101.5 cm) in men or greater than 35 inches (89 cm) in women is a marker for the metabolic syndrome.[438]

INSULIN SECRETION

Normal insulin secretory function is essential for maintaining normal glucose tolerance, and abnormal insulin secretion is invariably present in patients with T2DM. In this section, the physiology of normal insulin and the alterations that are present in persons with T2DM are reviewed.

Quantitation of Beta-Cell Function

The measurement of peripheral insulin concentrations by radioimmunoassay is still the most widely used method for quantifying beta-cell functions in vivo.[439] Although this approach provides valuable information, it is limited because 50% to 60% of the insulin produced by the pancreas is extracted by the liver without ever reaching the systemic circulation.[440,441] The standard radioimmunoassay for measuring insulin concentrations is also unable to distinguish between endogenous and exogenous insulin, making it ineffective as a measure of endogenous beta-cell reserve in the insulin-treated diabetic patient. Anti-insulin antibodies that may be present in patients treated with insulin interfere with the insulin radioimmunoassay, making insulin measurements in insulin-treated patients inaccurate. Conventional insulin radioimmunoassays are also unable to distinguish between levels of circulating proinsulin and true levels of circulating insulin.

Insulin is derived from a single-chain precursor, proinsulin.[442] Within the Golgi apparatus of the pancreatic beta cell, proinsulin is cleaved by convertases to form insulin, C peptide, and two pairs of basic amino acids. Insulin is subsequently released into the circulation at concentrations equimolar with those of C peptide.[443,444] In addition, small amounts of intact proinsulin and proinsulin conversion intermediates are released. Proinsulin and its related conversion intermediates can be detected in the circulation, where they constitute 20% of the total circulating insulin-like immunoreactivity.[445] In vivo, proinsulin has a biologic potency that is only about 10% of that of insulin,[446,447] and the potency of split proinsulin intermediates is between that of proinsulin and that of insulin.[448,449] C peptide has no known conclusive effects on carbohydrate metabolism,[450,451] although certain physiologic effects of C peptide have been proposed.[452] Unlike insulin, C peptide is not extracted by the liver[443,453,454] and is excreted almost exclusively by the kidneys. Its plasma half-life of approximately 30 minutes[455] contrasts sharply with that of insulin, which is approximately 4 minutes.

Because C peptide is secreted in equimolar concentrations with insulin and is not extracted by the liver, levels of C peptide can be used as a marker of beta-cell function. The use of plasma C-peptide levels as an index of beta-cell function depends on the critical assumption that the mean clearance rate of C peptide is constant over the range of C-peptide levels observed under normal physiologic conditions. This assumption has been shown to be valid for both dogs and humans,[441,456] and this approach can be used to derive rates of insulin secretion from plasma concentrations of C peptide under steady-state conditions.[456] However, because of the long plasma half-life of C peptide, under non–steady-state conditions (e.g., after stimulation of insulin secretion by glucose), peripheral plasma levels of C peptide do not change in proportion to the changing insulin secretion rate.[456,457] Therefore, under such conditions, insulin secretion rates are best calculated with use of the two-compartment model initially proposed by Eaton and coworkers.[458]

Modifications to the C peptide model of insulin secretion have been introduced. They combine the minimal model of insulin action with the two-compartment model of C-peptide kinetics and allow insulin secretion and insulin sensitivity to be derived after intravenous or oral administration of glucose.[459-462]

Signaling Pathways in the Beta Cell and Insulin Secretion

The signaling pathways in the pancreatic beta cell are involved in the stimulus-secretion coupling of insulin release. These pathways provide the mechanism whereby insulin secretion rates respond to changes in blood glucose concentrations (Fig. 31-13). Glucose enters the pancreatic beta cell by a process of facilitated diffusion mediated by the glucose transporter GLUT2. Although levels of GLUT2 on the beta-cell membrane are reduced in diabetic states for various reasons, it is not currently believed that this is a rate-limiting step in the regulation of insulin secretion.

The first rate-limiting step in this process is the phosphorylation of glucose to glucose 6-phosphate. This reaction is mediated by the enzyme glucokinase.[463,464] There is considerable evidence that glucokinase, by determining the rate of glycolysis, functions as the glucose sensor of the beta cell and that this is the primary mechanism by which the rate of insulin secretion adapts to changes in blood glucose. According to this view, as blood glucose levels increase, more glucose enters the beta cell, the rate of glycolysis increases, and the rate of insulin secretion increases. A fall in blood glucose levels results in a fall in the rate of glycolysis and a reduction in the rate of insulin secretion.

Glucose metabolism produces an increase in cytosolic ATP, the key signal that initiates insulin secretion by causing blockade of the K_{ATP} channel on the beta-cell membrane. Blockade of this channel induces membrane depolarization, which leads to an increase in cytosolic Ca^{2+} and insulin secretion. The biochemical events that link the increase in glycolysis to an increase in ATP are complex. Dukes and coworkers[465] proposed that glycolytic production of NADH during the oxidation of glyceraldehyde 3-phosphate is the key process because NADH is subsequently processed into ATP by mitochondria through the operation of specific shuttle systems.

The rate of pyruvate generation has also been proposed as an explanation for the link between glucose metabolism and increased insulin secretion.[466] According to this view, pyruvate generated by the glycolytic pathway enters the mitochondria and is metabolized further in the TCA cycle. Electron transfer from the TCA cycle to the respiratory chain by NADH and the reduced form of flavin adenine dinucleotide ($FADH_2$) promotes the generation of ATP, which is exported into the cytosol. The increase in ATP closes ATP-sensitive K^+ channels, which depolarizes the beta-cell membrane and opens the voltage-dependent Ca^{2+} channels, leading to an increase in intracellular Ca^{2+}. The increase in cytosolic Ca^{2+} is the main trigger for exocytosis,

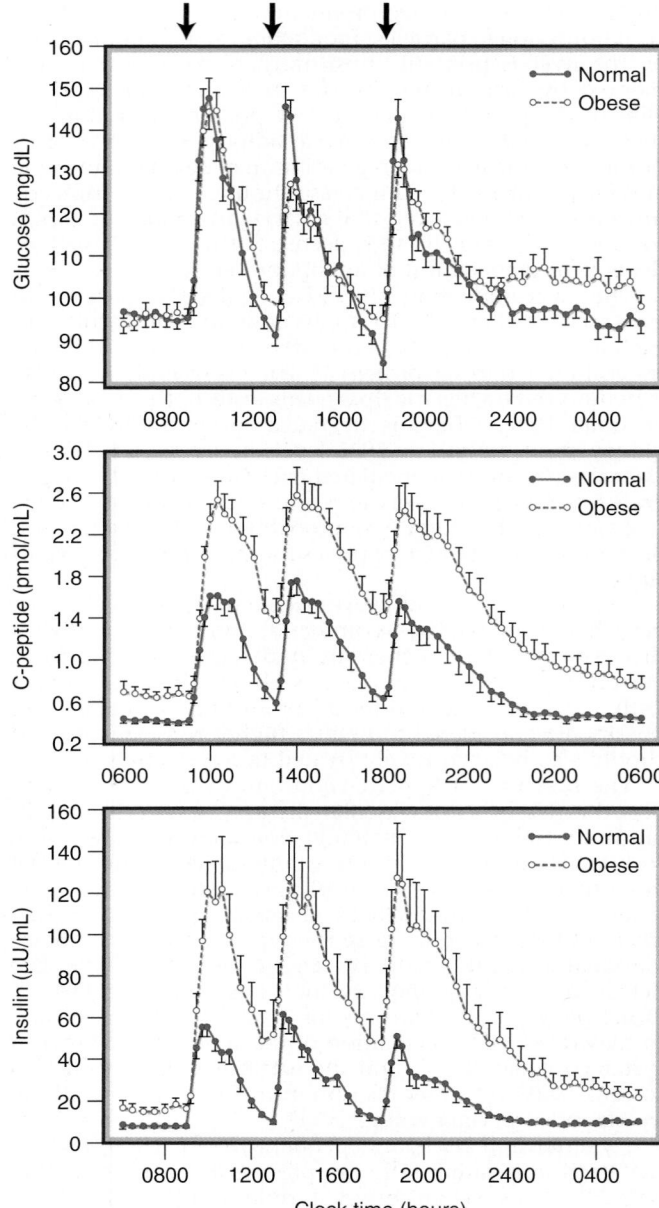

Figure 31-13 Mean 24-hour profiles of plasma concentrations of glucose *(top panel)*, C peptide *(middle panel)*, and insulin *(bottom panel)* in normal and obese subjects. The three arrows above the figure indicate the ingestion of the breakfast, lunch, and dinner meals, respectively. (From Polonsky KS, Given BD, van Cauter E. Twenty-four-hour profiles and pulsatile patterns of insulin secretion in normal and obese subjects. *J Clin Invest.* 1988;81:442-448.)

the process by which insulin-containing secretory granules fuse with the plasma membrane, leading to the release of insulin into the circulation. The increase in ATP not only closes K_{ATP} channels but also serves as a major permissive factor for movement of insulin granules and for priming of exocytosis.

Cyclic AMP also plays an important role in beta-cell signal transduction pathways. This second messenger is generated at the plasma membrane from ATP and potentiates glucose-stimulated insulin secretion, particularly in response to glucagon, GLP-1, and gastric inhibitory polypeptide (GIP; also known as glucose-dependent insulinotropic peptide). The cAMP-dependent pathways appear to be particularly important in the exocytotic machinery.

K_{ATP} channels play an essential role in beta-cell stimulus-secretion coupling; an excellent review was published by Aguilar-Bryan and colleagues.[467] K_{ATP} channels include sulfonylurea receptors (SURs) and potassium inward rectifiers (Kir6.1 and Kir6.2), which assemble to form a large octameric channel with a (SUR/Kir6.x) stoichiometry. In the pancreatic beta cell, the SUR1/Kir6.2 pairs constitute the K_{ATP} channel. K_{ATP} channels control the flux of potassium ions driven by an electrochemical potential. Opening of these channels can set the resting membrane potential of beta cells below the threshold for activation of voltage-gated Ca^{2+} channels when plasma glucose levels are low, thus reducing insulin secretion. Changes in the cytosolic concentrations of ATP and ADP lead to closure of the channels and depolarization of the beta-cell membrane. Mutations in both components of the beta-cell K_{ATP} (i.e., SUR1 and Kir6.2) have been shown to lead to hypersecretion of insulin, resulting clinically in either a recessive form of familial hyperinsulinemia or persistent hyperinsulinemic hypoglycemia of infancy.

Physiologic Factors Regulating Insulin Secretion

Carbohydrate Nutrients

The most important physiologic substance involved in the regulation of insulin release is glucose.[468-470] The effect of glucose on the beta cell is dose related. Dose-dependent increases in concentrations of insulin and C peptide and in rates of insulin secretion have been observed after oral and intravenous glucose loads, with 1.4 units of insulin, on average, being secreted in response to an oral glucose load as small as 12 g.[471-474] The insulin secretory response is greater after oral than after intravenous glucose administration.[475-477] Known as the *incretin effect*,[473,478] this enhanced response to oral glucose has been interpreted as an indication that absorption of glucose by way of the gastrointestinal tract stimulates the release of hormones and other mechanisms that ultimately enhance the sensitivity of the beta cell to glucose (see later discussion). In a study involving normal volunteers, glucose was infused at a rate designed to achieve levels previously attained after an oral glucose load. The amount of insulin secreted in response to the intravenous load was 26% less than that secreted in response to the oral load.[477]

Insulin secretion does not respond as a linear function of glucose concentration. The relationship of glucose concentration to the rate of insulin release follows a sigmoidal curve. The threshold corresponds to the glucose levels normally seen under fasting conditions, and the steep portion of the dose-response curve corresponds to the range of glucose levels normally achieved postprandially.[479-481] The sigmoidal nature of the dose-response curve has been attributed to a gaussian distribution of thresholds for stimulation among the individual beta cells.[481-483]

When glucose is infused intravenously at a constant rate, an initial biphasic secretory response is observed that consists of a rapid, early insulin peak followed by a second, more slowly rising peak.[468,474,475] The significance of the first-phase insulin release is unclear, but it might reflect the existence of a compartment of readily releasable insulin within the beta cell or a transient rise and fall of a metabolic signal for insulin secretion.[484] Despite early suggestions to the contrary,[485,486] it has been demonstrated that the first-phase response to intravenous glucose is highly reproducible within subjects.[487] After the acute response, a second phase of insulin release occurs that is directly related to the level of glucose elevation. In vitro studies of isolated islet cells and perfused pancreas have identified a third phase of insulin secretion that commences 1.5 to 3.0 hours after exposure to glucose and is characterized by a spontaneous decline in secretion to 15% to 25% of the amount released during peak secretion. This low level is subsequently maintained for longer than 48 hours.[488-491]

In addition to its acute secretagogue effects on insulin secretion, glucose has intermediate- and longer term effects that are physiologically and clinically relevant. In the intermediate term, exposure of the pancreatic beta cell to a high concentration of glucose primes its response to a subsequent glucose stimulus, leading to a shift to the left in the dose-response curve relating glucose and insulin secretion.[492,493] However, when pancreatic islets are exposed to high concentrations for prolonged periods, a reduction of insulin secretion is seen. Although all of the precise mechanisms responsible for these adverse effects, termed *glucotoxicity*, are not known, there is evidence that long-term exposure to high glucose reduces the expression of a number of genes that are critical to normal beta-cell function, including the insulin gene.[494,495]

Noncarbohydrate Nutrients

Amino acids have been shown to stimulate insulin release in the absence of glucose, the most potent secretagogues being the essential amino acids leucine, arginine, and lysine.[496,497] The effects of arginine and lysine on the beta cell appear to be more potent than those of leucine. The effects of amino acids on insulin secretion are potentiated by glucose.[498,499]

In contrast to amino acids, various lipids and their metabolites appear to have only minor effects on insulin release in vivo. Although carbohydrate-rich fat meals stimulate insulin secretion, carbohydrate-free fat meals have minimal effects on beta-cell function.[500] Ketone bodies and short- and long-chain fatty acids have been shown to stimulate insulin secretion acutely in islet cells and in human subjects.[501-505] The effects of elevated FFAs on the insulin secretory responses to glucose are related to the duration of the exposure. Zhou and Grill[506] first suggested that long-term exposure of pancreatic islets to FFAs inhibited glucose-induced insulin secretion and biosynthesis. This observation was confirmed in rats.[507] In humans, it was demonstrated that the insulin resistance induced by an acute (90-minute) elevation in FFAs was compensated by an appropriate increase in insulin secretion.[508] After chronic elevation of FFAs (48 hours), the beta-cell compensatory response for insulin resistance was not adequate. Additional studies demonstrated that the adverse effects of prolonged FFAs on glucose-induced insulin secretion are not seen in subjects with T2DM. From these results, it appears that elevated FFAs might contribute to the failure of beta-cell compensation for insulin resistance.

Hormonal Factors

The release of insulin from the beta cell after a meal is facilitated by a number of gastrointestinal peptide hormones, including GIP, cholecystokinin, and GLP-1.[478,509-516] These hormones are released from small intestinal endocrine cells postprandially and travel in the bloodstream to reach the beta cells, where they act through second messengers to increase the sensitivity of these islet cells to glucose. In general, these hormones are not themselves secretagogues, and their effects are evident only in the presence of hyperglycemia.[509-511] The release of these peptides might explain why the modest postprandial glucose levels achieved in normal subjects in vivo have such a dramatic effect on insulin production, whereas similar glucose concentrations in vitro elicit a much smaller response.[516] Similarly, this incretin effect could account for the greater beta-cell response observed after oral as opposed to intravenous glucose administration.

Whether impaired postprandial secretion of incretin hormones plays a role in the inadequate insulin secretory response to oral glucose and to meals in patients with IGT or diabetes is controversial,[517-524] but pharmacologic doses of these peptides might have future therapeutic benefit. Subcutaneous administration of GLP-1, the most potent of the incretin peptides, lowers glucose in patients with T2DM by stimulating endogenous insulin secretion and perhaps by inhibiting glucagon secretion and gastric emptying.[525,526] However, because of the short half-life of GLP-1, its longer-acting analogue, exendin-4, has greater therapeutic promise.[527] Treatment with supraphysiologic doses of GIP during hyperglycemia has been shown to augment insulin secretion in normal humans[528,529] but not in diabetics.[520,529] Although cholecystokinin has the ability to augment insulin secretion in humans, it is not firmly established whether it is an incretin at physiologic levels.[530-533] Its effects are also seen largely at pharmacologic doses.[534]

The postprandial insulin secretory response may also be influenced by other intestinal peptide hormones, including vasoactive intestinal polypeptide,[535] secretin,[536-539] and gastrin,[536,540] but the precise roles of these hormones remain to be elucidated.

The hormones produced by pancreatic alpha and beta cells also modulate insulin release. Whereas glucagon has a stimulatory effect on the beta cell,[541] somatostatin suppresses insulin release.[542] It is currently unclear whether these hormones reach the beta cell by traveling through the islet cell interstitium (thus exerting a paracrine effect) or through islet cell capillaries. Indeed, the importance of these two hormones in regulating basal and postprandial insulin levels under normal physiologic circumstances is in doubt. Paradoxically, the low insulin levels observed during prolonged periods of starvation have been attributed to the elevated glucagon concentrations seen in this setting.[500,543-546] Other hormones that exert a stimulatory effect on insulin secretion include growth hormone,[547] glucocorticoids,[548] prolactin,[549-551] placental lactogen,[552] and the sex steroids.[553]

Whereas all of the preceding hormones might stimulate insulin secretion indirectly by inducing a state of insulin resistance, some might also act directly on the beta cell, possibly to augment its sensitivity to glucose. Hyperinsulinemia is associated with conditions in which these hormones are present in excess, such as acromegaly, Cushing syndrome, and the second half of pregnancy. Furthermore, treatments with placental lactogen,[554] hydrocortisone,[555] and growth hormone[555,556] are all effective in reversing the reduction in insulin response to glucose that is observed in vitro after hypophysectomy. Although hyperinsulinemia after an oral glucose load has been observed in patients with hyperthyroidism,[557,558] the increased concentration of immunoreactive insulin in this setting may reflect elevations in serum proinsulin rather than a true increase in serum insulin.[559]

Neural Factors

The islets are innervated by the cholinergic and adrenergic limbs of the autonomic nervous system. Although both sympathetic stimulation and parasympathetic stimulation enhance secretion of glucagon,[560,561] the secretion of insulin is stimulated by vagal nerve fibers and inhibited by sympathetic nerve fibers.[560-565] Adrenergic inhibition of the beta cell appears to be mediated by the α-adrenoceptor, because its effect is attenuated by the α-antagonist phentolamine[561] and reproduced by the α_2-agonist clonidine.[566] There is also considerable evidence that many indirect effects of sympathetic nerve stimulation play a role in regulating beta-cell function through stimulation or inhibition of somatostatin, β_2-adrenoceptors, and the neuropeptides galanin and neuropeptide Y.[567]

Parasympathetic stimulation of islets results in stimulation of insulin, glucagon, and pancreatic polypeptide directly and through the neuropeptides vasoactive intestinal polypeptide, gastrin-releasing polypeptide, and pituitary adenylate cyclase-activating polypeptide.[567] In addition, sensory innervation of islets may play a role in tonic inhibition of insulin secretion through the neuropeptides calcitonin gene-related peptide[568-570] and, less clearly, substance P.[571,572]

The importance of the autonomic nervous system in regulating insulin secretion in vivo is unclear. The neural effects on beta-cell function cannot be entirely dissociated from the hormonal effects because some of the neurotransmitters of the autonomic nervous system are, in fact, hormones. Furthermore, the secretion of insulinotropic hormones such as GIP and GLP-1 postprandially has been shown to be under vagal[573,574] and adrenergic[575,576] control.

Temporal Pattern of Insulin Secretion

It has been estimated that 50% of the total insulin secreted by the pancreas in any 24-hour period is secreted under basal conditions, and the remainder is secreted in response to meals.[577,578] The estimated basal insulin secretion rates range from 18 to 32 units (0.7 to 1.3 mg) per 24 hours.[456,458,471,577] After meal ingestion, the insulin secretory response is rapid, and insulin secretion increases approximately fivefold over baseline to reach a peak within 60 minutes (Fig. 31-14; see Fig. 31-13). When study subjects consumed 20% of calories with breakfast and 40% with lunch and dinner, the amount of insulin secreted after each meal did not differ significantly. There was a rapid insulin secretory response to breakfast, with 71.6% ± 1.6% of the insulin secreted in the 4 hours after the meal being produced in the first 2 hours and the remainder in the next 2 hours. Insulin secretion did not decrease as rapidly after lunch and dinner, with, respectively, 62.8% ± 1.6% and 59.6% ± 1.4% of the total meal response secreted during the first 2 hours after the meal.

The normal insulin secretory profile is characterized by a series of insulin secretory pulses. After breakfast, 1.8 ± 0.2 secretory pulses were identified in normal volunteers, and the peaks of these pulses occurred 42.8 ± 3.4 minutes after the meal. Multiple insulin secretory pulses were also identified after lunch and dinner. After these meals, up to four pulses of insulin secretion were identified in both groups of subjects. In the 5-hour time interval between lunch and dinner, an average of 2.5 ± 0.3 secretory pulses were identified, and 2.6 ± 0.2 were identified in the same period after dinner.[578]

Pulses of insulin secretion that did not appear to be meal related were also identified. Between 11 PM and 6 AM and in the 3 hours before breakfast, on average 3.9 ± 0.3 secretory pulses were present in normal subjects. Therefore, over the 24-hour period of observation, a total of 11.1 ± 0.5 pulses were identified in normal subjects. Almost 90% (87% ± 3%) of postmeal pulses in insulin secretion, but only 47% ± 8% of non–meal-related pulses, were concomitant with a pulse in glucose.[578]

In vivo studies of beta-cell secretory function have demonstrated that insulin is released in a pulsatile manner. This

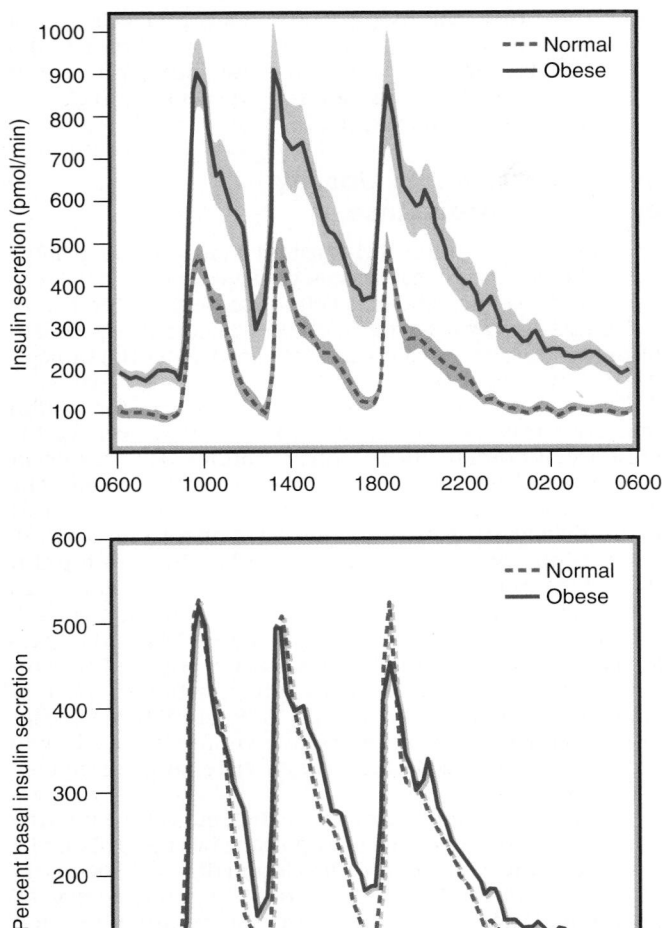

Figure 31-14 Mean 24-hour profiles of insulin secretion rates in normal and obese subjects *(top)*. The *shaded areas* represent ±1 standard error of the mean. The curves in the *lower panel* were derived by dividing the insulin secretion rate measured in each subject by the basal secretion rate derived in the same subject. Mean data for normal *(dashed line)* and obese *(solid line)* subjects are shown. (From Polonsky KS, Given BD, van Cauter E. Twenty-four-hour profiles and pulsatile patterns of insulin secretion in normal and obese subjects. *J Clin Invest.* 1988;81:442-448.)

behavior is characterized by rapid oscillations occurring every 8 to 15 minutes that are superimposed on slower (ultradian) oscillations occurring at a periodicity of 80 to 150 minutes.[579] The rapid oscillations persist in vitro and therefore are likely to be the result of metabolic pathways in the pancreatic beta cell that involve negative feedback loops with time lags.

Rapid Oscillations

The rapid oscillations of insulin are of small amplitude in the systemic circulation, averaging between 0.4 and 3.2 µU/mL in several published human studies.[580-582] Because these values are close to the limits of sensitivity of most standard insulin radioimmunoassays, the characterization

of these oscillations is subject to considerable pitfalls,[583] not the least of which is the need to differentiate between true oscillations of small amplitude and random assay noise. The latter problem has been overcome by the development of extremely sensitive enzyme-linked immunosorbent assays (ELISAs) that allow the detection of extremely small changes in peripheral insulin concentrations. The application of these assays in studies involving frequent sampling from the peripheral circulation has led to a series of studies of the role of these oscillations in the overall regulation of insulin secretion.[584-588]

These investigations suggested that the increases in overall insulin secretion seen in response to a variety of secretagogues in various physiologic and pathophysiologic states result from an increase in the amplitude of the bursts of insulin secretion. The researchers have proposed that 75% of insulin secretion is accounted for by secretory bursts and that the responses to GLP-1, sulfonylureas, and oral glucose are all mediated by an increase in the amplitude of insulin secretory pulses. Furthermore, consistent with observations made by O'Rahilly and colleagues,[589] relatives of patients with T2DM demonstrate a disorderly profile of the insulin secretory oscillations. A number of mathematical programs have been developed that allow these insulin secretory oscillations to be evaluated and studied.[590] The latest additions to the list are so-called approximate entropy *(ApEn)* and cross-approximate entropy *(cross-ApEn)*, which are statistics that measure temporal regularity of the oscillations in the insulin secretory profile.[591]

The low amplitude of the rapid oscillations in the systemic circulation contrasts sharply with observations in the portal vein, where pulse amplitudes of 20 to 40 µU/mL have been recorded in dogs.[592] Although the physiologic importance of these low-amplitude rapid pulses in the periphery is unclear, they are likely to be of physiologic importance in the portal vein. It is possible that the liver responds more readily to insulin delivered in a pulsatile fashion than to insulin delivered at a constant rate.[593-595]

Ultradian Oscillations

In contrast to the rapid oscillations, the slower (ultradian) oscillations are of much larger amplitude in the peripheral circulation. They are present under basal conditions but are amplified postprandially (Fig. 31-15), and they have been observed in subjects receiving intravenous glucose, suggesting that they are not generated by intermittent absorption of nutrients from the gut. Furthermore, they do not appear to be related to fluctuations in glucagon or cortisol levels,[488] and they are not regulated by neural factors, because these oscillations are also present in recipients of successful pancreas transplants.[596,597] Many of these ultradian insulin and C-peptide pulses are synchronous with pulses of similar oscillatory periods in glucose, raising the possibility that these oscillations are a product of the insulin-glucose feedback mechanism. Ultradian oscillations are self-sustained during constant glucose infusion at various rates; they are increased in amplitude after stimulation of insulin secretion without change in frequency, and there is a slight temporal advance of the glucose versus the insulin oscillation.

These findings suggest that the ultradian oscillations may be entirely accounted for by the major dynamic characteristics of the insulin-glucose feedback system, with no need to postulate the existence of an intrapancreatic pacemaker.[598] In support of this hypothesis, Sturis and colleagues[599] demonstrated that when glucose is administered in an oscillatory pattern, ultradian oscillations in plasma

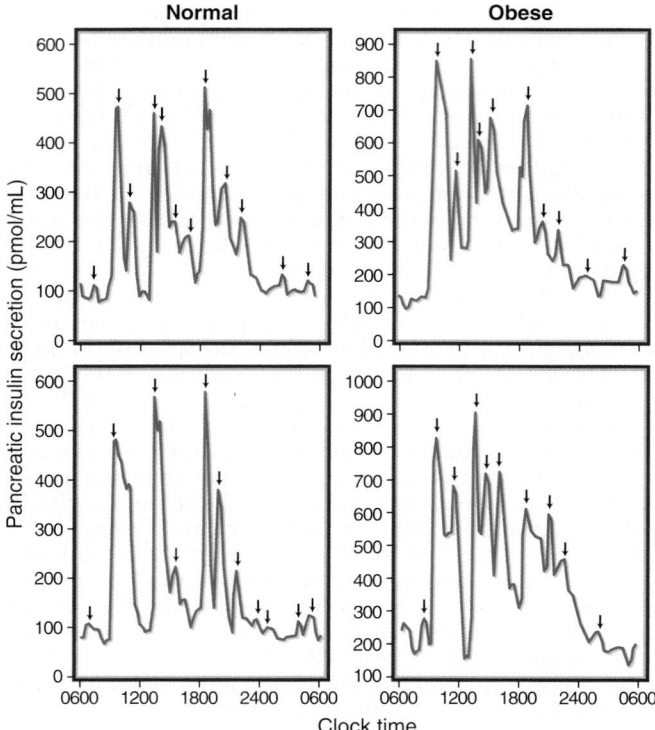

Figure 31-15 Patterns of insulin secretion in normal and obese subjects. Four representative 24-hour profiles are shown from two normal-weight subjects *(left)* and two obese subjects *(right)*. Meals were consumed at 0900, 1300, and 1800 hours. Statistically significant pulses of secretion are shown by the *arrows.* (From Polonsky KS, Given BD, van Cauter E. Twenty-four-hour profiles and pulsatile patterns of insulin secretion in normal and obese subjects. *J Clin Invest.* 1988;81:442-448.)

glucose and insulin secretion are generated that are 100% concordant with the oscillatory period of the exogenous glucose infusion. This close relationship between the ultradian oscillations in insulin secretion and similar oscillations in plasma glucose was further exemplified in a series of dose-response studies in which the largest-amplitude oscillations in insulin secretion were observed in those subjects exhibiting the largest amplitude glucose oscillations, which in turn were directly related to the infusion dose of glucose. It has been shown that, in normal humans, insulin is more effective in reducing plasma glucose levels when it is administered intravenously as a 120-minute oscillation than when it is delivered at a constant rate. These results indicate that the ultradian oscillations have functional significance.[599]

Circadian Oscillations

Circadian variations in the secretion of insulin have also been reported. When insulin secretory responses were measured for a 24-hour period during which subjects received three standard meals, the maximal postprandial responses were observed after breakfast.[578,580] These findings were mirrored by the results of studies in which subjects were tested for oral glucose tolerance at different times of the day and were found to exhibit maximal insulin secretory responses in the morning and lower responses in the afternoon and evening.[600,601] These diurnal differences were also noted in tests for intravenous glucose tolerance. Furthermore, although ultradian glucose and insulin oscillations are closely correlated during a constant 24-hour glucose infu-

sion, the nocturnal rise in mean glucose levels is not accompanied by a similar increase in the insulin secretory rate.[602] It has been postulated that these diurnal differences reflect diminished responsiveness of the beta cell to glucose in the afternoon and evening.[601]

Insulin Secretion in Obesity and Insulin Resistance

Obesity and other insulin-resistant states are associated with a substantially greater risk of developing T2DM. The ability of the pancreatic beta cell to compensate for insulin resistance determines whether blood glucose levels remain normal in insulin-resistant subjects or whether the subjects develop IGT or diabetes.

The nature of the beta cell's compensation for insulin resistance involves hypersecretion of insulin even in the presence of normal glucose concentrations. This can occur only if beta-cell sensitivity to glucose is increased. The increase in beta-cell sensitivity to glucose in obesity appears to be mediated by two factors. First, increased beta-cell mass is observed in obesity and other insulin-resistant states.[603] Second, insulin resistance appears to be associated with increased expression of hexokinase in the beta cell relative to the expression of glucokinase.[604] Because hexokinase has a significantly lower Michaelis constant (K_m) for glucose than glucokinase does, the functional effect of increased hexokinase expression is to shift the glucose–insulin secretion dose-response curve to the left, leading to increased insulin secretion across a wide range of glucose concentrations.

Assessment of the adequacy of the beta-cell compensation for insulin resistance is important because this is the major determinant of the development of diabetes. In insulin-resistant states, it is important to evaluate beta-cell function in relation to the degree of insulin resistance. Kahn and coworkers[605] studied the relationship between insulin sensitivity and beta-cell function in 93 relatively young, apparently healthy human subjects with varying degrees of obesity. A sensitivity index (SI) was calculated using the minimal model of Bergman as a measure of insulin sensitivity and was then compared with various measures of insulin secretion.[461,606] The relationship between the SI and the beta-cell measures was curvilinear and reciprocal for fasting insulin concentration ($p < 0.0001$), first-phase (acute) insulin response (AIR glucose; $p < 0.0001$), glucose potentiation slope ($n = 56$; $p < 0.005$), and beta-cell secretory capacity (AIR$_{max}$; $n = 43$; $p < 0.0001$). The curvilinear relationship between SI and the beta-cell measures could not be distinguished from a hyperbola (i.e., SI × beta-cell function = a constant). The nature of this relationship is consistent with a regulated feedback loop control system such that, for any difference in SI, a proportionate reciprocal difference occurs in insulin levels and responses in subjects with similar carbohydrate tolerance. Therefore, in human subjects with normal glucose tolerance and varying degrees of obesity, beta-cell function varies quantitatively with differences in insulin sensitivity. The increase in insulin secretion that is observed with a fall in SI should be viewed as the beta-cell compensation that allows normal glucose tolerance to be maintained in the presence of insulin resistance.

The insulin resistance of obesity is characterized by hyperinsulinemia. Hyperinsulinemia in this setting reflects a combination of increased insulin production and decreased insulin clearance, but most evidence suggests that increased insulin secretion is the predominant factor.[607,608] Both basal and 24-hour insulin secretory rates are three to four times higher in obese subjects and are

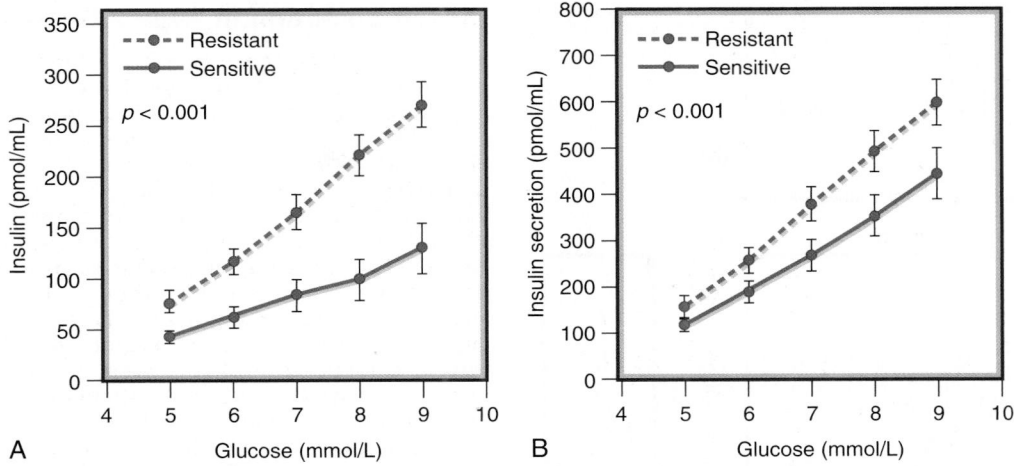

Figure 31-16 Plasma insulin concentrations (**A**) and insulin secretion rates (**B**) in response to molar increments in the plasma glucose concentration during a graded glucose infusion in insulin-resistant *(dotted line)* and insulin-sensitive *(solid line)* groups. (From Jones CNO, Pei D, Staris P, et al. Alterations in the glucose-stimulated insulin secretory dose-response curve and in insulin clearance in nondiabetic insulin-resistant individuals. *J Clin Endocrinol Metab.* 1997;82:1834-1838.)

strongly correlated with BMI. Insulin secretory responses to intravenous glucose have been studied in otherwise healthy insulin-resistant subjects and compared with the responses in insulin-sensitive subjects by means of a graded glucose infusion.

Figure 31-16 depicts insulin concentrations and insulin secretion rates at each level of plasma glucose achieved, outlining the respective dose-response relationships. Both insulin concentrations and insulin secretion rates are increased in insulin-resistant subjects as a result of a combination of increased insulin secretion and decreased insulin clearance. For each level of glucose, insulin secretion rates are higher in insulin-resistant than in insulin-sensitive subjects, reflecting an adaptive response of the beta cell to peripheral insulin resistance. Similar compensatory hyperinsulinemia has been demonstrated using other clinical techniques, such as the frequently sampled intravenous glucose tolerance test, in obese patients and in those with other insulin-resistant states, such as late pregnancy.[605,609]

The temporal pattern of insulin secretion is unaltered in obese subjects compared with normal subjects. Basal insulin secretion in obese subjects accounts for 50% of the total daily production of insulin, and secretory pulses of insulin occur every 1.5 to 2 hours.[580,607] However, the amplitude of these pulses postprandially is greater in obese subjects. Nevertheless, when these postprandial secretory responses are expressed as a percentage of the basal secretory rate, the postprandial responses in obese and normal subjects are identical.

Insulin Secretion in Subjects With Impaired Glucose Tolerance

It has been suggested that insulin secretion may be normal in subjects with IGT. However, substantial defects in insulin secretion have been demonstrated in people who have normal FPG and normal HbA$_{1c}$ concentrations, with glucose values greater than 140 mg/dL (7.8 mmol/L) 2 hours after oral ingestion of 75 g of glucose. Therefore, defects in insulin secretion can be detected before the onset of overt hyperglycemia.

Detailed study of insulin secretion in patients with IGT has demonstrated consistent quantitative and qualitative

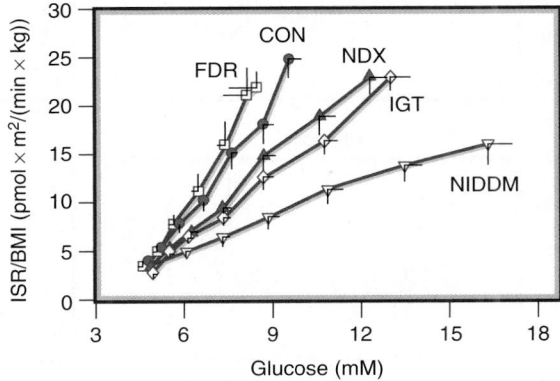

Figure 31-17 Dose-response relationship between glucose and insulin secretory rate (ISR) after an overnight fast in control subjects (CON), normoglycemic first-degree relatives (FDR) of subjects with a family history of non–insulin-dependent diabetes mellitus (NIDDM), subjects with a nondiagnostic oral glucose tolerance test (NDX), subjects with impaired glucose tolerance (IGT), and subjects with NIDDM. BMI, body mass index. (From Byrne MM, Sturis J, Sobel RJ, et al. Elevated plasma glucose 2 h postchallenge predicts defects in beta-cell function. *Am J Physiol.* 1996;270:E572-E579. Copyright 1996, the American Physiological Society.)

defects in this group. During OGTT, there is a delay in the peak insulin response.[143,610,611] The glucose–insulin secretion dose-response relationship is flattened and shifted to the right (Fig. 31-17), and first-phase insulin responses to an intravenous glucose bolus are consistently decreased in relation to ambient insulin sensitivity.[612,613]

The temporal pattern of insulin secretory responses is altered in IGT and is similar to but not as pronounced as that seen in diabetic subjects (see later discussion). There is a loss of coordinated insulin secretory responses during oscillatory glucose infusion, indicating that the ability of the beta cell to sense and respond appropriately to parallel changes in the plasma glucose level is impaired (Fig. 31-18). Abnormalities in rapid oscillations of insulin secretion have also been observed in first-degree relatives of patients with T2DM who have only mild IGT,[589] further suggesting that abnormalities in the temporal pattern of beta-cell

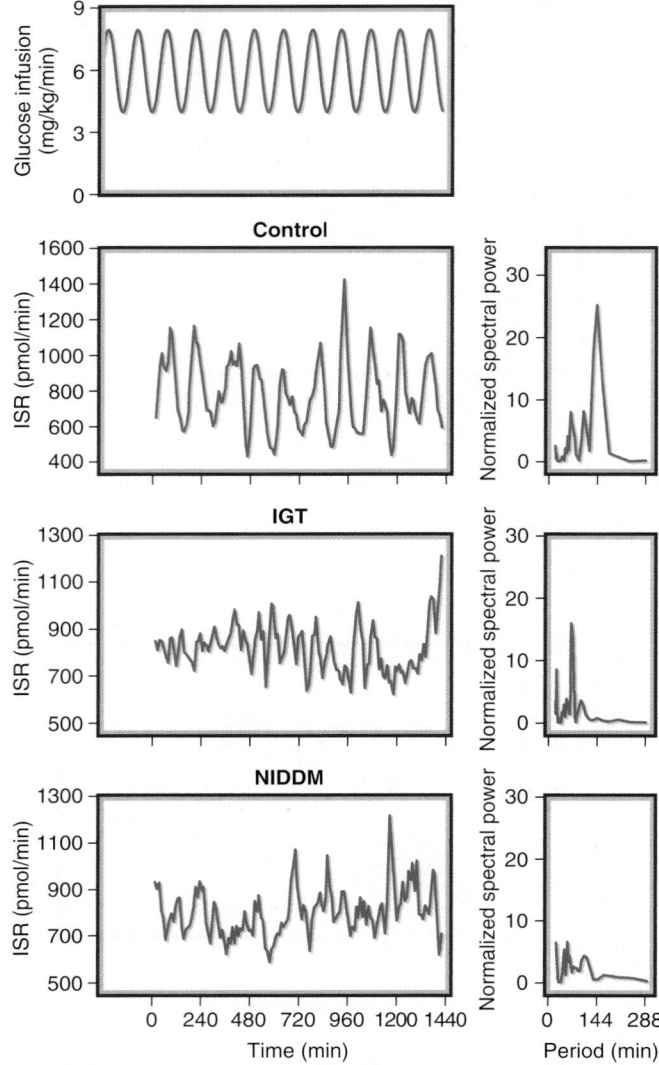

Figure 31-18 Oscillatory glucose infusions *(top panel)* were administered with a periodicity of 144 minutes to representative subjects with normal glucose tolerance (Control), impaired glucose tolerance (IGT), or type 2 diabetes (NIDDM). In the control subject, the insulin secretion rate (ISR) adjusts and responds to the 144-minute oscillations in glucose, resulting in sharp spectral peak at 144 minutes. In the other subjects, the ISR does not respond to the oscillatory glucose stimulus. Although oscillations in insulin secretion are evident, they are irregular, resulting in markedly reduced spectral peaks at 144 minutes and small-amplitude, high-frequency spectral peaks. These results are shown in the curves of normalized spectral power *(right column)* for each subject. (Modified from O'Meara NM, Sturis J, Van Cauter E, et al. Lack of control by glucose of ultradian insulin secretory oscillations in impaired glucose tolerance and in non-insulin-dependent diabetes mellitus. *J Clin Invest.* 1993;92:262-271.)

function may be an early manifestation of beta-cell dysfunction preceding the development of T2DM.

Because an elevation in serum proinsulin is seen in subjects with diabetes, the contribution of proinsulin to the hyperinsulinemia of IGT has been questioned. The hyperinsulinemia of IGT has not been accounted for by an increase in proinsulin, although elevations in fasting and stimulated proinsulin levels or proinsulin-to-insulin ratios have been found by many (although not all) investigators.[614-619] Correlation of elevated proinsulin levels in IGT as a predictor of future conversion to diabetes has also been observed.[620-622]

Insulin Secretion in Type 2 Diabetes Mellitus

Because of the presence of concomitant insulin resistance, patients with T2DM are often hyperinsulinemic, but the degree of hyperinsulinemia is inappropriately low for the prevailing glucose concentrations. Nevertheless, many of these patients have sufficient beta-cell reserve to maintain a euglycemic state by diet restriction with or without an oral agent. The beta-cell defect in patients with T2DM is characterized by an absent first-phase insulin and C-peptide response to an intravenous glucose load and a reduced second-phase response.[623] Although hyperglycemia can play a role in mediating these changes, the abnormal first-phase response to intravenous glucose persists in patients whose diabetic control has been greatly improved,[624,625] consistent with the idea that patients with T2DM have an intrinsic defect in the beta cell.

Furthermore, abnormalities in first-phase insulin secretion were observed in first-degree relatives of patients with T2DM who exhibited only mild IGT,[626] and an attenuated insulin response to oral glucose was observed in normoglycemic twins of patients with T2DM,[627] a group at high risk for T2DM and who can legitimately be classified as prediabetic.[628] This pattern of insulin secretion during the prediabetic phase was also seen in subjects with IGT who later developed T2DM[501,629,630] and in normoglycemic obese subjects with a recent history of gestational diabetes,[631] another group at high risk for T2DM.[632] Beta-cell abnormalities can therefore precede the development of overt T2DM by many years.

T2DM also affects proinsulin levels in serum. Increased levels of proinsulin are consistently seen in association with increases in the proinsulin-to-insulin molar ratio.[623] The amount of proinsulin produced in this setting appears to be related to the degree of glycemic control rather than the duration of the diabetic state, and in one series proinsulin levels contributed almost 50% of the total insulin immunoreactivity in T2DM patients who had marked hyperglycemia. In addition to intact proinsulin, the beta cell secretes one or more of the four major proinsulin conversion products (split 32,33-proinsulin, split 65,66-proinsulin, des-31,32-proinsulin, and des-64,65-proinsulin) into the circulation. These conversion products are produced within the secretory granules of the islet as a result of the activity of specific conversion enzymes at the two cleavage sites in proinsulin that link the C peptide to the A and B chains.[614-621]

The composition of the elevated proinsulin-like immunodeficiency in patients with T2DM compared with control subjects has not been fully characterized. Hales and colleagues[633] developed immunoradiometric assays for this purpose. In studies using these assays, split 32,33-proinsulin was reported to be the predominant proinsulin conversion product in the circulation, although des-31,32-proinsulin levels can also be elevated. Insulin, proinsulin, and conversion product concentrations were also measured with these assays 30 minutes after oral glucose administration in patients with T2DM. Insulin was reduced in all patients, with no overlap between patients and control subjects, and concentrations of proinsulin and conversion products were elevated in the diabetic patients. These data highlight the importance of the potentially confounding effects of proinsulin and proinsulin conversion products in the interpretation of circulating immunoreactive insulin in patients with T2DM and emphasize the need to measure the concentrations of the individual peptides.

Abnormalities in the temporal pattern of insulin secretion have also been demonstrated in patients with T2DM. In contrast to normal subjects, in whom equal amounts of

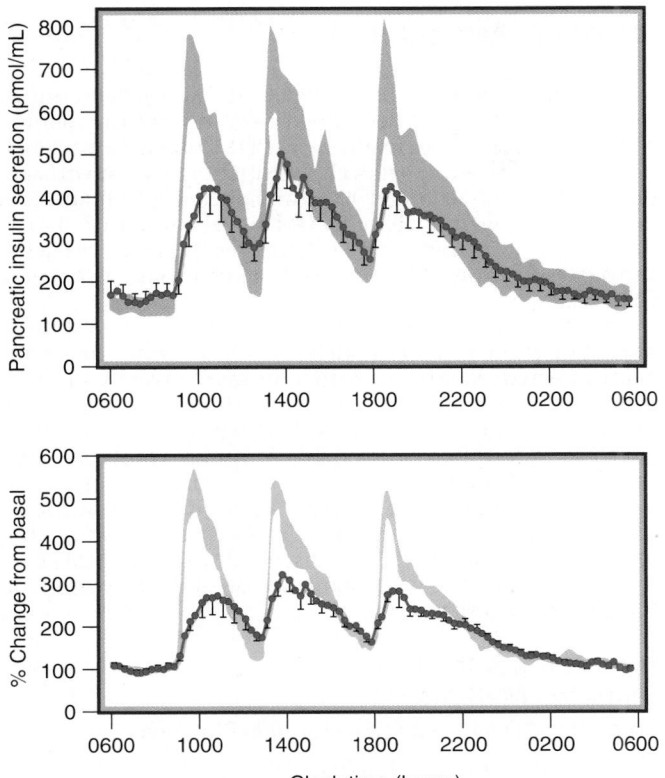

Figure 31-19 Mean rates of insulin secretion in type 2 diabetic patients compared with control subjects *(top panel)*. *Vertical bars* indicate standard error of the mean (SEM). The *shaded area* corresponds to 1 SEM above and below the mean in control subjects. The *curves* indicating percent change from basal secretion *(lower panel)* were derived by dividing, for each subject, the insulin secretion rate at each sampling time by the average fasting secretion rate measured between 6 AM and 9 AM in the same subject. (From Polonsky KS, Given BD, Hirsch LJ, et al. Abnormal patterns of insulin secretion in non-insulin-dependent diabetes mellitus. *N Engl J Med.* 1988;318: 1231-1239.)

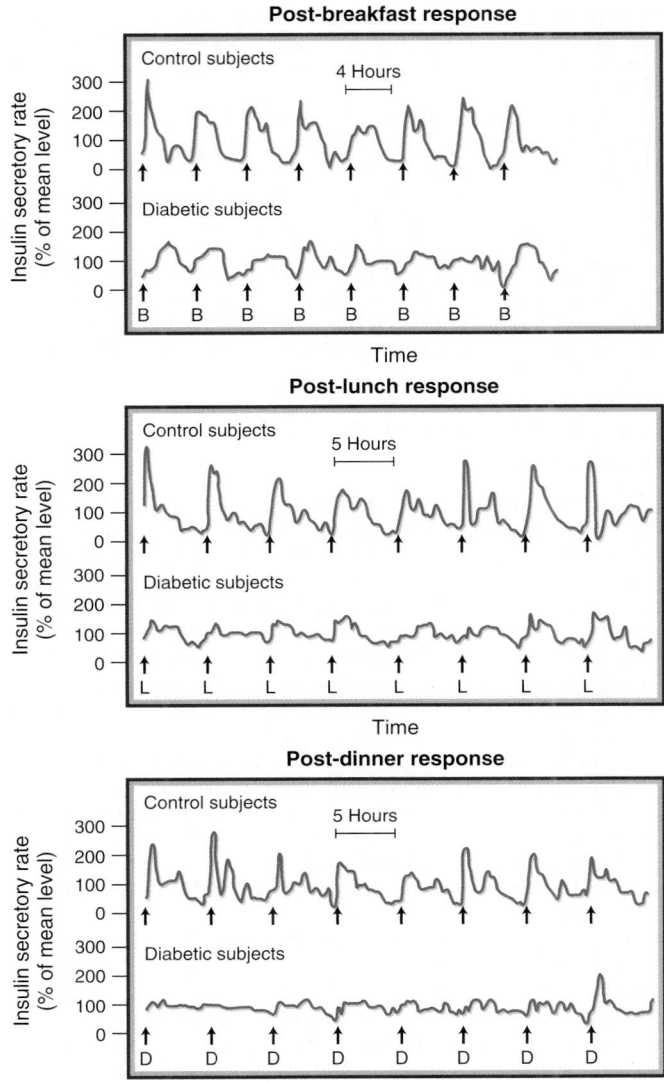

Figure 31-20 Temporal variations in rates of insulin secretion in control and diabetic subjects after breakfast, lunch, and dinner *(top, middle,* and *bottom panels,* respectively). In each subject, the secretion rates during the 30 minutes before the meal and the 4 hours after breakfast or the 5 hours after lunch or dinner were expressed as a percentage of the mean rate of insulin secretion during that interval. The curves were obtained by concatenating the resulting postmeal profiles in eight representative subjects. The times when the meals were served to the eight successive subjects in the series are indicated by *arrows*. (From Polonsky KS, Given BD, Hirsch LJ, et al. Abnormal patterns of insulin secretion in non-insulin-dependent diabetes mellitus. *N Engl J Med.* 1988;318:1231-1239.)

insulin are secreted basally and postprandially in a given 24-hour period, patients with T2DM secrete a greater proportion of their daily insulin under basal conditions (Fig. 31-19).[634] This reduction in the proportion of insulin secreted postprandially appears to be related in part to a reduction in the amplitude of the secretory pulses of insulin occurring after meals, rather than to a reduction in the number of pulses. In contrast to normal subjects, patients with T2DM have ultradian oscillations in insulin secretion that are less tightly coupled with oscillations in plasma glucose (Fig. 31-20). Similar findings were observed in patients with IGT studied under the same experimental conditions and in a further group of T2DM patients studied under fasting conditions. The rapid insulin pulses are also abnormal in patients with T2DM. The persistent regular rapid oscillations present in normal subjects are not observed. Instead, the cycles are shorter and irregular. Similar findings were observed in a group of first-degree relatives of patients with T2DM who had only mild IGT, suggesting that abnormalities in oscillatory activity may be an early manifestation of beta-cell dysfunction.[612]

The effects of therapy on beta-cell function in patients with T2DM have also been investigated. Although interpretation of the results in many instances is limited because beta-cell function was not always studied at comparable levels of glucose before and during therapy, the majority of the studies indicated that improvements in diabetic control are associated with an enhancement of beta-cell secretory activity. This increased endogenous production of insulin appears to be independent of the mode of treatment and is in particular associated with increases in the amount of insulin secreted postprandially.[625,635] The enhanced beta-cell secretory activity after meals reflects an increase in the amplitude of existing secretory pulses rather than an increased number of pulses. Despite improvements in glycemic control, beta-cell function is not normalized after therapy, suggesting that the intrinsic defect in the beta cell persists.

Treatment with the sulfonylurea glyburide increases the amount of insulin secreted in response to meals but does not correct the underlying abnormalities in the pattern of insulin secretion. In particular, the abnormalities in the pulsatile pattern of ultradian insulin secretory oscillations persist on treatment with glyburide despite the increased secretion of insulin.[636]

The effects on insulin secretion of improving insulin resistance in subjects with IGT through the use of the insulin-sensitizing agent troglitazone, a thiazolidinedione, have also been investigated. Troglitazone therapy improved insulin sensitivity, and this was associated with enhanced ability of the pancreatic beta cell to respond to a glucose stimulus, as judged by improvements in the dose-response relationships between glucose and insulin secretion as well as enhanced ability of the pancreatic beta cell to detect and respond to small oscillations in the plasma glucose concentration.[637]

Effects of Genetic Variants on Insulin Secretion

A number of the loci that have been associated with increased risk for T2DM appear to affect insulin secretion. Gene-phenotype studies have involved large numbers of subjects, and as a consequence, they have generally relied on simple measures of beta-cell function (e.g., the early insulin response to oral glucose). This approach has been very successful in identifying variants that primarily reduce insulin levels. More detailed phenotyping studies are now being undertaken in smaller groups of subjects to answer specific questions including the following:
1. Are the risk variants associated with altered clinical and physiologic findings before diabetes onset?
2. Is insulin secretion reduced equally in response to both oral and intravenous glucose?
3. Is the incretin effect reduced?
4. Are the dose-response relationships between glucose and insulin secretion altered?
5. Is there a concomitant change in insulin action?

Studies demonstrate that *KCNJ11* and *TCF7L2* are involved in the regulation of insulin secretion, but their clinical manifestations in humans are different, consistent with different mechanisms for their effects on the beta cell. Nondiabetic subjects with the *KCNJ11* T2DM-associated Lys-variant of E23K showed a significant reduction (approximately 40%) in insulin secretion after both oral and intravenous glucose, compared with subjects who did not carry this variant.[638] Hyperinsulinemic euglycemic clamps demonstrated that hepatic insulin sensitivity is increased in subjects with the Lys-variant, and as a result, normal glucose tolerance is maintained despite reduced insulin secretion. Therefore, the E23K variant appears to affect both insulin secretion and insulin action. The mechanisms responsible for the increase in insulin sensitivity are unclear. One possibility is that they represent a compensatory response to reduced insulin secretion. An increase in insulin sensitivity has also been observed in normoglycemic carriers of *HNF1A* mutations who have reduced insulin secretion.[639]

In contrast, carriers of risk variants in *TCF7L2* have a different phenotype, with normal insulin secretory responses to intravenous glucose including normal dose-response relationships between glucose and insulin secretion, reduced responses to oral glucose with a reduced incretin effect, and no change in insulin sensitivity. Concentrations of the two major incretins GLP-1 and GIP are normal after oral glucose administration, implicating resistance of the pancreatic beta cell to the stimulatory effects of one or both of these incretins. These results are consistent with those of Schafer and associates,[640] who also documented reduced responses to GLP-1.

RODENT MODELS

A number of spontaneous and genetically selected animal models of T2DM have been identified. Most of the models combine the two main features of T2DM: obesity-associated insulin resistance and beta-cell dysfunction with or without diminished beta-cell mass. As with diabetes in humans, the different rodent models of T2DM have similarities, but a number of overt and subtle differences make them useful surrogates for intensive study of the syndromes associated with T2DM.

An interesting observation is the striking sexual dimorphism in most rodent models of T2DM, with the male being affected exclusively, earlier, or more severely in most instances. This is not like the human situation. The advent of transgenic and knockout technology in mice has produced a wide range of models of insulin resistance and beta-cell dysfunction that result in hyperglycemia. It is beyond the scope of this chapter to review each of these, and the reader is referred to the primary literature for review of these animals. The discussion here is limited to the well-documented spontaneous or derived models of the disease in rodents.

Mouse Models of Type 2 Diabetes Mellitus

Leptin (*Lep*ob) and Leptin Receptor *(db)* Mutations

The *ob* mutation, now designated *Lep*ob, was first described in 1950,[641] but the gene mutation responsible for the syndrome was not described until the *ob* mutation was found to be located in the gene for leptin.[642] Mice homozygous for the *ob* mutation do not produce the satiety factor leptin and become markedly hyperphagic, obese, insulin resistant, and hyperinsulinemic. They have a multitude of other hypothalamic dysfunctions that render them hypometabolic, contribute to the obesity, and result in infertility.[643,644] Leptin treatment of these mice results in decreased food intake and reverses many of their other metabolic defects.[645-649] The *ob* mice develop obesity at weaning that becomes progressive because of hyperphagia. Insulin resistance is seen in muscle, adipose tissue, and liver, with a variety of signaling defects that are reversible with insulin administration.[650] The *ob* mouse becomes hyperglycemic and has a profound hyperinsulinemia associated with beta-cell hyperplasia, with up to a 10-fold increase in islet mass.[651,652]

Parabiotic experiments between *ob* and *db* mice suggested that the *db* mutation would be found in the receptor for *ob*. This was confirmed with the identification of multiple mutations in the leptin receptor in *db* mice.[653,654] Like *ob* mice, *db* mice are hyperphagic and begin to surpass their littermates in weight at weaning. They are progressively hyperinsulinemic, become hyperglycemic at 6 to 8 weeks and, because of a decline in beta-cell function,[655-658] become markedly hyperglycemic at 4 to 6 months. The reason for the more severe diabetes in *db* mice is not clear, but it may be related to background strain differences, because similar defects in insulin signaling are seen in this animal model as well.[659] Treatment of both *ob* and *db* mice with insulin-sensitizing agents such as thiazolidinediones reversed the insulin resistance and ameliorated or prevented the onset of diabetes.[660,661]

Agouti Mouse

In mice, dominant *yellow* mutations in the *agouti* gene produce obesity and hyperglycemia. Depending on the background strain, the *agouti* mutation has a variable phenotype. In susceptible strains, the onset of hyperinsulinemia begins at 6 weeks of age, and insulin levels continue to increase with age, along with beta-cell hyperplasia and hypertrophy.[662,663] The *agouti* mutation results in systemic production of a protein normally expressed in the skin, most frequently because of a retrotransposon insertion into the promoter region of the gene.[664] A number of genes, including the fatty acid synthase gene, have both insulin and agouti response elements; this results in a marked increase in expression and leads to increased hepatic fatty acid synthesis and enhanced fat deposition in adipocytes.[654,665,666] The hyperglycemia is postprandial, and the FPG levels are usually normal. The exact function of the *agouti* gene is unknown, but the animals are hyperphagic and show enhanced growth.

KK Mouse

KK mice were originally bred for enhanced size, but they are not as obese as most other obese mice (usually <60 g). Breeding of the KK mouse into various background strains has produced variable insulin resistance, hyperinsulinemia, and hyperglycemia. The most studied strain is the KKA^y, produced in Japan.[667] This mouse has markedly increased insulin levels (>1000 μU/mL) when fed a high-fat diet.[668,669] As the male mouse ages, glucose levels fall toward the normal range. The mutation responsible for the KK phenotype is unknown.

New Zealand Obese Mouse

New Zealand obese (NZO) mice were derived by inbreeding of abdominally obese outbred mice.[652,670-672] NZO neonates have high birth weights, and mice of both sexes are large and at weaning exhibit an elevated carcass fat content.[670] Approximately 40% to 50% of group-caged NZO males, but not females, develop T2DM between 12 and 20 weeks of age when maintained with a chow diet containing 4.5% fat.[673] Obesity in NZO mice is characterized by widespread accumulation of subcutaneous and visceral fat. The obesity in these mice is accompanied by IGT in males, associated with increased hepatic and peripheral insulin resistance. In contrast to those in *ob* and *db* mice, genes encoding certain gluconeogenic and glycolytic enzymes in the liver of NZO mice retain normal responsiveness to insulin, although there is evidence for an inappropriately active fructose-1,6-biphosphatase.[674-676] Defective beta-cell insulin secretion from NZO islets in vitro and in vivo has been described.[670] There appears be a defect in the glycolytic pathway in beta cells that leads to defective glucose-stimulated insulin release.[677]

The genetics of NZO mice show a polygenic disorder, and none of the allelic variants have been discovered. Complicating the analysis of the model is the susceptibility of the mice to autoimmune disorders, including a lupus-like syndrome[678,679] and insulin receptor autoantibodies.[680] There is also a maternal influence in the peripartum period in the development of the disorder, which may reflect substances in the maternal milk.[681]

Gold Thioglucose–Induced Diabetes

Gold thioglucose induces specific lesions in the ventromedial hypothalamus and induces an initial chronic hyperinsulinemia that leads to hypoglycemia, hyperphagia, obesity, and the development of insulin resistance and hyperglycemia.[682] This model has been used as an example of pancreatic dysfunction preceding the induction of insulin resistance as opposed to pancreatic compensation for insulin resistance.

Diabetes Induced by Fat Ablation

Three models of insulin-resistant diabetes have been created in which adipose tissue is genetically eliminated by overproduction of foreign genes using the fat-specific promoter aP2 (adipocyte protein 2). Expression of an attenuated diphtheria toxin in adipose tissue resulted in an age-dependent loss of fat, progressive insulin resistance, hyperinsulinemia, and significant diabetes.[683,684] Adipose-specific expression of a constitutively active form of the SREBP1c also resulted in fat ablation.[685] Lipoatrophy was induced by fat-specific overexpression of a dominant-negative form of the transcription factor A-ZIP/F.[686,687] The A-ZIP/F protein heterodimerizes with and inactivates basic zipper (bZIP) transcription factors, including AP1 and CCAAT/enhancer binding protein (CEBP) isoforms, probably disrupting normal fat development.

The lack of fat in the various models leads to hepatomegaly, insulin resistance with hyperinsulinemia, hypoleptinemia, and significant IGT and diabetes. These mice represent a model of human lipodystrophic diabetes and demonstrate the importance of fat in normal glucose homeostasis. It has been suggested that the lack of fat depots results in elevated fatty acid delivery to liver and muscle and the development of insulin resistance. The diabetes in these animals can be variously treated by thiazolidinediones,[683] leptin administration,[688] and fat transplantation.[687] Human lipodystrophy also responds to thiazolidinedione treatment,[689] suggesting that some of the effects of these compounds are not wholly dependent on adipose tissue.

C57BL/6J Mouse Fed a High-Fat Diet. Male C57BL/6J (also known as B6) mice that were fed a high-fat, high-carbohydrate diet (a so-called Western diet, 58% fat by kilocalories) developed hyperglycemia, hyperinsulinemia, hyperlipidemia, and increased adiposity.[690,691] Glucose-stimulated insulin secretion was blunted, and there was significant insulin resistance.[692,693] Despite obesity, plasma leptin levels in the Western diet–fed B6 mice were significantly lower than in control mice in the absence of hyperphagia.[690,694] The weight gain is related primarily to an increase in mesenteric adiposity, which makes this a good model for human adult-onset T2DM.

Rat Models of Type 2 Diabetes Mellitus
Zucker Diabetic Fatty Rat

The ortholog of the *db* mouse, the obese Zucker rat *(fa/fa)*, has a mutation in the leptin receptor that results in significant hyperphagia.[695] The *fa* mutation is different from the mutations in *db* in that it does not disrupt leptin receptor gene expression and does not affect ligand binding.[695,696] This mutation results in a constitutive intracellular signaling domain, which may induce a desensitization of the leptin signaling pathways.[697]

The selection of the inbred Zucker diabetic fatty (ZDF) rat strain used Zucker *(fa/fa)* rats that had progressed to a diabetic phenotype. Brother-sister matings resulted in a strain exhibiting development of diabetes in almost 100% of the male rats consuming a 5% fat diet.[698] Hyperglycemia begins to develop in males at 7 weeks of age, with serum glucose levels rising to 500 mg/dL by 12 weeks of age. The hyperinsulinemia precedes hyperglycemia with marked islet hyperplasia and dysmorphogenesis,[699] but by 19 weeks insulin levels drop concomitantly with islet atrophy, in part because of an imbalance of hyperplasia and apoptosis.[603] The islets of prediabetic ZDF rats secrete significantly more insulin in response to glucose, with elevated basal levels of insulin secretion and a leftward shift but a blunted glucose dose-response curve.[604,700] Islets of prediabetic male ZDF rats also have defects in the normal oscillatory pattern of insulin secretion.[701]

In contrast to the male ZDF rat, the female rat has significant insulin resistance but does not become diabetic unless given a proprietary high-fat diet (GMI 13004, developed by Genetic Models, Inc., Indianapolis, IN).[702] The high-fat diet appears to have a direct effect on the beta cell, because there is no change in peripheral insulin sensitivity (P. Hansen and C.F. Burant, unpublished observations). There is a decrease in peripheral triglyceride and FFA levels in the female rat after institution of the high-fat diet.

The underlying genetic defect that results in beta-cell failure in the ZDF rat is unknown. The beta-cell number and insulin content are not different from those in homozygous normal animals, but insulin promoter activity is doubled in the ZDF rat.[703] Insulin promoter mapping studies suggest that a critical region in the promoter of the insulin gene is affected. A number of other gene expression differences have been described in ZDF islets, including decreases in the expression of GLUT2[704,705]; increases in glucokinase and hexokinase activity[700]; decreases in mitochondrial metabolism[700]; accumulation of intraislet lipid and long-chain fatty acyl-CoA, which is associated with abnormal beta-cell secretion[701,706,707]; and increased accumulation of nitric oxide and ceramide,[708,709] which is associated with apoptosis. Other gene expression changes are also found in the prediabetic rat islet.[710] Which of these defects is important for the development of the diabetes is not clear.

The fixed genetic defect in the male animal leads to diabetes, but this defect also interacts with the insulin resistance, because treatment with insulin-sensitizing agents can prevent the onset of diabetes in male and female rats.[707,711] These agents are not effective in the male after establishment of diabetes; however, the female rat can respond to thiazolidinediones even after significant hyperglycemia.

Goto-Kakizaki Rat

The Goto-Kakizaki (GK) inbred rat strain was derived from outbred Wistar rats by selection for IGT.[712] Early in the development of diabetes, glucose and insulin are mildly elevated, but as the animals age, reduced beta-cell mass becomes evident, with markedly diminished insulin stores and abnormal secretory responses to glucose.[713,714] A number of biochemical defects have been described in the islets of these animals, including decreased energy production,[715-717] expression of proteins involved in insulin granule movement,[718] and decreased adenylate cyclase activity.[719] Defects in peripheral signaling include decreased maximal and submaximal insulin-stimulated IRS1 tyrosine phosphorylation, IRS1-associated PI3K activity, Akt activation in muscle,[720] defective regulation of protein phosphatase-1 and -2A, and mitogen-activated protein kinase activation by upstream insulin-signaling components in adipocytes.[721] Some of these defects may be a result of hyperglycemia, because they can be reversed by phlorizin-induced normalization of serum glucose.[720]

BHE/Cdb Rat

The Bureau of Home Economics (BHE/Cdb) rat is a subline of the parent BHE strain that was obtained by selection for hyperglycemia and dyslipidemia without obesity.[722]

Glucose-stimulated insulin secretion is markedly diminished in these rats, a trait that is maternally inherited.[723] A significant defect appears to be present in the liver. Increased gluconeogenesis and lipogenesis precede the hyperglycemia, which may be caused by defects in mitochondrial respiration associated with mitochondrial DNA mutations.[724,725]

Psammomys obesus (Sand Rat)

The sand rat (Psammomys obesus) is a nutritionally induced obesity model of T2DM. Genetically, the animal is in reality a gerbil, and it usually lives on a low-calorie vegetable diet.[726] When given a high-carbohydrate diet, the sand rat rapidly becomes hyperglycemic secondary to weight gain associated with significant insulin resistance[727] and enhanced hepatic glucose production.[728] When a relatively hypocaloric diet is restored, the metabolic syndrome reverts to normoglycemia. A subpopulation of the sand rat develops frank beta-cell failure and becomes ketotic.

Otsuka Long-Evans Tokushima Fatty Rat

The Otsuka Long-Evans Tokushima fatty (OLETF) rat strain was derived from the Long-Evans rat with polyuria, polydipsia, and mild obesity.[729] About 90% of the male animals become diabetic by 1 year of age. Statistical tests have determined that the locus containing the cholecystokinin A receptor is responsible for about 50% of the T2DM in the OLETF rats.[730] The receptor is disrupted in the OLETF rat because of a 165-bp deletion in exon 1.[731,732] Genetic segregation analysis has shown interaction with a second locus, Obd2, which acts in a synergistic fashion to result in NIDDM, and both of these loci are required in homozygous OLETF rats to cause elevated plasma glucose.[733]

The role of sex hormones is pronounced in this strain. Orchiectomy markedly reduces the incidence of diabetes in the male, and oophorectomy increases the rate of hyperglycemia to 30% in the female. Treatment of castrated males with testosterone restores the incidence of diabetes to 89%. The islets undergo a progressive inflammatory reaction with progressive fibrosis. This reaction is associated with the impairment of beta-cell function.[734] Obesity and insulin resistance appear to precede the development of beta-cell failure.[735] Studies have also shown that obesity is necessary for the development of T2DM in OLETF males and that insulin resistance may be closely related to fat deposition in the abdominal cavity.[736] Troglitazone and metformin have been used successfully to treat diabetes in the OLETF rat, and troglitazone completely prevents the morphologic and functional deterioration of the beta cells.[737]

Neonatal Streptozotocin

Two models have been described in which a single dose of the beta-cell toxin, streptozotocin, is given to 2-day-old female Wistar[738,739] or male Sprague-Dawley rats.[740,741] These animals have a transient hyperglycemia but develop IGT at 4 to 6 weeks of age. There is an initial reduction of beta-cell mass, but subsequent regeneration results in restoration of the beta-cell mass to a level approximately 50% lower than the normal adult level.

MANAGEMENT

Over the past 15 years, a conceptual transformation in the principles of management of T2DM has occurred.

Fundamentally, there has been a change in the level of concern about diabetes as a public health issue and in attitudes about its treatment. Dramatic advances in the spectrum of pharmacologic agents and monitoring technology available for the treatment of diabetes have made it possible to lower glucose levels safely to the near-normal range in most patients. Great strides have been made in establishing an evidence base for guidelines regarding glycemic control and efforts to reduce the risk of complications. Corporate and government health insurance providers have greatly improved the extent to which diabetes equipment and supplies are covered.

A comprehensive review of all the subtleties of diabetes management in the 21st century is beyond the scope of this chapter. Here, we deal with the salient features of the epidemiology of the complications of T2DM, diagnostic strategies, treatment guidelines, lifestyle interventions, and pharmacotherapy before turning briefly to a discussion of preventive measures for T2DM and its complications. An excellent source of information on these issues is the *Clinical Practice Recommendations* of the American Diabetes Association (ADA), which is published as the first supplement to the journal *Diabetes Care* each January and is available online.[742]

Scope of the Problem

As discussed previously, in the United States in 2014, nearly 30 million people had diabetes with over 25% undiagnosed. Since 2007, the prevalence has risen from 7.8% to 9.3%. The increasing burden of diabetes is driven by population aging; by population growth, particularly among ethnic groups with greater susceptibility to the disease; and by increases in rates of obesity as a consequence of increasingly sedentary lifestyles and greater consumption of simple sugars and calorie-dense foods. Furthermore, at least in the United States, opportunistic screening for diabetes in high-risk populations is recommended by professional societies and many insurers, and this has resulted in an increase in the proportion of people affected being diagnosed, from approximately 50% in the 1990s to over 70% today. The morbidity, mortality, and expense associated with diabetes are staggering.[3-5] In Western society, people with diabetes are three times more likely to be hospitalized than nondiabetic persons. In the United States, diabetes is the leading cause of blindness and accounts for more than 40% of new cases of end-stage renal disease. The risk of heart disease and stroke is two to four times higher, and the risk of lower-extremity amputation is approximately 20 times higher for people with diabetes than for those without diabetes. Life expectancy is reduced by approximately 10 years in people with diabetes, and although diabetes is the seventh leading cause of death in the United States, this figure is clearly an underestimate. Only about 35% to 40% of those who die with diabetes have the disease listed anywhere on the death certificate, and only 10% to 15% have it listed as the underlying cause of death.

Rates of complications in diabetes declined between 1990 and 2010 on the order of 50% or greater for MI, stroke, amputations, and death from hyperglycemic crisis; end-stage renal disease was reduced approximately 30%.[743] Our understanding of the natural history of diabetes is based on outcomes in patients diagnosed decades ago. Societal change, earlier diagnosis of diabetes, enhanced treatment of diabetes and its comorbid conditions, and intervention earlier in the course of complications results in substantial uncertainty about the future that patients diagnosed today will face. We believe that patients treated according to guidelines have an excellent prognosis in

2015. The major issues determining health outcomes today are socioeconomic and are related to access to care and health disparities.[744]

Glucose Treatment Guidelines
Study Results and Recommendations

Prospective, randomized clinical trials have documented improved rates of microvascular complications in patients with T2DM treated to lower glycemic targets. In the United Kingdom Prospective Diabetes Study (UKPDS),[745,746] patients with new-onset diabetes were treated with diet and exercise for 3 months, with an average reduction in HbA$_{1c}$ from approximately 9% to 7% (upper limit of normal is 6%). Those patients with FPG greater than 108 mg/dL (6 mmol/L) were then randomly assigned to two treatment policies. In the standard intervention, subjects continued the lifestyle intervention. Pharmacologic therapy was initiated only if the FPG reached 15 mmol/L (270 mg/dL) or the patient became symptomatic. In the more intensive treatment program, all patients were randomly assigned and treated with either sulfonylurea, metformin, or insulin as initial therapy, with the dose increased to try to achieve an FPG of less than 108 mg/dL. Combinations of agents were used only if the patient became symptomatic or FPG rose to greater than 270 mg/dL (15 mmol/L).

As a consequence of the design, although the HbA$_{1c}$ fell initially to about 6%, over the average 10 years of follow-up it rose to approximately 8%. The average HbA$_{1c}$ in the standard treatment group was approximately 1 percentage point higher. The risk of severe hypoglycemia was small (on the order of 1% to 5% per year in the insulin-treated group) and weight gain was modest; both were higher in patients randomly assigned to insulin and lower in those receiving metformin.[746] Associated with this improvement in glycemic control, there was a reduction in the risk of microvascular complications (retinopathy, nephropathy, and neuropathy) in the group receiving intensive treatment. Although there was a trend toward reduced rates of macrovascular events in the more intensively treated group, it did not reach statistical significance.[745]

Similar reductions in microvascular events were observed in another trial of entirely different design and much smaller size. In the Kumamoto study, Japanese patients of normal weight with T2DM receiving insulin were randomly assigned to standard treatment or an intensive program of insulin therapy designed to achieve normal glycemia. The control group maintained HbA$_{1c}$ values at approximately 9%, whereas the HbA$_{1c}$ in the intensive therapy group was reduced to approximately 7%, and the separation was maintained for 6 years. Again, there was a modest increased risk of hypoglycemia and weight gain, a reduction in microvascular complications, and a nonstatistically significant trend toward reduced rates of vascular end points.[747]

In 2008, three studies examining the effects of two levels of glycemic control on cardiovascular end points in T2DM were reported. Action to Control Cardiovascular Risk in Diabetes (ACCORD),[748] Action in Diabetes and Vascular Disease—Preterax and Diamicron Modified Release Controlled Evaluation (ADVANCE),[749] and the Veterans Affairs Diabetes Trial (VADT)[750] each randomized middle-aged and older individuals who were at high risk for cardiovascular events. ACCORD and VADT aimed for an HbA$_{1c}$ target of less than 6% using complex combinations of oral agents and insulin. ADVANCE aimed for an HbA$_{1c}$ target of 6.5% or less using a somewhat less intensive approach based on the addition of the sulfonylurea gliclazide. None of the trials demonstrated a statistically significant benefit on combined vascular end points. ACCORD demonstrated a 22% increase in total mortality rate, whereas VADT had numerically more deaths in the intensively treated group (hazard ratio, 1.07). Modest improvements in some microvascular end points in all three trials were demonstrated. In these studies, there were suggestions that people who were without clinical cardiovascular disease and had shorter duration of disease and lower baseline HbA$_{1c}$ demonstrated greater benefits from the more intensive glucose-lowering strategies.

Furthermore, a 10-year follow-up of the UKPDS cohort demonstrated that the relative benefit of more intensive management of glucose demonstrated at the end of the randomized portion of the trial was maintained, resulting in the emergence of statistically significant benefits on cardiovascular end points and total mortality rate.[751] Meta-analysis of cardiovascular outcomes in randomized trials suggested that an average HbA$_{1c}$ reduction of 0.9% correlates with a 17% reduction in nonfatal MI and a 15% reduction in coronary heart disease without significant effects on stroke or all-cause mortality rate; however, as mentioned previously, there is significant heterogeneity in the result with respect to mortality rate across trials, the cause of which is completely uncertain.[752]

Finally, two post hoc analyses in ACCORD have added further insights into the risk of fatality with intensive management. First, in an analysis of on-treatment HbA$_{1c}$, in the intensive treatment group, which did experience an overall increase in mortality rate, the increase was isolated to those who had on treatment average HbA$_{1c}$ greater than 7%. Thus, aiming for an HbA$_{1c}$ of less than 6% and achieving a target of less than 7% was not associated with excess mortality rate.[753] In the second analysis, the hemoglobin glycation index (HGI = observed HbA$_{1c}$ – predicted HbA$_{1c}$) was calculated using baseline HbA$_{1c}$ and fasting glucose. ACCORD participants in the top tertile of HGI (i.e., a higher HbA$_{1c}$ than would be predicted based on fasting glucose) had increased mortality rate and no benefit on the primary end point (the first occurrence of heart attack, stroke, or cardiovascular death). On the other hand, those in the lower and middle tertile of HGI had no increased mortality rate and an approximate 25% benefit on the primary end point. In ACCORD, HGI calculated at baseline identified subpopulations in ACCORD with harms or benefits from intensive glycemic control suggesting that HbA$_{1c}$ is not a one-size-fits-all indicator of blood glucose control, and failure to take this into account could result in suboptimal diabetes care.[754]

Blood Glucose Treatment Targets

Guidelines from the ADA and the American College of Endocrinology (ACE) are presented in Table 31-6. The ADA suggests that the goal of treatment in the management of diabetes should be an HbA$_{1c}$ value of less than 7% in general. Furthermore, the ADA suggests that lower targets may be pursued in selected patients, such as those with recent-onset disease, long life expectancy, and no significant cardiovascular disease, if they can be achieved without significant hypoglycemia or other adverse effects of treatment. Conversely, they recommend that less stringent HbA$_{1c}$ goals may be appropriate for patients with a history of severe hypoglycemia, limited life expectancy, advanced complications, and extensive comorbid conditions as well as in those who do not achieve HbA$_{1c}$ less than 7% despite diabetes self-management education and effective doses of insulin in combination therapy.[7] ACE has recommended an HbA$_{1c}$ goal that is less than or equal to 6.5%, again with language suggesting individualization of targets.[755]

Table 31-6

Glycemic Targets for Nonpregnant Adults

Parameter	Normal	ADA	ACE
Premeal PG (mg/dL)	<100 (mean ~90)	80-130*	<110
Postprandial PG (mg/dL)	<140	<180*†	<140
HbA$_{1c}$ (%)	4 to <5.7%	<7.0*	≤6.5**

ACE, American College of Endocrinology; ADA, American Diabetes Association; HbA$_{1c}$, glycosylated hemoglobin; PG, plasma glucose concentration.
*More or less stringent glycemic goals may be appropriate for individual patients. Goals should be individualized based on duration of diabetes, age/life expectancy, comorbid conditions, known cardiovascular disease or advanced microvascular complications, hypoglycemia unawareness, and individual patient considerations.
†Peak postprandial capillary plasma glucose. Postprandial glucose may be targeted if A$_{1c}$ goals are not met despite reaching preprandial glucose goals. Postprandial glucose measurements should be made 1-2 h after the beginning of the meal, generally peak levels in patients with diabetes.
**Individualize on the basis of age, comorbid conditions, duration of disease; in general ≤6.5 for most; closer to normal for healthy; less stringent for "less healthy."
Data from American Diabetes Association. Standards of medical care in diabetes—2015. *Diabetes Care.* 2015;38:s1-s93; Handelsman Y, Bloomgarden ZT, Grunberger G, et al. American Association of Clinical Endocrinologists and American College of Endocrinology—clinical practice guidelines for developing a diabetes mellitus comprehensive care plan—2015. *Endocr Pract.* 2015;21:1-87.

With respect to fasting, premeal, or postprandial targets, there is little support for any particular level of glycemic control in the management of T2DM because no large-scale outcome study has targeted particular levels of glucose with home glucose monitoring. The ADA target for fasting (and premeal) plasma glucose levels, 80 to 130 mg/dL, was developed based on an estimate of the range of average glucose values that would be associated with a low risk of hypoglycemia and an HbA$_{1c}$ of less than 7%.[7] The ACE fasting glucose target of less than 110 mg/dL is an effort to achieve normal levels of glycemia.[755] However, consistent fasting and premeal glucose levels lower than 110 mg/dL would be expected to be associated with an HbA$_{1c}$ of approximately 5.5%.[756]

The ADA treatment target for peak postprandial glucose levels is set at less than 180 mg/dL, in part because such levels would be associated with an HbA$_{1c}$ of approximately 7% and because nondiabetic persons who consume a large evening meal have been demonstrated to exhibit transient elevations of glucose to that level.[757] There are no published studies documenting safety or outcomes for a particular targeted level of postprandial blood glucose. However, there are effective HbA$_{1c}$-lowering agents that primarily target postprandial glucose levels, and monitoring of postprandial glucose levels may be necessary to optimize dose adjustment of these agents. Furthermore, some patients with diabetes have average FPG levels within their target range but an elevated HbA$_{1c}$. In these patients, monitoring and specific treatment of postprandial elevations can provide improvements in HbA$_{1c}$, perhaps with a lower risk of hypoglycemia and weight gain than has been associated with further lowering of fasting and premeal glucose levels.[758] The ACE has recommended a targeted 2-hour postprandial glucose concentration of less than 140 mg/dL (7.8 mmol/L) in an effort to achieve near-normal glycemia.[755] Consistent postprandial glucose values lower than 140 mg/dL would be associated with an average HbA$_{1c}$ of approximately 5%.[756]

Lifestyle Intervention

The components of lifestyle intervention include medical nutrition counseling, exercise recommendations, and comprehensive diabetes education with the purpose of changing the paradigm of care in diabetes from provider focused to patient focused. Arguably, since the turn of the 21st century, nothing has changed more fundamentally than the emphasis on lifestyle intervention. For decades, physicians and patients have paid lip service to the notion that lifestyle intervention is important. Now we have significant clinical trial evidence that each component of lifestyle intervention, when appropriately administered, can contribute to improved outcomes. Furthermore, since passage of the Balanced Budget Act of 1997 and complementary legislation in most state governments, lifestyle intervention has been a covered benefit for most insured people. Although full implementation of these regulations is still in progress, they have dramatically expanded the fraction of the population with diabetes who can acquire insurance coverage for these essential services.

Patient Education

Diabetes is a lifelong disease, and health care providers have almost no control over the extent to which patients adhere to the day-to-day treatment regimen. The appropriate role of the health care provider is to serve as a coach to the patient, who has primary responsibility for the delivery of daily care. As a result, health care providers must carefully engage patients as partners in the therapeutic process. It is critical for the health care professional to understand the context in which patients are taking care of their disease. A prescriptive approach, in which patients are told what to do, can work in some situations but fails more often than not because of unrecognized barriers to the execution of a particular plan. For long-term success, diabetes self-management education is critical.

Diabetes self-management education is the process of providing to the person with diabetes knowledge and skills needed to perform self-care, manage crises, and make lifestyle changes.[759] As a result of this process, the patient must become a knowledgeable and active participant in the management of his or her disease. To achieve this task, patients and providers work together in a long-term, ongoing process. Minimal diabetes education should be universally provided and individualized with emphasis on the core issues highlighted in Table 31-7. There are many more specialized topics relevant to almost all patients, such as how to adjust therapy when eating out or during travel, review of available local health care resources such as support groups, and insurance issues. Although there are only limited studies, they do provide support for the concept that diabetes education can be cost-effective and can improve outcomes.[760]

A team of providers is usually required to fully implement the process of diabetes self-management education, because the amount of information that needs to be exchanged is large and the needed range of expertise is broad. It is usually not possible to cover the recommended content fully in the context of several or even many brief encounters with a physician in an office setting. Potential providers in a team care approach include nurses, dietitians, exercise specialists, behavioral therapists, pharmacists, and other medical specialists including diabetologists or endocrinologists, podiatrists, medical subspecialists, obstetrician-gynecologists, psychiatrists, and surgeons. The potential role of the community in which the patient lives and works in the diabetes self-care process is enormous; family, friends, employers, and health insurance providers may all be involved. Each potential member of the team has a role to play in the process, which must be reviewed and assessed frequently (Table 31-8). The primary roles of the providers in this process are to supply guidance in goal setting to manage the risk of complications, suggest strategies for achieving goals and techniques to overcome barriers, provide training in skills, and help screen for complications. For this process to be a success, the patient must commit to the principles of self-care, participate fully in the development of a treatment plan, make ongoing decisions regarding self-care from day to day, and communicate honestly and with sufficient frequency with the team.

Fortunately, barriers to providing team care are becoming less daunting. Diabetes education programs are being rapidly established. The American Association of Diabetes Educators (telephone 800-TEAM-UP4) and the ADA (telephone 800-DIABETEs) can provide information regarding diabetes educators and education programs in the local area. A variety of novel approaches are under study including the use of telehealth capabilities, interactive gaming, and text messaging.

For team care to be most effective, communication, trust, and mutual respect are critical. However, in many

---

TABLE 31-7

Curricular Areas That Should Be Addressed in Diabetes Self-Management Education

- Describing the diabetes disease process and treatment options
- Incorporating nutritional management into lifestyle
- Incorporating physical activity into lifestyle
- Using medication(s) safely and for maximum therapeutic effectiveness
- Monitoring blood glucose and other parameters and interpreting and using the results for self-management decision making
- Preventing, detecting, and treating acute complications
- Preventing, detecting, and treating chronic complications
- Developing personal strategies to address psychosocial issues and concerns
- Developing personal strategies to promote health and behavior change

Modified from Haas L, Maryniuk M, Beck J, et al; 2012 Standards Revision Task Force. National standards for diabetes self-management education and support. *Diabetes Care.* 2014;37(Suppl 1):S144-S153.

TABLE 31-8

Team Care: Roles of the Players

Primary Care Provider

- To be a source of accurate information and to refer to and coordinate with other sources of information as necessary
- To provide guidance in developing goals of treatment
- To screen for complications and evaluate progress in meeting treatment goals
- To help develop strategies for achieving treatment goals and avoiding complications

Other Providers

- To be a source of accurate information, to communicate with the primary care provider, and to coordinate with other sources of information as necessary
- To provide guidance in developing goals of treatment and to help the primary care provider develop strategies to achieve treatment goals and avoid complications

Patient

- To commit to diabetes self-management (see Table 31-7)
- To be an active participant in the process
- To communicate with other team members when goals are not achieved or barriers or problems are encountered

Community

- To provide support to encourage ongoing diabetes self-care communities, the full benefit of consultation and ongoing care with diabetes educators, nurses, dietitians, pharmacists, and others is not achieved because of overly hierarchic approaches to care. Nonphysicians, including patients, ought to provide suggestions regarding medication and lifestyle adjustments and help in the process of identifying barriers to effective management such as lack of knowledge, lack of time, and lack of resources and strategies to overcome barriers.

Perhaps some of the most overlooked contributors to ineffective care in the setting of T2DM are the relatively common barriers created by psychiatric, neurocognitive function, and adjustment disorders, which are largely responsive to psychosocial therapies.[761]

Nutrition

With respect to self-management education, recent ADA statements document the effect of medical nutrition therapy and offer specific nutritional advice on diabetes-related outcomes (e.g., HbA$_{1c}$, weight, proteinuria).[7] These recommendations are summarized in Table 31-9. A comprehensive, individually negotiated nutrition program in which each patient's circumstances, preferences, and cultural background as well as the overall treatment program are considered is most likely to result in optimal outcomes. Because of the complexity of the medical and nutritional issues for most patients, it is recommended that a registered dietitian with specific skill and experience in implementing nutrition therapy in diabetes management work collaboratively with the patient and other health care team members to provide medical nutrition therapy.

Structured programs that emphasize lifestyle changes including education, reduced energy intake (and therefore often fat intake), conscious decisions regarding carbohydrate intake, regular physical activity, and recurring participant contact can produce long-term weight loss of 5% to 7% of starting weight and reduce the risk of developing diabetes. Everyone, especially family members of persons with T2DM, should be encouraged to engage in mindful eating and regular physical activity to decrease the risk of developing T2DM.

Physicians and other members of the health care team need to understand the major issues in diabetes and nutrition and to support the nutritional plan developed collaboratively. Individualized dietary advice can be developed by a physician from a brief diet history obtained by asking questions such as the following: What do you eat for breakfast? Lunch? Dinner? Do you have snacks between breakfast and lunch? Lunch and dinner? Dinner and bedtime? and What do you drink during the day? Ideally, this information should be obtained at each visit, with specific suggestions for changes that both patient and provider agree are important and achievable.

Easy issues to address include caloric beverages, which tend to elevate glucose levels dramatically and can usually be replaced quite painlessly by artificially sweetened alternatives. Juices are generally perceived as healthful but can significantly affect glycemic control and total calorie intake. Substituting low-fat products for higher-fat alternatives is often suggested but needs to be done with the recognition that these products are generally higher in carbohydrates. Fat-free and sugar-free foods need to be recognized as food that is not "free." Portion control and recipe modification are excellent techniques, particularly for meats and fried foods.

Adequate spacing between meals is usually good advice for patients with T2DM, because postprandial glucose levels typically peak 2 hours after a meal, when a snack would normally be taken. Eating approximately every 4 hours while awake is the most practical dietary plan for most overweight people. Frequent small meals have been shown to be of benefit when used in a controlled inpatient setting, but overweight patients who are encouraged to eat more frequently often overeat more frequently. At a minimum, avoiding high-calorie snacks is reasonable advice for most people with diabetes. A repeated diet history and additional modest changes negotiated every few weeks to months by all health care providers (i.e., doctor, nurse, or dietitian) allow assessment of whether previously agreed to changes were enacted, reinforcement of the importance of diet efforts, and slow enticement of patients into more healthful dietary choices.

In general, the critical nutrient for glycemic consistency is carbohydrate. Essentially every molecule of carbohydrate consumed is converted to glucose in the gut and requires the action of insulin to be cleared from the circulation. The carbohydrate-counting technique can be used in patients with T2DM to facilitate consistent carbohydrate intake or to allow insulin dose adjustment in response to changes in carbohydrates consumed.[762] Whereas the beta cell in T2DM has usually lost its responsiveness to glucose, the second phase of insulin secretion is largely spared in T2DM and is in part driven by amino acids and fatty acids. Therefore, including some protein and fat in each meal and snack is useful.

Dietary fat is the nutrient that is most closely associated in epidemiologic studies with the risk of developing T2DM. Although dietary fats clearly have an impact on total caloric intake (related to their caloric density) and on circulating lipids, they have a minimal impact on glycemia acutely. Fat intake is a contributor to obesity and is the critical nutrient for cardiovascular risk management. It is recommended that people with diabetes (and everyone in general) consume a diet that is modestly restricted in calories (if overweight) and contains less than 10% of total calories as saturated fat and less than 10% as polyunsaturated fat. Some advocate substituting foods high in monounsaturated fatty acids (i.e., seeds, nuts, avocado, olives, olive oil, and canola oil) for carbohydrate, but most patients do not find adequate variety in the monounsaturated fatty acid category and often overeat these high-calorie foods. Higher carbohydrate diets can raise postprandial glucose and triglycerides but are much less calorically dense than higher fat diets and have a higher thermic effect, both of which tend to promote weight loss.

Dietary protein similarly has a minimal impact on glucose levels, although amino acids do promote insulin secretion, which may be advantageous in patients with T2DM. Metabolism of protein results in the formation of acids and nitrogenous waste, which can lead to bone demineralization and glomerular hyperfiltration. At least 0.8 g of high-quality dietary protein per kilogram of body weight is generally recommended; restriction of protein intake to 10% to 20% of total calories minimizes potential adverse long-term effects of high protein intake.

The roles of vitamins, trace minerals, and nutritional supplements in the treatment of diabetes are poorly understood. Some clinicians are convinced of the utility of soluble fiber, magnesium, chromium, zinc, folic acid, pyridoxine, cyanocobalamin, vitamin A, vitamin C, vitamin E, vanadium, selenium, garlic, and other micronutrients. Clinical trial data to support their safety and efficacy are inconclusive at best. Many patients are convinced that nutritional supplementation is healthful, and it is often counterproductive to engage in scholarly discussion of the nature of the evidence base for their decision. At a minimum, discussion should include the documented

TABLE 31-9

Major Nutrition Recommendations for Diabetes

General

- Individuals who have prediabetes or diabetes should receive individualized medical nutrition therapy (MNT) as needed to achieve treatment goals, preferably provided by a registered dietitian familiar with the components of diabetes MNT.
- For individuals using fixed daily insulin doses, consistent carbohydrate intake with respect to time and amount can result in improved glycemic control and reduce hypoglycemia risk.
- A simple diabetes meal planning approach, such as portion control or healthful food choices, may be better suited to individuals with type 2 diabetes with health and numeracy literacy concerns. This strategy also may be effective for older adults.
- Because MNT can result in cost savings and improved outcomes, MNT should be covered by insurance and other payers.

Energy Balance, Overweight, and Obesity

- For overweight or obese adults with type 2 diabetes or at risk for diabetes, reducing energy intake while maintaining a healthful eating pattern is recommended to promote weight loss.
- Modest weight loss may provide clinical benefits in some individuals with diabetes, especially those early in the disease process. To achieve modest weight loss, intensive lifestyle interventions with ongoing support are recommended.

Eating Patterns and Macronutrient Distribution

- Evidence suggests that there is not an ideal percentage of calories from carbohydrate, protein, and fat for all people with diabetes; therefore, macronutrient distribution should be based on individualized assessment of current eating patterns, preferences, and metabolic goals.
- Carbohydrate amount and available insulin may be the most important factors influencing glycemic response after eating and should be considered when developing the eating plan.
- Monitoring carbohydrate intake, whether by carbohydrate counting or experience-based estimation, remains critical in achieving glycemic control.
- Carbohydrate intake from vegetables, fruits, whole grains, legumes, and dairy products should be advised over intake from other carbohydrate sources, especially those that contain added fats, sugars, or sodium.
- Substituting low glycemic-load foods for higher glycemic-load foods may modestly improve glycemic control.
- Individuals at high risk for type 2 diabetes should be encouraged to achieve the U.S. Department of Agriculture recommendation for dietary fiber (14 g fiber/1000 kcal) and to consume foods containing whole grains (one half of grain intake).
- Although substituting sucrose-containing foods for isocaloric amounts of other carbohydrates may have similar blood glucose effects, consumption should be minimized to avoid displacing nutrient-dense food choices.
- People with diabetes and those at risk should limit or avoid intake of sugar-sweetened beverages to reduce risk for weight gain and worsening of cardiometabolic risk profile.

Protein

- In individuals with type 2 diabetes, ingested protein appears to increase insulin response without increasing plasma glucose concentrations. Therefore, carbohydrate sources high in protein should not be used to treat or prevent hypoglycemia.

Dietary Fat Intake in Diabetes Management

- Evidence is inconclusive regarding an ideal amount of total fat for people with diabetes; therefore, goals should be individualized. Fat quality appears to be far more important than quantity.
- A Mediterranean-style eating pattern, rich in monounsaturated fatty acids, may benefit glycemic control and cardiovascular disease risk factors and can therefore be recommended as an effective alternative to a lower-fat, higher-carbohydrate eating pattern.
- Increased consumption of foods containing long-chain omega-3 fatty acids (eicosapentaenoic acid and docosahexaenoic acid), such as fatty fish, and omega-3 α-linolenic acid (ALA), is recommended.
- The consumption of fish (particularly fatty fish) at least two times (two servings) per week is recommended.
- The amount of dietary saturated fat, cholesterol, and *trans* fat recommended for people with diabetes is the same as that recommended for the general population.
- Evidence does not support recommending omega-3 supplements for people with diabetes for the prevention or treatment of cardiovascular events.

Micronutrients and Herbal Supplements

- There is no clear evidence of benefit from vitamin or mineral supplementation in people with diabetes who do not have underlying deficiencies.
- Routine supplementation with antioxidants, such as vitamins E and C and carotene, is not advised due to insufficient evidence of efficacy and concerns related to long-term safety.
- There is insufficient evidence to support the routine use of micronutrients such as chromium, magnesium, and vitamin D to improve glycemic control in people with diabetes.
- There is insufficient evidence to support the use of cinnamon or other herbs/supplements for the treatment of diabetes.
- It is recommended that individualized meal planning include optimization of food choices to meet recommended dietary allowance/dietary reference intake for all micronutrients.

Alcohol

- If adults with diabetes choose to drink alcohol, they should be advised to do so in moderation (no more than one drink per day for adult women and no more than two drinks per day for adult men).
- Alcohol consumption may place people with diabetes at an increased risk for delayed hypoglycemia, especially if taking insulin or insulin secretagogues. Education and awareness regarding the recognition and management of delayed hypoglycemia are warranted.

Sodium

- The recommendation for the general population to reduce sodium to less than 2300 mg/day is also appropriate for people with diabetes.
- For individuals with both diabetes and hypertension, further reduction in sodium intake should be individualized.

Modified from American Diabetes Association. Standards of medical care in diabetes—2015. *Diabetes Care.* 2015;38:s1-s93.

efficacy of more classic lifestyle and pharmacologic interventions and the idea that these efforts should not be left by the wayside when budget constraints affect potentially more effective interventions.[763]

Although a wide range of dietary recommendations have their proponents, few data support these suggestions from long-term outcome studies of prescribed diets. There are no consistent differences in weight loss or cardiovascular risk factors in up to 2 years of follow-up with low carbohydrate diets versus isoenergetic balanced weight loss diets.[764] That said, if a patient or practitioner wants to use a lower carbohydrate higher protein/fat reduced calorie diet, that is certainly a choice associated with short-term improvements in glycemia, cardiovascular risk markers, and weight. Arguably, the most validated meal plan is the so-called Mediterranean diet which in one large study was able to document reduced cardiovascular end points, fewer new cases of diabetes, and reduced cognitive decline.[765]

Weight loss is a goal of many patients with and without diabetes and certainly is associated with improvements in glycemic control, insulin resistance, circulating lipids, and blood pressure. As reviewed previously, numerous studies document that certain changes can result in modest weight loss that can be largely maintained with sustained effort. These changes include intensive lifestyle programs involving frequent contact with patients, individualized counseling, and education aimed at reducing calorie intake. Additional, complementary changes by the patient include regular physical activity and efforts to understand and control behaviors that result in overeating.

Exercise

There is a substantial body of literature supporting exercise as a modality of treatment in T2DM.[7] Exercise is perhaps the single most important lifestyle intervention in diabetes because it is associated with improved glycemic control, insulin sensitivity, cardiovascular fitness, and remodeling. Aerobic exercise and resistance (strength) training have positive impacts on glucose control. Improvements in glycemic control are usually apparent immediately and become maximal after a few weeks of consistent exercise. However, they may persist for only 3 to 6 days after cessation of training, hence the rationale for negotiating a minimum of three exercise sessions per week to maintain the benefit of the intervention.

The key concept is to promote an increase in activity using an approach similar to the one discussed for diet. Goals, methods, intensity, and frequency must be negotiated with patients with great sensitivity to recognizing barriers and helping patients discover solutions. The role of educators, exercise specialists, physical therapists, and social supports in this process is critical. The major role for the physician is to screen for complications (neuropathy, nephropathy, retinopathy, vascular disease) and discover ways for patients to be able to exercise safely. Exercise in the presence of uncontrolled diabetes, hypertension, retinopathy, nephropathy, neuropathy, and cardiovascular disease can create devastating problems. These obstacles can all be addressed creatively and should never present an insurmountable barrier to increasing physical activity.

Some authorities recommend that all patients older than 35 years have a stress test before initiating an exercise program. The utility of stress tests is potentially limited by their poor sensitivity and specificity. If the exercise program contemplated does not involve more strenuous activity (in intensity and duration) than the patient has engaged in recently but merely more frequent activity, screening cardiovascular stress testing is unlikely to be useful. However, when sedentary patients plan to embark on a program of strenuous exercise, stress testing may be prudent to evaluate for subclinical coronary disease. Patients at high risk for coronary artery disease should start with short periods of low-intensity exercise and increase the intensity and duration slowly as tolerated. Patients who develop symptoms of coronary ischemia, including dyspnea out of proportion with activity, should be referred for further evaluation and treatment. Even with negative results on stress testing, it is important to encourage patients not to overexert and to recognize exertional chest, jaw, or arm discomfort as well as palpitations and dyspnea as symptoms of cardiac dysfunction.

Over time, improved exercise tolerance should be viewed as a measure of improved cardiorespiratory function. For aerobic exercise to improve insulin sensitivity, glycemic control, and cardiovascular risk, the patient must engage in at least 150 minutes per week of moderate-intensity aerobic physical activity (50-70% of maximum heart rate) or 75 minutes per week of vigorous aerobic exercise (>70% of maximum heart rate). Exercise should be regular, at least every 48 hours. Patients with T2DM should be encouraged to perform resistance exercise targeting all major muscle groups at least two times a week. For the average patient with T2DM starting an exercise program, this equates to quite low-level activity initially, such as walking at a pace of 2 miles/hour. Initially, it may even be advantageous to negotiate once-weekly walks or shorter duration exercise sessions, or both, and proceed from there. Over time, patients are encouraged to pick up the pace as tolerated and to increase the duration and frequency of exercise sessions slowly to avoid overuse injuries. It is not unreasonable to suggest to patients that if they are going to incorporate exercise into their diabetes management program, they must think of exercise as a treatment that takes the place of a pill and requires adherence to produce benefit. All individuals should be encouraged to reduce sedentary time, particularly by breaking up extended amounts of time (>90 minutes) spent sitting.

Self-Monitoring of Blood Glucose

Self-monitoring of blood glucose (SMBG) has not been demonstrated in clinical trials to change outcomes in T2DM when evaluated in isolation.[7] However, many diabetes self-management programs have been demonstrated to help reduce complications. In all of these, SMBG is an integral part of the process, suggesting that SMBG is at least a component of effective therapy. The frequency and type of monitoring in diabetes therapy should be determined in consultation with the patient, taking into account the nature of the diabetes, the overall treatment plan and goals, and the patient's abilities. SMBG is particularly recommended for all patients with T2DM who are taking insulin or sulfonylureas because it allows patients to identify minimal or asymptomatic episodes of hypoglycemia.

Although severe hypoglycemia is relatively rare in T2DM, it can have devastating consequences, such as trauma or self-injury or change in the perceived ability of a patient to continue to live independently as a result of confusion or loss of consciousness. Also, it is essential to have patients critically assess the nature of any hypoglycemic symptoms that may occur. Many patients are fearful or overconcerned about hypoglycemia and routinely consume extra calories in response to a variety of life's circumstances, such as when they are hungry, sweaty, nervous, or upset. Monitoring studies document that most symptoms in patients with T2DM are not related to hypoglycemia and should not be treated with excessive calorie consumption.

Timing of SMBG varies depending on the diabetes therapy. It is important to advise patients to vary the time of the day at which blood glucose levels are checked. For some patients, the highest blood glucose of the day is the morning glucose, whereas for others the highest is before bed. Particularly in early diabetes, gestational diabetes, and well-controlled diabetes, monitoring 1 to 2 hours after meals allows patients to assess the effect of their lifestyle and pharmacologic efforts in controlling postprandial glucose levels, which are usually the only glycemic abnormality present. Monitoring (and thus targeting therapy) at just one time of day can leave the patient with a less than ideal overall response to therapy.

When glucose control is poor, having patients concentrate on premeal glucose levels is adequate. Once the premeal glucose levels reach the low 100s, many advocate that patients switch to checking 1- to 2-hour postprandial glucose levels; the latter approach amplifies the observed effect of diet on glycemic control and enables patients to see that moderate changes in meal plan, activity, and medications have a significant impact on glycemic control. Even after substantial inappropriate changes in food intake, activity, or timing or dose of medication, blood sugar values often return to near-normal levels overnight or by the time of the next meal.

The frequency of glucose monitoring needs to be matched to the individual patient's needs and treatment. Many clinicians ask patients to monitor at least once a day (at varying times before a meal, at bedtime, and at midsleep) as well as with hypoglycemic symptoms. Others ask patients receiving intensive insulin treatment to monitor with an intensity similar to that described for patients with T1DM: four times per day before meals; with weekly checks at least once after breakfast, lunch, dinner, and at midsleep; and with symptoms. Some ask for sets of glycemic readings more infrequently (e.g., fasting and 1 hour after the biggest meal). In the subset of patients who achieve stable blood glucose levels without significant hypoglycemia, it is usually appropriate to decrease the frequency of SMBG to a few times a week. It is critical that SMBG be frequent enough that both patient and provider have a good understanding of the adequacy of the treatment regimen and the stability of glycemic control.

It has been widely assumed that the benefits of SMBG stem from the effect of putting patients in a situation in which they can be in control of their own therapy. If patients are aware of the glycemic targets associated with the outcomes they seek to achieve, SMBG enables them to critically evaluate their response to therapy and assure themselves that they are reaching their goals. It is useful for patients to keep a daily diary of their SMBG results, so that they can assess their results periodically and can share them with the health care team. Many patients faithfully perform daily or more frequent SMBG, record the results as instructed, and discuss them with their health care team only at quarterly or semiannual visits even though their control is inadequate. Unless SMBG results are generally within agreed target ranges, they should be communicated and reviewed at least monthly with a member of the health care team by telephone, fax, mail, or e-mail or at an interim visit to trigger changes in therapy as the need arises. Unfortunately, such services usually are not reimbursed and can become an unsustainable burden on health care teams.

One of the most difficult areas in which to keep current is the area of available equipment and supplies, particularly for glucose monitoring. A useful resource in this regard is the annual *Consumer Guide*, which is published as the January issue of *Diabetes Forecast*, a magazine for laypeople with diabetes and their families.[766]

Pharmacotherapy for Type 2 Diabetes Mellitus

The revolution in the treatment of T2DM since 1995 in the United States has been driven by the release of several new classes of drugs that independently address different pathophysiologic mechanisms that contribute to the development of diabetes. The available oral antihyperglycemic agents can be divided by mechanism of action into several groups: insulin sensitizers with primary action in the liver, insulin sensitizers with primary action in peripheral tissues, insulin secretagogues, agents that slow the absorption of carbohydrates, insulins, agents that increase the activity of the incretin system, agents that increase glucose clearance into the urine, and novel agents whose influence on carbohydrate metabolism is still unclear. Insulin therapy in patients with T2DM effectively is a supplement to endogenous insulin secretion. The relative benefits of lifestyle intervention and the 13 classes of drugs available for the management of T2DM are shown in Table 31-10. This area has been the subject of extensive reviews.[7,755-767] In the following discussion, the principles outlined in these reviews are summarized, and limited additional references are provided.

Insulin Sensitizers With Predominant Action in the Liver

Metformin is the only biguanide available in the United States. Phenformin was removed from the U.S. market in the 1970s because of deaths associated with lactic acidosis. Phenformin and buformin remain available in some countries. Although metformin has been available in Europe for over 40 years, it has been approved in the United States only since 1995. The precise mechanism of action of metformin is still controversial.[768] Some studies suggest that it activates AMPK, an intracellular signal of depleted cellular energy stores that has been implicated in stimulation of skeletal muscle glucose uptake and inhibition of hepatic gluconeogenesis, whereas more recent studies implicate inhibiting mitochondrial glycerophosphate dehydrogenase as the primary action. The major clinical activity of metformin is to reduce hepatic gluconeogenesis and glucose production. It has more inconsistently improved insulin sensitivity in peripheral tissues. Because of its limited duration of action, it is usually taken at least twice daily, although a sustained-release formulation is available.

Because biguanides do not increase insulin levels, they are not associated with a significant risk of hypoglycemia. The most common adverse events are gastrointestinal: nausea, diarrhea, crampy abdominal pain, and dysgeusia. About one third of patients have some gastrointestinal distress, particularly early in their course of treatment. This distress can be minimized by starting with a low dose once daily with meals and titrating upward slowly (over weeks) to effective doses. Sustained-release metformin is associated with less frequent and less severe upper gastrointestinal symptoms, the more common of the adverse effects of metformin, but it can increase the frequency of diarrhea, a much less common adverse effect overall. Most patients note no adverse effects with metformin therapy, and at least 90% tolerate it adequately with long-term use. Perhaps as a result of clinical or subclinical gastrointestinal effects, metformin is associated with less weight gain than other antihyperglycemic agents, and in some studies it has been associated with a modest weight loss.

TABLE 31-10

Comparison of Therapies for Type 2 Diabetes

Class of Antihyperglycemic Therapy	Representative Agent(s)	Major Action	A_{1c} Lowering	Fasting/ Prandial Effect	Usual Dosing Frequency (times daily)	Route	Hypoglycemia	Weight Effect	CVD Risk Factor Benefits	Important Contraindications
Lifestyle	—	Broad	>1%	Both	—	—	No	Loss	Yes	—
Biguanide	Metformin	Liver sensitizer	>1%	Fasting	1-2	Oral	No	Neutral	Modest	Renal or hepatic failure
Sulfonylurea	Glimepiride, glipizide	Insulin secretagogue	>1%	Fasting	1-2	Oral	Yes	Gain	Negligible	—
Meglitinide	Repaglinide	Insulin secretagogue	>1%	Both	With meals	Oral	Yes	Gain	Negligible	—
Benzoic acid derived	Nateglinide	Insulin secretagogue	<1%	Prandial	With meals	Oral	Minimal	Minimal	Negligible	—
Basal insulin	NPH, glargine, detemir, degludec	Insulin supplement/ substitute	>1%	Fasting	1	Subcutaneous	Yes ++	Gain ++	Lowers TG	—
Prandial insulin	R, lispro, aspart, glulisine	Insulin supplement/ substitute	>1%	Prandial	With meals	Subcutaneous	Yes ++	Gain ++	Lowers TG	—
Thiazolidinediones	Pioglitazone, rosiglitazone	Peripheral sensitizer	>1%	Fasting	1	Oral	No	Gain ++	Variable—see text	Heart or liver failure
α-Glucosidase inhibitors	Acarbose, miglitol	Slows carbohydrate absorption	<1%	Prandial	With meals	Oral	No	Neutral	Negligible	—
Amylinomimetics	Pramlintide	Broad	<1%	Prandial	With meals	Subcutaneous	No	Loss	Negligible	—
GLP-1 receptor agonists	Exenatide, lixisenatide	Broad	~1%	Prandial	2	Subcutaneous	No	Loss	Modest with weight loss	Pancreatitis, renal failure
Long-acting GLP-1 receptor agonists	Liraglutide, exenatide OW, albiglutide, dulaglutide	Broad	>1%	Both	1 for liraglutide (others once weekly)	Subcutaneous	No	Loss	Lowers BP	Pancreatitis, medullary thyroid cancer
DPP-4 inhibitors	Sitagliptin, saxagliptin, linagliptin, alogliptin	Improve insulin/ glucagon secretion	<1%	Both	1	Oral	No	Neutral	Negligible	Pancreatitis
Bile-acid sequestrants	Colesevelam	Uncertain	<1%	Prandial	1-2	Oral	No	Neutral	Lowers LDL	Hypertriglyceridemia
Dopamine agonists	Bromocriptine	Uncertain	<1%	Fasting	1	Oral	No	Neutral	Modest	Migraine, lactation
SGLT2 inhibitors	Canagliflozin, dapagliflozin, empagliflozin	Promote glucosuria	>1%	Both	1	Oral	No	Loss	Lowers BP	Renal failure

BP, blood pressure; CVD, cardiovascular disease; DPP-4, dipeptidyl peptidase IV; GLP-1, glucagon-like peptide-1; LDL, low-density lipoprotein; NPH, neutral protamine Hagedorn; OW, once weekly; TG, triglycerides; SGLT2, sodium-glucose cotransporter 2;

Metformin has been said to cause lactic acidosis, which is quite rare and occurs almost exclusively in patients who are at high risk for development of the condition independent of metformin therapy.[769] The package insert states that metformin is contraindicated in patients with renal insufficiency (male patients with a serum creatinine concentration of 1.5 mg/dL or higher or female patients with 1.4 mg/dL or higher). The drug is cleared renally. Because there is a complex relationship between serum creatinine and renal function, reasonable practice might suggest that metformin can be used safely in patients with an estimated glomerular filtration rate (eGFR) based on the Modification of Diet in Renal Disease (MDRD) equation down to 30 mL/minute per 1.73 m², with dose reduction to a maximum daily dose of 1000 mg when the eGFR falls below about 50 mL/minute per 1.73 m² and avoidance when the eGFR is less than 30 mL/minute per 1.73 m².[770] Metformin is also contraindicated in patients with hepatic insufficiency and in the setting of alcohol abuse. Some patients taking metformin develop progressive vitamin B_{12} deficiency; supplementation with relatively high doses of vitamin B_{12} (e.g., 1000 µg daily) may be prudent.[771]

The glucose-lowering efficacy and the prevalence of adverse gastrointestinal effects of metformin increase proportionally in the dose range of 500 to 2000 mg/day. The maximal daily dose of 2550 mg does not generally provide additional benefit beyond that seen at 2000 mg daily. Newer formulations of metformin combined with various classes of oral antihyperglycemic agents have been developed to maximize glucose-lowering effectiveness with a single prescription through the synergy of two classes of agents with different actions.

Arguably, metformin has the best record among oral antihyperglycemic agents in outcome studies. In the UKPDS, among overweight subjects, those randomly assigned to metformin not only had improvements in microvascular complications similar to those of subjects randomly assigned to insulin and sulfonylurea but also demonstrated reduced rates of diabetes-related death and MI.[746] However, the validity of this observation has been challenged because of unusual responses in a subsequent subrandomization. The beneficial effect of metformin on macrovascular complications through mechanisms independent of glycemic control is certainly plausible and is supported by such observations as metformin-associated modest reductions in LDL, triglycerides, blood pressure, and procoagulant factors. The general recommendation is to initiate metformin therapy in all patients with T2DM absent contraindications at or near the time of diagnosis of diabetes.[767]

Insulin Sensitizers With Predominant Action in Peripheral Insulin-Sensitive Tissues

The thiazolidinedione class of drugs (TZDs or glitazones) has engendered great enthusiasm and controversy since the first agent, troglitazone, was approved in 1997. Rare fatal hepatotoxicity was associated with troglitazone, and it was withdrawn from the U.S. market in 2000, largely because the other TZDs (pioglitazone and rosiglitazone) were thought to be safer. These agents are believed to work through binding and modulation of the activity of a family of nuclear transcription factors termed *peroxisome proliferator-activated receptors* (PPARs). They are associated with slow improvement in glycemic control over weeks to months in parallel with an improvement in insulin sensitivity and a reduction in FFA levels.

Each of these agents varies in important ways with regard to potency, pharmacokinetics, metabolism, binding characteristics, and demonstrated lipid effects. At the same time, all are effective glucose-lowering agents that are generally well tolerated. The only significant early adverse effects are weight gain and fluid retention (and associated edema formation and hemodilution). There is no substantial evidence that these newer agents are associated with hepatotoxicity, but a record of safety has been established in appropriate patients. Patients should have liver function tests before beginning TZD therapy. TZDs are contraindicated in patients with active hepatocellular disease and in patients with unexplained serum alanine aminotransferase (ALT) levels greater than 2.5 times the upper limit of normal.

Pioglitazone and rosiglitazone are equally effective glucose-lowering agents with similar adverse effect profiles. They also provide equivalent improvements in markers of insulin resistance and inflammation. They differ with respect to lipid effects. In a head-to-head study among dyslipidemic patients, pioglitazone reduced triglycerides by approximately 20%, whereas rosiglitazone increased triglycerides on average by 5%. Pioglitazone is associated with a modestly greater improvement in HDL particle number and size and an improvement in LDL particle size and number. Rosiglitazone was associated with an increase in LDL particle number and improved LDL particle size.[772]

The promise of the thiazolidinedione class to reverse or prevent the negative cardiovascular associations of insulin resistance, in parallel with its demonstrated effect of improving insulin sensitivity, was suggested by a series of associations: reduced carotid intimal medial thickness, normalization of vascular endothelial function, improvements in dyslipidemia, lower blood pressure, and improved fibrinolytic and coagulation parameters. The PROactive (PROspective pioglitAzone Clinical Trial In macroVascular Events) Study was a randomized, double-blind, placebo-controlled trial in 5238 patients with T2DM and documented macrovascular disease. Subjects were randomized to placebo or to 45 mg/day of pioglitazone and otherwise treated according to guidelines for hyperglycemia and major cardiovascular risk factors. The primary end point was the time from randomization to a broad set of macrovascular end points. Pioglitazone was associated with a 10% reduction in the primary end point, but the reduction was not statistically significant. However, for the principal secondary end point, time from randomization to any cause of mortality rate, nonfatal MI (excluding silent MI), and stroke, pioglitazone therapy was associated with a 16% reduction, which was marginally statistically significant. Subsequent analysis and discussion of this technically negative and somewhat flawed trial has been extensive and supports the notion that pioglitazone therapy is associated with reductions in cardiovascular events that are largely accounted for by improvements in glycemia, lipids, and blood pressure. The benefits were in part mitigated by an increased incidence of heart failure, weight gain, and edema.[773]

The RECORD trial (rosiglitazone evaluated for cardiovascular outcomes in oral agent combination therapy for type 2 diabetes) was an open-label study that compared the effect of adding rosiglitazone versus either metformin or sulfonylurea to patients who had T2DM inadequately controlled with sulfonylurea or metformin. There was no difference in cardiovascular hospitalizations or death.[774] There has been a brewing controversy that perhaps rosiglitazone is associated with excess MI, with some calling for its withdrawal from the market.[775] Although there are no definitive data to prove this allegation, it has resulted in dramatic shifts in the marketplace away from rosiglitazone use.

A second attribute of the glitazones that has generated great enthusiasm is an improvement in insulin secretory dynamics in subjects with diabetes and IGT. More importantly, the ADOPT (A Diabetes Outcome Progression Trial) trial in patients with early diabetes demonstrated a lesser rate of secondary glycemic failure in patients treated with rosiglitazone, compared with metformin, and both showed a lesser failure rate than glyburide; these benefits were correlated with indices of beta-cell function.[776] Several trials have demonstrated the remarkable effectiveness of thiazolidinediones to delay or prevent the development of diabetes, with greater magnitude than has been reported for other antihyperglycemic agents.[7,767]

The glitazones have the best track record in regard to slowing the progressive nature of beta-cell deterioration, and this may have important implications for long-term prognosis. On the other hand, multiple adverse effects of the class have raised concerns; these effects include weight gain, fluid retention, and increased risk of bone fractures. Careful study indicates that the weight gain is a result of both fluid retention and subcutaneous (but not visceral) fat accumulation. There is, in fact, a reduction in visceral fat, hepatic fat, and intramyocellular fat. Therefore, it has been argued that the weight gain observed with glitazones may not have the same negative metabolic consequences that are generally ascribed to overweight and obesity. Nevertheless, weight gain is viewed negatively by most patients and practitioners. All patients prescribed glitazones should be counseled to redouble lifestyle efforts to minimize weight gain.

With regard to edema, with appropriate caution, almost no one should need to withdraw from therapy as a result of fluid retention. The patients most likely to experience edema are those treated with insulin and those with preexisting edema. Therefore, women, overweight patients, and patients with diastolic dysfunction or renal insufficiency are at greatest risk. It is prudent to teach patients with preexisting edema how to assess pitting pretibial edema at home and to suggest that they make a habit of checking nightly. If they note a pattern of increasing edema at home, patients can be instructed to restrict sodium intake, to start a diuretic, or to increase their diuretic dosage by some specified quantity on their own as needed.

In the previously edematous patient and in patients treated with insulin, it is prudent to initiate therapy with the lowest available dose of thiazolidinedione. In 1 to 3 months, if the glycemic response has been inadequate and significant edema has not developed, consider increasing the dose of thiazolidinedione further, with continued expectant home evaluation for edema. Most patients with mild edema respond to a thiazide diuretic or spironolactone. In patients with more extensive edema, combination therapy with a moderate-dose loop diuretic is sometimes required.[777] Anecdotal reports suggest that avoidance of nonsteroidal anti-inflammatory agents and dihydropyridine calcium channel blockers can reduce the frequency of edema as an adverse event. Fluid retention to the point of congestive heart failure and anasarca has been reported; in the PROactive and RECORD studies, an excess of approximately 2% of patients treated with high-dose glitazones required hospitalization for heart failure. In some patients, edema is refractory to diuretic therapy. Edema resolves with a reduction of thiazolidinedione dose in some patients, but some require drug withdrawal.

A more recent safety concern regarding thiazolidinediones is bone health. In pharmacoepidemiologic studies and in randomized, controlled trials, excess fractures have been reported, mainly in older women. Whereas distal sites were primarily affected in these studies, small randomized,

controlled trials have identified loss of bone density in the lumbar spine as well. Preclinical studies suggest that activation of PPARγ inhibits bone formation by diverting stem cells from the osteogenic to the adipocytic lineage. No data are available with respect to the prevention or management of thiazolidinedione-related bone loss, but prudent measures would include at a minimum an assessment of risk factors and appropriate bone density screening.[778]

Finally, pioglitazone has been implicated as causing bladder cancer as a result of inconsistent preclinical, clinical, and observational studies. In August 2014, a 10-year Kaiser Permanente Northern California study was announced suggesting no increased risk.[779] If pioglitazone is associated with bladder cancer, the absolute risk to an individual is very small. Current recommendations to avoid its use in patients with a history of bladder cancer, however, seem prudent.

Insulin Secretagogues

Currently available insulin secretagogues all bind to the SUR1, a subunit of the K_{ATP} potassium channel on the plasma membrane of pancreatic beta cells. The SUR1 subunit regulates the activity of the channel and also binds ATP and ADP, effectively functioning as a glucose sensor and trigger for insulin secretion. Sulfonylurea binding leads to closing of the channel, as do increases in intracellular ATP and decreases in ADP resulting from fuel metabolism. The membrane depolarization that ensues causes the opening of voltage-dependent L-type calcium channels. Subsequent calcium influx results in an increase in intracellular calcium, which leads to insulin secretion. Differences in pharmacokinetic and binding properties of the various insulin secretagogues result in the specific responses that each agent produces. The major differences among the insulin secretagogues seem to be related to duration of action and to subtle variations in hypoglycemic potential.

Sulfonylureas. The sulfonylureas have been available since the 1950s. They have a relatively slow onset and a variable duration of action. The numerous choices available (Table 31-11) can be divided into first- and second-generation agents. In general, the second-generation agents are more potent and, as a result, have fewer adverse effects and drug-drug interactions. Extended-release glipizide and glimepiride are preferred agents because they can be given once daily in most patients and involve a relatively low risk of hypoglycemia and weight gain. Gliclazide is not available in the United States but is a similarly preferred agent in much of the world. Nonetheless, glyburide is one of the most commonly prescribed insulin secretagogues, even in the face of concerns about its potential cardiovascular toxicity and higher risks of hypoglycemia compared with other secretagogues.[780]

An unusual characteristic of sulfonylureas is that the maximum marketed dose is two to four times higher than the maximum effective dose. There has been concern that sulfonylureas might cause increased arrhythmic cardiovascular events in patients with diabetes as a result of their activity on vascular and cardiac SUR2 receptors that blunts ischemic preconditioning, a protective autoregulatory mechanism in the heart. On the other hand, of the three recent cardiovascular outcome studies examining the effects of more intensive glycemic control on cardiovascular outcomes, only the ADVANCE trial, which employed the sulfonylurea gliclazide as its dominant strategy, did not exhibit any suggestion of cardiovascular toxicity[749] and the UKPDS similarly demonstrated the long-term safety of glyburide.[745]

TABLE 31-11
Characteristics of Sulfonylureas

Drug	Initial Daily Dose	Maximum Daily Dose	Equivalent Doses (mg)	Duration of Action	Comments
Acetohexamide	250 mg	1500 mg, div bid	500	Int: 12-18 hr	Metabolized by liver to active metabolite twice as potent as parent compound. Has diuretic activity. Has uricosuric activity.
Chlorpropamide	100 mg	750 mg (500 mg in older patients)	250	Very long: 60 hr	70% metabolized by liver to less active metabolites; 30% excreted intact by kidneys. Can potentiate ADH. Disulfiram-like reaction with alcohol occurs in almost 1/3 of patients.
Tolazamide	100 mg	1000 mg, div bid	250	Int: 12-24 hr	Metabolized by liver to less active and inactive products. Has diuretic activity.
Tolbutamide	250-500 mg or tid	3000 mg, div bid	1000	Short: 6-12 hr	Metabolized by liver to inactive product.
Glipizide	5 mg	40 mg, div bid	5	Int: 12-24 hr	Metabolized by liver to inactive products that are
Glipizide extended release	5 mg	20 mg qd	5	Long: >24 hr	excreted in the urine and, to a lesser extent, in the bile. Mild diuretic activity.
Glyburide	2.5 mg	20 mg, div bid	5	Int: 16-24 hr	Metabolized by liver to weakly active and inactive
Micronized glyburide	3 mg	6 mg bid	3	Shorter	products, excreted in urine and bile. Mild diuretic activity. Highest risk of hypoglycemia.
Glimepiride	1 mg	8 mg qd	2	Long: >24 hr	Metabolized to inactive metabolites by liver, excreted in urine and bile.

ADH, antidiuretic hormone; bid, twice a day; div, divided; int, intermediate; qd, every day; tid, three times a day.

Sulfonylureas are arguably the most cost-effective glucose-lowering agents. In general, limiting the dose to one fourth of the maximum marketed dose, unless higher doses are clearly demonstrated to provide significant benefits in glycemic control, minimizes costs and adverse events. Small doses of sulfonylurea (e.g., 0.5 to 1 mg of glimepiride or 2.5 mg of extended-release glipizide) are remarkably effective, particularly in patients receiving concomitant insulin-sensitizing therapy, and are almost uniformly well tolerated. The major opposition to early and frequent use of sulfonylureas relates to the generally modest weight gain and hypoglycemia but most specifically to the observation that they are associated with a higher rate of beta-cell failure, which may accelerate the time to requiring additional antihyperglycemic therapy.[776]

Glinides. Repaglinide is a member of the meglitinide family of insulin secretagogues, distinct from the sulfonylureas. It has a short half-life and a distinct SUR1 binding site. As a result of more rapid absorption, it produces a generally faster and briefer stimulus to insulin secretion. As a result, it is typically taken with each meal and provides better postprandial control and generally less hypoglycemia and weight gain than glyburide. Repaglinide does seem to have a long residence time on the SUR1 and a prolonged effect on FPG, even though its pharmacologic half-life is quite short. Repaglinide is available in 0.5-, 1-, and 2-mg tablets. The maximum dose is 4 mg with each meal. As with the sulfonylureas, there is only a modest glucose-lowering advantage of high doses compared with moderate doses of repaglinide.

Nateglinide is a derivative of phenylalanine and is structurally distinct from both sulfonylureas and the meglitinides. It has a quicker onset and a shorter duration of action than repaglinide. Its interaction with SUR1 is fleeting. As a result, its effect in lowering postprandial glucose is quite specific, and it has little effect in lowering FPG. This provides both advantages (less hypoglycemia) and disadvantages (less overall glucose-lowering effectiveness). Nateglinide is most appropriately used when FPG levels are modestly elevated in early diabetes or in combination with insulin sensitizers or long-acting evening insulin. Nateglinide is available as 120-mg tablets and is taken with each meal. A 60-mg tablet is available but is not generally used except in patients with minimal hyperglycemia.

The rationale for stimulating insulin secretion in a way that minimizes fasting hyperinsulinemia and maximizes postprandial control is compelling. Furthermore, these newer agents demonstrate little binding to the vascular smooth muscle and cardiac SUR2 receptors. However, the use in the United States of these newer glinide agents has been modest, in part because of the need for multiple daily doses, greater expense than with sulfonylureas, and lack of head-to-head comparative studies that demonstrate superiority over newer sulfonylureas, which are already perceived as having low potential for producing hypoglycemia and weight gain.

Carbohydrate Absorption Inhibitors: α-Glucosidase Inhibitors

α-Glucosidase inhibitors (AGIs) work to inhibit the terminal step of carbohydrate digestion at the brush border of the intestinal epithelium. As a result, carbohydrate absorption is shifted more distally in the intestine and is delayed, allowing the sluggish insulin secretory dynamics characteristic of T2DM to catch up with carbohydrate absorption.

The two currently available agents are acarbose and miglitol. Vogliobose is available in other countries. The use of AGIs in the United States has been limited by a number of factors, including the need to administer the medication at the beginning of each meal, flatulence as a common side effect, and only modest reductions in blood glucose levels. These factors should be balanced against the ability of AGIs to lower postprandial glucose, thereby improving glycemia without increasing weight or hypoglycemic risk. Even though they potentially lower glucose in everyone, the extent of the lowering is modest, calling into question the utility of these agents in light of the substantial expense and side effects. On the other hand, there is evidence that acarbose improves cardiovascular outcomes better than most antihyperglycemic agents.[781]

To maximize the potential for these agents to be well tolerated, start with a low dose (e.g., one fourth of the maximum dose) just once daily and increase over a period of weeks or months to one quarter to one half of the maximum dose with each meal.

Incretin-Related Therapies

The incretin effect describes the observation that oral glucose has a greater stimulatory effect on insulin secretion than does intravenous glucose at the same circulating glucose concentration. In humans, this effect seems to be primarily mediated by GLP-1 and GIP. GLP-1 is produced from the proglucagon gene in intestinal L cells and is secreted in response to nutrients. GLP-1 stimulates insulin secretion in a glucose-dependent fashion, inhibits inappropriate hyperglucagonemia, slows gastric emptying, reduces appetite and improves satiety, and has beta-cell proliferative, antiapoptotic, and differentiation effects at least in vitro and in preclinical models. GLP-1 has a very short half-life in plasma (1 to 2 minutes) due to amino-terminal degradation by the enzyme dipeptidyl peptidase 4 (DPP4). A variety of pharmacologic techniques have been developed to harness the potential of GLP-1 signaling to treat diabetes, including GLP-1 receptor agonists, which are peptides that produce increases of 10-fold or higher in GLP-1 activity, and DPP4 inhibitors, which are small-molecule inhibitors of the degradation of GLP-1 and GIP as well as other hormones.[782]

GLP-1 Receptor Agonists. Exendin-4 is a naturally occurring component of the saliva of the Gila monster (Heloderma suspectum) and shares 53% sequence identity with GLP-1; it is resistant to DPP4 degradation. Exenatide is synthetic exendin-4 and was the first GLP-1-based therapeutic agent to be approved for human use. When injected subcutaneously, it produces the effects listed earlier and has a peak of action and half-life of approximately 2 hours. With twice-daily injection within 1 hour before a meal, it produces a reduction of approximately 1% in HbA_{1c}, driven largely by a reduction in postprandial glucose along with modest weight loss (average, 5 to 10 lb/year). With prolonged use, weight loss has been associated with expected improvements in blood pressure and lipids. The most common adverse effect is nausea, which occurs in 40% to 50% of patients, usually early in the course of therapy. The nausea is mild to moderate in intensity and typically wanes over time. Nausea leads to withdrawal of therapy in about 5% of patients.

Newer, longer-acting GLP-1 receptor agonists include liraglutide, once-weekly exenatide, albiglutide, and dulaglutide.[783] In general, these longer-acting agents are associated with greater HbA_{1c}-lowering efficacy owing to more predominant effects on FPG than exenatide in the twice-daily formulation. They are also associated with fewer gastrointestinal adverse effects, probably because they seem to produce little or no gastric emptying effects. One could argue based on head-to-head studies that liraglutide and dulaglutide are similar in efficacy and minimally more effective than exenatide once weekly, which may be the best tolerated of the longer-acting GLP-1 receptor agonists, at least with respect to nausea. However, exenatide once weekly is associated with skin nodules at the site of injection. Albiglutide seems less effective than the other longer-acting agents. Liraglutide is administered once daily without any restriction as to timing or relation to meals. Once-weekly exenatide requires reconstitution and a somewhat larger bore needle for administration. Once-weekly albiglutide also requires reconstitution but has a smaller bore needle. Once-weekly dulaglutide does not require reconstitution; its pen-like device has a retracting needle and is clearly the least difficult once-weekly GLP-1 receptor agonist to use.

Weight loss is similar among the various GLP-1 receptor agonists, though perhaps less for albiglutide.[783] Hypoglycemia is not a direct effect of GLP-1 receptor agonists, but they can amplify the hypoglycemic effects of other agents. Therefore, for coadministration with secretagogues or insulin, it is recommended that the minimum dose of secretagogue be used when initiating GLP-1 receptor agonist therapy, uptitrating the secretagogue later if necessary. A 20% insulin dose reduction is prudent when initiating GLP-1 receptor agonists in insulin-treated patients with T2DM and HbA_{1c} less than 8%. A concern that emerged from postmarketing reports is pancreatitis. A causal link has not been proved, nor has a mechanism been established. Nevertheless, it is recommended that incretin-based therapy be avoided in those with a history of pancreatitis. Exenatide is renally cleared and is contraindicated in the setting of advanced kidney disease (eGFR <30 mL/minute per 1.73 m²). The other GLP-1 receptor agonists do not share this feature with exenatide. Nevertheless, cases of acute renal failure have been reported in association with GLP-1 receptor agonist therapy, usually in patients with chronic renal insufficiency who develop superimposed prerenal azotemia in the context of prolonged nausea, anorexia, and vomiting. To mitigate the risk of pancreatitis and renal failure, it is prudent to instruct patients treated with GLP-1 receptor agonists to hold their medication if they develop nausea, vomiting, or abdominal pain of more than a few hours' duration and to seek medical attention if they are unable to keep down fluids after 4 hours.

A new safety concern that arose in preclinical testing with these long-acting agents is medullary thyroid cancer. No signal exists for this problem with GLP-1–based therapy in humans, but there is a clear increase in the incidence of these tumors in rodents, although not in other animal models. GLP-1 plays a role in regulation of C cells in the rodent but apparently not in the human. Nevertheless, it is suggested that these agents be avoided in those with a personal or family history of medullary thyroid cancer.

DPP4 Inhibitors. Four DPP4 inhibitors—sitagliptin, saxagliptin, linagliptin, and alogliptin—are available in the United States and several others worldwide. These agents produce approximately twofold increases in fasting and postprandial GLP-1 and GIP levels, with subsequent HbA_{1c} reductions of approximately 0.7%. They are remarkably well tolerated, with an adverse effect profile similar to that of placebo. Specifically, they are not associated with nausea. Probably because of the lesser increase in GLP-1 activity than with the GLP-1 receptor agonists, there is no weight loss with DPP4 inhibitors; they tend to be weight neutral. Postmarketing cases of pancreatitis have been reported for the DPP4 inhibitors, and they are contraindicated for use in those with a prior history. Specificity for DPP4 appears to be crucial, because less specific inhibitors have demonstrated adverse effects on immune function and cancer growth in animal studies. Although the currently marketed DPP4 inhibitors are thought to be highly selective, continued long-term surveillance for unexpected adverse events is essential. Further, the biology of the agents is extremely complex owing to the multiple substrates and peptide fragments whose biology they affect.[784] In cardiovascular outcome trials, there was an increased risk for heart failure hospitalization with saxagliptin and a numerical imbalance for alogliptin; no increased risk was demonstrated for sitagliptin.[785] Whether this represents an important clinical distinction, the play of chance or differences in trial populations or conduct is unclear.

A nice feature of these agents is that they do not require titration. Linagliptin is only available in one tablet size. For the others, which are partially renally cleared, the usual

broad cardiovascular outcomes were improved 40% compared with placebo.[795] Recent studies suggest substantial efficacy in the setting of inadequate glycemic control on high-dose insulin therapy.[796]

Practical Aspects of Initiating and Progressively Managing Type 2 Diabetes Mellitus

A significant challenge in clinical decision making in diabetes is that the increased availability of therapeutic options for antihyperglycemic therapy is far ahead of adequate prospective outcome studies. Currently available clinical trial data have not identified the preferred agents in T2DM, either as initial therapy or in subsequent care. Each class of drugs and even individual agents within each class have advantages and limitations, and individual issues can significantly affect the appropriate choice of therapy in particular patients. Table 31-10 highlights some of the relative advantages and disadvantages of various agents and classes.

General Approach

A general approach in the absence of any patient-specific factors is suggested in the algorithm presented in Figure 31-21.[7,767] A growing body of experience suggests that the use of metformin as initial therapy in combination with diet, exercise, and a comprehensive diabetes education program can provide impressive lowering of glucose with essentially no risk of hypoglycemia. If the response is judged to be inadequate over 3 months, essentially any other agent can be added. There are six recommended second-line therapies: sulfonylurea, thiazolidinedione, DPP4 inhibitor, SGLT2 inhibitor, GLP-1 receptor agonist, and basal insulin. Each has its advantages and disadvantages. If HbA$_{1c}$ above target persists for an additional 3 months, adding virtually any agent not yet prescribed is acceptable. There is little rationale or data on the combination of GLP-1 receptor agonist with DPP4 inhibitors. Though there is great excitement about using GLP-1 receptor agonists with SGLT2 inhibitors, as both are associated with weight loss, no randomized controlled trial data are yet available. Certainly the other antihyperglycemic agent alternatives can be used, although they may provide no distinct advantage over these seven.

For patients whose glycemic control is farther than 1% from target, it is possible to use fixed-dose combination drugs at onset, and some advocate routine combination therapy. The combination of metformin and a DPP4 inhibitor is generally well tolerated, is not associated with weight gain or hypoglycemia, and has become quite popular. There are now more than a dozen fixed-dose combinations of two drugs from all five classes of oral agents on Figure 31-21; likewise, there are combinations of basal insulin and GLP-1 receptor agonists under development. Multiple daily injections of insulin plus metformin have been suggested as the final common therapy for most patients with diabetes who do not achieve adequate control otherwise for almost 2 decades. Only in this most recent guidance from the ADA and European Association for the Study of Diabetes (EASD) has basal insulin plus GLP-1 receptor agonists been recommended as an alternative based on greater efficacy and a lower risk of hypoglycemia and weight gain.[767,797]

The most critical issue in long-term glycemic management is that of continuously reassessing with patients the adequacy of their control, examining glucose monitoring logs and HbA$_{1c}$ values, and refining treatment regimens to achieve optimal control with the lowest doses of the fewest medications. Most patients in specialty care require two or more drugs to achieve recommended targets. In general, it is preferred to add agents if there was an improvement in control with the first agent selected and to continue to add agents as needed to achieve goals. Subsequent back-titration to optimize treatment is often possible after glycemic goals are achieved. The selection of initial therapy should be based on priorities mutually recognized by the patient and provider. When adding insulin in the management of inadequately controlled T2DM, some practitioners prefer to stop the oral antihyperglycemic agents and switch to insulin. Most continue the oral agents and add an evening dose of insulin. Classically, bedtime NPH insulin and, more recently, long-acting insulin analogues have been preferred for initiating insulin therapy. There are data suggesting that long-acting analogues can provide for lower morning glucose values with less nocturnal hypoglycemia or weight gain than NPH insulin, particularly in more overweight patients. Many patients eventually require more complex regimens, such as twice-daily injections or multiple-injection regimens, but insulin pump therapy is rarely used.

Some advocate starting multiple-injection therapy with rapid-acting insulin at each meal if adequate control is not achieved with basal insulin. Although the finding is not intuitive, recent data suggest that adding a single injection of rapid-acting insulin (at the morning meal or at the largest meal) to basal insulin titrated to provide for FPG control provides for a similar level of HbA$_{1c}$ as the multiple-injection regimen with less weight gain and hypoglycemia. As one progresses from an injection of basal insulin plus a single injection of rapid-acting insulin to higher-order regimens, it seems incumbent on the health care team to ensure that improved control develops or to simplify the regimen. Studies suggest that to achieve HbA$_{1c}$ levels lower than 7%, many patients require insulin doses on the order of 1 to 2 units/kg per day in addition to metformin. In the typical patient with insulin-resistant T2DM, there is usually little advantage to splitting basal insulin into two injections; in general, if a second injection is needed it should be prandial insulin.

It is important that both patient and health care provider agree on how to reach the goals of therapy. Therefore, biases and concerns of the patient should be addressed when trying to determine which agent should be prescribed. These biases can be elucidated in interviews with patients through discussions of various strategies.

Strategies

Minimal Cost Strategy. For a large fraction of patients, particularly those who are elderly, the cost of drugs is an overwhelming issue. Diet and exercise can be extremely effective and are almost cost-free. The least expensive drugs for the treatment of diabetes are the sulfonylureas, and metformin, thiazolidinediones, AGIs, and human insulin are relatively inexpensive. There can be marked differences in price by pharmacy, and websites are available to find the best prices.[798] Specifically with regard to human insulin, there is a store brand of human insulin (i.e., ReliOn), which is generally available for approximately one fourth the usual price of human insulin. Therefore, a minimum-cost strategy could start with a sulfonylurea or metformin or both and progress to the addition of bedtime NPH insulin. Although insulin is relatively inexpensive, at high doses (≥1 U/kg) the costs begin to rise and the benefits are modest, creating a rationale for adding a generic thiazolidinedione. Most pharmaceutical companies and some states and communities have programs to provide no-cost

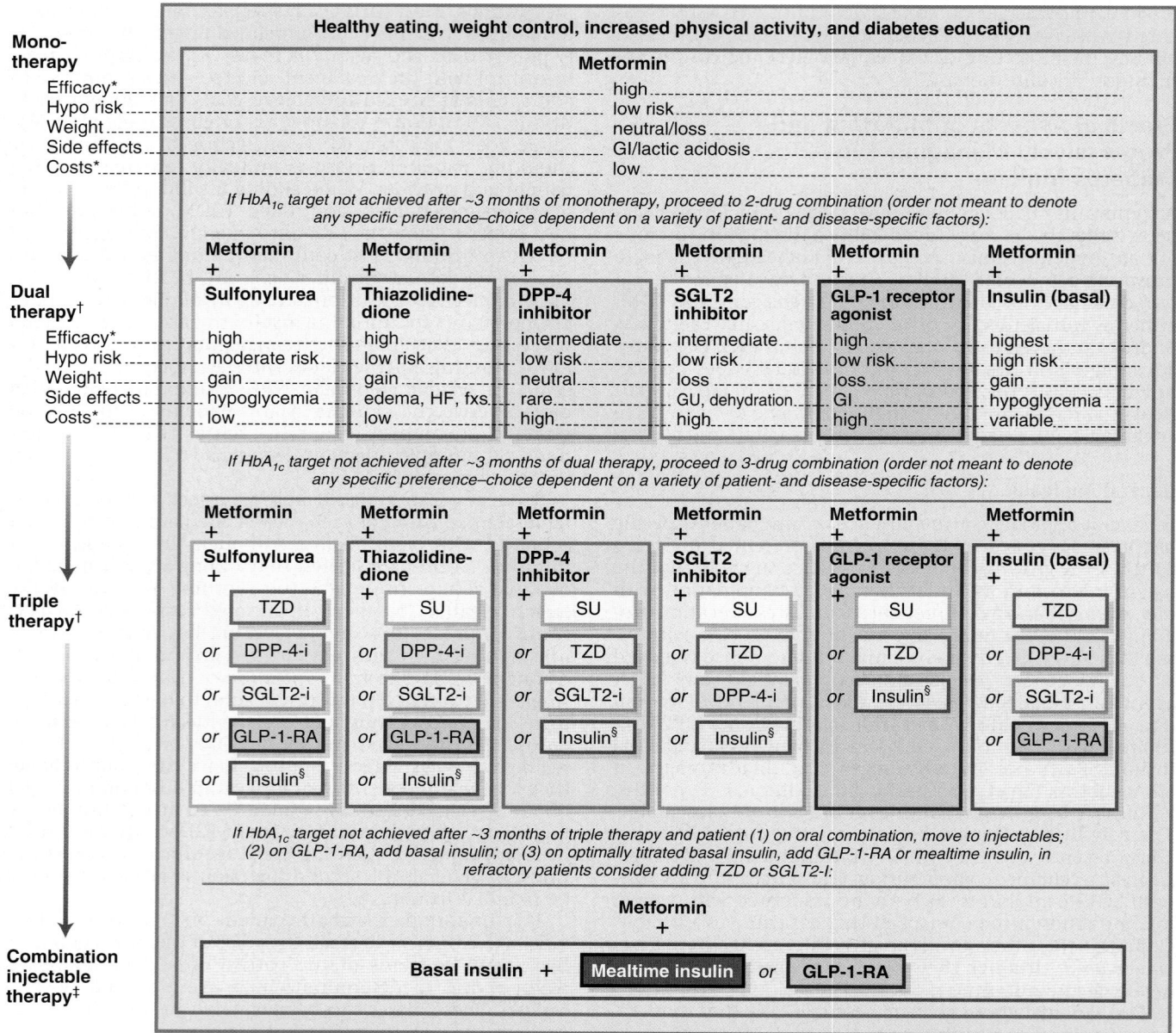

Figure 31-21 Antihyperglycemic therapy in type 2 diabetes: general recommendations of the ADA and EASD. The order in the chart was determined by historical availability and the route of administration, with injectables to the right; it is not meant to denote any specific preference. Potential sequences of antihyperglycemic therapy for patients with type 2 diabetes are displayed, with the usual transition moving vertically from top to bottom (although horizontal movement within therapy stages is also possible, depending on the circumstances). ADA, American Diabetes Association; EASD, European Association for the Study of Diabetes; DPP-4-i, DPP-4 inhibitor; fxs, fractures; GI, gastrointestinal; GLP, glucagon-like peptide; GLP-1-RA, GLP-1 receptor agonist; GU, genitourinary; HF, heart failure; Hypo, hypoglycemia; SGLT, sodium-glucose cotransporter; SGLT2-i, SGLT2 inhibitor; SU, sulfonylurea; TZD, thiazolidinedione. *See reference for description of efficacy categorization. †Consider starting dual therapy when HbA₁c is greater than 9%. ‡Consider starting with combination injectable therapy when blood glucose is higher than 300 to 350 mg/dL (16.7-19.4 mmol/L) or HbA₁c is greater than 10% to 12%, especially if symptomatic or catabolic features are present, in which case basal insulin plus mealtime insulin is the preferred initial regimen. §Usually a basal insulin. (Modified from Inzucchi SE, Bergenstal RM, Buse JB, et al. Management of hyperglycemia in type 2 diabetes, 2015: a patient-centered approach: update to a position statement of the American Diabetes Association and the European Association for the Study of Diabetes. *Diabetes Care.* 2015;38:140-149.)

or low-cost medications to the poor. Many websites offer this information.[799] For an increasing number of patients, the major driving force in their drug expenses is the number of prescriptions, because each is associated with a copayment. This provides another rationale for the use of combination agents.

Minimal Weight Gain Strategy. Weight gain associated with the treatment of diabetes is of concern to most clinicians and is often an overriding issue with patients. A strategy to minimize weight gain would emphasize diet and exer-

cise and would almost certainly employ metformin as initial therapy. GLP-1 receptor agonists and SGLT2 inhibitors are associated with moderate weight loss in most patients with long-term use, and they would almost always be used as second-line therapy if weight were truly the major consideration. AGIs, DPP4 inhibitors, colesevelam, and bromocriptine are all weight neutral. Currently there are no well-controlled studies that document the safety and efficacy of GLP-1 receptor agonists and SGLT2 inhibitors in combination.

Minimal Progressive Beta-Cell Loss Strategy. Progressive loss of beta-cell function is the hallmark of diabetes. It results in progressive deterioration of glycemic control and the eventual need for insulin treatment. Thiazolidinediones seem to be associated with the lowest rate of secondary failure and sulfonylurea with the highest, at least in comparison to metformin. Adoption of a strategy to minimize progressive beta-cell loss would lead to the use of a thiazolidinedione with metformin as initial therapies and the avoidance of secretagogues. GLP-1 receptor agonists and DPP4 inhibitors have been associated with improvements in beta-cell mass in rodent models, but this is completely unproved in humans.

Minimal Injection Strategy. Too many patients are determined to avoid insulin injections at any cost. The minimal injection strategy could involve the use of almost any combination of oral agents. Metformin and thiazolidinediones in combination with either sulfonylureas or DPP4 inhibitors have been best studied. Injected insulin or a GLP-1 receptor agonist would be added only if absolutely necessary. As dulaglutide once weekly GLP-1 receptor agonist therapy does not provide a visible needle as part of the injection device, some needle-phobic patients see it as an acceptable product. The strategy of using thiazolidinediones early in the course of diabetes, in the hope that this might reduce the rate of progressive beta-cell dysfunction, would be rational in this setting. It is important to try to dispel notions that insulin therapy is difficult, ominous, or fraught with peril by highlighting its efficacy and the great strides that have been made in insulin formulations and delivery devices. Most diabetic patients require insulin at some point in their lifetime. Quite a few patients who have resisted the use of insulin have not balked at GLP-1 receptor agonists. This suggests that, although patients may have identified the needle as the predominant barrier to insulin therapy, they really had other biases driving their fears.

Minimal Insulin Resistance Strategy. The possible atherogenic effects of insulin have been widely touted in the lay press and by marketing programs within the pharmaceutical industry. The relationship between circulating insulin levels and cardiovascular risk in nondiabetic populations is incontrovertible but is probably related to the presence of insulin resistance rather than the insulin concentrations per se. Furthermore, in essentially all studies of intensive management with insulin, improved outcomes were observed with insulin treatment. There are no clinical data to suggest that exogenous insulin is associated with adverse side effects or long-term complications beyond its hypoglycemic effects and the associated weight gain. A recent trial compared an insulin-providing strategy and an insulin-sparing strategy in high-risk patients in terms of mortality risk; there were essentially no differences in cardiovascular outcomes.[800] Adoption of a strategy to minimize insulin resistance would lead to the use of metformin and a thiazolidinedione before consideration of adding other agents.

Minimal Effort Strategy. Many patients are capable of making only a minimal effort with regard to their diabetes. Questioning patients about their pill-taking history and their realistic ability to comply with a prescribed frequency of therapy is important. The usual twice-daily therapy with metformin is a barrier to its use; sustained-release metformin would be an acceptable alternative. Taking a once-a-day sulfonylurea, DPP4 inhibitor, or thiazolidinedione requires the least effort by the patient. Combination products may have a role in this setting. The use of basal insulin or a once-daily or once-weekly GLP-1 receptor agonist is relatively well accepted by patients to whom this consideration is important. Developing strategies to improve adherence and increase motivation is a long-term goal in this population. There are devices under development for delivering exenatide in a subcutaneous implanted capsule every 6 months.[801]

Hypoglycemia Avoidance Strategy. Hypoglycemia avoidance is another important consideration for many patients. The AGIs and thiazolidinediones have been reported in small studies to reduce reactive hypoglycemia. Theoretically, GLP-1 receptor agonists, DPP4 inhibitors, and metformin should not be associated with hypoglycemia. Other oral agents could be added in any order, with the exception that insulin secretagogues would be added last, their dose minimized, and glyburide avoided. Nateglinide in particular among the secretagogues is associated with an exceptionally low risk of significant hypoglycemia. Basal insulin strategies seem to be associated with a lower risk of hypoglycemia than prandial insulin.[802]

Postprandial Targeting Strategy. Achieving postprandial glucose targets is generally associated with better control than just meeting premeal targets.[803] On the basis of epidemiologic studies, it has been suggested that postprandial plasma glucose (PPG) is more highly correlated with cardiovascular disease risk than FPG. However, correction for confounding variables such as components of the multiple metabolic syndrome has not been performed in these studies. Furthermore, there are no outcome studies that have demonstrated the superiority of these approaches in patients with T2DM.

Control of postprandial glycemia can be achieved only with specific lifestyle efforts and pharmacologic agents that target PPG. PPG monitoring is helpful in this regard because it reinforces the goals and is the most effective measure to assess the effectiveness of treatment. Nonpharmacologic techniques that can improve postprandial control include lowering the carbohydrate content of meals, adding fiber, substituting monounsaturated fats for carbohydrates, and encouraging physical activity after meals. The pharmacologic approach includes AGIs, exenatide twice daily, and rapid-acting insulin analogues. Nateglinide and repaglinide provide a theoretical advantage in this situation compared with other secretagogues, although formal head-to-head studies comparing these agents with glimepiride and sustained-release glipizide have not been completed.

Preventing Type 2 Diabetes Mellitus

The possibility that T2DM can be prevented in high-risk persons has been formally tested in a series of clinical trials reviewed elsewhere.[7] Lifestyle intervention seems to provide for a reduction of 30% to 60% in progression to diabetes over a 3- to 5-year time frame. These benefits seem to be sustained and best correlated with weight loss; however, the average sustained weight loss in these trials was modest, on the order of 5%. Metformin has likewise been associated with a somewhat more modest reduction in the progression of diabetes, although the benefit seemed to be similar to that of lifestyle intervention in those patients younger than 45 years of age, those with BMI greater than 35 kg/m^2, and those with an FPG level greater than 110 mg/dL. On average, metformin was generally without effect in patients older than 60 years of age, those with a BMI of less than 30 kg/m^2, and those with an FPG of less than 100 mg/dL. Acarbose has also been shown to reduce progression to diabetes, without evidence of diminished efficacy in different subgroups. The thiazolidinediones seem to be the most active antihyperglycemic agents tested for prevention, with efficacy as great as or greater than that of lifestyle intervention. However, concern regarding the long-term safety of thiazolidinediones in relation to effects on weight, heart, and bones has limited the enthusiasm for use of this class for prevention.

The success of the lifestyle interventions is impressive, demonstrating conclusively that with a variety of techniques it is possible for patients to achieve physiologically relevant changes in body weight. It is unknown whether lifestyle plus medications provides even greater benefit. The questions that arise are how to screen for people at risk and what intervention should be initiated in those with an interest in prevention. It seems reasonable to screen on the basis of current recommendations, as outlined earlier primarily for case finding, but also recognizing that patients with abnormal glucose values (HbA$_{1c}$ >5.7% and particularly ≥6%, FPG ≥100 mg/dL and particularly ≥110 mg/dL, or IGT) would be ideal candidates for preventive strategies. Certainly, high-risk persons should be counseled about nutritional approaches to achieve weight loss, instructed to increase physical activity, and observed prospectively to determine whether progression of hyperglycemia has occurred. Treatment for other cardiovascular risk factors should also be considered if they are present.

In the absence of outcome studies, it is difficult to strongly advocate for drug therapy to prevent diabetes, because significant diabetes complications are unlikely to develop in the short window of time during which glucose levels increase from an FPG of 100 to 126 mg/dL. On the other hand, metformin therapy seems innocuous enough, and its benefits are broad; therefore, consideration of metformin therapy in patients who are at particularly high risk is recommended.[7] An extension phase of the Diabetes Prevention Program that is under way should provide evidence concerning whether prevention or delay in the development of diabetes will prevent death or disability.

Future Directions

The present-day management of T2DM is significantly more effective and easier for patients than the situation that prevailed even in the 1990s. A better understanding of the barriers to effective diabetes management and how to overcome them would be of great benefit. Changes in the health care system in the United States promise to eradicate access to care as the major barrier to prevention of disabling complications. The epidemic in diabetes and obesity that is under way, coupled with the predicted early death and disability that follow, threatens to overwhelm health care systems globally. Screening for diabetes or prediabetes may be cost-saving.[804] Practical, cost-effective public health approaches to stem this tide are desperately needed.[805] Whether new blockbuster drugs exist in the pipeline of 180 novel pharmaceutical agents for the treatment of diabetes and its complications is uncertain.[806,807] Although the prognosis for people with diabetes has never been better, the major challenges that they face relate to the complexity and cost of care. The opportunities for therapies that broadly address the metabolic underpinnings and consequences of diabetes are enormous.

REFERENCES

1. Zimmet P, Alberti KG, Shaw J. Global and societal implications of the diabetes epidemic. *Nature.* 2001;414:782-787.
2. Shaw JE, Sicree RA, Zimmet PZ. Global estimates of the prevalence of diabetes for 2010 and 2030. *Diabetes Res Clin Pract.* 2010;87: 4-14.
3. International Diabetes Federation. *IDF Diabetes Atlas Update Poster.* 6th ed. Brussels, Belgium: International Diabetes Federation; 2014.
4. Centers for Disease Control and Prevention. *National Diabetes Statistics Report: Estimates of Diabetes and Its Burden in the United States, 2014.* Atlanta, GA: U.S. Department of Health and Human Services; 2014.
5. Zhuo X, Zhang P, Kahn HS, et al. Change in medical spending attributable to diabetes: national data from 1987 to 2011. *Diabetes Care.* 2015; 38:581-587.
6. Hamman RF, Bell RA, Dabelea D, et al., SEARCH for Diabetes in Youth Study Group. The SEARCH for Diabetes in Youth study: rationale, findings, and future directions. *Diabetes Care.* 2014;37(12): 3336-3344.
7. American Diabetes Association. Standards of medical care in diabetes—2015. *Diabetes Care.* 2015;38:s1-s93.
8. International Expert Committee. Report on the role of the A1C assay in the diagnosis of diabetes. *Diabetes Care.* 2009;32:1327-1334.
9. Kahn R, Alperin P, Eddy D, et al. Age at initiation and frequency of screening to detect type 2 diabetes: a cost-effectiveness analysis. *Lancet.* 2010;375:1365-1374.
10. Zhang X, Gregg EW, Williamson DF, et al. A1C level and future risk of diabetes: a systematic review. *Diabetes Care.* 2010;33:1665-1673.
11. Defronzo RA. Banting Lecture. From the triumvirate to the ominous octet: a new paradigm for the treatment of type 2 diabetes mellitus. *Diabetes.* 2009;58(4):773-795.
12. Almind K, Doria A, Kahn CR. Putting the genes for type II diabetes on the map. *Nat Med.* 2001;7:277-279.
13. Bell GI, Polonsky KS. Diabetes mellitus and genetically programmed defects in beta-cell function. *Nature.* 2001;414:788-791.
14. Taylor SI, Arioglu E. Genetically defined forms of diabetes in children. *J Clin Endocrinol Metab.* 1999;84:4390-4396.
15. Kahn CR, Flier JS, Bar RS, et al. The syndromes of insulin resistance and acanthosis nigricans: insulin-receptor disorders in man. *N Engl J Med.* 1976;294:739-745.
16. Donohue W. Leprechaunism: a euphemism for a rare familial disorder. *J Pediatr.* 1954;45:505-519.
17. Elders MJ, Schedewie HK, Olefsky J, et al. Endocrine-metabolic relationships in patients with leprechaunism. *J Natl Med Assoc.* 1982;74: 1195-1210.
18. Rosenberg AM, Haworth JC, Degroot GW, et al. A case of leprechaunism with severe hyperinsulinemia. *Am J Dis Child.* 1980;134: 170-175.
19. Rabson S, Mendenhall E. Familial hypertrophy of pineal body, hyperplasia of adrenal cortex and diabetes mellitus. *Am J Clin Pathol.* 1956;26:283-290.
20. Garg A. Lipodystrophies. *Am J Med.* 2000;108:143-152.
21. Vigouroux C, Magre J, Vantyghem MC, et al. Lamin A/C gene: sex-determined expression of mutations in Dunnigan-type familial partial lipodystrophy and absence of coding mutations in congenital and acquired generalized lipoatrophy. *Diabetes.* 2000;49:1958-1962.
22. Garg A. Acquired and inherited lipodystrophies. *N Engl J Med.* 2004; 350:1220-1234.
23. Magre J, Delepine M, Khallouf E, et al. Identification of the gene altered in Berardinelli-Seip congenital lipodystrophy on chromosome 11q13. *Nat Genet.* 2001;28:365-370.
24. Barroso I, Gurnell M, Crowley VE, et al. Dominant negative mutations in human PPARγ associated with severe insulin resistance, diabetes mellitus and hypertension. *Nature.* 1999;402:880-883.
25. Hegele RA, Pollex RL. Genetic and physiological insights into the metabolic syndrome. *Am J Physiol Regul Integr Comp Physiol.* 2005;289: R663-R669.
26. Moffett SP, Feingold E, Barmada MM, et al. The C161→T polymorphism in peroxisome proliferator-activated receptor gamma, but not P12A, is associated with insulin resistance in Hispanic and non-Hispanic white women: evidence for another functional variant in peroxisome proliferator-activated receptor gamma. *Metabolism.* 2005; 54:1552-1556.
27. Hattersley AT, Ashcroft FM. Activating mutations in Kir6.2 and neonatal diabetes: new clinical syndromes, new scientific insights and new therapy. *Diabetes.* 2005;54:2503-2513.
28. Haneda M, Polonsky KS, Bergenstal RM, et al. Familial hyperinsulinemia due to a structurally abnormal insulin: definition of an emerging new clinical syndrome. *N Engl J Med.* 1984;310:1288-1294.
29. Gruppuso PA, Gorden P, Kahn CR, et al. Familial hyperproinsulinemia due to a proposed defect in conversion of proinsulin to insulin. *N Engl J Med.* 1984;311:629-634.
30. Shibasaki Y, Kawakami T, Kanazawa Y, et al. Posttranslational cleavage of proinsulin is blocked by a point mutation in familial hyperproinsulinemia. *J Clin Invest.* 1985;76:378-380.
31. O'Rahilly S, Gray H, Humphreys PJ, et al. Brief report: impaired processing of prohormones associated with abnormalities of glucose homeostasis and adrenal function. *N Engl J Med.* 1995;333:1386-1390.
32. Ballinger SW, Shoffner JM, Hedaya EV, et al. Maternally transmitted diabetes and deafness associated with a 10.4 kb mitochondrial DNA deletion. *Nat Genet.* 1992;1:11-15.
33. Velho G, Byrne MM, Clement K, et al. Clinical phenotypes, insulin secretion, and insulin sensitivity in kindreds with maternally inherited diabetes and deafness due to mitochondrial tRNALeu(UUR) gene mutation. *Diabetes.* 1996;45:478-487.
34. Fajans SS, Bell GI, Polonsky KS. Molecular mechanisms and clinical pathophysiology of maturity-onset diabetes of the young. *N Engl J Med.* 2001;345:971-980.

35. Fajans SS, Bell GI. MODY: history, genetics, pathophysiology and clinical decision making. *Diabetes Care.* 2011;34:1878-1884.
36. Froguel P, Zouali H, Vionnet N, et al. Familial hyperglycemia due to mutations in glucokinase: definition of a subtype of diabetes mellitus. *N Engl J Med.* 1993;328:697-702.
37. Yamagata K, Furuta H, Oda N, et al. Mutations in the hepatocyte nuclear factor-4α gene in maturity-onset diabetes of the young (MODY1). *Nature.* 1996;384:458-460.
38. Yamagata K, Oda N, Kaisaki PJ, et al. Mutations in the hepatocyte nuclear factor-1α gene in maturity-onset diabetes of the young (MODY3). *Nature.* 1996;384:455-458.
39. Stoffers DA, Ferrer J, Clarke WL, et al. Early-onset type-II diabetes mellitus (MODY4) linked to IPF1. *Nat Genet.* 1997;17:138-139.
40. Horikawa Y, Iwasaki N, Hara N, et al. Mutation in hepatocyte nuclear factor-1β gene (TCF2) associated with MODY. *Nat Genet.* 1997;17:384-385.
41. Malecki MT, Jhala US, Antonellis A, et al. Mutations in NEUROD1 are associated with the development of type 2 diabetes mellitus. *Nat Genet.* 1999;23:323-328.
42. Njolstad PR, Sovik O, Cuesta-Munoz A, et al. Neonatal diabetes mellitus due to complete glucokinase deficiency. *N Engl J Med.* 2001;344:1588-1592.
43. Cereghini S. Liver-enriched transcription factors and hepatocyte differentiation. *FASEB J.* 1996;10:267-282.
44. Duncan SA, Navas MA, Dufort D, et al. Regulation of a transcription factor network required for differentiation and metabolism. *Science.* 1998;281:692-695.
45. Stoffel M, Duncan SA. The maturity-onset diabetes of the young (MODY1) transcription factor HNF4α regulates expression of genes required for glucose transport and metabolism. *Proc Natl Acad Sci U S A.* 1997;94:13209-13214.
46. Edlund H. Factors controlling pancreatic cell differentiation and function. *Diabetologia.* 2001;44:1071-1079.
47. Stoffers DA, Stanojevic V, Habener JF. Insulin promoter factor-1 gene mutation linked to early-onset type 2 diabetes mellitus directs expression of a dominant negative isoprotein. *J Clin Invest.* 1998;102:232-241.
48. Hani EH, Stoffers DA, Chevre JC, et al. Defective mutations in the insulin promoter factor-1 (IPF-1) gene in late-onset type 2 diabetes mellitus. *J Clin Invest.* 1999;104:R41-R48.
49. Kristinsson SY, Thorolfsdottir ET, Talseth B, et al. MODY in Iceland is associated with mutations in HNF-1α and a novel mutation in NeuroD1. *Diabetologia.* 2001;44:2098-2103.
50. Permutt MA, Hattersley AT. Searching for type 2 diabetes genes in the post-genome era. *Trends Endocrinol Metab.* 2000;11:383-393.
51. Grarup N, Sandholt CH, Hansen T, Pedersen O. Genetic susceptibility to type 2 diabetes and obesity: from genome wide association studies to rare variants and beyond. *Diabetologia.* 2014;57:1528-1541.
52. Florez JC. Clinical review: the genetics of type 2 diabetes—a realistic appraisal in 2008. *J Clin Endocrinol Metab.* 2008;93:4633-4642.
53. Doria A, Patti ME, Kahn CR. The emerging genetic architecture of type 2 diabetes. *Cell Metab.* 2008;8:186-200.
54. Perry JR, Frayling TM. New gene variants alter type 2 diabetes risk predominantly through reduced beta-cell function. *Curr Opin Clin Nutr Metab Care.* 2008;11:371-377.
55. Horikawa Y, Oda N, Cox NJ, et al. Genetic variation in the gene encoding calpain-10 is associated with type 2 diabetes mellitus. *Nat Genet.* 2000;26:163-175.
56. Song Y, Niu T, Manson JE, et al. Are variants in the CAPN10 gene related to risk of type 2 diabetes? A quantitative assessment of population and family-based association studies. *Am J Hum Genet.* 2004;74:208-222.
57. Gloyn AL, Weedon MN, Owen KR, et al. Large-scale association studies of variants in genes encoding the pancreatic beta-cell KATP channel subunits Kir6.2 (KCNJ11) and SUR1 (ABCC8) confirm that the KCNJ11 E23K variant is associated with type 2 diabetes. *Diabetes.* 2003;52:568-572.
58. Goll DE, Thompson VF, Li H, et al. The calpain system. *Physiol Rev.* 2003;83:731-801.
59. Sreenan SK, Zhou YP, Otani K, et al. Calpains play a role in insulin secretion and action. *Diabetes.* 2001;50:2013-2020.
60. Zhou YP, Sreenan S, Pan CY, et al. A 48-hour exposure of pancreatic islets to calpain inhibitors impairs mitochondrial fuel metabolism and the exocytosis of insulin. *Metabolism.* 2003;52:528-534.
61. Otani K, Han DH, Ford EL, et al. Calpain system regulates muscle mass and glucose transporter GLUT4 turnover. *J Biol Chem.* 2004;279:20915-20920.
62. Johnson JD, Han Z, Otani K, et al. RyR2 and calpain-10 delineate a novel apoptosis pathway in pancreatic islets. *J Biol Chem.* 2004;279:24794-24802.
63. Aguilar-Bryan L, Bryan J. Molecular biology of adenosine triphosphate-sensitive potassium channels. *Endocr Rev.* 1999;20:101-135.
64. Nielsen EM, Hansen L, Carstensen B, et al. The E23K variant of Kir6.2 associates with impaired post-OGTT serum insulin response and increased risk of type 2 diabetes. *Diabetes.* 2003;52:573-577.
65. Gloyn AL, Hashim Y, Ashcroft SJ, et al. Association studies of variants in promoter and coding regions of beta-cell ATP-sensitive K-channel genes SUR1 and Kir6.2 with type 2 diabetes mellitus (UKPDS 53). *Diabet Med.* 2001;18:206-212.
66. Hani EH, Boutin P, Durand E, et al. Missense mutations in the pancreatic islet beta cell inwardly rectifying K+ channel gene (KIR6.2/BIR): a meta-analysis suggests a role in the polygenic basis of type II diabetes mellitus in Caucasians. *Diabetologia.* 1998;41:1511-1515.
67. Love-Gregory L, Wasson J, Lin J, et al. E23K single nucleotide polymorphism in the islet ATP-sensitive potassium channel gene (Kir6.2) contributes as much to the risk of type II diabetes in Caucasians as the PPARγ Pro12Ala variant. *Diabetologia.* 2003;46:136-137.
68. 't Hart LM, van Haeften TW, Dekker JM, et al. Variations in insulin secretion in carriers of the E23K variant in the KIR6.2 subunit of the ATP-sensitive K(+) channel in the beta-cell. *Diabetes.* 2002;51:3135-3138.
69. Rosen ED, Kulkarni RN, Sarraf P, et al. Targeted elimination of peroxisome proliferator-activated receptor gamma in beta cells leads to abnormalities in islet mass without compromising glucose homeostasis. *Mol Cell Biol.* 2003;23:7222-7229.
70. Altshuler D, Hirschhorn JN, Klannemark M, et al. The common PPARγ Pro12Ala polymorphism is associated with decreased risk of type 2 diabetes. *Nat Genet.* 2000;26:76-80.
71. Love-Gregory LD, Wasson J, Ma J, et al. A common polymorphism in the upstream promoter region of the hepatocyte nuclear factor-4α gene on chromosome 20q is associated with type 2 diabetes and appears to contribute to the evidence for linkage in an Ashkenazi Jewish population. *Diabetes.* 2004;53:1134-1140.
72. Silander K, Mohlke KL, Scott LJ, et al. Genetic variation near the hepatocyte nuclear factor-4α gene predicts susceptibility to type 2 diabetes. *Diabetes.* 2004;53:1141-1149.
73. Weedon MN, Owen KR, Shields B, et al. Common variants of the hepatocyte nuclear factor-4α P2 promoter are associated with type 2 diabetes in the U.K. population. *Diabetes.* 2004;53:3002-3006.
74. Grant SF, Thorleifsson G, Reynisdottir I, et al. Variant of transcription factor 7-like 2 (TCF7L2) gene confers risk of type 2 diabetes. *Nat Genet.* 2006;38:320-323.
75. Florez JC, Jablonski KA, Bayley N, et al. TCF7L2 polymorphisms and progression to diabetes in the Diabetes Prevention Program. *N Engl J Med.* 2006;355:241-250.
76. Dupuis J, Langenberg C, Prokopenko I, et al. New genetic loci implicated in fasting glucose homeostasis and their impact on type 2 diabetes risk. *Nat Genet.* 2010;42:105-116.
77. Rung J, Cauchi S, Albrechtsen A, et al. Genetic variant near IRS1 is associated with type 2 diabetes, insulin resistance and hyperinsulinemia. *Nat Genet.* 2009;41:1110-1115.
78. Scott RA, Lagou V, Welch RP, et al. Large-scale association analyses identify new loci influencing glycemic traits and provide insight into the underlying biological pathways. *Nat Genet.* 2012;44:991-1005.
79. Manning AK, Hivert MF, Scott RA, et al. A genome-wide approach accounting for body mass index identifies genetic variants influencing fasting glycemic traits and insulin resistance. *Nat Genet.* 2012;44:659-669.
80. Parker SC, Stitzel ML, Taylor DL, et al. Chromatin stretch enhancer states drive cell-specific gene regulation and harbor human disease risk variants. *Proc Natl Acad Sci U S A.* 2013;110(44):17921-17926.
81. White MF, Kahn CR. The insulin signaling system. *J Biol Chem.* 1994;269:1-4.
82. Ward CW, Gough KH, Rashke M, et al. Systematic mapping of potential binding sites for Shc and Grb2 SH2 domains on insulin receptor substrate-1 and the receptors for insulin, epidermal growth factor, platelet-derived growth factor, and fibroblast growth factor. *J Biol Chem.* 1996;271:5603-5609.
83. Pessin JE, Saltiel AR. Signaling pathways in insulin action: molecular targets of insulin resistance. *J Clin Invest.* 2000;106:165-169.
84. McClain DA, Maegawa H, Thies RS, et al. Dissection of the growth versus metabolic effects of insulin and insulin-like growth factor-I in transfected cells expressing kinase-defective human insulin receptors. *J Biol Chem.* 1990;265:1678-1682.
85. McClain DA. Mechanism and role of insulin receptor endocytosis. *Am J Med Sci.* 1992;304:192-201.
86. Formisano P, Beguinot F. The role of protein kinase C isoforms in insulin action. *J Endocrinol Invest.* 2001;24:460-467.
87. Itani SI, Zhou Q, Pories WJ, et al. Involvement of protein kinase C in human skeletal muscle insulin resistance and obesity. *Diabetes.* 2000;49:1353-1358.
88. Peraldi P, Xu M, Spiegelman BM. Thiazolidinediones block tumor necrosis factor-α-induced inhibition of insulin signaling. *J Clin Invest.* 1997;100:1863-1869.
89. Goldstein BJ, Ahmad F, Ding W, et al. Regulation of the insulin signaling pathway by cellular protein-tyrosine phosphatases. *Mol Cell Biochem.* 1998;182:91-99.
90. Drake PG, Bevan AP, Burgess JW, et al. A role for tyrosine phosphorylation in both activation and inhibition of the insulin receptor tyrosine kinase in vivo. *Endocrinology.* 1996;137:4960-4968.

91. Elchebly M, Payette P, Michaliszyn E, et al. Increased insulin sensitivity and obesity resistance in mice lacking the protein tyrosine phosphatase-1B gene. *Science.* 1999;283:1544-1548.

92. Krook A, O'Rahilly S. Mutant insulin receptors in syndromes of insulin resistance. *Baillieres Clin Endocrinol Metab.* 1996;10:97-122.

93. Taylor SI, Arioglu E. Syndromes associated with insulin resistance and acanthosis nigricans. *J Basic Clin Physiol Pharmacol.* 1998;9:419-439.

94. White MF. The IRS-signaling system: a network of docking proteins that mediate insulin and cytokine action. *Recent Prog Horm Res.* 1998;53:119-138.

95. Previs SF, Withers DJ, Ren JM, et al. Contrasting effects of IRS-1 versus IRS-2 gene disruption on carbohydrate and lipid metabolism in vivo. *J Biol Chem.* 2000;275:38990-38994.

96. White MF. IRS proteins and the common path to diabetes. *Am J Physiol Endocrinol Metab.* 2002;283:E413-E422.

97. Czech MP, Corvera S. Signaling mechanisms that regulate glucose transport. *J Biol Chem.* 1999;274:1865-1868.

98. Kido Y, Nakae J, Accili D. Clinical review 125: the insulin receptor and its cellular targets. *J Clin Endocrinol Metab.* 2001;86:972-979.

99. Luiken JJ, Glatz JF, Bonen A. Fatty acid transport proteins facilitate fatty acid uptake in skeletal muscle. *Can J Appl Physiol.* 2000;25:333-352.

100. Kohn AD, Barthel A, Kovacina KS, et al. Construction and characterization of a conditionally active version of the serine/threonine kinase Akt. *J Biol Chem.* 1998;273:11937-11943.

101. Sarbassov DD, Guertin DA, Ali SM, et al. Phosphorylation and regulation of Akt/PKB by the rictor-mTOR complex. *Science.* 2005;307:1098-1101.

102. Cho H, Mu J, Kim JK, et al. Insulin resistance and a diabetes mellitus-like syndrome in mice lacking the protein kinase Akt2 (PKB beta). *Science.* 2001;292:1728-1731.

103. Zierath JR, Krook A, Wallberg-Henriksson H. Insulin action in skeletal muscle from patients with NIDDM. *Mol Cell Biochem.* 1998;182:153-160.

104. Krook A, Roth RA, Jiang XJ, et al. Insulin-stimulated Akt kinase activity is reduced in skeletal muscle from NIDDM subjects. *Diabetes.* 1998;47:1281-1286.

105. Kim YB, Nikoulina SE, Ciaraldi TP, et al. Normal insulin-dependent activation of Akt/protein kinase B, with diminished activation of phosphoinositide 3-kinase, in muscle in type 2 diabetes. *J Clin Invest.* 1999;104:733-741.

106. Zorzano A, Sevilla L, Tomas E, et al. Trafficking pathway of GLUT4 glucose transporters in muscle. *Int J Mol Med.* 1998;2:263-271.

107. Sakamoto K, Holman GD. Emerging role for AS160/TBC1D4 and TBC1D1 in the regulation of GLUT4 traffic. *Am J Physiol Endocrinol Metab.* 2008;295:E29-E37.

108. Stockli J, Meoli CC, Hoffman NJ, et al. The RabGAP TBC1D1 plays a central role in exercise-regulated glucose metabolism in skeletal muscle. *Diabetes.* 2015;64(6):1914-1922.

109. Davidson MB. Role of glucose transport and GLUT4 transporter protein in type 2 diabetes mellitus. *J Clin Endocrinol Metab.* 1993;77:25-26.

110. Garvey WT, Maianu L, Zhu JH, et al. Multiple defects in the adipocyte glucose transport system cause cellular insulin resistance in gestational diabetes: heterogeneity in the number and a novel abnormality in subcellular localization of GLUT4 glucose transporters. *Diabetes.* 1993;42:1773-1785.

111. Kennedy JW, Hirshman MF, Gervino EV, et al. Acute exercise induces GLUT4 translocation in skeletal muscle of normal human subjects and subjects with type 2 diabetes. *Diabetes.* 1999;48:1192-1197.

112. Nonogaki K. New insights into sympathetic regulation of glucose and fat metabolism. *Diabetologia.* 2000;43:533-549.

113. Moore MC, Connolly CC, Cherrington AD. Autoregulation of hepatic glucose production. *Eur J Endocrinol.* 1998;138:240-248.

114. Bavenholm PN, Pigon J, Ostenson CG, et al. Insulin sensitivity of suppression of endogenous glucose production is the single most important determinant of glucose tolerance. *Diabetes.* 2001;50:1449-1454.

115. Mitrakou A, Kelley D, Mokan M, et al. Role of reduced suppression of glucose production and diminished early insulin release in impaired glucose tolerance. *N Engl J Med.* 1992;326:22-29.

116. McCall RH, Wiesenthal SR, Shi ZQ, et al. Insulin acutely suppresses glucose production by both peripheral and hepatic effects in normal dogs. *Am J Physiol.* 1998;274:E346-E356.

117. Lewis GF, Vranic M, Giacca A. Glucagon enhances the direct suppressive effect of insulin on hepatic glucose production in humans. *Am J Physiol.* 1997;272:E371-E378.

118. Herzig S, Long F, Jhala US, et al. CREB regulates hepatic gluconeogenesis through the coactivator PGC-1. *Nature.* 2001;413:179-183.

119. Yoon JC, Puigserver P, Chen G, et al. Control of hepatic gluconeogenesis through the transcriptional coactivator PGC-1. *Nature.* 2001;413:131-138.

120. Koo SH, Flechner L, Qi L, et al. The CREB coactivator TORC2 is a key regulator of fasting glucose metabolism. *Nature.* 2005;437:1109-1111.

121. Cherrington AD, Edgerton D, Sindelar DK. The direct and indirect effects of insulin on hepatic glucose production in vivo. *Diabetologia.* 1998;41:987-996.

122. Chiasson JL, Liljenquist JE, Finger FE, et al. Differential sensitivity of glycogenolysis and gluconeogenesis to insulin infusions in dogs. *Diabetes.* 1976;25:283-291.

123. Rossetti L, Giaccari A, Barzilai N, et al. Mechanism by which hyperglycemia inhibits hepatic glucose production in conscious rats: implications for the pathophysiology of fasting hyperglycemia in diabetes. *J Clin Invest.* 1993;92:1126-1134.

124. Gasa R, Jansen PB, Berman HK, et al. Distinctive regulatory and metabolic properties of glycogen-targeting subunits of protein phosphatase-1 (PTG, GL, GM/RGl) expressed in hepatocytes. *J Biol Chem.* 2000;275:26396-26403.

125. Newgard CB, Brady MJ, O'Doherty RM, et al. Organizing glucose disposal: emerging roles of the glycogen targeting subunits of protein phosphatase-1. *Diabetes.* 2000;49:1967-1977.

126. Yeagley D, Guo S, Unterman T, et al. Gene- and activation-specific mechanisms for insulin inhibition of basal and glucocorticoid-induced insulin-like growth factor binding protein-1 and phosphoenolpyruvate carboxykinase transcription: roles of forkhead and insulin response sequences. *J Biol Chem.* 2001;276:33705-33710.

127. Jackson JG, Kreisberg JI, Koterba AP, et al. Phosphorylation and nuclear exclusion of the forkhead transcription factor FKHR after epidermal growth factor treatment in human breast cancer cells. *Oncogene.* 2000;19:4574-4581.

128. Hall RK, Yamasaki T, Kucera T, et al. Regulation of phosphoenolpyruvate carboxykinase and insulin-like growth factor-binding protein-1 gene expression by insulin: the role of winged helix/forkhead proteins. *J Biol Chem.* 2000;275:30169-30175.

129. Wolfrum C, Asilmaz E, Luca E, et al. Foxa2 regulates lipid metabolism and ketogenesis in the liver during fasting and in diabetes. *Nature.* 2004;432:1027-1032.

130. Asplin CM, Paquette TL, Palmer JP. In vivo inhibition of glucagon secretion by paracrine beta cell activity in man. *J Clin Invest.* 1981;68:314-318.

131. Shi ZQ, Wasserman D, Vranic M. Metabolic implications of exercise and physical fitness in physiology and diabetes. In: Porte D, Sherwin R, eds. *Ellenberg and Rifkin Diabetes Mellitus.* Norwalk, CT: Appleton & Lange; 1997:653-687.

132. Chen X, Iqbal N, Boden G. The effects of free fatty acids on gluconeogenesis and glycogenolysis in normal subjects. *J Clin Invest.* 1999;103:365-372.

133. Rebrin K, Steil GM, Mittelman SD, et al. Causal linkage between insulin suppression of lipolysis and suppression of liver glucose output in dogs. *J Clin Invest.* 1996;98:741-749.

134. Boden G. Fatty acids and insulin resistance. *Diabetes Care.* 1996;19:394-395.

135. Lewis GF, Vranic M, Giacca A. Role of free fatty acids and glucagon in the peripheral effect of insulin on glucose production in humans. *Am J Physiol.* 1998;275:E177-E186.

136. Lam TK, Pocai A, Gutierrez-Juarez R, et al. Hypothalamic sensing of circulating fatty acids is required for glucose homeostasis. *Nat Med.* 2005;11:320-327.

137. Minokoshi Y, Alquier T, Furukawa N, et al. AMP-kinase regulates food intake by responding to hormonal and nutrient signals in the hypothalamus. *Nature.* 2004;428:569-574.

138. Paolisso G, Tagliamonte MR, Rizzo MR, et al. Advancing age and insulin resistance: new facts about an ancient history. *Eur J Clin Invest.* 1999;29:758-769.

139. Himsworth H, Kerr RB. Insulin-sensitive and insulin-insensitive types of diabetes mellitus. *Clin Sci.* 1939;4:119-152.

140. Warram JH, Martin BC, Krowelski AS, et al. Slow glucose removal rate and hyperinsulinemia precede the development of type II diabetes in the offspring of diabetic parents. *Ann Intern Med.* 1990;113:909-915.

141. Lillioija S, Mott DM, Howard BV, et al. Impaired glucose tolerance as a disorder of insulin action: longitudinal and cross-sectional studies in Pima Indians. *N Engl J Med.* 1988;318:1217-1225.

142. Haffner SM, Stern MP, Dunn J, et al. Diminished insulin sensitivity and increased insulin response in nonobese, nondiabetic Mexican Americans. *Metabolism.* 1990;39:842-847.

143. Reaven GM, Bernstein R, Davis B, et al. Nonketotic diabetes mellitus: insulin deficiency or insulin resistance? *Am J Med.* 1976;60:80-88.

144. DeFronzo RA. The triumvirate: beta-cell, muscle, liver—a collusion responsible for NIDDM. Lilly Lecture 1987. *Diabetes.* 1988;37:667-687.

145. Groop L. Genetics of the metabolic syndrome. *Br J Nutr.* 2000;83(Suppl 1):S39-S48.

146. Lehtovirta M, Kaprio J, Forsblom C, et al. Insulin sensitivity and insulin secretion in monozygotic and dizygotic twins. *Diabetologia.* 2000;43:285-293.

147. Mayer EJ, Newman B, Austin MA, et al. Genetic and environmental influences on insulin levels and the insulin resistance syndrome: an analysis of women twins. *Am J Epidemiol.* 1996;143:323-332.

148. Hong Y, Pedersen NL, Brismar K, et al. Genetic and environmental architecture of the features of the insulin-resistance syndrome. *Am J Hum Genet.* 1997;60:143-152.

149. Fujioka S, Matsuzawa Y, Tokunaga K, et al. Contribution of intra-abdominal fat accumulation to the impairment of glucose and lipid metabolism in human obesity. *Metabolism.* 1987;36:54-59.

150. Brambilla P, Manzoni P, Sironi S, et al. Peripheral and abdominal adiposity in childhood obesity. *Int J Obes Relat Metab Disord.* 1994;18:795-800.

151. Berman DM, Rodriguez LM, Nicklas BJ, et al. Racial disparities in metabolism, central obesity, and sex hormone-binding globulin in postmenopausal women. *J Clin Endocrinol Metab.* 2001;86:97-103.

152. Hu FB, Manson JE, Stampfer MJ, et al. Diet, lifestyle, and the risk of type 2 diabetes mellitus in women. *N Engl J Med.* 2001;345:790-797.

153. Tuomilehto J, Lindstrom J, Eriksson G, et al. Prevention of type 2 diabetes mellitus by changes in lifestyle among subjects with impaired glucose tolerance. *N Engl J Med.* 2001;344:1343-1350.

154. Must A, Spadano J, Coakley EH, et al. The disease burden associated with overweight and obesity. *JAMA.* 1999;282:1523-1529.

155. Ornellas F, Mello VS, Mandarim-de-Lacerda CA, Aguila MB. Sexual dimorphism in fat distribution and metabolic profile in mice offspring from diet-induced obese mothers. *Life Sci.* 2013;93(12–14):454-463.

156. Klöting N, Fasshauer M, Dietrich A, et al. Insulin-sensitive obesity. *Am J Physiol Endocrinol Metab.* 2010;299(3):E506-E515.

157. Vidal-Puig A. Adipose tissue expandability, lipotoxicity and the metabolic syndrome. *Endocrinol Nutr.* 2013;60(Suppl 1):39-43.

158. Cefalu WT, Werbel S, Bell-Farrow AD, et al. Insulin resistance and fat patterning with aging: relationship to metabolic risk factors for cardiovascular disease. *Metabolism.* 1998;47:401-408.

159. Larsson B, Svardsudd K, Welin L, et al. Abdominal adipose tissue distribution, obesity, and risk of cardiovascular disease and death: 13 year follow up of participants in the study of men born in 1913. *Br Med J (Clin Res Ed).* 1984;288:1401-1404.

160. Despres JP, Tremblay A, Perusse L, et al. Abdominal adipose tissue and serum HDL-cholesterol: association independent from obesity and serum triglyceride concentration. *Int J Obes.* 1988;12:1-13.

161. Landin K, Krotkiewski M, Smith U. Importance of obesity for the metabolic abnormalities associated with an abdominal fat distribution. *Metabolism.* 1989;38:572-576.

162. Heitmann BL. The variation in blood lipid levels described by various measures of overall and abdominal obesity in Danish men and women aged 35-65 years. *Eur J Clin Nutr.* 1992;46:597-605.

163. Reeder BA, Senthilselvan A, Despres JP, et al. The association of cardiovascular disease risk factors with abdominal obesity in Canada. Canadian Heart Health Surveys Research Group. *Can Med Assoc J.* 1997;157(Suppl 1):S39-S45.

164. Lamarche B. Abdominal obesity and its metabolic complications: implications for the risk of ischaemic heart disease. *Coron Artery Dis.* 1998;9(8):473-481.

165. McLaughlin T, Lamendola C, Liu A, Abbasi F. Preferential fat deposition in subcutaneous versus visceral depots is associated with insulin sensitivity. *J Clin Endocrinol Metab.* 2011;96(11):E1756-E1760.

166. Evans DJ, Hoffmann RG, Kalkhoff RK, et al. Relationship of body fat topography to insulin sensitivity and metabolic profiles in premenopausal women. *Metabolism.* 1984;33:68-75.

167. Peiris AN, Mueller RA, Smith GA, et al. Splanchnic insulin metabolism in obesity: influence of body fat distribution. *J Clin Invest.* 1986;78:1648-1657.

168. Arner P, Hellstrom L, Wahrenberg H, et al. Beta-adrenoceptor expression in human fat cells from different regions. *J Clin Invest.* 1990;86:1595-1600.

169. Nicklas BJ, Rogus EM, Colman EG, et al. Visceral adiposity, increased adipocyte lipolysis, and metabolic dysfunction in obese postmenopausal women. *Am J Physiol.* 1996;270:E72-E78.

170. Mittelman SD, Van Citters GW, Kim SP, et al. Longitudinal compensation for fat-induced insulin resistance includes reduced insulin clearance and enhanced beta-cell response. *Diabetes.* 2000;49:2116-2125.

171. Lidell ME, Betz MJ, Enerback S. Brown adipose tissue and its therapeutic potential. *J Intern Med.* 2014;276(4):364-377.

172. Chondronikola M, Volpi E, Børsheim E, et al. Brown adipose tissue improves whole-body glucose homeostasis and insulin sensitivity in humans. *Diabetes.* 2014;63(12):4089-4099.

173. Dempersmier J, Sul HS. Shades of brown: a model for thermogenic fat. *Front Endocrinol (Lausanne).* 2015;6:71.

174. Olefsky JM, Revers RR, Prince M, et al. Insulin resistance in non-insulin dependent (type II) and insulin dependent (type I) diabetes mellitus. *Adv Exp Med Biol.* 1985;189:176-205.

175. Del Prato S, Leonetti F, Simonson DC, et al. Effect of sustained physiologic hyperinsulinaemia and hyperglycaemia on insulin secretion and insulin sensitivity in man. *Diabetologia.* 1994;37:1025-1035.

176. Ratzmann KP, Ruhnke R, Kohnert KD. Effect of pharmacological suppression of insulin secretion on tissue sensitivity to insulin in subjects with moderate obesity. *Int J Obes.* 1983;7:453-458.

177. Alemzadeh R, Langley G, Upchurch L, et al. Beneficial effect of diazoxide in obese hyperinsulinemic adults. *J Clin Endocrinol Metab.* 1998;83:1911-1915.

178. Chan JC, Malik V, Jia W, et al. Diabetes in Asia: epidemiology, risk factors, and pathophysiology. *JAMA.* 2009;301:2129-2140.

179. Iyer A, Fairlie DP, Prins JB, et al. Inflammatory lipid mediators in adipocyte function and obesity. *Nat Rev Endocrinol.* 2010;6:71-82.

180. Karastergiou K, Mohamed-Ali V. The autocrine and paracrine roles of adipokines. *Mol Cell Endocrinol.* 2010;318:69-78.

181. Howell JJ, et al. A growing role for mTOR in promoting anabolic metabolism. *Biochem Soc Trans.* 2013;41(4):906-912.

182. Tzatsos A, Kandror KV. Nutrients suppress phosphatidylinositol 3-kinase/Akt signaling via raptor-dependent mTOR-mediated insulin receptor substrate 1 phosphorylation. *Mol Cell Biol.* 2006;26:63-76.

183. Um SH, Frigerio F, Watanabe M, et al. Absence of S6K1 protects against age- and diet-induced obesity while enhancing insulin sensitivity. *Nature.* 2004;431:200-205.

184. Ron D, Walter P. Signal integration in the endoplasmic reticulum unfolded protein response. *Nat Rev Mol Cell Biol.* 2007;8:519-529.

185. Hotamisligil GS. Endoplasmic reticulum stress and the inflammatory basis of metabolic disease. *Cell.* 2010;140:900-917.

186. Schroder K, Tschopp J. The inflammasomes. *Cell.* 2010;140:821-832.

187. Shi H, Kokoeva MV, Inouye K, et al. TLR4 links innate immunity and fatty acid-induced insulin resistance. *J Clin Invest.* 2006;116:3015-3025.

188. Esser N, Paquot N, Scheen AJ. Anti-inflammatory agents to treat or prevent type 2 diabetes, metabolic syndrome and cardiovascular disease. *Expert Opin Investig Drugs.* 2015;24(3):283-307.

189. Scheer FA, Hilton MF, Mantzoros CS, Shea SA. Adverse metabolic and cardiovascular consequences of circadian misalignment. *Proc Natl Acad Sci U S A.* 2009;106(11):4453-4458.

190. Gustafson CL, Partch CL. Emerging models for the molecular basis of mammalian circadian timing. *Biochemistry.* 2015;54(2):134-149.

191. Buhr ED, Takahashi JS. Molecular components of the mammalian circadian clock. *Handb Exp Pharmacol.* 2013;217:3-27.

192. Knutson KL, Van Cauter E. Associations between sleep loss and increased risk of obesity and diabetes. *Ann N Y Acad Sci.* 2008;1129:287-304.

193. Reutrakul S, Van Cauter E. Interactions between sleep, circadian function, and glucose metabolism: implications for risk and severity of diabetes. *Ann N Y Acad Sci.* 2014;1311:151-173.

194. Maury E, Ramsey KM, Bass J. Circadian rhythms and metabolic syndrome: from experimental genetics to human disease. *Circ Res.* 2010;106:447-462.

195. Punjabi NM. Workshop Participants. Do sleep disorders and associated treatments impact glucose metabolism? *Drugs.* 2009;69(Suppl 2):13-27.

196. Marette A, Liu Y, Sweeney G. Skeletal muscle glucose metabolism and inflammation in the development of the metabolic syndrome. *Rev Endocr Metab Disord.* 2014;15(4):299-305.

197. Del Prato S, Bonadonna RC, Bonora E, et al. Characterization of cellular defects of insulin action in type 2 (non-insulin-dependent) diabetes mellitus. *J Clin Invest.* 1993;91:484-494.

198. Freymond D, Bogardus C, Okubo M, et al. Impaired insulin-stimulated muscle glycogen synthase activation in vivo in man is related to low fasting glycogen synthase phosphatase activity. *J Clin Invest.* 1988;82:1503-1509.

199. Charles MA, Eschwege E, Thibult N, et al. The role of non-esterified fatty acids in the deterioration of glucose tolerance in Caucasian subjects: results of the Paris Prospective Study. *Diabetologia.* 1997;40:1101-1106.

200. Paolisso G, Tataranni PA, Foley JE, et al. A high concentration of fasting plasma non-esterified fatty acids is a risk factor for the development of NIDDM. *Diabetologia.* 1995;38:1213-1217.

201. Garland PB, Newsholme EA, Randle PJ. Regulation of glucose uptake by muscle: 9. Effects of fatty acids and ketone bodies, and of alloxan-diabetes and starvation, on pyruvate metabolism and on lactate-pyruvate and L-glycerol 3-phosphate-dihydroxyacetone phosphate concentration ratios in rat heart and rat diaphragm muscles. *Biochem J.* 1964;93(3):665-678.

202. Roden M, Price TB, Perseghin G, et al. Mechanism of free fatty acid-induced insulin resistance in humans. *J Clin Invest.* 1996;97:2859-2865.

203. Jucker BM, Rennings AJ, Cline GW, et al. ^{13}C and ^{31}P NMR studies on the effects of increased plasma free fatty acids on intramuscular glucose metabolism in the awake rat. *J Biol Chem.* 1997;272:10464-10473.

204. Adams SH. Uncoupling protein homologs: emerging views of physiological function. *J Nutr.* 2000;130:711-714.

205. Rothman DL, Magnusson I, Cline G, et al. Decreased muscle glucose transport/phosphorylation is an early defect in the pathogenesis of non-insulin-dependent diabetes mellitus. *Proc Natl Acad Sci U S A.* 1995;92:983-987.

206. Price TB, Perseghin G, Duleba A, et al. NMR studies of muscle glycogen synthesis in insulin-resistant offspring of parents with non-insulin-dependent diabetes mellitus immediately after glycogen-depleting exercise. *Proc Natl Acad Sci U S A.* 1996;93:5329-5334.

207. Itani SI, Pories WJ, Macdonald KG, et al. Increased protein kinase C theta in skeletal muscle of diabetic patients. *Metabolism.* 2001;50:553-557.

208. Griffin ME, Marcucci MJ, Cline GW, et al. Free fatty acid-induced insulin resistance is associated with activation of protein kinase C theta and alterations in the insulin signaling cascade. *Diabetes.* 1999;48:1270-1274.

209. Hundal RS, Petersen KF, Mayerson AB, et al. Mechanism by which high-dose aspirin improves glucose metabolism in type 2 diabetes. *J Clin Invest.* 2002;109:1321-1326.

210. Pan DA, Lillioja S, Kriketos AD, et al. Skeletal muscle triglyceride levels are inversely related to insulin action. *Diabetes.* 1997;46:983-988.

211. Goodpaster BH, Thaete FL, Simoneau JA, et al. Subcutaneous abdominal fat and thigh muscle composition predict insulin sensitivity independently of visceral fat. *Diabetes*. 1997;46:1579-1585.

212. Perseghin G, Scifo P, De Cobelli F, et al. Intramyocellular triglyceride content is a determinant of in vivo insulin resistance in humans: a ^{1}H-^{13}C nuclear magnetic resonance spectroscopy assessment in offspring of type 2 diabetic parents. *Diabetes*. 1999;48:1600-1606.

213. Boesch C, Slotboom J, Hoppeler H, et al. In vivo determination of intra-myocellular lipids in human muscle by means of localized ^{1}H-MR-spectroscopy. *Magn Reson Med*. 1997;37(4):484-493.

214. Carlson LA, Ekelund LG, Froberg SO. Concentration of triglycerides, phospholipids and glycogen in skeletal muscle and of free fatty acids and beta-hydroxybutyric acid in blood in man in response to exercise. *Eur J Clin Invest*. 1971;1:248-254.

215. Laws A, Reaven GM. Effect of physical activity on age-related glucose intolerance. *Clin Geriatr Med*. 1990;6:849-863.

216. Gollnick PD, Saltin B. Significance of skeletal muscle oxidative enzyme enhancement with endurance training. *Clin Physiol*. 1982;2:1-12.

217. Turcotte LP, Richter EA, Kiens B. Increased plasma FFA uptake and oxidation during prolonged exercise in trained vs. untrained humans. *Am J Physiol*. 1992;262:E791-E799.

218. Romijn JA, Klein S, Coyle EF, et al. Strenuous endurance training increases lipolysis and triglyceride-fatty acid cycling at rest. *J Appl Physiol*. 1993;75:108-113.

219. Phillips SM, Green HJ, Tamopolsky MA, et al. Effects of training duration on substrate turnover and oxidation during exercise. *J Appl Physiol*. 1996;81:2182-2191.

220. Schenk S, Horowitz JF. Acute exercise increases triglyceride synthesis in skeletal muscle and prevents fatty acid-induced insulin resistance. *J Clin Invest*. 2007;117:1690-1698.

221. Stremmel W, Strohmeyer G, Borchard F, et al. Isolation and partial characterization of a fatty acid binding protein in rat liver plasma membranes. *Proc Natl Acad Sci U S A*. 1985;82:4-8.

222. Abumrad NA, el Maghrabi MR, Amri EZ, et al. Cloning of a rat adipocyte membrane protein implicated in binding or transport of long-chain fatty acids that is induced during preadipocyte differentiation: homology with human CD36. *J Biol Chem*. 1993;268:17665-17668.

223. Stahl A, Gimeno RE, Tartaglia LA, et al. Fatty acid transport proteins: a current view of a growing family. *Trends Endocrinol Metab*. 2001;12:266-273.

224. Binnert C, Koistinen HA, Martin G, et al. Fatty acid transport protein-1 mRNA expression in skeletal muscle and in adipose tissue in humans. *Am J Physiol*. 2000;279:E1072-E1079.

225. Veerkamp JH. Fatty acid transport and fatty acid-binding proteins. *Proc Nutr Soc*. 1995;54:23-37.

226. Schaap FG, van der Vusse GJ, Glatz JF. Fatty acid-binding proteins in the heart. *Mol Cell Biochem*. 1998;180:43-51.

227. Van Nieuwenhoven FA, Verstijnen CP, Abumrad NA, et al. Putative membrane fatty acid translocase and cytoplasmic fatty acid-binding protein are co-expressed in rat heart and skeletal muscles. *Biochem Biophys Res Commun*. 1995;207:747-752.

228. Linssen MC, Vork MM, de Jong YF, et al. Fatty acid oxidation capacity and fatty acid-binding protein content of different cell types isolated from rat heart. *Mol Cell Biochem*. 1990;98:19-25.

229. Binas B, Danneberg H, McWhir J, et al. Requirement for the heart-type fatty acid binding protein in cardiac fatty acid utilization. *FASEB J*. 1999;13:805-812.

230. Hotamisligil GS, Johnson RS, Distel RJ, et al. Uncoupling of obesity from insulin resistance through a targeted mutation in aP2, the adipocyte fatty acid binding protein. *Science*. 1996;274:1377-1379.

231. Simoneau JA, Veerkamp JH, Turcotte LP, et al. Markers of capacity to utilize fatty acids in human skeletal muscle: relation to insulin resistance and obesity and effects of weight loss. *FASEB J*. 1999;13:2051-2060.

232. McGarry JD. Glucose-fatty acid interactions in health and disease. *Am J Clin Nutr*. 1998;67(3 Suppl):500S-504S.

233. McGarry JD. Malonyl-CoA and satiety? Food for thought. *Trends Endocrinol Metab*. 2000;11:399-400.

234. Zammit VA, Price NT, Fraser F, et al. Structure-function relationships of the liver and muscle isoforms of carnitine palmitoyltransferase I. *Biochem Soc Trans*. 2001;29:287-292.

235. Minnich A, Tian N, Byan L, et al. A potent PPARα agonist stimulates mitochondrial fatty acid beta-oxidation in liver and skeletal muscle. *Am J Physiol*. 2001;280:E270-E279.

236. Power GW, Newsholme EA. Dietary fatty acids influence the activity and metabolic control of mitochondrial carnitine palmitoyltransferase I in rat heart and skeletal muscle. *J Nutr*. 1997;127:2142-2150.

237. Hildebrandt AL, Neufer PD. Exercise attenuates the fasting-induced transcriptional activation of metabolic genes in skeletal muscle. *Am J Physiol*. 2000;278:E1078-E1086.

238. Kim JY, Hickner RC, Cartright RL, et al. Lipid oxidation is reduced in obese human skeletal muscle. *Am J Physiol*. 2000;279:E1039-E1044.

239. Eaton S, Bartlett K, Pourfarzam M. Mammalian mitochondrial beta-oxidation. *Biochem J*. 1996;320:345-357.

240. Nada MA, Rhead WJ, Sprecher H, et al. Evidence for intermediate channeling in mitochondrial beta-oxidation. *J Biol Chem*. 1995;270:530-535.

241. Horowitz JF, Leone TC, Feng W, et al. Effect of endurance training on lipid metabolism in women: a potential role for PPARα in the metabolic response to training. *Am J Physiol*. 2000;279:E348-E355.

242. Porter RK. Mitochondrial proton leak: a role for uncoupling proteins 2 and 3? *Biochim Biophys Acta*. 2001;1504:120-127.

243. Bouillaud F, Couplan E, Pecqueur C, et al. Homologues of the uncoupling protein from brown adipose tissue (UCP1): UCP2, UCP3, BMCP1 and UCP4. *Biochim Biophys Acta*. 2001;1504:107-119.

244. Boss O, Muzzin P, Giacobino JP. The uncoupling proteins, a review. *Eur J Endocrinol*. 1998;139:1-9.

245. Schrauwen P, Hoppeler H, Billeter R, et al. Fiber type dependent upregulation of human skeletal muscle UCP2 and UCP3 mRNA expression by high-fat diet. *Int J Obes Relat Metab Disord*. 2001;25:449-456.

246. Tonkonogi M, Krook A, Walsh B, et al. Endurance training increases stimulation of uncoupling of skeletal muscle mitochondria in humans by non-esterified fatty acids: an uncoupling-protein-mediated effect? *Biochem J*. 2000;351:805-810.

247. Bao S, Kennedy A, Wojciechowski B, et al. Expression of mRNAs encoding uncoupling proteins in human skeletal muscle: effects of obesity and diabetes. *Diabetes*. 1998;47:1935-1940.

248. Schrauwen P, Xia J, Wakler K, et al. A novel polymorphism in the proximal UCP3 promoter region: effect on skeletal muscle UCP3 mRNA expression and obesity in male non-diabetic Pima Indians. *Int J Obes Relat Metab Disord*. 1999;23:1242-1245.

249. Schrauwen P, Hesselink MK. Oxidative capacity, lipotoxicity, and mitochondrial damage in type 2 diabetes. *Diabetes*. 2004;53:1412-1417.

250. Boirie Y. Insulin regulation of mitochondrial proteins and oxidative phosphorylation in human muscle. *Trends Endocrinol Metab*. 2003;14:393-394.

251. Pedersen BK, Steensberg A, Fischer C, et al. The metabolic role of IL-6 produced during exercise: is IL-6 an exercise factor? *Proc Nutr Soc*. 2004;63:263-267.

252. Puigserver P, Spiegelman BM. Peroxisome proliferator-activated receptor-γ coactivator 1α (PGC-1α): transcriptional coactivator and metabolic regulator. *Endocr Rev*. 2003;24:78-90.

253. Puigserver P, Wu Z, Park CW, et al. A cold-inducible coactivator of nuclear receptors linked to adaptive thermogenesis. *Cell*. 1998;92:829-839.

254. Mootha VK, Handschin C, Arow D, et al. Erralpha and Gabpa/b specify PGC-1α-dependent oxidative phosphorylation gene expression that is altered in diabetic muscle. *Proc Natl Acad Sci U S A*. 2004;101:6570-6575.

255. Mootha VK, Lindgren CM, Eriksson KF, et al. PGC-1α-responsive genes involved in oxidative phosphorylation are coordinately downregulated in human diabetes. *Nat Genet*. 2003;34:267-273.

256. Patti ME, Butte AJ, Crunkhorn S, et al. Coordinated reduction of genes of oxidative metabolism in humans with insulin resistance and diabetes: potential role of PGC1 and NRF1. *Proc Natl Acad Sci U S A*. 2003;100:8466-8471.

257. Kelley DE, He J, Menshikova EV, et al. Dysfunction of mitochondria in human skeletal muscle in type 2 diabetes. *Diabetes*. 2002;51:2944-2950.

258. Wisløff U, Najjar SM, Ellingsen O, et al. Cardiovascular risk factors emerge after artificial selection for low aerobic capacity. *Science*. 2005;307:418-420.

259. Korshunov SS, Skulachev VP, Starkov AA. High protonic potential actuates a mechanism of production of reactive oxygen species in mitochondria. *FEBS Lett*. 1997;416(1):15-18.

260. Muoio DM. Intramuscular triacylglycerol and insulin resistance: guilty as charged or wrongly accused? *Biochim Biophys Acta*. 2010;1801:281-288.

261. Schooneman MG, Vaz FM, Houten SM, Soeters MR. Acylcarnitines: reflecting or inflicting insulin resistance? *Diabetes*. 2013;62(1):1-8.

262. Wong KE, Mikus CR, Slentz DH, et al. Muscle-specific overexpression of PGC-1alpha does not augment metabolic improvements in response to exercise and caloric restriction. *Diabetes*. 2015;64(5):1532-1543.

263. Ruderman NB, Saha AK, Vavvas D, et al. Malonyl-CoA, fuel sensing, and insulin resistance. *Am J Physiol*. 1999;276:E1-E18.

264. McGarry JD. Malonyl-CoA and carnitine palmitoyltransferase I: an expanding partnership. *Biochem Soc Trans*. 1995;23:481-485.

265. Swanson ST, Foster DW, McGarry JD, et al. Roles of the N- and C-terminal domains of carnitine palmitoyltransferase I isoforms in malonyl-CoA sensitivity of the enzymes: insights from expression of chimaeric proteins and mutation of conserved histidine residues. *Biochem J*. 1998;335:513-519.

266. Kelley DE, Simoneau JA. Impaired free fatty acid utilization by skeletal muscle in non-insulin-dependent diabetes mellitus. *J Clin Invest*. 1994;94:2349-2356.

267. Kelley DE, Mandarino LJ. Hyperglycemia normalizes insulin-stimulated skeletal muscle glucose oxidation and storage in noninsulin-dependent diabetes mellitus. *J Clin Invest*. 1990;86:1999-2007.

268. Bavenholm PN, Pigon J, Saha AK, et al. Fatty acid oxidation and the regulation of malonyl-CoA in human muscle. *Diabetes.* 2000;49:1078-1083.
269. Jamil H, Madsen NB. Phosphorylation state of acetyl-coenzyme A carboxylase: I. Linear inverse relationship to activity ratios at different citrate concentrations. *J Biol Chem.* 1987;262:630-637.
270. Jamil H, Madsen NB. Phosphorylation state of acetyl-coenzyme A carboxylase: II. Variation with nutritional condition. *J Biol Chem.* 1987;262:638-642.
271. Winder WW, Wilson HA, Hardie DG, et al. Phosphorylation of rat muscle acetyl-CoA carboxylase by AMP-activated protein kinase and protein kinase A. *J Appl Physiol.* 1997;82:219-225.
272. Dean D, Daugaard JR, Young ME, et al. Exercise diminishes the activity of acetyl-CoA carboxylase in human muscle. *Diabetes.* 2000;49:1295-1300.
273. LaBarge S, Migdal C, Schenk S. Is acetylation a metabolic rheostat that regulates skeletal muscle insulin action? *Mol Cell.* 2015;38(4):297-303.
274. Lombard DB, Alt FW, Cheng HL, et al. Mammalian Sir2 homolog SIRT3 regulates global mitochondrial lysine acetylation. *Mol Cell Biol.* 2007;27(24):8807-8814.
275. Overmyer KA, Evans CR, Qi NR, et al. Maximal oxidative capacity during exercise is associated with skeletal muscle fuel selection and dynamic changes in mitochondrial protein acetylation. *Cell Metab.* 2015;21(3):468-478.
276. Gerich JE, Meyer C, Woerle HJ, et al. Renal gluconeogenesis: its importance in human glucose homeostasis. *Diabetes Care.* 2001;24:382-391.
277. Meyer C, Stumvoll M, Nadkami V, et al. Abnormal renal and hepatic glucose metabolism in type 2 diabetes mellitus. *J Clin Invest.* 1998;102:619-624.
278. Mittelman SD, Fu YY, Rebrin K, et al. Indirect effect of insulin to suppress endogenous glucose production is dominant, even with hyperglucagonemia. *J Clin Invest.* 1997;100:3121-3130.
279. Rothman DL, Magnusson I, Katz LD, et al. Quantitation of hepatic glycogenolysis and gluconeogenesis in fasting humans with ^{13}C NMR. *Science.* 1991;254:573-576.
280. Petersen KF, Price T, Cline GW, et al. Contribution of net hepatic glycogenolysis to glucose production during the early postprandial period. *Am J Physiol.* 1996;270:E186-E191.
281. Perriello G, Pampanelli S, Del Sindaco P, et al. Evidence of increased systemic glucose production and gluconeogenesis in an early stage of NIDDM. *Diabetes.* 1997;46:1010-1016.
282. DeFronzo RA, Bonadonna RC, Ferrannini E. Pathogenesis of NIDDM: a balanced overview. *Diabetes Care.* 1992;15:318-368.
283. DeFronzo RA, Simonson D, Ferrannini E. Hepatic and peripheral insulin resistance: a common feature of type 2 (non-insulin-dependent) and type 1 (insulin-dependent) diabetes mellitus. *Diabetologia.* 1982;23:313-319.
284. Bogardus C, Lillioja S, Howard BV, et al. Relationships between insulin secretion, insulin action, and fasting plasma glucose concentration in nondiabetic and noninsulin-dependent diabetic subjects. *J Clin Invest.* 1984;74:1238-1246.
285. Hother-Nielsen O, Beck-Nielsen H. Insulin resistance, but normal basal rates of glucose production in patients with newly diagnosed mild diabetes mellitus. *Acta Endocrinol (Copenh).* 1991;124:637-645.
286. Hother-Nielsen O, Beck-Nielsen H. On the determination of basal glucose production rate in patients with type 2 (non-insulin-dependent) diabetes mellitus using primed-continuous 3-^{3}H-glucose infusion. *Diabetologia.* 1990;33:603-610.
287. Firth R, Bell P, Rizza R. Insulin action in non-insulin-dependent diabetes mellitus: the relationship between hepatic and extrahepatic insulin resistance and obesity. *Metabolism.* 1987;36:1091-1095.
288. Groop LC, Bonadonna RC, Shank M, et al. Role of free fatty acids and insulin in determining free fatty acid and lipid oxidation in man. *J Clin Invest.* 1991;87:83-89.
289. Pigon J, Giacca A, Ostenson CG, et al. Normal hepatic insulin sensitivity in lean, mild noninsulin-dependent diabetic patients. *J Clin Endocrinol Metab.* 1996;81:3702-3708.
290. Stumvoll M, Nurjhan N, Perriello G, et al. Metabolic effects of metformin in non-insulin-dependent diabetes mellitus. *N Engl J Med.* 1995;333:550-554.
291. Lewis GF, Carpentier A, Vranic N, et al. Resistance to insulin's acute direct hepatic effect in suppressing steady-state glucose production in individuals with type 2 diabetes. *Diabetes.* 1999;48:570-576.
292. Staehr P, Hother-Nielsen O, Levin K, et al. Assessment of hepatic insulin action in obese type 2 diabetic patients. *Diabetes.* 2001;50:1363-1370.
293. Magnusson I, Rothman DL, Gerard DP, et al. Contribution of hepatic glycogenolysis to glucose production in humans in response to a physiological increase in plasma glucagon concentration. *Diabetes.* 1995;44:185-189.
294. Magnusson I, Rothman DL, Katz LD, et al. Increased rate of gluconeogenesis in type II diabetes mellitus: a ^{13}C nuclear magnetic resonance study. *J Clin Invest.* 1992;90:1323-1327.
295. Baron AD, Schaeffer L, Shragg P, et al. Role of hyperglucagonemia in maintenance of increased rates of hepatic glucose output in type II diabetics. *Diabetes.* 1987;36:274-283.
296. Rafacho A, Ortsäter H, Nadal A, Quesada I. Glucocorticoid treatment and endocrine pancreas function: implications for glucose homeostasis, insulin resistance and diabetes. *J Endocrinol.* 2014;223(3):R49-R62.
297. Gumbiner B, Mucha JF, Lindstrom JE, et al. Differential effects of acute hypertriglyceridemia on insulin action and insulin receptor autophosphorylation. *Am J Physiol.* 1996;270:E424-E429.
298. Saad MJ, Araki E, Miralpeix M, et al. Regulation of insulin receptor substrate-1 in liver and muscle of animal models of insulin resistance. *J Clin Invest.* 1992;90:1839-1849.
299. Zierath JR, Houseknecht KL, Gnudi L, et al. High-fat feeding impairs insulin-stimulated GLUT4 recruitment via an early insulin-signaling defect. *Diabetes.* 1997;46:215-223.
300. Anai M, Funaki M, Ogihara T, et al. Altered expression levels and impaired steps in the pathway to phosphatidylinositol 3-kinase activation via insulin receptor substrates 1 and 2 in Zucker fatty rats. *Diabetes.* 1998;47:13-23.
301. Krook A, Kawano Y, Song XM, et al. Improved glucose tolerance restores insulin-stimulated Akt kinase activity and glucose transport in skeletal muscle from diabetic Goto-Kakizaki rats. *Diabetes.* 1997;46:2110-2114.
302. Hotamisligil GS, Spiegelman BM. Tumor necrosis factor alpha: a key component of the obesity-diabetes link. *Diabetes.* 1994;43:1271-1278.
303. Miles PD, Romeo OM, Higo K, et al. TNF-α-induced insulin resistance in vivo and its prevention by troglitazone. *Diabetes.* 1997;46:1678-1683.
304. Hotamisligil GS, Peraldi P, Budavari A, et al. IRS-1-mediated inhibition of insulin receptor tyrosine kinase activity in TNF-α- and obesity-induced insulin resistance. *Science.* 1996;271:665-668.
305. Uysal KT, Wiesbrock SM, Marino MW, et al. Protection from obesity-induced insulin resistance in mice lacking TNF-α function. *Nature.* 1997;389:610-614.
306. The Diabetes Control and Complications Trial Research Group. The effect of intensive treatment of diabetes on the development and progression of long-term complications in insulin-dependent diabetes mellitus. *N Engl J Med.* 1993;329(14):977-986.
307. Turner RC. The U.K. Prospective Diabetes Study: a review. *Diabetes Care.* 1998;21(Suppl 3):C35-C38.
308. Sakul H, Pratley R, Cardon L, et al. Familiality of physical and metabolic characteristics that predict the development of non-insulin-dependent diabetes mellitus in Pima Indians. *Am J Hum Genet.* 1997;60:651-656.
309. Yki-Jarvinen H, Sahlin K, Ren JM, et al. Localization of rate-limiting defect for glucose disposal in skeletal muscle of insulin-resistant type I diabetic patients. *Diabetes.* 1990;39:157-167.
310. Kornfeld R. Studies on L-glutamine D-fructose 6-phosphate amidotransferase: I. Feedback inhibition by uridine diphosphate-N-acetylglucosamine. *J Biol Chem.* 1967;242:3135-3141.
311. Buse MG. Hexosamines, insulin resistance, and the complications of diabetes: current status. *Am J Physiol Endocrinol Metab.* 2006;290:E1-E8.
312. Marshall S, Bacote V, Traxinger RR. Discovery of a metabolic pathway mediating glucose-induced desensitization of the glucose transport system: role of hexosamine biosynthesis in the induction of insulin resistance. *J Biol Chem.* 1991;266:4706-4712.
313. Robinson KA, Weinstein ML, Lindenmayer GE, et al. Effects of diabetes and hyperglycemia on the hexosamine synthesis pathway in rat muscle and liver. *Diabetes.* 1995;44:1438-1446.
314. Hebert LF Jr, Daniels MC, Zhou J, et al. Overexpression of glutamine: fructose-6-phosphate amidotransferase in transgenic mice leads to insulin resistance. *J Clin Invest.* 1996;98:930-936.
315. Baron AD, Zhu JS, Zhu JH, et al. Glucosamine induces insulin resistance in vivo by affecting GLUT 4 translocation in skeletal muscle: implications for glucose toxicity. *J Clin Invest.* 1995;96:2792-2801.
316. Mallon PW, Cooper DA, Carr A. HIV-associated lipodystrophy. *HIV Med.* 2001;2(3):166-173.
317. Srinivasa S, Grinspoon SK. Metabolic and body composition effects of newer antiretrovirals in HIV-infected patients. *Eur J Endocrinol.* 2014;170(5):R185-R202.
318. Shevitz A, Wanke CA, Falutz J, et al. Clinical perspectives on HIV-associated lipodystrophy syndrome: an update. *AIDS.* 2001;15:1917-1930.
319. Purnell JQ, Zambon A, Knopp RH, et al. Effect of ritonavir on lipids and post-heparin lipase activities in normal subjects. *AIDS.* 2000;14:51-57.
320. Noor MA, Lo JC, Mulligan K, et al. Metabolic effects of indinavir in healthy HIV-seronegative men. *AIDS.* 2001;15:F11-F18.
321. Murata H, Hruz PW, Mueckler M. The mechanism of insulin resistance caused by HIV protease inhibitor therapy. *J Biol Chem.* 2000;275:20251-20254.
322. Shikuma CM, Hu N, Milne C, et al. Mitochondrial DNA decrease in subcutaneous adipose tissue of HIV-infected individuals with peripheral lipoatrophy. *AIDS.* 2001;15:1801-1809.
323. Caron M, Auclair M, Vigouroux C, et al. The HIV protease inhibitor indinavir impairs sterol regulatory element-binding protein-1 intranuclear localization, inhibits preadipocyte differentiation, and induces insulin resistance. *Diabetes.* 2001;50:1378-1388.

324. Dowell P, Flexner C, Kwiterovich PO, et al. Suppression of preadipocyte differentiation and promotion of adipocyte death by HIV protease inhibitors. *J Biol Chem.* 2000;275:41325-41332.

325. Carr A, Samaras K, Chisholm DJ, et al. Pathogenesis of HIV-1-protease inhibitor-associated peripheral lipodystrophy, hyperlipidaemia, and insulin resistance. *Lancet.* 1998;351:1881-1883.

326. Nolan D, Hammond E, Martin A, et al. Mitochondrial DNA depletion and morphologic changes in adipocytes associated with nucleoside reverse transcriptase inhibitor therapy. *AIDS.* 2003;17:1329-1338.

327. Milinkovic A, Martinez E. Current perspectives on HIV-associated lipodystrophy syndrome. *J Antimicrob Chemother.* 2005;56:6-9.

328. Grinspoon SK. Metabolic syndrome and cardiovascular disease in patients with human immunodeficiency virus. *Am J Med.* 2005; 118(Suppl 2):23S-28S.

329. Mauss S. HIV-associated and antiretroviral-induced hyperlipidaemia: an update. *J HIV Ther.* 2003;8:29-31.

330. Chuck SK, Penzak SR. Risk-benefit of HMG-CoA reductase inhibitors in the treatment of HIV protease inhibitor-related hyperlipidaemia. *Expert Opin Drug Saf.* 2002;1:5-17.

331. Knowler WC, Barrett-Connor E, Fowler SE, et al. Reduction in the incidence of type 2 diabetes with lifestyle intervention or metformin. *N Engl J Med.* 2002;346:393-403.

332. Kelley DE, Mandarino LJ. Fuel selection in human skeletal muscle in insulin resistance: a reexamination. *Diabetes.* 2000;49:677-683.

333. Long SD, O'Brien K, MacDonald KG Jr, et al. Weight loss in severely obese subjects prevents the progression of impaired glucose tolerance to type II diabetes: a longitudinal interventional study. *Diabetes Care.* 1994;17:372-375.

334. Wing RR, Venditti E, Jakicic JM, et al. Lifestyle intervention in overweight individuals with a family history of diabetes. *Diabetes Care.* 1998;21:350-359.

335. Kelley DE, Wing R, Buonocore C, et al. Relative effects of calorie restriction and weight loss in noninsulin-dependent diabetes mellitus. *J Clin Endocrinol Metab.* 1993;77(5):1287-1293.

336. Watts NB, Spanheimer RG, DiGirolamo M, et al. Prediction of glucose response to weight loss in patients with non-insulin-dependent diabetes mellitus. *Arch Intern Med.* 1990;150(4):803-806.

337. Rossmeislová L, Mališová L, Kračmerová J, Štich V. Adaptation of human adipose tissue to hypocaloric diet. *Int J Obes (Lond).* 2013; 37(5):640-650.

338. Cummings DE. Endocrine mechanisms mediating remission of diabetes after gastric bypass surgery. *Int J Obes (Lond).* 2009;33(Suppl 1): S33-S40.

339. Jackness C, Karmally W, Febres G, et al. Very low-calorie diet mimics the early beneficial effect of Roux-en-Y gastric bypass on insulin sensitivity and beta-cell function in type 2 diabetic patients. *Diabetes.* 2013;62(9):3027-3032.

340. Nesher R, Karl IE, Kipnis DM. Dissociation of effects of insulin and contraction on glucose transport in rat epitrochlearis muscle. *Am J Physiol.* 1985;249:C226-C232.

341. Wallberg-Henriksson H, Holloszy JO. Activation of glucose transport in diabetic muscle: responses to contraction and insulin. *Am J Physiol.* 1985;249:C233-C237.

342. Wallberg-Henriksson H, Constable SH, Young DA, et al. Glucose transport into rat skeletal muscle: interaction between exercise and insulin. *J Appl Physiol.* 1988;65:909-913.

343. Young DA, Wallberg-Henriksson H, Sleeper MD, et al. Reversal of the exercise-induced increase in muscle permeability to glucose. *Am J Physiol.* 1987;253:E331-E335.

344. Douen AG, Ramlal T, Rastogi S, et al. Exercise induces recruitment of the "insulin-responsive glucose transporter": evidence for distinct intracellular insulin- and exercise-recruitable transporter pools in skeletal muscle. *J Biol Chem.* 1990;265:13427-13430.

345. Goodyear LJ, Hirshman MF, King PA, et al. Skeletal muscle plasma membrane glucose transport and glucose transporters after exercise. *J Appl Physiol.* 1990;68:193-198.

346. Goodyear LJ, Giorgino F, Balon TW, et al. Effects of contractile activity on tyrosine phosphoproteins and PI3-kinase activity in rat skeletal muscle. *Am J Physiol.* 1995;268:E987-E995.

347. Lund S, Holman GD, Schmitz O, et al. Contraction stimulates translocation of glucose transporter GLUT4 in skeletal muscle through a mechanism distinct from that of insulin. *Proc Natl Acad Sci U S A.* 1995;92:5817-5821.

348. Zorzano A, Balon TW, Goodman MN, et al. Additive effects of prior exercise and insulin on glucose and AIB uptake by rat muscle. *Am J Physiol.* 1986;251:E21-E26.

349. Henriksen EJ, Bourey RE, Rodnick KJ, et al. Glucose transporter protein content and glucose transport capacity in rat skeletal muscles. *Am J Physiol.* 1990;259:E593-E598.

350. Gao J, Ren J, Gulve EA, et al. Additive effect of contractions and insulin on GLUT-4 translocation into the sarcolemma. *J Appl Physiol.* 1994;77: 1597-1601.

351. Lee AD, Hansen PA, Holloszy JO. Wortmannin inhibits insulin-stimulated but not contraction-stimulated glucose transport activity in skeletal muscle. *FEBS Lett.* 1995;361:51-54.

352. Yeh JI, Gulve EA, Rameh L, et al. The effects of wortmannin on rat skeletal muscle: dissociation of signaling pathways for insulin- and contraction-activated hexose transport. *J Biol Chem.* 1995;270:2107-2111.

353. Treadway JL, James DE, Burcel E, et al. Effect of exercise on insulin receptor binding and kinase activity in skeletal muscle. *Am J Physiol.* 1989;256:E138-E144.

354. Brozinick JT Jr, Etgen GJ Jr, Yaspelkis BB 3rd, et al. Contraction-activated glucose uptake is normal in insulin-resistant muscle of the obese Zucker rat. *J Appl Physiol.* 1992;73:382-387.

355. Azevedo JL Jr, Carey JO, Pories WJ, et al. Hypoxia stimulates glucose transport in insulin-resistant human skeletal muscle. *Diabetes.* 1995;44: 695-698.

356. Winder WW, Hardie DG. AMP-activated protein kinase, a metabolic master switch: possible roles in type 2 diabetes. *Am J Physiol.* 1999;277: E1-E10.

357. Hayashi T, Hirshman MF, Kurth EJ, et al. Evidence for 5′ AMP-activated protein kinase mediation of the effect of muscle contraction on glucose transport. *Diabetes.* 1998;47:1369-1373.

358. Merrill GF, Kurth EJ, Hardie DG, et al. AICA riboside increases AMP-activated protein kinase, fatty acid oxidation, and glucose uptake in rat muscle. *Am J Physiol.* 1997;273:E1107-E1112.

359. Bergeron R, Russell RR 3rd, Young LH, et al. Effect of AMPK activation on muscle glucose metabolism in conscious rats. *Am J Physiol.* 1999; 276:E938-E944.

360. Bergeron R, Previs SF, Cline GW, et al. Effect of 5-aminoimidazole-4-carboxamide-1-beta-D-ribofuranoside infusion on invivo glucose and lipid metabolism in lean and obese Zucker rats. *Diabetes.* 2001; 50(5):1076-1082.

361. Richter EA, Garetto LP, Goodman MN, et al. Muscle glucose metabolism following exercise in the rat: increased sensitivity to insulin. *J Clin Invest.* 1982;69:785-793.

362. Garetto LP, Richter EA, Goodman MN, et al. Enhanced muscle glucose metabolism after exercise in the rat: the two phases. *Am J Physiol.* 1984;246:E471-E475.

363. Cartee GD, Young DA, Sleeper MD, et al. Prolonged increase in insulin-stimulated glucose transport in muscle after exercise. *Am J Physiol.* 1989;256:E494-E499.

364. Richter EA, Young DA, Sleeper MD, et al. Effect of exercise on insulin action in human skeletal muscle. *J Appl Physiol.* 1989;66:876-885.

365. Hansen PA, Nolte LA, Chen MM, et al. Increased GLUT-4 translocation mediates enhanced insulin sensitivity of muscle glucose transport after exercise. *J Appl Physiol.* 1998;85:1218-1222.

366. Thorell A, Hirshman MF, Nygren J, et al. Exercise and insulin cause GLUT-4 translocation in human skeletal muscle. *Am J Physiol.* 1999; 277:E733-E741.

367. Zorzano A, Balon TW, Garetto LP, et al. Muscle α-aminoisobutyric acid transport after exercise: enhanced stimulation by insulin. *Am J Physiol.* 1985;248:E546-E552.

368. Wojtaszewski JF, Hansen BF, Kiens B, et al. Insulin signaling in human skeletal muscle: time course and effect of exercise. *Diabetes.* 1997;46: 1775-1781.

369. Oshida Y, Yamanouchi K, Hayamizu S, et al. Long-term mild jogging increases insulin action despite no influence on body mass index or VO$_2$ max. *J Appl Physiol.* 1989;66:2206-2210.

370. DeFronzo RA, Sherwin RS, Kraemer N. Effect of physical training on insulin action in obesity. *Diabetes.* 1987;36:1379-1385.

371. Helmrich SP, Rayland DR, Leung RW, et al. Physical activity and reduced occurrence of non-insulin-dependent diabetes mellitus. *N Engl J Med.* 1991;325:147-152.

372. Perseghin G, Price TB, Petersen KF, et al. Increased glucose transport-phosphorylation and muscle glycogen synthesis after exercise training in insulin-resistant subjects. *N Engl J Med.* 1996;335:1357-1362.

373. Ebeling P, Bourey R, Koranyi L, et al. Mechanism of enhanced insulin sensitivity in athletes: increased blood flow, muscle glucose transport protein (GLUT-4) concentration, and glycogen synthase activity. *J Clin Invest.* 1993;92:1623-1631.

374. Houmard JA, Egan PC, Neufer PD, et al. Elevated skeletal muscle glucose transporter levels in exercise-trained middle-aged men. *Am J Physiol.* 1991;261:E437-E443.

375. Hood DA. Invited review: contractile activity-induced mitochondrial biogenesis in skeletal muscle. *J Appl Physiol.* 2001;90:1137-1157.

376. Lin J, Wu H, Tarr PT, et al. Transcriptional co-activator PGC-1 alpha drives the formation of slow-twitch muscle fibres. *Nature.* 2002;418: 797-801.

377. Handschin C, Rhee J, Lin J, et al. An autoregulatory loop controls peroxisome proliferator-activated receptor γ coactivator 1α expression in muscle. *Proc Natl Acad Sci U S A.* 2003;100:7111-7116.

378. Michael LF, Wu Z, Cheatham RB, et al. Restoration of insulin-sensitive glucose transporter (GLUT4) gene expression in muscle cells by the transcriptional coactivator PGC-1. *Proc Natl Acad Sci U S A.* 2001;98: 3820-3825.

379. Nisoli E, Tonello C, Cardile A, et al. Calorie restriction promotes mitochondrial biogenesis by inducing the expression of eNOS. *Science.* 2005;310:314-317.

380. Wu H, Kanatous SB, Thurmond FA, et al. Regulation of mitochondrial biogenesis in skeletal muscle by CaMK. *Science.* 2002;296:349-352.
381. Puigserver P, Rhee J, Lin J, et al. Cytokine stimulation of energy expenditure through p38 MAP kinase activation of PPARγ coactivator-1. *Mol Cell.* 2001;8:971-982.
382. Cao W, Medvedev AV, Daniel KW, et al. β-Adrenergic activation of p38 MAP kinase in adipocytes: cAMP induction of the uncoupling protein 1 (UCP1) gene requires p38 MAP kinase. *J Biol Chem.* 2001;276:27077-27082.
383. Terada S, Tabata I. Effects of acute bouts of running and swimming exercise on PGC-1α protein expression in rat epitrochlearis and soleus muscle. *Am J Physiol Endocrinol Metab.* 2004;286:E208-E216.
384. Terada S, Goto M, Kato M, et al. Effects of low-intensity prolonged exercise on PGC-1 mRNA expression in rat epitrochlearis muscle. *Biochem Biophys Res Commun.* 2002;296:350-354.
385. Zong H, Ren JM, Young LH, et al. AMP kinase is required for mitochondrial biogenesis in skeletal muscle in response to chronic energy deprivation. *Proc Natl Acad Sci U S A.* 2002;99:15983-15987.
386. Stamler J, Vaccaro O, Neaton JD, et al. Diabetes, other risk factors, and 12-yr cardiovascular mortality for men screened in the Multiple Risk Factor Intervention Trial. *Diabetes Care.* 1993;16:434-444.
387. Haffner SM, Lehto S, Ronnemaa T, et al. Mortality from coronary heart disease in subjects with type 2 diabetes and in nondiabetic subjects with and without prior myocardial infarction. *N Engl J Med.* 1998;339:229-234.
388. Fontbonne AM, Eschwege EM. Insulin and cardiovascular disease. Paris Prospective Study. *Diabetes Care.* 1991;14:461-469.
389. Willeit J, Kiechl S, Egger G, et al. The role of insulin in age-related sex differences of cardiovascular risk profile and morbidity. *Atherosclerosis.* 1997;130(1–2):183-189.
390. Hu FB, Stampfer MJ, Soloman CG, et al. The impact of diabetes mellitus on mortality from all causes and coronary heart disease in women: 20 years of follow-up. *Arch Intern Med.* 2001;161:1717-1723.
391. Reaven GM. Role of insulin resistance in human disease. Banting Lecture 1988. *Nutrition.* 1997;13:65, discussion 64, 66.
392. Reaven GM. Role of insulin resistance in human disease (syndrome X): an expanded definition. *Annu Rev Med.* 1993;44:121-131.
393. Kahn R, Buse J, Ferrannini E, et al. The metabolic syndrome: time for a critical appraisal: Joint Statement from the American Diabetes Association and the European Association for the Study of Diabetes. *Diabetes Care.* 2005;28:2289-2304.
394. Siegel RD, Cupples A, Schaefer EJ, Wilson PW, et al. Lipoproteins, apolipoproteins, and low-density lipoprotein size among diabetics in the Framingham offspring study. *Metabolism.* 1996;45:1267-1272.
395. Davidson NO, Shelness GS. Apolipoprotein B: mRNA editing, lipoprotein assembly, and presecretory degradation. *Annu Rev Nutr.* 2000;20:169-193.
396. Lewis GF, Steiner G. Acute effects of insulin in the control of VLDL production in humans: implications for the insulin-resistant state. *Diabetes Care.* 1996;19:390-393.
397. Riches FM, Watts GF, Naoumova RP, et al. Hepatic secretion of very-low-density lipoprotein apolipoprotein B-100 studied with a stable isotope technique in men with visceral obesity. *Int J Obes Relat Metab Disord.* 1998;22:414-423.
398. Wang SL, Du EZ, Martin TD, et al. Coordinate regulation of lipogenesis, the assembly and secretion of apolipoprotein B-containing lipoproteins by sterol response element binding protein 1. *J Biol Chem.* 1997;272:19351-19358.
399. Moberly JB, Cole TG, Alpers DH, Schonfeld G. Oleic acid stimulation of apolipoprotein B secretion from HepG2 and Caco-2 cells occurs post-transcriptionally. *Biochim Biophys Acta.* 1990;1042:70-80.
400. Ellsworth JL, Erickson SK, Cooper AD. Very low and low density lipoprotein synthesis and secretion by the human hepatoma cell line Hep-G2: effects of free fatty acid. *J Lipid Res.* 1986;27:858-874.
401. Kobatake T, Matsuzawa Y, Tokunaga K, et al. Metabolic improvements associated with a reduction of abdominal visceral fat caused by a new α-glucosidase inhibitor, AO-128, in Zucker fatty rats. *Int J Obes.* 1989;13:147-154.
402. Matsuzawa Y, Shimomura I, Nakamura T, et al. Pathophysiology and pathogenesis of visceral fat obesity. *Diabetes Res Clin Pract.* 1994;24(Suppl):S111-S116.
403. Nguyen TT, Mijares AH, Johnson CM, et al. Postprandial leg and splanchnic fatty acid metabolism in nonobese men and women. *Am J Physiol.* 1996;271:E965-E972.
404. Gordon DA, Jamil H, Sharp D, et al. Secretion of apolipoprotein B-containing lipoproteins from HeLa cells is dependent on expression of the microsomal triglyceride transfer protein and is regulated by lipid availability. *Proc Natl Acad Sci U S A.* 1994;91:7628-7632.
405. Gordon DA, Jamil H. Progress towards understanding the role of microsomal triglyceride transfer protein in apolipoprotein-B lipoprotein assembly. *Biochim Biophys Acta.* 2000;1486:72-83.
406. Liao W, Kobayashi K, Chan L. Adenovirus-mediated overexpression of microsomal triglyceride transfer protein (MTP): mechanistic studies on the role of MTP in apolipoprotein B-100 biogenesis. *Biochemistry.* 1999;38:7532-7544.
407. Horowitz BS, Goldberg IJ, Merab J, et al. Increased plasma and renal clearance of an exchangeable pool of apolipoprotein A-I in subjects with low levels of high density lipoprotein cholesterol. *J Clin Invest.* 1993;91:1743-1752.
408. Lemieux I, Couillard C, Pascot A, et al. The small, dense LDL phenotype as a correlate of postprandial lipemia in men. *Atherosclerosis.* 2000;153:423-432.
409. Tan KC, Cooper MB, Ling KL, et al. Fasting and postprandial determinants for the occurrence of small dense LDL species in non-insulin-dependent diabetic patients with and without hypertriglyceridaemia: the involvement of insulin, insulin precursor species and insulin resistance. *Atherosclerosis.* 1995;113:273-287.
410. Austin MA, Selby JV. LDL subclass phenotypes and the risk factors of the insulin resistance syndrome. *Int J Obes Relat Metab Disord.* 1995;19(Suppl 1):S22-S26.
411. Stewart MW, Laker MF, Dyer RG, et al. Lipoprotein compositional abnormalities and insulin resistance in type II diabetic patients with mild hyperlipidemia. *Arterioscler Thromb.* 1993;13:1046-1052.
412. Alexander JK. Obesity and coronary heart disease. *Am J Med Sci.* 2001;321:215-224.
413. Laakso M, Edelman SV, Brechtel G, et al. Impaired insulin-mediated skeletal muscle blood flow in patients with NIDDM. *Diabetes.* 1992;41:1076-1083.
414. Steinberg HO, Brechtel G, Johnson A, et al. Insulin-mediated skeletal muscle vasodilation is nitric oxide dependent: a novel action of insulin to increase nitric oxide release. *J Clin Invest.* 1994;94:1172-1179.
415. Baron AD, Zhu JS, Marshall S, et al. Insulin resistance after hypertension induced by the nitric oxide synthesis inhibitor L-NMMA in rats. *Am J Physiol.* 1995;269:E709-E715.
416. Steinberg HO, Paradisi G, Hook G, et al. Free fatty acid elevation impairs insulin-mediated vasodilation and nitric oxide production. *Diabetes.* 2000;49:1231-1238.
417. Landsberg L. Insulin resistance, energy balance and sympathetic nervous system activity. *Clin Exp Hypertens A.* 1990;12(5):817-830.
418. Weidmann P, de Courten M, Bohlen L. Insulin resistance, hyperinsulinemia and hypertension. *J Hypertens Suppl.* 1993;11(Suppl 5):S27-S38.
419. Masuo K, Mikami H, Itoh M, et al. Sympathetic activity and body mass index contribute to blood pressure levels. *Hypertens Res.* 2000;23:303-310.
420. DeFronzo RA. Insulin and renal sodium handling: clinical implications. *Int J Obes.* 1981;5(Suppl 1):93-104.
421. DeFronzo RA, Goldberg M, Agus ZS. The effects of glucose and insulin on renal electrolyte transport. *J Clin Invest.* 1976;58:83-90.
422. DeFronzo RA, Cooke CR, Andres R, et al. The effect of insulin on renal handling of sodium, potassium, calcium, and phosphate in man. *J Clin Invest.* 1975;55:845-855.
423. Welborn TA, Breckenridge A, Rubinstein AH, et al. Serum-insulin in essential hypertension and in peripheral vascular disease. *Lancet.* 1966;1:1336-1337.
424. Gress TW, Nieto FJ, Shahar E, et al. Hypertension and antihypertensive therapy as risk factors for type 2 diabetes mellitus. Atherosclerosis Risk in Communities Study. *N Engl J Med.* 2000;342:905-912.
425. Yusuf S, Sleight P, Pogue J, et al. Effects of an angiotensin-converting-enzyme inhibitor, ramipril, on cardiovascular events in high-risk patients. The Heart Outcomes Prevention Evaluation Study Investigators. *N Engl J Med.* 2000;342:145-153.
426. Sebestjen M, Zegura B, Guzic-Salobir B, et al. Fibrinolytic parameters and insulin resistance in young survivors of myocardial infarction with heterozygous familial hypercholesterolemia. *Wien Klin Wochenschr.* 2001;113:113-118.
427. Juhan-Vague I, Alessi MC, Morange PE. Hypofibrinolysis and increased PAI-1 are linked to atherothrombosis via insulin resistance and obesity. *Ann Med.* 2000;32(Suppl 1):78-84.
428. Fujii S, Goto D, Zaman T, et al. Diminished fibrinolysis and thrombosis: clinical implications for accelerated atherosclerosis. *J Atheroscler Thromb.* 1998;5:76-81.
429. Sobel BE. The potential influence of insulin and plasminogen activator inhibitor type 1 on the formation of vulnerable atherosclerotic plaques associated with type 2 diabetes. *Proc Assoc Am Physicians.* 1999;111:313-318.
430. Festa A, D'Agostino R Jr, Mykkanen L, et al. Relative contribution of insulin and its precursors to fibrinogen and PAI-1 in a large population with different states of glucose tolerance. The Insulin Resistance Atherosclerosis Study (IRAS). *Arterioscler Thromb Vasc Biol.* 1999;19:562-568.
431. Lormeau B, Aurousseau MH, Valensi P, et al. Hyperinsulinemia and hypofibrinolysis: effects of short-term optimized glycemic control with continuous insulin infusion in type II diabetic patients. *Metabolism.* 1997;46:1074-1079.
432. Hamsten A, Eriksson P, Karpe F, et al. Relationships of thrombosis and fibrinolysis to atherosclerosis. *Curr Opin Lipidol.* 1994;5(5):382-389.
433. Grenett HE, Benza RL, Li XN, et al. Expression of plasminogen activator inhibitor type I in genotyped human endothelial cell cultures: genotype-specific regulation by insulin. *Thromb Haemost.* 1999;82:1504-1509.

434. Chomiki N, Henry M, Alessi MC, et al. Plasminogen activator inhibitor-1 expression in human liver and healthy or atherosclerotic vessel walls. *Thromb Haemost.* 1994;72:44-53.

435. Koistinen HA, Dusserre E, Ebeling P, et al. Subcutaneous adipose tissue expression of plasminogen activator inhibitor-1 (PAI-1) in nondiabetic and type 2 diabetic subjects. *Diabetes Metab Res Rev.* 2000;16:364-369.

436. Kruszynska YT, Yu JG, Olefsky JM, et al. Effects of troglitazone on blood concentrations of plasminogen activator inhibitor 1 in patients with type 2 diabetes and in lean and obese normal subjects. *Diabetes.* 2000;49:633-639.

437. Stunkard AJ. Current views on obesity. *Am J Med.* 1996;100:230-236.

438. Expert Panel on Detection, Evaluation and Treatment of High Blood Cholesterol in Adults. Executive Summary of the Third Report of the National Cholesterol Education Program (NCEP) Expert Panel on Detection, Evaluation and Treatment of High Blood Cholesterol in Adults (Adult Treatment Panel III). *JAMA.* 2001;285(19):2486-2497.

439. Yalow R, Berson S. Immunoassay of endogenous plasma insulin in man. *J Clin Invest.* 1960;39:1157-1175.

440. Polonsky K, Jaspan J, Emmanouel D, et al. Differences in the hepatic and renal extraction of insulin and glucagon in the dog: evidence for saturability of insulin metabolism. *Acta Endocrinol (Copenh).* 1983;102:420-427.

441. Polonsky K, Jaspan J, Pugh W, et al. Metabolism of C-peptide in the dog: in vivo demonstration of the absence of hepatic extraction. *J Clin Invest.* 1983;72:1114-1123.

442. Steiner DF, James DE. Cellular and molecular biology of the beta cell. *Diabetologia.* 1992;35(Suppl 2):S41-S48.

443. Melani F, Ryan WG, Rubenstein AH, et al. Proinsulin secretion by a pancreatic beta-cell adenoma: proinsulin and C-peptide secretion. *N Engl J Med.* 1970;283:713-719.

444. Horwitz D, Starr JI, Mako ME, et al. Proinsulin, insulin, and C-peptide concentrations in human portal and peripheral blood. *J Clin Invest.* 1975;55:1278-1283.

445. Melani F, Rubenstein A, Steiner D. Human serum proinsulin. *J Clin Invest.* 1970;49:497-507.

446. Bergenstal R, Cohen RM, Lever E, et al. The metabolic effects of biosynthetic human proinsulin in individuals with type I diabetes. *J Clin Endocrinol Metab.* 1984;58:973-979.

447. Revers R, Henry R, Schmeiser L, et al. The effects of biosynthetic human proinsulin on carbohydrate metabolism. *Diabetes.* 1984;33:762-770.

448. Peavy D, Brunner MR, Duckworth W, et al. Receptor binding and biological potency of several split forms (conversion intermediates) of human proinsulin: studies in cultured IM-9 lymphocytes and in vivo and in vitro in rats. *J Biol Chem.* 1985;260:13989-13994.

449. Gruppuso P, Frank B, Schwartz R. Binding of proinsulin and proinsulin conversion intermediates to human placental insulin-like growth factor 1 receptors. *J Clin Endocrinol Metab.* 1988;67:197.

450. Polonsky K, Rubenstein A. C-peptide as a measure of the secretion and hepatic extraction of insulin: pitfalls and limitations. *Diabetes.* 1984;33:486-494.

451. Wojcikowski C, Blackman J, Ostrega D, et al. Lack of effect of high-dose biosynthetic human C-peptide on pancreatic hormone release in normal subjects. *Metabolism.* 1990;39:827-832.

452. Wahren J, Ekberg K, Johansson J, et al. Role of C-peptide in human physiology. *Am J Physiol.* 2000;278:E759-E768.

453. Polonsky K, Pugh W, Jaspan JB, et al. C-peptide and insulin secretion: relationship between peripheral concentrations of C-peptide and insulin and their secretion rates in the dog. *J Clin Invest.* 1984;74:1821-1829.

454. Bratusch-Marrain P, Waldhausl WK, Gasic S, et al. Hepatic disposal of biosynthetic human insulin and porcine C-peptide in humans. *Metabolism.* 1984;33:151-157.

455. Faber O, Hagen C, Binder C, et al. Kinetics of human connecting peptide in normal and diabetic subjects. *J Clin Invest.* 1978;62:197-203.

456. Polonsky K, Licinio-Paixas J, Given BD, et al. Use of biosynthetic human C-peptide in the measurement of insulin secretion rates in normal volunteers and type I diabetic patients. *J Clin Invest.* 1986;77:98-105.

457. Shapiro E, Tillil H, Rubenstein H, et al. Peripheral insulin parallels changes in insulin secretion more closely than C-peptide after bolus intravenous glucose administration. *J Clin Endocrinol Metab.* 1988;67:1094-1099.

458. Eaton R, Allen RC, Schade DS, et al. Prehepatic insulin production in man: kinetic analysis using peripheral connecting peptide behavior. *J Clin Endocrinol Metab.* 1980;51:520-528.

459. Welch S, Gebhart SS, Bergman RN, et al. Minimal model analysis of intravenous glucose tolerance test-derived insulin sensitivity in diabetic subjects. *J Clin Endocrinol Metab.* 1990;71:1508-1518.

460. Breda E, Cavaghan MK, Toffolo G, et al. Oral glucose tolerance test minimal model indexes of beta-cell function and insulin sensitivity. *Diabetes.* 2001;50:150-158.

461. Bergman R, Phillips L, Cobelli C. Physiologic evaluation of factors controlling glucose tolerance in man: measurement of insulin sensitiv-

462. Caumo A, Bergman R, Cobelli C. Insulin sensitivity from meal tolerance tests in normal subjects: a minimal model index. *J Clin Endocrinol Metab.* 2000;85:4396-4402.

463. Davis EA, Cuesta-Munoz A, Raoul M, et al. Mutants of glucokinase cause hypoglycaemia and hyperglycaemia syndromes and their analysis illuminates fundamental quantitative concepts of glucose homeostasis. *Diabetologia.* 1999;42:1175-1186.

464. Matschinsky FM, Glaser B, Magnuson MA. Pancreatic beta-cell glucokinase: closing the gap between theoretical concepts and experimental realities. *Diabetes.* 1998;47:307-315.

465. Dukes ID, McIntyre MS, Mertz RJ, et al. Dependence on NADH produced during glycolysis for beta-cell glucose signaling. *J Biol Chem.* 1994;269:10979-10982.

466. Maechler P, Wollheim CB. Mitochondrial function in normal and diabetic beta-cells. *Nature.* 2001;414:807-812.

467. Aguilar-Bryan L, Bryan J, Nakazaki M. Of mice and men: K_{ATP} channels and insulin secretion. *Recent Prog Horm Res.* 2001;56:47-68.

468. Porte DJ, Pupo A. Insulin responses to glucose: evidence for a two-pooled system in man. *J Clin Invest.* 1969;48:2309-2319.

469. Chen M, Porte DJ. The effect of rate and dose of glucose infusion on the acute insulin response in man. *J Clin Endocrinol Metab.* 1976;42:1168-1175.

470. Ward W, Beard JC, Halter JB, et al. Pathophysiology of insulin secretion in non-insulin-dependent diabetes mellitus. *Diabetes Care.* 1984;7:491-502.

471. Waldhäus W, Bratusch-Marrain P, Gasic S, et al. Insulin production rate following glucose ingestion estimated by splanchnic C-peptide output in normal man. *Diabetologia.* 1979;17:221-227.

472. Eaton R, Allen R, Schade D. Hepatic removal of insulin in normal man: dose response to endogenous insulin secretion. *J Clin Endocrinol Metab.* 1983;56:1294-1300.

473. Nauck M, Homberger E, Siegel EG, et al. Incretin effects of increasing glucose loads in man calculated from venous insulin and C-peptide responses. *J Clin Endocrinol Metab.* 1986;63:492-498.

474. Tillil H, Shapiro ET, Miller MA, et al. Dose-dependent effects of oral and intravenous glucose on insulin secretion and clearance in normal humans. *Am J Physiol.* 1988;254:E349-E357.

475. Faber O, Madsbad S, Kehlet H, et al. Pancreatic beta cell secretion during oral and intravenous glucose administration. *Acta Med Scand Suppl.* 1979;624:61-64.

476. Madsbad S, Kehlet H, Hilsted J, et al. Discrepancy between plasma C-peptide and insulin response to oral and intravenous glucose. *Diabetes.* 1983;32:436-438.

477. Shapiro E, Tillil H, Miller MA, et al. Insulin secretion and clearance: comparison after oral and intravenous glucose. *Diabetes.* 1987;93:1120-1130.

478. Creutzfeldt W, Ebert R. New developments in the incretin concept. *Diabetologia.* 1985;28:565-576.

479. Pagliara A, Stillings SN, Hover B, et al. Glucose modulation of amino acid-induced glucagon and insulin release in the isolated perfused rat pancreas. *J Clin Invest.* 1974;54:819-832.

480. Gerich J, Charles M, Grodsky G. Characterization of the effects of arginine and glucose on glucagon and insulin release from the perfused rat pancreas. *J Clin Invest.* 1974;54:833-847.

481. Grodsky G. The kinetics of insulin release. In: Hasselblatt A, Bruchhausen F, eds. *Handbook of Experimental Pharmacology*, Vol. 32. Berlin, Germany: Springer-Verlag; 1975:1-19.

482. Salomon D, Meda P. Heterogeneity and contact-dependent regulation of hormone secretion by individual β cells. *Exp Cell Res.* 1986;162:507-520.

483. Schmitz O, Porksen N, Nyholm B, et al. Disorderly and nonstationary insulin secretion in relatives of patients with NIDDM. *Am J Physiol.* 1997;272:E218-E226.

484. Cerasi E, Luft R. The plasma insulin response to glucose infusion in healthy subjects and in diabetes mellitus. *Acta Endocrinol (Copenh).* 1967;55:278-304.

485. Smith C, Tam AC, Thomas JM, et al. Between and within subject variation of the first phase insulin response to intravenous glucose. *Diabetologia.* 1988;31:123-125.

486. Bardet S, Pasqual C, Maugendre D, et al. Inter and intra individual variability of acute insulin response during intravenous glucose tolerance tests. *Diabetes Metab.* 1989;15:224-232.

487. Rayman G, Clark P, Schneider AE, et al. The first phase insulin response to intravenous glucose is highly reproducible. *Diabetologia.* 1990;33:631-634.

488. Bolaffi J, Haldt A, Lewis LD, et al. The third phase of in vitro insulin secretion: evidence for glucose insensitivity. *Diabetes.* 1986;35:370-373.

489. Curry D. Insulin content and insulinogenesis by the perfused rat pancreas: effects of long term glucose stimulation. *Endocrinology.* 1986;118:170-175.

490. Hoenig M, MacGregor L, Matschinsky F. In vitro exhaustion of pancreatic β-cells. *Am J Physiol.* 1986;250:E502-E511.

ity and beta-cell glucose sensitivity from the response to intravenous glucose. *J Clin Invest.* 1981;68:1456-1467.

491. Grodsky G. A new phase of insulin secretion: how will it contribute to our understanding of β-cell function? *Diabetes.* 1989;38:673-678.

492. Cerasi E. Potentiation of insulin release by glucose in man. *Acta Endocrinol (Copenh).* 1975;79:511-534.

493. Grill V. Time and dose dependencies for priming effect of glucose on insulin secretion. *Am J Physiol.* 1981;240:E24-E31.

494. Poitout V, Robertson RP. Minireview: secondary beta-cell failure in type 2 diabetes—a convergence of glucotoxicity and lipotoxicity. *Endocrinology.* 2002;143:339-342.

495. Leahy JL. Natural history of beta-cell dysfunction in NIDDM. *Diabetes Care.* 1990;13:992-1010.

496. Levin S, Karam JH, Hane S, et al. Enhancement of arginine-induced insulin secretion in man by prior administration of glucose. *Diabetes.* 1971;20:171-176.

497. Fajans S, Floyd J. Stimulation of islet cell secretion by nutrients and by gastrointestinal hormones released during digestion. In: Steiner D, Freinkel N, eds. *Handbook of Physiology: Section 7. Endocrinology.* Washington, DC: American Physiological Society; 1972:473-493.

498. Ward W, Bolgiano DC, McKnight B, et al. Diminished β-cell secretory capacity in patients with non-insulin dependent diabetes mellitus. *J Clin Invest.* 1984;74:1318-1328.

499. Kadowaki T, Miyake Y, Hagura R, et al. Risk factors for worsening to diabetes in subjects with impaired glucose tolerance. *Diabetologia.* 1984;26:44-49.

500. Muller W, Faloona G, Unger R. The influence of the antecedent diet upon glucagon and insulin secretion. *N Engl J Med.* 1971;285:1450-1454.

501. Goberna R, Tamarit J Jr, Osorio J, et al. Action of β-hydroxybutyrate, acetoacetate and palmitate on the insulin release from the perfused isolated rat pancreas. *Horm Metab Res.* 1974;6:256-260.

502. Crespin S, Greenough D, Steinberg D. Stimulation of insulin secretion by long-chain free fatty acids. *J Clin Invest.* 1973;52:1979-1984.

503. Crespin S, Greenough W, Steinberg D. Stimulation of insulin secretion by infusion of fatty acids. *J Clin Invest.* 1969;48:1934-1943.

504. Paolisso G, Gambardella M, Amato L, et al. Opposite effects of short- and long-term fatty acid infusion on insulin secretion in healthy subjects. *Diabetologia.* 1995;38:1295-1299.

505. Boden G, Chen X. Effects of fatty acids and ketone bodies on basal insulin secretion in type 2 diabetes. *Diabetes.* 1999;48:577-583.

506. Zhou Y-P, Grill V. Long term exposure of rat pancreatic islets to fatty acids inhibits glucose-induced insulin secretion and biosynthesis through a glucose fatty acid cycle. *J Clin Invest.* 1994;93:870-876.

507. Mason T, Goh T, Tchipashvili V, et al. Prolonged elevation of plasma free fatty acids desensitizes the insulin secretory response to glucose in vivo in rats. *Diabetes.* 1999;48:524-530.

508. Carpentier A, Mittelman SD, Lamarche B, et al. Acute enhancement of insulin secretion by FFA in humans is lost with prolonged FFA elevation. *Am J Physiol.* 1999;276:E1055-E1066.

509. Dupre J, Ross SA, Watson D, et al. Stimulation of insulin secretion by gastric inhibitory polypeptide in man. *J Clin Endocrinol Metab.* 1973;37:826-828.

510. Andersen D, Elahi D, Brown JC, et al. Oral glucose augmentation of insulin secretion: interactions of gastric inhibitory polypeptide with ambient glucose and insulin levels. *J Clin Invest.* 1978;62:152-161.

511. Schmidt W, Siegel E, Creutzfeldt W. Glucagon-like peptide-2 stimulates insulin release from isolated rate pancreatic islets. *Diabetologia.* 1985;28:704-707.

512. Kreymann B, Williams G, Ghatei MA, et al. Glucagon-like peptide-1 7-36: a physiological incretin in man. *Lancet.* 1987;2:1300-1304.

513. Zawalich W, Diaz V. Prior cholecystokinin exposure sensitizes islets of Langerhans to glucose stimulation. *Diabetes.* 1987;36:118-227.

514. Zawalich W. Synergistic impact of cholecystokinin and gastric inhibitory polypeptide on the regulation of insulin secretion. *Metabolism.* 1988;37:778-781.

515. Weir G, Mojsovs S, Hendrick GK, et al. Glucagon-like peptide 1(7-37) actions on endocrine pancreas. *Diabetes.* 1989;38:338-342.

516. Rasmussen H, Zawalich KC, Ganesan S, et al. Physiology and pathophysiology of insulin secretion. *Diabetes Care.* 1990;13:655-666.

517. Fukase N, Manaka H, Sugiyama K, et al. Response of truncated glucagon-like peptide-1 and gastric inhibitory polypeptide to glucose ingestion in non-insulin dependent diabetes mellitus: effect of sulfonylurea therapy. *Acta Diabetol.* 1995;32:165-169.

518. Groop P. The influence of body weight, age and glucose tolerance on the relationship between GIP secretion and beta-cell function in man. *Scand J Clin Lab Invest.* 1989;49:367-379.

519. Creutzfeldt W, Ebert R, Nauck M, et al. Disturbances of the entero-insulin axis. *Scand J Gastroenterol.* 1983;83(Suppl):111-119.

520. Nauck M, Heimesaat MM, Orskov C, et al. Preserved incretin activity of glucagon-like peptide 1(7-36 amide) but not of synthetic human gastric inhibitory polypeptide in patients with type 2 diabetes mellitus. *J Clin Invest.* 1993;91:301-307.

521. Ahrén B, Larsson H, Holst J. Reduced gastric inhibitory polypeptide but normal glucagon-like peptide 1 response to oral glucose in postmenopausal women with impaired glucose tolerance. *Eur J Endocrinol.* 1997;137:127-131.

522. Rushakoff R, Goldfine ID, Beccaria LJ, et al. Reduced postprandial cholecystokinin (CCK) secretion in patients with noninsulin-dependent diabetes mellitus: evidence for a role for CCK in regulating postprandial hyperglycemia. *J Clin Endocrinol Metab.* 1993;76:489-493.

523. Meguro T, Shimosegawa T, Satoh A, et al. Gallbladder emptying and cholecystokinin and pancreatic polypeptide responses to a liquid meal in patients with diabetes mellitus. *J Gastroenterol.* 1997;32:628-634.

524. Hasegawa H, Shirohara H, Okabayashi Y, et al. Oral glucose ingestion stimulates cholecystokinin release in normal subjects and patients with non-insulin-dependent diabetes mellitus. *Metabolism.* 1996;45:196-202.

525. Nauck M, Wollschlager D, Werner J, et al. Effects of subcutaneous glucagon-like peptide 1 (GLP-1 (7-36 amide)) in patients with NIDDM. *Diabetologia.* 1996;39:1546-1553.

526. Creutzfeldt W, Kleine N, Willms B, et al. Glucagonostatic actions and reduction of fasting hyperglycemia by exogenous glucagon-like peptide I(7-36) amide in type I diabetic patients. *Diabetes Care.* 1996;19:580-586.

527. Young A, Gedulin BR, Bhavsar S, et al. Glucose-lowering and insulin-sensitizing actions of exendin-4: studies in obese diabetic *(ob/ob, db/db)* mice, diabetic fatty Zucker rats, and diabetic rhesus monkeys *(Macaca mulatta). Diabetes.* 1999;48:1026-1034.

528. Nauck M, Bartels E, Orskov C, et al. Additive insulinotropic effects of exogenous synthetic human gastric inhibitory polypeptide and glucagon-like peptide-1-(7-36) amide infused at near-physiological insulinotropic hormone and glucose concentrations. *J Clin Endocrinol Metab.* 1993;76:912-917.

529. Elahi D, McAloon-Dyke M, Fukagawa NK, et al. The insulinotropic actions of glucose-dependent insulinotropic polypeptide (GIP) and glucagon-like peptide-1 (7-37) in normal and diabetic subjects. *Regul Pept.* 1994;51:63-74.

530. Niederau C, Schwarzendrube J, Luthen R, et al. Effects of cholecysto-kinin receptor blockade in circulating concentrations of glucose, insulin, C-peptide, and pancreatic polypeptide after various meals in healthy human volunteers. *Pancreas.* 1992;7:1-10.

531. Fieseler P, Bridenbaugh S, Nustede R, et al. Physiological augmentation of amino acid-induced insulin secretion by GIP and GLP-I but not by CCK-8. *Am J Physiol.* 1995;268:E949-E955.

532. Reimers J, Nauck M, Creutzfeldt W, et al. Lack of insulinotropic effect of endogenous and exogenous cholecystokinin in man. *Diabetologia.* 1988;31:271-280.

533. Rushakoff R, Goldfine ID, Carter JD, et al. Physiological concentrations of cholecystokinin stimulate amino acid-induced insulin release in humans. *J Clin Endocrinol Metab.* 1987;65:395-401.

534. Ahrén B, Holst J, Efendic S. Antidiabetogenic action of cholecystokinin-8 in type 2 diabetes. *J Clin Endocrinol Metab.* 2000;85:1043-1048.

535. Schebalin M, Said S, Makhlouf G. Stimulation of insulin and glucagon secretion by vasoactive intestinal peptide. *Am J Physiol.* 1977;232:E197-E200.

536. Dupre J, Curtis JD, Unger RH, et al. Effects of secretin, pancreozymin, or gastrin on the response of the endocrine pancreas to administration of glucose or arginine in man. *J Clin Invest.* 1969;48:745-757.

537. Halter J, Porte DJ. Mechanisms of impaired acute insulin release in adult onset diabetes: studies with isoproterenol and secretin. *J Clin Endocrinol Metab.* 1978;46:952-960.

538. Glaser B, Shapiro B, Glowniak J, et al. Effects of secretin on the normal and pathological beta-cell. *J Clin Endocrinol Metab.* 1988;66:1138-1143.

539. Bertrand G, Puech R, Maisonnasse Y, et al. Comparative effects of PACAP and VIP on pancreatic endocrine secretions and vascular resistance in rat. *Br J Pharmacol.* 1996;117:764-770.

540. Rehfeld J, Stadil F. The effect of gastrin on basal- and glucose-stimulated insulin secretion in man. *J Clin Invest.* 1973;52:1415-1426.

541. Samols E, Marri G, Marks V. Promotion of insulin secretion by glucagon. *Lancet.* 1965;2:15-16.

542. Alberti K, Christensen NJ, Christensen SE, et al. Inhibition of insulin secretion by somatostatin. *Lancet.* 1973;2:1299-1301.

543. Aguilar-Parada E, Eisentraut A, Unger R. Effects of starvation on plasma pancreatic glucagon in normal man. *Diabetes.* 1969;18:717-723.

544. Marliss E, Aoki TT, Unger RH, et al. Glucagon levels and metabolic effects in fasting man. *J Clin Invest.* 1970;49:2256-2270.

545. Malaisse W, Malaisse L, Wright P. Effect of fasting upon insulin secretion in the rat. *Am J Physiol.* 1967;213:843-848.

546. Zawalich W, Dye ES, Pagliara AS, et al. Starvation diabetes in the rat: onset, recovery and specificity of reduced responsiveness of pancreatic β-cells. *Endocrinology.* 1979;104:1344-1351.

547. Felig P, Marliss E, Cahill JG. Metabolic response to human growth hormone during prolonged starvation. *J Clin Invest.* 1971;50:411-421.

548. Kalhan S, Adam P. Inhibitory effect of prednisone on insulin secretion in man: model for duplication of blood glucose concentration. *J Clin Endocrinol Metab.* 1975;41:600-610.

549. Landgraf R, Landgraf-Luers MM, Weissmann A, et al. Prolactin: a diabetogenic hormone. *Diabetologia.* 1977;13:99-104.

550. Gustafson A, Banasiak MF, Kalkhoff RK, et al. Correlation of hyperprolactinemia with altered plasma insulin and glucagon: similarity to effects of late human pregnancy. *J Clin Endocrinol Metab.* 1980;51:242-246.

551. Brelje T, Sorenson R. Nutrient and hormonal regulation of the threshold of glucose-stimulated insulin secretion in isolated rat pancreases. *Endocrinology.* 1988;123:1582-1590.

552. Beck P, Daughaday W. Human placental lactogen: studies of its acute metabolic effects and disposition in normal man. *J Clin Invest.* 1967; 46:103-110.

553. Ensinck J, Williams R. Hormonal and nonhormonal factors modifying man's response to insulin. In: Steiner D, Freinkel N, eds. *Handbook of Physiology: Section 7. Endocrinology.* Washington, DC: American Physiological Society; 1972:665-669.

554. Martin J, Friesen H. Effect of human placental lactogen on the isolated islets of Langerhans in vitro. *Endocrinology.* 1969;84:619-621.

555. Curry D, Bennett L. Dynamics of insulin release by perfused rat pancreases: effects of hypophysectomy, growth hormone, adrenocorticotropic hormone and hydrocortisone. *Endocrinology.* 1973;93:602-609.

556. Malaisse W, Malaisse-Lagae F, King S, et al. Effect of growth hormone on insulin secretion. *Am J Physiol.* 1968;215:423-428.

557. Randin J, Scazziga B, Jequier E, et al. Study of glucose and lipid metabolism by continuous indirect calorimetry in Graves' disease: effect of an oral glucose load. *J Clin Endocrinol Metab.* 1985;61:1165-1171.

558. Foss M, Paccola GM, Saad MJ, et al. Peripheral glucose metabolism in human hyperthyroidism. *J Clin Endocrinol Metab.* 1990;70:1167-1172.

559. Sestoft L, Heding L. Hypersecretion of proinsulin in thyrotoxicosis. *Diabetologia.* 1981;21:103-107.

560. Nishi S, Seino Y, Ishida H, et al. Vagal regulation of insulin, glucagon, and somatostatin secretion in vitro in the rat. *J Clin Invest.* 1987; 79:1191-1196.

561. Kurose T, Seino Y, Nishi S, et al. Mechanism of sympathetic neural regulation of insulin, somatostatin, and glucagon secretion. *Am J Physiol.* 1990;251:E220-E227.

562. Woods S, Porte DJ. Neural control of the endocrine pancreas. *Physiol Rev.* 1974;54:596-619.

563. Bloom SR, Edwards A. Certain pharmacological characteristics of the release of pancreatic glucagon in response to stimulation of the splanchnic nerves. *J Physiol (Lond).* 1975;280:25-35.

564. Porte D Jr, Girardier L, Seydoux J, et al. Neural regulation of insulin secretion in the dog. *J Clin Invest.* 1973;52:210-214.

565. Roy M, Lee KC, Jones MS, et al. Neural control of pancreatic insulin and somatostatin secretion. *Endocrinology.* 1984;115:770-775.

566. Skoglund G, Lundquist I, Ahren B. Selective α_2-adrenoceptor activation by clonidine: effects on $^{45}Ca^{2+}$ efflux and insulin secretion from isolated rat islets. *Acta Physiol Scand.* 1988;132:289-296.

567. Ahrén B. Autonomic regulation of islet hormone secretion: implications for health and disease. *Diabetologia.* 2000;43:393-410.

568. Pettersson M, Ahrén B. Calcitonin gene-related peptide inhibits insulin secretion: studies on ion fluxes and cyclic AMP in isolated rat islets. *Diabetes Res Clin Pract.* 1990;15:9-14.

569. Pettersson M, Ahrén B, Bottcher G, et al. Calcitonin gene-related peptide: occurrence in pancreatic islets in the mouse and the rat and inhibition of insulin secretion in the mouse. *Diabetologia.* 1986; 119:865-869.

570. Ahrén B, Mårtensson H, Nobin A. Effects of calcitonin gene-related peptide (CGRP) on islet hormone secretion in the pig. *Diabetologia.* 1987;30:354-359.

571. Lundquist I, Sundler F, Ahrén B, et al. Somatostatin, pancreatic polypeptide, substance P, and neurotensin: cellular distribution and effects on stimulated insulin secretion in the mouse. *Endocrinology.* 1979; 104:832-838.

572. Hermansen K. Effects of substance P and other peptides on the release of somatostatin, insulin and glucagon in vitro. *Endocrinology.* 1980; 107:256-261.

573. Larrimer J, Mazzaferri EL, Cataland S, et al. Effect of atropine on glucose-stimulated gastric inhibitory polypeptide. *Diabetes.* 1978;27: 638-642.

574. Rocca A, Brubaker P. Role of the vagus nerve in mediating proximal nutrient-induced glucagon-like peptide-1 secretion. *Endocrinology.* 1999;140:1687-1694.

575. Flaten O, Sand T, Myren J. β-Adrenergic stimulation and blockade of the release of gastric inhibitory polypeptide and insulin in man. *Scand J Gastroenterol.* 1982;17:283-288.

576. Claustre J, Brechet S, Plaisancie P, et al. Stimulatory effect of β-adrenergic agonists on ileal L cell secretion and modulation by α-adrenergic activation. *J Endocrinol.* 1999;162:271-278.

577. Kruszynska Y, Home PD, Hanning I, et al. Basal and 24-h C-peptide and insulin secretion rate in normal man. *Diabetologia.* 1987;30:16-21.

578. Polonsky KS, Given BD, Van Cauter E. Twenty-four-hour profiles and pulsatile patterns of insulin secretion in normal and obese subjects. *J Clin Invest.* 1988;81:442-448.

579. Polonsky KS. The beta-cell in diabetes: from molecular genetics to clinical research. Lilly Lecture 1994. *Diabetes.* 1995;44:705-717.

580. Lang DA, Matthews DR, Peto J, et al. Cyclic oscillations of basal plasma glucose and insulin concentrations in human beings. *N Engl J Med.* 1979;301:1023-1027.

581. Hansen BC, Jen KC, Belbez Pek S, et al. Rapid oscillations in plasma insulin, glucagon, and glucose in obese and normal weight humans. *J Clin Endocrinol Metab.* 1982;54:785-792.

582. Matthews DR, Lang DA, Burnett MA, et al. Control of pulsatile insulin secretion in man. *Diabetologia.* 1983;24:231-237.

583. O'Meara NM, Sturis J, Van Cauter E, et al. Lack of control by glucose of ultradian insulin secretory oscillations in impaired glucose tolerance and in non-insulin-dependent diabetes mellitus. *J Clin Invest.* 1993;92: 262-271.

584. Porksen N, Grafte B, Nyholm B, et al. Glucagon-like peptide 1 increases mass but not frequency or orderliness of pulsatile insulin secretion. *Diabetes.* 1998;47:45-49.

585. Porksen N, Nyholm B, Veldhuis JD, et al. In humans at least 75% of insulin secretion arises from punctuated insulin secretory bursts. *Am J Physiol.* 1997;273:E908-E914.

586. Porksen N, Hussain MA, Bianda TL, et al. IGF-I inhibits burst mass of pulsatile insulin secretion at supraphysiological and low IGF-I infusion rates. *Am J Physiol.* 1997;272:E352-E358.

587. Porksen NK, Munn SR, Steers JL, et al. Mechanisms of sulfonylurea's stimulation of insulin secretion in vivo: selective amplification of insulin secretory burst mass. *Diabetes.* 1996;45:1792-1797.

588. Porksen N, Munn S, Steers J, et al. Effects of glucose ingestion versus infusion on pulsatile insulin secretion: the incretin effect is achieved by amplification of insulin secretory burst mass. *Diabetes.* 1996;45: 1317-1323.

589. O'Rahilly S, Turner RC, Matthews DR. Impaired pulsatile secretion of insulin in relatives of patients with non-insulin-dependent diabetes. *N Engl J Med.* 1988;318:1225-1230.

590. Van Cauter E. Estimating false-positive and false-negative errors in analyses of hormonal pulsatility. *Am J Physiol.* 1988;254:E786-E794.

591. Pincus SM. Quantification of evolution from order to randomness in practical time series analysis. *Methods Enzymol.* 1994;240:68-89.

592. Jaspan JB, Lever E, Polonsky KS, et al. In vivo pulsatility of pancreatic islet peptides. *Am J Physiol.* 1986;251:E215-E226.

593. Matthews DR, Naylor BA, Jones RG, et al. Pulsatile insulin has greater hypoglycemic effect than continuous delivery. *Diabetes.* 1983;32: 617-621.

594. Bratusch-Marrain PR, Komjati M, Waldhausl WK. Efficacy of pulsatile versus continuous insulin administration on hepatic glucose production and glucose utilization in type I diabetic humans. *Diabetes.* 1986;35:922-926.

595. Ward GM, Walters JM, Aitken PM, et al. Effects of prolonged pulsatile hyperinsulinemia in humans: enhancement of insulin sensitivity. *Diabetes.* 1990;39:501-507.

596. Sonnenberg GE, Hoffmann RG, Johnson CP, et al. Low- and high-frequency insulin secretion pulses in normal subjects and pancreas transplant recipients: role of extrinsic innervation. *J Clin Invest.* 1992; 90:545-553.

597. Blackman JD, Polonsky KS, Jaspan JB, et al. Insulin secretory profiles and C-peptide clearance kinetics at 6 months and 2 years after kidney-pancreas transplantation. *Diabetes.* 1992;41:1346-1354.

598. Sturis J, Polonsky KS, Mosekilde E, et al. Computer model for mechanisms underlying ultradian oscillations of insulin and glucose. *Am J Physiol.* 1991;260:E801-E809.

599. Sturis J, Van Cauter E, Blackman JD, et al. Entrainment of pulsatile insulin secretion by oscillatory glucose infusion. *J Clin Invest.* 1991; 87:439-445.

600. Jarrett RJ, Baker IA, Keen H, et al. Diurnal variation in oral glucose tolerance: blood sugar and plasma insulin levels morning, afternoon, and evening. *Br Med J.* 1972;1:199-201.

601. Aparicio NJ, Puchulu FE, Gagliardino JJ, et al. Circadian variation of the blood glucose, plasma insulin and human growth hormone levels in response to an oral glucose load in normal subjects. *Diabetes.* 1974;23:132-137.

602. Van Cauter E, Desir D, Decoster C, et al. Nocturnal decrease in glucose tolerance during constant glucose infusion. *J Clin Endocrinol Metab.* 1989;69:604-611.

603. Pick A, Clark J, Kubstrup P, et al. Role of apoptosis in failure of beta-cell mass compensation for insulin resistance and beta-cell defects in the male Zucker diabetic fatty rat. *Diabetes.* 1998;47:358-364.

604. Cockburn BN, Ostrega DM, Sturis J, et al. Changes in pancreatic islet glucokinase and hexokinase activities with increasing age, obesity, and the onset of diabetes. *Diabetes.* 1997;46:1434-1439.

605. Kahn SE, Prigeon RL, McCulloch DK, et al. Quantification of the relationship between insulin sensitivity and beta-cell function in human subjects: evidence for a hyperbolic function. *Diabetes.* 1993;42: 1663-1672.

606. Toffolo G, Bergman RN, Finegood DT, et al. Quantitative estimation of beta cell sensitivity to glucose in the intact organism: a minimal model of insulin kinetics in the dog. *Diabetes.* 1980;29:979-990.

607. Polonsky KS, Given BD, Hirsch L, et al. Quantitative study of insulin secretion and clearance in normal and obese subjects. *J Clin Invest.* 1988;81:435-441.

608. Jones CN, Pei D, Staris P, et al. Alterations in the glucose-stimulated insulin secretory dose-response curve and in insulin clearance in nondiabetic insulin-resistant individuals. *J Clin Endocrinol Metab.* 1997;82: 1834-1838.

609. Buchanan TA, Metzger BE, Freinkel N, et al. Insulin sensitivity and B-cell responsiveness to glucose during late pregnancy in lean and

moderately obese women with normal glucose tolerance or mild gestational diabetes. *Am J Obstet Gynecol.* 1990;162:1008-1014.

610. Bergstrom RW, Wahl PW, Leonetti DL, et al. Association of fasting glucose levels with a delayed secretion of insulin after oral glucose in subjects with glucose intolerance. *J Clin Endocrinol Metab.* 1990;71:1447-1453.

611. Phillips DI, Clark PM, Hales CN, et al. Understanding oral glucose tolerance: comparison of glucose or insulin measurements during the oral glucose tolerance test with specific measurements of insulin resistance and insulin secretion. *Diabet Med.* 1994;11(3):286-292.

612. Byrne MM, Sturis J, Sobel RJ, et al. Elevated plasma glucose 2 h postchallenge predicts defects in beta-cell function. *Am J Physiol.* 1996;270:E572-E579.

613. Ahrén B, Pacini G. Impaired adaptation of first-phase insulin secretion in postmenopausal women with glucose intolerance. *Am J Physiol.* 1997;273:E701-E707.

614. Yoshioka N, Kuzuya T, Matsuda A, et al. Serum proinsulin levels at fasting and after oral glucose load in patients with type 2 (non-insulin-dependent) diabetes mellitus. *Diabetologia.* 1988;31:355-360.

615. Saad MF, Kahn SE, Nelson RG, et al. Disproportionately elevated proinsulin in Pima Indians with noninsulin-dependent diabetes mellitus. *J Clin Endocrinol Metab.* 1990;70:1247-1253.

616. Reaven GM, Chen YD, Hollenbeck CB, et al. Plasma insulin, C-peptide, and proinsulin concentrations in obese and nonobese individuals with varying degrees of glucose tolerance. *J Clin Endocrinol Metab.* 1993;76:44-48.

617. Larsson H, Ahren B. Relative hyperproinsulinemia as a sign of islet dysfunction in women with impaired glucose tolerance. *J Clin Endocrinol Metab.* 1999;84:2068-2074.

618. Snehalatha C, Ramachandran A, Satyavani K, et al. Specific insulin and proinsulin concentrations in nondiabetic South Indians. *Metabolism.* 1998;47:230-233.

619. Birkeland KI, Torjesen PA, Eriksson J, et al. Hyperproinsulinemia of type II diabetes is not present before the development of hyperglycemia. *Diabetes Care.* 1994;17:1307-1310.

620. Inoue I, Takahashi K, Katayama S, et al. A higher proinsulin response to glucose loading predicts deteriorating fasting plasma glucose and worsening to diabetes in subjects with impaired glucose tolerance. *Diabet Med.* 1996;13:330-336.

621. Kahn SE, Leonetti DL, Prigeon RL, et al. Proinsulin levels predict the development of non-insulin-dependent diabetes mellitus (NIDDM) in Japanese-American men. *Diabet Med.* 1996;13(9 Suppl 6):S63-S66.

622. Heine RJ, Nijpels G, Mooy JM. New data on the rate of progression of impaired glucose tolerance to NIDDM and predicting factors. *Diabet Med.* 1996;13(3 Suppl 2):S12-S14.

623. Porte D Jr. Clinical importance of insulin secretion and its interaction with insulin resistance in the treatment of type 2 diabetes mellitus and its complications. *Diabetes Metab Res Rev.* 2001;17:181-188.

624. Ferner RE, Ashworth L, Tronier B, et al. Effects of short-term hyperglycemia on insulin secretion in normal humans. *Am J Physiol.* 1986;250:E655-E661.

625. O'Meara NM, Shapiro ET, Van Cauter E, et al. Effect of glyburide on beta cell responsiveness to glucose in non-insulin-dependent diabetes mellitus. *Am J Med.* 1990;89:11S-16S, discussion 51S-53S.

626. O'Rahilly SP, Nugent Z, Rudenski AS, et al. Beta-cell dysfunction, rather than insulin insensitivity, is the primary defect in familial type 2 diabetes. *Lancet.* 1986;2:360-364.

627. Barnett AH, Spiliopoulos AJ, Pyke DA, et al. Metabolic studies in unaffected co-twins of non-insulin-dependent diabetics. *Br Med J (Clin Res Ed).* 1981;282:1656-1658.

628. Gerich JE. The genetic basis of type 2 diabetes mellitus: impaired insulin secretion versus impaired insulin sensitivity. *Endocr Rev.* 1998;19:491-503.

629. Kosaka K, Hagura R, Kuzuya T. Insulin responses in equivocal and definite diabetes, with special reference to subjects who had mild glucose tolerance but later developed definite diabetes. *Diabetes.* 1977;26:944-952.

630. Efendic S, Luft R, Wajngot A. Aspects of the pathogenesis of type 2 diabetes. *Endocr Rev.* 1984;5:395-410.

631. Ward WK, Johnston CL, Beard JC, et al. Insulin resistance and impaired insulin secretion in subjects with histories of gestational diabetes mellitus. *Diabetes.* 1985;34:861-869.

632. O'Sullivan JB. Body weight and subsequent diabetes mellitus. *JAMA.* 1982;248:949-952.

633. Clark PM, Levy JL, Cox L, et al. Immunoradiometric assay of insulin, intact proinsulin and 32-33 split proinsulin and radioimmunoassay of insulin in diet-treated type 2 (non-insulin-dependent) diabetic subjects. *Diabetologia.* 1992;35:469-474.

634. Polonsky KS, Given BD, Hirsch LJ, et al. Abnormal patterns of insulin secretion in non-insulin-dependent diabetes mellitus. *N Engl J Med.* 1988;318:1231-1239.

635. Block MB, Rosenfield RL, Mako ME, et al. Sequential changes in beta-cell function in insulin-treated diabetic patients assessed by C-peptide immunoreactivity. *N Engl J Med.* 1973;288:1144-1148.

636. Shapiro ET, Van Cauter E, Tillel H, et al. *J Clin Endocrinol Metab.* 1989;69(3):571-576.

637. Cavaghan MK, Ehrmann DA, Byrne MM, et al. Treatment with the oral antidiabetic agent troglitazone improves beta cell responses to glucose in subjects with impaired glucose tolerance. *J Clin Invest.* 1997;100:530-537.

638. Villareal DT, Koster JC, Robertson H, et al. Kir6.2 variant E23K increases ATP-sensitive K+ channel activitiy and is associated with impaired insulin release and enhanced insulin sensitivity in adults with normal glucose tolerance. *Diabetes.* 2009;58:1869-1878.

639. Stride A, Ellard S, Clark P, et al. β-Cell dysfunction, insulin sensitivity, and glycosuria precede diabetes in hepatocyte nuclear factor-1α mutation carriers. *Diabetes Care.* 2005;28:1751-1756.

640. Schafer SA, Tschritter O, Machicao F, et al. Impaired glucagon-like peptide-1-induced insulin secretion in carriers of transcription factor 7-like 2 (TCF7L2) gene polymorphisms. *Diabetologia.* 2007;50:2443-2450.

641. Ingalls AM, Dickie MM, Snell GD. Obese, a new mutation in the house mouse. *Obes Res.* 1996;4:101.

642. Zhang Y, Proenca R, Maffei M, et al. Positional cloning of the mouse obese gene and its human homologue. *Nature.* 1994;372:425-432.

643. Pelleymounter MA, Cullen MJ, Baker MB, et al. Effects of the obese gene product on body weight regulation in ob/ob mice. *Science.* 1995;269:540-543.

644. Halaas JL, Gajiwala KS, Maffei M, et al. Weight-reducing effects of the plasma protein encoded by the obese gene. *Science.* 1995;269:543-546.

645. Friedman JM, Halaas JL. Leptin and the regulation of body weight in mammals. *Nature.* 1998;395:763-770.

646. Friedman JM. Leptin and the regulation of body weight. *Harvey Lect.* 1999-2000;95:107-136.

647. Halaas JL, Boozer C, Blair-West J, et al. Physiological response to long-term peripheral and central leptin infusion in lean and obese mice. *Proc Natl Acad Sci U S A.* 1997;94:8878-8883.

648. Friedman JM. The alphabet of weight control. *Nature.* 1997;385:119-120.

649. Friedman JM. Leptin, leptin receptors and the control of body weight. *Eur J Med Res.* 1997;2:7-13.

650. Kerouz NJ, Horsch D, Pons S, et al. Differential regulation of insulin receptor substrates-1 and -2 (IRS-1 and IRS-2) and phosphatidylinositol 3-kinase isoforms in liver and muscle of the obese diabetic (ob/ob) mouse. *J Clin Invest.* 1997;100:3164-3172.

651. Genuth SM, Przybylski RJ, Rosenberg DM. Insulin resistance in genetically obese, hyperglycemic mice. *Endocrinology.* 1971;88:1230-1238.

652. Herberg L, Coleman DL. Laboratory animals exhibiting obesity and diabetes syndromes. *Metabolism.* 1977;26(1):59-99.

653. Lee GH, Proenca R, Montez JM, et al. Abnormal splicing of the leptin receptor in diabetic mice. *Nature.* 1996;379:632-635.

654. Chen H, Charlat O, Tartaglia LA, et al. Evidence that the diabetes gene encodes the leptin receptor: identification of a mutation in the leptin receptor gene in db/db mice. *Cell.* 1996;84:491-495.

655. Coleman DL, Hummel KP. Hyperinsulinemia in pre-weaning diabetes (db) mice. *Diabetologia.* 1974;10(Suppl):607-610.

656. Like AA, Chick WL. Studies in the diabetic mutant mouse. I. Light microscopy and radioautography of pancreatic islets. *Diabetologia.* 1970;6:207-215.

657. Lavine RL, Chick WL, Like AA, et al. Glucose tolerance and insulin secretion in neonatal and adult mice. *Diabetes.* 1971;20:134-139.

658. Like AA, Chick WL. Studies in the diabetic mutant mouse: II. Electron microscopy of pancreatic islets. *Diabetologia.* 1970;6:216-242.

659. Shargill NS, Tatoyan A, el-Rafai MF, et al. Impaired insulin receptor phosphorylation in skeletal muscle membranes of db/db mice: the use of a novel skeletal muscle plasma membrane preparation to compare insulin binding and stimulation of receptor phosphorylation. *Biochem Biophys Res Commun.* 1986;137:286-294.

660. Cantello BC, Cawthorne MA, Cottam GP, et al. [[omega-(heterocyclylamino)alkoxy]benzyl]-2,4-thiazolidinediones as potent antihyperglycemic agents. *J Med Chem.* 1994;37(23):3977-3985.

661. Lohray BB, Bhushan V, Rao BP, et al. Novel euglycemic and hypolipidemic agents: 1. *J Med Chem.* 1998;41:1619-1630.

662. Frigeri LG, Wolff GL, Robel G. Impairment of glucose tolerance in yellow (Avy/A) (BALB/c X VY) F-1 hybrid mice by hyperglycemic peptide(s) from human pituitary glands. *Endocrinology.* 1983;113:2097-2105.

663. Warbritton A, Gill AM, Yen TT, et al. Pancreatic islet cells in preobese yellow Avy/-mice: relation to adult hyperinsulinemia and obesity. *Proc Soc Exp Biol Med.* 1994;206:145-151.

664. Michaud EJ, Bultman SJ, Klebig ML, et al. A molecular model for the genetic and phenotypic characteristics of the mouse lethal yellow (Ay) mutation. *Proc Natl Acad Sci U S A.* 1994;91:2562-2566.

665. Claycombe KJ, Wang Y, Jones BH, et al. Transcriptional regulation of the adipocyte fatty acid synthase gene by agouti: interaction with insulin. *Physiol Genomics.* 2000;3:157-162.

666. Claycombe KJ, Wang Y, Jones BH, et al. Regulation of leptin by agouti. *Physiol Genomics.* 2000;2:101-105.

667. Kondo ZK, Nozawa K, Tomito T, et al. Inbred strains resulting from Japanese mice. *Bull Exp Anim.* 1957;5:107-116.

668. Iwatsuka H, Shino A, Suzuoki Z. General survey of diabetic features of yellow KK mice. *Endocrinol Jpn.* 1970;17:23-35.

669. Matsuo T, Shino A, Iwatsuka H, et al. Induction of overt diabetes in KK mice by dietary means. *Endocrinol Jpn.* 1970;17:477-488.

670. Veroni MC, Proietto J, Larkins RG. Evolution of insulin resistance in New Zealand obese mice. *Diabetes.* 1991;40:1480-1487.

671. Cameron DP, Opat F, Insch S. Studies of immunoreactive insulin secretion in NZO mice in vivo. *Diabetologia.* 1974;10(Suppl):649-654.

672. Bielschowsky M, Bielschowsky F. A new strain of mice with hereditary obesity. *Proc Univ Otago Med Sch.* 1953;31:29-31.

673. Leiter EH, Reifsnyder PC, Flurkey K, et al. NIDDM genes in mice: deleterious synergism by both parental genomes contributes to diabetogenic thresholds. *Diabetes.* 1998;47:1287-1295.

674. Thorburn A, Andrikopoulos S, Proietto J. Defects in liver and muscle glycogen metabolism in neonatal and adult New Zealand obese mice. *Metabolism.* 1995;44:1298-1302.

675. Andrikopoulos S, Proietto J. The biochemical basis of increased hepatic glucose production in a mouse model of type 2 (non-insulin-dependent) diabetes mellitus. *Diabetologia.* 1995;38:1389-1396.

676. Andrikopoulos S, Rosella G, Kacmarczyk SJ, et al. Impaired regulation of hepatic fructose-1,6-biphosphatase in the New Zealand obese mouse: an acquired defect. *Metabolism.* 1996;45:622-626.

677. Larkins RG, Simeonova L, Veroni MC. Glucose utilization in relation to insulin secretion in NZO and C57Bl mouse islets. *Endocrinology.* 1980;107:1634-1638.

678. Melez KA, Harrison LC, Gilliam JN, et al. Diabetes is associated with autoimmunity in the New Zealand obese (NZO) mouse. *Diabetes.* 1980;29:835-840.

679. Melez KA, Reeves JP, Steinberg AD. Regulation of the expression of autoimmunity in NZB × NZW F1 mice by sex hormones. *J Immunopharmacol.* 1978;1:27-42.

680. Harrison LC, Itin A. A possible mechanism for insulin resistance and hyperglycaemia in NZO mice. *Nature.* 1979;279:334-336.

681. Reifsnyder PC, Churchill G, Leiter EH. Maternal environment and genotype interact to establish diabesity in mice. *Genome Res.* 2000;10:1568-1578.

682. Blair SC, Caterson ID, Cooney GJ. Glucose and lipid metabolism in the gold-thioglucose injected mouse model of diabesity. In: Shafir E, ed. *Lessons from Animal Diabetes VI.* Boston, MA: Birkhauser; 1996:239-267.

683. Burant CF, Sreenan S, Hirano K, et al. Troglitazone action is independent of adipose tissue. *J Clin Invest.* 1997;100:2900-2908.

684. Ross SR, Graves RA, Choy L, et al. Transgenic mouse models of disease: altering adipose tissue function in vivo. *Ann N Y Acad Sci.* 1995;758:297-313.

685. Shimomura I, Hammer RE, Richardson JA, et al. Insulin resistance and diabetes mellitus in transgenic mice expressing nuclear SREBP-1c in adipose tissue: model for congenital generalized lipodystrophy. *Genes Dev.* 1998;12:3182-3194.

686. Reitman ML, Gavrilova O. A-ZIP/F-1 mice lacking white fat: a model for understanding lipoatrophic diabetes. *Int J Obes Relat Metab Disord.* 2000;24(Suppl 4):S11-S14.

687. Gavrilova O, Marcus-Samuels B, Graham D, et al. Surgical implantation of adipose tissue reverses diabetes in lipoatrophic mice. *J Clin Invest.* 2000;105:271-278.

688. Shimomura I, Hammer RE, Ikemoto S, et al. Leptin reverses insulin resistance and diabetes mellitus in mice with congenital lipodystrophy. *Nature.* 1999;401:73-76.

689. Arioglu E, Duncan-Marin J, Sebring N, et al. Efficacy and safety of troglitazone in the treatment of lipodystrophy syndromes. *Ann Intern Med.* 2000;133:263-274.

690. Surwit RS, Feinglos MN, Rodin J, et al. Differential effects of fat and sucrose on the development of obesity and diabetes in C57BL/6J and A/J mice. *Metabolism.* 1995;44:645-651.

691. Rebuffe-Scrive M, Surwit R, Feinglos M, et al. Regional fat distribution and metabolism in a new mouse model (C57BL/6J) of non-insulin-dependent diabetes mellitus. *Metabolism.* 1993;42:1405-1409.

692. Wencel HE, Smothers C, Opara ED, et al. Impaired second phase insulin response of diabetes-prone C57BL/6J mouse islets. *Physiol Behav.* 1995;57:1215-1220.

693. Lee SK, Opara EC, Surwit RS, et al. Defective glucose-stimulated insulin release from perifused islets of C57BL/6J mice. *Pancreas.* 1995;11:206-211.

694. Parekh PI, Petro AE, Tiller JM, et al. Reversal of diet-induced obesity and diabetes in C57BL/6J mice. *Metabolism.* 1998;47:1089-1096.

695. Phillips MS, Liu Q, Hammond HA, et al. Leptin receptor missense mutation in the fatty Zucker rat. *Nat Genet.* 1996;13:18-19.

696. Chua SC Jr, White DW, Wu-Peng XS, et al. Phenotype of fatty due to Gln269Pro mutation in the leptin receptor (Lepr). *Diabetes.* 1996;45:1141-1143.

697. White DW, Wang DW, Chua SC Jr, et al. Constitutive and impaired signaling of leptin receptors containing the Gln → Pro extracellular domain fatty mutation. *Proc Natl Acad Sci U S A.* 1997;94:10657-10662.

698. Peterson RG, Shaw WN, Neel M, et al. Zucker diabetic fatty rat as a model for non-insulin-dependent diabetes mellitus. *Inst Lab Anim Res News.* 1990;32:16-19.

699. Janssen SW, Hermus AR, Lange WP, et al. Progressive histopathological changes in pancreatic islets of Zucker diabetic fatty rats. *Exp Clin Endocrinol Diabetes.* 2001;109:273-282.

700. Zhou YP, Cockburn BN, Pugh W, et al. Basal insulin hypersecretion in insulin-resistant Zucker diabetic and Zucker fatty rats: role of enhanced fuel metabolism. *Metabolism.* 1999;48:857-864.

701. Unger RH. Lipotoxicity in the pathogenesis of obesity-dependent NIDDM: genetic and clinical implications. *Diabetes.* 1995;44:863-870.

702. Corsetti JP, Sparks JD, Peterson RG, et al. Effect of dietary fat on the development of non-insulin dependent diabetes mellitus in obese Zucker diabetic fatty male and female rats. *Atherosclerosis.* 2000;148(2):231-241.

703. Griffen SC, Wang J, German MS. A genetic defect in beta-cell gene expression segregates independently from the fa locus in the ZDF rat. *Diabetes.* 2001;50:63-68.

704. Johnson JH, Ogawa A, Chen L, et al. Underexpression of beta cell high K_m glucose transporters in noninsulin-dependent diabetes. *Science.* 1990;250:546-549.

705. Orci L, Ravazzola M, Baetens D, et al. Evidence that down-regulation of beta-cell glucose transporters in non-insulin-dependent diabetes may be the cause of diabetic hyperglycemia. *Proc Natl Acad Sci U S A.* 1990;87:9953-9957.

706. Lee Y, Hirose H, Zhou YT, et al. Increased lipogenic capacity of the islets of obese rats: a role in the pathogenesis of NIDDM. *Diabetes.* 1997;46:408-413.

707. Sreenan S, Keck S, Fuller T, et al. Effects of troglitazone on substrate storage and utilization in insulin-resistant rats. *Am J Physiol.* 1999;276:E1119-E1129.

708. Shimabukuro M, Ohneda M, Lee Y, et al. Role of nitric oxide in obesity-induced beta cell disease. *J Clin Invest.* 1997;100:290-295.

709. Shimabukuro M, Higa M, Zhou YT, et al. Lipoapoptosis in beta-cells of obese prediabetic fa/fa rats: role of serine palmitoyltransferase overexpression. *J Biol Chem.* 1998;273:32487-32490.

710. Tokuyama Y, Sturis J, DePaoli AM, et al. Evolution of beta-cell dysfunction in the male Zucker diabetic fatty rat. *Diabetes.* 1995;44:1447-1457.

711. Sreenan S, Sturis J, Pugh W, et al. Prevention of hyperglycemia in the Zucker diabetic fatty rat by treatment with metformin or troglitazone. *Am J Physiol.* 1996;271:E742-E747.

712. Goto Y, Kakizaki M, Masaki N. Spontaneous diabetes produced by selective breeding of normal Wistar rats. *Proc Jpn Acad.* 1975;51:80-85.

713. Movassat J, Saulnier C, Serradas P, et al. Impaired development of pancreatic beta-cell mass is a primary event during the progression to diabetes in the GK rat. *Diabetologia.* 1997;40:916-925.

714. Movassat J, Saulnier C, Portha B. Beta-cell mass depletion precedes the onset of hyperglycaemia in the GK rat, a genetic model of non-insulin-dependent diabetes mellitus. *Diabet Metab.* 1995;21:365-370.

715. Ostenson CG, Khan A, Abdel-Halim SM, et al. Abnormal insulin secretion and glucose metabolism in pancreatic islets from the spontaneously diabetic GK rat. *Diabetologia.* 1993;36:3-8.

716. Ostenson CG, Abdel-Halim SM, Rasschaert J, et al. Deficient activity of FAD-linked glycerophosphate dehydrogenase in islets of GK rats. *Diabetologia.* 1993;36:722-726.

717. Abdel-Halim SM, Guenifi A, Efendic S, et al. Both somatostatin and insulin responses to glucose are impaired in the perfused pancreas of the spontaneously noninsulin-dependent diabetic GK (Goto-Kakizaki) rats. *Acta Physiol Scand.* 1993;148:219-226.

718. Nagamatsu S, Nakamichi Y, Yamamura C, et al. Decreased expression of t-SNARE, syntaxin 1, and SNAP-25 in pancreatic beta-cells is involved in impaired insulin secretion from diabetic GK rat islets: restoration of decreased t-SNARE proteins improves impaired insulin secretion. *Diabetes.* 1999;48:2367-2373.

719. Guenifi A, Portela-Gomes GM, Grimelius L, et al. Adenylyl cyclase isoform expression in non-diabetic and diabetic Goto-Kakizaki (GK) rat pancreas: evidence for distinct overexpression of type-8 adenylyl cyclase in diabetic GK rat islets. *Histochem Cell Biol.* 2000;113:81-89.

720. Song XM, Kawano Y, Krook A, et al. Muscle fiber type-specific defects in insulin signal transduction to glucose transport in diabetic GK rats. *Diabetes.* 1999;48:664-670.

721. Begum N, Ragolia L. Altered regulation of insulin signaling components in adipocytes of insulin-resistant type II diabetic Goto-Kakizaki rats. *Metabolism.* 1998;47:54-62.

722. Berdanier CD. The BHE strain to rat: an example of the role of inheritance in determining metabolic controls. *Fed Proc.* 1976;35(11):2295-2299.

723. Berdanier CD, Tobin RB, DeVore V. Effects of age, strain, and dietary carbohydrate on the hepatic metabolism of male rats. *J Nutr.* 1979;109:261-271.

724. Mathews CE, McGraw RA, Dean R, et al. Inheritance of a mitochondrial DNA defect and impaired glucose tolerance in BHE/Cdb rats. *Diabetologia.* 1999;42:35-40.

725. McCusker RH, Deaver OE Jr, Berdanier CD. Effect of sucrose or starch feeding on the hepatic mitochondrial activity of BHE and Wistar rats. *J Nutr.* 1983;113:1327-1334.

726. Borenshtein D, Ofri R, Werman M, et al. Cataract development in diabetic sand rats treated with alpha-lipoic acid and its gamma-linolenic acid conjugate. *Diabetes Metab Res Rev*. 2001;17:44-50.

727. Ikeda Y, Olsen GS, Ziv E, et al. Cellular mechanism of nutritionally induced insulin resistance in *Psammomys obesus*: overexpression of protein kinase Cepsilon in skeletal muscle precedes the onset of hyperinsulinemia and hyperglycemia. *Diabetes*. 2001;50(3):584-592.

728. Kanety H, Moshe S, Shafrir E, et al. Hyperinsulinemia induces a reversible impairment in insulin receptor function leading to diabetes in the sand rat model of non-insulin-dependent diabetes mellitus. *Proc Natl Acad Sci U S A*. 1994;91:1853-1857.

729. Kawano K, Hirashima T, Mori S, et al. Spontaneous long-term hyperglycemic rat with diabetic complications. Otsuka Long-Evans Tokushima Fatty (OLETF) strain. *Diabetes*. 1992;41:1422-1428.

730. Moralejo DH, Ogino T, Zhu M, et al. A major quantitative trait locus co-localizing with cholecystokinin type A receptor gene influences poor pancreatic proliferation in a spontaneously diabetogenic rat. *Mamm Genome*. 1998;9(10):794-798.

731. Takiguchi S, Takata Y, Takahashi N, et al. A disrupted cholecystokinin A receptor gene induces diabetes in obese rats synergistically with *ODB1* gene. *Am J Physiol*. 1998;274:E265-E270.

732. Takiguchi S, Takata Y, Funakoshi A, et al. Disrupted cholecystokinin type-A receptor (CCKAR) gene in OLETF rats. *Gene*. 1997;197:169-175.

733. Hirashima T, Kawano K, Mori S, et al. A diabetogenic gene, ODB2, identified on chromosome 14 of the OLETF rat and its synergistic action with ODB1. *Biochem Biophys Res Commun*. 1996;224:420-425.

734. Shi K, Mizuno A, Sano T, et al. Sexual difference in the incidence of diabetes mellitus in Otsuka-Long-Evans-Tokushima-Fatty rats: effects of castration and sex hormone replacement on its incidence. *Metabolism*. 1994;43:1214-1220.

735. Ishida K, Mizuno A, Murakami T, et al. Obesity is necessary but not sufficient for the development of diabetes mellitus. *Metabolism*. 1996;45:1288-1295.

736. Okauchi N, Mizuno A, Zhu M, et al. Effects of obesity and inheritance on the development of non-insulin-dependent diabetes mellitus in Otsuka-Long-Evans-Tokushima fatty rats. *Diabetes Res Clin Pract*. 1995;29:1-10.

737. Kosegawa I, Chen S, Awata T, et al. Troglitazone and metformin, but not glibenclamide, decrease blood pressure in Otsuka Long Evans Tokushima fatty rats. *Clin Exp Hypertens*. 1999;21:199-211.

738. Triadou N, Portha B, Picon L, et al. Experimental chemical diabetes and pregnancy in the rat: evolution of glucose tolerance and insulin response. *Diabetes*. 1982;31:75-79.

739. Portha B, Picon L, Rosselin G. Chemical diabetes in the adult rat as the spontaneous evolution of neonatal diabetes. *Diabetologia*. 1979;17:371-377.

740. Kodama T, Iwase M, Nunoi K, et al. A new diabetes model induced by neonatal alloxan treatment in rats. *Diabetes Res Clin Pract*. 1993;20:183-189.

741. Iwase M, Nunoi K, Wakisaka M, et al. Spontaneous recovery from non-insulin-dependent diabetes mellitus induced by neonatal streptozotocin treatment in spontaneously hypertensive rats. *Metabolism*. 1991;40:10-14.

742. American Diabetes Association. Clinical Practice Recommendations. Available online at <http://professional.diabetes.org/CPR_search.aspx>.

743. Gregg EW, Li Y, Wang J, et al. Changes in diabetes-related complications in the United States, 1990-2010. *N Engl J Med*. 2014;370:1514-1523.

744. Grintsova O, Maier W, Mielck A. Inequalities in health care among patients with type 2 diabetes by individual socio-economic status (SES) and regional deprivation: a systematic literature review. *Int J Equity Health*. 2014;13:43.

745. U.K. Prospective Diabetes Study (UKPDS) Group. Intensive blood-glucose control with sulphonylureas or insulin compared with conventional treatment and risk of complications in patients with type 2 diabetes (UKPDS 33). *Lancet*. 1998;352:837-853.

746. U.K. Prospective Diabetes Study (UKPDS) Group. Effect of intensive blood-glucose control with metformin on complications in overweight patients with type 2 diabetes (UKPDS 34). *Lancet*. 1998;352:854-865.

747. Ohkubo Y, Kishikawa H, Araki E, et al. Intensive insulin therapy prevents the progression of diabetic microvascular complications in Japanese patients with non-insulin-dependent diabetes mellitus: a randomized prospective 6-year study. *Diabetes Res Clin Pract*. 1995;28:103-117.

748. Action to Control Cardiovascular Risk in Diabetes Study Group, Gerstein HC, Miller ME, Byington RP, et al. Effects of intensive glucose lowering in type 2 diabetes. *N Engl J Med*. 2008;358(24):2545-2559.

749. ADVANCE Collaborative Group, Patel A, MacMahon S, Chalmers J, et al. Intensive blood glucose control and vascular outcomes in patients with type 2 diabetes. *N Engl J Med*. 2008;358:2560-2572.

750. Duckworth W, Abraira C, Moritz T, et al. Intensive glucose control and complications in American veterans with type 2 diabetes. *N Engl J Med*. 2009;360:129-139.

751. Holman RR, Paul SK, Bethel MA, et al. 10-Year follow-up of intensive glucose control in type 2 diabetes. *N Engl J Med*. 2008;359:1577-1589.

752. Ray KK, Seshasai SR, Wijesuriya S, et al. Effect of intensive control of glucose on cardiovascular outcomes and death in patients with diabetes mellitus: a meta-analysis of randomised controlled trials. *Lancet*. 2009;373:1765-1772.

753. Riddle MC, Ambrosius WT, Brillon DJ, et al. Epidemiologic relationships between A1C and all-cause mortality during a median 3.4-year follow-up of glycemic treatment in the ACCORD trial. *Diabetes Care*. 2010;33:983-990.

754. Hempe JM, Liu S, Myers L, et al. The hemoglobin glycation index identifies subpopulations with harms or benefits from intensive treatment in the ACCORD trial. *Diabetes Care*. 2015;38:1067-1074.

755. Handelsman Y, Bloomgarden ZT, Grunberger G, et al. American Association of Clinical Endocrinologists and American College of Endocrinology—clinical practice guidelines for developing a diabetes mellitus comprehensive care plan, 2015. *Endocr Pract*. 2015;21:1-87.

756. Rohlfing CL, Wiedmeyer HM, Little RR, et al. Defining the relationship between plasma glucose and HbA$_{1c}$: analysis of glucose profiles and HbA$_{1c}$ in the Diabetes Control and Complications Trial. *Diabetes Care*. 2002;25:275-278.

757. Service FJ, Hall LD, Westland RE, et al. Effects of size, time of day and sequence of meal ingestion on carbohydrate tolerance in normal subjects. *Diabetologia*. 1983;25:316-321.

758. American Diabetes Association. Postprandial blood glucose. *Diabetes Care*. 2001;24:775-778.

759. Haas L, Maryniuk M, Beck J, et al. 2012 Standards Revision Task Force. National standards for diabetes self-management education and support. *Diabetes Care*. 2014;37(Suppl 1):S144-S153.

760. Boren SA, Fitzner KA, Panhalkar PS, et al. Costs and benefits associated with diabetes education: a review of the literature. *Diabetes Educ*. 2009;35:72-96.

761. Delamater AM, Jacobson AM, Anderson B, et al. Psychosocial therapies in diabetes: report of the Psychosocial Therapies Working Group. *Diabetes Care*. 2001;24:1286-1292.

762. Bergenstal RM, Johnson M, Powers MA, et al. Adjust to target in type 2 diabetes: comparison of a simple algorithm with carbohydrate counting for adjustment of mealtime insulin glulisine. *Diabetes Care*. 2008;31:1305-1310.

763. Nahas R, Moher M. Complementary and alternative medicine for the treatment of type 2 diabetes. *Can Fam Physician*. 2009;55:591-596.

764. Naude CE, Schoonees A, Senekal M, et al. Low carbohydrate versus isoenergetic balanced diets for reducing weight and cardiovascular risk: a systematic review and meta-analysis. *PLoS ONE*. 2014;9(7):e100652.

765. Martínez-González MA, Salas-Salvadó J, Estruch R, et al. Benefits of the Mediterranean diet: insights from the PREDIMED study. *Prog Cardiovasc Dis*. 2015;58(1):50-60.

766. Diabetes Forecast: The Healthy Living Magazine. Alexandria, VA: American Diabetes Association. Available at <www.forecast.diabetes.org>.

767. Inzucchi SE, Bergenstal RM, Buse JB, et al. Management of hyperglycemia in type 2 diabetes, 2015: a patient-centered approach: update to a position statement of the American Diabetes Association and the European Association for the Study of Diabetes. *Diabetes Care*. 2015;38:140-149.

768. Madiraju AK, Erion DM, Rahimi Y, et al. Metformin suppresses gluconeogenesis by inhibiting mitochondrial glycerophosphate dehydrogenase. *Nature*. 2014;510:542-546.

769. Salpeter SR, Greyber E, Pasternak GA, et al. Risk of fatal and nonfatal lactic acidosis with metformin use in type 2 diabetes mellitus. *Cochrane Database Syst Rev*. 2010;(4):CD002967.

770. George JT, McKay GA. Establishing pragmatic estimated glomerular filtration rate thresholds to guide metformin prescribing: careful assessment of risks and benefits is required. *Diabet Med*. 2008;25:636-637.

771. Liu Q, Li S, Quan H, Li J. Vitamin B12 status in metformin treated patients: systematic review. *PLoS ONE*. 2014;9(6):e100379.

772. Goldberg RB, Kendall DM, Deeg MA, et al. GLAI Study Investigators. A comparison of lipid and glycemic effects of pioglitazone and rosiglitazone in patients with type 2 diabetes and dyslipidemia. *Diabetes Care*. 2005;28:1547-1554.

773. Dormandy JA, Charbonnel B, Eckland DJ, et al. Secondary prevention of macrovascular events in patients with type 2 diabetes in the PROactive Study (PROspective pioglitAzone Clinical Trial In macroVascular Events): a randomised controlled trial. *Lancet*. 2005;366:1279-1289.

774. Home PD, Pocock SJ, Beck-Nielsen H, et al. RECORD Study Team. Rosiglitazone evaluated for cardiovascular outcomes in oral agent combination therapy for type 2 diabetes (RECORD): a multicentre, randomised, open-label trial. *Lancet*. 2009;373:2125-2135.

775. Graham DJ, Ouellet-Hellstrom R, Macurdy TE, et al. Risk of acute myocardial infarction, stroke, heart failure, and death in elderly Medicare patients treated with rosiglitazone or pioglitazone. *JAMA*. 2010;304:411-418.

776. Kahn SE, Haffner SM, Heise MA, et al. ADOPT Study Group. Glycemic durability of rosiglitazone, metformin, or glyburide monotherapy. *N Engl J Med*. 2006;355:2427-2443.

777. Karalliedde J, Buckingham RE. Thiazolidinediones and their fluid-related adverse effects: facts, fiction and putative management strategies. *Drug Saf.* 2007;30:741-753.

778. Riche DM, King ST. Bone loss and fracture risk associated with thiazolidinedione therapy. *Pharmacotherapy.* 2010;30(7):716-727.

779. Ryder RE. Pioglitazone has a dubious bladder cancer risk but an undoubted cardiovascular benefit. *Diabet Med.* 2015;32:305-313.

780. Riddle MC. Sulfonylureas differ in effects on ischemic preconditioning: is it time to retire glyburide? *J Clin Endocrinol Metab.* 2003; 88(2):528-530.

781. Hanefeld M, Schaper F. Acarbose: oral anti-diabetes drug with additional cardiovascular benefits. *Expert Rev Cardiovasc Ther.* 2008;6: 153-163.

782. Campbell JE, Drucker DJ. Pharmacology, physiology, and mechanisms of incretin hormone action. *Cell Metab.* 2013;17:819-837.

783. Trujillo JM, Nuffer W, Ellis SL. GLP-1 receptor agonists: a review of head-to-head clinical studies. *Ther Adv Endocrinol Metab.* 2015;6: 19-28.

784. Ussher JR, Drucker DJ. Cardiovascular actions of incretin-based therapies. *Circ Res.* 2014;114:1788-1803.

785. Green JB, Bethel MA, Armstrong PW, et al. Effect of sitagliptin on cardiovascular outcomes in type 2 diabetes. *N Engl J Med.* 2015; 373(3):232-242.

786. Tahrani AA, Barnett AH, Bailey CJ. SGLT inhibitors in management of diabetes. *Lancet Diabetes Endocrinol.* 2013;1:140-151.

787. Scheen AJ. Pharmacodynamics, efficacy and safety of sodium-glucose co-transporter type 2 (SGLT2) inhibitors for the treatment of type 2 diabetes mellitus. *Drugs.* 2015;75:33-59.

788. Peters AL, Buschur EO, Buse JB, et al. Euglycemic diabetic ketoacidosis: a potential complication of treatment with sodium-glucose cotransporter 2 inhibition. *Diabetes Care.* [Epub 2015 Jun 15].

789. Maiorino MI, Petrizzo M, Capuano A, et al. The development of new basal insulins: is there any clinical advantage with their use in type 2 diabetes? *Expert Opin Biol Ther.* 2014;14(6):799-808.

790. Kugler AJ, Fabbio KL, Pham DQ, Nadeau DA. Inhaled technosphere insulin: a novel delivery system and formulation for the treatment of types 1 and 2 diabetes mellitus. *Pharmacotherapy.* 2015;35:298-314.

791. Meah F, Juneja R. Insulin tactics in type 2 diabetes. *Med Clin North Am.* 2015;99:157-186.

792. Home P, Riddle M, Cefalu WT, et al. Insulin therapy in people with type 2 diabetes: opportunities and challenges? *Diabetes Care.* 2014; 37(6):1499-1508.

793. Ryan G, Briscoe TA, Jobe L. Review of pramlintide as adjunctive therapy in treatment of type 1 and type 2 diabetes. *Drug Des Devel Ther.* 2009;2:203-214.

794. Fonseca VA, Handelsman Y, Staels B. Colesevelam lowers glucose and lipid levels in type 2 diabetes: the clinical evidence. *Diabetes Obes Metab.* 2010;12:384-392.

795. Gaziano JM, Cincotta AH, O'Connor CM, et al. Randomized clinical trial of quick-release bromocriptine among patients with type 2 diabetes on overall safety and cardiovascular outcomes. *Diabetes Care.* 2010;33:1503-1508.

796. Roe ED, Chamarthi B, Raskin P. Impact of bromocriptin-QR on glycemic control and daily insulin requirement in type 2 diabetes mellitus whose dysglycemia is poorly controlled on high-dose insulin. *J Diabetes Res.* 2015;2015:834-903.

797. Eng C, Kramer CK, Zinman B, Retnakaran R. Glucagon-like peptide-1 receptor agonist and basal insulin combination treatment for the management of type 2 diabetes: a systematic review and meta-analysis. *Lancet.* 2014;384:2228-2234.

798. <http://www.goodrx.com/>.

799. Medicare.gov website. 6 Ways to Lower Drug Costs. Available at <http://www.medicare.gov/part-d/costs/coverage-gap/ways-to-lower-drug-costs.html>.

800. BARI 2D Study Group, Frye RL, August P, Brooks MM, et al. A randomized trial of therapies for type 2 diabetes and coronary artery disease. *N Engl J Med.* 2009;360(24):2503-2515.

801. Henry RR, Rosenstock J, Logan D, et al. Continuous subcutaneous delivery of exenatide via ITCA 650 leads to sustained glycemic control and weight loss for 48 weeks in metformin-treated subjects with type 2 diabetes. *J Diabetes Complications.* 2014;28(3):393-398.

802. Holman RR, Farmer AJ, Davies MJ, et al., 4-T Study Group. Three-year efficacy of complex insulin regimens in type 2 diabetes. *N Engl J Med.* 2009;361:1736-1747.

803. Buse JB, Hroscikoski M. The case for a role for postprandial glucose monitoring in diabetes management. *J Fam Pract.* 1998;47(5 Suppl): S29-S36.

804. Chatterjee R, Narayan KM, Lipscomb J, et al. Screening adults for pre-diabetes and diabetes may be cost-saving. *Diabetes Care.* 2010;33: 1484-1490.

805. Narayan KM, Gregg EW, Engelgau MM, et al. Translation research for chronic disease: the case of diabetes. *Diabetes Care.* 2000;23: 1794-1798.

806. 2014 Report: Medicines in Development for Diabetes. Available at: <http://www.phrma.org/research/medicines-development-diabetes>.

807. Bailey CJ. The current drug treatment landscape for diabetes and perspectives for the future. *Clin Pharmacol Ther.* 2015;98(2):170-184.

Type 1 Diabetes Mellitus

MARK A. ATKINSON*

KEY POINTS

- Type 1 diabetes mellitus (T1DM) is a disorder resulting from a chronic autoimmune destruction of the insulin-producing pancreatic beta cells.
- Throughout the globe, the incidence of T1DM is increasing at 3% to 5% per year.
- The disorder is clearly polygenic (over 40 loci impacting susceptibility identified to date), yet over half of disease susceptibility for T1DM is provided by the major histocompatibility complex (MHC).
- The pancreas of T1DM patients possesses an islet immune infiltrate derived from a variety of immunologic phenotypes, is reduced in size and weight, and is subject to unusual exocrine features.
- The long-held model describing the natural history of T1DM has been extensively readdressed, and there is a greater appreciation for the disorder's heterogeneity in pathogenesis and symptomatic presentation.
- The risk for the disease can be ascertained through a combination of immunologic, genetic, and metabolic markers of disease.
- Extensive efforts continue to be directed at preventing and reversing the disease, but although there has been progress toward this goal, at present there is no universally accepted means for doing so in a public health care setting.

- There is a growing appreciation that T1DM, rather than being a singular disease, may be a heterogeneous disorder with a common phenotype at clinical presentation/diagnosis.
- Significant advances in terms of disease management, afforded by technological innovations related to insulin analogues and more, set the foundation for marked reductions in hemoglobin A_{1c} (HbA_{1c}) and improved diabetes care.
- Numerous metrics (costs, patient outcomes, etc.) demonstrate that specialists (endocrinologists) provide more effective care for those with T1DM than nonspecialists.

Where to begin to tell the story of the disorder we now refer to as T1DM represents somewhat of a literary challenge. Does one begin with the earliest writings scripted thousands of years ago conveying the disease's symptoms, or is it more fitting to describe exciting works performed in the 1800s and early 1900s that defined both the anatomy of and physiologic roles for the pancreas and insulin-secreting beta cells?[1,2] Other pieces of literature initiate their narrative on T1DM by sharing an account of the fast-paced and ultimately Nobel Prize–winning efforts in the 1920s by Banting and Best,[3] when the ability to purify insulin from animal pancreata brought forward a means to sustain life to those who, in the absence of such an intervention, met an early demise.

However, we have elected to begin this chapter by building on the story of a German pathologist named Martin Schmidt who, in 1902, noted a small peri-islet cellular infiltrate on microscopic evaluation of the pancreas obtained at autopsy from a 10-year-old child with diabetes.[4] This effort represented a key early investigation seeking to better define the pathogenesis of the disorder, a process that was continued by many over the ensuing century. Works shortly thereafter by Shields Warren in the 1920s drew attention to the relationship between this infiltrate and the age of diabetes onset.[5] The term used to define this pancreatic feature, *insulitis*, was coined in 1940 by yet another pathologist, Hanns von Meyenburg.[6] Studies of pancreatic disease over ensuing decades taught us much regarding this inflammatory lesion, including its relative infrequency in older individuals diagnosed with the disease, its association with reduction in beta-cell mass, the identification of *pseudoatrophic* islets (i.e., islets devoid of insulin-containing cells), a preferential targeting of insulitis for beta cells containing insulin, and many other findings eventually deemed seminal.[7-11] These conditions, when joined together with immunologic and genetic studies of living patients in the 1970s, noting the presence

---

*John Buse was a coauthor of this chapter but has chosen to withdraw his name owing to his disagreement with Reed Elsevier's handling of "An open letter for the people in Gaza" (Manduca P, Chalmers I, Summerfield D, Gilbert M, Ang S. An open letter for the people in Gaza. Lancet. 2014;384(9941):397-398).

of self-reactive antibodies (i.e., autoantibodies) against islet cells in persons with T1DM and that disease susceptibility was associated with MHC molecules known to influence immune system functions, formed three lines of evidence pointing to an autoimmune basis for T1DM.[12,13] Built on this foundation, this chapter will share current views on the autoimmune nature of T1DM, including its natural history and pathogenesis, as well as consider how this information is vital to the optimal diagnosis and care of individuals with the disease.

DIAGNOSIS

A diagnosis of diabetes has historically included an elevated fasting blood glucose level, any glucose value higher than 200 mg/dL or 11 mmol/L with symptoms of hyperglycemia, or an abnormal 2-hour oral glucose tolerance test (OGTT).[14] American Diabetes Association (ADA) guidelines for the diagnosis of diabetes were modified in 2009 to include an HbA$_{1c}$ value greater than 6.5%.[15] Under certain settings (e.g., obesity, racial status other than Caucasian) and particularly among adults, the diagnosis of T1DM versus type 2 diabetes mellitus (T2DM) can prove quite challenging. At present, the best criterion for separating the two disorders resides in laboratory identification of any one of a number of islet cell autoantibodies (also known as T1DM-associated autoantibodies; i.e., anti-insulin autoantibodies [IAA], anti–glutamic acid decarboxylase [GADA], anti–insulinoma-associated antigen-2 [IA-2A], or zinc-transporter 8 [ZnT8A]). Literally hundreds of studies over the past 2 decades have suggested that the presence of these autoantibodies provides high sensitivity for diagnosing persons with T1DM.[16-18] Indeed, more than 90% of Caucasian children presenting with diabetes express at least one of these four T1DM-associated autoantibodies.[19] However, among African-American and Latino children and adolescents in the United States diagnosed with diabetes, almost one half lack any T1DM-associated autoantibody.[20-22] Many of these subjects representing ethnic minorities present clinically as if they have early-onset T2DM (e.g., mild ketosis, slow symptomatic onset), some have attendant risk factors such as obesity, and many lack human leukocyte antigen (HLA) alleles associated with T1DM. Further contributing to the overall setting of diagnostic complexity has been movement to increasingly diverse genetic admixtures due to geographic migration and social changes (e.g., interracial offspring).[23-25] Finally, in terms of specificity for disease, T1DM-associated autoantibodies are typically positive in less than 1% to 2% of control (i.e., non-T1DM) subjects, further validating their diagnostic utility.[26]

In childhood and adolescence, two peaks of T1DM presentation occur, one between 5 and 7 years of age, the other at or near puberty.[27] Although most autoimmune disorders disproportionately target females, T1DM affects males slightly more than females. The incidence of T1DM varies with seasonal changes and birth month. Incidence of T1DM diagnosis is higher in autumn and winter, whereas being born in the spring is associated with an increased likelihood for T1DM.[28,29] Interestingly, the development of T1DM-associated autoimmunity (i.e., the formation of islet autoantibodies) in the months to years prior to the onset of symptomatic T1DM also show a degree of seasonal synchronization.[30]

Although clearly beneficial to disease diagnosis, these T1DM-associated autoantibodies have also fueled much debate regarding the percentage of T1DM cases that are errantly misclassified as T2DM. Indeed, it is conceivable

that 5% to 15% of adults diagnosed with T2DM may have T1DM, given the frequency of T1DM-associated autoantibodies in populations diagnosed with T2DM.[31] This is, in effect, a problem in health care provider recognition of the potential for T1DM disease in adult populations combined with a lack of widespread screening for such autoantibodies in settings in which screening would seem warranted. If this assertion is correct, given the vastly greater number of persons diagnosed with T2DM (relative to that of T1DM), the number of actual T1DM cases in a given population may be vastly underestimated. This is therapeutically unfortunate because an accurate diagnosis of T1DM is vital for optimal care, avoiding complications, and correctly treating diabetic ketoacidosis (DKA) at diagnosis when it represents a key window for survival.[32]

Efforts to differentiate adult-onset T1DM from T2DM (Table 32-1) have also resulted in a series of proposed new disease classifications, most notably *ketosis prone diabetes* and *latent autoimmune disease of adults* (LADA).[33,34] However, the lack of firm diagnostic criteria has dramatically dampened enthusiasm for adopting these presumed new disease entities as novel categories for diabetes.[35] It is also important to note that T1DM patients can manifest insulin resistance, a feature most often associated with T2DM. Specifically, T1DM patients (including those who are autoantibody-positive) may present with diabetes characterized by high serum levels of fasting insulin or C-peptide but loss of stimulated insulin secretion.[36]

As noted previously, some Caucasian children (~10%) are devoid of a T1DM-associated autoantibody at disease diagnosis (i.e., time of hyperglycemic onset), raising questions as to whether such persons lost their autoantibody expression (or at least the ability to detect it with laboratory testing) by the time of diagnosis, or whether a diagnosis of T1DM is accurate.[16] The notion of autoantibody loss versus the presence of a different form of diabetes is also difficult to ascertain as many have HLA alleles associated with susceptibility for T1DM, are not insulin resistant, present with ketoacidosis, and with time, lose their C-peptide secretion. With appropriate laboratory testing, notation of such persons as T1DM patients negative for T1DM-associated autoantibodies can be an appropriate diagnosis. This said, advances in understanding the heretofore underappreciated disease classifications of monogenic diabetes, including those of maturity onset of diabetes in youth (MODY), warrant genetic testing of diabetes cases diagnosed in the very young (i.e., <1 year of age).[37]

ANIMAL MODELS

In relation to other autoimmune disorders, T1DM is somewhat unusual in the way its research has benefited from having a series of spontaneous animal models of the disease that can be subject to well-controlled investigations.[38-41] Indeed, these animal models have provided valuable clues toward the potential mechanisms of disease pathogenesis and allow for testing of therapies seeking to prevent or reverse the disorder. This said, as for most animal models of disease, only a limited number of therapeutic efforts have been effectively translated to humans, whereas in research settings one observes a clear clinical benefit (e.g., preserved C-peptide secretion), primary examples being anti-CD3 as well as a antithymocyte globulin plus granulocyte colony-stimulating factor (GCSF) combination.[39] Indeed, one of the primary concerns for animal models of T1DM, and the nonobese diabetic (NOD) mouse in particular, relates to the relative ease by which the disease can be prevented or reversed.[42-44] As for other

TABLE 32-1

Characteristic Comparison of Type 1 Versus Type 2 Diabetes

Characteristic	Type 1 Diabetes	Type 2 Diabetes
Nature *Very different*	Autoimmune disorder marked by destruction of insulin-producing beta cells and loss of insulin production	A disorder of insulin deficiency involving an interplay between both pancreatic and extrapancreatic contributions to disease
Symptoms *Partial overlap*	Rapid onset; very high to extremely high blood glucose levels; polyphagia; polydipsia, polyurea; ketoacidosis	Mild to moderate onset; modest to high elevations in blood glucose; mild polydipsia/polyurea; fatigue; visual changes/headache
Onset *Very different*	Sudden (symptoms for days to weeks)	Slower onset (symptoms for months to years)
Risk factors *Typically different but overlap*	Family history of autoimmune disease but in particular, T1D (10-fold increased risk versus general population)	Overweight/obese; poor diet; sedentary lifestyle; ethnicity (higher in African Americans, Hispanics); family history of T2D; history of gestational diabetes
Onset age *Typically different but overlap*	Typically early life through adolescence but can occur at any age	Typically adults but trending toward earlier age of onset
Treatment strategy *Typically different*	Absolute requirement for insulin (multiple daily injections or insulin pump); self-management lifestyle modification (monitor food types, exercise, etc.)	Dietary modifications and exercise alongside oral agents (for most); increasingly greater percentage of patients require insulin over time
Can it be prevented? *Very different*	Not at present (subject of major research efforts); future cases can be predicted by autoantibodies and genetics	Yes, for over half of potential cases, with dietary modifications and exercise
Can it be reversed? *Very different*	Not at present (subject of major research efforts)	No, but for a limited few; patients can see disease managed and risk for complications reduced through diet modifications, exercise; growing evidence for disease improvements through combination therapies
Complications *Mostly similar, but some variation*	Acute emergencies of hypoglycemia and ketoacidosis leading to hypoglycemic unawareness; chronic effects of hyperglycemia can lead to retinopathy, nephropathy, neuropathy, cardiovascular disease, etc.	Acute emergencies of hypoglycemia and ketoacidosis leading to hypoglycemic unawareness; chronic effects of hyperglycemia can lead to retinopathy, nephropathy, neuropathy, cardiovascular disease, etc.

limitations, animal models (unfortunately) also represent somewhat of an idealized situation characterized by features that are not reflective of the sociologic and lifestyle settings in humans, for example, limited genetic diversity through selective inbreeding, housing in highly controlled environments devoid of pathogens, uniform diets, and a number of other facets.

Despite these caveats, the two major spontaneous animal models of T1DM are remarkably similar to humans in a number of key pathogenic features. The most notable include the importance of MHC molecules for disease susceptibility and the presence of lymphocytic islet cell invasion followed by specific destruction of beta cells. Although multiple animal models for T1DM exist, our focus will be on the two most predominant models, the NOD mouse and BioBreeding (BB) rat.

Nonobese Diabetic Mice

The NOD mouse is, without question, the most intensively studied animal model for T1DM.[45] The frequency of diabetes among different colonies differs across the globe, ranging from 30% to 100% among female NOD mice, suggesting that housing conditions (i.e., environment) represent an important variable. Interestingly, unlike human T1DM that has a relatively equal distribution among genders, a strong female bias exists in NOD mice with respect to disease. Regarding the oft-noted hallmark facet of T1DM, that being insulitis, the NOD lesion appears much more intense and quantitatively obvious than in humans. Beginning at 3 to 4 weeks of age and continuing throughout their natural history, NOD mice see islet cell infiltration of so-called innate lymphoid cells, followed by a heterogeneous population of CD4 (T helper), CD8 (T cytotoxic), and CD11c (antigen presenting) cells and other

various cell phenotypes. Interestingly, with respect to T cells, a relative overrepresentation appears with respect to the number of cells bearing a T-cell receptor specific for a given beta-cell antigen, namely, insulin.[46] However, to be clear, there is considerable debate regarding the issue of whether any given beta-cell antigen is primary (i.e., the first, major driver of disease development in an autoimmune response), although a majority of studies have provided evidence for a central role of T-cell autoimmunity directed at insulin.[47] Yet, immunities against a variety of other beta-cell antigens including GAD,[48] islet-specific glucose-6 phosphate catalytic subunit-related protein (IGRP),[49] and chromogranin A[50] have been noted.

Studies of islet beta-cell mass indicate that both destruction and replication/regeneration are present months before the onset of diabetes,[51] although there is convincing evidence of an acceleration of beta-cell destruction at disease onset.[52-54] T cells, and not autoantibodies, appear to mediate beta-cell destruction. A seeming plethora of published studies have highlighted the notion of therapeutic beta-cell replication/regeneration in NOD mice or other rodent strains,[55-57] fueling hopes for such properties to represent a potential therapeutic target for reversing the disease in humans. However, recent convincing evidence exists to suggest that in terms of beta-cell replication, rodent models differ dramatically from human physiology, with beta-cell replication forming a rare event in humans from adolescence through adulthood.[58-60]

As with T1DM of humans, specific MHC class I and II molecules are central for disease pathogenesis.[61,62] The NOD mouse has genetic mutations that cause absence of the I-E class II MHC molecule (similar to the human MHC HLA-DR molecule) and an unusual I-A class II molecule (similar to human HLA-DQ).[63] The I-A molecule in the NOD mouse is termed I-Ag7, which designates a specific amino acid sequence. HLA class II molecules (in humans there are three—HLA-DP, HLA-DQ, and HLA-DR, described in detail later) function to bind peptides and present these peptides to the T-cell receptor of CD4-positive (helper) T lymphocytes. The MHC genes were termed *immune response genes* because common variations in their sequences (allelic variation) determine the peptides to which an individual mouse or person can mount a T-cell response. Hence, these molecules play a key role in controlling overall immune responses including those autoimmune in nature that result in beta-cell destruction. In addition to these class II molecules, many other genetic loci contribute to diabetes susceptibility, each with a relatively small contribution, each neither necessary nor sufficient for disease.[64-69] Therefore, inheritance of diabetes in the NOD mouse is polygenic. With respect to humoral immune responses, NOD mice, like humans, produce IAA before developing diabetes.[70] These autoantibodies usually appear between 6 and 8 weeks of age, with diabetes incidence usually peaking at approximately 18 weeks of age.

BioBreeding Rat

The BB rat was the first intensively studied animal model of T1DM. The diabetes in this model differs from human T1DM in that diabetes-prone BB rats have an autosomal recessive mutation that produces a severe T-cell lymphopenia.[71] Infection with a number of viruses, presumably activating innate immunity, can induce diabetes in a related strain of rat that does not have lymphopenia, termed the *BB diabetes-resistant* (BB-DR) rat. As in humans and the NOD mouse, the disease depends on specific MHC class II alleles (similar to human HLA-DR and HLA-DQ), in particular, RT1-U. Additional genes segregate to create diabetes susceptibility in these rat strains, but the number of genes is much lower than for NOD mice.[71-73] With respect to other hallmarks of T1DM, BB rats are not widely considered to possess autoantibodies against beta-cell antigens (including insulin), albeit the insulitis lesion is much more reminiscent of that observed in the human disorder.[74,75]

Induced Models of Type 1 Diabetes Mellitus

Diabetes, and even insulitis, can be induced in several strains of rodents by means of drugs that induce islet cell destruction and broadly activate immune responses, including those directed against beta-cell antigens. For example, the drug streptozotocin is directly toxic to islet beta cells. In high doses, it rapidly induces diabetes (i.e.,

hyperglycemia). In low doses, a more chronic diabetes (hyperglycemia) develops that is likely to have some immunologic derivation, meaning pathogenesis tied to immune responses against beta cells.[76,77] Administration of copolymer of polyinosinic and polycytidylic acids (poly-IC), a simple polynucleotide that activates production of interferon-α (IFN-α), when administered to a number of rat strains with the diabetes-susceptible RT1-U alleles, induces insulitis and diabetes.[78] This suggests that many animals are susceptible to diabetes or insulitis given a strong immunologic stimulus. Other examples of compounds used to induce diabetes include the toxin alloxan as well as viruses that target the pancreas, including islet cells.[79-83] Although each of these induced models of diabetes has proved valuable in studies of at least one facet of T1DM research, it must be emphasized that the vast predominance of interest by researchers has been directed at the aforementioned spontaneous models given their closer similarities (e.g., insulitis, autoantibodies, involvement of MHC) to the human disorder.

HISTOPATHOLOGY

As noted earlier, T1DM in humans is characterized by selective destruction of beta cells within the pancreatic islets.[84-87] Although certain exceptions exist, an overall assimilation of the literature would suggest that the presence of insulitis (Fig. 32-1) is largely limited to young donors (<14 years of age) with T1DM duration within 1 year of diagnosis and nondiabetic donors with multiple islet autoantibodies.[9,88-90] More specifically, T1DM patients with a disease onset at age 0 to 14 years and within 1 year of diagnosis show more inflamed islets (68%) and fewer islets with residual beta cells (39%) than in patients with onset at 15 to 39 years of age.[91] This finding suggests that a more vigorous autoimmune response occurs when disease develops in young children.

The immunotype of insulitic lesions has been reported in several studies with a predominance of CD8+ T lymphocytes and macrophages, but cells of other phenotypes are observed (CD4+, CD20+, and CD68+).[92-99] More recent studies have evaluated this concept as a function of age when younger age of onset is associated with higher levels of CD20+ B cells, CD45+ cells, and CD8+ T cells in insulitis lesions, alongside fewer insulin-positive islets.[100,101] Conversely, infiltrates with fewer CD20+ cells were observed in T1DM patients who were older at onset and associated with lower levels of CD45+ cells and CD8+ T cells, as well as more insulin-positive islets. These same studies also noted that

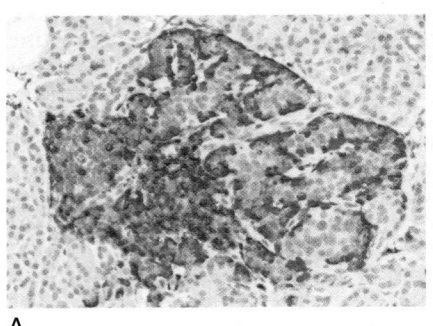

Islet cells in type 1 diabetes	Pancreas in type 1 diabetes
• Insulitis (mixed mononuclear, adjacent or within islet) • Loss of β cells (increase with disease duration) • Hyper-expression of class I MHC • β cell necrosis/apoptosis (?) • Diminished insulin in remaining β cells • β cell expression of interferon α	• Decreased overall weight • Atrophy of dorsal region • Exocrine atrophy • Hydrophic change (hypertrophy) (?) • Composed of pseudoatrophic (glucagon staining) islets in type 1A • Lobular loss of β cells • Heterogeneous lobular insulitis

A   B   C

Figure 32-1 Pathologic characteristics of the pancreas in type 1 diabetes mellitus (T1DM). **A,** Islet infiltrate (i.e., insulitis) seen in a patient with recent-onset T1DM. Immunohistochemistry shows the intra-islet presence of CD3-positive cells *(brown)* and glucagon-producing alpha cells *(pink)*. Histologic features of islet cells (**B**) and gross pathologic characteristics of the pancreas (**C**) associated with the natural history of T1DM (i.e., preonset, onset, post onset). MHC, major histocompatibility complex. (From Atkinson MA, Eisenbarth GS, Michels AW. Type 1 diabetes. *Lancet.* 2014;383:69-82, used with permission.)

islet CD8[+] T cells expressed T-cell receptors that bound MHC class I tetramers loaded with the beta-cell autoantigen IGRP and other target peptides in recent-onset T1DM patients.[101] These studies are also in agreement with recent findings that the T cells invading pancreatic islets are, in fact, directed at beta-cell antigens.[95] In contrast to long-standing dogma, the presence of insulitis in human T1DM is quantitatively limited, with an expert panel establishing a standardized definition for this lesion of three islets, containing more than 15 CD45[+] cells, in a pancreas.[102]

Somewhat surprisingly, inflammation is also present in pancreatic exocrine tissue in T1DM. Specifically, chronic inflammation, including enhanced CD8[+] T-cell infiltration (and, to a lesser degree, CD4[+] and CD11c[+] cells), is present in the exocrine pancreas in T1DM subjects.[103] Other studies report a similar propensity for neutrophil invasion of the pancreas (along with decreased peripheral neutrophil counts) in T1DM.[104] The propensity of this organ for inflammation/pancreatitis induced by multiple factors (e.g., hypertriglyceridemia, virus infection, drugs) could be a result of a susceptibility gene that affects tissue-based inflammation or other facets that have, in the past, been considered "leakiness."[105,106] Importantly, the inflammatory process in the exocrine pancreas appears to be subclinical, as most new-onset patients do not present with symptoms of pancreatic inflammation.

Recent studies assessing the persistence of insulin production in patients with long-standing T1DM (i.e., stimulated C-peptide production) have overturned the long-standing dogma that residual C-peptide secretion is rare.[107-109] Emerging histopathologic evidence supports this notion through the identification of insulin-positive islets, albeit extremely limited in number, in patients with long-standing T1DM.[11,110] The non–insulin-producing cells of the islets (i.e., alpha, delta, pancreatic polypeptide, etc.) remain in patients with long-standing T1DM, and these remaining islets, lacking insulitis and beta cells, are termed *pseudoatrophic*. This information sets the stage for another remarkable feature of the pancreas of patients with new-onset T1DM, namely, heterogeneity of islet lesions. Histopathologic examination of the same section of pancreas showed that a normal islet with no immune infiltrate can coexist with an islet containing beta cells with intense infiltration as well as a pseudoatrophic islet that has no infiltrate. This spottiness of the pathologic process is reminiscent of the destruction of areas of the skin in patients with vitiligo, in which melanocytes are destroyed in patches. Such heterogeneity of lesions may underlie the variable natural history of T1DM in which studies suggest the time period between initial beta-cell autoimmunity and overt symptoms can be one of months, or years, or even many decades.[111,112] Additionally, studies of pancreata from non-T1DM but autoantibody-positive subjects often show limited to no insulitis. Such information has been considered to support the notion that T1DM is a relapsing/remitting disease,[113] with waves of immunologic destruction.

The islets of T1DM patients as well as T1DM autoantibody-positive nondiabetic subjects overexpress class I HLA antigens, IFN-α, and potentially Fas molecules.[85,90,114,115] The specific means by which the immune system destroys beta cells is not known. Molecules such as Fas may be important as T cells expressing Fas ligand can induce apoptosis of beta cells.[116-118] This said, more enthusiasm surrounds the notion that cytokines (e.g., interleukin 1 [IL-1]) and CD8[+] cytotoxic lymphocytes are likely to be major contributors to beta-cell destruction.[119-125] With respect to the notion of what might induce these features, searches for viral particles and viral RNA within islets of patients with new-onset diabetes have largely been unrewarding, but newer technologies and concepts should facilitate additional studies, and it is likely that there is heterogeneity among patients.[125,126]

Finally, reduced pancreatic weights at autopsy or in organ donors have been demonstrated in recent-onset T1DM as well as in those with long-standing disease.[127,128] Reduced pancreas volume has also been shown in patients with T1DM through noninvasive imaging techniques.[129,130] The mechanisms underlying loss of pancreatic size or weight in T1DM are not well understood but have largely been hypothesized to result from loss of insulinotrophic effects on the exocrine pancreas as islets constitute only 1% to 2% of the entire pancreatic volume.[131]

GENETICS

It has long been recognized that diabetes is a heterogeneous group of metabolic disorders, with hyperglycemia representing a common feature. More recently, it has become increasingly apparent that T1DM is also heterogeneous as a disease entity. This conclusion is based on a series of observations including the age at disease onset, form of symptomatic presentation (i.e., rapid and ketotic versus mild without ketosis), pancreatic pathologic changes, form and number of autoantibodies, and certainly the notion of genetics.

Indeed, there are likely many genetic forms of T1DM, influenced to a major degree by the presence of specific forms of HLA class II molecules.[132] Beyond HLA, the form of T1DM is also influenced by the presence of abnormalities (immunologic, beta cell, etc.) fostered by the quantity and combinations of genes that influence these aberrancies. The number of specific genes that contribute to T1DM remains in flux, to some degree, as studies of loci validation in varying global populations are conducted.[133] However, current estimates provided by genome-wide association studies (GWAS) would suggest more than 40 such loci exist, the largest number thought to influence immune responses.[134] As far as how these genes influence T1DM as a collective, it is generally considered that specific combinations of HLA and non-HLA genes contribute to a loss of tolerance to self-antigens in beta cells, ultimately resulting in T1DM. Many of the HLA and non-HLA genes underlying T1DM susceptibility are similar in diverse countries, although specific alleles of those genes differ in their frequency.[135]

Beyond the polymorphisms seen in these HLA and non-HLA genes identified by GWAS, studies of genetics have also been extremely helpful in the identification and characterization of several monogenic forms of T1DM. Although these disorders continue to be classified as T1DM in most situations, increasing considerations are being given to whether such diseases should strictly be identified as *monogenic diabetes*.

Overview of Prevalence and Genetics

In the United States, the risk of childhood diabetes is approximately 1 in 300.[136] This risk is 15 times lower than the diabetes risk for a first-degree relative of a patient with T1DM (Table 32-2), which in turn is 150 times lower than the risk for a monozygotic twin of a patient with T1DM.[137,138] Although the risk of diabetes is much greater for relatives of patients with T1DM, it is important to realize that most persons (>85%) in whom T1DM develops do not have a first-degree relative with the disease. The incidence of sporadic cases results in part because almost 40% of persons

TABLE 32-2

Risk of Type 1 Diabetes Mellitus

Group	Childhood Annual Incidence
U.S. general population	0.3% (15-25/100,000)
Offspring	1%
Sibling	3.2% (through adolescence); 6% lifetime
Dizygotic twin	6%
Mother	2%
Father	4.6%
Both parents	~10%
Monozygotic twin	50%, but incidence varies with age of index twin

in the general population carry high-risk HLA alleles for T1DM (see "The Major Histocompatibility Complex" later).

The highest known incidence of T1DM is observed in Finland and Sardinia. Finland now has an annual incidence approaching 60 per 100,000 children.[139] Since the 1950s, the incidence has increased almost fivefold, suggesting a dramatic environmental change (either an increase of causative factors or a decrease of protective factors), and it is doubling in many Western countries, including the United States, every 10 to 15 years (Fig. 32-2). Of note, the increased T1DM incidence in many countries has not been linear but rather fluctuating over the past several decades.

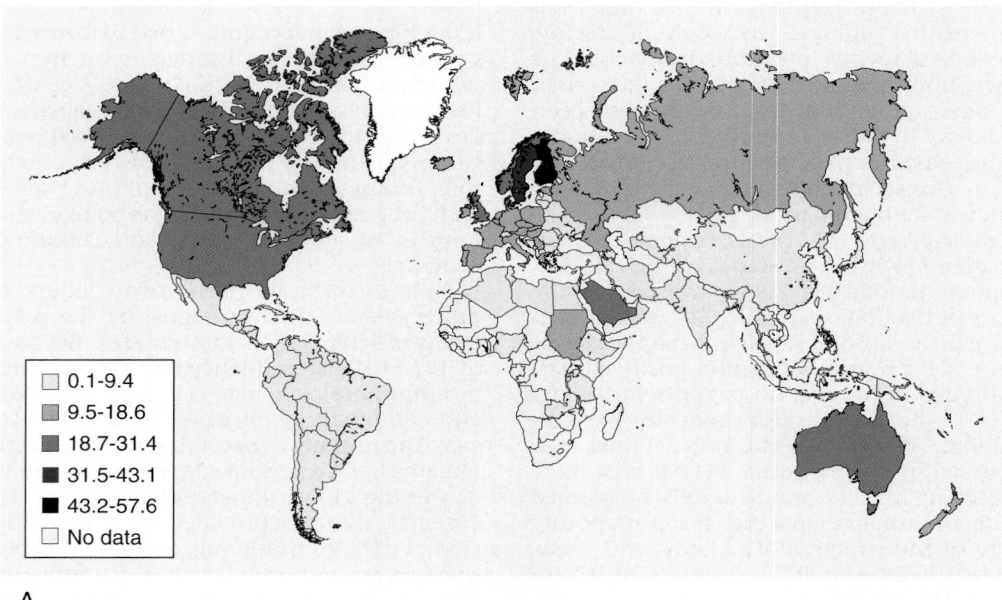

A

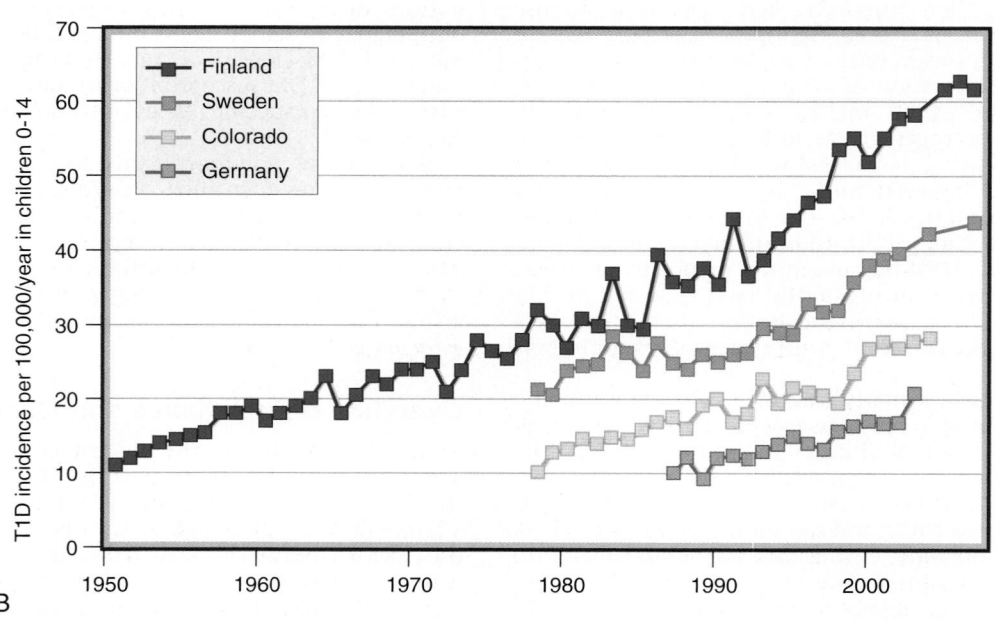

B

Figure 32-2 Incidence of type 1 diabetes (T1D) in children aged 0 to 14 years by geographic region and over time. **A,** Estimated global incidence of T1D, by region, in 2011. **B,** Time-based trends for the incidence of T1D in children ages 0 to 14 years in areas with high or high-intermediate rates of disease. (Redrawn from Atkinson MA, Eisenbarth GS, Michels AW. Type 1 diabetes. *Lancet.* 2014;383:69-82, used with permission.)

In contrast, the disorder is quite uncommon in China, India, and Venezuela (~0.1 per 100,000 per year).

Twin Studies

Twin studies of diabetes have made impressive contributions to our understanding of the disease. The study of monozygotic twins of patients with diabetes by Barnett and coworkers[140] contributed to the recognition of distinct forms of diabetes, initially termed *adult-onset* and *juvenile-onset*, later *insulin-dependent* and *non–insulin-dependent*, and now T1DM and T2DM.[133] The concordance rates for monozygotic and dizygotic twins provide important information regarding genetic factors contributing to a given disease, because monozygotic twins share all germline-inherited polymorphisms or mutations, whereas dizygotic twins are similar to siblings of patients with a disease and have only half of their genes in common. For a locus that contributes to disease in a recessive manner, only one quarter of dizygotic twins would be homozygous to a sibling with diabetes at that locus, but all monozygotic twins would be homozygous for all recessive loci of their diabetic twin. Although overall concordance rates of monozygotic twins for T1DM are calculated, it is likely that T1DM is heterogeneous and that groups of monozygotic twins have different genetic causes for their diabetes. With such genetic heterogeneity, one would expect different concordance rates for different genetic causes.

Redondo and coworkers[141] analyzed prospective follow-up data from a large series of initially discordant monozygotic twins from Great Britain combined with a series from the United States. Progression to diabetes was identical for both series of twins. There was no length of time of discordance beyond which a monozygotic twin of a patient with T1DM did not have a risk of developing the disease. Nevertheless, the hazard rate for development of diabetes decreased as the period of discordance increased. There was also a marked variation in the risk of diabetes relative to the age at which the disorder developed in the index twin. With long-term follow-up, the overall rate of concordance for monozygotic twins exceeds 50%.[142] However, if T1DM developed in the index twin after age 25 years, the concordance rate by life table analysis in Redondo's study was less than 10%. If diabetes developed in the index twin before age 5 years, the concordance rate was 70% after 40 years of follow-up. Therefore, environmental factors, random factors, and non–germline-inherited variations (e.g., imprinting, T-cell receptor polymorphisms, somatic mutations) likely contribute to lifetime diabetes risk.

An important unanswered question (given the limited number and size of research studies) is whether dizygotic twins of patients with T1DM have a diabetes risk greater than that of siblings. If the risk is identical, it suggests that environmental factors whose presence is time-dependent (e.g., uncommon infections) have little influence on the development of diabetes. Dizygotic twins differ from siblings in terms of a greater commonality of environment over time (e.g., common pregnancy). Interestingly, studies of dizygotic twins suggest that their risk of diabetes may not differ from that of siblings or, at most, may be increased by a factor of two compared with the 10-fold increase for monozygotic twins.[143]

Genetic factors influence not only the development of diabetes but also the expression of anti-islet autoantibodies. For identical twins, the expression of anti-islet autoantibodies is tightly linked to the eventual progression to overt diabetes, and true to form, monozygotic twins have a high prevalence of expression of these autoantibodies.[138] Dizygotic twins much less often express anti-islet autoantibodies, and the prevalence is similar to that of siblings.[144]

The Major Histocompatibility Complex

The most important loci determining the risk of T1DM reside within the MHC on chromosome 6p21 and, in particular, the HLA class II molecules (DR, DQ, and DP).[62,145-147] In addition, HLA class I loci (HLA-A, -B, and -C) influence disease, and it is likely that additional loci within or linked to the MHC influence immune function and contribute to risk.[148] The nomenclature for alleles of this region is somewhat daunting, but with definitions of several terms and a description of the basis for classification, it is comprehensible and quite important to understand.

As noted previously, the function of HLA molecules is to present peptides to T lymphocytes. Each molecule is made up of two chains, and each chain is encoded by a separate gene. These molecules are extremely polymorphic in amino acid sequence. Each polymorphic variant of each chain is designated with a gene locus name (e.g., DRB1) followed by an asterisk (*), followed by two digits referring to the serologic specificity (from the time in diagnostic history when typing was performed with antibodies), followed by two digits for the specific allele (now determined with DNA-based typing), followed by a single digit to distinguish silent nucleotide polymorphisms (nucleotide differences that do not change the amino acid sequence). For example, the designated allele DRB1*0405 has DR4 serologic specificity and is associated with high T1DM risk. For HLA-DR alleles, usually only the DRB chain is specified, because the DRA chain is not polymorphic. Likewise, for the class I molecules (A, B, and C), only a single chain is specified, because the other chain, β_2-microglobulin, is minimally polymorphic. There are hundreds of known alleles of DRB1. Each person inherits two DRB1 alleles, one from each parent.

Because HLA gene loci are in close proximity to each other on the sixth chromosome, a group of alleles is usually inherited as a unit, which is termed a *haplotype*. For example, the alleles A*0101, B*0801, DRB1*0301, and DQA1*0501,DQB1*0201 constitute a common haplotype associated with diabetes risk probably related to the presence of DRB1*0301. When specific alleles of different genes are nonrandomly associated with each other on a haplotype (e.g., A1, B8, and DR3), the alleles are said to be in linkage disequilibrium. Linkage disequilibrium is not the same as linkage, although to have linkage disequilibrium, genes must be linked. Genes are linked when they are close together on the same chromosome and thus transmitted from parent to child as a haplotype group. If alleles of linked genes are nonrandomly associated with each other in a population, they are in linkage disequilibrium.

Two MHC haplotypes, one inherited from each parent, constitute an individual's MHC genotype. This genotype ultimately determines the MHC-encoded risk of T1DM. For DQ molecules, both of the chains (DQA and DQB) are polymorphic. This adds an important level of diversity in that the protein chains encoded by the alleles of one haplotype can combine with the chains encoded by the other haplotype. For example, persons with the highest risk genotype DRB1*0301,DQA1*0501,DQB1*0201, and DRB1*0405,DQA1*0301,DQB1*0302 can produce four different DQ molecules: the expected DQA1*0501,DQB1*0201 and DQA1*0301,DQB1*0302 but also DQA1*0501, DQB1*0302 and DQA1*0301,DQB1*0201. Studies suggest that the DQA1*0501,DQB1*0302 combination determines enhanced diabetes risk for DR3/4 individuals. The DQ

TABLE 32-3

Diabetes Risk of Representative DR and DQ Haplotypes

DRB1	DQA1	DQB1
High Risk		
0401 or 0403 or 0405	0301	0302 (DQ8)
0301	0501	0201 (DQ2)
Moderate Risk		
0801	0401	0402
0404	0301	0302
0101	0101	0501
0901	0301	0303
Moderate Protection		
0403	0301	0302
0701	0201	0201
1101	0501	0301
Strong Protection		
1501	0102	0602 (DQ6)
1401	0101	0503
0701	0201	0303

molecule DQA1*0501,DQB1*0201 is also called DQ2, and DQA1*0301,DQB1*0302 is called DQ8. A common DQ molecule, DQA1*0102,DQB1*0602, provides dominant protection from T1DM and is termed *DQ6*. The major determinants of T1DM susceptibility are DR and DQ molecules, and specific alleles of both HLA-DR and -DQ can either increase or decrease the risk of diabetes. Table 32-3 summarizes the diabetes risk associated with a number of DR and DQ haplotypes.[149]

In a number of studies, children from the general population or relatives of patients with T1DM have been HLA typed.[70,150,151] The typing is relatively straightforward and is based on direct DNA sequencing of polymerase chain reaction (PCR)-amplified DNA fragments or DNA probes that hybridize specifically to different allelic sequences. In the United States, 2.4% of newborns have the highest risk DR-DQ genotype for T1DM, namely, DR3-DQ2 with DR4-DQ8 (DR3/4,DQ8/2 heterozygotes). Fifty percent of children younger than 10 years and approximately 30% of older children who develop T1DM have this highest risk genotype.

Approximately 1 of 16 children with the highest risk HLA genotype from the general population progresses to T1DM (compared with a population risk of 1 per 300). Alternatively, 15 of 16 children from the general population who are DQ8/DQ2 heterozygotes do not develop T1DM. Studies indicate that newborn siblings of patients with T1DM who have DQ2 and DQ8 have a risk of expressing islet autoantibodies exceeding 40% by age 6 years, and 50% of these newborns will develop diabetes by age 10 years. This suggests that a genetic risk, especially MHC encoded, is extremely high.[152]

Ninety-five percent of persons who develop T1DM have either DR3-DQ2 or DR4-DQ8, as does approximately 40% of the general population. The protective haplotype DRB1*1501,DQA1*0102,DQB1*0602 is present in 20% of the general population and in fewer than 3% of patients with T1DM. A DR allele, DRB1*1401, also appears to provide dominant protection.[153] There are additional high-risk haplotypes that are not common, such as DQA1*0401, DQB1*0402. It has been proposed as a simple rule that the presence of aspartic acid at position 57 of the DQβ chain and arginine at DQα 52 is associated with T1DM risk.[154]

There are many exceptions to this rule, and knowledge of the complete sequences (allele) rather than dependence on this rule is essential.

Insulin Locus

Although much of the attention toward T1DM genetics has resided on HLA, other loci have drawn attention for their potential contributions to disease. In 1984, Bell and colleagues[155] published their discovery that variations in the number of nucleotide repeat elements located 5′ of the insulin gene were associated with the development of T1DM. The longest group of repeats was associated with decreased diabetes risk.[156] In a mechanism potentially related to the aforementioned role of autoimmune regulator (AIRE) in the thymus, the protective insulin gene polymorphism is associated with greater insulin messenger ribonucleic acid (mRNA) expression within the thymus.[157,158] Indeed, for both the AIRE mutation of autoimmune polyendocrine syndrome type 1 (APS-1) and the effect of insulin gene mutations, the level of expression of insulin in the thymus may be critical.

PTPN22 Gene

PTPN22, a gene encoding a lymphoid-specific phosphatase that influences T-cell receptor signaling, is the third confirmed gene (versus mere loci) influencing T1DM risk.[159] This gene influences T-cell receptor signaling, and the polymorphism associated with diabetes (Trp for Arg) blocks binding to a signaling kinase molecule, CSK. Nevertheless, the relative risk associated with this polymorphism for T1DM and other autoimmune disorders, such as rheumatoid arthritis, is only 1.7. The variant associated with disease risk results in gain of function and decreased T-cell receptor signaling.[160]

Other Loci

In impressive collaborative form, more than a decade of international GWAS efforts led to the definition of many loci that contribute, to varying degrees but usually quite small, toward the development of T1DM.[161] For example, polymorphisms of the cytotoxic T-lymphocyte-associated protein 4 gene contribute to Graves disease and apparently to diabetes in some but not all populations, with relative risks less than 1.3.[162] A locus associated with the IL-2 receptor has a statistical association based on analysis of thousands of persons.[163] Sequencing in one region has also identified rare mutations of a gene influencing IFN-α induction.[164]

Monogenic Forms

The most common forms of diabetes, T1DM and T2DM, are polygenic, meaning the risk of developing these disorders is related to multiple genes. Environmental factors (discussed later) also play a part in the development of polygenic forms of diabetes. However, additional and rare forms of diabetes, termed *monogenic*, result from mutations in a single gene. Monogenic forms of diabetes account for about 1% to 5% of all cases of diabetes in young individuals. So far, more than 20 genes have been linked to monogenic diabetes. In most cases of monogenic diabetes, the gene mutation is inherited; in the remaining cases the gene mutation develops spontaneously. Neonatal diabetes (ND) and MODY are the two main forms of monogenic diabetes (Table 32-4). Cases of ND occur far less often than those of MODY. ND occurs in newborns and young infants,

TABLE 32-4
Characteristics of Monogenic Diabetes

Neonatal diabetes mellitus (NDM) (rare; occurs in about 1 of every 100,000 to 500,000 live births)
Permanent neonatal diabetes mellitus (PNDM) (50% of all cases of NDM)

Type of Diabetes	Gene or Syndrome	Affected Protein	How Common?	Typical Age at Onset	Type of Inheritance or Mutation	Causes Intrauterine Growth Restriction?	Transient or Permanent?	Treatment
PNDM	KCNJ11	Kir6.2	Most common type of PNDM	3 to 6 months	Autosomal dominant (10%) Spontaneous	Yes	Permanent (this gene also causes a transient form of NDM)	Treated with insulin in the past but often can be treated with oral sulfonylureas
PNDM	ABCC8	SUR1-sulfonylurea receptor 1	Rare	1 to 3 months	Autosomal dominant (12% of NDM cases) Spontaneous	No	Permanent (this gene also causes a transient form of NDM)	Treated with insulin in the past but often can be treated with oral sulfonylureas
PNDM	GCK	Glucokinase	Rare	1 week	Autosomal recessive	Yes	Permanent	Insulin
PNDM	IPF1; also known as PDX1	Insulin promoter factor 1	Rare	1 week	Autosomal recessive	Yes	Permanent	Treat to replace endocrine and exocrine pancreas functions
PNDM	PTF1A	Pancreas transcription factor 1 A	Rare	At birth	Autosomal recessive	Yes	Permanent	Treat to replace endocrine and exocrine pancreas functions
PNDM	FOXP3, IPEX syndrome	Forkhead box P3	Rare	Sometimes present at birth	X-linked	Yes	Permanent	Insulin
PNDM	EIF2AK3, Wolcott-Rallison syndrome	Eukaryotic translation initiation factor 2-alpha kinase 3	Rare	3 months	Autosomal recessive	Yes	Permanent	Insulin and treatment for associated conditions
Transient neonatal diabetes mellitus (TNDM) (50% of all cases of NDM)								
TNDM	ZAC/HYMAI	ZAC: pleomorphic adenoma gene-like 1 or PLAG1 HYMAI: hydatiform mole-associated and imprinted transcript	Most common form of NDM	Birth to 3 months	Autosomal dominant Spontaneous	Yes	Transient	Initially, treat with insulin; reduce dosage as needed; when diabetes recurs, treat with diet modification and physical activity; may also require insulin
TNDM	ABCC8	SUR1-sulfonylurea receptor 1	Rare	Birth to 6 months	Autosomal dominant Spontaneous	Varies	Transient (this gene also causes a permanent form of NDM)	Oral sulfonylureas
TNDM	KCNJ11	Kir6.2	Uncommon cause of TNDM but most common cause of PNDM	Birth to 6 months	Autosomal dominant Spontaneous	Yes	Transient (this gene also causes a permanent form of NDM)	Oral sulfonylureas
TNDM	HNF1 β (beta); also known as HNF1B	Hepatocyte nuclear factor 1B	Rare	Birth to 6 months	Autosomal dominant (60%) Spontaneous	Yes	Transient	Insulin

Continued

TABLE 32-4

Characteristics of Monogenic Diabetes—cont'd

Type of Diabetes	Gene or Syndrome	Affected Protein	How Common?	Typical Age at Onset	Type of Inheritance or Mutation	Causes Intrauterine Growth Restriction?	Transient or Permanent?	Treatment
Maturity-onset diabetes of the young (MODY) (1% to 5% of all cases of diabetes in the United States)								
MODY 1	HNF4A	Hepatocyte nuclear factor 4α (alpha)	Rare	Adolescence or early adulthood	Autosomal dominant	No	Permanent	For most, oral sulfonylureas; some patients may need insulin
MODY 2	GCK	Glucokinase	MODY 2 and MODY 3 account for about two thirds of all cases of MODY MODY 2 is the second most common form of MODY	Mild hyperglycemia may be present at birth; otherwise, early childhood	Autosomal dominant	Lower than normal birth weight can occur	Permanent	Diet modification and physical activity; medications usually not required; some patients do not require any treatment during childhood
MODY 3	TCF1	Hepatic nuclear factor 1α (alpha) or HNF1α (alpha) or HNF1A	MODY 3 is the most common form of MODY	Adolescence or early adulthood	Autosomal dominant	No	Permanent	Initially, treat with diet modification; can be treated with oral sulfonylureas; some patients may need insulin
MODY 4	IPF1; also known as PDX1	Insulin promoter factor 1	Rare	Early adulthood; can present later	Autosomal dominant	No	Permanent	Oral sulfonylureas; some patients may need insulin
MODY 5	TCF2	Hepatic nuclear factor 1β (beta) or HNF1B	Rare	Adolescence or early adulthood	Autosomal dominant	No	Permanent	Insulin; patients also may need treatment for related conditions such as kidney failure or cysts
MODY 6	NeuroD1, or BETA2	Neurogenic differentiation factor 1	Rare	In the fourth decade of life	Autosomal dominant	No	Permanent	Insulin

Adapted from *Monogenic Forms of Diabetes: Neonatal Diabetes Mellitus and Maturity-Onset Diabetes of the Young.* Bethesda, MD: The National Institute of Diabetes and Digestive and Kidney Diseases. Available at www.diabetes.niddk.nih.gov/dm/pubs/mody/.

whereas MODY usually occurs in children or adolescents, but may be mild or remain undetected until adulthood.

Genetic testing can diagnose most forms of monogenic diabetes. If genetic testing is not performed, people with monogenic diabetes may appear to have one of the polygenic forms of diabetes (i.e., T1DM or T2DM). When hyperglycemia is first detected in adulthood, T2DM is often diagnosed instead of monogenic diabetes. Importantly, some monogenic forms of diabetes can be treated with oral diabetes medications, whereas other forms require insulin injections. A correct diagnosis that allows the proper treatment to be selected should lead to better glucose control and improved health in the long term.

Neonatal Diabetes

ND is a monogenic form of diabetes that occurs in the first 6 months of life. It is a rare condition occurring in only 1 in 100,000 to 500,000 live births. Owing to lack of professional awareness (although at decreasing frequency) or lack of screening, ND can be mistaken for T1DM, a disorder that usually occurs later than the first 6 months of life. For approximately one half of those with ND, the condition is lifelong, yet for the remainder, the condition is transient and disappears during infancy but can reappear later in life (i.e., transient ND). Symptoms of ND mimic those of T1DM and include thirst, frequent urination, and dehydration. In severe cases, insulin deficiency can lead to ketoacidosis. In addition, fetuses with ND may not see normal growth in utero, with newborns being small for gestational age (i.e., intrauterine growth restriction). Following, some infants demonstrate protracted growth and weight gain, but appropriate therapy has the ability to improve and may in fact normalize growth and development.

Maturity-Onset Diabetes of the Young

MODY is a monogenic form of diabetes that usually first occurs during adolescence or early adulthood.[165] However, MODY sometimes remains undiagnosed until later in life. A number of different gene mutations have been shown to cause MODY (see Table 32-4).[166] It has been estimated that MODY accounts for about 1% to 5% of all cases of diabetes in the United States.[167] Beyond this, relatives of those with MODY are at increased risk for the disorder (e.g., children of a MODY parent have a 50% chance of inheriting the disease). MODY patients often are asymptomatic or demonstrate only mild hyperglycemia. MODY patients are generally not overweight. Although both T2DM and MODY can run in families, MODY pedigrees typically portray a family history of diabetes in multiple successive generations.

Autoimmune Polyendocrine Syndrome Type I (*AIRE* Gene Mutations)

APS-1 is rare (<500 cases worldwide), with an increased incidence in Finland and Sardinia and among Iranian Jews, but it has a worldwide occurrence. The disorders of the syndrome, such as T1DM, mucocutaneous candidiasis, hypoparathyroidism, Addison disease, and hepatitis (see Chapter 40 for a more detailed discussion beyond genetics herein), identify a unique syndrome, and patients with this group of disorders almost always have mutations (usually autosomal recessive) of the *AIRE* gene on chromosome 21, a gene that encodes a DNA-binding protein. Studies indicate that this gene may play an important role in maintaining self-tolerance as well as influence the expression of what immunologists term *peripheral antigens* (e.g., insulin) in the thymus. This notion becomes relevant in that it has been hypothesized that greater expression of insulin and other tissue-specific antigens leads to tolerance and disease suppression.[168] At the same time, the influence on insulin is not specific, as damage to the adrenal glands, parathyroid glands, and other organs underlie the major features of APS-1 and are why candidiasis infections predominate.

X-Linked Polyendocrinopathy, Immune Dysfunction, and Diarrhea (Scurfy Gene)

The syndrome of X-linked polyendocrinopathy, immune dysfunction, and diarrhea (*XPID*, also termed *IPEX*) is associated with overwhelming neonatal autoimmunity, and most children die in the first few days of life or in infancy.[169-172] In this syndrome, lymphocytes invade multiple organs. It is associated with insulitis and beta-cell destruction as well as lymphocytic intestinal inflammation with flattened villi and severe malabsorption. It is inherited as an X-linked recessive disease affecting only boys, with a frequent clinical history of lack of male births.

The disease results from mutations of the gene encoding forkhead box P3 (FOXP3), whose function as a transcription factor has been elucidated.[169,173,174] This gene functions as a master switch for regulatory (suppressor) CD4+/CD25+ T lymphocytes. Lack of such regulatory T cells leads to overwhelming autoimmunity. This is an important syndrome to recognize early as bone marrow transplantation, affording restoration of functional T-regulatory cells (even with partial chimerism), has proved to be therapeutic.

ENVIRONMENTAL FACTORS

Environmental factors have long been considered to have an important influence on the pathogenesis of T1DM. Consistent with this conclusion are the regional differences in disease rates based on geography, seasonality in its diagnosis, rising incidence trends, and variance among twins. However, despite decades of research, no single environmental agent has been identified that would universally explain these observations. Such a shortcoming was not for lack of trying as the identification of any such agent of influence is clearly made difficult due to facets of the disorder's pathogenesis (e.g., the long prodromal/prediabetic phase that often precedes T1DM, that 85% of new cases arise from the general population, the limited disease frequency of 1 in 300).

The fivefold increase in T1DM rates over the past half-century have been considered strong evidence that environmental factors related to diabetes risk have changed since the 1960s. Factors that increase diabetes risk may be increasing, or just as likely, factors that suppress the development of diabetes may be decreasing. In terms of this rising incidence, it is quite interesting that it is occurring at different rates globally as a function of age at onset. The increase in Finland has particularly occurred for children in whom the disease develops before age 5 years, yet in the United States, the recent Search for Diabetes in Youth Study (SEARCH) suggested the rise has been most rapid in teenagers.[175-177]

Models to Explain the Influence of Environment

Although the mechanisms by which environment influences T1DM are not known, numerous attempts have been made to develop hypothetical models to provide such an explanation. The accelerator and overload hypotheses suggest that environmental stresses, specifically childhood obesity for the former, increase insulin demand, thereby overloading the islet cells and accelerating beta-cell autoimmune damage.[178-180] In the Copenhagen model, beta-cell destruction is a result of interactions between the environment, immune system, and the beta cells themselves in genetically susceptible individuals.[181] The most often discussed model, the hygiene hypothesis, attributes the rising incidence of autoimmune disorders to the reduced or altered stimulation of the immune system by environmental factors.[182] Conversely, the fertile field hypothesis proposes that microbial infection induces a temporary state in which other antigens can more easily react to yield autoreactive T cells.[183] Also implicating the gut, the old friends hypothesis, which is based on the role of normal gastrointestinal microbes, implicates dietary exposure as a possible direct regulator of the immune system and of self-tolerance by altering gut microbiota and permeability.[184] Finally, the threshold hypothesis suggests that the etiologic influences of genetics and environment, when evaluated as intersecting and reciprocal odds-ratio–based trend lines, results in a method to define the attributable risk for T1DM.[185]

Beyond growth in the number of models, important intellectual changes have also occurred with respect to thoughts of how environment might influence disease development. Specifically, in part due to the widespread acceptance for a popular model of T1DM in which the notion of trigger was provided, most views aligned with this notion.[186] However, whereas it is true that the underlying genetic susceptibility to T1DM might allow for a triggering of anti–beta cell immunity by an environmental event, it is becoming increasingly considered that environmental agents may contribute far beyond an initial triggering and rather act throughout the natural history of T1DM development, for example, by modulating the ongoing autoimmune process (e.g., genes controlling immune regulation). With this, there is no shortage of potential environmental candidates (e.g., breastfeeding, antibiotics, cow milk consumption, viruses) that, either alone or in combination, may contribute to the disorder's pathogenesis. However, as a collective, most fall into the groups involving infection (viruses in particular), vaccination, and diet.

Candidate Environmental Factors

The best evidence, if not the only strong evidence, for a partial role for an environmental agent in T1DM involves congenital rubella infection. This event, but not noncongenital infection, greatly increases the development of T1DM.[187] The way in which this congenital infection increases diabetes development is currently unknown, with hypotheses ranging from molecular mimicry[188] to long-term alteration in T-cell function secondary to the congenital insult.[189]

However, without question, the most oft discussed agents associated with T1DM are the enteroviruses. Enteroviruses are small RNA viruses that often infect young children. Initial anecdotal reports that coxsackievirus (a form of enterovirus) infections might cause diabetes involved children who had severe infections and who died at disease onset.[190,191] These studies, however, preceded the realization that T1DM is not an acute disease, but one involving a chronic prediabetic period of autoimmunity. Thus, it is likely that viral infection at the onset of T1DM is most often incidental. At the time of presentation with diabetes, almost all children have a rising elevation in HbA_{1c}, reflecting what is likely months of hyperglycemia preceding diagnosis.[192,193]

The potential importance of enteroviral infection was emphasized by studies from Scandinavia in which enteroviral infection was evaluated during pregnancy and in infancy. Infection is usually detected by changes in antiviral antibodies or detection of enteroviral RNA by molecular techniques.[194] Although some studies have reported an increased incidence of enteroviral infection during pregnancy among mothers whose children later developed diabetes, others have not.[195,196] As infants with a genetic risk for the development of diabetes are followed from birth, it becomes possible to analyze prospectively the expression of enterovirus RNA. Enteroviral infection was found to be associated with the appearance of anti-islet autoantibodies in some regions (Finland)[195] but not in others (Colorado),[196] a finding that may be related to the frequency and timing of enteroviral infections in these two populations.

Other viruses are being evaluated for association with the triggering of autoimmunity. One study from Australia found an association with rotavirus infection,[197] a virus that commonly infects young children. Specifically, the study did not find an increase in rotavirus infection in children with T1DM compared with control subjects but rather found an association with increased anti-islet autoantibodies.

It has also been claimed that the timing of routine childhood vaccinations influences the development of T1DM.[198] This is an important health concern if parents alter their family's childhood vaccination schedule because of concern about development of T1DM. A series of studies have been performed addressing this notion,[199-201] yet none provided any evidence that childhood vaccinations influence the development of diabetes.

Perhaps only second to viral infections, the majority of investigations associating environment with T1DM relate to diet. Among the earliest was the hypothesis that early introduction of bovine milk increases the development of diabetes, based primarily on retrospective studies associating early or increased bovine milk ingestion (or less breastfeeding) with an increased risk of T1DM.[202] Several prospective studies in which infants were observed until the development of anti-islet autoantibodies failed to find an association or found only a weak association with either breastfeeding or bovine milk ingestion.[203-206] Pilot studies of an infant formula lacking bovine milk proteins have been initiated in Finland. Preliminary data suggest that such a restricted diet might produce a small decrease of cytoplasmic islet cell autoantibodies but not GAD65 autoantibodies.[207]

Studies from Germany and Denver provided evidence that early (<3 months) introduction of cereals may increase the development of islet autoimmunity.[208,209] Both vitamin D and ω-3 fatty acids, which can influence immune function, have also been associated with risk of T1DM.[210,211]

NATURAL HISTORY

Perhaps the most helpful and beneficial guide to studies pertaining to the natural history of T1DM was the model put forward in 1986 by the immediate past author of this chapter, the late Dr. George Eisenbarth.[212] In this model (Fig. 32-3), persons destined to develop T1DM were assumed to begin life with a full cadre of beta cells. However, a triggering insult, likely environmental, would initiate a process involving recruitment of antigen-presenting cells (APCs). APCs would sequester self-antigens released by injured beta cells, followed by their transport to pancreatic lymph nodes where they are subsequently presented to autoreactive T cells. These T cells, rogue constituents brought to life

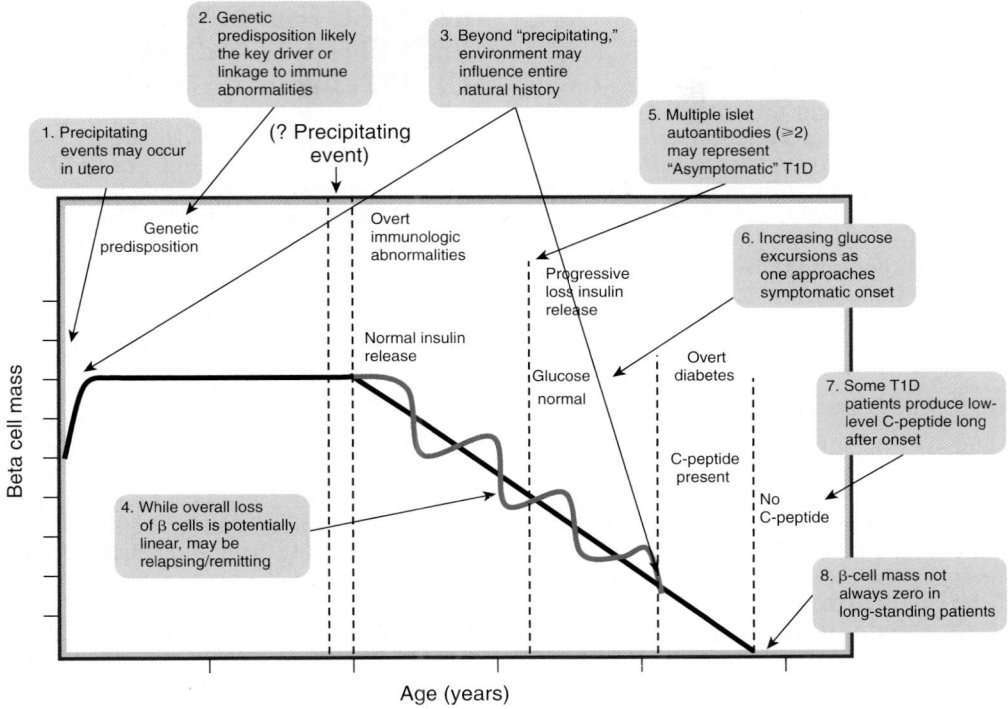

Figure 32-3 The natural history of type 1 diabetes (T1D)—a 25-year-old concept revisited. A re-creation of the model as originally proposed in 1986 is tracked by the black line. A number of additions and conjectures can be made to this model based on recent knowledge gains *(lavender line)*. (Redrawn from Atkinson MA, Eisenbarth GS, Michels AW. Type 1 diabetes. *Lancet.* 2014;383:69-82, used with permission.)

because of genetically driven failures of thymic deletion (i.e., central tolerance) combined with defects in mechanisms designed to induce peripheral immune tolerance, would come into play.[213] This toxic duo imparting lack of tolerance formation, again in the context of genetic susceptibility, would allow for migration of self-reactive T cells to islets, mediating beta-cell killing and promoting further inflammation.[214] When 85% to 90% of pancreatic beta cells meet their demise, symptoms of the disease appear. In the final stage of the model, the autoimmune process ends with the complete elimination of beta cells.

Although this model faithfully served as a guide for multiple decades and certainly the majority of its aspects hold true to this day, some constituents are under states of correction (e.g., the aforementioned notion that C-peptide production is lost in T1DM at onset[215]) or are still subject to intense investigation, facets that will be discussed throughout this chapter.

Genetic and Immunologic Heterogeneity by Age of Onset

T1DM can develop at any age, from the neonatal period to the last decades of life. Given that identical twins can become concordant more than 40 years after the first twin develops T1DM, not all age heterogeneity can be ascribed to different genetic syndromes.[144] Nevertheless, there is an overall correlation between the age at which diabetes develops in one twin or sibling and the age of development of diabetes in his or her relative. Children in whom T1DM develops at an early age more often are DR3/4,DQ8/2 heterozygotes. In addition, there is evidence that class I HLA alleles (or other non–class II genes within the HLA region)

can influence the age at diabetes onset; an example is the A24 allele.[216] At the other end of the age spectrum, there is evidence that the protective HLA allele DQA*10102, DQB1*0602 is not as protective for young adults as it is for children.[217]

The most characteristic difference related to age at diabetes onset is the presence of higher levels of IAA in children who develop the disease at an early age (e.g., <5 years).[218,219] The high levels and frequent positivity of IAA make measurement of these autoantibodies the best single marker for diabetes development in young children. In those children in whom autoantibodies arise during the first 3 years of life, IAA often appear first. In contrast, GAD65 autoantibodies are more often positive in adults who develop T1DM. The correlation of levels of IAA and age at diabetes onset may be related to faster progression to diabetes in children with higher levels.[220] However, such rapid progression occurs only if IAA are present with another anti-islet autoantibody (discussed in the next section).

Beta-Cell Mass Is Not Equal in All Individuals

Most historical models of T1DM have assumed a normal beta-cell mass at birth that declines once the autoimmune attack occurs (see Fig. 32-3). However, recent studies of cadaveric pancreata have shown that beta-cell mass in normal, nondiabetic humans varies threefold to fivefold, independent of adult age or body mass index, with beta-cell mass likely mostly determined in the first 2 decades of life.[221-223] This has important implications when one considers the starting point for declining beta-cell mass during autoimmune beta-cell destruction. Thus, an individual's timeline to diabetes onset could be determined not by the severity of the autoimmune attack but the starting point for beta-cell mass (see Fig. 32-3). The reasons for variation in beta-cell mass are unknown but could include the in utero environment, events during the first decade of life, and yet unknown genetic or environmental determinants. Further emphasizing the need to understand the timeline and determinants of human beta-cell mass are the afore-mentioned observations of a smaller pancreatic mass in individuals with new-onset T1DM.[127,128] These findings raise the possibility that determinants of both pancreatic mass and beta-cell mass might be impacted, because endo-crine islet cells and exocrine cells share a common embryo-logic heritage.

Metabolic Progression Before Hyperglycemia

The intravenous glucose tolerance test (GTT) aids in evalu-ating the time to onset of diabetes among persons express-ing anti-islet autoantibodies.[224] Most commonly, glucose is given at 0.5 g/kg over 5 minutes (maximum 35 g, 25 g/dL), and insulin levels are measured before and 1 and 3 minutes after the glucose infusion.[225,226] Most persons who are within 1 year of developing overt diabetes have no first-phase insulin secretion after intravenous glucose adminis-tration. A simpler measurement in someone progressing to T1DM is the HbA$_{1c}$, which in most prediabetic individuals increases progressively (although in the normal range) 1 or 2 years before overt hyperglycemia develops.

The diagnosis of T1DM usually relies on the presence of fasting hyperglycemia (≥126 mg/dL), but with prospective evaluation, many persons have diabetes determined by OGTT according to the 120-minute criterion (≥200 mg/dL), with a nondiagnostic fasting glucose level. Impaired fasting glucose (100 to 125 mg/dL) or impaired glucose tolerance (glucose at 120 minutes on OGTT, 140 to 199 mg/dL) is usually present within 6 months before the onset of overt diabetes.

C-Peptide Loss After Hyperglycemia

After diabetes is diagnosed, levels of C-peptide can be used to assess remaining beta-cell function. C-peptide levels are usually measured in the fasting state, after intravenous glucagon, or with a standard liquid meal. Such measure-ments are primarily of importance for trials of therapies to alleviate loss of insulin secretion after diagnosis. Determi-nation of the C-peptide concentration provides the best current measure for assessing the impact of new therapies. As shown in the Diabetes Control and Complications Trial (DCCT), a small amount of remaining C-peptide is associ-ated with impressive metabolic benefit.[227,228]

Transient Hyperglycemia

A significant number of children are evaluated by endocri-nologists for transient hyperglycemia. The usual history is one of severe stress associated with hyperglycemia that resolves within days to 1 month. Such children may be in the honeymoon phase of T1DM, or they may truly have a transient episode of hyperglycemia. Rarely, diabetes in children is misdiagnosed. Children without severe stress who have transient hyperglycemia or who have a relative with T1DM are more likely to have early T1DM. Absence of anti-islet autoantibodies and a normal intravenous GTT result strongly indicate transient hyperglycemia and not T1DM.[229] It is not known whether children with transient hyperglycemia are at increased risk for T2DM later in life.

IMMUNOTHERAPY FOR THE PREVENTION AND REVERSAL OF TYPE 1 DIABETES MELLITUS

The intersection of two independent events in the 1970s—the generalized acknowledgment that T1DM represents an autoimmune disease, alongside the development of immu-nosuppressive agents—led to decades of efforts directed toward immunotherapy as a means to either prevent T1DM (i.e., avert symptomatic onset) or once diagnosed, reverse it (commonly termed *intervention*). To be clear, studies attempting to prevent the development of T1DM involve treatment of persons at varying stages of disease risk based on a combination of genetic susceptibility, the number of T1DM-associated autoantibodies, and the degree to which glucose levels are elevated.[230,231] Although the populations subject to such procedures would differ, the common goal is to prevent further loss of beta-cell function.

At present, in a setting of either disease prevention or intervention, there is no proven safe and effective immu-notherapy for use in a general public health care setting that prevents T1DM or reverses the disease, as judged by preservation of C-peptide. However, in research settings, potentially promising candidates do exist for disease pre-vention (e.g., oral insulin, GAD vaccine) or intervention (e.g., anti-CD3, antithymocyte globulin plus GCSF, anti-CD2).[232-238] Indeed, dozens of clinical trials, ranging from small to large, have been completed in both settings, a limited number discussed later based on their proposed method of action.

Immunosuppression

The earliest studies of therapies to prevent beta-cell destruc-tion used immunosuppressive agents. Large intervention trials of cyclosporine indicated that this agent prevented further loss of C-peptide secretion and improved metabolic function while it was administered in recent-onset T1DM cases.[239-241] Cyclosporine therapy did not, however, main-tain a nondiabetic state when therapy was instituted after the onset of diabetes, and with discontinuation of the drug, patients rapidly lost C-peptide reserve. The combina-tion of inability to cure diabetes and toxicities associated with cyclosporine (in particular, nephrotoxicity and concern about increased risk of malignancy) ruled out its acceptance for use. Other immunosuppressive agents used in subsequent studies, such as prednisone and azathio-prine, demonstrated relatively little effect in disease intervention.[242-244] In the time since, a litany of agents (e.g., anti-CD20, antithymocyte globulin, mycophenolate plus anti-IL-2 receptor α-monoclonal antibody) thought to act at least in part via immune depletion, a form of immune suppression, have demonstrated mixed results in T1DM intervention efforts. Some provide no therapeutic benefit (i.e., preservation of C-peptide, reduced insulin needs, reduction in hypoglycemic events), whereas others have achieved at least one of these beneficial parameters, usually C-peptide preservation. However, even when efficacious, for the majority of subjects, the beneficial effect was not durable (i.e., 6 months to 1 year of benefit).[244-247] Therefore, at present, although T1DM is an immune-mediated disor-der, it is not treated with immunotherapeutic agents in clinical practice. This is not to say that hope is lost for such being the case in the future. Indeed, in recent times (e.g., 2000 to present), studies related to two forms of modified antibodies against the CD3 molecule have, without ques-tion, generated the most research interest and offer some degree of eventual optimism.

Throughout a number of phase I and phase II intervention studies, a single course of anti-CD3 therapy decreased the loss of C-peptide secretion over a 12- to 24-month period in new-onset patients.[235,248,249] However, phase III trials were not considered of therapeutic benefit to the extent that commercialization of these agents was to some degree disrupted. Concerns related to the activation of Epstein-Barr virus infection, the duration of C-peptide preservation, and the protocol by which the drugs are administered have further limited their development. This said, limited efforts continue to move anti-CD3 back into the therapeutic setting, including that of disease prevention.[236,249]

Immunologic Vaccination

In animal models (especially the NOD mouse), it is relatively easy to prevent T1DM.[39] Indeed, although somewhat dated, a widely recognized effort notes some 200 such means.[250] This said, animal models have allowed for the development of potentially the most exciting prevention or intervention modality, that being one of many forms of immunologic vaccination. Much of the excitement derives from the specificity of the therapy and the relatively low risk compared with immunosuppression. The basic concept behind most such therapies is the induction of lymphocytes that target a given beta-cell antigen and, on encountering the target antigen (e.g., insulin, GAD), produce cytokines that suppress autoimmunity and tissue destruction.[251,252]

Induction of a protective immune response may depend on the route of administration of the given antigen (e.g., oral, nasal, intradermal) or on the use of an altered antigen (e.g., altered peptide ligands). For example, insulin given either orally or by subcutaneous injection prevented diabetes in NOD mice.[253,254] Intact insulin is not necessary, because the insulin B chain and an immunodominant B(9-23) peptide of insulin were also effective.[255] The latter molecules have no insulin-like metabolic effect but are able to activate T lymphocytes that target insulin.

In terms of translation, the Diabetes Prevention Trial Type 1 (DPT-1) studied both oral insulin and parenteral injections of low doses of insulin. The results of the parenteral trial did not demonstrate a reduction in the risk of developing diabetes.[256] The oral trial did not document an overall benefit of insulin, but in the subgroup with higher levels of IAA at entry, a statistically significant delay in progression to diabetes was observed.[257] Because of this, the National Institutes of Health (NIH) TrialNet has coordinated a follow-up effort testing the efficacy of oral insulin to prevent T1DM in those having certain criteria related to age and IAA level. In addition, a pilot effort (Pre-POINT trial) led by investigators in Germany involving the administration of high-dose oral insulin in children at high genetic risk for T1DM with a family history of the disease reported that this form of therapy was capable of altering the anti-insulin immune response without inducing hypoglycemia.[258]

Targeting Mechanisms of Beta-Cell Death

As noted, studies of pancreatic disease suggest the most prominent cell found in human islets in settings of T1DM is the CD8+ cytotoxic T cell, which is also a likely candidate to aid in beta-cell killing because of its ability to recognize targets via antigen in the context of MHC class I, which is elevated in many islets in those with the disease.[259] Therapeutically, lymphocytes and memory lymphocytes of the adaptive immune response can be targeted by anti-T-cell drugs such as anti-CD3, anti-CD2 (LFA3-Ig), and certain costimulatory blockers.[260,261] Indeed, partial success of such compounds in recently diagnosed T1DM, defined by preservation of C-peptide production over several months to years, speaks toward an important role for such autoreactive lymphocytes in beta-cell destruction, at least late in the pathogenesis of this disease. Inflammatory cytokines are also known to harm islets, and therefore anti-inflammatory therapies targeting cytokines may hold promise, as observed in a trial blocking TNF.[262] These observations provide further support for the concept of combination therapies.

With the growing concept that multiple mechanisms likely contribute to the pathogenesis of T1DM, enthusiasm has increased for the concept of utilizing combination therapies to prevent or reverse the disease.[263] Examples of such combinations with respect to immune intervention would include an induction component using drugs targeting inflammation and T/B-cell memory as well as a maintenance component that could involve antigens to induce tolerance to beta cells. At the same time, emerging data have supported an increasing role for beta-cell stress and loss of function as potential contributing factors for T1DM development, and therefore, the notion of combination therapy involving the addition of drugs that stabilize and maintain beta cells/beta-cell function should be considered.[264]

PANCREAS AND ISLET CELL TRANSPLANTATION

Pancreatic transplantation for patients requiring a kidney transplant has become an accepted clinical procedure, but one that for a variety of reasons, particularly the shortage of organ donors, remains relatively rare.[265] Patients with a kidney transplant receive immunosuppressive drugs that, given the nature of clinical monitoring for said transplant (e.g., creatinine, albumin), allow for careful (i.e., tailored) drug delivery for optimal care. A number of studies suggest that improved results for pancreatic transplantation will occur in the setting of simultaneous pancreas and kidney (SPK) transplantation versus transplantation of pancreas alone.[266,267] Indeed, there is considerable debate concerning pancreas transplantation without transplantation of a kidney.[268] With a successful pancreas transplant, hyperglycemia is immediately reversed for most, and there is growing evidence of improved long-term outcomes.[265,269] Nevertheless, the surgery is extensive, and there are many potential complications associated with the transplant. Perhaps for these reasons, along with improvements in facets directed at improving diabetes management, it appears the procedure peaked in the mid- to late 2000s, with declines in the number of procedures performed in the United States thereafter.[270]

Beyond therapeutic interest in pancreatic transplantation, additional research has focused on the mechanisms of pancreas rejection for what it might reveal regarding the immunologic mechanisms of T1DM. In that regard, in T1DM patients provided with a pancreatic transplant, diabetes (i.e., a repeated need for exogenous insulin replacement therapy) can recur as a result of mechanisms considered attributable to either recurrent autoimmunity (as typified by the recurrence of T1DM-associated autoantibodies once lost) or, more often, allograft rejection.[271] It is difficult to monitor and determine which of these two forms of islet destruction are occurring with the development of hyperglycemia, and currently, there are no specific means in terms of treatment that would separate the two, albeit at least one study has provided evidence for recurrent autoimmunity manifest by the induction of islet autoantibodies prior to graft rejection.[272]

With respect to islet (versus pancreas) transplant, therapeutic hopes for this procedure have been high since the late 1960s when early pioneering approaches were developed for their isolation from whole pancreata. Yet until studies emanated from Edmonton, Canada, in the early 2000s, the results of islet transplantation were—with full transparency with regard to their efficacy—considered poor by many over a period of 2 decades. Indeed, fewer than 10% of patients with T1DM achieved insulin independence at 1 year.[273] In contrast, with autotransplantation of patients with pancreatitis, most patients become insulin independent and remain so.[273] To reverse this situation, the Edmonton group used meticulous islet isolation techniques, transplantation of islets from multiple pancreata, avoided the use of steroids, and utilized an immunosuppressive regimen involving the drug rapamycin. This so-called *Edmonton protocol* has subsequently been tested in a series of specialized centers throughout North America and Europe. It is clear that in many centers, albeit with varying degrees of success, islet cell transplant can prove effective (i.e., ~60% at 1 year), especially for patients with severe hypoglycemia when the goal is one of long-term prevention of severe hypoglycemic episodes. For most of the patients who achieve insulin independence, resumption of use of low doses of insulin is necessary within 2 years and by 5 years, the benefits of the form of therapy wane.[274] Even with these positive results, the number of islets available from cadaveric donors for transplantation is quite limited, and the toxicities of the drugs used probably exceed the level of benefit achieved except for those most subject to disease-associated complications (e.g., severe, recurrent hypoglycemia).[275] Further research to achieve tolerance without long-term immunosuppression is essential, as is continued development of systems allowing for xenogeneic transplantation.[276] Of immense promise for the future are therapies involving the use of surrogate beta cells (i.e., insulin producing, glucose responsive) produced from stem cells, either embryonic or induced in origin from a variety of tissues. In addition, the increasing use of long-term continuous glucose monitoring combined with improvements in modes of insulin delivery (e.g., analogues, pumps) or use of secondary agents in patients with T1DM will almost certainly raise the bar for consideration of the risks and benefits of both islet and pancreatic transplantation.

DISORDERS ASSOCIATED WITH IMMUNITY TO INSULIN/INSULIN RECEPTOR

Insulin Autoimmune Syndrome

The insulin autoimmune syndrome, also termed *Hirata syndrome*, is rare and is typically associated with hypoglycemia.[277] These patients have extremely high concentrations of autoantibodies reacting with human insulin in the absence of exogenous insulin therapy. It is thought that inappropriate (i.e., nonregulated by the prevailing glucose level) release of autoantibody-bound insulin produces the hypoglycemia. Interestingly and for reasons unknown, the disease occurs most commonly in persons of Asian descent.[278] Among 50 Japanese patients with the syndrome and possessing the typical polyclonal anti-IAA, 96% had

an HLA-DR4 allele and 84% possessed a DRB1*0406 allele.[279] In contrast, patients with monoclonal anti-IAA do not possess such a profound and specific HLA association.[280] Most patients with this disorder develop the disease in association with treatment of sulfhydryl-containing medications, in particular, methimazole, as well as α-lipoic acid.[281,282] Treatment usually consists of stopping these medications, and for more than 75% of the patients, the disease remits.[279]

Insulin Allergy

Mild immune reactivity against exogenously administered insulin is not an uncommon feature in T1DM management. Indeed, essentially all patients treated with recombinant human insulin produce anti-IAA.[283] The levels of these antibodies are relatively low, and they do not appear to interfere with insulin therapy for the vast majority of individuals, although there are reports correlating insulin antibodies with macrosomia.[284] In addition, most studies show no relationship between the presence of anti-insulin antibodies and complications associated with T1DM (e.g., retinopathy, neuropathy).[283] With the introduction of recombinant human insulin replacing animal insulins, symptomatic immune responses to insulin such as immediate hypersensitivity, delayed hypersensitivity, lipoatrophy, and lipohypertrophy have decreased.[285] Allergic reactions can occur with insulin analogues, modifications of recombinant human insulin devised to provide desired characteristics in terms of their therapeutic activities, although this is uncommon.[286] More common features include allergies to affiliated lubricants, preservatives, and plastics in bottles, stoppers, syringes, and needles. The usual mode of therapy for such situations consists of substituting the type or formulation of insulin, administration of oral antihistamines for immunoglobulin E–mediated local reactions, followed by insulin desensitization or addition of small amounts of glucocorticoids to the insulin injected for local delayed hypersensitivity reactions.[287]

Anti-insulin Receptor Autoantibodies

Anti-insulin receptor autoantibodies (i.e., type B insulin resistance) are associated with hypoglycemia, hypercatabolism, severe acanthosis nigricans, and insulin resistance.[288] It appears that anti-insulin receptor autoantibodies can act as either antagonists or agonists for this disease. This syndrome is quite rare, is often associated with non–organ-specific autoimmunity, and treatments usually involve various forms of immunosuppression (e.g., rituximab, steroids, intravenous immune globulin, cyclophosphamide), albeit with mixed success.[289,290]

CLINICAL PRESENTATION

The peak age for presentation of T1DM in children is at puberty. The symptoms and signs are related to the presence of hyperglycemia and the resulting effects on fluid and electrolyte balance; they include polyuria, polydipsia, polyphagia, weight loss, and blurred vision.[14] Because infection may have precipitated the initial presentation, symptoms of infection may also be present, such as fever, sore throat, cough, or dysuria. In children in particular, the onset of symptoms can occur over a brief period, and families may be able to date the onset with considerable accuracy. In older persons with T1DM, the onset of symptoms may be insidious over months, and many are mistakenly diagnosed as T2DM by screening during this asymptomatic period.

If onset of T1DM is associated with ketoacidosis, which is not uncommon, additional symptoms related to this acute metabolic complication of diabetes are also present. These symptoms can include abdominal pain, nausea, and vomiting. Variable effects on mental status may be seen, ranging from slight drowsiness to profound lethargy and even coma if the condition has been untreated for a significant period.

Laboratory Findings

Plasma glucose concentrations at presentation are elevated, usually in the range of 300 to 500 mg/dL. If the presentation is uncomplicated, the remainder of the fluid and electrolyte measurements may be completely normal. On the other hand, if diabetic ketoacidosis (DKA) is present, the measurements will reflect the presence of an acidosis as well as more severe dehydration. DKA is discussed more fully near the end of this chapter.

At presentation the C-peptide level (a surrogate marker for insulin secretion) is generally in the low normal range and declines over time. However, residual C-peptide may be detected throughout the natural history of diabetes. In reference laboratories, pancreatic autoantibodies are present in ~98% of individuals at diagnosis, but most commercial laboratories do not provide either the full spectrum of assays or equivalently sensitive or specific assays, resulting in both false negative and positive assays (discussed previously). Furthermore, antibody titers diminish over time and may be less prevalent in certain ethnicities.[292]

TREATMENT

Importance of Tight Glucose Control

The overriding principle in the treatment of most patients with T1DM is that a health care team that includes a physician, diabetes nurse educator, nutritionist, and other health care professionals as appropriate should work closely with the patient to achieve blood glucose concentrations as close to normal as possible, because these values are associated with a reduced risk of diabetic complications. Although studies in animal models[293-294] and epidemiologic studies[295-296] have suggested that tighter glucose control is associated with better long-term outcomes for the diabetic patient in terms of a reduced risk of complications, the most definitive study in this regard has been the DCCT, which was completed in 1993.[297] This landmark study involved a total of 1441 patients with T1DM—726 with no retinopathy at baseline (the primary prevention cohort) and 715 with mild retinopathy (the secondary intervention cohort)—who were randomly assigned to intensive therapy or conventional therapy.

Intensive therapy consisted of insulin administration by an external pump or by three or more daily insulin injections. The dosage was adjusted according to the results of self-monitoring of blood glucose performed at least four times per day as well as dietary intake and anticipated exercise. The goals of intensive therapy were to achieve blood glucose concentrations between 70 and 120 mg/dL before meals, values less than 180 mg/dL after meals, a weekly 3 AM measurement greater than 65 mg/dL, and an HbA_{1c} value within the normal range (≤6.05%). Patients in the intensive treatment group visited their centers each month and had more frequent contacts with a member of the health care team, usually weekly, to review and adjust their regimens.

Conventional therapy consisted of one or two daily injections of insulin, including mixed intermediate and rapid-acting insulins, daily self-monitoring of urine or blood glucose, and education about diet and exercise. The goals of conventional therapy included absence of symptoms of hyperglycemia; absence of ketonuria; maintenance of normal growth, development, and ideal body weight; and freedom from frequent severe hypoglycemia.

The entire cohort of patients was observed for a mean of 6.5 years, and 99% of the patients completed the study. Although only 5% of the subjects in the intensive treatment group were able to sustain the goal of a normal HbA_{1c} over time, they nevertheless did have significantly lower average values (approximately 7%) over time than the subjects in the conventional treatment group (approximately 9%). Average capillary blood glucose profiles in the intensive treatment group were 155 ± 30 mg/dL, compared with 231 ± 55 mg/dL in the conventional therapy group ($p < 0.0001$). These differences in glucose control formed the basis of analyses to determine the effects of lower levels of glycemia on diabetic complications.

When both the primary prevention and secondary intervention cohorts were considered, intensive therapy was shown to reduce the risk of proliferative or severe nonproliferative retinopathy by 47% and the need for treatment with photocoagulation by 56%. Intensive therapy reduced the mean adjusted risk of microalbuminuria (defined as urinary albumin excretion >40 mg/24 hours) by 34% in the primary prevention cohort and by 43% in the secondary intervention cohort. The risk of albuminuria was reduced by 56% in the secondary intervention cohort. Intensive therapy reduced the appearance of neuropathy by 69% in the primary prevention cohort and by 57% in the secondary intervention cohort.

Some have suggested a potential adverse effect of aggressive insulin therapy in exacerbating the predisposition to macrovascular disease in diabetes. In the DCCT study, intensive insulin therapy reduced the development of macrovascular disease by 41%, although the difference was not statistically significant.[298] Ninety-three percent of DCCT participants were monitored after the randomized portion of the trial in the Epidemiology of Diabetes Interventions and Complications (EDIC) study. Glycemic control in both groups drifted toward an HbA_{1c} value of slightly less than 8% within the first year or so after conclusion of the randomized trial. With 17 years of follow-up after randomization, despite similar glycemic control in both groups for 10 years, cardiovascular disease (defined as nonfatal myocardial infarction, stroke, death from cardiovascular disease, confirmed angina, or the need for coronary artery revascularization) was reduced by 42% and nonfatal myocardial infarction, stroke, and cardiovascular deaths were reduced by 57%.[299] After a mean of 27 years' follow-up of patients with type 1 diabetes, 6.5 years of initial intensive diabetes therapy was also associated with 33% reduction in all-cause mortality (absolute risk difference, 109 deaths per 100,000 patient-years) when compared to conventional therapy.[300]

Were there any adverse events associated with the intensive treatment regimen in the DCCT? The incidence of severe hypoglycemia was approximately three times higher in the intensive therapy group than in the conventional therapy group ($p < 0.001$). Some of the episodes of hypoglycemia were quite severe, resulting in motor vehicle accidents or need for hospitalization. Severe hypoglycemia occurred more often during sleep,[301] and approximately one third of the episodes that occurred while the patients were awake were not associated with warning symptoms. In intensively treated subjects, predictors of hypoglycemia included a history of severe hypoglycemia, longer duration of diabetes, higher baseline HbA_{1c}, and a lower recent HbA_{1c} value.

Weight gain also occurred in more of the intensively treated patients. Intensive therapy was associated with a 33% increase in risk of becoming overweight, defined as a body weight more than 120% above the ideal. Five years into the trial, patients being treated intensively had gained a mean of 4.6 kg more than patients receiving conventional therapy. Among subjects in the top quartile of weight gain, changes in plasma lipids, blood pressure, and body fat distribution were observed that were similar to those seen in cases of insulin resistance.[302]

Goals of Treatment

On the basis of the results just described, the authors of the DCCT study recommended that most patients with T1DM be treated with an intensive treatment regimen under the close supervision of a health care team consisting of a physician, nurses, nutritionist, and behavioral and exercise specialists as needed. More recent studies demonstrate that patients with type 1 diabetes who from diabetes onset achieve 25 year average A1C <7.6% are at very low risk of developing retinopathy requiring laser photocoagulation or persistent macroalbuminuria.[303] It may be appropriate to be more cautious about instituting intensive treatment regimens in populations such as children younger than 13 years of age, elderly people, and patients with advanced complications such as end-stage renal disease or significant cardiovascular or cerebrovascular disease.[304] It has also been reported that institution of aggressive insulin therapy in subjects with proliferative or severe nonproliferative retinopathy can lead to accelerated progression of retinopathy; treatment of the eye disease should be considered before an aggressive insulin regimen is started.[305] Patients who do not experience warning adrenergic symptoms of hypoglycemia (hypoglycemia unawareness) are at significantly greater risk for severe recurrent hypoglycemia, and this may prevent the safe institution of tight glucose control. The development of continuous glucose monitoring (CGM) may provide an additional level of safety in such individuals.[306]

Guidelines from the ADA[307] and the American College of Endocrinology (ACE)[308] are presented in Table 32-5. The

TABLE 32-5

Glycemic Targets for Nonpregnant Adults

Parameter	Normal	ADA	ACE
Premeal PG (mg/dL)	<100 (mean ~90)	80-130*	<110
Postprandial PG (mg/dL)	<140	<180*†	<140
HbA_{1c} (%)	4 to <5.7	<7.0*	≤6.5‡

*More or less stringent glycemic goals may be appropriate for individual patients. Goals should be individualized based on duration of diabetes, age/life expectancy, comorbid conditions, known CVD or advanced microvascular complications, hypoglycemia unawareness, and individual patient considerations.
†Peak postprandial capillary plasma glucose. Postprandial glucose may be targeted if A1C goals are not met despite reaching preprandial glucose goals. Postprandial glucose measurements should be made 1-2 h after the beginning of the meal, generally peak levels in patients with diabetes.
‡Individualize on the basis of age, comorbidities, duration of disease; in general ≤6.5 for most; closer to normal for healthy; less stringent for "less healthy."
ACE, American College of Endocrinology; ADA, American Diabetes Association; HbA_{1c}, glycosylated hemoglobin; PG, plasma glucose concentration.
Data from American Diabetes Association. Standards of medical care in diabetes—2015. *Diabetes Care.* 2015;38:s1-s93; Handelsman Y, Bloomgarden ZT, Grunberger G, et al. American Association of Clinical Endocrinologists and American College of Endocrinology—clinical practice guidelines for developing a diabetes mellitus comprehensive care plan—2015. *Endocr Pract.* 2015;21:1-87.

ADA suggests that the goal of treatment in the management of diabetes should be an HbA_{1c} value of less than 7% in general. Specifically in type 1 diabetes, A1C targets of <7.5% are suggested for youth (<18 years), <7.0% in adults, <7.5% in older adults who are healthy, <8.0% in older adults with complicating factors and intermediate health, and <8.5% in older adults with very complex medical problems and poor health.[292] Furthermore, the ADA suggests that lower targets can be pursued in selected patients, such as those with disease of recent onset, long life expectancy, and no significant cardiovascular disease, if they can be achieved without significant hypoglycemia or other adverse effects of treatment. Conversely, they recommend that less stringent HbA_{1c} goals "may be appropriate for patients with a history of severe hypoglycemia, limited life expectancy, advanced microvascular or macrovascular complications, and extensive comorbid conditions and those with long-standing diabetes in whom the general goal is difficult to attain despite diabetes self-management education, appropriate glucose monitoring, and effective doses of multiple glucose lowering agents including insulin."[307] The ACE has recommended a general HbA_{1c} goal of less than 6.5%.[308] It is recognized that to achieve glucose control at these levels in type 1 diabetes, patients need to monitor glucose frequently and to receive nutritional counseling and training in self-management of the insulin doses as well as problem solving to allow them to deal with the problems that they encounter in their daily lives.

Team Approach to Treatment

The DCCT trial validated the use of continuous subcutaneous insulin infusion (CSII) with an insulin pump and multiple daily injections (MDI), which are titrated based on frequent glucose monitoring. Several companies have developed continuous glucose sensors, and pramlintide, an amylin analogue, is the first fundamentally new treatment for patients with T1DM to become available since 1922. Because of the complex nature of modern intensive diabetes treatment regimens and the need for regular feedback and modification of the parameters of treatment, it has now become generally accepted that intensive insulin regimens can be instituted more effectively by a health care team than by a physician alone. Members of the team can include diabetes nurse educators, nutritionists, psychologists, medical social workers, and others, such as exercise physiologists, depending on the needs of a particular patient. A critical aspect of intensive diabetes treatment is the need for continuous monitoring of the effectiveness of specific components of the regimen with adjustments in response to changing life circumstances of the patient.

Pharmacokinetics of Available Insulin Preparations

In the past, insulin for human use was obtained from animal sources (i.e., cows and pigs). With advances in recombinant DNA technology, it is now possible to produce large quantities of insulin with an amino acid structure identical to that of human insulin or to modify the human amino acid sequence to produce desirable pharmacodynamic properties. The various formulations of insulin differ in the rapidity of their onset of action, the time from injection to peak action, and the duration of action, depending on the chemical nature of the particular insulin preparation. These data are summarized in Table 32-6. The available insulins can be divided on a pharmacokinetic basis into three broad categories: rapid-acting, intermediate, and long-acting.

TABLE 32-6

Pharmacokinetic Properties of Insulin Preparations

Preparation	Onset (hr)	Peak (hr)	Duration (hr)
Rapid-Acting			
Regular	0.5-1	2-4	6-8
Lispro	0.25	1	3-4
Aspart	0.25	1	3-4
Glulisine	0.25	1	3-4
Intermediate-Acting			
NPH	1-3	6-8	12-16
Long-Acting			
Glargine U-100	1	NA	29
Glargine U-300*	1	12-16	32-34
Detemin*	1	3-9	6-24

NPH, neutral protamine Hagedorn.
*May be 20%-30% less potent than glargine, requiring a higher dose to achieve similar efficacy.

Rapid-Acting Insulins

Rapid-acting insulins have an onset of action of 1 hour or less and are used to reduce the peak of glycemia that occurs after meal ingestion.

Regular Insulin. Regular insulin consists of zinc-insulin crystals dissolved in a clear fluid. After subcutaneous injection, regular insulin tends to dissociate from its normal hexameric form, first into dimers and then into monomers; only the monomeric and dimeric forms can pass through the endothelium into the circulation to any appreciable degree.[309] This feature determines the pharmacokinetic profile of regular insulin. The resulting relative delay in onset and duration of action of regular insulin limits its effectiveness in controlling postprandial glucose and results in dose-dependent pharmacokinetics, with a prolonged onset, peak, and duration of action with higher doses.

Insulin Analogues

Insulin Lispro. Insulin lispro, of recombinant DNA origin, is a human insulin analogue created by reversal of the amino acids at positions 28 and 29 on the human insulin B chain. Insulin lispro was the first insulin analogue to receive approval by the U.S. Food and Drug Administration. It is chemically Lys(B28),Pro(B29) insulin and is created in a special, nonpathogenic laboratory strain of *Escherichia coli* that has been genetically altered by the addition of the gene for insulin lispro.

The effect of this amino acid rearrangement is to reduce the capacity of the insulin to self-aggregate in subcutaneous tissues, resulting in behavior similar to that of monomeric insulin. This leads to lispro's more rapid absorption and shorter duration of action compared with regular insulin when given by subcutaneous injection. However, lispro is not intrinsically more active and on a molar basis is equipotent to human insulin. When they are given by intravenous injection, the pharmacokinetic profiles of lispro and human regular insulin are similar. Because of its rapid onset of action (within 5 to 15 minutes after administration) and peak action within 1 to 2 hours, lispro was the first insulin to mimic the time course of the increase in plasma glucose seen after ingestion of a carbohydrate-rich meal.

Insulin Aspart. Insulin aspart differs from human insulin by substitution of aspartic acid for proline in position B28.

Insulin Glulisine. Insulin glulisine involves substitution of lysine for the asparagine at position B3 and of glutamic acid for the lysine in position B29.

Advantages of Analogues. Lispro, aspart, and glulisine seem to have similar pharmacokinetics and clinical effects in the setting of T1DM. Although little difference is observed in most cases by either patients or providers, there certainly may be differences, at least in subsets of patients, which could be exploited to improve glycemic control.

In general, treatment with monomeric insulin analogues (lispro, aspart, and glulisine) is associated with a lower risk of hypoglycemia, particularly in sleep, than treatment with regular insulin. It is quite easy to document improved glycemic control in the postprandial state. Finally, patients may inject these insulin analogues immediately before or after meals instead of 30 to 60 minutes before meals, as is classically recommended with regular insulin, providing greater convenience. These features have been exploited in clinical trials to produce modest improvements in overall control with monomeric insulin analogues compared with regular insulin.

A variety of even more rapid-acting insulin formulations and delivery technologies is being developed. They may provide for greater advantage than available analogs.

Intermediate- and Long-Acting Insulins

Intermediate- and long-acting insulins have a significantly longer delay in their onset and duration of action. In the setting of T1DM, they should always be used in combination with a rapid-acting form of insulin. They are usually administered before bedtime and are titrated to produce normal glucose levels through the night and in the fasting state.

Neutral Protamine Hagedorn Insulin. Neutral protamine Hagedorn (NPH) insulin is a crystalline suspension of insulin with protamine and zinc, providing an intermediate-acting insulin with onset of action in 1 to 3 hours, duration of action up to 24 hours, and peak action from 6 to 8 hours. NPH insulin usually cannot be administered once daily in the setting of T1DM, at least in combination with rapid-acting monomeric analogue insulin. In the preanalogue era, NPH insulin was used successfully in combination with regular insulin, although this human insulin-based regimen has now been largely supplanted by analogue insulin because of a perceived lower risk of hypoglycemia.[310]

Insulin Glargine. Insulin glargine is a recombinant human insulin analogue that does provide 24-hour duration of action in most, but not all, patients with T1DM. It differs from human insulin in that the amino acid asparagine at position A21 is replaced by glycine, and two arginines are added to the carboxy (C)-terminus of the B chain. In the injection solution at pH 4, insulin glargine is completely soluble. However, it has low solubility at neutral pH.

After injection into the subcutaneous tissue, the acidic solution is neutralized, leading to the formation of microprecipitates from which small amounts of insulin glargine are slowly released; this results in absorption over a period of approximately 24 hours with no pronounced peak. Insulin glargine thus simulates the basal production of insulin. In other respects, its mechanism of action is similar to that of human insulin, and on a molar basis its glucose-lowering effects are similar to those of human insulin when given intravenously.

Because this insulin is provided in an acid vehicle, it cannot be mixed with other forms of insulin or intravenous fluids, and some patients have greater discomfort with injection at least some of the time. In general, glargine is less variably absorbed than NPH insulin, and in clinical trials in patients with T1DM it has been associated with a reduced risk of hypoglycemia, particularly nocturnal hypoglycemia.

In about 10% of patients, insulin glargine must be taken twice daily to provide 24-hour coverage of basal insulin needs. In a smaller percentage of patients, a modest peak in effect occurs 2 to 6 hours after injection and can result in nocturnal hypoglycemia.

Insulin Detemir. Insulin detemir differs from human insulin in that the threonine in position B30 has been eliminated and a C14 fatty acid chain has been attached to amino acid B29. It is unique among insulins of prolonged duration in that it is soluble both in the vial and under the skin. This may be the cause of its more consistent absorption after subcutaneous injection.[311] In comparison to NPH insulin in the setting of T1DM, detemir is associated with less weight gain (in some trials patients have experienced weight loss) and with reduced risk of hypoglycemia.[310]

Novel Basal Insulins

A variety of novel basal insulin formulations and analogs is being developed. Concentrated insulin glargine U-300, insulin degludec, and pegylated insulin lispro provide for extended durations of action and less within-day and day-to-day variability in pharmacodynamics and promise greater reductions in hypoglycemic risk, less weight gain, and potential improvements in glycemic control in the setting of type 1 diabetes treated with MDI regimens.[312]

Alternative Routes of Insulin Administration

Numerous alternative routes of insulin administration have been examined. The only commercially available formulation is an inhaled formulation of regular human insulin loaded in fumaryl diketopeperazine microparticles.[313] It produces peak insulin levels in ~20 minutes, with peak activity in 1 hour and a terminal half-life of 1 hour. In a subset of patients there has been great interest in inhaled insulin as a technique to avoid frequent injections, though basal insulin injections would still be required in type 1 diabetes. However, the current formulations require spirometry before initiation, at 6 months, and annually thereafter; are contraindicated in patients with asthma and COPD; provide precautions for patients with active lung cancer and smokers; are associated with cough, throat irritation, and throat pain in addition to the usual hypoglycemic risk; and are limited to 4-, 8-, and 12-unit doses. They have been shown to have limited efficacy when compared with injected analog insulin in the setting of type 1 diabetes.

Approaches to the Treatment of Type 1 Diabetes Mellitus

Levels of glucose control equivalent to those achieved in the intensive treatment group in the DCCT are not possible in most patients unless an MDI regimen combining rapid- and long-acting insulin or CSII is used. More important than the schedule and method of administration is the need for the patient to adjust the insulin dose depending on the self-monitored glucose levels, dietary intake, and physical activity. The reason is relatively simple. In patients with little or no endogenous insulin production, the exogenous insulin regimen needs to simulate the multiphasic profile of insulin secretory responses to meals and snacks that is present in normal subjects if levels of glycemia approaching normal are to be achieved.

A number of regimens have been used to achieve these ends. Three basic approaches are reviewed here, although other approaches may be effective in individual patients. Achieving the glycemic goals of therapy is far more important than the details of the insulin regimen. Nevertheless, one of the following general approaches to therapy is most likely to lead to the desired outcome.

Combination of Rapid-Acting and Intermediate-Acting Insulin with Breakfast and Dinner and Intermediate-Acting Insulin at Bedtime

The rationale for regimens that use rapid- and intermediate-acting insulin at breakfast and dinner is that the rapid-acting insulin limits the postprandial glucose rise after breakfast and dinner, the intermediate-acting insulin administered before breakfast limits glycemia in the afternoon, and the intermediate-acting insulin before dinner limits glycemia in the early hours of the morning. Although such a regimen may be sufficient to achieve glucose targets in some patients, in many persons the intermediate-acting insulin given before dinner is insufficient to control elevations in blood glucose commonly seen in the early morning (dawn phenomenon). Attempts to increase the dose of intermediate-acting insulin at dinner expose the patient to a greater risk of hypoglycemia in the middle of the night; hence, there is a need for a smaller dose at bedtime to provide sufficient insulin to restrain the dawn phenomenon the following morning while moderating the risk of nocturnal hypoglycemia. This three-injection regimen was the mainstay of therapy in the DCCT but has largely been supplanted by regimens that take greater advantage of the availability of insulin analogues.

Combination of Rapid-Acting Insulin Given with Meals and Long-Acting Insulin at Bedtime

The combination of rapid-acting insulin with meals and long-acting insulin at bedtime can also simulate the pattern of insulin production that occurs normally. Use of monomeric insulin analogues provides excellent meal coverage. Use of long-acting insulin at bedtime provides excellent control of the fasting plasma glucose level. This combination of rapid-acting monomeric insulin analogues with long-acting analogues has largely supplanted human insulin-based treatment regimens because it seems to be associated with less variability in glycemic control and with lower risks of hypoglycemia. When long-acting insulin is administered once a day in the evening, an unexplained and consistent rise in glucose can occur just before the evening injection of long-acting insulin because the analogue's duration is less than 24 hours. This is more common in patients who require low doses (<20 units) of long-acting analogue and arguably is more common with detemir than with glargine; it can be remedied by dosing the long-acting insulin twice daily.

Insulin Administration by an External Insulin Pump

An alternative method of delivering insulin is by an external mechanical pump. This approach involves administering a rapid-acting insulin preparation by CSII through a catheter that is usually inserted into the subcutaneous tissues of the anterior abdominal wall. The pump delivers insulin as a preprogrammed basal infusion in addition to patient-directed boluses given before meals or snacks or in response to elevations in the blood glucose concentration outside the desired range. With currently available pumps, the basal insulin infusion rate (usually about 1 U/hour) can be programmed either to continue at a constant rate over the 24-hour period or, more commonly, to increase and decrease at predetermined times of the day to prevent anticipated excursions in the blood glucose concentration (e.g., morning rises in glucose). Newer pumps allow multiple basal profiles to deal with recurrent patterns (e.g., menstruation, weekends, and activity). Protocols for insulin administration by the pump usually provide for approximately half of the insulin to be administered as a basal infusion and the remainder as premeal boluses.

Insulin administration by an external pump has some advantages over regimens that use multiple insulin injections. Only rapid-acting insulin is used in the insulin pump because of benefits versus human regular insulin with respect to hypoglycemia rates.[314] Consequently, adjustments to the basal insulin infusion rate or changes in the size and timing of the insulin boluses result in more rapid changes in the blood glucose concentration than are possible when adjustments are made to the dose of intermediate- or long-acting insulin. This leads to greater flexibility for the patient. Current pumps generally employ a bolus calculator that is able to recommend insulin doses based not only on the expected carbohydrate content of the meal and the premeal glucose but also on an estimate of current levels of subcutaneous insulin still available based on prior insulin boluses to avoid insulin stacking of doses when boluses are administered more frequently than the effective pharmacokinetics of the insulin administered. Though major clinical differences between analogue insulins in CSII have not been observed, in vitro, aspart and lispro may be more stable than glulisine and less likely to produce catheter occlusions.[314] Insulin pump therapy with analog insulin is superior to human insulin with respect to hypoglycemia and is associated with improved glycemic control and quality of life.[315]

There are also disadvantages of insulin pump therapy.[315] There is a significant initial cost of the pump itself, and the tubing, which needs to be changed every 24 to 72 hours, and other supplies are expensive. The risk of infection at the site of insulin administration is significant. Infections occur on average once per year per patient even in the best of practices; although they can usually be treated by changing the site of infusion and giving a short course of oral antibiotics, surgical drainage may be necessary if an abscess develops. In addition, because only rapid-acting insulin is used, pump failure as a result of mechanical malfunction or catheter-related problems can quickly result in severe hyperglycemia and even ketoacidosis. Patients treated with insulin pump therapy must monitor their glucose level frequently and must always be alert to the possibility of failure of the infusion system.

Controlled clinical trials have indicated that, on average, insulin pump therapy is associated with modest improvements in glycemic control compared with MDI regimens—on the order of 0.5% as assessed by HbA_{1c}. Some patients never achieve adequate control with MDI but experience dramatic improvements with pump therapy. Insulin pump therapy should be used only by candidates who are strongly motivated to improve glucose control and willing to work with their health care provider in assuming substantial responsibility for their day-to-day care. They must also understand and demonstrate use of the insulin pump and self-monitoring of blood glucose and be able to use the data obtained in an appropriate fashion.

Sensor-Augmented Pump Therapy and Low-Glucose Suspend

Recent studies have examined the use of sensor-augmented pump (SAP) therapy in patients with T1DM who have inadequate control with an MDI regimen.[316] SAP therapy integrates insulin pump therapy with a continuous glucose monitor that transmits to the pump and allows patients and clinicians to monitor treatment (insulin doses, carbohydrate intake, exercise) and response (glucose measured by the continuous monitor and by self-monitoring of blood glucose) through the use of Internet-based software. The Sensor-Augmented Pump Therapy for A1C Reduction (STAR-3) study was a 1-year, multicenter, randomized, controlled comparison of SAP versus MDI in 329 adults and 156 children with inadequately controlled T1DM previously treated in the investigator's practice for at least 6 months with MDI. Patients in both arms received recombinant insulin analogues and were supervised by expert clinical teams. HbA_{1c} was reduced from a baseline of 8.3% to 7.5% in the SAP group, compared with 8.1% in the MDI group ($p < 0.001$). There was no difference between the randomized therapies in the rates of severe hypoglycemia, ketoacidosis, or weight gain. This 0.6% relative difference is substantial and is of the same range required for approval of an antihyperglycemic medication. This is the first device that has been demonstrated to provide improvements in average glycemic control of that magnitude.

More recently, SAP therapy has been further enhanced with the availability of low-glucose suspend features that suspend insulin delivery when glucose levels reach a programmed lower limit or when hypoglycemia is predicted. This has been associated with lower rates of nocturnal and overall hypoglycemia.[315]

Algorithms of Insulin Administration

An essential component of intensive regimens of insulin replacement is the need to make regular adjustments to the insulin dose depending on the prevailing blood glucose concentration, planned activity, and food intake. Algorithms have been developed to guide these adjustments that aim to simulate the normal feedback control of insulin secretion, whereby hyperglycemia stimulates and hypoglycemia inhibits insulin secretion. They all involve frequent monitoring of the blood glucose concentration, usually four or more times per day, or the use of CGM technology; increases in the insulin dose if glucose levels are above the target upper level; reductions in the insulin dose if glucose levels are below the acceptable lower level; and techniques for adjusting insulin doses in relation to changes in diet. Several algorithms are available.[317-319]

Pramlintide

Amylin is a neuroendocrine hormone cosecreted with insulin by pancreatic beta cells. It was originally identified as a major constituent of pancreatic amyloid deposits. Its biologically active form is a 37–amino acid peptide that undergoes extensive post-translational processing, including C-terminal amidation and glycosylation. As would be expected, amylin deficiency develops in parallel with insulin deficiency in patients with T1DM. Amylin and insulin have complementary actions in regulating plasma glucose. Insulin can be thought of as regulating the rate of glucose disappearance from the circulation. Amylin is thought to exert its major antihyperglycemic actions through central mechanisms after binding to brain nuclei such as the nucleus accumbens, dorsal raphe, and area postrema, promoting satiety and reducing appetite. It also is thought to act via vagal efferents, mediating a decrease in the rate of gastric emptying and a suppression of glucagon secretion in a glucose-dependent fashion. Effectively, amylin plays a role in regulating the rate of glucose appearance from the gastrointestinal tract and the liver.[320]

However, amylin is relatively insoluble in aqueous solution and aggregates on plastic and glass. Pramlintide was developed as a soluble, nonaggregating, equipotent amylin analogue.[292] In 2005, pramlintide was approved for human use in the United States. As expected, when pramlintide is injected before meals, it slows gastric emptying, suppresses glucagon, and promotes satiety, with a subsequent reduction in the postprandial glucose level. In T1DM, pramlintide therapy is usually initiated at a dose of 15 μg before meals (0.025 mL or 2.5 units in a U-100 insulin syringe of the marketed pramlintide acetate 0.6 mg/dL). Slow titration from there to the usual dose in patients with T1DM (60 μg before meals) as tolerated is recommended to minimize nausea and insulin-induced hypoglycemia. The maximal labeled dose in the setting of T2DM is 120 μg before meals.

In T1DM, the addition of pramlintide can be expected to produce modest reductions in HbA$_{1c}$ (0.3 percentage points) and weight (1.5 kg), compared with placebo in controlled trials. Weight loss is more prevalent in overweight patients than in those with normal body weight, and it is generally independent of nausea. Severe insulin hypoglycemia can develop as a complication, particularly on initiation, because the effect of pramlintide on satiety can be robust, effectively stopping some patients from eating midmeal. To minimize this risk, it is suggested that patients reduce rapid-acting insulin at meals by approximately 50% on initiation of pramlintide; this is optimally accomplished by reducing the insulin-to-carbohydrate ratio and in many cases by administering pramlintide before the meal and insulin after the meal so that insulin dose reduction can be accomplished if the meal is not finished. Despite its role in glucagon regulation, pramlintide does not interfere with recovery from insulin-induced hypoglycemia.

Pramlintide is an agent whose role in the routine management of T1DM is evolving. The additional injections and expense certainly constitute a burden to patients and the health care system. Most patients note a dramatic improvement in postprandial glucose. Many find the appetite-suppressing effects quite helpful even in the absence of substantial weight gain. Some report an improvement in sense of well-being and energy. What is certain is that initiating and titrating pramlintide is complex and fraught with potential pitfalls. Perhaps more so than any other treatment for diabetes, it requires careful collaboration of patients and diabetes educators.

Use of Type 2 Diabetes Drugs in Type 1 Diabetes

The use of drugs primarily indicated for the management of type 2 diabetes in the setting of type 1 diabetes has become more common. In general the safety and benefits of these agents is not well established.[292] Metformin has been shown to produce some reduction in insulin dose and weight in the setting of type 1 diabetes. Glucagon-like peptide-1 (GLP-1) receptor agonists suppress the inappropriate rise in glucagon in the postprandial period as well as enhance satiety in the setting of type 1 diabetes and may reduce glycemic variability and promote weight loss. Sodium-glucose cotransporter 2 (SGLT2) inhibitors result in glycosuria and thus a non-insulin dependent clearance of glucose from the circulation with resulting improved glycemic control and weight loss. A recent report suggests that euglycemic DKA and ketosis may be more frequent in patients with type 1 or type 2 diabetes treated with SGLT2 inhibitors.[321] Thus any patient treated with SGLT2 inhibitors who experiences nausea, vomiting, or malaise, or who develops a metabolic acidosis, should be promptly evaluated for the presence of urine and/or serum ketones, even

if glucose levels are near normal. Thus SGLT2 inhibitors should only be used with great caution, extensive counseling, and close monitoring in the setting of type 1 diabetes.

Complications of Intensive Management
Hypoglycemia

The most serious complication of intensive regimens of insulin replacement is hypoglycemia, and this is usually the factor that limits patients' ability to achieve tight glucose control. In the DCCT, patients in the intensive treatment group had an approximately threefold greater risk of hypoglycemia than those in the conventional treatment group. Hypoglycemia can be life threatening, leading to motor vehicle accidents, serious falls with fractures, and seizures. Patients with T1DM have serious defects in mechanisms responsible for glucose counterregulation, and this is a major underlying reason for the predisposition to hypoglycemia. Glucose counterregulation is reviewed in detail in Chapter 33.

The risk of hypoglycemia can be reduced if all patients treated with intensive regimens of insulin replacement are carefully educated about recognizing the symptoms of hypoglycemia and about the measures that should be taken to prevent more serious hypoglycemia after symptoms are initially experienced. Certain patients, particularly those with long-standing diabetes and autonomic neuropathy, may not subjectively sense symptoms of hypoglycemia even in the presence of low glucose concentrations. Glycemic targets of therapy should be adjusted upward in these patients, because they are at particularly high risk for hypoglycemia. Similarly, patients with advanced end-stage microvascular or macrovascular diabetic complications, in whom the benefit of intensive glucose control is likely to be less, should not be exposed to the increased risk of hypoglycemia that is inherent in extremely intensive insulin-treatment regimens.

In addition to the availability of glucose tablets, hard candy, or other sources of a readily absorbable form of carbohydrate, almost all patients with T1DM should have emergency glucagon kits at home and at work, assuming that there are people in those settings who can be trained to use them. The administration of 0.5 to 1 mg of glucagon intramuscularly to a severely symptomatic person with hypoglycemia rapidly increases the plasma glucose concentration to an acceptable range and prevents the difficulties and dangers associated with attempting to get a stuporous or disoriented person to ingest glucose by mouth. Nevertheless, because of occasional failures of glucagon to reverse hypoglycemia fully, friends and family members should always be instructed to call for medical assistance as soon as the injection is provided.

Recurrent severe hypoglycemia is essentially a medical emergency. If the above measures are not successful in preventing severe hypoglycemia, CGM should be employed either alone or in the context of sensor-augmented insulin pump therapy, preferably with an automated low-glucose suspend feature. For the rare patient whose recurrent severe hypoglycemia persists, islet or pancreas transplant should be considered.[322]

Weight Gain

Improvement in glucose control with a reduction in glycosuria is invariably associated with weight gain as the leakage of calories into the urine is reduced or eliminated. In addition, increased food intake to treat or prevent hypoglycemia can contribute to weight gain. Insulin itself can stimulate appetite. As a result of the combination of all these effects, weight gain is common, particularly with intensive regimens of insulin replacement. As discussed earlier, weight gain can be minimized or partially reversed with the addition of pramlintide or with less well-validated therapies primarily indicated for type 1 diabetes such as metformin, GLP-1 receptor, or SGLT-2 inhibitors.[292]

Worsening of Retinopathy

The institution of regimens of tight glucose control has been reported to exacerbate underlying retinopathy. Therefore, if a patient with a serious background of proliferative retinopathy presents in poor glucose control, ophthalmologic treatment of the retinopathy should be considered before tight glucose control is instituted.

Insulin Allergy

Discussed earlier in this chapter, insulin allergy has become much less common with the use of human insulin. Most manifestations of allergic reactions to insulin consist of local wheal-and-flare reactions at the site of injection. The allergic reaction can be to the insulin itself or to other components of the insulin preparation, such as the protamine in NPH insulin, a component of the diluent or materials or coatings in the bottle or syringe. Switching insulin formulations or devices to administer insulin can result in resolution of the problem. Occasionally, more generalized allergic reactions occur, and even more rarely, anaphylactic reactions take place. In general, mild local allergic reactions to insulin can be treated with antihistamines. More severe reactions require desensitization or coadministration of glucocorticoids. Under close supervision of a physician with access to equipment for emergency resuscitation, a protocol is followed in which the patient is exposed to gradually increasing amounts of insulin administered according to a set schedule.[323]

ACUTE DIABETIC EMERGENCIES: DIABETIC KETOACIDOSIS

DKA is a life-threatening condition in which severe insulin deficiency leads to hyperglycemia, excessive lipolysis, and unrestrained fatty acid oxidation, producing the ketone bodies acetone, β-hydroxybutyrate, and acetoacetate. This results in metabolic acidosis, dehydration, and deficits in fluid and electrolytes. Excess secretion of primarily glucagon, as well as catecholamines, glucocorticoids, and growth hormone, in combination with insulin deficiency produces hyperglycemia by stimulating glycogenolysis and gluconeogenesis and impairing glucose disposal. DKA is a far more characteristic feature of T1DM than of T2DM, but it may be seen in persons with T2DM under conditions of stress such as occur with serious infections, trauma, and cardiovascular or other emergencies.

Clinical Presentation

Patients with uncontrolled diabetes present with nonspecific complaints. If the disease follows an indolent course over months to years, patients can manifest profound wasting, cachexia, and prostration similar in degree to those of patients with long-standing malignancy or chronic infection. With significant physical or emotional stress, sudden metabolic decompensation can occur. The cases of DKA that are misdiagnosed usually occur in patients with new-onset diabetes. Polyuria (or at least nocturia) and weight loss are almost always present, although they are often not reported by the patient. Any patient with severe illness (acute or chronic) or neurologic changes should have glucose and electrolytes measured.

In DKA, metabolic decompensation usually develops over a period of hours to a few days. Patients with DKA classically present with lethargy and a characteristic hyperventilation pattern with deep, slow breaths (Kussmaul respirations) associated with the fruity odor of acetone. They often complain of nausea and vomiting; abdominal pain is somewhat less frequent. The abdominal pain can be quite severe and may be associated with distention, ileus, and tenderness without rebound, but it usually resolves relatively quickly with therapy unless there is an underlying abdominal condition. Most patients are normotensive, tachycardic, and tachypneic and have signs of mild to moderate volume depletion. Hypothermia has been described in DKA, and patients with underlying infection might not manifest fever. Cerebral edema does occur, usually during therapy. Patients with DKA can have stupor and obvious profound dehydration, and they often demonstrate focal neurologic deficits such as Babinski reflexes, asymmetric reflexes, cranial nerve findings, paresis, fasiculations, and aphasia.

Laboratory Test Results and Differential Diagnosis
Laboratory Tests

Laboratory tests that are routinely monitored in the setting of DKA include hemoglobin, white blood cell and differential count, glucose, electrolytes, BUN, and creatinine. Changes in Na, K, Cl, P, BUN, and creatinine are also monitored.

The sine qua non of DKA is acidosis, and the serum bicarbonate (HCO_3^-) concentration is usually less than 10 mEq/L. The acidosis is caused by production and accumulation of ketones in the serum. Three ketones are produced in DKA: two ketoacids (β-hydroxybutyrate and acetoacetate) and the neutral ketone, acetone. Ketones can be detected in serum and urine using the nitroprusside reaction on diagnostic strips for use at the patient's bedside or in the clinical laboratory. This test detects acetoacetate more effectively than acetone and does not detect an increased concentration of β-hydroxybutyrate. Particularly in severe DKA, β-hydroxybutyrate is the predominant ketone, and it is possible, although unusual, to have a negative serum nitroprusside reaction in the presence of severe ketosis. However, under these circumstances the serum bicarbonate is still markedly reduced and the anion gap is increased, indicating metabolic acidosis. Home hand-held meters can measure β-hydroxybutyrate and can be useful in managing sick days, particularly in those with recurrent issues with DKA or ketosis.

The anion gap is a readily available index for unmeasured anions in the blood (normal, ≤14 mEq/L):

$$Anion\ gap = sodium - (chloride + bicarbonate)$$

Most patients with DKA present with an anion gap greater than 20 mEq/L, and some present with a gap greater than 40 mEq/L. However, patients occasionally have a hyperchloremic metabolic acidosis without a significant anion gap.[324]

Patients with DKA almost invariably have large amounts of ketones in their urine. The serum glucose in DKA is usually in the 500-mg/dL range. However, an entity known as euglycemic DKA has been described, particularly in patients who have decreased oral intake or are pregnant, in which the serum glucose is normal or near normal but the patient requires insulin therapy for clearance of ketoacidosis.[325] The arterial pH is commonly less than 7.3 and can be as low as 6.5. There is partial respiratory compensation with hypocarbia. Patients are often mildly hyperosmolar, although osmolality greater than 330 mOsm/kg is unusual without mental status changes.

Differential Diagnosis

Not all patients with hyperglycemia and an anion gap metabolic acidosis have DKA, and other causes of metabolic acidosis must be considered in these patients, particularly if the serum or urine ketone measurements are not elevated. The following causes of metabolic acidosis need to be considered in the differential diagnosis of DKA.

Lactic acidosis is the most common cause of metabolic acidosis in hospitalized patients and can be seen in patients with uncomplicated diabetes as well as those with DKA. Lactic acidosis usually occurs in the setting of decreased tissue oxygen delivery, which results in the nonoxidative metabolism of glucose to lactic acid. Lactic acidosis complicates other primary metabolic acidoses as a consequence of dehydration or shock, and assessing its relative contribution can be difficult. The presentation is identical to that of DKA. In pure lactic acidosis, the serum glucose and ketones should be normal and the serum lactate concentration should be greater than 5 mmol/L. The therapy for lactic acidosis is directed at the underlying cause and at optimization of tissue perfusion.[326]

Starvation ketosis is caused by inadequate carbohydrate availability, which results in physiologically appropriate lipolysis and ketone production to provide fuel substrates for muscle. The blood glucose concentration is usually normal. Although the urine can have large amounts of ketones, the blood rarely does. Arterial pH is normal, and the anion gap is at most mildly elevated.

Alcoholic ketoacidosis is a more severe form of starvation ketosis wherein the appropriate ketogenic response to poor carbohydrate intake is increased through as yet poorly defined effects of alcohol on the liver. Classically, these patients are long-standing alcoholics for whom ethanol has been the main caloric source for days to weeks. The ketoacidosis occurs when, for some reason, alcohol and caloric intake decrease. In isolated alcoholic ketoacidosis, the metabolic acidosis is usually mild to moderate. The anion gap is elevated. Serum and urine ketones are always present. However, alcoholic ketoacidosis produces an even higher ratio of β-hydroxybutyrate to acetoacetate than DKA does, and negative or weakly positive nitroprusside reactions are common. Respiratory alkalosis associated with delirium tremens, agitation, or pulmonary processes often normalizes the pH but should be evident with careful analysis of acid-base status. Usually, the patient is normoglycemic or hypoglycemic, although mild hyperglycemia is occasionally present. Patients who are significantly hyperglycemic should be treated as if they had DKA. The therapy for alcoholic ketoacidosis consists of thiamine, carbohydrates, fluids, and electrolytes, with special attention to the more severe consequences of alcohol toxicity, alcohol withdrawal, and chronic malnutrition. In more severely ill patients in whom alcoholic ketoacidosis is considered a possibility, there is usually another underlying illness such as pancreatitis, gastrointestinal bleeding, hepatic encephalopathy, delirium tremens, or infection complicated by concomitant lactic acidosis.[327,328]

Uremic acidosis is characterized by extremely large elevations in the BUN (often >200 mg/dL) and creatinine (>10 mg/dL) values with normoglycemia. The pH and anion gap are usually only mildly abnormal. The treatment is supportive, with careful attention to fluid and electrolytes until dialysis can be performed. Rhabdomyolysis is a cause of renal failure in which the anion gap can be significantly elevated and acidosis can be severe. There should be marked elevation of creatine phosphokinase and myoglobin. Mild rhabdomyolysis is not uncommon in DKA, but the presence of hyperglycemia and ketonemia leaves no doubt about the primary cause of the acidosis.[329]

Toxic ingestions can be differentiated from DKA by history and laboratory investigation. Salicylate intoxication produces an anion gap metabolic acidosis, usually with an accompanying respiratory alkalosis. The plasma glucose level is normal or low, the osmolality is normal, ketones are negative, and salicylates can be detected in the urine or blood. Salicylates can cause a false-positive glucose determination when the cupric sulfate method is used and a false-negative result when the glucose oxidase reaction is used. Methanol and ethylene glycol also produce an anion gap metabolic acidosis without hyperglycemia or ketones, but these toxins need to be kept in mind primarily because they produce an increase in the measured serum osmolality but not in the calculated serum osmolality—an osmolar gap. Their serum levels can also be measured. Isopropyl alcohol does not cause a metabolic acidosis but should be remembered because it is metabolized to acetone, which can produce a positive result in the nitroprusside reaction commonly used for the detection of ketoacids. These intoxications must be appropriately treated.[330-332] Rare cases of anion gap acidoses have been reported with other ingestions, including toluene, iron, hydrogen sulfide, nalidixic acid, papaverine, paraldehyde, strychnine, isoniazid, and outdated tetracycline. When DKA is considered, the diagnosis can be made quickly with routine laboratory tests. Measurements of blood and urine glucose and ketones can be obtained in minutes, using, respectively, glucose oxidase–impregnated strips and the nitroprusside reaction.

Osmolarity

The increase in osmolarity (in milliosmoles per liter [mOsm/L]) that occurs in DKA must be differentiated from the increase in osmolarity seen in hyperosmolar-hyperglycemic nonketotic (diabetic) coma (HHNC). The osmolarity can be measured by freezing point depression or estimated with the use of the following formula:

$$\text{Osmolarity} = (2 \times \text{sodium}) + (\text{glucose}/18) + (\text{BUN}/2.8) + (\text{ethanol}/4.6)$$

Patients with DKA not uncommonly present with hyperosmolarity and coma. In HHNC, the osmolarity is usually greater than 350 mOsm/L, and it can exceed 400 mOsm/L. The serum sodium and potassium levels can be high, normal, or low and do not reflect total-body levels, which are uniformly depleted. The glucose concentration is usually greater than 600 mg/dL, and levels higher than 1000 mg/dL are common. In pure HHNC, there is no significant metabolic acidosis or anion gap.

Patients often present with combinations of the preceding findings. HHNC can involve mild to moderate ketonemia and acidosis. Alcoholic ketoacidosis can contribute to either DKA or HHNC. Lactic acidosis is common in severe DKA and HHNC. Any patient with hyperglycemia greater than 250 mg/dL and an anion gap metabolic acidosis should be treated by the general principles outlined in the following section, with special consideration for other possible contributing metabolic acidoses.

Therapy

The optimal management of DKA has been a source of considerable controversy since the 1950s. Only recently have prospective studies of various therapeutic approaches been performed. The guidelines we propose rely heavily on prospective studies of DKA by Kitabchi and coworkers.[333,334] The general approach is to provide necessary fluids to restore the circulation, treat insulin deficiency with continuous insulin, treat electrolyte disturbances, observe the patient closely and carefully, and search for underlying causes of metabolic decompensation.

Fluids

Volume contraction is one of the hallmarks of DKA. It can contribute to acidosis through lactic acid production and decreased renal clearance of organic and inorganic acids. It contributes to hyperglycemia by decreasing renal clearance of glucose. Decreased tissue perfusion, if significant, causes insulin resistance by decreasing insulin delivery to the sites of insulin-mediated glucose disposal, namely muscle and adipose tissue, and through stimulation of catecholamine and glucocorticoid secretion. Fluid deficits on the order of 5 to 10 L are common in DKA. The urine produced during the osmotic diuresis of hyperglycemia is approximately half-normal with respect to sodium. Therefore, water deficits are in excess of sodium deficits. Historically, large quantities of isotonic intravenous fluids have been administered rapidly to patients in DKA. For patients with a history of congestive heart failure, chronic or acute renal failure, severe hypotension, or significant pulmonary disease, early invasive hemodynamic monitoring should be considered.

When there is physical evidence of dehydration (i.e., hypotension, decreased skin turgor, or dry mucous membranes), the general treatment is to administer 1 L of normal saline over the first hour and 200 to 500 mL/hour in subsequent hours until hypotension resolves and adequate circulation is maintained. If hypotension is severe, there is clinical evidence of hypoperfusion, and hypotension does not respond to crystalloid, therapy with colloid is considered, often in combination with invasive hemodynamic monitoring. If there is no hypotension and no concern about renal failure, 1 L of half-normal saline is administered over the first hour.

During that first hour, the laboratory data usually return and can be quite helpful in planning further therapy. Despite the excess of water losses over sodium, the measured sodium is usually low because of the osmotic effects of glucose. These osmotic effects can be corrected using a simple formula:

$$\text{Corrected sodium concentration} = \text{measured sodium} + 0.016 \times (\text{glucose} - 100)$$

Severe hypertriglyceridemia, which is common in severe diabetes, can cause a false decrease in the serum sodium concentration by approximately 1.0 mEq/L at a serum lipid concentration of 460 mg/dL.[323] An estimated water deficit can be calculated using the corrected sodium concentration:

$$\text{Water deficit (in liters)} = 0.6 \times \text{weight (in kg)} \times [(\text{sodium}/140) - 1]$$

Based on these formulas, a 70-kg patient with a measured sodium level of 140 mEq/L and a glucose concentration of 1000 mg/dL would have a calculated water deficit of 4.3 L. If the patient is normotensive after the first liter of fluids has been administered, it is reasonable to aim to replace urinary losses with one-half normal saline and to provide approximately one half of the water deficit (in this example, 2 L) as 5% dextrose over the first 12 to 24 hours and the remainder over the subsequent 24 hours. The plan for fluid therapy should be continuously reevaluated in light of the clinical and laboratory response of the patient. When the serum glucose level reaches 250 to 300 mg/dL, all fluids should contain 5% dextrose and therapy should be aimed at maintaining the serum glucose concentration in that range for 24 hours to allow slow equilibration of osmotically active substances across cell membranes.

The primary goal of fluid therapy is to maintain an adequate circulation, and the secondary goal is to maintain a brisk diuresis. Beyond that, pulmonary edema, hyperchloremic metabolic acidosis, and a rapid fall in the serum osmolality should be prevented by frequent monitoring of the patient and administration of glucose and electrolytes. It has been demonstrated that fluid administration and subsequent continued osmotic diuresis are responsible for a large portion of the initial decline in glucose during therapy.

Insulin

Insulin is the mainstay of therapy for DKA because DKA is essentially an insulin-deficient state. In the past, high doses of insulin (50 U/hour or more) were favored. In later studies, low-dose insulin therapy (0.1 U/kg/hour) has been shown to be as effective as higher doses in producing a decrease in serum glucose and clearance of ketones. Furthermore, low-dose therapy results in a reduction in the major morbidity of intensive insulin therapy, namely, hypoglycemia and hypokalemia.

Studies have also shown that intravenous insulin is significantly more effective than intramuscular or subcutaneous insulin in lowering the ketone body concentration over the first 2 hours of therapy. The subcutaneous route is probably inappropriate for the critically ill patient because of the possibility of tissue hypoperfusion and slower kinetics of absorption; however, one study documented that a subcutaneous rapid-acting insulin analogue administered every 1 to 2 hours was as safe and effective as intravenous regular insulin in the treatment of uncomplicated DKA.[335] Numerous studies attest to the efficacy of intramuscular therapy in severe DKA. If there is insufficient nursing monitoring or intravenous access to allow safe intravenous administration, intramuscular therapy is the route of choice.

It has been shown that a 10-U intravenous insulin priming dose given at the initiation of insulin therapy significantly improves the glycemic response to the first hour of therapy. The rationale is to saturate insulin receptors fully before beginning continuous therapy and to avoid the lag time that is necessary to achieve steady-state insulin levels. When insulin is mixed in normal saline, it does not seem to be necessary to add albumin to prevent insulin adsorption to the infusion set. However, the intravenous tubing should be flushed with the insulin infusate before use.

In the rare instances in which the glucose level does not decrease by at least 10% or 50 mg/dL in 1 hour, the insulin infusion rate should be increased by 50% to 100% and a second bolus of intravenous insulin should be administered. As the glucose level decreases, it is usually necessary to decrease the rate of infusion. After the glucose reaches approximately 250 mg/dL, it is prudent to decrease the insulin infusion rate and administer dextrose. It usually takes an additional 12 to 24 hours to clear ketones from the circulation after hyperglycemia is controlled. With resolution of ketosis, the rate of infusion approaches the physiologic range of 0.3 to 0.5 U/kg per day.

When the decision is made to feed the patient, intravenous or intramuscular therapy should be changed to subcutaneous therapy. Subcutaneous insulin should be administered before a meal, and the insulin drip should be discontinued approximately 30 minutes later. The glucose should be checked in 2 hours and at least every 4 hours afterward until a relatively stable insulin regimen is determined. Early conversion to oral feeding and subcutaneous insulin therapy is associated with a shorter hospital stay.

Potassium

Potassium losses during the development of DKA are usually quite high (3-10 mEq/kg) and are mediated by shifts to the extracellular space secondary to acidosis and protein catabolism compounded by hyperaldosteronism and osmotic diuresis. Although most patients with DKA or HHNC have a normal or even high serum potassium level at presentation, the initial therapy with fluids and insulin causes it to fall.

Our approach has been to monitor the electrocardiogram (ECG) for signs of hyperkalemia (peaked T wave, widening QRS complex) initially and to administer potassium if these signs are absent and the serum potassium level is less than 5.5 mEq/L. If the patient is oliguric, we do not administer potassium unless the serum concentration is less than 4 mEq/L or there are ECG signs of hypokalemia (U wave), and even then potassium is administered with extreme caution. With treatment of DKA, the potassium level always falls, usually reaching a nadir after several hours. We usually replace potassium at 10 to 20 mEq/hour (half as potassium chloride and half as potassium phosphate), monitor serum levels at least every 2 hours initially, and monitor ECG morphologic patterns. Occasionally, patients with DKA who have had protracted courses that include vomiting, hypokalemia, and acidosis require 40 to 60 mEq/hour by central line to prevent further decreases in the serum potassium concentration.

Phosphate

Like potassium, phosphate is depleted in patients with DKA. Although patients usually present with an elevated serum phosphate concentration, the serum level declines with therapy. No well-documented clinical significance of these findings has been determined and no benefit of phosphate administration has been demonstrated, but most authorities recommend phosphate therapy as before and monitoring for its possible complications, which include hypocalcemia and hypomagnesemia.

Bicarbonate

Serum bicarbonate is always low in DKA, but a true deficit is not present because the ketoacids and lactate anions are metabolized to bicarbonate during therapy. The use of bicarbonate in the treatment of DKA is highly controversial. No benefit of bicarbonate therapy has been demonstrated in clinical trials. In fact, in two trials, hypokalemia was more common in bicarbonate-treated patients. There are theoretical considerations against the use of bicarbonate. Cellular levels of 2,3-diphosphoglycerate are depleted in DKA, causing a shift in the oxyhemoglobin dissociation curve to the left and thus impairing tissue oxygen delivery. Acidemia has the opposite effect, and therefore acute reversal of acidosis could decrease tissue oxygen delivery. In addition, in vitro data suggest that pH is a regulator of cellular lactate metabolism, and correction of acidosis could increase lactate production. These observations are of questionable clinical relevance, however.

We reserve bicarbonate therapy for patients with severe acidosis (pH <6.9), patients with hemodynamic instability if the pH is less than 7.1, and patients with hyperkalemia with ECG findings. When bicarbonate is used, it should be used sparingly and considered a temporizing measure while definitive therapy with insulin and fluids is under way. Approximately 1 mEq/kg of bicarbonate is administered as a rapid infusion over 10 to 15 minutes, and further therapy is based on repeated arterial blood gas sampling every 30 to 120 minutes. Potassium therapy should be considered before treatment with bicarbonate is undertaken, because transient hypokalemia is not an uncommon complication of the administration of alkali.

Monitoring

It is possible to manage many cases of mild DKA without admitting the patient to the intensive care unit, depending on staff availability. We routinely admit patients with DKA to the intensive care unit if they have a pH of less than 7.3. If mental status is compromised, prophylactic intubation is considered, and nasogastric suctioning is always performed because of frequent ileus and danger of aspiration. If the patient cannot void at will, bladder catheterization is necessary to monitor urine output adequately. ECG monitoring is continuous, with hourly documentation of QRS intervals and T-wave morphologic appearance. Initially, serum glucose, electrolytes, BUN, creatinine, calcium, magnesium, phosphate, ketones, lactate, creatine phosphokinase, and liver function tests as well as urinalysis, ECG, upright chest radiograph, complete blood count, and arterial blood gas analyses are obtained. If there is any concern about possible toxic ingestions, toxicology screening is also performed. Subsequently, glucose and electrolytes are measured at least hourly; calcium, magnesium, and phosphate every 2 hours; and BUN, creatinine, and ketones every 6 to 24 hours.

It is often not necessary to monitor arterial blood gases routinely, because the bicarbonate level and the anion gap are relatively good indices of the response to therapy. Monitoring of venous pH has also been shown to reflect acidemia and response to therapy adequately. Usually, frequent blood work is necessary only for the first 12 hours or so. In the severely ill patient with obvious underlying disease, the course is often more protracted, and, particularly when venous access is a problem, early consideration should be given to placement of an arterial line. A flow sheet tabulating these findings as well as mental status, vital signs, insulin dose, fluid and electrolytes administered, and urine output allows easy analysis of response to therapy. After the acidosis begins to resolve and the response to therapy becomes predictable, it is reasonable to curtail laboratory testing. If the patient's cardiovascular status is unclear or troublesome, invasive hemodynamic monitoring is an appropriate guide for fluid therapy. The goals should be to achieve hemodynamic stability rapidly and to correct DKA fully in 12 to 36 hours.

Search for Underlying Causes

After the patient is stabilized, a careful history and physical examination is performed and a diagnostic strategy is developed that should be aimed at determining the precipitating event. In most inner-city practices, the most common cause of DKA is noncompliance with insulin therapy, which is usually easily treated. The second most common cause is infection, with viral syndromes, urinary tract infection, pelvic inflammatory disease, and pneumonia predominating. It is often difficult to determine initially whether the patient is infected. Fever is absent in a significant fraction of patients with diabetic emergencies. The white blood cell count is not uncommonly elevated in the range of 20,000/µL or higher, even in the absence of infection.[336] As a result, cultures should be performed for most patients, and if there is significant concern about infection, empiric broad antibiotic coverage should be considered pending microbiologic findings.

Special consideration should be given to ruling out meningitis in the patient with altered mental status. In this regard, most would perform lumbar puncture in all patients with meningismus and in patients with disproportionate mental status changes. If the index of suspicion is lower, the antibiotic therapy should be geared to cover bacterial meningitis, and a lumbar puncture should be performed if the mental status does not improve quickly with therapy. The cerebrospinal fluid glucose measurement is not particularly useful in determining whether the fluid is infected, and a level lower than 100 mg/dL is unusual when the serum glucose concentration is greater than 250 mg/dL.[337] The relative frequency of sinus infection (particularly with *Mucor*), foot infection, bacterial arthritis, cholecystitis, cellulitis, and necrotizing fasciitis should also be considered.

Pneumonia can be difficult to diagnose in patients with dehydration because the alveolar edema fluid that shows up as an infiltrate on chest radiographs is often not present but develops along with progressive hypoxia during hydration. To prevent this occurrence, we administer intravenous fluid judiciously to patients with suspected pneumonia. Pancreatitis and pregnancy are common precipitants and should be especially considered when assessing the abdominal pain that is almost ubiquitous at presentation. Abdominal guarding and tenderness associated with vomiting are common, and rebound is occasionally present. These symptoms and findings usually resolve quickly with therapy in the absence of intra-abdominal disease. The serum amylase is often elevated without pathologic significance, although lipase is usually more specific.[338] Acute myocardial infarction, stroke, and thromboembolic phenomena are frequent precipitants and complications of DKA. The more insulin resistant the patient seems to be, the more likely one is to find a precipitating cause. If a precipitating cause is found, treatment is essential if adequate metabolic control is to be achieved.

Complications and Prognosis

It should now be possible to treat almost all cases of DKA successfully. The most troublesome complication is cerebral edema. It is common particularly in children and can be fatal. In most reported series, specific causes could not be assigned, although aggressive hydration, particularly with hypotonic fluids, can contribute.[339] In 50% of patients who subsequently had a respiratory arrest, there were premonitory symptoms, and despite early intervention only half of them avoided severe or fatal brain damage.

Other complications of life-threatening severity that have been reported include the acute respiratory distress syndrome and bronchial mucus plugging.[340-342] Arterial and venous thromboembolic events are quite common. Standard prophylactic low-dose heparin is certainly reasonable in patients with DKA, but currently no indication exists

for full anticoagulation. Two studies show that specialists (endocrinologists) provide more cost-effective care than nonspecialists. Patients under the care of specialists have a shorter hospital stay, fewer medical procedures, and lower medical costs.[343,344]

REFERENCES

1. Neve ET. On the morbid anatomy of the pancreas. *Lancet.* 1891;138(3551):659-661.
2. Bayliss WM, Starling EH. The mechanism of pancreatic secretion. *J Physiol.* 1902;28:325-353.
3. Banting FG, Best CH. The internal secretion of the pancreas. *J Lab Clin Med.* 1922;7:251-266.
4. Schmidt MB. Über die Beziehung der Langerhans'schen Inseln des Pankreas zum Diabetes mellitus. *Münch Med Wochenschr.* 1902;49:51-54.
5. Warren S. The pathology of diabetes in children. *J Am Med Assoc.* 1927;88:99-101.
6. von Meyenburg H. Ueber "Insulitis" bei Diabetes. *Schweiz Med Wochenschr.* 1940;21:554-557.
7. Foulis AK, Stewart JA. The pancreas in recent-onset type 1 (insulin-dependent) diabetes mellitus: insulin content of islets, insulitis and associated changes in the exocrine acinar tissue. *Diabetologia.* 1984;26:456-461.
8. Atkinson MA, Gianani R. The pancreas in human type 1 diabetes: providing new answers to age-old questions. *Curr Opin Endocrinol Diabetes Obes.* 2009;16:279-285.
9. In't Veld P. Insulitis in human type 1 diabetes: the quest for an elusive lesion. *Islets.* 2011;3(4):131-138.
10. LeCompte PM, Legg MA. Insulitis (lymphocytic infiltration of pancreatic islets) in late-onset diabetes. *Diabetes.* 1972;21:762-769.
11. Gepts W. Pathologic anatomy of the pancreas in juvenile diabetes mellitus. *Diabetes.* 1965;14:619-633.
12. Bottazzo GF, Florin-Christensen A, Doniach D. Islet-cell antibodies in diabetes mellitus with autoimmune polyendocrine deficiencies. *Lancet.* 1974;2:1279-1283.
13. Bottazzo GF, Cudworth AG, Moul DJ, et al. Evidence for a primary autoimmune type of diabetes mellitus. *Br Med J.* 1978;2:1253-1255.
14. American Diabetes Association. Diagnosis and classification of diabetes mellitus. *Diabetes Care.* 2012;35(Suppl 1):S64-S71.
15. International Expert Committee report on the role of the A1C assay in the diagnosis of diabetes. *Diabetes Care.* 2009;32:1327-1334.
16. Ziegler AG, Hummel M, Schenker M, Bonifacio E. Autoantibody appearance and risk for development of childhood diabetes in offspring of parents with type 1 diabetes: the 2-year analysis of the German BABYDIAB Study. *Diabetes.* 1999;48:460-468.
17. Steck AK, Johnson K, Barriga KJ, et al. Age of islet autoantibody appearance and mean levels of insulin, but not GAD or IA-2 autoantibodies, predict age of diagnosis of type 1 diabetes: diabetes autoimmunity study in the young. *Diabetes Care.* 2011;34:1397-1399.
18. Orban T, Sosenko JM, Cuthbertson D, et al. Pancreatic islet autoantibodies as predictors of type 1 diabetes in the Diabetes Prevention Trial-Type 1. *Diabetes Care.* 2009;32:2269-2274.
19. Dabelea D, Pihoker C, Talton JW, et al. Etiological approach to characterization of diabetes type: the SEARCH for Diabetes in Youth Study. *Diabetes Care.* 2011;34:1628-1633.
20. Pinhas-Hamiel O, Dolan LM, Daniels SR, et al. Increased incidence of non-insulin-dependent diabetes mellitus among adolescents. *J Pediatr.* 1996;128:608-615.
21. Pinhas-Hamiel O, Dolan LM, Zeitler PS. Diabetic ketoacidosis among obese African-American adolescents with NIDDM. *Diabetes Care.* 1997;20:484-486.
22. Rosenbloom AL, House DV, Winter WE. Non-insulin dependent diabetes mellitus (NIDDM) in minority youth: research priorities and needs. *Clin Pediatr (Phila).* 1998;37:143-152.
23. Wilkin TJ. The accelerator hypothesis: a review of the evidence for insulin resistance as the basis for type I as well as type II diabetes. *Int J Obes (Lond).* 2009;33:716-726.
24. Soderstrom U, Aman J, Hjern A. Being born in Sweden increases the risk for type 1 diabetes—a study of migration of children to Sweden as a natural experiment. *Acta Paediatr.* 2012;101(1):73-77.
25. Puett RC, Lamichhane AP, Nichols MD, et al. Neighborhood context and incidence of type 1 diabetes: the SEARCH for Diabetes in Youth study. *Health Place.* 2012;18(4):911-916.
26. Zhang L, Eisenbarth GS. Prediction and prevention of type 1 diabetes mellitus. *J Diabetes.* 2011;3:48-57.
27. Harjutsalo V, Sjoberg L, Tuomilehto J. Time trends in the incidence of type 1 diabetes in Finnish children: a cohort study. *Lancet.* 2008;371:1777-1782.
28. Moltchanova EV, Schreier N, Lammi N, Karvonen M. Seasonal variation of diagnosis of type 1 diabetes mellitus in children worldwide. *Diabet Med.* 2009;26(7):673-678.

29. Kahn HS, Morgan TM, Case LD, et al. Association of type 1 diabetes with month of birth among U.S. youth: the SEARCH for Diabetes in Youth Study. *Diabetes Care.* 2009;32:2010-2015.
30. Kukko M, Kimpimaki T, Korhonen S, et al. Dynamics of diabetes-associated autoantibodies in young children with human leukocyte antigen-conferred risk of type 1 diabetes recruited from the general population. *J Clin Endocrinol Metab.* 2005;90:2712-2717.
31. Tuomi T. Type 1 and type 2 diabetes: what do they have in common? *Diabetes.* 2005;54(Suppl 2):S40-S45.
32. Usher-Smith JA, Thompson MJ, Sharp SJ, Walter FM. Factors associated with the presence of diabetic ketoacidosis at diagnosis of diabetes in children and young adults: a systematic review. *BMJ.* 2011; 343:d4092.
33. Leslie RD, Kolb H, Schloot NC, et al. Diabetes classification: grey zones, sound and smoke: action LADA 1. *Diabetes Metab Res Rev.* 2008;24: 511-519.
34. Naik RG, Brooks-Worrell BM, Palmer JP. Latent autoimmune diabetes in adults. *J Clin Endocrinol Metab.* 2009;94:4635-4644.
35. Gale EA. Latent autoimmune diabetes in adults: a guide for the perplexed. *Diabetologia.* 2005;48:2195-2199.
36. Palmer JP. C-peptide in the natural history of type 1 diabetes. *Diabetes Metab Res Rev.* 2009;25:325-328.
37. McDonald TJ, Colclough K, Brown R, et al. Islet autoantibodies can discriminate maturity-onset diabetes of the young (MODY) from type 1 diabetes. *Diabet Med.* 2011;28:1028-1033.
38. Mordes JP, Bortell R, Doukas J, et al. The BB/Wor rat and the balance hypothesis of autoimmunity. *Diabetes Metab Rev.* 1996;12:103-109.
39. Roep BO, Atkinson M, von Herrath M. Satisfaction (not) guaranteed: re-evaluating the use of animal models of type 1 diabetes. *Nat Rev Immunol.* 2004;4:989-997.
40. Thomas HE, Kay TW. Beta cell destruction in the development of autoimmune diabetes in the non-obese diabetic (NOD) mouse. *Diabetes Metab Res Rev.* 2000;16:251-261.
41. Wong FS, Janeway CA Jr. Insulin-dependent diabetes mellitus and its animal models. *Curr Opin Immunol.* 1999;11:643-647.
42. Reed JC, Herold KC. Thinking bedside at the bench: the NOD mouse model of T1DM. *Nat Rev Endocrinol.* 2015;11(5):308-314.
43. Tooley JE, Waldron-Lynch F, Herold KC. New and future immuno-modulatory therapy in type 1 diabetes. *Trends Mol Med.* 2012;18: 173-181.
44. Ben Nasr M, D'Addio F, Usuelli V, et al. The rise, fall, and resurgence of immunotherapy in type 1 diabetes. *Pharmacol Res.* 2015;98:31-38.
45. Eisenbarth G. Animal models of T1D: genetics and immunological function. In: Eisenbarth G, Lafferty K, eds. *T1D: Molecular, Cellular, and Clinical Immunology.* 2nd ed. New York, NY: Kluwer Academic; 2005: 91-116.
46. Bettini M, Blanchfield L, Castellaw A, et al. TCR affinity and tolerance mechanisms converge to shape T cell diabetogenic potential. *J Immunol.* 2014;193:571-579.
47. Nakayama M, Abiru N, Moriyama H, et al. Prime role for an insulin epitope in the development of type 1 diabetes in NOD mice. *Nature.* 2005;435:220-223.
48. Liu CP. Glutamic acid decarboxylase-specific CD4+ regulatory T cells. *Ann N Y Acad Sci.* 2006;1079:161-170.
49. Wang J, Tsai S, Shameli A, et al. In situ recognition of autoantigen as an essential gatekeeper in autoimmune CD8+ T cell inflammation. *Proc Natl Acad Sci U S A.* 2010;107:9317-9322.
50. Stadinski BD, Delong T, Reisdorph N, et al. Chromogranin A is an autoantigen in type 1 diabetes. *Nat Immunol.* 2010;11:225-231.
51. Sreenan S, Pick AJ, Levisetti M, et al. Increased beta-cell proliferation and reduced mass before diabetes onset in the nonobese diabetic mouse. *Diabetes.* 1999;48:989-996.
52. Dilts SM, Lafferty KJ. Autoimmune diabetes: the involvement of benign and malignant autoimmunity. *J Autoimmun.* 1999;12:229-232.
53. Shimada A, Charlton B, Taylor-Edwards C, Fathman CG. Beta-cell destruction may be a late consequence of the autoimmune process in nonobese diabetic mice. *Diabetes.* 1996;45:1063-1067.
54. Chatenoud L, Primo J, Bach JF. CD3 antibody-induced dominant self tolerance in overtly diabetic NOD mice. *J Immunol.* 1997;158:2947-2954.
55. Faleo G, Fotino C, Bocca N, et al. Prevention of autoimmune diabetes and induction of β-cell proliferation in NOD mice by hyperbaric oxygen therapy. *Diabetes.* 2012;61:1769-1778.
56. Soltani N, Qiu H, Aleksic M, et al. GABA exerts protective and regenerative effects on islet beta cells and reverses diabetes. *Proc Natl Acad Sci U S A.* 2011;108:11692-11697.
57. Campbell JE, Drucker DJ. Pharmacology, physiology, and mechanisms of incretin hormone action. *Cell Metab.* 2013;17:819-837.
58. Bonner-Weir S, Li W-C, Ouziel-Yahalom L, et al. β-Cell growth and regeneration: replication is only part of the story. *Diabetes.* 2010;59: 2340-2348.
59. Bender A, Stewart AF. Good news for the ageing beta cell. *Diabetologia.* 2014;57:265-269.
60. Mezza T, Kulkarni RN. The regulation of pre- and post-maturational plasticity of mammalian islet cell mass. *Diabetologia.* 2014;57: 1291-1303.
61. Hattori M, Buse JB, Jackson RA, et al. The NOD mouse: recessive diabetogenic gene in the major histocompatibility complex. *Science.* 1986; 231:733-735.
62. Noble JA, Valdes AM, Cook M, et al. The role of HLA class II genes in insulin-dependent diabetes mellitus: molecular analysis of 180 Caucasian, multiplex families. *Am J Hum Genet.* 1996;59:1134-1148.
63. Todd JA, Bell JI, McDevitt HO. HLA-DQ beta gene contributes to susceptibility and resistance to insulin-dependent diabetes mellitus. *Nature.* 1987;329:599-604.
64. Lyons PA, Hancock WW, Denny P, et al. The NOD Idd9 genetic interval influences the pathogenicity of insulitis and contains molecular variants of Cd30, Tnfr2, and Cd137. *Immunity.* 2000;13:107-115.
65. Mathews CE, Graser RT, Serreze DV, Leiter EH. Reevaluation of the major histocompatibility complex genes of the NOD-progenitor CTS/Shi strain. *Diabetes.* 2000;49:131-134.
66. Yui MA, Muralidharan K, Moreno-Altamirano B, et al. Production of congenic mouse strains carrying NOD-derived diabetogenic genetic intervals: an approach for the genetic dissection of complex traits. *Mamm Genome.* 1996;7(5):331-334.
67. Wicker LS, Miller BJ, Coker LZ, et al. Genetic control of diabetes and insulitis in the nonobese diabetic (NOD) mouse. *J Exp Med.* 1987;165: 1639-1654.
68. Wicker LS, Clark J, Fraser HI, et al. Type 1 diabetes genes and pathways shared by humans and NOD mice. *J Autoimmun.* 2005;25(Suppl): 29-33.
69. Wakeland EK. Hunting autoimmune disease genes in NOD: early steps on a long road to somewhere important (hopefully). *J Immunol.* 2014;193:3-6.
70. Yu L, Robles DT, Abiru N, et al. Early expression of antiinsulin autoantibodies of humans and the NOD mouse: evidence for early determination of subsequent diabetes. *Proc Natl Acad Sci U S A.* 2000;97: 1701-1706.
71. Achenbach P, Koczwara K, Knopff A, et al. Mature high-affinity immune responses to (pro)insulin anticipate the autoimmune cascade that leads to type 1 diabetes. *J Clin Invest.* 2004;114:589-597.
72. Awata T, Guberski DL, Like AA. Genetics of the BB rat: association of autoimmune disorders (diabetes, insulitis, and thyroiditis) with lymphopenia and major histocompatibility complex class II. *Endocrinology.* 1995;136:5731-5735.
73. Jacob HJ, Pettersson A, Wilson D, et al. Genetic dissection of autoimmune type I diabetes in the BB rat. *Nat Genet.* 1992;2:56-60.
74. Like AA, Appel MC, Rossini AA. Autoantibodies in the BB/W rat. *Diabetes.* 1982;31:816-820.
75. Logothetopoulos J, Valiquette N, Madura E, Cvet D. The onset and progression of pancreatic insulitis in the overt, spontaneously diabetic, young adult BB rat studied by pancreatic biopsy. *Diabetes.* 1984;33: 33-36.
76. Uchigata Y, Yamamoto H, Nagai H, Okamoto H. Effect of poly(ADP-ribose) synthetase inhibitor administration to rats before and after injection of alloxan and streptozotocin on islet proinsulin synthesis. *Diabetes.* 1983;32:316-318.
77. Tanaka S, Nakajima S, Inoue S, et al. Genetic control by I-A subregion in H-2 complex of incidence of streptozocin-induced autoimmune diabetes in mice. *Diabetes.* 1990;39:1298-1304.
78. Ellerman KE, Like AA. Susceptibility to diabetes is widely distributed in normal class IIu haplotype rats. *Diabetologia.* 2000;43:890-898.
79. Malaisse WJ, Malaisse-Lagae F, Sener A, Pipeleers DG. Determinants of the selective toxicity of alloxan to the pancreatic B cell. *Proc Natl Acad Sci U S A.* 1982;79:927-930.
80. Like AA, Rossini AA. Streptozotocin-induced pancreatic insulitis: new model of diabetes mellitus. *Science.* 1976;193:415-417.
81. von Herrath MG, Homann D, Gairin JE, Oldstone MB. Pathogenesis and treatment of virus-induced autoimmune diabetes: novel insights gained from the RIP-LCMV transgenic mouse model. *Biochem Soc Trans.* 1997;25:630-635.
82. Craighead JE, McLane MF. Diabetes mellitus: induction in mice by encephalomyocarditis virus. *Science.* 1968;162:913-914.
83. Ellerman KE, Richards CA, Guberski DL, et al. Kilham rat triggers T-cell-dependent autoimmune diabetes in multiple strains of rat. *Diabetes.* 1996;45:557-562.
84. Pipeleers D, Ling Z. Pancreatic beta cells in insulin-dependent diabetes. *Diabetes Metab Rev.* 1992;8(3):209-227.
85. Foulis A, Clark A. Pathology of the pancreas in diabetes mellitus. In: Kahn C, Weir G, eds. *Joslin's Diabetes Mellitus.* 13th ed. Philadelphia, PA: Lea & Febiger; 1994:265-281.
86. Doniach I, Morgan AG. Islets of Langerhans in juvenile diabetes mellitus. *Clin Endocrinol (Oxf).* 1973;2:233-248.
87. Gepts W, Lecompte PM. The pancreatic islets in diabetes. *Am J Med.* 1981;70:105-115.
88. In't Veld P, Lievens D, De Grijse J, et al. Screening for insulitis in adult autoantibody-positive organ donors. *Diabetes.* 2007;56(9):2400-2404.
89. Arif S, Leete P, Nguyen V, et al. Blood and islet phenotypes indicate immunological heterogeneity in type 1 diabetes. *Diabetes.* 2014;63: 3835-3845.

90. Foulis AK, Liddle CN, Farquharson MA, et al. The histopathology of the pancreas in type 1 (insulin-dependent) diabetes mellitus: a 25-year review of deaths in patients under 20 years of age in the United Kingdom. *Diabetologia.* 1986;29:267-274.

91. In't Veld P. Insulitis in human type 1 diabetes: a comparison between patients and animal models. *Semin Immunopathol.* 2014;36:569-579.

92. Willcox A, Richardson S, Bone A, et al. Analysis of islet inflammation in human type 1 diabetes. *Clin Exp Immunol.* 2009;155:173-181.

93. Hanafusa T, Imagawa A. Insulitis in human type 1 diabetes. *Ann N Y Acad Sci.* 2008;1150:297-299.

94. Itoh N, Hanafusa T, Miyazaki A, et al. Mononuclear cell infiltration and its relation to the expression of major histocompatibility complex antigens and adhesion molecules in pancreas biopsy specimens from newly diagnosed insulin-dependent diabetes mellitus patients. *J Clin Invest.* 1993;92:2313-2322.

95. Coppieters KT, Dotta F, Amirian N, et al. Demonstration of islet-autoreactive CD8 T cells in insulitic lesions from recent onset and long-term type 1 diabetes patients. *J Exp Med.* 2012;209:51-60.

96. Dotta F, Censini S, van Halteren A, et al. Coxsackie B4 virus infection of beta cells and natural killer cell insulitis in recent-onset type 1 diabetic patients. *Proc Natl Acad Sci U S A.* 2007;104:5115-5120.

97. Bottazzo GF, Dean BM, McNally JM, et al. In situ characterization of autoimmune phenomena and expression of HLA molecules in the pancreas in diabetic insulitis. *N Engl J Med.* 1985;313:353-360.

98. Hänninen A, Jalkanen S, Salmi M, et al. Macrophages, T cell receptor usage, and endothelial cell activation in the pancreas at the onset of insulin-dependent diabetes mellitus. *J Clin Invest.* 1992;90:1901-1910.

99. Somoza N, Vargas F, Roura-Mir C, et al. Pancreas in recent onset insulin-dependent diabetes mellitus. Changes in HLA, adhesion molecules and autoantigens, restricted T cell receptor V beta usage, and cytokine profile. *J Immunol.* 1994;153:1360-1377.

100. Stankov K, Benc D, Draskovic D. Genetic and epigenetic factors in etiology of diabetes mellitus type 1. *Pediatrics.* 2013;132:1112-1122.

101. Skowera A, Ladell K, McLaren JE, et al. Beta-cell-specific CD8 T cell phenotype in type 1 diabetes reflects chronic autoantigen exposure. *Diabetes.* 2015;64(3):916-925.

102. Campbell-Thompson ML, Atkinson MA, Butler AE, et al. The diagnosis of insulitis in human type 1 diabetes. *Diabetologia.* 2013;56:2541-2543.

103. Rodriguez-Calvo T, Ekwall O, Amirian N, et al. Increased immune cell infiltration of the exocrine pancreas: a possible contribution to the pathogenesis of type 1 diabetes. *Diabetes.* 2014;63:3880-3890.

104. Valle A, Giamporcaro GM, Scavini M, et al. Reduction of circulating neutrophils precedes and accompanies type 1 diabetes. *Diabetes.* 2013;62:2072-2077.

105. Vaarala O, Atkinson MA, Neu J. The "perfect storm" for type 1 diabetes: the complex interplay between intestinal microbiota, gut permeability, and mucosal immunity. *Diabetes.* 2008;57:2555-2562.

106. Bogdani M, Korpos E, Simeonovic CJ, et al. Extracellular matrix components in the pathogenesis of type 1 diabetes. *Curr Diab Rep.* 2014;14(12):552.

107. Oram RA, Jones AG, Besser RE, et al. The majority of patients with long-duration type 1 diabetes are insulin microsecretors and have functioning beta cells. *Diabetologia.* 2014;57(1):187-191.

108. Keenan HA, Sun JK, Levine J, et al. Residual insulin production and pancreatic ß-cell turnover after 50 years of diabetes: Joslin Medalist Study. *Diabetes.* 2010;59:2846-2853.

109. Liu EH, Digon BJ, Hirshberg B, et al. Pancreatic beta cell function persists in many patients with chronic type 1 diabetes, but is not dramatically improved by prolonged immunosuppression and euglycaemia from a beta cell allograft. *Diabetologia.* 2009;52:1369-1380.

110. Gepts W, De Mey J. Islet cell survival determined by morphology. An immunocytochemical study of the islets of Langerhans in juvenile diabetes mellitus. *Diabetes.* 1978;27(Suppl 1):251-261.

111. Atkinson MA, Eisenbarth GS. Type 1 diabetes: new perspectives on disease pathogenesis and treatment. *Lancet.* 2001;358:221-229.

112. Sosenko JM, Palmer JP, Greenbaum CJ, et al. Patterns of metabolic progression to type 1 diabetes in the Diabetes Prevention Trial-Type 1. *Diabetes Care.* 2006;29:643-649.

113. von Herrath M, Sanda S, Herold K. Type 1 diabetes as a relapsing-remitting disease? *Nat Rev Immunol.* 2007;7:988-994.

114. Foulis AK, Farquharson MA, Hardman R. Aberrant expression of class II major histocompatibility complex molecules by B cells and hyperexpression of class I major histocompatibility complex molecules by insulin containing islets in type 1 (insulin-dependent) diabetes mellitus. *Diabetologia.* 1987;30:333-343.

115. Huang X, Yuang J, Goddard A, et al. Interferon expression in the pancreases of patients with type I diabetes. *Diabetes.* 1995;44:658-664.

116. Amrani A, Verdaguer J, Thiessen S, et al. IL-1alpha, IL-1beta, and IFN-gamma mark beta cells for Fas-dependent destruction by diabetogenic CD4(+) T lymphocytes. *J Clin Invest.* 2000;105:459-468.

117. Itoh N, Imagawa A, Hanafusa T, et al. Requirement of Fas for the development of autoimmune diabetes in nonobese diabetic mice. *J Exp Med.* 1997;186:613-618.

118. Chervonsky AV, Wang Y, Wong FS, et al. The role of Fas in autoimmune diabetes. *Cell.* 1997;89:17-24.

119. Thomas HE, Kay TW. How beta cells die in type 1 diabetes. *Curr Dir Autoimmun.* 2001;4:144-170.

120. Marleau AM, Sarvetnick N. T cell homeostasis in tolerance and immunity. *J Leukoc Biol.* 2005;78:575-584.

121. Lo D. Immune regulation: susceptibility and resistance to autoimmunity. *Immunol Res.* 2000;21:239-246.

122. Wong FS, Janeway CA Jr. The role of CD4 vs. CD8 T cells in IDDM. *J Autoimmun.* 1999;13:290-295.

123. Lieberman SM, Takaki T, Han B, et al. Individual nonobese diabetic mice exhibit unique patterns of CD8+ T cell reactivity to three islet antigens, including the newly identified widely expressed dystrophia myotonica kinase. *J Immunol.* 2004;173:6727-6734.

124. Wong FS, Dittel BN, Janeway CA Jr. Transgenes and knockout mutations in animal models of type 1 diabetes and multiple sclerosis. *Immunol Rev.* 1999;169:93-104.

125. Ylipaasto P, Klingel K, Lindberg AM, et al. Enterovirus infection in human pancreatic islet cells, islet tropism in vivo and receptor involvement in cultured islet beta cells. *Diabetologia.* 2004;47:225-239.

126. Foulis AK, McGill M, Farquharson MA, Hilton DA. A search for evidence of viral infection in pancreases of newly diagnosed patients with IDDM. *Diabetologia.* 1997;40:53-61.

127. Williams AJ, Thrower SL, Sequeiros IM, et al. Pancreatic volume is reduced in adult patients with recently diagnosed type 1 diabetes. *J Clin Endocrinol Metab.* 2012;97(11):E2109-E2113.

128. Campbell-Thompson M, Wasserfall C, Montgomery EL, et al. Pancreas organ weight in individuals with disease-associated autoantibodies at risk for type 1 diabetes. *JAMA.* 2012;308:2337-2339.

129. Di Gialleonardo V, de Vries EF, Di Girolamo M, et al. Imaging of β-cell mass and insulitis in insulin-dependent (type 1) diabetes mellitus. *Endocr Rev.* 2012;33(6):892-919.

130. Gaglia JL, Guimaraes AR, Harisinghani M, et al. Noninvasive imaging of pancreatic islet inflammation in type 1A diabetes patients. *J Clin Invest.* 2011;121:442-445.

131. Henderson JR, Daniel PM, Fraser PA. The pancreas as a single organ: the influence of the endocrine upon the exocrine part of the gland. *Gut.* 1981;22:158-167.

132. Thorsby E. Invited anniversary review: HLA associated diseases. *Hum Immunol.* 1997;53:1-11.

133. Expert Committee on the Diagnosis and Classification of Diabetes Mellitus. American Diabetes Association: clinical practice recommendations 2002. *Diabetes Care.* 2002;25(Suppl 1):S1-S147.

134. Barrett JC, Clayton DG, Concannon P, et al. Genome-wide association study and meta-analysis find that over 40 loci affect risk of type 1 diabetes. *Nat Genet.* 2009;41:703-707.

135. Yu J, Shin CH, Yang SW, et al. Analysis of children with type 1 diabetes in Korea: high prevalence of specific anti-islet autoantibodies, immunogenetic similarities to Western populations with "unique" haplotypes, and lack of discrimination by aspartic acid at position 57 of DQB. *Clin Immunol.* 2004;113:318-325.

136. Rewers M, Norris J, Dabelea D. Epidemiology of type 1 diabetes mellitus. *Adv Exp Med Biol.* 2004;552:219-246.

137. Redondo M, Yu L, Hawa M, et al. Late progression to type 1 diabetes of discordant twins of patients with type 1 diabetes: combined analysis of two twin series (United States and United Kingdom) (abstract). *Diabetes.* 1999;48:780.

138. Kyvik KO, Green A, Beck-Nielsen H. Concordance rates of insulin dependent diabetes mellitus: a population based study of young Danish twins. *BMJ.* 1995;311:913-917.

139. Harjutsalo V, Sund R, Knip M, Groop PH. Incidence of type 1 diabetes in Finland. *JAMA.* 2013;310:427-428.

140. Barnett AH, Eff C, Leslie RD, Pyke DA. Diabetes in identical twins. A study of 200 pairs. *Diabetologia.* 1981;20:87-93.

141. Redondo MJ, Yu L, Hawa M, et al. Heterogeneity of type I diabetes: analysis of monozygotic twins in Great Britain and the United States. *Diabetologia.* 2001;44:354-362.

142. Redondo MJ, Jeffrey J, Fain PR, et al. Concordance for islet autoimmunity among monozygotic twins. *N Engl J Med.* 2008;359:2849-2850.

143. Kaprio J, Tuomilehto J, Koskenvuo M, et al. Concordance for type 1 (insulin-dependent) and type 2 (non-insulin-dependent) diabetes mellitus in a population-based cohort of twins in Finland. *Diabetologia.* 1992;35:1060-1067.

144. Redondo MJ, Fain PR, Krischer JP, et al. Expression of beta-cell autoimmunity does not differ between potential dizygotic twins and siblings of patients with type 1 diabetes. *J Autoimmun.* 2004;23:275-279.

145. Nepom GT, Kwok WW. Molecular basis for HLA-DQ associations with IDDM. *Diabetes.* 1998;47:1177-1184.

146. McDevitt HO. The role of MHC class II molecules in susceptibility and resistance to autoimmunity. *Curr Opin Immunol.* 1998;10:677-681.

147. Eisenbarth G. Genetic counseling for T1D. In: Lebovitz H, ed. *Therapy for Diabetes Mellitus and Related Disorders.* Alexandria, VA: American Diabetes Association; 2004.

148. Nakanishi K, Kobayashi T, Murase T, et al. Human leukocyte antigen-A24 and -QA1*0301 in Japanese insulin-dependent diabetes mellitus: independent contributions to susceptibility to the disease

and additive contributions to acceleration of beta-cell destruction. *J Clin Endocrinol Metab.* 1999;84:3721-3725.

149. Erlich H, Valdes AM, Noble J, et al. HLA DR-DQ haplotypes and geno-types and type 1 diabetes risk: analysis of the type 1 diabetes genetics consortium families. *Diabetes.* 2008;57:1084-1092.

150. Rewers M, Bugawan TL, Norris JM, et al. Newborn screening for HLA markers associated with IDDM: diabetes autoimmunity study in the young (DAISY). *Diabetologia.* 1996;39:807-812.

151. Kulmala P, Savola K, Reijonen H, et al. Genetic markers, humoral autoimmunity, and prediction of type 1 diabetes in siblings of affected children. Childhood Diabetes in Finland Study Group. *Diabetes.* 2000; 49:48-58.

152. Aly TA, Ide A, Jahromi MM, et al. Extreme genetic risk for type 1A diabetes. *Proc Natl Acad Sci U S A.* 2006;103:14074-14079.

153. Redondo MJ, Kawasaki E, Mulgrew CL, et al. DR- and DQ-associated protection from type 1A diabetes: comparison of DRB1*1401 and DQA1*0102-DQB1*0602*. *J Clin Endocrinol Metab.* 2000;85:3793-3797.

154. Morel PA, Dorman JS, Todd JA, et al. Aspartic acid at position 57 of the HLA-DQ beta chain protects against type I diabetes: a family study. *Proc Natl Acad Sci U S A.* 1988;85:8111-8115.

155. Bell GI, Horita S, Karam JH. A polymorphic locus near the human insulin gene is associated with insulin-dependent diabetes mellitus. *Diabetes.* 1984;33:176-183.

156. Bennett ST, Lucassen AM, Gough SC, et al. Susceptibility to human type 1 diabetes at IDDM2 is determined by tandem repeat variation at the insulin gene minisatellite locus. *Nat Genet.* 1995;9:284-292.

157. Pugliese A, Zeller M, Fernandez A Jr, et al. The insulin gene is tran-scribed in the human thymus and transcription levels correlated with allelic variation at the INS VNTR-IDDM2 susceptibility locus for type 1 diabetes. *Nat Genet.* 1997;15:293-297.

158. Vafiadis P, Bennett ST, Todd JA, et al. Insulin expression in human thymus is modulated by INS VNTR alleles at the IDDM2 locus. *Nat Genet.* 1997;15:289-292.

159. Bottini N, Musumeci L, Alonso A, et al. A functional variant of lym-phoid tyrosine phosphatase is associated with type I diabetes. *Nat Genet.* 2004;36:337-338.

160. Vang T, Miletic AV, Bottini N, Mustelin T. Protein tyrosine phospha-tase PTPN22 in human autoimmunity. *Autoimmunity.* 2007;40:453-461.

161. Concannon P, Rich SS, Nepom GT. Genetics of type 1A diabetes. *N Engl J Med.* 2009;360:1646-1654.

162. Larsen ZM, Kristiansen OP, Mato E, et al. IDDM12 (CTLA4) on 2q33 and IDDM13 on 2q34 in genetic susceptibility to type 1 diabetes (insulin-dependent). *Autoimmunity.* 1999;31:35-42.

163. Vella A, Cooper JD, Lowe CE, et al. Localization of a type 1 diabetes locus in the IL2RA/CD25 region by use of tag single-nucleotide poly-morphisms. *Am J Hum Genet.* 2005;76:773-779.

164. Nejentsev S, Walker N, Riches D, et al. Rare variants of IFIH1, a gene implicated in antiviral responses, protect against type 1 diabetes. *Science.* 2009;324:387-389.

165. Shields BM, Hicks S, Shepherd MH, et al. Maturity-onset diabetes of the young (MODY): how many cases are we missing? *Diabetologia.* 2010;53:2504-2508.

166. American Diabetes Association. Diagnosis and classification of diabetes mellitus. *Diabetes Care.* 2014;37(Suppl 1):S81-S90.

167. Permutt MA, Wasson J, Cox N. Genetic epidemiology of diabetes. *J Clin Invest.* 2005;115:1431-1439.

168. Anderson MS, Venanzi ES, Klein L, et al. Projection of an immunologi-cal self shadow within the thymus by the aire protein. *Science.* 2002; 298:1395-1401.

169. Clark LB, Appleby MW, Brunkow ME, et al. Cellular and molecular characterization of the scurfy mouse mutant. *J Immunol.* 1999;162:2546-2554.

170. Powell BR, Buist NR, Stenzel P. An X-linked syndrome of diarrhea, polyendocrinopathy, and fatal infection in infancy. *J Pediatr.* 1982;100:731-737.

171. Roberts J, Searle J. Neonatal diabetes mellitus associated with severe diarrhea, hyperimmunoglobulin E syndrome, and absence of islets of Langerhans. *Pediatr Pathol Lab Med.* 1995;15:477-483.

172. Cilio CM, Bosco S, Moretti C, et al. Congenital autoimmune diabetes mellitus. *N Engl J Med.* 2000;342:1529-1531.

173. Kanangat S, Blair P, Reddy R, et al. Disease in the scurfy (sf) mouse is associated with overexpression of cytokine genes. *Eur J Immunol.* 1996;26:161-165.

174. Fontenot JD, Gavin MA, Rudensky AY. Foxp3 programs the develop-ment and function of CD4+CD25+ regulatory T cells. *Nat Immunol.* 2003;4:330-336.

175. Gardner SG, Bingley PJ, Sawtell PA, et al. Rising incidence of insulin dependent diabetes in children aged under 5 years in the Oxford region: time trend analysis. The Bart's-Oxford Study Group. *BMJ.* 1997;315(7110):713-717.

176. Tuomilehto J, Karvonen M, Pitkaniemi J, et al. Record-high incidence of type I (insulin-dependent) diabetes mellitus in Finnish children. The Finnish Childhood Type I Diabetes Registry Group. *Diabetologia.* 1999;42:655-660.

177. Feltbower RG, McKinney PA, Bodansky HJ. Rising incidence of child-hood diabetes is seen at all ages and in urban and rural settings in Yorkshire, United Kingdom. *Diabetologia.* 2000;43:682-684.

178. Wilkin TJ. The accelerator hypothesis: weight gain as the missing link between type I and type II diabetes. *Diabetologia.* 2001;44(7):914-922.

179. Fourlanos S, Harrison LC, Colman PG. The accelerator hypothesis and increasing incidence of type 1 diabetes. *Curr Opin Endocrinol Diabetes Obes.* 2008;15:321-325.

180. Dahlquist G. Can we slow the rising incidence of childhood-onset autoimmune diabetes? The overload hypothesis. *Diabetologia.* 2006; 49:20-24.

181. Nerup J, Mandrup-Poulsen T, Helqvist S, et al. On the pathogenesis of IDDM. *Diabetologia.* 1994;37(Suppl 2):S82-S89.

182. Bach JF. Six questions about the hygiene hypothesis. *Cell Immunol.* 2005;233:158-161.

183. Cooke A. Review series on helminths, immune modulation and the hygiene hypothesis: how might infection modulate the onset of type 1 diabetes? *Immunology.* 2009;126:12-17.

184. von Herrath MG, Fujinami RS, Whitton JL. Microorganisms and auto-immunity: making the barren field fertile? *Nat Rev Microbiol.* 2003;1:151-157.

185. Wasserfall C, Nead K, Mathews C, Atkinson MA. The threshold hypothesis: solving the equation of nurture vs nature in type 1 diabe-tes. *Diabetologia.* 2011;54:2232-2236.

186. Eisenbarth GS. Type I diabetes mellitus. A chronic autoimmune dis-ease. *N Engl J Med.* 1986;314:1360-1368.

187. Shaver KA, Boughman JA, Nance WE. Congenital rubella syndrome and diabetes: a review of epidemiologic, genetic, and immunologic factors. *Am Ann Deaf.* 1985;130:526-532.

188. Ou D, Jonsen LA, Metzger DL, Tingle AJ. CD4+ and CD8+ T-cell clones from congenital rubella syndrome patients with IDDM recognize overlapping GAD65 protein epitopes. Implications for HLA class I and II allelic linkage to disease susceptibility. *Hum Immunol.* 1999;60:652-664.

189. Rabinowe SL, George KL, Loughlin R, et al. Congenital rubella. Mono-clonal antibody-defined T cell abnormalities in young adults. *Am J Med.* 1986;81:779-782.

190. Yoon JW, Austin M, Onodera T, Notkins AL. Isolation of a virus from the pancreas of a child with diabetic ketoacidosis. *N Engl J Med.* 1979;300:1173-1179.

191. Nigro G, Pacella ME, Patane E, Midulla M. Multi-system coxsackievirus B-6 infection with findings suggestive of diabetes mellitus. *Eur J Pediatr.* 1986;145:557-559.

192. Helminen O, Aspholm S, Pokka T, et al. HbA1c predicts time to diagnosis of type 1 diabetes in children at risk. *Diabetes.* 2015;64:1719-1727.

193. Sosenko JM, Palmer JP, Rafkin-Mervis L, et al. Group DPT-TS. Incident dysglycemia and progression to type 1 diabetes among participants in the Diabetes Prevention Trial-Type 1. *Diabetes Care.* 2009;32:1603-1607.

194. Robles DT, Eisenbarth GS. Type 1A diabetes induced by infection and immunization. *J Autoimmun.* 2001;16:355-362.

195. Lönnrot M, Korpela K, Knip M, et al. Enterovirus infection as a risk factor for beta-cell autoimmunity in a prospectively observed birth cohort: the Finnish Diabetes Prediction and Prevention Study. *Diabe-tes.* 2000;49:1314-1318.

196. Graves PM, Norris JM, Pallansch MA, et al. The role of enteroviral infections in the development of IDDM: limitations of current approaches. *Diabetes.* 1997;46:161-168.

197. Honeyman MC, Coulson BS, Stone NL, et al. Association between rotavirus infection and pancreatic islet autoimmunity in children at risk of developing type 1 diabetes. *Diabetes.* 2000;49:1319-1324.

198. Classen DC, Classen JB. The timing of pediatric immunization and the risk of insulin-dependent diabetes mellitus. *Infect Dis Clin Pract.* 1997;6:449-454.

199. Karvonen M, Cepaitis Z, Tuomilehto J. Association between type 1 diabetes and *Haemophilus influenzae* type b vaccination: birth cohort study. *BMJ.* 1999;318(7192):1169-1172.

200. Lindberg B, Ahlfors K, Carlsson A, et al. Previous exposure to measles, mumps, and rubella—but not vaccination during adolescence—correlates to the prevalence of pancreatic and thyroid autoantibodies. *Pediatrics.* 1999;104:e12.

201. Graves PM, Barriga KJ, Norris JM, et al. Lack of association between early childhood immunizations and beta-cell autoimmunity. *Diabetes Care.* 1999;22:1694-1697.

202. Akerblom HK, Savilahti E, Saukkonen TT, et al. The case for elimina-tion of cow's milk in early infancy in the prevention of type 1 diabetes: the Finnish experience. *Diabetes Metab Rev.* 1993;9:269-278.

203. Virtanen SM, Laara E, Hypponen E, et al. Cow's milk consumption, HLA-DQB1 genotype, and type 1 diabetes: a nested case-control study of siblings of children with diabetes. Childhood Diabetes in Finland Study Group. *Diabetes.* 2000;49:912-917.

204. Virtanen SM, Rasanen L, Aro A, et al. Infant feeding in Finnish children less than 7 yr of age with newly diagnosed IDDM. Child-hood Diabetes in Finland Study Group. *Diabetes Care.* 1991;14:415-417.

205. Couper JJ, Steele C, Beresford S, et al. Lack of association between duration of breast-feeding or introduction of cow's milk and development of islet autoimmunity. *Diabetes.* 1999;48:2145-2149.

206. Norris JM, Beaty B, Klingensmith G, et al. Lack of association between early exposure to cow's milk protein and beta-cell autoimmunity. Diabetes Autoimmunity Study in the Young (DAISY). *JAMA.* 1996; 276(8):609-614.

207. Akerblom HK, Virtanen SM, Ilonen J, et al. Dietary manipulation of beta cell autoimmunity in infants at increased risk of type 1 diabetes: a pilot study. *Diabetologia.* 2005;48:829-837.

208. Norris JM, Barriga K, Klingensmith G, et al. Timing of initial cereal exposure in infancy and risk of islet autoimmunity. *JAMA.* 2003; 290:1713-1720.

209. Ziegler AG, Schmid S, Huber D, et al. Early infant feeding and risk of developing type 1 diabetes-associated autoantibodies. *JAMA.* 2003;290: 1721-1728.

210. Norris JM, Yin X, Lamb MM, et al. Omega-3 polyunsaturated fatty acid intake and islet autoimmunity in children at increased risk for type 1 diabetes. *JAMA.* 2007;298:1420-1428.

211. Wenzlau JM, Juhl K, Yu L, et al. The cation efflux transporter ZnT8 (Slc30A8) is a major autoantigen in human type 1 diabetes. *Proc Natl Acad Sci U S A.* 2007;104:17040-17045.

212. Atkinson MA, George S. Eisenbarth, 1947-2012. *Diabetologia.* 2013;56: 435-438.

213. Bluestone JA, Herold K, Eisenbarth G. Genetics, pathogenesis and clinical interventions in type 1 diabetes. *Nature.* 2010;464:1293-1300.

214. Peakman M. Immunological pathways to beta-cell damage in type 1 diabetes. *Diabet Med.* 2013;30:147-154.

215. Atkinson MA, Eisenbarth GS, Michels AW. Type 1 diabetes. *Lancet.* 2014;383:69-82.

216. Fennessy M, Metcalfe K, Hitman GA, et al. A gene in the HLA class I region contributes to susceptibility to IDDM in the Finnish population. Childhood Diabetes in Finland (DiMe) Study Group. *Diabetologia.* 1994;37:937-944.

217. Kockum I, Sanjeevi CB, Eastman S, et al. Population analysis of protection by HLA-DR and DQ genes from insulin-dependent diabetes mellitus in Swedish children with insulin-dependent diabetes and controls. *Eur J Immunogenet.* 1995;22:443-465.

218. Vardi P, Ziegler AG, Mathews JH, et al. Concentration of insulin autoantibodies at onset of type I diabetes. Inverse log-linear correlation with age. *Diabetes Care.* 1988;11:736-739.

219. Arslanian SA, Becker DJ, Rabin B, et al. Correlates of insulin antibodies in newly diagnosed children with insulin-dependent diabetes before insulin therapy. *Diabetes.* 1985;34:926-930.

220. Eisenbarth GS, Gianani R, Yu L, et al. Dual-parameter model for prediction of type I diabetes mellitus. *Proc Assoc Am Physicians.* 1998;110: 126-135.

221. Butler PC, Meier JJ, Butler AE, Bhushan A. The replication of beta cells in normal physiology, in disease and for therapy. *Nat Clin Pract Endocrinol Metab.* 2007;3:758-768.

222. Gregg BE, Moore PC, Demozay D, et al. Formation of a human beta-cell population within pancreatic islets is set early in life. *J Clin Endocrinol Metab.* 2012;97:3197-3206.

223. Saisho Y, Butler AE, Manesso E, et al. Beta-cell mass and turnover in humans: effects of obesity and aging. *Diabetes Care.* 2013;36: 111-117.

224. Chase HP, Cuthbertson DD, Dolan LM, et al. First-phase insulin release during the intravenous glucose tolerance test as a risk factor for type 1 diabetes. *J Pediatr.* 2001;138:244-249.

225. Bingley PJ, Colman P, Eisenbarth GS, et al. Standardization of IVGTT to predict IDDM. *Diabetes Care.* 1992;15:1313-1316.

226. Bingley PJ. Interactions of age, islet cell antibodies, insulin autoantibodies, and first-phase insulin response in predicting risk of progression to IDDM in ICA+ relatives: the ICARUS data set. Islet Cell Antibody Register Users Study. *Diabetes.* 1996;45:1720-1728.

227. Epidemiology of severe hypoglycemia in the diabetes control and complications trial. The DCCT Research Group. *Am J Med.* 1991;90(4): 450-459.

228. Palmer JP, Fleming GA, Greenbaum CJ, et al. C-peptide is the appropriate outcome measure for type 1 diabetes clinical trials to preserve beta-cell function: report of an ADA workshop, 21-22 October 2001. *Diabetes.* 2004;53:250-264.

229. Ricker A, Herskowitz R, Wolfsdorf J, et al. Prognostic factors in children and young adults presenting with transient hyperglycemia or impaired glucose tolerance (abstract). *Diabetes.* 1986;35(Suppl 1):93A.

230. Sosenko JM, Skyler JS, Mahon J, et al. The application of the diabetes prevention trial-type 1 risk score for identifying a preclinical state of type 1 diabetes. *Diabetes Care.* 2012;35(7):1552-1555.

231. Sosenko JM, Skyler JS, Mahon J, et al. Use of the Diabetes Prevention Trial-Type 1 Risk Score (DPTRS) for improving the accuracy of the risk classification of type 1 diabetes. *Diabetes Care.* 2014;37: 979-984.

232. Vehik K, Cuthbertson D, Ruhlig H, et al. Long-term outcome of individuals treated with oral insulin: diabetes prevention trial-type 1 (DPT-1) oral insulin trial. *Diabetes Care.* 2011;34:1585-1590.

233. Hinke SA. Diamyd, an alum-formulated recombinant human GAD65 for the prevention of autoimmune diabetes. *Curr Opin Mol Ther.* 2008;10:516-525.

234. Hagopian W, Ferry RJ Jr, Sherry N, et al. Teplizumab preserves C-peptide in recent-onset type 1 diabetes: two-year results from the randomized, placebo-controlled Protege trial. *Diabetes.* 2013;62:3901-3908.

235. Herold KC, Gitelman SE, Ehlers MR, et al. Team AS. Teplizumab (anti-CD3 mAb) treatment preserves C-peptide responses in patients with new-onset type 1 diabetes in a randomized controlled trial: metabolic and immunologic features at baseline identify a subgroup of responders. *Diabetes.* 2013;62:3766-3774.

236. Herold KC, Gitelman SE, Willi SM, et al. Teplizumab treatment may improve C-peptide responses in participants with type 1 diabetes after the new-onset period: a randomised controlled trial. *Diabetologia.* 2013;56:391-400.

237. Haller MJ, Gitelman SE, Gottlieb PA, et al. Anti-thymocyte globulin/G-CSF treatment preserves β cell function in patients with established type 1 diabetes. *J Clin Invest.* 2015;125:448-455.

238. Orban T, Bundy B, Becker DJ, et al. Type 1 Diabetes TrialNet Abatacept Study Group. Costimulation modulation with abatacept in patients with recent-onset type 1 diabetes: follow-up 1 year after cessation of treatment. *Diabetes Care.* 2014;37(4):1069-1075.

239. Assan R, Feutren G, Debray-Sachs M, et al. Metabolic and immunological effects of cyclosporin in recently diagnosed type 1 diabetes mellitus. *Lancet.* 1985;1:67-71.

240. Chase HP, Butler-Simon N, Garg SK, et al. Cyclosporine A for the treatment of new-onset insulin-dependent diabetes mellitus. *Pediatrics.* 1990;85:241-245.

241. Stiller CR, Dupre J, Gent M, et al. Effects of cyclosporine immunosuppression in insulin-dependent diabetes mellitus of recent onset. *Science.* 1984;223:1362-1367.

242. Cook JJ, Hudson I, Harrison LC, et al. Double-blind controlled trial of azathioprine in children with newly diagnosed type I diabetes. *Diabetes.* 1989;38:779-783.

243. Silverstein J, Maclaren N, Riley W, et al. Immunosuppression with azathioprine and prednisone in recent-onset insulin-dependent diabetes mellitus. *N Engl J Med.* 1988;319:599-604.

244. Eisenbarth GS, Srikanta S, Jackson R, et al. Anti-thymocyte globulin and prednisone immunotherapy of recent onset type 1 diabetes mellitus. *Diabetes Res.* 1985;2:271-276.

245. Pescovitz MD, Greenbaum CJ, Krause-Steinrauf H, et al. Type 1 Diabetes TrialNet Anti-CD20 Study Group. Rituximab, B-lymphocyte depletion, and preservation of beta-cell function. *N Engl J Med.* 2009;361(22): 2143-2152.

246. Saudek F, Havrdova T, Boucek P, et al. Polyclonal anti-T-cell therapy for type 1 diabetes mellitus of recent onset. *Rev Diabet Stud.* 2004;1(2): 80-88.

247. Gottlieb PA, Quinlan S, Krause-Steinrauf H, et al. Type 1 Diabetes TrialNet MMF/DZB Study Group. Failure to preserve beta-cell function with mycophenolate mofetil and daclizumab combined therapy in patients with new-onset type 1 diabetes. *Diabetes Care.* 2010;33(4): 826-832.

248. Herold KC, Hagopian W, Auger JA, et al. Anti-CD3 monoclonal antibody in new-onset type 1 diabetes mellitus. *N Engl J Med.* 2002; 346:1692-1698.

249. Herold KC, Gitelman SE, Masharani U, et al. A single course of anti-CD3 monoclonal antibody hOKT3gamma1(Ala-Ala) results in improvement in C-peptide responses and clinical parameters for at least 2 years after onset of type 1 diabetes. *Diabetes.* 2005;54: 1763-1769.

250. Shoda LK, Young DL, Ramanujan S, et al. A comprehensive review of interventions in the NOD mouse and implications for translation. *Immunity.* 2005;23:115-126.

251. Muir A, Peck A, Clare-Salzler M, et al. Insulin immunization of non-obese diabetic mice induces a protective insulitis characterized by diminished intraislet interferon-gamma transcription. *J Clin Invest.* 1995;95:628-634.

252. Weiner H, Miller A, Khoury S, et al. Suppression of organ-specific autoimmune diseases by oral administration of auto antigens. Proceedings of the 8th International Congress on Immunology. Heidelberg: Springer-Verlag; 1992.

253. Zhang ZJ, Davidson L, Eisenbarth G, Weiner HL. Suppression of diabetes in nonobese diabetic mice by oral administration of porcine insulin. *Proc Natl Acad Sci U S A.* 1991;88:10252-10256.

254. Atkinson MA, Maclaren NK, Luchetta R. Insulitis and diabetes in NOD mice reduced by prophylactic insulin therapy. *Diabetes.* 1990;39: 933-937.

255. Daniel D, Wegmann DR. Protection of nonobese diabetic mice from diabetes by intranasal or subcutaneous administration of insulin peptide B-(9-23). *Proc Natl Acad Sci U S A.* 1996;93:956-960.

256. Diabetes Prevention Trial—Type 1 Diabetes Study Group. Effects of insulin in relatives of patients with type 1 diabetes mellitus. *N Engl J Med.* 2002;346(22):1685-1691.

257. Skyler JS, Krischer JP, Wolfsdorf J, et al. Effects of oral insulin in relatives of patients with type 1 diabetes: the Diabetes Prevention Trial—Type 1. *Diabetes Care.* 2005;28(5):1068-1076.

258. Bonifacio E, Ziegler AG, Klingensmith G, et al. Pre-POINT Study Group. Effects of high-dose oral insulin on immune responses in children at high risk for type 1 diabetes: the Pre-POINT randomized clinical trial. *JAMA*. 2015;313(15):1541-1549.

259. Richardson SJ, Willcox A, Bone AJ, et al. Immunopathology of the human pancreas in type-I diabetes. *Semin Immunopathol*. 2011;33:9-21.

260. Rigby MR, DiMeglio LA, Rendell MS, et al. Targeting of memory T cells with alefacept in new-onset type 1 diabetes (T1DAL study): 12 month results of a randomised, double-blind, placebo-controlled phase 2 trial. *Lancet Diabetes Endocrinol*. 2013;1:284-294.

261. Pope JE, Rampakakis E, Sampalis J. The durability of abatacept as a first and subsequent biologic and improvement in HAQ from a large multi-site real-world study. *Semin Arthritis Rheum*. 2015;44(5):499-505.

262. Nepom GT, Ehlers M, Mandrup-Poulsen T. Anti-cytokine therapies in T1D: concepts and strategies. *Clin Immunol*. 2013;149:279-285.

263. Schatz D, Gale EA, Atkinson MA. Why can't we prevent type 1 diabetes? Maybe it's time to try a different combination. *Diabetes Care*. 2003;26(12):3326-3328.

264. Ludvigsson J. Combination therapy for preservation of beta cell function in type 1 diabetes: new attitudes and strategies are needed! *Immunol Lett*. 2014;159:30-35.

265. Robertson RP, Sutherland DE, Kendall DM, et al. Metabolic characterization of long-term successful pancreas transplants in type I diabetes. *J Investig Med*. 1996;44(9):549-555.

266. Lehmann R, Graziano J, Brockmann J, et al. glycemic control in simultaneous islet-kidney versus pancreas-kidney transplantation in type 1 diabetes: a prospective 13-year follow-up. *Diabetes Care*. 2015;38:752-759.

267. Montiel-Casado MC, Perez-Daga JA, Aranda-Narvaez JM, et al. Pancreas graft survival in simultaneous pancreas-kidney versus pancreas-after-kidney and pancreas alone transplantations: a single institution experience. *Transplant Proc*. 2013;45:3609-3611.

268. Naftanel MA, Harlan DM. Pancreatic islet transplantation. *PLoS Med*. 2004;1:e58, quiz e75.

269. Robertson RP, Kendall D, Teuscher A, Sutherland D. Long-term metabolic control with pancreatic transplantation. *Transplant Proc*. 1994;26:386-387.

270. Redfield RR, Scalea JR, Odorico JS. Simultaneous pancreas and kidney transplantation: current trends and future directions. *Curr Opin Organ Transplant*. 2015;20:94-102.

271. Nakhleh RE, Gruessner RW, Swanson PE, et al. Pancreas transplant pathology. A morphologic, immunohistochemical, and electron microscopic comparison of allogeneic grafts with rejection, syngeneic grafts, and chronic pancreatitis. *Am J Surg Pathol*. 1991;15:246-256.

272. Pugliese A, Reijonen HK, Nepom J, Burke GW. Recurrence of autoimmunity in pancreas transplant patients: research update. *Diabetes Manag (Lond)*. 2011;1(2):229-238.

273. Shapiro AM, Lakey JR, Ryan EA, et al. Islet transplantation in seven patients with type 1 diabetes mellitus using a glucocorticoid-free immunosuppressive regimen. *N Engl J Med*. 2000;343:230-238.

274. Nanji SA, Shapiro AM. Advances in pancreatic islet transplantation in humans. *Diabetes Obes Metab*. 2006;8:15-25.

275. Toso C, Baertschiger R, Morel P, et al. Sequential kidney/islet transplantation: efficacy and safety assessment of a steroid-free immunosuppression protocol. *Am J Transplant*. 2006;6:1049-1058.

276. Tchorsh-Yutsis D, Hecht G, Aronovich A, et al. Pig embryonic pancreatic tissue as a source for transplantation in diabetes: transient treatment with anti-LFA1, anti-CD48, and FTY720 enables long-term graft maintenance in mice with only mild ongoing immunosuppression. *Diabetes*. 2009;58:1585-1594.

277. Uchigata Y, Kuwata S, Tsushima T, et al. Patients with Graves' disease who developed insulin autoimmune syndrome (Hirata disease) possess HLA-Bw62/Cw4/DR4 carrying DRB1*0406. *J Clin Endocrinol Metab*. 1993;77:249-254.

278. Uchigata Y, Hirata Y, Iwamoto Y. Insulin autoimmune syndrome (Hirata disease): epidemiology in Asia, including Japan. *Diabetol Int*. 2010;1:21-25.

279. Uchigata Y, Hirata Y. Insulin autoimmune syndrome (IAS, Hirata disease). In: Eisenbarth G, ed. *Molecular Mechanisms of Endocrine and Organ Specific Autoimmunity*. Austin, TX: RG Landes; 1999:133-148.

280. Uchigata Y, Tokunaga K, Nepom G, et al. Differential immunogenetic determinants of polyclonal insulin autoimmune syndrome (Hirata's disease) and monoclonal insulin autoimmune syndrome. *Diabetes*. 1995;44:1227-1232.

281. Gullo D, Evans JL, Sortino G, et al. Insulin autoimmune syndrome (Hirata disease) in European Caucasians taking alpha-lipoic acid. *Clin Endocrinol (Oxf)*. 2014;81:204-209.

282. Uchigata Y, Hirata Y, Iwamoto Y. Drug-induced insulin autoimmune syndrome. *Diabetes Res Clin Pract*. 2009;83:e19-e20.

283. Fineberg SE, Kawabata TT, Finco-Kent D, et al. Immunological responses to exogenous insulin. *Endocr Rev*. 2007;28:625-652.

284. Menon RK, Cohen RM, Sperling MA, et al. Transplacental passage of insulin in pregnant women with insulin-dependent diabetes mellitus. Its role in fetal macrosomia. *N Engl J Med*. 1990;323:309-315.

285. Schernthaner G. Immunogenicity and allergenic potential of animal and human insulins. *Diabetes Care*. 1993;16(Suppl 3):155-165.

286. Radermecker RP, Renard E, Scheen AJ. Circulating insulin antibodies: influence of continuous subcutaneous or intraperitoneal insulin infusion, and impact on glucose control. *Diabetes Metab Res Rev*. 2009;25:491-501.

287. Heinzerling L, Raile K, Rochlitz H, et al. Insulin allergy: clinical manifestations and management strategies. *Allergy*. 2008;63:148-155.

288. Taylor SI, Grunberger G, Marcus-Samuels B, et al. Hypoglycemia associated with antibodies to the insulin receptor. *N Engl J Med*. 1982;307:1422-1426.

289. Malek R, Chong AY, Lupsa BC, et al. Treatment of type B insulin resistance: a novel approach to reduce insulin receptor autoantibodies. *J Clin Endocrinol Metab*. 2010;95:3641-3647.

290. Dons RF, Havlik R, Taylor SI, et al. Clinical disorders associated with autoantibodies to the insulin receptor. Simulation by passive transfer of immunoglobulins to rats. *J Clin Invest*. 1983;72:1072-1080.

291. Reference deleted in review.

292. Chiang JL, Kirkman MS, Laffel LM, Peters AL. Type 1 Diabetes Sourcebook Authors. Type 1 diabetes through the life span: a position statement of the American Diabetes Association. *Diabetes Care*. 2014;37:2034-2054.

293. Engerman RL, Kern TS. Progression of incipient diabetic retinopathy during good glycemic control. *Diabetes*. 1987;36:808-812.

294. Cohen AJ, McGill PD, Rossetti RG, et al. Glomerulopathy in spontaneously diabetic rat. Impact of glycemic control. *Diabetes*. 1987;36:944-951.

295. Klein R, Klein BE, Moss SE, et al. Glycosylated hemoglobin predicts the incidence and progression of diabetic retinopathy. *JAMA*. 1988;260:2864-2871.

296. Chase HP, Jackson WE, Hoops SL, et al. Glucose control and the renal and retinal complications of insulin-dependent diabetes. *JAMA*. 1989;261:1155-1160.

297. The effect of intensive treatment of diabetes on the development and progression of long-term complications in insulin-dependent diabetes mellitus. The Diabetes Control and Complications Trial Research Group. *N Engl J Med*. 1993;329(14):977-986.

298. Effect of intensive diabetes management on macrovascular events and risk factors in the Diabetes Control and Complications Trial. *Am J Cardiol*. 1995;75(14):894-903.

299. Nathan DM, Cleary PA, Backlund JY, et al. Intensive diabetes treatment and cardiovascular disease in patients with type 1 diabetes. *N Engl J Med*. 2005;353:2643-2653.

300. Writing Group for the DCCT/EDIC Research Group, Orchard TJ, Nathan DM, Zinman B, et al. Association between 7 years of intensive treatment of type 1 diabetes and long-term mortality. *JAMA*. 2015;313:45-53.

301. The DCCT Research Group. Epidemiology of severe hypoglycemia in the diabetes control and complications trial. *Am J Med*. 1991;90:450-459.

302. Purnell JQ, Hokanson JE, Marcovina SM, et al. Effect of excessive weight gain with intensive therapy of type 1 diabetes on lipid levels and blood pressure: results from the DCCT. Diabetes Control and Complications Trial. *JAMA*. 1998;280:140-146.

303. Nordwall M, Abrahamsson M, Dhir M, et al. Impact of HbA1c, followed from onset of type 1 diabetes, on the development of severe retinopathy and nephropathy: the VISS Study (Vascular Diabetic Complications in Southeast Sweden). *Diabetes Care*. 2015;38:308-315.

304. Fullerton B, Jeitler K, Seitz M, et al. Intensive glucose control versus conventional glucose control for type 1 diabetes mellitus. *Cochrane Database Syst Rev*. 2014;(2):CD009122.

305. Blood glucose control and the evolution of diabetic retinopathy and albuminuria. A preliminary multicenter trial. The Kroc Collaborative Study Group. *N Engl J Med*. 1984;311(6):365-372.

306. Choudhary P, Ramasamy S, Green L, et al. Real-time continuous glucose monitoring significantly reduces severe hypoglycemia in hypoglycemia-unaware patients with type 1 diabetes. *Diabetes Care*. 2013;36:4160-4162.

307. American Diabetes Association. Standards of medical care in diabetes—2015. *Diabetes Care*. 2015;38:s1-s93.

308. Handelsman Y, Bloomgarden ZT, Grunberger G, et al. American Association of Clinical Endocrinologists and American College of Endocrinology—clinical practice guidelines for developing a diabetes mellitus comprehensive care plan—2015. *Endocr Pract*. 2015;21:1-87.

309. Hirsch IB. Intensive treatment of type 1 diabetes. *Med Clin North Am*. 1998;82:689-719.

310. Home P, Kurtzhals P. Insulin detemir: from concept to clinical experience. *Expert Opin Pharmacother*. 2006;7:325-343.

311. Heise T, Nosek L, Ronn BB, et al. Lower within-subject variability of insulin detemir in comparison to NPH insulin and insulin glargine in people with type 1 diabetes. *Diabetes*. 2004;53:1614-1620.

312. Maiorino MI, Petrizzo M, Capuano A, et al. The development of new basal insulins: is there any clinical advantage with their use in type 2 diabetes? *Expert Opin Biol Ther*. 2014;14(6):799-808.

313. Kugler AJ, Fabbio KL, Pham DQ, Nadeau DA. Inhaled technosphere insulin: a novel delivery system and formulation for the treatment of types 1 and 2 diabetes mellitus. *Pharmacotherapy.* 2015;35:298-314. http://www.accessdata.fda.gov/drugsatfda_docs/label/2008/021868 s016s017lbl.pdf.

314. Kerr D, Wizemann E, Senstius J, et al. Stability and performance of rapid-acting insulin analogs used for continuous subcutaneous insulin infusion: a systematic review. *J Diabetes Sci Technol.* 2013;7:1595-1606.

315. Pozzilli P, Battelino T, Danne T, et al. Continuous subcutaneous insulin infusion in diabetes: patient populations, safety, efficacy, and pharmacoeconomics. *Diabetes Metab Res Rev.* 2015. doi: 10.1002/dmrr.2653. [Epub ahead of print].

316. Bergenstal RM, Tamborlane WV, Ahmann A, et al. Effectiveness of sensor-augmented insulin-pump therapy in type 1 diabetes. *N Engl J Med.* 2010;363:311-320.

317. Bolderman KM. *Putting Your Patients on the Pump.* 2nd ed. Alexandria, VA: American Diabetes Association; 2013.

318. Kaufman FR. *Medical Management of Type 1 Diabetes.* 6th ed. Alexandria, VA: American Diabetes Association; 2012.

319. Wolfsdorf JI. *Intensive Diabetes Management.* 5th ed. Alexandria, VA: American Diabetes Association; 2012.

320. Young A. Clinical studies. *Adv Pharmacol.* 2005;52:289-320.

321. Peters AL, Buschur EO, Buse JB, et al. Euglycemic diabetic ketoacidosis: a potential complication of treatment with sodium-glucose cotransporter 2 inhibition. *Diabetes Care.* 2015. In press.

322. Choudhary P, Rickels MR, Senior PA, et al. Evidence-Informed Clinical Practice Recommendations for Treatment of Type 1 Diabetes Complicated by Problematic Hypoglycemia. *Diabetes Care.* 2015;38:1016-1029.

323. Jacquier J, Chik CL, Senior PA. A practical, clinical approach to the assessment and management of suspected insulin allergy. *Diabet Med.* 2013;30:977-985.

324. Kamel KS, Halperin ML. Acid-base problems in diabetic ketoacidosis. *N Engl J Med.* 2015;372:546-554.

325. Munro JF, Campbell IW, McCuish AC, Duncan LJ. Euglycaemic diabetic ketoacidosis. *Br Med J.* 1973;2:578-580.

326. Madias NE. Lactic acidosis. *Kidney Int.* 1986;29:752-774.

327. Fulop M. Alcoholism, ketoacidosis, and lactic acidosis. *Diabetes Metab Rev.* 1989;5:365-378.

328. Duffens K, Marx JA. Alcoholic ketoacidosis—a review. *J Emerg Med.* 1987;5:399-406.

329. Moller-Petersen J, Andersen PT, Hjorne N, Ditzel J. Nontraumatic rhabdomyolysis during diabetic ketoacidosis. *Diabetologia.* 1986;29:229-234.

330. Brenner BE, Simon RR. Management of salicylate intoxication. *Drugs.* 1982;24:335-340.

331. Turk J, Morrell L. Ethylene glycol intoxication. *Arch Intern Med.* 1986;146:1601-1603.

332. Rich J, Scheife RT, Katz N, Caplan LR. Isopropyl alcohol intoxication. *Arch Neurol.* 1990;47:322-324.

333. Kitabchi AE. Low-dose insulin therapy in diabetic ketoacidosis: fact or fiction? *Diabetes Metab Rev.* 1989;5:337-363.

334. Kitabchi AE, Umpierrez GE, Miles JM, Fisher JN. Hyperglycemic crises in adult patients with diabetes. *Diabetes Care.* 2009;32:1335-1343.

335. Umpierrez GE, Cuervo R, Karabell A, et al. Treatment of diabetic ketoacidosis with subcutaneous insulin aspart. *Diabetes Care.* 2004;27:1873-1878.

336. Burris AS. Leukemoid reaction associated with severe diabetic ketoacidosis. *South Med J.* 1986;79:647-648.

337. Powers WJ. Cerebrospinal fluid to serum glucose ratios in diabetes mellitus and bacterial meningitis. *Am J Med.* 1981;71:217-220.

338. Campbell IW, Duncan LJ, Innes JA, et al. Abdominal pain in diabetic metabolic decompensation. Clinical significance. *JAMA.* 1975;233:166-168.

339. Rosenbloom AL. Intracerebral crises during treatment of diabetic ketoacidosis. *Diabetes Care.* 1990;13:22-33.

340. Brun-Buisson CJ, Bonnet F, Bergeret S, et al. Recurrent high-permeability pulmonary edema associated with diabetic ketoacidosis. *Crit Care Med.* 1985;13:55-56.

341. Brandstetter RD, Tamarin FM, Washington D, et al. Occult mucous airway obstruction in diabetic ketoacidosis. *Chest.* 1987;91:575-578.

342. Hansen LA, Prakash UB, Colby TV. Pulmonary complications in diabetes mellitus. *Mayo Clin Proc.* 1989;64:791-799.

343. Levetan CS, Salas JR, Wilets IF, Zumoff B. Impact of endocrine and diabetes team consultation on hospital length of stay for patients with diabetes. *Am J Med.* 1995;99:22-28.

344. Levetan CS, Passaro MD, Jablonski KA, Ratner RE. Effect of physician specialty on outcomes in diabetic ketoacidosis. *Diabetes Care.* 1999;22:1790-1795.

CHAPTER 33

Complications of Diabetes Mellitus

MICHAEL BROWNLEE • LLOYD P. AIELLO • MARK E. COOPER • AARON I. VINIK • JORGE PLUTZKY • ANDREW J. M. BOULTON

KEY POINTS

- Microvascular complications are caused by chronic hyperglycemia, whereas macrovascular complications are caused by both chronic hyperglycemia and the consequences of insulin resistance. The effects of former high HbA$_{1c}$ levels can persist for years after HbA$_{1c}$ values have been lowered (hyperglycemic memory).
- Proliferative diabetic retinopathy (PDR) and macular edema both cause severe visual loss. Optimal treatment with panretinal photocoagulation reduces blindness from PDR by 98%. Treatment of macular edema with intraocular injection of agents that inhibit vascular endothelial growth factor A (anti-VEGF-A agents) causes long-term improvement in visual loss.
- Chronic diabetic kidney disease increases the risk of cardiovascular disease (CVD) and death. Optimal management includes early control of blood pressure using renin-angiotensin-aldosterone system blockade and other agents, control of hyperglycemia, and control of dyslipidemia.
- Diabetic neuropathies include distal symmetric polyneuropathy, mononeuropathies, and a variety of autonomic neuropathies. The cornerstone of treatment is blood glucose control. Specific antidepressants, anticonvulsants, and the γ-aminobutyric acid (GABA) analogue pregabalin are used to treat painful neuropathy. Loss of heart rate variability due to autonomic neuropathy increases the risk of cardiac events more than fourfold.
- Diabetes substantially increases risk of coronary disease, early and late post-MI (myocardial infarction) fatality rate, and risk of congestive heart failure (CHF), even after adjustment for other CVD risk factors. Hyperglycemia and insulin resistance interact with hypertension and dyslipidemia. Optimal treatment includes intensive lowering of low-density lipoprotein (LDL) cholesterol and blood pressure, and use of metformin. Coronary artery bypass grafting (CABG) provides better outcomes than percutaneous transluminal coronary angioplasty (PTCA) in diabetic patients. Angiotensin-converting enzyme (ACE) inhibitors reduce post-MI mortality risks.
- Diabetic foot ulcers are the major cause of nontraumatic leg amputation. Risk factors are sensory neuropathic loss of proprioception, motor neuropathic foot deformity, and peripheral vascular disease. Simple clinical interventions reduce amputation by up to 80%. Management involves pressure off-loading, parenteral antibiotics for infection, and ensuring adequate arterial inflow.

BIOCHEMISTRY AND MOLECULAR CELL BIOLOGY

All forms of diabetes, both inherited and acquired, are characterized by hyperglycemia, a relative or absolute lack of insulin, and the development of diabetes-specific microvascular disease in the retina, renal glomerulus, and peripheral nerve. Diabetes is also associated with accelerated atherosclerotic macrovascular disease affecting arteries that supply the heart, brain, and lower extremities.[1] Pathologically, this condition resembles macrovascular disease in nondiabetic patients, but it is more extensive and progresses more rapidly. As a consequence of its microvascular pathologic changes, diabetes mellitus is now the leading cause of new blindness in people 20 to 74 years of age and the leading cause of end-stage renal disease (ESRD).

People with diabetes mellitus are the fastest growing group of renal dialysis and transplant recipients. The life expectancy of patients with diabetic ESRD is only 3 or 4 years. More than 60% of diabetic patients are affected by neuropathy, which includes distal symmetric polyneuropathy, mononeuropathies, and a variety of autonomic neuropathies causing erectile dysfunction, urinary incontinence, gastroparesis, and nocturnal diarrhea. Because of accelerated lower extremity arterial disease in conjunction with neuropathy, diabetes mellitus accounts for 50% of all nontrauma amputations in the United States. The risk of cardiovascular complications is increased by twofold to sixfold in subjects with diabetes. Overall, life expectancy is about 7 to 10 years shorter than for people without diabetes mellitus because of diabetic complications.[2] In the past 2 decades the incidence of diabetes-related complications has declined substantially, but this decline is largely offset by the rising prevalence of diabetes.[3]

Large prospective clinical studies show a strong relationship between glycemia and diabetic microvascular complications in both type 1 diabetes mellitus (T1DM) and type 2 diabetes (T2DM).[4,5] There is a continuous, although not linear, relationship between the level of glycemia and the risk of development and progression of these complications (Fig. 33-1).[6,7] Hyperglycemia and the consequences of

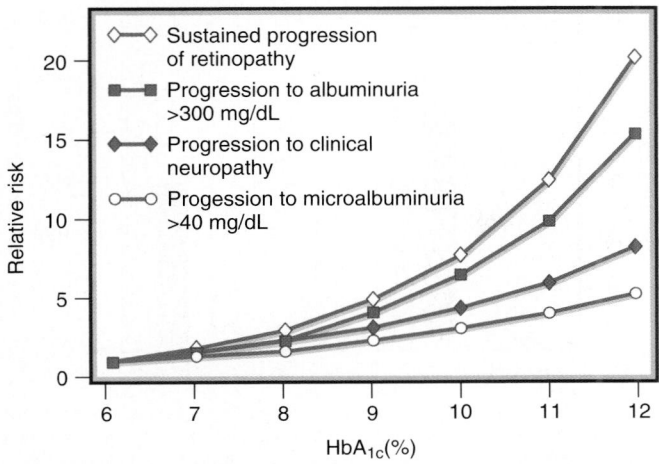

Figure 33-1 Relative risks for the development of diabetic complications at different mean levels of glycosylated hemoglobin (HbA$_{1c}$) obtained from the Diabetes Control and Complications Trial. (Adapted from Skyler J: Diabetic complications: the importance of glucose control. *Endocrinol Metab Clin North Am.* 1996;25:243-254.)

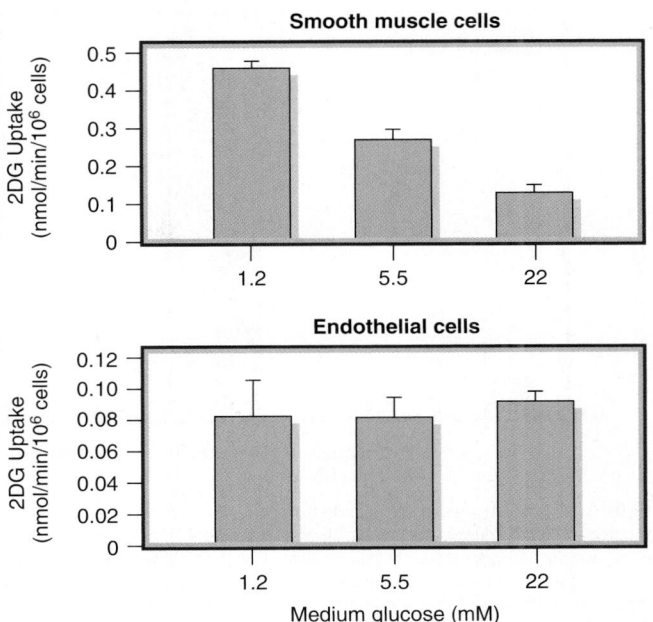

Figure 33-2 Lack of downregulation of glucose transport in cells affected by diabetic complications. *Upper panel* shows 2-deoxyglucose (2DG) uptake in vascular smooth muscle cells preexposed to 1.2, 5.5, or 22 mmol/L glucose. *Lower panel* shows 2DG uptake in bovine endothelial cells preexposed to 1.2, 5.5, or 22 mmol/L glucose. (From Kaiser N, Feener EP, Boukobza-Vardi N, et al. Differential regulation of glucose transport and transporters by glucose in vascular endothelial and smooth muscle cells. *Diabetes.* 1993;42:80-89.)

insulin resistance both appear to play important roles in the pathogenesis of macrovascular complications.[8-12]

Shared Pathophysiologic Features of Microvascular Complications

In the retina, glomerulus, and vasa nervorum, diabetes-specific microvascular disease is characterized by similar pathophysiologic features.

Requirement for Intracellular Hyperglycemia

Clinical and animal model data indicate that chronic hyperglycemia is the central initiating factor for all types of diabetic microvascular disease. The duration and magnitude of hyperglycemia are strongly correlated with the extent and rate of progression of diabetic microvascular disease. In the Diabetes Control and Complications Trial (DCCT), for example, T1DM patients whose intensive insulin therapy resulted in glycosylated hemoglobin (HbA$_{1c}$) levels 2% lower than those in patients receiving conventional insulin therapy had a 76% lower incidence of retinopathy, a 54% lower incidence of nephropathy, and a 60% reduction in neuropathy.[4,5] However, further analysis of the DCCT data showed that although intensive therapy reduced the risk of sustained retinopathy progression by 73% compared with standard treatment, HbA$_{1c}$ and duration of diabetes (glycemic exposure) explained only about 11% of the variation in retinopathy risk for the entire study population, suggesting that the remaining 89% of the variation in risk can be explained by aspects of glycemia not captured by HbA$_{1c}$.[13]

Although all diabetic cells are exposed to elevated levels of plasma glucose, hyperglycemic damage is limited to those cell types (e.g., endothelial cells) that develop intracellular hyperglycemia. Endothelial cells develop intracellular hyperglycemia because, unlike many other cells, they cannot downregulate glucose transport when exposed to extracellular hyperglycemia. As illustrated in Figure 33-2, vascular smooth muscle cells (VSMCs), which are not damaged by hyperglycemia, show an inverse relationship between extracellular glucose concentration and subsequent rate of glucose transport measured as 2-deoxyglucose uptake (see Fig. 33-2, upper part). In contrast, vascular endothelial cells show no significant change in subsequent

rate of glucose transport after exposure to elevated glucose concentrations (see Fig. 33-2, lower part).[14] That intracellular hyperglycemia is necessary and sufficient for the development of diabetic disease is further demonstrated by the fact that overexpression of glucose transporter 1 (GLUT1) in mesangial cells cultured in a normal glucose milieu mimics the diabetic phenotype, inducing the same increases in collagen type IV, collagen type I, and fibronectin gene expression as are observed in diabetic hyperglycemia (Fig. 33-3).[15] Similarly, diabetic mice with a podocyte-specific deletion of GLUT4 do not develop albuminuria and are protected from diabetes-induced hypertrophy, mesangial expansion, and albuminuria.[16]

Abnormal Cell Function

Early in the course of diabetes mellitus, before structural changes are evident, hyperglycemia causes abnormalities in blood flow and vascular permeability in the retina, glomerulus, and peripheral nerve vasa nervorum.[17,18] The increase in blood flow and intracapillary pressure is thought to reflect a hyperglycemia-induced decrease in nitric oxide (NO) production on the efferent side of capillary beds and possibly an increased sensitivity to angiotensin II. As a consequence of increased intracapillary pressure and endothelial cell dysfunction, retinal capillaries exhibit increased leakage of fluorescein, and glomerular capillaries have an elevated albumin excretion rate (AER). In both retina and glomerulus, crosstalk among different cell types plays a central role in pathogenesis. In the retina, different cell types in the neuroretina are critical. Deterioration of the inner blood-retinal barrier and consequent macular edema is characteristic of diabetic retinopathy. The neuronal guidance cue semaphorin 3A, induced in the early hyperglycemic phase of diabetes within the neuronal retina, precipitates the initial breakdown of endothelial barrier

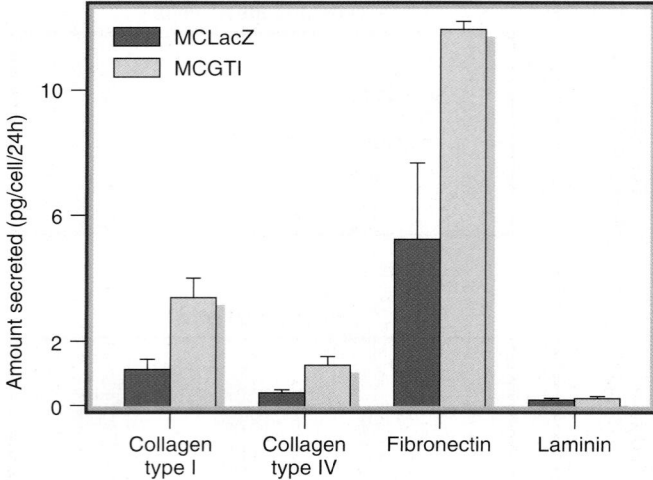

Figure 33-3 Overexpression of glucose transporter 1 (GLUT1) in mesangial cells cultured in normal glucose mimics the diabetic phenotype. Mesangial cells (MCs) were transfected with either β-galactosidase (LacZ) or GLUT1 (GT1). MCLacZ-expressing or MCGT1-expressing constructs were cultured in 5 mmol/L glucose, and the secreted amounts of the indicated matrix components were determined. (From Heilig CW, Concepcion LA, Riser BL, et al. Overexpression of glucose transporters in rat mesangial cells cultured in a normal glucose milieu mimics the diabetic phenotype. *J Clin Invest.* 1995;96:1802-1814.)

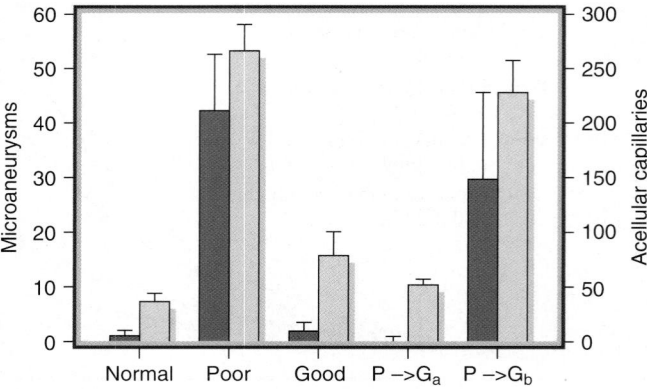

Figure 33-4 Development of retinopathy during posthyperglycemic normoglycemia (hyperglycemic memory). Quantitation of retinal microaneurysms and acellular capillaries in normal dogs (Normal), dogs with poor glycemic control for 5 years (Poor), dogs with good glycemic control for 5 years (Good), dogs with poor glycemic control for 2.5 years (P → G_a), and the same dogs after a subsequent 2.5 years of good glycemic control (P → G_b). Dark-colored bars indicate microaneurysms; light-colored bars indicate acellular capillaries. (Adapted from Engerman RL, Kern TS. Progression of incipient diabetic retinopathy during good glycemic control. *Diabetes.* 1987;36: 808-812.)

function via its cognate receptor neuropilin-1.[19] In retinal Müller cells, high glucose induces a time-dependent increase of endoplasmic reticulum stress, activating transcription factor 4 (ATF4) expression and inflammatory factor production.[20] Capillary pericytes also play a central role in endothelial cell survival and death.[21]

Growing evidence indicates that podocyte loss and epithelial dysfunction play important roles in diabetic kidney disease. Inflammation, cell hypertrophy, and dedifferentiation by the activation of classic pathways of regeneration further contribute to disease progression.[22] Emerging evidence indicates that endothelial-podocyte crosstalk across the glomerular filtration barrier may profoundly influence the function of both cell types.[23] One example is the impairment of endothelial thrombomodulin-dependent activated protein C (APC) formation by hyperglycemia. Loss of thrombomodulin-dependent APC formation interrupts crosstalk between the vascular compartment and podocytes, causing glomerular apoptosis and diabetic nephropathy.[24,25] In peripheral nerves, hyperglycemia induces abnormalities in both neurons, in Schwann cells, and in the vasa nervorum.[26]

Increased Vessel Wall Protein Accumulation

The common pathophysiologic feature of diabetic microvascular disease is progressive narrowing and eventual occlusion of vascular lumens, which results in inadequate perfusion and function of the affected tissues. Early hyperglycemia-induced microvascular hypertension and increased vascular permeability contribute to irreversible microvessel occlusion by three processes.

The first process is an abnormal leakage of periodic acid–Schiff (PAS)-positive, carbohydrate-containing plasma proteins, which are deposited in the capillary wall and can stimulate perivascular cells such as pericytes and mesangial cells to elaborate growth factors and extracellular matrix.

The second process is extravasation of growth factors, such as transforming growth factor-β1 (TGF-β1), which directly stimulates overproduction of extracellular matrix

components[27] and can induce apoptosis in certain complication-relevant cell types.

The third process is hypertension-induced stimulation of pathologic gene expression by endothelial cells and supporting cells, which include GLUT1, growth factors, growth factor receptors, extracellular matrix components, and adhesion molecules that can activate circulating leukocytes.[28] The observation that unilateral reduction in the severity of diabetic microvascular disease occurs on the side with ophthalmic or renal artery stenosis is consistent with this concept.[29,30]

Microvascular Cell Loss and Vessel Occlusion

The progressive narrowing and occlusion of diabetic microvascular lumens are also accompanied by microvascular cell loss. In the retina, diabetes mellitus induces programmed cell death of Müller cells and ganglion cells,[31] pericytes, and endothelial cells.[32] In the glomerulus, declining renal function is associated with widespread capillary occlusion and podocyte loss, but the mechanisms underlying glomerular cell loss are not yet known. In the vasa nervorum, degeneration of endothelial cells and pericytes occurs,[33] and these microvascular changes appear to precede the development of diabetic peripheral neuropathy.[34] The multifocal distribution of axonal degeneration in diabetes supports a causal role for microvascular occlusion, but hyperglycemia-induced decreases in neurotrophins might contribute by preventing normal axonal repair and regeneration.[35]

Development of Microvascular Complications During Posthyperglycemic Euglycemia

Another common feature of diabetic microvascular disease has been termed *hyperglycemic memory*, or the persistence or progression of hyperglycemia-induced microvascular alterations during subsequent periods of normal glucose homeostasis. The most striking example of this phenomenon is the development of severe retinopathy in histologically normal eyes of diabetic dogs, which occurred entirely during a 2.5-year period of normalized blood glucose that followed 2.5 years of hyperglycemia (Fig. 33-4).[36] Normal dogs were compared to diabetic dogs with either poor control (P) for 5 years, good control (G) for 5 years, or poor control for 2.5 years (P → Gₐ) followed by good control for the next 2.5 years (P → G_b). HbA_{1c} values for both the good control group and the P → G_b group were identical to those of the normal group. Hyperglycemia-induced increases in selected matrix gene transcription also persist for weeks after restoration of normoglycemia in vivo, and a less pronounced but qualitatively similar prolongation of hyperglycemia-induced increase in selected matrix gene transcription occurs in cultured endothelial cells.[37]

Data from the DCCT suggested that hyperglycemic memory occurs in patients. In the secondary intervention cohort, there was no difference in the incidence of sustained progression of retinopathy for the first 3 years, no difference in development of clinical albuminuria for 4 years, and no difference in the rate of change in creatinine clearance during the entire study. For neuropathy, the sural nerve sensory conduction velocity did not differ between the groups for 4 years, and intensive therapy did not slow the rate of decline of autonomic function at all.[4,38,39]

Data from the post-DCCT long-term follow-up study, the Epidemiology of Diabetes, Interventions, and Complications (EDIC) study, proved that the effects of former intensive and conventional therapy persist for at least 12 years. In the conventional therapy group, the effects of previous high HbA_{1c} on poststudy retinopathy, nephropathy, and CVD persisted as if there had been no improvement in HbA_{1c} at all. Atherosclerotic changes not even present at the end of the DCCT appeared subsequently in the previously higher HbA_{1c} group, followed by a twofold increase in heart attacks, strokes, and cardiovascular death, even though the HbA_{1c} level in these patients since the end of the DCCT was identical to that of the formerly intensive-control group during the entire time that these arterial changes developed (Fig. 33-5).[40,41] On the other hand, the beneficial effects of previous lower HbA_{1c} also persisted in the intensive treatment group after their HbA_{1c} went up, as if there had been no deterioration in their HbA_{1c}.

Therefore, the phenomenon of hyperglycemic memory presents a paradox: Patients in the DCCT with long-term exposure to a higher level of hyperglycemia became more susceptible to damage from subsequent lower levels of hyperglycemia than they were when they first started the trial. In contrast, lower levels of hyperglycemia made patients more resistant to damage from subsequent higher levels. Whether the effects of glucose control and hyperglycemic memory on atherosclerosis and cardiovascular events might also apply to patients with T2DM remains unresolved. The DCCT-EDIC experience also raises questions about the duration of drug exposure needed in order for the impact of specific antidiabetic agents and glucose-lowering strategies to be fully uncovered.

Genetic Determinants of Susceptibility to Microvascular Complications

Clinicians have long observed that different patients with similar duration and degree of hyperglycemia differ markedly in their susceptibility to microvascular complications. Such observations suggested that genetic differences exist that affected the pathways by which hyperglycemia damages microvascular cells. The leveling of risk of overt proteinuria after 30 years' duration of T1DM at 27% is evidence that only a subset of patients are susceptible to development of diabetic nephropathy.[42]

A role for a genetic determinant of susceptibility to diabetic nephropathy is most strongly supported by familial clustering, with an estimated heritability of at least 40%.[43] In two studies of families in which two or more siblings had T1DM, the risk of nephropathy in a diabetic sibling was 83% or 72% if the proband diabetic sibling had advanced diabetic nephropathy, but only 17% or 22% if the index patient did not have diabetic nephropathy (Fig. 33-6)[44,45] or retinopathy. The DCCT reported familial clustering for the risk of severe retinopathy as well, with an odds ratio of 5.4 in diabetic relatives of positive versus negative subjects from the conventional treatment group.[46] Diabetic retinopathy and coronary artery calcification, an indicator of subclinical atherosclerosis, also show familial clustering.

Numerous associations have been made between various genetic polymorphisms and the risk of diabetic complications. Examples include the 5′ insulin gene polymorphism,[47] the G2m²³⁺ immunoglobulin allotype,[48] ACE insertion/deletion polymorphisms,[49,50] HLA-DQB10201/0302 alleles,[51] polymorphisms of the aldose reductase gene,[52] and a polymorphic CCTTT(n) repeat of nitric oxide synthase 2A (NOS2A).[53] In all of these studies, there was

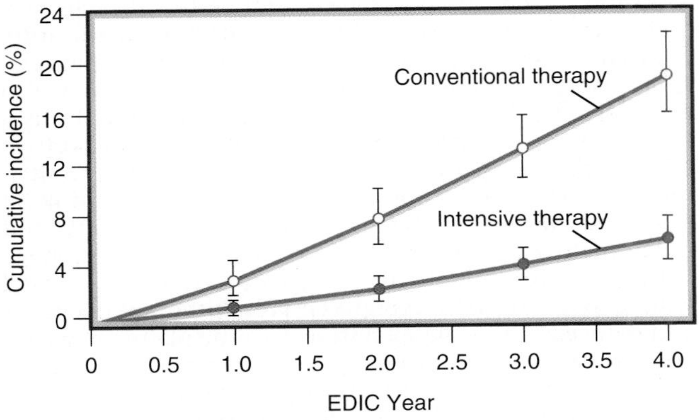

Figure 33-5 Cumulative incidence of further progression of retinopathy 4 years after the end of the Diabetes Control and Complications Trial. The median glycosylated hemoglobin level was 8.2% for the conventional therapy group and 7.9% for the intensive therapy group. EDIC, Epidemiology of Diabetes, Interventions, and Complications [Research Group]. (From Retinopathy and nephropathy in patients with type 1 diabetes four years after a trial of intensive therapy. The Diabetes Control and Complications Trial/Epidemiology of Diabetes Interventions and Complications Research Group. *N Engl J Med.* 2000;342:381-389.)

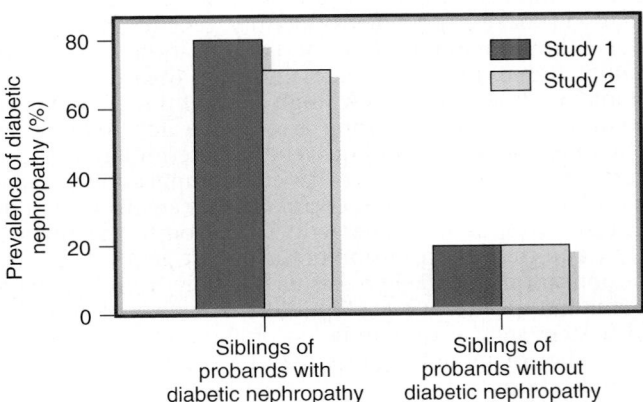

Figure 33-6 Familial clustering of diabetic nephropathy. Prevalence of diabetic nephropathy in two studies of diabetic siblings of probands with or without diabetic nephropathy. (Adapted from Seaquist ER, Goetz FC, Rich S, et al. Familial clustering of diabetic kidney disease: evidence for genetic susceptibility to diabetic nephropathy. *N Engl J Med.* 1989;320:1161-1165; Quinn M, Angelico MC, Warram JH, et al. Familial factors determine the development of diabetic nephropathy in patients with IDDM. *Diabetologia.* 1996;39:940-945.)

no indication that the polymorphic gene actually plays a functional role rather than simply being in linkage disequilibrium with the locus encoding the unidentified relevant genes.

A whole-genome linkage analysis using families of Pima Indians showed susceptibility loci for diabetic nephropathy on chromosomes 3, 7, and 20. Another linkage analysis using discordant sib-pairs of white families with T1DM identified a critical area on chromosome 3q. Evidence for linkage to kidney disease has been detected and replicated at several loci on chromosomes 3q (T1DM and T2DM nephropathy), 10q (diabetic and nondiabetic kidney disease), and 18q (T2DM nephropathy).[54]

Family-based studies of simple tandem repeat polymorphisms (STRPs) and single-nucleotide polymorphisms (SNPs) in 115 candidate genes for linkage and association with diabetic nephropathy in T1DM families of European descent showed a positive association with polymorphisms in 20 genes, including 12 that had not been studied previously. Three of these genes code for components of the extracellular matrix (COL4A1, LAMA4, and LAMC1), and two are involved in its metabolism (MMP9 and TIMP3). Five genes code for transcription factors or signaling molecules (HNF1B1/TCF2, NRP1, PRKCB1, SMAD3, and USF1). Three genes code for growth factors or growth factor receptors (IGF1, TGFBR2, and TGFBR3). The other genes (AGTR1, AQP1, BCL2, CAT, GPX1, LPL, and p22phox) code for a variety of products that are likely to be relevant in kidney function.[55]

An individual-based genetic association study of subjects from the DCCT/EDIC found that multiple variations in superoxide dismutase 1 (SOD1) were significantly associated with persistent microalbuminuria and severe nephropathy.[56] A combination of case-control association and functional studies demonstrated that the T allele of SNP rs1617640 in the promoter of the erythropoietin gene (EPO) was significantly associated with proliferative diabetic retinopathy (PDR) and ESRD in three European-American cohorts, suggesting that rs1617640 in the EPO promoter is significantly associated with PDR and ESRD.[57] In addition, a multicenter study based on 518 subjects with long-standing diabetes mellitus showed that three EPO SNPs were associated with overall diabetic retinopathy status in the combined T1DM and T2DM groups and in the T2DM-alone group.[58]

As genes are identified that affect susceptibility to diabetic complications, a new area of research has emerged that will make it possible to identify genetic modifiers of the clinical manifestations of complications. With the completion of the genetic map known as the International HapMap Project and new high-throughput genotyping technologies, this promising area of research holds great potential for understanding genetic determinants of the varying clinical severity of diabetic complications. These modifying genes are genetic variants that are distinct from disease-susceptibility genes and that modify the phenotypic and clinical expression of the disease genes.[59] Because complications are likely to result not only from hyperglycemia but also from a susceptibility to later pathophysiologic steps such as inflammation or aberrant angiogenesis, a number of modifier genes may be relevant to diabetic complications.

MicroRNAs and Diabetic Complications

Although polymorphisms in protein-coding genes were the initial focus of genetic studies, recent discoveries of noncoding regulatory RNAs have changed our understanding of how cells work. Although piwi-interacting RNAs (piRNAs), endogenous small interfering RNAs (siRNAs), intron-derived microRNAs (miRNAs), and a host of long noncoding RNAs all have regulatory roles, the best understood with respect to diabetic complications are the miRNAs, which regulate several key biologic pathways and cellular functions involved in diabetic complications. Among these are targets that regulate reactive oxygen species (ROS) levels, the underlying link between intracellular hyperglycemia and complications-causing pathways (described later under "Different Hyperglycemia-Induced Pathogenic Mechanisms Reflect a Single Upstream Process"). In whole retina, diabetes increases levels of the NFκB-responsive miRNAs miR-146, miR-155, miR-132, and miR-21.[60] However, in retinal microvessels, high glucose decreases miR-146a expression and increases fibronectin expression in endothelial cells. Similar changes are seen in the kidneys and hearts of type 1 and type 2 diabetic animals.[61] In diabetic mouse kidney cortex, levels of miR-192 are increased, and miR-192 knockdown prevents diabetes-induced proteinuria and renal fibrosis.[62] In contrast, the renal expression of miR-200a is reduced in mouse models with early and advanced diabetic nephropathy.[63] miR-200a downregulates the expression of TGF-β2 and the resulting overexpression of matrix proteins, and prevents TGF-β-dependent epithelial-mesenchymal transition (EMT), all hallmarks of diabetic nephropathy. TGF-β1 and TGF-β2 also downregulate expression of miR-200a, creating a positive feed-forward loop favoring continued renal damage.

In the kidney, diabetes also increases miR-29c, which induces cell apoptosis and increases extracellular matrix protein accumulation. Expression of miR-29c induces podocyte apoptosis. Knockdown of miR-29c prevents high glucose-induced cell apoptosis. Knockdown of miR-29c significantly reduces albuminuria and kidney mesangial matrix accumulation in db/db mice.[64]

MicroRNAs also function as a messenger in cell-to-cell communication. For example, miR-126 was identified as the predominantly expressed miR in endothelial microparticles (EMPs) released from apoptotic endothelial cells. Knockdown of miR-126 in EMPs abrogates EMP-mediated effects on human coronary artery endothelial cell migration and proliferation in vitro and reendothelialization in vivo. EMPs derived from glucose-treated endothelial cells contain significantly lower amounts of miR-126 and show reduced endothelial repair capacity in vitro and in vivo. Expression analysis of miR-126 in circulating microparticles from patients with stable coronary artery disease with and without diabetes mellitus revealed a significantly reduced miR-126 expression in circulating microparticles from diabetic patients.[65] Diabetic atherosclerosis may also be accelerated by microRNAs. MicroRNA 33 (miR-33) is a key negative regulator of reverse cholesterol transport. In mice placed on an atherogenic diet for 16 weeks and then made diabetic by streptozotocin injection, anti-miR-33 treatment decreases plaque macrophage content and inflammatory gene expression. The decreased macrophage content in anti-miR-33–treated diabetic mice is associated with a blunting of hyperglycemia-induced monocytosis and reduced monocyte recruitment to the plaque.[66] MicroRNAs may also play a role in the pathogenesis of diabetic cardiomyopathy. miR-451, which suppresses the LKB1/AMPK (liver kinase B1/adenosine monophosphate [AMP]-activated protein kinase) signaling pathway, is significantly increased in type 2 diabetic mouse hearts. Loss of miR-451 function ameliorated palmitate-induced lipotoxicity in neonatal rat cardiac myocytes. Similarly, high-fat-diet–induced cardiac hypertrophy and decreased contractile reserves are ameliorated in cardiomyocyte-specific miR-451 knockout mice compared with control mice.[67]

Most recently, differences in expression of a microRNA species were found to differentiate patients with over 50 years of T1DM and no microvascular complications from those with over 50 years of T1DM who had microvascular complications.[67a]

Progenitor Cells and Microvascular Complications

Proinflammatory processes initiated by marrow-derived cells are well known to play a major role in the pathogenesis of atherosclerosis. Recent evidence suggests that these cells may also play a critical role in the development of diabetic complications in the retina, kidney, and nerve.[68] Diabetic retinopathy and its pathognomonic hyperglycemia-induced loss of capillary endothelial cells and pericytes is associated with leukostasis.[21] A causal role and bone marrow origin of these cells are supported by the observation that diabetes-induced capillary degeneration, proinflammatory changes, and superoxide production in the retina are inhibited in diabetic animals in which iNOS (inducible nitric oxide synthase) or PARP1 (poly-ADP-ribose polymerase-1) was deleted from bone marrow cells only.[69] In kidneys from patients with diabetic nephropathy, the intensity of interstitial macrophage accumulation is proportional to the rate of subsequent decline in renal function.[70] In animal models, depletion of macrophages or suppression of macrophage recruitment by the kidney prevents experimental diabetic nephropathy.[70] Diabetes also causes impaired collateral blood vessel formation from bone marrow precursor cells (discussed later) and reduces the ability of cardiac stem cells (CSCs) to repair injured myocardium. Both diabetes and preconditioning CSCs in high glucose altered the proangiogenic capacity of CSCs. Increased expression of glyoxalase-1, an enzyme that prevents posttranslational modification of proteins by the glycolysis-derived α-oxoaldehyde, methylglyoxal (MG), restored the proangiogenic capacity of diabetic CSCs.[71]

Pathophysiologic Features of Macrovascular Complications

Unlike microvascular disease, which occurs only in patients with diabetes mellitus, macrovascular disease is thought to broadly resemble that found in subjects without diabetes, although even this general pathologic finding remains inconclusively established. However, subjects with diabetes have more rapidly progressive and extensive CVD, with a greater incidence of multivessel disease and a greater number of diseased vessel segments than nondiabetic persons.[72] Although dyslipidemia and hypertension occur with great frequency in T2DM populations, there is still excess risk in diabetic subjects after adjusting for these other risk factors.[73,74] Diabetes itself can confer 75% to 90% of the excess risk of coronary disease in these diabetic subjects, and it enhances the deleterious effects of the other major cardiovascular risk factors (Fig. 33-7).[75,76] A role for hyperglycemia in the pathogenesis of diabetic macrovascular disease is suggested by the observation that HbA$_{1c}$ is an independent risk factor for CVD[77] in T1DM, and correlational studies show that hyperglycemia is a continuous risk factor for macrovascular disease in T2DM as well.[78-82]

However, data from the United Kingdom Prospective Diabetes Study (UKPDS) show that hyperglycemia is not nearly as central a determinant of diabetic macrovascular disease as it is in microvascular disease. For microvascular disease end points, there is an almost 10-fold increase in risk as HbA$_{1c}$ increases from 5.5% to 9.5%, whereas over

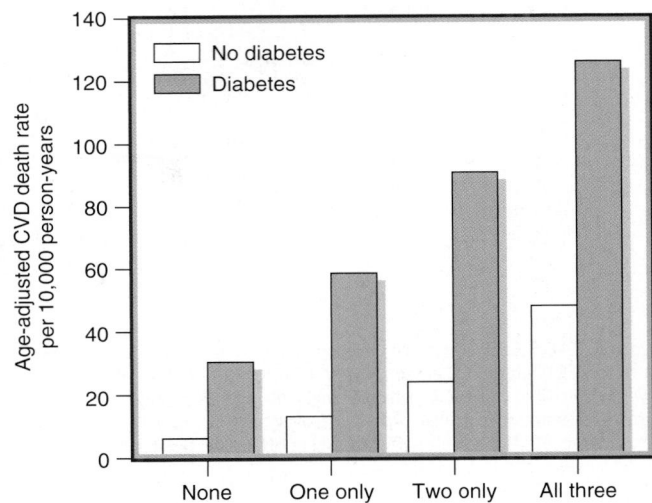

Figure 33-7 Adjusted death rates by number of cardiovascular disease (CVD) risk factors for diabetic and nondiabetic men. Subjects are participants from the Multiple Risk Factor Intervention Trial (MRFIT) study; risk factors are hypercholesterolemia, hypertension, and cigarette smoking. (From Stamler J, Vaccaro O, Neaton JD, et al. Diabetes, other risk factors, and 12-year cardiovascular mortality for men screened in the Multiple Risk Factor Intervention Trial. *Diabetes Care.* 1993;2:434-444.)

the same HbA$_{1c}$ range, macrovascular risk increases only about twofold.[4,5]

Insulin resistance occurs in most patients with T2DM and in two thirds of subjects with impaired glucose tolerance.[83] Both these groups have a significantly higher risk of developing CVD.[84-87] To isolate the effects of insulin resistance from those of hyperglycemia and diabetes, several studies have evaluated subjects with normal glucose tolerance. In T1DM, hyperglycemia itself causes secondary insulin resistance in almost all patients. In nonobese subjects without diabetes, insulin resistance predicted the development of CVD independently of other known risk factors.[88] In another group of subjects without diabetes or impaired glucose tolerance, those in the highest quintile of insulin resistance had a 2.5-fold increase in CVD risk compared with those in the lowest quintile.[89] These data indicate that insulin resistance itself promotes atherogenesis.

Insulin resistance is commonly associated with a proatherogenic dyslipidemia, with a characteristic lipoprotein profile that includes a high level of very low-density lipoprotein (VLDL) and low levels of high-density lipoprotein (HDL) and small, dense low-density lipoprotein (LDL). Both low HDL and small, dense LDL are independent risk factors for macrovascular disease. This profile arises as a direct result of increased net free fatty acid (FFA) release by insulin-resistant adipocytes (Fig. 33-8).[12] Increased FFA flux into hepatocytes stimulates VLDL secretion. In the presence of cholesteryl ester transfer protein, excess VLDL transfers significant amounts of triglyceride to HDL and LDL while depleting HDL and LDL of cholesteryl ester. The resultant triglyceride-enriched HDL carries less cholesteryl ester for reverse cholesterol transport to the liver, and loss of apolipoprotein 1A-1 (Apo1A-1) from these particles reduces the total concentration of HDL available for reverse cholesterol transport. The triglyceride-enriched, cholesteryl ester–depleted LDL is smaller and denser than normal LDL, allowing it to penetrate the vessel wall and be oxidized more easily.

Separately, VLDL hydrolysis by LPL can generate biologically active molecules, such as fatty acids, that activate nuclear receptors such as peroxisome proliferator-activated

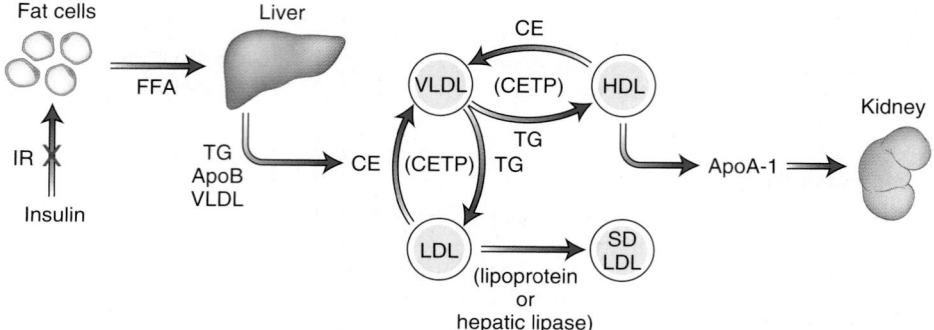

Figure 33-8 Schematic summary relating insulin resistance (IR) to the characteristic dyslipidemia of type 2 diabetes mellitus. IR at the adipocyte results in increased free fatty acid (FFA) release. Increased FFA flux stimulates secretion of very low density lipoprotein (VLDL), causing hypertriglyceridemia. VLDL stimulates a reciprocal exchange of triglyceride (TG) to cholesteryl ester (CE) from both high-density lipoprotein (HDL) and low-density lipoprotein (LDL), catalyzed by CE transfer protein (CETP). TG-enriched HDL dissociates from apolipoprotein (Apo) A-1, leaving less HDL for reverse cholesterol transport. TG-enriched LDL serves as a substrate for lipases that convert it to atherogenic small, dense (SD) LDL particles. (From Ginsberg HN. Insulin resistance and cardiovascular disease. *J Clin Invest.* 2000;106:453-458.)

receptor alpha (PPARα), thus modulating large transcriptional programs and exerting effects such as decreased endothelial inflammation.[2] Importantly, fatty acids generated in this way and their biologic effects must be distinguished from free fatty acids. In fact, when translational clinical studies consider free fatty acids, it is often after heparin infusion, which disrupts the fundamental physical interaction between LPL and VLDL on the endothelial surface, and subsequent uptake of hydrolyzed fatty acids. These endogenous PPAR ligands are also distinct from synthetic PPARα pharmacologic agents. The finding that LPL action on VLDL can activate PPARα has been reported in various settings and aligns closely with prior and new genetic evidence that genetic variants that increase LPL function, like loss of the LPL inhibitor apoCIII or LPL mutations with increased activity, result in lower triglycerides, higher HDLs, and less atherosclerosis.[4-7]

In vitro studies suggest that at the level of the vessel wall, insulin has both antiatherogenic and proatherogenic effects (Fig. 33-9).[90,91] One major antiatherogenic effect is the stimulation of endothelial NO production. NO released from endothelial cells is a potent inhibitor of platelet aggregation and adhesion to the vascular wall. Endothelial NO also controls the expression of genes involved in atherogenesis. It decreases expression of monocyte chemoattractant protein 1 (MCP-1) and of surface adhesion molecules such as CD11/CD18, P-selectin, vascular cell adhesion molecule 1 (VCAM-1), and intercellular adhesion molecule 1 (ICAM-1). Endothelial cell NO also reduces vascular permeability and decreases the rate of oxidation of LDL to its proatherogenic form. Finally, endothelial cell NO inhibits proliferation of VSMCs.[92] However, in diabetes, overproduction of ROS leads to oxidation of tetrahydrobiopterin (BH₄), the essential cofactor of endothelial nitric oxide synthase (eNOS). In BH₄ deficiency, oxygen reduction uncouples from NO synthesis, thereby converting eNOS to a superoxide-producing enzyme.[93]

Although this important antiatherogenic effect of insulin is blocked by diabetes-induced ROS, two major proatherogenic effects of insulin are not. Insulin both potentiates platelet-derived growth factor (PDGF)-induced VSMC proliferation and stimulates VSMC production of plasminogen activator inhibitor 1 (PAI-1).[94,95] Because the effects of insulin on smooth muscle cells are mediated by the signal transduction pathway involving Ras, Raf, MAPK (mitogen-activated protein kinase), and MEKK (MAPK/extracellular-signal–regulated kinase [ERK] kinase [MEK] kinase),[91,92] it has been proposed that pathway-selective

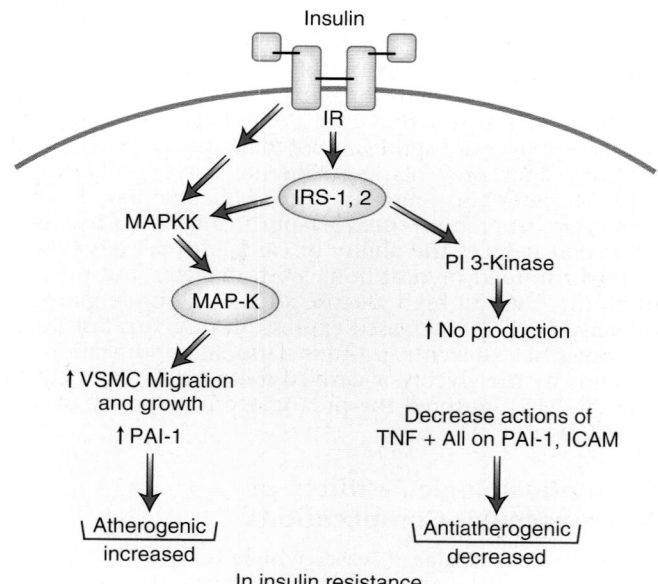

Figure 33-9 Schematic summary of proatherosclerotic and antiatherosclerotic actions of insulin on vascular cells. ICAM, intercellular adhesion molecule; IRS, insulin resistance syndrome; MAP-K, mitogen-activated protein kinase; MAPKK, MAPK kinase; PAI, plasminogen activator inhibitor; PI, phosphatidylinositol; TNF, tumor necrosis factor; VSMC, vascular smooth muscle cell. (Adapted from King G, Brownlee M. The cellular and molecular mechanisms of diabetic complications. *Endocrinol Metab Clin North Am.* 1996;2:255-270; Hsueh WA, Law RE. Cardiovascular risk continuum: implications of insulin resistance and diabetes. *Am J Med.* 1998;105:4S-14S.)

insulin resistance in arterial cells may contribute to diabetic atherosclerosis. Evidence of such selective vascular resistance to insulin has been demonstrated in the obese Zucker rat.[96]

Macrophages are a central element of atherogenesis. Some subpopulations of macrophages are proinflammatory, while others are anti-inflammatory. Macrophages isolated from two different mouse models of type 1 diabetes exhibit a proinflammatory phenotype. This inflammatory phenotype associates with increased expression of long-chain acyl-CoA synthetase 1 (ACSL1), an enzyme that catalyzes the thioesterification of fatty acids. Furthermore, myeloid-selective deletion of ACSL1 protects monocytes and macrophages from the inflammatory effects of diabetes. Myeloid-selective deletion of ACSL1 also prevents accelerated atherosclerosis in diabetic mice without affecting lesions in nondiabetic mice.[97] Monocytes from humans and mice with type 1 diabetes also exhibit increased ACSL1.

With hyperglycemia playing a smaller role in diabetic atherosclerosis, and fatty acid metabolism playing a larger role, it is not surprising that in subjects without diabetes or impaired glucose tolerance, after adjustment for 11 known cardiovascular risk factors, including LDL, triglycerides, HDL, systolic blood pressure (BP), and smoking, the most insulin-resistant subjects still have a twofold increase in the risk of CVD.[89] This observation suggests that a significant part of the increased CVD risk due to insulin resistance reflects a consequence of insulin resistance not previously identified as being proatherogenic. Increased flux of fatty acids from insulin-resistant adipose tissue to arterial cells both indirectly via endothelial catabolism of triglyceride-rich lipoproteins[98] or directly may be such a consequence. Another may be increased oxidation of FFAs by insulin-resistant aortic endothelial cells, which inactivates two important antiatherosclerotic enzymes: prostacyclin synthase and eNOS. This inactivation is reversed by inhibition of the rate-limiting enzyme of fatty acid oxidation, carnitine palmitoyltransferase I, through inhibition of FFA release from insulin-resistant adipose tissue and through reduction of superoxide levels.[99]

Although in T2DM the association of insulin resistance with CVD risk is clear, data concerning the relative role of hyperglycemia in promoting CVD in T1DM suggest a larger role. In T1DM, lowering of HbA$_{1c}$ levels with more intensive insulin treatment during the DCCT reduced both atherosclerosis surrogates during the trial and actual CVD events years after the trial had concluded. Intensive treatment reduced the risk of any CVD event by 42% and the risk of nonfatal MI, stroke, or death from CVD by 57%.[100] Consistent with this, in T1DM animal models hyperglycemia increases bone marrow production of neutrophils and monocytes, causing increased entry of these cells into early atherosclerotic lesions. Reduction of hyperglycemia by blocking renal glucose reabsorption with a sodium-glucose cotransporter 2 (SGLT2) inhibitor reduces monocytosis and monocyte entry into atherosclerotic lesions, thereby promoting lesion regression.[101,102]

Impaired Collateral Blood Vessel Formation From Bone Marrow Progenitor Cells

It has become apparent that diabetic complications result not only from damage to vascular cells but also from a defective repair process. Normally, in response to acute ischemia, new blood vessel growth rescues stunned areas of the heart or central nervous system, reducing morbidity and mortality risks. In response to chronic ischemia, collateral vessel development reduces the size and severity of subsequent infarction. In response to ischemia, circulating endothelial progenitor cells from the bone marrow promote the regeneration of blood vessels, acting in concert with cells and extracellular matrix at the site of injury. In experimental diabetes, however, these circulating endothelial progenitor cells are depleted and dysfunctional. As a result, diabetic animals have decreased vascular density after hind limb ischemia. Similarly, in human diabetes, endothelial progenitor cells are also depleted and dysfunctional.[103]

Clinically, diabetes is associated with poor outcomes after acute vascular occlusive events. This results in part from a failure to form adequate compensatory microvascu-

lature in response to ischemia. Posttranslational modification of proteins by the glycolysis-derived α-oxoaldehyde, methylglyoxal, appears to play a central role in this failure. High glucose induces a decrease in transactivation by the transcription factor hypoxia-inducible factor-1α (HIF-1α), which mediates production of hypoxia-stimulated chemokine and VEGF and the chemokine stromal cell-derived factor 1 (SDF-1; also known as CXCR12) by hypoxic tissue, and expression of the SDF-1 receptor (CXCR4) and eNOS in endothelial precursor cells in the bone marrow. Decreasing superoxide in diabetic mice, by transgenic expression of manganese superoxide dismutase (Mn-SOD) or by administration of a SOD mimetic, corrected postischemic defects in neovascularization, oxygen delivery, and chemokine expression, and normalized tissue survival. Decreased HIF-1α functional activity is specifically caused by impaired formation of the HIF-1α heterodimer with arylhydrocarbon receptor nuclear translocator (ARNT) and by impaired binding of the coactivator p300 to the HIF-1α–ARNT heterodimer. Hyperglycemia-induced covalent modification of p300 by the dicarbonyl metabolite methylglyoxal is responsible for this decreased association (Fig. 33-10). In diabetic mouse models of impaired angiogenesis and wound healing, decreasing mitochondrial formation of ROS normalizes both ischemia-induced new vessel formation and wound healing.[104,105]

Bone marrow–derived mesenchymal progenitor cells (BM-MPCs) are important for new blood vessel formation and demonstrate significant deficits in the context of diabetes. Two transcriptionally distinct subpopulations of homogeneous BM-MPCs have provasculogenic expression profiles, and these are selectively depleted in both T1DM and T2DM.[106]

Many diabetic patients who have impaired blood vessel growth after ischemic events also have increased retinal neovascularization (diabetic retinopathy). This diabetic paradox is at present poorly understood.[107,108] The question of how endothelial progenitor cell dysfunction can participate in diabetic retinopathy is especially intriguing, given the findings by Grant and colleagues[109] that bone marrow–derived endothelial progenitor cells play a role in a model of adult retinal revascularization. A plausible explanation may be that the cells responsible for increased VEGF production in the diabetic retina do not develop intracellular hyperglycemia and consequently do not develop HIF-1α dysfunction. They respond normally to ischemia, in contrast to ischemic tissue elsewhere in the body. VEGF is known to be significantly elevated in the ocular fluid of diabetic patients, but it has also been shown to be decreased in ischemic nonretinal tissues.[110] Because VEGF has a stimulatory effect on endothelial progenitor cell proliferation and is a potent stimulator of vasculogenesis,[111] retinal cells whose VEGF expression in response to ischemia is not affected by hyperglycemia may be sufficient to cause PDR.

Mechanisms of Hyperglycemia-Induced Damage

Murine models are valuable tools for defining the pathogenesis of diabetic complications. However, they have significant limitations, and it is important to recognize some of their limits.

No diabetic animal model, regardless of genetic background, recapitulates the structural and functional alterations of human complications. Rodent models do not develop proliferative retinopathy, renal interstitial fibrosis with heavy proteinuria and decreased GFR, or coronary atherosclerosis with complex plaque formation.

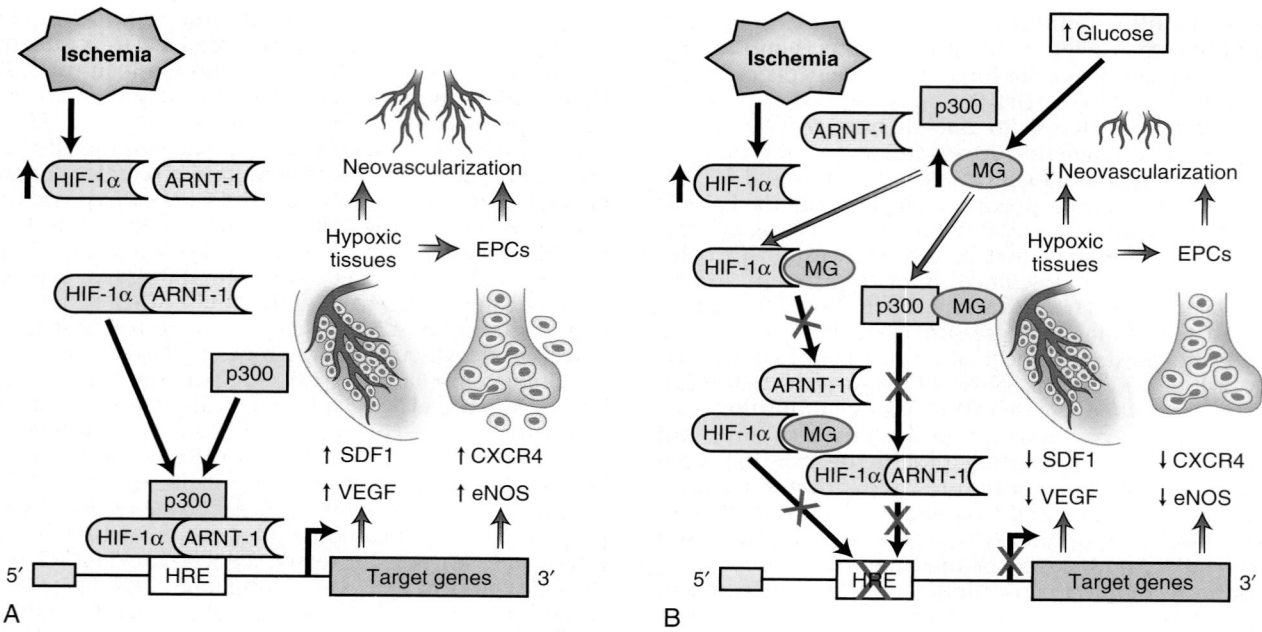

Figure 33-10 Ischemia-induced neovascularization in normal and high glucose. **A,** In the presence of normal glucose concentrations, ischemia-stabilized HIF-1α forms heterodimers with ARNT, which bind the coactivator p300. This complex binds to the hypoxia response element (HRE) and activates expression of genes required for neovascularization. **B,** High glucose–induced methylglyoxal (MG) modifies HIF-1α and p300, inhibiting complex binding to the HREs of genes required for neovascularization. ARNT, arylhydrocarbon receptor nuclear translocator; EPC, endothelial progenitor cells; eNOS, endothelial nitric oxide synthase; HIF-1α, hypoxia-inducible factor-1α; SDF1, stromal cell-derived factor 1; VEGF, vascular endothelial growth factor.

Consistent with this is the finding from a cross-species comparison of glomerular transcriptional networks from patients with diabetic nephropathy with those from three diabetic mouse models. This study showed that gene expression changes in these mouse models are similar to those in human nephropathy before the development of microalbuminuria, and therefore are most relevant to changes in very early human diabetic nephropathy.[112]

It is likely that in each diabetic complication, as with the different stages of atherosclerosis progressing from foam cells and fatty streaks to fibrous plaques and complicated lesions, dominant mechanisms differ for different stages. Most of the mechanistic data currently available come from studies of the early stages of each complication. More data about what molecular mechanisms are dominant in each complication target tissue at each pathologic stage are urgently needed.

In addition, only 33% to 50% of patients with poor glycemic control develop diabetic nephropathy, and a subset of patients with good glycemic control still develop diabetic nephropathy. Because rodents do not develop progressive complications resembling human diabetics, without data from human tissues, it is not possible to identify protective factors that allow a considerable percentage of patients with poor glycemic control to escape progression to ESRD.

Using primary human cells and mouse models, four major hypotheses about how hyperglycemia causes diabetic complications have generated a large amount of data as well as several clinical trials based on specific inhibitors of these mechanisms. From the late 1960s to 2000, there was no unifying hypothesis linking these four mechanisms together, nor was there an obvious connection between any of these mechanisms, each of which responds quickly to normalization of hyperglycemia, and the phenomenon of hyperglycemic memory (see earlier discussion).

Increased Polyol Pathway Flux

Aldose reductase [alditol:NADP$^+$ 1-oxidoreductase, EC 1.1.1.21] is a cytosolic, monomeric oxidoreductase that catalyzes the reduced nicotinamide adenine dinucleotide phosphate (NADPH)-dependent reduction of a wide variety of carbonyl compounds, including glucose. Triphosphopyridine nucleotide, the reduced form of NADP (NADPH), is the cofactor in this reaction and in the regeneration of glutathione by glutathione reductase. In the polyol pathway as originally proposed, sorbitol is oxidized to fructose by the enzyme sorbitol dehydrogenase, with nicotinamide adenine dinucleotide (NAD$^+$) reduced to NADH, and sorbitol then oxidized to fructose by the enzyme sorbitol dehydrogenase, with the pentose phosphate pathway generating the necessary NADPH (Fig. 33-11).

However, the amount of substrate converted to product per second (K_{cat}) of human aldose reductase for glucose is 0.15 [sec^{-1}]. K_{cat} values for most enzymes are between 1 and 10^4, although some have K_{cat} values orders of magnitude higher. Moreover, because the intracellular glucose concentration in capillary retinal endothelial cells incubated in 25 mM glucose is approximately 0.15 mM,[113] while the K_m of aldose reductase for glucose reported by Bohren and coworkers is 100 mM, and the K_{cat}/K_m is 1.3 [s^{-1} M^{-1}], the predicted rate of aldose reductase reduction of glucose to sorbitol in most kidney cells would be expected to be rather low. However, aldose reductase has high affinity and enzyme activity for a variety of other substrates, including several glycolytic intermediates such as glyceraldehyde 3-phosphate.[114]

In vivo studies of aldose reductase inhibition in a 5-year study in dogs showed that diabetic neuropathy was prevented, but aldose reductase inhibition failed to prevent retinopathy or capillary basement membrane thickening in the retina, kidney, or muscle.[115] In apolipoprotein E

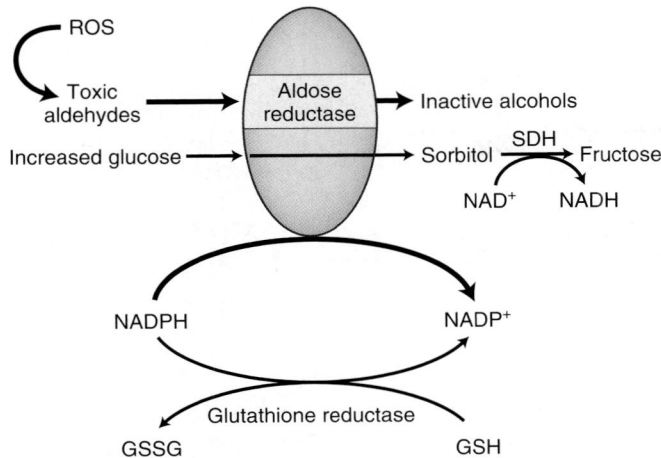

Figure 33-11 Aldose reductase and the polyol pathway. Aldose reductase reduces reactive oxygen species (ROS)-generated toxic aldehydes to inactive alcohols, and glucose to sorbitol, using triphosphopyridine nucleotide (NADPH), the reduced form of nicotinamide adenine dinucleotide phosphate (NADP+), as a cofactor. In cells in which aldose reductase activity is sufficient to deplete reduced glutathione (GSH), oxidative stress would be augmented. Sorbitol dehydrogenase (SDH) oxidizes sorbitol to fructose using nicotinamide adenine dinucleotide (NAD+) as a cofactor. GSSG, oxidized glutathione.

knockout mice, knockout of aldose reductase caused increased early lesion size in control and diabetic mice, rather than the expected decrease.[116]

Aldose reductase activity appears to be most significant for CVD, where in diabetic mice it perpetuates increased injury after MI, accelerates atherosclerotic lesion formation, and promotes restenosis via multiple mechanisms. Recent data show that in arteries of diabetic mice, aldose reductase drives hyperacetylation of Egr-1 with consequent upregulation of proinflammatory and prothrombotic signals.[117] Transgenic overexpression of aldose reductase in mouse cardiomyocytes contributes to heart failure and impaired recovery from ischemia with aging.[118]

Increased Intracellular Formation of Advanced Glycation End Products

Advanced Glycation End Products Are Formed From Intracellular Dicarbonyl Precursors. Advanced glycation end products (AGEs) are found in increased amounts in extracellular structures of diabetic retinal vessels[119-121] and renal glomeruli,[122-124] where they can cause damage by mechanisms described later in this section. These AGEs were originally thought to arise from nonenzymatic reactions between extracellular proteins and glucose. However, the rate of AGE formation from glucose is orders of magnitude slower than the rate of AGE formation from glucose-derived dicarbonyl precursors generated intracellularly, and it now seems likely that intracellular hyperglycemia is the primary initiating event in the formation of both intracellular and extracellular AGEs.[125] AGEs can arise from intracellular auto-oxidation of glucose to glyoxal,[126] decomposition of the Amadori product to 3-deoxyglucosone (perhaps accelerated by an amadoriase), and fragmentation of glyceraldehyde 3-phosphate to methylglyoxal (Fig. 33-12).[127] These reactive intracellular dicarbonyls react with amino groups of intracellular and extracellular proteins to form AGEs. Methylglyoxal and glyoxal are detoxified by the glyoxalase system.[127] All three AGE precursors are also substrates for other reductases.[128,129] In diabetic tissues where

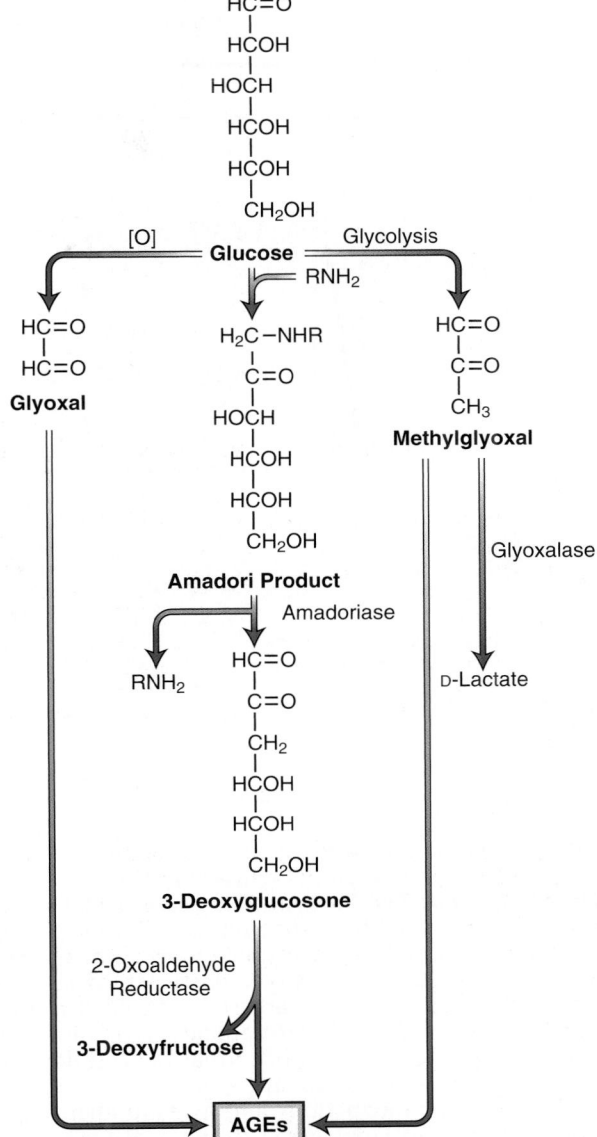

Figure 33-12 Potential pathways leading to the formation of advanced glycation end products (AGEs) from intracellular dicarbonyl precursors. Glyoxal arises from the auto-oxidation of glucose, 3-deoxyglucosone arises from decomposition of the Amadori product, and methylglyoxal arises from fragmentation of glyceraldehyde 3-phosphate. These reactive dicarbonyls react with amino groups of proteins to form AGEs. Methylglyoxal and glyoxal are detoxified by the glyoxalase system. (Adapted from Shinohara M, Thornalley PJ, Giardino I, et al. Overexpression of glyoxalase-I in bovine endothelial cells inhibits intracellular advanced glycation end-product formation and prevents hyperglycemia-induced increases in macromolecular endocytosis. *J Clin Invest.* 1998;101:1142-1147.)

complications occur, methylglyoxal accounts for almost all of the hyperglycemia-induced increase in reactive AGE precursors.[130]

Intracellular production of AGE precursors damages target cells by three general mechanisms (Fig. 33-13): intracellular proteins modified by AGEs have altered function. Extracellular matrix components modified by AGE precursors interact abnormally with other matrix components and with matrix receptors (integrins) on cells. Plasma proteins modified by AGE precursors bind to AGE receptors on cells such as macrophages, inducing receptor-mediated ROS production. This AGE-receptor ligation activates the

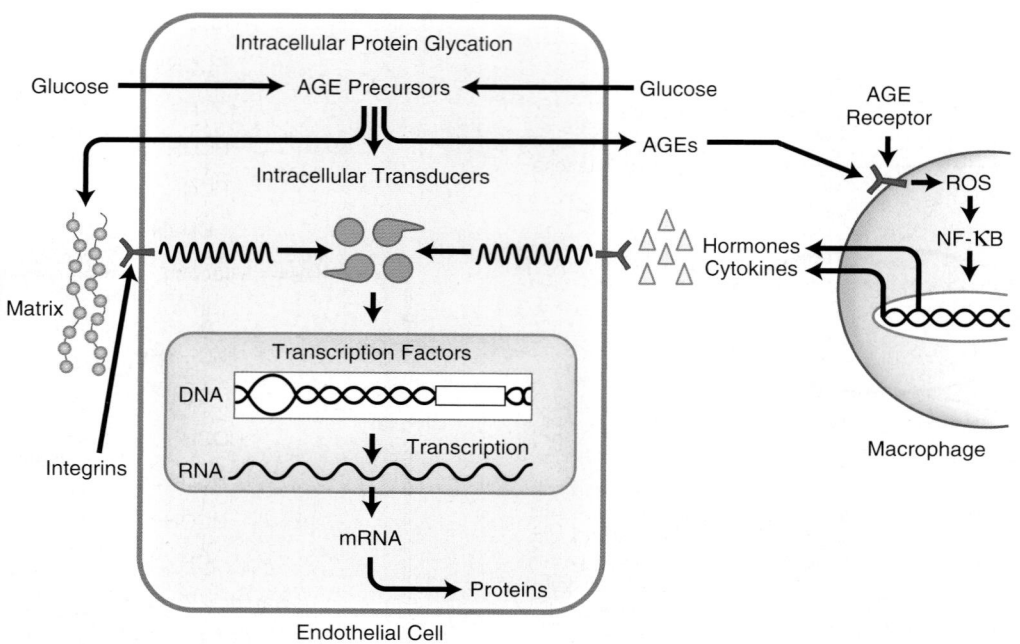

Figure 33-13 Potential mechanisms by which intracellular production of advanced glycation end-product (AGE) precursors damages vascular cells. First, intracellular protein modification alters protein function. Second, extracellular matrix modified by AGE precursors has abnormal functional properties. Third, plasma proteins modified by AGE precursors bind to AGE receptors on adjacent cells such as macrophages, thereby inducing receptor-mediated production of deleterious gene products such as cytokines. mRNA, messenger RNA; NFκB, nuclear factor-κB; ROS, reactive oxygen species. (Adapted from Brownlee M. Lilly Lecture 1993: glycation and diabetic complications. *Diabetes.* 1994;43:836-841.)

pleiotropic transcription factor nuclear factor-κB (NFκB), causing pathologic changes in gene expression.[131]

Advanced Glycation End Products Alter Intracellular Protein Function. It has recently been shown that AGE modification of intracellular proteins can regulate expression of genes involved in the pathogenesis of diabetic retinopathy. In diabetic retinal capillaries, the earliest morphologic changes are pericyte loss and acellular capillary formation. The primary pathologic processes of retinal pericyte loss and acellular capillary formation are regulated by complex context-dependent interactions among a number of pro-angiogenic and antiangiogenic factors,[132-134] including angiopoietin-2 (Ang-2). When insufficient levels of VEGF and other angiogenic signals are present, Ang-2 causes endothelial cell death and vessel regression.[135-137]

Diabetes induces a significant increase in retinal expression of Ang-2 in rats,[138] and diabetic Ang-2+/− mice have both decreased pericyte loss and reduced acellular capillary formation.[139] In retinal Müller cells, increased glycolytic flux causes increased methylglyoxal modification of the corepressor, mSin3A. Methylglyoxal modification of mSin3A results in increased Ang-2 expression. A similar mechanism involving methylglyoxal modification of other coregulator proteins may play a role in a variety of other diabetes-induced changes in gene expression.[140]

Diabetic painful neuropathy appears to result from abnormal function of the voltage-gated sodium channel Nav1.8, which is expressed exclusively in unmyelinated, small-diameter sensory neurons called C-fibers. Post-translational modification of Nav1.8 by methylglyoxal depolarizes sensory neurons, facilitating firing of these pain pathway neurons. In diabetic mice,[141] post-translation modification of Nav1.8 by methylglyoxal increased electrical excitability and facilitated firing of pain pathway neurons, which in turn facilitated neurosecretion of calcitonin gene-related peptide, increasing cyclooxygenase-2

(COX-2) expression. It also evokes thermal and mechanical hyperalgesia, which is reflected by increased blood flow in brain regions that are involved in pain processing.[141]

In diabetic mice with defective postischemia hind limb revascularization, overexpressing the methylglyoxal-metabolizing enzyme glyoxalase-1 (GLO1) exclusively in bone marrow cells (BMCs) is sufficient to restore BMC function and neovascularization of ischemic tissue in diabetes. GLO1-BMCs have superior migratory potential and increased viability compared with BMCs from wild-type diabetic mice.[142]

Methylglyoxal and the GLO1 system also play a central role in the pathogenesis of diabetic nephropathy. In nondiabetic mice, knockdown of Glo1 increases methylglyoxal modification of proteins and oxidative stress, causing alterations in kidney morphology indistinguishable from those caused by diabetes. In diabetic mice, Glo1 overexpression completely prevents diabetes-induced oxidative stress and kidney disease, despite unchanged levels of diabetic hyperglycemia. These data suggest that GLO1 activity regulates the sensitivity of the kidney to hyperglycemic-induced renal pathology.[143]

Advanced Glycation End Products Interfere with Normal Matrix-Matrix and Matrix-Cell Interactions. Methylglyoxal also leaks out of cells and is increased threefold to fivefold in the blood of diabetic patients, circulating at a concentration as high as 8 μmol/L.[144] Methylglyoxal at this level greatly enhances apoptosis caused by agents that induce oxidative stress and DNA damage.[145] Methylglyoxal also can act as an antiapoptotic modulator by direct modification of heat shock protein 27 (HSP27) at amino acid Arg-188, which allows HSP27 to repress cytochrome c–mediated caspase activation.[146]

AGE formation from circulating methylglyoxal and other AGE precursors alters the functional properties of several important matrix molecules. On type I collagen, this cross-linking induces an expansion of the molecular packing.[147] These AGE-induced cross-links alter the function of intact vessels. For example, AGEs decrease elasticity in large vessels from diabetic rats, even after vascular tone is abolished, and increase fluid filtration across the carotid artery.[148] AGE formation on type IV collagen from basement membrane inhibits lateral association of these molecules into a normal network-like structure by interfering with binding of the noncollagenous NC1 domain to the helix-rich domain.[149] AGE formation on laminin causes decreased polymer self-assembly, decreased binding to type IV collagen, and decreased binding of heparan sulfate proteoglycan, an important determinant of glomerular permselectivity.[150] In vitro AGE formation on intact glomerular basement membrane increases its permeability to albumin in a manner that resembles the abnormal permeability of diabetic nephropathy.[151,152]

AGE formation on extracellular matrix interferes not only with matrix-matrix interactions but also with matrix-cell interactions.[153] For example, AGE modification of the cell-binding domains of type IV collagen decreases endothelial cell adhesion, and AGE modification of a 6–amino acid growth-promoting sequence in the A chain of the laminin molecule markedly reduces neurite outgrowth.[154] AGE modification of vitronectin reduces cell attachment–promoting activity.[155] Increased modification of vascular basement membrane type IV collagen by methylglyoxal, at hot spot modification sites in the RGD and GFOGER integrin-binding sites of collagen, causes endothelial cell detachment and inhibition of angiogenesis.[156] In addition, matrix glycation impairs agonist-induced Ca^{2+} increases, and this may adversely affect regulatory functions of the endothelium.[157]

Advanced Glycation End Product Receptors Mediate Pathologic Changes in Gene Expression. Several cell-associated binding proteins for AGEs have been identified, including OST-48, 80K-H, galectin-3, macrophage scavenger receptor type II, and the AGE receptor RAGE.[158-162] Some of these are more likely to contribute to clearance of AGEs, whereas others, particularly RAGE,[163] cause sustained cellular perturbations mediated by ligand binding. In cell culture systems, these receptors appear to mediate long-term effects of AGEs on key cellular targets of diabetic complications such as macrophages, glomerular mesangial cells, and vascular endothelial cells. These effects include expression of cytokines and growth factors by macrophages and mesangial cells—interleukin 1 (IL-1), insulin-like growth factor type 1 (IGF-1), tumor necrosis factor-α (TNF-α), TGF-β, macrophage colony-stimulating factor (M-CSF), granulocyte-macrophage colony-stimulating factor (GM-CSF), and PDGF[164-178] and expression of procoagulatory or proinflammatory molecules by endothelial cells (i.e., thrombomodulin, tissue factor, and VCAM-1).[179-182] In addition, endothelial AGE receptor binding appears to mediate, in part, the hyperpermeability induced by diabetes, probably through the induction of VEGF.[183-185] RAGE deficiency attenuates the development of atherosclerosis in the diabetic apolipoprotein E (apoE)-null mouse model of accelerated atherosclerosis. Diabetic RAGE$^{-/-}$/apoE$^{-/-}$ mice had significantly reduced atherosclerotic plaque area. These beneficial effects on the vasculature were associated with attenuation of leukocyte recruitment; decreased expression of proinflammatory mediators, including the NKκB subunit p65, VCAM-1, and MCP-1; and reduced oxidative stress.[186]

More recent studies indicate that AGEs at the concentrations found in diabetic sera are not the major ligand for RAGE. Rather, several proinflammatory protein ligands have been identified that activate RAGE at low concentrations. These include several members of the S100 calgranulin family and high-mobility group box 1 (HMGB1), all of which are increased by diabetic hyperglycemia.[187] Ligation of these ligands with RAGE causes cooperative interaction with the innate immune system signaling molecule, toll-like receptor 4 (TLR4).[188] Expressions of RAGE, S100A8, S100A12, and HMGB1 are all increased by high levels of glucose in cell culture and in diabetic animals. This hyperglycemia-induced overexpression is mediated by ROS-induced increases of methylglyoxal, which increases binding of the transcription factors NFκB and activator protein 1 (AP1) to the promoters of RAGE and of RAGE ligands, respectively.[189]

Blockade of RAGE, a member of the pattern-recognition receptor class of the innate immune system, suppresses macrovascular disease in an atherosclerosis-prone type 1 diabetic mouse model in a glucose- and lipid-independent fashion.[190] Blockade of RAGE has also been shown to inhibit the development of diabetic vasculopathy,[191] nephropathy,[192] and periodontal disease[193] and to enhance wound repair in murine models via suppression of cytokines, TNF-α, IL-6, metalloproteinase 2 (MMP2), MMP3, and MMP9.[194] In the apoE-null mouse model of diabetic atherosclerosis, RAGE plays an important role in accelerated lesion formation and in lesion regression. Blockade of RAGE significantly reduced lesion size and structure and decreased parameters of inflammation as well as mononuclear phagocyte and smooth muscle cell activation.[190,195] Vascular endothelial cells and pericytes have been demonstrated to express two splice variants of full-length RAGE mRNA. One codes for an isoform that lacks the amino-terminal V-type immunoglobulin-like domain (N-truncated), and one codes for an isoform lacking the carboxy-terminal transmembrane domain (C-truncated). The C-truncated type lacks the transmembrane domain and is secreted extracellularly and detected in human serum as endogenous secretory RAGE (esRAGE). Circulating esRAGE levels are significantly lower in T1DM patients than in nondiabetic subjects, and plasma esRAGE levels are inversely correlated with carotid intima medial thickness (CIMT) and with increased risk of CVD.[196,197] High glucose–induced increased expression of RAGE is normalized by overexpression of GLO1, while knockdown of GLO1 in normal glucose mimicked the effect of high glucose,[189] implicating glycolysis-derived methylglyoxal as a key regulator of hyperglycemia-induced RAGE expression.

Activation of Protein Kinase C

Mechanism of Hyperglycemia-Induced Protein Kinase C Activation. The protein kinase C (PKC) family comprises at least 11 isoforms, 9 of which are activated by the lipid second-messenger, diacylglycerol (DAG). Intracellular hyperglycemia increases DAG content in cultured microvascular cells and in the retina and renal glomeruli of diabetic animals.[198-200] Intracellular hyperglycemia appears to increase DAG content primarily by increasing its de novo synthesis from the glycolytic intermediate glyceraldehyde 3-phosphate via reduction to glycerol 3-phosphate and stepwise acylation.[198,201] Increased de novo synthesis of DAG activates PKC in cultured vascular cells[200,202-204] and in retina and glomeruli of diabetic animals.[198,200,203] Increased DAG primarily activates the β and δ isoforms of PKC, but increases in other isoforms have also been found, such as PKC-α and -ε isoforms in the retina[205] and PKC-α and -δ isoforms in the glomerulus[206,207] of diabetic rats. DAG, its mimetics, the phorbol esters, and ROS all activate PKC isoforms by triggering the release of zinc ions from the cysteine-rich zinc finger of the regulatory domain. PKC isoforms can

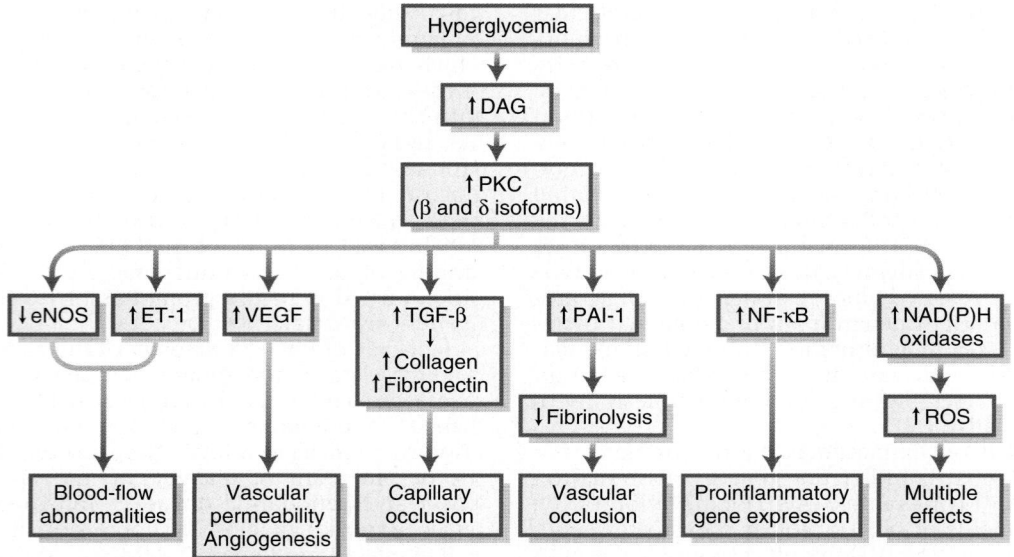

Figure 33-14 Potential consequences of hyperglycemia-induced protein kinase C (PKC) activation. Hyperglycemia increases diacylglycerol (DAG) content, which activates PKC, primarily the β and δ isoforms. Activated PKC has a number of pathogenic consequences. eNOS, endothelial nitric oxide synthase; ET-1, endothelin 1; NAD(P)H, nicotinamide adenine dinucleotide phosphate; NFκB, nuclear factor-κB; PAI, plasminogen activator inhibitor; ROS, reactive oxygen species; TGF, transforming growth factor; VEGF, vascular endothelial growth factor. (Adapted from Koya D, Jirousek MR, Lin YW, et al. Characterization of protein kinase C beta isoform activation on the gene expression of transforming growth factor-beta, extracellular matrix components, and prostanoids in the glomeruli of diabetic rats. *J Clin Invest.* 1997;100:115-126.)

also be activated through tyrosine phosphorylation in a manner unrelated to receptor-coupled hydrolysis of inositol phospholipids. The effect of hyperglycemia on PKC tyrosine phosphorylation has not yet been examined.[208,209]

Consequences of Hyperglycemia-Induced Protein Kinase C Activation. In early experimental diabetes, activation of PKC-β isoforms has been shown to mediate retinal and renal blood flow abnormalities,[210] perhaps by depressing NO production and increasing endothelin-1 activity (Fig. 33-14). In the diabetic retina, hyperglycemia persistently activates PKC and p38a MAPK to increase the expression of a previously unknown target of PKC signaling, Src homology-2 domain-containing phosphatase-1 (SHP-1), a protein tyrosine phosphatase. This signaling cascade leads to PDGF receptor-β dephosphorylation and a reduction in downstream signaling from this receptor, resulting in pericyte apoptosis.[211] Abnormal activation of PKC also has been implicated in the decreased glomerular production of NO induced by experimental diabetes[212] and in the decreased smooth muscle cell NO production induced by hyperglycemia.[213] PKC activation also mediates glucose-enhanced extracellular matrix accumulation in rat glomerular mesangial cells.[214] Hyperglycemia increases endothelin 1–stimulated MAPK activity in glomerular mesangial cells by activating PKC isoforms.[215] The increased endothelial cell permeability induced by high glucose concentrations in cultured cells is mediated by activation of PKC-α[216] and is independent of the intracellular calcium concentration–NO pathway.[217] Activation of PKC by elevated glucose levels also induces expression of the permeability-enhancing factor VEGF in smooth muscle cells.[218]

In addition to affecting hyperglycemia-induced abnormalities of blood flow and permeability, activation of PKC contributes to increased microvascular matrix protein accumulation by inducing the expression of TGF-β1, fibronectin, and α1 type IV collagen in cultured mesangial cells[214,219] and in glomeruli of diabetic rats.[212] Hyperglycemia-induced activation of PKC has also been implicated in the overexpression of the fibrinolytic inhibitor PAI-1[220] and in the activation of the pleiotrophic transcription factor NFκB in cultured endothelial cells and VSMC.[221,222] When PKC-β2 is selectively overexpressed in the myocardium of diabetic mice, expression of connective tissue growth factor (CTGF) and TGF-β1 increases, and the mice develop cardiomyopathy and cardiac fibrosis.[223]

In VSMC, activation of PKC by elevated glucose increases p38 MAPK activity and induces expression of the permeability-enhancing factor, VEGF.[219,224] PKC activation also activates various membrane-associated NAD(P)H-dependent oxidases.[225] Ex vivo treatment of human blood vessels from patients with diabetes and coronary artery disease (CAD) with a PKC inhibitor reduced diabetes-induced vascular superoxide production by NAD(P)H oxidases and superoxide-induced uncoupling of eNOS.[226] In normal subjects, the reduction in endothelium-dependent vasodilation induced by acute hyperglycemia is normalized by inhibition of PKC-β, consistent with prevention of hyperglycemia-induced eNOS uncoupling.[227]

PKC-β2 activation in mouse endothelial cells causes dysfunction and accelerates atherosclerosis by causing decreased insulin-stimulated Akt/eNOS activation and increased angiotensin-induced expression of the vasoconstrictor endothelin-1.[228]

Increased Hexosamine Pathway Flux

A fourth hypothesis about how hyperglycemia causes diabetic complications[229-232] states that glucose is shunted into the hexosamine pathway (Fig. 33-15). In this pathway, fructose 6-phosphate is diverted from glycolysis to provide substrates for reactions that require uridine diphosphate-*N*-acetylglucosamine (UDP-GlcNAc). Inhibition of glutamine: fructose-6-phosphate amidotransferase (GFAT), the rate-limiting enzyme in the conversion of glucose to glucosamine, blocks hyperglycemia-induced increases in the transcription of both TGF-α1[232] and TGF-β1.[230]

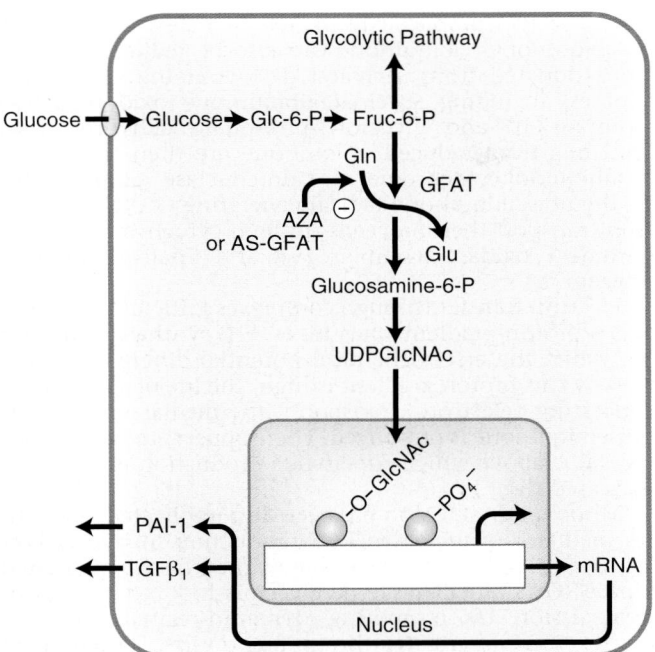

Figure 33-15 Schematic representation of the hexosamine pathway. The glycolytic intermediate, fructose 6-phosphate (Fruc-6-P), is converted to glucosamine 6-phosphate (Glc-6-P) by the enzyme glutamine:fructose-6-phosphate amidotransferase (GFAT). Increased donation of N-acetylglucosamine moieties to serine and threonine residues of transcription factors such as Sp1 increases production of such complication-promoting factors as plasminogen activator inhibitor 1 (PAI-1) and transforming growth factor-β1 (TGF-β1). AS-GFAT, antisense to GFAT; AZA, azaserine; GlcNAc, N-acetylglucosamine; mRNA, messenger RNA; UDP, uridine diphosphate. (Adapted from Du XL, Edelstein D, Rossetti L, et al. Hyperglycemia-induced mitochondrial superoxide overproduction activates the hexosamine pathway and induces plasminogen activator inhibitor-1 expression by increasing Sp1 glycosylation. *Proc Natl Acad Sci U S A.* 2000;97:12222-12226.)

The hexosamine pathway involves reversible posttranslational modification of Ser/Thr residues on proteins by N-acetylglucosamine, analogous to protein phosphorylation/dephosphorylation. Alternative splicing of the genes encoding the O-linked GlcNAc cycling enzymes O-GlcNAc transferase (OGT) and O-GlcNAcase (OGA) yields isoforms targeted to discrete sites in the nucleus, cytoplasm, and mitochondria. OGT and OGA also partner with cellular effectors and act in tandem with other post-translational modifications. The enzymes of O-GlcNAc cycling act preferentially on intrinsically disordered domains of target proteins impacting transcription, metabolism, apoptosis, organelle biogenesis, and transport.[233,234]

The mechanism by which increased flux through the hexosamine pathway mediates hyperglycemia-induced increases in gene transcription has not been clear, but the observation that Sp1 sites regulate hyperglycemia-induced activation of the PAI-1 promoter in VSMC[235] suggested that covalent modification of Sp1 by GlcNAc might explain the link between hexosamine pathway activation and hyperglycemia-induced changes in gene transcription. Glucosamine itself subsequently was shown to activate the PAI-1 promoter through Sp1 sites in glomerular mesangial cells.[236] Hyperglycemia has been shown to induce a 2.4-fold increase in hexosamine pathway activity in aortic endothelial cells, resulting in a 1.7-fold increase in Sp1 O-linked GlcNAc and a 70% to 80% decrease in Sp1 O-linked phosphothreonine and phosphoserine.[236] Concomitantly, hyperglycemia increased expression from an 85–base pair

truncated PAI-1 promoter luciferase reporter containing two Sp1 sites by 3.8-fold but failed to increase expression when the two Sp1 sites were mutated. In endothelial cells, signal transduction by the hexosamine pathway requires PKC-β1 and PKC-δ activation for regulation of the PAI-1 promoter.[237] GlcNAc modification of Sp1 also regulates glucose-responsive expression of the prosclerotic growth factor TGF-β1.

Because virtually every RNA polymerase II transcription factor examined has been found to be O-GlcNAcylated,[238] it is possible that reciprocal modification by O-GlcNAcylation and phosphorylation of transcription factors other than Sp1 function as a more generalized mechanism for regulating glucose-responsive gene transcription. In addition to transcription factors, many other nuclear and cytoplasmic proteins are dynamically modified by O-GlcNAc moieties and might exhibit reciprocal modification by phosphorylation in a manner analogous to Sp1. One example relevant to diabetic complications is the inhibition of eNOS activity by hyperglycemia-induced O-GlcNAcylation at the Akt site of the eNOS protein.[239]

Aberrant O-GlcNAc processing was recently shown to reduce mitochondrial protein expression and respiration. Significant decreases were observed in mitochondria-localized proteins involved in the respiratory chain and the tricarboxylic acid (TCA) cycle. Furthermore, mitochondrial morphology was altered in these cells. As a consequence of these changes, both cellular respiration and glycolysis were reduced in cells overexpressing GlcNAc cycling enzymes.[240]

The role of the hexosamine pathway in CVD has been reviewed recently.[241] Studies have linked chronically elevated O-GlcNAc levels to diabetic cardiovascular complications. Adverse cardiac effects of chronically increased O-GlcNAcylation include decreased contractile function, decreased mitochondrial function, and decreased autophagic signaling.

One of the most important emerging areas of hexosamine pathway investigation involves decreased contractility and altered calcium signaling. Decreased contractility appears to result from hyperglycemia-induced covalent modification of calcium/calmodulin-dependent protein kinase II (CaMKII) by O-GlcNAc. O-GlcNAc modification of CaMKII at Ser279 activates CaMKII autonomously, creating molecular memory even after Ca^{2+} concentration declines. CaMKII activation is seen in heart failure and can directly induce pathologic changes in ion channels, Ca^{2+} handling, and gene transcription. O-GlcNAc-modified CaMKII is increased in the heart of diabetic humans and rats.[242] Zetterqvist and coworkers showed that hyperglycemia activates the transcription factor NFAT (nuclear factor of activated T cells) in the arterial wall, inducing the expression of the proatherosclerotic protein osteopontin, and provided evidence that NFAT activation may be an important link between diabetes and atherogenesis.[243] Since hyperglycemia-induced increased GlcNAcylation activates calmodulin (CaM), this would explain increased NFAT nuclear import through activation of the phosphatase which dephosphorylates the amino termini of NFAT proteins, calcineurin (CN). Hyperglycemia-induced activation of the hexosamine pathway also increases activation of MMP2 and MMP9 in human coronary artery endothelial cells and in carotid plaques from patients with T2DM. O-GlcNAcylation of endothelial cell proteins is significantly increased.[244]

Hyperglycemia impairs cardiomyocyte calcium cycling through increased nuclear O-GlcNAcylation, which reduced sarcoplasmic reticulum Ca^{2+}-ATPase 2a (SERCA2a) mRNA and protein expression and decreased SERCA2a promoter activity.[245]

Different Hyperglycemia-Induced Pathogenic Mechanisms Reflect a Single Upstream Process

Although specific inhibitors of aldose reductase activity, AGE formation, and PKC activation ameliorate various diabetes-induced abnormalities in animal models, there has been no apparent common element linking the four mechanisms of hyperglycemia-induced damage discussed in the preceding section.[115,212,246-248] It has also been conceptually difficult to explain the phenomenon of hyperglycemic memory (discussed earlier) as a consequence of four processes that quickly normalize when euglycemia is restored. These issues were resolved by the discovery that each of the four different pathogenic mechanisms reflects a single hyperglycemia-induced process: overproduction of superoxide by the mitochondrial electron transport chain.[249,250]

Hyperglycemia increases ROS production in primary aortic endothelial cells and in a variety of other cell types damaged by diabetic hyperglycemia. To understand how this occurs, a brief overview of glucose metabolism is helpful. Intracellular glucose oxidation begins with glycolysis in the cytoplasm, which generates NADH and pyruvate. Cytoplasmic NADH can donate reducing equivalents to the mitochondrial electron transport chain via two shuttle systems, or it can reduce pyruvate to lactate, which exits the cell to provide substrate for hepatic gluconeogenesis. Pyruvate can also be transported into the mitochondria, where it is oxidized by the TCA cycle to produce CO_2, H_2O, four molecules of NADH, and one molecule of reduced flavin adenine dinucleotide ($FADH_2$). Mitochondrial NADH and $FADH_2$ provide energy for adenosine triphosphate (ATP) production via oxidative phosphorylation by the electron transport chain.

Electron flow through the mitochondrial electron transport chain is carried out by four inner membrane–associated enzyme complexes, plus cytochrome c and the mobile carrier, ubiquinone.[251] NADH derived from cytosolic glucose oxidation and mitochondrial TCA cycle activity donates electrons to NADH:ubiquinone oxidoreductase (complex I). Complex I ultimately transfers its electrons to ubiquinone. Ubiquinone can also be reduced by electrons donated from several $FADH_2$-containing dehydrogenases, including succinate:ubiquinone oxidoreductase (complex II) and glycerol-3-phosphate dehydrogenase. Electrons from reduced ubiquinone are then transferred to ubiquinol:cytochrome c oxidoreductase (complex III) by the ubisemiquinone radical-generating Q cycle.[252] Electron transport then proceeds through cytochrome c, cytochrome c oxidase (complex IV), and finally, molecular oxygen.

Electron transfer through complexes I, III, and IV generates a proton gradient that drives ATP synthase (complex V). When the electrochemical potential difference generated by this proton gradient is high, the life of superoxide-generating electron transport intermediates such as ubisemiquinone is prolonged. There appears to be a threshold value above which superoxide production is markedly increased (Fig. 33-16).[253]

Mitochondrial fission has been also implicated as a critical mediator of increased ROS production in hyperglycemic conditions.[254] It has been shown that the rho-associated kinase ROCK1 mediates hyperglycemia-induced mitochondrial fission by promoting dynamin-related protein-1 (Drp1) recruitment to the mitochondria. Deletion of ROCK1 in diabetic mice prevents mitochondrial fission, whereas mice with a constitutively active ROCK1 in podocytes exhibit increased mitochondrial fission. ROCK1 triggers mitochondrial fission by phosphorylating Drp1 at residue serine 600.[255] Interestingly, it has been shown that RhoA (the upstream activator of ROCK) can be directly activated by ROS in cells and that this requires two critical cysteine residues located in a unique redox-sensitive motif within the phosphoryl binding loop.[256] Excessive mitochondrial fission and a lack of fusion results in breakdown of the mitochondrial (mt) network, loss of the mtDNA, respiratory defects, and an increase in ROS.[257,258]

Investigators using inhibitors of both the shuttle that transfers cytosolic NADH into mitochondria and the transporter that transfers cytosolic pyruvate into the mitochondria showed that the TCA cycle is the source of

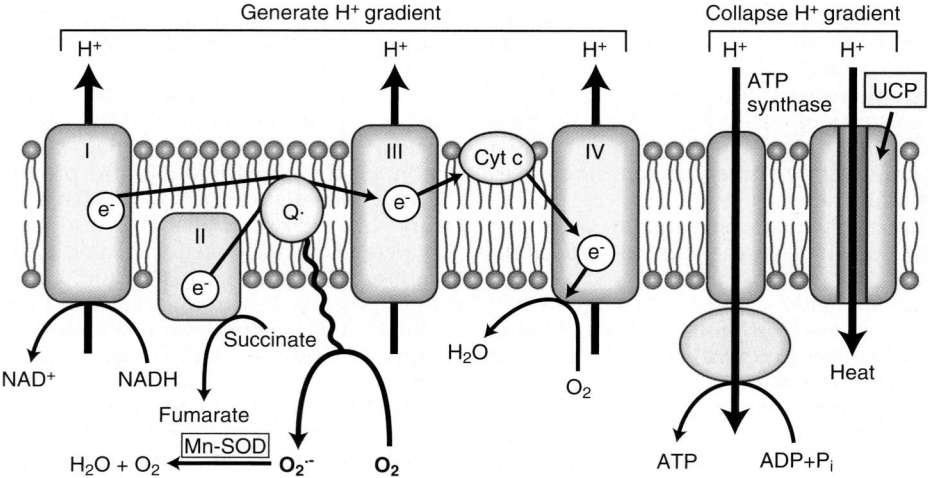

Figure 33-16 Production of superoxide by the mitochondrial electron transport chain. Increased hyperglycemia-derived electron donors from the tricarboxylic acid cycle (NADH and $FADH_2$) generate a high mitochondrial membrane potential ($\Delta\mu\ H^+$) by pumping protons across the mitochondrial inner membrane. This inhibits electron transport at complex III and increases the half-life of free radical intermediates of coenzyme Q, which reduce O_2 to superoxide. ADP, adenosine diphosphate; ATP, adenosine triphosphate; Cyt c, cytochrome c; Mn-SOD, manganese superoxide dismutase; NAD^+, nicotinamide adenine dinucleotide; NADH, reduced nicotinamide adenine dinucleotide; P_i, inorganic phosphate; UCP, uncoupling protein. (From Boss O, Hagen T, Lowell BB. Uncoupling proteins 2 and 3: potential regulators of mitochondrial energy metabolism. *Diabetes.* 2000;49:143-156.)

hyperglycemia-induced ROS in endothelial cells. Overexpression of uncoupling protein 1 (UCP-1), a specific protein uncoupler of oxidative phosphorylation capable of collapsing the proton electrochemical gradient,[259] also prevented the effect of hyperglycemia. These results demonstrated that hyperglycemia-induced intracellular ROS are produced by the proton electrochemical gradient generated by the mitochondrial electron transport chain. Overexpression of Mn-SOD, the mitochondrial form of this antioxidant enzyme,[249] prevents the increased ROS caused by hyperglycemia.

Prevention of mitochondrial superoxide production also completely prevents activation of the polyol pathway, AGE formation, PKC, and the hexosamine pathway (Fig. 33-17). In endothelial cells, PKC activates NFκB, a transcription factor that itself activates many proinflammatory genes in the vasculature. As expected, hyperglycemia-induced NFκB activation is also prevented by UCP-1 or Mn-SOD in cells and in animals.

In addition, diabetes-induced loss of vascular cyclic adenosine monophosphate (cAMP)-responsive element–binding protein (CREB) and enhanced expression of PDGFR-α in nonobese diabetic (NOD) mice are both reversed by treatment with an SOD mimetic,[260] and hyperglycemia-mediated interference with neuronal CREB and bcl-2 expression can be restored by treatment of the neurons in vitro with an SOD mimetic.[261]

Therefore, hyperglycemia-induced mitochondrial production of ROS is both necessary and sufficient for activation of each of these pathways.

Although historically viewed as purely harmful, recent evidence suggests that ROS function as important physiologic regulators of intracellular signaling pathways, ranging from the response to growth factor stimulation to the generation of the inflammatory response.[262,263] Thus, maintaining the functional integrity of cells in an organism where metabolic and hormonal profiles are continuously changing requires that ROS concentration and duration be closely integrated with tissue and whole-body physiology.[264]

After hyperglycemia induces mitochondrial ROS production, these ROS can activate a number of other superoxide production pathways that may amplify the original damaging effect of hyperglycemia (M. Brownlee, unpublished observations).

How does hyperglycemia-induced ROS activate AGE formation, PKC, the hexosamine pathway, and the polyol pathway? It does this by inhibiting activity of the key glycolytic enzyme, glyceraldehyde-3-phosphate dehydrogenase (GAPDH) (Fig. 33-18). When GAPDH activity is inhibited, the levels of all the glycolytic intermediates that are upstream of GAPDH increase. An increased level of the upstream glycolytic metabolite glyceraldehyde 3-phosphate activates two of the four pathways, because the major intracellular AGE precursor, methylglyoxal, and the activator of PKC, DAG, are both formed from glyceraldehyde 3-phosphate. Farther upstream, levels of the glycolytic metabolite fructose 6-phosphate increase, which increases flux through the hexosamine pathway, in which fructose 6-phosphate is converted by the enzyme GFAT to UDP-GlcNAc. Finally, inhibition of GAPDH also increases intracellular levels of the first glycolytic metabolite, glucose. This increases flux through the polyol pathway. Inhibition of GAPDH using DNA antisense activates each of the four pathways to the same extent as diabetes when glucose concentrations are physiologic.[265] Hyperglycemia-induced superoxide inhibits GAPDH activity indirectly by modifying the enzyme with polymers of adenosine diphosphate (ADP)-ribose.[266] Inhibition of mitochondrial superoxide

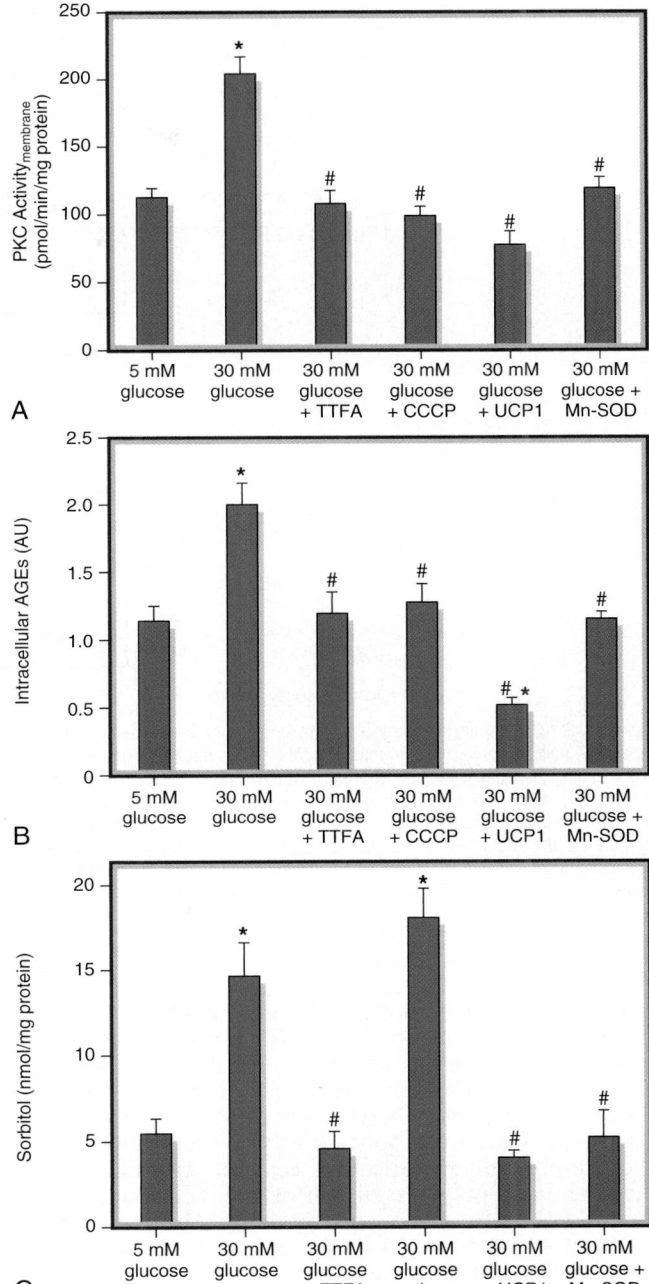

Figure 33-17 Effect of agents that alter mitochondrial electron transport chain function on the three main pathways of hyperglycemic damage. **A,** Hyperglycemia-induced protein kinase C (PKC) activation. **B,** Intracellular advanced glycation end-product (AGE) formation. **C,** Sorbitol accumulation. Cells were incubated in 5-mmol/L glucose, 30-mmol/L glucose alone, and 30-mmol/L glucose plus either agents that uncouple oxidative phosphorylation and reduce the high mitochondrial membrane potential (TTFA, CCCP, UCP-1) or manganese dismutase superoxide (Mn-SOD). CCCP, carbonyl cyanide *m*-chlorophenylhydrazone; TTFA, thenoyltrifluoroacetone; UCP-1, uncoupling protein 1; *, $p < 0.01$ compared to cells incubated in 5mM glucose; #, $p < 0.01$ compared to cells incubated in 30mM glucose. (From Nishikawa T, Edelstein D, Du XL, et al. Normalizing mitochondrial superoxide production blocks three pathways of hyperglycaemic damage. *Nature*. 2000;404:787-790.)

production with UCP-1 or Mn-SOD prevents both modification of GAPDH by ADP-ribose and reduction of its activity by hyperglycemia. Most importantly, both the modifications of GAPDH by ADP-ribose and the reduction of its activity by hyperglycemia are prevented by a specific

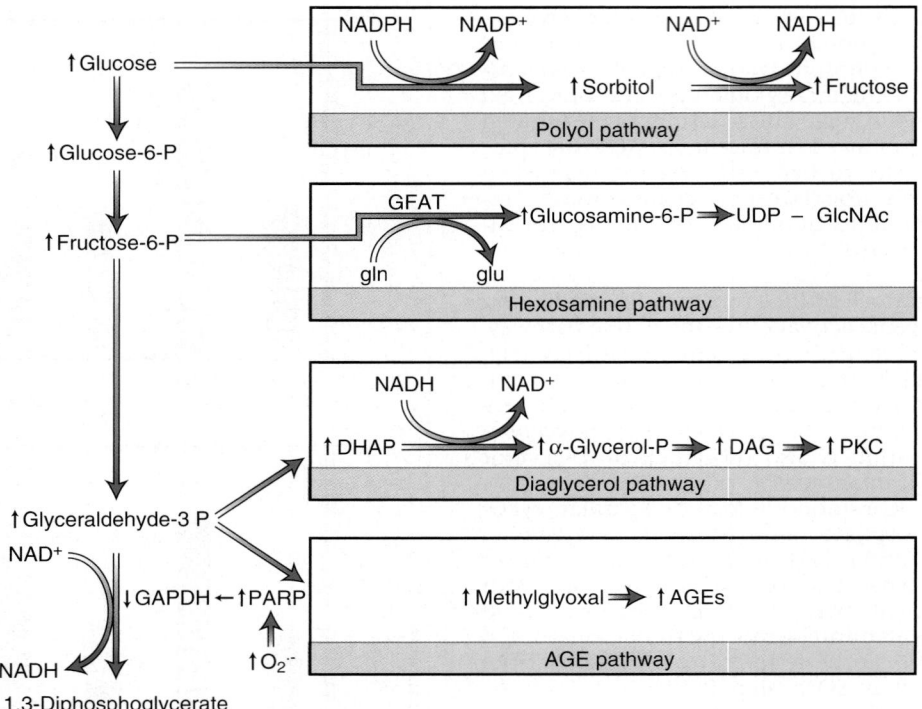

Figure 33-18 Potential mechanism by which hyperglycemia-induced mitochondrial superoxide overproduction activates four pathways of hyperglycemic damage. Excess superoxide partially inhibits the glycolytic enzyme glyceraldehyde-3-phosphate dehydrogenase (GAPDH) by activating PARP and causing ADP-ribosylation of GAPDH. Decreased GAPDH activity increases the concentrations of upstream metabolites and diverts them from glycolysis into pathways of glucose overutilization. This results in increased flux of triose phosphate to diacylglycerol (DAG), an activator of protein kinase C (PKC), and to methylglyoxal, the major intracellular advanced glycation end-product (AGE) precursor. Increased flux of fructose 6-phosphate to uridine diphosphate (UDP)-*N*-acetylglucosamine increases modification of proteins by hexosamine, and increased glucose flux through the polyol pathway consumes NADPH and depletes reduced glutathione (GSH). ADP, adenosine diphosphate; DHAP, dihydroxyacetone phosphate; GFAT, glutamine:fructose-6-phosphate amidotransferase; GlcNAc, *N*-acetylglucosamine; NAD+, nicotinamide adenine dinucleotide; NADH, reduced nicotinamide adenine dinucleotide; P, phosphate; PARP, poly(ADP-ribose) polymerase; NADPH, nicotinamide adenine dinucleotide phosphate.

inhibitor of the enzyme PARP. PARP is a nuclear DNA-repair enzyme that is activated by DNA double-strand breaks. Increased intracellular glucose generates increased ROS in the mitochondria, and these free radicals cause DNA double-strand breaks, thereby activating PARP (Fig. 33-19). Once activated, PARP splits the NAD+ molecule into its two component parts: nicotinic acid and ADP-ribose. PARP then generates polymers of ADP-ribose, which accumulate on GAPDH and other nuclear proteins. Although GAPDH is commonly thought to reside exclusively in the cytosol, it normally shuttles in and out of the nucleus, where it plays a critical role in DNA repair.[267] In addition, activation of PARP consumes NAD+, the cofactor necessary for activity of the sirtuin family of protein deacetylases.

A schematic summary showing the elements of the unified mechanism of hyperglycemia-induced cellular damage is shown in Figure 33-20. When intracellular hyperglycemia develops in target cells of diabetic complications, it causes increased mitochondrial production of ROS. The ROS causes double-strand breaks in nuclear DNA, which activates PARP. PARP then modifies GAPDH, reducing its activity. Decreased GAPDH activity activates the polyol pathway, increases intracellular AGE formation, activates PKC and subsequently NFκB, and activates hexosamine pathway flux. Additional recently described pathways of diabetic cellular damage activated by hyperglycemia-induced overproduction of ROS include homeobox-interacting protein kinase 2, which promotes renal fibrosis via p53, TGF-β, Wnt, the transcription factor NFATc3, implicated in diabetic atherosclerosis, the adapter protein

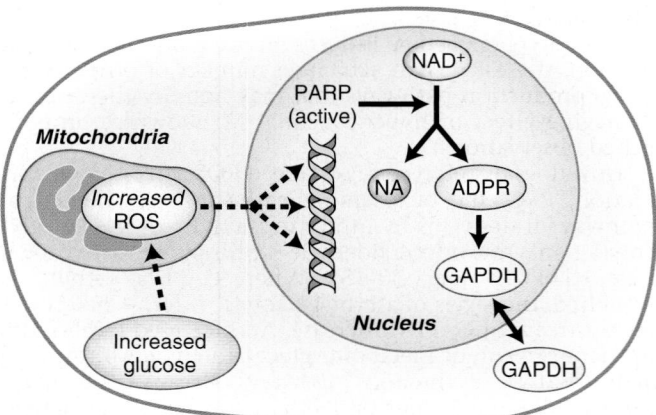

Figure 33-19 Schematic representation of the mechanism by which hyperglycemia-induced mitochondrial superoxide overproduction activates PARP and modifies GAPDH. Hyperglycemia-induced mitochondrial superoxide overproduction causes DNA strand breaks, thereby activating the nuclear DNA-repair enzyme, poly(ADP-ribose) polymerase (PARP). Activated PARP splits the NAD+ molecule into its two component parts: nicotinic acid (NA) and adenosine diphosphate–ribose (ADPR). PARP then generates polymers of ADP-ribose, which accumulate on glyceraldehyde-3-phosphate dehydrogenase, GAPDH, inactivating the enzyme. ROS, reactive oxygen species. (Adapted from Brownlee M. Banting Lecture 2004. The pathobiology of diabetic complications: a unifying mechanism. *Diabetes.* 2005;54:1615-1625.)

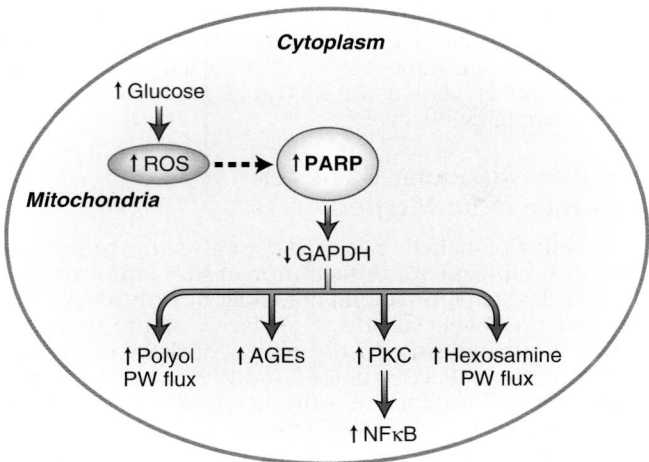

Figure 33-20 Unifying mechanism of hyperglycemia-induced cellular damage. Intracellular hyperglycemia causes increased mitochondrial production of reactive oxygen species (ROS). The ROS cause strand breaks in nuclear DNA, which activates poly(ADP-ribose) polymerase (PARP). PARP then modifies glyceraldehyde-3-phosphate dehydrogenase (GAPDH), thereby reducing its activity. Decreased GAPDH activity activates the polyol pathway, increases intracellular formation of advanced glycation end products (AGEs), activates protein kinase C (PKC) and subsequently nuclear factor-κB (NFκB), and activates hexosamine pathway (PW) flux. (Adapted from Brownlee M. Banting Lecture 2004. The pathobiology of diabetic complications: a unifying mechanism. *Diabetes.* 2005;54:1615-1625.)

p66shc, which causes cell cycle arrest and apoptosis, and osteopontin (OPN), a proinflammatory protein linked to vascular remodeling and calcification, especially in diabetic arteries. It has also been implicated in the pathogenesis of diabetic retinopathy and nephropathy in patients with type 2 diabetes. Serum OPN is a strong predictor of incipient diabetic nephropathy, a first-ever CVD event, and all-cause mortality in patients with T1DM.[268] Hyperglycemia effectively activates NFATc3 in the arterial wall and induces the expression of OPN.[269,270] OPN[−/−] knockout mice are protected from diabetes-induced albuminuria and renal damage, possibly by modulating podocyte signaling and motility.[271]

Overexpression of UCP-1 or Mn-SOD also prevents hyperglycemia-induced inhibition of the antiatherogenic enzyme, prostacyclin synthase.[272] In diabetes, inhibition of prostacyclin synthase causes accumulation of the precursor prostaglandin I_2 (PGI$_2$), which activates thromboxane receptors that trigger vasoconstriction, platelet aggregation, increased expression of leukocyte adhesion molecules, and apoptosis.[273]

Overexpression of Mn-SOD or UCP-1 also prevents inhibition of eNOS activity by hyperglycemia.[239] In streptozotocin-diabetic transgenic mice overexpressing human cytoplasmic Cu^{2+}/Zn^{2+}-SOD, albuminuria, glomerular hypertrophy, and glomerular content of TGF-β and α1 type IV collagen were all attenuated compared with wild-type littermates after 4 months of diabetes.[274] Overexpression of the human *SOD1* transgene in db/db diabetic mice similarly normalized the extensive expansion of the glomerular mesangial matrix that was otherwise evident by age 5 months in the nontransgenic db/db littermates.[275] Similarly, transgenic overexpression of the antioxidant enzymes Mn-SOD and catalase reduced ROS and prevented diabetes-induced abnormalities in cardiac contractility in an animal model of diabetic cardiomyopathy.[276,277] Mn-SOD overexpression in mice also prevented diabetic neuropathy and retinopathy.[278,279]

In cell culture and in mice overexpressing the mitochondrial antioxidant enzyme catalase, mitochondrial ROS in lesional macrophages amplify atherosclerotic lesion development by promoting NFκB-mediated entry of monocytes and other inflammatory processes.[280]

In humans, skin fibroblast gene expression profiles from two groups of T1DM patients—20 with very fast (fast-track) and 20 with very slow (slow-track) rates of development of diabetic nephropathy lesions—showed that the fast-track group has increased expression of oxidative phosphorylation genes, mitochondrial electron transport system complex III, and TCA-cycle genes. These associations are consistent with a central role for mitochondrial ROS production in the pathogenesis of diabetic nephropathy.[281]

Other cellular generators of superoxide are activated in many cell types damaged by hyperglycemia, including NADPH oxidases and uncoupled eNOS. However, in cells without mitochondrial genomes (ρ^0 cells), high glucose does not generate ROS,[272] suggesting that mitochondria ROS are required to activate these other sources of superoxide generation. Consistent with these data, while NADPH oxidase 4 (Nox4) is a source of renal ROS in a mouse model of diabetic nephropathy in ApoE(−/−) mice,[282] exogenous hydrogen peroxide acutely activates cellular superoxide production via Nox.[283,284] In mice, type 1 diabetes similarly upregulates left ventricular NADPH oxidase (Nox2), and increases systemic oxidative stress. This is significantly attenuated by the mitochondria-specific ROS scavenger coenzyme Q10 (CoQ10).[285]

Similarly, the active form of the enzyme eNOS, which normally exists as a head-to-tail homodimer, is converted to its monomeric, superoxide-generating form when its essential cofactor tetrahydrobiopterin (BH$_4$) is oxidized to BH$_2$ by ROS. Monomeric eNOS then acts as an NADPH oxidase, in which molecular oxygen rather than arginine becomes an electron acceptor.[286] This results in excess production of superoxide.

Dugan and associates[287] have suggested that diabetic nephropathy is caused by reduced, rather than increased, mitochondrial ROS production, based on their observation that AMPK activity, an activator of the cofactor proliferator-activated receptor γ coactivator 1α (PGC1α), which regulates mitochondrial biogenesis, is decreased in the diabetic kidney. PGC1 protein level and mitochondrial density were also decreased. These authors propose a model in which these observations reflect a feed-forward cycle initiated and maintained by decreased mitochondrial ROS. However, in human endothelial cells, silencing of AMPK causes increased, not decreased, ROS.[288] An alternate model of a feed-forward cycle involving decreased AMPK activity and decreased mitochondrial biogenesis caused by increased mitochondrial ROS is more consistent with these and other observations. In this model, ROS causes DNA strand breaks in the nucleus, resulting in activation of PARP. Active PARP degrades NAD$^+$ in the process of synthesizing ADP-ribose. Reduced content of NAD$^+$ inhibits the activity of the NAD$^+$-dependent protein deacetylase sirtuin 1 (SIRT1), which normally deacetylates and activates both PGC1α and LKB1, the kinase that activates AMPK. Thus, decreased SIRT1 activity would decrease activity of LKB1, PGC1α, and AMPK, as observed by Nishikawa and coworkers, but causing increased, not decreased, mitochondrial ROS production.[289] Consistent with this model, diabetic db/db mice with a conditional deletion of SIRT1 in podocytes developed more proteinuria and kidney injury compared with db/db control mice,[290] and PGC-1α knockout diabetic mice developed a more severe neuropathy, with mitochondrial degeneration and an increase in oxidative modification of intracellular proteins.[291]

Free Fatty Acid–Induced Proatherogenic Changes Are Also Caused by Mitochondrial Production of Reactive Oxygen Species

Insulin resistance causes increased FFA release from adipocytes. In macrovascular, but not microvascular, endothelial cells, the increased flux of FFA results in increased FFA oxidation by the mitochondria. Increased FFA oxidation also causes mitochondrial overproduction of ROS.

In the diabetic heart, increased fatty acid β-oxidation can saturate the mitochondria, leading to myocardial steatosis, which may lead to cell dysfunction and death.[292] FFAs are also the substrate for de novo ceramide biosynthesis. In rodent models of diabetes, increased myocardial ROS and ceramide content have been associated with cardiac dysfunction.[293] Ceramides generate increased ROS by directly inhibiting complex III of the mitochondrial electron transport chain, directly and indirectly promoting inflammation, autophagy, apoptosis, and insulin resistance.[294] In diabetic rat kidney cortical tubule mitochondria, the increased amounts and activities of selective fatty acid oxidation enzymes are associated with increased oxidative phosphorylation and increased ROS production with fatty acid substrates, whereas pyruvate oxidation is decreased and pyruvate-supported ROS production is unchanged. Mitochondrial fatty acid oxidation is the source of the increased net ROS production, and the site of electron leakage is located proximal to coenzyme Q at the electron transfer flavoprotein that shuttles electrons from acyl-CoA dehydrogenases to coenzyme Q.[295]

In arterial endothelial cells, this FFA-induced increase in ROS activates the same damaging pathways seen with high glucose: AGEs, PKC, the hexosamine pathway (GlcNAc), and NFκB. Together, they activate a variety of proinflammatory signals previously implicated in hyperglycemia-induced vascular damage (Fig. 33-21).

In addition, these ROS directly inactivate two important antiatherogenic enzymes, prostacyclin synthase and eNOS, independent of the pathways just discussed. In two insulin-resistant nondiabetic animal models, inhibition of either FFA release from adipocytes or FFA oxidation in arterial endothelium prevented the increased production of ROS and its damaging effects.[103]

Possible Molecular Basis for Hyperglycemic Memory

In the retina of diabetic rats with poor glycemic control for 2 months, subsequent normalization of HbA$_{1c}$ for 7 months lowered elevated retinal lipid peroxides by only about 50% and had no beneficial effects on levels of the oxidative marker 3-nitrotyrosine. In the retinas of diabetic animals with poor glycemic control for 6 months, subsequent normalization of HbA$_{1c}$ for 6 months had no effect on elevated retinal oxidative stress levels and only a small effect on elevated levels of 3-nitrotyrosine.[296]

Continued excess mitochondrial superoxide production or changes in antioxidant enzyme expression might explain these results and the occurrence of complications during posthyperglycemic normoglycemia. Alternatively, cumulative damage caused by excess ROS, or changes in expression of damage repair enzymes, could also explain hyperglycemia memory.

Although the molecular mechanisms underlying such very long term changes in gene expression in normoglycemic animals and humans have not yet been identified, induction of stable epigenetic changes such as DNA methylation and histone methylation and acetylation are likely candidates. Such changes can alter levels of gene expression for many years. Post-translational modifications of histones cause chromatin remodeling and changes in levels of gene expression.[297-299] Transient hyperglycemia, at a level sufficient to increase mitochondrial ROS production, induces long-lasting activating epigenetic changes (increased monomethylation of histone 3 lysine 4) in the proximal promoter of the NFκB subunit p65 in human aortic endothelial cells (16 hours' exposure) and in aortic cells in vivo in nondiabetic mice (6 hours' exposure). These epigenetic changes cause sustained increases in p65 gene expression and in the expression of p65-dependent proinflammatory genes. Both the epigenetic changes and the gene expression changes persist for at least 6 days of subsequent normal glycemia in cultured cells and for months in previously diabetic mice whose beta-cell function recovered.[300] Hyperglycemia-induced epigenetic changes and increased p65 expression are prevented by normalizing mitochondrial superoxide production or superoxide-induced methylglyoxal.[300] These results highlight the dramatic and long-lasting effects that short-term hyperglycemic spikes can have on vascular cells and suggest that transient spikes of hyperglycemia may be an HbA$_{1c}$-independent risk factor for diabetic complications. Demethylation of another histone lysine residue, histone 3 lysine 9, is also induced by hyperglycemia-induced overproduction of ROS. This reduces inhibition of p65 gene expression, and therefore acts synergistically with the activating methylation of histone 3 lysine 4 (Fig. 33-22).[300,301] Consistent with these observations, others have shown similar epigenetic changes in lymphocytes from patients with T1DM[302] and in VSMCs derived from db/db mice.[303,304]

Another component of epigenetic regulation is the action of epigenetic reader proteins that attach to histone-modified residues and facilitate the formation of transcriptional complexes. Recent work establishes that the bromodomain and extra-terminal (BET)-domain containing protein BRD4 is a novel determinant of cardiac hypertrophy and the p65 transcriptional cassette in endothelial

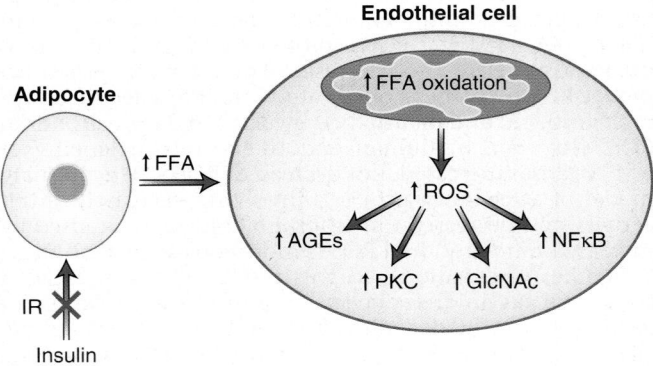

Endothelial cell

Adipocyte

↑FFA

↑FFA oxidation

↑ROS

↑AGEs   ↑NFκB

↑PKC   ↑GlcNAc

IR

Insulin

Figure 33-21 Schematic mechanism by which insulin resistance (IR) causes increased oxidation of free fatty acids (FFA) in arterial endothelial cells, which activates proatherogenic signals and inhibits key antiatherogenic enzymes. IR causes increased FFA release from adipocytes. In macrovascular endothelial cells, the increased flux of FFA results in increased FFA oxidation by the mitochondria, thereby causing mitochondrial overproduction of reactive oxygen species (ROS). FFA-induced increase in ROS activates advanced glycation end products (AGEs), protein kinase C (PKC), the hexosamine pathway (GlcNAc), and nuclear factor κB (NFκB), which together activate a variety of proinflammatory signals. In addition, ROS directly inactivate two important antiatherogenic enzymes, prostacyclin synthase and endothelial nitric oxide synthase (eNOS). GlcNAc, N-acetylglucosamine. (Adapted from Du X, Edelstein D, Obici S, et al. Insulin resistance reduces arterial prostacyclin synthase and eNOS activities by increasing endothelial fatty acid oxidation. *J Clin Invest.* 2006;116:1071-1080.)

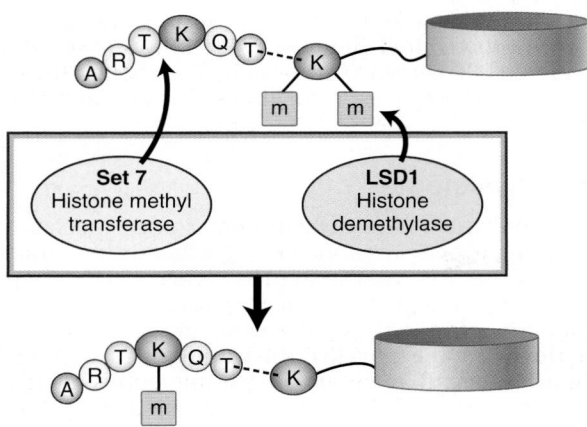

Figure 33-22 Hyperglycemia-induced activating modifications of histone 3 lysine 4 (monomethylation) and derepressing modifications of histone 3 lysine 9 (removal of two methyl groups) at the NFκB p65 proximal promoter. K is the symbol for the amino acid lysine. The chains of circled letters are the N-terminal tails of histone H3. (From Brasacchio D, Okabe J, Tikellis C, et al. Hyperglycemia induces a dynamic cooperativity of histone methylase and demethylase enzymes associated with gene-activating epigenetic marks that co-exist on the lysine tali. *Diabetes.* 2009;58:1229-1236; El-Osta A, Brasacchio D, Yao D, et al. Transient high glucose causes persistent epigenetic changes and altered gene expression during subsequent normoglycemia. *J Exp Med.* 2008;205:2409-2417.)

cells. These findings suggest that BET bromodomain inhibitors may be used to halt the progression of heart failure and coronary disease.[304a,304b]

Histone modifications and related histone methyltransferases and acetyltransferases have also been implicated in the regulation of inflammatory and profibrotic genes in renal and vascular cells under diabetic conditions.[305]

Chromatin immunoprecipitation linked to promoter tiling arrays to profile H3 lysine-9 acetylation (H3K9Ac), H3 lysine-4 trimethylation (H3K4Me3), and H3K9Me2 in blood monocytes and lymphocytes obtained from 30 DCCT conventional treatment group subjects versus 30 DCCT intensive treatment subjects show an association between HbA$_{1c}$ level and H3K9Ac. Monocytes from case subjects have statistically greater numbers of promoter regions with enrichment in H3K9Ac (active chromatin mark) compared with control subjects. Among the patients in the two groups combined, monocyte H3K9Ac was significantly associated with the mean HbA$_{1c}$ level during the DCCT and EDIC. The top hyperacetylated promoters include genes related to the NFκB inflammatory pathway and were enriched in genes related to diabetes complications.[306]

One of the best studied covalent modifications on DNA is 5-methylcytosine (5mC), a mark deposited by DNA methyltransferase (DNMT) enzymes. DNMTs can both introduce methylation marks (de novo methylation) and maintain them after the genome is replicated, making DNA methylation a long-term and potentially heritable mark. Conventionally, 5mC is associated with a transcriptionally repressed chromatin state. In adult zebrafish streptozocin treatment causes hyperglycemia. Following streptozocin withdrawal, blood glucose and serum insulin return to physiologic levels as a result of pancreatic beta-cell regeneration. However, caudal fin regeneration and skin wound healing remain impaired, and this impairment is transmissible to daughter cell tissue. In daughter tissue that was never exposed to hyperglycemia, CpG island methylation and genome-wide microarray expression analyses revealed the persistence of hyperglycemia-induced global DNA hypomethylation that correlates with aberrant gene expression for a subset of loci in this daughter tissue.[307] In zebrafish the ten-eleven translocation (TET) family of enzymes, which mediate DNA demethylation, are activated by hyperglycemia. In this model, hyperglycemia activation of ten-eleven translocase and hyperglycemia-induced DNA demethylation are prevented by inhibition of PARP, which prevented demethylation of specific loci and restored regenerative capacity to normal levels.[308] Because PARP1 is activated by ROS-mediated DNA double-strand breaks, this suggests that excess DNA double-strand breaks continue to occur during long periods of better glycemic control.

What could be responsible for such continued excess DNA strand breaks during periods of better glycemia? One possibility is continued overproduction of ROS, despite restoration of normal glycemia. Transient exposure to high glucose can cause persistent mitochondrial overproduction of ROS during subsequent prolonged periods of normal glucose through activation of a positive multicomponent feedback loop, which maintains persistent overproduction of oxygen free radicals for days of subsequent exposure to normal glucose concentrations.[309] Much has been learned since the original clinical description of hyperglycemic memory, but much more research remains to be done.

RETINOPATHY, MACULAR EDEMA, AND OTHER OCULAR COMPLICATIONS*

Diabetic retinopathy is a well-characterized sight-threatening chronic microvascular complication that eventually afflicts virtually all patients with diabetes mellitus.[86] Diabetic retinopathy is characterized by gradually progressive alterations in the retinal microvasculature, leading to areas of retinal nonperfusion, increased vascular permeability, and pathologic intraocular proliferation of retinal vessels. The complications associated with the increased vascular permeability, termed *macular edema,* and uncontrolled neovascularization, termed *proliferative diabetic retinopathy* (PDR), can result in severe and permanent vision loss if not treated in a timely and appropriate manner.

Despite decades of research, there is currently no known means of preventing diabetic retinopathy, and despite effective therapies, diabetic retinopathy remains the leading cause of new-onset blindness in working-age persons in most developed countries of the world.[86] With appropriate medical and ophthalmologic care, however, more than 90% of vision loss resulting from PDR can be prevented.[310] Thus, until a cure for diabetes is discovered, the primary clinical care emphasis for the prevention of vision loss is appropriately directed at early identification, accurate classification, and timely treatment of retinopathy.

The increased understanding of the mechanistic pathways underlying hyperglycemia-induced retinal changes has provided new targets against which novel therapies

---

*Portions of this section draw on, among others, Aiello LM, Cavallerano JD, Aiello LP. Diagnosis, management, and treatment of nonproliferative diabetic retinopathy and diabetic macular edema. In Albert DM, Jokobiec FA, eds. *Principles and Practice of Ophthalmology,* 2nd ed. Philadelphia, PA: WB Saunders, 2000:1900-1914; Aiello LP, Cavallerano J, Klein R. Diabetic eye disease. In DeGroot LJ, James JL, eds. *Endocrinology,* 5th ed. Philadelphia, PA: WB Saunders, 2005:1305-1317; Aiello LP, Gardner TW, King GL, et al. Diabetic retinopathy: technical review. American Diabetes Association. *Diabetes Care.* 1998;21:143-156; and Aiello LP, Cavallerano J. Diabetic retinopathy. In Johnstone MT, Veves A, eds. *Contemporary Cardiology: Diabetes and Cardiovascular Disease.* Totowa, NJ: Humana Press, 2001:385-398.

have been devised. These novel therapies, such as VEGF inhibitors, corticosteroids, and PKC-β inhibitors,[311-319] have been evaluated in clinical trials with promising results and have expanded the therapeutic options for patients with diabetic eye disease. In particular, multiple phase 3 clinical trials over the past 5 years have now established anti-VEGF therapy as the new standard of care for most eyes with visual impairment from center-involved diabetic macular edema (DME). Furthermore, the effect of select systemic medications such as ACE inhibitors and angiotensin II receptor blockers (ARBs) may affect the development and progression of diabetic retinopathy. These developments place further emphasis on the importance of adhering to lifelong routine ophthalmologic follow-up of the diabetic patient and optimization of associated systemic disorders.

Epidemiology and Impact

By 2035, it is estimated that 592 million persons worldwide will have diabetes.[320] Nearly 26 million Americans currently have diabetes mellitus, and of these, over 5 million remain unaware that they have the disease.[321] For the past 20 years, diabetic retinopathy has remained the leading cause of new cases of legal blindness among Americans between the ages of 20 and 74 years.[322] There is a higher risk of more frequent and severe ocular complications in T1DM.[323] Approximately 25% of patients with T1DM have retinopathy after 5 years, and this figure increases to 60% and 80% after 10 and 15 years, respectively. Because T2DM accounts for 90% to 95% of the diabetic population in the United States, type 2 disease accounts for a higher fraction of patients with vision loss. The most threatening form of retinopathy (PDR) is present in approximately 67% of T1DM patients who have had diabetes for 35 years.[324]

An estimated 700,000 persons have PDR, 130,000 with high-risk PDR, 500,000 with macular edema, and 325,000 with clinically significant macular edema (CSME) in the United States.[325-329] An estimated 63,000 cases of PDR, 29,000 cases of high-risk PDR, 80,000 cases of macular edema, 56,000 cases of CSME, and 12,000 to 24,000 new cases of legal blindness occur each year as a result of diabetic retinopathy.[325,326,330] Blindness has been estimated to be 25 times more common in persons with diabetes than in those without the disease.[331,332]

The 2010 National Health and Nutrition Examination Survey revealed that only 44.7% of Americans with DME were aware that diabetes had affected their eyes and that nearly 60% of these individuals had not had a dilated eye examination within the past year, suggesting both a lack of awareness among patients at risk for vision loss from diabetic eye complications and insufficient evaluation for many patients with vision-threatening retinopathy.[333]

The DCCT demonstrated that both the rate of development of any retinopathy and the rate of retinopathy progression once it was present were significantly reduced after 3 years of intensive insulin therapy.[334] Interestingly, the effect of reducing the HbA$_{1c}$ in this group from 9.1% for conventional treatment to the 7.3% for intensive treatment has resulted in a benefit maintained through 7 years of follow-up, even though the difference in mean HbA$_{1c}$ levels of the two former randomized treatment groups was only 0.4% at 1 year ($p < 0.001$), continued to narrow, and became statistically nonsignificant by 5 years (8.1% vs. 8.2%, $p = 0.09$). The further rate of progression of complications from their levels at the end of the DCCT remains less in the former intensive treatment group. Thus, the benefits of 6.5 years of intensive treatment extend well beyond the period of its most intensive implementation.[4,41,335,336] These remarkable benefits are continuing to accrue to this population.[337] Applying DCCT intensive insulin therapy to all persons in the United States with T1DM would result in a gain of 920,000 person-years of sight,[338] although the costs of intensive therapy are three times that of conventional therapy.[339]

Pathophysiology

A detailed discussion of the pathophysiologic mechanisms underlying diabetic retinopathy and other diabetes-related complications has been presented earlier in this chapter. The earliest histologic effects of diabetes mellitus in the eye include loss of retinal vascular pericytes (supporting cells for retinal endothelial cells), thickening of vascular endothelium basement membrane, and alterations in retinal blood flow (Fig. 33-23).[36,340-345] With increasing loss of retinal pericytes, the retinal vessel wall develops outpouchings (microaneurysms) and becomes fragile.

Clinically, microaneurysms and small retinal hemorrhages might not always be readily distinguishable and are usually evaluated together as "hemorrhages and microaneurysms" (Fig. 33-24A). Rheologic changes occur in diabetic retinopathy and result from increased platelet aggregation, integrin-mediated leukocyte adhesion, and endothelial damage.[346-348] Disruption of the blood-retina barrier can ensue, characterized by increased vascular permeability.[349,350] Subsequent leakage of blood and serum from the retinal vessels results in retinal hemorrhages, retinal edema, and hard exudates (see Fig. 33-24A and C). Vision loss can follow if the fovea is affected by the leakage.[351]

With time, increasing sclerosis and endothelial cell loss lead to narrowing of the retinal vessels, which decreases vascular perfusion and can ultimately lead to obliteration of the capillaries and small vessels (see Fig. 33-24B). The resulting retinal ischemia is a potent inducer of angiogenic growth factors. Several angiogenic growth factors have been isolated from eyes with diabetic retinopathy, including insulin-like growth factors, basic fibroblast growth factor (bFGF), hepatocyte growth factor (HGF), and VEGF.[352-355] These factors promote the development of new vessel growth and retinal vascular permeability.[356-360] Indeed, inhibition of molecules such as VEGF and their signaling pathways can suppress the development of retinal neovascularization and retinal vascular permeability.[357,361-365] Endogenous inhibitors of angiogenesis and vascular permeability such as pigment epithelial-derived factor (PEDF), and other VEGF independent pathways such as plasma kallikrein and erythropoietin have also been found in the eye, and these have physiologic and therapeutic potential.[57,366-368]

New vessels tend to grow in regions of strong vitreous adhesion to the retina, such as at the optic disc and major vascular arcades (see Fig. 33-24D and E). The posterior vitreous face also serves as a scaffold for pathologic neovascularization, and the new vessels commonly arise at the junctions between perfused and nonperfused retina. When the retina is severely ischemic, the concentration of angiogenic growth factors can reach sufficient concentration in the anterior chamber to cause abnormal new vessel proliferation on the iris and the anterior chamber angle.[354,369] Uncontrolled anterior segment neovascularization can result in neovascular glaucoma because the fibrovascular proliferation in the angle of the eye causes blockage of aqueous outflow through the trabecular meshwork.[370]

Proliferating new vessels in diabetic retinopathy are fragile and have a tendency to bleed, which results in preretinal and vitreous hemorrhages (see Fig. 33-24E and F). Although the presence of a large amount of blood in the

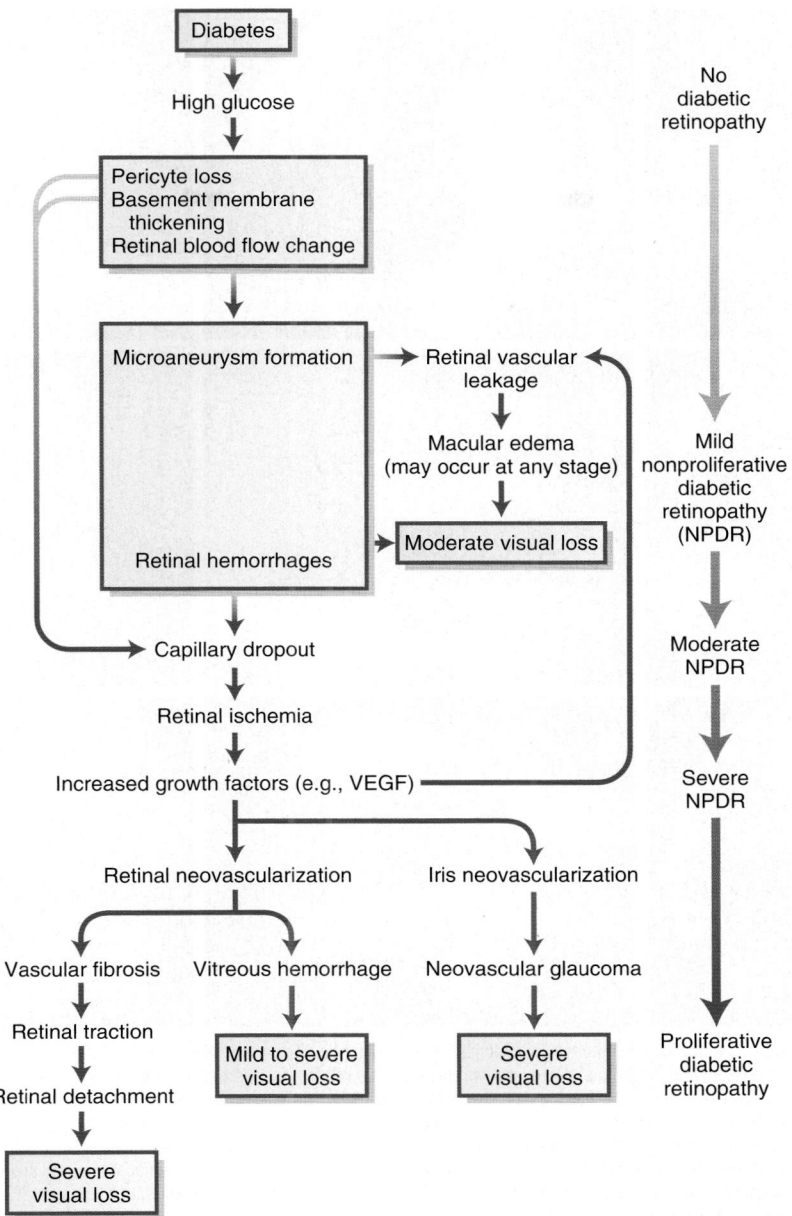

Figure 33-23 Pathogenesis of diabetic retinopathy. This schematic flow chart represents the major preclinical and clinical findings associated with the full spectrum of diabetic retinopathy and macular edema. VEGF, vascular endothelial growth factor.

preretinal space or vitreous cavity per se is not damaging to the retina, these intraocular hemorrhages often cause vision loss by blocking the visual axis. Vitreous hemorrhage can clear spontaneously without intervention, but eyes in which hemorrhage is nonclearing may need vitrectomy surgery in order to restore vision. Vitreous hemorrhage can also decrease the ability to visualize the retina and thereby limit the ability to adequately diagnose and treat other retinal disease. Membranes on the retinal surface can be induced by blood and result in wrinkling and traction on the retina. Although all retinal neovascularization given sufficient time eventually becomes quiescent, as with most scarring processes there is progressive fibrosis of the new vessel complexes that is associated with contraction. In the eye, such forces can exert traction on the retina, leading to tractional retinal detachment and retinal tears

that can result in severe and permanent vision loss if left untreated (see Fig. 33-24G and H).

In short, causes of vision loss from complications of diabetes mellitus include retinal ischemia involving the fovea, macular edema at or near the fovea, preretinal or vitreous hemorrhages, retinal detachment, and neovascular glaucoma. Vision loss can also result from more indirect effects of disease progression in diabetic patients, such as retinal vessel occlusion, accelerated atherosclerotic disease, and embolic phenomena.

Clinical Features

Risk Factors

Duration of diabetes is closely associated with the onset and severity of diabetic retinopathy. Diabetic retinopathy

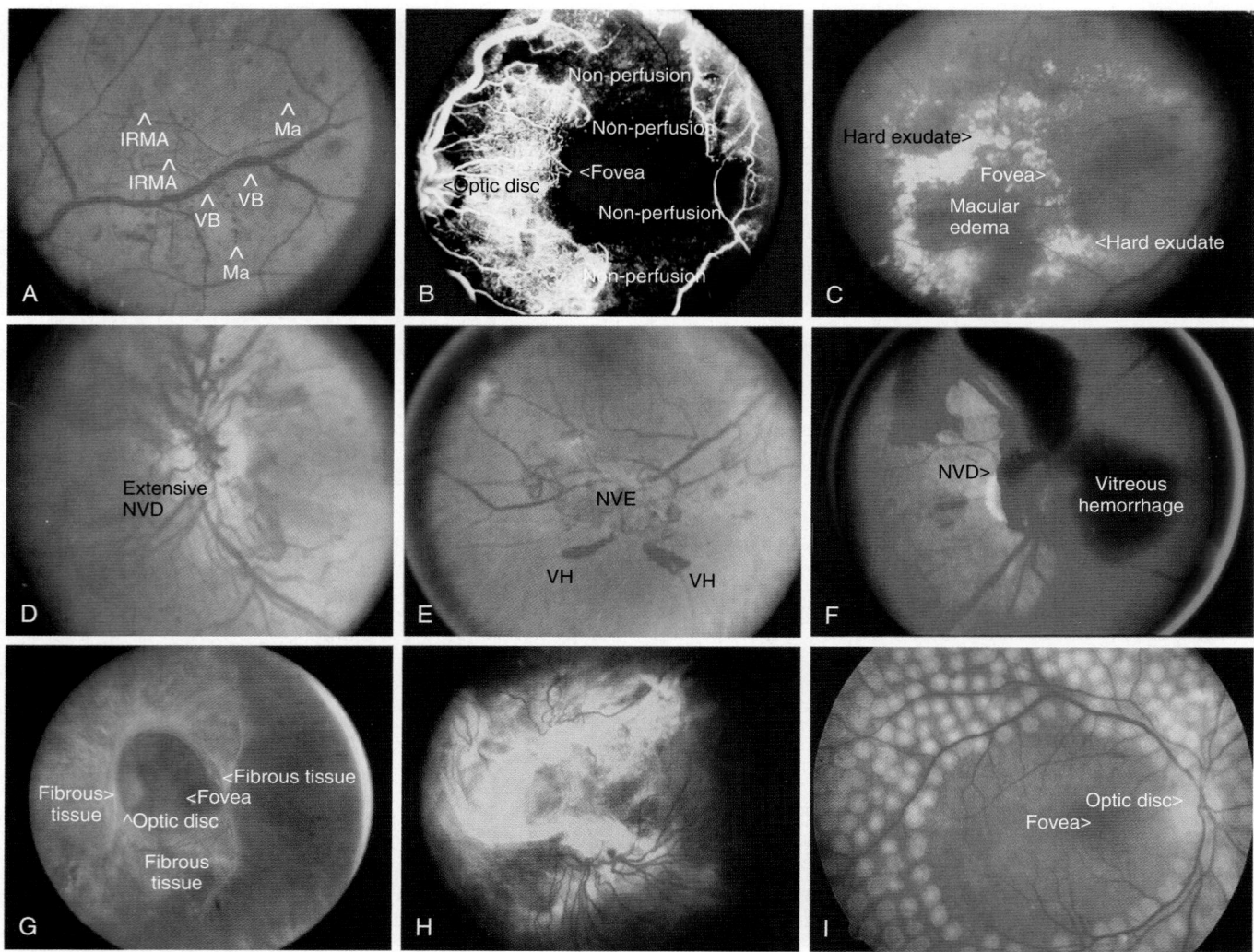

Figure 33-24 Clinical features of diabetic retinopathy: Some typical findings in human diabetic retinopathy. **A,** Findings in severe nonproliferative diabetic retinopathy, including microaneurysms (Ma), venous beading (VB), and intraretinal microvascular abnormalities (IRMA). **B,** Fluorescein angiogram showing marked capillary nonperfusion. **C,** Clinically significant macular edema with retinal thickening and hard exudates involving the fovea. **D,** Extensive neovascularization of the optic disc (NVD), illustrating high-risk proliferative diabetic retinopathy. **E,** Neovascularization elsewhere (NVE) and two small vitreous hemorrhages (VH), also illustrating high-risk proliferative diabetic retinopathy. **F,** Extensive vitreous hemorrhage arising from severe neovascularization of the disc (NVD). **G,** Severe fibrovascular proliferation surrounding the fovea. **H,** Traction retinal detachment from extensive fibrovascular proliferation. **I,** Scars from scatter (panretinal) laser photocoagulation. The macula, fovea, and optic disc are not treated to preserve central vision. Laser burns are evident as white retinal lesions. (Adapted from Aiello LP. Eye complications of diabetes. In Korenman SG, Kahn CR, eds. *Atlas of Clinical Endocrinology*. Vol 2: *Diabetes*. Philadelphia, PA: Blackwell Scientific, 1999.)

is rare in prepubescent patients with T1DM, but nearly all patients with T1DM and more than 60% of patients with T2DM develop some degree of retinopathy after 20 years.[86,324,371] In U.S. reports of patients with T2DM, approximately 20% had retinopathy at the time of diabetes diagnosis[371] and most had some degree of retinopathy over subsequent decades. In the UKPDS study of T2DM, 35% of female subjects and 39% of male subjects had some level of diabetic retinopathy at the time of diabetes diagnosis.[372]

Diabetic retinopathy is the most common cause of new-onset blindness among American adults aged 20 to 74 years. In the Wisconsin Epidemiologic Study of Diabetic Retinopathy, approximately 4% of patients younger than 30 years of age at diagnosis and nearly 2% of patients older than 30 years of age at diagnosis were legally blind. In the younger-onset group, 86% of blindness was attributable to diabetic retinopathy. In the older-onset group, in which other eye diseases were also common, 33% of the cases of

legal blindness were due to diabetic retinopathy.[324,371] Currently, diabetes is thought to account for 12,000 to 24,000 new cases of blindness in the United States each year.[330]

Lack of appropriate glycemic control is another significant risk factor for the onset and progression of diabetic retinopathy. The DCCT demonstrated a clear relationship between hyperglycemia and diabetic microvascular complications, including retinopathy, in 1441 patients with T1DM.[4,38,336,338,373]

In patients monitored for 4 to 9 years, the DCCT showed that intensive insulin therapy reduced or prevented the development of retinopathy by 27% as compared with conventional therapy. Additionally, intensive insulin therapy reduced the progression of diabetic retinopathy by 34% to 76% and had a substantial beneficial effect over the entire range of retinopathy severity. This improvement was achieved with an average 10% reduction in HbA_{1c} from 8% to 7.2%. These results underscore that although intensive therapy might not prevent retinopathy completely, it reduces the risk of retinopathy onset and progression.

Renal disease, as manifested by microalbuminuria and proteinuria, is yet another significant risk factor for onset and progression of diabetic retinopathy.[374,375] Hypertension is associated with PDR and is an established risk factor for the development of macular edema.[376] Additionally, elevated serum lipid levels are associated with extravasated lipid in the retina (hard exudates) and vision loss.[377]

Clinical Findings

Clinical findings associated with early and progressing diabetic retinopathy include hemorrhages or microaneurysms, cotton-wool spots, hard exudates, intraretinal microvascular abnormalities, and venous caliber abnormalities such as venous loops, venous tortuosity, and venous beading (see Fig. 33-24A and C). Microaneurysms are saccular outpouchings of the capillary walls that can leak fluid and result in intraretinal edema and hemorrhages. The intraretinal hemorrhages can be flame-shaped or dot-blot–like in appearance, reflecting the architecture of the layer of the retina in which they occur. Flame-shaped hemorrhages occur in inner retina closer to the vitreous, and dot-blot hemorrhages occur deeper in the retina. Intraretinal microvascular abnormalities are either new vessel growth within the retinal tissue itself or shunt vessels through areas of poor vascular perfusion. It is common for intraretinal microvascular abnormalities to be located adjacent to cotton-wool spots. Cotton-wool spots are caused by microinfarcts in the nerve fiber layer of the retina. Venous caliber abnormalities are generally a sign of severe retinal hypoxia. In some cases of extensive vascular loss, however, the retina might actually appear free of nonproliferative lesions. Such areas are termed *featureless retina* and are a sign of severe retinal hypoxia.

Vision loss from diabetic retinopathy generally results from persistent nonclearing vitreous hemorrhage, traction retinal detachment, or DME (see Figs. 33-23 and 33-24). Neovascularization with fibrous tissue contraction can distort the retina and lead to traction retinal detachment. The new vessels can bleed, causing preretinal or vitreous hemorrhage. The most common cause of vision loss from diabetes, however, is macular disease and macular edema. Macular edema is more likely to occur in patients with T2DM, which represents 90% to 95% of the diabetic population. In diabetic macular disease, macular edema involving the fovea or nonperfusion of the capillaries in the central macula is responsible for the loss of vision.

Classification Systems

Classification of Diabetic Retinopathy. Diabetic retinopathy is broadly classified into *nonproliferative diabetic retinopathy* (NPDR) and *proliferative diabetic retinopathy* (PDR) categories.[378,379] Macular edema can coexist with either group and is not used in the classification of level of retinopathy. The historical terms *background retinopathy* and *preproliferative diabetic retinopathy* have been replaced to reflect the specific characteristics and risk stratification of the prognostically important subgroups in NPDR (Table 33-1).

Generally, diabetic retinopathy progresses from no retinopathy through mild, moderate, severe, and very severe NPDR and eventually to PDR. The level of NPDR is determined by the extent and location of clinical manifestations of retinopathy. Mild NPDR is characterized by limited microvascular abnormalities such as hemorrhages or microaneurysms, cotton-wool spots, and increased vascular per-

meability. Moderate and severe NPDR is characterized by increasing severity of hemorrhages or microaneurysms, venous caliber abnormalities, intraretinal microvascular abnormalities, and vascular closure. The level of NPDR establishes the risk of progression to sight-threatening retinopathy and dictates appropriate clinical management and follow-up.

PDR is characterized by vasoproliferation of the retina and its complications, including new vessels on the optic disc (NVD), new vessels elsewhere on the retina (NVE), preretinal hemorrhage (PRH), vitreous hemorrhage, and fibrous tissue proliferation (FP). On the basis of the extent and location of these lesions, PDR is classified as *early PDR* or *high-risk PDR*. Larger areas of these complications as well as new vessels that are near the optic disc are associated with greater risks of vision loss.

Classification of Diabetic Macular Edema. DME can be present with any level of diabetic retinopathy. When edema involves or threatens the center of the macula, it is called *CSME*. CSME exists if there is retinal thickening at or within 500 μm of the fovea, hard exudates at or within 500 μm of the fovea with adjacent retinal thickening, or an area or areas of retinal thickening one disc area or more in size, any part of which is within 1500 μm of the fovea.[378,380,381] CSME is a clinical diagnosis that is not dependent on visual acuity or results of ancillary testing such as fluorescein angiography and can be present even when vision is 20/20 or better. The term *CSME* was first introduced in the Early Treatment Diabetic Retinopathy Study (ETDRS) to indicate an increased risk for moderate visual loss or doubling of the visual angle. Data from the ETDRS evaluating eyes with macular edema have shown that the presence or absence of thickening involving the center of the macula, now termed as *center-involved DME,* was significantly associated with short- and long-term visual acuity outcomes. In the ETDRS, eyes with center-involved DME had nearly a 10-fold greater risk for developing moderate visual loss compared to eyes without center involvement.

However, with the advent of ocular coherence tomography (OCT) and its objective quantitative measurement of retinal thickness, most clinical care and clinical trial end points have shifted to evaluating whether the center of the macula is involved or not. The identification of center-involved edema is critical because this generally will indicate onset of therapy. To date, if the center of the macula is not involved, there is often not compelling evidence that treatment is yet required. For these reasons, recent clinical studies have generally used the presence or absence of thickening of the central 1-mm-diameter retinal subfield as a threshold for treatment of eyes with DME.

International Classification of Diabetic Retinopathy. The American Academy of Ophthalmology initiated a project to establish a consensus International Classification of Diabetic Retinopathy and Diabetic Macular Edema in an effort to simplify classification and standardize communication among diabetes health care providers.[382,383] This international classification describes five clinical levels of diabetic retinopathy: no apparent retinopathy (no abnormalities), mild NPDR (microaneurysms only), moderate NPDR (more than microaneurysms only but less than severe NPDR), severe NPDR (any of the following: more than 20 intraretinal hemorrhages in each of four retinal quadrants, definite venous beading in two or more retinal quadrants, prominent intraretinal microvascular abnormalities in one or more retinal quadrants, and no PDR), and PDR (one or more of retinal neovascularization, vitreous hemorrhage, or preretinal hemorrhage). Table 33-2 compares levels of retinopathy in the international classification to those defined by the landmark ETDRS.

TABLE 33-1

Glossary and Abbreviations Pertinent to Diabetic Eye Disease

Term	Definition
Background diabetic retinopathy (BDR)	An outdated term referring to some stages of NPDR; not closely associated with disease progression; replaced by the various levels of NPDR
Clinically significant macular edema (CSME)	Thickening of the retina in the macular region of sufficient extent and location to threaten central visual function
Cotton-wool spot	A gray or white area lesion in the nerve fiber layer of the retina resulting from stasis of axoplasmic flow caused by microinfarcts of the retinal nerve fiber layer
Diabetes Control and Complications Trial (DCCT)	A multicenter, randomized clinical trial designed to address whether intensive insulin therapy could prevent or slow the progression of systemic complications of diabetes mellitus
Diabetic retinopathy (DR)	Retinal damage related to the underlying systemic disease of diabetes mellitus
Diabetic Retinopathy Study (DRS)	The first multicenter, randomized clinical trial to demonstrate the value of scatter (panretinal) photocoagulation in reducing the risk of vision loss among patients with all levels of diabetic retinopathy
Diabetic Retinopathy Vitrectomy Study (DRVS)	A multicenter clinical trial evaluating early vitrectomy for patients with very advanced diabetic retinopathy or nonresolving vitreous hemorrhage
Early Treatment Diabetic Retinopathy Study (ETDRS)	A multicenter, randomized clinical trial that addressed at what stage of retinopathy scatter (panretinal) photocoagulation was indicated, whether focal photocoagulation was effective for preventing moderate vision loss due to clinically significant macular edema, and whether aspirin therapy altered the progression of diabetic retinopathy
Focal or grid laser photocoagulation	A type of laser treatment whose main goal is to reduce vascular leakage, either by focal treatment of leaking retinal microaneurysms or by application of therapy in a grid-like pattern for patients with clinically significant macular edema
Hard exudate	Lipid accumulation within the retina as a result of increased vasopermeability
High-risk characteristic proliferative diabetic retinopathy (HRC-PDR)	Proliferative diabetic retinopathy of defined extent, location, or clinical findings that is particularly associated with severe vision loss
Microaneurysm	An early vascular abnormality consisting of an outpouching of the retinal microvasculature
Neovascular glaucoma (NVG)	Elevation of intraocular pressure caused by the development of neovascularization in the anterior segment of the eye
Neovascularization at the disc (NVD)	Retinal neovascularization occurring at or within 1500 µm of the optic disc
Neovascularization elsewhere (NVE)	Retinal neovascularization that is located more than 1500 µm away from the optic disc
Neovascularization of the iris (NVI)	Neovascularization occurring on the iris (rubeosis iridis), usually as a result of extensive retinal ischemia
No light perception (NLP)	The inability to perceive light
Nonproliferative diabetic retinopathy (NPDR)	Severities (mild, moderate, severe) of clinically evident diabetic retinopathy that precede the development of PDR
Preproliferative diabetic retinopathy (PPDR)	An outdated term referring to more advanced levels of NPDR; not closely associated with disease progression; replaced by the various levels of NPDR
Proliferative diabetic retinopathy (PDR)	An advanced level of diabetic retinopathy in which proliferation of new vessels or fibrous tissue occurs on or within the retina
Rubeosis iridis	Neovascularization of the iris

TABLE 33-2

Levels of Diabetic Retinopathy

International Classification Level	ETDRS Level
No apparent retinopathy	Level 10: DR absent
Mild NPDR	Level 20: very mild NPDR
Moderate NPDR	Levels 35, 43, and 47: moderate NPDR
Severe NPDR	Levels 53A-E: severe to very severe NPDR
PDR	Levels 61, 65, 71, 75, 81, 85: PDR, high-risk PDR, very severe or advanced PDR

DR, diabetic retinopathy; ETDRS, Early Treatment Diabetic Retinopathy Study; NPDR, nonproliferative diabetic retinopathy; PDR, proliferative diabetic retinopathy.
From Grading diabetic retinopathy from stereoscopic color fundus photographs—an extension of the modified Airlie House classification. ETDRS report number 10. Early Treatment Diabetic Retinopathy Study Research Group. *Ophthalmology.* 1991;98:786-806.

TABLE 33-3

International Classification of Diabetic Macular Edema (DME)

Disease Severity Level	Ophthalmic Findings (Retinal Thickening or Hard Exudates in Posterior Pole)	ETDRS Scale Equivalent
DME apparently absent	None apparent	
DME apparently present	Some apparent	
Mild DME	Some findings present but distant from center of the macula	DME but not CSME
Moderate DME	Findings approaching the center but not involving the center	CSME
Severe DME	Findings involving the center of the macula	CSME

CSME, clinically significant macular edema; ETDRS, Early Treatment Diabetic Retinopathy Study.

In regard to DME, the international classification identifies two broad categories: macular edema apparently absent (no apparent retinal thickening or hard exudates in the posterior pole) and macular edema apparently present (some apparent retinal thickening or hard exudates in the posterior pole). Macular edema is subclassified as mild (some retinal thickening or hard exudates in the posterior pole but distant from the center of the macula), moderate (retinal thickening or hard exudates approaching the center of the macula but not involving the center), or severe (retinal thickening or hard exudates involving the center of the macula). Table 33-3 compares levels of DME in the international classification to ETDRS levels of DME.

As compared with ETDRS retinopathy grading, the International Classification of Diabetic Retinopathy and Diabetic Macular Edema reduces the number of levels of diabetic retinopathy, simplifies descriptions of the categories, and describes the levels without relying on reference to the standard photographs of the Airlie House Classification of diabetic retinopathy. This approach makes clinical use easier and more uniform among practitioners not versed in the complexities of the ETDRS grading system. However, because of this simplification, the International Classification of Diabetic Retinopathy and Diabetic Macular Edema is not a replacement for ETDRS levels of diabetic retinopathy in large-scale clinical trials or studies for which precise retinopathy classification is required.

Other Ocular Manifestations of Diabetes

All structures of the eye are susceptible to complications of diabetes. The consequence of these changes can range from being unnoticed by both patient and physician, to symptomatic but not sight-threatening, to requiring evaluation to rule out potentially life-threatening underlying causes other than diabetes.

Mononeuropathies of the third, fourth, or sixth cranial nerves can arise in association with diabetes; mononeuropathy of the fourth cranial nerve is least likely associated with diabetes and warrants workup for other causes.[384-386] Nerve palsies present a significant diagnostic challenge because misdiagnosis can result in a life-threatening lesion remaining untreated. In one review of cranial nerve palsies treated in a diabetic patient population in 1967, 42% of mononeuropathies were not diabetic in origin.[385] This finding underscores the danger of routinely attributing mononeuropathies to the diabetic condition itself without carefully ruling out other potential causes. The percentage of all extraocular muscle palsies attributable to diabetes mellitus is estimated at 4.5% to 6%.[386] Mononeuropathies may be the initial presenting sign of new-onset diabetes, and diabetes should therefore be considered in the differential diagnosis of any mononeuropathy affecting the extraocular muscles, even in patients who do not claim a history of diabetes. Diabetes-induced third-, fourth-, and sixth-nerve palsies are usually self-limited and should resolve spontaneously in 2 to 6 months. Palsies can recur or subsequently develop in the contralateral eye.

The optic disc can be affected by diabetes in a variety of ways other than vasoproliferation. Diabetic papillopathy must be distinguished from other causes of disc swelling such as true papilledema from increased intracranial pressure, pseudopapilledema such as optic nerve head drusen, toxic optic neuropathies, neoplasms of the optic nerve, and hypertension.[387] Optic disc pallor can occur following spontaneous remission of proliferative retinopathy or remission following scatter (panretinal) laser photocoagulation (see Fig. 33-24I). Because diabetes poses an increased risk for developing open-angle glaucoma, the disc pallor following remission of retinopathy or laser photocoagulation must be considered when evaluating the optic nerve head for glaucoma.

A potentially serious diabetic ocular complication is neovascularization of the iris. Usually the new iris vessels are first observed at the pupillary border, followed by a fine network of vessels over the iris tissue progressing into the filtration angle of the eye. Closure of the angle by the fibrovascular network results in neovascular glaucoma.[388] Neovascular glaucoma is difficult to manage and requires aggressive treatment. Diabetes is the second leading cause of neovascular glaucoma, accounting for 32% of cases.[389] Neovascularization of the iris occurs in 4% to 7% of diabetic eyes and may be present in up to 40% to 60% of eyes with proliferative retinopathy.[390,391] When possible, scatter (panretinal) laser photocoagulation is the primary therapy for neovascularization of the iris, although other approaches such as goniophotocoagulation, topical or systemic antiglaucoma medications, and antiglaucomatous filtration surgery are available when needed.[392-394] Intravitreal administration of VEGF inhibitors has been tried in small-scale uncontrolled studies with remarkably rapid transient regression of the neovascularization.[395]

The cornea of the diabetic person is more susceptible to injury and slower to heal after injury than is the nondiabetic cornea.[387,396] The diabetic cornea is also more prone to infectious corneal ulcers, which can lead to rapid loss of vision, need for corneal transplant, or loss of the eye if it is not treated aggressively. Consequently, diabetic patients using contact lenses should exercise caution to avoid contact lens overwear and to maintain careful monitoring.

Open-angle glaucoma is 1.4 times more common in the diabetic population than in the nondiabetic population.[397] The prevalence of glaucoma increases with age and duration of diabetes, but medical therapy for open-angle glaucoma is generally effective. In a study of 76,318 women enrolled in the Nurses' Health Study, Pasquale and coworkers found that T2DM is associated with an increased risk of primary open-angle glaucoma in women.[398]

Diabetes effects on the crystalline lens can result in transient refractive changes, alterations in accommodative ability,[399] and cataracts. Refractive change can be significant and is related to fluctuation of blood glucose levels with osmotic lens swelling.[389] Cataracts can occur earlier in life and progress more rapidly in the presence of diabetes.[400,401] Cataracts are 1.6 times more common in people with diabetes than in those without diabetes.[400,401] In patients with earlier onset diabetes, duration of diabetes, retinopathy status, diuretic use, and HbA$_{1c}$ levels are risk factors.[402] In patients with later onset diabetes, age of the patient, lower intraocular pressure, smoking, and lower diastolic BP may be additional risk factors.[403,404] Diabetic patients undergoing simultaneous kidney and pancreas transplantation are at an increased risk of developing all types of cataracts, independent of the use of corticosteroids after transplantation.[405] Both phacoemulsification and extracapsular cataract extraction with intraocular lens implantation are appropriate surgical therapies. The principal determinant of postoperative vision and progression of retinopathy is related to the preoperative presence of DME and level of NPDR.[406,407]

Other findings with higher incidence among patients with diabetes include xanthelasma,[384] microaneurysms of the bulbar conjunctiva,[408] posterior vitreous detachment,[409] and the rare but often fatal orbital fungal infection *Mucorales* phycomycosis.[390,391] Prompt diagnosis and treatment of phycomycosis caused by *Mucor* species are crucial, although the survival rate remains at only 57%.[391,410]

Monitoring and Treatment of Diabetic Retinopathy

Appropriate clinical management of diabetic retinopathy has been defined by results of major randomized, multicenter clinical trials (Fig. 33-25): the Diabetic Retinopathy Clinical Research Network Protocol I,[411] Diabetic Retinopathy Study (DRS),[412] the ETDRS,[351] the Diabetic Retinopathy Vitrectomy Study (DRVS),[413] the DCCT,[414] and the UKPDS.[5] These studies have elucidated the progression rates of each level of diabetic retinopathy, guided follow-up intervals, and elucidated the proper delivery, timing, and resulting

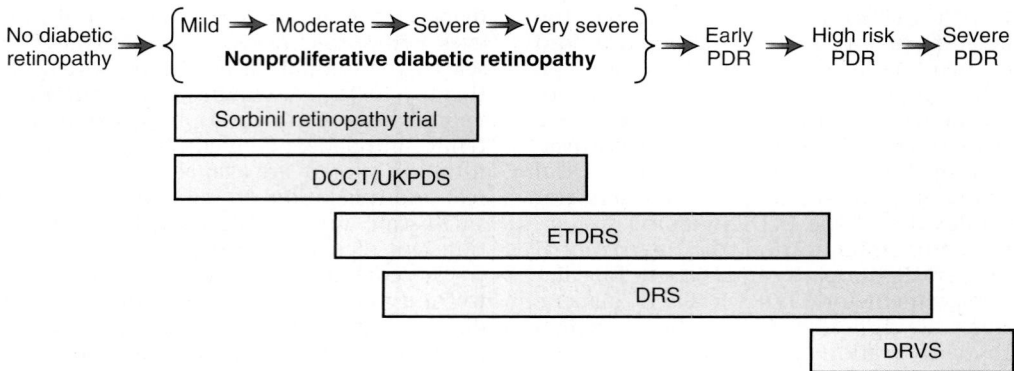

Figure 33-25 Schematic representation of the major multicenter clinical trials of diabetic retinopathy and the levels of diabetic retinopathy that they primarily addressed. DCCT, Diabetes Control and Complications Trial; DRS, Diabetic Retinopathy Study; DRVS, Diabetic Retinopathy Vitrectomy Study; ETDRS, Early Treatment Diabetic Retinopathy Study; PDR, proliferative diabetic retinopathy; UKPDS, United Kingdom Prospective Diabetes Study.

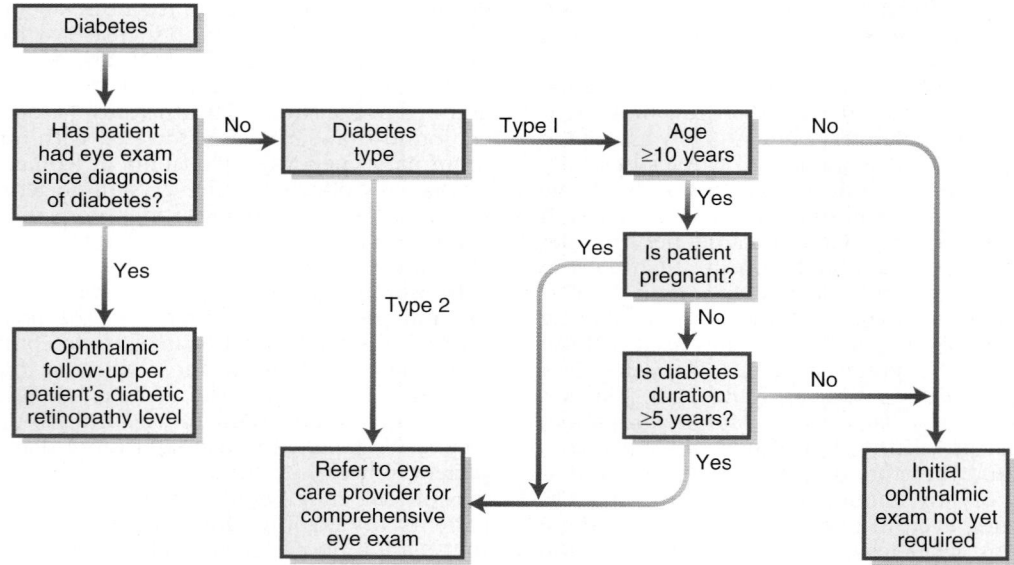

Figure 33-26 Schematic flow chart of major principles involved in determining the timing of initial ophthalmic examination after a diagnosis of diabetes mellitus. These are minimal recommended times. Ocular symptoms, complaints, or other associated medical issues can necessitate earlier evaluation. Guidelines are regularly reevaluated based on new study results.

effectiveness of glycemic control, laser photocoagulation surgery, and intravitreous anti-VEGF therapy (Figs. 33-26 to 33-29). They have also established recommendations for vitrectomy surgery.

Comprehensive Eye Examination

An accurate ocular examination detailing the extent and location of retinopathy-associated findings is critical for determining monitoring and treatment decisions in patients with diabetic retinopathy. As detailed later, most of the blindness associated with advanced stages of retinopathy can be averted with appropriate and timely diagnosis and therapy. Unfortunately, many diabetic patients do not receive adequate eye care at an appropriate stage in their disease.[415,416] In one study, 55% of patients with high-risk PDR or CSME had never had laser photocoagulation.[415] In fact, 11% of T1DM and 7% of T2DM patients with high-risk PDR necessitating prompt treatment had not been examined by an ophthalmologist within the past 2 years.[416]

The comprehensive eye examination is the mainstay of such evaluation and is necessary on a repetitive, lifelong basis for patients with diabetes.[378,417] Such an evaluation has four major components: history, examination, diagnosis, and treatment. Annual retinal evaluation to assess the presence and level of diabetic retinopathy and DME is essential to guide patient care. The fundamentals of a comprehensive eye examination for the nondiabetic patient have been detailed by the American Academy of Ophthalmology[417] and the American Optometric Association.[418] The examination of the patient with diabetes should be similar, with additional emphasis on portions of the examination that relate to problems particularly relevant to diabetes.

Dilated ophthalmic examination is superior to undilated evaluation because only 50% of eyes are correctly classified as to presence and severity of retinopathy through undilated pupils.[419,420] Appropriate ophthalmic evaluation entails pupillary dilation, slit-lamp biomicroscopy, examination of the retinal periphery with indirect ophthalmoscopy or mirrored contact lens, and sometimes

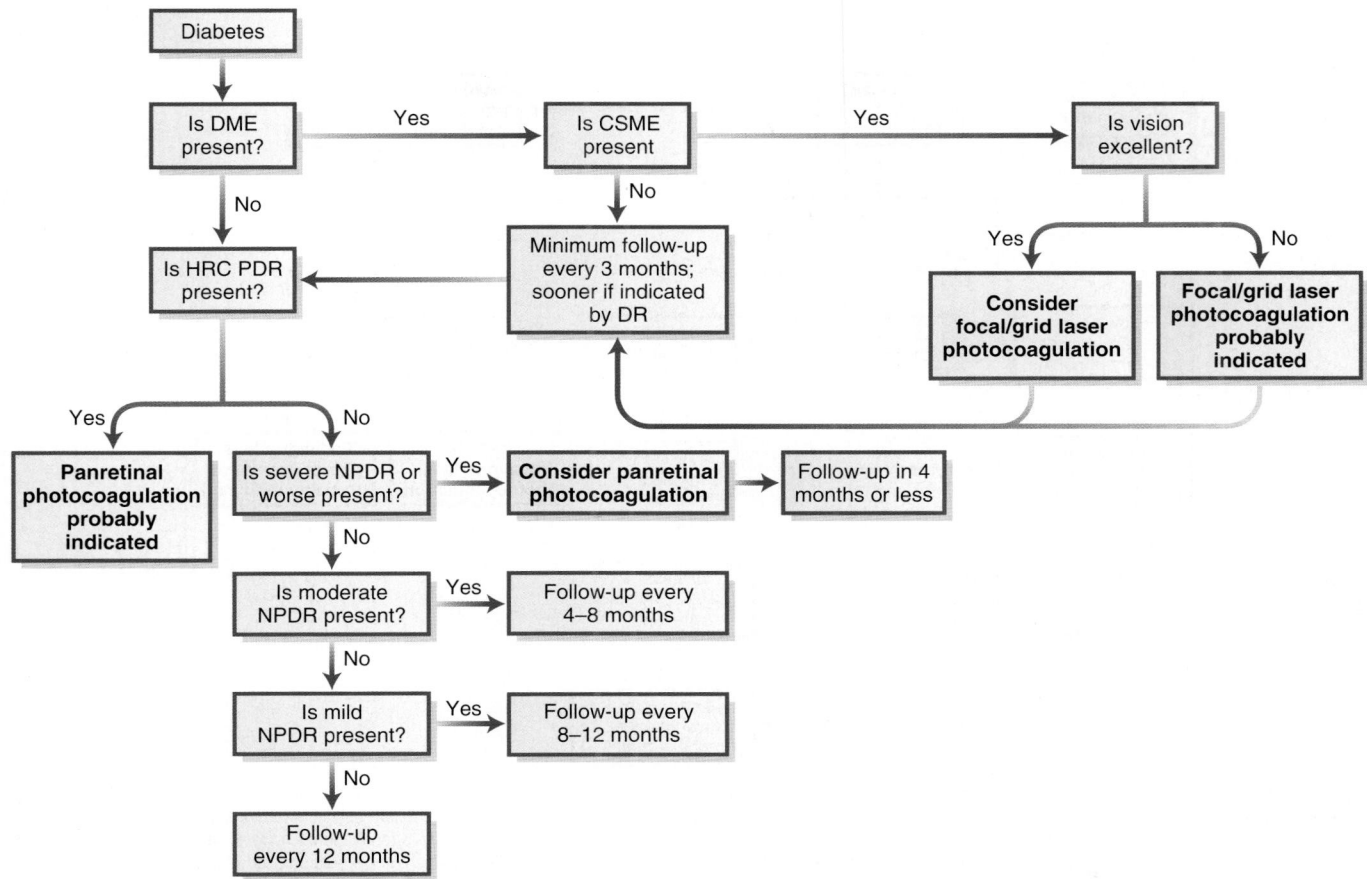

Figure 33-27 Diabetic retinopathy and macular edema examination and treatment flow chart: nonpregnant patients. The schematic flow chart presents major principles involved in determining routine ophthalmic follow-up and indications for treatment in nonpregnant patients with diabetes. These intervals are only general, minimal recommended frequencies. Ocular symptoms, complaints, or other associated ophthalmic or medical issues can necessitate earlier evaluation or an altered approach. Guidelines are regularly reevaluated based on new study results. CSME, clinically significant macular edema; DME, diabetic macular edema; DR, diabetic retinopathy; HRC PDR, high-risk characteristic proliferative diabetic retinopathy; NPDR, nonproliferative diabetic retinopathy; PDR, proliferative diabetic retinopathy.

gonioscopy.[417,418] Because of the complexities of the diagnosis and treatment of PDR and CSME, ophthalmologists with specialized knowledge and experience in the management of diabetic retinopathy are required to determine and provide appropriate surgical intervention.[421] Thus, it is recommended that all patients with diabetes should have dilated ocular examinations by an experienced eye care provider (ophthalmologist or optometrist), and diabetic patients should be under the direct or consulting care of an ophthalmologist experienced in the management of diabetic retinopathy at least by the time severe diabetic retinopathy or DME is present.[378] Retinal imaging that has demonstrated equivalency to dilated retinal fundus examination or the accepted standard of seven-standard-field stereoscopic retinal imaging when interpreted by a trained eye care provider can also be appropriate.[422,423] Furthermore, ocular telehealth programs for diabetic retinopathy that utilize validated means of retinal imaging have the potential to expand access to highly effective evidence-based diabetes eye care and provide cost-effective alternative methods of care.[424]

Initial Ophthalmic Evaluation

The recommendation for initial ocular examination in persons with diabetes is based on prevalence rates of retinopathy (see Fig. 33-26). Approximately 80% of T1DM patients have retinopathy after 15 years of disease, but only about 25% have any retinopathy after 5 years.[420] The prevalence of PDR is less than 2% at 5 years and 25% by 15 years. For T2DM, the onset date of diabetes is usually unknown, and more severe disease can be observed at diagnosis. Up to 3% of patients whose diabetes is first diagnosed after age 30 years (T2DM) have CSME or high-risk PDR at the time of initial diagnosis of diabetes.[425] Thus, in patients older than 10 years, initial ophthalmic examination is recommended beginning 5 years after the diagnosis of T1DM and on diagnosis of T2DM (see Fig. 33-26).[378,426]

Puberty and pregnancy can accelerate retinopathy progression. The onset of vision-threatening retinopathy is rare in children prior to puberty, regardless of the duration of diabetes[324,426-428]; however, significant retinopathy can arise within 6 years of disease if diabetes is diagnosed between the ages of 10 and 30 years.[325] Diabetic retinopathy can become particularly aggressive during pregnancy in patients with diabetes.[429,430] In the past, the prognosis for pregnancy in the diabetic patient with microvascular complications was so poor that pregnant diabetic patients were commonly advised to avoid or terminate pregnancies.[431] With recognition of the importance of glycemic control, many diabetic patients in the child-bearing age now experience safe pregnancy and childbirth with minimal risk to both the mother and the baby. There are excellent reviews on this subject.[432]

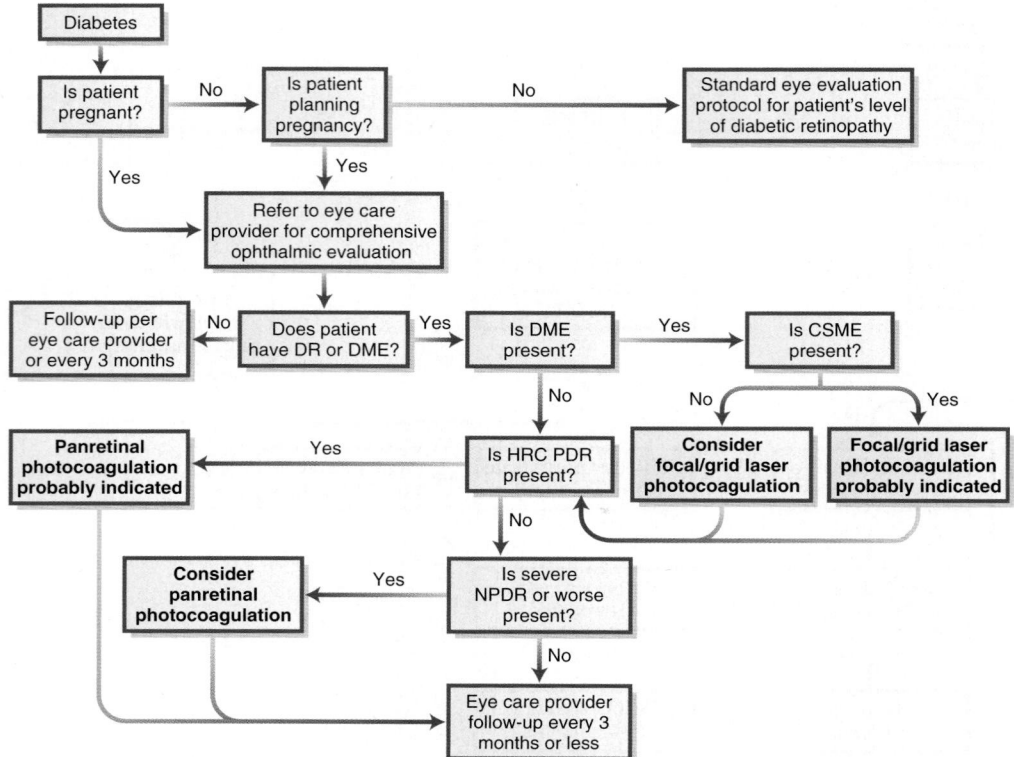

Figure 33-28 Diabetic retinopathy and macular edema examination and treatment flow chart: pregnant patients. The schematic flow chart shows major principles involved in determining routine ophthalmic follow-up and indications for treatment in pregnant patients with diabetes. These intervals are only general, minimal recommended frequencies. Ocular symptoms, complaints, or other associated ophthalmic or medical issues can necessitate earlier evaluation or an altered approach. Because retinopathy can progress rapidly in pregnant patients with diabetes, careful and more frequent evaluation is often indicated. Guidelines are regularly reevaluated based on new study results. CSME, clinically significant macular edema; DME, diabetic macular edema; DR, diabetic retinopathy; HRC PDR, high-risk characteristic proliferative diabetic retinopathy; NPDR, nonproliferative diabetic retinopathy.

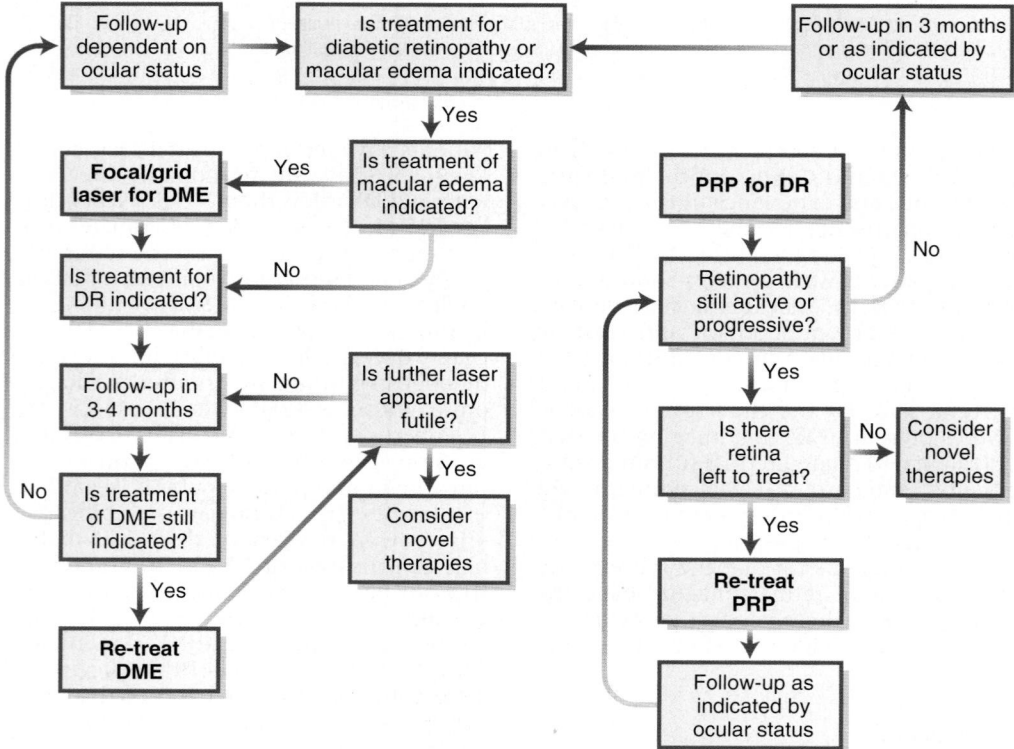

Figure 33-29 Photocoagulation flow chart. This schematic flow chart details general photocoagulation treatment approaches in patients with diabetic retinopathy or diabetic macular edema. These are only general guidelines, and actual treatment choices can be affected by numerous other factors, including findings in the same eye or in the contralateral eye and systemic issues. DR, diabetic retinopathy; DME, diabetic macular edema; PRP, scatter (panretinal) photocoagulation.

Ideally, patients with diabetes who are planning pregnancy should have a comprehensive eye examination within 1 year prior to conception (see Fig. 33-28). Patients who become pregnant should have a comprehensive eye examination in the first trimester of pregnancy. Close follow-up throughout pregnancy is indicated, with subsequent examinations determined by the findings present at the first-trimester examination.[378] This recommendation does not apply to women who develop gestational diabetes, because such women are not at increased risk of developing diabetic retinopathy.

Follow-Up Ophthalmic Examination

Follow-up ocular examination is determined from the risk of disease progression at any particular retinopathy level (see Fig. 33-27). NPDR is categorized into four levels of severity based on clinical findings compared to stereo fundus photographic standards: mild, moderate, severe, and very severe.[433] Progression of nonproliferative retinopathy to the visually threatening level of high-risk PDR is closely correlated with NPDR level (Table 33-4). Progression rates from each individual NPDR level to any other retinopathy level are also known. These are used to define standard minimal follow-up intervals as detailed in Figure 33-27 and Table 33-5. Because significant sight-threatening

retinopathy can initially occur with no or minimal symptoms, patients with no clinically evident diabetic retinopathy and no known ocular problems require annual comprehensive ophthalmic examinations even if they are totally asymptomatic.

Proliferative Diabetic Retinopathy. The extent and location of neovascularization determine the level of PDR.[434,435] PDR is best evaluated by dilated examination using slit-lamp biomicroscopy combined with indirect ophthalmoscopy or

TABLE 33-4		
Progression to PDR by Level of NPDR		
	Chance of High-Risk PDR (%)	
Retinopathy Level	**1 Year**	**5 Years**
Mild NPDR	1	16
Moderate NPDR	3-8	27-39
Severe NPDR	15	56
Very severe NPDR	45	71
PDR with fewer high-risk characteristics	22-46	64-75

NPDR, nonproliferative diabetic retinopathy; PDR, proliferative diabetic retinopathy.
From Aiello LP, Gardner TW, King GL, et al. Diabetic retinopathy: technical review. *Diabetes Care.* 1998;21:143-156.

TABLE 33-5							
Recommended General Management of Diabetic Retinopathy							
	Risk of Progression (%)		**Evaluation**		**Treatment**		
Level of DR	**To PDR (1 yr)**	**To High-Risk PDR (5 yr)**	**Color Photo**	**FA**	**Scatter Laser (PRP)**	**Focal Laser**	**Follow-up (mo)**
Mild NPDR							
All	5	15					
No ME			No	No	No	No	12
ME			Yes	Occ	No	No	4-6
CSME			Yes	Yes	No	Yes	2-4
Moderate NPDR							
All	12-27	33					
No ME			Yes	No	No	No	6-8
ME			Yes	Occ	No	Occ	4-6
CSME			Yes	Yes	No	Yes	2-4
Severe NPDR							
All	52	60					
No ME			Yes	No	Rarely	No	3-4
ME			Yes	Occ	Occ AF	Occ	2-3
CSME			Yes	Yes	Occ AF	Yes	2-3
Very Severe NPDR							
All	75	75					
No ME			Yes	No	Occ	No	2-3
ME			Yes	Occ	Occ AF	Occ	2-3
CSME			Yes	Yes	Occ AF	Yes	2-3
PDR < High Risk							
All	—	75					
No ME			Yes	No	Occ	No	2-3
ME			Yes	Occ	Occ AF	Occ	2-3
CSME			Yes	Yes	Occ AF	Yes	2-3
PDR with High-Risk Characteristics							
All	—	—					
No ME			Yes	No	Yes	No	2-3
ME			Yes	Yes	Yes	Usually	1-2
CSME			Yes	Yes	Yes	Yes	1-2

AF, after focal; CSME, clinically significant macular edema; FA, fluorescein angiography; ME macular edema; NPDR, nonproliferative diabetic retinopathy; Occ, occasionally; PDR, proliferative diabetic retinopathy.
Courtesy of Lloyd M. Aiello, MD, Joslin Diabetes Center, Boston, MA.

stereo fundus photography. Without photocoagulation, eyes with high-risk PDR have a 28% risk of severe vision loss within 2 years. This risk compares with a 7% risk of severe vision loss after 2 years for eyes with PDR but without high-risk characteristics.[434]

Severe vision loss is defined as best corrected acuity of 5/200 or worse on two consecutive visits 4 months apart. This represents vision loss substantially worse than the 20/200 or worse limit for legal blindness. The DRS demonstrated that scatter (panretinal) laser photocoagulation was effective in reducing the risk of severe vision loss from PDR by 50% or more. The ETDRS demonstrated that scatter (panretinal) laser photocoagulation applied when an eye approaches or just reaches high-risk PDR reduces the risk of severe vision loss to less than 4%. Prompt scatter photocoagulation is thus indicated for all patients with high-risk PDR, usually indicated for patients with PDR less than high risk, and may be advisable for patients with severe or very severe NPDR, especially in the setting of T2DM (see Fig. 33-27).[351,434-437] Recent progression of eye disease, status of the fellow eye, compliance with follow-up, concurrent health concerns such as hypertension or kidney disease, and other factors must be considered in determining if laser surgery should be performed in these patients. In particular, patients with T2DM should be considered for scatter photocoagulation before high-risk PDR develops because the risk of severe vision loss and the need for pars plana vitrectomy (PPV) can be reduced by 50% in these patients, especially when macular edema is present.[437]

In scatter photocoagulation, 1200 to 1800 laser burns are applied to the peripheral retinal tissue, actually focally destroying the outer photoreceptor and retinal pigment epithelium of the retina (see Fig. 33-24I). Large vessels are avoided, as are areas of preretinal hemorrhage. The treatment is thought to exert its effect by increasing oxygen delivery to the inner retina, decreasing viable hypoxic growth factor–producing cells, and increasing the relative perfusion per area of viable retina. The total treatment is usually applied over two or three sessions, spaced 1 to 2 weeks apart. Follow-up evaluation usually occurs at 3 months.

The response to scatter photocoagulation varies. The most desirable effect is to see a regression of the new vessels, although stabilization of the neovascularization with no further growth can result. This latter situation requires careful clinical monitoring. In some cases, new vessels continue to proliferate, requiring additional scatter photocoagulation (see Fig. 33-29). As discussed later, novel therapeutic approaches are now being used in some clinical settings, especially in cases where response to scatter photocoagulation is inadequate. Initial results from definitive multicenter randomized, controlled clinical trials will soon be reported, and additional clinical trials using these new therapeutic approaches continue to be performed.

The DRVS, completed in 1989, demonstrated that early PPV in persons with severe fibrovascular proliferation was more likely to result in better vision and less likely to result in poor vision, particularly in patients with T1DM.[413] PPV is surgery within the eye aimed primarily at removing abnormal fibrovascular tissue, alleviating retinal traction, allowing the retina to obtain a more anatomically normal position, and removing vitreous opacities such as vitreous hemorrhage. The actual outcome data from this study might not be entirely applicable today due to the dramatic advances in surgical techniques and the advent of laser endophotocoagulation that have occurred in the intervening years, although it is clear that PPV can save and restore vision in many cases of severe retinal disease not amenable or not responsive to laser photocoagulation.

Macular Edema. Untreated CSME is associated with an approximately 25% chance of moderate vision loss after 3 years (defined as at least doubling the visual angle; e.g., 20/40 reduced to 20/80).[351] Macular edema is best evaluated clinically by dilated examination using slit-lamp biomicroscopy or stereo fundus photography. The newer diagnostic ophthalmic imaging technique of optical coherence tomography (OCT) has provided a means to objectively quantify retinal thickening and is currently the objective method of choice. When used in conjunction with visual acuity measurement, OCT has been used to monitor response to treatment and help determine timing of intervention.[438,439] As discussed above, the current standard for macular edema evaluation focuses on determining the presence or absence of edema involving the center of the macula.

Current first-line therapy for most eyes with center-involved DME leading to visual impairment resulting in visual acuity of 20/32 or worse is intravitreal injections of VEGF inhibitors following a defined protocol such as that described by the Diabetic Retinopathy Clinical Research Network. Typically, injections are performed monthly with a loading dose of at least 4 to 6 injections. On average, 8 to 9 injections are performed in the first year of treatment. The average number of injections required to maintain the beneficial visual acuity gains declines substantially to 3 or 4 in the second year and 1 or 2 in the third year. Anti-VEGF intravitreal injections have been shown to reduce the risk of visual loss of two or more lines to less than 5%, with 50% or more of eyes substantially improving in visual acuity.

Focal laser photocoagulation may still be indicated for some patients with CSME (see Figs. 33-24C and 33-27) without center involvement or in eyes with good vision or in patients who cannot tolerate a regimen of intravitreal injections. The ETDRS demonstrated that focal laser photocoagulation for CSME reduced the 5-year risk of moderate vision loss by 50%, but 15% of patients continue to experience vision loss.[381] In focal laser photocoagulation, lesions from 500 to 3000 μm from the center of the macula that are contributing to thickening of the macular area are generally directly photocoagulated. These lesions are identified clinically or by fluorescein angiography and consist primarily of leaking microaneurysms. When leakage is diffuse or microaneurysms are extensive, photocoagulation may be applied to the macula in a grid configuration, avoiding the fovea region.

Although fluorescein angiography is useful for guiding therapy once CSME has been diagnosed, it is not required for the diagnosis of CSME or PDR because these findings should be clinically evident in most cases (Fig. 33-30). Fluorescein angiography is a valuable test for guiding treatment of CSME, identifying macular capillary nonperfusion, and evaluating unexplained vision loss. Because there are risks associated with fluorescein angiography, including nausea, urticaria, hives, and rarely death (1 in 222,000 patients) or severe medical sequelae (1 in 2000 patients),[440-442] fluorescein angiography is not part of the examination of an otherwise normal patient with diabetes, and the procedure is usually contraindicated in patients with known allergy to fluorescein dye or during pregnancy.

Follow-up evaluation of focal laser surgery generally occurs after 3 months (see Fig. 33-27). In the cases in which macular edema persists, further treatment may be necessary. In the presence of macular edema, patients with severe or very severe NPDR should be considered for anti-VEGF or laser treatment of macular edema whether or not the macular edema is center-involved because they are likely to require scatter laser photocoagulation in the near

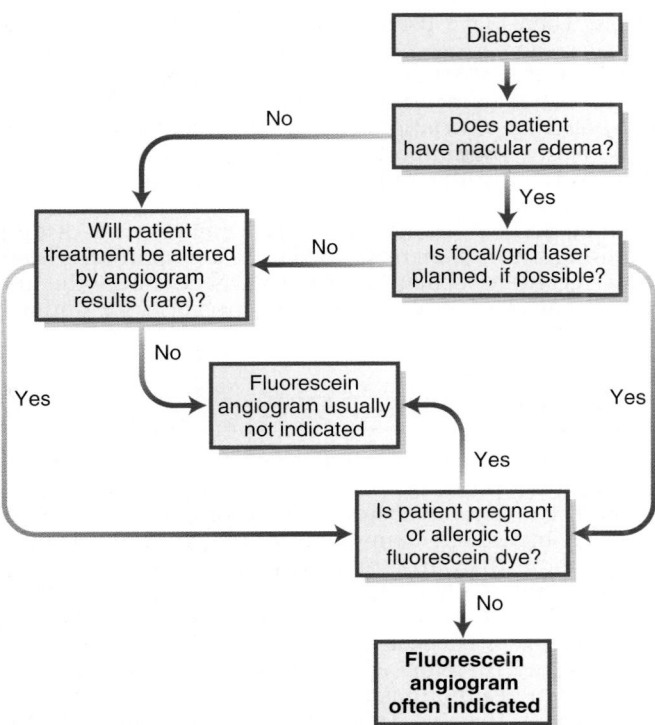

Figure 33-30 Fluorescein angiogram flow chart. The schematic flow chart details a general algorithm for appropriate use of fluorescein angiography in the ocular evaluation of patients with diabetes mellitus. In unusual cases, confounding factors can alter the appropriate approach.

future and because scatter photocoagulation, while beneficial for PDR, can exacerbate existing macular edema. As discussed below, novel therapeutic approaches are now being used in clinical settings to treat DME. However, the pathogenesis of DME is highly complex and a variable response to treatment modalities has been observed in many patients. These observations have prompted the investigation of varying drug dosages to identify the optimal treatment concentration and sustained drug delivery devices to limit repeated intraocular injections. Multicenter randomized, controlled clinical trials are under way for most of these new approaches.

Antiangiogenic Therapy

As mentioned in the earlier section, intravitreal injections of anti-VEGF agents have been shown to cause the regression of choroidal and retinal neovascularization and reduce the amount of vascular leakage. These compounds are injected into the vitreous cavity of the eye on a repetitive basis. Both aflibercept and ranibizumab have been FDA approved for the treatment of neovascular age-related macular degeneration, retinal vein occlusion, and DME. Bevacizumab has been widely used off-label in the treatment of neovascular age-related degeneration, retinal vein occlusion, and DME. Neovascular processes have been shown to be exquisitely sensitive to anti-VEGF agents, and eyes with severe neovascularization of the retina or anterior segment have dramatically and rapidly improved with anti-VEGF treatment.[363,443]

Results from a multicenter randomized controlled clinical trial evaluating intravitreal administration of ranibizumab either with immediate laser or with deferred laser have shown a marked benefit of anti-VEGF agents

compared to laser alone.[411] After 1 year, ranibizumab as applied in the trial resulted in a nine-letter mean gain ($p <$ 0.001) when combined either with prompt laser or deferral of laser for at least 24 weeks. This was more effective than prompt laser alone (three-letter gain) for the treatment of center-involving DME in eyes with central thickening and vision reduced to 20/32 to 20/320. The number of eyes gaining two or more lines of vision almost doubled in the anti-VEGF groups as compared with laser alone. Conversely, eyes losing two or more lines of vision were about one third as many in the anti-VEGF groups as compared to laser alone. These results have been shown to be sustained over 5 years even with a substantially decreased number of injections over years 2 to 5.[444,445]

No increased systemic events or serious ocular adverse events were attributed to the treatment other than the known small risk of endophthalmitis associated with intravitreal injections themselves. Much work is being done on drug delivery systems so as to eventually reduce the number of intravitreal injections required. Ongoing clinical trials continue to evaluate a variety of anti-VEGF agents to treat DME and PDR.

The ophthalmic use of corticosteroids administered either through the periocular or intravitreal routes for the treatment of DME gained widespread use due to early case reports and uncontrolled clinical trials documenting its rapid and often dramatic effect on retinal thickening. Two multicenter randomized prospective clinical trials were undertaken to address both the effectiveness and safety of both routes of steroid administration. Peribulbar steroid injections were found to have no significant benefit for the treatment of DME, but a beneficial effect of limiting retinopathy progression was observed.[446] The 3-year results of the multicenter randomized controlled trial comparing intravitreal steroids to focal laser therapy have shown that despite an initial rapid reduction in retinal thickness and improvement in vision with the intravitreal steroid injection, by 1 year the results were no better than laser photocoagulation, and after 2 years continuing to 3 years, the steroid was inferior to the laser treatment in both visual outcome and retinal thickness.[447,448]

Intravitreal steroid injection was associated with an approximately fourfold increase in the rate of intraocular pressure complications and fourfold increase in need for cataract surgery compared to laser treatment. As seen with peribulbar steroids, intravitreal steroid administration resulted in a 32% relative risk (RR) reduction for retinopathy progression. Interestingly, when used in combination with laser among patients who have already undergone cataract surgery prior to initiating anti-VEGF treatment, vision improvement may be comparable to anti-VEGF agents.[411] Currently, intravitreal steroid alone is not the preferred primary therapy for DME, but it may play a future role in treatment to limit retinopathy progression or in combination with laser among patients who cannot receive anti-VEGF agents or who are pseudophakic before treatment. However, development of cataracts and increases in intraocular pressure may limit its potential benefit.

Control of Systemic Disorders and Effect of Systemic Medications

In addition to the importance of intensive glycemic control in reducing the onset and progression of diabetic retinopathy as discussed earlier, it is critical for the optimal ocular health of diabetic patients that several other systemic considerations be optimized.

Patients with diabetes mellitus commonly suffer from concomitant hypertension. Patients with T1DM have a

17% prevalence of hypertension at baseline and a 25% incidence after 10 years.[448,449] There is a 38% to 68% prevalence in T2DM.[450-452] In most studies, hypertension is correlated to the duration of diabetes, higher HbA_{1c} level, presence of gross proteinuria, and male gender. Elevated BP exacerbates the development and progression of diabetic retinopathy. The risk of PDR is associated with the presence of hypertension at the baseline visit, higher glycosylated hemoglobin levels, and presence of more severe levels of retinopathy at the initial visit.[453] Patients with hypertension are more likely to develop retinopathy, diffuse macular edema, and more severe levels of retinopathy[454-456] and have more rapid progression of retinopathy when compared with diabetic patients who do not have hypertension.[456-458]

The large randomized, prospective UKPDS in 1148 patients with T2DM demonstrated a 34% ($p = 0.0004$) and 47% ($p < 0.004$) reduction in risk of diabetic retinopathy progression and moderate visual acuity loss, respectively, in patients assigned to intensive BP control.[459] These effects were independent of glycemic control, and the risk reductions were similar, regardless of whether the hypertension was controlled with an ACE inhibitor (captopril) or a beta blocker (atenolol). Overall, hypertension appears to be a significant risk factor in the development and progression of diabetic retinopathy and should be rigorously controlled. Until the results of specific trials investigating the BP levels required to minimize end organ damage in patients with diabetes are known,[460] target BP should most likely be maintained as low as safely possible.

Associations between renal and retinal angiopathy are numerous. Proteinuria or microalbuminuria is associated with retinopathy.[461-473] The presence and severity of diabetic retinopathy are indicators of the risk of gross proteinuria,[465,474] and conversely, proteinuria predicts PDR.[463,475,476] Half of all patients with T1DM with PDR and 10 or more years of diabetes have concomitant proteinuria.[461] In T1DM, the prevalence of PDR increases from 7% at onset of microalbuminuria to 29% 4 years after onset of albuminuria as compared with 3% and 8%, respectively, in patients without persistent microalbuminuria.[464] The Appropriate Blood Pressure Control in Diabetes (ABCD) Trial found both the severity and progression of retinopathy were associated with overt albuminuria.[477-479] The presence of gross proteinuria at baseline is associated with 95% increased risk of developing macular edema among patients with T1DM,[453] and dialysis can improve macular edema in diabetic patients with renal failure.[393]

Despite these associations, the frequent coexistence of retinal and renal microangiopathies and factors such as associated hypertension and disease duration can confound these results.[480] Overall, it is important to carefully consider the renal status of any patient with diabetes mellitus and to ensure that the patient is receiving optimal care in this regard. In addition, rapidly progressive retinopathy, especially in a patient with long history of diabetes mellitus and where retinopathy has been previously stable, should suggest the need for renal evaluation.

Low hematocrit was an independent risk factor in the ETDRS analysis of baseline risk factors for development of high-risk PDR and severe vision loss.[481] A cross-sectional study involving 1691 patients revealed a twofold increased risk of any retinopathy in patients with a hemoglobin level less than 12 g/dL as compared to those with a higher hemoglobin concentration using multivariate analyses controlling for serum creatinine, proteinuria, and other factors.[482] In patients with retinopathy, those with low hemoglobin levels have a fivefold increased risk of severe retinopathy compared with those with higher hemoglobin

levels. There have been limited reports of resolution of macular edema and hard exudate with improvement or stabilization of visual acuity in erythropoietin-treated patients after an increase in mean hematocrit.[483] In view of the potential association of low hematocrit and diabetic retinopathy, it is important to ensure that patients with diabetic retinopathy and anemia are receiving appropriate management.

In summary, diabetes is clearly a multisystem disease requiring a comprehensive medical team approach. Even with regard to ocular health, this necessitates the involvement of multiple health care specialists for optimal patient care.

DIABETIC NEPHROPATHY

Diabetic nephropathy remains a major cause of morbidity and death for persons with either T1DM or T2DM. In Western countries, diabetes is the leading single cause of ESRD.[484] Indeed, in many countries such as the United States, more than 50% of patients in renal replacement therapy programs have diabetes as the major cause of their renal failure.[485] However, the full impact of diabetic nephropathy is far greater.[486] Globally most patients with diabetes are in developing countries[487] that do not have the resources or health infrastructure to provide universal renal replacement therapy. Even in developed countries, for every 20 patients with diabetes and chronic kidney disease, less than one will survive to ESRD, succumbing instead to CVD, heart failure, or infection, to which the presence and severity of diabetic renal disease significantly contributes. For example, almost all of the excess in cardiovascular deaths in persons with diabetes younger than 50 years can be attributed to nephropathy.[488] Indeed, in T1DM subjects without nephropathy there is no evidence of premature death.[489] In patients with T2DM, microalbuminuria is associated with a twofold to fourfold increase in the risk of death. In patients with overt proteinuria and hypertension, the risk is even higher.[490] Consequently, the goal to reduce ESRD in patients with diabetes is only one component as part of the overall benefit in preventing diabetic kidney disease.

It is estimated that 25% to 40% of patients with T1DM and 5% to 40% of patients with T2DM ultimately develop diabetic kidney disease.[491,492] Up to 20% of patients with T2DM already have diabetic kidney disease when they are diagnosed with diabetes,[493] and a further 30% to 40% develop diabetic nephropathy, mostly within 10 years of diagnosis.[494] Although nephropathy appears be more common in T1DM, because of the large and increasing number of persons with T2DM,[495] more than 80% of diabetic patients in renal replacement programs have T2DM.

Natural History of Nephropathy in Type 1 Diabetes

Nephropathy and specifically proteinuria in the setting of diabetes have been known for more than 100 years, and the classic structural features of glomerulosclerosis were described more than 70 years ago.[496] However, it is only since the 1980s that the natural history of this condition has been extensively delineated. This is partly because significantly more patients are surviving to see the full presentation of this condition. For example, in 1971, the median survival time of patients with T1DM and overt nephropathy was 5 years, with less than 10% surviving more than 10 years.[497] Consequently, few patients were able to survive the course of their renal disease. By

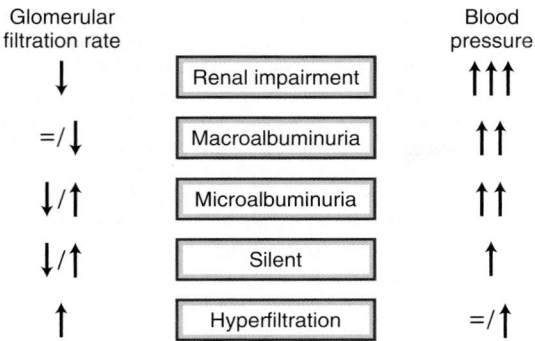

Glomerular filtration rate		Blood pressure
↓	Renal impairment	↑↑↑
=/↓	Macroalbuminuria	↑↑
↓/↑	Microalbuminuria	↑↑
↓/↑	Silent	↑
↑	Hyperfiltration	=/↑

Figure 33-31 The phases (natural history) of diabetic nephropathy.

comparison, in 1996, the median survival in an equivalent population was more than 17 years. Not surprisingly, nearly 10 times more patients with T1DM are now entering ESRD programs.

Diabetic nephropathy is characterized clinically as a triad of hypertension, proteinuria, and, ultimately, renal impairment.[498] The classic five stages of nephropathy as described by Mogensen and colleagues,[499] although not totally accurate, remain the best way of describing this condition (Fig. 33-31). This description relies on functional evaluation of the renal disease and is based on serial measurements of glomerular filtration rate (GFR) and albuminuria.

Stage 1: Hyperfiltration

The initial phase has been termed the *hyperfiltration* phase. It is associated with an elevation of GFR[500] and an increase in capillary glomerular pressure. Although invariably present in animal models of T1DM,[501] an elevation in GFR occurs in only a significant minority of type 1 diabetic patients. Hyperfiltration is considered to occur as a result of concomitant renal hypertrophy[502] as well as being partly due to a range of intrarenal hemodynamic abnormalities that occur in the diabetic milieu that contribute to glomerular hypertension.[503] The pathophysiology of renal hypertrophy associated with diabetes remains unexplained, although specific growth factors such as the growth hormone (GH)/IGF-1 system and TGF-β have been implicated.[504,505] Notably, there is not only glomerular but also tubular hypertrophy. Indeed, the tubular hypertrophy explains the increased kidney weight in diabetes because tubules make up more than 90% of the kidney weight.[506] In addition, increased salt reabsorption associated with proximal tubular hypertrophy can also contribute to glomerular hyperfiltration via tubuloglomerular feedback.[502]

The second explanation for the increase in GFR associated with diabetes relates to hemodynamic changes within the kidney. Although not directly tested in humans, micropuncture studies in rodents, particularly by Brenner's group in the 1980s, revealed that experimental diabetes was associated with a range of intrarenal hemodynamic changes.[503] Alongside hyperfiltration, there is an increase in effective renal plasma flow, and thus some investigators call this the *hyperperfusion-hyperfiltration* phase of diabetic nephropathy. At the same time, increased intraglomerular capillary pressure is increased, reflecting relative efferent versus afferent arteriolar vasoconstriction[503] with activation of the intrarenal renin-angiotensin system and reduced synthesis of the vasodilator NO.

The importance of this hyperfiltration phase as predicting and leading to diabetic nephropathy remains

controversial. Several groups have confirmed the initial relationship between elevated GFR and later development of proteinuria described by Mogensen and Christensen.[507] However, this has not been a universal finding. Nevertheless, subsequent studies with antihypertensive agents, and in particular agents that interrupt the renin-angiotensin system, have shown attenuation of some of these glomerular hemodynamic abnormalities. This provides justification to consider that at least some of these intrarenal hemodynamic changes in diabetes play a role in the development and progression of nephropathy.

Stage 2: The Silent Stage

The next stage is known as the *silent stage,* where, from a clinical point of view, there is no overt evidence of any form of renal dysfunction. Patients usually have normal GFR with no evidence of albuminuria. However, this phase is associated with significant structural changes including basement membrane thickening and mesangial expansion. Indeed, by performing detailed quantitative studies of renal morphology it is often possible to detect those who will develop renal damage.[508] This is a very important phase clinically because it is hoped that investigators will be able to develop new tests, such as biomarkers in plasma or urine or sophisticated assessments from renal biopsy material, to identify which patients will progress to more advanced renal disease. Because overall less than 40% of T1DM subjects will progress, it is critical that we detect those who are the potential progressors and could be candidates for early prevention and treatment strategies to avoid ESRD. As yet, no such surrogate markers or predictors have been identified at this silent phase of the disease.

Extensive studies using various plasma markers such as prorenin[509] or DNA studies to identify certain gene polymorphisms such as the ACE genotype[49] have been promising. The measurement of albumin fragments (ghost albumin) in the urine of patients with diabetes may be another, albeit unproven, approach.[510] Serial prospective ambulatory BP monitoring studies have also demonstrated modest rises in BP in patients in this silent phase up to 5 years before urinary albumin excretion begins to increase.[511] However, none of these markers has been proved to be sensitive or specific enough on further clinical evaluation for widespread clinical application.

This area of research has been recently reinvigorated with reports of effects of deletion of the key enzyme, ACE2,[512] and the impact of the new glucose-lowering drugs, the SGLT2 inhibitors, on intrarenal hemodynamics.[513]

Stage 3: Microalbuminuria

The third phase is known as *microalbuminuria* or the stage of *incipient nephropathy*. At this stage, often 5 to 15 years after the initial diagnosis of T1DM, the urinary albumin excretion rate has increased into the microalbuminuric range of 20 to 200 μg/minute or 30 to 300 mg/24 hours.[514] In the past, microalbuminuria was considered to be a predictor rather than a manifestation of diabetic kidney disease. Increasingly it has been appreciated, particularly when based on interpretation of renal morphologic studies, that in the microalbuminuric phase there is already widespread evidence of advanced glomerular structural changes.[515] Concomitant with these changes, systolic and diastolic BP are increased. Furthermore, the nocturnal dip in BP seen in normal persons is often lost with the development of microalbuminuria.[516] Renal function during this phase may be increased, normal, or reduced.

The best approach to screen for microalbuminuria remains controversial. The original studies used 24-hour or overnight urine sampling methods. However, a spot urine albumin-to-creatinine ratio in an early morning urine specimen has been validated and appears to be a practical option for routine clinical practice.[514] Because the onset of persistent microalbuminuria, if left untreated, is often a reliable harbinger of overt nephropathy,[507] it is incumbent on clinicians to perform serial measurements of this parameter and to repeat the measurement if there is an isolated elevation in urinary albumin excretion.

Studies suggest that in many patients with T1DM, microalbuminuria can be transient and can reverse to normoalbuminuria.[517] Thus, the onset of microalbuminuria does not irrevocably seal the fate of the patient. A study of 386 patients with persistent microalbuminuria showed that regression of microalbuminuria occurred in 58% of patients,[517] although other groups have reported much lower rates of this phenomenon.[518] Notably, in that study, microalbuminuria of short duration, optimal levels of HbA_{1c} (<8%), low systolic BP (<115 mm Hg), and low levels of both cholesterol and triglycerides were independently associated with the regression of microalbuminuria. Therefore, screening of diabetic patients for nephropathy is now recommended to include at least twice-annual measurements of urinary albumin concentrations in T1DM patients.

Stage 4: Macroalbuminuria

The next stage is the macroalbuminuria phase or overt nephropathy. This stage represents the phase that has been previously described as diabetic nephropathy and is highly predictive of subsequent renal failure if left untreated. It is characterized by a urinary albumin excretion rate greater than 300 mg/24 hours (200 µg/minute). This phase usually occurs after 10 to 15 years of diabetes, but the risk of overt renal disease never truly disappears and can appear after 40 or 50 years of T1DM.

There are at least two peaks of incidence of overt nephropathy, and this has been termed by some investigators as representing slow and fast trackers.[519] The key contributors of this marked variation in the timing of onset of proteinuria, independent of glycemia or BP control, remains elusive, although a range of genetic, molecular, and environmental factors have been proposed. In association with this increase in proteinuria, more than two thirds of patients have overt systemic hypertension.[520] During this phase, if left untreated, BP continues to rise, accelerating the decline in GFR, which promotes a further rise in BP, creating a vicious cycle of progressive renal impairment that ultimately leads to ESRD.

Stage 5: Uremia

The final uremic phase, which can occur in up to 40% of T1DM subjects, requires the institution of renal replacement therapy. As recently as the 1970s, patients with diabetes were not considered candidates for renal replacement therapy because of their abysmal prognosis. However, improvements in the management of CVD and renal replacement options have seen the survival on dialysis approach that of patients with renal disease from other causes. Many patients with diabetes and ESRD are also now considered candidates for renal transplantation, which is associated with better outcomes than remaining on dialysis. However, there is evidence that the renal lesions of diabetes often recur in the transplanted kidney, though the lead time to develop ESRD means that few kidneys are lost through recurrent disease.

Increasingly, single pancreas-kidney (SPK) and pancreas-after-kidney (PAK) transplantation have become therapeutic options for patients with T1DM and ESRD, and they appear to offer advantages over kidney-alone transplantation. In particular there is some evidence that maintaining euglycemia following pancreas transplantation can lead to resolution of many diabetes-related renal lesions such as mesangial expansion.[521] This reversal is often not apparent until after 10 years of euglycemia, emphasizing the slow turnover of matrix and the potential long-term effects of hyperglycemic memory in the kidney.

Natural History of Nephropathy in Type 2 Diabetes

The natural history of diabetic nephropathy in patients with T2DM is less well understood than in patients with T1DM. This partly reflects the fact that T2DM is largely a disease of an older population, with associated obesity, hypertension, and dyslipidemia and high rates of CVD that restrict the manifestation of diabetic renal disease. In addition, approximately 7% of patients with T2DM already have microalbuminuria at the time of diagnosis. This may be partly related to the fact that most of these patients have had untreated diabetes for 10 years (on average) before diagnosis. Within 5 years of a diagnosis of T2DM, up to 18% of patients have microalbuminuria, especially those with poor metabolic control and high BP levels. This has led some investigators to suggest that nephropathy in T2DM is different from that seen in patients with T1DM.

However, the natural history of nephropathy in T2DM has more similarities than differences from that seen in T1DM. Hyperfiltration does occur in T2DM,[522] although it has been reported to be less common than in T1DM. This observation must be interpreted with caution, because GFR normally declines with age, and hyperfiltration can still exist although the GFR remains in the normal adult range. Microalbuminuria also occurs in T2DM. However, the finding of microalbuminuria in T2DM might not be as specific for diabetic renal disease as described in the seminal studies in T1DM. In the context of a very high prevalence of CVD, microalbuminuria may be more closely associated with nonrenal events such as stroke and MI.[476] Furthermore, incipient or overt cardiac failure, urinary tract infection, and urinary obstruction (e.g., enlarged prostate) can also lead to microalbuminuria.[503]

Many patients with T2DM and microalbuminuria also progress to overt proteinuria. However, it is increasingly appreciated that the situation has become much more complex, and many groups have now described subjects with T1DM[523] as well as T2DM[524] who develop renal impairment in the absence of significant proteinuria. The exact explanation for this phenomenon is unknown, and ongoing studies are exploring if these patients have different renal morphologic changes from those with the more classic syndrome of diabetic nephropathy: overt proteinuria and declining GFR. Preliminary studies suggest a prominent vascular component for this form of nonproteinuric renal dysfunction. Nonetheless, it appears that the risk of ESRD in patients with T2DM and renal impairment is similar in the presence or absence of microalbuminuria, underlining the importance of an estimated GFR in the management of patients with T2DM. This has led to many of the national and international guidelines now recommending the inclusion of regular measurements of serum creatinine[525] and determination of estimated GFR using a variety of different formulas.

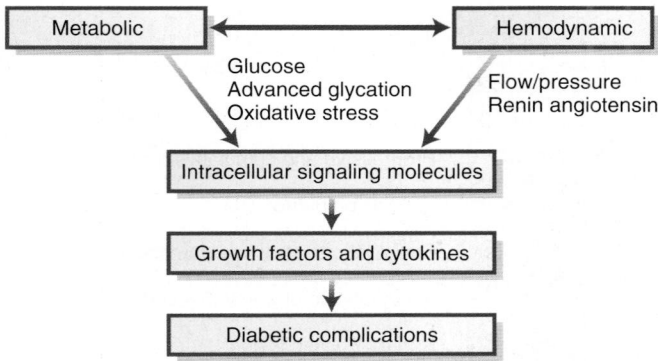

Figure 33-32 Interactions between metabolic and hemodynamic factors in promoting diabetic complications including nephropathy.

Pathogenesis

It is likely that many of the mechanisms implicated in diabetic microvascular complications, in general, play a central role in the development and progression of diabetic nephropathy (Fig. 33-32).[251] It is clearly evident that hyperglycemia is necessary for the initiation of renal injury, because patients without diabetes do not develop this type of nephropathy. Moreover, intensive therapy designed to achieve improved glycemic control is able to attenuate the development of nephropathy, as assessed by urinary albumin excretion, although it is not fully prevented.[335] However, it is now clear that other factors must also be involved because continuous florid hyperglycemia is not necessarily required for diabetic hyperfiltration and kidney growth to occur. Indeed, glomerular hyperfiltration and tubular hypertrophy can persist in patients with T1DM even after euglycemia is achieved through aggressive insulin therapy.[526]

Other pathways that may be involved in diabetic nephropathy include generation of mitochondrial ROS, accumulation of AGEs, and activation of intracellular signaling molecules such as PKC.[251] Many of the seminal studies performed in endothelial cells demonstrating a central role of mitochondrial ROS in activating pathways implicated in diabetic vascular complications have been reproduced in mesangial cells.[527] Advanced glycation, which occurs at an accelerated rate in diabetic patients, is a prominent phenomenon in the kidney. Not only is the kidney the major site for excretion of AGEs, but also many of the proteins with a long life, such as collagen, are extensively glycated in patients with diabetes.[528] Furthermore, various AGE receptors such as RAGE have been described in the kidney, which appear to play a role in mediating some of the deleterious effects of AGEs, such as stimulation of growth factor expression and induction of important phenotypic changes within certain renal cell populations to promote scarring.[192]

Preliminary studies using various approaches to inhibit renal AGE accumulation and action including a soluble RAGE (sRAGE). A range of pharmacologic agents have shown promising results, but clinical translation of these findings remains to be fully defined.[528] Selective PKC isoform inhibitors have been evaluated in small clinical trials but their role in renal disease remains to be confirmed.[316] Some exciting pilot studies evaluating a number of cytosolic sources of oxidative stress, such as NADPH oxidase, suggest that certain NADPH oxidase isoforms such as Nox4 may be excellent targets for new renoprotective therapies.[529] This is strengthened by the advent of orally bioavailable NADPH oxidase inhibitors,[282] which are now under clinical investigation.

In addition to the mechanisms described here, the diabetic kidney appears to be readily modulated by a range of vasoactive hormones. Indeed, it is increasingly appreciated that there may be important interactions between metabolic pathways and various hemodynamic factors including vasoactive hormones such as angiotensin II in mediating renal injury in diabetes (see Fig. 33-32).[530,531] Although many drugs that modulate hormone levels or action might not be specific for diabetic kidney disease, interruption of the renin-angiotensin system appears to be an excellent approach not only for reducing BP but also for correcting many of the cellular, biochemical, hemodynamic, and structural abnormalities seen in the diabetic kidney. These agents appear to be very powerful antiproteinuric agents, although the exact mechanism of action remains to be fully defined. Based on the discovery in the late 1990s that proteinuria in a range of nephropathies could occur as a result of molecular and structural abnormalities in a highly specialized structure known as the slit diaphragm within the glomerular epithelial cell (podocyte), a number of experimental studies, subsequently confirmed in humans, showed that depletion of one of these slit pore proteins, nephrin, could be attenuated or prevented by agents that interrupt the renin-angiotensin system.[532]

In addition to promoting glomerular nephrin depletion, angiotensin II also appears to have other actions that promote the development of proteinuria, including trophic effects on the kidney and increasing glomerular membrane pore size.[533] Although many investigators have focused on the renin-angiotensin system and, in particular, the vasoconstrictor angiotensin II, it is increasingly appreciated that other vasoconstrictors may be important. These include endothelin and a number of vasodilators such as nitric oxide, bradykinin, atrial natriuretic peptide, and vasodilative angiotensins, such as angiotensin 1-7.[534] This exploration of the role of vasoactive hormones and their respective receptors in the diabetic kidney is critical for designing new treatments for this condition, because these pathways are ideal targets for drug development. This point has already been demonstrated for agents that interrupt the renin-angiotensin system, including ACE inhibitors and ARBs.

Pathology

Diabetic renal disease was originally described as a glomerulopathy associated with diffuse or nodular glomerulosclerosis.[496] Subsequent studies using electron microscopy have revealed that glomerular basement membrane thickening and mesangial expansion are prominent glomerular abnormalities in diabetes[508] (Fig. 33-33). Indeed, prospective studies have shown that these changes predict to a certain degree the development of overt renal disease in patients with T1DM. However, fewer than one third of diabetic patients with microalbuminuria have the typical glomerulopathy described by Kimmelstiel and Wilson in 1936.[496,535] Although initial studies emphasized the mesangial cell changes in the glomerulus, glomerular epithelial cell abnormalities represent new areas of active research.[80] Podocyte dysfunction and subsequent apoptosis ultimately leading to depletion of podocytes within the glomerulus appears to play a pivotal role in the development of proteinuria in diabetes.

Although most of the focus has been on glomerular changes in the diabetic kidney, more recent studies have identified important changes in the other sites within the kidney, including the tubules, interstitium, medulla, and

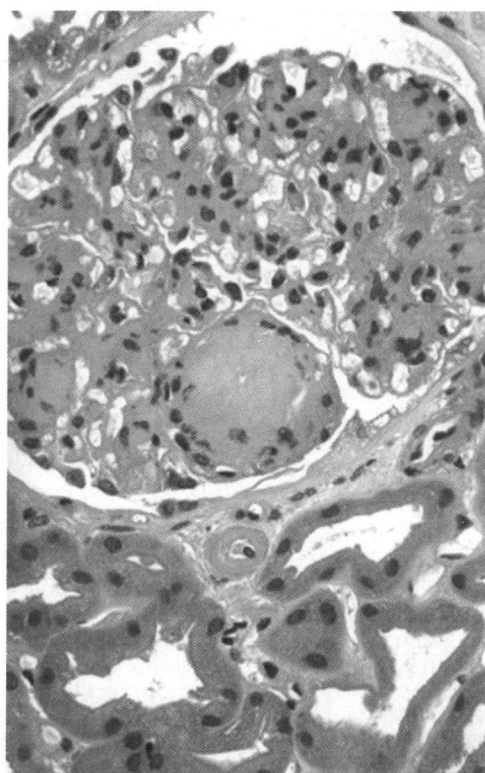

Glomerulopathy

Mesangial expansion

Glomerular hypertension

Diffuse thickening of the GBM

Broadening of foot processes

Podocyte loss

Reduced slit pore proteins

Glomerulomegaly

Kimmelstiel-Wilson lesion

Adhesions to Bowman's capsule

Neovascularization

Nodular and diffuse glomerulosclerosis

Tubulopathy

Tubular hyperplasia and hypertrophy

Progressive and cumulative atrophy

Thickening of the TBM

Epithelial mesenchymal transition

Accumulation of lysosomal bodies

Armani-Ebstein lesion

Reduced tubular brush border

Increased tubular salt reabsorption

Increased Na^+/H^+ antiporter activity

Impaired tubular acidification

Abnormal tubuloglomerular feedback

Decreased endocytosis of protein

Abnormal lysosomal processing

Impaired uptake of organic ions

Figure 33-33 Glomerular and tubular manifestations of diabetic nephropathy. GBM, glomerular basement membrane; TBM, tubular basement membrane.

papilla.[506] *Diabetic tubulopathy* is characterized by a variety of structural and functional changes, including tubulo-epithelial cell hypertrophy, tubular basement membrane thickening, epithelial-mesenchymal transition,[192] and the accumulation of glycogen (see Fig. 33-33). There is also an expansion of the interstitial space with infiltration of various cell types, including myofibroblasts and macrophages.

These tubular changes represent more than just the aftermath of diabetic nephropathy. The dysregulation of tubular functions in diabetes can precede or at least accompany the changes in the renal glomerulus and the onset of albuminuria.[535] Indeed, the functional and structural changes in the proximal tubule may be a key to the contributor to the development and progression of diabetic nephropathy.[506] For example, it has been suggested that tubuloglomerular feedback mechanisms can drive hyperfiltration associated with diabetes[502] and that tubular dysfunction can contribute to albuminuria due to defective uptake and lysosomal processing.[510] Indeed, renal function and prognosis correlate better with structural lesions in the tubules and cortical interstitium than with classic glomerular changes of diabetic nephropathy.

Renal Artery Stenosis

Because diabetic patients have, in general, an increased burden of atherosclerosis, they appear to have a higher risk of renal artery stenosis. However, although angiographic studies have demonstrated a high prevalence of renal artery stenosis in diabetic patients, these lesions are often of no hemodynamic significance. Nevertheless, a small subgroup will have a hemodynamically significant stenosis enhancing hypertension, increasing the risk of acute pulmonary edema, and inducing progressive renal impairment.[536] In such subjects, specific interventions such as

surgery or angioplasty need to be considered.[537] Furthermore, some patients have bilateral renal artery stenosis that, on commencement of an agent such as an ACE inhibitor, can lead to acute renal failure.[538] Fortunately, in most patients, if the renal failure is diagnosed early, cessation of the ACE inhibitor leads to rapid restoration of renal function in this situation.

Renal Papillary Necrosis

Renal papillary necrosis involves a severe destructive process, presumably as a result of ischemia to the medulla and papilla.[539] Beethoven's final illness might have been papillary necrosis in the context of diabetes.[540] The papilla is very sensitive to these ischemic changes because even in the normal setting it is exposed to a relatively hypoxic environment. Concomitant exacerbating factors include urinary tract infection and analgesic abuse. The importance of ischemia and possibly angiotensin II in this disorder has been suggested in experimental studies in transgenic rats that overexpress renin and angiotensin II in their kidney after induction of diabetes.[541] In these rats, diabetes was associated with development of papillary necrosis; development of papillary necrosis was prevented by blockade of the renin-angiotensin system. Clinically, papillary necrosis often manifests as flank pain, hematuria, and fever. Urinalysis reveals red and white blood cells, bacteria, and papillary fragments. Ureteric obstruction can occur as a result of these fragments and must be addressed as an emergency.

Renal Tubular Acidosis

A well-known functional abnormality associated with diabetic tubulopathy is *renal tubular acidosis*, manifesting as hyperkalemia and hyperchloremic metabolic acidosis.[542] This is thought to be a manifestation of hyporeninemic hypoaldosteronism associated with diabetes, resulting in proximal tubule ammonia production reduced to levels inadequate to buffer acid in the distal nephron. The precise causes of this abnormality remain to be established. In some patients there appears to be a defect in the conversion of prorenin to active renin.[543] It has also been suggested that damage to the tubular cells of the juxtaglomerular apparatus associated with diabetes can contribute to impaired renin release, possibly due to reduced renal prostaglandin production and elevated vasopressin levels.[544]

A major risk associated with hyporeninemic hypoaldosteronism is the development of life-threatening hyperkalemia. This is an increasingly important issue with the widespread use of ACE inhibitors and ARBs, often in combination, in this population. This is further exacerbated by the use of potassium-sparing diuretics (such as spironolactone) and beta blockers.

Other Renal Manifestations

Because many diabetic subjects have impaired renal function, they are at high risk for increased renal impairment from certain nephrotoxic agents. One of the most important risks relates to radiocontrast dyes.[545] Where possible, patients with diabetes and renal impairment should avoid imaging studies that involve contrast and, in particular, multiple studies performed in rapid succession. Where intravenous contrast forms an indispensable tool to management, low-osmolality, nonionic, or gadolinium-based contrast media may be less nephrotoxic in patients with

renal failure.[546] It is also critical to ensure that patients who require such procedures are well hydrated before, during, and after the procedure. The role of *N*-acetylcysteine, a thiol-containing antioxidant, shows promise to protect against contrast-induced nephropathy.[547] The oral hypoglycemic drug metformin should also be discontinued before contrast procedures to prevent life-threatening lactic acidosis.

Management

BP and glycemic control represent the major cornerstones for preventing and treating diabetic nephropathy (Figs. 33-34 and 33-35). In the early 1980s a number of Scandinavian researchers found that aggressive BP reduction reduces the rate of progression of diabetic nephropathy,[548,549] and in the 1990s other researchers found that intensified glycemic control has a similar benefit in both T1DM (DCCT)[335] and T2DM (UKPDS) diabetic subjects.[550] These findings have led to the view that optimization of BP and plasma glucose levels should be the mainstay of therapy for diabetic nephropathy.

Glycemic Control

The importance of glucose as a factor in the progression of diabetic kidney disease, as initially suggested from epidemiologic and preclinical studies, was clearly demonstrated in the DCCT study in patients with T1DM.[335] In both the primary and secondary prevention aim of the study, any decrease in HbA$_{1c}$ was strongly associated with a reduction in the risk of development of microalbuminuria as well as

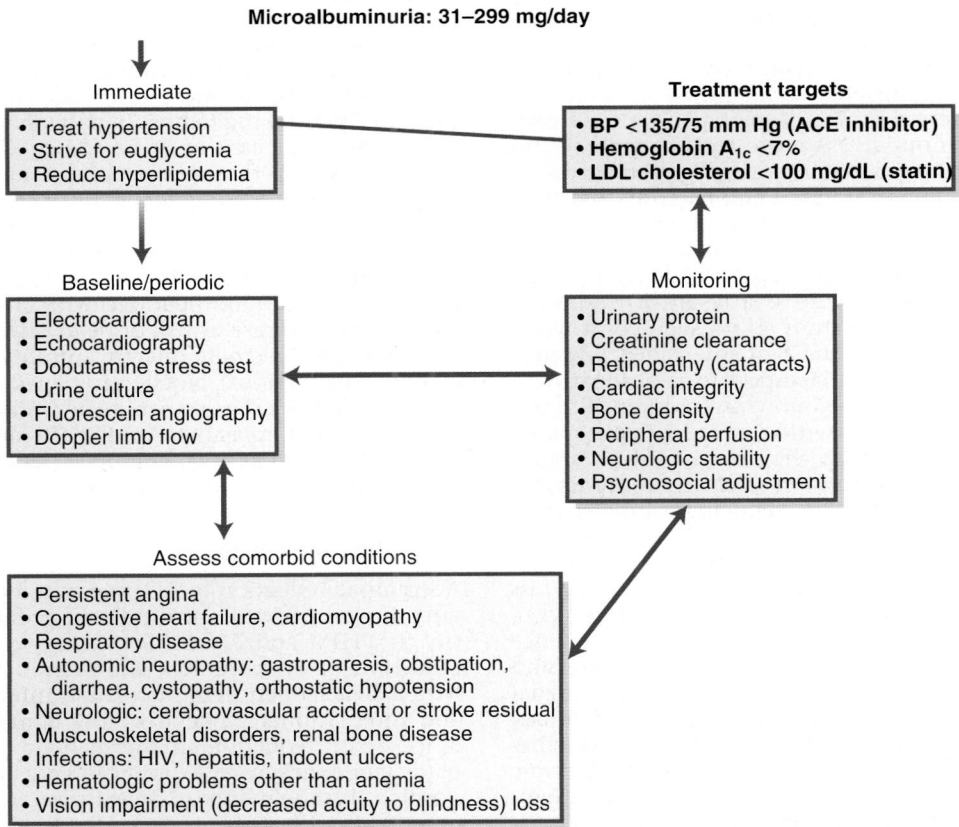

Figure 33-34 Flow chart illustrating the management of diabetic nephropathy before the onset of renal failure. ACE, angiotensin-converting enzyme; BP, blood pressure; HIV, human immunodeficiency virus; LDL, low-density lipoprotein.

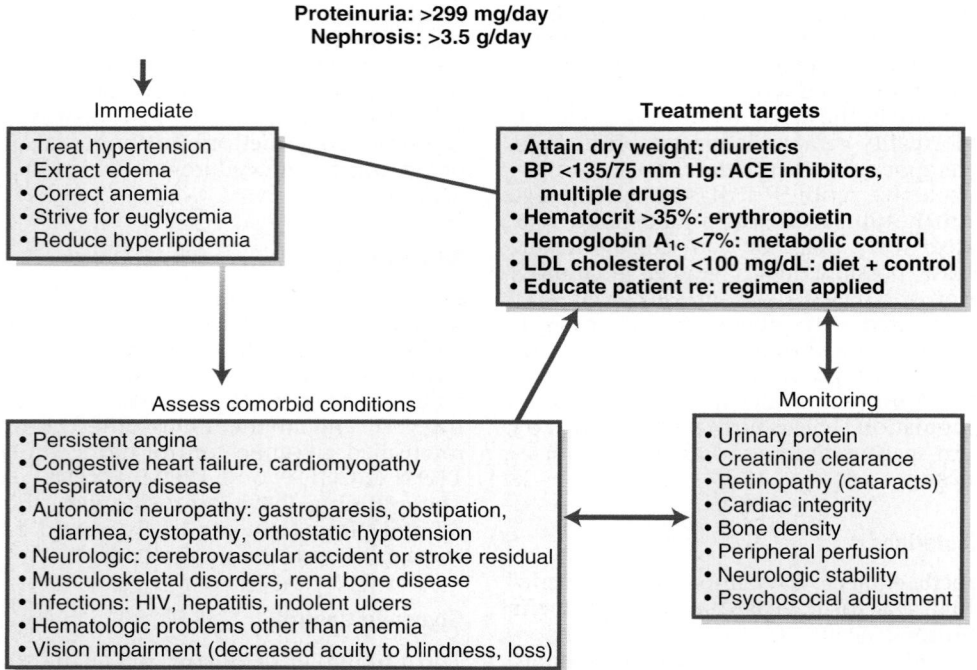

Figure 33-35 Flow chart illustrating the management of diabetic nephropathy after the onset of clinical proteinuria. ACE, angiotensin-converting enzyme; BP, blood pressure; HIV, human immunodeficiency virus; LDL, low-density lipoprotein.

a decrease in the risk of progression to overt nephropathy. The follow-up EDIC study has confirmed long-lasting benefits of this therapeutic approach. The UKPDS clearly demonstrated a role for intensified glycemic control in newly diagnosed T2DM subjects when treatment led to a reduction in HbA$_{1c}$ from 7.9 to 7.0%.[5] The ADVANCE study has demonstrated that a further reduction of HbA$_{1c}$ to an average of 6.5% was associated with a further reduction in renal events, as assessed by the development and progression of microalbuminuria.[551] A more recent report of this study[552] has demonstrated that intensified glycemic control reduced the development of ESRD, emphasizing that tight glycemic control continues to confer renal benefits even in the setting of more advanced renal disease. Thus, despite the ongoing controversy as to the appropriate HbA$_{1c}$ target to reduce macrovascular disease as a result of the recent findings from the ACCORD study,[553] no such controversy as to a possible deleterious effect of intensified glycemic control has been reported with respect to nephropathy.

It remains to be determined how useful intensification of glycemic control is in the setting of overt nephropathy as a last-ditch strategy to delay the onset of ESRD. Aggressive management of hypertension is clearly more important than glycemic control in reducing cardiovascular events and slowing renal disease progression at this stage of relatively advanced disease, although some studies suggest that poor glycemic control can accelerate the loss of renal function in diabetic nephropathy.[550] However, a number of large studies have failed to show any evidence that strict glycemic control per se retards renal progression once overt nephropathy is present.[554] In addition, as renal function fails, tight glycemic control becomes more hazardous, with an increased risk of hypoglycemia. Nonetheless, because there is sufficient evidence that glycemic control can reduce both macrovascular events and microvascular complications of diabetes at other sites, it is reasonable to suggest that optimization of metabolic control in patients with overt nephropathy remains worthwhile.

Similar benefits on renal disease in the context of T2DM are seen following optimization of glycemic control.[5] However, the choice of agent remains controversial. Certainly, several types of drugs are able improve glycemic control in the patients with T2DM; however, the particular advantages of one class over another for preventing and treating diabetic nephropathy remain to be established.

A number of differences in the side effect profiles should influence prescribing habits. In patients with renal impairment, particular care must be exercised in selecting and dosing oral diabetic therapy because an accumulation of either the drug or active metabolites can lead to hypoglycemia (e.g., with glyburide) and other serious adverse effects such as lactic acidosis (with metformin). Thiazolidinediones, such as pioglitazone and rosiglitazone, should be used with caution in patients with advanced nephropathy who have or are at risk of heart failure.

Other agents that directly inhibit glucose-induced changes in various biochemical pathways will likely become available. These include benfotiamine, a thiamine alternative that appears to inhibit the downstream effects of mitochondrial ROS generation,[555] and various antiglycation strategies,[556] as outlined previously.

Blood Pressure Control

A sustained reduction in BP appears to be the most important single intervention to prevent progressive nephropathy in T1DM and T2DM. For example, in the UKPDS, a reduction in BP from 154 to 144 mm Hg was associated with a 30% reduction in microalbuminuria.[459] All national and international guidelines now emphasize the importance of BP reduction in the diabetic patient. Although many guidelines suggest specific targets should be achieved, no such threshold appears to exist for any renal end point in patients with diabetes. In particular, the risk of progressive diabetic nephropathy continues to decrease, with BP reductions into the normal range and below, meaning that the lowest achievable BP is associated with the best clinical outcomes. This is particularly important in those with the greatest risk of renal damage, patients with overt nephropathy. In these patients, it has been suggested that optimal BP control is less than 125/75 mm Hg.[557] Indeed, in the recent subanalysis from the BP arm of the ADVANCE study, no BP threshold was detected. Specifically, in those subjects in whom achieved BP was reduced to levels even lower than currently recommended in national and international guidelines, there was a further decrease in renal events.[558] Thus, it is possible that if individuals can tolerate lower BPs without major side effects such as dizziness and syncope it may be worth considering treating some T2DM subjects to BP levels below those currently recommended.

There is good evidence that tight BP control, no matter how it was achieved, is associated with a significant reduction in the risk of microalbuminuria (primary prevention). Although BP reduction appears paramount, there is also evidence that ACE inhibitors[559] have renoprotective actions beyond their antihypertensive effects for primary prevention.[560-562] However, if treatment should commence in the normoalbuminuric stage, such a strategy would involve treating the majority of patients who are not at risk of nephropathy. Ideally, it would be useful to be able to identify patients, still normoalbuminuric, whose likelihood of progression is increased. As yet no such markers of predisposition to renal disease are available, although serum prorenin[509] and modest elevations in urinary albumin excretion albeit still within the normal range (borderline microalbuminuria)[517] might ultimately be such markers.

The issue of primary prevention has recently been readdressed in two studies in which subjects with normoalbuminuria were treated with agents that interrupt the renin-angiotensin system. In the first smaller trial, which included the performance of sequential renal biopsies, no benefit of early institution of either the ACE enalapril or the angiotensin II receptor antagonist losartan was observed, as defined not only as a lack of effect on albuminuria but also no significant retardation in progression of renal morphologic injury.[563] In the second, much larger trial known as the DIRECT study, the angiotensin II antagonist candesartan, despite some modest retinoprotective effects, had no major impact on reducing the new onset of microalbuminuria.[563]

In secondary prevention studies, the additional benefits achieved from blocking the renin-angiotensin system are clearer.[564] A meta-analysis incorporating the findings of more than 10 studies in patients with microalbuminuria has demonstrated the ability of ACE inhibitors not only to retard the development of overt proteinuria but also to decrease urinary albumin excretion by more than 30%. In some patients with microalbuminuria, ACE inhibition can reduce urinary albumin excretion into the normoalbuminuric range.[560] In patients with T1DM and overt proteinuria, aggressive BP reduction reduced proteinuria by up to 50% and retarded the rate of decline in renal function.[548,549]

Similar studies have been performed in T2DM patients. Two landmark trials, RENAAL (Reduction in Endpoints in patients with Non–insulin-dependent diabetes mellitus with the Angiotensin II Antagonist Losartan) and IDNT (Irbesartan in Diabetic Nephropathy Trial), examined the renoprotective effects of the ARBs losartan and irbesartan, respectively.[565,566] In both studies, when compared to various alternative antihypertensive agents such as calcium antagonists (but not ACE inhibitors), ARB treatment was associated with a reduction in end-stage renal failure, a greater than 30% decrease in proteinuria, and a major reduction in hospitalization for heart failure. As a result of these studies, ARBs are recommended as first-line treatment for BP reduction in T2DM patients with overt proteinuria.[567]

Although ACE inhibitors have not been as extensively studied in this population, the recently reported DETAIL (Diabetics Exposed to Telmisartan And EnalaprIL) trial suggested similar renoprotective actions of both drug classes.[568] Similar findings comparing the angiotensin II antagonist telmisartan to the ACE inhibitor, ramipril, are also reported in the much larger ONTARGET study, albeit that trial was not performed exclusively in diabetic subjects.[569] Thus, from a clinical perspective, no clear difference between these two drug classes has been identified. (The one exception is cough, which occurs in 5% to 30% of patients taking ACE inhibitors, depending on ethnicity [higher in Asian subjects].) In microalbuminuric T2DM subjects, ARBs have also been demonstrated to have a role. For example, in the IRMA2 (IRbesartan MicroAlbuminuria type 2) trial, irbesartan dose-dependently reduced the risk of development of macroproteinuria,[570] confirming the findings seen predominantly with ACE inhibitors in microalbuminuric T1DM subjects.[560]

Another approach to inhibit the renin-angiotensin system has involved the use of the recently introduced renin inhibitors such as aliskiren. For example, in the AVOID study in T2DM subjects[571] this agent appeared to have an additional effect on albuminuria when administered with the angiotensin II antagonist losartan. Unfortunately, as reported in the ALTITUDE study[572] aliskiren has failed to demonstrate superior cardiovascular or renal protection, and thus this approach of add-on renin inhibition is not recommended. Other approaches focusing on BP reduction continue to be examined in these populations. This includes mineralocorticoid receptor antagonists such as spironolactone[573] and the more selective agent eplerenone, which has fewer antiandrogenic side effects.[574] Furthermore, a number of agents, at various stages of preclinical and early clinical development, are under investigation, including endothelin antagonists and vasopeptidase (dual ACE/NEP) inhibitors.[575]

Other Approaches

Low-protein diets (0.75 g/kg per day) have been shown to retard the progression of renal disease, although the data are not totally convincing for diabetic nephropathy per se. A meta-analysis of five studies in T1DM subjects supported a minor renoprotective role for these diets,[576] but this has not been a universal finding.[577] There are even fewer data in T2DM subjects with overt nephropathy.[578] However, the expected benefits that can be achieved through protein restriction in patients with diabetic nephropathy are at best modest in comparison with adequate BP control and blockade of the renin-angiotensin system. Moreover, the nutritional impact of such interventions must be carefully considered, particularly in patients with brittle glycemic control.

The role of lipid-lowering agents as renoprotective drugs remains controversial. Although in rodents a large body of evidence suggests that lipids promote renal injury and that various lipid-lowering drugs reduce nephropathy, even in the setting of no or minimal effect on lipids,[579] the data in humans are variable.[580] However, in a study of fenofibrate in T2DM, there was an impressive reduction in albuminuria.[581] Furthermore, in the Heart Protection Study, simvastatin appeared to retard the decline in renal function, although this analysis was not confined to the diabetic subgroup.[582] Another group has also reported a potential renoprotective effect of a statin,[583] although this effect has not been observed in all studies. Nevertheless, because

CVD is so prominent in diabetic patients, particularly those with incipient or overt renal disease, lipid-lowering treatment should be considered in most patients independent of its putative renoprotective actions.[584]

Other approaches to consider include correction of anemia with agents such as erythropoietin.[585] The role of these agents as renoprotective drugs remains to be clarified,[586] but the potential benefits on general patient well-being and in reducing left ventricular hypertrophy[587] provide a rationale for using such agents judiciously in diabetic patients. However, the recently reported TREAT study, although focusing on cardiovascular events and mortality using the erythropoietin analogue darbopoietin, has not shown darbopoietin to be renoprotective, and the drug was unfortunately associated with a twofold increase in cerebrovascular events.[588]

Over the past few years, several clinical trials targeting diabetic nephropathy with novel agents have yielded disappointing results. For example, PKC-β inhibition with ruboxistaurin, which had renal benefits in experimental diabetes, failed to show any major benefits on albuminuria in T2DM subjects.[589] Another promising agent, sulodexide, postulated to restore the glomerular charge by repleting the loss of glycosaminoglycans[590] and thereby act as an antiproteinuric and ultimately renoprotective drug, also failed to demonstrate any evidence of renoprotection in several large trials. An endothelin antagonist, avosentan, was assessed in the ASCEND trial.[591] Although this drug was associated with impressive reductions in albuminuria, the associated side effect of fluid retention has reduced the current level of enthusiasm for this agent. However, another endothelin antagonist, avosentan, appears to have fewer side effects and is also antiproteinuric[592] and thus remains in clinical development. Finally, bardoxolone, an agonist of the transcription factor Nrf2, which appears to act as an antioxidant, has been investigated in T2DM subjects with impaired renal function. In the initial BEAM trial[593] an improvement in renal function was reported. However, recently a larger study in T2DM subjects with stage 4 chronic kidney disease was prematurely terminated because of increased cardiovascular events.[594]

Treatment of the Diabetic Uremic Patient

Renal impairment in a patient with diabetes necessitates changes in therapy. Often blood glucose control becomes more brittle because the half-life of insulin is prolonged and the renal response to hypoglycemia is impaired. High swinging blood glucose levels in a patient with nephropathy can often mistakenly lead to an increase in oral therapy. However, in patients with renal impairment, particular care must be exercised in the selection and dosing of oral hypoglycemic therapy. Nonsteroidal anti-inflammatory drugs (NSAIDs) and cyclooxgenase-2 (COX-2) inhibitors should be avoided when possible because their use is associated with inadequate BP control, often as a result of reduced efficacy of antihypertensive drug therapy. Patients at high risk for progressive deterioration in their renal function should be considered for an early referral to a nephrology service for management of renal failure (Fig. 33-36). This facilitates access to erythropoietin and control of calcium phosphate balance and to planning for renal replacement therapy with the preemptive placement of access catheters and lines. Delay in referral can result in a more precipitous start to renal replacement and usually a bad prognostic outcome.[595]

Many options are now available for the diabetic patient requiring renal replacement therapy.[596] These include home or facility hemodialysis, peritoneal dialysis, renal transplantation (cadaveric or living related), or combined

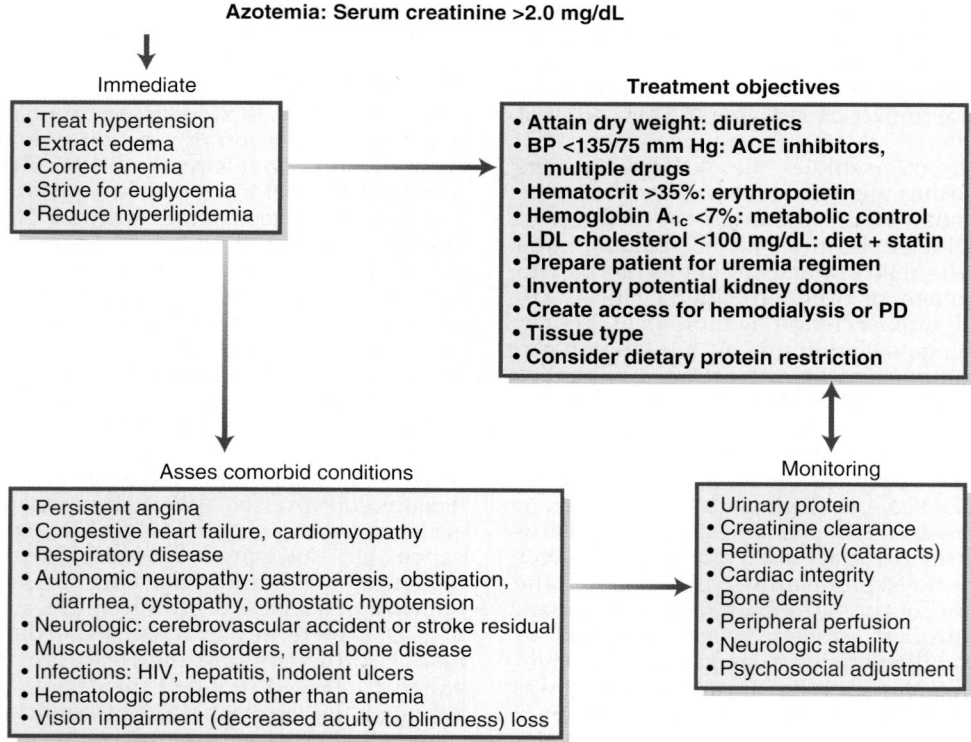

Azotemia: Serum creatinine >2.0 mg/dL

Immediate
- Treat hypertension
- Extract edema
- Correct anemia
- Strive for euglycemia
- Reduce hyperlipidemia

Treatment objectives
- **Attain dry weight: diuretics**
- **BP <135/75 mm Hg: ACE inhibitors, multiple drugs**
- **Hematocrit >35%: erythropoietin**
- **Hemoglobin A$_{1c}$ <7%: metabolic control**
- **LDL cholesterol <100 mg/dL: diet + statin**
- **Prepare patient for uremia regimen**
- **Inventory potential kidney donors**
- **Create access for hemodialysis or PD**
- **Tissue type**
- **Consider dietary protein restriction**

Asses comorbid conditions
- Persistent angina
- Congestive heart failure, cardiomyopathy
- Respiratory disease
- Autonomic neuropathy: gastroparesis, obstipation, diarrhea, cystopathy, orthostatic hypotension
- Neurologic: cerebrovascular accident or stroke residual
- Musculoskeletal disorders, renal bone disease
- Infections: HIV, hepatitis, indolent ulcers
- Hematologic problems other than anemia
- Vision impairment (decreased acuity to blindness) loss

Monitoring
- Urinary protein
- Creatinine clearance
- Retinopathy (cataracts)
- Cardiac integrity
- Bone density
- Peripheral perfusion
- Neurologic stability
- Psychosocial adjustment

Figure 33-36 Flow chart illustrating the management of diabetic nephropathy after onset of renal failure. ACE, angiotensin-converting enzyme; BP, blood pressure; HIV, human immunodeficiency virus; LDL, low-density lipoprotein; PD, peritoneal dialysis.

TABLE 33-6

Options in Therapy for End-Stage Renal Disease in Diabetic Patients

Variable	Peritoneal Dialysis	Hemodialysis	Kidney Transplantation
Extensive extrarenal disease	No limitation	No limitation except for hypotension	Excluded in cardiovascular insufficiency
Geriatric patients		No limitation	Arbitrary exclusion as determined by program
Complete rehabilitation	Rare, if ever	Very few patients	Common as long as graft functions
Death rate	Much higher than for nondiabetic patients	Much higher than for nondiabetic patients	About the same as for nondiabetic patients
First-year survival rate	~75%	~75%	>90%
Morbidity during first year	~15 days in hospital	~12 days in hospital	Weeks to months hospitalized
Survival to second decade	Almost never	<5%	~1 in 5
Progression of complications	Usual and unremitting; hyperglycemia and hyperlipidemia	Usual and unremitting; might benefit from metabolic control	Interdicted by functioning pancreas plus kidney; partially ameliorated by correction of azotemia
Special advantage	Can be self-performed; avoids swings in solute and level of intravascular volume	Can be self-performed; efficient extraction of solute and water in hours	Cures uremia; freedom to travel
Disadvantages	Peritonitis; hyperinsulinemia; hyperglycemia, hyperlipidemia; long hours of treatment; more days hospitalized than with either hemodialysis or transplantation	Blood access a hazard for clotting, hemorrhage, and infection; cyclic hypotension, weakness, aluminum toxicity, amyloidosis	Cosmetic disfigurement, hypertension, personal expense for cytotoxic drugs; induced malignancy; HIV (human immunodeficiency virus) transmission
Patient acceptance	Variable, usual compliance with passive tolerance for regimen	Variable; often noncompliant with dietary, metabolic, or antihypertensive components of regimen	Enthusiastic during periods of good renal allograft function; exalted when pancreas proffers euglycemia
Relative cost	Most expensive over long run	Less expensive than kidney transplantation in the first year; subsequent years more expensive	Pancreas plus kidney engraftment most expensive uremia therapy for diabetics; after first year, kidney transplantation alone is lowest cost option

pancreas-kidney transplantation. Most patients choose hemodialysis rather than peritoneal dialysis, although data conflict regarding which approach leads to better survival (Table 33-6). Some patients opt for withdrawal of treatment because their quality of life, with advanced CVD, visual impairment, and amputations, is poor.

The Burden of Nephropathy

One must never consider renal disease in a diabetic patient in isolation. Proteinuria per se is strongly associated with other complications such as macrovascular disease, heart failure, and retinopathy, and treatments directed toward one complication may be useful for the other complications. Indeed, intensified glycemic control has been shown to be particularly useful for other microvascular complications,[4] and the various antihypertensive regimens, particularly those using agents that interrupt the renin-angiotensin system, also confer important cardiovascular benefits such as reducing heart failure.[565] Thus, as clearly expounded in the Steno-2 study, the multifactorial approach in microalbuminuric subjects will not only lead to renal benefits but will also confer other advantages to the diabetic patient.[597] Because those with renal disease have the greatest risk for nonrenal complications, it stands to reason that they also are likely to have the greatest absolute benefit from risk-reduction strategies.

DIABETIC NEUROPATHIES

Diabetic neuropathies are a heterogeneous group of disorders that cause a wide range of clinical abnormalities. They are among the most common long-term complications of diabetes and are a significant cause of morbidity and fatality.[598,599] Estimates of the prevalence of neuropathy vary substantially, depending on specific diagnostic criteria.[600,601] In the United States, prevalence estimates have ranged from 5% to 100%.[598,600-603] In Pirart's classic study of a cohort of 4400 diabetic patients, prevalence was found to reach approximately 45% after 25 years.[604] Using this estimate, about 7 million persons in the United States alone have diabetic neuropathy, and about 2.7 million have painful neuropathy.[605] Furthermore, it is now evident that neuropathy can occur with impaired glucose tolerance[606] and with the metabolic syndrome in the absence of hyperglycemia.[607] It is the most common form of neuropathy in the developed countries of the world; it accounts for more hospitalizations than all the other diabetic complications combined; and it is responsible for 50% to 75% of nontrauma amputations.[602,603] Though rates of lower extremity amputation among Medicare-enrolled diabetics have decreased by 28.8% between 2000 and 2010,[608] the cost of caring for neuropathy complications has not decreased because of delay in diagnosis.[609] Diabetic peripheral neuropathy is also responsible for weakness and ataxia, with an estimated increase in likelihood of falling that is 15 times that of the unaffected population.[610,611]

Diabetic neuropathy is a set of clinical syndromes that affect distinct regions of the nervous system, singly or combined. Clinical signs and symptoms can be nonspecific and insidious, and progression can be slow. Neuropathy can be silent and go undetected while exercising its ravages, or it can manifest with clinical symptoms and signs that mimic those seen in many other diseases. It is, therefore, diagnosed by exclusion. Of patients attending a diabetes clinic, 25% volunteered symptoms, but 50% were found to have neuropathy after a simple clinical test such as eliciting the ankle reflex or vibration perception test. Unfortunately both endocrinologists and nonendocrinologists have not been trained to recognize the condition, and even when diabetic neuropathy is symptomatic, less than one third of physicians recognize the cause or discuss this with their patients.[612]

Almost 90% tested positive on sophisticated tests of autonomic function or peripheral sensation.[613] Neuropathy is grossly underdiagnosed by endocrinologists and nonendocrinologists.[612] Neurologic complications occur equally in T1DM and T2DM and additionally in various forms of acquired diabetes.[601]

The major morbidity associated with somatic neuropathy is foot ulceration, the precursor of gangrene and limb loss. Neuropathy increases the risk of amputation 1.7-fold overall, 12-fold if there is deformity (itself a consequence of neuropathy), and 36-fold if there is a history of previous ulceration.[614] There were about 65,700 amputations performed in the United States in 2006 secondary to diabetes,[615] and neuropathy is the major contributor in 87% of cases.[599] It has tremendous negative effects on the quality of life of persons with diabetes.[616] Once autonomic neuropathy is present, life can become quite dismal, and the mortality rate approximates 25% to 50% within 5 to 10 years.[617-620] The presence of neuropathy can severely affect quality of life, causing impaired activities of daily living, compromised physical functioning, and depression.[616,621] Impairment of physical functioning is associated with a 15-fold increase in the likelihood of falling and fractures, particularly in older diabetics.[622] Depression complicates the management of neuropathic pain and is a predictor of progression of neuropathy.[621]

Classification

Diabetic peripheral neuropathy (DPN) is a common late complication of diabetes. It results in a variety of syndromes for which there is no universally accepted classification. Such neuropathies are generally subdivided into focal/multifocal neuropathies, including diabetic amyotrophy, and symmetric polyneuropathies, including diabetic sensorimotor polyneuropathy (DSPN). The latter is the most common type, affecting about 30% of diabetic patients in hospital care and 25% of those in the community.[605,623] DPN has been recently defined as a symmetric, length-dependent DSPN attributable to metabolic and microvascular alterations as a result of chronic hyperglycemia exposure (diabetes) and cardiovascular risk covariates.[624] Its onset is generally insidious, and without treatment the course is chronic and progressive. The loss of small-fiber–mediated sensation results in the loss of thermal and pain perception, whereas large-fiber impairment results in loss of touch and vibration perception. Sensory-fiber involvement may also result in positive symptoms, such as paresthesias and pain. Nonetheless, up to 50% of neuropathic patients can be asymptomatic. DPN can be associated with the involvement of the autonomic nervous system (i.e., diabetic autonomic neuropathy that rarely causes severe symptoms),[625,626] but in its cardiovascular form is definitely associated with at least a threefold increased risk for death.[627-629] More recently, diabetic autonomic neuropathy or even autonomic imbalance between the sympathetic and the parasympathetic nervous systems has been implicated as a predictor of cardiovascular risk.[628,629]

Diabetic neuropathy is not a single entity but a number of different syndromes with subclinical or clinical manifestations, depending on the classes of nerve fibers involved. According to the San Antonio Convention,[630] the main groups of neurologic disturbances in diabetes mellitus include the following:
- Subclinical neuropathy, which is determined by abnormalities in electrodiagnostic and quantitative sensory testing
- Diffuse clinical neuropathy with distal symmetric sensorimotor and autonomic syndromes
- Focal syndromes

Subclinical neuropathy is diagnosed on the basis of abnormal electrodiagnostic tests with decreased nerve conduction velocity (NCV) or decreased amplitudes; abnormal quantitative sensory tests (QST) for vibration, tactile, thermal warming, and cooling thresholds; and quantitative autonomic function tests (QAFTs) revealing diminished heart rate variation with deep breathing, Valsalva maneuver, and postural testing. The importance of the skin biopsy as a diagnostic tool for diabetic polyneuropathy is now firmly established; it may be particularly useful in subjects with a small-fiber neuropathy phenotype.[607,631] The different clinical presentations of diabetic neuropathy are schematically illustrated in Figure 33-37.

Natural History

The natural history of neuropathies separates them into two distinct entities: those that progress gradually with increasing duration of diabetes and those that remit, usually completely. Sensory and autonomic neuropathies typically progress. Although the symptoms of mononeuropathies, radiculopathies, and acute painful neuropathies are severe, they are short-lived, and patients tend to recover.[632]

Progression of neuropathy is related to glycemic control in both T1DM and T2DM.[4,39] The most rapid deterioration of nerve function occurs soon after the onset of T1DM, and within 2 to 3 years the rate of progression slows. In contrast, in T2DM, slowing of NCVs may be one of the earliest neuropathic abnormalities and often is present even at diagnosis.[633] After diagnosis, slowing of NCV usually progresses at a steady rate of approximately 1 m/second per year, and the level of impairment is positively correlated with duration of diabetes. Although in most studies, symptomatic patients are more likely to have slower NCVs than patients without symptoms, NCVs do not relate to the severity of symptoms. In a long-term follow-up study of T2DM patients,[634] the prevalence of electrophysiologic abnormalities in the lower limb increased from 8% at baseline to 42% after 10 years.

A decrease in sensory and motor amplitudes, indicating axonal destruction, is more pronounced than the slowing of the NCVs. An increase of about 2 points in an 80-point clinical scale can be expected per year. These scales contain information on motor, sensory, and autonomic signs and symptoms. Using objective measures of sensory function, such as the vibration perception threshold test, the rate of decline in function has been reported to be 1 to 2 vibration units per year. However, this rate of evolution may be declining. For example, in a study of nerve growth factor (NGF), the vibration perception threshold in the placebo group was identical to that in the treatment group at the beginning of the study and at the end of 1 year.[635,636]

Host factors pertaining to general health and nerve nutrition are changing. This is particularly important in studies on the treatment of diabetic neuropathy, which have always relied on differences between drug treatment and placebo and have apparently been successful because of the decline in placebo-treated patients.[637] Based on the

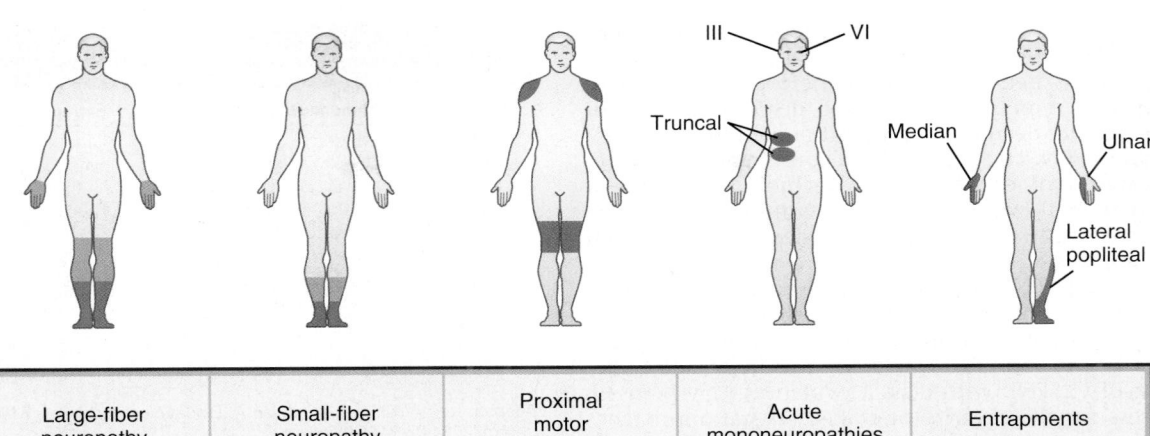

Large-fiber neuropathy	Small-fiber neuropathy	Proximal motor neuropathy	Acute mononeuropathies	Entrapments
Sensory loss: 0→+++ (touch, vibration) Pain: +→+++ Tendon reflex: N→↓↓↓ Motor deficit: 0→+++	Sensory loss: 0→+ (thermal, allodynia) Pain: +→+++ Tendon reflex: N→↓ Motor deficit: 0	Sensory loss: 0→+ Pain: +→+++ Tendon reflex: ↓↓ Proximal motor deficit: +→+++	Sensory loss: 0→+ Pain: +→+++ Tendon reflex: N Motor deficit: +→+++	Sensory loss in nerve distribution: +→+++ Pain: +→+ Tendon reflex: N Motor deficit: +→+++

Figure 33-37 Clinical presentations of diabetic neuropathies. (Modified from Pickup J, Williams G, eds. *Textbook of Diabetes*, Vol 1. Oxford, UK: Blackwell Scientific, 1997.)

earlier estimates of change, clinically meaningful loss of vibration perception and conduction velocity was estimated to take at least 3 years, dictating the need for studies to be carried out over a longer period.

It is also important to recognize that diabetic neuropathy is a disorder in which the prevailing abnormality is a loss of axons that electrophysiologically translates to a reduction in the amplitude and not the velocity of conduction. Changes in NCV might not be an appropriate means of monitoring progress or deterioration of nerve function. It has always been assumed that diabetes affects the longest fibers first—hence, the increased predisposition in taller persons.[638] Now it seems that small-fiber involvement can herald the onset of neuropathy and even diabetes. Small-fiber function is not detectable by standard electrophysiology and requires measurement of sensory, neurovascular, and autonomic thresholds and cutaneous nerve fiber density.[607,639-641] There are few data on the longitudinal trends in small-fiber dysfunction, although it appears that the nerve fiber loss in prediabetic neuropathy might respond to lifestyle changes.[642]

Much remains to be learned about the natural history of diabetic autonomic neuropathy. Karamitsos and colleagues[643] have reported that the progression of diabetic autonomic neuropathy is significant during the 2 years following its discovery. The mortality rate for patients with diabetic autonomic neuropathy has been estimated to be 44% within 2.5 years after diagnosis of symptomatic autonomic neuropathy in a group of T1DM patients.[617] A meta-analysis[644] revealed that the mortality rate after 5.8 years of diabetes with symptomatic autonomic neuropathy was 29%. In a meta-analysis of 12 published studies, reduced cardiovascular function as measured by heart rate variability was shown to be associated with an increased risk of silent MI.[620]

Similarly, a meta-analysis of prospective studies demonstrated increased mortality rate in patients with cardiac autonomic neuropathy, with the risk ratio increasing in direct proportion to the number of autonomic abnormalities.[619,620] The RR of mortality from 15 studies (N = 2900) was increased in patients with cardiac autonomic neuropa-

thy by 2.14 (95% confidence interval [CI], 1.83 to 2.51).[620] However, if cardiac autonomic neuropathy is defined by the presence of at least two abnormal autonomic function tests, this risk increased to 3.45 (95% CI, 2.66 to 4.47).[619] Probably the greatest justification for carrying out autonomic function tests resides in their predictive capacity for subsequent cardiovascular events and unexplained sudden death. In the ACCORD study, there was a significant increase in mortality rate in the intensively treated arm of glycemic control. Analysis of the hazard risk of mortality revealed an increase of up to 2.5 with loss of heart rate variability. If symptoms of neuropathy such as numbness were included, the risk rose to 4.33.[628] This is a cogent argument for identifying people at risk and tailoring the management of diabetes accordingly, as well as a serious consideration for study designs estimating cardiovascular risk or benefit for the future.

Clinical Presentation

An international consensus meeting on the outpatient diagnosis and management of diabetic neuropathy agreed on the following as a simple definition of diabetic neuropathy: "the presence of symptoms and/or signs of peripheral nerve dysfunction in people with diabetes after the exclusion of other causes."[645,646] It was also agreed that neuropathy cannot be diagnosed without a careful clinical examination; absence of symptoms cannot be equated with absence of neuropathy, because asymptomatic neuropathy is common. The American Diabetes Association (ADA) has endorsed these recommendations.[647] The importance of excluding nondiabetic causes was emphasized in the Rochester Diabetic Neuropathy Study, in which up to 10% of peripheral neuropathy in diabetic patients was deemed to be of nondiabetic cause.[601] Many conditions need to be excluded before the diagnosis of diabetic neuropathy can be made.[599] The Toronto Consensus panel was convened in 2009 and redefined minimal criteria for the diagnosis of typical diabetic neuropathy:[624]

1. Possible DSPN. The presence of symptoms or signs of DSPN may include the following: symptoms—decreased

sensation, positive neuropathic sensory symptoms (e.g., "asleep numbness," prickling or stabbing, burning or aching pain) predominantly in the toes, feet, or legs; or signs—symmetric decrease of distal sensation or unequivocally decreased or absent ankle reflexes.

2. Probable DSPN. The presence of a combination of symptoms and signs of neuropathy including any two or more of the following: neuropathic symptoms, decreased distal sensation, or unequivocally decreased or absent ankle reflexes.

3. Confirmed DSPN: The presence of an abnormality of nerve conduction and a symptom or symptoms, or a sign or signs, of neuropathy confirm DSPN. If nerve conduction is normal, a validated measure of small-fiber neuropathy (SFN) (with class 1 evidence) may be used. To assess for the severity of DSPN, several approaches can be recommended: for example, the graded approach outlined above; various continuous measures of sum scores of neurologic signs, symptoms, or nerve test scores; scores of function of activities of daily living; or scores of predetermined tasks or of disability.

4. Subclinical DSPN. The presence of no signs or symptoms of neuropathy are confirmed with abnormal nerve conduction or a validated measure of SFN (with class 1 evidence). Definitions 1, 2, or 3 can be used for clinical practice, and definitions 3 or 4 can be used for research studies.

5. Small-fiber neuropathy (SFN). SFN should be graded as follows: (1) possible: the presence of length-dependent symptoms and/or clinical signs of small-fiber damage; (2) probable: the presence of length-dependent symptoms, clinical signs of small-fiber damage, and normal sural nerve conduction; and (3) definite: the presence of length-dependent symptoms, clinical signs of small-fiber damage, normal sural nerve conduction, and altered intraepidermal nerve-fiber (IENF) density at the ankle and/or abnormal thermal thresholds at the foot.

Diabetic neuropathy is, however, woefully underdiagnosed by endocrinologists as well as nonendocrinologists. In the GOAL A_{1c} study,[611] the absence of neuropathy in 7000 patients could be adequately determined, but the presence of mild neuropathy was detected accurately only one third of the time, and accuracy of detection reached 75% only if neuropathy was severe. Clearly, there is a need for education on methods for detecting neuropathy.

The spectrum of clinical neuropathic syndromes described in patients with diabetes mellitus includes dysfunction of almost every segment of the somatic peripheral and autonomic nervous systems.[648] Each syndrome can be distinguished by its pathophysiologic, therapeutic, and prognostic features.

Focal Neuropathies

Mononeuropathies occur primarily in the older population. Their onset is usually acute and associated with pain, and their course is self-limited, resolving within 6 to 8 weeks. Mononeuropathies result from vascular obstruction after which adjacent neuronal fascicles take over the function of those infarcted.[649] Mononeuropathies must be distinguished from entrapment syndromes, which start slowly, progress, and persist without intervention (Table 33-7). Common entrapment sites in diabetic patients involve median, ulnar, and radial nerves; femoral nerves, lateral cutaneous nerves of the thigh, and peroneal nerves; and the medial and lateral plantar nerves.

Carpal tunnel syndrome occurs three times as often in persons with diabetes than in a normal, healthy population,[650,651] and its increased prevalence in diabetes may be

TABLE 33-7		
Mononeuritis and Entrapment Syndromes		
Feature	**Mononeuritis**	**Entrapment**
Onset	Sudden	Gradual
Nerves	Usually single but may be multiple	Single nerves exposed to trauma
Common nerves	C3, C6, C7, ulnar, median, peroneal	Median, ulnar, peroneal, medial and lateral plantar
Progression	Not progressive; resolves spontaneously	Progressive
Treatment	Symptomatic	Rest, splints, diuretics, steroid injections, surgery for paralysis

Adapted from Vinik A, Mehrabyan A. Diabetic neuropathies. *Med Clin North Am.* 2004;88:947-999.

related to diabetic cheiroarthropathy,[652] repeated undetected trauma (due to repetitive use of computer keyboards or power tools, piano playing, etc.), metabolic changes, or accumulation of fluid or edema within the confined space of the carpal tunnel.[648] It is found in up to one third of patients with diabetes.[653] If carpal tunnel syndrome is recognized, the diagnosis can be confirmed by electrophysiologic study, and therapy with surgical release is simple. The mainstays of nonsurgical treatment are resting of the wrist, aided by the placement of a wrist splint in a neutral position for day and night use, and the addition of anti-inflammatory medications. Surgical treatment consists of sectioning the volar carpal ligament.[654] The decision to proceed with surgery should be based on several considerations, including severity of symptoms, appearance of motor weakness, and failure of nonsurgical treatment.[655]

Diffuse Neuropathies

Proximal Motor Neuropathies. For many years, proximal neuropathy has been considered to be a component of diabetic neuropathy, although its pathogenesis was ill understood.[656] The condition has a number of synonyms: proximal neuropathy, femoral neuropathy, diabetic amyotrophy, and diabetic neuropathic cachexia.

Proximal motor neuropathy has certain common features. It primarily affects the elderly. Its onset, which can be gradual or abrupt, begins with pain in the thighs and hips or buttocks, followed by significant weakness of the proximal muscles of the lower limbs with inability to rise from the sitting position (positive Gower maneuver). The neuropathy begins unilaterally, spreads bilaterally, and coexists with DSPN and spontaneous muscle fasciculation. It can be provoked by percussion.

The condition is now recognized as secondary to a variety of causes that are unrelated to diabetes but have a greater incidence in patients with diabetes than in the general population. These include chronic inflammatory demyelinating polyneuropathy (CIDP), monoclonal gammopathy of unknown significance (MGUS), circulating monosialoganglioside (GM1) antibodies and antibodies to neuronal cells, and inflammatory vasculitis.[657,658]

The condition is readily recognizable clinically; there is prevailing weakness of the iliopsoas, obturator, and adductor muscles, together with relative preservation of function of the gluteus maximus and minimus and hamstrings.[659] Patients have great difficulty rising out of chairs unaided and often use their arms to assist themselves. Heel or toe standing is surprisingly good. In the classic form of diabetic amyotrophy, axonal loss is the predominant process, and

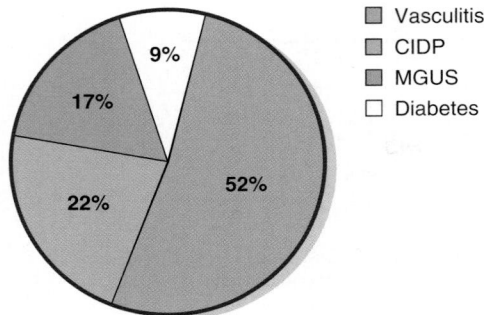

Figure 33-38 Obturator nerve biopsy findings and their frequencies. CIDP, chronic inflammatory demyelinating polyradiculoneuropathy; MGUS, monoclonal gammopathy of undetermined significance. (Adapted from Vinik A: Diagnosis and management of diabetic neuropathy. *Clin Geriatr Med.* 1999;15:293-319.)

the condition coexists with DSPN.[660] Electrophysiologic evaluation reveals lumbosacral plexopathy.[659]

If demyelination predominates and the motor deficit affects proximal and distal muscle groups, a diagnosis of CIDP, MGUS, or vasculitis should be considered.[661,662] It seems probable that these conditions occur more commonly in people with diabetes.[663,664] Vinik and colleagues[611,656-666] have pointed out that almost half the patients with proximal neuropathies have a vasculitis and all but 9% have CIDP, MGUS, or a ganglioside antibody syndrome.[667] Sharma examined more than 1000 patients with neurologic disorders and found that CIDP was 11 times more common in people with diabetes than in the nondiabetic population.[664]

Biopsy of the obturator nerve reveals demyelination, deposition of immunoglobulin, and inflammatory cell infiltrate of the vasa nervorum (Fig. 33-38).[668,669] Cerebrospinal fluid protein content is high, and there is an increase in the lymphocyte count. Treatment options include intravenous immunoglobulin (IVIG) for CIDP, plasma exchange for MGUS, steroids and azathioprine for vasculitis, and withdrawal from drugs or other agents that might have caused a vasculitis. It is important to divide proximal syndromes into these subcategories, because the CIDP variant responds dramatically to intervention,[661,670] whereas amyotrophy runs its own course over months to years. Until more evidence is available, they should be considered separate syndromes.

These conditions need to be distinguished from spinal stenosis syndromes (Fig. 33-39). In spinal stenosis, there is encroachment on nerve roots as they emerge from the spinal cord, and osteophytes can cause compression. With aging, there is hypertrophy of the ligamentum flavum and disk dehydration, and there may even be some form of arachnoiditis. When the compression involves the vascular system, claudication typically occurs on walking downhill, is relieved by bending forward, and originates at the watershed level between T12 and L1-L2. Nerve root compression is more typical at L5-S1, and in difficult cases it may be necessary to obtain a magnetic resonance image (MRI) of the lumbosacral spine. Diagnosis is critical, because therapy may range from simple physical therapy to surgical decompression if symptoms are severe or there is motor paralysis.

Distal Symmetric Polyneuropathy. DSPN is the most common and widely recognized form of diabetic neuropathy. The onset is usually insidious but occasionally is acute, occurring after stress or initiation of therapy for diabetes. DSPN may be sensory or motor and can involve small fibers, large fibers, or both.[671] Figure 33-40 is a simplified schematic

Spinal stenosis/claudication

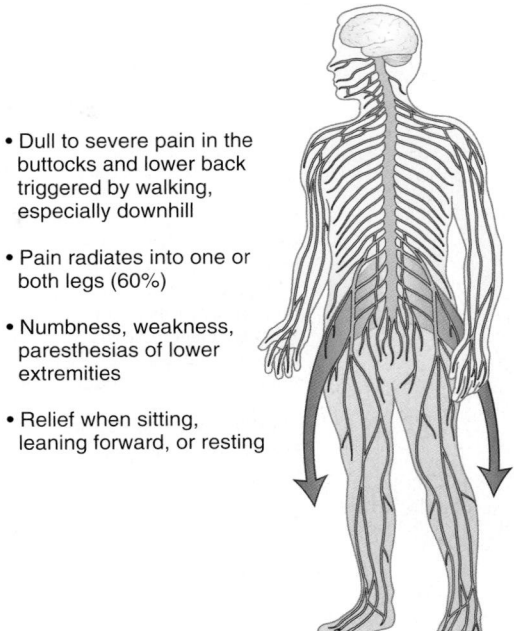

- Dull to severe pain in the buttocks and lower back triggered by walking, especially downhill

- Pain radiates into one or both legs (60%)

- Numbness, weakness, paresthesias of lower extremities

- Relief when sitting, leaning forward, or resting

Figure 33-39 Spinal stenosis syndromes.

A simplified view of the PNS

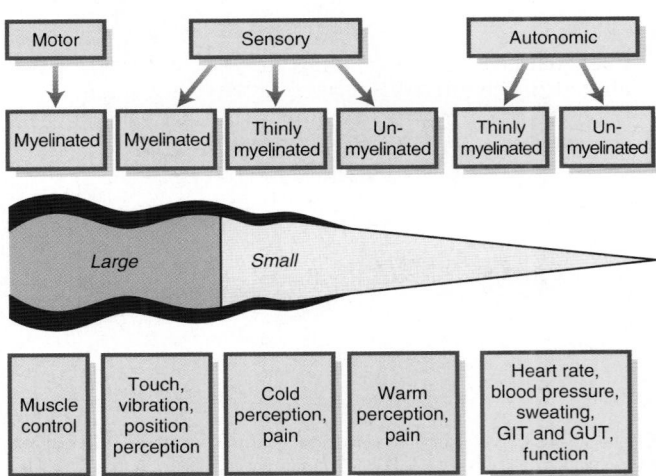

Figure 33-40 Simplified view of the peripheral nervous system (PNS). GIT, gastrointestinal tract; GUT, genitourinary tract. (From Vinik A, Ullal J, Parson H, et al. Diabetic neuropathies: clinical manifestations and current treatment options. *Nat Clin Pract Endocrinol Metab.* 2006;2:269-281.)

diagram of the fibers of the peripheral nervous system. Shown in Figure 33-41 is the usual clinical presentation of the large- and small-fiber neuropathies.

Dysfunction of the small nerve fibers usually occurs early and often is present without objective signs or electrophysiologic evidence of nerve damage. It is manifested early with symptoms of pain and hyperalgesia in the lower limbs, followed by a loss of thermal sensitivity and reduced sensation to light touch and pinprick.[648]

There is evidence that DSPN may be accompanied by loss of cutaneous nerve fibers that stain positive for the neuronal antigen protein gene product (PGP) 9.5[672]

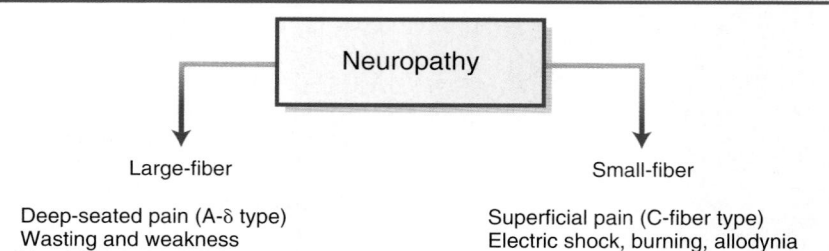

Distal symmetric diabetic neuropathies: subtypes

Neuropathy

Large-fiber

Deep-seated pain (A-δ type)
Wasting and weakness
Numbness, pins and needles,
   tingling, ataxia
Impaired vibration perception
Loss of position sense
Loss of reflexes
Impaired nerve conduction velocity

Interferes with normal life
Risk of falling and fractures

Small-fiber

Superficial pain (C-fiber type)
Electric shock, burning, allodynia
Autonomic dysfunction
Thermal imperception
Normal strength and reflexes
Electrophysiogically silent
Quantitative sensory testing
   and skin biopsies

Produces symptoms
Leads to morbidity and death

Figure 33-41 Differences in clinical presentations of large- and small-fiber neuropathies. (Adapted from Strotmeyer ES, Cauley JA, Schwartz AV, et al. Reduced peripheral nerve function is related to lower hip BMD and calcaneal QUS in older white and black adults: the Health, Aging, and Body Composition Study. *J Bone Miner Res.* 2006;21:1803-1810; Vinik A, Erbas T, Stansberry KB, Pittenger G. Small fiber neuropathy and neurovascular disturbances in diabetes mellitus. *Exp Clin Endocrinol Diabetes.* 2001;109:S451-S473.)

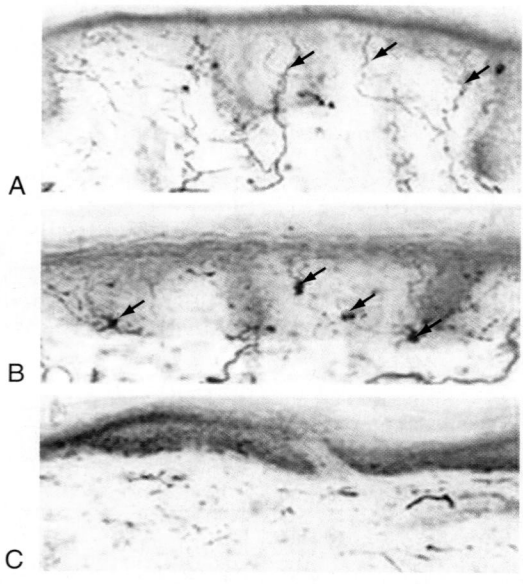

Figure 33-42 Loss of cutaneous nerve fibers that stain positive for the neuronal antigen protein gene product 9.5 (PGP 9.5) in sensory neuropathy. **A,** Normal epidermal fibers in the back. **B,** Slightly reduced density and swelling in the proximal thigh. **C,** Complete clearance in calf. (From McArthur JC, Stocks EA, Hauer P. Epidermal nerve fiber density: normative reference range and diagnostic efficiency. *Arch Neurol.* 1998;55:1513-1520.)

(Fig. 33-42) and by impaired neurovascular blood flow.[673] The importance of the skin biopsy as a diagnostic tool for diabetic peripheral neuropathy is increasingly being recognized.[607,631,639,674] This technique quantitates small epidermal nerve fibers through antibody staining of PGP 9.5.[668,675,676] It is minimally invasive (3-mm-diameter punch biopsies) but enables direct study of small fibers that cannot be evaluated by NCV studies (see Fig. 33-37). More recently, assessment of small nerve fiber function has been carried out using corneal confocal microscopy,[602,603] laser Doppler flare response to heat or acetylcholine, sudomotor responses to cholinergic or direct current stimulation,[600,601,612,677,678]

and contact heat evoked potentials (CHEPs).[613] However, the sensitivity and specificity of these techniques have not yet been established.

Pain in Diabetic Neuropathies

Overall, approximately 10% of patients with diabetes experience persistent pain from neuropathy.[679] Pain syndromes that last less than 6 to 12 months are classified as acute. These include the insulin neuritis syndrome, which occurs often at the beginning of therapy for diabetes and is self-limited. Pain syndromes lasting longer than 6 to 12 months are classified as chronic.[680] The pain may be ongoing, spontaneous, or hyperalgesic (increased response to a painful stimulus). It can be severe and is sometimes intractable.

Management of painful diabetic neuropathy, as well as other pain syndromes, is changing as research elucidates underlying pathophysiologic mechanisms. The complexities of pain syndromes and advances in basic pain research have contributed to an evolving concept of pain and strategies for its management. Experts in the neurology and the pain community define neuropathic pain as "pain arising as a direct consequence of a lesion or disease affecting the somatosensory system."[681]

Acute Painful Neuropathy

Some patients develop a predominantly small-fiber neuropathy, which is manifested by pain and paresthesias early in the course of diabetes (Fig. 33-43). It may be associated with the onset of insulin therapy and has been termed *insulin neuritis*.[682] By definition, it has been present for less than 6 months.

Symptoms often are exacerbated at night and are manifested in the feet more than the hands. Spontaneous episodes of pain can be severely disabling. The pain varies in intensity and character. In some patients, this pain has been variably described as burning, lancinating, stabbing, or sharp. Paresthesias or episodes of distorted sensation, such as pins and needles, tingling, coldness, numbness, or burning, often accompany the pain.[671] The lower legs may be exquisitely tender to touch, with any disturbance of the hair follicles resulting in excruciating pain. Because pain

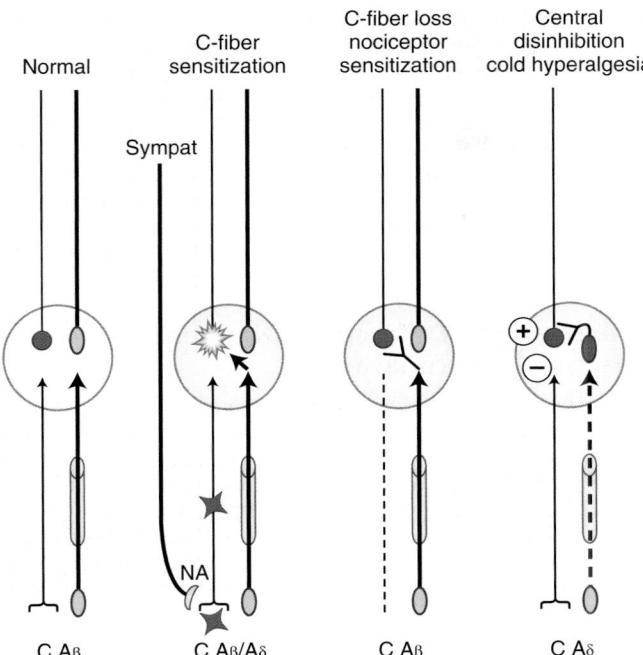

Figure 33-43 Schematic representation of the generation of pain. *Left panel,* Normal situation, no pain. Central terminals of unmyelinated primary C-afferents project into the dorsal horn and make contact with secondary pain-signaling neurons. Low-threshold mechanoreceptive primary Aβ-afferents project without synaptic transmission into the dorsal columns (not shown) and also contact secondary afferent dorsal horn neurons. *Center-left panel,* Peripheral sensitization and central sensitization processes in peripheral nociceptors (peripheral sensitization, star in the periphery) leading to spontaneous burning pain, static mechanical hyperalgesia, and heat hyperalgesia. This spontaneous activity in nociceptors induces secondary changes in central sensory processing, leading to spinal cord hyperexcitability (central sensitization, star in spinal cord) that causes input from mechanoreceptive Aβ fibers (light touching) and Aδ fibers (punctate stimuli) to be perceived as pain (dynamic and punctate mechanical allodynia). Moreover, afferent terminals in the periphery or afferent somata in the dorsal root ganglion acquire sensitivity to norepinephrine (noradrenaline, NA) through expression of A-receptors at their membrane. Activity in postganglionic sympathetic neurons (Sympat) is then capable of activating afferent neurons through the release of NA. *Center-right panel,* Synaptic reorganization after C-nociceptor degeneration. Nociceptor function may be selectively impaired and the fibers may degenerate after nerve lesion. Accordingly, the synaptic contacts between central nociceptor terminals and secondary nociceptive neurons are reduced. Central terminals from intact mechanoreceptive Aβ fibers start to sprout to form novel synaptic contacts with the free central nociceptive neurons. This anatomic reorganization in the dorsal horn causes input from mechanoreceptive Aβ fibers (light touching) to be perceived as pain (dynamic mechanical allodynia). In such patients, temperature sensation is profoundly impaired in areas of severe allodynia. *Right panel,* Central disinhibition and cold hyperalgesia. Normally, cold stimuli are conveyed by Aδ fibers and cold pain by C fibers. A selective damage of cold-sensitive Aδ fibers leads to a loss of central inhibition mediated by interneurons (disinhibition), resulting in cold hyperalgesia. (Adapted from Vinik A, Mehrabyan A. Diabetic neuropathies. *Med Clin North Am.* 2004;88:947-999.)

can be aggravated by repeated contact of the lower limbs with foreign objects, even basic daily activities such as sitting at a desk may be disrupted. Pain often occurs at the onset of the disease and is often worsened by initiation of therapy with insulin or sulfonylureas.[682] Gibbons and Freeman have written a concise review of the natural history, features, and outcome of insulin neuritis syndrome.[683]

Neuropathy may be associated with profound weight loss and severe depression that has been termed *diabetic neuropathic cachexia.*[684] This syndrome occurs predominantly in male patients and can develop at any time in the course of T1DM or T2DM. It is self-limited and invariably responds to simple symptomatic treatment. Conditions such as Fabry disease, amyloid, human immunodeficiency virus (HIV) infection, heavy metal poisoning (e.g., arsenic), and excess alcohol consumption should be excluded. Acute painful neuropathy does overlap with the idiopathic variety of acute painful small-fiber neuropathy that is also a diagnosis by exclusion.[685]

Chronic Painful Neuropathy

Chronic painful neuropathy is another variety of painful polyneuropathy. Onset is later, often years into the course of the diabetes; pain persists for longer than 6 months and becomes debilitating (see Fig. 33-41). This condition can result in tolerance to narcotics and analgesics, finally resulting in addiction. It is extremely resistant to all forms of intervention and is most frustrating to both patient and physician.

Pathophysiologic changes in the nervous system can produce symptoms defined as either negative (e.g., loss of sensory quality) or positive (e.g., spontaneous pain). Patients with neuropathic pain usually present with both positive and negative symptoms. Absence of pain sometimes is not from improvement in neuropathy but is rather a consequence of neuronal loss. Physicians must exclude progression of neuropathy when patients report loss of pain. Neuropathic pain can manifest as stimulus-independent pain or as stimulus-evoked or stimulus-dependent pain, whose underlying mechanisms are likely to differ. A simplified scheme of pain generation is shown in Figure 33-43.

Similarly, the mechanisms responsible for hyperalgesia and allodynia differ. Hyperalgesia is defined as an increased pain response to a normally painful stimulus. Allodynia occurs when pain is provoked by a stimulus that is not normally painful. This difference is related to the different nerve pathways implicated. For example, aberrations of the C and Aδ fibers can result in the burning and prickling sensations of stimulus-independent pain or of hyperalgesia. Under pathologic conditions, touch-sensitive Aβ fibers can cause stimulus-independent dysesthesias or paresthesias or stimulus-evoked allodynia.

Small-Fiber Neuropathies

Symptoms are prominent in small-fiber neuropathies. Pain is of the C-fiber type. It is burning and superficial and is associated with allodynia. Patients have defective autonomic function with decreased sweating, dry skin, impaired vasomotion and blood flow, and cold feet. There are abnormalities in thresholds for warm thermal perception, neurovascular function, pain, quantitative sudorimetry, and QAFTs. Late in the condition, hypoalgesia is present. However, there is remarkable intactness of reflexes and motor strength.

Clinical diagnosis is by reduced sensitivity to 1.0-g Semmes-Weinstein monofilament and a pricking sensation on the Wartenberg wheel or similar instrument. These neuropathies are electrophysiologically silent, but there is loss of cutaneous nerve fibers that stain for PGP 9.5. These may also be detected by evaluation of corneal confocal microscopy, laser Doppler flare reactions, sudomotor function tests, and CHEPs as outlined previously, but sensitivity and specificity of each remain to be defined.

Large-Fiber Neuropathies

Large-fiber neuropathies can involve sensory or motor nerves, or both. These tend to be the neuropathies of signs rather than symptoms. Large fibers subserve motor function, vibration perception, position sense, and cold thermal perception. Unlike the small nerve fibers, these are the myelinated, rapidly conducting fibers that begin in the toes and have their first synapse in the medulla oblongata. They tend to be affected first because of their length and the tendency in diabetes for nerves to die back. Because they are myelinated, they are the fibers represented in the electromyogram, and subclinical abnormalities in nerve function are readily detected. The symptoms may be minimal and include a sensation of walking on cotton, floors feeling strange, inability to turn the pages of a book, or inability to discriminate among coins by touch.

Clinical Presentation

Signs and symptoms of large-fiber neuropathy include impaired vibration perception (often the first objective evidence) and position sense, depressed tendon reflexes, and sensory ataxia (waddling like a duck). Aδ-fiber pain is deep-seated, gnawing, dull, like a toothache in the bones of the feet, or even crushing or cramplike pain. Signs in the distal lower extremities include wasting of the small muscles of the feet, with hammertoes (intrinsic minus feet and hands) and weakness of the feet; shortening of the Achilles tendon

with pes equinus; and increased blood flow (hot foot). Patients also have weakness in the hands.

Most patients with DSPN, however, have a mixed variety of neuropathy, with both large-fiber and small-fiber nerve damage. In the case of DSPN, a glove-and-stocking distribution of sensory loss is almost universal.[648] Early in the course of the neuropathic process, multifocal sensory loss also may be found. In some patients, severe distal muscle weakness can accompany the sensory loss, resulting in an inability to stand on the toes or heels. Some grading systems use this as a definition of severity.

Diagnosis and Differential Diagnosis of Peripheral Neuropathy

The diagnosis of diabetic neuropathy rests heavily on a careful history, for which a number of questionnaires have been developed by Young and colleagues[600,686,687] and others.[688,689] The initial neurologic evaluation should be directed toward detecting the specific part of the nervous system affected by diabetes (Fig. 33-44). Bedside neurologic examination is quick and easy but provides nominal or ordinal measures and contains substantial interindividual

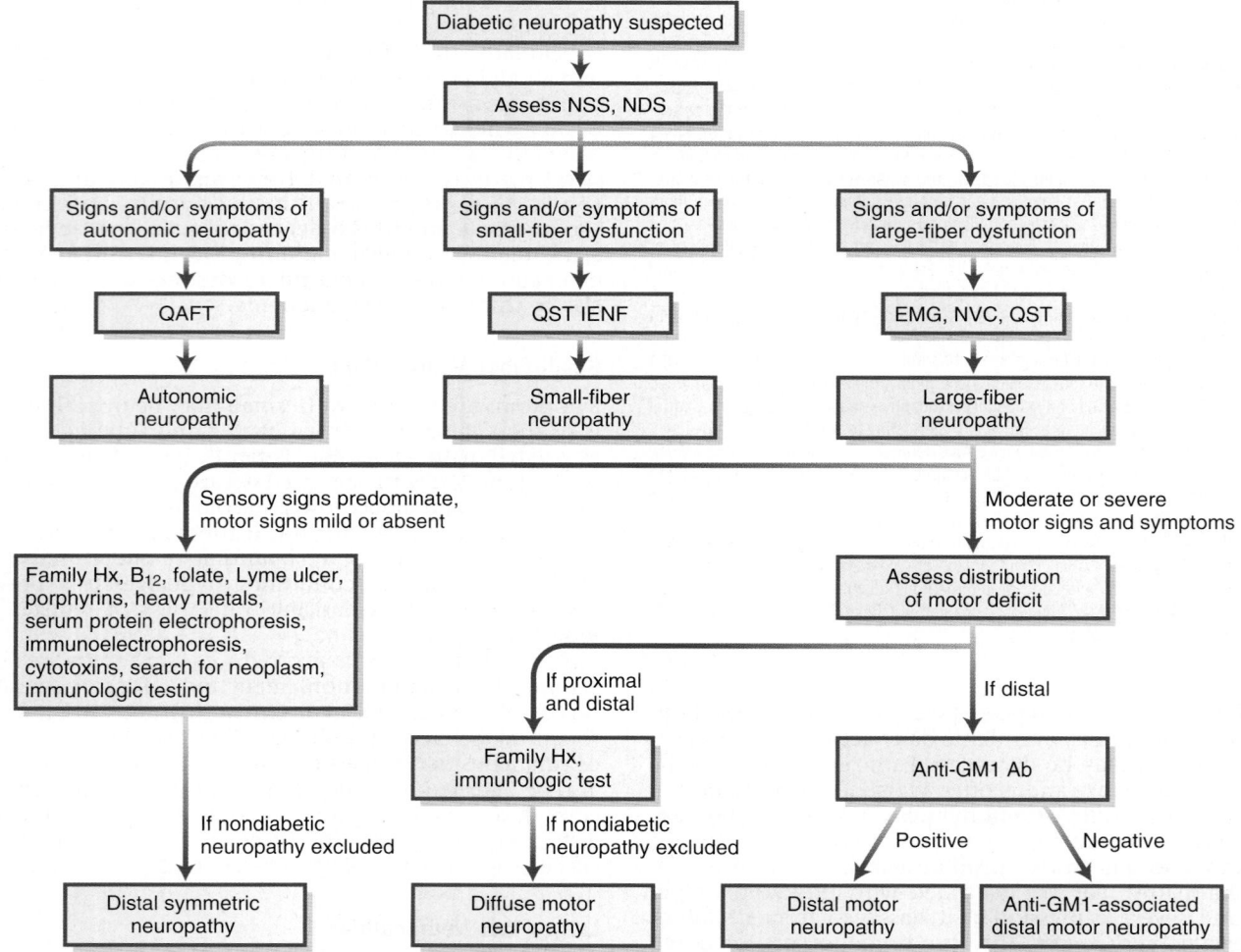

Figure 33-44 A diagnostic algorithm for assessing neurologic deficit and classification of neuropathic syndrome. Ab, antibody; EMG, electromyogram; GM1, monosialoganglioside; Hx, history; IENF, intraepidermal nerve fiber density; MGUS, monoclonal gammopathy of unknown significance; NCV, nerve conduction velocity; NDS, nerve disability (sensory and motor evaluation); NSS, neurologic symptom score; QAFT, quantitative autonomic function tests; QST, quantitative sensory tests. (Adapted from Vinik A, Mehrabyan A. Diabetic neuropathies. *Med Clin North Am.* 2004;88:947-999, used with permission.)

and intraindividual variation. For example, it is useless to measure vibration perception with a tuning fork other than one that has a frequency of 128 Hz. Similarly, use of a 10-g monofilament is good for predicting foot ulceration, as is the Achilles reflex, but both are insensitive to the early detection of neuropathy; a 1.0-g monofilament increases the sensitivity of detection from 60% to 90%.[690]

Sensory function must be evaluated on both sides of the feet and hands if one wants to be sure not to miss entrapment syndromes.[655] Tinel sign not only is useful for carpal tunnel problems but can also be applied to the ulnar notch, the head of the fibula, and below the medial tibial epicondyle for ulnar, peroneal, and medial plantar entrapments, respectively.[624] The 2009 conference of the American Academy of Neurology[647] recommended that at least one parameter from each of the following five categories be measured to classify diabetic neuropathy: symptom profiles, neurologic examination, QST, NCV study, and autonomic function testing. A number of simple symptom screening questionnaires are available to record symptom quality and severity. A simplified neuropathy symptom score that was used in the European prevalence studies could also be useful in clinical practice.[600,691] The Michigan Neuropathy Screening Instrument (MNSI) is a 15-item questionnaire that can be administered to patients as a screening tool for neuropathy.[689] Other similar symptom-scoring systems have also been described, such as the nerve impairment score of the lower limbs (NIS-LL).[692]

Simple visual analogue or verbal descriptive scales may be used to monitor patients' responses to treatment of their neuropathic symptoms.[693-695] However, it must always be remembered that identification of neuropathic symptoms is not useful as a diagnostic or screening tool in assessing diabetic neuropathy, as was shown by Franse and colleagues.[696] The QST and QAFT are objective indices of neurologic functional status. Combined, these tests cover vibratory, proprioceptive, tactile, pain, thermal, and autonomic function. A useful tool that evaluates quality of life in relation to health status and quantifies symptoms of small, large, and autonomic nervous system dysfunction has been validated and translated into 35 languages and is being used globally as an end point in studies on neuropathy.[697]

An international group of experts in diabetic neuropathy held a consensus meeting to develop guidelines for management of diabetic peripheral neuropathy by the practicing clinician.[630] This clinical staging is in general agreement with that proposed by Dyck[698] for use in both clinical practice and epidemiologic studies or controlled clinical trials. The clinical designation "no neuropathy" is equivalent to Dyck's N0 (no objective evidence of diabetic neuropathy) or N1a (no symptoms or signs but neuropathic test abnormalities). "Clinical neuropathy" is equivalent to N1b (test abnormalities plus neuropathic impairment on neurologic examination), N2a (symptoms, signs, and test abnormalities), and N2b (N2a plus significant ankle dorsiflexor weakness). "Late complications" is equivalent to Dyck N3 (disabling polyneuropathy).

There have been a number of other relevant reports, including two on measures for use in clinical trials to assess symptoms[699] and QST.[700] The strengths of QST are well documented,[700] but the limitations of QST are also clear. No matter what the instrument or procedure used, QST is only a semiobjective measure, because it is affected by the subject's attention, motivation, and cooperation and by anthropometric variables such as age, gender, body mass, and history of smoking and alcohol consumption.[701,702] Expectancy and subject bias are additional factors that can exert a powerful influence on QST findings.[703] Further, QST is sensitive to changes in structure or function along the entire neuroaxis from nerve to cortex; it is not a specific measure of peripheral nerve function.[704] The American Academy of Neurology reported on the use of QST for clinical and research purposes,[700] suggesting that it could be used as an ancillary test but was not sufficiently robust for routine clinical use.

Peripheral Testing Devices

A number of relatively inexpensive devices allow suitable assessment of somatosensory function, including vibration, thermal, light touch, and pain perception.[705] These types of instruments allow cutaneous sensory functions to be assessed noninvasively, and their measurements are correlated with specific neural fiber function.

The most widely used device in clinical practice is the Semmes-Weinstein monofilament.[706-708] The filament assesses pressure perception when gentle pressure is applied to the handle sufficient to buckle the nylon filament. Although filaments of many different sizes are available, the one that exerts 10 g of pressure is most commonly used to assess pressure sensation in the diabetic foot. It is also referred to as the 5.07 monofilament because, during calibration, the filaments are calibrated to exert a force measured in grams that is 10 times the log of the force exerted at the tip: hence, 5.07 exerts 10 g of force.

A number of cross-sectional studies have assessed the sensitivity of the 10 g,[709,710] although there is no consensus as to how many sites should be tested. The most common algorithm recommends four sites per foot, usually the hallux and the first, third, and fifth metatarsal heads.[707] However, there is little advantage to multiple site assessments.[705] There is also no universal agreement about what constitutes an abnormal result (one, two, three, or four abnormal findings from the sites tested). Despite these problems, the 10-g monofilament is widely used to clinically assess risk of foot ulceration; however, as we pointed out, one needs to use a monofilament of 1 g or less to detect neuropathy with a high sensitivity.[705] One final caution on the use of the filaments should be made[711]: filaments manufactured by certain companies do not actually buckle at 10 g of force. Indeed, several tested filaments buckled at less than 8 g. In our practice, we use 25-lb strain fishing line and cut it into 1000 pieces at a total cost of $10. We provide patients with these to test themselves at home, which assists in behavior modification. This has reduced the incidence of foot ulcers in our practice by more than 50%.[708]

The graduated Rydel-Seifer tuning fork is used in some centers to assess neuropathy.[712,713] This fork uses a visual optical illusion to allow the assessor to determine the intensity of residual vibration on a scale of 0 to 8 at the point of threshold (disappearance of sensation). Liniger and colleagues reported that results with this instrument correlated well with other QST measures.[712]

The tactile circumferential discriminator assesses the perception of calibrated change in the circumference of a probe (a variation of two-point discrimination).[714] Vileikyte and coworkers reported a 100% sensitivity in identifying patients at risk for foot ulceration.[715] This device also demonstrated good agreement with other measures of QST.

Neuropen is a clinical device that assesses pain using a pin (Neurotip) at one end of the pen and a 10-g monofilament at the other end. This was shown to be a sensitive device for assessing nerve function when compared with the simplified neuropathy disability score.[716]

CHEPs can be elicited by non-noxious heat or painful stimuli from the toe to the dorsum of the back with measurement of negative and positive amplitudes and latencies by recording impulses in the central nervous system. This promises to provide both temporal and spatial resolution of measures of nociception and has the unique ability to measure conduction in C and Aδ fibers, which are normally below the resolution of standard methods. CHEP coupled with functional MRI may lead to an improved understanding of nociceptive pathways and enhance the generation of new therapies directed at the pathways involved.[717,718]

CardiovascularTesting Devices

QAFT consists of a series of simple, noninvasive tests for detecting cardiovascular autonomic neuropathy.[719,720] These tests are based on detection of heart rate and BP responses to a series of maneuvers. Specific tests are used in evaluating disordered regulation of gastrointestinal, genitourinary, and sudomotor function and peripheral skin blood flow induced by autonomic diabetic neuropathy.[690]

Biopsy

Biopsy of nerve tissue may be helpful for excluding other causes of neuropathy and for determining predominant pathologic changes in patients with complex clinical findings as a means of dictating choice of treatment.[660,721]

The importance of the skin biopsy as a diagnostic tool for diabetic polyneuropathy is now firmly established[607,631]; it has some clinical advantages in diagnosing small-fiber neuropathies when all other measures are negative.[639,722] This technique quantitates small epidermal nerve fibers through antibody staining of the panaxonal marker PGP 9.5. It is minimally invasive (3-mm-diameter punch biopsies), yet enables a direct study of small fibers that cannot be evaluated by NCV studies. Intraepidermal nerve fiber density is reduced in approximately 88% of subjects with small-fiber neuropathy, compared with 10% of healthy control subjects.[723] Skin biopsy with intraepidermal nerve fiber density evaluation may be more sensitive than either clinical examination or quantitative sensory testing for detecting abnormalities in subjects with the small-fiber neuropathy phenotype. In a recent retrospective evaluation of 486 patients referred to neurology or neuromuscular disease clinics, skin biopsy showed a diagnostic efficiency of 88.4%, compared with 54.6% for clinical examination and 46.9% for QSTs.[724] The last evidence-based review on DSPN from the American Academy of Neurology concluded that skin biopsy is a validated technique for determining intraepidermal nerve fiber density and may be considered for the diagnosis of diabetic polyneuropathy, particularly small-fiber sensory neuropathy.[647]

Differential Diagnosis

Diabetes as the cause of neuropathy is diagnosed by excluding other causes of neuropathy.[648,725] Patients presenting with painful feet might have impaired glucose tolerance[726,727] or the metabolic syndrome.[728] Quantitation of intraepidermal nerve fiber density has also been used to demonstrate the ability to induce nerve regeneration and correlates with indices of neuropathy relevant to function of small unmyelinated C fibers.[729]

Nerve Conduction Studies

Whole-nerve electrophysiologic procedures (e.g., NCV, F waves, sensory amplitudes, and motor amplitudes) have emerged as important methods of tracing the onset and progression of peripheral neuropathy.[730] An appropriate battery of electrophysiologic tests supports the measurement of the speed of sensory and motor conduction, the amplitude of the propagating neural signal, the density and synchrony of muscle fibers activated by maximal nerve stimulation, and the integrity of neuromuscular transmission.[731,732] These are objective, parametric, noninvasive, and highly reliable measures. However, standard procedures, such as maximal NCV, reflect only a limited aspect of neural activity, and then only in a small subset of large-diameter and heavily myelinated axons. Even in large-diameter fibers, NCV testing is insensitive to many pathologic changes known to be associated with peripheral neuropathy.

However, a key role for electrophysiologic assessment is to rule out other causes of neuropathy or to identify neuropathies superimposed on peripheral neuropathy. Unilateral conditions, such as entrapments, are far more common in patients with diabetes than in healthy subjects.[651] The principal factors that influence the speed of NCV are the integrity and degree of myelination of the largest diameter fibers, the mean cross-sectional diameter of the responding axons, the representative internodal distance in the segment under study, and the microenvironment at the nodes, including the distribution of ion channels.[733] Demyelinating conditions affect conduction velocities, whereas diabetes primarily reduces amplitudes. NCV is only gradually diminished by peripheral neuropathy, with estimates of loss of approximately 0.5 m/second per year.[730] Therefore, the finding of a profound reduction in NCV in a diabetic patient strongly supports the occurrence of an alternative condition. For example, the odds of occurrence of chronic inflammatory demyelinating polyradiculoneuropathy was found to be 11 times higher among diabetic compared with nondiabetic patients.[734]

In a 10-year natural history study of 133 patients with newly diagnosed T2DM, NCV deteriorated in all six nerve segments evaluated, but the largest deficit was 3.9 m/second for the sural nerve (48.3 m/second slowed to 44.4 m/second); peroneal motor NCV was decreased by 3.0 m/second over the same period.[634] A similar slow rate of decline was demonstrated in the DCCT. A simple rule is that a decrease in HbA_{1c} of 1 percentage point improves conduction velocity by approximately 1.3 m/second.[735] There is, however, a strong correlation between myelinated fiber density and whole-nerve sural amplitude (r = 0.74; $p < 0.001$).[736]

Newly introduced means of evaluating small-fiber function include the use of corneal confocal microscopy, which allows the identification of unmyelinated axons in the cornea, and new sudomotor function devices. These completely noninvasive techniques offer the future potential of assessing nerve structure in vivo without the need for biopsy.[737] Data suggest that there is early loss of corneal fibers and reduction of their length, which may precede other measures of neuropathy and may predict the development of foot ulceration (Fig. 33-45).[738-740]

Sudomotor function testing involves measuring sweat gland nerve fiber function as a means to assess the peripheral autonomic nervous system. Sweat gland innervation is comprised of postganglionic, thinly myelinated or unmyelinated sympathetic C-fibers. Their similar nature to small sensory fibers allows sudomotor function tests to serve as surrogate measures of small-fiber function. Sudoscan, for example, which measures sudomotor function on the palms and soles, has been shown to have a sensitivity and specificity for DPN of 78% and 92%, respectively, and strongly correlates with the NIS-LL (Figs. 33-46 and

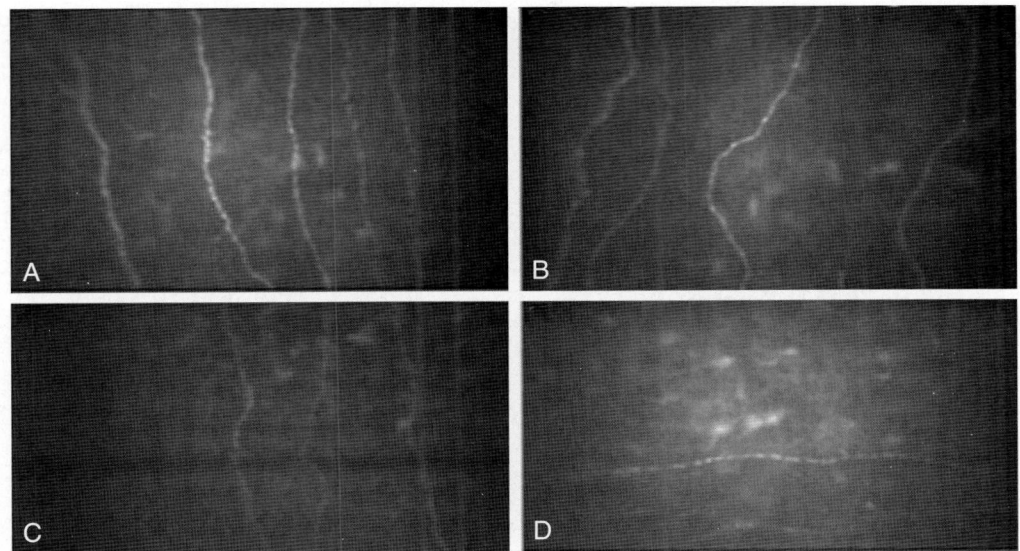

Figure 33-45 Comparison of corneal scans based on severity of neuropathy. **A,** Control. **B,** Diabetic with mild neuropathy. **C,** Diabetic with moderate neuropathy. **D,** Diabetic with severe neuropathy.

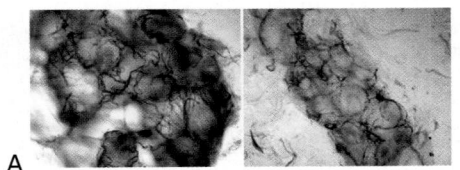

A

Degeneration of small C-fiber innervating sweat glands as observed in diabetes.

Application of a low voltage to electrodes on hands and feet to extract chlorides from the sweat.

Electrochemical reaction between the chlorides of the sweat and the stainless-steel electrodes creates a flow of ions.

Stratum corneum

Stainless steel sensor

Low voltage < 4V

ESC = Electrochemical sweat conductance

Low voltage < 4V

ESC ─ 100 μS

ESC ─ 100 μS

─ 0 μS

─ 0 μS

Sweat gland

Cl⁻ ions

Sympathetic C-fiber

B Subject with abnormal sweat function

C Subject with normal sweat function

Measurement of electrochemical sweat conductances, directly dependent on the glands' capability to transfer chlorides and reflecting small-C fiber status.

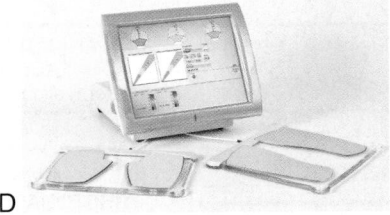

D

Figure 33-46 Sudoscan is a quick and simple method to measure nerve function. (**A** from Lauria G, Lombardi R. Skin biopsy: a new tool for diagnosing peripheral neuropathy. *BMJ.* 2007:334:1159-1162; **B** through **D** courtesy of Impeto Medical, Paris.)

33-47).[678] It also appears to be a promising tool in the diagnosis of suspected small-fiber neuropathies.[677]

Management

Once neuropathy has been diagnosed, therapy can be instituted with the goal of ameliorating symptoms and preventing the progression of neuropathy. Successful management

of these syndromes must be geared to individual pathogenic processes (Fig. 33-48).

Control of Hypergylcemia

Retrospective and prospective studies have suggested a relationship between hyperglycemia and the development and severity of diabetic neuropathy. Pirart[604] followed 4400

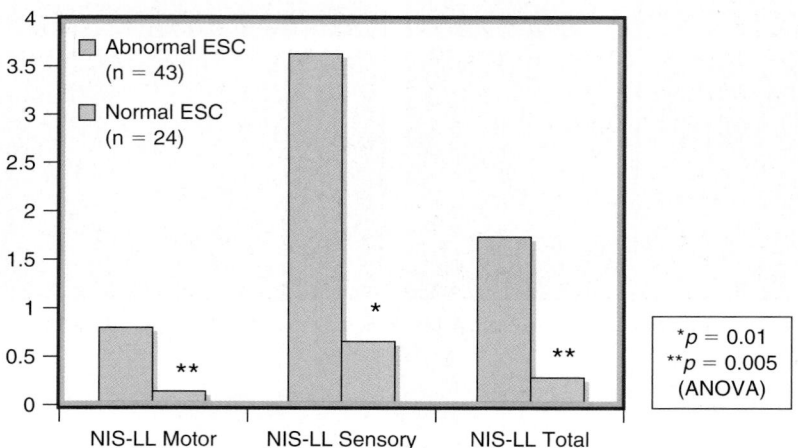

Figure 33-47 Mean NIS-LL (Neuropathy Impairment Score–Lower Legs) scores in diabetes mellitus patients with normal (≥60) vs. abnormal (<60) electrochemical sweat conductance (ESC) ($n = 67$). (From Casellini CM, Parson HK, Richardson MS, Nevoret ML, Vinik AI. Sudoscan, a noninvasive tool for detecting diabetic small fiber neuropathy and autonomic dysfunction. *Diabetes Technol Ther.* 2013;15(11):948-953.)

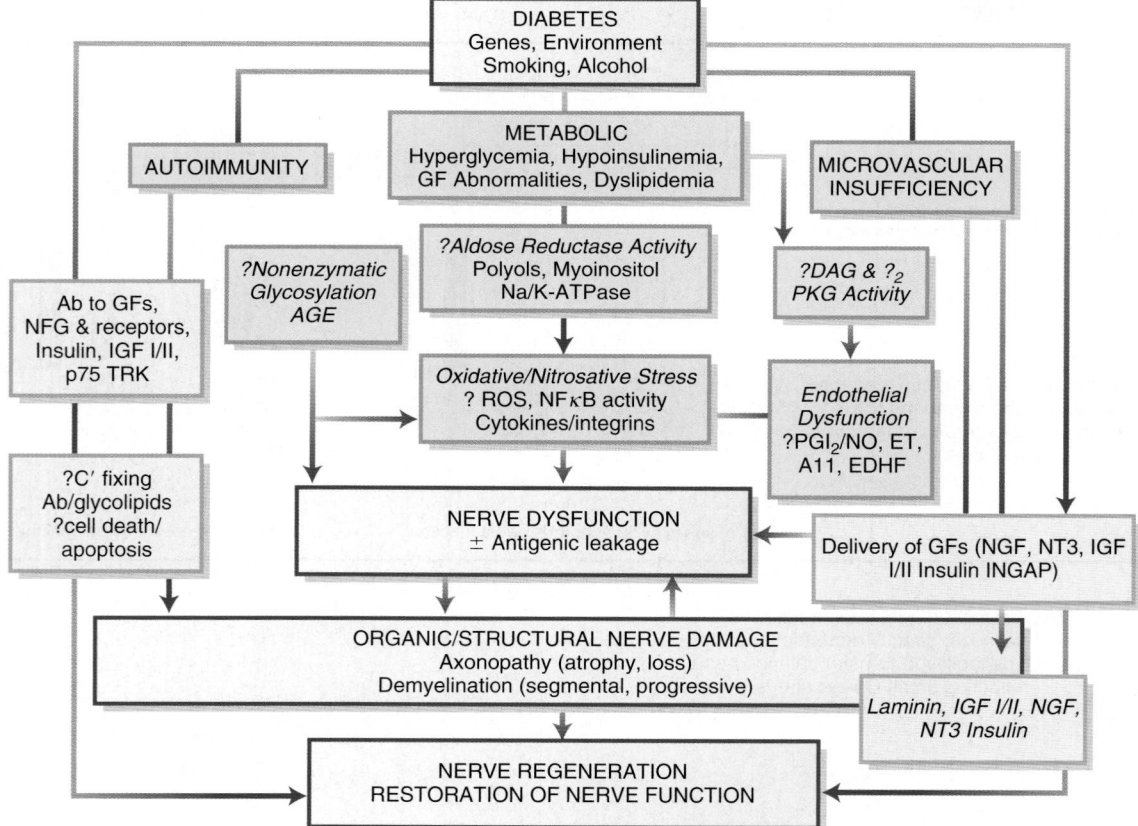

Figure 33-48 Pathogenesis of diabetic neuropathies. Ab, antibody; AGE, advanced glycation end products; ATPase, adenosine triphosphatase; C', complement; DAG, diacylglycerol; EDHF, endothelium-derived hyperpolarizing factor; ET, endothelin; GF, growth factor; IGF, insulin-like growth factor; NFκb, nuclear factor κB; NGF, nerve growth factor; NO, nitric oxide; NT3, neurotropin 3; PGI$_2$, prostaglandin I$_2$; PKC, protein kinase C; ROS, reactive oxygen species; TRK, tyrosine kinase. (From Vinik A, Ullal J, Parson HK, et al. Diabetic neuropathies; clinical manifestations and current treatment options. *Nat Clin Pract Endocrinol Metab.* 2006;2:269-81; used with permission.)

diabetic patients over 25 years and showed an increase in prevalence of clinically detectable diabetic neuropathy from 12% of patients at the time of diagnosis of diabetes to almost 50% after 25 years. The highest prevalence occurred among those patients with the poorest diabetic control.

The DCCT Research Group[4] reported significant effects of intensive insulin therapy on prevention of neuropathy. The prevalence rates for clinical or electrophysiologic evidence of neuropathy were reduced by 50% in those treated by intensive insulin therapy during 5 years. At that stage of the study, only 3% of the patients in the primary prevention cohort treated by intensive insulin therapy showed minimal signs of diabetic neuropathy, compared with 10% of those treated by the conventional regimen. In the secondary prevention cohort, intensive insulin therapy significantly reduced the prevalence of clinical neuropathy by 56% (7% in intensive insulin therapy group versus 16% in conventional therapy group). In the UKPDS, control of blood glucose was associated with improvement in vibration perception.[5,510,674] Similar to what was found in the DCCT, despite loss of diabetes control, with time nerve function improved in the formerly well-controlled group in what has now come to be known as legacy effect or good metabolic memory.[605,623]

The follow-up study to the DCCT, the EDIC study, has shown that, despite convergence of A_{1c} levels with time, the advantage accrued to the intensively controlled people during the course of the study persists. In the Steno trial,[741] a reduction of the odds ratio for the development of autonomic neuropathy to 0.32 was reported. This was a stepwise, progressive study that involved treatment of T2DM patients with hypotensive drugs, including ACE inhibitors, calcium-channel antagonists, hypoglycemic agents, aspirin, hypolipidemic agents, and antioxidants. These findings argue strongly for the multifactorial nature of neuropathy and for the need to address the multiple metabolic abnormalities.

Pharmacologic Therapy

Aldose Reductase Inhibitors. Aldose reductase inhibitors (ARIs) reduce the flux of glucose through the polyol pathway, inhibiting tissue accumulation of sorbitol and fructose and preventing reduction of redox potentials.

In a placebo-controlled, double-blind study of tolrestat, 219 diabetic patients with symmetric polyneuropathy, as defined by at least one pathologic cardiovascular reflex, were treated for 1 year.[742] Patients who received tolrestat showed significant improvement in autonomic function tests and in vibration perception, whereas placebo-treated patients showed deterioration in most of the parameters measured.[743]

There was a dose-dependent improvement in nerve fiber density, particularly in small unmyelinated nerve fibers, in a 12-month study of zenarestat.[744] This was accompanied by an increase in NCV, although the changes in NCV occurred at a dose of the drug that did not change the nerve fiber density. Impaired cardiac ejection fractions can be improved with zopolrestat.[745] Clinical improvement was reported for fidarestat and epalrestat in studies from Japan.[746,747]

The promise of the newer ARIs is being exploited by other companies, and encouraging results have been reported in a phase 2 study of the drug AS-3201 in the United States.[748] A 2-year, global phase 3 study of AS-3201 completed in 2013.[748a] However, it is also becoming clear that aldose reductase inhibition may be insufficient to achieve the desirable degree of metabolic enhancement

in patients with a multitude of biochemical abnormalities. Combinations of therapy with ARIs and antioxidants may become critical to curb the relentless progression of diabetic neuropathy. There is also support for the role of AGE/RAGE interaction in generating inflammation and oxidative and nitrosative stress and promising therapies with compounds that inhibit AGE accumulation and promote a reduction in the aggregation of amyloid fibrils in the nervous system. In addition, it has now been established that sRAGE may act as a decoy in which AGEs and other ligands preferentially bind to sRAGE, thereby precluding access to RAGE and resulting in a net decrease in the inflammation, oxidative, and nitrosative stress effects with salutary effects on the nervous system.[624]

α-Lipoic Acid. Lipoic acid (1,2-dithiolane-3-pentanoic acid), a derivative of octanoic acid, is present in food and is synthesized by the liver. It is a natural cofactor in the pyruvate dehydrogenase complex, where it binds acyl groups and transfers them from one part of the complex to another. α-Lipoic acid, which is also known as thioctic acid, has generated considerable interest as a thiol-replenishing and redox-modulating agent. It has been shown to be effective in ameliorating the somatic and autonomic neuropathies in patients with diabetes.[749-751] It is undergoing extensive trials in the United States and Europe.

γ-Linolenic Acid. Linoleic acid, an essential fatty acid, is metabolized to dihomo-γ-linolenic acid, which serves as an important constituent of neuronal membrane phospholipids and as a substrate for the formation of PGE, which appears to be important for preserving nerve blood flow. In diabetes, conversion of linoleic acid to γ-linolenic acid and subsequent metabolites is impaired, possibly contributing to the pathogenesis of diabetic neuropathy.[752] In a recent multicenter, double-blind, placebo-controlled trial, patients using γ-linolenic acid for 1 year showed significant improvements in clinical measures and on electrophysiologic testing.[753]

Protein Kinase C-β Inhibition. Neural vascular insufficiency has been proposed as a contributing factor to the development of diabetic neuropathy.[754] PKC activation is a critical step in the pathway to diabetic microvascular complications.[755] It is hyperactivated by hyperglycemia and disordered fatty acid metabolism, resulting in increased production of vasoconstrictive, angiogenic, and chemotactic cytokines including TGF-β, VEGF, endothelin, and ICAMs. Nonselective PKC inhibitors normalize hyperglycemia-induced decreases in endoneurial blood flow and abrogate the neuronal abnormalities seen in diabetic rodents.[621,694,756] Preclinical studies in animal diabetes models using ruboxistaurin mesylate (LY333531), a PKC-β inhibitor, have shown improvement in many diabetes-related changes in vascular function such as retinal blood flow[757] endoneurial blood flow, and NCV.[758]

Preliminary results of a multinational, randomized, double-blind, placebo-controlled phase 2 trial showed a statistically significant improvement in symptoms, measured by the Neuropathy Total Symptom Score 6 (NTSS-6), in ruboxistaurin-treated neuropathy groups compared with placebo treatment.[759] In patients with symptomatic neuropathy (NTSS-6 score >6) and a sural nerve action potential greater than 0 μV at baseline, a measure that has been shown to define a responsive subpopulation of peripheral neuropathy,[647] the frequency and intensity of symptoms and the change from baseline for vibratory detection threshold were statistically significantly improved in the treated groups. Vibratory detection threshold changes correlated well with the improvement in symptoms; the drug was well tolerated, and there were few adverse events.

Benfotiamine. Benfotiamine, a transketolase activator that reduces tissue AGEs, was shown to improve peroneal conduction velocity and vibration perception when combined with vitamins B_6 and B_{12}.[760-762] Further trials of benfotiamine administered alone have shown modest improvements of neuropathy; larger well-designed studies of benfotiamine are needed. Studies outlined previously on AGE/RAGE interactions support the notion that this pathway may contribute significantly to neuropathy and deficiencies in sRAGE may be the hallmark of severity of diabetic neuropathy.[763]

Metanx. Metanx is a product for management of endothelial dysfunction, containing L-methylfolate, pyridoxal 50-phosphate, and methylcobalamin. Metanx ingredients counteract eNOS uncoupling and oxidative stress in vascular endothelium and peripheral nerves. A 24-week placebo-controlled trial on the effects of Metanx on patients with established DPN was presented at the American Association of Clinical Endocrinologists annual meeting in 2011. The NTSS-6, which includes numbness, tingling, aching, burning, lancinating pain, and allodynia, improved significantly at week 16 ($p = 0.013$ vs. placebo) and week 24 ($p = 0.033$). Moreover, there were significant improvements in the mental health component of the SF-36 Role Emotional, Social Function, and Vitality. This response occurred with adverse events of less than 2%, mainly rash and gastrointestinal upset, which was no greater than occurred with placebo.[764]

Human Intravenous Immunoglobulin. Immune intervention with IVIG has become appropriate in some patients with forms of peripheral diabetic neuropathy associated with signs of antineuronal autoimmunity.[661,670] Treatment with immunoglobulin is well tolerated and is considered safe, especially with respect to viral transmission.[731] The major toxicity of IVIG has been an anaphylactic reaction, but the frequency of these reactions is now low and confined mainly to patients with immunoglobulin (usually IgA) deficiency. Patients may experience severe headache due to aseptic meningitis, which resolves spontaneously. In some instances, it may be necessary to combine treatment with prednisone or azathioprine. Relapses can occur, requiring repeated courses of therapy. However, new data support a predictive role of the presence of antineuronal antibodies on the later development of neuropathy[732]; they may not be innocent bystanders but neurotoxins.[765] Some patients, particularly those with autonomic neuropathy, antineuronal autoimmunity, and CIDP, may benefit from IVIG.[659,670] Others may benefit from the use of etanercept or azathioprine (Imuran).[766]

Neurotrophic Therapy

There is now considerable evidence in animal models of diabetes that decreased expression of NGF and its receptors, TrkA and p75, reduces retrograde axonal transport of NGF and diminishes support of small unmyelinated neurons and their neuropeptides, such as substance P and calcitonin gene–related peptide (CGRP), both potent vasodilators.[605,765,767,768] Furthermore, administration of recombinant human NGF (rhNGF) restores these neuropeptide levels.[769]

Although clinical trials with NGF have not been successful, it still holds promise for sensory and autonomic neuropathies.[636] The pathogenesis of diabetic neuropathy includes loss of vasa nervorum, so it is likely that appropriate application of vascular endothelial growth factor (VEGF) would reverse the dysfunction. Introduction of the *VEGF* gene into muscles of diabetic animals improved nerve function.[110] There are ongoing *VEGF* gene

studies with transfection of the gene into the muscle in humans.

Islet Neogenesis-Associated Protein. INGAP peptide comprises the core active sequence of islet neogenesis-associated protein (INGAP), a pancreatic cytokine that can induce new islet formation and restore euglycemia in diabetic rodents. Tam and colleagues[770] showed significant improvement in thermal hypoalgesia in diabetic mice after a 2-week treatment with INGAP peptide; humans have shown an increase in C-peptide secretion in T1DM patients and improvement in glycemic control in T2DM patients.[771] Nonetheless, information about its effect on DPN is still lacking.

Human Hepatocyte Growth Factor. Human trials are ongoing with this agent, which has been shown to be a potent angiogenic, antiapoptotic, and neurotropic factor. Because of the multiplicity of its actions, HGF is an intriguing candidate for targeting the complex pathogenesis of diabetic neuropathy.[772-777]

Pain Control

Control of pain constitutes one of the most difficult management issues in diabetic neuropathy. In essence, simple measures are tried first. If no distinction is made for pain syndromes, then the number (of patients) needed to (be) treat(ed) (NNT) to reduce pain by 50% is 1.4 for optimal-dose tricyclic antidepressants, 1.9 for dextromethorphan, 3.3 for carbamazepine, 3.4 for tramadol, 3.7 for gabapentin, 5.9 for capsaicin, 6.7 for selective serotonin reuptake inhibitors (SSRIs), and 10.0 for mexiletine.[778] If, however, pain is divided according to its derivation from different nerve fiber types (Aδ versus C fiber), from spinal cord, or from cerebral cortex, then different types of pain respond to different therapies (Fig. 33-49).

Effective pain treatment should achieve a favorable balance between pain relief and side effects without implying a maximum effect. The following general considerations in the pharmacotherapy of neuropathic pain require attention:

- The appropriate and effective drug has to be tried and identified in each patient by carefully titrating the dose based on efficacy and side effects.
- Lack of efficacy should be judged only after 2 to 4 weeks of treatment using an adequate dose.
- Because the evidence from clinical trials suggests only a maximal response of approximately 50% for any monotherapy, analgesic combinations may be useful.
- Potential drug interactions have to be considered, given the frequent use of polypharmacy in diabetic patients.

Analgesics are rarely of much benefit in the treatment of painful neuropathy, although they may be of some use on a short-term basis for some of the self-limited syndromes, such as painful diabetic third cranial nerve palsy. Narcotics are usually avoided in the setting of chronic pain because of the risk of addiction.

Calcitonin. In a placebo-controlled study, 10 patients with painful diabetic neuropathy were treated with 100 IU of calcitonin per day. About 39% of patients had near-complete relief of symptoms. The improvement was seen after only 2 weeks of treatment.[779]

C-Fiber Pain. Initially, when there is ongoing damage to the nerves, the patient experiences pain of the burning, lancinating, dysesthetic type, often accompanied by hyperalgesia and allodynia. Because the peripheral sympathetic nerve fibers are also small, unmyelinated C fibers, sympathetic blocking agents (clonidine) can lessen the pain. Loss of sympathetic regulation of sweat glands and arteriovenous shunt vessels in the foot creates a favorable

Pain targets

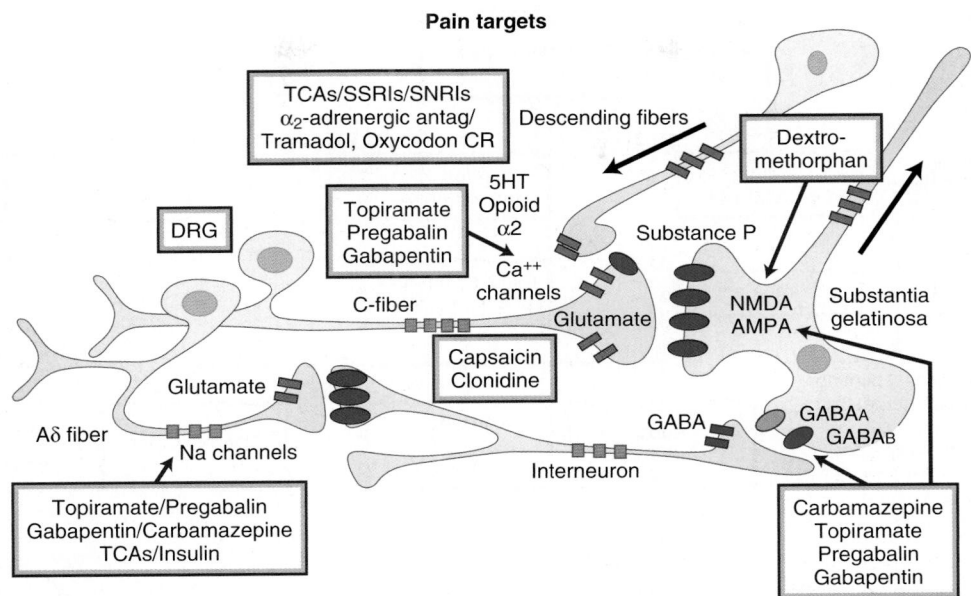

Figure 33-49 Pain response to various therapies. C fibers are modulated by sympathetic input with spontaneous firing of different neurotransmitters to the dorsal root ganglia, spinal cord, and cerebral cortex. Sympathetic blockers (e.g., clonidine) and depletion of axonal substance P used by C fibers as their neurotransmitter (e.g., by capsaicin) can relieve pain. In contrast, Aδ fibers use Na+ channels for conduction. Agents that inhibit Na+ exchange, such as antiepileptic drugs, tricyclic antidepressants (TCAs), and insulin, can ameliorate this form of pain. Anticonvulsants (carbamazepine, gabapentin, pregabalin, topiramate) potentiate the activity of γ-aminobutyric acid (GABA), inhibit Na+ and Ca2+ channels, and inhibit N-methyl-D-aspartate (NMDA) receptors and α-amino-3-hydroxy-5-methyl-4-isoxazole propionic acid (AMPA) receptors. Dextromethorphan blocks NMDA receptors in the spinal cord. TCAs, SSRIs (e.g., fluoxetine), and serotonin-norepinephrine reuptake inhibitors (SNRIs) inhibit serotonin and norepinephrine reuptake, enhancing their effect in endogenous pain-inhibitory systems in the brain. Tramadol is a central opioid analgesic. Antag, antagonists; CR, controlled release; 5HT, 5-hydroxytryptamine; DRG, dorsal root ganglia; SSRIs, selective serotonin reuptake inhibitors. (Adapted from Vinik AI, Ullal J, Parson H, et al. Diabetic neuropathies: clinical manifestations and current treatment options. *Nat Clin Pract Endocrinol Metab.* 2006;2:269-281.)

environment for bacteria to penetrate, multiply, and cause serious foot infections. These fibers use the neuropeptide substance P as their neurotransmitter, and agents that deplete axonal substance P (capsaicin) often lead to amelioration of the pain. However, when destruction of nerve tissue persists, the patient may become pain free with impaired warm temperature and pain thresholds. Disappearance of pain in these circumstances should be viewed as a warning that the neuropathy is progressing. Targeting higher levels of pain transmission also helps with C-fiber pain.[780,781]

Capsaicin. Capsaicin is extracted from chili peppers, and a simple, cheap mixture can be made by adding 1 to 3 teaspoons (15 to 45 mL) of cayenne pepper to a jar of cold cream and applying the cream to the area of pain. Capsaicin has high selectivity for a subset of sensory neurons that have been identified as unmyelinated C-fiber afferent or thin-myelinated (Aδ) fibers. Prolonged application of capsaicin depletes stores of substance P, and possibly other neurotransmitters, from sensory nerve endings. This reduces or abolishes the transmission of painful stimuli from the peripheral nerve fibers to the higher centers.[782] Care must be taken to avoid contact with the eyes and genitals, and gloves must be worn. Because of capsaicin's volatility, it is safer to cover affected areas with plastic wrap. There is initial exacerbation of symptoms followed by relief in 2 to 3 weeks.

Clonidine. There is an element of sympathetic-mediated C-fiber–type pain that can be overcome with clonidine (an α₂-adrenergic agonist) or phentolamine. Clonidine can be applied topically,[783] but the dose titration may be more

difficult. If clonidine fails, a trial of the local anesthetic agent, mexiletine, is warranted. If there is no response, treatment can continue as outlined in Figure 33-50.

Aδ-Fiber Pain. Aδ-fiber pain is a more deep-seated, dull, and gnawing ache that often does not respond to the previously described measures. A number of different agents have been used for the pain associated with these fibers with varying success.

Nerve Blocking. Lidocaine given by slow infusion has been shown to provide relief of intractable pain for 3 to 21 days. This form of therapy may be of most use in self-limited forms of neuropathy. If successful, therapy can be continued with oral mexiletine. Because of the cardiac conduction block reported with these drugs when given systemically, this is no longer done, and only the topical agents are still in use. These compounds target the pain caused by hyperexcitability of superficial free nerve endings.[785]

Tramadol and Dextromethorphan. There are two possible targeted therapies. Tramadol is a centrally acting, weak opioid analgesic that is used to treat moderate to severe pain. Tramadol was shown to be better than placebo in a randomized, controlled trial[786] of only 6 weeks' duration, but a subsequent follow-up study[787] suggested that symptomatic relief could be maintained for at least 6 months. Side effects are relatively common and are similar to those of other opioid drugs.

Tapentadol is a novel centrally active analgesic with a dual mode of action: μ-opioid receptor agonist and norepinephrine-reuptake inhibitor. The efficacy and tolerability of tapentadol extended release (ER) were evaluated

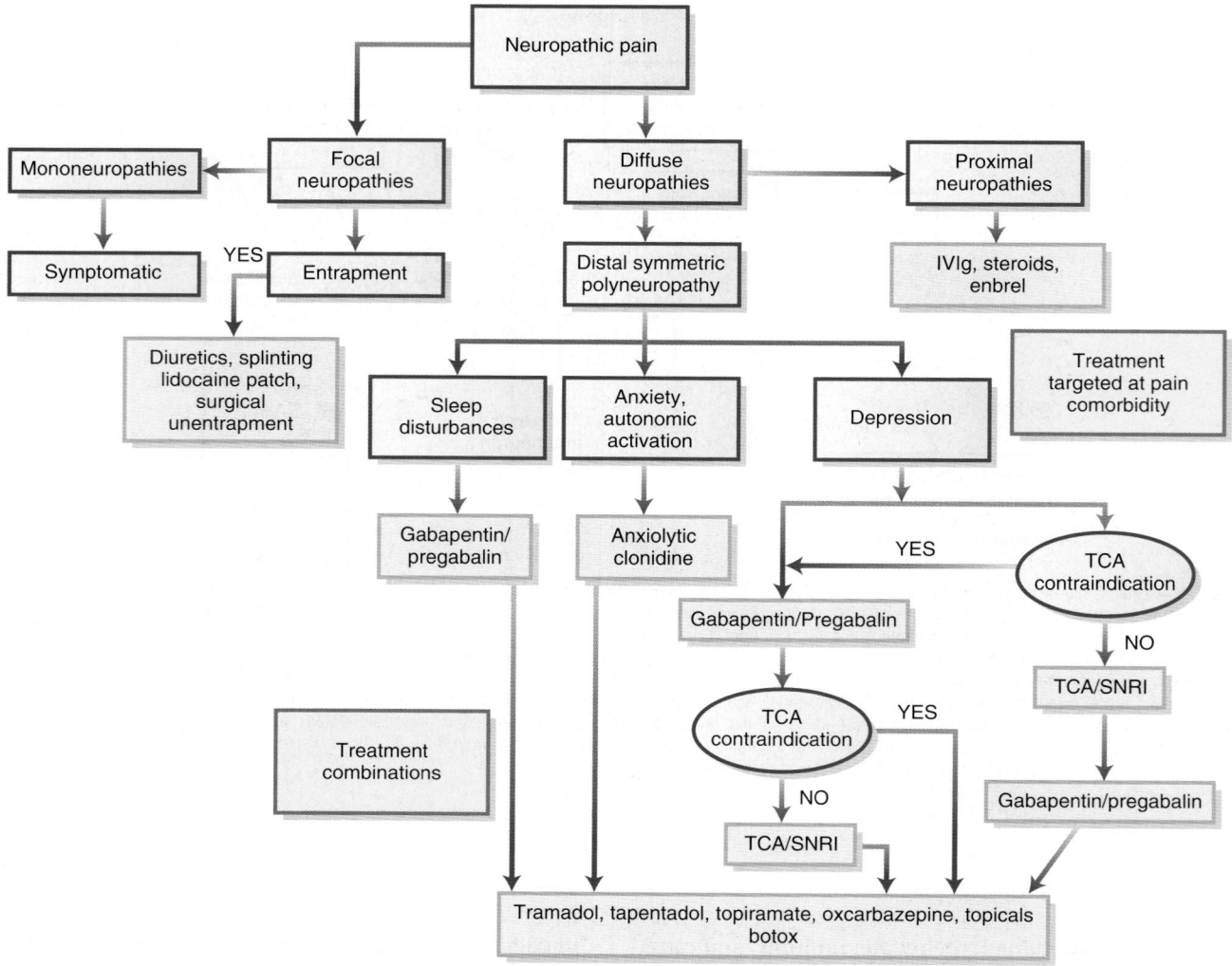

Figure 33-50 Treatment algorithm for neuropathic pain after exclusion of nondiabetic causes and stabilization of glycemic control. IVIg, intravenous immunoglobulin; SNR1, serotonin-noradrenaline reuptake inhibitors; TCA, tricyclic antidepressants. (Copyright © 2010, The Endocrine Society. From Vinik A. The approach to the management of the patient with neuropathic pain. *J Clin Endocrinol Metab.* 2010;95:4802-4811, used with permission.)

using pooled data from two randomized-withdrawal, placebo-controlled, phase 3 trials of similar design in patients with moderate to severe painful diabetic peripheral neuropathy (PDPN). From pretitration (baseline open-label) to the last week of double-blind treatment, 29% of patients in the placebo group (141/495) and 40% of patients in the tapentadol group (207/526) had at least a 50% improvement in pain intensity, giving an NNT of 9.2. Results support those of the individual studies and indicate that tapentadol ER was effective and well tolerated for managing moderate to severe, chronic, painful DPN.[788-790]

Another spinal cord target for pain relief is the excitatory glutaminergic N-methyl-D-aspartate (NMDA) receptor. Blockade of NMDA receptors is believed to be one mechanism by which dextromethorphan exerts analgesic efficacy.[791] The pharmacist can procure a sugar-free solution of dextromethorphan.

Antidepressants. Tricyclic antidepressants are an important component in the treatment of chronic pain syndromes. Imipramine, amitriptyline, and clomipramine induce a balanced reuptake inhibition of both norepinephrine and serotonin, whereas desipramine is a relatively selective norepinephrine reuptake inhibitor. The NNT for greater than 50% pain relief by tricyclic antidepressants is 2.4 (95% CI, 2.0 to 3.0).[792] Amitriptyline is frequently the drug of first choice, but it can alternatively be replaced by nortryptyline, which has less pronounced sedative and anticholinergic effects.

Antidepressants inhibit reuptake of norepinephrine or serotonin, or both. Their use is limited by anticholinergic effects, orthostatic hypotension, and sexual side effects that include decreased libido and erectile problems. Clinical trials have focused on interrupting pain transmission with antidepressant drugs that inhibit the reuptake of norepinephrine or serotonin. This central action accentuates the effects of these neurotransmitters in activation of endogenous pain-inhibitory systems in the brain that modulate pain-transmission cells in the spinal cord.[793] Side effects, including dysautonomia and dry mouth, can be troublesome. Switching to nortriptyline can lessen some of the anticholinergic effects of amitriptyline.

Antidepressants remain first-line agents in many centers, but consideration of their safety and tolerability is important to avoid adverse effects, a common result of treatment of neuropathic pain. Dosages must be titrated.[794] Among the norepinephrine reuptake inhibitors, desipramine, amitriptyline, and imipramine have been shown to be of benefit.[795,796]

SSRIs that have been used for neuropathic pain are paroxetine, fluoxetine, sertraline, and citalopram. Paroxetine appears to be associated with greater pain relief.[797] Fluoxetine failed a placebo-controlled trial.[793]

Recent interest has focused on antidepressants with dual selective inhibition of serotonin and norepinephrine (SNRIs), such as duloxetine and venlafaxine. Duloxetine has recently been approved for treatment of neuropathic pain in the United States. The efficacy and safety of duloxetine were evaluated in three controlled studies using doses of 60 and 120 mg/day over 12 weeks.[798] In all three studies, the average 24-hour pain intensity was significantly reduced with either dose, compared with placebo treatment. The response rates, defined as 50% or greater pain reduction, were 48.2% for the 120-mg/day dose, 47.2% for 60 mg/day, and 27.9% for placebo, giving an NNT of 4.9 (95% CI, 3.6 to 7.6) for 120 mg/day and 5.2 (95% CI, 3.8 to 8.3) for 60 mg/day.[798] Patients with higher pain intensity tend to respond better than those with lower pain levels.[799] The most frequent adverse effects are nausea, somnolence, dizziness, constipation, dry mouth, and reduced appetite. Physicians must be alert to suicidal ideation and exacerbation of autonomic symptoms as well as aggravation of depression in patients with bipolar tendencies. Venlafaxine (Effexor), another SNRI, has also shown efficacy in the treatment of painful diabetic neuropathy.[800]

Antiepileptic Drugs. For a detailed discussion of antiepileptic drug therapy for painful diabetic neuropathy, the reader is referred to the review by Vinik.[693,697]

Anticonvulsants have stood the test of time in the treatment of diabetic neuropathy.[801,802] Principal mechanisms of action include sodium channel blockade (felbamate, lamotrigine, oxcarbazepine, topiramate, zonisamide), potentiation of GABA activity (pregabalin, tiagabine, topiramate), calcium-channel blockade (felbamate, lamotrigine, topiramate, zonisamide), and antagonism of glutamate at NMDA receptors (felbamate) or α-amino-3-hydroxy-5-methyl-4-isoxazole propionic acid (AMPA) receptors (felbamate, topiramate).[803]

Pregabalin (Lyrica) is a GABA analogue with similar structure and actions to gabapentin, but it is a more specific α2-δ ligand with a higher binding affinity than gabapentin. The efficacy and safety of pregabalin were reported in a pooled analysis of seven studies over 5 to 13 weeks in 1510 patients with DPN. The response rates, defined as 50% or greater pain reduction, were 47% for a dosage of 600 mg/day, 39% for 300 mg/day, 27% for 150 mg/day, and 22% for placebo, giving NNTs of 4.0, 5.9, and 20.0, respectively.[804] Pregabalin treatment resulted in improved patient function/quality of life (QOL), as assessed by SF-36 scores, compared to placebo. Significant improvements over placebo were evident for the social functioning role–emotional, mental health, bodily pain, vitality, and general health domains of the SF-36. These findings demonstrated that in patients with chronic pain due to DPN or postherpetic neuralgia, pregabalin-mediated improvements in patient function/QOL are correlated with the extent of pain relief and are the result of a combination of pregabalin's effects on pain, sleep disturbance, and a direct effect on patient function itself.[805] The most frequent adverse effects from pregabalin were dizziness, somnolence, peripheral edema, headache, and weight gain.[693] Pregabalin is labeled a schedule V drug.[780]

Results of a phase 2 study of the new, highly specific α2-δ ligand molecule DS-5565 are anticipated to be released soon. Carbamazepine is useful for patients with shooting or electric shock–like pain. Several double-blind, placebo-controlled studies have demonstrated carbamazepine to be effective in the management of pain in diabetic neuropathy.[806] Toxic side effects can limit its use in some patients.

Phenytoin has long been used in the treatment of painful neuropathies. Double-blind, crossover studies have not demonstrated a therapeutic benefit of phenytoin compared with placebo in the treatment of diabetic neuropathy.[801] Phenytoin is associated with significant side effects, and it must be administered as often as three or four times daily. Some studies have reported positive findings, with 24% of patients indicating improvement,[807] but others have failed to show any benefit.[808] Also, side effects mitigate the use of phenytoin in people with diabetes. Its ability to suppress insulin secretion has resulted in precipitation of hyperosmolar diabetic coma. Valproic acid failed to prove superior to placebo on any outcome measures.[809]

Gabapentin is an effective anticonvulsant whose mechanism is not well understood, but it holds additional promise as an analgesic agent in cases of painful neuropathy.[810] In a multicenter study in the United States,[811] gabapentin monotherapy appeared to be efficacious for treatment of pain and sleep interference associated with diabetic peripheral neuropathy. It also exhibits positive effects on mood and quality of life.[812] Effective dosing can require 1800 to 3600 mg/day, and this is associated with untoward side effects. In a placebo-controlled trial, gabapentin-treated patients had significantly lower mean daily pain scores and improvement of all secondary efficacy parameters.[811] In another study on diabetic neuropathy, gabapentin was found to be equivalent to amitriptyline.[813] Gabapentin has the additional benefit of improving sleep,[811] which is often compromised in patients with chronic pain.[794] In the long term, it is known to produce weight gain, which can complicate diabetes management. Gabapentin has not been successful in all trials.[814]

Lamotrigine is an antiepileptic agent with at least two antinociceptive properties. In a randomized, placebo-controlled study, Eisenberg and colleagues[815] confirmed the efficacy of this agent in patients with neuropathic pain. However, titration needs to be inordinately slow to prevent Stevens-Johnson syndrome. Bradycardia has been reported. Lamotrigine caused a significant decrease in pain intensity in two controlled studies.[815,816] Two randomized, double-blind, placebo-controlled studies of lamotrigine in patients with painful diabetic neuropathy (each study with 360 subjects) revealed greater reduction in pain-intensity score among patients receiving lamotrigine 400 mg, compared with placebo.[817]

Topiramate is a fructose analogue that was initially examined because of its antidiabetic possibilities. A study using neuropathy end points with specificity for the nature and site of the pain was successful, but paresthesias were a side effect of the drug.[818] Topiramate also increased nerve fiber regeneration in the skin.[647] It therefore has the potential to relieve pain by altering the biology of the disease and has now been shown to increase intraepidermal nerve fiber density. Further trials are under way. One must start with no more than 15 mg/day, preferably at night, and then increase the dose only after the patient can tolerate the drug. A maximum of 200 mg was sufficient to induce nerve fiber recovery. In trials with topiramate, 50% of patients responded to treatment, compared with 34% of those patients receiving placebo; response was defined as a reduction of greater than 30% in pain score ($p < 0.004$). Topiramate also reduced pain intensity compared with placebo ($p < 0.003$) and improved sleep-disruption scores ($p < 0.02$).[818] It has also shown improvement in quality of life commensurate with its effects on small nerve fiber function contrasting with the large fiber effects of the PKC inhibitor.[618,628]

Pain symptoms in neuropathy significantly affect quality of life. Neuropathic pain therapy is challenging, and selection of pain medications and dosages must be individualized, with attention to potential side effects and drug interactions. Based on the information presented here, the scheme presented in Figure 33-50 is provided for decision making in the management of pain in people with diabetes.

Adjunct Management and Treatment of Complications

Although small-fiber neuropathy manifests as different forms of pain, large-fiber neuropathy is manifested by reduced vibration perception and position sense, weakness, muscle wasting, and depressed deep tendon reflexes. Diabetic patients with large-fiber neuropathies are uncoordinated and ataxic and are 17 times more likely to fall than their non-neuropathic counterparts.[819] Therefore, it is important to improve strength and balance in patients with large-fiber neuropathy. Patients can benefit from high-intensity strength training by increasing muscle strength and improving coordination and balance, thereby reducing fall and fracture risks.[820,821] Low-impact activities that emphasize muscle strength and coordination and challenge the vestibular system, such as Pilates, yoga, and tai chi, can also be particularly helpful. In addition, options to prevent and correct foot deformities are available, including orthotics, surgery, and reconstruction.

Prevention. Basic management of small-fiber neuropathies by the patient should be encouraged. These measures include foot protection and ulcer prevention by wearing padded socks; daily foot inspection using a mirror to examine the soles of the feet; selection of proper footwear; scrutiny of shoes for the presence of foreign objects that lodge themselves in closed shoes; and avoidance of sun-heated surfaces, hot bathwater, and sleeping with feet in front of a fireplace or heater. Patient education should reinforce these strategies and should also discourage soaking of the feet in water. Education also should promote foot care by encouraging use of emollient creams to help skin retain moisture and to prevent cracking and infection.

Stimulation. Transcutaneous nerve stimulation (electrotherapy) occasionally is helpful and certainly represents one of the more benign therapies for painful neuropathy.[822] Care should be taken to move the electrodes around to identify sensitive areas and obtain maximum relief. Static magnetic field therapy[823] has been reported to be of benefit, but it is difficult to blind such studies. Similarly, the use of infrared light has reportedly had benefit, but this remains to be proved.

A case series of patients with severe painful neuropathy unresponsive to conventional therapy suggested efficacy for the use of an implanted spinal cord stimulator.[682] However, this cannot be generally recommended except in very resistant cases, because it is invasive, expensive, and unproven in controlled studies. Even stochastic resonance therapy can improve sensation.[736,824] There is no support for the notion that surgical decompression can be used to treat common diabetic neuropathy.[825,826]

Management of Small-Fiber Neuropathies

Patients must be instructed on foot care including daily foot inspection. They must have a mirror in the bathroom for inspecting the soles of the feet. Providing patients with a monofilament for self-testing reduces the occurrence of ulcers.

All diabetic patients should wear padded socks. Shoes must fit well and have adequate support, and they must be inspected for the presence of foreign bodies (e.g., nails, pins) before donning.

Patients must exercise care with exposure to heat (no falling asleep in front of fires). Emollient creams should be used for the drying and cracking. After bathing, feet should be thoroughly dried and powdered between the toes. Nails should be cut transversely, preferably by a podiatrist.

Management of Large-Fiber Neuropathies

Patients with large-fiber neuropathies are uncoordinated and ataxic. As a result, they are more likely to fall than non-neuropathic age-matched persons.[827] High-intensity strength training in older people increases muscle strength in a variety of muscles. More importantly, the strength training results in improved coordination and balance that is quantifiable by backward tandem walking.[820,828] It has also been demonstrated that strength and rehabilitation training and simple walking exercise can markedly reduce the risk of falling.[628] Strength and balance training has widespread positive effects on physiologic function for patients with T2DM. It leads to decreased risk of falling, improved strength, and postural stability. In one study,[828] the training program also resulted in altered postural sway dynamics. The center of pressure (COP) output of the trained diabetic group became more similar to that seen in the age-matched control subjects. Therefore, it is vital for the patient to embark on a program of strength training and improvement of balance to include gait and strength training, tendon lengthening for Achilles tendon shortening, orthotics and proper shoes for the deformities, pain management as detailed earlier, bisphosphonates for osteopenia, and surgical reconstruction and full-length casting as necessary.

Autonomic Neuropathies

The autonomic nervous system (ANS) supplies all organs in the body and consists of an afferent and an efferent system, with long efferents in the vagus (cholinergic) system and short postganglionic unmyelinated fibers in the sympathetic (adrenergic) system. A third component is the neuropeptidergic system, with its neurotransmitters, substance P, vasoactive intestinal polypeptide (VIP), and CGRP, among others.

Diabetic autonomic neuropathy can cause dysfunction of every part of the body and often goes completely unrecognized by patient and physician alike because of its insidious onset and protean multiple-organ involvement. Alternatively, the appearance of complex and confusing symptoms in a single organ system as a result of diabetic autonomic neuropathy can cause profound symptoms and receive intense diagnostic and therapeutic attention. Subclinical involvement may be widespread, whereas clinical symptoms and signs may be focused within a single organ. The organ systems that most often exhibit prominent clinical autonomic signs and symptoms in diabetes include the ocular pupil, sweat glands, genitourinary system, gastrointestinal system, adrenal medullary system, and cardiovascular system (Table 33-8).

Involvement of the ANS can occur as early as the first year after diagnosis. Major manifestations are cardiovascular, gastrointestinal, and genitourinary system dysfunction.[648,829] Reduced exercise tolerance, edema, paradoxical supine or nocturnal hypertension, and intolerance to heat

TABLE 33-8
Clinical Manifestations of Autonomic Neuropathy

Cardiovascular

Alterations in skin blood flow
Cardiac denervation, painless myocardial infarction
Heat intolerance
Orthostatic hypotension
Tachycardia, exercise intolerance

Gastrointestinal

Constipation
Diarrhea
Esophageal dysfunction
Fecal incontinence
Gastroparesis diabeticorum

Genitourinary

Cystopathy
Erectile dysfunction
Neurogenic bladder
Retrograde ejaculation

Metabolic

Hypoglycemia unawareness
Hypoglycemia unresponsiveness

Pupillary

Argyll-Robertson pupil
Decreased diameter of dark-adapted pupil

Sweating Disturbances

Areas of symmetric anhidrosis
Gustatory sweating

---

due to defective thermoregulation are consequences of autonomic neuropathy.

Defective blood flow in the capillary circulation is found, with decreased responsiveness to mental arithmetic, cold pressor, hand grip, and heating.[673] The defect is associated with a reduction in the amplitude of vasomotion[819] that resembles premature aging.[673] There are differences in the glabrous and hairy skin circulations. In hairy skin, a functional defect is found before neuropathy develops,[830] and it is correctable with antioxidants.[831] The clinical counterpart is skin that is dry and cold, loses the ability to sweat, and develops fissures and cracks that are portals of entry for organisms, leading to infectious ulcers and gangrene. Silent MI, respiratory failure, amputations, and sudden death are hazards for diabetic patients with cardiac autonomic neuropathy.[644,832] There is now evidence that the greatest predictor of CVD as well as increased risk of death is autonomic nerve dysfunction,[826,833] and the increase in sudden death in the ACCORD study is likely due to the presence of autonomic dysfunction.[834] It has also become apparent that a combination of self-reported somatic neuropathy (i.e., numbness) combined with an index of loss in heart rate variability increases the risk of cardiac events and mortality by an RR of 4.5.[642] Therefore, it is vitally important to make this diagnosis early so that appropriate intervention can be instituted.[644,832,835,836] Furthermore, since the risk factors for CVD in the recent ADVANCE, ACCORD, and VADT trials have been established, the presence of autonomic dysfunction necessitates a modified approach to attempts at intensification of glycemic control. The ACE and ADA, therefore, have recently relaxed the recommended HbA$_{1c}$ goals, focusing on individualized glycemic control based on the risk to the patient.[423,837]

Disturbances in the ANS may be functional and include gastroparesis with hyperglycemia and ketoacidosis. In organic disturbances, nerve fibers are actually lost. This creates inordinate difficulties in diagnosing, treating, and prognosticating as well as establishing true prevalence rates. Tests of autonomic function typically stimulate entire reflex pathways. Furthermore, autonomic control for each organ system is usually divided between opposing sympathetic and parasympathetic innervations, so that heart rate acceleration, for example, could reflect either decreased parasympathetic or increased sympathetic nervous system stimulation.

Because many conditions affect the ANS and autonomic neuropathy is not unique to diabetes, the diagnosis of diabetic autonomic neuropathy rests with establishing the diagnosis and excluding other causes. The best studied tests, and those for which there are large databases and evidence to support their use in clinical practice, relate to the evaluation of cardiovascular reflexes. Evaluation of orthostasis is fairly straightforward and is readily done in clinical practice, and the same can be said for the establishment of the causes of gastrointestinal symptoms and erectile dysfunction. The evaluation of pupillary abnormalities, hypoglycemia unawareness and unresponsiveness, neurovascular dysfunction, and sweating disturbances is for the most part done only in research laboratories, requires specialized equipment and familiarity with the diagnostic procedures, and is best left in the hands of those who have a special interest in the area.

Tables 33-9 and 33-10 present the diagnostic tests that apply to the diagnosis of cardiovascular autonomic neuropathy. These tests can be used as a surrogate for the diagnosis of autonomic neuropathy of any system, because it is rare (although it does occur) to find involvement of any other division of the ANS in the absence of cardiovascular autonomic dysfunction. For example, if one entertains the possibility that the patient's erectile dysfunction is caused by autonomic neuropathy, then before embarking on a sophisticated and expensive evaluation of erectile status, one should measure the heart rate and its variability in response to deep breathing. If this measurement is normal, autonomic neuropathy is excluded as a cause of erectile dysfunction, and the cause should be sought elsewhere. Similarly, it is extremely unusual to find gastroparesis secondary to autonomic neuropathy in a patient with normal cardiovascular autonomic reflexes.

Prevention and Reversibility

It has now become clear that strict glycemic control[39] and stepwise progressive management of hyperglycemia, lipids, and BP, together with the use of antioxidants[750] and ACE inhibitors,[838] reduce the odds ratio for autonomic neuropathy to 0.32.[728] It has also been shown that mortality is a function of loss of beat-to-beat variability with MI. This can be reduced by 33% with acute administration of insulin.[839] Kendall and coworkers[840] reported that successful pancreas transplantation improves epinephrine response and normalizes hypoglycemia symptom recognition in patients with long-standing diabetes and established autonomic neuropathy. Burger's group[841] showed a reversible metabolic component in patients with early cardiac autonomic neuropathy (Table 33-11).

Management

Postural Hypotension. The syndrome of postural hypotension consists of posture-related dizziness and syncope (Fig. 33-51). Patients who have T2DM and orthostatic

TABLE 33-9
Differential Diagnosis of Diabetic Autonomic Neuropathy

Clinical Manifestations	Differential Diagnosis
Cardiovascular	
Cardiac denervation	Carcinoid syndrome
Exercise intolerance	Congestive heart disease
Orthostatic hypotension	Hyperadrenergic hypotension
Painless myocardial infarction	Hypovolemia
Tachycardia	Idiopathic orthostatic hypotension
	Multiple system atrophy with parkinsonism
	Panhypopituitarism
	Pheochromocytoma
	Orthostatic tachycardia
	Shy-Drager syndrome
Gastrointestinal	
Constipation	Bezoars
Diarrhea	Biliary disease
Esophageal dysfunction	Medications
Fecal incontinence	Obstruction
Gastroparesis diabeticorum	Psychogenic vomiting
	Secretory diarrhea (endocrine tumors)
Genitourinary	
Cystopathy	Alcohol abuse
Erectile dysfunction	Atherosclerotic vascular disease
Neurogenic bladder	Genital and pelvic surgery
Retrograde ejaculation	Medications
Neurovascular	
Dry skin	Amyloidosis
Gustatory sweating	Arsenic
Heat intolerance	Chagas disease
Impaired skin blood flow	
Metabolic	
Hypoglycemia-associated autonomic failure	Drugs that mask hypoglycemia
Hypoglycemia unawareness	Other cause of hypoglycemia
Hypoglycemia unresponsiveness	Intensive glycemic control
Pupillary	
Argyll-Robertson pupil	Syphilis
Decreased diameter of dark-adapted pupil	

TABLE 33-10
Diagnostic Tests for Cardiovascular Autonomic Neuropathy

Resting Heart Rate

Rate >100 beats/min is abnormal.

Beat-to-Beat Heart Rate Variation*

With the patient at rest and supine (no overnight coffee or hypoglycemic episodes), breathing 6 breaths/min, heart rate monitored by ECG or Anscore device, an HRV of >15 beats/min is normal and <10 beats/min is abnormal, E/I ratio of R-R intervals >1.17. All indices of HRV are age-dependent.[†]

Heart Rate Response to Standing*

During continuous ECG monitoring, the R-R interval is measured at beats 15 and 30 after standing. Normally, a tachycardia is followed by reflex bradycardia. The 30:15 ratio is normally >1.03.

Heart Rate Response to Valsalva Maneuver*

The subject forcibly exhales into the mouthpiece of a manometer to 40 mm Hg for 15 seconds during ECG monitoring. Healthy subjects develop tachycardia and peripheral vasoconstriction during strain and an overshoot bradycardia and rise in blood pressure with release. The ratio of longest to shortest R-R interval should be >1.2.

Systolic Blood Pressure Response to Standing

Systolic blood pressure is measured in the supine subject. The patient stands and the systolic blood pressure is measured after 2 min. Normal response is a fall of <10 mm Hg, borderline is a fall of 10-29 mm Hg, and abnormal is a fall of >30 mm Hg with symptoms.

Diastolic Blood Pressure Response to Isometric Exercise

The subject squeezes a handgrip dynamometer to establish a maximum. Grip is then squeezed at 30% maximum for 5 min. The normal response for diastolic blood pressure is a rise of >16 mm Hg in the other arm.

Electrocardiographic QT/QTc Intervals

The QTc (corrected QT interval on ECG) should be <440 ms.

Spectral Analysis

High-frequency peak ↓ (parasympathetic dysfunction)
Low-frequency peak ↓ (sympathetic dysfunction)
Low-frequency/high-frequency ratio ↓ (sympathetic imbalance)
Very-low-frequency peak ↓ (sympathetic dysfunction)

Neurovascular Flow

Noninvasive laser Doppler measures peripheral sympathetic responses to nociception.

*These tests can be performed quickly (<15 min) in the practitioner's office, with a central reference laboratory providing quality control and normative values, and are now readily available in most cardiology practices.
[†]Lowest normal value of expiration/inspiration (E/I) ratio by age is as follows: 20-24 yr, 1.17; 25-29 yr, 1.15; 30-34 yr, 1.13; 35-39 yr, 1.12; 40-44 yr, 1.10; 45-49 yr, 1.08; 50-54 yr, 1.07; 55-59 yr, 1.06; 60-64 yr, 1.04; 65-69 yr, 1.03; 70-75 yr, 1.02.
ECG, electrocardiogram; HRV, heart rate variation.

hypotension are hypovolemic and have sympathoadrenal insufficiency; both factors contribute to the pathogenesis of orthostatic hypotension.[842] Postural hypotension in the patient with diabetic autonomic neuropathy can present a difficult management problem. Increasing BP in the standing position to avoid symptoms often results in hypertension in the supine position. It is now recognized that symptoms of orthostasis can also result from inappropriate changes in heart rate without a fall in BP (i.e., orthostatic tachycardia or bradycardia without a fall in BP). Devices with algorithms for quantification of sympathetic or parasympathetic function allow the determination of ANS dysfunction in the arm,[627] which may provide a rationale for trying drugs that reduce either sympathetic or parasympathetic activity in these patients.

Supportive Garments. Whenever possible, attempts should be made to increase venous return from the periphery using total-body stockings. Leg compression alone is less effective, presumably reflecting the large capacity of the abdomen relative to the legs.[843] Patients should be instructed to put these garments on while lying down and not to remove them until returning to the supine position.

Drug Therapy. Some patients with postural hypotension benefit from treatment with 9-fluorohydrocortisone (Table 33-12). However, symptoms do not improve until edema occurs, and there is a significant risk of developing congestive heart failure (CHF) and hypertension. If 9-fluorohydrocortisone does not work satisfactorily, various adrenergic agonists and antagonists may be used.

If the adrenergic receptor status is known, therapy can be guided to the appropriate agent. Metoclopramide may be helpful in patients with dopamine excess or increased sensitivity to dopaminergic stimulation. Patients with α_2-adrenergic receptor excess might respond to the α_2-antagonist, yohimbine. Those few patients in whom β-adrenergic receptors are increased may be helped with propranolol. α_2-Adrenergic receptor deficiency can be

TABLE 33-11

Clinical Features, Diagnosis, and Treatment of Diabetic Autonomic Neuropathy

Symptoms	Tests	Treatments
Cardiac		
Resting tachycardia, exercise intolerance	HRV, MUGA thallium scan, MIBG scan	Graded supervised exercise, ACE inhibitors, β-blockers
Postural hypotension, dizziness, weakness, fatigue, syncope	HRV, supine and standing BP, catecholamines	Mechanical measures, clonidine, midodrine, octreotide, erythropoietin
Gastrointestinal		
Gastroparesis, erratic glucose control	Gastric emptying study, barium study	Frequent small meals, prokinetic agents (metoclopramide, domperidone, erythromycin)
Abdominal pain, early satiety, nausea, vomiting, bloating, belching	Endoscopy, manometry, electrogastrogram	Antibiotics, antiemetics, bulking agents, tricyclic antidepressants, pyloric botulinum toxin, gastric pacing
Constipation	Endoscopy	High-fiber diet, bulking agents, osmotic laxatives, lubricating agents
Diarrhea (often nocturnal alternating with constipation)		Soluble fiber, gluten and lactose restriction, anticholinergic agents, cholestyramine, antibiotics, somatostatin, pancreatic enzyme supplements
Sexual Dysfunction		
Erectile dysfunction	H&P, HRV, penile-brachial pressure index, nocturnal penile tumescence	Sex therapy, psychological counseling, phosphodiesterase inhibitors, PGE₁ injections, devices or prostheses
Vaginal dryness		Vaginal lubricants
Bladder Dysfunction		
Frequency, urgency, nocturia, urinary retention, incontinence	Cystometrogram, postvoid sonography	Bethanechol, intermittent catheterization
Sudomotor Dysfunction		
Anhidrosis, heat intolerance, dry skin, hyperhidrosis	Quantitative sudomotor axon reflex, sweat test, skin blood flow	Emollients and skin lubricants, scopolamine, glycopyrrolate, botulinum toxin, vasodilators
Pupillomotor and Visceral Dysfunction		
Blurred vision, impaired adaptation to ambient light, Argyll-Robertson pupil	Pupillometry, HRV	Care with driving at night
Impaired visceral sensation: silent MI, hypoglycemia unawareness		Recognition of unusual presentation of MI, control of risk factors, control of plasma glucose levels

ACE, acetylcholinesterase; BP, blood pressure; H&P, history and physical examination; HRV, heart rate variability; MI, myocardial infarction; MIBG, metaiodobenzylguanidine; MUGA, multigated angiography; PGE₁, prostaglandin E₁.

TABLE 33-12

Pharmacologic Treatment of Autonomic Neuropathy

Drug	Class	Dosage	Side Effects
Orthostatic Hypotension			
9α-Fluorohydrocortisone	Mineralocorticoid	0.5-2 mg/day	Congestive heart failure, hypertension
Clonidine	α₂-Adrenergic agonist	0.1-0.5 mg at bedtime	Hypotension, sedation, dry mouth
Octreotide	Somatostatin analogue	0.1-0.5 μg/kg per day	Injection site pain, diarrhea
Gastroparesis			
Metoclopramide	D₂ receptor antagonist	10 mg 30-60 min before meals and at bedtime	Galactorrhea, extrapyramidal symptoms
Domperidone	D₂ receptor antagonist	10-20 mg 30-60 min before meals and at bedtime	Galactorrhea
Erythromycin	Motilin receptor agonist	250 mg 30 min before meals	Abdominal cramp, nausea, diarrhea, rash
Levosulfide	D₂ receptor antagonist	25 mg tid	Galactorrhea
Diabetic Diarrhea			
Metronidazole	Broad-spectrum antibiotic	250 mg tid, minimum 3 wk	Orthostatic hypotension
Clonidine	α₂-Adrenergic agonist	0.1 mg bid or tid	Toxic megacolon
Cholestyramine	Bile acid sequestrant	4 g one to six times a day	Aggravates nutrient malabsorption (at higher doses)
Loperamide	Opiate-receptor agonist	2 mg qid	
Octreotide	Somatostatin analogue	50 μg tid	
Cystopathy			
Bethanechol	Acetylcholine receptor agonist	10 mg qid	
Doxazosin	α₁-Adrenergic antagonist	1-2 mg bid or tid	Hypotension, headache, palpitations
Erectile Dysfunction			
Sildenafil	GMP type 5 phosphodiesterase inhibitor	50 mg before sexual activity, only once per day	Hypotension and fatal cardiac event (with nitrate-containing drugs), headache, flushing, nasal congestion, dyspepsia, musculoskeletal pain, blurred vision

bid, twice a day; D₂, dopamine 2; GMP, guanosine monophosphate; qid, four times a day; tid, three times a day.

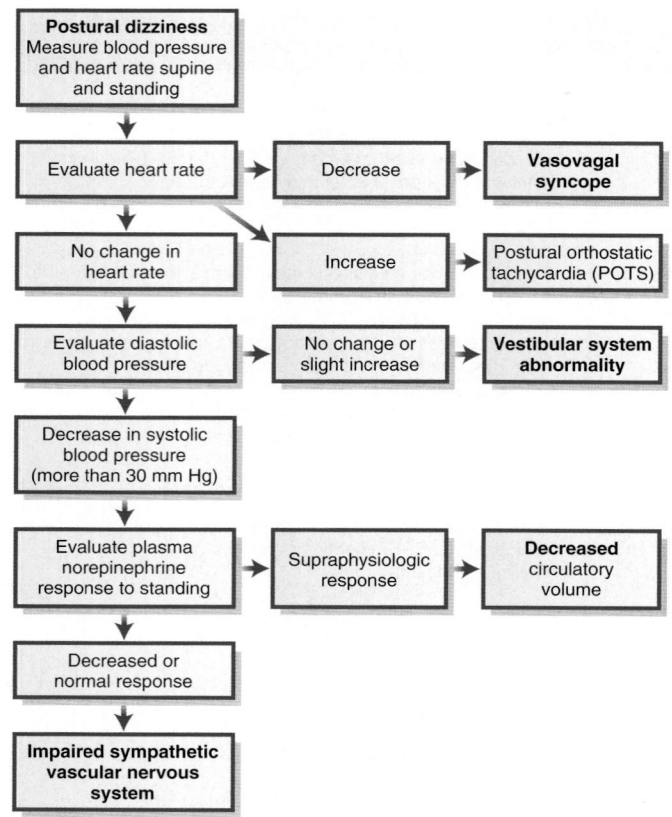

Figure 33-51 Evaluation of postural dizziness in diabetic patients. (Modified from Vinik A, Mehrabyan A. Diabetic neuropathies. *Med Clin North Am.* 2004;88:947-999.)

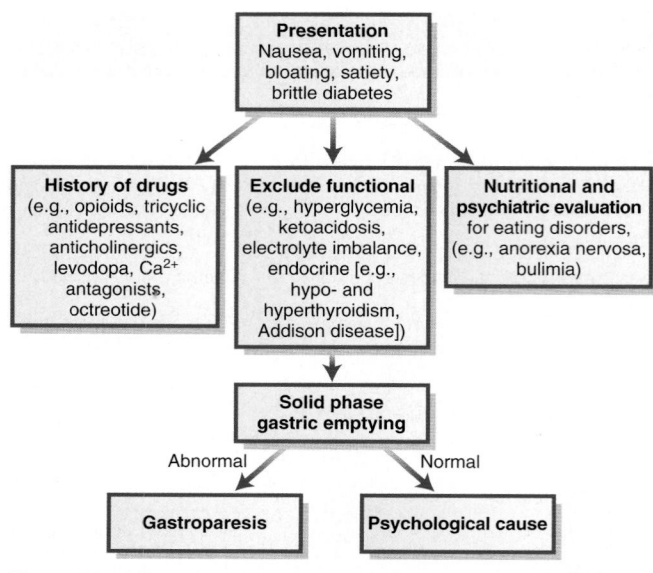

Figure 33-52 Evaluation of the patient with suspected gastroparesis. (Adapted from Vinik A, Mehrabyan A. Diabetic neuropathies. *Med Clin North Am.* 2004;88:947-999, used with permission.)

treated with the α_2-agonist clonidine, which in this setting can paradoxically increase BP. One should start with small doses and gradually increase the dose. If these measures fail, midodrine (an α_1-adrenergic agonist) or dihydroergotamine in combination with caffeine can help.

A particularly refractory form of postural hypotension occurs in some patients postprandially and may respond to therapy with octreotide given subcutaneously in the mornings.

Gastropathy. Gastrointestinal motor disorders (Fig. 33-52) are frequent and widespread in patients with T2DM regardless of symptoms,[844] and there is a poor correlation between symptoms and objective evidence of functional or organic defects. The first step in management of diabetic gastroparesis consists of multiple small feedings. The amount of fat should be decreased, because fat tends to delay gastric emptying. A low-fiber diet can also void bezoar formation. Maintenance of glycemic control is important.[845,846] Gastrokinetic drugs used to treat gastropathy include metoclopramide, erythromycin, and domperidone[847,848]; tachyphylaxis develops with all of these during prolonged administration. Erythromycin, given as a liquid or as a suppository, acts on the motilin receptor (the sweeper of the gut) and shortens gastric emptying time.[849] Several novel drugs including ghrelin (an orexigenic hormone) and ghrelin receptor agonists, motilin agonist (mitemcinal), 5HT4-receptor agonists, and a muscarinic antagonist are being investigated for their prokinetic effects. If medications fail and severe gastroparesis persists, jejunostomy placement into normally functioning bowel may be needed. Gastric electrical stimulation shows promise in treating refractory gastroparesis.

Enteropathy. Enteropathy involving the small bowel and colon can produce both chronic constipation and explosive diabetic diarrhea, making treatment of this particular complication difficult.

Antibiotics. Stasis of bowel contents with bacterial overgrowth can contribute to the diarrhea. Treatment with broad-spectrum antibiotics is the mainstay of therapy, including doxycycline or metronidazole. Metronidazole appears to be the most effective agent and should be continued for at least 3 weeks.

Cholestyramine. Retention of bile can occur and can be highly irritating to the gut. Chelation of bile salts with cholestyramine, 4 g mixed with fluid three times a day, can relieve symptoms.

Octreotide. Octreotide at a dose of 50 to 75 µg given subcutaneously twice a day inhibits the release of gastroenteropancreatic endocrine peptides, which may be responsible for diarrhea and electrolyte imbalance.

Diet. Patients with poor digestion can benefit from a gluten-free diet. Beware of certain fibers in the neuropathic patient that can lead to bezoar formation because of bowel stasis in gastroparetic or constipated patients. Most patients with constipation should respond to regular exercise, adequate hydration, and high-soluble fiber consumption supplemented with daily hydrophilic colloid.

Sexual Dysfunction

Male Sexual Dysfunction. Erectile dysfunction (ED) occurs in 50% to 75% of diabetic men, and it tends to occur at an earlier age than in the general population. The incidence of ED in diabetic men aged 20 to 29 years is 9% and increases to 95% by age 70 years. It may be the presenting symptom of diabetes. More than 50% of men who develop ED notice its onset within 10 years after the diagnosis of diabetes, but ED can precede the other complications of diabetes.

The etiology of ED in diabetes is multifactorial. Neuropathy, vascular disease, diabetes control, nutrition, endocrine disorders, psychogenic factors, and drugs used to treat diabetes and its complications play a role.[850,851] The diagnosis of the cause of ED is made by a logical, step-wise progression in all instances.[850,851] An approach to therapy has been presented and is discussed later in this chapter.[850]

Diagnosis. A thorough workup for impotence includes a medical and sexual history; physical and psychological evaluations; blood tests for diabetes and levels of testosterone, prolactin, and thyroid hormones; a test for nocturnal erections; assessments of penile, pelvic, and spinal nerve function; and measurements of penile blood supply and BP.

The health care provider should initiate questions that will help distinguish the various forms of organic ED from those that are psychogenic. The physical examination must include evaluations of the ANS, vascular supply, and hypothalamic-pituitary-gonadal axis.

Autonomic neuropathy causing ED is almost always accompanied by loss of ankle reflexes and absence or reduction of vibration sense over the large toes. More direct evidence of impairment of penile autonomic function can be obtained by demonstrating normal perianal sensation, assessing the tone of the anal sphincter during a rectal examination, and ascertaining the presence of an anal wink when the area of the skin adjacent to the anus is stroked or contraction of the anus when the glans penis is squeezed (bulbo-cavernosus reflex). These measurements are easily and quickly done at the bedside and reflect the integrity of sacral parasympathetic divisions.

Vascular disease is usually manifested by buttock claudication but may be caused by stenosis of the internal pudendal artery. A penile-brachial index of less than 0.7 indicates diminished blood supply. A venous leak manifests as unresponsiveness to vasodilators and needs to be evaluated by penile Doppler sonography.

To distinguish psychogenic from organic erectile dysfunction, nocturnal penile tumescence (NPT) can be tested. Normal NPT defines psychogenic ED, and a negative response to vasodilators implies vascular insufficiency. Application of NPT is not so simple. It is much like having a sphygmomanometer cuff inflate over the penis many times during the night while one is trying to have a normal night's sleep. The patient might have to take home the device and become familiar with it over several nights before a reliable estimate of the failure of NPT can be obtained.

Treatment. A number of treatment modalities are available, and each has positive and negative effects. Patients must be made aware of positive and negative aspects before a therapeutic decision is made. Before any form of treatment is considered, every effort should be made to have the patient withdraw from alcohol and eliminate smoking. If possible, drugs that are known to cause ED should be discontinued. Metabolic control should be optimized.

Relaxation of the corpus cavernosa smooth muscle cells is caused by NO and cGMP, and the ability to have and maintain an erection depends on the generation of NO. The peripherally acting phosphodiesterase inhibitors are the major oral medications for erectile dysfunction in diabetic patients. The PDE5 inhibitors block the action of phosphodiesterase and permit cGMP to accumulate. This class of agents consists of sildenafil, vardenafil, and tadalafil. These agents enhance blood flow to the corpora cavernosa with sexual stimulation and have been evaluated in diabetic patients with efficacy of about 70%. Generally, people with diabetes and ED require the maximum dose of each drug: sildenafil 100 mg, tadalafil 20 mg, and vardenafil 20 mg. Lower doses should be considered in patients with renal failure and hepatic dysfunction. The duration of the drug effect is 4 to 24 hours but may be prolonged. Before these drugs are prescribed, it is important to exclude ischemic heart disease. These drugs are absolutely contraindicated in patients being treated with nitroglycerine or other nitrate-containing drugs because severe hypotension and fatal cardiac events can occur.[781,852]

Direct injection of prostacyclin into the corpus cavernosum induces satisfactory erections in a significant number of men. Also, surgical implantation of a penile prosthesis may be appropriate. The less expensive type of prosthesis is a semirigid, permanently erect type that is embarrassing and uncomfortable for some patients. The inflatable type is three times more expensive and subject to mechanical failure, but it avoids the embarrassment caused by other devices.

Female Sexual Dysfunction. Women with diabetes mellitus can experience decreased sexual desire and more pain on sexual intercourse, but they are also at risk for decreased sexual arousal, with inadequate lubrication.[853] Diagnosis of female sexual dysfunction using vaginal plethysmography to measure lubrication and vaginal flushing has not been well established.

Cystopathy. In diabetic autonomic neuropathy, the motor function of the bladder is unimpaired, but afferent fiber damage results in diminished bladder sensation. The urinary bladder can be enlarged to more than three times its normal size. Patients are seen with bladders filled to their umbilicus, yet they feel no discomfort. Loss of bladder sensation occurs with diminished voiding frequency, and the patient is no longer able to void completely. Consequently, dribbling and overflow incontinence are common complaints. A postvoid residual of greater than 150 mL diagnoses cystopathy. Cystopathy can put patients at risk for urinary infections.

Patients with cystopathy should be instructed to palpate the bladder and, if they are unable to initiate micturition when their bladder is full, to use the Crede maneuver (massage or pressure on the lower portion of the abdomen just above the pubic bone) to start the flow of urine. The principal aim of the treatment should be to improve bladder emptying and to reduce the risk of urinary tract infection. Parasympathomimetics such as bethanechol are sometimes helpful, although often they do not help to fully empty the bladder. Extended sphincter relaxation can be achieved with an α_1-blocker, such as doxazosin.[648] Self-catheterization can be particularly useful in this setting, and the risk of infection generally is low.

Sweating Disturbances

Hyperhidrosis of the upper body, often related to eating (gustatory sweating), is a characteristic feature of autonomic neuropathy. Gustatory sweating accompanies the ingestion of certain foods, particularly spicy foods and cheeses. Gustatory sweating is more common than previously believed; topically applied—and possibly oral—glycopyrrolate (an antimuscarinic compound) is a very effective treatment in reducing both severity and frequency.[854,855] Symptoms are avoided by avoiding the inciting food.

Anhidrosis of the lower body is also common in autonomic neuropathy. Loss of lower body sweating can cause dry, brittle skin that cracks easily, predisposing the patient to ulcer formation that can lead to loss of a limb. Special attention must be paid to foot care.

Metabolic Dysfunction

Blood glucose concentration is normally maintained during starvation or increased insulin action by an asymptomatic parasympathetic response that includes bradycardia and mild hypotension, followed by a sympathetic response with glucagon and epinephrine secretion for short-term glucose counterregulation and growth hormone and cortisol for long-term regulation. The release of catecholamine alerts the patient to take the required measures to prevent coma due to low blood glucose. The inability to recognize the warning signs of impending neuroglycopenia is known as *hypoglycemic unawareness*. The failure of glucose counterregulation can be confirmed by the absence of glucagon and epinephrine responses to hypoglycemia induced by a standard controlled dose of insulin.[856]

In patients with T1DM, the glucagon response is impaired with diabetes duration of 1 to 5 years, and after 14 to 31 years of diabetes the glucagon response is almost undetectable. It is not present in those with autonomic neuropathy. However, a syndrome of hypoglycemic autonomic failure occurs with intensification of diabetes control and repeated episodes of hypoglycemia. The exact mechanism is not understood, but it does represent a real barrier to physiologic glycemic control. In the absence of severe autonomic dysfunction, hypoglycemic unawareness associated with hypoglycemia is at least in part reversible.

Patients with hypoglycemia unawareness and unresponsiveness pose a significant management problem for the physician. Although autonomic neuropathy can improve with intensive therapy and normalization of blood glucose, there is a risk to the patient, who may become hypoglycemic without being aware of it and who cannot mount a counterregulatory response. It is our recommendation that, if a pump is used, boluses of smaller than calculated amounts should be used. If intensive conventional therapy is used, long-acting insulin with very small boluses should be given. In general, to avoid insulin-induced hypoglycemia in these patients, treatment goals should be relaxed and should not aim for normal glucose and HbA_{1c} levels.[669] Continuous glucose monitors (CGMs) may decrease the number of hypoglycemic episodes, but their effect on hypoglycemia unawareness is uncertain.

Further complicating management in some diabetic patients is the development of a functional autonomic insufficiency associated with intensive insulin treatment, which resembles autonomic neuropathy in all relevant aspects. In these instances, it is prudent to relax therapy, as for the patient with bona fide autonomic neuropathy. If hypoglycemia occurs in these patients at a certain glucose level, it will take a lower glucose level to trigger the same symptoms in the next 24 to 48 hours. Avoidance of hypoglycemia for a few days results in recovery of the adrenergic response.

DIABETIC HEART DISEASE

Coronary Heart Disease

The past decades have witnessed substantial declines in coronary heart disease (CHD) mortality rates in the general population in the United States, but the improvement in CHD mortality rates has been significantly lower in diabetic men and women.[857] More than 90% of all patients with diabetes have T2DM, and it is this population (mostly middle-aged and elderly) that has been evaluated in most of the studies of CHD risk. In these studies, the excess morbidity and mortality rates associated with diabetes and elevated glucose remained even after adjustment for traditional CHD risk factors.

Effect of Diabetes on Risk of Coronary Heart Disease

The Framingham Study showed a twofold to threefold elevation in the risk of clinically evident atherosclerotic disease in patients with T2DM compared to those without diabetes.[858] Diabetic men in the Multiple Risk Factor Intervention Trial (MRFIT) had an absolute risk of CHD death more than three times higher than that of the nondiabetic cohort, even after adjustment for established risk factors.[73] Seminal work from Finland showed that patients with T2DM without a previous MI have a risk of MI over 7 years as high as that of nondiabetic patients with a history of MI (Fig. 33-53).[84] In this study, the case-fatality rate after MI was also substantially higher in patients with diabetes. In women, diabetes mitigates the cardioprotective effects of the premenopausal period, and women with diabetes had a CHD mortality rate as high as that of diabetic men.

The risk of cardiovascular fatality and events conferred by T2DM has been examined in several prospective and observational trials with varying populations of patients.[859-862] Prospective data from the Organization to Assess Strategies for Ischemic Syndromes (OASIS) registry was analyzed to determine the effect of diabetes on outcomes of patients with unstable angina and non–Q-wave MI.[859] Patients with diabetes had a significantly increased adjusted RR for total mortality (1.57; 95% CI, 1.38 to 1.81; $p < 0.001$), death due to CVD (1.49; 95% CI, 1.27 to 1.74; $p < 0.001$), new MI (1.34; 95% CI, 1.14 to 1.57; $p < 0.001$), stroke (1.45; 95% CI, 1.09 to 1.92; $p = 0.009$), and new CHF (1.41; 95% CI, 1.24 to 1.60; $p < 0.001$). Diabetic patients without prior CVD had the same event rates for all outcomes as nondiabetic patients with previous vascular disease.

In another prospective cohort trial,[860] the adjusted hazard ratio (HR) for overall mortality risk in diabetic patients ($n = 393$) after a first MI was 1.5 (95% CI, 1.1 to 2.0) compared with equivalent nondiabetic patients ($n = 1132$). The HR for cardiovascular mortality risk in diabetic patients was similar to that in nondiabetic patients who had experienced a previous MI. The risk of mortality from

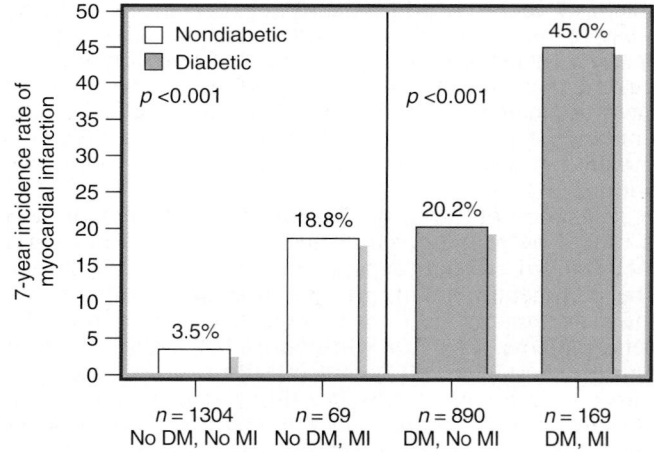

Figure 33-53 Marked increase in the risk of coronary artery disease in patients with type 2 diabetes mellitus (DM) compared with nondiabetic subjects, in a population-based study in Finland, over a 7-year follow-up period. Patients with diabetes who had no previous myocardial infarction (MI) had a risk of first MI approximately equal to that of nondiabetic subjects who had already sustained an MI. These data support recommendations from the American Diabetes Association to treat diabetic subjects as if they already have established coronary artery disease. (From Haffner SM, Lehto S, Ronnemaa T, et al. Mortality from coronary heart disease in subjects with type 2 diabetes and in nondiabetic subjects with and without prior myocardial infarction. *N Engl J Med.* 1998;339:229-234.)

all causes was significantly higher in women than in men (adjusted HR, 2.7 versus 1.3, $p = 0.01$).

In contrast to these findings, two large observational trials failed to find that diabetes conferred equivalent or greater risk of mortality than previous MI.[862,863] In the cross-sectional study, RR for all-cause mortality was 1.33 (95% CI, 1.14 to 1.55) for patients with MI compared to patients with T2DM. In the cohort study, patients with MI also had a significantly higher risk of all-cause death (adjusted RR, 1.35; 95% CI, 1.25 to 1.44), cardiovascular death (RR, 2.93; 95% CI, 2.54 to 3.41), and hospital admission for MI (RR, 3.1; 95% CI, 2.57 to 3.73). Based on these findings, the authors concluded that established CVD confers greater risk than diabetes.[861]

The risk of mortality conferred by diabetes was also assessed in the Atherosclerosis Risk in Communities (ARIC) study, a population-based cohort study that investigated the cause of atherosclerosis in a biracial population in the United States.[862] Patients with prior MI had an adjusted RR of 1.9 (95% CI, 1.35 to 2.56; $p < 0.001$) for fatal CHD or nonfatal MI and adjusted RR of 1.8 (95% CI, 1.22 to 2.72; $p = 0.003$) for fatal CHD or nonfatal MI, compared to the patients with diabetes and no previous MI. There was no significant difference in the risk of stroke in the two groups.

All of these studies demonstrated that diabetes alone results in a significantly increased risk of CVD. The strategy of considering diabetes as a CHD risk equivalent for purposes of assessing risk and defining a treatment regimen is appropriate.

The risk of CHD has also been evaluated in smaller subsets of patients with T1DM. In the Framingham Study, the cumulative CAD mortality rate in patients with T1DM was approximately four times that of nondiabetic patients by age 55 years.[863] As in patients with T2DM, the first deaths related to CAD in patients with T1DM occurred by the fourth decade of life, and the cumulative mortality rate increased at a similar rate in both groups in the subsequent 20 years. The rise in CAD mortality rate with age in patients with T1DM is substantially higher in those patients with nephropathy. In these patients, the risk of CAD can be as much as 15 times higher than in patients without persistent proteinuria. Therefore, persistent proteinuria is a strong predictor of the development of CAD in this population. These findings suggest that proteinuria is a marker of generalized vascular damage that predisposes to CVD.

Two prospective epidemiologic studies, the Pittsburgh Epidemiology of Diabetes Complications study (EDC)[864] and Eurodiab,[865] a multicenter, clinic-based study in Europe, confirmed the Framingham findings and reported an incidence of total coronary events of 16% over 10 years and 9% over 7 years of follow-up in patients with T1DM. These incidence rates presumably reflect patients in their late 30s, 10 years beyond baseline age in the studies. In EDC, the total incidence of CAD (including angina and ischemic electrocardiographic changes) was more than 2% per year for those older than 35 years. A more recent report, using 12-year follow-up data,[866] proposed that the annual rate of major CAD events (MI, fatal CAD, or revascularization) is 0.98% for those with diabetes duration of 20 to 30 years (average age, 28 to 38 years). The event rates are identical for both genders, consistent with a loss of the protection from CHD fatality in premenopausal women with diabetes.

The follow-up of the Diabetes UK cohort, a group of 23,751 subjects with insulin-treated diabetes diagnosed before the age of 30 years, also showed similar mortality rates for men and women, and the size of this cohort permitted robust gender-specific estimates of standardized mortality ratios (SMRs).[867] Among those aged 20 to 29

years, the SMRs for ischemic heart disease mortality were 11.8 in men and 44.8 in women; for those aged 30 to 39 years, the SMRs were 8.0 and 41.6, respectively. Other forms of CVD, such as hypertension, valvular disease, cardiomyopathy, heart failure, and stroke, were also increased.

Recent data further support and highlight the increased cardiovascular risk and overall mortality risk in patients with T1DM, which may be further heightened by the presence of renal dysfunction.[868]

It is unclear whether there has been any recent decline in mortality or morbidity rates from CHD associated with T1DM. The Pittsburgh EDC reported no difference in the cumulative incidence of CAD with 20, 25, or 30 years' disease duration according to year of diagnosis (1950 through 1980).[866] The benefits of improved diabetes care therefore do not appear to have reduced CAD mortality rates associated with T1DM.

Aggregation of Traditional Coronary Heart Disease Risk Factors in Diabetes

It is now well established that a number of traditional CHD risk factors (e.g., hypertension, dyslipidemia, obesity, insulin resistance) tend to occur together in patients with diabetes.[869] Approximately 50% of patients with diabetes have hypertension, and more than 30% have hypercholesterolemia at the time of diagnosis. As in nondiabetic patients, these risk factors independently predict the risk of CVD mortality.[73] However, even in the presence of one or more concomitant risk factors, diabetes increases the CVD death rate (Fig. 33-54). It also appears that diabetes interacts synergistically with other risk factors to more sharply increase risk as the number of total risk factors increases.

There are data suggesting that the cardiovascular risk associated with T2DM is a consequence of insulin resistance during the prediabetic state.[870] A population-based study of diabetes and CVD monitored Mexican-American and non–Latin American white subjects for 7 years. Those subjects who converted to diabetes from a prediabetic state and who were insulin resistant had higher BP, higher

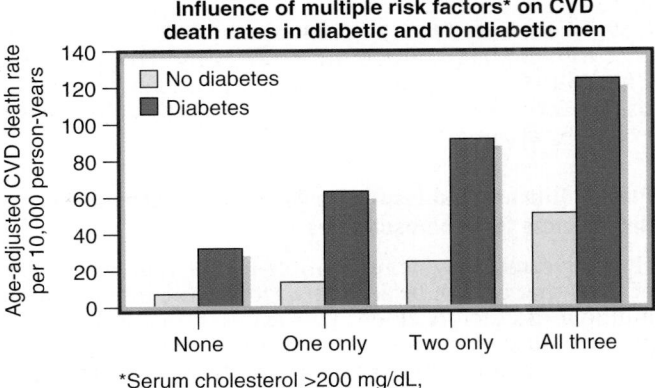

Figure 33-54 Age-adjusted cardiovascular disease (CVD) death rates by number of risk factors for men with and without diabetes at baseline screened for the Multiple Risk Factor Intervention Trial. In the presence of diabetes, the cardiovascular death rate steeply rises at any level of concomitant risk factors. SBP, systolic blood pressure. (From Stamler J, Vaccaro O, Neaton JD, et al. Diabetes, other risk factors, and 12-year cardiovascular mortality for men screened in the Multiple Risk Factor Intervention Trial. *Diabetes Care.* 1993;16:434-444.)

triglyceride levels, and lower HDL-cholesterol levels. These CVD risk factors suggest that the atherogenic changes seen during the prediabetic state are primarily associated with increased insulin resistance and that treatment strategies that increase insulin secretion in these patients can reduce cardiovascular risk.

Other studies have also concluded that impaired insulin sensitivity during the prediabetic state contributes to atherogenic risk.[871] Prediabetic subjects who were insulin resistant had higher levels of inflammatory markers (C-reactive protein, PAI-1, and fibrinogen) than converters with predominantly low insulin secretion or nonconverters. Therefore, a proinflammatory state can contribute to the atherogenic risk profile in prediabetic patients with increased insulin resistance. Evidence of inflammation is not seen in prediabetic patients with a primary defect in insulin secretion. Many aspects of the proatherogenic and proinflammatory state of prediabetes may derive from increased adiposity and in particular visceral fat.[872]

The UKPDS further confirmed the importance of risk factor aggregation in diabetic patients. In this large population of patients with newly diagnosed T2DM, the development of CAD during follow-up was significantly associated with increased concentrations of LDL-cholesterol, decreased concentrations of HDL-cholesterol, increased levels of HbA_{1c} and systolic BP, and a history of smoking measured at baseline.[873]

Given the multifactorial nature of atherogenic risk in patients with T2DM, it is reasonable to conclude that an aggressive multifactorial intervention could significantly reduce cardiovascular risk. The value of such a treatment regimen was tested in the Steno-2 study,[597] in which 160 patients with T2DM and microalbuminuria were randomized to receive either conventional treatment in accordance with national guidelines or intensive therapy that included behavior modification and targeted pharmacologic therapy for hyperglycemia, hypertension, dyslipidemia, and microalbuminuria along with secondary prevention of CVD with aspirin. Over a mean follow-up period of 7.8 years, patients who received intensive treatment had greater improvements in HbA_{1c}, BP, fasting serum cholesterol and triglyceride values, and urinary albumin excretion than patients receiving conventional therapy. The greater degree of improvement in risk factors with intensive therapy was also reflected in outcomes. Patients receiving intensive therapy had a significantly lower risk of CVD (HR 0.47; 95% CI, 0.24 to 0.73), nephropathy (HR 0.39; 95% CI, 0.17 to 0.87), retinopathy (HR 0.42; 95% CI, 0.21 to 0.86), and autonomic neuropathy (HR 0.37; 95% CI, 0.18 to 0.79). Overall, long-term intensive treatment of risk factors reduced the risk of CVD and microvascular events by about 50%.[597]

Plasma Glucose and Insulin Resistance as Independent Risk Factors for Atherosclerosis

Hyperglycemia may be responsible for the high excess risk of CHD that cannot be accounted for by the interaction of multiple risk factors alone. This association appears to be graded and continuous, without a clear threshold below which the relationship ends. One study showed that mortality rates from all causes, CVD, and ischemic heart disease increased progressively across quintiles of fasting blood glucose levels in patients with T2DM (Fig. 33-55).[874] Other data suggest a dose-response relationship between hyperglycemia and CVD mortality rate in diabetes, with patients with the highest levels of fasting blood glucose having a CVD mortality rate almost five times higher than patients with the two lowest levels combined.[875]

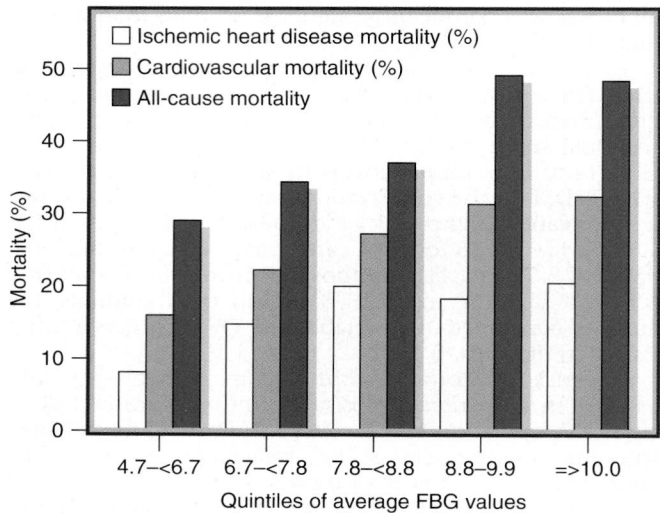

Figure 33-55 All-cause mortality, cardiovascular mortality, and ischemic heart disease mortality rates in patients with type 2 diabetes mellitus by quintiles of average fasting blood glucose (FBG) values. Cardiovascular mortality and all-cause mortality rates increase throughout the range of fasting plasma glucose in a graded fashion. (From Andersson DK, Svardsudd K. Long-term glycemic control relates to mortality in type II diabetes. *Diabetes Care*. 1995;18:1534-1543.)

In a more recent study of the relationship between blood glucose and cardiovascular fatality, 17,869 male civil servants enrolled in the Whitehall Study from 1967 to 1969 were monitored, and outcomes were correlated with baseline measurements of the 2-hour postload blood glucose (2hBG) level after a 50-g oral glucose load.[876] In these subjects, the HR for CHD mortality increased as a linear function of 2hBG for all values of 2hBG greater than 83 mg/dL. With 2hBG values between 83 and 200 mg/dL, the age-adjusted HR for CHD was 3.62 (95% CI, 2.3 to 5.6).

Tominaga and colleagues examined survival rates in a cohort of participants in a diabetes prevalence trial in Japan[877] and concluded that the risk of cardiovascular fatality is based on impaired glucose tolerance rather than impaired fasting glucose.

Further substantiation of the role of impaired glucose tolerance in cardiovascular mortality risk was provided by an analysis of data from the Diabetes Epidemiology: Collaborative Analysis of Diagnostic Criteria in Europe (DECODE) study.[878] In this study, more than 25,000 men and women were monitored for a mean of 7.3 years, and outcomes were correlated with measurements of fasting glucose and 2hBG after a 75-mg glucose load at baseline. The results indicated that the oral glucose tolerance test provides the best index of risk of mortality associated with impaired glucose tolerance.

The Nurses' Health Study also implicated the prediabetic state as a risk factor for CVD.[879] In this large cohort of women, 5894 developed diabetes over a 20-year follow-up. In this group, the age-adjusted RR for MI was 3.75 (95% CI, 3.10 to 4.53) in the period before diagnosis of diabetes and 4.57 (95% CI, 3.87 to 5.39) after diagnosis, compared with women who did not develop diabetes, even after adjustment for other cardiovascular risk factors. The risk of stroke was also increased before onset of diabetes.

The continuum of CVD risk with rising glucose levels has also been identified in patients with T1DM[880] and in subjects without clinically overt diabetes but with varying levels of glucose intolerance.[881] Hyperglycemia also has adverse effects on the vessel wall as judged by objective assessment of carotid intima medial thickness (CIMT).[8,882-884]

The Metabolic Syndrome

Definitions and Diagnosis

Almost all patients with diabetes and the concomitant CVD risk factors of hypertension, obesity, and dyslipidemia also have insulin resistance.[83] The clustering of these risk factors in a single patient has been termed the *metabolic syndrome*. Although there is general agreement on the components of the metabolic syndrome (i.e., obesity, hypertension, dyslipidemia, and dysfunctional glucose metabolism), the criteria for clinical diagnosis are still under discussion as is the clinical impact of identifying this clustering of risk factors. Separate sets of diagnostic criteria for the metabolic syndrome have been published by the National Cholesterol Education Program (NCEP) Adult Treatment Panel III (ATP III),[885] by the World Health Organization (WHO),[886] and by the International Diabetes Federation (IDF),[887] with there also being clinical overlap among these definitions and the designation of prediabetes.[888]

According to the NCEP guidelines,[885] the metabolic syndrome is based on the presence of three of the following five risk factors[885]:
- Abdominal obesity (waist circumference >40 inches in men and >35 inches in women)
- Plasma triglycerides 150 mg/dL or higher
- Plasma HDL-cholesterol less than 40 mg/dL in men, less than 50 mg/dL in women
- BP 130/85 mm Hg or higher
- Fasting plasma glucose 110 mg/dL or higher

The NCEP criteria give precedence to obesity as a contributor to the metabolic syndrome and apply cutpoints for triglycerides and HDL that are probably less stringent than would be used to identify a categorical risk factor, reflecting the fact that many marginal risk factors can result in a significant risk for CVD. The NCEP criteria do not require explicit demonstration of insulin resistance for diagnosis of the metabolic syndrome, and patients with diabetes are not excluded from the diagnosis.[886] There are modest differences between the NCEP criteria and those developed by the WHO[886] and the IDF.[887] One intriguing aspect of the IDF criteria is the recognition that individuals of Southeast Asian origins may have increased visceral adiposity with less waist circumference than what is observed in Western countries and hence the difference in waist circumference criteria for such individuals.

Epidemiology

The prevalence of the metabolic syndrome in the United States, as defined by the NCEP criteria, has been estimated from the National Health and Nutrition Examination Survey (NHANES) database.[889] Based on data from the third NHANES (1988-1994) survey, the overall age-adjusted prevalence of the metabolic syndrome was 23.7%. The prevalence increased with age, ranging from 6.7% in subjects aged 20 to 29 years to 43.5% in subjects aged 60 to 69 years. There were also differences in prevalence based on ethnicity, with the highest overall prevalence among Mexican Americans (31.9%).

The Metabolic Syndrome and Cardiovascular Disease

The impact of metabolic syndrome on incidence and mortality risk of CVD has been examined in several studies.[890-892] A Finnish prospective cohort study showed that the age-adjusted RR for CHD mortality was 2.96 (95% CI, 1.30 to 6.76), compared to patients without this condition. Similar increases in risk were also noted for CVD mortality (RR, 2.76; 95% CI, 1.45 to 5.24) and all-cause mortality (RR, 2.05; 95% CI, 1.31 to 3.21). Similar degrees of increase in risk with the metabolic syndrome were also seen when other diagnostic criteria were used.

In the United States, NHANES II studied the impact of the metabolic syndrome on CVD mortality.[893] The HRs for CHD mortality and CVD mortality were 1.65 (95% CI, 1.10 to 2.47; $p = 0.02$) and 1.56 (95% CI, 1.15 to 2.12; $p = 0.005$), respectively, compared to subjects without the metabolic syndrome.

The West of Scotland Coronary Prevention Study[892] also demonstrated increased risk of CHD in patients with the metabolic syndrome. In this study, elevated C-reactive protein was more common in subjects with the metabolic syndrome and added to the prognostic value for both CHD and diabetes.

A summary of all of the studies assessing the increased risk of mortality, CVD, and diabetes associated with the metabolic syndrome was published in 2005.[893] Studies that used NCEP and WHO diagnostic criteria for defining the metabolic syndrome were analyzed separately. For three studies that used the exact NCEP definition of the metabolic syndrome, the increased risk of all-cause mortality was not significant. For seven studies that used the NCEP definition, the RR for CVD was 1.65 (95% CI, 1.38 to 1.99). Inclusion of four other studies that used a modified NCEP definition did not appreciably change the RR. In four studies that used the NCEP definition, the RR for diabetes was 2.99 (95% CI, 1.96 to 4.57). For studies that used the most exact WHO definition of the metabolic syndrome, the fixed-effects estimates of RR were 1.37 (95% CI, 1.09 to 1.74) for all-cause mortality, 1.93 (95% CI, 1.39 to 2.67) for CVD, and 6.08 (95% CI, 4.76 to 7.76) for diabetes.

Clinical guidelines for diagnosis and management of the metabolic syndrome were addressed in 2005 in a joint statement by the American Heart Association and the National Heart, Lung, and Blood Institute (NHLBI) summarizing available steps for managing the risk factors associated with the metabolic syndrome.[894]

It has been hypothesized that hyperinsulinemia is the underlying link between hyperglycemia and CVD in these patients.[895] A number of studies have shown hyperinsulinemia to be an independent predictor of CVD risk. Furthermore, in patients spanning the spectrum of glucose tolerance, from normal to hyperglycemic to diabetic, insulin resistance positively correlates with atherosclerosis as assessed by CIMT.[896]

The San Antonio Heart Study, a population-based study of diabetes and CVD in Mexican Americans and non–Latin American whites, confirmed the relationship between insulin resistance or plasma insulin and CVD.[89]

The Role of Glycemic Control

The UKPDS confirmed the positive association between plasma glucose levels and CHD risk for HbA$_{1c}$ levels greater than 6.2% in patients with diabetes.[895] CHD risk increased by 11% with each percentage point elevation in HbA$_{1c}$ (Table 33-13). The question remains, however, whether intensive glycemic control can modify the cardiovascular risk profile of patients with diabetes.

Earlier studies, such as the DCCT and the smaller Veterans Affairs (VA) study, did not show a reduction in cardiovascular end points with intensive metabolic control. These studies had limitations, however. Although relatively large ($N = 1441$), the DCCT followed a relatively young (mean age, 27 years) population of patients with T1DM for

TABLE 33-13

Treatment Goals for Prevention of Coronary Heart Disease in Patients with Diabetes

Glycosylated hemoglobin (HbA_{1c}) ≤6.2%
Low-density lipoprotein cholesterol ≤100 mg/dL
Blood pressure ≤130/85 mm Hg
Aspirin 81-325 mg/day

more than 6 years. At the end of follow-up, few events had occurred.[4] Intensive therapy reduced the risk of CVD and peripheral vascular disease by 41% compared with conventional therapy, but the difference was not statistically significant. Similarly, in the VA study, intensive blood glucose control in patients with T2DM did not significantly reduce cardiovascular end points.[897] Both studies lacked adequate power to detect a difference in macrovascular events between treatment groups because of the small number of events in each group, small patient populations, and relatively short follow-up.

A 17-year follow-up of 1441 patients from the DCCT trial more unambiguously demonstrated the benefit of intensive glycemic control in T1DM.[898] This was part of the observational EDIC study. During follow-up, intensive treatment reduced the risk of CVD by 42% ($p = 0.02$) and the risk of nonfatal MI, stroke, or death from CVD by 57% ($p = 0.02$). After 11 years of follow-up, the treatment groups were virtually identical in terms of HbA_{1c}, BP, and lipid risk factors. Patients in the conventional treatment group had more albuminuria and microalbuminuria than intensively treated patients, but the differences in risk remained significant after adjustment for these factors. These findings indicate that intensive glycemic control reduced the long-term risk of CVD in patients with T1DM.

The UKPDS was larger and was adequately powered to detect a difference between groups in macrovascular events.[5] Intensive glycemic control trended toward demonstrating a lower rate of MI than conventional treatment ($p = 0.052$).[5] As in the DCCT, intensive therapy in the UKPDS significantly improved the rate of microvascular disease.

Despite the lack of overall efficacy of intensive treatment for management of macrovascular complications of diabetes in the UKPDS, there are indications that specific therapies may be effective.[5] In a retrospective analysis of an overweight subset ($n = 342$) of the UKPDS cohort who were treated with metformin, there were significant reductions in the occurrence of any diabetes-related end point (32%), diabetes-related death (42%), and all-cause mortality (36%), compared with conventionally treated patients.

Two studies have suggested that thiazolidinediones can prevent macrovascular events associated with T2DM. Because these drugs work by increasing insulin sensitivity rather than by increasing insulin levels, this finding is consistent with data showing that insulin resistance is positively correlated with cardiovascular outcomes (described earlier). Howard and colleagues demonstrated that 8 weeks of treatment with rosiglitazone 4 mg daily significantly reduced progression of thickening of the common carotid intima-media, a surrogate index of atherosclerotic disease progression, compared with placebo treatment in nondiabetic patients who had established CAD.[896] In the PROactive study (PROspective pioglitAzone Clinical Trial In macroVascular Events), 5238 patients with T2DM and evidence of macrovascular disease were randomized to receive or not receive pioglitazone in addition to glucose-lowering drugs and other medications, with the objective being

similar glucose control in both arms.[899] After a mean of 34.5 months, there was no significant difference in the two treatment groups in terms of the primary end point of the study, a composite of all-cause mortality, nonfatal MI, stroke, acute coronary syndrome, surgical intervention in the leg or coronary arteries, and amputation above the ankle. According to the investigators, this broad primary end point, which extended beyond the more standard, objective primary end point often employed in cardiovascular trials, was done to increase the chances of seeing benefit. In fact, improvements in peripheral vascular disease end points have been difficult to demonstrate, even in the presence of potent cardiovascular risk-reducing agents like statins. Of note, patients treated with pioglitazone had significantly lower risk for the secondary end point of composite all-cause mortality, nonfatal MI, and stroke (HR 0.84; 95% CI, 0.80 to 1.02; $p = 0.027$). Compared with placebo, pioglitazone also significantly reduced the need to add insulin to glucose-lowering regimens. Intravascular coronary ultrasound studies have also shown significant decreases in coronary atherosclerosis in response to pioglitazone.[900]

Despite the effect of thiazolidinediones in these studies, the putative beneficial effect of rosiglitazone on CVD was challenged by a meta-analysis conducted by Nissen and coworkers[900] that examined short-term trials designed to assess the effect of rosiglitazone on glycemic control and suggested that rosiglitazone was associated with a significant risk of excess MI. The studies in this meta-analysis did not examine cardiovascular events as primary end points, and the cardiovascular events were not adjudicated. In contrast, another meta-analysis, conducted by Lago and associates, examined only randomized clinical trials in which cardiovascular end points were prespecified as events of interest or in which such events were adjudicated. This examination did not show that either rosiglitazone or pioglitazone conferred an excess risk of cardiovascular death.[901] Subsequent studies have also suggested that rosiglitazone does not increase cardiovascular events, as also supported by an FDA consensus review panel.[902] Differences do exist between pioglitazone and rosiglitazone. Enthusiasm for the use of these agents has also been tempered by increased bone fractures and questions regarding bladder cancer.[903]

Three recent trials have examined whether lowering the target for glycemic control (to <7%) can reduce the risk for cardiovascular events. The ACCORD trial randomized patients with T2DM who had established CVD or multiple risk factors to a treatment-directed HbA_{1c} value lower than 7.0% or to standard therapy with an HbA_{1c} target value between 7.0% and 7.9%. Over 3.5 years of follow-up, total mortality rate was increased in the intensively treated group, and there was no significant reduction in cardiovascular events.[553] The Veterans Affairs Diabetes Trial (VADT) randomized patients to either intensive treatment (HbA_{1c}, 6.9%) or standard therapy (HbA_{1c}, 8.4%); it also did not demonstrate a reduction in cardiovascular events in the former group.[904] The ADVANCE trial randomly assigned patients to an intensively treated group attaining an HbA_{1c} of 6.5% or a standard-control group attaining an HbA_{1c} of 7.3%; it demonstrated a relative reduction of 10% in the combined outcome of major macrovascular and microvascular events, primarily due to a 21% reduction in nephropathy.[551] Taken together, these three studies do not support treatment to an HbA_{1c} value lower than the currently recommended 7.0% as a strategy to reduce cardiovascular events, despite the epidemiologic relationship between cardiovascular risk and HbA_{1c}.

The Bypass Angioplasty Revascularization Investigation 2 Diabetes (BARI 2D) trial randomized 2368 patients with

T2DM and CAD to either prompt revascularization or intensive medical therapy alone and to either insulin-sensitization or insulin-provision diabetes therapy. Randomization was stratified by the proposed revascularization method. The 5-year survival and major cardiovascular event rates were similar in all study subgroups except for those patients undergoing coronary artery bypass grafting (CABG), who had fewer major cardiovascular events after revascularization. There was less hypoglycemia and weight gain and greater apparent benefit from CABG in the insulin-sensitization group.

In response to the experience with rosiglitazone, the FDA instituted new safety hurdles that new antidiabetic drugs must meet in their approval process. As a result, a large amount of new data regarding cardiovascular effects of oral antidiabetic agents is now emerging or forthcoming. Dipeptidyl peptidase 4 (DPP4) inhibitors lower glucose by inhibiting degradation of the incretin GLP1. Two landmark trials testing the effects of saxagliptin and alogliptin on cardiovascular events have now been published. The Saxagliptin Assessment of Vascular Outcomes Recorded in Patients with Diabetes Mellitus (SAVOR)–Thrombolysis in Myocardial Infarction (TIMI) 53 (SAVOR-TIMI 53) trial established safety for this agent with no difference in cardiovascular events; a 27% increase in hospital admissions for heart failure was seen.[905] The Examination of Cardiovascular Outcomes with Alogliptin versus Standard of Care (EXAMINE) similarly established no cardiovascular hazard from the use of this DPP4.[906] Although EXAMINE investigators report that alogliptin has no impact on heart failure,[907] differences exist in the design and end point measurements in this trial as compared to SAVOR-TIMI 53.[908] There was a statistically significant increase in heart failure hospitalization among individuals with no history of heart failure at baseline. The FDA has elected to place a warning regarding heart failure in the label of both agents. Anticipated additional clinical trial data with other DPP4 inhibitors should help further address questions regarding DPP4 inhibitors and heart failure (Table 33-14), whereas studies with GLP1 agonists will shed light on whether any heart failure effects derive from the incretin axis itself as opposed to other substrates of the DPP4 enzyme. GLP1 agonists can promote weight loss and lower BP, which could underlie possible cardiovascular benefit.[909] Sodium-glucose cotransporter 2 (SGLT2) inhibitors, which block glucose absorption in the proximal tubule, also promote weight loss and lower BP and are also being investigated in large cardiovascular trials (see Table 33-14).[910]

All of these clinical trial efforts pursue a central but unresolved question in the field: is there an antidiabetic medication that can lower the known increased cardiovascular risk found in diabetes? The difficulties in establishing this seemingly straightforward proposition has been attributed to various factors: trial issues (too short, too small, poor design), offsetting effects of agents, pursuit of targets unlikely to yield benefit, or intervening in patients too late in their natural history. The latter notion is supported by signals in trials suggesting that subgroups with the shorter duration of diabetes do manifest cardiovascular benefit through tighter glucose control, whereas other work suggests those with less coronary calcification, which may also reflect a disease process of shorter duration, may benefit.[911,912] An alternative perspective on this broad dataset regarding therapeutic antidiabetic interventions to decrease cardiovascular risk is that HbA$_{1c}$ is lacking as a surrogate marker for cardiovascular outcomes. In terms of the effects of lowering glucose itself as a strategy for decreasing cardiovascular events, in ORIGIN, which employed insulin in patients with either prediabetes or early T2DM, achieving a fasting

TABLE 33-14

Major Recent and Ongoing Clinical Trials Testing Antidiabetic Agents in Cardiovascular Disease*

Trial	Drug	Sample Size	Stage
ORIGIN	Insulin glargine	12,500	Reported
TOSCA IT	Pioglitazone vs. sulfonylureas	3,371	Started 9/2008
TECOS	Sitagliptin	14,000	Started 12/2008; reported
ACE	Acarbose	7,500	Started 2/2009
TIDE	Rosiglitazone/ pioglitazone	16,000	Halted
EXAMINE	Alogliptin	5,400	Reported
CANVAS	Canagliflozin	4,500	Completed
T-emerge 8	Taspoglutide	2,000	Halted
AleCardio	Aleglitazar	7,000	Halted
SAVOR TIMI-53	Saxagliptin	16,500	Reported
ELIXA	Lixisenatide	6,000	Started 6/2010; reported
EXSCEL	Exenatide LAR	12,000	Started 6/2010
EMPA-REG Outcome	Empagliflozin	7,000	Started 7/2010
CAROLINA	Linagliptin	6,000	Started 10/2010
LEADER	Liraglutide	8,723	Started 8/2010
AlePrevent	Aleglitazar	19,000	Halted
REWIND	Dulaglutide	9,622	Started 7/2011
SUSTAIN 6	Semaglutide	3,260	Started 2/2013
DECLARE TIMI 58	Dapagliflozin	17,000	Started 4/2013
CARMELINA	Linagliptin	8,300	Started 7/2013
DEVOTE	Insulin degludec	7,500	Started 10/2013
MK-8835-004	Ertugliflozin	3,900	Started 11/2013
CANVAS-R	Canagliflozin	5,700	Started 12/2013
CREDENCE	Canagliflozin	3,700	Started 2/2014

*A listing is provided of recent large clinical trials evaluating the effects of different antidiabetic therapies on cardiovascular outcomes. Although prompted in part by the need to meet FDA-imposed safety hurdles, some of these studies were positioned to show cardiovascular benefit as a primary end point, which thus far has not been evident in any of these efforts.

plasma glucose of 95 versus 123 mg/dL had no effect on cardiovascular outcomes.[913]

Dyslipidemia and Its Treatment in Patients with Diabetes Mellitus

Dyslipidemia is the best characterized risk factor for increasing atherosclerosis in patients with T2DM. A number of features of dyslipidemia are uniquely associated with diabetes and appear to increase the predisposition to atherogenesis. Although patients with diabetes tend not to have marked elevations in plasma LDL-cholesterol levels, their LDL-cholesterol particles are generally smaller and more dense than typical LDL-cholesterol particles, a change that closely tracks hypertriglyceridemia. These small, dense LDL-cholesterol particles are more susceptible to oxidation, particularly in the setting of poor glucose control. Other evidence suggests that glycation of LDL may be enhanced in diabetes, impairing recognition of the lipoprotein by its hepatoreceptor and extending its half-life. Conversely, levels of the cardioprotective lipid fraction, HDL-cholesterol, are decreased in patients with diabetes. The HDL-cholesterol of these patients may also be less effective at protecting LDL-cholesterol from oxidative stress, one of the proposed mechanisms for the cardioprotective effect of HDL-cholesterol.[914]

Undoubtedly, the key feature of diabetic dyslipidemia is an increase in the production of VLDL by the liver in response to elevations in FFAs. Although insulin mediates the uptake of FFAs by striated muscle, reducing the levels presented to the liver, insulin resistance results in the opposite effect, increasing the levels of FFAs available to the liver. The metabolic syndrome, with its characteristic abdominal obesity, also increases the delivery of FFAs to the liver. In addition, reduced lipoprotein lipase activity in T2DM leads to an accumulation of triglyceride-rich lipoproteins in the plasma of these patients and may also result in decreased delivery of lipolytically derived, biologically active molecules. Triglyceride-rich lipoproteins also play a role in the reduced levels of HDL-cholesterol by increasing the transfer of cholesterol from these particles.

A number of landmark trials have proved that lowering lipid levels produces major clinical benefits in terms of reducing cardiovascular events in patients with and without a history of CHD at baseline. These findings have now been extended to the population of subjects with T2DM and dyslipidemia. For example, even though LDL levels are often within the average range in these patients, treatment with 3-hydroxy-3-methylglutaryl coenzyme A (HMG-CoA) reductase inhibitors (statins) has shown consistent improvement in outcomes among both nondiabetics and diabetics alike, with benefits seen in those with and without a prior history of heart disease.

In the Cholesterol and Recurrent Events (CARE) trial, diabetic patients with a prior cardiovascular event treated with pravastatin had a significant 25% reduction in the incidence of CHD death, nonfatal MI, CABG, and revascularization procedures.[9] In the Long-term Intervention with Pravastatin in Ischemic Disease (LIPID) study, patients with diabetes had a 19% reduction in major CHD (fatal CHD and nonfatal MI).[915] In a post hoc subgroup analysis of secondary prevention in a large cohort of patients with diabetes, impaired glucose tolerance, or normal glucose tolerance, simvastatin normalized associated elevations in total cholesterol and triglycerides across the range of glucose values.[916] Treatment also significantly reduced major coronary events and revascularizations in patients with diabetes and reduced major coronary events, revascularizations, and total and coronary mortality in patients with impaired glucose tolerance.

Several studies have further verified the use of statins in patients with diabetes and related conditions.[581,917-920] In the Heart Protection Study, a large ($N = 20{,}536$), randomized, placebo-controlled trial of the use of simvastatin 40 mg in high-risk patients, roughly 29% of the study participants had T2DM.[921] Over the 5-year course of the study, treatment with simvastatin resulted in a significant reduction in the occurrence of major vascular events in patients with T2DM who had previous MI or other CHD (33.4% vs. 37.8% in simvastatin- and placebo-treated patients, respectively), in diabetics with no prior CHD (13.8% vs. 18.6%), and in both categories combined (20.2% vs. 25.1%). Overall, the study also demonstrated a highly significant 12% RR reduction in all-cause mortality and an 18% RR reduction in coronary mortality among all subjects treated with simvastatin.

In terms of primary prevention, the Collaborative Atorvastatin Diabetes Study (CARDS) was a large ($N = 2838$), randomized, placebo-controlled trial that assessed the benefit of the lowest starting dose of atorvastatin (10 mg/day) for preventing acute CHD events, coronary revascularization, or stroke in patients with T2DM and no documented history of CVD and plasma LDL levels lower than 160 mg/dL.[922] The trial was terminated 2 years early because the prespecified efficacy criteria were met. After a median of 3.9 years' follow-up, patients treated with atorvastatin had an RR reduction for first cardiovascular event of 37% (95% CI, 52% to 17% reduction; $p = 0.001$), compared with placebo-treated patients. Assessed separately, acute CHD, coronary revascularizations, and stroke were significantly reduced, by 36%, 31%, and 48%, respectively. Based on these results, the CARDS investigators concluded that in patients with T2DM, a threshold LDL-cholesterol level should not be the sole determinant of whether a statin is prescribed. It is worth noting the reduction of stroke in CARDS given prior questions about whether LDL-lowering with statins might not reduce stroke to the same extent as they lower coronary heart disease. Such issues may stem from various factors, such as different kinds of strokes (hemorrhagic vs. atherosclerotic); statins are generally accepted as reducing cerebrovascular disease.[923]

A post hoc study compared major coronary events, total mortality, and revascularization rates in two subsets of patients who received simvastatin 20 to 40 mg/day for a median of 5.4 years in the Scandinavian Simvastatin Survival Study (4S).[917] Treatment with simvastatin resulted in a 52% RR reduction of major coronary events, a greater treatment effect than was seen in the patients with isolated high LDL-cholesterol. Reanalysis of the data after exclusion of the patients with diabetes did not substantially alter the findings.

The Treating to New Targets (TNT) study compared the effects of atorvastatin 10 mg or 80 mg daily for a median follow-up period of 4.9 years in patients with clinically evident CHD who also met the NCEP criteria for diagnosis of the metabolic syndrome.[918] The study included 778 patients with T2DM, who constituted 22% of the study population. Treatment with atorvastatin 80 mg was significantly more effective for reducing major cardiovascular events than atorvastatin 10 mg (HR = 0.71; 95% CI, 0.61 to 0.84; $p < 0.0001$), presumably due to the significantly greater reduction in LDL-cholesterol seen with the higher dosing of atorvastatin.

Data from the TNT study weigh in the ongoing controversies surrounding the revised cholesterol treatment guidelines provided by the American College of Cardiology and the American Heart Association.[924] These recommendations depart from prior guidelines, which were sponsored previously by the NHLBI, by focusing initiation of lipid-lowering therapy on four clinically defined patient groups who warranted either high-, moderate-, or low-intensity statin intervention while also abandoning use of LDL targets as a means of guiding therapy. Patients with diabetes were one of these four treatment groups, as supported by the data from primary and secondary prevention trials noted previously.

No longer using LDL targets to guide treatment has been especially controversial, especially given the subsequent reported IMPROVE-IT trial, which tested whether adding the nonstatin, LDL-lowering agent ezetimibe to stable statin therapy decreased cardiovascular events in patients with coronary heart disease. Indeed, in presented but not yet published results, it did, providing additional evidence that lowering LDL decreases cardiovascular events even with nonstatin therapy.[925] These results are potentially relevant in considering prior and future nonstatin therapies in reducing cardiovascular events in patients with diabetes.

In terms of other nonstatin therapies, the data with niacin have in general been disappointing, with no additional benefit seen when added to statins in several trials studying carotid intimal medial thickness or clinical outcomes.[919,926,927] Although the lower HDL levels found in patients with diabetes might make niacin an appealing treatment option, niacin's lack of proven efficacy noted here has combined with side effects of increasing insulin resistance, relatively poor tolerability, and questionable efficacy on clinical event reduction has limited its use. Recent genetic studies have demonstrated through analysis of mendelian randomization that variants associated with higher HDL levels often do not protect against CV events.[928] Current attention is focused on the concept that the key element in the inverse relationship between HDL and CV disease is HDL functionality, which may not be reflected in total HDL levels.[929] In contrast to these issues, genetic variants linked to triglyceride levels, like apolipoprotein CIII loss of function, do predict CV risk.[930,931]

Fibric acid derivatives have also been proposed as benefiting patients with diabetes given effects on the low HDL and high triglyceride levels found in diabetic dyslipidemia. In the VA High-Density Lipoprotein Cholesterol Intervention Trial (VA-HIT), men given gemfibrozil had lower rates of coronary events and strokes.[920] The suggestion that these effects were driven by benefits in the diabetic subgroup focused further attention on fibrates.

The Fenofibrate Intervention and Event Lowering in Diabetes (FIELD) study assessed the effect of long-term fenofibrate therapy on cardiovascular events in patients with T2DM.[581] Patients were randomized to receive either micronized fenofibrate 200 mg/day ($n = 4895$) or placebo ($n = 4900$). During 5-year follow-up, 5.9% of the placebo-treated patients and 5.2% of the fenofibrate-treated patients had a coronary event, a difference that was not statistically significant. Fenofibrate therapy significantly reduced total CVD events (HR, 0.89; 95% CI, 0.75 to 1.05; $p = 0.035$), progression of albuminuria, and the need for laser treatment of retinopathy. Statistical significance for the primary end point of the study might have been missed because a greater percentage of patients in the placebo group initiated statin therapy during the study period, thus masking the treatment effect.

The ACCORD trial addressed the use of fibrates in combination with statins in patients with T2DM. This trial investigated whether combination therapy with simvastatin plus fenofibrate, compared with simvastatin alone, would reduce cardiovascular events in diabetic patients at high risk for CVD. In this randomized clinical trial comparing fenofibrate to placebo in statin-treated patients, combination therapy did not reduce the rate of cardiovascular mortality, nonfatal MI, or nonfatal stroke, although other secondary parameters such as first MI were improved. In a prespecified subgroup with a high triglyceride ratio (triglycerides ≥ 204 mg/dL and HDL ≤ 34 mg/dL), fenofibrate was better than placebo in reducing the primary outcome. Similar patterns are seen in other fibrate trials, with benefit manifest in those with significantly elevated triglycerides and low HDL, which is the population in which the drugs would be used. At this time, there is no formal recommendation that these patients receive combination statin-fibrate therapy as an ingredient in risk factor reduction on the basis of T2DM alone.[932] In those with a significant history of CVD, elevated triglycerides, and low HDL, expert opinion may endorse fibrates as an adjunct to statin therapy as a reasonable if not yet definitively established therapeutic option. The importance of dyslipidemia as a contributor to cardiovascular risk in patients with diabetes was incorporated in the NCEP ATP III guidelines, which did include the presence of diabetes as equal to the risk of prior CHD.[885] According to the NCEP ATP III guidelines, diabetic patients are candidates for cholesterol-lowering therapy if the LDL-cholesterol level is higher than 3.36 mmol/L (130 mg/dL), with the goal of reducing LDL-cholesterol to less than 2.57 mmol/L (100 mg/dL),[887] although many clinicians consider it prudent to approach therapy more aggressively by instituting drug treatment if the LDL-cholesterol level is higher than 2.57 mmol/L

(100 mg/dL). Those guidelines were then modified to state that, when risk is very high, a goal of less than 70 mg/dL LDL-cholesterol is a reasonable clinical strategy, even when the high-risk patient has a baseline LDL-cholesterol level lower than 100 mg/dL.[933] Importantly, improved glycemic control and decreased insulin resistance, whether through drug therapy or improved lifestyle interventions and modest weight loss, can improve diabetic dyslipidemia.

Signature Features and Treatment of Hypertension in Diabetic Patients

It has been estimated that up to 50% of patients with newly diagnosed diabetes also have high BP. As with dyslipidemia, hypertension interacts with diabetes to amplify the risk of cardiac mortality (see Fig. 33-54). Although the cause of hypertension is multifactorial, the insulin-resistant state is one factor postulated to predispose patients to development of hypertension. In addition to its negative effects on the cardiovascular system, high BP is a key contributor to the development of microvascular disease in diabetes. Based on the guidelines of the Joint National Committee on Prevention, Detection, Evaluation, and Treatment of High Blood Pressure (JNC VII), BP should be reduced to less than 130/85 mm Hg in patients with diabetes.[934]

Results of the most recent clinical trials underscore the benefits of aggressive treatment of hypertension in patients with diabetes, although none of these studies achieved mean BP reductions to currently recommended targets. Use of a long-acting dihydropyridine calcium channel blocker in the Systolic Hypertension in Europe (Syst-Eur) study resulted in substantial reductions in rates of total mortality (55%), cardiovascular mortality (76%), and cardiovascular events (69%) in the diabetic subgroup, greater benefits than were seen in the subgroup without diabetes.

In the Heart Outcomes Prevention Evaluation (HOPE) study, in which almost 40% of patients had diabetes and one other cardiovascular risk factor, ramipril reduced the primary outcome by 24% and total mortality risk by 25%.[935] Even in normotensive patients with diabetes, some benefit was seen, with a 2- to 4-mm Hg drop in BP with ACE inhibitor therapy.

Other rigorously designed studies, such as the UKPDS[936] and the Hypertension Optimal Treatment (HOT) study,[937] suggested even greater benefits from tight BP control in patients with diabetes.

In the Losartan Intervention For Endpoint Reduction in Hypertension (LIFE) study, patients with diabetes, hypertension, and signs of left ventricular hypertrophy were randomly assigned to treatment with losartan-based ($n = 586$) or atenolol-based ($n = 609$) treatment for hypertension.[938] Despite similar BP reductions, losartan was more effective than atenolol for reducing rates of cardiovascular morbidity and mortality, mortality from CVD, and mortality from all causes. The ability of losartan to reduce events more effectively than atenolol may be related to the ability of ARBs to reverse left ventricular hypertrophy more effectively than beta blockers.

Although beta blockers are thought to worsen glycemic control in patients with diabetes, it is not clear whether this is a property of all members of this drug class or whether this property persists if beta blockers are given in combination with renin-angiotensin system inhibitors that are known to increase insulin sensitivity. In the Glycemic Effects in Diabetes Mellitus: Carvedilol-Metoprolol Comparison in Hypertensives (GENINI) trial, patients with documented T2DM and hypertension who were taking a stable dose of either an ARB or an ACE inhibitor were randomized to receive either carvedilol or metoprolol. Although the degree of BP control was similar with both beta blockers, HbA_{1c} and insulin resistance increased significantly with metoprolol but not with carvedilol. Therefore, carvedilol appears not to cause the adverse effects of metoprolol on glucose levels when used in combination with renin-angiotensin system inhibitors, although this conclusion needs to be tested in a longer-term outcome trial.

The investigators of the Antihypertensive and Lipid-Lowering Treatment to Prevent Heart Attack Trial (ALLHAT) compared outcomes during first-step treatment of hypertension in 31,512 patients with T2DM, impaired fasting glucose (IFG) levels, or normoglycemia with a calcium channel blocker (amlodipine 2.5 to 10 mg/day) or ACE inhibitor (lisinopril 10 to 40 mg/day) compared with a thiazide-type diuretic (chlorthalidone 12.5 to 25 mg/day).[938] There was no significant difference in the occurrence of the primary outcome (fatal CHD or nonfatal MI) in patients with T2DM treated with a calcium channel blocker or an ACE inhibitor compared with chlorthalidone. Patients with IFG treated with a calcium channel blocker had a significantly higher RR for the primary outcome than patients receiving chlorthalidone.

A major unresolved question has been whether treatment of hypertension to lower targets than currently recommended would reduce cardiovascular risk in patients with T2DM. Most trials establishing the remarkable benefit of BP lowering, regardless of the medications used, have studied subjects whose BP was higher than 140 mm Hg. In the ACCORD trial, two strategies of BP management were examined as to their efficacy in lowering cardiovascular risk. One group was randomized to a systolic BP lower than 120 mm Hg (intensive therapy), and the other group was treated to a systolic pressure lower than 140 mm Hg (standard therapy). Targeting the lower BP level did not reduce the rate of fatal and nonfatal cardiovascular events. Based on this result, there is no recommendation to treat patients with T2DM and hypertension to a systolic BP lower than the currently recommended target of 130 mm Hg to decrease cardiovascular events. However, further reduction may reduce the incidence of diabetic nephropathy.[558,939]

Acute Coronary Syndromes in Diabetes Mellitus

The case-fatality rate from MI is almost twice as high in patients with diabetes as in nondiabetic patients. This excess risk is seen both during the acute phase of MI and in the early and late postinfarction period. A number of mechanisms have been deemed to be responsible for worse outcomes in patients with diabetes, including the following:

- Increased risk of CHF due to maladaptive remodeling of the left ventricle[940-942]
- Increased risk of sudden death due to sympathovagal imbalance as a consequence of autonomic neuropathy[943-945]
- Increased likelihood of early reinfarction due to impaired fibrinolysis[946-948]
- Extensive underlying CAD[949,950]
- Changes in myocardial cell metabolism, including a shift from glucose oxidation to FFA oxidation, with less generation of ATP at any level of oxygen consumption[951,952]
- Associated cardiomyopathy[829]

Collective data provide strong evidence that a variety of treatment modalities can improve outcomes from MI in patients with diabetes. In terms of interventions, patients with diabetes experiencing an acute MI respond as favorably to fibrinolytic therapy as do nondiabetic patients.[52,949,950] Excellent glycemic control is an essential component of overall management. Glucose levels at hospital admission have been independently correlated with early and late fatality after MI in patients with and without diabetes mellitus.[953-956]

Studies such as the Diabetes and Insulin-Glucose Infusion in Acute Myocardial Infarction (DIGAMI) study have assessed the impact of intensive glycemic control in patients with diabetes during the acute phase of MI. Patients in this study were randomized to either intensive insulin therapy (insulin-glucose infusion for 24 hours, followed by subcutaneous insulin injection for 3 months) or standard glycemic control.[957] The intensive insulin regimen lowered blood glucose level during the first hour after admission and at discharge compared with conventional therapy. The 1-year mortality rate was significantly reduced with the insulin infusion group compared with the control group, a difference that was maintained after 3.4 years of follow-up.

DIGAMI 2, a prospective, randomized, open-label trial that followed up the DIGAMI trial, compared outcomes in patients with either T1DM or T2DM and failed to corroborate the earlier reported improvement in outcomes with intensive insulin treatment.[958] The lack of effect of long-term insulin treatment on outcomes may be at least partially explained by the fact that 14% of the patients in the conventional treatment group received insulin-glucose infusions in violation of the protocol, and as many as 41% had extra glucose injections. As a result, the blood glucose levels in all three groups were not significantly different after treatment.

Although the mechanisms responsible for the potential benefit shown in the original DIGAMI study are not entirely clear, experimental data suggest that strict glycemic control can improve myocardial cell metabolism by increasing the availability of glucose as a substrate for ATP generation and reducing the formation of FFAs, thereby shifting cardiac metabolism from FFA oxidation to glycolysis and glucose oxidation. Intensive glycemic control can also reverse the impaired fibrinolysis that is typically seen in patients with diabetes.

The CREATE-ECLA (Clinical Trial of Reviparin and Metabolic Modulation in Acute Myocardial Infarction Treatment Evaluation-Estudios Cardiologicos Latin America) randomized, controlled trial assigned 20,201 patients who presented with ST-segment elevation MI within 12 hours after onset of symptoms either to treatment with high-dose glucose-insulin-potassium (GIK) infusion (i.e., 25% glucose, 50 U/L regular insulin, and 80 mEq KCl) administered over 24 hours or to usual care.[959] Roughly 18% of the patients in both treatment arms had T2DM. After 30 days, there were no differences in the rate of occurrence of mortality, cardiac arrest, cardiogenic shock, or reinfarction in the two treatment groups.

Sulfonylureas have been implicated in an increased cardiovascular mortality rate, particularly in patients undergoing revascularization for acute MI.[960] The UKPDS did not show a deleterious effect of these agents on the incidence of sudden death or MI over 10 years of follow-up.[5] The sulfonylureas act through the sulfonylurea receptor component of ATP-sensitive potassium channels in the pancreatic beta cell. In the heart, ATP-sensitive potassium channels are involved in ischemic preconditioning and coronary vasodilation.[961-963] It is not clear whether the sulfonylureas modulate these channels in the heart or vascular system or whether they significantly increase risk in diabetic patients with an acute MI.

ACE inhibitors dramatically reduce the mortality rate after an MI in patients with diabetes, ostensibly through their effects to reduce infarct size and limit ventricular remodeling. In addition to these hemodynamic benefits, ACE inhibitors can also improve outcomes in diabetes by improving endothelial function,[964] improving fibrinolysis,[965] and decreasing insulin resistance.[966]

In a retrospective analysis of the Gruppo Italiano per lo Studio della Sopravvivenza nell'Infarto Miocardico (GISSI-3) study,[967] lisinopril administration within 24 hours after hospital admission substantially reduced both 6-week and 6-month mortality rates in patients with diabetes compared with the nondiabetic group. Similarly, a subgroup analysis from the Trandolapril Cardiac Evaluation Study (TRACE) showed that patients with diabetes suffering an anterior MII who were treated with trandolapril had greatly improved outcomes over 5 years compared with patients without diabetes, including an almost 50% reduction in the risk of sudden death, reinfarction, and progression of CHF.[968]

Beta blockers are now widely accepted for the treatment of acute coronary syndrome in patients with diabetes. Older, noncardioselective beta blockers might have adversely affected the lipid profile and inhibited the metabolic response to hypoglycemia, but more recent data with cardioselective beta blockers suggest that these agents have less negative effects on metabolic indices, perhaps because they increase peripheral blood flow and improve glucose delivery.[969,970] Clinical trial data confirm that beta blockers reduce the rates of mortality and reinfarction in patients with MI in the presence of diabetes. In fact, their effects in patients with diabetes appear to exceed those seen in nondiabetic patients. A large review of data from more than 45,000 patients, 26% of whom had diabetes, showed that beta-blocker therapy was associated with a lower 1-year mortality rate in patients with diabetes than in those without diabetes, with no evidence of an increase in diabetes-related complications.[971]

Postulated mechanisms for the benefit of beta blockers in patients with diabetes include dampening of the sympathetic nervous system overactivity that arises as a consequence of autonomic neuropathy. Beta blockers can also reduce FFA levels and thereby reduce myocardial oxygen requirements. Carvedilol, although not cardioselective, is a beta blocker that decreases insulin resistance and also has antioxidant effects, both of which may be of particular benefit in patients with T2DM.[972]

Aspirin is a cornerstone of therapy for the primary or secondary prevention of acute coronary syndrome in patients with T1DM and T2DM who do not have contraindications to its use. Aspirin significantly lowers the risk of MI without increasing the risk of vitreous or retinal bleeding, even in patients with retinopathy.[973] Enteric-coated aspirin, 81 to 325 mg/day, is currently recommended by the ADA.[974] The benefits of this therapy are likely to result from effects on the enhanced platelet aggregation that is evident in patients with either T1DM or T2DM.[975] Some controversy persists around the ideal dose of aspirin and whether enteric coating might interfere with aspirin's effects.[976]

Antiplatelet therapy with clopidogrel also benefits patients with diabetes. The CAPRIE trial compared outcomes in patients with non–ST-segment elevation MI treated with aspirin or with clopidogrel and included 3866 patients with diabetes.[977] Although the event rate was higher among the diabetic patients than in the overall study population, the response to treatment was also better. The event rate for the primary end point (vascular death, ischemic stroke, MI, or rehospitalization for ischemia or bleeding) was 17.7% for diabetic patients treated with aspirin and 15.6% for those randomized to clopidogrel, a significant RR reduction of 12.5%.

Newer adjunct therapies, such as the platelet glycoprotein IIb/IIIa receptor antagonists that antagonize platelet action, have also been assessed in diabetic patients who present with unstable angina or non–Q-wave infarction. Overall, these agents appear to work equally well, or perhaps slightly better, in patients with diabetes compared with nondiabetic patients. In the Platelet Receptor Inhibition in Ischemic Syndrome Management in Patients Limited by Unstable Signs and Symptoms (PRISM-PLUS) study, the addition of tirofiban to heparin therapy reduced the 7-day composite end point, compared with heparin alone. This effect was greater in patients with diabetes than in patients without diabetes.[978]

In one study of patients undergoing percutaneous transluminal coronary angioplasty (PTCA), glycoprotein IIb/IIIa antagonist therapy was associated with fewer acute events but a higher rate of target-vessel revascularization in the long term in the diabetic cohort compared with the nondiabetic cohort.[979] However, in another trial, in which stents were used, the rate of target vessel revascularization at 6 months was significantly decreased with the addition of a glycoprotein IIb/IIIa antagonist compared with placebo.[980]

Results of the Bypass Angioplasty Revascularization Investigation (BARI) showed that CABG provides better outcomes than PTCA in patients with diabetes, possibly because it addresses the extensive coronary vascular disease in these patients.[981] This study did not employ stents or glycoprotein IIb/IIIa inhibitors, two modalities that, when used together, appear to improve outcomes after PTCA in patients with diabetes.

Cardiomyopathy in Patients with Diabetes Mellitus

Diabetes is associated with a fourfold increase in the risk of CHF, even after adjustment for other cardiovascular risk factors such as age, BP, cholesterol level, obesity, and history of CAD.[982] Current nomenclature organizes heart failure into two broad categories: with preserved ejection fraction (HFpEF) and with reduction ejection fraction (HFrEF).[983] Patients with diabetes, who commonly present with either form, experience higher rates of CHF than do nondiabetic patients after an acute MI, regardless of the size of the infarct zone.[941,984] These findings suggest that diabetes itself causes deleterious effects on the myocardium, leading to poorer outcomes.

A number of key structural, functional, and metabolic factors in diabetes have been implicated in the increased risk of maladaptive remodeling that leads to CHF. For example, evidence of silent MI is found in up to 40% of patients with diabetes who present with a clinically apparent MI and can lead to unrecognized regional and global ventricular dysfunction.[967,985] As many as 50% of patients with diabetes and CAD have cardiac autonomic neuropathy, which is known to contribute to both systolic and diastolic dysfunction.[829] Like hypertension, diabetes can cause fibrosis of the myocardium and increased collagen deposition.[986,987] These effects are even more pronounced in patients with coexisting hypertension and diabetes and may contribute to the finding of diastolic dysfunction common in patients with diabetes.[988] Enhanced endothelial dysfunction in diabetes has also been described as a pathophysiologic pathway to impaired microvascular perfusion and ischemia.[989,990]

On a cellular level, both hyperglycemia and insulin resistance have direct negative effects on myocardial metabolism. Depression of myocardial GLUT4 levels in the setting of diabetes and ischemia inhibits glucose entry and glycolysis in the heart. As a result, intracellular metabolism shifts from glycolysis to FFA oxidation, thereby suppressing glycolytic ATP generation, a major source of energy under anaerobic (i.e., ischemic) conditions.[951] The production of oxygen free radicals can also be enhanced in this situation, further depressing myocardial contractile function.[990]

Collectively, these various abnormalities potentiate the characteristic left ventricular remodeling of diabetes, which is clinically manifested as serial wall motion changes, reduced regional ejection fraction, and increased end-diastolic and end-systolic volumes.[991,992]

THE DIABETIC FOOT

Of all the late complications of diabetes, foot problems are probably the most preventable. Joslin, who wrote in 1934 that "diabetic gangrene is not heaven-sent, but earth-born," was correct: the development of foot ulceration mostly results from the way we care for our patients or the way patients care for themselves.

Increasing interest in the diabetic foot has resulted in a better understanding of the factors that interact to cause ulceration and amputation. The neuropathic foot does not spontaneously ulcerate; insensitivity in combination with other factors, such as deformity and unperceived trauma (e.g., inappropriate footwear), leads to skin breakdown. Increased knowledge of this pathogenesis should permit the design of appropriate screening programs for risk and preventive education. Much progress has been made, but it has not yet resulted in a universal decrease in amputation rates. In the VA system, for example, amputation rates in diabetic patients[993] have not declined, although certain European countries have reported a significant reduction in amputation rates after implementation of foot screening and education programs.[994,995] Much research is still needed to implement strategies to reduce ulceration and amputation, and this is particularly required in the fields of behavioral and psychosocial aspects of the diabetic foot.[996]

Two major texts on the diabetic foot were published in the past decade.[997,998] The reader is referred to these sources together with other major recent review articles[999,1000] for more detailed discussion of this topic.

Epidemiology and Pathogenesis of Diabetic Foot Ulceration

Foot ulceration is common and occurs in both T1DM and T2DM. Approximately 5% to 10% of diabetic patients have had past or present foot ulceration, and 1% have undergone amputation.[997] Diabetes is the most common cause of nontraumatic lower limb amputation in the United States, and rates are 15 times greater than those in the nondiabetic population. More than 80% of amputations are preceded by foot ulcers. A large community-based study in the United Kingdom showed an annual incidence of ulceration of approximately 2%; this rose to 7% with known diabetic neuropathy and to as high as 50% with a past history of ulceration.[1001] The lifetime risk for development of a foot ulcer in a diabetic patient is estimated to be as high as 25%.[999]

Pathway to Ulceration

Foot ulceration results from the interaction of a number of component causes, none of which alone is sufficient to cause ulceration but which, when combined, complete the causal pathway to skin breakdown. Knowledge of these component causes and their potential to interact facilitates the design of preventive foot care programs.

Diabetic Neuropathy

All three components of neuropathy—sensory, motor, and autonomic—can contribute to ulceration in the foot. Chronic sensorimotor neuropathy is common, affecting at least one third of older patients in Western countries. Its onset is gradual and insidious, and symptoms may be so minimal that they go unnoticed. Although uncomfortable, painful, and paresthetic symptoms predominate in many patients, some never experience symptoms. Clinical examination usually reveals a sensory deficit in a glove-and-stocking distribution, with signs of motor dysfunction, such as small muscle wasting in the feet and absent ankle reflexes. Although a history of typical symptoms strongly suggests a diagnosis of neuropathy, absence of symptoms does not exclude the diagnosis and must never be equated with a lack of foot ulcer risk. Therefore, assessment of foot ulcer risk must always include a careful foot examination, whatever the history.

Sympathetic autonomic neuropathy affecting the lower limbs results in reduced sweating, dry skin, and development of cracks and fissures. In the absence of large-vessel arterial disease, there may be increased blood flow to the foot, with arteriovenous shunting leading to the warm but at-risk foot.

The importance of neuropathy as a contributory cause to foot ulceration has been confirmed. The risk in patients with neuropathy is sevenfold higher than in those without this complication of diabetes.[1001]

Peripheral Vascular Disease

Peripheral vascular disease in isolation rarely causes ulceration. However, the common combination of vascular disease with minor trauma can lead to ulceration. Minor injury and subsequent infection increase the demand for blood supply beyond the circulatory capacity, and ischemic ulceration and risk of amputation develop. Early identification of those patients who are at risk for peripheral vascular disease is essential, and appropriate investigation involving noninvasive studies, together with arteriography, often leads to bypass surgery to improve blood flow to the extremities. Distal bypass surgery is often performed, with good short-term but mixed long-term results in terms of limb salvage.[1002,1003] Doppler-derived ankle pressure can be misleadingly high in patients with long-standing diabetes. The presence or absence of a dorsalis pedis or posterior tibial pulse is the simplest and most reliable indicator of significant ischemia that can be elicited at the bedside.[1002]

Past Foot Ulceration or Foot Surgery

Foot ulceration is most common in patients with a history of similar problems. Even in experienced diabetic foot clinics, more than 50% of patients with new foot ulcers give a past ulcer history.

Other Diabetic Complications

Patients with retinopathy and renal dysfunction are at increased risk for foot ulceration. Among the diabetic patients at highest risk for ulceration are those on dialysis.[1004]

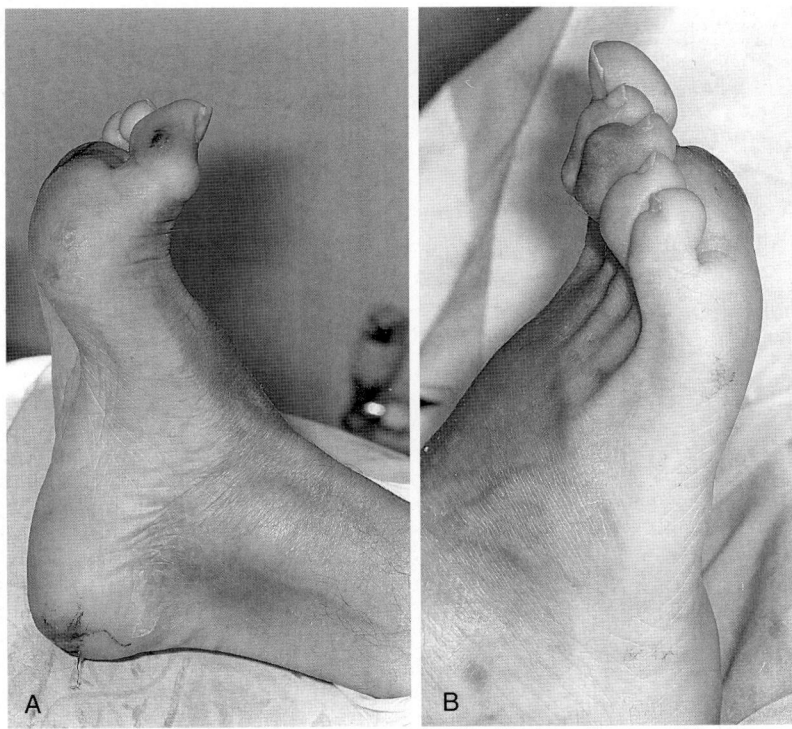

Figure 33-56 The high-risk neuropathic foot. **A** and **B,** Two lateral views of a patient with typical signs of a high-risk neuropathic foot. Notice the small-muscle wasting, clawing of the toes, and marked prominence of the metatarsal heads. At presentation with type 2 diabetes mellitus, this patient had severe neuropathy with foot ulceration on both the right foot (shown here) and the left foot. (From Andersson DK, Svardsudd K. Long-term glycemic control relates to mortality in type II diabetes. *Diabetes Care.* 1995;18:1534-1543.)

Callus, Deformity, and High Foot Pressures

Motor neuropathy, with imbalance of the flexor and extensor muscles in the foot, commonly results in foot deformity, with prominent metatarsal heads and clawing of the toes (Fig. 33-56). The combination of proprioceptive loss due to neuropathy and the prominence of metatarsal heads leads to increased pressures and loads under the diabetic foot. High pressures, together with dry skin, often result in the formation of callus under weight-bearing areas of the metatarsal heads. The presence of such plantar callus has been shown in cross-sectional and prospective studies to be a highly significant marker of foot ulcer risk. Conversely, removal of plantar callus is associated with a reduction in foot pressures and therefore a reduction in foot ulcer risk.[1005]

It is the combination of two or more of the earlier described risk factors that ultimately results in diabetic foot ulceration. In 1999, a North American/United Kingdom collaborative study[1006] assessed the risk factors that resulted in ulceration in more than 150 consecutive foot ulcer cases. From this study, a number of causal pathways were identified, but the most common triad of component causes—neuropathy, deformity, and trauma—was present in 63% of incident ulcers. Edema and ischemia were also common component causes.

Prevention of Foot Ulceration and Amputation

That diabetic foot ulceration is largely preventable is not disputed; small, mostly single-center studies have shown that relatively simple interventions can reduce amputations by up to 80%.[994,995] Therefore, strategies for early identification of patients at potential risk for ulceration are required, and education programs that can be adapted for widespread application need to be developed. Because foot ulcers precede most amputations, are among the most common causes of hospital admission for patients with diabetes, and account for much morbidity and even fatality, the widespread application of preventive foot care strategies is urgently required.

Patients with any type of diabetes require regular review and screening of the feet for evidence of risk factors for foot ulceration, irrespective of disease duration. At a minimum, such screening should be carried out annually. Of all the long-term complications of diabetes, foot problems and their risk factors are probably the easiest to detect. No expensive equipment is required, and the feet can be examined for evidence of neuropathic and vascular deficits in the office setting using simple equipment. Neuropathy, vascular disease, and even foot ulceration may be the presenting feature of T2DM, so there can be no exception to the rule of screening (Fig. 33-57).

In 2008, a task force of the ADA published a report on the components that should be included in the annual Comprehensive Diabetic Foot Examination (CDFE), which is summarized in Table 33-15.[1007] The most important message to practitioners is to have the patient remove shoes and socks and to look at the feet for risk factors such as presence of callus, deformity, muscle wasting, and dry skin, all of which are clearly visible on clinical inspection. A simple neurologic examination should include assessment of pressure perception using a 10-g monofilament; in a large U.K. community study,[1001] a simple clinical examination was the best predictor of foot ulcer risks. Absence of the ability to perceive pressure from a 10-g monofilament, inability to perceive a vibrating 128-Hz tuning fork

TABLE 33-15

Key Components of the Comprehensive Diabetic Foot Examination

Dermatologic

Skin status: color, thickness, dryness, cracking
Sweating
Infection: check between toes for fungal infection
Ulceration
Calluses/blistering: hemorrhage into callus?

Musculoskeletal

Deformity (e.g., claw toes, prominent metatarsal heads, Charcot joint)
Muscle wasting (guttering between metatarsals)
Assess whether shoes are appropriate for the feet (e.g., size, width)

Neurologic

Ability to perceive pressure from a 10-g monofilament plus one of the following:
　Vibration using 128-Hz tuning fork
　Pinprick sensation
　Ankle reflexes
　Vibratory perception threshold

Vascular

Foot pulses
Ankle-brachial index, if indicated

Adapted from Boulton AJM, Armstrong DG, Albert SG, et al. Comprehensive foot examination and risk assessment: a report of the Task Force of the Foot Care Interest Group of the American Diabetes Association, with endorsement by the American Association of Clinical Endocrinologists. *Diabetes Care.* 2008;31:1679-1686.

TABLE 33-16

Wagner Diabetic Foot Ulcer Classification System

Grade	Description
0	No ulcer, but high-risk foot (e.g., deformity, callus, insensitivity)
1	Superficial full-thickness ulcer
2	Deeper ulcer, penetrating tendons, no bone involvement
3	Deeper ulcer with bone involvement, osteitis
4	Partial gangrene (e.g., toes, forefoot)
5	Gangrene of whole foot

Modified from Oyibo S, Jude EB, Tarawneh I, et al. A comparison of two diabetic foot ulcer classification systems: the Wagner and the University of Texas wound classification systems. *Diabetes Care.* 2001;24:84-88.

takes responsibility for follow-up and care of the skin and nails and, together with the specialist nurse or diabetes educator, provides foot care education. The orthotist, or shoe fitter, is invaluable to advise about and sometimes design footwear to protect high-risk feet, and these members of the team should work closely with the diabetologist and the vascular and orthopedic surgeons. Patients with risk factors for ulceration require preventive foot care education and frequent review.[995,1005]

Classification of Foot Ulcers

Many different classification systems have been reported in the literature.[999,1005] The one developed by Wagner[1008] (Table 33-16) for grading diabetic foot ulcers has been widely used and accepted. More recently, the University of Texas (UT) group has developed an alternative classification system that, in addition to ulcer depth (as in the Wagner system), takes into account the presence or absence of infection and ischemia (Table 33-17).[614] A prospective study from 2001 assessed and compared these two wound classification systems and concluded that the UT scheme is a better predictor of outcome than the older Wagner system.[1008]

Management of Diabetic Foot Ulcers

Basic principles of wound healing apply equally to diabetic foot ulcers as to wounds in any other site or condition. Basically, a diabetic foot ulcer will heal if the following three conditions are satisfied:
- Arterial inflow is adequate.
- Infection is treated appropriately.
- Pressure is removed from the wound and the immediate surrounding area.

Although this approach might seem simplistic, failure of diabetic foot ulcers to heal is usually a result of failure to pay sufficient attention to one or more contributing conditions, including pressure on the wound, infection, ischemia, and inadequate débridement.

The most common cause of nonhealing of neuropathic foot ulcers is the failure to remove pressure from the wound and immediate surrounding area. Patients who are advised not to put pressure over an ulcer find it difficult to adhere to such advice if peripheral sensation is lost or reduced. Pain results in protection of an injured area; the lack of pain permits pressure to be put directly onto the ulcer and results in nonhealing. A patient with normal sensation and a foot wound will limp to avoid putting pressure on the wound because doing so is painful; hence, the observation is made initially in leprosy, and more recently in diabetic neuropathy, that a patient who walks on a plantar wound without limping must have neuropathy.

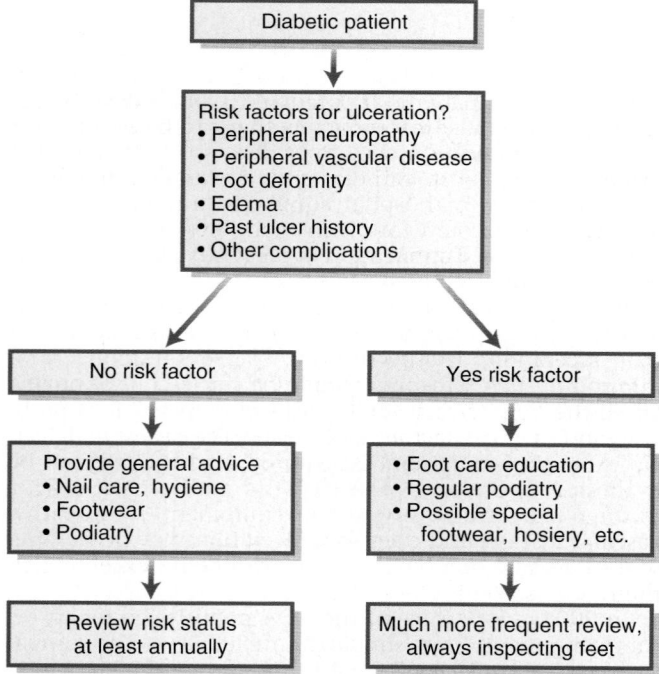

Figure 33-57 Simple algorithm for risk screening in the diabetic foot.

over the hallux, and absent ankle reflexes all have been shown to be predictors of foot ulceration.[1001,1005]

The Diabetic Foot Care Team

Patients identified as being at high risk for foot ulceration should be managed by a team of specialists with interest and expertise in the diabetic foot. The podiatrist usually

TABLE 33-17

University of Texas Wound Classification System

Stage	Grade 0	Grade 1	Grade 2	Grade 3
A	Preulcer or postulcer lesion; no skin break	Superficial ulcer	Deep ulcer to tendon or capsule	Wound penetrating bone or joint
B	+ Infection	+ Infection	+ Infection	+ Infection
C	+ Ischemia	+ Ischemia	+ Ischemia	+ Ischemia
D	+ Infection and ischemia	+ Infection and ischemia	+ Infection and ischemia	+ Infection and ischemia

Modified from Armstrong DG, Lavery LA, Harkless LB. Validation of a diabetic wound classification system. *Diabet Med.* 1998;14:855-859.

The effect of pressure relief on the histopathologic features of neuropathic ulcers was assessed in a randomized study.[1009] Patients with chronic neuropathic diabetic foot ulcers were randomly assigned to have a biopsy either at presentation or after 20 days of off-loading in a total-contact cast (TCC). Histologic features of chronic inflammation, with mononuclear infiltration, cellular debris, and scarce evidence of angiogenesis or granulation were seen in patients who underwent biopsy at presentation; granulation, neoangiogenesis, and a predominance of fibroblasts were seen in patients treated with TCC before biopsy. These important observations strongly suggest that repetitive pressure on a neuropathic wound contributes to the chronicity of the wound, whereas pressure relief results in the wound's appearing, in several respects, more like an acute wound in the reparative phase.

The next most common error is inappropriate management of infection. Topical applications are usually unhelpful, and if clinical infection is present, it must be treated appropriately (see later discussion).

Another common error is the failure to appreciate ischemic symptoms that are atypical due to altered pain sensation as a result of neuropathy. The most difficult ulcer to heal is the neuroischemic ulcer, and symptoms and even signs of ischemia may be altered in the diabetic state. Therefore, appropriate noninvasive investigation and arteriography are indicated for patients with a nonhealing diabetic foot ulcer if there is any question about the vascular status.

Inappropriate wound débridement is another reason for slow healing or nonhealing of a diabetic foot ulcer. When patients with neuropathy put pressure on active ulcer areas, the pressure leads to an often extensive buildup of callous tissue. Appropriate débridement and removal of all dead and macerated tissue is essential in the local treatment of a diabetic foot ulcer and has been shown to result in more rapid healing of ulcers compared with wounds that are inadequately débrided.

The principles of management of neuropathic and neuroischemic foot ulcers are considered in the following sections. Because it is not possible to provide complete details on the individual stages and grades of ulcers, we refer to both the UT and the Wagner grading systems.

Neuropathic Foot Ulcer Without Osteomyelitis (Wagner Grades 1, 2; University of Texas Grades 1a, 1b, 2a, 2b)

The most important feature in the management of neuropathic foot ulcers that typically occur under weight-bearing areas such as the metatarsal heads and great toe is the provision of adequate pressure relief. This is usually achieved by a cast such as a TCC or a removable Scotch cast boot.[999,1005]

The TCC has long been recognized as the gold standard for off-loading a foot wound and was confirmed as correct in a randomized, controlled trial in which Armstrong and colleagues compared three off-loading techniques and found that the TCC was associated with the shortest healing time.[1010] When any cast device is used, regular removal of the cast is essential, because regular débridement of the wound by a podiatrist is essential, and any casting device could injure insensitive skin, especially over bony prominences. For this reason, and because the TCC requires a specially trained casting technician to apply it, recent research has been directed toward alternative, irremovable devices that might be equally efficacious.

In the aforementioned trial by Armstrong's group,[1010] the removable cast walker (RCW) resulted in slower healing than the TCC, even though prior gait laboratory studies had suggested that they are equally efficacious at off-loading. The reason for this disparity was identified in an observational study of patients using RCWs in the treatment of their plantar neuropathic ulcers. Although patients were instructed to wear the RCW at all times, careful monitoring showed that RCWs were used for only 28% of all footsteps during a 24-hour period. It was therefore suggested that the RCW, which can be applied by any clinic personnel and does not require specialist training, might be rendered irremovable by wrapping it in casting material. A controlled trial showed that the irremovable RCW was as effective at healing neuropathic foot wounds as the TCC.[1011]

Theoretically, complete healing of all superficial and neuropathic ulcers should be possible without the need for amputation. In the treatment of neuropathic ulcers with a good peripheral circulation, antibiotics are not indicated unless there are clear clinical signs of infection, including prominent discharge, local erythema, and cellulitis. The presence of any of these features in Wagner grade 1 or 2 ulcers would warrant reclassification in the UT system from 1a or 2a to 1b or 2b. In such cases, deep wound swabs should be taken and broad-spectrum oral antibiotic treatment should be started with, for example, either an amoxicillin–clavulanic acid combination (Augmentin) or clindamycin. The antibiotic may need to be altered after sensitivity results become available.[1012]

Neuroischemic Ulcers (Wagner Grades 1, 2; University of Texas Grades 1c, 1d)

The principles of management of neuroischemic Wagner grade 1 and 2 ulcers are similar to those for neuropathic ulcers, with the following important exceptions. TCCs are not usually recommended for management of neuroischemic ulcers, although removable casts and pneumatic cast boots (Aircast) may be used in cases without infection. Antibiotic therapy is usually recommended for most neuroischemic ulcers. Investigation of the circulation is indicated, including noninvasive assessment and, if required, arteriography with appropriate subsequent surgical management or angioplasty.[1002]

Osteomyelitis (Wagner Grade 3; University of Texas Grades 3b, 3d)

Wagner or UT grade 3 ulcers are deeper and involve underlying bone, often with abscess formation. Osteomyelitis is a serious complication of foot ulceration and may be present in as many as 50% of diabetic patients with moderate to severe foot infections.[999] If the physician can probe down to bone in a deep ulcer, the presence of osteomyelitis is strongly suggested. Plain radiographs are indicated for any nonhealing foot ulcer and are useful in the diagnosis of osteomyelitis in more than two thirds of patients, although the radiologic changes may be delayed. In difficult cases, further investigation, such as MRI, bone scans, or an indium-111 (^{111}In)-labeled white blood cell scan can be useful in diagnosing bone infection.[1013]

Although the treatment of osteomyelitis is traditionally surgical and involves resection of the infected bone, there have been reports of successful long-term treatment with antibiotics effective against the underlying bacterium, most commonly *Staphylococcus aureus*. Therefore, agents such as clindamycin (which penetrates bone well) or flucloxacillin are often used. Most recently, a randomized controlled trial has confirmed that antibiotic therapy for 90 days was equally efficacious when compard to local surgery for diabetic foot osteomyelitis.[1014]

Gangrene (Wagner Grades 4, 5)

The presence of gangrene or areas of tissue death is always a serious sign in the diabetic foot. However, localized areas of gangrene, especially in the toes, that are without cellulitis, spreading infection, or discharge can occasionally be left to spontaneously autoamputate. The presence of more extensive gangrene requires urgent hospital admission; treatment of infection, often with multiple antibiotics; control of the diabetes, usually with intravenous insulin; and detailed vascular assessment. It is in this area that the team approach is most important, with close collaboration among the diabetes specialist, the vascular surgeon, and the radiologist.

Adjunct Treatments for Foot Ulcers

Platelet-Derived Growth Factors and Tissue-Engineered Skin

Genetically derived growth factors and novel bioengineered skin substitutes have been proposed as adjunctive treatments for diabetic foot ulcers. However, all of these new therapies are costly, as detailed in a recent systematic review and economic evaluation.[1015] This review covered treatments including Apligraf, a bilayered living human skin equivalent; Dermagraft, a human fibroblast-derived dermal substitute; and human PDGFs. Although the review did show some benefit for each of these agents, it is clear that they should be reserved only for those ulcers that fail to respond to the standard treatments noted earlier. Any new treatments should be seen not as a replacement but as an addition to good wound care, which must always include adequate off-loading and regular débridement.

Negative-Pressure Wound Therapy

Negative-pressure wound therapy, also known as vacuum-assisted closure, is increasingly used to treat large and complex diabetic foot wounds. The treatment appears to stimulate the development of granulation tissue in previously nonhealing wounds and can also be helpful in the postoperative management of diabetic foot wounds. Supportive data have been published from randomized, controlled trials in postoperative cases[1016] and in complex nonhealing diabetic foot ulcers.[1017]

Charcot Neuroarthropathy

Charcot neuroarthropathy is a rare and disabling condition that affects the joints and bones of the feet. Permissive features for the development of this condition include the presence of severe peripheral neuropathy and autonomic dysfunction with increased blood flow to the foot; the peripheral circulation is usually intact. In the Western world, diabetes is the most common cause of a Charcot foot, and increased awareness of this condition can enable earlier diagnosis and treatment to prevent severe deformity and disability.

The actual pathogenesis of the Charcot process is poorly understood; however, the patient with peripheral insensitivity and autonomic dysfunction with increased blood flow to the foot is vulnerable to trauma that the patient may not recall. Repetitive trauma results in increased blood flow through the bone, increased osteoclastic activity, and remodeling of bone. In certain cases, patients walk on a fracture, which leads to continuing destruction of bones and joints in that area. Recent evidence suggests that acute Charcot neuropathy may be triggered in the susceptible (i.e., neuropathic) individual by any event that leads to localized inflammation in the affected foot. This may trigger a vicious cycle in which there is increasing inflammation, increasing expression of RANKL (a member of the tumor necrosis factor superfamily), and increasing bone breakdown. The likely involvement of the RANKL/OPG pathway might lead to new possibilities for future treatments.[1018]

Charcot neuropathy is sometimes difficult to distinguish from osteomyelitis or an inflammatory arthropathy.[1013] However, a unilateral swollen, hot foot in a patient with neuropathy must be considered to be a Charcot foot until proved otherwise.

Charcot arthropathy can be diagnosed in most patients by plain radiography and a high index of suspicion. Radiographs may reveal bone and joint destruction, fragmentation, and remodeling, although in the early stages the radiographic finding may be normal. In such cases, the three-phase bisphosphonate bone scan shows increased bone uptake, although the ^{111}In-labeled bone scan will be negative in the absence of infection.

After diagnosis, management of the acute phase involves immobilization, usually in a TCC.[1019] Evidence suggests that treatment with bisphosphonates, which reduce osteoclastic activity, may reduce swelling, discomfort, and bone turnover markers, although larger trials are warranted in this area.[922,1018-1019]

Although Charcot neuroarthropathy is rare, it should be suspected in any patient with unexplained swelling and heat in a neuropathic foot. Early intervention with immobilization and possibly bisphosphonate treatment may halt progression that, in the untreated state, can lead to marked foot deformity and require local or major amputations.

ACKNOWLEDGMENTS

Dr. Brownlee would like to thank Ferdinando Giacco, PhD, for his help in preparing the section on biochemistry and molecular cell biology. Dr. Aiello would like to thank Jennifer K. Sun, MD, MPH, and Paolo Silva, MD, for their help in preparing the section on retinopathy, macular edema, and other ocular complications. Dr. Vinik would like to thank Marie-Laure Nevoret, MD, for her help in preparing the section on diabetic neuropathies. The authors gratefully acknowledge Richard W. Nesto, MD, for his contributions to the chapter in previous editions.

REFERENCES

1. Rask-Madsen C, King GL. Vascular complications of diabetes: mechanisms of injury and protective factors. *Cell Metab.* 2013;17(1):20-33.
2. Skyler JS. Diabetic complications. The importance of glucose control. *Endocrinol Metab Clin North Am.* 1996;25(2):243-254.
3. Gregg EW, Li Y, Wang J, et al. Changes in diabetes-related complications in the United States, 1990-2010. *N Engl J Med.* 2014;370(16):1514-1523.
4. Diabetes Control and Complications Trial Research Group. The effect of intensive treatment of diabetes on the development and progression of long-term complications in insulin-dependent diabetes mellitus. *N Engl J Med.* 1993;329:977-986.
5. UK Prospective Diabetes Study (UKPDS) Group. Intensive blood-glucose control with sulphonylureas or insulin compared with conventional treatment and risk of complications in patients with type 2 diabetes (UKPDS 33). *Lancet.* 1998;352:837-853.
6. Krolewski AS, Laffel LM, Krolewski M, et al. Glycosylated hemoglobin and the risk of microalbuminuria in patients with insulin-dependent diabetes mellitus. *N Engl J Med.* 1995;332:1251-1255.
7. Diabetes Control and Complications Trial Research Group. The absence of a glycemic threshold for the development of long-term complications: the perspective of the Diabetes Control and Complications Trial. *Diabetes.* 1996;45:1289-1298.
8. Wagenknecht LE, D'Agostino RB Jr, Haffner SM, et al. Impaired glucose tolerance, type 2 diabetes, and carotid wall thickness: the Insulin Resistance Atherosclerosis Study. *Diabetes Care.* 1998;21:1812-1818.
9. Goldberg RB, Mellies MJ, Sacks FM, et al. Cardiovascular events and their reduction with pravastatin in diabetic and glucose-intolerant myocardial infarction survivors with average cholesterol levels: subgroup analyses in the Cholesterol and Recurrent Events (CARE) trial. The Care Investigators. *Circulation.* 1998;98:2513-2519.
10. Haffner SM. The Scandinavian Simvastatin Survival Study (4S) subgroup analysis of diabetic subjects: implications for the prevention of coronary heart disease. *Diabetes Care.* 1997;20(4):469-471.
11. Ebara T, Conde K, Kako Y, et al. Delayed catabolism of apoB-48 lipoproteins due to decreased heparan sulfate proteoglycan production in diabetic mice. *J Clin Invest.* 2000;105(12):1807-1818.
12. Ginsberg HN. Insulin resistance and cardiovascular disease. *J Clin Invest.* 2000;106(4):453-458.
13. Lachin JM, Genuth S, Nathan DM, et al. DCCT/EDIC Research Group. Effect of glycemic exposure on the risk of microvascular complications in the diabetes control and complications trial—revisited. *Diabetes.* 2008;57(4):995-1001.
14. Kaiser N, Sasson S, Feener EP, et al. Differential regulation of glucose transport and transporters by glucose in vascular endothelial and smooth muscle cells. *Diabetes.* 1993;42(1):80-89.
15. Heilig CW, Concepcion LA, Riser BL, et al. Overexpression of glucose transporters in rat mesangial cells cultured in a normal glucose milieu mimics the diabetic phenotype. *J Clin Invest.* 1995;96(4):1802-1814.
16. Guzman J, Jauregui AN, Merscher-Gomez S, et al. Podocyte-specific GLUT4-deficient mice have fewer and larger podocytes and are protected from diabetic nephropathy. *Diabetes.* 2014;63(2):701-714.
17. Shore AC, Tooke JE, Pickup J, et al. Microvascular function and haemodynamic disturbances in diabetes mellitus and its complications. In: Pickup J, Williams G, eds. *Textbook of Diabetes*, Vol. 1. Oxford, England: Blackwell Scientific; 1997:1-43.
18. Kihara M, Schmelzer JD, Poduslo JF, et al. Aminoguanidine effects on nerve blood flow, vascular permeability, electrophysiology, and oxygen free radicals. *Proc Natl Acad Sci U S A.* 1991;88(14):6107-6111.
19. Cerani A, Tetreault N, Menard C, et al. Neuron-derived semaphorin 3A is an early inducer of vascular permeability in diabetic retinopathy via neuropilin-1. *Cell Metab.* 2013;18(4):505-518.
20. Zhong Y, Li J, Chen Y, et al. Activation of endoplasmic reticulum stress by hyperglycemia is essential for Muller cell-derived inflammatory cytokine production in diabetes. *Diabetes.* 2012;61(2):492-504.
21. Hammes HP, Feng Y, Pfister F, Brownlee M. Diabetic retinopathy: targeting vasoregression. *Diabetes.* 2011;60(1):9-16.
22. Reidy K, Kang HM, Hostetter T. Susztak K. Molecular mechanisms of diabetic kidney disease. *J Clin Invest.* 2014;124(6):2333-2340.
23. Siddiqi FS, Advani A. Endothelial-podocyte crosstalk: the missing link between endothelial dysfunction and albuminuria in diabetes. *Diabetes.* 2013;62(11):3647-3655.
24. Isermann B, Vinnikov IA, Madhusudhan T, et al. Activated protein C protects against diabetic nephropathy by inhibiting endothelial and podocyte apoptosis. *Nat Med.* 2007;13(11):1349-1358.
25. Brownlee M. Preventing kidney cell suicide. *Nat Med.* 2007;13(11):1284-1285.
26. Vincent AM, Callaghan BC, Smith AL, Feldman EL. Diabetic neuropathy: cellular mechanisms as therapeutic targets. *Nat Rev Neurol.* 2011;7(10):573-583.
27. Kopp JB, Factor VM, Mozes M, et al. Transgenic mice with increased plasma levels of TGF-beta 1 develop progressive renal disease. *Lab Invest.* 1996;74(6):991-1003.
28. Chien S, Li S, Shyy YJ. Effects of mechanical forces on signal transduction and gene expression in endothelial cells. *Hypertension.* 1998;31(1 Pt 2):162-169.
29. Walker JD, Viberti GC, Pickup J, Williams G. Pathophysiology of microvascular disease: an overview. In: Pickup J, Williams G, eds. *Textbook of Diabetes*, Vol. 1. Oxford, England: Blackwell Scientific; 1991:526-533.
30. Brownlee M, Rifkin H, Porte D Jr. Advanced products of nonenzymatic glycosylation and the pathogenesis of diabetic complications. In: Rifkin H, Porte D Jr, eds. *Diabetes Mellitus: Theory and Practice.* New York, NY: Elsevier; 1990:279-291.
31. Hammes HP, Federoff HJ, Brownlee M. Nerve growth factor prevents both neuroretinal programmed cell death and capillary pathology in experimental diabetes. *Mol Med.* 1995;1(5):527-534.
32. Mizutani M, Kern TS, Lorenzi M. Accelerated death of retinal microvascular cells in human and experimental diabetic retinopathy. *J Clin Invest.* 1996;97(12):2883-2890.
33. Giannini C, Dyck PJ. Ultrastructural morphometric features of human sural nerve endoneurial microvessels. *J Neuropathol Exp Neurol.* 1993;52(4):361-369.
34. Giannini C, Dyck PJ. Basement membrane reduplication and pericyte degeneration precede development of diabetic polyneuropathy and are associated with its severity. *Ann Neurol.* 1995;37(4):498-504.
35. Tomlinson DR, Fernyhough P, Diemel LT. Role of neurotrophins in diabetic neuropathy and treatment with nerve growth factors. *Diabetes.* 1997;46(Suppl 2):S43-S49.
36. Engerman RL, Kern TS. Progression of incipient diabetic retinopathy during good glycemic control. *Diabetes.* 1987;36(7):808-812.
37. Roy S, Sala R, Cagliero E, Lorenzi M. Overexpression of fibronectin induced by diabetes or high glucose: phenomenon with a memory. *Proc Natl Acad Sci U S A.* 1990;87(1):404-408.
38. Diabetes Control and Complications Trial Research Group. Effect of intensive therapy on the development and progression of diabetic nephropathy in the Diabetes Control and Complications Trial. *Kidney Int.* 1995;47:1703-1720.
39. Diabetes Control and Complications Trial Research Group. The effect of intensive diabetes therapy on the development and progression of neuropathy. *Ann Intern Med.* 1995;122(8):561-568.
40. Writing Team for the Diabetes Control and Complications/Trial Epidemiology of Diabetes Interventions and Complications Research Group. Sustained effect of intensive treatment of type 1 diabetes mellitus on development and progression of diabetic nephropathy: the Epidemiology of Diabetes Interventions and Complications EDIC study. *JAMA.* 2003;290(16):2159-2167.
41. Writing Team for the Diabetes Control and Complications Trial/Epidemiology of Diabetes Interventions and Complications Research Group. Effect of intensive therapy on the microvascular complications of type 1 diabetes mellitus. *JAMA.* 2002;287(19):2563-2569.
42. Krolewski AS, Warram JH, Freire MB. Epidemiology of late diabetic complications. A basis for the development and evaluation of preventive programs. *Endocrinol Metab Clin North Am.* 1996;25(2):217-242.
43. Wagenknecht LE, Bowden DW, Carr JJ, et al. Familial aggregation of coronary artery calcium in families with type 2 diabetes. *Diabetes.* 2001;50(4):861-866.
44. Seaquist ER, Goetz FC, Rich S, Barbosa J. Familial clustering of diabetic kidney disease. Evidence for genetic susceptibility to diabetic nephropathy. *N Engl J Med.* 1989;320(18):1161-1165.
45. Quinn M, Angelico MC, Warram JH, Krolewski AS. Familial factors determine the development of diabetic nephropathy in patients with IDDM. *Diabetologia.* 1996;39(8):940-945.
46. Diabetes Control and Complications Trial Research Group. Clustering of longterm complications in families with diabetes in the Diabetes Control and Complications Trial. *Diabetes.* 1997;46(11):1829-1839.
47. Raffel LJ, Vadheim CM, Roth MP, et al. The 5' insulin gene polymorphism and the genetics of vascular complications in type 1 (insulin-dependent) diabetes mellitus. *Diabetologia.* 1991;34(9):680-683.
48. Stewart LL, Field LL, Ross S, McArthur RG. Genetic risk factors in diabetic retinopathy. *Diabetologia.* 1993;36(12):1293-1298.
49. Marre M, Bernadet P, Gallois Y, et al. Relationships between angiotensin I converting enzyme gene polymorphism, plasma levels, and diabetic retinal and renal complications. *Diabetes.* 1994;43:384-388.
50. Marre M, Jeunemaitre X, Gallois Y, et al. Contribution of genetic polymorphism in the renin-angiotensin system to the development of renal complications in insulin-dependent diabetes: Genetique de la Nephropathie Diabetique (GENEDIAB) study group. *J Clin Invest.* 1997;99(7):1585-1595.
51. Agardh D, Gaur LK, Agardh E, et al. HLA-DQB1*0201/0302 is associated with severe retinopathy in patients with IDDM. *Diabetologia.* 1996;39(11):1313-1317.
52. Oates PJ, Mylari BL. Aldose reductase inhibitors: therapeutic implications for diabetic complications. *Exp Opin Invest Drugs.* 1999;8:2095-2119.
53. Warpeha KM, Xu W, Liu L, et al. Genotyping and functional analysis of a polymorphic (CCTTT)(n) repeat of NOS2A in diabetic retinopathy. *FASEB J.* 1999;13(13):1825-1832.

54. Satko SG, Freedman BI, Moossavi S. Genetic factors in end-stage renal disease. *Kidney Int Suppl.* 2005;94:S46-S49.

55. Ewens KG, George RA, Sharma K, et al. Assessment of 115 candidate genes for diabetic nephropathy by transmission/disequilibrium test. *Diabetes.* 2005;54(11):3305-3318.

56. Al-Kateb H, Boright AP, Mirea L, et al. Multiple superoxide dismutase 1/splicing factor serine alanine 15 variants are associated with the development and progression of diabetic nephropathy: the Diabetes Control and Complications Trial/Epidemiology of Diabetes Interventions and Complications Genetics study. *Diabetes.* 2008;57(1):218-228.

57. Tong Z, Yang Z, Patel S, et al. Promoter polymorphism of the erythropoietin gene in severe diabetic eye and kidney complications. *Proc Natl Acad Sci U S A.* 2008;105(19):6998-7003.

58. Abhary S, Abhary S, Burdon KP, et al. Association between erythropoietin gene polymorphisms and diabetic retinopathy. *Arch Ophthalmol.* 2010;128(1):102-106.

59. Haston CK, Hudson TJ. Finding genetic modifiers of cystic fibrosis. *N Engl J Med.* 2005;353(14):1509-1511.

60. Kato M, Castro NE, Natarajan R. MicroRNAs: potential mediators and biomarkers of diabetic complications. *Free Radic Biol Med.* 2013;64:85-94.

61. Feng B, Chen S, McArthur K, et al. miR-146a-mediated extracellular matrix protein production in chronic diabetes complications. *Diabetes.* 2011;60(11):2975-2984.

62. Putta S, Lanting L, Sun G, et al. Inhibiting microRNA-192 ameliorates renal fibrosis in diabetic nephropathy. *J Am Soc Nephrol.* 2012;23(3):458-469.

63. Wang B, Koh P, Winbanks C, et al. miR-200a prevents renal fibrogenesis through repression of TGF-beta2 expression. *Diabetes.* 2011;60(1):280-287.

64. Long J, Wang Y, Wang W, et al. MicroRNA-29c is a signature microRNA under high glucose conditions that targets Sprouty homolog 1, and its in vivo knockdown prevents progression of diabetic nephropathy. *J Biol Chem.* 2011;286(13):11837-11848.

65. Jansen F, Yang X, Hoelscher M, et al. Endothelial microparticle-mediated transfer of microRNA-126 promotes vascular endothelial cell repair via SPRED1 and is abrogated in glucose-damaged endothelial microparticles. *Circulation.* 2013;128(18):2026-2038.

66. Distel E, Barrett TJ, Chung K, et al. miR33 inhibition overcomes deleterious effects of diabetes mellitus on atherosclerosis plaque regression in mice. *Circ Res.* 2014;115(9):759-769.

67. Kuwabara Y, Horie T, Baba O, et al. MicroRNA-451 exacerbates lipotoxicity in cardiac myocytes and high-fat diet-induced cardiac hypertrophy in mice through suppression of the LKB1/AMPK pathway. *Circ Res.* 2015;116(2):279-288.

67a. Bhatt S, et al. Preserved DNA damage checkpoint pathway protects against complicaitons in long-standing type 1 diabetes. *Cell Metab.* 2015;22:239-252. <http://dx.doi.org/10.1016/j.cmet.2015.07.015>.

68. Kojima H, Kim J, Chan L. Emerging roles of hematopoietic cells in the pathobiology of diabetic complications. *Trends Endocrinol Metab.* 2014;25(4):178-187.

69. Li G, Veenstra AA, Talahalli RR, et al. Marrow-derived cells regulate the development of early diabetic retinopathy and tactile allodynia in mice. *Diabetes.* 2012;61(12):3294-3303.

70. Nguyen D, Ping F, Mu W, et al. Macrophage accumulation in human progressive diabetic nephropathy. *Nephrology.* 2006;11(3):226-231.

71. Molgat AS, Tilokee EL, Rafatian G, et al. Hyperglycemia inhibits cardiac stem cell-mediated cardiac repair and angiogenic capacity. *Circulation.* 2014;130(11 Suppl 1):S70-S76.

72. Granger CB, Califf RM, Young S, et al. Outcome of patients with diabetes mellitus and acute myocardial infarction treated with thrombolytic agents. The Thrombolysis and Angioplasty in Myocardial Infarction (TAMI) Study Group. *J Am Coll Cardiol.* 1993;21(4):920-925.

73. Stamler J, Vaccaro O, Neaton JD, Wentworth D. Diabetes, other risk factors, and 12-yr cardiovascular mortality for men screened in the Multiple Risk Factor Intervention Trial. *Diabetes Care.* 1993;16(2):434-444.

74. Fitzgerald AP, Jarrett RJ. Are conventional risk factors for mortality relevant in type 2 diabetes? *Diabet Med.* 1991;8(5):475-480.

75. Fuller JH, Shipley MJ, Rose G, et al. Coronary-heart-disease risk and impaired glucose tolerance. The Whitehall study. *Lancet.* 1980;1(8183):1373-1376.

76. Rosengren A, Welin L, Tsipogianni A, Wilhelmsen L. Impact of cardiovascular risk factors on coronary heart disease and mortality among middle aged diabetic men: a general population study. *BMJ.* 1989;299(6708):1127-1131.

77. Lehto S, Rönnemaa T, Pyörälä K, Laakso M. Poor glycemic control predicts coronary heart disease events in patients with type 1 diabetes without nephropathy. *Arterioscler Thromb Vasc Biol.* 1999;19(4):1014-1019.

78. Gerstein HC. Is glucose a continuous risk factor for cardiovascular mortality? *Diabetes Care.* 1999;22(5):659-660.

79. Gall MA, Borch-Johnsen K, Hougaard P, et al. Albuminuria and poor glycemic control predict mortality in NIDDM. *Diabetes.* 1995;44(11):1303-1309.

80. Kuusisto J, Mykkanen L, Pyorala K, Laakso M. NIDDM and its metabolic control predict coronary heart disease in elderly subjects. *Diabetes.* 1994;43:960-967.

81. Salomaa V, Riley W, Kark JD, et al. Non-insulin-dependent diabetes mellitus and fasting glucose and insulin concentrations are associated with arterial stiffness indexes. The ARIC Study. Atherosclerosis Risk in Communities Study. *Circulation.* 1995;91(5):1432-1443.

82. Laakso M, Kuusisto J. Epidemiological evidence for the association of hyperglycaemia and atherosclerotic vascular disease in non-insulin-dependent diabetes mellitus. *Ann Med.* 1996;28(5):415-418.

83. Bonora E, Kiechl S, Willeit J, et al. Prevalence of insulin resistance in metabolic disorders: the Bruneck study. *Diabetes.* 1998;47:1643-1649.

84. Haffner SM, Lehto S, Ronnemaa T, et al. Mortality from coronary heart disease in subjects with type 2 diabetes and in nondiabetic subjects with and without prior myocardial infarction. *N Engl J Med.* 1998;339:229-234.

85. Saydah SH, Miret M, Sung J, et al. Postchallenge hyperglycemia and mortality in a national sample of U.S. adults. *Diabetes Care.* 2001;24(8):1397-1402.

86. National Diabetes Data Group. *Diabetes in America.* 2nd ed. Bethesda, MD: National Institute of Diabetes and Digestive and Kidney Diseases; 1995.

87. DECODE Study Group, the European Diabetes Epidemiology Group. Glucose tolerance and cardiovascular mortality: comparison of fasting and 2-hour diagnostic criteria. *Arch Intern Med.* 2001;161(3):397-405.

88. Yip J, Facchini FS, Reaven GM. Resistance to insulin-mediated glucose disposal as a predictor of cardiovascular disease. *J Clin Endocrinol Metab.* 1998;83(8):2773-2776.

89. Hanley AJ, Williams K, Stern MP, et al. Homeostasis model assessment of IR in relation to the incidence of cardiovascular disease: the San Antonio Heart Study. *Diabetes Care.* 2002;25:1177-1184.

90. King G, Brownlee M. The cellular and molecular mechanisms of diabetic complications. *Endocrinol Metab Clin North Am.* 1996;2:255-270.

91. Hsueh WA, Law RE. Cardiovascular risk continuum: implications of insulin resistance and diabetes. *Am J Med.* 1998;105(1A):4S-14S.

92. Li H, Förstermann U. Nitric oxide in the pathogenesis of vascular disease. *J Pathol.* 2000;190(3):244-254.

93. Li H, Forstermann U. Pharmacological prevention of eNOS uncoupling. *Curr Pharm Des.* 2014;20(22):3595-3606.

94. Banskota NK, Taub R, Zellner K, King GL. Insulin, insulin-like growth factor I and platelet-derived growth factor interact additively in the induction of the protooncogene c-myc and cellular proliferation in cultured bovine aortic smooth muscle cells. *Mol Endocrinol.* 1989;8:1183-1190.

95. Stolar MW. Atherosclerosis in diabetes: the role of hyperinsulinemia. *Metab Clin Exp.* 1988;37(2 Suppl 1):1-9.

96. Jiang ZY, Lin YW, Clemont A, et al. Characterization of selective resistance to insulin signaling in the vasculature of obese Zucker (fa/fa) rats. *J Clin Invest.* 1999;104(4):447-457.

97. Kanter JE, Kramer F, Barnhart S, et al. Diabetes promotes an inflammatory macrophage phenotype and atherosclerosis through acyl-CoA synthetase 1. *Proc Natl Acad Sci U S A.* 2012;109(12):E715-E724.

98. Goldberg IJ, Bornfeldt KE. Lipids and the endothelium: bidirectional interactions. *Curr Atheroscler Rep.* 2013;15(11):365.

99. Du X, Edelstein D, Obici S, et al. Insulin resistance reduces arterial prostacyclin synthase and eNOS activities by increasing endothelial fatty acid oxidation. *J Clin Invest.* 2006;116(4):1071-1080.

100. Nathan DM, Cleary PA, Backlund J-YC, et al. Intensive diabetes treatment and cardiovascular disease in patients with type 1 diabetes. *N Engl J Med.* 2005;353(25):2643-2653.

101. Nagareddy PR, Murphy AJ, Stirzaker RA, et al. Hyperglycemia promotes myelopoiesis and impairs the resolution of atherosclerosis. *Cell Metab.* 2013;17(5):695-708.

102. Brownlee M. Hyperglycemia-stimulated myelopoiesis causes impaired regression of atherosclerosis in type 1 diabetes. *Cell Metab.* 2013;17(5):631-633.

103. Tepper OM, Galiano RD, Capla JM, et al. Human endothelial progenitor cells from type II diabetics exhibit impaired proliferation, adhesion, and incorporation into vascular structures. *Circulation.* 2002;106(22):2781-2786.

104. Thangarajah H, Yao D, Chang EI, et al. The molecular basis for impaired hypoxia-induced VEGF expression in diabetic tissues. *Proc Natl Acad Sci U S A.* 2009;106(32):13505-13510.

105. Ceradini DJ, Yao D, Grogan RH, et al. Decreasing intracellular superoxide corrects defective ischemia-induced new vessel formation in diabetic mice. *J Biol Chem.* 2008;283(16):10930-10938.

106. Januszyk M, Sorkin M, Glotzbach JP, et al. Diabetes irreversibly depletes bone marrow-derived mesenchymal progenitor cell subpopulations. *Diabetes.* 2014;63(9):3047-3056.

107. Duh E, Aiello LP. Vascular endothelial growth factor and diabetes: the agonist versus antagonist paradox. *Diabetes*. 1999;48(10):1899-1906.
108. Waltenberger J. Impaired collateral vessel development in diabetes: potential cellular mechanisms and therapeutic implications. *Cardiovasc Res*. 2001;49(3):554-560.
109. Grant MB, May WS, Caballero S, et al. Adult hematopoietic stem cells provide functional hemangioblast activity during retinal neovascularization. *Nat Med*. 2002;8(6):607-612.
110. Rivard A, Silver M, Chen D, et al. Rescue of diabetes-related impairment of angiogenesis by intramuscular gene therapy with adeno-VEGF. *Am J Pathol*. 1999;154(2):355-363.
111. Iwaguro H, Yamaguchi J, Kalka C, et al. Endothelial progenitor cell vascular endothelial growth factor gene transfer for vascular regeneration. *Circulation*. 2002;105(6):732-738.
112. Hodgin JB, Nair V, Zhang H, et al. Identification of cross-species shared transcriptional networks of diabetic nephropathy in human and mouse glomeruli. *Diabetes*. 2013;62(1):299-308.
113. Zhang JZ, Gao L, Widness M, et al. Captopril inhibits glucose accumulation in retinal cells in diabetes. *Invest Ophthalmol Vis Sci*. 2003;44(9):4001-4005.
114. Bohren KM, Grimshaw CE, Gabbay KH. Catalytic effectiveness of human aldose reductase. Critical role of C-terminal domain. *J Biol Chem*. 1992;267(29):20965-20970.
115. Engerman RL, Kern TS, Larson ME. Nerve conduction and aldose reductase inhibition during 5 years of diabetes or galactosaemia in dogs. *Diabetologia*. 1994;37(2):141-144.
116. Srivastava S, Vladykovskaya E, Barski OA, et al. Aldose reductase protects against early atherosclerotic lesion formation in apolipoprotein E-null mice. *Circ Res*. 2009;105(8):793-802.
117. Vedantham S, Thiagarajan D, Ananthakrishnan R, et al. Aldose reductase drives hyperacetylation of Egr-1 in hyperglycemia and consequent upregulation of proinflammatory and prothrombotic signals. *Diabetes*. 2014;63(2):761-774.
118. Son NH, Ananthakrishnan R, Yu S, et al. Cardiomyocyte aldose reductase causes heart failure and impairs recovery from ischemia. *PLoS ONE*. 2012;7(9):e46549.
119. Hammes HP, Martin S, Federlin K, et al. Aminoguanidine treatment inhibits the development of experimental diabetic retinopathy. *Proc Natl Acad Sci U S A*. 1991;88(24):11555-11558.
120. Stitt AW, Li YM, Gardiner TA, et al. Advanced glycation end products (AGEs) co-localize with AGE receptors in the retinal vasculature of diabetic and of AGE-infused rats. *Am J Pathol*. 1997;150(2):523-531.
121. Stitt AW, Moore JE, Sharkey JA, et al. Advanced glycation end products in vitreous: structural and functional implications for diabetic vitreopathy. *Invest Ophthalmol Vis Sci*. 1998;39(13):2517-2523.
122. Horie K, Miyata T, Maeda K, et al. Immunohistochemical colocalization of glycoxidation products and lipid peroxidation products in diabetic renal glomerular lesions. Implication for glycoxidative stress in the pathogenesis of diabetic nephropathy. *J Clin Invest*. 1997;100(12):2995-3004.
123. Nishino T, Horii Y, Shiiki H, et al. Immunohistochemical detection of advanced glycosylation end products within the vascular lesions and glomeruli in diabetic nephropathy. *Hum Pathol*. 1995;26(3):308-313.
124. Niwa T, Katsuzaki T, Miyazaki S, et al. Immunohistochemical detection of imidazolone, a novel advanced glycation end product, in kidneys and aortas of diabetic patients. *J Clin Invest*. 1997;99(6):1272-1280.
125. Degenhardt TP, Thorpe SR, Baynes JW. Chemical modification of proteins by methylglyoxal. *Cell Mol Biol*. 1998;44(7):1139-1145.
126. Wells-Knecht KJ, Zyzak DV, Litchfield JE, et al. Mechanism of autoxidative glycosylation: identification of glyoxal and arabinose as intermediates in the autoxidative modification of proteins by glucose. *Biochemistry*. 1995;34(11):3702-3709.
127. Thornalley PJ. The glyoxalase system: new developments towards functional characterization of a metabolic pathway fundamental to biological life. *Biochem J*. 1990;269(1):1-11.
128. Suzuki K, Koh YH, Mizuno H, et al. Overexpression of aldehyde reductase protects PC12 cells from the cytotoxicity of methylglyoxal or 3-deoxyglucosone. *J Biochem*. 1998;123(2):353-357.
129. Takahashi M, Fujii J, Teshima T, et al. Identity of a major 3-deoxyglucosone-reducing enzyme with aldehyde reductase in rat liver established by amino acid sequencing and cDNA expression. *Gene*. 1993;127(2):249-253.
130. Thornalley PJ, Battah S, Ahmed N, et al. Quantitative screening of advanced glycation endproducts in cellular and extracellular proteins by tandem mass spectrometry. *Biochem J*. 2003;375(Pt 3):581-592.
131. Chang EY, Szallasi Z, Acs P, et al. Functional effects of overexpression of protein kinase C-alpha, -beta, -delta, -epsilon, and eta in the mast cell line RBL-2H3. *J Immunol*. 1997;1159(6):2624-2632.
132. Carmeliet P. Angiogenesis in health and disease. *Nat Med*. 2003;9(6):653-660.
133. Hanahan D. Signaling vascular morphogenesis and maintenance. *Science (New York)*. 1997;277(5322):48-50.
134. Jain RK. Molecular regulation of vessel maturation. *Nat Med*. 2003;9(6):685-693.
135. Gale NW, Thurston G, Hackett SF. Angiopoietin-2 is required for postnatal angiogenesis and lymphatic patterning, and only the latter role is rescued by angiopoietin-1. *Dev Cell*. 2003;3(3):411-423.
136. Hackett SF, Wiegand S, Yancopoulos G, Campochiaro PA. Angiopoietin-2 plays an important role in retinal angiogenesis. *J Cell Physiol*. 2002;192(2):182-187.
137. Maisonpierre PC, Suri C, Jones PF, et al. Angiopoietin-2, a natural antagonist for Tie2 that disrupts in vivo angiogenesis. *Science (New York)*. 1997;277(5322):55-60.
138. Hammes H-P, Lin J, Wagner P, et al. Angiopoietin-2 causes pericyte dropout in the normal retina: evidence for involvement in diabetic retinopathy. *Diabetes*. 2004;53(4):1104-1110.
139. Hammes H-P, Lin J, Renner O, et al. Pericytes and the pathogenesis of diabetic retinopathy. *Diabetes*. 2002;51(10):3107-3112.
140. Yao D, Taguchi T, Matsumura T, et al. High glucose increases angiopoietin-2 transcription in microvascular endothelial cells through methylglyoxal modification of mSin3A. *J Biol Chem*. 2007;282(42):31038-31045.
141. Bierhaus A, Fleming T, Stoyanov S, et al. Methylglyoxal modification of Nav1.8 facilitates nociceptive neuron firing and causes hyperalgesia in diabetic neuropathy. *Nat Med*. 2012;18(6):926-933.
142. Vulesevic B, McNeill B, Geoffrion M, et al. Glyoxalase-1 overexpression in bone marrow cells reverses defective neovascularization in STZ-induced diabetic mice. *Cardiovasc Res*. 2014;101(2):306-316.
143. Giacco F, Du X, D'Agati VD, et al. Knockdown of glyoxalase 1 mimics diabetic nephropathy in nondiabetic mice. *Diabetes*. 2014;63(1):291-299.
144. McLellan AC, Thornalley PJ, Benn J, Sonksen PH. Glyoxalase system in clinical diabetes mellitus and correlation with diabetic complications. *Clin Sci (Lond.)*. 1994;87(1):21-29.
145. Godbout JP, Pesavento J, Hartman ME, et al. Methylglyoxal enhances cisplatin-induced cytotoxicity by activating protein kinase Cdelta. *J Biol Chem*. 2002;277(4):2554-2561.
146. Sakamoto H, Mashima T, Yamamoto K, Tsuruo T. Modulation of heat-shock protein 27 (Hsp27) anti-apoptotic activity by methylglyoxal modification. *J Biol Chem*. 2002;277(48):45770-45775.
147. Tanaka S, Avigad G, Brodsky B, Eikenberry EF. Glycation induces expansion of the molecular packing of collagen. *J Mol Biol*. 1988;203(2):495-505.
148. Huijberts MS, Wolffenbuttel BH, Boudier HA, et al. Aminoguanidine treatment increases elasticity and decreases fluid filtration of large arteries from diabetic rats. *J Clin Invest*. 1993;92(3):1407-1411.
149. Tsilibary EC, Charonis AS, Reger LA, et al. The effect of nonenzymatic glucosylation on the binding of the main noncollagenous NC1 domain to type IV collagen. *J Biol Chem*. 1988;263(9):4302-4308.
150. Charonis AS, Reger LA, Dege JE. Laminin alterations after in vitro nonenzymatic glycosylation. *Diabetes*. 1988;39:807-814.
151. Boyd-White J, Williams JC. Effect of cross-linking on matrix permeability. A model for AGE-modified basement membranes. *Diabetes*. 1996;45(3):348-353.
152. Cochrane SM, Robinson GB. In vitro glycation of glomerular basement membrane alters its permeability: a possible mechanism in diabetic complications. *FEBS Lett*. 1995;375(1-2):41-44.
153. Haitoglou CS, Tsilibary EC, Brownlee M, Charonis AS. Altered cellular interactions between endothelial cells and nonenzymatically glycosylated laminin/type IV collagen. *J Biol Chem*. 1992;267(18):12404-12407.
154. Federoff HJ, Lawrence D, Brownlee M. Nonenzymatic glycosylation of laminin and the laminin peptide CIKVAVS inhibits neurite outgrowth. *Diabetes*. 1993;42(4):509-513.
155. Hammes HP, Weiss A, Hess S, et al. Modification of vitronectin by advanced glycation alters functional properties in vitro and in the diabetic retina. *Lab Invest*. 1996;75(3):325-338.
156. Dobler D, Ahmed N, Song L, et al. Increased dicarbonyl metabolism in endothelial cells in hyperglycemia induces anoikis and impairs angiogenesis by RGD and GFOGER motif modification. *Diabetes*. 2006;55(7):1961-1969.
157. Bishara NB, Dunlop ME, Murphy TV, et al. Matrix protein glycation impairs agonist-induced intracellular Ca2+ signaling in endothelial cells. *J Cell Physiol*. 2002;193(1):80-92.
158. Li YM, Mitsuhashi T, Wojciechowicz D, et al. Molecular identity and cellular distribution of advanced glycation endproduct receptors: relationship of p60 to OST-48 and p90 to 80K-H membrane proteins. *Proc Natl Acad Sci U S A*. 1996;93(20):11047-11052.
159. Neeper M, Schmidt AM, Brett J, et al. Cloning and expression of a cell surface receptor for advanced glycosylation end products of proteins. *J Biol Chem*. 1992;267(21):14998-15004.
160. Schmidt AM, Mora R, Cao R, et al. The endothelial cell binding site for advanced glycation end products consists of a complex: an integral membrane protein and a lactoferrin-like polypeptide. *J Biol Chem*. 1994;269(13):9882-9888.
161. Schmidt AM, Vianna M, Gerlach M, et al. Isolation and characterization of two binding proteins for advanced glycosylation end products from bovine lung which are present on the endothelial cell surface. *J Biol Chem*. 1992;267(21):14987-14997.

162. Yang Z, Makita Z, Horii Y, et al. Two novel rat liver membrane proteins that bind advanced glycosylation endproducts: relationship to macrophage receptor for glucose-modified proteins. *J Exp Med.* 1991; 174(3):515-524.

163. Yan SF, Ramasamy R, Schmidt AM. The RAGE axis: a fundamental mechanism signaling danger to the vulnerable vasculature. *Circ Res.* 2010;106(5):842-853.

164. Abordo EA, Thornalley PJ. Synthesis and secretion of tumour necrosis factor-alpha by human monocytic THP-1 cells and chemotaxis induced by human serum albumin derivatives modified with methylglyoxal and glucose-derived advanced glycation endproducts. *Immunol Lett.* 1997;58(3):139-147.

165. Abordo EA, Westwood ME, Thornalley PJ. Synthesis and secretion of macrophage colony stimulating factor by mature human monocytes and human monocytic THP-1 cells induced by human serum albumin derivatives modified with methylglyoxal and glucose-derived advanced glycation endproducts. *Immunol Lett.* 1996;53(1):7-13.

166. Doi T, Vlassara H, Kirstein M, et al. Receptor-specific increase in extracellular matrix production in mouse mesangial cells by advanced glycosylation end products is mediated via platelet-derived growth factor. *Proc Natl Acad Sci U S A.* 1992;89(7):2873-2877.

167. Higashi T, Sano H, Saishoji T, et al. The receptor for advanced glycation end products mediates the chemotaxis of rabbit smooth muscle cells. *Diabetes.* 1997;46(3):463-472.

168. Horiuchi S, Higashi T, Ikeda K, et al. Advanced glycation end products and their recognition by macrophage and macrophage-derived cells. *Diabetes.* 1996;45(Suppl 3):S73-S76.

169. Kirstein M, Aston C, Hintz R, Vlassara H. Receptor-specific induction of insulin-like growth factor I in human monocytes by advanced glycosylation end product-modified proteins. *J Clin Invest.* 1992; 90(2):439-446.

170. Pugliese G, Pricci F, Romeo G, et al. Upregulation of mesangial growth factor and extracellular matrix synthesis by advanced glycation end products via a receptor-mediated mechanism. *Diabetes.* 1997;46(11):1881-1887.

171. Sano H, Higashi T, Matsumoto K, et al. Insulin enhances macrophage scavenger receptor-mediated endocytic uptake of advanced glycation end products. *J Biol Chem.* 1998;273(15):8630-8637.

172. Skolnik EY, Yang Z, Makita Z, et al. Human and rat mesangial cell receptors for glucose-modified proteins: potential role in kidney tissue remodelling and diabetic nephropathy. *J Exp Med.* 1991; 174(4):931-939.

173. Smedsrod B, Melkko J, Araki N, et al. Advanced glycation end products are eliminated by scavenger-receptor-mediated endocytosis in hepatic sinusoidal Kupffer and endothelial cells. *Biochemical Journal.* 1997;322:567-573.

174. Vlassara H, Brownlee M, Manogue KR, et al. Cachectin/TNF and IL-1 induced by glucose-modified proteins: role in normal tissue remodeling. *Science (New York).* 1988;240(4858):1546-1548.

175. Vlassara H, Li YM, Imani F, et al. Identification of galectin-3 as a high-affinity binding protein for advanced glycation end products (AGE): a new member of the AGE-receptor complex. *Mol Med (Cambridge, MA).* 1995;1(6):634-646.

176. Webster L, Abordo EA, Thornalley PJ, Limb GA. Induction of TNF alpha and IL-1 beta mRNA in monocytes by methylglyoxal- and advanced glycated endproduct-modified human serum albumin. *Biochem Soc Trans.* 1997;25(2):250S.

177. Westwood ME, Thornalley PJ. Induction of synthesis and secretion of interleukin 1 beta in the human monocytic THP-1 cells by human serum albumins modified with methylglyoxal and advanced glycation endproducts. *Immunol Lett.* 1996;50(1-2):17-21.

178. Yui S, Sasaki T, Araki N, et al. Induction of macrophage growth by advanced glycation end products of the Maillard reaction. *J Immunol (Baltimore, MD).* 1994;152(4):1943-1949.

179. Schmidt AM, Crandall J, Hori O, et al. Elevated plasma levels of vascular cell adhesion molecule-1 (VCAM-1) in diabetic patients with microalbuminuria: a marker of vascular dysfunction and progressive vascular disease. *Br J Haematol.* 1996;92(3):747-750.

180. Schmidt AM, Hori O, Chen JX, et al. Advanced glycation endproducts interacting with their endothelial receptor induce expression of vascular cell adhesion molecule-1 (VCAM-1) in cultured human endothelial cells and in mice. A potential mechanism for the accelerated vasculopathy of diabetes. *J Clin Invest.* 1995;96(3):1395-1403.

181. Sengoelge G, Födinger M, Skoupy S, et al. Endothelial cell adhesion molecule and PMNL response to inflammatory stimuli and AGE-modified fibronectin. *Kidney Int.* 1998;54(5):1637-1651.

182. Vlassara H, Fuh H, Donnelly T, Cybulsky M. Advanced glycation endproducts promote adhesion molecule (VCAM-1, ICAM-1) expression and atheroma formation in normal rabbits. *Mol Med (Cambridge, MA).* 1995;1(4):447-456.

183. Hirata C, Nakano K, Nakamura N, et al. Advanced glycation end products induce expression of vascular endothelial growth factor by retinal Muller cells. *Biochem Biophys Res Commun.* 1997;236(3):712-715.

184. Lu M, Kuroki M, Amano S, et al. Advanced glycation end products increase retinal vascular endothelial growth factor expression. *J Clin Invest.* 1998;101(6):1219-1224.

185. Wautier JL, Zoukourian C, Chappey O, et al. Receptor-mediated endothelial cell dysfunction in diabetic vasculopathy. Soluble receptor for advanced glycation end products blocks hyperpermeability in diabetic rats. *J Clin Invest.* 1996;97(1):238-243.

186. Soro-Paavonen A, Watson AMD, Li J, et al. Receptor for advanced glycation end products (RAGE) deficiency attenuates the development of atherosclerosis in diabetes. *Diabetes.* 2008;57(9):2461-2469.

187. Bierhaus A, Humpert PM, Morcos M, et al. Understanding RAGE, the receptor for advanced glycation end products. *J Mol Med (Berlin, Germany).* 2005;83(11):876-886.

188. Rong LL, Gooch C, Szabolcs M, et al. RAGE: a journey from the complications of diabetes to disorders of the nervous system: striking a fine balance between injury and repair. *Restor Neurol Neurosci.* 2005;23(5-6):355-365.

189. Yao D, Brownlee M. Hyperglycemia-induced reactive oxygen species increase expression of the receptor for advanced glycation end products (RAGE) and RAGE ligands. *Diabetes.* 2010;59(1):249-255.

190. Park L, Raman KG, Lee KJ, et al. Suppression of accelerated diabetic atherosclerosis by the soluble receptor for advanced glycation endproducts. *Nat Med.* 1998;4(9):1025-1031.

191. Kislinger T, Tanji N, Wendt T, et al. Receptor for advanced glycation end products mediates inflammation and enhanced expression of tissue factor in vasculature of diabetic apolipoprotein E-null mice. *Arterioscler Thromb Vasc Biol.* 2001;21(6):905-910.

192. Oldfield MD, Bach LA, Forbes JM, et al. Advanced glycation end products cause epithelial-myofibroblast transdifferentiation via the receptor for advanced glycation end products (RAGE). *J Clin Invest.* 2001;108:1853-1863.

193. Lalla E, Lamster IB, Feit M, et al. Blockade of RAGE suppresses periodontitis-associated bone loss in diabetic mice. *J Clin Invest.* 2000;105(8):1117-1124.

194. Goova MT, Li J, Kislinger T, et al. Blockade of receptor for advanced glycation end-products restores effective wound healing in diabetic mice. *Am J Pathol.* 2001;159(2):513-525.

195. Bucciarelli LG, Wendt T, Qu W, et al. RAGE blockade stabilizes established atherosclerosis in diabetic apolipoprotein E-null mice. *Circulation.* 2002;106(22):2827-2835.

196. Basta G, Sironi AM, Lazzerini G, et al. Circulating soluble receptor for advanced glycation end products is inversely associated with glycemic control and S100A12 protein. *J Clin Endocrinol Metab.* 2006; 91(11):4628-4634.

197. Naoto K, Munehide M, Hideaki K. Decreased endogenous secretory advanced glycation end product receptor in type 1 diabetic patients: its possible association with diabetic vascular complications. *Diabetes Care.* 2005;28:2716-2721.

198. Craven PA, Davidson CM, DeRubertis FR. Increase in diacylglycerol mass in isolated glomeruli by glucose from de novo synthesis of glycerolipids. *Diabetes.* 1990;39(6):667-674.

199. Inoguchi T, Battan R, Handler E, et al. Preferential elevation of protein kinase C isoform beta II and diacylglycerol levels in the aorta and heart of diabetic rats: differential reversibility to glycemic control by islet cell transplantation. *Proc Natl Acad Sci U S A.* 1992;89(22): 11059-11063.

200. Shiba T, Inoguchi T, Sportsman JR, et al. Correlation of diacylglycerol level and protein kinase C activity in rat retina to retinal circulation. *Am J Physiol.* 1993;265(5 Pt 1):E783-E793.

201. Inoguchi T, Xia P, Kunisaki M, et al. Insulin's effect on protein kinase C and diacylglycerol induced by diabetes and glucose in vascular tissues. *Am J Physiol.* 1994;267(3 Pt 1):E369-E379.

202. Ayo SH, Radnik R, Garoni JA, et al. High glucose increases diacylglycerol mass and activates protein kinase C in mesangial cell cultures. *Am J Physiol.* 1991;261(4 Pt 2):F571-F577.

203. Derubertis FR, Craven PA. Activation of protein kinase C in glomerular cells in diabetes. Mechanisms and potential links to the pathogenesis of diabetic glomerulopathy. *Diabetes.* 1994;43(1):1-8.

204. Xia P, Inoguchi T, Kern TS, et al. Characterization of the mechanism for the chronic activation of diacylglycerol-protein kinase C pathway in diabetes and hypergalactosemia. *Diabetes.* 1994;43(9): 1122-1129.

205. Koya D, King GL. Protein kinase C activation and the development of diabetic complications. *Diabetes.* 1998;47(6):859-866.

206. Kikkawa R, Haneda M, Uzu T, et al. Translocation of protein kinase C alpha and zeta in rat glomerular mesangial cells cultured under high glucose conditions. *Diabetologia.* 1994;37(8):838-841.

207. Koya D, Jirousek MR, Lin YW, et al. Characterization of protein kinase C beta isoform activation on the gene expression of transforming growth factor-beta, extracellular matrix components, and prostanoids in the glomeruli of diabetic rats. *J Clin Invest.* 1997;100(1): 115-126.

208. Knapp LT, Klann E. Superoxide-induced stimulation of protein kinase C via thiol modification and modulation of zinc content. *J Biol Chem.* 2000;275(31):24136-24145.

209. Konishi H, Tanaka M, Takemura Y, et al. Activation of protein kinase C by tyrosine phosphorylation in response to H_2O_2. *Proc Natl Acad Sci U S A.* 1997;94(21):11233-11237.

210. Ishii H, Jirousek MR, Koya D, et al. Amelioration of vascular dysfunctions in diabetic rats by an oral PKC beta inhibitor. *Science (New York)*. 1996;272(5262):728-731.

211. Geraldes P, Hiraoka-Yamamoto J, Matsumoto M, et al. Activation of PKC-delta and SHP-1 by hyperglycemia causes vascular cell apoptosis and diabetic retinopathy. *Nat Med*. 2009;15(11):1298-1306.

212. Craven PA, Studer RK, DeRubertis FR. Impaired nitric oxide-dependent cyclic guanosine monophosphate generation in glomeruli from diabetic rats. Evidence for protein kinase C-mediated suppression of the cholinergic response. *J Clin Invest*. 1994;93(1):311-320.

213. Ganz MB, Seftel A. Glucose-induced changes in protein kinase C and nitric oxide are prevented by vitamin E. *Am J Physiol Endocrinol Metab*. 2000;278(1):E146-E152.

214. Pugliese G, Pricci F, Pugliese F, et al. Mechanisms of glucose-enhanced extracellular matrix accumulation in rat glomerular mesangial cells. *Diabetes*. 1994;43(3):478-490.

215. Glogowski EA, Tsiani E, Zhou X, et al. High glucose alters the response of mesangial cell protein kinase C isoforms to endothelin-1. *Kidney Int*. 1999;55(2):486-499.

216. Hempel A, Maasch C, Heintze U, et al. High glucose concentrations increase endothelial cell permeability via activation of protein kinase C alpha. *Circ Res*. 1997;81(3):363-371.

217. Dang L, Seale JP, Qu X. High glucose-induced human umbilical vein endothelial cell hyperpermeability is dependent on protein kinase C activation and independent of the Ca2+-nitric oxide signalling pathway. *Clin Exp Pharmacol Physiol*. 2005;32(9):771-776.

218. Williams B, Gallacher B, Patel H, Orme C. Glucose-induced protein kinase C activation regulates vascular permeability factor mRNA expression and peptide production by human vascular smooth muscle cells in vitro. *Diabetes*. 1997;46(9):1497-1503.

219. Studer RK, Craven PA, DeRubertis FR. Role for protein kinase C in the mediation of increased fibronectin accumulation by mesangial cells grown in high-glucose medium. *Diabetes*. 1993;42(1):118-126.

220. Feener EP, Xia P, Inoguchi T, et al. Role of protein kinase C in glucose- and angiotensin II-induced plasminogen activator inhibitor expression. *Contrib Nephrol*. 1996;118:180-187.

221. Pieper GM, Riaz ul H. Activation of nuclear factor-kappaB in cultured endothelial cells by increased glucose concentration: prevention by calphostin C. *J Cardiovasc Pharmacol*. 1997;30(4):528-532.

222. Yerneni KK, Bai W, Khan BV, et al. Hyperglycemia-induced activation of nuclear transcription factor kappaB in vascular smooth muscle cells. *Diabetes*. 1999;48(4):855-864.

223. Way KJ, Isshiki K, Suzuma K, et al. Expression of connective tissue growth factor is increased in injured myocardium associated with protein kinase C beta2 activation and diabetes. *Diabetes*. 2002; 51(9):2709-2718.

224. Igarashi M, Wakasaki H, Takahara N, et al. Glucose or diabetes activates p38 mitogen-activated protein kinase via different pathways. *J Clin Invest*. 1999;103(2):185-195.

225. Fontayne A, Dang PM, Gougerot-Pocidalo MA, El-Benna J. Phosphorylation of p47phox sites by PKC alpha, beta II, delta, and zeta: effect on binding to p22phox and on NADPH oxidase activation. *Biochemistry*. 2002;41(24):7743-7750.

226. Guzik TJ, Mussa S, Gastaldi D, et al. Mechanisms of increased vascular superoxide production in human diabetes mellitus: role of NAD(P)H oxidase and endothelial nitric oxide synthase. *Circulation*. 2002; 105(14):1656-1662.

227. Beckman JA, Goldfine AB, Gordon MB, et al. Inhibition of protein kinase Cbeta prevents impaired endothelium-dependent vasodilation caused by hyperglycemia in humans. *Circ Res*. 2002;90(1):107-111.

228. Li Q, Park K, Li C, et al. Induction of vascular insulin resistance and endothelin-1 expression and acceleration of atherosclerosis by the overexpression of protein kinase C-beta isoform in the endothelium. *Circ Res*. 2013;113(4):418-427.

229. Daniels MC, Kansal P, Smith TM, et al. Glucose regulation of transforming growth factor-alpha expression is mediated by products of the hexosamine biosynthesis pathway. *Mol Endocrinol (Baltimore, MD)*. 1993;7(8):1041-1048.

230. Kolm-Litty V, Sauer U, Nerlich A, et al. High glucose-induced transforming growth factor beta1 production is mediated by the hexosamine pathway in porcine glomerular mesangial cells. *J Clin Invest*. 1998;101(1):160-169.

231. McClain DA, Paterson AJ, Roos MD, et al. Glucose and glucosamine regulate growth factor gene expression in vascular smooth muscle cells. *Proc Natl Acad Sci U S A*. 1992;89(17):8150-8154.

232. Sayeski PP, Kudlow JE. Glucose metabolism to glucosamine is necessary for glucose stimulation of transforming growth factor-alpha gene transcription. *J Biol Chem*. 1996;271(25):15237-15243.

233. Bond MR, Hanover JA. A little sugar goes a long way: the cell biology of O-GlcNAc. *J Cell Biol*. 2015;208(7):869-880.

234. Hardiville S, Hart GW. Nutrient regulation of signaling, transcription, and cell physiology by O-GlcNAcylation. *Cell Metab*. 2014;20(2): 208-213.

235. Chen YQ, Su M, Walia RR, et al. Sp1 sites mediate activation of the plasminogen activator inhibitor-1 promoter by glucose in vascular smooth muscle cells. *J Biol Chem*. 1998;273(14):8225-8231.

236. Goldberg HJ, Scholey J, Fantus IG. Glucosamine activates the plasminogen activator inhibitor 1 gene promoter through Sp1 DNA binding sites in glomerular mesangial cells. *Diabetes*. 2000;49(5): 863-871.

237. Goldberg HJ, Whiteside CI, Fantus IG. The hexosamine pathway regulates the plasminogen activator inhibitor-1 gene promoter and Sp1 transcriptional activation through protein kinase C-beta I and -delta. *J Biol Chem*. 2002;277(37):33833-33841.

238. Hart GW. Dynamic O-linked glycosylation of nuclear and cytoskeletal proteins. *Ann Rev Biochem*. 1997;66:315-335.

239. Du XL, Edelstein D, Dimmeler S, et al. Hyperglycemia inhibits endothelial nitric oxide synthase activity by posttranslational modification at the Akt site. *J Clin Invest*. 2001;108(9):1341-1348.

240. Tan EP, Villar MT, E L, et al. Altering O-linked beta-N-acetylglucosamine cycling disrupts mitochondrial function. *J Biol Chem*. 2014; 289(21):14719-14730.

241. Marsh SA, Collins HE, Chatham JC. Protein O-GlcNAcylation and cardiovascular (patho)physiology. *J Biol Chem*. 2014;289(50):34449-34456.

242. Erickson JR, Pereira L, Wang L, et al. Diabetic hyperglycaemia activates CaMKII and arrhythmias by O-linked glycosylation. *Nature*. 2013;502(7471):372-376.

243. Zetterqvist AV, Berglund LM, Blanco F, et al. Inhibition of nuclear factor of activated T-cells (NFAT) suppresses accelerated atherosclerosis in diabetic mice. *PLoS ONE*. 2014;8(6):e65020.

244. Federici M, Menghini R, Mauriello A, et al. Insulin-dependent activation of endothelial nitric oxide synthase is impaired by O-linked glycosylation modification of signaling proteins in human coronary endothelial cells. *Circulation*. 2002;106(4):466-472.

245. Clark RJ, McDonough PM, Swanson E, et al. Diabetes and the accompanying hyperglycemia impairs cardiomyocyte calcium cycling through increased nuclear O-GlcNAcylation. *J Biol Chem*. 2003; 278(45):44230-44427.

246. Brownlee M. Advanced protein glycosylation in diabetes and aging. *Ann Rev Med*. 1995;46:223-234.

247. Lee AY, Chung SK, Chung SS. Demonstration that polyol accumulation is responsible for diabetic cataract by the use of transgenic mice expressing the aldose reductase gene in the lens. *Proc Natl Acad Sci U S A*. 1995;92(7):2780-2784.

248. Sima AA, Prashar A, Zhang WX, et al. Preventive effect of long-term aldose reductase inhibition (ponalrestat) on nerve conduction and sural nerve structure in the spontaneously diabetic Bio-Breeding rat. *J Clin Invest*. 1990;85(5):1410-1420.

249. Nishikawa T, Edelstein D, Du XL, et al. Normalizing mitochondrial superoxide production blocks three pathways of hyperglycaemic damage. *Nature*. 2000;404(6779):787-790.

250. Brownlee M. Biochemistry and molecular cell biology of diabetic complications. *Nature*. 2001;414:813-820.

251. Wallace DC. Diseases of the mitochondrial DNA. *Ann Rev Biochem*. 1992;61:1175-1212.

252. Trumpower BL. The protonmotive Q cycle. Energy transduction by coupling of proton translocation to electron transfer by the cytochrome bc1 complex. *J Biol Chem*. 1990;265(20):11409-11412.

253. Korshunov SS, Skulachev VP, Starkov AA. High protonic potential actuates a mechanism of production of reactive oxygen species in mitochondria. *FEBS Lett*. 1997;416(1):15-18.

254. Yu T, Robotham JL, Yoon Y. Increased production of reactive oxygen species in hyperglycemic conditions requires dynamic change of mitochondrial morphology. *Proc Natl Acad Sci U S A*. 2006;103(8): 2653-2658.

255. Wang W, Wang Y, Long J, et al. Mitochondrial fission triggered by hyperglycemia is mediated by ROCK1 activation in podocytes and endothelial cells. *Cell Metab*. 2012;15(2):186-200.

256. Aghajanian A, Wittchen ES, Campbell SL, Burridge K. Direct activation of RhoA by reactive oxygen species requires a redox-sensitive motif. *PLoS ONE*. 2009;4(11):e8045.

257. Yaffe MP. The machinery of mitochondrial inheritance and behavior. *Science*. 1999;283(5407):1493-1497.

258. Bossy-Wetzel E, Barsoum MJ, Godzik A, et al. Mitochondrial fission in apoptosis, neurodegeneration and aging. *Curr Opin Cell Biol*. 2003; 15(6):706-716.

259. Casteilla L, Blondel O, Klaus S, et al. Stable expression of functional mitochondrial uncoupling protein in Chinese hamster ovary cells. *Proc Natl Acad Sci U S A*. 1990;87(13):5124-5128.

260. Haskins K, Bradley B, Powers K, et al. Oxidative stress in type 1 diabetes. *Ann N Y Acad Sci*. 2003;1005:43-54.

261. Pugazhenthi S, Nesterova A, Jambal P, et al. Oxidative stress-mediated down-regulation of bcl-2 promoter in hippocampal neurons. *J Neurochem*. 2003;84(5):982-996.

262. Finkel T. Signal transduction by reactive oxygen species. *J Cell Biol*. 2011;194(1):7-15.

263. Morimoto H, Iwata K, Ogonuki N, et al. ROS are required for mouse spermatogonial stem cell self-renewal. *Cell Stem Cell*. 2013;12(6): 774-786.

264. Liu J, Finkel T. Stem cells and oxidants: too little of a bad thing. *Cell Metab*. 2013;18(1):1-2.

265. Du X, Matsumura T, Edelstein D, et al. Inhibition of GAPDH activity by poly(ADP-ribose) polymerase activates three major pathways of hyperglycemic damage in endothelial cells. *J Clin Invest.* 2003;112(7):1049-1057.

266. Sawa A, Khan AA, Hester LD, Snyder SH. Glyceraldehyde-3-phosphate dehydrogenase: nuclear translocation participates in neuronal and nonneuronal cell death. *Proc Natl Acad Sci U S A.* 1997;94(21):11669-11674.

267. Schmitz HD. Reversible nuclear translocation of glyceraldehyde-3-phosphate dehydrogenase upon serum depletion. *Eur J Cell Biol.* 2001;80(6):419-427.

268. Gordin D, Forsblom C, Panduru NM, et al. Osteopontin is a strong predictor of incipient diabetic nephropathy, cardiovascular disease, and all-cause mortality in patients with type 1 diabetes. *Diabetes Care.* 2014;37(9):2593-2600.

269. Nilsson-Berglund LM, Zetterqvist AV, Nilsson-Ohman J, et al. Nuclear factor of activated T cells regulates osteopontin expression in arterial smooth muscle in response to diabetes-induced hyperglycemia. *Arterioscler Thromb Vasc Biol.* 2010;30(2):218-224.

270. Nilsson J, Nilsson LM, Chen YW, et al. High glucose activates nuclear factor of activated T cells in native vascular smooth muscle. *Arterioscler Thromb Vasc Biol.* 2006;26(4):794-800.

271. Kahles F, Findeisen HM, Bruemmer D. Osteopontin: a novel regulator at the cross roads of inflammation, obesity and diabetes. *Mol Metab.* 2014;3(4):384-393.

272. Brownlee M. The pathobiology of diabetic complications: a unifying mechanism. *Diabetes.* 2005;54(6):1615-1625.

273. Zou MH, Shi C, Cohen RA. High glucose via peroxynitrite causes tyrosine nitration and inactivation of prostacyclin synthase that is associated with thromboxane/prostaglandin H(2) receptor-mediated apoptosis and adhesion molecule expression in cultured human aortic endothelial cells. *Diabetes.* 2002;51(1):198-203.

274. Craven PA, Melhem MF, Phillips SL, DeRubertis FR. Overexpression of Cu2+/Zn2+ superoxide dismutase protects against early diabetic glomerular injury in transgenic mice. *Diabetes.* 2001;50(9):2114-2125.

275. DeRubertis FR, Craven PA, Melhem MF, Salah EM. Attenuation of renal injury in db/db mice overexpressing superoxide dismutase: evidence for reduced superoxide-nitric oxide interaction. *Diabetes.* 2004;53(3):762-768.

276. Shen X, Zheng S, Metreveli NS, Epstein PN. Protection of cardiac mitochondria by overexpression of MnSOD reduces diabetic cardiomyopathy. *Diabetes.* 2006;55(3):798-805.

277. Ye G, Metreveli NS, Donthi RV, et al. Catalase protects cardiomyocyte function in models of type 1 and type 2 diabetes. *Diabetes.* 2004;53(5):1336-1343.

278. Vincent AM, Russell JW, Sullivan KA, et al. SOD2 protects neurons from injury in cell culture and animal models of diabetic neuropathy. *Exp Neurol.* 2007;208(2):216-227.

279. Kowluru RA, Kowluru V, Xiong Y, Ho YS. Overexpression of mitochondrial superoxide dismutase in mice protects the retina from diabetes-induced oxidative stress. *Free Radic Biol Med.* 2006;41(8):1191-1196.

280. Wang Y, Wang GZ, Rabinovitch PS, Tabas I. Macrophage mitochondrial oxidative stress promotes atherosclerosis and nuclear factor-kappaB-mediated inflammation in macrophages. *Circ Res.* 2014;114(3):421-433.

281. Huang C, Kim Y, Caramori ML, et al. Diabetic nephropathy is associated with gene expression levels of oxidative phosphorylation and related pathways. *Diabetes.* 2006;55(6):1826-1831.

282. Jha JC, Gray SP, Barit D, et al. Genetic targeting or pharmacologic inhibition of NADPH oxidase nox4 provides renoprotection in long-term diabetic nephropathy. *J Am Soc Nephrol.* 2014;25(6):1237-1254.

283. Li WG, Miller FJ Jr, Zhang HJ, et al. H(2)O(2)-induced O(2) production by a non-phagocytic NAD(P)H oxidase causes oxidant injury. *J Biol Chem.* 2001;276(31):29251-29256.

284. Rathore R, Zheng YM, Niu CF, et al. Hypoxia activates NADPH oxidase to increase [ROS]i and [Ca2+]i through the mitochondrial ROS-PKCepsilon signaling axis in pulmonary artery smooth muscle cells. *Free Radic Biol Med.* 2008;45(9):1223-1231.

285. Huynh K, Kiriazis H, Du XJ, et al. Targeting the upregulation of reactive oxygen species subsequent to hyperglycemia prevents type 1 diabetic cardiomyopathy in mice. *Free Radic Biol Med.* 2013;60:307-317.

286. Cai S, Khoo J, Mussa S, et al. Endothelial nitric oxide synthase dysfunction in diabetic mice: importance of tetrahydrobiopterin in eNOS dimerisation. *Diabetologia.* 2005;48(9):1933-1940.

287. Dugan LL, You YH, Ali SS, et al. AMPK dysregulation promotes diabetes-related reduction of superoxide and mitochondrial function. *J Clin Invest.* 2013;123(11):4888-4899.

288. Wang S, Song P, Zou MH. AMP-activated protein kinase, stress responses and cardiovascular diseases. *Clin Sci.* 2012;122(12):555-573.

289. Nishikawa T, Brownlee M, Araki E. Mitochondrial reactive oxygen species in the pathogenesis of early diabetic nephropathy. *J Diabetes Invest.* 2015;6(2):137-139.

290. Liu R, Zhong Y, Li X, et al. Role of transcription factor acetylation in diabetic kidney disease. *Diabetes.* 2014;63(7):2440-2453.

291. Choi J, Chandrasekaran K, Inoue T, et al. PGC-1alpha regulation of mitochondrial degeneration in experimental diabetic neuropathy. *Neurobiol Dis.* 2014;64:118-130.

292. Boudina S, Abel ED. Diabetic cardiomyopathy, causes and effects. *Rev Endocr Metab Dis.* 2010;11(1):31-39.

293. van de Weijer T, Schrauwen-Hinderling VB, Schrauwen P. Lipotoxicity in type 2 diabetic cardiomyopathy. *Cardiovasc Res.* 2011;92(1):10-18.

294. Summers SA. Ceramides in insulin resistance and lipotoxicity. *Prog Lipid Res.* 2006;45(1):42-72.

295. Rosca MG, Vazquez EJ, Chen Q, et al. Oxidation of fatty acids is the source of increased mitochondrial reactive oxygen species production in kidney cortical tubules in early diabetes. *Diabetes.* 2012;61(8):2074-2083.

296. Kowluru RA. Effect of reinstitution of good glycemic control on retinal oxidative stress and nitrative stress in diabetic rats. *Diabetes.* 2003;52(3):818-823.

297. Vaissière T, Sawan C, Herceg Z. Epigenetic interplay between histone modifications and DNA methylation in gene silencing. *Mutat Res.* 2008;659(1-2):40-48.

298. Probst AV, Dunleavy E, Almouzni G. Epigenetic inheritance during the cell cycle. *Nat Rev Mol Cell Biol.* 2009;10(3):192-206.

299. Göndör A, Ohlsson R. Replication timing and epigenetic reprogramming of gene expression: a two-way relationship? *Nat Rev Genet.* 2009;10(4):269-276.

300. El-Osta A, Brasacchio D, Yao D, et al. Transient high glucose causes persistent epigenetic changes and altered gene expression during subsequent normoglycemia. *J Exp Med.* 2008;205(10):2409-2417.

301. Brasacchio D, Okabe J, Tikellis C, et al. Hyperglycemia induces a dynamic cooperativity of histone methylase and demethylase enzymes associated with gene-activating epigenetic marks that coexist on the lysine tail. *Diabetes.* 2009;58(5):1229-1236.

302. Miao F, Smith DD, Zhang L, et al. Lymphocytes from patients with type 1 diabetes display a distinct profile of chromatin histone H3 lysine 9 dimethylation: an epigenetic study in diabetes. *Diabetes.* 2008;57(12):3189-3198.

303. Villeneuve LM, Reddy MA, Lanting LL, et al. Epigenetic histone H3 lysine 9 methylation in metabolic memory and inflammatory phenotype of vascular smooth muscle cells in diabetes. *Proc Natl Acad Sci U S A.* 2008;105(26):9047-9052.

304. Reddy MA, Villeneuve LM, Wang M, et al. Role of the lysine-specific demethylase 1 in the proinflammatory phenotype of vascular smooth muscle cells of diabetic mice. *Circ Res.* 2008;103(6):615-623.

304a. Anand P, et al. BET bromodomains mediate transcriptional pause release in heart failure. *Cell.* 2013;154:569-582.

304b. Brown JD, et al. NF-kB directs dynamic super enhancer formation in inflammation and atherosclerosis. *Mol Cell.* 2014;56:219-231.

305. Reddy MA, Tak Park J, Natarajan R. Epigenetic modifications in the pathogenesis of diabetic nephropathy. *Semin Nephrol.* 2013;33(4):341-353.

306. Miao F, Chen Z, Genuth S, et al. Evaluating the role of epigenetic histone modifications in the metabolic memory of type 1 diabetes. *Diabetes.* 2014;63(5):1748-1762.

307. Olsen AS, Sarras MP Jr, Leontovich A, Intine RV. Heritable transmission of diabetic metabolic memory in zebrafish correlates with DNA hypomethylation and aberrant gene expression. *Diabetes.* 2012;61(2):485-491.

308. Dhliwayo N, Sarras MP Jr, Luczkowski E, et al. Parp inhibition prevents ten-eleven translocase enzyme activation and hyperglycemia-induced DNA demethylation. *Diabetes.* 2014;63(9):3069-3076.

309. Giacco F, Du X, Carratu A, et al. GLP-1 cleavage product reverses persistent ROS generation after transient hyperglycemia by disrupting an ROS-generating feedback loop. *Diabetes.* 2015;64:3273-3284.

310. Ferris FL. How effective are treatments for diabetic retinopathy? *JAMA.* 1993;269:1290-1291.

311. PKC-DRS Study Group. The effect of ruboxistaurin on visual loss in patients with moderately severe to very severe nonproliferative diabetic retinopathy: initial results of the PKC-DRS Multicenter Randomized Clinical Trial. *Diabetes.* 2005;54:2188-2197.

312. Strøm C, Sander B, Klemp K, et al. Effect of ruboxistaurin on blood-retinal barrier permeability in relation to severity of leakage in diabetic macular edema. *Invest Ophthalmol Vis Sci.* 2005;46:3855-3858.

313. Aiello LP, Clermont A, Arora V, et al. Inhibition of PKC-b by oral administration of ruboxistaurin (LY333531) mesylate is well-tolerated and ameliorates diabetes-induced retinal hemodynamic abnormalities in patients. *Invest Ophthalmol Vis Sci.* 2005;47:86-92.

314. PKC-DMES Study Group. Effect of ruboxistaurin, a PKCb isoform-selective inhibitor, in patients with diabetic macular edema: 30-month results of the randomized PKC-DMES clinical trial. *Arch Ophthalmol.* 2007;125:318-324.

315. PKC-DRS2 Study Group. Effect of ruboxistaurin on visual loss in patients with diabetic retinopathy. *Ophthalmology.* 2006;113:2221-2230.

316. Tuttle KR, Bakris GL, Toto RD, et al. The effect of ruboxistaurin on nephropathy in type 2 diabetes. *Diabetes Care.* 2005;28:2686-2690.

317. Cunningham ET, Adamis AP, Altaweel M, et al. and the Macugen Diabetic Retinopathy Study Group. A phase II randomized double-masked trial of pegaptanib, an anti-vascular endothelial growth

factor aptamer, for diabetic macular edema. *Ophthalmology*. 2005;46:3855-3858.

318. Chun DW, Heier JS, Topping TM, et al. A pilot study of multiple intravitreal injections of ranibizumab in patients with center-involving clinically significant diabetic macular edema. *Ophthalmology*. 2006;113:1706-1712.

319. Jager RD, Aiello LP, Patel SC, Cunningham ET. Risks of intravitreal injection: a comprehensive review. *Retina*. 2004;24:676-698.

320. Guariguata L, Whiting DR, Hambleton I, et al. Global estimates of diabetes prevalence for 2013 and projections for 2035. *Diabetes Res Clin Pract*. 2014;103(2):137-149.

321. Beckles GL, Chou CF. Diabetes: United States, 2006 and 2010. *MMWR Surveill Summ*. 2013;62(Suppl 3):99-104.

322. Kempen JH, O'Colmain BJ, Leske MC, et al. The prevalence of diabetic retinopathy among adults in the United States. *Arch Ophthalmol*. 2004;122(4):552-563.

323. Harris MI, Hadden WC, Knowler WC, Bennett PH. Prevalence of diabetes and impaired glucose tolerance and plasma glucose levels in US population aged 20-74 years. *Diabetes*. 1998;36:523-534.

324. Klein R, Klein BE, Moss SE, et al. The Wisconsin Epidemiologic Study of Diabetic Retinopathy: II. Prevalence and risk of diabetic retinopathy when age at diagnosis is less than 30 years. *Arch Ophthalmol*. 1984;102:520-536.

325. Klein R, Klein BE, Moss SE, Cruickshanks KJ. The Wisconsin Epidemiologic Study of Diabetic Retinopathy: XV. The long-term incidence of macular edema. *Ophthalmology*. 1995;102:7-16.

326. Javitt JC, Canner JK, Sommer A. Cost effectiveness of current approaches to the control of retinopathy in type 1 diabetics. *Ophthalmology*. 1989;96:255-264.

327. Javitt JC, Aiello LP, Bassi LJ, et al. Detecting and treating retinopathy in patients with type I diabetes mellitus: savings associated with improved implementation of current guidelines. American Academy of Ophthalmology. *Ophthalmology*. 1991;98:1565-1573.

328. Javitt JC, Aiello LP, Chiang Y, et al. Preventive eye care in people with diabetes is cost-saving to the federal government: implications for health-care reform. *Diabetes Care*. 1994;17:909-917.

329. Javitt JC, Aiello LP. Cost-effectiveness of detecting and treating diabetic retinopathy (see comments). *Ann Intern Med*. 1996;124(1 Pt 2):164-169.

330. Centers for Disease Control and Prevention. 2014 National Diabetes Statistics Report. National Estimate on Diabetes. Available at <http://www.cdc.gov/diabetes/pubs/statsreport14/national-diabetes-report-web.pdf>.

331. Kahn HA, Hiller R. Blindness caused by diabetic retinopathy. *Am J Ophthalmol*. 1974;78:58-67.

332. Palmberg PF. Diabetic retinopathy. *Diabetes*. 1977;26:703-709.

333. Bressler NM, Varma R, Doan QV, et al. Underuse of the health care system by persons with diabetes mellitus and diabetic macular edema in the United States. *JAMA Ophthalmol*. 2014;132(2):168-173.

334. Diabetes Control and Complications Trial Research Group. Design and methodologic considerations for the feasibility phase. *Diabetes*. 1986;35:530-545.

335. Diabetes Control and Complications Trial/Epidemiology of Diabetes Interventions and Complications Research Group. Retinopathy and nephropathy in patients with type 1 diabetes four years after a trial of intensive therapy. *N Engl J Med*. 2000;342:381-389.

336. Diabetes Control and Complications Trial Research Group. The relationship of glycemic exposure (HbA1c) to the risk of development and progression of retinopathy in the Diabetes Control and Complications trial. *Diabetes*. 1995;44:968-983.

337. Aiello LP. Diabetic retinopathy and other ocular findings in the diabetes control and complications trial/epidemiology of diabetes interventions and complications study. *Diabetes Care*. 2014;37:17-23.

338. Diabetes Control and Complications Trial Research Group. Lifetime benefits and costs of intensive therapy as practiced in the Diabetes Control and Complications Trial (see comments). *JAMA*. 1996;276(17):1409-1415. Published erratum appears in *JAMA*. 1997;278:25.

339. Diabetes Control and Complications Trial Research Group. Resource utilization and costs of care in the diabetes control and complications trial. *Diabetes Care*. 1995;18:1468-1478.

340. Cogan DG, Toussaint D, Kuwabara T. Retinal vascular patterns: IV. Diabetic retinopathy. *Arch Ophthalmol*. 1961;66:366-378.

341. Konno S, Feke GT, Yoshida A, et al. Retinal blood flow changes in type I diabetes: a long-term follow-up study. *Invest Ophthalmol Vis Sci*. 1996;37:1140-1148.

342. Grunwald JE, Riva CE, Sinclair SH, et al. Laser Doppler velocimetry study of retinal circulation in diabetes mellitus. *Arch Ophthalmol*. 1986;104:991-996.

343. Bursell SE, Clermont AC, Kinsley BT, et al. Retinal blood flow changes in patients with insulin-dependent diabetes mellitus and no diabetic retinopathy. *Am J Physiol*. 1996;270(1 Pt 2):R61-R70.

344. Sosula L, Beaumont P, Hollows FC, Jonson KM. Dilatation and endothelial proliferation of retinal capillaries in streptozotocin-diabetic rats: quantitative electron microscopy. *Invest Ophthalmol*. 1972;11:926-935.

345. Speiser P, Gittelsohn AM, Patz A. Studies on diabetic retinopathy: III. Influence of diabetes on intramural pericytes. *Arch Ophthalmol*. 1968;80:332-337.

346. Barouch FC, Miyamoto K, Allport JR, et al. Integrin-mediated neutrophil adhesion and retinal leukostasis in diabetes. *Invest Ophthalmol Vis Sci*. 2000;41:1153-1158.

347. Miyamoto K, Khosrof S, Bursell SE, et al. Vascular endothelial growth factor (VEGF)-induced retinal vascular permeability is mediated by intercellular adhesion molecule-1 (ICAM-1). *Am J Pathol*. 2000;156:1733-1739.

348. Miyamoto K, Khosrof S, Bursell SE, et al. Prevention of leukostasis and vascular leakage in streptozotocin-induced diabetic retinopathy via intercellular adhesion molecule-1 inhibition. *Proc Natl Acad Sci U S A*. 1999;96:10836-10841.

349. Stitt AW, Gardiner TA, Archer DB. Histological and ultrastructural investigation of retinal microaneurysm development in diabetic patients. *Br J Ophthalmol*. 1995;79:362-367.

350. Cunha-Vaz J, Faria DA Jr, Campos AJ. Early breakdown of the blood-retinal barrier in diabetes. *Br J Ophthalmol*. 1975;59:649-656.

351. Early Treatment Diabetic Retinopathy Study Research Group. Early photocoagulation for diabetic retinopathy. ETDRS Report No. 9. *Ophthalmology*. 1991;98(5 Suppl):766-785.

352. Meyer-Schwickerath R, Pfeiffer A, Blum WF, et al. Vitreous levels of the insulin-like growth factors I and II, and the insulin-like growth factor-binding proteins 2 and 3, increase in neovascular eye disease: studies in nondiabetic and diabetic subjects. *J Clin Invest*. 1993;92:2620-2625.

353. Nishimura M, Ikeda T, Ushiyama M, et al. Increased vitreous concentrations of human hepatocyte growth factor in proliferative diabetic retinopathy. *J Clin Endocrinol Metab*. 1999;84:659-662.

354. Aiello LP, Avery RL, Arrigg PG, et al. Vascular endothelial growth factor in ocular fluid of patients with diabetic retinopathy and other retinal disorders (see comments). *N Engl J Med*. 1994;331:1480-1487.

355. Adamis AP, Miller JW, Bernal MT, et al. Increased vascular endothelial growth factor levels in the vitreous of eyes with proliferative diabetic retinopathy. *Am J Ophthalmol*. 1994;118:445-450.

356. Aiello LP, Hata Y. Molecular mechanisms of growth factor action in diabetic retinopathy. *Curr Opin Endocrinol Diabetes*. 1999;6:146-156.

357. Aiello LP, Bursell SE, Clermont A, et al. Vascular endothelial growth factor-induced retinal permeability is mediated by protein kinase C in vivo and suppressed by an orally effective beta isoform-selective inhibitor. *Diabetes*. 1997;46:1473-1480.

358. Miller JW, Adamis AP, Aiello LP. Vascular endothelial growth factor in ocular neovascularization and proliferative diabetic retinopathy. *Diabetes Metab Rev*. 1997;13:37-50.

359. Okamoto N, Tobe T, Hackett SF, et al. Transgenic mice with increased expression of vascular endothelial growth factor in the retina: a new model of intraretinal and subretinal neovascularization (see comments). *Am J Pathol*. 1997;151:281-291.

360. Ozaki H, Hayashi H, Vinores SA, et al. Intravitreal sustained release of VEGF causes retinal neovascularization in rabbits and breakdown of the blood-retinal barrier in rabbits and primates. *Exp Eye Res*. 1997;64:505-517.

361. Aiello LP, Pierce EA, Foley ED, et al. Suppression of retinal neovascularization in vivo by inhibition of vascular endothelial growth factor (VEGF) using soluble VEGF-receptor chimeric proteins. *Proc Natl Acad Sci U S A*. 1995;92:10457-10461.

362. Robinson GS, Pierce EA, Rook SL, et al. Oligodeoxynucleotides inhibit retinal neovascularization in a murine model of proliferative retinopathy. *Proc Natl Acad Sci U S A*. 1996;93:4851-4856.

363. Adamis AP, Shima DT, Tolentino MJ, et al. Inhibition of vascular endothelial growth factor prevents retinal ischemia-associated iris neovascularization in a nonhuman primate. *Arch Ophthalmol*. 1996;114(1):66-71.

364. Danis RP, Bingaman DP, Jirousek M, Yang Y. Inhibition of intraocular neovascularization caused by retinal ischemia in pigs by PKC-β inhibition with LY333531. *Invest Ophthalmol Vis Sci*. 1998;39:171-179.

365. Ozaki H, Seo MS, Ozaki K, et al. Blockade of vascular endothelial cell growth factor receptor signaling is sufficient to completely prevent retinal neovascularization. *Am J Pathol*. 2000;156:697-707.

366. Duh EJ, Yang HS, Suzuma I, et al. Pigment epithelium–derived factor (PEDF) suppresses ischemia-induced retinal neovascularization and VEGF-induced migration and growth. *Invest Ophthalmol Vis Sci*. 2002;43(3):821-829.

367. Gao BB, Clermont A, Rook S, et al. Extracellular carbonic anhydrase mediates hemorrhagic retinal an cerebral vascular permeability through prekallikrein activation. *Nat Med*. 2007;13:181-188.

368. Phipps JA, Clermont AC, Sinha S, et al. Plasma kallikrein mediates angiotensin II type 1 receptor-stimulated retinal vascular permeability. *Hypertension*. 2009;53:175-181.

369. Tripathi RC, Li J, Tripathi BJ, et al. Increased level of vascular endothelial growth factor in aqueous humor of patients with neovascular glaucoma. *Ophthalmology*. 1998;105:232-237.

370. Tolentino MJ, Miller JW, Gragoudas ES, et al. Vascular endothelial growth factor is sufficient to produce iris neovascularization and

neovascular glaucoma in a nonhuman primate. *Arch Ophthalmol.* 1996;114:964-970.

371. Klein R, Klein BE, Moss SE, et al. The Wisconsin Epidemiologic Study of Diabetic Retinopathy: III. Prevalence and risk of diabetic retinopathy when age at diagnosis is 30 or more years. *Arch Ophthalmol.* 1984;102:527-532.

372. Kohner EM, Aldington SJ, Stratton IM, et al. United Kingdom Prospective Diabetes Study, 30: diabetic retinopathy at diagnosis of non–insulin-dependent diabetes mellitus and associated risk factors. *Arch Ophthalmol.* 1998;116:297-303.

373. Diabetes Control and Complications Trial Research Group. Progression of retinopathy with intensive versus conventional treatment in the Diabetes Control and Complications Trial. *Ophthalmology.* 1995;102:647-661.

374. Kroc Collaborative Study Group. Blood glucose control and the evolution of diabetic retinopathy and albuminuria: a preliminary multicenter trial. *N Engl J Med.* 1984;311:365-372.

375. Chase HP, Jackson WE, Hoops SL, et al. Glucose control and the renal and retinal complications of insulin-dependent diabetes. *JAMA.* 1989;261:1155-1160.

376. Krolewski AS, Canessa M, Warram JH, et al. Predisposition to hypertension and susceptibility to renal disease in insulin-dependent diabetes mellitus. *N Engl J Med.* 1988;318:140-145.

377. Chew EY, Klein ML, Ferris FL III, et al. Association of elevated serum lipid levels with retinal hard exudate in diabetic retinopathy. Early Treatment Diabetic Retinopathy Study (ETDRS) Report 22. *Arch Ophthalmol.* 1996;114:1079-1084.

378. Aiello LP, Gardner TW, King GL, et al. Diabetic retinopathy: technical review. *Diabetes Care.* 1998;21:143-156.

379. Diabetic Retinopathy Study Research Group. Four risk factors for severe visual loss in diabetic retinopathy. The Third Report from the Diabetic Retinopathy Study. *Arch Ophthalmol.* 1979;97:654-655.

380. Early Treatment Diabetic Retinopathy Study Research Group. Treatment techniques and clinical guidelines for photocoagulation of diabetic macular edema. Early Treatment Diabetic Retinopathy Study Report No. 2. *Ophthalmology.* 1987;94:761-774.

381. Early Treatment Diabetic Retinopathy Study Research Group. Photocoagulation for diabetic macular edema: Early Treatment Diabetic Retinopathy Study Report No. 4. *Int Ophthalmol Clin.* 1987;27:265-272.

382. Wilkinson CP, Ferris FL III, Klein RE, et al. Proposed International Clinical Diabetic Retinopathy and Diabetic Macular Edema Disease Severity Scales. *Ophthalmology.* 2003;110(9):1677-1682.

383. Chew EY. A simplified diabetic retinopathy scale. *Ophthalmology.* 2003;110(9):1675-1676.

384. Waite JH, Beetham WP. Visual mechanisms in diabetes mellitus: comparative study of 2002 diabetics and 437 nondiabetics for control. *N Engl J Med.* 1935;212:367-379.

385. Zorrilla E, Kozak GP. Ophthalmoplegia in diabetes mellitus. *Ann Intern Med.* 1967;67:968-976.

386. Rush JA, Younge BR. Paralysis of cranial nerves III, IV, and VI: cause and prognosis in 1000 cases. *Arch Ophthalmol.* 1981;99:76-79.

387. Khodadoust AA, Silverstein AM, Kenyon DR, Dowling JE. Adhesion of regenerating corneal epithelium: the role of basement membrane. *Am J Ophthalmol.* 1968;65:339-348.

388. Gartner S, Henkind P. Neovascularization of the iris (rubeosis iridis). *Surv Ophthalmol.* 1978;22:291-312.

389. Brown GC, Magargal LE, Schachat A, Shah H. Neovascular glaucoma: etiologic considerations. *Ophthalmology.* 1984;91:315-320.

390. Schwartz JN, Donnelly EH, Klintworth GK. Ocular and orbital phycomycosis. *Surv Ophthalmol.* 1977;22:3-28.

391. Blitzer A, Lawson W, Meyers BR, Biller HF. Patient survival factors in paranasal sinus mucormycosis. *Laryngoscope.* 1980;90:635-648.

392. Wand M, Dueker DK, Aiello LM, Grant WM. Effects of panretinal photocoagulation on rubeosis iridis, angle neovascularization, and neovascular glaucoma. *Am J Ophthalmol.* 1978;86:332-339.

393. Aiello LM, Wand M, Liang G. Neovascular glaucoma and vitreous hemorrhage following cataract surgery in patients with diabetes mellitus. *Ophthalmology.* 1983;90:814-820.

394. Simmons RJ, Dueker DK, Kimbrough RL, Aiello LM. Goniophotocoagulation for neovascular glaucoma. *Trans Am Acad Ophthalmol Otolaryngol.* 1977;83:80-89.

395. Mason JO 3rd, Albert MA Jr, Mays A, Vail R. Regression of neovascularization iris vessels by intravitreal injection of bevacizumab. *Retina.* 2006;26(7):839-841.

396. Hyndiuk RA, Kazarian EL, Schultz RO, Seideman S. Neurotrophic corneal ulcers in diabetes mellitus. *Arch Ophthalmol.* 1977;95:2193-2196.

397. Klein BE, Klein R, Moss SE. Intraocular pressure in diabetic persons. *Ophthalmology.* 1984;91:1356-1360.

398. Pasquale LR, Kang JH, Manson JE, et al. Prospective study of type 2 diabetes mellitus and risk of primary open-angle glaucoma in women. *Ophthalmology.* 2006;113:1081-1086.

399. Marmor MF. Transient accommodative paralysis and hyperopia in diabetes. *Arch Ophthalmol.* 1973;89:419-421.

400. Klein BE, Klein R, Moss SE. Prevalence of cataracts in a population-based study of persons with diabetes mellitus. *Ophthalmology.* 1985;92:1191-1196.

401. Ederer F, Hiller R, Taylor HR. Senile lens changes and diabetes in two population studies. *Am J Ophthalmol.* 1981;91:381-395.

402. Bursell SE, Baker RS, Weiss JN, et al. Clinical photon correlation spectroscopy evaluation of human diabetic lenses. *Exp Eye Res.* 1989;49:241-258.

403. Klein BE, Klein R, Moss SE. Incidence of cataract surgery in the Wisconsin Epidemiologic Study of Diabetic Retinopathy. *Am J Ophthalmol.* 1995;119:295-300.

404. Klein BE, Klein R, Wang Q, Moss SE. Older-onset diabetes and lens opacities: the Beaver Dam Eye Study. *Ophthalmic Epidemiol.* 1995;2:49-55.

405. Pai RP, Mitchell P, Chow VC, et al. Posttransplant cataract: lessons from kidney-pancreas transplantation (see comments). *Transplantation.* 2000;69:1108-1114.

406. Dowler JG, Hykin PG, Hamilton AM. Phacoemulsification versus extracapsular cataract extraction in patients with diabetes. *Ophthalmology.* 2000;107:457-462.

407. Borrillo JL, Mittra RA, Dev S, et al. Retinopathy progression and visual outcomes after phacoemulsification in patients with diabetes mellitus. *Trans Am Ophthalmol Soc.* 1999;97:435-445.

408. Funahashi T, Fink AI. The pathology of the bulbar conjunctiva in diabetes mellitus: I. Microaneurysms. *Am J Ophthalmol.* 1963;55:504-511.

409. Tagawa H, McMeel JW, Trempe CL. Role of the vitreous in diabetic retinopathy: II. Active and inactive vitreous changes. *Ophthalmology.* 1986;93:1188-1192.

410. Fleckner RA, Goldstein JH. Mucormycosis. *Br J Ophthalmol.* 1969;53:542-548.

411. Diabetic Retinopathy Clinical Research Network, Elman MJ, Aiello LP, et al. Randomized trial evaluating ranibizumab plus prompt or deferred laser or triamcinolone plus prompt laser for diabetic macular edema. *Ophthalmology.* 2010;117(6):1064-1077.e35.

412. Diabetic Retinopathy Study Research Group. Photocoagulation treatment of proliferative diabetic retinopathy: clinical application of Diabetic Retinopathy Study (DRS) findings, DRS Report No. 8. *Ophthalmology.* 1981;88:583-600.

413. Diabetic Retinopathy Vitrectomy Study Group. Two-year course of visual acuity in severe proliferative diabetic retinopathy with conventional management. Diabetic Retinopathy Vitrectomy Study (DRVS) Report No. 1. *Ophthalmology.* 1985;92:492-502.

414. Diabetes Control and Complications Trial Research Group. The effect of intensive diabetes treatment on the progression of diabetic retinopathy in insulin-dependent diabetes mellitus: the Diabetes Control and Complications Trial. *Arch Ophthalmol.* 1995;113:36-51.

415. Klein R, Klein BE, Moss SE, et al. The Wisconsin Epidemiologic Study of Diabetic Retinopathy: VI. Retinal photocoagulation. *Ophthalmology.* 1987;94:747-753.

416. Witkin SR, Klein R. Ophthalmologic care for persons with diabetes. *JAMA.* 1984;251:2534-2537.

417. American Academy of Ophthalmology. Comprehensive Adult Medical Eye Evaluation: Preferred Practice Pattern, 2010. PDF available for download at <http://www.aao.org/preferred-practice-pattern/comprehensive-adult-medical-eye-evaluation--october>.

418. American Optometric Association. Comprehensive Adult Eye and Vision Examination: Optometric Clinical Practice Guideline, 2005. PDF available at <http://www.aoa.org/documents/CPG-1.pdf>.

419. Klein R, Klein BE, Neider MW, et al. Diabetic retinopathy as detected using ophthalmoscopy, a nonmydriatic camera, and a standard fundus camera. *Ophthalmology.* 1985;92:485-491.

420. Moss SE, Klein R, Kessler SD, Richie KA. Comparison between ophthalmoscopy and fundus photography in determining severity of diabetic retinopathy. *Ophthalmology.* 1985;92:62-67.

421. Sussman EJ, Tsiaras WG, Soper KA. Diagnosis of diabetic eye disease. *JAMA.* 1982;247:3231-3234.

422. Cavallerano JD, Aiello LP, Cavallerano AA, et al. and the Joslin Vision Network Team. Nonmydriatic digital imaging alternative for annual retinal exam in persons with previously documented no or mild diabetic retinopathy. *Am J Ophthalmol.* 2005;140(4):667.

423. American Diabetes Association. Standards of medical care in diabetes—2014. *Diabetes Care.* 2014;37(Suppl 1):S14-S80.

424. Silva PS, Cavallerano JD, Aiello LM, Aiello LP. Telemedicine and diabetic retinopathy: moving beyond retinal screening. *Arch Ophthalmol.* 2011;129(2):236-242.

425. Klein R, Moss SE, Klein BE. New management concepts for timely diagnosis of diabetic retinopathy treatable by photocoagulation. *Diabetes Care.* 1987;10:633-638.

426. Krolewski AS, Warram JH, Rand LI, et al. Risk of proliferative diabetic retinopathy in juvenile-onset type I diabetes: a 40-year follow-up study. *Diabetes Care.* 1986;9:443-452.

427. Klein BE, Moss SE, Klein R. Is menarche associated with diabetic retinopathy? *Diabetes Care.* 1990;13:1034-1038.

428. Kostraba JN, Klein R, Dorman JS, et al. The epidemiology of diabetes complications study: IV. Correlates of diabetic background and proliferative retinopathy. *Am J Epidemiol.* 1991;133:381-391.

429. Sunness JS. The pregnant woman's eye. *Surv Ophthalmol.* 1988;32: 219-238.
430. Klein BE, Moss SE, Klein R. Effect of pregnancy on progression of diabetic retinopathy. *Diabetes Care.* 1990;13:34-40.
431. White P. Diabetes mellitus in pregnancy. *Clin Perinatol.* 1974;1: 331-347.
432. Best RM, Chakravarthy U. Diabetic retinopathy in pregnancy. *Br J Ophthalmol.* 1997;81:249-251.
433. Early Treatment Diabetic Retinopathy Study Research Group. Grading diabetic retinopathy from stereoscopic color fundus photographs—an extension of the modified Airlie House classification. ETDRS Report Number 10. *Ophthalmology.* 1991;98(5 Suppl):786-806.
434. Diabetic Retinopathy Study Research Group. Indications for photocoagulation treatment of diabetic retinopathy: Diabetic Retinopathy Study Report No. 14. *Int Ophthalmol Clin.* 1987;27:239-253.
435. Diabetic Retinopathy Study Research Group. Photocoagulation treatment of proliferative diabetic retinopathy: the second report of diabetic retinopathy study findings. *Ophthalmology.* 1978;85:82-106.
436. Early Treatment Diabetic Retinopathy Study Research Group. Photocoagulation for diabetic macular edema. Early Treatment Diabetic Retinopathy Study Report No. 1. *Arch Ophthalmol.* 1985;103:1796-1806.
437. Ferris F. Early photocoagulation in patients with either type 1 or type 2 diabetes. *Trans Am Ophthalmol Soc.* 1996;94:505-537.
438. Krzystolik MG, Strauber SF, Aiello LP, et al. Reproducibility of macular thickness and volume using Zeiss optical coherence tomography in patients with diabetic macular edema. *Ophthalmology.* 2007;114: 1520-1525.
439. Browning DJ, Glassman AR, Aiello LP, et al. Relationship between optical coherence tomography-measured central retinal thickness and visual acuity in diabetic macular edema. *Ophthalmology.* 2007; 114:525-536.
440. LaPiana FG, Penner R. Anaphylactoid reaction to intravenously administered fluorescein. *Arch Ophthalmol.* 1968;79:161-162.
441. Butner RW, McPherson AR. Adverse reactions in intravenous fluorescein angiography. *Ann Ophthalmol.* 1983;15:1084-1086.
442. Wittpenn JR, Rapoza P, Sternberg P, et al. Respiratory arrest following retrobulbar anesthesia. *Ophthalmology.* 1986;93:867-870.
443. Avery RL. Regression of retinal and iris neovascularization after intravitreal bevacizumab (Avastin) treatment. *Retina.* 2006;26:352-354.
444. Elman MJ, Bressler NM, Qin H, et al. Expanded 2-year follow-up of ranibizumab plus prompt or deferred laser or triamcinolone plus prompt laser for diabetic macular edema. *Ophthalmology.* 2011;118: 609-614.
445. Elman MJ, Qin H, Aiello LP, et al. Intravitreal ranibizumab for diabetic macular edema with prompt versus deferred laser treatment: three-year randomized trial results. *Ophthalmology.* 2012;119: 2312-2318.
446. Chew E, Strauber S, Beck R, et al. Randomized trial of peribulbar triamcinolone acetonide with and without focal photocoagulation for mild diabetic macular edema: a pilot study. *Ophthalmology.* 2007;114:1190-1196.
447. Diabetic Retinopathy Clinical Research Network. A randomized trial comparing intravitreal triamcinolone acetonide and focal/grid photocoagulation for diabetic macular edema. *Ophthalmology.* 2008;115: 1447-1449.
448. Beck RW, Edwards AR, Aiello LP, et al. Three-year follow-up of a randomized trial comparing focal/grid photocoagulation and intravitreal triamcinolone for diabetic macular edema. *Arch Ophthalmol.* 2009;127:245-251.
449. Klein R, Klein BE, Lee KE, et al. The incidence of hypertension in insulin-dependent diabetes. *Arch Intern Med.* 1996;156:622-627.
450. Thai Multicenter Research Group on Diabetes Mellitus. Vascular complications in non–insulin-dependent diabetics in Thailand. *Diabetes Res Clin Pract.* 1994;25:61-69.
451. Klein R, Klein BE, Moss SE, DeMets DL. Blood pressure and hypertension in diabetes. *Am J Epidemiol.* 1985;122:75-89.
452. Fujimoto WY, Leonetti DL, Kinyoun JL, et al. Prevalence of complications among second-generation Japanese-American men with diabetes, impaired glucose tolerance, or normal glucose tolerance. *Diabetes.* 1987;36:730-739.
453. Klein R, Klein BE, Moss SE, Cruickshanks KJ. The Wisconsin Epidemiologic Study of Diabetic Retinopathy: XVII. The 14-year incidence and progression of diabetic retinopathy and associated risk factors in type 1 diabetes (see comments). *Ophthalmology.* 1998;105: 1801-1815.
454. Zander E, Heinke P, Herfurth S, et al. Relations between diabetic retinopathy and cardiovascular neuropathy: a cross-sectional study in IDDM and NIDDM patients. *Exp Clin Endocrinol Diabetes.* 1997;105: 319-326.
455. Diabetes Drafting Group. Prevalence of small vessel and large vessel disease in diabetic patients from 14 centres: the World Health Organization Multinational Study of Vascular Disease in Diabetes. *Diabetologia.* 1985;28:615-640.
456. Agardh CD, Agardh E, Torffvit O. The association between retinopathy, nephropathy, cardiovascular disease, and long-term metabolic control in type 1 diabetes mellitus: a 5-year follow-up study of 442 adult patients in routine care. *Diabetes Res Clin Pract.* 1997;35: 113-121.
457. Lopes de Faria JM, Jalkh AE, Trempe CL, McMeel JW. Diabetic macular edema: risk factors and concomitants. *Acta Ophthalmol Scand.* 1999; 77:170-175.
458. Marshall G, Garg SK, Jackson WE, et al. Factors influencing the onset and progression of diabetic retinopathy in subjects with insulin-dependent diabetes mellitus. *Ophthalmology.* 1993;100:1133-1139.
459. UK Prospective Diabetes Study (UKPDS) Group. Tight blood pressure control and risk of macrovascular and microvascular complications in type 2 diabetes: UKPDS 38. *BMJ.* 1998;317:703-713.
460. Schrier RW, Estacio RO, Jeffers B. Appropriate Blood Pressure Control in NIDDM (ABCD) Trial. *Diabetologia.* 1996;39:1646-1654.
461. Klein R, Klein BE, Moss SE, et al. The Wisconsin Epidemiology Study of Diabetic Retinopathy: V. Proteinuria and retinopathy in a population of diabetic persons diagnosed prior to 30 years of age. In: Friedman EA, L'Esperance FA Jr, eds. *Diabetic Renal-Retinal Syndrome.* 3rd ed. Orlando, FL: Grune & Stratton; 1986:245-264.
462. Kullberg CE, Arnqvist HJ. Elevated long-term glycated haemoglobin precedes proliferative retinopathy and nephropathy in type 1 (insulin-dependent) diabetic patients. *Diabetologia.* 1993;36: 961-965.
463. Klein R, Moss SE, Klein BE. Is gross proteinuria a risk factor for the incidence of proliferative diabetic retinopathy? *Ophthalmology.* 1993;100:1140-1146.
464. Mathiesen ER, Ronn B, Storm B, et al. The natural course of microalbuminuria in insulin-dependent diabetes: a 10-year prospective study. *Diabet Med.* 1995;12:482-487.
465. Park JY, Kim HK, Chung YE, et al. Incidence and determinants of microalbuminuria in Koreans with type 2 diabetes. *Diabetes Care.* 1998;21:530-534.
466. Hasslacher C, Bostedt-Kiesel A, Kempe HP, Wahl P. Effect of metabolic factors and blood pressure on kidney function in proteinuric type 2 (non–insulin-dependent) diabetic patients. *Diabetologia.* 1993;36: 1051-1056.
467. Collins VR, Dowse GK, Plehwe WE, et al. High prevalence of diabetic retinopathy and nephropathy in Polynesians of Western Samoa. *Diabetes Care.* 1995;18:1140-1149.
468. Lee ET, Lee VS, Kingsley RM, et al. Diabetic retinopathy in Oklahoma Indians with NIDDM: incidence and risk factors. *Diabetes Care.* 1992;15:1620-1627.
469. Esmatjes E, Castell C, Gonzalez T, et al. Epidemiology of renal involvement in type II diabetics (NIDDM) in Catalonia. The Catalan Diabetic Nephropathy Study Group. *Diabetes Res Clin Pract.* 1996;32: 157-163.
470. Savage S, Estacio RO, Jeffers B, Schrier RW. Urinary albumin excretion as a predictor of diabetic retinopathy, neuropathy, and cardiovascular disease in NIDDM. *Diabetes Care.* 1996;19:1243-1248.
471. Fujisawa T, Ikegami H, Yamato E, et al. Association of plasma fibrinogen level and blood pressure with diabetic retinopathy, and renal complications associated with proliferative diabetic retinopathy, in type 2 diabetes mellitus. *Diabet Med.* 1999;16:522-526.
472. Cruickshanks KJ, Ritter LL, Klein R, Moss SE. The association of microalbuminuria with diabetic retinopathy. The Wisconsin Epidemiologic Study of Diabetic Retinopathy. *Ophthalmology.* 1993;100: 862-867.
473. Roy MS. Diabetic retinopathy in African Americans with type 1 diabetes—the New Jersey 725: II. Risk factors. *Arch Ophthalmol.* 2000;118:105-115.
474. Klein R, Klein BE, Moss SE, Cruickshanks KJ. Ten-year incidence of gross proteinuria in people with diabetes. *Diabetes.* 1995;44: 916-923.
475. Mogensen CE, Chachati A, Christensen CK, et al. Microalbuminuria: an early marker of renal involvement in diabetes. *Uremia Invest.* 1985;9:85-95.
476. Damsgaard EM, Froland A, Jorgensen OD, et al. Prognostic value of urinary albumin excretion rate and other risk factors in elderly diabetic patients and non-diabetic control subjects surviving the first 5 years after assessment. *Diabetologia.* 1993;36:1030-1036.
477. Villarosa IP, Bakris GL. The Appropriate Blood Pressure Control in Diabetes (ABCD) Trial. *J Hum Hypertens.* 1998;12:653-655.
478. Nelson RG, Knowler WC, Pettitt DJ, et al. Incidence and determinants of elevated urinary albumin excretion in Pima Indians with NIDDM. *Diabetes Care.* 1995;18:182-187.
479. Gomes MB, Lucchetti MR, Gazzola H, et al. Microalbuminuria and associated clinical features among Brazilians with insulin-dependent diabetes mellitus. *Diabetes Res Clin Pract.* 1997;35:143-147.
480. Microalbuminuria Collaborative Study Group. Predictors of the development of microalbuminuria in patients with type 1 diabetes mellitus: a seven-year prospective study (see comments). *Diabet Med.* 1999;16:918-925.
481. Davis MD, Fisher MR, Gangnon RE, et al. Risk factors for high-risk proliferative diabetic retinopathy and severe visual loss: Early Treatment Diabetic Retinopathy Study Report No. 18. *Invest Ophthalmol Vis Sci.* 1998;39:233-252.

482. Qiao Q, Keinanen-Kiukaanniemi S, Laara E. The relationship between hemoglobin levels and diabetic retinopathy. *J Clin Epidemiol.* 1997;50:153-158.
483. Friedman EA, Brown CD, Berman DH. Erythropoietin in diabetic macular edema and renal insufficiency. *Am J Kidney Dis.* 1995;26:202-208.
484. Gilbertson DT, Liu J, Xue JL, et al. Projecting the number of patients with end-stage renal disease in the United States to the year 2015. *J Am Soc Nephrol.* 2005;16:3736-3741.
485. U.S. Renal Data System. *USRDS 2006 Annual Data Report: Atlas of End-Stage Renal Disease in the United States.* Bethesda, MD: National Institutes of Health, National Institute of Diabetes and Digestive and Kidney Diseases; 2006.
486. Cooper ME, Jandeleit-Dahm K, Thomas MC. Targets to retard the progression of diabetic nephropathy. *Kidney Int.* 2005;68:1439-1445.
487. Atkins RC. The epidemiology of chronic kidney disease. *Kidney Int Suppl.* 2005;94:S14-S18.
488. Muhlhauser I, Sawicki PT, Blank M, et al. Reliability of causes of death in persons with type I diabetes. *Diabetologia.* 2002;45:1490-1497.
489. Groop PH, Thomas MC, Moran JL, et al. The presence and severity of chronic kidney disease predicts all-cause mortality in type 1 diabetes. *Diabetes.* 2009;58:1651-1658.
490. Stephenson JM, Kenny S, Stevens LK, et al. Proteinuria and mortality in diabetes: the WHO Multinational Study of Vascular Disease in Diabetes. *Diabet Med.* 1995;12:149-155.
491. Ismail N, Becker B, Strzelczyk P, et al. Renal disease and hypertension in non–insulin-dependent diabetes mellitus. *Kidney Int.* 1999;55:1-28.
492. Parving HH, Hommel E, Mathiesen E, et al. Prevalence of microalbuminuria, arterial hypertension, retinopathy and neuropathy in patients with insulin dependent diabetes. *Br Med J (Clin Res Ed).* 1988;296:156-160.
493. Standl E, Stiegler H. Microalbuminuria in a random cohort of recently diagnosed type 2 (non–insulin-dependent) diabetic patients living in the greater Munich area. *Diabetologia.* 1993;36:1017-1020.
494. Schmitz A, Vaeth M, Mogensen CE. Systolic blood pressure relates to the rate of progression of albuminuria in NIDDM. *Diabetologia.* 1994;37:1251-1258.
495. Zimmet P, Alberti KG, Shaw J. Global and societal implications of the diabetes epidemic. *Nature.* 2001;414:782-787.
496. Kimmelstiel P, Wilson C. Intercapillary lesions in the glomeruli in the kidney. *Am J Pathol.* 1936;12(1):83-97.
497. Ghavamian M, Gutch CF, Kopp KF, et al. The sad truth about hemodialysis in diabetic nephropathy. *JAMA.* 1972;222:1386-1389.
498. Cooper ME. Pathogenesis, prevention and treatment of diabetic nephropathy. *Lancet.* 1998;352:213-219.
499. Mogensen CE, Christensen CK, Vittinghus E. The stages in diabetic renal disease. With emphasis in the stage of incipient diabetic nephropathy. *Diabetes.* 1983;32(Suppl 2):64-78.
500. Cambien F. Application de la théorie de Rehberg a l'étude clinique des affections rénales et du diabète. *Annu Med.* 1934;35:273-299.
501. Allen TJ, Cooper ME, Lan HY. Use of genetic mouse models in the study of diabetic nephropathy. *Curr Diab Rep.* 2004;4(6):435-440.
502. Thomson SC, Vallon V, Blantz RC. Kidney function in early diabetes: the tubular hypothesis of glomerular filtration. *Am J Physiol Renal Physiol.* 2004;286:F8-F15.
503. Hostetter TH, Troy JL, Brenner BM. Glomerular hemodynamics in experimental diabetes mellitus. *Kidney Int.* 1981;19:410-415.
504. Sharma K, Jin Y, Guo J, et al. Neutralization of TGF-β by anti-TGF-β antibody attenuates kidney hypertrophy and the enhanced extracellular matrix gene expression in STZ-induced diabetic mice. *Diabetes.* 1996;45:522-530.
505. Segev Y, Landau D, Rasch R, et al. Growth hormone receptor antagonism prevents early renal changes in nonobese diabetic mice. *J Am Soc Nephrol.* 1999;10:2374-2381.
506. Thomas MC, Burns WC, Cooper ME. Tubular changes in early diabetic nephropathy. *Adv Chronic Kidney Dis.* 2005;12:177-186.
507. Mogensen CE, Christensen CK. Predicting diabetic nephropathy in insulin-dependent diabetic patients. *N Engl J Med.* 1984;311:89-93.
508. Mauer S, Steffes M, Ellis E, et al. Structural-functional relationships in diabetic nephropathy. *J Clin Invest.* 1984;74:1143-1155.
509. Allen TJ, Cooper ME, Gilbert RG, et al. Serum total renin is increased before microalbuminuria in diabetes (IDDM). *Kidney Int.* 1996;50:902-907.
510. Comper WD, Osicka TM, Clark M, et al. Earlier detection of microalbuminuria in diabetic patients using a new urinary albumin assay. *Kidney Int.* 2004;65:1850-1855.
511. Poulsen PL, Hansen KW, Mogensen CE. Ambulatory blood pressure in the transition from normo- to microalbuminuria. A longitudinal study in IDDM patients. *Diabetes.* 1994;43:1248-1253.
512. Tikellis C, Brown R, Head GA, et al. Angiotensin converting enzyme 2 and hyperfiltration associated with diabetes. *Am J Physiol Renal Physiol.* 2014;306(7):F773-F780.
513. Cherney DZ, Perkins BA, Soleymanlou N, et al. Renal hemodynamic effect of sodium-glucose cotransporter 2 inhibition in patients with type 1 diabetes mellitus. *Circulation.* 2014;129:587-597.

514. Mogensen CE, Keane WF, Bennett PH, et al. Prevention of diabetic renal disease with special reference to microalbuminuria. *Lancet.* 1995;346:1080-1084.
515. Steinke JM, Sinaiko AR, Kramer MS, et al. The early natural history of nephropathy in type 1 diabetes: III. Predictors of 5-year urinary albumin excretion rate patterns in initially normoalbuminuric patients. *Diabetes.* 2005;54:2164-2171.
516. Lurbe E, Redon J, Kesani A, et al. Increase in nocturnal blood pressure and progression to microalbuminuria in type 1 diabetes. *N Engl J Med.* 2002;347:797-805.
517. Perkins BA, Ficociello LH, Silva KH, et al. Regression of microalbuminuria in type 1 diabetes. *N Engl J Med.* 2003;348:2285-2293.
518. Hovind P, Tarnow L, Rossing P, et al. Predictors for the development of microalbuminuria and macroalbuminuria in patients with type 1 diabetes: inception cohort study. *BMJ.* 2004;328:1105.
519. Bilous RW, Mauer SM, Sutherland DE, et al. Mean glomerular volume and rate of development of diabetic nephropathy. *Diabetes.* 1989;38:1142-1147.
520. Parving HH, Andersen AR, Smidt VM, et al. Diabetic nephropathy and arterial hypertension. *Diabetologia.* 1983;24:10-12.
521. Fioretto P, Steffes MW, Sutherland DE, et al. Reversal of lesions of diabetic nephropathy after pancreas transplantation. *N Engl J Med.* 1998;339:69-75.
522. Vora JP, Leese GP, Peters JR, et al. Longitudinal evaluation of renal function in non-insulin dependent diabetic patients with early nephropathy. *J Diabetes Complications.* 1996;10:88-93.
523. Lane PH, Steffes MW, Mauer SM. Glomerular structure in IDDM women with low glomerular filtration rate and normal urinary albumin excretion. *Diabetes.* 1992;41:581-586.
524. Tsalamandris C, Allen TJ, Gilbert RE, et al. Progressive decline in renal function in diabetic patients with and without albuminuria. *Diabetes.* 1994;43:649-655.
525. American Diabetes Association. Standards of medical care in diabetes—2010. *Diabetes Care.* 2010;33(Suppl 1):S11-S61.
526. Wiseman MJ, Mangili R, Alberetto M, et al. Glomerular response mechanisms to glycemic changes in insulin-dependent diabetics. *Kidney Int.* 1987;31:1012-1018.
527. Kiritoshi S, Nishikawa T, Sonoda K, et al. Reactive oxygen species from mitochondria induce cyclooxygenase-2 gene expression in human mesangial cells: potential role in diabetic nephropathy. *Diabetes.* 2003;52:2570-2577.
528. Forbes JM, Cooper ME, Oldfield MD, et al. Role of advanced glycation end products in diabetic nephropathy. *J Am Soc Nephrol.* 2003;14:S254-S258.
529. Gorin Y, Block K, Hernandez J, et al. Nox4 NAD(P)H oxidase mediates hypertrophy and fibronectin expression in the diabetic kidney. *J Biol Chem.* 2005;280:39616-39626.
530. Cooper ME. Interaction of metabolic and haemodynamic factors in mediating experimental diabetic nephropathy. *Diabetologia.* 2001;44:1957-1972.
531. Thomas MC, Tikellis C, Burns WM, et al. Interactions between renin angiotensin system and advanced glycation in the kidney. *J Am Soc Nephrol.* 2005;16:2976-2984.
532. Cooper ME, Mundel P, Boner G. Role of nephrin in renal disease including diabetic nephropathy. *Semin Nephrol.* 2002;22:393-398.
533. Andersen S, Blouch K, Bialek J, et al. Glomerular permselectivity in early stages of overt diabetic nephropathy. *Kidney Int.* 2000;58:2129-2137.
534. Wassef L, Langham RG, Kelly DJ. Vasoactive renal factors and the progression of diabetic nephropathy. *Curr Pharm Des.* 2004;10:3373-3384.
535. Gilbert RE, Cooper ME. The tubulointerstitium in progressive diabetic kidney disease: More than an aftermath of glomerular injury? *Kidney Int.* 1999;56:1627-1637.
536. Gilbert RE, Cooper ME, Krum H. Drug administration in patients with diabetes mellitus. Safety considerations. *Drug Saf.* 1998;18(6):441-455.
537. Salifu MO, Haria DM, Badero O, et al. Challenges in the diagnosis and management of renal artery stenosis. *Curr Hypertens Rep.* 2005;7:219-227.
538. Hricik DE, Browning PJ, Kopelman R, et al. Captopril-induced functional renal insufficiency in patients with bilateral renal-artery stenoses or renal-artery stenosis in a solitary kidney. *N Engl J Med.* 1983;308:373-376.
539. Griffin MD, Bergstralhn EJ, Larson TS. Renal papillary necrosis—a sixteen-year clinical experience. *J Am Soc Nephrol.* 1995;6:248-256.
540. Davies PJ. Beethoven's nephropathy and death: discussion paper. *J R Soc Med.* 1993;86:159-161.
541. Kelly DJ, Wilkinson-Berka JL, Allen TJ, et al. A new model of diabetic nephropathy with progressive renal impairment in the transgenic (mRen-2)27 rat (tgr). *Kidney Int.* 1998;54:343-352.
542. DeFronzo RA. Hyperkalemia and hyporeninemic hypoaldosteronism. *Kidney Int.* 1980;17:118-134.
543. Lush DJ, King JA, Fray JC. Pathophysiology of low renin syndromes: sites of renal renin secretory impairment and prorenin overexpression. *Kidney Int.* 1993;43:983-999.

544. Nadler JL, Lee FO, Hsueh W, et al. Evidence of prostacyclin deficiency in the syndrome of hyporeninemic hypoaldosteronism. *N Engl J Med.* 1986;314:1015-1020.

545. Parfrey PS, Griffiths SM, Barrett BJ, et al. Contrast material-induced renal failure in patients with diabetes mellitus, renal insufficiency, or both. A prospective controlled study. *N Engl J Med.* 1989;320:143-149.

546. Weisberg LS, Kurnik PB, Kurnik BR. Risk of radiocontrast nephropathy in patients with and without diabetes mellitus. *Kidney Int.* 1994;45:259-265.

547. Tepel M, van der Giet M, Schwarzfeld C, et al. Prevention of radiographic-contrast-agent–induced reductions in renal function by acetylcysteine. *N Engl J Med.* 2000;343:180-184.

548. Mogensen CE. Long-term antihypertensive treatment inhibiting progression of diabetic nephropathy. *BMJ.* 1982;285:685-688.

549. Parving HH, Andersen AR, Smidt VM, et al. Effect of antihypertensive treatment on kidney function in diabetic nephropathy. *Br Med J.* 1987;294:1443-1447.

550. Björck S. Clinical trials in overt diabetic nephropathy. In: Mogensen CE, ed. *The Kidney and Hypertension in Diabetes Mellitus.* 3rd ed. London: Kluwer Academic; 1996:375-384.

551. ADVANCE Collaborative Group. Intensive blood glucose control and vascular outcomes in patients with type 2 diabetes. *N Engl J Med.* 2008;358:2560-2572.

552. Perkovic V, Heerspink HL, Chalmers J, et al. Intensive glucose control improves kidney outcomes in patients with type 2 diabetes. *Kidney Int.* 2013;83:517-523.

553. Action to Control Cardiovascular Risk in Diabetes Study Group. Effects of intensive glucose lowering in type 2 diabetes. *N Engl J Med.* 2008;358:2545-2559.

554. Parving HH. Renoprotection in diabetes: genetic and non-genetic risk factors and treatment. *Diabetologia.* 1998;41:745-759.

555. Babaei-Jadidi R, Karachalias N, Ahmed N, et al. Prevention of incipient diabetic nephropathy by high-dose thiamine and benfotiamine. *Diabetes.* 2003;52:2110-2120.

556. Thallas-Bonke V, Lindschau C, Rizkalla B, et al. Attenuation of extracellular matrix accumulation in diabetic nephropathy by the advanced glycation end product cross-link breaker ALT-711 via a protein kinase C-alpha-dependent pathway. *Diabetes.* 2004;53:2921-2930.

557. Chobanian AV, Bakris GL, Black HR, et al. Seventh report of the Joint National Committee on Prevention, Detection, Evaluation, and Treatment of High Blood Pressure. *Hypertension.* 2003;42(6):1206-1252.

558. de Galan BE, Perkovic V, Ninomiya T, et al. Lowering blood pressure reduces renal events in type 2 diabetes. *J Am Soc Nephrol.* 2009;20:883-892.

559. Strippoli G, Craig M, Craig J. Antihypertensive agents for preventing diabetic kidney disease. *Cochrane Database Syst Rev.* 2005;(4):CD004136.

560. ACE Inhibitors in Diabetic Nephropathy Trialist Group. Should all patients with type 1 diabetes mellitus and microalbuminuria receive angiotensin-converting enzyme inhibitors? A meta-analysis of individual patient data. *Ann Intern Med.* 2001;134:370-379.

561. EUCLID study group. Randomised placebo-controlled trial of lisinopril in normotensive patients with insulin-dependent diabetes and normoalbuminuria or microalbuminuria. *Lancet.* 1997;349:1787-1792.

562. Kvetny J, Gregersen G, Pedersen RS. Randomized placebo-controlled trial of perindopril in normotensive, normoalbuminuric patients with type 1 diabetes mellitus. *QJM.* 2001;94(2):89-94.

563. Mauer M, Zinman B, Gardiner R, et al. Renal and retinal effects of enalapril and losartan in type 1 diabetes. *N Engl J Med.* 2009;361:40-51.

564. Hommel E, Parving HH, Mathiesen E, et al. Effect of captopril on kidney function in insulin-dependent diabetic patients with nephropathy. *Br Med J.* 1986;293:467-470.

565. Brenner BM, Cooper ME, de Zeeuw D, et al. Effects of losartan on renal and cardiovascular outcomes in patients with type 2 diabetes and nephropathy. *N Engl J Med.* 2001;345:861-869.

566. Lewis EJ, Hunsicker LG, Clarke WR, et al. Renoprotective effect of the angiotensin-receptor antagonist irbesartan in patients with nephropathy due to type 2 diabetes. *N Engl J Med.* 2001;345:851-860.

567. Arauz-Pacheco C, Parrott MA, Raskin P. Treatment of hypertension in adults with diabetes. *Diabetes Care.* 2003;26(Suppl 1):S80-S82.

568. Barnett AH, Bain SC, Bouter P, et al. Angiotensin-receptor blockade versus converting-enzyme inhibition in type 2 diabetes and nephropathy. *N Engl J Med.* 2004;351:1952-1961.

569. Mann JF, Schmieder RE, McQueen M, et al. Renal outcomes with telmisartan, ramipril, or both, in people at high vascular risk (the ONTARGET study): a multicentre, randomised, double-blind, controlled trial. *Lancet.* 2008;372:547-553.

570. Parving HH, Lehnert H, Brochner-Mortensen J, et al. The effect of irbesartan on the development of diabetic nephropathy in patients with type 2 diabetes. *N Engl J Med.* 2001;345:870-878.

571. Parving HH, Persson F, Lewis JB, et al. Aliskiren combined with losartan in type 2 diabetes and nephropathy. *N Engl J Med.* 2008;358:2433-2446.

572. Parving HH, Brenner BM, McMurray JJ, et al. Cardiorenal end points in a trial of aliskiren for type 2 diabetes. *N Engl J Med.* 2012;367:2204-2213.

573. Schjoedt KJ, Rossing K, Juhl TR, et al. Beneficial impact of spironolactone in diabetic nephropathy. *Kidney Int.* 2005;68:2829-2836.

574. Epstein M. Aldosterone as a mediator of progressive renal disease: pathogenetic and clinical implications. *Am J Kidney Dis.* 2001;37:677-688.

575. Tikkanen I, Tikkanen T, Cao Z, et al. Combined inhibition of neutral endopeptidase with angiotensin converting enzyme or endothelin converting enzyme in experimental diabetes. *J Hypertens.* 2002;20:707-714.

576. Pedrini MT, Levey AS, Lau J, et al. The effect of dietary protein restriction on the progression of diabetic and nondiabetic renal diseases—a meta-analysis. *Ann Intern Med.* 1996;124:627-632.

577. Hansen HP, Tauber-Lassen E, Jensen BR, et al. Effect of protein restriction on prognosis in type 1 diabetic patients with diabetic nephropathy. *Kidney Int.* 2002;62:220-228.

578. Waugh NR, Robertson AM. Protein restriction for diabetic renal disease. *Cochrane Database Syst Rev.* 2000;(2):CD002181.

579. Jandeleit-Dahm K, Cao ZM, Cox AJ, et al. Role of hyperlipidemia in progressive renal disease: focus on diabetic nephropathy. *Kidney Int.* 1999;56:S31-S36.

580. Fried LF, Forrest KY, Ellis D, et al. Lipid modulation in insulin-dependent diabetes mellitus: effect on microvascular outcomes. *J Diabetes Complications.* 2001;15:113-119.

581. FIELD Study Investigators. Effects of long-term fenofibrate therapy on cardiovascular events in 9795 people with type 2 diabetes mellitus (the FIELD study): randomized controlled trial. *Lancet.* 2005;366:1849-1861.

582. Collins R, Armitage J, Parish S, et al. MRC/BHF Heart Protection Study of cholesterol-lowering with simvastatin in 5963 people with diabetes: a randomised placebo-controlled trial. *Lancet.* 2003;361:2005-2016.

583. Athyros VG, Papageorgiou AA, Elisaf M, et al. Statins and renal function in patients with diabetes mellitus. *Curr Med Res Opin.* 2003;19:615-617.

584. Colhoun HM, Betteridge DJ, Durrington PN, et al. Primary prevention of cardiovascular disease with atorvastatin in type 2 diabetes in the Collaborative Atorvastatin Diabetes Study (CARDS): multicentre randomised placebo-controlled trial. *Lancet.* 2004;364:685-696.

585. Thomas MC, Cooper ME, Tsalamandris C, et al. Anemia with impaired erythropoietin response in diabetic patients. *Arch Intern Med.* 2005;165:466-469.

586. Jungers P, Choukroun G, Oualim Z, et al. Beneficial influence of recombinant human erythropoietin therapy on the rate of progression of chronic renal failure in predialysis patients. *Nephrol Dial Transplant.* 2001;16(2):307-312.

587. Mix TC, Brenner RM, Cooper ME, et al. Rationale—Trial to Reduce Cardiovascular Events with Aranesp Therapy (TREAT): evolving the management of cardiovascular risk in patients with chronic kidney disease. *Am Heart J.* 2005;149:408-413.

588. Pfeffer MA, Burdmann EA, Chen CY, et al. A trial of darbepoetin alfa in type 2 diabetes and chronic kidney disease. *N Engl J Med.* 2009;361:2019-2032.

589. Tuttle KR, McGill JB, Haney DJ, et al. Kidney outcomes in long-term studies of ruboxistaurin for diabetic eye disease. *Clin J Am Soc Nephrol.* 2007;2:631-636.

590. Achour A, Kacem M, Dibej K, et al. One year course of oral sulodexide in the management of diabetic nephropathy. *J Nephrol.* 2005;18:568-574.

591. Wenzel RR, Littke T, Kuranoff S, et al. Avosentan reduces albumin excretion in diabetics with macroalbuminuria. *J Am Soc Nephrol.* 2009;20:655-664.

592. Kohan DE, Pritchett Y, Molitch M, et al. Addition of atrasentan to renin-angiotensin system blockade reduces albuminuria in diabetic nephropathy. *J Am Soc Nephrol.* 2011;22(4):763-772.

593. Pergola PE, Raskin P, Toto RD, et al. Bardoxolone methyl and kidney function in CKD with type 2 diabetes. *N Engl J Med.* 2011;365:327-336.

594. de Zeeuw D, Akizawa T, Audhya P, et al. Bardoxolone methyl in type 2 diabetes and stage 4 chronic kidney disease. *N Engl J Med.* 2013;369:2492-2503.

595. Jungers P, Zingraff J, Page B, et al. Detrimental effects of late referral in patients with chronic renal failure: a case-control study. *Kidney Int Suppl.* 1993;41:S170-S173.

596. Pirson Y. The diabetic patient with ESRD: how to select the modality of renal replacement. *Nephrol Dial Transplant.* 1996;11:1511-1513.

597. Gaede P, Vedel P, Larsen N, et al. Multifactorial intervention and cardiovascular disease in patients with type 2 diabetes. *N Engl J Med.* 2003;348:383-393.

598. Vinik AI, Mitchell BD, Leichter SB, et al. Epidemiology of the complications of diabetes. In: Leslie RDG, Robbins DC, eds. *Diabetes: Clinical Science in Practice.* Cambridge, UK: Cambridge University Press; 1995:221-287.

599. Vinik A, Mehrabyan A. Diabetic neuropathies. *Med Clin North Am.* 2004;88:947-999.

600. Young MJ, Boulton AJM, MacLeod AF, et al. A multicenter study of the prevalence of diabetic peripheral neuropathy in the United Kingdom hospital clinic population. *Diabetologia*. 1993;36:150-154.

601. Dyck PJ, Kratz KM, Karnes JL, et al. The prevalence by staged severity of various types of diabetic neuropathy, retinopathy, and nephropathy in a population-based cohort: The Rochester Diabetic Neuropathy Study. *Neurology*. 1993;43:817-824.

602. Holzer SE, Camerota A, Martens L, et al. Costs and duration of care for lower extremity ulcers in patients with diabetes. *Clin Ther*. 1998;20:169-181.

603. Caputo GM, Cavanagh PR, Ulbrecht JS, et al. Assessment and management of foot disease in patients with diabetes. *N Engl J Med*. 1994;331:854-860.

604. Pirart J. [Diabetes mellitus and its degenerative complications: a prospective study of 4,400 patients observed between 1947 and 1973. (3rd and last part) (author's transl)]. *Diabete Metab*. 1977;3(4):245-256.

605. Vinik A, Ullal J, Parson HK, Casellini CM. Diabetic neuropathies: clinical manifestations and current treatment options. *Nat Clin Pract Endocrinol Metab*. 2006;2:269-281.

606. Smith AG, Ramachandran P, Tripp S, Singleton JR. Epidermal nerve innervation in impaired glucose tolerance and diabetes-associated neuropathy. *Neurology*. 2001;57:1701-1704.

607. Pittenger GL, Ray M, Burcus NI, et al. Intraepidermal nerve fibers are indicators of small-fiber neuropathy in both diabetic and nondiabetic patients. *Diabetes Care*. 2004;27:1974-1979.

608. Belatti DA, Phisitkul P. Declines in lower extremity amputation in the US Medicare population, 2000-2010. *Foot Ankle Int*. 2013;34:923-931.

609. Driver VR, Fabbi M, Lavery LA, Gibbons G. The costs of diabetic foot: the economic case for the limb salvage team. *J Vasc Surg*. 2010;52:17S-22S.

610. Vinik AI. Diabetic neuropathy, mobility and balance. *Geriatr Times*. 2003;4:13-15.

611. Resnick HE, Stansberry KB, Harris TB, et al. Diabetes, peripheral neuropathy, and old age disability. *Muscle Nerve*. 2002;25:43-50.

612. Herman WH, Kennedy L. Underdiagnosis of peripheral neuropathy in type 2 diabetes. *Diabetes Care*. 2005;28:1480-1481.

613. Vinik A. Diabetic neuropathy: pathogenesis and therapy. *Am J Med*. 1999;107(2B):17S-26S.

614. Armstrong DG, Lavery LA, Harkless LB. Validation of a diabetic wound classification system. The contribution of depth, infection, and ischemia to risk of amputation. *Diabetes Care*. 1998;21(5):855-859.

615. Reiber GE, Boyco EJ, Smith DG. Lower extremity foot ulcers and amputations in diabetes. In: *Diabetes in America*. 2nd ed. Bethesda, MD: National Institute of Diabetes and Digestive and Kidney Diseases; 1995;409-428. Available at: <http://www.niddk.nih.gov/diabetes-america-2nd-edition.aspx>.

616. Vinik EJ, Hayes RP, Oglesby A, et al. The development and validation of the Norfolk QOL-DN, a new measure of patients' perception of the effects of diabetes and diabetic neuropathy. *Diabetes Technol Ther*. 2005;7:497-508.

617. Levitt NS, Stansberry KB, Wychanck S, Vinik AI. Natural progression of autonomic neuropathy and autonomic function tests in a cohort of IDDM. *Diabetes Care*. 1996;19:751-754.

618. Rathmann W, Ziegler D, Jahnke M, et al. Mortality in diabetic patients with cardiovascular autonomic neuropathy. *Diabet Med*. 1993;10:820-824.

619. Maser RE, Mitchell BD, Vinik AI, Freeman R. The association between cardiovascular autonomic neuropathy and mortality in individuals with diabetes: a meta-analysis. *Diabetes Care*. 2003;26:1895-1901.

620. Vinik AI, Maser RE, Mitchell BD, Freeman R. Diabetic autonomic neuropathy. *Diabetes Care*. 2003;26:1553-1579.

621. Vileikyte L, Peyrot M, Bundy C, et al. The development and validation of a neuropathy- and foot ulcer-specific quality of life instrument. *Diabetes Care*. 2003;26:2549-2555.

622. Strotmeyer ES, Cauley JA, Schwartz AV, et al. Reduced peripheral nerve function is related to lower hip BMD and calcaneal QUS in older white and black adults: the Health, Aging, and Body Composition Study. *J Bone Miner Res*. 2006;21:1803-1810.

623. Sadosky A, McDermott AM, Brandenburg NA, Strauss M. A review of the epidemiology of painful diabetic peripheral neuropathy, postherpetic neuralgia, and less commonly studied neuropathic pain conditions. *Pain Pract*. 2008;8:45-56.

624. Tesfaye S, Boulton AJ, Dyck PJ, et al. Diabetic neuropathies: update on definitions, diagnostic criteria, estimation of severity, and treatments. *Diabetes Care*. 2010;33:2285-2293.

625. Ziegler D. Painful diabetic neuropathy: treatment and future aspects. *Diabetes Metab Res Rev*. 2008;24(Suppl 1):S52-S57.

626. Boulton AJ, Malik RA, Arezzo JC, Sosenko JM. Diabetic somatic neuropathies. *Diabetes Care*. 2004;27:1458-1486.

627. Vinik AI, Ziegler D. Diabetic cardiovascular autonomic neuropathy. *Circulation*. 2007;115:387-397.

628. Vinik AI, Maser RE, Ziegler D. Neuropathy: the crystal ball for cardiovascular disease? *Diabetes Care*. 2010;33:1688-1690.

629. Vinik A, Maser R, Ziegler D. Autonomic imbalance: prophet of doom or scope for hope? *Diabet Med*. 2011;28(6):643-651.

630. American Diabetes Association American Academy of Neurology. Consensus statement; report and recommendations of the San Antonio conference on diabetic neuropathy. *Diabetes Care*. 1988;11(7):592-597.

631. Polydefkis M, Hauer P, Griffin JW, McArthur JC. Skin biopsy as a tool to assess distal small fiber innervation in diabetic neuropathy. *Diabetes Technol Ther*. 2001;3:23-28.

632. Watkins PJ. Progression of diabetic autonomic neuropathy. *Diabet Med*. 1993;10(Suppl 2):77S-78S.

633. Ziegler D, Cicmir I, Mayer P, et al. Somatic and autonomic nerve function during the first year after diagnosis of type 1 (insulin-dependent) diabetes. *Diabetes Res*. 1988;7:123-127.

634. Partanen J, Niskanen L, Lehtinen J, et al. Natural history of peripheral neuropathy in patients with non-insulin-dependent diabetes mellitus. *N Engl J Med*. 1995;333:89-94.

635. Apfel SC, Kessler JA, Adornato BT, et al. and the NGF Study Group. Recombinant human nerve growth factor in the treatment of diabetic polyneuropathy. *Neurology*. 1998;51:695-702.

636. Vinik AI. Treatment of diabetic polyneuropathy (DPN) with recombinant human nerve growth factor (rhNGF). *Diabetes*. 1999;48(Suppl 1):A54-A55.

637. Dyck PJ, Kratz KM, Lehman KA, et al. The Rochester Diabetic Neuropathy Study: design, criteria for types of neuropathy, selection bias, and reproducibility of neuropathic tests. *Neurology*. 1991;41:799-807.

638. Oh SJ. Clinical electromyography: nerve conduction studies. In: Oh SJ, ed. *Nerve Conduction in Polyneuropathies*. 2nd ed. Baltimore, MD: Williams & Wilkins; 1993:579-591.

639. Kennedy WR, Wendelschafer-Crabb G, Johnson T. Quantitation of epidermal nerves in diabetic neuropathy. *Neurology*. 1996;47:1042-1048.

640. Herrmann DN, Griffin JW, Hauer P, et al. Epidermal nerve fiber density and sural nerve morphometry in peripheral neuropathies. *Neurology*. 1999;53:1634-1640.

641. Vinik A, Erbas T, Park T, et al. Dermal neurovascular dysfunction in type 2 diabetes. *Diabetes Care*. 2001;24:1468-1475.

642. Smith AG, Russell J, Feldman EL, et al. Lifestyle intervention for pre-diabetic neuropathy. *Diabetes Care*. 2006;29:1294-1299.

643. Karamitsos DT, Didangelos TP, Athyros VG, et al. The natural history of recently diagnosed autonomic neuropathy over a period of 2 years. *Diabetes Res Clin Pract*. 1998;42:55-63.

644. Ziegler D. Diabetic cardiovascular autonomic neuropathy: prognosis, diagnosis and treatment. *Diabetes Metab Rev*. 1994;10:339-383.

645. England JD, Gronseth GS, Franklin G, et al. Practice parameter: evaluation of distal symmetric polyneuropathy: role of autonomic testing, nerve biopsy, and skin biopsy (an evidence-based review). Report of the American Academy of Neurology, American Association of Neuromuscular and Electrodiagnostic Medicine, and American Academy of Physical Medicine and Rehabilitation. *Neurology*. 2009;72:177-184.

646. Boulton AJ, Gries FA, Jervell JA. Guidelines for the diagnosis and outpatient management of diabetic peripheral neuropathy. *Diabet Med*. 1998;15:508-514.

647. Boulton AJ, Vinik AI, Arezzo JC, et al. Diabetic neuropathies: a statement by the American Diabetes Association. *Diabetes Care*. 2005;28:956-962.

648. Vinik AI, Holland MT, LeBeau JM, et al. Diabetic neuropathies. *Diabetes Care*. 1992;15:1926-1975.

649. Vinik AI. Suwanwalaikorn S. Autonomic neuropathy. In: DeFronzo RA, ed. *Current Therapy of Diabetes Mellitus*. St. Louis, MO: Mosby; 1997:165-176.

650. Karpitskaya Y, Novak CB, Mackinnon SE. Prevalence of smoking, obesity, diabetes mellitus, and thyroid disease in patients with carpal tunnel syndrome. *Ann Plast Surg*. 2002;48:269-273.

651. Perkins B, Olaleye D, Bril V. Carpal tunnel syndrome in patients with diabetic polyneuropathy. *Diabetes Care*. 2002;25:565-569.

652. Chaudhuri KR, Davidson AR, Morris IM. Limited joint mobiity and carpal tunnel syndrome in insulin dependent diabetes. *Br J Rheumatol*. 1989;28:191-194.

653. Wilbourn AJ. Diabetic entrapment and compression neuropathies. In: Dyck PJ, Thomas PK, eds. *Diabetic Neuropathy*. Philadelphia, PA: WB Saunders; 1999:481-508.

654. Dawson DM. Entrapment neuropathies of the upper extremities. *N Engl J Med*. 1993;329:2013-2018.

655. Vinik A, Mehrabyan A, Colen L, Boulton A. Focal entrapment neuropathies in diabetes. *Diabetes Care*. 2004;27:1783-1788.

656. Sima AAF, Sugimoto K. Experimental diabetic neuropathy: an update. *Diabetologia*. 1999;42:773-788.

657. Vinik AI, Pittenger GL, Milicevic Z, Cuca J. Autoimmune mechanisms in the pathogenesis of diabetic neuropathy. In: Eisenbarth RG, ed. *Molecular Mechanisms of Endocrine and Organ Specific Autoimmunity*. Georgetown, TX: Landes; 1998:217-251.

658. Steck AJ, Kappos L. Gangliosides and autoimmune neuropathies: classification and clinical aspects of autoimmune neuropathies. *J Neurol Neurosurg Psychiatry*. 1994;57(Suppl):26-28.

659. Sander HW, Chokroverty S. Diabetic amyotrophy: current concepts. *Semin Neurol.* 1996;16:173-178.

660. Said G, Goulon-Goreau C, Lacroix C, Moulonguet A. Nerve biopsy findings in different patterns of proximal diabetic neuropathy. *Ann Neurol.* 1994;35:559-569.

661. Krendel DA, Costigan DA, Hopkins LC. Successful treatment of neuropathies in patients with diabetes mellitus. *Arch Neurol.* 1995; 52:1053-1061.

662. Britland ST, Young RJ, Sharma AK, Clarke BF. Acute and remitting painful diabetic polyneuropathy: a comparison of peripheral nerve fibre pathology. *Pain.* 1992;48:361-370.

663. Stewart JD, MCKelvey R, Durcan L, et al. Chronic inflammatory demyelinating polyneuropathy (CIDP). *J Neurol Sci.* 1996;142: 59-64.

664. Sharma K, Ayyar D, Martinez-Arizala A, Bradley W. Diabetic demyelinating polyneuropathy responsive to intravenous immunoglobulin therapy. *Arch Neurol.* 2002;59:751-757.

665. Witzke KA, Vinik AI. Diabetic neuropathy in older adults. *Rev Endocr Metab Disord.* 2005;6:117-127.

666. Resnick H, Vinik A, Schwartz A, et al. Independent effects of peripheral nerve dysfunction on lower-extremity physical function in old age. *Diabetes Care.* 2000;23:1642-1647.

667. Milicevic Z, Newlon PG, Pittenger GL, et al. Anti-ganglioside GM1 antibody and distal symmetric "diabetic polyneuropathy" with dominant motor features. *Diabetologia.* 1997;40:1364-1365.

668. Griffin JW, McArthur JC, Polydefkis M. Assessment of cutaneous innervation by skin biopsies. *Curr Opin Neurol.* 2001;14:655-659.

669. Vinik A. Diagnosis and management of diabetic neuropathy. *Clin Geriatr Med.* 1999;15(5):293-319.

670. Barada A, Reljanovic M, Milicevic Z, et al. Proximal diabetic neuropathy-response to immunotherapy. *Diabetes.* 1999;48(Suppl 1):A148.

671. Bird SJ, Brown MJ. The clinical spectrum of diabetic neuropathy. *Semin Neurol.* 1996;16:115-122.

672. McArthur JC, Stocks EA, Hauer P, et al. Epidermal nerve fiber density: normative reference range and diagnostic efficiency. *Arch Neurol.* 1998;55:1513-1520.

673. Stansberry KB, Hill MA, Shapiro SA, et al. Impairment of peripheral blood flow responses in diabetes resembles an enhanced aging effect. *Diabetes Care.* 1997;20:1711-1716.

674. Hirai A, Yasuda H, Joko M, et al. Evaluation of diabetic neuropathy through the quantitation of cutaneous nerves. *J Neurol Sci.* 2000; 172:55-62.

675. Dalsgaard CJ, Rydh M, Haegerstrand A. Cutaneous innervation in man visualized with protein gene product 9.5 (PGP 9.5) antibodies. *Histochemistry.* 1989;92:385-390.

676. McCarthy BG, Hsieh ST, Stocks A, et al. Cutaneous innervation in sensory neuropathies: evaluation by skin biopsy. *Neurology.* 1995;45: 1848-1855.

677. Smith AG, Lessard M, Reyna S, et al. The diagnostic utility of Sudoscan for distal symmetric peripheral neuropathy. *J Diabetes Complications.* 2014;28(4):511-516.

678. Casellini CM, Parson HK, Richardson MS, et al. Sudoscan, a noninvasive tool for detecting diabetic small fiber neuropathy and autonomic dysfunction. *Diabetes Technol Ther.* 2013;15(11):948-953.

679. Low PA, Dotson RM. Symptomatic treatment of painful neuropathy. *JAMA.* 1998;280:1863-1864.

680. Vinik AI, Park TS, Stansberry KB, Pittenger GL. Diabetic neuropathies. *Diabetologia.* 2000;43:957-973.

681. Treede RD, Jensen TS, Campbell JN, et al. Neuropathic pain: redefinition and a grading system for clinical and research purposes. *Neurology.* 2008;70:1630-1635.

682. Tesfaye S, Malik R, Harris N, et al. Arterio-venous shunting and proliferating new vessels in acute painful neuropathy of rapid glycaemic control (insulin neuritis). *Diabetologia.* 1996;39:329-335.

683. Gibbons CH, Freeman R. Treatment-induced diabetic neuropathy: a reversible painful autonomic neuropathy. *Ann Neurol.* 2010;67: 534-541.

684. Van Heel DA, Levitt NS, Winter TA. Diabetic neuropathic cachexia: the importance of positive recognition and early nutritional support. *Int J Clin Pract.* 1998;52:591-592.

685. Holland NR, Crawford TO, Hauer P. Small-fiber sensory neuropathies: clinical course and neuropathology of idiopathic cases. *Ann Neurol.* 1998;44:47-59.

686. Dyck PJ. Detection, characterization and staging of polyneuropathy: assessed in diabetes. *Muscle Nerve.* 1988;11:21-32.

687. Vinik AI, Mitchell B. Clinical aspects of diabetic neuropathies. *Diabetes Metab Rev.* 1988;4:223-253.

688. Ziegler D, Hanefeld M, Ruhnau KJ, et al. Treatment of symptomatic diabetic peripheral neuropathy with the anti-oxidant alpha-lipoic acid. A 3-week multicentre randomized controlled trial (ALADIN Study). *Diabetologia.* 1995;38:1425-1433.

689. Feldman EL, Stevens MJ, Thomas PK, et al. A practical two-step quantitative clinical and electrophysiological assessment for the diagnosis and staging of diabetic neuropathy. *Diabetes Care.* 1994;17: 1281-1289.

690. Vinik AI, Newlon P, Milicevic Z, et al. Diabetic neuropathies: an overview of clinical aspects. In: LeRoith D, Taylor SI, Olefsky JM, eds. *Diabetes Mellitus: A Fundamental and Clinical Text.* Philadelphia, PA: Lippincot-Raven; 1996:737-751.

691. Cabezas-Cerrato J. The prevalence of diabetic neuropathy in Spain: a study in primary care and hospital clinic groups. *Diabetologia.* 1998; 41:1263-1269.

692. Bril V. NIS-LL: the primary measurement scale for clinical trial endpoints in diabetic peripheral neuropathy. *Eur Neurol.* 1999; 41(Suppl 1):8-13.

693. Vinik AI, Casellini CM. Guidelines in the management of diabetic nerve pain: clinical utility of pregabalin. *Diabetes Metab Syndr Obes.* 2013;6:57-78.

694. Hermenegildo C, Felipo V, Minana MD, et al. Sustained recovery of Na(+)-K(+)-ATPase activity in sciatic nerve of diabetic mice by administration of H7 or calphostin C, inhibitors of PKC. *Diabetes.* 1993; 42:257-262.

695. Cameron NE, Cotter MA, Basso M, Hohman TC. Comparison of the effects of inhibitors of aldose reductase and sorbitol dehydrogenase on neurovascular function, nerve conduction and tissue polyol pathway metabolites in streptozotocin-diabetic rats. *Diabetologia.* 1997;40:271-281.

696. Franse LV, Valk GD, Dekker JH, et al. Numbness of the feet is a poor indicator for polyneuropathy in type 2 diabetic patients. *Diabetes Care.* 2000;17:105-110.

697. Vinik A. Use of antiepileptic drugs in the treatment of chronic painful diabetic neuropathy. *J Clin Endocrinol Metab.* 2005;90:4936-4945.

698. Dyck PJ. Severity and staging of diabetic polyneuropathy. In: Gries FA, Cameron NE, Low PA, Ziegler D, eds. *Textbook of Diabetic Neuropathy.* Stuttgart, Germany: Thieme; 2003:170-175.

699. Apfel SC, Asbury A, Bril V, et al. Positive neuropathic sensory symptoms as endpoints in diabetic neuropathy trials (Abstract). *J Neurol Sci.* 2001;189:3-5.

700. Shy ME, Frohman EM, So Y, et al, Subcommittee of the American Academy of Neurology. Quantitative sensory testing: report on the Therapeutic and Technology Assessment Subcommittee of the American Academy of Neurology. *Neurology.* 2003;602:898-906.

701. Gerr F, Letz R. Covariates of human peripheral function: vibrotactile and thermal thresholds. *Neurotoxicol Teratol.* 1994;16:102-112.

702. Gelber DA, Pfeifer MA, Broadstone VL, et al. Components of variance for vibratory and thermal threshold testing in normal and diabetic subjects. *J Diabetes Complications.* 1995;9:170-176.

703. Dyck PJ, Dyck PJ, Larson TS, et al. Patterns of quantitative sensation testing of hypoesthesia and hyperalgesia are predictive of diabetic polyneuropathy: a study of three cohorts. Nerve growth factor study group. *Diabetes Care.* 2000;23(4):510-517.

704. Maser RE, Nielsen VK, Bass EB, et al. Measuring diabetic neuropathy. Assessment and comparison of clinical examination and quantitative sensory testing. *Diabetes Care.* 1989;12:270-275.

705. Vinik AI, Suwanwalaikorn S, Stansberry KB, et al. Quantitative measurement of cutaneous perception in diabetic neuropathy. *Muscle Nerve.* 1995;18:574-584.

706. Valk GD, de Sonnaville JJ, van Houtum WH, et al. The assessment of diabetic polyneuropathy in daily clinical practice: reproducibility and validity of Semmes Weinstein monofilaments examination and clinical neurological examination. *Muscle Nerve.* 1997;20:116-118.

707. Mayfield JA, Sugarman JR. The use of Semmes-Weinstein monofilament and other threshold tests for preventing foot ulceration and amputation in people with diabetes. *J Fam Pract.* 2000;49(Suppl): 517-529.

708. Bourcier ME, Ullal J, Parson HK, et al. Diabetic peripheral neuropathy: how reliable is a homemade 1-g monofilament for screening? *J Fam Pract.* 2006;55:505-508.

709. Kumar S, Fernando DJ, Veves A, et al. Semmes-Weinstein monofilaments: a simple, effective and inexpensive screening device for identifying diabetic patients at risk of foot ulceration. *Diabetes Res Clin Pract.* 1991;13:63-67.

710. Armstrong DG, Lavery LA, Vela SA, et al. Choosing a practical screening instrument to identify patients at risk for diabetic foot ulceration. *Arch Intern Med.* 1998;158:289-292.

711. Booth J, Young MJ. Differences in the performance of commercially available 10-g monofilaments. *Diabetes Care.* 2000;23:984-988.

712. Liniger C, Albeanu A, Bloise D, Assal JP. The tuning fork revisited. *Diabet Med.* 1990;7:859-864.

713. Shin JB, Seong YJ, Lee HJ, et al. Foot screening technique in diabetic populations. *J Korean Med Sci.* 2000;15:78-82.

714. Katoulis EC, Ebdon-Parry M, Lanshammar H, et al. Gait abnormalities in diabetic neuropathy. *Diabetes Care.* 1997;20:1904-1907.

715. Vileikyte L, Hutchings G, Hollis S, Boulton AJM. The tactile circumferential discriminator: a new simple screening device to identify diabetic patients at risk of foot ulceration. *Diabetes Care.* 1997;20: 623-626.

716. Paisley AN, Abbott CA, van Schie CHM, Boulton AJM. A comparison of the Neuropen against standard quantitative sensory threshold measures for assessing peripheral nerve function. *Diabet Med.* 2002; 19(5):400-405.

717. Parson HK, Nguyen VT, Orciga MA, et al. Contact heat-evoked potential stimulation for the evaluation of small nerve fiber function. *Diabetes Technol Ther.* 2013;15:150-157.
718. Zambreanu L, Wise RG, Brooks JC, et al. A role for the brainstem in central sensitisation in humans. Evidence from functional magnetic resonance imaging. *Pain.* 2005;114:397-407.
719. Hanson PH, Schumaker P, Debugne TH, Clerin M. Evaluation of somatic and autonomic small fibers neuropathy in diabetes. *Am J Phys Med Rehabil.* 1992;71:44-47.
720. Ducher M, Thivolet C, Cerutti C, et al. Noninvasive exploration of cardiac autonomic neuropathy. *Diabetes Care.* 1999;22:388-393.
721. Jaradeh SS, Prieto TE, Lobeck LJ. Progressive polyradiculoneuropathy in diabetes: correlation of variables and clinical outcome after immunotherapy. *J Neurol Neurosurg Psychiatry.* 1999;67:607-612.
722. Periquet MI, Novak V, Collins MP, et al. Painful sensory neuropathy: prospective evaluation using skin biopsy. *Neurology.* 1999;53:1641-1647.
723. Hlubocky A, Wellik K, Ross MA, et al. Skin biopsy for diagnosis of small fiber neuropathy: a critically appraised topic. *Neurologist.* 2010;16:61-63.
724. Devigoli G, Tugnoli V, Penza P, et al. The diagnostic criteria for small fibre neuropathy: from symptoms to neuropathology. *Brain.* 2008;131:1912-1925.
725. Krendel DA, Zacharias A, Younger DS. Autoimmune diabetic neuropathy. *Neurol Clin.* 1997;15:959-971.
726. Singleton JR, Smith AG, Bromberg MB. Painful sensory polyneuropathy associated with impaired glucose tolerance. *Muscle Nerve.* 2001;24:1225-1228.
727. Sumner CJ, Sheth S, Griffin JW, et al. The spectrum of neuropathy in diabetes and impaired glucose tolerance. *Neurology.* 2003;60:108-111.
728. Mehrabyan A, Pittenger G, Burcus N, et al. Polyneuropathy in patients with dysmetabolic syndrome and newly diagnosed. *Diabetes.* 2004;53(Suppl 2):A510.
729. Vinik A, Pittenger G, Anderson A, et al. Topiramate improves C-fiber neuropathy and features of the dysmetabolic syndrome in type 2 diabetes. *Diabetes.* 2003;52:A130.
730. Arezzo JC. The use of electrophysiology for the assessment of diabetic neuropathy. *Neurosci Res Communications.* 1997;21:13-22.
731. Suez D. Intravenous immunoglobulin therapy: indication, potential side effects and treatment guidelines. *J Intraven Nurs.* 1995;18(4):178-190.
732. Vinik AI, Anandacoomaraswamy D, Ullal J. Antibodies to neuronal structures: innocent bystanders or neurotoxins? *Diabetes Care.* 2005;28:2067-2072.
733. Arezzo JC, Zotova E. Electrophysiologic measures of diabetic neuropathy: mechanism and meaning. *Int Rev Neurobiol.* 2002;50:229-255.
734. Sharma K, Cross J, Farronay O, et al. Demyelinating neuropathy in diabetes mellitus. *Arch Neurol.* 2002;59:758-765.
735. Amthor KF, Dahl-Jorgensen K, Berg TJ, et al. The effect of 8 years of strict glycaemic control on peripheral nerve function in IDDM patients: the Oslo Study. *Diabetologia.* 1994;37:579-584.
736. Veves A, Malik RA, Lye RH, et al. The relationship between sural nerve morphometric findings and measures of peripheral nerve function in mild diabetic neuropathy. *Diabet Med.* 1991;8:917-921.
737. Quattrini C, Jeziorska M, Malik RA. Small fiber neuropathy in diabetes: clinical consequence and assessment. *Int J Low Extrem Wounds.* 2004;3(1):16-21.
738. Quattrini C, Tavakoli M, Jeziorska M, et al. Surrogate markers of small fiber damage in human diabetic neuropathy. *Diabetes.* 2007;56:2148-2154.
739. Tavakoli M, Quattrini C, Abbott C, et al. Corneal confocal microscopy: a novel noninvasive test to diagnose and stratify the severity of human diabetic neuropathy. *Diabetes Care.* 2010;33:1792-1797.
740. Tavakoli M, Marshall A, Pitceathly R, et al. Corneal confocal microscopy: a novel means to detect nerve fibre damage in idiopathic small fibre neuropathy. *Exp Neurol.* 2010;223:245-250.
741. Gaede P, Vedel P, Parving HH, Pedersen O. Intensified multifactorial intervention in patients with type 2 diabetes mellitus and microalbuminuria: the Steno type 2 randomized study. *Lancet.* 1999;353:617-622.
742. Boulton AJM, Levin S, Comstock J. A multicenter trial of the aldose reductase inhibitor, tolrestat, in patients with symptomatic diabetic neuropathy. *Diabetologia.* 1990;33:431-437.
743. Didangelos TP, Karamitsos DT, Athyros VG, Kourtoglou GI. Effect of aldose reductase inhibition on cardiovascular reflex tests in patients with definite diabetic autonomic neuropathy. *J Diabetes Complications.* 1998;12:201-207.
744. Daut RL, Cleeland CS, Flanery RC. Development of the Wisconsin Brief Pain Questionnaire to assess pain in cancer and other diseases. *Pain.* 1983;17:197-210.
745. Johnson BF, Law G, Nesto R, et al. Aldose reductase inhibitor zopolrestat improves systolic function in diabetics (Abstract). *Diabetes.* 1999;48(Suppl 1):A133.
746. Hotta N, Toyota T, Matsuoka K, et al., SNK-860 Diabetic Neuropathy Group. Clinical efficacy of fidarestat, a novel aldose reductase inhibitor, for diabetic peripheral neuropathy. *Diabetes Care.* 2001;24:1776-1782.
747. Hotta N, Akanuma Y, Kawamori R, et al. Long-term clinical effects of epalrestat, an aldose reductase inhibitor, on diabetic peripheral neuropathy: the 3-year, multicenter, comparative Aldose Reductase Inhibitor-Diabetes Complications Trial. *Diabetes Care.* 2006;29:1538-1544.
748. Bril V, Buchanan RA. Aldose reductase inhibition by AS-3201 in sural nerve from patients with diabetic sensorimotor polyneuropathy. *Diabetes Care.* 2004;27:2369-2375.
748a. Giannoukakis N. Evaluation of ranirestat for the treatment of diabetic neuropathy. *Expert Opin Drug Metab Toxicol.* 2014;10(7):1051-1059. doi: 10.1517/17425255.2014.916277; [Epub 2014 Apr 30].
749. Ziegler D, Schatz H, Conrad F, et al. Effects of treatment with the antioxidant alpha-lipoic acid on cardiac autonomic neuropathy in NIDDM patients. A 4-month randomized controlled multicenter trial (DEKAN Study). Deutsche Kardiale Autonome Neuropathie. *Diabetes Care.* 1997;20:369-373.
750. Ziegler D, Gries FA. Alpha-lipoic acid in the treatment of diabetic peripheral and cardiac autonomic neuropathy. *Diabetes.* 1997;46(Suppl 2):S62-S66.
751. Ziegler D, Hanefeld M, Ruhnau KJ, et al. Treatment of symptomatic diabetic polyneuropathy with the antioxidant alpha-lipoic acid: a 7-month multicenter randomized controlled trial (ALADIN III Study). ALADIN III Study Group. Alpha-lipoic acid in diabetic neuropathy. *Diabetes Care.* 1999;22:1296-1301.
752. Jamal GA. The use of gamma linolenic acid in the prevention and treatment of diabetic neuropathy. *Diabet Med.* 1994;11:145-149.
753. Keen H, Payan J, Allawi J, et al. Treatment of diabetic neuropathy with gamma-linolenic acid. The Gamma-Linolenic Acid Multicenter Trial Group. *Diabetes Care.* 1993;16(1):8-15.
754. Dyck PJ. Hypoxic neuropathy: does hypoxia play a role in diabetic neuropathy? The 1988 Robert Wartenberg lecture. *Neurology.* 1989;39:111-118.
755. Kles K, Vinik A. Pathophysiology and treatment of diabetic peripheral neuropathy: the case for diabetic neurovascular function as an essential component. *Curr Diabetes Rev.* 2006;2:131-145.
756. Hermenegildo C, Felipo V, Minana MD, Grisolia S. Inhibition of protein kinase C restores Na+,K(+)-ATPase activity in sciatic nerve of diabetic mice. *J Neurochem.* 1992;58:1246-1249.
757. Casellini CM, Barlow PM, Rice AL, et al. A 6-month, randomized, double-masked, placebo-controlled study evaluating the effects of the protein kinase c-{beta} inhibitor ruboxistaurin on skin microvascular blood flow and other measures of diabetic peripheral neuropathy. *Diabetes Care.* 2007;30:896-902.
758. Nakamura J, Koh N, Hamada Y, et al. Effect of a protein kinase C-B specific inhibitor on diabetic neuropathy in rats. *Diabetes.* 1998;47:A70.
759. Vinik A, Bril V, Kempler P, et al. the MBBQ Study. Treatment of symptomatic diabetic peripheral neuropathy with protein kinase Cβ inhibitor ruboxistaurin mesylate during a 1-year randomized, placebo-controlled, double-blind clinical trial. *Clin Ther.* 2005;27:1164s-1180s.
760. Stracke H, Lindemann A, Federlin K. A benfotiamine-vitamin B combination in treatment of diabetic polyneuropathy. *Exp Clin Endocrinol Diabetes.* 1996;104:311-316.
761. Stracke H, Gaus W, Achenbach U, et al. Benfotiamine in diabetic polyneuropathy (BENDIP): results of a randomised, double blind, placebo-controlled clinical study. *Exp Clin Endocrinol Diabetes.* 2008;116(10):600-605.
762. Haupt E, Ledermann H, Kopcke W. Benfotiamine in the treatment of diabetic polyneuropathy—a three-week randomized, controlled pilot study (BEDIP study). *Int J Clin Pharmacol Ther.* 2005;43:71-77.
763. Witzke K, Vinik A, Grant L, et al. Loss of RAGE defense: a cause of Charcot neuroarthropathy? *Diabetes Care.* 2011;34(7):1617-1621.
764. Fonseca V, Lavery L, Thethi T, et al. A 24-week, double-blind, placebo controlled, multicenter study of Metanx in patients with diabeteic peripheral neuropathy (abstract). American Association of Clinical Endocrinologists 2011 Annual Meeting, April 13-17, San Diego, CA, Abstract 212, 2011.
765. Diemel LT, Stevens JC, Willars GB, Tomlinson DR. Depletion of substance P and calcitonin gene-related peptide in sciatic nerve of rats with experimental diabetes: effects of insulin and aldose reductase inhibition. *Neurosci Lett.* 1992;137:253-256.
766. Anandacoomaraswamy D, Ullal J, Vinik AI. A 70-year-old male with peripheral neuropathy, ataxia and antigliadin antibodies shows improvement, but not ataxia, after intravenous immunoglobin and gluten-free diet. *J Multidisc Healthc.* 2008;1:93-96.
767. Hellweg R, Wohrle M, Hartung HD. Diabetes mellitus associated decrease in nerve growth factor levels is reversed by allogenetic pancreatic islet transplantation. *Neurosci Lett.* 1991;125:1-4.
768. Tomlinson DR, Fernyhough P, Diemel LT. Neurotrophins and peripheral neuropathy. *Philos Trans R Soc Lond B Biol Sci.* 1996;351:455-462.
769. Apfel SC, Kessler JA. Neurotropic factors in the therapy of peripheral neuropathy. *Baillieres Clin Neurol.* 1995;4(3):593-606.

770. Tam J, Rosenberg L, Maysinger D. INGAP peptide improves nerve function and enhances regeneration in streptozotocin-induced diabetic C57BL/6 mice. *FASEB J.* 2004;18:1767-1769.

771. Dungan KM, Buse JB, Ratner RE. Effects of therapy in type 1 and type 2 diabetes mellitus with a peptide derived from islet neogenesis associated protein (INGAP). *Diabetes Metab Res Rev.* 2009;25:558-565.

772. Bussolino F, Di Renzo MF, Ziche M, et al. Hepatocyte growth factor is a potent angiogenic factor which stimulates endothelial cell motility and growth. *J Cell Biol.* 1992;119:629-641.

773. Nakagami H, Kaneda Y, Ogihara T, Morishita R. Hepatocyte growth factor as potential cardiovascular therapy. *Expert Rev Cardiovasc Ther.* 2005;3:513-519.

774. Matsumoto K, Nakamura T. Emerging multipotent aspects of hepatocyte growth factor. *J Biochem.* 1996;119:591-600.

775. Jayasankar V, Woo YJ, Pirolli TJ, et al. Induction of angiogenesis and inhibition of apoptosis by hepatocyte growth factor effectively treats postischemic heart failure. *J Card Surg.* 2005;20:93-101.

776. Hashimoto N, Yamanaka H, Fukuoka T, et al. Expression of HGF and cMet in the peripheral nervous system of adult rats following sciatic nerve injury. *Neuroreport.* 2001;12(7):1403-1407.

777. Ajroud-Driss S, Christiansen M, Allen JA, Kessler JA. Phase 1/2 open-label dose-escalation study of plasmid DNA expressing two isoforms of hepatocyte growth factor in patients with painful diabetic peripheral neuropathy. *Mol Ther.* 2013;21(6):1279-1286.

778. Sindrup SH, Jensen TS. Efficacy of pharmacological treatments of neuropathic pain: an update and effect related to mechanism of drug action. *Pain.* 1999;83:389-400.

779. Zieleniewski W. Calcitonin nasal spray for painful diabetic neuropathy. *Lancet.* 1990;336:449.

780. Rosenstock J, Tuchman M, LaMoreaux L, Sharma U. Pregabalin for the treatment of painful diabetic peripheral neuropathy: a double-blind, placebo-controlled trial. *Pain.* 2004;110:628-638.

781. Goldstein DJ, Lu Y, Detke MJ, et al. Duloxetine vs. placebo in patients with painful diabetic neuropathy. *Pain.* 2005;116:109-118.

782. Rains C, Bryson HM. Topical capsaicin. A review of its pharmacological properties and therapeutic potential in post-herpetic neuralgia, diabetic neuropathy and osteoarthritis. *Drugs Aging.* 1995;7:317-328.

783. Bays-Smith MG, Max MB, Muir J, Kingman A. Transdermal clonidine compared to placebo in painful diabetic neuropathy using a two-stage "enriched enrollment" design. *Pain.* 1995;60:267-274.

784. Said G, Bigo A, Ameri A, et al. Uncommon early-onset neuropathy in diabetic patients. *J Neurol.* 1998;245:61-68.

785. Jarvis B, Coukell AJ. Mexiletine. A review of its therapeutic use in painful diabetic neuropathy. *Drugs.* 1998;56:691-707.

786. Harati Y, Gooch C, Swenson M. Double-blind randomized trial of tramadol for the treatment of the pain of diabetic neuropathy. *Neurology.* 1998;50:1842-1846.

787. Harati Y, Gooch C, Swenson M, et al. Maintenance of the long-term effectiveness of tramadol in treatment of the pain of diabetic neuropathy. *J Diabetes Complications.* 2000;14:65-70.

788. Schwartz S, Etropolski M, Shapiro DY, et al. Safety and efficacy of tapentadol ER in patients with painful diabetic peripheral neuropathy: results of a randomized-withdrawal, placebo-controlled trial. *Curr Med Res Opin.* 2011;27:151-162.

789. Vinik A, Shapiro D, Karcher K, et al. Patient global impression of change (PGIC) and brief pain inventory-short form (BPI-SF) assessments with tapentadol extended release (ER) for painful diabetic peripheral neuropathy (DPN). 72nd American Diabetes Association Scientific Sessions, June 8-12, 2012, Philadelphia, PA, 2012.

790. Schwartz S, Etropolski M, Shapiro D, et al. A pooled analysis evaluating efficacy and tolerability of tapentadol ER for chronic, painful diabetic peripheral neuropathy (DPN). 72nd American Diabetes Association Scientific Sessions, June 8-12, 2012, Philadelphia, PA, 2012.

791. Nelson KA, Park KM, Robinovitz E, et al. High-dose oral dextromethorphan versus placebo in painful diabetic neuropathy and postherpetic neuralgia. *Neurology.* 1997;48:1212-1218.

792. Cameron NE, Eaton SEM, Cotter MA, Tesfaye S. Vascular factors and metabolic interactions in the pathogenesis of diabetic neuropathy. *Diabetologia.* 2001;44:1973-1988.

793. Max M, Lynch S, Muir J. Effects of desipramine, amitriptyline and fluoxetine on pain in diabetic neuropathy. *N Engl J Med.* 1992;326:1250-1256.

794. Dworkin RH, Backonja M, Rowbotham MC, et al. Advances in neuropathic pain: diagnosis, mechanisms, and treatment recommendations. *Arch Neurol.* 2003;60:1524-1534.

795. McQuay H, Tramer M, Nye B, et al. A systematic review of antidepressants in neuropathic pain. *Pain.* 1996;68:227.

796. Joss JD. Tricyclic antidepressant use in diabetic neuropathy. *Ann Pharmacother.* 1999;33:996-1000.

797. Sindrup S, Gram L, Brosen K. The selective serotonin reuptake inhibitor paroxetine is effective in treatment of diabetic neuropathy symptoms. *Pain.* 1990;42:144.

798. Kajdasz DK, Iyengar S, Desaiah D, et al. Duloxetine for the management of diabetic peripheral neuropathic pain: evidence-based findings from post hoc analysis of three multicenter, randomized, double-blind, placebo-controlled, parallel-group studies. *Clin Ther.* 2007;29(Suppl):2536-2546.

799. Ziegler D, Pritchett YL, Wang F, et al. Impact of disease characteristics on the efficacy of duloxetine in diabetic peripheral neuropathic pain. *Diabetes Care.* 2007;30:664-669.

800. Rowbotham MC, Goli V, Kunz NR, Lei D. Venlafaxine extended release in the treatment of painful diabetic neuropathy: a double-blind, placebo-controlled study. *Pain.* 2004;110:697-706.

801. McQuay H, Carroll D, Jadad AR, et al. Anticonvulsant drugs for management of pain: a systematic review. *BMJ.* 1995;311:1047-1052.

802. Vinik AI. Advances in diabetes for the millennium: new treatments for diabetic neuropathies. *Med Gen Med.* 2004;6:13.

803. LaRoche SM, Helmers SL. The new antiepileptic drugs: scientific review. *JAMA.* 2004;291:605-614.

804. Freeman R, Durso-Decruz E, Emir B. Efficacy, safety, and tolerability of pregabalin treatment for painful diabetic peripheral neuropathy: findings from seven randomized, controlled trials across a range of doses. *Diabetes Care.* 2008;31:1448-1454.

805. Vinik A, Zlateva G, Cheung R, et al. Understanding the impact of pain response on changes in function, quality of life, and sleep interference in patients with painful diabetic peripheral neuropathy and post-herpetic neuralgia treated with pregabalin (abstract). American Pain Society 29th Annual Scientific Meeting, Baltimore, MD, 2010.

806. Jensen TS. Anticonvulsants in neuropathic pain: rationale and clinical evidence. *Eur J Pain.* 2002;6:61-68.

807. Chadda VS, Mathur MS. Double blind study of the effects of diphenylhydantoin sodium on diabetic neuropathy. *J Assoc Physicians India.* 1978;26:403-406.

808. Saudek CD, Werns S, Reidenberg MM. Phenytoin in the treatment of diabetic symmetrical polyneuropathy. *Clin Pharmacol Ther.* 1977;22:196-199.

809. Otto M, Bach FW, Jensen TS, Sindrup SH. Valproic acid has no effect on pain in polyneuropathy: a randomized, controlled trial. *Neurology.* 2004;62:285-288.

810. Gorson KC, Schott C, Herman R, et al. Gabapentin in the treatment of painful diabetic neuropathy: a placebo controlled, double blind, crossover trial. *J Neurol Neurosurg Psychiatry.* 1999;66:251-252.

811. Backonja M, Beydoun A, Edwards KR, et al. Gabapentin for the symptomatic treatment of painful neuropathy in patients with diabetes mellitus: a randomized controlled trial. *JAMA.* 1998;280:1831-1836.

812. Vinik A, Fonseca V, LaMoreaux L, et al. Neurontin (gabapentin, GBP) improves quality of life (QOL) in patients with painful diabetic peripheral neuropathy (Abstract). *Diabetes.* 1998;47(Suppl 1):A374.

813. Morello CM, Leckband SG, Stoner CP, et al. Randomized double-blind study comparing the efficacy of gabapentin with amitriptyline on diabetic peripheral neuropathy pain. *Arch Intern Med.* 1999;159:1931-1937.

814. DeToledo JC, Toledo C, DeCerce J, Ramsay RE. Changes in body weight with chronic, high-dose gabapentin therapy. *Ther Drug Monit.* 1997;19:394-396.

815. Eisenberg E, Lurie Y, Braker C, et al. Lamotrigine reduces painful diabetic neuropathy: a randomized, controlled study. *Neurology.* 2001;57:505-509.

816. Eisenberg E, Alon N, Ishay A, et al. Lamotrigine in the treatment of painful diabetic neuropathy. *Eur J Neurol.* 1998;5:167-173.

817. Vinik AI, Tuchman M, Safirstein B, et al. Lamotrigine for treatment of pain associated with diabetic neuropathy: results of two randomized, double-blind, placebo-controlled studies. *Pain.* 2007;128:169-179.

818. Raskin P, Donofrio PD, Rosenthal NR, et al. Topiramate vs placebo in painful diabetic neuropathy: analgesic and metabolic effects. *Neurology.* 2004;63:865-873.

819. Stansberry KB, Shapiro SA, Hill MA, et al. Impaired peripheral vasomotion in diabetes. *Diabetes Care.* 1996;19:715-721.

820. Nelson ME, Fiatarone MA, Morganti CM, et al. Effects of high-intensity strength training on multiple risk factors for osteoporotic fractures. A randomized controlled trial. *JAMA.* 1994;272:1909-1914.

821. Liu-Ambrose T, Khan KM, Eng JJ, et al. Resistance and agility training reduce fall risk in women aged 75 to 85 with low bone mass: a 6-month randomized, controlled trial. *J Am Geriatr Soc.* 2004;52:657-665.

822. Somers DL, Somers MF. Treatment of neuropathic pain in a patient with diabetic neuropathy using transcutaneous electrical nerve stimulation applied to the skin of the lumbar region. *Phys Ther.* 1999;79:767-775.

823. Weintraub M. Alternative medicine. Preliminary findings. *Am J Pain Manage.* 1998;8:12-16.

824. Cloutier R, Horr S, Niemi JB, et al. Prolonged mechanical noise restores tactile sense in diabetic neuropathic patients. *Int J Low Extrem Wounds.* 2009;8(1):6-10.

825. Chaudry V, Corse AM, Cornblath DR. Multifocal motor neuropathy: response to human immune globulin. *Ann Neurol.* 1993;33:237-242.

826. Cornblath DR, Vinik A, Feldman E, et al. Surgical decompression for diabetic sensorimotor polyneuropathy. *Diabetes Care.* 2007;30:421-422.

827. Cavanagh PR, Derr JA, Ulbrecht JS, et al. Problems with gait and posture in neuropathic patients with insulin-dependent diabetes mellitus. *Diabet Med.* 1992;9:469-474.

828. Morrison S, Colberg SR, Mariano M, et al. Balance training reduces falls risk in older individuals with type 2 diabetes. *Diabetes Care.* 2010;33:748-750.

829. Zola BE, Vinik AI. Effects of autonomic neuropathy associated with diabetes mellitus on cardiovascular function. *Coron Artery Dis.* 1992;3:33-41.

830. Stansberry KB, Peppard HR, Babyak LM, et al. Primary nociceptive afferents mediate the blood flow dysfunction in non-glabrous (hairy) skin of type 2 diabetes: a new model for the pathogenesis of microvascular dysfunction. *Diabetes Care.* 1999;22:1549-1554.

831. Haak ES, Usadel KH, Kohleisen M, et al. The effect of alpha-lipoic acid on the neurovascular reflex arc in patients with diabetic neuropathy assessed by capillary microscopy. *Microvasc Res.* 1999;58:28-34.

832. Valensi P. Diabetic autonomic neuropathy: what are the risks? *Diabets Metab.* 1998;24:66-72.

833. Dieleman JP, Kerklaan J, Huygen FJ, et al. Incidence rates and treatment of neuropathic pain conditions in the general population. *Pain.* 2008;137:681-688.

834. Ziegler D, Rathmann W, Dickhaus T, et al. Prevalence of polyneuropathy in pre-diabetes and diabetes is associated with abdominal obesity and macroangiopathy: the MONICA/KORA Augsburg Surveys S2 and S3. *Diabetes Care.* 2008;31:464-469.

835. Granberg V, Ejskjaer N, Peakman M, Sundkvist G. Autoantibodies to autonomic nerves associated with cardiac and peripheral autonomic neuropathy. *Diabetes Care.* 2005;28:1959-1964.

836. Mancia G, Paleari F, Parati G. Early diagnosis of diabetic autonomic neuropathy: present and future approaches. *Diabetologia.* 1997;40:482-484.

837. Garber AJ, Abrahamson MJ, Barzilay JI, et al. AACE comprehensive diabetes management algorithm 2013. *Endocr Pract.* 2013;19:327-336.

838. Athyros VG, Didangelos TP, Karamitsos DT, et al. Long-term effect of converting enzyme inhibition on circadian sympathetic and parasympathetic modulation in patients with diabetic autonomic neuropathy. *Acta Cardiol.* 1998;53:201-209.

839. Malmberg K, Norhammar A, Wedel H, Ryden L. Glycometabolic state at admission: important risk marker of mortality in conventionally treated patients with diabetes mellitus and acute myocardial infarction: long-term results from the Diabetes and Insulin-Glucose Infusion in Acute Myocardial Infarction (DIGAMI) study. *Circulation.* 1999;99:2626-2632.

840. Kendall DM, Rooney DP, Smets YF, et al. Pancreas transplantation restores epinephrine response and symptom recognition during hypoglycemia in patients with long-standing type I diabetes and autonomic neuropathy. *Diabetes.* 1997;46:249-257.

841. Burger AJ, Weinrauch LA, D'Elia JA, Aronson D. Effects of glycemic control on heart rate variability in type I diabetic patients with cardiac autonomic neuropathy. *Am J Cardiol.* 1999;84:687-691.

842. Laederach-Hofmann K, Weidmann P, Ferrari P. Hypovolemia contributes to the pathogenesis of orthostatic hypotension in patients with diabetes mellitus. *Am J Med.* 1999;106:50-58.

843. Denq JC, Opfer-Gehrking TL, Giuliani M, et al. Efficacy of compression of different capacitance beds in the amelioration of orthostatic hypotension. *Clin Auton Res.* 1997;7:321-326.

844. Annese V, Bassotti G, Caruso N, et al. Gastrointestinal motor dysfunction, symptoms, and neuropathy in noninsulin-dependent (type 2) diabetes mellitus. *J Clin Gastroenterol.* 1999;29:171-177.

845. Melga P, Mansi C, Ciuchi E, et al. Chronic administration of levosulpiride and glycemic control in IDDM patients with gastroparesis. *Diabetes Care.* 1997;20:55-58.

846. Stacher G, Schernthaner G, Francesconi M, et al. Cisapride versus placebo for 8 weeks on glycemic control and gastric emptying in insulin-dependent diabetes: a double blind cross-over trial. *J Clin Endocrinol Metab.* 1999;84:2357-2362.

847. Barone JA. Domperidone: a peripherally acting dopamine2-receptor antagonist. *Ann Pharmacother.* 1999;33:429-440.

848. Silvers D, Kipnes M, Broadstone V, et al. Domperidone in the management of symptoms of diabetic gastroparesis: efficacy, tolerability, and quality-of-life outcomes in a multicenter controlled trial. DOM-USA-5 Study Group. *Clin Ther.* 1998;20:438-453.

849. Erbas T, Varoglu E, Erbas B, et al. Comparison of metoclopramide and erythromycin in the treatment of diabetic gastroparesis. *Diabetes Care.* 1993;16:1511-1514.

850. Vinik AI, Richardson D. Erectile dysfunction in diabetes. *Diabetes Rev.* 1998;6:16-33.

851. Vinik AI, Richardson D. Erectile dysfunction in diabetes: pills for penile failure. *Clinica Diabetes.* 1998;16:108-119.

852. Rendell MS, Rajfer J, Wicker PA, Smith MD. Sildenafil Diabetes Study Group. Sildenafil for treatment of erectile dysfunction in men with diabetes: a randomized controlled trial. *JAMA.* 1999;281:421-426.

853. Enzlin P, Mathieu C, Vanderschueren D, Demyttenaere K. Diabetes mellitus and female sexuality: a review of 25 years' research. *Diabet Med.* 1998;15:809-815.

854. Shaw JE, Parker R, Hollis S, et al. Gustatory sweating in diabetes mellitus. *Diabet Med.* 1996;13:1033-1037.

855. Shaw JE, Abbott CA, Tindle K, et al. A randomised controlled trial of topical glycopyrrolate, the first specific treatment for diabetic gustatory sweating. *Diabetologia.* 1997;40:299-301.

856. Meyer C, Hering BJ, Grossmann R, et al. Improved glucose counterregulation and autonomic symptoms after intraportal islet transplants alone in patients with long-standing type I diabetes mellitus. *Transplantation.* 1998;66:233-240.

857. Gu K, Cowie CC, Harris MI. Diabetes and decline in heart disease mortality in US adults. *JAMA.* 1999;281:1291-1297.

858. Scott J, Huskisson EC. Graphic representation of pain. *Pain.* 1976;2:175-186.

859. Malmberg K, Yusuf S, Gerstein HC, et al. Impact of diabetes on long-term prognosis in patients with unstable angina and non-Q-wave myocardial infarction. *Circulation.* 2000;102:1014-1019.

860. Mukamal KJ, Nesto RW, Cohen MC, et al. Impact of diabetes on long-term survival after acute myocardial infarction. *Diabetes Care.* 2001;24:1422-1427.

861. Evans JM, Wang J, Morris AD. Comparison of cardiovascular risk between patients with type 2 diabetes and those who had a myocardial infarction: cross sectional and cohort studies. *BMJ.* 2002;324:939-943.

862. Lee CD, Folsom AR, Pankow JS, et al. Cardiovascular events in diabetic and nondiabetic adults with or without a history of myocardial infarction. *Circulation.* 2004;109:855-860.

863. Krolewski AS, Warram JH, Rand LI, et al. Epidemiologic approach to the etiology of type I diabetes mellitus and its complications. *N Engl J Med.* 1987;317:1390-1398.

864. Orchard TJ, Olson JC, Erbey JR, et al. Insulin resistance-related factors, but not glycemia, predict coronary artery disease in type 1 diabetes. *Diabetes Care.* 2003;26:1374-1379.

865. Soedamah-Muthu SS, Chaturvedi N, Toeller M, et al. EURODIAB Prospective Complications Study Group: risk factors for coronary heart disease in type 1 diabetic patients in Europe: The EURODIAB Prospective Complications Study. *Diabetes Care.* 2004;27:530-537.

866. Pambianco G, Costacou T, Ellis D, et al. The 30-year natural history of type 1 diabetes complications: the Pittsburgh Epidemiology of Diabetes Complications Study experience. *Diabetes.* 2006;55:1463-1469.

867. Laing SP, Swerdlow AJ, Slater SD, et al. Mortality from heart disease in a cohort of 23,000 patients with insulin-treated diabetes. *Diabetologia.* 2003;46:760-765.

868. Lind M, Svensson AM, Kosiborod M, et al. Glycemic control and excess mortality in type 1 diabetes. *N Engl J Med.* 2014;371:1972-1982.

869. Wilson PW, Kannel WB, Silbershatz H, et al. Clustering of metabolic factors and coronary heart disease. *Arch Intern Med.* 1999;159:1104-1109.

870. Haffner SM, Mykkanen L, Festa A, et al. Insulin-resistant prediabetic subjects have more atherogenic risk factors than insulin-sensitive prediabetic subjects. *Circulation.* 2000;101:975-980.

871. Festa A, Hanley AJG, Tracey RP, et al. Inflammation in the prediabetic state is related to increased insulin resistance rather than decreased insulin secretion. *Circulation.* 2003;108:1822-1830.

872. Lim S, Meigs JB. Links between ectopic fat and vascular disease in humans. *Arterioscler Thromb Vasc Biol.* 2014;34(9):1820-1826.

873. Turner RC. The UK Prospective Diabetes Study: a review. *Diabetes Care.* 1998;21(Suppl 3):C35-C38.

874. Andersson DK, Svardsudd K. Long-term glycemic control relates to mortality in type II diabetes. *Diabetes Care.* 1995;18:1534-1543.

875. Wei M, Gaskill SP, Haffner SM, et al. Effects of diabetes and level of glycemia on all-cause and cardiovascular mortality. The San Antonio Heart Study. *Diabetes Care.* 1998;21:1167-1172.

876. Brunner EJ, Shipley MJ, Witte DR, et al. Relation between blood glucose and coronary mortality over 33 years in the Whitehall study. *Diabetes Care.* 2006;29:26-31.

877. Tominaga M, Eguchi H, Manaka H, et al. Impaired glucose tolerance is a risk factor for cardiovascular disease but not impaired fasting glucose. *Diabetes Care.* 1999;22:920-924.

878. DECODE Study Group. Glucose tolerance and mortality: comparison of WHO and American Diabetic Association diagnostic criteria. *Lancet.* 1999;354:617-621.

879. Hu FB, Stampfner MJ, Haffner SM, et al. Elevated risk of cardiovascular disease prior to clinical diagnosis of type 2 diabetes. *Diabetes Care.* 2002;25:1129-1134.

880. Klein R, Klein BE, Moss SE. The Wisconsin Epidemiologic Study of Diabetic Retinopathy: XVI. The relationship of C-peptide to the incidence and progression of diabetic retinopathy. *Diabetes.* 1995;44:796-801.

881. Wingard DL, Barrett-Connor EL, Scheidt-Nave C, et al. Prevalence of cardiovascular and renal complications in older adults with normal or impaired glucose tolerance or NIDDM: a population-based study. *Diabetes Care.* 1993;16:1022-1025.

882. Folsom AR, Eckfeldt JH, Weitzman S, et al. Relation of carotid artery wall thickness to diabetes mellitus, fasting glucose and insulin, body

size, and physical activity. Atherosclerosis Risk in Communities (ARIC) Study Investigators. *Stroke.* 1994;25:66-73.

883. Temelkova-Kurktschiev TS, Koehler C, Leonhardt W, et al. Increased intimal-medial thickness in newly detected type 2 diabetes: risk factors. *Diabetes Care.* 1999;22:333-338.

884. Hanefeld M, Koehler C, Schaper F, et al. Postprandial plasma glucose is an independent risk factor for increased carotid intima-media thickness in non-diabetic individuals. *Atherosclerosis.* 1999;144:229-235.

885. National Cholesterol Education Program (NCEP). Expert Panel on the Detection, Evaluation, and Treatment of High Blood Cholesterol in Adults (Adult Treatment Panel III). Third report of the National Cholesterol Education Program (NCEP) Expert Panel on the Detection, Evaluation, and Treatment of High Blood Cholesterol in Adults (Adult Treatment Panel III) final report. *Circulation.* 2002;106(25):3143-3421.

886. Grundy SM, Brewer HB, Cleeman JI, et al. Definition of metabolic syndrome. Report of the National Heart, Lung, and Blood Institute/American Heart Association Conference on Scientific Issues Related to Definition. *Circulation.* 2004;109:433-438.

887. International Diabetes Foundation. The IDF worldwide definition of the metabolic syndrome. Available at <http://www.idf.org/metabolic-syndrome>.

888. American Diabetes Association. Standards of medical care in diabetes—2011. *Diabetes Care.* 2011;34(Suppl 1):S11-S61.

889. Ford ES, Giles WH, Dietz WH. Prevelence of the metabolic syndrome among US adults: findings from the Third National Health and Nutrition Examination Survey. *JAMA.* 2002;287:356-359.

890. Lakka HM, Laaksonen DE, Lakka TA, et al. The metabolic syndrome and total and cardiovascular disease mortality in middle-aged men. *JAMA.* 2002;288(21):2709-2716.

891. Malik S, Wong ND, Franklin SS, et al. Impact of the metabolic syndrome on mortality from coronary heart disease, cardiovascular disease, and all causes in United States adults. *Circulation.* 2004;110:1245-1250.

892. Sattar N, Gaw A, Scherbakova O, et al. Metabolic syndrome with and without C-reactive protein as a predictor of coronary heart disease and diabetes in the West of Scotland Coronary Prevention Study. *Circulation.* 2003;108:414-419.

893. Ford ES. Risk for all-cause mortality, cardiovascular disease, and diabetes associated with the metabolic syndrome. *Diabetes Care.* 2005;28:1769-1778.

894. Grundy SM, Cleeman JI, Daniels SR, et al. Diagnosis and management of the metabolic syndrome. An American Heart Association/National Heart, Lung, and Blood Institute scientific statement. *Circulation.* 2005;112:2735-2752.

895. Deedwania PC. The deadly quartet revisited. *Am J Med.* 1998;105:1S-3S.

896. Howard G, O'Leary DH, Zaccaro D, et al. Insulin sensitivity and atherosclerosis. The Insulin Resistance Atherosclerosis Study (IRAS) Investigators. *Circulation.* 1996;93:1809-1817.

897. Abraira C, Colwell J, Nuttall F, et al. Cardiovascular events and correlates in the Veterans Affairs Diabetes Feasibility Trial. Veterans Affairs Cooperative Study on Glycemic Control and Complications in Type II Diabetes. *Arch Intern Med.* 1997;157:181-188.

898. Diabetes Control and Complications Trial/Epidemiology of Diabetes Interventions and Complications (DCCT/EDIC) Study Research Group. Intensive diabetes treatment and cardiovascular disease in patients with type 1 diabetes. *N Eng J Med.* 2005;353:2643-2653.

899. Dormandy JA, Charbonnel B, Eckland DJA, et al. Secondary prevention of macrovascular events in patients with type 2 diabetes in the PROactive Study (PROspective pioglitAzone Clinical Trial In macroVascular Events): a randomized controlled trial. *Lancet.* 2005;366(9493):1279-1289.

900. Nissen SE, Nicholls SJ, Wolski K, et al. PERISCOPE Investigators. Comparison of pioglitazone vs glimepiride on progression of coronary atherosclerosis in patients with type 2 diabetes: the PERISCOPE randomized controlled trial. *JAMA.* 2008;299(13):1561-1573.

901. Lago RM, Singh PP, Nesto RW. Congestive heart failure and cardiovascular death in patients with prediabetes and type 2 diabetes given thiazolidinediones: a meta-analysis of randomised clinical trials. *Lancet.* 2007;370:1129-1136.

902. Mitka M. Panel recommends easing restrictions on rosiglitazone despite concerns about cardiovascular safety. *JAMA.* 2013;310:246-247.

903. Kung J, Henry RR. Thiazolidinedione safety. *Exp Opin Drug Saf.* 2012;11:565-579.

904. Duckworth W, Abraira C, Moritz T, et al. Glucose control and vascular complications in veterans with type 2 diabetes. *N Engl J Med.* 2009;360:129-139.

905. Scirica BM, Bhatt DL, Braunwald E, et al. SAVOR-TIMI 53 Steering Committee and Investigators. Saxagliptin and cardiovascular outcomes in patients with type 2 diabetes mellitus. *N Engl J Med.* 2013;369(14):1317-1326.

906. White WB, Cannon CP, Heller SR, et al. EXAMINE Investigators. Alogliptin after acute coronary syndrome in patients with type 2 diabetes. *N Engl J Med.* 2013;369(14):1327-1335.

907. Zannad F, Cannon CP, Cushman WC, et al. EXAMINE Investigators. Heart failure and mortality outcomes in patients with type 2 diabetes taking alogliptin versus placebo in EXAMINE: a multicentre, randomised, double-blind trial. *Lancet.* 2015;385:2067-2076.

908. Scirica BM, Braunwald E, Raz I, et al. Heart failure, saxagliptin, and diabetes mellitus: observations from the SAVOR-TIMI 53 randomized trial. *Circulation.* 2014;130:1579-1588.

909. Smilowitz NR, Donnino R. Schwartzbard A. Glucagon-like peptide-1 receptor agonists for diabetes mellitus: a role in cardiovascular disease. *Circulation.* 2014;129:2305-2312.

910. Inzucchi SE, Zinman B, Wanner C, et al. SGLT-2 inhibitors and cardiovascular risk: proposed pathways and review of ongoing outcome trials. *Diabetes Vasc Dis Res.* 2015;12:90-100.

911. Duckworth WC, Abraira C, Moritz TE, et al. The duration of diabetes affects the response to intensive glucose control in type 2 subjects: the VA Diabetes Trial. *J Diabetes Complications.* 2011;25:355-361.

912. Reaven PD, Moritz TE, Schwenke DC, et al. Veterans Affairs Diabetes Trial. Intensive glucose-lowering therapy reduces cardiovascular disease events in veterans affairs diabetes trial participants with lower calcified coronary atherosclerosis. *Diabetes.* 2009;58(11):2642-2648.

913. ORIGIN Trial Investigators, Bosch J, Gerstein HC, et al. n-3 fatty acids and cardiovascular outcomes in patients with dysglycemia. *N Engl J Med.* 2012;367(4):309-318.

914. Gowri MS, Van der Westhuyzen DR, Bridges SR, et al. Decreased protection by HDL from poorly controlled type 2 diabetic subjects against LDL oxidation may be due to the abnormal composition of HDL. *Arterioscler Thromb Vasc Biol.* 1999;19:2226-2233.

915. Long-Term Intervention with Pravastatin in Ischemic Disease (LIPID) Study Group. Prevention of cardiovascular events and death in pravastatin patients with coronary heart disease and a broad range of initial cholesterol levels. *N Engl J Med.* 1998;339:1349-1357.

916. Haffner SM, Alexander CM, Cook TJ, et al. Reduced coronary events in simvastatin-treated patients with coronary heart disease and diabetes or impaired glucose levels. *Arch Intern Med.* 1999;159:2661-2667.

917. Ballantyne CM, Olsson AG, Cook TJ, et al. Influence of low high-density lipoprotein cholesterol and elevated triglyceride on coronary heart disease events and response to simvastatin therapy in 4S. *Circulation.* 2001;104:3046-3051.

918. Deedwania P, Barter P, Carmena R, et al. Reduction of low-density lipoprotein cholesterol in patients with coronary heart disease and metabolic syndrome: analysis of the Treating to New Targets study. *Lancet.* 2006;368:919-928.

919. Taylor AJ, Sullenberger LE, Lee HJ, et al. Arterial Biology for the Investigation of the Treatment Effects of Reducing Cholesterol (ARBITER 2): a double-blind, placebo-controlled study of extended-release niacin on atherosclerosis progression in secondary prevention patients treated with statins. [Errata in *Circulation.* 2004;110:3615, *Circulation.* 2005;111:e446.]. *Circulation.* 2004;110(23):3512-3517.

920. Rubins HB, Robins SJ, Collins D, et al. Gemfibrozil for the secondary prevention of coronary heart disease in men with low levels of high-density lipoprotein cholesterol. Veterans Affairs High-Density Lipoprotein Cholesterol Intervention Trial Study Group. *N Engl J Med.* 1999;341:410-418.

921. Heart Protection Study Collaborative Group. MRC/BHF Heart protection study of cholesterol lowering with simvastatin in 20,536 high-risk individuals: a randomized, placebo-controlled study. *Lancet.* 2002;360:7-22.

922. Calhoun HM, Betteridge DJ, Durrington PN, et al. Primary prevention of cardiovascular disease with atorvastatin in type 2 diabetes in the Collaborative Atorvastatin Diabetes Study (CARDS): multicentre randomised placebo-controlled trial. *Lancet.* 2004;364:685-696.

923. Sarikaya H, Ferro J, Arnold M. Stroke prevention—medical and lifestyle measures. *Eur Neurol.* 2015;73:150-157.

924. Goff DC Jr, Lloyd-Jones DM, Bennett G, et al. 2013 ACC/AHA guideline on the assessment of cardiovascular risk: a report of the American College of Cardiology/American Heart Association Task Force on Practice Guidelines. *Circulation.* 2014;129:S49-S73.

925. Masana L, Pedro-Botet J, Civeira F. IMPROVE-IT clinical implications. Should the "high-intensity cholesterol-lowering therapy" strategy replace the "high-intensity statin therapy"? *Atherosclerosis.* 2015;240:161-162.

926. HPS2-THRIVE Collaborative Group, Landray MJ, Haynes R, et al. Effects of extended-release niacin with laropiprant in high-risk patients. *N Engl J Med.* 2014;371(3):203-212.

927. The AIM-HIGH Investigators. The role of niacin in raising high-density lipoprotein cholesterol to reduce cardiovascular events in patients with atherosclerotic cardiovascular disease and optimally treated low-density lipoprotein cholesterol, Rationale and study design. The atherothrombosis intervention in metabolic syndrome with low HDL/high triglycerides: impact on global health outcomes (AIM-HIGH). *Am Heart J.* 2011;161(3):471-477.

928. Voight BF, Peloso GM, Orho-Melander M, et al. Plasma HDL cholesterol and risk of myocardial infarction: a mendelian randomisation study. *Lancet.* 2012;380:572-580.

929. Rader DJ, Hovingh GK. HDL and cardiovascular disease. *Lancet.* 2014; 384:618-625.

930. Jorgensen AB, Frikke-Schmidt R, Nordestgaard BG, Tybjaerg-Hansen A. Loss-of-function mutations in APOC3 and risk of ischemic vascular disease. *N Engl J Med.* 2014;371:32-41.

931. TG and HDL Working Group of the Exome Sequencing Project, National Heart, Lung, and Blood Institute, Crosby J, Peloso GM, et al. Loss-of-function mutations in APOC3, triglycerides, and coronary disease. *N Engl J Med.* 2014;371(1):22-31.

932. Ginsberg HN, Elam MB, Lovato LC, et al. Effects of combination lipid therapy in type 2 diabetes mellitus. *N Engl J Med.* 2010;362: 1563-1574.

933. Grundy SM, Cleeman JI, Merz MB, et al. Implications of recent clinical trials for the National Cholesterol Education Program Adult Treatment Panel III Guidelines. *Circulation.* 2004;110:227-239.

934. Chobanian AV, Bakris GL, Black HR, et al. The Seventh Report of the Joint National Committee on Prevention, Detection, Evaluation, and Treatment of High Blood Pressure (JNC VII). *JAMA.* 2003;289(19): 2560-2572.

935. Heart Outcomes Prevention Evaluation Study Investigators. Effects of an angiotensin-converting enzyme inhibitor, ramipril, on cardiovascular events in high-risk patients. *N Engl J Med.* 2000;342:145-153.

936. UK Prospective Diabetes Study (UKPDS) Group. Efficacy of atenolol and captopril in reducing risk of macrovascular and microvascular complications in type 2 diabetes: UKPDS 39. *BMJ.* 1998;317: 713-720.

937. Hansson L, Zanchetti A, Carruthers SG, et al. Effects of intensive blood pressure lowering and low-dose aspirin in patients with hypertension: principal results of the Hypertension Optimal Treatment (HOT) randomised trial. HOT Study Group. *Lancet.* 1998;351: 1755-1762.

938. Whelton PK, Barzilay J, Cushman WC, et al. Clinical outcomes in antihypertensive treatment of type 2 diabetes, impaired fasting glucose concentration, and normoglycemia. *Arch Intern Med.* 2005; 165:1401-1409.

939. ACCORD Study Group, Cushman WC, Evans GW, et al. Effects of intensive blood-pressure control in type 2 diabetes mellitus. *N Engl J Med.* 2010;362(17):1575-1585.

940. Nesto RW, Zarich S. Acute myocardial infarction in diabetes mellitus: lessons learned from ACE inhibition. *Circulation.* 1998;97:12-15.

941. Jacoby RM, Nesto RW. Acute myocardial infarction in the diabetic patient: pathophysiology, clinical course and prognosis. *J Am Coll Cardiol.* 1992;20:736-744.

942. Iwasaka T, Takahashi N, Nakamura S, et al. Residual left ventricular pump function after acute myocardial infarction in NIDDM patients. *Diabetes Care.* 1992;15:1522-1526.

943. Bernardi L, Ricordi L, Lazzari P, et al. Impaired circadian modulation of sympathovagal activity in diabetes: a possible explanation for altered temporal onset of cardiovascular disease. *Circulation.* 1992; 86:1443-1452.

944. Zarich S, Waxman S, Freeman RT, et al. Effect of autonomic nervous system dysfunction on the circadian pattern of myocardial ischemia in diabetes mellitus. *J Am Coll Cardiol.* 1994;24:956-962.

945. Muller JE, Tofler GH, Stone PH. Circadian variation and triggers of onset of acute cardiovascular disease. *Circulation.* 1989;79:733-743.

946. Imperatore G, Riccardi G, Iovine C, et al. Plasma fibrinogen—a new factor of the metabolic syndrome: a population-based study. *Diabetes Care.* 1998;21:649-654.

947. Sobel BE, Woodcock-Mitchell J, Schneider DJ, et al. Increased plasminogen activator inhibitor type 1 in coronary artery atherectomy specimens from type 2 diabetic compared with nondiabetic patients: a potential factor predisposing to thrombosis and its persistence. *Circulation.* 1998;97:2213-2221.

948. Meigs JB, Mittleman MA, Nathan DM, et al. Hyperinsulinemia, hyperglycemia, and impaired hemostasis. The Framingham Offspring Study. *JAMA.* 2000;283:221-228.

949. Woodfield SL, Lundergan CF, Reiner JS, et al. Angiographic findings and outcome in diabetic patients treated with thrombolytic therapy for acute myocardial infarction: the GUSTO-I experience. *J Am Coll Cardiol.* 1996;28:1661-1669.

950. Mak KH, Moliterno DJ, Granger CB, et al. Influence of diabetes mellitus on clinical outcome in the thrombolytic era of acute myocardial infarction. GUSTO-I Investigators. Global Utilization of Streptokinase and Tissue Plasminogen Activator for Occluded Coronary Arteries. *J Am Coll Cardiol.* 1997;30(1):171-179.

951. Sun D, Nguyen N, DeGrado T, et al. Ischemia-induced translocation of the insulin-responsive glucose transporter GLUT4 in the plasma membrane of cardiac myocytes. *Circulation.* 1994;89:793-798.

952. Oliver M, Opie H. Effects of glucose and fatty acids on myocardial ischaemia and arrhythmias. *Lancet.* 1994;343:155-158.

953. Bellodi G, Manicardi V, Malavasi V, et al. Hyperglycemia and prognosis of acute myocardial infarction in patients without diabetes mellitus. *Am J Cardiol.* 1989;64:885-888.

954. Oswald GA, Smith CC, Betteridge DJ, et al. Determinants and importance of stress hyperglycaemia in non-diabetic patients with myocardial infarction. *BMJ.* 1986;293:917-922.

955. Fava S, Aquilina O, Azzopardi J, et al. The prognostic value of blood glucose in diabetic patients with acute myocardial infarction. *Diabetes Med.* 1996;13:80-83.

956. Capes SE, Hunt D, Malmberg K, et al. Stress hyperglycemia and increased risk of death after myocardial infarction in patients with and without diabetes: a systematic overview. *Lancet.* 2000;355: 773-778.

957. Malmberg K, Ryden L, Efendic S, et al. Randomized trial of insulin-glucose infusion followed by subcutaneous insulin treatment in diabetic patients with acute myocardial infarction (DIGAMI study): effects on mortality at 1 year. *J Am Coll Cardiol.* 1995;26:57-65.

958. Malmberg K, Ryden L, Wedel H, et al. Intense metabolic control by means of insulin in patients with diabetes mellitus and acute myocardial infarction (DIGAMI 2): effects on mortality and morbidity. *Eur Heart J.* 2005;26:650-661.

959. CREATE-ECLA Trial Group Investigators. Effect of glucose-insulin-potassium infusion on mortality in patients with ST-segment elevation myocardial infarction. *JAMA.* 2005;293:437-446.

960. Garratt KN, Brady PA, Hassinger NL, et al. Sulfonylurea drugs increase early mortality in patients with diabetes mellitus after direct angioplasty for acute myocardial infarction. *J Am Coll Cardiol.* 1999;33: 119-124.

961. Cleveland JC Jr, Meldrum DR, Cain BS, et al. Oral sulfonylurea hypoglycemic agents prevent ischemic preconditioning in human myocardium: two paradoxes revisited. *Circulation.* 1997;96:29-32.

962. Katsuda Y, Egashira K, Ueno H, et al. Glibenclamide, a selective inhibitor of ATP-sensitive K+ channels, attenuates metabolic coronary vasodilatation induced by pacing tachycardia in dogs. *Circulation.* 1995; 92:511-517.

963. Davis IIICA, Sherman AJ, Yaroshenko Y, et al. Coronary vascular responsiveness to adenosine is impaired additively by blockade of nitric oxide synthesis and a sulfonylurea. *Am J Cardiol.* 1998; 31:816-822.

964. O'Driscoll G, Green D, Maiorana A, et al. Improvement in endothelial function by angiotensin-converting enzyme inhibition in non-insulin-dependent diabetes mellitus. *J Am Coll Cardiol.* 1999;33: 1506-1511.

965. Vaughan DE, Rouleau JL, Ridker PM, et al. Effects of ramipril on plasma fibrinolytic balance in patients with acute anterior myocardial infarction. HEART Study Investigators. *Circulation.* 1997;96: 442-447.

966. Torlone E, Britta M, Rambotti AM, et al. Improved insulin action and glycemic control after long-term angiotensin-converting enzyme inhibition in subjects with arterial hypertension and type II diabetes. *Diabetes Care.* 1993;16:1347-1355.

967. Zuanetti G, Latini R, Maggioni A, et al. Effect of the ACE-inhibitor lisinopril on mortality in diabetic patients with acute myocardial infarction: the data from the GISSI-3 study. *Circulation.* 1997;96: 4239-4245.

968. Gustafsson I, Torp-Pedersen C, Kober L, et al. Effect of the angiotensin-converting enzyme inhibitor trandolapril on mortality and morbidity in diabetic patients with left ventricular dysfunction after acute myocardial infarction. Trace Study Group. *J Am Coll Cardiol.* 1999;34: 83-89.

969. Lakshman MR, Reda DJ, Materson BJ, et al. Diuretics and β-blockers do not have adverse effects at 1 year on plasma lipid and lipoprotein profiles in men with hypertension. Department of Veterans Affairs Cooperative Study Group on Antihypertensive Agents. *Arch Intern Med.* 1999;159:551-558.

970. Shorr RI, Ray WA, Daugherty JR, et al. Antihypertensives and the risk of serious hypoglycemia in older persons using insulin or sulfonylureas. *JAMA.* 1997;278:40-43.

971. Chen J, Marciniak TA, Radford MJ, et al. β-Blocker therapy for secondary prevention of myocardial infarction in elderly diabetic patients. Results from the National Cooperative Cardiovascular Project. *J Am Coll Cardiol.* 1999;34:1388-1394.

972. Giugliano D, Acampora R, Marfella R. Metabolic and cardiovascular effects of carvedilol and atenolol in non-insulin-dependent diabetes mellitus and hypertension. *Ann Intern Med.* 1997;126:955-959.

973. ETDRS Investigators. Aspirin effects on mortality and morbidity in patients with diabetes mellitus. Early Treatment Diabetic Retinopathy Study report 14. *JAMA.* 1992;268:1292-1300.

974. American Diabetes Association. Aspirin therapy in diabetes. *Diabetes Care.* 1997;20:772-773.

975. Davi G, Catalano I, Averna M, et al. Thromboxane biosynthesis and platelet function in type II diabetes mellitus. *N Engl J Med.* 1990; 322:1769-1774.

976. Grosser T, Fries S, Lawson JA, et al. Drug resistance and pseudoresistance: an unintended consequence of enteric coating aspirin. *Circulation.* 2013;127:377-385.

977. Hirsh J, Bhatt DL. Comparative benefits of clopidogrel and aspirin in high-risk patient populations: lessons from the CAPRIE and CURE studies. *Arch Intern Med.* 2004;164:2106-2110.

978. Platelet Receptor Inhibition in Ischemic Syndrome Management in Patients Limited by Unstable Signs and Symptoms (PRISM-PLUS) Study Investigators. Inhibition of the platelet glycoprotein IIb/IIIa receptor with tirofiban in unstable angina and non-Q-wave myocardial infarction. *N Engl J Med.* 1998;338:1488-1497.

979. EPILOG Investigators. Platelet glycoprotein IIb/IIIa receptor blockade and low-dose heparin during percutaneous coronary revascularization. *N Engl J Med.* 1997;336:1689-1696.

980. Lincoff AM, Califf RM, Moliterno DJ, et al. Complementary clinical benefits of coronary artery stenting and blockade of platelet glycoprotein IIb/IIIa receptors. Evaluation of Platelet IIb/IIIa Inhibition in Stenting Investigators. *N Engl J Med.* 1999;341:319-327.

981. Bypass Angioplasty Revascularization Investigation (BARI) Investigators. Comparison of coronary bypass surgery with angioplasty in patients with multivessel disease. *N Engl J Med.* 1996;335:217-225.

982. Kannel WB, Hjortland M, Castelli WP. Role of diabetes in congestive heart failure: the Framingham study. *Am J Cardiol.* 1974;34:29-34.

983. Seferovic PM, Paulus WJ. Clinical diabetic cardiomyopathy: a two-faced disease with restrictive and dilated phenotypes. *Eur Heart J.* 2015;36(27):1718-1727.

984. Aronson D, Rayfield E, Cheseboro J. Mechanisms determining course and outcome of diabetic patients who have had acute myocardial infarction. *Ann Intern Med.* 1997;126:296-306.

985. Cabin H, Roberts W. Quantitative comparison of extent of coronary narrowing and size of healed myocardial infarct in 33 necropsy patients with clinically recognized and in 28 with clinically unrecognized ("silent") previous acute myocardial infarction. *Am J Cardiol.* 1982;50:677-681.

986. van Hoeven KH, Factor SM. A comparison of the pathological spectrum of hypertensive, diabetic, and hypertensive-diabetic heart disease. *Circulation.* 1990;82:848-855.

987. Kawaguchi M, Techigawara M, Ishihata T, et al. A comparison of ultrastructural changes on endomyocardial biopsy specimens obtained from patients with diabetes mellitus with and without hypertension. *Heart Vessels.* 1997;12(6):267-274.

988. Paulus WJ, Tschope C. A novel paradigm for heart failure with preserved ejection fraction: comorbidities drive myocardial dysfunction and remodeling through coronary microvascular endothelial inflammation. *J Am Coll Cardiol.* 2013;62:263-271.

989. Nahser P, Brown R, Oskarsson H, et al. Maximal coronary flow reserve and metabolic coronary vasodilation in patients with diabetes mellitus. *Circulation.* 1995;91:635-640.

990. Depre C, Vanoverschelde JL, Taegtmeyer H. Glucose for the heart. *Circulation.* 1999;99:578-588.

991. Azzarelli A, Dini F, Cristofani R, et al. NIDDM as unfavorable factor to the postinfarction ventricular function in the elderly: echocardiography study. *Coron Artery Dis.* 1995;6:629-634.

992. Korup E, Dalsgaard D, Nyvad O, et al. Comparison of degrees of left ventricular dilation within three hours and up to six days after onset of first acute myocardial infarction. *Am J Cardiol.* 1997;80:449-453.

993. Mayfield JA, Reiber GE, Maynard C, et al. Trends in lower limb amputation in the Veterans Health Administration, 1989-1998. *J Rehabil Res Dev.* 2000;37:23-30.

994. van Houtum WH, Rauwerda JA, Ruwaard D, et al. Reduction in diabetes-related lower-extremity amputations in The Netherlands. *Diabetes Care.* 2004;27:1042-1046.

995. Krishnan S, Nash F, Baker N, et al. Reduction in diabetic amputations over 11 years in a defined UK population: benefits of multidisciplinary team work and continuous prospective audit. *Diabetes Care.* 2008;31:99-101.

996. Vileikyte L. Psychosocial and behavioral aspects of diabetic foot lesions. *Curr Diab Rep.* 2008;8:119-125.

997. Boulton AJM, Cavanagh PR, Rayman G, eds. *The Foot in Diabetes.* 4th ed. Chichester, UK: John Wiley & Sons; 2006.

998. Bowker JH, Pfeifer MA, eds. *Levin & O'Neal's The Diabetic Foot.* 7th ed. St. Louis, MO: Mosby; 2008.

999. The diabetic foot. *Diabetes Metab Res Rev.* 2012;28(Suppl 1):S1-S235.

1000. Boulton AJM. The diabetic foot. *Med Clin North Am.* 2013;97(5):775-992.

1001. Abbott CA, Carrington AL, Ashe H, et al. The North-West diabetes foot care study: incidence of, and risk factors for, new diabetic foot ulceration in a community-based cohort. *Diabet Med.* 2002;20:277-384.

1002. Jude EB, Eleftheriadou I, Tentolouris N. Peripheral arterial disease in diabetes: a review. *Diabet Med.* 2010;27:4-14.

1003. Albayati MA, Shearman CP. Peripheral arterial disease and bypass surgery in the diabetic lower limb. *Med Clin North Am.* 2013;97:821-834.

1004. Ndip A, Lavery LA, Lafontaine J, et al. High levels of foot ulceration and amputation risk in a multiracial cohort of diabetic patients on dialysis therapy. *Diabetes Care.* 2010;33:878-880.

1005. Boulton AJM. The diabetic foot: from art to science. *Diabetologia.* 2004;47:1343-1353.

1006. Reiber GE, Vileikyte L, Boyko EJ, et al. Causal pathways for incident lower extremity ulcers in patients with diabetes from two settings. *Diabetes Care.* 1999;22:157-162.

1007. Boulton AJM, Armstrong DG, Albert SG, et al. Comprehensive Foot Examination and Risk Assessment: a report of the Task Force of the Foot Care Interest Group of the American Diabetes Association, with endorsement by the American Association of Clinical Endocrinologists. *Diabetes Care.* 2008;31:1679-1686.

1008. Oyibo S, Jude EB, Tarawneh I, et al. A comparision of two diabetic foot ulcer classification systems: the Wagner and the University of Texas wound classification systems. *Diabetes Care.* 2001;24:84-88.

1009. Piaggesi A, Viacava P, Rizzo L, et al. Semi-quantitative analysis of the histopathological features of the neuropathic foot ulcer: effects of pressure relief. *Diabetes Care.* 2003;26:3123-3128.

1010. Armstrong DG, Nguyen HC, Lavery LA, et al. Off-loading the diabetic foot wound: a randomized clinical trial. *Diabetes Care.* 2001;24:1019-1022.

1011. Katz I, Harlan A, Miranda-Palma B, et al. A randomized trial of two irremovable offloading devices in the treatment of plantar neuropathic diabetic foot ulcers. *Diabetes Care.* 2005;28:555-559.

1012. Lipsky BA. New developments in diagnosing and treating diabetic foot infections. *Diabetes Metab Res Rev.* 2008;24(Suppl 1):S66-S71.

1013. Teh J, Berendt T, Lipsky BA. Rational imaging: investigating suspected bone infection in the diabetic foot. *BMJ.* 2010;340:415-417.

1014. Lazaro-Martinez JL, Aragon-Sanchez J, Garcia-Morales E. Antibiotics versus conservative surgery for treating diabetic foot osteomyelitis: a randomized comparative trial. *Diabetes Care.* 2014;37:789-795.

1015. Langer A, Rogowski W. Systematic review of economic evaluations of human cell-derived wound care products for the treatment of venous leg and diabetic foot ulcers. *BMC Health Serv Res.* 2009;9:115.

1016. Armstrong DG, Lavery LA. Negative pressure wound therapy after partial diabetic foot amputation: a multicentre, randomised controlled trial. *Lancet.* 2005;366:1704-1710.

1017. Blume PA, Walters J, Payne W, et al. Comparison of negative pressure wound therapy using vacuum-assisted closure with advanced moist wound therapy in the treatment of diabetic foot ulcers: a multicentre randomised controlled trial. *Diabetes Care.* 2008;31:631-636.

1018. Ndip A, Williams A, Jude EB, et al. The RANKL/RANK/OPG signalling pathway mediates medial arterial calcification in diabetic Charcot neuroarthropathy. *Diabetes.* 2011;60:2365-2369.

1019. Frykberg RG, ed. *The Diabetic Charcot Foot: Principles and Management.* Brooklandville, MD: Data Trace Publishing; 2010.

Hypoglycemia

PHILIP E. CRYER

KEY POINTS

- Hypoglycemia—a plasma glucose concentration low enough to cause symptoms or signs—is common in sulfonylurea-, glinide-, or insulin-treated diabetes but otherwise is uncommon.
- Hypoglycemia in diabetes is typically the result of the interplay of therapeutic hyperinsulinemia and compromised defenses against falling glucose levels resulting in hypoglycemia-associated autonomic failure (HAAF) including defective glucose counterregulation and impaired awareness of hypoglycemia.
- Induced by recent antecedent hypoglycemia, sleep, or prior exercise, an attenuated sympathoadrenal response to falling glucose levels, the key feature of HAAF, is reversible by short-term scrupulous avoidance of hypoglycemia.
- Iatrogenic hypoglycemia is associated with both morbidity as well as fatality in type 1 and type 2 diabetes.
- The practice of hypoglycemic risk reduction in persons with diabetes at risk of hypoglycemia includes addressing the issue, applying the principles of aggressive glycemic therapy, and considering the conventional risk factors and those indicative of HAAF.
- In the absence of diabetes, hypoglycemia in ill or medicated individuals can be caused by many drugs, critical illnesses, endocrine deficiencies, or non–islet cell tumors; in seemingly well individuals it may be caused by endogenous hyperinsulinism or by various accidental, surreptitious, or malicious mechanisms.
- The decision to evaluate a given nondiabetic person systematically—seeking evidence of endogenous insulin excess during hypoglycemia—is recommended only for persons in whom Whipple triad (symptoms, signs, or both consistent with hypoglycemia; a low reliably measured plasma glucose; and resolution of those symptoms or signs after the glucose concentrations is raised) can be documented.
- Short-term treatment of hypoglycemia includes oral carbohydrates or parenteral glucagon or glucose; long-term treatment requires correction of the hypoglycemic mechanism.

Glucose is an obligate metabolic fuel for the brain under physiologic conditions.[1-4] Because the brain cannot synthesize glucose, store more than a few minutes' supply as glycogen, or utilize physiologic concentrations of circulating fuels effectively, survival of the brain, and therefore the individual, requires a virtually continuous supply of glucose from the circulation.[1-4] Blood-to-brain glucose transport is a direct function of the arterial plasma glucose concentration and requires maintenance of the plasma glucose concentration within, or above, the physiologic range. Hypoglycemia causes functional brain failure, which is typically corrected after the plasma glucose concentration is raised.[5] Rarely, it causes a fatal cardiac arrhythmia or, if it is profound and prolonged, brain death.[5]

Given the survival value of maintenance of the plasma glucose concentration, it is not surprising that physiologic and behavioral mechanisms that normally prevent or rapidly correct hypoglycemia[4] have evolved. These mechanisms are so effective that hypoglycemia is an uncommon clinical event except in persons who use drugs that lower the plasma glucose concentration, such as insulin, sulfonylureas, or alcohol.[2,3]

A clinical practice guideline for the evaluation and management of hypoglycemic disorders has been published,[2] and the topic of hypoglycemia in diabetes has been reviewed in detail.[3]

PHYSIOLOGY OF DEFENSE AGAINST HYPOGLYCEMIA

Glucose Metabolism

Glucose is derived from three sources: intestinal absorption that occurs after digestion of dietary carbohydrates; *glycogenolysis*, which is the breakdown of glycogen, the polymerized storage form of glucose; and *gluconeogenesis*, which is the formation of glucose from precursors including lactate (and pyruvate), amino acids (especially alanine and glutamine), and to a lesser extent, glycerol. There are multiple fates of glucose transported into cells (external losses are normally negligible) (Fig. 34-1). Glucose may be stored as glycogen, or it may undergo glycolysis to pyruvate, which can be reduced to lactate, transaminated to form alanine, or converted to acetyl coenzyme A (CoA). Acetyl CoA in turn may be oxidized to carbon dioxide and water through the tricarboxylic acid cycle, converted to fatty acids that can be incorporated into triglycerides, oxidized, or utilized for synthesis of ketone bodies (acetoacetate, β-hydroxybutyrate) or cholesterol. Finally, glucose may be released into the circulation. Only liver and kidneys express

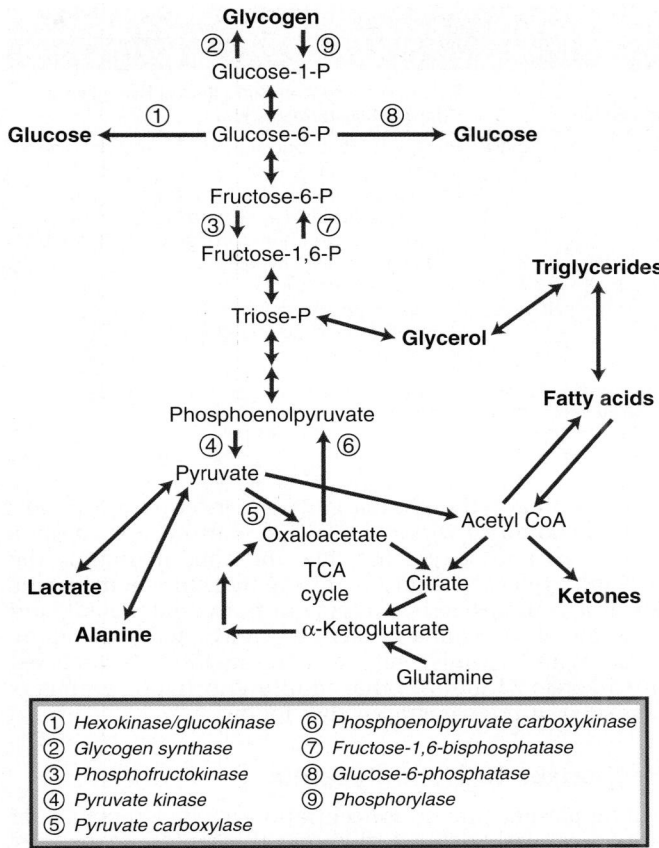

Figure 34-1 Schematic representation of glucose metabolism. CoA, coenzyme A; P, phosphate; TCA, tricarboxylic acid.

① Hexokinase/glucokinase
② Glycogen synthase
③ Phosphofructokinase
④ Pyruvate kinase
⑤ Pyruvate carboxylase
⑥ Phosphoenolpyruvate carboxykinase
⑦ Fructose-1,6-bisphosphatase
⑧ Glucose-6-phosphatase
⑨ Phosphorylase

TABLE 34-1

Systemic Glucose Balance* and Effects of Circulating Hormones on Endogenous Production and Use of Glucose

Source of Glucose Influx or Efflux	Hormonal Effects		
	Insulin	Glucagon	Epinephrine
Glucose Influx Into the Circulation			
Exogenous glucose delivery			
Endogenous glucose delivery			
In liver: glycogenolysis and gluconeogenesis	↓	↑	↑
In kidneys: gluconeogenesis	↓		↑
Glucose Efflux out of the Circulation			
Ongoing brain glucose utilization			
Variable glucose utilization by other tissues (e.g., muscle fat, liver, kidneys)	↑		↓

*Total glucose influx = total glucose efflux.

glucose-6-phosphatase, the enzyme necessary for the release of glucose into the circulation, at levels sufficient to permit substantial contributions to the systemic glucose pool. Many tissues express the enzymes required to synthesize and hydrolyze glycogen (glycogen synthase and phosphorylase, respectively). The liver and kidneys also express the enzymes necessary for gluconeogenesis, including the critical gluconeogenic enzymes pyruvate carboxylase, phosphoenolpyruvate carboxykinase, and fructose-1, 6-bisphosphatase.

The liver is the major source of net endogenous glucose production (through glycogenolysis and gluconeogenesis).[6] Conversely, the liver can be an organ of net glucose uptake. The kidneys also produce glucose (through gluconeogenesis) and utilize glucose.[7]

Muscle can take up and store glucose as glycogen, or it can metabolize glucose (through glycolysis) to pyruvate, which, among other fates, can be reduced to lactate or transaminated to form alanine. Lactate (and pyruvate) released from muscle can be transported to the liver and the kidneys, where it serves as a gluconeogenic precursor (the Cori or glucose-lactate cycle). Alanine, glutamine, and other amino acids can also flow from muscle to liver and kidneys, where they serve as gluconeogenic precursors. These constitute the glucose-alanine and glucose-glutamine cycles. Clearly, net new glucose formation is from precursors (e.g., amino acids) in which the carbons are not derived from glucose via these cycles. Although quantitatively less important than muscle, fat can also take up and metabolize glucose.

Glucose is essentially the sole metabolic fuel for the brain under physiologic conditions.[1] Glucose largely undergoes terminal oxidation in the brain. Although the adult human brain constitutes only about 2.5% of body weight, its oxidative metabolism accounts for approximately 25% of the basal metabolic rate and more than 50% of whole-body glucose utilization. The brain can utilize alternative fuels if their circulating levels rise high enough for them to enter the brain in quantity. For example, during extended fasting, markedly elevated circulating ketone levels can support the majority of the energy needs of the brain and reduce its utilization of glucose. Nonetheless, that is not a physiologic condition. Furthermore, ketogenesis is suppressed during episodes of insulin-mediated hypoglycemia. Again, the brain is critically dependent on a virtually continuous supply of glucose from the circulation.[1-4]

Systemic Glucose Balance

Normally, rates of endogenous glucose influx into the circulation and those of glucose efflux out of the circulation into tissues other than the brain are coordinately regulated—largely by the plasma glucose-lowering (regulatory) hormone insulin and the plasma glucose-raising (counterregulatory) hormones glucagon and epinephrine—such that systemic glucose balance is maintained, hypoglycemia (as well as hyperglycemia) is prevented, and a continuous supply of glucose to the brain is ensured (Table 34-1). This is accomplished despite wide variations in exogenous glucose influx (e.g., after meals versus during fasting) and in glucose efflux (e.g., during exercise versus rest). Hypoglycemia occurs when rates of glucose appearance in the circulation (the sum of endogenous glucose production and exogenous glucose delivery from ingested carbohydrates) fail to keep pace with rates of glucose disappearance from the circulation (the sum of ongoing glucose metabolism largely by the brain and of variable glucose utilization by tissues including muscle, fat, liver, and kidneys).

In healthy adults, the physiologic postabsorptive (fasting) plasma glucose concentration ranges from approximately 3.9 mmol/L (70 mg/dL) to 6.1 mmol/L (110 mg/dL), with a mean of about 5.0 mmol/L (90 mg/dL).[4] In the postabsorptive steady state, rates of glucose production and utilization average approximately 12 μmol/kg per minute (2.2 mg/kg per minute), with a range of 10 to 14 μmol/kg per minute (1.8 to 2.6 mg/kg per minute). These rates are as much as threefold higher in infants, at least in part because of their greater brain mass relative to body weight.

TABLE 34-2

Physiologic Responses to Decreasing Plasma Glucose Concentrations

Response	Glycemic Threshold* (mmol/L [mg/dL])	Physiologic Effects	Role in Prevention or Correction of Hypoglycemia (Glucose Counterregulation)
↓ Insulin	4.4-4.7 (80-85)	↑ R_a (↓ R_d)	Primary glucose regulatory factor, first defense against hypoglycemia
↑ Glucagon	3.6-3.9 (65-70)	↑ R_a	Primary glucose counterregulatory factor, second defense against hypoglycemia
↑ Epinephrine	3.6-3.9 (65-70)	↑ R_a, ↓ R_c	Involved, critical when glucagon is deficient, third defense against hypoglycemia
↑ Cortisol and growth hormone	3.6-3.9 (65-70)	↑ R_a, ↓ R_c	Involved, not critical
Symptoms	2.8-3.1 (50-55)	↑ Exogenous glucose	Prompt behavioral defense (food ingestion)
↓ Cognition	<2.8 (50)	—	(Compromises behavioral defense)

*Arterialized venous, not venous, plasma glucose concentrations.

R_a, rate of glucose appearance, glucose production by the liver and kidneys; R_c, rate of glucose clearance by insulin-sensitive tissues; R_d, rate of glucose disappearance, glucose utilization by insulin-sensitive tissues such as skeletal muscle (no direct effect on central nervous system glucose utilization).

The liver is the predominant source of endogenous glucose production in the postabsorptive state; the kidneys, which both utilize and produce glucose, contribute little to net glucose production. However, as in the liver, glucose production in the kidney is regulated; it is suppressed by insulin and stimulated by epinephrine but not by glucagon. As a result, net renal glucose production occurs under some conditions, including hypoglycemia.[8] Therefore, endogenous glucose production cannot be equated with hepatic glucose production.

Gluconeogenesis and glycogenolysis are important for maintenance of the plasma glucose concentration.[6] The glucose pool—namely, free glucose in the extracellular fluids and in the cells of certain tissues (primarily the liver)—is only about 83 to 111 mmol (15 to 20 g). Glycogen that can be mobilized to provide circulating glucose (e.g., hepatic glycogen) contains approximately 390 mmol (70 g) of glucose, with a range of about 135 to 722 mmol (25 to 130 g). Therefore, in an adult of average size, preformed glucose can provide less than an 8-hour supply, even at the diminished rate of glucose utilization that occurs in the postabsorptive state.

If fasting is prolonged to 24 to 48 hours, the plasma glucose concentration declines and then stabilizes; hepatic glycogen content falls to less than 55 mmol (10 g), and gluconeogenesis becomes the sole source of glucose production.[6] Because amino acids are the main gluconeogenic precursors that result in net glucose formation, muscle protein is degraded. Glucose utilization by muscle and fat virtually ceases. As lipolysis and ketogenesis accelerate and circulating ketone levels rise, ketones become a major fuel for the brain. Glucose utilization by the brain declines by about half; this reduces the rate of gluconeogenesis required to maintain the plasma glucose concentration and hence decreases protein wasting.

After a meal, glucose absorption into the circulation increases to more than twice the rate of postabsorptive endogenous glucose production, depending on the carbohydrate content of the meal, the rate of gastric transit, and the rate of digestion and absorption. As glucose is absorbed, endogenous glucose production is suppressed, and glucose utilization by muscle, fat, and liver accelerates. The exogenous glucose is assimilated and, after a small rise, the plasma glucose concentration returns to the postabsorptive level.

Exercise increases glucose utilization (by muscle) to rates that can be several times greater than those of the postabsorptive state. Endogenous glucose production normally accelerates to match use so that the plasma glucose concentration is maintained.

In summary, the plasma glucose concentration is normally maintained within a relatively narrow range despite wide variations in glucose flux and thus maintains the systemic glucose balance. This remarkable homeostatic feat is accomplished by an array of hormonal, neural, and substrate glucoregulatory factors.[4] Glucoregulatory failure resulting in hyperglycemia (diabetes mellitus) is discussed in Chapters 31 and 32; that resulting in hypoglycemia is discussed in the paragraphs that follow.

Responses to Hypoglycemia

Falling plasma glucose concentrations cause a sequence of responses, with defined glycemic thresholds, in healthy individuals (Table 34-2).[4,9-12] The first response is a decrease in insulin secretion. This decrease occurs as glucose levels decline within the physiologic range. Increased secretion of glucose counterregulatory hormones, including glucagon and epinephrine, occurs as glucose levels fall just below the physiologic range. Lower plasma glucose concentrations cause a more intense sympathoadrenal (sympathetic neural as well as adrenomedullary) response and symptoms. Even lower glucose levels cause cognitive dysfunction and additional manifestations of functional brain failure including seizure or coma.

Clinical Manifestations of Hypoglycemia

The symptoms and signs of hypoglycemia[12,13] are nonspecific. Clinical hypoglycemia—that sufficient to cause symptoms and signs[2]—is most convincingly documented by Whipple triad: (1) symptoms, signs, or both consistent with hypoglycemia; (2) a low reliably measured plasma glucose concentration; and (3) resolution of those symptoms and signs after the plasma glucose concentration is raised.

Neuroglycopenic symptoms are a direct result of brain glucose deprivation. They include cognitive impairments, behavioral changes, psychomotor abnormalities, and at lower glucose levels, seizure and coma.[2-4,12,13] Neurogenic (or autonomic) symptoms are largely the result of the perception of physiologic changes caused by the sympathoadrenal (particularly the sympathetic neural[13]) discharge triggered by hypoglycemia. They include adrenergic (catecholamine-mediated) symptoms such as palpitations, tremor, and anxiety/arousal and cholinergic (acetylcholine-mediated) symptoms such as sweating, hunger, and paresthesias. Central mechanisms may also be involved in the generation of some of these symptoms (e.g., hunger).[14] Subjective awareness of hypoglycemia is largely the result of the perception of neurogenic symptoms (Fig. 34-2).[12]

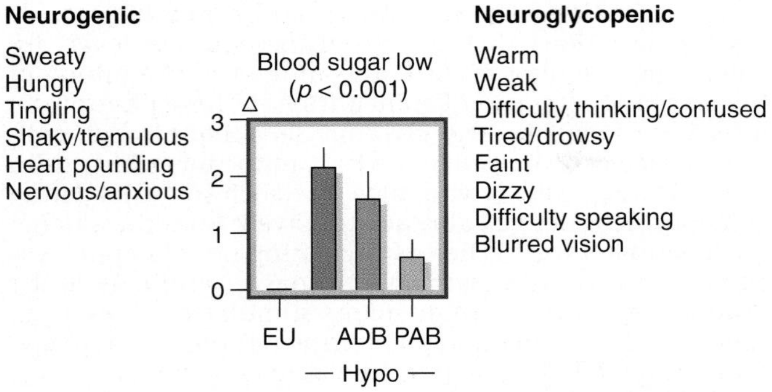

Neurogenic

Sweaty
Hungry
Tingling
Shaky/tremulous
Heart pounding
Nervous/anxious

Neuroglycopenic

Warm
Weak
Difficulty thinking/confused
Tired/drowsy
Faint
Dizzy
Difficulty speaking
Blurred vision

Blood sugar low
($p < 0.001$)

EU   ADB PAB
— Hypo —

Figure 34-2 Neurogenic (autonomic) and neuroglycopenic symptoms of hypoglycemia in healthy humans. Among the neurogenic symptoms, "sweaty," "hungry," and "tingling" are cholinergic and "shaky/tremulous," "heart pounding," and "nervous/anxious" are adrenergic. See text for discussion. Mean subject scores (± standard error) for awareness of hypoglycemia (low blood sugar) are shown during clamped euglycemia (EU) and during three conditions of hypoglycemia (Hypo): alone; with combined α- and β-adrenergic blockade by infused phentolamine and propranolol (ADB); and with combined α- and β-adrenergic blockade plus muscarinic cholinergic blockade by atropine (panautonomic blockade, PAB). (From Towler DA, Havlin CE, Craft S, et al. Mechanism of awareness of hypoglycemia: perception of neurogenic [predominantly cholinergic] rather than neuroglycopenic symptoms. *Diabetes Care.* 1993;42:1791-1798, used with permission of the American Diabetes Association.)

Signs of hypoglycemia include pallor and diaphoresis, which result from adrenergic cutaneous vasoconstriction and cholinergic activation of sweat glands, respectively.[2,3] Heart rates and systolic blood pressures are raised, but often not greatly. Neuroglycopenic manifestations are often observable.

Maintenance of Systemic Glucose Balance

Although obligatory glucose utilization, largely by the brain, is continuous, the delivery of exogenous glucose from dietary carbohydrates is intermittent. Systemic glucose balance (see Table 34-1) is normally maintained, and hypoglycemia and hyperglycemia are prevented, by dynamic, minute-to-minute regulation of endogenous glucose production from the liver and kidneys and of glucose utilization by tissues outside the central nervous system (CNS), such as muscle.[3,4] This regulation is exerted primarily by insulin, glucagon, and epinephrine[3,4] (Fig. 34-3; see also Table 34-2), although an array of hormones, neurotransmitters, and substrates is involved.[4]

The key physiologic defenses against falling plasma glucose concentrations are (1) a decrease in insulin, (2) an increase in glucagon, and, in the absence of the latter,

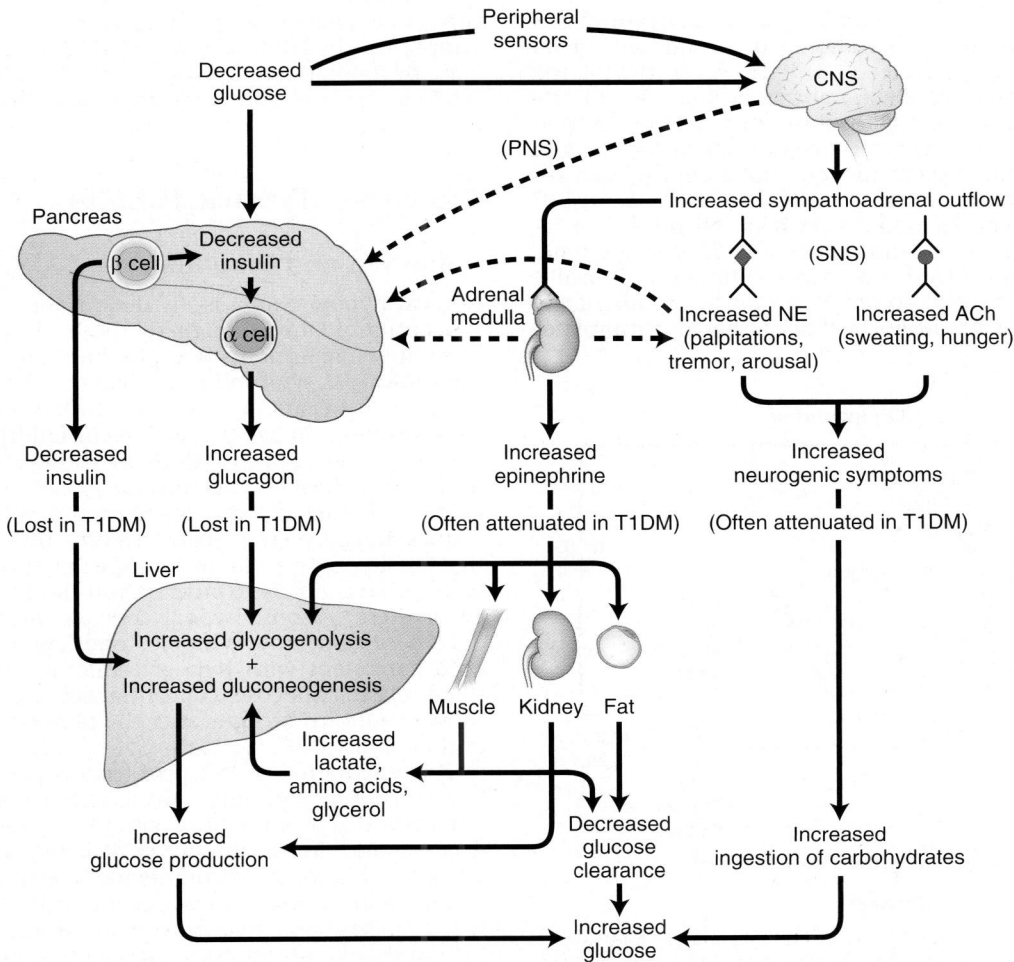

Figure 34-3 Physiologic and behavioral defenses against hypoglycemia in humans. ACh, acetylcholine; α cell, pancreatic islet alpha cells; β cell, pancreatic islet beta cells; CNS, central nervous system; NE, norepinephrine; PNS, parasympathetic nervous system; SNS, sympathetic nervous system; T1DM, type 1 diabetes. (From Cryer PE. Mechanisms of sympathoadrenal failure and hypoglycemia in diabetes. *J Clin Invest.* 2006;116:1470-1473, used with permission of the American Society for Clinical Investigation.)

(3) an increase in epinephrine.[3,4] The behavioral defense is carbohydrate ingestion prompted by symptoms that are largely sympathetic neural in origin (see Table 34-2 and Fig. 34-3).[3,4,13]

The first physiologic defense against hypoglycemia is a decrease in insulin secretion by the pancreatic islet beta cells. Signaled primarily by declining glucose levels at the beta cells, this response occurs as plasma glucose concentrations decline within the physiologic range[3,4] (see Table 34-2) and favors increased hepatic and renal glucose production with virtual cessation of glucose utilization by insulin-sensitive tissues such as muscle (see Fig. 34-3).[3,4]

The second physiologic defense against hypoglycemia is an increase in glucagon secretion by pancreatic islet alpha cells. This increase occurs as plasma glucose concentrations fall just below the physiologic range[3,4] (see Table 34-2) and stimulates hepatic glucose production, largely by stimulating glycogenolysis (see Fig. 34-3).[3,4] This response is signaled primarily by a decrease in intraislet insulin, perhaps among other beta-cell secretory products, in the setting of low alpha-cell glucose concentrations[3,4,15] (see Fig. 34-3) and only secondarily by increased autonomic nervous system (sympathetic, parasympathetic, adrenomedullary) inputs.[3,4,16]

The third physiologic defense against hypoglycemia, which becomes critical when glucagon is deficient, is an increase in adrenomedullary epinephrine secretion. Signaled via the CNS, it, too, occurs as plasma glucose concentrations fall just below the physiologic range[3,4] (see Table 34-2) and raises plasma glucose concentrations largely by β_2-adrenergic stimulation of hepatic and renal glucose production (see Fig. 34-3).[3,4] However, the plasma glucose-raising actions of epinephrine also involve limitation of glucose clearance by insulin-sensitive tissues, mobilization of gluconeogenic precursors such as lactate and amino acids from muscle and glycerol from fat, and α_2-adrenergic limitation of insulin secretion (Fig. 34-4).[3,4,17] Indeed, the adrenergic actions on beta-cell insulin secretion normally play an important role in the glycemic actions of epinephrine. α_2-Adrenergic limitation of insulin secretion permits the glycemic response; β_2-adrenergic stimulation alone has little effect because it also stimulates

insulin secretion.[4] On the other hand, some increase in insulin secretion—due to the rising glucose level, β_2-adrenergic stimulation, or both—limits the magnitude of the glycemic response to epinephrine.[17] These physiologic interactions explain why glycemic sensitivity to epinephrine is increased in patients who cannot increase insulin secretion (e.g., those with type 1 diabetes).[17] Circulating epinephrine is derived almost exclusively from the adrenal medulla in adults.[13] Whereas circulating norepinephrine is derived largely from sympathetic nerve terminals under resting conditions and in many stimulated states (e.g., exercise), the plasma norepinephrine response to hypoglycemia is derived largely from the adrenal medulla.[13]

These physiologic defenses against hypoglycemia typically abort episodes of declining plasma glucose concentrations and prevent clinical (i.e., symptomatic) hypoglycemia. If they do not, the lower plasma glucose concentration causes a more intense sympathoadrenal response, resulting in symptoms (see Table 34-2).[3,4] These symptoms, particularly the neurogenic symptoms, cause awareness of hypoglycemia that prompts the behavioral defense against hypoglycemia, ingestion of carbohydrates (see Fig. 34-3).[3,4]

The integrated physiology of glucose counterregulation[2-4] is further illustrated in Figure 34-5. Falling glucose levels within the pancreatic islet cells signal a decrease in insulin secretion and an increase in glucagon secretion. Falling glucose levels sensed in the periphery and in the CNS, acting through the hypothalamus, signal an increase in sympathoadrenal activity that results in an increase in adrenomedullary epinephrine secretion and in neurogenic symptoms, the latter largely resulting from increased sympathetic neural activity. Figure 34-5 includes a putative cerebral network that may modulate the hypothalamic response.

CLINICAL HYPOGLYCEMIA

Definition and Diagnosis

Clinical hypoglycemia is, by definition, a plasma glucose concentration low enough to cause symptoms or signs, including impairment of brain function.[2] The glycemic thresholds for symptoms and signs of hypoglycemia are dynamic; for example, they shift to lower plasma glucose concentrations in patients with recurrent hypoglycemia[18,19] and to higher concentrations in those with poorly controlled diabetes.[19,20] Therefore, it is not possible to state a single plasma glucose concentration that categorically defines hypoglycemia. Furthermore, the symptoms and signs of hypoglycemia are nonspecific,[2,3] and a low measured plasma glucose concentration can be artifactual.[2] For all of these reasons, hypoglycemia is most convincingly documented by the Whipple triad: symptoms, signs, or both consistent with hypoglycemia; a low reliably measured plasma glucose concentration; and resolution of those symptoms or signs after the plasma glucose concentration is raised.[2,3]

Documentation of Whipple triad is particularly important when hypoglycemia is suspected in a person who does not have diabetes mellitus, because hypoglycemic disorders are rare.[2] In the absence of diabetes, a thorough diagnostic evaluation is recommended only for patients in whom Whipple triad can be documented.[2] Ideally, patients with diabetes being treated with an insulin secretagogue or insulin should monitor their plasma glucose concentration whenever they suspect hypoglycemia.[2,3] However, that is sometimes not practical, and it often is not done. Nonetheless, the likelihood that a symptomatic episode is the result

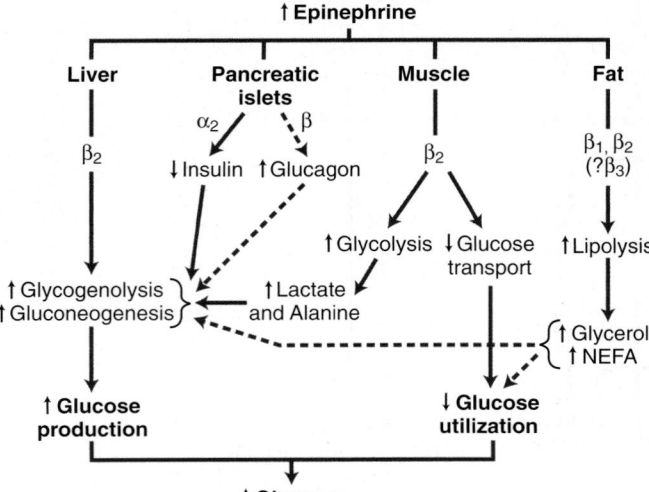

Figure 34-4 Schematic representation of the mechanisms of the hyperglycemic effect of epinephrine, mediated by α- and β-adrenergic stimulation. NEFA, nonesterified fatty acid. (From Cryer PE. Catecholamines, pheochromocytoma and diabetes. *Diabetes Rev.* 1993;1:309-317, used with permission of the American Diabetes Association.)

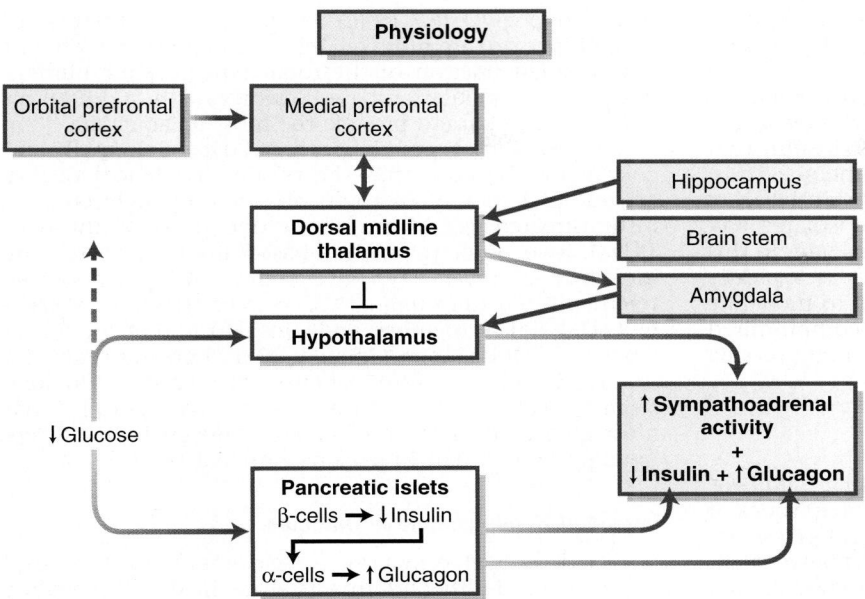

Figure 34-5 Schematic representation of the integrated mechanisms of the physiologic responses to hypoglycemia in humans: decrements in insulin secretion, increments in glucagon secretion, and increments in sympathoadrenal (adrenomedullary and sympathetic neural) activity. α-cells, pancreatic islet alpha cells; β-cells, pancreatic islet beta cells. (From Cryer PE. *Hypoglycemia in Diabetes: Pathophysiology, Prevalence and Prevention.* Alexandria, VA: American Diabetes Association; 2009, used with permission of the American Diabetes Association.)

of hypoglycemia is high, because hypoglycemia is common in such patients.[3]

General Mechanisms of Hypoglycemia

Hypoglycemia develops when glucose efflux out of the circulation exceeds glucose influx into the circulation. Glucose efflux is the sum of ongoing obligatory glucose utilization, largely by the brain, and regulated glucose utilization by insulin-sensitive tissues, and glucose influx is the sum of endogenous glucose production and exogenous glucose delivery from ingested carbohydrates (see Table 34-1). Although hypoglycemia can result from excessive glucose efflux, it is typically the result of glucose influx that is too low—either absolutely low or low relative to high rates of glucose efflux.

Clinical Classification of Hypoglycemia

Causes of hypoglycemia[2] are outlined in Table 34-3. Drugs are, by far, the most common cause of hypoglycemia. Such drugs include insulin secretagogues and insulin used to treat diabetes. Although persons with diabetes can suffer from the same hypoglycemic disorders as those without diabetes, their hypoglycemic episodes are usually the result of treatment of their diabetes.[2,3] Furthermore, the pathophysiology of hypoglycemia in diabetes is unique, and the diagnostic and management approaches are different from those for individuals without diabetes.[2,3] Therefore, hypoglycemia in persons with diabetes and hypoglycemia in those without diabetes are discussed separately in this chapter.

HYPOGLYCEMIA IN PERSONS WITH DIABETES

The Clinical Problem of Hypoglycemia in Diabetes

Iatrogenic hypoglycemia is the limiting factor in the glycemic management of diabetes.[3] It causes recurrent mor-

TABLE 34-3

Causes of Hypoglycemia in Adults

Ill or Medicated Individual

Drugs
Insulin or insulin secretagogue
Alcohol
Others (see Table 34-7)

Critical Illnesses
Hepatic, renal, or cardiac failure
Sepsis
Inanition

Hormonal Deficiency
Cortisol
Glucagon and epinephrine (in insulin-deficient diabetes mellitus)

Non–Islet Cell Tumor

Seemingly Well Individual

Endogenous Hyperinsulinism
Insulinoma
Functional beta-cell disorders (nesidioblastosis)
Noninsulinoma pancreatogenous hypoglycemia
Post–gastric bypass hypoglycemia
Autoimmune hypoglycemia
Antibody to insulin
Antibody to insulin receptor
Insulin secretagogue
Other

Accidental, Surreptitious, or Malicious Hypoglycemia

From Cryer PE, Axelrod L, Grossman AB, et al. Evaluation and management of adult hypoglycemic disorders: an Endocrine Society clinical practice guideline. *J Clin Endocrinol Metab.* 2009;94:709-728, used with permission of The Endocrine Society.

bidity in most persons with type 1 diabetes mellitus (T1DM) and in many of those with advanced type 2 diabetes mellitus (T2DM), and it is sometimes fatal. The barrier of hypoglycemia generally precludes maintenance of euglycemia over a lifetime of diabetes and thus full realization of the vascular benefits of glycemic control. Furthermore, hypoglycemia compromises physiologic and behavioral defenses against subsequent falling plasma glucose concentrations, resulting in a vicious cycle of recurrent hypoglycemia.

Hypoglycemia in diabetes is caused by pharmacokinetically imperfect treatment with an insulin secretagogue (such as a sulfonylurea or a glinide) or with insulin that results in episodes of therapeutic hyperinsulinemia. Thus, it is fundamentally iatrogenic. Episodes of substantial absolute therapeutic hyperinsulinemia can cause isolated episodes of hypoglycemia. However, as developed later in this chapter, recurrent hypoglycemia in diabetes is typically the result of the interplay of relative or mild to moderate absolute therapeutic hyperinsulinemia and compromised physiologic and behavioral defenses against falling plasma glucose concentrations.[3]

Frequency of Hypoglycemia in Diabetes

Hypoglycemia is a fact of life for people with T1DM.[3,21-25] The average patient suffers untold numbers of episodes of asymptomatic hypoglycemia (which are not benign because they impair defenses against subsequent hypoglycemia), approximately two episodes of symptomatic hypoglycemia per week (thousands of such episodes over a lifetime of diabetes), and roughly one episode per year of severe, at least temporarily disabling hypoglycemia, often with seizure or coma. This problem has not abated since it was highlighted by the report of the Diabetes Control and Complications Trial (DCCT)[21] in 1993. In 2007, the United Kingdom Hypoglycaemia Study Group (UKHSG) reported an incidence of severe hypoglycemia twice that reported in the DCCT among patients who had had T1DM for less than 5 years and five times the DCCT incidence among those with T1DM for more than 15 years in their population-based study.[24]

The overall incidence of hypoglycemia during treatment of T2DM with an insulin secretagogue, or even with insulin, is lower than that in patients with T1DM.[3,23,24,26-30] However, for pathophysiologic reasons discussed later, the incidence of hypoglycemia increases progressively over time as patients approach the absolute endogenous insulin-deficient end of the spectrum of T2DM.[3,24,26,27] Indeed, the incidence of hypoglycemia has been reported to be similar in patients with T2DM and in those with T1DM matched for duration of insulin therapy.[27] The UKHSG found a prevalence of severe hypoglycemia of 7% and an incidence of 10 episodes per 100 patient-years among patients with T2DM treated with insulin for less than 2 years; among those treated for longer than 5 years, these figures rose to 25% prevalence and 70 episodes per 100 patient-years.[24] The patterns for self-treated hypoglycemia were similar. Therefore, at least with current, less than euglycemic treatment goals, the frequency of iatrogenic hypoglycemia is relatively low during the first few years of treatment of T2DM with insulin but increases substantially in advanced T2DM, approaching the frequency among patients with T1DM.

Estimates of the incidence and prevalence of hypoglycemia in diabetes are generally underestimates because of the challenge of ascertainment.[3] Asymptomatic episodes will be missed unless they are incidentally detected by self-monitoring of blood glucose or by continuous glucose monitoring (CGM). Symptomatic episodes may not be recognized to be the result of hypoglycemia because the symptoms of hypoglycemia are nonspecific. Even if they are recognized, they may not be remembered[31,32] and reported at periodic patient contacts. Because they are dramatic events that are more likely to be reported (by the patient or an associate),[31,32] estimates of the frequency of severe hypoglycemia (that requiring the assistance of another person) are more reliable, although they represent only a small fraction of the total hypoglycemic burden. Prospective, population-based studies with a focus on hypoglycemia should provide the most reliable data.[24,25]

The prospective, population-based data of Donnelly and colleagues[23] indicate that the overall incidences of any episode of hypoglycemia and of severe hypoglycemia in insulin-treated T2DM are about one third of those in T1DM. Two other population-based studies reported the incidence of severe hypoglycemia requiring emergency treatment in insulin-treated T2DM to be 40%[28] and 100%[29] in T1DM. Taken together, and considering that the prevalence of T2DM is approximately 20-fold greater than that of T1DM and that most patients with T2DM ultimately require treatment with insulin, these data suggest that most episodes of iatrogenic hypoglycemia, including severe hypoglycemia, occur in persons with T2DM.

Impact of Hypoglycemia in Diabetes

Iatrogenic hypoglycemia causes recurrent physical and psychosocial morbidity and impairs glycemic defenses against subsequent hypoglycemia in many patients with diabetes.[3] The barrier of hypoglycemia generally precludes maintenance of euglycemia over a lifetime of diabetes.[3] Hypoglycemia often causes functional brain failure that is typically reversed after the plasma glucose concentration is raised.[5] Rarely, it causes sudden death, presumably the result of cardiac arrhythmia, or, if it is profound and prolonged, permanent brain dysfunction or death.[5]

At a minimum, an episode of symptomatic hypoglycemia is a nuisance and a distraction. It can impair judgment, behavior, and performance of physical tasks such as driving. It can cause a seizure or loss of consciousness. Transient neurologic deficits sometimes occur, but permanent neurologic damage is rare. Systematic long-term follow-up of the DCCT patients suggests that recurrent iatrogenic hypoglycemia does not cause chronic cognitive impairments in young adults,[33] but the possibility that it does so in young children[34,35] and the elderly[36] remains. Among other psychological disorders, fear of hypoglycemia can be a barrier to glycemic control.[37]

Iatrogenic hypoglycemia can be fatal.[5,38] That hypoglycemia could kill has been known since the discovery of insulin.[5] There are epidemiologic associations of hypoglycemia with death,[5] reports of excessive mortality rates during intensive glycemic therapy in randomized controlled trials of patients with T2DM[39,40] and intensive care unit patients,[41,42] and reports of iatrogenic hypoglycemia mortality rates in series of patients with diabetes.[33,43-49] Early reports indicated that 2% to 4% of persons with diabetes (mostly T1DM) died from hypoglycemia.[43-45] More recent reports indicated that 4%,[46] 6%,[33] 7%,[47] and 10%[48] of deaths of persons with T1DM were caused by hypoglycemia. Hypoglycemia at the time of death has been documented.[49] Deaths of up to 10% of patients with severe sulfonylurea-induced hypoglycemia have been reported.[50,51] Deaths of additional patients with T2DM, including those treated with insulin, have been attributed to hypoglycemia.[52] Thus, there are iatrogenic hypoglycemia mortality rates in both T1DM and T2DM.

Although prolonged, profound hypoglycemia can cause brain death, most instances of sudden hypoglycemic death are thought to be the result of cardiac arrhythmias triggered by an intense sympathoadrenal response to hypoglycemia.[3,5,53-56] These are mediated through β-adrenergic receptors.[56] Sudden death has been associated with QT interval prolongation and reduced baroreflex sensitivity in patients with classic diabetic autonomic neuropathy.[57-59] Adler and colleagues[60] demonstrated, in studies of nondiabetic individuals, that recent antecedent hypoglycemia causes reduced baroreflex sensitivity the following day. The induction of functional sympathetic failure by recent antecedent hypoglycemia as an additional, potentially fatal, feature of the concept of hypoglycemia-associated autonomic failure (HAAF) in diabetes[3] is discussed later in this chapter.

Clinical Definition and Classification of Hypoglycemia in Diabetes

The American Diabetes Association (ADA)/Endocrine Society (ES) Workgroup on Hypoglycemia[61] defined hypoglycemia in diabetes as "all episodes of abnormally low plasma glucose concentration that expose the individual to potential harm." That is broader than the recommended definition of clinical hypoglycemia in persons without diabetes (i.e., a plasma glucose concentration low enough to cause symptoms or signs[2]) because it includes asymptomatic episodes. The latter are not benign in persons with diabetes; they compromise defenses against subsequent hypoglycemia,[3] and they identify increased risk of imminent severe iatrogenic hypoglycemia.[62] Again, it is not possible to define a plasma glucose concentration that categorically defines hypoglycemia because the glycemic thresholds for responses to hypoglycemia are dynamic. They shift to lower plasma glucose concentrations in patients with recurrent hypoglycemia[18,19] and to higher plasma glucose concentrations in those with poorly controlled diabetes.[19,20]

The ADA/ES Workgroup recommended that people with diabetes (implicitly those treated with an insulin secretagogue or insulin) become concerned about the possibility of developing hypoglycemia at a self-monitored plasma glucose concentration of 3.9 mmol/L (70 mg/dL) or less.[61] Within the error of self-monitoring (or CGM), that conservative alert value approximates the lower limit of the nondiabetic postabsorptive plasma glucose range[4] and the normal glycemic thresholds for activation of physiologic glucose counterregulatory systems[4] (see Table 34-2); it is low enough to reduce glycemic defenses against subsequent hypoglycemia[63] in nondiabetic persons. Therefore, the recommended glucose alert level of 3.9 mmol/L (70 mg/dL) or less is data driven[64]; it usually gives the patient time to take action to prevent a clinical hypoglycemic episode, and it provides some margin for the limited accuracy of glucose monitoring devices at low plasma glucose concentrations. It has been implicitly endorsed by the U.S. Food and Drug Administration and the European Medicines Agency.

The recommended alert value does not, of course, mean that persons with diabetes should always self-treat for hypoglycemia at an estimated plasma glucose concentration of 3.9 mmol/L (70 mg/dL) or less.[64] Rather, they should consider actions ranging from repeating the measurement in the near term, through behavioral actions such as avoiding exercise or driving until the glucose level is raised, to carbohydrate ingestion and subsequent adjustments of the therapeutic regimen.

The ADA/ES Workgroup[61] also recommended a clinical classification of hypoglycemia in diabetes (Table 34-4).

Pathophysiology of Glucose Counterregulation in Diabetes

The pathophysiology of glucose counterregulation and its relationship to clinical hypoglycemia in diabetes have been

TABLE 34-4

Classification of Hypoglycemia in Diabetes

Clinical Classification	Definition
Severe hypoglycemia	An event requiring the assistance of another person to actively administer carbohydrate, glucagon, or other resuscitative actions. Plasma glucose measurements may not be available during such an event, but neurologic recovery attributable to the restoration of plasma glucose to a normal level is considered sufficient evidence that the event was induced by a low plasma glucose concentration.
Documented symptomatic hypoglycemia	An event during which typical symptoms of hypoglycemia are accompanied by a measured plasma glucose concentration of ≤70 mg/dL (3.9 mmol/L).
Asymptomatic hypoglycemia	An event not accompanied by typical symptoms of hypoglycemia but with a measured plasma glucose concentration of ≤70 mg/dL (3.9 mmol/L).
Probable symptomatic hypoglycemia	An event during which symptoms typical of hypoglycemia are not accompanied by a plasma glucose determination but were presumably caused by a plasma glucose concentration of ≤70 mg/dL (3.9 mmol/L).
Pseudohypoglycemia	An event during which the person with diabetes reports any of the typical symptoms of hypoglycemia and interprets those as indicative of hypoglycemia, with a measured plasma glucose concentration that is >70 mg/dL (3.9 mmol/L) but is approaching that level.

reviewed in detail[3] and are summarized in the paragraphs that follow (see earlier discussion and Figs. 34-3 and 34-5). Again, the key physiologic defenses against falling plasma glucose concentrations are a decrease in insulin, an increase in glucagon, and in the absence of the latter, an increase in epinephrine.[3,4] The behavioral defense is carbohydrate ingestion prompted by symptoms[12] that are largely sympathetic neural in origin.[3,4,13]

Insulin Excess

Episodes of therapeutic hyperinsulinemia, produced by treatment with an insulin secretagogue (a sulfonylurea or a glinide) or with insulin, are a prerequisite for the development of iatrogenic hypoglycemia. Marked absolute insulin excess can cause isolated episodes of hypoglycemia. However, iatrogenic hypoglycemia is typically the result of the interplay of relative or mild to moderate absolute therapeutic hyperinsulinemia and compromised physiologic and behavioral defenses against falling plasma glucose concentrations (Fig. 34-6).[3]

Defective Glucose Counterregulation and Hypoglycemia Unawareness

In established (absolute deficiency of endogenous insulin) T1DM, circulating (exogenous) insulin concentrations do not decrease as plasma glucose concentrations fall in response to therapeutic hyperinsulinemia.[3] That is the result of absolute beta-cell failure with no regulated endogenous insulin secretion. Therefore, the first physiologic defense against hypoglycemia[4] is lost. Furthermore, despite the presence of functional alpha cells, there is no increase in glucagon secretion (Fig. 34-7).[3,65] That, too, is the result

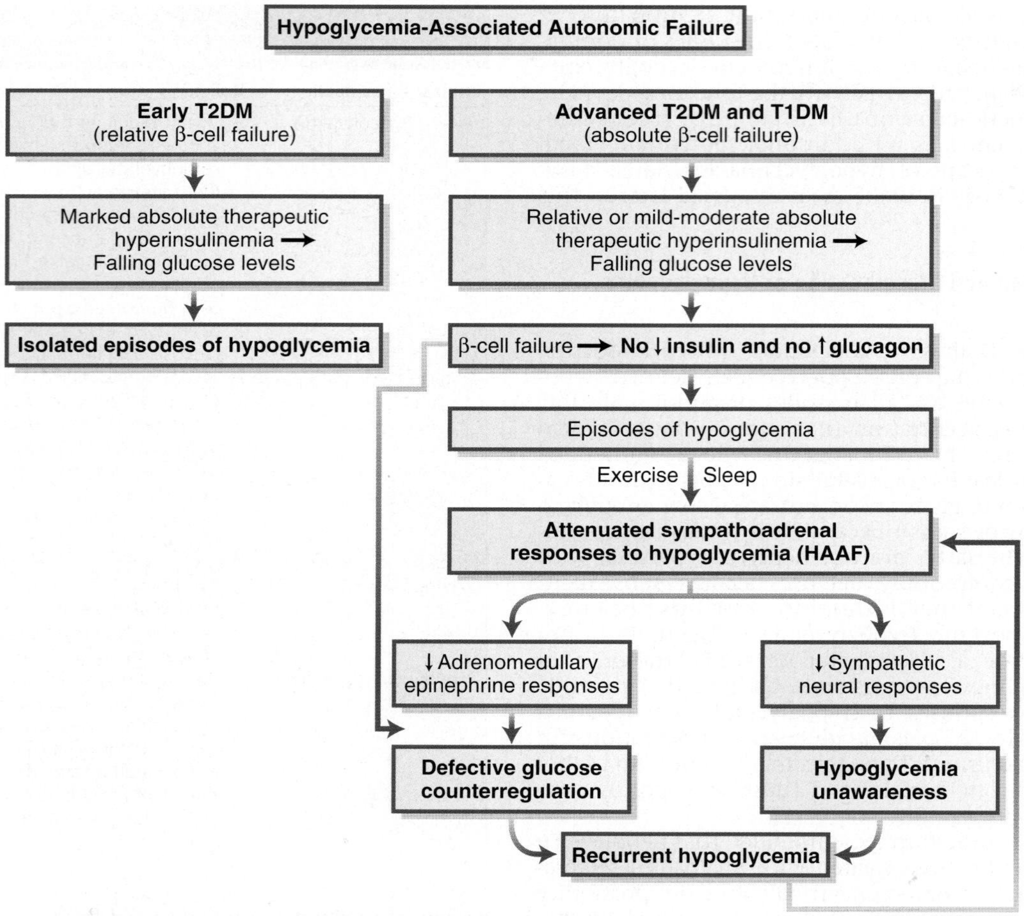

Hypoglycemia-Associated Autonomic Failure

Early T2DM (relative β-cell failure)	**Advanced T2DM and T1DM** (absolute β-cell failure)

Marked absolute therapeutic hyperinsulinemia → Falling glucose levels	Relative or mild-moderate absolute therapeutic hyperinsulinemia → Falling glucose levels

Isolated episodes of hypoglycemia

β-cell failure → **No ↓ insulin and no ↑ glucagon**

Episodes of hypoglycemia

Exercise ↓ Sleep

Attenuated sympathoadrenal responses to hypoglycemia (HAAF)

↓ Adrenomedullary epinephrine responses

↓ Sympathetic neural responses

Defective glucose counterregulation

Hypoglycemia unawareness

Recurrent hypoglycemia

Figure 34-6 Schematic representation of the concept of hypoglycemia-associated autonomic failure (HAAF) in diabetes and the pathogenesis of iatrogenic hypoglycemia including the clinical syndromes of defective glucose counterregulation and hypoglycemia unawareness. β-cell, pancreatic islet beta cells; T1DM, type 1 diabetes mellitus; T2DM, type 2 diabetes mellitus.

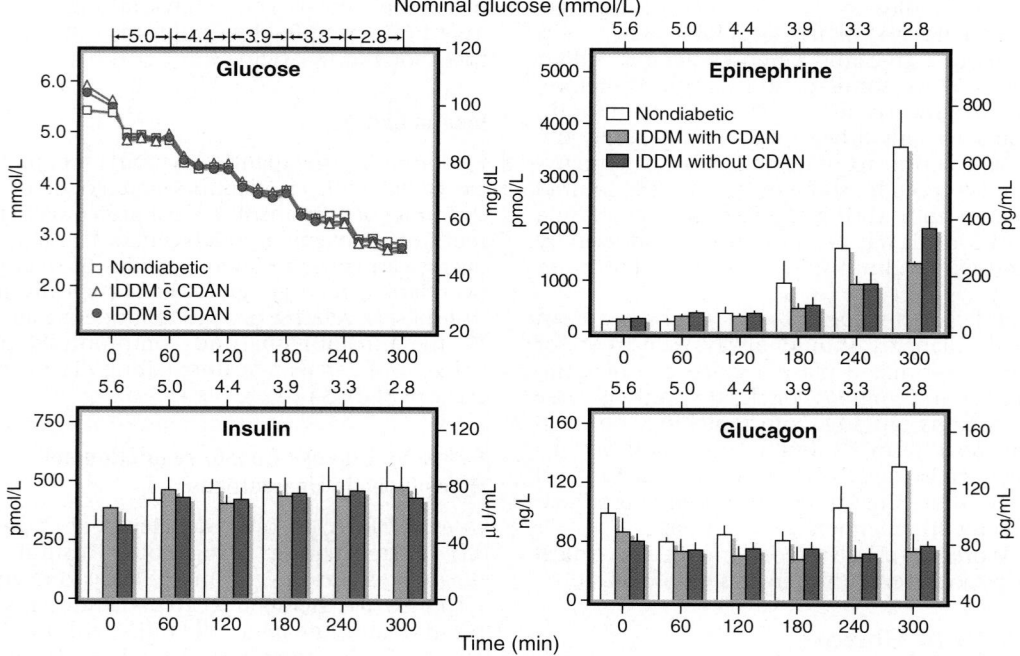

Figure 34-7 Mean (± standard error) plasma glucose, insulin, epinephrine, and glucagon concentrations during hyperinsulinemic stepped hypoglycemic glucose clamps in three groups of subjects: nondiabetic subjects (*open squares* and *columns*), people with type 1 diabetes (IDDM) who have classic diabetic autonomic neuropathy (CDAN; *open triangles* and *crosshatched columns*), and people with IDDM without CDAN (*closed circles* and *columns*). IDDM, insulin-dependent diabetes mellitus. (From Dagogo-Jack SE, Craft S, Cryer PE. Hypoglycemia-associated autonomic failure in insulin-dependent diabetes mellitus. *J Clin Invest.* 1993;91:819-828, used with permission of the American Society for Clinical Investigation.)

of beta-cell failure,[66] which causes loss of the decrement in insulin that normally signals an increase in alpha-cell glucagon secretion during hypoglycemia (see Figs. 34-3 and 34-5).[3,15] Therefore, the second physiologic defense against hypoglycemia[4] is also lost.

In addition, the increase in epinephrine secretion, the third physiologic defense against hypoglycemia,[4] is typically attenuated (see Fig. 34-7).[3,65] In the setting of absent insulin and glucagon responses, the attenuated epinephrine response causes the clinical syndrome of defective glucose counterregulation[3,65-68] (see Fig. 34-6), which is associated with a 25-fold[67] or greater[68] increased risk of severe hypoglycemia in T1DM. The attenuated epinephrine response is a marker of attenuation of the sympathoadrenal response (including the sympathetic neural response) that normally causes neurogenic symptoms that largely prompt the behavioral response leading to carbohydrate ingestion (see Figs. 34-3 and 34-5). This attenuated response (largely the attenuated sympathetic neural response) causes the clinical syndrome of hypoglycemia unawareness[3] (see Fig. 34-6), which is associated with a sixfold increased risk of severe hypoglycemia in T1DM.[69]

Although the term *hypoglycemia unawareness* is used widely, "impaired awareness of hypoglycemia"[69] is more precise because there is a spectrum ranging from partial to complete loss of symptoms. Attenuated sympathoadrenal responses to falling plasma glucose concentrations can be caused by recent antecedent hypoglycemia[3,65,70] (Figs. 34-8 and 34-9), prior exercise,[3,71] or sleep,[3,72,73] but the precise mechanism is not known.[66] (See later discussion of HAAF.)

Hypoglycemia unawareness is largely the result of reduced release of the sympathetic neurotransmitters norepinephrine and acetylcholine.[3,13] There is evidence of decreased β-adrenergic sensitivity, specifically reduced cardiac chronotropic sensitivity to isoproterenol, in affected patients.[74,75] However, vascular sensitivity to a β-adrenergic agonist was not found to be reduced in unaware patients.[76]

Reduced sensitivity to β-adrenergic signaling of neurogenic symptoms remains to be demonstrated in patients with unawareness, and it would be necessary to also postulate decreased cholinergic sensitivity to explain reduced cholinergic symptoms such as sweating.

In contrast to these compromised defenses in T1DM, defenses against hypoglycemia are intact early in the course of T2DM. However, they become compromised over time.[3,77] In advanced T2DM (i.e., with absolutely deficient endogenous insulin), insulin and glucagon responses to falling plasma glucose concentrations are lost and sympathoadrenal responses to hypoglycemia are reduced by recent antecedent hypoglycemia, as is observed in T1DM.[3,77]

In summary, the pathophysiology of glucose counterregulation is the same in T1DM and T2DM but with different time courses.[3,65,66,77] The pathogenesis of an episode of iatrogenic hypoglycemia involves therapeutic hyperinsulinemia resulting in falling plasma glucose concentrations. With absence of appropriate decrements in insulin and of increments in glucagon, hypoglycemia occurs. That, in turn, causes attenuated sympathoadrenal responses to subsequent falling glucose levels and recurrent episodes of hypoglycemia (see Fig. 34-6). Because beta-cell failure, which causes loss of both insulin and glucagon responses, occurs rapidly in T1DM but slowly in T2DM, the syndromes of defective glucose counterregulation and hypoglycemia unawareness develop early in T1DM but later in T2DM. That temporal pattern of compromised glycemic defenses explains why iatrogenic hypoglycemia becomes progressively more frequent as patients approach the insulin-deficient end of the spectrum of T2DM.[24]

Hypoglycemia-Associated Autonomic Failure in Diabetes

The concept of HAAF in diabetes posits that recent antecedent hypoglycemia (see Figs. 34-8 and 34-9),[3,65,70] prior exercise,[3,71] or sleep[3,72,73] can cause both defective glucose

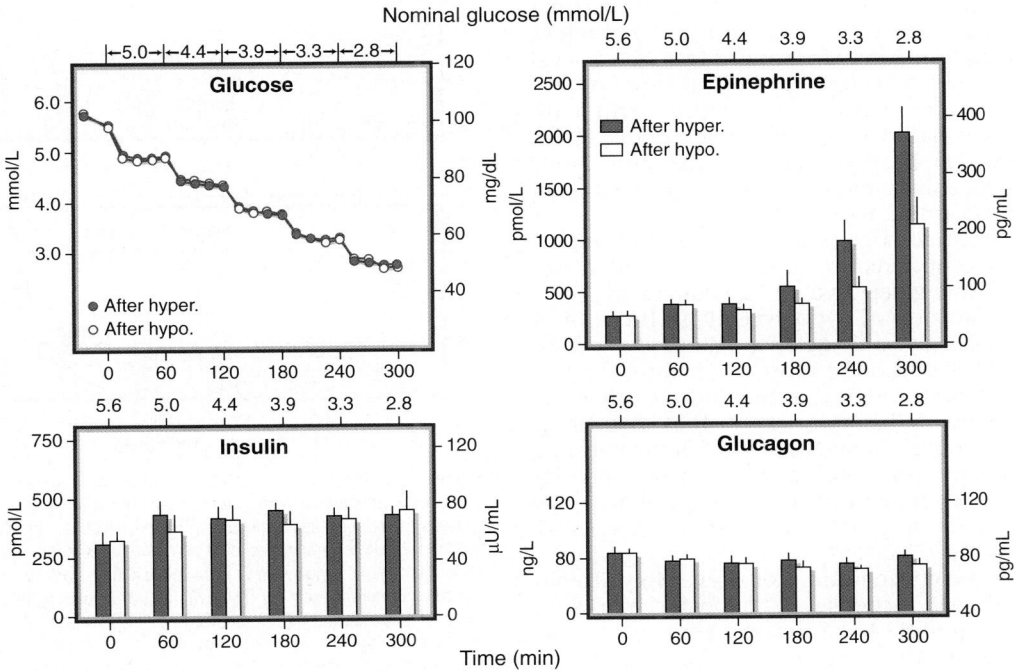

Figure 34-8 Mean (± standard error) plasma glucose, insulin, epinephrine, and glucagon concentrations during hyperinsulinemic stepped hypoglycemic glucose clamps in patients with type 1 (insulin-dependent) diabetes without classical diabetic autonomic neuropathy on mornings after afternoon hyperglycemia (After hyper.; *closed circles* and *columns*) and on mornings after afternoon hypoglycemia (After hypo.; *open circles* and *columns*). (From Dagogo-Jack SE, Craft S, Cryer PE. Hypoglycemia-associated autonomic failure in insulin-dependent diabetes mellitus. *J Clin Invest.* 1993;91:819-828, used with permission of the American Society for Clinical Investigation.)

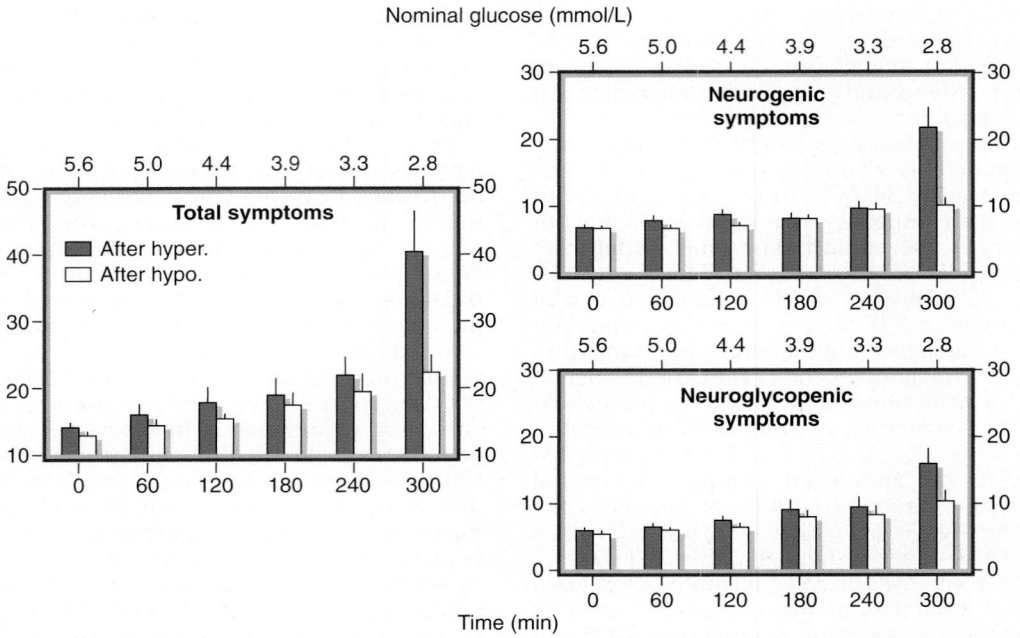

Figure 34-9 Mean (± standard error) total, neurogenic, and neuroglycopenic symptom scores during hyperinsulinemic stepped hypoglycemic glucose clamps in patients with type 1 (insulin-dependent) diabetes mellitus without classical diabetic autonomic neuropathy on mornings after afternoon hyperglycemia (After hyper., *closed columns*) and on mornings after afternoon hypoglycemia (After hypo., *open columns*). (From Dagogo-Jack SE, Craft S, Cryer PE. Hypoglycemia-associated autonomic failure in insulin-dependent diabetes mellitus. *J Clin Invest*. 1993;91:819-828, used with permission of the American Society for Clinical Investigation.)

counterregulation and hypoglycemia unawareness during subsequent hypoglycemia. The mechanisms are, respectively, attenuation of the epinephrine response (in the setting of absent insulin and glucagon responses) and attenuation of the sympathoadrenal (including the sympathetic neural) response and the resulting neurogenic symptom responses. The development of these defects sets up a vicious cycle of recurrent hypoglycemia (see Fig. 34-6). HAAF is a functional form of autonomic failure, distinct from classic diabetic autonomic neuropathy. Nonetheless, an attenuated sympathoadrenal response to a given level of hypoglycemia, the key feature of HAAF, is more prominent in patients with autonomic neuropathy.[78,79] In addition to its role in the pathogenesis of hypoglycemia, HAAF has cardiovascular implications because, like autonomic neuropathy, it reduces baroreflex sensitivity[60] and may predispose patients to cardiac arrhythmias.

Recent antecedent hypoglycemia, even asymptomatic nocturnal hypoglycemia, reduces epinephrine and symptomatic responses to a given level of subsequent hypoglycemia,[80] reduces detection of hypoglycemia in the clinical setting,[81] and reduces glycemic defense against hyperinsulinemia[65] in T1DM. Perhaps the most compelling support for the clinical relevance of HAAF is the finding, originally from three independent laboratories,[82-85] that as little as 2 to 3 weeks of scrupulous avoidance of hypoglycemia reverses hypoglycemia unawareness (Fig. 34-10) and improves the attenuated epinephrine component of defective glucose counterregulation in most affected patients. HAAF also occurs in advanced T2DM.[3,77]

There are three recognized causes of a reversibly attenuated sympathoadrenal response to hypoglycemia and, therefore, three forms of HAAF.[3] Antecedent hypoglycemia–related HAAF[3,65,70] led to the concept.[3,65,70] Exercise-related HAAF[3,71] is exemplified by late postexercise hypoglycemia, which typically occurs 6 to 15 hours after strenuous exercise and is often nocturnal.[86,87] Sleep-related HAAF[3,72,73] is the result of further attenuation of the sympathoadrenal

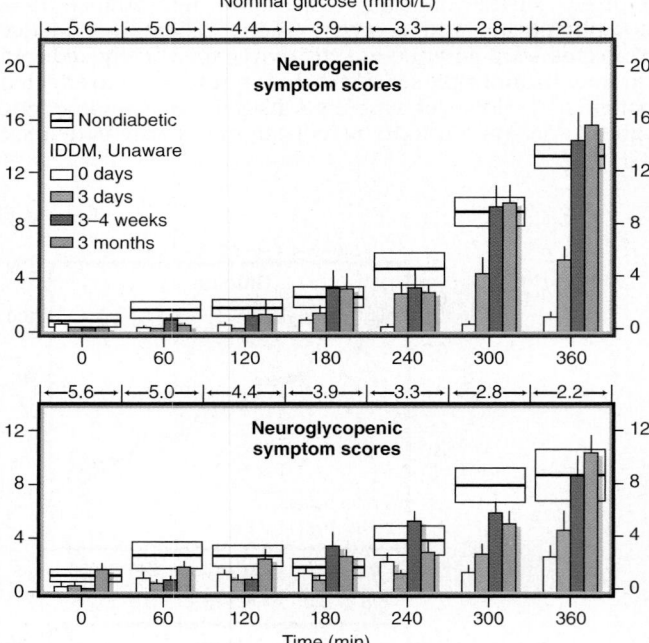

Figure 34-10 Mean (± standard error) neurogenic and neuroglycopenic symptom scores during hyperinsulinemic stepped hypoglycemic glucose clamps in nondiabetic subjects *(rectangles)* and in people with type 1 diabetes (IDDM) selected for clinical hypoglycemia unawareness studied at various time points during scrupulous avoidance of iatrogenic hypoglycemia: at baseline (0 days), after 3 days, after 3 to 4 weeks, and after 3 months (see key in figure). IDDM, insulin-dependent diabetes mellitus. (From Dagogo-Jack S, Rattarasarn C, Cryer PE. Reversal of hypoglycemia unawareness, but not defective glucose counterregulation, in IDDM. *Diabetes*. 1994;43:1426-1434, used with permission of the American Diabetes Association.)

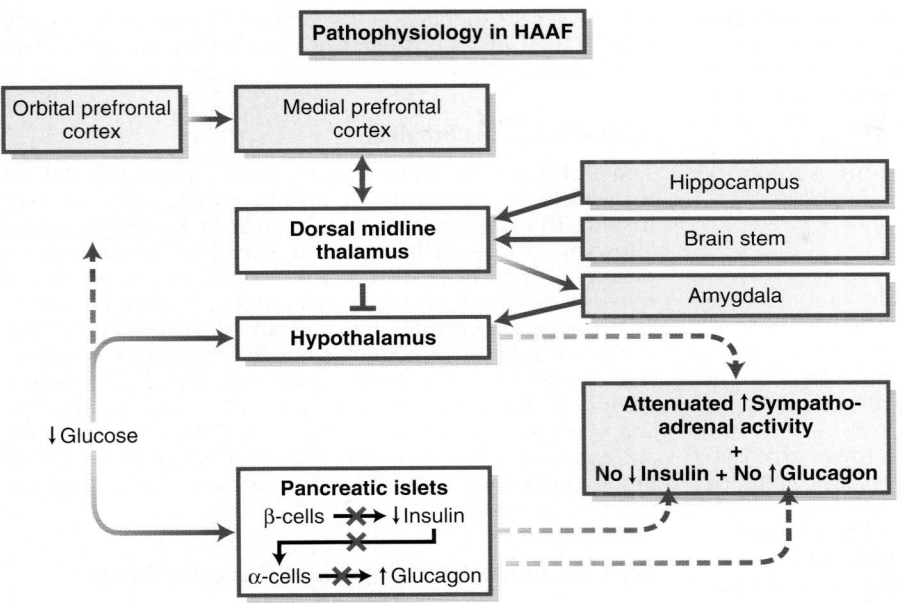

Figure 34-11 Schematic representation of the integrated mechanisms of hypoglycemia-associated autonomic failure (HAAF) in diabetes. Compare with Figure 34-5 and see text for discussion. α-cells, pancreatic islet alpha cells; β-cells, pancreatic islet beta cells. (From Cryer PE. The barrier of hypoglycemia in diabetes. *Diabetes.* 2008;57:3169-3176; and Cryer PE. *Hypoglycemia in Diabetes: Pathophysiology, Prevalence and Prevention.* Alexandria, VA: American Diabetes Association; 2009, used with permission of the American Diabetes Association.)

response to hypoglycemia during sleep. Sleeping patients with T1DM are much less likely to be awakened by hypoglycemia than nondiabetic individuals,[73] probably because of their attenuated sympathoadrenal responses. There may well be additional, unrecognized causes of HAAF, and there may also be a structural (neuropathic) component.[3]

The integrated pathophysiologic mechanisms of HAAF are illustrated in Figure 34-11. Loss of insulin and glucagon responses to falling plasma glucose concentrations caused by therapeutic hyperinsulinemia is the result of beta-cell failure in T1DM and advanced T2DM.[3,66] Neither can be attributed to loss of islet autonomic innervation, because low glucose concentrations decrease insulin secretion and increase glucagon secretion in patients with a transplanted (i.e., denervated) pancreas,[88] in dogs with a denervated pancreas,[89] and in isolated perfused pancreas and perifused islets. The mechanism of the attenuated sympathoadrenal response is not known, but it must involve the brain or the afferent or efferent components of the sympathoadrenal system.[3,66] The proposed mechanisms include the systemic mediator, brain fuel transport, brain metabolism, and cerebral network hypotheses.[3,66,90-94] There is considerable evidence against the first two of these proposed mechanisms.[3,66] Among many potential mechanisms,[90,91] an effect of lactate on brain metabolism has been studied.[95-98]

Much of the fundamental research into the mechanism of HAAF has focused on the hypothalamus, the central integrator of the sympathoadrenal response to hypoglycemia. It is conceivable, however, that the changes in the hypothalamic/sympathoadrenal response reflect modulation by higher brain centers.[3,66,92-94] For example, measurements of regional cerebral blood flow using oxygen-15–labeled water and positron emission tomography indicate that hypoglycemia increases synaptic activity in widespread but interconnected brain regions in humans[92] and that recent antecedent hypoglycemia both reduces sympathoadrenal and symptomatic responses (a model of HAAF) and increases synaptic activation in the dorsal midline thalamus (and only in that brain region) during subsequent hypoglycemia.[93,94] Therefore, it has been suggested that there may be a cerebral network that results in thalamic inhibition of hypothalamic activity in HAAF.[93,94] Such a putative cerebral network is included in Figure 34-11, although it remains theoretical.

TABLE 34-5
Risk Factors for Hypoglycemia in Diabetes

Conventional Risk Factors: Absolute or Relative Insulin Excess
Insulin or insulin secretagogue doses are excessive, ill-timed, or of the wrong type
Exogenous glucose delivery is decreased (e.g., after missed meals, during the overnight fast)
Glucose utilization is increased (e.g., during exercise)
Endogenous glucose production is decreased (e.g., after alcohol ingestion)
Sensitivity to insulin is increased (e.g., after weight loss, with improved fitness or improved glycemic control, in the middle of the night)
Insulin clearance is decreased (e.g., with renal failure)
Risk Factors for Hypoglycemia-Associated Autonomic Failure (HAAF)
Absolute endogenous insulin deficiency
A history of severe hypoglycemia, hypoglycemia unawareness, or both and recent antecedent hypoglycemia, prior exercise, or sleep
Aggressive glycemic therapy per se (lower HbA$_{1c}$ levels, lower glycemic goals, or both)

HbA$_{1c}$, glycosylated hemoglobin.

Risk Factors for Hypoglycemia in Diabetes

The risk factors for iatrogenic hypoglycemia[3,99] (Table 34-5) follow directly from the pathophysiology of glucose counterregulation in diabetes and are based on the tenet that iatrogenic hypoglycemia is typically the result of the interplay of relative or absolute therapeutic insulin excess and compromised physiologic and behavioral defenses against falling plasma glucose concentrations (i.e., HAAF) in T1DM and advanced T2DM, as discussed earlier.

Absolute or Relative Insulin Excess

The conventional risk factors for hypoglycemia in diabetes[3,99] (see Table 34-5) are based on the premise that absolute or relative insulin excess is the sole determinant of risk. Absolute therapeutic insulin excess occurs when doses of insulin or insulin secretagogue are excessive, ill-timed, or of the wrong type or when the clearance of insulin is decreased (as in renal failure). Relative insulin excess occurs when exogenous glucose delivery is reduced, glucose utilization is increased, endogenous glucose production is decreased, or sensitivity to insulin is increased. Persons with diabetes and their caregivers must consider these risk factors, including each of the examples listed in Table 34-5, when iatrogenic hypoglycemia is recognized to be a problem. However, these factors explain only a minority of episodes.[100]

Risk Factors for HAAF

The risk factors for HAAF[3,35,99-106] (see Table 34-5) include the following:
1. Absolute endogenous insulin deficiency[3,99,101-105]
2. A history of severe iatrogenic hypoglycemia, hypoglycemia unawareness, or both and recent antecedent hypoglycemia, prior exercise, or sleep[3,35,99,102-104]
3. Aggressive glycemic therapy per se (i.e., lower glycosylated hemoglobin [HbA$_{1c}$] levels, lower glycemic goals, or both)[3,30,99,102-106]

As discussed earlier, the degree of beta-cell failure determines the extent to which insulin levels will not decrease and glucagon levels will not increase as glucose levels fall in response to therapeutic hyperinsulinemia. The importance of loss of a decrease in insulin as glucose levels decline in response to therapeutic hyperinsulinemia is underscored by the fact that patients with type 1 diabetes and some degree of preserved insulin secretion have a lower incidence of hypoglycemia.[107] A history of severe hypoglycemia indicates (and that of hypoglycemia unawareness implies) recent antecedent hypoglycemia. Like prior exercise or sleep, recent antecedent hypoglycemia causes attenuated sympathoadrenal and symptomatic responses to subsequent hypoglycemia, the key feature of HAAF. Studies of intensive glycemic therapy that included a control group treated to a higher HbA$_{1c}$ level have consistently reported higher rates of hypoglycemia in the group treated to a lower HbA$_{1c}$ level in T1DM[21,22,108] and in T2DM.[30,39,109,110] Therefore, aggressive glycemic therapy is a risk factor for hypoglycemia. That does not mean, however, that one cannot both improve glycemic control and minimize the risk of hypoglycemia in many patients[3,99] (see later discussion).

Prevention of Hypoglycemia in Diabetes

Hypoglycemia risk factor reduction[3,99] (Table 34-6) is an empiric approach to minimizing the risk of iatrogenic hypoglycemia while maintaining or improving glycemic control in persons with diabetes. It involves four steps: acknowledge the problem; apply the principles of aggressive glycemic therapy,[3,99,111,112] consider the conventional risk factors, and consider the risk factors for HAAF (see Table 34-5).

Acknowledge the Problem

The problem of hypoglycemia should be addressed, at least in persons treated with an insulin secretagogue or with insulin, in every patient contact. Acknowledging the issue allows the caregiver to move on, if hypoglycemia is not a problem, or to deal with it and keep it in perspective, if hypoglycemia is a problem. Some patients are reluctant to raise the issue, but their concerns about the reality, or even the possibility, of hypoglycemia can be a barrier to glycemic control.[113,114] If possible, close associates of the patient should be asked whether they have observed clues to episodes not recognized by the patient. Even if no concerns are expressed, review of the record of self-monitoring of blood glucose (or CGM data) may disclose that hypoglycemia is a problem.

Apply the Principles of Aggressive Glycemic Therapy

These principles[3,99,111,112] include diabetes self-management by a well-informed patient, frequent self-monitoring of blood glucose levels (and in some instances CGM), flexible and appropriate insulin and other drug regimens, individualized glycemic goals, and ongoing professional guidance and support (see Table 34-6).

As the therapeutic regimen becomes progressively more complex—early in T1DM and later in T2DM—successful glycemic management becomes progressively more dependent on the many decisions and the skills of a well-informed person with diabetes. Therefore, patient education and empowerment are fundamentally important. Patients treated with insulin secretagogues or insulin need to know the common symptoms of hypoglycemia, their individual most meaningful symptoms, and how to treat (and not overtreat) an episode. They need to know the relevant conventional risk factors for hypoglycemia, including the temporal patterns of the glucose-lowering actions of their individual secretagogue or insulin preparations and the effects of missed meals, the overnight fast, exercise, and alcohol ingestion. They also need to know that increasing episodes of hypoglycemia signal an increased likelihood of future, often more severe, hypoglycemia.[30,62,102-104] Close associates also need to know how to recognize hypoglycemia, to understand why a neuroglycopenic patient may become uncooperative, and to know when and how to administer glucagon. Finally, patients need to learn to apply the data from their self-monitoring of blood glucose concentrations (or from CGM) toward the goal of minimizing hypoglycemia (as well as hyperglycemia). Structured education focused on avoidance of hypoglycemia can restore awareness of hypoglycemia and reduce the incidence of severe hypoglycemia without deterioration of glycemic control.[115-117]

Frequent self-monitoring also becomes vital to diabetes self-management as the therapeutic regimen becomes more complex, early in T1DM and later in T2DM. Ideally, patients should monitor their glucose level whenever they suspect hypoglycemia. That would confirm or refute an episode and help the patients learn their individual key symptoms and might lead to regimen adjustments. It is important for patients with hypoglycemia unawareness to monitor glucose levels before performing critical tasks such as driving. Unfortunately, conventional blood glucose monitoring, in which a measurement is obtained at one point in time, does not indicate whether the glucose level

---

TABLE 34-6

Hypoglycemia Risk Factor Reduction*

1. Acknowledge the problem.
2. Apply the principles of aggressive glycemic therapy.
   Diabetes self-management (patient education and empowerment)
   Frequent self-monitoring of blood glucose (and in some instances continuous glucose sensing)
   Flexible and appropriate insulin (and other drug) regimens
   Individualized glycemic goals
   Ongoing professional guidance and support
3. Consider the conventional risk factors for hypoglycemia.*
4. Consider the risk factors for HAAF.*

*See Table 34-5.
HAAF, hypoglycemia-associated autonomic failure in diabetes.

is falling, stable, or rising. That shortcoming is being addressed by evolving technologies for CGM.[118-122]

Typically coupled with continuous subcutaneous insulin infusion (CSII), CGM has been reported to reduce the incidence of severe hypoglycemia.[120] When used with a CSII pump with a low glucose suspend function—which stops infusing insulin for up to 2 hours when the CGM detects glucose levels that have fallen to a preselected low value—it can reduce the frequency of hypoglycemia.[121,122]

Therapeutic hyperinsulinemia, a prerequisite for iatrogenic hypoglycemia, can occur during treatment with an insulin secretagogue (such as a sulfonylurea or a glinide) or with insulin. Early in its course, T2DM may respond to drugs that do not raise insulin levels at normal or low plasma glucose concentrations and therefore should not, and probably do not,[123] cause hypoglycemia. Such drugs include the biguanide metformin, SGLT2 (sodium-glucose cotransporter 2) inhibitors, thiazolidinediones, α-glucosidase inhibitors, glucagon-like peptide 1 (GLP-1) receptor agonists, and dipeptidyl peptidase intravenous (DPP-IV) inhibitors. All of these drugs require endogenous insulin secretion to lower plasma glucose concentrations, and insulin secretion declines appropriately as glucose levels fall into the normal range. That is true even for the GLP-1 receptor agonists and DPP-IV inhibitors, which enhance glucose-stimulated insulin secretion (among other actions). Nonetheless, all six categories of drugs increase the risk of hypoglycemia if used with an insulin secretagogue or insulin.

Among the commonly prescribed sulfonylureas, hypoglycemia is more often associated with the longer-acting glyburide (glibenclamide) than with the shorter-acting glimepiride.[124] In a therapeutic regimen involving multiple daily injections of insulin, the use of long-acting insulin analogues (e.g., glargine, detemir) rather than NPH (neutral protamine Hagedorn) insulin as the basal insulin preparation reduces at least the incidence of nocturnal hypoglycemia, and perhaps that of total and symptomatic hypoglycemia, in T1DM and T2DM.[125-127] The newer longer acting basal insulins degludec[128,129] and LY2605541[130,131] are associated with less nocturnal hypoglycemia than glargine in T1DM and T2DM. The use of a rapid-acting insulin analogue (e.g., lispro, aspart, glulisine) as the prandial insulin reduces the incidence of nocturnal hypoglycemia at least in T1DM.[125,127] Approaches to the prevention of nocturnal hypoglycemia, in addition to the use of insulin analogues, include attempts to produce sustained delivery of exogenous carbohydrate or sustained endogenous glucose production throughout the night.[132] Closed-loop insulin replacement[133] has been shown to reduce nocturnal hypoglycemia in T1DM.[134]

As reviewed in detail elsewhere,[5] there is compelling evidence from randomized controlled trials that tight glycemic control partially prevents or delays microvascular complications (retinopathy, nephropathy, neuropathy) in T1DM[21] and T2DM.[135,136] As reviewed there[5] and developed earlier in this chapter, there is also compelling evidence that tight glycemic control increases hypoglycemic morbidity and mortality risks. Thus, it follows that the selection of a glycemic goal should be linked to the risk of hypoglycemia.[5] A reasonable glycemic goal is the lowest HbA$_{1c}$ that does not cause severe hypoglycemia and preserves awareness of hypoglycemia, preferably with little or no symptomatic or even asymptomatic hypoglycemia, at a given stage in the evolution of the individual's diabetes.[5] That might be accomplished with a normal HbA$_{1c}$ if glycemic control were achieved with lifestyle, with medical or surgical weight loss, or with drugs that do not cause hypoglycemia (i.e., drugs other than a sulfonylurea, a glinide,

or insulin). A somewhat higher HbA$_{1c}$ might well be necessary if glycemic control were achieved with the latter drugs. Nonetheless, there is substantial long-term microvascular benefit from reduction of HbA$_{1c}$ from high to lower, even if not optimal, levels.[137]

Finally, because the glycemic management of diabetes is empiric, caregivers should work with each patient to find the most effective and safest regimen at a given point in the course of that patient's diabetes.

Consider the Conventional Risk Factors

The conventional risk factors are those that result in relative, as well as absolute, insulin excess (see Table 34-5). In addition to insulin secretagogue doses, timing, and type, they include conditions in which exogenous glucose delivery or endogenous glucose production is decreased, glucose utilization or sensitivity to insulin is increased, or insulin clearance is decreased.

Consider the Risk Factors for HAAF

The risk factors indicative of HAAF (see Table 34-5) include the degree of endogenous insulin deficiency; a history of severe hypoglycemia, hypoglycemia unawareness, or both and recent antecedent hypoglycemia, prior exercise, or sleep; and aggressive glycemic therapy per se. An episode of severe hypoglycemia is a clinical red flag. Unless the cause is easily remediable, it should prompt consideration of a fundamental change in the therapeutic regimen. Without such a change, the risk of a subsequent episode of severe hypoglycemia is high.[3,62,102-104] In a patient with hypoglycemia unawareness, patient reeducation[115-117] and a 2- to 3-week period of scrupulous avoidance of hypoglycemia is advisable and can be expected to restore awareness.[82-85] This approach usually requires somewhat higher glycemic goals in the short term. A history of late postexercise hypoglycemia, nocturnal hypoglycemia, or both should prompt appropriately timed regimen adjustments to provide more carbohydrate intake, less insulin action, or both.

Treatment of Hypoglycemia in Diabetes

Most episodes of symptomatic hypoglycemia or of asymptomatic hypoglycemia detected by self-monitoring or CGM are effectively self-treated by ingestion of glucose tablets or carbohydrates.[138] A reasonable dose is 20 g of glucose.[138] Clinical improvement should occur in 15 to 20 minutes. The temptation to overtreat is understandable but should be avoided. With ongoing hyperinsulinemia, the glycemic response to oral glucose is transient, typically lasting less than 2 hours (Fig. 34-12).[138] Therefore, ingestion of a snack or meal shortly after the glucose level is raised is usually advisable.

In a patient who is unable or unwilling (because of neuroglycopenia) to take carbohydrate orally, parenteral therapy is necessary. Glucagon, in a dose of 1.0 mg in adults, can be injected subcutaneously or intramuscularly by an associate of the patient. Administration of glucagon can be lifesaving, but it often causes substantial, albeit transient, hyperglycemia (see Fig. 34-12), and it can cause nausea and even vomiting. Smaller doses of glucagon (e.g., 150 μg), repeated if necessary, have been found to be effective without side effects.[139] For the prompt treatment of episodes of severe iatrogenic hypoglycemia and particularly for inclusion, with insulin, in a bihormonal artificial pancreas, a glucagon analogue that is stable in solution and that retains the rapid plasma glucose-raising action[140] is needed.

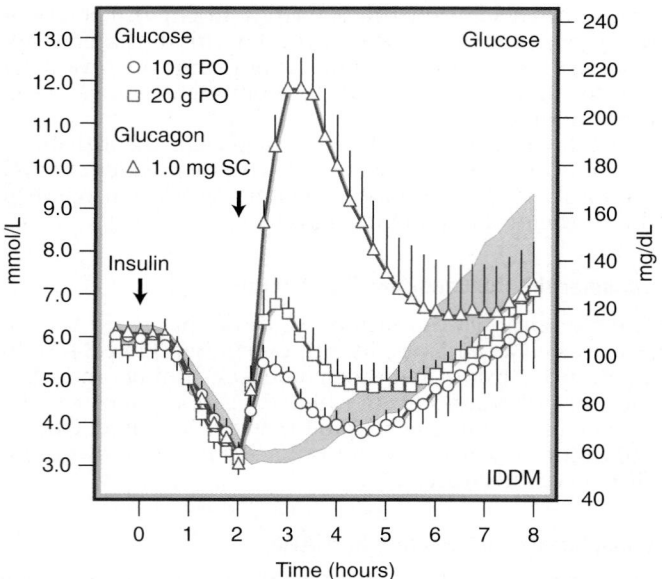

Figure 34-12 Mean (± standard error) plasma glucose concentrations during hypoglycemia produced by subcutaneous insulin injection in people with type 1 diabetes in response to 10 g *(circles)* or 20 g *(squares)* of oral (PO) glucose or 1.0 mg of subcutaneous (SC) glucagon *(triangles)*, compared with placebo *(shaded area)*. IDDM, insulin-dependent diabetes mellitus. (From Wiethop BV, Cryer PE. Alanine and terbutaline in treatment of hypoglycemia in IDDM. *Diabetes Care.* 1993;16:1131-1136, used with permission of the American Diabetes Association.)

Because it acts by stimulating glycogenolysis, glucagon is ineffective in glycogen-depleted individuals (e.g., after a binge of alcohol ingestion). Although it is not an issue in T1DM or advanced T2DM, glucagon stimulates insulin secretion. Indeed, glucagon has been reported to cause hypoglycemia in nondiabetic individuals (see later discussion). Glucagon can be administered intravenously by medical personnel, but in that setting IV glucose is the standard parenteral therapy. A common initial dose is 25 g.[138] The glycemic response to IV glucose is, of course, transient in the setting of ongoing hyperinsulinemia. Therefore, IV glucose administration often needs to be followed by glucose infusion and, once it is practical, by carbohydrate feeding.

The duration of an episode of severe hypoglycemia is a function of its cause. An episode caused by a rapid-acting insulin secretagogue or insulin analogue will be relatively brief. That caused by a long-acting insulin secretagogue or insulin analogue can result in prolonged hypoglycemia requiring hospitalization.

HYPOGLYCEMIA IN PERSONS WITHOUT DIABETES

The Decision to Evaluate for Hypoglycemia

Although hypoglycemia is common in persons with diabetes,[3] it is a distinctly uncommon clinical event in persons who do not have diabetes[2] because of the effectiveness of the normal physiologic and behavioral defenses against falling plasma glucose concentrations.[4] Therefore, in the absence of diabetes, a thorough evaluation for hypoglycemia is recommended only for patients in whom Whipple triad (symptoms, signs, or both consistent with hypoglycemia; a low reliably measured plasma glucose concentration; and resolution of those symptoms or signs after the

plasma glucose concentration is raised[2,3]) can be documented. In the absence of such documentation, evaluation for hypoglycemia may expose the patient to unnecessary evaluation, costs, and potential harm without expectation of benefit.[2]

Plasma glucose concentrations used to document Whipple triad must be measured with a reliable laboratory method and not with a blood glucose self-monitor. A reliably measured low plasma glucose concentration obtained in the absence of recognized symptoms or signs should not be ignored. However, such a finding raises the possibility of "pseudohypoglycemia," an artifact of continued glucose metabolism by the formed elements of the blood after the blood sample is drawn.[2] This may occur if the sample is collected in a container that does not include an inhibitor of glycolysis and separation of the plasma or serum from the formed elements is delayed, particularly in the setting of erythrocytosis, leukocytosis, or thrombocytosis.

Venous sampling is standard in the clinical setting, but it is the arterial plasma glucose concentration that fuels the brain.[4] Arteriovenous plasma glucose concentration differences are negligible in the postabsorptive state, but antecubital venous glucose levels are as much as one third lower than arterial glucose levels when insulin secretion is increased (e.g., after an oral glucose load) stimulating glucose extraction across the forearm.[141] Because of the provision of alternative fuels (specifically ketones) to the brain, plasma glucose concentrations lower than the overnight fasted physiologic range occur in healthy individuals, especially women and children, during extended fasting.[4] Finally, the glycemic thresholds of responses to hypoglycemia shift to lower plasma glucose concentrations in patients with recurrent hypoglycemia.[18,19] For all of these reasons, it is important to document Whipple triad before concluding that a hypoglycemic disorder exists in a person without diabetes.[2] On the other hand, a reliably measured, unequivocally normal plasma glucose concentration (e.g., >3.9 mmol/L [70 mg/dL]) during a symptomatic episode provides strong evidence that the symptoms were not the result of hypoglycemia.[2]

Clinical Classification of Hypoglycemic Disorders

The traditional classification of hypoglycemic disorders in nondiabetic persons, as either postabsorptive (fasting) or postprandial (reactive) hypoglycemias, has been supplanted by a clinical categorization. This distinguishes a patient who has a relevant disease or treatment from a patient who is otherwise seemingly well (see Table 34-3).[2,142] The presence of postprandial symptoms without Whipple triad, previously called "reactive hypoglycemia," is now considered a functional disorder in which symptoms are not due to hypoglycemia and for which an oral glucose tolerance test is not indicated.[2]

Ill or Medicated Individual

Drugs are the most common cause of hypoglycemia.[2,143-149] In addition to insulin secretagogues and insulin (discussed earlier), offending drugs include alcohol[144-145] among many others (Table 34-7).[147-149] Drugs, often in the setting of critical illnesses including renal failure, are the most common cause of hypoglycemia in hospitals.[143] Again, insulin or insulin secretagogues are common offending drugs,[143,150] particularly if they are administered when enteral or parenteral nutrition is interrupted.

Ethanol inhibits gluconeogenesis. Clinical alcohol-induced hypoglycemia typically follows a binge of alcohol

TABLE 34-7

Drugs, Other Than Antihyperglycemic Agents and Alcohol, Reported to Cause Hypoglycemia*

Moderate Quality of Evidence

Cibenzoline
Gatifloxacin
Pentamidine
Quinine
Indomethacin
Glucagon (during endoscopy)

Low Quality of Evidence

Chloroquinoxaline sulfonamide
Artesunate/artemisinin/artemether
Insulin-like growth factor type 1
Lithium
Propoxyphene/dextropropoxyphene

Very Low Quality of Evidence

>25 Cases Identified

Angiotensin-converting enzyme inhibitors
Angiotensin receptor antagonists
β-Adrenergic receptor antagonists
Levofloxacin
Mifepristone
Disopyramide
Trimethoprim-sulfamethoxazole
Heparin
6-Mercaptopurine

<25 Cases Identified
See Murad et al, 2009[147]

*From Cryer PE, Axelrod L, Grossman AB, et al. Evaluation and management of adult hypoglycemic disorders: an Endocrine Society clinical practice guideline. *J Clin Endocrinol Metab.* 2009;94:709-728; and based on Murad MH, Coto-Yglesias F, Wang AT, et al. Drug-induced hypoglycemia: a systematic review. *J Clin Endocrinol Metab.* 2009;94:741-745, with permission of the Endocrine Society.

consumption during which the person eats little food (i.e., in the setting of glycogen depletion).[145] Alcohol-induced hypoglycemia can be fatal, but with restoration of euglycemia and supportive care, recovery is the rule. Ethanol is usually measurable in blood at the time of presentation.

Hypoglycemia sometimes occurs in patients with critical illnesses (see Table 34-3).[2] Hepatogenous hypoglycemia occurs most commonly when destruction of the liver is rapid and massive (e.g., in toxic hepatitis). It is unusual in common forms of cirrhosis or hepatitis, although glucose metabolism is measurably altered in uncomplicated viral hepatitis.[151] Hypoglycemia is also unusual in metastatic liver disease despite extensive hepatic replacement.[152] The pathogenesis of hypoglycemia in some patients with renal failure is unknown and likely multifactorial; it has been attributed to drugs, sepsis, or inanition.[143,153-155] Reduced renal clearance of insulin and reduced renal glucose production might be relevant factors. However, renal transplantation did not correct hypoglycemia in patients with glucose-6-phosphatase deficiency.[156]

The pathogenesis of the hypoglycemia occasionally seen in patients with severe cardiac failure is also not understood. The finding of elevated blood lactate levels associated with hypoglycemia[157] raises the possibility of inhibited gluconeogenesis. Sepsis is a relatively common cause of hypoglycemia.[143,144,158] Increased glucose utilization (by skeletal muscle and by macrophage-rich tissues such as liver, spleen, and lung), which is thought to be cytokine-mediated and is matched initially by increased glucose production, characterizes experimental sepsis.[159-161] The

later decline in glucose production, which in the setting of persistently high glucose utilization results in hypoglycemia, is not the result of glucose counterregulatory failure; rather, it is caused by decreased responsiveness to appropriate glucose counterregulatory signals (i.e., low insulin and high glucagon and epinephrine levels).[162] Finally, hypoglycemia can be caused by inanition.[163] A plausible suggestion is that glucose becomes the sole oxidative fuel in the setting of total body fat depletion, and the resulting high rates of glucose utilization exceed the capacity to produce glucose because of a limited supply of gluconeogenic precursors (e.g., amino acids). Postabsorptive hypoglycemia (with low circulating alanine concentrations) has been reported in patients with profound muscle atrophy[164,165]; hypoglycemia is presumably the result of substrate limitation of gluconeogenesis in such patients.

With the notable exception of HAAF in patients with T1DM and advanced T2DM[3] (discussed earlier), hormone deficiencies resulting in hypoglycemia are not common. Postabsorptive hypoglycemia, typically after a period of caloric deprivation caused by an intercurrent illness, can occur in patients with deficient secretion of cortisol, growth hormone, or both, particularly infants and young children.[166-168] Glycemic intolerance of fasting is largely corrected by glucocorticoid replacement; growth hormone replacement has a lesser effect.[167,168] Because cortisol normally supports gluconeogenesis by increasing gluconeogenic enzyme activities and mobilizing gluconeogenic precursors,[167,169] the hypoglycemic mechanism is thought to be reduced glucose production in the setting of glycogen deficiency. Nonetheless, most adults with deficiencies of these hormones do not experience hypoglycemia. Indeed, plasma glucose concentrations and rates of endogenous glucose production after overnight fasting have been reported to be indistinguishable from normal values in short-term glucocorticoid-withdrawn patients with hypopituitarism never treated with growth hormone.[170] Hypoglycemia has been reported in adrenocorticotropic hormone (ACTH)-deficient adults when glucose utilization or loss was increased (as during exercise or pregnancy, respectively)[171] or when glucose production is impaired (as after alcohol ingestion).[172]

Non–islet cell tumor hypoglycemia (NICTH) is rare. The tumors are usually, but not invariably, large, clinically apparent, and mesenchymal in origin. NICTH is often the result of overproduction of incompletely processed pro–insulin-like growth factor 2 (pro-IGF-2),[173-176] but hypoglycemia attributed to overproduction of insulin-like growth factor 1 (IGF-1) has also been reported.[177] The pro-IGF-2 binds poorly to its binding proteins and therefore more freely enters tissue spaces, where its insulin-like actions cause hypoglycemia. Concentrations of plasma free IGF-2 (or IGF-1[177]) are elevated,[174] but these measurements are not widely available. Because of suppression of growth hormone secretion and the resulting low IGF-1 levels, the ratio of plasma IGF-2 to IGF-1 is elevated in pro-IGF-2–mediated hypoglycemia. Plasma total IGF-2 levels may be within the normal range, but the ratio of pro-IGF-2 to IGF-2 may be elevated.[175] Endogenous insulin secretion is suppressed appropriately during hypoglycemia in NICTH. Treatment of the tumor is seldom curative but may alleviate hypoglycemia. Treatment with a glucocorticoid, growth hormone, or both is sometimes effective.

Seemingly Well Individual

In seemingly well individuals with no evidence of drug, critical illness, hormone deficiency, or non–islet cell tumor as a cause of their hypoglycemia, the differential diagnosis narrows to two categories: accidental, surreptitious, or even malicious hypoglycemia and endogenous hyperinsulinism (see Table 34-3).[2,178,179] Consideration of the former possibility should precede a systematic assessment of the latter. Medical, pharmacy, and hospital errors can result in hypoglycemia and do occur. Surreptitious hypoglycemia[178-182] is more common in people with knowledge of, and access to, glucose-lowering medications. Malicious hypoglycemia[178,179] can be accomplished by administration of an insulin secretagogue or insulin.

Insulinomas (insulin-secreting pancreatic beta-cell tumors) are the prototypical, but not the only, cause of endogenous hyperinsulinemic hypoglycemia.[2,142,178,183-186] Patients with an insulinoma typically present with a history of episodes of neuroglycopenia occurring in the postabsorptive (fasting) state. However, an appreciable subset of patients (6% in one series[183]) report symptoms exclusively in the postprandial state. Insulinomas are rare; an incidence of 1 in 250,000 patient-years has been reported.[187] Fewer than 10% of the patients have malignant insulinomas, multiple insulinomas, or the multiple endocrine neoplasia type 1 (MEN1) syndrome.[187] Long-term survival is the rule after successful surgical removal of an insulinoma.[187]

Some patients (4% of one series[188]) with fasting endogenous hyperinsulinemic hypoglycemia do not have an insulinoma but have diffuse islet involvement with islet hypertrophy, sometimes with hyperplasia, and enlarged and hyperchromatic beta-cell nuclei.[188-198] This condition is often termed *nesidioblastosis*, although the histologic finding of islets budding from pancreatic ducts is not invariably present.[188,189] Such patients are clinically indistinguishable from those with an insulinoma.[188-191] Other patients have the noninsulinoma pancreatogenous hypoglycemia syndrome (NIPHS)[192-195] or post–gastric bypass hypoglycemia.[196-206]

NIPHS[192-195] is characterized by spells of neuroglycopenia caused by endogenous hyperinsulinemic hypoglycemia occurring typically, but not invariably, after a meal. NIPHS is less common than insulinoma.[2] Because the syndrome is diffuse, anatomic tumor imaging studies are uniformly negative. Given documented postprandial hyperinsulinemic hypoglycemia, documentation of diffuse beta-cell hyperfunction depends on a positive selective arterial calcium stimulation test. The findings from that test can be used to guide partial pancreatectomy if empiric medical therapy (e.g., diet, an α-glucosidase inhibitor, diazoxide, octreotide) fails. In one relatively large surgical series most patients improved but recurrence of symptoms was the rule and some patients were not helped after partial pancreatectomy.[194]

Some patients who have undergone Roux-en-Y gastric bypass develop postprandial endogenous hyperinsulinemic hypoglycemia several months after the surgery.[196-206] Affected patients have accelerated absorption of ingested glucose that triggers a large insulin secretory response that is mediated, at least in part, by a robust increase in GLP-1.[199-203] Post–gastric bypass hypoglycemia is rare, reported to occur in 0.2% of operated patients.[204] Partial pancreatectomy may be required if empiric medical therapy fails; again, the results are mixed.[205] Indeed, bypass reversal has been reported to reduce, but not eliminate, symptomatic hypoglycemia.[206]

Autoimmune hypoglycemia caused by an antibody to insulin is rare.[207,208] Affected individuals often have a history of other autoimmune disorders. Hypoglycemia occurs in the late postprandial period as insulin, which is secreted in response to the meal, and when bound to the circulating antibody, dissociates from the antibody in an unregulated fashion. A clue to the diagnosis is the finding of very high measured plasma insulin levels during hypoglycemia. The diagnosis is made by the finding of high-titer serum insulin antibodies. There is no consistently effective therapy. A similar disorder has been reported in patients with a high-capacity insulin-binding monoclonal paraprotein.[209]

Accidental or surreptitious ingestion of an insulin secretagogue causes endogenous hyperinsulinemic hypoglycemia indistinguishable from that caused by an insulinoma aside from the presence of a measurable oral hypoglycemic agent in the circulation at the time of hypoglycemia.[2]

Very rare causes of insulin-related hypoglycemia have been linked to a mutation of the insulin receptor,[210] to exercise-induced hyperinsulinemia,[211] or to an agonist antibody to the insulin receptor.[212] In the latter case, endogenous insulin secretion is suppressed appropriately, and inappropriately high insulin levels are thought to result from blockade of receptor-mediated insulin clearance by the antibody. Finally, although seemingly convincing cases of ectopic insulin secretion have been reported (e.g., by Seckl and colleagues[213]), the condition must be extraordinarily rare.

Diagnostic Approach

Patients with a hypoglycemic disorder may present in a number of different ways including with a history of symptomatic episodes compatible with hypoglycemia, a serendipitously measured low plasma glucose concentration, or a familial syndrome that includes a hypoglycemic disorder (e.g., MEN1).[2,142,178] A careful history of any spells—including the specific symptoms, their timing in relation to meals, their duration, and any factors that aggravate or alleviate them—is important for the formulation of a diagnostic plan. A history that includes neuroglycopenia is particularly compelling.[2] Again, documentation of Whipple triad establishes that a hypoglycemic disorder exists.[2] The diagnostic strategy recommended in the Endocrine Society clinical practice guideline[2] is described here.

First, review the history, physical findings, and all available laboratory data seeking clues to specific disorders such as drugs, critical illnesses, hormone deficiencies, or non–islet cell tumors (see Table 34-3) and pursue those.[2] This approach will identify the cause of hypoglycemia in most instances. Again, drugs[2,143-150] are, by far, the most common cause of hypoglycemia (see Table 34-7).

If the cause of a hypoglycemic disorder is not evident (i.e., in a seemingly healthy individual), measure plasma glucose, insulin, C-peptide, proinsulin, and β-hydroxybutyrate concentrations and screen for oral hypoglycemic agents during an episode of spontaneous hypoglycemia, and observe the plasma glucose response to IV injection of 1.0 mg of glucagon.[2] Also, measure insulin antibodies.[2]

Failure of insulin secretion to fall to very low rates as plasma glucose concentrations fall to hypoglycemic levels is the key pathophysiologic feature of endogenous hyperinsulinism. Hypoglycemia is the result of low rates of glucose production rather than high rates of glucose utilization.[214] Plasma insulin, C-peptide, and proinsulin concentrations may not always be high relative to normal values obtained under euglycemic conditions, but they are essentially always inappropriately high relative to the low plasma glucose concentrations.[2,142,178] The traditional critical diagnostic criteria (assuming Whipple triad is documented) are plasma insulin concentrations equal to or greater than 18 pmol/L (≥3 μU/mL), plasma C-peptide concentrations of 0.2 nmol/L (0.6 ng/mL) or higher, and plasma proinsulin concentrations of 5.0 pmol/L or higher when plasma glucose concentrations are less than

TABLE 34-8

Patterns of Findings During Fasting or After a Mixed Meal in Normal Individuals* and in Individuals With Hyperinsulinemic (or IGF-Mediated) Hypoglycemia or Hypoglycemia Caused by Other Mechanisms

Symptoms, Signs, or Both	Glucose (mg/dL)	Insulin (μU/mL)	C-Peptide (nmol/L)	Proinsulin (pmol/L)	β-Hydroxybutyrate (mmol/L)	Glucose Increase After Glucagon (mg/dL)	Circulating Oral Hypoglycemic Agent	Antibody to Insulin	Diagnostic Interpretation
No	<55	<3	<0.2	<5	<2.7	<25	No	No	Normal
Yes	<55	≫3	<0.2	<5	≤2.7	>25	No	Neg (Pos)	Exogenous insulin
Yes	<55	≥3	≥0.2	≥5	≤2.7	>25	No	Neg	Insulinoma, NIPHS, PGBH
Yes	<55	≥3	≥0.2	≥5	≤2.7	>25	Yes	Neg	Oral hypoglycemic agent
Yes	<55	≫3	≫0.2†	≫5†	≤2.7	>25	No	Pos	Insulin autoimmune
Yes	<55	<3	<0.2	<5	≤2.7	>25	No	Neg	IGF‡
Yes	<55	<3	<0.2	<5	>2.7	<25	No	Neg	Not insulin- or IGF-mediated

*Normal individuals are those with no symptoms or signs despite relatively low plasma glucose concentrations (i.e., those in whom Whipple triad is not documented).
†Concentrations of free C-peptide and proinsulin are low.
‡Increased pro-IGF-2, free IGF-2, and IGF-2/IGF-1 ratio.
IGF, insulin-like growth factor; NIPHS, noninsulinoma pancreatogenous hypoglycemia; PGBH, post–gastric bypass hypoglycemia.
From Cryer PE, Axelrod L, Grossman AB, et al. Evaluation and management of adult hypoglycemic disorders: an Endocrine Society clinical practice guideline. *J Clin Endocrinol Metab.* 2009;94:709-728, used with permission of the Endocrine Society. Data from Service[142] and Placzkowski and associates.[183] See discussion of Guettier and associates[186] for independent data.

3.0 mmol/L (<55 mg/dL) (Table 34-8). These data, first published in 1995,[142] reassessed in 2009,[183] and incorporated into the Endocrine Society clinical practice guideline on adult hypoglycemic disorders,[2] were independently reassessed in 2013.[186] Notably, however, the extent to which the unaffected subjects had low plasma glucose concentrations at the time of insulin, C-peptide, and proinsulin sampling is not made clear.[186] The insulin criterion of 18 pmol/L or higher (≥3 μU/mL) was generally supported: 93% sensitivity with 95% to 100% specificity[183] and 98% sensitivity with 60% specificity.[186] The C-peptide criterion of 0.2 nmol/L or higher (≥0.6 ng/mL) was not: sensitivity at 100% or lower with specificity of 60% to 78%[183] versus sensitivity at 100% but specificity only 10%[186]; raising the criterion to 0.8 nmol/L or higher (≥2.3 ng/mL) lowered sensitivity to 84% but raised specificity to 76%.[186] The proinsulin criterion of 5 pmol/L or higher provided 100% sensitivity in both series but with specificity of 68% to 78%[183] and 41%[186]; raising the criterion to 27 pmol/L or higher still provided 100% sensitivity but with 100% specificity.[186] Plasma β-hydroxybutyrate concentrations equal to or lower than 2.7 mmol/L and an increase in the plasma glucose concentration of more than 1.4 mmol/L (>25 mg/dL) over the low value over 30 minutes after glucagon injection provide evidence of biologic actions of inappropriately high insulin (or IGF) levels, with suppression of lipolysis and ketogenesis and preservation of hepatic glycogen stores, respectively. The patterns of findings in patients with a hypoglycemic disorder and in those with hyperinsulinemic (or IGF-mediated) hypoglycemia are summarized in Table 34-8. Occasionally, a patient with an insulinoma may not fulfill these criteria even during a 72-hour fast,[215] and a few have plasma insulin levels lower than 18 pmol/L (<3 μU/mL) during hypoglycemia, but at least in some series[216] plasma C-peptide and proinsulin levels are elevated in such patients.

If Whipple triad has not been documented and the measurements described have not been obtained during an episode of spontaneous hypoglycemia, an attempt should be made to recreate the circumstances in which symptomatic hypoglycemia is likely to occur.[2] This can be accomplished by withholding food in a patient with a history suggestive of fasting hypoglycemia or by providing a mixed meal likely to cause a symptomatic episode in a patient with a history suggestive of postprandial hypoglycemia. Failing these relatively informal procedures, a patient with a history suggestive of fasting hypoglycemia should undergo a prolonged supervised fast.[2] The fast should be continued until Whipple triad is documented (or until a plasma glucose concentration of <3.0 mmol/L [<55 mg/dL] is reached if Whipple triad was unequivocally documented previously[215]) unless a progressive increase in plasma β-hydroxybutyrate levels signals a negative fast. Serial plasma glucose concentrations should be measured with a precise method, not with a point-of-care glucose monitor. About two thirds of patients with an insulinoma meet the diagnostic criteria during a fast of less than 24 hours; most, but not all, do so in less than 48 hours.[215] Therefore, the diagnostic fast can be initiated, and often completed,[183] in the outpatient setting and continued in the inpatient setting if necessary. On the other hand, a patient with a history suggestive of postprandial hypoglycemia should undergo a mixed meal test conducted over 5 hours. Standards for interpretation of the findings of the mixed meal test have not been established; current usage[2] is to apply the criteria developed under fasting conditions.[142] Detailed suggestions for performance of a prolonged supervised fast and of a mixed meal test have been published.[2]

A patient with documented Whipple triad; inappropriately high levels of insulin, C-peptide, and proinsulin and no detectable circulating oral hypoglycemic agent; suppressed β-hydroxybutyrate levels; a brisk glycemic response to IV glucagon during fasting (or even postprandial[183]) hypoglycemia; and no circulating insulin antibody may well have an insulinoma. However, as noted earlier, there are other causes of hyperinsulinemic hypoglycemia (see Tables 34-3 and 34-8). Therefore, the next step is to attempt to localize an insulinoma.[2]

Computed tomography (CT), magnetic resonance imaging (MRI), and transabdominal ultrasonography detect approximately 75% of insulinomas.[183,217,218] They also detect metastases in the minority of patients who have a malignant insulinoma. Somatostatin receptor scintigraphy is somewhat less sensitive.[219] Endoscopic pancreatic

TABLE 34-9

Causes of Hypoglycemia Unique to, or Typically With Onset in, Infancy and Childhood

Intolerance of Fasting

Preterm or small-for-gestational-age infants
Hypopituitarism, adrenal hypoplasia, congenital adrenal hyperplasia
Ketotic hypoglycemia of childhood

Hyperinsulinism

Infant of a diabetic mother
Maternal drugs (sulfonylurea, β_2-adrenergic agonist)
Congenital hyperinsulinism, insulinoma
Others: Rh incompatibility, Beckwith-Wiedemann syndrome, exchange transfusions, perinatal stress

Enzyme Defects

Carbohydrate metabolism: glycogen storage disease types I, III, and VI; glycogen synthase deficiency; fructose-1,6-bisphosphatase deficiency; fructose-1-phosphate aldolase deficiency; galactose-1-phosphate uridyltransferase deficiency
Protein metabolism: branched-chain α-keto acid dehydrogenase complex deficiency
Fat metabolism: fatty acid oxidation defects including deficiencies in the carnitine cycle, the β-oxidation spiral, the electron transport system, and the ketogenesis sequence

ultrasonography (EUS), with the option of fine-needle aspiration of a detected tumor, has a sensitivity of greater than 90%.[220,221] With the combination of noninvasive imaging and, if necessary, EUS, preoperative localization of insulinomas has become the rule.[183] Given the promise of positron emission tomography with radiotracers such as fluorine-18–labeled dihydroxyphenylalanine,[222] noninvasive localization of insulinomas may become the preferred approach. If anatomic localization of insulinoma is negative or equivocal, selective pancreatic arterial calcium injections, with an end point of at least a twofold[223,224] increase (or perhaps a greater than fivefold increase with contemporary assays[225]) in hepatic venous insulin levels over baseline, regionalize insulinomas with high sensitivity.[225,226] Although this invasive procedure is seldom necessary in patients with an insulinoma, it is the procedure of choice for confirming NIPHS[192-195] and hypoglycemia occurring after Roux-en-Y gastric bypass (Table 34-9).[196-206] Finally, intraoperative pancreatic ultrasonography almost invariably localizes tumors that are not apparent even to the experienced pancreatic surgeon.

Treatment of Hypoglycemia Disorders

Prevention of ongoing or recurrent hypoglycemia requires treatment that corrects or circumvents the hypoglycemic mechanism.[2] Obviously, treatment should be tailored to the specific hypoglycemic disorder identified. Offending drugs can be discontinued or their dosage reduced. Critical illnesses can often be treated. Deficient hormones, such as cortisol, can be replaced. Reduction of non–islet cell tumor mass with surgery, irradiation, or chemotherapy may alleviate hypoglycemia even if the tumor cannot be cured. Treatment with a glucocorticoid, growth hormone, or even octreotide may alleviate hypoglycemia in such patients. Surgical resection of a benign insulinoma is typically curative. In unresectable disease empirical treatments (diet, diazoxide, octreotide) can be tried; there has been progress with chemotherapy.[227,228] Diet, including frequent feedings, an α-glucosidase inhibitor, diazoxide, or octreotide, can be tried in patients with NIPHS or post–gastric bypass hypoglycemia, but partial pancreatectomy may be required.

Treatment of autoimmune hypoglycemia (with a glucocorticoid or another immunosuppressive medication) is problematic, but the disorder is sometimes self-limited. Failing these treatments, frequent feedings during the day and bedtime administration of large doses of uncooked cornstarch or even overnight intragastric glucose infusion may be necessary.

HYPOGLYCEMIA IN INFANCY AND CHILDHOOD

The fetus receives a continuous supply of glucose from the maternal circulation. Plasma glucose concentrations decline after birth as the neonate makes the transition to endogenous glucose production. Because mobilizable glycogen stores are limited and feeding is intermittent, the newborn is largely dependent on gluconeogenesis initially. In the setting of relatively low plasma glucose concentrations, the normal combination of hypoinsulinemia and activated glucose counterregulatory systems favors not only gluconeogenesis but also lipolysis and eventually ketogenesis. Impairment of these glucoregulatory mechanisms can cause transient or persistent neonatal hypoglycemia. Enzymatic defects can cause hypoglycemia in infants that persists into childhood.[229,230]

As in adults,[2] a diagnosis of clinical hypoglycemia should include symptoms and signs, but those are quite nonspecific in a neonate, and it is not possible to state a single low plasma glucose concentration that categorically defines neonatal hypoglycemia.[229,230] A cutoff value of 2.6 mmol/L (47 mg/dL)[231] seems reasonable, but compelling evidence is lacking.[230]

Hypoglycemia in children can be caused by the same mechanisms as in adults[2] (see Table 34-3), including drugs and critical illnesses. For example, 18% of children receiving resuscitative care were found to be hypoglycemic.[232] Of the 10 who died, 5 were hypoglycemic. Nonetheless, several hypoglycemic disorders are unique to, or have their onset in, infancy and childhood.[229,230] In general, those hypoglycemic disorders can be classified as intolerance of fasting, hyperinsulinism, and enzyme defects (see Table 34-9).

Intolerance of Fasting

At least in the absence of seizure or coma, neonatal hypoglycemia is usually transient. It is particularly common in preterm or small-for-gestational-age infants and is thought to result from incomplete development of gluconeogenic mechanisms.[233] Deficiency of cortisol can be congenital and can cause hypoglycemia through mechanisms discussed earlier.

The syndrome of ketotic hypoglycemia of childhood, which typically has its onset between ages 2 and 5 years and remits spontaneously before age 10 years, may represent those children who are least tolerant of fasting, because hypoglycemia occurs when feeding is interrupted, usually during an intercurrent illness. It appears to involve diminished mobilization of gluconeogenic precursors.[234]

Hyperinsulinism

Maternal diabetes is a common cause of transient neonatal hypoglycemia.[230] Infants of diabetic mothers have been hyperglycemic in utero in proportion to the mother's hyperglycemia. Presumably because of chronic stimulation of fetal insulin secretion in utero and the failure of insulin to fall normally as glucose levels decline shortly after birth, transient neonatal hypoglycemia develops. Affected infants are typically macrosomic. Transient hyperinsulinemia also causes transient neonatal hypoglycemia under other conditions listed in Table 34-9. As in adults, hyperinsulinemic hypoglycemia can be accidental, surreptitious, or even malicious, and postprandial hypoglycemia analogous to that occurring after gastric bypass can follow Nissen fundoplication.

Congenital hyperinsulinism[235-238] is the most common cause of nontransient neonatal hypoglycemia, although it occurs in only 1 of every 30,000 to 50,000 live births. Hypoglycemia may persist from the neonatal period or become apparent during the first year of life. (Patients in that age range rarely harbor an insulinoma; however, an insulinoma is occasionally found in children who develop endogenous hyperinsulinemic hypoglycemia after the first year of life.) The need for very high glucose infusion rates is a diagnostic clue.

Glucose-stimulated insulin secretion normally involves increased glucose transport into beta cells, glucokinase-mediated phosphorylation of glucose, glucose metabolism resulting in an increase in the ratio of adenosine triphosphate (ATP) to the diphosphate (ADP), closure of membrane ATP-gated potassium (K_{ATP}) channels and their SUR1 and Kir6.2 subunits, membrane depolarization, calcium influx, and exocytosis of insulin. Several inherited abnormalities of these cellular mechanisms are now known to cause congenital hyperinsulinism and hypoglycemia in neonates and infants.[235-238]

Congenital hyperinsulinism has been associated with mutations of an increasing array of genes[235-238] including the sulfonylurea receptor-1 (SUR1, encoded by *ABCC8*), the potassium inward rectifying channel (Kir6.2, encoded by *KCNJ11*), glucokinase (GK, encoded by *GCK*), glutamate dehydrogenase (GDH, encoded by *GLUD1*), short-chain 3-hydroxyacyl-CoA dehydrogenase (SCHAD encoded by *HADH*), ectopic expression on beta-cell plasma membranes of *SLD16A1*, which encodes monocarboxylate transporter 1 (MCT1) and mutations of *HNF4A* and *HNF1A*.

Many patients with hyperinsulinemic hypoglycemia respond to the K_{ATP} channel opener diazoxide,[239] others to octreotide.[240]

Inactivating SUR1 or Kir6.2 mutations, typically recessively inherited, are the most common and most severe causes of congenital hyperinsulinism. They result in reduced K_{ATP} channel activity and, consequently, increased constitutive insulin secretion. Therefore, affected patients do not respond to treatment with the K_{ATP} channel opener, diazoxide, which normally suppresses insulin secretion. (Patients with dominantly inherited mutations do retain responsiveness to diazoxide.) Approximately half of patients with these mutations have diffuse islet involvement; for those who do not have a sustained response to medical therapy (e.g., frequent feedings, diazoxide, octreotide), near-total pancreatectomy is required. Other affected patients have focal lesions that are the result of loss of heterozygosity involving a paternally derived mutation of the *ABCC8* or *KCNJ11* gene and a specific loss of maternal alleles of the imprinted chromosome region 11p15. The focal lesion is curable by surgical resection. It can often be detected noninvasively with [^{18}F]-dihydroxyphenylalanine positron emission tomography.[241]

Activating, dominantly inherited mutations of the glutamate dehydrogenase gene cause the hyperinsulinemia and hyperammonemia syndrome, the second most common form of congenital hyperinsulinism. Hypoglycemia typically develops after several months of life and is responsive to diazoxide. Activating, dominantly inherited muta-

tions of the glucokinase gene cause varying degrees of hypoglycemia that may respond to diazoxide but may require pancreatectomy. Recessively inherited mutations of the SCHAD gene result in hypoglycemia that is generally responsive to diazoxide. In addition to hyperinsulinemic hypoglycemia, biochemical markers include increased levels of plasma 3-hydroxybutyrylcarnitine and increased urinary 3-hydroxy-glutarate. Dominantly inherited mutations of the monocarboxylate transporter-1 gene (*SLC16A1*), resulting in increased pyruvate transport into beta cells and hyperinsulinism, have been associated with exercise-induced hypoglycemia.

Clinical manifestations, including low plasma glucose concentrations and inappropriately high levels of plasma insulin and C-peptide coupled with low plasma β-hydroxybutyrate levels and a brisk glycemic response to administered glucagon—all analogous to hyperinsulinemic hypoglycemia in adults[2]—characterize congenital hyperinsulinism in neonates and infants.[235-238] As in adults with endogenous hyperinsulinism,[2] plasma insulin concentrations are not invariably 18 pmol/L or higher (≥3 μU/mL) during hypoglycemia in patients with congenital hyperinsulinism,[238] although hyperinsulinism is often documented by serial insulin measurements and by inclusion of C-peptide measurements during hypoglycemia. Therefore, the pattern of clinical hypoglycemia with low β-hydroxybutyrate levels and a brisk glycemic response to glucagon needs to be considered. Genetic testing for many mutations is available commercially. Finally, an association of hypertrophic cardiomyopathy and congenital hyperinsulinism has been recognized.[242]

Activating mutations in the postreceptor insulin signaling pathway (e.g., in the *AKT2* gene[243,244]) results in hypoinsulinemic hypoglycemia that resembles hyperinsulinemic hypoglycemia aside from evidence of reduced insulin secretion.

Given the array of potential causes of hypoglycemia in neonates and infants, the differential diagnosis is facilitated by an array of measurements during hypoglycemia when the precise hypoglycemic mechanism is obscure.[245] In addition to glucose, insulin, C-peptide, and β-hydroxybutyrate levels (and the glycemic response to glucagon), such measurements should include plasma bicarbonate, ammonia, lactate, nonesterified fatty acid (NEFA), growth hormone, and cortisol levels. A plasma acylcarnitine profile and measurement of urine organic acids are also needed but do not have to be obtained during hypoglycemia.

Enzyme Defects

Hypoglycemia that develops in infancy and persists into adult life with effective therapy can be caused by enzymatic defects in carbohydrate, protein, or fat metabolism (see Table 34-9).[229] Hypoglycemia usually becomes apparent later in infancy as the intervals between feedings become longer.

Glycogen storage disease (GSD) type Ia (von Gierke disease) is caused by mutations in *G6PC*, the gene that encodes glucose-6-phosphatase. It occurs in approximately 1 of every 100,000 live births.[246] The absence of glucose-6-phosphatase activity results in low rates of endogenous glucose production and severe fasting hypoglycemia[246] with no glycemic response to administered glucagon. Clinical findings include failure to thrive, hepatomegaly (due to both glycogen and fat accumulation), hypertriglyceridemia, accelerated lipolysis and ketogenesis, and lactic acidosis with hyperuricemia. With the exception of hepatomegaly, these abnormalities can be reversed by effective prevention of hypoglycemia with frequent feedings during waking hours and continuous intragastric glucose infusion during sleep or bedtime administration of large doses of uncooked cornstarch. Liver transplantation corrects hypoglycemia and the associated metabolic abnormalities.[247] Late complications include progressive renal disease and hepatic adenomas. GSD type Ib is caused by mutations in *G6PT1*, the glucose-6-phosphate transporter. The diagnosis of GSD type Ia and type Ib is confirmed by mutation analysis of *G6PC* and *G6PT1*. Hypoglycemia is less prominent in GSD type III (amylo-1,6-glucosidase deficiency due to mutations in *AGL*), GSD type VI (glycogen phosphorylase deficiency due to mutations in *PYGL*), and GSD type IX (phosphorylase kinase deficiency due to mutations in *PHKA2*). Hypoglycemia can also be caused by glycogen synthase deficiency (GSD type 0), which results from mutations in *GYS2* and does not cause hepatomegaly.

Hypoglycemia can also be caused by enzymatic defects in gluconeogenesis, including fructose-1,6-bisphosphatase, phosphoenolpyruvate carboxykinase, and pyruvate carboxylase deficiencies.[229] In patients with a mutation in the glucose transporter 1 (GLUT1) gene, plasma glucose concentrations are normal but brain glucose levels are low, causing neuroglycopenia.[248] Hypoglycemia has been attributed to GLUT2 deficiency in the Fanconi-Bickel syndrome. Postprandial, rather than postabsorptive, hypoglycemia occurs in galactosemia and in hereditary fructose intolerance (fructose-1-phosphate aldolase deficiency).

Deficiencies of enzymes involved in protein metabolism (see Table 34-9) that can cause fasting hypoglycemia include branched-chain ketoaciduria (maple syrup urine disease). The pathogenesis of hypoglycemia is unclear but includes defective gluconeogenesis.

Several defects that ultimately impair fatty acid oxidation result in hypoglycemia with hypoketonemia during extended fasting.[249] Mitochondrial fatty acid oxidation and ketogenesis require transport of fatty acids across the plasma membrane, formation of fatty acyl-CoA derivatives, and transport of those derivatives into mitochondria. Because the inner mitochondrial membranes are not permeable to long-chain (as opposed to medium-chain and short-chain) fatty acyl-CoA esters, the long-chain fatty acyl-CoA esters are transesterified to fatty acylcarnitines at the outer surface of the membranes (by carnitine palmitoyltransferase 1, CPT1), transported across the membranes (by a translocase), and reconverted to the fatty acyl-CoA esters (by carnitine palmitoyltransferase 2, CPT2) at the inner surface of the membranes. Then, they can be oxidized or converted to ketones. Insulin decreases fat oxidation and ketogenesis by decreasing lipolysis and by increasing lipogenesis and the formation of malonyl CoA, which inhibits CPT1. Conversely, low insulin levels favor fatty acid oxidation and ketogenesis. High glucagon levels do so by decreasing malonyl CoA; catecholamines do so largely by stimulating lipolysis. Any defect in this complex sequence (see Table 34-9) decreases fatty acid oxidation (and ketogenesis) and reciprocally increases glucose oxidation, resulting in hypoketonemic postabsorptive hypoglycemia. Reduced plasma carnitine levels (20% to 50% of normal) are the rule in these disorders, but extremely low carnitine levels characterize the carnitine transport defect, a true carnitine deficiency state that is responsive to carnitine supplementation.[250] The diagnosis of specific fatty acid oxidation defects is typically accomplished by blood acylcarnitine profiling,[245] although molecular diagnosis is increasingly possible.

There are many fatty acid oxidation disorders that result in hypoketonemic hypoglycemia.[229,249] The most common is medium-chain acyl-CoA dehydrogenase (MCAD) deficiency. Because affected patients can become symptomatic—fatigue, vomiting, seizure, coma—before becoming hypoglycemic, a normal acylcarnitine profile should be documented before a diagnostic fast is performed in such infants. Other fatty oxidation disorders include very long-, long-, and short-chain acyl-CoA dehydrogenase defects as well as defects in electron transfer (glutaric acidemia type 2), 3-hydroxy-3-methylglutaryl coenzyme A (HMG-CoA) synthase deficiency, and HMG-CoA lyase deficiency. Defects in carnitine transport and in the carnitine cycle that cause hypoketonemic hypoglycemia include primary carnitine deficiency due to autosomal recessive mutations in the carnitine transporter (*OCTN2*). Others are CPT1 deficiency, carnitine acylcarnitine translocase (*CACT*) deficiency, and CPT2 deficiency. Treatment includes frequent feedings and a low-fat diet rich in medium-chain triglycerides[251] in CPT1 deficiency and carnitine supplementation in primary carnitine deficiency.

In summary, neonatal hypoglycemia with suppressed levels of NEFAs and β-hydroxybutyrate suggest hyperinsulinism, and that with high NEFA but low β-hydroxybutyrate suggests a defect in fatty acid oxidation or ketogenesis. Hypoglycemia with high lactate levels suggests a defect in gluconeogenesis or glucose release. High concentrations of both NEFA and β-hydroxybutyrate suggest a defect in glucose production or release including deficiency of cortisol, although NEFA and ketone levels need not be elevated in patients with hypopituitarism.

ACKNOWLEDGMENTS

The author's original work cited in this chapter has been supported, in part, by U.S. Public Health Service, National Institutes of Health grants R37 DK27085, M01 RR00036 (now UL1 RR24992), P60 DK20579, and T32 DK07120 and fellowship and grant awards from the American Diabetes Association. The author is grateful for the contributions of postdoctoral fellows and the skilled nursing, technical, dietary, and data management statistical assistance of the staff of the Washington University General Clinical Research Center. Ms. Janet Dedeke prepared this manuscript.

This chapter was written after the author chaired a panel that developed *Evaluation and Management of Adult Hypoglycemic Disorders*, an Endocrine Society clinical practice guideline,[2] and shortly after publication of the second edition of the author's book, *Hypoglycemia in Diabetes: Pathophysiology, Prevalence and Prevention*.[3] Therefore, much of the conceptual and interpretive content here is the same, as is no small part of the phraseology.

DISCLOSURES

The author has served as a consultant to several pharmaceutical or device firms including Amgen Inc., Johnson & Johnson, MannKind Corp., Marcadia Biotech, Medtronic MiniMed Inc., Merck and Co., Novo Nordisk A/S, Takeda Pharmaceuticals North America, and TolerRx Inc. in recent years.

REFERENCES

1. Clark DD, Sokoloff L. Circulation and energy metabolism of the brain. In: Siegel G, Agranoff B, Albers RW, Molinoff P, eds. *Basic Neurochemistry: Molecular, Cellular and Medical Aspects.* 5th ed. New York, NY: Raven Press; 1994:645-680.
2. Cryer PE, Axelrod L, Grossman AB, et al. Evaluation and management of adult hypoglycemic disorders: an Endocrine Society clinical practice guideline. *J Clin Endocrinol Metab.* 2009;94:709-728.

3. Cryer PE. *Hypoglycemia in Diabetes: Pathophysiology, Prevalence and Prevention.* 2nd ed. Alexandria, VA: American Diabetes Association; 2012.

4. Cryer PE. The prevention and correction of hypoglycemia. In: Jefferson LS, Cherrington AD, eds. *Handbook of Physiology. Section 7: The Endocrine System. Volume II: The Endocrine Pancreas and Regulation of Metabolism.* New York, NY: Oxford University Press; 2001:1057-1092.

5. Cryer PE. Glycemic goals in diabetes: the trade-off between glycemic control and iatrogenic hypoglycemia. *Diabetes.* 2014;63(7):2188-2195.

6. Boden G. Gluconeogenesis and glycogenolysis in health and diabetes. *J Investig Med.* 2004;52:375-378.

7. Stumvoll M, Chintalapudi U, Perriello G, et al. Uptake and release of glucose by the human kidney. *J Clin Invest.* 1995;96:2528-2533.

8. Woerle HJ, Meyer C, Popa EM, et al. Renal compensation for impaired hepatic glucose release during hypoglycemia in type 2 diabetes: further evidence for hepatorenal reciprocity. *Diabetes.* 2003;52:1386-1392.

9. Schwartz NS, Clutter WE, Shah SD, et al. Glycemic thresholds for activation of glucose counterregulatory systems are higher than the threshold for symptoms. *J Clin Invest.* 1987;79:777-781.

10. Mitrakou A, Ryan C, Veneman T, et al. Hierarchy of glycemic thresholds for counterregulatory hormone secretion, symptoms, and cerebral dysfunction. *Am J Physiol Endocrinol Metab.* 1991;260:E67-E74.

11. Fanelli C, Pampanelli S, Epifano L, et al. Relative roles of insulin and hypoglycaemia on induction of neuroendocrine responses to, symptoms of, and deterioration of cognitive function in hypoglycaemia in male and female humans. *Diabetologia.* 1994;37:797-807.

12. Towler DA, Havlin CE, Craft S, et al. Mechanism of awareness of hypoglycemia. Perception of neurogenic (predominantly cholinergic) rather than neuroglycopenic symptoms. *Diabetes.* 1993;42:1791-1798.

13. DeRosa MA, Cryer PE. Hypoglycemia and the sympathoadrenal system: neurogenic symptoms are largely the result of sympathetic neural, rather than adrenomedullary, activation. *Am J Physiol Endocrinol Metab.* 2004;287:E32-E41.

14. Schultes B, Oltmanns KM, Kern W, et al. Modulation of hunger by plasma glucose and metformin. *J Clin Endocrinol Metab.* 2003;88:1133-1141.

15. Raju B, Cryer PE. Loss of the decrement in intraislet insulin plausibly explains loss of the glucagon response to hypoglycemia in insulin-deficient diabetes. *Diabetes.* 2005;54:757-764.

16. Taborsky GJ Jr, Ahrén B, Havel PJ. Autonomic mediation of glucagon secretion during hypoglycemia: implications for impaired alpha-cell responses in type 1 diabetes. *Diabetes.* 1998;47:995-1005.

17. Berk MA, Clutter WE, Skor D, et al. Enhanced glycemic responsiveness to epinephrine in insulin-dependent diabetes mellitus is the result of the inability to secrete insulin. *J Clin Invest.* 1985;75:1842-1851.

18. Mitrakou A, Fanelli C, Veneman T, et al. Reversibility of unawareness of hypoglycemia in patients with insulinomas. *N Engl J Med.* 1993;329:834-839.

19. Amiel SA, Sherwin RS, Simonson DC, et al. Effect of intensive insulin therapy on glycemic thresholds for counterregulatory hormone release. *Diabetes.* 1988;37:901-907.

20. Boyle PJ, Schwartz NS, Shah SD, et al. Plasma glucose concentrations at the onset of hypoglycemic symptoms in patients with poorly controlled diabetes and in nondiabetics. *N Engl J Med.* 1988;318:1487-1492.

21. The Diabetes Control and Complications Trial Research Group. The effect of intensive treatment of diabetes on the development and progression of long-term complications in insulin-dependent diabetes mellitus. *N Engl J Med.* 1993;329:977-986.

22. Reichard P, Pihl M. Mortality and treatment side-effects during long-term intensified conventional insulin treatment in the Stockholm Diabetes Intervention Study. *Diabetes.* 1994;43:313-317.

23. Donnelly LA, Morris AD, Frier BM, et al. Frequency and predictors of hypoglycaemia in type 1 and insulin-treated type 2 diabetes: a population-based study. *Diabet Med.* 2005;22:749-755.

24. U.K. Hypoglycaemia Study Group. Risk of hypoglycaemia in types 1 and 2 diabetes: effects of treatment modalities and their duration. *Diabetologia.* 2007;50:1140-1147.

25. The Diabetes Control and Complications Trial Research Group. Hypoglycemia in the Diabetes Control and Complications Trial. *Diabetes.* 1997;46:271-286.

26. United Kingdom Prospective Diabetes Study Group. United Kingdom Prospective Diabetes Study 24: a 6-year, randomized, controlled trial comparing sulfonylurea, insulin, and metformin therapy in patients with newly diagnosed type 2 diabetes that could not be controlled with diet therapy. *Ann Intern Med.* 1998;128:165-175.

27. Hepburn DA, MacLeod KM, Pell AC, et al. Frequency and symptoms of hypoglycaemia experienced by patients with type 2 diabetes treated with insulin. *Diabet Med.* 1993;10:231-237.

28. Holstein A, Plaschke A, Egberts EH. Clinical characterisation of severe hypoglycaemia: a prospective population-based study. *Exp Clin Endocrinol Diabetes.* 2003;111:364-369.

29. Leese GP, Wang J, Broomhall J, et al. DARTS/MEMO Collaboration. Frequency of severe hypoglycemia requiring emergency treatment in type 1 and type 2 diabetes: a population-based study of health service resource use. *Diabetes Care.* 2003;26:1176-1180.

30. Wright AD, Cull CA, Macleod KM, et al. for the UKPDS Group. Hypoglycaemia in type 2 diabetic patients randomized to and maintained on monotherapy with diet, sulfonylurea, metformin, or insulin for 6 years from diagnosis. UKPDS73. *J Diabetes Complications.* 2006;20:395-401.

31. Pramming S, Thorsteinsson B, Bendtson I, et al. Symptomatic hypoglycaemia in 411 type 1 diabetic patients. *Diabet Med.* 1991;8:217-222.

32. Pedersen-Bjergaard U, Pramming S, Thorsteinsson B. Recall of severe hypoglycaemia and self-estimated state of awareness in type 1 diabetes. *Diabetes Metab Res Rev.* 2003;19:232-240.

33. Diabetes Control and Complications Trial/Epidemiology of Diabetes Interventions and Complications Study Research Group. Long-term effect of diabetes and its treatment on cognitive function. *N Engl J Med.* 2007;356:1842-1852.

34. Lin A, Northam EA, Rankins D, et al. Neuropsychological profile of young people with type 1 diabetes 12 yr after disease onset. *Pediatr Diabetes.* 2010;11:235-243.

35. Arbeláez AM, Semenkovich K, Hershey T. Glycemic extremes in youth with T1DM: the structural and functional integrity of the developing brain. *Pediatr Diabetes.* 2013;14:541-553.

36. Yaffe K, Falvey CM, Hamilton N, et al. for the Health ABC Study. Association between hypoglycemia and dementia in a biracial cohort of older adults with diabetes mellitus. *JAMA Intern Med.* 2013;173:1300-1306.

37. Jacobson AM. The psychological care of patients with insulin-dependent diabetes mellitus. *N Engl J Med.* 1996;334:1249-1253.

38. Cryer PE. Death during intensive glycemic therapy of diabetes: mechanisms and implications. *Am J Med.* 2011;124:993-996.

39. The Action to Control Cardiovascular Risk in Diabetes Study Group. Effects of intensive glucose lowering in type 2 diabetes. *N Engl J Med.* 2008;358:2545-2559.

40. The ORIGIN Trial Investigators. Does hypoglycemia increase the risk of cardiovascular events? A report from the ORIGIN trial. *Eur Heart J.* 2013;34:3137-3144.

41. The NICE-SUGAR Study Investigators. Hypoglycemia and risk of death in critically ill patients. *N Engl J Med.* 2012;367:1108-1118.

42. Macrae D, Grieve R, Allen E, et al. for the CHiP Investigators. A randomized trial of hyperglycemic control in pediatric intensive care. *N Engl J Med.* 2014;370:107-118.

43. Deckert T, Poulsen JE, Larsen M. Prognosis of diabetics with diabetes onset before the age of thirty-one. I: survival, causes of death, and complications. *Diabetologia.* 1978;14:363-370.

44. Tunbridge WM. Factors contributing to deaths of diabetics under fifty years of age. *Lancet.* 1981;2:569-572.

45. Laing SP, Swerdlow AJ, Slater SD, et al. The British Diabetic Association Cohort Study. I: all-cause mortality in patients with insulin-treated diabetes mellitus. *Diabet Med.* 1999;16:459-465.

46. Patterson CC, Dahlquist G, Harjutsalo V, et al. Early mortality in the EURODIAB population-based cohorts of type 1 diabetes diagnosed in childhood since 1989. *Diabetologia.* 2007;50:2439-2442.

47. Feltbower RG, Bodansky HJ, Patterson CC, et al. Acute complications and drug misuse are important causes of death for children and young adults with type 1 diabetes: results from the Yorkshire Register of diabetes in children and young adults. *Diabetes Care.* 2008;31:922-926.

48. Skrivarhaug T, Bangstad HJ, Stene LC, et al. Long-term mortality in a nationwide cohort of childhood-onset type 1 diabetic patients in Norway. *Diabetologia.* 2006;49:298-305.

49. Tanenberg RJ, Newton CA, Drake AJIII. Confirmation of hypoglycemia in the "dead-in-bed" syndrome, as captured by a retrospective continuous glucose monitoring system. *Endocr Pract.* 2010;16:244-248.

50. Gerich JE. Oral hypoglycemic agents. *N Engl J Med.* 1989;321:1231-1245.

51. Holstein A, Egberts EH. Risk of hypoglycaemia with oral antidiabetic agents in patients with type 2 diabetes. *Exp Clin Endocrinol Diabetes.* 2003;111:405-414.

52. Bonds DE, Miller ME, Bergenstal RM, et al. The association between symptomatic severe hypoglycaemia and mortality in type 2 diabetes: retrospective epidemiological analysis of the ACCORD study. *BMJ.* 2010;340:b4909.

53. Frier BM, Schernthaner G, Heller SR. Hypoglycemia and cardiovascular risks. *Diabetes Care.* 2011;34(Suppl 2):S132-S137.

54. Nordin C. The proarrhythmic effect of hypoglycemia: evidence for increased risk from ischemia and bradycardia. *Acta Diabetol.* 2014;51:5-14.

55. Chow E, Bernjak A, Williams S, et al. Risk of cardiac arrhythmias during hypoglycemia in patients with type 2 diabetes and cardiovascular risk. *Diabetes.* 2014;63(5):1738-1747.

56. Reno CM, Daphna-Iken D, Chen YS, et al. Severe hypoglycemia-induced lethal cardiac arrhythmias are mediated by sympathoadrenal activation. *Diabetes.* 2013;62:3570-3581.

57. Murphy NP, Ford-Adams ME, Ong KK, et al. Prolonged cardiac repolarisation during spontaneous nocturnal hypoglycaemia in children and adolescents with type 1 diabetes. *Diabetologia.* 2004;47:1940-1947.

58. Gill GV, Woodward A, Casson IF, et al. Cardiac arrhythmia and nocturnal hypoglycaemia in type 1 diabetes: the "dead in bed" syndrome revisited. *Diabetologia.* 2009;52:42-45.
59. Ewing DJ, Neilson JM. QT interval length and diabetic autonomic neuropathy. *Diabet Med.* 1990;7:23-26.
60. Adler GK, Bonyhay I, Failing H, et al. Antecedent hypoglycemia impairs autonomic cardiovascular function: implications for rigorous glycemic control. *Diabetes.* 2009;58:360-366.
61. American Diabetes Association and Endocrine Society Workgroup on Hypoglycemia. Hypoglycemia in diabetes. *Diabetes Care.* 2013;36:1384-1395.
62. Cox DJ, Gonder-Frederick L, Ritterband L, et al. Prediction of severe hypoglycemia. *Diabetes Care.* 2007;30:1370-1373.
63. Davis SN, Shavers C, Mosqueda-Garcia R, et al. Effects of differing antecedent hypoglycemia on subsequent counterregulation in normal humans. *Diabetes.* 1997;46:1328-1335.
64. Cryer PE. Preventing hypoglycaemia: what is the appropriate glucose alert value? *Diabetologia.* 2009;52:35-37.
65. Dagogo-Jack SE, Craft S, Cryer PE. Hypoglycemia-associated autonomic failure in insulin-dependent diabetes mellitus: recent antecedent hypoglycemia reduces autonomic responses to, symptoms of, and defense against subsequent hypoglycemia. *J Clin Invest.* 1993;91:819-828.
66. Cryer PE. Mechanisms of hypoglycemia-associated autonomic failure in diabetes. *N Engl J Med.* 2013;369:362-372.
67. White NH, Skor DA, Cryer PE, et al. Identification of type I diabetic patients at increased risk for hypoglycemia during intensive therapy. *N Engl J Med.* 1983;308:485-491.
68. Bolli GB, De Feo P, De Cosmo S, et al. A reliable and reproducible test for adequate glucose counterregulation in type I diabetes mellitus. *Diabetes.* 1984;33:732-737.
69. Geddes J, Schopman JE, Zammitt NN, et al. Prevalence of impaired awareness of hypoglycaemia in adults with type 1 diabetes. *Diabet Med.* 2008;25:501-504.
70. Heller SR, Cryer PE. Reduced neuroendocrine and symptomatic responses to subsequent hypoglycemia after 1 episode of hypoglycemia in nondiabetic humans. *Diabetes.* 1991;40:223-226.
71. Ertl AC, Davis SN. Evidence for a vicious cycle of exercise and hypoglycemia in type 1 diabetes mellitus. *Diabetes Metab Res Rev.* 2004;20:124-130.
72. Jones TW, Porter P, Sherwin RS, et al. Decreased epinephrine responses to hypoglycemia during sleep. *N Engl J Med.* 1998;338:1657-1662.
73. Banarer S, Cryer PE. Sleep-related hypoglycemia-associated autonomic failure in type 1 diabetes: reduced awakening from sleep during hypoglycemia. *Diabetes.* 2003;52:1195-1203.
74. Berlin I, Grimaldi A, Payan C, et al. Hypoglycemic symptoms and decreased beta-adrenergic sensitivity in insulin-dependent diabetic patients. *Diabetes Care.* 1987;10:742-747.
75. Fritsche A, Stefan N, Häring H, et al. Avoidance of hypoglycemia restores hypoglycemia awareness by increasing beta-adrenergic sensitivity in type 1 diabetes. *Ann Intern Med.* 2001;134:729-736.
76. De Galan BE, De Mol P, Wennekes L, et al. Preserved sensitivity to beta2-adrenergic receptor agonists in patients with type 1 diabetes mellitus and hypoglycemia unawareness. *J Clin Endocrinol Metab.* 2006;91:2878-2881.
77. Segel SA, Paramore DS, Cryer PE. Hypoglycemia-associated autonomic failure in advanced type 2 diabetes. *Diabetes.* 2002;51:724-733.
78. Bottini P, Boschetti E, Pampanelli S, et al. Contribution of autonomic neuropathy to reduced plasma adrenaline responses to hypoglycemia in IDDM: evidence for a nonselective defect. *Diabetes.* 1997;46:814-823.
79. Meyer C, Grossmann R, Mitrakou A, et al. Effects of autonomic neuropathy on counterregulation and awareness of hypoglycemia in type 1 diabetic patients. *Diabetes Care.* 1998;21:1960-1966.
80. Fanelli CG, Paramore DS, Hershey T, et al. Impact of nocturnal hypoglycemia on hypoglycemic cognitive dysfunction in type 1 diabetes. *Diabetes.* 1998;47:1920-1927.
81. Ovalle F, Fanelli CG, Paramore DS, et al. Brief twice-weekly episodes of hypoglycemia reduce detection of clinical hypoglycemia in type 1 diabetes mellitus. *Diabetes.* 1998;47:1472-1479.
82. Fanelli CG, Epifano L, Rambotti AM, et al. Meticulous prevention of hypoglycemia normalizes the glycemic thresholds and magnitude of most of neuroendocrine responses to, symptoms of, and cognitive function during hypoglycemia in intensively treated patients with short-term IDDM. *Diabetes.* 1993;42:1683-1689.
83. Cranston I, Lomas J, Maran A, et al. Restoration of hypoglycaemia awareness in patients with long-duration insulin-dependent diabetes. *Lancet.* 1994;344:283-287.
84. Fanelli C, Pampanelli S, Epifano L, et al. Long-term recovery from unawareness, deficient counterregulation and lack of cognitive dysfunction during hypoglycaemia, following institution of rational, intensive insulin therapy in IDDM. *Diabetologia.* 1994;37:1265-1276.
85. Dagogo-Jack S, Rattarasarn C, Cryer PE. Reversal of hypoglycemia unawareness, but not defective glucose counterregulation, in IDDM. *Diabetes.* 1994;43:1426-1434.
86. MacDonald MJ. Postexercise late-onset hypoglycemia in insulin-dependent diabetic patients. *Diabetes Care.* 1987;10:584-588.
87. Tansey MJ, Tsalikian E, Beck RW, et al. Diabetes Research in Children Network (DirecNet) Study Group. The effects of aerobic exercise on glucose and counterregulatory hormone concentrations in children with type 1 diabetes. *Diabetes Care.* 2006;29:20-25.
88. Diem P, Redmon JB, Abid M, et al. Glucagon, catecholamine and pancreatic polypeptide secretion in type I diabetic recipients of pancreas allografts. *J Clin Invest.* 1990;86:2008-2013.
89. Sherck SM, Shiota M, Saccomando J, et al. Pancreatic response to mild non-insulin-induced hypoglycemia does not involve extrinsic neural input. *Diabetes.* 2001;50:2487-2496.
90. Beall C, Ashford ML, McCrimmon RJ. The physiology and pathophysiology of the neural control of the counterregulatory response. *Am J Physiol Regul Integr Comp Physiol.* 2012;302:R215-R223.
91. Chan O, Sherwin R. Influence of VMH fuel sensing on hypoglycemic responses. *Trends Endocrinol Metab.* 2013;24:616-624.
92. Teves D, Videen TO, Cryer PE, et al. Activation of human medial prefrontal cortex during autonomic responses to hypoglycemia. *Proc Natl Acad Sci U S A.* 2004;101:6217-6221.
93. Arbelaez AM, Powers WJ, Videen TO, et al. Attenuation of counterregulatory responses to recurrent hypoglycemia by active thalamic inhibition: a mechanism for hypoglycemia-associated autonomic failure. *Diabetes.* 2008;57:470-475.
94. Arbeláez AM, Rutlin JR, Hershey T, et al. Thalamic activation during slightly subphysiological glycemia in humans. *Diabetes Care.* 2012;35:2570-2574.
95. De Feyter HM, Mason GF, Shulman GI, et al. Increased brain lactate concentrations without increased lactate oxidation during hypoglycemia in type 1 diabetic individuals. *Diabetes.* 2013;62:3075-3080.
96. Herzog RI, Jiang L, Herman P, et al. Lactate preserves neuronal metabolism and function following antecedent recurrent hypoglycemia. *J Clin Invest.* 2013;123:1988-1998.
97. Chan O, Paranjape SA, Horblitt A, et al. Lactate-induced release of GABA in the ventromedial hypothalamus contributes to counterregulatory failure in recurrent hypoglycemia and diabetes. *Diabetes.* 2013;62:4239-4246.
98. Arbeláez AM, Cryer PE. Lactate and the mechanism of hypoglycemia-associated autonomic failure in diabetes. *Diabetes.* 2013;62:3999-4001.
99. Cryer PE, Davis SN, Shamoon H. Hypoglycemia in diabetes. *Diabetes Care.* 2003;26:1902-1912.
100. The DCCT Research Group. Epidemiology of severe hypoglycemia in the Diabetes Control and Complications Trial. *Am J Med.* 1991;90:450-459.
101. Fukuda M, Tanaka A, Tahara Y, et al. Correlation between minimal secretory capacity of pancreatic beta-cells and stability of diabetic control. *Diabetes.* 1988;37:81-88.
102. Davis TME, Brown SGA, Jacobs IG, et al. Determinants of severe hypoglycemia complicating type 2 diabetes: the Fremantle Diabetes Study. *J Clin Endocrinol Metab.* 2010;95:2240-2247.
103. Mühlhauser I, Overmann H, Bender R, et al. Risk factors of severe hypoglycaemia in adult patients with type I diabetes: a prospective population based study. *Diabetologia.* 1998;41:1274-1282.
104. Allen C, LeCaire T, Palta M, et al. Risk factors for frequent and severe hypoglycemia in type 1 diabetes. *Diabetes Care.* 2001;24:1878-1881.
105. Steffes MW, Sibley S, Jackson M, et al. Beta-cell function and the development of diabetes-related complications in the diabetes control and complications trial. *Diabetes Care.* 2003;26:832-836.
106. Lüddeke HJ, Sreenan S, Aczel S, et al. PREDICTIVE—a global, prospective observational study to evaluate insulin detemir treatment in types 1 and 2 diabetes: baseline characteristics and predictors of hypoglycaemia from the European cohort. *Diabetes Obes Metab.* 2007;9:428-434.
107. Lachin JM, McGee P, Palmer JP, DCCT/EDIC Research Group. Impact of C-peptide preservation on metabolic and clinical outcomes in the Diabetes Control and Complications Trial. *Diabetes.* 2014;63:739-748.
108. Egger M, Davey Smith G, Stettler C, et al. Risk of adverse effects of intensified treatment in insulin-dependent diabetes mellitus: a meta-analysis. *Diabet Med.* 1997;14:919-928.
109. ADVANCE Collaborative Group. Intensive blood glucose control and vascular outcomes in patients with type 2 diabetes. *N Engl J Med.* 2008;358:2560-2572.
110. Duckworth W, Abraira C, Moritz T, et al. Veterans Affairs Diabetes Therapy Investigators. Glucose control and vascular complications in veterans with type 2 diabetes. *N Engl J Med.* 2009;360:129-139.
111. Rossetti P, Porcellati F, Bolli GB, et al. Prevention of hypoglycemia while achieving good glycemic control in type 1 diabetes: the role of insulin analogs. *Diabetes Care.* 2008;31(Suppl 2):S113-S120.
112. Heller SR. Minimizing hypoglycemia while maintaining glycemic control in diabetes. *Diabetes.* 2008;57:3177-3183.
113. Gonder-Frederick LA, Fisher CD, Ritterband LM, et al. Predictors of fear of hypoglycemia in adolescents with type 1 diabetes and their parents. *Pediatr Diabetes.* 2006;7:215-222.

114. Nordfeldt S, Ludvigsson J. Fear and other disturbances of severe hypoglycaemia in children and adolescents with type 1 diabetes mellitus. *J Pediatr Endocrinol Metab.* 2005;18:83-91.

115. Hopkins D, Lawrence I, Mansell P, et al. Improved biomedical and psychological outcomes 1 year after structured education in flexible insulin therapy for people with type 1 diabetes: the U.K. DAFNE experience. *Diabetes Care.* 2012;35:1638-1642.

116. Leelarathna L, Little SA, Walkinshaw E, et al. Restoration of self-awareness of hypoglycaemia in adults with longstanding type 1 diabetes. *Diabetes Care.* 2013;36:4063-4070.

117. de Zoysa N, Rogers H, Stadler M, et al. A psychoeducational program to restore hypoglycemia awareness: the DAFNE-HART pilot study. *Diabetes Care.* 2014;37:863-866.

118. Deiss D, Hartmann R, Schmidt J, et al. Results of a randomised controlled cross-over trial on the effect of continuous subcutaneous glucose monitoring (CGMS) on glycaemic control in children and adolescents with type 1 diabetes. *Exp Clin Endocrinol Diabetes.* 2006;114:63-67.

119. Juvenile Diabetes Research Foundation Continuous Glucose Monitoring Study Group. Continuous glucose monitoring and intensive treatment of type 1 diabetes. *N Engl J Med.* 2008;359:1464-1476.

120. Choudhary P, Ramasamy S, Green L, et al. Real-time continuous glucose monitoring significantly reduces severe hypoglycemia in hypoglycemia-unaware patients with type 1 diabetes. *Diabetes Care.* 2013;36:4160-4162.

121. Ly TT, Nicolas JA, Retterath A, et al. Effect of sensor-augmented insulin pump therapy and automated insulin suspension vs standard insulin pump therapy on hypoglycemia in patients with type 1 diabetes: a randomized clinical trial. *JAMA.* 2013;310:1240-1247.

122. Bergenstal RM, Klonoff DC, Garg SK, et al. for the ASPIRE In-Home Study Group. Threshold-based insulin pump interruption for reduction of hypoglycemia. *N Engl J Med.* 2013;369:224-232.

123. Bolen S, Feldman L, Vassy J, et al. Systematic review: comparative effectiveness and safety of oral medications for type 2 diabetes mellitus. *Ann Intern Med.* 2007;147:386-399.

124. Gangji AS, Cukierman T, Gerstein HC, et al. A systematic review and meta-analysis of hypoglycemia and cardiovascular events: a comparison of glyburide with other secretagogues and with insulin. *Diabetes Care.* 2007;30:389-394.

125. Hirsch IB. Insulin analogues. *N Engl J Med.* 2005;352:174-183.

126. Horvath K, Jeitler K, Berghold A, et al. Long-acting insulin analogues versus NPH insulin (human isophane insulin) for type 2 diabetes mellitus. *Cochrane Database Syst Rev.* 2007;(2):CD005613.

127. Gough SC. A review of human and analogue insulin trials. *Diabetes Res Clin Pract.* 2007;77:1-15.

128. Heller S, Buse J, Fisher M, et al. on behalf of the BEGIN Basal-Bolus Type 1 Trial Investigators. Insulin degludec, an ultra-longacting basal insulin, versus insulin glargine in basal-bolus treatment with mealtime insulin aspart in type 1 diabetes. *Lancet.* 2012;379:1489-1497.

129. Garber AJ, King AB, Del Prato S, et al. on behalf of the NN1250-3582 (BEGIN BB T2D) Trial Investigators. Insulin degludec, an ultra-longacting basal insulin, versus insulin glargine in basal-bolus treatment with mealtime insulin aspart in type 2 diabetes. *Lancet.* 2012;379:1498-1507.

130. Rosenstock J, Bergenstal RM, Blevins TC, et al. Better glycemic control and weight loss with the novel long-acting basal insulin LY2605541 compared with insulin glargine in type 1 diabetes: a randomized, crossover study. *Diabetes Care.* 2013;36:522-528.

131. Bergenstal RM, Rosenstock J, Arakaki RF, et al. A randomized, controlled study of once-daily LY2605541, a novel long-acting basal insulin, versus insulin glargine in basal insulin-treated patients with type 2 diabetes. *Diabetes Care.* 2012;35:2140-2147.

132. Raju B, Arbelaez AM, Breckenridge SM, et al. Nocturnal hypoglycemia in type 1 diabetes: an assessment of preventive bedtime treatments. *J Clin Endocrinol Metab.* 2006;91:2087-2092.

133. Radziuk J. The artificial pancreas. *Diabetes.* 2012;61:2221-2224.

134. Phillip M, Battelino T, Atlas E, et al. Nocturnal glucose control with an artificial pancreas at a diabetes camp. *N Engl J Med.* 2013;368:824-833.

135. United Kingdom Prospective Diabetes Study Group. Intensive blood-glucose control with sulphonylureas or insulin compared with conventional treatment and risk of complications in patients with type 2 diabetes. UKPDS 33. *Lancet.* 1998;352:837-853.

136. United Kingdom Prospective Diabetes Study Group. Effect of intensive blood-glucose control with metformin on complications in overweight patients with type 2 diabetes. UKPDS 34. *Lancet.* 1998;352:854-865.

137. Lachin JM, Genuth S, Nathan DM, et al. DCCT/EDIC Research Group. Effect of glycemic exposure on the risk of microvascular complications in the diabetes control and complications trial—revisited. *Diabetes.* 2008;57:995-1001.

138. Wiethop BV, Cryer PE. Alanine and terbutaline in treatment of hypoglycemia in IDDM. *Diabetes Care.* 1993;16:1131-1136.

139. Haymond MW, Schreiner B. Mini-dose glucagon rescue for hypoglycemia in children with type 1 diabetes. *Diabetes Care.* 2001;24:643-645.

140. Chabenne J, Chabenne MD, Zhao Y, et al. A glucagon analogue chemically stabilized for immediate treatment of life-threatening hypoglycemia. *Mol Metab.* 2014;3(3):293-300.

141. Jackson RA, Peters N, Advani U, et al. Forearm glucose uptake during the oral glucose tolerance test in normal subjects. *Diabetes.* 1973;22:442-458.

142. Service FJ. Hypoglycemic disorders. *N Engl J Med.* 1995;332:1144-1152.

143. Fischer KF, Lees JA, Newman JH. Hypoglycemia in hospitalized patients: causes and outcomes. *N Engl J Med.* 1986;315:1245-1250.

144. Malouf R, Brust JC. Hypoglycemia: causes, neurological manifestations, and outcome. *Ann Neurol.* 1985;17:421-430.

145. Marks V, Teale JD. Drug-induced hypoglycemia. *Endocrinol Metab Clin North Am.* 1999;28:555-577.

146. Park-Wyllie LY, Juurlink DN, Kopp A, et al. Outpatient gatifloxacin therapy and dysglycemia in older adults. *N Engl J Med.* 2006;354:1352-1361.

147. Murad MH, Coto-Yglesias F, Wang AT, et al. Drug-induced hypoglycemia: a systematic review. *J Clin Endocrinol Metab.* 2009;94:741-745.

148. Ben Salem C, Fathallah N, Hmouda H, Bouraoui K. Drug-induced hypoglycemia. *Drug Saf.* 2011;34:21-45.

149. Chou H-W, Wang J-L, Chang C-H, et al. Risk of severe dysglycemia among diabetic patients receiving levofloxacin, ciprofloxacin, or moxifloxacin in Taiwan. *Clin Infect Dis.* 2013;57:971-980.

150. Cohen MR, Proulx SM, Crawford SY. Survey of hospital systems and common serious medication errors. *J Healthc Risk Manag.* 1998;18(1):16-27.

151. Felig P, Brown WV, Levine RA, et al. Glucose homeostasis in viral hepatitis. *N Engl J Med.* 1970;283:1436-1440.

152. Younus S, Soterakis J, Sossi AJ, et al. Hypoglycemia secondary to metastases to the liver: a case report and review of the literature. *Gastroenterology.* 1977;72:334-337.

153. Haviv YS, Sharkia M, Safadi R. Hypoglycemia in patients with renal failure. *Ren Fail.* 2000;22:219-223.

154. Garber AJ, Bier DM, Cryer PE, et al. Hypoglycemia in compensated chronic renal insufficiency: substrate limitation of gluconeogenesis. *Diabetes.* 1974;23:982-986.

155. Rutsky EA, McDaniel HG, Tharpe DL, et al. Spontaneous hypoglycemia in chronic renal failure. *Arch Intern Med.* 1978;138:1364-1368.

156. Chen YT, Burchell A, et al. Glycogen storage diseases. In: Scriver CR, Beaudet AL, Sly WS, eds. *The Metabolic and Molecular Bases of Inherited Disease.* 7th ed. New York, NY: McGraw Hill; 1995:935-965.

157. Medalle R, Webb R, Waterhouse C. Lactic acidosis and associated hypoglycemia. *Arch Intern Med.* 1971;128:273-278.

158. Miller SI, Wallace RJ Jr, Musher DM, et al. Hypoglycemia as a manifestation of sepsis. *Am J Med.* 1980;68:649-654.

159. Maitra SR, Wojnar MM, Lang CH. Alterations in tissue glucose uptake during the hyperglycemic and hypoglycemic phases of sepsis. *Shock.* 2000;13:379-385.

160. Sakurai Y, Zhang XJ, Wolfe RR. TNF directly stimulates glucose uptake and leucine oxidation and inhibits FFA flux in conscious dogs. *Am J Physiol.* 1996;270:E864-E872.

161. Metzger S, Nusair S, Planer D, et al. Inhibition of hepatic gluconeogenesis and enhanced glucose uptake contribute to the development of hypoglycemia in mice bearing interleukin-1beta-secreting tumor. *Endocrinology.* 2004;145:5150-5156.

162. Hargrove DM, Lang CH, Bagby GJ, et al. Epinephrine-induced increase in glucose turnover is diminished during sepsis. *Metabolism.* 1989;38:1070-1076.

163. Wharton B. Hypoglycaemia in children with kwashiorkor. *Lancet.* 1970;1:171-173.

164. Bruce AK, Jacobsen E, Dossing H, et al. Hypoglycaemia in spinal muscular atrophy. *Lancet.* 1995;346:609-610.

165. Ørngreen MC, Zacho M, Hebert A, et al. Patients with severe muscle wasting are prone to develop hypoglycemia during fasting. *Neurology.* 2003;61:997-1000.

166. Goodman HG, Grumbach MM, Kaplan SL. Growth and growth hormone. II: a comparison of isolated growth-hormone deficiency and multiple pituitary-hormone deficiencies in 35 patients with idiopathic hypopituitary dwarfism. *N Engl J Med.* 1968;278:57-68.

167. Haymond MW, Karl I, Weldon VV, et al. The role of growth hormone and cortisone on glucose and gluconeogenic substrate regulation in fasted hypopituitary children. *J Clin Endocrinol Metab.* 1976;42:846-856.

168. Wolfsdorf JI, Sadeghi-Nejad A, Senior B. Hypoketonemia and age-related fasting hypoglycemia in growth hormone deficiency. *Metabolism.* 1983;32:457-462.

169. Frizzell RT, Campbell PJ, Cherrington AD. Gluconeogenesis and hypoglycemia. *Diabetes Metab Rev.* 1988;4:51-70.

170. Boyle PJ, Cryer PE. Growth hormone, cortisol, or both are involved in defense against, but are not critical to recovery from, hypoglycemia. *Am J Physiol.* 1991;260:E395-E402.

171. Smallridge RC, Corrigan DF, Thomason AM, et al. Hypoglycemia in pregnancy: occurrence due to adrenocorticotropic hormone and growth hormone deficiency. *Arch Intern Med.* 1980;140:564-565.

172. Steer P, Marnell R, Werk EE Jr. Clinical alcohol hypoglycemia and isolated adrenocorticotrophic hormone deficiency. *Ann Intern Med.* 1969;71:343-348.

173. Fukuda I, Hizuka N, Ishikawa Y, et al. Clinical features of insulin-like growth factor-II producing non-islet-cell tumor hypoglycemia. *Growth Horm IGF Res.* 2006;16:211-216.

174. Daughaday WH. Hypoglycemia due to paraneoplastic secretion of insulin-like growth factor-I. *J Clin Endocrinol Metab.* 2007;92:1616.

175. Miraki-Moud F, Grossman AB, Besser M, et al. A rapid method for analyzing serum pro-insulin-like growth factor-II in patients with non-islet cell tumor hypoglycemia. *J Clin Endocrinol Metab.* 2005;90: 3819-3823.

176. Dynkevich Y, Rother KI, Whitford I, et al. Tumors, IGF-2, and hypoglycemia: insights from the clinic, the laboratory, and the historical archive. *Endocr Rev.* 2013;34:798-826.

177. Nauck MA, Reinecke M, Perren A, et al. Hypoglycemia due to paraneoplastic secretion of insulin-like growth factor-I in a patient with metastasizing large-cell carcinoma of the lung. *J Clin Endocrinol Metab.* 2007;92:1600-1605.

178. Guettier JM, Gorden P. Hypoglycemia. *Endocrinol Metab Clin North Am.* 2006;35:753-766.

179. Marks V, Teale JD. Hypoglycemia: factitious and felonious. *Endocrinol Metab Clin North Am.* 1999;28:579-601.

180. Service FJ, Palumbo PJ. Factitial hypoglycemia: three cases diagnosed on the basis of insulin antibodies. *Arch Intern Med.* 1974;134:336-340.

181. Giurgea I, Ulinski T, Touati G, et al. Factitious hyperinsulinism leading to pancreatectomy: severe forms of Munchausen syndrome by proxy. *Pediatrics.* 2005;116:e145-e148.

182. Manning PJ, Espiner EA, Yoon K, et al. An unusual cause of hyperinsulinaemic hypoglycaemia syndrome. *Diabet Med.* 2003;20:772-776.

183. Placzkowski KA, Vella A, Thompson GB, et al. Secular trends in the presentation and management of functioning insulinoma at the Mayo Clinic, 1987-2007. *J Clin Endocrinol Metab.* 2009;94:1069-1073.

184. Toaiari M, Davì MV, Dalle Carbonare L, et al. Presentation, diagnostic features and glucose handling in a monocentric series of insulinomas. *J Endocrinol Invest.* 2013;36:753-758.

185. Sakurai A, Yamazaki M, Suzuki S, et al. Clinical features of insulinoma in patients with multiple endocrine neoplasia type 1: analysis of the database of the MEN Consortium of Japan. *Endocr J.* 2012;59: 859-866.

186. Guettier J-M, Lungu A, Goodling A, et al. The role of proinsulin and insulin in the diagnosis of insulinoma: a critical evaluation of the Endocrine Society clinical practice guideline. *J Clin Endocrinol Metab.* 2013;98:4752-4758.

187. Service FJ, McMahon MM, O'Brien PC, et al. Functioning insulinoma—incidence, recurrence, and long-term survival of patients: a 60-year study. *Mayo Clin Proc.* 1991;66:711-719.

188. Anlauf M, Wieben D, Perren A, et al. Persistent hyperinsulinemic hypoglycemia in 15 adults with diffuse nesidioblastosis: diagnostic criteria, incidence, and characterization of beta-cell changes. *Am J Surg Pathol.* 2005;29:524-533.

189. Klöppel G, Anlauf M, Raffel A, et al. Adult diffuse nesidioblastosis: genetically or environmentally induced? *Hum Pathol.* 2008;39:3-8.

190. Kaczirek K, Soleiman A, Schindl M, et al. Nesidioblastosis in adults: a challenging cause of organic hyperinsulinism. *Eur J Clin Invest.* 2003; 33:488-492.

191. Witteles RM, Straus FH II, Sugg SL, et al. Adult-onset nesidioblastosis causing hypoglycemia: an important clinical entity and continuing treatment dilemma. *Arch Surg.* 2001;136:656-663.

192. Service FJ, Natt N, Thompson GB, et al. Noninsulinoma pancreatogenous hypoglycemia: a novel syndrome of hyperinsulinemic hypoglycemia in adults independent of mutations in Kir6.2 and SUR1 genes. *J Clin Endocrinol Metab.* 1999;84:1582-1589.

193. Starke A, Saddig C, Kirch B, et al. Islet hyperplasia in adults: challenge to preoperatively diagnose non-insulinoma pancreatogenic hypoglycemia syndrome. *World J Surg.* 2006;30:670-679.

194. Vanderveen KA, Grant CS, Thompson GB, et al. Outcomes and quality of life after partial pancreatectomy for noninsulinoma pancreatogenous hypoglycemia from diffuse islet cell disease. *Surgery.* 2010;148: 1237-1246.

195. Won JG, Tseng HS, Yang AH, et al. Clinical features and morphological characterization of 10 patients with noninsulinoma pancreatogenous hypoglycaemia syndrome (NIPHS). *Clin Endocrinol (Oxf).* 2006;65: 566-578.

196. Service GJ, Thompson GB, Service FJ, et al. Hyperinsulinemic hypoglycemia with nesidioblastosis after gastric-bypass surgery. *N Engl J Med.* 2005;353:249-254.

197. Patti ME, McMahon G, Mun EC, et al. Severe hypoglycaemia post-gastric bypass requiring partial pancreatectomy: evidence for inappropriate insulin secretion and pancreatic islet hyperplasia. *Diabetologia.* 2005;48:2236-2240.

198. Goldfine A, Mun E, Patti M. Hyperinsulinemic hypoglycemia following gastric bypass surgery for obesity. *Curr Opin Endocrinol Diabetes.* 2006;13:419-424.

199. Goldfine AB, Mun EC, Devine E, et al. Patients with neuroglycopenia after gastric bypass surgery have exaggerated incretin and insulin secretory responses to a mixed meal. *J Clin Endocrinol Metab.* 2007;92: 4678-4685.

200. Meier JJ, Butler AE, Galasso R, et al. Hyperinsulinemic hypoglycemia after gastric bypass surgery is not accompanied by islet hyperplasia or increased beta-cell turnover. *Diabetes Care.* 2006;29:1554-1559.

201. Vella A, Service FJ. Incretin hypersecretion in post-gastric bypass hypoglycemia: primary problem or red herring? *J Clin Endocrinol Metab.* 2007;92:4563-4565.

202. Ritz P, Hanaire H. Post-bypass hypoglycaemia: a review of current findings. *Diabetes Metab.* 2011;37:274-281.

203. Salehi M, Gastaldelli A, D'Alessio DA. Blockade of glucagon-like peptide 1 receptor corrects postprandial hypoglycemia after gastric bypass. *Gastroenterology.* 2014;146:669-680.

204. Marsk R, Jonas E, Rasmussen F, Näslund E. Nationwide cohort study of post-gastric bypass hypoglycaemia including 5,040 patients undergoing surgery for obesity in 1986-2006 in Sweden. *Diabetologia.* 2010; 53:2307-2311.

205. Mathavan VK, Arregui M, Davis C, et al. Management of postgastric bypass noninsulinoma pancreatogenous hypoglycemia. *Surg Endosc.* 2010;24:2547-2555.

206. Campos GM, Ziemelis M, Paparodis R, et al. Laparoscopic reversal of Roux-en-Y gastric bypass: technique and utility for treatment of endocrine complications. *Surg Obes Relat Dis.* 2014;10(1):36-43.

207. Lupsa BC, Chong AY, Cochran EK, et al. Autoimmune forms of hypoglycemia. *Medicine.* 2009;88:141-153.

208. Basu A, Service FJ, Yu L, et al. Insulin autoimmunity and hypoglycemia in seven white patients. *Endocr Pract.* 2005;11:97-103.

209. Halsall DJ, Mangi M, Soos M, et al. Hypoglycemia due to an insulin binding antibody in a patient with an IgA-kappa myeloma. *J Clin Endocrinol Metab.* 2007;92:2013-2016.

210. Højlund K, Hansen T, Lajer M, et al. A novel syndrome of autosomal-dominant hyperinsulinemic hypoglycemia linked to a mutation in the human insulin receptor gene. *Diabetes.* 2004;53:1592-1598.

211. Meissner T, Friedmann B, Okun JG, et al. Massive insulin secretion in response to anaerobic exercise in exercise-induced hyperinsulinism. *Horm Metab Res.* 2005;37:690-694.

212. Arioglu E, Andewelt A, Diabo C, et al. Clinical course of the syndrome of autoantibodies to the insulin receptor (type B insulin resistance): a 28-year perspective. *Medicine (Baltimore).* 2002;81:87-100.

213. Seckl MJ, Mulholland PJ, Bishop AE, et al. Hypoglycemia due to an insulin-secreting small-cell carcinoma of the cervix. *N Engl J Med.* 1999;341:733-736.

214. Rizza RA, Haymond MW, Verdonk CA, et al. Pathogenesis of hypoglycemia in insulinoma patients: suppression of hepatic glucose production by insulin. *Diabetes.* 1981;30:377-381.

215. Service FJ, Natt N. The prolonged fast. *J Clin Endocrinol Metab.* 2000; 85:3973-3974.

216. Vezzosi D, Bennet A, Fauvel J, et al. Insulin, C-peptide and proinsulin for the biochemical diagnosis of hypoglycaemia related to endogenous hyperinsulinism. *Eur J Endocrinol.* 2007;157:75-83.

217. Noone TC, Hosey J, Firat Z, et al. Imaging and localization of islet-cell tumours of the pancreas on CT and MRI. *Best Pract Res Clin Endocrinol Metab.* 2005;19:195-211.

218. Grossman AB, Reznek RH. Commentary: imaging of islet-cell tumours. *Best Pract Res Clin Endocrinol Metab.* 2005;19:241-243.

219. Virgolini I, Traub-Weidinger T, Decristoforo C. Nuclear medicine in the detection and management of pancreatic islet-cell tumours. *Best Pract Res Clin Endocrinol Metab.* 2005;19:213-227.

220. Joseph AJ, Kapoor N, Simon EG, et al. Endoscopic ultrasonography—a sensitive tool in the preoperative localization of insulinoma. *Endocr Pract.* 2013;19:602-608.

221. Camera L, Paoletta S, Mollica C, et al. Screening of pancreaticoduodenal endocrine tumours in patients with MEN 1: multidetector-row computed tomography vs. endoscopic ultrasound. *Radiol Med.* 2011; 116:595-606.

222. Kauhanen S, Seppänen M, Minn H, et al. Fluorine-18-L-dihydroxyphenylalanine (18F-DOPA) positron emission tomography as a tool to localize an insulinoma or beta-cell hyperplasia in adult patients. *J Clin Endocrinol Metab.* 2007;92:1237-1244.

223. Brown CK, Bartlett DL, Doppman JL, et al. Intraarterial calcium stimulation and intraoperative ultrasonography in the localization and resection of insulinomas. *Surgery.* 1997;122:1189-1193, discussion 1193-1194.

224. Doppman JL, Miller DL, Chang R, et al. Insulinomas: localization with selective intraarterial injection of calcium. *Radiology.* 1991;178:237-241.

225. Wiesli P, Brändle M, Schmid C, et al. Selective arterial calcium stimulation and hepatic venous sampling in the evaluation of hyperinsulinemic hypoglycemia: potential and limitations. *J Vasc Interv Radiol.* 2004;15(11):1251-1256.

226. Jackson JE. Angiography and arterial stimulation venous sampling in the localization of pancreatic neuroendocrine tumours. *Best Pract Res Clin Endocrinol Metab.* 2005;19:229-239.

227. Liu E, Marincola P, Öberg K. Everolimus in the treatment of patients with advanced pancreatic neuroendocrine tumors: latest findings and interpretations. *Therap Adv Gastroenterol.* 2013;6(5):412-419.

228. Bernard V, Lombard-Bohas C, Taquet M-C, et al. Efficacy of everolimus in patients with metastatic insulinoma and refractory hypoglycemia. *Eur J Endocrinol*. 2013;168:665-674.

229. Hoe FM. Hypoglycemia in infants and children. *Adv Pediatr*. 2008; 55:367-384.

230. Rozance PJ. Update on neonatal hypoglycemia. *Curr Opin Endocrinol Diabetes Obes*. 2014;21:45-50.

231. Harris DL, Weston PJ, Harding JE. Incidence of neonatal hypoglycemia in babies identified as at risk. *J Pediatr*. 2012;161:787-791.

232. Losek JD. Hypoglycemia and the ABC's (sugar) of pediatric resuscitation. *Ann Emerg Med*. 2000;35:43-46.

233. Haymond MW, Karl IE, Pagliara AS. Increased gluconeogenic substrates in the small-for-gestational-age infant. *N Engl J Med*. 1974;291: 322-328.

234. Haymond MW, Karl IE, Pagliara AS. Ketotic hypoglycemia: an amino acid substrate limited disorder. *J Clin Endocrinol Metab*. 1974;38: 521-530.

235. Sperling MA. New insights and new conundrums in neonatal hypoglycemia: enigmas wrapped in mystery. *Diabetes*. 2013;62:1373-1375.

236. Kapoor RR, Flanagan SE, Arya VB, et al. Clinical and molecular characterization of 300 patients with congenital hyperinsulinism. *Eur J Endocrinol*. 2013;168:557-564.

237. Snider KE, Becker S, Boyajian L, et al. Genotype and phenotype correlations in 417 children with congenital hyperinsulinism. *J Clin Endocrinol Metab*. 2013;98:E355-E363.

238. Arya VB, Flanagan SE, Kumaran A, et al. Clinical and molecular characterization of hyperinsulinaemic hypoglycaemia in infants born small-for-gestational age. *Arch Dis Child Fetal Neonatal Ed*. 2013; 98(4):F356-F358.

239. Hu S, Xu Z, Yan J, et al. The treatment effect of diazoxide on 44 patients with congenital hyperinsulinism. *J Pediatr Endocrinol Metab*. 2012;25:1119-1122.

240. Le Quan Sang K-H, Arnoux J-B, Mamoune A, et al. Successful treatment of congenital hyperinsulinism with long-acting octreotide. *Eur J Endocrinol*. 2012;166:333-339.

241. Blomberg BA, Moghbel MC, Saboury B, et al. The value of radiologic interventions and 18F-DOPA PET in diagnosing and localizing focal congenital hyperinsulinism: systemic review and meta-analysis. *Mol Imaging Biol*. 2013;15:97-105.

242. Huang T, Kelly A, Becker SA, et al. Hypertrophic cardiomyopathy in neonates with congenital hyperinsulinism. *Arch Dis Child Fetal Neonatal Ed*. 2013;98:F351-F354.

243. Hussain K, Challis B, Rocha N, et al. An activating mutation of AKT2 and human hypoglycemia. *Science*. 2011;334:474.

244. Arya VB, Flanagan SE, Schober E, et al. Activating AKT2 mutation: hypoinsulinemic hypoketotic hypoglycemia. *J Clin Endocrinol Metab*. 2014;99:391-394.

245. Santra S, Hendriksz C. How to use acylcarnitine profiles to help diagnose inborn errors of metabolism. *Arch Dis Child Educ Pract Ed*. 2010; 95:151-156.

246. Weghuber D, Mandl M, Krssák M, et al. Characterization of hepatic and brain metabolism in young adults with glycogen storage disease type 1: a magnetic resonance spectroscopy study. *Am J Physiol Endocrinol Metab*. 2007;293:E1378-E1384.

247. Karaki C, Kasahara M, Sakamoto S, et al. Glycemic management in living donor liver transplantation for patients with glycogen storage disease type 1b. *Pediatr Transplant*. 2012;16:465-470.

248. Rotstein M, Engelstad K, Yang H, et al. Glut1 deficiency: inheritance pattern determined by haploinsufficiency. *Ann Neurol*. 2010;68: 955-958.

249. Spiekerkoetter U, Mayatepek E. Update on mitochondrial fatty acid oxidation disorders. *J Inherit Metab Dis*. 2010;33:467-468.

250. Nezu J, Tamai I, Oku A, et al. Primary systemic carnitine deficiency is caused by mutations in a gene encoding sodium ion-dependent carnitine transporter. *Nat Genet*. 1999;21:91-94.

251. Bougnères PF, Saudubray JM, Marsac C, et al. Fasting hypoglycemia resulting from hepatic carnitine palmitoyl transferase deficiency. *J Pediatr*. 1981;98:742-746.

CHAPTER 35

Neuroendocrine Control of Energy Stores

ROGER D. CONE • JOEL K. ELMQUIST

KEY POINTS

- The hypothalamus and brainstem contain key circuits regulating food intake and energy expenditure, and coordinate these activities to achieve energy homeostasis.
- Important nuclei in the hypothalamus involved in energy homeostasis include the arcuate nucleus, the ventral medial nucleus, the dorsal medial nucleus, the paraventricular nucleus, the lateral hypothalamus, and the perifornical hypothalamus; important brainstem nuclei include the dorsal motor nucleus of the vagus and the nucleus of the solitary tract.
- In the past two decades, characterization of the basis of obesity in monogenic obesity strains in the ob, db, and AY mice led to our current understanding of the importance of leptin as an adipostatic factor, and to the role of the central melanocortin circuits in the control of energy homeostasis.
- Brain regions such as the VMH, along with key leptin and melanocortin circuits, also play a role in the central control of glucose homeostasis.
- Gut peptides involved in satiety and hunger include cholecystokinin (CCK), peptide YY (PYY), ghrelin, preproglucagon-derived peptides, and amylin.
- Food and drug rewards share some common neural substrates. If rational strategies to combat obesity are to be developed, then an increased understanding of the molecular mechanisms of the rewarding aspects of feeding behavior is required.
- A wide variety of disorders of hypothalamic and neuroendocrine function are known to produce obesity, including Frölich syndrome, craniopharyngioma, endocrine disorders such as Cushing disease, and various genes.

HISTORICAL PERSPECTIVE

Obesity and diabetes are major health issues facing society. Fortunately, since the turn of the new century several key molecules including hormones and receptors controlling energy homeostasis have been identified. Indeed, we now have a broad understanding of the key sites in the central nervous system (CNS) through which key metabolic signals exert their effects. For example, key components of the central control of energy balance are located in the hypothalamus. In the 21st century it is taken for granted that the hypothalamus is required for coordinated control of food intake and energy homeostasis. The intimate interaction of the hypothalamus and the pituitary gland has been appreciated for some time. However, understanding the primary role of the hypothalamus in controlling long-term energy stores, and thus adipose mass, is relatively recent. For example, at the end of the 19th century clinicians including Alfred Fröhlich described an adiposogenital dystrophic condition in patients with pituitary tumors. This condition became known as Fröhlich syndrome and was characterized by pituitary tumors associated with excessive subcutaneous fat and hypogonadism.[1,2] However, whether the cause of this syndrome was due to injury to the pituitary gland or to the overlying hypothalamus was extremely controversial. Several groups, including Cushing and his colleagues, argued that the syndrome was due to disruption of the pituitary gland.[3-5] However, Aschner demonstrated in dogs that mere removal of the pituitary gland without damage to the overlying hypothalamus did not result in obesity.[6] The most definitive evidence of the vital role of the hypothalamus was provided by Hetherington and Ranson when they demonstrated that destruction of the medial basal hypothalamus without damage to the pituitary gland could result in morbid obesity and neuroendocrine derangements in a very similar fashion to the patients reported by Frölich.[7] These and subsequent studies firmly established that an intact hypothalamus is required for normal energy and glucose homeostasis.

Following the discoveries that hypothalamic lesions could cause obesity, it also became apparent that lesions in other regions, such as the lateral hypothalamus, could cause leanness. Based on these results, it was suggested that a feeding center was located in the lateral hypothalamus and a satiety center in the ventromedial hypothalamus.[8] As a result of these and other studies, the importance of the hypothalamus as an integrator and effector of energy balance and neuroendocrine function was generally accepted. Humans and other mammals have a remarkable ability to match caloric intake and expenditure, leading to relative stability of body weight and adipose mass over long periods. Based on this observation, Kennedy[9] proposed a mechanism of body weight regulation in which a signal related to energy stores elicited compensatory changes in food intake and energy expenditure, with the result being maintenance of adipose mass at a presumed set-point.

This view was supported by studies in rodents showing that weight gain from forced overfeeding resulted in a compensatory decrease in voluntary food intake, increased energy expenditure, and eventual restoration of body weight to the previous level, whereas starvation or lipectomy stimulated feeding and decreased energy expenditure in order to restore body weight and adipose mass to a previous set-point.[10-12] However, the signal(s) mediating the potential interaction between adipose tissue and the brain were not known. Studies by Hervey[13-15] offered important insights into potential signals linking energy stores with energy homeostatic mechanisms. He showed that parabiosis between obese rats with VMH lesions and normal (non-lesioned) rats led to starvation and weight loss in the latter. In contrast, the VMH-lesioned rats gained weight when parabiosed with lean rats or other VMH-lesioned rats. Results of these studies were thought to indicate that obese VMH-lesioned rats produced a circulating satiety factor leading to inhibition of feeding in nonlesioned parabiotic rats. In contrast, the lack of response in VMH-lesioned rats was consistent with the existence of a satiety center proposed in earlier studies.[8]

The ensuing model from these landmark studies received support following the discovery of recessive mutations in the *obese* and *diabetic* mice, *ob* and *db*, both of which led to hyperphagia, decreased energy expenditure, and morbid obesity.[16] Parabiosis of lean (wild-type) and *ob/ob* mice suppressed weight gain in *ob/ob* mice, whereas parabiosis of wild-type and *db/db* mice caused profound hypophagia and weight loss in the former.[17-19] These results led to the prediction that the *ob* locus produced a circulating satiety factor, whereas the *db* locus encoded a component required for the response mechanism to the satiety factor. Predictions based on parabiosis studies were confirmed by the cloning of *ob* and *db* genes in the mid-1990s.[20-22] The hormone product of the *ob* gene was named *leptin* (from the Greek root *leptos*, meaning thin) because it potently inhibited feeding, body weight, and adipose mass when injected into leptin-deficient mice, and had partial activity when injected into normal mice.[23-26]

In addition to the *ob* and *db* mouse strains, the *lethal yellow agouti* (A^Y) mouse had long been known to express an obesity syndrome. Just as molecular cloning of the *ob* and *db* loci led to the discovery of the primary adipostatic factor and its receptor, cloning and characterization of the agouti gene[27-29] has led to characterization of one of the important CNS circuits involved in regulating energy homeostasis, the central melanocortin system.[30,31] These and related discoveries over the past 15 years have taken the understanding of energy homeostasis from the level of gross anatomy to the beginnings of a cellular and molecular basis for the neuroendocrine control of energy stores, the topic of this chapter (Fig. 35-1).

CIRCUITS REGULATING ENERGY BALANCE

Key circuits regulating energy homeostasis and food intake reside in hypothalamic brain regions (Fig. 35-2). The hypothalamus is essential for life and is an evolutionarily highly conserved region of the mammalian brain, being the ultimate brain structure that allows mammals to maintain homeostasis. Destruction of the hypothalamus is not compatible with life.[32] Hypothalamic control of homeostasis stems from the ability of hypothalamic neurons to orchestrate behavioral, autonomic, and behavioral responses. This control is derived from the anatomic connections (both inputs and outputs) of the hypothalamus.

The hypothalamus receives sensory inputs from the external environment and information regarding the internal environment. In addition, several hormones known to be key in regulating food intake and metabolism (e.g., glucocorticoids, estrogen, leptin, ghrelin) directly act on neurons in the hypothalamus. The hypothalamus integrates all of this information and in turn provides motor outputs to key regulatory sites including the anterior pituitary gland, the posterior pituitary gland, the cerebral cortex, premotor and motor neurons in the brainstem and spinal cord, and autonomic (parasympathetic and sympathetic) preganglionic neurons. The hypothalamic outputs to these effector sites ultimately result in coordinated endocrine, behavioral, and autonomic responses that maintain homeostasis in several physiologic systems, including energy balance. Within the hypothalamus, several hypothalamic sites are thought to be key in regulating energy homeostasis (see Fig. 35-1). The primary group comprises sites located in the medial hypothalamus, including the arcuate nucleus, the ventral medial nucleus, the dorsal medial nucleus, and the paraventricular nucleus. In addition, the lateral hypothalamus (LHA and perifornical hypothalamus) is key in regulating food intake and energy homeostasis.

In addition to the hypothalamus, circuits in the brainstem are involved in the coordinated control of food intake as well.[33-36] For example, the brainstem also receives a wide variety of signals from visceral organs including the gastrointestinal (GI) tract, which sends signals from the visceral sensory afferents that converge on the dorsal vagal complex (DVC). The DVC comprises the nucleus of the solitary tract (nucleus tractus solitarius [NTS]), the dorsal motor nucleus of the vagus (DMV) (vagal motor neurons), and the area postrema (AP). Sensory afferent signals carried by the glossopharyngeal and vagus nerves include indications of taste, gastric stretch, and levels of glucose and lipids in the liver and portal vein. Afferent terminals carrying this information innervate the NTS. This information is relayed to multiple sites including the DMV that are parasympathetic preganglionic neurons. The vagal motor neurons in turn innervate and provide parasympathetic input to the entire GI tract, including the pancreas.

In addition, key sensory inputs to the NTS from the GI tract and taste information are directly relayed to the paraventricular, dorsomedial, and arcuate nuclei of the hypothalamus and the LHA; the central nucleus of the amygdala and bed nucleus of the stria terminalis; and the parabrachial nucleus.[32,37] The parabrachial nucleus then projects to the thalamus, the cerebral cortex, the amygdala, and several hypothalamic sites.[32] Notably, recent data have demonstrated that key hypothalamic neurons regulating feeding, such as the agouti-related peptide (AgRP) neurons of the arcuate nucleus, also innervate the parabrachial nucleus.[38-43] Thus, the parabrachial nucleus serves as a key weigh station integrating inputs from the brainstem and hypothalamus as it relates to the regulation of energy balance.

The AP is a circumventricular organ that lies directly above the NTS. Unlike the NTS, which lies inside the blood-brain barrier, and thus is not in direct contact with circulating factors and hormones, neurons in the AP sit outside the blood-brain barrier.[44] Neurons in the AP likely respond to circulating gut hormones (e.g., CCK, glucagon-like peptide-1 [GLP-1]) and relay those signals into the NTS and the parabrachial nucleus.[35-37,45-48]

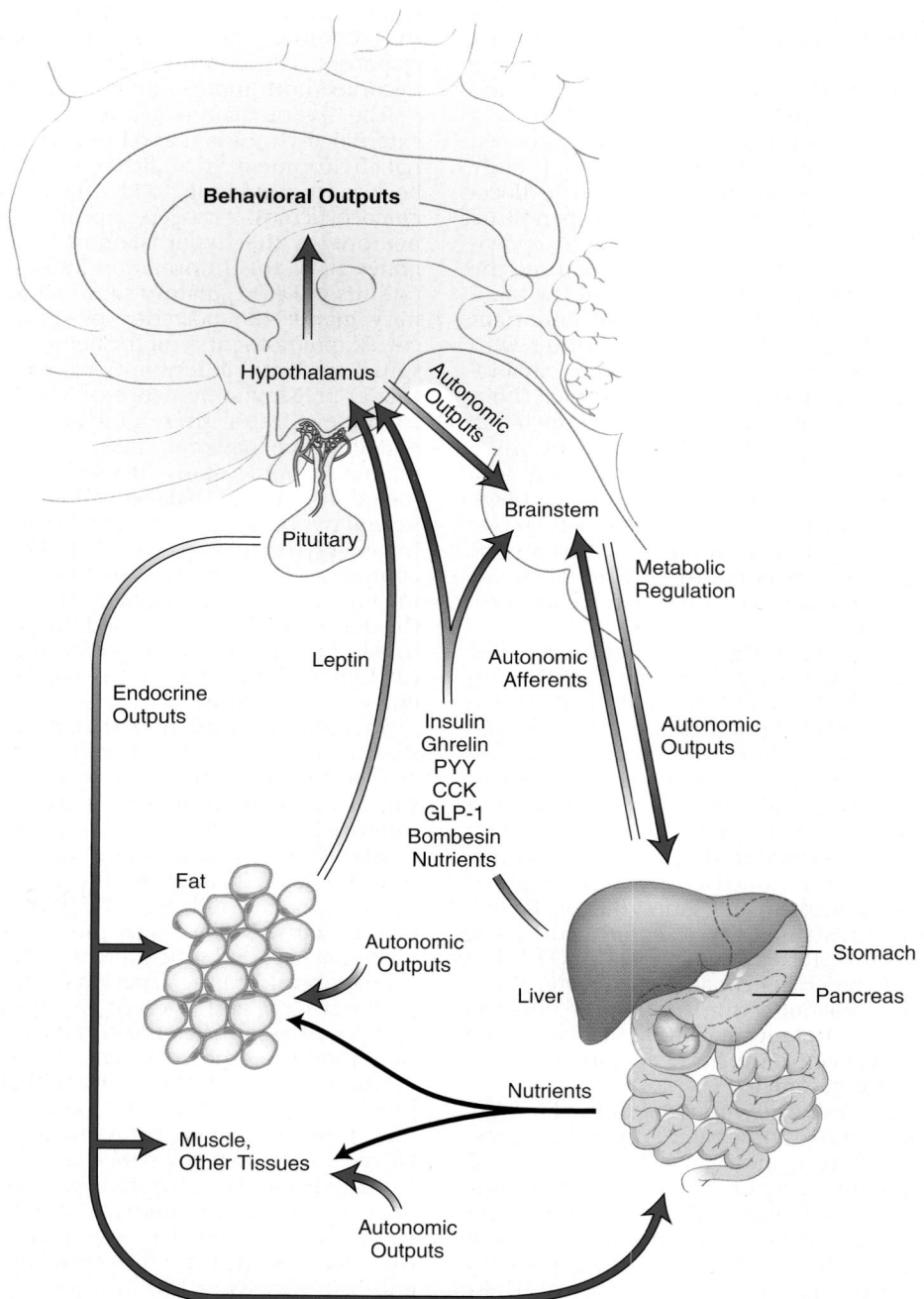

Figure 35-1 Regulation of energy homeostasis by the brain-gut-adipose axis. CCK, cholecystokinin; GLP-1, glucagon-like peptide 1; PYY, peptide YY.

Ventromedial Hypothalamic Neuron Control of Glucose and Energy Homeostasis

As noted earlier, several regions of the brain have been identified as physiologically important regulators of energy balance. They include neurons in the VMH nucleus.[49-51] The VMH has historically been linked to the regulation of body weight based on the classic lesion studies that led to the view that the VMH was a satiety center. Over the years this model fell out of favor, in part, because of uncertainty regarding the exact nature of the obesity-inducing lesions. However, several studies have reestablished that the VMH is a physiologically important site regulating body weight homeostasis. This work has focused on the role of steroido-

genic factor 1 (SF1), which is an orphan nuclear receptor transcription factor. Notably, SF1 is expressed by neurons exclusively in the VMH.[52] Mice lacking SF1 do not develop an intact VMH and display late-onset obesity.[53-55] Notably, leptin receptors are abundantly expressed in the VMH,[56] as are MC3Rs,[57] and selective deletion of leptin receptors from SF1 neurons produces obesity.[51] Thus, the VMH is a critical site in the brain regulating body weight.

VMH neurons can also regulate insulin sensitivity in peripheral tissues including skeletal muscle, white adipose tissue, and brown adipose tissue (BAT). Leptin action in the VMH significantly increases glucose uptake in the skeletal muscle and BAT, suggesting that leptin acts on VMH neurons to enhance peripheral insulin sensitivity.[58-61] In

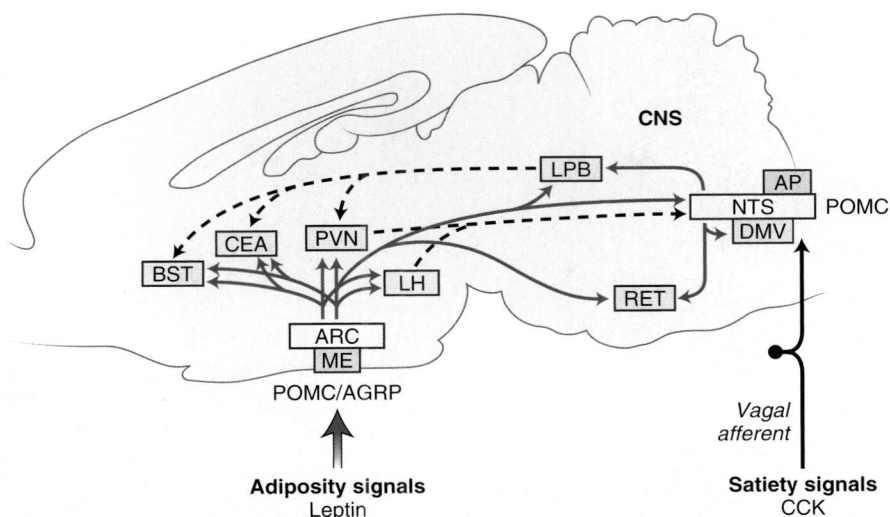

Figure 35-2 Brain structures involved in energy homeostasis. Receipt of long-term adipostatic signals and acute satiety signals by neurons in arcuate nucleus and brainstem, respectively. Pale blue boxes indicate nuclei containing pro-opiomelanocortin (POMC) neurons; tan boxes indicate nuclei containing melanocortin-4 receptor (MC4R) neurons that may serve to integrate adipostatic and satiety signals; and darker blue boxes show some circumventricular organs involved in energy homeostasis. Magenta arrows designate a subset of projections of POMC neurons; blue arrows show a subset of projections of agouti-related peptide (AGRP neurons). AP, area postrema; ARC, arcuate nucleus; BST, bed nucleus of the stria terminalis; CCK, cholecystokinin; CEA, central nucleus of the amygdala; CNS, central nervous system; DMV, dorsal motor nucleus of the vagus; LH, lateral hypothalamic area; LPB, lateral parabrachial nucleus; ME, median eminence; NTS, nucleus tractus solitarius; PVN, paraventricular nucleus of the hypothalamus; RET, reticular formation. (Modified from Fan W, Ellacott KL, Halatchev IG, et al. Cholecystokinin-mediated suppression of feeding involves the brainstem melanocortin system. *Nat Neurosci.* 2004;7:335-336.)

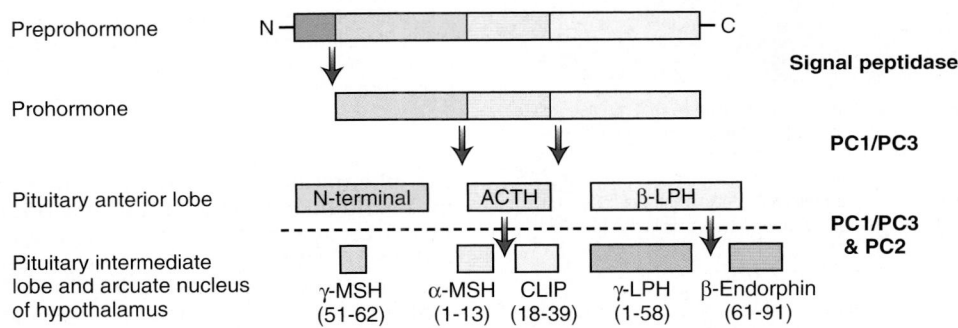

Figure 35-3 Organization of pro-opiomelanocortin (POMC), the precursor hormone of corticotropin (ACTH, adrenocorticotropic hormone), β-lipoprotein (β-LPH), and related peptides. The precursor protein contains a leader sequence (signal peptide), followed by a long fragment that includes sequence 51-62, corresponding to γ-melanocyte-stimulating hormone (γ-MSH). This fragment is cleaved at Lys-Arg bonds to form corticotropin 1-39, which in turn includes the sequences for α-MSH (corticotropin 1-13) and corticotropin-like intermediate lobe peptide (CLIP; corticotropin 18-39) and a sequence corresponding to β-LPH (1-91) that includes γ-LPH (1-58) and β-endorphin (61-91). The β-endorphin sequence also includes a sequence corresponding to met-enkephalin. The precursor molecule in the anterior lobe of the pituitary is processed predominantly to corticotropin and β-LPH. In the intermediate pituitary lobe (in the rat), corticotropin and β-LPH are further processed to α-MSH and a β-endorphin–like material. In all extrapituitary tissues, post-translational processing of the prohormone resembles that in the intermediate lobe. Hypothalamic processing is similar but not identical to that in the intermediate lobe. In the latter, β-endorphin and α-MSH are present predominantly in their acetylated forms. C, carboxy-terminal; PC, prohormone-converting enzyme. (Courtesy of Dr. Malcolm Low, University of Michigan, Ann Arbor, MI.)

addition, mice lacking leptin receptors in SF1 neurons in the VMH develop insulin resistance.[50] In contrast, selective deletion of suppressor of cytokine signaling 3 (SOCS3, a negative regulator of leptin signaling) in SF1 neurons prevents insulin resistance induced by high fat feeding.[62]

The Arcuate Nucleus Is a Key Node of Hypothalamic Control of Energy Balance

The arcuate nucleus is probably the best characterized hypothalamic nucleus involved in the control of energy balance. Specifically, pro-opiomelanocortin (POMC) neurons and agouti related protein (AgRP) neurons that reside within the arcuate nucleus are required for regulating energy homeostasis, food intake, and glucose homeostasis. POMC is a multifunctional propeptide that is differentially processed into key peptides in different tissues[63] (Fig. 35-3). In the brain, melanocortin peptides including α-melanocyte-stimulating hormone (α-MSH) are key products that regulate food intake and energy homeostasis. α-MSH is the agonist for the MC4R, which is established as key in regulating food intake, energy homeostasis, and glucose homeostasis in both mice and humans.[63,64] Uniquely, an endogenous MC4R antagonist exists (AgRP) and is coexpressed with neuropeptide Y (NPY) and GABA in a second distinct class of neurons in the arcuate nucleus of the hypothalamus.

Supportive of a key role of the arcuate nucleus in regulating food intake and energy homeostasis, leptin deficiency (*ob/ob* mice) and fasting, which lowers leptin levels, result in decreased POMC expression and increased AgRP and NPY expression.[65,66] POMC and NPY/AgRP neurons are located in the arcuate nucleus (Figs. 35-4 and 35-5) and

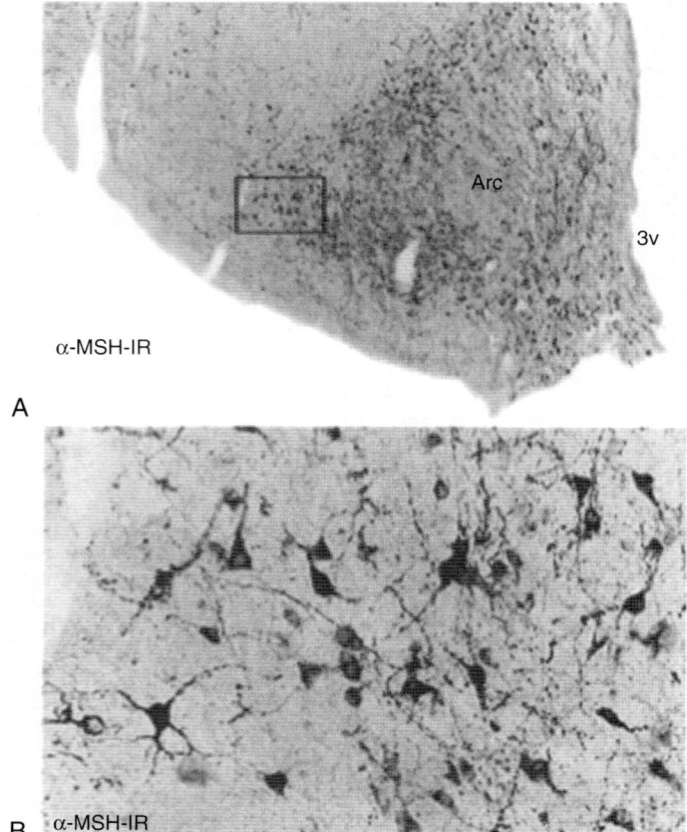

Figure **35-4** **A** and **B,** Photomicrographs demonstrate that α-melanocyte-stimulating hormone–immunoreactive (α-MSH-IR) neurons are present in the human hypothalamus. The neurons are found in the arcuate nucleus of the hypothalamus (Arc; infundibular nucleus). 3v, third ventricle. (Modified from Elias CF, Saper CB, Maratos-Flier E, et al. Chemically defined projections linking the mediobasal hypothalamus and the lateral hypothalamic area. *J Comp Neurol.* 1998;402:442-459.)

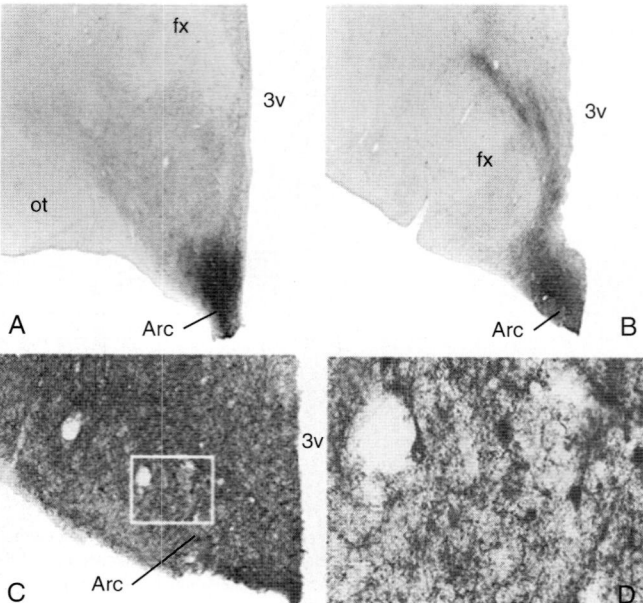

Figure **35-5** Photomicrographs demonstrate that agouti-related peptide–immunoreactive (AgRP-IR) neurons are present in the human hypothalamus. **A** and **B,** Two rostral to caudal low-power photomicrographs demonstrate that AgRP-IR neurons localize to the arcuate nucleus of the hypothalamus (Arc; infundibular nucleus). In B, immunoreactive fibers are also observed streaming dorsally out of the arcuate nucleus. **C** and **D,** AgRP-IR neurons are observed in the arcuate nucleus. D is a higher magnification of boxed area in C. 3v, third ventricle; fx, fornix; ot, olfactory tubercle. (Modified from Elias CF, Saper CB, Maratos-Flier E, et al. Chemically defined projections linking the mediobasal hypothalamus and the lateral hypothalamic area. *J Comp Neurol.* 1998;402:442-459.)

are directly regulated by leptin, ghrelin, glucose, and other metabolic signals. For example, leptin directly depolarizes (activates) POMC neurons and hyperpolarizes (inhibits) AgRP/NPY neurons,[67,68] and deletion of leptin receptors selectively in POMC neurons produces mild obesity.[69] Studies have reinforced the notion that AgRP neurons are key regulators of food intake. Notably, complete ablation of AgRP neurons results in anorexia.[40,70-72] In addition, acute optogenetic or chemogenetic activation of AgRP neurons increases food intake and body weight.[42,73-75] Importantly, the NPY/AgRP neurons provide direct inhibitory input to the adjacent POMC neurons, and thus the orexigenic NPY/AgRP and anorexigenic POMC neurons of the arcuate nucleus are coordinately regulated by a wide variety of hormones, drugs, and perhaps nutrients (Fig. 35-6B).[49,51] In addition to leptin, other key metabolic signals act directly on POMC and AgRP neurons in the arcuate nucleus. For example, ghrelin directly depolarizes AgRP/NPY neurons.[76]

Another key regulator of energy balance is the central serotonin (5-HT) system. The central serotonin system is complex and includes 14 different 5-HT receptors (5-HTRs).[77,78] These efforts have pinpointed that serotonin and dexfenfluramine act predominantly via central 5-HT$_{2C}$Rs[79-81] and downstream melanocortin pathways to suppress feeding, thus reducing body weight.[78,82-86] Moreover, the anorexic properties of fenfluramine depend in part on MC4Rs.[84,87] Fenfluramine was used in combination with phentermine (Fen/Phen) to successfully reduce food intake and body weight in humans, prior to removal from the market as a result of heart valve disorders. The approval of the 5-HT$_{2C}$R agonist Belviq (lorcaserin) by the U.S. Food and Drug Administration (FDA) in 2012 highlights the persistent interest in central 5-HT$_{2C}$Rs as a target to treat obesity.[88]

The precise mechanisms and neural pathways underlying the ability of serotonin to regulate energy balance and glucose homeostasis via actions on melanocortin neurons have also been reported. Evidence from several groups suggests that hypothalamic POMC neurons are physiologically important targets of serotonin to regulate energy homeostasis. For example, POMC neurons coexpress 5-HT$_{2C}$Rs.[83] In addition, serotonin directly activates POMC neurons[83] and inhibits NPY/AgRP neurons[84]; serotonin activates POMC neurons via 5-HT$_{2C}$R-mediated mechanisms.[83,89,90] In addition, 5-HT$_{2C}$R agonists stimulate POMC mRNA expression in the arcuate nucleus.[86,91]

Finally, mice in which expression of the 5-HT$_{2C}$R is disrupted globally but the receptor is re-expressed only in POMC neurons do not develop the hyperphagia and obesity characteristic of global 5-HT$_{2C}$R deficiency.[85,90] Thus, it is likely that serotonin and antiobesity drugs exert their effects in part by activating 5-HT$_{2C}$Rs expressed by POMC neurons in the arcuate nucleus of the hypothalamus.

Melanocortin-4 Receptors Regulate Energy and Glucose Homeostasis

Several pieces of evidence definitively demonstrate the role for MC4Rs in the regulation of energy homeostasis. For

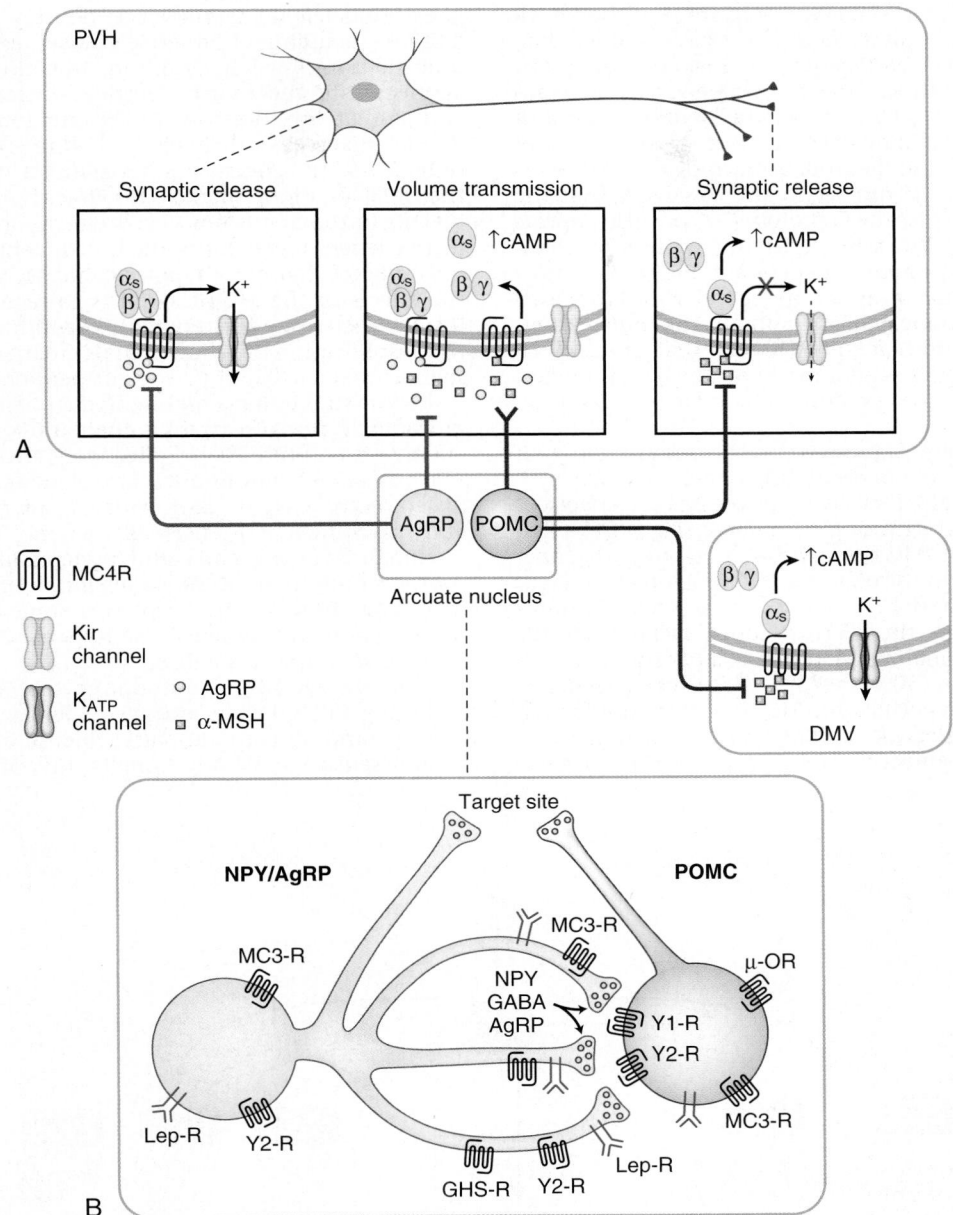

Figure 35-6 A, Divergent signaling modalities for the MC4R. Earlier models of α-MSH and AgRP action suggested competitive binding of these peptides to individual MC4R sites through volume release onto shared MC4R sites to stimulate or inhibit, respectively, G protein signaling and intracellular cAMP levels. Existing neuroanatomic data characterizing POMC and AgRP neuronal projections show that α-MSH may act independently of AgRP at many sites in the central nervous system. The ability of AgRP to act independently of α-MSH as a potent hyperpolarizing agonist, via regulation of Kir7.1, suggests the likely existence of independent AgRP sites of action *(left square).* Another MC4R signaling pathway, involving cAMP/K+-dependent activation of K$_{ATP}$ channels and α-MSH-induced hyperpolarization, has been demonstrated in MC4R neurons in the DMV in the brainstem *(bottom right).*[98] **B,** Regulation of the arcuate nucleus of the hypothalamus by various hormones and neuropeptides. NPY/AgRP and POMC neurons within the arcuate nucleus form a coordinately regulated network due to dense NPY/AgRP fibers that project to POMC cell bodies. Some receptors for the large numbers of hormones and neuropeptides known to regulate the network are indicated. AgRP, agouti-related peptide; ATP, adenosine triphosphate; cAMP, cyclic adenosine monophosphate; DMV, dorsal motor nucleus of the vagus; GABA, γ-aminobutyric acid; GHS, growth-hormone secretagogue receptor; Lep, leptin; MC3, melanocortin-3; MC4R, melanocortin-4 receptor; α-MSH, α-melanocyte-stimulating hormone; NPY, neuropeptide Y; μ-OR, μ-opiate receptor; POMC, pro-opiomelanocortin; PVH, paraventricular nucleus of the hypothalamus; R, receptor; GLP-1, glucagon-like peptide 1. (A modified from Ghamari-Langroudi M, Digby GJ, Sebag JA, et al. G-protein-independent coupling of MC4R to Kir7.1 in hypothalamic neurons. *Nature.* 2015;520:94-98; B modified from Cowley MA, Smart JL, Rubinstein M, et al. Leptin activates anorexigenic POMC neurons through a neural network in the arcuate nucleus. *Nature.* 2001;411:480-484.)

example, ectopic expression of MC4R antagonists in the brain induces obesity and diabetes.[30,64] In addition, MC4R deletion in mice produces obesity,[31] and humans with MC4R mutations display obesity.[92-95] Indeed, estimates suggest that 5% of cases of severe early-onset obesity are the result of MC4R mutations, making this the most common genetic obesity syndrome. The high prevalence of melanocortin obesity syndrome (~1/1500) results from the fact that this receptor acts like a rheostat on energy storage and that haploinsufficency resulting from one null or hypomorphic mutation causes morbid early-onset obesity with a penetrance of around 70%. Much remains to be learned about how the MC4R regulates the activity of the neurons in which it is expressed. In the paraventricular nucleus of the hypothalamus (PVH), MC4R agonists depolarize and increase firing of a variety of neuronal subtypes,[96,97] whereas in the DMV, activation of the MC4R hyperpolarizes and inhibits neurons.[98] Early models had also proposed that the endogenous agonist and antagonist of the MC4R, α-MSH and AgRP, respectively, may act competitively to bind to and determine the relative amount of activation of the MC4R; however, a more nuanced view of the neuroanatomy and neuropharmacology of MC4R is developing (see Fig. 35-6B). With the discovery that the MC4R not only activates the G protein GαS but also appears to directly regulate inwardly rectifying potassium channels, Kirs, in a G protein–independent manner, it now appears that AgRP may function independently as a biased agonist. Neuroanatomic data also support the independent action of these peptides at some sites, in that in the PVH, AgRP-positive synapses predominate at MC4R cell bodies, whereas POMC synapses predominate at spines and distal dendrites.[99,100]

MC4Rs are widely expressed in the brain, many of which could play a role in regulating energy balance.[101-103] The sites in the brain that mediate the varied effects of MC4R agonists are beginning to emerge (Fig. 35-7). Evidence suggests that MC4Rs expressed by hypothalamic neurons contribute to the effects of MC4R agonists to regulate energy homeostasis.[104,105] For example, selective restoration of MC4Rs in the PVH in mice lacking MC4Rs everywhere else normalizes food intake and reduces excessive body weight by 50% to 75%.[105] However, evidence suggests that extrahypothalamic MC4Rs contribute to melanocortin action to decrease adipose mass, food intake, and increase energy expenditure. For example, MC4R messenger ribonucleic acid (mRNA) is densely expressed in the DMV,[101] including cholinergic parasympathetic preganglionic neurons.[102,103] In addition, injections of the MC4R agonists into the fourth ventricle decreases food intake, and similar injections of MC4R antagonists dose dependently increase food intake.[106,107] Interestingly, injections of both MC4R agonists and antagonists into the region of the DMV alter food intake. This effect is likely mediated by MC4Rs in the brainstem as it occurs at doses that are ineffective when injected into the fourth ventricle. These findings suggest that extrahypothalamic MC4Rs contribute to the effects of the MC4R agonists to regulate food intake, insulin secretion, and energy expenditure. This includes the amplification of satiety signals emanating from the gut such as that mediated by the gut peptide CCK.[108]

Recent studies have highlighted a potentially important physiologic role of extrahypothalamic MC4Rs to regulate energy expenditure.[109,110] Collectively, these studies suggest that MC4Rs in autonomic control neurons modestly reduced body weight gain without altering food intake and was sufficient to normalize energy expenditure and attenuate hyperglycemia and hyperinsulinemia. In contrast, restoration of MC4R expression in brainstem neurons including those in the DMV was sufficient to attenuate hyperinsulinemia, whereas the hyperglycemia and energy balance were not normalized.

Deleting MC4Rs in autonomic (cholinergic) neurons including SPNs lowers energy expenditure, resulting in obesity, and directly impairs glucose homeostasis and insulin sensitivity.[110] Additionally, loss of MC4Rs in SPNs

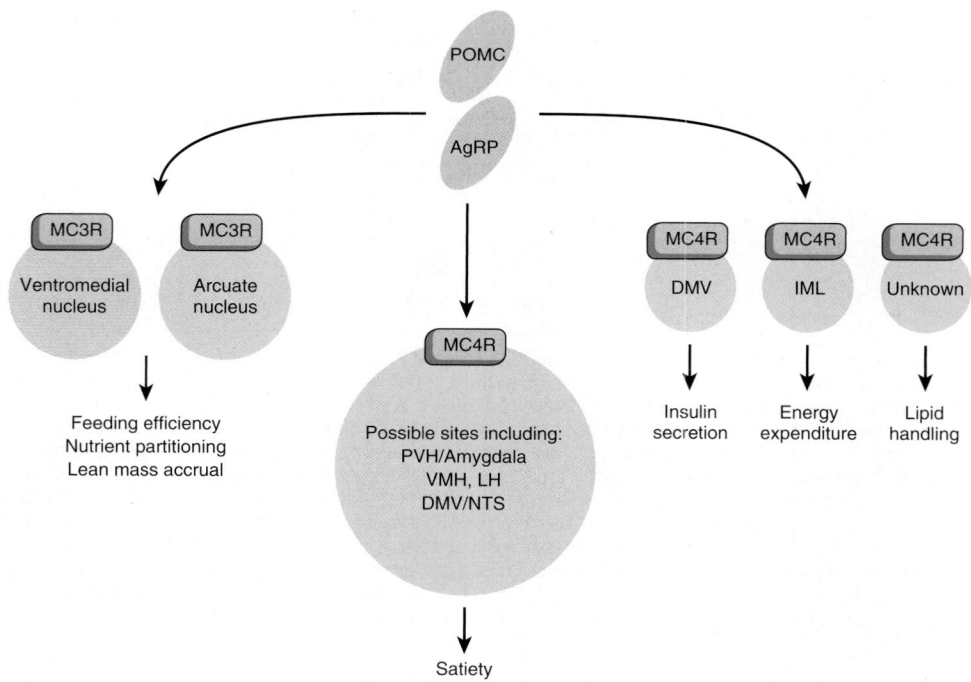

Figure 35-7 Central nervous system (CNS) melanocortin action. The pro-opiomelanocortin (POMC) neurons of the arcuate nucleus produce melanocortin-receptor agonists, whereas agouti-related peptide (AgRP)-producing neurons antagonize melanocortin action. The two predominant CNS melanocortin receptors, MC3R and MC4R, mediate distinct effects. MC3R is expressed at high levels in the arcuate nucleus and ventromedial nucleus and mainly controls the conversion of food to fat, nutrient partitioning, and buildup of lean mass, whereas MC4R predominantly mediates effects on food intake. The specific neurons that express MC4R are unclear; however, genetic data suggest important roles for the paraventricular hypothalamic (PVH) nucleus and amygdala MC4R in these effects, whereas other data, including pharmacologic data, suggest roles for MC4R at other sites such as the ventromedial hypothalamic (VMH) nucleus, lateral hypothalamus (LH), dorsal motor nucleus of the vagus (DMV), and nucleus tractus solitarius (NTS) as well as the lateral parabrachial nucleus. In addition to mediating metabolic effects attributable to body weight, MC4R mediates the control of insulin secretion through the DMV and energy expenditure through the intermediolateral cell column (IML) of the spinal cord. MC4R also contributes to lipid handling in the body, but the MC4R-expressing site or sites that mediate these effects remain undefined. (From Myers MG, Olson DP. Central nervous system control of metabolism. *Nature.* 2012;491:357-363.)

amplifies high-fat-diet–induced obesity and dampens "browning or beiging" of white adipose tissue[111] following exposure to a high-fat diet. This deletion also blunts cold-induced thermogenesis in BAT and maintenance of core body temperature. In contrast, deleting MC4Rs in parasympathetic preganglionic neurons (vagal motor neurons) causes hyperinsulinemia and insulin resistance but does not significantly impact energy balance. Collectively, these results suggest that MC4Rs expressed by autonomic neurons regulate energy expenditure and hepatic glucose production. Recent data also suggest the existence of a leptin-melanocortin axis in the gut,[112] and functional MC4R has also been demonstrated in the majority of mouse and human colonic enteroendocrine L cells.[113] Although the physiologic role of MC4R in enteroendocrine cells remains unknown, stimulation of the receptor ex vivo and in vivo results in release of the gut peptides PYY and GLP-1.[113,114] A related melanocortin receptor, the MC3R, is expressed in largely nonoverlapping sites in the CNS from the MC4R, and also plays a role in energy homeostasis. In the mouse, this receptor is most highly expressed in the POMC and AgRP neurons of the arcuate nucleus, the VMH, dopaminergic neurons of the ventral tegmental area, and the medial habenula.[57,115] Although haploinsufficiency does not produce a phenotype, homozygous deletion of the receptor causes an unusual syndrome,[116,117] with phenotypes including increased adipose mass, decreased lean mass, reduced fast-induced refeeding,[118] elevated basal and fasting-induced corticosterone,[118] and defects in circadian rhythms and meal entrainment.[119,120] The MC3R is also expressed presynaptically on AgRP terminals and acts as an inhibitory autoreceptor on the POMC-MC4R circuitry.[67] A syndrome resulting from MC3R mutations in humans has not yet been definitively identified.

The Lateral Hypothalamus Links Coordinated Food Intake Control and Arousal

The lateral hypothalamus includes the LHA and perifornical hypothalamus. This region of the brain has long been suggested to play a key role in the regulation of ingestive behavior since the early lesion studies of Anand and Brobeck.[121] In the 1990s, two neuropeptides were discovered that are expressed by neurons in the lateral hypothalamus. These metabolically regulated peptides are melanin-concentrating hormone (MCH) and the orexins (also known as hypocretins).[122-125] MCH and orexin are expressed by distinct subsets of intermingled neurons in the LHA.[126,127] However, both populations broadly innervate the entire neuraxis including monosynaptic projections to other hypothalamic sites, the cerebral cortex, the amygdala, the brainstem, and the spinal cord.[122,128] The expression patterns of the receptors for both peptides are also widespread.[129-131]

Current data support the view that these LHA neuropeptides play a key role in regulating food intake, adipose mass, and glucose homeostasis. For example, injection of MCH into the brain increases food intake.[123] Mice lacking MCH (knockouts) are hypophagic and lean, and mice that overexpress MCH are obese and hyperleptinemic.[132,133] In addition, mice lacking MCH and leptin are leaner compared to mice that lack leptin but express MCH.[134] The role of orexins in regulating food intake is complex, but it is clear that orexins are required for normal energy balance.[135,136] For example, central injections of orexin peptides increase feeding behavior.[124,137] However, the best characterized role for orexins is in the regulation of state control and the maintenance of wakefulness,[138,139] because it has been demonstrated that defective orexin

signaling causes narcolepsy in mice, dogs, and humans. Other studies have recently demonstrated the ability of orexin neurons to sense changing levels of glucose (see discussion later).

The exact sites targeted by MCH and orexin neurons to induce feeding remain to be determined, and this is an area of active investigation. However, both MCH and orexin neurons have very similar and widespread projection patterns that include the hypothalamus, the brainstem, the cerebral cortex, and the spinal cord. Targets in the brainstem include motor systems and cranial nerve motor nuclei that underlie behaviors such as chewing, licking, and swallowing.[48,140] The MCH and orexin neurons also innervate the sympathetic and parasympathetic preganglionic nuclei in the medulla and the spinal cord, suggesting that both may be key in regulating the autonomic nervous system. Finally, a key target for both MCH and orexin neurons in coordinating feeding behavior may be their reciprocal connections with the nucleus accumbens.[141-145] The nucleus accumbens is known to be critical in mediating rewarding components of several stimuli, including drugs of abuse, and potentially the rewarding aspects of feeding. Although still being investigated, it is likely that MCH and orexin neurons may be able to enhance the hedonic value of food.[48,141,142,146,147] Regardless of the specific sites that mediate these effects, it is clear that MCH and orexin neurons are ideally positioned to regulate complex behavior, endocrine function, and autonomic outflow, all of which are key for coordinated control of energy balance.

CENTRAL NERVOUS SYSTEM CONTROL OF THERMOGENESIS

Coordinated energy homeostasis necessarily includes a balance between energy intake and energy expenditure. Energy expenditure is often grouped into three categories: energy required for basal metabolism, energy required for voluntary and involuntary physical activity, and the thermic effect of food. The latter, often referred to as *diet-induced thermogenesis* (DIT), is estimated at 8% to 10% of total expenditure and is defined as the increased energy expenditure in response to energy intake.[148] This process is under the control of the sympathetic nervous system, and energy expenditure is increased by stimulation of β-adrenergic receptors. In rodents, the major tissue mediating this response is BAT, which contains adipocytes with dense collections of mitochondria.[149] In addition, the brown adipocytes express uncoupling protein 1 (UCP1), which uncouples mitochondrial respiration and thus induces energy expenditure and heat. In humans the key tissue mediating energy expenditure in response to changing energy intake remains to be determined but likely includes skeletal muscle.[149] Traditionally, it was thought that BAT in humans was found in infants but was only minimally present in adults. However, the discovery of brown fat depots in some adults as a result of [18F]-fluorodeoxyglucose (18FDG) positron emission tomography–computed tomography (PET-CT) imaging for malignancies has reactivated the field.[150] Regardless, it is clear that the sympathetic nervous system is required for coordinated control of energy expenditure and resistance to diet-induced obesity. For example, mice lacking β-adrenergic receptors (triple knockouts) develop severe obesity when placed on a high-fat diet.[151] Thus, coordinated control of the sympathetic nervous system is required for control of DIT.

As noted earlier, the CNS integrates metabolic information into a coordinated set of endocrine, autonomic, and behavioral responses to maintain homeostasis.[32,152,153] Key mediators of these responses are parasympathetic and sympathetic preganglionic neurons (PGNs and SPNs) in the brainstem and spinal cord.[32,154] SPNs extend from the upper thoracic to the upper lumbar segments of the spinal cord and are found within the interomediolateral cell column (IML). Different rostral-caudal levels of the IML provide innervation to different target organs and thus mediate distinct autonomic responses. For example, SPNs in the upper thoracic levels of the IML are thought to be important for control of the heart and cardiovascular system. Additionally, SPNs in the T6-T12 level of the IML provide innervation of the adrenal gland and endocrine pancreas.[152,155-159]

In addition to the autonomic preganglionic neurons themselves, a key component of the central autonomic control system is direct (monosynaptic) descending innervation from key regulatory groups in the hypothalamus and brainstem.[32,160,161] The projection to the SPNs in the spinal cord is composed of inputs from the arcuate nucleus/retrochiasmatic area, the paraventricular nucleus, and the lateral hypothalamus.[152,161-167] Major projections also arise from the brainstem and include inputs from the raphe pallidus (RPa), catecholaminergic cells in the A5 group of the pons, and C1 cells in the rostral ventral lateral medulla that are critical in maintaining sympathetic tone in the cardiovascular system.[168-171] Thus, there is a relatively circumscribed distribution of neurons providing descending input to SPNs that regulate the cardiovascular system, energy expenditure, adrenal catecholamine secretion, and the endocrine pancreas.

As noted, in rodents the central melanocortin circuitry is known to regulate energy expenditure in addition to its effects on food intake. For example, it has been demonstrated that MC4R blockade in mice prevents DIT[172] and blocks the upregulation of BAT activity.[173] In addition, blocking MC4R signaling prevents upregulation of expression of uncoupling proteins normally seen when mice are placed on a high-fat diet.[174] The sites mediating the effects of MC4R agonists on energy expenditure are still not definitively identified. However, a site of MC4R action relevant to the control of energy expenditure may be the SPNs, which express MC4Rs.[102] Notably, these neurons receive direct inputs from leptin-responsive POMC neurons.[175] Thus, MC4Rs expressed by SPNs in the spinal cord may contribute to melanocortin's effects on energy expenditure. Supportive of this model, selective deletion or re-expression of MC4R expression in cholinergic neurons produces mice that display alterations in the ability to regulate energy expenditure.[109,110] Specifically, these mice are sensitive to diet-induced obesity and fail to upregulate energy expenditure when exposed to a high-fat diet and display a deficit in the ability to "beige" white adipose tissue.[111] Moreover, the mice display cold intolerance and fail to upregulate a thermogenic transcriptional program in BAT.[110]

Recently, evidence has also suggested that the effects on energy expenditure by MC4R agonists are mediated by MC4R-bearing neurons in the RPa in the brainstem.[176,177] Neurons in the RPa innervate SPNs in the IML.[178,179] In addition, RPa neurons are activated by thermogenic stimuli and have been shown to control BAT thermogenesis.[180,181] Of note, injections of MC4R agonists into the RPa increase sympathetic nerve activity to BAT.[177] Thus, MC4R expressing neurons in the raphe nucleus may also be key in the ability of melanocortin receptor agonists to increase energy expenditure.

HORMONAL AND NUTRITIONAL REGULATORS OF ENERGY BALANCE CIRCUITS

Adipostatic Factors

Leptin Is the Prototypical Regulator of Energy Homeostasis

Discovery of the molecular basis for several obesity syndromes, prominent among them the hormone leptin[22] and its receptor,[21] has rapidly and dramatically increased our understanding of the pathophysiology of obesity and related disorders. Leptin, the product of the *ob* gene,[22] is produced by white adipose tissue and affects feeding behavior, thermogenesis, and neuroendocrine status. Leptin protein is highly conserved throughout mammalian evolution, as demonstrated by mouse and human leptin being 84% homologous. Leptin has also been identified in fish and birds but appears much less conserved. This protein comprises 167 amino acids and 16 kDa and circulates in the blood at concentrations proportional to the amount of fat depots. Leptin circulates in the bloodstream both as a free protein but also bound to a soluble isoform of its receptor (Ob-Re). Leptin is secreted primarily from the adipocyte; however, minor levels of regulated leptin expression also occur in other sites, such as skeletal muscle, placenta, and stomach.[182,183]

Total lack of leptin or leptin signaling in rodents and humans causes morbid obesity that is accompanied by a wide array of neuroendocrine abnormalities. Replacement with exogenous leptin normalizes these abnormalities.[23,24,26,184] Starvation, a time of low energy stores, leads to a fall in serum leptin levels and has profound effects on several neuroendocrine systems, including activation of the hypothalamic-pituitary-adrenal (HPA) axis, inhibition of the growth hormone and thyroid axes, and inhibition of reproductive function.[189-187] Therefore, lack of leptin has many physiologic responses that are also found in a state of starvation. Interestingly, many of these starvation-induced endocrine and autonomic changes are blocked or blunted by pretreatment with systemic leptin.[185] The dose needed to reverse these abnormalities is lower than that needed to induce weight loss in normal rodents. These observations have led to the suggestion that circulating leptin may have evolved to signal the brain that energy stores are sufficient and that a lack of leptin may be responsible for multiple neuroendocrine abnormalities caused by starvation.[188,189] Soon after the discovery of leptin it was clear that most of the varied effects of leptin are mediated by the brain. Over the past few years, studies have begun to unravel some of the complex circuitry involved in leptin signaling.[49]

Distribution of Leptin Receptors

Within the brain (past the blood-brain barrier), leptin binds to specific receptors in the hypothalamus and brainstem. The *long-form* leptin receptor (OB-Rb) is a member of the cytokine-receptor superfamily.[20,21,190] The leptin receptor binds Janus kinases (JAK), tyrosine kinases involved in intracellular cytokine signaling. Activation of JAK leads to phosphorylation of members of the signal transduction and transcription (STAT) family of proteins. In turn, these STAT proteins activate transcription of leptin target genes.

The long-form leptin receptor is required for normal energy homeostasis as mutations of this gene result in the obese phenotype of the *db/db* mouse and the Zucker rat.[20,191,192] Leptin receptors are highly expressed by several hypothalamic nuclei within the medial basal hypothalamus.[56,193-198] This includes the arcuate, dorsomedial, ventromedial, and ventral premammillary nuclei. Interestingly, leptin receptors are expressed in several extrahypothalamic sites including the NTS (where vagal afferents terminate), the substantia nigra, and the ventral tegmental area.

The role of extrahypothalamic leptin receptors is evolving, but evidence is accumulating that leptin has important sites of action within the brainstem. For example, leptin administration increased STAT-3 phosphorylation in several extrahypothalamic sites including the parabrachial nucleus, dorsal raphe, and NTS.[199] Moreover, administration of leptin into the fourth ventricle and into the DVC significantly reduced food intake.[33,140,200-202]

The Role of Insulin and Glucose in the Regulation of Energy Homeostasis

The concept that the CNS plays a primary role in the control of insulin action and glucose homeostasis is actually a very old one. It originated with observations published in 1849 by physiologist Claude Bernard. He suggested that the CNS regulates blood glucose levels following his famous experiments that demonstrated that "piqure" of the floor of the fourth ventricle of rabbits produced increases in blood glucose that was measured by glucose levels in the urine.[4,203] Remarkably, he concluded that the effect was mediated by stimulation of the autonomic input to the liver. Later lesion studies of the hypothalamus also disassociated actions of insulin independent of food intake.[4] These early observations fit remarkably well with more recent findings that have predicted that similar to obesity, diabetes may be viewed as a disorder with underlying defects in the CNS (Fig. 35-8).[204-208]

Insulin Action in the Brain

In addition to its well-known role in increasing glucose uptake in tissues such as muscle and fat, insulin also has actions on the brain to regulate energy balance.[209] Insulin receptors are expressed in the brain, and injections of insulin into the brain reduce food intake.[209,210] In addition, deletion of insulin receptors specifically from neurons results in mild obesity.[211] More recently, the role of insulin action in the CNS has been investigated in the context of regulation of glucose homeostasis. For example, downregulation of insulin receptors affects glucose homeostasis, including glucose production by the liver.[212] Thus, insulin action in the brain may be key in coordinated physiologic responses to changing levels of metabolic fuels. Multiple additional actions of insulin in the brain have been characterized using site-specific deletion of the insulin receptor gene, including effects on HPA axis function[213] and even hypothalamic development.[214] However, it should be noted that the physiologic significance of central insulin action in acute regulation of glucose homeostasis in humans, especially glucose production by the liver, is still debated.[215-218]

Glucose Levels Are Sensed by Neurons in the Brain

Changing levels of blood glucose are sensed by several distinct populations of neurons in the brain. This idea was first suggested by classic experiments[219] that demonstrated that some neurons are activated by rising concentrations of glucose but that other classes of neurons are inhibited by rising glucose. This model has evolved such that several contemporary models predict that neurons that are activated by rising glucose respond and behave very similarly

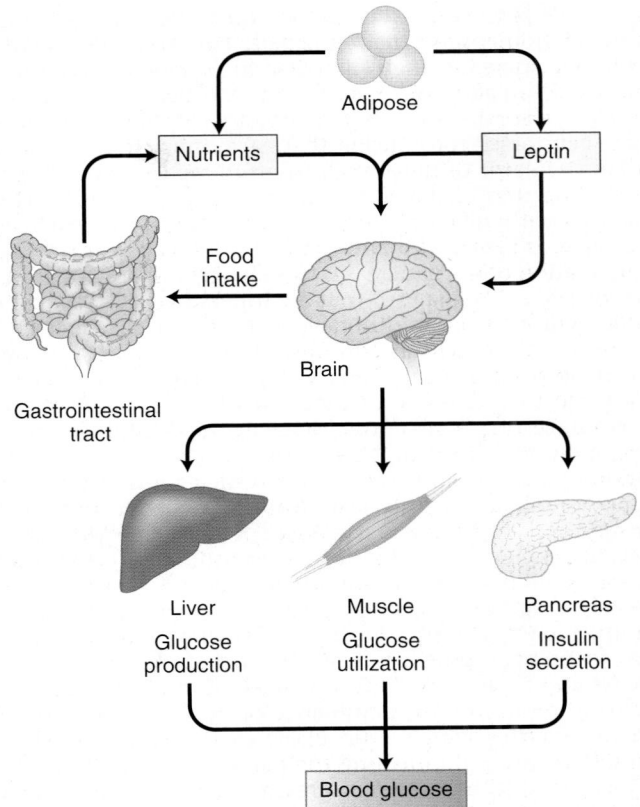

Figure 35-8 Model of central nervous system (CNS) regulation of glucose homeostasis. The CNS integrates signals from both long-term energy stores (e.g., leptin) and short-term availability (nutrients; e.g., free fatty acids) and orchestrates responses that coordinate hepatic glucose production, peripheral glucose uptake, and insulin secretion to maintain glucose homeostasis. (Redrawn from Morton GJ, Schwartz MW. Leptin and the central nervous system control of glucose metabolism. *Physiol Rev.* 2011;91:389-411, Fig. 1.)

to beta cells of the endocrine pancreas.[220-222] The chemical identity and location of these glucose sensing neurons are still to be determined. For example, several populations of glucose-sensitive neurons have been described in the hypothalamus. However, it is clear neurons in the brainstem also sense glucose and are capable of inducing coordinated responses to falling levels of glucose.[223-225]

The cellular mechanisms underlying glucose-mediated neuronal excitation likely involve a rise in adenosine triphosphate (ATP), resulting from an increase in glucose metabolism, promoting the closure of K_{ATP} potassium channels.[222] In contrast, the mechanisms underlying the ability of neurons to be inhibited by rises in glucose (or conversely to be activated by falling glucose) are not as clearly defined but may involve the TASK subfamily of two-pore potassium channels as mediating the glucose-activated inhibitory current in orexin neurons.[226] Collectively, these observations have led to predictions that changes in glucose levels alter the electrical activity of specific neurons that in turn lead to changes in feeding behavior and glucose production. These models also predict that dysregulation of nutrient sensing in the CNS may contribute to the metabolic alterations characteristic of diabetes and obesity.

Pro-opiomelanocortin Neurons Sense Changes in Glucose Concentration

Consistent with the demonstration that metabolic cues such as leptin and glucose directly act on POMC neurons, a key role of the central melanocortin system in regulating glucose homeostasis has emerged. For example, POMC neurons increase their activity in response to rising glucose.[222] In addition, mice lacking MC4Rs are hyperinsulinemic prior to the onset of obesity.[31,204] Reported data have reinforced the concept that vagal input to the liver is a key regulator of hepatic glucose production, potentially including that mediated by melanocortin agonists.[227] The parasympathetic (cholinergic) innervation to the pancreas and liver is provided by the DMV.[159,228,229] The sympathetic innervation of the pancreas is from postganglionic neurons in the celiac ganglia[158,230] that are innervated by preganglionic neurons from midthoracic levels of the spinal cord.

In addition, central administration of MC4R agonists decrease plasma insulin levels in lean and obese mice.[204] This effect was blocked by blockade of α-adrenergic receptors, suggesting that central MC4R agonists inhibit insulin secretion by activating the sympathetic nervous system. Additionally, administration of MC4R agonists increases glucose tolerance, and lean MC4R knockout mice are insulin resistant prior to the onset of obesity.[204] Moreover, MC4R-deficient humans are hyperinsulinemic, more so than would be expected from their degree of obesity alone. Notably, subjects as young as 12 months old are hyperinsulinemic.[92,93] The sites in the CNS mediating these effects are to be determined, but MC4Rs are expressed by both PGNs and SPNs.[102,103] Thus, it is likely that MC4R agonists exert a tonic inhibitory influence on insulin secretion by increasing the sympathetic input to the pancreas while simultaneously diminishing the parasympathetic input.[204]

As noted, the activity of orexin neurons of the lateral hypothalamus is altered by changing levels of blood glucose. Specifically, orexin neurons are activated by physiologically relevant decreases in glucose concentrations.[226,231-234] Though still evolving, orexin neurons may be key in coordinating endocrine and autonomic responses to falling glucose levels. It is also likely that orexin neurons may represent one of the populations of glucose-inhibited neurons in the lateral hypothalamus that respond to physiologic falls in glucose levels with an increase in activity.[221,235] Moreover, because of its unique anatomic and physiologic properties, the central orexin system may be required to link glucose sensing with wakefulness (i.e., hypoglycemic unawareness) and coordinated autonomic responses.

Satiety and Hunger Factors
Role of the Brainstem in Satiety and Hunger

The brainstem is classically understood as the center for detection and response to hunger and satiety signals. The NTS is the primary site for innervation by vagal afferents from the gut.[36,236-240] The afferent branches deriving from different aspects of the GI tract map viscerotopically along the NTS, from its rostral to caudal aspect.[241] Rostrally, the NTS is a bilaterally symmetric nucleus, which merges into a single medial body at its caudal extent, called the *commissural NTS*.[32] Vagal afferents deriving input from the upper GI tract are responsive to three basic stimuli: gastric and duodenal distention or contraction, chemical contents of the lumen, and gut peptides and neurotransmitters released from the stomach and duodenum in response to nutrients.[236] In the rat, vagal afferents responding to gastric and duodenal distention tend to map to the medial and commissural divisions of the NTS.[242,243] Vagal afferents responsive to the gut peptide CCK also map to the caudal NTS.[244] The DMV, located just ventral to the NTS, is the primary site of motor efferents to the gut and is densely innervated by NTS fibers. Together these cell groups, with

the AP, a circumventricular organ, form the DVC and serve as the neuroanatomic substrate for the vagovagal reflex.

Gut Peptides Involved in Satiety and Hunger

In addition to signals from gut distention, gut peptides stimulated by meal intake mediate satiety through centers in the brainstem. Signals received by the brainstem are then thought to interact primarily with long-term weight regulation centers via neural connections to the hypothalamus to regulate total daily intake by adjusting meal size, number, or both.

We now also must consider gut factors that stimulate food intake. Chapter 38 examines GI hormones in detail, focusing on their peripheral actions. Here we consider their central actions. As discussed later, newer data also suggest that a subset of these GI hormones may also act directly on hypothalamic control centers.

Cholecystokinin. Produced by the GI tract in response to meal ingestion, CCK's diverse actions include stimulation of pancreatic enzyme secretion and intestinal motility, inhibition of gastric motility, and acute inhibition of feeding. Early experiments administering CCK peripherally supported a role for increased CCK levels in the early termination of a meal.[245,246] The finding that repeated injections of CCK lead to reduced meal size without a change in body weight, due to a compensatory increase in meal frequency, argued against CCK acting as a signal regulating long-term energy stores.[247,248]

Two subtypes of the CCK receptor belonging to the G protein–coupled family of receptors have been described: CCKA and CCKB. Studies using CCK receptor–specific antagonists as well as surgical or chemical vagotomy have demonstrated that the satiety effects of CCK are specifically mediated via CCKA receptors on afferent vagal nerves.[249-255]

This interaction between acute vagal input from CCKA receptors and meal termination involves activation of cells in the NTS and AP, modulated by neural connections from the hypothalamus receiving inputs from insulin and leptin. Peripheral administration of CCK potently activates large numbers of neurons in both the NTS and AP (Fig. 35-9). Furthermore, central administration of insulin and leptin potentiates the satiety-inducing effects of peripherally administered CCK[256-260] and leads to sustained weight loss with repeated injections that is greater than injection of the agents separately.[261] However, more remains to be learned regarding the neuroanatomic substrate underlying this convergence of long-term and short-term information. Although basomedial hypothalamic cell groups involved in leptin signaling are densely innervated by catecholaminergic neurons from the brainstem, a 2003 report demonstrates that norepinephrine is not required for CCK-induced reduction of feeding, because the dopamine β-hydroxylase knockout mouse is still responsive to CCK-induced satiety.[262] The central melanocortin system may be one element of this integration of satiety with long-term energy homeostasis, because MC4R blockade in the brainstem appears to inhibit the satiating activity of peripherally administered CCK.[108]

In addition to its function in the induction of satiety through vagally mediated signaling, a small body of literature supports a central role for CCK action in regulation of feeding. Immunohistochemistry of the brain and spinal cord shows that the CCKA and CCKB receptors are widely distributed in the CNS, including in the arcuate nucleus[263] and other hypothalamic regions.[263,264] Intracerebroventricular (ICV) administration of CCK to mice[265] inhibits food intake that is reversible by prior administration of a CCKA

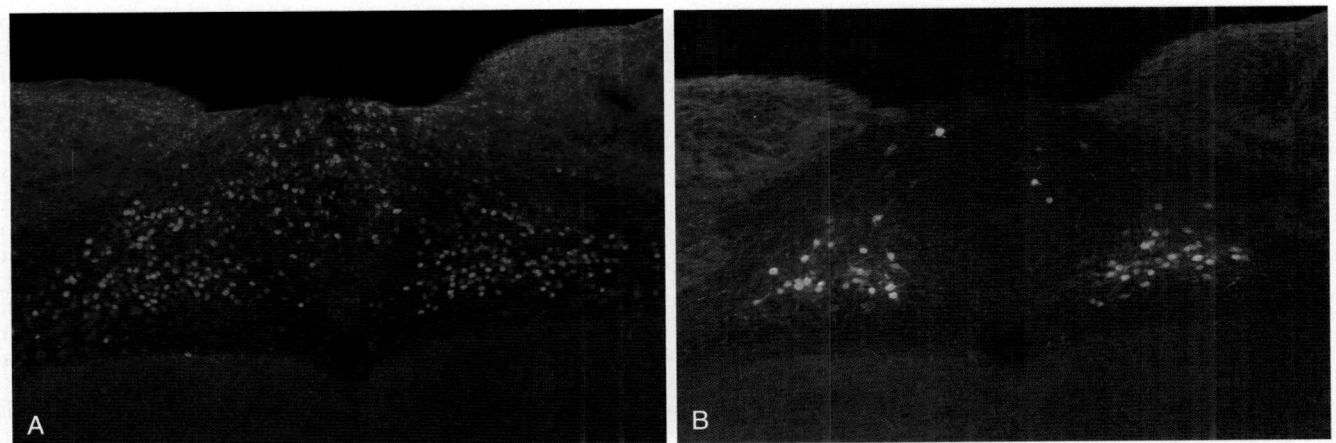

Figure 35-9 Brainstem neurons activated by satiety. **A,** Neurons activated by intraperitoneal administration of 10 µg/kg cholecystokinin (CCK) in the nucleus tractus solitarius (NTS) of the mouse. Neurons visualized by immunohistochemical reaction against Fos, a marker of neuronal activation. **B,** Neurons in the NTS activated by CCK encompass a variety of different neurochemical subtypes, such as glucagon-like peptide 1 (GLP1)-positive neurons, and the pro-opiomelanocortin (POMC)-positive neurons. POMC neurons are visualized through immunohistochemical detection of green fluorescent protein (GFP) in tissue from a transgenic mouse in which GFP is expressed under the control of the POMC promoter. (From Cowley MA, Smart JL, Rubinstein M, et al. Leptin activates anorexigenic POMC neurons through a neural network in the arcuate nucleus. *Nature.* 2001;411:480-484; photographs provided by Dr. Kate L.J. Ellacott, Vanderbilt University School of Medicine, Nashville, TN.)

receptor antagonist. The significance of these hypothalamic-arcuate CCK receptors to weight regulation in the free feeding state is not known.

Peptide YY. PYY, a peptide related to NPY and pancreatic peptide (PP), is postprandially released by endocrine cells in the ileum and colon.[266] PYY is found in vivo in both a full length 36–amino acid form and a 34–amino acid form, designated PYY(3-36), in approximately a 2:1 to 1:1 molar ratio.[267] PYY is a potent agonist of both Y1 and Y2 receptors, whereas PYY(3-36) is a Y2-specific agonist, with approximately a 1000 times greater affinity for the Y2 versus Y1 receptor.[268] Y1- and Y2-preferring binding sites are located in the AP and in the DVC (NTS and DMV). Peripheral administration of PYY (300 mg/kg) in the rat induces c-fos in the AP, as well as in the medial and commissural NTS, the latter being the same region of the NTS known to express POMC.[269] Infusion of PYY within the physiologic range has numerous effects, including inhibition of gastric emptying,[270] gastric acid secretion,[271] and pancreatic exocrine secretion.[271] Evidence shows that these actions of PYY appear to be mediated by PYY action directly on the DVC as well as on gastric mucosal enterochromaffin-like cells (for review see Yang[272]). Both Y1 and Y2 receptors are found within the DVC.[273] For example, PYY appears to inhibit gastric acid secretion primarily through vagal innervation of the gastric fundus.[274] The ability of low-dose PYY and PYY(3-36) to inhibit the activity of DMV efferents appears to be Y2-mediated, whereas Y1 agonists appear to stimulate these cells.[272]

Peripheral administration of PYY(3-36) in pharmacologic doses appears to have an anorexigenic effect in rodents as well as humans,[275-281] thus suggesting that the peptide also functions as a satiety factor. The mechanisms underlying the action of PYY(3-36) in reduction of food intake have not been fully elucidated. Intraperitoneal administration of PYY(3-36) was found to activate 12% to 13% of arcuate POMC neurons, as assayed by increase in expression of c-fos.[275,282] However, vagotomy also blocks PYY(3-36)-induced inhibition of feeding.[283] A direct hypothalamic site of action has been challenged by several studies. Inhibition of feeding by PYY(3-36) persists in the MC4R knockout mouse[277] and in obese agouti mice.[284] Thus, release of melanocortin peptides derived from POMC and their subsequent activation of the MC4R, a well-

characterized anorexigenic pathway, does not appear to be required for the inhibition of feeding by PYY(3-36). Furthermore, PYY appears to induce conditioned taste aversion in rodents and nausea in some human studies, suggesting an aversive effect of the peptide likely to involve brainstem sites such as the AP.

Despite the short-acting anorexic effects of the peptide in most experimental models, two knockout studies have demonstrated that removal of the gene encoding the peptide produces obese hyperinsulinemic mice,[285,286] suggesting that the peptide may also play an important role in the regulation of long-term energy stores. One study shows the peptide may be specifically involved in the satiating effects of protein in the diet.[285]

Ghrelin. Ghrelin is the endogenous ligand for the growth hormone secretagogue receptor (GHSR).[287,288] Ghrelin is an acylated 28–amino acid peptide predominantly secreted by the stomach and regulated by ingestion of nutrients[289-292] with potent effects on appetite.[291,292] Ghrelin levels are markedly reduced with meal ingestion in both rodents and humans but rebound to baseline before the next meal or increase after an overnight fast[290-292] (Fig. 35-10). In rodents, this was demonstrated to be a nutrient-specific effect because a similar volume of saline infused into the stomach did not affect ghrelin levels.[291] GHSR has been demonstrated on arcuate NPY/AgRP-containing neurons,[293] and pharmacologic doses of ghrelin injected peripherally or into the hypothalamus activate c-fos and Egr1 solely in arcuate NPY neurons in rats[294] and stimulate food intake and obesity, in part by stimulating NPY and AgRP expression,[295-300] which antagonizes leptin's anorexic effect.[299]

This orexigenic action occurs in rodents even with peripheral administration of ghrelin that matches fasting levels.[301] Stimulation of appetite and food intake during an infusion of ghrelin over 4.5 hours in humans has also been demonstrated.[302] Additionally, ghrelin may also effect gastric emptying. This study establishes that, similar to rodents, ghrelin can stimulate appetite and food intake in humans when given in a supraphysiologic dose, but a role for physiologic changes in ghrelin levels or signaling in human energy homeostasis remains unknown.

Ghrelin's characteristics make it unique among the gut-derived signals. Unlike other signals involved with energy

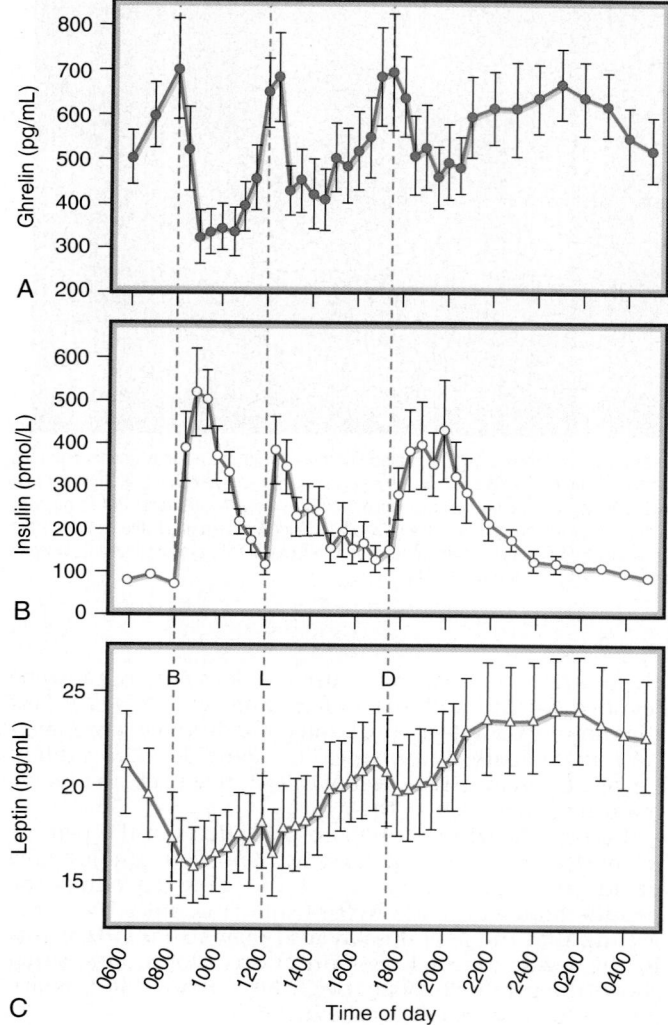

Figure 35-10 Average plasma ghrelin, insulin, and leptin concentrations during a 24-hour period in 10 human subjects consuming breakfast (B), lunch (L), and dinner (D) at the times indicated (0800, 1200, and 1730 hours, respectively). (From Cummings DE, Purnell JQ, Frayo RS, et al. A preprandial rise in plasma ghrelin levels suggests a role in meal initiation in humans. *Diabetes.* 2001;50:1714-1719.)

sion only in arcuate NPY/AgRP neurons, not in other hypothalamic or brainstem sites,[305] and ablation of the arcuate nucleus blocks the actions of ghrelin administration on feeding but not elevation of growth hormone.[306] For example, reexpression of ghrelin receptors only in AgRP neurons in mice lacking ghrelin receptors everywhere else is sufficient to restore the ability of exogenous ghrelin administration to increase food intake.[307] Consistent with a role of the AgRP/NPY neuron in mediating the effects of ghrelin administration to increase food intake, stimulation of food intake by ghrelin administration is blocked by administration of NPY/Y1 and Y5 antagonists,[299] and reduced in the NPY[-/-] mouse. Administration of the melanocortin agonist MTII blocks further stimulation of weight gain by GHRP-2 in the NPY[-/-] mouse.[308]

Peripheral ghrelin may access the arcuate nucleus via vagal afferents; because GHSR is expressed on vagal afferents, ghrelin suppresses firing of vagal nerves, and surgical or chemical vagotomy blocks stimulation of feeding and c-fos activation in the arcuate nucleus by peripheral but not central ghrelin administration.[309] Peripheral ghrelin may largely suppress brainstem satiety centers, thus explaining the lack of c-fos activation at these sites. However, reexpression of ghrelin receptors only in brainstem neurons (including those in the NTS) in mice lacking ghrelin receptors everywhere else is not sufficient to restore the ability of exogenous ghrelin administration to increase food intake.[307,310]

Despite the significant amount of data suggesting that activation of ghrelin receptors increases food intake, much work remains to establish the physiologic role of ghrelin in regulating energy balance and feeding. Indeed, recent genetic evidence suggests that ghrelin may play a modest role in regulating feeding and body weight but rather may be key in regulating blood glucose levels in the context of chronic caloric restriction.[311] Ghrelin is a unique hormone; it requires the addition of an eight-carbon fatty acid (octanoate) side chain in order to have agonist activity at the ghrelin receptor.[312-314] The enzyme that catalyzes the addition of the octanoyl group is ghrelin *O*-acyltransferase (GOAT).[314] Neither genetic deletion of GOAT[315] or ablation of ghrelin-producing cells[316] results in major changes in food intake and body weight. However, mice lacking GOAT expression or ghrelin cells display profound hypoglycemia in response to chronic caloric restriction. These and other findings have questioned the physiologic importance of ghrelin and its receptor in regulating energy balance but have highlighted an unexpected role in regulating blood glucose levels during periods of severe calorie restriction.[311]

Preproglucagon-Derived Peptides. Current strategies for the treatment of type 2 diabetes mellitus are not optimally effective, and even multiple drug combinations often fail to normalize glycemia in a sustained manner in many subjects. Hence, there remains intense interest in new therapies that safely and effectively lower blood glucose in diabetic subjects. Recently, strategies mimicking the actions of the incretin class of hormones are being used to treat type 2 diabetes and obesity.[317,318] Incretins are hormones that are released by oral ingestion of nutrients to increase insulin secretion. The prototypical incretin hormone is GLP-1, which is derived from the proglucagon gene. The proglucagon-derived peptides are generated in the A cells of the pancreas (principally glucagon), the L cells of the intestine (GLP-1, GLP-2, and glicentin), and the brain (glucagon, GLP-1, GLP-2).[317,318]

As outlined in detail in Chapter 38, GLP-1 receptor agonists induce multiple desirable antidiabetic and anti-obesity actions, and protease-resistant long-acting GLP-1

homeostasis, ghrelin secretion is inhibited in response to meals, and instead of acting as a satiety signal (like CCK or PYY(3-36)), ghrelin stimulates appetite, potentially through arcuate signaling. These properties have led to the prediction that ghrelin is a candidate meal-initiating signal.[292] In addition, fasting ghrelin levels have now been shown to be inversely proportional to body weight[303] and to be higher in underweight subjects with anorexia nervosa and cardiac cachexia compared to control subjects.[289,304] Downregulation of ghrelin in obese subjects suggests an adaptive response to the obese state, whereas a rise in levels in weight-reduced subjects is compatible with a counterregulatory role to restore fat depots. These properties inversely parallel those of insulin, which is stimulated by meals, inhibits food intake when injected by ICV route, circulates in the fasting state in direct proportion to body weight, and whose secretion is decreased following weight loss.

With regard to mechanism of action, much evidence indicates the melanocortin system is central to ghrelin's pharmacologic effects to regulate food intake. Finally, peripheral administration of ghrelin activates c-fos expres-

analogues are currently available for the treatment of type 2 diabetes.[317,318] The first of these drugs, Byetta (exenatide), is a potent GLP-1 receptor agonist and mimics GLP-1 enhancing glucose-dependent insulin secretion by slowing gastric emptying, inhibiting gastric acid secretion, and reducing food intake. The latter effect may be due to action on circuits in the brain involved in the control of energy homeostasis (see later).

GLP-1 and GLP-1R Neurons in the Central Nervous System. Despite recent intense interest in GLP-1 and related peptides, it is less appreciated that GLP-1 is an endogenous neuropeptide expressed by neurons in the CNS. The CNS actions are not well understood. Given the increasing use in diabetes treatment of GLP-1 analogues and DPP4 inhibitors that block GLP-1 degradation and the FDA approval in 2014 of liraglutide for the treatment of obesity, understanding central actions of GLP-1 is important for predicting the biologic consequences of sustained GLP-1 administration.

Initial interest in the CNS actions of GLP-1 stemmed from the observation that GLP-1 inhibits food intake.[319-323] In humans, peripheral GLP-1 administration to normal and diabetic subjects induces satiety and reduces food intake in short-term studies.[324-327] Chronic continuous GLP-1 administration to human diabetic subjects is associated with modest weight loss.[328] The effects of GLP-1 on appetite may be mediated in part via inhibition of gastric emptying and may also reflect direct effects of GLP-1 on satiety, and induction of taste aversion.[46,329-333] GLP-1 appears to directly activate POMC neurons in the mouse, and GLP-1R is required for the weight loss activity of liraglutide in this system.[334]

The CNS expression of GLP-1 is very restricted and includes a population of neurons within the caudal NTS. Caudal NTS neurons receive and process viscerosensory information from thoracic and abdominal viscera. The NTS is reciprocally connected with various brain areas, including hypothalamic areas thought to regulate feeding.[32,335] Additionally, the NTS is located adjacent to a circumventricular organ, the AP, and the NTS contains fenestrated capillaries, potentially allowing circulating peptides access to the nucleus. Thus, neurons in the NTS (including GLP-1 cells) process information arising from a variety of neural and humoral sources. GLP-1 neurons are in a prime position to rapidly modify ingestive behavior in direct response to either transiently altered levels of metabolic cues such as leptin or glucose as well as neural modulators from other brain sites including POMC neurons in the arcuate nucleus. For example, the adipocyte-derived hormone leptin communicates the status of energy stores to the brain. The vast majority of work investigating the neural circuits that mediate leptin action has focused on the hypothalamus. However, increasing evidence implicates a significant role for extrahypothalamic sites of leptin action.[33,140] For example, intravenous leptin increases neuronal activation (induces Fos-like immunoreactivity) in regions of the hindbrain, including GLP-1 neurons in the NTS,[336] as well as POMC neurons in some cases.[337]

In addition to the varied inputs, GLP-1 neurons in the NTS also have a widespread projection pattern in the brain.[338] This includes direct innervations of several hypothalamic nuclei, including the PVH, LHA, and arcuate nucleus, and the GLP-1 receptor mRNA has been found within these areas.[339] The location of GLP-1 neurons in the NTS and their diffuse projection pattern suggest that GLP-1 neurons are ideally situated to integrate key signals and regulate complex physiologic processes.

Amylin. Amylin, or islet amyloid polypeptide (IAPP), is a 37–amino acid polypeptide that co-localizes with insulin in beta cells in the pancreas. In humans, IAPP in the pancreas can form amyloid fibrils and is thought to play a role in the decline in islet cell function that accompanies type 2 diabetes.[340,341] In addition, amylin has been shown to impair gastric motility and have effects independent of insulin on energy homeostasis mediated through hypothalamic signaling.

Amylin is cosecreted with insulin in response to nutrient intake and insulin secretagogues.[342,343] Amylin readily enters the brain, and high-affinity amylin-binding sites have been found in several brain regions including the hypothalamus and arcuate nucleus.[344,345] Both peripheral and ICV infusions of amylin inhibit food intake acutely and, during chronic infusion, lead to a sustained reduction in body weight.[344-349] This anorectic effect has been shown by Rushing and associates to be blocked by coadministration of the amylin antagonist AC187 centrally and for AC187 to result in a significant increase in body adiposity when infused by ICV route over 14 days compared to control animals.[349] Studies of coadminstration of amylin with other GI hormones has shown that the acute satiety effects of amylin are equipotent to CCK[350] and additive when peripherally coinjected with either CCK[351] or insulin.[352] The precise central neuroendocrine mechanism mediating amylin's anorexic effects has yet to be elucidated. The diverse CNS binding of amylin suggests that multiple sites may have roles in the anorectic effects of amylin, but the inhibition of appetite with ICV administration and demonstrated binding in the arcuate nucleus suggests that the hypothalamus may be an important site of amylin action.

Bariatric Surgery and the Role of the Gastrointestinal System in the Control of Energy Homeostasis

No pharmacologic treatment has yet been devised that is capable of resetting the adipostat—that is, treatment that allows significant long-term weight loss to be maintained. In contrast, certain types of bariatric surgeries, such as the Roux-en-Y gastric bypass (RYGB) and vertical sleeve gastrectomy (described in Chapter 36), appear to not only cause significant weight loss but also allow this weight loss to be maintained for many years (Fig. 35-11). Furthermore, improvement in diabetes following these procedures is often seen before significant weight loss occurs and is sustained in a significant percentage of patients. Both these findings imply that the procedures are having a profound impact on the neuroendocrine control of long-term energy stores. The fact that bariatric surgery appears capable of creating a new stable weight set-point suggests that hormonal or vagal and nutritional signals from the gut may indeed have a more profound impact on long-term energy homeostasis than previously thought. An important field of research has emerged that is attempting to identify the peripheral and central changes that produce weight loss and improve glucose control following these procedures, with the ultimate goal being to reproduce the response to surgery using a nonsurgical approach. For example, circulating GLP-1 is elevated following sleeve gastrectomy[353,354] and RYGB,[354-360] as are bile acids. Notwithstanding the lack of effect of GLP-1R deletion on weight loss or glucose responsiveness in a vertical sleeve gastrectomy model in the mouse,[361] data in rodent and human bariatric surgery support a role for both of these factors in efficacy of the procedures.[362] In terms of central homeostatic circuits, a role for melanocortin signaling in the efficacy of RYGB is supported by the findings that MC4R deletion significantly blunts weight loss in response to RYGB in mice.[363,364]

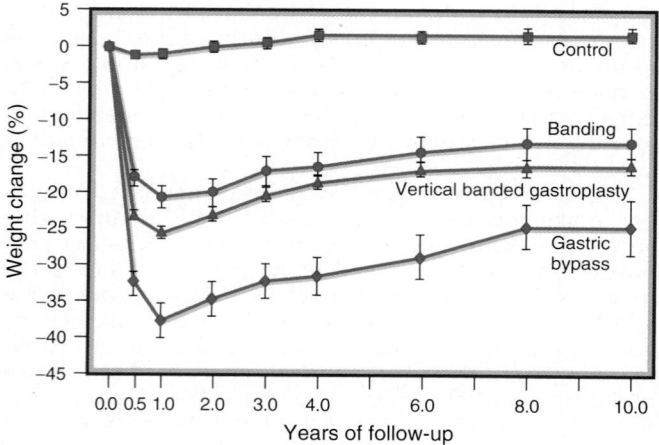

Figure 35-11 Apparent alteration of the adipostatic set-point after bariatric surgery. (Modified from Sjostrom L, Lindroos AK, Peltonen M, et al, Swedish Obese Subjects Study Scientific Group. Lifestyle, diabetes, and cardiovascular risk factors 10 years after bariatric surgery. *N Engl J Med.* 2004;351:2683-2693.)

Steroid Hormones

In addition to their pleiotropic effects, gonadal steroids also play a key role in regulating energy balance and glucose homeostasis.[365-369] For example, estrogens exert antiobesity and antidiabetic effects, and lower levels of estrogens in postmenopausal women are associated with an increased risk for developing obesity.[370-372] Ovariectomy (OVX) in animals with reduced estrogen signaling causes them to develop obesity and hyperadiposity.[373-375] Although OVX induces increase in food intake, the hyperphagia does not account for all of the obesity.[376] Further, OVX causes rats to gain weight to a similar extent when they are pair-fed to estradiol-treated rats,[377,378] suggesting that endogenous estrogens regulate body weight homeostasis primarily by modulating energy expenditure. Consistently, a recent study showed that OVX decreases energy expenditure but has no effect on food intake in mice.[379] However, estradiol replacement was shown to decrease food intake and increase energy expenditure in rodents,[380] indicating that exogenous estrogens may promote a negative energy balance by influencing both energy intake and energy expenditure. Importantly, estrogens are also thought to play a role in regulating fat distribution.[366-369] For example, female humans and rodents distribute relatively more fat in subcutaneous depot, whereas males have more fat stored in visceral depot, which is more likely to cause metabolic syndromes, such as insulin resistance.[381-383] Estrogen appears to account for this sexual dimorphism.[366-369]

ERα mediates many of the estrogenic effects on body weight homeostasis. For example, female mice with a targeted deletion (knockout [KO]) in the ERα gene (ERαKO) develop obesity and hyperadiposity, primarily because of decreased energy expenditure.[384] Although no hyperphagia is observed in ERαKO mice,[384-386] ERα is clearly required to mediate the normal satiation process because estradiol-induced hypophagia and CCK-induced satiation in wild-type mice are blocked in ERαKO mice.[386]

ERα is expressed in brain regions implicated in the regulation of energy balance. These include the arcuate, paraventricular, and ventral medial nuclei in the hypothalamus and key brainstem sites such as the NTS.[387,388] In 2007 the role of estrogens and ERα in the VMH in the regulation of energy balance was reexamined using the ERα silencing approach.[389] Knockdown of ERα in the VMH produced mice that are less sensitive to estradiol-induced weight loss and develop the obesity characteristic of increased visceral fat.[389] The obesity syndrome is likely caused by decreased physical activity and impaired DIT, whereas food intake of these animals is not directly affected.[389]

Deletion of ERα in VMH SF1 neurons in female mice does not affect food intake but significantly reduces basal metabolic rate and DIT. This ultimately leads to obesity and increased adipose tissue deposition.[365,390] Interestingly, a significant increase in visceral fat deposition (versus subcutaneous fat deposition) was observed selectively in female mice. The decreased energy expenditure and increased visceral fat distribution in mice lacking ERα in VMH neurons presumably result from decreased sympathetic tone.[365,390] Collectively, these results support the hypothesis that ERα signaling in VMH neurons plays an important role in regulating energy expenditure and fat distribution.

A 2009 study demonstrated that hypothalamic expression of NPY and AgRP in mice is tightly regulated across the estrus cycle, with the lowest levels during the estrus that coincides with the plasma estrogen peak and feeding nadir.[391] Central estradiol administration suppresses fasting-induced activation of NPY/AgRP neurons and blunts the refeeding response.[391] Importantly, the cyclic changes in food intake and estradiol-induced anorexia are blunted in mice with ablated NPY/AgRP neurons.[391] This study indicates that NPY/AgRP neurons are functionally required for the cyclic changes in feeding across the estrous cycle. Surprisingly, these authors also found that ERα is not expressed in NPY/AgRP neurons,[391] suggesting that estrogen may regulate these neurons indirectly via presynaptic neurons that express ERα.

One likely mediator is expressed by POMC neurons, which reside adjacent to NPY/AgRP neurons. POMC neurons coexpress ERα[365,392,393] and estrogens regulate excitability of POMC neurons. The number of excitatory synaptic inputs to arcuate POMC neurons rises as mice enter proestrus when estrogen levels are high.[380,394] Further, central estradiol administration rapidly increases the excitatory synapses on POMC neurons.[380,394] The synaptic changes in POMC neurons are tightly paralleled with the effects of estradiol on food intake and body weight.[380] Similarly, estradiol administration in hypothalamic slices activates POMC neurons by rapidly uncoupling GABA_B receptors from the G protein–gated inwardly rectifying K$^+$ channels.[395] Notably, female mice lacking ERα only in POMC neurons develop hyperphagia.[54,55,89,396-419] These observations suggest that estrogen signals in POMC neurons are physiologically relevant in the regulation of food intake.[365]

Hypothalamic Inflammation

Although this chapter has been focused on the interaction between hormones and hypothalamic neuronal circuits involved in the regulation of energy homeostasis, it is important to keep in mind the presence of large numbers of macroglia (astrocytes, oligodendrocytes, tanacytes) and microglia in the CNS that can also play a regulatory role in homeostasis. Recently, it has been demonstrated that high-fat diet and obesity can cause hypertrophy, hyperplasia, and an activated state of glial cells in the rodent CNS[420-424] and in the hypothalamus in particular (Fig. 35-12).[425] For example, findings published in 2015 show that activation of astrocytes specifically in the arcuate nucleus of the mouse appear to inhibit AgRP neurons and food intake, via increased gliotransmission and subsequent activation of adenosine A1 receptors on AgRP neurons.[426] These findings suggest three routes to the control of AgRP and food intake,

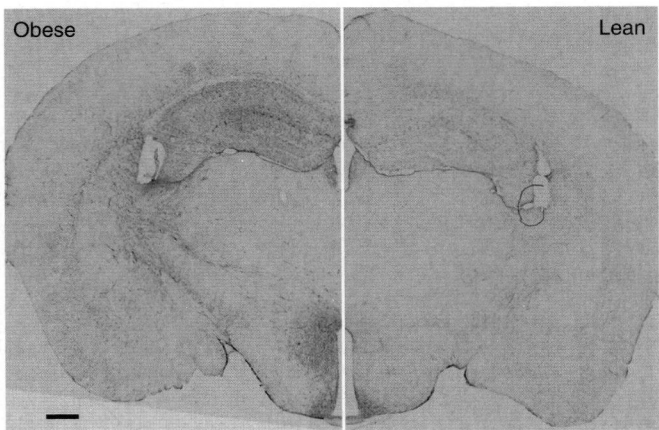

Figure 35-12 Hypothalamic gliosis in obese mice. Increased expression of glial-fibrillary acidic protein (GFAP) is seen in both hypothalamic and extrahypothalamic regions in obese compared with lean animals. A side-by-side comparison of GFAP immunoreactivity across an entire brain slice reveals an increased expression in the multiple brain regions in the diet-induced obese animals including the arcuate nucleus, paraventricular nucleus, hippocampus, medial habenula, internal capsule, and reticular thalamic nuclei. Scale bar = 500 μm. (Modified from Buckman LB, Thompson MM, Moreno HN, et al. Regional astrogliosis in the mouse hypothalamus in response to obesity. *J Comp Neurol.* 2013;521:1322-1333, Fig. 8.)

control via peripheral hormones like leptin and ghrelin, control via glutamatergic and other neuronal inputs, and control via local glial cells.[427] Activation of microglia in response to overnutrition and obesity has been demonstrated as well.[428] Importantly, evidence of gliosis in humans as a function of elevated body mass index has also been demonstrated using neuroimaging.[422,429]

INTERSECTION OF ENERGY BALANCE AND REWARD CIRCUITS

A relatively recent and novel concept to emerge is that that food and drug rewards share some common neural substrates.[48,430-437] This is potentially quite important as it is logical to predict that if rational strategies to combat obesity are to be developed, then an increased understanding of the molecular mechanisms of the rewarding aspects of feeding behavior is required.[48,430,437,438] Motivation and reward have been studied in the context of drug addiction.[439-441]

The nucleus accumbens and its dopamine inputs have been strongly implicated in mediating several rewarding stimuli.[439,442] Although dopamine is widely accepted to be involved in reward processes, it has become clear that the relationship between dopamine and reward is complex.[48] For example, lesions of the nucleus accumbens do reduce food intake[443] and the ability to display operant conditioning in response to food.[444] However, evidence has demonstrated a dopamine component of food reward. For example, mice lacking the ability to produce dopamine normally die of starvation but will resume feeding after reintroduction of dopamine into the striatum.[445,446]

Additional evidence has suggested that key metabolic cues act directly on dopamine neurons in the midbrain. For example, midbrain dopamine neurons express leptin and ghrelin receptors.[438,447-449] Interestingly, Fulton and colleagues demonstrated that leptin also affects brain self–stimulation,[450] suggesting that leptin has the ability to affect CNS circuits classically involved in reward. Taken together, these findings suggest that alterations of cues such as leptin and ghrelin may not only affect hypothalamic pathways but may also act directly on midbrain dopamine neurons. Although this field of study is still evolving, these findings lead to a model with potentially broad implications. These models could provide a mechanism for signals regulating food intake to intersect with brain circuitry critical in the regulation of motivated behaviors. Moreover, dysregulation of these pathways may be relevant to the pathophysiology of obesity as well as eating disorders such as anorexia nervosa.[430,432,436,438,451,452]

MONOGENIC DISORDERS OF ENERGY HOMEOSTASIS

A wide variety of disorders of hypothalamic and neuroendocrine function are known to produce obesity. For example, as discussed in the historical introduction to this chapter, insults to the function of the basal hypothalamus, including Fröhlich syndrome and craniopharyngioma, are known to cause obesity, as are endocrine disorders such as Cushing disease. However, in the past 2 decades there have been multiple genes discovered that are causative in human obesity disorders, including *LEP, LEPR, POMC, MC4R, PCSK1, GNAS, SH2B1, BDNF, TRKB,* and *SIM1*.[453] These mendelian disease genes appear to act primarily in the hypothalalamus. Furthermore, genome-wide association studies have identified close to 100 single nucleotide polymorphisms significantly associated with body mass index, and these are predominantly located in or near genes thought to act primarily in the CNS.[454] These studies have provided mechanistic insights into the control of energy homeostasis in humans, and syndromes involving leptin and melanocortin signaling are discussed here.

Leptin and Leptin Receptor Deficiency in Humans

Despite being extremely rare, leptin deficiency[455] and leptin receptor defects[456] in humans are quite illustrative of the physiologic importance of this hormone. For example, serum leptin levels in humans are generally proportional to adipose mass.[187,457] Thus, the vast majority of obese humans may be considered to be leptin-resistant rather than leptin deficient.[64,186,458] Despite rapid increases in our understanding of obesity and leptin action, the molecular basis of leptin resistance remains poorly understood.

Clinical studies have now demonstrated that leptin treatment is safe and well tolerated and clearly effective in individuals with congenital leptin deficiency[184] and in patients who are very low in adipose tissue.[459,460] For example, doses of methionyl-leptin were given to subjects with congenital deficiency that resulted in leptin levels 10% of that predicted based on body fat. Leptin in this study was well tolerated and resulted in dramatic declines in appetite, body weight, and food intake.[184] In addition, administration of recombinant leptin to women with hypothalamic amenorrhea due to strenuous exercise training and very low body fat normalized several endocrine indices of reproductive function and bone density.[460] Unfortunately, in individuals with common obesity, leptin had only very modest effects on appetite and body weight.[461]

A recent concept that has emerged is that leptin has potent effects on whole-body glucose and lipid homeostasis independent of its effects on body weight.[49,208,462-465]

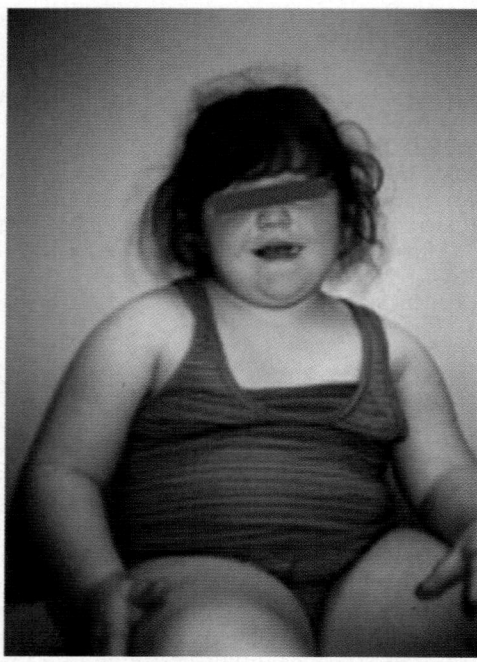

Figure 35-13 A monogenic neuroendocrine obesity syndrome of adrenocortico-tropic hormone insufficiency, obesity, and red hair resulting from a null mutation in the pro-opiomelanocortin gene. (Photograph courtesy of Dr. A. Gruters, Charité-Universitätsmedzin, Berlin, Germany.)

These studies of leptin action may be relevant to models linking diabetes and hypothalamic resistance to metabolic cues. Leptin deficiency, as seen in lipodystrophic mice and humans, induces severe insulin resistance. This extreme resistance is corrected by leptin replacement.[466-468] This effect can be explained by actions of leptin in the arcuate nucleus of the hypothalamus. Restoration of leptin receptors only in the arcuate nucleus in mice lacking leptin receptors everywhere had remarkably improved glucose homeostasis.[464,465,469-471] Thus, leptin action in the arcuate nucleus is sufficient to mediate the antidiabetic actions of leptin.

Obesity Resulting From Defective Melanocortin Signaling

Evidence that the melanocortin obesity syndrome can occur in humans resulted from the astute recognition of an agouti-mouse–like syndrome in two families, resulting from null mutations in the *POMC* gene[472] (Fig. 35-13). These patients have a rare syndrome that includes ACTH insufficiency, red hair, and obesity, resulting from the lack of ACTH peptide in the serum and a lack of melanocortin peptides in skin and brain, respectively. These data demonstrated, for the first time, that the central melanocortin circuitry subserves energy homeostasis in humans as it does in the mouse. Shortly thereafter, heterozygous frameshift mutations in the human *MC4R* were reported, associated with nonsyndromic obesity in two separate families.[94,95] Additional reports,[93,473,474] provide a clearer picture of the frequency and diversity of *MC4R* mutations and show that haploinsufficiency of the MC4R in humans is the most common monogenic cause of severe obesity at the present time, accounting for up to 5% of cases. Two 2003 reports provide a detailed clinical picture of the syndrome.[92,475] Remarkably, the syndrome is virtually identical to that reported for the mouse,[31,178,214] with increased adipose

mass, increased linear growth and lean mass, hyperinsulinemia greater than that seen in matched obese control subjects, and severe hyperphagia. MC4R haploinsufficient adults have been demonstrated to exhibit reduced sympathetic tone, as indicated by reduced 24-hour urinary norepinephrine levels, and to be mildly hypotensive.[476] In this same study, investigators administered a melanocortin peptide agonist, LY2112688, to healthy volunteers, and demonstrated a mild pressor response, and this target-based pressor response has thus far stymied the development of MC4R agonists for the treatment of obesity.

REFERENCES

1. Bramwell B. *Intracranial Tumours*. Edinburgh, UK: Pentland; 1888.
2. Fröhlich A. Ein fall von tumor der hypophysis cerebri ohne akromegalie. *Wien Klin Rundsch*. 1901;15:883.
3. Crowe SJ, Cushing H, Homans J. Experimental hypophysectomy. *Bull Johns Hopkins Hosp*. 1910;21:127.
4. Stevenson JAF. Neural control of food and water intake. In: Haymaker W, Anderson E, Nauta WJH, eds. *The Hypothalamus*. Springfield, IL: Charles C Thomas; 1969:524-621.
5. Elmquist JK, Elias CF, Saper CB. From lesions to leptin: hypothalamic control of food intake and body weight. *Neuron*. 1999;22(2):221-232.
6. Aschner B. Uber die funktion der hypophyse. *Pflugers Arch Physiol*. 1912;146:1.
7. Hetherington AW, Ranson SW. Hypothalamic lesions and adiposity in the rat. *Anat Rec*. 1940;78:149-172.
8. Stellar E. The physiology of motivation. *Physiol Rev*. 1954;61:5-22.
9. Kennedy GC. The role of depot fat in the hypothalamic control of food intake in the rat. *Proc R Soc Lond B Biol Sci*. 1953;140(901):578-596.
10. Harris RB, Kasser TR, Martin RJ. Dynamics of recovery of body composition after overfeeding, food restriction or starvation of mature female rats. *J Nutr*. 1986;116(12):2536-2546.
11. Harris RB. Role of set-point theory in regulation of body weight. *FASEB J*. 1990;4(15):3310-3318.
12. Faust IM, Johnson PR, Hirsch J. Surgical removal of adipose tissue alters feeding behavior and the development of obesity in rats. *Science*. 1977;197(4301):393-396.
13. Hervey GR. The effects of lesions in the hypothalamus in parabiotic rats. *J Physiol*. 1959;145(2):336-352.
14. Hervey GR. Physiological mechanisms for the regulation of energy balance. *Proc Nutr Soc*. 1971;30(2):109-116.
15. Parameswaran SV, Steffens AB, Hervey GR, de Ruiter L. Involvement of a humoral factor in regulation of body weight in parabiotic rats. *Am J Physiol*. 1977;232(5):R150-R157.
16. Ingalls AM, Dickie MM, Snell GD. Obese, a new mutation in the house mouse. *J Hered*. 1950;41:317-318.
17. Coleman DL, Hummel KP. Effects of parabiosis of normal with genetically diabetic mice. *Am J Physiol*. 1969;217(5):1298-1304.
18. Coleman DL. Obese and diabetes: two mutant genes causing diabetes-obesity syndromes in mice. *Diabetologia*. 1978;14:141-148.
19. Coleman DL. Effects of parabiosis of obese with diabetes and normal mice. *Diabetologia*. 1973;9:294-298.
20. Lee GH, Proenca R, Montez JM, et al. Abnormal splicing of the leptin receptor in diabetic mice. *Nature*. 1996;379(6566):632-635.
21. Tartaglia LA, Dembski M, Weng X, et al. Identification and expression cloning of a leptin receptor, OB-R. *Cell*. 1995;83(7):1263-1271.
22. Zhang Y, Proenca R, Maffei M, et al. Positional cloning of the mouse obese gene and its human homologue. *Nature*. 1994;372:425-432.
23. Campfield LA, Smith FJ, Guisez Y, et al. Recombinant mouse OB protein: evidence for a peripheral signal linking adiposity and central neural networks. *Science*. 1995;269(5223):546-549.
24. Halaas J, Gajiwala K, Maffei M, et al. Weight-reducing effects of the plasma protein encoded by the obese gene. *Science*. 1995;269(5223):543-546.
25. Halaas JL, Boozer C, Blair-West J, et al. Physiological response to long-term peripheral and central leptin infusion in lean and obese mice. *Proc Natl Acad Sci U S A*. 1997;94:8878-8883.
26. Pelleymounter MA, Cullen MJ, Baker MB, et al. Effects of the obese gene product on body weight regulation in ob/ob mice [see comments]. *Science*. 1995;269(5223):540-543.
27. Miller MW, Duhl DMJ, Vrieling H, et al. Cloning of the mouse agouti gene predicts a novel secreted protein ubiquitously expressed in mice carrying the lethal yellow (A^y) mutation. *Genes Dev*. 1993;7:454-467.
28. Bultman SJ, Michaud EJ, Woychik R. Molecular characterization of the mouse agouti locus. *Cell*. 1992;71(7):1195-1204.
29. Lu D, Willard D, Patel IR, et al. Agouti protein is an antagonist of the melanocyte-stimulating hormone receptor. *Nature*. 1994;371:799-802.
30. Fan W, Boston BA, Kesterson RA, et al. Role of melanocortinergic neurons in feeding and the agouti obesity syndrome. *Nature*. 1997;385:165-168.

31. Huszar D, Lynch CA, Fairchild-Huntress V, et al. Targeted disruption of the melanocortin-4 receptor results in obesity in mice. *Cell.* 1997; 88:131-141.

32. Saper CB. Central autonomic system. In: Paxinos G, ed. *The Rat Nervous System.* San Diego, CA: Academic Press; 1995:107-135.

33. Grill HJ, Schwartz MW, Kaplan JM, et al. Evidence that the caudal brainstem is a target for the inhibitory effect of leptin on food intake. *Endocrinology.* 2002;143(1):239-246.

34. Morton GJ, Kaiyala KJ, Fisher JD, et al. Identification of a physiological role for leptin in the regulation of ambulatory activity and wheel running in mice. *Am J Physiol Endocrinol Metab.* 2011;300(2):E392-E401.

35. Moran TH, Ladenheim EE. Adiposity signaling and meal size control. *Physiol Behav.* 2011;103(1):21-24.

36. Moran TH. Gut peptides in the control of food intake. *Int J Obes (Lond).* 2009;33(Suppl 1):S7-S10.

37. Herbert H, Moga MM, Saper CB. Connections of the parabrachial nucleus with the nucleus of the solitary tract and the medullary reticular formation in the rat. *J Comp Neurol.* 1990;293(4):540-580.

38. Wu Q, Clark MS, Palmiter RD. Deciphering a neuronal circuit that mediates appetite. *Nature.* 2012;483(7391):594-597.

39. Wu Q, Palmiter RD. GABAergic signaling by AgRP neurons prevents anorexia via a melanocortin-independent mechanism. *Eur J Pharmacol.* 2011;660(1):21-27.

40. Wu Q, Boyle MP, Palmiter RD. Loss of GABAergic signaling by AgRP neurons to the parabrachial nucleus leads to starvation. *Cell.* 2009; 137(7):1225-1234.

41. Betley JN, Cao ZF, Ritola KD, Sternson SM. Parallel, redundant circuit organization for homeostatic control of feeding behavior. *Cell.* 2013; 155(6):1337-1350.

42. Atasoy D, Betley JN, Su HH, Sternson SM. Deconstruction of a neural circuit for hunger. *Nature.* 2012;488(7410):172-177.

43. Shah BP, Vong L, Olson DP, et al. MC4R-expressing glutamatergic neurons in the paraventricular hypothalamus regulate feeding and are synaptically connected to the parabrachial nucleus. *Proc Natl Acad Sci U S A.* 2014;111(36):13193-13198.

44. Broadwell RD, Brightman MW. Entry of peroxidase into neurons of the central and peripheral nervous systems from extracerebral and cerebral blood. *J Comp Neurol.* 1976;166(3):257-283.

45. Billig I, Yates BJ, Rinaman L. Plasma hormone levels and central c-Fos expression in ferrets after systemic administration of cholecystokinin. *Am J Physiol Regul Integr Comp Physiol.* 2001;281(4):R1243-R1255.

46. Rinaman L. A functional role for central glucagon-like peptide-1 receptors in lithium chloride-induced anorexia. *Am J Physiol.* 1999;277(5 Pt 2):R1537-R1540.

47. Yamamoto H, Kishi T, Lee CE, et al. Glucagon-like peptide-1-responsive catecholamine neurons in the area postrema link peripheral glucagon-like peptide-1 with central autonomic control sites. *J Neurosci.* 2003;23(7):2939-2946.

48. Saper CB, Chou TC, Elmquist JK. The need to feed: homeostatic and hedonic control of eating. *Neuron.* 2002;36(2):199-211.

49. Elmquist JK, Coppari R, Balthasar N, et al. Identifying hypothalamic pathways controlling food intake, body weight, and glucose homeostasis. *J Comp Neurol.* 2005;493(1):63-71.

50. Bingham NC, Anderson KK, Reuter AL, et al. Selective loss of leptin receptors in the ventromedial hypothalamic nucleus results in increased adiposity and a metabolic syndrome. *Endocrinology.* 2008; 149(5):2138-2148.

51. Dhillon H, Zigman JM, Ye C, et al. Leptin directly activates SF1 neurons in the VMH, and this action by leptin is required for normal body-weight homeostasis. *Neuron.* 2006;49(2):191-203.

52. Ikeda Y, Luo X, Abbud R, et al. The nuclear receptor steroidogenic factor 1 is essential for the formation of the ventromedial hypothalamic nucleus. *Mol Endocrinol.* 1995;9(4):478-486.

53. Majdic G, Young M, Gomez-Sanchez E, et al. Knockout mice lacking steroidogenic factor 1 are a novel genetic model of hypothalamic obesity. *Endocrinology.* 2002;143(2):607-614.

54. Kim KW, Sohn JW, Kohno D, et al. SF-1 in the ventral medial hypothalamic nucleus: a key regulator of homeostasis. *Mol Cell Endocrinol.* 2011;336(1-2):219-223.

55. Kim KW, Zhao L, Donato J Jr, et al. Steroidogenic factor 1 directs programs regulating diet-induced thermogenesis and leptin action in the ventral medial hypothalamic nucleus. *Proc Natl Acad Sci U S A.* 2011;108(26):10673-10678.

56. Elmquist JK, Bjorbaek C, Ahima RS, et al. Distributions of leptin receptor mRNA isoforms in the rat brain. *J Comp Neurol.* 1998;395(4): 535-547.

57. Roselli-Rehfuss L, Mountjoy KG, Robbins LS, et al. Identification of a receptor for gamma melanotropin and other proopiomelanocortin peptides in the hypothalamus and limbic system. *Proc Natl Acad Sci U S A.* 1993;90(19):8856-8860.

58. Minokoshi Y, Haque MS, Shimazu T. Microinjection of leptin into the ventromedial hypothalamus increases glucose uptake in peripheral tissues in rats. *Diabetes.* 1999;48(2):287-291.

59. Shiuchi T, Haque MS, Okamoto S, et al. Hypothalamic orexin stimulates feeding-associated glucose utilization in skeletal muscle via sympathetic nervous system. *Cell Metab.* 2009;10(6):466-480.

60. Haque MS, Minokoshi Y, Hamai M, et al. Role of the sympathetic nervous system and insulin in enhancing glucose uptake in peripheral tissues after intrahypothalamic injection of leptin in rats. *Diabetes.* 1999;48(9):1706-1712.

61. Gutierrez-Juarez R, Obici S, Rossetti L. Melanocortin-independent effects of leptin on hepatic glucose fluxes. *J Biol Chem.* 2004;279(48): 49704-49715.

62. Zhang R, Dhillon H, Yin H, et al. Selective inactivation of Socs3 in SF1 neurons improves glucose homeostasis without affecting body weight. *Endocrinology.* 2008;149(11):5654-5661.

63. Cone RD. Anatomy and regulation of the central melanocortin system. *Nat Neurosci.* 2005;8(5):571-578.

64. Barsh GS, Farooqi IS, O'Rahilly S. Genetics of body-weight regulation. *Nature.* 2000;404(6778):644-651.

65. Schwartz MW, Seeley RJ, Woods SC, et al. Leptin increases hypothalamic pro-opiomelanocortin mRNA expression in the rostral arcuate nucleus. *Diabetes.* 1997;46(12):2119-2123.

66. Stephens TW, Basinski M, Bristow PK, et al. The role of neuropeptide Y in the antiobesity action of the obese gene product. *Nature.* 1995; 377(6549):530-532.

67. Cowley MA, Smart JL, Rubinstein M, et al. Leptin activates anorexigenic POMC neurons through a neural network in the arcuate nucleus. *Nature.* 2001;411(6836):480-484.

68. Spanswick D, Smith MA, Groppi VE, et al. Leptin inhibits hypothalamic neurons by activation of ATP-sensitive potassium channels. *Nature.* 1997;390(6659):521-525.

69. Balthasar N, Coppari R, McMinn J, et al. Leptin receptor signaling in POMC neurons is required for normal body weight homeostasis. *Neuron.* 2004;42(6):983-991.

70. Gropp E, Shanabrough M, Borok E, et al. Agouti-related peptide-expressing neurons are mandatory for feeding. *Nat Neurosci.* 2005; 8(10):1289-1291.

71. Luquet S, Perez FA, Hnasko TS, Palmiter RD. NPY/AgRP neurons are essential for feeding in adult mice but can be ablated in neonates. *Science.* 2005;310(5748):683-685.

72. Wu Q, Howell MP, Cowley MA, Palmiter RD. Starvation after AgRP neuron ablation is independent of melanocortin signaling. *Proc Natl Acad Sci U S A.* 2008;105(7):2687-2692.

73. Krashes MJ, Koda S, Ye C, et al. Rapid, reversible activation of AgRP neurons drives feeding behavior in mice. *J Clin Invest.* 2011;121(4): 1424-1428.

74. Aponte Y, Atasoy D, Sternson SM. AGRP neurons are sufficient to orchestrate feeding behavior rapidly and without training. *Nat Neurosci.* 2011;14(3):351-355.

75. Yang Y, Atasoy D, Su HH, Sternson SM. Hunger states switch a flip-flop memory circuit via a synaptic AMPK-dependent positive feedback loop. *Cell.* 2011;146(6):992-1003.

76. Cowley MA, Smith RG, Diano S, et al. The distribution and mechanism of action of ghrelin in the CNS demonstrates a novel hypothalamic circuit regulating energy homeostasis. *Neuron.* 2003;37(4): 649-661.

77. Bello NT, Liang NC. The use of serotonergic drugs to treat obesity—is there any hope? *Drug Des Devel Ther.* 2011;5:95-109.

78. Garfield AS, Heisler LK. Pharmacological targeting of the serotonergic system for the treatment of obesity. *J Physiol.* 2009;587(Pt 1):49-60.

79. Nonogaki K, Strack AM, Dallman MF, Tecott LH. Leptin-independent hyperphagia and type 2 diabetes in mice with a mutated serotonin 5-HT2C receptor gene. *Nat Med.* 1998;4(10):1152-1156.

80. Tecott LH, Sun LM, Akana SF, et al. Eating disorder and epilepsy in mice lacking 5-HT2c serotonin receptors. *Nature.* 1995;374(6522):542-546.

81. Vickers SP, Clifton PG, Dourish CT, Tecott LH. Reduced satiating effect of d-fenfluramine in serotonin 5-HT(2C) receptor mutant mice. *Psychopharmacology (Berl).* 1999;143(3):309-314.

82. Heisler LK, Cowley MA, Kishi T, et al. Central serotonin and melanocortin pathways regulating energy homeostasis. *Ann N Y Acad Sci.* 2003;994:169-174.

83. Heisler LK, Cowley MA, Tecott LH, et al. Activation of central melanocortin pathways by fenfluramine. *Science.* 2002;297(5581):609-611.

84. Heisler LK, Jobst EE, Sutton GM, et al. Serotonin reciprocally regulates melanocortin neurons to modulate food intake. *Neuron.* 2006;51(2): 239-249.

85. Xu Y, Jones JE, Kohno D, et al. 5-HT2CRs expressed by pro-opiomelanocortin neurons regulate energy homeostasis. *Neuron.* 2008;60(4):582-589.

86. Zhou L, Sutton GM, Rochford JJ, et al. Serotonin 2C receptor agonists improve type 2 diabetes via melanocortin-4 receptor signaling pathways. *Cell Metab.* 2007;6(5):398-405.

87. Xu Y, Jones JE, Lauzon DA, et al. A serotonin and melanocortin circuit mediates D-fenfluramine anorexia. *J Neurosci.* 2010;30(44):14630-14634.

88. Colman E, Golden J, Roberts M, et al. The FDA's assessment of two drugs for chronic weight management. *N Engl J Med.* 2012;367(17): 1577-1579.

89. Sohn JW, Xu Y, Jones JE, et al. Serotonin 2C receptor activates a distinct population of arcuate pro-opiomelanocortin neurons via TRPC channels. *Neuron.* 2011;71(3):488-497.

90. Xu Y, Berglund ED, Sohn JW, et al. 5-HT2CRs expressed by pro-opiomelanocortin neurons regulate insulin sensitivity in liver. *Nat Neurosci.* 2010;13(12):1457-1459.

91. Lam DD, Przydzial MJ, Ridley SH, et al. Serotonin 5-HT2C receptor agonist promotes hypophagia via downstream activation of melanocortin 4 receptors. *Endocrinology.* 2008;149(3):1323-1328.

92. Farooqi IS, Keogh JM, Yeo GS, et al. Clinical spectrum of obesity and mutations in the melanocortin 4 receptor gene. *N Engl J Med.* 2003; 348(12):1085-1095.

93. Farooqi IS, Yeo GS, Keogh JM, et al. Dominant and recessive inheritance of morbid obesity associated with melanocortin 4 receptor deficiency. *J Clin Invest.* 2000;106(2):271-279.

94. Yeo GS, Farooqi IS, Aminian S, et al. A frameshift mutation in MC4R associated with dominantly inherited human obesity [letter]. *Nat Genet.* 1998;20(2):111-112.

95. Vaisse C, Clement K, Guy-Grand B, Froguel P. A frameshift mutation in human MC4R is associated with a dominant form of obesity. *Nat Genet.* 1998;20(2):113-114.

96. Ghamari-Langroudi M, Srisai D, Cone RD. Multinodal regulation of the arcuate/paraventricular nucleus circuit by leptin. *Proc Natl Acad Sci U S A.* 2011;108(1):355-360.

97. Ghamari-Langroudi M, Vella KR, Srisai D, et al. Regulation of thyrotropin-releasing hormone-expressing neurons in paraventricular nucleus of the hypothalamus by signals of adiposity. *Mol Endocrinol.* 2010;24(12):2366-2381.

98. Sohn JW, Harris LE, Berglund ED, et al. Melanocortin 4 receptors reciprocally regulate sympathetic and parasympathetic preganglionic neurons. *Cell.* 2013;152(3):612-619.

99. Bouyer K, Simerly RB. Neonatal leptin exposure specifies innervation of presympathetic hypothalamic neurons and improves the metabolic status of leptin-deficient mice. *J Neurosci.* 2013;33(2):840-851.

100. Atasoy D, Betley JN, Li WP, et al. A genetically specified connectomics approach applied to long-range feeding regulatory circuits. *Nat Neurosci.* 2014;17(12):1830-1839.

101. Mountjoy KG, Mortrud MT, Low MJ, et al. Localization of the melanocortin-4 receptor (MC4-R) in neuroendocrine and autonomic control circuits in the brain. *Mol Endocrinol.* 1994;8(10):1298-1308.

102. Kishi T, Aschkenasi CJ, Lee CE, et al. Expression of melanocortin 4 receptor mRNA in the central nervous system of the rat. *J Comp Neurol.* 2003;457(3):213-235.

103. Liu H, Kishi T, Roseberry AG, et al. Transgenic mice expressing green fluorescent protein under the control of the melanocortin-4 receptor promoter. *J Neurosci.* 2003;23(18):7143-7154.

104. Cowley MA, Pronchuk N, Fan W, et al. Integration of NPY, AGRP, and melanocortin signals in the hypothalamic paraventricular nucleus: evidence of a cellular basis for the adipostat. *Neuron.* 1999;24(1): 155-163.

105. Balthasar N, Dalgaard LT, Lee CE, et al. Divergence of melanocortin pathways in the control of food intake and energy expenditure. *Cell.* 2005;123(3):493-505.

106. Grill HJ, Ginsberg AB, Seeley RJ, Kaplan JM. Brainstem application of melanocortin receptor ligands produces long-lasting effects on feeding and body weight. *J Neurosci.* 1998;18(23):10128-10135.

107. Williams DL, Kaplan JM, Grill HJ. The role of the dorsal vagal complex and the vagus nerve in feeding effects of melanocortin-3/4 receptor stimulation. *Endocrinology.* 2000;141(4):1332-1337.

108. Fan W, Ellacott KL, Halatchev IG, et al. Cholecystokinin-mediated suppression of feeding involves the brainstem melanocortin system. *Nat Neurosci.* 2004;7(4):335-336.

109. Rossi J, Balthasar N, Olson D, et al. Melanocortin-4 receptors expressed by cholinergic neurons regulate energy balance and glucose homeostasis. *Cell Metab.* 2011;13(2):195-204.

110. Berglund ED, Liu T, Kong X, et al. Melanocortin 4 receptors in autonomic neurons regulate thermogenesis and glycemia. *Nat Neurosci.* 2014;17(7):911-913.

111. Nedergaard J, Cannon B. The browning of white adipose tissue: some burning issues. *Cell Metab.* 2014;20(3):396-407.

112. Iqbal J, Li X, Chang BH, et al. An intrinsic gut leptin-melanocortin pathway modulates intestinal microsomal triglyceride transfer protein and lipid absorption. *J Lipid Res.* 2010;51(7):1929-1942.

113. Panaro BL, Tough IR, Engelstoft MS, et al. The melanocortin-4 receptor is expressed in enteroendocrine L cells and regulates the release of peptide YY and glucagon-like peptide 1 in vivo. *Cell Metab.* 2014; 20(6):1018-1029.

114. Chen KY, Muniyappa R, Abel BS, et al. RM-493, a melanocortin-4 receptor (MC4R) agonist, increases resting energy expenditure in obese individuals. *J Clin Endocrinol Metab.* 2015;100(4):1639-1645.

115. Lippert RN, Ellacott KL, Cone RD. Gender-specific roles for the melanocortin-3 receptor in the regulation of the mesolimbic dopamine system in mice. *Endocrinology.* 2014;155(5):1718-1727.

116. Butler AA, Kesterson RA, Khong K, et al. A unique metabolic syndrome causes obesity in the melanocortin-3 receptor-deficient mouse. *Endocrinology.* 2000;141(9):3518-3521.

117. Chen AS, Marsh DJ, Trumbauer ME, et al. Inactivation of the mouse melanocortin-3 receptor results in increased fat mass and reduced lean body mass. *Nat Genet.* 2000;26(1):97-102.

118. Renquist BJ, Murphy JG, Larson EA, et al. Melanocortin-3 receptor regulates the normal fasting response. *Proc Natl Acad Sci U S A.* 2012; 109(23):E1489-E1498.

119. Sutton GM, Perez-Tilve D, Nogueiras R, et al. The melanocortin-3 receptor is required for entrainment to meal intake. *J Neurosci.* 2008; 28(48):12946-12955.

120. Begriche K, Girardet C, McDonald P, Butler AA. Melanocortin-3 receptors and metabolic homeostasis. *Prog Mol Biol Transl Sci.* 2013;114: 109-146.

121. Anand BK, Brobeck JR. Localization of a "feeding center" in the hypothalamus of the rat. *Proc Soc Exp Biol Med.* 1951;77:323-324.

122. Bittencourt JC, Presse F, Arias C, et al. The melanin-concentrating hormone system of the rat brain: an immuno- and hybridization histochemical characterization. *J Comp Neurol.* 1992;319(2):218-245.

123. Qu D, Ludwig DS, Gammeltoft S, et al. A role for melanin-concentrating hormone in the central regulation of feeding behaviour. *Nature.* 1996;380(6571):243-247.

124. Sakurai T, Amemiya A, Ishii M, et al. Orexins and orexin receptors: a family of hypothalamic neuropeptides and G protein-coupled receptors that regulate feeding behavior. *Cell.* 1998;92(4):573-585.

125. de Lecea L, Kilduff TS, Peyron C, et al. The hypocretins: hypothalamus-specific peptides with neuroexcitatory activity. *Proc Natl Acad Sci U S A.* 1998;95(1):322-327.

126. Elias CF, Saper CB, Maratos-Flier E, et al. Chemically defined projections linking the mediobasal hypothalamus and the lateral hypothalamic area. *J Comp Neurol.* 1998;402(4):442-459.

127. Broberger C, De Lecea L, Sutcliffe JG, Hokfelt T. Hypocretin/orexin- and melanin-concentrating hormone-expressing cells form distinct populations in the rodent lateral hypothalamus: relationship to the neuropeptide Y and agouti gene-related protein systems. *J Comp Neurol.* 1998;402(4):460-474.

128. Peyron C, Tighe DK, van den Pol AN, et al. Neurons containing hypocretin (orexin) project to multiple neuronal systems. *J Neurosci.* 1998;18(23):9996-10015.

129. Marcus JN, Aschkenasi CJ, Lee CE, et al. Differential expression of orexin receptors 1 and 2 in the rat brain. *J Comp Neurol.* 2001; 435(1):6-25.

130. Saito Y, Cheng M, Leslie FM, Civelli O. Expression of the melanin-concentrating hormone (MCH) receptor mRNA in the rat brain. *J Comp Neurol.* 2001;435(1):26-40.

131. Kilduff TS, de Lecea L. Mapping of the mRNAs for the hypocretin/orexin and melanin-concentrating hormone receptors: networks of overlapping peptide systems. *J Comp Neurol.* 2001;435(1):1-5.

132. Shimada M, Tritos NA, Lowell BB, et al. Mice lacking melanin-concentrating hormone are hypophagic and lean. *Nature.* 1998; 396(6712):670-674.

133. Ludwig DS, Tritos NA, Mastaitis JW, et al. Melanin-concentrating hormone overexpression in transgenic mice leads to obesity and insulin resistance. *J Clin Invest.* 2001;107(3):379-386.

134. Segal-Lieberman G, Bradley RL, Kokkotou E, et al. Melanin-concentrating hormone is a critical mediator of the leptin-deficient phenotype. *Proc Natl Acad Sci U S A.* 2003;100(17):10085-10090.

135. Willie JT, Chemelli RM, Sinton CM, Yanagisawa M. To eat or to sleep? Orexin in the regulation of feeding and wakefulness. *Annu Rev Neurosci.* 2001;24:429-458.

136. Hara J, Beuckmann CT, Nambu T, et al. Genetic ablation of orexin neurons in mice results in narcolepsy, hypophagia, and obesity. *Neuron.* 2001;30(2):345-354.

137. Clegg DJ, Air EL, Woods SC, Seeley RJ. Eating elicited by orexin-a, but not melanin-concentrating hormone, is opioid mediated. *Endocrinology.* 2002;143(8):2995-3000.

138. Chemelli RM, Willie JT, Sinton CM, et al. Narcolepsy in orexin knock-out mice: molecular genetics of sleep regulation. *Cell.* 1999;98(4): 437-451.

139. Lin L, Faraco J, Li R, et al. The sleep disorder canine narcolepsy is caused by a mutation in the hypocretin (orexin) receptor 2 gene [see comments]. *Cell.* 1999;98(3):365-376.

140. Grill HJ, Kaplan JM. The neuroanatomical axis for control of energy balance. *Front Neuroendocrinol.* 2002;23(1):2-40.

141. Pissios P, Frank L, Kennedy AR, et al. Dysregulation of the mesolimbic dopamine system and reward in MCH-/- mice. *Biol Psychiatry.* 2008; 64(3):184-191.

142. Georgescu D, Sears RM, Hommel JD, et al. The hypothalamic neuropeptide melanin-concentrating hormone acts in the nucleus accumbens to modulate feeding behavior and forced-swim performance. *J Neurosci.* 2005;25(11):2933-2940.

143. Chaudhury D, Walsh JJ, Friedman AK, et al. Rapid regulation of depression-related behaviours by control of midbrain dopamine neurons. *Nature.* 2013;493(7433):532-536.

144. Lutter M, Krishnan V, Russo SJ, et al. Orexin signaling mediates the antidepressant-like effect of calorie restriction. *J Neurosci.* 2008;28(12): 3071-3075.

145. Louis GW, Leinninger GM, Rhodes CJ, Myers MG Jr. Direct innervation and modulation of orexin neurons by lateral hypothalamic LepRb neurons. *J Neurosci.* 2010;30(34):11278-11287.

146. Domingos AI, Sordillo A, Dietrich MO, et al. Hypothalamic melanin concentrating hormone neurons communicate the nutrient value of sugar. *eLife*. 2013;2:e01462.

147. Nestler EJ, Carlezon WA Jr. The mesolimbic dopamine reward circuit in depression. *Biol Psychiatry*. 2006;59(12):1151-1159.

148. Rothwell NJ. CNS regulation of thermogenesis. *Crit Rev Neurobiol*. 1994;8(1-2):1-10.

149. Lowell BB, Bachman ES. Beta-adrenergic receptors, diet-induced thermogenesis, and obesity. *J Biol Chem*. 2003;278(32):29385-29388.

150. Cypess AM, Lehman S, Williams G, et al. Identification and importance of brown adipose tissue in adult humans. *N Engl J Med*. 2009;360(15):1509-1517.

151. Bachman ES, Dhillon H, Zhang CY, et al. betaAR signaling required for diet-induced thermogenesis and obesity resistance. *Science*. 2002;297(5582):843-845.

152. Jansen AS, Nguyen XV, Karpitskiy V, et al. Central command neurons of the sympathetic nervous system: basis of the fight-or-flight response. *Science*. 1995;270(5236):644-646.

153. Loewy AD. Forebrain nuclei involved in autonomic control. *Prog Brain Res*. 1991;87:253-268.

154. Loewy AD, Spyer KM. *Central Regulation of Autonomic Functions*. New York, NY: Oxford University Press; 1990:xii, 390.

155. Strack AM, Sawyer WB, Platt KB, Loewy AD. CNS cell groups regulating the sympathetic outflow to adrenal gland as revealed by transneuronal cell body labeling with pseudorabies virus. *Brain Res*. 1989;491(2):274-296.

156. Strack AM, Sawyer WB, Marubio LM, Loewy AD. Spinal origin of sympathetic preganglionic neurons in the rat. *Brain Res*. 1988;455(1):187-191.

157. Strack AM, Sawyer WB, Hughes JH, et al. A general pattern of CNS innervation of the sympathetic outflow demonstrated by transneuronal pseudorabies viral infections. *Brain Res*. 1989;491(1):156-162.

158. Jansen AS, Hoffman JL, Loewy AD. CNS sites involved in sympathetic and parasympathetic control of the pancreas: a viral tracing study. *Brain Res*. 1997;766(1-2):29-38.

159. Rinaman L, Miselis RR. The organization of vagal innervation of rat pancreas using cholera toxin-horseradish peroxidase conjugate. *J Auton Nerv Syst*. 1987;21(2-3):109-125.

160. Saper CB, Loewy AD, Swanson LW, Cowan WM. Direct hypothalamo-autonomic connections. *Brain Res*. 1976;117(2):305-312.

161. Loewy AD, McKellar S, Saper CB. Direct projections from the A5 catecholamine cell group to the intermediolateral cell column. *Brain Res*. 1979;174(2):309-314.

162. Cechetto DF, Saper CB. Neurochemical organization of the hypothalamic projection to the spinal cord in the rat. *J Comp Neurol*. 1988;272(4):579-604.

163. Loewy AD, Burton H. Nuclei of the solitary tract: efferent projections to the lower brain stem and spinal cord of the cat. *J Comp Neurol*. 1978;181(2):421-449.

164. Loewy AD. Descending pathways to sympathetic and parasympathetic preganglionic neurons. *J Auton Nerv Syst*. 1981;3(2-4):265-275.

165. Loewy AD. Descending pathways to the sympathetic preganglionic neurons. *Prog Brain Res*. 1982;57:267-277.

166. Tucker DC, Saper CB. Specificity of spinal projections from hypothalamic and brainstem areas which innervate sympathetic preganglionic neurons. *Brain Res*. 1985;360(1-2):159-164.

167. Tucker DC, Saper CB, Ruggiero DA, Reis DJ. Organization of central adrenergic pathways: I. Relationships of ventrolateral medullary projections to the hypothalamus and spinal cord. *J Comp Neurol*. 1987;259(4):591-603.

168. Chan RK, Sawchenko PE. Spatially and temporally differentiated patterns of c-fos expression in brainstem catecholaminergic cell groups induced by cardiovascular challenges in the rat. *J Comp Neurol*. 1994;348(3):433-460.

169. Morrison SF, Milner TA, Reis DJ. Reticulospinal vasomotor neurons of the rat rostral ventrolateral medulla: relationship to sympathetic nerve activity and the C1 adrenergic cell group. *J Neurosci*. 1988;8(4):1286-1301.

170. Haselton JR, Guyenet PG. Electrophysiological characterization of putative C1 adrenergic neurons in the rat. *Neuroscience*. 1989;30(1):199-214.

171. Reis DJ, Ruggiero DA, Morrison SF. The C1 area of the rostral ventrolateral medulla oblongata. A critical brainstem region for control of resting and reflex integration of arterial pressure. *Am J Hypertens*. 1989;2(12 Pt 2):363S-374S.

172. Butler AA, Marks DL, Fan W, et al. Melanocortin-4 receptor is required for acute homeostatic responses to increased dietary fat. *Nat Neurosci*. 2001;4(6):605-611.

173. Yasuda T, Masaki T, Kakuma T, Yoshimatsu H. Hypothalamic melanocortin system regulates sympathetic nerve activity in brown adipose tissue. *Exp Biol Med (Maywood)*. 2004;229(3):235-239.

174. Voss-Andreae A, Murphy JG, Ellacott KL, et al. Role of the central melanocortin circuitry in adaptive thermogenesis of brown adipose tissue. *Endocrinology*. 2007;148(4):1550-1560.

175. Elias CF, Lee C, Kelly J, et al. Leptin activates hypothalamic CART neurons projecting to the spinal cord. *Neuron*. 1998;21(6):1375-1385.

176. Morrison SF. Central pathways controlling brown adipose tissue thermogenesis. *News Physiol Sci*. 2004;19:67-74.

177. Fan W, Voss-Andreae A, Cao WH, Morrison SF. Regulation of thermogenesis by the central melanocortin system. *Peptides*. 2005;26(10):1800-1813.

178. Loewy AD. Raphe pallidus and raphe obscurus projections to the intermediolateral cell column in the rat. *Brain Res*. 1981;222(1):129-133.

179. Bacon SJ, Zagon A, Smith AD. Electron microscopic evidence of a monosynaptic pathway between cells in the caudal raphe nuclei and sympathetic preganglionic neurons in the rat spinal cord. *Exp Brain Res*. 1990;79(3):589-602.

180. Bamshad M, Song CK, Bartness TJ. CNS origins of the sympathetic nervous system outflow to brown adipose tissue. *Am J Physiol*. 1999;276(6 Pt 2):R1569-R1578.

181. Morrison SF. Differential control of sympathetic outflow. *Am J Physiol Regul Integr Comp Physiol*. 2001;281(3):R683-R698.

182. Wang J, Liu R, Hawkins M, et al. A nutrient-sensing pathway regulates leptin gene expression in muscle and fat. *Nature*. 1998;393(6686):684-688.

183. Masuzaki H, Ogawa Y, Sagawa N, et al. Nonadipose tissue production of leptin: leptin as a novel placenta-derived hormone in humans. *Nat Med*. 1997;3(9):1029-1033.

184. Farooqi IS, Jebb SA, Langmack G, et al. Effects of recombinant leptin therapy in a child with congenital leptin deficiency. *N Engl J Med*. 1999;341(12):879-884.

185. Ahima RS, Prabakaran D, Mantzoros C, et al. Role of leptin in the neuroendocrine response to fasting. *Nature*. 1996;382(6588):250-252.

186. Spiegelman BM, Flier JS. Obesity and the regulation of energy balance. *Cell*. 2001;104(4):531-543.

187. Frederich RC, Hamann A, Anderson S, et al. Leptin levels reflect body lipid content in mice: evidence for diet-induced resistance to leptin action. *Nat Med*. 1995;1(12):1311-1314.

188. Ahima RS, Saper CB, Flier JS, Elmquist JK. Leptin regulation of neuroendocrine systems. *Front Neuroendocrinol*. 2000;21(3):263-307.

189. Flier JS. Clinical review 94: what's in a name? In search of leptin's physiologic role. *J Clin Endocrinol Metab*. 1998;83(5):1407-1413.

190. Tartaglia LA. The leptin receptor. *J Biol Chem*. 1997;272(10):6093-6096.

191. Chen H, Charlat O, Tartaglia LA, et al. Evidence that the diabetes gene encodes the leptin receptor: identification of a mutation in the leptin receptor gene in db/db mice. *Cell*. 1996;84(3):491-495.

192. White DW, Wang DW, Chua SC Jr, et al. Constitutive and impaired signaling of leptin receptors containing the Gln –> Pro extracellular domain fatty mutation. *Proc Natl Acad Sci U S A*. 1997;94(20):10657-10662.

193. Mercer JG, Hoggard N, Williams LM, et al. Coexpression of leptin receptor and prepro-neuropeptide Y mRNA in arcuate nucleus of mouse hypothalamus. *J Neuroendocrinol*. 1996;8(10):733-735.

194. Mercer JG, Hoggard N, Williams LM, et al. Localization of leptin receptor mRNA and the long form splice variant (Ob-Rb) in mouse hypothalamus and adjacent brain regions by in situ hybridization. *FEBS Lett*. 1996;387(2-3):113-116.

195. Fei H, Okano HJ, Li C, et al. Anatomic localization of alternatively spliced leptin receptors (Ob-R) in mouse brain and other tissues. *Proc Natl Acad Sci U S A*. 1997;94(13):7001-7005.

196. Schwartz MW, Seeley RJ, Campfield LA, et al. Identification of targets of leptin action in rat hypothalamus. *J Clin Invest*. 1996;98(5):1101-1106.

197. Cheung CC, Clifton DK, Steiner RA. Proopiomelanocortin neurons are direct targets for leptin in the hypothalamus. *Endocrinology*. 1997;138(10):4489-4492.

198. Scott MM, Lachey JL, Sternson SM, et al. Leptin targets in the mouse brain. *J Comp Neurol*. 2009;514(5):518-532.

199. Hosoi T, Kawagishi T, Okuma Y, et al. Brain stem is a direct target for leptin's action in the central nervous system. *Endocrinology*. 2002;143(9):3498-3504.

200. Finn PD, Cunningham MJ, Rickard DG, et al. Serotonergic neurons are targets for leptin in the monkey. *J Clin Endocrinol Metab*. 2001;86(1):422-426.

201. Mercer JG, Moar KM, Hoggard N. Localization of leptin receptor (Ob-R) messenger ribonucleic acid in the rodent hindbrain. *Endocrinology*. 1998;139(1):29-34.

202. Mercer JG, Moar KM, Findlay PA, et al. Association of leptin receptor (OB-Rb), NPY and GLP-1 gene expression in the ovine and murine brainstem. *Regul Pept*. 1998;75-76:271-278.

203. Bernard C. Chiens rendus diabetiques. *C R Soc Biol (Paris)*. 1849;1:60.

204. Fan W, Dinulescu DM, Butler AA, et al. The central melanocortin system can directly regulate serum insulin levels. *Endocrinology*. 2000;141:3072-3079.

205. Obici S, Rossetti L. Minireview: nutrient sensing and the regulation of insulin action and energy balance. *Endocrinology*. 2003;144(12):5172-5178.

206. Obici S, Feng Z, Morgan K, et al. Central administration of oleic acid inhibits glucose production and food intake. *Diabetes*. 2002;51(2):271-275.

207. Schwartz MW. Progress in the search for neuronal mechanisms coupling type 2 diabetes to obesity. *J Clin Invest.* 2001;108(7):963-964.
208. Elmquist JK, Marcus JN. Rethinking the central causes of diabetes. *Nat Med.* 2003;9(6):645-647.
209. Schwartz MW, Woods SC, Porte D Jr, et al. Central nervous system control of food intake. *Nature.* 2000;404(6778):661-671.
210. Woods SC, Lotter EC, McKay LD, Porte D Jr. Chronic intracerebroventricular infusion of insulin reduces food intake and body weight of baboons. *Nature.* 1979;282(5738):503-505.
211. Bruning JC, Gautam D, Burks DJ, et al. Role of brain insulin receptor in control of body weight and reproduction. *Science.* 2000;289(5487):2122-2125.
212. Obici S, Feng Z, Karkanias G, et al. Decreasing hypothalamic insulin receptors causes hyperphagia and insulin resistance in rats. *Nat Neurosci.* 2002;5(6):566-572.
213. Chong AC, Vogt MC, Hill AS, et al. Central insulin signaling modulates hypothalamus-pituitary-adrenal axis responsiveness. *Mol Metab.* 2015;4(2):83-92.
214. Vogt MC, Paeger L, Hess S, et al. Neonatal insulin action impairs hypothalamic neurocircuit formation in response to maternal high-fat feeding. *Cell.* 2014;156(3):495-509.
215. Buettner C, Patel R, Muse ED, et al. Severe impairment in liver insulin signaling fails to alter hepatic insulin action in conscious mice. *J Clin Invest.* 2005;115(5):1306-1313.
216. Okamoto H, Obici S, Accili D, Rossetti L. Restoration of liver insulin signaling in Insr knockout mice fails to normalize hepatic insulin action. *J Clin Invest.* 2005;115(5):1314-1322.
217. Edgerton DS, Lautz M, Scott M, et al. Insulin's direct effects on the liver dominate the control of hepatic glucose production. *J Clin Invest.* 2006;116(2):521-527.
218. Ramnanan CJ, Edgerton DS, Cherrington AD. Evidence against a physiologic role for acute changes in CNS insulin action in the rapid regulation of hepatic glucose production. *Cell Metab.* 2012;15(5):656-664.
219. Oomura Y, Ono T, Ooyama H, Wayner MJ. Glucose and osmosensitive neurones of the rat hypothalamus. *Nature.* 1969;222(190):282-284.
220. Levin BE. Metabolic sensing neurons and the control of energy homeostasis. *Physiol Behav.* 2006;89(4):486-489.
221. Levin BE, Routh VH, Kang L, et al. Neuronal glucosensing: what do we know after 50 years? *Diabetes.* 2004;53(10):2521-2528.
222. Ibrahim N, Bosch MA, Smart JL, et al. Hypothalamic proopiomelanocortin neurons are glucose responsive and express K(ATP) channels. *Endocrinology.* 2003;144(4):1331-1340.
223. DiRocco RJ, Grill HJ. The forebrain is not essential for sympathoadrenal hyperglycemic response to glucoprivation. *Science.* 1979;204(4397):1112-1114.
224. Ritter S, Bugarith K, Dinh TT. Immunotoxic destruction of distinct catecholamine subgroups produces selective impairment of glucoregulatory responses and neuronal activation. *J Comp Neurol.* 2001;432(2):197-216.
225. Ritter S, Dinh TT, Zhang Y. Localization of hindbrain glucoreceptive sites controlling food intake and blood glucose. *Brain Res.* 2000;856(1-2):37-47.
226. Burdakov D, Jensen LT, Alexopoulos H, et al. Tandem-pore K+ channels mediate inhibition of orexin neurons by glucose. *Neuron.* 2006;50(5):711-722.
227. Obici S, Feng Z, Tan J, et al. Central melanocortin receptors regulate insulin action. *J Clin Invest.* 2001;108(7):1079-1085.
228. Fox EA, Powley TL. Tracer diffusion has exaggerated CNS maps of direct preganglionic innervation of pancreas. *J Auton Nerv Syst.* 1986;15(1):55-69.
229. Loewy AD, Franklin MF, Haxhiu MA. CNS monoamine cell groups projecting to pancreatic vagal motor neurons: a transneuronal labeling study using pseudorabies virus. *Brain Res.* 1994;638(1-2):248-260.
230. Berthoud HR, Fox EA, Powley TL. Localization of vagal preganglionics that stimulate insulin and glucagon secretion. *Am J Physiol.* 1990;258(1 Pt 2):R160-R168.
231. Cai XJ, Widdowson PS, Harrold J, et al. Hypothalamic orexin expression: modulation by blood glucose and feeding. *Diabetes.* 1999;48(11):2132-2137.
232. Griffond B, Risold PY, Jacquemard C, et al. Insulin-induced hypoglycemia increases preprohypocretin (orexin) mRNA in the rat lateral hypothalamic area. *Neurosci Lett.* 1999;262(2):77-80.
233. Moriguchi T, Sakurai T, Nambu T, et al. Neurons containing orexin in the lateral hypothalamic area of the adult rat brain are activated by insulin-induced acute hypoglycemia. *Neurosci Lett.* 1999;264(1-3):101-104.
234. Scott MM, Marcus JN, Elmquist JK. Orexin neurons and the TASK of glucosensing. *Neuron.* 2006;50(5):665-667.
235. Oomura Y, Yoshimatsu H. Neural network of glucose monitoring system. *J Auton Nerv Syst.* 1984;10(3-4):359-372.
236. Schwartz GJ. The role of gastrointestinal vagal afferents in the control of food intake: current prospects. *Nutrition.* 2000;16(10):866-873.
237. Moran TH. Gut peptides in the control of food intake: 30 years of ideas. *Physiol Behav.* 2004;82(1):175-180.
238. Moran TH, Gao S. Looking for food in all the right places? *Cell Metab.* 2006;3(4):233-234.
239. Grill HJ, Hayes MR. The nucleus tractus solitarius: a portal for visceral afferent signal processing, energy status assessment and integration of their combined effects on food intake. *Int J Obes.* 2009;33(Suppl 1):S11-S15.
240. Grill HJ, Hayes MR. Hindbrain neurons as an essential hub in the neuroanatomically distributed control of energy balance. *Cell Metab.* 2012;16(3):296-309.
241. Altschuler SM, Bao XM, Bieger D, et al. Viscerotopic representation of the upper alimentary tract in the rat: sensory ganglia and nuclei of the solitary and spinal trigeminal tracts. *J Comp Neurol.* 1989;283(2):248-268.
242. Raybould HE, Gayton RJ, Dockray GJ. CNS effects of circulating CCK8: involvement of brainstem neurones responding to gastric distension. *Brain Res.* 1985;342(1):187-190.
243. Zhang X, Fogel R, Renehan WE. Relationships between the morphology and function of gastric- and intestine-sensitive neurons in the nucleus of the solitary tract. *J Comp Neurol.* 1995;363:37-52.
244. Rinaman L, Verbalis JG, Stricker EM, Hoffman GE. Distribution and neurochemical phenotypes of caudal medullary neurons activated to express cFos following peripheral administration of cholecystokinin. *J Comp Neurol.* 1993;338(4):475-490.
245. Gibbs J, Falasco JD, McHugh PR. Cholecystokinin-decreased food intake in rhesus monkeys. *Am J Physiol.* 1976;230(1):15-18.
246. Gibbs J, Young RC, Smith GP. Cholecystokinin decreases food intake in rats. *J Comp Physiol Psychol.* 1973;84(3):488-495.
247. Crawley JN, Beinfeld MC. Rapid development of tolerance to the behavioural actions of cholecystokinin. *Nature.* 1983;302(5910):703-706.
248. West D, Fey D, Woods S. Cholecystokinin persistently suppresses meal size but not food intake in free-feeding rats. *Am J Physiol.* 1984;246:R776-R787.
249. Smith GP, Jerome C, Cushin BJ, et al. Abdominal vagotomy blocks the satiety effect of cholecystokinin in the rat. *Science.* 1981;213(4511):1036-1037.
250. South EH, Ritter RC. Capsaicin application to central or peripheral vagal fibers attenuates CCK satiety. *Peptides.* 1988;9(3):601-612.
251. Hewson G, Leighton GE, Hill RG, Hughes J. The cholecystokinin receptor antagonist L364,718 increases food intake in the rat by attenuation of the action of endogenous cholecystokinin. *Br J Pharmacol.* 1988;93(1):79-84.
252. Dourish CT, Ruckert AC, Tattersall FD, Iversen SD. Evidence that decreased feeding induced by systemic injection of cholecystokinin is mediated by CCK-A receptors. *Eur J Pharmacol.* 1989;173(2-3):233-234.
253. Dourish C, Rycroft W, Iversen S. Postponement of satiety by blockade of brain cholecystokinin (CCKB) receptors. *Science.* 1989;245:1509-1511.
254. Reidelberger RD, O'Rourke MF. Potent cholecystokinin antagonist L 364718 stimulates food intake in rats. *Am J Physiol.* 1989;257(6 Pt 2):R1512-R1518.
255. Gutzwiller JP, Drewe J, Ketterer S, et al. Interaction between CCK and a preload on reduction of food intake is mediated by CCK-A receptors in humans. *Am J Physiol Regul Integr Comp Physiol.* 2000;279(1):R189-R195.
256. Riedy CA, Chavez M, Figlewicz DP, Woods SC. Central insulin enhances sensitivity to cholecystokinin. *Physiol Behav.* 1995;58(4):755-760.
257. Figlewicz DP, Sipols AJ, Seeley RJ, et al. Intraventricular insulin enhances the meal-suppressive efficacy of intraventricular cholecystokinin octapeptide in the baboon. *Behav Neurosci.* 1995;109(3):567-569.
258. Matson CA, Wiater MF, Kuijper JL, Weigle DS. Synergy between leptin and cholecystokinin (CCK) to control daily caloric intake. *Peptides.* 1997;18(8):1275-1278.
259. Matson CA, Ritter RC. Long-term CCK-leptin synergy suggests a role for CCK in the regulation of body weight. *Am J Physiol.* 1999;276:R1038.
260. Emond M, Schwartz GJ, Ladenheim EE, Moran TH. Central leptin modulates behavioral and neural responsivity to CCK. *Am J Physiol.* 1999;276(5 Pt 2):R1545-R1549.
261. Matson CA, Reid DF, Cannon TA, Ritter RC. Cholecystokinin and leptin act synergistically to reduce body weight. *Am J Physiol.* 2000;278:R882.
262. Cannon CM, Palmiter RD. Peptides that regulate food intake: norepinephrine is not required for reduction of feeding induced by cholecystokinin. *Am J Physiol Regul Integr Comp Physiol.* 2003;284(6):R1384-R1388.
263. Lodge DJ, Lawrence AJ. Comparative analysis of the central CCK system in Fawn Hooded and Wistar Kyoto rats: extended localisation of CCK-A receptors throughout the rat brain using a novel radioligand. *Regul Pept.* 2001;99(2-3):191-201.
264. Mercer LD, Beart PM. Histochemistry in rat brain and spinal cord with an antibody directed at the cholecystokinin A receptor. *Neurosci Lett.* 1997;225(2):97-100.
265. Hirosue Y, Inui A, Teranishi A, et al. Cholecystokinin octapeptide analogues suppress food intake via central CCK-A receptors in mice. *Am J Physiol.* 1993;265(3 Pt 2):R481-R486.

266. Adrian TE, Ferri GL, Bacarese-Hamilton AJ, et al. Human distribution and release of a putative new gut hormone, peptide YY. *Gastroenterology*. 1985;89:1070-1077.

267. Grandt D, Schimiczek M, Beglinger C, et al. Two molecular forms of peptide YY (PYY) are abundant in human blood: characterization of a radioimmunoassay recognizing PYY 1-36 and PYY 3-36. *Regul Pept*. 1994;51(2):151-159.

268. Grandt D, Schimiczek M, Struk K, et al. Characterization of two forms of peptide YY, PYY(1-36) and PYY(3-36), in the rabbit. *Peptides*. 1994; 15(5):815-820.

269. Bonaz B, Taylor I, Tache Y. Peripheral peptide YY induces c-fos-like immunoreactivity in the rat brain. *Neurosci Lett*. 1993;163:77-80.

270. Allen JM, Fitzpatrick ML, Yeats JC, et al. Effects of peptide YY and neuropeptide Y on gastric emptying in man. *Digestion*. 1984;30(4): 255-262.

271. Adrian TE, Savage AP, Sagor GR, et al. Effect of peptide YY on gastric, pancreatic, and biliary function in humans. *Gastroenterology*. 1985; 89(3):494-499.

272. Yang H. Central and peripheral regulation of gastric acid secretion by peptide YY. *Peptides*. 2002;23:349-358.

273. Dumont Y, Fournier A, St-Pierre S, Quirion R. Autoradiographic distribution of [125I]Leu31, Pro34PYY and [125I]PYY3-36 binding sites in the rat brain evaluated with two newly developed Y1 and Y2 receptor radioligands. *Synapse*. 1996;22(2):139-158.

274. Lloyd KC, Amirmoazzami S, Friedik F, et al. Candidate canine enterogastrones: acid inhibition before and after vagotomy. *Am J Physiol*. 1997;272(5 Pt 1):G1236-G1242.

275. Batterham RL, Cowley MA, Small CJ, et al. Gut hormone PYY(3-36) physiologically inhibits food intake. *Nature*. 2002;418(6898):650-654.

276. Adams SH, Won WB, Schonhoff SE, et al. Effects of peptide YY[3-36] on short-term food intake in mice are not affected by prevailing plasma ghrelin levels. *Endocrinology*. 2004;145(11):4967-4975.

277. Challis BG, Coll AP, Yeo GS, et al. Mice lacking pro-opiomelanocortin are sensitive to high-fat feeding but respond normally to the acute anorectic effects of peptide-YY(3-36). *Proc Natl Acad Sci U S A*. 2004; 101(13):4695-4700.

278. Chelikani PK, Haver AC, Reidelberger RD. Intravenous infusion of peptide YY(3-36) potently inhibits food intake in rats. *Endocrinology*. 2005;146(2):879-888.

279. Cox JE, Randich A. Enhancement of feeding suppression by PYY(3-36) in rats with area postrema ablations. *Peptides*. 2004;25(6):985-989.

280. Pittner RA, Moore CX, Bhavsar SP, et al. Effects of PYY[3-36] in rodent models of diabetes and obesity. *Int J Obes Relat Metab Disord*. 2004; 28(8):963-971.

281. Moran TH, Smedh U, Kinzig KP, et al. Peptide YY(3-36) inhibits gastric emptying and produces acute reductions in food intake in rhesus monkeys. *Am J Physiol Regul Integr Comp Physiol*. 2005;288(2):R384-R388.

282. Halatchev IG, Ellacott KL, Fan W, Cone RD. Peptide YY3-36 inhibits food intake in mice through a melanocortin-4 receptor-independent mechanism. *Endocrinology*. 2004;145(6):2585-2590.

283. Abbott CR, Monteiro M, Small CJ, et al. The inhibitory effects of peripheral administration of peptide YY(3-36) and glucagon-like peptide-1 on food intake are attenuated by ablation of the vagal-brainstem-hypothalamic pathway. *Brain Res*. 2005;1044(1):127-131.

284. Martin NM, Small CJ, Sajedi A, et al. Pre-obese and obese agouti mice are sensitive to the anorectic effects of peptide YY(3-36) but resistant to ghrelin. *Int J Obes Relat Metab Disord*. 2004;28(7):886-893.

285. Batterham RL, Heffron H, Kapoor S, et al. Critical role for peptide YY in protein-mediated satiation and body-weight regulation. *Cell Metab*. 2006;4(3):223-233.

286. Boey D, Lin S, Karl T, et al. Peptide YY ablation in mice leads to the development of hyperinsulinaemia and obesity. *Diabetologia*. 2006;49: 1360-1370.

287. Kojima M, Hosoda H, Date Y, et al. Ghrelin is a growth-hormone-releasing acylated peptide from stomach. *Nature*. 1999;402:656-660.

288. Kojima M, Hosoda H, Matsuo H, Kangawa K. Ghrelin: discovery of the natural endogenous ligand for the growth hormone secretagogue receptor. *Trends Endocrinol Metab*. 2001;12:118-122.

289. Ariyasu H, Takaya K, Tagami T, et al. Stomach is a major source of circulating ghrelin, and feeding state determines plasma ghrelin-like immunoreactivity levels in humans. *J Clin Endocrinol Metab*. 2001; 86(10):4753-4758.

290. Tschop M, Wawarta R, Riepl RL, et al. Post-prandial decrease of circulating human ghrelin levels. *J Endocrinol Invest*. 2001;24(6):RC19-RC21.

291. Tschop M, Smiley DL, Heiman ML. Ghrelin induces adiposity in rodents. *Nature*. 2000;407:908-913.

292. Cummings DE, Purnell JQ, Frayo RS, et al. A preprandial rise in plasma ghrelin levels suggest a role in meal initiation in humans. *Diabetes*. 2001;50:1714-1719.

293. Willesen M, Kristensen P, Romer J. Co-localization of growth hormone secretagogue receptor and NPY mRNA in the arcuate nucleus of the rat. *Neuroendocrinology*. 1999;70(5):306-316.

294. Hewson AK, Dickson SL. Systemic administration of ghrelin induces Fos and Egr-1 proteins in the hypothalamic arcuate nucleus of fasted and fed rats. *J Neuroendocrinol*. 2000;12:1047-1049.

295. Kamegai J, Tamura H, Shimizu T, et al. Central effect of ghrelin, an endogenous growth hormone secretagogue, on hypothalamic peptide gene expression. *Endocrinology*. 2000;141:4797-4800.

296. Kamegai J, Tamura H, Shimizu T, et al. Chronic central infusion of ghrelin increases hypothalamic neuropeptide Y and Agouti-related protein mRNA levels and body weight in rats. *Diabetes*. 2001;50(11):2438-2443.

297. Asakawa A, Inui A, Kaga T, et al. Ghrelin is an appetite-stimulatory signal from stomach with structural resemblance to motilin. *Gastroenterology*. 2001;120:337-345.

298. Nakazato M, Murakami N, Date Y, et al. A role for ghrelin in the central regulation of feeding. *Nature*. 2001;409:194-198.

299. Shintani M, Ogawa Y, Ebihara K, et al. Ghrelin, an endogenous growth hormone secretagogue, is a novel orexigenic peptide that antagonizes leptin action through the activation of hypothalamic neuropeptide Y/Y1 receptor pathway. *Diabetes*. 2001;50:227-232.

300. Wren AM, Small CJ, Ward HL, et al. The novel hypothalamic peptide ghrelin stimulates food intake and growth hormone secretion. *Endocrinology*. 2000;141:4325-4328.

301. Wren AM, Small CJ, Abbott CR, et al. Ghrelin causes hyperphagia and obesity in rats. *Diabetes*. 2001;50(11):2540-2547.

302. Wren AM, Seal LJ, Cohen MA, et al. Ghrelin enhances appetite and increases food intake in humans. *J Clin Endocrinol Metab*. 2001;86(12): 5992.

303. Tschop M, Weyer C, Tataranni PA, et al. Circulating ghrelin levels are decreased in human obesity. *Diabetes*. 2001;50:707-709.

304. Nagaya N, Uematsu M, Kojima M, et al. Chronic administration of ghrelin improves left ventricular dysfunction and attenuates development of cardiac cachexia in rats with heart failure. *Circulation*. 2001;104(12):1430-1435.

305. Wang L, Saint-Pierre DH, Tache Y. Peripheral ghrelin selectively increases Fos expression in neuropeptide Y-synthesizing neurons in mouse hypothalamic arcuate nucleus. *Neurosci Lett*. 2002;325(1): 47-51.

306. Tamura H, Kamegai J, Shimizu T, et al. Ghrelin stimulates GH but not food intake in arcuate nucleus ablated rats. *Endocrinology*. 2002;143(9): 3268-3275.

307. Wang Q, Liu C, Uchida A, et al. Arcuate AgRP neurons mediate orexigenic and glucoregulatory actions of ghrelin. *Mol Metab*. 2014;3(1): 64-72.

308. Tschop M, Statnick MA, Suter TM, Heiman ML. GH-releasing peptide-2 increases fat mass in mice lacking NPY: indication for a crucial mediating role of hypothalamic agouti-related protein. *Endocrinology*. 2002; 143(2):558-568.

309. Date Y, Murakami N, Toshinai K, et al. The role of the gastric afferent vagal nerve in ghrelin-induced feeding and growth hormone secretion in rats. *Gastroenterology*. 2002;123(4):1120-1128.

310. Scott MM, Perello M, Chuang JC, et al. Hindbrain ghrelin receptor signaling is sufficient to maintain fasting glucose. *PLoS ONE*. 2012; 7(8):e44089.

311. Goldstein JL, Zhao TJ, Li RL, et al. Surviving starvation: essential role of the ghrelin-growth hormone axis. *Cold Spring Harb Symp Quant Biol*. 2011;76:121-127.

312. Hosoda H, Kojima M, Matsuo H, Kangawa K. Ghrelin and des-acyl ghrelin: two major forms of rat ghrelin peptide in gastrointestinal tissue. *Biochem Biophys Res Commun*. 2000;279(3):909-913.

313. Hosoda H, Kojima M, Mizushima T, et al. Structural divergence of human ghrelin. Identification of multiple ghrelin-derived molecules produced by post-translational processing. *J Biol Chem*. 2003;278(1): 64-70.

314. Yang J, Brown MS, Liang G, et al. Identification of the acyltransferase that octanoylates ghrelin, an appetite-stimulating peptide hormone. *Cell*. 2008;132(3):387-396.

315. Li RL, Sherbet DP, Elsbernd BL, et al. Profound hypoglycemia in starved, ghrelin-deficient mice is caused by decreased gluconeogenesis and reversed by lactate or fatty acids. *J Biol Chem*. 2012;287(22):17942-17950.

316. McFarlane MR, Brown MS, Goldstein JL, Zhao TJ. Induced ablation of ghrelin cells in adult mice does not decrease food intake, body weight, or response to high-fat diet. *Cell Metab*. 2014;20(1):54-60.

317. Drucker DJ. The biology of incretin hormones. *Cell Metab*. 2006; 3(3):153-165.

318. Drucker DJ, Nauck MA. The incretin system: glucagon-like peptide-1 receptor agonists and dipeptidyl peptidase-4 inhibitors in type 2 diabetes. *Lancet*. 2006;368(9548):1696-1705.

319. Thiele TE, Van Dijk G, Campfield LA, et al. Central infusion of GLP-1, but not leptin, produces conditioned taste aversions in rats. *Am J Physiol*. 1997;272(2 Pt 2):R726-R730.

320. Thiele TE, Seeley RJ, D'Alessio D, et al. Central infusion of glucagon-like peptide-1-(7-36) amide (GLP-1) receptor antagonist attenuates lithium chloride-induced c-Fos induction in rat brainstem. *Brain Res*. 1998;801(1-2):164-170.

321. Tang-Christensen M, Larsen PJ, Goke R, et al. Central administration of GLP-1-(7-36) amide inhibits food and water intake in rats. *J Physiol*. 1996;271:848-856.

322. Turton MD, O'Shea D, Gunn I, et al. A role for glucagon-like peptide-1 in the central regulation of feeding. *Nature*. 1996;379:69-72.

323. McMahon LR, Wellman PJ. PVN infusion of GLP-1-(7-36) amide suppresses feeding but does not induce aversion or alter locomotion in rats. *Am J Physiol*. 1998;274(1 Pt 2):R23-R29.

324. Flint A, Raben A, Astrup A, Holst JJ. Glucagon-like peptide 1 promotes satiety and suppresses energy intake in humans. *J Clin Invest*. 1998; 101(3):515-520.

325. Gutzwiller JP, Drewe J, Goke B, et al. Glucagon-like peptide-1 promotes satiety and reduces food intake in patients with diabetes mellitus type 2. *Am J Physiol*. 1999;276(5 Pt 2):R1541-R1544.

326. Toft-Nielsen MB, Madsbad S, Holst JJ. Continuous subcutaneous infusion of glucagon-like peptide 1 lowers plasma glucose and reduces appetite in type 2 diabetic patients. *Diabetes Care*. 1999;22(7): 1137-1143.

327. Verdich C, Flint A, Gutzwiller JP, et al. A meta-analysis of the effect of glucagon-like peptide-1 (7-36) amide on ad libitum energy intake in humans. *J Clin Endocrinol Metab*. 2001;86:4382-4389.

328. Zander M, Madsbad S, Madsen JL, Holst JJ. Effect of 6-week course of glucagon-like peptide 1 on glycaemic control, insulin sensitivity, and beta-cell function in type 2 diabetes: a parallel-group study. *Lancet*. 2002;359(9309):824-830.

329. Nakabayashi H, Nishizawa M, Nakagawa A, et al. Vagal hepatopancreatic reflex effect evoked by intraportal appearance of tGLP-1. *Am J Physiol*. 1996;271(5 Pt 1):E808-E813.

330. Imeryuz N, Yegen BC, Bozkurt A, et al. Glucagon-like peptide-1 inhibits gastric emptying via vagal afferent-mediated central mechanisms. *Am J Physiol*. 1997;273(4 Pt 1):G920-G927.

331. Lachey JL, D'Alessio DA, Rinaman L, et al. The role of central glucagon-like peptide-1 in mediating the effects of visceral illness: differential effects in rats and mice. *Endocrinology*. 2005;146(1):458-462.

332. Rinaman L. Interoceptive stress activates glucagon-like peptide-1 neurons that project to the hypothalamus. *Am J Physiol*. 1999;277(2 Pt 2):R582-R590.

333. Rinaman L, Rothe EE. GLP-1 receptor signaling contributes to anorexigenic effect of centrally administered oxytocin in rats. *Am J Physiol Regul Integr Comp Physiol*. 2002;283(1):R99-R106.

334. Secher A, Jelsing J, Baquero AF, et al. The arcuate nucleus mediates GLP-1 receptor agonist liraglutide-dependent weight loss. *J Clin Invest*. 2014;124(10):4473-4488.

335. Sawchenko PE, Swanson LW. The organization of forebrain afferents to the paraventricular and supraoptic nuclei of the rat. *J Comp Neurol*. 1983;218:121-144.

336. Elias CF, Kelly JF, Lee CE, et al. Chemical characterization of leptin-activated neurons in the rat brain. *J Comp Neurol*. 2000;423(2): 261-281.

337. Ellacott KL, Halatchev IG, Cone RD. Characterization of leptin-responsive neurons in the caudal brainstem. *Endocrinology*. 2006; 147(7):3190-3195.

338. Larsen PJ, Tang-Christensen M, Holst JJ, Orskov C. Distribution of glucagon-like peptide-1 and other preproglucagon-derived peptides in the rat hypothalamus and brainstem. *Neuroscience*. 1997;77:257-270.

339. Merchenthaler I, Lane M, Shughrue P. Distribution of pre-pro-glucagon and glucagon-like peptide-1 receptor messenger RNAs in the rat central nervous system. *J Comp Neurol*. 1999;403(2):261-280.

340. Kahn SE, Andrikopoulos S, Verchere CB. Islet amyloid: a long-recognized but underappreciated pathological feature of type 2 diabetes. *Diabetes*. 1999;48(2):241-253.

341. Hoppener JW, Ahren B, Lips CJ. Islet amyloid and type 2 diabetes mellitus. *N Engl J Med*. 2000;343(6):411-419.

342. Hartter E, Svoboda T, Ludvik B, et al. Basal and stimulated plasma levels of pancreatic amylin indicate its co-secretion with insulin in humans. *Diabetologia*. 1991;34(1):52-54.

343. Butler PC, Chou J, Carter WB, et al. Effects of meal ingestion on plasma amylin concentration in NIDDM and nondiabetic humans. *Diabetes*. 1990;39(6):752-756.

344. Banks WA, Kastin AJ, Maness LM, et al. Permeability of the blood-brain barrier to amylin. *Life Sci*. 1995;57(22):1993-2001.

345. Beaumont K, Kenney MA, Young AA, Rink TJ. High affinity amylin binding sites in rat brain. *Mol Pharmacol*. 1993;44(3):493-497.

346. Morley JE, Flood JF. Amylin decreases food intake in mice. *Peptides*. 1991;12(4):865-869.

347. Arnelo U, Blevins JE, Larsson J, et al. Effects of acute and chronic infusion of islet amyloid polypeptide on food intake in rats. *Scand J Gastroenterol*. 1996;31(1):83-89.

348. Rushing PA, Hagan MM, Seeley RJ, et al. Amylin: a novel action in the brain to reduce body weight. *Endocrinology*. 2000;141(2):850-853.

349. Rushing PA, Hagan MM, Seeley RJ, et al. Inhibition of central amylin signaling increases food intake and body adiposity in rats. *Endocrinology*. 2001;142(11):5035.

350. Reidelberger RD, Arnelo U, Granqvist L, Permert J. Comparative effects of amylin and cholecystokinin on food intake and gastric emptying in rats. *Am J Physiol Regul Integr Comp Physiol*. 2001;280(3):R605-R611.

351. Bhavsar S, Watkins J, Young A. Synergy between amylin and cholecystokinin for inhibition of food intake in mice. *Physiol Behav*. 1998; 64(4):557-561.

352. Rushing PA, Lutz TA, Seeley RJ, Woods SC. Amylin and insulin interact to reduce food intake in rats. *Horm Metab Res*. 2000;32(2):62-65.

353. Chambers AP, Jessen L, Ryan KK, et al. Weight-independent changes in blood glucose homeostasis after gastric bypass or vertical sleeve gastrectomy in rats. *Gastroenterology*. 2011;141(3):950-958.

354. Peterli R, Wolnerhanssen B, Peters T, et al. Improvement in glucose metabolism after bariatric surgery: comparison of laparoscopic Roux-en-Y gastric bypass and laparoscopic sleeve gastrectomy: a prospective randomized trial. *Ann Surg*. 2009;250(2):234-241.

355. le Roux CW, Aylwin SJ, Batterham RL, et al. Gut hormone profiles following bariatric surgery favor an anorectic state, facilitate weight loss, and improve metabolic parameters. *Ann Surg*. 2006;243(1): 108-114.

356. Patriti A, Facchiano E, Gulla N, et al. Gut hormone profiles following bariatric surgery favor an anorectic state, facilitate weight loss, and improve metabolic parameters. *Ann Surg*. 2007;245(1):157-158.

357. Salehi M, Prigeon RL, D'Alessio DA. Gastric bypass surgery enhances glucagon-like peptide 1-stimulated postprandial insulin secretion in humans. *Diabetes*. 2011;60(9):2308-2314.

358. Korner J, Bessler M, Inabnet W, et al. Exaggerated glucagon-like peptide-1 and blunted glucose-dependent insulinotropic peptide secretion are associated with Roux-en-Y gastric bypass but not adjustable gastric banding. *Surg Obes Relat Dis*. 2007;3(6):597-601.

359. Korner J, Inabnet W, Febres G, et al. Prospective study of gut hormone and metabolic changes after adjustable gastric banding and Roux-en-Y gastric bypass. *Int J Obes*. 2009;33(7):786-795.

360. Valderas JP, Irribarra V, Rubio L, et al. Effects of sleeve gastrectomy and medical treatment for obesity on glucagon-like peptide 1 levels and glucose homeostasis in non-diabetic subjects. *Obes Surg*. 2011;21(7): 902-909.

361. Wilson-Perez HE, Chambers AP, Ryan KK, et al. Vertical sleeve gastrectomy is effective in two genetic mouse models of glucagon-like peptide 1 receptor deficiency. *Diabetes*. 2013;62(7):2380-2385.

362. Ryan KK, Tremaroli V, Clemmensen C, et al. FXR is a molecular target for the effects of vertical sleeve gastrectomy. *Nature*. 2014;509(7499): 183-188.

363. Hatoum IJ, Stylopoulos N, Vanhoose AM, et al. Melanocortin-4 receptor signaling is required for weight loss after gastric bypass surgery. *J Clin Endocrinol Metab*. 2012;97(6):E1023-E1031.

364. Zechner JF, Mirshahi UL, Satapati S, et al. Weight-independent effects of Roux-en-Y gastric bypass on glucose homeostasis via melanocortin-4 receptors in mice and humans. *Gastroenterology*. 2013;144(3):580-590.

365. Xu Y, Nedungadi TP, Zhu L, et al. Distinct hypothalamic neurons mediate estrogenic effects on energy homeostasis and reproduction. *Cell Metab*. 2011;14(4):453-465.

366. Frank A, Brown LM, Clegg DJ. The role of hypothalamic estrogen receptors in metabolic regulation. *Front Neuroendocrinol*. 2014;35(4): 550-557.

367. Fuente-Martin E, Garcia-Caceres C, Morselli E, et al. Estrogen, astrocytes and the neuroendocrine control of metabolism. *Rev Endocr Metab Disord*. 2013;14(4):331-338.

368. Brown LM, Clegg DJ. Estrogen and leptin regulation of endocrinological features of anorexia nervosa. *Neuropsychopharmacology*. 2013; 38(1):237.

369. Clegg DJ. Minireview: the year in review of estrogen regulation of metabolism. *Mol Endocrinol*. 2012;26(12):1957-1960.

370. Carr MC. The emergence of the metabolic syndrome with menopause. *J Clin Endocrinol Metab*. 2003;88(6):2404-2411.

371. Flegal KM, Carroll MD, Ogden CL, Johnson CL. Prevalence and trends in obesity among US adults, 1999-2000. *JAMA*. 2002;288(14): 1723-1727.

372. Freedman DS, Khan LK, Serdula MK, et al. Trends and correlates of class 3 obesity in the United States from 1990 through 2000. *JAMA*. 2002;288(14):1758-1761.

373. Drewett RF. Oestrous and dioestrous components of the ovarian inhibition on hunger in the rat. *Anim Behav*. 1973;21(4):772-780.

374. Blaustein JD, Gentry RT, Roy EJ, Wade GN. Effects of ovariectomy and estradiol on body weight and food intake in gold thioglucose-treated mice. *Physiol Behav*. 1976;17(6):1027-1030.

375. Wallen WJ, Belanger MP, Wittnich C. Sex hormones and the selective estrogen receptor modulator tamoxifen modulate weekly body weights and food intakes in adolescent and adult rats. *J Nutr*. 2001;131(9): 2351-2357.

376. Wallen K. Sex and context: hormones and primate sexual motivation. *Horm Behav*. 2001;40(2):339-357.

377. Roy EJ, Wade GN. Role of food intake in estradiol-induced body weight changes in female rats. *Horm Behav*. 1977;8(3):265-274.

378. Mueller GP. Attenuated pituitary beta-endorphin release in estrogen-treated rats. *Proc Soc Exp Biol Med*. 1980;165(1):75-81.

379. Rogers NH, Perfield JW 2nd, Strissel KJ, et al. Reduced energy expenditure and increased inflammation are early events in the development of ovariectomy-induced obesity. *Endocrinology*. 2009;150(5): 2161-2168.

380. Gao Q, Mezei G, Nie Y, et al. Anorectic estrogen mimics leptin's effect on the rewiring of melanocortin cells and Stat3 signaling in obese animals. *Nat Med*. 2007;13(1):89-94.

381. Bjorntorp P. Neuroendocrine factors in obesity. *J Endocrinol*. 1997; 155(2):193-195.

382. Bjorntorp P. Hormonal control of regional fat distribution. *Hum Reprod.* 1997;12(Suppl 1):21-25.

383. Bjorntorp P. Body fat distribution, insulin resistance, and metabolic diseases. *Nutrition.* 1997;13(9):795-803.

384. Heine PA, Taylor JA, Iwamoto GA, et al. Increased adipose tissue in male and female estrogen receptor-alpha knockout mice. *Proc Natl Acad Sci U S A.* 2000;97(23):12729-12734.

385. Ohlsson C, Hellberg N, Parini P, et al. Obesity and disturbed lipoprotein profile in estrogen receptor-alpha-deficient male mice. *Biochem Biophys Res Commun.* 2000;278(3):640-645.

386. Geary N. Estradiol, CCK and satiation. *Peptides.* 2001;22(8):1251-1263.

387. Osterlund M, Kuiper GG, Gustafsson JA, Hurd YL. Differential distribution and regulation of estrogen receptor-alpha and -beta mRNA within the female rat brain. *Brain Res Mol Brain Res.* 1998;54(1):175-180.

388. Merchenthaler I, Lane MV, Numan S, Dellovade TL. Distribution of estrogen receptor alpha and beta in the mouse central nervous system: in vivo autoradiographic and immunocytochemical analyses. *J Comp Neurol.* 2004;473(2):270-291.

389. Musatov S, Chen W, Pfaff DW, et al. Silencing of estrogen receptor alpha in the ventromedial nucleus of hypothalamus leads to metabolic syndrome. *Proc Natl Acad Sci U S A.* 2007;104(7):2501-2506.

390. Davis KE, D Neinast M, Sun K, et al. The sexually dimorphic role of adipose and adipocyte estrogen receptors in modulating adipose tissue expansion, inflammation, and fibrosis. *Mol Metab.* 2013;2(3):227-242.

391. Olofsson LE, Pierce AA, Xu AW. Functional requirement of AgRP and NPY neurons in ovarian cycle-dependent regulation of food intake. *Proc Natl Acad Sci U S A.* 2009;106(37):15932-15937.

392. Miller MM, Tousignant P, Yang U, et al. Effects of age and long-term ovariectomy on the estrogen-receptor containing subpopulations of beta-endorphin-immunoreactive neurons in the arcuate nucleus of female C57BL/6J mice. *Neuroendocrinology.* 1995;61(5):542-551.

393. de Souza FS, Nasif S, Lopez-Leal R, et al. The estrogen receptor alpha colocalizes with proopiomelanocortin in hypothalamic neurons and binds to a conserved motif present in the neuron-specific enhancer nPE2. *Eur J Pharmacol.* 2011;660(1):181-187.

394. Gao Q, Horvath TL. Cross-talk between estrogen and leptin signaling in the hypothalamus. *Am J Physiol Endocrinol Metab.* 2008;294(5):E817-E826.

395. Malyala A, Zhang C, Bryant DN, et al. PI3K signaling effects in hypothalamic neurons mediated by estrogen. *J Comp Neurol.* 2008;506(6):895-911.

396. Aad G, Abbott B, Abdallah J, et al. Measurement of the W+ W- cross section in sqrt(s) = 7 TeV pp collisions with ATLAS. *Phys Rev Lett.* 2011;107(4):041802.

397. Aad G, Abbott B, Abdallah J, et al. Search for a heavy particle decaying into an electron and a muon with the ATLAS detector in sqrt[s] = 7 TeV pp collisions at the LHC. *Phys Rev Lett.* 2011;106(25):251801.

398. Aad G, Abbott B, Abdallah J, et al. Measurement of dijet azimuthal decorrelations in pp collisions at sqrt(s) = 7 TeV. *Phys Rev Lett.* 2011;106(17):172002.

399. Aad G, Abbott B, Abdallah J, et al. Search for supersymmetry using final states with one lepton, jets, and missing transverse momentum with the ATLAS detector in radicals = 7 TeV pp collisions. *Phys Rev Lett.* 2011;106(13):131802.

400. Beguin C, Potuzak J, Xu W, et al. Differential signaling properties at the kappa opioid receptor of 12-epi-salvinorin A and its analogues. *Bioorg Med Chem Lett.* 2012;22(2):1023-1026.

401. Cai C, Che J, Xu L, et al. Tumor endothelium marker-8 based decoys exhibit superiority over capillary morphogenesis protein-2 based decoys as anthrax toxin inhibitors. *PLoS ONE.* 2011;6(6):e20646.

402. Donato J Jr, Cravo RM, Frazao R, et al. Leptin's effect on puberty in mice is relayed by the ventral premammillary nucleus and does not require signaling in Kiss1 neurons. *J Clin Invest.* 2011;121(1):355-368.

403. Dowshen N, Forke CM, Johnson AK, et al. Religiosity as a protective factor against HIV risk among young transgender women. *J Adolesc Health.* 2011;48(4):410-414.

404. Gautron L, Sakata I, Udit S, et al. Genetic tracing of Nav1.8-expressing vagal afferents in the mouse. *J Comp Neurol.* 2011;519(15):3085-3101.

405. Khanicheh E, Mitterhuber M, Kinslechner K, et al. Factors affecting the endothelial retention of targeted microbubbles: influence of microbubble shell design and cell surface projection of the endothelial target molecule. *J Am Soc Echocardiogr.* 2012;25(4):460-466.

406. Liu HZ, Wang YJ, Xu L, Li SM. Investigation into the potential of electroporation facilitated topical delivery of cyclosporin a. *PDA J Pharm Sci Technol.* 2010;64(3):191-199.

407. Liu Y, Lv L, Xiao W, et al. Leptin activates STAT3 and ERK1/2 pathways and induces endometrial cancer cell proliferation. *J Huazhong Univ Sci Technolog Med Sci.* 2011;31(3):365-370.

408. Marston OJ, Garfield AS, Heisler LK. Role of central serotonin and melanocortin systems in the control of energy balance. *Eur J Pharmacol.* 2011;660(1):70-79.

409. Morin A, Kaufmann KW, Fortenberry C, et al. Computational design of an endo-1,4-beta-xylanase ligand binding site. *Protein Eng Des Sel.* 2011;24(6):503-516.

410. Nohara K, Zhang Y, Waraich RS, et al. Early-life exposure to testosterone programs the hypothalamic melanocortin system. *Endocrinology.* 2011;152(4):1661-1669.

411. Peterson EA, Andrews PS, Be X, et al. Discovery of triazine-benzimidazoles as selective inhibitors of mTOR. *Bioorg Med Chem Lett.* 2011;21(7):2064-2070.

412. Sandoval DA, Ryan KK, de Kloet AD, et al. Female rats are relatively more sensitive to reduced lipid versus reduced carbohydrate availability. *Nutr Diabetes.* 2012;2:e27.

413. Selcher JC, Xu W, Hanson JE, et al. Glutamate receptor subunit GluA1 is necessary for long-term potentiation and synapse unsilencing, but not long-term depression in mouse hippocampus. *Brain Res.* 2012;1435:8-14.

414. Sergouniotis PI, Davidson AE, Mackay DS, et al. Recessive mutations in KCNJ13, encoding an inwardly rectifying potassium channel subunit, cause leber congenital amaurosis. *Am J Hum Genet.* 2011;89(1):183-190.

415. Sun C, Yang H, Yuan Y, et al. Controlling assembly of paired gold clusters within apoferritin nanoreactor for in vivo kidney targeting and biomedical imaging. *J Am Chem Soc.* 2011;133(22):8617-8624.

416. Tezuka A, Yamamoto H, Yokoyama J, et al. The MC1R gene in the guppy *(Poecilia reticulata)*: genotypic and phenotypic polymorphisms. *BMC Res Notes.* 2011;4(1):31.

417. Vastermark A, Schioth HB. The early origin of melanocortin receptors, agouti-related peptide, agouti signalling peptide, and melanocortin receptor-accessory proteins, with emphasis on pufferfishes, elephant shark, lampreys, and amphioxus. *Eur J Pharmacol.* 2011;660(1):61-69.

418. Whitby RJ, Stec J, Blind RD, et al. Small molecule agonists of the orphan nuclear receptors steroidogenic factor-1 (SF-1, NR5A1) and liver receptor homologue-1 (LRH-1, NR5A2). *J Med Chem.* 2011;54(7):2266-2281.

419. Xu W, Morishita W, Buckmaster PS, et al. Distinct neuronal coding schemes in memory revealed by selective erasure of fast synchronous synaptic transmission. *Neuron.* 2012;73(5):990-1001.

420. Horvath TL, Sarman B, Garcia-Caceres C, et al. Synaptic input organization of the melanocortin system predicts diet-induced hypothalamic reactive gliosis and obesity. *Proc Natl Acad Sci U S A.* 2010;107(33):14875-14880.

421. Buckman LB, Ellacott KL. The contribution of hypothalamic macroglia to the regulation of energy homeostasis. *Front Syst Neurosci.* 2014;8:212.

422. Thaler JP, Yi CX, Schur EA, et al. Obesity is associated with hypothalamic injury in rodents and humans. *J Clin Invest.* 2012;122(1):153-162.

423. Fuente-Martin E, Garcia-Caceres C, Diaz F, et al. Hypothalamic inflammation without astrogliosis in response to high sucrose intake is modulated by neonatal nutrition in male rats. *Endocrinology.* 2013;154(7):2318-2330.

424. Garcia-Caceres C, Yi CX, Tschop MH. Hypothalamic astrocytes in obesity. *Endocrinol Metab Clin North Am.* 2013;42(1):57-66.

425. Buckman LB, Thompson MM, Moreno HN, Ellacott KL. Regional astrogliosis in the mouse hypothalamus in response to obesity. *J Comp Neurol.* 2013;521(6):1322-1333.

426. Yang L, Qi Y, Yang Y. Astrocytes control food intake by inhibiting AGRP neuron activity via adenosine A1 receptors. *Cell Rep.* 2015;11(5):798-807.

427. Bingham NC, Cone RD. Regulation of orexigenic AgRP neurons: a third way? *Trends Endocrinol Metab.* 2015;26(7):339-340.

428. Tapia-Gonzalez S, Garcia-Segura LM, Tena-Sempere M, et al. Activation of microglia in specific hypothalamic nuclei and the cerebellum of adult rats exposed to neonatal overnutrition. *J Neuroendocrinol.* 2011;23(4):365-370.

429. Drake C, Boutin H, Jones MS, et al. Brain inflammation is induced by co-morbidities and risk factors for stroke. *Brain Behav Immun.* 2011;25(6):1113-1122.

430. Liu C, Lee S, Elmquist JK. Circuits controlling energy balance and mood: inherently intertwined or just complicated intersections? *Cell Metab.* 2014;19(6):902-909.

431. Kelley AE, Bakshi VP, Haber SN, et al. Opioid modulation of taste hedonics within the ventral striatum. *Physiol Behav.* 2002;76(3):365-377.

432. Kumar J, Chuang JC, Na ES, et al. Differential effects of chronic social stress and fluoxetine on meal patterns in mice. *Appetite.* 2013;64:81-88.

433. Chuang JC, Sakata I, Kohno D, et al. Ghrelin directly stimulates glucagon secretion from pancreatic alpha-cells. *Mol Endocrinol.* 2011;25(9):1600-1611.

434. Fujikawa T, Chuang JC, Sakata I, et al. Leptin therapy improves insulin-deficient type 1 diabetes by CNS-dependent mechanisms in mice. *Proc Natl Acad Sci U S A.* 2010;107(40):17391-17396.

435. Perello M, Sakata I, Birnbaum S, et al. Ghrelin increases the rewarding value of high-fat diet in an orexin-dependent manner. *Biol Psychiatry.* 2010;67(9):880-886.

436. Lutter M, Sakata I, Osborne-Lawrence S, et al. The orexigenic hormone ghrelin defends against depressive symptoms of chronic stress. *Nat Neurosci.* 2008;11(7):752-753.
437. Elmquist J, Zigman J, Lutter M. Molecular determinants of energy homeostasis. *Am J Psychiatry.* 2006;163(7):1137.
438. Chuang JC, Perello M, Sakata I, et al. Ghrelin mediates stress-induced food-reward behavior in mice. *J Clin Invest.* 2011;121(7):2684-2692.
439. Nestler EJ. Is there a common molecular pathway for addiction? *Nat Neurosci.* 2005;8(11):1445-1449.
440. Berke JD, Hyman SE. Addiction, dopamine, and the molecular mechanisms of memory. *Neuron.* 2000;25(3):515-532.
441. Laakso A, Mohn AR, Gainetdinov RR, Caron MG. Experimental genetic approaches to addiction. *Neuron.* 2002;36(2):213-328.
442. Wise RA. Brain reward circuitry: insights from unsensed incentives. *Neuron.* 2002;36(2):229-240.
443. Ikemoto S, Panksepp J. Dissociations between appetitive and consummatory responses by pharmacological manipulations of reward-relevant brain regions. *Behav Neurosci.* 1996;110(2):331-345.
444. Balleine B, Killcross S. Effects of ibotenic acid lesions of the nucleus accumbens on instrumental action. *Behav Brain Res.* 1994;65(2):181-193.
445. Szczypka MS, Kwok K, Brot MD, et al. Dopamine production in the caudate putamen restores feeding in dopamine-deficient mice. *Neuron.* 2001;30(3):819-828.
446. Szczypka MS, Mandel RJ, Donahue BA, et al. Viral gene delivery selectively restores feeding and prevents lethality of dopamine-deficient mice. *Neuron.* 1999;22(1):167-178.
447. Figlewicz DP, Evans SB, Murphy J, et al. Expression of receptors for insulin and leptin in the ventral tegmental area/substantia nigra (VTA/SN) of the rat. *Brain Res.* 2003;964(1):107-115.
448. Zigman JM, Jones JE, Lee CE, et al. Expression of ghrelin receptor mRNA in the rat and the mouse brain. *J Comp Neurol.* 2006;494(3):528-548.
449. Figlewicz DP. Adiposity signals and food reward: expanding the CNS roles of insulin and leptin. *Am J Physiol Regul Integr Comp Physiol.* 2003;284(4):R882-R892.
450. Fulton S, Woodside B, Shizgal P. Modulation of brain reward circuitry by leptin. *Science.* 2000;287(5450):125-128.
451. Zigman JM, Elmquist JK. Minireview: from anorexia to obesity—the yin and yang of body weight control. *Endocrinology.* 2003;144(9):3749-3756.
452. Vialou V, Cui H, Perello M, et al. A role for DeltaFosB in calorie restriction-induced metabolic changes. *Biol Psychiatry.* 2011;70(2):204-207.
453. Farooqi IS, O'Rahilly S. Genetic factors in human obesity. *Obes Rev.* 2007;8(Suppl 1):37-40.
454. Locke AE, Kahali B, Berndt SI, et al. Genetic studies of body mass index yield new insights for obesity biology. *Nature.* 2015;518(7538):197-206.
455. Montague CT, Farooqi IS, Whitehead JP, et al. Congenital leptin deficiency is associated with severe early-onset obesity in humans. *Nature.* 1997;387(6636):903-908.
456. Clement K, Vaisse C, Lahlou N, et al. A mutation in the human leptin receptor gene causes obesity and pituitary dysfunction. *Nature.* 1998;392(6674):398-401.
457. Considine RV, Sinha MK, Heiman ML, et al. Serum immunoreactive-leptin concentrations in normal-weight and obese humans. *N Engl J Med.* 1996;334(5):292-295.
458. Friedman JM. Leptin, leptin receptors, and the control of body weight. *Nutr Rev.* 1998;56(2 Pt 2):s38-s46, discussions 54-75.
459. Chan JL, Mantzoros CS. Role of leptin in energy-deprivation states: normal human physiology and clinical implications for hypothalamic amenorrhoea and anorexia nervosa. *Lancet.* 2005;366(9479):74-85.
460. Welt CK, Chan JL, Bullen J, et al. Recombinant human leptin in women with hypothalamic amenorrhea. *N Engl J Med.* 2004;351(10):987-997.
461. Heymsfield SB, Greenberg AS, Fujioka K, et al. Recombinant leptin for weight loss in obese and lean adults: a randomized, controlled, dose-escalation trial. *JAMA.* 1999;282(16):1568-1575.
462. Morton GJ, Schwartz MW. Leptin and the central nervous system control of glucose metabolism. *Physiol Rev.* 2011;91(2):389-411.
463. German JP, Thaler JP, Wisse BE, et al. Leptin activates a novel CNS mechanism for insulin-independent normalization of severe diabetic hyperglycemia. *Endocrinology.* 2011;152(2):394-404.
464. Bjorbaek C, Kahn BB. Leptin signaling in the central nervous system and the periphery. *Recent Prog Horm Res.* 2004;59:305-331.
465. Huo L, Gamber K, Greeley S, et al. Leptin-dependent control of glucose balance and locomotor activity by POMC neurons. *Cell Metab.* 2009;9(6):537-547.
466. Shimomura I, Hammer RE, Ikemoto S, et al. Leptin reverses insulin resistance and diabetes mellitus in mice with congenital lipodystrophy. *Nature.* 1999;401(6748):73-76.
467. Ebihara K, Ogawa Y, Masuzaki H, et al. Transgenic overexpression of leptin rescues insulin resistance and diabetes in a mouse model of lipoatrophic diabetes. *Diabetes.* 2001;50(6):1440-1448.
468. Oral EA, Simha V, Ruiz E, et al. Leptin-replacement therapy for lipodystrophy. *N Engl J Med.* 2002;346(8):570-578.
469. Coppari R, Ichinose M, Lee CE, et al. The hypothalamic arcuate nucleus: a key site for mediating leptin's effects on glucose homeostasis and locomotor activity. *Cell Metab.* 2005;1(1):63-72.
470. Morton GJ, Gelling RW, Niswender KD, et al. Leptin regulates insulin sensitivity via phosphatidylinositol-3-OH kinase signaling in mediobasal hypothalamic neurons. *Cell Metab.* 2005;2(6):411-420.
471. Goncalves GH, Li W, Garcia AV, et al. Hypothalamic agouti-related peptide neurons and the central melanocortin system are crucial mediators of leptin's antidiabetic actions. *Cell Rep.* 2014;7(4):1093-1103.
472. Krude H, Biebermann H, Luck W, et al. Severe early-onset obesity, adrenal insufficiency and red hair pigmentation caused by POMC mutations in humans. *Nat Genet.* 1998;19:155-157.
473. Hinney A, Schmidt A, Nottebom K, et al. Several mutations in the melanocortin-4 receptor gene including a nonsense and a frameshift mutation associated with dominantly inherited obesity in humans. *J Clin Endocrinol Metab.* 1999;84(4):1483-1486.
474. Vaisse C, Clement K, Durand E, et al. Melanocortin-4 receptor mutations are a frequent and heterogenous cause of morbid obesity. *J Clin Invest.* 2000;106(2):253-262.
475. Branson R, Potoczna N, Kral JG, et al. Binge eating as a major phenotype of melanocortin 4 receptor gene mutations. *N Engl J Med.* 2003;348(12):1096-1103.
476. Greenfield JR, Miller JW, Keogh JM, et al. Modulation of blood pressure by central melanocortinergic pathways. *N Engl J Med.* 2009;360(1):44-52.

Obesity

SAMUEL KLEIN • JOHANNES A. ROMIJN

KEY POINTS

- The relationship between body mass index (BMI) and health risk is influenced by body fat distribution, age, concomitant medical illness, weight gain, aerobic fitness, and ethnicity.
- Energy homeostasis involves complex molecular and physiologic processes and constant communication within and among multiple organs.
- Body size is determined by a complex interaction among genetic, environmental, endocrine, neurologic, psychological, behavioral, and developmental factors.
- The Prader-Willi syndrome is characterized by chronic hunger with excessive eating and life-threatening obesity, cognitive disabilities, short stature, and secondary hypogonadism.
- A large number of human genes have been identified that show variations in DNA sequences that might contribute to obesity.
- Currently available weight-loss treatments include dietary intervention, increased physical activity, behavior modification, pharmacotherapy, and surgery.

Obesity is a chronic and stigmatizing disease that is causally related to serious medical illnesses, impaired quality of life, and considerable economic burden due to increased health care costs and loss of productivity.[1,2] This chapter addresses the important clinical and pathophysiologic issues in obesity.

DEFINITION OF OBESITY

Body Mass Index

Although obesity represents an unhealthy excess in body fat mass, the current practical definition of obesity is determined by an assessment of BMI. BMI is calculated by dividing a person's weight (in kilograms) by height (in meters squared); alternatively, the weight (in pounds) multiplied by 704 and divided by height (in inches squared) can be used. Table 36-1 summarizes the classification of weight status by BMI proposed by the major national and international health organizations.[3-6] These guidelines were based largely on the relationship between BMI and mortality rate, not the relationship between BMI and body fat mass. Even though there is a curvilinear relation between BMI and percent body fat mass,[7] there is considerable variability in this relationship, and some people can have a normal amount of body fat but an obese BMI value because of increased muscle mass, whereas others can have excessive body fat but a lean BMI value because of decreased muscle mass.

Data from large epidemiologic studies[8,9] have demonstrated a J-shaped relationship between BMI and mortality rate (Fig. 36-1). Men and women with a BMI between 25.0 and 29.9 kg/m² are considered to be overweight, and those with a BMI greater than 30.0 kg/m² are considered to be obese. The severity of obesity is further stratified by subclassifications: class I obesity (BMI 30.0-34.9 kg/m²), class II obesity (BMI 35.0-39.9 kg/m²), and class III obesity (BMI ≥40 kg/m²). In addition, *morbid obesity* is a term used to define patients who meet criteria for bariatric surgery (BMI ≥40 kg/m², or BMI 35.0-39.9 kg/m² and one or more severe obesity-related medical complications, such as hypertension, type 2 diabetes mellitus (T2DM), heart failure, or sleep apnea). A careful review of the data from the National Health and Nutrition Examination Survey (NHANES) collected between 1971 and 2000 questions the notion that overweight is associated with increased mortality risk.[9] These data found that persons who were overweight or even had class I obesity did not have a significant increase in mortality risk.

The relationship between BMI and disease risk differs from the relationship between BMI and mortality risk. Therefore, overweight can be a risk factor for certain medical conditions without being a risk factor for mortality. The prevalence of obesity-related diseases, such as T2DM, begins to increase at BMI values lower than 25.0 kg/m² (Fig. 36-2). Therefore, if the risk for T2DM were used to define overweight and obesity, the relationship curve

TABLE 36-1

Weight Classification by Body Mass Index (BMI)

Weight Classification	Obesity Class	BMI (kg/m²)	Risk of Disease
Underweight		<18.5	Increased
Normal weight		18.5-24.9	Normal
Overweight		25.0-29.9	Increased
Obesity	I	30.0-34.9	High
	II	35.0-39.9	Very high
Extreme obesity	III	≥40.0	Extremely high

Data from the National Institutes of Health, National Heart, Lung, and Blood Institute. Clinical guidelines on the identification, evaluation, and treatment of overweight and obesity in adults: the evidence report. *Obes Res.* 1998;6(Suppl 2):51S-209S.

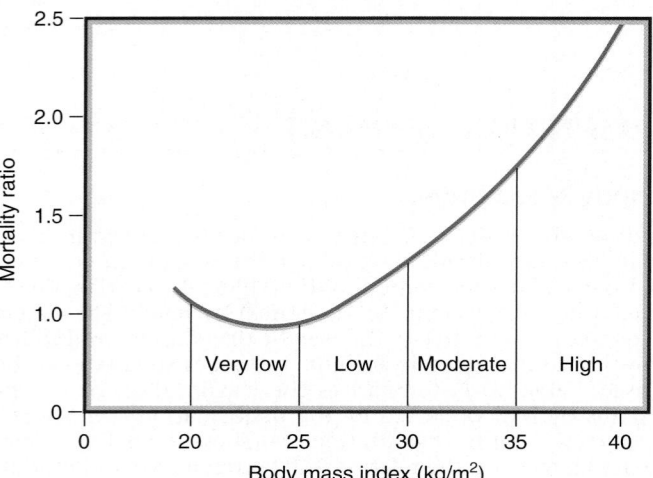

Figure 36-1 Relationship between body mass index and cardiovascular mortality risk in men and women in the United States who never smoked and had no preexisting illness. The vertical lines group underweight and lean subjects *(left side)* and overweight and obese subjects *(right side)* according to body mass index. (Based on data from Les EA, Garfunkel L. Variation in mortality by weight among 750,000 men and women. *J Chron Dis.* 1987;32:563, as adapted by Bray GA. Obesity: basic considerations and clinical approaches. *Dis Mon.* 1989;18:449.)

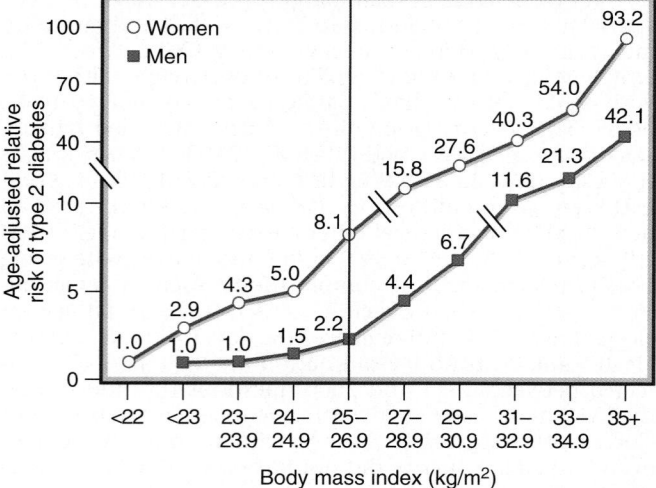

Figure 36-2 Relationship between body mass index and type 2 diabetes in men and women in the United States. The vertical line separates underweight and lean subjects *(left side)* from overweight and obese subjects *(right side)*. The data demonstrate that the risk of diabetes begins to increase at the upper end of the lean body mass index category. (Adapted from Colditz GA, Willett WC, Rotnitzky A, et al. Weight gain as a risk factor for clinical diabetes mellitus in women. *Ann Intern Med.* 1995;122:481-486; and Chan JM, Rimm EB, Colditz GA, et al. Obesity, fat distribution, and weight gain as risk factors for clinical diabetes in men. *Diabetes Care.* 1994;17:961-969.)

would be shifted to the left, and the cutoff BMI values would be lower.

Factors Affecting Body Mass Index–Related Risk

The relationship between BMI and health risk is influenced by body fat distribution, age, concomitant medical illness, weight gain, aerobic fitness, and ethnicity.

Body Fat Distribution

Obese persons with excess abdominal fat are at higher risk for diabetes, hypertension, dyslipidemia, and ischemic heart disease than obese persons whose fat is located predominantly in the lower body.[10] Those with increased lower body fat mass are protected from metabolic complications.[11-13] Waist circumference is highly correlated with abdominal fat mass and is often used as a surrogate marker for abdominal (upper body) obesity. Waist circumference is an important predictor of health outcomes in adult men and women of all age groups and ethnicities, including Caucasians, African Americans, Asians, and Hispanics. The relationship between waist circumference and clinical outcome is strongest for diabetes risk, and waist circumference is an independent and better predictor of diabetes than BMI.[14] The recommended waist circumference thresholds for increased cardiometabolic risk is 40 inches (102 cm) in men and 35 inches (88 cm)[4] in women; these cutoff values were derived from waist circumference values that correlated with a BMI of 30 kg/m² or greater.[15] However, these values are based on populations of European origin and might not be appropriate for non-Europeans.

Asian populations tend to have a higher percentage of body fat for the same BMI value and an increased prevalence of cardiovascular risk factors at lower BMI values compared with Caucasians.[16-18] Moreover, at any given waist circumference, the relative risk of mortality is higher in Asians than in African Americans or Europeans.[19] The World Health Organization (WHO) has indicated that waist circumference thresholds denoting increased risk in the Asian population should be 90 cm for men and 80 cm for women.[20] Different levels have been suggested in Japan and China, with cutoff values of 85 cm for men and 80 cm for women, and slightly lower values have been suggested in India.[21]

Age

The threshold BMI value associated with increasing relative risk of mortality increases with advancing age.[9,22]

Concomitant Medical Illness

In patients with certain medical conditions, being overweight or obese is associated with lower mortality rates than for similar patients with normal BMI values. This BMI paradox is associated with (1) cardiovascular disease (myocardial infarction,[23] congestive heart failure,[24] hypertension and coronary heart disease [CHD],[25] coronary artery bypass graft surgery,[26] heart transplant[27]); (2) renal disease (end-stage renal disease)[28]; (3) hip fractures[29]; (4) rheumatoid arthritis[30]; and (5) tuberculosis.[31]

Weight Gain

Another factor that modifies the risk of obesity-related complications is weight gain during adulthood. In both men and women, weight gain of 5 kg or more since the ages of 18 to 20 years increases the risk of developing diabetes, hypertension, and CHD, and the risk of disease increases with the amount of weight gained.[32-37]

Aerobic Fitness

The risk of developing obesity-associated diabetes or cardiovascular disease can be modified by aerobic fitness. In a cohort of more than 8000 men who were monitored for an average of 6 years, the incidences of diabetes[38] and cardiovascular fatality[39] were lower in those who were fit, as defined by maximal ability to consume oxygen during exercise, compared with those who were unfit across a range of body adiposity.

Ethnicity

BMI-associated health risk is also influenced by ethnicity.[40] At the same BMI values, Asian-Pacific populations are at increased risk for the development of diabetes and cardiovascular disease than Caucasians. Accordingly, WHO has proposed maintaining the current BMI cutoff points as international classifications in Southeast Asian populations but reducing the BMI cutoffs for potential public health action to 17.5 to 22.9 kg/m² as normal weight, 23.0 to 27.4 kg/m² as overweight, and 27.5 kg/m² or more as obese.[20]

PHYSIOLOGY OF ENERGY HOMEOSTASIS

Energy homeostasis, which can be defined as the balance between energy intake and energy expenditure and energy needed for organ growth and development in children and adolescents, involves complex molecular and physiologic processes and constant communication within and among multiple organs, particularly adipose tissue, skeletal muscle, the gastrointestinal tract, liver, pancreas, and the central nervous system. The homeostatic control of energy homeostasis relies on physiologic integration of biologic signals from these different organs as well as nutrient-related signals, postprandial neural and hormonal influences, and stimuli related to hedonic, situational, or stress-related circumstances. A complex physiologic system regulates energy homeostasis by integrating signals from peripheral organs with central coordination in the brain.[41] The hypothalamus functions as the main cerebral center in which these anorexigenic and orexigenic signals converge.[42]

A balanced interaction between two sets of neurons occurs within the arcuate nucleus of the hypothalamus. Activation of neurons secreting neuropeptide Y (NPY) and agouti-related protein (AgRP) has an orexigenic effect and promotes food intake, whereas that of neurons secreting pro-opiomelanocortin (POMC) and cocaine- and amphetamine-regulated transcript (CART) has an anorexigenic effect. The NPY/AgRP neurons also inhibit POMC/CART neurons through γ-aminobutyric acid (GABA). The orexigenic and anorexigenic signals from the NPY/AgRP and POMC/CART neurons are sent to other brain nuclei, ultimately resulting in alterations in food intake and energy expenditure. The system is very complex and involves interactions among various areas of the brain.

The endocannabinoid system is also involved in the regulation of food intake, particularly the cannabinoid 1 (CB₁) receptors (encoded by *CNR1*) and their endogenous ligands, anandamide (*N*-arachidonoyl-ethanolamine) and 2-arachidonoylglycerol. Absence of CB₁ receptors in mice with a disrupted CB₁ gene causes hypophagia and leanness.[43] Administration of cannabinoids increases food intake and promotes body-weight gain, and treatment with selective CB₁ receptor antagonists decreases food intake and body weight in obese mice.[44] Randomized controlled trials (RCTs) in obese people have shown that treatment with a CB₁ receptor antagonist decreases body weight.[45,46] Therefore, these studies demonstrated that the cannabinoid system has an important role in the regulation of ingestive behavior in animals and humans.[47]

The major peripheral organs participating in the regulation of food intake are the stomach, gut, pancreas, and adipose tissue.[42] The stomach and the duodenum secrete the orexigenic peptide ghrelin, which increases before eating and decreases after feeding. Many so-called satiety signals are transmitted to the brain via vagal afferent fibers from the gut that synapse in the nucleus tractus solitarius (NTS) in the hindbrain, which participates in gustatory, satiety, and visceral sensation. For instance, oral taste receptor cells generate information that is transmitted to the NTS by afferent sensory fibers. Insulin, secreted by the pancreas, has an anorexigenic effect through the arcuate nucleus. The PYY(3-36) form of peptide YY is secreted by the gastrointestinal tract after food ingestion and might also be anorexigenic.[48] Glucagon-like peptide-1 (GLP-1) is derived from preproglucagon and secreted in response to food ingestion by the proximal gastrointestinal tract. It exerts pleiotropic effects, including slight anorexic effects.[49] Satiety is also mediated by other gut proteins, such as cholecystokinin (CCK). Leptin, secreted by the adipose tissue, also serves as an anorexigenic signal.

PATHOGENESIS

Energy Balance

Obesity is caused by an excessive intake of calories in relation to energy expenditure over a long period of time. Large increases in body fat can result from even small, but chronic, differences between energy intake and energy expenditure. For example, consuming an additional 10 kcal every day will lead to approximately 1 lb of eventual weight gain, when body weight reaches a new steady state and energy intake equals energy expenditure.[50] It will take about 1 year to achieve 50% and approximately 3 years to achieve 95% of this increase in body weight. Consuming an extra candy bar (~220 kcal) as a snack every day will result in a gain of approximately 11 lb (5 kg) in 1 year and approximately 22 lb (10 kg) in 3 years.

Genes and Environment

Body size is determined by a complex interaction among genetic, environmental, endocrine, neurologic, psychological, behavioral, and developmental factors. The marked increase in the prevalence of obesity since the 1980s must have resulted largely from alterations in nongenetic factors that increase energy intake and reduce physical activity. For example, more meals are now eaten outside the home, there is greater availability of convenience and snack foods, serving sizes are larger, and daily physical activity has decreased because of sedentary lifestyle and work activities.

Environmental Effects in High-Risk Populations

Dramatic examples of the influence of environment on body weight have been reported globally. These examples illustrate that persons of certain genetic backgrounds are especially prone to gain weight and develop obesity-related diseases when exposed to a modern lifestyle.

Since the 1950s, striking changes in the lifestyle of Pima Indians living in Arizona have led to an epidemic of obesity and diabetes in this population.[51] The diet of these urbanized Pimas is much higher in fat (50% of energy as fat) than the traditional Pima diet (15% of energy as fat). In addition, urbanized Pimas are much more sedentary than the Pimas who remained in the Sierra Madre Mountains of northern Mexico and were isolated from Western influences. These rural Pimas eat a traditional diet and are physically active as farmers and sawmill workers; they have a much lower incidence of obesity and diabetes than their Arizona kindred. The Aborigines of northern Australia are another high-risk population whose weight and health status has been compromised by exposure to a modern environment. Urbanized Aborigines are heavier than their hunter-gatherer kindred, who are usually very lean (BMI < 20.0 kg/m²), and they have a high prevalence of T2DM and hypertriglyceridemia.[52] The traditional hunter-gatherer lifestyle of the Aborigines involves a low-fat, low-calorie diet of wild game, fish, and plants and a high level of physical activity. In one study, short-term (7 weeks) reexposure to the traditional lifestyle resulted in weight loss and significant improvements or normalization of glucose tolerance and fasting blood glucose, insulin, and triglyceride concentrations in urbanized Aborigines with T2DM and hypertriglyceridemia.[53]

Influences of Childhood and Parental Obesity

The risk of becoming an obese adult is increased both by having been obese as a child and by having had at least one obese parent. The risk of adult obesity increases with increasing age and with the severity of obesity in childhood. For example, the risk of being obese at 21 to 29 years of age ranged from 8% for persons who were obese at 1 to 2 years of age and had nonobese parents to 79% for persons who were obese at 10 to 14 years of age and had at least one obese parent.[54] Although persons who were obese at 1 to 2 years of age and had lean parents did not have an increased risk of obesity in adulthood, persons who became obese after 6 years of age had a greater than 50% chance of becoming obese adults.

Genetics and Obesity

Monogenic Causes of Obesity

Only a small percentage of obese people have a primary genetic cause for their obesity. Hundreds of people have been identified whose obesity is the consequence of single-gene mutations, such as leptin, leptin receptor, prohormone convertase 1, POMC, melanocortin 3 and 4 receptors, neurotrophin receptor TrkB (tyrosine receptor kinase B), and SIM1 (single-minded homolog 1).[55]

Leptin Gene Mutation. The pathophysiologic relevance of leptin was established in two extremely obese cousins with hyperphagia who belonged to a consanguineous family of Pakistani origin.[56] These cousins were homozygous for a single nucleotide deletion at position 398 of the leptin gene. This mutation resulted in a frameshift of the leptin-coding region and premature termination of leptin synthesis. The parents of the cousins were heterozygous for this mutation.

Another mutation, involving a homozygous single-nucleotide transversion in the leptin gene that resulted in a substitution of Trp for Arg in the mature peptide and low serum leptin levels, was discovered in three extremely obese persons, including one adult man and one adult woman, both of whom were hyperinsulinemic.[57] The man exhibited hypothalamic hypogonadism and dysfunction of the sympathetic nervous system, and the woman had primary amenorrhea.

Leptin treatment has successfully reversed the obesity of leptin-deficient patients. Treatment with recombinant human leptin resulted in a weight loss of 1 to 2 kg/month over a 12-month period. Loss of fat mass accounted for 95% of this weight loss.[58]

The possibility that leptin levels are reduced in obesity has been investigated in large groups of subjects. However, serum leptin levels increase exponentially with fat mass, suggesting that most obese persons are resistant or insensitive to body weight regulation by endogenous leptin.[59]

Leptin Receptor Mutation. Three extremely obese sisters from a consanguineous family were found to have markedly high serum leptin levels and to be homozygous for a single-nucleotide substitution at the splice site of exon 16 of the leptin receptor gene.[60] This mutation resulted in a truncated protein that lacked both the transmembrane and the intracellular domains of the receptor. The sisters displayed hypogonadotropic hypogonadism, failure of pubertal development, growth delay, and secondary hypothyroidism. This finding confirms the endocrine abnormalities in leptin-deficient subjects and implies a role for leptin and its receptor in the central regulation of energy balance and hypothalamic endocrine functions in humans.

Prohormone Convertase 1 Gene Mutation. Prohormone convertase 1 (also known as proprotein convertase 1, prohormone convertase 3, and neuroendocrine convertase 1) is an enzyme, encoded by the *PCSK1* gene, that cleaves POMC and is involved in processing proinsulin and proglucagon in pancreatic islets. Melanocortins, including α-melanocortin–stimulating hormone, are formed through the processing of POMC by PCSK1. A mutation in *PCSK1* was identified in a 43-year-old obese woman with a history of severe childhood obesity.[61] This woman had impaired glucose tolerance, postprandial hypoglycemia, low plasma cortisol levels, and hypogonadotropic hypogonadism. In addition, she had increased plasma concentrations of proinsulin and POMC but very low plasma insulin concentrations. She was a compound heterozygote for two mutations in the *PCSK1* gene, which resulted in loss of the autocatalytic cleavage ability of *PCSK1*. A second patient has also been described.[62] Therefore, reduced production of melanocortin might have been responsible for obesity in these patients.

Pro-opiomelanocortin Gene Mutation. A mutation in the POMC gene was described in two obese children with hyperphagia.[63] The children also had red hair pigmentation and were deficient in adrenocorticotropic hormone (ACTH). The mutations resulted in complete loss of the ability to synthesize α-melanocortin–stimulating hormone and ACTH. The red hair pigmentation and obesity are believed to be due to deficiency of α-melanocortin–stimulating hormone.

Melanocortin 4 Receptor Mutation. Although they are rare, mutations in the melanocortin 4 receptor (MC4R) are the most common monogenic cause of obesity.[64] Moreover, MC4R mutations are characterized by both dominant and recessive modes of inheritance, in contrast to the other monogenic forms of obesity, which have recessive modes of inheritance. In children with MC4R mutations, the degree of obesity and hyperphagia correlates with the extent of impairment of MC4R signaling. However, adult carriers of the mutations cannot be phenotypically distinguished from other obese subjects.[65]

Mutation of the Neurotrophin Receptor TrkB. The survival and differentiation of neurons in the peripheral nervous system are dependent on neurotrophic factors, which are secreted by the target tissues. Neurotrophin signaling occurs through the specific activation of receptor tyrosine kinases of the Trk family. An 8-year-old boy with a complex developmental syndrome and severe obesity was found to be heterozygous for a de novo missense mutation resulting in a Tyr722Cys substitution in the neurotrophin receptor TrkB. This mutation markedly impaired receptor autophosphorylation and signaling to mitogen-activated protein kinase. Mutation of *NTRK2*, the gene encoding for TrkB, seems to result in a unique human syndrome of hyperphagic obesity.[66]

Obesity in Pleiotropic Syndromes. About 30 mendelian disorders have been described in which obesity is a clinical feature; often, this obesity is associated with mental retardation, dysmorphic features, and organ-specific developmental abnormalities—the pleiotropic syndromes. Positional genetic techniques have led to the identification of different mutations underlying these syndromes. However, in most cases these genes encode for proteins whose functions are unresolved.[67]

Obesity Syndromes Due to Chromosomal Rearrangements

Prader-Willi Syndrome. The Prader-Willi syndrome is characterized by chronic hunger with excessive eating and life-threatening obesity, cognitive disabilities, short stature, and secondary hypogonadism. It is the most common syndromic cause of obesity, occurring in 1 of every 25,000 births.[68] In these patients, the paternal segment of chromosome 15q11.2-q12 is absent. The omission can result from deletion of the paternal segment (75%) or from loss of the entire paternal chromosome 15, with the presence of two maternal homologs (uniparental maternal disomy). The role of the genes encoded by the paternal segment and the mechanisms by which they cause the obesity syndrome have not been resolved.[68]

SIM1 Gene Mutation. A de novo balanced translocation between chromosomes 1 and 6 was found in a severely obese girl who weighed 47 kg at 67 months of age.[69] The mutation caused a disruption in *SIM1,* the human homolog of the *Drosophila* single-minded *(sim)* gene that regulates neurogenesis. *SIM1* encodes a transcription factor involved in the formation of the paraventricular and supraoptic nuclei. It is likely that this abnormality altered energy balance in this patient by stimulating food intake, because measured resting energy expenditure was normal.

Polygenic Causes of Obesity

Obesity is likely to result from the interaction of many different gene-gene and gene-environment interactions. In contrast to the small number of single-gene mutations that are rare causes of obesity, a large number of human genes have been identified that show variations in DNA sequences that might contribute to obesity.[70]

The use of the genome-wide association approach has identified over 80 loci with robust associations but usually with only modest contributions to overall genetic susceptibility to obesity or high BMI. It is a challenge to determine how these results fit into current models of the genetic architecture and pathophysiology of obesity, because no existing hypothesis explains all the data.

The first major breakthrough provided by genome-wide association studies was the discovery of the fat mass and obesity-associated gene *(FTO)* as a potential obesity gene. *FTO* encodes a 2-oxoglutarate–dependent nucleic acid demethylase. Studies of wild-type mice indicate that Fto messenger RNA (mRNA) is most abundant in the brain, particularly in hypothalamic nuclei governing energy balance, and that Fto mRNA levels in the arcuate nucleus are regulated by feeding and fasting.[71] Data from several studies have documented a strong association between fat mass or BMI and a single-nucleotide polymorphism (SNP) in *FTO* in both childhood and adult obesity. The association of this variant with BMI was replicated in 13 cohorts containing more than 38,000 subjects. Sixteen percent of the adults were homozygous for this particular SNP; they weighed about 3 kg more than the subjects without this SNP and had a 1.67-fold increased risk of obesity.[72] Another SNP, rs1121980, in the first intron of the *FTO* gene, is also strongly associated with severe adult obesity (odds ratio, 1.55) in French individuals of European ancestry.[73] The same report also showed associations of SNPs in the *FTO* gene with obesity in three additional cohorts including children or adults.[74] Three of the four most significantly associated SNPs (rs17817449, rs3751812, and rs1421085) are putatively functional. Although SNP rs9939609 in the *FTO* gene is strongly associated with T2DM, this allele is also strongly associated with an increased BMI.[72] Therefore, the association between this *FTO* SNP and T2DM was abolished by adjustment for BMI, suggesting that the risk of diabetes was due to the increase in BMI.

ENERGY METABOLISM

Total daily energy expenditure (TEE) comprises resting energy expenditure (REE), which accounts for approximately 70% of TEE; energy expended by physical activity (approximately 20% of TEE); and the thermic effect of food (TEF), which accounts for approximately 10% of TEE. REE represents the energy expended for normal cellular and organ function under postabsorptive resting conditions. Energy expended in physical activity includes the energy costs of both volitional activity, such as exercise, and nonvolitional activity, such as spontaneous muscle contractions, maintaining posture, and fidgeting. The TEF represents the energy expended in digestion, absorption, and sympathetic nervous system activation after ingestion of a meal.

Cross-sectional studies have investigated whether alterations in energy metabolism are involved in obesity. Obese persons usually have greater rates of REE than lean persons of the same height because obese persons have greater lean and adipose tissue cell mass.[75] Defects in REE or TEE have not been detected in patients with diet-resistant obesity—that is, those who maintain their weight despite the claim of strict adherence to a low-calorie diet (LCD).[76,77] Instead, such patients appear to underestimate their food intake and actually consume twice as many calories as they record in food-intake diaries. During non–weight-bearing activity (e.g., cycling), obese persons expend the same amount of energy as lean persons to perform the same amount of work.[78] However, during weight-bearing activities, obese persons expend more energy than lean ones, because more work is required to carry their greater body weight. Evidence from studies in obese and lean subjects matched for either fat mass or lean body mass suggests that obese subjects have a small (approximately 75 kcal/day) but potentially important reduction in TEF. This reduction in TEF might arise from the insulin resistance and blunted sympathetic nervous system activity that occur in obesity.[79]

Although extensive research has failed to reveal significant defects in the energy metabolism of persons who are already obese, the possibility remains that inherent abnormalities in energy metabolism contribute to the subsequent development of obesity. However, data from most studies do not support the involvement of a defect in metabolic rate in the development of obesity. In one longitudinal study, daily TEE at 3 months of age was 21% lower in infants who later became overweight compared with those who maintained a normal weight,[80] but a larger subsequent study did not confirm this finding.[81] In a longitudinal study of 126 Pima Indians, those in the lowest tertile of REE at baseline had the highest cumulative incidence of a 10-kg weight gain after 1 to 4 years.[82] In contrast, the Baltimore Longitudinal Study on Aging, which followed 775 men for an average of 10 years, did not detect a relationship between initial REE and weight change.[83] However, currently available research technology is unable to detect small but chronic defects in energy metabolism that may be clinically important. In addition, it is difficult to establish a causal relationship between energy expenditure and the development of obesity because energy metabolism measurements capture only a brief point in time and therefore may not reveal abnormalities that emerge during specific life stages.

When energy intake exceeds energy expenditure, weight gain occurs, but the amount of weight gained varies among individuals. Genetic factors can influence the amount of weight gained with overfeeding. Data from a study that fed monozygotic twins an extra 1000 kcal/day for 84 days found considerable variability in weight gained among twins but that members of each twin pair gained similar amounts of weight.[84] In another study, increase in body fat after 8 weeks of overfeeding was inversely related to changes in nonvolitional energy expenditure (e.g., fidgeting).[85] Therefore, in some persons, nonvolitional energy expenditure during periods of overingestion could be a mechanism that limits weight gain through the dissipation of excess ingested energy.

Diet-induced weight loss decreases REE, which promotes weight regain. This observation underlies the set-point theory, which posits that body weight is predetermined such that weight loss (or gain) promotes a decrease (or increase) in metabolic rate that acts to restore body weight to a preset level. In both lean and obese persons, hypocaloric feeding reduces REE by 15% to 30%. This reduction in REE cannot be completely accounted for by the accompanying decrease in body size or lean body mass and is considered a normal part of the physiologic adaptation to energy restriction.[86]

The reduction in REE that occurs during negative energy balance is transient and does not persist during maintenance of a lower body weight. As reported in several studies, long-term maintenance of weight loss is not associated with an abnormal decrease in REE or TEE when adjustments are made for changes in body composition.[87,88] In a meta-analysis of 15 studies, the REE of subjects who were formerly obese was found to be similar to that of subjects who were never obese.[89] Although the decrease in energy metabolism with weight loss is largely appropriate for the concomitant changes in body composition, this decrease might nonetheless promote weight regain.

ADIPOSE TISSUE AND TRIGLYCERIDE METABOLISM

Triglycerides stored within adipose tissue constitute the body's major energy reserve (Table 36-2). Triglycerides are a much more compact fuel than glycogen because of the energy density and hydrophobic nature of fat. Triglycerides

TABLE 36-2
Endogenous Fuel Stores in a Man Weighing 70 Kg

	Mass	
Fuel Source	Grams	Kcal
Adipose Tissue		
Triglyceride	13,000	120,000
Liver		
Glycogen	100	400
Triglyceride	50	450
Muscle		
Glycogen	500	2000
Triglyceride	300	2700
Blood		
Glucose	15	60
Triglyceride	4	35
Free fatty acids	0.5	5

yield 9.3 kcal/g on oxidation and are compactly stored as oil inside the fat cell, accounting for 85% of adipocyte weight. Glycogen, in contrast, yields only 4.1 kcal/g on oxidation and is stored intracellularly as a gel containing approximately 2 g of water for every 1 g of glycogen.

Adipose tissue is an effective storage mechanism for transportable fuel that allows mobility and survival when food is scarce. During starvation, the duration of survival is determined by the size of the adipose tissue mass. Lean persons die after only approximately 60 days of starvation, when more than 35% of body weight is lost.[90] Obese persons have tolerated much longer therapeutic fasts, even for more than 1 year, without adverse effects. In the longest reported fast, a 207-kg man ingested only acaloric fluids, vitamins, and minerals for 382 days and lost 126 kg, or 61% of his initial weight.[91]

Triglyceride Storage

The major function of adipocytes is the storage of triglycerides for future use as energy substrate. Lipogenesis from glucose makes only a limited contribution to triglyceride storage in the adipocyte.[92] Most of the triglyceride in adipocytes is derived from chylomicrons and very low density lipoprotein (VLDL) triglycerides that originate, respectively, from dietary and hepatic sources. These plasma triglycerides are hydrolyzed by lipoprotein lipase (LPL), a key regulator of fat cell triglyceride uptake from circulating triglycerides. LPL is synthesized by adipocytes and transported to the endoluminal surface of endothelial cells. The interaction of LPL with chylomicrons and VLDL releases fatty acids from plasma triglycerides, which are then taken up by local adipocytes. Plasma free fatty acids themselves can also be taken up by adipose tissue, independently of LPL.

Insulin and cortisol are the principal hormones involved in regulation of LPL activity and expression.[93] The activity of LPL within individual tissues is a key factor in partitioning triglycerides among different body tissues. Insulin influences this partitioning through its stimulation of LPL activity in adipose tissue.[94] Insulin also promotes triglyceride storage in adipocytes through other mechanisms, including inhibition of lipolysis, stimulation of adipocyte differentiation, and escalation of glucose uptake. The importance of cortisol in fat distribution is supported by the clinical appearance of patients with Cushing syndrome.

The obesity-promoting effect of cortisol can involve a synergistic effect of cortisol and insulin on the induction of LPL in adipose tissue, as has been demonstrated in vitro. Testosterone, growth hormone, catecholamines, tumor necrosis factor (TNF), and other related cytokines inhibit LPL activity.[93]

Lipolysis

The balance between triglyceride storage and lipolysis is regulated by complex hormonal and neuronal mechanisms. To become available as energy substrate, triglycerides stored within adipocytes must be hydrolyzed by hormone-sensitive lipase (HSL) and adipose triglyceride lipase (ATL) into fatty acids. These fatty acids can be released from adipocytes into the circulation. The circulating half-life of plasma fatty acids is only 3 to 4 minutes. During resting conditions, fatty acid release by adipose tissue exceeds the rate of fatty acid oxidation.[95] The excess availability of fatty acids in plasma provides a ready supply of oxidizable substrate to respond to sudden changes in energy requirements, such as are induced by exercise. The plasma fatty acids that escape immediate oxidation are usually reesterified to triglyceride in adipose tissue, muscle, or liver. These fatty acids are the major precursors of hepatic VLDL triglyceride synthesis.[96] In turn, VLDL triglycerides are secreted by the liver and redistributed throughout the body, depending on tissue-specific factors, such as the activity of LPL. These observations imply that there is continuous redistribution of triglycerides between adipose tissue and the rest of the body.

There is considerable variation within and between subjects in the rate of lipolysis and, consequently, in the level of fatty acids in plasma. Insulin and catecholamines are the major circulating hormones that influence lipolysis in adipocytes. Insulin inhibits lipolysis through its effect on HSL, whereas catecholamines stimulate lipolysis. Small changes in the plasma concentrations of insulin and catecholamines have major effects on lipolytic rate. Half-maximal suppression of lipolysis occurs at postabsorptive insulin levels, and maximal suppression of lipolysis occurs at insulin levels within the range observed after a regular meal.[97] Minor increases in resting catecholamine levels stimulate lipolysis. Other factors also modulate the rate of lipolysis. For example, growth hormone and cortisol stimulate lipolysis. In general, the effects of these other factors are less potent than the effects of insulin and catecholamines.

In contrast to the tight feedback regulation of insulin secretion by glucose levels, insulin and catecholamine concentrations are not regulated by lipolysis or fatty acid levels. Although free fatty acid levels affect glucose-stimulated insulin release, there is no feedback between insulin release and rate of lipolysis. The wide physiologic variations in plasma free fatty acid concentrations among subjects can be explained, in part, by the finely tuned dose-response effects of insulin and catecholamines on lipolysis, in combination with the absence of tight feedback regulation of insulin and catecholamine levels by free fatty acids.

Basal plasma fatty acid concentrations are often increased in obese persons, particularly those with abdominal obesity. An increased rate of free fatty acid release into plasma because of an increased rate of lipolysis from upper-body subcutaneous fat is responsible for the higher levels of circulating fatty acids.[98,99] The excess free fatty acid availability in plasma might lead to increased hepatic free fatty acid uptake, intrahepatic triglyceride content, VLDL triglyceride synthesis and secretion, intramuscular triglyceride formation, and insulin resistance.

TABLE 36-3
Adipocyte-Secreted Proteins

Category	Protein
Hormones	Leptin, resistin, angiotensinogen, adiponectin, estrogens, visfatin, angiopoietin 4
Cytokines	Interleukins 1, 6, 8, 10, monocyte chemoattractant protein 1, interferon-γ, tumor necrosis factor-α
Extracellular matrix proteins	Various subtypes of collagen-α1, various metalloproteinases, fibronectin, osteonectin, laminin, entactin, thrombospondin 1 and 2
Complement factors	Adipsin, complement C3, factor B
Enzymes	Cholesterol ester transfer protein, lipoprotein lipase
Acute phase response proteins	Alpha-1-acid glycoprotein, haptoglobin
Other	Fatty acids, plasminogen activator inhibitor 1, prostacyclin

ADIPOSE TISSUE AS AN ENDOCRINE AND IMMUNE ORGAN

Traditionally, adipocytes have been viewed as energy depots that store triglycerides during feeding and release fatty acids during fasting to provide fuel for other tissues. However, adipose tissue secretes numerous proteins that have important physiologic functions (Table 36-3). These factors participate in autocrine and paracrine regulation within adipose tissue, and, as circulating hormones, they can affect the functions of distant organs such as muscle, pancreas, liver, and the central nervous system.

The function of adipose tissue as an endocrine organ has important implications for understanding the pathophysiologic relationship between excess body fat and pathologic states such as insulin resistance and T2DM.[100,101] Not all products released by adipose tissue are produced by adipocytes. Other cells contained within the adipose tissue, including endothelial cells, immune cells, and adipocyte precursor cells, can also participate in endocrine functions. Selected proteins produced by adipose tissue are reviewed next.

Leptin

Adipocytes produce leptin and secrete it into the bloodstream. Leptin has pleiotropic effects on food intake, hypothalamic neuroendocrine regulation, reproductive function, and energy expenditure.[102,103] There is a direct relationship between plasma leptin concentrations and BMI or body fat percentage.[104] However, there can be considerable variability in leptin concentrations among persons with the same BMI, suggesting that leptin production is also regulated by factors other than adipose tissue mass. Leptin levels decrease rapidly within 12 hours after the start of starvation. Conversely, leptin levels increase in response to overfeeding.[105] Therefore, plasma leptin concentrations reflect adipose tissue mass and are influenced by energy balance. Leptin is a bidirectional signal that switches physiologic regulation between fed and starved states. Plasma leptin concentrations increase with increasing fat mass and decrease rapidly during early fasting. The relative importance of the central versus peripheral effects of leptin in body weight regulation in most obese persons is still unclear.[106]

Resistin

Resistin is another signaling polypeptide secreted by adipocytes.[107] Resistin levels are increased in mice with diet-induced and genetic forms of obesity and insulin resistance. Administration of recombinant resistin to normal mice leads to impaired glucose tolerance and insulin action. Neutralization of resistin levels leads to reduced hyperglycemia in obese, insulin-resistant mice, in part by improving insulin sensitivity. Based on these findings, it has been proposed that resistin is a hormone that links obesity to diabetes by inducing insulin resistance.

Adiponectin

Adiponectin is the most abundant secretory protein produced by adipocytes. In contrast to other secretory products of adipocytes, the plasma concentrations of adiponectin are decreased in obesity and insulin resistance. There is a close association between hypoadiponectinemia, insulin resistance, and hyperinsulinemia.[108] Conversely, adiponectin expression increases with improved insulin sensitivity and weight loss.[109] Interventions that improve insulin sensitivity, such as weight loss or treatment with thiazolidinediones, are associated with increased adipose tissue adiponectin gene expression and plasma concentrations.[110] Moreover, administration of recombinant adiponectin exerts glucose-lowering effects and ameliorates insulin resistance in mouse models of obesity or diabetes.[111] These data suggest that decreased plasma levels of adiponectin contribute to some of the metabolic complications associated with obesity.

Estrogens

Adipose tissue has P450 aromatase activity. This enzyme is important for transforming androstenedione into estrone. Estrone is the second major circulating estrogen in premenopausal women and the most important estrogen in postmenopausal women.[101] The conversion rate of androstenedione into estrone increases with age and obesity, and it is higher in women with lower-body obesity than in those with upper-body obesity. In addition to a role in endocrine regulation, the effects of P450 aromatase on estrogen metabolism might also have a role in autocrine and paracrine action, because estrogen receptors are present in adipose tissue.

Selected Cytokines

Tumor Necrosis Factor-α

Adipocytes secrete TNF-α, and TNF-α expression is increased in the enlarged adipocytes of obese subjects.[112] However, plasma TNF-α levels are generally at or below the detection limit of available assays, which suggests that the TNF-α produced in adipose tissue has paracrine, rather than endocrine, functions. The multiple effects of TNF-α on adipocytes include impairment of insulin signaling. Therefore, it has been proposed that TNF-α may partially contribute to insulin resistance in obesity.[100]

Interleukin 6

Adipose tissue interleukin 6 (IL-6) secretion may account for 30% of circulating IL-6.[113,114] Obesity is associated with increased plasma IL-6 concentrations, which may contribute to systemic inflammation and insulin resistance. Insulin sensitivity is inversely related to plasma IL-6 levels,[115] and IL-6 directly impairs insulin signaling.[116]

Administration of IL-6 to human subjects induces dose-dependent increases in fasting blood glucose, probably by stimulating release of glucagon and other counterregulatory hormones or by inducing peripheral resistance to insulin action, or both.[117]

ADIPOCYTE BIOLOGY

White Adipose Tissue

Obesity is associated with an increased number of adipocytes. A lean adult has about 35 billion adipocytes, each containing approximately 0.4 to 0.6 µg of triglyceride; an extremely obese adult can have four times as many adipocytes (125 billion), each containing twice as much lipid (0.8 to 1.2 µg of triglyceride).[118]

Understanding of adipocyte differentiation is largely derived from studies conducted in preadipocytes in culture.[119,120] The current concept is that adipocytes are derived from fibroblast precursor cells after the concerted actions of extracellular signals and intrinsic transcription factors and coactivators.

The cornerstone of obesity therapy is to increase the use of endogenous fat stores as fuel by reducing energy intake below energy expenditure. The composition of weight loss induced by calorie restriction is approximately 75% to 85% fat and 15% to 25% fat-free mass (FFM).[121]

The distribution of fat loss is characterized by regional heterogeneity.[122,123] Relative losses of intra-abdominal fat are greater than the relative losses of subcutaneous and total body fat masses. A decrease in the size (triglyceride content) of existing adipocytes accounts for most, if not all, of the fat loss.[124] In humans, there is also evidence that the number of adipocytes is reduced with large, long-term fat loss.[125] However, it is possible that this perception of decreased fat cell number is false owing to inability of standard cell counting techniques to detect adipocytes that have undergone marked shrinkage.

There are two possible mechanisms through which weight loss could eliminate fat cells: dedifferentiation (the morphologic and biochemical reversion of mature adipocytes to preadipocytes) and apoptosis. Adipocyte dedifferentiation has been observed in vitro, but there is no evidence that it occurs in vivo.[126] Adipocyte apoptosis has been induced in vitro,[127] and it has been demonstrated to occur in vivo in some patients with cancer.[128] To date, it is not known whether diet-mediated weight loss induces adipocyte apoptosis.

Brown Adipose Tissue

The recent identification of brown adipose tissue (BAT) in humans has greatly stimulated the interest in BAT biology. BAT is structurally different from white adipose tissue; it contains multilocular fat vacuoles and large mitochondria and is intensively innervated by sympathetic nerves.[129] In humans, biopsies of areas of uncoupling protein 1 (UCP1) activity identified by positron emission tomography provided histologic confirmation of the presence of supraclavicular BAT.[130,131] UCP1 activity was stimulated by cold exposure.[132] Another study in humans documented a very strong seasonal variation in the presence of BAT.[133] In rodents, BAT is very important for nonshivering thermogenesis. The uncoupling of phosphorylation in BAT results from the activity of UCP1 within the inner mitochondrial membrane, which exhausts the electrochemical gradient needed for oxidative phosphorylation by creating a proton leak. BAT consequently affects energy expenditure by producing heat from uncoupled phosphorylation.[129]

It is possible that altered regulation of BAT activity is involved in the pathogenesis of obesity. Several studies showed that human BAT activity is negatively associated with age, obesity, and type 2 diabetes.[134] Conversely, weight loss after bariatric surgery is associated with increased BAT activity.[135] Nonetheless, at present these observational studies do not provide adequate evidence of a causal relation between BAT activity and fat mass in people.

PREVALENCE OF OBESITY

The global prevalence of obesity in children and adults has continued to increase from 1980 to 2013 in both developed and developing countries. Island nations in the Pacific and the Caribbean and countries in the Middle East and Central America have the highest prevalence rates of obesity.[136] The prevalence of obesity in adults in the United States has more than doubled, from 13% to 32%, since 1960,[137] but there has been no significant change in obesity prevalence in the period between 2003 and 2004 and 2011 and 2012.[138]

Data from the 2011-2012 NHANES found 35% of adults (age ≥ 20 years) in the United States were obese.[138] Although the overall prevalence of obesity did not differ between men and women, it was much higher in non-Hispanic black women (57%) than men (37%). In addition, the prevalence of obesity was higher among non-Hispanic black (48%), Hispanic (43%), and non-Hispanic white (33%) adults than among non-Hispanic Asian adults (11%).

In children, the diagnosis of obesity is based on data from National Center for Health Statistics growth charts; the BMI normal range changes with age and is different in boys and girls. In infants (birth to 36 months), *obesity* is defined as weight in the 95th percentile or greater for length and sex. In children and adolescents (age 2-20 years), obesity is defined as a BMI in the 95th percentile or greater for age and sex. Data from the 2011-2012 NHANES found that 17% of youth (age 2-19 years) in the United States are considered obese.[138] Diseases commonly associated with obesity in adults, such as T2DM, hypertension, hyperlipidemia, gallbladder disease, nonalcoholic steatohepatitis (NASH), sleep apnea, and orthopedic complications, are now increasingly observed in children.[139]

METABOLICALLY NORMAL OBESITY

Obesity is commonly associated with alterations in metabolic function—namely, insulin resistance, diabetes, dyslipidemia (increased serum triglyceride and decreased serum high-density lipoprotein cholesterol [HDL-C]), and increased blood pressure. However, 2% to 50% of obese adults are classified as metabolically normal, depending on the criteria used to define metabolic normality, and the sex and age of the study cohort.[140-145,146] Approximately 25% of obese adults are metabolically normal based on insulin sensitivity as measured by the hyperinsulinemic euglycemic clamp technique.[140,141] In addition, NHANES data covering 1994 to 2004 indicated that 32% of obese adults were metabolically normal, defined as having no more than one cardiometabolic abnormality (i.e., blood pressure, a homeostasis model assessment of insulin resistance [HOMA-IR] value, and concentrations of plasma glucose, triglyceride, HDL-C, and C-reactive protein).[142]

Obese persons who are metabolically normal (also called uncomplicated obesity, metabolically benign obesity, and metabolically healthy obesity) have a similar percentage of

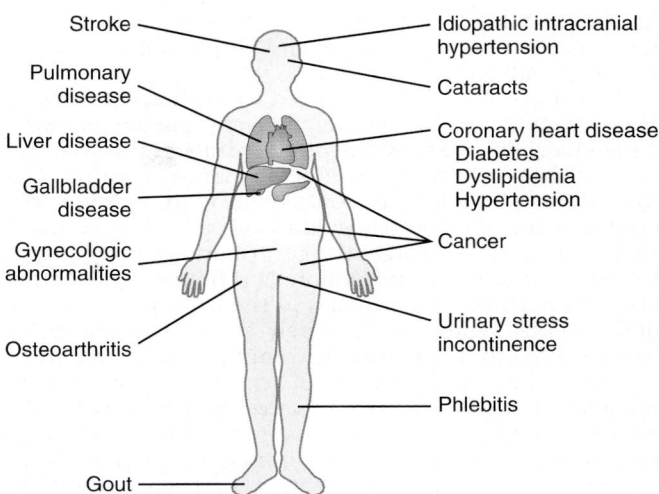

Figure 36-3 Medical complications associated with obesity.

body fat but less visceral and liver fat than metabolically abnormal obese persons, and have normal insulin sensitivity, blood pressure, lipid profile, and inflammatory profile (plasma C-reactive protein).[140-145] Metabolically normal obese adults are at lower risk of developing diabetes or cardiovascular disease than metabolically abnormal obese adults but are at higher risk for these diseases than metabolically normal subjects of normal weight.[147-150]

CLINICAL FEATURES AND COMPLICATIONS OF OBESITY

Obesity causes many serious medical complications that impair quality of life and lead to increased morbidity and premature death (Fig. 36-3).

Endocrine and Metabolic Diseases
The Dysmetabolic Syndrome
In the dysmetabolic syndrome, also known as metabolic syndrome, insulin-resistance syndrome, or syndrome X, the specific phenotype of upper-body (or abdominal) obesity is associated with a cluster of metabolic risk factors for CHD. Features of this syndrome include insulin resistance with associated hyperinsulinemia, impaired glucose tolerance, impaired insulin-mediated glucose disposal, and T2DM; dyslipidemia, characterized by hypertriglyceridemia and low serum HDL-C levels; and hypertension. Other metabolic risk factors, including increased serum levels of apolipoprotein B; small, dense low-density lipoprotein (LDL) particles; and plasminogen activator inhibitor 1 (PAI1, encoded by *SERPINE1*) with impaired fibrinolysis, have also been associated with abdominal obesity.[151] The dysmetabolic syndrome usually occurs in persons with frank obesity, but it has also been reported in normal-weight persons who presumably have an increased amount of abdominal fat.[152]

The dysmetabolic syndrome was originally identified and defined on the basis of epidemiologic associations. The underlying pathogenesis and the interrelationships among the individual features have not been completely elucidated. Insulin resistance has been hypothesized to be the common underlying pathogenic mechanism.[153] However, according to a factor analysis of data obtained from nondiabetic subjects in the Framingham Offspring Study, insulin resistance may not be the only precedent condition, and more than one independent physiologic process may be involved.[154]

Abdominal obesity is associated with insulin resistance. However, it is unclear whether visceral (omental and mesenteric) or subcutaneous deposits of abdominal fat are more closely related to insulin resistance, because data from different studies are contradictory. In addition, visceral fat mass often correlates with subcutaneous fat mass, so it is difficult to separate the contribution of each depot to insulin resistance. Furthermore, it is not known whether visceral fat actually participates in the pathogenesis of the dysmetabolic syndrome or merely serves as a marker of increased risk for the metabolic complications of obesity.[155]

The ectopic distribution of excess triglycerides in nonadipose tissue is also closely correlated with the metabolic complications of obesity. Insulin resistance to glucose metabolism in skeletal muscle is correlated with the intramyocellular concentration of triglyceride.[156] In addition, excessive intrahepatic triglyceride content is associated with a constellation of cardiometabolic abnormalities, including T2DM, dyslipidemia (high plasma triglyceride, low plasma HDL-C, or both), hypertension, the dysmetabolic syndrome, CHD, and multiorgan insulin resistance.[157-159] It is unlikely that intracellular triglycerides themselves are involved in the pathogenesis of insulin resistance, but they may be a marker of toxic fatty acid–derived metabolites or a general process that impairs insulin signaling.[160]

Type 2 Diabetes Mellitus

The marked increase in the prevalence of obesity has played an important role in the 25% increase in the prevalence of diabetes that has occurred in the United States over the past 25 years.[161] According to data from NHANES III, two thirds of the men and women in the United States with diagnosed T2DM have a BMI of 27.0 kg/m² or greater.[137] The risk of diabetes increases linearly with BMI; for example, the prevalence of diabetes in NHANES III increased from 2% in those with a BMI of 25.0 to 29.9 kg/m², to 8% with a BMI of 30 to 34.9 kg/m², and to 13% with a BMI greater than 35 kg/m².[161] In the Nurses' Health Study, the risk of diabetes began to increase when BMI exceeded the normal value of 22 kg/m² (see Fig. 36-2).[34,162] In addition, the risk of diabetes increases with increases in abdominal fat mass, waist circumference, waist-to-hip ratio, waist-to-thigh ratio, and waist-to-height ratio at any given BMI value.[163-165] The risk of diabetes also increases with weight gain during adulthood. Among men and women aged 35 to 60 years, the risk of diabetes was three times greater in those who had gained 5 to 10 kg since the age of 18 to 20 years, compared with those who had maintained their weight within 2 kg of their earlier value.[34,35]

Dyslipidemia

Obesity is associated with several serum lipid abnormalities, including hypertriglyceridemia, reduced HDL-C levels, and an increased fraction of small, dense LDL particles.[166-168] This association is especially strong in persons with abdominal obesity.[168] The serum lipid abnormalities associated with obesity are important risk factors for CHD.[169,170]

Cardiovascular Disease
Hypertension

There is a linear relationship between hypertension and BMI.[171,172] In NHANES III, the age-adjusted prevalence rates of hypertension (defined as a systolic blood pressure ≥140 mm Hg, a diastolic blood pressure ≥90 mm Hg, or use of antihypertensive medication) in obese men and women were 42% and 38%, respectively. These rates are more than twice as high as those in lean men and women (approximately 15%).[168] The risk of hypertension also increases with weight gain. Among subjects in the Framingham Study, there was a 6.5–mm Hg increase in blood pressure with every 10% increase in body weight.[173]

Coronary Heart Disease

The risk of CHD is increased in obese persons, particularly in those with increased abdominal fat distribution and in those who gained weight during young adulthood. Moreover, CHD risk starts to increase at the normal BMI levels of 23.0 kg/m² in men and 22.0 kg/m² in women.[174] In the Nurses' Health Study, the risk of fatal and nonfatal myocardial infarctions was greater in women who had the lowest BMI but the highest waist-to-hip circumference ratio than it was in women with the highest BMI but the lowest waist-to-hip circumference ratio.[175] At any BMI level, the risk of CHD increases with the presence of increased abdominal fat. The risk of fatal and nonfatal myocardial infarction also increases when 5 kg or more is gained after 18 years of age.[176]

Obesity-related CHD risk factors—particularly hypertension, dyslipidemia, impaired glucose tolerance, and diabetes—are largely responsible for the increase in CHD. However, even after adjusting for other known risk factors, several long-term epidemiologic studies still found that overweight and obesity increased the risk of CHD.[176] As a result, the American Heart Association recently classified obesity as a major preventable risk factor for CHD.[177,178]

Cerebrovascular and Thromboembolic Disease

The risk of fatal and nonfatal ischemic stroke is approximately twice as great in obese as in lean persons and increases progressively with increasing BMI.[179,180] The risks of venous stasis, deep vein thrombosis, and pulmonary embolism are also increased in obesity, particularly in persons with abdominal obesity.[181] Lower-extremity venous disease can result from increased intra-abdominal pressure, impaired fibrinolysis, and the increase in inflammatory mediators.[182,183]

Pulmonary Disease
Restrictive Lung Disease

Obesity increases the pressure placed on the chest wall and thoracic cage, which restricts pulmonary function by decreasing respiratory compliance, increasing the work of breathing, restricting ventilation (measured as decreased total lung capacity, decreased forced vital capacity, and decreased maximal ventilatory ventilation), and limiting ventilation of lung bases.[184]

Obesity-Hypoventilation Syndrome

In obesity-hypoventilation syndrome, the partial pressure of carbon dioxide (P_{CO_2}) is higher than 50 mm Hg because of decreased ventilatory responsiveness to hypercapnia or hypoxia (or both) and an inability of respiratory muscles to meet the increased ventilatory demand imposed by the mechanical effects of obesity. There is an elevation of alveolar ventilation because of shallow and inefficient ventilation related to decreased tidal volume, inadequate inspiratory strength, and elevation of the diaphragm.

Symptoms increase when patients are lying down because of increased abdominal pressure on the diaphragm. The resulting increase in intrathoracic pressure further compromises lung function and respiratory capacity.

The pickwickian syndrome is a severe form of the obesity-hypoventilation syndrome. Named after an obese character in Charles Dickens' *The Pickwick Papers,* this syndrome involves extreme obesity, irregular breathing, somnolence, cyanosis, secondary polycythemia, and right ventricular dysfunction.

Obstructive Sleep Apnea

In obstructive sleep apnea, excessive episodes of apnea and hypopnea during sleep are caused by partial or complete upper airway obstruction despite persistent respiratory efforts. Daytime sleepiness and cardiopulmonary dysfunction result from the interruption in nighttime sleep and arterial hypoxemia. In general, patients with sleep apnea are characterized by a BMI greater than 30.0 kg/m^2, excess abdominal fat, and a large neck girth (>17 inches in men, >16 inches in women).[185-187]

Musculoskeletal Disease
Gout

Hyperuricemia and gout are associated with obesity.[188,189]

Osteoarthritis

The risk of osteoarthritis, particularly in weight-bearing joints, is increased in overweight and obese persons. The knees are most often involved because much more body weight is exerted across the knees than across the hips during weight-bearing activity.[190] There is a stronger relationship between body size and osteoarthritis in women than in men; in women, even small increases in body weight can promote osteoarthritis. In a study of twins, symptomatic or asymptomatic lower-extremity osteoarthritis was found in persons who were only 3 to 5 kg heavier than their twin sibling.[191] However, metabolic dysfunction is also associated with osteoarthritis, and the number of metabolic syndrome components increases the risk of both occurrence and progression of knee osteoarthritis.[192]

Cancer

Overweight and obesity increase the risk of cancer. Based on data from a prospective study in more than 900,000 U.S. adults,[193] it was estimated that overweight and obesity could account for 14% of all deaths from cancer in men and 20% of such deaths in women. Obesity is associated with higher rates of death due to cancers of the gastrointestinal tract (liver, pancreas, stomach, esophagus, colon and rectum, and gallbladder), and kidney, multiple myeloma, and non-Hodgkin lymphoma, as well as prostate cancer in men and uterus, cervix, ovary, and postmenopausal breast cancer in women.[193] The risks of breast and endometrial cancer fatality increase with both obesity and weight gain after age 18 years.[194] The risk of breast cancer increases with increasing BMI in postmenopausal women; in premenopausal women, increased BMI may actually protect against breast cancer.[195,196]

Genitourinary Disease in Women

Obese women are often affected by irregular menses, amenorrhea, and infertility.[197] Pregnant obese women are at increased risks for gestational diabetes and hypertension[198] and delivery complications,[199] and their babies are at increased risk for congenital malformations.[200] The risk of urinary incontinence is also increased in obese women.[201] In extremely obese patients, incontinence typically resolves after considerable weight loss, such as that achieved by bariatric surgery.[202]

Neurologic Disease

Obesity increases the incidence of ischemic stroke. Obesity is also associated with idiopathic intracranial hypertension (IIH), also known as *pseudotumor cerebri*. This syndrome is manifested by headache, vision abnormalities, tinnitus, and sixth cranial nerve paresis. Although the prevalence of IIH increases with increasing BMI, the risk is increased even in persons who are only 10% above ideal body weight.[203,204] The observation that weight loss in extremely obese patients with IIH decreases intracranial pressure and resolves most associated clinical signs and symptoms suggests there is a causal relationship between obesity and IIH.[205,206]

Cataracts

Overweight and obesity are associated with an increased prevalence of cataracts.[207] Moreover, persons with abdominal obesity are at greater risk than those with lower-body obesity, suggesting that insulin resistance may be involved in the pathogenesis of cataract formation.

Gastrointestinal Disease
Gastroesophageal Reflux Disease

A higher incidence of reflux symptoms in obese compared with lean persons has been found in most[208,209] large epidemiologic studies and meta-analyses.[210,211] The relationship between increasing BMI and gastroesophageal reflux disease is greater in women than men, possibly because of increased circulating estrogen in women, which increases acid reflux.[212]

Gallstones

The risk of symptomatic gallstones increases linearly with BMI.[37,213] The Nurses' Health Study found that the annual incidence of symptomatic gallstones was 1% in women with a BMI greater than 30.0 kg/m^2 and 2% in women with a BMI greater than 45.0 kg/m^2.[213] The risk of gallstones increases during weight loss, particularly if the weight loss is rapid. This increased risk is related to increased bile cholesterol supersaturation, enhanced cholesterol crystal nucleation, and decreased gallbladder contractility.[214]

If the rate of weight loss exceeds 1.5 kg (or about 1.5% of body weight) per week, the risk of gallstone formation increases exponentially.[215] Among obese patients who underwent rapid weight loss with a very low calorie (600 kcal/day) and low-fat (1 to 3 g/day) diet[216,217] or with gastric surgery,[218] the incidence of new gallstones was approximately 25% and 35%, respectively. Gallstone formation is also promoted by the low-fat content of a very low-calorie diet (VLCD), because more than 4 to 10 g of fat in a meal is needed to stimulate maximal gallbladder contractility.[219] Therefore, increasing the fat content of a VLCD can prevent the development of new gallstones.[220] Increasing dietary fat content might not be as important in preventing gallstones in patients consuming an LCD rather than a VLCD. Administration of ursodeoxycholic acid (600 mg/day) during weight loss markedly decreases gallstone formation.[221]

Pancreatitis

Obese patients would be expected to be at increased risk for gallstone pancreatitis because of their increased prevalence of gallstones. However, few studies have addressed this issue. Several studies showed that overweight and obese patients with pancreatitis had a higher risk of local complications, severe pancreatitis, and death than lean patients.[222] It has been hypothesized that the increased deposition of fat in the peripancreatic and retroperitoneal spaces predisposes obese patients to develop peripancreatic fat necrosis and subsequent local and systemic complications.

Liver Disease

Obesity is associated with a spectrum of liver abnormalities known as nonalcoholic fatty liver disease (NAFLD), which is characterized by an increase in intrahepatic triglyceride content (i.e., steatosis) with or without inflammation and fibrosis (i.e., steatohepatitis). NAFLD has become an important public health problem because of its high prevalence, potential progression to severe liver disease, and association with serious cardiometabolic abnormalities, including T2DM, the dysmetabolic syndrome, and CHD.[157] The prevalence rate of NAFLD increases with increasing BMI.[223] The prevalence rates of steatosis and steatohepatitis are approximately 15% and 3%, respectively, in nonobese persons; 65% and 20% in persons with class I or II obesity (BMI 30.0 to 39.9 kg/m²); and 85% and 40% in extremely obese patients (BMI >40 kg/m²).[224-227] The relationship between BMI and NAFLD is influenced by racial or ethnic background and by genetic variation in specific genes.[228-230]

The presence of NAFLD is an important marker of metabolic dysfunction in obese persons, independent of BMI, percent body fat, or visceral fat mass.[231-235] NAFLD is associated with insulin resistance in liver, skeletal muscle, and adipose tissue[231,236,237]; with increased hepatic de novo lipogenesis[238,239]; and with increased VLDL-triglyceride secretion rate.[232] However, it is not clear whether the relationship between NAFLD and metabolic abnormalities is causal or simply an association. In fact, steatosis is not always associated with insulin resistance. Overexpression of hepatic diacylglycerol acyltransferase (DGAT),[240] blockade of hepatic VLDL secretion,[241] and pharmacologic blockade of beta oxidation[242] in mice cause hepatic steatosis but not hepatic or skeletal muscle insulin resistance. Steatosis in patients with familial hypobetalipoproteinemia, which is caused by genetic deficiency of apolipoprotein B synthesis and decreased VLDL secretion rate, is not accompanied by hepatic or peripheral insulin resistance.[243] This dissociation between steatosis and insulin resistance suggests that other factors associated with steatosis (e.g., inflammation, circulating adipokines, endoplasmic reticulum stress) or other unidentified metabolites affect insulin sensitivity.

BENEFITS OF INTENTIONAL WEIGHT LOSS

Effect on Morbidity

Intentional weight loss improves many of the medical complications associated with obesity. Many of these beneficial effects have a dose-dependent relationship with the amount of weight lost, and they begin after a small weight loss of only 2% of initial body weight. In addition, weight loss can decrease the risk of developing new obesity-related diseases.

Type 2 Diabetes Mellitus

Weight loss in obese patients with T2DM can improve beta-cell function, insulin sensitivity, and glycemic control. Short-term calorie restriction itself, with minimal changes in body weight, rapidly improves hepatic insulin sensitivity within 48 hours.[244] Subsequent weight loss further improves glycemic control and insulin-mediated glucose uptake by skeletal muscle.[245-247] Significant long-term improvements in fasting blood glucose, insulin, and hemoglobin A_{1c} (HbA_{1c}) concentrations and the need for diabetes medications begin after about a 5% weight loss and improve progressively with greater weight loss.[248,249] Remission of T2DM can occur with large amounts of weight loss. For example, approximately 15% weight loss after treatment with a VLCD for 8 weeks[250] or approximately 20% to 30% weight loss induced by bariatric surgery[251,252] caused complete remission in 73% to 100% of obese patients with T2DM.

Moderate weight loss and increased physical activity can prevent the development of new cases of diabetes in high-risk people.[253-255] Data reported from the Finnish Diabetes Prevention Study and the U.S. Diabetes Prevention Program demonstrated that changes in lifestyle resulting in a modest (5%) weight loss decreased the incidence of diabetes after 3 to 4 years by 58% in subjects with impaired glucose tolerance.[254,255]

Data from several studies suggest weight loss is more difficult in obese patients with T2DM than in those without diabetes.[256,257] Moreover, successful weight loss may be inversely related to the duration and severity of diabetes.[258] The reasons obese patients with diabetes are less responsive to weight-loss therapy are not known but may involve the energy-conserving effects of improved glycemic control (e.g., reduced glycosuria) and the tendency for weight gain associated with most drug treatments for diabetes.

Nonalcoholic Fatty Liver Disease

Calorie restriction with subsequent weight loss is an effective therapy for obese patients with NAFLD. A marked decrease in intrahepatic triglyceride content and improvement in hepatic insulin sensitivity occur very rapidly, within 48 hours after calorie restriction (approximately 1100 kcal/day) is initiated.[244] Progressive weight loss causes a progressive reduction in intrahepatic triglyceride content.[259,260] A weight loss of 5% to 10% improves liver biochemistries and liver histologic findings (steatosis, inflammation, ballooning, and NASH activity score).[261] Data from a 5-year longitudinal study raised concern that weight loss induced by bariatric surgery can actually worsen NAFLD by increasing hepatic fibrosis.[262] However, data from most surgical series demonstrate that weight loss induced by bariatric surgery decreases the cellular factors involved in the pathogenesis of hepatic inflammation and fibrogenesis[263] and improves the histologic findings of steatosis, inflammation, and fibrosis.[264]

Dyslipidemia

Progressive weight loss causes a progressive decrease in serum triglyceride and LDL-C concentrations and progressive increase in serum HDL-C concentration, and significant changes in triglycerides can occur with only a 2% to 4% weight loss.[249,265] The therapeutic effect of weight loss is usually greater for serum triglyceride and HDL-C concentrations than for LDL-C concentrations.[249] Serum HDL-C concentrations decrease during active weight loss but tend to increase once weight loss stabilizes.[266] The macronutrient composition of the diet can also affect the lipid profile in response to weight loss; low-carbohydrate diets tend to cause greater improvements in serum triglyceride and HDL-C concentrations, whereas low-fat diets tend to cause a greater improvement in LDL-C concentrations.[267,268]

Hypertension

Systolic and diastolic blood pressures decrease with weight loss, independent of sodium restriction.[269] In the Trials of Hypertension Prevention Phase II (TOHP II), approximately 1200 overweight and obese patients were randomly assigned to a dietary weight loss intervention or usual care.[270] The study showed a dose-response relationship between weight loss and change in blood pressure at 36 months. During the first 6 months, patients who successfully lost weight experienced a marked reduction in blood pressure. However, among patients who regained most or all of their lost weight, blood pressure steadily increased to near-baseline values.

The marked weight loss induced by gastric surgery improves or completely resolves hypertension in about two thirds of extremely obese hypertensive patients.[271] However, data from the SOS (Swedish Obese Subjects) study indicated that the beneficial effect of weight loss on blood pressure might not persist.[272] Much of the improvement in blood pressure observed at 1 and 2 years after gastric surgery disappeared by 3 years, and both systolic and diastolic pressures increased over the next 5 years. These findings imply that the current energy balance and the direction of weight change are important in blood pressure control.

A decreased incidence of hypertension with weight loss has been reported by several large, prospective, epidemiologic and intervention studies. For example, TOHP II found that persons who maintained a weight loss of at least 4.5 kg at 36 months had a 65% decrease in the risk of hypertension compared with control group participants who gained 1.8 kg.[270] The Nurses' Health Study observed a direct correlation between the risk of developing hypertension and changes in body weight among normotensive women who were observed for 12 to 15 years. With weight loss of 5.0 to 9.9 kg, the risk of developing hypertension decreased by 15%; with a loss of 10 kg or more, it decreased by 26%.[36]

Cardiovascular Disease

Modest weight loss can simultaneously affect the entire cluster of cardiovascular risk factors associated with obesity. In the Framingham Offspring Study, a weight loss of 5 lb (2.25 kg) or more over 16 years was associated with reductions of 48% (in men) and 40% (in women) in the sum of these risk factors (defined as the highest quintile of systolic blood pressure, serum triglyceride, serum total cholesterol, fasting blood glucose, and BMI and the lowest quintile of HDL-C).[273]

Improvements in cardiovascular structure and function associated with weight loss include reductions in blood volume and hemodynamic demands on the heart, left ventricular mass and chamber size, and septal wall thickness.[274] Such improvements in cardiac function may be responsible for the reduced frequency of chest pain and dyspnea reported by patients who lost weight after bariatric surgery.[275] Weight loss can also delay the progression of, and even reduce, markers of atherosclerosis, assessed by evaluating carotid-intima media thickness.[276,277]

Pulmonary Disease

Weight loss improves pulmonary function, obstructive sleep apnea, and the obesity-hypoventilation syndrome. Changes in the apnea-hypopnea index (AHI) were related in a dose-response fashion to changes in body weight. Data from a 4-year longitudinal study found that a 10% weight loss was associated with a 26% decrease, whereas a 10% weight gain was associated with a 32% increase in the AHI.[278] Moderate (~10%) weight loss at 1 year, induced by intensive lifestyle intervention, in obese subjects with T2DM had beneficial effects on the AHI that persisted at 4 years, despite an almost 50% weight regain.[279] These data demonstrate that the effect of lifestyle intervention on AHI is not entirely due to weight loss.

Reproductive and Urinary Tract Function in Women

Marked weight loss (>20% of initial body weight) has been shown to correct urinary overflow incontinence,[201] resolve amenorrhea, and improve fertility.

Effect on Mortality

The effect of intentional weight loss on mortality was addressed in three studies that obtained baseline data between 1959 and 1960 and monitored the participants for an average of 12 years.[280-282] The composite results of these studies suggested that intentional, and possibly transient, weight loss increases survival among overweight and obese persons who have T2DM. Data from two large trials demonstrated that weight loss induced by bariatric surgery improves long-term survival in morbidly obese patients.[283,284] A total of 10,000 obese subjects who underwent bariatric surgery and a matched cohort of obese subjects who did not have surgery were monitored for up to 15 years. Subjects who had surgery lost between 14% and 25% of body weight, whereas the average weight change among control subjects was less than 2%. The overall mortality rate, particularly deaths from diabetes, heart disease, and cancer, was 20% to 40% lower in patients who had surgery than in those who did not have surgery.

OBESITY THERAPY

Many obese persons can achieve short-term weight loss by dieting alone, but successful long-term weight maintenance is much more difficult to achieve. Weight cycling and yo-yo dieting are popular terms used to describe repetitive cycles of weight loss and subsequent regain.[285] Although some adverse consequences have been associated with weight cycling,[286] available data on the health effects of weight cycling are inconclusive and should not deter obese persons from attempting to lose weight.[285] Currently available weight-loss treatments include dietary intervention, increased physical activity, behavior modification, pharmacotherapy, and surgery.

Dietary Intervention

For most obese persons, negative energy balance is more readily achieved by decreasing food intake than by increasing physical activity. Therefore, dietary intervention is the cornerstone of weight-loss therapy. Weight-loss diets typically involve modifications of energy content and macronutrient composition. However, the degree of weight loss achieved depends primarily on the energy content rather than the relative macronutrient composition of the diet.

Energy Content

Weight-loss diets can be classified according to their energy content. A balanced-deficit diet of conventional foods usually contains less than 1500 kcal/day and an appropriate balance of macronutrients. LCDs contain 800 to 1500 kcal/day and are consumed as liquid formula, nutritional bars, conventional food, or a combination of these items. VLCDs contain less than 800 kcal/day and are usually high in protein (70 to 100 g/day) and low in fat (<15 g/day). Such diets may be consumed as a commercially prepared liquid formula and may include nutritional bars. VLCDs consumed as conventional foods (mostly lean meat, fish, or fowl) are known as *protein-sparing modified fasts*.

According to the treatment guidelines issued by the U.S. National Institutes of Health (NIH),[4] persons who are overweight (BMI 25.0 to 29.9 kg/m²) and have two or more cardiovascular disease risk factors and persons who have class I obesity (BMI 30.0 to 34.9 kg/m²) should decrease their daily energy intake by approximately 500 kcal. This deficit in energy intake will promote a weight loss of approximately 0.5 lb (0.23 kg) per week and result in reduction of initial weight by about 5% at 6 months. The NIH guidelines recommend a more aggressive energy deficit of 500 to 1000 kcal/day for persons with more severe obesity (BMI ≥ 35.0 kg/m²). This will produce a weight loss of approximately 1 lb/week and result in an approximate 10% weight loss at 6 months.

Total daily energy requirements can be estimated by using standard equations[287,288] or by using the Body Weight Simulator developed at the NIH[289]; all are based on the patient's size, age, sex, and activity level. However, the use of standard equations and even the Body Weight Simulator is cumbersome, the estimates of total daily energy requirements are imprecise, and the ability to formulate a diet that has a precise energy content is poor. The simple diet guidelines outlined in Table 36-4 are suggested as an alternative to developing a specific energy-deficit diet based on the patient's daily energy requirements. Patients who follow these guidelines typically lose weight. Because many patients do not fully adhere to their prescribed diet, the energy content of the diet should be regularly adjusted according to the patient's weight loss response.

More than 30 prospective RCTs have investigated the effectiveness of LCDs for weight loss.[5] The composite results of these trials indicate that a 1000- to 1500-kcal/day LCD induces a weight loss of about 8% after 16 to 26 weeks of treatment. However, these results may not be typical for LCDs prescribed in routine clinical practice, because the trial participants volunteered to enroll in a weight-loss study and most study protocols included some form of behavior modification therapy.

VLCDs induce a weight loss of about 15% to 20% in 12 to 16 weeks of treatment, but this loss is not usually maintained.[290,291] In fact, several randomized trials have shown that weight regain is greater after VLCD than after LCD therapy.[292-295] Therefore, 1 year after treatment, weight loss with a VLCD is often similar to that obtained with an LCD. In addition, there is greater risk of medical complications associated with VLCD therapy, such as hypokalemia, dehydration, and gallstone formation. Therefore, patients treated with a VLCD require closer medical supervision than those treated with an LCD.

Macronutrient Composition

Altering the macronutrient composition of the diet does not induce weight loss unless total energy intake is reduced. Low-fat diets have traditionally been prescribed for weight loss, because dietary fat increases the palatability and energy density (kcal/g) of food. The results of epidemiologic and diet intervention studies suggest that increased dietary fat intake is associated with increases in total energy intake and body weight.[296-298]

Some of the weight-loss effects of a low-fat diet may be related to the effect of dietary fat on energy density. Because the energy density of fat is so high, there is a high correlation between dietary fat content and diet energy density. According to short-term studies lasting up to 14 days, energy intake is regulated according to the weight of ingested food rather than its fat or energy content.[299-301] For example, the weight of food ingested was the same when lean and obese subjects were given either an ad libitum high-fat/high-energy-density (1.5 kcal/g) diet or a low-fat/low-energy-density (0.7 kcal/g) diet.[299] As a result, energy intake on the high-fat/high-energy-density diet (3000 kcal/day) was almost double the intake on the low-fat/low-energy-density diet (1570 kcal/day). In other studies, the weight of food ingested remained the same when subjects were given liquid diets that had the same energy density but varied in fat content (20% to 60%)[300] and when energy density was varied but fat content remained constant.[301] Providing low-energy dense foods has also been shown to enhance weight loss in longer-term, 1-year weight-loss trials.[302,303]

The weight-loss efficacy of low-carbohydrate diets has been evaluated in a series of RCTs. Several short-term (approximately 12 weeks) trials (e.g., Yang and Van Itallie[304]) have compared the effects of low-carbohydrate and high-carbohydrate diets on weight loss when energy intake was kept constant. These studies found weight loss during the first 4 weeks is greater with a low-carbohydrate diet despite equal energy intake but that weight loss between 6 and 12 weeks is the same with either diet, suggesting that, even when energy intake is the same, low-carbohydrate diets induce greater initial decline in body weight due to fluid losses. Five of six RCTs conducted in adults[305-310] found that subjects consuming a low-carbohydrate diet (approximately 25% to 40% carbohydrate) achieved greater weight loss at 6 months[305-307] but not at 12 months,[305,309,310] compared with those consuming a low-fat diet (approximately 25% to 30% fat and 55% to 60% carbohydrate). The data from these studies also found greater improvements in serum triglyceride and HDL-C, but not in serum LDL-C, in the low-carbohydrate versus the low-fat group. The decrease in body weight associated with a low-carbohydrate diet can be completely explained by a decrease in total energy intake.[311] However, the mechanism responsible for decreased energy consumption when dietary carbohydrates are restricted but fats and proteins are unlimited is not known. It could be that it is simply easier to follow and

TABLE 36-4	
Suggested Energy Composition of Initial Reduced-Calorie Diet	
Body Weight (lb)	**Suggested Energy Intake (kcal/day)**
150-199	1200
200-249	1500
250-299	1800
300-349	2000
≥350	2500

comply with a low-carbohydrate diet than a low-fat diet, and requires less behavioral counseling. For example, a multicenter, 2-year RCT found weight loss was the same at 3, 6, 12, and 24 months in obese subjects randomized to low-carbohydrate or low-fat diet therapy, when both diets were accompanied by intensive behavioral therapy.[267]

Data from a 2-year study found that a calorie-restricted Mediterranean diet—one that is rich in vegetables and low in red meat (with poultry and fish replacing beef and lamb), with up to 35% of calories from fat, primarily from olive oil and nuts—is just as effective as a low-fat, unrestricted-calorie diet and resulted in greater weight loss than conventional low-fat, restricted-calorie diet therapy.[312] Another randomized trial evaluated four diets that varied in the percentage of calories from fat, carbohydrate, and protein and found that all diets achieved the same weight loss, with maximum weight loss at 1 year and subsequent weight regain thereafter.[313] In summary, these data demonstrate that different dietary approaches can be used to achieve moderate weight loss in obese patients and that rigid prescription of a conventional low-fat diet is unwarranted.

Physical Activity

Metabolic Rate

Although there is a profound increase in energy expenditure during an actual episode of exercise, the addition of regular exercise to a weight-loss program has negligible effects on REE. In a meta-analysis of prospective RCTs that assigned obese subjects to treatment with diet alone or diet plus exercise, the addition of exercise did not circumvent the expected decline in REE when REE was adjusted for body mass.[314]

Body Composition

The composition of weight loss can be influenced by the addition of exercise to a diet program. Pooled data from two meta-analyses found that exercise can reduce the loss of FFM that occurs with weight loss.[315] When diet-induced weight loss was approximately 10 kg, regular exercise of low or moderate intensity reduced the percentage of weight lost as FFM from approximately 25% to 12%. Although the difference in weight lost as FFM was large on a percentage basis, it nonetheless represented only a small (approximately 1 kg) difference in the absolute amount of FFM lost. This preservation of FFM with exercise might not necessarily reflect preservation of muscle protein; instead, it may involve increased retention of body water and muscle glycogen. Indeed, nitrogen balance studies have not been able to detect any nitrogen-sparing effect of exercise during diet-induced weight loss in women.[316]

Diabetes and Coronary Heart Disease

Endurance exercise increases insulin sensitivity[317] and is associated with decreased risks of developing diabetes[318,38] and of dying from cardiovascular disease.[39]

Weight Loss

Increasing physical activity alone is not an effective strategy for promoting initial weight loss. Most studies have shown that moderate endurance exercise (e.g., brisk walking for 45 to 60 minutes, four times a week, for up to 1 year) usually induces only minor weight loss.[314] In obese persons, the energy deficit created by exercise is usually much less and requires more effort than the energy deficit created by a reduced-calorie diet. For example, to achieve a 300-kcal deficit an obese patient would have to walk or run approximately 3 miles or not eat a 2-oz bag of potato chips.

Although exercise alone is not an effective strategy for inducing initial weight loss, it has been proposed that increasing physical activity is an important component of successful long-term weight management. Several large-scale, cross-sectional case studies have shown that obese subjects who were successful in maintaining weight loss for 1 year or longer engaged in regular exercise.[319,320] Retrospective analyses of data from prospective randomized studies found that subjects treated with diet plus exercise who continued to exercise sustained significantly larger long-term weight losses than subjects who stopped exercising or subjects treated with diet alone.[321] The amount of exercise that is associated with weight-loss maintenance is considerable and requires expending approximately 2500 kcal/week.[322,323] This level of energy expenditure can be accomplished through vigorous activity (aerobics, cycling, or jogging) for approximately 30 min/day or more moderate activity (brisk walking) for 60 to 75 min/day. However, when the data are analyzed on an intention-to-treat basis, most prospective randomized trials do not find a statistically significant effect of exercise on the long-term maintenance of weight loss, presumably because adherence to the exercise program is often poor. Therefore, it is possible that the putative long-term beneficial effects of exercise on weight maintenance could reflect a selection bias: people who are able to maintain an aggressive physical activity program are those who are also able to maintain dietary compliance. In some people, exercise training results in compensatory mechanisms, such as increased energy intake or reduced activity during the rest of the day, that attenuate weight loss.

Behavior Modification

Principles

Behavior-modification therapy attempts to enable obese patients to recognize and subsequently alter eating and activity habits that promote their obesity. Behavior modification is derived from the classic conditioning principle that behavior is often triggered by an antecedent event. The association between the antecedent event (e.g., watching television) and the behavior (e.g., eating) is strengthened by repetition: the more often the two are paired, the stronger the association between them becomes.

Behavior modification for the treatment of obesity usually involves multiple strategies to modify eating and activity habits. These strategies include stimulus control (avoiding the cues that prompt eating), self-monitoring (keeping daily records of food intake and physical activity), problem-solving skills (developing a systematic manner of analyzing a problem and identifying possible solutions), cognitive restructuring (thinking in a positive manner), social support (cooperation from family members and friends in altering lifestyle behavior), and relapse prevention (methods to promote recovery from bouts of overeating or weight regain).

Effectiveness

Treatment by a comprehensive group behavior therapy approach typically results in the loss of about 9% of initial weight in 20 to 26 weeks.[324] After treatment ends, weight regain is commonly observed. During the year after treatment, patients usually regain about 30% to 35% of their lost weight; however, most patients sustain clinically significant weight loss of more than 5% of initial body weight.[325] Increasing the duration of behavior therapy programs has only marginally improved total weight loss, but it probably prevents the weight regain that usually occurs after treatment is stopped.[326]

Pharmacotherapy

Conventional lifestyle (diet, physical activity and behavioral education) therapy is associated with a high rate of recidivism. Therefore, the most important goal of pharmacotherapy is to maintain long-term weight loss. Pharmacotherapy should not be considered a short-term approach for weight loss, because patients who lose weight with drug therapy usually regain weight when the therapy is discontinued.[327,328] Some obese patients do not respond to drug therapy, and long-term success is unlikely if weight loss does not occur within the first 4 weeks of drug treatment.

Weight loss usually begins to plateau at around 6 months of treatment and weight begins to increase after 1 year.[327,328] This observation implies that the efficacy of weight loss medications declines with time or that obesity is a progressive disease, or both. Treatment outcome is less successful when pharmacotherapy is administered alone than when pharmacotherapy is administered as part of a comprehensive weight-loss program that includes diet, exercise, and behavior modification (Fig. 36-4).[329] Therefore, the use of obesity pharmacotherapy alone exposes patients to the full risks of the drug without the full medical benefits of more comprehensive treatment.

Table 36-5 lists the drugs currently approved by the U.S. Food and Drug Administration (FDA) for the treatment of obesity. All currently approved weight-loss drugs act as anorexiants with the exception of orlistat, which inhibits the absorption of dietary fat. Anorexiant medications enhance satiation (level of fullness during consumption of a meal, which influences the amount of food consumed), satiety (level of hunger after consumption of a meal, which influences the frequency of eating), or both. Four anorexiant drugs have been withdrawn from the market because of the increased incidence of valvular heart disease (fenfluramine and dexfenfluramine),[330] hemorrhagic stroke (phenylpropanolamine),[331] and cardiovascular events (sibutramine)[332] associated with their use.

Weight-loss pharmacotherapy is approved for patients who have no contraindications to therapy and who have a BMI greater than 30.0 kg/m² or a BMI between 27.0 and 29.9 kg/m² and an obesity-related medical condition.[333] The most commonly prescribed weight loss medication is phentermine. Orlistat, lorcaserin, and phentermine-topiramate are the only medications approved by the FDA for long-term use in the management of obesity. However, lorcaserin and phentermine-topiramate are not marketed in Europe because of safety concerns of the European Medicines Agency.

Phentermine

Phentermine stimulates the release of norepinephrine, and to a lesser extent serotonin (5-HT, 5-hydroxytryptamine) and dopamine, from nerve terminals. Only one RCT, published in 1968, evaluated the effect of at least 8 months of phentermine therapy on body weight.[334] In that study, 108 obese women were randomized to receive an LCD and treatment with either daily phentermine (30 mg/day), daily phentermine every other month alternating with daily placebo every other month, or daily placebo for 36 weeks. Of the 64 subjects who completed the study, those randomized to either continuous or every-other-month phentermine therapy achieved the same 13% weight loss, which was greater than the 5% weight loss observed in the placebo group. In a more recent trial, subjects who completed 28 weeks of therapy with one half (15 mg/day) or one fourth (7.5 mg/day) the usual dose of phentermine had a 7.4% and 6.7% weight loss, respectively, compared with 2.3% weight loss in the placebo group.[335] The most common side effects of phentermine are dry mouth, insomnia, and constipation. Although all sympathomimetic agents can increase blood pressure and heart rate, these abnormalities usually do not occur with phentermine therapy in the presence of weight loss.

Orlistat

Orlistat is synthesized from lipstatin, a product of *Streptomyces toxytricini* mold that inhibits most mammalian lipases.[336] Orlistat binds to lipases in the gastrointestinal tract and thereby blocks the digestion of dietary triglycerides. This inhibition of fat digestion reduces micelle formation and, consequently, the absorption of long-chain fatty acids, cholesterol, and certain fat-soluble vitamins. The degree of fat malabsorption is directly related in a

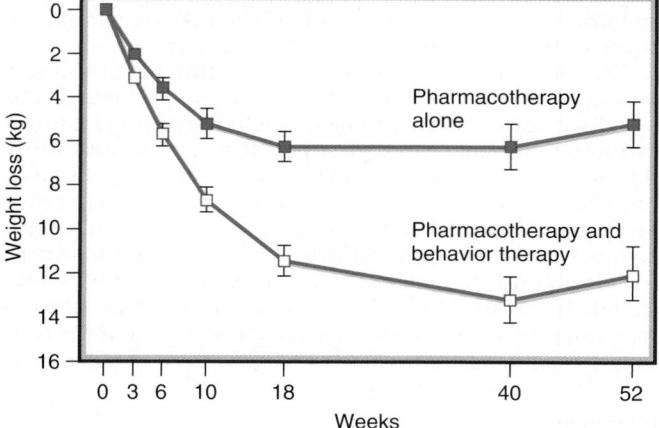

Figure 36-4 Weight loss in obese subjects treated with anorexiant medication alone, group behavioral therapy alone, or medication plus group behavioral therapy. These data demonstrate that greater weight loss is achieved when antiobesity medications are used in conjunction with lifestyle modification than when they are used alone. (Adapted from Wadden TA, Berkowitz RI, Womble LG, et al. Randomized trial of lifestyle modification and pharmacotherapy for obesity. *N Engl J Med.* 2005; 353:2111-2120.)

TABLE 36-5		
Drugs Approved by the U.S. Food and Drug Administration for the Treatment of Obesity		
Year Approved	**Generic Name**	**Trade Name**
1959	Phendimetrazine tartrate	Bontril, Plergine, Prelu-2, X-Trozine
1959	Phentermine	Ionamine, Adipex-P, Fastin, Oby-trim
1959	Diethylpropion hydrochloride	Tenuate, Tenuate Dospan
1960	Benzphetamine HCl	Didrex
1973	Mazindol	Sanorex, Mazanor
1999	Orlistat	Xenical, Ally (over the counter)
2012	Phentermine-topiramate extended release	Qsymia
2013	Lorcaserin	Belviq

curvilinear fashion to the dose of orlistat administered.[337] Excretion of about 30% of ingested triglycerides, which is near the maximum plateau value, occurs at a dose of 360 mg/day (120 mg three times daily with meals). Orlistat has no effect on systemic lipases because less than 1% of the administered dose is absorbed.[338]

Data from two meta-analyses[339,340] showed that subjects treated with orlistat lost about 3% (3 kg) more weight than those randomized to placebo at 1 year of therapy. In addition, about twice as many subjects randomized to orlistat lost at least 5% or at least 10% of their initial body weight, compared with those randomized to placebo. In a 4-year RCT, weight loss was 5% greater (11% versus 6%) at 1 year and 3% greater (7% versus 4%) at 4 years for those treated with orlistat compared with placebo.[341]

The results of several RCTs suggest that orlistat administration is associated with a reduction of serum LDL-C that is independent of the effect of weight loss alone. Even after adjusting for percent weight loss, these studies found that subjects treated with orlistat sustained a greater reduction in serum LDL-C concentrations than those treated with placebo.[342,343] The mechanism responsible for this effect may be related to orlistat-induced inhibition of dietary cholesterol absorption.[344]

The most common side effects associated with orlistat therapy are gastrointestinal complaints. Approximately 70% to 80% of subjects treated with orlistat experienced one or more gastrointestinal events, compared with 50% to 60% of those treated with placebo.[327,342,343,345-347] These gastrointestinal events were induced by fat malabsorption, usually occurred within the first 4 weeks of treatment, and were of mild or moderate intensity. Subjects rarely reported more than two episodes despite continued orlistat treatment. Orlistat treatment can also affect fat-soluble vitamin status and the absorption of some lipophilic medications.[348-350] Therefore, it is recommended that all patients treated with orlistat also receive a daily multivitamin supplement and that orlistat not be taken for at least 2 hours before or after the ingestion of vitamin supplements or lipophilic drugs.

Lorcaserin

Lorcaserin is a selective 5-HT2C receptor agonist that is thought to decrease food intake through the central POMC system. The recommended dose is 10 mg twice a day; if a patient has not lost at least 5% of baseline body weight by 12 weeks, it is recommended to discontinue drug treatment. The results from two RCTs in subjects without diabetes[351,352] and one RCT in subjects with T2DM[353] demonstrated that the 1-year placebo-subtracted weight loss was only 2% to 4%, which did not meet the FDA-proposed guidelines, but did meet the FDA criteria for adequate categorical (≥5%) weight loss. The most frequent adverse effects of lorcaserin in these studies were headache, dry mouth, dizziness, and nausea. There was no difference in the development of cardiac valvulopathy between drug-treated and placebo-treated subjects at 1 or 2 years. This cardiac safety profile supports the selectivity of lorcaserin for the 5-HT2C receptor, because the activation of the 5-HT2B receptors expressed on cardiac valvular interstitial cells was likely responsible for the valvulopathy induced by two previous weight loss drugs, fenfluramine and dexfenfluramine.

Phentermine and Topiramate Extended Release

Phentermine/topiramate extended release (ER) is a combination of phentermine and topiramate, an anticonvulsant. These two agents were combined in an effort to get synergistic weight loss while using lower doses than usually required for each drug alone, in an effort to reduce the adverse side effects of each medication when given at their normal full dose. Four different doses of phentermine and ER topiramate are available: (1) starting dose (3.75 mg/23 mg), (2) recommended dose (7.5 mg/46 mg), (3) transition dose (11.25 mg/69 mg), and (4) top dose (15 mg/92 mg). If less than 3% weight loss after 12 weeks does not occur with the recommended dose, it is advised to discontinue or advance to top dose by providing the transition dose for 2 weeks. If less than 5% weight loss is achieved after 12 weeks on the full dose, treatment should be stopped by taking the medication every other day for 1 week and then discontinue completely.

Phentermine-topiramate ER has been evaluated in two large RCTs.[354,355] Weight loss at 1 year demonstrated a dose-response relationship and was similar in both studies. In an intention-to-treat analysis after 1 year of therapy, the placebo-subtracted weight loss was approximately 9% for the top dose and approximately 6.5% for the recommended dose. A third study evaluated the potential weight loss efficacy at 2 years of therapy.[356] In that study, 78% of participants from one of the 1-year RCTs continued to receive their blinded treatment for an additional year and demonstrated that the weight loss achieved at the end of year 1 was maintained through year 2.

The most common adverse effects of phentermine-topiramate ER were dry mouth, dizziness, dysgeusia, constipation, insomnia, and paresthesia. In addition, cognitive impairment (attention or memory deficits) can occur, and there is a potential risk of fetal toxicity in pregnant women treated with topiramate (topiramate monotherapy exposure during pregnancy is associated with twofold to fivefold increased prevalence of oral clefts). Acute myopia and secondary angle closure glaucoma can also occur.

Diabetes Medications That Cause Weight Loss

Diabetes therapy usually results in weight gain.[357] However, several medications used to treat diabetes, including metformin, GLP-1 agonists, amylin, and sodium glucose cotransporter 2 (SGLT2) inhibitors cause weight loss.

The data from most studies on the effect of metformin on body weight indicated that metformin does not cause weight gain and that treatment with metformin reduces the amount of weight that is gained with other diabetes medications.[358] However, the effect of metformin on body weight in patients with diabetes is modest. For example, 10-year follow-up data from the U.K. Prospective Diabetes Study (UKPDS) found that subjects randomized to metformin therapy gained about 1.5 kg, compared with a gain of 2 kg in those treated with diet, 4 kg with glibenclamide, and 6 kg with insulin.[357] Subjects enrolled in the Diabetes Progression Outcomes Trial were randomized to monotherapy with either metformin, glyburide, or rosiglitazone for 4 years; those treated with metformin lost an average of 3 kg, whereas the glyburide and rosiglitazone groups gained an average of 1.5 kg and 5 kg, respectively.[359] The weight loss effect of metformin has also been studied in nondiabetic obese subjects. A systematic review of RCTs of metformin (duration 15 days to 1 year) in subjects without diabetes or polycystic ovary syndrome found that weight loss was usually small (≤2 kg) and insufficient to consider metformin as an effective obesity therapy.[360]

Treatment of diabetes with short- or long-acting GLP-1 agonists is usually accompanied by a decrease in body weight. A meta-analysis of 21 RCTs evaluated the effect of treatment with short-acting (exenatide) and once-daily (liraglutide) GLP-1 agonists on body weight in diabetic subjects who were treated for at least 12 weeks.[361] The data show that GLP-1 agonists caused a mean reduction in BMI of 0.4 kg/m² compared with placebo. These results are similar to those reported in another meta-analysis of 29 RCTs of at least 12 weeks' duration, which showed that treatment with exenatide in combination with other oral agents or treatment with liraglutide alone resulted in a 1.4-kg weight loss compared with placebo and a 4.8-kg weight differential compared with insulin.[362] In addition, compared with placebo therapy, liraglutide added to metformin and rosiglitazone therapy resulted in a weight loss of 1 kg (with 1.2 mg/day of liraglutide) or 2 kg (with 1.8 mg/day of liraglutide) at 6 months in obese diabetic subjects.[363] Liraglutide also causes a dose-dependent weight loss in obese patients who do not have diabetes: liraglutide given as 1.2, 1.8, 2.4, or 3.0 mg/day caused a 2- to 4-kg greater weight loss than placebo therapy and a 1- to 2-kg greater weight loss than orlistat therapy.[364]

Pramlintide, a synthetic analogue of human amylin, causes greater weight loss than placebo treatment in obese subjects with and without diabetes. In one 16-week RCT, pramlintide therapy resulted in a 3.7% placebo-corrected reduction in body weight.[365] In a second 4-month RCT, conducted in nondiabetic obese subjects, pramlintide resulted in a dose-dependent weight loss of 4.5 to 8 kg, compared with a 2.5-kg weight loss in the placebo group.[366]

SGLT2 inhibitors reduce renal glucose absorption in the proximal convoluted tubule, which causes urinary glucose excretion and 2% decrease in body weight compared with placebo therapy.[367]

Surgical Therapy
Indications

Gastrointestinal surgery is the most effective therapy for achieving major weight loss in extremely obese patients. In 1991, guidelines for the surgical treatment of obesity were established by an NIH Consensus Conference.[368] According to these guidelines, eligible candidates for surgery include patients with a BMI of 40 kg/m² or more and those with a BMI of 35.0 to 39.9 kg/m² with one or more severe medical complications of obesity (e.g., hypertension, heart failure, T2DM, sleep apnea). Additional eligibility criteria are the inability to maintain weight loss with conventional therapy, acceptable operative risks, absence of active substance abuse, and ability to comply with the long-term treatment and follow-up required. Approval to lower the BMI requirement for laparoscopic adjustable gastric banding to include patients with a BMI of 30.0-34.9 kg/m² with one or more severe medical complications of obesity was established by the FDA in 2011.

Types of Procedures

There are currently five different standard bariatric surgery procedures: (1) laparoscopic adjustable gastric banding, (2) Roux-en-Y gastric bypass (RYGB), (3) sleeve gastrectomy, (4) biliopancreatic diversion, and (5) biliopancreatic diversion with duodenal switch (Fig. 36-5).[369] Laparoscopic adjustable gastric banding involves placing a silicone ring with an inflatable inner tube around the upper stomach, just distal to the gastroesophageal junction. The inner tube

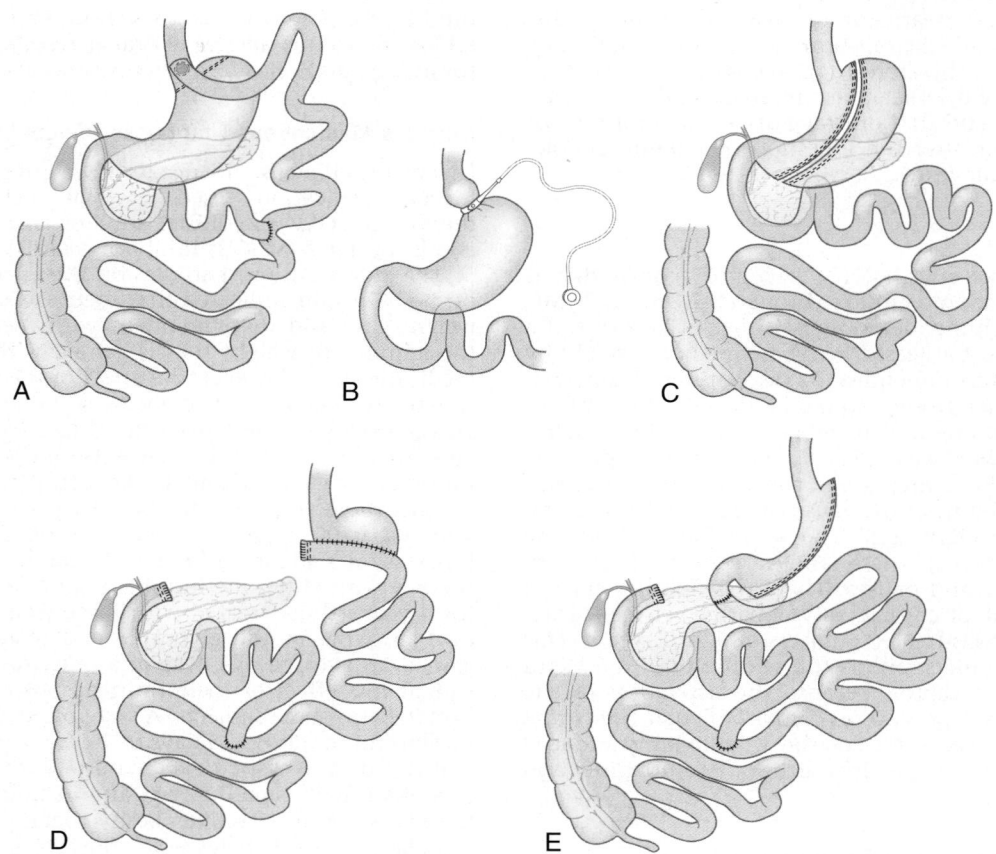

Figure 36-5 Schematic diagrams of Roux-en-Y gastric bypass (**A**), laparoscopic adjustable gastric banding (**B**), sleeve gastrectomy (**C**), biliopancreatic diversion (**D**), and biliopancreatic diversion with duodenal switch (**E**). (From Bradley D, Magkos F, Klein S. Effects of bariatric surgery on glucose homeostasis and type 2 diabetes. *Gastroenterology.* 2012;143:897-912).

is connected to a subcutaneous port, which is used to inject or withdraw saline to adjust the band diameter. Typically, six adjustments are made in the first year after band placement, as needed to enhance weight loss. RYGB involves the creation of a small gastric pouch (<30 mL) that is connected to a segment of jejunum, which has been transected at 30 to 75 cm from the ligament of Treitz, to form a Roux-en-Y limb. Bowel continuity is restored via an anastomosis between the Roux limb and the excluded biliopancreatic limb approximately 75 to 150 cm distal to the gastrojejunostomy. Sleeve gastrectomy involves dividing the stomach along its vertical length, removing approximately 75% of the stomach, and creating a banana-shaped sleeve. Biliopancreatic diversion involves a horizontal gastrectomy, leaving behind 200 to 500 mL of stomach, which is anastomosed to the small intestine, 250 cm from the ileocecal valve. The excluded biliopancreatic limb is anastomosed to the ileum, 50 cm from the ileocecal valve. The distal 50-cm common channel is where digestive secretions from the biliopancreatic limb mix with the ingested food delivered by the alimentary limb. Biliopancreatic diversion with duodenal switch involves constructing a 150- to 200-mL vertical sleeve gastrectomy with preservation of the pylorus and formation of a duodenal-ileal anastomosis. The excluded biliopancreatic limb is anastomosed to the ileum, 100 cm from the ileocecal valve, where digestive secretions and nutrients mix. Both biliopancreatic diversion and biliopancreatic diversion with duodenal switch cause considerable malabsorption.

Weight Loss

The weight loss efficacy of surgery varies according to the procedure. In general, laparoscopic adjustable gastric banding causes approximately a 20% weight loss, both RYGB and sleeve gastrectomy a 30% weight loss, and both biliopancreatic diversion and biliopancreatic diversion with duodenal switch a 35% weight loss. In addition, not all patients lose a lot of weight, and some patients who lose weight initially regain most or all of their lost weight over time.[370]

Effect of Bariatric Surgery on Type 2 Diabetes

Bariatric surgery–induced weight loss is extraordinarily effective in both preventing[371] and treating[251,372-375] T2DM. In a nonrandomized, prospective, controlled study, bariatric surgery appeared to be markedly more effective than usual care to prevent T2DM in obese subjects with a BMI of 34 kg/m² or more: 6.8 versus 28.4 cases per 1000 person-years.[251] Data from a series of RCTs have demonstrated that weight loss induced by bariatric surgery results in much better glucose control than conventional treatment with lifestyle intervention and drug therapy.[251,372-374] Moreover, bariatric surgery results in remission of T2DM in most patients. Longer duration of T2DM, inadequate postoperative weight loss, more severe diabetes requiring insulin therapy before surgery, and older age decrease the odds of achieving diabetes remission after surgery.[376-379]

The precise rate of remission is affected by the criteria used to define *remission*. No uniform definition of diabetes remission has been used routinely in bariatric surgery studies. Remission has most often been defined as the withdrawal of all diabetes medications, in conjunction with a normal fasting plasma glucose concentration (ranging from <100 to <126 mg/dL), or a normal HbA$_{1c}$ (ranging from <6% to <7%). Differences in the definition of remission among studies will obviously result in differences in estimated remission rates.[380,381] Moreover, diabetes

relapse occurs after 5 or more years in about half of the patients who achieved an early remission within 2 years after surgery.[382-384] The precise reasons for recurrence of diabetes are not known but are likely related to recidivism of weight loss because relapse or worsening of T2DM is associated with weight regain.[384]

Procedures that involve anatomic diversion of the upper gastrointestinal tract (e.g., RYGB and biliopancreatic diversion) have greater therapeutic effects in patients with diabetes than those that maintain intestinal continuity (e.g., laparoscopic adjustable gastric banding and sleeve gastrectomy). Several observations from clinical studies have led to the concept that bypassing the upper gastrointestinal tract has additional benefits on glucose homeostasis beyond weight loss alone. For example, the rates of remission of diabetes are greater in patients who have had RYGB surgery or biliopancreatic diversion, compared with those who have had banding procedures or sleeve gastrectomy,[372,375,384] and greater improvement in oral glucose tolerance associated with an increased GLP-1 response to feeding occurs after a 10-kg weight loss induced by RYGB surgery than after calorie restriction alone.[385-387]

Selected Complications

Perioperative Mortality and Morbidity. The overall early and late mortality rate is about 0% to 2%; the risk of complications and death is influenced by the type of procedure, experience of the surgeon, presence of a competent bariatric surgery team and hospital, and medical status of the patient. Approximately three fourths of the deaths that occur are caused by anastomotic leaks and peritonitis, and one fourth are caused by pulmonary embolism. Most complications that occur with any gastrointestinal surgical procedure also occur after bariatric surgery, including atelectasis, pneumonia, deep vein thrombosis, pulmonary embolism, anastomotic leak with peritonitis, wound infection, gastrointestinal bleeding, and internal hernias. In addition, dumping syndrome can occur in a subset of patients after RYGB surgery, which can usually be controlled with dietary management.

Postprandial Hypoglycemia. Severe postprandial hypoglycemia with hyperinsulinemia has been described as a rare complication of RYGB surgery.[388,389] Patients with this condition present with repeated episodes of profound symptomatic postprandial neuroglycopenia associated with endogenous hyperinsulinemia. The pathophysiologic mechanisms leading to endogenous hyperinsulinemic hypoglycemia after RYGB surgery are not clear but could be related to an inappropriately enlarged beta-cell mass or function or to abnormalities in the central nervous system response to a decrease in blood glucose concentrations.

TREATMENT GUIDELINES

The goal of weight management therapy in obese patients with T2DM is to improve or eliminate obesity- and diabetes-related health risk factors for future disease, improve or eliminate current obesity- and diabetes-related medical comorbid conditions, and improve physical function and quality of life. Weight management is a key component in the treatment of overweight or obese patients with T2DM. Even a moderate weight loss of 5% of initial body weight improves glycemic control and reduces the need for hypoglycemic medication. Moreover, moderate weight loss also improves other diabetes-related risk factors for CHD. However, successful weight management is more difficult to achieve in obese patients with T2DM than in

TABLE 36-6

Suggested Weight-Loss Treatment Options Based on BMI and Risk Factors

BMI (kg/m²)	Conventional Therapy*	Pharmacotherapy†	Surgery‡
25.0-26.9	With CHD risk factors or obesity-related disease	No	No
27.0-29.9	With CHD risk factors or obesity-related disease	With obesity-related disease	No
30.0-34.9	Yes	Yes	LAGB With obesity-related disease
35.0-39.9	Yes	Yes	With obesity-related disease
≥40	Yes	Yes	Yes

*Conventional therapy comprises diet, physical activity, and behavior therapy.
†Pharmacotherapy should be considered only for patients who are unable to achieve adequate weight loss with available conventional therapy and who do not have any absolute contraindications for drug therapy.
‡Bariatric surgery should be considered only for patients who are unable to lose weight with available conventional therapy and who do not have any absolute contraindications for surgery.
BMI, body mass index; CHD, coronary heart disease, LAGB, laparoscopic adjustable gastric banding.

those without diabetes, and treatment of diabetes itself is often associated with an increase in body weight. Therefore, therapeutic lifestyle intervention, weight loss medications, diabetes medications that are associated with the least amount of weight gain, and bariatric surgery should all be considered as part of the potential therapeutic options for obese patients with T2DM.

A guide to the management of overweight and obesity in adults was recently developed by the Obesity Society, the American College of Cardiology, and the American Heart Association Task Force on Practice Guidelines.[390] An overview of the general treatment guidelines is shown in Table 36-6. An effective treatment plan must consider the patient's willingness to undergo therapy, ability to comply with specific treatment approaches, access to skilled caregivers, and financial considerations. The therapeutic approach should also approach obesity as a chronic disease and incorporate a chronic disease model into treatment.

REFERENCES

1. Klein S, Wadden T, Sugerman HJ. American Gastroenterological Association technical review: clinical issues in obesity. *Gastroenterology.* 2002;123:882-932.
2. Lehnert T, Sonntag D, Konnopka A, et al. Economic costs of overweight and obesity. *Best Pract Res Clin Endocrinol Metab.* 2013;27:105-115.
3. World Health Organization. *Obesity: Preventing and Managing the Global Epidemic.* Report of a WHO Consultation on Obesity. Geneva, Switzerland: WHO; 1998.
4. National Institutes of Health, National Heart, Lung, and Blood Institute. Clinical guidelines on the identification, evaluation, and treatment of overweight and obesity in adults: the evidence report. *Obes Res.* 1998;6(Suppl 2):51S-209S.
5. U.S. Department of Health and Human Services. Nutrition and overweight. In: *Healthy People 2010.* Washington, DC: U.S. Government Printing Office; 2000.
6. U.S. Department of Agriculture and U.S. Department of Health and Human Services. *Nutrition and Your Health: Dietary Guidelines for Americans.* 5th ed. Home and Garden Bulletin no. 232. Washington, DC: U.S. Government Printing Office; 2000.
7. Gallagher D, Heymsfield SB, Heo M, et al. Health percentage body fat ranges: an approach for developing guidelines based on body mass index. *Am J Clin Nutr.* 2000;72:694-701.
8. Calle EE, Thun MJ, Petrelli JM, et al. Body-mass index and mortality in a prospective cohort of U.S. adults. *N Engl J Med.* 1999;341:1097-1105.
9. Flegal KM, Graubard BI, Williamson DF, et al. Excess deaths associated with underweight, overweight, and obesity. *JAMA.* 2005;293:1861-1867.
10. Kissebah AH, Videlingum N, Murray R, et al. Relation of body fat distribution to metabolic complications of obesity. *J Clin Endocrinol Metab.* 1982;54:254-260.
11. Snijder MB, Dekker JM, Visser M, et al. Trunk fat and leg fat have independent and opposite associations with fasting and postload glucose levels: the Hoorn study. *Diabetes Care.* 2004;27(2):372-377.
12. Jensen MD. Gender differences in regional fatty acid metabolism before and after meal ingestion. *J Clin Invest.* 1995;96:2297-2303.
13. Guo ZK, Hensrud DD, Johnson CM, et al. Regional postprandial fatty acid metabolism in different obesity phenotypes. *Diabetes.* 1999;48:1586-1592.
14. Wang Y, Rimm EB, Stampfer MJ, et al. Comparison of abdominal adiposity and overall obesity in predicting risk of type 2 diabetes among men. *Am J Clin Nutr.* 2005;81:555-563.
15. Lean ME, Han TS, Morrison CE. Waist circumference as a measure for indicating need for weight management. *BMJ.* 1995;311:158-161.
16. Deurenberg-Yap M, Chew SK, Lin VF, et al. Relationships between indices of obesity and its co-morbidities in multi-ethnic Singapore. *Int J Obes Relat Metab Disord.* 2001;25:1554-1562.
17. Deurenberg-Yap M, Schmidt G, van Staveren WA, et al. The paradox of low body mass index and high body fat percentage among Chinese, Malays and Indians in Singapore. *Int J Obes Relat Metab Disord.* 2000;24:1011-1017.
18. Wu CH, Heshka S, Wang J, et al. Truncal fat in relation to total body fat: influences of age, sex, ethnicity and fatness. *Int J Obes (Lond).* 2007;31:1384-1391.
19. Koster A, Leitzmann MF, Schatzkin A, et al. Waist circumference and mortality. *Am J Epidemiol.* 2008;167:1465-1475.
20. World Health Organization. WHO expert consultation: appropriate body-mass index for Asian populations and its implications for policy and intervention strategies. *Lancet.* 2004;363:157-163.
21. Alberti KG, Eckel RH, Grundy SM, et al. Harmonizing the metabolic syndrome: a joint interim statement of the International Diabetes Federation Task Force on Epidemiology and Prevention; National Heart, Lung, and Blood Institute; American Heart Association; World Heart Federation; International Atherosclerosis Society; and International Association for the Study of Obesity. *Circulation.* 2009;120:1640-1645.
22. Andres R, Elahi D, Tobin JD, et al. Impact of age on weight goals. *Ann Intern Med.* 1985;103(6 Pt 2):1030.
23. Kragelund C, Hassager C, Hildebrandt P, et al. TRACE study group: impact of obesity on long-term prognosis following acute myocardial infarction. *Int J Cardiol.* 2005;98:123-131.
24. McAuley P, Myers J, Abella J, et al. Body mass, fitness and survival in veteran patients: another obesity paradox? *Am J Med.* 2007;120:518-524.
25. Uretsky S, Messerli FH, Bangalore S, et al. Obesity paradox in patients with hypertension and coronary artery disease. *Am J Med.* 2007;120:863-870.
26. Oreopoulos A, Padwal R, Norris CM, et al. Effect of obesity on short- and long-term mortality postcoronary revascularization: a meta-analysis. *Obesity (Silver Spring).* 2008;16:442-450.
27. Mano A, Fujita K, Uenomachi K, et al. Body mass index is a useful predictor of prognosis after left ventricular assist system implantation. *J Heart Lung Transplant.* 2009;28:428-433.
28. Lea JP, Crenshaw DO, Onufrak SJ, et al. Obesity, end-stage renal disease, and survival in an elderly cohort with cardiovascular disease. *Obesity (Silver Spring).* 2009;17:2216-2222.
29. Beck TJ, Petit MA, Wu G, et al. Does obesity really make the femur stronger? BMD, geometry, and fracture incidence in the Women's Health Initiative—Observational Study. *J Bone Miner Res.* 2009;24:1369-1379.
30. Van der Helm-van Mil AH, van der Kooij SM, Allaart CF, et al. A high body mass index has a protective effect on the amount of joint destruction in small joints in early rheumatoid arthritis. *Ann Rheum Dis.* 2008;67:769-774.
31. Leung CC, Lam TH, Chan WM, et al. Lower risk of tuberculosis in obesity. *Arch Intern Med.* 2007;167:1297-1304.
32. Willett WC, Manson JE, Stampfer MJ, et al. Weight, weight change, and coronary heart disease in women: risk within the "normal" weight range. *JAMA.* 1995;273:461-465.

33. Hall KD, Sacks G, Chandramohan D, et al. Quantification of the effect of energy imbalance on body weight. *Lancet.* 2011;378:826-837.

34. Colditz GA, Willett WC, Rotnitzky A, Manson JE. Weight gain as a risk factor for clinical diabetes mellitus in women. *Ann Intern Med.* 1995; 122:481-486.

35. Chan JM, Rimm EB, Colditz GA, et al. Obesity, fat distribution, and weight gain as risk factors for clinical diabetes in men. *Diabetes Care.* 1994;17:961-969.

36. Huang Z, Willett WC, Manson JE, et al. Body weight, weight change, and risk for hypertension in women. *Ann Intern Med.* 1998;128:81-88.

37. Maclure KM, Hayes KC, Colditz GA, et al. Weight, diet, and risk of symptomatic gallstones in middle-aged women. *N Engl J Med.* 1989; 321:563-569.

38. Wei M, Gibbons L, Mitchell T, et al. The association between cardiorespiratory fitness and impaired fasting glucose and type 2 diabetes mellitus in men. *Ann Intern Med.* 1999;130:89-96.

39. Lee CD, Blair SN, Jackson AS. Cardiorespiratory fitness, body composition, and all-cause and cardiovascular disease mortality in men. *Am J Clin Nutr.* 1999;69:373-380.

40. McKeigue P, Shah B, Marmont MG. Relation of central obesity and insulin resistance with high diabetes prevalence and cardiovascular risk in South Asians. *Lancet.* 1991;337:382-386.

41. Morton GJ, Cummings DE, Baskin DG, et al. Central nervous system control of food intake and body weight. *Nature.* 2006;443:289-295.

42. Badman MK, Flier JF. The gut and energy balance: visceral allies in the obesity wars. *Science.* 2005;307:1909-1914.

43. Cota D, Marsicano G, Tschöp M, et al. The endogenous cannabinoid system affects energy balance via central orexigenic drive and peripheral lipogenesis. *J Clin Invest.* 2003;112:423-431.

44. Ravinet C, Arnone M, Delgorge C, et al. Anti-obesity effect of SR141716, a CB1 receptor antagonist, in diet-induced obese mice. *Am J Physiol Regul Integr Comp Physiol.* 2003;284:R345-R353.

45. Pi-Sunyer FX, Aronne LJ, Heshmati HM, et al. Effect of rimonabant, a cannabinoid-1 receptor blocker, on weight and cardiometabolic risk factors in overweight or obese patients—RIO-North America: a randomized controlled trial. *JAMA.* 2006;295:761-775.

46. Despres JP, Golay A, Sjostrom L. Effects of rimonabant on metabolic risk factors in overweight patients with dyslipidemia. Rimonabant in Obesity-Lipids Study Group. *N Engl J Med.* 2005;353:2121-2134.

47. Vickers SP, Kennett GA. Cannabinoids and the regulation of ingestive behaviour. *Curr Drug Targets.* 2005;6:215-223.

48. McGowan BM, Bloom SR. Peptide YY and appetite control. *Curr Opin Pharmacol.* 2004;4:583-588.

49. Deacon CF. Therapeutic strategies based on glucagon-like peptide 1. *Diabetes.* 2004;53:2181-2189.

50. Rosenbaum M, Leibel RL, Hirsch J. Obesity. *N Engl J Med.* 1997;337:396-408.

51. Pratley RE. Gene-environment interactions in the pathogenesis of type 2 diabetes mellitus: lessons learned from the Pima Indians. *Proc Nutr Soc.* 1998;57:175-181.

52. O'Dea K, White N, Sinclair A. An investigation of nutrition-related risk factors in an isolated Aboriginal community in northern Australia: advantages of a traditionally-orientated life style. *Med J Aust.* 1988; 148:177-180.

53. O'Dea K. Marked improvement in carbohydrate and lipid metabolism in diabetic Australian Aborigines after temporary reversion to traditional lifestyle. *Diabetes.* 1984;33:596-603.

54. Whitaker RC, Wright JA, Pepe MS, et al. Predicting obesity in young adulthood from childhood and parental obesity. *N Engl J Med.* 1997; 337:869-873.

55. Rankinen T, Zuberi A, Chagnon YC, et al. The human obesity gene map: the 2005 update. *Obesity.* 2006;14:529.

56. Montague CT, Farooqi IS, Whitehead JP, et al. Congenital leptin deficiency is associated with severe early-onset obesity in humans. *Nature.* 1997;387:903-908.

57. Strobel A, Issad T, Camoin L, et al. A leptin missense mutation associated with hypogonadism and morbid obesity. *Nat Genet.* 1998;18:213-215.

58. Farooqi IS, Jebb SA, Langmack G, et al. Effects of recombinant leptin therapy in a child with congenital leptin deficiency. *N Engl J Med.* 1999;341:879-884.

59. Consadine RV, Sinha MK, Heiman ML, et al. Serum immunoreactive-leptin concentrations in normal-weight and obese humans. *N Engl J Med.* 1996;334:292-295.

60. Clement K, Vaisse C, Lahlou N, et al. A mutation in the human leptin receptor gene causes obesity and pituitary dysfunction. *Nature.* 1998; 392:398-401.

61. Jackson RS, Creemers JW, Ohagi S, et al. Obesity and impaired prohormone processing associated with mutations in the human prohormone convertase 1 gene. *Nat Genet.* 1997;16:303-306.

62. Jackson RS, Creemers JWM, Farooqi IS, et al. Small intestinal dysfunction accompanies the complex endocrinopathy of human proprotein convertase 1 deficiency. *J Clin Invest.* 2003;112:1550-1560.

63. Krude H, Biebermann H, Luck W, et al. Severe early-onset obesity, adrenal insufficiency and red hair pigmentation caused by POMC mutations in humans. *Nat Genet.* 1998;19:155-157.

64. Farooqi IS, Yeo GS, Keogh JM, et al. Dominant and recessive inheritance of morbid obesity associated with melanocortin 4 receptor deficiency. *J Clin Invest.* 2000;106:271-279.

65. Farooqi IS, Keogh JM, Giles SH, et al. Clinical spectrum of obesity and mutations in the melanocortin 4 receptor gene. *N Engl J Med.* 2003; 348:1085-1095.

66. Yeo GS, Connie Hung CC, Rochford J, et al. A de novo mutation affecting human TrkB associated with severe obesity and developmental delay. *Nat Neurosci.* 2004;7:1187-1189.

67. Farooqi IS, O'Rahilly S. Monogentic obesity in humans. *Annu Rev Med.* 2005;56:443-458.

68. Goldstone AP. Prader-Willi syndrome: advances in genetics, pathophysiology and treatment. *Trends Endocrinol Metab.* 2004;15:12-20.

69. Holder JL Jr, Butte NF, Zinn AR. Profound obesity associated with a balanced translocation that disrupts the SIM1 gene. *Hum Mol Genet.* 2000;9(1):101-108.

70. Speliotes EK, Willer CJ, Berndt SI, et al. Association analyses of 249,796 individuals reveal 18 new loci associated with body mass index. *Nat Genet.* 2010;42:937-948.

71. Gerken T, Girard CA, Tung YC, et al. The obesity-associated FTO gene encodes a 2-oxoglutarate-dependent nucleic acid demethylase. *Science.* 2007;318:1469-1472.

72. Frayling TM, Timpson NJ, Weedon MN, et al. A common variant in the FTO gene is associated with body mass index and predisposes to childhood and adult obesity. *Science.* 2007;316:889-894.

73. Dina C, Meyre D, Gallina S, et al. Variation in FTO contributes to childhood obesity and severe adult obesity. *Nat Genet.* 2007;39:724-726.

74. Scuteri A, Sanna S, Chen WM, et al. Genome-wide association scan shows genetic variants in the FTO gene are associated with obesity-related traits. *PLoS Genet.* 2007;3:e115.

75. Ravussin E, Burnand B, Schutz Y, et al. Twenty-four-hour energy expenditure and resting metabolic rate in obese, moderately obese, and control subjects. *Am J Clin Nutr.* 1982;35:566-573.

76. Skov AR, Toubro S, Buemann B, et al. Normal levels of energy expenditure in patients with reported "low metabolism." *Clin Physiol.* 1997;17:279-285.

77. Lichtman SW, Pisarka K, Berman ER, et al. Discrepancy between self-reported and actual caloric intake and exercise in obese subjects. *N Engl J Med.* 1992;327:1893-1898.

78. Segal KR, Presta E, Gutin B. Thermic effect of food during graded exercise in normal weight and obese men. *Am J Clin Nutr.* 1984;40:95-100.

79. de Jonge L, Bray GA. The thermic effect of food and obesity: a critical review. *Obesity Res.* 1997;5:622-631.

80. Roberts SB, Savage J, Coward WA, et al. Energy expenditure and intake from infants born to lean and overweight mothers. *N Engl J Med.* 1988;318:461-466.

81. Stunkard AJ, Berkowitz RI, Stallings VA, et al. Energy intake, not energy output, is a determinant of body size in infants. *Am J Clin Nutr.* 1999; 69:524-530.

82. Ravussin E, Lillioja S, Knowler WC, et al. Reduced rate of energy expenditure as a risk factor for body-weight gain. *N Engl J Med.* 1988; 318:467-472.

83. Seidell JC, Muller DC, Sorkin JD, et al. Fasting respiratory exchange ratio and resting metabolic rate as predictors of weight gain: the Baltimore Longitudinal Study on Aging. *Int J Obes Relat Metab Disord.* 1992;16:667-674.

84. Bouchard C, Tremblay A, Despres JP, et al. The response to long-term overfeeding in identical twins. *N Engl J Med.* 1990;322:1477-1482.

85. Levine JA, Eberhardt NL, Jensen MD. Role of nonexercise activity thermogenesis in resistance to fat gain in humans. *Science.* 1999; 282:212-214.

86. Wadden TA, Foster GD, Letizia KA, et al. Long-term effects of dieting on resting metabolic rate in obese outpatients. *JAMA.* 1990;264:707-711.

87. Amatruda JM, Statt MC, Welle SL. Total resting energy expenditure in obese women reduced to ideal body weight. *J Clin Invest.* 1993;92:1236-1242.

88. Weinsier RL, Nagy TR, Hunter GR, et al. Do adaptive changes in metabolic rate favor weight regain in weight-reduced individuals? An examination of the set-point theory. *Am J Clin Nutr.* 2000;72:1088-1094.

89. Astrup A, Gotzsche PC, van de Werken K, et al. Meta-analysis of resting metabolic rate in formerly obese subjects. *Am J Clin Nutr.* 1999;69:1117-1122.

90. Leiter LA, Marliss EB. Survival during fasting may depend on fat as well as protein stores. *JAMA.* 1982;248:2306-2307.

91. Stewart WK, Fleming LW. Features of a successful therapeutic fast of 382 days duration. *Postgrad Med J.* 1973;49:203-209.

92. Angel A, Bray GA. Synthesis of fatty acids and cholesterol by the liver, adipose tissue and intestinal mucosa from obese and control subjects. *Eur J Clin Invest.* 1979;9:355-362.

93. Ramsay TG. Fat cells. *Endocrinol Metab Clin North Am.* 1996;25:847-870.

94. Simsolo RB, Ong JM, Saffari B, et al. Effect of improved diabetes control on the expression of lipoprotein lipase in human adipose tissue. *J Lipid Res.* 1992;33:89-95.

95. Heiling VJ, Miles JM, Jensen MD. How valid are isotopic measurements of fatty acid oxidation? *Am J Physiol.* 1991;261:E572-E577.

96. Leweis GF. Fatty acid regulation of very low density lipoprotein production. *Curr Opin Lipidol.* 1997;8:146-153.

97. Jensen MD. Diet effects on fatty acid metabolism in lean and obese subjects. *Am J Clin Nutr.* 1998;67:531S-534S.

98. Jensen MD, Haymond MW, Rizza RA, et al. Influence of body fat distribution on free fatty acid metabolism in obesity. *J Clin Invest.* 1989; 83:12168-12173.

99. Martin ML, Jensen MD. Effects of body fat distribution on regional lipolysis in obesity. *J Clin Invest.* 1991;88:609-613.

100. Kahn BB, Flier JS. Obesity and insulin resistance. *J Clin Invest.* 2000; 106:473-481.

101. Wajchenberg BL. Subcutaneous and visceral adipose tissue: their relation to the metabolic syndrome. *Endocr Rev.* 2000;21:697-738.

102. Friedman JM. Obesity in the new millennium. *Nature.* 2000;404: 632-634.

103. Lee Y, Wang MY, Wang ZW, et al. Liporegulation in diet-induced obesity: the antisteatotic role of hyperleptinemia. *J Biol Chem.* 2001; 276:5629-5635.

104. Considine RV, Sinha MK, Heiman ML, et al. Serum immunoreactive leptin concentrations in normal weight and obese humans. *N Engl J Med.* 1996;334:292-295.

105. Kolaczynsky JW, Ohammesian JP, Considine RV, et al. Response of leptin to short-term and prolonged overfeeding in humans. *J Clin Endocrinol Metab.* 1996;81:4162-4165.

106. Flier JS. Clinical review 94: what's in a name? In search of leptin's physiologic role. *J Clin Endocrinol Metab.* 1998;83:1407-1413.

107. Steppan CM, Bailey ST, Bhat S, et al. The hormone resistin links obesity to diabetes. *Nature.* 2001;409:307-312.

108. Weyer C, Funahashi T, Tanaka S, et al. Hypoadiponectinemia in obesity and type 2 diabetes: close association with insulin resistance and hyperinsulinemia. *J Clin Endocrinol Metab.* 2001;86:1930-1935.

109. Yang WS, Lee WJ, Funahashi T, et al. Weight reduction increases plasma levels of an adipose-derived anti-inflammatory protein, adiponectin. *J Clin Endocrinol Metab.* 2001;86:3815-3819.

110. Yu JG, Javorschi S, Hevener AL, et al. The effect of thiazolidinediones on plasma adiponectin levels in normal, obese, and type 2 diabetic subjects. *Diabetes.* 2002;51:2968-2974.

111. Berg AH, Combs TP, Scherer PE. ACRP30/adiponectin: an adipokine regulating glucose and lipid metabolism. *Trends Endocrinol Metab.* 2002;13:84-89.

112. Peraldi P, Spiegelman B. TNF-α and insulin resistance: summary and future prospects. *Mol Cell Biochem.* 1998;182:169-171.

113. Mohamed-Ali V, Pinkney JH, Coppack SW. Adipose tissue as an endocrine and paracrine organ. *Int J Obes Relat Metab Disord.* 1998;22: 1145-1158.

114. Bastard JP, Jardel C, Bruckert E, et al. Elevated levels of interleukin 6 are reduced in serum and subcutaneous adipose tissue of obese women after weight loss. *J Clin Endocrinol Metab.* 2000;85:3338-3342.

115. Bastard JP, Maachi M, Van Nhieu JT, et al. Adipose tissue IL-6 content correlates with resistance to insulin activation of glucose uptake both in vivo and in vitro. *J Clin Endocrinol Metab.* 2002;87:2084-2089.

116. Senn JJ, Klover PJ, Nowak IA, et al. Interleukin-6 induces cellular insulin resistance in hepatocytes. *Diabetes.* 2002;51:3391-3399.

117. Tsigos C, Papanicolaou DA, Kyrou I, et al. Dose-dependent effects of recombinant human interleukin-6 on glucose regulation. *J Clin Endocrinol Metab.* 1997;82:4167-4170.

118. Hirsch J, Knittle JL. Cellularity of obese and non-obese human adipose tissue. *Fed Proc.* 1970;29:1516-1521.

119. Ntambi JM, Kim Y-C. Adipocyte differentiation and gene expression. *J Nutr.* 2000;130:3122S-3126S.

120. Shimomura I, Hammer RE, Richardson JA, et al. Insulin resistance and diabetes mellitus in transgenic mice expressing nuclear SREBP-1c in adipose tissue: model for congenital generalized lipodystrophy. *Genes Dev.* 1998;12:3182-3194.

121. Ballor DL, Poehlman ET. Exercise-training enhances fat-free mass preservation during diet-induced weight loss: a meta-analytical finding. *Int J Obes Relat Metab Disord.* 1994;18:35-40.

122. Ross R, Rissanen J, Pedwell H, et al. Influence of diet and exercise on skeletal muscle and visceral adipose tissue in men. *J Appl Physiol.* 1996; 81:2445-2455.

123. Smith SR, Zachwieja JJ. Visceral adipose tissue: a critical review of intervention strategies. *Int J Obes Relat Metab Disord.* 1999;23: 329-335.

124. Knittle JL, Ginsberg-Fellner F. Effect of weight reduction on in vitro adipose tissue lipolysis and cellularity in obese adolescents and adults. *Diabetes.* 1972;21:754-761.

125. Naslund I, Hallgren P, Sjostrom L. Fat cell weight and number before and after gastric surgery for morbid obesity in women. *Int J Obes.* 1988;12:191-197.

126. Prins JB, O'Rahilly S. Regulation of adipose cell number in man. *Clin Sci.* 1997;92:3-11.

127. Prins JB, Walker NL, Winterford CM, et al. Apoptosis of human adipocyte in vitro. *Biochem Biophys Res Commun.* 1994;201:500-507.

128. Prins JB, Walker NL, Winterford CM, et al. Human adipocyte apoptosis occurs in malignancy. *Biochem Biophys Res Commun.* 1994;205: 625-630.

129. Cannon B, Nedergaard J. Brown adipose tissue: function and physiological significance. *Physiol Rev.* 2004;84:277-359.

130. Virtanen KA, Lidell ME, Orava J, et al. Functional brown adipose tissue in healthy adults. *N Engl J Med.* 2009;360:1518-1525.

131. Cypess AM, Lehman S, Williams G, et al. Identification and importance of brown adipose tissue in adult humans. *N Engl J Med.* 2009; 360:1509-1517.

132. van Marken Lichtenbelt WD, Vanhommerig JW, Smulders NM, et al. Cold-activated brown adipose tissue in healthy men. *N Engl J Med.* 2009;360:1500-1508.

133. Au-Yong IT, Thorn N, Ganatra R, et al. Brown adipose tissue and seasonal variation in people. *Diabetes.* 2009;58:2583-2587.

134. Lee P, Swarbrick MM, Ho KK. Brown adipose tissue in adult humans: a metabolic renaissance. *Endocr Rev.* 2013;34:413-438.

135. Vijgen GH, Bouvy ND, Teule GJ, et al. Increase in brown adipose tissue activity after weight loss in morbidly obese subjects. *J Clin Endocrinol Metab.* 2012;97:E1229-E1233.

136. Ng M, Fleming T, Robinson M, et al. Global, regional, and national prevalence of overweight and obesity in children and adults during 1980-2013: a systematic analysis for the Global Burden of Disease Study 2013. *Lancet.* 2014;384(9945):766-781.

137. Flegal KM, Carroll MD, Kuczmarski RJ, et al. Overweight and obesity in the United States: prevalence and trends, 1960-1994. *Int J Obes Relat Metab Disord.* 1998;22:39-47.

138. Ogden CL, Carroll MD, Kit BK, Flegal KM. Prevalence of childhood and adult obesity in the United States, 2011-2012. *JAMA.* 2014;311: 806-814.

139. Barlow SE, Dietz WH. Obesity evaluation and treatment: Expert Committee recommendations. The Maternal and Child Health Bureau, Health Resources and Services Administration and the Department of Health and Human Services. *Pediatrics.* 1998;102(3):E29.

140. Brochu M, Tchernof A, Dionne IJ, et al. What are the physical characteristics associated with a normal metabolic profile despite a high level of obesity in postmenopausal women? *J Clin Endocrinol Metab.* 2001;86:1020-1025.

141. Ferrannini E, Natali A, Bell P, et al. Insulin resistance and hypersecretion in obesity. European Group for the Study of Insulin Resistance (EGIR). *J Clin Invest.* 1997;100:1166-1173.

142. Wildman RP, Muntner P, Reynolds K, et al. The obese without cardiometabolic risk factor clustering and the normal weight with cardiometabolic risk factor clustering: prevalence and correlates of 2 phenotypes among the US population (NHANES 1999-2004). *Arch Intern Med.* 2008;168:1617-1624.

143. Calori G, Lattuada G, Piemonti L, et al. Prevalence, metabolic features, and prognosis of metabolically healthy obese Italian individuals: the Cremona Study. *Diabetes Care.* 2011;34(1):210-215.

144. Stefan N, Häring H-U, Hu FB, Schulze MB. Metabolically healthy obesity: epidemiology, mechanisms, and clinical implications. *Lancet Diabetes Endocrinol.* 2013;1(2):152-162.

145. van Vliet-Ostaptchouk JV, Nuotio ML, Slagter SN, et al. The prevalence of metabolic syndrome and metabolically healthy obesity in Europe: a collaborative analysis of ten large cohort studies. *BMC Endocr Disord.* 2014;14(1):9.

146. Karelis AD, Faraj M, Bastard JP, et al. The metabolically healthy but obese individual presents a favorable inflammation profile. *J Clin Endocrinol Metab.* 2005;90:4145-4150.

147. Meigs JB, Wilson PW, Fox CS, et al. Body mass index, metabolic syndrome, and risk of type 2 diabetes or cardiovascular disease. *J Clin Endocrinol Metab.* 2006;91:2906-2912.

148. Kramer CK, Zinman B, Retnakaran R. Are metabolically healthy overweight and obesity benign conditions?A systematic review and meta-analysis. *Ann Intern Med.* 2013;159:758-769.

149. Appleton SL, Seaborn CJ, Visvanathan R, et al. Diabetes and cardiovascular disease outcomes in the metabolically healthy obese phenotype: a cohort study. *Diabetes Care.* 2013;36:2388-2394.

150. Hamer M, Stamatakis E. Metabolically healthy obesity and risk of all-cause and cardiovascular disease mortality. *J Clin Endocrinol Metab.* 2012;97(7):2482-2488.

151. Lemieux I, Pascot A, Couillard C, et al. Hypertriglyceridemic waist: a marker of the atherogenic metabolic triad (hyperinsulinemia; hyperapolipoprotein B; small, dense LDL) in men? *Circulation.* 2000;102: 179-184.

152. Ruderman N, Chisholm D, Pi-Sunyer X, et al. The metabolically obese, normal-weight individual revisited. *Diabetes.* 1998;47:699-713.

153. Reaven GM. Role of insulin resistance in human disease. *Diabetes.* 1988;37:1595-1607.

154. Meigs JB, D'Agostino RB, Wilson WF, et al. Risk variable clustering in the insulin resistance syndrome. *Diabetes.* 1997;46:1594-1600.

155. Frayn KN. Visceral fat and insulin resistance: causative or correlative? *Br J Nutr.* 2000;83(Suppl 1):S71-S77.

156. Krssak M, Petersen KF, Dresner A, et al. Intramyocellular lipid concentrations are correlated with insulin sensitivity in humans: a 1H NMR spectroscopy study. *Diabetologia.* 1999;42:113-116.

157. Marchesini G, Bugianesi E, Forlani G, et al. Nonalcoholic fatty liver, steatohepatitis, and the metabolic syndrome. *Hepatology.* 2003;37:917-923.

158. Adams LA, Lymp JF, St Sauver J, et al. The natural history of nonalcoholic fatty liver disease: a population-based cohort study. *Gastroenterology.* 2005;129:113-121.

159. Perry RJ, Samuel VT, Petersen KF, Shulman GI. The role of hepatic lipids in hepatic insulin resistance and type 2 diabetes. *Nature.* 2014;5(510):84-91.

160. Fabbrini E, Sullivan S, Klein S. Obesity and nonalcoholic fatty liver disease: biochemical, metabolic and clinical implications. *Hepatology.* 2010;51:679-689.

161. Cowie CC, Rust KF, Ford ES, et al. Full accounting of diabetes and pre-diabetes in the U.S. population in 1988-1994 and 2005-2006. *Diabetes Care.* 2009;32:287-294.

162. Colditz GA, Willett WC, Stampfer MJ, et al. Weight as a risk factor for clinical diabetes in women. *Am J Epidemiol.* 1990;132:501-513.

163. Ohlson LO, Larsson B, Svardsudd K, et al. The influence of body fat distribution on the incidence of diabetes mellitus. *Diabetes.* 1985;34:1055-1058.

164. Lundgren H, Bengtsson C, Blohme G, et al. Adiposity and adipose tissue distribution in relation to incidence of diabetes in women: results from a prospective population study in Gothenburg, Sweden. *Int J Obes.* 1989;13:413-423.

165. Li C, Ford ES, Zhao G, et al. Waist-to-thigh ratio and diabetes among US adults: the Third National Health and Nutrition Examination Survey. *Diabetes Res Clin Pract.* 2010;89:79-87.

166. Reaven GM, Chen YDI, Jeppesen J, et al. Insulin resistance and hyperinsulinemia in individuals with small, dense, low density lipoprotein particles. *J Clin Invest.* 1993;92:141-146.

167. Terry RB, Wood PD, Haskell WL, et al. Regional adiposity pattern in relation to lipids, lipoprotein cholesterol, and lipoprotein subfraction mass in men. *J Clin Endocrinol Metab.* 1989;68:191-199.

168. Brown CD, Higgins M, Donato KA, et al. Body mass index and the prevalence of hypertension and dyslipidemia. *Obes Res.* 2000;8:605-619.

169. Assmann G, Schulte H. Relation of high-density lipoprotein cholesterol and triglycerides to incidence of atherosclerotic coronary artery disease (the PROCAM experience). *Am J Cardiol.* 1992;70:733-737.

170. Lamarche B, Lemieux I, Despres JP. The small, dense LDL phenotype and the risk of coronary heart disease: epidemiology, pathophysiology and therapeutic aspects. *Diabetes Metab.* 1999;25:199-211.

171. Hubert HB, Feinleib M, McNamara PM, et al. Obesity as an independent risk factor for cardiovascular disease: a 26-year follow-up of participants in the Framingham Heart Study. *Circulation.* 1983;67:968-977.

172. Stamler R, Stamler J, Riedlinger WF, et al. Weight and blood pressure: findings in hypertension screening of 1 million Americans. *JAMA.* 1978;240:1607-1609.

173. Kannel W, Brand N, Skinner J, et al. The relation of adiposity to blood pressure and development of hypertension. The Framingham Study. *Ann Intern Med.* 1967;67:48-59.

174. Stamler J, Wentworth D, Neaton JD. Is relationship between serum cholesterol and risk of premature death from coronary disease continuous or graded? Findings in 356,222 primary screenees of the Multiple Risk Factor Intervention Trial (MRFIT). *JAMA.* 1986;256:2823-2828.

175. Rexrode KM, Carey VJ, Hennekens CH, et al. Abdominal adiposity and coronary heart disease in women. *JAMA.* 1998;280:1843-1848.

176. Manson JE, Willett WC, Stampfer MJ, et al. Body weight and mortality among women. *N Engl J Med.* 1995;333:677-685.

177. Eckel RH, Krauss RM. American Heart Association call to action: obesity as a major risk factor for coronary heart disease. *Circulation.* 1998;97:2099-2100.

178. Krause RM, Eckel RH, Howard B, et al. AHA dietary guidelines revision 2000: a statement for healthcare professionals from the nutrition committee of the American Heart Association. *Circulation.* 2000;102:2296-2311.

179. Walker SP, Rimm EB, Ascherio A, et al. Body size and fat distribution as predictors of stroke among U.S. men. *Am J Epidemiol.* 1996;144:1143-1150.

180. Rexrode KM, Hennekens CH, Willett WC, et al. A prospective study of body mass index weight change, and risk of stroke in women. *JAMA.* 1997;277:1539-1545.

181. Hansson PO, Eriksson H, Welin L, et al. Smoking and abdominal obesity: risk factors for venous thromboembolism among middle-aged men. "The study of men born in 1913." *Arch Intern Med.* 1999;159:1886-1890.

182. Sugerman HJ, Windsor ACJ, Bessos MK, et al. Abdominal pressure, sagittal abdominal diameter and obesity co-morbidity. *J Int Med.* 1997;241:71-79.

183. Visser M, Bouter LM, McQuillan GM, et al. Elevated C-reactive protein levels in overweight and obese adults. *JAMA.* 1999;282:2131-2135.

184. Strohl KP, Strobel RJ, Parisi RA. Obesity and pulmonary function. In: Bray GA, Bouchard C, James WPT, eds. *Handbook of Obesity.* New York, NY: Marcel Dekker; 1998:725-739.

185. Vgontzas AN, Tan TL, Bixler EO, et al. Sleep apnea and sleep disruption in obese patients. *Arch Intern Med.* 1994;154:1705-1711.

186. Davies RJ, Stradling JR. The relationship between neck circumference, radiographic pharyngeal anatomy, and the obstructive sleep apnoea syndrome. *Eur Respir J.* 1990;3:509-514.

187. Katz I, Stradling J, Slutsky AS, et al. Do patients with obstructive sleep apnea have thick necks? *Am Rev Respir Dis.* 1990;141:1228-1231.

188. Roubenoff R, Klag MJ, Mead LA, et al. Incidence and risk factors for gout in white men. *JAMA.* 1991;266:3004-3007.

189. Cigolini M, Targher G, Tonoli M, et al. Hyperuricaemia: relationships to body fat distribution and other components of the insulin resistance syndrome in 38-year-old healthy men and women. *Int J Obes Relat Metab Disord.* 1995;19:92-96.

190. Felson DT, Anderson JJ, Naimark A, et al. Obesity and knee osteoarthritis: the Framingham Study. *Ann Intern Med.* 1988;109:18-24.

191. Cicuttini FM, Baker JR, Spector TD. The association of obesity with osteoarthritis of the hand and knee in women: a twin study. *J Rheumatol.* 1996;23:1221-1226.

192. Yoshimura N, Muraki S, Oka H, et al. Accumulation of metabolic risk factors such as overweight, hypertension, dyslipidaemia, and impaired glucose tolerance raises the risk of occurrence and progression of knee osteoarthritis: a 3-year follow-up of the ROAD study. *Osteoarthritis Cartilage.* 2012;20(11):1217-1226.

193. Calle EE, Rodriguez C, Walker-Thurmond K, et al. Overweight, obesity and mortality from cancer in a prospectively studied cohort of U.S. adults. *N Engl J Med.* 2003;348:1625-1638.

194. Huang Z, Hankinson SE, Colditz GA, et al. Dual effects of weight and weight gain on breast cancer risk. *JAMA.* 1997;278:1407-1411.

195. Renehan AG, Tyson M, Egger M, et al. Body-mass index and incidence of cancer: a systematic review and meta-analysis of prospective observational studies. *Lancet.* 2008;16(371):569-578.

196. Willett WC, Browne ML, Bain C, et al. Relative weight and risk of breast cancer among premenopausal women. *Am J Epidemiol.* 1985;122:731-740.

197. Grodstein F, Goldman MB, Cramer DW. Body mass index and ovulatory infertility. *Epidemiology.* 1994;5:247-250.

198. Johnson SR, Kolberg BH, Varner MW, et al. Maternal obesity and pregnancy. *Surg Gynecol Obstet.* 1987;164:431-437.

199. Garbaciak JA Jr, Richter M, Miller S, Barton JJ. Maternal weight and pregnancy complications. *Am J Obstet Gynecol.* 1985;152(2):238-245.

200. Prentice A, Goldberg G. Maternal obesity increases congenital malformations. *Nutr Rev.* 1996;54:146-152.

201. Dwyer PL, Lee ETC, Hay DM. Obesity and urinary incontinence in women. *Br J Obstet Gynaecol.* 1988;95:91-96.

202. Bump RC, Sugerman HJ, Fantl JA, et al. Obesity and lower urinary tract function in women: effect of surgically induced weight loss. *Am J Obstet Gynecol.* 1992;167:392-399.

203. Durcan FJ, Corbett JJ, Wall M. The incidence of pseudotumor cerebri: population studies in Iowa and Louisiana. *Arch Neurol.* 1988;45:875-877.

204. Giuseffi V, Wall M, Siegel PZ, et al. Symptoms and disease associations in idiopathic intracranial hypertension (pseudotumor cerebri): a case-control study. *Neurology.* 1991;41:239-244.

205. Sugerman HJ, Felton WL, Sismanis A, et al. Effects of surgically induced weight loss on pseudotumor cerebri in morbid obesity. *Neurology.* 1995;45:1655-1659.

206. Sugerman HJ, Felton WL III, Sismanis A, et al. Gastric surgery for pseudotumor cerebri associated with severe obesity. *Ann Surg.* 1999;229:634-642.

207. Glynn RJ, Christen WG, Manson JE, et al. Body mass index: an independent predictor of cataract. *Arch Ophthalmol.* 1995;113:1131-1137.

208. Romero Y, Cameron AJ, Locke GR III, et al. Familial aggregation of gastroesophageal reflux in patients with Barrett's esophagus and esophageal adenocarcinoma. *Gastroenterology.* 1997;113:1449-1456.

209. Locke GR, Talley NJ, Fett SL, et al. Risk factors associated with symptoms of gastroesophageal reflux. *Am J Med.* 1999;106:642-649.

210. Corley DA, Kubo A. Body mass index and gastroesophageal reflux disease: a systematic review and meta-analysis. *Am J Gastroenterol.* 2006;101(11):2619-2628.

211. Hampel H, Abraham N, El-Serag H. Meta-analysis: obesity and the risk for gastroesophageal reflux disease and its complications. *Ann Intern Med.* 2005;143:199.

212. Corley D, Kubo A, Nilsson M, et al. Obesity and estrogen as risk factors for gastroesophageal reflux symptoms. *JAMA.* 2003;290:66-72.

213. Stampfer MJ, Maclure KM, Colditz GA, et al. Risk of symptomatic gallstones in women. *Am J Clin Nutr.* 1992;55:652-658.

214. Hay DW, Carey MC. Pathophysiology and pathogenesis of cholesterol gallstone formation. *Semin Liver Dis.* 1990;10:159-170.

215. Weinsier RL, Wilson LJ, Lee J. Medically safe rate of weight loss for the treatment of obesity: a guideline based on risk of gallstone formation. *Am J Med.* 1995;98:115-117.

216. Broomfield PH, Chopra R, Sheinbaum RC, et al. Effects of ursodeoxycholic acid and aspirin on the formation of lithogenic bile gallstones during loss of weight. *N Engl J Med.* 1988;319:1567-1572.
217. Shiffman ML, Kaplan GD, Brinkman-Kaplan V, et al. Prophylaxis against gallstone formation with ursodeoxycholic acid in patients participating in a very-low-calorie diet program. *Ann Intern Med.* 1995;122:899-905.
218. Wattchow DA, Hall JC, Whiting MJ, et al. Prevalence and treatment of gallstones after gastric bypass surgery for morbid obesity. *Br Med J (Clin Res Ed).* 1983;286(6367):763.
219. Stone BG, Ansel HJ, Peterson FJ, et al. Gallbladder emptying stimuli in obese and normal weight subjects. *Hepatology.* 1990;12:795-798.
220. Festi D, Colecchia A, Orsini M, et al. Gallbladder motility and gallstone formation in obese patients following very low calorie diets: use it (fat) to lose it (well). *Int J Obes.* 1998;22:592-600.
221. Shoheiber O, Biskupiak JE, Nash DB. Estimation of the cost savings resulting from the use of ursodiol for the prevention of gallstones in obese patients undergoing rapid weight reduction. *Int J Obes Relat Metab Disord.* 1997;21:1038-1045.
222. Funnell IC, Bornman PC, Weakley SP. Obesity: an important prognostic factor in acute pancreatitis. *Br J Surg.* 1993;80:484-486.
223. Ruhl CE, Everhart JE. Determinants of the association of overweight with elevated serum alanine aminotransferase activity in the United States. *Gastroenterology.* 2003;124:71-79.
224. Marcos A, Fisher RA, Ham JM, et al. Selection and outcome of living donors for adult to adult right lobe transplantation. *Transplantation.* 2000;69:2410-2415.
225. Hilden M, Christoffersen P, Juhl E, et al. Liver histology in a "normal" population: examinations of 503 consecutive fatal traffic casualties. *Scand J Gastroenterol.* 1977;12:593-597.
226. Lee RG. Nonalcoholic steatohepatitis: a study of 49 patients. *Hum Pathol.* 1989;20:594-598.
227. Gholam PM, Kotler DP, Flancbaum LJ. Liver pathology in morbidly obese patients undergoing Roux-en-Y gastric bypass surgery. *Obes Surg.* 2002;12:49-51.
228. Petersen KF, Dufour S, Feng J, et al. Increased prevalence of insulin resistance and nonalcoholic fatty liver disease in Asian-Indian men. *Proc Natl Acad Sci U S A.* 2006;103:18273-18277.
229. Romeo S, Kozlitina J, Xing C, et al. Genetic variation in PNPLA3 confers susceptibility to nonalcoholic fatty liver disease. *Nat Genet.* 2008;40:1461-1465.
230. Browning JD, Szczepaniak LS, Dobbins R, et al. Prevalence of hepatic steatosis in an urban population in the United States: impact of ethnicity. *Hepatology.* 2004;40:1387-1395.
231. Korenblat KM, Fabbrini E, Mohammed BS, et al. Liver, muscle, and adipose tissue insulin action is directly related to intrahepatic triglyceride content in obese subjects. *Gastroenterology.* 2008;134:1369-1375.
232. Fabbrini E, Mohammed BS, Magkos F, et al. Alterations in adipose tissue and hepatic lipid kinetics in obese men and women with nonalcoholic fatty liver disease. *Gastroenterology.* 2008;134:424-431.
233. Deivanayagam S, Mohammed BS, Vitola BE, et al. Nonalcoholic fatty liver disease is associated with hepatic and skeletal muscle insulin resistance in overweight adolescents. *Am J Clin Nutr.* 2008;88:257-262.
234. Fabbrini E, deHaseth D, Deivanayagam S, et al. Alterations in fatty acid kinetics in obese adolescents with increased intrahepatic triglyceride content. *Obesity (Silver Spring).* 2009;17(1):25-29.
235. Fabbrini E, Magkos F, Mohammed BS, et al. Intrahepatic fat, not visceral fat, is linked with metabolic complications of obesity. *Proc Natl Acad Sci U S A.* 2009;106:15430-15435.
236. Gastaldelli A, Cusi K, Pettiti M, et al. Relationship between hepatic/visceral fat and hepatic insulin resistance in nondiabetic and type 2 diabetic subjects. *Gastroenterology.* 2007;133:496-506.
237. Seppala-Lindroos A, Vehkavaara S, Hakkinen AM, et al. Fat accumulation in the liver is associated with defects in insulin suppression of glucose production and serum free fatty acids independent of obesity in normal men. *J Clin Endocrinol Metab.* 2002;87:3023-3028.
238. Diraison F, Moulin P, Beylot M. Contribution of hepatic de novo lipogenesis and reesterification of plasma non esterified fatty acids to plasma triglyceride synthesis during non-alcoholic fatty liver disease. *Diabetes Metab.* 2003;29:478-485.
239. Donnelly KL, Smith CI, Schwarzenberg SJ, et al. Sources of fatty acids stored in liver and secreted via lipoproteins in patients with nonalcoholic fatty liver disease. *J Clin Invest.* 2005;115:1343-1351.
240. Monetti M, Levin MC, Watt MJ, et al. Dissociation of hepatic steatosis and insulin resistance in mice overexpressing DGAT in the liver. *Cell Metab.* 2007;6:69-78.
241. Minehira K, Young SG, Villanueva CJ, et al. Blocking VLDL secretion causes hepatic steatosis but does not affect peripheral lipid stores or insulin sensitivity in mice. *J Lipid Res.* 2008;49:2038-2044.
242. Grefhorst A, Hoekstra J, Derks TG, et al. Acute hepatic steatosis in mice by blocking beta-oxidation does not reduce insulin sensitivity of very-low-density lipoprotein production. *Am J Physiol Gastrointest Liver Physiol.* 2005;289:G592-G598.
243. Amaro A, Fabbrini E, Kars M, et al. Dissociation between intrahepatic triglyceride content and insulin sensitivity in subjects with familial hypobetalipoproteinemia. *Gastroenterology.* 2010;139:149-153.
244. Kirk E, Reeds DN, Finck BN, et al. Dietary fat and carbohydrates differentially alter insulin sensitivity during caloric restriction. *Gastroenterology.* 2009;136(5):1552-1560.
245. Petersen KF, Dufour S, Befroy D, et al. Reversal of nonalcoholic hepatic steatosis, hepatic insulin resistance, and hyperglycemia by moderate weight reduction in patients with type 2 diabetes. *Diabetes.* 2005;54:603-608.
246. Hughes TA, Gwynne JT, Switzer BR, et al. Effects of caloric restriction and weight loss on glycemic control, insulin release and resistance, and atherosclerotic risk in obese subjects with type II diabetes mellitus. *JAMA.* 1984;77:7-17.
247. Markovic TP, Jenkins AB, Campbell LV, et al. The determinants of glycemic responses to diet restriction and weight loss in obesity and NIDDM. *Diabetes Care.* 1998;21:687-694.
248. Wing RR, Koeske R, Epstein LH, et al. Long-term effects of modest weight loss in type II diabetic patients. *Arch Intern Med.* 1987;147:1749-1753.
249. Wing RR, Lang W, Wadden TA, Look AHEAD Research Group, et al. Benefits of modest weight loss in improving cardiovascular risk factors in overweight and obese individuals with type 2 diabetes. *Diabetes Care.* 2011;34(7):1481-1486.
250. Lim EL, Hollingsworth KG, Aribisala BS, et al. Reversal of type 2 diabetes: normalisation of beta cell function in association with decreased pancreas and liver triacylglycerol. *Diabetologia.* 2011;54:2506-2514.
251. Dixon JB, O'Brien PE, Playfair J, et al. Adjustable gastric banding and conventional therapy for type 2 diabetes: a randomized controlled trial. *JAMA.* 2008;299:316-323.
252. Pories WJ, Swanson MS, MacDonald KG, et al. Who would have thought it? An operation proves to be the most effective therapy for adult-onset diabetes mellitus. *Ann Surg.* 1995;222:339-350, discussion 350-352.
253. Pan XR, Li GW, Hu YH, et al. Effects of diet and exercise in preventing NIDDM in people with impaired glucose tolerance: the Da Qing IGT and Diabetes Study. *Diabetes Care.* 1997;20:537-544.
254. Tuomilehto J, Lindstrom J, Eriksson JG, Finnish Diabetes Prevention Study Group, et al. Prevention of type 2 diabetes mellitus by changes in lifestyle among subjects with impaired glucose tolerance. *N Engl J Med.* 2001;344:1343-1350.
255. Knowler WC, Barrett-Connor E, Fowler SE, Diabetes Prevention Program Research Group, et al. Reduction in the incidence of type 2 diabetes with lifestyle intervention or metformin. *N Engl J Med.* 2002;346:393-403.
256. Wing RR, Marcus MD, Epstein LH, et al. Type II diabetic subjects lose less weight than their overweight nondiabetic spouses. *Diabetes Care.* 1987;10:563-566.
257. Khan MA, St Peter JV, Breen GA, et al. Diabetes disease stage predicts weight loss outcomes with long-term appetite suppressants. *Obes Res.* 2000;8:43-48.
258. U.K. Prospective Diabetes Study (UKPDS) Group. Intensive blood-glucose control with sulphonylureas or insulin compared with conventional treatment and risk of complications in patients with type 2 diabetes (UKPDS 33). *Lancet.* 1998;352:837-853.
259. Lazo M, Solga SF, Horska A, Fatty Liver Subgroup of the Look AHEAD Research Group, et al. Effect of a 12-month intensive lifestyle intervention on hepatic steatosis in adults with type 2 diabetes. *Diabetes Care.* 2010;33:2156-2163.
260. Larson-Meyer DE, Newcomer BR, Heilbronn LK, et al. Effect of 6-month calorie restriction and exercise on serum and liver lipids and markers of liver function. *Obesity (Silver Spring).* 2008;16:1355-1362.
261. Promrat K, Kleiner DE, Niemeier HM, et al. Randomized controlled trial testing the effects of weight loss on nonalcoholic steatohepatitis. *Hepatology.* 2010;51:121-129.
262. Mathurin P, Hollebecque A, Arnalsteen L, et al. Prospective study of the long-term effects of bariatric surgery on liver injury in patients without advanced disease. *Gastroenterology.* 2009;137:532-540.
263. Klein S, Mittendorfer B, Eagon JC, et al. Gastric bypass surgery improves metabolic and hepatic abnormalities associated with nonalcoholic fatty liver disease. *Gastroenterology.* 2006;130:1564-1572.
264. Dixon JB, Bhathal PS, Hughes NR, et al. Nonalcoholic fatty liver disease: improvement in liver histological analysis with weight loss. *Hepatology.* 2004;39:1647-1654.
265. Dattilo AM, Kris-Etherton PM. Effects of weight reduction on blood lipids and lipoproteins: a meta-analysis. *Am J Clin Nutr.* 1992;56:320-328.
266. Wadden TA, Anderson DA, Foster GD. Two-year changes in lipids and lipoproteins associated with the maintenance of a 5% to 10% reduction in initial weight: some findings and some questions. *Obes Res.* 1999;7:170-178.
267. Foster GD, Wyatt HR, Hill JO, et al. Effects of low-carbohydrate and low-fat diets on body weight and coronary heart disease risk factors: a two-year, multi-center randomized trial. *Ann Intern Med.* 2010;153:147-157.

268. Krauss RM, Blanche PJ, Rawlings RS, et al. Separate effects of reduced carbohydrate intake and weight loss on atherogenic dyslipidemia. *Am J Clin Nutr.* 2006;83(5):1025-1031.

269. The Trials of Hypertension Prevention Collaborative Research Group. Effects of weight loss and sodium reduction intervention on blood pressure and hypertension incidence in overweight people with high-normal blood pressure. The Trials of Hypertension Prevention, phase II. *Arch Intern Med.* 1997;157:657-667.

270. Stevens VJ, Obarzanek E, Cook NR, et al. Long-term weight loss and changes in blood pressure: results of the Trials of Hypertension Prevention, phase II. *Ann Intern Med.* 2001;134:1-11.

271. Carson JL, Ruddy ME, Duff AE, et al. The effect of gastric bypass surgery on hypertension in morbidly obese patients. *Arch Intern Med.* 1994;154:193-200.

272. Sjöström CD, Peltonen M, Wedel H, et al. Differentiated long-term effects of intentional weight loss on diabetes and hypertension. *Hypertension.* 2000;36:20-25.

273. Wilson PW, Kannel WB, Silbershatz H, et al. Clustering of metabolic factors and coronary heart disease. *Arch Intern Med.* 1999;159:1104-1109.

274. MacMahon SW, Wilcken D, MacDonald GJ. The effect of weight reduction on left ventricular mass. *N Engl J Med.* 1986;314:334-339.

275. Karason K, Lindroos AK, Stenlof K, et al. Relief of cardiorespiratory symptoms and increased physical activity after surgically induced weight loss: results from the Swedish Obese Subjects study. *Arch Intern Med.* 2000;160:1797-1802.

276. Karason K, Wikstrand J, Sjostrom L, Wendelhag I. Weight loss and progression of early atherosclerosis in the carotid artery: a four-year controlled study of obese subjects. *Int J Obes Relat Metab Disord.* 1999;23:948-956.

277. de las Fuentes L, Waggoner AD, Mohammed BS, et al. Effect of moderate diet-induced weight loss and regain on cardiovascular structure and function. *J Am Coll Cardiol.* 2009;54:2376-2381.

278. Peppard PE, Young T, Palta M, et al. Longitudinal study of moderate weight change and sleep-disordered breathing. *JAMA.* 2000;284:3015-3021.

279. Kuna ST, Reboussin DM, Borradaile KE, Sleep AHEAD Research Group of the Look AHEAD Research Group, et al. Long-term effect of weight loss on obstructive sleep apnea severity in obese patients with type 2 diabetes. *Sleep.* 2013;36:641-649.

280. Williamson DF, Pamuk E, Thun M, et al. Prospective study of intentional weight loss and mortality in never-smoking overweight U.S. white women aged 40-64 years. *Am J Epidemiol.* 1995;14:1128-1141.

281. Williamson DF, Pamuk E, Thun M, et al. Prospective study of intentional weight loss and mortality in overweight weight white men aged 40-64 years. *Am J Epidemiol.* 1999;149:491-503.

282. Williamson DF, Thompson TJ, Thun M, et al. Intentional weight loss and mortality among overweight individuals with diabetes. *Diabetes Care.* 2000;23:1499-1504.

283. Sjöström CD, Narbro K, Sjöström CD, et al. Effects of bariatric surgery on mortality in Swedish obese subjects. *N Engl J Med.* 2007;357:741-752.

284. Adams TD, Gress RE, Smith SC, et al. Long-term mortality after gastric bypass surgery. *N Engl J Med.* 2007;357:753-761.

285. National Task Force on the Prevention and Treatment of Obesity. Weight cycling. *JAMA.* 1994;272:1196-1202.

286. Lissner L, Odell PM, D'Agostino RB, et al. Variability of body weight and health outcomes in the Framingham population. *N Eng J Med.* 1991;324:1839-1844.

287. Mifflin MD, St Jeor ST, Hill LA, et al. A new predictive equation for resting energy expenditure in healthy individuals. *Am J Clin Nutr.* 1990;51(2):241-247.

288. World Health Organization. *WHO/FAO/UNO Report: Energy and Protein Requirements.* WHO Technical Report Series, No. 724. Geneva, Switzerland: WHO; 1985.

289. National Institutes of Health. Body Weight Simulator. Accessed at <http://bwsimulator.niddk.nih.gov>.

290. Wing RR, Marcus MD, Salata R, et al. Effects of a very-low-calorie diet on long-term glycemic control in obese type 2 diabetic subjects. *Arch Intern Med.* 1991;151:1334-1340.

291. Torgerson JS, Lissner L, Lindross AK, et al. VLCD plus dietary and behavioral support versus support alone in the treatment of severe obesity: a randomised two-year clinical trial. *Int J Obes Relat Metab Disord.* 1997;21:987-994.

292. Wadden TA, Foster GD, Letizia KA. One-year behavioral treatment of obesity: comparison of moderate and severe caloric restriction and the effects of weight maintenance therapy. *J Consult Clin Psychol.* 1994; 62:165-171.

293. Wadden TA, Stunkard AJ. A controlled trial of very-low-calorie diet, behavior therapy, and their combination in the treatment of obesity. *J Consult Clin Psychol.* 1986;4:482-488.

294. Miura J, Arai K, Ohno M, et al. The long term effectiveness of combined therapy by behavior modification and very low calorie diet: 2 year follow-up. *Int J Obes.* 1989;13:73-77.

295. Ryttig KR, Flaten H, Rossner S. Long-term effects of a very low calorie diet (Nutrilett) in obesity treatment: a prospective, randomized, comparison between VLCD and a hypocaloric diet + behavior modification and their combination. *Int J Obes Relat Metab Disord.* 1997;21:574-579.

296. Bray GA, Popkin BM. Dietary fat intake does affect obesity! *Am J Clin Nutr.* 1998;68:1157-1173.

297. Yu-Poth S, Zhao G, Etherton T, et al. Effects of the National Cholesterol Education Program's Step I and Step II dietary intervention programs on cardiovascular disease risk factors: a meta-analysis. *Am J Clin Nutr.* 1999;69:632-646.

298. Astrup A, Grunwald GK, Melanson EL, et al. The role of low-fat diets in body weight control: a meta-analysis of ad libitum dietary intervention studies. *Int J Obes Relat Metab Disord.* 2000;24:1545-1552.

299. Duncan KH, Bacon JA, Weinsier RL. The effects of high and low energy density diets on satiety, energy intake, and eating time of obese and nonobese subjects. *Am J Clin Nutr.* 1983;37:763-767.

300. Stubbs RJ, Harbron CG, Murgatroyd PR, et al. Covert manipulation of dietary fat and energy density: effect on substrate flux and food intake in men eating ad libitum. *Am J Clin Nutr.* 1995;62:316-329.

301. Bell EA, Castellanos VH, Pelkman CL, et al. Energy density of foods affects energy intake in normal-weight women. *Am J Clin Nutr.* 1998; 67:412-420.

302. Ello-Martin JA, Roe LS, Ledikwe JH, et al. Dietary energy density in the treatment of obesity: a year-long trial comparing 2 weight-loss diets. *Am J Clin Nutr.* 2007;85(6):1465-1477.

303. Rolls BJ, Roe LS, Beach AM, Kris-Etherton PM. Provision of foods differing in energy density affects long-term weight loss. *Obes Res.* 2005;13(6):1052-1060.

304. Yang M-U, Van Itallie TB. Composition of weight lost during short-term weight reduction. *J Clin Invest.* 1976;58:722-730.

305. Foster GD, Wyatt HR, Hill JO, et al. A randomized trial of a low-carbohydrate diet for obesity. *N Engl J Med.* 2003;348:2082-2090.

306. Samaha FF, Iqbal N, Seshadri P, et al. A low-carbohydrate as compared with a low-fat diet in severe obesity. *N Engl J Med.* 2003;348:2074-2081.

307. Brehm BJ, Seeley RJ, Daniels SR, et al. A randomized trial comparing a very low carbohydrate diet and a calorie-restricted low fat diet on body weight and cardiovascular risk factors in healthy women. *J Clin Endocrinol Metab.* 2003;88:1617-1623.

308. Yancy WS, Olsen MK, Guyton JR, et al. A low-carbohydrate, ketogenic diet versus a low-fat diet to treat obesity and hyperlipidemia. *Ann Intern Med.* 2004;140:769-777.

309. Stern L, Iqbal N, Seshadri P, et al. The effects of low-carbohydrate versus conventional weight loss diets in severely obese adults: one-year follow up of a randomized trial. *Ann Intern Med.* 2004;140:778-785.

310. Dansinger ML, Gleason JA, Griffith JL, et al. Comparison of the Atkins, Ornish, Weight Watchers, and Zone diets for weight loss and heart disease risk reduction: a randomized trial. *JAMA.* 2005;293:43-53.

311. Boden G, Sargrad K, Homko C, et al. Effect of a low-carbohydrate diet on appetite, blood glucose levels, and insulin resistance in obese patients with type 2 diabetes. *Ann Intern Med.* 2005;142:403-411.

312. Shai I, Schwarzfuchs D, Henkin Y, Dietary Intervention Randomized Controlled Trial (DIRECT) Group, et al. Weight loss with a low-carbohydrate, Mediterranean, or low-fat diet. *N Engl J Med.* 2008;359:229-241.

313. Sacks FM, Bray GA, Carey VJ, et al. Comparison of weight-loss diets with different compositions of fat, protein, and carbohydrates. *N Engl J Med.* 2009;360:859-873.

314. Ballor DL, Poehlman ET. A meta-analysis of the effects of exercise and/or dietary restriction on resting metabolic rate. *Eur J Appl Physiol Occup Physiol.* 1995;71:535-542.

315. Garrow JS, Summerbell CD. Meta-analysis: effect of exercise, with or without dieting, on the body composition of overweight subjects. *Eur J Clin Nutr.* 1995;49:1-10.

316. Warwick PM, Garrow JS. The effect of addition of exercise to a regime of dietary restriction on weight loss, nitrogen balance, resting metabolic rate and spontaneous physical activity in three obese women in a metabolic ward. *Int J Obes Relat Metab Disord.* 1981;5:25-32.

317. Holloszy JO, Schultz J, Kusnierkiewicz J, et al. Effects of exercise on glucose tolerance and insulin resistance. *Acta Med Scand.* 1986;711:55-65.

318. Helmrich SP, Ragland DR, Leung RW, Paffenbarger RS Jr. Physical activity and reduced occurrence of non-insulin-dependent diabetes mellitus. *N Engl J Med.* 1991;325(3):147-152.

319. Klem ML, Wing RR, McGuire MT, et al. A descriptive study of individuals successful at long-term maintenance of substantial weight loss. *Am J Clin Nutr.* 1997;66:239-246.

320. Kayman S, Bruvold W, Stern JS. Maintenance and relapse after weight loss in women: behavioral aspects. *Am J Clin Nutr.* 1990;52:800-807.

321. Hill JO, Schlundt DG, Sbrocco T, et al. Evaluation of an alternating-calorie diet with and without exercise in the treatment of obesity. *Am J Clin Nutr.* 1989;50:248-254.

322. Schoeller DA, Shay K, Kushner RF. How much physical activity is needed to minimize weight gain in previously obese women? *Am J Clin Nutr.* 1997;66:551-556.

323. Jakicic JM, Wing RR, Winters D. Effects of intermittent exercise and use of home exercise equipment on adherence, weight loss, and fitness in overweight women. *JAMA.* 1999;282:1554-1560.

324. Wadden TA, Sarwer DB, Berkowitz RI. Behavioural treatment of the overweight patient. *Bailliere's Clin Endocrin Metab.* 1999;13:93-107.

325. Wadden TA, Foster GD. Behavioral treatment of obesity. *Med Clin North Am.* 2000;84:441-461.

326. Perri MG, Nezu AM, Viegener BJ. *Improving the Long-Term Management of Obesity: Theory, Research and Clinical Guidelines.* New York, NY: John Wiley and Sons; 1992.

327. Sjostrom L, Rissanen A, Andersen T, et al. Randomised placebo-controlled trial of orlistat for weight loss and prevention of weight regain in obese patients. *Lancet.* 1998;352:167-172.

328. Weintraub M, Sundaresan PR, Schuster B, et al. Long-term weight control study V (weeks 190 to 210): follow-up of participants after cessation of medication. *Clin Pharmacol Ther.* 1992;51:615-618.

329. Wadden TA, Berkowitz RI, Womble LG, et al. Randomized trial of lifestyle modification and pharmacotherapy for obesity. *N Engl J Med.* 2005;353:2111-2120.

330. Khan MA, Herzog CA, St. Peter JV, et al. The prevalence of cardiac valvular insufficiency assessed by transthoracic echocardiography in obese patients treated with appetite-suppressant drugs. *N Engl J Med.* 1998;339:713-718.

331. Kernan WN, Viscoli CM, Brass LM, et al. Phenylpropanolamine and the risk of hemorrhagic stroke. *N Engl J Med.* 2000;343:1826-1832.

332. James WP, Caterson ID, Coutinho W, SCOUT Investigators, et al. Effect of sibutramine on cardiovascular outcomes in overweight and obese subjects. *N Engl J Med.* 2010;363(10):905-917.

333. National Institutes of Health; National Heart, Lung, and Blood Institute; North American Association for the Study of Obesity. *Practical Guide to the Identification, Evaluation, and Treatment of Overweight and Obesity in Adults.* NIH Publication No. 00-4084. Bethesda, MD: National Institutes of Health; 2000.

334. Munro JF, MacCuish AC, Wilson EM, Duncan LJP. Comparison of continuous and intermittent anorectic therapy in obesity. *Br Med J.* 1968;1:352-356.

335. Aronne LJ, Wadden TA, Peterson C, et al. Evaluation of phentermine and topiramate versus phentermine/topiramate extended-release in obese adults. *Obesity.* 2013;21:2163-2171.

336. Hadvary P, Lengsfield H, Wolfer H. Inhibition of pancreatic lipase in vitro by the covalent inhibitor tetrahydrolipstatin. *Biochem J.* 1998;256:357-361.

337. Zhi J, Melia AT, Guerciolini R, et al. Retrospective population-based analysis of the dose-response (fecal fat excretion) relationship of orlistat in normal and obese volunteers. *Clin Pharmacol Ther.* 1994;56:82-86.

338. Zhi J, Melia AT, Funk C, et al. Metabolic profiles of minimally absorbed orlistat in obese/overweight volunteers. *J Clin Pharmacol.* 1996;36:1006-1011.

339. Padwal R, Li SK, Lau DC. Long-term pharmacotherapy for overweight and obesity: a systematic review and meta-analysis of randomized controlled trials. *Int J Obes Relat Metab Disord.* 2003;27:1437-1446.

340. Li Z, Maglione M, Tu W, et al. Meta-analysis: pharmacologic treatment of obesity. *Ann Intern Med.* 2005;142:532-546.

341. Torgerson JS, Hauptman J, Boldrin MN, et al. XENical in the Prevention of Diabetes in Obese Subjects (XENDOS) study: a randomized study of orlistat as an adjunct to lifestyle changes for the prevention of type 2 diabetes in obese patients. *Diabetes Care.* 2004;27:155-161.

342. Sjöström L, Rissanen A, Andersen T, et al. Randomised placebo-controlled trial of orlistat for weight loss and prevention of weight regain in obese patients. *Lancet.* 1998;352:167-172.

343. Davidson MH, Hauptman J, DiGirolamo M, et al. Weight control and risk factor reduction in obese subjects treated for 2 years with orlistat. *JAMA.* 1999;281:235-242.

344. Mittendorfer B, Ostlund R, Patterson BW, et al. Orlistat inhibits dietary cholesterol absorption. *Obes Res.* 2001;9:599-604.

345. Rössner S, Sjöström L, Noack R, et al. Weight loss, weight maintenance, and improved cardiovascular risk factors after 2 years treatment with orlistat for obesity. *Obes Res.* 2000;8:49-61.

346. Finer N, James WP, Kopelman PG, et al. One-year treatment of obesity: a randomized, double-blind, placebo-controlled, multicentre study of orlistat, a gastrointestinal lipase inhibitor. *Int J Obes Relat Metab Disord.* 2000;24:306-313.

347. Hollander PA, Elbein SC, Hirsch IB, et al. Role of orlistat in the treatment of obese patients with type 2 diabetes. *Diabetes Care.* 1998;21:1288-1294.

348. Zhi J, Melia AT, Kross-Twardy SG, et al. The effect of orlistat, an inhibitor of dietary fat absorption, on the pharmacokinetics of beta-carotene in healthy volunteers. *J Clin Pharmacol.* 1996;36:152-159.

349. Melia AT, Kross-Twardy SG, Zhi J. The effect of orlistat, an inhibitor of dietary fat absorption, on the absorption of vitamins A and E in healthy volunteers. *J Clin Pharmacol.* 1996;36:647-653.

350. Colman E, Fossler M. Reduction in blood cyclosporin concentrations by orlistat. *N Engl J Med.* 2000;342:1141-1142.

351. Smith SR, Weissman NJ, Anderson CM, et al. Multicenter, placebo-controlled trial of lorcaserin for weight management. *N Engl J Med.* 2010;363:245-256.

352. Fidler MC, Sanchez M, Raether B, et al. A one-year randomized trial of lorcaserin for weight loss in obese and overweight adults: the BLOSSOM trial. *J Clin Endocrinol Metab.* 2011;96:3067-3077.

353. O'Neil PM, Smith SR, Weissman NJ, et al. Randomized placebo-controlled clinical trial of lorcaserin for weight loss in type 2 diabetes mellitus: the BLOOM-DM study. *Obesity (Silver Spring).* 2012;20:1426-1436.

354. Allison DB, Gadde KM, Garvey WT, et al. Controlled-release phentermine/topiramate in severely obese adults: a randomized controlled trial (EQUIP). *Obesity.* 2012;20:330-342.

355. Gadde KM, Allison DB, Ryan DH, et al. Effects of low-dose, controlled-release, phentermine plus topiramate combination on weight and associated comorbidities in overweight and obese adults (CONQUER): a randomized, placebo-controlled, phase 3 trial. *Lancet.* 2011;377:1341-1352.

356. Garvey WT, Ryan DH, Look M, et al. Two-year sustained weight loss and metabolic benefits with controlled-release phentermine/topiramate in obese and overweight adults (SEQUEL): a randomized, placebo-controlled, phase 3 extension study. *Am J Clin Nutr.* 2012;95(2):297-308.

357. U.K. Prospective Diabetes Study Group. Effect of intensive blood glucose control with metformin on complications in overweight patients with type 2 diabetes (UKPDS 34). *Lancet.* 1998;352:854-865.

358. Golay A. Metformin and body weight. *Int J Obes (Lond).* 2008;32:61-72.

359. Kahn SE, Haffner SM, Heise MA, et al. Glycemic durability of rosiglitazone, metformin, or glyburide monotherapy. *N Engl J Med.* 2006;355:2427-2443.

360. Levri KM, Slaymaker E, Last A, et al. Metformin as treatment for overweight and obese adults: a systematic review. *Ann Fam Med.* 2005;3:457-461.

361. Monami M, Marchionni N, Mannucci E. Glucagon-like peptide-1 receptor agonists in type 2 diabetes: a meta-analysis of randomized clinical trials. *Eur J Endocrinol.* 2009;160:909-917.

362. Amori RE, Lau J, Pittas AG. Efficacy and safety of incretin therapy in type 2 diabetes: systematic review and meta-analysis. *JAMA.* 2007;298:194-206.

363. Zinman B, Gerich J, Buse JB, et al. Efficacy and safety of the human glucagon-like peptide-1 analog liraglutide in combination with metformin and thiazolidinedione in patients with type 2 diabetes (LEAD-4 Met+TZD). *Diabetes Care.* 2009;32:1224-1230.

364. Astrup A, Rössner S, Van Gaal L, et al. NN8022-1807 Study Group. Effects of liraglutide in the treatment of obesity: a randomised, double-blind, placebo-controlled study. *Lancet.* 2009;374:1606-1616.

365. Aronne L, Fujioka K, Aroda V, et al. Progressive reduction in body weight after treatment with the amylin analog pramlintide in obese subjects: a phase 2, randomized, placebo-controlled, dose-escalation study. *J Clin Endocrinol Metab.* 2007;92:2977-2983.

366. Smith SR, Aronne LJ, Burns CM, et al. Sustained weight loss following 12-month pramlintide treatment as an adjunct to lifestyle intervention in obesity. *Diabetes Care.* 2008;31:1816-1823.

367. Vasilakou D, Karagiannis T, Athanasiadou E, et al. Sodium-glucose cotransporter 2 inhibitors for type 2 diabetes: a systematic review and meta-analysis. *Ann Intern Med.* 2013;159(4):262-274.

368. Consensus Development Conference Panel. NIH conference: gastrointestinal surgery for severe obesity. *Ann Intern Med.* 1991;115(12):956-961.

369. Bradley D, Magkos F, Klein S. Effects of bariatric surgery on glucose homeostasis and type 2 diabetes. *Gastroenterology.* 2012;143:897-912.

370. Courcoulas AP, Christian NJ, Belle SH, et al. Longitudinal Assessment of Bariatric Surgery (LABS) Consortium. Weight change and health outcomes at 3 years after bariatric surgery among individuals with severe obesity. *JAMA.* 2013;310(22):2416-2425.

371. Carlsson LM, Peltonen M, Ahlin S, et al. Bariatric surgery and prevention of type 2 diabetes in Swedish obese subjects. *N Engl J Med.* 2012;367:695-704.

372. Schauer PR, Kashyap SR, Wolski K, et al. Bariatric surgery versus intensive medical therapy in obese patients with diabetes. *N Engl J Med.* 2012;366:1567-1576.

373. Mingrone G, Panunzi S, De Gaetano A, et al. Bariatric surgery versus conventional medical therapy for type 2 diabetes. *N Engl J Med.* 2012;366:1577-1585.

374. Ikramuddin S, Korner J, Lee WJ, et al. Roux-en-Y gastric bypass vs intensive medical management for the control of type 2 diabetes, hypertension, and hyperlipidemia: the Diabetes Surgery Study randomized clinical trial. *JAMA.* 2013;309:2240-2249.

375. Buchwald H, Estok R, Fahrbach K, et al. Weight and type 2 diabetes after bariatric surgery: systematic review and meta-analysis. *Am J Med.* 2009;122:248-256.

376. Schauer PR, Burguera B, Ikramuddin S, et al. Effect of laparoscopic Roux-en Y gastric bypass on type 2 diabetes mellitus. *Ann Surg.* 2003;238(4):467-484.

377. Kadera BE, Lum K, Grant J, et al. Remission of type 2 diabetes after Roux-en-Y gastric bypass is associated with greater weight loss. *Surg Obes Relat Dis.* 2009;5:305-309.

378. Hamza N, Abbas MH, Darwish A, et al. Predictors of remission of type 2 diabetes mellitus after laparoscopic gastric banding and bypass. *Surg Obes Relat Dis.* 2011;7:691-696.
379. Chikunguwo SM, Wolfe LG, Dodson P, et al. Analysis of factors associated with durable remission of diabetes after Roux-en-Y gastric bypass. *Surg Obes Relat Dis.* 2010;6:254-259.
380. Blackstone R, Bunt JC, Cortes MC, et al. Type 2 diabetes after gastric bypass: remission in five models using HbA1c, fasting blood glucose, and medication status. *Surg Obes Relat Dis.* 2012;8:548-555.
381. Pournaras DJ, Aasheim ET, Sovik TT, et al. Effect of the definition of type II diabetes remission in the evaluation of bariatric surgery for metabolic disorders. *Br J Surg.* 2012;99:100-103.
382. Sjostrom L, Lindroos AK, Peltonen M, et al. Lifestyle, diabetes, and cardiovascular risk factors 10 years after bariatric surgery. *N Engl J Med.* 2004;351:2683-2693.
383. Arterburn DE, Bogart A, Sherwood NE, et al. A multisite study of long-term remission and relapse of type 2 diabetes mellitus following gastric bypass. *Obes Surg.* 2013;23(1):93-102.
384. Brethauer SA, Aminian A, Romero-Talamás H, et al. Can diabetes be surgically cured? Long-term metabolic effects of bariatric surgery in obese patients with type 2 diabetes mellitus. *Ann Surg.* 2013;258(4):628-636.
385. Laferrère B, Teixeira J, McGinty J, et al. Effect of weight loss by gastric bypass surgery versus hypocaloric diet on glucose and incretin levels in patients with type 2 diabetes. *J Clin Endocrinol Metab.* 2008;93:2479-2485.
386. Vidal J, Nicolau J, Romero F, et al. Long-term effects of Roux-en-Y gastric bypass surgery on plasma glucagon-like peptide-1 and islet function in morbidly obese subjects. *J Clin Endocrinol Metab.* 2009;94:884-891.
387. Salinari S, Bertuzzi A, Asnaghi S, et al. First-phase insulin secretion restoration and differential response to glucose load depending on the route of administration in type 2 diabetic subjects after bariatric surgery. *Diabetes Care.* 2009;32:375-380.
388. Service GJ, Thompson GB, Service FJ, et al. Hyperinsulinemic hypoglycemia with nesidioblastosis after gastric bypass surgery. *N Engl J Med.* 2005;353:249-254.
389. Patti ME, McMahon G, Mun EC, et al. Severe hypoglycaemia post-gastric bypass requiring partial pancreatectomy: evidence for inappropriate insulin secretion and pancreatic islet hyperplasia. *Diabetologia.* 2005;48:2236-2240.
390. Jensen MD, Ryan DH, Donato KA, et al. Guidelines (2013) for the management of overweight and obesity in adults. *Obesity.* 2014;22(Suppl 2):S1-S410.

CHAPTER 37

Disorders of Lipid Metabolism

CLAY F. SEMENKOVICH • ANNE C. GOLDBERG • IRA J. GOLDBERG

KEY POINTS

- Abnormalities of lipid metabolism cause heart disease, pancreatitis, vitamin deficiencies, and gallstones.
- Endocrine disorders such as diabetes and obesity have protean effects on lipid metabolism.
- Lowering low-density lipoprotein (LDL) with statins decreases vascular disease and prolongs life.
- Extreme elevations of triglycerides should be treated to avoid pancreatitis.
- Moderate elevations of triglycerides may be associated with vascular disease, but optimal treatment for this condition is unknown.
- Pharmacologic elevation of high-density lipoprotein (HDL) is not clearly beneficial.
- Substantial additional lowering of LDL beyond that seen with statins can be achieved by inhibiting proprotein convertase subtilisin/kexin type 9 (PCSK9).

LIPID BIOCHEMISTRY AND METABOLISM

Endocrine disorders have important effects on serum and tissue lipids, making the mechanisms underlying primary and secondary disorders of lipid metabolism relevant to clinicians as well as basic scientists. Some primary disorders of lipid metabolism, such as familial hypercholesterolemia (FH), are uncommon but important to understand. The LDL receptor pathway altered in FH helps explain genetic predispositions to heart disease; the mechanism of action of statin drugs, which decrease the risk of vascular events and prolong life;[1,2] and the mechanism of action of PCSK9 inhibitors, which strikingly lower lipid levels even in the setting of statin treatment.[3] The quintessential secondary disorder of lipid metabolism is that seen in diabetes, a disease so frequently characterized by abnormalities of fat that lipids have been implicated in its pathogenesis.

Lipids are ubiquitous. They constitute the physical bilayer that allows the formation of cell membranes, which are required for specialized organelles inside the cell and for regulating transport between the extracellular and intracellular environments. They circulate in the blood, with fatty acids and triglycerides providing an energy source to tissues such as heart and skeletal muscle and non-nutritive sterols providing substrates for hormone production by gonads and adrenals. Their specialized functions include the development of surfactant in lung to maintain patency of alveoli, formation of bile to facilitate excretion of a variety of metabolites, and constitution of myelin throughout the nervous system to ensure the fidelity of nerve transmission. Lipids are also signaling molecules, serving as targets of lipid kinases that perpetuate signaling cascades, substrates for cyclooxygenases and related enzymes that generate prostaglandins, and ligands for nuclear receptors such as the peroxisome proliferator-activated receptors (PPARs). The broad spectrum of lipid functions results in part from their biophysical characteristics.

Simple and Complex Lipids

Lipids owe their functional versatility to their hydrophobic structure. Because of the presence of fairly long carbon chains, lipids tend to associate with each other and have limited or no solubility in water. Fatty acids and cholesterol are simple lipids, whereas triglycerides and phospholipids are complex lipids (Fig. 37-1).

Fatty Acids

Chemical structures for the fatty acids are determined by the number of carbon atoms and the number of double bonds (see Fig. 37-1A). For example, stearic acid has 18 carbon atoms and is saturated, meaning that it has no double bonds; this is designated by the abbreviation C18:0. The 18-carbon monounsaturated fatty acid oleic acid (C18:1) has one double bond, and the polyunsaturated fatty acid linoleic acid (C18:2) has two double bonds.

Linoleic acid and arachidonic acid (C20:4) are ω-6 fatty acids, meaning that a double bond is present at the sixth carbon from the end of the molecule farthest from the carboxy (COOH)-terminal. Fish oils, which lower lipids, are ω-3 fatty acids, with a double bond present at the third carbon from the end opposite the COOH-terminal. Saturated fatty acids and some unsaturated fatty acids such as oleic acid are nonessential (i.e., they can be synthesized). Most ω-6 and ω-3 fatty acids are essential; they cannot be

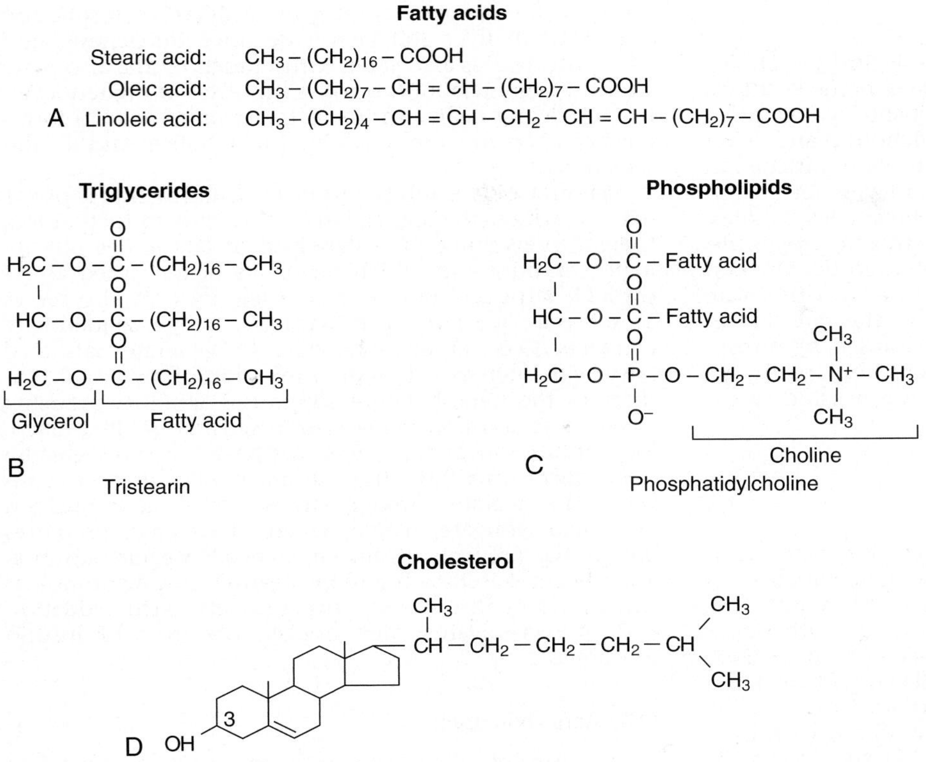

Fatty acids

Stearic acid: $CH_3 - (CH_2)_{16} - COOH$

Oleic acid: $CH_3 - (CH_2)_7 - CH = CH - (CH_2)_7 - COOH$

A Linoleic acid: $CH_3 - (CH_2)_4 - CH = CH - CH_2 - CH = CH - (CH_2)_7 - COOH$

Figure 37-1 Structures of common lipids, exemplified by the stearic, oleic, and linoleic fatty acids (**A**), the triglyceride tristearin (**B**), the phospholipid phosphatidylcholine (**C**), and cholesterol (**D**).

TABLE 37-1
Major Fatty Acids

Chemical Designation	Common Name	Common Food
Saturated Fatty Acids (No Double Bonds)		
C12:0	Lauric	Coconut oil
C14:0	Myristic	Coconut oil, butter fat
C16:0	Palmitic	Butter, cheese, meat
C18:0	Stearic	Beef, chocolate
Monounsaturated Fatty Acids (One Double Bond)		
C18:1	Oleic	Olive and canola oils
Polyunsaturated Fatty Acids (Two or More Double Bonds)		
Omega-6 Fatty Acids		
C18:2	Linoleic	Sunflower, corn, soybean, and safflower oils
C20:4	Arachidonic	
Omega-3 Fatty Acids		
C18:3	α-Linolenic	Canola, flaxseed, and soybean oils
C20:5	Eicosapentaenoic (EPA)	Salmon, cod, mackerel, tuna
C22:6	Docosahexaenoic (DHA)	Salmon, cod, mackerel, tuna

synthesized and are usually required for health, especially during development and in times of physiologic stress. Table 37-1 shows major food sources of fatty acids.

Triglycerides

The structure of tristearin, a triglyceride with three molecules of stearic acid connected to a glycerol molecule by means of ester linkages, is shown in Figure 37-1B. Other triglycerides have a similar structure with alternative fatty acids esterified to the glycerol backbone.

Most of the mass of adipose tissue in the body is composed of triglycerides; triglycerides that circulate in the blood mostly reflect the fatty acid composition of adipose tissue triglycerides, and both sources reflect dietary fatty acid composition. Butter in Western diets consists of similar amounts of palmitate and oleate with a lesser amount of stearate; adipose tissue and circulating triglycerides in persons eating Western diets contain mostly palmitate and oleate. Olive oil in Mediterranean diets is predominantly oleate with much less palmitate, so fat and circulating triglycerides in people eating a Mediterranean diet are enriched in oleic acid. Extremely high levels of triglycerides in the blood predispose to pancreatitis.

Phospholipids

The chemical structure for a generic phosphatidylcholine, a type of phospholipid, is shown in Figure 37-1C. As with triglycerides, phospholipids have a glycerol backbone to which fatty acids are esterified at the first two alcohols. The characteristics of these fatty acids are important for determining cell membrane shape and function.[4] The third alcohol is esterified to a phosphate moiety linked to another molecule, such as choline, ethanolamine, or serine.

The presence of long-chain fatty acids comprising hydrophobic regions and the charged species at the end of the molecule make phospholipids perfect for generating cell membranes and lipoprotein surface components: the bilayer is oriented so that the hydrophobic regions point toward each other, and the hydrophilic regions interact with the aqueous environment. Phospholipids are distributed asymmetrically in cell membranes, with choline-containing lipids directed toward the outer surface and amine-containing lipids directed toward the cytoplasmic surface. Appearance of the aminophospholipid phosphatidylserine on the cell surface initiates blood clotting and marks apoptotic cells for phagocytosis.

Cholesterol

The structure of cholesterol is shown in Figure 37-1D. The presence of cholesterol in the plasma membrane is critical for maintaining membrane fluidity, probably by disrupting the interactions between phosphatidylcholine and other molecules. The concentration of cholesterol is enriched in the plasma membrane, with much lower levels detected in the membranes of most intracellular organelles. Cholesterol is necessary for the synthesis of estrogen, progestins, androgens, aldosterone, vitamin D, glucocorticoids, and bile acids. Cholesterol deficiency is associated with severe developmental defects, as manifested in the rare Smith-Lemli-Optiz syndrome, which is likely caused by disruption of the Hedgehog signal transduction pathway.[5] Cholesterol excess is associated with gallstones and vascular disease.

Fatty Acid Metabolism

Fatty Acid Biosynthesis

In humans eating a typical Western diet, the overall contribution of de novo lipogenesis to lipid metabolism is small because the ingestion of exogenous fat is sufficient to suppress the energy-requiring process of synthesizing fats from carbohydrates. However, high-carbohydrate diets, especially those containing fructose,[6] substantially increase lipogenesis in liver and adipose tissue of humans.

Most tissues carry out fatty acid biosynthesis to at least a small degree regardless of nutritional status. Several of the key steps in fatty acid biosynthesis, presented in Figure 37-2, also have major effects on systemic metabolism. Citrate derived from the tricarboxylic acid (TCA) cycle is converted to acetyl coenzyme A (acetyl CoA) in the cytoplasm by the action of adenosine triphosphate (ATP) citrate lyase. Acetyl CoA is then converted to malonyl CoA by acetyl CoA carboxylase (ACC), which exists in two iso-

forms: ACC1 (encoded by the gene *ACACA*) is cytosolic and important in liver and fat for de novo lipogenesis, and ACC2 *(ACACB)* is associated with mitochondria, also plays a role in liver metabolism, and is expressed at highest levels in muscle and heart. Antisense targeting of ACC isoforms has been shown to improve lipid metabolism and insulin sensitivity.[7]

Malonyl CoA inhibits carnitine palmitoyltransferase 1 (CPT1), which transports fatty acids into mitochondria, thereby preventing the catabolism of fats under physiologic conditions in which energy is being stored as fat through fatty acid biosynthesis. Malonyl CoA also serves as substrate for fatty acid synthase, which sequentially connects two carbon fragments to generate saturated fatty acids such as palmitate. Inhibition of fatty acid synthase in the hypothalamus suppresses appetite, inducing weight loss and improving insulin sensitivity.[8] Pharmacologic inhibition of fatty acid synthase improves glucose metabolism and fatty liver in mice.[9] Palmitate is converted to stearate through the action of a long-chain fatty acid elongase, which, when inactivated, promotes obesity but prevents insulin resistance.[10] Stearate is subsequently converted to oleate by stearoyl-CoA desaturase 1, which, when inactivated, increases fatty acid oxidation and protects against diet-induced obesity and insulin resistance.[11]

Fatty Acid Oxidation

Metabolism of fatty acids provides more energy than metabolism of carbohydrates or proteins. Fatty acids undergo the process of β-oxidation in mitochondria (see Fig. 37-2). They are transported across (or diffuse across) the plasma membrane, converted to acyl-CoA species by acyl-CoA synthase, and then translocated to the mitochondrial matrix by CPT1 and CPT2. β-Oxidation removes two carbon fragments through the sequential actions of

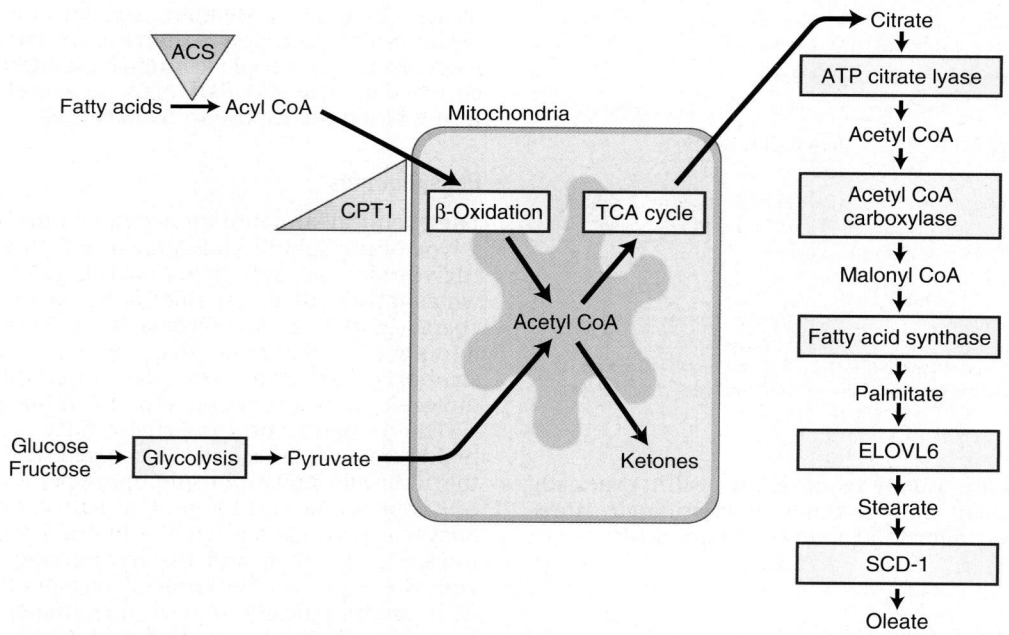

Figure 37-2 Fatty acid metabolism. Fatty acids are substrates for acyl-CoA synthase (ACS), which generates CoA moieties that are transported into mitochondria by carnitine palmitoyltransferase 1 (CPT1). Here, β-oxidation generates acetyl CoA, which can also be generated from glycolysis *(bottom left)*. Acetyl CoA can be used to produce ketones, or it may enter the TCA cycle, leading to production of citrate; in the cytoplasm, citrate is a substrate for ATP citrate lyase, which produces acetyl CoA. The acetyl CoA serves as a substrate for de novo synthesis of fatty acids, as depicted on the right side of the figure. ATP, adenosine triphosphate; CoA, coenzyme A; ELOVL6, elongation of very long chain fatty acid protein 6; SCD-1, stearoyl-CoA desaturase 1; TCA, tricarboxylic acid.

acyl-CoA dehydrogenases (e.g., medium-chain acyl-CoA dehydrogenase [MCAD] and very long chain acyl-CoA dehydrogenase [VLCAD]), enoyl-CoA hydratase, hydroxy-CoA dehydrogenase, and thiolase. This process generates reduced nicotinamide adenine dinucleotide (NADH) and reduced flavin adenine dinucleotide (FADH), which participate in electron transport to yield ATP. After multiple cycles, acetyl CoA is produced, which is a substrate for the TCA cycle and for ketogenesis.

Ketogenesis is necessary for life during times of nutritional deprivation. Extreme production of ketones occurs in the setting of insulin deficiency and represents a threat to life. 3-Hydroxy-3-methylglutaryl coenzyme A (HMG-CoA) synthase (rate-limiting in mitochondria) converts acetyl CoA to hydroxymethylglutaryl CoA, which is converted to acetoacetate by HMG-CoA lyase. Acetoacetate is either reduced to β-hydroxybutyrate or converted to acetone.

Defects in fatty acid oxidation are among the most common inborn errors of metabolism. Presentations include nonketotic hypoglycemia, liver dysfunction, and cardiomyopathy.[12]

Triglyceride and Phospholipid Metabolism

Dietary fat consists of triglycerides and phospholipids, which are digested in the stomach and proximal small intestine. Triglycerides are broken down into component fatty acids in part through the action of pancreatic lipase, which is activated by bile acids. Bile salts form micelles that acquire fatty acids and interact with the unstirred water layer of the intestine, where fatty acids are absorbed. Long-chain fatty acids are taken up by enterocytes, re-esterified into triglycerides, and exported into the lymph as lipoproteins. Medium-chain (≤C10) fatty acids directly enter the portal vein to access the liver.

Lipolysis of Triglyceride Stores in Adipose Tissue

The greatest triglyceride mass resides in adipose tissue, and turnover of energy stores at this site has important effects on lipid metabolism, normal physiology, and human health. Increased lipolysis in adipose tissue of the obese results in elevated circulating levels of free fatty acids, which may cause dysfunction in pancreatic beta cells, liver, skeletal muscle, and heart. Healthy subjects whose parents have type 2 diabetes mellitus have impaired insulin-mediated suppression of circulating fatty acids,[13] suggesting that an early defect in adipose tissue fatty acid metabolism contributes to the evolution of diabetes.

Release of free fatty acids and glycerol from adipose tissue is controlled by a variety of hormones, many of which act through G protein–coupled receptors. The most robust mediators of fatty acid release are catecholamines, which bind to β-adrenergic receptors, activating stimulatory G proteins (G_s) that prompt an increase in the activity of cyclic adenosine monophosphate and protein kinase A. Glucagon, adrenocorticotropic hormone, α-melanocyte-stimulating hormone, and thyroid-stimulating hormone also induce lipolysis through activity of G_s proteins. Adenosine suppresses lipolysis by binding to receptors that activate inhibitory G proteins (G_i). Niacin, which suppresses lipolysis, binds to the G protein receptor GPR109A, but this interaction does not mediate the effects of this vitamin on lipid metabolism.[14] A major mediator of lipolytic inhibition is insulin, which activates the insulin receptor-signaling cascade and suppresses lipolysis at many steps, one of which includes a decrease in protein kinase A activity.

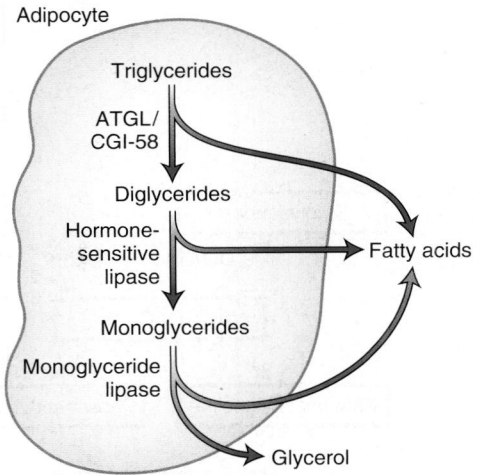

Figure 37-3 Lipolysis in adipocytes. Stored triglycerides are metabolized to yield the fatty acids that circulate in plasma through the action of three distinct lipases with separate substrate specificities. Triglycerides are acted on by adipose triglyceride lipase (ATGL) in complex with the coactivator protein CGI-58 to yield diglycerides, which are acted on by hormone-sensitive lipase to yield monoglycerides. The monoglycerides, in turn, are acted on by monoglyceride lipase to yield glycerol. Lipid droplet proteins modulate this lipolytic process.

At least three enzymes and two accessory proteins are required for the normal process of hormone-induced lipolysis in adipose tissue.[15] Stored triglycerides are acted on by the enzyme, adipose triglyceride lipase (encoded by *PNPLA2*), which requires the coactivator protein CGI-58. Diglycerides are hydrolyzed by hormone-sensitive lipase, yielding monoglycerides that are metabolized by monoglyceride lipase. This process cannot occur unless perilipin, a protein that coats small lipid droplets, is phosphorylated by protein kinase A. This process is depicted schematically in Figure 37-3. Human mutations in adipose triglyceride lipase or CGI-58 are responsible for two variants of neutral lipid storage disease that are characterized by hepatic steatosis, lipid accumulation in muscle tissues, neurologic problems, and, in one variant, skin defects.

Triglyceride and Phospholipid Synthesis and Tissue Delivery of Lipids

Triglyceride Synthesis. Key steps in triglyceride synthesis have major effects on systemic metabolism. Most triglycerides are synthesized through the glycerol phosphate pathway (Fig. 37-4, top portion) by a sequence of acylations. Another pathway, the monoacylglycerol pathway, is believed to be active only in the small intestine. Glycerol-3-phosphate is acted on by one of the glycerol-3-phosphate acyltransferases (GPATs) to generate lysophosphatidic acid. An important isoform is GPAT1, which is thought to compete with CPT1 for fatty acyl CoA molecules inside the cell, with GPAT1 prevailing when energy is to be stored and CPT1 dominant when energy is required. The next acylation is mediated by acylglycerol-3-phosphate acyltransferases (AGPATs) and generates phosphatidic acid. Human mutations in AGPAT2 are responsible for the disease known as *congenital generalized lipodystrophy*.

Phosphatidic acid represents an important branch point in lipid metabolism. It serves as substrate for synthesis of either cytidine diphosphate diacylglycerol (CDP-DAG, the precursor for molecules such as phosphatidylinositol) or diacylglycerol (DAG). Synthesis of DAG requires a phosphatase activity provided by lipins.[16] These proteins have complicated effects on insulin sensitivity and metabolism.

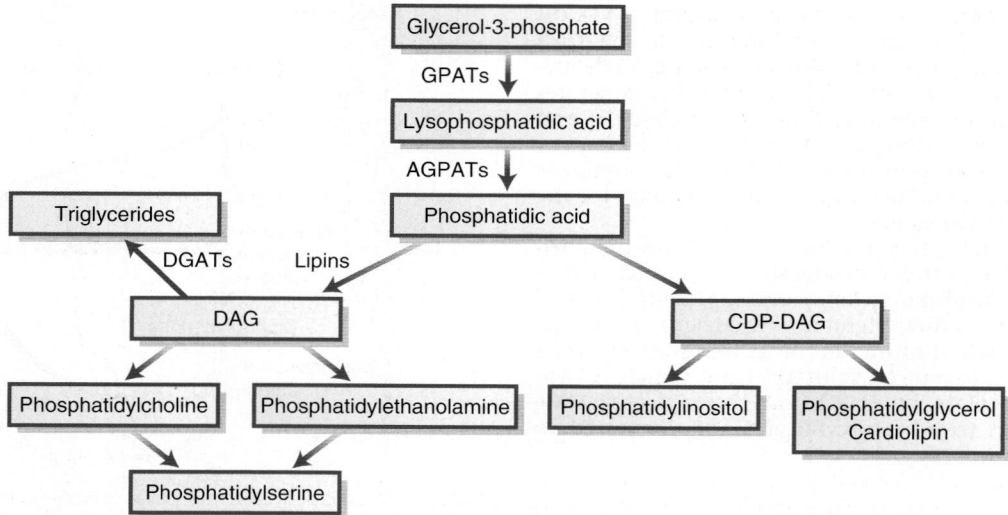

Figure 37-4 Phospholipid and triglyceride synthesis. Glycerol-3-phosphate is converted by glycerol-3-phosphate acyltransferases (GPATs) to lysophosphatidic acid, which is converted to phosphatidic acid by acylglycerol-phosphate acyltransferases (AGPATs). Phosphatidic acid can be converted to cytidine diphosphate diacylglycerol (CDP-DAG), to fuel one arm of phospholipid synthesis, or to diacylglycerol (DAG), which is a substrate for another arm of phospholipid synthesis and for acyl-CoA:diacylglycerol acyltransferases (DGATs), which generate triglycerides.

DAG can serve as a signaling molecule and as substrate for synthesis of either triglycerides or common phospholipids. The acylation of DAG to form triglycerides is catalyzed by acyl-CoA:diacylglycerol acyltransferases (DGATs). Inactivation of DGAT1 renders mice resistant to diet-induced obesity.[17]

Phospholipid Synthesis. As shown in the bottom portion of Figure 37-4, phospholipid synthesis is intimately related to triglyceride synthesis. Generation of one of the most important phospholipids, phosphatidylcholine, occurs mostly through the Kennedy pathway, which utilizes choline as an initial substrate and DAG at the final step. Mammalian liver is also able to generate phosphatidylcholine from phosphatidylethanolamine through successive methylations. Both phosphatidylcholine and phosphatidylethanolamine can be converted to phosphatidylserine.

Lipoprotein Lipase. Most lipids are delivered to peripheral tissues such as muscle and fat through the activity of lipoprotein lipase (LPL). LPL, which is rate-limiting for clearance of plasma triglycerides and essential for generation of HDL particles,[18] hydrolyzes triglycerides (and, to a lesser extent, phospholipids) in circulating triglyceride-rich lipoproteins to allow peripheral sites such as adipose tissue and muscle access to preformed fatty acids. Much of this lipid flux is controlled by insulin, which increases LPL in fat and decreases LPL in muscle. Exercise tends to have the opposite effect,[19] ensuring appropriate energy supplies are available to meet metabolic demands.

Free fatty acids released from lipoproteins by the action of LPL presumably diffuse into resident cells in the local tissues, where they are converted to acyl CoA species and either stored as triglycerides or subjected to fatty acid oxidation. This hydrolytic release reaction occurs at the capillary endothelium. LPL is not synthesized in endothelial cells but is produced in adipocytes, cardiac myocytes, and skeletal myocytes and then secreted and targeted to the luminal surface of the endothelium through mechanisms that are poorly understood. At the endothelium, LPL and triglyceride-rich lipoproteins bind to glycosylphosphatidylinositol-anchored high-density lipoprotein–binding protein 1 (GPIHBP1). GPIHBP1 is believed to serve as a platform for lipolysis in the plasma.[20]

Cholesterol Metabolism

In adults, dietary cholesterol is not required because many tissues are capable of cholesterol synthesis. However, most diets include animal products, the source of cholesterol. Plants do not have cholesterol, but their membranes contain phytosterols, which are structurally similar to cholesterol and are useful in the dietary treatment of hypercholesterolemia because they compete with cholesterol for absorption. The liver and intestine are quantitatively the most important sites for cholesterol metabolism in humans, although a very small amount of cholesterol is also lost through the normal turnover of skin.

Cholesterol Absorption, Synthesis, and Excretion

Cholesterol is absorbed through a process that requires the formation of bile salt micelles. The efficiency of absorption varies widely in humans. There is a gradient of absorption through the intestine that is greatest in the proximal small intestine and least in the ileum. This gradient parallels the expression of Niemann-Pick C1–like 1 (NPC1L1), a transmembrane protein with a sterol-sensing domain that is involved in cholesterol absorption.[21] NPC1L1 is the target of ezetimibe, a drug that lowers cholesterol and has been shown to decrease heart disease (see later discussion). NPC1L1 also absorbs phytosterols such as sitosterol. Sterols are pumped out of the enterocyte and into the intestinal lumen by two ATP-binding cassette (ABC) transporters, ABCG5 and ABCG8. Human mutations in these transporters cause the rare disorder sitosterolemia,[22] characterized by increased absorption and circulating levels of sitosterol and cholesterol, xanthomas, and heart disease (see later discussion).

Figure 37-5A illustrates cholesterol synthesis. Acetate is converted to HMG-CoA. The latter is a substrate for HMG-CoA reductase, the enzyme that is rate-limiting for cholesterol biosynthesis and is inhibited by statin drugs. Cells exquisitely regulate cholesterol acquisition.[23] When levels are low, mechanisms are activated to increase cholesterol biosynthesis and import cholesterol from the extracellular environment. Statins, by lowering cholesterol and

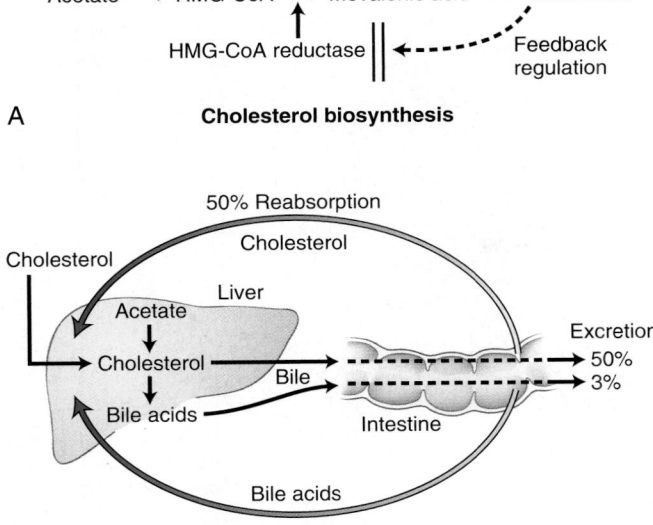

A **Cholesterol biosynthesis**

B **Enterohepatic circulation of cholesterol and bile acids**

Figure 37-5 A, Cholesterol biosynthesis. 3-Hydroxy-3-methylglutaryl coenzyme A (HMG-CoA) reductase is the rate-limiting enzyme regulating cholesterol biosynthesis. The enzyme is downregulated by excess cholesterol in the cell. **B,** Enterohepatic circulation of cholesterol and bile acids. Approximately 50% of cholesterol and 97% of bile acids are reabsorbed from the intestine and recirculated to the liver. (**A,** Modified from Brown MS, Goldstein JL. A receptor-mediated pathway for cholesterol homeostasis. *Science.* 1986;232:34-47.)

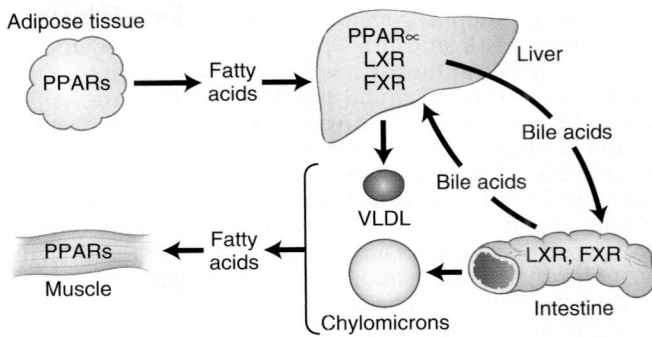

Figure 37-6 Nuclear receptors in lipid metabolism. Peroxisome proliferator-activated receptors (PPARs) are active in adipose tissue, which is a source of fatty acids that are transported to liver, where PPARα, the liver X receptors (LXR), and farnesoid X receptor (FXR) are active. Bile acids produced by the liver participate in an enterohepatic circulation with the intestine, another site of LXR and FXR expression. Very low density lipoprotein (VLDL), produced by liver, and chylomicrons, from intestine, are metabolized to release fatty acids that fuel muscle (another site of PPAR expression) and may be stored by adipose tissue.

preventing cholesterol biosynthesis, work predominantly by increasing liver uptake of cholesterol from the plasma through the LDL receptor (see later discussion) and promoting its excretion. Free cholesterol in cells is esterified to form cholesteryl esters for storage. This esterification reaction is carried out by acyl CoA:cholesterol acyltransferases (ACATs). These endoplasmic reticulum enzymes exist in two forms: ACAT1 is present in macrophages and has been implicated in atherosclerosis, and ACAT2 is present in liver and intestine and is implicated in cholesterol absorption. Nonspecific ACAT inhibition in humans does not affect serum lipids and does not have beneficial effects on atherosclerosis.[24]

Cholesterol, which is non-nutritive and cannot be catabolized to carbon dioxide and water, is either secreted into the bile as free cholesterol (about half of which is reabsorbed) or converted to bile acids for secretion into bile. Most bile acids are reabsorbed in the terminal ileum. This enterohepatic circulation of cholesterol and bile acids is shown in Figure 37-5B. The rate-limiting enzyme for bile acid synthesis is cholesterol 7α-hydroxylase, which is under feedback regulation by bile acids. Interruption of the enterohepatic circulation of bile acids through the use of bile acid sequestrants (BAS) increases bile acid synthesis, lowers plasma cholesterol, and decreases vascular disease events. At least in mice, evidence suggests that cholesterol can be excreted directly by enterocytes (independent of the biliary system) through an active metabolic process termed transintestinal cholesterol excretion (TICE).[25]

NUCLEAR RECEPTORS AND LIPID METABOLISM

Nuclear receptors, usually transcription factors with ligand-binding and DNA-binding domains, affect lipid metabo-

lism. Classic hormones that interact with nuclear receptors and have important lipid effects include thyroid hormone, glucocorticoids, estrogen, and testosterone.

Thyroid hormone regulates cholesterol metabolism through direct effects on the gene for a transcription factor that controls LDL-receptor expression, sterol regulatory element–binding protein 2 (SREBP2).[26] This role explains why lipid levels tend to be high in hypothyroid patients and low with hyperthyroidism. Glucocorticoids have robust effects on multiple aspects of lipid metabolism, inducing expression of HMG-CoA reductase to promote cholesterol synthesis, increasing expression of fatty acid synthase to promote fatty acid synthesis, and decreasing LPL to impair clearance of circulating lipids. Accordingly, hyperlipidemia is seen commonly in the setting of glucocorticoid treatment, and insulin resistance induced by glucocorticoids amplifies the hyperlipidemia. Estrogens and selective estrogen receptor modulators such as raloxifene lower cholesterol[27] by inducing LDL-receptor activity; they tend to increase triglyceride levels, especially when higher oral doses are administered. Derivatives of cholesterol can serve as selective estrogen-receptor modulators (SERMs) to affect the vasculature.[28] Androgens, by activating the androgen receptor, decrease levels of HDL.[29]

Aside from classic hormones and their receptors, other nuclear receptors affect lipid metabolism after interacting with several types of metabolic by-products. These receptors include the PPARs, the liver X receptors (LXRs), and the farnesoid X receptor (FXR). A schematic view of the roles of these receptors in lipid metabolism is presented in Figure 37-6.

There are three known types of PPARs: α, γ, and δ. PPARα promotes fatty acid oxidation as well as ketogenesis and is induced by starvation. It is expressed at highest levels in tissues that are adapted to metabolize fats, such as liver and skeletal muscle, but is also present at numerous other sites. In humans, pharmacologic activation of PPARα with fibrates lowers triglycerides and increases HDL. Fatty acids interact with the receptor, but a phosphatidylcholine species was identified as an endogenous ligand for PPARα.[30]

Whereas PPARα facilitates energy utilization, PPARγ activates genes that promote energy storage. It is expressed at highest levels in adipose tissue and is also found in macrophages, where it may help coordinate the complex relationship between inflammation and metabolism. Ether lipids, phospholipids generated in peroxisomes, appear to be endogenous ligands for PPARγ.[31,32] Pharmacologic activation of PPARγ in humans with thiazolidinediones results in insulin sensitization and weight gain. The latter effect occurs because this nuclear receptor promotes adipogenesis as well as fluid retention through effects on the kidney. Thiazolidinedione treatment in humans tends to lower triglycerides and increase HDL, probably by modulating insulin signaling, but the impact of these agents on atherosclerosis is unclear. Dual agonists for PPARα and PPARγ were shown to lower hemoglobin A_{1c} as well as serum lipids in humans but also increased all-cause mortality rate.

PPARδ has important effects in tissues such as skeletal muscle, and its activation may mimic the effects of exercise. Agents targeting this receptor in humans appear to show benefit, in part by increasing fatty acid oxidation.[33]

LXRs and FXR are also involved in lipid metabolism. LXRα and LXRβ are activated by oxysterols (modified derivatives of cholesterol) to increase the conversion of cholesterol into bile acids, increase bile acid excretion, and decrease cholesterol absorption.[34] LXR activation inhibits cholesterol uptake by inducing the degradation of the LDL receptor.[35] LXRs also induce fatty acid and triglyceride synthesis. FXR is activated by bile acids to stimulate bile acid secretion as well as reabsorption. Administration of a BAS to humans with diabetes lowers blood sugar, which may be a consequence of effects on FXR as well as activation of the G protein–coupled receptor TGR5 to increase glucagon-like peptide 1 by the intestine.[36]

Additional nuclear receptors also play important roles in lipogenesis—the process of converting carbohydrates to triglycerides rather than glycogen. Carbohydrate response element–binding protein (ChREBP) may control as much as 50% of this process. It responds to carbohydrate excess by transactivating a series of glycolytic and lipogenic genes. SREBP1 is also critical for this process.[37]

PLASMA LIPOPROTEINS, APOLIPOPROTEINS, RECEPTORS, AND OTHER PROTEINS

Physiologic requirements at sites remote from the source of external lipids (i.e., the gut) have resulted in selective pressure to develop a system capable of moving nutrients, vitamins, structural components, and proteins with specialized functions through the plasma compartment. The effectors of this system are lipoproteins, spherical particles that circulate in the blood. Appropriate concentrations of lipoproteins are essential for health. When certain lipoproteins are present at high levels in the circulation, cardiovascular disease and pancreatitis may result. When other lipoproteins are absent or present at very low levels, vitamin deficiency syndromes and cardiovascular disease may develop. The roles of the various lipoproteins are discussed in detail in the following sections.

Major Lipoproteins

A prototypical lipoprotein is shown in Figure 37-7. The fundamental structure of a lipoprotein exploits the biochemical characteristics of its components. The surface consists of charged molecules that interact with the aqueous environment, such as phospholipids and free cholesterol. Amphipathic proteins (with hydrophilic as well as hydrophobic domains), known as *apolipoproteins* (or simply *apoproteins*), are also present on the surface, with their hydrophilic domains oriented toward the plasma and

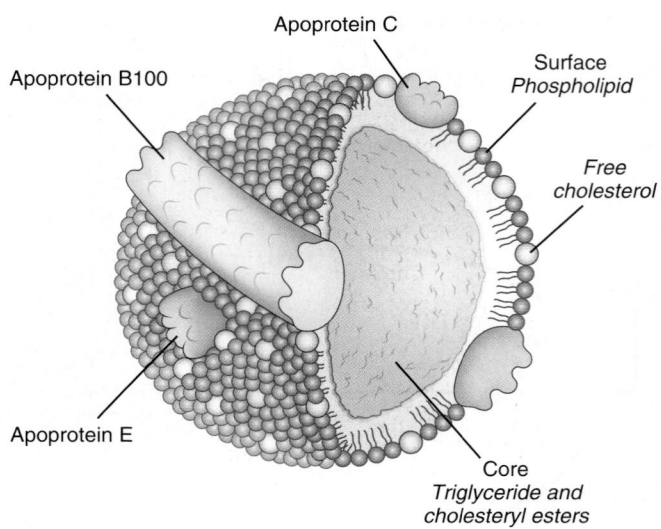

Figure 37-7 General structure of lipoproteins: schematic representation of a very low density lipoprotein (VLDL) particle.

their hydrophobic domains toward the core of the particle. Apolipoproteins direct lipoproteins toward their appropriate sites of metabolism. The lipoprotein core consists of neutral (uncharged) lipids such as triglycerides and cholesteryl esters.

Lipoprotein movement through the plasma compartment is dynamic. Humans spend most of their lives in the postprandial state. Eating is associated with generation of lipoproteins, induction of enzymes that metabolize those lipoproteins, interactions among lipoproteins in the plasma involving the exchange of both lipid and protein components, rapid alterations of lipoprotein size as large particles are metabolized to smaller ones, genesis of new lipoproteins in the circulation as excess surface components of shrinking particles are extruded, and movement of critical nutrients and vitamins into tissues. Clinical assessment of disease risk is based on fasting measurements, but most lipid metabolism that causes disease occurs in the fed state.

The major classes of lipoproteins are listed in Table 37-2. Their original identification was accomplished based on migration in an ultracentrifuge, and classes were defined based on density. An alternative original classification scheme, which is no longer useful, involved electrophoretic mobility in agarose gels. Chylomicrons, chylomicron remnants, and very low density lipoproteins (VLDLs) are rich in triglycerides. Intermediate-density lipoproteins (IDLs), LDLs, and lipoprotein(a), or Lp(a), are rich in cholesterol. HDLs are enriched in phospholipids. Triglyceride-rich lipoproteins such as chylomicrons are large and generally insoluble, which accounts for the cloudy appearance of plasma when it is obtained in nonfasting subjects or in fasting subjects with some types of hyperlipidemias. Table 37-2 provides general ranges for particle size, which differs substantially among lipoproteins and within each class. Certain lipoprotein subtypes, such as small dense LDL, may promote cardiovascular disease and are more likely to occur with insulin resistance.

Chylomicrons originate in the gut. They are lighter than water and float to the top of a plasma sample. The particles are cleared fairly rapidly after a meal and should be absent after an overnight fast. Their distinguishing apolipoprotein is apoB48, which is the only form of apolipoprotein B

TABLE 37-2

Major Classes of Plasma Lipoproteins

Type	Density (g/mL)	Origin	Major Lipids	Major Apolipoproteins	Size (nm)
Chylomicrons	<0.95	Intestine	85% Triglyceride	B48, AI, AIV, E, CI, CII, CIII	~100-500
Chylomicron remnants	<1.006	Derived from chylomicrons	60% Triglyceride 20% Cholesterol	B48, E	~80-125
VLDL	<1.006	Liver	55% Triglyceride 20% Cholesterol	B100, E, CI, CII, CIII	30-80
IDL	1.006-1.019	Derived from VLDL	35% Cholesterol 25% Triglyceride	B100, E	25-35
LDL	1.019-1.063	Derived from IDL	60% Cholesterol 5% Triglyceride	B100	18-25
HDL	1.063-1.21	Liver, intestine, plasma	25% Phospholipid 20% Cholesterol 5% Triglyceride	AI, AII, CI, CII, CIII, E	5-12
Lp(a)	1.05-1.09	Liver	60% Cholesterol 5% Triglyceride	B100, apo(a)	~30

apo, apolipoprotein; IDL, intermediate-density lipoprotein; LDL, low-density lipoprotein; Lp(a), lipoprotein(a); VLDL, very low density lipoprotein.

produced by intestinal cells in humans. Chylomicrons acquire apoC and apoE molecules by interacting with HDL particles, a process that promotes chylomicron metabolism and conversion to chylomicron remnants. Chylomicron remnants, also characterized by the presence of apoB48, are cleared rapidly from the plasma. Remnant particles may promote ischemic heart disease, particularly in obesity.[38]

VLDL particles are of hepatic origin. Smaller than chylomicrons, their distinguishing apolipoprotein is apoB100, the form of apoB produced by the liver. VLDLs also carry apoC molecules that modulate the conversion of VLDLs to IDLs, which are VLDL remnants and are thought to be atherogenic. IDL particles contain apoB100 and apoE, and they are converted to LDL, which is characterized by carrying essentially only apoB100 as an apolipoprotein. LDL, known as "bad cholesterol," is the major carrier of cholesterol in most humans, and its measurement forms the basis for coronary heart disease (CHD) risk stratification and treatment goals. For most clinical laboratories, LDL results represent both IDL and LDL particles.

HDL particles have a complex biology. They can be generated by liver and intestine or assembled in the plasma as a consequence of the metabolism of other lipoproteins. They are arbitrarily divided into HDL_2 (less dense, at 1.063 to 1.125 g/mL), which typically contains apoAI as well as apoCs, and HDL_3 (more dense, at 1.125 to 1.21 g/mL), which typically contains apoAI, apoAII, and apoCs. There is also a minor subclass known as HDL_1 that carries a large percentage of plasma apoE. HDL is known as "good cholesterol" and high levels are associated with low cardiovascular risk, but it is not known if HDL plays a direct role in atherosclerosis. Concentrations of HDL may not be helpful in determining risk. Instead, a functional assay, cholesterol efflux capacity, may be a useful biomarker for vascular disease. This activity, reflecting the movement of labeled cholesterol from a cultured macrophage cell line to apoB-depleted plasma, is inversely associated with cardiovascular events.[39]

Lp(a), produced by the liver, consists of an LDL particle in which the apolipoprotein apo(a) has been covalently linked to apoB100. Apo(a) has substantial protein homology to plasminogen, required for the endogenous thrombolytic response, and it exists in isoforms based on kringle repeats (named after a type of pastry). Isoforms with fewer repeats, and therefore lower mass, tend to circulate at higher concentrations. Higher levels increase the risk of myocardial infarction and aortic valve calcification.[40,41]

Major Apolipoproteins

The chromosomal location, size, sites of synthesis, and major functions of important apolipoproteins are summarized in Table 37-3.

Apolipoproteins AI, AII, AIV, and AV

ApoAI is the most abundant apolipoprotein in HDL. It is synthesized by the liver and intestine and is known to activate the enzyme lecithin:cholesterol acyltransferase (LCAT), which transfers a fatty acid from lecithin to the free hydroxyl group on cholesterol to generate cholesteryl ester. This activity is involved in the maturation of HDL particles, which begin as lipid-poor discs containing apoAI and then acquire free cholesterol; they convert this cholesterol to cholesteryl ester through the activity of LCAT and expand into spheres as cholesteryl ester is stuffed into the growing core. ApoAI is important for mediating the efflux of cholesterol from peripheral tissues, an important step in the process of reverse cholesterol transport.[42] Human genetic mutations in apoAI cause low levels of HDL and corneal opacities. ApoAI is considered to be an antiatherogenic protein, but genetic defects in apoAI are not consistently associated with coronary artery disease. Its presence may be important in the setting of an atherosclerotic environment with elevated levels of atherogenic lipoproteins.

ApoAII is present with apoAI in some HDL particles. Synthesized mostly in the liver, it has been implicated in the activation of hepatic lipase, an enzyme involved in lipoprotein processing, including HDL metabolism, and in the inhibition of LCAT. ApoAII may disrupt the ability of HDL to promote reverse cholesterol transport, but the genetic absence of this protein in humans does not seem to be associated with a phenotype.[43]

ApoAIV originates in the gut, and its secretion is induced by the consumption of a high-fat meal. It may affect food intake in mice, but information in humans is not available.

ApoAV is encoded by a locus near the apoAIV gene in the apoAI/CIII/AIV/AV gene cluster on chromosome 11. It is produced by liver and circulates at low concentrations in association with VLDL particles in humans. ApoAV is involved in the hydrolysis of triglyceride-rich lipoproteins by LPL, its expression in mice is inversely related to triglyceride levels, and it promotes lipoprotein clearance by hepatic proteoglycans.[44]

TABLE 37-3

Major Apolipoproteins

Apolipoprotein (Chromosome No.)	Molecular Weight (kDa)	Synthesis	Functions
AI (11)	~29	Liver, intestine	Structural protein (HDL) Cofactor for LCAT Crucial role in reverse cholesterol transport Ligand for ABC-A1 and SR-BI
AII (1)	~17 (dimer)	Liver	Inhibits apoE binding to receptors Activates hepatic lipase Inhibits LCAT
AIV (11)	~45	Intestine	Potential satiety factor Activator of LCAT Facilitates lipid secretion from intestine
AV (11)	39	Liver	Activator of LPL-mediated lipolysis Might inhibit hepatic VLDL synthesis
B100 (2)	~500	Liver	Structural protein (VLDL and LDL) Ligand for LDL receptor
B48 (2)	~200	Intestine	Structural protein (chylomicrons)
CI (19)	6.6	Liver	Modulates remnant binding to receptors Activates LCAT
CII (19)	8.9	Liver	Cofactor for LPL
CIII (11)	8.8	Liver	Modulates remnant binding to receptors Inhibitor of LPL
E (19)	~34	Liver, brain, skin, testes, spleen	Ligand for LDL and remnant receptors Local lipid redistribution Reverse cholesterol transport (HDL with apoE)
apo(a) (6)	~400-800	Liver	Modulates thrombosis/fibrinolysis

ABCA1, adenosine triphosphate–binding cassette transporter A1; apo, apolipoprotein; HDL, high-density lipoprotein; LCAT, lecithin:cholesterol acyltransferase; LDL, low-density lipoprotein; LPL, lipoprotein lipase; SR-B1, scavenger receptor class B type 1; VLDL, very low density lipoprotein.

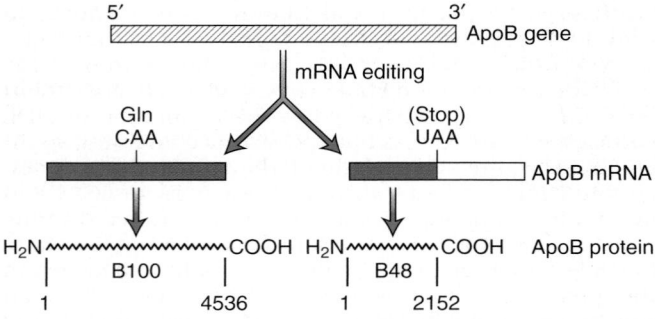

Figure 37-8 Synthesis of apolipoprotein B100 and apoB48 by a messenger RNA (mRNA) editing mechanism. In the human intestine, a specific cytosine (C) is changed to a uracil (U) in the apoB mRNA. This change results in a stop codon and the formation of apoB48, which contains only the first 2152 amino acids of the full-length apoB100 (4536 amino acids). COOH, carboxy-terminus; Gln, glutamine; H₂N, amino-terminus.

Apolipoprotein B

There are two forms of this apolipoprotein, apoB100 and apoB48, which are derived from a single gene by a unique mechanism that involves RNA editing (Fig. 37-8). In both liver and intestinal cells, the same messenger RNA is transcribed, but an editing protein complex interacts with the message only in the intestine (in humans) to change the cytosine at nucleotide position 6666 to a uracil.[45] This enzymatic effect converts a glutamine codon to a stop codon, resulting in an intestinal protein that is approximately 48% of the length of apoB100—hence, the name apoB48.

ApoB48, in essence a truncated form of apoB100, thus originates in the gut, where it is important for the assembly of chylomicrons.[46] There are one or two B48 molecules on each chylomicron, where they provide structural support to the particle. The COOH-terminus of apoB100, missing in apoB48, determines interaction with the LDL receptor, so apoB48 does not appear to be involved in the clearance of gut-derived lipoproteins.

ApoB100 originates in the liver, where it is cotranslationally associated with lipids to coordinate the formation of VLDL particles. VLDL assembly and export, which affect the levels of circulating atherogenic lipoproteins, are determined not by transcriptional control of the apoB gene but by a unique mechanism involving stabilization of the apoB protein by lipid. VLDL production is shown in Figure 37-9. Assembly is thought to involve two distinct processes. First, as the apoB message is translated on the rough endoplasmic reticulum, it binds to lipids that are provided by microsomal triglyceride transfer protein (MTP, the target of a new medication, see later). This protein heterodimerizes with protein disulfide isomerase, which remodels the apoB protein by rearranging the positions of disulfide bonds in the molecule to accommodate incoming lipid. Most of this lipid originates in adipose tissue, where triglyceride lipolysis releases free fatty acids that are transported to the liver. Phospholipids and cholesterol also associate with apoB at this step. If sufficient lipids are not available in the liver, apoB (which is constitutively produced) is ubiquitinated and degraded in the proteasome. Second, maturing VLDL particles fuse with additional lipid droplets in the Golgi apparatus, a process facilitated by apoE. The triglyceride-rich particles are then secreted into the space of Disse. Because these particles carry the apolipoproteins that determine VLDL binding to liver receptors, it might be expected that they would be taken up immediately and never access the circulation. This does not occur, probably because high concentrations of phosphatidylethanolamine in nascent VLDL obscure receptor binding sites. These sites are revealed in the circulation as phospholipids are removed. Transfer of apolipoproteins from other lipoproteins in the circulation also modifies VLDL structure to promote metabolism in the periphery.

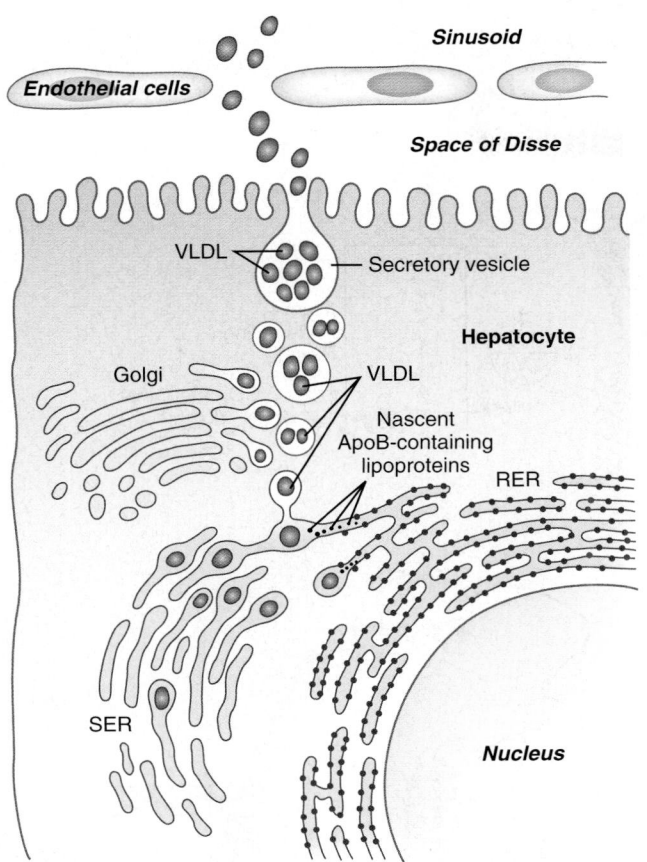

Figure 37-9 Very low density lipoprotein (VLDL) biosynthesis by hepatocytes. The nascent apolipoprotein B (apoB)-containing apolipoproteins synthesized by the rough endoplasmic reticulum (RER) are thought to combine with lipids in the smooth endoplasmic reticulum (SER). The VLDLs are processed in the Golgi apparatus and accumulate in large secretory vesicles. They are then released into the space of Disse and enter the plasma. (Modified from Alexander CA, Hamilton RL, Havel RJ. Subcellular localization of B apoprotein of plasma lipoproteins in rat liver. *J Cell Biol.* 1976;69:241-263; by copyright permission of the Rockefeller University Press.)

Increased VLDL production, fueled by the increased availability of lipid, is predominantly responsible for the dyslipidemia seen with obesity and diabetes. Hepatitis C, a major cause of human liver disease, circulates in VLDL particles, and this virus assimilates the VLDL assembly machinery. There is one copy of apoB100 on each VLDL particle, and this relationship is retained as these lipoproteins are metabolized to IDL and then to LDL. Therefore, measurements of apoB100 in the plasma reflect particle number, and higher levels of apoB are associated with cardiovascular disease. The complete absence of apoB, which occurs in the rare human disorder abetalipoproteinemia, is not caused by mutations in apoB but by defects in MTP.[47] Patients with this disease have severe neurologic deficits, probably reflecting vitamin E deficiency, because triglyceride-rich lipoproteins transport this lipid-soluble vitamin. Very low, but not absent, apoB, which occurs in the human disorder hypobetalipoproteinemia, is caused by mutations in apoB. These individuals present with low levels of cholesterol and triglycerides and appear to be healthy. A mutation at amino acid residue 3500 of the apoB100 protein, within the COOH-terminal region of the molecule that mediates binding to the LDL receptor, causes familial defective apoB100. These individuals have high levels of LDL cholesterol, mimicking the presentation of FH.[48]

Apolipoproteins CI, CII, and CIII

These small apolipoproteins are encoded by loci residing at two different locations in the genome. ApoCI and apoCII are transcribed from a site on chromosome 19 near the apoE gene. The apoCIII gene is a component of the apoAI/CIII/AIV/AV cluster on chromosome 11. ApoCs, which can be exchanged freely among lipoprotein particles, are important for triglyceride metabolism because their presence either interferes with the recognition of apoE by lipoprotein receptors or displaces apoE from lipoproteins (both of which would increase triglycerides by impairing their clearance). The function of apoCII is more complex than that of CI and CIII. High levels in mice cause elevated triglycerides by displacing apoE, but normal levels of apoCII are required for normal lipid clearance because this apolipoprotein is a cofactor for the enzyme LPL. Mutations of apoCII in humans cause severe hypertriglyceridemia, mimicking LPL deficiency.

ApoCIII may be particularly relevant to human health. Its levels are increased in the setting of many dyslipidemias, and most lipid-lowering medications lower apoCIII levels. A mutation in the apoCIII gene causing lower apoCIII levels is associated with an improved lipid profile and less atherosclerosis,[49] suggesting that therapies targeted at apoCIII might provide clinical benefit. In patients with extremely high triglycerides due to the familial chylomicronemia syndrome (see later discussion), inhibiting the apoCIII mRNA results in substantial triglyceride lowering.[50]

Apolipoprotein E

ApoE biology is more complex than that of other apolipoproteins. The highest level of apoE expression is found in liver, with the second highest in brain. Many other cell types synthesize the protein, including macrophages. In brain, astrocytes and microglial cells make apoE, but it can also be produced by injured neurons. ApoE circulates in plasma as a part of every lipoprotein with the probable exception of LDL. Its principal function involves interactions with the two major receptors mediating the clearance of plasma lipoproteins, the LDL receptor and the LDL receptor–related protein (i.e., LRP1, also known as the chylomicron remnant receptor). Therefore, it is apoE that is primarily responsible for the clearance of intestinal-derived lipoproteins after a meal and for the clearance of VLDL and IDL particles before they are converted to LDL.

There are three major apoE isoforms: E2, E3, and E4. They are encoded, respectively, by alleles referred to as ε2, ε3, and ε4, which exist because of charge differences caused by variations in amino acids at residues 112 and 158 in the protein. ApoE3 is considered to be the normal isoform; it has a cysteine at residue 112 and an arginine at 158. ApoE2 has cysteines at both 112 and 158, and apoE4 has an arginine at both 112 and 158. These variations have structural and functional consequences (Fig. 37-10). The protein has two domains: an amino (NH_2)-terminus interacts with lipoprotein receptors, and a COOH-terminus interacts with lipids (Fig. 37-10A). In apoE4, the isoform associated with disease, these domains interact; this does not occur with apoE3 (Fig. 37-10B).

Comprehensive data (>86,000 individuals for lipids, >37,000 for coronary events) link apoE allele and genotype frequencies, lipid levels, and coronary risk.[51] Allele frequencies in healthy adults are 7% for ε2, 82% for ε3, and 11% for ε4. Genotype frequencies are 0.7% for ε2/ε2, 11.6% for ε2/ε3, 2.2% for ε2/ε4, 62.3% for ε3/ε3 (the most abundant genotype), 21.3% for ε3/ε4, and 1.9% for ε4/ε4. There is a

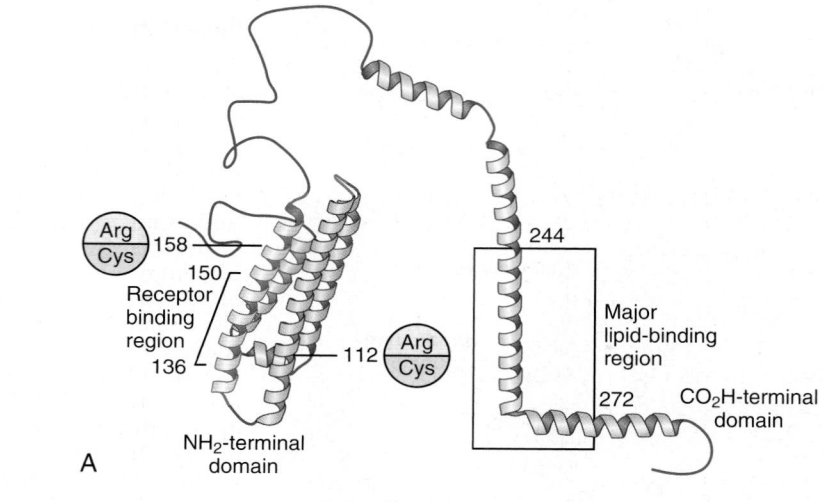

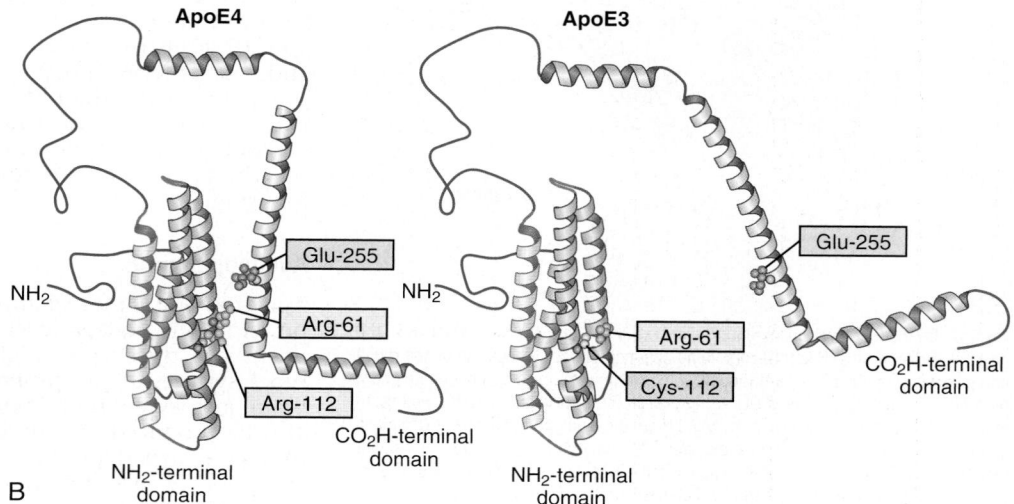

Figure 37-10 A, The amino (NH₂)-terminal domain of apoprotein E is composed of a four-helix bundle. A region of random structure encompassing residues 165 to 200 forms a connector or hinge region linked to the carboxy (CO₂H-terminal domain. There are two major functional regions. Residues 136 to 150 *(yellow helix)* encompass the receptor-binding region; residues 240 to 260 in the carboxy-terminal domain encompass the lipid-binding region. **B,** ApoE4 displays the unique property of domain interaction that distinguishes it from apoE3 (Arg61 in the amino-terminal domain interacts with Glu255 in the carboxy-terminal domain). Arg, arginine; Cys, cysteine; Glu, glutamic acid.

linear relationship between the genotype and both LDL cholesterol level and coronary risk, from least to most, as follows: ε2/ε2 < ε2/ε3 < ε2/ε4 < ε3/ε3 < ε3/ε4 < ε4/ε4. Compared to the reference group (ε3/ε3), the presence of the ε2 allele decreases coronary risk by about 20%, and the presence of the ε4 allele slightly increases risk. These observations are interesting for two reasons. First, ε2/ε2 individuals, although they are protected from CHD on a population basis, are at risk for dysbetalipoproteinemia. In the setting of appropriate additional conditions, about 5% of ε2/ε2 individuals will develop this disorder, which is associated with aggressive vascular disease. Second, the E2 protein binds less well to the LDL receptor than E3 and E4 do. This suggests that LDL cholesterol in patients with the E2 protein should be higher (because it is less likely to be cleared by this receptor), yet the opposite is observed. These data suggest that other receptor-mediated processes, such as those mediated by heparan sulfate proteoglycans (HSPG), may be critical for clearance of apoE-containing lipoproteins.[52]

ApoE is involved in Alzheimer disease. Risk of this neurodegenerative disease increases approximately threefold in those with one ε4 allele and 12-fold in those with two ε4 alleles.[53] The presence of an ε2 allele is protective. These relationships hold for both early- and late-onset Alzheimer disease. There are HDL-like lipoproteins in the central nervous system (CNS), and apoE-mediated delivery of cholesterol is important for normal synaptic function. The relation of lipid metabolism to Alzheimer disease is incompletely understood, but some evidence suggests that deposition of amyloid-β (the major constituent of the plaques that characterize the disease) begins sooner in the brains of those with the E4 protein. Because people with the ε4 allele are also more likely to have atherosclerosis, CNS vascular disease may help explain why this apoE variant is involved in neurodegeneration.

Major Receptors Involved in Lipid Metabolism
Low-Density Lipoprotein Receptor Gene Family

Including distant relatives, the LDL receptor family contains at least 10 members. The two most important ones for systemic lipid metabolism are the LDL receptor and LRP1. The LDL receptor recognizes apoB100 as well as apoE, whereas LRP1 recognizes apoE but not apoB100. Other core family members (those that share considerable structural homology) include the VLDL receptor (VLDLR), the apolipoprotein E receptor 2 (apoER2 or LRP8), LRP4, LRP1B, and megalin (LRP2, also known as gp330 and as the major Heymann nephritis antigen).

Three family members lack some of the structural features of the others. They are sortilin-related receptor L1 (LR11/SORL1), LRP5, and LRP6. Aside from the LDL receptor and LRP1, these receptors appear to be most important for brain development, synaptic function, and neuroprotection, making them relevant to Alzheimer disease.[54] LRP5 and LRP6 are involved in endocrine disease. Both are coreceptors for a family of G protein–coupled receptors known as "frizzled receptors." Frizzled receptors bind the Wnt molecule to induce an important signaling cascade upstream of the transcription factor β-catenin. Genetic variants in LRP5 are associated with obesity,[55] and a human mutation in LRP6 results in the metabolic syndrome and coronary artery disease.[56] Loss-of-function mutations in LRP5 or LRP6 cause osteoporosis in humans. These observations suggest that insulin resistance, coronary disease, and osteoporosis, common comorbid conditions in patients, may be related to abnormal Wnt signaling.

Low-Density Lipoprotein Receptor. The LDL receptor is a large (160 kDa) glycoprotein expressed on most cells. Because it recognizes apoB100 as well as apoE, it is involved in the uptake of LDL, chylomicron remnants, VLDL, and IDL. Most HDL particles do not have apoE and therefore do not interact with this receptor or the LRP. The discovery of this receptor in the 1970s by Brown and Goldstein was important because its deficiency explained a human disease (FH), its physiologic regulation explained the mechanism of action of drugs that lower cholesterol, and its biology defined receptor-mediated endocytosis as a paradigm for providing cells with critical components from the external environment.[57]

Domains shared with other members of this receptor family comprise the LDL receptor. These include the ligand-binding domain, the epidermal growth factor (EGF) precursor domain, the O-linked sugar domain at the cell surface, the membrane-spanning domain, and the cytoplasmic domain at the COOH-terminus (Fig. 37-11). In the ligand-binding domain, there are seven repeats of approximately 40 amino acids, each containing six cysteines that form three disulfide bonds within the repeat to stabilize the structure. Each repeat also includes negatively charged amino acids that interact with positive charged residues on apoB and apoE and with calcium ions that allow the repeat to bind to the ligand. The EGF precursor domain consists of three EGF-like repeats (see Fig. 37-11) with a structure known as a β-propeller located between repeats B and C. The O-linked sugar domain is the site at which carbohydrate moieties attach to the molecule, and this is followed by a short sequence that traverses the membrane. The cytoplasmic domain consists of 50 residues that include an NPXY (asparagine, proline, any amino acid, tyrosine) targeting sequence where adapter proteins dock, which leads to receptor clustering in coated pits.

Coated pits are specialized regions of the cell surface that are characterized by the presence of the protein complex clathrin. When LDL receptors bind lipoproteins, they migrate to coated pits, and clathrin directs the receptors to a cell membrane region that folds inward, creating an intracellular vesicle or endosome (Fig. 37-12). Endosomes become acidic, which prompts the lipoprotein to be displaced from the LDL receptor by the β-propeller of the EGF precursor domain.[58] The unoccupied receptor recycles back to the cell surface. In the presence of PCSK9 (see later discussion), the LDL receptor conformation is altered, promoting its degradation and preventing its recycling to the cell surface.[59]

Lipoproteins are degraded in lysosomes. Lysosomal lipids appear to affect longevity in model organisms.[60] Cholesterol is transported out of the lysosomes through

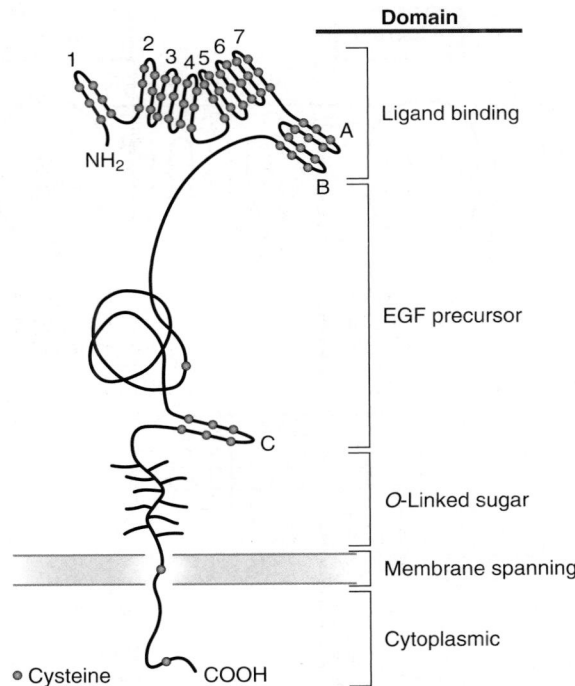

Figure 37-11 Functional domains of the low-density lipoprotein receptor. Numbers 1 through 7 indicate repeats in the ligand-binding domain. A, B, and C are epidermal growth factor (EGF)-like repeats in the EGF precursor domain. See text for complete description.

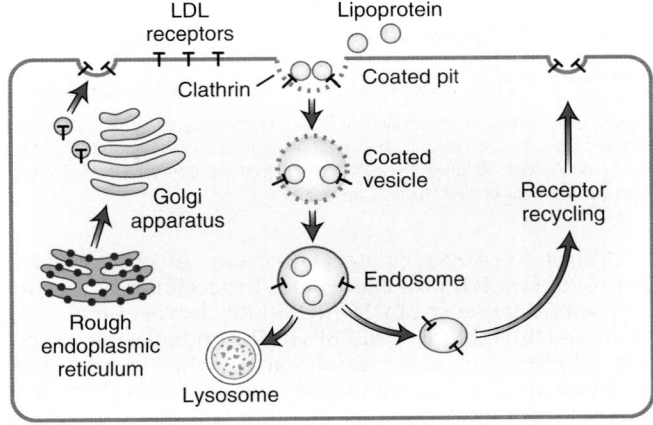

Figure 37-12 Low-density lipoprotein (LDL) receptor pathway. LDL interacts with receptors on the cell surface. The complex enters the coated pit and is internalized. The coated vesicle loses its clathrin coat and becomes an endosome, the site of lipoprotein and receptor dissociation. The receptors recycle to the cell surface, and the lipoproteins are degraded. Alternatively, new receptors are synthesized in the rough endoplasmic reticulum and transported to the cell surface. (Modified from Brown MS, Goldstein JL. A receptor-mediated pathway for cholesterol homeostasis. *Science.* 1986;232:34-47; and Myant NB. *Cholesterol Metabolism, LDL, and the LDL Receptor.* San Diego: Academic Press; 1990.)

the action of two proteins, Niemann-Pick C1 and C2 (NPC1 and NPC2), which are mutated in the human disease Niemann-Pick type C. Accumulation of cholesterol and other lipids characterizes this disorder. It is believed that NPC2, which is soluble, binds cholesterol after lipoprotein hydrolysis in the lysosome and moves this sterol to the membrane-associated NPC1 for subsequent release to the cell, where it serves structural and regulatory functions.

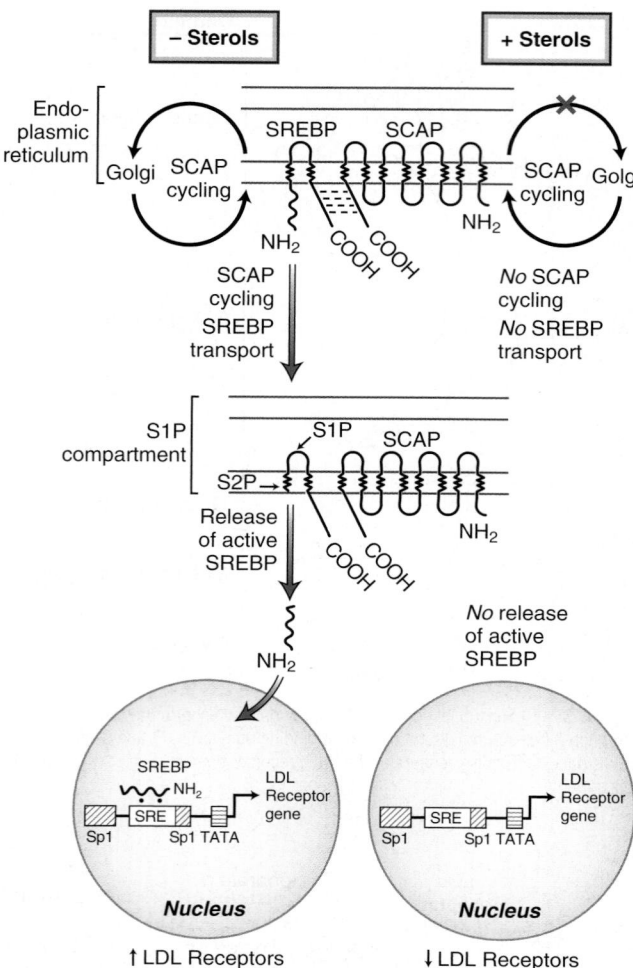

Figure 37-13 Low-density lipoprotein (LDL) receptor gene regulation. S1P, site-1 protease; S2P, site-2 protease; SCAP, SREBP cleavage–activating protein; SRE, sterol regulatory element; SREBP, sterol regulatory element–binding protein; TATA, indicates the TATA box or core promoter sequence.

One of the key regulatory functions of cholesterol is control of LDL receptor expression. Intracellular sterol concentrations are sensed by SCAP (SREBP cleavage–activating protein), which binds to SREBPs in the endoplasmic reticulum. SREBPs are transcription factors that control LDL receptor expression as well as the expression of other genes important for lipid metabolism. SREBP2 is most important for LDL receptor transcription; its NH_2-terminus contains a leucine zipper–type transcription factor structure that binds to a sterol regulatory element in the promoter of the LDL receptor gene. When cells are sterol-depleted (Fig. 37-13, left side), SCAP migrates to the Golgi apparatus, where sugar moieties attached to the protein are modified. This allows SCAP to transport SREBPs to the S1P compartment. There, two proteases, site-1 protease (S1P) and site-2 protease (S2P), sequentially act on SREBPs to release their NH_2-terminus, which migrates to the nucleus and binds to the sterol regulatory element in the promoter region of lipid genes such as the LDL receptor, increasing transcription and subsequent levels of functional proteins. In the presence of sterols (see Fig. 37-13, right side), SCAP does not cycle to the Golgi structure, it cannot move SREBPs to the S1P compartment, and SREBPs are not cleaved to allow their transcription factor to migrate to the nucleus.

LDL Receptor–Related Protein 1. LRP1 is also known as the apoE receptor or the chylomicron remnant receptor. LRP1

roughly consists of the equivalent of four LDL receptors with a multiplicity of ligand-binding domains. It is critical for normal development, because inactivation of LRP1 (but not of the LDL receptor) is lethal in mice. The major cell types in which LRP1 is expressed are hepatocytes, neurons (where it participates in critical functions), and syncytio-trophoblasts in the placenta. Multiple different ligands bind to LRP1 and participate in nutrient flow as well as signaling. These ligands include amyloid precursor protein (relevant in Alzheimer disease because it is processed to form the amyloid-β of plaques), bacterial by-products, tissue plasminogen activator (which interacts with LRP1 to modulate physiology in the setting of brain ischemia), plasminogen activator inhibitors, and α_2-macroglobulin (which plays multiple roles in inflammation, in part by inactivating matrix metalloproteinases). Given the promiscuity of LRP1 binding, it is not surprising it is linked with receptor-associated protein, a small protein that is involved in intracellular LRP1 processing and occupies the LRP1 binding sites during transport to the cell surface.

LRP1 binds apoE but not apoB100. Therefore, it mediates the metabolism of the major apoE-containing lipoproteins, including chylomicron remnants and IDL (VLDL remnants), but is not involved in LDL metabolism. The interaction between LRP1 and lipoproteins is more complex than that between LDL and the LDL receptor. Multiple apoE molecules are required for LRP1 binding, and this interaction requires an initial binding of the lipoprotein to HSPG on the cell surface. Other moieties on apoE-containing lipoproteins also are believed to facilitate the binding process. LPL, which metabolizes chylomicrons and VLDL particles, adheres to particles after mediating the release of fatty acids and other substitutents at the endothelium. Lipoprotein-bound LPL molecules (as well as hepatic lipase) are thought to interact with LRP1 and to facilitate the uptake of remnants by the liver.

Pattern Recognition Receptors

One of the most serious consequences of abnormal lipid metabolism is atherosclerosis, which requires the delivery of excess lipids to blood vessels. This process involves the innate immune system and at least two broad types of receptors—scavenger receptors and toll-like receptors (TLRs)—that preferentially recognize patterns instead of discrete species.

Scavenger Receptors. The discovery of scavenger receptors was prompted by the observation that macrophages can bind and internalize modified forms of LDL but not native LDL. There are now thought to be 10 classes of these receptors[61] that are generally characterized by the ability to bind altered (e.g., oxidized, acetylated) LDL or other polyanionic ligands. Class A and class B receptors may be particularly important.

Class A receptors include scavenger receptor A (SR-A types 1 and 2, which consists of alternative splice variants), macrophage receptor with collagenous structure (MARCO), scavenger receptor A 5 (SCARA5), and scavenger receptor with C-type lectin domain (SRCL-I/II, also referred to as CL-P1). SR-A, the first to be discovered, binds a wide variety of ligands (including bacterial by-products), activates stress signaling pathways including mitogen-activated protein kinases, and is believed to be involved in atherosclerosis, the clearance of apoptotic cells, and Alzheimer disease.

Class B receptors include CD36 and scavenger receptor class B (SR-BI [called CLA-1 in humans]). These receptors bind modified LDL, but unlike the other classes of scavenger receptors, they also bind VLDL, native LDL, and HDL. CD36 is expressed on a wide variety of cell types, including monocytes, macrophages, adipocytes, platelets, endothelial cells, hepatocytes, microglial cells, and the tongue, where it detects dietary fat. In addition to lipoproteins, long-chain fatty acids are ligands for CD36.[62] The tissue distribution of SR-BI is more limited, with expression on hepatocytes, monocyte/macrophages, and steroidogenic tissues. Given the panoply of ligands that bind to scavenger receptors and their effects on innate immunity, their roles in lipid metabolism and atherosclerosis may be complex.

Toll-like Receptors. The TLR family comprises key effectors of the innate immune system that are required for host defense mechanisms against simple pathogens. Their activation has been implicated in many chronic inflammatory diseases, including atherosclerosis. Some scavenger receptors such as CD36 may be coreceptors for TLRs. TLRs are found on myeloid cells such as monocyte/macrophages but also on the gut epithelium; they bind ligands such as lipopolysaccharide (TLR4) and glycolipids found in bacteria (TLR2). TLR4 is also known to bind saturated fatty acids, an interaction that is believed to be involved in insulin resistance in mammals.[63] TLR2 mediates monocyte activation by apoCIII on triglyceride-rich lipoproteins.[64]

Other Enzymes and Transfer Proteins Mediating Lipid Metabolism

Hepatic Lipase

Primarily a phospholipase with some triglyceride lipase activity, hepatic lipase is made in hepatocytes and is found mostly on endothelial cells in the liver and on HSPG in the space of Disse. It is also found in steroidogenic tissues but is not synthesized at those sites. Unlike LPL, which is mostly present at tissues remote from the liver to ensure the peripheral delivery of lipids and vitamins, hepatic lipase coordinates lipoprotein metabolism centrally. Its functions include the conversion of IDL to LDL, the conversion of HDL_2 to HDL_3, and probably the final metabolism of chylomicron remnants to facilitate their uptake by LRP1. Unlike LPL, hepatic lipase does not require a cofactor such as apoCII, but both enzymes are displaced from their endothelial sites of activity by injection of heparin (postheparin lipase activity). High levels of hepatic lipase decrease HDL concentrations, whereas high levels of LPL increase HDL.

Endothelial Lipase

Evolutionarily related to hepatic lipase and LPL, endothelial lipase is a phospholipase with almost no triglyceride lipase activity. It is expressed at high levels in embryonic endothelial cells, with expression declining during maturation. Considerable levels are found in adult tissues that include the thyroid, lung, liver, placenta, and gonads (with expression in those tissues reflecting the endothelium and not parenchymal cells). In mice, overexpression decreases HDL and inactivation increases HDL. Endothelial lipase is expressed in aorta, where it may increase with atherosclerosis. Human loss-of-function mutations are associated with increased HDL cholesterol levels.[65]

Proprotein Convertase Subtilisin/Kexin Type 9

PCSK9 is a secreted protease that promotes the degradation of the LDL receptor, but its catalytic activity is not required for receptor degradation. Mostly expressed in liver, intestine, and kidney, PCSK9 was found to be important in lipid metabolism when missense mutations (subsequently determined to be gain-of-function mutations) in its gene were determined to be associated with hypercholesterolemia and coronary artery disease.[66] Overexpression of PCSK9 in mice decreases LDL-receptor protein. Human loss-of-function mutations in PCSK9 are associated with low levels of LDL and decreased risk of vascular disease.[67,68] Antibodies to PCSK9 may be useful for treatment in humans (see discussion later).

Lipoprotein-Associated Phospholipase A_2

Phospholipases hydrolyze the ester bond at the sn2 position of phospholipids, usually resulting in the release of a fatty acid and lysophosphatidylcholine, which can induce inflammation. This type of enzyme was originally identified as a component of snake venom, and many distinct classes of phospholipases have subsequently been characterized. For most, membrane phospholipids are the substrate. Lipoprotein-associated phospholipase A_2 (Lp-PLA$_2$) is an exception because it can hydrolyze substrate in the aqueous phase. Lp-PLA$_2$ binds to LDL as well as HDL lipoproteins and is a biomarker for coronary artery disease.[69] Inhibition of this enzyme decreases the expansion of the lipid core of atherosclerotic plaques in humans.[70] However, administration of an oral inhibitor of Lp-PLA2 did not decrease cardiovascular end points in large clinical trials.[71,72]

Cholesteryl Ester Transfer Protein

Cholesteryl ester transfer protein (CETP) promotes the exchange between lipoproteins of two classes of neutral lipids: cholesteryl esters and triglycerides. HDL cholesteryl esters are transferred to VLDL, IDL, and chylomicron remnants; in return, triglycerides from VLDL, IDL, and remnants are transferred to HDL. Humans and other primates have CETP activity; the transfer of cholesteryl ester from HDL to apoB-containing lipoproteins ultimately leads to most of their cholesterol burden being carried by LDL, and this is thought to result in atherosclerosis. Rodents and dogs do not have CETP. Most of their cholesterol is carried in HDL; levels of LDL are low, and these animals are resistant to atherosclerosis. Such observations have led to the notion of inhibiting CETP activity as a treatment for atherosclerosis in humans. One CETP inhibitor was shown to increase HDL cholesterol and lower LDL cholesterol in humans, but it also increased mortality rate,[73] perhaps due to off-target effects including increased levels of aldosterone. Another CETP inhibitor selectively increased HDL but had no impact on cardiovascular events.[74]

Lecithin:Cholesterol Acyltransferase

LCAT is an enzyme synthesized mostly in the liver; it circulates in the plasma associated with HDL particles and, to a lesser extent, with LDL particles. LCAT is activated by several apolipoproteins (apoAI and others) and uses the phospholipid lecithin (phosphatidylcholine) and free cholesterol as substrates to generate lysolecithin (lysophosphatidylcholine) and cholesteryl ester. Most of the cholesteryl esters in lipoproteins are derived from LCAT activity. Rare human mutations in LCAT result in low HDL levels in the setting of a range of disorders, including fish-eye disease (in which activity is deficient on HDL particles but continues on LDL particles) and a more severe presentation with corneal clouding (resulting from free cholesterol in the cornea), hemolytic anemia, and renal failure. The role of LCAT in atherosclerosis is uncertain. Although LCAT deficiency might be expected to promote atherosclerosis because of low HDL levels, studies of humans with

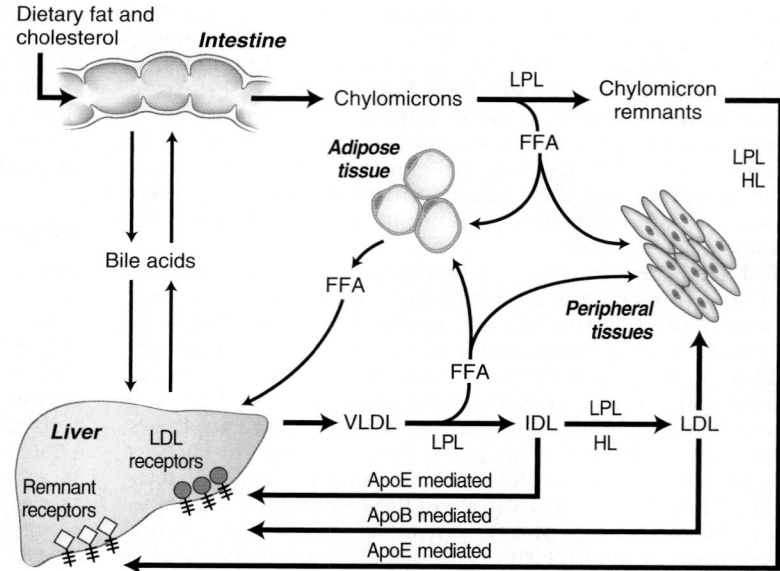

Figure 37-14 General scheme summarizing the major pathways involved in the metabolism of chylomicrons synthesized by the intestine and very low density lipoprotein (VLDL) synthesized by the liver. ApoB, apolipoprotein B; ApoE, apolipoprotein E; FFA, free fatty acid; HL, hepatic lipase; IDL, intermediate-density lipoprotein; LPL, lipoprotein lipase. (Modified from Mahley RW. Biochemistry and physiology of lipid and lipoprotein metabolism. In: Becker KL, ed. *Principles and Practice of Endocrinology and Metabolism*, 2nd ed. Philadelphia: JB Lippincott; 1995:1369-1378.)

loss-of-function LCAT mutations suggest that these individuals are not at increased risk for atherosclerosis.[75]

INTEGRATIVE PHYSIOLOGY OF LIPID METABOLISM

Lipid metabolism is characterized by a dynamic flux of multiple lipid species from the external environment to the liver, from the liver to peripheral tissues, from peripheral tissues back to the liver, and eventually back to the external environment through the excretion of bile acids. Integrated views of the major pathways involved are shown in Figures 37-14 and 37-15.

Exogenous Lipid Transport

Dietary fat and cholesterol (see Fig. 37-14, top left) absorbed by the duodenum and proximal jejunum are used to generate chylomicrons that are secreted at the lateral borders of enterocytes and enter mesenteric lymphatics. They access the plasma via the thoracic duct and are rapidly metabolized by LPL to yield chylomicron remnants. These are taken up by remnant receptors (LRP1/HSPG) and by LDL receptors in the liver. Free fatty acids liberated by the action of LPL are available to adipose tissue for storage and to other tissues (e.g., skeletal muscle, heart) for use as energy substrates.

Endogenous Lipid Transport

Lipid derived from remnants and from lipolysis of adipose tissue is reassembled in the liver (see Fig. 37-14, bottom left) as VLDL particles, which are secreted into the plasma. Abnormal lipid metabolism in insulin resistance is mediated in large part by overproduction of VLDL, an event that occurs through disruption of signaling downstream of the insulin receptor and the insulin receptor substrate (IRS) adapter proteins. VLDL particles are metabolized by LPL to yield IDL particles, which are metabolized by LPL and hepatic lipase to yield LDL particles. Thus, LDL is derived from VLDL, which helps explain why treatment to lower triglycerides (carried by VLDL) is frequently associated with

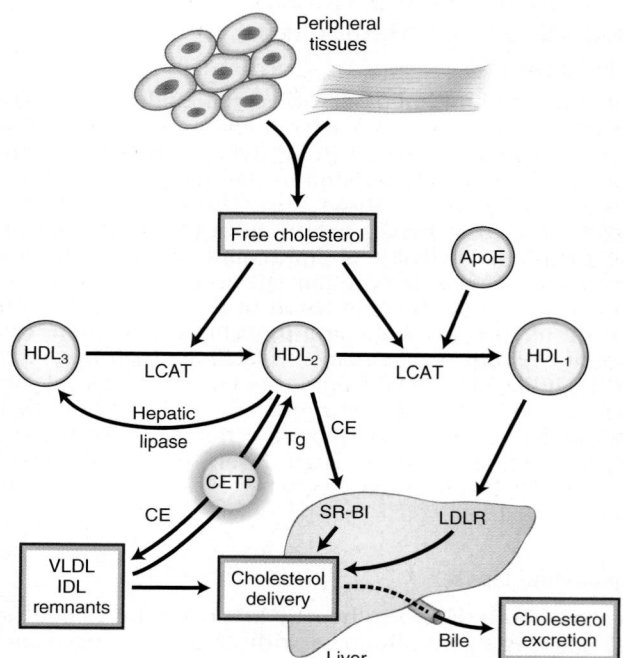

Figure 37-15 Role of high-density lipoprotein (HDL) in the redistribution of lipids from cells with excess cholesterol to cells requiring cholesterol or to the liver for excretion. The reverse cholesterol transport pathway is indicated by arrows (net transfer of cholesterol from cells to HDL, then to LDL and liver). ApoE, apolipoprotein E; CE, cholesteryl ester; CETP, cholesteryl ester transfer protein; IDL, intermediate-density lipoprotein; LCAT, lecithin:cholesterol acyltransferase; LDLR, low-density lipoprotein receptor; SR-BI, scavenger receptor class B, type 1; Tg, triglyceride; VLDL, very low density lipoprotein.

at least transient increases in LDL. IDL can be taken up by the liver through an apoE-dependent process, and LDL is taken up by the liver through the binding of apoB100 to LDL receptors. Small VLDL particles, IDL particles, and LDL particles may be taken up by peripheral tissues to deliver nutrients, cholesterol, and fat-soluble vitamins. When present in excess, each of these lipoproteins may be atherogenic.

Reverse Cholesterol Transport and Dysfunctional HDL

Cholesterol cannot be metabolized by peripheral tissues and must be returned to the liver for excretion. This process, known as *reverse cholesterol transport*, is dependent on HDL and its precursors and is depicted in Figure 37-15. Excess cholesterol in tissues can be effluxed either to lipid-poor apoAI, mediated by the protein transporter ABCA1 (adenosine triphosphate–binding cassette transporter 1), or to nascent HDL particles, mediated by ABCG1. Efflux from cultured cells to human plasma as a biomarker of cardiovascular risk[39] is thought to mostly reflect the activity of ABCA1. There is also evidence that cholesterol can be acquired by HDL without the assistance of transporters by following a concentration gradient at the cell surface. LCAT esterifies HDL-associated cholesterol to form cholesteryl ester and induce the maturation of HDL. HDL particles have three pathways for transporting sterols to the liver. First, they can directly bind to SR-BI (CLA-1) at the liver, which induces cholesteryl ester delivery through a mechanism involving lateral lipid transfer and not receptor internalization. Second, cholesteryl esters can be transferred to apoB-containing lipoproteins by CETP, and these particles can deliver cholesterol to the liver through the LDL receptor. Third, a small portion of HDL can acquire apoE and bind to the liver LDL receptor. Once in the liver, cholesterol is converted to bile acids for excretion.

HDL2 particles are partially depleted of cholesteryl esters and enriched in triglycerides through the activity of CETP, which renders them suitable as substrates for hepatic lipase. Hepatic lipase hydrolyzes the triglyceride-enriched HDL2 particles and regenerates HDL3, yielding particles that are again suited to accept cholesterol from peripheral cells.

Because cholesterol is the principal component of atherosclerotic plaque, it is reasonable to pursue the notion that atherosclerosis could be treated by promoting the efflux of cholesterol from lesions. HDL participates in this process, but static levels of HDL cholesterol are poor predictors of reverse cholesterol transport. Measurements of the rate of flux of cholesterol from the periphery to the liver, which may be possible in humans, would represent a better predictor of beneficial therapies. In vitro HDL efflux capacity represents an initial step toward assessing reverse cholesterol transport.[39] The presence of high levels of HDL particles that have been modified to prevent their capacity to promote cholesterol efflux would not be expected to decrease vascular risk. Such dysfunctional particles may explain why some HDL-elevating interventions have not been associated with decreased cardiovascular disease.

In addition to participating in reverse cholesterol transport, HDL has other properties that could be impaired by a variety of processes leading to a dysfunctional particle. They include the induction of endothelial nitric oxide synthase, the transport of proteins involved in the acute phase response and inflammation, and the suppression of thrombosis through induction of prostacyclin (which decreases thrombin production via the protein C pathway and decreases platelet activation).

OVERVIEW OF HYPERLIPIDEMIA AND DYSLIPIDEMIA

Two major clinical disorders are associated with common lipoprotein disorders. Very elevated triglyceride levels are a risk factor for development of pancreatitis. Elevated cholesterol due to greater concentrations of LDL and remnant lipoproteins and reduced levels of HDL promote atherosclerosis. Clinicians are often faced with evaluation and treatment of patients who have hypertriglyceridemia, hypercholesterolemia, combined hyperlipidemia due to elevated cholesterol and triglycerides, and low HDL syndromes. A summary of the primary and secondary causes of each condition is presented in Table 37-4.

Plasma lipid levels are highly dependent on lifestyle; for example, the high-fat, high-cholesterol diets eaten in Western societies raise plasma cholesterol, and vigorous exercise lowers both atherogenic particles and triglycerides.

TABLE 37-4
Differential Diagnosis of Hyperlipidemia and Dyslipidemia

Hypertriglyceridemia	Hypercholesterolemia	Increased Cholesterol and Triglycerides	Low HDL
Primary Disorders			
LPL deficiency ApoCII deficiency Familial hypertriglyceridemia Dysbetalipoproteinemia	Familial hypercholesterolemia Familial defective apoB100 Polygenic hypercholesterolemia Sitosterolemia	Familial combined hyperlipidemia Dysbetalipoproteinemia	Familial hypoalphalipoproteinemia ApoAI mutations LCAT deficiency ABCA1 deficiency
Secondary Disorders			
Diabetes mellitus Hypothyroidism High-carbohydrate diets Renal failure Obesity/insulin resistance Estrogens Ethanol Beta blockers Protease inhibitors Glucocorticoids Retinoids Bile acid–binding resins Antipsychotics Lipodystrophies Thiazides	Hypothyroidism Obstructive liver disease Nephrotic syndrome Thiazides	Diabetes mellitus Hypothyroidism Glucocorticoids Immunosuppressives Protease inhibitors Nephrotic syndrome Lipodystrophies	Anabolic steroids Retinoids HIV infection Hepatitis C infection

ABCA1, adenosine triphosphate–binding cassette transporter 1; apo, apolipoprotein; HDL, high-density lipoprotein; LCAT, lecithin:cholesterol acyltransferase; LPL, lipoprotein lipase.

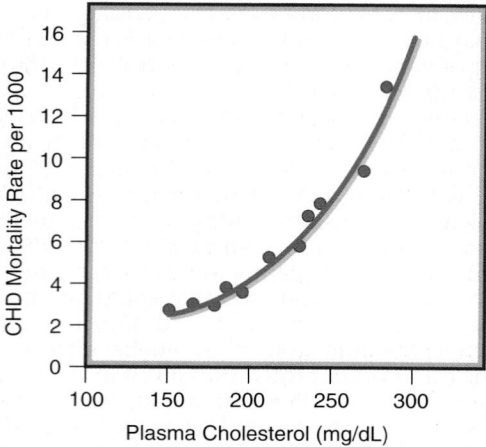

Figure 37-16 Relation between plasma cholesterol levels and coronary heart disease (CHD) mortality rate in the Multiple Risk Factor Intervention Trial. (Modified from Stamler J, Wentworth D, Neaton JD. Is relationship between serum cholesterol and risk of premature death from coronary heart disease continuous and graded? Findings in 356,222 primary screenees of the Multiple Risk Factor Intervention Trial [MRFIT]. *JAMA.* 1986;256:2823-2828; Copyright © 1986, by the American Medical Association.)

TABLE 37-5

Criteria for Diagnosis of the Metabolic Syndrome

Measure*	Categorical Threshold
Waist circumference	*Whites, African Americans, Latin Americans:* Men, ≥40 in; women, ≥35 in *Asians:* Men, ≥35 in; women, ≥32 in
Elevated triglycerides	≥150 mg/dL *or* On drug treatment for elevated triglycerides
Reduced HDL-C	Men, <40 mg/dL; women, <50 mg/dL *or* On drug treatment for reduced HDL-C
Elevated blood pressure	≥130 mm Hg systolic or ≥85 mm Hg diastolic *or* On antihypertensive drug treatment
Elevated fasting glucose	≥100 mg/dL *or* On drug treatment for elevated glucose

*Three of the five measures are required for diagnosis.
HDL-C, high-density lipoprotein cholesterol.
Adapted from Grundy SM, Cleeman JI, Daniels SR, et al. Diagnosis and management of the metabolic syndrome: an American Heart Association/National Heart, Lung, and Blood Institute scientific statement. *Circulation.* 2005;112:2735-2752.

For this reason, normal blood concentrations—those that are within 2 standard deviations of the mean—vary among countries and over time. For Western adults, cholesterol concentrations higher than 240 mg/dL (6.2 mmol/L) or triglyceride concentrations higher than 150 mg/dL (1.7 mmol/L) constitute high-risk hyperlipidemia. The overriding influences of diet and lifestyle on plasma cholesterol were illustrated by studies of ethnic Japanese populations. Plasma cholesterol was markedly increased in Japanese-Americans and was associated with a more westernized food intake.[76] Because serum total cholesterol levels correlate with the risk for CHD over a broad range (Fig. 37-16), normal levels are often defined as those associated with minimal cardiovascular risk rather than population averages, suggesting that most of those in the developed world have lipid levels that put them at risk for heart disease.

The National Cholesterol Education Program (NCEP) created a standard for cholesterol levels and pioneered a practical approach to treatment by dividing the population according to cardiac risk, based on the presence of vascular disease or other cardiac risk factors. In 2001, the NCEP classified plasma cholesterol levels lower than 200 mg/dL as desirable, those between 200 and 240 mg/dL as borderline high, and levels greater than 240 mg/dL as high.[77] (Because plasma lipid levels increase with age, values in children are lower.[78]) Total cholesterol concentrations between 170 and 200 mg/dL are considered borderline high, and levels greater than 200 mg/dL are high. Triglyceride levels greater than 500 mg/dL carry a risk of pancreatitis, and those greater than 150 mg/dL are considered elevated. The Endocrine Society used different definitions in 2012,[79] in part influenced by clinical data that severe hypertriglyceridemia is associated with pancreatitis with triglyceride levels of greater than 2000 mg/dL.

Hyperlipidemias are caused by increased concentrations of plasma lipoproteins. Although the clinical diagnosis is made solely on the basis of circulating lipids, the diseases are classified by abnormalities of lipoproteins (see Table 37-2) and are often referred to as *hyperlipoproteinemias.* As noted earlier, lipoproteins differ in their physiologic functions, metabolic pathways, and pathologic significance.

The NCEP also recognized the existence of the metabolic syndrome, a common condition linked to insulin resistance but without a unifying mechanistic cause. The presence of at least three of the five features described in Table 37-5 is sufficient to make the diagnosis. This condition is clearly associated with increased risk of vascular disease and development of type 2 diabetes and is equivalent to what was previously referred to as *prediabetes.*[80] Evaluation and therapy for the metabolic syndrome should be directed at individual components including hypertriglyceridemia and low HDL cholesterol (HDL-C).

HYPERTRIGLYCERIDEMIA

Fasting Hyperchylomicronemia

The most dramatic example of severe hypertriglyceridemia is that of fasting hyperchylomicronemia. This can result from a primary defect in chylomicron metabolism, or it can occur secondary to increased VLDL and saturation of LPL actions to metabolize triglycerides into free fatty acids and generate remnant lipoproteins that are amenable to uptake by the liver through pathways mediated by the LDL receptor, LRP1, and proteoglycans. LPL saturation occurs when triglyceride levels exceed about 500 mg/dL. Therefore, familial hypertriglyceridemia, familial combined hyperlipidemia, and dysbetalipoproteinemia can manifest with fasting hyperchylomicronemia. One common cause of such exacerbations is out-of-control diabetes leading to increased adipose intracellular lipolysis, return of fatty acids to the liver, greater secretion of VLDL triglyceride, and saturation of LPL. Several dietary and environmental factors also modulate triglyceride production. The most dramatic is alcohol, a major substrate for triglyceride production. In addition, diets that are rich in free carbohydrates, and especially simple sugars, induce triglyceride production. Fructose also increases de novo production of lipids in the liver but has less effect on circulating triglycerides.

Defective clearance of plasma lipids is a major cause of fasting hyperchylomicronemia. Patients with genetic defects leading to this condition are often referred to as having *familial chylomicronemia syndrome* (FCS). Genetic defects in LPL commonly cause FCS; the lack of normal

LPL prevents chylomicron clearance. LPL deficiency usually, but not always, manifests in childhood. The symptoms vary from difficulty feeding young infants to frank pancreatitis, which is sometimes mistaken as appendicitis. The plasma is often milky, and whole blood may have a pinkish, "cream of tomato soup" hue. The trigger level of triglyceride elevation leading to pancreatitis is variable; some patients have triglycerides in excess of 10,000 mg/dL with no symptoms, whereas others develop pancreatitis at much lower triglyceride levels, but usually in excess of 2000 mg/dL. However, patients presenting with pancreatitis have often avoided eating and the first measured sample may not reflect the peak triglyceride levels. Several additional mutations in proteins required for normal LPL actions also cause FCS (see later).

The pathophysiology of the relationship between hyperchylomicronemia and pancreatitis is unknown. Lipid-rich blood may sludge, leading to pancreatic ischemia. The small amount of lipases that normally leak from the acinar cells may lead to exuberant local lipolysis, creation of toxic local concentrations of free fatty acids and lysolecithin, a toxic lipid produced from phosphatidylcholine, and further acinar cell damage to adjacent cells.[81] Insults to the acinar cells such as that provided by alcohol can fan this process.

Although most patients with severe hyperchylomicronemia who do not develop pancreatitis are asymptomatic, a few with extreme levels exceeding 10,000 mg/dL develop the hyperchylomicronemia syndrome. These patients have dyspnea and confusion that may be indistinguishable from early dementia. Presumably this is the result of reduced blood flow or defective oxygen delivery.

The marked increase in blood triglyceride concentration can lead to accumulation of triglycerides in several organs and can be observed in the blood. The latter is best appreciated by examining the blood directly, allowing the red blood cells to settle, and observing a creamy layer on the plasma, or by noting the pinkish discoloration of the blood on funduscopic examination, known as *lipemia retinalis* (Fig. 37-17B). Eruptive xanthomas, as shown in Figure 37-17G, are 2- to 5-mm papules with a yellow center surrounded by erythema. They are caused by triglyceride-enriched skin macrophages. These lesions are sometimes confused with acne or folliculitis. For unclear reasons, eruptive xanthomas are most commonly found on the buttocks, extensor surfaces of the arms, and the back. Enlargement of the liver and spleen is not uncommon and is thought to be caused by triglyceride accumulation in these organs.

Aside from the severe hypertriglyceridemia, other laboratory indices are sometimes abnormal. Plasma sodium is reduced; liver transaminases are sometimes elevated. Despite the presence of pancreatitis, amylase may be normal due to an assay artifact; serum lipase is a more reliable indicator in this setting. Often the clinical laboratory will note the severe lipemia and fail to report measurements of routine chemistries due to the turbidity of the serum. If these other measurements are required, plasma can be centrifuged, the chylomicron layer removed, and the remaining plasma examined.

Fasting hyperchylomicronemia in adults is frequently accompanied by comorbid conditions such as uncontrolled diabetes and excessive alcohol intake.

Lipoprotein Lipase Deficiency

Almost every racial group has been reported to have patients with genetic defects in LPL,[82] and a founder mutation makes the defect especially common among French Canadians. Approximately half of the cases of severe primary hypertriglyceridemia are the result of LPL defects. Most LPL enzyme deficiencies are caused by inactive LPL protein. However, lack of protein production has also been reported, and because LPL might have receptor functions that do not require catalytic function, patients with these defects may have a more severe phenotype.

Although genetic LPL deficiency has been reported to manifest in adulthood, most cases of severe hyperchylomicronemia in adulthood are associated with partial LPL deficiency or other causes. In adults, the most important of these causes are type 2 diabetes and obesity, because insulin resistance is associated with defective clearance of lipoproteins.[83] Postprandial lipemia is a prominent feature of diabetes.[84] A thorough history of triglyceride-raising medications should be taken (see later discussion).

Regulation of LPL is complicated, and defects in its actions are associated with genetic or acquired abnormalities that are exclusive of genetic defects in the LPL molecule. Defective apoCII, the obligate cofactor for LPL, leads to deficient LPL activity.[85] Two molecular defects initially found in mice are the cause of occasional severe human hypertriglyceridemia. GPIHBP (discussed earlier) is a molecule expressed by endothelial cells whose deficiency leads to defective association of LPL with its binding site on the capillary lumen and defective intravascular lipolysis.[86] In one report, 20% of patients with FCS had GPIHBP mutations.[87] Lipase maturation factor 1 (LMF1) is an intracellular protein that is required for correct intracellular folding and activation of LPL.[88] Mutations in LPL, GPIHBP, and LMF1 all lead to reduced postheparin LPL activity; mutated apoCII does not, but serum from these patients fails to maximally activate LPL.

LPL deficiency also occurs as a secondary phenomenon. Autoimmune conditions can be associated with defective triglyceride catabolism due to inhibition of LPL, apoCII, or heparin. Antibodies against heparin are thought to prevent normal LPL association with the endothelial surface. In addition, patients with vascular disease or generalized intravascular reactions to transfusions or chemotherapy can occasionally develop defects in LPL. Transient episodes of fasting hyperchylomicronemia have been attributed to viral infections and to excessive fat/calorie intake after fasting.

Postprandial Hyperlipidemia

Although plasma lipid levels are usually measured after an overnight fast, chylomicron remnants are associated with vascular disease in a number of animal models and with genetic or dietary causes of hyperlipidemia. This has led to a widely accepted hypothesis that remnant lipoproteins are an overlooked cause of human vascular disease. Postprandial lipidemia, measured as triglyceride increase, is associated with greater risk of heart disease.[89] However, postprandial triglyceride elevations are also correlated with fasting triglycerides and reduced HDL levels, so the use of postprandial measurements in clinical practice is not currently recommended.

Diagnostic Evaluation of Severe Hypertriglyceridemia

Assessment of underlying medical conditions, consideration of age at onset, and, in some cases, biochemical evaluation of LPL are required. Conditions that cause fasting hypertriglyceridemia (discussed later) can lead to severe hypertriglyceridemia when exacerbated by diet, drugs, or other conditions such as diabetes or pregnancy.

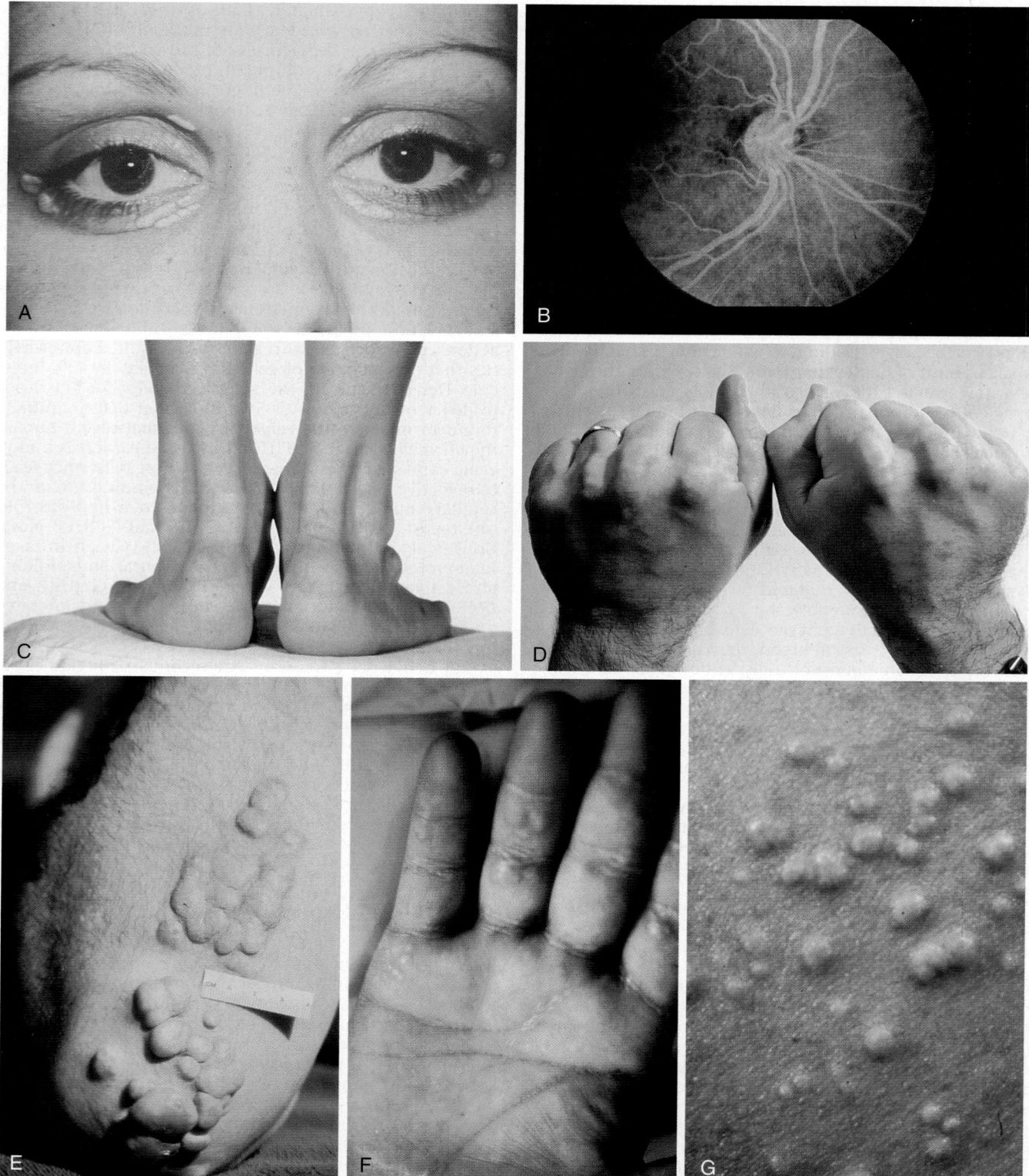

Figure 37-17 Physical examination findings associated with hyperlipidemia. **A,** Xanthelasma. **B,** Lipemia retinalis. **C,** Achilles tendon xanthomas. Notice the marked thickening of the tendons. **D,** Tendon xanthomas. **E,** Tuberous xanthomas. **F,** Palmar xanthomas. **G,** Eruptive xanthomas. (**A** and **B,** Courtesy of Dr. Mark Dresner and Hospital Practice [May 1990, p 15]; **C** through **F,** courtesy of Dr. Tom Bersot; **G,** Courtesy of Dr. Alan Chait.)

Genetic LPL deficiency is diagnosed by both the clinical setting and biochemical deficiency of LPL activity in post-heparin blood; LPL deficiency is more typically associated with younger age at onset, especially onset in childhood. A family history of low HDL is the most common lipid abnormality in heterozygous carriers.[90] LPL variants are also a determinant of HDL levels within the general population. A family history of French Canadian ancestry is suggestive. Although a presumptive diagnosis can be made on clinical grounds, it is sometimes useful for genetic reasons and treatment approach to confirm the diagnosis of LPL deficiency.

More than 100 mutations of the LPL gene have been described, and for this reason biochemical rather than genetic evaluation is still performed. Fasting patients are given an intravenous injection of 60 units/kg of heparin, which releases LPL into the bloodstream. Ten minutes later, a sample of postheparin blood is obtained and stored on ice, after which the plasma is frozen and sent to a lipid specialty laboratory for analysis. Heparin species are calibrated by their anticoagulant activity, and their ability to release LPL into the plasma varies, so a normal control postheparin plasma obtained with use of the same heparin is needed. Hepatic lipase (see later discussion) is also routinely measured in these samples. Postheparin samples should not clot. If they do, it may be an indicator of a defective injection or antibodies to heparin (e.g., in the case of a patient with an autoimmune disease). Postheparin plasma is not usually obtained during an acute episode of pancreatitis. Patients with a history of bleeding disorders or recent use of anticoagulant or antiplatelet drugs should be studied with caution, if at all. Deficiency of apoCII, the LPL activator, and inhibitors of LPL such as antibodies can be detected by mixing the patient's serum with a standard human or bovine source of LPL and then assessing activity.

Moderate Fasting Hypertriglyceridemia Due to Elevated Very Low Density Lipoprotein

Less dramatic elevations of triglyceride are not a cause of acute symptoms. They are of concern if serum triglycerides begin to exceed 500 mg/dL. Otherwise, the major issue is the relationship of triglycerides to cardiovascular disease. Triglyceride levels of 150 to 500 mg/dL are considered to be abnormal. Genome-wide association studies (GWAS)[91] and the observation that reduced triglyceride levels associated with genetic mutations in apoCIII, a protein that might inhibit LPL actions and also reduce uptake of triglyceride-rich lipoproteins by the liver, suggest an atherogenic role of triglycerides. The NCEP categorizes triglyceride levels of 200 to 499 mg/dL as high and those of 150 to 199 mg/dL as borderline high.[77] Several different clinical conditions lead to fasting hypertriglyceridemia. Familial combined hyperlipidemia is associated with increased apoB production, and at different times and in different family members it can manifest with hypertriglyceridemia (increased VLDL), increased cholesterol (LDL), or both. This disorder is associated with increased risk of vascular disease,[92] but its specific role is clouded by its presence in patients with other risk factors associated with the metabolic syndrome. The concomitant insulin resistance, obesity, and/or overt diabetes in many hypertriglyceridemic patients make it difficult to isolate one specific cause of this metabolic disturbance. In contrast, it has been suggested that isolated triglyceride elevations do not lead to more vascular disease. In the presence of the metabolic syndrome, triglyceride elevations probably predispose to vascular disease through unclear mechanisms.

Some cases of isolated hypertriglyceridemia have been associated with hepatic overproduction of bile acids in the setting of impaired intestinal absorption of bile acids.[93] This is analogous to the hypertriglyceridemia associated with use of bile acid–binding resins and reduced bile interaction with the liver FXR receptor.[94] There is uncertainty as to whether the large, triglyceride-rich VLDLs seen in this and similar clinical circumstances are atherogenic.

Dysbetalipoproteinemia is caused by a homozygous mutation in apoE, apoE2/E2, leading to defective clearance of chylomicron and small VLDL remnants (see earlier discussion). These patients, with a prevalence of approximately 1 of every 10,000 in the general population, present with elevated triglyceride and cholesterol due to defective lipid clearance of remnant lipoproteins. Patients with dysbetalipoproteinemia sometimes have tuberous and palmar xanthomas and a propensity to peripheral vascular disease (see later discussion).

Heterozygous LPL deficiency can be relatively common in some populations. As these individuals age or if the LPL deficiency is superimposed on other conditions that tend to elevate triglycerides, hypertriglyceridemia may be uncovered.

Genetic hypoalphalipoproteinemia syndromes are invariably associated with moderate hypertriglyceridemia. These syndromes include LCAT deficiency, Tangiers disease, and apoAI Milano variant. A reduced apoCII reservoir on HDL may be responsible.

Secondary Causes of Hypertriglyceridemia

Diabetes Mellitus. Diabetes mellitus is the most prominent cause of hypertriglyceridemia, which is found in up to one third of all patients with type 2 diabetes. Insulin reduces fatty acid flux from adipose tissue, reduces liver apoB production, inhibits de novo triglyceride synthesis, and optimizes LPL production. Kinetic studies in humans show that in patients with diabetes both increased triglyceride secretion and reduced clearance of triglyceride from the bloodstream often occur in concert.[95] Diabetes is also associated with increased postprandial lipemia. The most common diabetic dyslipidemia is moderate hypertriglyceridemia and low HDL. The reduced HDL results from greater exchange of VLDL triglyceride for HDL cholesterol, hydrolysis of the triglyceride-rich HDL by hepatic lipase, and more rapid clearance of the smaller HDL from the circulation. Defective lipolysis might also reduce the amount of cholesterol contributed to HDL from triglyceride-rich lipoproteins. CETP also enhances transfer of triglyceride to LDL, allowing these lipoproteins to be converted to smaller, denser forms that may be more atherogenic. This lipoprotein phenotype is also commonly found in nonhyperglycemic patients with metabolic syndrome. Although most patients with diabetes do not have increased LDL, some do, and LDL reduction will occur with improved diabetes control. As stated earlier, diabetes is associated with severe fasting chylomicronemia. Although many such patients also have an underlying dyslipidemia (e.g., due to heterozygous LPL deficiency), others do not have a defined lipid disorder.

Patients with type 1 diabetes in poor control also develop hypertriglyceridemia. However, because insulin stimulates HDL production, patients in good control sometimes develop high levels of HDL. However, limited data suggest that insulin-induced increases in HDL do not prevent cardiovascular disease.

Renal Failure. Renal failure is also associated with hypertriglyceridemia and low HDL levels. The reasons for this are not clear, but it may reflect underlying insulin resistance and defects in lipolysis of plasma triglycerides.

Hypertriglyceridemia in nephrotic syndrome has been linked to increased circulating levels of the LPL inhibitor angiopoietin-like protein 4.[96]

Drugs. Various drugs can elevate triglycerides. Diabetes, obesity, and renal disease are common causes of fasting hypertriglyceridemia. The most common drugs associated with hypertriglyceridemia are estrogen-like compounds, thiazides, beta blockers, protease inhibitors, glucocorticoids, immunosuppressives, retinoids (isotretinoin, Accutane), bile acid–binding resins, and newer antipsychotic medications.

Oral estrogen therapy increases plasma triglyceride levels as a result of greater liver production of VLDL, but combined estrogen-progestin therapy does not raise triglycerides and is sometimes associated with reduced LDL.[97] In the setting of an underlying hypertriglyceridemia, severe hyperchylomicronemia and pancreatitis can occur in patients taking oral estrogen alone or birth control pills, or during oocyte induction for fertility. For this reason, triglyceride levels should be measured in women before estrogen therapy or estrogen-inducing therapy is initiated. Transdermal estrogen administration, which does not lead to high liver exposure, does not result in triglyceride elevation.[98] Tamoxifen, a SERM, can cause severe hypertriglyceridemia and pancreatitis,[99] but raloxifene, another SERM, does not raise triglycerides.[100]

Diet and Alcohol. Diets lead to marked changes in plasma triglyceride levels. Most lipoprotein profiles use fasting blood to avoid the postprandial increase in triglycerides that represent both dietary fat and de novo triglyceride production by the liver. Liver production of triglyceride is especially robust after the intake of simple sugars such as those found in sweetened foods (especially beverages including high fructose corn syrup) and other carbohydrates (bread, pasta, rice, and potatoes). Excessive intake of simple carbohydrates usually leads to moderate hypertriglyceridemia, but it can also exacerbate underlying genetic hypertriglyceridemias. Fat intake, especially in the setting of triglyceride levels greater than 500 mg/dL, can cause severe hyperchylomicronemia.

A major clinical cause of hypertriglyceridemia is alcohol intake. Sensitivity to the triglyceride-raising effects of alcohol is variable, but removal of alcohol from the diet of hypertriglyceridemic patients is often curative. Alcohol has many effects on lipid metabolism, including inducing de novo fatty acid synthesis and inhibiting fatty acid oxidation in the liver.[101] A common clinical conundrum is deciding whether hypertriglyceridemia alone is responsible for pancreatitis in an alcohol-using patient. Subjects with dysbetalipoproteinemia are particularly sensitive to the effects of alcohol consumption because the alcohol-induced overproduction of VLDL and subsequent production of remnant particles occur in the setting of impaired remnant clearance. Because alcohol also raises HDL, the presence of elevated triglycerides without reduced HDL is a clinical clue that an alcohol effect may be contributing to the lipid disorder.

Diagnostic Evaluation of Moderate Hypertriglyceridemia

A search for associated disorders, review of medication use, and delineation of dietary choices are appropriate. If both triglycerides and cholesterol are elevated, a search for the underlying lipoprotein disorder is sometimes useful. By ultracentrifugation, dysbetalipoproteinemia due to the presence of cholesterol-enriched VLDL can be differentiated from that of familial combined hyperlipidemia: The usual ratio of VLDL triglyceride to cholesterol of approximately 5 is reduced to 3 or less in dysbetalipoproteinemia. ApoE genotyping is also useful. Cholesterol-enriched VLDL is also found in patients with hypothyroidism, renal failure, or hepatic lipase deficiency.

HYPERCHOLESTEROLEMIA WITHOUT HYPERTRIGLYCERIDEMIA

Because all lipoproteins contain cholesterol, dramatic increases in triglycerides will invariably also lead to elevated blood cholesterol values. However, the ratio of triglyceride to cholesterol will be greater than 5. Disorders associated with primarily increased cholesterol are discussed in this section. The clinical presentation of hypercholesterolemia is limited. Although patients with severe disease occasionally present with cosmetic concerns or orthopedic issues associated with tendon xanthomas, hypercholesterolemia is usually clinically occult and uncovered by blood testing during routine assessment or in the setting of vascular disease.

Genetic Familial Hypercholesterolemia

The centrality of the LDL receptor to the understanding of cholesterol metabolism was uncovered through investigations by the Brown and Goldstein laboratory (discussed earlier) into the cause of FH. This relatively common cause of severe hypercholesterolemia results from one of many defects in production of the LDL receptor leading to impaired function or production of the LDL receptor protein.[102] Patients with FH (most with heterozygous forms of the disease) have cholesterol levels that exceed 300 mg/dL. Homozygous presentations of the disease include cholesterol levels that are approximately twice this value. The heterozygous form may be as common as 1 in 200[103] in the general population and is a major cause of early-onset coronary artery disease. In addition, homozygous and some other severe forms of LDL receptor deficiency are associated with aortic valve calcification and stenosis.[104]

For unknown reasons, elevated LDL cholesterol leads to cholesterol deposition on tendons. Tendon xanthomas like those seen in Figure 37-17C and D occur in approximately 75% of FH patients. They are most common on the Achilles tendon. On inspection, a loss of the usual bowlike shape of the tendon occurs, or a bump or generalized thickening of the tendon is apparent. The irregularity of the tendon can also be detected by palpation. This physical finding is sometimes similar to that results from tendon rupture. If the tendon is abnormal, a history of athletic injury should be sought. Xanthomas also occur on extensor tendons of the hands, but less frequently, and are best appreciated on the knuckles of a clenched fist. Xanthomas of the Achilles tendon can cause recurrent episodes of Achilles tendinitis. Some xanthomas are subtle and are apparent only as a thickening of the tendon or a small bump at the insertion of the tendon into muscle. Patients with FH also have xanthelasmas (Fig. 37-17A) and premature corneal arcus (i.e., in persons younger than 40 years of age), but these findings can also occur in patients without FH. Many affected subjects have no physical findings. Premature coronary artery disease is common but variable. Some FH patients develop coronary disease in the third or fourth decade of life, especially if they also have reduced HDL cholesterol levels or associated risk due to cigarette smoking. Even before the introduction of statin therapy, some patients (especially women) never developed clinical vascular disease.

Homozygosity for FH is not common but is likely to occur more frequently than previously appreciated.[105] These subjects come to clinical attention early in life because of the appearance of tendon and planar xanthomas as well as tuberous xanthomas (Fig. 37-17E), marked hypercholesterolemia apparent at birth, premature coronary disease, or aortic valve disease. Typical plasma cholesterol concentrations range from 15.5 mmol/L (600 mg/dL) to 25.9 mmol/L (1000 mg/dL), and LDL cholesterol (LDL-C) concentrations range from 500 to 950 mg/dL.[106] Symptomatic coronary disease can occur before age 10 years. If not treated, these homozygous persons usually die from myocardial infarction by age 20 years. Aortic valve disease in homozygotes can be valvular or supravalvular.[104] The diagnosis of homozygous FH should be suspected in any child with extremely high plasma cholesterol (typically >500 mg/dL) or the xanthomas characteristic of FH. Both parents are obligate heterozygotes and should manifest the phenotype of heterozygous FH. However, ongoing study of the biology of the LDL receptor and its interaction with PCSK9 (see earlier discussion) in its degradation has shown that individuals with defects in both LDL receptors and PCSK9 can have normal plasma LDL levels.[102]

Familial Defective Apolipoprotein B100

Defects in LDL binding to normal LDL receptors also lead to elevated plasma cholesterol. The ligands for the LDL receptor are apoB100 and apoE. Familial defective apoB100 increases LDL and has a phenotype that is indistinguishable from that of FH, including increased susceptibility to CHD. The substitution of glutamine for arginine at amino acid 3500, which reduces LDL binding to the LDL receptor, accounts for most cases of familial defective apoB100, although other defects have also been reported. Often the LDL elevations are less severe, a reflection of a partial defect in receptor binding attributed to the mutation or the continued ability of apoE to mediate lipoprotein uptake.

Rare Mutations Associated With Elevated LDL Levels

Several rare, isolated causes of hypercholesterolemia have been reported. Mutations in *LDLRAP1*, the gene encoding a putative adaptor protein (ARH) that is required for internalization of LDL bound by the LDL receptor on the surface of hepatocytes, cause autosomal recessive hypercholesterolemia. Mutations in ARH associated with autosomal recessive hypercholesterolemia have been reported mostly in Italians (Sardinia) and Lebanese.

Autosomal dominant hypercholesterolemia caused by a mutation in the gene encoding cholesterol 7α-hydroxylase has been reported.[107] The hypercholesterolemia is caused by defective cholesterol conversion to cholic acid.

Mutation of PCSK9 (see earlier discussion) leads to alterations in LDL receptor expression because this enzyme modulates intracellular LDL degradation.[108] Gain-of-function mutations reduce LDL receptor numbers and lead to defective LDL clearance by the liver. Because PCSK9 promotes LDL receptor degradation,[109] inhibitors of this protein are being studied as a therapy for hypercholesterolemia.[3] As noted earlier, loss-of-function mutations in PSCK9 are associated with low levels of total cholesterol and LDL-C and decreased risk of coronary artery disease.[67]

Elevated Plasma Lipoprotein(a)

Apo(a), a protein of unknown function that shares high sequence homology with plasminogen, associates with apoB to produce an LDL termed Lp(a). Some but not all studies suggest that elevated plasma Lp(a) concentrations are associated with an increased risk of coronary disease.[110] Lp(a) was initially thought not to be a cardiovascular risk factor in Africans or African Americans.[111] Patients with high levels of Lp(a) are more likely to clot bypass grafts and stents. Unlike LDL, which confers risk as a continuous function of plasma level, risk is found only in individuals with the highest levels of Lp(a).

Plasma Lp(a) levels are to a great extent determined genetically. Lp(a) particles contain a variable number of a protein repeat known as a kringle. Smaller Lp(a) particles, with fewer kringle repeats, are usually produced at higher levels. For this reason, some have suggested that it is Lp(a) size, rather than plasma level, that confers vascular risk. Renal failure leads to elevations of Lp(a) levels.

Polygenic Hypercholesterolemia

Most patients with elevated LDL cholesterol do not have FH, and even cholesterol levels above 300 mg/dL are not usually associated with xanthomas or defects in the LDL receptor. If, as is conventional for other laboratory values, hypercholesterolemia is defined as a cholesterol value that exceeds the 95th percentile for the population, only 1 in 25 of these patients should have FH. Although diet and lifestyle influence LDL, the genetic and environmental factors associated with most elevated LDL cholesterol levels are unknown, and therefore this type of hypercholesterolemia is referred to as polygenic. Nonetheless, the increased cholesterol levels are associated with a higher risk of coronary artery disease.

Increased LDL levels can be a result of defective LDL clearance with normal LDL receptors, a more subtle regulation of the receptor, or increased LDL production. This last type occurs in the setting of familial combined hyperlipoproteinemia (see later discussion), which can manifest as primary elevations of LDL. Greater LDL production due to greater absorption of gut cholesterol, abnormalities in the regulation of lipid-regulated nuclear transcription factors, or gain-of-function abnormalities in cholesterol and apoB lipoprotein assembly pathways are all possible but poorly defined.

Lipoprotein(X)

Obstructive liver disease sometimes leads to a marked increase in plasma cholesterol. In part, this is the result of increased LDL, presumably due to a defect in LDL receptors. In addition, free cholesterol circulates in association with albumin, a particle referred to as *Lp(X)*. This is caused by a deficiency in the cholesterol esterifying enzyme, LCAT. The clinical setting suggests the diagnosis. In addition, an abnormal ratio of free to total cholesterol (or cholesteryl ester) can be determined by the laboratory. The relationship of Lp(X) to vascular disease is unclear.

Sitosterolemia

In this rare disorder, dietary sitosterol and other plant sterols, which are not normally absorbed in significant quantities in the intestine, are absorbed in large amounts, resulting in their accumulation in the plasma and in peripheral tissues and causing premature atherosclerosis.[112] The molecular cause is a mutation in the genes encoding ABCG8 and ABCG5, which are responsible for resecretion of absorbed plant sterols. Patients develop tendon xanthomas in childhood and have normal to high plasma levels of LDL; the differential diagnosis includes FH and cerebrotendinous xanthomatosis. The diagnosis can be confirmed by gas-liquid chromatography of plasma lipids, which demonstrates the high levels of plant sterols. Therapy consists of restriction of plant sterols in the diet and treatment with ezetimibe (see later), which inhibits absorption of dietary sterols.[113]

Cerebrotendinous Xanthomatosis

Cerebrotendinous xanthomatosis is a rare disorder of sterol metabolism that is associated with neurologic disease, tendon xanthomas, and cataracts in young adults. Neurologic manifestations include cerebellar ataxia, dementia, spinal cord paresis, and subnormal intelligence. Premature atherosclerosis is common. Osteoporosis has been reported and is presumably caused by alterations in vitamin D metabolism. The disorder results from mutations that cause deficiencies of 27-hydroxylase, a key enzyme in cholesterol oxidation and bile acid synthesis, leading to high plasma levels of cholesterol and cholestanol, with subsequent accumulation of these sterols in tendons and in tissues of the nervous system. Chenodeoxycholic acid is indicated for treatment.

Hypothyroidism and Elevated Cholesterol

All patients with significant hyperlipidemia should be screened for hypothyroidism, because thyroid hormone deficiency causes hypercholesterolemia, and low levels of thyroid hormone predispose to statin-induced myositis.[114] Although hypothyroidism usually increases LDL-C due to reduced LDL clearance, it can also be associated with high plasma triglyceride levels. Levels of HDL-C are usually unchanged or slightly lower in hypothyroidism and may be reduced in hyperthyroidism. Subclinical hypothyroidism is a cause of hypercholesterolemia that sometimes responds to thyroid hormone replacement.[115]

Diagnostic Evaluation of Isolated Hypercholesterolemia

A lipoprotein assessment is appropriate and, if the cholesterol level is higher than 300 mg/dL, a search for signs of FH is needed. The diagnosis of heterozygous FH is suggested by the presence of high plasma levels of total cholesterol and LDL-C, normal plasma triglycerides, tendon xanthomas, and a family history of premature coronary disease. Heterozygous FH should be suspected in any person with premature heart disease. In one study it accounted for 4% of men who survived myocardial infarction before 60 years of age.[116] The diagnosis of FH is primarily clinical, but genetic testing is available through many laboratories. Such testing may be helpful for assessing risk in family members and in genetic counseling.

Increased High-Density Lipoprotein

Occasionally, patients with hypercholesterolemia have elevations primarily of HDL, with normal levels of LDL. Usually, this pattern is found in families with little cardiovascular disease, and high HDL syndromes are associated with longevity.[117] Conventional risk factor analysis and ratios of total cholesterol to HDL suggest that patients with high HDL have reduced risk of cardiovascular disease. However, GWAS failed to link genetic factors that elevate HDL with reduced vascular disease.[118] This has led to a reevaluation of the HDL hypothesis.[119]

Newer information suggests that there are subgroups of these patients with a less sanguine prognosis. These rela-

tively unusual patients are insufficiently represented in population studies to assess coronary risk. Isolation of HDL from patients with cardiovascular disease and high levels of HDL led to the observation that these HDLs do not have anti-inflammatory properties.[120] Atherogenic HDL has been detected in patients with systemic lupus erythematosus.[121] Therefore, there are clinical circumstances in which HDL may be dysfunctional (see earlier discussion).

Genetic Disorders Causing Increased High-Density Lipoprotein

CETP deficiency is a hereditary syndrome in which plasma HDL-C levels are increased because of diminished activity of plasma CETP. The disorder is not uncommon in the Japanese population. Its features include marked elevations of plasma HDL-C in homozygotes (usually >100 mg/dL). Despite the elevated HDL-C levels, the effect on coronary disease risk of CETP gene mutations is unclear. Heterozygotes have moderately elevated HDL-C levels. The lower activity of CETP results in diminished transfer of cholesteryl esters from HDL to apoB-containing lipoproteins. As a result, more cholesteryl esters are found in HDL, and the ratio of total cholesterol to HDL-C is markedly reduced. CETP is most active in the setting of hypertriglyceridemia, so, in addition to reducing HDL cholesterol, it provides a mechanism for reduction of triglyceride through HDL metabolism. Perhaps for this reason, studies in mice, which normally do not have significant plasma CETP activity, have shown reduced apoB-containing lipoproteins and reduced atherosclerosis with addition of a CETP transgene. Therefore, the effect of CETP on vascular disease varies as a function of the underlying plasma lipid profile. As noted earlier, the first CETP inhibitor tested clinically failed in a trial because the drug increased cardiovascular events despite elevating HDL. This result was attributed by some increased aldosterone production, leading to hypertension. Drugs without this side effect are being studied, but results will be difficult to interpret because some of these agents also decrease LDL.[122] Several other pharmacologic agents are associated with increased plasma HDL. The antiatherogenic capacity of HDL produced in these circumstances is unknown. HDL induction occurs with the use of oral estrogens, alcohol intake, phenytoin (Dilantin), phenobarbital, and insulin therapy in some patients with type 1 diabetes.

Endothelial lipase deficiency is caused by defects in the third member of the lipase gene family, endothelial lipase. As described earlier, loss-of-function mutations in this lipase are associated with increased HDL levels.

ELEVATED TRIGLYCERIDES AND CHOLESTEROL

Elevated triglyceride and cholesterol levels can be caused by increased VLDL and LDL, combined hyperlipidemia, or the presence of increased circulating remnant lipoproteins (dysbetalipoproteinemia). These are indistinguishable by routine laboratory examination, but treatment approaches differ somewhat.

Combined Hyperlipidemia

Combined hyperlipidemia is a common disorder associated with elevations of plasma cholesterol and triglyceride levels and increased susceptibility to coronary disease. Lipoprotein isolation reveals increased LDL and VLDL. Kinetic analysis has associated this pattern primarily with overproduction, rather than defective clearance, of apoB lipoproteins. When it occurs within families, it is termed *familial combined hyperlipidemia*. These individuals, who do not necessarily have other causes for lipid abnormalities, characteristically come from families with various hyperlipidemias that include increased isolated triglycerides or increased isolated LDL. Moreover, the abnormal lipoprotein pattern (increased triglycerides, cholesterol, or both) can vary over time in an individual.

Regulation of apoB production involves a number of steps (see earlier discussion), and understanding of this physiology explains some of the association of combined hyperlipidemia with other diseases. Increased fatty acid return to the liver and reduced insulin action prevent degradation of newly synthesized apoB. Therefore, it is not surprising that both metabolic syndrome and type 2 diabetes are commonly found with combined hyperlipidemias. Although the genetics of this disorder have been investigated, the coexistence of this lipoprotein pattern with insulin resistance and obesity syndromes has been a confounder. Therefore, although alterations in a number of genes associated with lipid metabolism, such as LPL and apoCIII, have been observed, a firm genetic marker is not currently available.

Familial Dysbetalipoproteinemia (Type III Hyperlipoproteinemia)

Familial dysbetalipoproteinemia (formerly known as type III hyperlipoproteinemia) is an uncommon disorder of lipoprotein metabolism that is characterized by moderate to severe hypertriglyceridemia and hypercholesterolemia caused by the accumulation of cholesterol-rich remnant particles in the plasma. Premature peripheral vascular disease and coronary artery disease are common. The cause is mutations in the apoE gene that result in defective binding of apoE to lipoprotein receptors. The disorder is associated with the apoE2 isoform and in most instances is inherited as an autosomal recessive trait. Because the phenotypic expression of the disorder is limited to approximately 1% of the patients with the apoE2/E2 phenotype, other genetic or environmental factors must also be operative. The hyperlipidemia is caused by a defect in clearance of remnant lipoproteins whose liver uptake requires apoE interaction with the LDL receptor, LRP1, and HSPG (see earlier discussion). The remnants that accumulate have lost much of their triglyceride through LPL-mediated triglyceride hydrolysis and therefore are cholesterol rich. The predominant remnant particles, termed *β-VLDL*, can be identified by abnormal migration on gel electrophoresis or by abnormal lipid content.

Dysbetalipoproteinemia is usually diagnosed in adulthood and is rarely detected in persons younger than 20 years of age. The disorder is more common in men than in women. It is characterized by moderately severe elevations in plasma triglyceride and cholesterol levels; typically, these values both range from 300 to 400 mg/dL. Concentrations of HDL-C are normal. Xanthomas are present in more than half of affected subjects. Palmar xanthomas, which are planar xanthomas in the palmar creases (see Fig. 37-17F), are pathognomonic for this disorder. Tuberous or tuboeruptive xanthomas (see Fig. 37-17E) are also common but are less specific for this disorder. Tendon xanthomas and xanthelasma occur in some patients. Unlike FH, in which peripheral vascular disease is uncommon, premature peripheral vascular disease occurs in addition to premature coronary artery disease in patients with dysbetalipoproteinemia. Coexisting metabolic conditions

that exacerbate the phenotype of dysbetalipoproteinemia, such as obesity, alcohol consumption, diabetes mellitus, and hypothyroidism, are often present.

In addition to homozygosity for the apoE2 isoform, some mutations in the apoE gene are known to lead to the dysbetalipoproteinemia phenotype in an autosomal dominant fashion. The phenotype manifests at an early age without exacerbating factors.

Hepatic Lipase Deficiency

Hepatic lipase deficiency is a rare disorder associated with lack of heparin-releasable hepatic lipase activity in the plasma. Because this enzyme mediates the final step of conversion of IDL to LDL and is involved in chylomicron remnant clearance, its deficiency causes a phenotype that is similar to that found with dysbetalipoproteinemia—namely, elevated levels of plasma cholesterol (250 to 1500 mg/dL) and triglycerides (395 to 8200 mg/dL). Patients also have palmar and tuboeruptive xanthomas, premature arcus corneae, and premature coronary artery disease. Because hepatic lipase also mediates HDL metabolism, HDL levels are not decreased. The demonstration of hepatic lipase deficiency requires in vitro assays of hepatic lipase activity in postheparin plasma or DNA analysis to identify mutations.

Nephrotic Syndrome

Hyperlipidemia almost always accompanies the nephrotic syndrome. Total cholesterol, VLDL, LDL-C, total triglycerides, and plasma apoB may all be elevated. Nephrotic syndrome increases liver production of apoB-containing lipoproteins, leading to increased plasma LDL or VLDL, or both. This may be a response to hypoalbuminemia and an associated generalized increase in liver protein secretion.

Protease Inhibitor Use in Human Immunodeficiency Virus Infection

Treatments for human immunodeficiency virus (HIV) infection often cause hyperlipidemia, lipodystrophy, and insulin resistance. Hypertriglyceridemia is the most common lipid abnormality, although increases in LDL are also found. These effects were initially thought to result from the use of protease inhibitors, but other agents, such as reverse transcriptase inhibitors, can cause dyslipidemia. The metabolic syndrome is not uniformly induced by all drugs; older agents such as ritonavir are more likely to have metabolic side effects. The cause of this syndrome is unclear but may be related to greater liver production of apoB lipoproteins and triglycerides.

Immunosuppressive Regimens

Patients undergoing transplantation who require a number of medications commonly present with hypertriglyceridemia with or without hypercholesterolemia. Glucocorticoids more often raise triglycerides, cyclosporine raises cholesterol, and rapamycin increases both cholesterol and triglycerides.

Diagnostic Evaluation of Elevated Triglycerides and Cholesterol

Appropriate assessment usually requires that clinicians determine whether the hyperlipidemia is primarily a genetic disorder or is secondary to another systemic disease. The clinical setting and accompanying drug therapies must be considered. In some situations, an evaluation for dysbetalipoproteinemia is useful. In other cases, empiric treatment is reasonable (see later discussion). The presence of cholesterol-enriched β-VLDL is determined by a direct measurement of the VLDL-C level to detect cholesterol-rich remnant particles. The directly measured ratio of VLDL-C to plasma triglycerides (in milligrams per deciliter) is a useful screen. In dysbetalipoproteinemia, this ratio is usually greater than 0.3 (when hyperlipidemia is present), whereas the normal ratio is typically about 0.2 (i.e., the VLDL-C concentration is about 20% of the plasma triglyceride level). Patients with suspected dysbetalipoproteinemia can be evaluated for apoE2 homozygosity by apoE genotyping of DNA.

HYPOCHOLESTEROLEMIA

Secondary causes that can lead to very low levels of apoB-containing lipoproteins and low cholesterol levels include malabsorption, sepsis, liver failure, and malnutrition. There are also genetic conditions that cause low cholesterol.

Familial Hypobetalipoproteinemia

Familial hypobetalipoproteinemia is defined as apoB and LDL-C levels below the 5th percentile. Hypobetalipoproteinemia is not associated with a phenotype and leads to a reduced risk for cardiovascular disease. Possible causes of this syndrome include mutations leading to truncation of apoB and mutations in PCSK9 presumably leading to increased numbers of LDL receptors. PCSK9 loss-of-function mutations occur in as many as 2% of African Americans but are rare in persons of European descent. Other patients have a defect in angiopoietin-like protein 3.[123] Patients with hypobetalipoproteinemia have an increased risk of hepatic steatosis.

Abetalipoproteinemia

Abetalipoproteinemia is a rare autosomal recessive disorder caused by a deficiency in MTP (see discussion earlier), which results in a virtual absence of apoB-containing lipoproteins in the plasma. Abetalipoproteinemia occurs in fewer than 1 in 10⁶ persons and has the same phenotype as homozygous hypobetalipoproteinemia, including malabsorption of fat and fat-soluble vitamins from the intestine, which can lead to neurologic disease related to vitamin E deficiency. The disorder is usually detected in infancy because of fat malabsorption associated with marked decreases in plasma cholesterol and triglyceride levels.

Chylomicron Retention Syndrome

Anderson disease, or chylomicron retention syndrome, is a rare condition that is phenotypically similar to abetalipoproteinemia. Subjects with Anderson disease cannot secrete chylomicrons from the intestine. Eight mutations in the *SAR1B* gene (formerly *SARA2*) have been linked to Anderson disease. This gene encodes SAR1B, a protein that is important in the transport of chylomicrons through the secretory pathway in enterocytes.

Familial Hypoalphalipoproteinemia

Although low HDL in the general population is correlated with greater coronary artery disease, genetic disorders leading to very low plasma levels of HDL have variable and sometimes undefined coronary risk. In part, this might result from the rarity of some of these diseases. For this reason, the approach to the disorders is often unclear.

Apolipoprotein AI Mutations

Mutations in the apoAI gene can decrease HDL formation and result in low plasma HDL-C levels. ApoAI deficiency can be caused by point mutations in the apoAI gene or by deletions or gene rearrangements at the apoAI/CIII/AIV/AV gene locus. ApoAI deficiency typically results in plasma HDL-C levels lower than 0.3 mmol/L (10 mg/dL). Some apoAI variants activate LCAT poorly (see later discussion). The molecular diagnosis is made by protein analysis showing an altered apoAI size or by genetic sequencing. Some apoAI variants are associated with amyloidosis.

The apoAI Milano variant (apoAI_{Milano}) is caused by a substitution of cysteine for arginine at amino acid 173. This results in low plasma HDL-C levels without premature CHD. Therefore, this HDL is hypothesized to be antiatherogenic and has been used in a human clinical trial.[124]

Lecithin:Cholesterol Acyltransferase Deficiency

LCAT deficiency leads to low HDL as a consequence of defective conversion of cholesterol to cholesteryl ester. In a phenotypically appropriate patient, measurement of the ratio of free cholesterol to cholesteryl ester is diagnostic; normally free cholesterol is approximately 30% of the total, but this percentage increases to more than 90% in LCAT deficiency. LCAT activity measurements and sequencing can also be performed. LCAT deficiency leads to striking corneal arcus (sometimes leading to marked visual impairment), normochromic anemia, and, occasionally, renal failure in young adults. Renal biopsies show characteristic foam cells. Despite their very low HDL levels, the risk of coronary disease in patients with LCAT deficiency is not pronounced; this may reflect the low levels of LDL that are also found in many of these patients.

A variant of LCAT deficiency, called *fish-eye disease*, is also caused by mutations of the LCAT gene. The phenotype is less severe than that seen in complete LCAT deficiency.[125] Fish-eye disease is characterized by low plasma HDL-C levels and corneal opacities; anemia and renal disease do not occur. The phenotypic differences between LCAT deficiency and fish-eye disease have been attributed to whether mutations in the LCAT gene encode variants that fail to esterify cholesterol of both HDL and apoB-containing lipoproteins (LCAT deficiency) or of HDL only (fish-eye disease).

Adenosine Triphosphate–Binding Cassette Transporter A1 Deficiency

The ABCA1 transporter is essential to complete synthesis of mature HDL by the liver and the small intestine. A number of mutations in this receptor are associated with hypoalphalipoproteinemia. Because the number of genetic mutations is great, assays often study fibroblast "unloading" of cholesterol to apoAI to show the defect.

Tangier disease is the most flagrant example of a defect in ABCA1. These patients, originally from Tangier Island in the Chesapeake Bay, had hypocholesterolemia resulting from a marked decrease in plasma HDL as well as low LDL and the striking physical finding of orange tonsils. The orange tonsils are thought to result from defective reverse cholesterol transport from macrophages of the reticuloendothelial system, with the color probably caused by carotenoids. The risk of cardiovascular disease with this syndrome is uncertain.

OVERVIEW OF ATHEROGENESIS

Atherosclerosis and its clinical presentation as coronary artery disease, stroke, and peripheral vascular disease is likely to be the product of several pathophysiologic changes. Depending on the patient and setting, arterial disease results from a varying reaction to lipid infiltration, arterial damage, and macrophage inflammation. Population, genetic, and therapeutic data suggest that atherosclerosis is frequently caused by cholesterol deposition within the arterial wall. As described earlier, a number of genetic hyperlipidemic disorders are associated with premature atherosclerosis. Reductions of blood cholesterol by diet, surgical ileal bypass, statins, and other cholesterol-lowering therapies have convincingly shown that cholesterol reduction will reduce the incidence of major cardiovascular events, especially myocardial infarction, need for revascularization, and stroke. Most striking is the observation that the majority of patients with coronary artery disease will have reduced disease (i.e., regression) with statin therapy.[126] This cholesterol hypothesis is further supported by a wealth of animal data: altering blood lipid levels by diet or genetic modification causes atherosclerosis-free animals to develop disease, and reduction of cholesterol leads to regression.

In animals and humans, vascular disease is not universal, even among those individuals with marked hypercholesterolemia. Similarly, patients with low cholesterol are not assured of being protected from the disease. It is estimated that about 50% of all atherosclerosis is attributable to hyperlipidemia and other known cardiac risk factors.[127]

In contrast, approaches to atherosclerosis treatment directed toward several nonlipid causes have not been successful. Use of vitamin E and antibiotics has not altered cardiovascular event rates. Although low-dose aspirin has some anti-inflammatory properties, its reduction of cardiovascular events is most likely secondary to effects on coagulation rather than direct effects on atherosclerosis. Trials are in progress to test the hypothesis that decreasing inflammation impacts cardiovascular event rates.

There are a number of clinical situations in which cholesterol reduction has failed to alter vascular disease. Most notably, statin-mediated cholesterol reduction appears to be ineffective in end-stage renal disease. In contrast, cardiovascular events in patients with less severe renal disease are reduced by treatment with statin/ezetimibe.[128] Other inflammatory diseases (e.g., collagen-vascular diseases) that are associated with cardiac events have not yet been shown to respond to cholesterol-lowering therapies.

Cholesterol-Induced Atherosclerosis

More than 100 years ago, pathologists identified cholesterol as a major component of atherosclerosis. This poorly metabolized lipid is found both associated with matrix and within arterial cells. Macrophages and smooth muscle cells are converted into foam cells, so called because of their intracellular foamy lipid. In addition, there are often acellular lipid-rich areas, a variable amount of overlying collagen-rich connective tissue, and regions where the atherosclerotic plaque has ruptured. The process begins with lipid infiltration into the arterial wall.[129,130]

Unresolved pathogenic issues include the following: (1) How does lipid enter the artery? (2) What pathways lead to excess lipid uptake by foam cells? (3) What processes cause rupture and thrombosis?

Infiltration of lipoproteins into the artery wall is likely to be a normal and continuous process. Larger particles, such as chylomicrons, are likely to be excluded by the endothelial barrier. LDL can leave the circulation via channels between cells, along the continuous transendothelial movement of cell-free plasma, or via interaction with specific receptors. Once in the subendothelial space, lipoproteins must accumulate to cause disease. It is theorized that positive charges on apoB interact with negatively charged proteoglycans to promote lipoprotein retention. Both apoB100 in LDL and VLDL, apoB48 in chylomicron remnants, and apoE in several classes of lipoproteins have proteoglycan-binding sequences.[131] Another possibility is that, within the artery, lipoproteins fuse to form large aggregates that are unable to disassociate and reenter the circulation. Lipoprotein uptake into cells is usually well controlled, because excess cellular cholesterol downregulates LDL receptors. Therefore, aberrant lipoprotein receptor regulation may be a factor, or LDL (and remnants) may enter cells by non–cholesterol-regulated pattern recognition receptors (see earlier discussion).

Cholesterol-containing lipoproteins can become inflammatory. Enzymes within the artery might induce alterations in the protein and lipid content of LDL that convert these particles into more inflammatory oxidized LDL.

Unstable Plaque and Regression

The atherogenic process occurs within the artery wall. Initially, it was thought that the lumen was progressively narrowed by the accumulation of macrophages, the proliferation of smooth muscle cells, and the deposition of cholesterol. In fact, the truly dangerous lesion (the culprit lesion) may not cause marked luminal narrowing.[132] As atherosclerosis progresses, there is a compensatory expansion of the lumen that maintains an almost constant lumen size. As the lesion develops within the intima, the complication of rupture of the overlying intima or endothelial erosion leads to exposure of the lesional contents to platelets, initiating thrombosis. It is the acute thrombosis that is responsible for infarctions in most patients. Rupture or erosion occurs where the fibrous cap covering the underlying thrombogenic lipid is thin.

The surfaces of complicated lesions can become thrombogenic as endothelial cells are lost or the fibrous cap ruptures and the subendothelial space is exposed. Platelets can adhere to this exposed surface, promoting thrombus formation. In these unstable plaques, blood actually dissects into the artery wall, leading to the formation of a large thrombus. Calcification is also a feature of late lesions. Advanced lesions can weaken the elasticity and integrity of the artery wall, potentially creating an aneurysm of the vessel. As clinical trial data have shown, removal or reduction of the atherogenic stimulus can result in plaque regression and stabilization, leaving a remnant devoid of lipid that resembles a wound scar and is less likely to serve as a nidus for thrombus formation.

Atherosclerosis usually develops in the setting of hypercholesterolemia. Observations first made in animals and now confirmed in humans indicate that this process can be reversed if plasma cholesterol reduction is intensive.[133]

EVIDENCE SUPPORTING TREATMENT OF LIPID DISORDERS

Cholesterol and Cardiovascular Disease

Despite a very significant decrease in the incidence of vascular disease, cardiovascular diseases including CHD and cerebrovascular disease remain the major causes of death in the United States for both men and women.[134] The major risk factors are age, elevated LDL-C, reduced HDL-C, smoking, hypertension, insulin resistance with or without overt diabetes mellitus, and a family history of premature CHD. Modifiable risk factors account for most of the excess CHD risk. Although a number of new risk factors have been proposed to increase the accuracy of predicting risk of CHD events, only four conditions—dyslipidemia, hypertension, cigarette smoking, and diabetes—account for increased CHD risk in 80% to 90% of patients.[135,136]

Understanding of the relationship of cholesterol and lipids to atherosclerosis has evolved over the past century and especially over the past 60 years.[137] The *lipid hypothesis*, which postulates that increased plasma cholesterol concentrations increase the risk of CHD, that diets high in fat (especially saturated fat of animal origin) and cholesterol increase plasma cholesterol levels, and that lowering of cholesterol levels would decrease the risk of atherosclerotic vascular disease, was not accepted for many years. Data from population studies, animal studies, cell culture experiments, and, eventually, clinical trials of lipid-lowering interventions have made the treatment of hyperlipidemia an accepted strategy for decreasing cardiovascular risk.[138,139]

Epidemiologic Evidence

A number of studies have demonstrated a relationship between plasma cholesterol levels and the risk of CHD. Analysis of cholesterol levels of men who were screened for the Multiple Risk Factor Intervention Trial (see Fig. 37-16) showed that there is increased risk at total cholesterol levels greater than 5.2 mmol/L (200 mg/dL).[140] Multiple studies have demonstrated the relationship between cardiovascular risk factors, dietary cholesterol and saturated fats, and the incidence of CHD, providing solid epidemiologic data for the lipid hypothesis. Epidemiologic and clinical studies involving lifestyle changes have led to a variety of recommendations for diet and exercise approaches to decreasing cardiovascular risk.[141]

Clinical Trials

Lowering cholesterol decreases the risk of CHD, as has been shown in many human clinical trials. In all groups examined, including patients with and without preexisting CHD over a range of initial plasma cholesterol levels, the results have demonstrated that sufficient lowering of plasma cholesterol levels reduces the risk of CHD regardless of the baseline cholesterol level.

Clinical trial data of lipid-modifying therapies include trials of both primary and secondary prevention, with measurements of clinical events and surrogate measurements such as carotid intima media thickness, quantitative coronary angiography, and intravascular ultrasound and a variety of therapies including diet, partial ileal bypass, nicotinic acid, fibric acid derivatives, BAS, HMG-CoA reductase inhibitors, ω-3 fatty acids, LDL apheresis, and combinations of drugs. The most rigorous evidence is that of randomized controlled trials with cardiovascular events as the end point.

Before 1984, a number of clinical trials demonstrated the benefits of cholesterol lowering in both primary and secondary prevention settings using several medications, but they did not convince the medical profession that lowering of cholesterol was beneficial. In 1984, the large, randomized, placebo-controlled, Coronary Primary Prevention Trial demonstrated that cholesterol lowering with

the BAS cholestyramine decreased the risk of nonfatal myocardial infarction and cardiac death in men with high cholesterol levels.[142] However, the study did not have adequate statistical power to show an effect on mortality, and there remained concerns that cholesterol lowering did not decrease overall mortality rate. Other studies in the 1980s showed that use of cholesterol-lowering medications could decrease the progression of coronary atherosclerosis as demonstrated by coronary angiography, including the Cholesterol Lowering Atherosclerosis Study (CLAS)[143] and the Familial Atherosclerosis Treatment Study (FATS).[144]

The Scandinavian Simvastatin Survival Study (4S),[145] a randomized, placebo-controlled trial using simvastatin in men and women with preexisting coronary artery disease and high LDL-C levels (190 mg/dL), evaluated total and cardiovascular mortality rates. It demonstrated a decrease in both cardiovascular and total mortality rates and provided compelling evidence of the benefit of cholesterol reduction. The 4S study finally convinced many researchers and practitioners of the value of lipid lowering, at least for secondary prevention. Cholesterol and Recurrent Events (CARE), another secondary prevention event trial done in patients with a history of myocardial infarction and baseline LDL-C levels of 115 to 175 mg/dL, showed a decrease in event rate with pravastatin treatment.[146] In the Heart Protection Study, simvastatin decreased the first major vascular event by 24% in high-risk patients, even when LDL-C cholesterol was lower than 3.0 mmol/L (116 mg/dL).[147] Evidence for even lower LDL-C targets came from the Pravastatin or Atorvastatin Evaluation and Infection Therapy (PROVE-IT) study, which showed a benefit of atorvastatin (80 mg/day) compared with pravastatin (40 mg/day) in patients with acute coronary syndromes,[148] and from the Treating to New Target (TNT) study comparing different dosages of atorvastatin (80 mg/day vs. 10 mg/day) in patients with stable coronary disease.[149]

Clinical trials of primary prevention such as the West of Scotland study,[150] the Air Force/Texas Coronary Atherosclerosis Protection (AFCAPS/TexCAPS) study,[151] and the Collaborative Atorvastatin Diabetes Study (CARDS)[152] demonstrated the benefits of lowering LDL-C to reduce coronary artery disease events in patients without a history of CHD who had, respectively, high LDL-C levels (with no prior myocardial infarction), low HDL-C levels (in both men and women), and type 2 diabetes. Additional evidence for the use of statins in primary prevention of cardiovascular events came from the Justification for the Use of Statins in Prevention: an Intervention Trial Evaluating Rosuvastatin (JUPITER) study, in which men and women with LDL-C levels of 108 mg/dL at baseline were randomly assigned to receive either rosuvastatin or placebo. The trial was terminated early when there was a highly significant decrease in cardiovascular events in the statin-treated group.[153]

Meta-analyses of clinical trials demonstrate that statins reduce risk of cardiovascular events in most groups of patients, including men and women, with and without coronary artery disease, with diabetes, with hypertension, and regardless of baseline LDL cholesterol.[154,155]

Although the beneficial effect of cholesterol lowering through LDL-C reduction is well established, evidence for the benefit of lowering triglycerides or raising HDL-C levels, or both, is not strong. Data are most significant in studies of the fibric acid gemfibrozil and of niacin; niacin also lowers LDL-C levels at high doses. The Helsinki Heart Study[156] and the Veterans Affairs–High-Density Lipoprotein Cholesterol Intervention Trial (VA-HIT)[157] both used gemfibrozil, the former for primary prevention and the latter for secondary prevention, and in both studies the greatest benefit was in men with high triglyceride and low HDL-C levels. Studies with other fibrates, such as fenofibrate, have yielded results without unequivocal statistical significance.[158] In the lipid treatment arm of the ACCORD (Action to Control Cardiovascular Risk in Diabetes) trial in type 2 diabetes, fenofibrate was added to statin therapy in patients with an average triglyceride level of 162. There was no overall benefit, although a subgroup of patients with higher triglycerides and reduced HDL had reduced cardiovascular events.[159] A trial is under way to assess the effects of fenofibrate in subjects who have hypertriglyceridemia in the range that appears to benefit from this treatment. The niacin arm of the Coronary Drug Project showed a decrease in nonfatal myocardial infarctions in men with coronary artery disease during the 6-year trial and a decrease in total mortality rate in the 9 years after the study.[160] However, more recent trials of niacin in subjects whose LDL was already markedly reduced by statins, the AIM-HIGH and HPS2-THRIVE (Treatment of HDL to Reduce the Incidence of Vascular Events) studies, have failed to show additional benefit.[161,162]

Although event trials provide the best evidence, studies using carotid intima medial thickness, coronary artery angiography, or coronary intravascular ultrasound have provided useful information. Trials with statins have shown an effect on the progression of atherosclerosis. In an uncontrolled study, rosuvastatin was associated with a reduction of total atheroma volume by 6.8% as determined by intravascular ultrasound (A Study to Evaluate the Effect of Rosuvastatin on Intravascular Ultrasound-Derived Coronary Atheroma Burden: ASTEROID).[133] In the Reversal of Atherosclerosis with Aggressive Lipid Lowering (REVERSAL) study, treatment with atorvastatin 80 mg/day (treatment LDL-C, 79 mg/dL) was associated with no progression of coronary artery disease compared with pravastatin 40 mg/day (treatment LDL-C, 110 mg/dL), which led to progression of disease.[163]

Clinical event trial data for combination therapy of hyperlipidemia are minimal, but surrogate end point studies using coronary angiography have suggested benefit of combination therapy. Studies using a BAS and niacin, a statin and niacin, or triple therapy with a statin, niacin, and BAS have shown decreased progression of atherosclerosis.[143,144,164,165] Some of these imaging studies of combination therapy included niacin and indicated benefit, but as noted earlier, adding niacin in the setting of LDL reduction achieved with statins has not shown benefit in outcome trials.[161,162]

The large beneficial effect of cholesterol lowering, particularly with statins, on rates of cardiovascular events for both primary and secondary prevention and in a wide variety of patients, has continued to inform committees writing guidelines for the treatment of hyperlipidemia.[138,139,166]

Although decreasing LDL-C reduces CHD risk by 30% to 50% in statin studies, there is still significant residual risk, especially in patients with established vascular disease, many of whom have events despite achieving LDL-C levels of 70 to 80 mg/dL, raising the issue of how to decrease this residual risk. Other questions include: How early in life should therapy be started for primary prevention? Will longer duration of therapy lead to better outcomes? What is the benefit of lowering triglycerides or raising HDL-C? What biomarkers are best to screen and monitor in at-risk patients? Can other mediators of atherosclerosis be manipulated? How can lifestyle changes be accomplished? Ongoing trials address some of these questions.

TREATMENT OF LIPID DISORDERS

Rationale for Treating Hyperlipidemia

Clinical trials have clearly demonstrated the benefit of LDL-C reduction.[154,155] The benefit of treating moderate elevations of triglycerides is less clear.[167] Treatment of severe hypertriglyceridemia is indicated to reduce the risk of pancreatitis. Optimal management of risk factors reduces the risk of atherosclerotic clinical events. However, in the United States, the 5-year incidence of myocardial infarction or cardiac death from a first heart attack remains high, with rates that can exceed 50% depending on age, race, and gender.[134]

Data from the INTERHEART study, a case-control study spanning 52 countries, suggest that optimization of nine easily measured and potentially modifiable risk factors could result in a 90% reduction in the risk of an initial acute myocardial infarction. The effect of these risk factors is consistent in men and women across different geographic regions and ethnic groups. The nine risk factors are cigarette smoking, abnormal blood lipid levels, hypertension, diabetes, abdominal obesity, lack of physical activity, low daily fruit and vegetable consumption, alcohol overconsumption, and a psychosocial index (reflecting depression, interpersonal stress at work or home, financial stress, major life events, and lack of control).[168]

Approach to the Hyperlipidemic Patient

The initial evaluation consists of a history and physical examination, including assessment of CHD risk factors (Table 37-6) and measurement of plasma lipids. Exclusion of secondary causes of lipid disorders (see earlier discussion) is important. Obesity is an independent risk factor for CHD not included as a traditional risk factor, although it is reflected in the waist circumference measurement that is used to define the metabolic syndrome (see Table 37-5). Obesity aggravates dyslipidemia, hypertension, and insulin resistance and is a target of therapy regardless of the severity of traditional CHD risk factors. Particular emphasis should be placed on obtaining a detailed history of all first-degree relatives to identify cholesterol disorders or premature CHD.

Physical Examination

The examination should emphasize the cardiovascular system, manifestations of hyperlipidemia, and disorders causing secondary lipid abnormalities. Several unique clinical findings are illustrated in Figure 37-17.

TABLE 37-6
Traditional Risk Factors for Atherosclerotic Cardiovascular Disease
Age
Sex
Total cholesterol
HDL cholesterol
Systolic blood pressure
Use of antihypertensive therapy
Diabetes mellitus
Current smoking

HDL, high-density lipoprotein.
Data from Goff DC Jr, Lloyd-Jones DM, Bennett G, et al. 2013 ACC/AHA guideline on the assessment of cardiovascular risk: a report of the American College of Cardiology/American Heart Association Task Force on Practice Guidelines. *J Am Coll Cardiol*. 2014;63:2935-2959.

Xanthelasmas (see Fig. 37-17A), a type of xanthoma, are raised, yellowish macules that typically appear around the medial canthus. Involvement can extend to the eyelids or skin immediately below the eye. They occur in patients with FH, familial defective apoB100, or dysbetalipoprotein-emia. They occasionally occur in patients with normal cholesterol levels. Xanthelasmas typically regress with cholesterol lowering and may be treated effectively in the setting of normal cholesterol levels with cholesterol-lowering drugs.

Lipemia retinalis (see Fig. 37-17B), a condition in which lipemic blood causes opalescence of retinal arterioles, can be observed during funduscopic examination. It is typically seen only when the triglyceride levels are 22.6 mmol/L (2000 mg/dL) or higher.

Tendon xanthomas (see Fig. 37-17C and D) are nodular deposits of cholesterol that accumulate in tissue macro-phages in the Achilles and other tendons, including the extensor tendons in the hands, knees, and elbows. Tendon xanthomas are often present in patients with FH or familial defective apoB100 and sometimes in those with dysbetali-poproteinemia. As discussed earlier, the Achilles tendon should be palpated for assessment of thickness and contour.

Tuberous or tuboeruptive xanthomas (see Fig. 37-17E) develop in areas that are susceptible to trauma, such as the elbows and knees. They range from pea-sized to lemon-sized and can be seen in dysbetalipoproteinemia and FH. Palmar xanthomas (see Fig. 37-17F) are found in the palmar and digital creases of the hands. This type of xanthoma is almost pathognomonic for high plasma levels of β-VLDL and dysbetalipoproteinemia. Eruptive xanthomas (see Fig. 37-17G) appear as small, yellowish, round papules that contain a pale center and an erythematous base. Their distribution includes the abdominal wall, back, buttocks, and other pressure contact areas. They are caused by accumulation of triglyceride in dermal histiocytes and typically occur when the plasma triglyceride level is 11.3 to 22.6 mmol/L (1000 to 2000 mg/dL) or higher. They can disappear rapidly with lowering of the plasma triglyceride concentration.

Screening for Secondary Disorders

The history and physical examination should be directed toward uncovering secondary disorders of lipid metabolism and identifying agents including medications that could cause hyperlipidemia. Minimal studies should include fasting blood glucose, glycosylated hemoglobin, renal and hepatic function tests, urinary protein, and thyroid-stimulating hormone.

Measurement of Plasma Lipids

Ideally, plasma lipids should be measured at least twice under fasting steady-state conditions before therapeutic decisions are made. Plasma lipids are usually measured after a 12-hour fast due to postprandial fluctuations of triglycerides. Because cholesterol is a minor component of chylomicrons, total plasma cholesterol can be measured in either a fasting or a nonfasting state. Plasma lipid measurements are usually reliable if done within the first 24 hours after an acute myocardial infarction.[169]

Most clinical laboratories measure plasma levels of total triglycerides, total cholesterol, and HDL-C; the last analysis is performed after apoB-containing lipoproteins are removed from the plasma. The plasma LDL-C concentration is then calculated from these measurements by the Friedewald formula:

$$\text{LDL cholesterol} = \text{total cholesterol} - \text{HDL} - \text{VLDL}$$

where VLDL is calculated as triglycerides divided by 5. This formula assumes that cholesterol content of VLDL is about 20% of the plasma triglyceride level. It is reliable only when triglycerides are 4.5 mmol/L (400 mg/dL) or less. LDL-C concentrations calculated by this formula may be inaccurate in the presence of severe hypertriglyceridemia or when the triglyceride-to-cholesterol ratio of VLDL differs from the usual 4:1 ratio (as occurs in dysbetalipoprotein-emia). Specialized laboratories can directly assay different lipoproteins by ultracentrifugation or nuclear magnetic resonance techniques. Direct measurement of LDL-C is also available in many clinical laboratories.

Non-HDL cholesterol (total cholesterol minus HDL cho-lesterol) is a measure of atherogenic lipoproteins that is useful when triglycerides are elevated and when patients are not fasting.

A triglyceride level higher than 11.3 mmol/L (1000 mg/dL) usually signifies the presence of two or more abnormalities of lipid metabolism (e.g., estrogen therapy in the presence of underlying familial hypertriglyceridemia). Elevated plasma triglyceride levels can fluctuate markedly in a single person over short periods. The fluctuation occurs because the LPL-mediated clearance mechanisms for triglyceride-rich particles become saturated at plasma tri-glyceride concentrations of approximately 5.6 mmol/L (500 mg/dL), and above this level plasma triglyceride con-centrations largely reflect dietary fat intake. Therefore, tri-glyceride levels can rise precipitously as dietary fat intake increases and can fall rapidly with dietary fat restriction.

A complete plasma lipid profile (total cholesterol, LDL-C, HDL-C, and triglycerides) should be measured in all adults 20 years of age and older. It is reasonable to assess tradi-tional atherosclerotic cardiovascular disease (ASCVD) risk factors every 4 to 6 years in adults 20 to 79 years of age who are free from ASCVD. In adults aged 40 to 79 without ASCVD, 10-year ASCVD risk can be estimated every 4 to 6 years. If the patient does not have an indication for LDL-lowering therapy, data support screening every 4 to 6 years between ages 40 and 75.[170] Triglycerides should be measured in all patients with pancreatitis.

Lipid screening in children is controversial.[171,172] The National Lipid Association Expert Panel recommended screening all children between the ages of 9 and 11 and as young as 2 years of age in the presence of known family history of hyperlipidemia or vascular disease.[173] This approach is similar to that of a National Heart, Lung, and Blood Institute Expert Panel, which also included screening all children between ages 9 and 11 and again between ages 17 and 21 with earlier lipid testing in some children because of high-risk conditions or family history of premature coro-nary artery disease.[174]

Patient Selection and Treatment Goals

Prevention of ASCVD is the primary goal of the 2013 Amer-ican College of Cardiology (ACC)/American Heart Associa-tion (AHA) Guidelines. These guidelines address risk assessment,[170] lifestyle modifications,[141] evaluation and treatment of obesity,[175] and evaluation and management of blood cholesterol.[138]

The 2013 ACC/AHA cholesterol guidelines define four groups qualifying for statin therapy: patients with clinical ASCVD, patients with LDL cholesterol 190 mg/dL or higher, patients with diabetes, and patients with a calcu-lated ASCVD risk of 7.5% or more (Table 37-7). For patients without clinical ASCVD or LDL 190 mg/dL or higher, the guidelines advise calculating risk for ASCVD based on age, sex, ethnicity, total and HDL cholesterol, systolic blood pressure (treated or untreated), presence of diabetes mellitus, and current smoking status. A risk calculator with the guidelines applies to U.S. populations.[176] Different risk scoring systems may be appropriate for diverse populations and regions.[139]

Hyperlipidemia treatment in patients with established CHD is considered secondary prevention, whereas treatment in those who do not have known disease is primary

TABLE 37-7
ACC/AHA 2013 Statin Benefit Groups

Benefit Group	Management
Clinical atherosclerotic cardiovascular disease (ASCVD)	Age < 75 without contraindications: high-intensity statin Age > 75 or with contraindications: moderate-intensity statin
LDL-C > 190 mg/dL, age > 21 years	High-intensity statin Can consider nonstatin drug if further LDL-C reduction is desirable
Primary prevention: diabetes: age 40-75 years, LDL-C 70-189 mg/dL	Moderate-intensity statin If 10-year ASCVD risk is ≥7.5%, consider high-intensity statin
Primary prevention: no diabetes*: ≥7.5% 10-year ASCVD risk,[†] age 40-75 years, LDL-C 70-189 mg/dL	Moderate- to high-intensity statin

*Requires risk discussion between clinician and patient before statin initiation.
[†]Statin therapy may be considered if risk decision is uncertain after use of ASCVD risk calculator.
LCL-C, low-density lipoprotein cholesterol.
Data from Stone NJ, Robinson JG, Lichtenstein AH, et al. 2013 ACC/AHA guideline on the treatment of blood cholesterol to reduce atherosclerotic cardiovascular risk in adults: a report of the American College of Cardiology/American Heart Association Task Force on Practice Guidelines. *J Am Coll Cardiol.* 2014;63:2889-2934.

prevention. When lipid-lowering therapy for primary prevention should be initiated is an unresolved question. There are no reliable biomarkers or imaging techniques that predict first events in people with dyslipidemia. Studies of high-risk groups for primary prevention have provided some guidance. The JUPITER trial[153] showed a statistically significant reduction in total mortality ($p < 0.02$) in men aged 50 years and older and women 60 years and older, many of whom would not have fit the NCEP Adult Treatment Panel III guidelines for therapy. Treatment of hypercholesterolemia in persons older than 85 years is of unclear benefit, but CHD accounts for a high percentage of deaths in this age group, and there are survival benefits of treatment in elderly patients up to the age of 85 years who have known CHD. Guidelines for treatment of patients with type 2 diabetes mellitus take into account their increased risk of cardiovascular events. Patients with established vascular disease and diabetes mellitus are considered to be at very high risk.[177]

Severe hypertriglyceridemia (>11.3 mmol/L [1000 mg/dL]) should be treated aggressively because pancreatitis associated with these levels can be fatal.[167]

The 2013 ACC/AHA cholesterol guidelines used clinical trial data to identify individuals for whom there is substantial evidence of the benefit of therapy. The guidelines do not specify treatment thresholds or goals of therapy, but other guidelines have included treatment goals as well as other risk scoring systems and calculators (Table 37-8).[138,139,178,179] The International Atherosclerosis Society recommends optimal levels of non-HDL cholesterol in addition to LDL cholesterol.

Some patients with LDL-C levels below previous treatment thresholds benefit from statin treatment. Therefore,

TABLE 37-8
Comparison of Dyslipidemia Guidelines

Risk Category	Treatment Intensity or Goals		
	ACC/AHA*	IAS[†]	ESC/EAS[‡]
Secondary prevention/ high or very high risk	Clinical ASCVD: Lifestyle + high-intensity statin (LDL-C reduction ≥50%)	ASCVD: Lifestyle + medication (statin + other) Optimal LDL-C < 70 mg/dL (1.8 mmol/L) and non-HDL-C < 100 mg/dL (2.6 mmol/L)	Very high risk (CAD, CKD, DM) or SCORE ≥10% (country specific) and baseline LDL-C level: lifestyle + medication Goal LDL-C < 70 mg/dL (1.8 mmol/L)
Primary prevention	LDL-C ≥ 190 mg/dL (rule out secondary causes): lifestyle + high-intensity statin (add nonstatin if insufficient response) Diabetes mellitus without ASCVD, LDL-C < 190 mg/dL: perform risk calculation Moderate- to high-intensity statin ASCVD risk ≥7.5% Risk discussion with patient Moderate- to high-intensity statin	Lifestyle + medication adjusted for lifetime risk Optimal LDL-C < 100 mg/dL (2.6 mmol/L) or non-HDL-C < 130 mg/dL (3.4 mmol/L)	High risk: SCORE ≥5 to <10% and baseline LDL-C level: lifestyle + or – medication Goal LDL-C < 100 mg/dL (2.5 mmol/L) Moderate risk SCORE level >1 to ≤5% and baseline LDL-C: Lifestyle + or – medication Goal LDL-C < 115 mg/dL (3.0 mmol/L)
Other considerations	Evaluate triglycerides > 500 mg/dL	FH, hypertriglyceridemia	FH, combined hyperlipidemia, CKD, transplantation, PAD, autoimmune disorders, stroke, elderly

*ACC/AHA data from American College of Cardiology/American Heart Association, Stone NJ, Robinson JG, Lichtenstein AH, et al. ACC/AHA guideline on the treatment of blood cholesterol to reduce atherosclerotic cardiovascular risk in adults: a report of the American College of Cardiology/American Heart Association Task Force on Practice Guidelines. *J Am Coll Cardiol.* 2014;63:2889-2934.
[†]IAS data from International Atherosclerosis Society Position Paper: Global recommendations for the management of dyslipidemia—full report. *J Clin Lipidol.* 2014;8:29-60.
[‡]ESC/EAS data from European Society of Cardiology/European Atherosclerosis Society. *Eur Heart J.* 2011;32:1769-1818. Available at www.escardio.org/guidelines.
ACC/AHA, American College of Cardiology/American Heart Association; ASCVD, atherosclerotic cardiovascular disease; ESC/EAS, European Society of Cardiology/European Atherosclerosis Society.
CAD, coronary artery disease; CKD: chronic kidney disease; DM, diabetes mellitus; FH, familial hypercholesterolemia; HDL-C, high-density lipoprotein cholesterol; IAS, International Atherosclerosis Society; LCL-C, low-density lipoprotein cholesterol; PAD, peripheral arterial disease; SCORE, Systematic Coronary Risk Estimation.

treat-to-target approaches may not capture all patients who would benefit from therapy. Data from multiple sources suggest that LDL levels lower than those identified as treatment goals decrease the risk of atherosclerosis.[180,181] Cardiovascular outcome trials using PCSK9 antibodies, which can reduce LDL-C to very low levels, may lead to recommendations for LDL-C levels below current goals.

Specific Therapies

Specific therapies include lifestyle changes (diet, weight management, and exercise recommendations) and drug therapy.[138]

Lifestyle Treatment

Lifestyle changes including dietary intervention, moderate exercise, and weight loss are first-line therapies for hyperlipidemia (Table 37-9) and may be sufficient for mild dyslipidemias in low-risk patients. All other treatments should build on therapeutic lifestyle changes.[139] In patients with established CHD, drug therapy should be instituted with diet therapy. Most patients will have a 10% to 15% decrease in LDL-C levels with diet; this may be adequate in low-risk patients for primary prevention. Hypertriglyceridemia often responds to decreased intake of fat, simple sugars, alcohol, and calories. Response to lipid-lowering drugs may be disappointing in patients who do not follow dietary recommendations.

Dietary changes are best when individualized and instituted gradually. Involvement of family members is important. The DASH (Dietary Approaches to Stop Hypertension) or Mediterranean diets are appropriate. Patients with elevated triglycerides also need to restrict simple sugars and alcohol. Patients with the chylomicronemia syndrome

TABLE 37-9
Lifestyle Recommendations to Reduce Cardiovascular Risk

Modality	Intervention
Diet	Follow a dietary pattern high in vegetables, fruits, whole grains, poultry, fish, low-fat dairy products, legumes, nontropical vegetable oils and nuts Limit red meat, sweets, and sugar-sweetened beverages Limit saturated fat to 5-6% of total calories Limit calories from trans fats
Physical activity	Engage in aerobic physical activity 3 to 4 sessions per week of moderate- to vigorous-intensity physical activity averaging 40 minutes per session
Weight management	For obese patients (BMI ≥ 30) or overweight patients (BMI ≥ 25) who have additional risk factors, sustained weight loss of 3-5% or greater reduces ASCVD risk Consultation with a registered dietitian may be helpful to plan, start, and maintain a diet that promotes weight loss and restricts intake of saturated fats

ASCVD, atherosclerotic cardiovascular disease; BMI, body mass index.
Data from Eckel RH, Jakicic JM, Ard JD, et al. 2013 AHA/ACC guideline on lifestyle management to reduce cardiovascular risk: a report of the American College of Cardiology American/Heart Association Task Force on Practice Guidelines. *J Am Coll Cardiol.* 2014;63:2960-2984; Jensen MD, Ryan DH, Apovian CM, et al. 2013 AHA/ACC/TOS guideline for the management of overweight and obesity in adults: a report of the American College of Cardiology/American Heart Association Task Force on Practice Guidelines and the Obesity Society. *J Am Coll Cardiol.* 2014;63:2985-3023.

may initially require a diet with less than 10% of calories from fat to decrease chylomicron production. The response to very low fat diets may be disappointing in patients with impaired glucose tolerance unless the diet is hypocaloric.

Daily moderate exercise, such as walking, may help reduce triglyceride levels. Exercise may be particularly useful in obese, insulin-resistant patients with high triglyceride levels, low HDL-C, and moderately elevated LDL-C. Weight loss is beneficial, and an exercise program combined with a moderately hypocaloric diet may lead to significant improvements in lipid levels as well as glucose tolerance. Modest weight loss may improve dyslipidemia as well as glucose tolerance and blood pressure in patients with the metabolic syndrome.

The effects of various types of dietary fats have been studied extensively.[182] Current recommendations[141] are to restrict intake of saturated fats and trans fats and to substitute complex carbohydrates, polyunsaturated fats, and monounsaturated fats. Saturated fats elevate plasma cholesterol levels by decreasing receptor-mediated clearance of LDL. High levels of cholesterol intake raise plasma cholesterol by reducing receptor-mediated catabolism of LDL and by increasing LDL synthesis. Trans fats are unsaturated fatty acids with at least one *trans* double bond; they are produced when liquid vegetable oils are partially hydrogenated to produce semisolid fats used in margarines and shortening. Trans fats raise LDL-C and reduce HDL-C and have been implicated in cardiovascular disease.

Fish oils are rich in eicosapentaenoic (EPA) or docosahexaenoic acid (DHA) (see Table 37-1). Daily doses of 4 g of EPA plus DHA lower VLDL and treat hypertriglyceridemia. It is not clear that fish oil supplementation in the current era is effective for primary prevention of CHD.[183] Observational data suggest that fish intake is associated with decreased cardiovascular risk. In those with and without known CHD, many experts recommend eating two servings of oily fish weekly. Taking fish oil capsules that provide 1 g/day of EPA plus DHA daily is reasonable for those not interested in consuming fish.

Other dietary components can influence plasma lipid levels. For example, soluble fibers such as psyllium or oat bran, which can bind bile acids in the gut and promote net cholesterol excretion, decrease LDL-C modestly (about 5% to 10%). Margarines made with sitostanol or sitosterol, plant sterols that inhibit cholesterol absorption, reduce serum cholesterol by about 10%. The combination of plant sterols, soluble fiber, and restriction of saturated fat and cholesterol can reduce LDL-C levels by about 30%.[184]

Team management that includes nutritionists and dietitians is likely to enhance dietary therapies.

Drug Treatment

Table 37-10 lists drugs that interfere with bile acid absorption from the gut (BAS), inhibit cholesterol synthesis in cells (HMG-CoA reductase inhibitors), or block cholesterol absorption from the gut (ezetimibe). These agents work mainly by inducing LDL-receptor expression in hepatocytes. Niacin, fibrates, and ω-3 fatty acids either inhibit VLDL production or enhance clearance of triglyceride-rich particles. Drugs that decrease production of VLDL cholesterol by the liver include the apolipoprotein B antisense oligonucleotide, mipomersen, and the MTP inhibitor, lomitapide.

The best drugs for lowering LDL-C are the HMG-CoA reductase inhibitors lovastatin, pravastatin, simvastatin, fluvastatin, atorvastatin, pitavastatin, and rosuvastatin; the BAS resins cholestyramine, colestipol, and colesevelam; the cholesterol absorption inhibitor ezetimibe; and nicotinic

TABLE 37-10
Drugs Used to Treat Hyperlipidemia

Class and Drugs Available	Dosage	Major Lipoprotein Decreased	Mechanism
Bile Acid Sequestrants			
Cholestyramine	4-12 g bid	LDL	Increase sterol excretion and LDL clearance
Colestipol	5-15 g bid		
Colesevelam	3.75-4.375 g qd		
Nicotinic Acid			
Niacin (crystalline)	1-3 g qd	VLDL (LDL)	Decrease VLDL production
Niaspan (extended-release niacin)	500-2000 mg qd		
Fibric Acid Derivatives			
Gemfibrozil	600 mg bid	VLDL (LDL)	Decrease VLDL production; enhance LPL action
Fenofibrate*	30-200 mg qd		
HMG-CoA Reductase Inhibitors			
Lovastatin	10-80 mg qd	LDL	Decrease cholesterol synthesis; increase LDL receptor–mediated removal of LDL
Pravastatin	10-40 mg qd		
Simvastatin	5-80 mg qd[†]		
Fluvastatin	20-80 mg qd		
Atorvastatin	10-80 mg qd		
Rosuvastatin	5-40 mg qd		
Pitavastatin	1-4 mg qd		
Intestinal Cholesterol Absorption Inhibitor			
Ezetimibe	10 mg qd	LDL	Inhibits cholesterol absorption
Omega-3 Fatty Acids			
Lovaza (1-g capsule contains EPA and DHA)	4 g qd	VLDL	Inhibits VLDL production
Vascepa (1-g capsule contains EPA)	4 g qd		
Epanova (1-g capsule contains EPA and DHA free fatty acids)	2-4 gd		
Apo B Antisense Oligonucleotide			
Mipomersen	200 mg once a week subcutaneous injection	VLDL, LDL, Lp(a)	Inhibits synthesis of apolipoprotein B
Microsomal Triglyceride Transfer Protein Inhibitor			
Lomitapide	5 mg to 60 mg qd	VLDL, LDL, Lp(a)	Inhibits microsomal triglyceride transfer protein

*There are several different preparations of fenofibrate with different doses.
[†]Simvastatin 80 mg is not recommended.
bid, twice a day; EPA, highly concentrated ethyl esters of eicosapentaenoic acid; DHA, docosahexaenoic acid; HMG-CoA, 3-hydroxy-3-methylglutaryl coenzyme A; LDL, low-density lipoproteins; Lp(a), lipoprotein(a); LPL, lipoprotein lipase; qd, every day; VLDL, very low density lipoprotein.

acid (also called niacin). Mipomersen and lomitapide are used in patients with the severely elevated LDL levels seen in homozygous FH. Nicotinic acid, gemfibrozil, and fenofibrate are useful for hypertriglyceridemia. For elevated LDL-C combined with mild to moderate (<500 mg/dL) elevations of triglycerides, the statins, nicotinic acid, fenofibrate, or gemfibrozil may provide acceptable results. Omega-3 fatty acids can also lower triglycerides. In cases of severe hypercholesterolemia (e.g., FH) or when the goal is to attain very low levels of LDL-C, combinations of agents may be required.

HMG-CoA Reductase Inhibitors (Statins). Introduced in 1987, HMG-CoA reductase inhibitors have been extensively studied for both primary and secondary prevention of cardiovascular events. Meta-analyses suggest a 20% decrease in the relative risk of major cardiovascular event rates for every millimole (about 40 mg/dL) decrease in LDL cholesterol.[154,155] The 2013 ACC/AHA guidelines categorize statins as high, moderate, and low intensity based on usual LDL-C reductions (Table 37-11).

Statin inhibition of cholesterol biosynthesis upregulates LDL receptors, enhances LDL clearance, reduces lipoprotein release from the liver, and may decrease triglycerides

TABLE 37-11
High-, Moderate-, and Low-Intensity Statin Therapy

High-Intensity Statin Therapy	Moderate-Intensity Statin Therapy	Low-Intensity Statin Therapy
Daily dose lowers LDL-C on average by approximately ≥50%:*	Daily dose lowers LDL-C on average, by approximately 30% to <50%:*	Daily dose lowers LDL-C, on average, by <30%:*
Atorvastatin 40-80 mg	Atorvastatin 10-20 mg	Simvastatin 10 mg
Rosuvastatin 20-40 mg	Rosuvastatin 5-10 mg	Pravastatin 10-20 mg
	Simvastatin 20-40 mg	Lovastatin 20 mg
	Pravastatin 40-80 mg	Fluvastatin 20-40 mg
	Lovastatin 40 mg	Pitavastatin 1 mg
	Fluvastatin 40 mg bid	
	Pitavastatin 2-4 mg	

*Note that individual responses vary.
bid, twice a day; LDL-C, low-density lipoprotein cholesterol.
Data from Robinson JG, Lichtenstein AH, et al. ACC/AHA guideline on the treatment of blood cholesterol to reduce atherosclerotic cardiovascular risk in adults: a report of the American College of Cardiology/American Heart Association Task Force on Practice Guidelines. *J Am Coll Cardiol.* 2014;63:2889-2934.

by enhancing VLDL clearance and decreasing lipoprotein production.

Statins are useful in all types of hyperlipidemias in which LDL-C is elevated, but they are less effective in homozygous LDL-receptor deficiency. They are particularly useful for patients with vascular disease and those with very high levels of LDL-C (e.g., FH, combined hyperlipidemia), and they are the drugs of choice for lowering LDL-C as secondary prevention. Several statins are approved for use in children and adolescents with FH and in others with high LDL-C levels or a significant family history of premature coronary artery disease.

Table 37-12 lists expected effects of various statins on LDL-C. They reduce LDL-C by 20% to 60%, increase HDL-C by 2% to 16%, and reduce triglycerides by 7% to 37%, depending on the drug, the dosage, and, in the case of triglycerides, baseline levels. Effects also vary among patients, with greater or lesser degrees of LDL-C reduction even at the same dose. For each statin, doubling of the dose typically produces an additional 6% reduction of LDL-C.[185] LDL-C lowering is seen within 1 to 2 weeks after the start of therapy and is stable in about 4 to 6 weeks. Pitavastatin, atorvastatin, and rosuvastatin have long half-lives, about 12 hours, 14 hours, and 21 hours, respectively. The other statins have half-lives of about 2 to 3 hours. Fluvastatin and lovastatin are available in extended-release preparations. Atorvastatin and fluvastatin have minimal renal clearance and may be more suitable for patients with significant renal insufficiency.

Lovastatin is best given with food, usually with the evening meal, but other statins can be given with or without food at any time of the day. Several statins are available as generic drugs in the United States. Table 37-13 shows specific features of available statins.

Most common side effects are abdominal pain, constipation, flatulence, nausea, headache, fatigue, diarrhea, and muscle complaints. Except for musculoskeletal symptoms, most side effects are infrequent and occur in only about 5% of patients. Adverse effects tend to correlate with drug dose.

Liver toxicity is not common with statin use. Hepatic aminotransferase elevation is usually mild and does not require discontinuation of the statin. It may be dose dependent, as demonstrated in clinical trials that showed rates of persistent elevations of liver aminotransferase greater than three times the upper limit of normal occurring in 0.1% to 1.9% of patients, depending on the statin and the dose.

Only about 1% of patients have aminotransferase increases to greater than three times the upper limit of normal, and the elevation often decreases even if patients continue on the statin.[186] A common cause is hepatic steatosis, which responds to weight loss. Statins can be used cautiously in the presence of liver disease that is not decompensated. Nonalcoholic hepatic steatosis is not a contraindication.[187] Hepatic transaminases should be obtained at baseline and during treatment if there is a clinical indication for their measurement.[138] The requirement for routine monitoring of hepatic transaminases was removed from statin labeling by the U.S. Food and Drug Administration (FDA) in 2012. If aminotransferases remain greater than three times the upper limit of normal,

TABLE 37-12
Typical LDL-C Reductions (% Change from Baseline) by Statin Dose

Treatment	5 mg	10 mg	20 mg	40 mg	80 mg
Rosuvastatin	−40	−46	−52	−55	—
Atorvastatin	—	−37	−43	−48	−51
Simvastatin	−26	−30	−38	−41	−47
Lovastatin	—	−21	−27	−31	−40
Pravastatin	—	−20	−24	−30	−36
Fluvastatin	—	—	−22	−25	−35
Pitavastatin	—	—	(1 mg) −32	(2 mg) −36	(4 mg) −43
Ezetimibe 10 mg plus variable simvastatin	—	−45	−52	−55	−60

LDL-C, low-density lipoprotein cholesterol; —, data not available.
Data from Hou R, Goldberg AC. Lowering low-density lipoprotein cholesterol: statins, ezetimibe, bile acid sequestrants, and combinations—comparative efficacy and safety. *Endocrinol Metab Clin North Am.* 2009;38:79-97; Livalo package insert. Available from http://www.kowapharma.com/documents/LIVALO_PI _CURRENT.pdf.

TABLE 37-13
Features of Individual Statins

Drug	Pharmacologic Considerations	Safety Issues
Fluvastatin	Synthetic drug; minimal renal excretion	Can interact with warfarin, phenytoin, glyburide, diclofenac, fluconazole, ketoconazole
Pravastatin	Derived from fermentation product of *Aspergillus terreus;* dose reduction in renal insufficiency	Drug interaction with cyclosporine
Lovastatin	First statin marketed in United States; isolated from a strain of *A. terreus;* food intake increases absorption	Interactions with CYP3A4 substrates
Simvastatin	Synthetic derivative of fermentation product of *A. terreus;* dose reduction in severe renal insufficiency	Interactions with CYP3A4 substrates
Atorvastatin	Synthetic drug; <2% excreted in urine; half-life 14 hours	Interacts with CYP3A4 substrates; increases digoxin levels
Rosuvastatin	Synthetic compound; active metabolite is formed by CYP2C9	Can increase INR when used with warfarin—monitor INR; dose reduction in renal insufficiency, Asian patients, and elderly patients
Pitavastatin	Dose reduction in severe renal failure	Drug interaction with cyclosporine, erythromycin, rifampin

CYP2C9 and CYP3A4, cytochrome P450 isoenzymes 2C9 and 3A4; INR, international normalized ratio.
Data from Hou R, Goldberg AC. Lowering low-density lipoprotein cholesterol: statins, ezetimibe, bile acid sequestrants, and combinations—comparative efficacy and safety. *Endocrinol Metab Clin North Am.* 2009;38:79-97; Livalo package insert. Available from http://www.kowapharma.com/documents/LIVALO_PI _CURRENT.pdf.

consider changing to a different statin and identify other contributing conditions or drugs. Irreversible liver damage resulting from statins is extremely rare, with a liver failure rate of 1 case per 1 million person-years of use.[187]

Muscle-related complaints occur in about 10% of people taking statins. Several large randomized, placebo-controlled clinical trials have not shown differences in rates of myalgias and creatine kinase elevations between statin-treated and placebo groups, but muscle complaints are a common reason for statin discontinuation by patients.[188] Other disorders must be excluded, such as hypothyroidism, vitamin D deficiency, rheumatologic conditions, and perhaps depression. Inhibition of statin catabolism is associated with increased myopathy risk. Drugs metabolized through the cytochrome P450 (CYP) system, such as ketoconazole, itraconazole, clarithromycin, and erythromycin, increase statin plasma levels. Other drugs that increase the risk of statin myopathy include gemfibrozil, cyclosporine, digoxin, verapamil, diltiazem, amiodarone, colchicine, and protease inhibitors. The most serious potential side effect is rhabdomyolysis leading to myoglobinuria and renal failure. Rhabdomyolysis is rare and is more likely in patients with renal insufficiency, advanced age, other comorbid conditions, or polypharmacy and during perioperative periods. Routine surveillance of creatine kinase levels is not useful in most patients. Management of dyslipidemia in patients with muscle-related complaints is challenging and may include using a different statin, decreasing the dosing frequency, or resorting to other LDL-lowering drugs.[138]

Statins modestly increase the incidence of diabetes.[189] The risk is estimated to range from 0.1 (with moderate-intensity statin) to 0.3 (with high-intensity statin) excess case per 100 people treated for 1 year. The benefit of treatment for cardiovascular risk reduction outweighs the excess risk of diabetes in all but those at lowest ASCVD risk. Attention to diet, exercise, and weight can mitigate the diabetes risk.

Statin-treated patients with complaints about confusion or memory loss should be appropriately evaluated for causes of these symptoms.[138]

There is no evidence that statins cause direct adverse effects on renal function beyond that due to rhabdomyolysis. Statins are contraindicated during pregnancy and nursing and in patients with significant hepatic dysfunction.

Bile Acid Sequestrants. The BAS have been used since the 1970s. Cholestyramine, colestipol, and colesevelam are available in the United States. BAS have been shown to reduce cardiovascular events in clinical trials.[142,190]

They work by binding negatively charged bile acids and bile salts in the small intestine to interrupt the enterohepatic circulation of bile acids and increase the conversion of cholesterol into bile. Decreased hepatocyte cholesterol content increases LDL receptors. Cholesterol synthesis also increases, which promotes VLDL secretion. This limits the LDL-lowering effect and raises triglyceride levels.

BAS reduce LDL-C and total cholesterol; HDL-C may increase modestly. As monotherapy, BAS lower LDL-C by 5% to 30% in a dose-dependent manner. Colesevelam has greater bile acid–binding capacity and affinity than cholestyramine or colestipol and is used at lower doses. LDL-C reduction is typically 15% at 3.8 g/day (six 625-mg tablets) and 18% at 4.3 g/day (seven 625-mg tablets).[191,192]

BAS are most useful in patients with elevated LDL-C levels as their major lipid abnormality. They can be combined with statins or niacin to achieve greater LDL-C reduction in patients with severe LDL-C elevations, or they can be used alone for initial therapy in low-risk patients and in patients who cannot tolerate statins. BAS lower fasting blood glucose and hemoglobin A_{1c} levels in patients with diabetes.[193] Effects are seen with the addition of colesevelam to sulfonylurea, metformin, or insulin.

The BAS are neither absorbed nor metabolized and therefore have essentially no systemic exposure. They are extremely safe and can be used in women not using contraception. Gastrointestinal disturbances are common and include constipation, nausea, bloating, abdominal pain, flatulence, and aggravation of hemorrhoids. Initiation with low doses, patient education, and use of stool softeners or psyllium can increase compliance. Cholestyramine and colestipol can affect the absorption of a wide variety of drugs. When used with these agents, other drugs should be taken either 1 to 2 hours before or 4 to 6 hours after the BAS. Colesevelam is better tolerated and does not bind most drugs, with the exceptions of verapamil and thyroxine.[193,194]

These drugs should not be used in patients with severe constipation or bowel or biliary obstruction, nor those taking complicated medical regimens. They worsen hypertriglyceridemia and therefore should not be used in patients with severe hypertriglyceridemia or dysbetalipoproteinemia. Despite a theoretical concern about absorption of fat-soluble vitamins, vitamin K deficiency and bleeding are rare.

Niacin. Nicotinic acid, or niacin, is a B-complex vitamin that was found to lower plasma cholesterol in humans in 1955. Its mechanism of action is not completely understood, but it decreases triglyceride synthesis, leading to decreased VLDL secretion. How niacin elevates HDL is unclear.

Niacin affects multiple lipoproteins and is the most effective drug currently available to raise HDL-C. At doses of 500 to 2000 mg/day, niacin lowers triglycerides by 10% to 30% and increases HDL-C by 10% to 40%. Doses of 1500 to 2000 mg/day decrease LDL-C by 10% to 20%. Niacin also lowers Lp(a) by up to 25%. It is useful for patients with combined hyperlipidemia and low HDL. It is not the best LDL-lowering agent, but it may be helpful in certain circumstances such as statin intolerance or when cost is a limiting factor (crystalline niacin is inexpensive). As noted earlier, older studies suggested benefits in clinical trials,[143,144,164,165] but in the current era niacin added to statins (e.g., to raise HDL-C) does not decrease rick of cardiovascular events.[161,162]

Cutaneous flushing, most notable with the first doses, is the most common side effect. It occurs 15 to 60 minutes after ingestion, lasts 15 to 30 minutes, and may be related to release of dermal prostaglandin D_2. Ingestion with food and taking aspirin (preferably 325 mg) 30 to 60 minutes in advance of niacin minimizes flushing. Starting low and gradually increasing the dose improves tolerability. Repeated and consistent dosing is associated with tolerance to the flushing syndrome. A severe flush can sometimes be stopped by the ingestion of an 81-mg aspirin tablet dissolved in water.[195] Crystalline niacin should always be given with meals. Prescription extended-release niacin (Niaspan) may be better tolerated than crystalline niacin. It is usually initiated with 500 mg at bedtime for 1 month and then titrated over 8 to 12 weeks to the maximum dose of 2000 mg/day. Niaspan can be given with meals if patients awaken with flushing in the middle of the night. Alcoholic beverages potentiate flushing.

Hepatotoxicity is the most serious side effect. Some over-the-counter sustained-release preparations have been associated with severe liver toxicity, so crystalline (non–timed-release) nonprescription preparations should be used, and patients should not change brands after being titrated to high doses. Extended-release niacin available by prescription was not associated with significant liver toxicity in clinical trials. Nausea, fatigue, and malaise may be signs of hepatotoxicity.

Worsening of glucose tolerance and hyperuricemia may also occur. Niacin can be used safely in patients with glucose intolerance or diabetes mellitus, especially in those treated with glucose-lowering agents. Initiation of niacin may increase glucose, but glycemic control usually returns to pretreatment levels.[196] Niacin should be used with caution in patients who have a history of gout. It is contraindicated in those with active peptic ulcer disease. Rare side effects include blurred vision and a reversible condition known as *cystoid macular edema*. Myopathy is rare with niacin alone or in combination with statins. Niacin is contraindicated during pregnancy.

It is useful to check transaminases, glucose, and uric acid at baseline and during dose titration. Patients taking niacin should be monitored at 4- to 6-month intervals for signs of hepatic toxicity. Niacin can be discontinued temporarily if transaminases rise significantly. Retitration is possible once enzyme levels return to normal.

Fibrates. In the Helsinki Heart Study (primary prevention) and the VA-HIT (secondary prevention), the use of the fibrate gemfibrozil reduced fatal and nonfatal CHD events and did not increase mortality from noncardiac causes.[156,157] In the Fenofibrate Intervention and Event Lowering in Diabetes (FIELD) study, fenofibrate probably decreased cardiac events but not cardiovascular or total mortality rates in patients with type 2 diabetes.[158]

These drugs activate PPARα (see earlier discussion), which increases fatty acid oxidation, increases LPL, decreases apoCIII, and increases apoAI as well as apoAII, lowering triglycerides (by 30% to 50%) and raising HDL (by 10% to 20% in those with elevated triglycerides). Fibrates may lower LDL-C modestly, but they are most commonly used for severe hypertriglyceridemia and combined hyperlipidemia. Fenofibrate may be taken once daily. Gemfibrozil is given twice a day with meals.

Side effects may include gastrointestinal discomfort, rash, and pruritus. The risk of gallstones may be increased. Liver transaminases may increase, particularly with fenofibrate. Fenofibrate should be avoided in patients with renal insufficiency, which predisposes to myopathy. The combination of gemfibrozil and most statins is associated with an increased risk of myopathy due to increased statin blood levels. Fenofibrate does not interfere with statin metabolism and is preferred in fibrate/statin combination regimens.[197] Because of the effects on protein binding, warfarin doses may need to be adjusted when fibrate therapy is started. Fibrates are contraindicated in patients with liver or gallbladder disease. Gemfibrozil may be used beginning in the second trimester in pregnant women with severely elevated triglycerides who are at risk for pancreatitis.

Fenofibrate decreased the progression of retinopathy in patients with diabetes in substudies of the FIELD and ACCORD trials.[198,199]

Ezetimibe. Ezetimibe inhibits cholesterol absorption (see earlier discussion). It is mostly used in combination with statins to further lower LDL-C. Its use with simvastatin provided greater benefits than simvastatin alone in patients with acute coronary syndromes in the IMPROVE-IT study presented in late 2014.[200]

The drug interacts with the NPC1L1 transporter[21] to decrease intestinal cholesterol absorption, leading to decreased hepatic cholesterol and increased LDL receptors, clearance of LDL-C from the plasma, and consequent reduction of plasma LDL-C. Naturally occurring mutations of NPC1L1 lower LDL-C and reduce the risk of coronary disease.[201]

Ezetimibe alone lowers LDL-C by 14% to 25%. It lowers LDL-C by an additional 15% to 20% when combined with any statin at any dose. Ezetimibe can be useful in patients who are intolerant of statins. Absorption is not affected by food.

Side effects include diarrhea and possibly myalgias. Myopathy is rare and is not clearly related to the medication. Ezetimibe can increase cyclosporine levels. Fibrates can increase the levels of ezetimibe, a finding with unknown clinical significance. Ezetimibe monotherapy does not significantly increase hepatic aminotransferases, but elevations may occur when ezetimibe is combined with a statin. This effect has not been related to any clinical significance.

Ezetimibe is contraindicated in pregnancy and in severe liver dysfunction.

Omega-3 Fatty Acids. Fish-derived ω-3 fatty acids (EPA and DHA) improve plasma lipids and may decrease the risk of sudden death through antiarrhythmic effects.[202] The Japan EPA Lipid Intervention Study (JELIS) showed that combined treatment with a statin plus EPA (1.8 g/day) in patients with CHD reduced major coronary events by 19% compared with a statin alone.[203] As noted earlier, a primary prevention study in Italy did not demonstrate benefit.[182]

Omega-3 fatty acids decrease triglyceride secretion from the liver, through unclear mechanisms. EPA and DHA lower triglycerides by 20% to 50% depending on the baseline levels. There is minimal effect on HDL-C. LDL-C may increase as VLDL is converted to LDL. Approximately 3 to 4 g/day of EPA plus DHA is required to lower triglycerides.

Over-the-counter preparations have variable quantities of EPA and DHA. Prescription formulations of ω-3 fatty acid are available and have been indicated for triglyceride levels higher than 500 mg/dL. One preparation contains EPA and DHA: four tablets contain about 3.6 g of ω-3 acid ethyl esters and can lower triglyceride levels by 30% to 40%. Other preparations contain only EPA or contain unesterified EPA and DHA. Unlike fibrates, EPA and DHA do not affect statin metabolism, and they do not increase the risk of myopathy. Side effects with ω-3 fatty acids include eructation, diarrhea, and abdominal discomfort. There is potential for increased bleeding, but this has not been seen in clinical trials.

Combination Therapies

Combination therapy is indicated for patients with severe lipid elevations and those who have an insufficient response to monotherapy.[138] Patients with FH or familial combined hyperlipidemia are at particularly increased risk and may require LDL-C reductions that cannot be achieved with a single agent. LDL-C levels lower than 70 mg/dL can be difficult to achieve with a single drug. Higher statin doses may be associated with increased side effects. If the highest tolerated statin dose does not produce adequate LDL-C reduction, adding an agent from a different class may produce the desired result. Statins, ezetimibe, and BAS work through different mechanisms and can be more effective in combination than when used alone. Data on clinical outcomes with combination therapy are limited.

Combination Therapy for Reduction of Low-Density Lipoprotein Cholesterol

Statin Plus Bile Acid Sequestrants. All three BAS have been studied in combination with statins. The decreases in LDL-C range from 24% to 60%. For example, colesevelam 3.8 g/day plus atorvastatin 10 mg/day and atorvastatin

80 mg alone each lower LDL-C by about 50%, a result that is relevant for those who cannot tolerate higher statin doses. Drugs from both classes decrease CHD event rates. Cholestyramine and colestipol can interfere with the absorption of statins. Colesevelam does not affect statin absorption. The statin-colesevelam combination may not be ideal for patients with high triglycerides but may be useful in type 2 diabetes mellitus because colesevelam reduces glycemia.

Statin Plus Ezetimibe. Ezetimibe added to a statin may further reduce LDL-C, by 20% or more, and reduce triglycerides by 7% to 13%. Ezetimibe added to a low-dose statin given two to three times per week can improve tolerance. Combination pills containing simvastatin and ezetimibe as well as atorvastatin and ezetimibe are available. The most common side effects reflect those of the individual drugs. The combination of ezetimibe and simvastatin has been shown to decrease cardiovascular events in patients with renal disease[128] and in those with acute coronary syndrome.[204]

Adding ezetimibe to a statin is the preferred approach for treatment of FH.[105]

Statin Plus Niacin. Adding niacin to a statin can lower LDL-C by 10% to 20% in addition to beneficial effects on triglycerides. When used in combination with a statin, the maximum dose of niacin should be 2000 mg/day. Fixed-dose combinations of extended-release niacin with lovastatin (Advicor) and simvastatin (Simcor) are available.

Side effects of the combination of niacin with a statin are the same as those with niacin alone. Flushing is the most common reason for drug discontinuation.

Bile Acid Sequestrants Plus Niacin. Before the availability of statins, BAS plus niacin were used to lower LDL-C in high-risk patients. The availability of colesevelam and extended-release niacin has made this combination tolerable and useful for many patients who are unable to use statins.

Ezetimibe Plus Bile Acid Sequestrants. Ezetimibe inhibits cholesterol absorption, and BAS resins enhance cholesterol excretion through conversion to bile acids, so the combination can have additive effects. It is useful for those patients who cannot take statins.

Three-Drug Combinations. Three medications can be useful in high-risk patients who have very high levels of LDL-C, such as patients with FH who have baseline LDL-C levels greater than 250 mg/dL. Combinations of a statin plus niacin plus BAS or ezetimibe have been used.[205]

Four-Drug Combinations. Four drugs may be necessary in patients with FH. Various combinations of a statin, BAS, niacin, and ezetimibe have been used in practice, but clinical studies are lacking.

Combination Therapy for Other Hyperlipidemias

Statin Plus Fibrate. The combination of a statin plus a fibrate can be used in patients requiring treatment for elevated triglycerides and elevated LDL-C, which may be useful for patients with metabolic syndrome, diabetes, or other forms of mixed dyslipidemia.

Risk of myopathy, including rhabdomyolysis, is increased with the combination of most statins with gemfibrozil, because the latter drug interferes with the glucuronidation of statins, leading to higher serum levels of the statin drug.[206] Rhabdomyolysis is about 15 times less likely with fenofibrate combined with statins (0.58 per 1 million prescriptions) than with gemfibrozil plus statins (8.6 per 1 million prescriptions).[197]

Statin-fibrate combinations should be avoided in patients with renal insufficiency, congestive heart failure, severe debility, or other conditions that affect medication clearance. Side effects include mild gastrointestinal discomfort, rash, and pruritus. Mild aminotransferase eleva-tions occur in 5% of the patients and return to normal after drug discontinuation.

Other Combinations. Triple-drug therapy with a statin, ezetimibe, and fenofibrate may help to obtain adequate reductions of both triglyceride levels and LDL-C without using very high statin doses. When triglyceride levels are decreased with a fibrate, LDL-C may increase. If statins are not tolerated and triglycerides well controlled, BAS could be added. Ezetimibe may lower LDL-C in combination with a fibrate when triglyceride levels are not optimal. Adding ω-3 fatty acids can be helpful if triglycerides are not well controlled. For markedly elevated triglyceride levels, it may be necessary to combine a fibrate with niacin or with ω-3 fatty acids, or both.

Surgical Treatment and Other Modalities

Partial ileal bypass surgery has been used to reduce lipid levels in patients with severe hypercholesterolemia who cannot tolerate lipid-lowering drugs. This surgical therapy reduces total cholesterol by 20% to 25% and causes regression of atherosclerotic lesions.[207] Liver transplantation and portacaval shunting have been used as experimental therapies for homozygous FH. LDL apheresis can be used to lower atherogenic lipids in patients who cannot achieve lipid lowering despite combination therapy; it is the primary treatment modality for those with no LDL receptor function.

Specific Disorders and Therapy

Treatment for Chylomicronemia Syndrome. Patients with chylomicronemia syndrome usually present with acute pancreatitis and severe hypertriglyceridemia. They should be treated with total fat restriction until the triglycerides fall to less than 11.3 mmol/L (1000 mg/dL), after which a fat-restricted diet (e.g., <10% of calories) can be instituted. The goal is to maintain triglycerides lower than 11.3 mmol/L (1000 mg/dL) and preferably lower than 4.5 mmol/L (400 mg/dL). Diet and modification of glycemia, alcohol consumption, or offending medications are useful. Medium-chain triglyceride oils can be provided for cooking. A fibrate or niacin is usually required to control triglycerides. Therapy with orlistat to block fat absorption may be beneficial, because it mimics a low-fat diet.[208] In the setting of pancreatitis risk, a low-fat/low-carbohydrate liquid formula diet may be indicated.

A gene therapy treatment for LPL deficiency is available in Europe. Alipogene tiparvovec or AAV1-LPL^{S447X} is a viral vector containing the LPL gene that is administered via multiple intramuscular injections. It has shown promise in decreasing pancreatitis episodes due to severe hypertriglyceridemia.[209]

Treatment for Familial Hypercholesterolemia. Guidelines for FH patients are available.[105,173] Treatment is multifactorial. Risk factors, such as smoking, should be addressed. Treatment of heterozygous FH includes a diet low in total and saturated fats and cholesterol, but effects on cholesterol are modest (5% to 15%). Adequate cholesterol lowering can occasionally be achieved with a single potent statin. However, combinations of two or three drugs are often needed. The usual approach includes a potent statin plus either a BAS or ezetimibe or both. The addition of niacin is also helpful. Ileal bypass surgery is an option, but it is used rarely. LDL apheresis is appropriate for those who cannot tolerate lipid-lowering drugs.

The age at which drug treatment should begin in heterozygous FH is controversial, but starting treatment at younger ages may have a favorable impact during early stages of lesion development. Statins are approved for the treatment of children with heterozygous FH who are 8 years of age (pravastatin) or 10 years of age (other agents) or older. Factors such as the age at onset of coronary disease in parents and grandparents and the presence of other risk factors should be considered.

High doses of atorvastatin or rosuvastatin combined with ezetimibe have been useful in homozygotes but do not provide sufficient lowering of LDL-C. The therapy of choice is LDL apheresis, which is performed every 1 to 3 weeks. Liver transplantation, which provides functional LDL receptors, has also been used.

Two new therapies are available for treatment of homozygous FH. Mipomersen is an apoB antisense oligonucleotide approved in the United States for the treatment of homozygous FH. It prevents apoB translation, which decreases apoB levels and LDL-C.[210] It lowers LDL-C patients with homozygous and heterozygous FH.[211,212] Pyrexia, body aches, and reactions at the injection site are the most common side effects. Liver fat may increase. Lomitapide is an inhibitor of MTP approved in the United States and European Union for the treatment of homozygous FH. MTP (see earlier discussion) is required for VLDL assembly. It may decrease LDL-C by 50% in homozygous FH.[213] Side effects include diarrhea, elevated hepatic transaminases, and increased hepatic fat. In a long-term study in homozygous FH, lomitapide decreased LDL-C by 50% during the initial phase of the study and 31% at 78 weeks of treatment. Hepatic fat initially increased but then stabilized.[214]

Treatment of familial defective apoB100 is similar to that of heterozygous FH and consists of a low-fat, low-cholesterol diet and a combination drug regimen. Family members at risk should also be screened for the dominant mutation.

Treatment for Familial Combined Hyperlipidemia. Weight reduction and dietary treatment can help correct metabolic abnormalities, such as obesity and insulin resistance, that contribute to the hyperlipidemia. Drug therapy should be directed at the predominant lipid abnormality. Statins are most appropriate for most patients. Fibrates can lower triglycerides and raise HDL-C levels, and they reduce the incidence of coronary events in insulin-resistant hypertriglyceridemic patients with low HDL-C levels. Patients with low HDL-C should be treated with statins. Because familial combined hyperlipidemia is associated with premature CHD, affected family members should be identified.

Treatment for Metabolic Syndrome. All patients with a diagnosis of the metabolic syndrome should be informed of their increased risk of developing cardiovascular disease and type 2 diabetes mellitus. Weight loss and increased physical activity are the best therapy and may be the only therapy that many of these patients require. All patients should be assessed according to existing guidelines for treatment of high triglyceride levels, low HDL, hypertension, and hyperglycemia. Aspirin therapy may be indicated because of the prothrombotic state.[215]

Treatment for Dysbetalipoproteinemia. Because dysbetalipoproteinemia is influenced by coexisting metabolic conditions, a vigorous effort should be made to identify and treat obesity, diabetes mellitus, and hypothyroidism and to reduce alcohol consumption. Lipid abnormalities can often be resolved without the use of drug therapies. Dysbetalipoproteinemia is associated with hypothyroidism in particular and responds dramatically to thyroid hormone replacement therapy. Diet therapy should be aimed at restricting total fat, saturated fat, cholesterol, and, if appropriate, calories. If diet and treatment of coexisting metabolic conditions are unsatisfactory, drug therapy should

be initiated using niacin, fibric acid derivatives, or statins, all of which are effective for this disorder. Combination therapy may be required. Because the disorder is associated with premature vascular disease, first-degree relatives should be screened for the presence of apoE2 (see earlier discussion).

Treatment for Elevated Plasma Lipoprotein(a). There are no outcome trials of lowering Lp(a). Niacin appears to lower plasma Lp(a) levels, but LDL-C in patients with elevated Lp(a) should be treated appropriately and risk factors for CHD addressed. Apheresis lowers Lp(a) and has been used in those with elevated Lp(a) and progressive CHD.[216] Mipomersen, lomitapide, and antibodies to PCSK9 each lower Lp(a) in addition to lowering LDL-C.

Treatment for Low Levels of High-Density Lipoproteins. Patients with familial hypoalphalipoproteinemia can have normal or modestly increased plasma cholesterol but very low HDL-C, resulting in a predisposition to CHD. Such patients can have high ratios of total cholesterol to HDL-C (e.g., >10) despite having a normal plasma cholesterol level. Of the available drugs, niacin results in the largest increase in HDL-C. Fibrates do not increase HDL-C in patients with normal triglycerides. Statins lower total cholesterol and represent the most efficacious way to lower the ratio of total cholesterol to HDL-C. Statins decrease clinical events in patients with low HDL-C.[151] As noted earlier, pharmacologic therapies for raising HDL levels, notably niacin and inhibition of CETP, have not yet shown efficacy in cardiovascular outcome trials. It is possible that such therapies could be guided with a biomarker such as HDL cholesterol efflux capacity.[39]

Drugs in Development

Loss-of-function mutations involving PCSK9 decrease risk of cardiovascular disease.[67] Monoclonal antibodies to PCSK9 produce up to 70% reductions of LDL-C in statin-treated patients, and they appear to be well tolerated.[217] Two PCSK9 inhibitors, evolocumab and alirocumab, are under review by the FDA, and several others are in development.

Inhibition of CETP (see earlier discussion) continues to be tested in clinical trials. Effective agents may decrease LDL-C in addition to elevating HDL-C. Infusion of ApoA1 to improve HDL, antisense inhibition of apoC3 to lower triglycerides, and inhibition of diacylglycerol acyl transferase (DGAT) are being pursued.[218]

REFERENCES

1. Baigent C, Keech A, Kearney PM, et al. Efficacy and safety of cholesterol-lowering treatment: prospective meta-analysis of data from 90,056 participants in 14 randomised trials of statins. *Lancet.* 2005;366: 1267-1278.
2. Taylor F, Huffman MD, Macedo AF, et al. Statins for the primary prevention of cardiovascular disease. *Cochrane Database Syst Rev.* 2013; (1):CD004816.
3. Dadu RT, Ballantyne CM. Lipid lowering with PCSK9 inhibitors. *Nat Rev Cardiol.* 2014;11:563-575.
4. Pinot M, Vanni S, Pagnotta S, et al. Lipid cell biology. Polyunsaturated phospholipids facilitate membrane deformation and fission by endocytic proteins. *Science.* 2014;345:693-697.
5. Cooper MK, Wassif CA, Krakowiak PA, et al. A defective response to Hedgehog signaling in disorders of cholesterol biosynthesis. *Nat Genet.* 2003;33:508-513.
6. Stanhope KL, Schwarz JM, Keim NL, et al. Consuming fructose-sweetened, not glucose-sweetened, beverages increases visceral adiposity and lipids and decreases insulin sensitivity in overweight/obese humans. *J Clin Invest.* 2009;119:1322-1334.
7. Savage DB, Choi CS, Samuel VT, et al. Reversal of diet-induced hepatic steatosis and hepatic insulin resistance by antisense oligonucleotide inhibitors of acetyl-CoA carboxylases 1 and 2. *J Clin Invest.* 2006;116: 817-824.

8. Chakravarthy MV, Zhu Y, Lopez M, et al. Brain fatty acid synthase activates PPARalpha to maintain energy homeostasis. *J Clin Invest.* 2007;117:2539-2552.

9. Wu M, Singh SB, Wang J, et al. Antidiabetic and antisteatotic effects of the selective fatty acid synthase (FAS) inhibitor platensimycin in mouse models of diabetes. *Proc Natl Acad Sci U S A.* 2011;108: 5378-5383.

10. Matsuzaka T, Shimano H, Yahagi N, et al. Crucial role of a long-chain fatty acid elongase, Elovl6, in obesity-induced insulin resistance. *Nat Med.* 2007;13:1193-1202.

11. Ntambi JM, Miyazaki M, Stoehr JP, et al. Loss of stearoyl-CoA desaturase-1 function protects mice against adiposity. *Proc Natl Acad Sci U S A.* 2002;99:11482-11486.

12. Shekhawat PS, Matern D, Strauss AW. Fetal fatty acid oxidation disorders, their effect on maternal health and neonatal outcome: impact of expanded newborn screening on their diagnosis and management. *Pediatr Res.* 2005;57:78R-86R.

13. Brassard P, Frisch F, Lavoie F, et al. Impaired plasma nonesterified fatty acid tolerance is an early defect in the natural history of type 2 diabetes. *J Clin Endocrinol Metab.* 2008;93:837-844.

14. Lauring B, Taggart AK, Tata JR, et al. Niacin lipid efficacy is independent of both the niacin receptor GPR109A and free fatty acid suppression. *Sci Transl Med.* 2012;4(148):148ra115.

15. Zechner R, Zimmermann R, Eichmann TO, et al. FAT SIGNALS—lipases and lipolysis in lipid metabolism and signaling. *Cell Metab.* 2012;15:279-291.

16. Csaki LS, Dwyer JR, Fong LG, et al. Lipins, lipinopathies, and the modulation of cellular lipid storage and signaling. *Prog Lipid Res.* 2013;52:305-316.

17. Chen HC, Farese RV Jr. Inhibition of triglyceride synthesis as a treatment strategy for obesity: lessons from DGAT1-deficient mice. *Arterioscler Thromb Vasc Biol.* 2005;25:482-486.

18. Coleman T, Seip RL, Gimble JM, et al. COOH-terminal disruption of lipoprotein lipase in mice is lethal in homozygotes, but heterozygotes have elevated triglycerides and impaired enzyme activity. *J Biol Chem.* 1995;270:12518-12525.

19. Seip RL, Angelopoulos TJ, Semenkovich CF. Exercise induces human lipoprotein lipase gene expression in skeletal muscle but not adipose tissue. *Am J Physiol.* 1995;268:E229-E236.

20. Young SG, Zechner R. Biochemistry and pathophysiology of intravascular and intracellular lipolysis. *Genes Dev.* 2013;27:459-484.

21. Altmann SW, Davis HR Jr, Zhu LJ, et al. Niemann-Pick C1-like 1 protein is critical for intestinal cholesterol absorption. *Science.* 2004; 303:1201-1204.

22. Berge KE, Tian H, Graf GA, et al. Accumulation of dietary cholesterol in sitosterolemia caused by mutations in adjacent ABC transporters. *Science.* 2000;290:1771-1775.

23. Brown MS, Goldstein JL. Cholesterol feedback: from Schoenheimer's bottle to Scap's MELADL. *J Lipid Res.* 2009;50(Suppl):S15-S27.

24. Nissen SE, Tuzcu EM, Brewer HB, et al. Effect of ACAT inhibition on the progression of coronary atherosclerosis. *N Engl J Med.* 2006;354: 1253-1263.

25. Tietge UJ, Groen AK. Role the TICE? Advancing the concept of transintestinal cholesterol excretion. *Arterioscler Thromb Vasc Biol.* 2013;33: 1452-1453.

26. Shin DJ, Osborne TF. Thyroid hormone regulation and cholesterol metabolism are connected through sterol regulatory element-binding protein-2 (SREBP-2). *J Biol Chem.* 2003;278:34114-34118.

27. Kauffman RF, Bensch WR, Roudebush RE, et al. Hypocholesterolemic activity of raloxifene (LY139481): pharmacological characterization as a selective estrogen receptor modulator. *J Pharmacol Exp Ther.* 1997; 280:146-153.

28. Umetani M, Domoto H, Gormley AK, et al. 27-Hydroxycholesterol is an endogenous SERM that inhibits the cardiovascular effects of estrogen. *Nat Med.* 2007;13:1185-1192.

29. Wu FC, von Eckardstein A. Androgens and coronary artery disease. *Endocr Rev.* 2003;24:183-217.

30. Chakravarthy MV, Lodhi IJ, Yin L, et al. Identification of a physiologically relevant endogenous ligand for PPARalpha in liver. *Cell.* 2009;138: 476-488.

31. Lodhi IJ, Yin L, Jensen-Urstad AP, et al. Inhibiting adipose tissue lipogenesis reprograms thermogenesis and PPARgamma activation to decrease diet-induced obesity. *Cell Metab.* 2012;16:189-201.

32. Lodhi IJ, Semenkovich CF. Peroxisomes: a nexus for lipid metabolism and cellular signaling. *Cell Metab.* 2014;19:380-392.

33. Riserus U, Sprecher D, Johnson T, et al. Activation of peroxisome proliferator-activated receptor (PPAR)delta promotes reversal of multiple metabolic abnormalities, reduces oxidative stress, and increases fatty acid oxidation in moderately obese men. *Diabetes.* 2008;57: 332-339.

34. Shulman AI, Mangelsdorf DJ. Retinoid x receptor heterodimers in the metabolic syndrome. *N Engl J Med.* 2005;353:604-615.

35. Zelcer N, Hong C, Boyadjian R, Tontonoz P. LXR regulates cholesterol uptake through Idol-dependent ubiquitination of the LDL receptor. *Science.* 2009;325:100-104.

36. Sonne DP, Hansen M, Knop FK. Bile acid sequestrants in type 2 diabetes: potential effects on GLP1 secretion. *Eur J Endocrinol.* 2014;171: R47-R65.

37. Xu X, So JS, Park JG, Lee AH. Transcriptional control of hepatic lipid metabolism by SREBP and ChREBP. *Semin Liver Dis.* 2013;33:301-311.

38. Varbo A, Benn M, Smith GD, et al. Remnant cholesterol, low-density lipoprotein cholesterol, and blood pressure as mediators from obesity to ischemic heart disease. *Circ Res.* 2015;116(4):665-673.

39. Rohatgi A, Khera A, Berry JD, et al. HDL cholesterol efflux capacity and incident cardiovascular events. *N Engl J Med.* 2014;371:2383-2393.

40. Kamstrup PR, Tybjaerg-Hansen A, Steffensen R, Nordestgaard BG. Genetically elevated lipoprotein(a) and increased risk of myocardial infarction. *JAMA.* 2009;301:2331-2339.

41. Thanassoulis G, Campbell CY, Owens DS, et al. Genetic associations with valvular calcification and aortic stenosis. *N Engl J Med.* 2013;368: 503-512.

42. Hellerstein M, Turner S. Reverse cholesterol transport fluxes. *Curr Opin Lipidol.* 2014;25(1):40-47.

43. Deeb SS, Takata K, Peng RL, et al. A splice-junction mutation responsible for familial apolipoprotein A-II deficiency. *Am J Hum Genet.* 1990;46:822-827.

44. Gonzales JC, Gordts PL, Foley EM, Esko JD. Apolipoproteins E and AV mediate lipoprotein clearance by hepatic proteoglycans. *J Clin Invest.* 2013;123:2742-2751.

45. Anant S, Davidson NO. Identification and regulation of protein components of the apolipoprotein B mRNA editing enzyme. A complex event. *Trends Cardiovasc Med.* 2002;12:311-317.

46. Shelness GS, Ledford AS. Evolution and mechanism of apolipoprotein B-containing lipoprotein assembly. *Curr Opin Lipidol.* 2005;16: 325-332.

47. Berriot-Varoqueaux N, Aggerbeck LP, Samson-Bouma M, Wetterau JR. The role of the microsomal triglyceride transfer protein in abetalipoproteinemia. *Annu Rev Nutr.* 2000;20:663-697.

48. Innerarity TL, Mahley RW, Weisgraber KH, et al. Familial defective apolipoprotein B-100: a mutation of apolipoprotein B that causes hypercholesterolemia. *J Lipid Res.* 1990;31:1337-1349.

49. Pollin TI, Damcott CM, Shen H, et al. A null mutation in human APOC3 confers a favorable plasma lipid profile and apparent cardioprotection. *Science.* 2008;322:1702-1705.

50. Gaudet D, Brisson D, Tremblay K, et al. Targeting APOC3 in the familial chylomicronemia syndrome. *N Engl J Med.* 2014;371:2200-2206.

51. Bennet AM, Di Angelantonio E, Ye Z, et al. Association of apolipoprotein E genotypes with lipid levels and coronary risk. *JAMA.* 2007;298: 1300-1311.

52. Williams KJ. Molecular processes that handle—and mishandle—dietary lipids. *J Clin Invest.* 2008;118:3247-3259.

53. Kim J, Basak JM, Holtzman DM. The role of apolipoprotein E in Alzheimer's disease. *Neuron.* 2009;63:287-303.

54. Lane-Donovan C, Philips GT, Herz J. More than cholesterol transporters: lipoprotein receptors in CNS function and neurodegeneration. *Neuron.* 2014;83:771-787.

55. Guo YF, Xiong DH, Shen H, et al. Polymorphisms of the low-density lipoprotein receptor-related protein 5 (LRP5) gene are associated with obesity phenotypes in a large family-based association study. *J Med Genet.* 2006;43:798-803.

56. Mani A, Radhakrishnan J, Wang H, et al. LRP6 mutation in a family with early coronary disease and metabolic risk factors. *Science.* 2007; 315:1278-1282.

57. Brown MS, Goldstein JL. A receptor-mediated pathway for cholesterol homeostasis. *Science.* 1986;232:34-47.

58. Rudenko G, Henry L, Henderson K, et al. Structure of the LDL receptor extracellular domain at endosomal pH. *Science.* 2002;298:2353-2358.

59. Leren TP. Sorting an LDL receptor with bound PCSK9 to intracellular degradation. *Atherosclerosis.* 2014;237:76-81.

60. Folick A, Oakley HD, Yu Y, et al. Aging. Lysosomal signaling molecules regulate longevity in *Caenorhabditis elegans. Science.* 2015;347: 83-86.

61. Prabhudas M, Bowdish D, Drickamer K, et al. Standardizing scavenger receptor nomenclature. *J Immunol.* 2014;192:1997-2006.

62. Abumrad NA, Davidson NO. Role of the gut in lipid homeostasis. *Physiol Rev.* 2012;92:1061-1085.

63. Shi H, Kokoeva MV, Inouye K, et al. TLR4 links innate immunity and fatty acid-induced insulin resistance. *J Clin Invest.* 2006;116:3015-3025.

64. Kawakami A, Osaka M, Aikawa M, et al. Toll-like receptor 2 mediates apolipoprotein CIII-induced monocyte activation. *Circ Res.* 2008;103: 1402-1409.

65. Edmondson AC, Brown RJ, Kathiresan S, et al. Loss-of-function variants in endothelial lipase are a cause of elevated HDL cholesterol in humans. *J Clin Invest.* 2009;119:1042-1050.

66. Abifadel M, Varret M, Rabes JP, et al. Mutations in PCSK9 cause autosomal dominant hypercholesterolemia. *Nat Genet.* 2003;34:154-156.

67. Cohen JC, Boerwinkle E, Mosley TH Jr, Hobbs HH. Sequence variations in PCSK9, low LDL, and protection against coronary heart disease. *N Engl J Med.* 2006;354:1264-1272.

68. Kathiresan S. A PCSK9 missense variant associated with a reduced risk of early-onset myocardial infarction. *N Engl J Med.* 2008;358:2299-2300.
69. Packard CJ, O'Reilly DS, Caslake MJ, et al. Lipoprotein-associated phospholipase A2 as an independent predictor of coronary heart disease. West of Scotland Coronary Prevention Study Group. *N Engl J Med.* 2000;343:1148-1155.
70. Serruys PW, Garcia-Garcia HM, Buszman P, et al. Effects of the direct lipoprotein-associated phospholipase A(2) inhibitor darapladib on human coronary atherosclerotic plaque. *Circulation.* 2008;118:1172-1182.
71. O'Donoghue ML, Braunwald E, White HD, et al. Effect of darapladib on major coronary events after an acute coronary syndrome: the SOLID-TIMI 52 randomized clinical trial. *JAMA.* 2014;312:1006-1015.
72. White HD, Held C, Stewart R, et al. Darapladib for preventing ischemic events in stable coronary heart disease. *N Engl J Med.* 2014;370:1702-1711.
73. Barter PJ, Caulfield M, Eriksson M, et al. Effects of torcetrapib in patients at high risk for coronary events. *N Engl J Med.* 2007;357:2109-2122.
74. Schwartz GG, Olsson AG, Abt M, et al. Effects of dalcetrapib in patients with a recent acute coronary syndrome. *N Engl J Med.* 2012;367:2089-2099.
75. Calabresi L, Baldassarre D, Castelnuovo S, et al. Functional lecithin:cholesterol acyltransferase is not required for efficient atheroprotection in humans. *Circulation.* 2009;120:628-635.
76. Kato H, Tillotso J, Nichaman MZ, et al. Epidemiologic studies of coronary heart-disease and stroke in Japanese men living in Japan, Hawaii and California—serum-lipids and diet. *Am J Epidemiol.* 1973;97:372-385.
77. Third Report of the National Cholesterol Education Program (NCEP). Expert Panel on Detection, Evaluation, and Treatment of High Blood Cholesterol in Adults (Adult Treatment Panel III) final report. *Circulation.* 2002;106(25):3143-3421.
78. Kavey RE, Daniels SR, Lauer RM, et al. American Heart Association guidelines for primary prevention of atherosclerotic cardiovascular disease beginning in childhood. *J Pediatr.* 2003;142:368-372.
79. Berglund L, Brunzell JD, Goldberg AC, et al. Evaluation and treatment of hypertriglyceridemia: an Endocrine Society clinical practice guideline. *J Clin Endocrinol Metab.* 2012;97:2969-2989.
80. Haffner SM, Stern MP, Hazuda HP, et al. Cardiovascular risk factors in confirmed prediabetic individuals. Does the clock for coronary heart disease start ticking before the onset of clinical diabetes? *JAMA.* 1990;263:2893-2898.
81. Tsuang W, Navaneethan U, Ruiz L, et al. Hypertriglyceridemic pancreatitis: presentation and management. *Am J Gastroenterol.* 2009;104:984-991.
82. Merkel M, Eckel RH, Goldberg IJ. Lipoprotein lipase: genetics, lipid uptake, and regulation. *J Lipid Res.* 2002;43:1997-2006.
83. Wilson DE, Hata A, Kwong LK, et al. Mutations in exon 3 of the lipoprotein lipase gene segregating in a family with hypertriglyceridemia, pancreatitis, and non-insulin-dependent diabetes. *J Clin Invest.* 1993;92:203-211.
84. Ginsberg HN. Diabetic dyslipidemia: basic mechanisms underlying the common hypertriglyceridemia and low HDL cholesterol levels. *Diabetes.* 1996;45(Suppl 3):S27-S30.
85. Connelly PW, Maguire GF, Little JA. Apolipoprotein CIISt. Michael. Familial apolipoprotein CII deficiency associated with premature vascular disease. *J Clin Invest.* 1987;80(6):1597-1606.
86. Beigneux AP, Franssen R, Bensadoun A, et al. Chylomicronemia with a mutant GPIHBP1 (Q115P) that cannot bind lipoprotein lipase. *Arterioscler Thromb Vasc Biol.* 2009;29:956-962.
87. Chokshi N, Blumenschein SD, Ahmad Z, Garg A. Genotype-phenotype relationships in patients with type I hyperlipoproteinemia. *J Clin Lipidol.* 2014;8:287-295.
88. Peterfy M, Ben-Zeev O, Mao HZ, et al. Mutations in LMF1 cause combined lipase deficiency and severe hypertriglyceridemia. *Nat Genet.* 2007;39:1483-1487.
89. Nordestgaard BG, Benn M, Schnohr P, Tybjaerg-Hansen A. Nonfasting triglycerides and risk of myocardial infarction, ischemic heart disease, and death in men and women. *JAMA.* 2007;298:299-308.
90. Wilson DE, Emi M, Iverius PH, et al. Phenotypic expression of heterozygous lipoprotein lipase deficiency in the extended pedigree of a proband homozygous for a missense mutation. *J Clin Invest.* 1990;86:735-750.
91. Do R, Willer CJ, Schmidt EM, et al. Common variants associated with plasma triglycerides and risk for coronary artery disease. *Nat Genet.* 2013;45:1345-1352.
92. Austin MA, McKnight B, Edwards KL, et al. Cardiovascular disease mortality in familial forms of hypertriglyceridemia: a 20-year prospective study. *Circulation.* 2000;101:2777-2782.
93. Duane WC. Abnormal bile acid absorption in familial hypertriglyceridemia. *J Lipid Res.* 1995;36:96-107.
94. Watanabe M, Houten SM, Wang L, et al. Bile acids lower triglyceride levels via a pathway involving FXR, SHP, and SREBP-1c. *J Clin Invest.* 2004;113:1408-1418.
95. Taskinen MR, Adiels M, Westerbacka J, et al. Dual metabolic defects are required to produce hypertriglyceridemia in obese subjects. *Arterioscler Thromb Vasc Biol.* 2011;31:2144-2150.
96. Clement LC, Mace C, Avila-Casado C, et al. Circulating angiopoietin-like 4 links proteinuria with hypertriglyceridemia in nephrotic syndrome. *Nat Med.* 2014;20:37-46.
97. Wolfe BM, Barrett PH, Laurier L, Huff MW. Effects of continuous conjugated estrogen and micronized progesterone therapy upon lipoprotein metabolism in postmenopausal women. *J Lipid Res.* 2000;41:368-375.
98. Sanada M, Tsuda M, Kodama I, et al. Substitution of transdermal estradiol during oral estrogen-progestin therapy in postmenopausal women: effects on hypertriglyceridemia. *Menopause.* 2004;11:331-336.
99. Elisaf MS, Nakou K, Liamis G, Pavlidis NA. Tamoxifen-induced severe hypertriglyceridemia and pancreatitis. *Ann Oncol.* 2000;11:1067-1069.
100. Mosca L, Harper K, Sarkar S, et al. Effect of raloxifene on serum triglycerides in postmenopausal women: influence of predisposing factors for hypertriglyceridemia. *Clin Ther.* 2001;23:1552-1565.
101. Frohlich JJ. Effects of alcohol on plasma lipoprotein metabolism. *Clin Chim Acta.* 1996;246:39-49.
102. Soutar AK, Naoumova RP. Mechanisms of disease: genetic causes of familial hypercholesterolemia. *Nat Clin Pract Cardiovasc Med.* 2007;4:214-225.
103. Benn M, Watts GF, Tybjaerg-Hansen A, Nordestgaard BG. Familial hypercholesterolemia in the Danish general population: prevalence, coronary artery disease, and cholesterol-lowering medication. *J Clin Endocrinol Metab.* 2012;97:3956-3964.
104. Kawaguchi A, Miyatake K, Yutani C, et al. Characteristic cardiovascular manifestation in homozygous and heterozygous familial hypercholesterolemia. *Am Heart J.* 1999;137:410-418.
105. Cuchel M, Bruckert E, Ginsberg HN, et al. Homozygous familial hypercholesterolaemia: new insights and guidance for clinicians to improve detection and clinical management. A position paper from the Consensus Panel on Familial Hypercholesterolaemia of the European Atherosclerosis Society. *Eur Heart J.* 2014;35:2146-2157.
106. Raal FJ, Santos RD. Homozygous familial hypercholesterolemia: current perspectives on diagnosis and treatment. *Atherosclerosis.* 2012;223:262-268.
107. Pullinger CR, Eng C, Salen G, et al. Human cholesterol 7alpha-hydroxylase (CYP7A1) deficiency has a hypercholesterolemic phenotype. *J Clin Invest.* 2002;110:109-117.
108. Maxwell KN, Fisher EA, Breslow JL. Overexpression of PCSK9 accelerates the degradation of the LDLR in a post-endoplasmic reticulum compartment. *Proc Natl Acad Sci U S A.* 2005;102:2069-2074.
109. Grefhorst A, McNutt MC, Lagace TA, Horton JD. Plasma PCSK9 preferentially reduces liver LDL receptors in mice. *J Lipid Res.* 2008;49:1303-1311.
110. Jacobson TA. Lipoprotein(a), cardiovascular disease, and contemporary management. *Mayo Clin Proc.* 2013;88:1294-1311.
111. Guyton JR, Dahlen GH, Patsch W, et al. Relationship of plasma lipoprotein Lp(a) levels to race and to apolipoprotein B. *Arteriosclerosis.* 1985;5:265-272.
112. Berge KE. Sitosterolemia: a gateway to new knowledge about cholesterol metabolism. *Ann Med.* 2003;35:502-511.
113. Salen G, von Bergmann K, Lutjohann D, et al. Ezetimibe effectively reduces plasma plant sterols in patients with sitosterolemia. *Circulation.* 2004;109:966-971.
114. Thompson PD, Clarkson P, Karas RH. Statin-associated myopathy. *JAMA.* 2003;289:1681-1690.
115. Diekman T, Lansberg PJ, Kastelein JJ, Wiersinga WM. Prevalence and correction of hypothyroidism in a large cohort of patients referred for dyslipidemia. *Arch Intern Med.* 1995;155:1490-1495.
116. Goldstein JL, Schrott HG, Hazzard WR, et al. Hyperlipidemia in coronary heart disease. II. Genetic analysis of lipid levels in 176 families and delineation of a new inherited disorder, combined hyperlipidemia. *J Clin Invest.* 1973;52:1544-1568.
117. Barzilai N, Atzmon G, Schechter C, et al. Unique lipoprotein phenotype and genotype associated with exceptional longevity. *JAMA.* 2003;290:2030-2040.
118. Voight BF, Peloso GM, Orho-Melander M, et al. Plasma HDL cholesterol and risk of myocardial infarction: a mendelian randomisation study. *Lancet.* 2012;380:572-580.
119. Hewing B, Moore KJ, Fisher EA. HDL and cardiovascular risk: time to call the plumber? *Circ Res.* 2012;111:1117-1120.
120. Navab M, Anantharamaiah GM, Reddy ST, Fogelman AM. Apolipoprotein A-I mimetic peptides and their role in atherosclerosis prevention. *Nat Clin Pract Cardiovasc Med.* 2006;3:540-547.
121. McMahon M, Grossman J, FitzGerald J, et al. Proinflammatory high-density lipoprotein as a biomarker for atherosclerosis in patients with systemic lupus erythematosus and rheumatoid arthritis. *Arthritis Rheum.* 2006;54:2541-2549.
122. Nicholls SJ, Brewer HB, Kastelein JJ, et al. Effects of the CETP inhibitor evacetrapib administered as monotherapy or in combination with statins on HDL and LDL cholesterol: a randomized controlled trial. *JAMA.* 2011;306:2099-2109.

123. Musunuru K, Pirruccello JP, Do R, et al. Exome sequencing, ANGPTL3 mutations, and familial combined hypolipidemia. *N Engl J Med.* 2010; 363:2220-2227.
124. Nissen SE, Tsunoda T, Tuzcu EM, et al. Effect of recombinant ApoA-I Milano on coronary atherosclerosis in patients with acute coronary syndromes: a randomized controlled trial. *JAMA.* 2003;290:2292-2300.
125. Kuivenhoven JA, Pritchard H, Hill J, et al. The molecular pathology of lecithin:cholesterol acyltransferase (LCAT) deficiency syndromes. *J Lipid Res.* 1997;38:191-205.
126. Nicholls SJ, Ballantyne CM, Barter PJ, et al. Effect of two intensive statin regimens on progression of coronary disease. *N Engl J Med.* 2011;365:2078-2087.
127. Wilson PW, D'Agostino RB, Levy D, et al. Prediction of coronary heart disease using risk factor categories. *Circulation.* 1998;97:1837-1847.
128. Baigent C, Landray MJ, Reith C, et al. The effects of lowering LDL cholesterol with simvastatin plus ezetimibe in patients with chronic kidney disease (Study of Heart and Renal Protection): a randomised placebo-controlled trial. *Lancet.* 2011;377:2181-2192.
129. Page IH. Atherosclerosis: an introduction. *Circulation.* 1954;10:1-27.
130. Moore KJ, Tabas I. Macrophages in the pathogenesis of atherosclerosis. *Cell.* 2011;145:341-355.
131. Goldberg IJ, Kako Y, Lutz EP. Responses to eating: lipoproteins, lipolytic products and atherosclerosis. *Curr Opin Lipidol.* 2000;11: 235-241.
132. Virmani R, Kolodgie FD, Burke AP, et al. Lessons from sudden coronary death: a comprehensive morphological classification scheme for atherosclerotic lesions. *Arterioscler Thromb Vasc Biol.* 2000;20:1262-1275.
133. Nissen SE, Nicholls SJ, Sipahi I, et al. Effect of very high-intensity statin therapy on regression of coronary atherosclerosis: the ASTEROID trial. *JAMA.* 2006;295:1556-1565.
134. Mozaffarian D, Benjamin EJ, Go AS, et al. Heart disease and stroke statistics—2015 update: a report from the American Heart Association. *Circulation.* 2015;131(4):e23-e322.
135. Greenland P, Knoll MD, Stamler J, et al. Major risk factors as antecedents of fatal and nonfatal coronary heart disease events. *JAMA.* 2003;290:891-897.
136. Khot UN, Khot MB, Bajzer CT, et al. Prevalence of conventional risk factors in patients with coronary heart disease. *JAMA.* 2003;290: 898-904.
137. Steinberg D, Gotto AM Jr. Preventing coronary artery disease by lowering cholesterol levels: fifty years from bench to bedside. *JAMA.* 1999; 282:2043-2050.
138. Stone NJ, Robinson JG, Lichtenstein AH, et al. 2013 ACC/AHA guideline on the treatment of blood cholesterol to reduce atherosclerotic cardiovascular risk in adults: a report of the American College of Cardiology/American Heart Association Task Force on Practice Guidelines. *J Am Coll Cardiol.* 2014;63:2889-2934.
139. An International Atherosclerosis Society Position Paper: global recommendations for the management of dyslipidemia—full report. *J Clin Lipidol.* 2014;8:29-60.
140. Stamler J, Wentworth D, Neaton JD. Is relationship between serum cholesterol and risk of premature death from coronary heart disease continuous and graded? Findings in 356,222 primary screenees of the Multiple Risk Factor Intervention Trial (MRFIT). *JAMA.* 1986;256: 2823-2828.
141. Eckel RH, Jakicic JM, Ard JD, et al. 2013 AHA/ACC guideline on lifestyle management to reduce cardiovascular risk: a report of the American College of Cardiology/American Heart Association Task Force on Practice Guidelines. *J Am Coll Cardiol.* 2014;63:2960-2984.
142. The Lipid Research Clinics Coronary Primary Prevention Trial results. I. Reduction in incidence of coronary heart disease. *JAMA.* 1984;251: 351-364.
143. Blankenhorn DH, Nessim SA, Johnson RL, et al. Beneficial effects of combined colestipol-niacin therapy on coronary atherosclerosis and coronary venous bypass grafts. *JAMA.* 1987;257:3233-3240.
144. Brown G, Albers JJ, Fisher LD, et al. Regression of coronary artery disease as a result of intensive lipid-lowering therapy in men with high levels of apolipoprotein B. *N Engl J Med.* 1990;323:1289-1298.
145. Randomised trial of cholesterol lowering in 4444 patients with coronary heart disease: the Scandinavian Simvastatin Survival Study (4S). *Lancet.* 1994;344(8934):1383-1389.
146. Sacks FM, Pfeffer MA, Moye LA, et al. The effect of pravastatin on coronary events after myocardial infarction in patients with average cholesterol levels. Cholesterol and Recurrent Events Trial investigators. *N Engl J Med.* 1996;335:1001-1009.
147. Heart Protection Study Collaborative Group. MRC/BHF Heart Protection Study of cholesterol lowering with simvastatin in 20,536 high-risk individuals: a randomised placebo-controlled trial. *Lancet.* 2002; 360(9326):7-22.
148. Cannon CP, Braunwald E, McCabe CH, et al. Intensive versus moderate lipid lowering with statins after acute coronary syndromes. *N Engl J Med.* 2004;350:1495-1504.
149. LaRosa JC, Grundy SM, Waters DD, et al. Intensive lipid lowering with atorvastatin in patients with stable coronary disease. *N Engl J Med.* 2005;352:1425-1435.
150. Shepherd J, Cobbe SM, Ford I, et al. Prevention of coronary heart disease with pravastatin in men with hypercholesterolemia. West of Scotland Coronary Prevention Study Group. *N Engl J Med.* 1995;333: 1301-1307.
151. Downs JR, Clearfield M, Weis S, et al. Primary prevention of acute coronary events with lovastatin in men and women with average cholesterol levels: results of AFCAPS/TexCAPS. Air Force/Texas Coronary Atherosclerosis Prevention Study. *JAMA.* 1998;279:1615-1622.
152. Colhoun HM, Betteridge DJ, Durrington PN, et al. Primary prevention of cardiovascular disease with atorvastatin in type 2 diabetes in the Collaborative Atorvastatin Diabetes Study (CARDS): multicentre randomised placebo-controlled trial. *Lancet.* 2004;364:685-696.
153. Ridker PM, Danielson E, Fonseca FA, et al. Rosuvastatin to prevent vascular events in men and women with elevated C-reactive protein. *N Eng J Med.* 2008;359:2195-2207.
154. Baigent C, Blackwell L, Emberson J, et al. Efficacy and safety of more intensive lowering of LDL cholesterol: a meta-analysis of data from 170,000 participants in 26 randomised trials. *Lancet.* 2010;376: 1670-1681.
155. Mihaylova B, Emberson J, Blackwell L, et al. The effects of lowering LDL cholesterol with statin therapy in people at low risk of vascular disease: meta-analysis of individual data from 27 randomised trials. *Lancet.* 2012;380:581-590.
156. Frick MH, Elo O, Haapa K, et al. Helsinki Heart Study: primary-prevention trial with gemfibrozil in middle-aged men with dyslipidemia. Safety of treatment, changes in risk factors, and incidence of coronary heart disease. *N Engl J Med.* 1987;317:1237-1245.
157. Rubins HB, Robins SJ, Collins D, et al. Gemfibrozil for the secondary prevention of coronary heart disease in men with low levels of high-density lipoprotein cholesterol. Veterans Affairs High-Density Lipoprotein Cholesterol Intervention Trial Study Group. *N Engl J Med.* 1999; 341:410-418.
158. Keech A, Simes RJ, Barter P, et al. Effects of long-term fenofibrate therapy on cardiovascular events in 9795 people with type 2 diabetes mellitus (the FIELD study): randomised controlled trial. *Lancet.* 2005; 366:1849-1861.
159. Ginsberg HN, Elam MB, Lovato LC, et al. Effects of combination lipid therapy in type 2 diabetes mellitus. *N Engl J Med.* 2010;362: 1563-1574.
160. Canner PL, Berge KG, Wenger NK, et al. Fifteen year mortality in Coronary Drug Project patients: long-term benefit with niacin. *J Am Coll Cardiol.* 1986;8:1245-1255.
161. Boden WE, Probstfield JL, Anderson T, et al. Niacin in patients with low HDL cholesterol levels receiving intensive statin therapy. *N Engl J Med.* 2011;365:2255-2267.
162. Landray MJ, Haynes R, Hopewell JC, et al. Effects of extended-release niacin with laropiprant in high-risk patients. *N Engl J Med.* 2014;371: 203-212.
163. Nissen SE, Tuzcu EM, Schoenhagen P, et al. Effect of intensive compared with moderate lipid-lowering therapy on progression of coronary atherosclerosis: a randomized controlled trial. *JAMA.* 2004;291: 1071-1080.
164. Kane JP, Malloy MJ, Ports TA, et al. Regression of coronary atherosclerosis during treatment of familial hypercholesterolemia with combined drug regimens. *JAMA.* 1990;264:3007-3012.
165. Brown BG, Zhao XQ, Chait A, et al. Simvastatin and niacin, antioxidant vitamins, or the combination for the prevention of coronary disease. *N Engl J Med.* 2001;345:1583-1592.
166. Catapano AL, Reiner Z, De Backer G, et al. ESC/EAS Guidelines for the management of dyslipidaemias The Task Force for the management of dyslipidaemias of the European Society of Cardiology (ESC) and the European Atherosclerosis Society (EAS). *Atherosclerosis.* 2011;217:3-46.
167. Miller M, Stone NJ, Ballantyne C, et al. Triglycerides and cardiovascular disease: a scientific statement from the American Heart Association. *Circulation.* 2011;123:2292-2333.
168. Yusuf S, Hawken S, Ounpuu S, et al. Effect of potentially modifiable risk factors associated with myocardial infarction in 52 countries (the INTERHEART study): case-control study. *Lancet.* 2004;364:937-952.
169. Henkin Y, Crystal E, Goldberg Y, et al. Usefulness of lipoprotein changes during acute coronary syndromes for predicting postdischarge lipoprotein levels. *Am J Cardiol.* 2002;89:7-11.
170. Goff DC Jr, Lloyd-Jones DM, Bennett G, et al. 2013 ACC/AHA guideline on the assessment of cardiovascular risk: a report of the American College of Cardiology/American Heart Association Task Force on Practice Guidelines. *J Am Coll Cardiol.* 2014;63:2935-2959.
171. Psaty BM, Rivara FP. Universal screening and drug treatment of dyslipidemia in children and adolescents. *JAMA.* 2012;307:257-258.
172. Gillman MW, Daniels SR. Is universal pediatric lipid screening justified? *JAMA.* 2012;307:259-260.
173. Goldberg AC, Hopkins PN, Toth PP, et al. Familial hypercholesterolemia: screening, diagnosis and management of pediatric and adult patients: clinical guidance from the National Lipid Association Expert Panel on Familial Hypercholesterolemia. *J Clin Lipidol.* 2011;5:S1-S8.
174. Expert panel on integrated guidelines for cardiovascular health and risk reduction in children and adolescents: summary report. *Pediatrics.* 2011;128(Suppl 5):S213-S256.

175. Jensen MD, Ryan DH, Apovian CM, et al. 2013 AHA/ACC/TOS guideline for the management of overweight and obesity in adults: a report of the American College of Cardiology/American Heart Association Task Force on Practice Guidelines and the Obesity Society. *J Am Coll Cardiol.* 2014;63:2985-3023.

176. American Heart Association/American College of Cardiology. CV Risk Calculator (downloadable spreadsheet): 2013 Prevention Guidelines Tools. Available at: <http://my.americanheart.org/professional/StatementsGuidelines/Prevention-Guidelines_UCM_457698_Sub HomePage.jsp>.

177. Grundy SM, Cleeman JI, Merz CN, et al. Implications of recent clinical trials for the National Cholesterol Education Program Adult Treatment Panel III guidelines. *Circulation.* 2004;110:227-239.

178. Catapano AL, Reiner Z, De Backer G, et al. ESC/EAS Guidelines for the management of dyslipidaemias: the Task Force for the management of dyslipidaemias of the European Society of Cardiology (ESC) and the European Atherosclerosis Society (EAS). *Atherosclerosis.* 2011; 217(Suppl 1):S1-S44.

179. Anderson TJ, Gregoire J, Hegele RA, et al. 2012 update of the Canadian Cardiovascular Society guidelines for the diagnosis and treatment of dyslipidemia for the prevention of cardiovascular disease in the adult. *Can J Cardiol.* 2013;29:151-167.

180. Boekholdt SM, Hovingh GK, Mora S, et al. Very low levels of atherogenic lipoproteins and the risk for cardiovascular events: a meta-analysis of statin trials. *J Am Coll Cardiol.* 2014;64:485-494.

181. Ference BA, Yoo W, Alesh I, et al. Effect of long-term exposure to lower low-density lipoprotein cholesterol beginning early in life on the risk of coronary heart disease: a Mendelian randomization analysis. *J Am Coll Cardiol.* 2012;60:2631-2639.

182. Van Horn L, McCoin M, Kris-Etherton PM, et al. The evidence for dietary prevention and treatment of cardiovascular disease. *J Am Diet Assoc.* 2008;108:287-331.

183. Risk and Prevention Study Collaborative Group, Roncaglioni MC, Tombesi M, Avanzini F, et al. n-3 fatty acids in patients with multiple cardiovascular risk factors. *N Engl J Med.* 2013;368(19): 1800-1808.

184. Jenkins DJ, Kendall CW, Marchie A, et al. Effects of a dietary portfolio of cholesterol-lowering foods vs lovastatin on serum lipids and C-reactive protein. *JAMA.* 2003;290:502-510.

185. Knopp RH. Drug treatment of lipid disorders. [see comment]. *N Engl J Med.* 1999;341:498-511.

186. Kashani A, Phillips CO, Foody JM, et al. Risks associated with statin therapy: a systematic overview of randomized clinical trials. *Circulation.* 2006;114:2788-2797.

187. Cohen DE, Anania FA, Chalasani N. An assessment of statin safety by hepatologists. *Am J Cardiol.* 2006;97:77C-81C.

188. Cohen JD, Brinton EA, Ito MK, Jacobson TA. Understanding Statin Use in America and Gaps in Patient Education (USAGE): an Internet-based survey of 10,138 current and former statin users. *J Clin Lipidol.* 2012; 6:208-215.

189. Sattar N, Preiss D, Murray HM, et al. Statins and risk of incident diabetes: a collaborative meta-analysis of randomised statin trials. *Lancet.* 2010;375:735-742.

190. Watts GF, Lewis B, Brunt JN, et al. Effects on coronary artery disease of lipid-lowering diet, or diet plus cholestyramine, in the St Thomas' Atherosclerosis Regression Study (STARS) [see comment]. *Lancet.* 1992; 339:563-569.

191. Davidson MH, Dicklin MR, Maki KC, Kleinpell RM. Colesevelam hydrochloride: a non-absorbed, polymeric cholesterol-lowering agent. *Expert Opin Investig Drugs.* 2000;9:2663-2671.

192. Insull W Jr, Toth P, Mullican W, et al. Effectiveness of colesevelam hydrochloride in decreasing LDL cholesterol in patients with primary hypercholesterolemia: a 24-week randomized controlled trial. *Mayo Clin Proc.* 2001;76:971-982.

193. Zieve FJ, Kalin MF, Schwartz SL, et al. Results of the glucose-lowering effect of WelChol study (GLOWS): a randomized, double-blind, placebo-controlled pilot study evaluating the effect of colesevelam hydrochloride on glycemic control in subjects with type 2 diabetes. *Clin Ther.* 2007;29:74-83.

194. Donovan JM, Stypinski D, Stiles MR, et al. Drug interactions with colesevelam hydrochloride, a novel, potent lipid-lowering agent. *Cardiovasc Drugs Ther.* 2000;14:681-690.

195. Brown WV, Goldberg AC, Guyton JR, Knopp RH. The use of niacin. *J Clin Lipidol.* 2009;3:65-69.

196. Zhao XQ, Morse JS, Dowdy AA, et al. Safety and tolerability of simvastatin plus niacin in patients with coronary artery disease and low high-density lipoprotein cholesterol (the HDL Atherosclerosis Treatment Study). *Am J Cardiol.* 2004;93:307-312.

197. Jones PH, Davidson MH. Reporting rate of rhabdomyolysis with fenofibrate + statin versus gemfibrozil + any statin. *Am J Cardiol.* 2005; 95:120-122.

198. Keech AC, Mitchell P, Summanen PA, et al. Effect of fenofibrate on the need for laser treatment for diabetic retinopathy (FIELD study): a randomised controlled trial. *Lancet.* 2007;370:1687-1697.

199. Chew EY, Ambrosius WT, Davis MD, et al. Effects of medical therapies on retinopathy progression in type 2 diabetes. *N Engl J Med.* 2010; 363:233-244.

200. American Heart Association Scientific Sessions, November 2014. IMPROVE-IT trial. Available at: <http://my.americanheart.org/idc/groups/ahamah-public/@wcm/@sop/@scon/documents/download able/ucm_469669.pdf>.

201. Stitziel NO, Won HH, Morrison AC, et al. Inactivating mutations in NPC1L1 and protection from coronary heart disease. *N Engl J Med.* 2014;371:2072-2082.

202. Kris-Etherton PM, Harris WS, Appel LJ. Fish consumption, fish oil, omega-3 fatty acids, and cardiovascular disease. *Circulation.* 2002;106: 2747-2757.

203. Yokoyama M, Origasa H, Matsuzaki M, et al. Effects of eicosapentaenoic acid on major coronary events in hypercholesterolaemic patients (JELIS): a randomised open-label, blinded endpoint analysis. *Lancet.* 2007;369:1090-1098.

204. Americanheart.org. Data available at: <http://my.americanheart.org/idc/groups/ahamah-public/@wcm/@sop/@scon/documents/downloadable/ucm_469669.pdf>.

205. Huijgen R, Abbink EJ, Bruckert E, et al. Colesevelam added to combination therapy with a statin and ezetimibe in patients with familial hypercholesterolemia: a 12-week, multicenter, randomized, double-blind, controlled trial. *Clin Ther.* 2010;32:615-625.

206. Bottorff MB. Statin safety and drug interactions: clinical implications. *Am J Cardiol.* 2006;97:27C-31C.

207. Buchwald H, Varco RL, Matts JP, et al. Effect of partial ileal bypass surgery on mortality and morbidity from coronary heart disease in patients with hypercholesterolemia. Report of the Program on the Surgical Control of the Hyperlipidemias (POSCH). *N Engl J Med.* 1990;323:946-955.

208. Goldberg IJ. Hypertriglyceridemia: impact and treatment. *Endocrinol Metab Clin North Am.* 2009;38:137-149.

209. Gaudet D, Methot J, Dery S, et al. Efficacy and long-term safety of alipogene tiparvovec (AAV1-LPLS447X) gene therapy for lipoprotein lipase deficiency: an open-label trial. *Gene Ther.* 2013;20:361-369.

210. Kastelein JJ, Wedel MK, Baker BF, et al. Potent reduction of apolipoprotein B and low-density lipoprotein cholesterol by short-term administration of an antisense inhibitor of apolipoprotein B. *Circulation.* 2006;114:1729-1735.

211. Raal FJ, Santos RD, Blom DJ, et al. Mipomersen, an apolipoprotein B synthesis inhibitor, for lowering of LDL cholesterol concentrations in patients with homozygous familial hypercholesterolaemia: a randomised, double-blind, placebo-controlled trial. *Lancet.* 2010;375: 998-1006.

212. Stein EA, Dufour R, Gagne C, et al. Apolipoprotein B synthesis inhibition with mipomersen in heterozygous familial hypercholesterolemia: results of a randomized, double-blind, placebo-controlled trial to assess efficacy and safety as add-on therapy in patients with coronary artery disease. *Circulation.* 2012;126:2283-2292.

213. Cuchel M, Bloedon LT, Szapary PO, et al. Inhibition of microsomal triglyceride transfer protein in familial hypercholesterolemia. *N Engl J Med.* 2007;356:148-156.

214. Cuchel M, Meagher EA, du Toit Theron H, et al. Efficacy and safety of a microsomal triglyceride transfer protein inhibitor in patients with homozygous familial hypercholesterolaemia: a single-arm, open-label, phase 3 study. *Lancet.* 2013;381:40-46.

215. Grundy SM, Cleeman JI, Daniels SR, et al. Diagnosis and management of the metabolic syndrome: an American Heart Association/National Heart, Lung, and Blood Institute Scientific Statement. *Circulation.* 2005;112:2735-2752.

216. Leebmann J, Roeseler E, Julius U, et al. Lipoprotein apheresis in patients with maximally tolerated lipid-lowering therapy, lipoprotein(a)-hyperlipoproteinemia, and progressive cardiovascular disease: prospective observational multicenter study. *Circulation.* 2013; 128:2567-2576.

217. Stein EA, Raal F. Reduction of low-density lipoprotein cholesterol by monoclonal antibody inhibition of PCSK9. *Annu Rev Med.* 2014;65: 417-431.

218. Rached FH, Chapman MJ, Kontush A. An overview of the new frontiers in the treatment of atherogenic dyslipidemias. *Clin Pharmacol Ther.* 2014;96:57-63.

CHAPTER 38

Gastrointestinal Hormones and Gut Endocrine Tumors

ADRIAN VELLA*

KEY POINTS

- Endocrine tumors originating from islet or enteroendocrine cells present either with symptoms due to their location in the pancreas or intestine or, more commonly, with symptoms arising from dysregulated secretion of bioactive hormones.
- The historical classification of enteroendocrine cells is based principally on the phenotype ascribed to the production of one or more peptide hormones. However, enteroendocrine cell subpopulations exhibit multiple plurihormonal phenotypes.
- The secretion of one or more peptide hormones resulting in the production of symptoms attributable to hormone excess facilitates the diagnosis of a hormone-secreting endocrine tumor.
- Insulinomas are the most common functioning islet cell tumor and are characterized by hypoglycemia, which is usually precipitated by exercise or fasting.
- A large number of peptides are synthesized in and secreted by endocrine cells of the pancreas and gastrointestinal tract. Many of these peptides circulate as hormones, but they also function as paracrine modulators or neurotransmitters in the gut and in the central and peripheral nervous systems.

Endocrine tumors originating from islet or enteroendocrine cells present with symptoms caused by their location in the pancreas or intestine or, more commonly, with symptoms arising from dysregulated secretion of bioactive hormones. In this chapter, we discuss the development of endocrine cell lineages during organogenesis in both the endocrine pancreas and the intestine and review the biologic actions of peptide hormones produced in pancreatic and intestinal endocrine cells and enteric nerves. The physiology of many of these peptides is incompletely understood and is the subject of active investigation. However, several clinical syndromes are attributable to functioning enteroendocrine tumors in the gastrointestinal tract or the pancreas.

ENDOCRINE CELL DEVELOPMENT IN THE PANCREAS

The endocrine and exocrine parts of the pancreas develop from the primitive foregut endoderm, a process that begins with the evagination of the embryonic foregut into ventral and dorsal buds at 28 days' gestation in humans and at embryonic day 8 (E8) in mice. Rotation of the stomach and duodenum during development results in simultaneous rotation of the ventral bud, which fuses with the dorsal bud to give rise to the primitive pancreas. The ventral bud develops into the posterior portion of the pancreatic head, including the uncinate process, while the remaining pancreas is derived from the dorsal bud. The rotation of the ventral bud gives rise to considerable variation in the duct system of the pancreas, including the presence of accessory ducts. In mice, a complex, treelike, epithelium-lined ductal system develops within the pancreatic diverticula, with glucagon-immunoreactive cells detected as early as E9.5, followed by detection of cells containing insulin at E10.5. Stem cells that give rise to terminally differentiated endocrine and exocrine acinar cells are thought to reside within the islets and in ductal epithelium. Indeed, complexes of insulin-producing cells (or at least staining for insulin) in the pancreatic ducts are considered to be the hallmark of nesidioblastosis.[1]

In humans, islet formation begins at gestational week 12 with the aggregation of polyclonal endocrine cells. Between weeks 13 and 16, small aggregates of endocrine cells arise from the pancreatic duct and develop their own blood supply. By weeks 17 to 20, fewer islets are observed in contact with the ducts, and a mantle of non-beta endocrine cells forms around the beta cells. Between gestational weeks 21 and 26, a continual increase in the proportion of islet tissue and in the average size of the islets is observed, with occasional non-beta cells in the center of the islet, a morphologic appearance that is characteristic of the postnatal islet. At birth, the endocrine pancreas accounts for 1% to 2% of the entire pancreatic cell mass.

Although genetic studies in mice have yielded valuable insights into the ontogeny of islet development, the relative order of appearance of unique populations of hormone-producing islet endocrine cells is different in humans

---

*Daniel J. Drucker was a coauthor of this chapter but has chosen to withdraw his name owing to his disagreement with Reed Elsevier's handling of "An open letter for the people in Gaza" (Manduca P, Chalmers I, Summerfield D, Gilbert M, Ang S. An open letter for the people in Gaza. *The Lancet.* 2014;384(9941):397-398. doi:10.1016/S0140-6736(14)61044-8.)

TABLE 38-1

Effects of Disruption of Genes Important for Development of Pancreatic Endocrine Cells

Gene	Phenotype in Homozygous (–/–) Mutant Mice
Arx	Failure to develop glucagon-positive alpha cells
FoxM1	Impaired beta-cell replication
Glis3	Impaired islet and beta-cell development
Hes1	Increased glucagon-positive alpha cells, pancreatic hypoplasia
Hlxb9	Dorsal lobe agenesis, small islets, reduced beta cells
Isl1	Loss of differentiated islet cells
Myt1	Abnormal islet cell development
Nkx2.2	Absent mature beta cells, reduced alpha and pancreatic polypeptide (PP) cells
Nkx6.1	Reduced beta cell precursors
NeuroD	Reduced beta cells, arrested islet morphogenesis
Ngn3	Absent islet cells and defective enteroendocrine cell formation
Nkx6	Impaired alpha-cell development
Pax4	Absent islet beta and delta cells
Pax6	Absent islet alpha cells
Pbx1	Marked reduction in islet alpha and beta cells
Pdx1	Pancreatic agenesis
Sox4	Defective islet development

and mice. Somatostatin- and pancreatic polypeptide (PP)-positive cells are detected at 7 weeks' gestation in the human pancreas, scattered among ductal cells. One week later, glucagon cells appear, and by 9 to 10 weeks' gestation, insulin-producing cells are detectable. In mice, both insulin- and glucagon-expressing cells are first detected between days E9.5 and E10.5, and somatostatin and PP are expressed by E15.5. Although cells coexpressing insulin and glucagon are detected during early islet development, cell lineage studies employing specific transgenes that mark or ablate islet cell precursors suggest that the alpha- and beta-cell lineages arise independently during ontogeny in the mouse.[2] Peptide YY (PYY) co-localizes with each of the four main islet hormones in the developing pancreas, but genetic evidence for an essential role of a PYY-producing precursor cell in pancreatic endocrine development has not been developed.

Delineation of the genetic determinants that regulate the developmental formation and organization of pancreatic endocrine cell populations has been facilitated by studies of mice with disruption of candidate regulatory genes, principally islet transcription factors (Table 38-1). The homeobox transcription factor Pdx1 is required for transcription of multiple beta-cell genes, including those for insulin and glucokinase in the adult beta cell, and for developmental formation of the entire pancreas.[3] Similarly, the homeodomain transcription factor Prox1 controls pancreatic morphogenesis and formation of islet cell precursors after E13.5. Mice homozygous for a null mutation in *Pdx1* fail to develop a pancreas, whereas restricted inactivation of Pdx1 in the murine beta cell produces insulin deficiency and diabetes. Pancreatic agenesis has also been reported in human subjects homozygous for a loss-of-function PDX1 mutation,[4] and subjects heterozygous for PDX1 develop a form of maturity-onset diabetes of the young (MODY4). A similar phenotype (isolated pancreatic agenesis) has been identified in individuals with loss-of-function mutations in the genes encoding pancreas-specific transcription factor 1a[5] and GATA6.[6]

Targeted disruption of the LIM domain *Isl1* gene in mice results in abnormal development of the dorsal pancreatic mesenchyme and abnormal differentiation of islet cells. A heterozygous human *ISL1* mutation has been reported in a single patient with type 2 diabetes. Mutations in the *Pax4*

and *Pax6* genes produce profound abnormalities in developmental formation of murine pancreatic endocrine cells.[7] Binding sites for the MODY genes *PDX1*, *HNF1A*, and *HNF4A* have been identified in the PAX4 promoter, suggesting that MODY genes may be upstream regulators of genes critical for islet cell formation and islet function in the pancreas. Single-nucleotide polymorphisms in *PAX4* occur more commonly in some subjects with MODY, and a human kindred with aniridia and a *PAX6* mutation exhibited impaired glucose tolerance associated with evidence for impaired processing of proinsulin.[8] Although islet function has not been extensively studied in humans with *PAX6* mutations, subjects harboring a PAX6 SNP rs685428 AG (in the noncoding region) exhibit reduced islet *PAX6* and *PCSK1* expression, a lower proinsulin/insulin ratio, decreased arginine-stimulated insulin levels, and reduced circulating levels of gastric inhibitory polypeptide (GIP) and glucagon. Nevertheless, the risk of developing diabetes was not increased in subjects with this allele.[9]

Genes encoding members of the Notch receptor family, their ligands, and downstream targets are essential for developmental formation of the endocrine pancreas (see Table 38-1). Targeted inactivation of genes in the Notch signaling pathway markedly perturbs the normal development and differentiation of pancreatic endocrine cells. Mice lacking neurogenin 3 (Ngn3, also designated Neurog3), a basic helix-loop-helix (bHLH) transcription factor, fail to develop pancreatic endocrine cells and die from diabetes postnatally, whereas overexpression of Ngn3 produces accelerated differentiation of pancreatic endocrine cells. These findings, taken together with the loss of Isl1, Pax4, Pax6, and NeuroD expression in *Ngn3*[−/−] mice, implicate Ngn3 as a key upstream regulator of pancreatic endocrine cell development.

NEUROD1 is a bHLH transcription factor that plays an important role in the development of the endocrine pancreas. Mice lacking this gene fail to develop mature islets, with severe insulin deficiency and death within the first few days of life. Heterozygous loss-of-function mutations in *NEUROD1* have been identified as a very rare cause of MODY and late-onset diabetes in humans.[10] Homozygous mutations in this gene have also been associated with permanent neonatal diabetes mellitus. Unlike other MODY genes, variation in *NEUROD1* does not appear to play a role in the pathogenesis of type 2 diabetes.[11,12] Common genetic variation in this locus was reported to predispose to type 1 diabetes, but testing in larger cohorts has shown no association with the disease.[13]

The transcription factor Arx is expressed in an Ngn3-dependent manner, and targeted inactivation of the *Arx* gene results in hypoglycemia and neonatal lethality, with a failure to develop islet alpha cells.[14] Similarly, the Nkx transcription factor family appears to be essential for the formation of beta and alpha cell lineages in the mouse.[15] Targeted deletion of the *Nkx2.2* gene produced murine islets expressing ghrelin,[16] and subsequent studies demonstrated that ghrelin is produced within a subset of normal islet alpha cells and in a small proportion of newly identified ghrelin-producing epsilon cells.[16] Research into the identification of upstream control mechanisms and downstream targets that promote islet cell formation, growth, and differentiation is proceeding rapidly and informing scientists and clinicians about the genetic determinants regulating the growth of endocrine cells.[17,18] Studies have used the power of modern genetics to identify gene mutations in individuals with neonatal diabetes; 75% of the mutations identified in genes do not encode for transcription factors, and 25% of the mutations correspond to genes controlling transcription and often development of the endocrine or entire pancreas.[19] Table 38-1 summarizes the genetic mutations associated with abnormal formation of pancreatic endocrine cells in the mouse.

ENDOCRINE CELL DEVELOPMENT IN THE INTESTINE

Stem cells associated with the intestinal epithelium differentiate into four cell lineages: enterocytes, Paneth cells, goblet cells, and enteroendocrine cells. In mice, the bHLH gene *Atoh1* (formerly designated *Math1*) is a critical regulator of intestinal secretory cell lineages. Deletion of *Atoh1* results in failure to develop goblet, Paneth, or enteroendocrine cell lineages.[20] The enteroendocrine cell population comprises less than 1% of all intestinal epithelial cells but represents the largest mass of endocrine cells in the body. Compared with pancreatic endocrine cell development, much less is known about the molecular control of enteroendocrine cell formation and differentiation. Numerous enteroendocrine cell types have been identified that can be classified based on morphologic criteria and expression of one or more secretory products. In the stomach, gastrin cells first appear in the duodenum; they localize to the antrum and pylorus in adult gastric mucosa. In the small bowel, a secretin-precursor cell appears to be important for enteroendocrine cell lineage formation. In the murine colon, PYY is the first detectable hormone marking the appearance of enteroendocrine cells; it is coexpressed in most endocrine cells in the large intestine as they first differentiate. Gene expression profiling of individual enteroendocrine cell populations reveals that most cells are plurihormonal and exhibit surprisingly few unique differences in expression of transcription factors across the small and large intestines.

The Notch signaling pathway is essential for developmental formation of enteroendocrine cells. Activation of the Notch pathway in mice results in increased expression of the bHLH transcriptional repressor Hes1, which functionally antagonizes bHLH genes that regulate cellular differentiation. Mice deficient in *Hes1* demonstrate premature cellular differentiation and severe pancreatic hypoplasia due to depletion of pancreatic epithelial precursors.[21] These mice also demonstrate excessive differentiation of multiple endocrine cell types in the developing stomach and gut, suggesting that Hes1 is a negative regulator of endodermal endocrine differentiation. Ngn3 is expressed at early time points during gut development and is essential for development of enteroendocrine cells in the small intestine[22] and stomach.[23] Notch1 and Ngn3 act upstream of BETA2/NeuroD, which is also important for differentiation of endocrine cells in the intestine (Table 38-2).[24]

Mice homozygous for a null mutation in the *Pdx1* gene demonstrate poorly differentiated duodenal intestinal epithelium with absence of Brunner glands and a deficiency of gastrin cells in the stomach. Just distal to the abnormal epithelium, the number of enteroendocrine cells is reduced. In contrast, expression of Pdx1 in gut epithelial cells redirects cell lineage toward an enteroendocrine phenotype. Inactivation of BETA2/NeuroD in mice results in absence of secretin- and cholecystokinin (CCK)-producing enteroendocrine cells.[24] The complexity of lineage relationships between gut endocrine cell populations is further illustrated by studies in mice with targeted ablation of secretin-producing cells. These mice exhibit almost complete elimination of enteroendocrine cell populations producing CCK, PYY, and glucagon and a reduction in cells producing GIP, somatostatin, and serotonin.[25] Similarly

TABLE 38-2

Consequences of Disruption of Genes Important for Development of Enteroendocrine Cells

Gene	Phenotype in Homozygous (–/–) Mutant Mice
Hes1	Enhanced numbers of enteroendocrine cells
Insm1	Defective enteroendocrine cell differentiation
NeuroD	Absent secretin and CCK lineages
Ngn3	Absent enteroendocrine cell development in the small intestine
Nkx2.2	Abnormal allocation of gut endocrine cell lineages
Pax4	Reduced endocrine cell lineages in duodenum and stomach
Pax6	Reduced number of GIP + K cells, antral gastrin and somatostatin cells, and L cells
Pdx1	Reduced enteroendocrine cells in stomach and duodenum
Ihh	Reduced enteroendocrine cells in duodenum

CCK, cholecystokinin; GIP, gastric inhibitory polypeptide.

combined deletion of *Foxa1* and *Foxa2* from the gut results in reduction of selected endocrine cell lineages.

Members of the *Pax* gene family are also essential for the formation of enteroendocrine cells (see Table 38-2). In mice, targeted disruption of *Pax4* markedly reduces the number of murine duodenal cells immunopositive for serotonin, secretin, GIP, PYY, and CCK and decreases the number of somatostatin- and serotonin-positive cells in the stomach. Complete disruption of the *Pax6* locus more selectively reduces the number of duodenal cells expressing GIP and CCK[26] and decreases the number of gastrin- and somatostatin-immunopositive cells in the stomach, whereas Sey-Neu mice that express a dominant negative mutant *Pax6* allele demonstrate markedly reduced levels of *Gcg* messenger RNA (mRNA) transcripts in the small and large intestines, with almost complete depletion of enteroendocrine cells exhibiting glucagon-like peptide 1 (GLP-1) and glucagon-like peptide 2 (GLP-2) immunoreactivity (Fig. 38-1).[27] Nkx2.2 appears to control the expression of Pax6, and *Nkx2*-null mice exhibit significant reductions in expression of CCK, gastrin, glucagon, GIP, neurotensin, and somatostatin.[28] The historical classification of enteroendocrine cells is based principally on the phenotype ascribed to the production of one or more peptide hormones. However, enteroendocrine cell subpopulations exhibit multiple plurihormonal phenotypes, necessitating reconsideration of earlier concepts. Insights gained from the differentiation of progenitor stem cells into functioning islets will also help inform our understanding of the development of enteroendocrine cells.[29]

PANCREATIC AND GUT HORMONES

Amylin

Amylin, also known as islet amyloid–associated peptide, is a 37–amino acid hormone produced in islet beta cells and in scattered endocrine cells in the stomach and the proximal small intestine. Exogenous administration of amylin inhibits gastric emptying and glucagon secretion in rodents and humans. Excess amylin secretion and deposition in the endocrine pancreas has been implicated as a potential pathogenic feature in some subjects with type 2 diabetes, and transgenic mice engineered to overexpress human amylin develop islet amyloid and impaired insulin secretion after a high-fat feeding.[30] Amylin exerts its actions through interaction with the calcitonin receptor in the presence of a receptor activity–modifying protein (RAMP). Mice deficient in amylin display modest perturbations in islet function and enhanced glucose clearance after a

+/+   −/−

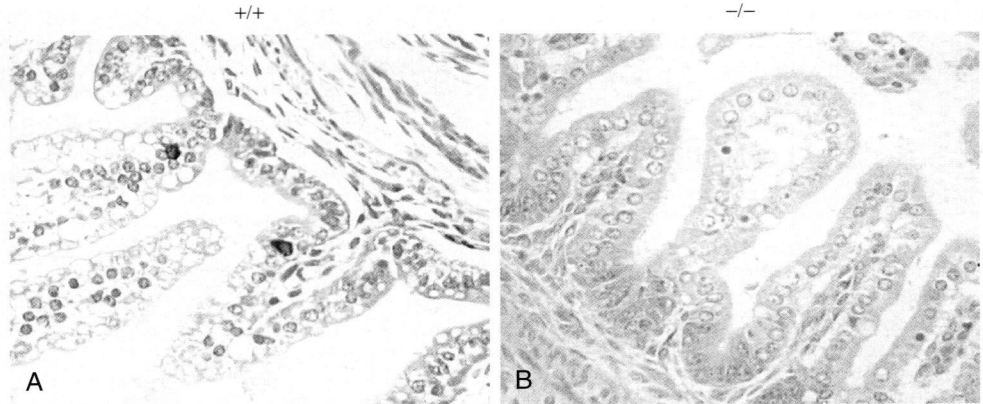

Figure 38-1 A, *Pax6* is an essential requirement for glucagon-immunopositive enteroendocrine cell formation in the murine intestine. **B,** *Pax6* Sey-Neu mutant mice (−/−) exhibit markedly reduced numbers of glucagon-immunopositive cells in the small and large intestine.

glucose challenge. The role of gut-derived amylin in human physiology has not been clearly established, but the amylin analogue pramlintide is approved for the adjunctive treatment of type 1 and type 2 diabetes with concomitant insulin administration.[31] It delays gastric emptying in a dose-dependent manner through vagally mediated mechanisms. Intriguingly, there seems to be a differential dose-response relationship to pramlintide in amylin-deficient (type 1 diabetes) states compared to amylin-sufficient (type 2 diabetes) states, with gastrointestinal symptoms that are more prominent in the former at lower doses. Although amylin expression has been detected in pancreatic and gut endocrine tumors, a specific syndrome attributable to amylin overexpression has not been delineated.

Apelin

Apelin is a 36–amino acid peptide originally purified from bovine stomach extracts that was determined to be the endogenous ligand for the orphan G protein–coupled receptor APJ (now designated APLNR).[32] Apelin and its receptor are widely expressed in peripheral tissues, such as the lung, heart, and mammary gland, and in the central nervous system (CNS); in the gastrointestinal tract, apelin is most abundant in the stomach.[33] Apelin promotes cardiomyogenesis during development and produces vasodilator and inotropic actions in the adult cardiovascular system.[34] The apelin system shares significant similarities with the renin-angiotensin system, and the two systems may have antagonistic and overlapping roles. Apelin is downregulated in left ventricular dysfunction, exerts cardioprotective and vasodilatory actions in preclinical and clinical studies, and functions as an adipokine, enhancing insulin action in mouse models of insulin resistance.[35] The apelin receptor functions as a coreceptor for human immunodeficiency virus (HIV) in vitro, and apelin-related peptides act as antagonists of HIV infection.[34]

Calcitonin Gene–Related Peptide

Calcitonin gene–related peptide (CGRP) is a member of a larger family of peptides that includes calcitonin, amylin, and adrenomedullin. In humans, distinct genes *CALCA* and *CALCB* encode calcitonin and CGRP and give rise to two 37–amino acid, carboxy-terminal–amidated neuropeptides designated α-CGRP and β-CGRP. These neuropeptides share considerable amino acid sequence homology, with a difference of only three amino acids in humans. α-CGRP is expressed predominantly in primary afferent sensory neurons arising from the spinal cord, whereas β-CGRP is

TABLE 38-3

Location of Enteroendocrine Cells and Their Associated Peptide Hormones in the Gastrointestinal Tract

Hormones	Enteroendocrine Cell	Location
Somatostatin	D cells	Stomach, duodenum, small intestine, colon
Gastrin, TRH	G cells	Stomach and duodenum
CCK	I cells	Duodenum and jejunum
GIP	K cells	Duodenum and proximal jejunum
GLP-1, GLP-2, PYY	L cells	Ileum, colon, and rectum
Motilin	M cells	Duodenum and proximal jejunum
Neurotensin	N cells	Small intestine, especially ileum
Secretin	S cells	Duodenum and proximal jejunum

CCK, cholecystokinin; GIP, gastric inhibitory polypeptide; GLP, glucagon-like peptide; PYY, peptide YY; TRH, thyrotropin-releasing hormone.

expressed in enteric neurons. Two calcitonin/CGRP seven-transmembrane domain, G protein–coupled receptors[36] interact with a family of RAMPs; coexpression of calcitonin receptor–like receptor with RAMP1 results in ligand specificity for CGRP, whereas expression of the same receptor with RAMP2 results in specificity for adrenomedullin.[37]

CGRP immunoreactivity has been localized to enteroendocrine cells in the human rectum and to endocrine cells and neurons in the small intestine. Intestinal CGRP is released in response to glucose and by gastric acid secretion. CGRP produces marked vasodilatation in the stomach, splanchnic, and peripheral circulation through stimulation of nitric oxide release. CGRP also inhibits gastric acid and pancreatic exocrine secretion, probably through stimulation of somatostatin release. Although focal CGRP positivity has been detected in some human carcinoid and pancreatic endocrine tumors, its utility as a tumor marker has not been firmly established.

Cholecystokinin

CCK was first characterized as a factor that stimulates gallbladder contraction. The *CCK* gene is expressed in open-type enteroendocrine cells in the proximal small intestine (Table 38-3) and in nerve fibers branching to the gastric and colonic myenteric plexus and submucosal plexus, where CCK acts as a neurotransmitter. CCK-immunoreactive peptides are found in the cerebral cortex and in the limbic system, as well as in pituitary corticotrophs, C cells of the thyroid, adrenal medulla, and acrosome of the developing and mature spermatozoa. The *CCK* gene encodes a

94–amino acid prohormone that is post-translationally processed in a tissue-specific fashion into multiple molecular forms, including CCK-83, CCK-58, CCK-39, CCK-33, CCK-22, CCK-8, and CCK-5, all sharing a common carboxy-terminus. The major active form, CCK-8, is an octapeptide containing a sulfated tyrosine residue and an amidated carboxy-terminal phenylalanine residue. CCK-33 appears to be the predominant circulating form in human plasma.[38]

CCK binds with high affinity to CCKAR, a seven-transmembrane domain, G protein–coupled receptor expressed in pancreatic acinar cells, gallbladder, smooth muscle, chief and D cells of the gastric mucosa, and the central and peripheral nervous systems. In the stomach, CCK inhibits proximal gastric motility while increasing the force of antral and pyloric contractions. CCK also regulates meal-stimulated pancreatic enzyme secretion and gallbladder contraction, and CCK action mediates fat-stimulated GLP-1 secretion in human subjects.[39]

CCK exhibits trophic effects on pancreatic acini in rats. Experimental manipulations that increase levels of circulating CCK, such as treatment with soybean trypsin inhibitor or long-term pancreatobiliary diversion, result in pancreatic growth and premalignant changes. Elevated circulating levels of CCK also enhanced the development of preneoplastic acinar lesions induced by azaserine, a pancreatic carcinogen in rats. In contrast, the Otsuka Long-Evans Tokushima Fatty (OLETF) rat fails to express a functional CCKAR and exhibits reduced pancreatic size.[40] The CCKB receptor (CCKBR) mediates the trophic actions of progastrin in murine normal and neoplastic gut.[41] Although CCK/gastrin receptors are expressed in early pancreatic intraepithelial neoplasia lesions and in human pancreatic cancer, the importance of CCK receptor signaling for tumor promotion or growth remains uncertain.[42]

Exogenous administration of CCK decreases the size of spontaneously ingested meals, whereas CCKAR antagonists increase appetite and delay gastric emptying in humans. A human subject with autoimmune polyglandular syndrome type 1 exhibited severe diarrhea and malabsorption associated with reduced numbers of enteroendocrine cells and CCK deficiency.[43] CCK secretion in response to oral nutrient ingestion probably regulates nutrient absorption and postprandial satiety, and CCK-8 regulates hepatic glucose production through a CNS-dependent CCKAR mechanism that may be defective in the setting of obesity-induced insulin resistance.[44] Nevertheless, CCK receptors do not appear to be essential for weight regulation in vivo because mice with targeted disruption of Cckar and Cckbr exhibit normal food intake and weight gain well into adult life—underlining in part the multiple redundancies of the mechanisms mediating satiation.[45]

Galanin

Galanin was initially isolated from porcine intestine as a 29–amino acid, carboxy-terminal–amidated neuropeptide. In humans, the two molecular forms of galanin are 19 and 30 amino acids long. Galanin is expressed in the central and peripheral nervous systems, in the pituitary, and in the neural structures of the gut, pancreas, thyroid, and adrenal gland. In the intestine, galanin immunoreactivity is detected predominantly within enteric neurons located in the myenteric and submucosal plexus that innervate the mucosa and the circular and longitudinal smooth muscle layers. Galanin is released by enteric neurons in response to intestinal distention, chemical stimulation of the mucosa, and electrical stimulation of periarterial nerves and extrinsic sympathetic neurons.

At least three galanin receptor subtypes have been identified: GALR1, GALR2, and GALR3; they are widely expressed in gastric and intestinal smooth muscle cells, in the pancreas, and in the CNS.[46] Galanin regulates food intake, memory and cognition, and antinociception, and it modulates multiple neuroendocrine systems in the pituitary, pancreas, and gut. Galanin exhibits potent anticonvulsant activity in experimental rodent models of seizure disorders,[47] and it likely acts through modulation of glutamate release. Galanin may also act as a neuroprotective factor, and galanin knockout mice exhibit enhanced sensitivity to neuronal injury.[48] Although $Galr1^{-/-}$ mice exhibit increased anxiety and abnormal nociceptive sensitivity, mice with inactivation of $Galr2$ are normal and do not exhibit defects in classic phenotypes ascribed to galanin.

Galanin knockout mice that have reduced levels of prolactin and complete failure of lactation exemplify the importance of galanin in pituitary lactotroph biology. Although galanin can inhibit GIP- and GLP-1-induced proinsulin gene transcription and insulin secretion, galanin knockout mice exhibit paradoxically impaired insulin secretion but infusion of galanin in diabetic and nondiabetic humans has no effect on plasma glucose concentrations.[49,50] Galanin also inhibits pancreatic exocrine secretion and intestinal ion transport, and it induces contraction and relaxation of intestinal smooth muscle. In humans, intravenous administration of galanin delays gastric emptying and prolongs colonic transit times. Although galanin expression has been detected in hypothalamic, pituitary, and adrenal tumors, galanin immunopositivity in pancreatic or gut endocrine tumor cells is rare.

Gastric Inhibitory Polypeptide

GIP, also called glucose-dependent insulinotropic polypeptide, is a 42–amino acid peptide secreted by enteroendocrine K cells located in the duodenum and proximal jejunum. GIP levels rise immediately after nutrient ingestion, leading to modest inhibitory effects on gastric acid secretion and gastrointestinal motility. The precise role of GIP as an enterogastrone remains controversial, because supraphysiologic concentrations of GIP are required to inhibit gastric acid secretion and gastric emptying in humans.

The actions of GIP on the pancreatic beta cell are primarily those of an incretin, a gut-derived peptide that stimulates insulin secretion in the setting of raised plasma glucose levels after oral nutrient ingestion. GIP receptor knockout mice exhibit impaired oral glucose tolerance and enhanced susceptibility to diabetes after high-fat feeding.[51] GIP receptors are expressed on adipocytes, where they modulate lipid accumulation. Transient blockade of GIP receptor signaling with GIP antagonists or genetic elimination of the GIP receptor in mice reduces fat storage in adipocytes and may contribute to improved insulin sensitivity through reduction of body weight and adipokine expression.[52]

GIP is an essential determinant of bone resorption in rodents, but the role of GIP in the control of bone turnover in human subjects remains uncertain. Experimental and clinical diabetes is associated with defective GIP action and reduced insulinotropic activity of exogenous GIP. The reduced insulinotropic activity of GIP in diabetic subjects can be partially reversed by a brief period of insulin administration.[53] GIP-secreting endocrine tumors are rare, but gut-derived GIP may contribute to the development of food-induced Cushing syndrome in a subset of patients with adrenal adenomas that express the GIP receptor.[54] The suitability of GIP analogues or GIP-based co-agonists for the treatment of diabetes and obesity remains a subject of active investigation.[55]

Gastrin

A single mRNA transcript encodes a preprogastrin precursor of 101 amino acids that undergoes post-translational processing into many biologically active molecular forms of circulating gastrin, including G-34, G-17, and G-14. Gastrin is produced predominantly in G cells located in the gastric antrum and duodenal bulb, but gastrin immunoreactivity has also been detected in the central and peripheral nervous systems, pituitary, adrenal gland, genital tract, respiratory tract, and tumors. The fetal endocrine pancreas produces large amounts of amidated gastrin, suggesting a possible role of gastrin in pancreatic development. However, gastrin-deficient mice do not demonstrate overt abnormalities in pancreatic islet morphologic structure.

G cells are open-type endocrine cells that are subject to regulation by luminal contents in addition to humoral and neural influences. The effects of gastrin on acid secretion are mediated by the fully processed amidated forms of gastrin (G-17 and G-34) at CCKBRs (formerly known as gastrin/CCK2 receptors) located on the enterochromaffin-like (ECL) cells of the oxyntic mucosa. Gastrin stimulates histamine synthesis and release from ECL cells; histamine then induces acid secretion by binding to the histamine H_2 receptor located on the basolateral aspect of the parietal cell. Gastrin also stimulates acid secretion from parietal cells through the CCKBR.

The actions of progastrin and glycine-extended gastrin are less completely defined but involve regulation of the growth and differentiation of the gastrointestinal tract. Amidated gastrin has trophic effects on the oxyntic mucosa of the stomach, where it stimulates proliferation of gastric stem cells and ECL cells, resulting in increased parietal and ECL mass. Glycine-extended gastrin exerts trophic effects on the colonic mucosa and stimulates growth of a diverse number of human cancers. Transgenic mice expressing progastrin or glycine-extended gastrin exhibit increased colonic proliferation and mucosal thickness and are more prone to formation of aberrant crypt foci after treatment with azoxymethane, whereas inactivation of the gastrin gene results in reduced basal rates of colonic proliferation.[56] The proliferative actions of progastrin in the normal gut and in colonic neoplasms require a functional CCKBR.[41]

Gastrin induces proliferation of colon cancer cell lines expressing the CCKBR, but most colon cancers and normal colonic epithelium do not normally express this receptor. A truncated gastrin-binding receptor has been described in some colon cancer cell lines, and a constitutively active CCKBR mutant, called CCK2i4svR, that confers ligand-independent growth to transfected cells has been identified in human colorectal and pancreatic cancers.[57,58] CCKAR and CCKBR are capable of forming homodimers and heterodimers, and heterodimerization appears to modulate the sensitivity to agonist-induced cell growth.[59]

The trophic effects of gastrin prompted studies of gastrin-neutralizing antisera for the potential treatment of intestinal neoplasia.[60] Conversely, G-17 has been shown to reduce cell proliferation and induce apoptosis in human colon cancer cells expressing the CCKBR.[61] Gastrin is mitogenic for rodent and human pancreatic islet and ductal cells that have been cultured in vitro or propagated in immunodeficient, nonobese diabetic (NOD), severe combined immunodeficient (SCID) mice.[62] Treatment of mice with gastrin and epidermal growth factor or gastrin plus GLP-1 ameliorates type 1 diabetes in NOD mice, and gastrin modulates islet neogenesis in preclinical studies. Nevertheless, the use of proton pump inhibitors to increase gastrin levels in human subjects with type 2 diabetes has yielded inconsistent results in studies examining insulin secretion and glucose control.[63,64]

Gastrin-Releasing Peptide and Related Peptides

The bombesin family of peptides was originally isolated from frog skin and includes bombesin, gastrin-releasing peptide (GRP, the mammalian homolog of bombesin), neuromedin B, and neuromedin C. GRP is a 27–amino acid peptide; neuromedin B and neuromedin C are decapeptides. These peptides share an identical carboxy-terminal α-amidated heptapeptide sequence that is essential for biologic activity. GRP is expressed in the central, peripheral, and enteric nervous systems; the reproductive tract; and the lung, where it acts as a neurotransmitter. Neuromedin B is expressed predominantly in the brain and the gastrointestinal tract. Within the intestine, GRP and neuromedin B are localized to neurons in the submucosal and myenteric plexus of the stomach, small intestine, and colon. GRP-containing neurons are also distributed throughout the human pancreas. Bombesin and GRP stimulate smooth muscle cell contraction in the stomach, intestine, and gallbladder. GRP stimulates the release of CCK, gastrin, GIP, glucagon, GLP-1, GLP-2, motilin, PP, PYY, and somatostatin in some species.

Three GRP receptor subtypes that are seven-transmembrane domain, G protein–coupled receptors that bind bombesin-like peptides have been cloned. They include a GRP-preferring subtype (expressed throughout the intestine), a neuromedin B–preferring subtype (expressed in the esophageal and intestinal muscularis), and a third subtype designated bombesin receptor subtype 3, which preferentially binds GRP over neuromedin B and is expressed in testes and small cell lung cancer. GRP regulates appetite, memory, inflammatory responses, and thermoregulation and suppresses appetite after intracerebroventricular or systemic administration. Mice with knockout of the GRP-preferring receptor exhibit defective control of food intake and increased body weight gain.[65] GRP stimulates pancreatic growth in part through a CCK-dependent mechanism. The expression of GRP in human tumors with neuroendocrine properties (e.g., small cell carcinoma, medullary thyroid carcinoma) and its autocrine and endocrine effects on cell growth suggest that GRP may contribute to regulation of tumor cell growth.[66] GRP exhibits angiogenic properties, and GRP antagonists reduce tumor growth and angiogenesis in vivo.[67] The widespread expression of multiple GRP receptor subtypes in human tumors has fueled investigation of whether GRP antagonists or ligand conjugates can be used to target cancer cells for therapeutic or imaging purposes.[68,69]

Ghrelin

Ghrelin, a motilin-related peptide, is a 28–amino acid growth hormone–releasing factor that originally was purified from rat stomach. It stimulates growth hormone release through the growth hormone secretagogue receptor (GHSR). Fasting increases gastric ghrelin gene expression, and ghrelin exhibits gastric prokinetic activity and orexigenic activity after intracerebroventricular or peripheral administration through the ghrelin receptor expressed in hypothalamic nuclei. Control of ghrelin acylation is regulated by ghrelin O-acyl transferase (GOAT), which is regulated by nutrient availability, requires specific dietary lipids as acylation substrates, and links the availability of medium-chain fatty acids to control of energy expenditure and body fat mass.[70] Ghrelin and GOAT are essential for maintaining glucose levels in response to starvation via induction of growth hormone secretion.[71]

Ghrelin expression is induced by stressors, and ghrelin may play a role in the murine anxiogenic stress response in a corticotropin-releasing factor–dependent manner. Most rat and human gut endocrine cells that express ghrelin are localized to the stomach, with a small number of ghrelin-positive cells identified in the small and large intestine.[72] The GHSR also is expressed in the gut, but the function of the intestinal ghrelin-GHSR axis remains poorly understood. Ghrelin agonists directly increase the rate of gastric emptying and postprandial glycemic excursion in people with diabetes,[73,74] and ghrelin agonists have been explored for the treatment of gastroparesis.[75] Bioactive ghrelin is acylated, and circulating immunoreactive ghrelin represents a mixture of the free acylated form and molecules bound to higher-molecular-weight proteins.[72]

Circulating levels of ghrelin in human subjects increase and fall before and after food ingestion, respectively, consistent with a role for ghrelin in appetite regulation. Ghrelin can increase appetite through a direct central effect even after partial gastrectomy or esophagogastrectomy.[76,77] Many hormonal mediators regulate plasma levels of ghrelin, including PYY(3-36), which suppresses appetite in association with a reduction in circulating ghrelin. Diet-induced weight loss is associated with a compensatory increase in circulating ghrelin, but some patients with weight loss after gastric bypass surgery fail to upregulate plasma levels of ghrelin—this heterogeneity is likely attributable to differences between bariatric surgical procedures—patients who undergo Roux-en-Y gastric bypass are able to increase concentrations of acylated ghrelin in response to prolonged fasting. In contrast, after sleeve gastrectomy—which entails resection of the ghrelin-secreting portion of the stomach, there is no such increase. Whether these changes in ghrelin secretion contribute to differences in weight loss after bariatric surgery remains to be ascertained[78-81] especially given the suggestion that intact vagal innervation is required for an effect on appetite.[82]

Ghrelin exhibits several actions beyond control of appetite, including regulation of insulin sensitivity and hepatic glucose output and regulation of immature Leydig cell proliferation. Ghrelin action in the CNS increases food intake, most likely through activation of neurons containing neuropeptide Y (NPY)/agouti-related peptide. Central ghrelin infusion also enhances glucose uptake in peripheral adipose tissue. Ghrelin is expressed in pancreatic islet alpha cells and may regulate glucose-induced insulin secretion; however, human studies show only modest effects of ghrelin on glucose homeostasis.[83] Ghrelin exhibits effects on cardiovascular function, including vasodilation, inhibition of a proinflammatory response in endothelial cells, and improvement of left ventricular contractility and exercise capacity in human subjects with left ventricular failure.[84] Ghrelin agonists have been explored for the treatment of anorexia or cachexia, whereas ongoing efforts continue to assess the utility of blocking ghrelin or inhibiting GOAT for the treatment of obesity.[85]

Glucagon, Glucagon-like Peptide 1, and Glucagon-like Peptide 2

The proglucagon gene is expressed in the pancreatic alpha cell, the intestinal L cell, and specialized regions of the brain, primarily neurons in the brainstem and, to a lesser extent, in the hypothalamus. In mammals, a single proglu-cagon precursor is differentially processed to yield multiple proglucagon-derived peptides, including glucagon in the islet alpha cell and glicentin, oxyntomodulin, GLP-1, GLP-2, and several spacer or intervening peptides in the gut enteroendocrine L cell. GLP-1 (liberated by prohormone convertase 1) may be produced in islet alpha cells after islet or pancreatic inflammation or injury, whereas glucagon, liberated by prohormone convertase 2, may be synthesized in gastric or intestinal endocrine cells in settings characterized by pancreatic or intestinal resection or injury.[86]

Pancreatic glucagon is a 29–amino acid peptide that regulates plasma glucose levels through effects on gluconeogenesis and glycogenolysis. Glucagon excess represents one of the hallmark metabolic derangements that contribute to hyperglycemia in type 1 and type 2 diabetes.[87] Conversely, increased glucagon secretion functions as the primary counterregulatory mechanism to restore normal levels of plasma glucose in the setting of hypoglycemia, and individuals who are prone to frequent episodes of hypoglycemia may use glucagon injections for emergency management of severe hypoglycemia. The physiologic importance of glucagon action has been examined after genetic or transient interruption of glucagon receptor expression. Glucagon receptor knockout mice exhibit modest fasting hypoglycemia, pancreatic alpha cell hyperplasia, and markedly elevated levels of circulating glucagon and GLP-1.[88] Similarly, reduction of hepatic glucagon receptor mRNA transcripts in rodents markedly lowers blood glucose, improves insulin secretion, and increases levels of circulating GLP-1 in rodents with experimental diabetes. Although glucagon receptor antagonists reduce glycemia in subjects with type 2 diabetes, modest elevations in transaminase and lipid levels raise questions about the risk/benefit ratio of blocking glucagon action in human diabetics.[89]

GLP-1 secreted from the gut endocrine cell enhances glucose disposal after nutrient ingestion by stimulation of insulin and inhibition of glucagon secretion.[90] Preclinical studies demonstrate that GLP-1 inhibits food intake, stimulates pancreatic islet neogenesis and proliferation, and inhibits beta-cell apoptosis, biologic actions that facilitate long-term control of nutrient homeostasis (Fig. 38-2). The physiologic importance of endogenous GLP-1 has been

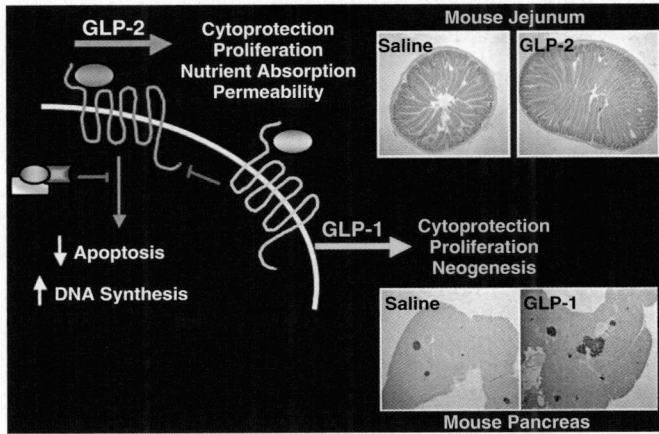

Figure 38-2 Molecular mechanisms of glucagon-like peptide (GLP) action. The GLP-1 receptor expressed on islet beta cells promotes growth and cytoprotection, leading to expansion of beta-cell mass. The GLP-2 receptor, expressed on human gut endocrine cells, enteric neurons, and myofibroblasts, indirectly activates pathways coupled to control of mucosal permeability, cell proliferation, and apoptosis, leading to expansion of the surface area of the small bowel mucosal epithelium.

studied using the GLP-1 receptor antagonist exendin(9-39) and *Glp1r*$^{-/-}$ mice. Exendin(9-39) deteriorates glycemic control, increases insulin and decreases glucagon levels, and accelerates gastric emptying while decreasing gastric compliance in rodents and humans.[91,92] Similarly, *Glp1r*$^{-/-}$ mice exhibit defective glucose-stimulated insulin secretion, glucose intolerance, and enhanced susceptibility to islet injury. These findings illustrate the essential importance of endogenous GLP-1 in the control of islet hormone secretion and gut motility. Of note, these effects are exaggerated in patients after Roux-en-Y gastric bypass—perhaps due to underlying differences in the degree of postprandial elevation of GLP-1.[93] Several GLP-1 receptor agonists have been approved for the treatment of type 2 diabetes including small peptides with short circulating half-lives (exenatide, lixisenatide) and an acylated human GLP-1 analogue with more prolonged pharmacokinetics (liraglutide). Several GLP-1 receptor agonists are suitable for once weekly administration (exenatide once weekly, albiglutide, dulaglutide); all of these agents are associated with weight loss or prevention of weight gain in randomized clinical trials of subjects with type 2 diabetes.[94] The principal side effects associated with the use of GLP-1 receptor agonists are gastrointestinal, predominantly nausea. Antibodies against exenatide or lixisenatide are detected in about 40% to 70% of treated patients but do not seem to correlate with therapeutic outcome. Liraglutide appears to be slightly more effective in controlling blood glucose, compared with twice-daily exenatide, lixisenatide, or albiglutide.[95] Most once-weekly GLP-1 receptor agonists appear to be better tolerated than the shorter-acting agonists. Whether better tolerability reflects gastrointestinal tachyphylaxis to sustained GLP-1 receptor agonism or differences in pharmacokinetics remains to be ascertained.[96]

GLP-2 is a 33–amino acid peptide cosecreted with GLP-1, oxyntomodulin, and glicentin from enteroendocrine cells in a nutrient-dependent manner. GLP-2 inhibits both centrally induced antral motility and meal-stimulated gastric acid secretion. GLP-2 exhibits trophic actions in the small intestine and colon (see Fig. 38-2) through stimulation of crypt cell proliferation and reduction of apoptosis within the crypt and villus compartments.[97] GLP-2 also enhances intestinal epithelial barrier function and stimulates gut blood flow and intestinal nutrient absorption.[98] Preclinical studies demonstrate that GLP-2 prevents injury and enhances repair, regeneration, and function in the gastrointestinal epithelium.[98,99] Teduglutide, a degradation-resistant human GLP-2 receptor agonist, reduces requirements for parenteral nutrition support and is approved for treatment of human subjects with short bowel syndrome.[100]

The actions of GLP-1 and GLP-2 are transduced through distinct receptors, and both peptides are rapidly cleaved at the position 2 alanine by dipeptidyl peptidase 4 (DPP4). Genetic elimination of DPP4 action in rodents increased the levels of GIP and GLP-1, enhanced glucose-stimulated insulin secretion, and lowered blood glucose levels.[101] Conversely, chemical inhibitors of DPP4 lowered glucose and hemoglobin A_{1c} values in preclinical models and in humans with type 2 diabetes.[94] Several DPP4 inhibitors (e.g., sitagliptin, vildagliptin, saxagliptin, alogliptin, linagliptin) are approved for the treatment of type 2 diabetes. They increase insulin and suppress postprandial glucagon secretion but do not produce changes in gastrointestinal motility, satiety, or body weight.[94,102] Incretin signaling is necessary for the glucose lowering of DPP-4 inhibitors.[103]

In contrast to GLP-1 and GLP-2, the biologic actions of the proglucagon-derived peptides glicentin and oxyntomodulin are less well established. Glicentin is trophic for the gut mucosal epithelium, whereas oxyntomodulin

inhibits short-term food intake and pentagastrin-stimulated gastric acid secretion in vitro and in vivo. Oxyntomodulin administered three times daily for 4 weeks reduced body weight in overweight and obese human subjects.[104] Although distinct G protein–coupled receptors for glucagon, GLP-1, and GLP-2 have been characterized, separate receptors that mediate the actions of glicentin and oxyntomodulin have not been identified, and the anorectic action of oxyntomodulin requires a functional GLP-1 receptor.[105] Oxyntomodulin simultaneously activates both glucagon and GLP-1 receptors, and oxyntomodulin mimetics resulted in enhanced weight loss in preclinical models compared with the actions of GLP-1 receptor agonists alone.[106] Multiple co-agonists targeting the glucagon, GLP-1, or GIP receptors exhibit enhanced activity on appetite and weight loss and are being explored for the treatment of human subjects with diabetes and obesity.[55]

Motilin

Motilin is a 22–amino acid peptide originally isolated from porcine intestine. Motilin immunoreactivity has been detected in open-type enteroendocrine epithelial M cells located predominantly in the duodenum and proximal jejunum. Secretion of motilin occurs in a cyclic manner during the interdigestive state between meals. The presence of nutrients in the duodenum suppresses the endogenous release of motilin in dogs and humans. Duodenal alkalinization, sham feeding, gastric distention, and administration of opioid agonists promote motilin secretion. A putative motilin receptor has been cloned that exhibits 52% amino acid identity with the human receptor for growth hormone secretagogues. The motilin receptor is expressed in many regions of the gastrointestinal tract, predominantly in smooth muscle and enteric neurons, and it binds the macrolide antibiotic erythromycin.[107]

Motilin induces phase III contractions in the stomach, an effect that can be abolished by food ingestion, duodenal acidification, somatostatin, pentagastrin, and CCK. Atropine and 5-hydroxytryptamine antagonists also abolish phase III contractions, emphasizing the importance of the cholinergic and serotoninergic neuronal pathways. Motilin stimulates gastric and pancreatic enzyme secretion and induces contraction of the gallbladder, sphincter of Oddi, and lower esophageal sphincter. Administration of motilin induces nausea and inhibits gastric emptying in human subjects, and erythromycin-related antibiotics exhibit functional antagonist and prokinetic activity through the motilin receptor.[108]

Neuropeptide Y

NPY is primarily synthesized and secreted by neurons in the central and peripheral nervous systems. In the brain, NPY is expressed in the hypothalamus, where it exhibits extremely potent effects on nutrient intake, and in the cortex, hippocampus, basal forebrain striation, limbic structures, amygdala, and brainstem. In the peripheral nervous system, NPY expression occurs predominantly in sympathetic neurons and in the myenteric and submucous plexuses of the enteric nervous system. NPY and vasoactive intestinal peptide (VIP) are often coexpressed in enteric neurons. NPY is synthesized in and released from pancreatic islet cells, and it inhibits glucose-stimulated insulin secretion through the Y1 receptor. Elevated circulating NPY levels are observed after sympathetic nervous system activation and in patients with pancreatic endocrine tumors and carcinoid tumors or neurogenic tumors, including neuroblastomas and pheochromocytomas.

NPY exerts its actions through at least four receptor subtypes, including the Y1 and Y2 receptors, which bind NPY and PYY with similar affinities, and the Y3 receptor, which exhibits a preference for NPY over PYY. Increased hypothalamic NPY is a potent stimulator of food intake in rodents, but NPY antagonists have not proved useful for the treatment of human obesity. NPY is also produced in adipocytes, where it promotes adipogenesis. NPY actions in the cardiovascular system include stimulation of vascular smooth muscle cell growth and neointima formation through Y1 and Y1 receptors, and its angiogenic effects are mediated through Y2 and Y5 receptor activation.[109] NPY and PYY are targets for amino-terminal degradation by the enzyme DPP4, leading to the generation of NPY(3-36) and PYY(3-36), peptides that exhibit preferential binding to the Y2 receptor. In the gastrointestinal tract, NPY reduces fluid and electrolyte secretion and inhibits gastric and small intestinal motility. Intravascular administration of NPY is associated with marked vasoconstriction of the splanchnic circulation, independent of α- or β-adrenergic signaling.

Neurotensin

Neurotensin is a 13–amino acid peptide originally detected in bovine hypothalamus. Neurotensin-related peptides include neuromedin N (a 6–amino acid, neurotensin-like peptide coencoded in proneurotensin), xenin, and xenopsin. In the gastrointestinal tract, processing favors the generation of neurotensin in N cells of the ileum and in enteric neurons. Neurotensin also is produced in the central and peripheral nervous systems, heart, adrenals, pancreas, and respiratory tract. Neurotensin secretion is stimulated by luminal nutrients, especially lipids, but not by amino acids or carbohydrates. GRP also stimulates neurotensin release, and somatostatin exerts an inhibitory effect.

At least three neurotensin receptors or neurotensin-binding proteins have been identified. NTS1 and NTS2 belong to the G protein–coupled receptor family, whereas NTS3 represents a structurally unrelated protein with neurotensin-binding properties.[110] NTS1 is expressed in the brain and intestine, whereas NTS2 and NTS3 are expressed exclusively in the brain. Neurotensin administration to rats augments the adaptive response to small bowel resection in the intestinal remnant, and neurotensin stimulates growth of the colonic epithelium in vivo. Neurotensin also inhibits postprandial gastric acid secretion and pancreatic exocrine secretion, stimulates colonic motility, and inhibits gastric and small intestinal motility. Neurotensin facilitates fatty acid uptake in the proximal small intestine and induces histamine release from mast cells. Neurotensin receptor expression has been detected in a subset of human colon and pancreatic ductal cancers, and neurotensin is trophic for some pancreatic and colon cancer cells in vitro. Experiments using neurotensin antagonists or knockout mice have suggested a role for neurotensin in pain perception or nociception, and reduction of neurotensin action improves survival in preclinical models of sepsis.[111]

Pituitary Adenylate Cyclase–Activating Peptide

Pituitary adenylate cyclase–activating peptide (PACAP), VIP, and growth hormone–releasing factor (GHRH, somatocrinin) are structurally related members of the glucagon/secretin superfamily.[112] PACAP-immunoreactive nerve fibers are distributed along the gastrointestinal tract from the esophagus to the colon. Both bioactive forms, PACAP-38 and PACAP-27, are detected in many tissues, and PACAP-38 is usually the predominant peptide. PACAP stimulates histamine release from the stomach; increases the secretion

of pancreatic fluid, protein, and bicarbonate; and stimulates insulin and glucagon secretion and catecholamine release. It reduces blood pressure and causes vasodilation, which may limit its therapeutic utility. PACAP-deficient mice exhibit defective glucagon responses to insulin-induced hypoglycemia. PACAP signaling in gastric ECL cells may also constitute an important component of the neural regulation of gastric acid secretion.

PACAP exerts neuroprotective actions in the CNS and peripheral nervous system, likely related to stimulation of cyclic adenosine monophosphate (cAMP) accumulation. PACAP may also play a role in the central control of ventilation; PACAP-deficient mice experience prolonged apneas, atrioventricular block, and an increased incidence of sudden death. PACAP modulates platelet function, and PACAP overexpression may be associated with increased platelet cAMP accumulation and defective platelet aggregation.[113] Three PACAP receptors (designated PAC1, VPAC1, and VPAC2) have been cloned, and they bind PACAP and VIP with different affinities. Consistent with the putative importance of PACAP for islet function, PAC1 receptor knockout mice exhibit defective glucose-stimulated insulin secretion. PACAP exhibits vasodilatory effects in the pulmonary vasculature, whereas PAC1 receptor–deficient mice exhibit pulmonary artery hypertension and right ventricular failure. PACAP also regulates normal megakaryopoiesis through the VPAC1 receptor. Whether DPP4 inhibition modulates the actions of PACAP(1-38) in vivo remains uncertain.

Peptide YY

PYY, NPY, and PP are members of the pancreatic polypeptide family. These peptides consist of 36 amino acids, contain several tyrosine residues, and share considerable amino acid identity with amidated carboxy-terminal ends. Although these peptides likely share a common ancestry, they exhibit unique actions and patterns of tissue-specific expression, with PYY and PP acting as hormones and NPY acting primarily as a neurotransmitter.

PYY is expressed in the fetal and adult gastrointestinal tract in enteroendocrine cells. Distinct enteroendocrine subpopulations have been identified that express PYY alone or express both PYY and GLP-1 in the small bowel, colon, and rectum.[114] Immunoreactive PYY has been detected in the developing endocrine pancreas and in a subpopulation of glucagon-producing alpha cells in mature islets. PYY is secreted as a 36–amino acid peptide, and it circulates as two molecular forms, PYY(1-36) and PYY(3-36), an amino-terminally truncated form. Luminal nutrients, CCK, GRP, and vagal tone regulate PYY secretion.

PYY exerts its actions in part through the NPY Y1 and Y2 receptors. Whereas PYY(1-36) binds both Y1 and Y2 receptors, PYY(3-36) is selective for the Y2 receptor. PYY demonstrates inhibitory effects on gastrointestinal secretion, motility, and blood flow. In the stomach, PYY functions as an enterogastrone, inhibiting gastric acid secretion and gastric emptying. PYY also increases intestinal transit times by inhibiting motility of the small and large intestine. The role of PYY as an intestinal epithelial growth factor remains unclear, but some studies have demonstrated an intestinotrophic effect of PYY in rodents. In the pancreas, PYY(1-36) and PYY(3-36) inhibit pancreatic exocrine secretion.

Administration of PYY(3-36) to rodents and to normal and obese humans potently inhibited food intake in short-term studies, and PYY(3-36) produced a conditioned taste aversion in some but not all studies in rodents. Functional magnetic resonance imaging (MRI) studies demonstrated that infusion of PYY(3-36) in humans produces changes in neural activity within corticolimbic and higher cortical areas and in homeostatic brain regions that mimic neuronal activity pursuant to meal ingestion.[115] Obese humans exhibit attenuated release of PYY(3-36), and alterations in these signals may lead to increased hunger or reduced satiety in response to meal ingestion. Whether prolonged PYY(3-36) administration can produce weight loss in obese humans has not been determined.

PYY concentrations after bariatric surgery rise to a degree proportional to the rate of distal delivery of calories so that procedures that do not change gastric emptying such as adjustable gastric banding do not change PYY, whereas procedures such as Roux-en-Y gastric bypass raise PYY concentrations after a meal challenge. Nevertheless, selective administration of a Y2 receptor–selective antagonist had no effect on the magnitude of weight loss achieved following gastric bypass surgery in mice.[116]

Pancreatic Polypeptide

PP was isolated from chicken pancreatic extracts as a by-product of insulin purification. Most PP is expressed in pancreatic endocrine cells located predominantly in the periphery of islets in the pancreatic head and uncinate process. Elevated plasma levels of PP have been detected in patients with gastrointestinal endocrine tumors, and PP may be used as a tumor marker in appropriate clinical scenarios. Nutrients, hormones, neurotransmitters, gastric distention, insulin-induced hypoglycemia, and direct vagal nerve stimulation regulate PP secretion, whereas hyperglycemia, bombesin, and somatostatin inhibit PP secretion. The PP response to sham feeding has been used as a test of vagal integrity given that vagal cholinergic stimulation promotes PP secretion.[117]

The actions of PP are mediated by the Y4 receptor, a G protein–coupled receptor linked to inhibition of cAMP accumulation.[118] The human Y4 receptor is expressed in the stomach, small intestine, colon, pancreas, prostate, enteric nervous system, and certain CNS neurons. Exogenous administration of PP reduces CCK-induced gastric acid secretion and increases intestinal transit times by reducing gastric emptying and upper intestinal motility. PP also inhibits postprandial exocrine pancreas secretion through a vagus-dependent pathway. Transgenic mice that overexpress PP exhibit reduced weight gain, reduced rate of gastric emptying, and decreased fat mass, and long-acting PP analogues are being explored for the treatment of human obesity.[119] The biologic actions of PP in the gastrointestinal tract and pancreas are in part centrally mediated, and intracisternal injections of PP cause increased gastric acid secretion, increased gastric motility, and reduced pancreatic secretion. Administration of PP inhibits gastric emptying and reduces food intake in human subjects over a 24-hour study period.[120]

Secretin

Secretin is a 27–amino acid peptide that is synthesized predominantly in the brain and gastrointestinal tract. In the gut, secretin is produced by the enteroendocrine S cell in the duodenum and proximal jejunum. Gastric acid, bile salts, and luminal nutrients stimulate secretin, and somatostatin inhibits its release. Secretin stimulates pancreatic and biliary bicarbonate and water secretion and regulates pancreatic enzyme secretion; however, secretin knockout mice exhibit normal pancreatic development and adaptive responses to protease inhibition. Secretin also stimulates the gastric secretion of pepsinogen and inhibits lower esophageal sphincter tone, postprandial gastric emptying, gastrin release, and gastric acid secretion. Although secretin is expressed in the fetal endocrine pancreas, its function in islet biology remains uncertain. Only a single secretin receptor has been isolated and characterized. Secretin has been proposed as a treatment for autism, but clinical trial results have not been consistently positive.[121]

Somatostatin

Somatostatin, originally isolated as a hypothalamic growth hormone release–inhibiting factor, is expressed in the intestine and pancreas. Post-translational processing of prosomatostatin liberates somatostatin-14 and somatostatin-28, biologically active peptides corresponding to the carboxy-terminal 14 and 28 amino acids of prosomatostatin. Somatostatin-28 is the predominant molecular form liberated by enteroendocrine D cells, whereas somatostatin-14 is the predominant species liberated by D cells in the stomach and pancreas.

Five somatostatin receptor subtypes (SSTR1 through SSTR5) have been identified and are expressed in a tissue-specific manner.[122] SSTR2 modulates islet hormone secretion, whereas SSTR4 regulates inflammatory responses.[123] Variants in the SSTR2 gene have been linked to increased risk of glucose intolerance. Somatostatin actions usually are inhibitory; somatostatin inhibits the secretion of growth hormone and thyrotropin in the pituitary and inhibits secretion of insulin, glucagon, and PP in the endocrine pancreas. In the gastrointestinal tract, somatostatin inhibits the secretion of a broad range of gut peptides. Somatostatin inhibits pancreatic exocrine secretion and acts in a paracrine manner on G cells, ECL cells, and parietal cells to inhibit gastric acid secretion. In the brain, somatostatin regulates metabolism of amyloid-β peptide, a primary pathogenic agent of Alzheimer disease, by modulating proteolytic degradation catalyzed by neprilysin.[124]

The inhibitory properties of somatostatin make it suitable for the treatment of conditions characterized by excess hormone secretion. Although the circulating half-life of native somatostatin is short, longer-acting synthetic somatostatin analogues such as octreotide and lanreotide are useful in the treatment of neuroendocrine tumors, acromegaly, and portal hypertension.[125] Octreotide and lanreotide are octapeptides that bind the SSTR2 and SSTR5 receptors, which are commonly expressed in neuroendocrine tumors. A meta-analysis of clinical trials using these analogues for treatment of acromegaly demonstrated that the efficacy of long-acting release (LAR) octreotide is greater than that of sustained-release (SR) lanreotide among subjects unselected for prior somatostatin analogue responsiveness.[126] Pasireotide is a newer somatostatin analogue that has high affinity to SSTR1 through SSTR5, with greatest affinity for SSTR5, suggesting that this compound might be useful in the treatment for neuroendocrine tumors that have failed to respond to octreotide or lanreotide.[127]

Somatostatin analogues are also employed for the treatment of portal hypertension and gastrointestinal bleeding. Tumor-associated somatostatin receptor expression forms the basis for the radiolabeled octreotide scan, a test used for the detection of a broad spectrum of human neoplasms. Somatostatin-deficient mice exhibit normal growth but have defects in sexually dimorphic hepatic gene expression.

Tachykinins

The family of tachykinins includes substance P, neurokinin A, and neurokinin B, all of which share a common carboxy-terminal pentapeptide sequence essential for biologic action. Two genes encode these tachykinins: a tachykinin precursor 1 gene *(TAC1)* encodes substance P and neurokinin A, and a tachykinin 3 gene *(TAC3)* encodes neurokinin B. Tachykinins are synthesized within neurons localized to the submucous and myenteric plexuses, extrinsic sensory fibers, and enterochromaffin cells in the gut epithelium. Tachykinins are also widely distributed throughout the central and peripheral nervous systems, respiratory tract, skin, sensory organs, and urogenital tract. Four tachykinin receptors have been cloned: NK1 (TACR1), NK2 (TACR2), NK3 (TACR3), and a putative NK4 that appears to be a variant of the NK3 receptor rather than a distinct tachykinin receptor subtype. These receptors bind tachykinin peptides with different affinities. NK1 receptors preferentially bind substance P, NK2 receptors preferentially bind neurokinin A, and NK3 and NK4 receptors preferentially bind neurokinin B.[128]

Tachykinins produce a broad range of biologic actions, including regulation of inflammation and vasomotor and gastrointestinal motor activity. Germline mutations in neurokinin B *(TAC3)* or its receptor *(TACR3)* have been identified in families with hypogonadotropic hypogonadism, implicating the neurokinin B axis as a critical regulator of human reproduction.[129] The ability of tachykinins to induce vasodilatation or vasoconstriction appears to be species specific and vascular bed specific. Tachykinins exhibit direct and indirect effects on intestinal smooth muscle contractile activity. Activation of NK1 receptors on the interstitial cells of Cajal and NK2 receptors on intestinal smooth muscle cells directly promotes peristalsis, whereas activation of NK3 receptors on enteric neurons exerts a prokinetic effect that is indirectly mediated through cholinergic stimulation of enteric smooth muscle cells.

The NK1 and NK3 receptors can inhibit intestinal motility by inducing the release of inhibitory molecules such as nitric oxide and VIP from inhibitory neurons. NK2 receptors can inhibit intestinal motility by stimulation of sympathetic ganglia or activation of nonadrenergic inhibitory mechanisms. NK2 receptor antagonists reduce or prevent trinitrobenzenesulfonic acid (TNBS)-induced weight loss and intestinal injury, and an NK1 receptor antagonist exhibits protective effects in acetic acid–induced colitis and in colitis induced by the *Clostridium difficile* toxin. Tachykinins are commonly produced by gut carcinoids and may be responsible for mediating some of the clinical manifestations associated with these tumors. There is considerable interest in determining whether blockade of NK1 and NK2 receptors may represent a therapeutic approach for the treatment of asthma. Similarly, the NK1 and NK3 receptors are targets for development of therapeutic agents that modulate gut motility and pain, potentially in the setting of irritable bowel syndrome.[130]

Thyrotropin-Releasing Hormone

Originally isolated as a hypothalamic regulatory peptide, thyrotropin-releasing hormone (TRH) is expressed throughout the gastrointestinal tract, including the stomach, colon, and pancreas. In the pancreas, TRH is most abundantly expressed during perinatal development. Prepro-TRH is synthesized by islet beta cells, G cells in the stomach, and neurons composing the myenteric plexus of the esophagus, stomach, and intestine. In the stomach, histamine and serotonin stimulate and endogenous opioids inhibit TRH release. TRH acts through two related G protein–coupled receptors, TRHR1 and TRHR2. TRH suppresses pentagastrin-stimulated gastric acid secretion, and chronic administration of TRH induces pancreatic hyperplasia and inhibits amylase release. Centrally administered TRH modulates pancreatic blood flow and gastric mucosal permeability. TRH also attenuates CCK-induced gallbladder smooth muscle contraction and inhibits cholesterol synthesis within the intestinal mucosa.

Vasoactive Intestinal Peptide

VIP is a 28–amino acid member of a peptide superfamily that includes PACAP, peptide histidine isoleucine, and peptide histidine methionine, which are neurotransmitters and neuromodulators of the enteric nervous system. The *VIP* gene is widely expressed in the central and peripheral nervous systems. Receptors for VIP and PACAP belong to the same family of G protein–coupled receptors. The adenylate cyclase–activating polypeptide 1 (pituitary) receptor type 1 (ADCYAP1R1) binds PACAP(1-27) and PACAP(1-38) with the same affinity, but it is unable to bind VIP. VIP receptor 1 (VIPR1) and VIPR2 recognize both VIP and PACAP.[131]

In the digestive tract, VIP functions as an inhibitory neurotransmitter that induces relaxation of vascular and nonvascular smooth muscle. VIP mediates relaxation of the lower esophageal sphincter, sphincter of Oddi, and anal sphincter. VIPergic innervation along the intestine plays an important role in the nonadrenergic, noncholinergic inhibition of smooth muscle contraction leading to the relaxation phase of peristalsis, in part through a nitric oxide–dependent mechanism. VIP-deficient mice exhibit anatomic abnormalities of the intestine, with thickening of the muscularis propria, focal loss of the myenteric plexus, and impaired gastrointestinal transit.[132] In humans, VIP and PACAP may be co-localized to some neuronal subpopulations, and co-released as neurotransmitters, leading to nitric oxide regeneration. VIP inhibits gastric acid secretion but stimulates biliary water and bicarbonate, pancreatic enzyme, and intestinal chloride secretion. VIP may also regulate pancreatic release of insulin and glucagon, and it exerts either trophic or growth inhibitory effects on both normal and neoplastic cells.[133] In the lung, VIP functions as a bronchodilator through the VIPR2. Consistent with the importance of the ADCYAP1R1 for control of pulmonary artery pressure,[134] VIP reduced mean pulmonary artery pressure, increased cardiac output, and increased mixed venous oxygen saturation in eight human subjects with pulmonary hypertension.[135]

Miscellaneous Gut Endocrine Peptides

In addition to the peptide hormones outlined previously and summarized in Table 38-4, several other gut endocrine peptides exist. Chromogranins and secretogranins are a family of secretory proteins that are found in secretory vesicles of endocrine cells and neurons. Chromogranin A (CgA), a protein belonging to this family of peptides, induces the formation of mobile secretory granules and is secreted into the circulation by several neuroendocrine tumors, especially small gastrinomas and pheochromocytomas. Circulating levels of CgA directly correlate with tumor burden, making this a well-suited marker for assessing treatment response. CgA likely helps to regulate blood pressure, because elimination of CgA expression in a knockout mouse led to decreased size and number of chromaffin granules and hypertension, whereas transgenic expression of human CgA or exogenous injection of human catestatin, a CgA-derived cholinergic antagonist, restored normal blood pressure in CgA knockout mice.[136]

Opioid peptides regulate intestinal motility and inhibit gastric acid secretion. Neuromedin B and its receptor are

TABLE 38-4

Summary of Gastrointestinal-Derived Hormones

Hormone	Cell or Tissue of Origin	Related Peptides	Actions	Secretory Stimuli
Amylin	Pancreatic beta cell, endocrine cells of stomach and small intestine	Calcitonin, CGRP, adrenomedullin	Inhibits gastric emptying Inhibits arginine-stimulated and postprandial glucagon secretion Inhibits insulin secretion Satiety factor	Cosecreted with insulin in response to oral nutrient ingestion
CGRP	α-CGRP is expressed predominantly in afferent sensory nerves from the spinal cord β-CGRP is expressed in enteric neurons and enteroendocrine cells of the rectum	Calcitonin, amylin, adrenomedullin	Produces marked vasodilation in the splanchnic and peripheral circulation by stimulating nitric oxide release Inhibits gastric acid and pancreatic exocrine secretion Induces intestinal smooth muscle relaxation	Glucose and gastric acid secretion
CCK	Enteroendocrine I cells and enteric nerves, CNS, pituitary corticotrophs, C cells of the thyroid, adrenal medulla, and the acrosome of developing and mature spermatozoa		Inhibits proximal gastric motility while increasing antral and pyloric contractions Regulates meal-stimulated pancreatic enzyme secretion and gallbladder contraction Trophic effects on pancreatic acini in rats Postprandial satiety In the brain, CCK affects memory, sleep, sexual behavior, and anxiety	Oral nutrient ingestion Several intestine-derived hormones, including GRP and bombesin Activation of β-adrenergic receptors
Galanin	CNS and PNS, pituitary, neural structures of the gut, pancreas, thyroid, and adrenal gland		In the brain, regulation of food intake, memory and cognition, and antinociception Inhibits pancreatic exocrine secretion and intestinal ion transport Induces both contraction and relaxation of intestinal smooth muscle, depending on the species examined Delays gastric emptying and prolongs colonic transit times Inhibits secretion of insulin, PYY, gastrin, somatostatin, enteroglucagon, neurotensin, and PP	Intestinal distention Chemical stimulation of the intestinal mucosa Electrical stimulation of periarterial nerves Extrinsic sympathetic neurons
GIP	Neuroendocrine K cells in the duodenum and proximal jejunum		Inhibits gastric acid secretion and GI motility Increases insulin release and regulates glucose and lipid metabolism Exerts anabolic actions in bone	Oral nutrient ingestion, especially long-chain fatty acids
Gastrin	Predominantly enteroendocrine G cells of the stomach and duodenal bulb, CNS and PNS, pituitary, adrenal gland, genital tract, respiratory tract, fetal pancreas		Induces gastric acid secretion Amidated gastrins are trophic to the oxyntic mucosa of the stomach Progastrin and glycine-extended gastrin induce colonic epithelial proliferation	Luminal contents, especially partially digested aromatic amino acids, small peptides, calcium, coffee, and ethanol Humoral and neural influences, including the vagus nerve, β-adrenergic and GABA neurons, and GRP
GRP and related peptides	CNS, enteric nervous system, reproductive tract, and the lungs, where it acts as a neurotransmitter; GRP neurons are also distributed throughout the human pancreas	Bombesin, neuromedin B, neuromedin C	Stimulates smooth muscle contraction in the stomach, intestine, and gallbladder Stimulates release of CCK, gastrin, GIP, glucagon, GLP-1, GLP-2, motilin, PP, PYY, and somatostatin Stimulates gastric acid secretion via direct effect on G cells In the brain, regulates appetite, memory, thermogenesis, and cardiac function Stimulates pancreatic growth In the lungs, growth factor for normal and neoplastic tissue	Cholinergic stimulation
Ghrelin	CNS, stomach, small intestine, colon	Motilin	Stimulates GH release Stimulates gastric kinetic activity Orexigenic activity Stimulates energy production and signals hypothalamic regulatory nuclei that control energy homeostasis	Fasting
Glucagon	Pancreatic alpha cell, CNS		Primary counterregulatory mechanism to restore plasma glucose levels in hypoglycemia by increasing gluconeogenesis, glycogenolysis, and protein-lipid flux in the liver and periphery GI smooth muscle relaxation	Neural and humoral factors released in response to hypoglycemia

TABLE 38-4

Summary of Gastrointestinal-Derived Hormones—cont'd

Hormone	Cell or Tissue of Origin	Related Peptides	Actions	Secretory Stimuli
GLP-1	Enteroendocrine L cells located in the ileum and colon, CNS		Enhances glucose disposal after nutrient ingestion by inhibiting gastric emptying, stimulating insulin secretion, and inhibiting glucagon secretion Inhibits food intake Stimulates pancreatic islet neogenesis and proliferation Inhibits sham feeding–induced gastric acid secretion	Oral nutrient ingestion, especially carbohydrates and fat-rich meals Vagal nerve, GRP, and GIP ACh and neuromedin C Somatostatin inhibits secretion
GLP-2	Enteroendocrine L cells located in the ileum and colon, CNS		Induces small intestinal and colonic mucosal growth by stimulating crypt cell proliferation and inhibiting apoptosis Inhibits centrally induced antral motility and meal-stimulated gastric acid secretion Enhances intestinal epithelial barrier function Stimulates intestinal hexose transport Inhibits short-term control of food intake	Oral nutrient ingestion, especially carbohydrates and fat-rich meals Vagus nerve, GRP, and GIP ACh and neuromedin C Somatostatin inhibits secretion
Motilin	Brain, bronchoepithelial cells, and enteroendocrine M cells located in the duodenum and proximal jejunum	Ghrelin	Induces phase III contractions in the stomach Stimulates gastric and pancreatic enzyme secretion Induces contraction of the gallbladder, sphincter of Oddi, and LES	Duodenal alkalinization, sham feeding, gastric distention; opioid agonists promote secretion Unlike most GI hormones, motilin is suppressed in the presence of duodenal nutrients
NPY	CNS and PNS, pancreatic islet cells	PYY and PP	Potent stimulator of oral nutrient intake Inhibits glucose-stimulated insulin secretion Reduces GI fluid and electrolyte secretion Inhibits gastric and small intestine motility Induces market vasoconstriction of the splanchnic circulation	Oral nutrient ingestion Activation of the sympathetic nervous system
NT	N cells located in the small intestine mucosa, especially the ileum; CNS and PNS, including the enteric nervous system; heart, adrenal gland, pancreas, and respiratory tract	Neuromedin N, xenin, and xenopsin	Stimulates growth of the colonic epithelium Inhibits postprandial gastric acid secretion and pancreatic exocrine secretion Stimulates colonic motility but inhibits gastric and small intestine motility Facilitates fatty acid uptake in the proximal and small intestine and induces histamine release from mast cells Trophic in some pancreatic and colon cancer cell lines in vitro	Luminal nutrients, especially lipids, but not amino acids or carbohydrates GRP and bombesin Somatostatin inhibits secretion
PP	Major site of expression is pancreatic endocrine cells located in periphery of islets in pancreatic head and uncinate process	NPY and PYY	Reduces CCK-induced gastric acid secretion Increases intestinal transit times by reducing gastric emptying and upper intestinal motility Inhibits postprandial exocrine pancreas secretion via vagal-dependent pathway	Stimulated by nutrients, hormones, neurotransmitters, gastric distention, insulin-induced hypoglycemia, and direct vagal nerve stimulation Hyperglycemia, bombesin, and somatostatin inhibit secretion
PYY	Enteroendocrine cells, developing endocrine pancreas, subpopulation of pancreatic alpha cells in mature islets	NPY and PP	Enterogastrone inhibits gastric acid secretion and gastric motility Increases intestinal transit time by reducing intestinal motility Inhibits pancreatic exocrine secretion Role as an intestinal epithelial growth factor remains controversial Peripheral vasoconstriction and reduced mesenteric and pancreatic vascular blood flow	After oral nutrient ingestion, early secretion is mediated by the vagus nerve and hormonal influences; later, secretion occurs as a result of direct L-cell stimulation Bile acids and fatty acids Amino acids administered intracolonically Activation of CNS
PACAP	Brain, respiratory tract, and enteric nervous system	VIP, PHI, and PHM	Stimulates histamine release from the stomach Increases secretion of pancreatic fluid, protein, and bicarbonate Stimulates insulin and catecholamine release Neural regulation of gastric acid secretion	

Continued

TABLE 38-4

Summary of Gastrointestinal-Derived Hormones—cont'd

Hormone	Cell or Tissue of Origin	Related Peptides	Actions	Secretory Stimuli
Secretin	CNS, fetal endocrine pancreas, and enteroendocrine S cells located in the duodenum and proximal jejunum		Principal hormonal stimulant of pancreatic and biliary bicarbonate and water excretion Regulates pancreatic enzyme secretion Stimulates gastric secretion of pepsinogen Inhibits LES tone, postprandial gastric emptying, gastrin release, and gastric acid secretion	Gastric acid, bile salts, and luminal nutrients, especially fatty acids, peptides, and ethanol Somatostatin inhibits secretion
Somatostatin	CNS, pancreatic delta cells, enteroendocrine D cells		Inhibits secretion of islet hormones, including insulin, glucagon, and PP Inhibits secretion of gut peptides, including gastrin, secretin, VIP, CCK, GLP-1, and GLP-2 Inhibits pancreatic exocrine secretion Acts in a paracrine manner on G cells, enterochromaffin-like cells, and parietal cells to inhibit gastric acid secretion Reduces splanchnic blood flow, intestinal motility, and carbohydrate absorption while increasing water and electrolyte absorption	Luminal nutrients Gastrin, CCK, bombesin, GLP-1, and GIP Neural influences, including PACAP, VIP, and β-adrenergic agonists stimulate while ACh inhibits secretion
Tachykinins	Throughout the CNS and PNS, including the respiratory tract, skin, sensory organs, and urogenital tract; in the GI tract, neurons localized in the submucous and myenteric plexuses, extrinsic sensory fibers, and enterochromaffin cells in the gut epithelium	Substance P, neurokinin A, and neurokinin B	Regulate vasomotor and GI smooth muscle contractility Chemotaxis and activation of immune cells, mucous secretion, water absorption and secretion Role in visceral inflammation, hyperreflexia, and hyperalgesia	Direct or indirect activation of neurons
TRH	CNS and enteric nervous system, colon, G cells of the stomach, pancreatic islet beta cells		Suppresses pentagastrin-stimulated gastric acid secretion Chronic administration induces pancreatic hyperplasia and inhibits amylase release Attenuates CCK-induced gallbladder smooth muscle contraction Inhibits cholesterol synthesis within the intestinal mucosa	In the stomach, histamine and serotonin stimulate and endogenous opioids inhibit secretion
VIP	Widely expressed in the CNS and PNS including the enteric nervous system	PACAP, PHI, and PHM	Induces relaxation of vascular and nonvascular smooth muscle Mediates relaxation of the LES, sphincter of Oddi, and anal sphincter Regulates relaxation-associated gut contraction and may be involved with reflex vasodilation in the small intestine Inhibits gastric acid secretion Stimulates biliary water, bicarbonate, pancreatic enzyme, and intestinal chloride secretion	Mechanical stimulation Activation of the CNS and PNS

ACh, acetylcholine; CCK, cholecystokinin; CGRP, calcitonin gene–related peptide; CNS, central nervous system; GABA, γ-aminobutyric acid; GH, growth hormone; GI, gastrointestinal; GIP, gastric inhibitory polypeptide; GLP, glucagon-like peptide; GRP, gastrin-releasing peptide; LES, lower esophageal sphincter; NPY, neuropeptide Y; NT, neurotensin; PACAP, pituitary adenylate cyclase–activating peptide; PHI, peptide histidine isoleucine; PHM, peptide histidine methionine; PNS, peripheral nervous system; PP, pancreatic polypeptide; PYY, peptide YY; TRH, thyrotropin-releasing hormone; VIP, vasoactive intestinal peptide.

expressed in the gut, where they activate pathways coupled to epithelial mitogenesis. Neuromedin U is a neurotransmitter that is expressed in the enteric nervous system, where it regulates intestinal motility and ion secretion. Several hormones are secreted by the gastrointestinal tract directly into the lumen, where they modulate the secretion and release of other hormones. Guanylin and uroguanylin stimulate water, bicarbonate, and chloride secretion by the intestine and kidney while inhibiting sodium reabsorption.[137] Guanylin may also regulate cell proliferation in the colon; guanylin$^{-/-}$ mice have increased epithelial cell migration and colonocyte proliferation. A missense mutation in the coding region of the GUCY2C guanylate cyclase C gene, resulting in enhanced receptor signaling, increased cyclic guanosine monophosphate, and excessive chloride and water secretion from enterocytes, has been described in a large family with autosomal dominant familial diarrhea.[138] Other luminally secreted peptides include sorbin, a 153–amino acid peptide involved with monitoring fluid and sodium fluxes in the duodenum, and monitor peptide, which is a 61–amino acid peptide that stimulates CCK release. Xenin-25 is a 25–amino acid neurotensin-related peptide produced by a subset of K cells in the intestine. Its functions are uncertain, although in animals it decreases food ingestion and alters gastrointestinal motility. In humans, it appears to act as a weak insulin secretagogue and delays gastric emptying.[139]

PANCREATIC AND GUT ENDOCRINE TUMORS

The ontogeny of pancreatic and gut endocrine cells provides some insight into the molecular pathophysiology of pancreatic endocrine tumors. Although gastrin is not normally produced in human adult islets of Langerhans, the finding of gastrinomas arising from adult endocrine pancreas may reflect the dedifferentiation of neoplastic endocrine tumor cells that recapitulates, in part, patterns of islet gene expression observed during embryonic development. Similarly, the observation that pancreatic and gut endocrine tumors are frequently plurihormonal is consistent with studies demonstrating co-localization of peptide hormones in fetal and adult endocrine cells in the pancreas and gut. Finally, in disorders such as multiple endocrine neoplasia type 1 (MEN1), a single genetic defect is associated with the presence of multiple synchronous or asynchronous tumors which, when functional, secrete different hormones (e.g., gastrin and insulin).

Although pancreatic endocrine tumors frequently manifest as sporadic, isolated lesions, genetic alterations detected in tumors from patients with familial syndromes may also be detected in sporadic tumors. MEN1; phakomatoses such as von Hippel-Lindau disease, von Recklinghausen disease, or neurofibromatosis type 1; and tuberous sclerosis represent the common familial syndromes associated with pancreatic endocrine tumors. Defects in distinct tumor suppressor genes account for the phenotypic manifestations and development of tumors in these syndromes (Table 38-5). Loss of heterozygosity at 10q has been detected in sporadic pancreatic endocrine tumors, with cellular rather than nuclear localization of PTEN (phosphatase and tensin homolog, deleted on chromosome 10) detected in a substantial proportion of malignant pancreatic endocrine tumors.[140] Similarly, loss of heterozygosity at the 11q13 MEN1 locus has been detected in sporadic pancreatic endocrine tumors, and alterations in loci of the CDKN2A (formerly called p16 or MTS1), SMAD4 (formerly DP64), and ERBB2 (also called HER2 or Neu) genes have also been reported.

Mutations in MEN1, the gene encoding menin, give rise to the MEN1 syndrome, which is associated with an increased incidence of endocrine dysfunction due to cellular hyperplasia and excess secretion or the presence of discrete functioning tumors in the pancreas, pituitary, parathyroid, and gut and carcinoids in the stomach. In addition, the condition is associated with thymic carcinoma and large, bilateral nonfunctioning adrenal tumors.[141] The MEN1 gene encodes a 610–amino acid nuclear protein that interacts with the amino-terminus of the JunD transcription factor, presumably resulting in derepressed cell growth. Menin regulates cell growth through control of histone methylation and regulation of cyclin-dependent kinase (CDK) inhibitors. Menin functions as a molecular adaptor linking the mixed-lineage leukemia (MLL) histone methyltransferase with lens epithelium–derived growth factor (LEDGF). LEDGF is a chromatin-associated protein that is required for both MLL-dependent transcription and leukemic transformation; menin mutations in MEN1 patients abrogate interaction with LEDGF, thereby compromising MLL- or menin-dependent functions.[142] About 10% of all MEN1 germline mutations arise de novo. The utility of genetic testing for patients with possible MEN1 syndrome remains unclear because of the large number of heterogeneous mutations identified in the menin gene. The likelihood of detecting MEN1 mutations correlates directly with the number of MEN1-related tumors in the index case at presentation.[143] The reduced cost and widespread availability of whole genome sequencing suggests that genetic counseling and discussion of genetic testing options is prudent for MEN1 patients.

A search for clinical manifestations of diseases associated with these genetic syndromes is an important component in the initial diagnosis and ongoing management of patients with pancreatic endocrine tumors. Careful phenotype-genotype analyses have ascertained that facial angiofibromas, collagenomas, lipomas, leiomyomas, and adrenocortical tumors may be seen with increased frequency in patients with MEN1.[144] Moreover, somatic mutations of the menin gene have been described in isolated cases of gastrinoma, insulinoma, and gut endocrine tumors.[144]

The secretion of one or more peptide hormones resulting in the production of symptoms attributable to hormone excess, such as hypoglycemia, peptic ulcers, hyperglycemia, and a skin rash, or profuse watery diarrhea in patients with insulinoma, gastrinoma, glucagonoma, or VIPoma, respectively, facilitates the diagnosis of a hormone-secreting endocrine tumor. Somatostatinoma and glucagonoma are associated with the development of type 2 diabetes due to impaired insulin action (glucagon) and reduced insulin secretion (somatostatin). Subjects with somatostatin excess may also develop steatorrhea and gallstones. In some instances, pancreatic or gut endocrine tumors may not be associated with clinically or biochemically detectable hormone excess and development of a recognizable syndrome. Because nonfunctioning pancreatic endocrine tumors may escape clinical detection, they often are larger and more frequently malignant at the time of diagnosis. The term *nonfunctioning* may be a misnomer, because these tumors frequently produce peptide hormones (Fig. 38-3) whose biologic actions are less clinically apparent. In some instances, tumor-associated defects in posttranslational processing may preclude the efficient synthesis and secretion of peptide hormones. The histologic appearance of such tumors is often a poor guide to their behavior because most tumors appear to be well differentiated. Extrapancreatic spread is at present the best guide to the malignant potential or otherwise of such tumors. Factors affecting prognosis include liver metastases, incomplete resection of the primary tumor, and poorly differentiated tumor cells. Measurement of the Ki-67 labeling index (i.e., number of cells staining for Ki-67 on immunohistochemistry) is a useful marker of mitotic activity, with a labeling index of less than 5% suggesting benign behavior.[145,146] Loss of heterozygosity or inactivation of the PHLDA (Pleckstrin homology-like domain family A member 2) gene is associated with disease progression and poor prognosis in pancreatic endocrine tumors.[147]

TABLE 38-5		
Genetic Diseases Associated With the Development of Pancreatic or Gut Endocrine Tumors		
Gene	**Disease**	**Phenotype**
Menin	MEN1	Parathyroid, pituitary, and pancreatic endocrine tumors
VHL	von Hippel-Lindau syndrome	Pancreatic endocrine tumors, hemangiomas, and multiple neoplasms
NF1	Neurofibromatosis	Neurofibromas, pheochromocytomas
TSC1/2	Tuberous sclerosis	Pancreatic endocrine tumors, hamartomas

MEN1, multiple endocrine neoplasia type 1; NF1, neurofibromin 1; TSC1/2, tuberous sclerosis genes 1 and 2; VHL, von Hippel-Lindau tumor suppressor gene.

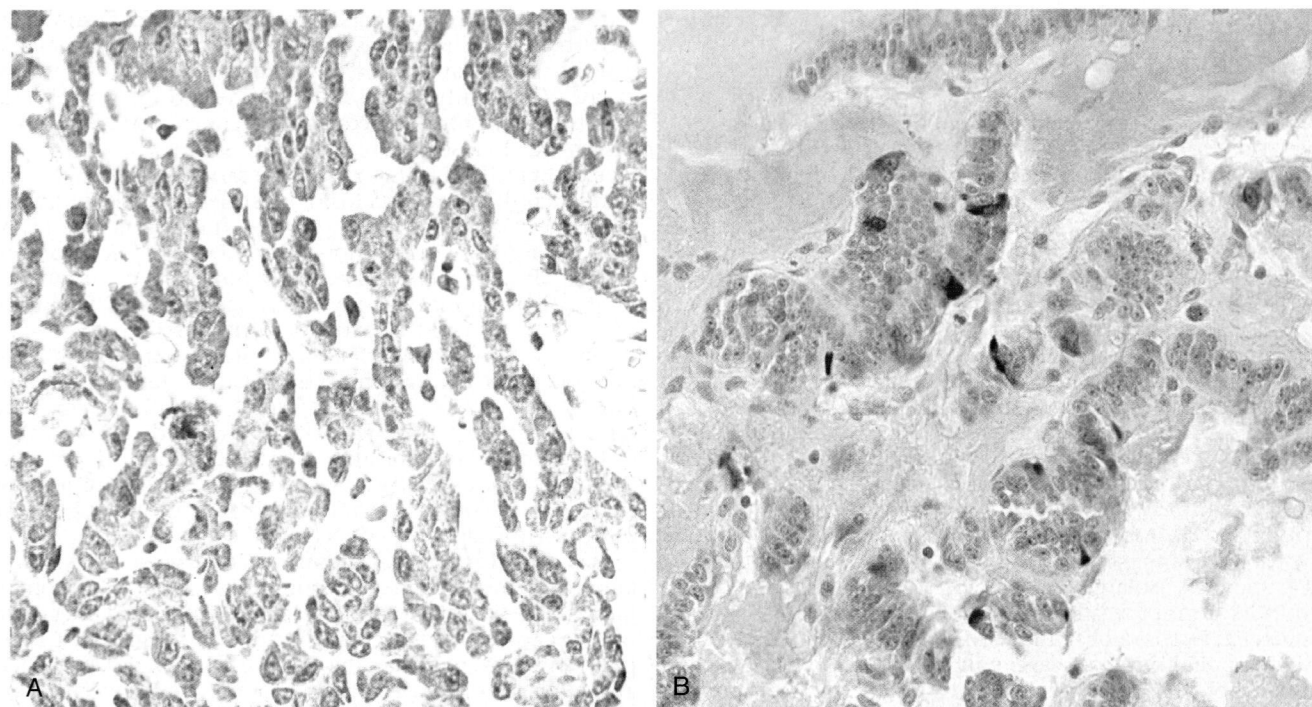

Figure 38-3 Clinically nonfunctioning tumors often are found to express one or more peptide hormones after immunocytochemical analyses. Histologic sections from the identical nonfunctioning human pancreatic endocrine tumor exhibit immunopositivity for glucagon (**A**) and pancreatic polypeptide (**B**).

The use of somatostatin receptor scintigraphy and measurement of gene products commonly expressed in endocrine cells, such as chromogranin, PP, neuron-specific enolase, or glycoprotein hormone subunits, may be useful as an adjunct for monitoring the tumor response to therapy. Widespread expression of receptors for somatostatin and multiple peptide hormone G protein–coupled receptors, including the GLP-1 receptor,[148] has stimulated efforts to develop novel radiolabeled peptide ligands for the localization and treatment of endocrine and nonendocrine neoplasms.

Despite the large number and complexity of endocrine cell populations in the human small bowel, gut endocrine tumors, including ileal carcinoids, are uncommon. Similarly, peptide hormone–secreting carcinoid tumors arising from the colon are much less common than colonic adenocarcinomas. The molecular basis for the infrequent malignant transformation of human gut endocrine cells remains incompletely understood. Mutations in the regenerating islet-derived 1α gene (REG1A) have been identified in a subset of patients with ECL cell tumors and associated hypergastrinemia, but the contribution of this genetic mutation to transformation of these cells remains unclear. The clinical presentation, diagnosis, and treatment of several more common pancreatic and gut endocrine tumors are discussed later, and treatment is reviewed elsewhere.[149-151] Surgical resection remains the principal goal and therapeutic strategy, because chemotherapeutic regimens have had only modest success in patients with malignant tumors. Embolization of large, functional metastatic tumors also plays an important part in the treatment of symptomatic disease.

Insulinomas

The first insulinoma was described by Wilder and colleagues in 1927[152] in an orthopedic surgeon who experi-enced neuroglycopenic symptoms during prolonged fasting when in the operating room. He was found to have a widely metastatic neuroendocrine tumor at laparotomy and extracts from the tumor tissue caused hypoglycemia in rabbits. Insulinomas are the most common functioning islet cell tumors, and they are characterized by hypoglycemia that often is precipitated by exercise or fasting. A subset of insulinomas is characterized by postprandial hypoglycemia. As many as 25% of insulinoma patients report both fasting and postprandial hypoglycemia, emphasizing that the timing of hypoglycemia can be a poor guide to the underlying hypoglycemic disorder.[153] More than 80% are solitary, benign tumors with an indolent course. Patients may tolerate symptoms of hypoglycemia for years before seeking medical attention; in a large series the average duration of preceding symptoms was approximately 2 years. Surgical enucleation is the treatment of choice, and cure should be expected in patients without the MEN1 syndrome. In these patients, the recurrence rate is low, often less than 10%. Recurrence can occur at the site of original enucleation (implying fracture during surgery or incomplete resection) or can occur due to the development of an asynchronous lesion at a site separate from the original presenting tumor. Insulinomas that accompany MEN1 tend to occur at an earlier age. Although they account for about one third of pancreatic islet cell tumors seen in MEN1 patients, they occur more often before 40 years of age and are the most common tumor seen before age 20. Insulinomas may be the first manifestation of MEN1; however, if MEN1 is suspected, an evaluation of parathyroid function is indicated in such circumstances.

In contrast to the single adenoma found in most patients with sporadic insulinoma, many patients with MEN1 have multicentric benign disease and a higher incidence of recurrence (>20%). When possible, distal subtotal pancreatic resection to the level of the portal vein combined with enucleation of tumors in the head of the pancreas (guided by intraoperative ultrasonography for safe removal) is thought to be the optimal treatment—in part to preserve pancreatic function and to facilitate early detection of recurrent disease using conventional imaging and endoscopic ultrasound. Preservation of endocrine and exocrine pancreatic function is not always possible in these situations. Insulinomas may be malignant (about 5%), defined by the presence of local invasion or lymph node or distal organ metastases.[153] Resection of hepatic metastases may provide effective palliation and probably will prolong survival, depending on the extent of resectable tumor burden. Palliative resection should be considered only when at least 90% of the tumor bulk can be excised. The success rate for identification of insulin-secreting pancreatic endocrine tumors with noninvasive testing such as computed tomography (CT) and transabdominal ultrasound has remained constant at about 75%. However, with the implementation of endoscopic ultrasound and selective arterial calcium stimulation testing, preoperative localization rates have significantly improved.[153]

Gastrinoma

In 1955, Zollinger and Ellison described two patients with intractable peptic ulcer disease and pancreatic islet cell tumors.[154] Subsequent studies demonstrated elevated levels of circulating gastrin associated with gastric acid hypersecretion in patients with Zollinger-Ellison syndrome.

Although the gastrin gene is not normally expressed in the adult pancreas, gastrinomas commonly arise from within the pancreas and manifest as solitary adenoma, microadenoma, metastatic endocrine carcinoma, or endocrine cell hyperplasia. Gastrinoma and insulinoma represent the two most common pancreatic endocrine tumors. Between 20% and 40% of gastrin-secreting tumors arise from the duodenum. Most (75%) are sporadic, but about 25% are associated with the MEN1 syndrome. Sporadic duodenal gastrinomas are frequently small, commonly located in the proximal duodenum, and associated with regional lymph node metastases in 60% of patients.[155] Patients presenting with gastrinoma as a component of the MEN1 syndrome may develop pituitary (60%) and adrenal (45%) dysfunction and carcinoid tumors (30%).[156] A substantial proportion of MEN1 patients also present with benign skin lesions, such as angiofibromas and collagenomas.[157] Patients with MEN1-related duodenal gastrinomas frequently exhibit hyperplastic foci of gastrin-immunopositive cells in the adjacent duodenal tissue. Sporadic gastrinomas may contain menin gene mutations. MEN1 patients tend to be younger at the time of tumor diagnosis than those without MEN1. Sporadic tumors are most often solitary and malignant; MEN1-associated tumors are usually multiple but may be more localized at the time of diagnosis.

Based on the presence of metastases at the time of diagnosis, about 50% to 60% of gastrinomas are malignant, perhaps because of the long delay between initial clinical presentation and diagnosis of Zollinger-Ellison syndrome. Nevertheless, gastrin-secreting tumors are often slow growing and associated with prolonged survival despite complications arising from intestinal ulceration. Loss of heterozygosity at 1q or on the X chromosome may be associated with a more aggressive clinical presentation.

Clinical manifestations of gastrinomas are usually related to excessive gastric acid secretion, resulting in severe refractory peptic ulceration complicated by hemorrhage, perforation, and stricture. Many patients report symptoms for 5 to 6 years before the diagnosis of Zollinger-Ellison syndrome is established.[156] Abdominal pain, diarrhea, and heartburn are common presenting symptoms, with diarrhea and pain observed in more than 70% of patients with Zollinger-Ellison syndrome. The diarrhea results in part from fat malabsorption due to degradation of pancreatic lipase by excess gastric acid. Small bowel inflammation and impaired nutrient absorption may also arise from excess gastric acid. Antisecretory therapy usually abolishes the diarrhea and diminishes many clinical features of Zollinger-Ellison syndrome. Although much less common, tumors may also secrete CCK and present with diarrhea, weight loss, and gallstones, mimicking some of the features associated with gastrinomas.

The diagnosis of gastrinoma is based on the detection of elevated fasting circulating gastrin levels (>200 pg/mL) and gastric acid hypersecretion whether by direct measurement (basal acid output > 15 mEq/hour with an intact stomach or > 5 mEq/hour after ulcer surgery) in patients off all acid antisecretory medication or by observation of peptic ulceration. Measurement of circulating gastrin using commercially available assays may yield misleading or inconclusive results because of problems with assay specificity and aberrant processing of gastrin by some tumors.[158] Although many patients with Zollinger-Ellison syndrome have serum gastrin values that exceed 500 pg/mL, a secretin stimulation test may be performed when the serum gastrin levels are in the range of 200 to 500 pg/mL to confirm the diagnosis. Provocative testing requires overnight fasting and the intravenous administration of secretin 0.4 μg/kg over 1 minute (2 units/kg bolus) followed by serial measurement of circulating gastrin levels at 2, 5, 10, 15, and 20 minutes. A rise in the serum gastrin level of more than 200 pg/mL within 15 minutes or a doubling of the fasting gastrin level strongly suggests the presence of a gastrinoma. Secretin receptor expression in tumors correlates with the gastrin response to secretin infusion, and calcium infusion testing may be useful in patients with an equivocal secretin test result.[159] Provocative testing may be useful in distinguishing gastrinomas from other causes of ulcerogenic hypergastrinemia, such as gastric outlet obstruction, retained antrum after a Billroth II gastrectomy, antral G-cell hyperplasia, and *Helicobacter pylori* infection, which demonstrate a flat gastrin response to secretin. Difficulty in obtaining clinical supplies of secretin has precluded routine use of the secretin test, and intravenous calcium administration has been successfully used to stimulate gastrin secretion in several cases. More than 90% of patients have prominent gastric folds at the time of endoscopy, consistent with the trophic effect of gastrin on the stomach mucosa. Assays of serum calcium and parathyroid hormone levels (note that hypercalcemia per se can raise gastrin levels), baseline pituitary function tests, and imaging studies should be considered to rule out the MEN1 syndrome.

Localization of small primary tumors or endocrine hyperplasia can be difficult. Conventional endoscopy or an upper gastrointestinal series occasionally can be used to directly visualize duodenal lesions, but tumors are often confined to the submucosa, making detection and biopsy challenging. Radiolabeled octreotide scanning may be useful for detecting the primary tumor and metastases. MRI or CT can be informative, but the primary tumor may not be detected with these modalities alone. Endoscopic ultrasonography has been used for tumor localization with increasing success; less commonly, angiography with selective venous sampling may be helpful in localizing occult tumors. Primary tumors may be localized to lymph nodes, and ectopic gastrinomas have been found in sites such as the ovary.

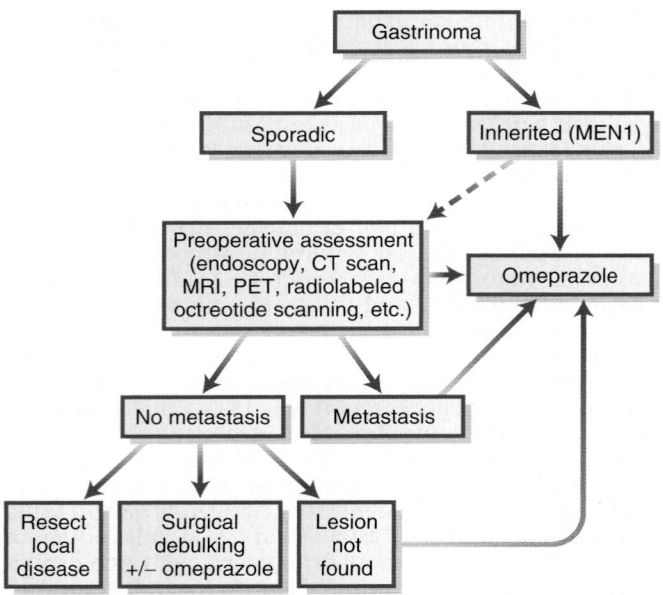

Figure 38-4 Treatment algorithm for the management of a patient with gastrinoma. In some circumstances, patients with familial gastrinoma may also be candidates for surgical resection if disease is highly limited *(dotted line)*. CT, computed tomography; MEN1, multiple endocrine neoplasia type 1; MRI, magnetic resonance imaging; PET, positron emission tomography.

Initial treatment of patients with gastrinoma is directed at pharmacologic reduction of gastric acid secretion and the treatment of complications (such as perforation). Although H_2-blockers have been used with some success, H^+/K^+-adenosine triphosphatase inhibitors such as omeprazole have become the treatment of choice because of their longer duration of action. Doses should be titrated to keep the H^+ ion output to less than 10 mEq/hour (5 mEq/hour in patients with prior acid-reducing surgery) for the hour before the next dose of the drug is received.

As outlined in Figure 38-4, except in the presence of unresectable disease, all patients with sporadic gastrinoma should undergo surgical exploration with the intent of curative surgical resection. Exploration should include a combination of duodenal palpation, endoscopic transillumination, intraoperative ultrasonography, and duodenotomy. In up to 20% of patients undergoing surgical exploration, the primary tumor remains undetected at laparotomy despite meticulous exploration of the abdominal cavity. Total gastrectomy should be performed only rarely in patients with severe ulcer disease refractory to medical therapy in which the primary tumor cannot be resected. Primary surgery usually is not indicated in patients with gastrinoma and MEN1 syndrome because they often have multiple small pancreatic tumors that are not amenable to surgical resection.

Glucagonomas

Most glucagonomas are pancreatic in origin. Approximately 80% of tumors occur sporadically, with the remainder associated with the MEN1 syndrome. About 75% of glucagonomas are malignant and have metastasized by the time of diagnosis. The clinical presentation reflects the various actions of the proglucagon-derived peptides and depends on the profile of the peptides liberated due to tumor-specific differences in the post-translational processing of proglucagon. A hallmark of this syndrome is necrolytic migratory erythema, a rash that usually begins in the groin and perineum as a raised, erythematous patch with occasional bullae that may also involve the lower extremities and perioral area. The exact cause of the rash remains unknown, but elevated plasma glucagon levels and deficiencies of zinc, amino acids, and fatty acids may represent contributing factors.

Patients with glucagonomas may exhibit weight loss, abdominal pain, diabetes, stomatitis, glossitis, cheilitis, nail dystrophy, thromboembolic events, anemia, hypoaminoacidemia, and neuropsychiatric symptoms. The triad of hyperglucagonemia, necrolytic migratory erythema, and a pancreatic tumor is seen in a few cases. Intestinal obstructive symptoms and increased intestinal transit times have been reported and may reflect tumor-specific liberation of GLP-1 and GLP-2, peptides with antimotility and intestinotrophic properties, respectively.[160]

The diagnosis may be confirmed by measurement of significantly elevated levels of plasma glucagon in association with a pancreatic mass. Extremely high levels of glucagon are more often seen with the classic glucagonoma syndrome, whereas more modest elevations of glucagon are detected in the setting of plurihormonal tumors. In contrast to insulinomas, glucagonomas are often large and more easily localized with imaging modalities. Somatostatin receptor scintigraphy is effective in detecting metastatic disease that most commonly involves the liver, lymph nodes, adrenal glands, or vertebrae. Therapy with a somatostatin analogue may be useful in the setting of metastatic disease by reducing levels of circulating glucagon through action at the SSTR2 receptor, improving the rash and promoting weight gain. The rash may also respond to selective nutrient supplementation. Somatostatin analogues may reduce glucagon secretion and tumor-associated symptoms, but effects on tumor growth are often modest. Patients with unresectable or recurrent disease may be treated with chemotherapy or with the selective use of arterial embolization.

Somatostatinomas

Somatostatinomas are rare tumors that arise in the pancreas and the duodenum. Most clinical symptoms observed in the originally described somatostatinoma syndrome reflect the inhibitory properties of somatostatin on digestive organs. A classic triad involving mild diabetes mellitus, steatorrhea, and cholelithiasis is observed in a minority of patients and is caused by reduced insulin secretion, reduced biliary and pancreatic secretions, and inhibition of gallbladder motility. More prominent symptoms seen with duodenal tumors include weight loss, postprandial fullness and abdominal pain, cholelithiasis, anemia, and hypochlorhydria. Many patients present with nonspecific symptoms so that extensive hepatic metastases are present at the time of diagnosis.

Duodenal tumors often are associated with neurofibromatosis type 1 or, less commonly, with von Hippel-Lindau syndrome, and they may be associated with pheochromocytomas. Most duodenal tumors are not associated with symptoms of classic somatostatinoma syndrome, and they may manifest with mechanical symptoms. Pancreatic tumors usually occur sporadically or as part of the MEN1 syndrome and are most commonly located in the head of the pancreas. The diagnosis is confirmed by the presence of markedly elevated levels of plasma somatostatin. Conventional and endoscopic ultrasonography and CT may be used to localize the duodenal tumors (Fig. 38-5). In the small proportion of patients with localized disease, surgical resection can be curative. Patients with incurable or recurrent disease can be treated with chemotherapy.

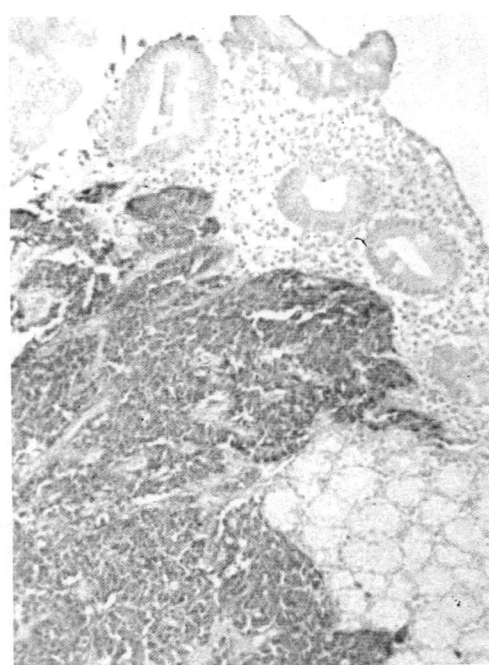

Figure 38-5 Somatostatin immunoreactivity in a human duodenal D-cell tumor. This low-power micrograph illustrates the diffuse somatostatin immunoreactivity. Brunner glands and the partly eroded mucosa are seen to the lower right and upper right, respectively, of the immunopositive endocrine tumor.

Vasoactive Intestinal Peptide–Secreting Tumors

The VIPoma syndrome is also known as pancreatic cholera, Verner-Morrison syndrome, or the watery diarrhea, hypokalemia, and achlorhydria (WDHA) syndrome. Approximately 90% of individuals with a VIPoma present with a pancreatic endocrine tumor that secretes VIP and, often, prostaglandins. The remaining tumors arise outside the pancreas, usually involving the sympathetic chain or adrenal medulla. VIPomas may manifest as sporadic tumors or as part of the MEN1 syndrome.

Clinical manifestations include intermittent, severe watery diarrhea that contains large quantities of potassium, bicarbonate, and chloride. Patients may exhibit signs and symptoms of hypokalemia, metabolic acidosis, and dehydration. Hypotension may result from dehydration and the vasodilator effects of VIP. The secretory diarrhea does not respond to antidiarrheal medications. Gastric analysis usually reveals hypochlorhydria or achlorhydria, although an appropriate increase in acid secretion is observed in response to a pentagastrin challenge. Glucose intolerance may reflect hypokalemia and decreased insulin action. Cutaneous flushing of the head and trunk, usually during a bout of diarrhea, may be observed in 15% of patients and may be associated with a patchy, erythematous rash.

The diagnosis of VIPoma is challenging because of the intermittent nature of the symptoms. A history of recurrent, severe diarrhea and elevated fasting levels of plasma VIP (>200 pg/mL) should prompt a search for a pancreatic tumor. Increased circulating levels of peptide histidine methionine, PP, neurotensin, and prostaglandins have also been detected in patients with VIP-producing tumors.

Initial treatment of patients with the VIPoma syndrome involves aggressive fluid and electrolyte replacement. Somatostatin analogues may be used preoperatively to control the diarrhea by lowering circulating VIP levels and directly inhibiting intestinal secretion. Definitive treatment requires surgical resection of the tumor, which is commonly located in the body or tail of the pancreas. Although tumors are usually solitary, 60% are malignant at the time of diagnosis; 75% metastasize to the liver and regional lymph nodes, but distant metastases also occur. If a pancreatic tumor cannot be identified, exploration of the retroperitoneum, including the adrenal glands and sympathetic chains, is indicated. If no pancreatic tumor is identified, some patients may elect to be closely monitored, but others opt for an 80% distal pancreatectomy. The latter strategy may be beneficial for the 10% to 20% of symptomatic patients with diffuse islet cell hyperplasia.

Miscellaneous Gut Hormone–Producing Tumors

Pancreatic endocrine tumors are rare but may secrete parathyroid hormone, growth hormone–releasing hormone, and adrenocorticotropic hormone, leading to development of hypercalcemia, acromegaly, and Cushing syndrome, respectively. A large number of peptide hormones may be produced by pancreatic endocrine tumor cells, including PYY, calcitonin, neurotensin, melanocyte-stimulating hormone, corticotropin-releasing hormone, NPY, neuromedin B, CGRP, GRP, and motilin. In some cases, the hormone precursors are produced but the correctly processed intact hormone is not secreted by the tumor. Accordingly, excessive production of many of these hormones may not always be associated with characteristic signs and symptoms. Similarly, carcinoid tumors of the gastrointestinal tract often stain for multiple peptide hormones in the absence of a recognizable clinical syndrome.

A large number of peptides are synthesized in and secreted by endocrine cells of the pancreas and gastrointestinal tract. Many of these peptides circulate as hormones, but they also function as paracrine modulators or neurotransmitters in the gut and in the central and peripheral nervous systems. Although some biologic actions have been delineated for many of these peptides, it seems likely that new peptides, receptors, and biologic functions will continue to be characterized. These discoveries may provide opportunities for better understanding the pathophysiology, diagnosis, and treatment of endocrine disease.

REFERENCES

1. Rumilla KM, Erickson LA, Service FJ, et al. Hyperinsulinemic hypoglycemia with nesidioblastosis: histologic features and growth factor expression. *Mod Pathol*. 2009;22:239-245.
2. Herrera PL. Adult insulin- and glucagon-producing cells differentiate from two independent cell lineages. *Development*. 2000;127:2317-2322.
3. Habener JF, Kemp DM, Thomas MK. Minireview: transcriptional regulation in pancreatic development. *Endocrinology*. 2005;146:1025-1034.
4. Stoffers DA, Zinkin NT, Stanojevic V, et al. Pancreatic agenesis attributable to a single nucleotide deletion in the human IPF1 gene coding sequence. *Nat Genet*. 1997;15:106-110.
5. Weedon MN, Cebola I, Patch AM, et al. Recessive mutations in a distal PTF1A enhancer cause isolated pancreatic agenesis. *Nat Genet*. 2014;46:61-64.
6. Lango Allen H, Flanagan SE, Shaw-Smith C, et al. GATA6 haploinsufficiency causes pancreatic agenesis in humans. *Nat Genet*. 2012;44:20-22.
7. Dohrmann C, Gruss P, Lemaire L. Pax genes and the differentiation of hormone-producing endocrine cells in the pancreas. *Mech Dev*. 2000;92:47-54.
8. Wen JH, Chen YY, Song SJ, et al. Paired box 6 (PAX6) regulates glucose metabolism via proinsulin processing mediated by prohormone convertase 1/3 (PC1/3). *Diabetologia*. 2009;52:504-513.
9. Ahlqvist E, Turrini F, Lang ST, et al. A common variant upstream of the PAX6 gene influences islet function in man. *Diabetologia*. 2012;55:94-104.

10. Malecki MT, Jhala US, Antonellis A, et al. Mutations in NEUROD1 are associated with the development of type 2 diabetes mellitus. *Nat Genet*. 1999;23:323-328.
11. Rubio-Cabezas O, Minton JA, Kantor I, et al. Homozygous mutations in NEUROD1 are responsible for a novel syndrome of permanent neonatal diabetes and neurological abnormalities. *Diabetes*. 2010;59:2326-2331.
12. Flannick J, Beer NL, Bick AG, et al. Assessing the phenotypic effects in the general population of rare variants in genes for a dominant Mendelian form of diabetes. *Nat Genet*. 2013;45:1380-1385.
13. Vella A, Howson JMM, Barratt BJ, et al. Lack of association of the Ala(45)Thr polymorphism and other common variants of the NeuroD gene with type 1 diabetes. *Diabetes*. 2004;53:1158-1161.
14. Collombat P, Mansouri A, Hecksher-Sorensen J, et al. Opposing actions of Arx and Pax4 in endocrine pancreas development. *Genes Dev*. 2003;17:2591-2603.
15. Henseleit KD, Nelson SB, Kuhlbrodt K, et al. NKX6 transcription factor activity is required for alpha- and beta-cell development in the pancreas. *Development*. 2005;132:3139-3149.
16. Prado CL, Pugh-Bernard AE, Elghazi L, et al. Ghrelin cells replace insulin-producing beta cells in two mouse models of pancreas development. *Proc Natl Acad Sci U S A*. 2004;101:2924-2929.
17. Oliver-Krasinski JM, Stoffers DA. On the origin of the beta cell. *Genes Dev*. 2008;22:1998-2021.
18. Sugiyama T, Benitez CM, Ghodasara A, et al. Reconstituting pancreas development from purified progenitor cells reveals genes essential for islet differentiation. *Proc Natl Acad Sci U S A*. 2013;110:12691-12696.
19. Flanagan SE, De Franco E, Lango Allen H, et al. Analysis of transcription factors key for mouse pancreatic development establishes NKX2-2 and MNX1 mutations as causes of neonatal diabetes in man. *Cell Metab*. 2014;19:146-154.
20. Yang Q, Bermingham NA, Finegold MJ, Zoghbi HY. Requirement of Math1 for secretory cell lineage commitment in the mouse intestine. *Science*. 2001;294:2155-2158.
21. Jensen J, Pedersen EE, Galante P, et al. Control of endodermal endocrine development by Hes-1. *Nat Genet*. 2000;24:36-44.
22. Jenny M, Uhl C, Roche C, et al. Neurogenin3 is differentially required for endocrine cell fate specification in the intestinal and gastric epithelium. *EMBO J*. 2002;21:6338-6347.
23. Lee CS, Perreault N, Brestelli JE, Kaestner KH. Neurogenin 3 is essential for the proper specification of gastric enteroendocrine cells and the maintenance of gastric epithelial cell identity. *Genes Dev*. 2002;16:1488-1497.
24. Naya FJ, Huang HP, Qiu Y, et al. Diabetes, defective pancreatic morphogenesis, and abnormal enteroendocrine differentiation in beta2/neuroD-deficient mice. *Genes Dev*. 1997;11:2323-2334.
25. Rindi G, Ratineau C, Ronco A, et al. Targeted ablation of secretin-producing cells in transgenic mice reveals a common differentiation pathway with multiple enteroendocrine cell lineages in the small intestine. *Development*. 1999;126:4149-4156.
26. Larsson LI, St-Onge L, Hougaard DM, et al. Pax 4 and 6 regulate gastrointestinal endocrine cell development. *Mech Dev*. 1998;79:153-159.
27. Hill ME, Asa SL, Drucker DJ. Essential requirement for Pax6 in control of enteroendocrine proglucagon gene transcription. *Mol Endocrinol*. 1999;13:1474-1486.
28. Desai S, Loomis Z, Pugh-Bernard A, et al. Nkx2.2 regulates cell fate choice in the enteroendocrine cell lineages of the intestine. *Dev Biol*. 2008;313:58-66.
29. Pagliuca FW, Melton DA. How to make a functional beta-cell. *Development*. 2013;140:2472-2483.
30. Hull RL, Andrikopoulos S, Verchere CB, et al. Increased dietary fat promotes islet amyloid formation and beta-cell secretory dysfunction in a transgenic mouse model of islet amyloid. *Diabetes*. 2003;52:372-379.
31. Schmitz O, Brock B, Rungby J. Amylin agonists: a novel approach in the treatment of diabetes. *Diabetes*. 2004;53(Suppl 3):S233-S238.
32. Tatemoto K, Hosoya M, Habata Y, et al. Isolation and characterization of a novel endogenous peptide ligand for the human APJ receptor. *Biochem Biophys Res Commun*. 1998;251:471-476.
33. Wang G, Anini Y, Wei W, et al. Apelin, a new enteric peptide: localization in the gastrointestinal tract, ontogeny, and stimulation of gastric cell proliferation and of cholecystokinin secretion. *Endocrinology*. 2004;145:1342-1348.
34. Kleinz MJ, Davenport AP. Emerging roles of apelin in biology and medicine. *Pharmacol Ther*. 2005;107:198-211.
35. Dray C, Knauf C, Daviaud D, et al. Apelin stimulates glucose utilization in normal and obese insulin-resistant mice. *Cell Metab*. 2008;8:437-445.
36. Wimalawansa SJ. Calcitonin gene-related peptide and its receptors: molecular genetics, physiology, pathophysiology, and therapeutic potentials. *Endocr Rev*. 1996;17:533-585.
37. McLatchie LM, Fraser NJ, Main MJ, et al. RAMPs regulate the transport and ligand specificity of the calcitonin-receptor-like receptor. *Nature*. 1998;393:333-339.
38. Rehfeld JF, Sun G, Christensen T, Hillingso JG. The predominant cholecystokinin in human plasma and intestine is cholecystokinin-33. *J Clin Endocrinol Metab*. 2001;86:251-258.
39. Beglinger S, Drewe J, Schirra J, et al. Role of fat hydrolysis in regulating glucagon-like peptide-1 secretion. *J Clin Endocrinol Metab*. 2010;95:879-886.
40. Moran TH, Katz LF, Plata-Salaman CR, Schwartz GJ. Disordered food intake and obesity in rats lacking cholecystokinin A receptors. *Am J Physiol*. 1998;274:R618-R625.
41. Jin G, Ramanathan V, Quante M, et al. Inactivating cholecystokinin-2 receptor inhibits progastrin-dependent colonic crypt fission, proliferation, and colorectal cancer in mice. *J Clin Invest*. 2009;119:2691-2701.
42. Smith JP, Solomon TE. Cholecystokinin and pancreatic cancer: the chicken or the egg? *Am J Physiol Gastrointest Liver Physiol*. 2014;306:G91-G101.
43. Hogenauer C, Meyer RL, Netto GJ, et al. Malabsorption due to cholecystokinin deficiency in a patient with autoimmune polyglandular syndrome type I. *N Engl J Med*. 2001;344:270-274.
44. Cheung GW, Kokorovic A, Lam CK, et al. Intestinal cholecystokinin controls glucose production through a neuronal network. *Cell Metab*. 2009;10:99-109.
45. Begg DP, Woods SC. The endocrinology of food intake. *Nat Rev Endocrinol*. 2013;9:584-597.
46. Branchek TA, Smith KE, Gerald C, Walker MW. Galanin receptor subtypes. *Trends Pharmacol Sci*. 2000;21:109-117.
47. Haberman RP, Samulski RJ, McCown TJ. Attenuation of seizures and neuronal death by adeno-associated virus vector galanin expression and secretion. *Nat Med*. 2003;9:1076-1080.
48. Elliott-Hunt CR, Marsh B, Bacon A, et al. Galanin acts as a neuroprotective factor to the hippocampus. *Proc Natl Acad Sci U S A*. 2004;101:5105-5110.
49. Ahren B, Pacini G, Wynick D, et al. Loss-of-function mutation of the galanin gene is associated with perturbed islet function in mice. *Endocrinology*. 2004;145:3190-3196.
50. Mazziotti G, Bonadonna S, Doga M, et al. Biochemical evaluation of patients with active acromegaly and type 2 diabetes mellitus: efficacy and safety of the galanin test. *Neuroendocrinology*. 2008;88:299-304.
51. Miyawaki K, Yamada Y, Yano H, et al. Glucose intolerance caused by a defect in the entero-insular axis: a study in gastric inhibitory polypeptide receptor knockout mice. *Proc Natl Acad Sci U S A*. 1999;96:14843-14847.
52. Miyawaki K, Yamada Y, Ban N, et al. Inhibition of gastric inhibitory polypeptide signaling prevents obesity. *Nat Med*. 2002;8:738-742.
53. Hojberg PV, Vilsboll T, Rabol R, et al. Four weeks of near-normalisation of blood glucose improves the insulin response to glucagon-like peptide-1 and glucose-dependent insulinotropic polypeptide in patients with type 2 diabetes. *Diabetologia*. 2009;52:199-207.
54. Lacroix A, Ndiaye N, Tremblay J, Hamet P. Ectopic and abnormal hormone receptors in adrenal Cushing's syndrome. *Endocr Rev*. 2001;22:75-110.
55. Finan B, Ma T, Ottaway N, et al. Unimolecular dual incretins maximize metabolic benefits in rodents, monkeys, and humans. *Sci Transl Med*. 2013;5:209ra151.
56. Dockray GJ, Varro A, Dimaline R, Wang T. The gastrins: their production and biological activities. *Annu Rev Physiol*. 2001;63:119-139.
57. Hellmich MR, Rui XL, Hellmich HL, et al. Human colorectal cancers express a constitutively active cholecystokinin-B/gastrin receptor that stimulates cell growth. *J Biol Chem*. 2000;275:32122-32128.
58. Olszewska-Pazdrak B, Townsend CM Jr, Hellmich MR. Agonist-independent activation of Src tyrosine kinase by a cholecystokinin-2 (CCK2) receptor splice variant. *J Biol Chem*. 2004;279:40400-40404.
59. Cheng ZJ, Harikumar KG, Holicky EL, Miller LJ. Heterodimerization of type A and B cholecystokinin receptors enhance signaling and promote cell growth. *J Biol Chem*. 2003;278:52972-52979.
60. Ferrand A, Wang TC. Gastrin and cancer: a review. *Cancer Lett*. 2006;238:15-29.
61. Muerkoster S, Isberner A, Arlt A, et al. Gastrin suppresses growth of CCK2 receptor expressing colon cancer cells by inducing apoptosis in vitro and in vivo. *Gastroenterology*. 2005;129:952-968.
62. Suarez-Pinzon WL, Lakey JR, Brand SJ, Rabinovitch A. Combination therapy with epidermal growth factor and gastrin induces neogenesis of human islet beta-cells from pancreatic duct cells and an increase in functional beta-cell mass. *J Clin Endocrinol Metab*. 2005;90:3401-3409.
63. Singh PK, Hota D, Dutta P, et al. Pantoprazole improves glycemic control in type 2 diabetes: a randomized, double-blind, placebo-controlled trial. *J Clin Endocrinol Metab*. 2012;97:E2105-E2108.
64. Hove KD, Brons C, Faerch K, et al. Effects of 12 weeks' treatment with a proton pump inhibitor on insulin secretion, glucose metabolism and markers of cardiovascular risk in patients with type 2 diabetes: a randomised double-blind prospective placebo-controlled study. *Diabetologia*. 2013;56:22-30.
65. Ladenheim EE, Hampton LL, Whitney AC, et al. Disruptions in feeding and body weight control in gastrin-releasing peptide receptor deficient mice. *J Endocrinol*. 2002;174:273-281.

66. Zhou J, Chen J, Mokotoff M, Ball ED. Targeting gastrin-releasing peptide receptors for cancer treatment. *Anticancer Drugs*. 2004;15: 921-927.

67. Martinez A, Zudaire E, Julian M, et al. Gastrin-releasing peptide (GRP) induces angiogenesis and the specific GRP blocker 77427 inhibits tumor growth in vitro and in vivo. *Oncogene*. 2005;24:4106-4113.

68. Patel O, Clyde D, Chang M, et al. Pro-GRP-derived peptides are expressed in colorectal cancer cells and tumors and are biologically active in vivo. *Endocrinology*. 2012;153:1082-1092.

69. Zhang X, Cai W, Cao F, et al. 18F-labeled bombesin analogs for targeting GRP receptor-expressing prostate cancer. *J Nucl Med*. 2006;47(3): 492-501.

70. Kirchner H, Gutierrez JA, Solenberg PJ, et al. GOAT links dietary lipids with the endocrine control of energy balance. *Nat Med*. 2009;15: 741-745.

71. Zhao TJ, Liang G, Li RL, et al. Ghrelin O-acyltransferase (GOAT) is essential for growth hormone-mediated survival of calorie-restricted mice. *Proc Natl Acad Sci U S A*. 2010;107:7467-7472.

72. Kojima M, Kangawa K. Ghrelin: structure and function. *Physiol Rev*. 2005;85:495-522.

73. Shin A, Camilleri M, Busciglio I, et al. The ghrelin agonist RM-131 accelerates gastric emptying of solids and reduces symptoms in patients with type 1 diabetes mellitus. *Clin Gastroenterol Hepatol*. 2013; 11:1453-1459.

74. Shin A, Camilleri M, Busciglio I, et al. Randomized controlled phase Ib study of ghrelin agonist, RM-131, in type 2 diabetic women with delayed gastric emptying: pharmacokinetics and pharmacodynamics. *Diabetes Care*. 2013;36:41-48.

75. McCallum RW, Lembo A, Esfandyari T, et al. Phase 2b, randomized, double-blind 12-week studies of TZP-102, a ghrelin receptor agonist for diabetic gastroparesis. *Neurogastroenterol Motil*. 2013;25:e705-e717.

76. Adachi S, Takiguchi S, Okada K, et al. Effects of ghrelin administration after total gastrectomy: a prospective, randomized, placebo-controlled phase II study. *Gastroenterology*. 2010;138:1312-1320.

77. Yamamoto K, Takiguchi S, Miyata H, et al. Randomized phase II study of clinical effects of ghrelin after esophagectomy with gastric tube reconstruction. *Surgery*. 2010;148:31-38.

78. Cummings DE, Weigle DS, Frayo RS, et al. Plasma ghrelin levels after diet-induced weight loss or gastric bypass surgery. *N Engl J Med*. 2002; 346:1623-1630.

79. Lee WJ, Chen CY, Chong K, et al. Changes in postprandial gut hormones after metabolic surgery: a comparison of gastric bypass and sleeve gastrectomy. *Surg Obes Relat Dis*. 2011;7(6):683-690.

80. Malin SK, Samat A, Wolski K, et al. Improved acylated ghrelin suppression at 2 years in obese patients with type 2 diabetes: effects of bariatric surgery vs standard medical therapy. *Int J Obes*. 2014;38:364-370.

81. Yousseif A, Emmanuel J, Karra E, et al. Differential effects of laparoscopic sleeve gastrectomy and laparoscopic gastric bypass on appetite, circulating acyl-ghrelin, peptide YY3-36 and active GLP-1 levels in non-diabetic humans. *Obes Surg*. 2014;24:241-252.

82. le Roux CW, Neary NM, Halsey TJ, et al. Ghrelin does not stimulate food intake in patients with surgical procedures involving vagotomy. *J Clin Endocrinol Metab*. 2005;90:4521-4524.

83. Tong J, Prigeon RL, Davis HW, et al. Physiologic concentrations of exogenously infused ghrelin reduces insulin secretion without affecting insulin sensitivity in healthy humans. *J Clin Endocrinol Metab*. 2013;98:2536-2543.

84. Nagaya N, Moriya J, Yasumura Y, et al. Effects of ghrelin administration on left ventricular function, exercise capacity, and muscle wasting in patients with chronic heart failure. *Circulation*. 2004;110:3674-3679.

85. Allas S, Abribat T. Clinical perspectives for ghrelin-derived therapeutic products. *Endocr Dev*. 2013;25:157-166.

86. Ellingsgaard H, Hauselmann I, Schuler B, et al. Interleukin-6 enhances insulin secretion by increasing glucagon-like peptide-1 secretion from L cells and alpha cells. *Nat Med*. 2011;17:1481-1489.

87. Unger RH, Cherrington AD. Glucagonocentric restructuring of diabetes: a pathophysiologic and therapeutic makeover. *J Clin Invest*. 2012; 122:4-12.

88. Gelling RW, Du XQ, Dichmann DS, et al. Lower blood glucose, hyperglucagonemia, and pancreatic alpha cell hyperplasia in glucagon receptor knockout mice. *Proc Natl Acad Sci U S A*. 2003;100: 1438-1443.

89. Bagger JI, Knop FK, Holst JJ, Vilsboll T. Glucagon antagonism as a potential therapeutic target in type 2 diabetes. *Diabetes Obes Metab*. 2011;13:965-971.

90. Drucker DJ. The biology of incretin hormones. *Cell Metab*. 2006;3: 153-165.

91. Deane AM, Nguyen NQ, Stevens JE, et al. Endogenous glucagon-like peptide-1 slows gastric emptying in healthy subjects, attenuating postprandial glycemia. *J Clin Endocrinol Metab*. 2010;95:215-221.

92. Schirra J, Nicolaus M, Roggel R, et al. Endogenous glucagon-like peptide 1 controls endocrine pancreatic secretion and antro-pyloro-duodenal motility in humans. *Gut*. 2006;55:243-251.

93. Shah M, Law JH, Micheletto F, et al. Contribution of endogenous glucagon-like peptide 1 to glucose metabolism after Roux-en-Y gastric bypass. *Diabetes*. 2014;63:483-493.

94. Lovshin JA, Drucker DJ. Incretin-based therapies for type 2 diabetes mellitus. *Nat Rev Endocrinol*. 2009;5:262-269.

95. Buse JB, Rosenstock J, Sesti G, et al. Liraglutide once a day versus exenatide twice a day for type 2 diabetes: a 26-week randomised, parallel-group, multinational, open-label trial (LEAD-6). *Lancet*. 2009; 374:39-47.

96. Umapathysivam MM, Lee MY, Jones KL, et al. Comparative effects of prolonged and intermittent stimulation of the glucagon-like peptide 1 receptor on gastric emptying and glycemia. *Diabetes*. 2014;63: 785-790.

97. Drucker DJ, Erlich P, Asa SL, Brubaker PL. Induction of intestinal epithelial proliferation by glucagon-like peptide 2. *Proc Natl Acad Sci U S A*. 1996;93:7911-7916.

98. Estall JL, Drucker DJ. Tales beyond the crypt: glucagon-like peptide-2 and cytoprotection in the intestinal mucosa. *Endocrinology*. 2005;146: 19-21.

99. Jeppesen PB, Sanguinetti EL, Buchman A, et al. Teduglutide (ALX-0600), a dipeptidyl peptidase IV resistant glucagon-like peptide 2 analogue, improves intestinal function in short bowel syndrome patients. *Gut*. 2005;54:1224-1231.

100. Drucker DJ, Yusta B. Physiology and pharmacology of the enteroendocrine hormone glucagon-like peptide-2. *Annu Rev Physiol*. 2014;76: 561-583.

101. Marguet D, Baggio L, Kobayashi T, et al. Enhanced insulin secretion and improved glucose tolerance in mice lacking CD26. *Proc Natl Acad Sci U S A*. 2000;97:6874-6879.

102. Vella A, Bock G, Giesler PD, et al. Effects of dipeptidyl peptidase-4 inhibition on gastrointestinal function, meal appearance, and glucose metabolism in type 2 diabetes. *Diabetes*. 2007;56:1475-1480.

103. Hansotia T, Baggio LL, Delmeire D, et al. Double incretin receptor knockout (DIRKO) mice reveal an essential role for the enteroinsular axis in transducing the glucoregulatory actions of DPP-IV inhibitors. *Diabetes*. 2004;53:1326-1335.

104. Wynne K, Park AJ, Small CJ, et al. Subcutaneous oxyntomodulin reduces body weight in overweight and obese subjects: a double-blind, randomized, controlled trial. *Diabetes*. 2005;54:2390-2395.

105. Baggio LL, Huang Q, Brown TJ, Drucker DJ. Oxyntomodulin and glucagon-like peptide-1 differentially regulate murine food intake and energy expenditure. *Gastroenterology*. 2004;127:546-558.

106. Day JW, Ottaway N, Patterson JT, et al. A new glucagon and GLP-1 co-agonist eliminates obesity in rodents. *Nat Chem Biol*. 2009;5: 749-757.

107. Feighner SD, Tan CP, McKee KK, et al. Receptor for motilin identified in the human gastrointestinal system. *Science*. 1999;284:2184-2188.

108. Chapman MJ, Nguyen NQ, Deane AM. Gastrointestinal dysmotility: evidence and clinical management. *Curr Opin Clin Nutr Metab Care*. 2013;16:209-216.

109. Pons J, Lee EW, Li L, Kitlinska J. Neuropeptide Y: multiple receptors and multiple roles in cardiovascular diseases. *Curr Opin Investig Drugs*. 2004;5:957-962.

110. Vincent JP, Mazella J, Kitabgi P. Neurotensin and neurotensin receptors. *Trends Pharmacol Sci*. 1999;20:302-309.

111. Piliponsky AM, Chen CC, Nishimura T, et al. Neurotensin increases mortality and mast cells reduce neurotensin levels in a mouse model of sepsis. *Nat Med*. 2008;14:392-398.

112. Vaudry D, Gonzalez BJ, Basille M, et al. Pituitary adenylate cyclase-activating polypeptide and its receptors: from structure to functions. *Pharmacol Rev*. 2000;52:269-324.

113. Freson K, Hashimoto H, Thys C, et al. The pituitary adenylate cyclase-activating polypeptide is a physiological inhibitor of platelet activation. *J Clin Invest*. 2004;113:905-912.

114. Habib AM, Preston E, Davenport A. Risk factors for developing encapsulating peritoneal sclerosis in the icodextrin era of peritoneal dialysis prescription. *Nephrol Dial Transplant*. 2010;25(5):1633-1638.

115. Batterham RL, Ffytche DH, Rosenthal JM, et al. PYY modulation of cortical and hypothalamic brain areas predicts feeding behaviour in humans. *Nature*. 2007;450:106-109.

116. Ye J, Hao Z, Mumphrey MB, et al. GLP-1 receptor signaling is not required for reduced body weight after RYGB in rodents. *Am J Physiol*. 2014;306:R352-R362.

117. Balaji NS, Crookes PF, Banki F, et al. A safe and noninvasive test for vagal integrity revisited. *Arch Surg*. 2002;137:954-958, discussion 958-959.

118. Michel MC, Beck-Sickinger A, Cox H, et al. XVI. International Union of Pharmacology recommendations for the nomenclature of neuropeptide Y, peptide YY, and pancreatic polypeptide receptors. *Pharmacol Rev*. 1998;50:143-150.

119. Hameed S, Dhillo WS, Bloom SR. Gut hormones and appetite control. *Oral Dis*. 2009;15:18-26.

120. Batterham RL, Le Roux CW, Cohen MA, et al. Pancreatic polypeptide reduces appetite and food intake in humans. *J Clin Endocrinol Metab*. 2003;88:3989-3992.

121. Unis AS, Munson JA, Rogers SJ, et al. A randomized, double-blind, placebo-controlled trial of porcine versus synthetic secretin for reducing symptoms of autism. *J Am Acad Child Adolesc Psychiatry*. 2002;41: 1315-1321.

122. Low MJ. Clinical endocrinology and metabolism. The somatostatin neuroendocrine system: physiology and clinical relevance in gastrointestinal and pancreatic disorders. *Best Pract Res Clin Endocrinol Metab.* 2004;18:607-622.

123. Helyes Z, Pinter E, Sandor K, et al. Impaired defense mechanism against inflammation, hyperalgesia, and airway hyperreactivity in somatostatin 4 receptor gene-deleted mice. *Proc Natl Acad Sci U S A.* 2009;106:13088-13093.

124. Saito T, Iwata N, Tsubuki S, et al. Somatostatin regulates brain amyloid beta peptide Abeta42 through modulation of proteolytic degradation. *Nat Med.* 2005;11:434-439.

125. van der Hoek J, Hofland LJ, Lamberts SW. Novel subtype specific and universal somatostatin analogues: clinical potential and pitfalls. *Curr Pharm Des.* 2005;11:1573-1592.

126. Freda PU, Katznelson L, van der Lely AJ, et al. Long-acting somatostatin analog therapy of acromegaly: a meta-analysis. *J Clin Endocrinol Metab.* 2005;90:4465-4473.

127. Bousquet C, Lasfargues C, Chalabi M, et al. Clinical review: current scientific rationale for the use of somatostatin analogs and mTOR inhibitors in neuroendocrine tumor therapy. *J Clin Endocrinol Metab.* 2012;97:727-737.

128. Page NM. New challenges in the study of the mammalian tachykinins. *Peptides.* 2005;26:1356-1368.

129. Topaloglu AK, Reimann F, Guclu M, et al. TAC3 and TACR3 mutations in familial hypogonadotropic hypogonadism reveal a key role for neurokinin B in the central control of reproduction. *Nat Genet.* 2009;41:354-358.

130. Holzer P, Holzer-Petsche U. Tachykinin receptors in the gut: physiological and pathological implications. *Curr Opin Pharmacol.* 2001;1:583-590.

131. Harmar AJ, Fahrenkrug J, Gozes I, et al. Pharmacology and functions of receptors for vasoactive intestinal peptide and pituitary adenylate cyclase-activating polypeptide: IUPHAR review 1. *Br J Pharmacol.* 2012;166:4-17.

132. Lelievre V, Favrais G, Abad C, et al. Gastrointestinal dysfunction in mice with a targeted mutation in the gene encoding vasoactive intestinal polypeptide: a model for the study of intestinal ileus and Hirschsprung's disease. *Peptides.* 2007;28:1688-1699.

133. Gozes I, Furman S. Clinical endocrinology and metabolism. Potential clinical applications of vasoactive intestinal peptide: a selected update. *Best Pract Res Clin Endocrinol Metab.* 2004;18:623-640.

134. Otto C, Hein L, Brede M, et al. Pulmonary hypertension and right heart failure in pituitary adenylate cyclase-activating polypeptide type I receptor-deficient mice. *Circulation.* 2004;110:3245-3251.

135. Petkov V, Mosgoeller W, Ziesche R, et al. Vasoactive intestinal peptide as a new drug for treatment of primary pulmonary hypertension. *J Clin Invest.* 2003;111:1339-1346.

136. Mahapatra NR, O'Connor DT, Vaingankar SM, et al. Hypertension from targeted ablation of chromogranin A can be rescued by the human ortholog. *J Clin Invest.* 2005;115:1942-1952.

137. Forte LR Jr. Uroguanylin and guanylin peptides: pharmacology and experimental therapeutics. *Pharmacol Ther.* 2004;104:137-162.

138. Fiskerstrand T, Arshad N, Haukanes BI, et al. Familial diarrhea syndrome caused by an activating GUCY2C mutation. *N Engl J Med.* 2012;366:1586-1595.

139. Wice BM, Reeds DN, Tran HD, et al. Xenin-25 amplifies GIP-mediated insulin secretion in humans with normal and impaired glucose tolerance but not type 2 diabetes. *Diabetes.* 2012;61:1793-1800.

140. Perren A, Komminoth P, Saremaslani P, et al. Mutation and expression analyses reveal differential subcellular compartmentalization of PTEN in endocrine pancreatic tumors compared to normal islet cells. *Am J Pathol.* 2000;157:1097-1103.

141. Chandrasekharappa SC, Guru SC, Manickam P, et al. Positional cloning of the gene for multiple endocrine neoplasia-type 1. *Science.* 1997;276:404-407.

142. Yokoyama A, Cleary ML. Menin critically links MLL proteins with LEDGF on cancer-associated target genes. *Cancer Cell.* 2008;14:36-46.

143. Ellard S, Hattersley AT, Brewer CM, Vaidya B. Detection of an MEN1 gene mutation depends on clinical features and supports current referral criteria for diagnostic molecular genetic testing. *Clin Endocrinol.* 2005;62:169-175.

144. Schussheim DH, Skarulis MC, Agarwal SK, et al. Multiple endocrine neoplasia type 1: new clinical and basic findings. *Trends Endocrinol Metab.* 2001;12:173-178.

145. McCall CM, Shi C, Cornish TC, et al. Grading of well-differentiated pancreatic neuroendocrine tumors is improved by the inclusion of both Ki67 proliferative index and mitotic rate. *Am J Surg Pathol.* 2013;37:1671-1677.

146. Khan MS, Luong TV, Watkins J, et al. A comparison of Ki-67 and mitotic count as prognostic markers for metastatic pancreatic and midgut neuroendocrine neoplasms. *Br J Cancer.* 2013;108:1838-1845.

147. Ohki R, Saito K, Chen Y, et al. PHLDA3 is a novel tumor suppressor of pancreatic neuroendocrine tumors. *Proc Natl Acad Sci U S A.* 2014;111:E2404-E2413.

148. Christ E, Wild D, Forrer F, et al. Glucagon-like peptide-1 receptor imaging for localization of insulinomas. *J Clin Endocrinol Metab.* 2009;94:4398-4405.

149. Warner RR. Enteroendocrine tumors other than carcinoid: a review of clinically significant advances. *Gastroenterology.* 2005;128:1668-1684.

150. de Herder WW, Lamberts SW. Clinical endocrinology and metabolism. Gut endocrine tumours. *Best Pract Res Clin Endocrinol Metab.* 2004;18(4):477-495.

151. Fendrich V, Waldmann J, Bartsch DK, Langer P. Surgical management of pancreatic endocrine tumors. *Nat Rev Clin Oncol.* 2009;6:419-428.

152. Wilder RM, Allan FN, Power MH, Robertson HE. Carcinoma of the islands of the pancreas. *JAMA.* 1927;89:348-355.

153. Placzkowski KA, Vella A, Thompson GB, et al. Secular trends in the presentation and management of functioning insulinoma at the Mayo Clinic, 1987-2007. *J Clin Endocrinol Metab.* 2009;94:1069-1073.

154. Zollinger RM, Ellison EH. Primary peptic ulcerations of the jejunum associated with islet cell tumors of the pancreas. *Ann Surg.* 1955;142:709-723, discussion, 724-708.

155. Zogakis TG, Gibril F, Libutti SK, et al. Management and outcome of patients with sporadic gastrinoma arising in the duodenum. *Ann Surg.* 2003;238:42-48.

156. Gibril F, Schumann M, Pace A, Jensen RT. Multiple endocrine neoplasia type 1 and Zollinger-Ellison syndrome: a prospective study of 107 cases and comparison with 1009 cases from the literature. *Medicine.* 2004;83:43-83.

157. Asgharian B, Turner ML, Gibril F, et al. Cutaneous tumors in patients with multiple endocrine neoplasm type 1 (MEN1) and gastrinomas: prospective study of frequency and development of criteria with high sensitivity and specificity for MEN1. *J Clin Endocrinol Metab.* 2004;89:5328-5336.

158. Rehfeld JF, Gingras MH, Bardram L, et al. The Zollinger-Ellison syndrome and mismeasurement of gastrin. *Gastroenterology.* 2011;140:1444-1453.

159. Berna MJ, Hoffmann KM, Long SH, et al. Serum gastrin in Zollinger-Ellison syndrome: II. Prospective study of gastrin provocative testing in 293 patients from the National Institutes of Health and comparison with 537 cases from the literature. Evaluation of diagnostic criteria, proposal of new criteria, and correlations with clinical and tumoral features. *Medicine.* 2006;85:331-364.

160. Brubaker PL, Drucker DJ, Asa SL, et al. Prolonged gastrointestinal transit in a patient with a glucagon-like peptide (GLP)-1- and -2-producing neuroendocrine tumor. *J Clin Endocrinol Metab.* 2002;87:3078-3083.

Section IX

Polyendocrine and Neoplastic Disorders

CHAPTER 39

Multiple Endocrine Neoplasia

STEPHEN J. MARX • SAMUEL A. WELLS, JR.

KEY POINTS

- Each multiple endocrine neoplasia (MEN) syndrome shows characteristic hormone-secreting tumors in a case or in a family. They are rare. Each also has some nonhormonal expressions.
- The main hormonal tumors in MEN type 1 (MEN1) are parathyroid, pancreatico-duodenal neuroendocrine, anterior pituitary, and foregut carcinoid. The main hormonal tumors in MEN type 2 (MEN2) are thyroid C-cell, adrenomedullary chromaffin, and parathyroid tumors.
- Management is often different and more difficult in a MEN tumor than for the same sporadic tumor.
- The differences from sporadic tumor are generally attributable to younger age at onset in MEN and to tumor multiplicity in MEN.
- The specific phenotype and the familial involvement helped the previous identification of the main gene (*MEN1* gene in MEN1 or *RET* gene in MEN2) mutated in the germline. Mutation of either of these main genes in somatic tissue causes a high proportion of common endocrine tumors in that tissue.
- Germline testing of *MEN1* or *RET* mutation is the main method for carrier identification. Testing for characteristic clinical traits is an alternative method.
- Early carrier identification can lead to early thyroidectomy for prevention or cure of medullary thyroid cancer in MEN2A. Carrier identification in MEN1 does not lead to tumor prevention but gives useful information to patients and caregivers.
- The *RET* gene encodes the RET protein; the *MEN1* gene encodes the menin protein. Much about the RET pathway is understood. This information helps development of drugs for therapy. Not enough is understood of the menin pathway to be useful in drug development.

INTRODUCTION TO MULTIPLE ENDOCRINE NEOPLASIA SYNDROMES

The MEN syndromes offer special chances for gene discovery and for insights into the pathogenesis of all endocrine tumors. This possibility has drawn disproportionate attention to them since their first recognition. The MEN syndromes were described in the early 1900s[1] and subsequently were classified into two principal categories, MEN1 and MEN2. They were named *multiple endocrine neoplasia* or *multiple endocrine adenomatosis* syndromes because they caused tumors in two or more types of hormone-secreting organs and consequently produced syndromes of multiple hormone excess.

From 1950 to 1980, advances in the fields of steroid and peptide hormone assays, imaging and histopathology, and connections of genes to cancers led to a fuller delineation of these syndromes. These technologies assisted the recognition that a recurring spectrum of endocrine tumors occurred in certain sporadic cases and in certain families. Furthermore, unique sets of hormones were associated with specific tumors, cell types, and clinical syndromes. Hormone measurements were used to identify specific neoplasms with the hope that earlier recognition and management would improve the course. Prominent among these hormones are parathyroid hormone to identify parathyroid tumors, prolactin to identify adenomas of the pituitary, gastrin and insulin to identify pancreaticoduodenal tumors, catecholamines or their metabolites to identify adrenal medullary tumors, and calcitonin (CTN) to identify C-cell hyperplasia (CCH) or C-cell neoplasia.

During this same period, at least six MEN syndromes with several subvariants were described: MEN1, MEN2, von Hippel-Lindau (VHL) disease, neurofibromatosis type 1 (NF1), Carney complex (CNC), and McCune-Albright syndrome (MAS).[2-8] The first five of these are transmitted in the germline with autosomal dominant transmission; the sixth (MAS) develops as a result of very early embryonic somatic mutations leading to tumors in multiple cell types but without transmission to offspring. Each of these syndromes meets the definition of MEN with the potential for production of multiple hormones. Special methods were developed to manage the multifocal tumors of each organ.[9] What was not completely recognized at the time of their early description is that each of these syndromes also causes nonendocrine neoplasias, and, in some cases, the nonendocrine manifestations cause the chief morbidity. This chapter will not provide an in-depth review of the management of nonendocrine manifestations. The current phase in our understanding of these syndromes focuses on the main gene mutated in each disease; this phase began in the 1980s and continues today. The one main gene for each of the six MEN syndromes has been identified, and this finding has answered some important questions and led to major changes in management. New identification of an MEN-related gene led rapidly to gene sequencing to detect germline mutations in affected patients and in relatives. Mutation testing for *RET* had a large impact on management in young members of MEN2 families; such impact did not derive from testing of other MEN genes, because the tumors and precursor cells associated with the other genes are not easily amenable to ablation and replacement and because the benefits of ablating target organs prior to presentation of clinical abnormalities have not been established. Gene sequencing has provided molecular evidence that most of the clinical variants of each syndrome are in fact initiated by mutations of a single gene. The only exceptions to this at present are MEN1 and CNC, in which a second or even more gene(s) at a distinct chromosomal locus remain to be identified. In two other syndromes, VHL and MEN2, specific mutations of the causative genes define unique clinical variants, making genetic information useful for predicting the phenotype. For most of these disorders, mutations of the same gene have been found in sporadic tumors of the same tissue type, indicating a broader importance for these genes beyond rare syndromes and extending to common endocrine and nonendocrine neoplasia. Examples include the identification of somatic mutations of *MEN1* in a high percentage of common pancreatic islet tumors, *VHL* mutations in sporadic renal cell carcinoma, and somatic mutations of *RET* in sporadic medullary thyroid cancers (MTCs).

The genetic and molecular abnormalities in these tumor syndromes are representative of the abnormalities found in all human neoplasia: MEN1, VHL, CNC, and NF1 are caused by inactivating mutations of a growth suppressor gene (tumor suppressor), and MAS and MEN2 are caused by activating mutations of a growth promoter gene (oncogene). In at least one of these syndromes, MEN2, the identification of the molecular defect has helped to lead to the development of pharmacologic agents that may blunt the mutated signal transduction abnormalities and has led to human clinical trials to reverse malignant tumor growth. Thus, current progress in understanding these disorders results from the premise that the pathogenesis of MEN is a special case of the pathogenesis of neoplasia more generally.

Progress has been extremely rapid during the current the era of gene discovery, and further exciting discoveries are expected shortly. Still, a number of important questions remain: How do the molecular defects cause transformation, sometimes benign and sometimes malignant? What is the mechanism of cell or tissue specificity? Is hyperplasia a necessary precursor? Are there signaling events that can be used as therapeutic targets?

MULTIPLE ENDOCRINE NEOPLASIA TYPE 1 SYNDROME

MEN1 (Online Mendelian Inheritance of Men [OMIM] 131100) is defined as a disease presenting with tumors of two of the following three cell types: parathyroid, duodeno-pancreatic endocrine, and pituitary. Although there were earlier descriptions,[10] the syndrome was recognized as a clinical and familial syndrome separately by Moldawer and associates[3] and by Wermer[4] in 1954 (thus the eponym *Wermer syndrome*). MEN2 was recognized as distinct from MEN1 in 1968.[6] In previous years, MEN1 patients presented with advanced manifestations of parathyroid, pancreatic islet, or pituitary neoplasia (or some combination of these) in the third and fourth decades of life. However, improved carrier ascertainment and improved tumor surveillance have now resulted in earlier identification and earlier treatment of its hormonal and nonhormonal expressions.

The most common mode of presentation for MEN1 currently results from evaluations in a previously identified kindred; less often, a patient with newly diagnosed advanced disease may be the propositus of a new kindred or a sporadic case. MEN1 remains the most challenging of the MEN syndromes. The many affected tissues cause morbidity and complexity and expense in diagnosis and treatment. It is important for the clinician to recognize the high probability of eventual recurrent or new neoplasms in many affected organ systems and to balance this likelihood against the potential effects of a deficiency syndrome from complete organ removal. Furthermore, even with satisfactory control of symptoms from hormone excess, patients have a high likelihood of eventual MEN1-related cancer. Although life expectancy may be long, the ultimate cause of death has been reported as due to MEN1 in 30% to 70% of cases.[9,11,12]

In this chapter, the discussion of MEN1 will first consider tumor expression, then tumor management, and last, molecular genetics. Data on the molecular pathway from the direct actions of the *MEN1* gene to clinical manifestations have not yet been sufficient to apply to management. However, in the subsequent sections on MEN2, data on molecular genetics will be covered early because information about both the *RET* gene and its molecular pathway has achieved a central role in management.

Tumor Expression and Management

Parathyroid Tumors in Multiple Endocrine Neoplasia Type 1

Hyperparathyroidism (HPT) is the most common hormonal manifestation of MEN1 (Table 39-1).[5,13-17] Prospective tumor surveillance in members of MEN1 families has shown HPT as early as age 8 years,[13-15,18-22] and by age 40 years about 95% of MEN1 carriers have been hyperparathyroid.[13,23] Nevertheless, because MEN1 is uncommon (the population prevalence is about 1 in 30,000), it accounts for only about 1% to 3% of all cases of primary HPT.[13]

Expressions of Parathyroid Tumors. HPT in MEN1 is most commonly asymptomatic; symptomatic expressions include hypercalcemia, urolithiasis, parathyroid hormone (PTH)-induced bone abnormalities, musculoskeletal complaints, weakness, and alterations of mental status. These features are similar to those associated with other forms of primary HPT (see Chapter 28).

HPT in MEN1 differs in some ways from that caused by a sporadic adenoma. First is a different epidemiology. HPT in MEN1 has an earlier age of onset (typically 25 years vs. 55 years)[15,16] (Fig. 39-1) and lack of gender imbalance (1:1 vs. 3:1 female-to-male ratio). Earlier onset implies that it can last longer. In particular, bone mass among women with MEN1-related HPT is often decreased when these women are in their 20s and 30s.[24,25] Second is a different parathyroid pathology; unlike solitary adenoma, enlargement, albeit highly asymmetric, of 3 to 4 parathyroid glands is usually present at the time of parathyroid exploration in MEN1 (Fig. 39-2).[26,27] Third, the distributions of outcomes of parathyroid surgery differ. The presence of multiglandular disease and the resulting need to examine each gland during an initial operation result in a higher postoperative rate of hypoparathyroidism and a lower rate of euparathyroidism.[26] Successful subtotal parathyroidectomy is also followed within 10 years by recurrent HPT in half of MEN1 cases.[28,29] In fact, true recurrent HPT after surgery for common HPT is unusual, and recurrence should suggest the possibility of unrecognized MEN1. True recurrent HPT, as with other tumor recurrences in MEN1, could arise theoretically from a small remnant of tumor tissue or from a new tumor clone arising in residual normal tissue. Fourth, HPT in MEN1 almost never progresses to parathyroid cancer, even though untreated HPT lasts longer in MEN1 than in sporadic cases.[30]

There are several characteristics of hyperfunctioning parathyroid cells in MEN1 that can have mechanistic

TABLE 39-1

Features of Multiple Endocrine Neoplasia Type 1 in Adults

Tumor Type	Estimated Average Penetrance
Endocrine Features	
Parathyroid	
Adenoma	95%
Pancreaticoduodenal	
Gastrinoma	40%
Insulinoma	10%
Nonfunctioning,* including pancreatic polypeptidoma†	20%
Other: glucagonoma, VIPoma, etc.	each <1%
Foregut Carcinoid	
Thymic carcinoid nonfunctioning	2%
Bronchial carcinoid nonfunctioning	4%
Gastric enterochromaffin-like tumor nonfunctioning	10%
Anterior Pituitary	
Prolactinoma	25%
Other	
Nonfunctioning	10%
Growth hormone + prolactin, Growth hormone	5%
ACTH	2%
Thyrotropin	5%
Adrenal	
Cortex	
Nonfunctioning	30%
Functioning or cancer	2%
Medulla: pheochromocytoma	<1%
Nonendocrine Features	
Angiofibroma	85%
Collagenoma	70%
Lipoma	30%
Leiomyoma	5%
Meningioma	5%

Italics indicate tumor types with substantial (>20% of cases) malignant potential.

*Many nonfunctioning MEN1 tumors synthesize a peptide hormone or other factors (such as small amine) but do not oversecrete enough to produce a hormonal expression.

†Omits nearly 100% prevalence of nonfunctioning and clinically silent tumors, some of which are detected incidental to pancreaticoduodenal surgery in MEN1.

ACTH, adrenocorticotropic hormone; MEN, multiple endocrine neoplasia; VIP, vasoactive intestinal peptide.

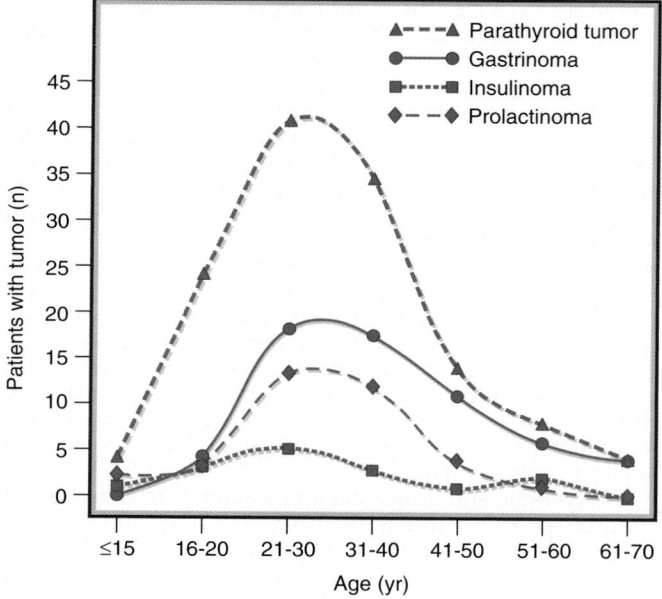

Figure 39-1 Age at onset for endocrine tumor expressions in multiple endocrine neoplasia type 1 (MEN1). Data from retrospective analysis of multiple tumor expressions in 130 inpatients with MEN1 during 15 years. Age of tumor onset was defined as the earlier of age at first symptom or age at first abnormal test result. (Modified from Marx S, Spiegel AM, Skarulis MC, et al. Multiple endocrine neoplasia type 1: clinical and genetic topics. *Ann Intern Med.* 1998;129:484-494.)

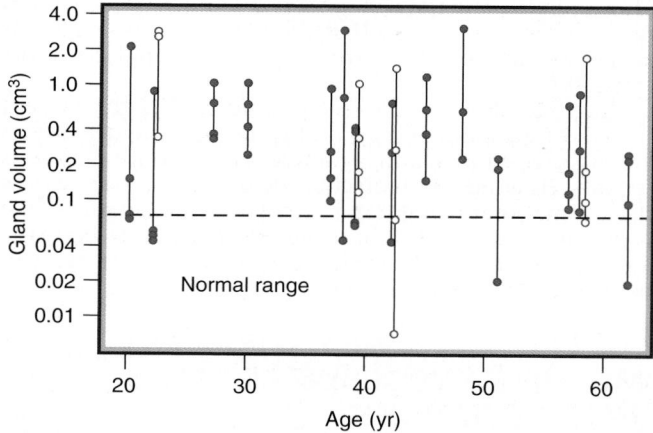

Figure 39-2 Parathyroid gland sizes at initial parathyroidectomy for 18 cases with familial multiple endocrine neoplasia type 1. The mean ratio of largest versus smallest tumor at one operation is 9:1. Volumes of all glands at one operation are connected by a *vertical line*. Adjacent symbols are highlighted by *open circles. Dashed horizontal line* is upper limit of normal gland volume (0.075 cm³, equivalent to 75-mg mass). (Modified from Marx SJ, Menczel J, Campbell G, et al. Heterogeneous size of the parathyroid glands in familial multiple endocrine neoplasia type 1. *Clin Endocrinol [Oxf].* 1991;35:521-526.)

implications. First, most or all parathyroid glands have been overgrown by one or a few neoplastic clones by the time of parathyroid surgery in MEN1 (Fig. 39-3).[31] Second, a circulating growth factor is specific to the plasma of MEN1 patients and mitogenic toward normal parathyroid cells in vitro (see later).[32]

Management of Parathyroid Tumors

Decision for Surgery. Surgery is the treatment of choice for HPT in MEN1, although the timing and the type of operation remain variable. Parathyroid surgery is definitely indicated in an MEN1 patient with a moderately elevated PTH and other moderately advanced features of HPT, such as an albumin-adjusted serum calcium level higher than 3.0 mmol/L (12.0 mg/dL), kidney stones, or PTH-induced bone disease.

Prospective surveillance for HPT in MEN1 families has led to systematic identification of affected members, including some as young as ages 8 to 15 years, with minimal elevations of serum calcium and PTH concentration. The optimal management of young patients with mild HPT is

not clear. The common surgical indication of age below 50 cannot be applied to all cases of HPT in MEN1.[33] Early parathyroid surgery in MEN1 has been advocated by some, believing that HPT should always be treated as early as possible or that normalization of the serum calcium concentration might lead to a reduction of gastrin secretion and, possibly, lowered pancreatic islet cell growth or transformation, or both.[13] An opposite approach is to delay surgery, thereby assuring an easier parathyroidectomy and perhaps decreasing the ultimate number of parathyroid operations during a lifetime. Although parathyroidectomy can decrease gastrin secretion by gastrinoma in MEN1 (Fig. 39-4), there is no evidence that this intervention prevents

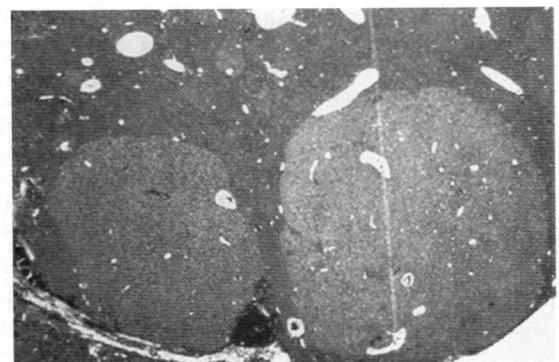

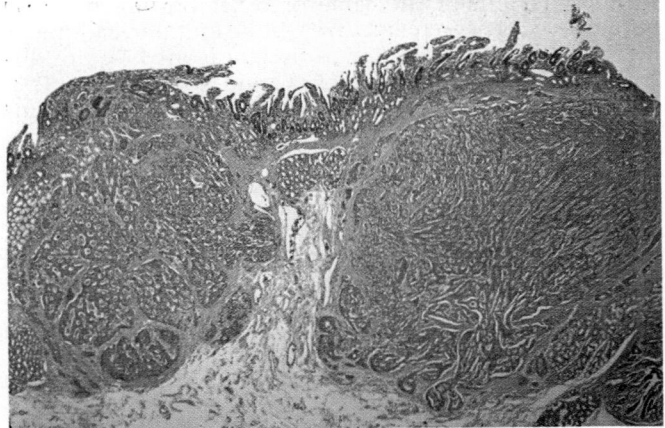

Figure 39-3 Tumor multiplicity within a tissue in multiple endocrine neoplasia type 1 (MEN1). *Top*, Hypercellular parathyroid gland from patient with MEN1. The gland is totally replaced by diffuse sheets of chief cells and two discrete nodules of chief cells. It suggests three or more abnormal parathyroid clones. This image could reflect three or more second hits to the normal copy of the *MEN1* gene in three different clone precursor cells and thus growth of three or more independent clones. An alternative pathogenesis could be stepwise evolution from one clone, that is, third hits to genes other than *MEN1*. *Bottom*, Duodenal mucosa from a second MEN1 patient, showing two large submucosal microgastrinomas. Each tumor was positive for gastrin immunostain and negative for other peptide hormones. Possible development of these two adjacent tumors could have followed mechanisms suggested for the two parathyroid nodules at the top. (Microphotographs from I. Lubensky, National Institutes of Health, Bethesda, MD.)

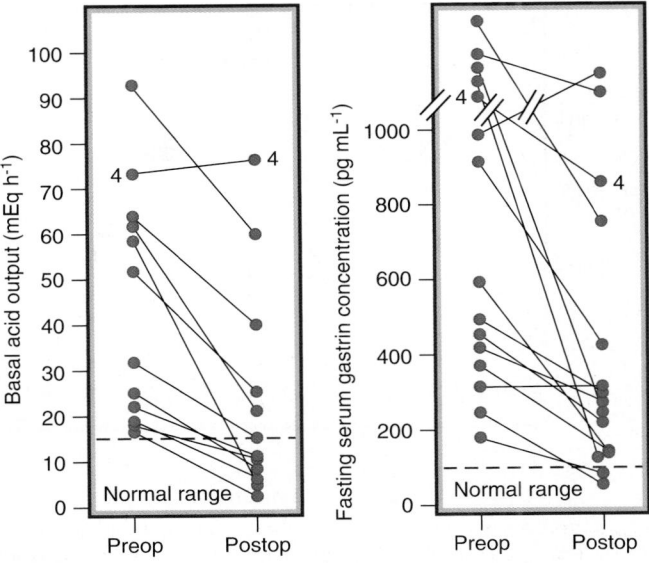

Figure 39-4 Remission of Zollinger-Ellison syndrome after parathyroidectomy in patients with both multiple endocrine neoplasia type 1 and Zollinger-Ellison syndrome. Basal acid output and fasting serum gastrin are shown. All patients became normocalcemic except for one (case 4), who remained hypercalcemic. (From Jensen RT. Management of the Zollinger-Ellison syndrome in patients with multiple endocrine neoplasia type 1. *J Intern Med.* 1998;243:477-488.)

or slows gastrin-cell transformation.[34] For this reason, and because drug control of gastric acid oversecretion is usually excellent, the coexistence of a gastrinoma is not a sufficient indication for parathyroidectomy in MEN1, except in the rare case in which medical control of Zollinger-Ellison syndrome (ZES) is prohibitively difficult.

Preoperative and Intraoperative Assessment of Parathyroid Tumors. Noninvasive imaging (ultrasonography, technetium-99m sestamibi, computed tomography [CT] scan, magnetic resonance imaging [MRI], or combinations) is being performed with increasing frequency before parathyroid surgery.[35] The major justification for the added costs of these procedures in sporadic HPT is to perform a unilateral or even more limited neck exploration, thereby reducing operative morbidity, time, and cost.[36] In MEN1 the likely presence of multiple parathyroid tumors makes it necessary to perform an exploration for four or more tumors at initial surgery, thereby eliminating one major rationale for preoperative imaging. Furthermore, imaging rarely shows all of the overactive parathyroid glands in MEN1. A separate, and less frequent, concern is that if four glands are overactive in MEN1, then there is a fourfold greater possibility than in solitary adenoma that one tumor has an abnormal location. A much stronger case can be made for the use of

noninvasive and carefully selected invasive procedures (guided fine-needle aspiration [FNA] for PTH assay, CT, selective arteriography, and selective venous sampling for PTH) in MEN1 patients before reoperation.[37,38]

Several intraoperative tools can increase the likelihood of successful parathyroid surgery. Rapid online assay of PTH can be done at 5-minute intervals, with a turnaround time of 10 minutes for each result.[39-41] A substantial PTH fall from baseline predicts that no hyperfunctioning parathyroid tissue remains (Fig. 39-5). These tests are even more likely to be helpful during parathyroid reoperations in MEN1, because the numbers and locations of tumors during a second operation are particularly hard to predict. Rarely, this test can give a false-positive signal if a "sleeping parathyroid" has been suppressed but awakens immediately after surgery.[42] Intraoperative PTH assay and ultrasonography may be useful as a backup option at initial parathyroid surgery, particularly in any patient expected to have multiple parathyroid tumors (as in MEN1). Sensitive ultrasound transducers routinely can image parathyroid tumors intraoperatively in difficult locations, such as within the thyroid gland and within scar from prior surgery.[35]

Removal of Parathyroid Tumors. The standard surgical approach for initial parathyroidectomy in MEN1 is removal of 3.5 glands and conservation of approximately 50 mg of the most normal-appearing gland, attached to its vascular pedicle in the neck. Because eventual parathyroid reoperation in MEN1 is likely, the recording of careful operative notes and diagrams and the marking of remaining tissue with nonresorbable materials enhance the likelihood of success in subsequent operations.

An alternative approach is attempted complete removal of all parathyroid tissue from the neck and immediate autotransplantation of small fragments to pockets in the nondominant forearm.[43] This strategy is dependent on the likelihood of achieving a high rate of graft success. This technique does not prevent recurrent HPT but can simplify its management. For example, a PTH concentration in the venous effluent of the graft greater than in the effluent

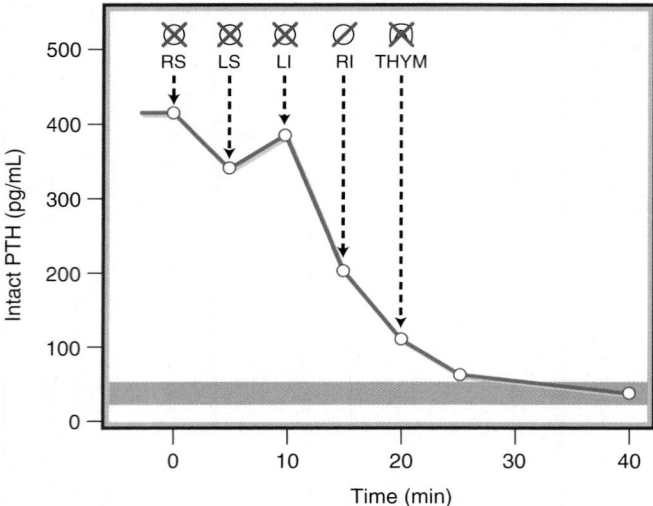

Figure 39-5 Intact parathyroid hormone (PTH) by rapid assay during parathyroid surgery. Normal range is indicated by *shading*. The patient had multiple endocrine neoplasia type 1 and primary hyperparathyroidism without prior parathyroidectomy. Three and one half similarly enlarged parathyroid glands (0.8-1.6 g; normal is <0.08 g) and the accessible portions of the thymus (THYM) were removed at the times indicated; the thymus contained no identified parathyroid tumor. A rapid fall of PTH below a cutoff criterion indicates that little or no hyperfunctioning parathyroid tumor remains. Removal of the first two parathyroid tumors was not followed by a fall in PTH. The PTH assay result for each time point was available within several minutes to help establish the time at which no hyperfunctioning parathyroid tumor remained and thereby contribute to serial decisions about extending or ending the operation. I, inferior; L, left; R, right; S, superior. (From SK Libutti, HR Alexander, and A Remaley, National Institutes of Health, Bethesda, MD.)

from the contralateral arm confirms graft function; still, this does not prove graft hyperfunction, and it does not exclude the presence or hyperfunction of other parathyroid tissue in the neck or chest. Lastly, surgical removal of parathyroid tissue from the forearm graft bed during the likely second or third operation is technically easier than a neck reexploration. Cryopreservation of viable parathyroid tumor fragments is a useful option in MEN1, given the high rate of postoperative hypoparathyroidism in MEN1. Cryopreservation permits a late parathyroid autograft.[43] Parathyroid cryopreservation in the United States is discouraged by regulatory considerations.

Partial thymectomy can be done through the cervical incision.[44] This procedure not only results in subtotal removal of intrathymic parathyroid tissue but also can remove thymic carcinoid tissue, an issue discussed later in this chapter. The best time for this is during the initial neck operation because scar tissue can hinder a subtotal transcervical thymectomy at reoperation. Thymic carcinoid can occasionally occur after transcervical thymectomy either because it may already have been established or because removal of the entire thymus is not possible by this approach.

Parathyroid surgery in the patient with MEN1 requires judgment, familiarity with neck anatomy, and experience. An excellent outcome is more likely when initial or reoperative procedures are performed by an experienced endocrine surgery team.

Pancreaticoduodenal Neuroendocrine Tumors

Neoplasia of the pancreaticoduodenal neuroendocrine cells is the second most common endocrine manifestation of MEN1 and eventually occurs in about 60% of MEN1 patients (see Table 39-1). Also, multiple clinically silent

pancreaticoduodenal macroadenomas may be recognized at surgery or autopsy in nearly 100% of MEN1 patients older than 40 years.[45,46] Gastric carcinoid tumors are described in a separate section (see "Foregut Carcinoid Tumors"). The pancreaticoduodenal tumors are multiple, can oversecrete various hormones, and can become malignant. It is notable that in this era of excellent pharmacotherapy for gastric hyperacidity, about one sixth of MEN1 patients with gastrinoma can die from metastatic gastrinoma but rarely from hypergastrinemia-induced metabolic complications.[47]

Although the MEN1 patient can show symptoms or signs caused by one pancreaticoduodenal hormone, there are often several associated and asymptomatic tumors with production of the same or other hormones or no hormone.[48,49] The frequency of peptide immunostaining in MEN1 pancreatic islet tumors is glucagon 35%, insulin 25%, pancreatic polypeptide 25%, and no hormone 10%; gastrin staining is rare.[48-50] There are no data on the comparable frequency in duodenal gastrinomas.

Interpretation of pancreatic islet histologic features in MEN1 has changed over the decades. Early studies emphasized hyperplastic processes and budding of islet cells from ducts (termed *nesidioblastosis*).[51] Such features have now been reinterpreted as nonspecific in MEN1. The overriding and important islet lesion in MEN1, now termed *multifocal microadenoma*, is a monoclonal or oligoclonal process (see Fig. 39-3).[52,53] Molecular evidence for a hyperplastic precursor stage to tumor in MEN1 is also accumulating. Hyperplastic foci of gastrin cells are seen by light microscopy in the duodenum of gastrinoma specimens from MEN1 but not from sporadic gastrinoma.[54] Furthermore, heterozygous knockout of the *MEN1* gene in the mouse provides a good model of human MEN1; multiple giant hyperplastic islets are striking and precede insulinoma in this model, suggesting that subtle islet hyperplasia is an undetected islet tumor precursor lesion also in MEN1 of humans.[55] Because MEN1 cases often have multiple islet macroadenomas, some with differing hormonal properties, tumor imaging has roles different from those in sporadic islet tumors. Sensitive new imaging methods such as endoscopic ultrasound and gallium-68 DOTATATE PET (positron emission tomography) scan may achieve roles that remain to be defined.[56]

Rarely, pancreaticoduodenal neuroendocrine tumors occur in several members of a family without other features of MEN1; these tumors have been insulinomas[57] or glucagonomas.[57b] Nonfunctioning pancreatic islet tumors and pheochromocytoma can also appear uncommonly in a familial setting as expressions of VHL syndrome.[58]

Gastrinoma

Expressions of Gastrinoma. Gastrinoma is the second most common endocrine tumor and is the most common cause of severe symptoms and signs in MEN1. The symptoms and signs reflect two processes: (1) malignancy and (2) gastrin induction of excessive acid secretion by the stomach. Gastrinomas are found in about 40% of adults with MEN1 (see Table 39-1).[13,15,34] ZES is defined here as symptoms or signs of gastric acid hypersecretion caused by a gastrin-secreting pancreaticoduodenal neuroendocrine tumor or tumors. Among all patients with ZES, MEN1 is found often, on the order of 25% in large series.[59] MEN1 in most of these patients is readily recognizable from personal and family history. In contrast, among carefully defined sporadic ZES cases without obvious MEN1, occult MEN1 is much less frequent, a conclusion based on family history, long-term follow-up, and mutational analysis of the *MEN1* gene.[60]

Symptoms of ZES include diarrhea, esophageal reflux, and those associated with peptic ulceration. Symptoms can antedate recognition of fasting hypergastrinemia. At one extreme, ulcer perforation can be caused infrequently by hypergastrinemia, even without prior symptoms.[61] The laboratory diagnosis of gastrinoma is mainly by finding an elevated serum gastrin level. Other causes of elevated gastrin (false-positive results) that must be differentiated from gastrinoma include hypochlorhydria, including that resulting from autoimmunity or from pharmacologic agents that inhibit peptic acid secretion.[62,63] HPT in MEN1 often exacerbates hypergastrinemia (see earlier) (see Fig. 39-4).

Recognition of elevated gastrin or acid-related symptoms (peptic pain or diarrhea) should be followed by assessment of the gastric acid secretion rate without acid-blocking drugs; the normal rate is less than 15 mEq/hour (or less than 5 mEq/hour after acid-reducing surgery).[64] The diagnosis of gastrinoma can also be confirmed by measuring the serum gastrin response to intravenous synthetic secretin. A gastrin increase of more than 114 pmol/L (200 pg/mL) diagnoses gastrinoma. This test differentiates gastrinoma from other hypergastrinemic states, such as retained gastric antrum, massive small bowel resection, gastric outlet obstruction, or *H. pylori* infection. Gastric endoscopy and ultrasound are advisable at the initial evaluation for ZES in MEN1 and allow assessment of associated peptic ulcerations, gastric carcinoids, duodenal gastrinomas, and Barrett esophagus.[64] Other imaging should also be used to search for gastric carcinoids, which are common in MEN1 (see later).

Like parathyroid adenomas, gastrinomas have two features that are relatively specific for MEN1. One is earlier age of onset than sporadic tumors. On the average, gastrinoma begins 10 years earlier with MEN1 than without it, a lesser age differential than the 30 years of difference for HPT.[65] The second is multifocal tumor: the gastrinomas in MEN1 are often small, multiple, and intraduodenal (see Fig. 39-3).[66] The duodenal predominance differs only modestly from that in sporadic gastrinoma.[66] Gastrinomas in MEN1 have a high propensity to metastasize to local nodes.[34] High-grade aggressive behavior, including distant spread to the liver and occasionally other tissues, also occurs in about 20% of cases. Diffuse hepatic metastases are particularly ominous, predicting a 5-year survival rate of only 50%.[63] The prognosis of gastrinoma in MEN1 is similar to that in sporadic cases.[63] No early features have allowed reliable prediction of which gastrinomas will behave aggressively.[67]

Therapy for Gastrinoma. Most centers have reported a virtually zero success rate for surgical cure of gastrinoma in MEN1, even though one third of gastrinoma patients without MEN1 are cured by surgery.[68] Unique characteristics of gastrinoma in MEN1 that contribute to the low rate of curative resection are the multiplicity of small tumors and the frequency of local metastases. The largest tumor was not a gastrinoma in 40% of operations for gastrinoma in MEN1. Extreme approaches, mainly pancreaticoduodenectomy, have been suggested,[69] but long-term benefit is unproved and the associated potential for surgically induced morbidity seems unacceptable. Several academic centers have reported frequent surgical cure of gastrinoma by pancreaticoduoden in MEN1.[70-74] Other groups have not reported similar success rates despite the use of similar approaches.[66] Differences in criteria for cure and in selection of patients, such as age, can contribute to the differences in outcome.

The development of H_2 histamine receptor antagonists (cimetidine and ranitidine) and proton pump inhibitors (PPIs; omeprazole and other members of this class) makes it possible to perform a pharmacologic gastrectomy for ZES.[75] The PPIs are even more effective than the H_2 receptor antagonists. If compliance is good, the need for surgical total gastrectomy is eliminated.[76,77] Side effects, including those from achlorhydria, are mild. Gastric carcinoids develop in rats given large doses of PPIs.[78] Gastric carcinoids are also seen in MEN1[79]; however, the PPIs do not seem to exacerbate them in MEN1. There remains disagreement about whether the PPIs worsen enterochromaffin-like cell hyperplasia in sporadic ZES.[80,81] The somatostatin analogue octreotide inhibits partially the secretion of both gastrin and gastric acid,[82] and it is under evaluation for a role in malignant gastrinoma.[83] In addition, the gastrin-lowering effect of somatostatin analogues might account for their effective suppression of gastric carcinoid mass in MEN1.[84]

Although medical acid pump blocker therapy for ZES in MEN1 is effective and preferred, the need for lifetime medical therapy, the recognition that small duodenal gastrinomas cause a high percentage of cases, and the poor outcome (50% 5-year survival rate) in patients with hepatic metastasis lead to frequent reexamination of treatment choices.

Insulinoma. Insulinoma is the second most common hormone-secreting pancreaticoduodenal neuroendocrine tumor in MEN1, with an overall lifetime prevalence of 10% among adults with MEN1 (see Table 39-1).[15,16] By coincidence, MEN1 also accounts for approximately 10% of all patients with insulinoma.[85] The clinical features and diagnostic criteria are the same in MEN1 and sporadic cases: glucopenic symptoms and fasting hypoglycemia with high insulin, C peptide, or proinsulin (see Chapter 34). Insulinoma syndrome in MEN1 is usually caused by a single dominant and benign pancreatic islet tumor, although simultaneous nonhypersecreting islet tumors that stain for insulin or another gut hormone are common in MEN1. The main insulinoma is generally 1 to 2 cm in diameter and is located anywhere in the pancreas. Removal of the main insulinoma is usually curative.[16] Rarely, more than one tumor causes the insulinoma syndrome in MEN1 at one time or sequentially. The postoperative recurrence rate of insulinoma may be higher in MEN1 than in sporadic cases. Recurrent insulinoma in MEN1 might arise after 10% of operations, the same as the overall frequency of insulinoma in unoperated MEN1 cases.

Preferred treatment is surgical removal of the insulinoma. Other incidental pancreatic islet macroadenomas should also be removed, mainly because of the possibility that one might become malignant. Somatostatin receptor scintigraphy (SRS) can give 30% to 60% true-positive images.[86] Radiolabeled exendin-4 analogues bind to cell surface receptors for glucagon-like peptide-1; they are being explored for imaging of insulinomas.[87] When surgery is performed with guidance only by intraoperative ultrasonography,[88,89] the success rate should be satisfactory, although no large series has yet documented this in insulinoma of MEN1. In some centers, routine distal pancreatectomy is performed as an adjunct in MEN1 for prevention of other tumors.

No matter how sensitive, current imaging methods for a mass do not establish an islet tumor to be an insulinoma in MEN1, mainly because of tumor multiplicity. Several techniques, based on insulin radioimmunoassay, can be useful for localization of an insulinoma in patients with MEN1. These include infusion of calcium into selectively catheterized pancreatic arteries with measurement of insulin in right or left hepatic venous effluent.[90] Identification of an insulin peak after an intra-arterial calcium infusion localizes the insulinoma to the distribution of the infused artery. Other tests that have been useful include rapid intraoperative insulin and glucose levels in serum[91] or intraoperative insulin levels in fine-needle aspirates of a pancreatic tumor.[92]

Metastatic insulinoma causing hypoglycemia should be treated surgically for palliation, but operative strategies are not likely to be curative.[93,94] Hypoglycemia caused by unlocated or metastatic insulinoma can be controlled with diazoxide[94]; somatostatin analogues are less effective.[95]

Tumors Secreting Glucagon, Vasoactive Intestinal Peptide, or Other Hormones

Glucagonoma. The glucagonoma syndrome consists of hyperglycemia, anorexia, glossitis, anemia, diarrhea, venous thrombosis, and a characteristic skin rash termed *necrolytic migratory erythema* (see Chapter 38). Glucagonoma syndrome is rare in MEN1,[96] although one third of MEN1 pancreaticoduodenal neuroendocrine tumors immunostain for glucagon.[48] Glucagonoma is usually large and metastatic at presentation. Palliation is often possible with surgery or another ablative procedure (see later). Some patients have responded partially to the somatostatin analogue octreotide, although an initial response has not predicted a long-term response.[97]

VIPoma. Although the most common cause of diarrhea in MEN1 is gastrinoma, a separate diarrheal syndrome is caused by oversecretion of vasoactive intestinal peptide (VIP) and is termed *WDHA* (watery diarrhea, hypokalemia, and achlorhydria) or *VIPoma syndrome*[98] (see Chapter 38). In MEN1 it is rare and can occur with pancreaticoduodenal neuroendocrine tumor.[96] Half of such tumors also cause hypercalcemia, perhaps by cosecreting PTH-related peptide[99]; of course, coexistent primary HPT is common in patients with MEN1. The tumor is usually malignant, large, and metastatic at presentation. Treatment considerations are the same as with glucagonoma (see later).

Growth Hormone–Releasing Hormone Oversecretion. Oversecretion of growth hormone–releasing hormone (GHRH) is a rare manifestation of a pancreaticoduodenal neuroendocrine tumor; however, half of such rare cases are found with MEN1 (see later).[100] GHRH oversecretion can also occur with bronchial carcinoid in MEN1.[101]

Other Ectopic Hormones. Other peptides that may rarely be oversecreted by pancreaticoduodenal neuroendocrine tumors in MEN1 include adrenocorticotropic hormone (ACTH), PTH-related peptide,[99] somatostatin,[102] and CTN.[103] The last can cause confusion with thyroidal C-cell cancer, but serum CTN levels are generally much higher in C-cell cancer than in MEN1 cancers.

Nonfunctional Tumors.

One third of pancreaticoduodenal neuroendocrine tumors in MEN1 immunostain mainly for pancreatic polypeptide; similar percentages immunostain mainly for insulin or for glucagon.[48,49] Pancreaticoduodenal neuroendocrine tumors in MEN1 commonly also oversecrete pancreatic polypeptide.[104,105] Oversecretion of pancreatic polypeptide is not associated with any identifiable hormonal syndrome. Like other nonfunctional pancreaticoduodenal neuroendocrine tumors in MEN1, these tumors are often large, malignant, and metastatic at presentation.[96]

Nonfunctional tumor is an abused but convenient term. In the context of MEN1, it is applied to pancreaticoduodenal neuroendocrine tumors, anterior pituitary tumors, or foregut carcinoids that do not immunostain for the common hormones of that tissue or that immunostain for one or more hormones but do not hypersecrete that hormone. Most pancreaticoduodenal tumors in MEN1 fit this definition,[48,49] and most never become a clinical problem. Of course, one oversecreting tumor is sufficient to dominate the clinical features. If a nonfunctioning tumor becomes malignant, its lack of symptomatic

hormone hypersecretion can allow progression to an advanced stage before recognition. About 5% of islet or duodenal tumors in MEN1 immunostain for somatostatin without clinical expression; these tumors rarely metastasize.[102]

Staging of Pancreaticoduodenal Neuroendocrine Tumors.

Appropriate management of pancreaticoduodenal neuroendocrine tumor or tumors in MEN1 is challenging because of the multicentric nature of the tumors and the need to decide between surgical and other approaches. A pancreaticoduodenal tumor causing a hormone excess state in MEN1 is likely to be accompanied by separate nonfunctional tumor(s). Some of the experience acquired with imaging of sporadic tumors of the same types cannot be generalized to MEN1 tumors. Accurate localization of tumor and, in particular, identification of metastatic disease is critical for preoperative decision making. The multicentricity and variable size of these tumors stretch the limitations of radiologic techniques that have difficulty imaging tumors smaller than 1 cm in diameter. And their rarity has prevented organization of controlled trials.

SRS (such as ^{111}In-octreotide or ^{68}Ga-DOTATATE scan) enhanced by single photon emission CT (SPECT) is a generally useful method for imaging pancreaticoduodenal neuroendocrine and foregut neuroendocrine tumors.[56,106,107] It can image the primary tumor and local or distant metastases.[108-112] It is particularly useful for multiple gastrinomas in MEN1,[110,111] and it has replaced most angiographic procedures in MEN1-associated gastrinoma.[56,112,113] SRS fails to image one third of lesions identified at surgery even in sporadic gastrinoma.[112] The yield of SRS with sporadic insulinoma is somewhat lower than with other pancreatic islet tumors, with 30% to 60% true positives.[86] Abdominal imaging by CT, particularly helical CT,[114,115] combined with early-phase images after contrast agent injection or MRI provides enhanced sensitivity for detection of small lesions and is complementary to SRS.[56,116] ^{11}C-5-Hydroxytryptophan PET scanning is a relatively new method being explored for insulinoma, and ^{18}F-DOPA PET is generally more sensitive than SRS, but neither has been explored in MEN1.[117,118]

No imaging technique used for evaluation of MEN1 pancreaticoduodenal tumors is completely satisfactory. Endoscopic ultrasonography with or without needle aspiration of a pancreatic mass is useful for characterizing pancreaticoduodenal abnormalities but is a technically demanding and expensive option for the foreseeable future.[119,120] It can image many small tumors that might not warrant any intervention. With the exception of endoscopic ultrasonography, the current preoperative imaging methods are not able to image tumors confined to the pancreas and smaller than 1.5 cm in diameter. They also fail to identify metastases in 25% of cases and the extent of tumor multiplicity in MEN1 cases.[107] In contrast, intraoperative ultrasonography is a useful tool for localizing some small tumors not detectable by the eye or fingers of the surgeon. This technique has become the primary approach for diagnosis of small insulinomas in most medical centers, although experience has been limited to sporadic tumors.[86,121]

Functional (i.e., insulin-specific) testing can be useful to assess insulinoma because, unlike other pancreaticoduodenal neuroendocrine tumors in MEN1, insulinoma may be symptomatic when it is small and solitary (see earlier).

Serum markers in MEN1, mainly chromogranin A, provide useful diagnostic tools in monitoring mass of a pancreaticoduodenal tumor but not the emergence of a small tumor.[122] Chromogranin A has not been helpful in insulinoma, perhaps because of the small tumor mass.[123] Chromogranin A and gastrin as possible tumor markers also have not been reliable indices of gastrinoma extent or progression.[124]

Treatment of Pancreaticoduodenal Neuroendocrine Tumors.

Many aspects of treatment specific to gastrinomas and insulinoma in MEN1 have already been described. Treatment of these and other pancreaticoduodenal neuroendocrine tumors in MEN1 is controversial and guided in part by staging procedures and local preferences. The main controversies are highlighted in the following paragraphs.

Is Tumor Size Important? Metastasis has been associated with gastrinomas more than 3 cm in diameter. This association has led some to recommend resection for all pancreaticoduodenal tumors larger than 2.5 cm.[125] Another analysis of this strategy suggested a failure to prevent later emergence of hepatic metastases.[126] Some others have not found a relation of tumor size and metastasis and do not use a size criterion for surgery.[127]

Should All Pancreaticoduodenal Neuroendocrine Tumors in MEN1 Be Removed? There is no consensus on this point. In MEN1, for every identifiable pancreatic tumor there are likely to be several smaller unidentified tumors that coexist or emerge at a later date. Improvements in pancreatic surgical technique, however, have made it possible to excise smaller lesions surgically, although the benefit from doing this is less clear. Certainly there is no compelling evidence to suggest that surgical removal of small tumors, unless they produce a hormonal syndrome, improves overall outcome. Some urge removal of all detectable macroadenomas if removal would not be dangerous.[128] Others urge a large size cutoff (2.5-3 cm in diameter) for removal. Pylorus-sparing total duodenectomy for ZES in MEN1 is under evaluation in a few academic centers; its strength is removal of all nonmetastatic duodenal gastrinomas; its limitations are its not addressing pancreatic tumors and its undocumented rate of long-term metabolic consequence.[74]

Should Metastatic Pancreaticoduodenal Cancer Be Debulked? Total pancreatectomy with a high rate of complications has been used for very large tumors.[129] Many methods are under exploration for resecting or otherwise palliating pancreaticoduodenal neuroendocrine cancer.[130,131] Results are too preliminary to justify endorsing any of these.

Should Medications Be Used to Control Tumor Progression? Pancreaticoduodenal neuroendocrine tumors are usually well differentiated and quite resistant to chemotherapy. Several regimens have been tried including streptozotocin, doxorubicin, and interferon, but there is no proof of long-term efficacy.[132-135] Octreotide has been effective in inhibiting hormone secretion by benign and malignant pancreaticoduodenal neuroendocrine tumors[82,136-138]; however, it has not been effective by itself in blocking growth of these tumors except to a small degree for malignant gastrinoma.[83,139] Lanreotide, another somatostatin analogue, prolonged the interval to tumor progression in metastatic enteropancreatic neuroendocrine tumors, particularly in pancreatic islet cancers.[140] Inhibitors of mammalian target of rapamycin (mTOR) or tyrosine kinase give benefit in sporadic advanced islet neoplasia.[141,142] The preceding trials have focused on the more common sporadic neuroendocrine tumors, and generally excluded MEN1. Multidrug regimens need further evaluation.

Somatostatin Analogue Linked to a Radioisotope. Because of their selectivity for certain tumors, somatostatin analogues have been explored as vehicles to deliver a toxic radioactive isotope to that tumor. The best results seem to be from lutetium-177 bound to octreotate.[143] However, controlled studies have not yet been done. These drugs are currently under investigation in the United States.

Pituitary Tumor or Adrenal Cortical Tumor

Anterior pituitary tumor occurs in about one third of MEN1 patients.[13,16,143] The frequency of MEN1 in cases of apparently sporadic pituitary tumor is probably less than 5%, although estimates vary widely to as high as 15% with prolactinoma.[144,145] The distributions of hormones hypersecreted are similar to those in non-MEN1 pituitary tumors: prolactin 60%, growth hormone with or without prolactin 15%, nonsecreting 25%, and ACTH 5%; thyrotropin or gonadotropins is rare.[13,146] Pituitary mass effects can be the principal problem.[147] In fact, pituitary tumors in MEN1 have been larger and less responsive to treatment than those without MEN1.[146] Pituitary tumor can occur early in MEN1 and is occasionally the first recognized feature.[146-148] Rarely, two independent pituitary tumors have been suggested.[149,150]

Prolactinoma. Prolactinoma is the most common pituitary tumor in MEN1 and the third most common endocrine tumor in MEN1 after parathyroid tumors and gastrinomas (see Table 39-1). The general properties are similar to those of sporadic prolactinoma (see Chapter 9); MEN1 prolactinoma may be even larger.[146,151] Dopamine agonists (e.g., cabergoline, bromocriptine, quinagolide) are the preferred treatment.[152,153] A reduction in side effects and greater potency make cabergoline the current treatment of choice and have improved patient compliance. In patients who escape the growth-inhibitory effects of these dopamine agonists or who are noncompliant, transsphenoidal surgery combined with radiation therapy is usually effective.

Tumors That Produce Growth Hormone or Growth Hormone–Releasing Hormone. The clinical features of growth hormone excess are similar in cases with and without MEN1.[154] There are two different etiologic mechanisms with different treatment implications. The majority of MEN1 pituitary adenomas arises clonally from inactivation of both alleles of the *MEN1* gene in a tumor precursor cell.[155] Other genes such as *AIP* or *GNAS* (encodes the α-subunit of the stimulatory G protein) may be implicated outside MEN1.[156] The alternate mechanism of pituitary GH tumorigenesis is secondary to overproduction of GHRH by pancreatic islet or carcinoid tumor.[100,157-159] The resulting secondary pituitary tumor is a polyclonal or hyperplastic process, which responds poorly to therapy directed only at the pituitary; removal of the primary GHRH-producing tumor is essential. Although acromegaly secondary to GHRH is rare in sporadic or MEN1 cases,[157] among cases with GHRH tumors, a disproportionate fraction have had MEN1. Thus, measurement of serum GHRH in MEN1 acromegalic patients seems worthwhile. GH-producing pituitary tumors also produce GHRH locally, but this has not interfered with the interpretation of serum GHRH levels.[159,160]

Treatment for acromegaly with MEN1 is the same as that without MEN1 (see Chapter 9). Surgery is usually the first choice, but the development of other pharmacologic therapies including long-acting somatostatin receptor antagonists or growth hormone receptor antagonists can provide effective, albeit expensive, control.[161,162] In patients with large tumors causing mass effects or those in whom growth hormone effects are not controlled by surgery or pharmacologic therapy, radiation using an external beam, gamma knife, or proton beam is an alternative (see Chapter 9).

Corticotropin Hypersecretion. Hypercortisolism in MEN1 can be caused by a pituitary tumor producing ACTH, uncommonly by ectopic production of ACTH from a carcinoid or an islet tumor, by ectopic production of ACTH-releasing hormone, by corticotropin-releasing hormone (CRH), or by adrenal tumor. Therapy should be directed initially to treat the ACTH- or CRH-producing primary tumor. When therapy directed toward the primary source is not successful, corticosteroid production can be controlled by bilateral adrenalectomy or medical therapy (see Chapter 15).

Primary Adrenocortical Hyperfunction. One or both adrenal glands are enlarged in up to 40% of MEN1 patients.[163,164] This enlargement, most often discovered during pancreatic imaging, is generally clinically silent and rarely requires treatment. The silent enlargement represents a presumably polyclonal or hyperplastic process of unknown cause, and it rarely behaves as a neoplasm. MEN1 cases have been identified occasionally with primary hypercortisolism, hyperaldosteronism, or adrenocortical cancer.[165] Adrenocortical tumor seems more often to be malignant in MEN1 than in sporadic cases.[166,167]

Foregut Carcinoid Tumors

Carcinoid tumor is recognized in 5% to 15% of MEN1 patients.[13] Although sporadic carcinoid is derived mainly from midgut and hindgut, MEN1 carcinoid is primarily found in derivatives of the foregut (thymus, bronchus, stomach, etc.). Certain carcinoid tumors, unlike any other manifestation of MEN1, have a strong sex-specific distribution. In MEN1, thymic carcinoid is found mainly in male patients and with clustering in some families, and bronchial carcinoid is found with less gender bias mainly in female patients.[168-172] The average age of carcinoid recognition in MEN1 is 45 years,[170] later than that of other MEN1 tumors. This later age might reflect the lack of compression-induced symptoms and the lack of a hormone oversecretion syndrome with most MEN1 carcinoids.

Thymic carcinoid in MEN1 is usually found at an already advanced stage as a large invasive mass. Much less commonly it is recognized during chest imaging or during thymectomy adjunctive to parathyroidectomy. Thymic carcinoid is more often malignant (about 70%) than bronchial carcinoid (about 20%) in MEN1.[173,174] The latter has a more indolent course.[171] MEN1 thymic or bronchial carcinoids rarely oversecrete ACTH, CTN, or GHRH; similarly, they rarely oversecrete serotonin or histamine and rarely cause the carcinoid syndrome. Most can thus be considered clinically as nonfunctioning. Mediastinal or bronchial carcinoids are best imaged by CT; however, SRS and new PET ligands sometimes give positive results.[175]

Gastric carcinoid has been recognized more recently but is less well characterized in MEN1. It is a tumor of enterochromaffin-like cells. Large gastric carcinoids can cause a hormonal syndrome from serotonin and histamine secretion in MEN1.[176] In up to 15% of MEN1 patients they have been recognized incidentally during endoscopy. The overall malignancy rate seems low.[177] At early stages they can regress after treatment with somatostatin analogues.[137]

Carcinoid occurs occasionally in several members of a small family without other manifestations of MEN1.[178,179] The cause of familial isolated carcinoids is under study.[180-182b]

Miscellaneous Tumors of MEN1

Miscellaneous Endocrine Tumors in MEN1

Pheochromocytoma. Pheochromocytoma is a rare feature in MEN1. There have been about 10 reported cases.[164,183] Most have been unilateral and chemically silent; one was malignant. In two tumors, 11q13 loss of heterozygosity (LOH) was documented,[184] making it likely that all or most of these rare pheochromocytomas in MEN1 are true clonal expressions from biallelic *MEN1* gene inactivation. This cause is supported by pheochromocytoma being even more frequent in mouse MEN1 than human MEN1.[55]

Thyroid Follicular Neoplasm. Thyroid follicular neoplasm has been associated with MEN1 since the earliest reviews. This association is likely related to the high incidence of thyroid follicular neoplasms in the general population (unrelated to MEN1) and their incidental discovery during the inevitable neck exploration for parathyroid disease in MEN1. Further support for a coincidental association is the rare identification of *MEN1* gene mutations in sporadic thyroid follicular tumors.[185]

Miscellaneous Nonendocrine Tumors. MEN1 has nonendocrine tumors that vary from rare to common, with some offering possible use in the diagnosis of MEN1 carriers.

Lipoma. The association of lipoma with MEN1 has been known since the 1960s.[5] MEN1 lipomas are generally dermal, small, and sometimes multiple. Their frequency in MEN1 is about 30% versus 5% in control subjects without MEN1.[186] This frequency in normal subjects has limited their use for MEN1 carrier ascertainment.

Angiofibromas. Angiofibromas are acneiform papules on the face that do not regress and that can extend across the vermilion border of the lips (Fig. 39-6). They have been found in 85% of MEN1 patients, but none have been found in control subjects.[186,187] Half of MEN1 patients have five or more.

Collagenoma. Collagenomas are whitish macular and rarely pedunculated lesions about the trunk, sparing the face and neck. Collagenoma was observed in 70% of MEN1 patients but in none of the control subjects.[187] The MEN1 lipomas, angiofibromas, and collagenomas show loss of one copy of 11q13.[188] Thus, it is likely that these are clonal neoplasms and caused by inactivation of the (first and then) second copy of the *MEN1* gene.

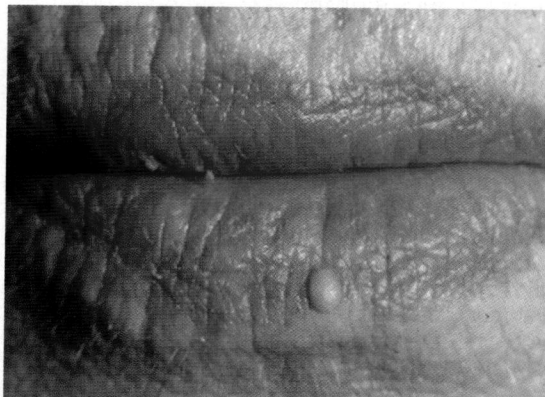
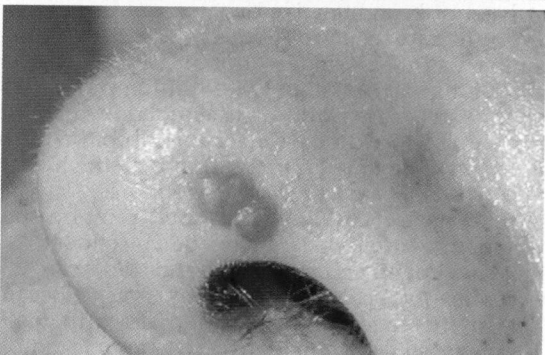

Figure 39-6 Facial angiofibroma in patients with multiple endocrine neoplasia type 1. A small, light pink lesion on the vermilion border of the lip *(top)* and a large, reddish angiofibroma on the nose *(bottom)* are shown. Typical lesions are smaller than these and multiple and might require biopsy for confirmation. (From T Darling and M Turner, National Institutes of Health, Bethesda, MD.)

Spinal Cerebellar Ependymoma. Spinal cerebellar ependymoma has been seen in four MEN1 patients.[189] There are no studies to determine whether 11q13 LOH or other *MEN1* gene abnormalities are present.

Malignant Melanoma. Malignant melanoma has occurred in at least seven MEN1 patients, but direct involvement of the *MEN1* gene has not been tested.[190]

Leiomyoma (of Esophagus, Lung, Rectum, or Uterus). Leiomyoma has been reported in several MEN1 patients.[191,192] Identification of 11q13 LOH established that esophageal and uterine leiomyoma are specific to MEN1 patients.[193] In contrast, *MEN1* inactivation was not implicated in sporadic uterine leiomyoma.

Meningioma (Cranial). A large prospective series reported meningioma in 8% of MEN1 patients. These tumors are mostly small and incidental and would not be recognized without direct imaging.[194] A large and locally aggressive meningioma was seen in one MEN1 patient who had prior radiation to a pituitary tumor (SJM, personal observation). This tumor showed biallelic inactivation of *MEN1*.

Barrett Esophagus. The frequency of the presumably premalignant Barret esophagus was increased fivefold in cases with MEN1 and ZES compared to that in cases with ZES alone.[195] This finding may relate to a long interval with uncontrolled excess of stomach acid.

MEN1-like Phenotypes
Phenocopies and Differential Diagnosis of Multiple Endocrine Neoplasia Type 1

When MEN1 occurs in its typical and full forms, it is easily diagnosed. However, presentation as a single apparently sporadic tumor, as familial isolated hyperparathyroidism (FIH), or as atypical combinations presents the clinician with difficult challenges to diagnosis and understanding.

Varying Penetrance of Tumors by Tissue or by Age

MEN1 is the most heterogeneous of all multiple neoplasia syndromes. The many tumors of MEN1 have a wide range of penetrance (see Table 39-1). If the organ is paired and the penetrance is high, the tumors are generally bilateral (e.g., parathyroid adenomas); if the tumor is rare in MEN1, its random occurrence is generally unilateral even in a paired organ (e.g., pheochromocytoma). Naturally, the apparent penetrance of any tumor type is heavily dependent upon the scrutiny that the organ is given. Thus, the frequent facial angiofibromas of MEN1 were not recognized until 1997.[186] When symptoms alone are the main basis for disease recognition, the first feature of MEN1 in adolescents is not HPT but rather prolactinoma or insulinoma.[196]

For each tumor type, penetrance necessarily increases with age (see Fig. 39-1). Overall, the penetrance for MEN1 reaches nearly 100% by age 50 years,[15] but occasional obligate *MEN1* mutation carriers have not shown any tumor beyond age 70 years.[189] Earliest penetrance and earliest preventable morbidity must be considered in decisions about when to begin tumor surveillance in a known carrier.[189b] The earliest ages for identification of specific tumor expression in MEN1 have been as follows: prolactinoma at age 5 years,[148] insulinoma at age 6 years,[197] HPT at age 8 years,[15] and gastrinoma at age 12 years.[198] The information about tumor morbidity for most of these young patients is incomplete; thus, more information is needed before it is possible to improve the recommendations about age at which to begin carrier ascertainment, tumor surveillance, and possibly intervention.

Familial Variation in Phenotype

Clustering of clinical subvariants of MEN1, similar to that seen for MEN2 (see later), has been evaluated. Preliminary analyses in small MEN1 families suggested clusters of ACTH-producing pituitary tumors, insulinomas,[199,200] intestinal carcinoids,[176] thymic carcinoids,[201] or aggressive gastrinomas.[173] Identification of a specific *MEN1* mutation or a modifier locus that correlates with a specific clinical variant in multiple kindreds would be most meaningful. Subsequent analysis has failed to identify such a relationship (see later), increasing the likelihood of random clustering of traits in most of these families.

Prolactinoma Variant of MEN1

The prolactinoma variant of MEN1 is defined in a family with high penetrance for HPT and prolactinoma but low penetrance for gastrinoma (typically 90%, 50%, and 5%, respectively, among adults). Three such families have been reported, each with eight or more affected members.[202] The largest has more than 100 affected members. Because their ancestors colonized the Burin Peninsula of Newfoundland, Canada, their trait has been termed *MEN1*$_{Burin}$. Several smaller families seem similar but cannot be categorized because of their small size. Foregut carcinoid tumors seemed prominent (10-15%) in MEN1$_{Burin}$. Their *MEN1* mutations have not been unusual.

Isolated Hyperparathyroidism Variant of MEN1

HPT is the most common clinical feature of MEN1 and may begin at a relatively young age. It would therefore not be surprising to identify isolated HPT in small families with otherwise occult MEN1, particularly those with a disproportionate number of young members. Larger families (four or more affected members) have been identified with FIH and an identifiable *MEN1* mutation but still could represent a random part of the normal spectrum of MEN1 expression.[203] Eventually, most would probably develop other clinical features of MEN1.[85] Two FIH families with *MEN1* mutation have been particularly large, with 11 and 14 hyperparathyroid members, raising the likelihood that in some families, isolated HPT can exist and continue as the only manifestation of *MEN1* mutation.[203,204] Though these patients by definition have *MEN1* mutation, *MEN1* mutation is rare among all families with FIH (see later).[205]

Sporadic Tumor or Tumors

MEN1 can occur without a recognized or even recognizable family history of MEN1. When sporadic patients present with two or more typical tumors, some meet the definition criteria for MEN1[206]; for others, the suspicion of MEN1 is high. The prevalence of *MEN1* mutation is 7% to 70% in tumor-specific subgroups, depending on the specific tumors (see later discussion).[207] When the sporadic case manifests with tumor in only one tissue, the suspicion and the true frequency of *MEN1* mutation are low. The frequency of occult MEN1 with sporadic tumor in one tissue can be estimated as follows: HPT, 2%,[208] gastrinoma, 5%,[60] prolactinoma, 5%.[144,145,209] Factors that increase the likelihood of MEN1 in these settings are suggestive features in the family, earlier onset, and tumor multiplicity in the same tissue. Diffuse or multifocal hyperplasia of the islets or nesidioblastosis is rare and sometimes seen as a consequence of gastric bypass surgery.[210] Isolated alpha-cell disease of the islets with glucagon cell hyperplasia with multiple glucagonomas is sporadic and very rare[211] and has no documented association with germline MEN1 mutation.

Familial Isolated Endocrine Tumors Not From the *MEN1* Gene

Familial Isolated Hyperparathyroidism. When HPT is familial and isolated to this tissue, the main possibilities include occult MEN1 (see earlier), familial hypocalciuric hypercalcemia (FHH) (OMIM 145980 HHC1), hyperparathyroidism–jaw tumor syndrome (HPT-JT) (OMIM 145002), MEN2A, and so-called true FIH[205] (OMIM 145000). FHH, with a frequency similar to that of MEN1, is an autosomal dominant disorder characterized by lifelong hypercalcemia with normal urine calcium excretion (i.e., relative hypocalciuria).[212,213] PTH levels and parathyroid gland mass are normal or minimally increased.[214,215] After subtotal parathyroidectomy, the residual parathyroid tissue directs persistent hypercalcemia. The parathyroid dysfunction is not monoclonal but polyclonal.[216] A remarkably high rate of persistence after subtotal parathyroidectomy and a low morbidity rate without surgery justify efforts to avoid parathyroid surgery in FHH. Useful diagnostic features of FHH are the low ratio of renal calcium clearance to creatinine clearance (in the presence of hypercalcemia), normal PTH level despite hypercalcemia, and the onset of hypercalcemia in young relatives, even before age 1 year.

Two thirds of FHH index cases have an identifiable inactivating mutation of the calcium-sensing receptor gene (*CASR*).[217] One family with a missense mutation of *CASR* had features more like typical HPT.[218] Two large prospective studies of FIH found unexpected germline mutation of *CASR* in 15% of families. These families were small (mainly with two or three affected members), and no family had typical clinical features of FHH.[205,219] A minority of kindreds with FHH have heterozygous mutation in *GNA11* (OMIM 145981 HHC2) or *AP2S1* (OMIM 600740 HHC3).[220,221] These two genes have not been shown to cause a phenotype different from the *CASR*.

HPT-JT is a syndrome of HPT, jaw tumors, and renal lesions.[222] Transmission is autosomal dominant. The most common and sometimes the only feature is HPT.[223] The HPT typically involves one parathyroid gland at a time, and there is a uniquely high malignant potential in the parathyroid tumor; 15% of patients have parathyroid cancer.[205,224] Germline *HRPT2* mutation is also found in most seemingly sporadic parathyroid cancers, suggesting an occult familial process.[225] The associated jaw tumors (in 25%) are ossifying or cementifying fibromas.[226] Unlike the jaw tumors of HPT, they are not osteoclast-rich or influenced by the parathyroid status. The associated renal lesions (in 5%) are multiple renal cysts, hamartomas, or Wilms tumor.[227] Uterine tumors are common and can impair fertility.[228] *HRPT2* mutation has been found in 5% to 10% of kindreds with FIH.[205,219,229] Occult MEN2A, theoretically another cause of FIH, has not been identified in the form of FIH.[230,231]

Many small kindreds with two or three affected members receive a diagnosis of FIH.[85,232,233] For years FIH was not pursued as a syndrome because of its bland features and the belief that most kindreds had occult MEN1. Analyses of collected kindreds with FIH have recently found occult MEN1, FHH, or HPT-JT in the minority.[85] Probably mutation in undiscovered genes will account for most kindreds with FIH. One such gene seems to be on chromosome 2 by genetic linkage analysis.[219]

Familial Isolated Pituitary Tumor. Familial isolated tumor of the anterior pituitary (OMIM 102200) has been recognized in several small and a few large families.[234,235] The tumors are usually somatotropinomas or prolactinomas. In some families, somatotropinoma is the main expression. In theory, familial isolated tumor of the anterior pituitary could be an expression of occult MEN1. To date, however, no family with familial isolated somatotropinoma has had a *MEN1* mutation (see later). About 15% of these families harbor mutations of the *AIP* gene, which coincidentally is very near the *MEN1* gene also at 11q13.[236] A lower fraction characterized by onset of gigantism in childhood had mutation of *GPR101*.[235]

Other Familial Endocrine Tumors

Isolated Chromaffin Tumor. Chromaffin tumor refers to adrenal pheochromocytoma and to extra-adrenal paraganglioma. Isolated chromaffin tumor occurs in some families. Most family clusters are caused by more than four genes that encode proteins in the mitochondrial succinate dehydrogenase complex (*SDHB, SDHC, SDHD, SDH5*).[237] This topic is covered in more detail in Chapter 16.

Isolated Carcinoid Tumor. Carcinoid tumor clustering in families is statistically significant. However, few families have been described, and most have fewer than five affected members. The tumors seem distributed between foregut and hindgut. None has been associated with *MEN1* mutation. In fact, no single gene or gene locus has been implicated.

The Normal *MEN1* Gene and Normal Menin Protein

Larsson and colleagues[238] showed in 1988 that the *MEN1* gene mapped to chromosome band 11q13 and that it probably caused tumor by a loss of function (see the following).[239,240] However, almost a full decade passed before the *MEN1* gene there was identified.[241]

The *MEN1* gene is 10 kb in extent and encodes transcripts of 2.7 and 3.1 kb.[242] The transcripts are expressed in all or most tissues and with little cell cycle dependence.[243] They encode a 610–amino acid protein termed *menin*. Rat, mouse, zebra fish, snail, *Drosophila*, and human menins are highly homologous.[244] Menin is absent in yeasts and roundworms.

Menin has two nuclear localization signals near the carboxy-terminus that are likely to be responsible for its predominantly nuclear compartmentalization.[243]

Because menin has an amino acid sequence without any homologues in the genome, its sequence alone is also not informative about mechanism of action. The principal method applied to searching for its molecular pathway has been that of menin partnering to proteins or chromatin. Approximately 25 protein partners for menin have been identified, but only a few have been reproduced in other laboratories. The first interacting protein partner identified for menin was selectively junD but not other members of the activator protein-1 (AP1) transcription factor family including fos, fra, or other jun proteins.[245,246] The menin-junD interaction can confer upon junD unique effects by which junD differs from other members of the AP1 transcription family. For example, junD has several actions opposite to those of c-jun, and in the absence of menin binding to it, junD behaves more like c-jun.[247] The importance of the menin-junD interaction for the development of MEN1 is unclear. Homozygous knockout of junD in the mouse resulted in no identifiable abnormality of tissues involved in MEN1.[248] Other studies have identified COMPASS (a mixed-lineage leukemia [MLL]-containing complex), SMAD3, PEM, NM23, nuclear factor κB, and several other proteins that potentially interact with menin. Each interacting partner has unknown importance.[249] Hundreds of chromatin binding sites for menin have been identified but no specific DNA recognition element. At present no one of the menin partners has been convincingly shown to be critical in MEN1 tumorigenesis. The most attention has been committed to junD and MLL, and these studies have been reviewed elsewhere. The crystal structure of menin indicated a large shallow groove that could simultaneously hold junD and MLL.[250]

Abnormal *MEN1* Gene: Tumorigenesis Roles of the *MEN1* Gene

The first DNA-based discoveries in MEN1 suggested that the *MEN1* gene was a tumor suppressor[238-240] (see Chapter 4); these observations were supported by subsequent studies (see later).

Two-Step Inactivation of the *MEN1* Gene

Complete inactivation of the *MEN1* gene's function requires, in addition to the inherited or somatically acquired first hit (inactivating mutation), a second hit at the same genetic locus that finishes the inactivation of both copies of the *MEN1* gene. Inactivation of the second allele can be by mutation or other (epigenetic) means such as promoter methylation.[251] A two-hit model for tumorigenesis was developed by Alfred Knudson[239,240] in 1971 to account for epidemiologic observations in retinoblastoma. In comparison with sporadic cases, some hereditary tumors occurred earlier and in multiple sites (see Chapter 4). This can now be generalized to say that in a hereditary tumor, the germline mutation is obligatorily present in every cell. Thus, the earliest step in the precursor cell for sporadic tumorigenesis caused by the *MEN1* gene is bypassed in the hereditary form. All cells in susceptible tissues are thus primed for somatic mutations at the second or normal copy of the tumorigenic gene, to cause early and multiple tumors. Surprisingly, aspects of this model can also be extended to stepwise tumorigenesis by an oncogene such as *RET*, in which a second hit at the *RET* gene is not required (see later).

Somatic Point Mutations (First Hits) of the *MEN1* Gene in Sporadic Tumors.
MEN1 is one of the most commonly mutated genes in sporadic endocrine tumors. Among sporadic tumors, the frequency of *MEN1* mutation is 10% to 30% in parathyroid adenomas.[252-255] A few other genes including *CDKI* genes are mutated less frequently in sporadic parathyroid adenoma[256-258]; in particular, the *ZFX* gene is mutated in 6%.[259] MEN1 is mutated in 25% in gastrinomas,[260-262] 10% to 20% in insulinomas,[263] 50% in VIPomas,[264] and 25% to 35% in bronchial carcinoids.[265] MEN1 is mutated in 20% of adrenocortical cancers.[266] Some other sporadic endocrine tumors show a lower frequency of *MEN1* somatic mutation: 0% to 5% in anterior pituitary tumor,[267-270] 0% in non–C-cell thyroid tumor,[185] 0% in benign adrenocortical neoplasm,[264,271] 0% in uremic secondary HPT,[272] and 0% in parathyroid cancer.[273] Sporadic nonendocrine tumors have undergone little evaluation; the *MEN1* mutation frequency was 2 in 19 in angiofibromas,[274] 1 in 6 in lipomas,[274] 0% in lung cancer other than carcinoid,[275] 1% in malignant melanoma,[276] and 0% in leukemia.[277]

The First Step (First Hit) Can Be in the Germline or in Somatic Tissue.
Virtually all germline or somatic first hits at the *MEN1* gene have been small mutations, involving one or several bases.[278,279] The mutations are broadly distributed across the *MEN1* open reading frame, so much so that half of newly ascertained index cases are still found to have a novel mutation. At the same time, the other half show recurring mutations. These are equally distributed in the germline between cause by common ancestry (founder effect)[280-284] and cause by a hot spot for new mutation.[278]

Accumulated patterns of germline and somatic first-hit *MEN1* mutations have further supported the two-hit gene inactivation hypothesis for tumorigenesis by the *MEN1* gene (Fig. 39-7). Three fourths of *MEN1* first-hit mutations predict premature truncation of the menin protein. Although the biologic functions of menin are not established, such truncation mutations would probably cause menin inactivation or even absence. For example, all truncation-type *MEN1* mutations cause loss of the most carboxy-terminal nuclear localization signal (see Fig. 39-7) and could thus compromise the nuclear localization of menin.[243] The remainder predict missense or replacement of one to three amino acids. The functional consequences of any one missense mutation are uncertain and even hard to distinguish from a rare benign polymorphism; however, their frequent occurrence specifically in MEN1 and their absence in normal subjects established that all or most are deleterious mutations.

The Second Hit in *MEN1* Tumorigenesis.
The second hit is usually a large chromosomal or subchromosomal rearrangement (mutation), causing a deletion that includes the remaining normal *MEN1* gene. Another potential mechanism for creating a mutant second copy is deletion of DNA spanning all or part of the normal copy and then duplication of the DNA from the mutant chromosome 11, called *gene conversion*. In either case, the result is that neither copy of the *MEN1* gene remains normal. LOH or loss of alleles at the affected locus is usually inherent in this process and can provide evidence that gene inactivation has occurred in that chromosomal segment. Other rare mechanisms for the second hit include small mutations (one to three bases) or promoter methylation.[251] The second hit is always in somatic tissue and almost always occurs postnatally.

Loss of Heterozygosity About the Locus of the *MEN1* Gene.
LOH about 11q13 has been used mainly to deduce loss of the normal copy of the *MEN1* gene (i.e., the second hit in tumorigenesis). In MEN1, 11q13 LOH was found for almost 100% of parathyroid tumors,[31,285] gastrinoma and other pancreatic islet tumors,[51,52] gastric carcinoid,[286] anterior pituitary tumors,[155] and mesenchymal tumors (lipoma, angiofibroma, collagenoma, and leiomyoma).[188,191,193] These prevalences are higher than those for detected first hits as small mutations of *MEN1* in the same tumors (see earlier); thus, undetetected mutations of *MEN1* may initiate some tumors. Surprisingly, thymic carcinoid tumor and adrenocortical tumor in MEN1 have not shown 11q13 LOH.[163,287] This finding has led to speculation that the normal *MEN1* copy can be inactivated by other mechanisms, such as promoter methylation, that would not cause LOH.

Among sporadic endocrine tumors of the type found in MEN1, some but not all have frequent 11q13 LOH. The frequencies of 11q13 LOH in these tumors have been as follows: sporadic primary hyperparathyroid 30% to 40%,[252,253,288,289] uremic parathyroid 0% to 5%,[288,290-292] parathyroid cancer 0%,[273] gastrinoma 25% to 70%,[53,260] insulinoma 30%,[53] bronchial and other foregut carcinoid 40% to 70%,[265] and anterior pituitary 5% to 10%.[156,267-270,293] In the adrenal cortex, 11q13 LOH was less common in benign than in malignant tumors (20% and 80%, respectively).[264,271] Assessment of 11q13 LOH is not useful in clinical practice as it does not help in staging or in germline diagnosis; however, it has been used in research as an indicator of an underlying first hit in a tumor suppressor gene at that locus.

11q13 LOH has also been used as an indicator of tissue monoclonality or oligoclonality. Because 11q13 LOH is a DNA rearrangement, it can be detected only if it is present in the DNA of most or a substantial minority of cells in a

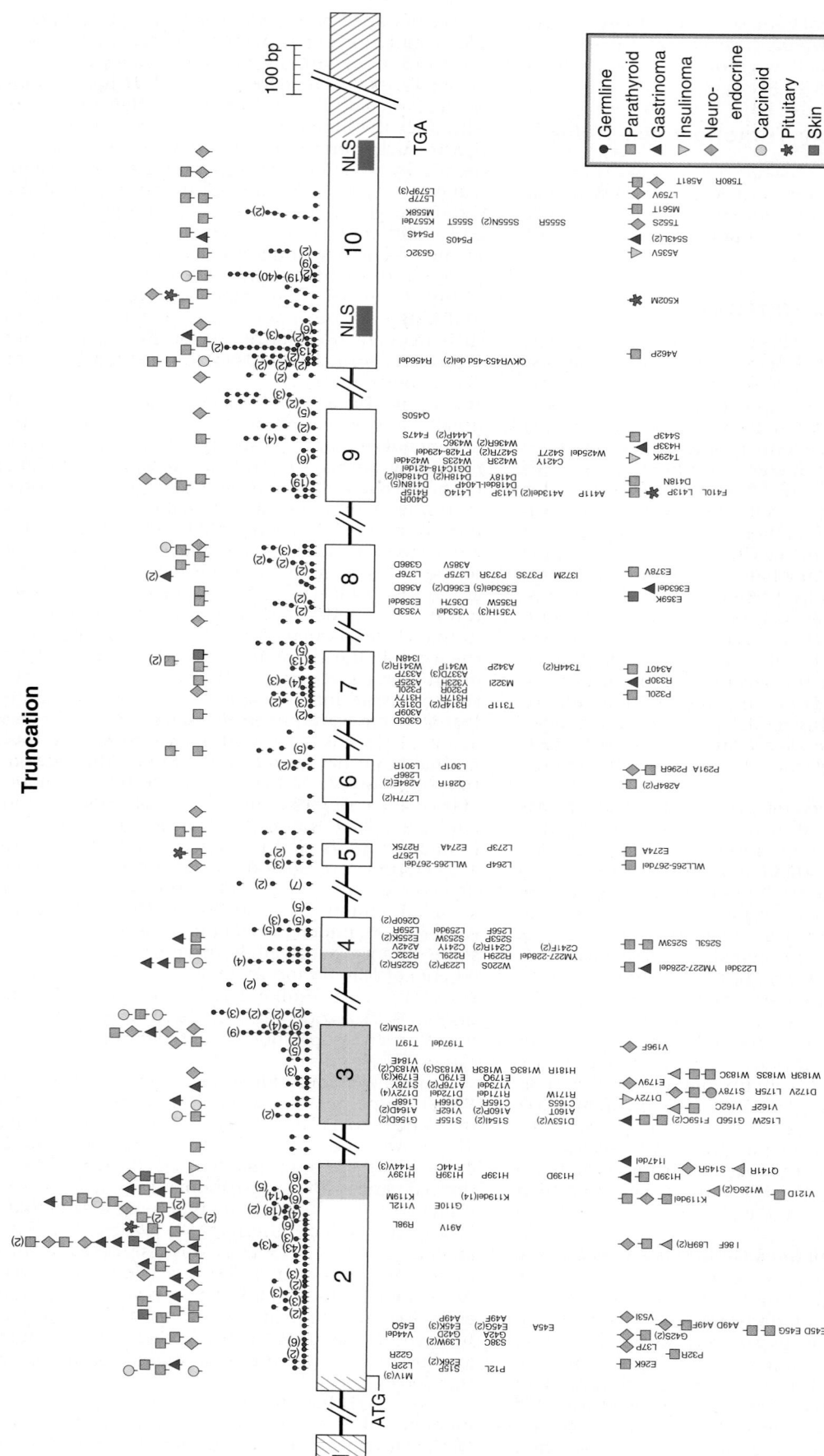

Figure 39-7 Germline and somatic mutations of the *MEN1* gene. Unique germline *MEN1* mutations in families, sporadic cases, and nonhereditary tumors. This figure shows 670 unique mutations identified as of 2006. Repeating mutations within the germline or somatic category (common ancestry versus hot spots for mutation) are shown only once, with a small number in parentheses to indicate total occurrences. Germline mutations are shown as *black lollipops* or as code about the messenger ribonucleic acid (mRNA). Somatic *MEN1* mutations in diverse tumors are shown separately as flags along the upper and lower border and as code. *MEN1* mRNA is diagrammed with exons numbered; untranslated regions are *crosshatched*. Truncating mutations (frameshift mutations, splice error, and nonsense [stop codon] mutations) account for 75% of all mutations. Codon change mutations (missense mutations or small in-frame deletions) are shown below with their three-letter amino acid code. *Gray shading* about exon 3 represents the main zone of menin interaction with JunD. Several large deletions, probably of the entire *MEN1* gene, are not shown.[252] MEN, multiple endocrine neoplasia; NLS, nuclear localization sequence.

specimen. Thus, the nuclei are deduced to be monoclonal or oligoclonal descendants from one or a few precursor cells with that rearrangement or mutation. Early studies of MEN1 parathyroid glands by light microscopy suggested oncogenesis through a polyclonal hyperplastic process, an observation supported by the finding in MEN1 plasma of a factor mitogenic for parathyroid cells.[32] The subsequent finding of nearly universal 11q13 LOH in MEN1 parathyroids[241,242,285] established that monoclonal or oligoclonal growth was predominant and that tumorigenesis in MEN1 was by loss of MEN1 gene function.

Hyperplasia and DNA Repair. Other than the first hit, the earliest tissue-level effects toward tumorigenesis in MEN1 are not well defined, nor are many intermediate steps. Although a widespread role for hyperplasia prior to neoplasia has been seen in MEN2 and many hereditary neoplasias, hyperplasia has been subtle or unrecognized as a tumor precursor in MEN1 tissues. A related progression has been identified from gastrin cell hyperplasia to microtumor as a precursor to gastrinoma in MEN1 but not in sporadic gastrinoma.[54] In addition, the mouse MEN1 knockout model for MEN1 has striking giant hyperplastic islets as a precursor for insulinoma,[55] suggesting that more subtle hyperplasia might have gone unrecognized in human MEN1. If there is a role for hyperplasia, it would be uncertain whether this is an expression of inactivation of one MEN1 allele alone or further processes. MEN1 plasma contains a growth factor that promotes mitogenesis in normal parathyroid cells and could contribute to hyperplasia.[32,294] Considering the overriding roles of MEN1 gene inactivation and of clonal growth, it is not certain whether the growth factor is a contributor to or a consequence of oncogenesis in MEN1.

Clonal cell proliferation has been identified in mesenchymal perivascular tissues about MEN1 angiofibromas[295]; this could represent a precursor stage of that tumor.[296]

Other unknown genes can be implicated in MEN1 tumor evolution through gene loss of function (tumor suppressor gene) or gene gain of function (oncogene).[295-305] Genome instability has been suggested in studies of MEN1 lymphocytes and fibroblasts.[302,303] Also MEN1 leukocytes show a subtle deficiency in repair of DNA damage.[304] Menin null cells of the mouse show a defect in repair of DNA, damaged selectively by ionizing radiation.[305]

MEN1 Mutations and Tumor Phenotypes

There have been no clear relations of MEN1 genotype with phenotype, unlike the situation in MEN2 (see later). The truncating MEN1 mutations cause the same diverse types of tumor expression as the missense mutations, and expression does not differ between amino-terminal and carboxy-terminal mutations. The distribution of somatic mutations about the open reading frame is similar to that of germline mutations (see Fig. 39-7) and seems almost random. There appears to be a deficiency of missense mutations near the carboxy-terminus and a cluster of missense mutations between amino acids 100 and 200. Otherwise, there is no clear clustering of missense mutations that could point to a zone of menin protein susceptible to change of function.

The prolactinoma variant of MEN1, one of the clinical variants described before in three unrelated kindreds, was associated with three different MEN1 mutations that were similar to mutations in typical MEN1.[306] MEN1 mutation has been found in 20% or less of tested families with isolated hyperparathyroidism (FIH).[203,204] Two of the largest MEN1 mutation-positive families with isolated HPT had similarly located missense mutations (E255K and Q260P).[203,307] However, MEN1 mutations in 14 other kindreds with FIH show no patterns of similarity.[205]

A MEN1 mutation has not been found with familial isolated anterior pituitary tumor, although more than 100 such families have been evaluated.[269,270,293,308] Thus, most kindreds with isolated pituitary tumor, like most with FIH, represent MEN1 phenocopies; that is, they are probably caused by mutation in genes (such as the AIP or GRP101 gene) other than MEN1.[234,235] There has also been no relationship between a specific somatic MEN1 mutation and tumor type. Tumor testing for somatic MEN1 mutation has not shown prognostic or staging value when evaluated in sporadic gastrinomas of varying aggressiveness.[260]

Germline Mutation of a Cyclin-Dependent Kinase Inhibitor Gene or Other Gene as a Rare Cause of MEN1

Inactivation of certain other tumor suppressor genes, alone or in combination, can cause specific endocrine tumors in mice. In particular, mice with homozygous knockout of both p18INK4c and p27KIP1 develop neoplasia in at least eight types of tissues, including tumors of parathyroid, pituitary, pancreas islet, and duodenum (as in MEN1); in addition, they develop C-cell cancers and pheochromocytoma (as in MEN2).[309] The knocked-out genes encode members of the two cyclin-dependent kinase inhibitor (CDKI) families that participate in the cell cycling pathway and include retinoblastoma and cyclin D1.[306] Rats with homozygous inactivation of p27 show a similar spectrum of tumors comprising MEN1 and MEN2.[309] Less than 20 human index cases and several of their relatives exhibited MEN1-like tumors from inactivation of one copy of p27.[309,310] This form has been termed MEN4 (OMIM 610755). Based on this limited number of cases, the spectrum of MEN4 is indistinguishable from MEN1, and it has not yet been found to include its rodent counterparts of C-cell neoplasia or pheochromocytoma. Similar mutations in three other CDKI genes (p15, p18, and p21) and similar clinical features have also been seen in rare cases and families.[306] The similar features from mutation of MEN1 or several of the CDKI genes suggest that they share an overlapping pathway. For example, menin might activate the promoter of a CDKI gene and thereby function as a growth suppressor.[311]

Testing for Carrier State or for Tumor Emergence in MEN1

The Carrier of the MEN1 Syndrome

We define the MEN1 carrier as a person who carries the susceptibility to express the MEN1 syndrome. The carrier can be defined as affected if he or she expresses at least one component of MEN1. Alternately, the carrier can be silent, meaning he or she expresses no feature of MEN1. The carrier may occasionally remain silent into the eighth decade; such an individual is not considered to have MEN1, although the susceptibility likely persists indefinitely. These definitions are not dependent on carriage of MEN1 gene mutation. Other genes such as a CDKI and even other unknown processes could cause the subject to be a MEN1 carrier. Conversely, one who has a pathologic mutation of the MEN1 gene is necessarily a carrier of the MEN1 syndrome.

Screening and Counseling for Multiple Endocrine Neoplasia Type 1

A screening program for MEN1 patients should routinely meet three main objectives: identify MEN1 carriers, identify MEN1 tumors particularly at a treatable stage, and be cost effective (Fig. 39-8).[312] The term *screening* has been applied to several processes in the setting of MEN1. Herein, a distinction is made between testing for carrier ascertainment and periodic testing for emergence of new tumor or surveillance of known tumors in a known carrier. Note that when carrier testing with DNA (mutation or haplotype test) is not possible, streamlined and periodic tumor surveillance becomes the preferred method for carrier ascertainment.

Encounters for carrier ascertainment often involve counseling of the patient. In addition to standard genetics topics, counseling in MEN1 addresses two different faces of MEN1: an endocrinopathy with good but complex management options and a cancer syndrome with limited management options. An MEN1 information web page can help in orientation.[313] In general, compliance with a simple and regular tumor surveillance protocol is high (Table 39-2); complicated, expensive, and erratic efforts are associated with lower compliance.

Benefits and Limitations of Carrier Ascertainment

The benefits of this type of analysis are several. First is the secure proof of the MEN1 carrier state in a person with a

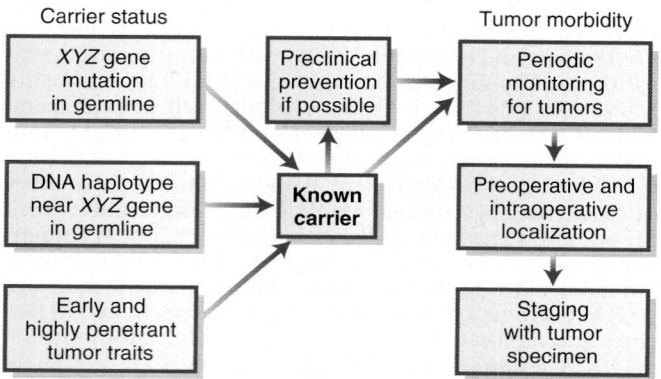

Figure 39-8 Test categories and test methods in a hereditary tumor syndrome. Tests of the germline carrier status *(left)* are largely distinguished from tests of tumor status *(right)*. When DNA testing is not informative, carrier status can be tested by streamlined surveillance of tumors *(lower left)*.

TABLE 39-2
Representative Protocol of Tests and Schedules to Survey for Tumor Emergence in a Carrier of Multiple Endocrine Neoplasia Type 1

Tumor	Age to Begin Testing (yr)	Biochemical Tests Annually	Imaging Tests Every 3-5 yr
Anterior pituitary	5	Prolactin; IGF-1	MRI
Foregut carcinoid	20	NA*	CT
Gastrinoma	20	Gastrin	None
Insulinoma	5	Fasting glucose	None
Other pancreatico-duodenal tumors	15	^{111}In-DTPA octreotide†; CT or MRI	
Parathyroid adenoma	8	Calcium, PTH	None

*Robust test with serum not available. Chromogranin A has not been proved to screen for small tumors.
†Stomach best evaluated for carcinoids (ECLomas) incidental to gastric endoscopy. Thymus removed partially at parathyroidectomy in MEN1.
CT, computed tomography; DTPA, diethylenetriaminepentaacetic acid; ECL, enterochromaffin-like; IGF-1, insulin-like growth factor 1; MRI, magnetic resonance imaging; NA, not available; PTH, parathyroid hormone.

mutation, along with the equally important benefit of the potential to exclude the MEN1 carrier state by a normal sequence analysis when another affected member of the kindred has an identified mutant *MEN1* gene sequence. This type of information can assist in decisions about family planning, future medical needs, and so forth. Second, the information from an index case, if shared, can be helpful to relatives unaware or uncertain of their status. In particular, after a germline *MEN1* mutation is first identified, the information may be shared with a laboratory and with relatives, and DNA-based information may be used to develop an accurate shortcut test for that mutation in relatives (see later). Third, the information is useful to the physician. It assists in further plans about counseling and tumor surveillance. Occasionally, it is important in a decision about surgery, as in a case of apparently sporadic gastrinoma.

What the MEN1 carrier ascertainment test does not do is also important. MEN1 carrier ascertainment, unlike similar testing for MEN2, does not routinely lead to a recommendation for medical or surgical intervention. MEN1 cancers, in contrast to MTC in the thyroid, arise in tissues that cannot easily be ablated. This lack of mutation-guided intervention makes mutation testing at early ages in MEN1 less urgent than in MEN2. One approach is to recommend DNA testing in children of gene carriers at age 5 years, the youngest age at which a morbid and possibly treatable MEN1-related tumor (prolactinoma) has been identified.[148] An alternative, based on the fact that MEN1 morbidity is rare before the age of 20 years, is to delay carrier ascertainment until the child can make a mature decision about a test that could affect availability of insurance or job opportunities.

No identifiable *MEN1* mutation is found in 10% to 30%[207,314-316] of typical MEN1 kindreds, although most are believed to harbor *MEN1* mutations not detected by the most common DNA sequencing strategies. Carrier ascertainment in such kindreds can be established by 11q13 haplotype analysis or by streamlined tumor surveillance (see later) (see Fig. 39-8). Overall, the potential for benefit from the *MEN1* mutation test is generally proportional to the likelihood of finding a *MEN1* mutation. Thus, obvious benefit is possible for an index case with familial or sporadic MEN1 or with a state that resembles MEN1 but does not quite meet the usual definitions. For example, a *MEN1* germline mutation was found in each of four patients with sporadic HPT and carcinoid tumor.[208] The likelihood of benefit in a case of atypical MEN1 is generally much lower and varies greatly with the specific tumor(s) identified. For example, the likelihood of finding a *MEN1* germline mutation in a case of sporadic HPT (without special features such as youth or multigland disease) is probably less than 5%.

Germline DNA: Mutation or Haplotype Ascertainment

The following sections cover carrier ascertainment by mutation testing, haplotype testing, and tumor surveillance. The general principles of alternative ascertainment methods, with slight modification, are applicable to MEN2 and to many hereditary syndromes (see Fig. 39-8).

Germline DNA mutation analysis can identify or rule out most *MEN1* mutation carriers by a test applied only one time during the life span. This test is available through several commercial and academic laboratories.[312] The usual tissue surrogate for germline DNA is blood leukocytes; MEN1-associated tumor is satisfactory for this because any identified mutation could have occurred somatically. The *MEN1* mutation test is based on polymerase chain reaction amplification of the nine translated exons (the open reading frame) and the intron-exon boundaries. Laboratories use modestly differing protocols.

MEN1 germline mutations have been detected in 60% to 100% of well-defined MEN1 families.[306,312-315] The wide variability in mutation detection rate is explained partly by family selection but more likely by differences in laboratory detection methods. Genetic linkage analysis previously mapped all well-characterized MEN1 kindreds to 11q13, making it likely that mutation of the *MEN1* gene causes almost all familial MEN1.[309,316] Three atypical MEN1 families have not been linked to 11q13.[308,317,318] Failure to identify a *MEN1* mutation could be explained by the presence of mutations involving 5′ or 3′ untranslated or central intronic regions, sequences that are not normally examined, or by a large *MEN1* deletion that results in no abnormal polymerase chain reaction product.[279] Mutation at another gene, such as a member of the *CDKI* gene family, is also occasionally possible.

The germline *MEN1* mutation detection rate has been lower (10-80%) in sporadic than in familial MEN1,[191,281] probably because of differences in selection of patients. The *MEN1* germline mutation rate has been high (about 75%) in sporadic cases with HPT and ZES,[306] but it is far lower (about 7%) in sporadic cases with HPT and acromegaly.[207,319] For the same reason, the *MEN1* mutation detection rate has also been low (0-30%) in sporadic cases with atypical MEN1, a truly broad category without a consensus definition.[320] Most *MEN1* mutations are familial, but about 10% arise de novo.

When *MEN1* mutation cannot be detected in the germline DNA of a MEN1 index case, ascertainment of the carrier state in relatives is more difficult. Carrier ascertainment can still be based on streamlined periodic tumor surveillance in a relative (see later) or on haplotype analysis (similar to genetic linkage analysis) in a kindred (see Fig. 39-8). With three or more affected relatives, haplotype or linkage analysis for the MEN1 trait may sometimes be done with high degrees of confidence[321]; however, few laboratories are doing these analyses.

Carrier Ascertainment for Multiple Endocrine Neoplasia Type 1 by Streamlined Surveillance for Tumors: An Alternative to DNA Testing

In kindreds with no identifiable *MEN1* mutation and no possibility of 11q13 haplotype analysis, it is necessary to base assignment of the carrier status on the clinical identification of a frequent tumor of MEN1 (see Fig. 39-8). Streamlined periodic surveillance for tumors by biochemical tests should be offered to asymptomatic offspring of known carriers every 3 to 5 years. HPT is the most common and usually the earliest manifestation of MEN1, and therefore its recognition is central to this carrier-ascertainment strategy. The preferred parathyroid tumor surveillance test is the ionized calcium test, beginning at the age of 8 years or later. A serum PTH assay should be performed at the same time. If the ionized calcium test is unavailable, an albumin-adjusted calcium test is suitable and is also preferable to measuring total serum calcium.

Five years is a suggested starting age for prolactinoma surveillance, based on the occurrence of a morbid macro-prolactinoma in a child of that age with MEN1.[148] Because serum prolactin rises with stress, avoidance of phlebotomy stress in a child can require an indwelling venous catheter and three blood samples at 20-minute intervals.[322] Gastrinoma surveillance can be introduced during adulthood because of the generally later age of onset of ZES in MEN1 (see Fig. 39-1). Only rarely is gastrinoma the first clinical tumor to occur in MEN1.[64] Surveillance for cutaneous manifestations of MEN1, collagenomas or facial angiofibromas, may be promising but has not yet been explored in children.[186] False-positive test results are often found in MEN1 tumor surveillance through the assays of prolactin (caused by stress, pregnancy, or psychotropic medications) or gastrin (caused mainly by hypochlorhydria, including that resulting from inhibitors of gastric acid secretion). Rarely can one be misled by a sporadic but common endocrine tumor (such as parathyroid adenoma or pituitary tumor) that could occur in a family member who is not an MEN1 carrier.[323]

Periodic Surveillance for Tumors After Proving the MEN1 Carrier State

When the MEN1 carrier status has been identified by any method, it is appropriate to focus continued and increased attention on the carrier with the goal of identifying and treating neoplastic manifestations at an appropriate stage (see Table 39-2). Surveillance for parathyroid tumor, prolactinoma, and insulinoma can begin in proven carriers at age 5 to 8 years; surveillance for gastrinoma, other islet tumors, and foregut carcinoids should be delayed until after the age of 15 to 20 years.[324] Cost-effective surveillance combines a carefully obtained history focused on clinical symptoms associated with these tumors, limited hormonal and serum chemistry analysis, and carefully defined (i.e., selective and less frequent) use of imaging (see Table 39-2).[206]

Some have recommended more extensive surveillance measures that include measurement of pancreatic polypeptide,[105,108] chromogranin A, proinsulin, or cortisol. Furthermore, a meal-stimulated test was developed in the hope of increasing the MEN1-related diagnostic information from pancreatic polypeptide and other markers.[104,123,325] Although a case can be made that these tests can result in earlier tumor recognition, it is unclear whether such detection has been validated and whether it might result in benefit to the patient.[29]

MULTIPLE ENDOCRINE NEOPLASIA TYPE 2 SYNDROME

Beginning more than 50 years ago, a series of independent, seemingly unrelated clinical and basic science discoveries provided the basis for the characterization of the type 2 MEN syndromes: MEN2A, MEN2B, and familial medullary thyroid carcinoma (FMTC). In 1959, Hazard, Hawk, and Crile identified MTC as a specific clinicopathologic entity, but it was not until 7 years later that Williams described that MTC derived from the neural crest C cells in the thyroid gland.[326,327] In 1962, Copp and Cheney discovered the polypeptide hormone CTN, which lowers blood calcium.[328] Although they hypothesized that the parathyroid cells secreted CTN, Hirsch and associates subsequently demonstrated that the thyroid gland produced the hormone.[329] Tashjian and Melvin discovered that the thyroid C cells secrete CTN, and they, and subsequently others, showed that intravenously administered calcium, or pentagastrin, or both together, are potent CTN secretagogues.[330,331] Although 75% of MTCs occur sporadically 25% present in a familial pattern. In 1968 Steiner and associates described a kindred with MTC, pheochromocytomas, HPT, and Cushing syndrome.[6] They named the disease complex MEN2, and we now know it as MEN2A (OMIM 171400, incidence 1 : 1,973,500). Since the original description of MEN2A it has been recognized that two diseases, Hirschsprung disease (HD) and cutaneous lichen amyloidosis (CLA), also occur as part of the syndrome. In 1966 Williams described a syndrome of endocrine tumors associated with multiple mucosal neuromas, similar to von Recklinghausen disease, and 2 years later Schimke and colleagues described a similar entity of bilateral pheochromocytomas, MTC, and multiple mucosal neuromas, a disorder we now know as MEN2B (OMIM 162300, incidence 1 : 38,750,000).[327,332] In 1986 Farndon and associates described a large family with MTC without other endocrine tumors. This endocrinopathy is FMTC (OMIM 155240), and it appears to be closely related to, if not an integral part of, MEN2A.[333]

At the Seventh International Workshop on MEN a group of experienced clinicians developed the first guidelines for managing patients with MEN1 and MEN2.[206] The guidelines for MEN2 were based on the disease phenotypes associated with specific *RET* mutations and recommended ages at which thyroidectomy should be performed in patients who had inherited a *RET* mutation. Subsequently, as more *RET* mutations were discovered it became clear that the original guidelines needed modification. Recently, several professional associations published guidelines for managing patients with sporadic and hereditary MTC.[334-336]

Whereas the MEN2A and MEN2B syndromes are well characterized, such has not been the case with FMTC. Originally there were strict criteria for the diagnosis of FMTC: more than 10 family members with MTC, multiple carriers or affected family members over 50 years of age, and an adequate medical history to exclude the presence of pheochromocytomas and HPT.[206] At present, there are only three such reported families that meet these criteria; however, there are many other families or single individuals with germline *RET* mutations who have only MTC but have not been evaluated over time for the development of pheochromocytomas.[337-339] Currently, most clinical investigators consider FMTC a part of MEN2A and not a freestanding syndrome.

In the recent American Thyroid Association (ATA) revised guidelines for the management of MTC it is recommended that there be two classes of MEN2: MEN2A and MEN2B. Within MEN2A, which accounts for 95% of MEN2 cases, there are four variants: classical MEN2A, MEN2A with HD, MEN2A with CLA, and FMTC. It was also recommended that the aggressiveness of the MTC should be based on the specific *RET* mutation and the clinical experience of patients with these mutations. Thus, patients with *RET M918T* mutations are in the highest risk category (HST), patients with *RET C634* and *A883F* mutations are in the high-risk category (H), and patients with other *RET* mutations are in the moderate category (MOD).

The Molecular Basis for Medullary Thyroid Carcinoma

Structure and Function of the Normal *RET* Proto-oncogene

In 1985 Takahashi and colleagues reported a novel human transforming hybrid oncogene, which they named *RET* (*RE*arranged during *T*ransfection).[340] The *RET* oncogene, derived from a recombination event of two unrelated DNA sequences that were transfected into cultured cells, encodes a fusion protein comprising an amino-terminal region linked to a tyrosine kinase. *RET* is located in the pericentromeric region of chromosome 10q11.2 and spans 21 exons, including more than 60 kb of genomic DNA.[10,341] *RET* is highly conserved and homologues have been found in lower vertebrates and *Drosophila*.[342]

The RET protein structure consists of three domains: (1) an extracellular ligand-binding segment containing four cadherin-like repeats, a calcium-binding site, and a cysteine-rich region important for receptor dimerization; (2) a hydrophobic transmembrane domain; and (3) an internal catalytic core containing two tyrosine kinase subdomains (TK1 and TK2) that are involved in the activation of several intracellular signal transduction pathways (Fig. 39-9). Alternate 3′ splicing of RET produces three isoforms with either 9, 43, or 51 amino acids at the carboxy-terminus, referred to as RET9, RET43, and RET51. The two major isoforms, RET9 and RET51, have markedly different associated signaling complexes, suggesting different physiologic functions.[343-345]

RET plays a central role in various intracellular signaling cascades that regulate cellular differentiation, proliferation, migration, and survival. A tripartite cell-surface complex is needed for RET signaling: one of four glial cell line–derived neurotrophic factor (GDNF) family ligands (GFLs)—GDNF, neurturin, artemin, or persephin—binds RET in conjunction with one of four glycosylphosphatidylinositol-anchored coreceptors, designated GDNF-family α-receptors (GFRαs): GFRα1, GFRα2, GFRα3, and GFRα4.[346] GDNF primarily associates with GFRα1, whereas neurturin, artemin, and persephin preferentially bind GFRα2, GFRα3, and GFRα4, respectively. All GDNF family members have similar downstream signaling pathways, because all GFRαs bind and activate the same tyrosine kinase and induce phosphorylation of the same four key RET receptors: Y905, Y1015, Y1062, and Y1096.[347-351]

Ligand stimulation leads to activation of the RET receptor with dimerization and subsequent autophosphorylation of intracellular tyrosine residues, which serve as docking sites for various adaptor proteins. At least 18 specific phosphorylation sites have been identified, most of which are shown in Figure 39-9.

The normal RET extracellular cysteine residues are involved in the formation of intramolecular disulfide bonds, which are necessary for maintaining the tertiary structure of the extracellular domain. RET cysteine mutants induce constitutive disulfide-linked dimerization of RET molecules.[352]

RET is expressed in cells derived from the neural crest (including thyroid C cells, adrenal medullary cells, and neural cells, including parasympathetic and sympathetic ganglion cells), the branchial arches (parathyroid cells), and the urogenital system. RET plays a central role in the development of the kidney and the enteric nervous system, as evidenced by the similar phenotype of renal and neural abnormalities in mouse embryos or newborns with deficiencies of RET.[10,341,353-357]

Cloning of the *RET* Proto-oncogene and Its Role in Sporadic and Hereditary Medullary Thyroid Carcinoma

The first step in cloning the mutated *RET* proto-oncogene was the demonstration through linkage analysis that a putative genetic marker for MEN2A mapped to a small region on chromosome 10q11.2.[358,359] Subsequently, it was shown that *RET* germline mutations on chromosome 10 were associated with MEN2A, FMTC, and MEN2B.[360-363] Almost all of the *RET* mutations causing the MEN2 syndromes are missense point mutations occurring in a confined segment either in the extracellular domain of *RET* (exons 10 and 11) or in the tyrosine kinase domain (exons 13-16). Approximately half of the patients with sporadic MTC have somatic *RET* mutations, most often of codon M918T.[364,365] It was recently discovered in patients with sporadic MTC that 20% to 80% of their MTCs without *RET*

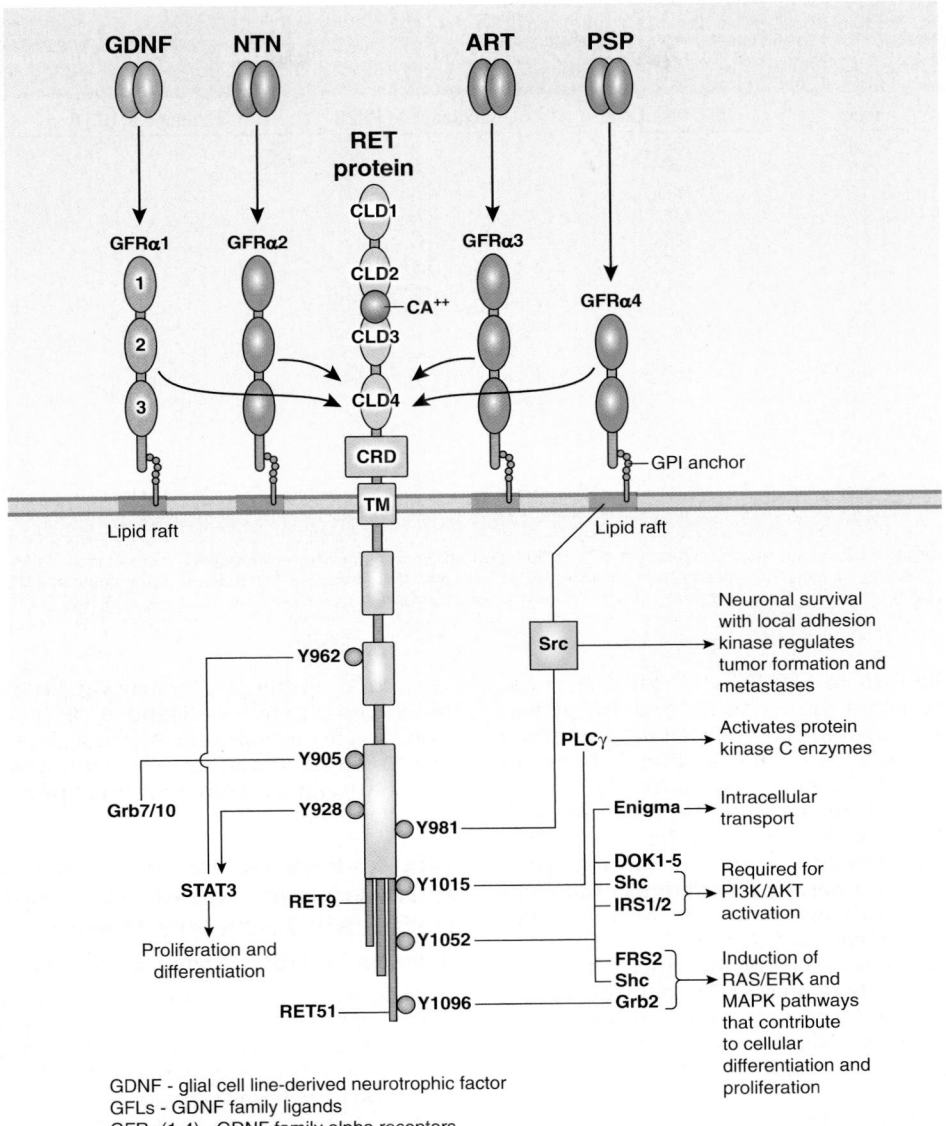

Figure 39-9 Molecular pathways activated by the *RET* proto-oncogene. ART, artemin; CLD, cadhedrin-like domain repeats; CRD, cysteine-rich domain; DOK, docking protein; FRS2, fibroblast growth factor receptor substrate 2; GPI, glycophosphatidylinositol; Grb, granzyme B; IRS1/2, internal resolution sites 1/2; NTN, neurturin; PCLγ, phospholipase C gamma; PSP, persephin; Shc, sarc homology; Src, sarc; STAT, signal transducer and activator of transcription; TM, transmembrane; Y752, Y1096, tyrosine docking sites. (Modified from Wells SA, Santoro M. Targeting the *RET* pathway in thyroid cancer. *Clin Cancer Res.* 2009;15:7119-7123.)

mutations have somatic mutations of *HRAS, KRAS,* or rarely *NRAS* oncogenes.[366-368]

The finding that dominant activating mutations of the *RET* proto-oncogene cause the MEN2 syndromes was unexpected, because most inherited tumor syndromes previously described were associated with tumor suppressor genes or mismatch repair genes. To date there have been over 100 *RET* mutations, duplications, insertions, or deletions in patients with hereditary MTC. The most common *RET* germline mutations associated with MEN2A and MEN2B are shown in Table 39-3, and the complete list of *RET* mutations reported in patients with MEN2A and MEN2B is found in the online supplemental information for this chapter. The ATA risk categories (HST, H, and MOD) for mutations associated with MEN2A are also shown in Table 39-3. A complete tabulation of all reported *RET* mutations associated with the MEN2 syndromes can be found in the online supplemental information (e-Table 39-4) and at the Human Gene Mutation Database at the Institute of Medical Genetics,[369] the Online Mendelian Inheritance in Man website,[370] the Johns Hopkins University School of Medicine, and the continually updated AURP website.[371,372]

The mutations for MEN2A are mostly located in the extracellular, cysteine-rich region of exon 10 (including codons 609, 611, 618, and 620) and exon 11 (including codons 630 and 634). Approximately 85% of the mutations associated with MEN2A involve *RET* codon 634, and approximately half of those are *C634R RET* mutations. The reason for the prevalence of codon 634 mutations in MEN2A is unknown. Unusual variants on this theme, including a 12–base pair duplication in the cysteine-rich extracellular domain of RET that introduces an additional in-frame cysteine as well as dual de novo mutations that mutate Cys 634 as well as Ala 640 on the same *RET* allele, have been reported in MEN2A.[373,374]

TABLE 39-3

Relationship of Common *RET* Mutations to Risk of Aggressive MTC in MEN2A and MEN2B and to the Incidence of PHEO, HPTH, CLA, and HD in MEN2A

RET Mutation*	Exon	MTC Risk Level	Incidence of PHEO	Incidence of HPTH	CLA	HD
G533C	8	MOD	+	nil	N	N
C609F/G/R/S/Y	10	MOD	+/++	+	N	Y
C611F/G/S/Y/W	10	MOD	+/++	+	N	Y
C618F/R/S	10	MOD	+/++	+	N	Y
C620F/R/S	10	MOD	+/++	+	N	Y
C630R/Y	11	MOD	+/++	+	N	N
D631Y	11	MOD	+++	nil	N	N
C634F/G/R/S/W/Y	11	H	+++	++	Y	N
K666E	11	MOD	+	nil	N	N
E768D	13	MOD	nil	nil	N	N
L790F	13	MOD	+	nil	N	N
V804L	14	MOD	+	+	N	N
V804M	14	MOD	+	+	Y	N
A883F	15	H	+++	nil	N	N
S891A	15	MOD	+	+	N	N
R912P	16	MOD	nil	nil	N	N
M918T	16	HST	+++	nil	N	N

*The references for each of the *RET* mutations can be found in e-Table 39-4 (available online), in which all reported *RET* mutations in MTC are listed.
CLA, cutaneous lichen amyloidosis; H, high; HD, Hirschsprung disease; HPTH, hyperparathyroidism; HST, highest; MOD, moderate; MTC, medullary thyroid carcinoma; N, negative occurrence; PHEO, pheochromocytoma; Y, positive occurrence; +, ~ (approximately) 10%; ++, ~20-30%; +++, ~50%.

Unlike the mechanism in MEN2A, the MEN2B mutations in the kinase domain cause constitutive RET activation in a monomeric form of RET, thereby altering substrate specificity, presumably due to a conformational change in the binding pocket of the kinase. Approximately 95% of mutations causing MEN2B are in codon 918 (exon 16), and 5% are located in codon 883 (exon 15). There have been four reports of patients with an atypical MEN2B syndrome who were found to have double *RET* mutations in tandem on the same allele, involving codon V804M and either codon Y806C, S904C, E805K, or Q718R.[375-378]

The *RET* proto-oncogene is central not only to the development of sporadic and hereditary MTC but also to the genesis of other malignant and nonmalignant diseases as well. Chromosomal translocations activating *RET* occur in 20% to 30% of patients with papillary thyroid carcinoma and are also seen, but much less frequently, in patients with lung adenocarcinoma and chronic myelomonocytic leukemia.[379-381] Also, inactivating mutations throughout *RET* occur in patients with sporadic and hereditary HD.[382,383]

Histopathology of Medullary Thyroid Carcinoma

During embryogenesis the ultimobranchial bodies migrate from the neural crest and become entrapped within the middle and upper poles of the thyroid lobes as the lateral thyroid complex closes. There they give rise to the C cells, which are more numerous in males compared to females.[384] Thus, MTC is a neuroendocrine tumor, but it is more commonly classified as a thyroid tumor because of its anatomic location.

Macroscopically, MTC is firm and red to whitish tan in color. Sporadic MTC is usually solitary and involves one thyroid lobe, whereas in hereditary MTC the tumor is bilateral and multicentric. On histologic examination the MTC cells are round, polyhedral, or spindle shaped. If MTC is stained with Congo red and viewed under polarized light an amyloid-like material, representing full-length CTN, is almost always present[385] (Fig. 39-10). The MTC cells express cytokeratins, mainly CK7 and CK18, TTF-1, and chromogranin A, but the most important diagnostic markers are CTN and carcinoembryonic antigen (CEA). Immunohisto-chemical staining of CTN may vary in intensity and extent, but in its absence a diagnosis of MTC should be questioned. The immunohistochemical reactivity of CTN is often reduced in undifferentiated tumors, whereas staining for CEA is almost always strongly positive.[386]

Clinical Expression and Genotype-Phenotype Correlation of Patients With Sporadic and Hereditary Medullary Thyroid Carcinoma

Sporadic Medullary Thyroid Carcinoma

In approximately 75% of patients with MTC, the tumors are sporadic and 50% of them have somatic *RET* mutations, most often involving codon M918T. The MTCs housing the M918T mutation, compared to the MTCs with other *RET* mutations, are more aggressive clinically and are associated with a poorer prognosis.[387,388] It was recently discovered that somatic mutations of *KRAS, HRAS*, or rarely *NRAS* are present in 20% to 80% of sporadic MTCs without somatic *RET* mutations.[366-368]

Sporadic MTC presents as a thyroid nodule between the fourth and sixth decades of life, and at the time of diagnosis 70% of patients have cervical metastases and 10% have distant metastases.[337] On multivariate analysis only age and disease stage at diagnosis are significant independent prognostic factors.[389] The 10-year survival rates for patients with stages I, II, III, and IV MTC are 100%, 93%, 71%, and 21%, respectively.[390]

Hereditary Medullary Thyroid Carcinoma

Classical MEN2A. Classical MEN2A is the most common of the four MEN2A variants. Virtually all patients develop MTC and lesser numbers develop pheochromocytomas or HPT, the frequency depending on the specific *RET* mutation. For example, *RET* codon 634 mutations in exon 11 are associated with a 50% penetrance of pheochromocytoma, whereas a much lower penetrance is seen in patients with exon 10 *RET* mutations in codons 609 (4-26%), 611 (10-25%), 618 (12-23%), and 620 (13-24%).[391,392] The pheochromocytomas are usually multicentric and associated with a diffuse nodular adrenal medullary hyperplasia. They

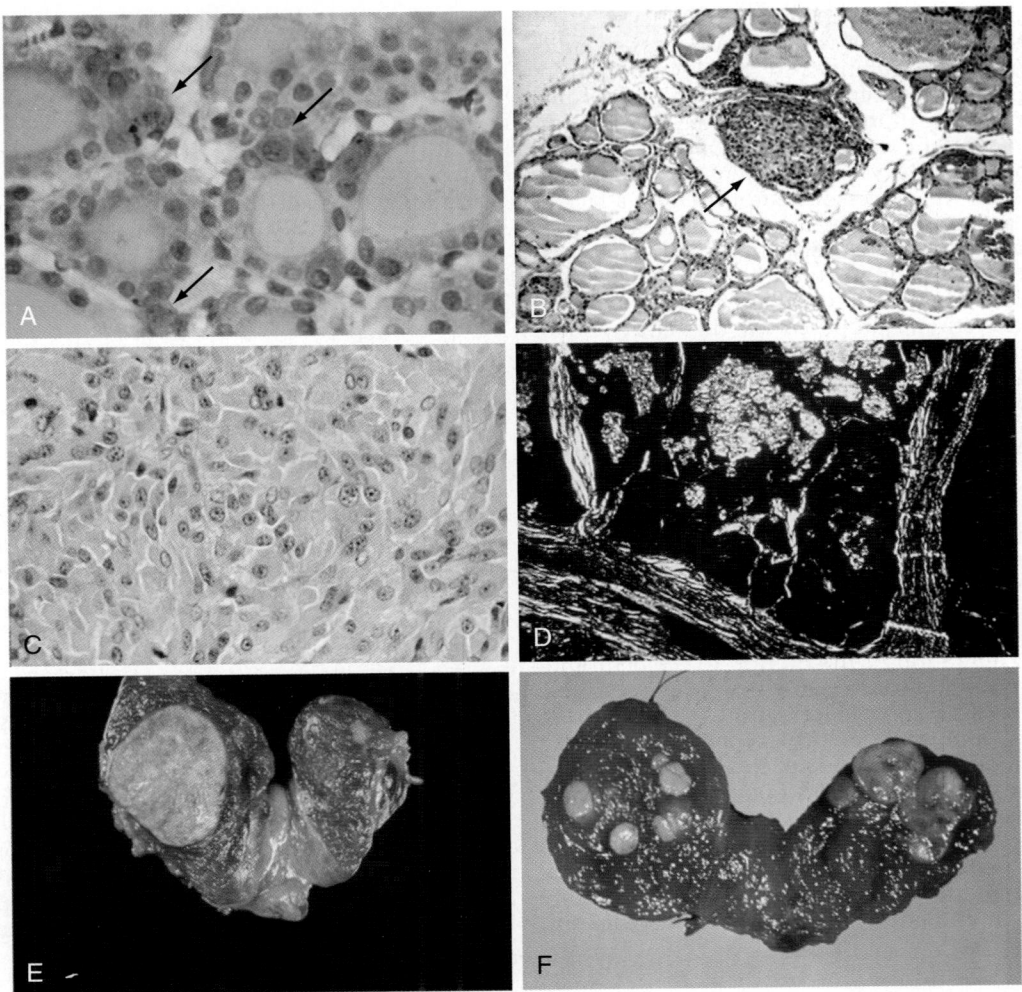

Figure 39-10 Histology of C-cell disorders: **A,** Parafollicular C-cells stained with an anti-carcinoembryonic antigen (anti-CEA) antibody *(arrows)* (original magnification ×40). **B,** Focus of C-cell hyperplasia (hematoxylin-eosin stain, original magnification ×20). **C,** Medullary thyroid carcinoma (MTC) (hematoxylin-eosin stain, original magnification ×40). **D,** Medullary thyroid carcinoma showing positive staining for amyloid-like material, which actually represents calcitonin fibrils (Congo red stain, viewed under polarized light; original magnification ×20). **E** and **F,** Coronal sections of thyroid glands of two patients with multiple endocrine neoplasia type 2A (MEN2A). Note location of multiple foci of MTC *(pale structures)* in the upper and middle portion of each thyroid lobe.

are almost always benign and confined to the adrenal gland. Patients with MEN2A and a unilateral pheochromocytoma usually develop a contralateral pheochromocytoma within 10 years. Prior to the development of biochemical and genetic tests to establish the diagnosis of hereditary MTC, pheochromocytoma, instead of MTC, was the most common cause of death.[393] The HPT in patients with classical MEN2A is usually mild and asymptomatic. The individual parathyroid glands may be either enlarged or of normal size. A *RET* codon 634 mutation is associated with a moderate penetrance of HPT (up to 30%), and *RET* mutations in codons 609, 611, 618, and 620 are associated with penetrance between 2% and 12%.[392,394]

MEN2A and Cutaneous Lichen Amyloidosis. CLA is characterized by dermatologic lesions in the scapular region of the back corresponding to dermatomes T2 to T6.[395] The classical symptom is intense pruritus that improves with sun exposure and worsens during periods of stress. Repetitive scratching causes the skin to become rough and hyperpigmented. The inciting lesion appears to be notalgia paresthetica, a sensory neuropathy involving the dorsal spinal nerves.[396] The CLA may present at a young age in an otherwise normal appearing patient, thus serving as a precur-

sor of MEN2A.[395,396] CLA occurs almost exclusively in patients with a codon 634 mutation, although it has been reported in a patient with a codon 804 mutation.[397,398] In one study CLA, or regional pruritus without CLA, occurred in 36% of patients with the *RET* codon 634 mutation.[396] CLA may also occur as an isolated sporadic or familial entity, in which the skin lesions are generalized, rather than intrascapular, and patients have neither *RET* mutations nor MTC.[399]

MEN2A and Hirschsprung Disease. Inactivating mutations occur throughout the *RET* proto-oncogene in 50% of patients with hereditary HD and in 15% to 20% of patients with sporadic HD.[382] Over 100 *RET* mutations have been described in HD, including microdeletions and insertions, nonsense or missense point mutations, splicing mutations, and larger deletions encompassing segments of the *RET* gene.[382,400,401] HD also occurs in 7% of patients with MEN2A who have *RET* point mutations in exon 10 codons 609 (15%), 611 (5%), 618 (30%), or 620 (50%).[402] Conversely, 2% to 5% of patients with HD have MEN2A.[403] The HD is almost always apparent shortly after birth, but it may not manifest until later in life. Patients with HD and exon 10 *RET* mutations should be evaluated for MEN2A. It seems paradoxical that MEN2A and HD occur together, because the *RET* mutations associated with HD are "loss of function," whereas the *RET* mutations in MEN2A are "gain of function." The generally accepted explanation for this dual occurrence is that constitutive activation of RET is sufficient to trigger neoplastic transformation of the C cells and adrenal chromaffin cells yet insufficient to generate a trophic response in the precursor neurons due to a lack of expression of the RET protein at the cell surface.[404,405]

Familial Medullary Thyroid Carcinoma. FMTC is characterized by the presence of *RET* germline mutations in subjects who develop only MTC. The variant includes families who meet the original strict criteria proposed for this entity, small families of at least two generations with at least 2 but fewer than 10 subjects with *RET* germline mutations, small families of fewer than 2 members with *RET* germline mutations, and single individuals with *RET* germline mutations.[206]

MEN2B. MEN2B accounts for 5% of patients with MEN2. The MTC often presents in infancy and is highly aggressive. Approximately 75% of patients with MEN2B are sporadic and present as de novo *RET* mutations. Most patients with MEN2B have *RET M918T* mutations in exon 16, and most of the remainder have *RET A883F* mutations in exon 15.[364,406] Recent reports suggest that patients with the A883F mutation have a less aggressive MTC compared to those with the M918T mutation.[407] In addition to pheochromocytomas, which develop in 50% of cases, patients have a characteristic physical appearance with a typical facies, ophthalmologic abnormalities (thickened and everted eyelids, mild ptosis, and prominent corneal nerves), and skeletal malformations (marfanoid body habitus, narrow long facies, pes cavus, pectus excavatum, high-arched palate, scoliosis, and slipped capital femoral epiphysis) (Fig. 39-11). Patients also have a generalized ganglioneuromatosis throughout the aerodigestive tract and are almost always symptomatic with intermittent diarrhea and constipation (Fig. 39-12). Some patients require surgery early in life because of the gastrointestinal malfunction.[408,409] It is important to establish the diagnosis of MEN2B at an early age when there is a possibility that thyroidectomy will be curative.

It is estimated that in 10% of patients with MEN2A the disease also arises de novo. In all founder cases of MEN2A and MEN2B studied thus far, the de novo mutation arises from the paternally inherited allele. Also, of the 43 founder cases with MEN2B, 28 were female and 15 were male, a finding that appears unlikely to be due to chance.[409] The reason for this distorted sex ratio is unknown.[410,411]

Secretory Products of Medullary Thyroid Carcinoma

The C cells of the thyroid gland secrete several hormones or biogenic amines, the most significant of which are CTN and CEA. These agents serve as tumor markers, as their serum concentrations are directly related to the C-cell mass. Intravenously administered calcium ion and pentagastrin given alone or together are potent secretagogues for CTN but not for CEA.

Calcitonin

CTN is a 32–amino acid monomeric peptide that results from cleavage and post-translational processing of procalcitonin. Currently, most clinical laboratories use immunochemiluminometric assays (ICMAs) that are highly specific for monomeric CTN. In the normal state serum CTN levels are higher in men than women, most likely because of a larger C-cell mass in men compared to women.[384] In one study the 95th percentile for serum CTN levels was 5.2 pg/mL and 121.7 pg/mL in women and men, respectively. Serum CTN levels are much higher in infants, with a

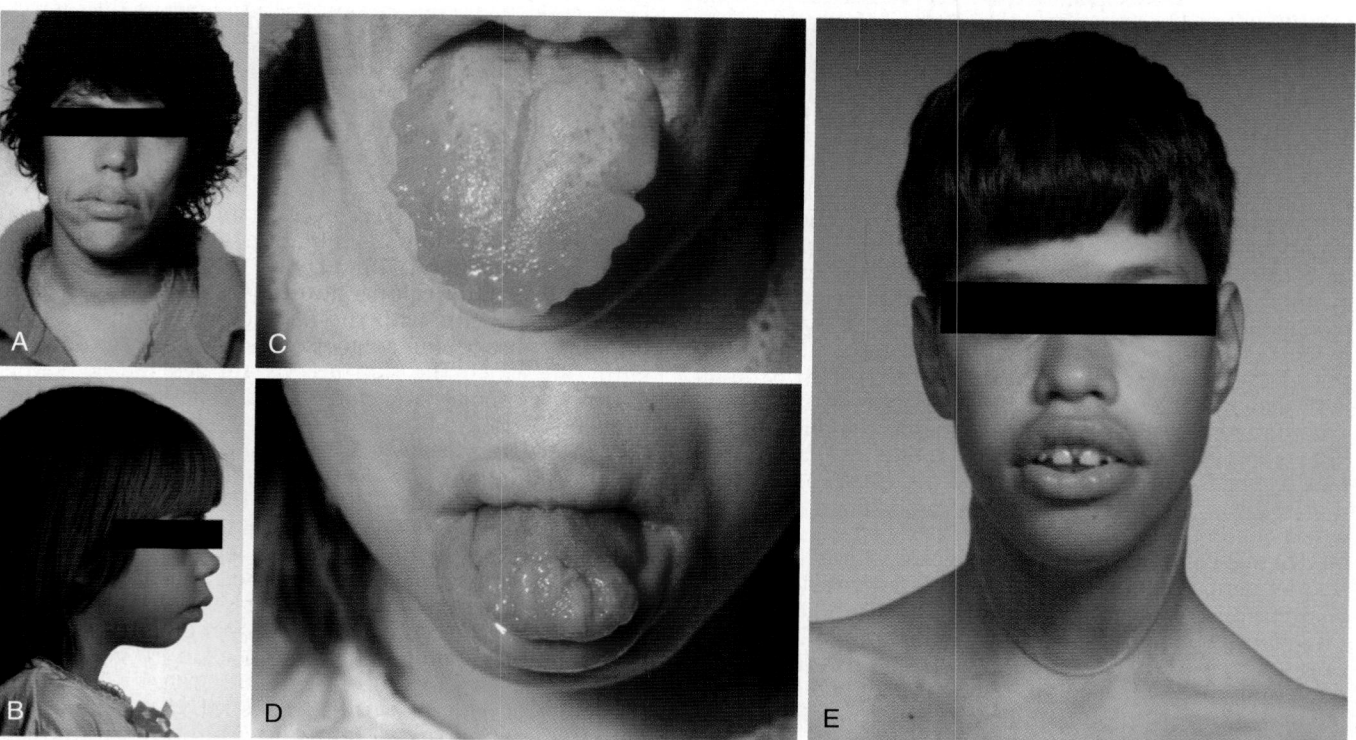

Figure 39-11 Facial appearance of three patients with multiple endocrine neoplasia type 2B (MEN2B) (**A**, **B**, and **E**). Note characteristic mucosal neuromas on the tongues (**C** and **D**) of the mother and daughter shown in **A** and **B**, respectively.

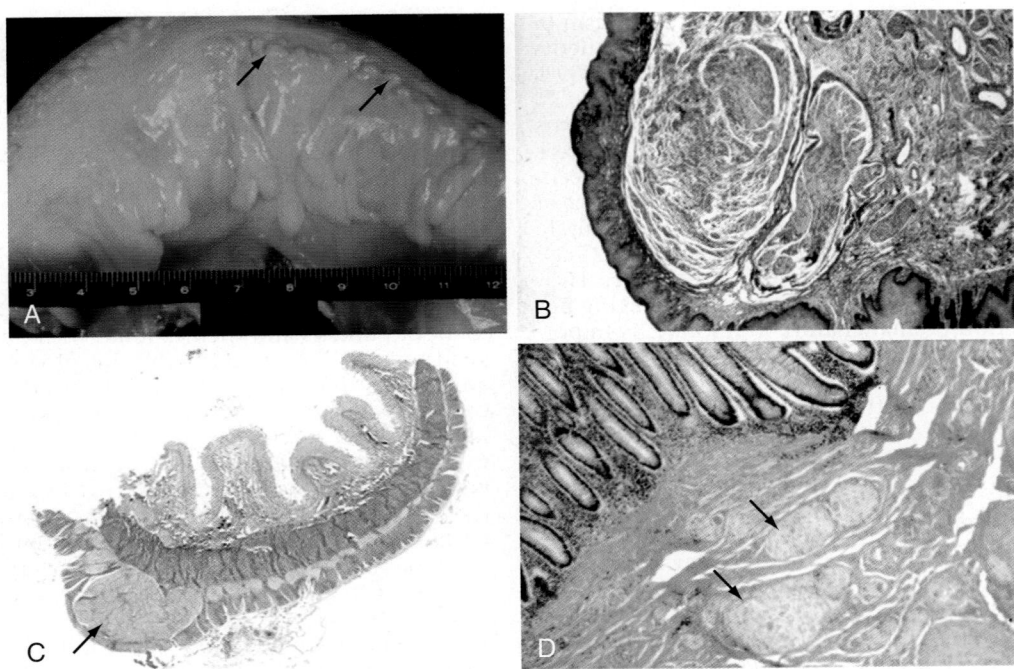

Figure 39-12 Pathologic specimens of the colon in patients with multiple endocrine neoplasia type 2B (MEN2B). **A,** Masses of hypertrophied ganglia cells in the large bowel wall *(arrows).* **B,** Mucosal neuroma of the tongue (hematoxylin-eosin stain; original magnification ×10). **C,** Cross section of large bowel wall shown in **A** with mass of subserosal ganglia cells *(arrow)* (Masson trichrome stain; original magnification ×2). **D,** Section of bowel wall showing enlarged myenteric plexus *(arrows)* (hematoxylin-eosin stain; original magnification ×40).

reference range of 40 pg/mL in children younger than 6 months of age and less than 15 pg/mL in children between 6 months and 3 years of age.[384] Regardless of age, it is important that clinicians use the same assay to evaluate patients over time. The administration of provocative agents, calcium ion and pentagastrin, may increase the sensitivity of the CTN assay; however, there has been controversy regarding whether one of the secretagogues is a more potent CTN stimulant than the other.[412] Following the introduction of ICMAs for measuring CTN many clinicians no longer use provocative testing and rely on basal serum CTN levels alone to establish the diagnosis of MTC and to evaluate patients following thyroidectomy or during treatment for advanced disease.

Measurement of Serum Calcitonin. Currently almost all commercial firms use ICMAs to measure serum CTN levels. The assays are highly specific for monometric CTN, and cross-activity with procalcitonin and other CTN-related peptides is largely eliminated.[413,414] Serum CTN levels may also be increased in patients with chronic renal failure, HPT, thyroiditis, and various malignancies.[415-421] Heterophilic antibodies (human antibodies with a broad reactivity with antibodies of other animal species) have been shown to cause falsely elevated or lowered serum CTN levels.[422] The *hook effect* refers to low analyte levels in the immunoassay resulting from very high levels of CTN, which affects the binding capacity of the antibody. Such a situation occurs most commonly in patients with widely disseminated MTC. Although the hook effect is less likely to occur with ICMAs it should remain a concern in the clinic when there is an inordinately low serum CTN level in patients with advanced stages of MTC.

Carcinoembryonic Antigen

The determination of serum CEA levels is not useful in the early diagnosis of MTC, primarily because it is not a specific marker for MTC and it is a less sensitive tumor marker compared to serum CTN. False elevation of serum CEA may result from tobacco smoking, chronic inflammatory diseases, and various malignancies. Increased serum levels of CTN and CEA indicate disease progression. Occasionally, however, patients with progressive MTC have increasing serum CEA levels and stable or declining serum CTN levels, an indication of a poorly differentiated MTC.[386] Rarely patients with advanced MTC have normal levels of serum CTN and CEA, which may also indicate tumor dedifferentiation. Such patients have intermediate or, more commonly, rapid disease progression, leading to death within a year or two after diagnosis.[423]

The Clinical Diagnosis of Medullary Thyroid Carcinoma

Almost all patients with MTC, whether sporadic or familial, present with a palpable thyroid nodule, which either they or their physicians detected on visual observation or physical examination. Less often, a member of a family with MEN2A or MEN2B who is at direct risk for inheriting a mutated *RET* allele is identified by direct DNA testing.

Fine-Needle Aspiration Biopsy

The MTC cells are usually discohesive and spindle-shaped, plasmacytoid, or epithelioid. The diagnosis of MTC can be verified by immunolocalization of CTN, chromogranin, or CEA. The immunochemical reactivity of CTN may vary in intensity and is frequently reduced in undifferentiated tumors, whereas staining for CEA is usually strongly positive.[386] FNA biopsy is an accurate method of establishing the histologic diagnosis of thyroid cancer. In a review of cytopathologic examination in 34 cases of MTC, 28 were diagnosed correctly as MTC, whereas 6 were misdiagnosed as either suspicious for MTC ($n = 2$), follicular neoplasm ($n = 3$), or desmoid tumor.[424] In another study of 91 patients with MTC, FNA findings were diagnostic of MTC in 89% of cases.[425]

On open biopsy the MTC is usually firm and appears red or tan. Sporadic tumors are usually solitary, whereas hereditary tumors are most often bilateral and multicentric. In hereditary MTC CCH precedes the development of MTC. The entity CCH is a misnomer and a more accurate descriptor would be C-cell carcinoma in situ, or C-cell neoplasia. CCH also occurs in conditions such as HPT, lymphocytic thyroiditis, renal insufficiency, and aging but does not represent a premalignant condition. It is important to distinguish CCH from microcarcinomas (MTCs less than 1 cm without capsular invasion). Microcarcinomas occur in 30% of patients with MTC and increase in aggressiveness (lymph node metastases and lower cure rates) with increasing tumor size (2-10 mm).[426]

Measurement of Basal Serum Calcitonin Levels

The practice of measuring basal serum CTN levels to detect MTC in patients with thyroid nodules has been widely accepted in Europe. In this screening approach (abnormal basal serum CTN >20 pg/mL) MTC was detected in 0.40% of 10,864 patients with nodular thyroid disease. Compared to FNA of nodules, a positive CTN measurement had a higher diagnostic sensitivity and specificity.[427] In another study of 5817 patients basal serum CTN levels were above 20 pg/mL in 66 patients. Nine patients had basal serum CTN levels above 100 pg/mL, and each had histologically confirmed MTC at thyroidectomy. In the remaining 57 patients serum CTN levels were elevated above 100 pg/mL following pentagastrin stimulation in 4 of 8 patients with basal serum CTN levels between 50 and 100 pg/mL and in 8 of 49 patients with basal serum CTN levels between 20 and 50 pg/mL. Following thyroidectomy in the 12 patients with stimulated CTN levels over 100 pg/mL, 6 had CCH and 6 had MTC.[428] The place of basal serum CTN determination in patients with thyroid nodules has been controversial but generally has not been adopted by clinicians in the United States, Canada, and other countries, primarily because of concerns of cost effectiveness.[429,430] All patients with presumed sporadic MTC should have *RET* mutation analysis, as approximately 7% of them will have *RET* germline mutations.[431,432] This result has important implications, not only for screening these patients for pheochromocytoma but also for advising their first-degree relatives to undergo genetic counseling and genetic testing.

Direct DNA Analysis to Detect Mutations in the *RET* Proto-oncogene

Currently, 63 laboratories internationally perform direct DNA analysis for *RET* mutations by direct sequence analysis with or without the addition of target mutation analysis for selected hot spots.[433] Prenatal diagnosis is offered in 18 laboratories. Screening is relatively simple in families with hereditary MTC in which the germline mutation is known, as a targeted approach can be used to detect the specific mutated *RET* allele. In new families, in which the specific *RET* mutation is unknown, the usual strategy is to sequence first the most commonly mutated cysteine codons in exons 10 and 11 (C609, C611, C618, C620, 630, and C634) as well as codon mutations in exons 13, 14, 15, and 16. Some laboratories include exon 8.[433]

Other laboratories use a two-tiered approach, starting with analysis of the most commonly mutated *hot spot exons*. However, tiered approaches are at risk of failing to detect rare *RET* double or multiple mutations, which may be associated with an unusual clinical phenotype, compared to that seen with the corresponding single *RET* mutations. This has been reported in several kindreds from Brazil, featuring coincident Y791F and C634Y *RET* mutations.[434,435] Considering the markedly reduced cost of sequencing, it may soon be practical to sequence the entire *RET* coding region as the first step in diagnosis.

Genetic Counseling

Genetic counselors have an important role in the management of patients and their families with hereditary cancer syndromes. Whereas formerly, the physician alone gave advice and informed patients of treatment options based on available data, contemporary screening programs involving predictive genetic testing require a broader explanatory interface between medical personnel and the patient. Genetic counselors fill this role and are usually the first interface with the family members to explain the nature of their disease, including patterns of inheritance, the process and technique of genetic testing, the relationship between genotype and phenotype, and possible therapeutic options.

It is important to explain the implications of a given genetic test to the patient and also to tell him or her that family members may be at risk for developing the disease. In most cases the patient will inform family members of their risk; however, there are situations in which the patient might not, and this omission presents a problem for the doctor and the doctor's duty to warn those who might be at risk for foreseeable harm. This issue is complex and has been debated in the courts, thus emphasizing the importance of providing genetic information to patients in the setting of genetic counseling. In situations, especially in the pediatric population, in which there is uncertainty about the correct course of action, physicians should ask advice from their institution's ethics committee or seek legal counsel. Experts in the field have reviewed issues related to informed consent in the new age of personalized genetic medicine.[436,437]

Considering reproductive options, prenatal testing and preimplantation testing are available to women with MEN2.[438-440] Prenatal testing can be performed in the first trimester by chorionic villus sampling or in the second trimester by amniocentesis. Also, a technique of high-resolution melting genotype analysis was recently used to detect a *RET C634Y* mutation in a fetus by detecting the mutation in the serum of a normal mother whose husband had the *C634Y* mutation.[441] Preimplantation genetic diagnosis involves polymerase chain reaction analysis of one or two cells removed from the eight-cell blastocyst to determine if a *RET* mutation is present. Embryos without *RET* mutations are then implanted back into the mother.[442] In practice there is little evidence that patients have availed themselves of this technology, perhaps because there is the perception that the MTC can be managed by timely surgical intervention. Also, preimplantation genetic diagnosis and in vitro fertilization are costly and usually not covered by insurance.

Preoperative imaging is indicated in patients who present with extensive disease or distant metastases or signs or symptoms suggestive of distant metastases. In a study of 300 patients evaluated prior to initial thyroidectomy for MTC, distant metastases were not detected when the basal serum CTN level was below 500 ng/L.[443] Ultrasound examination of the neck is the most useful preoperative imaging study in patients with primary MTC. Although no single imaging study provides optimal total body imaging, contrast-enhanced CT scanning is most useful in detecting lung and mediastinal metastases, CT scanning or contrast enhanced MRI is the most sensitive method to detect liver metastases, and axial MRI or bone scintigraphy is the most useful method to detect bone metastases.[444]

The Management of the Tumors Associated With MEN2A and MEN2B

Medullary Thyroid Carcinoma

The treatment of MTC varies depending on the clinical setting. In patients who present with a newly detected thyroid nodule, confirmed to be MTC on FNA, and no evidence of regional or distant metastases, the first step is a physical examination with ultrasound evaluation of the neck. Hereditary MTC must be excluded by family history and direct DNA testing for germline *RET* mutations. In patients with MEN2A and MEN2B, the presence of a pheochromocytoma must be excluded prior to any interventional studies.

In patients presenting with a MTC nodule in the thyroid the initial treatment is total thyroidectomy. The majority of patients will have metastases to lymph nodes in the neck either detected preoperatively by physical examination or ultrasound of the neck or found following pathologic examination of the resected thyroid and soft tissue specimens.[445,446] Some surgeons place an emphasis on these examinations in addition to the preoperative serum levels of CTN and CEA, as there is a relation between the levels of these markers and the extent of lymph node metastases. There are rarely lymph node metastases in patients with serum CTN levels less than 20 pg/mL (normal reference range 10 pg/mL); however, with levels exceeding 20, 50, 200, and 500 pg/L metastases begin to appear in the ipsilateral central and lateral neck, the contralateral central neck, the contralateral lateral neck, and the upper mediastinum, respectively. Half of the patients treated with bilateral compartment-oriented neck dissection will be cured biochemically (basal serum CTN <10 pg/mL) when the preoperative serum CTN is less than 1000 pg/mL; however, serum CTN levels from 1000 to 2000, from 2000 to 10,000, and above 10,000 pg/mL are associated with biochemical cures of 10%, 6%, and 0%, respectively.[443] Preoperative serum CEA levels are also useful in predicting the likelihood of lymph node metastases and surgical cure, but less so than serum CTN levels.[447] Patients who are cured biochemically following thyroidectomy have a 5- to 7.5-year risk of recurrence of 3% to 10% and a 10-year survival rate of 98%.[390,448]

Occasionally, the diagnosis of MTC is established following hemithyroidecomy. The opposite lobe should be removed in all patients with hereditary MTC and in those with sporadic MTC if the serum CTN is elevated or there is imaging evidence of residual MTC.[449]

It is important to note that clearance of lymph nodes and other structures in the neck is associated with significant complications, including lymphatic leakage, hypoparathyroidism, and damage to the spinal accessory nerve with associated shoulder dysfunction.[450,451] The parathyroid glands are frequently injured or resected during total thyroidectomy, and the surgeon should be experienced in not only identifying the parathyroid glands but in assuring that their function is preserved. If parathyroid glands cannot be spared during thyroidectomy or if their viability is questioned, they should be transplanted to the sternocleidomastoid muscle in patients with sporadic MTC or MEN2B. In patients with MEN2A the parathyroids should be grafted to a heterotopic site such as the brachioradialis muscle in the forearm.[452]

In the postoperative period patients are evaluated for hypocalcemia. Oral calcium and calcitriol are given to patients who develop symptomatic hypocalcemia. Almost all patients can be weaned from this medication over a few weeks; however, rarely a patient may require permanent replacement therapy. Patients also require replacement therapy with levothyroxine sufficient to maintain serum thyroid-stimulating hormone (TSH) levels in the euthyroid range.

Prophylactic Thyroidectomy in Children With Hereditary Medullary Thyroid Carcinoma

Hereditary MTC progresses from CCH, to MTC, and to regional and then distant metastases over several months to years, depending on the specific *RET* mutation. The management of patients with hereditary MTC provides an unusual opportunity in which an organ at risk for cancer can be resected before cancer develops or while it is still confined to the organ. Ideally, prophylactic surgery in patients with hereditary cancer syndromes should meet the following criteria: (1) the genetic mutation causing the malignancy is characterized by complete or near complete penetrance, (2) there is a highly reliable test for detecting the mutated allele, (3) the organ at risk is expendable, or if not expendable, there is therapy to replace the organ's function, and (4) there is a reliable test to determine if the operation has been curative. Many hereditary cancer syndromes meet some, but not all, of these criteria, whereas MEN2A and MEN2B meet all of them.

The goal of thyroid surgery is to remove the thyroid before MTC develops or while it is still confined to the gland. The most critical factor in attaining that goal is determining the age at which the thyroid should be removed. The term *prophylactic thyroidectomy* is a misnomer as the resected thyroid gland of very young children often shows CCH or small foci of MTC. The term *prophylactic thyroidectomy* is in common usage, however, and in the present context we use it to describe removal of a thyroid gland that appears normal microscopically or shows early manifestations of a C-cell disorder confined to the thyroid gland.

Prophylactic Thyroidectomy in Children With MEN2A. Prior to the introduction of genetic testing to detect *RET* mutations in youngsters with MEN2A, measurement of serum CTN levels either basally or following provocative testing was used to detect the presence of a C-cell disorder. At the time, this diagnostic method was very useful; however, there were two problems. There were no standard guidelines regarding the timing of thyroidectomy based on serum CTN levels. Thus, in some children the resected thyroid gland was normal, as was later genetic testing. Also, children who consistently tested negative required repetitive annual testing, often over several years, and with time some discontinued testing, because of frustration with the repetitive testing and the anxiety that a test might be positive. This was unfortunate because the children were at substantial risk for returning in the future with clinically evident MTC.[453] Because of this, rather than embark on a protocol of annual testing that might last for years, some parents and their child elected to proceed with a thyroidectomy, reasoning that it would be indicated at some time in the future.

With the advent of direct DNA analysis to detect *RET* germline mutations, the diagnostic focus shifted. It soon became evident, however, that there was great variability in the time of MTC onset, not only among, but within, families having the same *RET* germline mutation (excluding those with *RET 634* or *RET 918* codon mutations in which predictably MTCs develop at a young age). Although a patient's *RET* mutation alone gave a general idea of the time range of MTC onset, the serum CTN level proved to pinpoint more precisely the timing of thyroidectomy. It is difficult to recommend a definitive basal, or stimulated, serum CTN value when thyroidectomy should be recommended, because guidelines vary from clinic to clinic. Currently, the combination of genetic testing and serum CTN measurement serves as the basis for timing thyroidectomy.

In the recently revised ATA guidelines for the management of patients with MTC it was recommended that children with MEN2A be classified according to the aggressiveness and age of onset of their MTC. Therefore, patients with *RET* germline mutations in codons 634 and 883 are at high (H) risk for developing an aggressive MTC early in life, and they should be managed by annual clinical examination and measurement of serum CTN levels beginning at 3 years of age. Most of these children will require surgery at or before 5 years of age. Patients with MEN2A and other *RET* germline mutations should have an annual clinical examination and serum CTN measurements beginning at 5 years of age. In many of these children the evaluation will be prolonged if their annual evaluations and serum CTN levels remain within the normal range for years. It is important that the child, the child's parents, the pediatrician, and the surgeon meet annually to discuss the results of testing and decide on a treatment plan.

Prophylactic Thyroidectomy for Children With MEN2B. Patients with MEN2B caused by the *M918T RET* mutation have highly aggressive MTC (ATA category HST). A distinction should be made between the 25% of patients who present with a known family history of MEN2B and the 75% who have de novo *RET* mutations. Children with known hereditary MEN2B should have direct DNA analysis at birth or soon thereafter. Thyroidectomy is indicated in the first year of life, perhaps even the first months of life, the exact timing to be determined by the pediatrician, the surgeon, and the child's parents. There are complicating factors associated with thyroidectomy in very young children. The serum CTN levels are very high in the first months of life and of little use in timing thyroidectomy. More important, the parathyroid glands are very small and hard to identify, creating a significant risk of permanent hypoparathyroidism, a serious complication in a young child who will need replacement therapy for life. In the absence of suspicious

lymph nodes the central zone of the neck should be left unresected at total thyroidectomy. Regardless of the surgical procedure there should be a liberal approach to grafting resected or damaged parathyroid glands into the sternocleidomastoid muscle.

In children with MEN2B and de novo *RET* mutations the diagnosis is rarely made before a thyroid nodule is evident. Unwary clinicians rarely make a diagnosis of MEN2B before it is clinically apparent and incurable. However, when the diagnosis is made early because of the recognized phenotype instead of by the presence of a thyroid nodule, children are younger and have lower serum CTN levels, smaller thyroid nodules, and a lower incidence of extrathyoidal extension of the MTC, regional and distant metastases. Moreover, such children are more often cured biochemically following thyroidectomy.[454,455] Regardless of the age at diagnosis children should be treated by total thyroidectomy and compartment-oriented lymphadenectomy, depending on the sites involved.

Children with MEN2B and *A883F RET* germline mutations have a less aggressive MTC and are managed by annual evaluation, including neck ultrasound and serum CTN levels beginning at 3 years of age. Few patients have been described with double *RET* mutations involving codon *V804M* and either codon Y806C, S904C, E805K, or Q781R, and it appears that they should be treated as MEN2A patients in the MOD category.

Pheochromocytomas

Pheochromocytomas present at around 40 years of age, somewhat earlier than in patients with sporadic pheochromocytoma.[456] The diagnosis is made concurrently with MTC in 30% to 70% of cases. Less often, a pheochromocytoma is the first manifestations of MEN2.[456] Patients with MEN2 and pheochromocytomas have an associated adrenal medullary hyperplasia, which is often evident on radiographic imaging as thickening of the gland (Fig. 39-13). The adrenal medullary hyperplasia is similar to CCH, but it is not a premalignant condition.

There is substantial morbidity associated with performing a thyroidectomy, or any interventional procedure, in a patient with a pheochromocytoma. Also, pregnant women with a pheochromocytoma are at substantial risk for hypertensive crisis during delivery. The standard diagnostic test for pheochromocytoma is measurement of plasma-free or urinary-fractionated metanephrines, or both. Either CT or

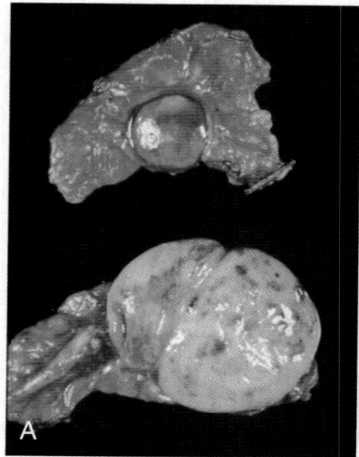
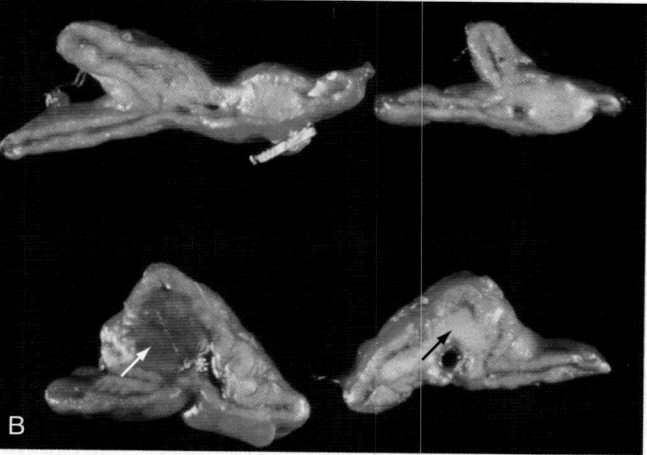

Figure 39-13 Pheochromocytomas: **A,** Bilateral pheochromocytomas in the left adrenal gland *(top)* and the right adrenal gland *(bottom).* Also notice the multiple pheochromocytomas in the bottom adrenal gland. **B,** Foci of adrenal medullary hyperplasia in adrenal gland *(black arrow)* and pheochromocytoma *(white arrow).*

MRI will confirm the presence and anatomic location of pheochromocytoma(s). In patients with both an MTC and a pheochromocytoma, almost always the pheochromocytoma should be removed prior to thyroidectomy.

Prior to surgery, it is critical that patients be prepared with the α-adrenergic blocker phenoxybenzamine, which is usually given in a dose of 10 mg orally twice a day for 10 to 14 days preoperatively. Higher doses, up to 80 mg twice daily, may be needed to ensure blood pressure control. Patients with pheochromocytomas are volume constricted and should be observed for the development of postural hypotension during phenoxybenzamine treatment. Most patients can be prepared on an outpatient basis; however, if blood pressure proves to be labile, hospitalization may be required. β-Adrenergic blockade is usually unnecessary unless it is difficult to control the hypertension or the patient develops a tachyarrhythmia. If β-blockade is administered, it should be undertaken only after α-blockade; otherwise, patients may develop severe hypertension due to unopposed vasoconstriction. Before anesthetic induction, a radial artery catheter is placed and a urinary bladder catheter is inserted. A pulmonary artery catheter for central monitoring is usually unnecessary unless the patient has cardiac disease. During manipulation of the pheochromocytoma intraoperatively, there may be episodes of hypertension, which are best controlled with sodium nitroprusside or esmolol. The patient may experience hypotension after resection of the pheochromocytoma, but this is easily managed pharmacologically. There must be adequate glucocorticoid coverage intraoperatively and postoperatively. Following discharge it is critical that patients subjected to bilateral adrenalectomy have information on their person that they have no adrenal glands and must have glucocorticoid and mineralocorticoid replacement if they are subject to serious injury or illness.

Whether to perform a unilateral or bilateral adrenalectomy depends on the extent of disease at the time of diagnosis. Bilateral adrenalectomy is indicated in patients with bilateral pheochromocytomas; however, there has been controversy regarding the management of patients with a single pheochromocytoma. Most surgeons perform a unilateral adrenalectomy for a solitary pheochromocytoma, because it may be years before a contralateral pheochromocytoma develops, if it will at all. The argument for a bilateral adrenalectomy in patients with a unilateral pheochromocytoma relates to the likelihood that they will develop a second pheochromocytoma in the future and the reduced risks associated with a single operation. This preference is offset by the substantial risk associated with Addison disease following bilateral adrenalectomy.[457] The operative procedure of choice is laparoscopic or retroperitoneoscopic adrenalectomy.[458] More recently some surgeons have performed subtotal adrenalectomy in an attempt to preserve adrenal cortical tissue; however, there is a 20% risk of recurrent pheochromocytoma in the adrenal remnant within 20 years after subtotal adrenalectomy.[459]

Children with MEN2 in the ATA H and HST categories develop pheochromocytomas as early as 8 and 12 years of age, respectively, and in the ATA MOD category as early as 19 years of age.[460-462] Thus, it is recommended that screening for pheochromocytoma should begin at 11 years of age in children in the ATA HST and ATA H categories and at 19 years of age in children in the ATA MOD category.

Hyperparathyroidism

HPT also presents around 40 years of age, although the age of onset may be earlier because the majority of patients are asymptomatic.[463] For practical reasons, screening for HPT (measuring serum calcium levels, with or without intact PTH levels) should be done concurrently with screening for pheochromocytomas. The HPT that develops in patients with MEN2A is milder than that occurring in patients with MEN1 or sporadic HPT. From one to four parathyroid glands may be enlarged (Fig. 39-14). Resection of only enlarged parathyroid glands with concurrent PTH monitoring to assure that all hyperfunctioning tissue is removed has become the treatment of choice for patients with MEN2A and HPT. Removal of 3½ glands or total parathyroidectomy with ectopic parathyroid transplantation are other options. It is not uncommon for patients with

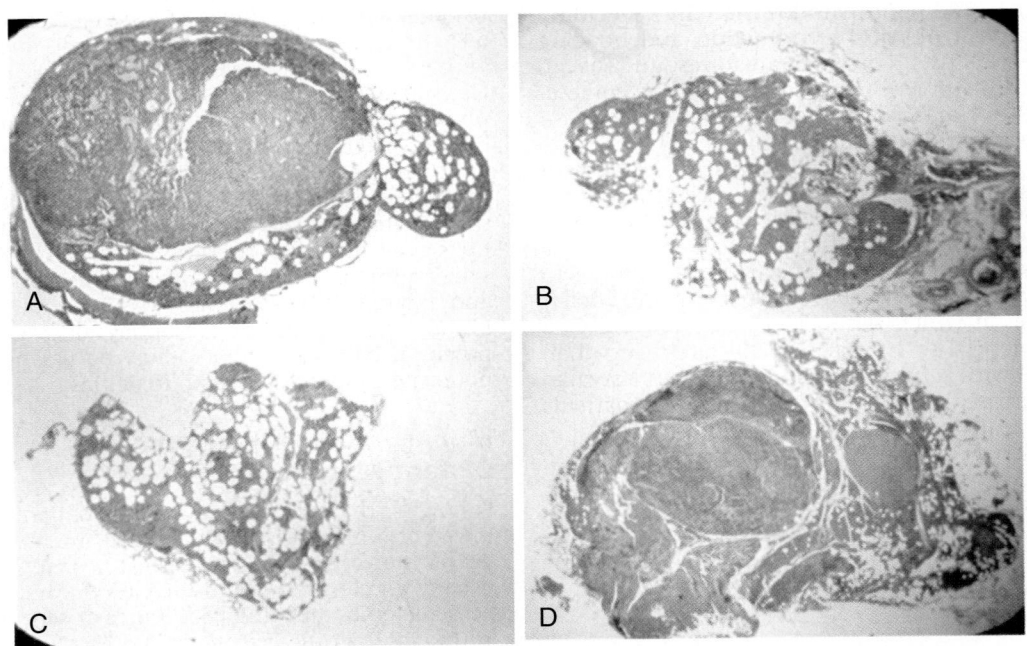

Figure 39-14 Parathyroid glands: **A,** right upper; **B,** right lower; **C,** left upper; **D,** left lower. Microscopically, the parathyroid glands in panels **A** and **D** are consistent with parathyroid adenomas, whereas the parathyroid glands in panels **B** and **C** appear histologically normal. However, each parathyroid gland was grossly enlarged.

MEN2A to develop HPT following thyroidectomy for MTC. Preoperative localization should be attempted with sestamibi scanning, ultrasound, and CT. The repeat neck exploration is often difficult because of scarring and distorted anatomy from prior surgery. If there is documentation that three parathyroid glands have been removed, the remaining large gland should be resected and a portion of it transplanted to a heterotopic site. If only one enlarged parathyroid is identified and the number of remaining glands is in question, a portion of the enlarged gland could be cryopreserved, although this technique is practiced infrequently.[464] If the HPT cannot be cured, or if patients are not candidates for parathyroid exploration, medical therapy with calcimimetics should be considered.[465]

Evaluation of Patients Following Thyroidectomy for Medullary Thyroid Carcinoma

It is important to evaluate patients postoperatively to determine if they have been cured of MTC. The American Joint Committee for Cancer tumor-node-metastasis staging system, primarily based on pathologic analysis and preoperative imaging studies, provides useful information regarding patient prognosis (see Table 39-2). The system, however, does not include preoperative and postoperative CTN and CEA levels. If the surgeon removes all thyroid tissue during total thyroidectomy the serum CTN level should be undetectable.[466] The serum CTN level normalizes over time depending on the absence or presence of residual normal thyroid tissue or MTC. Some investigators have proposed that serum CTN measured at 3 months after thyroidectomy is the optimal time to establish a postoperative baseline value.[467] An undetectable serum CTN level following stimulation with calcium or pentagastrin or both indicates a curative thyroidectomy; however, a more commonly used, albeit less strict, guideline for biochemical cure is a basal serum CTN level less than 10 pg/mL.[468] There is a substantial overlap in the serum CTN levels of patients with locally persistent or recurrent MTC and patients with distant metastases; generally, however, elevated serum CTN levels less than 150 pg/mL are associated with local-regional disease.[467] Evaluation of patients who have serum CTN levels exceeding 150 pg/mL following thyroidectomy should begin with a physical examination and imaging procedures, the most useful of which are ultrasound (neck), CT (lung), and MRI (liver). Bone scintigraphy is complementary to MRI for axial skeletal lesions but superior for the detection of peripheral lesions.[444]

In patients with documented recurrent or distant disease, imaging procedures should be repeated every 3 months to determine if the metastatic sites have changed significantly, according to the Response Evaluation Criteria in Solid Tumors (RECIST).[469] Also, a particularly useful technique in the evaluation of patients postoperatively is determining the rates at which serum levels of CTN and CEA double over time.[470] The 10-year survival rate is less than 10% in patients with serum CTN doubling times less than 6 months, compared to approximately 40% in patients with doubling times between 6 and 24 months. The doubling times of serum CTN and CEA are strongly correlated in the large majority of patients; however, in the minority they are discordant and less useful in determining prognosis.[471]

Treatment of Patients With Local or Regional Metastases

Repeat operation should be considered in patients with persistent or recurrent MTC localized to the neck, even though the majority of them will not be cured. In about 30% of patients the serum CTN levels will be reduced to the normal range, in which case the prognosis is relatively good with prevention of recurrence in the neck and durable reductions in the serum CTN levels.[472] Compared to the primary procedure, repeat neck operations are more difficult, as there is much scarring and distortion of normal anatomy. Before embarking on a lengthy and complicated operative procedure one should exclude the presence of distant metastases. Because imaging procedures do not always identify distant metastases, especially if they are small, clinicians have explored other localization techniques, such as selective venous sampling with measurement of neck and hepatic vein CTN levels compared to peripheral vein levels and laparoscopic evaluation of the liver. The latter procedure has been most useful as approximately 20% of patients have small liver metastases demonstrated on laparoscopy that were not evident on imaging procedures.[473]

It was initially thought that radioactive iodine (RAI) taken up in nearby normal follicular cells would destroy MTC cells in a postoperative thyroid remnant by way of a *bystander effect*. However, in a study comparing patients with MTC treated by total thyroidectomy and the subsequent administration of RAI compared to no RAI, there was no difference in disease-specific survival.[474]

In patients with residual MTC following total thyroidectomy there have been no randomized, controlled trials comparing repeat neck operations to other forms of therapy. This is especially true of external beam radiotherapy (EBRT) to the neck, which is commonly applied in this clinical setting despite there being little evidence of its efficacy. For example, an analysis of Surveillance, Epidemiology, and End Results (SEER) data showed no survival benefit of EBRT in patients with MTC and positive lymph nodes.[475] The goal of treatment, however, has not been to improve survival but to reduce the incidence of local recurrence. Thus, postoperative EBRT has been reserved mostly for patients without distant metastases who are likely to develop locally recurrent MTC following thyroidectomy. The rate of local control depends on the amount of residual MTC following thyroidectomy, being virtually 100% in patients with no evidence of residual disease, compared to 65% in those with microscopic disease and 25% in those with gross residual disease.[476] The typical EBRT dose (60-66 Gy delivered to the thyroid bed over 6 weeks using 4-6 mV photons) should be sufficient to eradicate microscopic disease. Higher doses are administered to patients with gross residual disease. Intensity-modulated radiotherapy is indicated in patients with recurrent MTC adjacent to the spinal cord or other vital structures. Substantial acute toxicity is associated with the administration of EBRT, primarily skin erythema and desquamation, mucositis, esophagitis, and laryngeal edema. Late toxicities may include neck fibrosis, hoarseness, and esophageal stricture. Thus, the potential benefits of EBRT must be balanced against the potential acute and chronic toxicities.

Management of Patients With Distant Metastases

Following thyroidectomy for MTC, patients should be followed at 6-month intervals during the first year and then yearly thereafter. The first indicator of recurrent disease is usually an elevated serum CTN level. Metastatic MTC can be detected by imaging procedures at serum CTN levels of 150 to 400 pg/mL, is evident in 50% of patients with CTN levels of 5000 pg/mL, and is almost always present at CTN levels of 20,000 pg/mL.[477]

The specific treatment varies depending on the site of the metastases. Other than to the soft tissues of the neck region, MTC spreads first to liver and bone. Liver metastases occur in 45% of patients with advanced MTC and may be associated with pain and diarrhea. It may be possible to resect large solitary liver metastases; however, most metastases are small and disseminated throughout the liver, in which case percutaneous ethanol ablation, radiofrequency ablation, or systemic therapy are more effective treatments.

Unsuspected bone metastases may be found on anatomic or functional imaging. Patients may be symptomatic and present with painful bone metastases or fractures. Intravenous bisphosphonates (zoledronic acid or pamidronate), or the receptor activator for nuclear factor κB ligand (RANKL) inhibitor, denosumab, have been effective treatments for patients with painful bony metastases; however, they are associated with side effects including hypocalcemia and, uncommonly, osteonecrosis of the mandible and atypical subtrochanteric fractures.[478] Bone fractures should be treated with stabilization and thermoablation (radiofrequency or cryoblation), cement injection, or EBRT.[478] Patients with acute symptoms of spinal cord compression must be treated emergently with corticosteroid administration, surgical stabilization, and EBRT.[479]

Less commonly, MTC metastasizes to lung, brain, or skin. Lung metastases are usually multiple and not amenable to surgical resection, unless they invade an airway or blood vessel. Metastases in the trachea or a major bronchus may be treated with laser or photodynamic therapy. Metastases to the brain or skin may also be treated by palliative surgical resection, but symptom relief is short lived and patients usually succumb to disease shortly after diagnosis.[480]

There is a role for palliation in some patients with advanced MTC. Patients who present with aggressive MTC extending beyond the thyroid capsule into the soft tissues involving the trachea, esophagus, and recurrent laryngeal nerves (with or without distant metastases) are difficult to cure, and the goal of surgery is more palliative with attention to minimizing complications. The surgeon must decide on the extent of dissection considering possible postoperative rehabilitation, quality of life, and life expectancy. The management decision involves discussions with other medical disciplines and especially the patient. Some patients live for years with advanced disease and function reasonably well. Sometimes it is best to do nothing.

Hormonally Active Metastases

Patients with a large MTC tumor burden and markedly elevated serum CTN levels often have diarrhea that is resistant to conventional therapies. The cause of the diarrhea is unclear, but it can be debilitating in terms of quality of life and nutrition. Antimotility agents such as loperamide and codeine are often used as initial therapy. Somatostatin analogues have had minimal efficacy. In some patients tumor debulking or chemoembolization may provide relief.

The MTC cells also may secrete ACTH or CRH, resulting in Cushing syndrome. Approximately 3% of all cases of ectopic Cushing syndrome are due to MTC. Patients with the syndrome are often debilitated due to hypokalemia, diabetes, hypertension, and gastritis. Patients should be treated despite a poor prognosis. Ketoconazole, mifepristone, metyrapone, and mitotane have shown efficacy in some patients. If these therapies are not effective, bilateral adrenalectomy may be indicated. The tyrosine kinase inhibitors (TKIs) recently introduced to treat patients with metastatic MTC have also shown efficacy in the treatment of the associated Cushing syndrome.[481,482]

Systemic Therapy

Until recently the administration of chemotherapy, with either single agents or combination therapy, was front-line therapy for patients with metastatic MTC, even though it was characterized by low response rates of short duration and substantial toxicity.[483,484]

Over the past 2 decades the treatment of patients with metastatic MTC has shifted to the use of TKIs, which have shown significant therapeutic efficacy in phase II and phase III clinical trials. The initial clinical studies with the TKI, imatinib mesylate, demonstrated remarkable efficacy in patients with chronic myelogenous leukemia, in that 87% of patients were in complete cytologic remission 60 months after initiation of treatment. It was assumed and hoped that TKIs, which targeted specific oncogenes, would prove equally beneficial in other liquid and solid tumors.[485] Such was not the case in patients with advanced MTC. In phase II and III clinical studies of various TKIs, including axitinib, cabozantinib, gefitinib, imatinib, motesanib, sorafenib, sunitinib, and vandetanib, there were some impressive responses, including prolonged periods of stable disease; however, responses were mostly transient and patients' tumors progressed because of drug resistance.[486-496] On the basis of prospective, randomized, double-blinded, phase III randomized trials, two TKIs, vandetanib and cabozantinib, demonstrated significant progression-free survival (PFS) and were recently approved by the U.S. Food and Drug Administration (FDA) and European Medicines Agency (EMA) for the treatment of patients with advanced systemic progressive MTC.[488,496]

In the vandetanib trial (NCT00322452) 331 patients with metastatic MTC were randomized 2:1 to vandetanib (300 mg/day) or placebo. Patients who progressed on the placebo could be crossed over to vandetanib at the time of tumor progression. Partial responses were observed in 45% of the patients randomized to vandetanib, and many patients were able to resume a normal quality of life. The median PFS was 19.3 months in the placebo arm, compared to a predicted median PFS of 30.5 months in the vandetanib arm (HR:0.46; $p < 0.0001$). Patients with and without *RET* mutations responded to vandetanib, but the response rate was higher in those with *RET* mutations. Adverse events included diarrhea, fatigue, rash, hypertension, and prolongation of the QTc interval. Only 12% of patients discontinued the drug due to toxicity, and 35% required dose reductions. The FDA included a black box warning regarding the QTc toxicity, and the EMA approval was conditional, based on the need for additional data regarding the response of patients with no *RET* mutations.[496]

In a second phase III prospective, randomized, double-blinded trial (NCT00704730), cabozantinib (175 mg/day) was administered 2:1 compared to placebo in 330 patients with progressive metastatic MTC.[488] Patients randomized to placebo were not allowed to cross over to cabozantinib. The PFS was 4.0 months in the placebo, compared to 11.2 months with cabozantinib (hazard ratio 0.28, $p < 0.0001$). There were significant side effects with the drug, including diarrhea, abdominal pain, fatigue, hypertension, and palmoplantar erythrodysesthesia, such that 16% of the patients discontinued the drug due to toxicity and 79% of patients required dose reductions. There was also an important warning with cabozantinib regarding the possible development of gastrointestinal fistulas and life-threatening bleeding. The toxicity is most likely partly due to the dose of cabozantinib, as 60 mg/day has been the starting dose in subsequent clinical trials with other malignancies.

Vandetanib and cabozantinib now serve as front-line therapy for patients with advanced progressive MTC. Although both drugs have shown improved PFS compared to placebo, neither has shown improved overall survival, and they are not likely to do so, because of the crossover arm from placebo in the vandetanib trial, and the likelihood that patients on the cabozantinib trial, and the vandetanib trial for that matter, will be treated with other TKIs when they fail therapy with these drugs. The experience with vandetanib and cabozantinib has been seen with other TKIs used to treat other malignancies and speaks to a general issue with TKIs that most patients develop resistance to the drugs and their disease progresses. It is unlikely that a single TKI will be curative in patients with metastatic MTC and the current focus is on developing effective combinatorial therapy, which will depend on an understanding of mechanisms of tumor resistance and defining vulnerable molecular targets other than *RET*.

REFERENCES

1. Erdheim J. Zur normalen und pathologischen histologie der glandula thyreoidea, parathyreoidea und hypophysis. *Beitr Pathol Anat.* 1903; 33:158-263.
2. Underdahl LO, Woolner LB, Black BM. Multiple endocrine adenomas; report of 8 cases in which the parathyroids, pituitary and pancreatic islets were involved. *J Clin Endocrinol Metab.* 1953;13:20-47.
3. Moldawer MP, Nardi GL, Raker JW. Concomitance of multiple adenomas of the parathyroids and pancreatic islets with tumor of the pituitary: a syndrome with a familial incidence. *Am J Med Sci.* 1954; 228:190-206.
4. Wermer P. Genetic aspects of adenomatosis of endocrine glands. *Am J Med.* 1954;16:363-371.
5. Ballard HS, Fame B, Hartsock RJ. Familial multiple endocrine adenoma-peptic ulcer complex. *Medicine (Baltimore).* 1964;43:481-516.
6. Steiner AL, Goodman AD, Powers SR. Study of a kindred with pheochromocytoma, medullary thyroid carcinoma, hyperparathyroidism and Cushing's disease: multiple endocrine neoplasia, type 2. *Medicine (Baltimore).* 1968;47:371-409.
7. Melvin KE, Tashjian AH Jr, Miller HH. Studies in familial (medullary) thyroid carcinoma. *Recent Prog Horm Res.* 1972;28:399-470.
8. Sipple J. The association of pheochromocytoma with carcinoma of the thyroid gland. *Am J Med.* 1961;31:163-166.
9. Marx SJ. Multiplicity of hormone-secreting tumors: common themes about cause, expression, and management. *J Clin Endocrinol Metab.* 2013;98(8):3139-3148.
10. Zordan P, Tavella S, Brizzolara A, et al. The immediate upstream sequence of the mouse Ret gene controls tissue-specific expression in transgenic mice. *Int J Mol Med.* 2006;18:601-608.
11. Dean PG, van Heerden JA, Farley DR, et al. Are patients with multiple endocrine neoplasia type I prone to premature death? *World J Surg.* 2000;24:1437-1441.
12. Goudet P, Murat A, Binquet C, et al. Risk factors and causes of death in MEN1 disease. A GTE (Groupe d'Etude des Tumeurs Endocrines) cohort study among 758 patients. *World J Surg.* 2010;34(2):249-255.
13. Marx S. Multiple endocrine neoplasia type 1. In: Bilezekian JP, Marcus R, Levine MA, eds. *The Parathyroids: Basic and Clinical Concepts.* 2nd ed. San Diego, CA: Academic Press; 2001:535-584.
14. Marx SJ, Vinik AI, Santen RJ, et al. Multiple endocrine neoplasia type I: assessment of laboratory tests to screen for the gene in a large kindred. *Medicine (Baltimore).* 1986;65:226-241.
15. Benson L, Ljunghall S, Akerstrom G, Oberg K. Hyperparathyroidism presenting as the first lesion in multiple endocrine neoplasia type 1. *Am J Med.* 1987;82:731-737.
16. Trump D, Farren B, Wooding C, et al. Clinical studies of multiple endocrine neoplasia type 1 (MEN1). *QJM.* 1996;89(9):653-669.
17. Marx S, Spiegel AM, Skarulis MC, et al. Multiple endocrine neoplasia type 1: clinical and genetic topics. *Ann Intern Med.* 1998;129: 484-494.
18. Jackson CE, Boonstra CE. The relationship of hereditary hyperparathyroidism to endocrine adenomatosis. *Am J Med.* 1967;43:727-734.
19. Johnson GJ, Summerskill WH, Anderson VE, Keating FR Jr. Clinical and genetic investigation of a large kindred with multiple endocrine adenomatosis. *N Engl J Med.* 1967;277:1379-1385.
20. Craven DE, Goodman D, Carter JH. Familial multiple endocrine adenomatosis. Multiple endocrine neoplasia, type I. *Arch Intern Med.* 1972;129:567-569.
21. Snyder N 3rd, Scurry MT, Deiss WP. Five families with multiple endocrine adenomatosis. *Ann Intern Med.* 1972;76:53-58.
22. Jung RT, Grant AM, Davie M, et al. Multiple endocrine adenomatosis (type I) and familial hyperparathyroidism. *Postgrad Med J.* 1978;54: 92-94.
23. Eberle F, Grun R. Multiple endocrine neoplasia, type I (MEN I). *Ergeb Inn Med Kinderheilkd.* 1981;46:76-149.
24. Burgess JR, David R, Greenaway TM, et al. Osteoporosis in multiple endocrine neoplasia type 1: severity, clinical significance, relationship to primary hyperparathyroidism, and response to parathyroidectomy. *Arch Surg.* 1999;134:1119-1123.
25. Eller-Vainicher C, Chiodini I, Battista C, et al. Sporadic and MEN1-related primary hyperparathyroidism: differences in clinical expression and severity. *J Bone Miner Res.* 2009;24:1404-1410.
26. Rizzoli R, Green J 3rd, Marx SJ. Primary hyperparathyroidism in familial multiple endocrine neoplasia type I. Long-term follow-up of serum calcium levels after parathyroidectomy. *Am J Med.* 1985;78:467-474.
27. Marx SJ, Menczel J, Campbell G, et al. Heterogeneous size of the parathyroid glands in familial multiple endocrine neoplasia type 1. *Clin Endocrinol (Oxf).* 1991;35:521-526.
28. Hellman P, Skogseid B, Oberg K, et al. Primary and reoperative parathyroid operations in hyperparathyroidism of multiple endocrine neoplasia type 1. *Surgery.* 1998;124:993-999.
29. de Laat JM, Pieterman CR, Weijmans M, et al. Low accuracy of tumor markers for diagnosing pancreatic neuroendocrine tumors in multiple endocrine neoplasia type 1 patients. *J Clin Endocrinol Metab.* 2013; 98:4143-4151.
30. Agha A, Carpenter R, Bhattacharya S, et al. Parathyroid carcinoma in multiple endocrine neoplasia type 1 (MEN1) syndrome: two case reports of an unrecognised entity. *J Endocrinol Invest.* 2007;30:145-149.
31. Friedman E, Sakaguchi K, Bale AE, et al. Clonality of parathyroid tumors in familial multiple endocrine neoplasia type 1. *N Engl J Med.* 1989;321:213-218.
32. Brandi ML, Aurbach GD, Fitzpatrick LA, et al. Parathyroid mitogenic activity in plasma from patients with familial multiple endocrine neoplasia type 1. *N Engl J Med.* 1986;314:1287-1293.
33. Bilezikian JP, Brandi ML, Eastell R, et al. Guidelines for the management of asymptomatic primary hyperparathyroidism: summary statement from the Fourth International Workshop. *J Clin Endocrinol Metab.* 2014;99:3561-3569.
34. Jensen RT. Management of the Zollinger-Ellison syndrome in patients with multiple endocrine neoplasia type 1. *J Intern Med.* 1998;243: 477-488.
35. Shawker T. Ultrasound evaluation of primary hyperparathyroidism. *Ultrasound Q.* 2000;16:73-87.
36. Udelsman R, Lin Z, Donovan P. The superiority of minimally invasive parathyroidectomy based on 1650 consecutive patients with primary hyperparathyroidism. *Ann Surg.* 2011;253:585-591.
37. Thompson GB, Grant CS, Perrier ND, et al. Reoperative parathyroid surgery in the era of sestamibi scanning and intraoperative parathyroid hormone monitoring. *Arch Surg.* 1999;134(7):699-704, discussion 704-705.
38. Jaskowiak N, Norton JA, Alexander HR, et al. A prospective trial evaluating a standard approach to reoperation for missed parathyroid adenoma. *Ann Surg.* 1996;224(3):308-320, discussion 320-321.
39. Irvin GL 3rd, Molinari AS, Figueroa C, Carneiro DM. Improved success rate in reoperative parathyroidectomy with intraoperative PTH assay. *Ann Surg.* 1999;229(6):874-878, discussion 878-879.
40. Tonelli F, Spini S, Tommasi M, et al. Intraoperative parathormone measurement in patients with multiple endocrine neoplasia type I syndrome and hyperparathyroidism. *World J Surg.* 2000;24(5):556-562, discussion 562-563.
41. Libutti SK, Alexander HR, Bartlett DL, et al. Kinetic analysis of the rapid intraoperative parathyroid hormone assay in patients during operation for hyperparathyroidism. *Surgery.* 1999;126(6):1145-1150, discussion 1150-1151.
42. Yavuz S, Simonds WF, Weinstein LS, et al. Sleeping parathyroid tumor: rapid hyperfunction after removal of the dominant tumor. *J Clin Endocrinol Metab.* 2012;97:1834-1841.
43. Feldman AL, Sharaf RN, Skarulis MC, et al. Results of heterotopic parathyroid autotransplantation: a 13-year experience. *Surgery.* 1999; 126:1042-1048.
44. Powell AC, Alexander HR, Pingpank JF, et al. The utility of routine transcervical thymectomy for multiple endocrine neoplasia 1-related hyperparathyroidism. *Surgery.* 2008;144(6):878-883, discussion 883-884.
45. Majewski JT, Wilson SD. The MEA-I syndrome: an all or none phenomenon? *Surgery.* 1979;86:475-484.
46. Skogseid B, Oberg K, Eriksson B, et al. Surgery for asymptomatic pancreatic lesion in multiple endocrine neoplasia type I. *World J Surg.* 1996;20(7):872-876, discussion 877.
47. Yu F, Venzon DJ, Serrano J, et al. Prospective study of the clinical course, prognostic factors, causes of death, and survival in patients with long-standing Zollinger-Ellison syndrome. *J Clin Oncol.* 1999; 17:615-630.
48. Kloppel G, Willemer S, Stamm B, et al. Pancreatic lesions and hormonal profile of pancreatic tumors in multiple endocrine neoplasia

type I. An immunocytochemical study of nine patients. *Cancer.* 1986;57:1824-1832.

49. Le Bodic MF, Heymann MF, Lecomte M, et al. Immunohistochemical study of 100 pancreatic tumors in 28 patients with multiple endocrine neoplasia, type I. *Am J Surg Pathol.* 1996;20:1378-1384.

50. Pipeleers-Marichal M, Somers G, Willems G, et al. Gastrinomas in the duodenums of patients with multiple endocrine neoplasia type 1 and the Zollinger-Ellison syndrome. *N Engl J Med.* 1990;322:723-727.

51. Ariel I, Kerem E, Schwartz-Arad D, et al. Nesidiodysplasia—a histologic entity? *Hum Pathol.* 1988;19:1215-1218.

52. Lubensky IA, Debelenko LV, Zhuang Z, et al. Allelic deletions on chromosome 11q13 in multiple tumors from individual MEN1 patients. *Cancer Res.* 1996;56:5272-5278.

53. Debelenko LV, Zhuang Z, Emmert-Buck MR, et al. Allelic deletions on chromosome 11q13 in multiple endocrine neoplasia type 1-associated and sporadic gastrinomas and pancreatic endocrine tumors. *Cancer Res.* 1997;57:2238-2243.

54. Anlauf M, Perren A, Meyer CL, et al. Precursor lesions in patients with multiple endocrine neoplasia type 1-associated duodenal gastrinomas. *Gastroenterology.* 2005;128:1187-1198.

55. Crabtree JS, Scacheri PC, Ward JM, et al. A mouse model of multiple endocrine neoplasia, type 1, develops multiple endocrine tumors. *Proc Natl Acad Sci U S A.* 2001;98:1118-1123.

56. Yang J, Kan Y, Ge BH, et al. Diagnostic role of gallium-68 DOTATOC and gallium-68 DOTATATE PET in patients with neuroendocrine tumors: a meta-analysis. *Acta Radiol.* 2014;55:389-398.

57. Maioli M, Ciccarese M, Pacifico A, et al. Familial insulinoma: description of two cases. *Acta Diabetol.* 1992;29(1):38-40.

57b. Sipos B, Sperveslage J, Anlauf M, et al. Glucagon cell hyperplasia and neoplasia with and without glucagon receptor mutations. *J Clin Endocrinol Metab.* 2015;100(5):E783-E788.

58. Lubensky IA, Pack S, Ault D, et al. Multiple neuroendocrine tumors of the pancreas in von Hippel-Lindau disease patients: histopathological and molecular genetic analysis. *Am J Pathol.* 1998;153:223-231.

59. Farley DR, van Heerden JA, Grant CS, et al. The Zollinger-Ellison syndrome. A collective surgical experience. *Ann Surg.* 1992;215:561-569, discussion 569-570.

60. Serrano J. Occurrence of multiple endocrine neoplasia type 1 (MEN1) gene mutations in Zollinger Ellison syndrome (ZES) (abstract). *Gastroenterology.* 1998;114:G2022.

61. Waxman I, Gardner JD, Jensen RT, Maton PN. Peptic ulcer perforation as the presentation of Zollinger-Ellison syndrome. *Dig Dis Sci.* 1991;36:19-24.

62. Metz D. Multiple endocrine neoplasia type 1: clinical features and management. In: Bilezekian J, Levine MA, Marx SJ, eds. *The Parathyroids.* New York, NY: Raven Press; 1994:591-646.

63. Gibril F, Schumann M, Pace A, Jensen RT. Multiple endocrine neoplasia type 1 and Zollinger-Ellison syndrome: a prospective study of 107 cases and comparison with 1009 cases from the literature. *Medicine (Baltimore).* 2004;83:43-83.

64. Benya RV, Metz DC, Venzon DJ, et al. Zollinger-Ellison syndrome can be the initial endocrine manifestation in patients with multiple endocrine neoplasia-type I. *Am J Med.* 1994;97:436-444.

65. Roy PK, Venzon DJ, Shojamanesh H, et al. Zollinger-Ellison syndrome. Clinical presentation in 261 patients. *Medicine (Baltimore).* 2000;79:379-411.

66. Norton JA, Fraker DL, Alexander HR, et al. Surgery to cure the Zollinger-Ellison syndrome. *N Engl J Med.* 1999;341:635-644.

67. Gibril F, Venzon DJ, Ojeaburu JV, et al. Prospective study of the natural history of gastrinoma in patients with MEN1: definition of an aggressive and a nonaggressive form. *J Clin Endocrinol Metab.* 2001;86:5282-5293.

68. Ruszniewski P, Podevin P, Cadiot G, et al. Clinical, anatomical, and evolutive features of patients with the Zollinger-Ellison syndrome combined with type I multiple endocrine neoplasia. *Pancreas.* 1993;8(3):295-304.

69. Stadil F, Bardram L, Gustafsen J, Efsen F. Surgical treatment of the Zollinger-Ellison syndrome. *World J Surg.* 1993;17:463-467.

70. Thompson NW. Current concepts in the surgical management of multiple endocrine neoplasia type 1 pancreatic-duodenal disease. Results in the treatment of 40 patients with Zollinger-Ellison syndrome, hypoglycaemia or both. *J Intern Med.* 1998;243:495-500.

71. Tonelli F, Fratini G, Nesi G, et al. Pancreatectomy in multiple endocrine neoplasia type 1-related gastrinomas and pancreatic endocrine neoplasias. *Ann Surg.* 2006;244:61-70.

72. Bartsch DK, Fendrich V, Langer P, et al. Outcome of duodenopancreatic resections in patients with multiple endocrine neoplasia type 1. *Ann Surg.* 2005;242:757-764, discussion 764-766.

73. Lopez CL, Falconi M, Waldmann J, et al. Partial pancreaticoduodenectomy can provide cure for duodenal gastrinoma associated with multiple endocrine neoplasia type 1. *Ann Surg.* 2013;257:308-314.

74. Imamura M, Komoto I, Ota S, et al. Biochemically curative surgery for gastrinoma in multiple endocrine neoplasia type 1 patients. *World J Gastroenterol.* 2011;17:1343-1353.

75. Frucht H, Maton PN, Jensen RT. Use of omeprazole in patients with Zollinger-Ellison syndrome. *Dig Dis Sci.* 1991;36:394-404.

76. Maton PN. Review article: the management of Zollinger-Ellison syndrome. *Aliment Pharmacol Ther.* 1993;7:467-475.

77. Maton PN. Omeprazole. *N Engl J Med.* 1991;324:965-975.

78. Jensen R. Gastrinoma as a model for prolonged hypergastrinemia. In: Walsh J, ed. *Gastrin.* New York, NY: Raven Press; 1993:373-393.

79. Solcia E, Capella C, Fiocca R, et al. Gastric argyrophil carcinoidosis in patients with Zollinger-Ellison syndrome due to type 1 multiple endocrine neoplasia. A newly recognized association. *Am J Surg Pathol.* 1990;14:503-513.

80. Maton PN, Lack EE, Collen MJ, et al. The effect of Zollinger-Ellison syndrome and omeprazole therapy on gastric oxyntic endocrine cells. *Gastroenterology.* 1990;99:943-950.

81. Cadiot G, Lehy T, Ruszniewski P, et al. Gastric endocrine cell evolution in patients with Zollinger-Ellison syndrome. Influence of gastrinoma growth and long-term omeprazole treatment. *Dig Dis Sci.* 1993;38:1307-1317.

82. Gyr K. Human pharmacological effects of SMS 201-995 on gastric secretion. *Scan J Gastroenterol Suppl.* 1986;119:96-102.

83. Shojamanesh H, Gibril F, Louie A, et al. Prospective study of the antitumor efficacy of long-term octreotide treatment in patients with progressive metastatic gastrinoma. *Cancer.* 2002;94:331-343.

84. Tomassetti P, Migliori M, Caletti GC, et al. Treatment of type II gastric carcinoid tumors with somatostatin analogues. *N Engl J Med.* 2000;343:551-554.

85. Marx SJ, Spiegel AM, Levine MA, et al. Familial hypocalciuric hypercalcemia: the relation to primary parathyroid hyperplasia. *N Engl J Med.* 1982;307:416-426.

86. Proye C, Malvaux P, Pattou F, et al. Noninvasive imaging of insulinomas and gastrinomas with endoscopic ultrasonography and somatostatin receptor scintigraphy. *Surgery.* 1998;124:1134-1143, discussion 1143-1144.

87. Xu Y, Pan D, Xu Q, et al. Insulinoma imaging with glucagon-like peptide-1 receptor targeting probe (18)F-FBEM-Cys (39)-exendin-4. *J Cancer Res Clin Oncol.* 2014;140:1479-1488.

88. Norton JA, Cromack DT, Shawker TH, et al. Intraoperative ultrasonographic localization of islet cell tumors. A prospective comparison to palpation. *Ann Surg.* 1988;207:160-168.

89. Boukhman MP, Karam JM, Shaver J, et al. Localization of insulinomas. *Arch Surg.* 1999;134:818-822, discussion 822-823.

90. Doppman JL, Chang R, Fraker DL, et al. Localization of insulinomas to regions of the pancreas by intra-arterial stimulation with calcium. *Ann Intern Med.* 1995;123:269-273.

91. Proye C, Pattou F, Carnaille B, et al. Intraoperative insulin measurement during surgical management of insulinomas. *World J Surg.* 1998;22:1218-1224.

92. Libutti SK, et al. Unpublished observations. Bethesda, MD: National Institutes of Health.

93. Stefanini P, Carboni M, Patrassi N, Basoli A. Beta-islet cell tumors of the pancreas: results of a study on 1,067 cases. *Surgery.* 1974;75:597-609.

94. Goode PN, Farndon JR, Anderson J, et al. Diazoxide in the management of patients with insulinoma. *World J Surg.* 1986;10:586-592.

95. Lamberts SW, Pieters GF, Metselaar HJ, et al. Development of resistance to a long-acting somatostatin analogue during treatment of two patients with metastatic endocrine pancreatic tumours. *Acta Endocrinol (Copenh).* 1988;119:561-566.

96. Levy-Bohbot N, Merle C, Goudet P, et al. Prevalence, characteristics and prognosis of MEN 1-associated glucagonomas, VIPomas, and somatostatinomas: study from the GTE (Groupe des Tumeurs Endocrines) registry. *Gastroenterol Clin Biol.* 2004;28:1075-1081.

97. Gorden P, Comi RJ, Maton PN, Go VL. NIH conference. Somatostatin and somatostatin analogue (SMS 201-995) in treatment of hormone-secreting tumors of the pituitary and gastrointestinal tract and non-neoplastic diseases of the gut. *Ann Intern Med.* 1989;110:35-50.

98. Park SK, O'Dorisio MS, O'Dorisio TM. Vasoactive intestinal polypeptide-secreting tumours: biology and therapy. *Baillieres Clin Gastroenterol.* 1996;10:673-696.

99. Wu TJ, Lin CL, Taylor RL, et al. Increased parathyroid hormone-related peptide in patients with hypercalcemia associated with islet cell carcinoma. *Mayo Clin Proc.* 1997;72:1111-1115.

100. Liu SW, van de Velde CJ, Heslinga JM, et al. Acromegaly caused by growth hormone-relating hormone in a patient with multiple endocrine neoplasia type I. *Jpn J Clin Oncol.* 1996;26:49-52.

101. Ezzat S, Asa SL, Stefaneanu L, et al. Somatotroph hyperplasia without pituitary adenoma associated with a long standing growth hormone-releasing hormone-producing bronchial carcinoid. *J Clin Endocrinol Metab.* 1994;78:555-560.

102. Garbrecht N, Anlauf M, Schmitt A, et al. Somatostatin-producing neuroendocrine tumors of the duodenum and pancreas: incidence, types, biological behavior, association with inherited syndromes, and functional activity. *Endocr Relat Cancer.* 2008;15:229-241.

103. Fleury A, Flejou JF, Sauvanet A, et al. Calcitonin-secreting tumors of the pancreas: about six cases. *Pancreas.* 1998;16:545-550.

104. Skogseid B, Oberg K, Benson L, et al. A standardized meal stimulation test of the endocrine pancreas for early detection of pancreatic endocrine tumors in multiple endocrine neoplasia type 1 syndrome: five years experience. *J Clin Endocrinol Metab.* 1987;64:1233-1240.

105. Mutch MG, Frisella MM, DeBenedetti MK, et al. Pancreatic polypeptide is a useful plasma marker for radiographically evident pancreatic islet cell tumors in patients with multiple endocrine neoplasia type 1. *Surgery.* 1997;122:1012-1019, discussion 1019-1020.

106. Garin E, Le Jeune F, Devillers A, et al. Predictive value of 18F-FDG PET and somatostatin receptor scintigraphy in patients with metastatic endocrine tumors. *J Nucl Med.* 2009;50:858-864.

107. Skogseid B, Oberg K, Akerstrom G, et al. Limited tumor involvement found at multiple endocrine neoplasia type I pancreatic exploration: can it be predicted by preoperative tumor localization? *World J Surg.* 1998;22:673-677, discussion 677-678.

108. Pisegna JR, Doppman JL, Norton JA, et al. Prospective comparative study of ability of MR imaging and other imaging modalities to localize tumors in patients with Zollinger-Ellison syndrome. *Dig Dis Sci.* 1993;38:1318-1328.

109. Frilling A, Malago M, Martin H, Broelsch CE. Use of somatostatin receptor scintigraphy to image extrahepatic metastases of neuroendocrine tumors. *Surgery.* 1998;124:1000-1004.

110. Cadiot G, Bonnaud G, Lebtahi R, et al. Usefulness of somatostatin receptor scintigraphy in the management of patients with Zollinger-Ellison syndrome. Groupe de Recherche et d'Etude du Syndrome de Zollinger-Ellison (GRESZE). *Gut.* 1997;41:107-114.

111. Yim JH, Siegel BA, DeBenedetti MK, et al. Prospective study of the utility of somatostatin-receptor scintigraphy in the evaluation of patients with multiple endocrine neoplasia type 1. *Surgery.* 1998;124:1037-1042.

112. Alexander HR, Fraker DL, Norton JA, et al. Prospective study of somatostatin receptor scintigraphy and its effect on operative outcome in patients with Zollinger-Ellison syndrome. *Ann Surg.* 1998;228:228-238.

113. Doppman JL, Miller DL, Chang R, et al. Gastrinomas: localization by means of selective intraarterial injection of secretin. *Radiology.* 1990;174:25-29.

114. Legmann P, Vignaux O, Dousset B, et al. Pancreatic tumors: comparison of dual-phase helical CT and endoscopic sonography. *AJR Am J Roentgenol.* 1998;170:1315-1322.

115. Sheridan MB, Ward J, Guthrie JA, et al. Dynamic contrast-enhanced MR imaging and dual-phase helical CT in the preoperative assessment of suspected pancreatic cancer: a comparative study with receiver operating characteristic analysis. *AJR Am J Roentgenol.* 1999;173:583-590.

116. Ichikawa T, Peterson MS, Federle MP, et al. Islet cell tumor of the pancreas: biphasic CT versus MR imaging in tumor detection. *Radiology.* 2000;216:163-171.

117. Koopmans KP, Neels OC, Kema IP, et al. Improved staging of patients with carcinoid and islet cell tumors with 18F-dihydroxy-phenylalanine and 11C-5-hydroxy-tryptophan positron emission tomography. *J Clin Oncol.* 2008;26:1489-1495.

118. Orlefors H, Sundin A, Garske U, et al. Whole-body (11)C-5-hydroxy-tryptophan positron emission tomography as a universal imaging technique for neuroendocrine tumors: comparison with somatostatin receptor scintigraphy and computed tomography. *J Clin Endocrinol Metab.* 2005;90:3392-3400.

119. Bansal R, Tierney W, Carpenter S, et al. Cost effectiveness of EUS for preoperative localization of pancreatic endocrine tumors. *Gastrointest Endosc.* 1999;49:19-25.

120. Suits J, Frazee R, Erickson RA. Endoscopic ultrasound and fine needle aspiration for the evaluation of pancreatic masses. *Arch Surg.* 1999;134:639-642, discussion 642-643.

121. Hiramoto JS, Feldstein VA, LaBerge JM, Norton JA. Intraoperative ultrasound and preoperative localization detects all occult insulinomas. *Arch Surg.* 2001;136:1020-1025, discussion 1025-1026.

122. Granberg D, Stridsberg M, Seensalu R, et al. Plasma chromogranin A in patients with multiple endocrine neoplasia type 1. *J Clin Endocrinol Metab.* 1999;84:2712-2717.

123. Nobels FR, Kwekkeboom DJ, Coopmans W, et al. Chromogranin A as serum marker for neuroendocrine neoplasia: comparison with neuron-specific enolase and the alpha-subunit of glycoprotein hormones. *J Clin Endocrinol Metab.* 1997;82:2622-2628.

124. Goebel SU, Serrano J, Yu F, et al. Prospective study of the value of serum chromogranin A or serum gastrin levels in the assessment of the presence, extent, or growth of gastrinomas. *Cancer.* 1999;85:1470-1483.

125. Weber HC, Venzon DJ, Lin JT, et al. Determinants of metastatic rate and survival in patients with Zollinger-Ellison syndrome: a prospective long-term study. *Gastroenterology.* 1995;108:1637-1649.

126. Cadiot G, Vuagnat A, Doukhan I, et al. Prognostic factors in patients with Zollinger-Ellison syndrome and multiple endocrine neoplasia type 1. Groupe d'Etude des Neoplasies Endocriniennes Multiples (GENEM and groupe de Recherche et d'Etude du Syndrome de Zollinger-Ellison (GRESZE). *Gastroenterology.* 1999;116:286-293.

127. Lowney JK, Frisella MM, Lairmore TC, Doherty GM. Pancreatic islet cell tumor metastasis in multiple endocrine neoplasia type 1: correlation with primary tumor size. *Surgery.* 1998;124:1043-1048, discussion 1048-1049.

128. Wiedenmann B, Jensen RT, Mignon M, et al. Preoperative diagnosis and surgical management of neuroendocrine gastroenteropancreatic tumors: general recommendations by a consensus workshop. *World J Surg.* 1998;22:309-318.

129. Lairmore TC, Chen VY, DeBenedetti MK, et al. Duodenopancreatic resections in patients with multiple endocrine neoplasia type 1. *Ann Surg.* 2000;231:909-918.

130. Carty SE, Jensen RT, Norton JA. Prospective study of aggressive resection of metastatic pancreatic endocrine tumors. *Surgery.* 1992;112:1024-1031, discussion 1031-1032.

131. Kim YH, Ajani JA, Carrasco CH, et al. Selective hepatic arterial chemoembolization for liver metastases in patients with carcinoid tumor or islet cell carcinoma. *Cancer Invest.* 1999;17:474-478.

132. Eriksson B, Oberg K, Alm G, et al. Treatment of malignant endocrine pancreatic tumours with human leucocyte interferon. *Lancet.* 1986;2:1307-1309.

133. Frank M, Klose KJ, Wied M, et al. Combination therapy with octreotide and alpha-interferon: effect on tumor growth in metastatic endocrine gastroenteropancreatic tumors. *Am J Gastroenterol.* 1999;94:1381-1387.

134. Moertel CG, Lefkopoulo M, Lipsitz S, et al. Streptozocin-doxorubicin, streptozocin-fluorouracil or chlorozotocin in the treatment of advanced islet-cell carcinoma. *N Engl J Med.* 1992;326:519-523.

135. Pisegna JR, Slimak GG, Doppman JL, et al. An evaluation of human recombinant alpha interferon in patients with metastatic gastrinoma. *Gastroenterology.* 1993;105:1179-1183.

136. Maton PN, Gardner JD, Jensen RT. Use of long-acting somatostatin analog SMS 201-995 in patients with pancreatic islet cell tumors. *Dig Dis Sci.* 1989;34:28S-39S.

137. Tomassetti P, Migliori M, Corinaldesi R, Gullo L. Treatment of gastroenteropancreatic neuroendocrine tumours with octreotide LAR. *Aliment Pharmacol Ther.* 2000;14:557-560.

138. Wymenga AN, Eriksson B, Salmela PI, et al. Efficacy and safety of prolonged-release lanreotide in patients with gastrointestinal neuroendocrine tumors and hormone-related symptoms. *J Clin Oncol.* 1999;17:1111.

139. di Bartolomeo M, Bajetta E, Buzzoni R, et al. Clinical efficacy of octreotide in the treatment of metastatic neuroendocrine tumors. A study by the Italian Trials in Medical Oncology Group. *Cancer.* 1996;77:402-408.

140. Caplin ME, Pavel M, Cwikla JB, et al. Lanreotide in metastatic enteropancreatic neuroendocrine tumors. *N Engl J Med.* 2014;371:224-233.

141. Yao JC, Shah MH, Ito T, et al. Everolimus for advanced pancreatic neuroendocrine tumors. *N Engl J Med.* 2011;364:514-523.

142. Raymond E, Dahan L, Raoul JL, et al. Sunitinib malate for the treatment of pancreatic neuroendocrine tumors. *N Engl J Med.* 2011;364:501-513.

143. Van Essen M, Krenning EP, De Jong M, et al. Peptide receptor radionuclide therapy with radiolabelled somatostatin analogues in patients with somatostatin receptor positive tumours. *Acta Oncol.* 2007;46:723-734.

144. Corbetta S, Pizzocaro A, Peracchi M, et al. Multiple endocrine neoplasia type 1 in patients with recognized pituitary tumours of different types. *Clin Endocrinol (Oxf).* 1997;47:507-512.

145. Tortosa F, Chico A, Rodriguez-Espinosa J, et al. Prevalence of MEN1 in patients with prolactinoma. MEN1 Study Group of the Hospital de la Santa Creu i Sant Pau of Barcelona. *Clin Endocrinol (Oxf).* 1999;50:272.

146. Verges B, Boureille F, Goudet P, et al. Pituitary disease in MEN type 1 (MEN1): data from the France-Belgium MEN1 multicenter study. *J Clin Endocrinol Metab.* 2002;87:457-465.

147. Carty SE, Helm AK, Amico JA, et al. The variable penetrance and spectrum of manifestations of multiple endocrine neoplasia type 1. *Surgery.* 1998;124:1106-1113, discussion 1113-1114.

148. Stratakis CA, Schussheim DH, Freedman SM, et al. Pituitary macroadenoma in a 5-year-old: an early expression of multiple endocrine neoplasia type 1. *J Clin Endocrinol Metab.* 2000;85:4776-4780.

149. Sahdev A, Jager R. Bilateral pituitary adenomas occurring with multiple endocrine neoplasia type one. *AJNR Am J Neuroradiol.* 2000;21:1067-1069.

150. Trouillas J, Labat-Moleur F, Sturm N, et al. Pituitary tumors and hyperplasia in multiple endocrine neoplasia type 1 syndrome (MEN1): a case-control study in a series of 77 patients versus 2509 non-MEN1 patients. *Am J Surg Pathol.* 2008;32:534-543.

151. O'Brien T, O'Riordan DS, Gharib H, et al. Results of treatment of pituitary disease in multiple endocrine neoplasia, type I. *Neurosurgery.* 1996;39:273-278, discussion 278-279.

152. Bevan JS, Webster J, Burke CW, Scanlon MF. Dopamine agonists and pituitary tumor shrinkage. *Endocr Rev.* 1992;13:220-240.

153. Weil C. The safety of bromocriptine in long-term use: a review of the literature. *Curr Med Res Opin.* 1986;10:25-51.

154. Stewart PM. Current therapy for acromegaly. *Trends Endocrinol Metab.* 2000;11:128-132.

155. Weil RJ, Vortmeyer AO, Huang S, et al. 11q13 allelic loss in pituitary tumors in patients with multiple endocrine neoplasia syndrome type 1. *Clin Cancer Res.* 1998;4:1673-1678.

156. Thakker RV, Pook MA, Wooding C, et al. Association of somatotrophinomas with loss of alleles on chromosome 11 and with gsp mutations. *J Clin Invest.* 1993;91:2815-2821.

157. Asa SL, Singer W, Kovacs K, et al. Pancreatic endocrine tumour producing growth hormone-releasing hormone associated with multiple endocrine neoplasia type I syndrome. *Acta Endocrinol (Copenh).* 1987; 115:331-337.

158. Sano T, Yamasaki R, Saito H, et al. Growth hormone-releasing hormone (GHRH)-secreting pancreatic tumor in a patient with multiple endocrine neoplasia type I. *Am J Surg Pathol.* 1987;11: 810-819.

159. Thorner MO, Frohman LA, Leong DA, et al. Extrahypothalamic growth-hormone-releasing factor (GRF) secretion is a rare cause of acromegaly: plasma GRF levels in 177 acromegalic patients. *J Clin Endocrinol Metab.* 1984;59:846-849.

160. Oka H, Kameya T, Sato Y, et al. Significance of growth hormone-releasing hormone receptor mRNA in non-neoplastic pituitary and pituitary adenomas: a study by RT-PCR and in situ hybridization. *J Neurooncol.* 1999;41(3):197-204.

161. Newman CB, Melmed S, Snyder PJ, et al. Safety and efficacy of long-term octreotide therapy of acromegaly: results of a multicenter trial in 103 patients: a clinical research center study. *J Clin Endocrinol Metab.* 1995;80:2768-2775.

162. Trainer PJ, Drake WM, Katznelson L, et al. Treatment of acromegaly with the growth hormone-receptor antagonist pegvisomant. *N Engl J Med.* 2000;342:1171-1177.

163. Skogseid B, Larsson C, Lindgren PG, et al. Clinical and genetic features of adrenocortical lesions in multiple endocrine neoplasia type 1. *J Clin Endocrinol Metab.* 1992;75:76-81.

164. Waldmann J, Bartsch DK, Kann PH, et al. Adrenal involvement in multiple endocrine neoplasia type 1: results of 7 years prospective screening. *Langenbecks Arch Surg.* 2007;392:437-443.

165. Houdelette P, Chagnon A, Dumotier J, Marthan E. [Malignant adrenocortical tumor as a part of Wermer's syndrome. Apropos of a case]. *J Chir (Paris).* 1989;126(6-7):385-387.

166. Gatta-Cherifi B, Chabre O, Murat A, et al. Adrenal involvement in MEN1. Analysis of 715 cases from the Groupe d'etude des Tumeurs Endocrines database. *Eur J Endocrinol.* 2012;166:269-279.

167. Simonds WF, Varghese S, Marx SJ, Nieman LK. Cushing's syndrome in multiple endocrine neoplasia type 1. *Clin Endocrinol (Oxf).* 2012;76: 379-386.

168. Abe T, Yoshimoto K, Taniyama M, et al. An unusual kindred of the multiple endocrine neoplasia type 1 (MEN1) in Japanese. *J Clin Endocrinol Metab.* 2000;85:1327-1330.

169. Harpole DH Jr, Feldman JM, Buchanan S, et al. Bronchial carcinoid tumors: a retrospective analysis of 126 patients. *Ann Thorac Surg.* 1992;54:50-54, discussion 54-55.

170. Teh BT, Zedenius J, Kytola S, et al. Thymic carcinoids in multiple endocrine neoplasia type 1. *Ann Surg.* 1998;228:99-105.

171. de Laat JM, Pieterman CR, van den Broek MF, et al. Natural course and survival of neuroendocrine tumors of thymus and lung in MEN1 patients. *J Clin Endocrinol Metab.* 2014;99:3325-3333.

172. Teh BT. Thymic carcinoids in multiple endocrine neoplasia type 1. *J Intern Med.* 1998;243:501-504.

173. Burgess JR, Greenaway TM, Parameswaran V, et al. Enteropancreatic malignancy associated with multiple endocrine neoplasia type 1: risk factors and pathogenesis. *Cancer.* 1998;83:428-434.

174. Gould PM, Bonner JA, Sawyer TE, et al. Bronchial carcinoid tumors: importance of prognostic factors that influence patterns of recurrence and overall survival. *Radiology.* 1998;208:181-185.

175. Musi M, Carbone RG, Bertocchi C, et al. Bronchial carcinoid tumours: a study on clinicopathological features and role of octreotide scintigraphy. *Lung Cancer.* 1998;22:97-102.

176. Norton JA, Melcher ML, Gibril F, Jensen RT. Gastric carcinoid tumors in multiple endocrine neoplasia-1 patients with Zollinger-Ellison syndrome can be symptomatic, demonstrate aggressive growth, and require surgical treatment. *Surgery.* 2004;136:1267-1274.

177. Bordi C, Falchetti A, Azzoni C, et al. Aggressive forms of gastric neuroendocrine tumors in multiple endocrine neoplasia type I. *Am J Surg Pathol.* 1997;21:1075-1082.

178. Anderson RE. A familial instance of appendiceal carcinoid. *Am J Surg.* 1966;111:738-740.

179. Yeatman TJ, Sharp JV, Kimura AK. Can susceptibility to carcinoid tumors be inherited? *Cancer.* 1989;63:390-393.

180. Babovic-Vuksanovic D, Constantinou CL, Rubin J, et al. Familial occurrence of carcinoid tumors and association with other malignant neoplasms. *Cancer Epidemiol Biomarkers Prev.* 1999;8:715-719.

181. Hemminki K, Li X. Familial carcinoid tumors and subsequent cancers: a nation-wide epidemiologic study from Sweden. *Int J Cancer.* 2001; 94:444-448.

182. Oliveira AM, Tazelaar HD, Wentzlaff KA, et al. Familial pulmonary carcinoid tumors. *Cancer.* 2001;91:2104-2109.

182b. Sei Y, Zhao X, Forbes J, et al. A hereditary form of small intestinal carcinoid associated with a germline mutation in inositol polyphosphate multikinase. *Gastroenterology.* 2015;149:67-78.

183. Denes J, Swords F, Rattenberry E, et al. Heterogeneous genetic background of the association of pheochromocytoma/paraganglioma and pituitary adenoma—results from a large patient cohort. *J Clin Endocrinol Metab.* 2015;100(3):E531-E541.

184. Cote G. *The spectrum of mutations in the MEN1 variant syndromes.* Abstract OR43-1. New Orleans, LA: Program and Abstracts of the Endocrine Society; 1998:106.

185. Nord B, Larsson C, Wong FK, et al. Sporadic follicular thyroid tumors show loss of a 200-kb region in 11q13 without evidence for mutations in the MEN1 gene. *Genes Chromosomes Cancer.* 1999;26:35-39.

186. Darling TN, Skarulis MC, Steinberg SM, et al. Multiple facial angiofibromas and collagenomas in patients with multiple endocrine neoplasia type 1. *Arch Dermatol.* 1997;133:853-857.

187. Asgharian B, Turner ML, Gibril F, et al. Cutaneous tumors in patients with multiple endocrine neoplasm type 1 (MEN1) and gastrinomas: prospective study of frequency and development of criteria with high sensitivity and specificity for MEN1. *J Clin Endocrinol Metab.* 2004; 89:5328-5336.

188. Pack S, Turner ML, Zhuang Z, et al. Cutaneous tumors in patients with multiple endocrine neoplasia type 1 show allelic deletion of the MEN1 gene. *J Invest Dermatol.* 1998;110:438-440.

189. Giraud S, Choplin H, Teh BT, et al. A large multiple endocrine neoplasia type 1 family with clinical expression suggestive of anticipation. *J Clin Endocrinol Metab.* 1997;82:3487-3492.

189b. Goudet P, Dalac A, Le Bras M, et al. MEN1 disease occurring before 21 years old: a 160-patient cohort study from the Groupe d'étude des Tumeurs Endocrines. *J Clin Endocrinol Metab.* 2015;100:1568-1577.

190. Nord B, Platz A, Smoczynski K, et al. Malignant melanoma in patients with multiple endocrine neoplasia type 1 and involvement of the MEN1 gene in sporadic melanoma. *Int J Cancer.* 2000;87:463-467.

191. Dackiw AP, Cote GJ, Fleming JB, et al. Screening for MEN1 mutations in patients with atypical endocrine neoplasia. *Surgery.* 1999;126:1097-1103, discussion 1103-1104.

192. Vortmeyer AO, Lubensky IA, Skarulis M, et al. Multiple endocrine neoplasia type 1: atypical presentation, clinical course, and genetic analysis of multiple tumors. *Mod Pathol.* 1999;12:919-924.

193. McKeeby JL, Li X, Zhuang Z, et al. Multiple leiomyomas of the esophagus, lung, and uterus in multiple endocrine neoplasia type 1. *Am J Pathol.* 2001;159:1121-1127.

194. Asgharian B, Chen YJ, Patronas NJ, et al. Meningiomas may be a component tumor of multiple endocrine neoplasia type 1. *Clin Cancer Res.* 2004;10:869-880.

195. Hoffmann KM, Gibril F, Entsuah LK, et al. Patients with multiple endocrine neoplasia type 1 with gastrinomas have an increased risk of severe esophageal disease including stricture and the premalignant condition, Barrett's esophagus. *J Clin Endocrinol Metab.* 2006;91: 204-212.

196. Shepherd JJ. The natural history of multiple endocrine neoplasia type 1. Highly uncommon or highly unrecognized? *Arch Surg.* 1991;126: 935-952.

197. Kontogeorgos G, Kapranos N, Tzavara I, et al. Monosomy of chromosome 11 in pituitary adenoma in a patient with familial multiple endocrine neoplasia type 1. *Clin Endocrinol (Oxf).* 2001;54:117-120.

198. Robert T, Jensen MD. Senior Investigator. Bethesda, Md: National Institute of Diabetes, and Digestive, and Kidney Diseases, National Institutes of Health.

199. Gaitan D, Loosen PT, Orth DN. Two patients with Cushing's disease in a kindred with multiple endocrine neoplasia type I. *J Clin Endocrinol Metab.* 1993;76:1580-1582.

200. Skogseid B, Eriksson B, Lundqvist G, et al. Multiple endocrine neoplasia type 1: a 10-year prospective screening study in four kindreds. *J Clin Endocrinol Metab.* 1991;73:281-287.

201. Lim LC, Tan MH, Eng C, et al. Thymic carcinoid in multiple endocrine neoplasia 1: genotype-phenotype correlation and prevention. *J Intern Med.* 2006;259:428-432.

202. Hao W, Skarulis MC, Simonds WF, et al. Multiple endocrine neoplasia type 1 variant with frequent prolactinoma and rare gastrinoma. *J Clin Endocrinol Metab.* 2004;89:3776-3784.

203. Kassem M, Kruse TA, Wong FK, et al. Familial isolated hyperparathyroidism as a variant of multiple endocrine neoplasia type 1 in a large Danish pedigree. *J Clin Endocrinol Metab.* 2000;85:165-167.

204. Carrasco CA, Gonzalez AA, Carvajal CA, et al. Novel intronic mutation of MEN1 gene causing familial isolated primary hyperparathyroidism. *J Clin Endocrinol Metab.* 2004;89:4124-4129.

205. Simonds WF, James-Newton LA, Agarwal SK, et al. Familial isolated hyperparathyroidism: clinical and genetic characteristics of 36 kindreds. *Medicine (Baltimore).* 2002;81:1-26.

206. Brandi ML, Gagel RF, Angeli A, et al. Guidelines for diagnosis and therapy of MEN type 1 and type 2. *J Clin Endocrinol Metab.* 2001;86: 5658-5671.

207. Ozawa A, Agarwal SK, Mateo CM, et al. The parathyroid/pituitary variant of multiple endocrine neoplasia type 1 usually has causes other than p27Kip1 mutations. *J Clin Endocrinol Metab.* 2007;92:1948-1951.

208. Uchino S, Noguchi S, Sato M, et al. Screening of the MEN1 gene and discovery of germ-line and somatic mutations in apparently sporadic parathyroid tumors. *Cancer Res.* 2000;60:5553-5557.
209. Andersen HO, Jorgensen PE, Bardram L, Hilsted L. Screening for multiple endocrine neoplasia type 1 in patients with recognized pituitary adenoma. *Clin Endocrinol (Oxf).* 1990;33:771-775.
210. Kloppel G, Anlauf M, Raffel A, et al. Adult diffuse nesidioblastosis: genetically or environmentally induced? *Hum Pathol.* 2008;39:3-8.
211. Henopp T, Anlauf M, Schmitt A, et al. Glucagon cell adenomatosis: a newly recognized disease of the endocrine pancreas. *J Clin Endocrinol Metab.* 2009;94:213-217.
212. Marx SJ, Attie MF, Levine MA, et al. The hypocalciuric or benign variant of familial hypercalcemia: clinical and biochemical features in fifteen kindreds. *Medicine (Baltimore).* 1981;60:397-412.
213. Law WM Jr, Heath H 3rd. Familial benign hypercalcemia (hypocalciuric hypercalcemia). Clinical and pathogenetic studies in 21 families. *Ann Intern Med.* 1985;102:511-519.
214. Firek AF, Kao PC, Heath H 3rd. Plasma intact parathyroid hormone (PTH) and PTH-related peptide in familial benign hypercalcemia: greater responsiveness to endogenous PTH than in primary hyperparathyroidism. *J Clin Endocrinol Metab.* 1991;72:541-546.
215. Thorgeirsson U, Costa J, Marx SJ. The parathyroid glands in familial hypocalciuric hypercalcemia. *Hum Pathol.* 1981;12:229-237.
216. Marx SJ. Clinical review 109: contrasting paradigms for hereditary hyperfunction of endocrine cells. *J Clin Endocrinol Metab.* 1999;84:3001-3009.
217. Brown EM, Pollak M, Hebert SC. The extracellular calcium-sensing receptor: its role in health and disease. *Annu Rev Med.* 1998;49:15-29.
218. Warner JV, Nyholt DR, Busfield F, et al. Familial isolated hyperparathyroidism is linked to a 1.7 Mb region on chromosome 2p13.3-14. *J Med Genet.* 2006;43:e12.
219. Warner J, Epstein M, Sweet A, et al. Genetic testing in familial isolated hyperparathyroidism: unexpected results and their implications. *J Med Genet.* 2004;41:155-160.
220. Nesbit MA, Hannan FM, Howles SA, et al. Mutations affecting G-protein subunit alpha11 in hypercalcemia and hypocalcemia. *N Engl J Med.* 2013;368:2476-2486.
221. Nesbit MA, Hannan FM, Howles SA, et al. Mutations in AP2S1 cause familial hypocalciuric hypercalcemia type 3. *Nat Genet.* 2013;45:93-97.
222. Jackson CE, Norum RA, Boyd SB, et al. Hereditary hyperparathyroidism and multiple ossifying jaw fibromas: a clinically and genetically distinct syndrome. *Surgery.* 1990;108:1006-1012, discussion 1012-1013.
223. Teh BT, Farnebo F, Twigg S, et al. Familial isolated hyperparathyroidism maps to the hyperparathyroidism-jaw tumor locus in 1q21-q32 in a subset of families. *J Clin Endocrinol Metab.* 1998;83:2114-2120.
224. Streeten EA, Weinstein LS, Norton JA, et al. Studies in a kindred with parathyroid carcinoma. *J Clin Endocrinol Metab.* 1992;75:362-366.
225. Shattuck TM, Valimaki S, Obara T, et al. Somatic and germ-line mutations of the HRPT2 gene in sporadic parathyroid carcinoma. *N Engl J Med.* 2003;349:1722-1729.
226. Szabo J, Heath B, Hill VM, et al. Hereditary hyperparathyroidism-jaw tumor syndrome: the endocrine tumor gene HRPT2 maps to chromosome 1q21-q31. *Am J Hum Genet.* 1995;56:944-950.
227. Teh BT, Farnebo F, Kristofferson U, et al. Autosomal dominant primary hyperparathyroidism and jaw tumor syndrome associated with renal hamartomas and cystic kidney disease: linkage to 1q21-q32 and loss of the wild type allele in renal hamartomas. *J Clin Endocrinol Metab.* 1996;81:4204-4211.
228. Bradley KJ, Hobbs MR, Buley ID, et al. Uterine tumours are a phenotypic manifestation of the hyperparathyroidism-jaw tumour syndrome. *J Intern Med.* 2005;257:18-26.
229. Simonds WF, Robbins CM, Agarwal SK, et al. Familial isolated hyperparathyroidism is rarely caused by germline mutation in HRPT2, the gene for the hyperparathyroidism-jaw tumor syndrome. *J Clin Endocrinol Metab.* 2004;89:96-102.
230. Keiser HR, Beaven MA, Doppman J, et al. Sipple's syndrome: medullary thyroid carcinoma, pheochromocytoma, and parathyroid disease. Studies in a large family. NIH conference. *Ann Intern Med.* 1973;78:561-579.
231. Schuffenecker I, Virally-Monod M, Brohet R, et al. Risk and penetrance of primary hyperparathyroidism in multiple endocrine neoplasia type 2A families with mutations at codon 634 of the RET proto-oncogene. Groupe D'etude des Tumeurs a Calcitonine. *J Clin Endocrinol Metab.* 1998;83:487-491.
232. Huang SM, Duh QY, Shaver J, et al. Familial hyperparathyroidism without multiple endocrine neoplasia. *World J Surg.* 1997;21:22-28, discussion 29.
233. Watanabe T, Tsukamoto F, Shimizu T, et al. Familial isolated hyperparathyroidism caused by single adenoma: a distinct entity different from multiple endocrine neoplasia. *Endocr J.* 1998;45:637-646.
234. Daly AF, Jaffrain-Rea ML, Ciccarelli A, et al. Clinical characterization of familial isolated pituitary adenomas. *J Clin Endocrinol Metab.* 2006;91:3316-3323.
235. Trivellin G, Daly AF, Faucz FR, et al. Gigantism and acromegaly due to Xq26 microduplications and GPR101 mutation. *N Engl J Med.* 2014;371:2363-2374.
236. Vierimaa O, Georgitsi M, Lehtonen R, et al. Pituitary adenoma predisposition caused by germline mutations in the AIP gene. *Science.* 2006;312:1228-1230.
237. Welander J, Andreasson A, Juhlin CC, et al. Rare germline mutations identified by targeted next-generation sequencing of susceptibility genes in pheochromocytoma and paraganglioma. *J Clin Endocrinol Metab.* 2014;99:E1352-E1360.
238. Larsson C, Skogseid B, Oberg K, et al. Multiple endocrine neoplasia type 1 gene maps to chromosome 11 and is lost in insulinoma. *Nature.* 1988;332:85-87.
239. Knudson AG Jr. Mutation and cancer: statistical study of retinoblastoma. *Proc Natl Acad Sci U S A.* 1971;68:820-823.
240. Knudson AG. Hereditary cancer: two hits revisited. *J Cancer Res Clin Oncol.* 1996;122:135-140.
241. Chandrasekharappa SC, Guru SC, Manickam P, et al. Positional cloning of the gene for multiple endocrine neoplasia-type 1. *Science.* 1997;276:404-407.
242. Guru SC, Olufemi SE, Manickam P, et al. A 2.8-Mb clone contig of the multiple endocrine neoplasia type 1 (MEN1) region at 11q13. *Genomics.* 1997;42:436-445.
243. Guru SC, Goldsmith PK, Burns AL, et al. Menin, the product of the MEN1 gene, is a nuclear protein. *Proc Natl Acad Sci U S A.* 1998;95:1630-1634.
244. Manickam P, Vogel AM, Agarwal SK, et al. Isolation, characterization, expression and functional analysis of the zebrafish ortholog of MEN1. *Mamm Genome.* 2000;11(6):448-454.
245. Agarwal SK, Guru SC, Heppner C, et al. Menin interacts with the AP1 transcription factor JunD and represses JunD-activated transcription. *Cell.* 1999;96:143-152.
246. Gobl AE, Berg M, Lopez-Egido JR, et al. Menin represses JunD-activated transcription by a histone deacetylase-dependent mechanism. *Biochim Biophys Acta.* 1999;1447:51-56.
247. Knapp JI, Heppner C, Hickman AB, et al. Identification and characterization of JunD missense mutants that lack menin binding. *Oncogene.* 2000;19:4706-4712.
248. Thepot D, Weitzman JB, Barra J, et al. Targeted disruption of the murine junD gene results in multiple defects in male reproductive function. *Development.* 2000;127:143-153.
249. Agarwal S. MEN1 gene: mutation and pathophysiology. *Ann d'Endocrinol.* 2006;67(Suppl 4):IS12-IS13.
250. Huang J, Gurung B, Wan B, et al. The same pocket in menin binds both MLL and JUND but has opposite effects on transcription. *Nature.* 2012;482:542-546.
251. Cavallari I, Silic-Benussi M, Rende F, et al. Decreased expression and promoter methylation of the menin tumor suppressor in pancreatic ductal adenocarcinoma. *Genes Chromosomes Cancer.* 2009;48(5):383-396.
252. Carling T, Correa P, Hessman O, et al. Parathyroid MEN1 gene mutations in relation to clinical characteristics of nonfamilial primary hyperparathyroidism. *J Clin Endocrinol Metab.* 1998;83:2960-2963.
253. Farnebo F, Kytola S, Teh BT, et al. Alternative genetic pathways in parathyroid tumorigenesis. *J Clin Endocrinol Metab.* 1999;84:3775-3780.
254. Farnebo F, Teh BT, Kytola S, et al. Alterations of the MEN1 gene in sporadic parathyroid tumors. *J Clin Endocrinol Metab.* 1998;83:2627-2630.
255. Heppner C, Kester MB, Agarwal SK, et al. Somatic mutation of the MEN1 gene in parathyroid tumours. *Nat Genet.* 1997;16:375-378.
256. Cromer MK, Starker LF, Choi M, et al. Identification of somatic mutations in parathyroid tumors using whole-exome sequencing. *J Clin Endocrinol Metab.* 2012;97:E1774-E1781.
257. Newey PJ, Nesbit MA, Rimmer AJ, et al. Whole-exome sequencing studies of nonhereditary (sporadic) parathyroid adenomas. *J Clin Endocrinol Metab.* 2012;97:E1995-E2005.
258. Gluick T, Yuan Z, Libutti SK, Marx SJ. Mutations in CDKN2C (p18) and CDKN2D (p19) may cause sporadic parathyroid adenoma. *Endocr Relat Cancer.* 2013;20:L27-L29.
259. Arnold A, Soong CP. New role for ZFX in oncogenesis. *Cell Cycle.* 2014;13:3465-3466.
260. Goebel SU, Heppner C, Burns AL, et al. Genotype/phenotype correlation of multiple endocrine neoplasia type 1 gene mutations in sporadic gastrinomas. *J Clin Endocrinol Metab.* 2000;85:116-123.
261. Wang EH, Ebrahimi SA, Wu AY, et al. Mutation of the MENIN gene in sporadic pancreatic endocrine tumors. *Cancer Res.* 1998;58:4417-4420.
262. Zhuang Z, Vortmeyer AO, Pack S, et al. Somatic mutations of the MEN1 tumor suppressor gene in sporadic gastrinomas and insulinomas. *Cancer Res.* 1997;57:4682-4686.
263. Gortz B, Roth J, Krahenmann A, et al. Mutations and allelic deletions of the MEN1 gene are associated with a subset of sporadic endocrine pancreatic and neuroendocrine tumors and not restricted to foregut neoplasms. *Am J Pathol.* 1999;154:429-436.
264. Gortz B, Roth J, Speel EJ, et al. MEN1 gene mutation analysis of sporadic adrenocortical lesions. *Int J Cancer.* 1999;80:373-379.

265. Debelenko LV, Brambilla E, Agarwal SK, et al. Identification of MEN1 gene mutations in sporadic carcinoid tumors of the lung. *Hum Mol Genet.* 1997;6:2285-2290.

266. Assie G, Letouze E, Fassnacht M, et al. Integrated genomic characterization of adrenocortical carcinoma. *Nat Genet.* 2014;46:607-612.

267. Prezant TR, Levine J, Melmed S. Molecular characterization of the MEN1 tumor suppressor gene in sporadic pituitary tumors. *J Clin Endocrinol Metab.* 1998;83:1388-1391.

268. Schmidt MC, Henke RT, Stangl AP, et al. Analysis of the MEN1 gene in sporadic pituitary adenomas. *J Pathol.* 1999;188:168-173.

269. Tanaka C, Kimura T, Yang P, et al. Analysis of loss of heterozygosity on chromosome 11 and infrequent inactivation of the MEN1 gene in sporadic pituitary adenomas. *J Clin Endocrinol Metab.* 1998;83: 2631-2634.

270. Zhuang Z, Ezzat SZ, Vortmeyer AO, et al. Mutations of the MEN1 tumor suppressor gene in pituitary tumors. *Cancer Res.* 1997;57: 5446-5451.

271. Heppner C, Reincke M, Agarwal SK, et al. MEN1 gene analysis in sporadic adrenocortical neoplasms. *J Clin Endocrinol Metab.* 1999; 84:216-219.

272. Tahara H, Imanishi Y, Yamada T, et al. Rare somatic inactivation of the multiple endocrine neoplasia type 1 gene in secondary hyperparathyroidism of uremia. *J Clin Endocrinol Metab.* 2000;85: 4113-4117.

273. Imanishi Y, Palanisamy N, Tahara H, et al. Molecular pathogenetic analysis of parathyroid carcinoma (abstract). *J Bone Miner Res.* 1999;14(Suppl 1):S421.

274. Boni R, Vortmeyer AO, Pack S, et al. Somatic mutations of the MEN1 tumor suppressor gene detected in sporadic angiofibromas. *J Invest Dermatol.* 1998;111:539-540.

275. Debelenko LV, Swalwell JI, Kelley MJ, et al. MEN1 gene mutation analysis of high-grade neuroendocrine lung carcinoma. *Genes Chromosomes Cancer.* 2000;28:58-65.

276. Boni R, Vortmeyer AO, Huang S, et al. Mutation analysis of the MEN1 tumour suppressor gene in malignant melanoma. *Melanoma Res.* 1999;9:249-252.

277. Thieblemont C, Pack S, Sakai A, et al. Allelic loss of 11q13 as detected by MEN1-FISH is not associated with mutation of the MEN1 gene in lymphoid neoplasms. *Leukemia.* 1999;13:85-91.

278. Agarwal SK, Debelenko LV, Kester MB, et al. Analysis of recurrent germline mutations in the MEN1 gene encountered in apparently unrelated families. *Hum Mutat.* 1998;12:75-82.

279. Owens M, Ellard S, Vaidya B. Analysis of gross deletions in the MEN1 gene in patients with multiple endocrine neoplasia type 1. *Clin Endocrinol (Oxf).* 2008;68:350-354.

280. Teh BT, Kytola S, Farnebo F, et al. Mutation analysis of the MEN1 gene in multiple endocrine neoplasia type 1, familial acromegaly and familial isolated hyperparathyroidism. *J Clin Endocrinol Metab.* 1998;83: 2621-2626.

281. Poncin J, Abs R, Velkeniers B, et al. Mutation analysis of the MEN1 gene in Belgian patients with multiple endocrine neoplasia type 1 and related diseases. *Hum Mutat.* 1999;13:54-60.

282. Mutch MG, Dilley WG, Sanjurjo F, et al. Germline mutations in the multiple endocrine neoplasia type 1 gene: evidence for frequent splicing defects. *Hum Mutat.* 1999;13:175-185.

283. Mayer K, Ballhausen W, Rott HD. Mutation screening of the entire coding regions of the TSC1 and the TSC2 gene with the protein truncation test (PTT) identifies frequent splicing defects. *Hum Mutat.* 1999;14:401-411.

284. Olufemi SE, Green JS, Manickam P, et al. Common ancestral mutation in the MEN1 gene is likely responsible for the prolactinoma variant of MEN1 (MEN1Burin) in four kindreds from Newfoundland. *Hum Mutat.* 1998;11:264-269.

285. Thakker RV, Bouloux P, Wooding C, et al. Association of parathyroid tumors in multiple endocrine neoplasia type 1 with loss of alleles on chromosome 11. *N Engl J Med.* 1989;321:218-224.

286. Debelenko LV, Emmert-Buck MR, Zhuang Z, et al. The multiple endocrine neoplasia type I gene locus is involved in the pathogenesis of type II gastric carcinoids. *Gastroenterology.* 1997;113:773-781.

287. Teh BT, McArdle J, Chan SP, et al. Clinicopathologic studies of thymic carcinoids in multiple endocrine neoplasia type 1. *Medicine (Baltimore).* 1997;76:21-29.

288. Farnebo F, Farnebo LO, Nordenstrom J, Larsson C. Allelic loss on chromosome 11 is uncommon in parathyroid glands of patients with hypercalcaemic secondary hyperparathyroidism. *Eur J Surg.* 1997;163: 331-337.

289. Tahara H, Smith AP, Gas RD, et al. Genomic localization of novel candidate tumor suppressor gene loci in human parathyroid adenomas. *Cancer Res.* 1996;56:599-605.

290. Shan L, Nakamura Y, Murakami M, et al. Clonal emergence in uremic parathyroid hyperplasia is not related to MEN1 gene abnormality. *Jpn J Cancer Res.* 1999;90:965-969.

291. Arnold A, Brown MF, Urena P, et al. Monoclonality of parathyroid tumors in chronic renal failure and in primary parathyroid hyperplasia. *J Clin Invest.* 1995;95:2047-2053.

292. Falchetti A, Bale AE, Amorosi A, et al. Progression of uremic hyperparathyroidism involves allelic loss on chromosome 11. *J Clin Endocrinol Metab.* 1993;76:139-144.

293. Tanaka C, Yoshimoto K, Yamada S, et al. Absence of germ-line mutations of the multiple endocrine neoplasia type 1 (MEN1) gene in familial pituitary adenoma in contrast to MEN1 in Japanese. *J Clin Endocrinol Metab.* 1998;83:960-965.

294. Zimering MB, Katsumata N, Sato Y, et al. Increased basic fibroblast growth factor in plasma from multiple endocrine neoplasia type 1: relation to pituitary tumor. *J Clin Endocrinol Metab.* 1993;76: 1182-1187.

295. Vortmeyer AO, Boni R, Pack SD, et al. Perivascular cells harboring multiple endocrine neoplasia type 1 alterations are neoplastic cells in angiofibromas. *Cancer Res.* 1999;59:274-278.

296. Deng G, Lu Y, Zlotnikov G, et al. Loss of heterozygosity in normal tissue adjacent to breast carcinomas. *Science.* 1996;274:2057-2059.

297. Jakobovitz O, Nass D, DeMarco L, et al. Carcinoid tumors frequently display genetic abnormalities involving chromosome 11. *J Clin Endocrinol Metab.* 1996;81:3164-3167.

298. Shen WT, Sturgeon C, Clark OH, et al. Should pheochromocytoma size influence surgical approach? A comparison of 90 malignant and 60 benign pheochromocytomas. *Surgery.* 2004;136:1129-1137.

299. Kytola S, Makinen MJ, Kahkonen M, et al. Comparative genomic hybridization studies in tumours from a patient with multiple endocrine neoplasia type 1. *Eur J Endocrinol.* 1998;139:202-206.

300. Franklin DS, Godfrey VL, O'Brien DA, et al. Functional collaboration between different cyclin-dependent kinase inhibitors suppresses tumor growth with distinct tissue specificity. *Mol Cell Biol.* 2000;20: 6147-6158.

301. Pestell RG, Albanese C, Reutens AT, et al. The cyclins and cyclin-dependent kinase inhibitors in hormonal regulation of proliferation and differentiation. *Endocr Rev.* 1999;20:501-534.

302. Scappaticci S, Fossati GS, Valenti L, et al. A search for double minute chromosomes in cultured lymphocytes from different types of tumors. *Cancer Genet Cytogenet.* 1995;82:50-53.

303. Sakurai A, Katai M, Itakura Y, et al. Premature centromere division in patients with multiple endocrine neoplasia type 1. *Cancer Genet Cytogenet.* 1999;109:138-140.

304. Ikeo Y, Sakurai A, Suzuki R, et al. Proliferation-associated expression of the MEN1 gene as revealed by in situ hybridization: possible role of the menin as a negative regulator of cell proliferation under DNA damage. *Lab Invest.* 2000;80:797-804.

305. Kottemann MC, Bale AE. Characterization of DNA damage-dependent cell cycle checkpoints in a menin-deficient model. *DNA Repair (Amst).* 2009;8:944-952.

306. Agarwal SK, Kester MB, Debelenko LV, et al. Germline mutations of the MEN1 gene in familial multiple endocrine neoplasia type 1 and related states. *Hum Mol Genet.* 1997;6:1169-1175.

307. Teh BT, Esapa CT, Houlston R, et al. A family with isolated hyperparathyroidism segregating a missense MEN1 mutation and showing loss of the wild-type alleles in the parathyroid tumors. *Am J Hum Genet.* 1998;63:1544-1549.

308. Larsson C, Calender A, Grimmond S, et al. Molecular tools for presymptomatic testing in multiple endocrine neoplasia type 1. *J Intern Med.* 1995;238:239-244.

309. Pellegata NS, Quintanilla-Martinez L, Siggelkow H, et al. Germ-line mutations in p27Kip1 cause a multiple endocrine neoplasia syndrome in rats and humans. *Proc Natl Acad Sci U S A.* 2006;103: 15558-15563.

310. Agarwal SK, Mateo CM, Marx SJ. Rare germline mutations in cyclin-dependent kinase inhibitor genes in multiple endocrine neoplasia type 1 and related states. *J Clin Endocrinol Metab.* 2009;94:1826-1834.

311. Milne TA, Hughes CM, Lloyd R, et al. Menin and MLL cooperatively regulate expression of cyclin-dependent kinase inhibitors. *Proc Natl Acad Sci U S A.* 2005;102:749-754.

312. Roijers JF, de Wit MJ, van der Luijt RB, et al. Criteria for mutation analysis in MEN 1-suspected patients: MEN 1 case-finding. *Eur J Clin Invest.* 2000;30:487-492.

313. National Institute of Diabetes and Digestive and Kidney Diseases. Multiple Endocrine Neoplasia Type 1. Available at <http://endocrine.niddk.nih.gov/pubs/men1/men1.aspx>.

314. Lemos MC, Thakker RV. Multiple endocrine neoplasia type 1 (MEN1): analysis of 1336 mutations reported in the first decade following identification of the gene. *Hum Mutat.* 2008;29:22-32.

315. Tham E, Grandell U, Lindgren E, et al. Clinical testing for mutations in the MEN1 gene in Sweden: a report on 200 unrelated cases. *J Clin Endocrinol Metab.* 2007;92:3389-3395.

316. Courseaux A, Grosgeorge J, Gaudray P, et al. Definition of the minimal MEN1 candidate area based on a 5-Mb integrated map of proximal 11q13. *Genomics.* 1996;37:345-353.

317. Giraud S, Zhang CX, Serova-Sinilnikova O, et al. Germ-line mutation analysis in patients with multiple endocrine neoplasia type 1 and related disorders. *Am J Hum Genet.* 1998;63:455-467.

318. Stock JL, Warth MR, Teh BT, et al. A kindred with a variant of multiple endocrine neoplasia type 1 demonstrating frequent expression of pituitary tumors but not linked to the multiple endocrine neoplasia type

1 locus at chromosome region 11q13. *J Clin Endocrinol Metab*. 1997; 82:486-492.

319. Hai N, Aoki N, Shimatsu A, et al. Clinical features of multiple endocrine neoplasia type 1 (MEN1) phenocopy without germline MEN1 gene mutations: analysis of 20 Japanese sporadic cases with MEN1. *Clin Endocrinol (Oxf)*. 2000;52:509-518.

320. Bassett JH, Forbes SA, Pannett AA, et al. Characterization of mutations in patients with multiple endocrine neoplasia type 1. *Am J Hum Genet*. 1998;62:232-244.

321. Waterlot C, Porchet N, Bauters C, et al. Type 1 multiple endocrine neoplasia (MEN1): contribution of genetic analysis to the screening and follow-up of a large French kindred. *Clin Endocrinol (Oxf)*. 1999; 51:101-107.

322. Grayson RH, Halperin JM, Sharma V, et al. Changes in plasma prolactin and catecholamine metabolite levels following acute needle stick in children. *Psychiatry Res*. 1997;69:27-32.

323. Burgess JR, Nord B, David R, et al. Phenotype and phenocopy: the relationship between genotype and clinical phenotype in a single large family with multiple endocrine neoplasia type 1 (MEN 1). *Clin Endocrinol (Oxf)*. 2000;53:205-211.

324. Goncalves TD, Toledo RA, Sekiya T, et al. Penetrance of functioning and nonfunctioning pancreatic neuroendocrine tumors in multiple endocrine neoplasia type 1 in the second decade of life. *J Clin Endocrinol Metab*. 2014;99:E89-E96.

325. Oberg K, Skogseid B. The ultimate biochemical diagnosis of endocrine pancreatic tumours in MEN-1. *J Intern Med*. 1998;243:471-476.

326. Hazard JB, Hawk WA, Crile G Jr. Medullary (solid) carcinoma of the thyroid; a clinicopathologic entity. *J Clin Endocrinol Metab*. 1959; 19(1):152-161.

327. Williams ED. Histogenesis of medullary carcinoma of the thyroid. *J Clin Pathol*. 1966;19:114-118.

328. Copp DH, Cheney B. Calcitonin-a hormone from the parathyroid which lowers the calcium-level of the blood. *Nature*. 1962;193: 381-382.

329. Hirsch PF, Gauthier GF, Munson PL. Thyroid hypocalcemic principle and recurrent laryngeal nerve injury as factors affecting the response to parathyroidectomy in rats. *Endocrinology*. 1963;73:244-252.

330. Tashjian AH Jr, Melvin EW. Medullary carcinoma of the thyroid gland. Studies of thyrocalcitonin in plasma and tumor extracts. *N Engl J Med*. 1968;279(6):279-283.

331. Wells SA Jr, Baylin SB, Linehan WM, et al. Provocative agents and the diagnosis of medullary carcinoma of the thyroid gland. *Ann Surg*. 1978;188:139-141.

332. Schimke RN, Hartmann WH, Prout TE, Rimoin DL. Syndrome of bilateral pheochromocytoma, medullary thyroid carcinoma and multiple neuromas. A possible regulatory defect in the differentiation of chromaffin tissue. *N Engl J Med*. 1968;279:1-7.

333. Farndon JR, Leight GS, Dilley WG, et al. Familial medullary thyroid carcinoma without associated endocrinopathies: a distinct clinical entity. *Br J Surg*. 1986;73:278-281.

334. Kloos RT, Eng C, Evans DB, et al. Medullary thyroid cancer: management guidelines of the American Thyroid Association. *Thyroid*. 2009;19:565-612.

335. Chen H, Sippel RS, O'Dorisio MS, et al. The North American Neuroendocrine Tumor Society consensus guideline for the diagnosis and management of neuroendocrine tumors: pheochromocytoma, paraganglioma, and medullary thyroid cancer. *Pancreas*. 2010;39: 775-783.

336. Tuttle RM, Ball DW, Byrd D, et al. Medullary carcinoma. *J Natl Compr Canc Netw*. 2010;8(5):512-530.

337. Boccia LM, Green JS, Joyce C, et al. Mutation of RET codon 768 is associated with the FMTC phenotype. *Clin Genet*. 1997;51:81-85.

338. Siggelkow H, Melzer A, Nolte W, et al. Presentation of a kindred with familial medullary thyroid carcinoma and Cys611Phe mutation of the RET proto-oncogene demonstrating low grade malignancy. *Eur J Endocrinol*. 2001;144:467-473.

339. Jimenez C, Dang GT, Schultz PN, et al. A novel point mutation of the RET protooncogene involving the second intracellular tyrosine kinase domain in a family with medullary thyroid carcinoma. *J Clin Endocrinol Metab*. 2004;89:3521-3526.

340. Takahashi M, Ritz J, Cooper GM. Activation of a novel human transforming gene, ret, by DNA rearrangement. *Cell*. 1985;42:581-588.

341. Pachnis V, Mankoo B, Costantini F. Expression of the c-ret proto-oncogene during mouse embryogenesis. *Development*. 1993;119: 1005-1017.

342. Hahn M, Bishop J. Expression pattern of *Drosophila* RET suggests a common ancestral origin between the metamorphosis precursors in insect endoderm and the vertebrate enteric neurons. *Proc Natl Acad Sci U S A*. 2001;98:1053-1058.

343. Carter MT, Yome JL, Marcil MN, et al. Conservation of RET proto-oncogene splicing variants and implications for RET isoform function. *Cytogenet Cell Genet*. 2001;95:169-176.

344. Myers SM, Eng C, Ponder BA, Mulligan LM. Characterization of RET proto-oncogene 3' splicing variants and polyadenylation sites: a novel C-terminus for RET. *Oncogene*. 1995;11:2039-2045.

345. Borrello MG, Mercalli E, Perego C, et al. Differential interaction of enigma protein with the two RET isoforms. *Biochem Biophys Res Commun*. 2002;296:515-522.

346. Tsui-Pierchala BA, Ahrens RC, Crowder RJ, et al. The long and short isoforms of Ret function as independent signaling complexes. *J Biol Chem*. 2002;277:34618-34625.

347. Lin LF, Doherty DH, Lile JD, et al. GDNF: a glial cell line-derived neurotrophic factor for midbrain dopaminergic neurons. *Science*. 1993; 260:1130-1132.

348. Kotzbauer PT, Lampe PA, Heuckeroth RO, et al. Neurturin, a relative of glial-cell-line-derived neurotrophic factor. *Nature*. 1996;384:467-470.

349. Baloh RH, Tansey MG, Lampe PA, et al. Artemin, a novel member of the GDNF ligand family, supports peripheral and central neurons and signals through the GFRalpha3-RET receptor complex. *Neuron*. 1998;21(6):1291-1302.

350. Milbrandt J, de Sauvage FJ, Fahrner TJ, et al. Persephin, a novel neurotrophic factor related to GDNF and neurturin. *Neuron*. 1998;20: 245-253.

351. Airaksinen MS, Titievsky A, Saarma M. GDNF family neurotrophic factor signaling: four masters, one servant? *Mol Cell Neurosci*. 1999;13: 313-325.

352. Arighi E, Borrello MG, Sariola H. RET tyrosine kinase signaling in development and cancer. *Cytokine Growth Factor Rev*. 2005;16(4-5): 441-467.

353. Santoro M, Rosati R, Grieco M, et al. The ret proto-oncogene is consistently expressed in human pheochromocytomas and thyroid medullary carcinomas. *Oncogene*. 1990;5:1595-1598.

354. Pausova Z, Soliman E, Amizuka N, et al. Role of the RET proto-oncogene in sporadic hyperparathyroidism and in hyperparathyroidism of multiple endocrine neoplasia type 2. *J Clin Endocrinol Metab*. 1996;81:2711-2718.

355. Tsuzuki T, Takahashi M, Asai N, et al. Spatial and temporal expression of the ret proto-oncogene product in embryonic, infant and adult rat tissues. *Oncogene*. 1995;10:191-198.

356. Schuchardt A, D'Agati V, Larsson-Blomberg L, et al. Defects in the kidney and enteric nervous system of mice lacking the tyrosine kinase receptor Ret. *Nature*. 1994;367:380-383.

357. Manie S, Santoro M, Fusco A, Billaud M. The RET receptor: function in development and dysfunction in congenital malformation. *Trends Genet*. 2001;17:580-589.

358. Mathew CG, Chin KS, Easton DF, et al. A linked genetic marker for multiple endocrine neoplasia type 2A on chromosome 10. *Nature*. 1987;328:527-528.

359. Simpson NE, Kidd KK, Goodfellow PJ, et al. Assignment of multiple endocrine neoplasia type 2A to chromosome 10 by linkage. *Nature*. 1987;328:528-530.

360. Donis-Keller H, Dou S, Chi D, et al. Mutations in the RET proto-oncogene are associated with MEN 2A and FMTC. *Hum Mol Genet*. 1993;2:851-856.

361. Mulligan LM, Eng C, Healey CS, et al. Specific mutations of the RET proto-oncogene are related to disease phenotype in MEN 2A and FMTC. *Nat Genet*. 1994;6:70-74.

362. Carlson KM, Dou S, Chi D, et al. Single missense mutation in the tyrosine kinase catalytic domain of the RET protooncogene is associated with multiple endocrine neoplasia type 2B. *Proc Natl Acad Sci U S A*. 1994;91:1579-1583.

363. Hofstra RM, Landsvater RM, Ceccherini I, et al. A mutation in the RET proto-oncogene associated with multiple endocrine neoplasia type 2B and sporadic medullary thyroid carcinoma. *Nature*. 1994;367: 375-376.

364. Eng C, Smith DP, Mulligan LM, et al. Point mutation within the tyrosine kinase domain of the RET proto-oncogene in multiple endocrine neoplasia type 2B and related sporadic tumours. *Hum Mol Genet*. 1994;3:237-241.

365. Marsh DJ, Learoyd DL, Andrew SD, et al. Somatic mutations in the RET proto-oncogene in sporadic medullary thyroid carcinoma. *Clin Endocrinol (Oxf)*. 1996;44:249-257.

366. Moura MM, Cavaco BM, Pinto AE, Leite V. High prevalence of RAS mutations in RET-negative sporadic medullary thyroid carcinomas. *J Clin Endocrinol Metab*. 2011;96:E863-E868.

367. Boichard A, Croux L, Al Ghuzlan A, et al. Somatic RAS mutations occur in a large proportion of sporadic RET-negative medullary thyroid carcinomas and extend to a previously unidentified exon. *J Clin Endocrinol Metab*. 2012;97:E2031-E2035.

368. Ciampi R, Mian C, Fugazzola L, et al. Evidence of a low prevalence of RAS mutations in a large medullary thyroid cancer series. *Thyroid*. 2013;23:50-57.

369. The Human Gene Mutation Database at the Institute of Medical Genetics in Cardiff, UK. Available at <http://www.hgmd.org/>.

370. National Center for Biotechnology Information. Online Mendelian Inheritance in Man. Available at <http://www.ncbi.nlm.nih.gov/omim>.

371. AURP Laboratories website. Available at >http://www.arup.utah.edu/database.MEN2/MEN2_welcome.php>.

372. Margraf RL, Crockett DK, Krautscheid PM, et al. Multiple endocrine neoplasia type 2 RET protooncogene database: repository of

MEN2-associated RET sequence variation and reference for genotype/phenotype correlations. *Hum Mutat.* 2009;30:548-556.

373. Hoppner W, Ritter MM. A duplication of 12 bp in the critical cysteine rich domain of the RET proto-oncogene results in a distinct phenotype of multiple endocrine neoplasia type 2A. *Hum Mol Genet.* 1997;6: 587-590.

374. Tessitore A, Sinisi AA, Pasquali D, et al. A novel case of multiple endocrine neoplasia type 2A associated with two de novo mutations of the RET protooncogene. *J Clin Endocrinol Metab.* 1999;84:3522-3527.

375. Miyauchi A, Futami H, Hai N, et al. Two germline missense mutations at codons 804 and 806 of the RET proto-oncogene in the same allele in a patient with multiple endocrine neoplasia type 2B without codon 918 mutation. *Jpn J Cancer Res.* 1999;90:1-5.

376. Menko FH, van der Luijt RB, de Valk IA, et al. Atypical MEN type 2B associated with two germline RET mutations on the same allele not involving codon 918. *J Clin Endocrinol Metab.* 2002;87:393-397.

377. Yamaguchi R, Hirano T, Ootsuyama Y, et al. Increased 8-hydroxyguanine in DNA and its repair activity in hamster and rat lung after intratracheal instillation of crocidolite asbestos. *Jpn J Cancer Res.* 1999;90: 505-509.

378. Nakao KT, Usui T, Ikeda M, et al. Novel tandem germline RET proto-oncogene mutations in a patient with multiple endocrine neoplasia type 2B: report of a case and a literature review of tandem RET mutations with in silico analysis. *Head Neck.* 2013;35:E363-E368.

379. Santoro M, Melillo RM, Fusco A. RET/PTC activation in papillary thyroid carcinoma: European Journal of Endocrinology Prize Lecture. *Eur J Endocrinol.* 2006;155:645-653.

380. Kohno T, Ichikawa H, Totoki Y, et al. KIF5B-RET fusions in lung adenocarcinoma. *Nat Med.* 2012;18:375-377.

381. Ballerini P, Struski S, Cresson C, et al. RET fusion genes are associated with chronic myelomonocytic leukemia and enhance monocytic differentiation. *Leukemia.* 2012;26:2384-2389.

382. Attie T, Pelet A, Edery P, et al. Diversity of RET proto-oncogene mutations in familial and sporadic Hirschsprung disease. *Hum Mol Genet.* 1995;4:1381-1386.

383. Amiel J, Sproat-Emison E, Garcia-Barcelo M, et al. Hirschsprung disease, associated syndromes and genetics: a review. *J Med Genet.* 2008;45:1-14.

384. Guyetant S, Rousselet MC, Durigon M, et al. Sex-related C cell hyperplasia in the normal human thyroid: a quantitative autopsy study. *J Clin Endocrinol Metab.* 1997;82:42-47.

385. Khurana R, Agarwal A, Bajpai VK, et al. Unraveling the amyloid associated with human medullary thyroid carcinoma. *Endocrinology.* 2004; 145:5465-5470.

386. Mendelsohn G, Wells SA Jr, Baylin SB. Relationship of tissue carcinoembryonic antigen and calcitonin to tumor virulence in medullary thyroid carcinoma. An immunohistochemical study in early, localized, and virulent disseminated stages of disease. *Cancer.* 1984;54:657-662.

387. Zedenius J, Wallin G, Hamberger B, et al. Somatic and MEN 2A de novo mutations identified in the RET proto-oncogene by screening of sporadic MTC:s. *Hum Mol Genet.* 1994;3:1259-1262.

388. Elisei R, Cosci B, Romei C, et al. Prognostic significance of somatic RET oncogene mutations in sporadic medullary thyroid cancer: a 10-year follow-up study. *J Clin Endocrinol Metab.* 2008;93:682-687.

389. Kebebew E, Ituarte PH, Siperstein AE, et al. Medullary thyroid carcinoma: clinical characteristics, treatment, prognostic factors, and a comparison of staging systems. *Cancer.* 2000;88:1139-1148.

390. Modigliani E, Cohen R, Campos JM, et al. Prognostic factors for survival and for biochemical cure in medullary thyroid carcinoma: results in 899 patients. The GETC Study Group. Groupe d'etude des tumeurs a calcitonine. *Clin Endocrinol (Oxf).* 1998;48:265-273.

391. Imai T, Uchino S, Okamoto T, et al. High penetrance of pheochromocytoma in multiple endocrine neoplasia 2 caused by germ line RET codon 634 mutation in Japanese patients. *Eur J Endocrinol.* 2013;168: 683-687.

392. Frank-Raue K, Rybicki LA, Erlic Z, et al. Risk profiles and penetrance estimations in multiple endocrine neoplasia type 2A caused by germline RET mutations located in exon 10. *Hum Mutat.* 2011;32:51-58.

393. Lips CJ, Landsvater RM, Hoppener JW, et al. Clinical screening as compared with DNA analysis in families with multiple endocrine neoplasia type 2A. *N Engl J Med.* 1994;331:828-835.

394. Herfarth KK, Bartsch D, Doherty GM, et al. Surgical management of hyperparathyroidism in patients with multiple endocrine neoplasia type 2A. *Surgery.* 1996;120:966-973, discussion 973-974.

395. Nunziata V, Giannattasio R, Di Giovanni G, et al. Hereditary localized pruritus in affected members of a kindred with multiple endocrine neoplasia type 2A (Sipple's syndrome). *Clin Endocrinol (Oxf).* 1989;30: 57-63.

396. Verga U, Fugazzola L, Cambiaghi S, et al. Frequent association between MEN 2A and cutaneous lichen amyloidosis. *Clin Endocrinol (Oxf).* 2003;59:156-161.

397. Ceccherini I, Romei C, Barone V, et al. Identification of the Cys634 → Tyr mutation of the RET proto-oncogene in a pedigree with multiple endocrine neoplasia type 2A and localized cutaneous lichen amyloidosis. *J Endocrinol Invest.* 1994;17(3):201-204.

398. Rothberg AE, Raymond VM, Gruber SB, Sisson J. Familial medullary thyroid carcinoma associated with cutaneous lichen amyloidosis. *Thyroid.* 2009;19:651-655.

399. Hofstra RM, Sijmons RH, Stelwagen T, et al. RET mutation screening in familial cutaneous lichen amyloidosis and in skin amyloidosis associated with multiple endocrine neoplasia. *J Invest Dermatol.* 1996;107: 215-218.

400. Romeo G, Ronchetto P, Luo Y, et al. Point mutations affecting the tyrosine kinase domain of the RET proto-oncogene in Hirschsprung's disease. *Nature.* 1994;367:377-378.

401. Edery P, Lyonnet S, Mulligan LM, et al. Mutations of the RET proto-oncogene in Hirschsprung's disease. *Nature.* 1994;367:378-380.

402. Mulligan LM, Eng C, Attie T, et al. Diverse phenotypes associated with exon 10 mutations of the RET proto-oncogene. *Hum Mol Genet.* 1994; 3:2163-2167.

403. Sijmons RH, Hofstra RM, Wijburg FA, et al. Oncological implications of RET gene mutations in Hirschsprung's disease. *Gut.* 1998;43: 542-547.

404. Asai N, Jijiwa M, Enomoto A, et al. RET receptor signaling: dysfunction in thyroid cancer and Hirschsprung's disease. *Pathol Int.* 2006;56: 164-172.

405. Chappuis-Flament S, Pasini A, De Vita G, et al. Dual effect on the RET receptor of MEN 2 mutations affecting specific extracytoplasmic cysteines. *Oncogene.* 1998;17:2851-2861.

406. Smith DP, Houghton C, Ponder BA. Germline mutation of RET codon 883 in two cases of de novo MEN 2B. *Oncogene.* 1997;15:1213-1217.

407. Jasim S, Ying AK, Waguespack SG, et al. Multiple endocrine neoplasia type 2B with a RET proto-oncogene A883F mutation displays a more indolent form of medullary thyroid carcinoma compared with a RET M918T mutation. *Thyroid.* 2011;21:189-192.

408. Cohen MS, Phay JE, Albinson C, et al. Gastrointestinal manifestations of multiple endocrine neoplasia type 2. *Ann Surg.* 2002;235:648-654, discussion 654-655.

409. Waguespack SG, Rich TA, Perrier ND, et al. Management of medullary thyroid carcinoma and MEN2 syndromes in childhood. *Nat Rev Endocrinol.* 2011;7:596-607.

410. Carlson KM, Bracamontes J, Jackson CE, et al. Parent-of-origin effects in multiple endocrine neoplasia type 2B. *Am J Hum Genet.* 1994;55: 1076-1082.

411. Schuffenecker I, Ginet N, Goldgar D, et al. Prevalence and parental origin of de novo RET mutations in multiple endocrine neoplasia type 2A and familial medullary thyroid carcinoma. Le Groupe d'Etude des Tumeurs a Calcitonine. *Am J Hum Genet.* 1997;60:233-237.

412. Lorenz K, Elwerr M, Machens A, et al. Hypercalcitoninemia in thyroid conditions other than medullary thyroid carcinoma: a comparative analysis of calcium and pentagastrin stimulation of serum calcitonin. *Langenbecks Arch Surg.* 2013;398:403-409.

413. Becker KL, Nylen ES, White JC, et al. Clinical review 167: procalcitonin and the calcitonin gene family of peptides in inflammation, infection, and sepsis: a journey from calcitonin back to its precursors. *J Clin Endocrinol Metab.* 2004;89:1512-1525.

414. Whang KT, Steinwald PM, White JC, et al. Serum calcitonin precursors in sepsis and systemic inflammation. *J Clin Endocrinol Metab.* 1998; 83:3296-3301.

415. Borchhardt KA, Horl WH, Sunder-Plassmann G. Reversibility of "secondary hypercalcitoninemia" after kidney transplantation. *Am J Transplant.* 2005;5:1757-1763.

416. Bevilacqua M, Dominguez LJ, Righini V, et al. Dissimilar PTH, gastrin, and calcitonin responses to oral calcium and peptones in hypocalciuric hypercalcemia, primary hyperparathyroidism, and normal subjects: a useful tool for differential diagnosis. *J Bone Miner Res.* 2006;21: 406-412.

417. Schuetz M, Duan H, Wahl K, et al. T lymphocyte cytokine production patterns in Hashimoto patients with elevated calcitonin levels and their relationship to tumor initiation. *Anticancer Res.* 2006;26: 4591-4596.

418. Pratz KW, Ma C, Aubry MC, et al. Large cell carcinoma with calcitonin and vasoactive intestinal polypeptide-associated Verner-Morrison syndrome. *Mayo Clin Proc.* 2005;80:116-120.

419. Sim SJ, Glassman AB, Ro JY, et al. Serum calcitonin in small cell carcinoma of the prostate. *Ann Clin Lab Sci.* 1996;26:487-495.

420. Machens A, Haedecke J, Holzhausen HJ, et al. Differential diagnosis of calcitonin-secreting neuroendocrine carcinoma of the foregut by pentagastrin stimulation. *Langenbecks Arch Surg.* 2000;385:398-401.

421. Toledo SP, Lourenco DM Jr, Santos MA, et al. Hypercalcitoninemia is not pathognomonic of medullary thyroid carcinoma. *Clinics (Sao Paulo).* 2009;64:699-706.

422. Preissner CM, Dodge LA, O'Kane DJ, et al. Prevalence of heterophilic antibody interference in eight automated tumor marker immunoassays. *Clin Chem.* 2005;51:208-210.

423. Frank-Raue K, Machens A, Leidig-Bruckner G, et al. Prevalence and clinical spectrum of nonsecretory medullary thyroid carcinoma in a series of 839 patients with sporadic medullary thyroid carcinoma. *Thyroid.* 2013;23:294-300.

424. Chang TC, Wu SL, Hsiao YL. Medullary thyroid carcinoma: pitfalls in diagnosis by fine needle aspiration cytology and relationship of

cytomorphology to RET proto-oncogene mutations. *Acta Cytol.* 2005; 49:477-482.

425. Papaparaskeva K, Nagel H, Droese M. Cytologic diagnosis of medullary carcinoma of the thyroid gland. *Diagn Cytopathol.* 2000;22:351-358.

426. Machens A, Dralle H. Biological relevance of medullary thyroid microcarcinoma. *J Clin Endocrinol Metab.* 2012;97:1547-1553.

427. Elisei R, Bottici V, Luchetti F, et al. Impact of routine measurement of serum calcitonin on the diagnosis and outcome of medullary thyroid cancer: experience in 10,864 patients with nodular thyroid disorders. *J Clin Endocrinol Metab.* 2004;89:163-168.

428. Costante G, Meringolo D, Durante C, et al. Predictive value of serum calcitonin levels for preoperative diagnosis of medullary thyroid carcinoma in a cohort of 5817 consecutive patients with thyroid nodules. *J Clin Endocrinol Metab.* 2007;92:450-455.

429. Daniels GH. Screening for medullary thyroid carcinoma with serum calcitonin measurements in patients with thyroid nodules in the United States and Canada. *Thyroid.* 2011;21:1199-1207.

430. Cheung K, Roman SA, Wang TS, et al. Calcitonin measurement in the evaluation of thyroid nodules in the United States: a cost-effectiveness and decision analysis. *J Clin Endocrinol Metab.* 2008;93:2173-2180.

431. Romei C, Cosci B, Renzini G, et al. RET genetic screening of sporadic medullary thyroid cancer (MTC) allows the preclinical diagnosis of unsuspected gene carriers and the identification of a relevant percentage of hidden familial MTC (FMTC). *Clin Endocrinol (Oxf).* 2011;74: 241-247.

432. Elisei R, Romei C, Cosci B, et al. RET genetic screening in patients with medullary thyroid cancer and their relatives: experience with 807 individuals at one center. *J Clin Endocrinol Metab.* 2007;92:4725-4729.

433. Gene Tests: Medical Genetics Information Resource database online, 2012. Available at <http://www.genetest.org>.

434. Cerutti JM, Maciel RM. An unusual genotype-phenotype correlation in MEN 2 patients: should screening for RET double germline mutations be performed to avoid misleading diagnosis and treatment? *Clin Endocrinol (Oxf).* 2013;79:591-592.

435. Valente FO, Dias da Silva MR, Camacho CP, et al. Comprehensive analysis of RET gene should be performed in patients with multiple endocrine neoplasia type 2 (MEN 2) syndrome and no apparent genotype-phenotype correlation: an appraisal of p.Y791F and p.C634Y RET mutations in five unrelated Brazilian families. *J Endocrinol Invest.* 2013;36:975-981.

436. Rosenthal MS, Diekema DS. Pediatric ethics guidelines for hereditary medullary thyroid cancer. *Int J Pediatr Endocrinol.* 2011;2011:847603.

437. Committee on Bioethics, American Academy of Pediatrics. Informed consent, parental permission, and assent in pediatric practice. *Pediatrics.* 1995;95(2):314-317.

438. Martinelli P, Maruotti GM, Pasquali D, et al. Genetic prenatal RET testing and pregnancy management of multiple endocrine neoplasia type II A (MEN2A): a case report. *J Endocrinol Invest.* 2004;27:357-360.

439. Offit K, Kohut K, Clagett B, et al. Cancer genetic testing and assisted reproduction. *J Clin Oncol.* 2006;24:4775-4782.

440. Offit K, Sagi M, Hurley K. Preimplantation genetic diagnosis for cancer syndromes: a new challenge for preventive medicine. *JAMA.* 2006;296: 2727-2730.

441. Macher HC, Martinez-Broca MA, Rubio-Calvo A, et al. Non-invasive prenatal diagnosis of multiple endocrine neoplasia type 2A using COLD-PCR combined with HRM genotyping analysis from maternal serum. *PLoS ONE.* 2012;7:e51024.

442. Lietman SA. Preimplantation genetic diagnosis for hereditary endocrine disease. *Endocr Pract.* 2011;17(Suppl 3):28-32.

443. Machens A, Dralle H. Biomarker-based risk stratification for previously untreated medullary thyroid cancer. *J Clin Endocrinol Metab.* 2010; 95:2655-2663.

444. Giraudet AL, Vanel D, Leboulleux S, et al. Imaging medullary thyroid carcinoma with persistent elevated calcitonin levels. *J Clin Endocrinol Metab.* 2007;92:4185-4190.

445. Weber T, Schilling T, Frank-Raue K, et al. Impact of modified radical neck dissection on biochemical cure in medullary thyroid carcinomas. *Surgery.* 2001;130:1044-1049.

446. Moley JF, DeBenedetti MK. Patterns of nodal metastases in palpable medullary thyroid carcinoma: recommendations for extent of node dissection. *Ann Surg.* 1999;229:880-887, discussion 887-888.

447. Machens A, Ukkat J, Hauptmann S, Dralle H. Abnormal carcinoembryonic antigen levels and medullary thyroid cancer progression: a multivariate analysis. *Arch Surg.* 2007;142:289-293, discussion 294.

448. Franc S, Niccoli-Sire P, Cohen R, et al. Complete surgical lymph node resection does not prevent authentic recurrences of medullary thyroid carcinoma. *Clin Endocrinol (Oxf).* 2001;55:403-409.

449. Miyauchi A, Matsuzuka F, Hirai K, et al. Prospective trial of unilateral surgery for nonhereditary medullary thyroid carcinoma in patients without germline RET mutations. *World J Surg.* 2002;26:1023-1028.

450. Roh JL, Kim DH, Park CI. Prospective identification of chyle leakage in patients undergoing lateral neck dissection for metastatic thyroid cancer. *Ann Surg Oncol.* 2008;15:424-429.

451. Sobol S, Jensen C, Sawyer W 2nd, et al. Objective comparison of physical dysfunction after neck dissection. *Am J Surg.* 1985;150(4): 503-509.

452. Olson JA Jr, DeBenedetti MK, Baumann DS, Wells SA Jr. Parathyroid autotransplantation during thyroidectomy. Results of long-term follow-up. *Ann Surg.* 1996;223:472-478, discussion 478-480.

453. Bihan H, Baudin E, Meas T, et al. Role of prophylactic thyroidectomy in RET 790 familial medullary thyroid carcinoma. *Head Neck.* 2012; 34:493-498.

454. Wray CJ, Rich TA, Waguespack SG, et al. Failure to recognize multiple endocrine neoplasia 2B: more common than we think? *Ann Surg Oncol.* 2008;15:293-301.

455. Brauckhoff M, Machens A, Lorenz K, et al. Surgical curability of medullary thyroid cancer in multiple endocrine neoplasia 2B: a changing perspective. *Ann Surg.* 2014;259:800-806.

456. Pomares FJ, Canas R, Rodriguez JM, et al. Differences between sporadic and multiple endocrine neoplasia type 2A phaeochromocytoma. *Clin Endocrinol (Oxf).* 1998;48:195-200.

457. Lairmore TC, Ball DW, Baylin SB, Wells SA Jr. Management of pheochromocytomas in patients with multiple endocrine neoplasia type 2 syndromes. *Ann Surg.* 1993;217(6):595-601, discussion 601-603.

458. Miccoli P, Materazzi G, Brauckhoff M, et al. No outcome differences between a laparoscopic and retroperitoneoscopic approach in synchronous bilateral adrenal surgery. *World J Surg.* 2011;35:2698-2702.

459. Brauckhoff M, Dralle H. [Function-preserving adrenalectomy for adrenal tumors]. *Chirurg.* 2012;83(6):519-527.

460. Machens A, Brauckhoff M, Holzhausen HJ, et al. Codon-specific development of pheochromocytoma in multiple endocrine neoplasia type 2. *J Clin Endocrinol Metab.* 2005;90:3999-4003.

461. Nguyen L, Niccoli-Sire P, Caron P, et al. Pheochromocytoma in multiple endocrine neoplasia type 2: a prospective study. *Eur J Endocrinol.* 2001;144:37-44.

462. Rowland KJ, Chernock RD, Moley JF. Pheochromocytoma in an 8-year-old patient with multiple endocrine neoplasia type 2A: implications for screening. *J Surg Oncol.* 2013;108:203-206.

463. Kraimps JL, Denizot A, Carnaille B, et al. Primary hyperparathyroidism in multiple endocrine neoplasia type IIa: retrospective French multicentric study. Groupe d'Etude des Tumeurs a Calcitonine (GETC, French Calcitonin Tumors Study Group), French Association of Endocrine Surgeons. *World J Surg.* 1996;20:808-812, discussion 812-813.

464. Agarwal A, Waghray A, Gupta S, et al. Cryopreservation of parathyroid tissue: an illustrated technique using the Cleveland Clinic protocol. *J Am Coll Surg.* 2013;216:e1-e9.

465. Peacock M, Bilezikian JP, Klassen PS, et al. Cinacalcet hydrochloride maintains long-term normocalcemia in patients with primary hyperparathyroidism. *J Clin Endocrinol Metab.* 2005;90:135-141.

466. Engelbach M, Gorges R, Forst T, et al. Improved diagnostic methods in the follow-up of medullary thyroid carcinoma by highly specific calcitonin measurements. *J Clin Endocrinol Metab.* 2000;85:1890-1894.

467. Elisei R, Pinchera A. Advances in the follow-up of differentiated or medullary thyroid cancer. *Nat Rev Endocrinol.* 2012;8:466-475.

468. Pellegriti G, Leboulleux S, Baudin E, et al. Long-term outcome of medullary thyroid carcinoma in patients with normal postoperative medical imaging. *Br J Cancer.* 2003;88:1537-1542.

469. Eisenhauer EA, Therasse P, Bogaerts J, et al. New response evaluation criteria in solid tumours: revised RECIST guideline (version 1.1). *Eur J Cancer.* 2009;45:228-247.

470. Barbet J, Campion L, Kraeber-Bodere F, Chatal JF. Prognostic impact of serum calcitonin and carcinoembryonic antigen doubling-times in patients with medullary thyroid carcinoma. *J Clin Endocrinol Metab.* 2005;90:6077-6084.

471. Giraudet AL, Al Ghulzan A, Auperin A, et al. Progression of medullary thyroid carcinoma: assessment with calcitonin and carcinoembryonic antigen doubling times. *Eur J Endocrinol.* 2008;158(2):239-246.

472. Fialkowski E, DeBenedetti M, Moley J. Long-term outcome of re-operations for medullary thyroid carcinoma. *World J Surg.* 2008;32: 754-765.

473. Tung WS, Vesely TM, Moley JF. Laparoscopic detection of hepatic metastases in patients with residual or recurrent medullary thyroid cancer. *Surgery.* 1995;118:1024-1029, discussion 1029-1030.

474. Meijer JA, Bakker LE, Valk GD, et al. Radioactive iodine in the treatment of medullary thyroid carcinoma: a controlled multicenter study. *Eur J Endocrinol.* 2013;168:779-786.

475. Martinez SR, Beal SH, Chen A, et al. Adjuvant external beam radiation for medullary thyroid carcinoma. *J Surg Oncol.* 2010;102:175-178.

476. Fife KM, Bower M, Harmer CL. Medullary thyroid cancer: the role of radiotherapy in local control. *Eur J Surg Oncol.* 1996;22:588-591.

477. Machens A, Schneyer U, Holzhausen HJ, Dralle H. Prospects of remission in medullary thyroid carcinoma according to basal calcitonin level. *J Clin Endocrinol Metab.* 2005;90:2029-2034.

478. Wexler JA. Approach to the thyroid cancer patient with bone metastases. *J Clin Endocrinol Metab.* 2011;96:2296-2307.

479. Quan GM, Pointillart V, Palussiere J, Bonichon F. Multidisciplinary treatment and survival of patients with vertebral metastases from thyroid carcinoma. *Thyroid.* 2012;22:125-130.

480. Santarpia L, El-Naggar AK, Sherman SI, et al. Four patients with cutaneous metastases from medullary thyroid cancer. *Thyroid.* 2008;18: 901-905.

481. Baudry C, Paepegaey AC, Groussin L. Reversal of Cushing's syndrome by vandetanib in medullary thyroid carcinoma. *N Engl J Med.* 2013;369:584-586.
482. Fox E, Widemann BC, Chuk MK, et al. Vandetanib in children and adolescents with multiple endocrine neoplasia type 2B associated medullary thyroid carcinoma. *Clin Cancer Res.* 2013;19:4239-4248.
483. Bajetta E, Rimassa L, Carnaghi C, et al. 5-Fluorouracil, dacarbazine, and epirubicin in the treatment of patients with neuroendocrine tumors. *Cancer.* 1998;83:372-378.
484. Orlandi F, Caraci P, Berruti A, et al. Chemotherapy with dacarbazine and 5-fluorouracil in advanced medullary thyroid cancer. *Ann Oncol.* 1994;5:763-765.
485. Druker BJ, Guilhot F, O'Brien SG, et al. Five-year follow-up of patients receiving imatinib for chronic myeloid leukemia. *N Engl J Med.* 2006;355:2408-2417.
486. Cohen EE, Rosen LS, Vokes EE, et al. Axitinib is an active treatment for all histologic subtypes of advanced thyroid cancer: results from a phase II study. *J Clin Oncol.* 2008;26:4708-4713.
487. de Groot JW, Zonnenberg BA, van Ufford-Mannesse PQ, et al. A phase II trial of imatinib therapy for metastatic medullary thyroid carcinoma. *J Clin Endocrinol Metab.* 2007;92:3466-3469.
488. Elisei R, Schlumberger MJ, Muller SP, et al. Cabozantinib in progressive medullary thyroid cancer. *J Clin Oncol.* 2013;31:3639-3646.
489. Frank-Raue K, Fabel M, Delorme S, et al. Efficacy of imatinib mesylate in advanced medullary thyroid carcinoma. *Eur J Endocrinol.* 2007;157:215-220.
490. Kurzrock R, Sherman SI, Ball DW, et al. Activity of XL184 (cabozantinib), an oral tyrosine kinase inhibitor, in patients with medullary thyroid cancer. *J Clin Oncol.* 2011;29:2660-2666.
491. Lam ET, Ringel MD, Kloos RT, et al. Phase II clinical trial of sorafenib in metastatic medullary thyroid cancer. *J Clin Oncol.* 2010;28:2323-2330.
492. Nguyen CT, Fu AZ, Gilligan TD, et al. Defining the optimal treatment for clinical stage I nonseminomatous germ cell testicular cancer using decision analysis. *J Clin Oncol.* 2010;28:119-125.
493. Pennell NA, Daniels GH, Haddad RI, et al. A phase II study of gefitinib in patients with advanced thyroid cancer. *Thyroid.* 2008;18:317-323.
494. Robinson BG, Paz-Ares L, Krebs A, et al. Vandetanib (100 mg) in patients with locally advanced or metastatic hereditary medullary thyroid cancer. *J Clin Endocrinol Metab.* 2010;95:2664-2671.
495. Wells SA Jr, Gosnell JE, Gagel RF, et al. Vandetanib for the treatment of patients with locally advanced or metastatic hereditary medullary thyroid cancer. *J Clin Oncol.* 2010;28:767-772.
496. Wells SA Jr, Robinson BG, Gagel RF, et al. Vandetanib in patients with locally advanced or metastatic medullary thyroid cancer: a randomized, double-blind phase III trial. *J Clin Oncol.* 2012;30:134-141.

CHAPTER 40

The Immunoendocrinopathy Syndromes

JENNIFER M. BARKER • MARK S. ANDERSON • PETER A. GOTTLIEB

KEY POINTS

- Endocrine diseases may occur together, and understanding of these associations can lead to earlier diagnosis of additional disorders.
- Many autoimmune endocrine diseases have genetic risk at overlapping genetic loci, explaining, in part, their concurrence in individuals.
- Elucidation of the causes of these rare disorders has led to fundamental insights into the functioning of the immune system in autoimmunity.
- Studies of these disorders have uncovered the genetic basis for these rare syndromes and have helped to define important immune pathways.
- The search for means to define endocrine autoimmunity and disease states has led to the development of new assays that have become the cornerstone of endocrine autoimmune testing.
- Recommended testing for these related disorders is discussed in this chapter.

Since Addison's initial description of primary adrenal insufficiency in a patient with two autoimmune disorders (vitiligo and the hyperpigmentation of Addison disease), the immunoendocrinopathy syndromes have contributed to the understanding of both endocrinology and immunology (Fig. 40-1). Understanding the pathogenesis of the polyendocrine syndromes continues to expand. In particular, shared genetic loci underlying disease susceptibility, potential environmental factors, and organ-specific autoantigens targeted by the immune system are being defined. Recent advances include the development of more reliable T-cell and other immunologic assays, further refinement in predictive models of disease, and continued unraveling of the genetic factors underlying disease susceptibility.

Most autoimmune endocrine disorders (e.g., type 1 diabetes, autoimmune thyroid disease) occur in isolation. Two distinct autoimmune polyendocrine syndromes with characteristic groupings of manifestations are readily recognized. *Autoimmune polyendocrine syndrome type I* (APS-I) is a rare disorder with autosomal recessive inheritance that is caused by defects in the *autoimmune regulator (AIRE)* gene. In contrast, *autoimmune polyendocrine syndrome type II* (APS-II) is more common but less well defined and includes overlapping groups of disorders. A unifying characteristic within APS-II is the strong association with polymorphic genes of the human leukocyte antigen (HLA) region located on the short arm of chromosome 6 (band 6p21.3). In addition to HLA, many other genetic loci are likely to contribute to susceptibility to APS-II. For purposes of simplicity in this chapter, APS-II encompasses what some clinicians divide into APS-II (Addison disease plus type 1 diabetes or thyroid autoimmunity), APS-III (thyroid autoimmunity plus other autoimmune diseases, not Addison disease or type 1 diabetes), and APS-IV (two or more other organ-specific autoimmune disorders).

APS-II has also been known by various other names, including Schmidt syndrome, polyglandular autoimmune disease, polyglandular failure syndrome, organ-specific autoimmune disease, and polyendocrinopathy diabetes. Such diverse names reflect the large number of studies and case reports of this syndrome and its historical importance. Each of these other names has some shortcomings, such as failure to include the fact that both hyperfunction and hypofunction of endocrine glands can occur or failure to recognize that nonendocrine disorders such as pernicious anemia and celiac disease are parts of the syndrome. Studies of patients with APS-II were instrumental in identifying the autoimmune bases of several diseases and developing autoantibody assays such as those for type 1 diabetes and cytoplasmic islet cell antibodies.

Other rare autoimmune endocrine disorders have contributed to understanding of the development of autoimmunity. For example, the rare disorder immunodysregulation polyendocrinopathy enteropathy X-linked syndrome (IPEX) is caused by a mutation of the *forkhead box P3 (FOXP3)* gene. *FOXP3* plays a central role in the development and function of regulatory CD4+ T cells that function to maintain tolerance to self. It has become increasingly recognized that these T cells play a key role in the pathogenesis of many autoimmune diseases, and therapies targeting these cells will likely be developed and tested. A

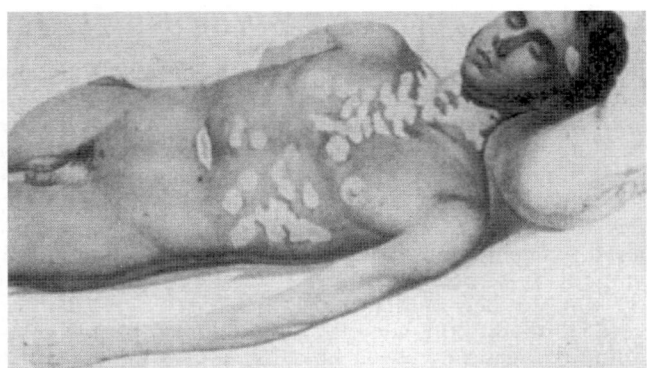

Figure 40-1 This illustration accompanied Addison's initial description of primary adrenal insufficiency (Addison disease). (From Addison T. *On the Constitutional and Local Effects of Disease of the Supra-renal Capsules.* London, UK: Samuel Highley; 1855.)

thorough understanding of these rare and often genetically simple disorders provides insight into the development of syndromes that are characterized by polygenic inheritance and that affect a larger group of patients.

AUTOIMMUNITY PRIMER

An understanding of the pathophysiology of autoimmune disease requires a basic knowledge of the immunologic mechanisms that underlie tolerance (the ability to differentiate self from nonself). Autoimmunity develops when the mechanisms of immune tolerance break down. It can occur centrally at the level of the generative organs (e.g., thymus, bone marrow) or peripherally in the target organs or lymphoid tissues. T lymphocytes and autoantibodies produced by B cells are two arms of the immune system that differ fundamentally in their recognition of target antigens. Autoantibodies react with intact molecules (including both soluble and cell surface molecules) and usually interact with conformational determinants of the autoantigen. In contrast, T lymphocytes recognize peptide fragments of autoantigens, often 8 to 12 amino acids in length, that are presented on the surface of another cell by molecules of the major histocompatibility complex (MHC).

Histocompatibility molecules interact with T-cell receptors when bound with an antigenic peptide. These molecules resemble a hot dog in a bun, with the antigenic peptide (the hot dog) bound in the groove of the histocompatibility molecule (the bun). Histocompatibility molecules are extremely polymorphic, with different amino acids lining the peptide-binding groove. These variable amino acids determine which peptides are bound and presented to T lymphocytes.

T cells differ based on multiple cell surface molecules, and these molecules determine their function in the immune system. T cells interact with other cells within and outside the immune system. CD4+ T cells typically react with peptides that are derived from proteins in extracellular compartments that are bound and acquired by class II histocompatibility molecules (HLA-DP, HLA-DQ, or HLA-DR in humans), expressed on antigen-presenting cells (APCs) such as macrophages, dendritic cells, and B lymphocytes. CD8+ T cells react with peptides bound by class I histocompatibility molecules (HLA-A, HLA-B, and HLA-C). Class I molecules are present on the surface of almost all nucleated cells. The antigen peptide in this case is derived from proteins expressed endogenously and is presented in a complex by class I HLA by the target cell itself. Recognition of the antigenic peptide by CD8+ T cells typically leads to the release of cytotoxic chemicals that kill the target cell.

The T-cell response depends on the context in which the antigen is presented. The simple expression of histocompatibility molecules and recognition of antigen by a T cell are not sufficient for T-cell activation. This context is at least partially determined by the interaction of cell surface molecules on both the T cell and the APC. Interaction among the MHC, the peptide, and the T-cell receptor *(signal one)* is critical to the activation process; other molecules then help to define the nature of the immune response *(signal two)*. The context in which the antigens are presented is critical for the determination of this response. Cell surface molecules and receptors, cytokines, and chemokines form the context in which the antigen is presented. Based on this context, the cell can become activated, tolerized, or anergic (immune unresponsive). For example, the APC cell surface molecule CD80 or CD86 engages the CD28 receptor on the T cell and amplifies signal one, which leads to T-cell activation. When a T cell recognizes an antigen in the context of the MHC and does not receive the appropriate second signal, anergy results.

Tolerance induction is a staged process that begins in the thymus during T-cell maturation. This process depends in part on the presence of *peripheral antigens* in the thymus. Peripheral antigens are self-antigens (e.g., insulin) normally expressed in tissues outside the immune system that are expressed at low levels in the thymus. Developing T cells that react strongly to these peripheral molecules in the context of the MHC are deleted in the thymus and are thus removed from the T-cell repertoire. Study of *AIRE* gene knockout mice has supported the importance of these phenomena in the development of autoimmunity. These mice have low levels of expression of peripheral antigens in the thymus and develop lymphocytic infiltrates in multiple organs (see later).[1,2]

Peripheral tolerance is an important mechanism for tolerance induction after T cells have matured in the thymus. Anergic and regulatory T cells are integral in the development of tolerance for naïve T cells. A major population of T-regulatory cells carry the cell surface markers CD4 and CD25 and express FOXP3. The function of the population of CD4+/CD25high cells involves an active suppressive activity and relies on the transcription factor FOXP3. Deletion of this transcription factor leads to fulminant autoimmunity in neonates (e.g., neonatal type 1 diabetes and enteropathy), often resulting in death within the first year of life (the IPEX syndrome; see later).

Cognate help is the process by which B cells are activated by CD4+ T cells that are responding to the same antigen. CD4+ T cells activate B cells to produce the humoral immune response. This occurs after the CD4+ T cell engages an antigen in the context of the MHC on the cell surface of a B cell. The cytokines (interleukin [IL]-4, IL-5, and IL-6) produced by the CD4+ T cells induce the maturation of a B cell. Depending on the cytokine milieu, the B cell will switch from producing immunoglobulin M (IgM) to IgG, IgE, or IgA. The development of B-cell tolerance is partially dependent on this linked recognition: autoreactive B-cell clones that do not have a CD4+ T cell that can bind with the antigen in its MHC groove will not normally be activated. Thus, in most cases the generation of autoantibodies by B cells is also linked to an autoreactive T cell specific for the same self-antigen. Growing evidence supports the role of autoreactive B cells as critical APCs to autoreactive T cells, creating a positive feedback loop in the expansion and maintenance of the autoimmune process.

NATURAL HISTORY OF AUTOIMMUNE DISORDERS

The natural history of autoimmune disorders can be divided into a series of stages beginning with genetic susceptibility, followed by triggering of autoimmunity (e.g., dietary gliadin exposure in celiac disease), active autoimmunity preceding clinical manifestations (e.g., progressive glandular destruction), and, finally, overt disease. This is a theoretical construct that may be useful for understanding factors involved with the development of autoimmunity and disease, but of necessity it is simplified and does not reflect the potential relapsing-remitting nature of autoimmunity (Fig. 40-2).

Genetic Associations

Although there is familial aggregation of APS-II and its component disorders, there is no simple pattern of inheritance (Table 40-1). Susceptibility is probably determined by multiple genetic loci (with HLA having the strongest effect) interacting with environmental factors. Autoimmune diseases share common genetic risk factors, including HLA, the MHC class I–related gene A *(MICA)*, the gene for lymphoid tyrosine phosphatase *(PTPN22)*, the cytotoxic T lymphocyte–associated antigen 4 (CTLA4), and the gene for NACHT leucine-rich repeat protein 1 (NLRP1, or NALP1). In addition, genetic susceptibility for some autoimmune diseases has been linked to polymorphisms that are organ specific; for example, polymorphisms in the

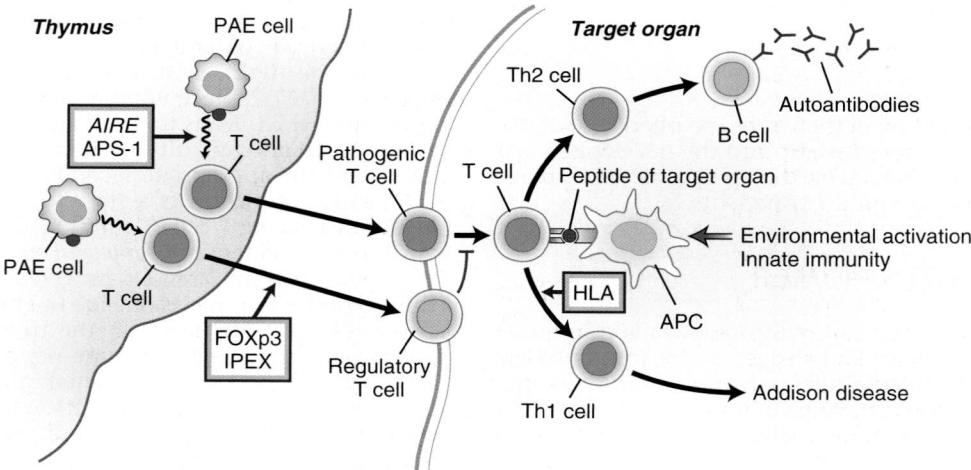

Figure 40-2 Model of the pathogenesis of autoimmunity in polyendocrine disorders. The development of autoimmune disease is determined by a group of T cells that recognize one or more organ-specific epitomes. Peptides are presented in the human leukocyte antigen (HLA) molecule and are recognized by the T-cell receptor. Recognition of self molecules depends on the maturation of the T cell, a process that begins in the thymus and continues in the periphery. The transcription factor FOXp3 stimulates the development of CD4+/CD25+ regulatory T cells. B cells produce autoantibodies under the stimulation of T cells. AIRE, autoimmune regulator; APC, antigen-presenting cell; APS-1, autoimmune polyendocrine syndrome 1; IPEX, immune dysregulation, polyendocrinopathy, enteropathy, X-linked; PAE, peripheral antigen-expressing cell; Th1, type 1 helper T cell; Th2, type 2 helper T cell. (From Eisenbarth GS, Gottlieb PA. Autoimmune polyendocrine syndromes. *N Engl J Med.* 2004;350:2068-2079.)

TABLE 40-1

Genetic Associations With Autoimmune Disease

Gene	Proposed Mechanism of Action	Polymorphism/Mutation	Disease	Inheritance
HLA	Antigen presentation	DR3-DQ2/DR4-DQ8 DR3-DQ2 DR3-DQ2/DRB1*0404-DQ8 DR3-DQ2/DR4-DQ8 DR3 DR5	Type 1 diabetes Celiac disease Addison disease Graves disease Hypothyroidism	Multigenic
MICA	Priming of naïve T cells	5, 5.1 4, 5.1 5.1	Type 1 diabetes Celiac disease Addison disease	Multigenic
PTPN22	T-cell receptor signaling pathway through interaction with regulatory kinases	Tryptophan substitution for arginine at position 620	Type 1 diabetes SLE RA Graves disease Hypothyroidism Vitiligo	Multigenic
CTLA4	Receptor on activated CD4+ and CD8+ T cells; decreases T-cell activation	CT60 CT60; +49A/G CT60; +49A/G ++49A/G ++49A/G	Type 1 diabetes Graves disease Hypothyroidism Celiac disease Addison disease	Multigenic
AIRE	"Peripheral" antigen presentation in the thymus	Multiple reported mutations	APS-I	Autosomal recessive
FOXP3	Transcription factor important for maturation of CD4+/CD25+ regulatory T cells	Multiple reported mutations	IPEX	X-linked

AIRE, autoimmune regulator; *APS-I,* autoimmune polyendocrine syndrome type I; *CTLA4,* cytotoxic T lymphocyte–associated antigen 4; *FOXP3,* forkhead box protein 3; *HLA,* human leukocyte antigen; IPEX, immunodysregulation polyendocrinopathy enteropathy X-linked syndrome; *MICA,* MHC class I-related gene A; *PTPN22,* the gene for lymphoid tyrosine phosphatase; RA, rheumatoid arthritis; SLE, systemic lupus erythematosus.

variable nucleotide tandem repeat (VNTR) upstream from the insulin gene have been associated with risk for type 1 diabetes.[3]

Genes located on the MHC found on chromosome 6 have been implicated in the pathogenesis of organ-specific autoimmune diseases. These genes are in strong linkage disequilibrium with each other and encode proteins that are important in the function of the immune system. Foremost in importance for the genetics of organ-specific autoimmune diseases are class I and class II HLA genes. Molecular HLA genotyping has revealed many subtypes of the older, serologically defined alleles, and the unique genetic sequence encoding each polymorphic chain of the histocompatibility molecules is now given a unique identifying number. A case in point is the DQ molecule, which is the histocompatibility molecule most strongly associated with endocrine autoimmunity. A number is assigned for each unique α- and β-chain sequence. Examples are DQA1*0501 for the α chain and DQB1*0201 for the β chain of the DQ molecule (also termed DQ2) commonly encoded on DR3 (DRB1*0301) haplotypes. A haplotype consists of a series of alleles of different genes on a contiguous region of a chromosome (e.g., DQA1 and DQB1 alleles) that are inherited together. A genotype is the combination of the haplotypes of both chromosomes. Fine mapping of the HLA has shown remarkable conservation of the HLA-A1/B8/DR3 haplotype such that a region of approximately 2.9 megabases is invariable. Conservation of large areas suggests that these areas of the genome have been inherited without recombination and are in very tight linkage disequilibrium. This greatly complicates the ability to identify which, if any, of the genes within the area of conservation are associated with disease and must be accounted for when assessing susceptibility to disease in this region.

Part of the overlapping risk for autoimmune disease is related to shared genetic susceptibility, especially within the HLA. For example, the highest risk HLA genotype for type 1 diabetes is DR3-DQ2, DR4-DQ8 (DQ8 = DQA1*0301-DQB1*0302). The importance of this HLA genotype in the development of type 1 diabetes is highlighted by the observation that children who inherited the same DR3-DQ2, DR4-DQ8 as a sibling with type 1 diabetes are at greater than 75% risk for development of autoimmunity by age 12 years and at greater than 50% risk of developing diabetes by 12 years.[4] A specific DR4 subtype of this gene, DRB1*0404, shows a strong association with Addison disease.[5,6] The DR3-DQ2 haplotype is associated with celiac disease both in the presence[7] and in the absence[8] of type 1 diabetes. This haplotype has been associated with autoimmune thyroid disease,[9] although conflicting reports exist.[10]

Whereas some HLA alleles increase disease risk, others are associated with protection from disease. For example, the DQ alleles DQA1*0102-DQB1*0602 (usually associated with DR2) confer strong protection from type 1A diabetes in a dominant fashion[11] but also confer susceptibility to another autoimmune disorder, multiple sclerosis. Furthermore, this protection is not general to endocrine autoimmunity, because no protection from Addison disease is afforded by DQB1*0602. DP is another gene within the MHC, and its 0402 polymorphism has been shown to be associated with a decreased risk for type 1 diabetes in subjects with the highest risk HLA genotype for type 1 diabetes (DR3/DR4).[12] Observations such as these suggest that, as more is learned about the genetic influence of disease, researchers will be able to combine different genotypes and refine prediction of autoimmune disease.

MICA produces a protein that is expressed in the thymus and in naïve CD8+ T cells. Polymorphisms of MICA have been associated with type 1 diabetes,[13] celiac disease,[14] and Addison disease.[15] A particular polymorphism of MICA, denoted 5.1, results from the insertion of a single base pair. This insertion produces a premature stop codon and a truncated protein. This particular polymorphism has been shown to influence the risk for Addison disease in subjects with autoimmunity associated with Addison disease.

Genes outside the MHC have also been implicated in the pathogenesis of autoimmune disease. For example, the PTPN22 gene encodes lymphoid tyrosine phosphatase (LYP) protein. LYP, through interactions with regulatory kinases such as CSK, appears to act as an inhibitor of the signal cascade downstream from the T-cell receptor. A specific polymorphism associated with a tryptophan substitution for arginine at position 620 (R620W) blocks LYP's interaction with CSK.[16] Recent work has suggested that this allele may increase the development of autoreactive B cells[16,17] and affect intracellular signaling pathways in both T and B cells.[18] This polymorphism has been associated with type 1 diabetes,[19] rheumatoid arthritis,[20] systemic lupus erythematosus (SLE),[21] Graves disease,[22] and vitiligo[23] and is weakly associated with Addison disease.[24] Furthermore, this disease-associated allele has also been associated with SLE, rheumatoid arthritis, type 1 diabetes, and autoimmune hypothyroidism in families with several members affected by more than one autoimmune disease.[24]

CTLA4 is expressed on activated CD4+ and CD8+ T cells, where it is hypothesized to act as a negative regulator.[25] Several polymorphisms within the CTLA4 gene have been associated with autoimmune diseases. One polymorphism associated with AT repeats has been shown to reduce the inhibitory function of CTLA4 in subjects with Graves disease.[26] A single nucleotide polymorphism in the 3' untranslated region, denoted CT60, has been associated with Graves disease[27] and autoimmune hypothyroidism.[28] An additional polymorphism, denoted +49A/G, has been associated with celiac disease in the Dutch population,[29] with autoimmune thyroid disease,[30] and with Addison disease.[31]

NALP1 regulates the innate immune system. After the initial observation that this gene was associated with the risk of vitiligo[32] and other related autoimmune diseases, it was associated with Addison disease and type 1 diabetes.[33]

Organ-specific genetic polymorphisms have been associated with the development of specific autoimmune diseases. For example, polymorphisms of the variable number of tandem repeats (VNTR) upstream of the insulin gene have been associated with the development of type 1 diabetes. Higher numbers of tandem repeats are associated with increased production of insulin in the thymus and protection from type 1 diabetes.[3] Similarly, polymorphisms of the thyroglobulin gene are associated with autoimmune thyroid disease.[34]

Single-gene defects such as AIRE and FOXP3 cause multiorgan autoimmunity and are discussed in sections devoted to those topics. Analysis of mutations of the AIRE gene indicates that it generally does not play a role in APS-II or sporadic Addison disease, with 1 (1.1%) of 90 patients with Addison disease (non–APS-I) and 1 (0.2%) of 576 control subjects having AIRE mutations.[31]

Environmental Triggers

Although genetics is known to play an important role in the development of autoimmunity, it does not tell the whole story. For example, the highest risk HLA genotype for type 1 diabetes (DR3-DQ2, DR4-DQ8) is associated with a risk of 1 in 20 for the development of diabetes.[35] Although this is greater than the general population prevalence rate of 1 in 200 by the age of 20 years, it is certainly not a 100% risk. Therefore, other factors (genetic and environmental) must be involved in the initiation of autoimmunity. Some theorize that these factors may be environmental triggers.

For one disease, celiac disease, the underlying environmental trigger has been identified: gluten. Through studies such as the Diabetes Autoimmunity Study in the Young (DAISY), BabyDiab, and Celiac Disease Autoimmunity Research (CEDAR), the timing of first exposure to cereal has been identified as a risk factor for the development of diabetes and celiac disease autoimmunity. Infants exposed at a very young age to cereal developed diabetes and celiac-associated autoimmunity at a greater rate than those who had cereal introduced at a later date.[36-38] In epidemiologic studies, cod liver oil consumption has been associated with a decreased risk for type 1 diabetes. Cod liver oil contains ω-3 polyunsaturated fats and vitamin D. In prospective studies, there is some suggestion that lower consumption of ω-3 polyunsaturated fats is associated with an increased risk for autoimmunity associated with type 1 diabetes.[39] Further investigation may identify additional environmental associations. Changes in our diet, our food composition, and use of medicines such as antibiotics have the potential to change our gut flora and microbiome. Animal studies suggest that changes in the gut microbiome can affect disease in these models of autoimmunity.[40,41] Human evidence is being sought to determine whether the interaction between the microbiome and innate immunity is leading to increased inflammation and setting the stage for increased frequencies of all autoimmune disorders that have recently been observed.[42,43]

Virus and other infections have been considered as a cause of autoimmunity and have been shown to cause the development of type 1 diabetes when infection occurs in utero for rubella, for example. Examination of pancreata from individuals with prediabetes (autoantibodies) or those with diabetes has provided evidence consistent with viral infection of the organ.[44,45] Association is not causality and further experiments are needed to determine whether this finding is an important component of how either autoimmunity is initiated or propagated.

Immunologic therapies, especially in patients with an autoimmune disease, can induce autoimmunity. A remarkable example is the treatment of patients with multiple sclerosis with an anti-CD52 monoclonal antibody. One third of 27 patients given the monoclonal antibody developed antithyrotropin receptor autoantibodies and hyperthyroidism.[46] Interferon-α (IFN-α) therapy for hepatitis has been associated with thyroid autoimmunity[47] and type 1 diabetes.[48] Severe hypoglycemia associated with insulin autoantibodies in the absence of insulin administration, termed *Hirata disease*, is associated with methimazole treatment of Graves disease. The development of Hirata disease in these patients is associated with HLA-Bw62/Cw4/DR4 with a specific DRB1 allele (DRB1*0406).[49]

Development of Organ-Specific Autoimmunity

Autoantibodies highly specific for a given disorder are present before disease onset. Each specific autoantibody reacts with only a single autoantigen, although autoantigens may be present in multiple tissues. The targets of autoantibodies appear to be unrelated except that for organ-specific autoimmunity they are usually expressed in specific cells and cellular sites. Anti-islet antibodies include antibodies to glutamic acid decarboxylase (GAD), islet cell antibody (ICA) 512 (also termed *insulinoma antigen-2* [IA-2]), insulin, and the most recently discovered, ZnT8.[50] Celiac disease is associated with antibodies against tissue transglutaminase (tTG). Addison disease is associated with antibodies against 21-hydroxylase.

Given that the antibodies can be identified before the development of organ dysfunction, they can be used to screen subjects who are at high risk for development of autoimmune disease to identify risk for additional autoimmune diseases. This approach has been employed in studies such as TrialNet for Type 1 Diabetes to screen first-degree relatives of patients with type 1 diabetes for diabetes-related autoantibodies. In this and other cohorts, risk for development of diabetes increases with the number of autoantibodies and their persistence.

Organ-specific autoantibodies (identified with appropriate assays) are rarely present (approximately 1 in 100) in the general population and identify a subset of people who are at greater risk for clinical disease. These autoantibodies may be expressed for years before the disease develops, and additional autoantibodies can develop over time. The pace at which disease develops is highly variable. For example, children as young as 1 year of age can present with type 1 diabetes. In contrast, a subset of subjects (5% to 10%) with type 2 diabetes diagnosed in adulthood have autoimmunity as the underlying cause. This may be due in part to genetics, because subjects who develop autoimmune diabetes at an older age have a higher proportion of the protective diabetes allele DQB1 *0602, although even in adults DQB1*0602 provides dramatic protection.[51]

In contrast, less is known concerning the specificity of pathogenic T cells. Given the observation that cross-reactive recognition by pathogenic T-cell clones may be determined by as few as four properly spaced amino acids of a nonapeptide and the estimate that each T-cell receptor might react with a million different peptides, there is considerable potential for patterns of autoimmunity to be determined by cross-reactive T cells. An important development has been the discovery in the thymus and other lymphoid tissues of peripheral antigen-expressing cells that express autoantigens such as insulin. Minute quantities of such molecules in the thymus can contribute to tolerance. Insulin messenger RNA (mRNA) in the thymus is regulated by genetic polymorphisms of the insulin gene associated with diabetes risk.[3] There is also evidence that stromal and lymphoid cells (CD11c⁺) in the spleen, lymph nodes, and circulation express multiple similar antigens.[52]

Failure of Gland

Organ dysfunction develops over time and can include a period of intermediate function that may be characterized by increased levels of the stimulatory hormones (e.g., thyroid-stimulating hormone, corticotropin [ACTH]) with normal levels of certain hormones (triiodothyronine, thyroxine, and cortisol). Once a significant portion of the gland has been destroyed, overt disease is then present.

AUTOIMMUNE POLYENDOCRINE SYNDROME TYPE I

Clinical Features

Table 40-2 compares the features of APS-I with those of APS-II. Table 40-3 shows the clinical features and recommended follow-up for patients with APS-I. Note some of the distinctions in the pattern of disease features of the two syndromes, in particular the propensity for hypoparathyroidism and candidiasis in APS-I, which is virtually absent in APS-II. Likewise, celiac disease is frequently observed in APS-II but is not seen in APS-I.

APS-I (Mendelian Inheritance in Man [MIM] 240300), also known as *autoimmune polyendocrinopathy-candidiasis-ectodermal dystrophy* (APECED), is characterized by the classic triad of mucocutaneous candidiasis, autoimmune hypoparathyroidism, and Addison disease, which form three of the most common components of the disorder. Patients with APS-I are at risk for the development of autoimmune diseases affecting almost every organ. More than 140 patients have been reported, including subjects in two large series from Finland[53-55] and the United States.[56]

In a series of 89 Finnish patients described by Perheentupa, all had chronic candidiasis at some time, 86% had hypoparathyroidism, and 79% had Addison disease. Gonadal failure (72% in women, 26% in men) and hypoplasia of the dental enamel (77% of patients) were also frequent findings. Other manifestations that occurred less often included alopecia (40%), vitiligo (26%), intestinal malabsorption (18%), type 1 diabetes (23%), pernicious anemia (31%), chronic active hepatitis (17%), and hypothyroidism (18%).[53] The incidence rates for many of these disorders peak in the first or second decade of life, and the disease continues to develop over decades (Fig. 40-3). Therefore, reported prevalence rates of component disorders are highly dependent on the age at which follow-up ended.

APS-I is characteristically recognized in early childhood. Infants can present with chronic or recurrent

TABLE 40-2
Contrasting Features of Autoimmune Polyendocrine Syndrome

Feature	APS-I	APS-II
Inheritance pattern	Autosomal recessive (only siblings affected)	Polygenic (multiple generations affected)
Associated gene	*AIRE* gene mutation	*HLA-DR3* and *DR-4* associated
Gender association	Equal gender incidence	Female preponderance
Age at onset	Onset in infancy	Peak onset 20 to 60 years
Clinical features	Mucocutaneous candidiasis	Type 1 diabetes
	Hypoparathyroidism	Autoimmune thyroid disease
	Addison disease	Addison disease
Diagnostic antibodies	Anti-interferon	

APS, autoimmune polyendocrine syndrome.

TABLE 40-3
Clinical Features and Recommended Follow-up for APS-I and APS-II

Component Disease	Frequency at Age 40 Yr (%)	Recommended Evaluation
Autoimmune Polyendocrine Syndrome Type I		
Addison disease	79	Sodium, potassium, ACTH, cortisol, plasma renin activity, 21-hydroxylase autoantibodies
Diarrhea	18	History
Ectodermal dysplasia	50-75	Physical examination
Hypoparathyroidism	86	Serum calcium, phosphate, PTH
Hepatitis	17	Liver function test
Hypothyroidism	18	TSH; thyroid peroxidase and/or thyroglobulin autoantibodies
Male hypogonadism	26	FSH/LH
Mucocutaneous candidiasis	100	Physical examination
Obstipation	21	History
Ovarian failure	72	FSH/LH
Pernicious anemia	31	CBC, vitamin B_{12} levels
Splenic atrophy	15	Blood smear for Howell-Jolly bodies; platelet count; ultrasound if positive
Type 1 diabetes	23	Glucose, hemoglobin A_{1c}, diabetes-associated autoantibodies (insulin, GAD65, IA-2)
Autoimmune Polyendocrine Syndrome Type II*		
Addison disease	0.5	21-Hydroxylase autoantibodies
		ACTH stimulation testing if positive
Alopecia		Physical examination
Autoimmune hypothyroidism	15-30	TSH; thyroid peroxidase and/or thyroglobulin autoantibodies
Celiac disease	5-10	Transglutaminase autoantibodies; small intestine biopsy if positive
Cerebellar ataxia	Rare[†]	Dictated by signs and symptoms of disease
Chronic inflammatory demyelinating polyneuropathy	Rare[†]	Dictated by signs and symptoms of disease
Hypophysitis	Rare[†]	Dictated by signs and symptoms of disease
Idiopathic heart block	Rare[†]	Dictated by signs and symptoms of disease
IgA deficiency	0.5	IgA level
Myasthenia gravis	Rare[†]	Dictated by signs and symptoms of disease
Myocarditis	Rare[†]	Dictated by signs and symptoms of disease
Pernicious anemia	0.5-5	Anti–parietal cell autoantibodies
		CBC, vitamin B_{12} levels if positive
Serositis	Rare[†]	Dictated by signs and symptoms of disease
Stiff-man syndrome	Rare[†]	Dictated by signs and symptoms of disease
Vitiligo	1-9	Physical examination

*In the population with type 1 diabetes.
[†]Rare reported disorders in subjects with APS-II.
ACTH, adrenocorticotropic hormone; APS, autoimmune polyendocrine syndrome; CBC, complete blood count; FSH, follicle-stimulating hormone; GAD, glutamic acid decarboxylase; IA-2, insulinoma antigen 2; IgA, immunoglobulin A; LH, luteinizing hormone; PTH, parathyroid hormone; TSH, thyroid-stimulating hormone.

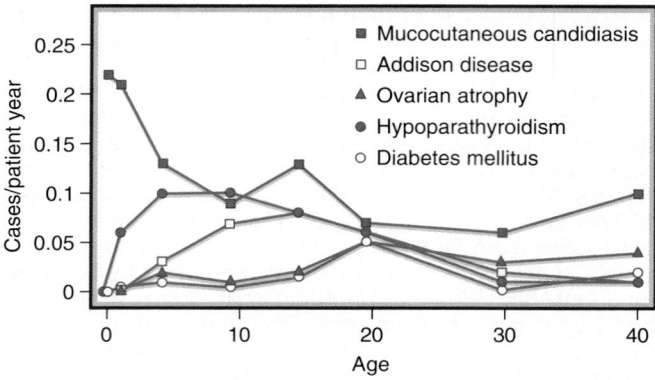

Figure 40-3 Incidence of disease development by age in patients with autoimmune polyendocrine syndrome type I (APS-I). (From Perheentupa J. APS-I/APECED: the clinical disease and therapy. *Endocrinol Metab Clin North Am.* 2002;31:295-320.)

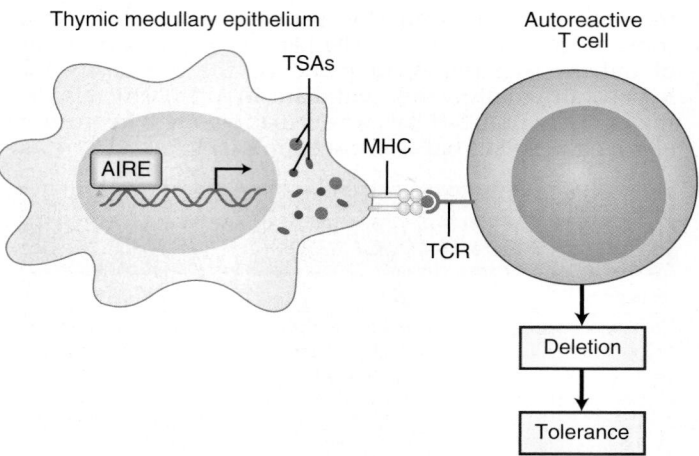

Figure 40-4 The autoimmune regulator (AIRE) gene functions to maintain tolerance by promoting the display of self-antigens in the thymus. Shown is an AIRE-expressing thymic medullary epithelial cell on the left. AIRE operates in the nucleus to promote the expression of thousands of different tissue-specific self-antigens (TSAs) that include many endocrine organ-specific proteins such as insulin. Peptide fragments of these TSAs are displayed on major histocompatibility complex (MHC) molecules to help promote the deletion of autoreactive T cells *(right)* that can be generated in the thymus from random gene rearrangement of the T-cell receptor (TCR). Such T cells are deleted when they encounter their antigen-MHC in the thymus and thus immune tolerance is maintained.

mucocutaneous candidiasis in the first year of life, followed by hypoparathyroidism and Addison disease, but new components can develop at any age. Decades can elapse between the diagnosis of one disorder and the onset of another in the same patient. Consequently, lifelong follow-up is important to allow early detection of additional components.

Recurrent candidiasis commonly affects the mouth and nails and, less frequently, the skin and esophagus.[53] Chronic oral candidiasis can result in atrophic disease with areas suggestive of leukoplakia. If this develops, the patient is at significant risk for carcinoma of the oral mucosa (with its high mortality rate).

Ectodermal dystrophy is another component of the syndrome (manifested by pitted nails, keratopathy, and enamel hypoplasia) and cannot be attributed to hypoparathyroidism. Enamel hypoplasia can precede the onset of hypoparathyroidism and, despite adequate replacement therapy, can also affect teeth forming after the onset of hypoparathyroidism.[57]

Friedman and colleagues[58] reported the frequent occurrence of asplenism and cholelithiasis as additional features of APS-I. Splenic atrophy may also cause immune deficiency. Although the cause of this part of the disorder is unknown, it is relatively common: up to 15% of patients are asplenic.[53] The presence of Howell-Jolly bodies on peripheral blood smear is suggestive of asplenia. If asplenia is identified, immunization with polyvalent pneumococcal vaccine should be administered, and follow-up antibody titers should be obtained. If an adequate response is not produced, daily prophylactic antibiotics may be necessary.

Malabsorption with steatorrhea is of uncertain origin, is usually intermittent, and may be exacerbated by hypocalcemia. Bereket and associates[59] reported a case in which patchy intestinal lymphangiectasia was discovered by endoscopically directed biopsy. Pancreatic insufficiency has been treated with cyclosporine.[60] Autoantibodies (e.g., tryptophan hydroxylase, histidine decarboxylase) reacting with intestinal endocrine cells (enterochromaffin, cholecystokinin, and enterochromaffin-like) occur and are associated with loss of endocrine cells on biopsy and with gastrointestinal dysfunction.[61,62]

Genetics

APS-I is inherited in a classic mendelian autosomal recessive fashion and is caused by mutations in the *AIRE* gene, located on the short arm of chromosome 21 (near markers D21s49 and D21s171 on 21p22.3).[63] The gene encodes a

transcriptional regulator protein that is highly expressed in antigen-presenting epithelial cells in the thymus and in a small subset of cells in lymphoid tissues.[2,64] It has been localized to the nucleus, and mutations have been demonstrated to be associated with decreased transcription of reporter products.[65,66] A mouse model of APS-I has been generated and *Aire* knockout mice also spontaneously develop autoimmune features. Detailed analyses of antigen-presenting epithelial cells in the thymus of *Aire* knockout mice has shown that these cells have decreased expression of peripheral *tissue-specific self-antigens* (TSAs) and that Aire promotes the expression of thousands of such self-antigens in these cells.[2] Furthermore, autoreactive T cells with specificity to these TSAs can escape thymic deletion when Aire is defective and promote autoimmunity.[67-69] Thus, Aire appears to act as a transcriptional activator that promotes the expression of a wide array of TSAs in the thymus to promote central tolerance (Fig. 40-4).

Multiple mutations of *AIRE* have been identified in subjects with APS-I. The frequency of specific mutations varies in different populations. For example, in Sardinia, a deletion of amino acid 257 is present in 90% of mutated alleles. A 136–base pair deletion in exon 8 is present in 71% of British alleles and in 56% of alleles in the United States. Analysis of haplotypes indicates that this deletion has arisen on many occasions.

Most cases of APS-I are associated with autosomal recessive inheritance patterns. A rare kindred of patients from Italy have a mutation of the AIRE protein G228W that, when present in the heterozygous state, is associated with autoimmunity, thus fitting an autosomal dominant inheritance pattern.[70] In a mouse model of this mutation, the expression of TSAs in the thymus was decreased, compared with the control model, suggesting a mechanism for this observed inheritance pattern.[71]

Diagnosis

The diagnosis of APS-I is highly likely when two or more of the primary component disorders (i.e., mucocutaneous candidiasis, hypoparathyroidism, and Addison disease) are present. Siblings of an affected patient should be considered affected even if only one of these disorders is present. Sequence analysis of *AIRE* for mutations may be helpful in identifying subjects with APS-I. Any patient with any of the component disorders deserves careful follow-up to watch for the development of additional disease.

Autoantibodies against IFN-α and IFN-ω have been identified in almost 100% of subjects with APS-I, regardless of age at screening.[72] The autoantibody has been found in subjects with many different mutations of the *AIRE* gene; it is not present in other autoimmune diseases, and it has been proposed to use this autoantibody to screen subjects with multiple autoimmune diseases for APS-I. It is unclear if antibodies to these type 1 IFNs are of any clinical consequence as APS-I subjects do not have an increased propensity for viral infections.[53] In contrast, it has also been shown that many APS-I subjects also harbor autoantibodies to IL-17A, IL-17F, and IL-22.[73,74] These are key cytokines for the function of the Th17 T-cell subset, and recent work has demonstrated that loss of function of these cytokines, as in patients with mutations in the IL-17 receptor, is associated with increased susceptibility to *Candida albicans* infections.[75] Thus, it appears that the *Candida* susceptibility in APS-I may be due to an autoimmune response against this effector cytokine family.

Therapy and Follow-up

The treatment of adrenal insufficiency and hypoparathyroidism is the same as that discussed in other chapters with the caveat that malabsorption can complicate treatment. The therapy for mucocutaneous candidiasis has been improved with the use of orally active antifungal drugs such as fluconazole and ketoconazole. Infection often recurs when the drug is discontinued or the dosage is decreased. Patients must be monitored carefully, because ketoconazole can inhibit adrenal and gonadal steroid synthesis and can precipitate adrenal failure. It is also associated with transient elevation of liver enzyme levels and, occasionally, with hepatitis. Fluconazole is associated with a lower frequency of hepatitis and does not inhibit steroidogenesis when given in the recommended doses.

Autoantibodies associated with multiple autoimmune diseases have been reported. Antiparathyroid and antiadrenal antibodies have been reported. Whereas 21-hydroxylase appears to be the major autoantigen in isolated Addison disease and in Addison disease associated with APS-II, autoantibodies against 17α-hydroxylase and cytochrome P450 side-chain cleavage enzyme (CYP11A1) have also been reported in Addison disease associated with APS-I.[76] There have been reports of antibodies to tryptophan hydroxylase in intestinal disease, tyrosine hydroxylase in alopecia areata, L-amino acid decarboxylase in hepatitis and vitiligo, and phenylalanine hydroxylase[77,78] and antibodies reacting with hair follicles.[79] Tuomi and coworkers originally observed that many more APS-I patients (41%) express anti-GAD65 autoantibodies than become diabetic, suggesting that reactivity to this single autoantigen has low predictive value in this population.[80] Recently, antibodies against NALP5 were identified in 49% of patients with APS-I and hypoparathyroidism, compared with none of those with APS-I but no hypoparathyroidism.[81] Screening for autoantibodies associated with additional autoimmune diseases may be useful in patients with APS-I.

Screening to allow the early detection of new disorders before overt symptoms and signs develop is recommended, including autoantibody studies, electrolytes, calcium and phosphorus levels, thyroid and liver function tests, blood smear, and plasma vitamin B_{12}. Patients at risk for adrenal failure can be screened by measurement of basal ACTH and supine plasma renin activity, followed by dynamic testing as appropriate. Evaluation for asplenism[58] with abdominal ultrasonography and blood smear examination for Howell-Jolly bodies is warranted, with pneumococcal vaccination and appropriate antibiotic coverage for affected patients.

There are case reports of severely affected patients who have benefited from immunosuppressive therapy. For example, Ward and colleagues[60] treated a 13-year-old patient who had keratoconjunctivitis, hepatitis, and severe pancreatic insufficiency. Treatment with cyclosporine was associated with normalization of stool fat (from 31.5 to 2.5 g/day).

AUTOIMMUNE POLYENDOCRINE SYNDROME TYPE II

Clinical Features

APS-II (MIM 269200) is defined by the occurrence in the same patient of two or more of the following: primary adrenal insufficiency (Addison disease), Graves disease, autoimmune thyroiditis, type 1A diabetes mellitus, primary hypogonadism, myasthenia gravis, and celiac disease. Vitiligo, alopecia, serositis, and pernicious anemia also occur with increased frequency in patients with this syndrome and in their family members (see Table 40-3). APS-II is more common than APS-I. It occurs more often in female than in male patients, often has its onset in adulthood, and exhibits familial aggregation (see Table 40-2).

When one of the component disorders is present, an associated disorder occurs more commonly than in the general population. Furthermore, circulating organ-specific autoantibodies are often present even in the absence of overt clinical disease. For example, in subjects with type 1 diabetes, there is a 15% to 20% risk of hypothyroidism, a 5% to 10% risk of celiac-related autoimmunity, and a 1.5% risk of adrenal autoimmunity. The risk of autoimmunity is greater in relatives of patients with APS-II. In our assessment of APS-II families with Addison disease, up to 15% of relatives were found to have 21-hydroxylase autoantibodies (Addison disease–associated autoantibodies), anti-islet autoantibodies, or tTG autoantibodies (celiac disease–associated autoantibodies). The initial lesion and precipitating events that result in the syndrome are unknown, but immunogenetic and immunologic similarities are present with regard to both the time course and the pathogenesis of each of the component disorders.

Because of the chronic development of organ-specific autoimmunity, patients with the syndrome and their families should have repeated endocrinologic evaluations over time. In a family in which the syndrome has been documented, relatives should be advised of the early symptoms and signs of the principal component diseases (a list is available from the Barbara Davis Center for Diabetes website[82]). Relatives of patients with multiple disorders should have a medical history, physical examination, and screening every 3 to 5 years, with measurement of anti-islet autoantibodies, a sensitive thyrotropin assay, and measurement of serum vitamin B_{12} levels. If there are any symptoms or signs or if 21-hydroxylase autoantibodies are present, the patient should have annual assays of basal ACTH levels with Cortrosyn stimulation testing.

Among 224 patients with Addison disease and APS-II reported by Neufeld and colleagues,[56] type 1 diabetes and autoimmune thyroid disease were the most common coexisting conditions (52% and 69% of patients, respectively). Other components were less common, including vitiligo (5%) and gonadal failure (4%). In an Italian cohort of over 600 patients, the majority of patients with Addison disease (86.7%, after exclusion of subjects with APS-I) had additional autoimmunity diseases, most frequently thyroid disease (56%) and diabetes (12%). A significant proportion of subjects exhibited thyroid- (16%) and diabetes- (8.8%) related autoimmunity without yet developing disease over average follow-up of 10 years.[83] Therefore, careful monitoring of patients with Addison disease for additional autoimmune diseases including thyroid, type 1A diabetes, and premature ovarian insufficiency is warranted.

Among patients with type 1A diabetes, thyroid autoimmunity and celiac disease coexist with sufficient frequency to justify screening. Thyroid peroxidase autoantibodies are present in 10% to 20% of children with type 1 diabetes; this incidence is higher in female patients and increases in all patients with age and with diabetes duration. A significant fraction of patients with type 1 diabetes and thyroid peroxidase autoantibodies develop thyroid disease. One study showed that after follow-up for more than 15 years, 80% of patients with thyroid peroxidase autoantibodies and type 1 diabetes became hypothyroid.[84] However, several studies have shown that a subset of patients with negative autoantibodies develop thyroid disease. Therefore, patients with type 1 diabetes should be screened annually for thyrotropin levels, which is a cost-effective approach.

With the identification of tTG as the major endomysial autoantigen of celiac disease, radioimmunoassays were developed and demonstrated that 10% to 12% of patients with type 1 diabetes have tTG autoantibodies.[7] The prevalence of tTG autoantibodies was higher in diabetic patients with HLA-DQ2; one third of DQ2-homozygous subjects were found to express anti-tTG antibody, reflective of the influence of HLA-DQ2 in the development of both type 1 diabetes and celiac disease. Seventy percent of those with high-titer antibody who underwent biopsy were subsequently found to have the disease.[85] Celiac disease may be identified at onset of type 1 diabetes. However, it can develop in patients with long-standing diabetes as well and in at least one cohort has been shown to be increased in patients with adult onset type 1 diabetes compared with childhood onset.[86] If left untreated, symptomatic celiac disease is also associated with an increased risk of gastrointestinal malignancy, especially lymphoma. Survival analysis in patients with type 1 diabetes and celiac disease shows an increase in mortality rate in patients with type 1 diabetes and celiac disease duration of greater than 15 years.[87] Frequency and method of screening remain areas of debate. At the very least, providers should be aware of the association and have a low threshold for screening with tTG antibodies. If the results are positive and are confirmed on repeat assay, small bowel biopsy to document celiac disease is warranted, with institution of a gluten-free diet if the disease is present. Many patients have asymptomatic celiac disease that is nevertheless associated with osteopenia and impaired growth.

Diagnosis

The diagnosis of APS-II requires an understanding of the risk for additional autoimmune diseases in patients with a single autoimmune endocrine disorder. A thorough history and physical examination may identify symptoms or signs of an additional autoimmune disorder. Screening for disease can include screening for markers of the autoimmune diseases (organ-specific autoantibodies) and assays of glandular function (e.g., thyrotropin levels).

Improved assays for several organ-specific autoantibodies have been developed since the cloning of specific autoantigens and the development of assays that use recombinant antigens. These radioimmunoassays are superior to assays based on immunofluorescence with tissue sections, such as ICA testing. The most notable finding is the identification of multiple autoantigens targeted even in single autoimmune disorders. Most of the endocrine autoantigens are hormones (e.g., insulin) or enzymes associated with differentiated endocrine function: thyroid peroxidase in thyroiditis; GAD, carboxypeptidase H, and ICA 512/IA-2 in type 1 diabetes; 17α-hydroxylase and 21-hydroxylase in Addison disease; and the parietal cell enzyme H^+/K^+-adenosine triphosphatase in pernicious anemia.

In type 1 diabetes, the four most informative assays identify autoantibodies reacting with insulin, GAD65, ICA512/IA-2, and ZnT8.[50] Similarly, a radioassay for autoantibodies against the enzyme 21-hydroxylase in Addison disease has been developed and provides excellent disease specificity and sensitivity. Adrenal autoantibodies reacting with recombinant 21-hydroxylase usually precede the development of Addison disease. Screening with 21-hydroxylase autoantibodies may identify patients with antibodies but have normal production of cortisol in response to ACTH. Annual screening with a basal level of corticotropin with follow-up cosyntropin stimulation testing is an effective strategy for identifying adrenal insufficiency in patients with 21-hydroxylase autoantibodies.

Typically, autoantibodies mark the presence of or risk for autoimmune disease caused by T-cell–mediated glandular destruction. However, autoantibodies may also be pathogenic. A hallmark of pathogenic autoantibodies is the existence of a neonatal form of the disorder, secondary to transplacental passage of the autoantibody. Examples include neonatal Graves disease (anti–thyrotropin-receptor autoantibodies) and neonatal myasthenia gravis (anti–acetylcholine-receptor autoantibodies).

Therapy

Treatment of the individual diseases of the polyendocrine autoimmune syndrome is discussed in other chapters. Therapeutic considerations related specifically to APS-II are discussed here.

Many of the component disorders of the syndrome have a long prodromal phase and are associated with the expression of autoantibodies before the manifestation of overt disease. Therefore, people at risk for autoimmune diseases can be identified prior to the clinical onset of disease, and if the right treatment were identified, disease may be preventable. This is particularly important for type 1A diabetes but is also likely to apply to Addison disease and hypogonadism.

Prevention strategies have been extensively evaluated in patients with type 1 diabetes. Prevention of disease can occur at multiple time points along the natural history of evolving beta-cell dysfunction. Treatments targeted at patients with genetic risk without evidence for autoimmunity will expose people who will never get disease to an intervention (primary prevention). Therefore, any intervention must be safe and easily administered. Prevention trials in patients with diabetes-related autoantibodies prior to abnormalities of glucose metabolism (secondary prevention) can employ agents with higher risks of adverse events. Tertiary prevention of diabetes employs immune-modulating agents for the preservation of the beta-cell mass with the hopes of inducing a prolonged C-peptide production.

Primary prevention of type 1 diabetes targets infants at the highest risk for the development of type 1 diabetes on the basis of family history or specific HLA genotypes. Infants must be negative for diabetes-related autoantibodies. Interventions have focused on dietary manipulations including gluten-free diets, docosahexaenoic acid (DHA) supplementation, and elemental formulas lacking bovine insulin. To date, the interventions have not prevented the development of diabetes-related autoantibodies or diabetes in large-scale clinical trials.[88]

Secondary prevention of type 1 diabetes has been antigen specific (insulin and GAD65) and antigen nonspecific (nicotinamide). These studies have targeted subjects with positive diabetes-related autoantibodies prior to the development of diabetes. Some studies have included patients with abnormalities of glucose metabolism such as impaired first-phase insulin response and impaired glucose tolerance.

A large National Institutes of Health (NIH) trial, the Diabetes Prevention Trial—Type 1 (DPT-1), directly tested oral and parenteral insulin for prevention of diabetes. DPT-1 had two arms: intravenous-subcutaneous for those at high risk (risk of diabetes > 50% within 5 years) and oral insulin for those at moderate risk (risk of diabetes 25% to 50% within 5 years). Neither parenteral[89] nor oral[90] insulin slowed progression to diabetes. However, in a subgroup analysis of subjects in the DPT-1 oral trial, a treatment effect was noted for those who had the higher insulin autoantibody levels at diagnosis,[90] and further trials are under way. In preclinical Addison disease, a short course of glucocorticoids appeared to suppress the expression of adrenal autoantibodies and prevent progressive adrenal destruction.[91] Studies of immune-modulating agents (abatacept and teplizumab) in patients with diabetes-related autoantibodies and abnormalities of glucose metabolism are currently under way.

Because of the autoimmune nature of these disorders, several studies have evaluated the use of immunosuppressive and immune-modulating drugs. Drugs such as cyclosporine have preserved some residual insulin secretion. However, because cyclosporine is nephrotoxic and potentially oncogenic, more generalized use is precluded. Newer immunosuppressive agents (e.g., sirolimus) are being studied, and biologics such as anti-CD20 antibody (rituximab), abatacept, and nonmitogenic CD3 antibodies have been shown to prolong C-peptide production and to result in a decreased insulin dose through the first year of diabetes, compared with control subjects.[92-96]

Thyroxine therapy can precipitate a life-threatening addisonian crisis in a patient with untreated adrenal insufficiency and hypothyroidism. Therefore, it is necessary to evaluate adrenal function in all hypothyroid patients in whom the syndrome is suspected before instituting such therapy. A decreasing insulin requirement in a patient with insulin-dependent diabetes mellitus can be one of the earliest indications of adrenal insufficiency, occurring before the development of hyperpigmentation or electrolyte abnormalities.

OTHER POLYENDOCRINE DEFICIENCY AUTOIMMUNE SYNDROMES

Rare polyendocrine syndromes are listed in Table 40-4.

TABLE 40-4
Rare Polyendocrine Disorders

Disorder	Clinical Features	Cause
Hirata disease (insulin resistance syndrome)	Hypoglycemia	Insulin autoantibodies Associated with methimazole
IPEX	Type 1 diabetes Enteropathy	Mutations of *FOXP3*
Kearns-Sayre syndrome	Hypoparathyroidism Primary gonadal failure Nonautoimmune diabetes Hypopituitarism	Deletions of mitochondrial DNA
POEMS	Polyneuropathy Organomegaly Diabetes Primary gonadal failure	Plasma cell dyscrasia with production of M protein and cytokines
Thymic tumors	Myasthenia gravis Red blood cell hypoglobulinemia Autoimmune thyroid disease Adrenal insufficiency	Thymomas
Type B insulin resistance	Severe insulin resistance	Insulin receptor autoantibodies
Wolfram syndrome	Diabetes insipidus Nonautoimmune diabetes Bilateral optic atrophy Sensorineural deafness	Mutations of *WSF1*, which encodes wolframin

IPEX, immunodysregulation polyendocrinopathy enteropathy X-linked syndrome; POEMS, plasma cell dyscrasia with polyneuropathy, organomegaly, endocrinopathy, m protein, and skin changes.

Immunodysregulation Polyendocrinopathy Enteropathy X-Linked Syndrome

IPEX (MIM 340790, MIM 300292), first described in 1982, is a rare, X-linked recessive disorder that is characterized by immune dysregulation and results in multiple autoimmune diseases and early death (Fig. 40-4). It is caused by mutations of the *FOXP3* gene. Clinical characteristics include very early onset type 1A diabetes, severe enteropathy resulting in failure to thrive, and dermatitis, generally resulting in death within the first couple of years of life unless definitive treatment is pursued. Other reported abnormalities include atopy, thrombocytopenia, hemolytic anemia, hypothyroidism, lymphadenopathy, nephropathy, and alopecia (2012 review).[97] Immunologic evaluation shows elevated immunoglobulin E and eosinophilia in addition to the abnormalities associated with the component disorders.

The identification of *FOXP3* as the gene associated with IPEX was aided by the scurfy mouse model. The scurfy mouse exhibits characteristics similar to those seen in children affected with IPEX. The gene associated with this disorder in the scurfy mouse was found to be a DNA binding protein with characteristics of a transcription factor.[98] Clues about the function of this gene included the observations that implantation of thymus from a scurfy mouse into immune-incompetent mice transfers the disease, but transplantation of thymus into immune-competent mice does not transfer disease, and injections of normal T cells can rescue the phenotype, suggesting that a regulatory cell is involved in the pathogenesis of this disorder. Linkage analysis demonstrated that a 17-centimorgan (cM) stretch of the X chromosome (Xp11.1-q13.3) is associated with IPEX, and mutations within the *FOXP3* gene have been identified in most of the families studied thus far.[99] *FOXP3* encodes a protein that is a member of the forkhead class of winged helix transcription factors (forkhead box protein 3). *FOXP3* has been shown to be expressed in CD4+/CD25+ regulatory T cells.[100] These T cells can suppress activation of other T cells.[100] Therefore, mutations in *FOXP3* result in inability to generate regulatory T cells and the development of IPEX. Patients with mutations throughout the *FOXP3* gene have been described. In general, milder phenotypes are associated with point mutations or small deletions that do not result in a total lack of *FOXP3*. However, significant variability in phenotype within a single mutation suggests that other genes or environmental exposures may play an important role in the development of the disorder.

Treatment options are targeted to the underlying disorders. At the time of diagnosis, infants may be so affected by the enteropathy that they require bowel rest and parenteral nutrition. Diabetes is managed with insulin therapy. Immunosuppression with calcineurin inhibitors has been used in the initial, stabilization phase of treatment. Definitive treatment is with hematopoietic stem cell transplantation (HSCT). HSCT results in reversal of the enteropathy and other autoimmune components.[101] Generally, established type 1 diabetes and thyroid disease do not resolve. However, some reports document reversal of type 1 diabetes in patients who have received the conditioning immunotherapy and HSCT.[102] An additional case report shows reconstitution of the gut immune system may occur later than reconstitution of the bone marrow.[103] Novel approaches to insert a functional *FOXP3* gene into lymphocytes as gene therapy in addition to or eventually in place of HSCT are being developed as well.[104,105]

Over the past several years, disorders with similar clinical characteristics as IPEX but without mutations in *FOXP3* have been identified. In these disorders, mutations in *IL2RA, STAT5b, STAT-1,* and *ITCH* result in abnormalities of regulatory T-cell function, emphasizing the important role of these cell populations in the maintenance of immune tolerance.

Anti–Insulin Receptor Autoantibodies

In this rarely reported disorder (<100 patients), also known as *type B insulin resistance* or *acanthosis nigricans*, insulin resistance is caused by the presence of anti–insulin receptor antibodies and anti-insulin antibodies.[106] Approximately one third of patients with these antibodies have an associated autoimmune illness such as SLE or Sjögren syndrome. Arthralgia, vitiligo, alopecia, autoimmune thyroid disease, secondary amenorrhea, and family history of autoimmunity have also been reported. Autoimmune thyroid disease has been described in two such patients, one with hypothyroidism and the other with antithyroid antibodies. Antinuclear antibodies, an elevated erythrocyte sedimentation rate, hyperglobulinemia, leukopenia, and hypocomplementemia are common.[107]

The major clinical manifestations are related to the anti–insulin receptor antibodies. Insulin resistance is profound, and up to 175,000 U of insulin given intravenously per day may be ineffective in lowering the elevated glucose. Despite hyperglycemia and marked insulin resistance, ketoacidosis is uncommon. The course of the diabetes is variable, and several patients have had spontaneous remissions. Other patients have had severe hypoglycemia (perhaps related to the insulin-like effects of anti–insulin receptor antibodies demonstrable in vitro).[108] The acanthosis nigricans, which is caused by hypertrophy and folding of otherwise histologically normal skin, appears to be related to the insulin-resistant state. Other forms of marked insulin resistance in the absence of antireceptor antibodies are also associated with acanthosis nigricans. A treatment regimen developed at NIH that includes rituximab that targets B lymphocytes with cyclophosphamide and pulse corticosteroids has been used successfully to treat this rare disorder.[108,109]

POEMS Syndrome

The components of the multisystem disorder POEMS (*p*lasma cell dyscrasia with polyneuropathy, *o*rganomegaly, *e*ndocrinopathy, *m*onoclonal plasma cell disorder, and *s*kin changes), also known as Crow-Fukase syndrome (MIM 192240), consist of diabetes mellitus (3-36% of patients), primary gonadal failure (55-89% of patients), plasma cell dyscrasia, sclerotic bone lesions, and neuropathy.[110] Patients usually present with severe progressive sensorimotor polyneuropathy, hepatosplenomegaly, lymphadenopathy, and hyperpigmentation. On evaluation, they are found to have plasma cell dyscrasia and sclerotic bone lesions. Patients present in the fifth to sixth decades of life and have a median survival time after diagnosis of 14 years.[110,111]

The pathophysiology of POEMS is poorly understood. There is evidence implicating cytokines such as IL-1A, IL-6, and TNF-α in addition to the M protein in the pathogenesis of this disorder. In several studies, elevated levels of vascular endothelial growth factor (VEGF) correlated with the disease state, and treatment with immunosuppressive agents reduced the symptoms of the disease and the levels of VEGF, suggesting that this growth factor plays a role in the disease.[112,113] A therapeutic trial of an anti-VEGF antibody would provide more definitive evidence for this hypothesis.

Algorithms have been proposed for the treatment of POEMS.[111] Important features of treatment include extensive baseline evaluation, ongoing monitoring for component disorders, systemic therapy for the plasma cell disorder, and radiation at the site of identified bone lesions. The diabetes mellitus responds to small, subcutaneous doses of insulin.

Kearns-Sayre Syndrome

The rare Kearns-Sayre syndrome (MIM 530000), also known as oculocraniosomatic disease or oculocraniosomatic neuromuscular disease with ragged red fibers, is characterized by myopathic abnormalities leading to ophthalmoplegia and progressive weakness in association with several endocrine abnormalities, including hypoparathyroidism, primary gonadal failure, diabetes mellitus, and hypopituitarism.[114] Crystalline mitochondrial inclusions are found in muscle biopsy specimens, and such inclusions have also been observed in the cerebellum. The relation between the mitochondrial disorders and endocrinologic abnormalities is not known. Antiparathyroid antibodies have not been described; however, antibodies to the anterior pituitary gland and striated muscle have been found, and the disease may have autoimmune components. Other abnormalities include retinitis pigmentosa and heart block. Deletions in mitochondrial DNA have been associated with Kearns-Sayre syndrome.[115] These mutations usually occur sporadically and are not associated with a familial syndrome.

Thymic Tumors

The thymus is a complex tissue with a specialized endocrine epithelium that synthesizes a variety of biologically active peptides involved in the control of T-cell maturation. This epithelium is derived from the neural crest and contains complex gangliosides that react with monoclonal antibody (A2B5) and tetanus toxin in a manner similar to that of pancreatic islets.

The illnesses associated with thymomas are similar to those seen in APS-II,[116] although the incidence of specific disorders is different. In one review of patients with thymoma, myasthenia gravis was found to occur in 44% of the patients, red blood cell aplasia in approximately 20%, hypoglobulinemia in 6%, autoimmune thyroid disease in 2%, and adrenal insufficiency in 1 of 423 patients (0.24%). The incidence of autoimmune thyroid disease reported in patients with thymoma is probably an underestimate, given the incidence of unsuspected thyroid disease in patients with myasthenia gravis. Mucocutaneous candidiasis in adults is also associated with thymomas. Interestingly, recent work suggests that an alteration in the proper expression of AIRE and peripheral antigens may be part of the explanation of the autoimmunity that arises in these patients.[117]

Wolfram Syndrome

Wolfram syndrome (MIM 222300, chromosome 4; MIM 598500, mitochondrial) is a rare autosomal recessive disease that is also called DIDMOAD (*d*iabetes *i*nsipidus, *d*iabetes *m*ellitus, progressive bilateral *o*ptic *a*trophy, and sensorineural *d*eafness). In addition, neurologic and psychiatric disturbances are prominent in most patients and can cause severe disability. Atrophic changes in the brain have been found on magnetic resonance imaging.[118] Segregation analysis of the mutations found in familial and sporadic cases of Wolfram syndrome led to the identification of wolframin, a 100-kDa transmembrane protein encoded by *WFS1*, a gene located at 4p16.1.116. Genotype and phenotype analyses have identified the severe phenotype (defined as the development of neurologic disease within the first decade) in patients with truncated proteins and mutations in the carboxy-terminus of the protein.[119]

Wolframin has been localized to the endoplasmic reticulum[120] and is found in neuronal and neuroendocrine tissue.[121] Its expression induces ion channel activity with a resultant increase in intracellular calcium and may play an important role in intracellular calcium homeostasis.[122] Functional studies have shown that reported *WFS1* mutations lead to decreased stability of the protein wolframin.[123] Linkage to other loci in addition to *WFS1* may explain the variability in phenotype seen in this disorder.

Wolfram syndrome appears to be a slowly progressive neurodegenerative process, and there is also (nonautoimmune) selective destruction of the pancreatic beta cells, recently associated in a stem-cell model with increased endoplasmic reticulum stress in the pancreatic beta cell.[124] This association is probably a result of the expression pattern of *WFS1*. Diabetes mellitus with an onset in childhood is usually the first manifestation. Diabetes mellitus and optic atrophy are present in all reported cases, but expression of the other features is variable. Duration of diabetes is linked to the development of microvascular complications.[123] Additional endocrinologic diseases, such as ACTH deficiency and growth hormone deficiency, have been reported.[123] In one case report, two related children with Wolfram syndrome had megaloblastic and sideroblastic anemia that responded to treatment with thiamine. Furthermore, thiamine treatment was associated with a marked decrease in insulin requirements.[125]

Omenn Syndrome

Omenn syndrome (MIM 603554) is a primary immunodeficiency syndrome with autoimmune manifestations affecting mainly the skin and gastrointestinal tract. Mutations associated with decreased recombination of the T-cell receptor have been described. One study showed that the levels of *AIRE* gene expression were decreased in the thymus of two affected patients and that this was associated with decreased expression of peripheral antigens compared with control subjects.[111]

Chromosomal Disorders

Down syndrome, or trisomy 21 (MIM 190685), is associated with the development of type 1 diabetes mellitus, thyroiditis, and celiac disease. Patients with Turner syndrome are at increased risk for the development of thyroid disease and celiac disease. It is recommended to screen patients with trisomy 21 and Turner syndrome for associated autoimmune diseases on a regular basis.

CONCLUSION

Through the study of rare disorders such as APS-I and IPEX, the processes of thymic expression of peripheral antigens and development of regulatory T cells are beginning to be defined. This understanding provides invaluable insight into the development of the normal immune system and the mistakes that can occur and lead to autoimmunity. Lessons learned from these rare diseases will help to better define the pathophysiology of more common autoimmune endocrine disorders, possibly leading to the development of immunologic methods for the prevention and treatment of these disorders.

REFERENCES

1. Ramsey C, Winqvist O, Puhakka L, et al. Aire deficient mice develop multiple features of APECED phenotype and show altered immune response. *Hum Mol Genet.* 2002;11:397-409.
2. Anderson MS, Venanzi ES, Klein L, et al. Projection of an immunological self shadow within the thymus by the Aire protein. *Science.* 2002;298:1395-1401.
3. Pugliese A, Zeller M, Fernandez A Jr, et al. The insulin gene is transcribed in the human thymus and transcription levels correlated with allelic variation at the INS VNTR-IDDM2 susceptibility locus for type 1 diabetes. *Nat Genet.* 1997;15:293-297.
4. Aly TA, Ide A, Jahromi MM, et al. Extreme genetic risk for type 1A diabetes. *Proc Natl Acad Sci U S A.* 2006;103:14074-14079.
5. Yu L, Brewer KW, Gates S, et al. DRB1*04 and DQ alleles: expression of 21-hydroxylase autoantibodies and risk of progression to Addison's disease. *J Clin Endocrinol Metab.* 1999;84:328-335.
6. Myhre AG, Undlien DE, Lovas K, et al. Autoimmune adrenocortical failure in Norway autoantibodies and human leukocyte antigen class II associations related to clinical features. *J Clin Endocrinol Metab.* 2002;87:618-623.
7. Bao F, Yu L, Babu S, et al. One third of HLA DQ2 homozygous patients with type 1 diabetes express celiac disease-associated transglutaminase autoantibodies. *J Autoimmun.* 1999;13(1):143-148.
8. Hoffenberg EJ, MacKenzie T, Barriga KJ, et al. A prospective study of the incidence of childhood celiac disease. *J Pediatr.* 2003;143:308-314.
9. Levin L, Ban Y, Concepcion E, et al. Analysis of HLA genes in families with autoimmune diabetes and thyroiditis. *Hum Immunol.* 2004;65:640-647.
10. Ban Y, Davies TF, Greenberg DA, et al. The influence of human leucocyte antigen (HLA) genes on autoimmune thyroid disease (AITD): results of studies in HLA-DR3 positive AITD families. *Clin Endocrinol.* 2002;57:81-88.
11. Baisch JM, Weeks T, Giles R, et al. Analysis of HLA-DQ genotypes and susceptibility in insulin-dependent diabetes mellitus. *N Engl J Med.* 1990;322:1836-1841.
12. Baschal EE, Aly TA, Babu SR, et al. HLA-DPB1*0402 protects against type 1A diabetes autoimmunity in the highest risk DR3-DQB1*0201/DR4-DQB1*0302 DAISY population. *Diabetes.* 2007;56:2405-2409.
13. Zake LN, Ghaderi M, Park YS, et al. MHC class I chain-related gene alleles 5 and 5.1 are transmitted more frequently to type 1 diabetes offspring in HBDI families. *Ann N Y Acad Sci.* 2002;958:309-311.

14. Bilbao JR, Martin-Pagola A, Vitoria JC, et al. HLA-DRB1 and MHC class 1 chain-related A haplotypes in Basque families with celiac disease. *Tissue Antigens.* 2002;60(1):71-76.

15. Park YS, Sanjeevi CB, Robles D, et al. Additional association of intra-MHC genes, MICA and D6S273, with Addison's disease. *Tissue Antigens.* 2002;60:155-163.

16. Menard L, Saadoun D, Isnardi I, et al. The PTPN22 allele encoding an R620W variant interferes with the removal of developing autoreactive B cells in humans. *J Clin Invest.* 2011;121:3635-3644.

17. Habib T, Funk A, Rieck M, et al. Altered B cell homeostasis is associated with type I diabetes and carriers of the PTPN22 allelic variant. *J Immunol.* 2012;188:487-496.

18. Cerosaletti K, Buckner JH. Protein tyrosine phosphatases and type 1 diabetes: genetic and functional implications of PTPN2 and PTPN22. *Rev Diabet Stud.* 2012;9(4):188-200.

19. Bottini N, Musumeci L, Alonso A, et al. A functional variant of lymphoid tyrosine phosphatase is associated with type I diabetes. *Nat Genet.* 2004;36:337-338.

20. van Oene M, Wintle RF, Liu X, et al. Association of the lymphoid tyrosine phosphatase R620W variant with rheumatoid arthritis, but not Crohn's disease, in Canadian populations. *Arthritis Rheum.* 2005; 52:1993-1998.

21. Orozco G, Sanchez E, Gonzalez-Gay MA, et al. Association of a functional single-nucleotide polymorphism of PTPN22, encoding lymphoid protein phosphatase, with rheumatoid arthritis and systemic lupus erythematosus. *Arthritis Rheum.* 2005;52:219-224.

22. Velaga MR, Wilson V, Jennings CE, et al. The codon 620 tryptophan allele of the lymphoid tyrosine phosphatase (LYP) gene is a major determinant of Graves' disease. *J Clin Endocrinol Metab.* 2004;89: 5862-5865.

23. Canton I, Akhtar S, Gavalas NG, et al. A single-nucleotide polymorphism in the gene encoding lymphoid protein tyrosine phosphatase (PTPN22) confers susceptibility to generalised vitiligo. *Genes Immun.* 2005;6:584-587.

24. Criswell LA, Pfeiffer KA, Lum RF, et al. Analysis of families in the multiple autoimmune disease genetics consortium (MADGC) collection: the PTPN22 620W allele associates with multiple autoimmune phenotypes. *Am J Hum Genet.* 2005;76:561-571.

25. Vaidya B, Pearce S. The emerging role of the CTLA-4 gene in autoimmune endocrinopathies. *Eur J Endocrinol.* 2004;150:619-626.

26. Takara M, Kouki T, DeGroot LJ. CTLA-4 AT-repeat polymorphism reduces the inhibitory function of CTLA-4 in Graves' disease. *Thyroid.* 2003;13:1083-1089.

27. Ban Y, Concepcion ES, Villanueva R, et al. Analysis of immune regulatory genes in familial and sporadic Graves' disease. *J Clin Endocrinol Metab.* 2004;89:4562-4568.

28. Ban Y, Tozaki T, Taniyama M, et al. Association of a CTLA-4 3′ untranslated region (CT60) single nucleotide polymorphism with autoimmune thyroid disease in the Japanese population. *Autoimmunity.* 2005;38:151-153.

29. van Belzen MJ, Mulder CJ, Zhernakova A, et al. CTLA4 +49 A/G and CT60 polymorphisms in Dutch coeliac disease patients. *Eur J Hum Genet.* 2004;12:782-785.

30. Ban Y, Davies TF, Greenberg DA, et al. Analysis of the CTLA-4, CD28, and inducible costimulator (ICOS) genes in autoimmune thyroid disease. *Genes Immun.* 2003;4:586-593.

31. Vaidya B, Imrie H, Geatch DR, et al. Association analysis of the cytotoxic T lymphocyte antigen-4 (CTLA-4) and autoimmune regulator-1 (AIRE-1) genes in sporadic autoimmune Addison's disease. *J Clin Endocrinol Metab.* 2000;85:688-691.

32. Jin Y, Mailloux CM, Gowan K, et al. NALP1 in vitiligo-associated multiple autoimmune disease. *N Engl J Med.* 2007;356:1216-1225.

33. Magitta NF, Boe Wolff AS, Johansson S, et al. A coding polymorphism in NALP1 confers risk for autoimmune Addison's disease and type 1 diabetes. *Genes Immun.* 2009;10:120-124.

34. Tomer Y, Greenberg DA, Concepcion E, et al. Thyroglobulin is a thyroid specific gene for the familial autoimmune thyroid diseases. *J Clin Endocrinol Metab.* 2002;87:404-407.

35. Lambert AP, Gillespie KM, Thomson G, et al. Absolute risk of childhood-onset type 1 diabetes defined by human leukocyte antigen class II genotype: a population-based study in the United Kingdom. *J Clin Endocrinol Metab.* 2004;89:4037-4043.

36. Norris JM, Barriga K, Hoffenberg EJ, et al. Risk of celiac disease autoimmunity and timing of gluten introduction in the diet of infants at increased risk of disease. *JAMA.* 2005;293:2343-2351.

37. Norris JM, Barriga K, Klingensmith G, et al. Timing of initial cereal exposure in infancy and risk of islet autoimmunity. *JAMA.* 2003; 290:1713-1720.

38. Ziegler AG, Schmid S, Huber D, et al. Early infant feeding and risk of developing type 1 diabetes-associated autoantibodies. *JAMA.* 2003; 290:1721-1728.

39. Norris JM, Yin X, Lamb MM, et al. Omega-3 polyunsaturated fatty acid intake and islet autoimmunity in children at increased risk for type 1 diabetes. *JAMA.* 2007;298:1420-1428.

40. Hara N, Alkanani AK, Ir D, et al. The role of the intestinal microbiota in type 1 diabetes. *Clin Immunol.* 2013;146:112-119.

41. Wen L, Ley RE, Volchkov PY, et al. Innate immunity and intestinal microbiota in the development of type 1 diabetes. *Nature.* 2008;455: 1109-1113.

42. Endesfelder D, zu Castell W, Ardissone A, et al. Compromised gut microbiota networks in children with anti-islet cell autoimmunity. *Diabetes.* 2014;63:2006-2014.

43. Dunne JL, Triplett EW, Gevers D, et al. The intestinal microbiome in type 1 diabetes. *Clin Exp Immunol.* 2014;177:30-37.

44. Kondrashova A, Hyoty H. Role of viruses and other microbes in the pathogenesis of type 1 diabetes. *Int Rev Immunol.* 2014;33:284-295.

45. Schneider DA, von Herrath MG. Potential viral pathogenic mechanism in human type 1 diabetes. *Diabetologia.* 2014;57:2009-2018.

46. Coles AJ, Wing M, Smith S, et al. Pulsed monoclonal antibody treatment and autoimmune thyroid disease in multiple sclerosis. *Lancet.* 1999;354:1691-1695.

47. Gisslinger H, Gilly B, Woloszczuk W, et al. Thyroid autoimmunity and hypothyroidism during long-term treatment with recombinant interferon-alpha. *Clin Exp Immunol.* 1992;90:363-367.

48. Bosi E, Minelli R, Bazzigaluppi E, et al. Fulminant autoimmune type 1 diabetes during interferon-alpha therapy: a case of Th1-mediated disease? *Diabet Med.* 2001;18(4):329-332.

49. Uchigata Y, Kuwata S, Tsushima T, et al. Patients with Graves' disease who developed insulin autoimmune syndrome (Hirata disease) possess HLA-Bw62/Cw4/DR4 carrying DRB1*0406. *J Clin Endocrinol Metab.* 1993;77:249-254.

50. Wenzlau JM, Moua O, Sarkar SA, et al. SlC30A8 is a major target of humoral autoimmunity in type 1 diabetes and a predictive marker in prediabetes. *Ann N Y Acad Sci.* 2008;1150:256-259.

51. Lohmann T, Sessler J, Verlohren HJ, et al. Distinct genetic and immunological features in patients with onset of IDDM before and after age 40. *Diabetes Care.* 1997;20(4):524-529.

52. Gardner JM, Devoss JJ, Friedman RS, et al. Deletional tolerance mediated by extrathymic Aire-expressing cells. *Science.* 2008;321:843-847.

53. Perheentupa J. APS-I/APECED: the clinical disease and therapy. *Endocrinol Metab Clin North Am.* 2002;31:295-320, vi.

54. Ahonen P, Myllarniemi S, Sipila I, et al. Clinical variation of autoimmune polyendocrinopathy-candidiasis-ectodermal dystrophy (APECED) in a series of 68 patients. *N Engl J Med.* 1990;322:1829-1836.

55. Perheentupa J, Miettinen A. Autoimmune polyendocrinopathy-candidiasis-ectodermal dystrophy. In: Eisenbarth GS, ed. *Endocrine and Organ Specific Autoimmunity.* Austin, TX: RG Landes; 1999:19-40.

56. Neufeld M, Maclaren NK, Blizzard RM. Two types of autoimmune Addison's disease associated with different polyglandular autoimmune (PGA) syndromes. *Medicine.* 1981;60:355-362.

57. Walls AW, Soames JV. Dental manifestations of autoimmune hypoparathyroidism. *Oral Surg Oral Med Oral Pathol.* 1993;75:452-454.

58. Friedman TC, Thomas PM, Fleisher TA, et al. Frequent occurrence of asplenism and cholelithiasis in patients with autoimmune polyglandular disease type I. *Am J Med.* 1991;91:625-630.

59. Bereket A, Lowenheim M, Blethen SL, et al. Intestinal lymphangiectasia in a patient with autoimmune polyglandular disease type I and steatorrhea. *J Clin Endocrinol Metab.* 1995;80:933-935.

60. Ward L, Paquette J, Seidman E, et al. Severe autoimmune polyendocrinopathy-candidiasis-ectodermal dystrophy in an adolescent girl with a novel AIRE mutation: response to immunosuppressive therapy. *J Clin Endocrinol Metab.* 1999;84:844-852.

61. Gianani R, Eisenbarth GS. Autoimmunity to gastrointestinal endocrine cells in autoimmune polyendocrine syndrome type I. *J Clin Endocrinol Metab.* 2003;88:1442-1444.

62. Hogenauer C, Meyer RL, Netto GJ, et al. Malabsorption due to cholecystokinin deficiency in a patient with autoimmune polyglandular syndrome type I. *N Engl J Med.* 2001;344:270-274.

63. Aaltonen J, Bjorses P, Sandkuijl L, et al. An autosomal locus causing autoimmune disease: autoimmune polyglandular disease type I assigned to chromosome 21. *Nat Genet.* 1994;8:83-87.

64. Gardner JM, Metzger TC, McMahon EJ, et al. Extrathymic Aire-expressing cells are a distinct bone marrow-derived population that induce functional inactivation of CD4(+) T cells. *Immunity.* 2013;39: 560-572.

65. Bjorses P, Halonen M, Palvimo JJ, et al. Mutations in the AIRE gene: effects on subcellular location and transactivation function of the autoimmune polyendocrinopathy-candidiasis-ectodermal dystrophy protein. *Am J Hum Genet.* 2000;66:378-392.

66. Halonen M, Kangas H, Ruppell T, et al. APECED-causing mutations in AIRE reveal the functional domains of the protein. *Hum Mutat.* 2004; 23:245-257.

67. DeVoss J, Hou Y, Johannes K, et al. Spontaneous autoimmunity prevented by thymic expression of a single self-antigen. *J Exp Med.* 2006; 203:2727-2735.

68. Anderson MS, Venanzi ES, Chen Z, et al. The cellular mechanism of Aire control of T cell tolerance. *Immunity.* 2005;23:227-239.

69. Liston A, Lesage S, Wilson J, et al. Aire regulates negative selection of organ-specific T cells. *Nat Immunol.* 2003;4:350-354.

70. Cetani F, Barbesino G, Borsari S, et al. A novel mutation of the autoimmune regulator gene in an Italian kindred with autoimmune polyendocrinopathy-candidiasis-ectodermal dystrophy, acting in a

dominant fashion and strongly cosegregating with hypothyroid autoimmune thyroiditis. *J Clin Endocrinol Metab*. 2001;86:4747-4752.

71. Su MA, Giang K, Zumer K, et al. Mechanisms of an autoimmunity syndrome in mice caused by a dominant mutation in Aire. *J Clin Invest*. 2008;118:1712-1726.

72. Meager A, Visvalingam K, Peterson P, et al. Anti-interferon autoantibodies in autoimmune polyendocrinopathy syndrome type 1. *PLoS Med*. 2006;3:e289.

73. Kisand K, Boe Wolff AS, Podkrajsek KT, et al. Chronic mucocutaneous candidiasis in APECED or thymoma patients correlates with autoimmunity to Th17-associated cytokines. *J Exp Med*. 2010;207:299-308.

74. Puel A, Doffinger R, Natividad A, et al. Autoantibodies against IL-17A, IL-17F, and IL-22 in patients with chronic mucocutaneous candidiasis and autoimmune polyendocrine syndrome type I. *J Exp Med*. 2010; 207:291-297.

75. Puel A, Cypowyj S, Bustamante J, et al. Chronic mucocutaneous candidiasis in humans with inborn errors of interleukin-17 immunity. *Science*. 2011;332:65-68.

76. Uibo R, Aavik E, Peterson P, et al. Autoantibodies to cytochrome P450 enzymes P450scc, P450c17, and P450c21 in autoimmune polyglandular disease types I and II and in isolated Addison's disease. *J Clin Endocrinol Metab*. 1994;78:323-328.

77. Ekwall O, Hedstrand H, Haavik J, et al. Pteridin-dependent hydroxylases as autoantigens in autoimmune polyendocrine syndrome type I. *J Clin Endocrinol Metab*. 2000;85:2944-2950.

78. Husebye ES, Boe AS, Rorsman F, et al. Inhibition of aromatic L-amino acid decarboxylase activity by human autoantibodies. *Clin Exp Immunol*. 2000;120:420-423.

79. Hedstrand H, Perheentupa J, Ekwall O, et al. Antibodies against hair follicles are associated with alopecia totalis in autoimmune polyendocrine syndrome type I. *J Invest Dermatol*. 1999;113:1054-1058.

80. Tuomi T, Bjorses P, Falorni A, et al. Antibodies to glutamic acid decarboxylase and insulin-dependent diabetes in patients with autoimmune polyendocrine syndrome type I. *J Clin Endocrinol Metab*. 1996; 81:1488-1494.

81. Alimohammadi M, Bjorklund P, Hallgren A, et al. Autoimmune polyendocrine syndrome type 1 and NALP5, a parathyroid autoantigen. *N Engl J Med*. 2008;358:1018-1028.

82. Barbara Davis Center for Diabetes. Available at: <www.barbaradaviscenter.org>.

83. Betterle C, Scarpa R, Garelli S, et al. Addison's disease: a survey on 633 patients in Padova. *Eur J Endocrinol*. 2013;169:773-784.

84. Umpierrez GE, Latif KA, Murphy MB, et al. Thyroid dysfunction in patients with type 1 diabetes: a longitudinal study. *Diabetes Care*. 2003;26:1181-1185.

85. Hoffenberg EJ, Bao F, Eisenbarth GS, et al. Transglutaminase antibodies in children with a genetic risk for celiac disease. *J Pediatr*. 2000;137: 356-360.

86. Tiberti C, Panimolle F, Bonamico M, et al. Long-standing type 1 diabetes: patients with adult-onset develop celiac-specific immunoreactivity more frequently than patients with childhood-onset diabetes, in a disease duration-dependent manner. *Acta Diabetol*. 2014;51:675-678.

87. Mollazadegan K, Sanders DS, Ludvigsson J, et al. Long-term coeliac disease influences risk of death in patients with type 1 diabetes. *J Intern Med*. 2013;274:273-280.

88. Knip M, Akerblom HK, Becker D, et al. Hydrolyzed infant formula and early beta-cell autoimmunity: a randomized clinical trial. *JAMA*. 2014; 311:2279-2287.

89. The Diabetes Prevention Trial—Type 1 Diabetes Study Group. Effects of insulin in relatives of patients with type 1 diabetes mellitus. *N Engl J Med*. 2002;346(22):1685-1691.

90. Skyler JS, Krischer JP, Wolfsdorf J, et al. Effects of oral insulin in relatives of patients with type 1 diabetes: The Diabetes Prevention Trial—Type 1. *Diabetes Care*. 2005;28:1068-1076.

91. De Bellis A, Bizzarro A, Rossi R, et al. Remission of subclinical adrenocortical failure in subjects with adrenal autoantibodies. *J Clin Endocrinol Metab*. 1993;76:1002-1007.

92. Pescovitz MD, Torgerson TR, Ochs HD, et al. Effect of rituximab on human in vivo antibody immune responses. *J Allergy Clin Immunol*. 2011;128(6):1295-1302.

93. Orban T, Bundy B, Becker DJ, et al. Costimulation modulation with abatacept in patients with recent-onset type 1 diabetes: follow-up 1 year after cessation of treatment. *Diabetes Care*. 2014;37:1069-1075.

94. Rigby MR, DiMeglio LA, Rendell MS, et al. Targeting of memory T cells with alefacept in new-onset type 1 diabetes (T1DAL study): 12 month results of a randomised, double-blind, placebo-controlled phase 2 trial. *Lancet Diabetes Endocrinol*. 2013;1(4):284-294.

95. Lebastchi J, Deng S, Lebastchi AH, et al. Immune therapy and beta-cell death in type 1 diabetes. *Diabetes*. 2013;62:1676-1680.

96. Herold KC, Gitelman SE, Willi SM, et al. Teplizumab treatment may improve C-peptide responses in participants with type 1 diabetes after the new-onset period: a randomised controlled trial. *Diabetologia*. 2013;56:391-400.

97. d'Hennezel E, Bin Dhuban K, Torgerson T, Piccirillo CA. The immunogenetics of immune dysregulation, polyendocrinopathy, enteropathy, X-linked (IPEX) syndrome. *J Med Genet*. 2012;49:291-302.

98. Godfrey VL, Wilkinson JE, Russell LB. X-linked lymphoreticular disease in the scurfy (sf) mutant mouse. *Am J Pathol*. 1991;138: 1379-1387.

99. Chatila TA, Blaeser F, Ho N, et al. JM2, encoding a fork head-related protein, is mutated in X-linked autoimmunity-allergic disregulation syndrome. *J Clin Invest*. 2000;106:R75-R81.

100. Walker MR, Kasprowicz DJ, Gersuk VH, et al. Induction of FoxP3 and acquisition of T regulatory activity by stimulated human CD4+CD25- T cells. *J Clin Invest*. 2003;112:1437-1443.

101. Zhan H, Sinclair J, Adams S, et al. Immune reconstitution and recovery of FOXP3 (forkhead box P3)-expressing T cells after transplantation for IPEX (immune dysregulation, polyendocrinopathy, enteropathy, X-linked) syndrome. *Pediatrics*. 2008;121:e998-e1002.

102. Baud O, Goulet O, Canioni D, et al. Treatment of the immune dysregulation, polyendocrinopathy, enteropathy, X-linked syndrome (IPEX) by allogeneic bone marrow transplantation. *N Engl J Med*. 2001;344:1758-1762.

103. Gambineri E, Ciullini Mannurita S, Robertson H, et al. Gut immune reconstitution in immune dysregulation, polyendocrinopathy, enteropathy, X-linked syndrome after hematopoietic stem cell transplantation. *J Allergy Clin Immunol*. 2015;135(1):260-262.

104. Passerini L, Rossi Mel E, Sartirana C, et al. CD4(+) T cells from IPEX patients convert into functional and stable regulatory T cells by FOXP3 gene transfer. *Sci Transl Med*. 2013;5(215):215ra174.

105. Passerini L, Sio FR, Porteus MH, et al. Gene/cell therapy approaches for immune dysregulation polyendocrinopathy enteropathy X-linked syndrome. *Curr Gene Ther*. 2014;14(6):422-428.

106. Kahn CR, Flier JS, Bar RS, et al. The syndromes of insulin resistance and acanthosis nigricans. Insulin-receptor disorders in man. *N Engl J Med*. 1976;294:739-745.

107. Flier JS, Bar RS, Muggeo M, et al. The evolving clinical course of patients with insulin receptor autoantibodies: spontaneous remission or receptor proliferation with hypoglycemia. *J Clin Endocrinol Metab*. 1978;47:985-995.

108. Malek R, Chong AY, Lupsa BC, et al. Treatment of type B insulin resistance: a novel approach to reduce insulin receptor autoantibodies. *J Clin Endocrinol Metab*. 2010;95:3641-3647.

109. Manikas ED, Isaac I, Semple RK, et al. Successful treatment of type B insulin resistance with rituximab. *J Clin Endocrinol Metab*. 2015; 100(5):1719-1722.

110. Dispenzieri A, Kyle RA, Lacy MQ, et al. POEMS syndrome: definitions and long-term outcome. *Blood*. 2003;101:2496-2506.

111. Latov N. Diagnosis and treatment of chronic acquired demyelinating polyneuropathies. *Nat Rev Neurol*. 2014;10:435-446.

112. Soubrier M, Dubost JJ, Serre AF, et al. Growth factors in POEMS syndrome: evidence for a marked increase in circulating vascular endothelial growth factor. *Arthritis Rheum*. 1997;40:786-787.

113. Watanabe O, Maruyama I, Arimura K, et al. Overproduction of vascular endothelial growth factor/vascular permeability factor is causative in Crow-Fukase (POEMS) syndrome. *Muscle Nerve*. 1998;21: 1390-1397.

114. Harvey JN, Barnett D. Endocrine dysfunction in Kearns-Sayre syndrome. *Clin Endocrinol*. 1992;37:97-103.

115. De Block CE, De Leeuw IH, Maassen JA, et al. A novel 7301-bp deletion in mitochondrial DNA in a patient with Kearns-Sayre syndrome, diabetes mellitus, and primary amenorrhoea. *Exp Clin Endocrinol Diabetes*. 2004;112:80-83.

116. Combs RM. Malignant thymoma, hyperthyroidism and immune disorder. *South Med J*. 1968;61:337-341.

117. Cheng MH, Fan U, Grewal N, et al. Acquired autoimmune polyglandular syndrome, thymoma, and an AIRE defect. *N Engl J Med*. 2010; 362:764-766.

118. Rando TA, Horton JC, Layzer RB. Wolfram syndrome: evidence of a diffuse neurodegenerative disease by magnetic resonance imaging. *Neurology*. 1992;42:1220-1224.

119. Smith CJ, Crock PA, King BR, et al. Phenotype-genotype correlations in a series of Wolfram syndrome families. *Diabetes Care*. 2004;27: 2003-2009.

120. Takeda K, Inoue H, Tanizawa Y, et al. WFS1 (Wolfram syndrome 1) gene product: predominant subcellular localization to endoplasmic reticulum in cultured cells and neuronal expression in rat brain. *Hum Mol Genet*. 2001;10:477-484.

121. Hofmann S, Philbrook C, Gerbitz KD, et al. Wolfram syndrome: structural and functional analyses of mutant and wild-type wolframin, the WFS1 gene product. *Hum Mol Genet*. 2003;12:2003-2012.

122. Osman AA, Saito M, Makepeace C, et al. Wolframin expression induces novel ion channel activity in endoplasmic reticulum membranes and increases intracellular calcium. *J Biol Chem*. 2003;278:52755-52762.

123. Medlej R, Wasson J, Baz P, et al. Diabetes mellitus and optic atrophy: a study of Wolfram syndrome in the Lebanese population. *J Clin Endocrinol Metab*. 2004;89:1656-1661.

124. Shang L, Hua H, Foo K, et al. Beta-cell dysfunction due to increased ER stress in a stem cell model of Wolfram syndrome. *Diabetes*. 2014; 63:923-933.

125. Borgna-Pignatti C, Marradi P, Pinelli L, et al. Thiamine-responsive anemia in DIDMOAD syndrome. *J Pediatr*. 1989;114:405-410.

Endocrinology of HIV/AIDS

STEVEN K. GRINSPOON

KEY POINTS

- In patients infected with human immunodeficiency virus (HIV) adrenal dysfunction is common. Specific protease inhibitors, including ritonavir, may reduce metabolism of inhaled and injected steroids.
- Hypogonadism is often seen among HIV-infected patients, is frequently associated with low or normal gonadotropins, and should be assessed using a specific free testosterone assay, given increases in sex hormone–binding globulin in this population.
- Fracture prevalence is increased among HIV-infected patients and is multifactorial in nature, potentially related to increases in bone turnover, vitamin D deficiency, and gonadal dysfunction.
- Cardiovascular disease is increased among HIV-infected patients and relates to increases in traditional risk factors as well as nontraditional risk factors including immunologic and inflammatory factors.
- Endocrine management of insulin resistance, diabetes mellitus, and dyslipidemia, common among HIV-infected patients, may reduce cardiovascular disease risk in this population.
- AIDS (acquired immunodeficiency syndrome) wasting, characterized by sarcopenia, should be distinguished from HIV lipodystrophy, characterized by subcutaneous fat loss.
- Endocrine strategies may be used to treat sarcopenia in AIDS wasting (testosterone and growth hormone) or to reduce visceral fat (growth hormone–releasing hormone) in HIV lipodystrophy.
- Medications used in the treatment of HIV disease have numerous endocrine and metabolic effects, including effects on steroid metabolism, gonadal function, vitamin D synthesis, renal phosphate excretion, glucose uptake, and very low density lipoprotein metabolism.

HIV disease affects up to 34 million patients worldwide and over 1.4 million in the United States. In many parts of the world, for example, in sub-Saharan Africa, HIV remains epidemic, with an estimated 23.5 million people infected.[1] In addition, the number of HIV-infected patients is growing rapidly in Asia and other parts of the world. Endocrine dysfunction is common among HIV-infected patients. Adrenal, gonadal, thyroid, bone, and metabolic abnormalities have all been reported. HIV itself, related infectious organisms, immune activation, cytokines, and antiretroviral medications may all affect endocrine function. Endocrine disorders in HIV disease, for example, hypogonadism, adrenal insufficiency, diabetes, and bone loss, may cause significant morbidity and are thus important to diagnose. Interactions between antiretroviral therapy (ART) and specific medication may also contribute to endocrine disturbances. Endocrine strategies may improve quality of life and long-term survival through effects on critical metabolic and body composition parameters, including loss of muscle mass (sarcopenia) in AIDS wasting, fat redistribution with loss of peripheral and abdominal subcutaneous fat, and relative or absolute gains in central (visceral) adiposity among some patients. However, diagnosis and treatment may be difficult because of varying nutritional conditions and effects of the varied medications used to treat HIV disease. As HIV patients live longer as a result of the success of antiretroviral medications, adverse effects resulting from these very medications and HIV-related immune dysfunction have resulted in increased cardiovascular risk and metabolic changes that require intervention and long-term management by the endocrine specialist. This chapter will review the prevalence, mechanisms, and optimal treatment strategies for endocrine abnormalities in HIV-infected patients.

ADRENAL FUNCTION

Adrenal dysfunction may be suspected in the patient with advanced HIV disease because of fatigue, hyponatremia, and other features of adrenal insufficiency. Although clinical adrenal dysfunction is relatively rare among patients with AIDS, subtle impairments in adrenal reserve may be seen in this population. Adrenal dysfunction most often is caused by destruction of adrenal tissue by cytomegalovirus (CMV) in patients with advanced HIV disease but may also be caused by medications, hypothalamic/pituitary disease from opportunistic infection, idiopathic inflammation or tissue destruction, or in rare cases, by cortisol resistance. In addition, some features of Cushing syndrome may be seen among HIV-infected patients with fat redistribution, but true Cushing disease is rare.

Adrenal Insufficiency

Biochemical evidence of adrenal insufficiency is relatively common among hospitalized AIDS patients, with 17% of 74 hospitalized AIDS patients screened by cosyntropin test demonstrating inadequate adrenal stimulation (1 hour cortisol < 18 µg/dL) in an early study. In contrast, fewer patients, 4%, demonstrate clinical symptoms of adrenal insufficiency.[2] Among patients with clinical symptoms and signs of adrenal insufficiency, including hyponatremia, a higher percentage, up to 30%, may demonstrate inadequate reserve using cosyntropin testing.[3]

Adrenal insufficiency occurring in the context of advanced HIV disease is most often caused by tissue destruction of the adrenal glands from opportunistic infections. CMV adrenalitis is the most common cause, seen in approximately 40% to 90% of patients with CMV infections at autopsy. However, adrenocortical destruction caused by CMV is usually less than 50% and therefore unlikely to cause adrenal insufficiency,[4] and CMV disease is rare with well-preserved immune function in patients on newer potent antiretroviral therapies. Other organisms and processes that have been associated with adrenal destruction in HIV disease include *Mycobacterium tuberculosis*, *Mycobacterium avium-intracellulare* (MAI), *Cryptococcus*, and hemorrhage. Additionally, pituitary/hypothalamic destruction resulting in secondary adrenal insufficiency may be caused in rare instances by opportunistic infection (e.g., toxoplasmosis, *Cryptococcus*, and CMV). Idiopathic adenohypophyseal necrosis is also observed in a minority of patients, approximately 10% at autopsy, and may be related to a direct effect of HIV.[5]

Glucocorticoid Excess: Adrenal Shunting and Cortisol Resistance

Increased cortisol levels may also be seen in HIV-infected patients. More commonly, increased cortisol levels are seen as a stress response, in association with low weight or increasing degree of illness. Intra-adrenal shunting toward cortisol synthesis, potentially as a result of 17,20-lyase dysfunction, has been suggested by studies demonstrating a reduced dehydroepiandrosterone (DHEA)/cortisol ratio on cosyntropin testing.[6] Cytokine modulation of the hypothalamic-pituitary-adrenal (HPA) axis may also contribute to increased cortisol levels. Interleukin 1 (IL-1), produced in the median eminence, has been shown to increase corticotropin-releasing hormone (CRH) and adrenocorticotropic hormone (ACTH) secretion in vitro and in animal studies. Increased IL-1 secretion from infected monocytes in the median eminence is thus another possible cause of increased cortisol secretion in HIV-infected patients. In turn, higher cortisol levels and greater diurnal variation may reduce T-cell immune activation.[7] Glucocorticoid resistance has also been shown in rare patients with advanced HIV disease, who demonstrate addisonian symptoms, including hyperpigmentation, in the setting of hypercortisolism and increased ACTH.

Medication Effects

Medications may contribute to adrenal insufficiency in HIV patients (Table 41-1). Ketoconazole, an antifungal agent, inhibits side-chain cleavage enzyme and 11β-hydroxylase. These effects are not generally seen with fluconazole, itraconazole, and more recently introduced imidazole derivatives. Phenytoin, opiates, and rifampin, among other drugs, affect cortisol metabolism. For example, adrenal insufficiency may be precipitated by the use of rifampin for treatment of tuberculosis in patients with reduced adrenal reserve. Megestrol acetate, a potent synthetic progestational derivative used as an appetite stimulant, has glucocorticoid properties and decreases ACTH. Abrupt withdrawal of megestrol acetate may precipitate adrenal insufficiency, and such patients should be tested for adrenal insufficiency and receive physiologic glucocorticoid administration as needed after megestrol withdrawal. In addition, megestrol acetate can decrease gonadal function, which should also be monitored during and after therapy. Cases of Cushing syndrome have been described with the concomitant use of fluticasone and ritonavir, via inhibition of CYP3A4 by ritonavir and resultant reduction in metabolism of fluticasone. This combination of medications can result in symptoms of severe cortisol excess and potential severe adrenal insufficiency with discontinuation of fluticasone.[8] Such patients demonstrate very low measured cortisol and ACTH levels, despite symptoms of hypercortisolemia, due to suppression of the endogenous HPA axis by increased concentrations of circulating fluticasone. After discontinuation of the fluticasone, long-term physiologic steroid replacement is necessary until the HPA axis recovers. In addition, adrenal insufficiency has been reported in approximately 5% of patients receiving intra-articular steroids while on protease inhibitors (PIs), particularly ritonavir, with increasing risk seen among those with more than two injections within the prior 6 months.[9]

Clinical Assessment

HIV-infected patients with symptoms of adrenal insufficiency and particularly those with hyponatremia and risk factors for adrenal insufficiency, e.g., known disseminated CMV or recent use of megestrol acetate, should be evaluated. Evaluation of the cortisol axis should proceed as in other patients with suspected adrenal dysfunction. Cosyntropin testing is usually an adequate first step, except in those patients in whom hypothalamic or pituitary insufficiency of recent onset is suspected. In such patients, use of morning cortisol levels, metyrapone, or insulin tolerance testing may be necessary, if there are no contraindications. After adrenal insufficiency is documented, ACTH testing and appropriate imaging are used to localize the defect. In patients with clinical symptoms of adrenal insufficiency and elevated cortisol levels, cortisol resistance may be present and the diagnosis may be made by glucocorticoid receptor studies in blood monocytes. Conversely, in patients with symptoms of adrenal excess and low cortisol and ACTH levels, exogenous steroid use or interactions with ART should be suspected.

GONADAL FUNCTION

Male Gonadal Dysfunction

Gonadal dysfunction is common among HIV-infected men with weight loss and advanced illness. Initial studies indicated biochemical hypogonadism in approximately 50% of men with AIDS, in association with increased disease severity. Among HIV-infected men with low weight, hypogonadism was seen in 20%.[10] More recent studies suggest a lower prevalence of hypogonadism of approximately 9% to 16%.[11-13] The mechanisms of hypogonadism in HIV-infected patients may relate to severe illness or effects of undernutrition on gonadotropin secretion, medication effects, or more rarely, tissue destruction from opportunistic infections. Most often, hypogonadism is secondary in

TABLE 41-1

Major Endocrine and Metabolic Effects of Medications Used in the Treatment of HIV

Endocrine/Metabolic System	Interacting Medication	Mechanism	Effect
Adrenal	Ritonavir	CYP3A4 inhibitor that decreases metabolism of fluticasone and potentially other steroids	Cushing stigmata with reduced ACTH/cortisol
	Ketoconazole	11β-Hydroxylase inhibition	Adrenal insufficiency
	Megestrol acetate	Synthetic progestational agent with glucocorticoid properties	Adrenal insufficiency
	Rifampin	Increased cortisol metabolism	Adrenal insufficiency
Gonadal	Megestrol acetate	Decreased gonadotropins	Hypogonadism
	Ketoconazole	Inhibits side-chain cleavage enzyme	Hypogonadism
	Protease inhibitors	Variable effects to cause hyperprolactinemia directly or via dopamine antagonism	Potential hypogonadism
	Anabolic steroids	Decreased gonadotropins	Hypogonadism
Thyroid	Rifampin	Increased hepatic clearance of thyroid hormone	Reduced thyroxine levels
	Interferon	Autoimmune thyroiditis	Variable effects on thyroid function
Fluid and electrolytes	Trimethoprim	Structural similarities to amiloride with inhibition of tubular potassium secretion	Hyperkalemia
	Tenofovir	Fanconi-like syndrome, phosphate wasting	Hypokalemia
Calcium	Protease inhibitors	Variable effects to inhibit 1α-hydroxylation of 25-hydroxyvitamin D	Hypocalcemia
	Rifabutin	Induces cytochrome P450 and alters vitamin D metabolism	Vitamin D deficiency
	Foscarnet	Complexes with calcium	Decreased ionized calcium, magnesium
	Pentamidine	Renal magnesium wasting	Hypocalcemia
	Ketoconazole	Inhibits 1,25-dihydroxyvitamin D synthesis	Hypocalcemia
Bone	Tenofovir	Phosphate wasting and tubulopathy	Bone loss
	Efavirenz	Vitamin D deficiency	Bone loss
Glucose	Protease inhibitors	Variable effects to inhibit GLUT4-mediated glucose transport	Hyperglycemia
	NRTIs	Variable effects to inhibit mitochondrial DNA polymerase gamma	Hyperglycemia
	Pentamidine	Islet cell inflammation and insulin release	Hypoglycemia and subsequent hyperglycemia
Body composition	Protease inhibitors	Variable effects to inhibit SREBP-1 and PPARγ signaling in subcutaneous fat	Subcutaneous fat loss
	NRTIs	Variable effects to inhibit mitochondrial DNA polymerase gamma in subcutaneous fat	Subcutaneous fat loss
Lipids	Protease inhibitors	Variable effects to decrease lipoprotein lipase-mediated clearance of VLDL and TG	Hypertriglyceridemia
	Anabolic steroids	Possible effects on hepatic lipase and LCAT	Low HDL

ACTH, adrenocorticotropic hormone (corticotropin); GLUT4, glucose transporter type 4; HDL, high-density lipoprotein; HIV, human immunodeficiency virus; LCAT, lecithin:cholesterol acyltransferase; NRTI, nucleoside reverse transcriptase inhibitor; PPAR, peroxisome proliferator-activated receptor; SREB-1, sterol regulatory element–binding protein 1; TG, triglyceride; VLDL, very low density lipoprotein.

nature, with low or inappropriately normal gonadotropin levels, as seen in 91% of patients with reduced free testosterone levels during initiation of highly active antiretroviral therapy (HAART) in the Swiss HIV cohort.[14] Primary hypogonadism is seen less often and may be caused by cytokine effects on the testes, including effects of tumor necrosis factor (TNF) to inhibit steroidogenesis via effects on the side-chain cleavage enzyme and of IL-1 to inhibit Leydig cell steroidogenesis and luteinizing hormone binding to the Leydig cell. Indeed, among young men, median age 45 years, using an early morning total testosterone as a test to define hypogonadism in a large Italian cohort, Rochira and associates demonstrated that gonadotropins were elevated in 16% of patients studied[12] (Fig. 41-1). In addition, opportunistic infections of the testes have rarely been reported and up to 25% of HIV-infected patients with AIDS will demonstrate testicular involvement of widespread opportunistic infection or systemic neoplasms, including CMV, toxoplasmosis, Kaposi sarcoma (KS), and testicular lymphoma, though there are few data to suggest that primary hypogonadism develops in all such cases.

In addition, a number of medications may affect the hypothalamic-pituitary-gonadal (HPG) axis. Ketoconazole inhibits side-chain cleavage enzyme and other critical enzymes in testicular steroidogenesis. Megestrol acetate is used to increase appetite, but as a synthetic progestational agent it suppresses gonadotropin secretion and results in hypogonadism. Opiate therapy affects gonadotropin-releasing hormone (GnRH) secretion and may result in hypogonadotropic hypogonadism.

More recently, increased prolactin levels and gynecomastia have been demonstrated among HIV-infected patients. In a case-control study, gynecomastia was seen in 1.8% of 2275 consecutively screened HIV-infected patients and was associated with hypogonadism, hepatitis C, and degree of lipoatrophy (subcutaneous fat loss associated with potent ART). Thyroid-stimulating hormone (TSH, thyrotropin) levels were increased, although the proportion with hypothyroidism was not different.[15] Hyperprolactinemia has been reported in 21% of HIV-infected men with stable HIV disease and was significantly associated with opioid use and increased CD4 count but not with changes in body composition or gynecomastia.[16] Increased prolactin levels in association with galactorrhea have also been described among patients treated with PIs. The mechanism of this effect is unclear and may relate to a direct stimulation of prolactin secretion by specific PIs or effects on the P450 system to potentiate the dopamine antagonistic effect of other drugs.[17] Dopamine agonists should be used cautiously among HIV-infected men receiving PIs because of the potential for interactions.

Sex hormone–binding globulin (SHBG) levels are increased in 30% to 55% of HIV-infected patients. Therefore,

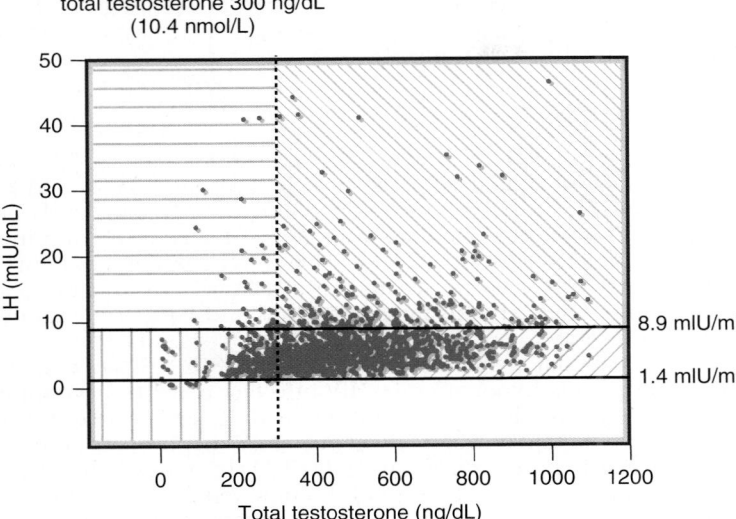

Figure 41-1 Gonadal status according to serum total testosterone threshold of 300 ng/dL and luteinizing hormone (LH) normal range. (From Rochira V, Zirilli L, Orlando G, et al. Premature decline of serum total testosterone in HIV-infected men in the HAART-era. *PLoS One*. 2011;6:e28512, Fig. 2.)

use of bioavailable or free testosterone is recommended to diagnose hypogonadism, because use of total testosterone assays may underestimate the prevalence of true hypogonadism in this population. As a caveat, analogue assays of free testosterone may not be independent of SHBG and should not be used. In contrast, determination of free testosterone by equilibrium dialysis or calculation by an accepted equation are more useful strategies to detect hypogonadism among the HIV population. For example, Monroe and colleagues conducted a large study in the Multicenter AIDS Cohort Study (MACS), comparing normal-weight HIV-infected and well-matched uninfected patients in the current era of ART. In this study, total testosterone levels were similar in HIV-infected versus non–HIV-infected, but free testosterone calculated using the Vermeulen equation was significantly lower in the HIV-infected patients. Reliance on total testosterone alone would have missed 33% of patients with hypogonadism.[11] Use of total testosterone or free testosterone analogue radioimmunoassay to diagnose hypogonadism among HIV-infected patients is associated with poor sensitivities of 25% and 33%, respectively.[13]

In patients in whom acute and chronic illness may contribute to hypogonadism, retesting of gonadal function by measuring an early morning bioavailable testosterone level is recommended upon resolution of the illness, as endogenous function may return with improved health. In patients who remain hypogonadal, administration of physiologic testosterone replacement after appropriate diagnostic workup for the cause of hypogonadism is appropriate. In contrast to the potential utility of specific anabolic steroids in the treatment of weight loss in AIDS wasting (see "Treatment of AIDS Wasting and Loss of Lean Body Mass"), no role has been demonstrated for the use of anabolic steroids alone or in combination with testosterone for the treatment of hypogonadism per se in HIV-infected men.

Female Gonadal Dysfunction

Amenorrhea is seen in approximately 25% of HIV-infected women and may be caused by the reduction of gonadotro-

pin production associated with the stress of illness. In contrast, anovulation may be seen in up to 50% of HIV-infected women in association with reduced CD4 counts. Among anovulatory HIV-infected women, changes in menstrual function are three times as likely compared to normally ovulating patients. Early menopause has been reported in up to 8% of HIV-infected women.[18]

Androgen levels are often reduced in HIV-infected women. In one study, androgen levels, assessed with the use of a free testosterone assay, were reduced below the level seen in age-matched healthy women in over 50% of HIV-infected women with significant weight loss and in over one third of HIV-infected women without weight loss.[19] The mechanisms of androgen deficiency in HIV disease may be caused in part by intra-adrenal shunting toward cortisol production and away from androgen production, particularly in women with significant weight loss[6] (see "Adrenal Function").

THYROID FUNCTION

Altered thyroid function tests (TFTs) are common in HIV-infected patients. Thyroid-binding globulin (TBG) levels are increased in HIV-infected patients and correlate inversely with CD4 counts.[20] Abnormal thyroid function test results may be caused by the stress of illness in patients with advanced disease or concomitant disorders, as found in other patients with euthyroid sick syndrome. However, among adults, some studies have shown that reverse triiodothyronine (rT$_3$) levels do not rise in association with decreasing T$_3$ levels, as one would expect in nonthyroidal illness.[3] Patients with progressive HIV disease therefore exhibit decreased T$_3$ levels, increased TBG, and decreased rT$_3$ levels with increasing illness.

In addition to the euthyroid sick syndrome, large screening studies have demonstrated an increased prevalence of primary hypothyroidism in HIV-infected patients. Recent studies have investigated the prevalence of thyroid dysfunction in the current era of HAART. In one study of 1565 HIV-infected patients, the prevalence of overt hypothyroidism was 2.5% and of overt hyperthyroidism 1%. A higher percentage of patients demonstrated subclinical hypothyroidism (4%) and abnormal thyroid test results associated with nonthyroidal illness (17%). Conversely, 76% of patients demonstrated normal thyroid function tests. HIV therapy and specific antiretroviral medications were not associated with thyroid dysfunction.[21] Among 2437 HIV-infected patients, Nelson and coworkers demonstrated prevalence rates of hyperthyroidism and hypothyroidism each to be 1%.[22] Use of specific antiretroviral agents, including PIs and efavirenz were associated with thyroid dysfunction, but this has not been a consistent finding among studies.

Increased TSH has been demonstrated in young children with average age 1.5 years and failure to thrive. Thyroxine (T_4) levels were normal, but thyrotropin-releasing hormone testing showed exaggerated TSH responses, and growth rates increased in response to thyroid hormone.[23] Fundaro and associates demonstrated increased antithyroglobulin antibodies in 34% of symptomatic HIV-infected children.[24] Increased TSH levels were found in 28% of HIV-infected children, particularly those with severe immunosuppression. In contrast, a larger study in perinatally infected children demonstrated reduced total T_3, total T_4, and free T_4 and increased rT_3, TBG, and TSH, with negative autoantibodies, suggesting a euthyroid sick pattern, particularly in those with severe immunosuppression. HIV-infected children with failure to thrive should be screened for true hypothyroidism, but more often the thyroid function tests will reflect nonthyroidal illness and the severity of immune compromise.[25]

Recently, thyroid dysfunction has been described with an immune reconstitution syndrome in which autoimmune thyroid disease occurs in association with use of potent ART and improved immune function, typically 12 to 36 months after ART is initiated.[26] Graves disease is most often reported in this context. The estimated prevalence for immune reconstitution thyroid disease with initiation of HAART was 3% for women and 0.2% for men.[27] Graves disease has also been described after IL-2 therapy in HIV-infected patients.[28]

In addition to autoimmune causes, thyroid disease related to anatomic replacement and infection of the thyroid has been reported in HIV-infected patients. *Pneumocystis* thyroiditis has been reported to cause a painful thyroiditis-like picture, with hyperthyroidism followed by hypothyroidism, decreased uptake on scanning, and a firm but tender gland. *Pneumocystis* thyroiditis may result from the use of inhaled pentamidine, which is associated with extrapulmonary *Pneumocystis* infections.

CMV, MAI, *Cryptococcus*, and KS have been demonstrated in the thyroid on autopsy but have not been related to clinical thyroid disease among patients with AIDS. Clinically apparent thyroidal abscesses from *Aspergillus* and *Rhodococcus equi* have been reported. Hypothalamic/pituitary replacement from opportunistic infections, such as toxoplasmosis and CMV, has also been reported to cause secondary hypothyroidism.

Medications may affect thyroid function. Rifampin influences hepatic clearance of T_4, and interferon is associated with an increased incidence of autoimmune hypothyroidism.

FLUID BALANCE AND ELECTROLYTES

Disorders of fluid balance and electrolytes are common among patients with AIDS. Hyponatremia may be seen in upward of 50% of patients and is most often related to the syndrome of inappropriate secretion of antidiuretic hormone (SIADH). Hyperkalemia is also frequently reported and may be seen in association with various drugs, such as trimethoprim. More rarely, hyperkalemia may be associated with adrenal insufficiency.

Sodium

Hyponatremia (sodium < 130 mmol/L) is seen in 40% to 60% of hospitalized patients with AIDS and 20% of outpatients. SIADH (volume-replete patients with low levels of serum sodium, and inappropriately elevated levels of urine osmolarity) is seen in 23% to 47% of hyponatremic patients. SIADH may be caused by various infections and tumors and is treated with fluid restriction and hypertonic saline if severe.

Adrenal insufficiency is documented in 30% of volume-depleted, hyponatremic HIV-infected patients.[29] Volume depletion (diarrhea, vomiting) with excessive free water and impaired water clearance (HIV nephropathy) may cause hyponatremia among ill HIV-infected patients, especially those in the hospital. Volume repletion is the treatment. Hyporeninemic hypoaldosteronism,[30] more typically associated with hyperkalemia, may be another cause of hyponatremia and is treated with mineralocorticoids. The use of medications such as vidarabine, miconazole, and pentamidine is associated with hyponatremia of unknown cause. Hypernatremia may be caused by foscarnet-induced nephrogenic diabetes insipidus.

Potassium

Hyperkalemia occurs in 20% to 53% of AIDS patients on trimethoprim because of structural similarities to amiloride and inhibition of tubular potassium excretion.[31] Other potential causes include pentamidine-associated tubular nephropathy, HIV-nephropathy (glomerular sclerosis), primary adrenal insufficiency, and, rarely, hyporeninemic hypoaldosteronism. Physiologic studies investigating potassium balance in HIV-infected patients also suggest an inadequate aldosterone response to hyperkalemia in HIV-infected patients. A Fanconi-like syndrome with tubular dysfunction, phosphate wasting, and hypokalemia has been described with the use of tenofovir and more rarely with adefovir, cidofovir, and didanosine.[32]

CALCIUM HOMEOSTASIS AND BONE CHANGES

Calcium Homeostasis

Hypocalcemia is common in HIV-infected patients. Hypocalcemia, based on albumin-adjusted total calcium levels, was demonstrated in 6.5% of a large cohort of HIV-infected patients with AIDS. Calcium levels decreased progressively with stage of disease. Among patients with hypocalcemia, 48% were vitamin D deficient, and the expected increase in parathyroid hormone (PTH) levels was lacking in the majority.[33] Jaeger and colleagues also demonstrated decreased PTH secretion in severely immunocompromised patients with AIDS, but the mechanism is unknown.[34] In addition, decreased PTH levels may occur in the setting of hypomagnesemia during severe illness or in association with renal magnesium wasting. Vitamin D deficiency may be caused by malabsorption from AIDS enteropathy or by specific effects of antiretroviral drugs (e.g., inhibition of 1α-hydroxylation of 25-hydroxyvitamin D by PIs).[35] Severe vitamin D deficiency of nutritional origin has also been described in HIV-infected children. Recently, Earle and coworkers described three cases of Fanconi syndrome in HIV-infected adults, characterized by excess phosphate excretion and osteomalacia in the context of tenofovir and cedofovir administration.[36] Osteomalacia was also associated with use of rifabutin for MAI in an HIV-infected patient. Rifabutin induces cytochrome P450, which may affect vitamin D metabolism. Other drugs that induce P450 could have a similar effect. A number of drugs may affect calcium homeostasis (see Table 41-1). Foscarnet complexes with calcium to decrease ionized calcium levels and may also induce severe hypomagnesemia. Pentamidine therapy has been associated with renal magnesium wasting and severe hypomagnesemia, which may, in turn, cause hypocalcemia, through decreased PTH release and resistance to circulating PTH. Ketoconazole inhibits 1,25-dihydroxyvitamin D synthesis. Among patients with HIV disease, hypercalcemia can be caused by excessive 1,25-dihydroxyvitamin D production in the setting of granulomatous disease (tuberculosis) or lymphoma; by local osteoclastic bone resorption from disseminated CMV; or by human T-cell lymphotropic virus 1 (HTLV-1)-related activation of parathyroid hormone–related protein (PTHrP). Immune reconstitution–associated hypercalcemia has been described in the setting of ART initiation among patients with known tuberculosis, in whom immune reconstitution results in increased granulomatous activity and 1,25-dihydroxyvitamin D production.[37]

Bone Loss: Prevalence, Etiologic Factors, and Treatment Strategies

Studies performed recently in the current era of ART give an estimate of the prevalence and risk factors for progression of bone loss among HIV-infected patients. Bonjoch and associates investigated 671 HIV-infected patients and demonstrated osteopenia in 47.5% and osteoporosis in 23%.[38] Progression rates to osteopenia and osteoporosis were 12.5% and 15.6% over 2.5 years of follow-up and 18% and 29% over 5 years of follow-up. In this large cohort, factors associated with progression of bone loss were age, male sex, lower BMI, PI use, and tenofovir use.[38] Significant bone loss has also been shown among postmenopausal HIV-infected women, with time since menopause and traditional risk factors most significantly associated with bone loss. In a longitudinal analysis of postmenopausal HIV-infected women, Yin and coworkers demonstrated increased markers of bone resorption and annualized bone loss in HIV-infected women versus non–HIV-infected control subjects (Fig. 41-2).[39]

Specific antiretroviral strategies may affect bone in the HIV population. Studies demonstrate that switching to a tenofovir-based regimen is associated with bone loss and increased bone turnover[40,41] (Fig. 41-3). Strong evidence for an effect of tenofovir is shown in studies in which patients at risk for HIV are given single agent tenofovir for preexposure prophylaxis. In these patients, bone loss averaged approximately 1% compared to control subjects over 2 years of follow-up. Larger effects might be seen in less healthy HIV-infected patients with other comorbid contributors.[42]

Recent data suggest that immunologic factors including T-cell activation,[43] low CD4 cell count,[44] and coinfection with hepatitis B and C are strongly related to reduced bone density, particularly among women.[45] These data suggest the need to assess and follow bone density in HIV-infected patients with specific risk factors, for example, older age, long-term ART use, low body mass index (BMI), hypogonadism, hepatitis, low CD4 count, and tenofovir use.

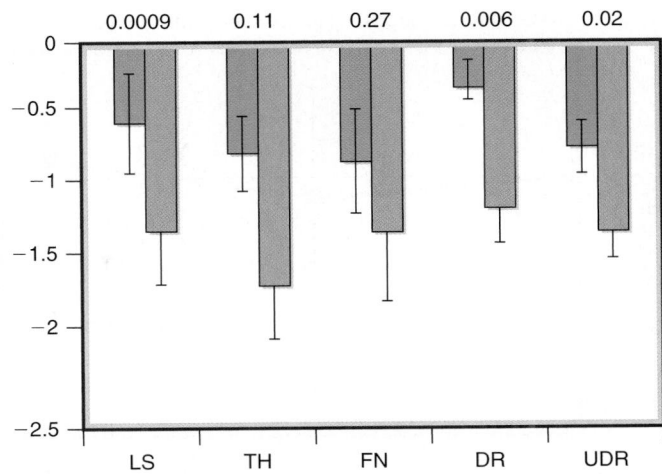

Figure 41-2 Annualized percentage change in bone mineral density (BMD) in human immunodeficiency virus (HIV)-negative ($n = 55$; *teal bars*) and HIV-positive ($n = 73$; *purple bars*) women. P values are adjusted for BMD at baseline visit. DR, distal radius; FN, femoral neck; LS, lumbar spine; TH, total hip; UDR, ultradistal radius. (From Yin MT, Zhang CA, McMahon DJ, et al. Higher rates of bone loss in postmenopausal HIV-infected women: a longitudinal study. *J Clin Endocrinol Metab.* 2012;97: 554-562, Fig. 2, used with permission.)

Endocrine factors may contribute to reduced bone density in HIV-infected patients, including hypogonadism, relative GH deficiency, and vitamin D deficiency. GH pulse area determined from overnight frequent sampling was reduced in patients with central fat accumulation and correlated significantly with vertebral bone density.[46] This relationship may explain in part the inverse association between increased visceral fat and reduced bone density in HIV-infected patients.[47] Vitamin D deficiency is common among HIV-infected patients. In a study of ambulatory clinic patients in London, the prevalence of 25-hydroxyvitamin D deficiency (<20 ng/mL) and severe 25-hydroxyvitamin D deficiency (<10 ng/mL) was 58.5% and 12.6%, respectively.[48] In a large cohort of 2044 consecutively followed HIV patients in Brussels, the prevalence of severe vitamin D deficiency using the 10-ng/mL cutoff was 32.4%.[49] Among HIV-infected patients in the study, advanced disease (CD4 < 200 cells/mm³) and current use of efavirenz were significantly associated with severe vitamin D deficiency.[49] In carefully conducted case matching studies the odds ratio (OR) for vitamin D deficiency in HIV versus non–HIV-infected patients tended to be increased at 1.46, though this did not reach statistical significance.[50] Tenofovir may increase PTH and bone turnover, potentially related to effects on proximal tubule phosphate reabsorption or other effects. PIs may also inhibit 1α-hydroxylase and result in vitamin D deficiency.[35]

Studies in HIV-infected patients receiving HAART have investigated markers of bone resorption and formation and found evidence of increased bone turnover.[51] Tebas and colleagues evaluated serum and urine bone markers in 73 HIV-positive patients receiving PI therapy.[52] Increased serum bone alkaline phosphatase and urine N-telopeptide were found to be inversely correlated with bone mineral density T- and Z-scores measured by dual energy x-ray absorptiometry (DXA), suggesting an increased rate of bone turnover among HIV-infected patients receiving PI therapy.[52] Recent data investigating the receptor activator for nuclear factor κB ligand (RANKL) system demonstrate reduced soluble RANKL in HIV-infected patients,[53,54] arguing against activation of this system as a mechanism

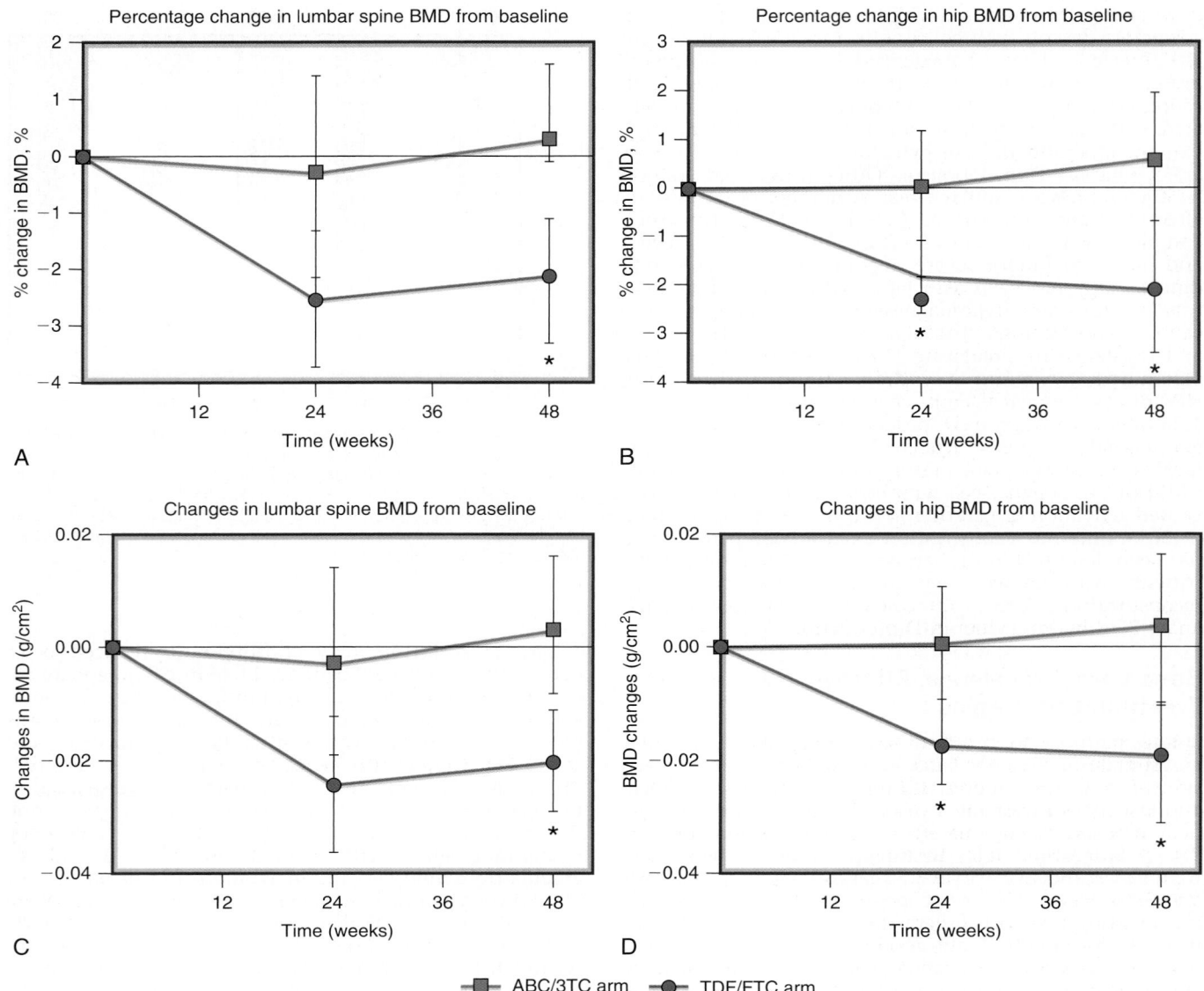

Figure 41-3 Changes from baseline in hip and lumbar spine BMD. Percentage and absolute mean changes from baseline in lumbar spine (**A**, **C**) and hip (**B**, **D**) bone mass density as measured by dual energy x-ray absorptiometry (DXA). ABC/3TC, abacavir/lamivudine; BMD, bone mineral density; TDF/FTC, tenofovir/emtricitabine. Error bars show 95% confidence intervals. (From Rasmussen TA, Jensen D, Tolstrup M, et al. Comparison of bone and renal effects in HIV-infected adults switching to abacavir or tenofovir based therapy in a randomized trial. *PLoS One.* 2012;7:e32445, Fig. 2.)

for increased bone turnover in HIV-infected patients. In contrast, increased osteoprotegerin was shown among HIV-infected women with low bone density, suggesting a compensatory increase in the context of low bone density and high bone resorption rates.[55]

A number of recent studies have examined fracture rates among HIV-infected patients. In a U.S.-based data registry study, the overall fracture prevalence was 2.87 versus 1.77 per 100 persons for HIV versus non–HIV-infected patients.[56] In a large cohort study performed in Europe, significantly increased adjusted hazard ratios for hip and major fracture were 4.7 and 1.8, with an increased relative risk of fracture among older HIV-infected patients in the study[57] (Fig. 41-4). In a Veterans Administration (VA) cohort of men, Womack and coworkers demonstrated that increased fragility fractures were strongly associated with higher frailty score, low BMI, alcohol-related diagnoses, white race, proton pump inhibitor use, and PI use.[58] In a study limited to women, lifetime fragility fractures were significantly

more common in HIV-infected versus non–HIV-infected women (OR 1.7 95%, confidence interval [CI] 1.1-2.6).[59] Use of the FRAX (Fracture Risk Assessment Tool) score to predict fragility fracture has shown relative poor sensitivity but good specificity among HIV-infected patients.[60] In partial contrast to the data on bone density, data from nonrandomized longitudinal cohorts demonstrate that overall use of PIs, nucleoside reverse transcriptase inhibitors (NRTIs), and non-NRTIs (NNRTIs) is associated with reduced fracture rates, whereas the effects of individual drugs vary. Low CD4 count, hepatitis, and diabetes are independently related to increased fracture risk.[61] These data suggest that overall effects of ART may be to improve bone through effects on improving immune function and virologic factors, but adverse effects of specific ART agents on bone may also be important.[62]

Limited data are available on treatment strategies for bone loss in HIV-infected patients. Among patients with idiopathic bone loss and high bone turnover, recent studies

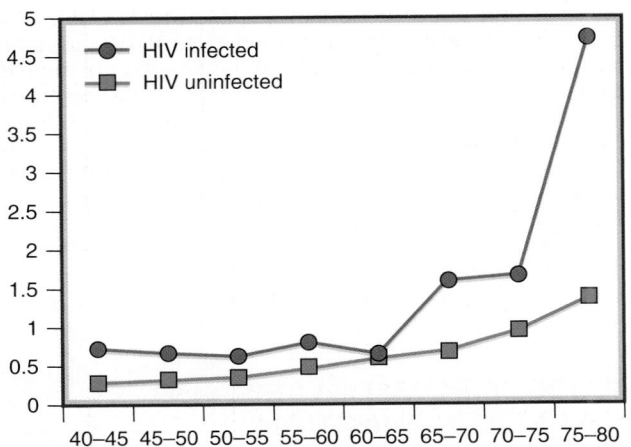

Figure 41-4 Age-specific fracture incidence rates (per 100 person-years) in human immunodeficiency virus (HIV)-infected versus uninfected patients. (From Guerri-Fernandez R, Vestergaard P, Carbonell C, et al. HIV infection is strongly associated with hip fracture risk, independently of age, gender, and comorbidities: a population-based cohort study. *J Bone Miner Res.* 2013;28:1259-1263, Fig. 1, used with permission.)

suggest that alendronate is effective in increasing bone density among HIV-infected patients, with studies demonstrating increases in lumbar spine bone density from 3.4% to 5.2% over 42 weeks and good safety tolerability, albeit in relatively small numbers of patients.[63,64] Use of longer acting bisphosphonates (e.g., zoledronate) showed even greater changes in spinal bone density of 8.9% over 2 years in a randomized, placebo-controlled study.[65] Importantly, significant differences persisted for bone density and bone turnover between groups 5 years after the final dose, suggesting potent, persistent effects after short-term dosing (Fig. 41-5).[66] Although studies suggest a high prevalence of vitamin D deficiency in HIV and an effect of vitamin D supplementation on PTH and bone turnover markers, data demonstrating an effect of vitamin D supplementation on bone density in HIV-infected adults with vitamin D deficiency are not available. Among men with AIDS wasting, testosterone at high doses (200 mg/week) has been shown to increase bone density.[67]

Bone Metabolism in HIV-Infected Children

Reduced bone density has also been reported in HIV-infected children. O'Brien and associates demonstrated reduced total-body bone density in perinatally infected girls at age 9 in association with increased *N*-telopeptide and PTH levels.[68] In a 2013 study, HIV-infected children age 12 to 13 years had a greater prevalence of low bone density compared to HIV-exposed but uninfected children, though these differences were attenuated after height and weight adjustment, suggesting that delays in growth may account for differences in bone density.[69] Among young HIV-infected adults age 20 to 25 years, Tanner stage 5, infected either perinatally or during adolescence, volumetric bone density as well as cortical and trabecular thickness on high-resolution peripheral quantitative computed tomography (HR-pQCT) was reduced, suggesting lower peak bone mass among HIV-infected patients.[70] In contrast to increased markers of resorption, reduced osteocalcin levels have been reported in HIV-infected children, suggesting reduced bone formation and a relative discrepancy between increased resorption and reduced formation in this group.[71] Similar to data in adults, bone density is

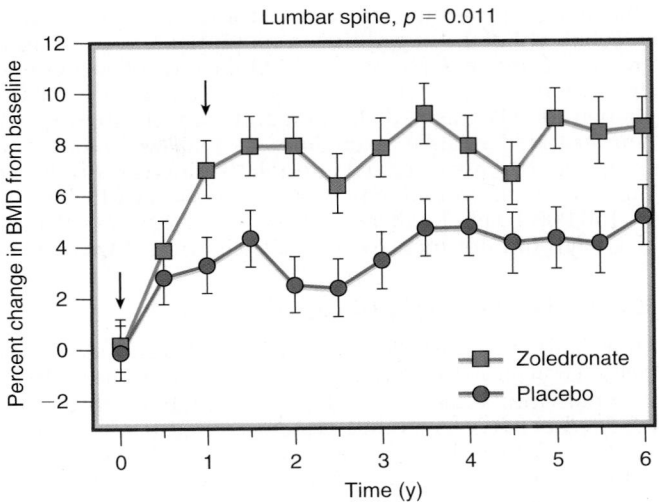

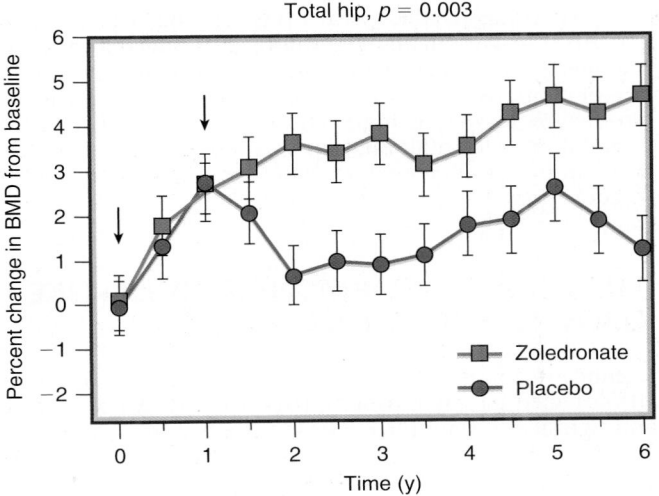

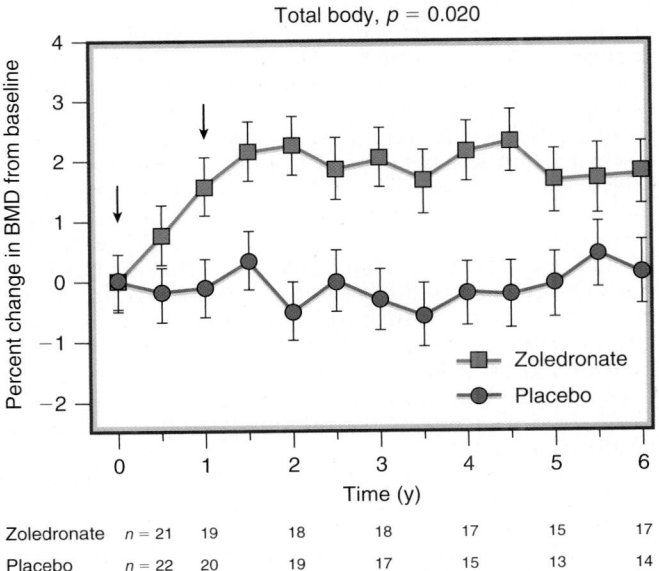

Zoledronate	n = 21	19	18	18	17	15	17
Placebo	n = 22	20	19	17	15	13	14

Figure 41-5 The effects of two annual doses of 4 mg zoledronate or placebo (indicated by *arrows*) on bone mineral density (BMD) at the lumbar spine, total hip, and total body. Data are mean (SE) percentage change from baseline. *P* values are for the time × treatment interaction. SE, standard error. (From Bolland MJ, Grey A, Horne AM, et al. Effects of intravenous zoledronate on bone turnover and bone density persist for at least five years in HIV-infected men. *J Clin Endocrinol Metab.* 2012;97:1922-1928, Fig. 3, used with permission.)

related to insulin-like growth factor 1 (IGF-1) in HIV-infected children, suggesting a potential effect of low growth hormone (GH) on bone.[72] Mora and colleagues followed bone density longitudinally over 1 year to compare changes in HIV-infected children and control subjects and demonstrated relative reductions in total body but not spinal bone density accrual and relative increases in bone turnover.[73] Among children, supplementation with vitamin D (100,000 IU cholecalciferol every 2 months and calcium [1 g/day]) did not increase bone density over 2 years.[74]

Avascular Necrosis of Bone

Miller and coworkers demonstrated a 4.4% prevalence of avascular necrosis (AVN) among 339 asymptomatic HIV-infected individuals.[75] A significant relationship was reported between AVN and prior use of systemic corticosteroids. Other potential factors significantly associated with an increased risk of AVN included the presence of anticardiolipin antibodies as well as routine bodybuilding and its associated mechanical stress. Alcohol use may also be a factor associated with AVN among HIV-infected patients.[76] In a recent analysis among HIV-infected patients, osteonecrosis of the bone was associated with exposure to one or more ART drugs and high triglyceride and cholesterol levels, as well as high serum IgE.[77] A role for altered coagulation and inflammation was also suggested by the observation of increased D-dimer among patients with osteonecrosis.[78]

THE GROWTH HORMONE/INSULIN-LIKE GROWTH FACTOR 1 AXIS

Significant abnormalities in the GH/IGF-1 axis occur in HIV-infected patients. Among patients with AIDS wasting and significant weight loss, GH levels are increased in association with reduced IGF-1 levels, a pattern typical of GH resistance seen with malnutrition. In contrast, in the setting of visceral fat accumulation, frequent sampling of GH levels over 24 hours has suggested a different pattern.[79] Mean overnight GH and GH pulse amplitude were decreased in this setting, whereas pulse frequency was not different compared to age-matched and BMI-matched nonlipodystrophic HIV and non–HIV-infected patients. Reduced GH levels were strongly predicted by increased visceral fat in the patients. A role for suppression of GH release by free fatty acids (FFAs) was suggested by experiments in which acipimox, a nicotinic acid derivative that blocks peripheral tissue lipolysis and lowers FFA levels, was administered. Peak GH response to GH–releasing hormone (GHRH) was increased in response to acipimox, in inverse association to the change in FFA.[80] Physiologic studies of GH in HIV-infected patients suggest a schema whereby increased somatostatin tone, reduced ghrelin, and increased lipolysis contribute to reduced GH secretion in viscerally obese HIV-infected patients with lipodystrophic changes in fat distribution.[80]

GH deficiency is a potential cause of growth failure in HIV-infected children, and treatment with GH results in improved auxologic parameters in such children.[81] Increased IGF-binding protein 3 (IGFBP3) proteolysis and reduced IGF-1, IGFBP3, and acid-labile subunit of the IGFBP3 ternary complex are demonstrated among HIV-infected children with failure to thrive.[82] IGF-1 and IGFBP3 responses to GH may be impaired in HIV-infected children, suggesting a degree of GH insensitivity in this population. These responses may improve with weight gain and

improved immune function in response to HAART.[83] GH deficiency may also disrupt normal thymic development in HIV-infected children. GH has been used to increase height in HIV-infected children with normal GH responses to stimulatory testing.[81] Among HIV-infected children, reduced GH secretion is associated with excess visceral adiposity. Among adults, GH is Food and Drug Administration (FDA) approved for the treatment of AIDS wasting. In addition, a GHRH analogue, tesamorelin, is FDA approved to reduce excess visceral fat accumulation in HIV lipodystrophy (see discussion under "Treatment of Metabolic and Body Composition Changes in HIV-Infected Patients").

GLUCOSE HOMEOSTASIS AND PANCREATIC FUNCTION

Disorders of glucose homeostasis were relatively infrequent prior to the institution of potent ART but may result from use of specific antiretroviral agents and are commonly seen in association with dyslipidemia and fat redistribution in the current era of HAART (see "Metabolic and Body Composition Changes in HIV-Infected Patients"). The pancreas is a frequent target of opportunistic infections and malignancies in patients with HIV disease. However, clinical endocrine dysfunction rarely results, except in cases of massive pancreatic replacement from lymphoma or KS. For example, opportunistic infections of the pancreas are seen on postmortem examination but are rarely clinically relevant. More commonly, pancreatitis and hypoglycemia follow use of certain drugs, such as pentamidine, didanosine, or zalcitabine. Hypoglycemia can result from pentamidine administration secondary to islet cell inflammation and insulin release, especially in the context of high-dose therapy and azotemia. Subsequently, chronic hyperglycemia from pancreatic B cell destruction may follow pentamidine use. Megestrol acetate use has been associated with new-onset diabetes mellitus (DM) because of its potent glucocorticoid action. Pancreatitis is common among patients with HIV and most often related to a drug effect, i.e., pentamidine, trimethoprim-sulfamethoxazole, didanosine, and zalcitabine. In a large study of almost 6000 patients followed for 23,460 person-years at the Johns Hopkins HIV Clinic, the incidence of acute pancreatitis was 5.1/1000 person-years between 2001 and 2006. Low CD4 count, aerosolized pentamidine, and female gender were associated with pancreatitis. In contrast, specific antiretroviral medications were not.[84] In the EuroSIDA study, a lower incidence of pancreatitis was seen since 2001, 1.27/1000 person-years, and again low CD4 count was predictive. Similar to the data from the Hopkins cohort, no association was seen between cumulative exposure to ART and exposure to didanosine and stavudine, NRTIs that have been associated with pancreatitis.[85] Amylase levels may also be elevated in HIV-infected patients secondary to macroamylasemia and salivary amylase.

METABOLIC AND BODY COMPOSITION CHANGES IN HIV-INFECTED PATIENTS

HIV-infected patients demonstrate a number of changes in body composition and metabolism. These changes are present to varying degrees among HIV-infected patients and are multifactorial in nature related in part to the HIV virus itself, inflammation, specific antiretroviral drugs, and the interplay of these factors.[86,87] Of importance, some of these changes may contribute to increased cardiovascular disease (CVD) and respond to changes in ART, lifestyle modification (LSM), and specific pharmacologic strategies (e.g., to improve lipids or insulin sensitivity).

The AIDS Wasting Syndrome and Loss of Lean Body Mass

Wasting was initially a common feature of progressive HIV disease, which was known originally as "slim disease." The AIDS wasting syndrome is currently defined by weight less than 90% ideal body weight or weight loss greater than 10% over 3 months. It is characterized by a disproportionate loss of lean body mass, with a relative sparing of body fat, particularly in men. In women, fat mass may be lost disproportionately with disease progression. The loss of lean body mass occurs early and may antedate weight loss. Muscle wasting, weakness, and increased resting energy expenditure of 8% to 9% are also features of this disease. Macallan and associates demonstrated that energy expenditure fell during periods of rapid weight loss but less than the decrease in caloric intake.[88] Cytokines associated with severe illness may increase energy expenditure and decrease appetite. In addition, chronic weight loss may be associated with gastrointestinal disease, including malabsorption. Weight loss is a significant predictor of mortality rate in HIV infection, with BMI less than 18.4 kg/m^2 associated with a 2.2-fold increase in mortality rate and BMI less than 16.0 kg/m^2 associated with a 4.4-fold increase in mortality rate.[89] Hypogonadism is observed in 30% to 50% of men with AIDS wasting and may contribute to loss of lean body mass[90] (see "Gonadal Function").

In contrast to the traditional paradigm of wasting, recent data suggest HIV disease may be associated with overweight and obesity, particularly in developed countries with emerging obesity epidemics. In one study, performed at a large urban clinic for HIV-infected patients located in the southern United States, the prevalence of underweight was less than 10% and the prevalence of overweight and obesity was 44% despite high viral load at ART initiation.[91] With ART, 20% of patients increased from normal to overweight or overweight to obese (Fig. 41-6).[91] Subjects with more severe immune dysfunction and using boosted PIs tended to gain the most weight with ART.

Changes in Fat Mass and Distribution

The most commonly seen change in body composition among HIV-infected patients is loss of abdominal and peripheral subcutaneous fat, including loss of subcutaneous fat in the face.[92] Other changes that may also be seen include relative preservation of central fat, with relative accumulation of excess visceral fat and excess upper trunk fat.[92,93] In addition, ectopic fat collections can be seen, including in the dorsocervical area. Increased fat deposition in the liver and muscle is also seen and is associated with insulin resistance. In prospective studies of antiretroviral-naïve patients beginning treatment, including an NRTI and PI, initial gains in both peripheral subcutaneous and central fat depots are seen with reversal of the catabolic wasting state in association with control of viral infection. These changes are followed by subsequent decreases in peripheral fat and relative preservation and even absolute gains in central fat. Recent data from the Study of Fat Redistribution and Metabolic Change in HIV Infection (FRAM study) demonstrate that increases in visceral fat and reductions in limb fat are independently associated with increased mortality rate in HIV-infected patients (Fig. 41-7).[94]

The cause of relative central fat accumulation remains unknown. For example, it remains unknown whether this is a direct effect of specific antiretroviral drugs and whether abnormal nutrient partitioning to relatively preserved central adipose stores, less affected by NRTI administration and mitochondrial toxicity, may contribute. In contrast, a number of mechanisms have been shown to contribute to the fat loss seen peripherally. NRTIs can inhibit mitochondrial DNA polymerase gamma and contribute to mitochondrial dysfunction. Use of specific NRTIs, including older NRTIs such as stavudine, has been associated with apoptosis of fat and reduced mitochondrial DNA in vitro and in vivo, as well as reduced expression of lipid metabolism genes, and clinically with reduced subcutaneous fat and lipoatrophy.[95,96] PIs may have direct effects on adipogenesis (via inhibition of nuclear localization of sterol regulatory element–binding protein 1 [SREBP1] and reduction in peroxisome proliferator-activated receptor-γ [PPARγ] expression).[97] NRTIs and PIs have been associated with increased lipolysis in vivo and in vitro.

Recent evidence suggests that genetic polymorphisms may predispose to changes in body composition and metabolic alterations in HIV-infected patients receiving ART. Such findings could indicate a gene-environment interaction contributing to such changes. For example, single nucleotide polymorphisms in the resistin gene were seen to predict the development of dyslipidemia, insulin resistance, and limb fat loss in response to a specific antiretroviral regimen.[98] In the same study, polymorphisms in the hemachromatosis gene and specific mitochondrial gene haplotypes were also associated with increased limb fat loss.[99] Specific haplotypes of the Fas gene (APOC3), PPAR gene, and adrenergic receptor have also been associated with the development of lipoatrophy.[100]

Other studies suggest early molecular changes in the fat of patients with subsequent peripheral adipose tissue loss. Kratz and colleagues showed that reduced expression of messenger RNA (mRNA) encoding lipoprotein lipase and the transcription factors SREBP1, PPARγ, and CCAAT/enhancer binding protein C/EBPα in thigh subcutaneous fat were associated with the loss of fat, before it became evident clinically, whereas increased levels of mRNA

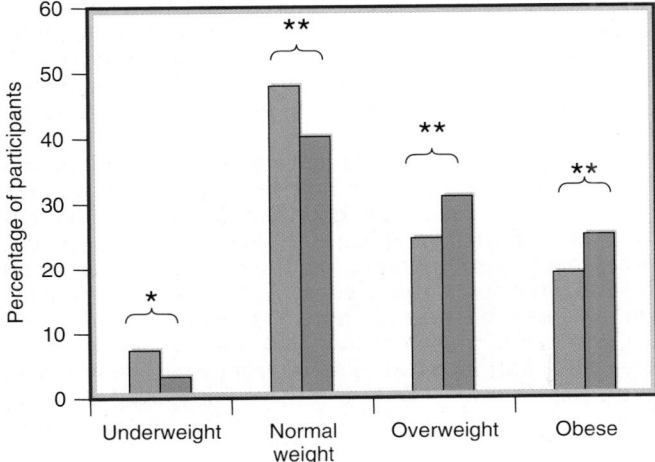

Figure 41-6 Proportion of study sample by body mass index (BMI) category at antiretroviral therapy initiation vs. 2 years on therapy among treatment-naïve human immunodeficiency virus (HIV)-infected patients at the University of Alabama at Birmingham 1917 HIV/AIDS Clinic, 2000-2008. Purple bars = therapy initiation; teal bars = 24 months. * = $p < 0.05$; ** = $p < 0.01$. (From Tate T, Willig AL, Willig JH, et al. HIV infection and obesity: where did all the wasting go? *Antivir Ther.* 2012;17:1281-1289, Fig. 2A, used with permission.)

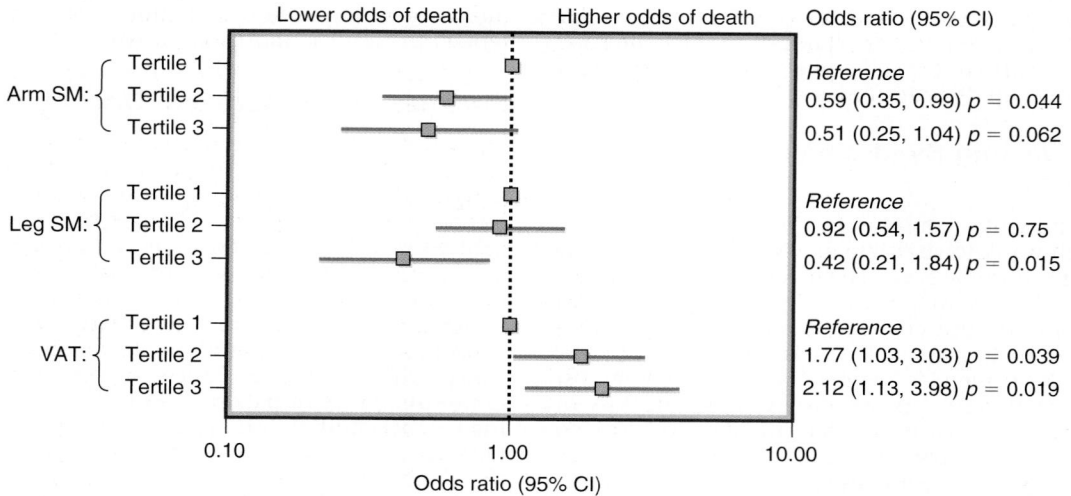

Figure 41-7 Multivariable adjusted associations of magnetic resonance imaging–measured skeletal muscle and adipose tissue with 5-year mortality rate in human immunodeficiency virus (HIV)-infected FRAM participants. The x-axis is on $\log_{10}$ scale. Estimates from multivariable adjusted models controlling for age, sex, race, traditional cardiovascular disease risk factors, HIV-related factors, C-reactive protein, fibrinogen, eGFR cys (estimated glomerular filtration rate using cystatin C), albuminuria, arm SM, leg SM, and VAT. Reference category is tertile 1, those with the lowest amount of muscle or adipose tissue. CI, confidence interval; SM, skeletal muscle; VAT, visceral adipose tissue. (From Scherzer R, Heymsfield SB, Lee D, et al. Decreased limb muscle and increased central adiposity are associated with 5-year all-cause mortality in HIV infection. *AIDS.* 2011;25(11):1405-1414, Fig. 1, used with permission.)

encoding hydroxysteroid 11β-dehydrogenase 1 and the transcription factor C/EBPβ were found in adipose tissue from patients with preservation of subcutaneous fat mass.[101]

Changes in fat distribution have been most widely recognized since the introduction of HAART, but abnormal fat distribution can be seen in antiretroviral-naïve patients, suggesting that viral factors also may contribute. In this regard, recent data suggest that adipose tissue dysfunction may be related to a viral accessory protein, Vpr, which may simultaneously coactivate the glucocorticoid receptor and repress PPARγ.[102]

The changes in fat distribution seen among HIV-infected patients bear some similarities to those in Cushing syndrome, with dorsocervical fat accumulation and centripetal fat distribution. However, more specific stigmata of true Cushing syndrome, including proximal muscle weakness, facial plethora, thin skin, bruising, and violaceous striae, have not been seen, and thus these changes constitute a pseudo-Cushing syndrome.[103] Miller and coworkers observed normal cortisol levels and adequate suppression in response to dexamethasone among HIV-infected patients with cushingoid features.[103] Yanovski and associates compared HIV-infected patients with PI-associated lipodystrophic changes in fat to control patients and those with true Cushing syndrome.[104] In contrast to patients with true Cushing syndrome, patients with PI-associated lipodystrophy demonstrated normal diurnal variation in cortisol levels. Twenty-four-hour urine free cortisol levels were reduced and 17-hydroxysteroid levels were increased compared to levels in control subjects. Among HIV-infected patients with changes in fat distribution, increased 11β-hydroxysteroid dehydrogenase expression in subcutaneous adipose tissue (SAT) has been demonstrated in association with an increased ratio of urinary cortisol to cortisone metabolites and may also contribute to increased cortisol production.[105] In addition, as noted earlier, viral proteins may activate the glucocorticoid receptor in specific fat depots.[102]

Other abnormalities of steroid metabolism have been noted in association with changes in fat distribution. In a longitudinal evaluation, the development of lipodystrophy was associated with reduced DHEA, increased cortisol/

DHEA ratio, and increased interferon-alpha (IFN-α).[106] Increased cortisol regeneration from affected fat depots may contribute to insulin resistance and further fat redistribution.

Lipid Abnormalities

Lipid abnormalities are highly prevalent among HIV-infected patients, particularly those with changes in fat distribution and increased visceral fat and upper trunk fat. Hypertriglyceridemia has long been associated with HIV infection, was observed prior to the introduction of potent ART, and is related in part to increased very low density lipoprotein (VLDL) secretion and decreased clearance.[107] The cause of these changes is not known but may relate to the effects of viral infection itself, microbial translocation via lipopolysaccharide (LPS),[108] altered cytokines including IFN-α,[109] or increased apolipoprotein E.[110] In longitudinal studies, reduction in high-density lipoprotein (HDL), total cholesterol, and LDL cholesterol has been observed with seroconversion. With antiretroviral treatment, cholesterol and LDL rise to preinfection levels but low HDL levels persist.[111]

Among HIV-infected patients receiving combination ART including a PI, hypercholesterolemia (>240 mg/dL), hypertriglyceridemia (>200 mg/dL), and low HDL (<35 mg/dL) were reported in 27%, 40%, and 27%, respectively, compared to corresponding percentages of 8%, 15%, and 26% in previously untreated patients.[112] Among patients with changes in fat distribution, 57% demonstrated hypertriglyceridemia and 46% low HDL in comparison to an age- and BMI-matched cohort from the Framingham Offspring Study.[113] Recent studies also suggest more atherogenic small dense LDL among HIV-infected patients with lipodystrophy.[114] In addition, investigators have demonstrated increased triglyceride enrichment of LDL and impaired hepatic lipase, suggesting impaired lipoprotein processing, further contributing to atherogenic dyslipidemia.[115]

Dyslipidemia among HIV-infected patients may result from the effects of antiretroviral drugs, including specific PIs, which have been shown to increase triglyceride levels.

Use of PIs may also be associated with an atherogenic dyslipidemia and an increase in small dense LDL,[116] increased apolipoprotein C-III and apolipoprotein E, and decreased proteosomal degradation of apolipoprotein B.[117,118] Mulligan and colleagues demonstrated that changes in lipid levels occur within 3 months of PI therapy.[119] Hypertriglyceridemia is most severe among patients treated with ritonavir or the ritonavir/saquinavir combination. Among the currently approved PIs, atazanavir is least often associated with hyperlipidemia.[120] Lipid changes appear to be less and improve with use of atazanavir, in contrast to other PIs.[121] NNRTIs may raise total cholesterol and non-HDL cholesterol but also raise HDL cholesterol.[122]

Hyperglycemia and Insulin Resistance

Insulin resistance and DM are relatively common among HIV-infected patients. In an early longitudinal study, DM was 3.1 times more likely to develop in HIV-infected patients receiving combination ART than in control subjects.[123] More recent studies confirm increased risk of DM prior to 2000 but found equivalent rates among HIV-infected and non–HIV-infected patients in the era of modern ART with agents less likely to contribute to glucose abnormalities.[124] These estimates suggest a peak incidence of 23.2/1000 patient-years immediately prior to 2000 that has decreased to less than 10/1000 patient-years, with no difference between subjects naïve to and those using ART (Fig. 41-8).[125] Increased BMI, lipodystrophy, low CD4 counts, and exposure to specific, older ART medications including stavudine and indinavir are predictive of DM in the HIV population.[124] HIV-infected patients with impaired glucose tolerance demonstrate hyperinsulinemia, suggesting insulin resistance contributes to the development of impaired glucose homeostasis in this population.

Hemoglobin A_{1c} has been shown to underestimate levels of blood glucose in HIV-infected patients, particularly those with increased mean corpuscular volume resulting from specific ART agents. In one study, use of an A_{1c} cutoff of 5.8% optimized the area under the curve for the diagnosis of DM and increased sensitivity from 40.9% to 88.8%, while simultaneously decreasing specificity from 97.5% to 77.5% compared to use of a cutoff of 6.5%.[126]

Insulin resistance among HIV-infected patients may be caused by the abnormal fat distribution itself (e.g., increased central adiposity, loss of peripheral subcutaneous fat, and associated molecular changes). These changes include altered cytokines (e.g., low adiponectin, increased resistin, or elevated TNF) or changes in other processes such as mitochondrial dysfunction, increased lipolysis, increased proteolysis, increased expression of suppressor of cytokine signaling 1 (SOCS1),[127] and increased accumulation of fat in the muscle and liver. Increased inflammation after initiation of ART is associated with development of DM among HIV-infected patients,[128] and metabolic changes may result from persistent microbial translocation across the gastrointestinal barrier resulting in increased levels of LPS in the blood, despite viral suppression.[129] Metabolic abnormalities in HIV have been shown to be associated with increased levels of retinol-binding protein 4 (RB4), which may further contribute to insulin resistance.[130] Rarely, insulin receptor autoantibodies may develop among HIV-infected patients experiencing an immune reconstitution syndrome during ART initiation.[131] In addition, significant evidence suggests direct effects of specific antiretrovirals to reduce insulin sensitivity. PIs have been

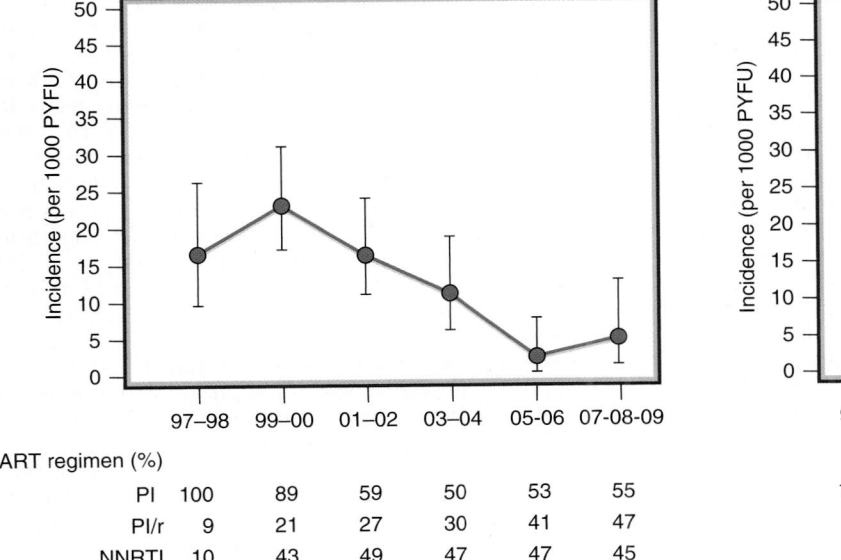

ART regimen (%)	97–98	99–00	01–02	03–04	05-06	07-08-09
PI	100	89	59	50	53	55
PI/r	9	21	27	30	41	47
NNRTI	10	43	49	47	47	45
Stavudine	69	66	46	25	13	7
Indinavir	47	35	19	12	5	3
Didanosine	31	36	35	31	24	15

A

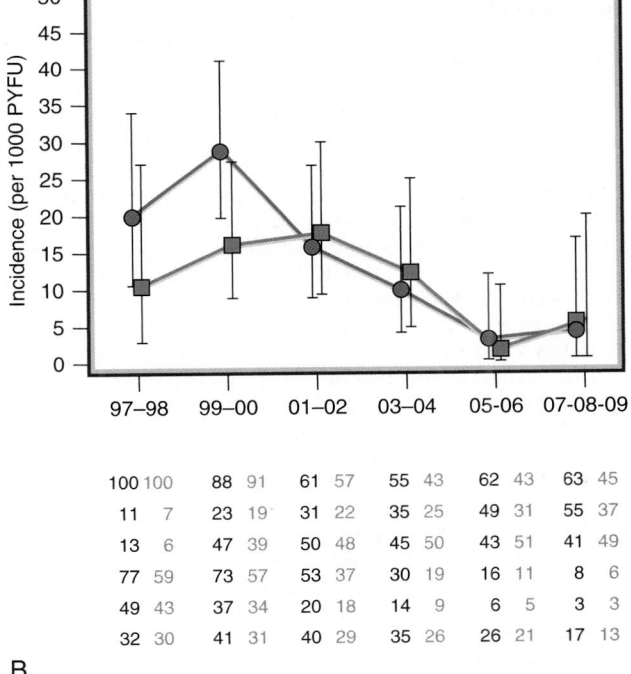

	97–98		99–00		01–02		03–04		05-06		07-08-09	
PI	100	100	88	91	61	57	55	43	62	43	63	45
PI/r	11	7	23	19	31	22	35	25	49	31	55	37
NNRTI	13	6	47	39	50	48	45	50	43	51	41	49
Stavudine	77	59	73	57	53	37	30	19	16	11	8	6
Indinavir	49	43	37	34	20	18	14	9	6	5	3	3
Didanosine	32	30	41	31	40	29	35	26	26	21	17	13

B

Figure 41-8 Calendar incidence of new-onset diabetes and antiretroviral exposure in the ANRS CO8 APROCO-COPILOTE cohort. Diabetes incidence per 1000 PYFU over the period from 1997 to 2009 is indicated for two groups: **A**, all included patients and **B**, patients who had never previously been treated with ART prior to PI initiation (ART-naïve, teal line) or patients who had previously been treated with ART (non-naïve, purple line). The percentages of patients receiving various drugs during follow-up are presented below the graphs (in graph B, gray lettering corresponds to ART-naïve patients). Vertical lines indicate 95% confidence intervals. ART, antiretroviral therapy; NNRTI, nonnucleoside analogue reverse transcriptase inhibitor; PI, protease inhibitor; PI/r, ritonavir-boosted PI; PYFU, person-years of follow-up. (From Capeau J, Bouteloup V, Katlama C, et al. Ten-year diabetes incidence in 1046 HIV-infected patients started on a combination antiretroviral treatment. *AIDS*. 2012;26:303-314, Fig. 1, used with permission.)

shown to decrease glucose uptake by inhibiting the transport function of GLUT4 (glucose transporter type 4) in vitro[132] and have been shown to reduce insulin sensitivity in vivo.[133] Effects to decrease beta cell apoptosis and compromise insulin secretion have also been postulated.[134] NRTIs are associated with insulin resistance, which may be a direct effect, potentially related to mitochondrial toxicity[135] or through effects on subcutaneous fat.[96] For more details of the metabolic effects of specific ART agents, see Table 41-1. The specific manifestations and course of DM in HIV patients have not been well studied, but initial studies suggest an increased risk of albuminuria in HIV-infected patients, particularly those with increased viral load, independent of blood pressure.[136]

Treatment of Metabolic and Body Composition Changes in HIV-Infected Patients

There are a number of options available for the treatment of body composition and metabolic abnormalities in HIV-infected patients.

Treatment of AIDS Wasting and Loss of Lean Body Mass

Testosterone has been used successfully to increase lean body mass in men with AIDS wasting. Randomized studies of intramuscular testosterone for hypogonadal men with AIDS wasting suggest a beneficial effect of testosterone administration on lean body mass (2.0 kg over 6 months) and improved quality of life.[137] Although a limited number of studies have shown a benefit of anabolic steroids in HIV-infected patients with wasting, these agents potently suppress endogenous gonadal function and may thus cause hypogonadism. Methyltestosterone and anabolic steroids may cause problems with the liver including peliosis hepatitis, worsening liver function, and potentially malignancy. In addition, high-dose oxandrolone suppressed endogenous testosterone levels, significantly increased transaminase levels, and increased LDLs.[138] Recently, nandrolone (100 mg intramuscularly every other week) was shown to be effective in increasing weight and lean body mass in HIV-infected women with weight loss.[139] Anabolic steroids are associated with decreased HDL and other side effects, including effects on the liver, and hold no advantage over natural testosterone in the treatment of hypogonadism associated with AIDS-related weight loss. Short-term use of anabolic steroids may be considered in eugonadal patients with severe wasting, but may be associated with adverse effects and should generally be avoided. DHEA may be used to improve mood and depression among HIV-infected patients with subsyndromal depression and dysthymia,[140] but the use of DHEA has not been standardized particularly with respect to dose, duration of treatment, and clinical end points, and thus it remains investigational.

A number of studies have investigated androgen administration to HIV-infected women with low weight. These studies have investigated testosterone using a transdermal patch designed to deliver low physiologic doses of 150 to 300 µg/day. Among studies using the 150-µg/day dose, functional capacity and strength significantly improved with a trend toward increased lean body mass over 6 months. Hirsutism was not seen, and virilization did not occur. An 18-month randomized, placebo-controlled study conducted among relatively androgen-deficient HIV-infected women demonstrated that 300 µg/day increased lean body mass and bone density at the hip and improved depression indices without aggravation of lipid or glucose parameters.[141] Preliminary studies have investigated the effects of DHEA on androgen levels in HIV-infected

premenopausal women, but the clinical utility of this strategy in HIV-infected women remains unknown.

Megestrol acetate is a synthetic progestational agent with glucocorticoid-like properties. Randomized studies in the literature show that megestrol acetate increases weight 3 to 4 kg over 12 weeks with an increase in caloric intake.[142,143] However, the change in weight is almost entirely fat mass without an increase in lean body mass. In addition, megestrol acetate, because of its glucocorticoid-like properties, is associated with a number of side effects, including hypogonadism and hyperglycemia, and abrupt withdrawal can precipitate adrenal crisis. In children, megestrol acetate promotes weight gain without improving linear growth.[144]

A number of other agents have been used in the setting of AIDS wasting. Thalidomide blocks the action of TNF-α and decreases esophageal ulcers in AIDS patients. Clinical studies demonstrate a modest beneficial short-term effect of thalidomide on weight indices but significant associated adverse effects, including rash and fever. Human chorionic gonadotropin results in increased testosterone levels and may have independent effects to inhibit KS. No data are available from randomized, controlled studies to determine effects on wasting in humans.

In addition, patients with AIDS wasting may demonstrate a typical pattern of nutrition-related GH resistance (see "The Growth Hormone/Insulin-like Growth Factor 1 Axis"). These patients exhibit elevated GH levels but decreased IGF-1, the primary hormone mediating the action of GH on muscle, suggesting GH resistance.[145,146] GH has been used in HIV-infected patients to increase lean body mass in sarcopenic patients with AIDS wasting. Among patients with AIDS wasting, high-dose, supraphysiologic GH (0.1 mg/kg/day) has been investigated. Relatively small but significant effects on weight (1.6 kg) were seen over 3 months in a placebo-controlled study.[147] GH administration at 0.1 mg/kg has also been shown to increase work output during treadmill exercise[147] and quality of life as well as peripheral muscle oxygen extraction and utilization in patients with AIDS wasting.[148] These studies suggest that large doses of GH may be necessary to significantly increase lean mass in patients with AIDS wasting and nutritionally mediated resistance to GH. However, high-dose GH is associated with side effects including hyperglycemia and fluid retention[149] and is not well tolerated in the long term. For these reasons, caution should be used with respect to long-term high doses of GH for treatment of AIDS wasting, because this treatment may cause acute and chronic side effects of GH excess. At high doses, GH was shown to increase thymic mass and circulating CD4 cells in one study[150] and to induce HIV-1 specific T-cell responses at low doses (0.7 mg/day) in patients on effective ART,[151] but further studies are needed to investigate the effects of GH on the immune axis.

A multidisciplinary approach to the AIDS wasting syndrome is most useful. Optimization of ART is paramount in conjunction with provision of adequate nutrition and protein intake. However, even in this context, weight and muscle loss may occur, because of the highly catabolic nature of the disease. In such cases, endocrine evaluation should include assessment of gonadal function, which will often be reduced. GH levels are increased in AIDS wasting, but supraphysiologic administration, as approved by the FDA, can further increase lean body mass. This strategy is best reserved for severe wasting refractory to other treatments. Other therapeutic strategies that increase weight by stimulating appetite, including megestrol acetate, are not associated with gain in lean body mass and may be associated with side effects. In the current era of HAART, lipoatrophy, usually associated with antiretroviral use, should be distinguished from traditional wasting. Whereas true AIDS wasting involves sarcopenia and requires anabolic strategies to increase muscle mass, the presence of severe lipoatrophy suggests the need for strategies to spare fat loss.

Strategies for Treating Lipoatrophy and Subcutaneous Fat Loss

Antiretroviral switching to less toxic NRTIs or PIs may be useful for improving changes in fat distribution and hyperlipidemia.[152] For example, one study demonstrated that switching off lopinavir/ritonavir to atazanavir/ritonavir improved glucose trafficking into muscle, reduced triglyceride levels (by 182 mg/dL on average), and decreased visceral fat by 25%.[121] Other studies have demonstrated significant increases in SAT and reductions in visceral adipose tissue (VAT) after switching to a nonthymidine analogue-based ART strategy.[153] LSM and resistance training is unlikely to reverse the loss of subcutaneous fat often seen in HIV-infected patients receiving ART.

Treatments for Visceral Fat Accumulation

LSM, in combination with exercise, may improve lipid levels and visceral adiposity among HIV-infected patients.[154] Progressive resistance training (PRT) may also significantly improve glucose homeostasis in HIV-infected patients through a reduction in muscle adiposity.[155] Recent studies of LSM in HIV-infected patients modeled after the Diabetes Prevention Program demonstrate effects of LSM to improve cardiorespiratory fitness and raise levels of HDL and C-reactive protein (CRP)[156] but did not show significant effects on body composition.

Limited data are now available on the use of testosterone among relatively androgen-deficient HIV-infected men with abdominal fat accumulation (waist-to-hip ratio > 0.95 or waist circumference > 100 cm).[157] Ten grams of topical testosterone daily did not improve visceral fat mass, but reduced overall trunk fat by 15% relative to placebo over 24 weeks. Significant effects on glucose and insulin were not seen. Effects of high-dose testosterone and anabolic steroids on lipid parameters may limit utility of this class of drugs to reduce visceral fat in HIV-infected patients. Moreover, recent studies among older male non–HIV-infected patients suggest that testosterone use may be associated with increased CVD events.[158,159] Use of testosterone among HIV-infected men should be limited to those with documented hypogonadism, among whom treatment may improve lean body mass and bone.

GH has also been used to reduce visceral fat in HIV-infected patients with central fat accumulation. Lo and coworkers investigated low-dose, long-term GH over 18 months in HIV-infected patients with central fat accumulation and deficient responses to GHRH-arginine testing. Low-dose GH was shown to reduce VAT by 9% over 18 months, simultaneously lowering blood pressure and triglyceride level. Even with low-dose GH, however, 2-hour glucose increased, demonstrating that GH is potentially useful in decreasing central fat accumulation but is hard to titrate in a population with significant insulin resistance.[160] Largely because of its ability to aggravate glucose, GH was not approved by the FDA for HIV lipodystrophy.

In contrast, GH secretagogues have been used successfully to increase lean body mass and reduce visceral and truncal fat, without significant effects on glucose. In the combined analysis of two large, randomized, placebo-controlled phase III trials of over 800 patients, GHRH(1-44) (tesamorelin) reduced VAT by 15.4% relative to placebo in HIV-infected patients with central fat accumulation. Improvements were noted in triglyceride level, equal to 43 mg/dL, total cholesterol, and cholesterol-to-HDL ratio. Further improvements in body composition were seen over 12 months (Fig. 41-9).[161] Interestingly, no clinically significant effect to reduce SAT was seen, and thus GHRH(1-44) was selective for VAT. Use of GHRH(1-44) was associated with physiologic increases in IGF-1 levels and was not associated with increased glucose or insulin levels, in contrast to low-dose GH. Larger reductions in visceral fat were associated with improvements in lipid and glucose levels, as well as adiponectin, suggesting metabolic improvements

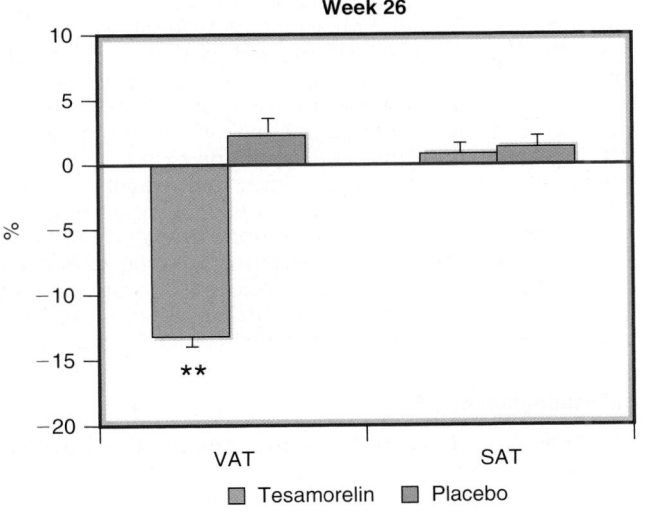

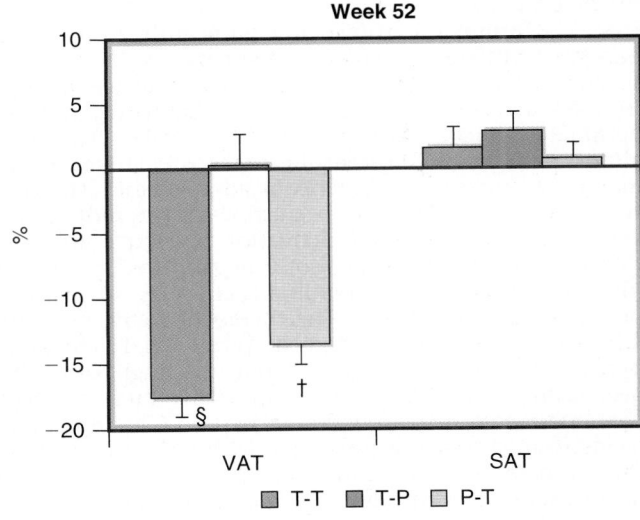

Figure 41-9 Percent change from baseline in VAT and SAT at 26 (**A**) and 52 (**B**) weeks. Data are mean ± SEM. **, $p < 0.001$ vs. placebo; §, $p < 0.001$ vs. baseline and vs. T-P; †, $p < 0.001$ vs. baseline; SAT, subcutaneous adipose tissue; SEM, standard error of the mean; T-T, tesamorelin for initial 26 weeks and subsequent 26 weeks; T-P, tesamorelin for initial 26 weeks and placebo for subsequent 26 weeks; P-T, placebo for initial 26 weeks and tesamorelin for subsequent 26 weeks; VAT, visceral adipose tissue. (From Falutz J, Mamputu JC, Potvin D, et al. Effects of tesamorelin (TH9507), a growth hormone-releasing factor analog, in human immunodeficiency virus-infected patients with excess abdominal fat: a pooled analysis of two multicenter, double-blind placebo-controlled phase 3 trials with safety extension data. *J Clin Endocrinol Metab.* 2010;95:4291-4304, Fig. 2, used with permission.)

with VAT reduction.[162] Recently GHRH(1-44) was also shown to improve liver fat in association with visceral fat, suggesting beneficial effects on other ectopic fat depots.[163] Discontinuation of both GH and GHRH resulted in reaccumulation of visceral fat back to baseline levels, demonstrating that the effects of these agents do not outlast the treatment period.[164-166] GHRH(1-44) was approved by the FDA for the treatment of central fat accumulation in HIV-infected patients in 2010.

Insulin-Sensitizing Strategies

Significant insulin resistance occurs among HIV-infected patients, in association with use of specific antiretroviral agents, changes in fat distribution, and other factors. Metformin is particularly appropriate for use in patients with significant truncal adiposity and increased FFA concentrations, in whom insulin resistance is in part attributable to increased hepatic glucose production. In addition, metformin has a modestly favorable effect on lipids. In patients with hyperlipidemia, metformin has been demonstrated to decrease triglyceride and LDL levels without adversely affecting other parameters. The modest 10% to 20% reduction in plasma triglyceride levels is thought to be caused by decreased hepatic VLDL production.

The effects of metformin have been investigated in HIV-infected patients with central fat accumulation and insulin resistance. Using a dose of 500 mg orally twice a day in a randomized, placebo-controlled 12-week study,[167] Hadigan and associates demonstrated that administration of low-dose metformin over 12 weeks significantly reduced insulin resistance, diastolic blood pressure, tissue plasminogen activator (tPA), and plasminogen activator inhibitor (PAI) concentrations and tended to reduce abdominal visceral fat, thus improving the CVD risk profile of such patients.[167,168] The effects of metformin were sustained over 9 months.[169] Other studies of metformin in HIV-infected patients also demonstrate general improvements in markers of insulin sensitivity but less consistent effects on abdominal fat.[170] In a randomized trial, the effects of metformin and PRT were compared to metformin alone, and the addition of PRT to metformin further improved central adiposity, blood pressure, and insulin resistance.[171] Compared to LSM, metformin was shown to significantly reduce coronary artery calcium in HIV-infected patients.[156]

The loss of subcutaneous fat in HIV-infected patients may further contribute to insulin resistance by limiting peripheral glucose and triglyceride uptake. Therefore, attention has focused on insulin-sensitizing strategies that may act to increase subcutaneous adipogenesis. The thiazolidinediones (TZDs) have been shown to promote adipogenesis, primarily through activation of PPARγ. Although the TZDs have effects on both hepatic and peripheral insulin resistance, the dominant effect is to improve peripheral glucose uptake. The therapeutic efficacy of the TZDs has been questioned among non–HIV-infected patients, in whom rosiglitazone, but not pioglitazone, has been associated with increased mortality rate.[172] Weight has reported to increase in response to TZDs, in contrast to metformin, which is associated with weight loss. Nonetheless, based on the known effects of TZDs to stimulate insulin sensitivity through PPARγ and promote adipogenesis, this strategy has been investigated in HIV-infected patients with subcutaneous fat loss and insulin resistance.

In a 3-month randomized, placebo-controlled study involving 28 patients selected based on insulin resistance, rosiglitazone was shown to improve insulin sensitivity, adiponectin, FFA, and subcutaneous fat mass.[173] In contrast, an effect of rosiglitazone on subcutaneous fat was not shown over 48 weeks in patients with lipoatrophy, selected for fat loss but not for insulin resistance.[174] Adiponectin levels significantly increased and resisting levels decreased in response to rosiglitazone among HIV-infected patients. Rosiglitazone may be effective in increasing subcutaneous fat in selected subpopulations of HIV-infected patients, particularly those with insulin resistance,[175] but significant adverse effects on lipid levels, particularly LDL, suggest that pioglitazone may be better in this regard. Slama and colleagues investigated pioglitazone among HIV-infected patients with confirmed lipoatrophy in a large, randomized placebo-controlled trial.[176] Pioglitazone increased peripheral fat and improved HDL levels, suggesting the potential utility among HIV-infected patients with insulin resistance and fat atrophy. Overall, the glitazones contrast with metformin in terms of effects on lipid and body composition but demonstrate similar effects to improve glucose in HIV-infected patients (Fig. 41-10).[177]

Recently, attention has focused on mitochondrial function, which is significantly affected by NRTI therapy in HIV-infected patients. Mallon and associates have shown that simultaneous use of NRTIs may reduce effects of TZD agents to promote subcutaneous adipogenesis in HIV-infected patients with lipoatrophy by limiting effects of rosiglitazone to increase adipose expression of PPARγ.[178] In addition, therapies for mitochondrial dysfunction, including increasing glutathione with cysteine and glycine supplementation, have been shown to improve mitochondrial fat and carbohydrate oxidation and insulin sensitivity in small studies among HIV-infected patients.[179] L-Acetylcarnitine was shown to decrease intramyocellular lipid accumulation and to increase percentage of leg fat while decreasing FFA in an open label study[180] and then was shown to increase T-cell mitochondrial DNA but to have no effect on body composition and metabolic indices in a second randomized study.[181] Studies to date using strategies to improve mitochondrial function are small, and further research is needed in this area.

Leptin Treatment for Metabolic Dysregulation Among HIV-Infected Patients With Lipoatrophy

Leptin levels are low in association with fat loss and lipoatrophy in HIV-infected patients. Initial small studies of leptin administration to HIV-infected patients with lipoatrophy and reduced leptin levels demonstrated significant improvements in insulin sensitivity, HDL, and triglyceride and reduced truncal and visceral fat.[182,183] Among patients with mixed lipoatrophy and lipohypertrophy, but low leptin levels, leptin administration improved total cholesterol and non-HDL cholesterol as well as glucose parameters but not HDL or triglyceride or lipid kinetics.[184] Because leptin reduces appetite, administration may be associated with weight loss. Further studies are needed to understand the clinical potential of leptin to improve metabolic parameters and fat redistribution among HIV-infected patients.

Lipid Management

See "Strategies for Hyperlipidemia Among HIV-Infected Patients."

CARDIOVASCULAR DISEASE IN HIV-INFECTED PATIENTS

CVD is increased among HIV-infected patients. Traditional risk factors for CVD in HIV-infected patients include

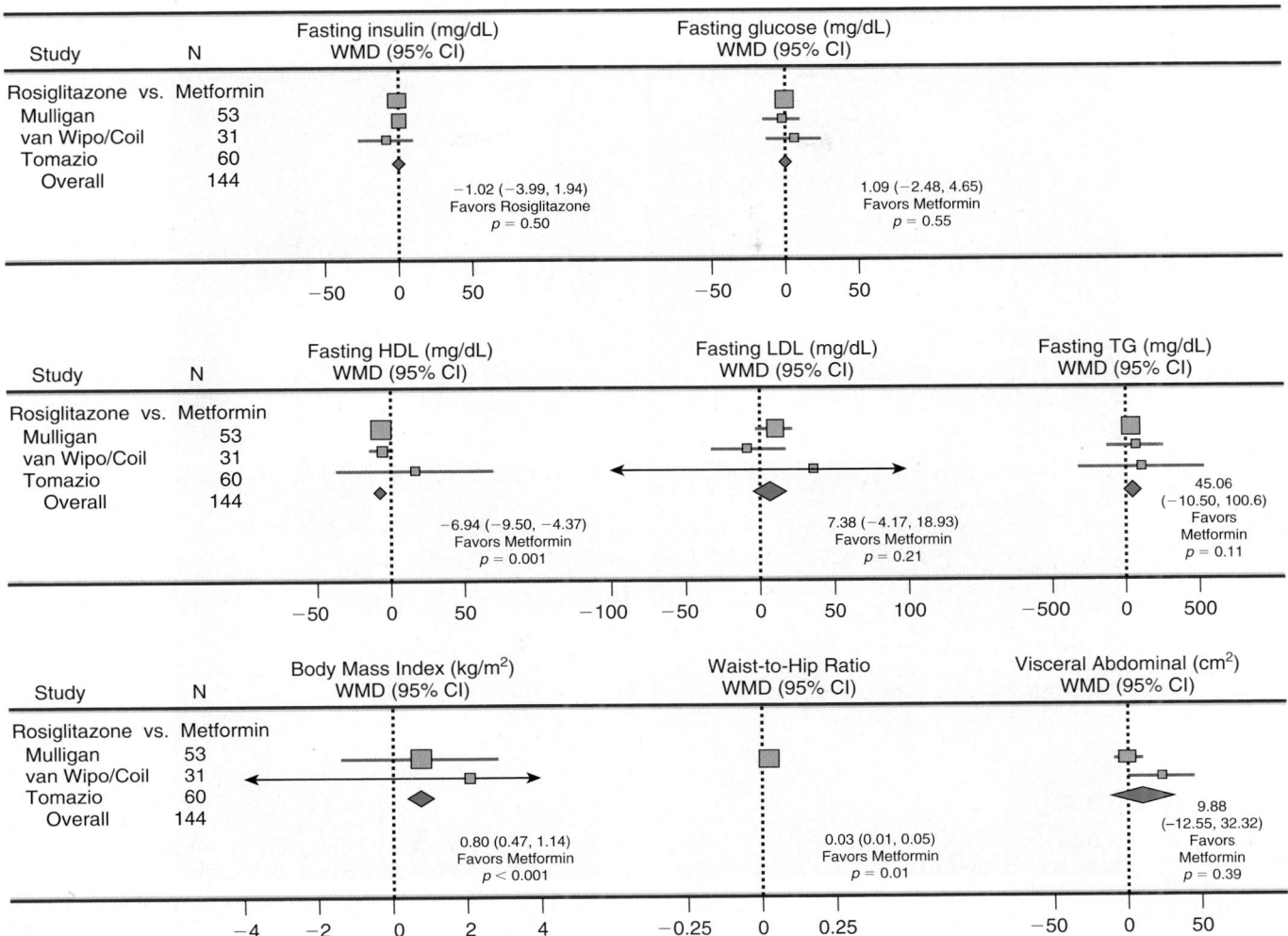

Figure 41-10 Effects of rosiglitazone vs. metformin on insulin sensitivity, lipid profiles, and morphology in patients with human immunodeficiency virus (HIV)-associated lipodystrophy syndrome. CI, confidence interval; HDL, high-density lipoprotein; LDL, low-density lipoprotein; TG, triglyceride; WMD, weighted mean difference. (From Sheth SH, Larson RJ. The efficacy and safety of insulin-sensitizing drugs in HIV-associated lipodystrophy syndrome: a meta-analysis of randomized trials. *BMC Infect Dis.* 2010;10:183, Fig. 4.)

increased smoking rates, insulin resistance, atherogenic dyslipidemia, truncal adiposity, hypertension (HTN), impaired fibrinolysis, and increased PAI-I and tPA levels, as well as reduced adiponectin and increased CRP levels. DM is a risk equivalent in HIV-infected patients conferring an increase in relative risk (RR) of coronary heart disease equivalent to 2.41.[185] Over 40% of HIV-infected subjects meet the definition of the metabolic syndrome, and predicted myocardial infarction (MI) rates are increased in this subgroup.[186]

Abnormalities in surrogate markers, including carotid intima-media thickness (CIMT) and endothelial function, suggest increased CVD in HIV-infected patients. Abnormal endothelial function correlates with dyslipidemia, including increased chylomicrons, VLDLs, and intermediate-density lipoproteins and reduced HDL. Recently, significant evidence for subclinical atherosclerosis has been demonstrated using coronary computed tomography in HIV-infected patients. Lo and coworkers demonstrated an increased prevalence of coronary plaque among asymptomatic HIV-infected patients compared to well-matched non–HIV-infected patients (59% vs. 34%).[187] Follow-up studies confirmed that the plaque in HIV-infected patients is more often noncalcified,[188] with vulnerable plaque features, including low attenuation fatty lesions and eccentric positive remodeling.[189] Using fluorodeoxyglucose positron emission tomography (FDG-PET) to assess the degree of inflammation at the vascular surface, Subramanian and associates demonstrated increased arterial inflammation (Fig. 41-11),[190] even among those with minimal traditional cardiovascular risk indices. Increased immune activation indices correlated with the arterial inflammation, independent of traditional risk factors, suggesting an important role for nontraditional risk factors, including immune activation, in the accelerated atherogenesis observed in HIV-infected patients. In particular, markers of monocyte activation, including soluble CD163 and CD14,[191,192] and bacterial translocation[193] have been associated with atherosclerotic indices, including intima-media thickness and noncalcified coronary plaque among HIV-infected patients. In contrast, traditional risk factors cluster with coronary calcium among such patients[191] and may underestimate atherosclerotic burden.[194] Genetic polymorphisms and mRNA expression of CCR5 (chemokine receptor type 5) and oxidative stress markers may also be associated with increased atherosclerosis among HIV-infected patients.[195,196] Immune activation may contribute to the increased prevalence of inflamed vulnerable plaque with high-risk

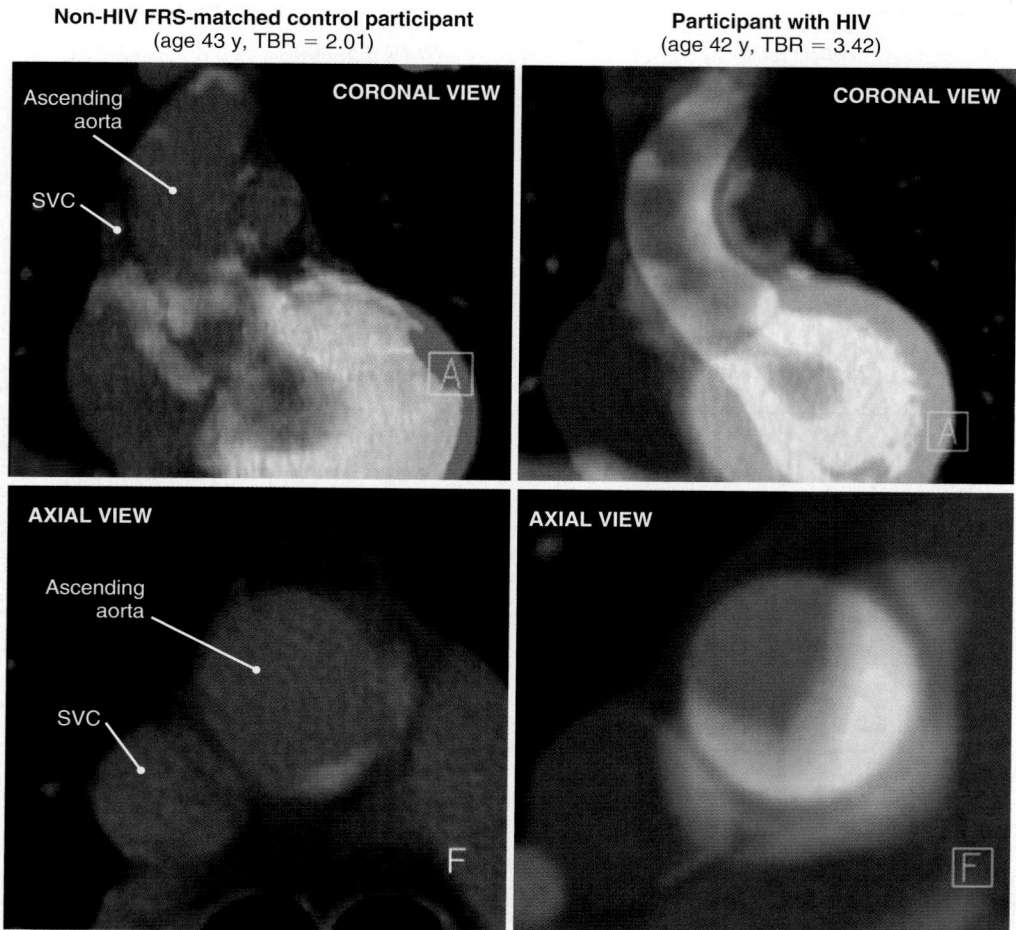

Figure 41-11 Representative ^{18}F-FDG-PET/CT imaging of the aorta. There is increased aortic PET-FDG uptake (red coloration) in a participant infected with HIV compared with a non-HIV FRS-matched control participant. Neither participant had known heart disease. For each participant, the FRS was low with a score of 2 and calcium was not present on the cardiac CT scan. Neither participant was receiving a statin. A indicates anterior-posterior orientation, and F indicates foot-head orientation. CT, computed tomography; ^{18}F-FDG-PET, [^{18}F]fluoro-2-deoxy-D-glucose positron emission tomography; FRS, Framingham risk score; HIV, human immunodeficiency virus; SVC, superior vena cava; TBR, target-to-background ratio. (From Subramanian S, Tawakol A, Burdo TH, et al. Arterial inflammation in patients with HIV. *JAMA.* 2012;308:379-386, Fig. 2, used with permission.)

morphologic findings, which in turn may contribute to the increased risk of sudden cardiac death among HIV-infected patients.[197]

A number of studies suggest increased MI rates in HIV patients. Initial studies suggested dyslipidemia from ART was a major factor contributing to increased CVD risk in HIV-infected patients. In a large prospective study of 23,468 patients, the covariate-adjusted risk was 1.26 per each additional year of antiretroviral exposure. Other risk factors included male sex, diabetes, older age, previous MI, HTN, and dyslipidemia.[198] Controlling for dyslipidemia significantly reduced the effects of HAART exposure, suggesting that dyslipidemia may contribute to excess CVD in HIV-infected patients.

In contrast, more contemporary studies suggest other factors beyond traditional risks may contribute to increased CVD rates in HIV. In a large study of patients in a major U.S. health care center, Triant and colleagues demonstrated a relative risk of 1.75 (95% CI, 1.51-2.02; $p < 0.0001$) for increased MI in HIV versus non–HIV-infected patients in a model accounting for age, gender, and race[199] (Fig. 41-12). Increased rates of traditional risk factors, including DM (11.5 vs. 6.6%, HIV-infected vs. non–HIV-infected), HTN (21.2 vs. 15.9%), and dyslipidemia (23.3 vs. 17.6%) were

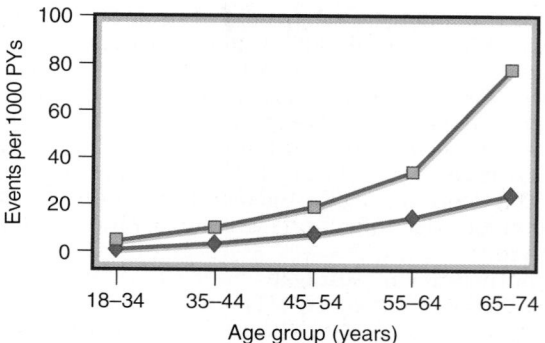

Figure 41-12 Myocardial infarction rates by age group. *Top line (squares)* indicates patients diagnosed with human immunodeficiency virus (HIV) disease. *Bottom line (diamonds)* indicates patients not diagnosed with HIV disease. Data shown include both genders. Rates represent number of events per 1000 person-years (PYs) as determined by International Classification of Diseases (ICD) coding. (From Triant VA, Lee H, Hadigan C, Grinspoon SK. Increased acute myocardial infarction rates and cardiovascular risk factors among patients with human immunodeficiency virus disease. *J Clin Endocrinol Metab.* 2007;92:2506-2512, Fig. 1B, used with permission.)

seen, and each contributed to the increase in MI rates (RRs of 1.62, 1.98, and 3.03, respectively, for each risk factor). However, regression modeling, accounting for HTN, DM, and dyslipidemia, demonstrated that these three risk factors contributed to only 25% of the excess risk in HIV-versus non–HIV-infected patients, suggesting that other factors might contribute. Freiberg and associates demonstrated an increased hazard ratio of 1.48 for MI among a large cohort of HIV-infected men in the VA system, controlling for Framingham Risk Factors.[199a] Smoking rates are increased and may contribute to increased CVD risk in HIV patients.

Recent studies also suggest that inflammation may play an important role in increased CVD risk among HIV-infected patients. Increased CRP levels are observed among HIV-infected patients and predict increased MI rates.[200] The SMART (Strategies for Management of Antiretroviral Therapy) Study Group demonstrated an increased rate of cardiovascular events among patients randomized to interrupted therapy with less strict goals for control of immune function.[201] Indeed, a 2014 study suggests that low CD4 and nadir CD4 are important contributing factors to CVD among HIV-infected patients, suggesting an important role for immune dysfunction.[202]

HIV-infected women are also at risk for increased CVD. In large cohort studies, the relative risk of MI and stroke is more increased in HIV-infected women compared to non–HIV-infected female control subjects (RR 2.98 for acute MI) than among HIV-infected men compared to non–HIV-infected male control subjects (RR 1.40 for acute MI).[199] Increased waist-to-hip ratio, visceral adiposity, CRP, IL-6, triglyceride, and LDL and reduced HDL and adiponectin have been demonstrated in HIV-infected women compared to age- and BMI-matched control subjects. Central adiposity was significantly predictive of abnormal CVD risk indices, including newer inflammatory indices.[203] In addition, studies suggest a marked increase in immune activation indices among HIV-infected female patients, including markers of monocyte activation, in association with non-calcified plaque.[204]

Strategies for Hyperlipidemia Among HIV-Infected Patients

Treatment for hyperlipidemia among HIV-infected patients is indicated to reduce cardiovascular risk and should proceed according to standard National Cholesterol Education Program (NCEP) guidelines. Severe hypertriglyceridemia should be treated to reduce the risk of pancreatitis. An initial option in patients with severe elevations in triglyceride levels is to switch treatment to a PI less likely to cause dyslipidemia. Triglyceride levels are reduced approximately 20% by diet[205] and 30% by exercise[206] in HIV-infected patients. Neither diet nor exercise is likely to normalize triglyceride levels in the HIV population with severe dyslipidemia. Fenofibrate resulted in a 40% reduction in triglyceride levels and a 14% reduction in total cholesterol levels over 3 months in HIV-infected patients with hypertriglyceridemia.[207] Lesser but nonetheless beneficial effects may be seen with gemfibrozil or other fibrate derivatives. Niacin also significantly reduces triglyceride level, but may worsen glucose tolerance in HIV-infected patients, although such changes in glucose may only be transient.[208] In addition, niacin may be difficult to use because of its associated flushing and potential liver abnormalities. In a large randomized 24-week controlled trial of diet and exercise with either fenofibrate, niacin, or both, maximal reduction in triglyceride (−52%) was seen with combination drug therapy plus diet and exercise, whereas HDL increased

most with niacin and diet and exercise. Flushing was reported by 35% to 40% of niacin-treated subjects.[209] Recent studies also suggest the efficacy of omega-3 polyunsaturated fatty acids, which were shown to reduce triglyceride levels by 25.5% and be well tolerated in a randomized, placebo-controlled study.[210] In a study investigating combined therapy, triglyceride levels were reduced by 65.5% among hypertriglyceridemic HIV-infected patients receiving simultaneous fenofibrate and fish oil.[211] Comparing fish oil to gemfibrozil, fibrates, and atorvastatin in hypertriglyceridemic HIV-infected patients, fish oil was shown to decrease triglyceride by 45 mg/dL, whereas fibrates (−66 mg/dL), but not atorvastatin (−39 mg/dL), were more effective in this regard.[212]

The 3-hydroxy-3-methylglutaryl coenzyme A (HMG-CoA) reductase inhibitors are most useful for lowering cholesterol levels in HIV-infected patients but are less effective in lowering triglyceride levels. For example, pravastatin combined with dietary advice reduced total cholesterol levels by 17% over 24 weeks without effects on triglyceride levels.[213] The combination of gemfibrozil and atorvastatin resulted in a 30% reduction in cholesterol and 60% reduction in triglyceride in HIV-infected patients[205] and may be useful in HIV-infected patients with combined hyperlipidemia. When using the combination of HMG-CoA reductase inhibitors and fibric acid derivatives, the risk of rhabdomyolysis increases. In addition, data suggest that the PIs can themselves affect metabolism of the HMG-CoA reductase inhibitors. In this regard ritonavir was shown to increase simvastatin levels by 3059% and atorvastatin levels by 79%.[214] Use of simvastatin should be avoided in patients receiving PI therapy. In an analysis of almost 900 HIV-infected patients in the Kaiser Permanente system, use of statins was shown to lower LDL by 25.6% versus 28.3% in HIV-versus non–HIV-infected patients, whereas use of gemfibrozil lowered triglyceride by 44.2% versus 59.3% in HIV- and non–HIV-infected patients. Effects of statins on LDL did not vary by antiretroviral treatment class, whereas effects of gemfibrozil were less in HIV-infected patients receiving PIs and best among those patients receiving therapy with NNRTIs. Safety of the statins, including atorvastatin, pravastatin, and lovastatin were good, with few cases of myositis. The relative potency of each statin on LDL was generally similar, with reductions ranging from −26.4% with atorvastatin to −23.6% with pravastatin.[215] Rosuvastatin must be used at lower doses due to potential interaction with darunavir but has been shown to lower LDL by 28% at 10 mg/day in placebo-controlled trials.[216] New drugs, such as pitavastatin, may have the fewest interactions with ART, because they are glucuronidated and do not affect CYP3A metabolism. Ezetimibe is well tolerated in combination with statins in patients with HIV and further lowers LDL (additional 14% reduction).[217] Effects of statins on clinical events have not yet been investigated in large randomized controlled trials, but cohort studies suggest a potential benefit on overall mortality rate among HIV-infected patients treated with ART with virologic suppression,[218] and preliminary studies suggest effects to improve atherosclerotic indices, such as carotid intima-media thickness and coronary plaque.[219,220]

Anti-inflammatory Strategies for Cardiovascular Disease in HIV

Initial studies are now investigating effects of anti-inflammatory strategies to improve endothelial function and reduce arterial inflammation. Such strategies include use of pentoxifylline and methotrexate, but safety and efficacy of these agents in the HIV population remain unclear. Use of statins may also be beneficial as an anti-inflammatory strategy, as they may lower CRP and have pleiotropic effects on monocyte activation.

ACKNOWLEDGMENT

The author would like to thank Jinhee K. Oh for her help in preparing this chapter.

REFERENCES

1. AVERT. Worldwide HIV & AIDS Statistics. Available at <http://www.avert.org/worldstats.htm>.
2. Membreno L, Irony I, Dere W, et al. Adrenocortical function in acquired immune deficiency syndrome. *J Clin Endocrinol Metab*. 1987;65:482-487.
3. Grinspoon SK, Bilezikian JB. HIV disease and the endocrine system. *N Engl J Med*. 1992;327:1360-1365.
4. Glasgow BJ, Steinsapir KD, Anders K, Layfield LJ. Adrenal pathology in the acquired immune deficiency syndrome. *Am J Clin Pathol*. 1985;84:594-597.
5. Ferreiro J, Vinters HV. Pathology of the pituitary gland in patients with the acquired immune deficiency syndrome. (AIDS). *Pathology*. 1988;20:211-215.
6. Grinspoon S, Corcoran C, Stanley T, et al. Mechanisms of androgen deficiency in human immunodeficiency virus-infected women with the wasting syndrome. *J Clin Endocrinol Metab*. 2001;86:4120-4126.
7. Patterson S, Moran P, Epel E, et al. Cortisol patterns are associated with T cell activation in HIV. *PLoS ONE*. 2013;8:e63429.
8. Foisy MM, Yakiwchuk EM, Chiu I, Singh AE. Adrenal suppression and Cushing's syndrome secondary to an interaction between ritonavir and fluticasone: a review of the literature. *HIV Med*. 2008;9:389-396.
9. Hyle EP, Wood BR, Backman ES, et al. High frequency of hypothalamic-pituitary-adrenal axis dysfunction after local corticosteroid injection in HIV-infected patients on protease inhibitor therapy. *J Acquir Immune Defic Syndr*. 2013;63:602-608.
10. Rietschel P, Corcoran C, Stanley T, et al. Prevalence of hypogonadism among men with weight loss related to human immunodeficiency virus infection who were receiving highly active antiretroviral therapy. *Clin Infect Dis*. 2000;31:1240-1244.
11. Monroe AK, Dobs AS, Palella FJ, et al. Morning free and total testosterone in HIV-infected men: implications for the assessment of hypogonadism. *AIDS Res Ther*. 2014;11:6.
12. Rochira V, Zirilli L, Orlando G, et al. Premature decline of serum total testosterone in HIV-infected men in the HAART-era. *PLoS ONE*. 2011;6:e28512.
13. Moreno-Perez O, Escoin C, Serna-Candel C, et al. The determination of total testosterone and free testosterone (RIA) are not applicable to the evaluation of gonadal function in HIV-infected males. *J Sex Med*. 2010;7:2873-2883.
14. Wunder DM, Bersinger NA, Fux CA, et al. Hypogonadism in HIV-1-infected men is common and does not resolve during antiretroviral therapy. *Antivir Ther*. 2007;12:261-265.
15. Biglia A, Blanco JL, Martinez E, et al. Gynecomastia among HIV-infected patients is associated with hypogonadism: a case-control study. *Clin Infect Dis*. 2004;39:1514-1519.
16. Collazos J, Ibarra S, Martinez E, Mayo J. Serum prolactin concentrations in patients infected with human immunodeficiency virus. *HIV Clin Trials*. 2002;3:133-138.
17. Hutchinson J, Murphy M, Harries R, Skinner CJ. Galactorrhoea and hyperprolactinaemia associated with protease-inhibitors. *Lancet*. 2000;356:1003-1004.
18. Clark RA, Mulligan K, Stamenovic E, et al. Frequency of anovulation and early menopause among women enrolled in selected adult AIDS clinical trials group studies. *J Infect Dis*. 2001;184:1325-1327.
19. Grinspoon S, Corcoran C, Miller K, et al. Body composition and endocrine function in women with acquired immunodeficiency syndrome wasting [published erratum appears in *J Clin Endocrinol Metab*. 1997;82(10):3360]. *J Clin Endocrinol Metab*. 1997;82:1332-1337.
20. Bourdoux PP, De Wit SA, Servais GM, et al. Biochemical thyroid profile in patients infected with the human immunodeficiency virus. *Thyroid*. 1991;1:147-149.
21. Madge S, Smith CJ, Lampe FC, et al. No association between HIV disease and its treatment and thyroid function. *HIV Med*. 2007;8:22-27.
22. Nelson M, Powles T, Zeitlin A, et al. Thyroid dysfunction and relationship to antiretroviral therapy in HIV-positive individuals in the HAART era. *J Acquir Immune Defic Syndr*. 2009;50:113-114.
23. Rana S, Nunlee-Bland G, Valyasevi R, Iqbal M. Thyroid dysfunction in HIV-infected children: is L-thyroxine therapy beneficial? *Pediatr AIDS HIV Infect*. 1996;7:424-428.
24. Fundaro C, Olivieri A, Rendeli C, et al. Occurrence of anti-thyroid autoantibodies in children vertically infected with HIV-1. *J Pediatr Endocrinol Metab*. 1998;11:745-750.
25. Chiarelli F, Galli L, Verrotti A, et al. Thyroid function in children with perinatal human immunodeficiency virus type 1 infection. *Thyroid*. 2000;10:499-505.
26. Hoffmann CJ, Brown TT. Thyroid function abnormalities in HIV-infected patients. *Clin Infect Dis*. 2007;45:488-494.
27. Chen F, Day SL, Metcalfe RA, et al. Characteristics of autoimmune thyroid disease occurring as a late complication of immune reconstitution in patients with advanced human immunodeficiency virus (HIV) disease. *Medicine (Baltimore)*. 2005;84:98-106.
28. Jimenez C, Moran SA, Sereti I, et al. Graves' disease after interleukin-2 therapy in a patient with human immunodeficiency virus infection. *Thyroid*. 2004;14:1097-1102.
29. Tang WW, Kaptein E, Feinstein EI, Massry SG. Hyponatremia in hospitalized patients with the acquired immunodeficiency syndrome (AIDS) and the AIDS-related complex. *Am J Med*. 1993;94:169-174.
30. Kalin MF, Poretsky L, Seres DS, Zumoff B. Hyporeninemic hypoaldosteronism associated with acquired immune deficiency syndrome. *Am J Med*. 1987;82:1035-1038.
31. Choi MJ, Fernandez PC, Patnaik A, et al. Brief report: trimethoprim-induced hyperkalemia in a patient with AIDS. *Ann Intern Med*. 1993;328:703-706.
32. Mathew G, Knaus SJ. Acquired Fanconi's syndrome associated with tenofovir therapy. *J Gen Intern Med*. 2006;21:C3-C5.
33. Kuehn EW, Anders HJ, Bogner JR, et al. Hypocalcaemia in HIV infection and AIDS. *J Intern Med*. 1999;245:69-73.
34. Jaeger P, Otto S, Speck RF, et al. Altered parathyroid gland function in severely immunocompromised patients infected with human immunodeficiency virus. *J Clin Endocrinol Metab*. 1994;79:1701-1705.
35. Cozzolino M, Vidal M, Arcidiacono MV, et al. HIV-protease inhibitors impair vitamin D bioactivation to 1,25-dihydroxyvitamin D. *AIDS*. 2003;17:513-520.
36. Earle KE, Seneviratne T, Shaker J, Shoback D. Fanconi's syndrome in HIV+ adults: report of three cases and literature review. *J Bone Miner Res*. 2004;19:714-721.
37. Tsao YT, Wu CC, Chu P. Immune reconstitution syndrome-induced hypercalcemic crisis. *Am J Emerg Med*. 2011;29:e243-e246.
38. Bonjoch A, Figueras M, Estany C, et al. High prevalence of and progression to low bone mineral density in HIV-infected patients: a longitudinal cohort study. *AIDS*. 2010;24:2827-2833.
39. Yin MT, Zhang CA, McMahon DJ, et al. Higher rates of bone loss in postmenopausal HIV-infected women: a longitudinal study. *J Clin Endocrinol Metab*. 2012;97:554-562.
40. Cotter AG, Vrouenraets SM, Brady JJ, et al. Impact of switching from zidovudine to tenofovir disoproxil fumarate on bone mineral density and markers of bone metabolism in virologically suppressed HIV-1 infected patients; a substudy of the PREPARE study. *J Clin Endocrinol Metab*. 2013;98:1659-1666.
41. Rasmussen TA, Jensen D, Tolstrup M, et al. Comparison of bone and renal effects in HIV-infected adults switching to abacavir or tenofovir based therapy in a randomized trial. *PLoS ONE*. 2012;7:e32445.
42. Liu AY, Vittinghoff E, Sellmeyer DE, et al. Bone mineral density in HIV-negative men participating in a tenofovir pre-exposure prophylaxis randomized clinical trial in San Francisco. *PLoS ONE*. 2011;6:e23688.
43. Gazzola L, Bellistri GM, Tincati C, et al. Association between peripheral T-lymphocyte activation and impaired bone mineral density in HIV-infected patients. *J Transl Med*. 2013;11:51.
44. Casado JL, Banon S, Andres R, et al. Prevalence of causes of secondary osteoporosis and contribution to lower bone mineral density in HIV-infected patients. *Osteoporos Int*. 2014;25:1071-1079.
45. Lawson-Ayayi S, Cazanave C, Kpozehouen A, et al. Chronic viral hepatitis is associated with low bone mineral density in HIV-infected patients, ANRS CO 3 Aquitaine cohort. *J Acquir Immune Defic Syndr*. 2013;62:430-435.
46. Koutkia P, Canavan B, Breu J, Grinspoon S. Effects of growth hormone-releasing hormone on bone turnover in human immunodeficiency virus-infected men with fat accumulation. *J Clin Endocrinol Metab*. 2005;90:2154-2160.
47. Huang JS, Rietschel P, Hadigan CM, et al. Increased abdominal visceral fat is associated with reduced bone density in HIV-infected men with lipodystrophy. *AIDS*. 2001;15:975-982.
48. Gedela K, Edwards SG, Benn P, Grant AD. Prevalence of vitamin D deficiency in HIV-positive, antiretroviral treatment-naive patients in a single centre. *Int J STD AIDS*. 2013;25(7):488-492.
49. Theodorou M, Serste T, Van Gossum M, Dewit S. Factors associated with vitamin D deficiency in a population of 2044 HIV-infected patients. *Clin Nutr*. 2014;33:274-279.
50. Sherwood JE, Mesner OC, Weintrob AC, et al. Vitamin D deficiency and its association with low bone mineral density, HIV-related factors, hospitalization, and death in a predominantly black HIV-infected cohort. *Clin Infect Dis*. 2012;55:1727-1736.
51. Aukrust P, Haug CJ, Ueland T, et al. Decreased bone formative and enhanced resorptive markers in human immunodeficiency virus

infection: indication of normalization of the bone-remodeling process during highly active antiretroviral therapy. *J Clin Endocrinol Metab.* 1999;84:145-150.

52. Tebas P, Powderly WG, Claxton S, et al. Accelerated bone mineral loss in HIV-infected patients receiving potent antiretroviral therapy. *AIDS.* 2000;14:F63-F67.

53. Hwang JJ, Wei J, Abbara S, et al. Receptor activator of nuclear factor-kappaB ligand (RANKL) and its relationship to coronary atherosclerosis in HIV patients. *J Acquir Immune Defic Syndr.* 2012;61:359-363.

54. Kelesidis T, Kendall MA, Yang OO, et al. Perturbations of circulating levels of RANKL-osteoprotegerin axis in relation to lipids and progression of atherosclerosis in HIV-infected and -uninfected adults: ACTG NWCS 332/A5078 Study. *AIDS Res Hum Retroviruses.* 2013;29:938-948.

55. Dolan SE, Huang JS, Killilea KM, et al. Reduced bone density in HIV-infected women. *AIDS.* 2004;18:475-483.

56. Triant VA, Brown TT, Lee H, Grinspoon SK. Fracture prevalence among human immunodeficiency virus (HIV)-infected versus non-HIV-infected patients in a large U.S. healthcare system. *J Clin Endocrinol Metab.* 2008;93:3499-3504.

57. Guerri-Fernandez R, Vestergaard P, Carbonell C, et al. HIV infection is strongly associated with hip fracture risk, independently of age, gender, and comorbidities: a population-based cohort study. *J Bone Miner Res.* 2013;28:1259-1263.

58. Womack JA, Goulet JL, Gibert C, et al. Physiologic frailty and fragility fracture in HIV-infected male veterans. *Clin Infect Dis.* 2013;56:1498-1504.

59. Prior J, Burdge D, Maan E, et al. Fragility fractures and bone mineral density in HIV positive women: a case-control population-based study. *Osteoporos Int.* 2007;18:1345-1353.

60. Pepe J, Isidori AM, Falciano M, et al. The combination of FRAX and ageing male symptoms scale better identifies treated HIV males at risk for major fracture. *Clin Endocrinol (Oxf).* 2012;77:672-678.

61. Young B, Dao CN, Buchacz K, et al. Increased rates of bone fracture among HIV-infected persons in the HIV Outpatient Study (HOPS) compared with the US general population, 2000-2006. *Clin Infect Dis.* 2011;52:1061-1068.

62. Mundy LM, Youk AO, McComsey GA, Bowlin SJ. Overall benefit of antiretroviral treatment on the risk of fracture in HIV: nested case-control analysis in a health-insured population. *AIDS.* 2012;26:1073-1082.

63. Mondy K, Powderly WG, Claxton SA, et al. Alendronate, vitamin D, and calcium for the treatment of osteopenia/osteoporosis associated with HIV infection. *J Acquir Immune Defic Syndr.* 2005;38:426-431.

64. McComsey GA, Kendall MA, Tebas P, et al. Alendronate with calcium and vitamin D supplementation is safe and effective for the treatment of decreased bone mineral density in HIV. *AIDS.* 2007;21:2473-2482.

65. Bolland MJ, Grey AB, Horne AM, et al. Annual zoledronate increases bone density in highly active antiretroviral therapy-treated human immunodeficiency virus-infected men: a randomized controlled trial. *J Clin Endocrinol Metab.* 2007;92:1283-1288.

66. Bolland MJ, Grey A, Horne AM, et al. Effects of intravenous zoledronate on bone turnover and bone density persist for at least five years in HIV-infected men. *J Clin Endocrinol Metab.* 2012;97:1922-1928.

67. Fairfield WP, Finkelstein JS, Klibanski A, Grinspoon SK. Osteopenia in eugonadal men with acquired immune deficiency syndrome wasting syndrome. *J Clin Endocrinol Metab.* 2001;86:2020-2026.

68. O'Brien KO, Razavi M, Henderson RA, et al. Bone mineral content in girls perinatally infected with HIV. *Am J Clin Nutr.* 2001;73:821-826.

69. DiMeglio LA, Wang J, Siberry GK, et al. Bone mineral density in children and adolescents with perinatal HIV infection. *AIDS.* 2013;27:211-220.

70. Yin MT, Lund E, Shah J, et al. Lower peak bone mass and abnormal trabecular and cortical microarchitecture in young men infected with HIV early in life. *AIDS.* 2014;28:345-353.

71. Zamboni G, Antoniazzi F, Bertoldo F, et al. Altered bone metabolism in children infected with human immunodeficiency virus. *Acta Paediatr.* 2003;92:12-16.

72. Stagi S, Bindi G, Galluzzi F, et al. Changed bone status in human immunodeficiency virus type 1 (HIV-1) perinatally infected children is related to low serum free IGF-I. *Clin Endocrinol (Oxf).* 2004;61:692-699.

73. Mora S, Zamproni I, Beccio S, et al. Longitudinal changes of bone mineral density and metabolism in antiretroviral-treated human immunodeficiency virus-infected children. *J Clin Endocrinol Metab.* 2004;89:24-28.

74. Arpadi SM, McMahon DJ, Abrams EJ, et al. Effect of supplementation with cholecalciferol and calcium on 2-y bone mass accrual in HIV-infected children and adolescents: a randomized clinical trial. *Am J Clin Nutr.* 2012;95:678-685.

75. Miller KD, Masur H, Jones EC, et al. High prevalence of osteonecrosis of the femoral head in HIV-infected adults. *Ann Intern Med.* 2002;137:17-25.

76. Lawson-Ayayi S, Bonnet F, Bernardin E, et al. Avascular necrosis in HIV-infected patients: a case-control study from the Aquitaine Cohort, 1997-2002, France. *Clin Infect Dis.* 2005;40:1188-1193.

77. Mazzotta E, Agostinone A, Rosso R, et al. Osteonecrosis in human immunodeficiency virus (HIV)-infected patients: a multicentric case-control study. *J Bone Miner Metab.* 2011;29:383-388.

78. Morse CG, Dodd LE, Nghiem K, et al. Elevations in D-dimer and C-reactive protein are associated with the development of osteonecrosis of the hip in HIV-infected adults. *AIDS.* 2013;27:591-595.

79. Rietschel P, Hadigan C, Corcoran C, et al. Assessment of growth hormone dynamics in human immunodeficiency virus- related lipodystrophy. *J Clin Endocrinol Metab.* 2001;86:504-510.

80. Koutkia P, Meininger G, Canavan B, et al. Metabolic regulation of growth hormone by free fatty acids, somatostatin, and ghrelin in HIV-lipodystrophy. *Am J Physiol Endocrinol Metab.* 2004;286:E296-E303.

81. Pinto G, Blanche S, Thiriet I, et al. Growth hormone treatment of children with human immunodeficiency virus-associated growth failure. *Eur J Pediatr.* 2000;159:937-938.

82. Frost RA, Nachman SA, Lang CH, Gelato MC. Proteolysis of insulin-like growth factor-binding protein-3 in human immunodeficiency virus-positive children who fail to thrive. *J Clin Endocrinol Metab.* 1996;81:2957-2962.

83. Van Rossum AM, Gaakeer MI, Verweel S, et al. Endocrinologic and immunologic factors associated with recovery of growth in children with human immunodeficiency virus type 1 infection treated with protease inhibitors. *Pediatr Infect Dis J.* 2003;22:70-76.

84. Riedel DJ, Gebo KA, Moore RD, Lucas GM. A ten-year analysis of the incidence and risk factors for acute pancreatitis requiring hospitalization in an urban HIV clinical cohort. *AIDS Patient Care STDS.* 2008;22:113-121.

85. Smith CJ, Olsen CH, Mocroft A, et al. The role of antiretroviral therapy in the incidence of pancreatitis in HIV-positive individuals in the EuroSIDA study. *AIDS.* 2008;22:47-56.

86. Grinspoon SK, Grunfeld C, Kotler DP, et al. State of the science conference: initiative to decrease cardiovascular risk and increase quality of care for patients living with HIV/AIDS: executive summary. *Circulation.* 2008;118:198-210.

87. Grunfeld C, Kotler DP, Arnett DK, et al. Contribution of metabolic and anthropometric abnormalities to cardiovascular disease risk factors. *Circulation.* 2008;118:e20-e28.

88. Macallan DE, Noble C, Baldwin C, et al. Energy expenditure and wasting in human immunodeficiency virus infection. *N Engl J Med.* 1995;333:83-88.

89. Thiebaut R, Malvy D, Marimoutou C, Davis F. Anthropometric indices as predictors of survival in AIDS adults. Aquitaine cohort, France, 1985-1997. Groupe d'Epidemiologie Clinique du Sida en Aquitaine (GECSA). *Eur J Epidemiol.* 2000;16:633-639.

90. Grinspoon S, Corcoran C, Lee K, et al. Loss of lean body and muscle mass correlates with androgen levels in hypogonadal men with acquired immunodeficiency syndrome and wasting. *J Clin Endocrinol Metab.* 1996;81:4051-4058.

91. Tate T, Willig AL, Willig JH, et al. HIV infection and obesity: where did all the wasting go? *Antivir Ther.* 2012;17:1281-1289.

92. Bacchetti P, Gripshover B, Grunfeld C, et al. Fat distribution in men with HIV infection. *J Acquir Immune Defic Syndr.* 2005;40:121-131.

93. Joy T, Keogh HM, Hadigan C, et al. Relationship of body composition to body mass index in HIV-infected patients with metabolic abnormalities. *J Acquir Immune Defic Syndr.* 2008;47:174-184.

94. Scherzer R, Heymsfield SB, Lee D, et al. Decreased limb muscle and increased central adiposity are associated with 5-year all-cause mortality in HIV infection. *AIDS.* 2011;25(11):1405-1414.

95. Shikuma CM, Hu N, Milne C, et al. Mitochondrial DNA decrease in subcutaneous adipose tissue of HIV-infected individuals with peripheral lipoatrophy. *AIDS.* 2001;15:1801-1809.

96. Mallon PW, Unemori P, Sedwell R, et al. In vivo, nucleoside reverse-transcriptase inhibitors alter expression of both mitochondrial and lipid metabolism genes in the absence of depletion of mitochondrial DNA. *J Infect Dis.* 2005;191:1686-1696.

97. Caron M, Auclair M, Vigouroux C, et al. The HIV protease inhibitor indinavir impairs sterol regulatory element-binding protein-1 intranuclear localization, inhibits preadipocyte differentiation, and induces insulin resistance. *Diabetes.* 2001;50:1378-1388.

98. Ranade K, Geese WJ, Noor M, et al. Genetic analysis implicates resistin in HIV lipodystrophy. *AIDS.* 2008;22:1561-1568.

99. Hulgan T, Tebas P, Canter JA, et al. Hemochromatosis gene polymorphisms, mitochondrial haplogroups, and peripheral lipoatrophy during antiretroviral therapy. *J Infect Dis.* 2008;197:858-866.

100. Zanone Poma B, Riva A, Nasi M, et al. Genetic polymorphisms differently influencing the emergence of atrophy and fat accumulation in HIV-related lipodystrophy. *AIDS.* 2008;22:1769-1778.

101. Kratz M, Purnell JQ, Breen PA, et al. Reduced adipogenic gene expression in thigh adipose tissue precedes human immunodeficiency virus-associated lipoatrophy. *J Clin Endocrinol Metab.* 2008;93:959-966.

102. Agarwal N, Iyer D, Patel SG, et al. HIV-1 Vpr induces adipose dysfunction in vivo through reciprocal effects on PPAR/GR co-regulation. *Sci Transl Med.* 2013;5:213ra164.

103. Miller KK, Daly PA, Sentochnik D, et al. Pseudo-Cushing's syndrome in human immunodeficiency virus-infected patients. *Clin Infect Dis.* 1998;27:68-72.

104. Yanovski JA, Miller KD, Kino T, et al. Endocrine and metabolic evaluation of human immunodeficiency virus-infected patients with evidence of protease inhibitor-associated lipodystrophy. *J Clin Endocrinol Metab*. 1999;84:1925-1931.

105. Sutinen J, Kannisto K, Korsheninnikova E, et al. In the lipodystrophy associated with highly active antiretroviral therapy, pseudo-Cushing's syndrome is associated with increased regeneration of cortisol by 11beta-hydroxysteroid dehydrogenase type 1 in adipose tissue. *Diabetologia*. 2004;47:1668-1671.

106. Christeff N, De Truchis P, Melchior JC, et al. Longitudinal evolution of HIV-1-associated lipodystrophy is correlated to serum cortisol:DHEA ratio and IFN-alpha. *Eur J Clin Invest*. 2002;32:775-784.

107. Hellerstein MK, Grunfeld C, Wu K, et al. Increased de novo hepatic lipogenesis in human immunodeficiency virus infection. *J Clin Endocrinol Metab*. 1993;76:559-565.

108. Timmons T, Shen C, Aldrovandi G, et al. Microbial translocation and metabolic and body composition measures in treated and untreated HIV infection. *AIDS Res Hum Retroviruses*. 2014;30:272-277.

109. Grunfeld C, Pang M, Doerrler W, et al. Lipids, lipoproteins, triglyceride clearance, and cytokines in human immunodeficiency virus infection and the acquired immunodeficiency syndrome. *J Clin Endocrinol Metab*. 1992;74:1045-1052.

110. Grunfeld C, Doerrler W, Pang M, et al. Abnormalities of apolipoprotein E in the acquired immunodeficiency syndrome. *J Clin Endocrinol Metab*. 1997;82:3734-3740.

111. Riddler SA, Smit E, Cole SR, et al. Impact of HIV infection and HAART on serum lipids in men. *JAMA*. 2003;289:2978-2982.

112. Friis-Moller N, Weber R, Reiss P, et al. Cardiovascular disease risk factors in HIV patients: association with antiretroviral therapy. Results from the DAD study. *AIDS*. 2003;17:1179-1193.

113. Hadigan C, Meigs JB, Corcoran C, et al. Metabolic abnormalities and cardiovascular disease risk factors in adults with human immunodeficiency virus infection and lipodystrophy. *Clin Infect Dis*. 2001;32:130-139.

114. Srisawasdi P, Suwalak T, Sukasem C, et al. Small-dense LDL cholesterol/large-buoyant LDL cholesterol ratio as an excellent marker for indicating lipodystrophy in HIV-infected patients. *Am J Clin Pathol*. 2013;140:506-515.

115. Gillard BK, Raya JL, Ruiz-Esponda R, et al. Impaired lipoprotein processing in HIV patients on antiretroviral therapy: aberrant high-density lipoprotein lipids, stability, and function. *Arterioscler Thromb Vasc Biol*. 2013;33:1714-1721.

116. Schmitz M, Michl GM, Walli R, et al. Alterations of apolipoprotein B metabolism in HIV-infected patients with antiretroviral combination therapy. *J Acquir Immune Defic Syndr*. 2001;26:225-235.

117. Bonnet E, Ruidavets JB, Tuech J, et al. Apoprotein c-III and E-containing lipoparticles are markedly increased in HIV-infected patients treated with protease inhibitors: association with the development of lipodystrophy. *J Clin Endocrinol Metab*. 2001;86:296-302.

118. Liang JS, Distler O, Cooper DA, et al. HIV protease inhibitors protect apolipoprotein B from degradation by the proteasome: a potential mechanism for protease inhibitor-induced hyperlipidemia. *Nat Med*. 2001;7:1327-1331.

119. Mulligan K, Grunfeld C, Tai VW, et al. Hyperlipidemia and insulin resistance are induced by protease inhibitors independent of changes in body composition in patients with HIV infection. *J Acquir Immune Defic Syndr*. 2000;23:35-43.

120. Wood R, Phanuphak P, Cahn P, et al. Long-term efficacy and safety of atazanavir with stavudine and lamivudine in patients previously treated with nelfinavir or atazanavir. *J Acquir Immune Defic Syndr*. 2004;36:684-692.

121. Stanley TL, Joy T, Hadigan CM, et al. Effects of switching from lopinavir/ritonavir to atazanavir/ritonavir on muscle glucose uptake and visceral fat in HIV-infected patients. *AIDS*. 2009;23:1349-1357.

122. Rhoads MP, Lanigan J, Smith CJ, Lyall EG. Effect of specific ART drugs on lipid changes and the need for lipid management in children with HIV. *J Acquir Immune Defic Syndr*. 2011;57:404-412.

123. Brown TT, Cole SR, Li X, et al. Antiretroviral therapy and the prevalence and incidence of diabetes mellitus in the multicenter AIDS cohort study. *Arch Intern Med*. 2005;165:1179-1184.

124. Rasmussen LD, Mathiesen ER, Kronborg G, et al. Risk of diabetes mellitus in persons with and without HIV: a Danish nationwide population-based cohort study. *PLoS ONE*. 2012;7:e44575.

125. Capeau J, Bouteloup V, Katlama C, et al. Ten-year diabetes incidence in 1046 HIV-infected patients started on a combination antiretroviral treatment. *AIDS*. 2012;26:303-314.

126. Eckhardt BJ, Holzman RS, Kwan CK, et al. Glycated hemoglobin A(1c) as screening for diabetes mellitus in HIV-infected individuals. *AIDS Patient Care STDS*. 2012;26:197-201.

127. Carper MJ, Cade WT, Cam M, et al. HIV-protease inhibitors induce expression of suppressor of cytokine signaling-1 in insulin-sensitive tissues and promote insulin resistance and type 2 diabetes mellitus. *Am J Physiol Endocrinol Metab*. 2008;294:E558-E567.

128. Brown TT, Tassiopoulos K, Bosch RJ, et al. Association between systemic inflammation and incident diabetes in HIV-infected patients after initiation of antiretroviral therapy. *Diabetes Care*. 2010;33:2244-2249.

129. Pedersen KK, Pedersen M, Troseid M, et al. Microbial translocation in HIV infection is associated with dyslipidemia, insulin resistance, and risk of myocardial infarction. *J Acquir Immune Defic Syndr*. 2013;64:425-433.

130. Han SH, Chin BS, Lee HS, et al. Serum retinol-binding protein 4 correlates with obesity, insulin resistance, and dyslipidemia in HIV-infected subjects receiving highly active antiretroviral therapy. *Metabolism*. 2009;58:1523-1529.

131. Mohammedi K, Roussel R, El Dbouni O, et al. Type B insulin resistance syndrome associated with an immune reconstitution inflammatory syndrome in an HIV-infected woman. *J Clin Endocrinol Metab*. 2011;96:E653-E657.

132. Murata H, Hruz PW, Mueckler M. The mechanism of insulin resistance caused by HIV protease inhibitor therapy. *J Biol Chem*. 2000;275:20251-20254.

133. Noor MA, Seneviratne T, Aweeka FT, et al. Indinavir acutely inhibits insulin-stimulated glucose disposal in humans: a randomized, placebo-controlled study. *AIDS*. 2002;16:F1-F8.

134. Zhang S, Carper MJ, Lei X, et al. Protease inhibitors used in the treatment of HIV+ induce beta-cell apoptosis via the mitochondrial pathway and compromise insulin secretion. *Am J Physiol Endocrinol Metab*. 2009;296:E925-E935.

135. Fleischman A, Johnsen S, Systrom DM, et al. Effects of a nucleoside reverse transcriptase inhibitor, stavudine, on glucose disposal and mitochondrial function in muscle of healthy adults. *Am J Physiol Endocrinol Metab*. 2007;292:E1666-E1673.

136. Kim PS, Woods C, Dutcher L, et al. Increased prevalence of albuminuria in HIV-infected adults with diabetes. *PLoS ONE*. 2011;6:e24610.

137. Grinspoon S, Corcoran C, Askari H, et al. Effects of androgen administration in men with the AIDS wasting syndrome. A randomized, double-blind, placebo-controlled trial. *Ann Intern Med*. 1998;129:18-26.

138. Grunfeld C, Kotler DP, Dobs A, et al. Oxandrolone in the treatment of HIV-associated weight loss in men: a randomized, double-blind, placebo-controlled study. *J Acquir Immune Defic Syndr*. 2006;41:304-314.

139. Mulligan K, Zackin R, Clark RA, et al. Effect of nandrolone decanoate therapy on weight and lean body mass in HIV-infected women with weight loss: a randomized, double-blind, placebo-controlled, multicenter trial. *Arch Intern Med*. 2005;165:578-585.

140. Rabkin JG, McElhiney MC, Rabkin R, et al. Placebo-controlled trial of dehydroepiandrosterone (DHEA) for treatment of nonmajor depression in patients with HIV/AIDS. *Am J Psychiatry*. 2006;163:59-66.

141. Dolan Looby SE, Collins M, Lee H, Grinspoon S. Effects of long-term testosterone administration in HIV-infected women: a randomized, placebo-controlled trial. *AIDS*. 2009;23:951-959.

142. Von Roenn JH, Armstron D, Kotler DP, et al. Megesterol acetate in patients with AIDS-related cachexia. *Ann Intern Med*. 1994;121:393-399.

143. Oster MH, Enders SR, Samuels SJ, et al. Megesterol acetate in patients with AIDS and cachexia. *Ann Intern Med*. 1994;121:400-408.

144. Clarick RH, Hanekom WA, Yogev R, Chadwick EG. Megestrol acetate treatment of growth failure in children infected with human immunodeficiency virus. *Pediatrics*. 1997;99:354-357.

145. Grinspoon S, Corcoran C, Stanley T, et al. Effects of androgen administration on the growth hormone-insulin-like growth factor I axis in men with acquired immunodeficiency syndrome wasting. *J Clin Endocrinol Metab*. 1998;83:4251-4256.

146. Frost RA, Fuhrer J, Steigbigel R, et al. Wasting in the acquired immune deficiency syndrome is associated with multiple defects in the serum insulin-like growth factor system. *Clin Endocrinol (Oxf)*. 1996;44:501-514.

147. Schambelan M, Mulligan K, Grunfeld C, et al. Recombinant human growth hormone in patients with HIV-associated wasting. A randomized, placebo-controlled trial. Serostim Study Group. *Ann Intern Med*. 1996;125:873-882.

148. Esposito JG, Thomas SG, Kingdon L, Ezzat S. Growth hormone treatment improves peripheral muscle oxygen extraction-utilization during exercise in patients with human immunodeficiency virus-associated wasting: a randomized controlled trial. *J Clin Endocrinol Metab*. 2004;89:5124-5131.

149. Moyle GJ, Daar ES, Gertner JM, et al. Growth hormone improves lean body mass, physical performance, and quality of life in subjects with HIV-associated weight loss or wasting on highly active antiretroviral therapy. *J Acquir Immune Defic Syndr*. 2004;35:367-375.

150. Napolitano LA, Schmidt D, Gotway MB, et al. Growth hormone enhances thymic function in HIV-1-infected adults. *J Clin Invest*. 2008;118:1085-1098.

151. Herasimtchuk AA, Hansen BR, Langkilde A, et al. Low-dose growth hormone for 40 weeks induces HIV-1-specific T cell responses in patients on effective combination anti-retroviral therapy. *Clin Exp Immunol*. 2013;173:444-453.

152. Carr A, Workman C, Smith DE, et al. Abacavir substitution for nucleoside analogs in patients with HIV lipoatrophy: a randomized trial. *JAMA*. 2002;288:207-215.

153. Tebas P, Zhang J, Hafner R, et al. Peripheral and visceral fat changes following a treatment switch to a non-thymidine analogue or a nucleoside-sparing regimen in HIV-infected subjects with peripheral lipoatrophy: results of ACTG A5110. *J Antimicrob Chemother*. 2009;63: 998-1005.

154. Jones SP, Doran DA, Leatt PB, et al. Short-term exercise training improves body composition and hyperlipidaemia in HIV-positive individuals with lipodystrophy. *AIDS*. 2001;15:2049-2051.

155. Driscoll SD, Meininger GE, Ljunquist K, et al. Differential effects of metformin and exercise on muscle adiposity and metabolic indices in human immunodeficiency virus-infected patients. *J Clin Endocrinol Metab*. 2004;89:2171-2178.

156. Fitch K, Abbara S, Lee H, et al. Effects of lifestyle modification and metformin on atherosclerotic indices among HIV-infected patients with the metabolic syndrome. *AIDS*. 2012;26:587-597.

157. Bhasin S, Parker RA, Sattler F, et al. Effects of testosterone supplementation on whole body and regional fat mass and distribution in human immunodeficiency virus-infected men with abdominal obesity. *J Clin Endocrinol Metab*. 2007;92:1049-1057.

158. Bhasin S, Storer TW, Berman N, et al. The effects of supraphysiologic doses of testosterone on muscle size and strength in normal men. *N Engl J Med*. 1996;335:1-7.

159. Vigen R, O'Donnell CI, Baron AE, et al. Association of testosterone therapy with mortality, myocardial infarction, and stroke in men with low testosterone levels. *JAMA*. 2013;310:1829-1836.

160. Lo J, You SM, Canavan B, et al. Low-dose physiological growth hormone in patients with HIV and abdominal fat accumulation: a randomized controlled trial. *JAMA*. 2008;300:509-519.

161. Falutz J, Mamputu JC, Potvin D, et al. Effects of tesamorelin (TH9507), a growth hormone-releasing factor analog, in human immunodeficiency virus-infected patients with excess abdominal fat: a pooled analysis of two multicenter, double-blind placebo-controlled phase 3 trials with safety extension data. *J Clin Endocrinol Metab*. 2010;95: 4291-4304.

162. Stanley TL, Falutz J, Marsolais C, et al. Reduction in visceral adiposity is associated with an improved metabolic profile in HIV-infected patients receiving tesamorelin. *Clin Infect Dis*. 2012;54:1642-1651.

163. Stanley TL, Feldpausch MN, Oh J, et al. Effect of tesamorelin on visceral fat and liver fat in HIV-infected patients with abdominal fat accumulation: a randomized clinical trial. *JAMA*. 2014;312: 380-389.

164. Kotler DP, Muurahainen N, Grunfeld C, et al. Effects of growth hormone on abnormal visceral adipose tissue accumulation and dyslipidemia in HIV-infected patients. *J Acquir Immune Defic Syndr*. 2004;35:239-252.

165. Kotler DP, Muurahainen N, Grunfeld C, et al. Effects of growth hormone on visceral adipose tissue and dyslipidemia in HIV, an erratum. *J Acquir Immune Defic Syndr*. 2006;43:378-380.

166. Falutz J, Allas S, Mamputu JC, et al. Long-term safety and effects of tesamorelin, a growth hormone-releasing factor analogue, in HIV patients with abdominal fat accumulation. *AIDS*. 2008;22:1719-1728.

167. Hadigan C, Corcoran C, Basgoz N, et al. Metformin in the treatment of HIV lipodystrophy syndrome: a randomized controlled trial. *JAMA*. 2000;284:472-477.

168. Hadigan C, Meigs JB, Rabe J, et al. Increased PAI-1 and tPA antigen levels are reduced with metformin therapy in HIV-infected patients with fat redistribution and insulin resistance. *J Clin Endocrinol Metab*. 2001;86:939-943.

169. Hadigan C, Rabe J, Grinspoon S. Sustained benefits of metformin therapy on markers of cardiovascular risk in human immunodeficiency virus-infected patients with fat redistribution and insulin resistance. *J Clin Endocrinol Metab*. 2002;87:4611-4615.

170. Mulligan K, Yang Y, Wininger DA, et al. Effects of metformin and rosiglitazone in HIV-infected patients with hyperinsulinemia and elevated waist to hip ratio. *AIDS*. 2007;21:47-57.

171. Driscoll SD, Meininger GE, Lareau MT, et al. Effects of exercise training and metformin on body composition and cardiovascular indices in HIV infected patients. *AIDS*. 2004;18:465-473.

172. Nissen SE, Wolski K. Effect of rosiglitazone on the risk of myocardial infarction and death from cardiovascular causes. [See comment]. *N Engl J Med*. 2007;356:2457-2471.

173. Hadigan C, Yawetz S, Thomas A, et al. Metabolic effects of rosiglitazone in HIV lipodystrophy: a randomized controlled trial. *Ann Intern Med*. 2004;140:786-794.

174. Carr A, Workman C, Carey D, et al. No effect of rosiglitazone for treatment of HIV-1 lipoatrophy: randomized, double-blind, placebo-controlled trial. *Lancet*. 2004;363:429-438.

175. van Wijk JP, de Koning EJ, Cabezas MC, et al. Comparison of rosiglitazone and metformin for treating HIV lipodystrophy: a randomized trial. *Ann Intern Med*. 2005;143:337-346.

176. Slama L, Lanoy E, Valantin MA, et al. Effect of pioglitazone on HIV-1-related lipodystrophy: a randomized double-blind placebo-controlled trial (ANRS 113). *Antivir Ther*. 2008;13:67-76.

177. Sheth SH, Larson RJ. The efficacy and safety of insulin-sensitizing drugs in HIV-associated lipodystrophy syndrome: a meta-analysis of randomized trials. *BMC Infect Dis*. 2010;10:183.

178. Mallon PW, Sedwell R, Rogers G, et al. Effect of rosiglitazone on peroxisome proliferator-activated receptor gamma gene expression in human adipose tissue is limited by antiretroviral drug-induced mitochondrial dysfunction. *J Infect Dis*. 2008;198:1794-1803.

179. Nguyen D, Hsu JW, Jahoor F, Sekhar RV. Effect of increasing glutathione with cysteine and glycine supplementation on mitochondrial fuel oxidation, insulin sensitivity, and body composition in older HIV-infected patients. *J Clin Endocrinol Metab*. 2014;99:169-177.

180. Benedini S, Perseghin G, Terruzzi I, et al. Effect of L-acetylcarnitine on body composition in HIV-related lipodystrophy. *Horm Metab Res*. 2009; 41:840-845.

181. Milazzo L, Menzaghi B, Caramma I, et al. Effect of antioxidants on mitochondrial function in HIV-1-related lipoatrophy: a pilot study. *AIDS Res Hum Retroviruses*. 2010;26:1207-1214.

182. Mulligan K, Khatami H, Schwarz JM, et al. The effects of recombinant human leptin on visceral fat, dyslipidemia, and insulin resistance in patients with human immunodeficiency virus-associated lipoatrophy and hypoleptinemia. *J Clin Endocrinol Metab*. 2009;94: 1137-1144.

183. Lee JH, Chan JL, Sourlas E, et al. Recombinant methionyl human leptin therapy in replacement doses improves insulin resistance and metabolic profile in patients with lipoatrophy and metabolic syndrome induced by the highly active antiretroviral therapy. *J Clin Endocrinol Metab*. 2006;91:2605-2611.

184. Sekhar RV, Jahoor F, Iyer D, et al. Leptin replacement therapy does not improve the abnormal lipid kinetics of hypoleptinemic patients with HIV-associated lipodystrophy syndrome. *Metabolism*. 2012;61: 1395-1403.

185. Worm SW, De Wit S, Weber R, et al. Diabetes mellitus (DM), pre-existing coronary heart diseased (CHD) and the risk of subsequent CHD events in HIV-infected patients: The D:A:D Study. *Circulation*. 2009;119:805-811.

186. Hadigan C, Meigs JB, Wilson PW, et al. Prediction of coronary heart disease risk in HIV-infected patients with fat redistribution. *Clin Infect Dis*. 2003;36:909-916.

187. Lo J, Abbara S, Shturman L, et al. Increased prevalence of subclinical coronary atherosclerosis detected by coronary computed tomography angiography in HIV-infected men. *AIDS*. 2010;24:243-253.

188. Post WS, Budoff M, Kingsley L, et al. Associations between HIV infection and subclinical coronary atherosclerosis. *Ann Intern Med*. 2014; 160:458-467.

189. Zanni MV, Abbara S, Lo J, et al. Increased coronary atherosclerotic plaque vulnerability by coronary computed tomography angiography in HIV-infected men. *AIDS*. 2013;27(8):1263-1272.

190. Subramanian S, Tawakol A, Burdo TH, et al. Arterial inflammation in patients with HIV. *JAMA*. 2012;308:379-386.

191. Burdo TH, Lo J, Abbara S, et al. Soluble CD163, a novel marker of activated macrophages, is elevated and associated with noncalcified coronary plaque in HIV-infected patients. *J Infect Dis*. 2011;204: 1227-1236.

192. Barbour JD, Jalbert EC, Chow DC, et al. Reduced CD14 expression on classical monocytes and vascular endothelial adhesion markers independently associate with carotid artery intima media thickness in chronically HIV-1 infected adults on virologically suppressive antiretroviral therapy. *Atherosclerosis*. 2014;232:52-58.

193. Kelesidis T, Kendall MA, Yang OO, et al. Biomarkers of microbial translocation and macrophage activation: association with progression of subclinical atherosclerosis in HIV-1 infection. *J Infect Dis*. 2012;206: 1558-1567.

194. Parra S, Coll B, Aragones G, et al. Nonconcordance between subclinical atherosclerosis and the calculated Framingham risk score in HIV-infected patients: relationships with serum markers of oxidation and inflammation. *HIV Med*. 2010;11:225-231.

195. Fernandez-Sender L, Alonso-Villaverde C, Rull A, et al. A possible role for CCR5 in the progression of atherosclerosis in HIV-infected patients: a cross-sectional study. *AIDS Res Ther*. 2013;10:11.

196. Parra S, Marsillach J, Aragones G, et al. Paraoxonase-1 gene haplotypes are associated with metabolic disturbances, atherosclerosis, and immunologic outcome in HIV-infected patients. *J Infect Dis*. 2010;201: 627-634.

197. Tseng ZH, Secemsky EA, Dowdy D, et al. Sudden cardiac death in patients with human immunodeficiency virus infection. *J Am Coll Cardiol*. 2012;59:1891-1896.

198. Friis-Moller N, Sabin CA, Weber R, et al. Combination antiretroviral therapy and the risk of myocardial infarction. *N Engl J Med*. 2003;349: 1993-2003.

199. Triant VA, Lee H, Hadigan C, Grinspoon SK. Increased acute myocardial infarction rates and cardiovascular risk factors among patients with human immunodeficiency virus disease. *J Clin Endocrinol Metab*. 2007;92:2506-2512.

199a. Freiberg MS, Chang CH, Kuller LH, et al. HIV infection and the risk of acute myocardial infarction. *JAMA Intern Med*. 2013;173(8): 614-622.

200. Triant VA, Meigs JB, Grinspoon SK. Association of C-reactive protein and HIV infection with acute myocardial infarction. *J Acquir Immune Defic Syndr.* 2009;51:268-273.

201. El-Sadr WM, Lundgren JD, Neaton JD, et al. CD4+ count-guided interruption of antiretroviral treatment. *N Engl J Med.* 2006;355:2283-2296.

202. Silverberg MJ, Leyden WA, Xu L, et al. Immunodeficiency and risk of myocardial infarction among HIV-positive individuals with access to care. *J Acquir Immune Defic Syndr.* 2014;65:160-166.

203. Dolan SE, Hadigan C, Killilea KM, et al. Increased cardiovascular disease risk indices in HIV-infected women. *J Acquir Immune Defic Syndr.* 2005;39:44-54.

204. Fitch K, Srinivasa S, Abbara S, et al. Noncalcified coronary atherosclerotic plaque and immune activation in HIV-infected women. *J Infect Dis.* 2013;208(11):1737-1746.

205. Henry K, Melroe H, Huebesch J, et al. Atorvastatin and gemfibrozil for protease-inhibitor-related lipid abnormalities. *Lancet.* 1998;352:1031-1032.

206. Yarasheski KE, Tebas P, Stanerson B, et al. Resistance exercise training reduces hypertriglyceridemia in HIV-infected men treated with antiviral therapy. *J Appl Physiol.* 2001;90:133-138.

207. Badiou S, De Boever M, Dupuy AM, et al. Fenofibrate improves the atherogenic lipid profile and enhances LDL resistance to oxidation in HIV-positive adults. *Atherosclerosis.* 2004;172:273-279.

208. Dube MP, Wu JW, Aberg JA, et al. Safety and efficacy of extended-release niacin for the treatment of dyslipidaemia in patients with HIV infection: AIDS Clinical Trials Group Study A5148. *Antivir Ther.* 2006;11:1081-1089.

209. Balasubramanyam A, Coraza I, Smith EO, et al. Combination of niacin and fenofibrate with lifestyle changes improves dyslipidemia and hypoadiponectinemia in HIV patients on antiretroviral therapy: results of "heart positive," a randomized, controlled trial. *J Clin Endocrinol Metab.* 2011;96:2236-2247.

210. De Truchis P, Kirstetter M, Perier A, et al. Reduction in triglyceride level with N-3 polyunsaturated fatty acids in HIV-infected patients taking potent antiretroviral therapy: a randomized prospective study. *J Acquir Immune Defic Syndr.* 2007;44:278-285.

211. Gerber JG, Kitch DW, Fichtenbaum CJ, et al. Fish oil and fenofibrate for the treatment of hypertriglyceridemia in HIV-infected subjects on antiretroviral therapy: results of ACTG A5186. *J Acquir Immune Defic Syndr.* 2008;47:459-466.

212. Munoz MA, Liu W, Delaney JA, et al. Comparative effectiveness of fish oil versus fenofibrate, gemfibrozil, and atorvastatin on lowering triglyceride levels among HIV-infected patients in routine clinical care. *J Acquir Immune Defic Syndr.* 2013;64:254-260.

213. Moyle GJ, Lloyd M, Reynolds B, et al. Dietary advice with or without pravastatin for the management of hypercholesterolaemia associated with protease inhibitor therapy. *AIDS.* 2001;15:1503-1508.

214. Fichtenbaum CJ, Gerber JG. Interactions between antiretroviral drugs and drugs used for the therapy of the metabolic complications encountered during HIV infection. *Clin Pharmacokinet.* 2002;41:1195-1211.

215. Silverberg MJ, Leyden W, Hurley L, et al. Response to newly prescribed lipid-lowering therapy in patients with and without HIV infection. *Ann Intern Med.* 2009;150:301-313.

216. Eckard AR, Jiang Y, Debanne SM, et al. Effect of 24 weeks of statin therapy on systemic and vascular inflammation in HIV-infected subjects receiving antiretroviral therapy. *J Infect Dis.* 2014;209:1156-1164.

217. Chow D, Chen H, Glesby MJ, et al. Short-term ezetimibe is well tolerated and effective in combination with statin therapy to treat elevated LDL cholesterol in HIV-infected patients. *AIDS.* 2009;23:2133-2141.

218. Moore RD, Bartlett JG, Gallant JE. Association between use of HMG CoA reductase inhibitors and mortality in HIV-infected patients. *PLoS ONE.* 2011;6:e21843.

219. Calza L, Manfredi R, Colangeli V, et al. Two-year treatment with rosuvastatin reduces carotid intima-media thickness in HIV type 1-infected patients receiving highly active antiretroviral therapy with asymptomatic atherosclerosis and moderate cardiovascular risk. *AIDS Res Hum Retroviruses.* 2013;29:547-556.

220. Lo J, Lu JT, Ihenachor EJ, et al. Effects of statin therapy on coronary artery plaque volume and high-risk plaque morphology in HIV-infected patients with subclinical atherosclerosis: a randomised, double-blind, placebo-controlled trial. *Lancet HIV.* 2015;2(2):e52-e63.

CHAPTER 42

The Long-Term Endocrine Sequelae of Multimodality Cancer Therapy

ROBERT D. MURRAY

KEY POINTS

- With increasing survival from cancer the adverse sequelae of the tumor, and treatment thereof, on multiple organ systems have increasingly been recognized. The endocrine system is one of the most frequent organ systems to be affected, with over 40% of childhood cancer survivors showing one or more abnormalities.
- Dependent on the insult(s) received during multimodality cancer therapy, endocrine late-occurring effects may encompass abrogated growth, skeletal disproportion, precocious puberty, hypopituitarism, gonadal dysfunction, subfertility, transient and permanent thyroid dysfunction, benign and malignant thyroid nodules, hyperparathyroidism, osteoporosis, and avascular necrosis.
- The potential for development of adverse endocrine sequelae is relatively predictable from the tumor site and the components of cancer therapies utilized to induce remission. It is therefore imperative to establish the individual chemotherapeutic medications received, fields that are exposed to radiation, and cumulative dosages delivered.
- Time scales over which endocrine anomalies occur are dependent upon the insult received and the tissue affected, necessitating monitoring over a long duration of time. For example, gonadal dysfunction and thyroiditis are not infrequent during active cancer treatment, whereas hyperparathyroidism develops following exposure of the glands to radiation therapy after a latency period usually in excess of 2 decades.
- Bone disease characterized by osteoporosis and avascular necrosis is observed with chemotherapeutic regimens containing high-dose glucocorticoids. Loss of bone mass, osteoporosis, and fractures are also observed with endocrine manipulation (androgen deprivation therapy, aromatase inhibitors [AIs]). Individuals undergoing these therapies should be assessed at baseline and prophylactic therapy introduced in those at greatest risk. In other settings bone mass is relatively well preserved.
- In addition to traditional chemotherapeutic regimens and conformal radiotherapy, more recently introduced antineoplastic agents including immune-modulating therapies and tyrosine kinase inhibitors (TKIs) have been increasingly implicated in the cause of endocrine dysfunction.

Over the past 4 decades cure rates for childhood malignancies have improved at a remarkable pace. Overall 5-year survival rates have improved from less than 30% in the late 1960s to 78% in 2000,[1] with 73% expected to survive at least 10 years[2,3] (Fig. 42-1). Survival from adult cancers has lagged behind, but significant inroads have been made. For example, progress made in treatment of Hodgkin disease, which affects predominantly a young adult population, has resulted in long-term survival rates of 70% to 90% using combination chemotherapy, radiotherapy, or both.[4,5] With increasing survivorship from both childhood and adult cancers the long-term detrimental effects of multimodality cancer therapy on multiple organ systems has been recognized.[6] The long-term adverse sequelae are likely to gain increasing importance due to the significant demands on health service resources by these individuals. Within the United Kingdom it is estimated that around 2 million (3%) of the population is living with a diagnosis of cancer. Of these, 1.2 million had their initial cancer diagnosis more than 5 years ago.[7] It is predicted that the number of cancer survivors in the United Kingdom will increase by 1 million per decade from 2010 to 2040, reflecting an increase in both cancer incidence and survival rates, as well as an aging population.[7,8]

Concentrating on the endocrine system alone, at least one long-term endocrine sequela is prevalent in 43% of unselected long-term childhood cancer survivors.[9] Data from adult survivors has been less forthcoming as survival has, until recently, been of much shorter duration than achieved in childhood cancers. Endocrine late effects include disturbances of growth and puberty, hypothalamic-pituitary dysfunction, primary hypogonadism, subfertility, thyroid dysfunction, benign and malignant thyroid nodules, hyperparathyroidism, and reduced bone mass.

GROWTH

Table 42-1 outlines the primary effects of multimodality cancer therapy on growth. Initial evidence for the impact of irradiation on growth velocity and final height was derived from animal studies and growth data in children

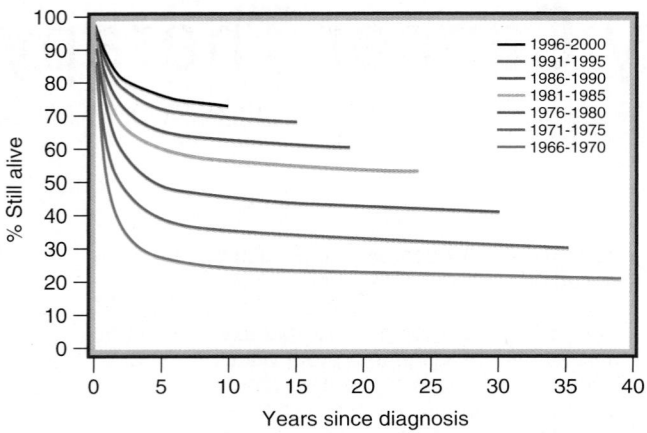

Figure 42-1 Survival of childhood cancer patients diagnosed 1966-2000, by period of diagnosis. (Stiller CA. *Childhood Cancer in Britain: Incidence, Survival, Mortality.* Oxford, UK: Oxford University Press; 2007:166, Fig. 5.14, by permission of Oxford University Press.)

who received cranial irradiation for a variety of malignant and nonmalignant conditions. Cranial irradiation of 2-day-old rats leads to a dose-dependent reduction in growth[10] with reduction in the size of the pituitary gland. The mechanism of growth disturbance was, however, unclear as insulin-like growth factor 1 (IGF-1) levels remained similar to control rats and no increase in growth was observed after treatment with bovine growth hormone (GH). The severity of growth retardation was greatest in rats receiving cranial irradiation in the first few days of life, with a degree of tolerance developing by the end of the first postnatal week.[11]

Early observations in humans noted somatic growth to be retarded in children irradiated for brain tumors[12,13] and acute leukemia.[14,15] The Childhood Cancer Survivors Study is a multicenter questionnaire-based study of individuals within the United States who have survived at least 5 years following childhood cancer. A subanalysis of survivors of brain tumors within this cohort reveals 40% of patients to have a final height below the 10th percentile.[16] In these individuals who have undergone multimodality cancer therapy for childhood malignancy the exact contribution of the endocrine perturbations to the growth failure is difficult to disentangle from the additional effects of chemotherapy, corticosteroid therapy, spinal irradiation, graft-versus-host disease (GVHD), poor nutritional status, and the acute illness itself.[17,18] Endocrine disturbances, including radiation-induced hypothyroidism, precocious puberty, and GH insufficiency, have an adverse impact on growth. The importance of cranial or craniospinal irradiation on growth is clear from studies of survivors of childhood acute leukemia and brain tumors.[15,19] The degree of height loss

TABLE 42-1

Overview of the Primary Effects of Multimodality Cancer Therapy on Growth and Hypothalamic-Pituitary Function in Cancer Survivors

Physiologic System	Insult	Pathology	Comments
Growth	Cranial XRT	Impaired GH secretion Precocious puberty	All insults culminate in reduced height velocity and final height. There are no robust data supporting a direct action of chemotherapy on growth. The ultimate impact on height is dependent on age at XRT, dosage, and schedule. Puberty occurs earlier, spinal growth is more attenuated, and GHD is more prevalent if XRT occurs at a younger age, in fewer fractions, and at higher dosage.
	Spinal XRT	Impaired spinal growth Disproportion	
	Chemotherapy	?Potentiation of XRT effects ?Direct effect on growth plate	
Growth hormone and IGF-1 axis	Cranial XRT	GHD (a) Childhood: reduced growth velocity. (b) Transition: impaired somatic development (c) Adult: impaired quality of life, adverse body composition and vascular risk profile	Cranial XRT doses as low as 18 Gy given during childhood result in GHD in around a third of individuals by 5 yr after treatment, whereas doses of 30-40 Gy result in GHD in 60-100% of patients by 5 yr.[4] Prevalence of GHD is dependent on age at irradiation, fractionation schedule, and dose.
Hypothalamic-pituitary axis	Cranial XRT	LH/FSH deficiency ACTH deficiency TSH deficiency Hyperprolactinemia	Additional anterior pituitary hormone deficits are generally observed with XRT doses >30 Gy and are dependent on dose, fractionation schedule, and time since XRT.[4] In most cases the progression of hormone loss follows the pattern GH → LH/FSH → ACTH → TSH. Other than GHD, additional deficits are unusual within the first 2 years following XRT except with exposure to very high doses. Transient hyperprolactinemia is frequently observed following XRT, resolving over the following few years.
Hypothalamic-pituitary axis	Cranial XRT	Early/precocious puberty	Early puberty is a consequence of disinhibition of cortical influences on the GnRH pulse generator. The earlier the age at XRT (25-50 Gy), the earlier puberty occurs.[8] Early puberty effectively foreshortens the time available for growth-promoting interventions when growth is impaired.

Superscript numbers in table indicate references found at the end of this chapter.
ACTH, adrenocorticotropic hormone; FSH, follicle-stimulating hormone; GH, growth hormone; GHD, growth hormone deficiency; GnRH, gonadotropin-releasing hormone; IGF-1, insulin-like growth factor 1; LH, luteinizing hormone; TSH, thyroid-stimulating hormone; XRT, radiation therapy.

correlates inversely to age at irradiation, the most profound reduction in final height occurring in the youngest at irradiation,[18] and to irradiation dosage, there being greater height loss even with small increases in overall dosage (e.g., 18 Gy vs. 24 Gy).[15] Growth is frequently observed to be reduced during intensive therapy of acute lymphoblastic leukemia (ALL) followed by normal growth thereafter.[19,20] It must be emphasized, therefore, that GH insufficiency is not present in all patients with growth failure,[14] and GH replacement therapy may, therefore, not be indicated.

Spinal irradiation administered prior to puberty significantly impairs spinal growth.[21,22] Leg-length standard deviation scores (SDS) in patients who receive cranial and craniospinal irradiation are equivalent, whereas spinal growth is impaired primarily in the latter patients.[21] The impairment of spinal growth results in disproportion, reflected by an increase in the leg length/sitting height ratio. The impact on the skeleton of spinal irradiation correlates with age; the younger the individual is at the time of irradiation, the greater is the impairment of spinal growth and the greater the degree of disproportion.[21,22] This observation simply reflects the fact that the younger the patient when an insult to growth occurs then the greater the loss in growth potential. Notably, a degree of disproportion has been observed in children who receive a combination of cranial irradiation and chemotherapy for acute leukemia[15]; most likely it relates to disturbance of puberty or a direct effect of the chemotherapy. The effect of cytotoxic chemotherapy on growth remains contentious, but there is a suggestion that subsequent growth may be attenuated.[15] Additionally, chemotherapy has been shown to potentiate the growth impairment resulting from craniospinal irradiation.[17,18] Although the pathophysiologic mechanism by which chemotherapy adversely influences growth is unclear, a reduction in growth factors including IGF-1, increased sensitivity of bone to irradiation damage, and a direct action on the growth plate have been postulated.

Height loss correlates negatively with the age of onset of puberty.[23] Radiation doses of less than 50 Gy during childhood may result in early or precocious puberty,[24] whereas higher doses more frequently result in gonadotropin deficiency. The impact of early puberty in a child is to reduce the time available for growth. When the child is additionally GH insufficient the available time for intervention with GH therapy will also be foreshortened, thereby restricting the therapeutic efficacy of this intervention. For this reason children with early puberty are treated with a combination of gonadotropin-releasing hormone (GnRH) analogues with or without GH replacement. Studies examining the effect of GnRH analogues on final height in GH-insufficient children treated with cranial irradiation have generally reported improvements in auxologic outcome.[25] The majority of studies have been nonrandomized and open label, and they compare patients treated with GnRH analogues with those who did not receive this intervention. The decision to initiate GnRH analogues is frequently based on the child having a poorer final height prediction. Direct comparison of GnRH-treated and -untreated individuals have therefore almost certainly underestimated the beneficial impact of GnRH analogues on final height.

Despite the multiple insults on growth in cancer survivors, the importance of GH status is exemplified by the greater loss of final height in patients with impaired GH secretion compared with those with normal GH secretion who have undergone otherwise similar treatment regimens.[23] Normal growth and peak GH responses are frequently observed in long-term survivors of ALL who receive cranial irradiation doses of less than 24 Gy.[26,27] Higher irradiation doses result in progressive impairment of the GH axis with height loss correlating negatively with the peak GH response to stimulation.[23]

GH replacement therapy is able to increase growth velocity in children with radiation-induced GH insufficiency.[18] Most studies have shown improvements in height velocity, but height data have been conflicting. Early studies showed disappointingly small differences in the height loss prevented by the use of GH replacement and much less than observed in children treated for idiopathic growth hormone deficiency (GHD).[18,23,28-30] A number of factors contribute to the failure of GH to fully redeem the loss of height resulting from multimodality cancer therapy including chemotherapy, spinal irradiation, precocious puberty, a prolonged interval between irradiation and initiation of GH therapy, and inadequate GH schedules.[18,23] The predominant factor likely relates to the interval between hypothalamic-pituitary irradiation and initiation of GH therapy. Because the risk of recurrence of childhood brain tumors is relatively low more than 2 years out from treatment, and there is no evidence that GH increases the risk of recurrence of brain tumors,[31-34] it is reasonable to consider GH replacement at this time. The approach of clinicians is variable, with some offering GH replacement only to children who demonstrate a reduced peak GH response to stimulation in association with a reduced height velocity, whereas others offer GH replacement on the basis of the biochemistry alone with the aim of preventing height loss that, once established, may not be fully remediable. When growth velocity and GH stimulation tests are normal at 2 years after treatment, growth should be monitored at least every 6 months, and the GH stimulation tests should be repeated annually. Use of GH therapy to promote growth in children who have received spinal irradiation can exacerbate disproportion.[18] Whereas the long bones respond appropriately, the irradiated spine is relatively resistant to the growth-promoting effects of GH. In this scenario, growth should be monitored using leg-length velocity, because spinal growth is abrogated.

THE HYPOTHALAMIC-PITUITARY AXIS

Deficiency of one or more anterior pituitary hormones is a consequence of treatment with external beam radiation when the hypothalamic-pituitary axis falls within the field of irradiation (see Table 42-1).[35] GH is almost exclusively the first axis to be affected.[36] Prospective studies from treatment of pituitary adenoma[37] and nasopharyngal carcinoma[36] show that gonadotropin or adrenocorticotropic hormone (ACTH, corticotropin) deficiency evolves next, with thyroid-stimulating hormone (TSH, thyrotropin) deficiency being relatively infrequent. A similar temporal pattern is observed independent of whether radiation exposure occurs during childhood or adult life. To date there are no reported cases of the development of diabetes insipidus as a consequence of cranial irradiation, in either children or adults, at any radiation dosage used.[36,38,39]

The site of radiation damage to the hypothalamic-pituitary axis remains a matter of conjecture. With radiation doses less than 50 Gy, hypothalamic-pituitary hormone deficits are attributable to the cumulative damage from the delayed neurotoxic effects of irradiation on the hypothalamus and secondary pituitary atrophy. Higher radiation doses are thought to cause concurrent damage directly at the level of the pituitary. There are a number of lines of support for this consensus. Patients treated for pituitary adenoma with insertion of yttrium-90 implants

(500-1500 Gy) show a lower prevalence of combined ACTH and TSH deficits[40] compared with conventional external beam radiation (37.5-42.5 Gy)[37]; the likely explanation for this observation is that the field of exposure during conventional irradiation includes the hypothalamus, which is relatively spared with beta emissions from yttrium-90. Evidence of hyperprolactinemia after irradiation is suggestive of a reduction in prolactin inhibitory factors from the hypothalamus with relative preservation of the lactotrophs.[41] A frequent observation following irradiation of the hypothalamic-pituitary axis is of a delayed TSH response to thyrotropin-releasing hormone (TRH) in the absence of overt hypothyroidism, further suggestive of hypothalamic dysfunction.[41] Greater impairment of GH response to the insulin tolerance test (ITT) in comparison with growth hormone–releasing hormone (GHRH) adds further weight to the notion of a hypothalamic site of damage.[42] Nonetheless, GH profiles in irradiated individuals show preservation of GH pulsatility, despite a significant reduction in pulse amplitude.[43] GH pulse generation is dependent on GHRH, supporting a concept that radiation-induced hypopituitarism likely results from combined hypothalamic and pituitary damage, with compensatory overdrive of the remaining pituicytes by hypothalamic hormones to try to maintain the normal hormonal milieu.

The pathophysiologic mechanism responsible for radiation-induced hypothalamic damage is unclear and may reflect either vascular or direct neuronal damage. Hypothalamic blood flow declines with time following irradiation; however, there is no change in the hypothalamic/occipital blood flow ratio between 6 months and 5 years following irradiation.[44] This finding is in contrast to the progressive endocrine dysfunction, suggesting the nature of the damage to be predominantly neuronal.

Although an association between the development of hypopituitarism and chemotherapy has been suggested,[45] no robust relationship has been established.[46,47] In particular, no individual class of chemotherapeutic agent has been implicated. It is possible that the poor reproducibility and variable potency of different secretagogues used in endocrine stimulation tests may provide a more appropriate explanation for occasional individuals being falsely diagnosed as GH deficient.[48,49] There is stronger evidence, however, that cytotoxic drugs may increase the incidence of radiation-induced hypopituitarism.[17,18,50] A number of chemotherapeutic agents modulate antidiuretic hormone (ADH) release from the posterior pituitary, resulting in the syndrome of inappropriate ADH secretion (SIADH). Cisplatin, cyclophosphamide, melphalan, vinblastine, and vincristine have all been implicated, but by no means is this a comprehensive list.

Growth Hormone Deficiency
Childhood Growth Hormone Deficiency

Isolated GHD is commonly the only hormonal sequela of neuroendocrine injury following irradiation of the hypothalamic-pituitary axis with doses less than 40 Gy. Based on animal models GHD has been attributed to selective radiosensitivity of the somatotropic axis.[51,52] Long-term data reveal nearly all children irradiated with doses in excess of 30 Gy develop blunted GH responses to provocation,[53,54] whereas only around a third of patients treated with lower doses show impaired GH release. Although infrequent, isolated GHD in children has been described with radiation doses as low as 10 Gy used in total-body irradiation.[55] The severity and speed of onset of GHD in childhood as a result of irradiation are dose-dependent.[56,57] Blunting of GH responses to provocative tests may occur

as early as 12 months after high-dose irradiation (40-60 Gy) for brain tumors.[58,59] Progressive impairment in GH production occurs with time since treatment,[58,60] necessitating prolonged follow-up and regular assessment of hypothalamic-pituitary function. The prevalence of GHD is also influenced by how the dose is delivered. In children treated for acute leukemia with a cranial irradiation dose of 25 Gy delivered in 10 fractions, a greater proportion develop GHD when compared with those who received 24 Gy in 20 fractions,[61] highlighting the importance of dose fractionation. Abrogated GH responses are more likely to occur if irradiation is administered at a younger age, suggesting that the younger hypothalamic-pituitary axis is more susceptible to radiation-induced damage.[56]

A threshold effect has been proposed for the hypothalamic-pituitary axis; irradiation dosages above 24 to 25 Gy result in impaired GH secretion, and lower doses have a negligible effect on the axis.[56,62] In keeping with this, normal growth is frequently observed in long-term survivors of ALL who receive cranial irradiation doses lower than 24 Gy.[26,27] In children, regimens used in treatment of acute leukemia involving cranial irradiation doses of 24 Gy for central nervous system (CNS) prophylaxis can result in impaired spontaneous and stimulated GH secretion.[14,63] Within this population a continuum between retention of normal GH secretion and severe GHD is observed. Spontaneous GH secretion shows a reduction in both daytime and nocturnal GH secretion, with a reduction in GH pulse amplitude[14,43,63,64] (Fig. 42-2). Normal pulsatile characteristics are, however, maintained.[43] In those individuals showing the greatest reduction in spontaneous GH secretion there is loss of the normal GH diurnal rhythm and a fall in IGF-1 levels below the reference range.[63] At the other end of the continuum a subgroup of children are described in whom the impact of irradiation on the hypothalamic-pituitary axis is minimal, leading to failure of the expected increase in GH secretion only at puberty when demands are increased.[65,66] The reduction in spontaneous GH secretion is purported to occur before attenuation of the peak GH response to stimulation[63]—a phenomenon termed *neurosecretory dysfunction*. Neurosecretory dysfunction of the GH axis is best understood when put in context alongside the growth data. Growth velocity is normal prepubertally, but an attenuated growth spurt is observed during puberty[65] when GH secretion is normally amplified twofold to threefold.[67,68] This phenomenon likely represents inability of the hypothalamic GH control mechanisms to respond to the pubertal rise in endogenous sex steroids. Notably, although individual stimulated GH values are normal when defining GH neurosecretory dysfunction, group mean values are reduced compared with control data.[66] This change suggests that neurosecretory dysfunction may more factually represent decompensation of a partially damaged hypothalamic-pituitary axis. It is likely therefore that the term *neurosecretory dysfunction* has in part been created by difficulties in defining a normal GH axis using pharmacologic stimulation tests.

Prophylactic cranial irradiation in children with ALL has been undertaken on the premise of reducing the rates of CNS relapse. In an attempt to minimize the adverse effects on GH secretion and neuropsychological function prophylactic cranial irradiation dosage was reduced from 24 Gy to 18 Gy. This reduction in dosage does not result in a greater incidence of CNS relapse.[69] Cranial irradiation doses of 18 Gy were, therefore, subsequently introduced in the 1980s, and then later abandoned completely in favor of high-dose intravenous methotrexate or intrathecal chemotherapy. Although significantly attenuated stimulated GH responses are infrequently observed following 18-Gy

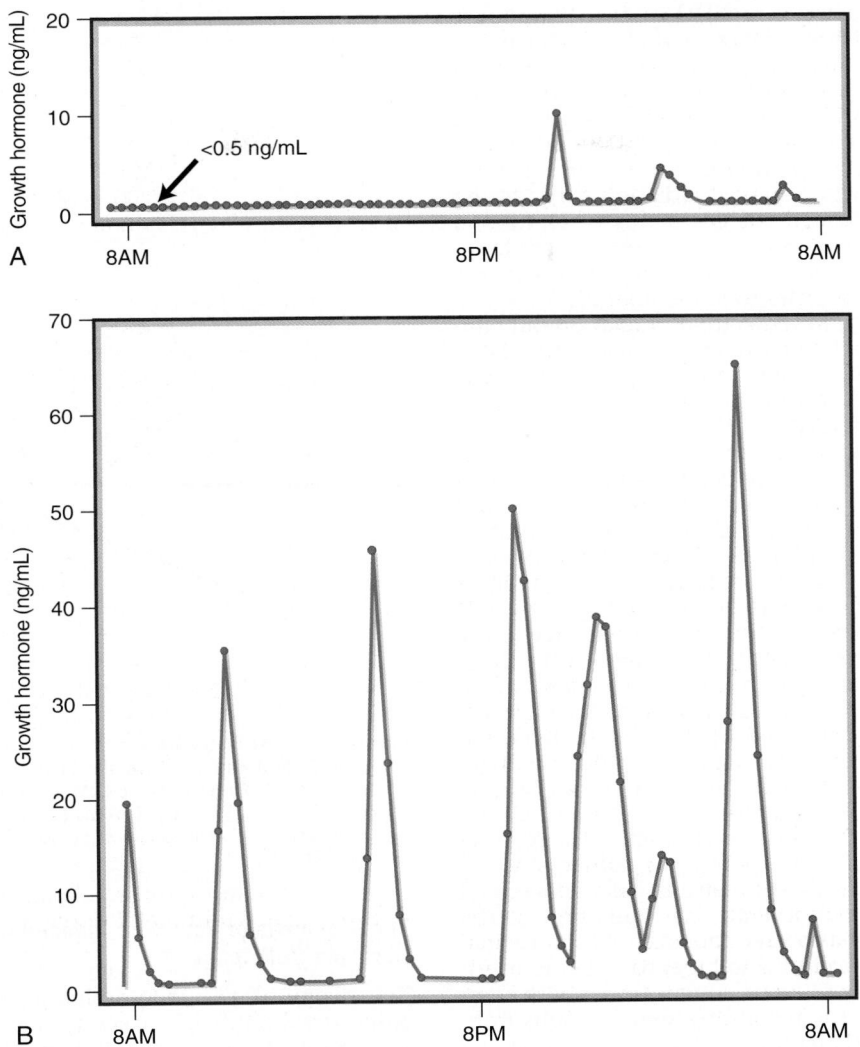

Figure 42-2 Spontaneous pulsatile growth hormone secretion in a patient with acute lymphoblastic leukemia (ALL) who received prophylactic intrathecal methotrexate and cranial irradiation with 24 Gy (**A**) and in a representative normal child (**B**). (From Blatt J, Bercu BB, Gillin JC, et al. Reduced pulsatile growth hormone secretion in children after therapy for acute lymphoblastic leukemia. *J Pediatr.* 1984;104:182-186.)

cranial irradiation, the pubertal increase in spontaneous GH secretion may be attenuated[70] in association with randomization of GH pulsatility.[70] The randomized bursts are explained by a reduction in somatostatin tone, as is similarly observed in rats with focused lesions in the median eminence that reduce somatostatin tone.[71]

Adult Growth Hormone Deficiency

Following cranial irradiation the importance of GHD in adults is twofold. First, GHD almost exclusively occurs before deficits in the additional anterior pituitary hormone axes, and therefore GHD acts as a marker that damage to the additional hypothalamic-pituitary axes may ensue.[36] Second, with recognition of the beneficial effects of GH replacement in adults[72-74] consideration should be given to replacement therapy, particularly when quality of life is significantly impaired.[75,76] The underlying cancer diagnosis and duration of remission must, however, be taken into account before embarking upon this course of management.

Similar to observations in children, the occurrence of adult GHD following irradiation is dependent on a number of variables. After a dose of 37.5 to 45.0 Gy to the hypothalamic-pituitary axis, mean peak GH levels following insulin-induced hypoglycemia were observed to decrease over the first 5 to 6 years and plateau thereafter.[77] Blunting of GH responses to stimulation are reported as early as 12 months after high-dose radiation (50-70 Gy) therapy of nasopharyngeal carcinomas.[78] In addition to length of follow-up, the peak GH response to stimulation correlates with the radiation dosage received by the hypothalamic-pituitary axis.[60] Development of GHD, defined by a peak GH response of less than 2 µg/L (5 mU/L), will occur in patients with preirradiation peak GH responses of 12 µg/L (30 mU/L), 8 µg/L (20 mU/L), and 4 µg/L (10 mU/L) at a mean of 4 years, 3 years, and 1 year, respectively.[77] Thus, if the basal peak GH response is in excess of 20 µg/L (50 mU/L) prior to radiotherapy, it is unlikely that severe GHD will occur within 5 years.[77]

Adult Survivors of Childhood Cancer. Adult survivors of childhood cancer who have received irradiation to the hypothalamic-pituitary axis during their childhood cancer treatment frequently exhibit impaired GH secretion. Assessment of GH status in young adult survivors of ALL who received cranial irradiation of 18 to 25 Gy revealed a third of patients to have severe GHD (peak GH response <3 μg/L) and a further third to have partial GHD (peak GH response 3-7 μg/L).[62] Almost all patients with impaired GH secretion received 24 to 25 Gy, supporting a threshold effect of the irradiation dosage on the GH axis.[62] Impaired GH secretion during adult life, following childhood irradiation of the hypothalamic-pituitary axis, is more likely to be observed in those who received radiation early during childhood.[62] Late assessment of GH status of childhood brain tumor survivors (40-50 Gy) in adult, or predominantly adult, cohorts reveals the vast majority of patients to have blunted GH responses to stimulation.[60]

In adults who have received cranial irradiation but who retain normal individual, but attenuated mean, stimulated GH responses, a similar phenomenon to the described GH neurosecretory dysfunction of puberty is not observed.[79] When the GH axis of these individuals is placed under stress during prolonged fasting, spontaneous GH secretion increases appropriately.[79,80] A number of qualitative changes in the GH profiles of these adults are observed[79,81] and reflect those observed in adults with severe GHD.[43] Profiles show elevated nadir and interpeak GH levels, reduced peak GH, reduced pulsatile GH, and a decrease in the ratio of pulsatile area under the curve (AUC) to the total AUC GH secretion.[79,81] The diurnal rhythm, pulse frequency, pulse duration, and interpulse interval are unaffected. In those individuals with severe GHD an increase in approximate entropy (irregularity and unpredictability of fluctuations) is observed, consistent with perturbation of the hypothalamic control of GH release.[43] Mechanistically these changes are attributable to a reduction in somatostatin tone leading to higher nadir GH levels and reduced peak levels. GHRH activity is essential to GH pulse generation,[82,83] suggesting that irradiation damage is not purely the consequence of hypothalamic damage to GHRH neurons. The reduced GH secretion following low-dose (<40 Gy) irradiation of the hypothalamic-pituitary axis can, therefore, be postulated to occur as a combination of a mild hypothalamic insult and direct damage to the pituitary somatotrophs with compensatory overdrive of the remaining somatotrophs from the hypothalamic GHRH neurons.[53,79]

Survivors of Cancer Treated in Adult Life. Radiation-induced GHD is recognized to occur following treatment of brain tumors and sinonasal carcinomas during adult life. Some of the most robust data come from individuals who have received high-dose radiation (45-60 Gy) for stage I (T1 N0 M0) or stage II (T1 N1 M0) nasopharyngeal carcinoma. These tumors receive the majority of their radiation through opposing lateral facial fields, which include the pituitary gland and frequently the basal hypothalamus (Fig. 42-3). When investigated for hypothalamic-pituitary dysfunction on the premise of putative symptoms of hormonal dysfunction after at least 5 years without recurrence, almost all of these individuals show impaired stimulated GH responses.[41,84] When irradiated during adult life, age and gender have no measurable effect on the risk of developing GHD.[36]

Only limited data are available for GH status following irradiation of nonpituitary brain tumors. The prevalence of severe GHD at 5 years after treatment is reportedly around 30%.[45,85] Prospective assessment of pituitary function following irradiation of nasopharyngeal carcinoma shows mean stimulated GH levels to fall from as early as 1 year.[36] At 5 years after radiotherapy 60% to 65% of individuals would be expected to show abrogated GH levels (<20 mU/L, 6.7 μg/L).[36] Similar radiation doses to the hypothalamic-pituitary axis administered during childhood would, however, be expected to result in an earlier onset of GHD and a greater prevalence of GHD.[59,86,87]

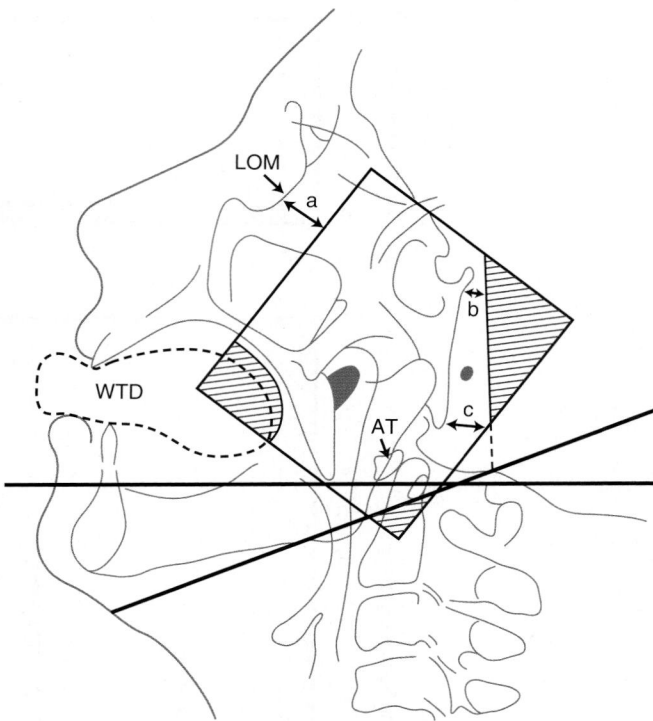

Figure 42-3 Lateral facial field used during radiotherapy of nasopharyngeal carcinoma. The shielded areas are shown shaded. Distances shown are 1.5 cm (*a* and *c*) and 0.75 cm (*b*). AT, atlantoid tubercle; LOM, lateral orbital margin; WTD, wax tongue depressor. (From Lam KS, Wang C, Yeung RT, et al. Hypothalamic hypopituitarism following cranial irradiation for nasopharyngeal carcinoma. *Clin Endocrinol (Oxf).* 1986;24:643-651.)

The Diagnosis of Radiation-Induced Growth Hormone Deficiency

The diagnosis of radiation-induced GHD in children is suspected when height velocity SDS remains below normal after completion of cancer therapy. The diagnosis can then be confirmed or refuted biochemically using appropriate GH stimulation tests. In the absence of a pathophysiologic marker equivalent to growth, the diagnosis of radiation-induced adult GHD becomes dependent exclusively on the prevailing biochemistry. In general, biochemical evaluation of GH status in both children and adults is undertaken as it would be in other diseases causative of GHD. Because radiation-induced GHD is frequently isolated, the diagnosis can robustly be achieved only through the use of two provocative tests of GH reserve.[88,89] The ITT is generally considered the gold standard test for the diagnosis of GHD in adults at risk of hypopituitarism.[89,90] In children profound hypoglycemia during the ITT has led to deaths and irreversible neurologic damage,[91] and therefore the test should be performed only in centers experienced in the use of this test in children. In addition to cranial irradiation, individuals requiring assessment of their GH status may have received anthracycline therapy as part of their treatment regimen. Anthracycline therapy has been implicated in the development of cardiomyopathies,[92-94] which can decompensate during times of significant stress on the cardiovascular system. Although no data exist for decompensation occurring during assessment of the hypothalamic-pituitary axis using the ITT, an alternative stimulation test should be used where echocardiographic evidence for significant anthracycline cardiac damage exists.

Debate has risen as to whether all GH stimulation tests, when abrogated, appropriately represent a state of GHD.

Following irradiation of the hypothalamic-pituitary axis it is notable that the peak GH response to the ITT is often more attenuated than when using the arginine,[95] GHRH plus arginine,[96,97] or GHRH tests.[42] Following radiotherapy the peak GH response to the ITT falls significantly within the first 5 years, with less change over the subsequent 10 years.[96] In contrast, the peak GH response to the GHRH plus arginine test shows little change in the first 5 years, with a more significant fall occurring over the following 10 years.[96,98,99] Thus, the evolution in GH responsiveness to provocative tests is stimulus dependent and suggests initial hypothalamic damage followed by later somatotroph dysfunction. The GHRH plus arginine test may be unreliable in characterizing GH status in the first 5 years after radiotherapy.

In irradiated individuals showing discordant responses, characterized by a subnormal response to the ITT (peak GH < 5 μg/L), but a normal or less attenuated response to the GHRH plus arginine test, spontaneous GH release is reliably reduced only in those patients who failed the GHRH test (peak GH < 16.5 μg/L).[81] When only the response to the ITT is impaired, spontaneous GH secretion is normal.[81] In patients with impaired responses to the ITT, however, IGF-1 levels are reduced to a similar extent in patients with both reduced and normal spontaneous GH secretion.[81] This observation questions the validity of defining GH status by a measurement of 24-hour GH secretion.[100] The diagnosis of GHD in these individuals thus remains complex, and it is not clear which test most accurately reflects a state of GHD.

Growth Hormone Replacement in Adult Cancer Survivors

Long-term survivors of cancer who have been rendered GH deficient by multimodality cancer therapy exhibit a clinical picture identical to that of GH-deficient adults with primary hypothalamic-pituitary disease: increased fat mass; reduced lean body mass, strength, exercise tolerance, and bone mass; an adverse lipid profile; and impaired quality of life.[101,102] The pattern of impairment of quality of life in GH-deficient adult cancer survivors is identical to that of patients with primary pituitary disease, the domain relating to vitality showing the greatest impairment.[103] The extent to which GHD contributes to the abnormalities observed in adult cancer survivors is difficult to disentangle from the direct effects of the primary tumor, treatment modalities used to induce remission, limited exercise, and poor nutritional status.

There are no data specific to the use of GH replacement during transition with radiation-induced GHD; however, it is intuitive to surmise that the beneficial effects of GH replacement in these individuals would be similar to those in GHD hypopituitary adults of other causes.[104,105] Before committing an individual who received childhood GH replacement for radiation-induced GHD to transitional GH replacement it is essential to reassess the GH axis. This necessity is derived from the fact that all degrees of GHD are treated during childhood and only those with severe GHD qualify for treatment as an adult. Furthermore, the reproducibility of GH stimulation tests is poor, and reassessment of GH status in childhood brain tumor survivors shows only around 60% retest as severely GH deficient after reaching final height.[106] GH doses used to treat GHD adults during transition should be aimed at normalizing the IGF-1 level in contrast to the weight-based regimens used during childhood.[107]

Low-dose GH replacement in adult GH-deficient survivors of childhood cancer leads to small improvements in body composition and serum lipids; a significant improvement in quality of life; and increased spinal bone mineral density (BMD).[102,108] As yet there are no data available on the effect of GH on fracture rates of these individuals. Previous spinal irradiation impairs the osteo-anabolic effects of low-dose GH replacement on bone accretion.[108] Improvements in quality of life occur in all domains; however, similar to patients with primary pituitary diseases the greatest improvement occurs in vitality.[103] In adult survivors of childhood cancer the minor changes in body composition, lipid profile, and bone mass following GH replacement suggests GHD may not be a major etiologic factor in their pathogenesis. The converse appears to be true for quality-of-life status in these individuals, and this improvement should be the primary indication for initiation of GH replacement therapy.

Several lines of evidence suggest a link between the GH axis and development of various cancers. Epidemiologic data suggest a link between both prostate cancer and premenopausal breast cancer and that of circulating serum IGF-1 levels. Those individuals with IGF-1 values in the upper reaches of the normative range have an increased relative risk compared with those in the lowest quartile.[109,110] Patients with active acromegaly show an increased risk of colonic polyps and carcinoma[111]; and in vitro data show that GH and IGF-1 promote leukemic blast cell replication.[112] Given these data, concerns over the potential of GH replacement to induce recurrence or increase relapse rates of patients in remission from malignant disease have been raised. Reassuringly, no increase in recurrence rates of childhood brain tumors or acute leukemias are observed with GH replacement therapy[32,34,113,114]; and analysis by brain tumor subtype has shown no diagnostic subgroup to be at increased risk of recurrence.[34,113] No trend in the relative risk of recurrence with cumulative duration of GH treatment is observed, adding further support to the safety of GH replacement in these individuals.[32] Second tumors are a frequent consequence of cranial irradiation; however, data to date show no increase in these tumors in patients who receive GH replacement.[114,115] Residual abnormalities on computed tomography are not a contraindication to treatment of childhood brain tumor survivors.[34] Continued neurologic surveillance imaging is warranted in these individuals, based on the limited power of studies to date.

Cranial Irradiation and Additional Anterior Pituitary Hormone Deficits

Although low-dose radiation most frequently results in isolated GHD, damage to additional anterior pituitary hormone axes as a consequence of hypothalamic-pituitary irradiation is well recognized.[58,116,117] Similar to children who develop GHD, the vulnerability to more extensive hypothalamic-pituitary dysfunction following irradiation during childhood is dependent on age at irradiation[50,56,87,118]; time since treatment[41,85,119]; irradiation dose, fractionation, and time allowed between fractions for tissue repair[35,38,39,41,46,85]; and the margins of the irradiation field.[41] During adult life, gender, age of irradiation, and adjuvant chemotherapy do not predict development of hypopituitarism.[85] The greater the dose of irradiation, the more likely the patient will develop deficits and the earlier these deficiencies will occur.[35] For example, when treating tumors of the pituitary gland or anatomically related lesions during adult life the 5-year cumulative risk of TSH deficiency increases from 10% to 52% with dose escalation from 20 Gy delivered in 8 fractions to 42 to 45 Gy delivered in 15 fractions, respectively[38] (Fig. 42-4). Modern radiation schedules generally do not use more than 2 Gy per fraction with no more than 5 fractions per week. An

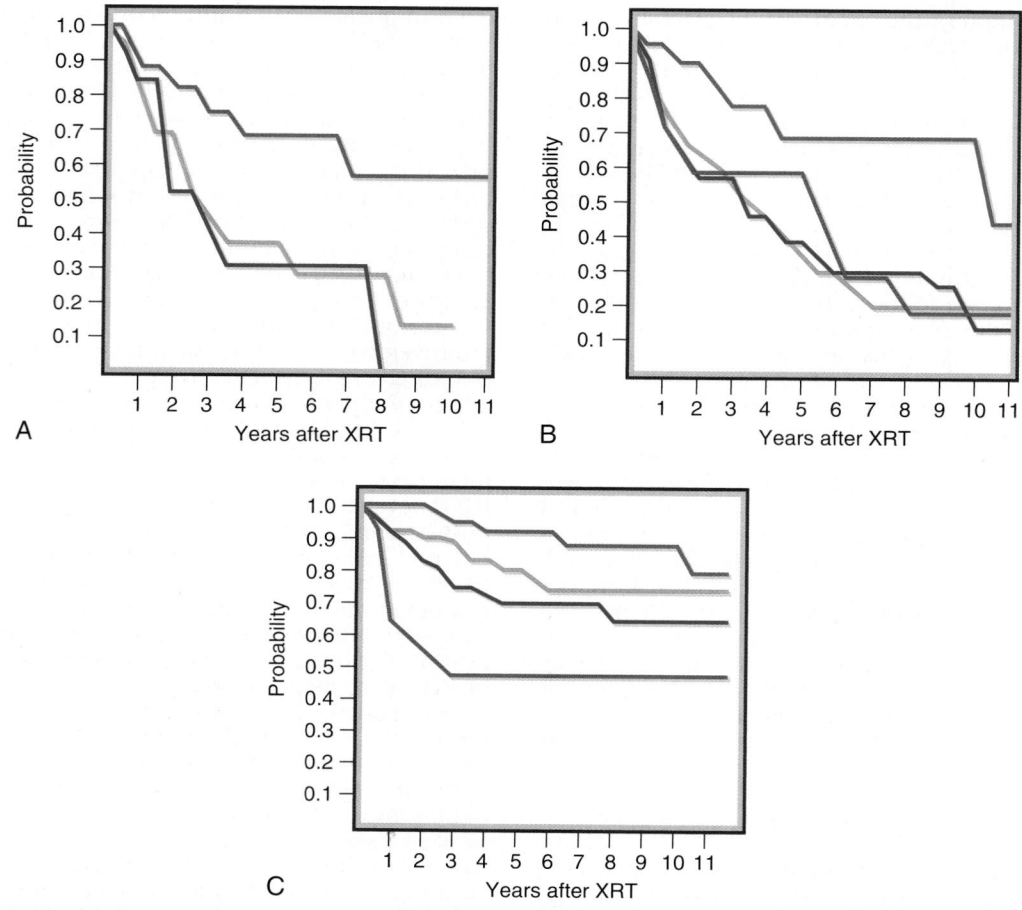

Figure 42-4 The probability that secretion of gonadotropin (**A**), adrenocorticotropic hormone (ACTH) (**B**), and thyroid-stimulating hormone (TSH) (**C**) will remain normal up to 11 years after radiotherapy using three or four dosing regimens, shown by the colored lines. Blue line, 20 Gy in 8 fractions; green line, 42-45 Gy in 15 fractions; magenta line, 40 Gy in 15 fractions; yellow line, 35-37 Gy in 15 fractions; XRT, radiation therapy. (From Littley MD, Shalet SM, Beardwell CG, et al. Radiation-induced hypopituitarism is dose-dependent. *Clin Endocrinol (Oxf)*. 1989;31:363-373.)

increase in the fractionation size leads to relatively more injury to late responding (neuronal) tissues compared with early responding (tumoral) tissues.[120] Notably, the presence of a pituitary lesion or previous surgery in the region of the hypothalamic-pituitary axis increases susceptibility to irradiation-induced damage as the axis may already be compromised to some extent.[37,45,121] Overall, however, the relative frequencies of deficiencies affecting the various anterior pituitary hormones is similar to those following irradiation of pituitary tumors,[36,37] with GH, gonadotropins, ACTH, and TSH being affected in descending order of frequency (Fig. 42-5).

As with GHD, much of the data concerning irradiation-induced hypopituitarism characterized in adults result from the long-term sequelae of cranial irradiation administered in treatment of childhood cancers. Deficiency of the gonadotropins, ACTH, and TSH in adulthood following cranial irradiation of 18 to 25 Gy administered during treatment of childhood ALL is relatively infrequent. Irradiation doses used in childhood for the treatment of CNS relapses of ALL, brain tumor, and soft tissue sarcomas of the head and neck (35-60 Gy), however, require closer observation for long-term pituitary hormone dysfunction. Hypopituitarism consequent to irradiation used during adulthood to treat tumors anatomically distant to the pituitary gland is best exemplified by data derived from brain tumors[85,122] and sinonasal carcinomas.[36,123,124] Radiation doses used in treatment of these tumors is generally in excess of 40 to 50 Gy. Following irradiation therapy of sinonasal disease, deficiency of one or more pituitary hormones is reported to occur in 60% to 80% of individuals with long-term follow-up.[36,41,46,123,125]

Gonadotropins

Gonadotropin deficiency following cranial irradiation occurs in a continuum from impaired luteinizing hormone (LH) or follicle-stimulating hormone (FSH) responses to GnRH while maintaining normal sex steroids, to that of severe deficiency of both gonadotropins and sex steroids. In the first year following irradiation of the hypothalamic-pituitary axis in men with nasopharyngeal carcinoma a rise in basal and stimulated FSH is observed with no change in either LH or testosterone levels.[36,78] After the first year a progressive decline in both the FSH and LH occurs.[36,78] Studies in humans and primates suggest that these changes reflect an initial decline in pulse frequency of hypothalamic GnRH, followed by a progressive reduction in GnRH pulse amplitude.[126,127] In the majority of cases in which the gonadotropins have been affected by irradiation, levels continue to lie within the normative range. In men this is usually accompanied by a testosterone level that lies in the lower reaches of the normative range or only slightly below. In women the failure of adequate pulsatile gonadotropin secretion leads to failure of egg development or ovulation, initially at intermittent cycles; oligomenorrhea

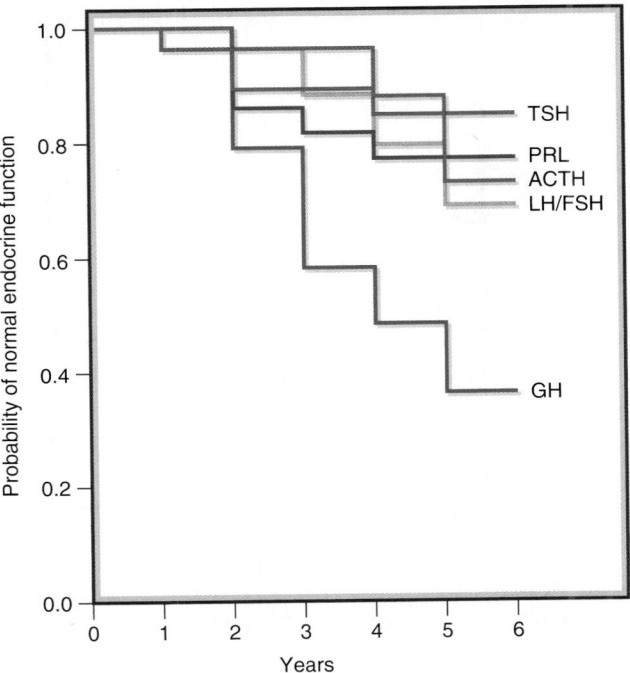

Figure 42-5 Cumulative probability of retaining normal endocrine function following irradiation of the hypothalamic-pituitary axis during treatment of nasopharyngeal carcinoma. ACTH, adrenocorticotropic hormone; FSH, follicle-stimulating hormone; LH, luteinizing hormone; PRL, prolactin; TSH, thyroid-stimulating hormone. (From Lam KS, Tse VK, Wang C, et al. Effects of cranial irradiation on hypothalamic-pituitary function: a 5-year longitudinal study in patients with nasopharyngeal carcinoma. *Q J Med.* 1991;286:165-176.)

ensues before the onset of amenorrhea and estrogen deficiency. Symptoms of gonadotropin deficiency frequently bring to attention the possibility of evolving hypopituitarism if these individuals are not undergoing regular endocrine screening.[41] In postmenopausal women gonadotropin deficiency is silent and may only be recognized biochemically by failure of physiologic elevation of these hormones. Care must be taken in assessing radiation-induced gonadotropin deficiency due to the not infrequent presence of concurrent hyperprolactinemia.[36,41,84]

Gonadotropin deficiency is uncommon when radiation doses to the hypothalamic-pituitary axis are below 40 Gy, with a remarkable increase in incidence following more intensive schedules. Following irradiation for brain tumors[45,47,85] (40-70 Gy) or nasopharyngeal carcinomas[36,39,125] gonadotropin deficiency is reported in around 30% of individuals 5 years after exposure. A similar proportion of women and men are affected.[36,47] Repeated infusion of GnRH may induce LH and FSH pulsatility, suggesting predominantly hypothalamic damage, with the prospect of restoring fecundity.[128]

In addition to gonadotropin deficiency cranial irradiation doses of less than 50 Gy can result in precocious or early puberty in children.[24,129] Both genders are affected equally with irradiation doses employed in the treatment of brain tumors (25-50 Gy),[24] whereas lower doses used for prophylaxis in treatment of acute lymphocytic leukemia (18-25 Gy) result in a predominance of precocious puberty in girls.[130] A linear relationship between age at irradiation and age at onset of puberty is observed. For cranially irradiated children, the onset of puberty occurs at a mean of 8.51 years in girls and 9.21 years in boys plus 0.29 year for every year of age at irradiation.[24] The mechanism responsible for early puberty is thought to result from disinhibition of

cortical influences on the hypothalamus, allowing GnRH pulse frequency and amplitude to increase prematurely. It has been postulated that the cortical restraint on the onset of puberty is more easily disrupted in girls than boys by any insult, including irradiation.

Adrenocorticotropic Hormone

Impaired cortisol reserve as a consequence of ACTH deficiency is less common than both GH and gonadotropin deficiency following irradiation of the hypothalamic-pituitary axis. When present it is a relatively late occurrence and there is almost exclusively evidence for additional anterior pituitary hormone deficits.[36,41,47] Occasionally ACTH deficiency may occur before gonadotropin deficiency[37] and may rarely be the first hormone deficiency to occur.[36] ACTH deficiency is uncommon with radiation doses less than 40 to 50 Gy[131] and is virtually absent with doses less than 24 Gy.[55,132] Following irradiation of brain tumors distant to the hypothalamic-pituitary axis in adult life approximately 20% of patients are reported to be ACTH deficient.[45,85] The 5-year prevalence of biochemical ACTH deficiency following treatment of nasopharyngeal carcinomas is reportedly up to 27% of patients, though many individuals show only borderline subnormal results.[36,39,125]

Normal or slightly exaggerated cortisol responses to corticotropin-releasing hormone (CRH)[47] are also described following cranial irradiation for brain tumors. Individuals who retain normal cortisol response to stimulation show activation of the hypothalamic-pituitary-adrenal axis.[133] Integrated 24-hour cortisol levels and cortisol production rates are increased by 14% and 20%, respectively. Cortisol half-life, pulsatility, and diurnal rhythmicity are unchanged.[133] It is reasonable to assume the increase in cortisol secretion reflects underlying activation of the CRH-ACTH axis. The pathophysiologic mechanism pertaining to these observations remains unclear, though it has been speculated that chronic stress or a local radiation-induced inflammatory response may play a role.

Thyroid-Stimulating Hormone

Central hypothyroidism is most classically represented by low free thyroid hormones in association with an inappropriately low TSH level. In most cases the TSH level lies below, or in the lower reaches of, the normative range. The infrequent contribution of immunoreactive, but bioinactive, TSH in irradiated individuals with central hypothyroidism can lead to TSH values that are in the upper reaches of the normative range or mildly elevated.[134]

A delayed TSH response to TRH and a diminished nocturnal TSH surge are reported to occur in children, adult survivors of childhood cancer, and adults who have received cranial irradiation.[41,78,84,135,136] These qualitative changes are suggestive of dysfunction of the hypothalamic control of the thyroid axis. It has been proposed that they may represent a diagnosis of hidden central hypothyroidism and that TSH secretion may be compromised even before the somatotropic axis.[136] Despite a relatively high proportion of individuals displaying these qualitatively abnormal TSH responses (~30%) following cranial radiotherapy, free thyroxine (T$_4$) levels are generally normal, and few individuals go on to develop overt secondary hypothyroidism.[36,78] The latter observations suggest that the TSH anomalies are functional and do not represent hidden central hypothyroidism.[135] Notably, however, the majority of patients who develop overt hypothyroidism do show a delayed or decreased TSH response to TRH. To date there is no convincing evidence to support the routine use of the

TRH test or assessment of TSH surge to improve the diagnostic sensitivity and specificity of central hypothyroidism.

Deficiency of TSH occurs late and is infrequently seen within the first 2 to 3 years after radiotherapy, even when the hypothalamic-pituitary axis is exposed to high-dose radiation.[36] The prevalence of central hypothyroidism in children exposed to cranial irradiation (35-45 Gy) in treatment of nonpituitary brain tumors is in the region of 3% to 6%,[131,137] and central hypothyroidism is virtually absent after prophylactic cranial irradiation used in treatment of acute leukemia.[138-140]

In adults treated for sinonasal disease the 5- and 10-year actuarial risk of clinical central hypothyroidism following irradiation (40-70 Gy) is in the region of 3% and 13%[141] and 9% and 22% for subclinical (biochemical) hypothyroidism, respectively.[141] Nine percent of adults irradiated with a median biologic effective dose (BED) of 54 Gy for nonpituitary brain tumors show biochemical evidence of central hypothyroidism 3 years after therapy.[85] A dose-dependent increase in the incidence of central hypothyroidism is observed over the dose range of 40 to 70 Gy.[141] There is no detectable effect of dose fractionation, age, or gender on development of TSH deficiency in irradiated adults.[141] Adjuvant chemotherapy does not predispose to development of radiation-induced central hypothyroidism.[141]

Hyperprolactinemia

In adults mild hyperprolactinemia is observed in a minority of patients following low-dose irradiation of the hypothalamic-pituitary axis.[38] When higher irradiation doses are used in the treatment of nasopharyngeal carcinoma and brain tumors, hyperprolactinemia is seen more frequently.[36,39,41,47,84,85] Prolactin levels are rarely elevated more than three to four times the upper limit of the normative range.[36,85] The pattern of development shows a gender dichotomy, being elevated more often in women but only infrequently in men,[36,41,47] and hyperprolactinemia is more likely if irradiation occurs during adult cancer therapy than if it occurs during childhood.[47,53] The hyperprolactinemia not infrequently returns to baseline values over the following few years (Fig. 42-6). When symptomatic in women the irradiation-induced hyperprolactinemia may lead to oligomenorrhea and galactorrhea.[36] Men are rarely symptomatic. Individuals with low serum prolactin levels, generally associated with panhypopituitarism, have additionally been described.[85]

GONADAL FUNCTION

Table 42-2 outlines the primary effects of multimodality cancer therapy on the reproductive system. Multimodality treatment regimens employed in the treatment of cancer damage the gonadal axis directly at the level of the gonad and centrally at the hypothalamus and pituitary, as previously discussed. Damage to the gonads and damage to central structures are not mutually exclusive and it is not uncommon for an individual who has received multimodality cancer therapy to have involvement at both levels. Damage to the gonads can occur from irradiation exposure and cytotoxic chemotherapy. Irradiation of the gonads occurs during treatment of gonadal tumors, testicular relapses of hematologic malignancies, and soft tissue sarcomas of the pelvis; during total-body irradiation (TBI) in preparation for bone marrow transplantation (BMT); and from scatter during spinal irradiation for certain brain and relapsed hematologic malignancies. Damage from cyto-

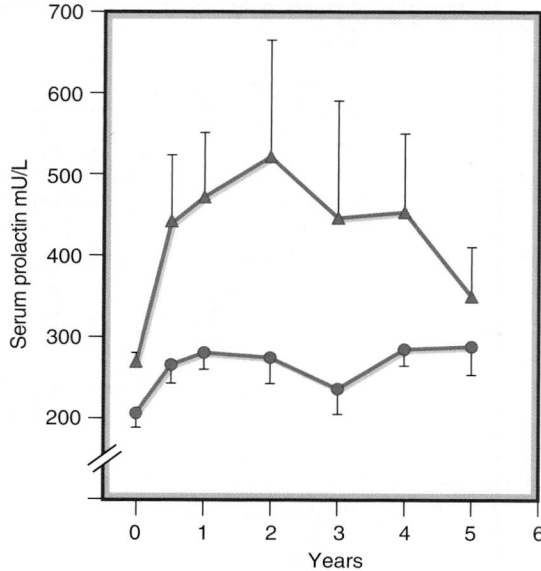

Figure 42-6 Mean serum prolactin concentration (mU/L) of adult men (●) and women (▲) with time following radiotherapy to the hypothalamic-pituitary axis. Error bars represent ±SEM (standard error of the mean). (From Littley MD, Shalet SM, Beardwell CG, et al. Hypopituitarism following external radiotherapy for pituitary tumours in adults. *Q J Med.* 1989;70:145-160, used with permission.)

toxic chemotherapy is most frequently described following alkylating agents, including cyclophosphamide, chlorambucil, and mustine. However, nitrosoureas, procarbazine, vinblastine, cytosine arabinoside, and cisplatin have also been incriminated.[142]

In children, it has been suggested that the chances of maintaining or recovering gonadal function following multimodality cancer therapy are greater for girls than for boys.[143,144] In unselected female childhood cancer survivors around 6% to 7% developed ovarian failure within 5 years of diagnosis. Of the patients with ovarian failure, over 50% received ovarian irradiation in excess of 10 Gy.[145] Female 5-year childhood cancer survivors who continued to menstruate at age 21 years display a risk of entering the menopause fourfold greater than expected by age 21 to 25 years, and around 40% have entered menopause by age 31 years compared with 5% of the general population.[146] Independent risk factors for development of ovarian failure include increasing age, exposure to ovarian irradiation, and treatment with alkylating agents, particularly procarbazine or cyclophosphamide.[145,146] The direct and synergistic effect of taxanes, tyrosine-kinase inhibitors, and monoclonal antibodies on gonadal function are not yet clear.

Male Gonadal Function and Cancer Therapy
Radiation and the Testis

The testis is one of the most radiosensitive tissues in the body. A dichotomy between damage to the germinal epithelium and the Leydig cells is observed; very low doses of radiation can cause significant impairment of spermatogenesis, whereas sex hormone production is impaired only with high radiation doses. As a consequence, puberty generally progresses normally in male children, and secondary sexual characteristics are maintained in the majority of adults who received radiation to the testis. Testicular volumes are small, reflecting damage to the germinal epithelium,[132] and should not be relied upon for staging puberty. In contrast to most other tissues, dose fractionation increases the degree of gonadal toxicity.

TABLE 42-2

Overview of the Effects of Multimodality Cancer Therapy on the Reproductive System of Cancer Survivors

Physiologic System	Insult	Pathology	Comments
Male reproductive system	Local XRT, spinal XRT, and TBI	Oligospermia, azoospermia Subfertility, sterility Leydig cell insufficiency	Primary insult to germ cells of testis—azoospermia occurring within 2 months from XRT doses as low as 2 Gy. Recovery occurs at mean of 30 months and >5 yr following 2-3 or 4-6 Gy, respectively.[10] Impaired spermatogenesis leads to small testis, which should not be used to stage puberty. Leydig cell function is rarely compromised with doses <20 Gy. Puberty progresses normally and secondary sexual characteristics are maintained, despite subfertility.
Ovarian function	Local XRT, spinal XRT, and TBI	Transient amenorrhea Premature ovarian failure Subfertility, sterility Estrogen deficiency	Insult reflects damage to a fixed pool of oocytes. Impact of XRT on ovarian function is age- and dose-dependent.[14] XRT doses >6 Gy result in a premature menopause in women over 40 yr of age; however, in young women a dose of 20 Gy leads to premature ovarian failure in only ~50%. Recovery is infrequent, usually transient, and occurs almost exclusively in younger women. Concurrent estrogen deficiency results in failure of puberty to progress.
Uterine function	Pelvic XRT	Immature uterus Failure to carry a child	Irradiation (20-30 Gy) of the uterus during childhood results in impaired growth, reduced uterine blood flow, and failure of the endometrium to respond to estrogen and progesterone. The younger the patient at XRT, the greater the impact. With egg donation, the impaired uterine function reduces the likelihood of carrying a child through pregnancy.
Male reproductive system	Chemotherapy	Oligospermia, azoospermia Subfertility, sterility Leydig cell insufficiency	Gonadal toxic agents include the alkylating agents procarbazine, cisplatin, vinblastine, and cytosine. Damage depends on the cumulative dosage. Multiagent chemotherapy is generally more gonadotoxic than single-agent therapy. Primary insult is to the germ cells with high-dose therapy additionally resulting in compensated hypogonadism.[18] Recovery frequently occurs; speed of recovery depends on the regimen administered.
Ovarian function	Chemotherapy	Transient amenorrhea Premature ovarian failure Subfertility, sterility Estrogen deficiency	Insult reflects damage to a fixed pool of oocytes. Ovarian toxicity occurs with similar agents to testis. Impact of chemotherapy on ovarian function is dependent on age and the cumulative dose.[20] Recovery of ovarian function is frequently observed, but these individuals may undergo a premature menopause.

Superscript numbers in table indicate references found at the end of this chapter.
TBI, total-body irradiation; XRT, radiation therapy.

The effect of single-fraction low-dose radiotherapy on spermatogenesis is well documented (Fig. 42-7). The most immature cells, spermatogonia, are the most radiosensitive, with doses as low as 0.1 Gy causing a significant reduction in sperm count and morphologic changes in the spermatozoa. Higher doses of 2 to 3 Gy are required to kill spermatocytes, leading to a reduction in spermatid number. Doses of 4 to 6 Gy significantly reduce the number of spermatozoa, implying direct damage to the spermatids.[147] A fall in the number of spermatozoa is seen 60 to 70 days following damage to immature cells from irradiation doses of up to 3 Gy. At higher doses the reduction in sperm count occurs earlier, reflecting damage to the spermatids. Doses of less than 0.8 Gy tend to result in oligospermia and doses higher than 0.8 Gy azoospermia. At the doses discussed recovery of spermatogenesis occurs from proliferation of surviving stem cells. Complete recovery of the germinal epithelia and achievement of premorbid sperm counts occurs 9 to 18 months, 30 months, and 5 years or more following radiation doses of less than 1 Gy, 2 to 3 Gy, and higher than 4 Gy, respectively.[147-149] The majority of testicular radiation exposure occurs as a consequence of fractionated irradiation, which is significantly more toxic to the germinal epithelium. Fractionated radiotherapy doses of less than 0.2 Gy have no significant effect on spermatogenesis, doses of 0.2 to 0.7 Gy cause a dose-dependent increase in FSH and transient reduction in spermatogenesis that recovers within 12 to 24 months,[150] and doses of 2.0 to 3.0 Gy frequently result in azoospermia with recovery of spermatogenesis often delayed for 10 years or more.

At the irradiation doses discussed, Leydig cell function is relatively spared, the vast majority of patients having normal testosterone levels, albeit frequently at the cost of elevated LH levels. With time the elevated LH level returns to normal. During adulthood irradiation doses of 20 to 30 Gy used for carcinoma in situ in the contralateral testis following unilateral orchidectomy result in overt Leydig cell insufficiency,[151] characterized by a fall in testosterone and a compensatory increase in LH levels. The fall in testosterone, however, is not so great as to require replacement therapy in the majority of adults. In contrast, there is a suggestion that individuals who have undergone a similar treatment regimen for testicular cancer during childhood may be more vulnerable to Leydig cell damage and frequently require testosterone replacement as an adult. It is noteworthy that an irradiation dose of 20 to 30 Gy will completely ablate the germinal epithelium.

Chemotherapy and the Testis

The adverse impact of chemotherapeutic agents on the testis is directed primarily at the germinal epithelium, with

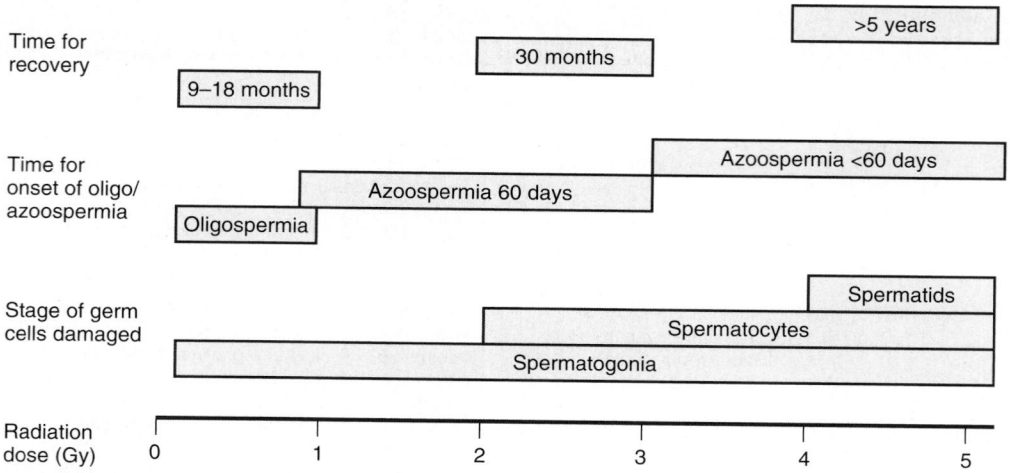

Figure 42-7 Impairment of spermatogenesis following single-dose irradiation: The effect of radiation dose on stage of germ cell damage and time for onset and recovery from germ cell damage. (Adapted from data of Rowley MJ, Leach DR, Warner GA, et al. Effect of graded doses of ionizing radiation on the human testis. *Radiat Res.* 1974;59:665-678; and Howell SJ, Shalet SM. Effect of cancer therapy on pituitary-testicular axis. *Int J Androl.* 2002;25:269-276.)

evidence for Leydig cell dysfunction usually limited to a raised LH level with normal or low normal testosterone levels.[142] The extent of damage and potential for recovery of spermatogenesis is dependent on the chemotherapeutic agents used and the cumulative dosage.[143,152] It has been suggested that the adult testis is more susceptible to damage than the prepubertal testis. However, few studies suggest a relationship between age and risk of gonadal failure.[143,152] In general, combination chemotherapy is more toxic than use of single agents, and the induced azoospermia is less likely to recover.

Insight into testicular function following chemotherapy comes mainly from studies of cyclophosphamide and combination chemotherapy regimens used in treatment of lymphoma and testicular tumors. In men treated with cyclophosphamide as monotherapy approximately 45% show evidence of testicular dysfunction, with the incidence of gonadal dysfunction correlating with the cumulative dosage.[143] Over 80% of postpubertal men who received a total dose of more than 300 mg/kg show evidence of testicular dysfunction.[143] The use of the combination chemotherapy regimens incorporating alkylating agents, such as MVPP (mustine, vinblastine, procarbazine, prednisolone), in treatment of Hodgkin disease renders almost all men azoospermic after the first cycle, and less than a quarter will have a normal sperm count 5 years after receiving six or more cycles.[144,152-154] Regimens comprising nonalkylating chemotherapy (i.e., ABVD; doxorubicin [Adriamycin], bleomycin, vinblastine, dacarbazine) infrequently result in germinal epithelial failure; however, if this does occur, recovery is relatively rapid.[152,154] In the treatment of metastatic testicular cancer, despite rendering the majority of patients azoospermic following use of CVB (cisplatin, vinblastine, bleomycin), the outlook for fertility is relatively good, with 50% of men having a normal sperm count 3 years following this schedule. In general, standard combination chemotherapy regimens used in the treatment of leukemia spare spermatogenesis in the vast majority of individuals, with only 10% to 20% showing persistent gonadal damage.[155,156] Newer regimens for the treatment of lymphoma and testicular tumors have a better outlook for testicular function owing to an absence of procarbazine and lower doses of alkylating agents used.

Although subnormal testosterone levels (<7 nmol/L) are infrequent, there is irrefutable evidence for a subtler impact

of chemotherapy on Leydig cell function.[157] The most frequent abnormalities of Leydig cell function are an elevated basal and GnRH-stimulated LH level in the setting of a normal or low-normal testosterone level. Physiologically LH pulse amplitude is increased while pulse frequency remains unaltered. The compensatory increase in LH means testosterone replacement is rarely necessary. In men treated with high-dose chemotherapy for Hodgkin disease approximately 30% have an elevated LH level in association with a testosterone level in the lower half of the normal range or frankly subnormal, and a further 7% show an isolated raised LH level.[157] These biochemical abnormalities support the hypothesis that a significant proportion of men treated with cytotoxic chemotherapy have mild testosterone deficiency. Studies of testosterone replacement in these individuals with elevated LH and testosterone levels within the lower reaches of the normative range have failed to show significant benefits to date.[158]

Preservation of Male Fertility and Sex Hormone Replacement

Discussions as to strategies for preservation of fertility need to be discussed with the patient and undertaken as early as possible prior to commencement of cancer therapy. At present, sperm cryopreservation is the only option for fertility preservation that is widely accepted and available for postpubertal men.[159] All other techniques remain in the realms of research (Table 42-3).

Men at risk of azoospermia due to their impending treatment schedule can have sperm cryopreserved for future use. This procedure is relatively simple and part of standard practice but is of no value in prepubertal males. Sperm storage is most effective when the sperm concentration, motility, and morphologic features are not affected by the primary disease process. A significant proportion of men with lymphoma, leukemia, and testicular tumors are oligospermic or have impaired semen quality at presentation.[160-162] For prepubertal boys there has been interest in harvesting testicular tissue or spermatogonial stem cells, which can then be cryopreserved and stored for future use. Reimplantation of this tissue into the testis after attainment of remission from cancer and completion of puberty could result in restoration of spermatogenesis.[163,164] In vitro maturation of spermatogonial stem

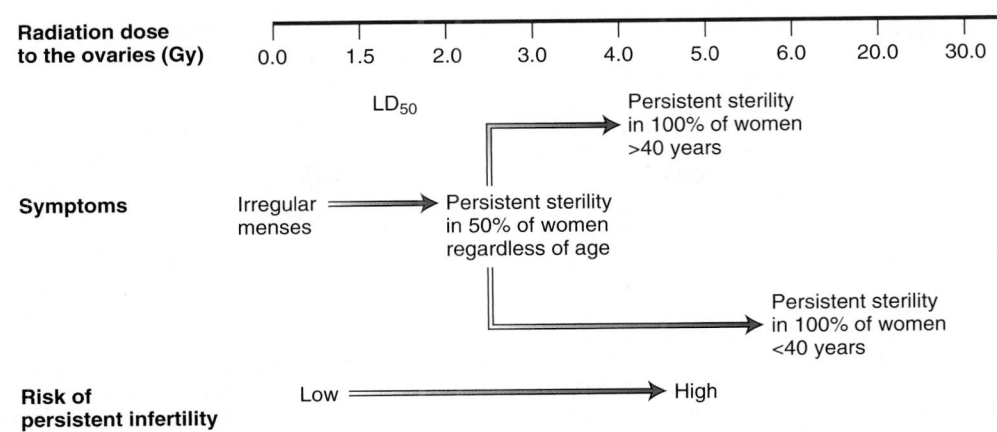

Figure 42-8 The relationship between radiation dosage to the ovaries and ovarian function. LD$_{50}$, lethal dose that will result in sterility of 50% of the tested group. (From Nakayama K, Milbourne A, Schover LR, et al. Gonadal failure after treatment of hematologic malignancies: from recognition to management for health-care providers. *Nat Clin Pract Oncol.* 2008;5;78-89.)

TABLE 42-3
Methods of Preserving Fertility in Men and Women Prior to Cancer Therapy

Type of Method	Methods Used in Men	Methods Used in Women
Current clinical practice	Semen cryopreservation (ejaculation or electrical stimulation) Microsurgical aspiration Testicular biopsy	Embryo cryopreservation Oocyte cryopreservation Oophoropexy
Experimental procedures	Germ cell cryopreservation Testicular tissue cryopreservation In vitro maturation of stem cells	Ovarian cortex cryopreservation Ovarian cryopreservation In vitro maturation of primordial follicles In vitro maturation of immature oocytes Ovarian transplantation (from monozygotic twin)

cells is a further investigational method that has been examined in animals. Unfortunately, these investigational methods may be the only option for prepubertal boys, and they should be discussed when available. After chemotherapy an increase in genetic abnormalities is observed in the spermatozoa. Concerns over the potential transmissibility of genetic anomalies, however, have not materialized. Suppression of the gonadal axis with GnRH analogues prior to cancer therapy has shown gonadal protection in animal models,[165] but there is no convincing evidence to date for benefit in either sex in the human.[166,167]

Men with overt hypogonadism should have testosterone replacement instituted to improve body composition, prevent osteoporosis, and maintain sexual function and well-being.[168,169] In pubertal boys who fail to progress through puberty due to overt testosterone deficiency, testosterone replacement will need to be titrated to bring the individual through puberty and maintain body composition and well-being thereafter. In men with compensated hypogonadism secondary to cytotoxic chemotherapy sexual function has been found to be impaired[170] along with slight reduction in bone mass and subtle body composition changes.[171] It is unclear whether these changes are secondary to the mild Leydig cell insufficiency or the primary tumor and treatment thereof. Testosterone replacement in these individuals has not resulted in a significant improvement in bone mass, body composition, serum lipids, sexual function, or quality of life with the exception of a reduction in physical fatigue and low-density lipoprotein (LDL) cholesterol.[158]

Female Gonadal Function and Cancer Therapy
Radiation and the Female Reproductive Tract

The ovaries are irradiated in the management of pelvic tumors and lymphoma, during the spinal component of craniospinal irradiation, and during TBI preconditioning prior to BMT. The effect of irradiation and chemotherapy on the ovary can best be explained by loss of oocytes from a fixed population that, once destroyed, cannot be replaced. The natural history of the healthy ovary is for oocyte numbers to fall exponentially with aging. Ovaries of older women are therefore much more sensitive to radiation-induced damage, and a dose of 6 Gy is liable to result in a permanent menopause in women aged 40 years or older. In contrast, in young women it is estimated that 20 Gy over a 6-week period will result in permanent sterility in around 50%[172] (Fig. 42-8). Higher doses inevitably result in ovarian failure irrespective of age. In childhood, the median lethal dose (LD$_{50}$) of the oocyte has been estimated to be 4 Gy[173,174] and may present as failure to enter or complete puberty or may appear later in life with a premature menopause. Ovarian recovery following childhood irradiation has been reported but is often temporary, with the onset of secondary amenorrhea usually ensuing within the following few years.

Pelvic irradiation during childhood that involves the uterus within the irradiation field leads to changes that result in failure to carry a child. In those patients who do conceive, the risk of miscarriage and low-birth-weight infants is greatly increased.[175] An irradiation dose of 20 to 30 Gy during childhood leads to a reduction in adult uterine length and failure of the endometrium to respond to physiologic estrogen and progesterone therapy.[176] Uterine blood flow is reduced in the postirradiation uterine arteries on Doppler ultrasound. An adequate blood flow is essential to uterine function, particularly endometrial proliferation, implantation, and successful continuation of pregnancy. It is unlikely that an adult who has received a significant radiation dose to the uterus during childhood would be able to carry a child to term. Uterine irradiation impacts not only on patients who retain normal ovarian function but also on those who request in vitro fertilization with donor oocytes for concomitant ovarian failure.

Chemotherapy and the Ovary

Ovarian damage presents clinically with amenorrhea with or without symptoms of estrogen deficiency or failure to progress through puberty. Hormonally, the gonadotropins may be grossly elevated with an unrecordable estradiol level, or there may be moderate elevation of the gonadotropins in association with a midfollicular estradiol level. Similar to irradiation-induced ovarian damage, the susceptibility of the ovary to chemotherapeutic damage, speed of onset of amenorrhea, and potential for recovery are dependent on age and cumulative dosage.[143,177] Smaller doses of chemotherapy are thus required with increasing age to induce ovarian failure.

In women with breast cancer treated with multiagent chemotherapy including cyclophosphamide the average dose of cyclophosphamide to induced amenorrhea in women in their 20s, 30s, and 40s is 20.4, 9.3, and 5.2 g, respectively.[178] Intuitively, prepubertal and pubertal girls would be assumed to be at lower risk of ovarian damage; however, clinical and morphologic studies reveal that they are not totally resistant to cytotoxic ovarian damage, although it occurs infrequently. Following treatment of Hodgkin disease with the alkylating combination chemotherapy regimens MVPP, MOPP (mustine, vincristine, procarbazine, prednisolone), or ChlVPP (chlorambucil, vinblastine, procarbazine, prednisolone) 15% to 62% of survivors develop amenorrhea.[177,179,180] In those over 35 years of age amenorrhea is almost inevitable. In many the onset is abrupt, but in others there is progression to oligomenorrhea with later development of a premature menopause. In contrast, ABVD is much less gonadotoxic.[181] Treatment of acute leukemias with standard regimens results in persistent ovarian failure in fewer than 20% of survivors.[145,182]

Assessment and Preservation of Female Fertility

Strategies aimed at prevention of gonadal damage have led to the use of chemotherapeutic regimens, such as ABVD for the treatment of Hodgkin disease, that have equivalent cure rates but significantly less impact on gonadal function. There remains some risk to gonadal function, however, with almost all cancer therapies, and discussions as to strategies for preservation of fertility need to be undertaken as early as possible in the management algorithm. At present, embryo and oocyte cryopreservation are the only options for fertility preservation in women that are widely accepted and available. Both require hormonal ovarian stimulation. All other techniques to improve outcomes remain predominantly in the realms of research (see Table 42-3).

A large number of cytotoxic agents have been implicated as teratogenic to the fetus, and it is therefore important that during cancer therapy women use appropriate contraception until remission is achieved. In women who retain normal ovulatory cycles after having received cytotoxic chemotherapy and who spontaneously conceive no evidence of an increase in birth defects has been detected. Recovery of ovarian function in amenorrheic women and the possibility of a premature menopause in women retaining a normal cycle are difficult to predict accurately following an insult to the gonads received during multimodality cancer therapy. The use of transvaginal ultrasound to accurately quantitate ovarian volume and antral follicle count, along with measurement of inhibin B and antimüllerian hormone (AMH) have been proposed as guides of future reproductive potential following cancer therapy.[183,184] Both inhibin B and AMH are secreted by

granulosa cells, and thus concentrations decline with depletion of follicles. Further work is required to optimize the predictive models.

Preservation of fertility in women who are to undergo intense treatment likely to result in infertility is a significant research growth area. Treatment of Hodgkin disease frequently includes local irradiation of involved lymph nodes, including those along the iliac vessels. The ovaries lie adjacent to the iliac vessels and will receive a dose of approximately 35 Gy, inevitably resulting in premature ovarian failure. Oophoropexy to remove the ovaries from the irradiation field, combined with shielding, can reduce the dose of irradiation received by the ovaries to less than 6 Gy, thereby reducing the incidence of amenorrhea by around 50%.[185,186] The exact reduction in risk of amenorrhea as a consequence of oophoropexy is controversial and needs to be assessed in the context of disease extent, patient age, and surgical expertise. Both oocytes and embryos can be frozen. Embryo storage requires the patient to be in a stable relationship and undergo controlled stimulation of the ovary for several weeks, along with regular ultrasonograph monitoring and aspiration of follicles. This technique is time-consuming when there is a pressing need to start treatment, is invasive, does not permit natural conception, and is not applicable to prepubertal girls. Pregnancy rates approximate to 15% to 30% per cycle with thawed embryos. Over the past decade stimulatory regimens using AIs combined with standard fertility drugs have been developed for use in women with estrogen-sensitive cancers.[187-189] These regimens enable ovarian stimulation while maintaining estrogen levels near physiologic.[188,189] Outcomes, in terms of number of embryos and pregnancies, appear equivalent to traditional regimens. Oocyte cryopreservation is considered for patients without a partner; it requires stimulation of the ovaries and retrieval of the oocytes. Success rates have improved significantly in specialist reproductive centers, so this procedure should be considered where available.[190]

Ovarian suppression with GnRH analogues has not reliably been shown to improve fertility outcomes in women and requires further study. Interest has remained in cryopreservation of ovarian cortical strips rich in primordial follicles that can later be thawed and grafted back into the patient at the original site (orthotopic) or elsewhere (heterotopic).[191,192] This technique is available to both prepubertal and mature women. Several large centers are now storing ovarian strips, and to date over 20 live births following orthotopic regrafting in women surviving cancer have been reported.[193-195] Theoretical concerns remain as to whether cancer cells may be transferred back to the recipient; however, this has not been described in humans to date. Only time will tell if this technique will further improve fertility prospects of women who undergo multimodality cancer therapy.

In women under the age of 50 years who have developed gonadal failure the impact is twofold—fertility and sex steroid production. Sex steroid replacement is recommended to alleviate symptoms of hot flushes, mood changes, and vaginal dryness, as well as to prevent loss of bone mass.[151] The impact of sex steroid replacement on cardiovascular events remains controversial in patients below the age of 50 years in light of recent data showing an increase in vascular events in postmenopausal women treated with hormone replacement therapy (HRT).[196,197] Reassuringly, after stratification of the Women's Health Initiative study data by age, the relative risk of cardiovascular disease was not increased in those aged 50 to 55 years.[198] The use of HRT in postmenopausal women has been associated with an increased risk of breast cancer.[196]

It is probable that this latter risk equates to lifetime exposure to estrogens, and therefore, continuing estrogen replacement until age 50 in these individuals should not convey an excess risk. Exposure of the breast to radiation scatter during mantle irradiation in Hodgkin disease[199,200] or TBI prior to BMT[201] is associated with an increased risk of breast cancer. Whether estrogen replacement amplifies this risk further is not yet known.

Radioiodine Therapy and the Gonadal Axis

Although radioiodine doses used in treatment of hyperthyroidism have minimal, if any, effect on gonadal function, the effect on gonadal and reproductive function is an important consideration when treating differentiated thyroid carcinoma (DTC) as a consequence of the high and often repeated administrations.

In women, transient absence of menstrual periods occurs in 8% to 27% of women in the first year after radioactive iodine for DTC,[202,203] particularly when treating women closer to the age of menopause. In the first year after radioiodine therapy, several studies have reported increased rates of spontaneous and induced abortions.[202] Radioiodine treatment for DTC is, however, not associated with a significantly increased risk of long-term infertility, miscarriage, induced abortions, stillbirths, offspring neonatal fatality, or congenital defects.[202-205] Radioiodine-treated women may experience their menopause at a slightly younger age than untreated women.[202,205] There is otherwise little observational evidence to suggest important adverse effects of radioiodine treatment on gonadal function, fertility, or pregnancy outcomes beyond 12 months.

Doses of radioiodine used in treatment of thyrotoxicosis result in only minimal and transient changes in the germinal epithelium and Leydig cell function in men.[206] Reassuringly, there is no significant variation in sperm concentration or percentage of normal forms. Following therapy for DTC in men with single high-dose therapy, FSH levels frequently increase at 6 months, following which a decline is observed, with all subjects showing normal values by 18 months.[207-210] Similarly, inhibin B levels fall significantly at 3 to 6 months after treatment but normalize by 18 months,[209] reflecting transient damage to spermatogenesis. Increases in LH are much less frequent and when present return to normal levels by 12 months.[207,209] Testosterone levels remain normal. A greater proportion of patients experience elevated gonadotropins after cumulative radioiodine activities of greater than 14 GBq.[207] At these doses short-term oligospermia is common,[207] though there is little evidence for long-term infertility.[208,210]

PRIMARY THYROID DISEASE

The effects of multimodal cancer therapy on the thyroid are summarized in Table 42-4. The recognition of the adverse effects of head and neck irradiation, particularly for secondary cancers, has led to the demise of radiation therapy for benign diseases, including acne vulgaris, goiter, tuberculous adenitis, thymic enlargement, and tonsillar hyperplasia. Use of low-dose (2-7 Gy) radiation therapy for benign disease was common in the United States from the 1930s through the 1950s. Since the 1960s exposure of the thyroid and parathyroid glands to radiation has occurred almost exclusively during treatment of malignant disease, most commonly during neck irradiation in Hodgkin disease and sinonasal carcinomas; craniospinal irradiation of certain brain tumors; TBI before BMT; and from unavoidable scatter during treatment of primary brain tumors.

Thyroid tissue is among the most radiosensitive tissues in the body. Following irradiation the prevalence of both thyroid dysfunction and formation of thyroid nodules increases significantly.[211-213] The absolute incidence of thyroid disorders following radiation, however, is not clear cut owing to differences in radiation dose and schedules (duration and fractionation); previous thyroid surgery; volume of thyroid irradiated; duration of follow-up; definition of thyroid disorders (clinical vs. biochemical hypothyroidism); and effects of adjuvant therapies.[214] This uncertainty is reflected in a survey among radiation oncologists who estimated the risk of clinical hypothyroidism after administration of 50 Gy to the whole thyroid as between 2% and 50%.[215] Damage to the thyroid from irradiation is proposed to result from direct thyroid cell injury, immune-mediated damage, and damage to small thyroid arterioles.[214]

Thyroid Dysfunction
Hypothyroidism

The first reports of the development of hypothyroidism as a consequence of irradiation for head and neck cancers

---

TABLE 42-4

Overview of the Effects of Multimodality Cancer Therapy on the Thyroid and Parathyroid Glands of Cancer Survivors

Physiologic System	Insult	Pathology	Comments
Thyroid nodules	Neck XRT or TBI	Malignant nodules	Risk is significantly increased following neck XRT (RR ~15).[22] Incidence increases from 5-10 yr after XRT. Possible "cell kill" effect at doses above 30 Gy.[23] Risk is significantly greater in children compared with adults and in females compared with males.[23]
		Benign nodules	There is increased prevalence of all benign thyroid disease.[22] Palpable nodules occur in 20-30% patients who received neck XRT. Prevalence depends on time since XRT, female gender, and XRT dose.
Thyroid dysfunction	Neck XRT or TBI	Hypothyroidism	Frank or compensated hypothyroidism occurs in 20-30% of patients who receive TBI and in 30-50% of those who received neck irradiation (30-50 Gy).[22] Hypothyroidism generally occurs within 5 yr of XRT. Thyroxine therapy should be instituted early because of the hypothesis that an elevated TSH may drive early thyroid cancers.
		Hyperthyroidism	Graves disease is reported to occur at increased frequency (RR ~8).[22]
Parathyroid	Neck XRT	Late-onset hyperparathyroidism	Latency period is 25-47 yr. Dose dependency has been observed.[24]

Superscript numbers in table indicate references found at the end of this chapter.
RR, relative risk; TBI, total-body irradiation; TSH, thyroid-stimulating hormone; XRT, radiation therapy.

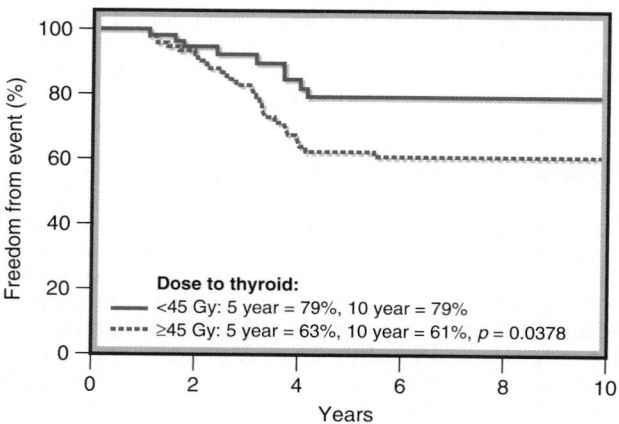

Figure 42-9 Probability of remaining free from hypothyroidism in patients following irradiation therapy during treatment of extracranial head and neck malignancies. Patients are divided according to the radiation dosage received to the neck. (From Bhandare N, Kennedy L, Malyapa RS, et al. Primary and central hypothyroidism after radiotherapy for head-and-neck tumors. *Int J Radiat Oncol Biol Phys.* 2007;68:1131-1139; used with permission.)

were published in the 1960s.[216,217] Hypothyroidism is the most common late sequela of irradiation of the thyroid and may be overt or subclinical. Neck irradiation in treatment of adult sinonasal disease results in a 5-year actuarial risk of clinical and subclinical primary hypothyroidism of 32% and 29%, respectively,[141] with little change in prevalence thereafter (Fig. 42-9).[141] Thus, in the long term, biochemical evidence for primary hypothyroidism is present in up to 60% of patients receiving high-dose radiation (30-70 Gy) to the neck for sinonasal disease or Hodgkin lymphoma.* A similar incidence is observed following craniospinal irradiation for primary brain tumors during childhood.[47] Interestingly, although the thyroid does not lie directly within the field of irradiation administered during cranial irradiation for brain tumors, there is an increased incidence of subsequent hypothyroidism.[223]

At least half the cases of hypothyroidism occur within the first 5 years following radiation,[†] with peak incidence at 2 to 3 years.[‡] Conversely, the latency period may be prolonged.[212,213] A dose-dependent increase is observed in the incidence of clinical primary hypothyroidism.[§] Dose is additionally inversely associated with the latency period to the development of thyroid dysfunction[224] such that postradiation hypothyroidism can occur within the first 6 months following high-dose therapy.[218] Fractionation of the dose, in contrast to other radiosensitive organs, has minimal impact on development of hypothyroidism.[218] Up to 20% of cases of subclinical hypothyroidism may show improvement or resolution of elevated TSH levels.[223,224]

Within adults exposed to neck irradiation no effect of age[141,219,221,227] or gender[219,221,226,227] on the development of thyroid dysfunction is observed. A higher proportion of individuals irradiated in childhood, however, develop thyroid dysfunction when compared with those irradiated during adult life.[220,226] Within childhood an inverse relationship is observed between age at irradiation and the development of hypothyroidism.[213,225,228] Importantly, the risk of developing primary hypothyroidism is dependent on the proportion of the gland exposed to irradiation, with primary hypothyroidism occurring infrequently when

---

*References 125,213,214,218-222.
[†]References 213,218,221,222,224,225.
[‡]References 218,221,222,224,225.
[§]References 141,213,222,224,226.

less than 50% of the gland is irradiated.[141,226] In keeping with this latter observation, hypothyroidism is more common in patients who have undergone a surgical hemithyroidectomy as part of their cancer therapy prior to irradiation.[229,230]

Treatment of both subclinical and overt hypothyroidism should be undertaken early with levothyroxine aiming to place the TSH value in the lower reaches of the normative range. In the majority of cases, patients presenting with subclinical hypothyroidism are likely to progress to overt hypothyroidism with time, and therefore, early intervention is warranted. Furthermore, even mildly elevated TSH values may convey an elevated risk of both benign and malignant thyroid nodules in the irradiated thyroid[231] that can be abrogated by levothyroxine replacement. Use of levothyroxine to suppress TSH prior to radiation has been proposed as a potential method to reduce thyroid cell turnover and thereby ameliorate irradiation-induced thyroid damage. To date this strategy has not proved to be efficacious.[232]

Hyperthyroidism

In addition to hypothyroidism, Graves disease,[222,233] Graves ophthalmopathy,[211,222,233] and thyroiditis[212,222] occur with increased prevalence following neck irradiation. The relative risk of hyperthyroidism following neck irradiation is 5- to 20-fold[213,222,233] and shows a similar temporal distribution to that of radiation-induced hypothyroidism.[213,222] The actuarial risk of Graves disease thus equates to around 2% to 3% at 10 years after radiation.[222,233] Radiation-induced hyperthyroidism is dose-dependent,[213] with prevalence increasing with time since treatment.[213] Age at irradiation and gender have no effect on the development of Graves disease.[222] Graves ophthalmopathy following head and neck irradiation is indistinguishable clinically from that occurring in nonirradiated individuals,[233] and it is seen in both the euthyroid and the hyperthyroid states.[222]

Effects of Chemotherapy

Although adjuvant chemotherapy has been suggested to cause thyroid dysfunction or influence the development of hypothyroidism following irradiation,[222,223,225] this has not been conclusively demonstrated.* Both interferon and interleukin 2 increase the risk of developing autoimmune hypothyroidism.[234,235] This condition is usually transient, though a small proportion of patients may remain hypothyroid in the long term. A number of chemotherapeutic agents affect thyroid function tests by modulating thyroid hormone binding; 5-fluorouracil increases total triiodothyronine (T_3) and T_4, but patients remain euthyroid with normal TSH and free T_4 levels; asparaginase decreases production of hepatic thyroid-binding globulin (TBG) and total T_4 levels through its widespread effects on protein and DNA synthesis.

Thyroid Nodules

In 1950 Duffy and Fitzgerald raised the possibility that irradiation of the thymus gland during infancy was an etiologic factor in the future development of thyroid carcinoma. In their series 9 of 28 cases of childhood thyroid carcinoma had been exposed to low-dose neck radiation.[236] Since that time a number of epidemiologic studies have conclusively established an association between exposure to external irradiation of the thyroid and development of

---

*References 141,213,219,221,223,227.

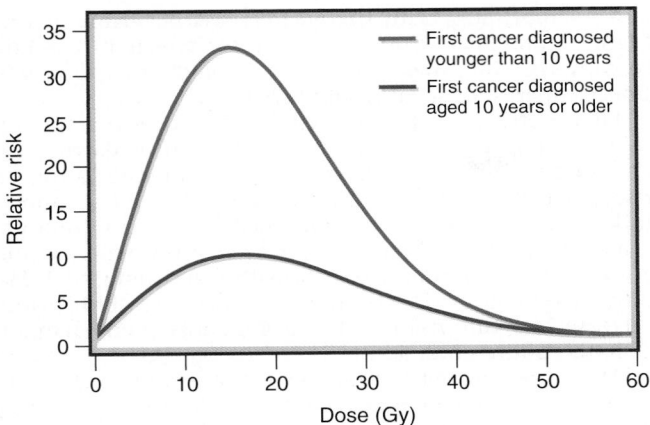

Figure 42-10 Thyroid cancer risk by radiation dose according to age at diagnosis of first cancer. (From Sigurdson AJ, Ronckers CM, Mertens AC, et al. Primary thyroid cancer after a first tumour in childhood (the Childhood Cancer Survivor Study): a nested case-control study. *Lancet.* 2005;365:2014-2023.)

both benign thyroid neoplasia and DTC.[200,237-240] Occurrence of radiation-induced thyroid nodules is uncommon in the first 5 years following exposure, with the peak incidence of excess risk occurring 15 to 20 years after radiotherapy.[213,237,239,241] Twenty years following exposure the excess relative risk decreases; however, the excess absolute risk continues to increase for at least 40 years.[238] The dose-response relationship approximates linearity from 0.1 Gy to a few grays,[237] with the relative risk per gray for both carcinoma and adenoma being in the region of fourfold to eightfold.[237] Risk increases with higher doses but at a more gradual rate. Early data suggested that the risk of developing thyroid cancer was linearly associated with dose; however, more recent data confirm this to be true only for radiation doses up to 20 to 29 Gy[242] (Fig. 42-10). At doses greater than 30 Gy a fall in the dose response has been observed and is consistent with a cell-killing effect of radiation at high doses.[242] The cumulative risk in individuals receiving greater than 5 Gy is estimated to be in the region of 4% to 6% at 25 to 30 years,[237,239] with relative risk calculated to be 15 to 50 times that in the nonirradiated population.[200,214,239] In contrast to other radiosensitive endocrine glands, fractionation of the dose seems to have little effect on reducing the incidence of nodules.[237] The use of adjuvant chemotherapy has yet to be shown to have an independent effect or demonstrable influence on the incidence of radiation-induced nodules.[237,239,242] A similar gender dimorphism is observed to that of spontaneous tumors in nonirradiated individuals. Tumor development is significantly greater when irradiation occurs at a younger age[239,242-244] and reflects the greater susceptibilty of growing tissues to radiation-induced damage. When exposure occurs during treatment of childhood malignancy the risk of developing thyroid carcinoma is greater in those with a primary diagnosis of either neuroblastoma or Wilms tumor,[239] suggestive of an underlying predisposition of these individuals to tumor development.

Around two thirds of thyroid nodules occurring following radiation are benign, and one third are malignant. The distribution of thyroid carcinoma histologic subtypes following irradiation is not dissimilar to that observed in the general population, with the majority being papillary and a lesser proportion follicular carcinomas.[213,237-239,241] These radiation-induced tumors do not seem to act differently from spontaneous tumors,[244,245] though regional lymph node metastases are reported to occur at a higher frequency (up to 30%) than that seen in nonirradiated individuals.[238,241] A number of RET/PTC rearrangements have been shown to be more frequent in radiation-induced thyroid tumors.[246,247]

The use of routine ultrasound scans to monitor the thyroid glands of patients who have received neck irradiation remains controversial. Thyroid ultrasound may be an overly sensitive screening tool owing to the low specificity, in that the clinical relevance of lesions detected is unclear.[248] To place this in perspective, thyroid ultrasound of children administered radiation for Hodgkin disease has been reported as abnormal in all cases, with focal lesions in over 40%.[249] Once palpable or ultrasound-characterized thyroid nodules are elucidated, fine-needle aspiration for cytologic evaluation should be performed. Cytologic evaluation may, however, prove difficult because of the presence of radiation-induced cellular atypia,[250] and there should therefore be a low threshold for undertaking a diagnostic lobectomy.

HYPERPARATHYROIDISM

Early studies of the effects of irradiation in animal models revealed parathyroid tumors to occur in 8% of irradiated rats compared with none in nonirradiated control rats.[251] A putative association between radiation and development of hyperparathyroidism in humans was first hypothesized in 1975 by Rosen and associates, who described the development of radiation dermatitis, a sublingual salivary gland pleomorphic adenoma, and hyperparathyroidism in a young woman treated with face and neck radiation for hirsutism.[252] A number of series followed in which low-dose radiation used in treatment of benign conditions was correlated to the occurrence of hyperparathyroidism (see Table 42-4). In studies from the late 1970s and early 1980s, the prevalence of previous low-dose (<8 Gy) head and neck radiation in patients diagnosed with surgically proven or biochemical hyperparathyroidism has been found to be significantly higher (11%-30%) than in control populations (0%-8%) without hyperparathyroidism.[253-257] Later studies are unlikely to be able to confirm this observation because of the reduced use of low-dose radiation therapy for treatment of benign disease since the 1950s. Furthermore, in patients who have received low-dose neck irradiation the prevalence of hyperparathyroidism is found to be 1% to 11%, significantly greater than that found in background population data and matched control groups.[253,258-260] The relative risk of hyperparathyroidism increases by 0.11 per cGy.[260] The presence of a dose relationship between irradiation and development of hyperparathyroidism supports the previous observational data of a causal association. Radiation-induced hyperparathyroidism follows a benign and indolent course, with many patients remaining clinically asymptomatic.[253,256]

The majority of studies relate to radiation administered during childhood or adolescence. Middle-aged individuals who receive low-dose irradiation to the neck show a prevalence of hyperparathyroidism of less than 5% when assessed 25 years later, the vast majority of whom do not require operative intervention.[261] Few robust data are available regarding the occurrence of hyperparathyroidism after high-dose neck radiation has been used in treatment of malignant diseases, though recently an association has been described.[262,263] Notably, in those individuals who developed hyperparathyroidism the estimated irradiation dose at the thyroid was only 0.9 to 13.2 Gy. It has been hypothesized that a "cell kill" effect of higher irradiation doses may prevent development of hyperparathyroidism.

Monitoring of calcium and parathyroid hormone (PTH) levels in the first 36 months following high-dose neck irradiation shows increasing PTH levels in the setting of normal calcium levels,[264] without the development of hyperparathyroidism.

The latency period from low-dose radiation to the development of hyperparathyroidism is prolonged, and although cases have been reported as early as 5 years following radiation, most cases occur 24 to 45 years later.* A longer latency period has been suggested to occur in younger individuals,[255,262] though age at irradiation does not significantly affect the overall incidence of hyperparathyroidism.[258,260] In nonirradiated populations there is a gender dichotomy, with females showing a higher incidence of hyperparathyroidism. This dichotomy holds true for irradiated individuals, and a similar gender distribution[253] and relative risk of radiation-induced hyperparathyroidism are present in males and females.[258] Irradiation-induced hyperparathyroidism may be the result of either adenoma or hyperplasia. Single adenomas are around twofold more frequent when compared with hyperplasia and multiple gland involvement.[238,255,257,260] Histologic appearance usually confirms a predominance of chief cells,[256,257] but cases with a high proportion of oxyphil cells have been described in hyperfunctioning adenoma and hyperplasia.[256,257] This latter observation is difficult to reconcile because oxyphil cells are generally held to be nonfunctioning. Although cases of parathyroid carcinoma following neck irradiation have been described,[265] they are infrequent and surprisingly have not been observed in the larger series.[253,254]

The frequency of synchronous benign nodules or nonmedullary carcinoma of the thyroid is at least two to three times higher in individuals with radiation-induced hyperparathyroidism compared with nonirradiated patients.† The association between radiation-induced thyroid and parathyroid disease is the likely consequence of sensitivity of both endocrine organs to irradiation; however, a genetic predisposition to radiation-induced tumorigenesis cannot be excluded.

BONE HEALTH

Both patients actively undergoing cancer therapies and long-term survivors are variably at risk of adverse bone health, which can be manifest as low bone mass, increased fractures, and avascular necrosis. The cause is generally multifactorial with contributions from a catabolic illness, poor nutrition, reduced weight-bearing exercise, endocrine deficiencies, therapeutic inhibition of the sex steroids, radiotherapy, chemotherapy, and glucocorticoid therapy. The risk to bone health may vary, even following treatment for the same tumor, depending on the protocol used, and may also vary during an individual treatment regimen.

Cytotoxic chemotherapeutic agents have direct and indirect effects on bone metabolism. Multiagent chemotherapy acts directly to reduce osteoblast proliferation and function in vitro and in vivo.[268,269] Some of the most robust data are derived from patients receiving high-dose methotrexate therapy, which has been shown to have adverse effects on bone in both adults and children. Methotrexate decreases bone formation by reducing numbers of stromal progenitor cells; decreasing osteogenesis and increasing adipogenesis differentiation from mesenchymal stem cells; and promoting osteoclast formation.[270-272] In children methotrexate increases bone pain, osteopenia,

and fracture rates, with the greatest risk occurring at the highest cumulative doses.[273,274] Indirect effects of chemotherapy on bone mass are related to endocrine dysfunction, primarily gonadal insufficiency.

Glucocorticoids administered during cancer therapy for their immunosuppressant, antiedema, antileukemic, or antiemetic effects have direct effects on bone, resulting in reduced bone formation and increased bone resorption. Indirect adverse effects of glucocorticoids occur through impaired gonadal function, decreased intestinal calcium absorption, steroid-induced myopathy, and reduced 1,25-dihydroxyvitamin D_3 synthesis.[275] Reduced BMD and increased fracture risk occur in a dose-dependent manner in both children and adults.[276,277]

There are no robust data to suggest a direct action of radiotherapy on bone mass; however, radiotherapy is documented to have a number of effects on bone (as discussed earlier). During childhood, radiotherapy impairs growth of the irradiated bone. There is also evidence of resistance of irradiated bone to the osteoanabolic effects of GH. Indirect effects of radiotherapy through endocrine dysfunction can predispose to low bone mass.

Childhood Cancer Survivors

Adolescent and adult childhood cancer survivors have variably been reported to have reduced bone mass. Data from brain tumor survivors from the Childhood Cancer Survivors Study suggested a 25-fold relative risk of osteoporosis.[9] Survivors of childhood leukemia and lymphoma also show reduced bone mass,[278,279] although low bone mass has not been universal to all studies,[280,281] and very low BMD appears to be relatively uncommon.[282,283] When present, low bone mass has been found to be most frequently associated with high-dose cranial or craniospinal irradiation and GHD.[279,282] It is important to note that fracture risk is elevated twofold to sixfold in children treated for ALL and appears greatest during and following the early intensive phases of treatment.[284,285] Independently of bone mass, avascular necrosis is emerging as a significant cause of skeletal morbidity in children treated for ALL since the introduction of dexamethasone as the standard glucocorticoid used in treatment regimens.[286,287]

Although low bone mass is unlikely to be a common long-term sequela of childhood cancer therapy, it is important to assess risk for each individual. This enables identification of those individuals most at risk and who warrant further investigation and follow-up. When significant risk factors are present, in the absence of fractures, a dual-energy x-ray absorptiometry (DXA) scan should be performed to establish a baseline for disease monitoring. Interpretation of DXA during childhood should be undertaken cautiously as bone mass is dependent on age, height, and pubertal staging. Given these variables, the threshold of BMD below which fracture risk is increased is not known for childhood cancer survivors. A diagnosis of osteoporosis should therefore not be made on the basis of densitometric criteria alone during childhood and adolescence and more appropriately requires the presence of a clinically significant fracture history in combination with low bone mineral content or density (Z-score < −2.0, adjusted for age, gender, and body size).[288]

Bone mass of childhood cancer survivors improves through adolescence and young adult life,[282] likely reflecting improvements in general health, nutrition, and pubertal progression when delayed. Hormone deficiencies (GH, sex steroids) contribute significantly to low bone mass. Earlier recognition of hormone deficiencies and implementation of replacement therapy over the past 2 to 3 decades

---

*References 238,253-255,258,259,265.
†References 238,256,258,259,265-267.

has greatly improved, impacting positively on bone health. In the absence of fractures most childhood cancer survivors with low bone mass should be managed by lifestyle interventions, including improving nutrition and weight-bearing exercise. Vitamin D status should be optimized. Repeat DXA scans should be performed at an appropriate interval of 2 to 4 years, depending on the magnitude of the deficit in bone acquisition. If repeat fragility fractures occur, a DXA scan should be performed, lifestyle measures instituted, and vitamin D status optimized. Pharmacologic intervention should be considered when fragility fractures occur in conjunction with low bone mass. Bisphosphonates, either oral or intravenous, are generally considered first-line therapy. In children, most experience has been gained using pamidronate. Teriparatide is contraindicated in patients who have received radiotherapy to bone because of a theoretical possibility of increasing the risk of osteosarcoma.[289] At present there is insufficient experience with denosumab used to reduce fragility fractures in childhood cancer survivors to recommend its use.

Adult Cancer Survivors

The adverse skeletal effects of AIs and androgen deprivation therapy (ADT) are well recognized as the predominant causes of significant bone loss in adult cancer survivors. A twofold to fourfold increased risk of osteoporosis is also observed following BMT,[287,290,291] whereas survivors of lymphoma, leukemia, and testicular cancer have normal bone mass.[292-294] Most studies in patients treated in adulthood suggest chemotherapy has minimal impact on bone mass.

In the absence of endocrine dysfunction (AIs, ADT, gonadal failure, etc.) clinically significant bone disease is uncommon in adult cancer survivors. Multiple risk factors are, however, present in a large proportion of cancer survivors. It is therefore important to recognize and screen at-risk individuals, as effective strategies for fracture prevention are available. Osteoporosis is defined by a T-score of less than −2.5 on DXA bone densitometry. However, isolated measurements correlate poorly with fracture risk of an individual. This observation in part relates to the fact that DXA values can be influenced by a number of variables including height, BMI, degenerative skeletal changes, and previous vertebral fractures. Furthermore, causes of secondary osteoporosis including glucocorticoid therapy and previous cancer therapy modify the relationship between fractures and bone density. In an attempt to more accurately assess fracture risk in an individual the World Health Organization (WHO) fracture risk assessment tool (FRAX) should be used.[295] This tool is, however, not applicable below age 40 years.

In patients in whom the FRAX tool suggests the 10-year fracture risk is elevated, lifestyle interventions should be implemented, and vitamin D levels optimized. Lifestyle interventions should include weight-bearing exercise, dietary advice as to calcium intake, and avoidance of smoking and alcohol. Consideration must be given to pharmacologic treatments in patients with fragility fractures or elevated FRAX score. In the United Kingdom the FRAX tool is linked to the National Osteoporosis Guideline Group (NOGG), which provides intervention thresholds for an individual based on the provided data. The final decision to initiate therapeutic intervention, however, lies with the clinician. Pharmaceutical intervention is initiated with oral or intravenous bisphosphonate therapy, the choice depending on patient and physician preference. There are insufficient data to recommend use of denosumab in this setting.

Androgen Deprivation Therapy

Appropriate use of ADT in advanced or aggressive prostate cancer can improve overall survival. ADT is, however, associated with a number of adverse sequelae including loss of bone and muscle mass, fatigue, sweats and hot flashes, metabolic syndrome (weight gain, insulin resistance), impaired cognition, gynecomastia, and sexual dysfunction. There has remained concern as to whether these changes culminate, in the long-term, in an increase in cardiovascular morbidity and mortality risks.

Prospective studies of bone mass in patients receiving ADT show a fall in BMD of 5% to 10% during the first year of treatment.[296,297] Epidemiologic data support a significant increase in fracture rates, with a relative risk of 20% to 50%.[298,299] Preventive therapy to reduce bone loss and fractures has therefore been examined in a number of studies. There are no randomized studies of the beneficial effects of calcium and vitamin D supplementation in this setting; however, it would appear reasonable to ensure men on ADT are receiving at least 1200 mg of calcium, either from diet or supplements, and 800 to 1000 units of supplemental vitamin D. There are a number of randomized studies examining the impact of bisphosphonate therapy on bone mass when used concomitantly with ADT. In general, bisphosphonates have led to either preservation of bone mass or small increases, studies using alendronate or zoledronate showing the greatest effect.[300,301] A recent systematic review and meta-analysis of bisphosphonate use in men on ADT showed a significant effect in preventing osteoporosis and fractures.[302] The humanized monoclonal antibody to receptor activator of nuclear factor-κB ligand (RANKL), denosumab, in a large randomized study of men on ADT increased BMD at the lumbar spine (5.6% at 24 months), femoral neck, and radius. Additionally, denosumab reduced the incidence of new vertebral fractures at 36 months (relative risk 0.38).[303] The selective estrogen receptor modulators (SERMs), raloxifene and toremifene, reduce bone loss of men on ADT at the lumbar spine and hip.[304,305] Toremifene has also been shown to reduce new vertebral fractures by around 50%. There are therefore several therapeutic options to consider to prevent bone loss in men on ADT. A baseline DXA scan should be obtained, with follow-up imaging after 12 months in these high-risk individuals to enable assessment of fracture risk.[306] In addition to calcium and vitamin D supplementation, when the 10-year risk of hip fracture exceeds 3% on the WHO FRAX tool, men on ADT should receive denosumab (60 mg subcutaneously, every 6 months), zoledronate (5 mg intravenously, annually), or alendronate (70 mg orally, weekly).

During the first 12 months of ADT, on average patients experience an approximate 2% increase in weight, about 9% increase in fat mass, and a 3% fall in lean body mass.[307] Triglyceride and high-density lipoprotein (HDL) levels increase, and insulin sensitivity is reduced.[307,308] The risk of developing diabetes is increased by 30% to 40%.[309,310] Although there are relatively good epidemiologic data to suggest the metabolic changes culminate in an increased risk of both arterial and venous vascular events,[309-311] the impact on vascular mortality risk is less well established.[312] Adverse vascular outcomes appear more frequent in patients receiving GnRH agonists compared with orchidectomized patients[309] or those receiving the GnRH antagonist, degarelix.[313] Management of diabetes, weight gain, and elevated triglycerides in men on ADT is the same as for individuals not on these drugs should they fulfill criteria for intervention. There is a suggestion that exercise can alleviate some of the adverse metabolic sequelae and help maintain muscle mass,[314,315] though it is uncertain to what degree. A further promising intervention is that of metformin, though there is insufficient evidence for routine use to improve metabolic manifestations.[314] Lifestyle advice concerning exercise should be given to all individuals receiving ADT. A program of resistance exercise can additionally improve fatigue associated with ADT.[316]

Vasomotor flushing can be a significant negative influence on quality of life. Gabapentin at 900 mg daily, venlafaxine 75 mg daily, medroxyprogesterone acetate 20 mg daily, and cyproterone acetate 100 mg daily have all shown benefit.[317,318] Several small uncontrolled trials of acupuncture have also shown decreases in vasomotor symptoms. The incidence of gynecomastia can be as high as 85% on ADT but is reduced by prophylactic tamoxifen or single-fraction radiation (10-15 Gy).[319,320] Alternatively, these therapies can effectively be used should troublesome gynecomastia occur during androgen deprivation.[321]

Aromatase Inhibitors

The aromatase enzyme complex (CYP19) is critical within the steroid biosynthetic pathway for conversion of androgen precursors into estradiol. Aromatase is present in the ovary, adipose tissue, muscle, brain, breast, and bone. Inhibition of this enzyme complex with clinically available AIs leads to profound estrogen deficiency, both systemically and within the tissues, including the bone microenvironment. Studies of in vivo aromatase inhibition with all three currently available AIs (anastrozole, letrozole, and exemestane) in postmenopausal women have demonstrated greater than 98% suppression of enzyme activity.[322] Physiologically, estrogens decrease bone resorption by inhibiting differentiation of early osteoblastic and osteoclastic precursors. This action is accomplished primarily through suppression of RANKL and induction of osteoprotegerin[323,324] (Fig. 42-11). Conversely, estrogen deficiency results in decreased cell death in osteoclasts and osteocytes, activation of the RANKL system, and increases in osteoclastogenesis.

Use of AIs in patients with estrogen receptor–positive breast cancer is associated with improved long-term outcomes. Current guidelines would suggest the use of an AI as monotherapy for 5 years, or subsequent to tamoxifen therapy, as standard adjuvant therapy for postmenopausal women with hormone receptor–positive invasive breast cancer.[325] Nearly 50% of women who start an AI will complain of early-onset new vasomotor or joint symptoms, often leading to treatment discontinuation.[326,327] A more serious problem has been that the profound estrogen depletion induced by these drugs leads to significant loss of bone mass, with resultant osteoporosis and fracture. Bone loss is greater in sites with higher trabecular bone content, such as the spine, rather than those with a higher proportion of cortical bone, as in the hip. The adverse effects on bone are particularly problematic in postmenopausal women, premenopausal women rendered estrogen deficient by chemotherapy, and those who have received steroids in their treatment regimen. It should be recognized that both glucocorticoid and AIs can predispose to development of fractures at a higher bone mass, as delineated by DXA, than traditionally accepted in postmenopausal osteoporosis (T-score < –2.5). Over the first 12 to 24 months following initiation of AIs, bone mass falls by 3% to 5% at the spine and 2% to 5% at the hip.[322,328,329] Notably, it is unusual for an individual with normal bone mass at initiation of AIs to become osteoporotic. The reported fall in bone mass and concurrent change in bone quality translate into a significantly higher fracture rate compared with untreated patients or those who are receiving tamoxifen.[328,330,331] Estimates of fracture rates vary widely between studies and with duration of follow-up. Interpretation of these studies is complicated by comparison with tamoxifen in the majority of studies, which has a protective effect on bone mass and fracture incidence.[332] Long-term studies of fracture rates at 5 years in patients taking AIs are 40% to 50% greater when compared with those taking tamoxifen.[333-335] Fracture rates also exceed those in control populations but to a lesser degree.[336] Six months after discontinuation of AIs the accelerated bone loss is reversed, and the fracture risk is normalized.[337,338]

Bisphosphonate therapy prevents loss of bone mass through potent inhibition of osteoclast action, the primary cause of bone loss in estrogen deficiency. Intuitively, therefore, bisphosphonates appear to be an appropriate intervention to abrogate AI-induced loss of bone mass. Studies of oral risedronate and ibandronate as adjuvant therapy to the use of AI in breast cancer at 12 months show improvements in BMD of 2% to 3% at the lumbar spine and 0.4% to 2.0% at the hip compared with baseline values.[339,340]

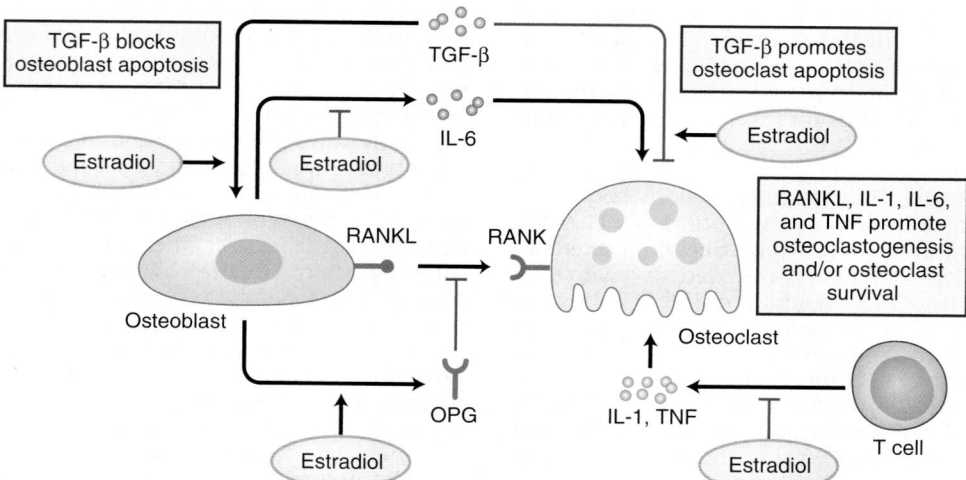

Figure 42-11 Effects of estradiol on bone cell function. Estradiol stimulates transforming growth factor-β (TGF-β) actions on both osteoclasts and osteoblasts, while inhibiting the apoptotic effects of interleukin 6 (IL-6) and T-cell production of IL-1 and tumor necrosis factor (TNF). Therefore, in an estrogen-deficient state, there are more active, longer living osteoclasts, whereas osteoblasts have shorter survival. OPG, osteoprotegerin; RANK, receptor activator of nuclear factor κB; RANKL, RANK ligand. (Redrawn from Coleman RE, Rathbone E, Brown JE. Management of cancer treatment-induced bone loss. Nat Rev Rheum. 2013;9(6):365-374.)

Intravenous zoledronate 4 mg every 6 months for up to 5 years maintains BMD above baseline at the spine and hip, equating to 6% to 8% greater BMD than with unopposed AI therapy.[341,342] To date, a reduction in fracture incidence has not been demonstrated with the use of bisphosphonates because of inadequate power of studies for this end point. Bisphosphonates commenced concurrently with AI prevent loss of BMD to a greater extent than delaying treatment until BMD decreases significantly or fractures occur.[342] No difference in fracture reduction between these two treatment strategies has, however, been shown. Similar effects on BMD to those of bisphosphonates are seen with the monoclonal RANKL antibody, denosumab.[343,344] Studies of teriparatide in the setting of AI-induced loss of bone mass have been limited by the fact that most patients have received radiation therapy as part of their treatment regimen, a relative contraindication to use of teriparatide.

A number of guidelines have been published to aid management of AI-induced loss of bone mass and are for the most part consistent.[345-347] All postmenopausal women require assessment at the time of commencing AI therapy to establish their risk of osteoporosis and fracture. Patients should be given lifestyle advice including undertaking regular weight-bearing exercise, smoking cessation, and reducing alcohol intake. Vitamin D and calcium supplementation containing at least 800 units of cholecalciferol should be commenced. A baseline DXA bone densitometry scan should be obtained, and fracture risk should be assessed using the WHO FRAX tool.[295] All osteoporotic women should receive adjuvant bisphosphonate therapy. Women with osteopenia should receive adjuvant bisphosphonates when additional risk factors for fracture are present. Osteopenic women with no additional risk factors should undergo a further DXA scan in 12 to 24 months, and bisphosphonates should be commenced if the T-score worsens to below −2.0 or annual bone loss exceeds 4% to 5%.

THE METABOLIC SYNDROME AND VASCULAR RISK

Epidemiologic data show childhood cancer survivors to have excess morbidity and mortality risks for at least 10 to 15 years, with survivors of more than 5 years showing an approximately 10-fold higher mortality rate.[348,349] After exclusion of deaths relating to recurrence or progression of the primary tumor, mortality rates remain elevated, with a standardized mortality rate for cardiac and cerebrovascular disease increased fivefold to eightfold.[348,349] An increased risk of late-occurring stroke among childhood survivors of Hodgkin disease, leukemia, and brain tumors is observed when compared with sibling controls,[350,351] with the relative risk estimated at 4.3, 6.4, and 29.0, respectively.[350,351] Examination of demographic and treatment variables reveals the increase in vascular disease to be highest in patients who received chest and spinal irradiation[348] or anthracycline therapy.[352] The relative importance of these mechanisms in placing childhood survivors of cancer at increased risk of vascular disease is unclear. Abnormalities of left ventricular function are observed in individuals treated with anthracyclines,[92,94,353,354] with total cumulative dose being the most significant risk factor for anthracycline late-onset cardiomyopathy.[92,94,353] Anthracycline cardiac toxicity fails to explain the increased vascular morbidity in patients who do not receive this class of drug.

Derangements in both traditional and nontraditional cardiovascular risk factors, consistent with the metabolic syndrome, are prevalent in childhood cancer survivors and can be proposed to have a putative role in predisposition to atherothrombosis. Abnormalities of body composition in childhood survivors of cancer are well documented. The prevalence of obesity is significantly increased,[355-360] with the distribution of excess fat mass located predominantly in the central compartment.[361] During childhood, obesity is observed to develop between time of treatment and attainment of final height,[356,362,363] and cranial irradiation has been implicated in its development.[363] The greatest degree of obesity is observed in those who are treated at the youngest age.[356]

Fasting glucose and insulin are elevated in long-term survivors of childhood cancer[359] and recipients of bone marrow transplants during childhood.[364] Prospective data concerning glucose tolerance show the recorded frequency of hyperinsulinemia, impaired glucose tolerance, and diabetes to be significantly elevated at 18%.[365] Dyslipidemia is an important determinant of vascular disease. Childhood cancer survivors show adverse lipid profiles characterized by increased LDL, apolipoprotein B, total cholesterol/HDL ratio, and trigycerides accompanied by decreased HDL levels.[359,361,364] Blood pressure abnormalities have also been reported in survivors of childhood cancers (brain tumors) in some[361] but not all studies.[358,359,365] Insulin resistance in cancer survivors is associated with obesity, subnormal HDL levels, and hypertriglyceridemia, consistent with a diagnosis of metabolic syndrome.

Nontraditional risk factors, including von Willebrand factor (vWf), plasminogen activator inhibitor-1 (PAI-1), and C-reactive protein (CRP) plasma levels, are elevated in cancer survivors,[366] but data in this area are limited, and therefore concrete conclusions cannot be made. Direct confirmation of premature vascular disease can be acquired from imaging of the great arteries. In studies of young adult survivors of Hodgkin disease who received neck irradiation the incidence of abnormal carotid scans (26% vs. 3%) and intima-media thickness (IMT) is increased compared with control subjects.[367] Long-term survivors of childhood brain tumors also show an increased IMT of the carotid bulb.[361]

BONE MARROW TRANSPLANTATION

Survival from childhood and adult hematologic malignancies has been improved by the development of effective procedures for BMT, used primarily to treat poor prognosis and relapsed leukemias, lymphoma, and myeloma. BMT encompasses allogeneic and autologous transplantation of stem cells from the bone marrow or peripheral blood. The complex treatment regimens employed prior to and during BMT to achieve such remarkable cure rates entail usage of combination chemotherapy, frequently encompassing high-dose alkylating agents, TBI, and immunosuppressive agents. The relative frequency of long-term adverse sequelae of these regimens is greater than might be predicted from the individual components, suggesting synergism between the toxic effects of treatment modalities on normal tissues.

Growth and Growth Hormone

Children who receive TBI as part of the preparative regimen show significant impairment of height velocity and height SDS.[368-373] Interpretation of the effect of TBI on height velocity is complicated by the frequent concomitant use of cranial irradiation before progression to BMT.[372,374] Both height and height velocity are impaired to a greater extent by the combination of cranial irradiation and TBI compared with TBI alone.[369,371-373] Single-fraction TBI (sfTBI) leads to greater impairment of growth than if TBI is fractionated (fTBI).[369,370,375] The adverse effect of TBI on growth is demonstrable within the first year following BMT in patients who additionally received cranial irradiation, but in the absence of cranial irradiation it may be delayed several years.[371] Mean relative change in height SDS between BMT and final height of children who received both cranial irradiation and sfTBI, sfTBI alone, fTBI, and no irradiation are in the region of –2.0, –1.4, –0.9, and –0.1, respectively.[376] Importantly, the degree of height loss consequent to TBI is greater in cases in which the radiation is administered at a younger age.[372,373]

TBI, in the absence of cranial radiation, results in GH insufficiency (peak GH level to stimulation < 20 mU/L [6.7 µg/L]) in 7% to 66% of recipients of children undergoing BMT, and when assessed in only those children with growth failure, then 60% to 95% are GH insufficient.* The wide prevalence of GH insufficiency results from significant differences in study designs and patient populations. Evidence from comparison of patients who receive sfTBI with those who receive fTBI suggests that fractionation of the radiation dose reduces the risk of developing GH insufficiency.[370] In the setting of impaired GH secretion secondary to TBI, GH replacement therapy significantly improves height velocity.[369,371,379] In contrast to observations in children, the irradiation dosage employed during TBI (10-13.2 Gy) prior to BMT has not been shown to cause GHD when delivered during adult life.[132]

There are a number of skeletal sequelae in addition to reduced final height that may be present in the adult survivor of childhood BMT. Spinal disproportion has been reported to occur as a consequence of TBI received during childhood,[374,379] suggestive of a greater inhibitory effect of TBI on the spine compared with the long bones. Spinal irradiation, corticosteroid therapy, sex steroid deficiency, and childhood GH insufficiency[108,380] are associated with reduced bone acquisition during childhood. There are no data on peak bone mass in adult survivors of childhood BMT, although the impaired bone acquisition is likely to result in lower than genetic peak bone mass, in the long term placing these individuals at risk of osteoporosis and fragility fractures. In young adult recipients of BMT, BMD is transiently reduced at the spine and hip, which tends to improve over the subsequent 2 years.[381]

Hypopituitarism

Although there is a large amount of available data concerning the GH axis following childhood BMT, there are far fewer data on the additional anterior pituitary axes. Abnormalities of the cortisol axis are reported in up to 24% of patients when assessed using the metyrapone test, but all of the patients were asymptomatic.[375] This finding likely reflects the test employed, which is plagued by false-positive results even in normal healthy individuals. When assessed using the ITT, the cortisol axis is normal in all[368,370,371] or almost all patients.[55,377] When cortisol responses have been subnormal, the patients have either been taking or recently taken corticosteroids for graft-versus-host disease (GVHD).[377] If present, cortisol deficiency usually presents late (5-10 years after irradiation). The true prevalence of cortisol deficiency in adult long-term survivors of malignancy who received a BMT during childhood is unclear. There are few data concerning prolactin levels in recipients of BMT; however, elevated levels are usually infrequent, mild, and asymptomatic.[55,132] TBI (10-13.2 Gy) prior to BMT, but delivered during adult life, has not been shown to cause hypopituitarism.[132]

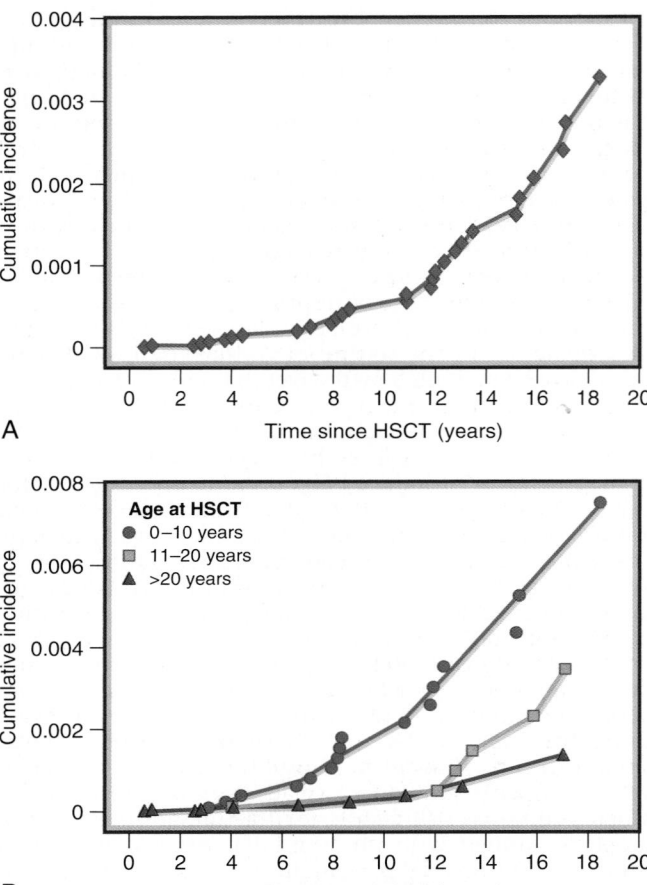

Figure 42-12 A, Cumulative incidence of thyroid cancer after hematopoietic stem cell transplant (HSCT). **B,** Cumulative incidence of thyroid cancer by age at transplantation. (From Cohen A, Rovelli A, Merlo DF, et al. Risk for secondary thyroid carcinoma after hematopoietic stem-cell transplantation: an EBMT Late Effects Working Party Study. *J Clin Oncol.* 2007;25:2449-2454.)

Primary Thyroid Disorders

Thyroid function is abnormal in a significant percentage of both childhood and adult survivors of BMT. As with the wide prevalence of GH insufficiency following childhood TBI, similar data are described for thyroid dysfunction (5%-43%).* Subclinical hypothyroidism is much more frequently observed than overt hypothyroidism.[132,382] Thyroiditis and hyperthyroidism have also been described to occur following exposure of the thyroid to TBI.[382,383] Thyroid dysfunction develops more frequently in patients who received sfTBI compared with those who received fTBI[55,374,377] and is more frequent in patients who received BMT at a younger age.[382] Although the frequency of abnormal thyroid function tests is relatively high, transient increases in TSH that resolve during follow-up are relatively common.[374,377,382]

Where the thyroid has been exposed to irradiation it is at greater risk of developing both benign thyroid nodules and carcinoma.[237-239] The standard incidence ratio (SIR) for development of thyroid carcinoma after BMT with TBI preconditioning is around sevenfold to eightfold higher than in the general population[384] (Fig. 42-12). The risk is significantly greater when irradiation occurs at a younger age[384,385] (see Fig. 42-12). The latency period from BMT to diagnosis of thyroid carcinoma is usually in excess of 5 years, but cases are reported within the first few years following TBI.[384-386] Almost all cases present subclinically.[386] Histologically, the majority of cases are papillary, with the additional cases being follicular.[384,386] TSH is a trophic factor for thyroid cell growth, and in established differentiated thyroid cancer suppression of TSH with levothyroxine reduces recurrence and mortality rates. In patients who have received TBI the elevated TSH in subclinical hypothyroidism is thought to be an etiologic factor in the development of thyroid carcinoma, and it is therefore recommended that these patients receive levothyroxine replacement. Given the potential transient nature of subclinical hypothyroidism after BMT, a significant proportion of patients will be able to discontinue the levothyroxine at a later date. There are no data on the success of levothyroxine withdrawal following earlier treatment of subclinical hypothyroidism resulting from TBI.

Gonadal Failure

The ovaries are exquisitely sensitive to radiation damage. TBI (10-15 Gy) used in combination with gonadotoxic chemotherapy almost invariably results in ovarian failure[55,132,387] (Fig. 42-13). Ovarian failure during childhood results in either delayed or failed progression through puberty[368,375] and renders almost all postpubertal women amenorrheic.[375,387] Characteristically, gonadotropin levels are elevated and estradiol levels are low.[55,368,374,375] Short-term ovarian recovery is recognized to occur in the first few

years following regimens inclusive of TBI[387] (see Fig. 42-13). Recovery occurs in at least 50% of prepubertal girls who receive high-dose chemotherapy and hyperfractionated TBI such as to allow progression of puberty and spontaneous menstruation.[388,389] With advancing age at treatment, recovery is increasingly infrequent.[387] Rarely, ovarian recovery can occur after a significant period of amenorrhea. It has been suggested that fTBI may be less damaging to the ovaries than sfTBI.[377] Young female survivors of BMT during adolescence or young adult life experience significant symptoms of estrogen deficiency including hot flushes, night sweats, and vaginal dryness.[390] They additionally express concerns over infertility, amenorrhea, and femininity. Libido is impaired in the majority, and coitus becomes painful, with difficulty achieving orgasm.[390,391] The consequence of direct radiation damage to the uterus alongside estrogen deficiency results in poor development of the uterus, which may not enlarge appropriately in response to estrogen replacement therapy.[368]

Estrogen replacement therapy significantly improves the symptoms of estrogen deficiency in the majority of hypogonadal young women[25] and should also be considered to maintain bone mass and potentially improve long-term vascular outcomes. There are no comparative data on sexual health in survivors of childhood BMT taking estrogen replacement therapy and normal individuals. Breast cancer risk is elevated in survivors of BMT (SIR 2.2), with risk increasing with duration of survival, younger age at transplantation, and TBI.[201] There are no data on whether estrogen replacement further elevates the risk of breast cancer. Intuitively it is appropriate to replace estrogen to physiologic levels, which would be unlikely to increase risk above that of women who retain normal ovarian function. All women who have received TBI during BMT, regardless of estrogen replacement status, should be enrolled in a breast cancer screening program.

In boys the germinal epithelium is significantly more sensitive to irradiation than the Leydig cells. As a consequence testosterone production is generally maintained, and puberty progresses normally.[55,372,389] Testicular volumes are small, reflecting the damage to the germinal epithelium.[55] Biochemically, FSH is elevated in the majority (68%-90%) of peripubertal and pubertal boys,[55,375] and LH elevated in 40% to 50%,[55,375] whereas testosterone levels are infrequently low (0%-16%).[55,132,375] There are no robust data documenting sperm counts during adult life to determine what proportion of boys receiving BMT would be spontaneously fertile or fertile with the help of assisted fertility techniques. Severe oligospermia or azoospermia, associated with testicular volumes below the normal range, and normal testosterone levels are expected following TBI during adult life.[132] Sterility is not universal,[132] and patients should be advised with respect to contraception. Adult males commonly report an adverse impact on long-term sexual functioning after BMT, though to a lesser degree than females.[391]

Effects of Chemotherapy-Only Preparatory Regimens

Children who undergo BMT having received only chemotherapy during their preparative regimen, without preceding irradiation, experience no adverse effects on height and height velocity SDS.[368,371,376] In fact, catch-up growth after BMT is a frequent observation in these individuals,[368,370] and final height is not significantly affected.[376] GH stimulation tests in these children who are growing normally after preconditioning with chemotherapy alone show appropriate responses.[370,392] Impaired stimulated GH responses have

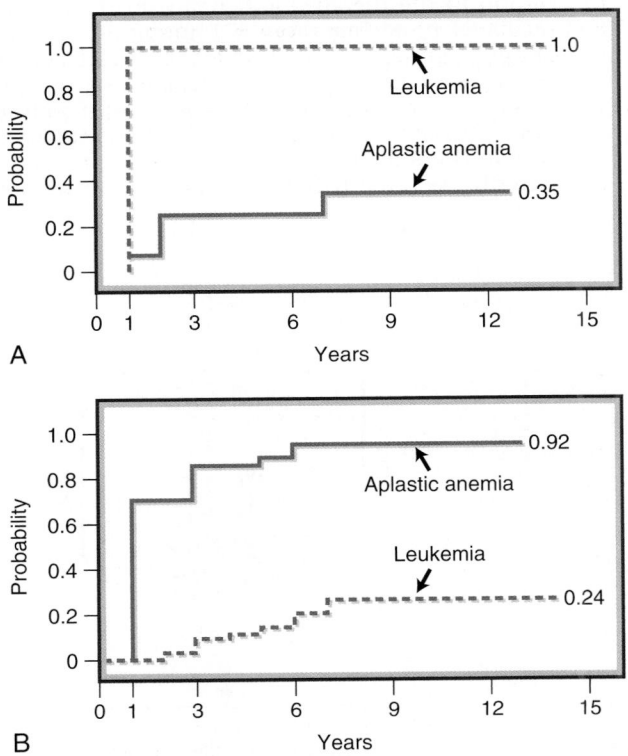

Figure 42-13 A, The probability of developing ovarian failure as determined by the first elevated LH/FSH levels beginning at 1 year following hematopoietic stem cell transplantation. **B,** The probability of recovery of normal ovarian function as determined by first normal LH/FSH levels from 1 year following transplantation. FSH, follicle-stimulating hormone; LH, luteinizing hormone. (From Sanders JE, Buckner CD, Amos D, et al. Ovarian function following marrow transplantation for aplastic anemia or leukemia. *J Clin Oncol.* 1988;6:813-818.)

been reported occasionally following chemotherapy-alone preparatory regimens administered during childhood.[371,393] The class of drugs involved and mechanisms for this result remain unclear. Whether the abrogated GH responses relate to inadequate or inappropriate assessment of the GH axis is also unclear. The cortisol axis and thyroid function in childhood are unaffected in patients receiving chemotherapy alone for preconditioning.[368,370,371,382,392] The relative risk for development of thyroid cancer in BMT regimens that do not include TBI is not significantly elevated.[384,386]

Permanent gonadal damage is uncommon in children, with the majority of patients progressing through puberty spontaneously.[368] Gonadotoxic agents including cyclophosphamide, busulphan, and cytarabine (Ara-C) have a dose-dependent toxic effect on the male germinal epithelium, with a high incidence of transient or permanent oligo- or azospermia.[388] Mild Leydig cell dysfunction, characterized by compensated hypergonadotropic hypogonadism, is frequently observed, but puberty is usually completed without the need for testosterone replacement therapy.[388]

Most adult females are rendered amenorrheic with elevated gonadotropins when using cyclophosphamide-based preparatory regimens.[383,387,394] Return of menses and normalization of the gonadotropins occurs in the majority, with a median duration of 6 months[387] (see Fig. 42-11). The likelihood of ovarian recovery is age-related, with younger individuals having the more promising outlook.[387,394] Many individuals will, however, have received gonadotoxic treatments prior to going forward with BMT, and the cumulative effect of these therapies will have significant impact on recovery rates.[394] Recovery of reproductive function in older individuals (>25 years) is more likely to be transient, though frequently menses can be present for several years before the onset of a premature menopause.[387]

TARGETED THERAPIES

Increasing understanding of cellular physiology and pathologic mechanisms has allowed specific targeting of disease, including cancer. Monoclonal antibodies provide the opportunity for highly selective modulation of disease and are associated with typical side effects that are usually characteristic of the class of drug. Activation of cellular signaling pathways via tyrosine kinases provides a target through which to inhibit growth factor receptors. Use of TKIs has found utility in treatment of a number of cancers.

Immune-Modulating Therapies
Monoclonal Antibodies to CTLA4

The cytotoxic T-lymphocyte–associated antigen 4 (CTLA4) present on T cells inhibits T-cell activation and proliferation, thereby limiting the immune response. In the setting of cancer CTLA4 induces a degree of T-cell immune tolerance to cancer cells.[395] Inhibition of CTLA4 leads to immune activation and augmentation of an immune-mediated antitumoral response (Fig. 42-14). Two monoclonal antibodies to CTLA4, ipilimumab and tremelimumab, have been used in clinical trials of malignant diseases including melanoma, renal cell carcinoma, small cell and non–small cell lung cancer, prostate cancer, and pancreatic adenocarcinoma. Ipilimumab has been licensed for use in treating metastatic melanoma following two phase III clinical trials in patients with unresectable/metastatic malignant melanoma that showed significantly improved overall patient survival.[396,397] Ipilimumab doses used in studies have ranged between 0.3 and 10 mg/kg. Significant, objective clinical responses, and an overall survival benefit, were demonstrated with a dose of 3 mg/kg,[397] higher doses resulting in significantly greater side effects. In contrast to ipilimumab, the pivotal phase III trial of tremelimumab in unresectable melanoma showed negative results on tumor control.[398]

In addition to the therapeutic benefits of ipilimumab, CTLA4-mediated protection from autoimmunity is abrogated, leading to immune-related adverse events. The most common immune-related adverse events are enterocolitis, hepatitis, rashes, and vitiligo.[399,400] The most common endocrinopathies are hypophysitis with hypopituitarism (0%-17%) and thyroiditis (3%-6%).[396,397,401] The frequency of hypophysitis reported between studies has been wide,

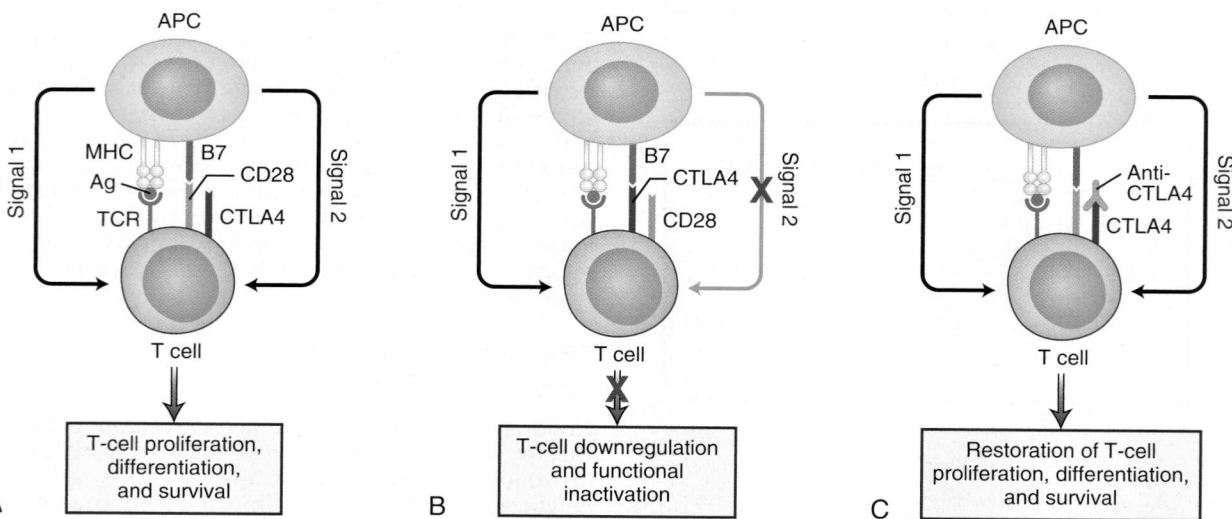

Figure 42-14 Mechanism of action of CTLA4 inhibitor. **A,** Activation of T cells requires two signals; presentation of antigen to TCR by MHC and interaction between co-stimulatory molecule B7 and CD28. **B,** T-cell activation upregulates CTLA4, which binds to B7 with greater affinity than CD28 and blocks signal 2, thus downregulating the T cell. **C,** Anti-CTLA4 antibodies bind and block CTLA4, thus allowing resumption of signal 2 and restoration of T-cell activation. Ag, antigen; APC, antigen-presenting cell; B7, peripheral membrane protein; CD, cluster of differentiation; CTLA4, cytotoxic T-lymphocyte antigen 4; MHC, major histocompatibility complex; TCR, T-cell receptor. (From Juszczak A, Gupta A, Karavitaki N, et al. Ipilimumab: a novel immunomodulating therapy causing autoimmune hypophysitis: a case report and review. *Eur J Endo.* 2012;167:1-5.)

but in more recent larger series is 8% to 13%.[402,403] The higher incidence in more recent studies likely represents increased recognition of this side effect. Clinically, presentation of hypophysitis is nonspecific with headache, asthenia, fatigue, malaise, pyrexia, nausea, and loss of libido. Visual-field defects are infrequent as pituitary enlargement on magnetic resonance imaging is usually modest. The onset of hypophysitis is reported most frequently at a median time of 9 to 11 weeks after initiating ipilimumab therapy.[397,401,403] Pituitary hormone deficiencies relating to hypophysitis are variable; however, ACTH and TSH deficiencies are most frequent, with gonadotropin deficiency in men also being common. Less data are available concerning the GH axis. Diabetes insipidus has been reported but is rare.[404] Prolactin levels may be either elevated or low. Imaging of the pituitary is variable with a spectrum from normal appearance to that of an enlarged gland with homogeneous increase in contrast enhancement and stalk thickening.[401,405] Rapid and timely diagnosis of this immune-related side effect is essential to avoid potentially fatal adrenal crises as a consequence of secondary adrenal insufficiency. Management is with high-dose steroids and appropriate HRT. The high-dose glucocorticoids are slowly tapered, depending upon clinical and laboratory responses. Clinical improvement generally occurs within a few days. In the longer term improvements are observed in pituitary imaging and resolution of hormone deficits following high-dose glucocorticoid therapy, but the ACTH deficiency is rarely reversible,[403-405] requiring potentially lifelong glucocorticoid replacement therapy.

Monoclonal Antibodies to PD1

Immune activation is also observed when employing drugs targeting the programmed death-1 (PD1) pathway. PD1 is a key immune regulatory receptor expressed by activated T cells. It has two ligands: PD1-L1 is expressed by cancer cells and tumor-infiltrative macrophages, and PD1-L2 is expressed by antigen-presenting cells. Activation of the PD1 receptor by its ligands leads to inhibition of cytokine production and T-cell cytolytic activity. Nivolumab is a monoclonal antibody to PD1 aimed at preventing activation of the PD1 receptor, thereby increasing immune function and antitumoral immunity. In a phase I study of 296 patients with advanced cancer only one case of hypophysitis was reported.[406] In phase I studies of lambrolizumab, a further monoclonal antibody to PD1, no cases of pituitary dysfunction were described.[407] The more peripheral action of these drugs to activate immunity appears to significantly reduce the risk of endocrine autoimmunity.

Tyrosine Kinase Inhibitors

Activation of a multitude of cellular signaling pathways is dependent on the transfer of phosphate, from adenosine triphosphate (ATP) to the catalytic domain of tyrosine kinase molecules within growth factor receptors. Many of these pathways are critical to cell survival and proliferation. TKIs are small molecules that act as ATP analogues, preventing ATP activation of tyrosine kinases and thereby inhibiting cell signaling pathways. TKIs have been developed specifically to inhibit critical cell proliferation pathways within cancers.[408,409] Targeted pathways include breakpoint cluster region proto-oncogene ABL1 fusion protein (BCR-ABL); epidermal growth factor receptor (EGFR); vascular endothelial growth factor receptor (VEGFR); platelet-derived growth factor receptor (PDGFR)-α; mitogen-activated protein kinase (MAPK); and v-raf murine sarcoma viral oncogene homologue B1 (BRAF).[408] Notably,

all TKIs currently in clinical use have varying affinity for the previous tyrosine kinases, but in addition can have actions on tyrosine kinases involved in other cellular processes. Over the past decade TKIs have established themselves within both first- and second-line therapy for solid and hematologic malignancies.

The most robust data concerning thyroid dysfunction comes from patients receiving sunitinib. Estimates of the incidence of hypothyroidism range from 7% to 85%.[408-411] Not all cases are mild, with reports of both severe hypothyroidism and myxedema.[412] Sunitinib is administered as 4 weeks "on" and 2 weeks "off." TSH levels are seen to rise during the "on" phases and regress toward normal during the "off" phase. The risk of significant hypothyroidism appears to worsen with duration of treatment or, alternately, the number of cycles of sunitinib received.[413,414] The time of onset is thus variable, with cases occurring up to 94 months after commencing treatment. Given these variables, the long-term cumulative incidence of hypothyroidism with sunitinib is not known. Similarly to sunitinib, sorafenib, cabozantinib, pazopanib, axitinib, nilotinib, and dasatinib have all been implicated in causing primary hypothyroidism, though less frequently.[410,415-418] For sorafenib the median time to development of hypothyroidism was 20 months. There are no data to inform whether the thyroid can recover function should sunitinib be withdrawn; however, despite small numbers recovery of thyroid function has been observed on withdrawal of sorafenib. In many cases hypothyroidism is preceded by a suppressed TSH level, suggesting the possibility of a thyroiditis. This has been observed with sunitinib, sorafenib, and axitinib.[413,414,419,420] In this setting, scintigraphic studies in patients treated with sorafenib have suggested a destructive thyroiditis.[419] It has been proposed that the described thyroiditis and development of hypothyroidism result from capillary dysfunction due to inhibition of VEGFR[421,422] and subsequent ischemic thyroiditis. Alternate hypotheses include a direct toxic effect of TKIs on thyrocytes, impaired iodine uptake, and reduced thyroid peroxidase activity.[413,423]

In thyroidectomized or hypothyroid patients significant increases, and less frequently decreases, in TSH and appropriate adjustments in levothyroxine dosage are required on commencing imatinib, sorafenib, axitinib, pazopanib, carbozantinib, motesanib, and vandetanib.[410,415-417,424-427] This suggests a separate action on thyroid hormone metabolism to that observed with sunitinib. Requisite increases in levothyroxine dose can be as much as 50%. Notably, in patients with a normal thyroid gland both imatinib and vandetanib do not cause hyper- or hypothyroidism.[427,428] These changes may in part relate to anorexia, weight loss, and diarrhea, which are common side effects of TKI; however, this is unlikely to be the full explanation. The decrease in T_3/T_4 and T_3/rT_3 ratios observed with sorafinib and sunitinib suggests the possibility of enhanced deactivation of thyroid hormones via enhanced type 3 deiodinase activity.[421,429] A number of TKIs inhibit monocarboxylate transporter 8 (MCT8), the predominant thyroid hormone transport protein, reducing thyroid hormone uptake into the tissues.[430] Additionally, should MCT8 be inhibited within the gut, levothyroxine absorption could potentially be reduced.

The occurrence of hyperthyroidism, other than in the setting of thyroiditis, is less well established. Within the German cohort study, however, around 3% of patients receiving either sunitinib or sorafenib are receiving antithyroid drugs.[431] This would suggest a putative increase in hyperthyroidism in these patients. Given the frequent abnormalities of thyroid function occurring in patients receiving TKIs, it would appear only appropriate for these individuals to undergo regular monitoring of their thyroid function tests on a monthly basis for 4 to 6 months, and extending to every 2 months thereafter.

REFERENCES

1. Stiller CA. Population based survival rates for childhood cancer in Britain, 1980-91. *BMJ.* 1994;309:1612-1616.
2. Stiller CA, Kroll ME, Pritchard-Jones K. Population survival from childhood cancer in Britain during 1978-2005 by eras of entry to clinical trials. *Ann Oncol.* 2012;23:2464-2469.
3. Stiller CA. *Childhood Cancer in Britain: Incidence, Survival, Mortality.* Oxford, UK: Oxford University Press; 2007.
4. Roy P, Vaughan Hudson G, Vaughan Hudson B, et al. Long-term survival in Hodgkin's disease patients. A comparison of relative survival in patients in trials and those recorded in population-based cancer registries. *Eur J Cancer.* 2000;36:384-389.
5. Urba WJ, Longo DL. Hodgkin's disease. *N Engl J Med.* 1992;326:678-687.
6. Leung W, Hudson MM, Strickland DK, et al. Late effects of treatment in survivors of childhood acute myeloid leukemia. *J Clin Oncol.* 2000; 18:3273-3279.
7. Department of Health, Macmillan Cancer Support. *NHS Improvement: The National Cancer Survivorship Initiative Vision.* London, UK: NHS; 2010 Available at: <www.ncsi.org/uk/wp-content/uploads/NCSI-Vision-Document.pdf>.
8. Maddams J, Utley M, Moller H. Projections of cancer prevalence in the United Kingdom, 2010-2040. *Br J Cancer.* 2012;107:1195-1202.
9. Gurney JG, Kadan-Lottick NS, Packer RJ, et al. Endocrine and cardiovascular late effects among adult survivors of childhood brain tumors: Childhood Cancer Survivor Study. *Cancer.* 2003;97:663-673.
10. Mosier HD Jr, Jansons RA. Stunted growth in rats following x-irradiation of the head. *Growth.* 1967;31(2):139-148.
11. Yamazaki JN, Bennett LR, Mc Fall RA, Clemente CD. Brain radiation in newborn rats and differential effects of increased age. I. Clinical observations. *Neurology.* 1960;10:530-536.
12. Onoyama Y, Abe M, Takahashi M, et al. Radiation therapy of brain tumors in children. *Radiology.* 1975;115:687-693.
13. Bamford FN, Jones PM, Pearson D, et al. Residual disabilities in children treated for intracranial space-occupying lesions. *Cancer.* 1976; 37:1149-1151.
14. Kirk JA, Raghupathy P, Stevens MM, et al. Growth failure and growth-hormone deficiency after treatment for acute lymphoblastic leukaemia. *Lancet.* 1987;1:190-193.
15. Davies HA, Didcock E, Didi M, et al. Disproportionate short stature after cranial irradiation and combination chemotherapy for leukaemia. *Arch Dis Child.* 1994;70:472-475.
16. Gurney JG, Ness KK, Stovall M, et al. Final height and body mass index among adult survivors of childhood brain cancer: Childhood Cancer Survivor Study. *J Clin Endocrinol Metab.* 2003;88(10):4731-4739.
17. Olshan JS, Gubernick J, Packer RJ, et al. The effects of adjuvant chemotherapy on growth in children with medulloblastoma. *Cancer.* 1992;70:2013-2017.
18. Ogilvy-Stuart AL, Shalet SM. Growth and puberty after growth hormone treatment after irradiation for brain tumours. *Arch Dis Child.* 1995;73:141-146.
19. Robison LL, Nesbit ME Jr, Sather HN, et al. Height of children successfully treated for acute lymphoblastic leukemia: a report from the Late Effects Study Committee of Childrens Cancer Study Group. *Med Pediatr Oncol.* 1985;13:14-21.
20. Shalet SM, Price DA, Beardwell CG, et al. Normal growth despite abnormalities of growth hormone secretion in children treated for acute leukemia. *J Pediatr.* 1979;94:719-722.
21. Shalet SM, Gibson B, Swindell R, Pearson D. Effect of spinal irradiation on growth. *Arch Dis Child.* 1987;62:461-464.
22. Wallace WH, Shalet SM, Morris-Jones PH, et al. Effect of abdominal irradiation on growth in boys treated for a Wilms' tumor. *Med Pediatr Oncol.* 1990;18:441-446.
23. Adan L, Souberbielle JC, Blanche S, et al. Adult height after cranial irradiation with 24 Gy: factors and markers of height loss. *Acta Paediatr.* 1996;85(9):1096-1101.
24. Ogilvy-Stuart AL, Clayton PE, Shalet SM. Cranial irradiation and early puberty. *J Clin Endocrinol Metab.* 1994;78:1282-1286.
25. Gleeson HK, Stoeter R, Ogilvy-Stuart AL, et al. Improvements in final height over 25 years in growth hormone (GH)-deficient childhood survivors of brain tumors receiving GH replacement. *J Clin Endocrinol Metab.* 2003;88:3682-3689.
26. Swift PG, Kearney PJ, Dalton RG, et al. Growth and hormonal status of children treated for acute lymphoblastic leukaemia. *Arch Dis Child.* 1978;53:890-894.
27. Cicognani A, Cacciari E, Vecchi V, et al. Differential effects of 18- and 24-Gy cranial irradiation on growth rate and growth hormone release in children with prolonged survival after acute lymphocytic leukemia. *Am J Dis Child.* 1988;142:1199-1202.
28. Clayton PE, Shalet SM, Price DA. Growth response to growth hormone therapy following craniospinal irradiation. *Eur J Pediatr.* 1988;147:597-601.
29. Adan L, Sainte-Rose C, Souberbielle JC, et al. Adult height after growth hormone (GH) treatment for GH deficiency due to cranial irradiation. *Med Pediatr Oncol.* 2000;34:14-19.
30. Leung W, Rose SR, Zhou Y, et al. Outcomes of growth hormone replacement therapy in survivors of childhood acute lymphoblastic leukemia. *J Clin Oncol.* 2002;20:2959-2964.
31. Sklar CA, Mertens AC, Mitby P, et al. Risk of disease recurrence and second neoplasms in survivors of childhood cancer treated with growth hormone: a report from the Childhood Cancer Survivor Study. *J Clin Endocrinol Metab.* 2002;87:3136-3141.
32. Swerdlow AJ, Reddingius RE, Higgins CD, et al. Growth hormone treatment of children with brain tumors and risk of tumor recurrence. *J Clin Endocrinol Metab.* 2000;85:4444-4449.
33. Ogilvy-Stuart AL. Safety of growth hormone after treatment of a childhood malignancy. *Horm Res.* 1995;44(Suppl 3):73-79.
34. Ogilvy-Stuart AL, Ryder WD, Gattamaneni HR, et al. Growth hormone and tumour recurrence. *BMJ.* 1992;304:1601-1605.
35. Shalet SM. Radiation and pituitary dysfunction. *N Engl J Med.* 1993; 328:131-133.
36. Lam KS, Tse VK, Wang C, et al. Effects of cranial irradiation on hypothalamic-pituitary function: a 5-year longitudinal study in patients with nasopharyngeal carcinoma. *Q J Med.* 1991;78:165-176.
37. Littley MD, Shalet SM, Beardwell CG, et al. Hypopituitarism following external radiotherapy for pituitary tumours in adults. *Q J Med.* 1989;70:145-160.
38. Littley MD, Shalet SM, Beardwell CG, et al. Radiation-induced hypopituitarism is dose-dependent. *Clin Endocrinol (Oxf).* 1989;31:363-373.
39. Pai HH, Thornton A, Katznelson L, et al. Hypothalamic/pituitary function following high-dose conformal radiotherapy to the base of skull: demonstration of a dose-effect relationship using dose-volume histogram analysis. *Int J Radiat Oncol Biol Phys.* 2001;49:1079-1092.
40. Jadresic A, Jimenez LE, Joplin GF. Long-term effect of 90Y pituitary implantation in acromegaly. *Acta Endocrinol (Copenh).* 1987;115:301-306.
41. Lam KS, Ho JH, Lee AW, et al. Symptomatic hypothalamic-pituitary dysfunction in nasopharyngeal carcinoma patients following radiation therapy: a retrospective study. *Int J Radiat Oncol Biol Phys.* 1987;13:1343-1350.
42. Schmiegelow M, Lassen S, Poulsen HS, et al. Growth hormone response to a growth hormone-releasing hormone stimulation test in a population-based study following cranial irradiation of childhood brain tumors. *Horm Res.* 2000;54:53-59.
43. Darzy KH, Pezzoli SS, Thorner MO, Shalet SM. The dynamics of growth hormone (GH) secretion in adult cancer survivors with severe GH deficiency acquired after brain irradiation in childhood for nonpituitary brain tumors: evidence for preserved pulsatility and diurnal variation with increased secretory disorderliness. *J Clin Endocrinol Metab.* 2005;90:2794-2803.
44. Chieng PU, Huang TS, Chang CC, et al. Reduced hypothalamic blood flow after radiation treatment of nasopharyngeal cancer: SPECT studies in 34 patients. *AJNR Am J Neuroradiol.* 1991;12(4):661-665.
45. Schneider HJ, Rovere S, Corneli G, et al. Endocrine dysfunction in patients operated on for non-pituitary intracranial tumors. *Eur J Endocrinol.* 2006;155:559-566.
46. Bhandare N, Kennedy L, Malyapa RS, et al. Hypopituitarism after radiotherapy for extracranial head and neck cancers. *Head Neck.* 2008; 30:1182-1192.
47. Constine LS, Woolf PD, Cann D, et al. Hypothalamic-pituitary dysfunction after radiation for brain tumors. *N Engl J Med.* 1993;328:87-94.
48. Hoeck HC, Vestergaard P, Jakobsen PE, Laurberg P. Test of growth hormone secretion in adults: poor reproducibility of the insulin tolerance test. *Eur J Endocrinol.* 1995;133:305-312.
49. Rahim A, Toogood AA, Shalet SM. The assessment of growth hormone status in normal young adult males using a variety of provocative agents. *Clin Endocrinol (Oxf).* 1996;45:557-562.
50. Bhandare N, Kennedy L, Malyapa RS, et al. Hypopituitarism after radiotherapy for extracranial head and neck cancers in pediatric patients. *Am J Clin Oncol.* 2008;31:567-572.
51. Robinson IC, Fairhall KM, Hendry JH, Shalet SM. Differential radiosensitivity of hypothalamo-pituitary function in the young adult rat. *J Endocrinol.* 2001;169:519-526.
52. Hochberg Z, Kuten A, Hertz P, et al. The effect of single-dose radiation on cell survival and growth hormone secretion by rat anterior pituitary cells. *Radiat Res.* 1983;94:508-512.
53. Darzy KH, Shalet SM. Hypopituitarism following radiotherapy. *Pituitary.* 2009;12:40-50.
54. Clayton PE, Shalet SM. Dose dependency of time of onset of radiation-induced growth hormone deficiency. *J Pediatr.* 1991;118:226-228.
55. Ogilvy-Stuart AL, Clark DJ, Wallace WH, et al. Endocrine deficit after fractionated total body irradiation. *Arch Dis Child.* 1992;67:1107-1110.

56. Shalet SM, Beardwell CG, Pearson D, Jones PH. The effect of varying doses of cerebral irradiation on growth hormone production in childhood. *Clin Endocrinol (Oxf)*. 1976;5:287-290.

57. Shalet SM, Beardwell CG, Twomey JA, et al. Endocrine function following the treatment of acute leukemia in childhood. *J Pediatr*. 1977;90:920-923.

58. Shalet SM, Beardwell CG, Morris-Jones PH, Pearson D. Pituitary function after treatment of intracranial tumours in children. *Lancet*. 1975;2:104-107.

59. Duffner PK, Cohen ME, Voorhess ML, et al. Long-term effects of cranial irradiation on endocrine function in children with brain tumors. A prospective study. *Cancer*. 1985;56:2189-2193.

60. Schmiegelow M, Lassen S, Poulsen HS, et al. Cranial radiotherapy of childhood brain tumours: growth hormone deficiency and its relation to the biological effective dose of irradiation in a large population based study. *Clin Endocrinol (Oxf)*. 2000;53:191-197.

61. Shalet SM, Beardwell CG, Jones PH, Pearson D. Growth hormone deficiency after treatment of acute leukaemia in children. *Arch Dis Child*. 1976;51:489-493.

62. Brennan BM, Rahim A, Mackie EM, et al. Growth hormone status in adults treated for acute lymphoblastic leukaemia in childhood. *Clin Endocrinol (Oxf)*. 1998;48:777-783.

63. Blatt J, Bercu BB, Gillin JC, et al. Reduced pulsatile growth hormone secretion in children after therapy for acute lymphoblastic leukemia. *J Pediatr*. 1984;104:182-186.

64. Spoudeas HA, Hindmarsh PC, Matthews DR, Brook CG. Evolution of growth hormone neurosecretory disturbance after cranial irradiation for childhood brain tumours: a prospective study. *J Endocrinol*. 1996;150:329-342.

65. Moell C, Garwicz S, Westgren U, Wiebe T. Disturbed pubertal growth in girls treated for acute lymphoblastic leukemia. *Pediatr Hematol Oncol*. 1987;4:1-5.

66. Moell C, Garwicz S, Westgren U, et al. Suppressed spontaneous secretion of growth hormone in girls after treatment for acute lymphoblastic leukaemia. *Arch Dis Child*. 1989;64:252-258.

67. Giustina A, Veldhuis JD. Pathophysiology of the neuroregulation of growth hormone secretion in experimental animals and the human. *Endocr Rev*. 1998;19:717-797.

68. Rose SR, Municchi G, Barnes KM, et al. Spontaneous growth hormone secretion increases during puberty in normal girls and boys. *J Clin Endocrinol Metab*. 1991;73:428-435.

69. Nesbit ME Jr, Sather HN, Robison LL, et al. Presymptomatic central nervous system therapy in previously untreated childhood acute lymphoblastic leukaemia: comparison of 1800 rad and 2400 rad. A report for Children's Cancer Study Group. *Lancet*. 1981;1:461-466.

70. Crowne EC, Moore C, Wallace WH, et al. A novel variant of growth hormone (GH) insufficiency following low dose cranial irradiation. *Clin Endocrinol (Oxf)*. 1992;36:59-68.

71. Willoughby JO, Terry LC, Brazeau P, Martin JB. Pulsatile growth hormone, prolactin, and thyrotropin secretion in rats with hypothalamic deafferentation. *Brain Res*. 1977;127:137-152.

72. Jorgensen JO, Pedersen SA, Thuesen L, et al. Beneficial effects of growth hormone treatment in GH-deficient adults. *Lancet*. 1989;1:1221-1225.

73. Salomon F, Cuneo RC, Hesp R, Sonksen PH. The effects of treatment with recombinant human growth hormone on body composition and metabolism in adults with growth hormone deficiency. *N Engl J Med*. 1989;321:1797-1803.

74. Carroll PV, Christ ER, Bengtsson BA, et al. Growth hormone deficiency in adulthood and the effects of growth hormone replacement: a review. Growth Hormone Research Society Scientific Committee. *J Clin Endocrinol Metab*. 1998;83:382-395.

75. Murray RD, Skillicorn CJ, Howell SJ, et al. Dose titration and patient selection increases the efficacy of GH replacement in severely GH deficient adults. *Clin Endocrinol (Oxf)*. 1999;50:749-757.

76. Drake WM, Coyte D, Camacho-Hubner C, et al. Optimizing growth hormone replacement therapy by dose titration in hypopituitary adults. *J Clin Endocrinol Metab*. 1998;83:3913-3919.

77. Toogood AA, Ryder WD, Beardwell CG, Shalet SM. The evolution of radiation-induced growth hormone deficiency in adults is determined by the baseline growth hormone status. *Clin Endocrinol (Oxf)*. 1995;43:97-103.

78. Lam KS, Tse VK, Wang C, et al. Early effects of cranial irradiation on hypothalamic-pituitary function. *J Clin Endocrinol Metab*. 1987;64:418-424.

79. Darzy KH, Pezzoli SS, Thorner MO, Shalet SM. Cranial irradiation and growth hormone neurosecretory dysfunction: a critical appraisal. *J Clin Endocrinol Metab*. 2007;92:1666-1672.

80. Darzy KH, Murray RD, Gleeson HK, et al. The impact of short-term fasting on the dynamics of 24-hour growth hormone (GH) secretion in patients with severe radiation-induced GH deficiency. *J Clin Endocrinol Metab*. 2006;91:987-994.

81. Darzy KH, Thorner MO, Shalet SM. Cranially irradiated adult cancer survivors may have normal spontaneous GH secretion in the presence of discordant peak GH responses to stimulation tests (compensated GH deficiency). *Clin Endocrinol (Oxf)*. 2009;70:287-293.

82. Ho PJ, Kletter GB, Hopwood NJ, et al. Somatostatin withdrawal alone is an ineffective generator of pulsatile growth hormone release in man. *Acta Endocrinol (Copenh)*. 1993;129:414-418.

83. Veldhuis JD, Anderson SM, Shah N, et al. Neurophysiological regulation and target-tissue impact of the pulsatile mode of growth hormone secretion in the human. *Growth Horm IGF Res*. 2001;11(Suppl A):S25-S37.

84. Lam KS, Wang C, Yeung RT, et al. Hypothalamic hypopituitarism following cranial irradiation for nasopharyngeal carcinoma. *Clin Endocrinol (Oxf)*. 1986;24:643-651.

85. Agha A, Sherlock M, Brennan S, et al. Hypothalamic-pituitary dysfunction after irradiation of nonpituitary brain tumors in adults. *J Clin Endocrinol Metab*. 2005;90:6355-6360.

86. Brauner R, Rappaport R, Prevot C, et al. A prospective study of the development of growth hormone deficiency in children given cranial irradiation, and its relation to statural growth. *J Clin Endocrinol Metab*. 1989;68:346-351.

87. Samaan NA, Schultz PN, Yang KP, et al. Endocrine complications after radiotherapy for tumors of the head and neck. *J Lab Clin Med*. 1987;109:364-372.

88. Shalet SM, Toogood A, Rahim A, Brennan BM. The diagnosis of growth hormone deficiency in children and adults. *Endocr Rev*. 1998;19:203-223.

89. Consensus guidelines for the diagnosis and treatment of adults with growth hormone deficiency: summary statement of the Growth Hormone Research Society Workshop on Adult Growth Hormone Deficiency. *J Clin Endocrinol Metab*. 1998;83(2):379-381.

90. Ho KK. Consensus guidelines for the diagnosis and treatment of adults with GH deficiency II: a statement of the GH Research Society in association with the European Society for Pediatric Endocrinology, Lawson Wilkins Society, European Society of Endocrinology, Japan Endocrine Society, and Endocrine Society of Australia. *Eur J Endocrinol*. 2007;157:695-700.

91. Shah A, Stanhope R, Matthew D. Hazards of pharmacological tests of growth hormone secretion in childhood. *BMJ*. 1992;304:173-174.

92. Lipshultz SE, Lipsitz SR, Sallan SE, et al. Chronic progressive cardiac dysfunction years after doxorubicin therapy for childhood acute lymphoblastic leukemia. *J Clin Oncol*. 2005;23:2629-2636.

93. Kremer LC, van Dalen EC, Offringa M, Voute PA. Frequency and risk factors of anthracycline-induced clinical heart failure in children: a systematic review. *Ann Oncol*. 2002;13:503-512.

94. Kremer LC, van der Pal HJ, Offringa M, et al. Frequency and risk factors of subclinical cardiotoxicity after anthracycline therapy in children: a systematic review. *Ann Oncol*. 2002;13:819-829.

95. Lissett CA, Saleem S, Rahim A, et al. The impact of irradiation on growth hormone responsiveness to provocative agents is stimulus dependent: results in 161 individuals with radiation damage to the somatotropic axis. *J Clin Endocrinol Metab*. 2001;86:663-668.

96. Darzy KH, Aimaretti G, Wieringa G, et al. The usefulness of the combined growth hormone (GH)-releasing hormone and arginine stimulation test in the diagnosis of radiation-induced GH deficiency is dependent on the post-irradiation time interval. *J Clin Endocrinol Metab*. 2003;88:95-102.

97. Bjork J, Link K, Erfurth EM. The utility of the growth hormone (GH) releasing hormone-arginine test for diagnosing GH deficiency in adults with childhood acute lymphoblastic leukemia treated with cranial irradiation. *J Clin Endocrinol Metab*. 2005;90:6048-6054.

98. Achermann JC, Brook CG, Hindmarsh PC. The GH response to low-dose bolus growth hormone-releasing hormone (GHRH(1-29)NH2) is attenuated in patients with longstanding post-irradiation GH insufficiency. *Eur J Endocrinol*. 2000;142:359-364.

99. Ham JN, Ginsberg JP, Hendell CD, Moshang T Jr. Growth hormone releasing hormone plus arginine stimulation testing in young adults treated in childhood with cranio-spinal radiation therapy. *Clin Endocrinol (Oxf)*. 2005;62:628-632.

100. Hoffman DM, O'Sullivan AJ, Baxter RC, Ho KK. Diagnosis of growth-hormone deficiency in adults. *Lancet*. 1994;343:1064-1068.

101. Murray RD, Brennan BM, Rahim A, Shalet SM. Survivors of childhood cancer: long-term endocrine and metabolic problems dwarf the growth disturbance. *Acta Paediatr Suppl*. 1999;88:5-12.

102. Murray RD, Darzy KH, Gleeson HK, Shalet SM. GH-deficient survivors of childhood cancer: GH replacement during adult life. *J Clin Endocrinol Metab*. 2002;87:129-135.

103. Mukherjee A, Tolhurst-Cleaver S, Ryder WD, et al. The characteristics of quality of life impairment in adult growth hormone (GH)-deficient survivors of cancer and their response to GH replacement therapy. *J Clin Endocrinol Metab*. 2005;90:1542-1549.

104. Attanasio AF, Shavrikova E, Blum WF, et al. Continued growth hormone (GH) treatment after final height is necessary to complete somatic development in childhood-onset GH-deficient patients. *J Clin Endocrinol Metab*. 2004;89:4857-4862.

105. Shalet SM, Shavrikova E, Cromer M, et al. Effect of growth hormone (GH) treatment on bone in postpubertal GH-deficient patients: a 2-year randomized, controlled, dose-ranging study. *J Clin Endocrinol Metab*. 2003;88:4124-4129.

106. Gleeson HK, Gattamaneni HR, Smethurst L, et al. Reassessment of growth hormone status is required at final height in children treated with growth hormone replacement after radiation therapy. *J Clin Endocrinol Metab.* 2004;89:662-666.

107. Clayton PE, Cuneo RC, Juul A, et al. Consensus statement on the management of the GH-treated adolescent in the transition to adult care. *Eur J Endocrinol.* 2005;152:165-170.

108. Murray RD, Adams JE, Smethurst LE, Shalet SM. Spinal irradiation impairs the osteo-anabolic effects of low-dose GH replacement in adults with childhood-onset GH deficiency. *Clin Endocrinol (Oxf).* 2002;56:169-174.

109. Chan JM, Stampfer MJ, Giovannucci E, et al. Plasma insulin-like growth factor-I and prostate cancer risk: a prospective study. *Science.* 1998;279:563-566.

110. Hankinson SE, Willett WC, Colditz GA, et al. Circulating concentrations of insulin-like growth factor-I and risk of breast cancer. *Lancet.* 1998;351:1393-1396.

111. Jenkins PJ, Fairclough PD, Richards T, et al. Acromegaly, colonic polyps and carcinoma. *Clin Endocrinol (Oxf).* 1997;47:17-22.

112. Estrov Z, Meir R, Barak Y, et al. Human growth hormone and insulin-like growth factor-1 enhance the proliferation of human leukemic blasts. *J Clin Oncol.* 1991;9:394-399.

113. Chung TT, Drake WM, Evanson J, et al. Tumour surveillance imaging in patients with extrapituitary tumours receiving growth hormone replacement. *Clin Endocrinol (Oxf).* 2005;63:274-279.

114. Wang ZF, Chen HL. Growth hormone treatment and risk of recurrence or development of secondary neoplasms in survivors of pediatric brain tumors. *J Clin Neurosci.* 2014;21:2155-2159.

115. Patterson BC, Chen Y, Sklar CA, et al. Growth hormone exposure as a risk factor for the development of subsequent neoplasms of the central nervous system: a report from the Childhood Cancer Survivor Study. *J Clin Endocrinol Metab.* 2014;99:2030-2037.

116. Harrop JS, Davies TJ, Capra LG, Marks V. Hypothalamic-pituitary function following successful treatment of intracranial tumours. *Clin Endocrinol (Oxf).* 1976;5:313-321.

117. Perry-Keene DA, Connelly JF, Young RA, et al. Hypothalamic hypopituitarism following external radiotherapy for tumours distant from the adenohypophysis. *Clin Endocrinol (Oxf).* 1976;5:373-380.

118. Brauner R, Czernichow P, Rappaport R. Greater susceptibility to hypothalamopituitary irradiation in younger children with acute lymphoblastic leukemia. *J Pediatr.* 1986;108:332.

119. Kanumakala S, Warne GL, Zacharin MR. Evolving hypopituitarism following cranial irradiation. *J Paediatr Child Health.* 2003;39:232-235.

120. Withers HR. Biology of radiation oncology. In: Tobias JS, Thomas PR, eds. *Current Radiation Oncology.* London, UK: Edward Arnold; 1994: 5-23.

121. Brada M, Rajan B, Traish D, et al. The long-term efficacy of conservative surgery and radiotherapy in the control of pituitary adenomas. *Clin Endocrinol (Oxf).* 1993;38:571-578.

122. Madaschi S, Fiorino C, Losa M, et al. Time course of hypothalamic-pituitary deficiency in adults receiving cranial radiotherapy for primary extrasellar brain tumors. *Radiother Oncol.* 2011;99:23-28.

123. Snyers A, Janssens GO, Twickler MB, et al. Malignant tumors of the nasal cavity and paranasal sinuses: long-term outcome and morbidity with emphasis on hypothalamic-pituitary deficiency. *Int J Radiat Oncol Biol Phys.* 2009;73:1343-1351.

124. Woo E, Lam K, Yu YL, et al. Temporal lobe and hypothalamic-pituitary dysfunctions after radiotherapy for nasopharyngeal carcinoma: a distinct clinical syndrome. *J Neurol Neurosurg Psychiatry.* 1988;51:1302-1307.

125. Samaan NA, Vieto R, Schultz PN, et al. Hypothalamic, pituitary and thyroid dysfunction after radiotherapy to the head and neck. *Int J Radiat Oncol Biol Phys.* 1982;8:1857-1867.

126. Gross KM, Matsumoto AM, Southworth MB, Bremner WJ. Evidence for decreased luteinizing hormone-releasing hormone pulse frequency in men with selective elevations of follicle-stimulating hormone. *J Clin Endocrinol Metab.* 1985;60:197-202.

127. Wildt L, Hausler A, Marshall G, et al. Frequency and amplitude of gonadotropin-releasing hormone stimulation and gonadotropin secretion in the rhesus monkey. *Endocrinology.* 1981;109:376-385.

128. Hall JE, Martin KA, Whitney HA, et al. Potential for fertility with replacement of hypothalamic gonadotropin-releasing hormone in long term female survivors of cranial tumors. *J Clin Endocrinol Metab.* 1994;79:1166-1172.

129. Brauner R, Rappaport R. Precocious puberty secondary to cranial irradiation for tumors distant from the hypothalamo-pituitary area. *Horm Res.* 1985;22:78-82.

130. Leiper AD, Stanhope R, Kitching P, Chessells JM. Precocious and premature puberty associated with treatment of acute lymphoblastic leukaemia. *Arch Dis Child.* 1987;62:1107-1112.

131. Livesey EA, Hindmarsh PC, Brook CG, et al. Endocrine disorders following treatment of childhood brain tumours. *Br J Cancer.* 1990;61: 622-625.

132. Littley MD, Shalet SM, Morgenstern GR, Deakin DP. Endocrine and reproductive dysfunction following fractionated total body irradiation in adults. *Q J Med.* 1991;78:265-274.

133. Darzy KH, Shalet SM. Absence of adrenocorticotropin (ACTH) neurosecretory dysfunction but increased cortisol concentrations and production rates in ACTH-replete adult cancer survivors after cranial irradiation for nonpituitary brain tumors. *J Clin Endocrinol Metab.* 2005;90:5217-5225.

134. Lee KO, Persani L, Tan M, et al. Thyrotropin with decreased biological activity, a delayed consequence of cranial irradiation for nasopharyngeal carcinoma. *J Endocrinol Invest.* 1995;18:800-805.

135. Darzy KH, Shalet SM. Circadian and stimulated thyrotropin secretion in cranially irradiated adult cancer survivors. *J Clin Endocrinol Metab.* 2005;90:6490-6497.

136. Rose SR, Lustig RH, Pitukcheewanont P, et al. Diagnosis of hidden central hypothyroidism in survivors of childhood cancer. *J Clin Endocrinol Metab.* 1999;84:4472-4479.

137. Oberfield SE, Allen JC, Pollack J, et al. Long-term endocrine sequelae after treatment of medulloblastoma: prospective study of growth and thyroid function. *J Pediatr.* 1986;108:219-223.

138. Mohn A, Chiarelli F, Di Marzio A, et al. Thyroid function in children treated for acute lymphoblastic leukemia. *J Endocrinol Invest.* 1997;20: 215-219.

139. Carter EP, Leiper AD, Chessells JM, Hurst A. Thyroid function in children after treatment for acute lymphoblastic leukaemia. *Arch Dis Child.* 1989;64:631.

140. Voorhess ML, Brecher ML, Glicksman AS, et al. Hypothalamic-pituitary function of children with acute lymphocytic leukemia after three forms of central nervous system prophylaxis. A retrospective study. *Cancer.* 1986;57:1287-1291.

141. Bhandare N, Kennedy L, Malyapa RS, et al. Primary and central hypothyroidism after radiotherapy for head-and-neck tumors. *Int J Radiat Oncol Biol Phys.* 2007;68:1131-1139.

142. Howell SJ, Shalet SM. Effect of cancer therapy on pituitary-testicular axis. *Int J Androl.* 2002;25:269-276.

143. Rivkees SA, Crawford JD. The relationship of gonadal activity and chemotherapy-induced gonadal damage. *JAMA.* 1988;259:2123-2125.

144. Ortin TT, Shostak CA, Donaldson SS. Gonadal status and reproductive function following treatment for Hodgkin's disease in childhood: the Stanford experience. *Int J Radiat Oncol Biol Phys.* 1990;19:873-880.

145. Chemaitilly W, Mertens AC, Mitby P, et al. Acute ovarian failure in the Childhood Cancer Survivor Study. *J Clin Endocrinol Metab.* 2006;91: 1723-1728.

146. Byrne J, Fears TR, Gail MH, et al. Early menopause in long-term survivors of cancer during adolescence. *Am J Obstet Gynecol.* 1992;166: 788-793.

147. Rowley MJ, Leach DR, Warner GA, Heller CG. Effect of graded doses of ionizing radiation on the human testis. *Radiat Res.* 1974;59: 665-678.

148. Shalet SM. Effect of irradiation treatment on gonadal function in men treated for germ cell cancer. *Eur Urol.* 1993;23:148-151, discussion 152.

149. Pedrick TJ, Hoppe RT. Recovery of spermatogenesis following pelvic irradiation for Hodgkin's disease. *Int J Radiat Oncol Biol Phys.* 1986;12: 117-121.

150. Centola GM, Keller JW, Henzler M, Rubin P. Effect of low-dose testicular irradiation on sperm count and fertility in patients with testicular seminoma. *J Androl.* 1994;15:608-613.

151. Mulder JE. Benefits and risks of hormone replacement therapy in young adult cancer survivors with gonadal failure. *Med Pediatr Oncol.* 1999;33:46-52.

152. van der Kaaij MA, Heutte N, Le Stang N, et al. Gonadal function in males after chemotherapy for early-stage Hodgkin's lymphoma treated in four subsequent trials by the European Organisation for Research and Treatment of Cancer: EORTC Lymphoma Group and the Groupe d'Etude des Lymphomes de l'Adulte. *J Clin Oncol.* 2007;25:2825-2832.

153. Whitehead E, Shalet SM, Blackledge G, et al. The effects of Hodgkin's disease and combination chemotherapy on gonadal function in the adult male. *Cancer.* 1982;49:418-422.

154. Viviani S, Santoro A, Ragni G, et al. Gonadal toxicity after combination chemotherapy for Hodgkin's disease. Comparative results of MOPP vs ABVD. *Eur J Cancer Clin Oncol.* 1985;21:601-605.

155. Wallace WH, Shalet SM, Lendon M, Morris-Jones PH. Male fertility in long-term survivors of childhood acute lymphoblastic leukaemia. *Int J Androl.* 1991;14:312-319.

156. Waxman J, Terry Y, Rees LH, Lister TA. Gonadal function in men treated for acute leukaemia. *Br Med J (Clin Res Ed).* 1983;287: 1093-1094.

157. Howell SJ, Radford JA, Ryder WD, Shalet SM. Testicular function after cytotoxic chemotherapy: evidence of Leydig cell insufficiency. *J Clin Oncol.* 1999;17:1493-1498.

158. Howell SJ, Radford JA, Adams JE, et al. Randomized placebo-controlled trial of testosterone replacement in men with mild Leydig cell insufficiency following cytotoxic chemotherapy. *Clin Endocrinol (Oxf).* 2001;55:315-324.

159. Loren AW, Mangu PB, Beck LN, et al. Fertility preservation for patients with cancer: American Society of Clinical Oncology clinical practice guideline update. *J Clin Oncol.* 2013;31:2500-2510.

160. Blackhall FH, Atkinson AD, Maaya MB, et al. Semen cryopreservation, utilisation and reproductive outcome in men treated for Hodgkin's disease. *Br J Cancer.* 2002;87:381-384.

161. Botchan A, Hauser R, Gamzu R, et al. Sperm quality in Hodgkin's disease versus non-Hodgkin's lymphoma. *Hum Reprod.* 1997;12:73-76.

162. Hallak J, Kolettis PN, Sekhon VS, et al. Cryopreservation of sperm from patients with leukemia: is it worth the effort? *Cancer.* 1999;85:1973-1978.

163. Ogawa T, Dobrinski I, Avarbock MR, Brinster RL. Transplantation of male germ line stem cells restores fertility in infertile mice. *Nat Med.* 2000;6:29-34.

164. Radford J, Shalet S, Lieberman B. Fertility after treatment for cancer. Questions remain over ways of preserving ovarian and testicular tissue. *BMJ.* 1999;319:935-936.

165. Ward JA, Robinson J, Furr BJ, et al. Protection of spermatogenesis in rats from the cytotoxic procarbazine by the depot formulation of Zoladex, a gonadotropin-releasing hormone agonist. *Cancer Res.* 1990;50:568-574.

166. Johnson DH, Linde R, Hainsworth JD, et al. Effect of a luteinizing hormone releasing hormone agonist given during combination chemotherapy on posttherapy fertility in male patients with lymphoma: preliminary observations. *Blood.* 1985;65:832-836.

167. Blumenfeld Z, Avivi I, Linn S, et al. Prevention of irreversible chemotherapy-induced ovarian damage in young women with lymphoma by a gonadotrophin-releasing hormone agonist in parallel to chemotherapy. *Hum Reprod.* 1996;11:1620-1626.

168. Bhasin S, Storer TW, Berman N, et al. Testosterone replacement increases fat-free mass and muscle size in hypogonadal men. *J Clin Endocrinol Metab.* 1997;82:407-413.

169. Behre HM, Kliesch S, Leifke E, et al. Long-term effect of testosterone therapy on bone mineral density in hypogonadal men. *J Clin Endocrinol Metab.* 1997;82:2386-2390.

170. Howell SJ, Radford JA, Smets EM, Shalet SM. Fatigue, sexual function and mood following treatment for haematological malignancy: the impact of mild Leydig cell dysfunction. *Br J Cancer.* 2000;82:789-793.

171. Howell SJ, Radford JA, Adams JE, Shalet SM. The impact of mild Leydig cell dysfunction following cytotoxic chemotherapy on bone mineral density (BMD) and body composition. *Clin Endocrinol (Oxf).* 2000;52:609-616.

172. Lushbaugh CC, Casarett GW. The effects of gonadal irradiation in clinical radiation therapy: a review. *Cancer.* 1976;37:1111-1125.

173. Wallace WH, Shalet SM, Hendry JH, et al. Ovarian failure following abdominal irradiation in childhood: the radiosensitivity of the human oocyte. *Br J Radiol.* 1989;62:995-998.

174. Wallace WH, Thomson AB, Saran F, Kelsey TW. Predicting age of ovarian failure after radiation to a field that includes the ovaries. *Int J Radiat Oncol Biol Phys.* 2005;62:738-744.

175. Li FP, Gimbrere K, Gelber RD, et al. Outcome of pregnancy in survivors of Wilms' tumor. *JAMA.* 1987;257:216-219.

176. Critchley HO, Wallace WH, Shalet SM, et al. Abdominal irradiation in childhood; the potential for pregnancy. *Br J Obstet Gynaecol.* 1992;99:392-394.

177. Andrieu JM, Ochoa-Molina ME. Menstrual cycle, pregnancies and offspring before and after MOPP therapy for Hodgkin's disease. *Cancer.* 1983;52:435-438.

178. Koyama H, Wada T, Nishizawa Y, et al. Cyclophosphamide-induced ovarian failure and its therapeutic significance in patients with breast cancer. *Cancer.* 1977;39:1403-1409.

179. Mackie EJ, Radford M, Shalet SM. Gonadal function following chemotherapy for childhood Hodgkin's disease. *Med Pediatr Oncol.* 1996;27:74-78.

180. Whitehead E, Shalet SM, Blackledge G, et al. The effect of combination chemotherapy on ovarian function in women treated for Hodgkin's disease. *Cancer.* 1983;52:988-993.

181. Santoro A, Bonadonna G, Valagussa P, et al. Long-term results of combined chemotherapy-radiotherapy approach in Hodgkin's disease: superiority of ABVD plus radiotherapy versus MOPP plus radiotherapy. *J Clin Oncol.* 1987;5:27-37.

182. Wallace WH, Shalet SM, Tetlow LJ, Morris-Jones PH. Ovarian function following the treatment of childhood acute lymphoblastic leukaemia. *Med Pediatr Oncol.* 1993;21:333-339.

183. Bath LE, Wallace WH, Shaw MP, et al. Depletion of ovarian reserve in young women after treatment for cancer in childhood: detection by anti-Mullerian hormone, inhibin B and ovarian ultrasound. *Hum Reprod.* 2003;18:2368-2374.

184. Anderson RA, Themmen AP, Al-Qahtani A, et al. The effects of chemotherapy and long-term gonadotrophin suppression on the ovarian reserve in premenopausal women with breast cancer. *Hum Reprod.* 2006;21:2583-2592.

185. Haie-Meder C, Mlika-Cabanne N, Michel G, et al. Radiotherapy after ovarian transposition: ovarian function and fertility preservation. *Int J Radiat Oncol Biol Phys.* 1993;25:419-424.

186. Williams RS, Littell RD, Mendenhall NP. Laparoscopic oophoropexy and ovarian function in the treatment of Hodgkin disease. *Cancer.* 1999;86:2138-2142.

187. Azim AA, Costantini-Ferrando M, Oktay K. Safety of fertility preservation by ovarian stimulation with letrozole and gonadotropins in patients with breast cancer: a prospective controlled study. *J Clin Oncol.* 2008;26:2630-2635.

188. Azim AA, Costantini-Ferrando M, Lostritto K, Oktay K. Relative potencies of anastrozole and letrozole to suppress estradiol in breast cancer patients undergoing ovarian stimulation before in vitro fertilization. *J Clin Endocrinol Metab.* 2007;92:2197-2200.

189. Oktay K, Hourvitz A, Sahin G, et al. Letrozole reduces estrogen and gonadotropin exposure in women with breast cancer undergoing ovarian stimulation before chemotherapy. *J Clin Endocrinol Metab.* 2006;91:3885-3890.

190. Rudick B, Opper N, Paulson R, et al. The status of oocyte cryopreservation in the United States. *Fertil Steril.* 2010;94:2642-2646.

191. Radford JA, Lieberman BA, Brison DR, et al. Orthotopic reimplantation of cryopreserved ovarian cortical strips after high-dose chemotherapy for Hodgkin's lymphoma. *Lancet.* 2001;357:1172-1175.

192. Falcone T, Attaran M, Bedaiwy MA, Goldberg JM. Ovarian function preservation in the cancer patient. *Fertil Steril.* 2004;81:243-257.

193. Donnez J, Dolmans MM, Demylle D, et al. Livebirth after orthotopic transplantation of cryopreserved ovarian tissue. *Lancet.* 2004;364:1405-1410.

194. Meirow D, Levron J, Eldar-Geva T, et al. Pregnancy after transplantation of cryopreserved ovarian tissue in a patient with ovarian failure after chemotherapy. *N Engl J Med.* 2005;353:318-321.

195. Oktay K, Turkcuoglu I, Rodriguez-Wallberg KA. Four spontaneous pregnancies and three live births following subcutaneous transplantation of frozen banked ovarian tissue: what is the explanation? *Fertil Steril.* 2011;95(2):804.

196. Rossouw JE, Anderson GL, Prentice RL, et al. Risks and benefits of estrogen plus progestin in healthy postmenopausal women: principal results from the Women's Health Initiative randomized controlled trial. *JAMA.* 2002;288(3):321-333.

197. Hulley S, Grady D, Bush T, et al. Randomized trial of estrogen plus progestin for secondary prevention of coronary heart disease in postmenopausal women. Heart and Estrogen/progestin Replacement Study (HERS) Research Group. *JAMA.* 1998;280(7):605-613.

198. Rossouw JE, Prentice RL, Manson JE, et al. Postmenopausal hormone therapy and risk of cardiovascular disease by age and years since menopause. *JAMA.* 2007;297:1465-1477.

199. Alm El-Din MA, El-Badawy SA, Taghian AG. Breast cancer after treatment of Hodgkin's lymphoma: general review. *Int J Radiat Oncol Biol Phys.* 2008;72:1291-1297.

200. Sankila R, Garwicz S, Olsen JH, et al. Risk of subsequent malignant neoplasms among 1,641 Hodgkin's disease patients diagnosed in childhood and adolescence: a population-based cohort study in the five Nordic countries. Association of the Nordic Cancer Registries and the Nordic Society of Pediatric Hematology and Oncology. *J Clin Oncol.* 1996;14:1442-1446.

201. Friedman DL, Rovo A, Leisenring W, et al. Increased risk of breast cancer among survivors of allogeneic hematopoietic cell transplantation: a report from the FHCRC and the EBMT-Late Effect Working Party. *Blood.* 2008;111(2):939-944.

202. Sawka AM, Lakra DC, Lea J, et al. A systematic review examining the effects of therapeutic radioactive iodine on ovarian function and future pregnancy in female thyroid cancer survivors. *Clin Endocrinol (Oxf).* 2008;69:479-490.

203. Vini L, Hyer S, Al-Saadi A, et al. Prognosis for fertility and ovarian function after treatment with radioiodine for thyroid cancer. *Postgrad Med J.* 2002;78:92-93.

204. Bal C, Kumar A, Tripathi M, et al. High-dose radioiodine treatment for differentiated thyroid carcinoma is not associated with change in female fertility or any genetic risk to the offspring. *Int J Radiat Oncol Biol Phys.* 2005;63:449-455.

205. Manuel Garcia-Quiros Munoz J, Martin Hernandez T, Torres Cuadro A, et al. [Age of menopause in patients with differentiated thyroid cancer treated with radioiodine]. *Endocrinol Nutr.* 2010;57:105-109.

206. Ceccarelli C, Canale D, Battisti P, et al. Testicular function after 131I therapy for hyperthyroidism. *Clin Endocrinol (Oxf).* 2006;65:446-452.

207. Rosario PW, Barroso AL, Rezende LL, et al. Testicular function after radioiodine therapy in patients with thyroid cancer. *Thyroid.* 2006;16:667-670.

208. Hyer S, Vini L, O'Connell M, et al. Testicular dose and fertility in men following I(131) therapy for thyroid cancer. *Clin Endocrinol (Oxf).* 2002;56:755-758.

209. Wichers M, Benz E, Palmedo H, et al. Testicular function after radioiodine therapy for thyroid carcinoma. *Eur J Nucl Med.* 2000;27:503-507.

210. Pacini F, Gasperi M, Fugazzola L, et al. Testicular function in patients with differentiated thyroid carcinoma treated with radioiodine. *J Nucl Med.* 1994;35:1418-1422.

211. Nelson DF, Reddy KV, O'Mara RE, Rubin P. Thyroid abnormalities following neck irradiation for Hodgkin's disease. *Cancer.* 1978;42:2553-2562.

212. Fleming ID, Black TL, Thompson EI, et al. Thyroid dysfunction and neoplasia in children receiving neck irradiation for cancer. *Cancer.* 1985;55:1190-1194.

213. Sklar C, Whitton J, Mertens A, et al. Abnormalities of the thyroid in survivors of Hodgkin's disease: data from the Childhood Cancer Survivor Study. *J Clin Endocrinol Metab.* 2000;85:3227-3232.

214. Jereczek-Fossa BA, Alterio D, Jassem J, et al. Radiotherapy-induced thyroid disorders. *Cancer Treat Rev.* 2004;30:369-384.

215. Shakespeare TP, Dwyer M, Mukherjee R, et al. Estimating risks of radiotherapy complications as part of informed consent: the high degree of variability between radiation oncologists may be related to experience. *Int J Radiat Oncol Biol Phys.* 2002;54:647-653.

216. Einhorn J, Wikholm G. Hypothyroidism after external irradiation to the thyroid region. *Radiology.* 1967;88:326-328.

217. Markson JL, Flatman GE. Myxoedema after deep x-ray therapy to the neck. *Br Med J.* 1965;1:1228-1230.

218. Colevas AD, Read R, Thornhill J, et al. Hypothyroidism incidence after multimodality treatment for stage III and IV squamous cell carcinomas of the head and neck. *Int J Radiat Oncol Biol Phys.* 2001;51: 599-604.

219. Smith RE Jr, Adler AR, Clark P, et al. Thyroid function after mantle irradiation in Hodgkin's disease. *JAMA.* 1981;245:46-49.

220. Shalet SM, Rosenstock JD, Beardwell CG, et al. Thyroid dysfunction following external irradiation to the neck for Hodgkin's disease in childhood. *Clin Radiol.* 1977;28:511-515.

221. Mercado G, Adelstein DJ, Saxton JP, et al. Hypothyroidism: a frequent event after radiotherapy and after radiotherapy with chemotherapy for patients with head and neck carcinoma. *Cancer.* 2001;92:2892-2897.

222. Hancock SL, Cox RS, McDougall IR. Thyroid diseases after treatment of Hodgkin's disease. *N Engl J Med.* 1991;325:599-605.

223. Ogilvy-Stuart AL, Shalet SM, Gattamaneni HR. Thyroid function after treatment of brain tumors in children. *J Pediatr.* 1991;119:733-737.

224. Constine LS, Donaldson SS, McDougall IR, et al. Thyroid dysfunction after radiotherapy in children with Hodgkin's disease. *Cancer.* 1984; 53:878-883.

225. Paulino AC. Hypothyroidism in children with medulloblastoma: a comparison of 3600 and 2340 cGy craniospinal radiotherapy. *Int J Radiat Oncol Biol Phys.* 2002;53:543-547.

226. Glatstein E, McHardy-Young S, Brast N, et al. Alterations in serum thyrotropin (TSH) and thyroid function following radiotherapy in patients with malignant lymphoma. *J Clin Endocrinol Metab.* 1971;32: 833-841.

227. Bethge W, Guggenberger D, Bamberg M, et al. Thyroid toxicity of treatment for Hodgkin's disease. *Ann Hematol.* 2000;79:114-118.

228. Green DM, Brecher ML, Yakar D, et al. Thyroid function in pediatric patients after neck irradiation for Hodgkin disease. *Med Pediatr Oncol.* 1980;8:127-136.

229. Thorp MA, Levitt NS, Mortimore S, Isaacs S. Parathyroid and thyroid function five years after treatment of laryngeal and hypopharyngeal carcinoma. *Clin Otolaryngol Allied Sci.* 1999;24:104-108.

230. Biel MA, Maisel RH. Indications for performing hemithyroidectomy for tumors requiring total laryngectomy. *Am J Surg.* 1985; 150:435-439.

231. Constine LS. What else don't we know about the late effects of radiation in patients treated for head and neck cancer? *Int J Radiat Oncol Biol Phys.* 1995;31:427-429.

232. Bantle JP, Lee CK, Levitt SH. Thyroxine administration during radiation therapy to the neck does not prevent subsequent thyroid dysfunction. *Int J Radiat Oncol Biol Phys.* 1985;11:1999-2002.

233. Loeffler JS, Tarbell NJ, Garber JR, Mauch P. The development of Graves' disease following radiation therapy in Hodgkin's disease. *Int J Radiat Oncol Biol Phys.* 1988;14:175-178.

234. Koh LK, Greenspan FS, Yeo PP. Interferon-alpha induced thyroid dysfunction: three clinical presentations and a review of the literature. *Thyroid.* 1997;7:891-896.

235. Krouse RS, Royal RE, Heywood G, et al. Thyroid dysfunction in 281 patients with metastatic melanoma or renal carcinoma treated with interleukin-2 alone. *J Immunother Emphasis Tumor Immunol.* 1995; 18:272-278.

236. Duffy BJ Jr, Fitzgerald PJ. Cancer of the thyroid in children: a report of 28 cases. *J Clin Endocrinol Metab.* 1950;10:1296-1308.

237. de Vathaire F, Hardiman C, Shamsaldin A, et al. Thyroid carcinomas after irradiation for a first cancer during childhood. *Arch Intern Med.* 1999;159:2713-2719.

238. De Jong SA, Demeter JG, Jarosz H, et al. Thyroid carcinoma and hyperparathyroidism after radiation therapy for adolescent acne vulgaris. *Surgery.* 1991;110:691-695.

239. Tucker MA, Jones PH, Boice JD Jr, et al. Therapeutic radiation at a young age is linked to secondary thyroid cancer. The Late Effects Study Group. *Cancer Res.* 1991;51:2885-2888.

240. Rubino C, Adjadj E, Guerin S, et al. Long-term risk of second malignant neoplasms after neuroblastoma in childhood: role of treatment. *Int J Cancer.* 2003;107:791-796.

241. Black P, Straaten A, Gutjahr P. Secondary thyroid carcinoma after treatment for childhood cancer. *Med Pediatr Oncol.* 1998;31:91-95.

242. Sigurdson AJ, Ronckers CM, Mertens AC, et al. Primary thyroid cancer after a first tumour in childhood (the Childhood Cancer Survivor Study): a nested case-control study. *Lancet.* 2005;365:2014-2023.

243. Hancock SL, McDougall IR, Constine LS. Thyroid abnormalities after therapeutic external radiation. *Int J Radiat Oncol Biol Phys.* 1995;31: 1165-1170.

244. Inskip PD. Thyroid cancer after radiotherapy for childhood cancer. *Med Pediatr Oncol.* 2001;36:568-573.

245. Acharya S, Sarafoglou K, LaQuaglia M, et al. Thyroid neoplasms after therapeutic radiation for malignancies during childhood or adolescence. *Cancer.* 2003;97:2397-2403.

246. Klugbauer S, Lengfelder E, Demidchik EP, Rabes HM. A new form of RET rearrangement in thyroid carcinomas of children after the Chernobyl reactor accident. *Oncogene.* 1996;13:1099-1102.

247. Klugbauer S, Lengfelder E, Demidchik EP, Rabes HM. High prevalence of RET rearrangement in thyroid tumors of children from Belarus after the Chernobyl reactor accident. *Oncogene.* 1995;11:2459-2467.

248. Roman SA. Endocrine tumors: evaluation of the thyroid nodule. *Curr Opin Oncol.* 2003;15:66-70.

249. Shafford EA, Kingston JE, Healy JC, et al. Thyroid nodular disease after radiotherapy to the neck for childhood Hodgkin's disease. *Br J Cancer.* 1999;80:808-814.

250. Carr RF, LiVolsi VA. Morphologic changes in the thyroid after irradiation for Hodgkin's and non-Hodgkin's lymphoma. *Cancer.* 1989;64:825-829.

251. Berdjis CC. Parathyroid diseases and irradiation. *Strahlentherapie.* 1972;143(1):48-62.

252. Rosen IB, Strawbridge HG, Bain J. A case of hyperparathyroidism associated with radiation to the head and neck area. *Cancer.* 1975;36: 1111-1114.

253. Rao SD, Frame B, Miller MJ, et al. Hyperparathyroidism following head and neck irradiation. *Arch Intern Med.* 1980;140:205-207.

254. Christensson T. Hyperparathyroidism and radiation therapy. *Ann Intern Med.* 1978;89:216-217.

255. Fiorica V, Males JL. Hyperparathyroidism after radiation of the head and neck: a case report and review of the literature. *Am J Med Sci.* 1979;278:223-228.

256. Russ JE, Scanlon EF, Sener SF. Parathyroid adenomas following irradiation. *Cancer.* 1979;43:1078-1083.

257. Netelenbos C, Lips P, van der Meer C. Hyperparathyroidism following irradiation of benign diseases of the head and neck. *Cancer.* 1983;52: 458-461.

258. Cohen J, Gierlowski TC, Schneider AB. A prospective study of hyperparathyroidism in individuals exposed to radiation in childhood. *JAMA.* 1990;264:581-584.

259. Palmer JA, Mustard RA, Simpson WJ. Irradiation as an etiologic factor in tumours of the thyroid, parathyroid and salivary glands. *Can J Surg.* 1980;23:39-42.

260. Schneider AB, Gierlowski TC, Shore-Freedman E, et al. Dose-response relationships for radiation-induced hyperparathyroidism. *J Clin Endocrinol Metab.* 1995;80:254-257.

261. Hedman I, Fjalling M, Lindberg S, et al. An assessment of the risk of developing hyperparathyroidism and thyroid disorders subsequent to neck irradiation in middle-aged women. *J Surg Oncol.* 1985;29: 78-81.

262. McMullen T, Bodie G, Gill A, et al. Hyperparathyroidism after irradiation for childhood malignancy. *Int J Radiat Oncol Biol Phys.* 2009;73: 1164-1168.

263. Karstrup S, Hegedus L, Sehested M. Hyperparathyroidism after neck irradiation for Hodgkin's disease. *Acta Med Scand.* 1984;215:287-288.

264. Holten I, Petersen LJ. Early changes in parathyroid function after high-dose irradiation of the neck. *Cancer.* 1988;62:1476-1478.

265. Christmas TJ, Chapple CR, Noble JG, et al. Hyperparathyroidism after neck irradiation. *Br J Surg.* 1988;75:873-874.

266. Tsunoda T, Mochinaga N, Eto T, Maeda H. Hyperparathyroidism following the atomic bombing in Nagasaki. *Jpn J Surg.* 1991;21:508-511.

267. Stephen AE, Chen KT, Milas M, Siperstein AE. The coming of age of radiation-induced hyperparathyroidism: evolving patterns of thyroid and parathyroid disease after head and neck irradiation. *Surgery.* 2004;136:1143-1153.

268. Davies JH, Evans BA, Jenney ME, Gregory JW. Effects of chemotherapeutic agents on the function of primary human osteoblast-like cells derived from children. *J Clin Endocrinol Metab.* 2003;88:6088-6097.

269. Crofton PM, Ahmed SF, Wade JC, et al. Effects of intensive chemotherapy on bone and collagen turnover and the growth hormone axis in children with acute lymphoblastic leukemia. *J Clin Endocrinol Metab.* 1998;83:3121-3129.

270. Georgiou KR, Scherer MA, Fan CM, et al. Methotrexate chemotherapy reduces osteogenesis but increases adipogenic potential in the bone marrow. *J Cell Physiol.* 2012;227:909-918.

271. King TJ, Georgiou KR, Cool JC, et al. Methotrexate chemotherapy promotes osteoclast formation in the long bone of rats via increased pro-inflammatory cytokines and enhanced NF-kappaB activation. *Am J Pathol.* 2012;181:121-129.

272. Fan C, Georgiou KR, King TJ, Xian CJ. Methotrexate toxicity in growing long bones of young rats: a model for studying cancer chemotherapy-induced bone growth defects in children. *J Biomed Biotechnol.* 2011;2011:903097.

273. Ragab AH, Frech RS, Vietti TJ. Osteoporotic fractures secondary to methotrexate therapy of acute leukemia in remission. *Cancer.* 1970;25:580-585.

274. Ecklund K, Laor T, Goorin AM, et al. Methotrexate osteopathy in patients with osteosarcoma. *Radiology.* 1997;202:543-547.

275. Leonard MB. Glucocorticoid-induced osteoporosis in children: impact of the underlying disease. *Pediatrics.* 2007;119(Suppl 2):S166-S174.

276. van Staa TP, Cooper C, Leufkens HG, Bishop N. Children and the risk of fractures caused by oral corticosteroids. *J Bone Miner Res.* 2003;18:913-918.

277. Compston J. Management of glucocorticoid-induced osteoporosis. *Nat Rev Rheumatol.* 2010;6:82-88.

278. Gilsanz V, Carlson ME, Roe TF, Ortega JA. Osteoporosis after cranial irradiation for acute lymphoblastic leukemia. *J Pediatr.* 1990;117:238-244.

279. Nysom K, Molgaard C, Holm K, et al. Bone mass and body composition after cessation of therapy for childhood cancer. *Int J Cancer Suppl.* 1998;11:40-43.

280. Henderson RC, Madsen CD, Davis C, Gold SH. Bone density in survivors of childhood malignancies. *J Pediatr Hematol Oncol.* 1996;18:367-371.

281. Muszynska-Roslan K, Panasiuk A, Latoch E, et al. Little evidence of low bone mass in acute lymphoblastic leukemia survivors. *J Clin Densitom.* 2012;15(1):108-115.

282. Gurney JG, Kaste SC, Liu W, et al. Bone mineral density among long-term survivors of childhood acute lymphoblastic leukemia: results from the St. Jude Lifetime Cohort Study. *Pediatr Blood Cancer.* 2014;61:1270-1276.

283. Henderson RC, Madsen CD, Davis C, Gold SH. Longitudinal evaluation of bone mineral density in children receiving chemotherapy. *J Pediatr Hematol Oncol.* 1998;20:322-326.

284. Hogler W, Wehl G, van Staa T, et al. Incidence of skeletal complications during treatment of childhood acute lymphoblastic leukemia: comparison of fracture risk with the General Practice Research Database. *Pediatr Blood Cancer.* 2007;48:21-27.

285. van der Sluis IM, van den Heuvel-Eibrink MM, Hahlen K, et al. Altered bone mineral density and body composition, and increased fracture risk in childhood acute lymphoblastic leukemia. *J Pediatr.* 2002;141:204-210.

286. Elmantaser M, Stewart G, Young D, et al. Skeletal morbidity in children receiving chemotherapy for acute lymphoblastic leukaemia. *Arch Dis Child.* 2010;95:805-809.

287. Baker KS, Gurney JG, Ness KK, et al. Late effects in survivors of chronic myeloid leukemia treated with hematopoietic cell transplantation: results from the Bone Marrow Transplant Survivor Study. *Blood.* 2004;104:1898-1906.

288. Rauch F, Plotkin H, DiMeglio L, et al. Fracture prediction and the definition of osteoporosis in children and adolescents: the ISCD 2007 Pediatric Official Positions. *J Clin Densitom.* 2008;11:22-28.

289. Tastekin N, Zateri C. Probable osteosarcoma risk after prolonged teriparatide treatment: comment on the article by Saag et al. *Arthritis Rheum.* 2010;62(6):1837, author reply 1837-1838.

290. Baker KS, Ness KK, Weisdorf D, et al. Late effects in survivors of acute leukemia treated with hematopoietic cell transplantation: a report from the Bone Marrow Transplant Survivor Study. *Leukemia.* 2010;24:2039-2047.

291. Majhail NS, Ness KK, Burns LJ, et al. Late effects in survivors of Hodgkin and non-Hodgkin lymphoma treated with autologous hematopoietic cell transplantation: a report from the Bone Marrow Transplant Survivor Study. *Biol Blood Marrow Transplant.* 2007;13:1153-1159.

292. Greenfield DM, Walters SJ, Coleman RE, et al. Prevalence and consequences of androgen deficiency in young male cancer survivors in a controlled cross-sectional study. *J Clin Endocrinol Metab.* 2007;92:3476-3482.

293. Brown JE, Ellis SP, Silcocks P, et al. Effect of chemotherapy on skeletal health in male survivors from testicular cancer and lymphoma. *Clin Cancer Res.* 2006;12:6480-6486.

294. Murugaesu N, Powles T, Bestwick J, et al. Long-term follow-up of testicular cancer patients shows no predisposition to osteoporosis. *Osteoporos Int.* 2009;20:1627-1630.

295. Kanis JA, Johnell O, Oden A, et al. FRAX and the assessment of fracture probability in men and women from the UK. *Osteoporos Int.* 2008;19:385-397.

296. Goldray D, Weisman Y, Jaccard N, et al. Decreased bone density in elderly men treated with the gonadotropin-releasing hormone agonist decapeptyl (D-Trp6-GnRH). *J Clin Endocrinol Metab.* 1993;76:288-290.

297. Daniell HW, Dunn SR, Ferguson DW, et al. Progressive osteoporosis during androgen deprivation therapy for prostate cancer. *J Urol.* 2000;163:181-186.

298. Smith MR, Lee WC, Brandman J, et al. Gonadotropin-releasing hormone agonists and fracture risk: a claims-based cohort study of men with nonmetastatic prostate cancer. *J Clin Oncol.* 2005;23:7897-7903.

299. Shahinian VB, Kuo YF, Freeman JL, Goodwin JS. Risk of fracture after androgen deprivation for prostate cancer. *N Engl J Med.* 2005;352:154-164.

300. Smith MR, Eastham J, Gleason DM, et al. Randomized controlled trial of zoledronic acid to prevent bone loss in men receiving androgen deprivation therapy for nonmetastatic prostate cancer. *J Urol.* 2003;169:2008-2012.

301. Klotz LH, McNeill IY, Kebabdjian M, et al. A phase 3, double-blind, randomised, parallel-group, placebo-controlled study of oral weekly alendronate for the prevention of androgen deprivation bone loss in nonmetastatic prostate cancer: the Cancer and Osteoporosis Research with Alendronate and Leuprolide (CORAL) study. *Eur Urol.* 2013;63:927-935.

302. Serpa Neto A, Tobias-Machado M, Esteves MA, et al. Bisphosphonate therapy in patients under androgen deprivation therapy for prostate cancer: a systematic review and meta-analysis. *Prostate Cancer Prostatic Dis.* 2012;15:36-44.

303. Smith MR, Egerdie B, Hernandez Toriz N, et al. Denosumab in men receiving androgen-deprivation therapy for prostate cancer. *N Engl J Med.* 2009;361:745-755.

304. Smith MR, Fallon MA, Lee H, Finkelstein JS. Raloxifene to prevent gonadotropin-releasing hormone agonist-induced bone loss in men with prostate cancer: a randomized controlled trial. *J Clin Endocrinol Metab.* 2004;89:3841-3846.

305. Smith MR, Morton RA, Barnette KG, et al. Toremifene to reduce fracture risk in men receiving androgen deprivation therapy for prostate cancer. *J Urol.* 2010;184:1316-1321.

306. Mohler JL, Armstrong AJ, Bahnson RR, et al. Prostate cancer, version 3: featured updates to the NCCN guidelines. *J Natl Compr Canc Netw.* 2012;10(9):1081-1087.

307. Smith MR, Finkelstein JS, McGovern FJ, et al. Changes in body composition during androgen deprivation therapy for prostate cancer. *J Clin Endocrinol Metab.* 2002;87:599-603.

308. Smith MR, Lee H, Nathan DM. Insulin sensitivity during combined androgen blockade for prostate cancer. *J Clin Endocrinol Metab.* 2006;91:1305-1308.

309. Keating NL, O'Malley AJ, Smith MR. Diabetes and cardiovascular disease during androgen deprivation therapy for prostate cancer. *J Clin Oncol.* 2006;24:4448-4456.

310. Keating NL, O'Malley AJ, Freedland SJ, Smith MR. Diabetes and cardiovascular disease during androgen deprivation therapy: observational study of veterans with prostate cancer. *J Natl Cancer Inst.* 2010;102:39-46.

311. Tsai HK, D'Amico AV, Sadetsky N, et al. Androgen deprivation therapy for localized prostate cancer and the risk of cardiovascular mortality. *J Natl Cancer Inst.* 2007;99:1516-1524.

312. Punnen S, Cooperberg MR, Sadetsky N, Carroll PR. Androgen deprivation therapy and cardiovascular risk. *J Clin Oncol.* 2011;29:3510-3516.

313. Albertsen PC, Klotz L, Tombal B, et al. Cardiovascular morbidity associated with gonadotropin releasing hormone agonists and an antagonist. *Eur Urol.* 2014;65:565-573.

314. Nobes JP, Langley SE, Klopper T, et al. A prospective, randomized pilot study evaluating the effects of metformin and lifestyle intervention on patients with prostate cancer receiving androgen deprivation therapy. *BJU Int.* 2012;109:1495-1502.

315. Segal RJ, Reid RD, Courneya KS, et al. Resistance exercise in men receiving androgen deprivation therapy for prostate cancer. *J Clin Oncol.* 2003;21:1653-1659.

316. Baumann FT, Zopf EM, Bloch W. Clinical exercise interventions in prostate cancer patients—a systematic review of randomized controlled trials. *Support Care Cancer.* 2012;20:221-233.

317. Loprinzi CL, Dueck AC, Khoyratty BS, et al. A phase III randomized, double-blind, placebo-controlled trial of gabapentin in the management of hot flashes in men (N00CB). *Ann Oncol.* 2009;20:542-549.

318. Irani J, Salomon L, Oba R, et al. Efficacy of venlafaxine, medroxyprogesterone acetate, and cyproterone acetate for the treatment of vasomotor hot flushes in men taking gonadotropin-releasing hormone analogues for prostate cancer: a double-blind, randomised trial. *Lancet Oncol.* 2010;11:147-154.

319. Tyrrell CJ, Payne H, Tammela TL, et al. Prophylactic breast irradiation with a single dose of electron beam radiotherapy (10 Gy) significantly reduces the incidence of bicalutamide-induced gynecomastia. *Int J Radiat Oncol Biol Phys.* 2004;60:476-483.

320. Boccardo F, Rubagotti A, Battaglia M, et al. Evaluation of tamoxifen and anastrozole in the prevention of gynecomastia and breast pain induced by bicalutamide monotherapy of prostate cancer. *J Clin Oncol.* 2005;23:808-815.

321. Di Lorenzo G, Perdona S, De Placido S, et al. Gynecomastia and breast pain induced by adjuvant therapy with bicalutamide after radical prostatectomy in patients with prostate cancer: the role of tamoxifen and radiotherapy. *J Urol.* 2005;174:2197-2203.

322. Lonning PE, Geisler J, Krag LE, et al. Effects of exemestane administered for 2 years versus placebo on bone mineral density, bone biomarkers, and plasma lipids in patients with surgically resected early breast cancer. *J Clin Oncol.* 2005;23:5126-5137.

323. Di Gregorio GB, Yamamoto M, Ali AA, et al. Attenuation of the self-renewal of transit-amplifying osteoblast progenitors in the murine bone marrow by 17 beta-estradiol. *J Clin Invest.* 2001;107:803-812.

324. Jilka RL, Takahashi K, Munshi M, et al. Loss of estrogen upregulates osteoblastogenesis in the murine bone marrow. Evidence for autonomy from factors released during bone resorption. *J Clin Invest.* 1998;101:1942-1950.

325. Burstein HJ, Prestrud AA, Seidenfeld J, et al. American Society of Clinical Oncology clinical practice guideline: update on adjuvant endocrine therapy for women with hormone receptor-positive breast cancer. *J Clin Oncol.* 2010;28:3784-3796.

326. Crew KD, Greenlee H, Capodice J, et al. Prevalence of joint symptoms in postmenopausal women taking aromatase inhibitors for early-stage breast cancer. *J Clin Oncol.* 2007;25:3877-3883.

327. Henry NL, Giles JT, Ang D, et al. Prospective characterization of musculoskeletal symptoms in early stage breast cancer patients treated with aromatase inhibitors. *Breast Cancer Res Treat.* 2008; 111:365-372.

328. Chien AJ, Goss PE. Aromatase inhibitors and bone health in women with breast cancer. *J Clin Oncol.* 2006;24:5305-5312.

329. Eastell R, Hannon RA, Cuzick J, et al. Effect of an aromatase inhibitor on BMD and bone turnover markers: 2-year results of the Anastrozole, Tamoxifen, Alone or in Combination (ATAC) trial (18233230). *J Bone Miner Res.* 2006;21:1215-1223.

330. Baum M, Buzdar A, Cuzick J, et al. Anastrozole alone or in combination with tamoxifen versus tamoxifen alone for adjuvant treatment of postmenopausal women with early-stage breast cancer: results of the ATAC (Arimidex, Tamoxifen Alone or in Combination) trial efficacy and safety update analyses. *Cancer.* 2003;98:1802-1810.

331. Thurlimann B, Keshaviah A, Coates AS, et al. A comparison of letrozole and tamoxifen in postmenopausal women with early breast cancer. *N Engl J Med.* 2005;353:2747-2757.

332. Cooke AL, Metge C, Lix L, et al. Tamoxifen use and osteoporotic fracture risk: a population-based analysis. *J Clin Oncol.* 2008;26: 5227-5232.

333. Howell A, Cuzick J, Baum M, et al. Results of the ATAC (Arimidex, Tamoxifen, Alone or in Combination) trial after completion of 5 years' adjuvant treatment for breast cancer. *Lancet.* 2005;365:60-62.

334. Coombes RC, Kilburn LS, Snowdon CF, et al. Survival and safety of exemestane versus tamoxifen after 2-3 years' tamoxifen treatment (Intergroup Exemestane Study): a randomised controlled trial. *Lancet.* 2007;369:559-570.

335. Coates AS, Keshaviah A, Thurlimann B, et al. Five years of letrozole compared with tamoxifen as initial adjuvant therapy for postmenopausal women with endocrine-responsive early breast cancer: update of study BIG 1-98. *J Clin Oncol.* 2007;25:486-492.

336. Mincey BA, Duh MS, Thomas SK, et al. Risk of cancer treatment-associated bone loss and fractures among women with breast cancer receiving aromatase inhibitors. *Clin Breast Cancer.* 2006;7:127-132.

337. Eastell R, Adams J, Clack G, et al. Long-term effects of anastrozole on bone mineral density: 7-year results from the ATAC trial. *Ann Oncol.* 2011;22:857-862.

338. Coleman RE, Banks LM, Girgis SI, et al. Reversal of skeletal effects of endocrine treatments in the Intergroup Exemestane Study. *Breast Cancer Res Treat.* 2010;124:153-161.

339. Lester JE, Dodwell D, Purohit OP, et al. Prevention of anastrozole-induced bone loss with monthly oral ibandronate during adjuvant aromatase inhibitor therapy for breast cancer. *Clin Cancer Res.* 2008; 14:6336-6342.

340. Van Poznak C, Hannon RA, Mackey JR, et al. Prevention of aromatase inhibitor-induced bone loss using risedronate: the SABRE trial. *J Clin Oncol.* 2010;28:967-975.

341. Brufsky AM, Bosserman LD, Caradonna RR, et al. Zoledronic acid effectively prevents aromatase inhibitor-associated bone loss in postmenopausal women with early breast cancer receiving adjuvant letrozole: Z-FAST study 36-month follow-up results. *Clin Breast Cancer.* 2009;9: 77-85.

342. Brufsky AM, Harker WG, Beck JT, et al. Final 5-year results of Z-FAST trial: adjuvant zoledronic acid maintains bone mass in postmenopausal breast cancer patients receiving letrozole. *Cancer.* 2012;118: 1192-1201.

343. Ellis GK, Bone HG, Chlebowski R, et al. Randomized trial of denosumab in patients receiving adjuvant aromatase inhibitors for non-metastatic breast cancer. *J Clin Oncol.* 2008;26:4875-4882.

344. Ellis GK, Bone HG, Chlebowski R, et al. Effect of denosumab on bone mineral density in women receiving adjuvant aromatase inhibitors for non-metastatic breast cancer: subgroup analyses of a phase 3 study. *Breast Cancer Res Treat.* 2009;118:81-87.

345. Hillner BE, Ingle JN, Chlebowski RT, et al. American Society of Clinical Oncology 2003 update on the role of bisphosphonates and bone health issues in women with breast cancer. *J Clin Oncol.* 2003;21: 4042-4057.

346. Reid DM, Doughty J, Eastell R, et al. Guidance for the management of breast cancer treatment-induced bone loss: a consensus position statement from a UK Expert Group. *Cancer Treat Rev.* 2008;34(Suppl 1): S3-S18.

347. Gralow JR, Biermann JS, Farooki A, et al. NCCN Task Force Report: Bone Health in Cancer Care. *J Natl Compr Canc Netw.* 2009;7(Suppl 3): S1-S32, quiz S33-S35.

348. Mertens AC, Yasui Y, Neglia JP, et al. Late mortality experience in five-year survivors of childhood and adolescent cancer: the Childhood Cancer Survivor Study. *J Clin Oncol.* 2001;19:3163-3172.

349. Moller TR, Garwicz S, Barlow L, et al. Decreasing late mortality among five-year survivors of cancer in childhood and adolescence: a population-based study in the Nordic countries. *J Clin Oncol.* 2001;19: 3173-3181.

350. Bowers DC, McNeil DE, Liu Y, et al. Stroke as a late treatment effect of Hodgkin's disease: a report from the Childhood Cancer Survivor Study. *J Clin Oncol.* 2005;23:6508-6515.

351. Bowers DC, Liu Y, Leisenring W, et al. Late-occurring stroke among long-term survivors of childhood leukemia and brain tumors: a report from the Childhood Cancer Survivor Study. *J Clin Oncol.* 2006;24: 5277-5282.

352. Green DM, Hyland A, Chung CS, et al. Cancer and cardiac mortality among 15-year survivors of cancer diagnosed during childhood or adolescence. *J Clin Oncol.* 1999;17:3207-3215.

353. Adams MJ, Lipshultz SE. Pathophysiology of anthracycline- and radiation-associated cardiomyopathies: implications for screening and prevention. *Pediatr Blood Cancer.* 2005;44:600-606.

354. Hamada H, Ohkubo T, Maeda M, Ogawa S. Evaluation of cardiac reserved function by high-dose dobutamine-stress echocardiography in asymptomatic anthracycline-treated survivors of childhood cancer. *Pediatr Int.* 2006;48:313-320.

355. Meacham LR, Gurney JG, Mertens AC, et al. Body mass index in long-term adult survivors of childhood cancer: a report of the Childhood Cancer Survivor Study. *Cancer.* 2005;103:1730-1739.

356. Didi M, Didcock E, Davies HA, et al. High incidence of obesity in young adults after treatment of acute lymphoblastic leukemia in childhood. *J Pediatr.* 1995;127:63-67.

357. Nysom K, Holm K, Michaelsen KF, et al. Degree of fatness after treatment for acute lymphoblastic leukemia in childhood. *J Clin Endocrinol Metab.* 1999;84:4591-4596.

358. Haddy TB, Mosher RB, Reaman GH. Hypertension and prehypertension in long-term survivors of childhood and adolescent cancer. *Pediatr Blood Cancer.* 2007;49:79-83.

359. Talvensaari KK, Lanning M, Tapanainen P, Knip M. Long-term survivors of childhood cancer have an increased risk of manifesting the metabolic syndrome. *J Clin Endocrinol Metab.* 1996;81:3051-3055.

360. Oeffinger KC, Mertens AC, Sklar CA, et al. Obesity in adult survivors of childhood acute lymphoblastic leukemia: a report from the Childhood Cancer Survivor Study. *J Clin Oncol.* 2003;21:1359-1365.

361. Heikens J, Ubbink MC, van der Pal HP, et al. Long term survivors of childhood brain cancer have an increased risk for cardiovascular disease. *Cancer.* 2000;88:2116-2121.

362. Sainsbury CP, Newcombe RG, Hughes IA. Weight gain and height velocity during prolonged first remission from acute lymphoblastic leukaemia. *Arch Dis Child.* 1985;60:832-836.

363. Sklar CA, Mertens AC, Walter A, et al. Changes in body mass index and prevalence of overweight in survivors of childhood acute lymphoblastic leukemia: role of cranial irradiation. *Med Pediatr Oncol.* 2000; 35:91-95.

364. Taskinen M, Saarinen-Pihkala UM, Hovi L, Lipsanen-Nyman M. Impaired glucose tolerance and dyslipidaemia as late effects after bone-marrow transplantation in childhood. *Lancet.* 2000;356:993-997.

365. Neville KA, Cohn RJ, Steinbeck KS, et al. Hyperinsulinemia, impaired glucose tolerance, and diabetes mellitus in survivors of childhood cancer: prevalence and risk factors. *J Clin Endocrinol Metab.* 2006;91: 4401-4407.

366. Nuver J, Smit AJ, Sleijfer DT, et al. Microalbuminuria, decreased fibrinolysis, and inflammation as early signs of atherosclerosis in long-term survivors of disseminated testicular cancer. *Eur J Cancer.* 2004;40: 701-706.

367. King LJ, Hasnain SN, Webb JA, et al. Asymptomatic carotid arterial disease in young patients following neck radiation therapy for Hodgkin lymphoma. *Radiology.* 1999;213:167-172.

368. Liesner RJ, Leiper AD, Hann IM, Chessells JM. Late effects of intensive treatment for acute myeloid leukemia and myelodysplasia in childhood. *J Clin Oncol.* 1994;12:916-924.

369. Huma Z, Boulad F, Black P, et al. Growth in children after bone marrow transplantation for acute leukemia. *Blood.* 1995;86:819-824.

370. Brauner R, Fontoura M, Zucker JM, et al. Growth and growth hormone secretion after bone marrow transplantation. *Arch Dis Child.* 1993;68: 458-463.

371. Giorgiani G, Bozzola M, Locatelli F, et al. Role of busulfan and total body irradiation on growth of prepubertal children receiving bone marrow transplantation and results of treatment with recombinant human growth hormone. *Blood.* 1995;86:825-831.

372. Cohen A, Rovelli A, Van-Lint MT, et al. Final height of patients who underwent bone marrow transplantation during childhood. *Arch Dis Child.* 1996;74:437-440.

373. Holm K, Nysom K, Rasmussen MH, et al. Growth, growth hormone and final height after BMT. Possible recovery of irradiation-induced growth hormone insufficiency. *Bone Marrow Transplant.* 1996;18: 163-170.

374. Leiper AD, Stanhope R, Lau T, et al. The effect of total body irradiation and bone marrow transplantation during childhood and adolescence on growth and endocrine function. *Br J Haematol.* 1987;67: 419-426.

375. Sanders JE, Pritchard S, Mahoney P, et al. Growth and development following marrow transplantation for leukemia. *Blood.* 1986;68: 1129-1135.

376. Cohen A, Rovelli A, Bakker B, et al. Final height of patients who underwent bone marrow transplantation for hematological disorders during childhood: a study by the Working Party for Late Effects-EBMT. *Blood.* 1999;93:4109-4115.

377. Thomas BC, Stanhope R, Plowman PN, Leiper AD. Endocrine function following single fraction and fractionated total body irradiation for bone marrow transplantation in childhood. *Acta Endocrinol (Copenh).* 1993;128:508-512.

378. Wingard JR, Plotnick LP, Freemer CS, et al. Growth in children after bone marrow transplantation: busulfan plus cyclophosphamide versus cyclophosphamide plus total body irradiation. *Blood.* 1992;79: 1068-1073.

379. Papadimitriou A, Urena M, Hamill G, et al. Growth hormone treatment of growth failure secondary to total body irradiation and bone marrow transplantation. *Arch Dis Child.* 1991;66:689-692.

380. Kaufman JM, Taelman P, Vermeulen A, Vandeweghe M. Bone mineral status in growth hormone-deficient males with isolated and multiple pituitary deficiencies of childhood onset. *J Clin Endocrinol Metab.* 1992; 74:118-123.

381. Gandhi MK, Lekamwasam S, Inman I, et al. Significant and persistent loss of bone mineral density in the femoral neck after haematopoietic stem cell transplantation: long-term follow-up of a prospective study. *Br J Haematol.* 2003;121:462-468.

382. Ishiguro H, Yasuda Y, Tomita Y, et al. Long-term follow-up of thyroid function in patients who received bone marrow transplantation during childhood and adolescence. *J Clin Endocrinol Metab.* 2004;89: 5981-5986.

383. Tauchmanova L, Selleri C, Rosa GD, et al. High prevalence of endocrine dysfunction in long-term survivors after allogeneic bone marrow transplantation for hematologic diseases. *Cancer.* 2002;95:1076-1084.

384. Cohen A, Rovelli A, Merlo DF, et al. Risk for secondary thyroid carcinoma after hematopoietic stem-cell transplantation: an EBMT Late Effects Working Party Study. *J Clin Oncol.* 2007;25:2449-2454.

385. Bhatia S, Louie AD, Bhatia R, et al. Solid cancers after bone marrow transplantation. *J Clin Oncol.* 2001;19:464-471.

386. Cohen A, Rovelli A, van Lint MT, et al. Secondary thyroid carcinoma after allogeneic bone marrow transplantation during childhood. *Bone Marrow Transplant.* 2001;28:1125-1128.

387. Sanders JE, Buckner CD, Amos D, et al. Ovarian function following marrow transplantation for aplastic anemia or leukemia. *J Clin Oncol.* 1988;6:813-818.

388. Cohen A, Rovelli R, Zecca S, et al. Endocrine late effects in children who underwent bone marrow transplantation: review. *Bone Marrow Transplant.* 1998;21(Suppl 2):S64-S67.

389. Sarafoglou K, Boulad F, Gillio A, Sklar C. Gonadal function after bone marrow transplantation for acute leukemia during childhood. *J Pediatr.* 1997;130:210-216.

390. Cust MP, Whitehead MI, Powles R, et al. Consequences and treatment of ovarian failure after total body irradiation for leukaemia. *BMJ.* 1989; 299:1494-1497.

391. Watson M, Wheatley K, Harrison GA, et al. Severe adverse impact on sexual functioning and fertility of bone marrow transplantation, either allogeneic or autologous, compared with consolidation chemotherapy alone: analysis of the MRC AML 10 trial. *Cancer.* 1999;86: 1231-1239.

392. Lahteenmaki PM, Chakrabarti S, Cornish JM, Oakhill AH. Outcome of single fraction total body irradiation-conditioned stem cell transplantation in younger children with malignant disease—comparison with a busulphan-cyclophosphamide regimen. *Acta Oncol.* 2004;43: 196-203.

393. Rose SR, Schreiber RE, Kearney NS, et al. Hypothalamic dysfunction after chemotherapy. *J Pediatr Endocrinol Metab.* 2004;17:55-66.

394. Tauchmanova L, Selleri C, De Rosa G, et al. Gonadal status in reproductive age women after haematopoietic stem cell transplantation for haematological malignancies. *Hum Reprod.* 2003;18:1410-1416.

395. Thompson CB, Allison JP. The emerging role of CTLA-4 as an immune attenuator. *Immunity.* 1997;7:445-450.

396. Robert C, Thomas L, Bondarenko I, et al. Ipilimumab plus dacarbazine for previously untreated metastatic melanoma. *N Engl J Med.* 2011;364: 2517-2526.

397. Hodi FS, O'Day SJ, McDermott DF, et al. Improved survival with ipilimumab in patients with metastatic melanoma. *N Engl J Med.* 2010;363: 711-723.

398. Ribas A, Kefford R, Marshall MA, et al. Phase III randomized clinical trial comparing tremelimumab with standard-of-care chemotherapy in patients with advanced melanoma. *J Clin Oncol.* 2013;31:616-622.

399. Torino F, Barnabei A, Paragliola RM, et al. Endocrine side-effects of anti-cancer drugs: mAbs and pituitary dysfunction: clinical evidence and pathogenic hypotheses. *Eur J Endocrinol.* 2013;169:R153-R164.

400. Juszczak A, Gupta A, Karavitaki N, et al. Ipilimumab: a novel immunomodulating therapy causing autoimmune hypophysitis: a case report and review. *Eur J Endocrinol.* 2012;167:1-5.

401. Min L, Vaidya A, Becker C. Association of ipilimumab therapy for advanced melanoma with secondary adrenal insufficiency: a case series. *Endocr Pract.* 2012;18:351-355.

402. Ryder M, Callahan M, Postow MA, et al. Endocrine-related adverse events following ipilimumab in patients with advanced melanoma: a comprehensive retrospective review from a single institution. *Endocr Relat Cancer.* 2014;21:371-381.

403. Min L, Hodi FS, Giobbie-Hurder A, et al. Systemic high-dose corticosteroid treatment does not improve the outcome of ipilimumab-related hypophysitis: a retrospective cohort study. *Clin Cancer Res.* 2015;21(4):749-755.

404. Dillard T, Yedinak CG, Alumkal J, Fleseriu M. Anti-CTLA-4 antibody therapy associated autoimmune hypophysitis: serious immune related adverse events across a spectrum of cancer subtypes. *Pituitary.* 2010; 13:29-38.

405. Blansfield JA, Beck KE, Tran K, et al. Cytotoxic T-lymphocyte-associated antigen-4 blockage can induce autoimmune hypophysitis in patients with metastatic melanoma and renal cancer. *J Immunother.* 2005;28:593-598.

406. Topalian SL, Hodi FS, Brahmer JR, et al. Safety, activity, and immune correlates of anti-PD-1 antibody in cancer. *N Engl J Med.* 2012;366: 2443-2454.

407. Hamid O, Robert C, Daud A, et al. Safety and tumor responses with lambrolizumab (anti-PD-1) in melanoma. *N Engl J Med.* 2013;369: 134-144.

408. Hamnvik OP, Larsen PR, Marqusee E. Thyroid dysfunction from antineoplastic agents. *J Natl Cancer Inst.* 2011;103:1572-1587.

409. Illouz F, Braun D, Briet C, et al. Endocrine side-effects of anti-cancer drugs: thyroid effects of tyrosine kinase inhibitors. *Eur J Endocrinol.* 2014;171:R91-R99.

410. Motzer RJ, Hutson TE, Cella D, et al. Pazopanib versus sunitinib in metastatic renal-cell carcinoma. *N Engl J Med.* 2013;369:722-731.

411. Rini BI, Tamaskar I, Shaheen P, et al. Hypothyroidism in patients with metastatic renal cell carcinoma treated with sunitinib. *J Natl Cancer Inst.* 2007;99:81-83.

412. Chen SY, Kao PC, Lin ZZ, et al. Sunitinib-induced myxedema coma. *Am J Emerg Med.* 2009;27(3):370.e1-370.e3.

413. Mannavola D, Coco P, Vannucchi G, et al. A novel tyrosine-kinase selective inhibitor, sunitinib, induces transient hypothyroidism by blocking iodine uptake. *J Clin Endocrinol Metab.* 2007;92: 3531-3534.

414. Desai J, Yassa L, Marqusee E, et al. Hypothyroidism after sunitinib treatment for patients with gastrointestinal stromal tumors. *Ann Intern Med.* 2006;145:660-664.

415. Elisei R, Schlumberger MJ, Muller SP, et al. Cabozantinib in progressive medullary thyroid cancer. *J Clin Oncol.* 2013;31:3639-3646.

416. Kim TD, Schwarz M, Nogai H, et al. Thyroid dysfunction caused by second-generation tyrosine kinase inhibitors in Philadelphia chromosome-positive chronic myeloid leukemia. *Thyroid.* 2010;20: 1209-1214.

417. Motzer RJ, Escudier B, Tomczak P, et al. Axitinib versus sorafenib as second-line treatment for advanced renal cell carcinoma: overall survival analysis and updated results from a randomised phase 3 trial. *Lancet Oncol.* 2013;14:552-562.

418. Tamaskar I, Bukowski R, Elson P, et al. Thyroid function test abnormalities in patients with metastatic renal cell carcinoma treated with sorafenib. *Ann Oncol.* 2008;19:265-268.

419. Iavarone M, Perrino M, Vigano M, et al. Sorafenib-induced destructive thyroiditis. *Thyroid.* 2010;20:1043-1044.

420. Ohba K, Takayama T, Matsunaga H, et al. Inappropriate elevation of serum thyrotropin levels in patients treated with axitinib. *Thyroid.* 2013;23:443-448.

421. Kappers MH, van Esch JH, Smedts FM, et al. Sunitinib-induced hypothyroidism is due to induction of type 3 deiodinase activity and thyroidal capillary regression. *J Clin Endocrinol Metab.* 2011;96: 3087-3094.

422. Makita N, Miyakawa M, Fujita T. Iiri T. Sunitinib induces hypothyroidism with a markedly reduced vascularity. *Thyroid.* 2010;20:323-326.

423. Wong E, Rosen LS, Mulay M, et al. Sunitinib induces hypothyroidism in advanced cancer patients and may inhibit thyroid peroxidase activity. *Thyroid.* 2007;17:351-355.

424. Gupta-Abramson V, Troxel AB, Nellore A, et al. Phase II trial of sorafenib in advanced thyroid cancer. *J Clin Oncol.* 2008;26: 4714-4719.

425. Schneider TC, Abdulrahman RM, Corssmit EP, et al. Long-term analysis of the efficacy and tolerability of sorafenib in advanced radio-iodine refractory differentiated thyroid carcinoma: final results of a phase II trial. *Eur J Endocrinol.* 2012;167:643-650.

426. Sherman SI, Wirth LJ, Droz JP, et al. Motesanib diphosphate in progressive differentiated thyroid cancer. *N Engl J Med.* 2008;359:31-42.

427. Brassard M, Neraud B, Trabado S, et al. Endocrine effects of the tyrosine kinase inhibitor vandetanib in patients treated for thyroid cancer. *J Clin Endocrinol Metab.* 2011;96:2741-2749.

428. Dora JM, Leie MA, Netto B, et al. Lack of imatinib-induced thyroid dysfunction in a cohort of non-thyroidectomized patients. *Eur J Endocrinol.* 2008;158:771-772.

429. Abdulrahman RM, Verloop H, Hoftijzer H, et al. Sorafenib-induced hypothyroidism is associated with increased type 3 deiodination. *J Clin Endocrinol Metab.* 2010;95:3758-3762.

430. Braun D, Kim TD, le Coutre P, et al. Tyrosine kinase inhibitors non-competitively inhibit MCT8-mediated iodothyronine transport. *J Clin Endocrinol Metab.* 2012;97:E100-E105.

431. Feldt S, Schussel K, Quinzler R, et al. Incidence of thyroid hormone therapy in patients treated with sunitinib or sorafenib: a cohort study. *Eur J Cancer.* 2012;48:974-981.

CHAPTER 43

Neuroendocrine Gastrointestinal and Lung Tumors (Carcinoid Tumors), the Carcinoid Syndrome, and Related Disorders

KJELL ÖBERG

KEY POINTS

- The World Health Organization (WHO) classification system (2010) in neuroendocrine tumors (NET-G1, NET-G2) and neuroendocrine carcinoma (NEC-G3) is informative for the clinical management of neuroendocrine intestinal and lung tumors (carcinoids).
- The most important circulating biomarkers are chromogranin A (general) and urinary 5-hydroxyindoleacetic acid (5-HIAA).
- The carcinoid syndrome includes the following: flushing, diarrhea, right-sided heart fibrosis, and bronchial wheezing.
- Molecular imaging ^{111}In-DTPA-Phe octreotide (Octreoscan) and more recently ^{68}Ga-DOTA-octreotate positron emission tomography (PET) scanning are important procedures for staging of the disease as well determining possible therapy with peptide receptor radiotherapy (PRRT).
- First-line therapy for low proliferating small intestinal neuroendocrine tumors (NET-G1) are somatostatin analogues.
- Chemotherapy is reserved for NET-G2 mostly in the lung (atypical carcinoids).
- Peptide receptor radiotherapy could be considered for both NET-G1 and NET-G2.

The first clinical and histopathologic description of carcinoid tumor was made by Otto Lubarsch in 1888.[1] He was impressed by the multicentric origin of carcinoid tumors of the gastrointestinal (GI) tract, their lack of gland formation, and their lack of similarity with the usual adenocarcinoma of the alimentary system.

The term *Karzinoide* was introduced in 1907 by the pathologist Siegfried Oberndorfer[2] as a descriptive name for what he considered to be a benign type of neoplasm of the ileum, which could nevertheless behave like a carcinoma. It was subsequently generally accepted that the carcinoid tumor was a very slow growing and benign neoplasm with no potential for invasiveness and no tendency to give rise to metastases. This myth of benignity has survived to the present, even though in 1949 Pearson and Fitzgerald[3] described a large series of metastasizing carcinoid tumors.

Carcinoid tumors have subsequently been reported in a wide range of organs, but they most commonly involve the lungs and GI tract. Carcinoid tumors of the thymus, ovaries, testes, heart, and middle ear have also been described. The clinically well-known *carcinoid syndrome* was described by Thorson and associates[4] in 1954; 1 year earlier, Lembeck[5] had extracted serotonin from a carcinoid tumor.

PHYLOGENESIS AND EMBRYOLOGY

Carcinoid tumors are derived from neuroendocrine cells, and Gosset and Masson[6] in 1914 were the first to point out the neuroendocrine properties of carcinoid tumors. Masson[7] later described the remarkable affinity for silver salts displayed by intracytoplasmic granules in tumor cells and noted that carcinoid tumors originate from enterochromaffin cells, the Kulchitsky cells in the crypts of Lieberkühn in the intestinal epithelium. Furthermore, he suggested that the tumors were of endocrine origin (Fig. 43-1).

The mammalian GI tract and pancreas contain 14 endocrine cell types, which initially were believed to originate from the neuroectoderm. This observation gave rise to the *APUD concept* (*a*mine *p*recursor *u*ptake and *d*ecarboxylation) because of the ability of these cells to take up and

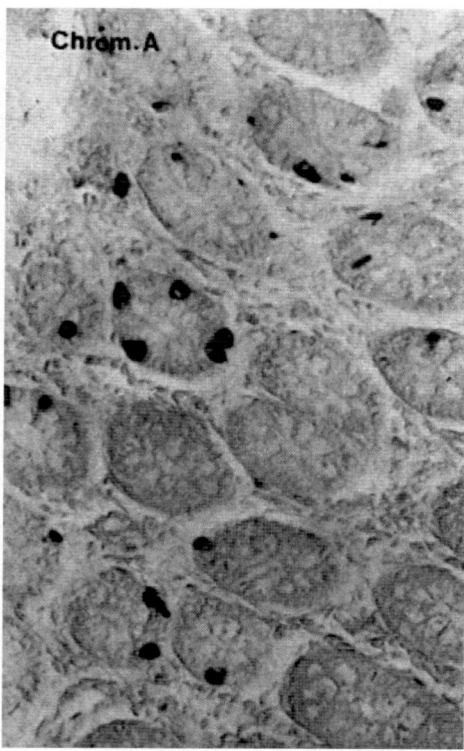

Figure 43-1 Normal human intestine stained with chromogranin A (Chrom. A) to delineate neuroendocrine cells. The cells are scattered in the intestinal mucosa.

decarboxylate amino acid precursors of biogenic amines such as serotonin and catecholamines.[8] The APUD concept was later revised by others, who postulated that these endocrine cells might also be derived from mesoderm and endoderm.[9] The neuronal phenotype is clearly seen when culturing carcinoid tumor cells in vitro. The enterochromaffin cells, from which many carcinoid tumors derive, have the property of producing and secreting amines (such as serotonin) and polypeptides (such as neurokinin A and substance P).

Carcinoid tumors might also originate from other neuroendocrine cells, such as the enterochromaffin-like (ECL) cells of the gut and endocrine cells in the bronchi. The tumors derived from these cells can produce a wide range of hormones, such as gastrin, gastrin-releasing peptide (GRP), ghrelin, calcitonin, pancreatic polypeptide, adrenocorticotropic hormone (ACTH), corticotropin-releasing hormone (CRH), and growth hormone–releasing hormone (GHRH), as well as somatostatin, glucagon, and calcitonin gene–related peptide (CGRP).[10] A common secretory product from all types of carcinoid tumors is the glycoprotein chromogranin A (CgA)—the most important general tumor marker in these patients (see later).

MOLECULAR GENETICS

Despite advances in the diagnosis, localization, and treatment of carcinoid tumors, no etiologic factor associated with the development of these tumors has been identified. Little is known about molecular genetic changes underlying tumorigenesis. Sporadic foregut carcinoids as well as the familial-type multiple endocrine neoplasia type 1 (MEN1) often display allelic losses at chromosome 11q13, and somatic *MEN1* gene mutations have been reported in

one third of sporadic foregut tumors.[11] In contrast with foregut carcinoids, molecular and cytogenetic data for midgut carcinoids are quite limited, and these tumors are not included in MEN1 syndrome. Deletions of chromosomes 18q and 18p have been reported in 38% and 33%, respectively, of GI carcinoids.[12]

In one publication, deletions on chromosome 18 were found in 88% of midgut carcinoid tumors, but the *SMAD4/DPC4* locus was not deleted.[13] In addition to the consistent finding of deletions on chromosome 18, multiple deletions on other chromosomes (4, 5, 7, 9, 14, 20) were noticed in single tumors. The region telomeric to *SMAD4/DPC4/DCC* loci must be further explored for possible losses of a tumor suppressor gene in this area. Gene expression arrays in carcinoid tumors have demonstrated upregulation of the *RET* proto-oncogene, but no mutations have been detected so far. Reports indicate that the Notch signaling pathway is a significant regulator of neuroendocrine differentiation and serotonin production in GI carcinoid tumors.[14,15] The Wnt signaling pathway as well as transforming growth factor beta (TGF-β) signaling are upregulated in carcinoid tumors.[16]

CLASSIFICATION

In 1963, Williams and Sandler reported a relationship between the embryonic origin of carcinoid tumors and the histologic, biochemical, and, to some extent, clinical features of the tumors.[17] Three distinct groups were formed (Table 43-1): foregut carcinoids (i.e., intrathoracic, gastric, and duodenal carcinoids), midgut carcinoids (carcinoids of the small intestine, appendix, and proximal colon), and hindgut carcinoids (carcinoid tumors of the distal colon and rectum).

Although this original classification has been useful in the clinical assessment of patients with carcinoid tumors, it has demonstrated significant shortcomings. As a result,

TABLE 43-1

Classification of Carcinoid Tumors

	Foregut	Midgut	Hindgut
Histopathology			
	Argyrophilic CgA positive NSE positive	Argentaffin positive CgA positive NSE positive	Argyrophilic SVP-2 positive CgA positive, NSE positive
Molecular Genetics			
	Chromosome 11q13 deletion	Chromosome 18q, 18p deletion	Unknown
Secretory Products			
	CgA, 5-HT, 5-HTP, histamine, ACTH, GHRH, CGRP, somatostatin, AVP, glucagon, gastrin, NKA, substance P, neurotensin, GRP	CgA, 5-HT, NKA, substance P, prostaglandin E_1 and F_2, bradykinin	PP, YY, somatostatin
Carcinoid Syndrome			
	Present (30%)	Present (70%)	Absent

ACTH, adrenocorticotropic hormone; AVP, arginine vasopressin; CgA, chromogranin A; CGRP, calcitonin gene–releasing peptide; GRP, gastrin-releasing peptide; 5-HT, 5-hydroxytryptamine; 5-HTP, 5-hydroxytryptophan; NKA, neurokinin; NSE, neuron-specific enolase; PP, pancreatic peptide; YY, peptide YY; SVP-2, synaptic vesicle protein 2.

a new classification system (WHO classification 2010) has emerged that takes into account not only the site of origin but also variations in the histopathologic characteristics of carcinoid tumors.[18] In this revised system, typical tumors are classified as NET-G1 tumors, which show a characteristic growth pattern (Fig. 43-2). These tumors are usually slow growing, with low proliferation capacity (proliferation index < 2%). They are usually confined to the mucosa and submucosa and are less than 1 to 2 cm in diameter (classical midgut carcinoid). NET-G2 tumors show widely invasive growth and a high proliferation index (PI 2% to 20%). Poorly differentiated carcinomas (NET-G3) are large tumors with metastases and a proliferation index greater than 20% (Table 43-2). The European Neuroendocrine Tumor Society (ENETS) has proposed a new tumor-node-metastasis (TNM) classification and grading system, which is widely used in the clinic.[19]

The neuroendocrine lung tumors are divided into typical carcinoids, atypical carcinoids, large cell neuroendocrine carcinomas, and small cell lung carcinomas. The difference between the typical and atypical carcinoid is based on histopathologic features, with higher proliferation and necrosis found in the atypical carcinoid.[20] The incidence of carcinoid tumors is similar in Western countries and is estimated to be 2.8 to 4.5 per 100,000 people (Surveillance, Epidemiology, and End Results [SEER] database)[21] (Fig. 43-3). Because many carcinoid tumors are indolent, the true incidence may be higher. In particular, appendiceal carcinoids have not been included in many studies, but a higher incidence of 8.2 per 100,000 was found in an autopsy study when appendiceal carcinoids were included.[22] The incidence of patients with a carcinoid syndrome is about 0.5 per 100,000.[23] Data from the United States, based on results from the End Results Group and the Third National Cancer Survey, 1950 to 1969 and 1969 to 1971, respectively, found that the stomach was the most common site of carcinoid tumors, followed by the rectum, ileum, lungs, and bronchi.[25]

An analysis done in the SEER program of the National Cancer Institute between 1973 and 2000 reported an increase in the percentage of pulmonary and gastric carcinoids and a decrease in the percentage of appendiceal carcinoids.[21] Age-specific incidence rates showed a peak between 65 and 75 years (7.5-9.5/100,000), with a male predominance. In persons younger than 50 years, a female predominance has been observed both for appendiceal and lung carcinoids.[24] Analyses of the SEER database show an incidence of 5.2/100,000 and a prevalence of 35/100,000, indicating a significant increase since 2000.[21,25]

BIOCHEMISTRY

The production of hormones is a highly organized function of carcinoid cells. In 1953, Lembeck isolated serotonin from a carcinoid tumor; since then, the carcinoid syndrome has been related to serotonin overproduction.[5] The biosynthesis of serotonin and its metabolic degradation are outlined in Figure 43-4.

Carcinoid tumors of the midgut and foregut regions with metastatic disease secrete serotonin and show elevated urinary excretion of 5-HIAA in 76% and 30%, respectively.[26] Carcinoid tumors arising from the foregut, however, commonly have low levels of L-amino acid decarboxylase, which converts 5-hydroxytryptophan (5-HTP) to serotonin. Thus, these tumors secrete primarily 5-HTP.[27,28]

For many years, it was believed that the entire carcinoid syndrome could be explained by the secretion of these biologically active amines. However, further studies have indicated that serotonin is mainly involved in the pathogenesis of diarrhea and that other biologically active substances play a more important part in the carcinoid flush and bronchoconstriction.

Oates and associates[29] proposed that *kallikrein*, an enzyme found in carcinoid tumors, is released in association with flush and stimulates plasma kininogen to liberate lysyl-bradykinin and bradykinin. These biologically active substances cause vasodilation, hypotension, tachycardia, and edema.[29-31] Furthermore, prostaglandins (E_1, E_2, F_1, F_2) might also play a role in the carcinoid syndrome.[32] Gastric

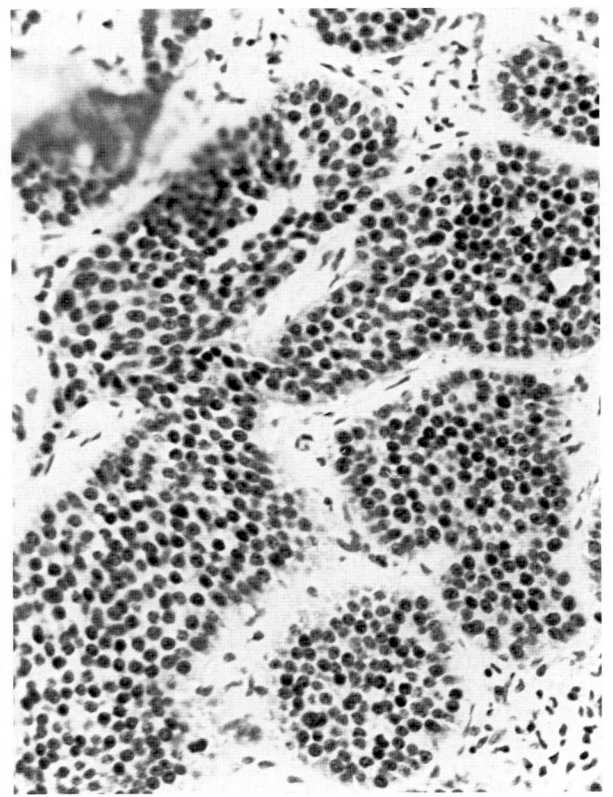

Figure 43-2 Histopathology of a classic well-differentiated midgut carcinoid tumor.

TABLE 43-2						
World Health Organization Classification of Neuroendocrine Tumors						
WHO 1980	**WHO 2000**	**Histologic Differentiation**	**Size**	**Metastases**	**WHO 2010**	**Ki-67 Index (%)**
Carcinoid(s)	WDET	Well	≤1-2 cm	−	NET-G1	≤2
	WDEC	Well	>2 cm	+	NET-G2	3-20
	PDEC	Poorly	Any	+	NEC-G3	>20
		Small or large cell phenotype				

NEC, neuroendocrine carcinoma; NET, neuroendocrine tumor; PDEC, poorly differentiated endocrine carcinoma; WDEC, well-differentiated endocrine carcinoma; WDET, well-differentiated endocrine tumor; WHO, World Health Organization.

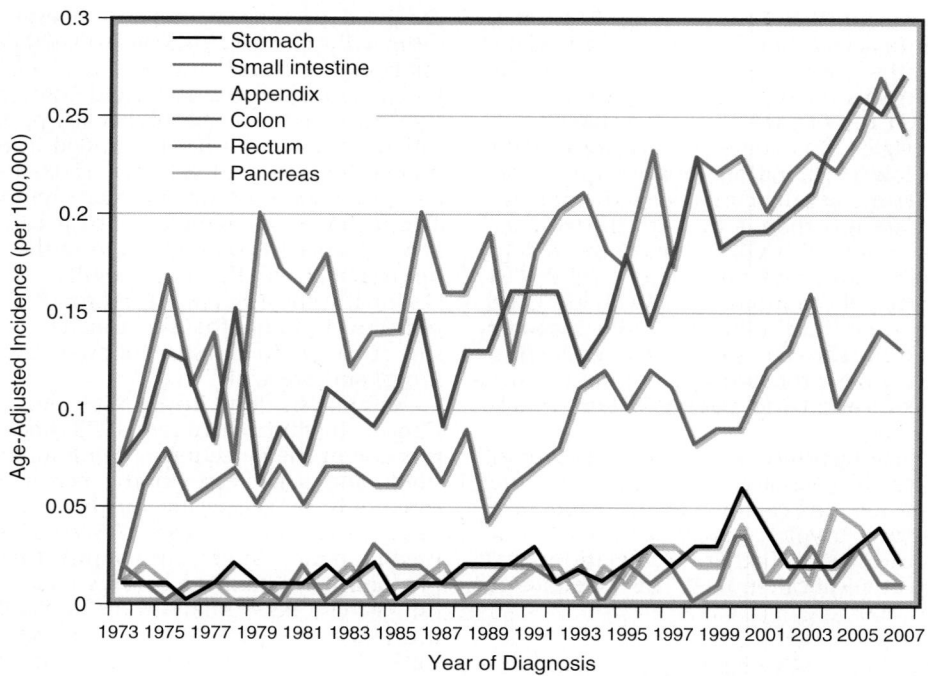

Figure 43-3 Age-adjusted incidence of gastroenteropancreatic neuroendocrine tumors by primary site (SEER 9 registry). Notice the significant increase during the past decades. SEER, Surveillance, Epidemiology, and End Results.

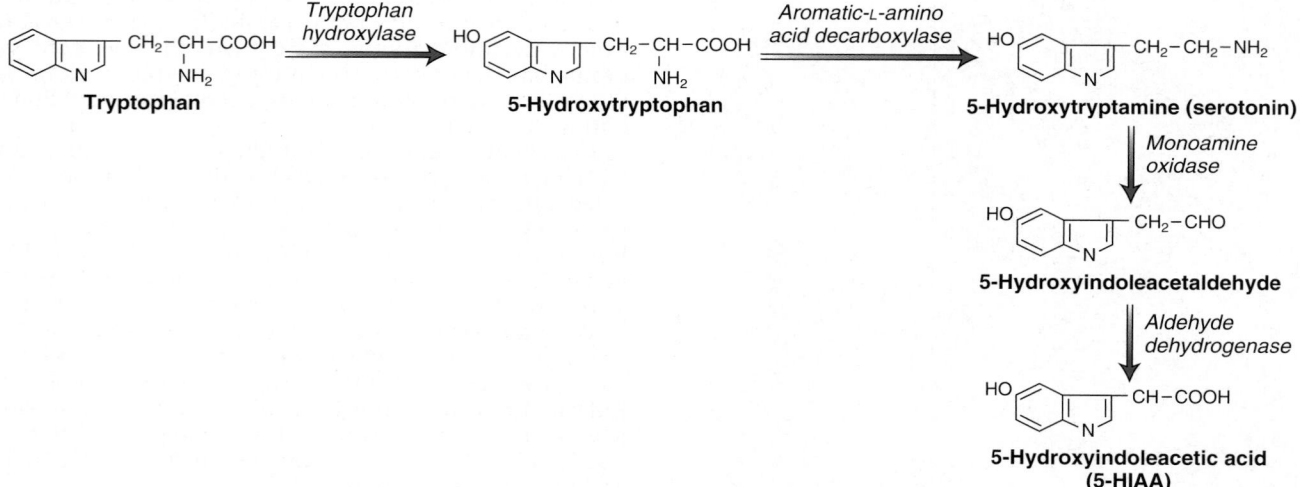

Figure 43-4 Biosynthesis and metabolism of 5-hydroxytryptamine (5-HT) (serotonin).

Substance P	Arg-Pro-Lys-Pro-Gln-Gln-Phe-Phe-Gly-Leu-Met-NH2
Neurokinin A	His-Lys-Thr-Asp-Ser-Phe-Val-Gly-Leu-Met-NH2
Neurokinin B	Asp-Met-His-Asp-Phe-Val-Gly-Leu-Met-NH2
Eledoisin	Pyr-Pro-Ser-Lys-Asp-Ala-Phe-Ile-Gly-Leu-Met-NH2
Kassinin	Asp-Val-Pro-Lys-Ser-Asp-Glu-Phe-Val-Gly-Leu-Met-NH2
Physalemin	Pyr-Ala-Asp-Pro-Asn-Lys-Phe-Tyr-Gly-Leu-Met-NH2
Neuropeptide K	Arg-His-Lys-Thr-Asp-Ser-Phe-Val-Gly-Leu-Met-NH2

^{1}-Lys-His-Ser-Ile-Gln-Gly-His-Gly-Tyr-Leu-Ala-Lys

Asp-Ala-Asp-Ser-Ser-Ile-Glu-Lys-Gln-Val-Ala-Leu-Leu^1

Figure 43-5 The tachykinin family of peptides shares the same carboxy-terminus. Neuropeptide K is a prohormone containing neurokinin A, which can be spliced off.

carcinoids and lung carcinoids have been found to contain and secrete histamine, which might be responsible for the characteristic bright red flush seen in these patients.[33-35] Metabolites of histamine are often present in high concentration in the urine from these patients. Dopamine and norepinephrine have also been found in carcinoid tumors.[36]

The occurrence of *substance P* in carcinoid tumors was first demonstrated by Håkansson and coworkers in 1977.[37] Substance P belongs to a family of polypeptides that share the same carboxy-terminus and are called *tachykinins* (Fig. 43-5). A number of tachykinin-related peptides have been isolated from carcinoid tumors, such as neurokinin A, neuropeptide K, and eledoisin. During stimulation of flush in patients with midgut carcinoids, multiple forms of tachykinins are released to the circulation (Fig. 43-6).[38-40]

Many different polypeptides (e.g., insulin, gastrin, somatostatin, S100 protein, polypeptide YY, pancreatic polypeptide, human chorionic gonadotropin α-subunit [hCG-α], motilin, calcitonin, vasoactive intestinal polypeptide [VIP], and endorphins) have been demonstrated in carcinoid tumors by immunohistochemical staining and sometimes in tumor extracts.[10] Ectopic ACTH or CRH production may be found in foregut carcinoids; in particular, patients with bronchial or thymic carcinoids seem susceptible to Cushing syndrome.[41] Patients with carcinoid tumors of the foregut type might also present with acromegaly due to ectopic secretion of GHRH from the tumor.[42] Duodenal carcinoids as part of von Recklinghausen disease can secrete somatostatin.[43]

The *chromogranin/secretogranin* family consists of CgA, CgB (sometimes called *secretogranin I*), secretogranin II (sometimes called *CgC*), and some other members. CgA was first isolated in 1965 as a water-soluble protein present in chromaffin cells from bovine adrenal medulla.[44] Its immunoreactivity has been found in all parts of the GI tract and pancreas and has also been isolated from all endocrine glands.[45]

CgA is an acidic glycoprotein of 439 amino acids with a molecular weight of 48 kDa. It can be spliced into smaller fragments at dibasic cleavage sites, generating multiple bioactive fragments such as vasostatins, chromostatin, and pancreastatin (Fig. 43-7).[45-49]

Amines and hormones are stored intracellularly in two types of vesicles: large dense-core vesicles and small synaptic-like vesicles. These vesicles release amines and hormones on stimulation. Large dense-core vesicles contain the hormones and one or more members of the chromogranin/secretogranin family of proteins.[46,50] Both amines and peptides are coreleased (Fig. 43-8).

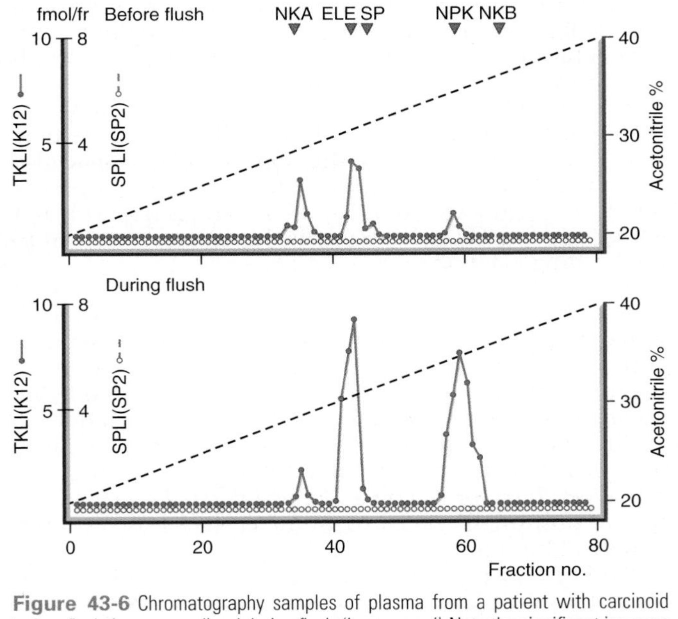

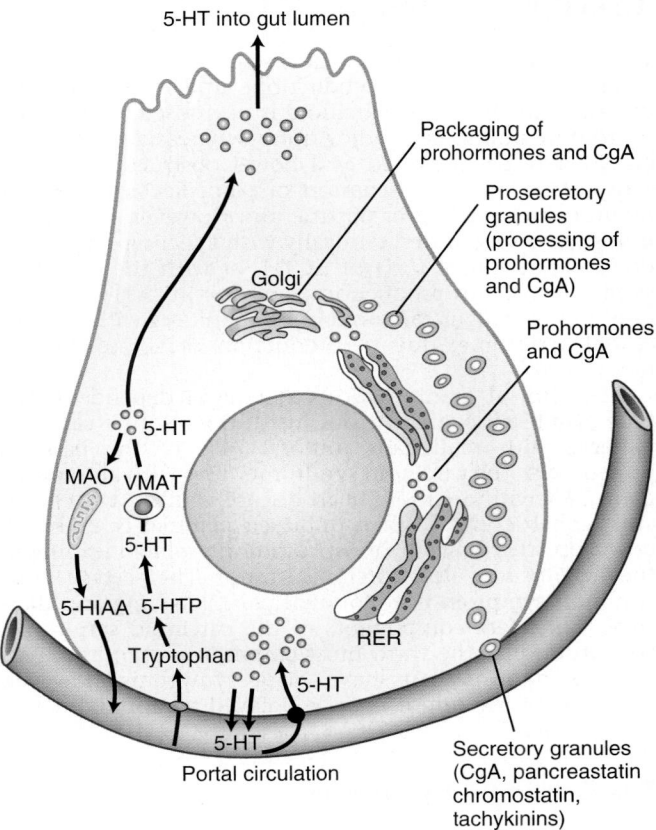

Figure 43-8 Schematic drawing of an enterochromaffin cell. The initial step in 5-hydroxytryptamine (5-HT) synthesis is carrier transport of the amino acid tryptophan from blood into the cell across the cell membrane. Intracellular tryptophan is first converted to 5-hydroxytryptophan (5-HTP), which in turn is converted to 5-HT and stored in secretory granules. The transport of 5-HT into granules requires vesicular monoamine transporters (VMATs). Via the basal lateral membrane, 5-HT can be released into the circulation. There is also a membrane pump mechanism in the cell membrane responsible for amine reuptake. A minor part of 5-HT can also be released into the gut lumen. Monoamine oxidase (MAO) degrades 5-HT to 5-hydroxyindoleacetic acid (5-HIAA). Peptide prohormones are synthesized in the rough endoplasmic reticulum (RER) together with chromogranin A (CgA) and other granule proteins. The products are transported to the Golgi apparatus for packaging into prosecretory granules. On stimulation, the secretory products are released from the granules by exocytosis.

Figure 43-6 Chromatography samples of plasma from a patient with carcinoid before flush *(upper panel)* and during flush *(lower panel)*. Note the significant increase in eledoisin-like peptide as well as in neuropeptide K. ELE, eledoisin; NKA, neurokinin A; NKB, neurokinin B; NPK, neuropeptide K; SP, substance P; SPLI(SP2), substance P–like immunoreactivity; TKLI(K12), tachykinin-like immunoreactivity.

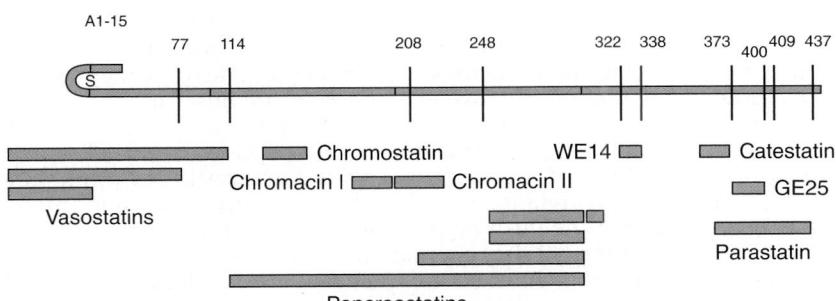

Figure 43-7 The glycoprotein chromogranin A and related peptides, including GE25 and WE14.

The physiologic function of CgA is not fully elucidated. Its ubiquitous presence in neuroendocrine tissues and its cosecretion with peptide hormones and amines indicate a storage role of the peptide within the secretory granule.[45,46,50] It also acts as a prohormone that can generate bioactive smaller fragments. CgA is an important tissue and serum marker for different types of carcinoid tumors, including those of the foregut, midgut, and hindgut (see Table 43-1 and later discussion).

CLINICAL PRESENTATION

The clinical presentation of carcinoid tumors depends on localization, hormone production, and extent of the disease. Usually, a lung carcinoid is diagnosed incidentally on routine pulmonary radiography, whereas a midgut carcinoid may be identified as a bowel obstruction or as a cause of abdominal discomfort or pain. Rectal carcinoids might cause bleeding or obstruction. However, lung carcinoids can also manifest clinically with Cushing syndrome, due to secretion of CRH or ACTH, or with the carcinoid syndrome, due to production of serotonin, 5-HTP, or histamine.[51] A midgut carcinoid often manifests with the carcinoid syndrome, due to production of serotonin and tachykinins.

The clinical manifestations at referral depend on the type of referral center. At our institution, which cares for patients with malignant tumors, 74% of the patients present with the carcinoid syndrome, 13% with abdominal pain, 12% with carcinoid heart disease, and 2% with bronchial constriction.[25] When unbiased material is analyzed, bowel obstruction is the most common problem leading to the diagnosis of ileal carcinoid tumor. The second most common symptom is abdominal pain. Flushing and diarrhea, which are components of the carcinoid syndrome, constitute only the third most common presentation.[52-54] Because many patients have vague symptoms, however, diagnosis of the tumor may be delayed by approximately 2 to 3 years.[23]

The Carcinoid Syndrome

In 1954, Thorson and coworkers for the first time described the carcinoid syndrome as having the following features: malignant carcinoid of the small intestine with metastasis to the liver, valvular disease of the right side of the heart (pulmonary stenosis and tricuspid insufficiency without septal defect), peripheral vasomotor symptoms, bronchial constriction, and an unusual type of cyanosis.[4] One year later, Dr. William Bean[55] gave this colorful description of the carcinoid syndrome: "This witch's brew of unlikely signs and symptoms, intriguing to the most fastidious connoisseur of clinical esoterica—the skin underwent rapid and extreme changes—resembling in clinical miniature the fecal phantasmagoria of the aurora borealis."

The syndrome is thus well characterized and includes flushing, diarrhea, right-sided heart failure, and sometimes bronchial constriction and increased urinary levels of 5-HIAA.[56,57] This is the classic carcinoid syndrome, but some patients display only one or two of the features. Other symptoms related to the syndrome are weight loss, sweating, and pellagra-like skin lesions.

Development of the carcinoid syndrome is a function of tumor mass, extent and localization of metastases, and localization of the primary tumor. The syndrome is most common in tumors originating in the small intestine and proximal colon; 40% to 60% of patients with these tumors experience the syndrome.[25,53,56,57] The disorders are less common in patients with bronchial carcinoids and do not occur in patients with rectal carcinoids.[51,58,59] The syndrome rarely occurs in patients with midgut carcinoids and a small tumor burden, such as only regional lymph node metastases.[54] Patients with the full syndrome usually have multiple liver metastases. The association with hepatic metastases is due to efficient inactivation by the liver of amines and peptides released into the portal circulation. The venous drainage of liver metastases is directly into the systemic circulation and bypasses hepatic inactivation.[60]

Other carcinoid tumors likely to be associated with the carcinoid syndrome in the absence of liver metastases are ovarian carcinoids and bronchial carcinoids, which release mediators directly into the systemic rather than the portal circulation. Retroperitoneal metastases from classic midgut carcinoids also release mediators directly into the circulation and might cause the carcinoid syndrome without any liver metastases.[56,57]

Flushing

Four types of flushing have been described in the literature: erythematous, violaceous, prolonged, and bright red.[56,57]

The first and best known type is the sudden, diffuse, erythematous flush, usually affecting the face, neck, and upper chest (i.e., the normal flushing area) (Fig. 43-9). This type of flush is commonly of short duration, lasting from 1 to 5 minutes, and is related to early-stage midgut carcinoids. Patients usually experience a sensation of warmth during flushing and sometimes heart palpitations. This type of flushing is reported in 20% to 70% of patients with midgut carcinoid at onset of the disease.[23,56,58]

The second type is the violaceous flush, which affects the same area of the body. It has roughly the same time course or sometimes lasts a little longer. Patients may also have facial telangiectasia. This flush occurs during the later stages of midgut carcinoid (Fig. 43-10) and is normally not felt by patients because they have become accustomed to the flushing reaction.

The third type is prolonged flushing that usually lasts a couple of hours but can last up to several days. This flush sometimes involves the whole body and is associated with profuse lacrimation, swelling of the salivary gland, hypotension, and facial edema (Fig. 43-11). These symptoms are usually associated with malignant bronchial carcinoids.

The fourth type of flushing is a bright red, patchy flush, seen in patients with chronic atrophic gastritis and ECL cell hyperplasia, or ECLoma (derived from ECL cells). This type of flushing is related to an increased release of histamine and histamine metabolites.

Flushes may be spontaneous or may be precipitated by stress (physical and mental); infection; alcohol; certain foods (spicy); or drugs, such as by injections of catecholamines, calcium, or pentagastrin (see later). The pathophysiology of flushing in the carcinoid syndrome is not yet elucidated.[61-63] It was previously believed to be totally related to excess production of serotonin or serotonin metabolites.[62] However, several patients with high levels of plasma serotonin did not have any flushing, nor did a serotonin antagonist (e.g., methysergide, cyproheptadine, or ketanserin) have any effect on the flushing.[61,64]

In a study from our own group in which we measured the release of tachykinins, neuropeptide K, and substance P during flushing provoked by pentagastrin or alcohol, a clear correlation was found between the onset and intensity of the flushing reaction and the release of tachykinins (see Fig. 43-6). Furthermore, when the release of tachykinins was blocked by prestimulatory administration of octreotide, little or no flushing was observed in the same

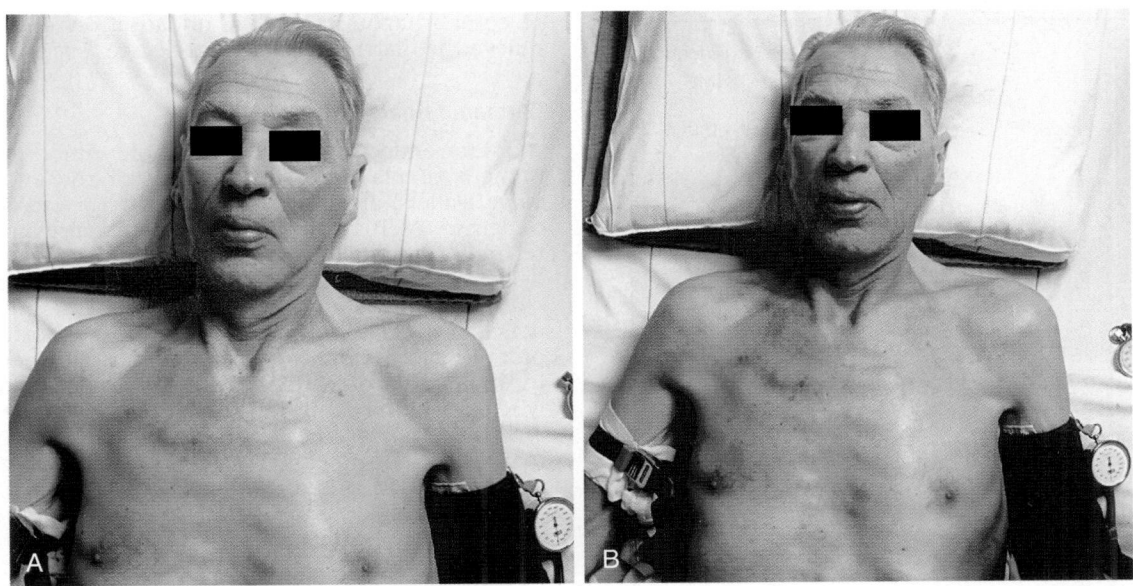

Figure 43-9 Carcinoid syndrome before and after provocation. **A,** Before flush provocation. **B,** The same patient after pentagastrin-stimulated flush.

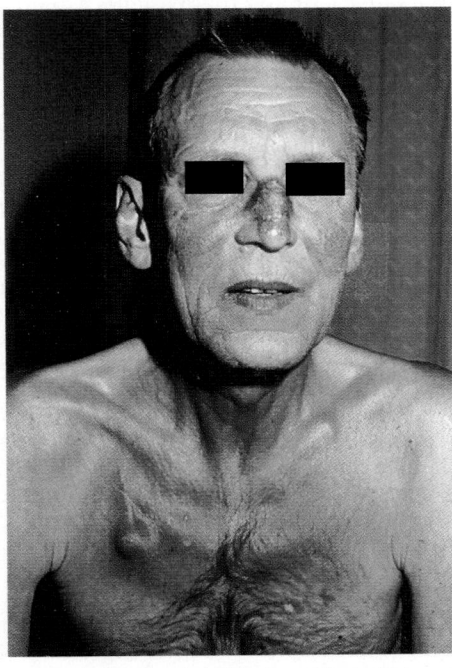

Figure 43-10 Long-lasting chronic flushing in a patient with long-standing carcinoid disease. Note the telangiectases.

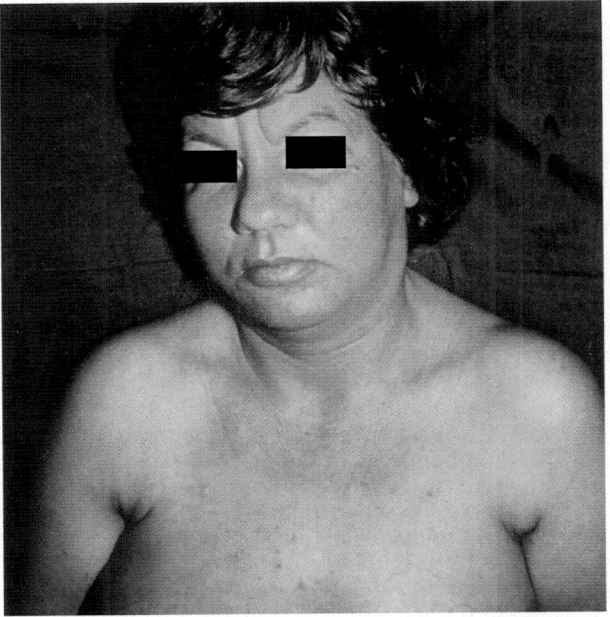

Figure 43-11 This patient has lung carcinoid and carcinoid syndrome with severe, long-standing flushing, lacrimation, and a swollen face.

patient (Fig. 43-12).[38-40] Other mediators of the flushing reaction may be kallikrein and bradykinins, which are released during provoked flushing.[29-31]

Histamine may be a mediator of the flushes seen in lung carcinoids and in gastric carcinoids (ECLomas).[33-35] Tachykinins, bradykinins, and histamines are well-known vasodilators, and somatostatin analogues might alleviate flushing by reducing circulating levels of these agents (see later).[38-40,63-68] Furschgott and Zawadski have suggested that flushing is caused by an indirect vasodilation mediated by endothelium-derived relaxing factor (EDRF) or by nitric oxide released by 5-HTP during platelet activation.[69]

The facial flushing associated with carcinoid tumors should be distinguished from idiopathic flushing and menopausal hot flushes. Patients with idiopathic flushes usually have a long history of flushing starting early in life and sometimes with a family history without occurrence of a tumor. Menopausal hot flushes usually involve the whole body and are accompanied by intense sweating. Postmenopausal women in whom a true carcinoid syndrome is developing can differentiate between the two types of flushes.

Diarrhea

Diarrhea occurs in 30% to 80% of patients with the carcinoid syndrome.[23,25,56,57] Its pathophysiology is poorly understood but is probably multifactorial. The diarrhea is

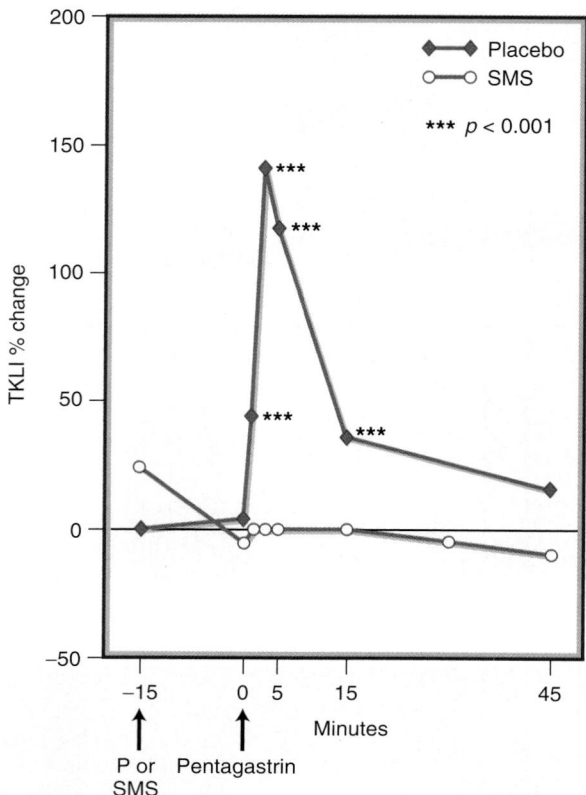

Figure 43-12 Tachykinin levels (TKLI) after stimulation with pentagastrin in patients with classic midgut carcinoids. Pretreatment for 15 minutes with somatostatin (SMS) causes inhibition of tachykinin release and inhibition of the flush reaction (*open circles*. P, placebo.

often accompanied by abdominal cramping, and endocrine, paracrine, and mechanical factors contribute to this condition. A variety of tumor products, including serotonin, tachykinins, histamines, kallikrein, and prostaglandins, can stimulate peristalsis, electromechanical activity, and tone in the intestine.[63,70-72] Secretory diarrhea can occur with fluid and electrolyte imbalance. Malabsorption can result from intestinal resections, from lymphangiectasia, secondary to mesenteric fibrosis, from bacterial overgrowth, and secondary to a tumor partially obstructing the small bowel or rapid intestinal transit. Increased secretion by the small bowel, malabsorption, or accelerated transit can overwhelm the normal storage and absorptive capacity of proximal colon and result in diarrhea, which may be aggravated if the reabsorptive function of the colon is impaired.

In a study of patients with elevated serotonin levels and the carcinoid syndrome, transit time in the small bowel and colon was significantly decreased in comparison with that of normal subjects.[73] The volume of the ascending colon was significantly smaller than that in normal subjects, and the postprandial colonic tone was markedly increased. This indicates that in patients in whom the carcinoid syndrome is associated with diarrhea, major alterations in gut motor function occur that affect both the small intestine and the colon. Many patients with carcinoid tumors have undergone wide resection of the small intestine, and they may be affected by the symptoms of short-bowel syndrome.

Serotonin is believed to be responsible for the diarrhea in the carcinoid syndrome by its effects on gut motility and intestinal electrolyte and fluid secretion.[57,70-72] Serotonin

receptor antagonists, such as ondansetron and ketanserin, relieve the diarrhea to a certain degree.[70,74-76]

Carcinoid Heart Disease

A unique endocrine effect of carcinoid tumors is the development of plaquelike thickenings of the endocardium, valve leaflets, atria, and ventricles in 10% to 20% of the patients.[77,78] This fibrotic involvement causes stenosis and regurgitation of the blood flow. Findings of new collagen beneath the endothelium of the endocardium is almost pathognomonic for carcinoid heart disease.[77-79] The incidence of these lesions depends on the diagnostic methodology. Echocardiography can demonstrate early lesions in about 70% of patients with the carcinoid syndrome, whereas routine clinical examinations detect them in only 30% to 40%.[77,78,80] These figures have significantly dropped to 5% to 10%, probably because of earlier diagnosis and the use of biologic antitumor treatments such as somatostatin analogues and α-interferons. Both of these agents control the hormonal release and excess that are thought to be involved in the fibrotic process.

In a study performed in 1987,[23] 40% of patients with carcinoid tumors died of cardiac complications related to the carcinoid disease. Data from 2008 reveal that this complication is a rare event and that patients usually die of the effects of a progressive tumor.[25]

The precise mechanism behind the fibrosis in the right side of the heart has not been determined yet, but it occurs mainly in patients with liver metastases who usually also have the carcinoid syndrome.[77,78] Substances inducing fibrosis are believed to be released directly into the right side of the heart and are then neutralized or degraded as they pass through the pulmonary circulation, because few patients present with similar lesions of the left side of the heart.[77,78] However, patients with lung carcinoids occasionally display the same fibrotic changes in the left side of the heart. Histologically, the plaque-like thickenings in the endocardium consist of myofibroblasts and fibroblasts embedded in a stroma that is rich in mucopolysaccharides and collagen.[77]

We have previously shown that the TGF-β family of growth factors is upregulated in carcinoid fibrous plaques on the right side of the heart.[81] The TGF-β family of growth factors is known to stimulate matrix formation and collagen deposition. The substances that induce TGF-β locally in the heart are not known, but serotonin, tachykinins, and insulin-like growth factor 1 (IGF-1) may be mediators.[77,82]

A correlation has been found between circulating levels of serotonin and tachykinins and the degree and frequency of carcinoid heart lesions. The weight-reducing drugs fenfluramine and dexfenfluramine appear to interfere with normal serotonin metabolism and have been associated with valvular lesions identical to those seen in carcinoid heart disease.[83,84] However, treatment resulting in decreased urinary 5-HIAA excretion does not result in regression of cardiac lesions.[85] Two animal studies indicate that serotonin might play a significant role in the development of carcinoid heart disease. Serotonin is also known to induce TGF-β₁ in in vitro experiments.[86-88] Connective tissue growth factor (CTGF) is produced by carcinoid tumor cells, and increased expression is found in patients with advanced fibrosis. CTGF is known to stimulate TGF-β.[89]

Bronchial Constriction

A true asthma episode is rare in patients with the carcinoid syndrome.[23,56,57] The causative agents of bronchial constriction are not known, but tachykinins and bradykinins have been suggested as mediators.[90,91] These agents can constrict smooth muscle in the respiratory tract and can also cause local edema in the airways.

Other Manifestations of the Carcinoid Syndrome

Fibrotic complications other than heart lesions may be found in patients with carcinoid tumors. They include intra-abdominal and retroperitoneal fibroses, occlusion of the mesenteric arteries and veins, Peyronie disease, and carcinoid arthropathy.[56,57]

Intra-abdominal fibrosis can lead to intestinal adhesions and bowel obstruction and is a more common cause of bowel obstruction than is the primary carcinoid tumor itself.[54,92,93] Retroperitoneal fibrosis can result in obstruction of the ureter that impairs kidney function, which sometimes requires treatment with ureteral stents.

Narrowing and occlusion of arteries and veins by fibrosis are potentially life-threatening. Ischemic loops of the bowel might have to be removed, and this procedure ultimately causes short-bowel syndrome.[54,93]

Other rare features of the syndrome are pellagra-like skin lesions with hyperkeratosis and pigmentation, myopathy, and sexual dysfunction.[57]

Carcinoid Crisis

Carcinoid crisis has become rare since the introduction of treatment with somatostatin analogues.[94] It might occur spontaneously or during induction of anesthesia, embolization procedures, chemotherapy, or infection. Carcinoid crisis is a clinical condition characterized by severe flushing, diarrhea, hypotension, hyperthermia, and tachycardia. Without treatment, patients might die during the crisis.[94-96]

Intravenous (IV) or subcutaneous somatostatin analogues (or both) are given before, during, and after surgery to prevent the development of carcinoid crisis.[94,96-98] Patients with metastatic lung carcinoids are particularly difficult to treat during crisis. IV infusions of octreotide at doses of 50 to 100 μg/hour, supplemented with histamine H_1-receptor and H_2-receptor blockers and IV sodium chloride, are recommended.[99]

Other Clinical Manifestations of Carcinoid Tumors

Ectopic secretion of CRH and ACTH from pulmonary carcinoid tumors and thymic carcinoids accounts for 1% of all cases of Cushing syndrome.[41,100] Acromegaly due to ectopic secretion of GHRH has also been reported in foregut carcinoids.[42,101] Gastric carcinoid tumors make up less than 1% of gastric neoplasms. They can be separated into three distinct groups or types on the basis of clinical and histologic characteristics and originate from gastric ECL cells.[102] Type 1 is associated with chronic atrophic gastritis type A (80%). Type 2 is associated with Zollinger-Ellison syndrome as part of MEN1 syndrome (6%). Type 3 represents sporadic gastric carcinoids occurring without hypergastrinemia and pursue a more malignant course, with 50% to 60% developing metastases.[102,103]

About 80% of gastric carcinoids are associated with chronic atrophic gastritis type A, and more than 50% of patients with these carcinoids also have pernicious anemia. These tumors are more common in women than in men and are usually identified endoscopically during diagnostic evaluation for anemia or abdominal pain.[102,104] They are often multifocal and localized in the gastric fundus area,

and they are derived from ECL cells. Patients have hypochlorhydria and hypergastrinemia. Gastrin hypersecretion has been postulated to result in hyperplasia of the ECL cells, which might later develop into carcinoid tumors.[105,106] Hyperplasia of ECL cells has been noticed in patients on long-standing proton-pump inhibitor therapy.[107,108]

DIAGNOSIS

The diagnosis of a suspected carcinoid tumor must take into consideration molecular genetics, tumor biology, histopathology, biochemistry, and localization. The diagnosis of a carcinoid tumor may be suspected from clinical symptoms suggesting the carcinoid syndrome or from the presence of other clinical symptoms, or it can be made in relatively asymptomatic patients from the histopathologic findings at surgery or after liver biopsy for unknown hepatic lesions.

In one study involving 154 consecutive patients with GI carcinoids found at surgery, 60% were asymptomatic.[109] In patients with symptomatic tumors, the time from onset of symptoms until diagnosis is often delayed 1 to 2 years.[23] The current tumor biology program includes growth factors (platelet-derived growth factor, epidermal growth factor, IGF-1, TGF)[110] and proliferation factors (measurements of the nuclear antigen Ki-67) as a proliferation index. Such an index correlates with tumor aggressiveness and survival.[111,112] Adhesion molecules such as CD-44, particularly exon-V6 and exon-V9, have been related to improved survival.[113] Determination of the expression of angiogenic factors basic fibroblast growth factor (b-FGF) and vascular endothelial growth factor (VEGF) should also be included in a tumor biology program. Somatostatin analogues are cornerstones in the treatment of the carcinoid syndrome; therefore, determination of the different subtypes of somatostatin receptors (SSTR1 to SSTR5) with specific antibodies is warranted.[114,115] Rare cases with familial carcinoids should be analyzed with respect to loss of heterozygosity on chromosome 11q13 and chromosome 18.

Histopathologic Diagnosis

The histopathologic diagnosis of carcinoids is based on immunohistochemistry using antibodies against CgA, synaptophysin, and neuron-specific enolase. These immunohistochemical stains have replaced the old silver stains, the argyrophil stains by Grimelius and Sevier-Munger. The argentaffin stain by Masson to demonstrate content of serotonin has also been replaced by immunocytochemistry with serotonin antibodies.[10] These neuroendocrine markers can be supplemented by specific immunocytochemistry to different hormones such as substance P, gastrin, and ACTH. The WHO classification forms the basis for therapeutic decisions (see earlier) and therefore determination of Ki-67 (MIB-1) for analysis of cell proliferation is mandatory. Antibodies to TTF-1 and CDX-2 give good information on the localization of the primary tumor in patients with unknown primary tumors.[116]

Biochemical Diagnosis

In patients with flushing and other manifestations of the carcinoid syndrome, the diagnosis can be established by measuring the urinary excretion of 5-HIAA because levels are invariably elevated under these circumstances.[117] Patients with carcinoid tumors usually have urinary 5-HIAA levels of 100 to 3000 μmol/24 hours (15 to 60 mg/24 hours) (reference range: <50 μmol/24 hours [10 mg/24 hours]).

Assays for urinary 5-HIAA include high-pressure liquid chromatography (HPLC) with electrochemical detection and colorimetric and fluorescence methods.[118] Various foods and drugs can interfere with the measurement of urinary 5-HIAA, and patients should avoid these agents during the 24-hour sampling (Table 43-3).[119] Normally, two 24-hour urine collections are recommended. In a study of patients with malignant midgut carcinoid tumors, 60% to 73% presented with increased urinary 5-HIAA levels,[25,56,57] with a specificity of almost 100%.

TABLE 43-3
Factors That Interfere With Determination of Urinary 5-HIAA

Foods	Drugs
Factors That Produce False-Positive Results	
Avocado	Acetaminophen
Banana	Acetanilid
Chocolate	Caffeine
Coffee	Fluorouracil
Eggplant	Guaifenesin
Pecan	L-Dopa
Pineapple	Melphalan
Plum	Mephenesin
Tea	Methamphetamine
Walnuts	Methocarbamol
	Methysergide maleate
	Phenmetrazine
	Reserpine
	Salicylates
Factors That Cause False-Negative Results	
None	Corticotropin
	p-Chlorophenylalanine
	Chlorpromazine
	Heparin
	Imipramine
	Isoniazid
	Methenamine mandelate
	Methyldopa
	Monoamine oxidase inhibitors
	Phenothiazine
	Promethazine

5-HIAA, 5-hydroxyindoleacetic acid.

Today, measurement of urinary 5-HIAA for diagnosis of carcinoid tumor is the predominant biochemical analytic procedure. However, urinary and platelet measurements of serotonin itself can give additional information. In some studies, platelet serotonin levels were more sensitive than urinary 5-HIAA and urinary serotonin levels and were not affected by the patient's diet, as are 5-HIAA levels.

In a comparative study of 44 consecutive patients with carcinoid tumor, the platelet serotonin, urinary 5-HIAA, and urinary serotonin levels were measured. In foregut carcinoids the sensitivities were 50%, 29%, and 55%, respectively. For midgut carcinoids, the sensitivities were 100%, 92%, and 82%, respectively, and for hindgut carcinoids they were 20%, 0%, and 60%, respectively.[120]

A method to determine 5-HIAA in serum has been developed and is under clinical evaluation.[121] Elevations of 5-HIAA can occur in malabsorption states and a number of other conditions. Foregut carcinoids tend to produce an atypical carcinoid syndrome with increased plasma 5-HTP, but not serotonin, because they lack the appropriate decarboxylase that results in normal urinary 5-HIAA.[27,36] However, some of the 5-HTP is decarboxylated in the intestine and other tissues, and many of these patients have slightly elevated urinary 5-HT or 5-HIAA levels.

Attempts have been made to identify more specific and sensitive serum markers for carcinoid tumors that might allow earlier diagnosis. One such marker is CgA. It has been shown that CgA and CgB are more abundant than CgC in human neuroendocrine tissues.[45,46,121] In 44 patients with carcinoid tumors, CgA was increased in 99%, CgB in 88%, and CgC in only 6% (Fig. 43-13).[122] It has been proposed that CgA levels in plasma might reflect tumor size. In a study of 75 patients with midgut carcinoids and the carcinoid syndrome, CgA was elevated in 87% of carcinoid patients. Furthermore, a correlation between levels of plasma chromogranin and extent of disease was found ($p < 0.0001$).[25] In the same study, urinary 5-HIAA was elevated in 76% of midgut carcinoids, and there were no correlations with tumor size or extent of disease.

CgA is a more sensitive marker than urinary 5-HIAA in detecting carcinoid tumors, but because CgA is released and secreted from various types of neuroendocrine tumors, the specificity is lower.[122-125] Therefore, in a workup of

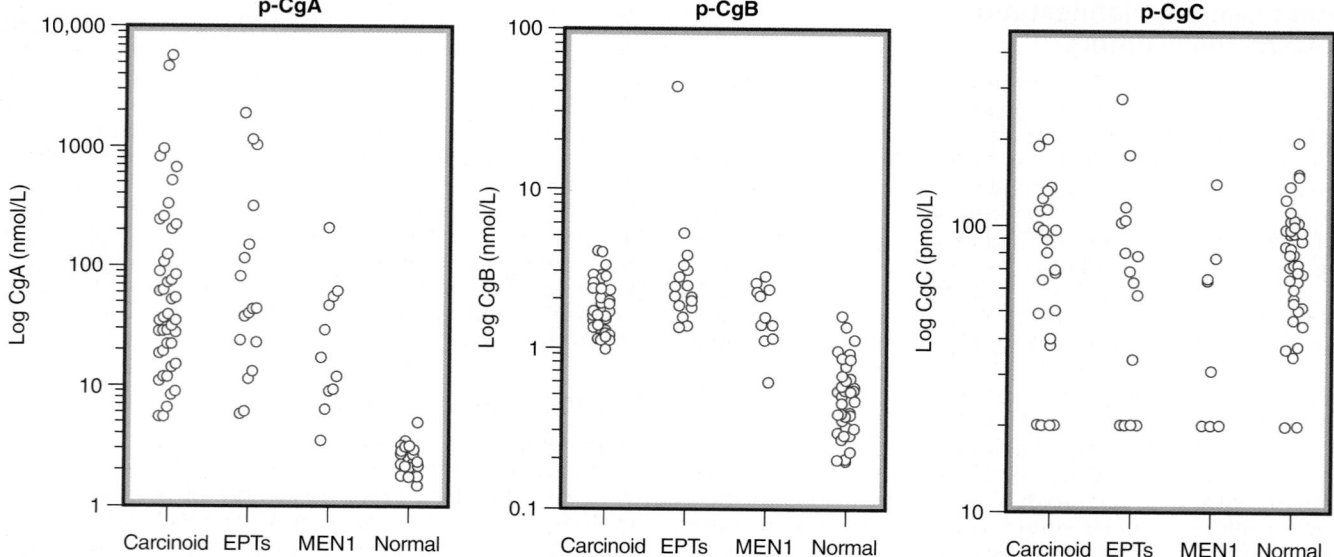

Figure 43-13 Plasma (p) levels of chromogranin A (CgA), CgB, and CgC in patients with various neuroendocrine tumors. EPTs, endocrine pancreatic tumors; MEN1, multiple endocrine neoplasia type 1.

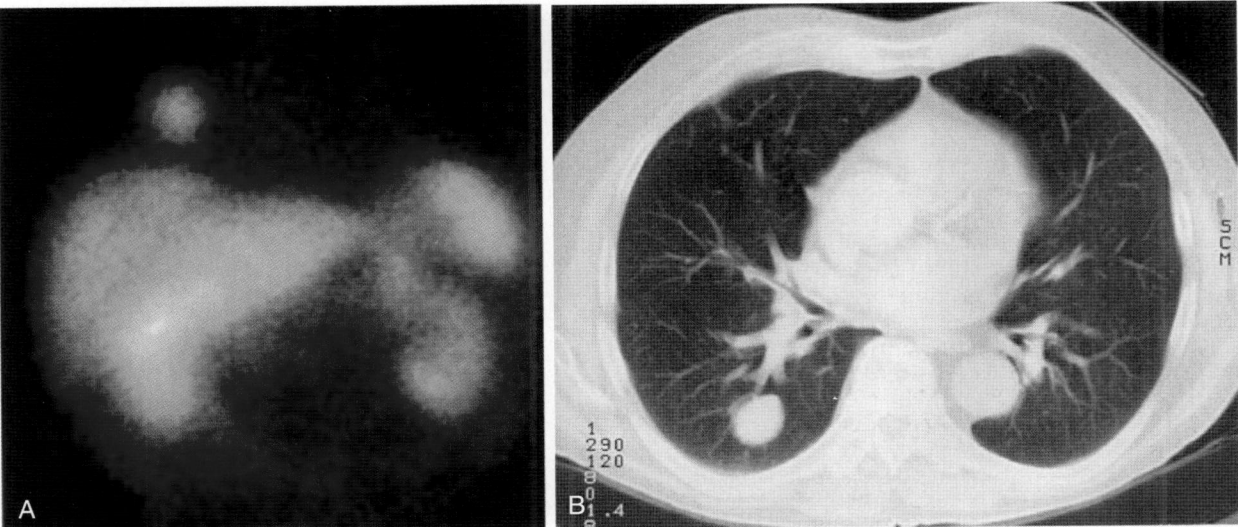

Figure 43-14 Bronchial carcinoid. **A,** Somatostatin-receptor scintigraphy in a patient with a bronchial carcinoid. **B,** Computed tomography scan in the same patient.

patients with the carcinoid syndrome, one should combine the determination of plasma CgA with urinary 5-HIAA or serotonin. Plasma neuron-specific enolase shows a lower sensitivity and specificity than does plasma CgA.[122] Serum hCG-α has been reported to be increased in 60% of patients with foregut carcinoid tumors and in 50% of those with hindgut carcinoids but only 11% in those patients with midgut carcinoids and the carcinoid syndrome. Plasma neuropeptide K levels have been reported to be elevated in 46% of patients with midgut carcinoids, whereas only 9% of patients with foregut carcinoids displayed elevated levels.[123,126] Plasma substance P has a sensitivity of 32% and a specificity of 85%.[25,38-40] Pancreatic polypeptide levels are also elevated in about one third of patients with midgut carcinoids and in as many with foregut carcinoids.[127,128]

During therapy with somatostatin analogues, neither plasma CgA nor urinary 5-HIAA is a reliable marker of tumor size because somatostatin inhibits the synthesis and release of the hormones without changes in tumor size.

Localization Procedures

Numerous imaging techniques, including endoscopy, barium enema, chest radiography, ultrasonography, computed tomography (CT), magnetic resonance imaging (MRI), and angiography, have been used to determine the location of the primary tumor as well as the metastases in patients with carcinoid tumors. In more recent years, somatostatin-receptor scintigraphy (SRS) and iodinated meta-iodobenzylguanidine (^{131}I-MIBG) scanning have been used to localize and stage the disease.[127-130] Bronchial carcinoids are usually detected by chest radiography, CT, or, occasionally, bronchoscopy.[131] The primary midgut tumor is usually small and difficult to localize with traditional diagnostic methods such as barium enema, CT scan, or MRI. Some of these tumors can be localized by angiography, capsule endoscopy, or SRS. Liver metastases are usually detected by CT or MRI. At present, CT or MRI and SRS are the primary diagnostic modalities for tumor staging (Fig. 43-14).

A more sensitive method is PET using ^{11}C-5-HTP, the precursor of serotonin synthesis (Fig. 43-15).[132,133] This isotope accumulates in carcinoid tumors, and with the development of PET cameras, tumors as small as 0.5 cm in

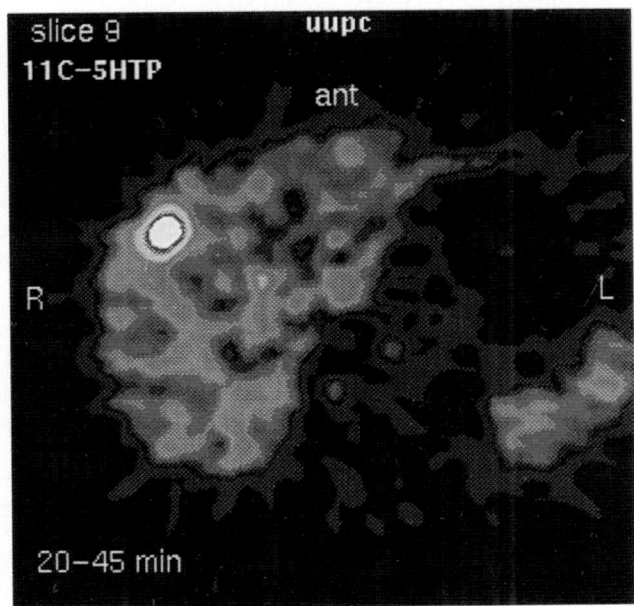

Figure 43-15 Positron emission tomography (PET) scan with ^{11}C-5-hydroxytryptophan. Note the metastasis in the liver.

diameter can be detected.[132] During treatment, a close relation has been found among changes in the PET scan, transport rate constant, and urinary 5-HIAA, suggesting that PET scanning may be useful in monitoring the results of therapy. PET scanning using ^{18}F-fluorodeoxyglucose (FDG-PET) is not useful in detecting low-proliferating neuroendocrine tumors, but it can be beneficial in identifying poorly differentiated anaplastic tumors.

Carcinoid tumors contain high-affinity receptors for somatostatin in 80% to 100% of cases.[114,115,134] The receptors are present in both the primary tumor and metastases. Five subtypes of somatostatin receptors have been cloned (SSTR1 to SSTR5), and somatostatin receptor type 2 is the predominant subtype expressed in carcinoid tumors.

The most commonly available somatostatin analogue, *octreotide,* binds with high affinity to SSTR2 and with lower affinity to SSTR3 and SSTR5.[135-137] SRS with ^{111}In-DTPA-Phe-octreotide (Octreoscan) has been reported to detect carcinoids with a sensitivity of 80% to 90% in patients.[137,138] Many studies have demonstrated that SRS has greater sensitivity for localizing carcinoids compared with conventional imaging studies.[138-142] False-positive scans can be encountered in patients with granulomas (e.g., sarcoidosis, tuberculosis), activated lymphocytes (lymphomas, chronic infection), thyroid diseases (goiter, thyroiditis), endocrine pancreatic tumors, and other endocrine tumors. Because of its high sensitivity and ability to image, whole-body SRS should be the initial imaging procedure to localize and establish the stage of the disease. Bone metastases, which are common with carcinoid tumors, are efficiently detected by SRS, which is as sensitive as traditional bone scanning with technetium.[140,143,144] In addition, ^{68}Ga-DOTA-octreotate PET scanning has been developed, showing higher sensitivity than Octreoscan[145] (Fig. 43-16).

Scintigraphy with ^{123}I-MIBG has been applied in patients with midgut carcinoids with a sensitivity of about 50%, which is lower than that for SRS (80% to 90%). However, it can pick up carcinoids in patients who are sensitive to therapy with ^{123}I-MIBG.[146] The current imaging workup is summarized by Van Essen and coworkers.[147]

A diagnostic algorithm is outlined in Figure 43-17.

TREATMENT

Treatment of carcinoid tumors with the carcinoid syndrome requires a multimodal approach, including symptomatic control as well as tumor reduction. Most patients with the carcinoid syndrome have metastatic disease. The therapeutic goals are to ameliorate and improve clinical symptoms, abrogate the tumor growth, improve quality of life, and if possible, prolong overall survival.

Symptomatic control of the carcinoid syndrome includes lifestyle changes, diet supplementation, and specific medical treatment that reduces the clinical symptoms related to the different components of the carcinoid syndrome. Avoiding stress, both psychological and physical,

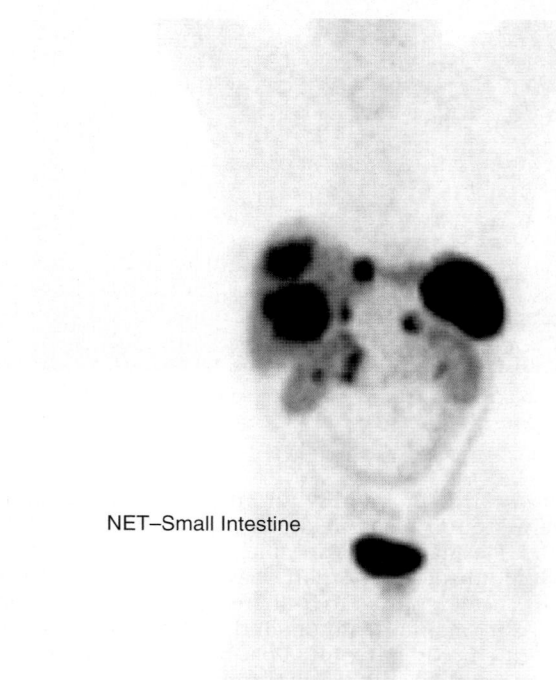

NET—Small Intestine

Figure 43-16 ^{68}Ga-DOTA-octreotate PET/CT scan of a patient with carcinoid tumors. Notice liver and lymph node metastases. CT, computed tomography; NET, neuroendocrine tumor; PET, positron emission tomography.

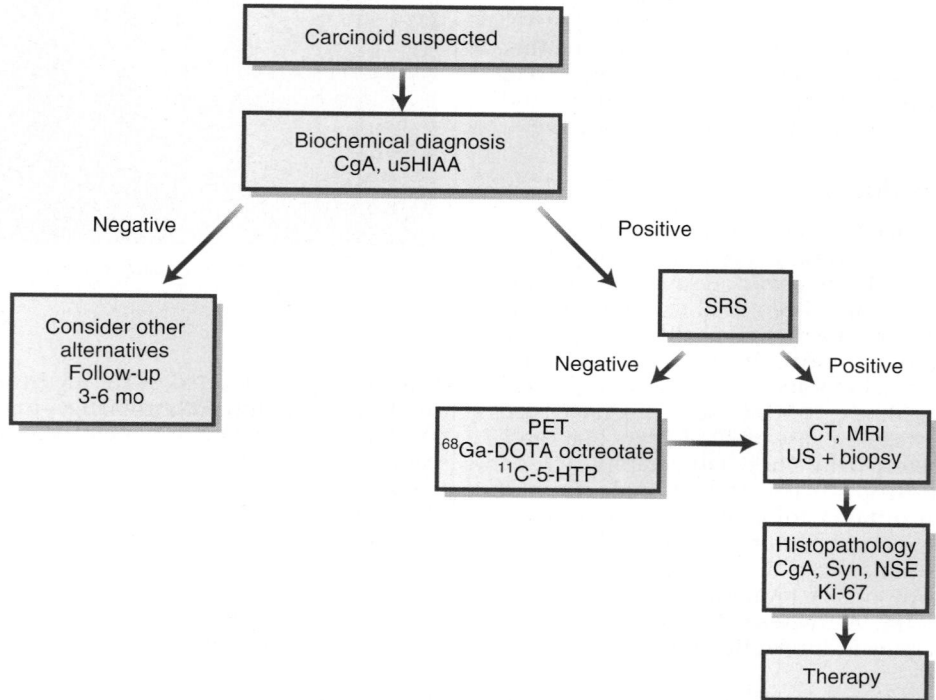

Figure 43-17 Diagnostic algorithm for small intestinal neuroendocrine tumors (carcinoids). CgA, chromogranin A; ^{11}C-5-HTP, ^{11}C-5-hydroxytryptophan; CT, computed tomography; 5-HIAA, 5-hydroxyindoleacetic acid; MRI, magnetic resonance imaging; NSE, neuron-specific enolase; PET, positron emission tomography; SRS, somatostatin-receptor scintigraphy; Syn, synaptophysin; US, ultrasound.

as well as substances such as alcohol, spicy foods, and medications that precipitate a flushing reaction might be sufficient in early cases.[57]

Production of serotonin by the tumor consumes tryptophan. Normally, about 1% of body tryptophan is used for production of serotonin; in carcinoid tumors, however, as much as 60% of the available tryptophan may be consumed for the synthesis of serotonin, and this can result in tryptophan and niacin deficiencies. Therefore, supplemental niacin to prevent the development of pellagra has been recommended over the years. Many patients have undergone resection of the terminal ileum, which can result in vitamin B_{12} and folic acid deficiencies. Supplementation is needed in these patients.

Heart failure due to carcinoid heart disease can require diuretics or angiotensin-converting enzyme (ACE) inhibitors. A few patients need bronchodilators such as salbutamol, which interacts with α-adrenergic receptors and does not induce flushing. The diarrhea seen in the carcinoid syndrome might be controlled by loperamide or diphenoxylate.[148] If patients still have the carcinoid syndrome, they receive somatostatin analogue treatment, which has replaced most of the earlier types of serotonin and serotonin receptor inhibitors. Serotonin inhibitors (e.g., para-chlorophenylalanine and α-methyldopa), which inhibit serotonin synthesis, and serotonin receptor antagonists (e.g., cyproheptadine, methysergide, and ketanserin) are not used routinely clinically.

These earlier treatments had limited efficacy in terms of inhibiting flushing and diarrhea and were accompanied by significant side effects. Telotristat etiprate, an inhibitor of the enzyme tryptophan hydroxylase, reduces the serotonin levels. In one study the compound reduced bowel movements by 44% and urinary 5-HIAA levels by 75%. The patients experienced a significant improvement.[147] A combination of histamine H_1 and H_2 receptor antagonists is effective in the carcinoid syndrome that is caused by foregut carcinoids due to concomitant secretion of histamine and serotonin. Prednisolone in doses of 15 to 30 mg/day gives occasional relief in some cases with severe flushing and diarrhea.[148]

Somatostatin Analogues

Although natural somatostatin-14 reduces symptoms in patients with the carcinoid syndrome,[67] its use is limited by its short half-life (~2.5 minutes). During the past 2 decades, synthetic somatostatin analogues (octapeptides) have been developed for clinical use. Octreotide is the most commonly available drug; other analogues are lanreotide and vapreotide.[149-151]

The somatostatin analogues used in clinical practice (octreotide, lanreotide) (Fig. 43-18) bind to receptors SSTR1 and SSTR5 and, with lower affinity, to SSTR3. They exert their cellular action through interaction with specific cell and transmembrane receptors belonging to the superfamily of G protein–coupled membrane receptors. They inhibit adenylate cyclase activity, activate phosphotyrosine phosphatases (PTPs), and modulate mitogen-activated protein kinases (MAPKs).[135,152-154] Receptor subtypes 2 and 5 modulate K^+ and Ca^{2+} fluxes in the cell.[148] Activation of all these pathways results in inhibition of known growth factor production and release and has antiproliferative effects.[154-157]

SSTR3 is known to mediate PTP-dependent apoptosis accompanied by activation of TP53 and BAX.[158] Four of the five somatostatin receptor subtypes (SSTR2 to SSTR5) undergo rapid internalization after ligand binding, which has been explored by tumor-targeted radioactive somatostatin analogue therapy.[152,154,159]

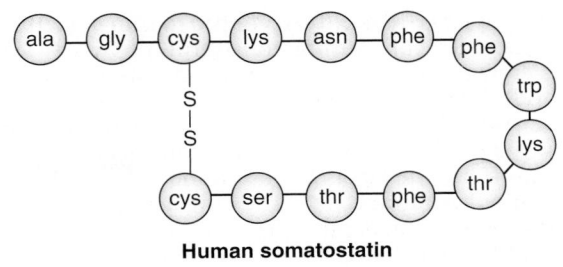
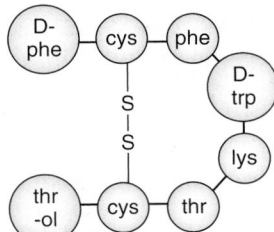
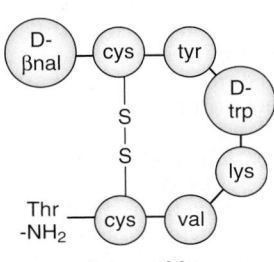

Figure 43-18 Molecular structure of human somatostatin-14, octreotide acetate, and lanreotide.

An antiproliferative effect has been reported, probably through a combination of SSTR2 and SSTR5 activities, which inhibits MAPK and K^+ and Ca^{2+} fluxes leading to cell cycle arrest[154-157]; the precise antitumor mechanism, however, is not known.

It is now known that different subtypes of somatostatin receptors (SSTR1 and SSTR5) form heterodimers with dopamine receptor D_2. This cross-talk modulates the intracellular signal and gives a fine tuning of the mediated effects.[160]

All five subtypes of somatostatin receptors are expressed in carcinoid tumors; they are expressed in various combinations, although some tumors express all five subtypes.[115,152,161,162] The receptors are expressed not only on tumor cells but also in peritumoral veins.[163] Antiangiogenesis might be another antitumor mechanism of somatostatin analogues.[164]

Subcutaneous administration of octreotide and lanreotide every 8 to 12 hours can control the clinical symptoms in about 60% to 70% of patients with the carcinoid syndrome; these agents are considered the drugs of choice.[97,165-169] Octreotide and lanreotide decrease serotonin and urinary 5-HIAA levels as well as plasma tachykinin and CgA levels. The recommended dose for octreotide is 100 to 150 µg two or three times a day, a standard treatment for controlling clinical symptoms.[97] However, some patients require higher doses, up to a total of 3000 µg/day, to control the clinical symptoms and tumor growth, particularly during long-term therapy.

Tachyphylaxis (reduced sensitivity) to somatostatin analogues can develop during long-term therapy.[154] Long-acting, slow-release formulations of octreotide acetate and lanreotide have been developed, and doses of octreotide LAR of 20 to 30 mg given once a month or Somatuline Autogel 90 to 120 mg once a month control clinical symptoms and hormone levels in 50% to 60% of patients with the carcinoid syndrome.[170-172] The long-acting formulations of somatostatin analogues have clearly improved the quality of life of patients by reducing the number of injections and provide more stable control of clinical symptoms.[171] A new somatostatin analogue (SOM230) binding to SSTR1, SSTR2, SSTR3, and SSTR5 has come into some clinical trials in carcinoid tumors. In a Phase II study of carcinoid patients refractory to octreotide, the number of bowel movements and flushing episodes was reduced in one third of the patients.[173]

High-dose therapy with lanreotide (12 mg/day) and octreotide (3 mg/day) has increased the percentage of patients demonstrating a significant reduction in tumor size (12% versus 5% for the standard dose).[174-177] Induction of apoptosis has been reported during high-dose therapy,[178] possibly mediated through activation of SSTR3. Ultra-high-dose octreotide has generated significant antitumor responses in patients resistant to standard dose therapy.[179] A prospective randomized study in midgut carcinoids (PROMID) demonstrated a significantly longer time to progression for octreotide LAR compared to placebo.[180] These data have changed the U.S. National Comprehensive Cancer Network (NCCN) guidelines for treatment of carcinoid tumors. All types of carcinoid tumors, irrespective of functionality, can now be treated with octreotide. The early results indicating an antitumor effect of somatostatin analogues is further supported by a 2014 study (CLARINET).[183] Lanreotide significantly prolongs progression-free survival time in nonfunctioning neuroendocrine tumors.[181]

For patients at risk for carcinoid crisis, somatostatin analogue therapy is the treatment of choice. Carcinoid crisis is a life-threatening complication of the carcinoid syndrome and can occur spontaneously or may be associated with stress and anesthesia, chemotherapy, and infections (see earlier). Patients usually experience severe flushing, diarrhea, abdominal pain, and hypotension. Continuous infusion with somatostatin analogues, 50 to 100 µg/hour, is recommended and usually alters the life-threatening condition. It is also recommended that patients be given subcutaneous somatostatin analogues before surgery or other stressful situations.

Side effects of somatostatin analogue therapy have generally not been serious and occur in 20% to 40% of patients. They include pain at the injection site, gas formation, diarrhea, and abdominal cramping. Significant long-term side effects include gallstone formation, sludge in the gallbladder, steatorrhea, deterioration of glucose tolerance, and hypocalcemia.[97,170,171] The incidence of gallstones in patients treated over the long term has varied from 5% to 70%, and the incidence of symptomatic gallstones requiring surgical treatment is less than 10%.[182]

Interferons

Interferon-α (IFN-α)—alone or in combination with a somatostatin analogue—is effective in the treatment of the carcinoid syndrome. Symptomatic and biochemical control may be obtained in 40% to 50% of patients with the recommended doses of 3 to 5 million units of recombinant interferon alfa-2a or interferon alfa-2b three to five times per week subcutaneously.[183-189] Significant tumor reduction is reported in 10% to 20% of the patients.[183,189]

IFN-α exerts a direct effect on the tumor cells by blocking cell division in the G_1/S phase, by inhibiting protein and hormone synthesis, and by reducing angiogenesis through inhibition of angiogenic factors b-FGF and VEGF. It has also an indirect effect through stimulation of the immune system, particularly T cells and natural killer cells.[190-192] Response to IFN-α can be predicted by analyzing induction of 2′,5′-oligoadenylate synthetase or protein kinase p68 (PKR), enzymes involved in cell cycle regulation and protein synthesis.[193,194] Long-acting formulations of IFN-α are now available (pegylated interferons) that can be applied at doses of 80 to 150 µg/week subcutaneously.

Treatment with IFN-α induces an intratumoral fibrosis that is not picked up by regular CT scanning or ultrasonography; therefore, tumor size may remain unchanged.[195] The side effects of α-interferons are more pronounced than with somatostatin analogues and include chronic fatigue syndrome, anemia, leukopenia, and thrombocytopenia as well as the development of autoimmune reactions in 10% to 15% of the patients.[184,196] Most of the side effects are dose-dependent and can be managed by individualizing the dose.

Patients with the carcinoid syndrome who have not responded to octreotide or IFN-α alone may be given a combination of both agents. Such combinations have generated symptomatic control in 70% of patients and stabilization of tumor growth in 40% to 50% of patients.[197,198] The combination also offers better tolerance of α-interferons when somatostatin analogues are added. Moreover, somatostatin analogue treatment is hampered by development of tachyphylaxis with time, which means less sensitivity to the somatostatin analogue, necessitating escalating doses and, finally, withdrawal of the compound for several months, when IFN-α therapy can continue. Conversely, IFN-α can be withdrawn and the somatostatin analogue can be continued if severe side effects to IFN-α (mainly chronic fatigue syndrome or mental depression) develop.[199]

Chemotherapy

Most agree that patients with classic midgut carcinoids and the carcinoid syndrome, in which tumors show low proliferation capacity, should not receive chemotherapy. The results in various studies have been disappointing: response rates are not more than 5% to 10%, are short lived, and are accompanied by considerable side effects.[200,201] The combination of streptozotocin and 5-fluorouracil, which has demonstrated antitumor effect in endocrine pancreatic tumors, has not shown similar effects in classic midgut carcinoids.[202] In foregut carcinoids, which usually manifest a more malignant behavior, however, cytotoxic treatment may be attempted. Such combinations include streptozotocin plus 5-fluorouracil, doxorubicin, cisplatin plus etoposide, and dacarbazine plus 5-fluorouracil.[203-205] Temozolamide has significant efficacy in foregut carcinoids.[206] All of these cytotoxic treatments can be combined with a somatostatin analogue.

Other Agents

Tyrosine kinase receptors (platelet-derived growth factor receptor [PDGFR] α/β, epidermal growth factor receptor [EGFR], VEGFR) are expressed in carcinoid tumor cells as well as in the stroma cells. Therefore, treatment with tyrosine kinase receptor inhibitors has been attempted with objective response rates of about 10% to 15%.[207] Mammalian target of rapamycin (mTOR) inhibitors are new drugs that block the mTOR signaling pathway, which is activated in many tumors. Everolimus alone or in combination with octreotide has generated 15% to 20% objective responses.[208,209]

Surgery

Because most tumors in patients with the carcinoid syndrome are malignant at the time of clinical presentation, surgical cure is seldom obtained. Resection of local disease or regional nodular metastatic disease can cure some patients; however, even if radical surgery cannot be performed, debulking procedures and bypass should always be considered and can be performed at any time during the course of treatment.[54,93,209]

A more proactive attitude among surgeons has emerged, and currently wider resections and debulking procedures are being performed.[54,210,211] In contrast to other metastatic tumors to the liver, in which liver transplantation has generally given poor results, an interest in liver transplantation is increasing for patients with metastatic carcinoids.[212,213] In a review of 103 patients with malignant neuroendocrine tumors, including both carcinoids and pancreatic endocrine tumors, 5- and 2-year survival rates were 16% and 47%, respectively; however, recurrence-free survival rate was less than 24%.[212] Liver transplantation might be considered in younger patients (<50 years of age) with a life-threatening uncontrolled carcinoid syndrome during medical therapy or tumor-targeted radioactive treatment without known metastatic spread outside the liver (Milan criteria). However, a study from our group challenges the results of liver transplantation, with a 5-year survival time in patients younger than 55 years without surgery of 92 ± 9 months compared with transplanted patients fulfilling the Milan criteria showing a 5-year survival time of 97 ± 6 months.[214]

Another means of tumor reduction is hepatic artery embolization, which not only improves the carcinoid syndrome in about 50% of the patients but also reduces the tumor size in as many. The therapeutic effect may last for 9 to 12 months, and the procedure can be repeated.[215,216] Chemoembolization, simultaneous embolization with surgical gel (Gelfoam), and chemotherapy (doxorubicin, mitomycin C, cisplatin, 5-fluorouracil), or IFN-α has resulted in symptomatic improvement in a significant number of patients with the carcinoid syndrome.[217,218] However, hepatic artery occlusion or embolization can result in serious side effects (nausea, vomiting, liver pain, fever) and major complications (hepatorenal syndrome, sepsis, gallbladder perforation, and intestinal necrosis). Complications are seen in 5% to 7% of patients.[216-218]

Other cytoreductive treatments include cryotherapy and radiofrequency ablation.[219] However, these procedures are limited to patients with smaller tumor burden, tumors less than 5 cm in diameter, and a limited number of metastases.

Irradiation

External irradiation has demonstrated limited efficacy and is used mainly to palliate symptoms related to bone and brain metastases.[220,221] MIBG is taken up by carcinoids and is concentrated. The possibility of radiolabeled MIBG therapy has been evaluated in a limited number of patients. The response rate has been reported to be about 30% with ^{125}I-MIBG or ^{131}I-MIBG.[222,223,224]

Somatostatin analogue–based tumor-targeted radioactive treatment has been applied using ^{111}In-DTPA-octreotide. Symptomatic improvement is reported in about 40% of the patients and tumor stabilization in about 30%.[219] Indium-111 (^{111}In) is a weak irradiator (Auger electrons) and seems to have been replaced by yttrium-90 (^{90}Y) and lutetium-177 (Lu[177]) (α- and β-emitters).

Studies with ^{90}Y-DOTA-octreotide have been reported with promising results.[225,226,227] A relatively new isotope, Lu[177]-DOTA-octreotate (α-emitter), has come into clinical use with further improved results. Significant tumor reduction occurs in 30% to 40% of patients with advanced disease. However, it is more effective for small tumors. It is an attractive mode of treatment because the radioactive ligand, after binding to the receptor, is internalized and transported to the cell nucleus, causing DNA damage.[221] Because tumor cells usually have higher-density somatostatin receptors (SSTR2 and SSTR5) than do surrounding normal tissues, the treatment might be better tolerated.

In liver-dominant disease radioembolization might be a valid alternative using ^{90}Y microspheres in the form of glass or resin beads injected into the hepatic artery.[228] The current treatment of metastatic carcinoid tumor is summarized in an algorithm (Fig. 43-19).

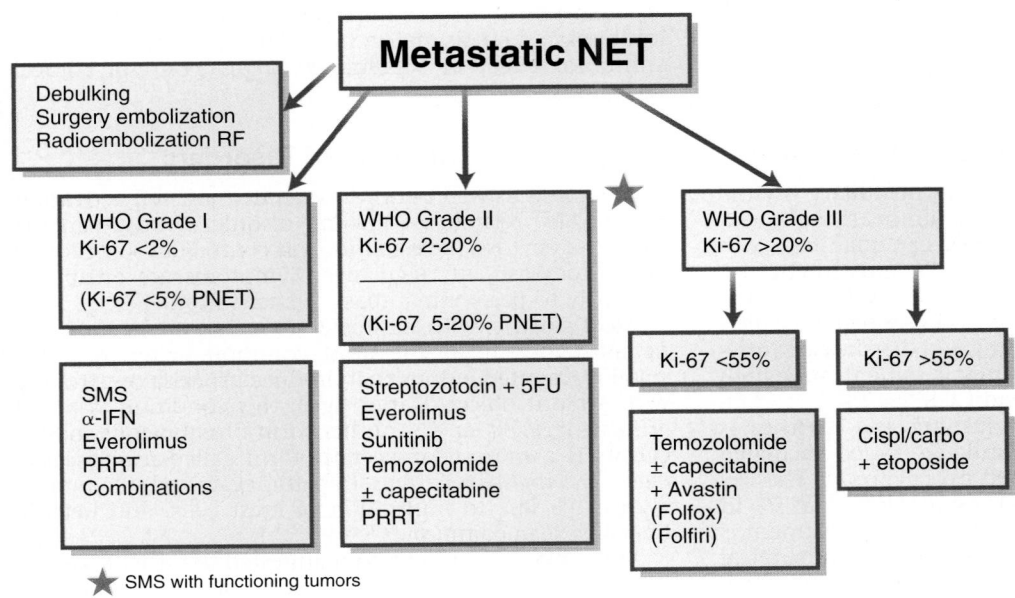

Figure 43-19 Treatment algorithm for metastatic neuroendocrine tumor (NET). Cispl/carbo, cisplatin/carboplatin; IFN, interferon; PNET, primitive neuroectodermal tumor; PRRT, peptide receptor radiotherapy; SMS, somatostatin; RF, radiofrequency; WHO, World Health Organization.

PROGNOSIS

Clinically, the carcinoid syndrome is generally a manifestation of advanced disease. Carcinoids from various sites differ not only in the percentage developing the carcinoid syndrome but also in their aggressiveness. Survival rates for patients with various carcinoids depend on the site, the extent of the tumor, and tumor biology. In patients with only localized disease, the 5-year survival rate for midgut carcinoids is about 65%, not essentially higher than that for patients with regional metastases. In patients with distant metastases, the 5-year survival rate is reduced to 39%.[10,19,20,23,25] The relative 5-, 10-, and 15-year survival rates for midgut carcinoids were 67%, 54%, and 44%, respectively.[229] The 5- and 10-year survival rates for typical bronchial carcinoid are 95% and 80%. Atypical lung carcinoids have significantly shorter survival, only 50% 5-year survival rate.[18]

One of the main determinants of survival in carcinoid patients is the presence of metastases. Female gender and a younger age are associated with a better prognosis. Other factors that correlate with lower survival rates are high CgA level at diagnosis and high proliferation index (Ki-67).[34,111] During the 1990s, there was a reduced incidence of death from carcinoid heart disease, possibly a result of earlier diagnosis, active surgery, and the introduction of somatostatin analogues and α-interferons. In an earlier study performed by our group, 30% of the patients died of carcinoid heart complications.[22] In a more recent 2008 study, this rate was reduced to less than 10%.[25] Clinically significant carcinoid heart disease is now rare. Between 5% and 10% of patients with carcinoids are at an increased risk for developing simultaneous adenocarcinoma of the large intestine. The occurrence of a second malignancy is associated with a worse prognosis.[20,23] In two studies (in 2011 and 2014) comparing almost 900 patients with midgut or hindgut tumors, survival correlated with the WHO grading system as well with the TNM staging. For grade 1 (G1) the 10-year survival rate was 80%, for G2 tumor 50% to 66%, and for G3 tumor 35%; for stage I and II tumors survival rate was 100%, stage III 85%, and stage IV 35%.[216,230]

Significant negative prognostic factors for overall survival were old age at diagnosis, carcinoid heart disease, liver tumor load, high WHO grade, and peritoneal carcinomatosis.[228,231] Locoregional surgery had a positive impact on survival.[228]

OTHER FLUSHING DISORDERS

Medullary Thyroid Carcinoma and VIPoma

Other neuroendocrine tumors, such as medullary thyroid carcinoma (MTC) and VIP-producing tumors (ganglioneuroma, endocrine pancreatic tumors), can manifest with flushing syndromes (Fig. 43-20).[230,232] Patients might also have diarrhea, particularly those with VIP-producing tumors, which are accompanied by a severe secretory diarrhea. In patients with MTC, flushing and diarrhea are infrequent symptoms and are seen mainly in patients with high circulating levels of calcitonin and CGRP.

The mechanism behind the flushing and diarrhea is unknown, but it has been postulated to be mediated through prostaglandins stimulated by calcitonin. The frequency of flushing and diarrhea is usually less than 5% in patients with advanced metastatic MTC.[230,233] Treatment is directed against tumor growth and can consist of surgical resection, embolization of liver metastases, and cytotoxic

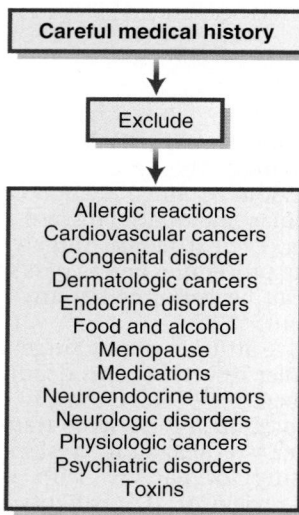

Figure 43-20 Evaluation of flushing disorders. (From Yale SH, Vasudeva S, Mazza JJ, et al. Disorders of flushing. *Compr Ther.* 2005;31(1):59-71.)

treatment (doxorubicin-based combination therapies). Somatostatin analogue therapy can alleviate the diarrhea. Therapy with tyrosine kinase inhibitor vandetanib can reduce these symptoms and present an antitumor effect.[234]

VIPoma or WDHA (*w*atery *d*iarrhea, *h*ypokalemia, and *a*chlorhydria) syndrome (Verner-Morrison syndrome) is associated with severe secretory diarrhea (up to 15 L/day), and some patients also display a continuous whole-body violaceous flushing and hypotension.[232,235] The syndrome also includes achlorhydria, hypokalemia, and metabolic acidosis and is related to overproduction of VIP and a related peptide-peptide histidine methionine. These patients have tumors in the pancreas, lung, or sympathetic ganglia.[232,235]

The diagnosis is confirmed by measuring plasma VIP, which usually exceeds 70 pmol/L.[236]

Treatment is directed against the tumor and hormone excess. Administration of somatostatin analogues by either subcutaneous or IV infusion in the worst cases can control clinical symptoms.[237] Cytotoxic treatment with streptozotocin-based combinations, 5-fluorouracil, or doxorubicin is recommended for malignant cases.[197] Inhibitors, such as mTor (everolimus), demonstrate an antitumor effect in VIPomas with reduction of clinical symptoms.[237]

Mastocytosis and Related Disorders

Mastocytosis as well as other systemic mast cell activation is clinically related to flushing disorders. Most patients with mastocytosis have an indolent course, but some forms of mastocytosis are aggressive. Symptoms are attributed primarily to paroxysmal mast cell activation.[238,239]

Most patients with mastocytosis have evidence of cutaneous involvement, the most common being multiple, small pigmented lesions that produce urticaria on stroking with a blunt object (Darier sign); this condition is called *urticaria pigmentosa*.[240] Another form of cutaneous mastocytosis is a more telangiectatic form called *telangiectasia macularis eruptiva persistans*. Hepatomegaly and splenomegaly can be due to infiltration of mast cells, and hepatic fibrosis is also common.[241,242]

Bone involvement can be manifested by either osteoporosis or osteosclerosis.[243] Systemic mastocytosis can also involve the GI tract with mucosal nodules in the ileum, stomach, and large bowel.[244]

Hematologic abnormalities are nonspecific, with marked mast cell infiltration of the bone, anemia, leukocytosis, sometimes lymphadenopathy, and eosinophilia.[245] In a subgroup of patients, the mastocytosis is secondary to primary hematologic disorders, usually myeloproliferative or myelodysplastic disease.[246,247] Mast cell leukemia has been reported in rare cases.[248] Some cases with FIP1-like 1/ PDGFR-α *(FIP1L1-PDGFRA)* gene arrangement overlap to chronic eosinophilic leukemia. They also manifest elevated serum tryptase levels.[230] A majority (>80%) of patients with systemic mastocytosis have activating c-kit mutation in the mast cell.[228,232,249]

Clinical signs of systemic mastocytosis include flushing, tachycardia, hypotension, and sometimes nausea, vomiting, and diarrhea. This syndrome resembles the carcinoid syndrome. Histamine is a potent vasodilator and is released from mast cells. Other mediators of the syndrome are the release of prostaglandin D_2, tryptase, and heparin.[250] Prostaglandin D_2 is a more potent mediator than is histamine.

The diagnosis is made by measurement of histamine and histamine metabolites in the urine.[250,251] Quantification of histamine metabolites (N-methylhistamine and methylimidazole acetic acid) appears to be more sensitive for overproduction of histamine in patients with mastocytosis.[251] Measurement of endogenous production of prostaglandin D_2 can be assessed by quantifying the major urinary metabolite (9α-hydroxy-11,15-dioxo-2,3,18,19-tetranorprost-5-ene-1,20-dioic acid).[252] However, these measurements can be done only in specialized laboratories. Measurement of the tryptase release is easier to perform, and increased quantities of this granule-associated enzyme tryptase can be detected by immunoassay.[253] Bone marrow analysis of CD25 cells might support the diagnosis of mast cell disease.[254]

Treatment depends on the severity of the disease. As in the treatment of allergic anaphylaxis, epinephrine is effective in reversing the hypotension associated with mast cell mediator release[255]; thus, these patients should have constant access to epinephrine in the form of subcutaneous injection or inhalation. Chronic therapy to prevent acute attacks includes antihistamine therapy combined with inhibition of prostaglandin biosynthesis. Blockade of both histamine H_1 and H_2 receptors is required to prevent the vasodilator effect of histamine.[99,254]

Nonsteroidal anti-inflammatory drugs (NSAIDs) inhibit the cyclooxygenase enzyme that catalyzes the formation of prostaglandins. Aspirin has been used, but some patients cannot tolerate it because of side effects in the gut and allergic reactions.[256] In patients resistant to both antihistamines and NSAIDs, IFN-α has been attempted with a reduction in mast cell numbers as well as excretion of mast cell mediators. Treatment with IFN-α is still considered experimental.[254,257] A subset of patients who carry the *FIP1L1-PDGFRA* oncogene will achieve complete clinical, histologic, and molecular remission with imatinib mesylate therapy, in contrast to those with c-kit D816V-mutation.[254]

REFERENCES

1. Lubarsch O. Ueber den primaren Krebs des Ileum, nebst Bemerkungen über das gleichzeitige Vorkommen von Krebs und Tuberkuolose. *Virchow Archiv Pathol Anatom Physiol Klin Med.* 1867;111:280-317.
2. Oberndorfer S. Karzenoide Tumoren des Dünndarms. *Frankf Zschr Pathol.* 1907;1:426-430.
3. Pearson CM, Fitzgerald PJ. Carcinoid tumors—a re-emphasis of their malignant nature: review of 140 cases. *Cancer.* 1949;2(6):1005-1026.
4. Thorson A, Biorck G, Bjorkman G, Waldenstrom J. Malignant carcinoid of the small intestine with metastases to the liver, valvular disease of the right side of the heart (pulmonary stenosis and tricuspid regurgitation without septal defects), peripheral vasomotor symptoms, bronchoconstriction, and an unusual type of cyanosis; a clinical and pathologic syndrome. *Am Heart J.* 1954;47(5):795-817.
5. Lembeck F. 5-Hydroxytryptamine in carcinoid tumor. *Nature.* 1953;172:910-911.
6. Gosset A, Masson P. Tumeurs endocrines de l'appendice. *Presse Med.* 1914;25:237-239.
7. Masson P. Carcinoid (argentaffin-cell tumors) and nerve hyperplasia of appendicular mucosa. *Am J Pathol.* 1928;4:181-212.
8. Pearse AG. The cytochemistry and ultrastructure of polypeptide hormone-producing cells of the APUD series and the embryologic, physiologic and pathologic implications of the concept. *J Histochem Cytochem.* 1969;17(5):303-313.
9. Andrew A. The APUD concept: where has it led us? *Br Med Bull.* 1982;38(3):221-225.
10. Wilander E, Lundqvist M, Oberg K. Gastrointestinal carcinoid tumours. Histogenetic, histochemical, immunohistochemical, clinical and therapeutic aspects. *Prog Histochem Cytochem.* 1989;19(2):1-88.
11. Debelenko LV, Brambilla E, Agarwal SK, et al. Identification of MEN1 gene mutations in sporadic carcinoid tumors of the lung. *Hum Mol Genet.* 1997;6(13):2285-2290.
12. Zhao J, de Krijger RR, Meier D, et al. Genomic alterations in well-differentiated gastrointestinal and bronchial neuroendocrine tumors (carcinoids): marked differences indicating diversity in molecular pathogenesis. *Am J Pathol.* 2000;157(5):1431-1438.
13. Lollgen RM, Hessman O, Szabo E, et al. Chromosome 18 deletions are common events in classical midgut carcinoid tumors. *Int J Cancer.* 2001;92(6):812-815.
14. Gartner W, Mineva I, Daneva T, et al. A newly identified RET proto-oncogene polymorphism is found in a high number of endocrine tumor patients. *Hum Genet.* 2005;117(2–3):143-153.
15. Nakakura EK, Sriuranpong VR, Kunnimalaiyaan M, et al. Regulation of neuroendocrine differentiation in gastrointestinal carcinoid tumor cells by notch signaling. *J Clin Endocrinol Metab.* 2005;90(7):4350-4356.
16. Grande E, Capdevila J, Berruiso J, et al. Gastroenteropancreatic neuroendocrine tumor cancer stem cells: do they exist? *Cancer Metastasis Rev.* 2012;31(1–2):47-53.
17. Williams ED, Sandler M. The classification of carcinoid tumours. *Lancet.* 1963;1:238-239.
18. Bosnen F, Carneiro F, Hruban RM, et al. *WHO-Classification of Tumors of the Digestive System.* Lyon, France: IARC Press; 2010.
19. Rindi G, Kloppel G, Couvelard A, et al. TNM staging of midgut and hindgut (neuro) endocrine tumors: a consensus proposal including a grading system. *Virchows Arch.* 2007;451:757-762.
20. Travis WD, Rush W, Flieder DB, et al. Survival analysis of 200 pulmonary neuroendocrine tumors with clarification of criteria for atypical carcinoid and its separation from typical carcinoid. *Am J Surg Pathol.* 1998;22(8):934-944.
21. Lawrence B, Gustafsson BI, Chan A, et al. The epidemiology of gastroenteropancreatic neuroendocrine tumors. *Endocrinol Metab Clin North Am.* 2011;40(1):1-18.
22. Berge T, Linell F. Carcinoid tumours. Frequency in a defined population during a 12-year period. *Acta Pathol Microbiol Scand [A].* 1976;84(4):322-330.
23. Norheim I, Oberg K, Theodorsson-Norheim E, et al. Malignant carcinoid tumors. An analysis of 103 patients with regard to tumor localization, hormone production, and survival. *Ann Surg.* 1987;206(2):115-125.
24. Quaedvlieg PF, Visser O, Lamers CB, et al. Epidemiology and survival in patients with carcinoid disease in The Netherlands. An epidemiological study with 2391 patients. *Ann Oncol.* 2001;12(9):1295-1300.
25. Yao JC, Hassan M, Phan A, et al. One hundred years after "carcinoid": epidemiology of and prognostic factors for neuroendocrine tumors in 35,825 cases in the United States. *J Clin Oncol.* 2008;26(18):3063-3072.
26. Janson ET, Holmberg L, Stridsberg M, et al. Carcinoid tumors: analysis of prognostic factors and survival in 301 patients from a referral center. *Ann Oncol.* 1997;8(7):685-690.
27. Sandler M, Scheuer PJ, Wat PJ. 5-Hydroxytryptophan-secreting bronchial carcinoid tumour. *Lancet.* 1961;2(7211):1067-1069.
28. Oates JA, Sjoerdsma A. A unique syndrome associated with secretion of 5-hydroxytryptophan by metastatic gastric carcinoids. *Am J Med.* 1962;32:333-342.
29. Oates JA, Melmon K, Sjoerdsma A, et al. Release of a kinin peptide in the carcinoid syndrome. *Lancet.* 1964;1(7332):514-517.
30. Lucas KJ, Feldman JM. Flushing in the carcinoid syndrome and plasma kallikrein. *Cancer.* 1986;58(10):2290-2293.
31. Gustafsen J, Boesby S, Nielsen F, Giese J. Bradykinin in carcinoid syndrome. *Gut.* 1987;28(11):1417-1419.
32. Metz SA, McRae JR, Robertson RP. Prostaglandins as mediators of paraneoplastic syndromes: review and up-date. *Metabolism.* 1981;30(3):299-316.

33. Roberts LJ 2nd, Bloomgarden ZT, Marney SR Jr, et al. Histamine release from a gastric carcinoid: provocation by pentagastrin and inhibition by somatostatin. *Gastroenterology.* 1983;84(2):272-275.

34. Gilligan CJ, Lawton GP, Tang LH, et al. Gastric carcinoid tumors: the biology and therapy of an enigmatic and controversial lesion. *Am J Gastroenterol.* 1995;90(3):338-352.

35. Todd TR, Cooper JD, Weisberg D, et al. Bronchial carcinoid tumors: twenty years' experience. *J Thorac Cardiovasc Surg.* 1980;79(4):532-536.

36. Kema IP, de Vries EG, Slooff MJ, et al. Serotonin, catecholamines, histamine, and their metabolites in urine, platelets, and tumor tissue of patients with carcinoid tumors. *Clin Chem.* 1994;40(1):86-95.

37. Håkansson R, Bergmark S, Brodin E, et al. Substance-P-like immuno-reactivity in intestinal carcinoid tumors. In: von Euler U, Pernow B, eds. *Substance-P.* New York: Raven; 1977:55-58.

38. Norheim I, Theodorsson-Norheim E, Brodin E, Oberg K. Tachykinins in carcinoid tumors: their use as a tumor marker and possible role in the carcinoid flush. *J Clin Endocrinol Metab.* 1986;63(3):605-612.

39. Theodorsson-Norheim E, Norheim I, Oberg K, et al. Neuropeptide K: a major tachykinin in plasma and tumor tissues from carcinoid patients. *Biochem Biophys Res Commun.* 1985;131(1):77-83.

40. Conlon JM, Deacon CF, Richter G, et al. Measurement and partial characterization of the multiple forms of neurokinin A-like immuno-reactivity in carcinoid tumours. *Regul Pept.* 1986;13(2):183-196.

41. Becker M, Aron DC. Ectopic ACTH syndrome and CRH-mediated Cushing's syndrome. *Endocrinol Metab Clin North Am.* 1994;23(3):585-606.

42. Melmed S. Medical progress: acromegaly. *N Engl J Med.* 2006;355(24):2558-2573.

43. Mao C, Shah A, Hanson DJ, Howard JM. Von Recklinghausen's disease associated with duodenal somatostatinoma: contrast of duodenal versus pancreatic somatostatinomas. *J Surg Oncol.* 1995;59(1):67-73.

44. Banks P, Helle K. The release of protein from the stimulated adrenal medulla. *Biochem J.* 1965;97(3):40C-41C.

45. Fischer-Colbrie R, Hagn C, Schober M. Chromogranins A, B, and C: widespread constituents of secretory vesicles. *Ann N Y Acad Sci.* 1987;493:120-134.

46. Iacangelo AL, Eiden LE, Chromogranin A. Current status as a precursor for bioactive peptides and a granulogenic/sorting factor in the regulated secretory pathway. *Regul Pept.* 1995;58(3):65-88.

47. Tatemoto K, Efendic S, Mutt V, et al. Pancreastatin, a novel pancreatic peptide that inhibits insulin secretion. *Nature.* 1986;324(6096):476-478.

48. Angeletti RH, Mints L, Aber C, Russell J. Determination of residues in chromogranin A-(16-40) required for inhibition of parathyroid hormone secretion. *Endocrinology.* 1996;137(7):2918-2922.

49. Aardal S, Helle KB, Elsayed S, et al. Vasostatins, comprising the N-terminal domain of chromogranin A, suppress secretion in isolated human blood vessel segments. *J Neuroendocrinol.* 1993;5(4):405-412.

50. Wiedenmann B, Huttner WB. Synaptophysin and chromogranins/secretogranins: widespread constituents of distinct types of neuroendocrine vesicles and new tools in tumor diagnosis. *Virchows Arch.* 1989;58(2):95-121.

51. Harpole DH Jr, Feldman JM, Buchanan S, et al. Bronchial carcinoid tumors: a retrospective analysis of 126 patients. *Ann Thorac Surg.* 1992;54(1):50-54, discussion 54-55.

52. Barclay TH, Schapira DV. Malignant tumors of the small intestine. *Cancer.* 1983;51(5):878-881.

53. Moertel CG, Sauer WG, Dockerty MB, Baggenstoss AH. Life history of the carcinoid tumor of the small intestine. *Cancer.* 1961;14:901-912.

54. Makridis C, Oberg K, Juhlin C, et al. Surgical treatment of mid-gut carcinoid tumors. *World J Surg.* 1990;14(3):377-383, discussion 384-385.

55. Bean WB, Olch D, Weinberg HB. The syndrome of carcinoid and acquired valve lesions of the right side of the heart. *Circulation.* 1955;12(1):1-6.

56. Grahame-Smith DG. The carcinoid syndrome. *Am J Cardiol.* 1968;21(3):376-387.

57. Feldman JM. Carcinoid tumors and syndrome. *Semin Oncol.* 1987;14(3):237-246.

58. Smith RA. Bronchial carcinoid tumours. *Thorax.* 1969;24(1):43-50.

59. Caldarola VT, Jackman RJ, Moertel CG, Dockerty MB. Carcinoid tumors of the rectum. *Am J Surg.* 1964;107:844-849.

60. Levin R, Elsas L, Duvall C, et al. Malignant carcinoid tumors with and without flushing. *JAMA.* 1963;186:905-907.

61. Matuchansky C, Launay JM. Serotonin, catecholamines, and spontaneous midgut carcinoid flush: plasma studies from flushing and non-flushing sites. *Gastroenterology.* 1995;108(3):743-751.

62. Robertson JI, Peart WS, Andrews TM. The mechanism of facial flushes in the carcinoid syndrome. *Q J Med.* 1962;31:103-123.

63. Makridis C, Theodorsson E, Akerstrom G, et al. Increased intestinal non-substance P tachykinin concentrations in malignant midgut carcinoid disease. *J Gastroenterol Hepatol.* 1999;14(5):500-507.

64. Creutzfeldt W, Stockmann F. Carcinoids and carcinoid syndrome. *Am J Med.* 1987;82(5B):4-16.

65. Emson PC, Gilbert RF, Martensson H, Nobin A. Elevated concentrations of substance P and 5-HT in plasma in patients with carcinoid tumors. *Cancer.* 1984;54(4):715-718.

66. Schaffalitzky De Muckadell OB, Aggestrup S, Stentoft P. Flushing and plasma substance P concentration during infusion of synthetic substance P in normal man. *Scand J Gastroenterol.* 1986;21(4):498-502.

67. Frolich JC, Bloomgarden ZT, Oates JA, et al. The carcinoid flush. Provocation by pentagastrin and inhibition by somatostatin. *N Engl J Med.* 1978;299(19):1055-1057.

68. Nawa H, Doteuchi M, Igano K, et al. Substance K: a novel mammalian tachykinin that differs from substance P in its pharmacological profile. *Life Sci.* 1984;34(12):1153-1160.

69. Furschgott R, Zawadski JU. The obligatory role of endothelial cells in the relaxation of arterial smooth muscle by acetylcholine. *Nature.* 1980;288:373-376.

70. Jensen RT. Overview of chronic diarrhea caused by functional neuro-endocrine neoplasms. *Semin Gastrointest Dis.* 1999;10(4):156-172.

71. Donowitz M, Binder HJ. Jejunal fluid and electrolyte secretion in carcinoid syndrome. *Am J Dig Dis.* 1975;20(12):1115-1122.

72. Debongnie JC, Phillips SF. Capacity of the human colon to absorb fluid. *Gastroenterology.* 1978;74(4):698-703.

73. von der Ohe MR, Camilleri M, Kvols LK, Thomforde GM. Motor dysfunction of the small bowel and colon in patients with the carcinoid syndrome and diarrhea. *N Engl J Med.* 1993;329(15):1073-1078.

74. Wymenga AN, de Vries EG, Leijsma MK, et al. Effects of ondansetron on gastrointestinal symptoms in carcinoid syndrome. *Eur J Cancer.* 1998;34(8):1293-1294.

75. Wilde MI, Markham A. Ondansetron: a review of its pharmacology and preliminary clinical findings in novel applications. *Drugs.* 1996;52(5):773-794.

76. Gustafsen J, Lendorf A, Raskov H, Boesby S. Ketanserin versus placebo in carcinoid syndrome. A clinical controlled trial. *Scand J Gastroenterol.* 1986;21(7):816-818.

77. Lundin L, Norheim I, Landelius J, et al. Carcinoid heart disease: relationship of circulating vasoactive substances to ultrasound-detectable cardiac abnormalities. *Circulation.* 1988;77(2):264-269.

78. Roberts WC, Sjoerdsma A. The cardiac disease associated with the carcinoid syndrome (carcinoid heart disease). *Am J Med.* 1964;36:5-34.

79. Ferrans VJ, Roberts WC. The carcinoid endocardial plaque; an ultrastructural study. *Hum Pathol.* 1976;7(4):387-409.

80. Lundin L, Landelius J, Andren B, Oberg K. Transoesophageal echocardiography improves the diagnostic value of cardiac ultrasound in patients with carcinoid heart disease. *Br Heart J.* 1990;64(3):190-194.

81. Waltenberger J, Lundin L, Oberg K, et al. Involvement of transforming growth factor-beta in the formation of fibrotic lesions in carcinoid heart disease. *Am J Pathol.* 1993;142(1):71-78.

82. Robiolio PA, Rigolin VH, Wilson JS, et al. Carcinoid heart disease. Correlation of high serotonin levels with valvular abnormalities detected by cardiac catheterization and echocardiography. *Circulation.* 1995;92(4):790-795.

83. Connolly HM, Crary JL, McGoon MD, et al. Valvular heart disease associated with fenfluramine-phentermine. *N Engl J Med.* 1997;337(9):581-588.

84. Khan MA, Herzog CA, St Peter JV, et al. The prevalence of cardiac valvular insufficiency assessed by transthoracic echocardiography in obese patients treated with appetite-suppressant drugs. *N Engl J Med.* 1998;339(11):713-718.

85. Pellikka PA, Tajik AJ, Khandheria BK, et al. Carcinoid heart disease. Clinical and echocardiographic spectrum in 74 patients. *Circulation.* 1993;87(4):1188-1196.

86. Musunuru S, Carpenter JE, Sippel RS, et al. A mouse model of carcinoid syndrome and heart disease. *J Surg Res.* 2005;126(1):102-105.

87. Gustafsson BI, Tommeras K, Nordrum I, et al. Long-term serotonin administration induces heart valve disease in rats. *Circulation.* 2005;111(12):1517-1522.

88. Jian B, Xu J, Connolly J, et al. Serotonin mechanisms in heart valve disease I: serotonin-induced up-regulation of transforming growth factor-beta1 via G-protein signal transduction in aortic valve interstitial cells. *Am J Pathol.* 2002;161(6):2111-2121.

89. Kidd M, Modlin IM, Shapiro MD, et al. CTGF, intestinal stellate cells and carcinoid fibrogenesis. *World J Gastroenterol.* 2007;13(39):5208-5216.

90. Hua X, Lundberg JM, Theodorsson-Norheim E, Brodin E. Comparison of cardiovascular and bronchoconstrictor effects of substance P, substance K and other tachykinins. *Naunyn Schmiedebergs Arch Pharmacol.* 1984;328(2):196-201.

91. Gardner B, Dollinger M, Silen W, et al. Studies of the carcinoid syndrome: its relationship to serotonin, bradykinin, and histamine. *Surgery.* 1967;61(6):846-852.

92. Vinik AI, McLeod MK, Fig LM, et al. Clinical features, diagnosis, and localization of carcinoid tumors and their management. *Gastroenterol Clin North Am.* 1989;18(4):865-896.

93. Andaker L, Lamke LO, Smeds S. Follow-up of 102 patients operated on for gastrointestinal carcinoid. *Acta Chir Scand.* 1985;151(5):469-473.

94. Kvols LK, Martin JK, Marsh HM, Moertel CG. Rapid reversal of carcinoid crisis with a somatostatin analogue. *N Engl J Med.* 1985;313(19):1229-1230.
95. Vaughan DJ, Brunner MD. Anesthesia for patients with carcinoid syndrome. *Int Anesthesiol Clin.* 1997;35(4):129-142.
96. Veall GR, Peacock JE, Bax ND, Reilly CS. Review of the anaesthetic management of 21 patients undergoing laparotomy for carcinoid syndrome. *Br J Anaesth.* 1994;72(3):335-341.
97. Harris AG, Redfern JS. Octreotide treatment of carcinoid syndrome: analysis of published dose-titration data. *Aliment Pharmacol Ther.* 1995;9(4):387-394.
98. Kvols LK. Therapy of the malignant carcinoid syndrome. *Endocrinol Metab Clin North Am.* 1989;18(2):557-568.
99. Roberts LJ 2nd, Marney SR Jr, Oates JA. Blockade of the flush associated with metastatic gastric carcinoid by combined histamine H1 and H2 receptor antagonists. Evidence for an important role of H2 receptors in human vasculature. *N Engl J Med.* 1979;300(5):236-238.
100. Limper AH, Carpenter PC, Scheithauer B, Staats BA. The Cushing syndrome induced by bronchial carcinoid tumors. *Ann Intern Med.* 1992;117(3):209-214.
101. Carroll DG, Delahunt JW, Teague CA, et al. Resolution of acromegaly after removal of a bronchial carcinoid shown to secrete growth hormone releasing factor. *Aust N Z J Med.* 1987;17(1):63-67.
102. Rindi G, Bordi C, Rappel S, et al. Gastric carcinoids and neuroendocrine carcinomas: pathogenesis, pathology, and behavior. *World J Surg.* 1996;20(2):168-172.
103. Granberg D, Wilander E, Stridsberg M, et al. Clinical symptoms, hormone profiles, treatment, and prognosis in patients with gastric carcinoids. *Gut.* 1998;43(2):223-228.
104. Thomas RM, Baybick JH, Elsayed AM, Sobin LH. Gastric carcinoids. An immunohistochemical and clinicopathologic study of 104 patients. *Cancer.* 1994;73(8):2053-2058.
105. Sjoblom SM, Sipponen P, Karonen SL, Jarvinen HJ. Mucosal argyrophil endocrine cells in pernicious anaemia and upper gastrointestinal carcinoid tumours. *J Clin Pathol.* 1989;42(4):371-377.
106. Solcia E, Fiocca R, Villani L, et al. Morphology and pathogenesis of endocrine hyperplasias, precarcinoid lesions, and carcinoids arising in chronic atrophic gastritis. *Scand J Gastroenterol.* 1991;180:146-159.
107. Havu N. Enterochromaffin-like cell carcinoids of gastric mucosa in rats after life-long inhibition of gastric secretion. *Digestion.* 1986;35(Suppl 1):42-55.
108. Rindi G, Luinetti O, Cornaggia M, et al. Three subtypes of gastric argyrophil carcinoid and the gastric neuroendocrine carcinoma: a clinicopathologic study. *Gastroenterology.* 1993;104(4):994-1006.
109. Thompson GB, van Heerden JA, Martin JK Jr, et al. Carcinoid tumors of the gastrointestinal tract: presentation, management, and prognosis. *Surgery.* 1985;98(6):1054-1063.
110. Chaudhry A, Oberg K, Gobl A, et al. Expression of transforming growth factors beta 1, beta 2, beta 3 in neuroendocrine tumors of the digestive system. *Anticancer Res.* 1994;14(5B):2085-2091.
111. Chaudhry A, Oberg K, Wilander E. A study of biological behavior based on the expression of a proliferating antigen in neuroendocrine tumors of the digestive system. *Tumour Biol.* 1992;13(1–2):27-35.
112. von Herbay A, Sieg B, Schurmann G, et al. Proliferative activity of neuroendocrine tumours of the gastroenteropancreatic endocrine system: DNA flow cytometric and immunohistological investigations. *Gut.* 1991;32(8):949-953.
113. Granberg D, Wilander E, Oberg K, Skogseid B. Prognostic markers in patients with typical bronchial carcinoid tumors. *J Clin Endocrinol Metab.* 2000;85(9):3425-3430.
114. Patel YC, Srikant CB. Somatostatin receptors. *Trends Endocrinol Metab.* 1997;8(10):398-405.
115. Schaer JC, Waser B, Mengod G, Reubi JC. Somatostatin receptor subtypes sst1, sst2, sst3 and sst5 expression in human pituitary, gastroentero-pancreatic and mammary tumors: comparison of mRNA analysis with receptor autoradiography. *Int J Cancer.* 1997;70(5):530-537.
116. Saqi A, Alexis D, Remotti F, et al. Usefulness of CDx2 and TTF1 in differentiating gastrointestinal from pulmonary carcinoids. *Am J Clin Pathol.* 2005;123:394-404.
117. Feldman JM. Urinary serotonin in the diagnosis of carcinoid tumors. *Clin Chem.* 1986;32(5):840-844.
118. Mailman RB, Kilts CD. Analytical considerations for quantitative determination of serotonin and its metabolically related products in biological matrices. *Clin Chem.* 1985;31(11):1849-1854.
119. Nuttall KL, Pingree SS. The incidence of elevations in urine 5-hydroxyindoleacetic acid. *Ann Clin Lab Sci.* 1998;28(3):167-174.
120. De Vries EG, Kema IP, Slooff MJ, et al. Recent developments in diagnosis and treatment of metastatic carcinoid tumours. *Scand J Gastroenterol.* 1993;200:87-93.
121. Tohmola N, Itkonen O, Sane T, et al. Analytical and preanalytical validation of a new mass spectrometric serum 5-hydroxyindoleacetic acid assay as neuroendocrine tumor marker. *Clin Chim Acta.* 2014;428:38-43.
122. Stridsberg M, Oberg K, Li Q, et al. Measurements of chromogranin A, chromogranin B (secretogranin I), chromogranin C (secretogranin II) and pancreastatin in plasma and urine from patients with carcinoid tumours and endocrine pancreatic tumours. *J Endocrinol.* 1995;144(1):49-59.
123. Nobels FR, Kwekkeboom DJ, Coopmans W, et al. Chromogranin A as serum marker for neuroendocrine neoplasia: comparison with neuron-specific enolase and the alpha-subunit of glycoprotein hormones. *J Clin Endocrinol Metab.* 1997;82(8):2622-2628.
124. Baudin E, Gigliotti A, Ducreux M, et al. Neuron-specific enolase and chromogranin A as markers of neuroendocrine tumours. *Br J Cancer.* 1998;78(8):1102-1107.
125. Oberg K, Stridsberg M. Chromogranins as diagnostic and prognostic markers in neuroendocrine tumours. *Adv Exp Med Biol.* 2000;482:329-337.
126. Grossmann M, Trautmann ME, Poertl S, et al. Alpha-subunit and human chorionic gonadotropin-beta immunoreactivity in patients with malignant endocrine gastroenteropancreatic tumours. *Eur J Clin Invest.* 1994;24(2):131-136.
127. Feldman JM, O'Dorisio TM. Role of neuropeptides and serotonin in the diagnosis of carcinoid tumors. *Am J Med.* 1986;81(6B):41-48.
128. Oberg K, Grimelius L, Lundqvist G, Lorelius LE. Update on pancreatic polypeptide as a specific marker for endocrine tumours of the pancreas and gut. *Acta Med Scand.* 1981;210(3):145-152.
129. Mani S, Modlin IM, Ballantyne G, et al. Carcinoids of the rectum. *J Am Coll Surg.* 1994;179(2):231-248.
130. Krenning EP, Kwekkeboom DJ, Oei HY, et al. Somatostatin-receptor scintigraphy in gastroenteropancreatic tumors. An overview of European results. *Ann N Y Acad Sci.* 1994;733:416-424.
131. Westlin JE, Janson ET, Arnberg H, et al. Somatostatin receptor scintigraphy of carcinoid tumours using the [111In-DTPA-D-Phe1]-octreotide. *Acta Oncol (Stockholm).* 1993;32(7–8):783-786.
132. Taal BG, Hoefnagel CA, Valdes Olmos RA, Boot H. Combined diagnostic imaging with 131I-metaiodobenzylguanidine and 111In-pentetreotide in carcinoid tumours. *Eur J Cancer.* 1996;32A(11):1924-1932.
133. Nessi R, Basso Ricci P, Basso Ricci S, et al. Bronchial carcinoid tumors: radiologic observations in 49 cases. *J Thorac Imaging.* 1991;6(2):47-53.
134. Orlefors H, Sundin A, Garske U, et al. Whole-body (11)C-5-hydroxy-tryptophan positron emission tomography as a universal imaging technique for neuroendocrine tumors: comparison with somatostatin receptor scintigraphy and computed tomography. *J Clin Endocrinol Metab.* 2005;90(6):3392-3400.
135. Eriksson B, Bergstrom M, Orlefors H, et al. Use of PET in neuroendocrine tumors. In vivo applications and in vitro studies. *Q J Nucl Med.* 2000;44(1):68-76.
136. Reubi JC, Kvols LK, Waser B, et al. Detection of somatostatin receptors in surgical and percutaneous needle biopsy samples of carcinoids and islet cell carcinomas. *Cancer Res.* 1990;50(18):5969-5977.
137. Reisine T, Bell GI. Molecular biology of somatostatin receptors. *Endocr Rev.* 1995;16(4):427-442.
138. Patel YC, Srikant CB. Subtype selectivity of peptide analogs for all five cloned human somatostatin receptors (hsstr 1-5). *Endocrinology.* 1994;135(6):2814-2817.
139. Kubota A, Yamada Y, Kagimoto S, et al. Identification of somatostatin receptor subtypes and an implication for the efficacy of somatostatin analogue SMS 201-995 in treatment of human endocrine tumors. *J Clin Invest.* 1994;93(3):1321-1325.
140. Janson ET, Westlin JE, Eriksson B, et al. [111In-DTPA-D-Phe1]octreotide scintigraphy in patients with carcinoid tumours: the predictive value for somatostatin analogue treatment. *Eur J Endocrinol.* 1994;131(6):577-581.
141. Kisker O, Weinel RJ, Geks J, et al. Value of somatostatin receptor scintigraphy for preoperative localization of carcinoids. *World J Surg.* 1996;20(2):162-167.
142. Lebtahi R, Cadiot G, Delahaye N, et al. Detection of bone metastases in patients with endocrine gastroenteropancreatic tumors: bone scintigraphy compared with somatostatin receptor scintigraphy. *J Nucl Med.* 1999;40(10):1602-1608.
143. Nilsson O, Kolby L, Wangberg B, et al. Comparative studies on the expression of somatostatin receptor subtypes, outcome of octreotide scintigraphy and response to octreotide treatment in patients with carcinoid tumors. *Br J Cancer.* 1998;77(4):632-637.
144. Gibril F, Doppman JL, Reynolds JC, et al. Bone metastases in patients with gastrinomas: a prospective study of bone scanning, somatostatin receptor scanning, and magnetic resonance image in their detection, frequency, location, and effect of their detection on management. *J Clin Oncol.* 1998;16(3):1040-1053.
145. Janson ET, Gobl A, Kalkner KM, Oberg K. A comparison between the efficacy of somatostatin receptor scintigraphy and that of in situ hybridization for somatostatin receptor subtype 2 messenger RNA to predict therapeutic outcome in carcinoid patients. *Cancer Res.* 1996;56(11):2561-2565.
146. Gabriel M, Decristoforo C, Kendler D, et al. 68Ga-DOTA-Tyr3-octreotide PET in neuroendocrine tumors: comparison with somatostatin receptor scintigraphy and CT. *J Nucl Med.* 2007;48(4):508-518.

147. van Essen M, Sundin A, Krenning EP, Kwekkeboom DJ. Neuroendocrine tumours: the role of imaging for diagnosis and therapy. *Nat Rev Endocrinol.* 2014;10:102-114.

148. Kaltsas G, Korbonits M, Heintz E, et al. Comparison of somatostatin analog and meta-iodobenzylguanidine radionuclides in the diagnosis and localization of advanced neuroendocrine tumors. *J Clin Endocrinol Metab.* 2001;86(2):895-902.

149. Gregor M. Therapeutic principles in the management of metastasising carcinoid tumors: drugs for symptomatic treatment. *Digestion.* 1994; 55(Suppl 3):60-63.

150. Pavel M, Hörsch D, Caplin M, et al. Telotristat etiprate for carcinoid syndrome: a single-arm phase 2 trial. *J Clin Endocrinol Metab.* 2015;[Epub ahead of print].

151. Bauer W, Briner U, Doepfner W, et al. SMS 201-995: a very potent and selective octapeptide analogue of somatostatin with prolonged action. *Life Sci.* 1982;31(11):1133-1140.

152. Murphy WA, Heiman ML, Lance VA, et al. Octapeptide analogs of somatostatin exhibiting greatly enhanced in vivo and in vitro inhibition of growth hormone secretion in the rat. *Biochem Biophys Res Commun.* 1985;132(3):922-928.

153. Cai RZ, Szoke B, Lu R, et al. Synthesis and biological activity of highly potent octapeptide analogs of somatostatin. *Proc Natl Acad Sci U S A.* 1986;83(6):1896-1900.

154. Patel YC. Somatostatin and its receptor family. *Front Neuroendocrinol.* 1999;20(3):157-198.

155. Coy DH, Taylor JE. Receptor-specific somatostatin analogs: correlations with biological activity. *Metabolism.* 1996;45(8 Suppl 1): 21-23.

156. Scarpignato C, Pelosini I. Somatostatin analogs for cancer treatment and diagnosis: an overview. *Chemotherapy.* 2001;47(Suppl 2):1-29.

157. Buscail L, Esteve JP, Saint-Laurent N, et al. Inhibition of cell proliferation by the somatostatin analogue RC-160 is mediated by somatostatin receptor subtypes SSTR2 and SSTR5 through different mechanisms. *Proc Natl Acad Sci U S A.* 1995;92(5):1580-1584.

158. Cordelier P, Esteve JP, Bousquet C, et al. Characterization of the antiproliferative signal mediated by the somatostatin receptor subtype sst5. *Proc Natl Acad Sci U S A.* 1997;94(17):9343-9348.

159. Cattaneo MG, Amoroso D, Gussoni G, et al. A somatostatin analogue inhibits MAP kinase activation and cell proliferation in human neuroblastoma and in human small cell lung carcinoma cell lines. *FEBS Lett.* 1996;397(2–3):164-168.

160. Sharma K, Patel YC, Srikant CB. Subtype-selective induction of wild-type p53 and apoptosis, but not cell cycle arrest, by human somatostatin receptor 3. *Mol Endocrinol.* 1996;10(12):1688-1696.

161. Hofland LJ, van Koetsveld PM, Waaijers M, et al. Internalization of the radioiodinated somatostatin analog [125I-Tyr3]octreotide by mouse and human pituitary tumor cells: increase by unlabeled octreotide. *Endocrinology.* 1995;136(9):3698-3706.

162. Rocheville M, Lange DC, Kumar U, et al. Receptors for dopamine and somatostatin: formation of hetero-oligomers with enhanced functional activity. *Science.* 2000;288(5463):154-157.

163. Janson ET, Stridsberg M, Gobl A, et al. Determination of somatostatin receptor subtype 2 in carcinoid tumors by immunohistochemical investigation with somatostatin receptor subtype 2 antibodies. *Cancer Res.* 1998;58(11):2375-2378.

164. Reubi JC, Kappeler A, Waser B, et al. Immunohistochemical localization of somatostatin receptors sst2A in human tumors. *Am J Pathol.* 1998;153(1):233-245.

165. Denzler B, Reubi JC. Expression of somatostatin receptors in peritumoral veins of human tumors. *Cancer.* 1999;85(1):188-198.

166. Fassler J, Hughes J, Cataland S, et al. Somatostatin analogue: an inhibitor of angiogenesis? *Biomed Res.* 1988;II(Suppl):181-185.

167. Lamberts SW, van der Lely AJ, de Herder WW, Hofland LJ. Octreotide. *N Engl J Med.* 1996;334(4):246-254.

168. Kvols LK, Moertel CG, O'Connell MJ, et al. Treatment of the malignant carcinoid syndrome. Evaluation of a long-acting somatostatin analogue. *N Engl J Med.* 1986;315(11):663-666.

169. Oberg K, Norheim I, Lundqvist G, Wide L. Treatment of the carcinoid syndrome with SMS 201-995, a somatostatin analogue. *Scand J Gastroenterol.* 1986;119:191-192.

170. Scarpignato C. Somatostatin analogues in the management of endocrine tumors of the pancreas. In: Mignon M, Jensen RT, eds. *Endocrine Tumors of the Pancreas.* Basel: Karger; 1995:385-414.

171. Lamberts SW, Krenning EP, Reubi JC. The role of somatostatin and its analogs in the diagnosis and treatment of tumors. *Endocr Rev.* 1991; 12(4):450-482.

172. Ruszniewski P, Ducreux M, Chayvialle JA, et al. Treatment of the carcinoid syndrome with the long-acting somatostatin analogue lanreotide: a prospective study in 39 patients. *Gut.* 1996;39(2):279-283.

173. Wymenga AN, Eriksson B, Salmela PI, et al. Efficacy and safety of prolonged-release lanreotide in patients with gastrointestinal neuroendocrine tumors and hormone-related symptoms. *J Clin Oncol.* 1999; 17(4):1111.

174. Rubin J, Ajani J, Schirmer W, et al. Octreotide acetate long-acting formulation versus open-label subcutaneous octreotide acetate in malignant carcinoid syndrome. *J Clin Oncol.* 1999;17(2):600-606.

175. Kvols LK, Oberg KE, O'Dorisio TM, et al. Pasireotide (SOM230) shows efficacy and tolerability in the treatment of patients with advanced neuroendocrine tumors refractory or resistant to octreotide LAR: results from a phase II study. *Endocr Relat Cancer.* 2012;19:657-666.

176. Faiss S, Wiedenmann B. Dose-dependent and antiproliferative effects of somatostatin. *J Endocrinol Invest.* 1997;20:68-70.

177. Eriksson B, Renstrup J, Imam H, Oberg K. High-dose treatment with lanreotide of patients with advanced neuroendocrine gastrointestinal tumors: clinical and biological effects. *Ann Oncol.* 1997;8(10): 1041-1044.

178. Anthony L, Johnson D, Hande K, et al. Somatostatin analogue phase I trials in neuroendocrine neoplasms. *Acta Oncol (Stockholm).* 1993; 32(2):217-223.

179. Eriksson B, Janson ET, Bax ND, et al. The use of new somatostatin analogues, lanreotide and octastatin, in neuroendocrine gastrointestinal tumours. *Digestion.* 1996;57(Suppl 1):77-80.

180. Imam H, Eriksson B, Lukinius A, et al. Induction of apoptosis in neuroendocrine tumors of the digestive system during treatment with somatostatin analogs. *Acta Oncol (Stockholm).* 1997;36(6):607-614.

181. Welin SV, Janson ET, Sundin A, et al. High-dose treatment with a long-acting somatostatin analogue in patients with advanced midgut carcinoid tumours. *Eur J Endocrinol.* 2004;151(1):107-112.

182. Arnold R, Miller H, Schade-Brittinger C, et al. Placebo-controlled, double-blind, prospective randomized study of the effect of octreotide LAR in the control of tumor growth in patients with metastatic neuroendocrine midgut tumors: a report from the PROMID Study Group. *J Clin Oncol.* 2009;27:4656-4663.

183. Caplin M, Ruzniewski P, Pavel M, et al. A randomize double-blind placebo-controlled study of lanreotide antiproliferative response in patients with gastroenteropancreatic neuroendocrine tumors. Abstract presented at the European Society for Medical Oncology (ESMO) meeting. Amsterdam: 2013.

184. Oberg K, Norheim I, Lind E, et al. Treatment of malignant carcinoid tumors with human leukocyte interferon: long-term results. *Cancer Treat Rep.* 1986;70(11):1297-1304.

185. Oberg K, Eriksson B. The role of interferons in the management of carcinoid tumors. *Acta Oncol (Stockholm).* 1991;30(4):519-522.

186. Nobin A, Lindblom A, Mansson B, Sundberg M. Interferon treatment in patients with malignant carcinoids. *Acta Oncol (Stockholm).* 1989; 28(3):445-449.

187. Hanssen LE, Schrumpf E, Jacobsen MB, et al. Extended experience with recombinant alpha-2b interferon with or without hepatic artery embolization in the treatment of midgut carcinoid tumours. A preliminary report. *Acta Oncol (Stockholm).* 1991;30(4):523-527.

188. Oberg K, Eriksson B, Janson ET. The clinical use of interferons in the management of neuroendocrine gastroenteropancreatic tumors. *Ann N Y Acad Sci.* 1994;733:471-478.

189. Hanssen LE, Schrumpf E, Kolbenstvedt AN, et al. Treatment of malignant metastatic midgut carcinoid tumours with recombinant human alpha2b interferon with or without prior hepatic artery embolization. *Scand J Gastroenterol.* 1989;24(7):787-795.

190. Moertel CG, Rubin J, Kvols LK. Therapy of metastatic carcinoid tumor and the malignant carcinoid syndrome with recombinant leukocyte A interferon. *J Clin Oncol.* 1989;7(7):865-868.

191. Fleischmann D, Fleischmann C. Mechanism of interferon's antitumor actions. In: Baron S, Coppenhaver D, Dianzani F, eds. *Interferon: Principles and Medical Application.* Galveston, TX: University of Texas Medical Branch; 1992:299-310.

192. Oberg K. The action of interferon alpha on human carcinoid tumours. *Semin Cancer Biol.* 1992;3(1):35-41.

193. Grander D, Sangfelt O, Erickson S. How does interferon exert its cell growth inhibitory effect? *Eur J Haematol.* 1997;59(3):129-135.

194. Hobeika AC, Subramaniam PS, Johnson HM. IFNalpha induces the expression of the cyclin-dependent kinase inhibitor p21 in human prostate cancer cells. *Oncogene.* 1997;14(10):1165-1170.

195. Grander D, Oberg K, Lundqvist ML, et al. Interferon-induced enhancement of 2',5'-oligoadenylate synthetase in mid-gut carcinoid tumours. *Lancet.* 1990;336(8711):337-340.

196. Zhou Y, Gobl A, Wang S, et al. Expression of p68 protein kinase and its prognostic significance during IFN-alpha therapy in patients with carcinoid tumours. *Eur J Cancer.* 1998;34(13):2046-2052.

197. Andersson T, Wilander E, Eriksson B, et al. Effects of interferon on tumor tissue content in liver metastases of human carcinoid tumors. *Cancer Res.* 1990;50(11):3413-3415.

198. Ronnblom LE, Alm GV, Oberg KE. Autoimmunity after alpha-interferon therapy for malignant carcinoid tumors. *Ann Intern Med.* 1991;115(3): 178-183.

199. Tiensuu Janson EM, Ahlstrom H, Andersson T, Oberg KE. Octreotide and interferon alfa: a new combination for the treatment of malignant carcinoid tumors. *Eur J Cancer.* 1992;28A(10):1647-1650.

200. Frank M, Klose KJ, Wied M, et al. Combination therapy with octreotide and alpha-interferon: effect on tumor growth in metastatic endocrine gastroenteropancreatic tumors. *Am J Gastroenterol.* 1999;94(5): 1381-1387.

201. Oberg K. Interferon in the management of neuroendocrine GEP-tumors: a review. *Digestion.* 2000;62(Suppl 1):92-97.

202. Oberg K. The use of chemotherapy in the management of neuroendocrine tumors. *Endocrinol Metab Clin North Am.* 1993;22(4):941-952.
203. Rougier P, Ducreux M. Systemic chemotherapy of advanced digestive neuroendocrine tumours. *Ital J Gastroenterol Hepatol.* 1999;31(Suppl 2):S202-S206.
204. Engstrom PF, Lavin PT, Moertel CG, et al. Streptozocin plus fluorouracil versus doxorubicin therapy for metastatic carcinoid tumor. *J Clin Oncol.* 1984;2(11):1255-1259.
205. Moertel CG, Kvols LK, O'Connell MJ, Rubin J. Treatment of neuroendocrine carcinomas with combined etoposide and cisplatin. Evidence of major therapeutic activity in the anaplastic variants of these neoplasms. *Cancer.* 1991;68(2):227-232.
206. Di Bartolomeo M, Bajetta E, Bochicchio AM, et al. A phase II trial of dacarbazine, fluorouracil and epirubicin in patients with neuroendocrine tumours. A study by the Italian Trials in Medical Oncology (I.T.M.O.) Group. *Ann Oncol.* 1995;6(1):77-79.
207. Bajetta E, Rimassa L, Carnaghi C, et al. 5-Fluorouracil, dacarbazine, and epirubicin in the treatment of patients with neuroendocrine tumors. *Cancer.* 1998;83(2):372-378.
208. Ekeblad S, Sundin A, Janson ET, et al. Temozolomide as monotherapy is effective in treatment of advanced malignant neuroendocrine tumors. *Clin Cancer Res.* 2007;13(10):2986-2991.
209. Yao JC. Neuroendocrine tumors. Molecular targeted therapy for carcinoid and islet-cell carcinoma. *Best Pract Res Clin Endocrinol Metab.* 2007;21(1):163-172.
210. Yao JC, Phan AT, Chang DZ, et al. Efficacy of RAD001 (everolimus) and octreotide LAR in advanced low- to intermediate-grade neuroendocrine tumors: results of a phase II study. *J Clin Oncol.* 2008;26(26):4311-4318.
211. Pavel ME, Hainsworth JD, Baudin E, et al. Everolimus plus octreotide long-acting repeatable for the treatment of advanced neuroendocrine tumours associated with carcinoid syndrome (RADIANT-2): a randomised, placebo-controlled, phase 3 study. *Lancet.* 2011;378:2005-2012.
212. Wangberg B, Westberg G, Tylen U, et al. Survival of patients with disseminated midgut carcinoid tumors after aggressive tumor reduction. *World J Surg.* 1996;20(7):892-899, discussion 899.
213. Norlen O, Stalberg P, Oberg K, et al. Long-term results of surgery for small intestinal neuroendocrine tumors at a tertiary referral center. *World J Surg.* 2012;36(6):1419-1431.
214. Lehnert T. Liver transplantation for metastatic neuroendocrine carcinoma: an analysis of 103 patients. *Transplantation.* 1998;66(10):1307-1312.
215. Anthuber M, Jauch KW, Briegel J, et al. Results of liver transplantation for gastroenteropancreatic tumor metastases. *World J Surg.* 1996;20(1):73-76.
216. Norlen O, Daskalakis K, Oberg K, et al. Indication for liver transplantation in young patients with small intestinal NETs is rare? *World J Surg.* 2014;38:742-747.
217. Drougas JG, Anthony LB, Blair TK, et al. Hepatic artery chemoembolization for management of patients with advanced metastatic carcinoid tumors. *Am J Surg.* 1998;175(5):408-412.
218. Eriksson BK, Larsson EG, Skogseid BM, et al. Liver embolizations of patients with malignant neuroendocrine gastrointestinal tumors. *Cancer.* 1998;83(11):2293-2301.
219. Kim YH, Ajani JA, Carrasco CH, et al. Selective hepatic arterial chemoembolization for liver metastases in patients with carcinoid tumor or islet cell carcinoma. *Cancer Invest.* 1999;17(7):474-478.
220. Diamandidou E, Ajani JA, Yang DJ, et al. Two-phase study of hepatic artery vascular occlusion with microencapsulated cisplatin in patients with liver metastases from neuroendocrine tumors. *AJR Am J Roentgenol.* 1998;170(2):339-344.
221. Seifert JK, Cozzi PJ, Morris DL. Cryotherapy for neuroendocrine liver metastases. *Semin Surg Oncol.* 1998;14(2):175-183.
222. Schupak KD, Wallner KE. The role of radiation therapy in the treatment of locally unresectable or metastatic carcinoid tumors. *Int J Radiat Oncol Biol Phys.* 1991;20(3):489-495.
223. Kimmig BN. Radiotherapy for gastroenteropancreatic neuroendocrine tumors. *Ann N Y Acad Sci.* 1994;733:488-495.
224. Hoefnagel CA, den Hartog Jager FC, Taal BG, et al. The role of I-131-MIBG in the diagnosis and therapy of carcinoids. *Eur J Nucl Med.* 1987;13(4):187-191.
225. Taal BG, Hoefnagel CA, Valdes Olmos RA, et al. Palliative effect of metaiodobenzylguanidine in metastatic carcinoid tumors. *J Clin Oncol.* 1996;14(6):1829-1838.
226. Krenning EP, Valkema R, Kooij PP, et al. Scintigraphy and radionuclide therapy with [indium-111-labelled-diethyl triamine penta-acetic acid-D-Phe1]-octreotide. *Ital J Gastroenterol Hepatol.* 1999;31(Suppl 2):S219-S223.
227. Kwekkeboom DJ, de Herder WW, Kam BL, et al. Treatment with the radiolabeled somatostatin analog [177 Lu-DOTA 0,Tyr3]octreotate: toxicity, efficacy, and survival. *J Clin Oncol.* 2008;26(13):2124-2130.
228. Kennedy AS, Dezarn WA, McNeillie P, et al. Radioembolization for unresectable neuroendocrine hepatic metastases using resin 90Y-microspheres: early results in 148 patients. *Am J Clin Oncol.* 2008;31:271-279.
229. Kwekkeboom DJ, de Herder WW, van Eijck CH, et al. Peptide receptor radionuclide therapy in patients with gastroenteropancreatic neuroendocrine tumors. *Semin Nucl Med.* 2010;40:78-88.
230. Jann H, Roll S, Couvelard A, et al. Neuroendocrine tumors of midgut and hindgut origin: tumor-node-metastasis classification determines clinical outcome. *Cancer.* 2011;117:3332-3341.
231. Zar N, Garmo H, Holmberg L, et al. Long-term survival of patients with small intestinal carcinoid tumors. *World J Surg.* 2004;28(11):1163-1168.
232. Williams ED. Medullary carcinoma of the thyroid. *J Clin Pathol.* 1996;20:395-398.
233. Verner JV, Morrison AB. Islet cell tumor and a syndrome of refractory watery diarrhea and hypokalemia. *Am J Med.* 1958;25(3):374-380.
234. Gray TK, Bieberdorf FA, Fordtran JS. Thyrocalcitonin and the jejunal absorption of calcium, water, and electrolytes in normal subjects. *J Clin Invest.* 1973;52(12):3084-3088.
235. Long RG, Bryant MG, Mitchell SJ, et al. Clinicopathological study of pancreatic and ganglioneuroblastoma tumours secreting vasoactive intestinal polypeptide (VIPomas). *Br Med J.* 1981;282(6278):1767-1771.
236. Krejs GJ, Fordtran JS, Fahrenkrug J, et al. Effect of VIP infusion in water and ion transport in the human jejunum. *Gastroenterology.* 1980;78(4):722-727.
237. Maton PN, Gardner JD, Jensen RT. Use of long-acting somatostatin analog SMS 201-995 in patients with pancreatic islet cell tumors. *Dig Dis Sci.* 1989;34(3 Suppl):28S-39S.
238. Friedman BS, Metcalfe DD. Mastocytosis. *Prog Clin Biol Res.* 1989;297:163-173.
239. Metcalfe DD. Classification and diagnosis of mastocytosis: current status. *J Invest Dermatol.* 1991;96(3):2S-4S.
240. Soter NA. The skin in mastocytosis. *J Invest Dermatol.* 1991;96(3):32S-38S, discussion 38S-39S.
241. Mican JM, Di Bisceglie AM, Fong TL, et al. Hepatic involvement in mastocytosis: clinicopathologic correlations in 41 cases. *Hepatology.* 1995;22(4 Pt 1):1163-1170.
242. Metcalfe DD. The liver, spleen, and lymph nodes in mastocytosis. *J Invest Dermatol.* 1991;96(3):45S-46S.
243. Sostre S, Handler HL. Bony lesions in systemic mastocytosis: scintigraphic evaluation. *Arch Dermatol.* 1977;113(9):1245-1247.
244. Ammann RW, Vetter D, Deyhle P, et al. Gastrointestinal involvement in systemic mastocytosis. *Gut.* 1976;17(2):107-112.
245. Czarnetzki BM, Kolde G, Schoemann A, et al. Bone marrow findings in adult patients with urticaria pigmentosa. *J Am Acad Dermatol.* 1988;18(1 Pt 1):45-51.
246. Travis WD, Li CY, Yam LT, et al. Significance of systemic mast cell disease with associated hematologic disorders. *Cancer.* 1988;62(5):965-972.
247. Hutchinson RM. Mastocytosis and co-existent non-Hodgkin's lymphoma and myeloproliferative disorders. *Leuk Lymphoma.* 1992;7(1-2):29-36.
248. Travis WD, Li CY, Hoagland HC, et al. Mast cell leukemia: report of a case and review of the literature. *Mayo Clin Proc.* 1986;61(12):957-966.
249. Valent P, Akin C, Sperr WR, et al. Mastocytosis: pathology, genetics, and current options for therapy. *Leuk Lymphoma.* 2005;46(1):35-48.
250. Roberts LJ 2nd, Oates JA. Biochemical diagnosis of systemic mast cell disorders. *J Invest Dermatol.* 1991;96(3):19S-24S, discussion 25S.
251. Keyzer JJ, de Monchy JG, van Doormaal JJ, van Voorst Vader PC. Improved diagnosis of mastocytosis by measurement of urinary histamine metabolites. *N Engl J Med.* 1983;309(26):1603-1605.
252. Awad JA, Morrow JD, Roberts LJ 2nd. Detection of the major urinary metabolite of prostaglandin D2 in the circulation: demonstration of elevated levels in patients with disorders of systemic mast cell activation. *J Allergy Clin Immunol.* 1994;93(5):817-824.
253. Schwartz LB, Metcalfe DD, Miller JS, et al. Tryptase levels as an indicator of mast-cell activation in systemic anaphylaxis and mastocytosis. *N Engl J Med.* 1987;316(26):1622-1626.
254. Pardanani A. Systemic mastocytosis: bone marrow pathology, classification, and current therapies. *Acta Haematol.* 2005;114(1):41-51.
255. Turk J, Oates JA, Roberts LJ 2nd. Intervention with epinephrine in hypotension associated with mastocytosis. *J Allergy Clin Immunol.* 1983;71(2):189-192.
256. Butterfield JH, Kao PC, Klee GC, Yocum MW. Aspirin idiosyncrasy in systemic mast cell disease: a new look at mediator release during aspirin desensitization. *Mayo Clin Proc.* 1995;70(5):481-487.
257. Czarnetzki BM, Algermissen B, Jeep S, et al. Interferon treatment of patients with chronic urticaria and mastocytosis. *J Am Acad Dermatol.* 1994;30(3):500-501.

Index

Page numbers followed by "*f*" indicate figures, and "*t*" indicate tables.

A

AANAT. *see* Arylalkylamine
    N-acetyltransferase (AANAT)
Aarskog syndrome, growth retardation due
    to, 1008
ABCC8 gene, neonatal diabetes and, 1390
Aberrant hormone synthesis, RAIU in, 364
Abetalipoproteinemia, 1684
Abnormal bleeding, with intrauterine
    progestins, 675-676
Abscesses, pituitary, 247
Abuse, psychosocial dwarfism and, 166
ACA. *see* Affordable Care Act (ACA)
Academic medical centers, 75
Acanthosis nigricans, 36
Acarbose, for type 2 diabetes mellitus,
    1435-1436
Accessory gland dysfunction, male infertility
    due to, 727
Accountable Care Organizations (ACOs), 70
    increase in value, 71-73, 71*t*
Accuracy, in analytic validation, 97-98, 98*f*
ACE inhibitors
    for diabetes mellitus, 1557
    for diabetic nephropathy, 1523
Acetylation, skeletal muscle fatty acid
    metabolism and, 1403
Acetylcholine, GH secretion and, 143
Acetyl-CoA carboxylase (ACC), skeletal
    muscle fatty acid metabolism and,
    1402-1403
Achlorhydria, with hypothyroidism, 419
Achondroplasia, 1006
    growth curves for, 966
    growth retardation due to, 1006
Acne
    with contraceptive implants, 677
    in puberty, 1086-1088
    testosterone replacement therapy and,
      772
ACOs. *see* Accountable Care Organizations
    (ACOs)
Acquired disorders
    androgen resistance syndromes and, 760
    primary hypogonadism due to, 743-744,
      747
    secondary hypogonadism due to, 750-754,
      758-759
Acquired immunodeficiency syndrome
    (AIDS)
    adrenal function of, 1776-1777
      adrenal insufficiency, 1777, 1780
      adrenal shunting, 1777
      clinical assessment of, 1777
      cortisol resistance, 1777
      glucocorticoid excess, 1777
      impaired adrenal reserve, 1776
      medication effects in, 1777, 1778*t*
    body composition changes in, 1784-1790,
      1785*f*
      treatment for, 1788-1790
    bone changes in
      avascular necrosis of bone, 1784
      bone loss, 1781-1783, 1781*f*-1783*f*
      bone metabolism in children with,
        1783-1784
      calcium homeostasis in, 1780-1781
    cardiovascular disease in, 1790-1794,
      1791*f*-1792*f*
      anti-inflammatory strategies for,
        1793-1794

Acquired immunodeficiency syndrome
    (AIDS) *(Continued)*
    cardiovascular risk in, 1786*f*, 1792-1793
    changes in fat mass and distribution in,
      1785-1786, 1786*f*
    endocrinology of, 1776-1798
    fluid balance and electrolytes in, 1780
    glucose homeostasis and pancreatic
      function in, 1784
    gonadal function, 1777-1779, 1779*f*
      female, 1779
      male, 1777-1779
    growth hormone/insulin-like growth
      factor 1 axis in, 1784
    growth retardation due to, 1004
    hyperglycemia in, 1787-1788, 1787*f*
    hyperlipidemia in, strategies for, 1793
    insulin resistance and, 1404
    insulin resistance in, 1787-1788, 1787*f*
      treatment for, 1790, 1791*f*
    lipid abnormalities in, 1786-1787
    menstrual cycle in, 1779
    metabolic changes in, 1784-1790, 1785*f*
      treatment for, 1788-1790
    SIADH due to, 318
    thyroid function in, 1779-1780
Acquired primary adrenal insufficiency, 525,
    525*t*
Acrocyanosis, with hypothalamic disease,
    167
Acromegaloidism, 271
Acromegaly, 268-285
    clinical features of, 271-274, 272*t*, 273*f*
      gigantism as, 271-272
    diagnosis of, 276
      differential, 276
      GH and IGF-1 measurement in, 276,
        277*f*-278*f*
    endocrine hypertension due to, 583
    and GH, 1041
    GHRH hypersecretion and, 163
    growth hormone and tumor formation in,
      274-276, 275*t*
      endocrine complications in, 275
      morbidity and mortality in, 275-276,
        276*f*
    incidence of, 268
    pathogenesis of, 268-271, 269*f*
      extrapituitary, 270-271
      pituitary, 268-269, 270*f*, 271*t*
    screening tests for, 235*t*
    treatment for, 276-285, 1731
      aims of, 276-278
      choice of, 282-285, 285*f*, 286*t*, 287*f*
      medical management as, 280-282,
        281*f*-285*f*
      radiation therapy as, 279-280, 279*f*
      surgical management as, 278-279,
        278*f*-279*f*, 278*t*
Acrosomal cap, 698
Acrosome reaction, of sperm, 698
ACTH. *see* Adrenocorticotropic hormone
    (ACTH)
ACTH-secreting tumors, 285-287
    assessment of surgical outcome in, 287
    medical treatment for, 287
    silent corticotroph adenoma and, 287
Activation function 1 (AF1), 44
    of androgen receptor, 933
Activation function 2 (AF2), of androgen
    receptor, 933

Activin receptor (ActR), 28-29
Activins, 28-29, 207-208, 208*f*
    in female reproductive axis, 590-591
    FSH regulation by, 596
    ovary production of, 609-610, 609*f*
    in pubertal growth spurt, 1101-1103
Acute coronary syndromes, with diabetes
    mellitus, 1556-1557
Acute illness, secondary hypogonadism due
    to, 757
Acute infectious thyroiditis, 442-443, 443*t*
    clinical manifestations of, 443
    incidence of, 443
Acute painful neuropathy, 1530-1531, 1531*f*
ADA. *see* American Diabetes Association
    (ADA)
ADD. *see* Attention deficit disorder (ADD)
Addison disease, 524-525, 525*t*
Adenohypophysiotropic hormones, 181
Adenohypophysis, 114, 115*f*
Adenoma, hyperplasia *vs.*, 1280
Adenomatous nodules, 454
Adenomatous polyposis coli (APC), 1339
Adenosine monophosphate-activated
    protein kinase (AMPK)
    acute exercise and, 1405
    in glucose metabolism, 1396
    insulin sensitizers and, 1425
Adenosine triphosphate (ATP)-sensitive
    potassium channel(s) (K$_{ATP}$ channels)
    beta-cell and, 1409
    neonatal diabetes and, 1390
Adenosine triphosphate-binding cassette
    transporter A1 (ABCA1) deficiency,
    familial hypoalphalipoproteinemia
    with, 1684
Adenylate cyclase, vasopressin and, 303-304
Adenylyl cyclase, 32, 33*f*
Aδ-fiber, neuropathies of, pain control for,
    1539-1542
ADHR. *see* Autosomal dominant
    hypophosphatemic rickets (ADHR)
Adipocytes
    adiponectin, 1639*t*, 1640
    cytokines, 1639*t*, 1640
    estrogens, 1639*t*, 1640
    leptin, 1639, 1639*t*
    resistin, 1639*t*, 1640
Adipocytokines, in hypothyroidism, 423
Adipokines, 19-20
Adiponectin
    adipocyte secretion of, 1639*t*, 1640
    in hypothyroidism, 423
Adipose tissue. *see also* Brown adipose tissue
    (BAT)
    biology of, 1640-1641
      brown tissue, 1640-1641
      white tissue, 1640
    as endocrine and immune organ,
      1639-1640, 1639*t*
    GH action in, 977
    insulin resistance and, 1398
    lipolysis of triglyceride stores in, 1663,
      1663*f*
    obesity and, 1638-1639, 1638*t*
Adipostatic factors, 1616-1617
Adluminal compartment, 696
Adolescence
    characteristics of, 1097
    DSD presentation during, 951
    growth of, 1089-1095